18th Edition

HARRISON'S™
PRINCIPLES OF
INTERNAL MEDICINE

EDITORS OF PREVIOUS EDITIONS

T. R. Harrison
Editor-in-Chief, Editions 1, 2, 3, 4, 5

W. R. Resnick
Editor, Editions 1, 2, 3, 4, 5

M. M. Wintrobe
Editor, Editions 1, 2, 3, 4, 5
Editor-in-Chief, Editions 6, 7

G. W. Thorn
Editor, Editions 1, 2, 3, 4, 5, 6, 7
Editor-in-Chief, Edition 8

R. D. Adams
Editor, Editions 2, 3, 4, 5, 6, 7, 8, 9, 10

P. B. Beeson
Editor, Editions 1, 2

I. L. Bennett, Jr.
Editor, Editions 3, 4, 5, 6

E. Braunwald
Editor, Editions 6, 7, 8, 9, 10,
12, 13, 14, 16, 17
Editor-in-Chief, Editions 11, 15

K. J. Isselbacher
Editor, Editions 6, 7, 8, 10, 11, 12, 14
Editor-in-Chief, Editions 9, 13

R. G. Petersdorf
Editor, Editions 6, 7, 8, 9, 11, 12
Editor-in-Chief, Edition 10

J. D. Wilson
Editor, Editions 9, 10, 11, 13, 14
Editor-in-Chief, Edition 12

J. B. Martin
Editor, Editions 10, 11, 12, 13, 14

A. S. Fauci
Editor, Editions 11, 12, 13, 15, 16
Editor-in-Chief, Editions 14, 17

R. Root
Editor, Edition 12

D. L. Kasper
Editor, Editions 13, 14, 15, 17
Editor-in-Chief, Edition 16

S. L. Hauser
Editor, Editions 14, 15, 16, 17

D. L. Longo
Editor, Editions 14, 15, 16, 17
Editor-in-Chief, Edition 18

J. L. Jameson
Editor, Editions 15, 16, 17

J. Lozcalzo
Editor, Edition 17

18th Edition

HARRISON'S™ PRINCIPLES OF INTERNAL MEDICINE

EDITORS

Dan L. Longo, MD
Professor of Medicine, Harvard Medical School; Senior Physician, Brigham and Women's Hospital; Deputy Editor, New England Journal of Medicine, Boston, Massachusetts

Dennis L. Kasper, MD
William Ellery Channing Professor of Medicine, Professor of Microbiology and Molecular Genetics, Harvard Medical School; Director, Channing Laboratory, Department of Medicine, Brigham and Women's Hospital, Boston, Massachusetts

J. Larry Jameson, MD, PhD
Robert G. Dunlop Professor of Medicine; Dean, University of Pennsylvania School of Medicine; Executive Vice-President of the University of Pennsylvania for the Health System, Philadelphia, Pennsylvania

Anthony S. Fauci, MD
Chief, Laboratory of Immunoregulation; Director, National Institute of Allergy and Infectious Diseases, National Institutes of Health, Bethesda, Maryland

Stephen L. Hauser, MD
Robert A. Fishman Distinguished Professor and Chairman, Department of Neurology, University of California, San Francisco, San Francisco, California

Joseph Loscalzo, MD, PhD
Hersey Professor of the Theory and Practice of Medicine, Harvard Medical School; Chairman, Department of Medicine; Physician-in-Chief, Brigham and Women's Hospital, Boston, Massachusetts

VOLUME II

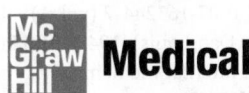

New York Chicago San Francisco Lisbon London Madrid Mexico City
Milan New Delhi San Juan Seoul Singapore Sydney Toronto

Note: Dr. Fauci's work as editor and author was performed outside the scope of his employment as a U.S. government employee. This work represents his personal and professional views and not necessarily those of the U.S. government.

Harrison's ™
PRINCIPLES OF INTERNAL MEDICINE
Eighteenth Edition

2 3 4 5 6 7 8 9 10 DOW/DOW 15 14 13 12

Two Volume Set ISBN 978-0-07174889-6; MHID 0-07-174889-X
Volume 1 ISBN 978-0-07-163244-7; MHID 0-07-163244-1
Volume 2 ISBN 978-0-07-174887-2; MHID 0-07-174887-3
DVD ISBN 978-0-07-174888-9; MHID 0-07-174888-1

FOREIGN LANGUAGE EDITIONS
Arabic (13e): McGraw-Hill Libri Italia srl (1996)
Albanian(17e): Tabernakul Publishing, Skopje, Macedonia
Chinese Long Form (15e): McGraw-Hill International Enterprises, Inc., Taiwan
Chinese Short Form (15e): McGraw-Hill Education (Asia), Singapore
Croatian (16e): Placebo, Split, Croatia
French (16e): Medecine-Sciences Flammarion, Paris, France
German (17e): ABW Wissenschaftsverlagsgesellschaft GmbH, Berlin, Germany
Greek (17e): Parissianos, S.A., Athens, Greece
Italian (17e): The McGraw-Hill Companies, Srl, Milan, Italy
Japanese (17e): MEDSI-Medical Sciences International Ltd, Tokyo, Japan
Korean (17e): McGraw-Hill Korea, Inc., Seoul, Korea
Macedonian (17e): Tabernakul Publishing, Skopje, Macedonia
Polish (17e): Czelej Publishing Company, Lubin, Poland
Portuguese (17e): McGraw-Hill Interamericana Editores, SA de C.V. Mexico City, Mexico
Romanian (17e): Editura All, Bucharest, Romania
Serbian (15e): Publishing House Romanov, Bosnia & Herzegovina, Republic of Serbska
Spanish (17e): McGraw-Hill Interamericana Editores, SA de C.V. Mexico City, Mexico
Turkish (17e): Nobel Tip Kitabevleri, Ltd., Istanbul, Turkey
Vietnamese (15e): McGraw-Hill Education (Asia), Singapore

This book was set in Minion Pro by Cenveo Publisher Services. The editors were James F. Shanahan and Kim J. Davis. The production managers were Phil Galea and John Williams; production assistance was provided by Rajni Pisharody at Cenveo Publisher Services. The index was prepared by Susan Hunter and Ann Blum. The text designer was Alan Barnett; cover design was by Anthony Landi. RR Donnelley was printer and binder.

Library of Congress Cataloging-in-Publication Data

Harrison's principles of internal medicine.—18th ed. / editors, Dan L. Longo … [et al.]. p. ; cm.
Includes bibliographical references and index.
ISBN 978-0-07-174889-6 (set)—ISBN 978-0-07-163244-7 (vol. 1)—ISBN 978-0-07-174887-2 (vol. 2)
1. Internal medicine. I. Longo, Dan L. (Dan Louis), 1949- II. Harrison, Tinsley Randolph, 1900-1978. III. Title: Principles of internal medicine.
[DNLM: 1. Internal Medicine. WB 115 H322 2011]
RC46.H333 2008
616—dc22 2008053547

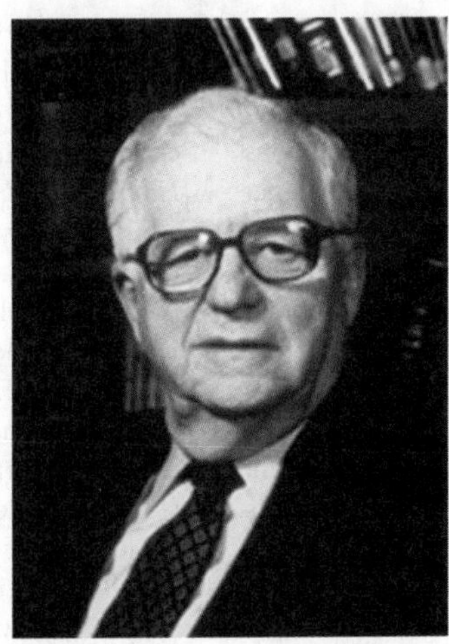

Dedication: Eugene Braunwald

This edition of *Harrison's Principles of Internal Medicine*, the 18th edition, is respectfully and warmly dedicated to our colleague, teacher, mentor, and friend, Eugene Braunwald. Dr. Braunwald has been a fixture on the editorial board of this book since 1967, when the 6th edition was being planned—a period of more than 40 years. No one has served the book so long or with as much distinction. He was an inexhaustible source of ideas and innovations throughout his period of service, for which we and the former editors are most grateful.

Of course, his work on this book was only a small fraction of his prodigious intellectual output. He graduated first in his class from New York University (NYU) School of Medicine, spent two years in internal medicine training at Mount Sinai Hospital, returned to NYU for a year as a research fellow with Andre Cournand (who would later win the Nobel Prize for inventing cardiac catheterization), spent two years as a Clinical Associate at the National Heart Institute, and then completed his final year of internal medicine training on the Osler service at Johns Hopkins. After completing his training, he returned to the National Heart Institute as a tenured senior investigator in 1958 at 29 years of age, becoming Chief of the Cardiology Branch in 1959 and Clinical Director of the institute in 1966. He published about 370 papers during his 10 years at the National Institutes of Health, many of which were seminal findings that became an essential part of the fabric of our cardiovascular knowledge base. In 1968, he was enticed into becoming the founding Chairman of the Department of Medicine at a new medical school, University of California, San Diego (UCSD). During his four years there, he demonstrated that he was not only a creative scientist but an innovative medical educator, administrator, and academic leader. In 1972, he was recruited to be the Hersey Professor of the Theory and Practice of Medicine (the oldest endowed chair in medicine) at Harvard Medical School and Chairman of the Department of Medicine at the Peter Bent Brigham Hospital, a position he held for 24 years. He is now the Distinguished Hersey Professor and the Chairman of the Thrombolysis in Myocardial Infarction (TIMI) Study Group, a cooperative research organization that has completed nearly 60 (and counting) prospective randomized trials that have defined the elements of the optimal care of patients with acute coronary syndromes.

His research has spanned many dimensions of cardiology, in scope and over time. In the earliest phase, he focused on valvular heart disease, which was much more prevalent than it is today because of the late effects of poorly treated rheumatic fever in the preantibiotic era. Among his accomplishments were the very first recordings in humans of the pressure gradient across a stenotic mitral valve and the effects of valvulotomy on hemodynamics; the development of transseptal left heart catheterization, then a breakthrough in the measurement of left heart function in vivo, and now used to treat mitral valve disease, to perform electrophysiology and ablation procedures in the left atrium and to provide access for assist devices; demonstration of the reversibility of high pulmonary vascular resistance by mitral valve replacement in patients with mitral stenosis (high pulmonary vascular resistance had been used to disqualify patients from the operation); and demonstration of the dire prognosis of patients with aortic stenosis when they develop symptoms of heart failure, syncope, or angina (which led to earlier surgical intervention).

Working closely with his surgical colleague at the National Institutes of Health, Glenn Andrew Morrow, he identified a previously unknown disease entity: hypertrophic cardiomyopathy. Based on pressure recordings that showed an unexplained dynamic pressure gradient between the left ventricle and the aorta in the presence of a normal aortic valve, they proposed that the obstruction to left ventricular outflow was caused by left ventricle contraction itself; hypertrophic heart muscle during contraction blocked the flow of blood from the ventricle to the aorta. Hypertrophic cardiomyopathy is now known to be the most common Mendelian inherited heart disease (1 in 500 births). The Braunwald team described the fascinating physiologic changes associated with the condition in detail, including the diagnostic sign of the *reduction* in pulse pressure following a premature contraction instead of the expected potentiation of pulse pressure. They developed treatments (beta blockers and myotomy/myectomy) that are still the cornerstones of therapy 40 years later.

Dr. Braunwald defined fundamental features of the pathophysiology and treatment of heart failure. He and his colleagues documented that normal human heart muscle follows Starling's law (the greater the tension on the muscle, the stronger its contraction) and that left ventricular end-diastolic pressure was a key determinant of stroke volume, stroke work, and stroke power. They showed that these properties were seriously altered in the failing heart, with the length-tension curves shifting dramatically to the left (that is, for any particular amount of stretch on the muscle, contraction extent and velocity were reduced). They also demonstrated the improvement in cardiac function caused by drugs that reduce afterload, including beta blockers and angiotensin-converting enzyme inhibitors or receptor antagonists—treatments that extend the lives of patients with failing hearts. We measure left ventricular ejection fraction today as a method of assessing cardiac function based on concepts and techniques the Braunwald team pioneered.

His work on myocardial ischemia and infarction has formed the basis for current (and likely future) management strategies of this most common disease. It was his work that defined the basic determinants of myocardial oxygen consumption: tension development, contractility, and heart rate account for 92% of consumed oxygen. This finding led directly to the observation that the size of an infarct could be profoundly altered by a number of physiologic and pharmacologic interventions that modify myocardial oxygen consumption and interventions that restore coronary perfusion, especially if implemented within three hours of occlusion. The formation of the Thrombolysis in Myocardial Infarction (TIMI) study group has led to widespread changes in practice and has saved untold numbers of lives. In addition to exploring thrombolytic therapy in its early days, the group has proved the value of early invasive intervention for unstable angina, aggressive lipid-lowering strategies after a heart attack to prevent recurrence and death, and the use of antiplatelet agents and other anticoagulants as adjuncts to coronary artery stenting to prevent restenosis, among others.

His administrative accomplishments are legion. He has served as head of major organizations since he was 31 years old. As the first Chairman of Medicine at UCSD, he took the department from a concept to a leading center in four years, recruiting 75 faculty members and establishing a first-rate training program. Under his leadership, the Brigham and Women's Hospital Department of Medicine grew dramatically, recruited outstanding physician/scientists whose work has influenced every corner of internal medicine, and trained two generations of academic researchers who either stayed on at one or more of the Harvard hospitals or went to other universities and exerted a major influence in academic medicine.

His educational impact extends well beyond the worldwide influence of his mentorship to hundreds of physician scientists and medical educators and his enormous contributions to the cardiology, pulmonology, and renal sections of twelve editions of *Harrison's Principles of Internal Medicine.* Teaching has always been a high priority for him. At UCSD, he helped to establish an educational program in which physicians taught the basic sciences so that the clinical relevance of the information would always be at hand. He created the cardiology textbook *Heart Disease* (now known as *Braunwald's Heart Disease*), wrote a major fraction of its chapters, and has shepherded the book through seven editions.

He has been elected President of nearly every organization to which he belongs. He has published nearly 1300 papers. He is a member of the United States National Academy of Sciences and its Institute of Medicine. A list of his awards and honorary degrees would exceed the length of this dedication. Eugene Braunwald is one of the leading lights in the history of medicine. His indelible impact on the institutions he has led, the practice of cardiology, medical education, this textbook, and the many individuals whom he has trained will continue to be felt in future generations. We therefore dedicate this edition of *Harrison's Principles of Internal Medicine* to him with respect, admiration, and heartfelt gratitude.

THE EDITORS

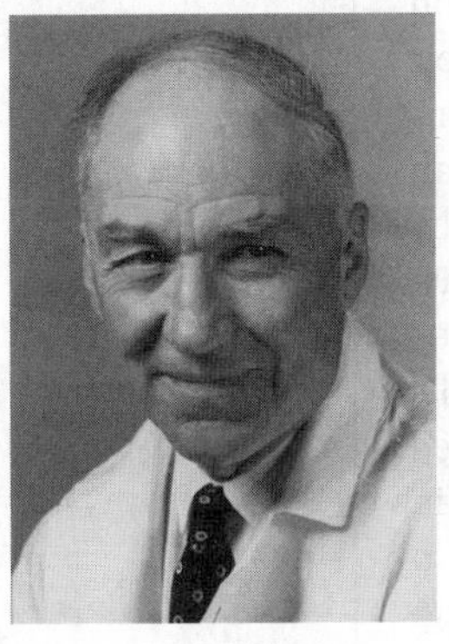

In Memoriam: Raymond D. Adams (1911–2008)

Ray Adams's tenure as editor of *Harrison's Principles of Internal Medicine* began with the second edition, published in 1954; he then remained on the editorial board for more than three decades. Dr. Adams was born in Portland, Oregon and graduated from the University of Oregon and Duke University Medical School. After a discouraging foray into a psychoanalytic career, he found his calling when appointed to the Neurology and Neuropathology Service at Boston City Hospital and then, in 1951, as Chief of the Neurology Service at Massachusetts General Hospital. His contributions to neurology and medicine were prodigious, grounded in a fastidious approach to clinicopathologic correlation. There are few areas of neurology in which he did not have an impact. He identified immune mechanisms and the cause of disability in multiple sclerosis and Guillain-Barré syndrome; clarified nutritional, alcoholic, syphilitic, and metabolic disorders of the nervous system; performed careful studies of embolic stroke and anoxic brain disease; focused attention on mental retardation and language disability as core problems in neurology; and described many muscle diseases. Ray Adams was also an extraordinary clinician and teacher who trained generations of physician-scientists. Today they represent an important part of his legacy. The excellence of *Harrison's* owes much to Dr. Adams, and his commitment to education continues to be reflected in the pages of each new edition.

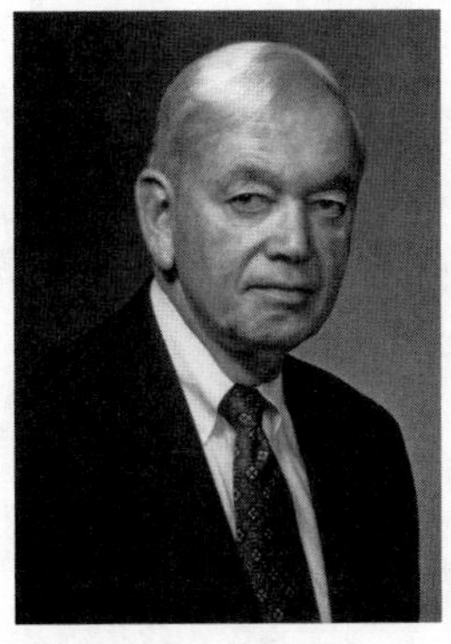

In Memoriam: Robert G. Petersdorf (1926–2006)

An editor of *Harrison's Principles of Internal Medicine* from 1968 through 1990, Robert G. Petersdorf was for many years one of the most powerful figures in American medicine and an internationally recognized expert and educator in infectious diseases. He gained prominence in 1961 through his classic study of fever of unknown origin, conducted at Yale in collaboration with Paul Beeson. During his distinguished career, Dr. Petersdorf held key positions at several institutions, including Chair of the Department of Medicine at the University of Washington in Seattle, President of Brigham and Women's Hospital in Boston, and Vice Chancellor for Health Sciences and Dean of the School of Medicine at the University of California, San Diego. He served from 1986 to 1994 as President of the Association of American Medical Colleges, where he advocated for better communication between the medical community and Congress, for increased enrollment of underrepresented minorities in medical schools, and for greater numbers of primary care doctors in general internal medicine and family practice. As a central figure in the training of many leaders in American medicine, Dr. Petersdorf was described as blunt and demanding but also very kind; a colleague recalled that he constantly reminded students to listen to the patient, who, he maintained, "was always right." Dr. Petersdorf's efforts through seven editions of *Harrison's* were instrumental in establishing the book's pivotal role in the education of students, residents, and practitioners of medicine.

The Editors

NOTICE

COVER ILLUSTRATIONS (VOLUME II)

Background Image: A stylized scanning electron microscope image of *Mycobacterium tuberculosis.* This bacterium causes most cases of tuberculosis. *(Credit: MedicalRF.com)*

Top Panel: The coronary vessels of the heart. *(Credit: © MedicalRF.com/Corbis)*

Center Panel: MRI scan of the brain. *(Credit: © Image Source/Corbis)*

Bottom Panel: Arthritic ankle, x-ray. Colored profile x-ray of the ankle of a 66-year-old male with osteoarthritis. *(Credit: © Dr. P. Marazzi/Science Photo Library/Corbis.)*

CONTENTS

CONTENTS

CONTENTS

CONTENTS

CONTENTS

PART 12: Critical Care Medicine

SECTION 1 Respiratory Critical Care

SECTION 2 Shock and Cardiac Arrest

SECTION 3 Neurologic Critical Care

SECTION 4 Oncologic Emergencies

PART 13: Disorders of the Kidney and Urinary Tract

PART 14: Disorders of the Gastrointestinal System

SECTION 1 Disorders of the Alimentary Tract

SECTION 2 Disorders of Bone and Mineral Metabolism

SECTION 3 Disorders of Intermediary Metabolism

PART 17: Neurologic Disorders

SECTION 1 Diagnosis of Neurologic Disorders

SECTION 2 Diseases of the Central Nervous System

SUMMARIES OF CHAPTERS e1 TO e57

Chapter e1 Primary Care in Low- and Middle-Income Countries

This chapter looks first at the nature of the health challenges in low- and middle-income countries that underlie the health divide. It then outlines the values and principles of a primary health care approach with a focus on primary care services. Next, the chapter reviews the experience of low- and middle-income countries in addressing health challenges through primary care and a primary health care approach. Finally, the chapter identifies how current challenges and global context provide an agenda and opportunities for the renewal of primary health care and primary care.

Chapter e2 Complementary, Alternative, and Integrative Medicine

Complementary and alternative medicine (CAM) refers to a group of diverse medical and health care systems, practices, and products that are not considered part of conventional or allopathic medicine or that have historic origins outside mainstream medicine. Most of these practices are used together with conventional therapies and therefore have been called *complementary* to distinguish them from *alternative* practices, which are those used instead of standard care. *Integrative medicine* refers to a style of practice that places strong emphasis on a holistic approach to patient care, focusing on reduced use of technology and preventive strategies for maintenance of health.

Chapter e3 The Economics of Medical Care

This chapter attempts to explain to physicians how economists think about physicians and medical care. Economists' mode of thinking has shaped health care policy and institutions and, thus, the environment for in which physicians practice. As a result, it may be useful physicians to understand some aspects of this way of thinking even if at times it may seem foreign or uncongenial.

Chapter e4 Racial and Ethnic Disparities in Health Care

This chapter provides an overview of racial and ethnic disparities in health and health care, identifies root causes, and provides key recommendations to address them at both the clinical and health system level.

Chapter e5 Ethical Issues in Clinical Medicine

This chapter discusses fundamental and ethical guidelines, patients who lack decision-making capacity, decisions and life-sustaining interventions, conflicts of interest, and just allocation of resources. The chapter helps the physician to follow two fundamental but frequently conflicting ethical principles: respecting patient autonomy and acting in the patient's best interest.

Chapter e6 Neoplasia During Pregnancy

This chapter looks at the complex problem of cancer in a pregnant woman, covering topics such as cervical cancer, breast cancer, and melanoma during pregnancy. The chapter examines the possible influence of the pregnancy on the natural history of the cancer, the effects of the diagnostic and staging procedures, and the treatments of the cancer on both the mother and the developing fetus. These issues may lead to dilemmas: what is best for the mother may be harmful to the fetus, and what is best for the fetus may be harmful to the mother.

Chapter e7 Atlas of Rashes Associated With Fever

Given the extremely broad differential diagnosis, the presentation of a patient with fever and rash often poses a thorny diagnostic challenge for even the most astute and experienced clinician. Rapid narrowing of the differential by prompt recognition of a rash's key features can result in appropriate and sometimes life-saving therapy. This atlas presents high-quality images of a variety of rashes that have an infectious etiology and are commonly associated with fever.

Chapter e8 Video Library of Gait Disorders

Problems with gait and balance are major causes of falls, accidents, and resulting disability, especially in later life, and are often harbingers of neurologic disease. Early diagnosis is essential, especially for treatable conditions, as it may permit the institution of prophylactic measures to prevent dangerous falls, and also to reverse or ameliorate the underlying cause. In this video, examples of gait disorders due to Parkinson's disease, other extrapyramidal disorders, and ataxias, as well as other common gait disorders, are presented.

Chapter e9 Memory Loss

This chapter discusses the formation of both long- and short-term memories. Long-term memory is divided into declarative and nondeclarative memory; the former is further subdivided into episodic and semantic memories. Short-term, or working, memory relies on different regions of the brain and lesions that disrupt their structure or function can be devastating.

Chapter e10 Primary Progressive Aphasia, Memory Loss, and Other Focal Cerebral Disorders

Language and memory are essential human functions. For the experienced clinician, the recognition of different types of language and memory disturbances often provides essential clues to the anatomic localization and diagnosis of neurologic disorders. This video illustrates classic disorders of language and speech (including the aphasias), memory (the amnesias), and other disorders of cognition that are commonly encountered in clinical practice.

Chapter e11 Video Library of Neuro-Ophthalmology

The proper control of eye movements requires the coordinated activity of many different anatomic structures in the peripheral and central nervous system, and in turn manifestations of a diverse array of neurologic and medical disorders are revealed as disorders of eye movement. In this remarkable video collection, an introduction to distinctive eye movement disorders encountered in the context of neuromuscular, paraneoplastic, demyelinating, neurovascular and neurodegenerative disorders is presented.

Chapter e12 Atlas of Oral Manifestations of Disease

The health status of the oral cavity is linked to cardiovascular disease, diabetes, and other systemic illnesses. Thus, examining the oral cavity for signs of disease is a key part of the physical exam. This atlas presents numerous outstanding clinical photographs illustrating many of the conditions affecting the teeth, periodontal tissues, and oral mucosa.

Chapter e13 Approach to the Patient With a Heart Murmur

This chapter provides comprehensive coverage of heart murmurs (systolic, diastolic, and continuous), their major attributes, and their response to bedside maneuvers, detected by auscultation.

Chapter e14 Atlas of Urinary Sediments and Renal Biopsies

This chapter illustrates key diagnostic features of selected diseases in renal biopsy using light microscopy, immunofluorescence, and electron microscopy. Common urinalysis findings are also documented.

Chapter e15 Fluid and Electrolyte Imbalances and Acid-Base Disturbances: Case Examples

Acid-base, fluid, and electrolyte disorders can be intimidating to trainees and practicing physicians alike. The real-life clinical vignettes in this chapter have been chosen to reinforce selected concepts covered in the relevant chapters. These are short, directed discussions, focused on key issues in diagnosis and/or therapy.

Chapter e16 Atlas of Skin Manifestations of Internal Disease

This atlas provides pictures of a selected group of inflammatory skin eruptions and neoplastic conditions illustrating (1) common skin diseases and lesions, (2) nonmelanoma skin cancer, (3) melanoma and pigmented lesions, (4) infectious disease and the skin, (5) immunologically mediated skin disease, and (6) skin manifestations of internal disease.

Chapter e17 Atlas of Hematology and Analysis of Peripheral Blood Smears

This atlas gives many examples of both normal and abnormal blood smears and a guide to blood smear interpretation. A normal peripheral blood smear is shown, as are normal granulocytes, monocytes, eosinophils, basophils, plasma cells, and bone marrow.

Chapter e18 Mitochondrial DNA and Heritable Traits and Diseases

The structure and function of mitochondrial DNA (mtDNA) are discussed in depth in this chapter, which includes the proposition that the total cumulative burden of somatic mtDNA mutations acquired with age may contribute to aging and common age-related disturbances.

Chapter e19 Systems Biology in Health and Disease

This chapter presents new concepts related to the complex molecular and genetic systems that underlie all human disease. Using the evolving approaches of systems biology, interaction models of human disease that include the molecular networks specific to the disease, as well as those molecular networks that define generic mechanisms common to all disease (e.g., fibrosis and inflammation), are presented. Environmental factors that influence the behavior of these networks and their effects on the pathophenotype (e.g., epigenesis or posttranslational modification of the proteome) are included in this new disease paradigm.

Chapter e20 Thymoma

This chapter begins with a brief overview of the composition and function of the thymus and lists the various abnormalities that can occur and discusses the clinical presentation and differential diagnosis of thymoma as well as staging, pathology and etiology, and treatment.

Chapter e21 Less Common Hematologic Malignancies

This chapter focuses on the more unusual forms of hematologic malignancy, covering diseases such as hairy cell leukemia, mediastinal large B cell lymphoma, and Langerhans' cell histiocytosis.

Chapter e22 Laboratory Diagnosis of Infectious Diseases

This chapter documents the evolution of methods used in the clinical microbiology laboratory to detect and identify viral, bacterial, fungal, and parasitic agents and to determine the antibiotic susceptibility of bacterial and fungal pathogens.

Chapter e23 Infectious Complications of Burns

This chapter details the consequences of breaches in the skin barrier from burns, which may cause massive destruction of the integument as well as derangements in humoral and cellular immunity, permitting the development of infection caused by environmental opportunists and components of the host's skin flora.

Chapter e24 Infectious Complications of Bites

This chapter discusses breaches in the skin from bites and scratches that represent a form of immunocompromise and predispose the patient to infection. The treatment section covers wound management, antibiotic therapy for established infection and for prophylactic purposes, and rabies and tetanus prophylaxis.

Chapter e25 Laboratory Diagnosis of Parasitic Infections

This chapter emphasizes the importance of the history and epidemiology of a patient's illness. Tables provide clear information on the geographic distribution, transmission, anatomic locations, and methods employed for the diagnosis of flatworm, roundworm, and protozoal infections.

Chapter e26 Pharmacology of Agents Used to Treat Parasitic Infections

This chapter deals exclusively with the pharmacologic properties of the agents used to treat infections due to parasites. Specific treatment recommendations for the parasitic diseases of humans are listed in the chapters on those diseases. Information on these agents' major toxicities, spectrum of activity, and safety for use during pregnancy and lactation is presented in Chapter 208.

Chapter e27 Atlas of Blood Smears of Malaria and Babesiosis

This chapter provides both thin and thick blood films for *Plasmodium falciparum*, *P. vivax*, *P. ovale*, and *P. malariae*. The thick film allows detection of densities as low as 50 parasites per microliter, with great sensitivity; the thin film is better for speciation and provides useful prognostic information in severe falciparum malaria. One thin blood film showing trophozoites of *Babesia* is included.

Chapter e28 Atlas of Electrocardiography

The electrocardiograms in this atlas supplement those illustrated in Chapter 228. The interpretations emphasize findings of specific teaching value.

Chapter e29 Atlas of Noninvasive Cardiac Imaging

This chapter provides "real-time" image clips as they are viewed in clinical practice, as well as additional static images. Noninvasive cardiac imaging is essential to the diagnosis and management of patients with known or suspected cardiovascular disease. This atlas supplements Chapter 229, which describes the principles and clinical applications of these important techniques.

Chapter e30 Atlas of Cardiac Arrhythmias

The electrocardiograms in this atlas supplement those illustrated in Chapters 232 and 233. The interpretations emphasize findings of specific teaching value.

Chapter e31 Cardiac Manifestations of Systemic Disease

This chapter covers the common systemic disorders that have associated cardiac manifestations, such as diabetes mellitus, hyper- and hypothyroidism, and systemic lupus erythematosus.

Chapter e32 Atlas of Atherosclerosis

This atlas consists of six videos that highlight some of the current understanding of atherosclerosis. Topics include pulse pressure, plaque instability, rudiments of the clinically important lipoproteins, formation and complications of atherosclerotic plaques, mechanisms of atherogenesis, and metabolic derangements that underlie the metabolic syndrome.

Chapter e33 Atlas of Percutaneous Revascularization

This atlas presents seven case studies illustrating the use of percutaneous coronary intervention in a variety of commonly encountered clinical and anatomic situations, such as chronic total occlusion of a coronary artery, bifurcation disease, acute STEMI, saphenous vein graft disease, left main coronary artery disease, multivessel disease, and stent thrombosis.

Chapter e34 Atlas of Chest Imaging

This atlas is a collection of interesting chest radiographs and CT scans illustrative of specific major findings that are categorized by those of volume loss, loss of parenchyma, interstitial processes, alveolar processes, bronchiectasis, pleural abnormalities, nodules and masses, and pulmonary vascular abnormalities.

Chapter e35 Interstitial Cystitis/Painful Bladder Syndrome

This chapter covers interstitial cystitis/painful bladder syndrome, a chronic condition that occurs primarily in women and is characterized by pain perceived to be from the urinary bladder, urinary urgency and frequency, and nocturia.

Chapter e36 Video Atlas of Gastrointestinal Endoscopy

Gastrointestinal endoscopy is an increasingly important method for diagnosis and treatment of disease. This atlas demonstrates endoscopic findings in a variety of gastrointestinal infectious, inflammatory, vascular, and neoplastic conditions. Cancer screening and prevention are common indications for gastrointestinal endoscopy, and the premalignant conditions of Barrett's esophagus and colonic polyps are illustrated. Endoscopic treatment modalities for gastrointestinal bleeding, polyps, and biliary stones are demonstrated in video clips.

Chapter e37 The Schilling Test

While not available commercially in the United States for the last few years, the Schilling test is performed to determine the cause for cobalamin malabsorption. Since understanding the physiology and pathophysiology of cobalamin absorption is very valuable for enhancing one's understanding of aspects of gastric, pancreatic, and ileal function, discussion of the Schilling test is provided as supplemental information to Chapter 294.

Chapter e38 Atlas of Liver Biopsies

Included in this atlas of liver biopsies are examples of common morphologic features of acute and chronic liver disorders, some involving the lobular areas (e.g., the lobular inflammatory changes of acute hepatitis, apoptotic hepatocyte degeneration in acute and chronic hepatitis, virus antigen localization in hepatocyte cytoplasm and/or nuclei, viral inclusion bodies, copper or iron deposition, other inclusion bodies), and others involving the portal tracts (e.g., the portal mononuclear infiltrate that expands and spills over beyond the border of periportal hepatocytes in chronic hepatitis C, autoimmune hepatitis, and liver allograft rejection) or centrizonal areas (e.g., acute acetaminophen hepatotoxicity).

Chapter e39 Primary Immunodeficiencies Associated With (or Secondary to) Other Diseases

There are an increasing number of conditions in which a primary immunodeficiency (PID) has been described as one facet of a more complex disease setting. It is essential to consider associated diseases when a PID is identified as the primary manifestation and, conversely, not neglect the potentially harmful consequences of a PID that could be masked by other manifestations of a particular syndrome. This chapter provides descriptions of these syndromes in which the PID is classified according to the arm of the immune system that is affected.

Chapter e40 Atlas of the Vasculitic Syndromes

Diagnosis of the vasculitic syndromes is usually based upon characteristic histologic or arteriographic findings in a patient who has clinically compatible features. The images provided in this atlas highlight some of the characteristic histologic and radiographic findings that may be seen in the vasculitic diseases. These images demonstrate the importance that tissue histology may have in securing the diagnosis of vasculitis, the utility of diagnostic imaging in the vasculitic diseases, and the improvements in the care of vasculitis patients that have resulted from radiologic innovations.

Chapter e41 Atlas of Clinical Manifestations of Metabolic Diseases

This atlas provides a visual survey of selected metabolic disorders with references to the topics elsewhere in the text. The emerging field of *metabolomics* is based on the premise that the identification and measurement of metabolic products will enhance our understanding of physiology and disease. Over the years, the classification of metabolic diseases has extended beyond traditional pathways involved in fuel metabolism to include disorders such as lysosomal storage diseases or connective tissue diseases.

Chapter e42 The Neurologic Screening Exam

Knowledge of the basic neurologic examination is an essential clinical skill. A simple neurologic screening examination—assessment of mental status, cranial nerves, motor system, sensory system, coordination, and gait—can be reliably performed in 3-5 minutes. Although the components of the examination may appear daunting at first, skills usually improve rapidly with repetition and practice. In this video, the technique of performing a simple and efficient screening examination is presented.

Chapter e43 Video Atlas of the Detailed Neurologic Examination

The comprehensive neurologic examination is an irreplaceable tool for the efficient diagnosis of neurologic disorders. Mastery of its details requires knowledge of normal nervous system anatomy and physiology, combined with personal experience performing orderly and systematic examinations on large numbers of patients and healthy individuals. In the hands of a great clinician, the neurologic examination also becomes a thing of beauty—the pinnacle of the art of medicine. In this video, the most commonly used components of the examination are presented in detail, with a particular emphasis on those elements that are most helpful for assessment of common neurologic problems.

Chapter e44 Atlas of Neuroimaging

This atlas comprises 29 cases to assist the clinician caring for patients with neurologic symptoms. The majority of the images are MRIs; other techniques used are MR and conventional angiography and CT scans. Many neurologic diseases are illustrated, such as tuberculosis of the central nervous system (CNS), neurosyphilis, CNS aspergillosis, neurosarcoid, middle cerebral artery stenosis, CNS vasculitis, Huntington's disease, and acute transverse myelitis.

Chapter e45 Electrodiagnostic Studies of Nervous System Disorders: EEG, Evoked Potentials, and EMG

This chapter covers the two main techniques for electrodiagnosis of neurologic symptoms: electroencephalogram (EEG) and the electromyogram (EMG). Evoked potentials (sensory, cognitive, and motor) are also covered.

Chapter e46 Technique of Lumbar Puncture

This chapter covers the procedure of lumbar puncture (LP) in detail (with illustrations), from indications for imaging and laboratory studies prior to LP, analgesia, positioning, and the procedure itself (including dealing with complications that may arise during LP). Also included is a section on the main complication of LP—the post-LP headache—and its causes and therapy and strategies to avoid it.

Chapter e47 Special Issues in Inpatient Neurologic Consultation

Inpatient neurologic consultations usually involve questions about specific disease processes or prognostication after various cerebral injuries. Common reasons for neurologic consultation include stroke, seizures, altered mental status, headache, and management of coma and other neurocritical care conditions. This chapter focuses on additional common reasons for consultation that are not addressed elsewhere in the text.

Chapter e48 Neuropsychiatric Illnesses in War Veterans

Neuropsychiatric sequelae are common in combat veterans. Although psychiatric and neurologic problems have been well documented in veterans of prior wars, the conflicts in Iraq and Afghanistan have been unique in terms of the level of commitment by the U.S. Department of Defense, Department of Veterans Affairs, and Veterans Health Administration to support research as the wars have unfolded, and to utilize that knowledge to guide population-level screening, evaluation, and treatment initiatives.

These conflicts, like previous ones, have produced hundreds of thousands of combat veterans, many of whom have received or will need care in government and civilian medical facilities. Two conditions in particular have been labeled the signature injuries related to these wars: post-traumatic stress disorder (PTSD) and mild traumatic brain injury (mTBI)—also known as concussion. Although particular emphasis will be given in this chapter to PTSD and concussion/mTBI, it is important to understand that service in all wars is associated with a number of health concerns that coexist and overlap, and a multidisciplinary patient-centered approach to care is necessary.

Chapter e49 Heavy Metal Poisoning

This chapter provides specific information about the four main heavy metals that pose a significant threat to health via occupational and environmental exposures: lead, mercury, arsenic, and cadmium. A table clearly details the main sources, metabolism, toxic effects produced, diagnosis, and appropriate therapy for poisoning from these metals.

Chapter e50 Poisoning and Drug Overdosage

This chapter provides comprehensive coverage of the dose-related adverse effects following exposure to chemicals, drugs, or other xenobiotics. The section on diagnosis gives thorough coverage of the physical examination, laboratory assessment, electrocardiographic and radiologic studies, and *toxicologic analysis.* The treatment section gives detailed coverage of the general principles of care, supportive care, prevention of poison absorption, enhancement of poison elimination, administration of antidotes, and prevention of reexposure.

Chapter e51 Altitude Illness

Altitude illness can be benign, occurring as acute mountain sickness, or life-threatening, manifesting as high-altitude pulmonary edema or high-altitude cerebral edema. This chapter details the clinical presentation and pathophysiology of altitude illness, providing strategies for its prevention and treatment. The chapter also discusses other problems unrelated to altitude illness (especially neurologic abnormalities) that may be caused by hypoxia at high altitudes. Finally, in line with the increasing popularity of travel to high-altitude locations, the chapter considers the special issues that must be taken into account when travelers have common preexisting conditions, such as hypertension, asthma, and coronary artery disease.

Chapter e52 Hyperbaric and Diving Medicine

This chapter describes the physical and pharmacologic mechanisms by which hyperbaric oxygen may modulate certain disease processes, and reviews the evidence in support of its use for specific clinical indications. Particular examples include selected problem wounds, delayed tissue injury after radiotherapy, and carbon monoxide poisoning. There is an overview of the highly specialized field of diving medicine, which includes a brief summary of key elements in pathophysiology, diagnosis, and treatment of decompression sickness.

Chapter e53 The Clinical Laboratory in Modern Health Care

The clinical laboratory plays a critical role in modern health care. This chapter describes the rationale for ordering laboratory tests, the use of critical values, the principles of laboratory-based diagnosis and reference range establishment, sources of error in the testing process, specific issues related to genetic testing, and the regulatory environment in which clinical laboratories operate in the United States.

Chapter e54 Clinical Procedure Tutorial: Central Venous Catheter Placement

Chapter e55 Clinical Procedure Tutorial: Thoracentesis

Chapter e56 Clinical Procedure Tutorial: Abdominal Paracentesis

Chapter e57 Clinical Procedure Tutorial: Endotracheal Intubation

Clinical procedures are an important component of medical student and resident training, and some are required for board and hospital certification. In these new *Harrison's* e-chapters, video tutorials are presented for performing abdominal paracentesis, thoracentesis, endotracheal intubation, and central venous catheter placement. These videos have been created specifically for *Harrison's*. Each includes the indications, contraindications, equipment, potential complications, and related patient safety considerations. Additional video tutorials covering clinical procedures such as breast biopsy, IV line insertion, phlebotomy, arterial line insertion, arthrocentesis, bone marrow biopsy, lumbar puncture, pelvic examination, thyroid aspiration, basic suturing, and urethral catheterization are available to subscribers of *Harrison's Online* and AccessMedicine (available at *www.accessmedicine.com*).

CONTRIBUTORS

James L. Abbruzzese, MD
Professor and Chair, Department of GI Medical Oncology; M.G. and Lillie Johnson Chair for Cancer Treatment and Research, University of Texas, MD Anderson Cancer Center, Houston, Texas [99]

Jamil Aboulhosn, MD
Assistant Professor, Departments of Medicine and Pediatrics, David Geffen School of Medicine, University of California, Los Angeles, Los Angeles, California [236]

John C. Achermann, MD, PhD
Wellcome Trust Senior Fellow, UCL Institute of Child Health, University College London, London, United Kingdom [349]

John W. Adamson, MD
Clinical Professor of Medicine, Department of Hematology/Oncology, University of California, San Diego, San Diego, California [57, 103]

Anthony A. Amato, MD
Professor of Neurology, Harvard Medical School; Department of Neurology, Brigham and Women's Hospital, Boston, Massachusetts [384, 385, 387]

Michael J. Aminoff, MD, DSc
Professor of Neurology, University of California, San Francisco School of Medicine, San Francisco, California [22, 23, e45]

Neil M. Ampel, MD
Professor of Medicine, University of Arizona, Tucson, Arizona [200]

Kenneth C. Anderson, MD
Kraft Family Professor of Medicine, Harvard Medical School; Chief, Jerome Lipper Multiple Myeloma Center, Dana-Farber Cancer Institute, Boston, Massachusetts [111, 113]

Elliott M. Antman, MD
Professor of Medicine, Harvard Medical School; Brigham and Women's Hospital; Boston, Massachusetts [243, 245]

Frederick R. Appelbaum, MD
Director, Division of Clinical Research, Fred Hutchinson Cancer Research Center, Seattle, Washington [114]

Gordon L. Archer, MD
Professor of Medicine and Microbiology/Immunology; Senior Associate Dean for Research and Research Training, Virginia Commonwealth University School of Medicine, Richmond, Virginia [133]

Cesar A. Arias, MD, PhD
Assistant Professor, University of Texas Medical School, Houston, Texas; Director, Molecular Genetics and Antimicrobial Resistance Unit, Universidad El Bosque, Bogotá, Colombia [137]

Wiebke Arlt, MD, DSc, FRCP, FMedSci
Professor of Medicine, Centre for Endocrinology, Diabetes and Metabolism, School of Clinical and Experimental Medicine, University of Birmingham; Consultant Endocrinologist, University Hospital Birmingham, Birmingham, United Kingdom [342]

Valder R. Arruda, MD, PhD
Associate Professor of Pediatrics, University of Pennsylvania School of Medicine; Division of Hematology, The Children's Hospital of Philadelphia, Philadelphia, Pennsylvania [116]

Arthur K. Asbury, MD, FRCP
Van Meter Professor Emeritus of Neurology, University of Pennsylvania School of Medicine, Philadelphia, Pennsylvania [23]

John R. Asplin, MD
Medical Director, Litholink Corporation; Chicago, Illinois [287]

John C. Atherton, MD, FRCP
Nottingham Digestive Diseases Centre Biomedical Research Unit (NDDC BRU), University of Nottingham and Nottingham University Hospitals NHS Trust, Nottingham, United Kingdom [151]

Evelyn Attia, MD
Professor of Clinical Psychiatry, Columbia College of Physicians and Surgeons; Weill Cornell Medical College, New York, New York [79]

Paul S. Auerbach, MD, MS
Redlich Family Professor, Department of Surgery, Division of Emergency Medicine, Stanford University School of Medicine, Palo Alto, California [396]

K. Frank Austen, MD
AstraZeneca Professor of Respiratory and Inflammatory Diseases; Director, Inflammation and Allergic Diseases Research Section, Harvard Medical School; Brigham and Women's Hospital, Boston, Massachusetts [317]

Eric H. Awtry, MD
Assistant Professor of Medicine, Boston University School of Medicine; Inpatient Clinical Director, Section of Cardiology, Boston Medical Center Boston, Massachusetts [240, e31]

Bruce R. Bacon, MD
James F. King, MD Endowed Chair in Gastroenterology; Professor of Internal Medicine, St. Louis University Liver Center, St. Louis University School of Medicine, St. Louis, Missouri [308, 309]

Lindsey R. Baden, MD
Associate Professor of Medicine, Harvard Medical School; Dana-Farber Cancer Institute, Brigham and Women's Hospital, Boston, Massachusetts [178]

John R. Balmes, MD
Professor of Medicine, San Francisco General Hospital, San Francisco, California [256]

Manisha Balwani, MD, MS
Assistant Professor, Department of Genetics and Genomic Sciences, Mount Sinai School of Medicine of New York University, New York, New York [358]

Peter A. Banks, MD
Professor of Medicine, Harvard Medical School; Senior Physician, Division of Gastroenterology, Brigham and Women's Hospital, Boston, Massachusetts [312, 313]

Robert L. Barbieri, MD
Kate Macy Ladd Professor of Obstetrics, Gynecology and Reproductive Biology, Harvard Medical School; Chairperson, Department of Obstetrics and Gynecology, Brigham and Women's Hospital, Boston, Massachusetts [7]

Joanne M. Bargman, MD, FRCPC
Professor of Medicine, University of Toronto; Staff Nephrologist, University Health Network; Director, Home Peritoneal Dialysis Unit and Co-Director, Renal Rheumatology Lupus Clinic, University Health Network, Toronto, Ontario, Canada [280]

Tamar F. Barlam, MD
Associate Professor of Medicine, Boston University School of Medicine, Boston, Massachusetts [121, 146]

Peter J. Barnes, DM, DSc, FMedSci, FRS
Head of Respiratory Medicine, Imperial College, London, United Kingdom [254]

Richard J. Barohn, MD
Chairman, Department of Neurology; Gertrude and Dewey Ziegler Professor of Neurology, University of Kansas Medical Center, Kansas City, Kansas [384]

Miriam J. Baron, MD
Assistant Professor of Medicine, Harvard Medical School; Associate Physician, Brigham and Women's Hospital, Boston, Massachusetts [127]

Rebecca M. Baron, MD
Assistant Professor, Harvard Medical School; Associate Physician, Department of Pulmonary and Critical Care Medicine, Brigham and Women's Hospital, Boston, Massachusetts [258]

John G. Bartlett, MD
Professor of Medicine and Chief, Division of Infectious Diseases, Department of Medicine, Johns Hopkins School of Medicine, Baltimore, Maryland [258]

Robert C. Basner, MD
Professor of Clinical Medicine, Division of Pulmonary, Allergy, and Critical Care Medicine, Columbia University College of Physicians and Surgeons, New York, New York [Appendix]

Buddha Basnyat, MD, MSc, FACP, FRCP(E)
Principal Investigator, Oxford University Clinical Research Unit-Patan Academy of Health Sciences; Medical Director, Nepal International Clinic, Kathmandu, Nepal [e51]

Shari S. Bassuk, ScD
Epidemiologist, Division of Preventive Medicine, Brigham and Women's Hospital, Boston, Massachusetts [348]

John F. Bateman, PhD
Director, Cell Biology, Development and Disease, Murdoch Childrens Research Institute, Parkville, Victoria, Australia [363]

David W. Bates, MD, MSc
Professor of Medicine, Harvard Medical School; Chief, General Internal Medicine and Primary Care Division, Brigham and Women's Hospital; Medical Director, Clinical and Quality Analysis, Partners HealthCare System, Inc., Boston, Massachusetts [10]

Robert P. Baughman, MD
Department of Internal Medicine, University of Cincinnati Medical Center, Cincinnati, Ohio [329]

M. Flint Beal, MD
Chairman of Neurology and Neuroscience; Neurologist-in-Chief, New York Presbyterian Hospital; Weill Cornell Medical College, New York, New York [366, 376]

Laurence H. Beck, Jr., MD, PhD
Assistant Professor of Medicine, Boston University School of Medicine, Boston, Massachusetts [285]

Nicholas J. Beeching, MA, BM BCh, FRCP, FRACP, FFTM RCPS (Glasg), DCH, DTM&H
Senior Lecturer (Clinical) in Infectious Diseases, Liverpool School of Tropical Medicine; Clinical Lead, Tropical and Infectious Disease Unit, Royal Liverpool University Hospital; Honorary Consultant, Health Protection Agency; Honorary Civilian Consultant in Infectious Diseases, Army Medical Directorate, Liverpool, United Kingdom [157]

Robert S. Benjamin, MD
P.H. and Fay E. Robinson Distinguished Professor and Chair, Department of Sarcoma Medical Oncology, University of Texas MD Anderson Cancer Center, Houston, Texas [98]

Michael H. Bennett, MD, MBBS
Conjoint Associate Professor in Anesthesia and Hyperbaric Medicine; Faculty of Medicine, University of New South Wales; Senior Staff Specialist, Department of Diving and Hyperbaric Medicine, Prince of Wales Hospital, Sydney, Australia [e52]

Edward J. Benz, Jr., MD
Richard and Susan Smith Professor of Medicine, Professor of Pediatrics, Professor of Genetics, Harvard Medical School; President and CEO, Dana-Farber Cancer Institute; Director, Dana-Farber/Harvard Cancer Center (DF/HCC), Boston, Massachusetts [104]

Jean Bergounioux, MD, PhD
Pediatric Intensive Care Unit, Hôpital Necker-Enfants Malades, Paris, France [154]

Joseph R. Betancourt, MD, MPH
Associate Professor of Medicine, Harvard Medical School; Director, The Disparities Solutions Center, Massachusetts General Hospital, Boston, Massachusetts [e4]

Atul K. Bhan, MBBS, MD
Professor of Pathology, Harvard Medical School; Director of Immunopathology, Department of Pathology, Massachusetts General Hospital, Boston, Massachusetts [e38]

Shalender Bhasin, MD
Professor of Medicine; Section Chief, Division of Endocrinology, Diabetes and Nutrition, Boston University School of Medicine, Boston, Massachusetts [346]

Deepak L. Bhatt, MD, MPH
Associate Professor of Medicine, Harvard Medical School; Chief of Cardiology, VA Boston Healthcare System; Director, Integrated Interventional Cardiovascular Program, Brigham and Women's Hospital and VA Boston Healthcare System; Senior Investigator, TIMI Study Group, Boston, Massachusetts [246, e33]

David R. Bickers, MD
Carl Truman Nelson Professor and Chair, Department of Dermatology, College of Physicians and Surgeons, Columbia University Medical Center; Dermatologist-in-Chief, New York Presbyterian Hospital, New York, New York [56]

Henry J. Binder, MD
Professor Emeritus of Medicine; Senior Research Scientist, Yale University, New Haven, Connecticut [294, e37]

William R. Bishai, MD, PhD
Professor and Co-Director, Center for Tuberculosis Research, Department of Medicine, Division of Infectious Diseases, Johns Hopkins University School of Medicine, Baltimore, Maryland [138]

Bruce R. Bistrian, MD, PhD
Professor of Medicine, Harvard Medical School; Chief, Clinical Nutrition, Beth Israel Deaconess Medical Center, Boston, Massachusetts [76]

Martin J. Blaser, MD
Frederick H. King Professor of Internal Medicine; Chair, Department of Medicine; Professor of Microbiology, New York University School of Medicine, New York, New York [151, 155]

Gijs Bleijenberg, PhD
Professor; Head, Expert Centre for Chronic Fatigue, Radboud University Nijmegen Medical Centre, Nijmegen, Netherlands [389]

Clara D. Bloomfield, MD
Distinguished University Professor; William G. Pace, III Professor of Cancer Research; Cancer Scholar and Senior Advisor, The Ohio State University Comprehensive Cancer Center; Arthur G. James Cancer Hospital and Richard J. Solove Research Institute, Columbus, Ohio [109]

Richard S. Blumberg, MD
Chief, Division of Gastroenterology, Brigham and Women's Hospital, Boston, Massachusetts [295]

Jean L. Bolognia, MD
Professor of Dermatology, Yale University School of Medicine, New Haven, Connecticut [53]

Joseph V. Bonventre, MD, PhD
Samuel A. Levine Professor of Medicine, Harvard Medical School; Chief, Renal Division; Chief, BWH HST Division of Bioengineering, Brigham and Women's Hospital, Boston, Massachusetts [279]

George J. Bosl, MD
Professor of Medicine, Weill Cornell Medical College; Chair, Department of Medicine; Patrick M. Byrne Chair in Clinical Oncology, Memorial Sloan-Kettering Cancer Center, New York, New York [96]

Richard C. Boucher, MD
Kenan Professor of Medicine, Pulmonary and Critical Care Medicine; Director, Cystic Fibrosis/Pulmonary Reseach and Treatment Center, University of North Carolina at Chapel Hill, Chapel Hill, North Carolina [259]

Eugene Braunwald, MD, MA (Hon), ScD (Hon) FRCP
Distinguished Hersey Professor of Medicine, Harvard Medical School; Founding Chairman, TIMI Study Group, Brigham and Women's Hospital, Boston, Massachusetts [36, 239, 244]

Irwin M. Braverman, MD
Professor of Dermatology, Yale University School of Medicine, New Haven, Connecticut [53]

Otis W. Brawley, MD
Chief Medical Officer, American Cancer Society Professor of Hematology, Oncology, Medicine, and Epidemiology, Emory University, Atlanta, Georgia [82]

Joel G. Breman, MD, DTPH
Scientist Emeritus, Fogarty International Center, National Institutes of Health, Bethesda, Maryland [210, e27]

George J. Brewer, MD
Morton S. and Henrietta K. Sellner Professor Emeritus of Human Genetics; Emeritus Professor of Internal Medicine, University of Michigan Medical School, Senior Vice President for Research and Development, Adeona Pharmaceuticals, Inc., Ann Arbor, Michigan [360]

Josephine P. Briggs, MD
Director, National Center for Complementary and Alternative Medicine, National Institutes of Health, Bethesda, Maryland [e2]

F. Richard Bringhurst, MD
Associate Professor of Medicine, Harvard Medical School; Physician, Massachusetts General Hospital, Boston, Massachusetts [352]

Steven M. Bromley, MD
Clinical Assistant Professor of Neurology, Department of Medicine, New Jersey School of Medicine and Dentistry–Robert Wood Johnson Medical School, Camden, New Jersey [29]

Kevin E. Brown, MD, MRCP, FRCPath
Consultant Medical Virologist, Virus Reference Department, Health Protection Agency, London, United Kingdom [184]

Robert H. Brown, Jr., MD, PhD
Chairman, Department of Neurology, University of Massachusetts Medical School, Worchester, Massachusetts [374, 387]

Amy E. Bryant, PhD
Research Scientist, Veterans Affairs Medical Center, Boise, Idaho; Affiliate Assistant Professor, University of Washington School of Medicine, Seattle, Washington [142]

Christopher M. Burns, MD
Assistant Professor, Department of Medicine, Section of Rheumatology, Dartmouth Medical School; Dartmouth Hitchcock Medical Center, Lebanon, New Hampshire [359]

David M. Burns, MD
Professor Emeritus, Department of Family and Preventive Medicine, University of California, San Diego School of Medicine, San Diego, California [395]

Stephen B. Calderwood, MD
Morton Swartz MD Academy Professor of Medicine (Microbiology and Molecular Genetics), Harvard Medical School; Chief, Division of Infectious Diseases, Massachusetts General Hospital, Boston, Massachusetts [128]

Michael V. Callahan, MD, DTM&H (UK), MSPH
Clinical Associate Physician, Division of Infectious Diseases, Massachusetts General Hospital, Boston, Massachusetts; Program Manager, Biodefense, Defense Advanced Research Project Agency (DARPA), United States Department of Defense, Washington, DC [18]

Michael Camilleri, MD
Atherton and Winifred W. Bean Professor; Professor of Medicine and Physiology, Mayo Clinic College of Medicine, Rochester, Minnesota [40]

Christopher P. Cannon, MD
Associate Professor of Medicine, Harvard Medical School; Senior Investigator, TIMI Study Group, Brigham and Women's Hospital, Boston, Massachusetts [244]

Jonathan Carapetis, PhD, MBBS, FRACP, FAFPHM
Director, Menzies School of Health Research, Charles Darwin University, Darwin, Australia [322]

Kathryn M. Carbone, MD
Deputy Scientific Director, Division of Intramural Research, National Institute of Dental and Craniofacial Research, Bethesda, Maryland [194]

Brian I. Carr, MD, PhD, FRCP
Professor of Oncology and Hepatology, IRCCS De Bellis Medical Research Institute, Castellana Grotte, Italy [92]

Arturo Casadevall, MD, PhD
Chair, Department of Microbiology and Immunology, Albert Einstein College of Medicine, Bronx, New York [202]

Agustin Castellanos, MD
Professor of Medicine, and Director, Clinical Electrophysiology, Division of Cardiology, University of Miami Miller School of Medicine, Miami, Florida [273]

Bartolome R. Celli, MD
Lecturer on Medicine, Harvard Medical School; Staff Physician, Division of Pulmonary and Critical Care Medicine, Brigham and Women's Hospital, Boston, Massachusetts [269]

Murali Chakinala, MD
Associate Professor of Medicine, Division of Pulmonary and Critical Care Medicine, Washington University School of Medicine, St. Louis, Missouri [234]

Anil Chandraker, MD, FASN, FRCP
Associate Professor of Medicine, Harvard Medical School; Medical Director of Kidney and Pancreas Transplantation; Assistant Director, Schuster Family Transplantation Research Center, Brigham and Women's Hospital; Children's Hospital, Boston, Massachusetts [282]

Stanley W. Chapman, MD
Professor of Medicine, University of Mississippi Medical Center, Jackson, Mississippi [201]

Panithaya Chareonthaitawee, MD
Associate Professor of Medicine, Mayo Clinic College of Medicine, Rochester, Minnesota [229, e29]

Lan X. Chen, MD, PhD
Penn Presbyterian Medical Center, Philadelphia, Pennsylvania [333]

Yuan-Tsong Chen, MD, PhD
Distinguished Research Fellow, Institute of Biomedical Sciences, Academia Sinica, Taiwan [362]

Glenn M. Chertow, MD, MPH
Norman S. Coplon/Satellite Healthcare Professor of Medicine; Chief, Division of Nephrology, Stanford University School of Medicine, Palo Alto, California [281]

John S. Child, MD, FACC, FAHA, FASE
Streisand Professor of Medicine and Cardiology, Geffen School of Medicine, University of California, Los Angeles (UCLA); Director, Ahmanson-UCLA Adult Congenital Heart Disease Center; Director, UCLA Adult Noninvasive Cardiodiagnostics Laboratory, Ronald Reagan-UCLA Medical Center; Los Angeles, California [236]

Augustine M. K. Choi, MD
Parker B. Francis Professor of Medicine, Harvard Medical School; Chief, Division of Pulmonary and Critical Care Medicine, Brigham and Women's Hospital, Boston, Massachusetts [251, 253, 268]

Irene Chong, MRCP, FRCR
Clinical Research Fellow, Royal Marsden NHS Foundation Trust, London and Sutton, United Kingdom [93]

Raymond T. Chung, MD
Associate Professor of Medicine, Harvard Medical School; Director of Hepatology; Vice Chief, Gastrointestinal Unit, Massachusetts General Hospital, Boston, Massachusetts [310]

Fredric L. Coe, MD
Professor of Medicine, University of Chicago, Chicago, Illinois [287]

Jeffrey I. Cohen, MD
Chief, Medical Virology Section, Laboratory of Clinical Infectious Diseases, National Institutes of Health, Bethesda, Maryland [181, 191]

Ronit Cohen-Poradosu, MD
Senior Physician, Department of Clinical Microbiology and Infectious Diseases, Hadassah Hebrew Medical Center, Jerusalem, Israel [164]

Francis S. Collins, MD, PhD
Director, National Institutes of Health, Bethesda, Maryland [83]

Wilson S. Colucci, MD
Thomas J. Ryan Professor of Medicine, Boston University School of Medicine; Chief of Cardiovascular Medicine, Boston Medical Center, Boston, Massachusetts [240, e31]

Darwin L. Conwell, MD
Associate Professor of Medicine, Harvard Medical School; Associate Physician, Division of Gastroenterology, Brigham and Women's Hospital, Boston, Massachusetts [312, 313]

Michael J. Corbel, PhD, DSc, FRCPath
Head, Division of Bacteriology, National Institute for Biological Standards and Control, Hertfordshire, United Kingdom [157]

William Edward Corcoran, V, MD
Clinical Instructor, Harvard Medical School; Cardiothoracic Fellow, Department of Anesthesiology, Perioperative, and Pain Medicine, Brigham and Women's Hospital, Boston, Massachusetts [e54]

Kathleen E. Corey, MD, MPH
Clinical and Research Fellow, Harvard Medical School; Fellow, Gastrointestinal Unit, Massachusetts General Hospital, Boston, Massachusetts [43]

Lawrence Corey, MD
Professor of Medicine and Laboratory Medicine and Head, Virology Division, Department of Laboratory Medicine, University of Washington; Head, Program in Infectious Diseases, Fred Hutchinson Cancer Research Center, Seattle, Washington [179]

Felicia Cosman, MD
Professor of Clinical Medicine, Columbia University College of Physicians and Surgeons, New York [354]

Mark A. Creager, MD
Professor of Medicine, Harvard Medical School; Simon C. Fireman Scholar in Cardiovascular Medicine; Director, Vascular Center, Brigham and Women's Hospital, Boston, Massachusetts [248, 249]

Leslie J. Crofford, MD
Gloria W. Singletary Professor of Internal Medicine; Chief, Division of Rheumatology, University of Kentucky, Lexington, Kentucky [335]

Jennifer M. Croswell, MD, MPH
Acting Director, Office of Medical Applications of Research, National Institutes of Health, Bethesda, Maryland [82]

Philip E. Cryer, MD
Irene E. and Michael M. Karl Professor of Endocrinology and Metabolism in Medicine, Washington University School of Medicine; Physician, Barnes-Jewish Hospital, St. Louis, Missouri [345]

David Cunningham, MD, FRCP
Professor of Cancer Medicine, Royal Marsden NHS Foundation Trust, London and Sutton, United Kingdom [93]

John J. Cush, MD
Director of Clinical Rheumatology, Baylor Research Institute, Dallas, Texas [331]

Charles A. Czeisler, MD, PhD, FRCP
Baldino Professor of Sleep Medicine; Director, Division of Sleep Medicine, Harvard Medical School; Chief, Division of Sleep Medicine, Department of Medicine, Brigham and Women's Hospital, Boston, Massachusetts [27]

Marinos C. Dalakas, MD, FAAN
Professor of Neurology, Department of Pathophysiology, National University of Athens Medical School, Athens, Greece [388]

Josep Dalmau, MD, PhD
ICREA Research Professor, Institute for Biomedical Investigations, August Pi i Sunyer (IDIBAPS)/Hospital Clinic, Department of Neurology, University of Barcelona, Barcelona, Spain; Adjunct Professor of Neurology University of Pennsylvania, Philadelphia, Pennsylvania [101]

Daniel F. Danzl, MD
University of Louisville, Department of Emergency Medicine, Louisville, Kentucky [19]

Robert B. Daroff, MD
Professor and Chair Emeritus, Department of Neurology, Case Western Reserve University School of Medicine; University Hospitals–Case Medical Center, Cleveland, Ohio [21]

Charles E. Davis, MD
Professor of Pathology and Medicine, Emeritus, University of California, San Diego School of Medicine; Director Emeritus, Microbiology, University of California, San Diego Medical Center, San Diego, California [e25]

Stephen N. Davis, MBBS, FRCP
Theodore E. Woodward Professor and Chairman, Department of Medicine, University of Maryland School of Medicine; Physician-in-Chief, University of Maryland Medical Center, Baltimore, Maryland [345]

Lisa M. DeAngelis, MD
Professor of Neurology, Weill Cornell Medical College; Chair, Department of Neurology, Memorial Sloan-Kettering Cancer Center, New York, New York [379]

John Del Valle, MD
Professor and Senior Associate Chair of Medicine, Department of Internal Medicine, University of Michigan School of Medicine, Ann Arbor, Michigan [293]

Marie B. Demay, MD
Professor of Medicine, Harvard Medical School; Physician, Massachusetts General Hospital, Boston, Massachusetts [352]

Bradley M. Denker, MD
Associate Professor, Harvard Medical School; Physician, Department of Medicine, Brigham and Women's Hospital; Chief of Nephrology, Harvard Vanguard Medical Associates, Boston, Massachusetts [44]

David W. Denning, MB BS, FRCP, FRCPath
Professor of Medicine and Medical Mycology; Director, National Aspergillosis Centre, The University of Manchester and Wythenshawe Hospital, Manchester, United Kingdom [204]

Robert J. Desnick, MD, PhD
Dean for Genetics and Genomics; Professor and Chairman, Department of Genetics and Genomic Sciences, Mount Sinai School of Medicine of New York University, New York, New York [358]

Richard A. Deyo, MD, MPH
Kaiser Permanente Professor of Evidence-Based Family Medicine, Department of Family Medicine, Department of Medicine, Department of Public Health and Preventive Medicine, Center for Research in Occupational and Environmental Toxicology, Oregon Health and Science University; Clinical Investigator, Kaiser Permanente Center for Health Research, Portland, Oregon [15]

Betty Diamond, MD
The Feinstein Institute for Medical Research, North Shore LIJ Health System; Center for Autoimmunity and Musculoskeletal Diseases, Manhasset, New York [318]

Jules L. Dienstag, MD
Carl W. Walter Professor of Medicine and Dean for Medical Education, Harvard Medical School; Physician, Gastrointestinal Unit, Department of Medicine, Massachusetts General Hospital, Boston, Massachusetts [304, 305, 306, 310, e38]

William P. Dillon, MD
Elizabeth Guillaumin Professor of Radiology, Neurology and Neurosurgery; Executive Vice-Chair, Department of Radiology and Biomedical Imaging, University of California, San Francisco, San Francisco, California [368, e44]

Charles A. Dinarello, MD
Professor of Medicine, Division of Infectious Diseases, University of Colorado School of Medicine, Aurora, Colorado [16]

Raphael Dolin, MD
Maxwell Finland Professor of Medicine (Microbiology and Molecular Genetics), Harvard Medical School; Beth Israel Deaconess Medical Center; Brigham and Women's Hospital, Boston, Massachusetts [178, 186, 187]

Richard L. Doty, PhD
Professor, Department of Otorhinolaryngology: Head and Neck Surgery; Director, Smell and Taste Center, University of Pennsylvania School of Medicine, Philadelphia, Pennsylvania [29]

Neil J. Douglas, MD, MB ChB, DSc, Hon MD, FRCPE
Professor of Respiratory and Sleep Medicine, University of Edinburgh, Edinburgh, Scotland, United Kingdom [265]

Daniel B. Drachman, MD
Professor of Neurology and Neuroscience, W. W. Smith Charitable Trust Professor of Neuroimmunology, Department of Neurology, Johns Hopkins School of Medicine, Baltimore, Maryland [386]

David F. Driscoll, PhD
Associate Professor of Medicine, University of Massachusetts Medical School, Worchester, Massachusetts [76]

Thomas D. DuBose, Jr., MD, MACP
Tinsley R. Harrison Professor and Chair, Internal Medicine; Professor of Physiology and Pharmacology, Department of Internal Medicine, Wake Forest University School of Medicine, Winston-Salem, North Carolina [47, e15]

J. Stephen Dumler, MD
Professor, Division of Medical Microbiology, Department of Pathology, Johns Hopkins University School of Medicine, Baltimore, Maryland [174]

Andrea Dunaif, MD
Charles F. Kettering Professor of Endocrinology and Metabolism; Vice-Chair for Research, Department of Medicine, Northwestern University Feinberg School of Medicine, Chicago, Illinois [6]

Samuel C. Durso, MD, MBA
Mason F. Lord Professor of Medicine; Director, Division of Geriatric Medicine and Gerontology, Johns Hopkins University School of Medicine, Baltimore, Maryland [32, e12]

Janice Dutcher, MD
Department of Oncology, New York Medical College, Montefiore, Bronx, New York [276]

Mark S. Dworkin, MD, MPH&TM
Associate Professor, Division of Epidemiology and Biostatistics, University of Illinois at Chicago School of Public Health, Chicago, Illinois [172]

Johanna Dwyer, DSc, RD
Professor of Medicine (Nutrition), Friedman School of Nutrition Science and Policy, Tufts University School of Medicine; Director, Frances Stern Nutrition Center, Tufts Medical Center, Boston, Massachusetts [73]

Jeffery S. Dzieczkowski, MD
Physician, St. Alphonsus Regional Medical Center; Medical Director, Coagulation Clinic, Saint Alphonsus Medical Group, International Medicine and Travel Medicine, Boise, Idaho [113]

Kim A. Eagle, MD
Albion Walter Hewlett Professor of Internal Medicine; Director, Cardiovascular Center, University of Michigan Health System, Ann Arbor, Michigan [8]

Robert H. Eckel, MD
Professor of Medicine, Division of Endocrinology, Metabolism and Diabetes, Division of Cardiology; Professor of Physiology and Biophysics, Charles A. Boettcher, II Chair in Atherosclerosis, University of Colorado School of Medicine, Anschutz Medical Campus, Director Lipid Clinic, University of Colorado Hospital, Aurora, Colorado [242]

John E. Edwards, Jr., MD
Chief, Division of Infectious Diseases, Harbor/University of California, Los Angeles (UCLA) Medical Center, Torrance, California; Professor of Medicine, David Geffen School of Medicine at UCLA, Los Angeles, California [198, 203]

David A. Ehrmann, MD
Professor of Medicine, The University of Chicago, Chicago, Illinois [49]

Andrew J. Einstein, MD, PhD
Assistant Professor of Clinical Medicine, Columbia University College of Physicians and Surgeons; Department of Medicine, Division of Cardiology, Department of Radiology, Columbia University Medical Center and New York-Presbyterian Hospital, New York, New York [Appendix]

Ezekiel J. Emanuel, MD, PhD
Chief, Department of Clinical Bioethics, National Institutes of Health, Bethesda, Maryland [9]

Joey D. English, MD
Assistant Clinical Professor, Department of Neurology, Univeristy of California, San Francisco, San Francisco, California [370]

John W. Engstrom, MD
Betty Anker Fife Distinguished Professor of Neurology; Neurology Residency Program Director; Clinical Chief of Service, University of California, San Francisco, San Francisco, California [15, 375]

Moshe Ephros, MD
Senior Lecturer, Faculty of Medicine, Technion—Israel Institute of Technology; Pediatric Infectious Disease Unit, Carmel Medical Center; Haifa, Israel [160]

Jonathan A. Epstein, MD, DTMH
William Wikoff Smith Professor of Medicine; Chairman, Department of Cell and Developmental Biology; Scientific Director, Cardiovascular Institute, University of Pennsylvania, Philadelphia, Pennsylvania [224]

Tim Evans, MD, PhD
Assistant Director-General, Information, Evidence, and Research, World Health Organization, Geneva, Switzerland [e1]

Christopher Fanta, MD
Associate Professor of Medicine, Harvard Medical School; Member, Pulmonary and Critical Care Division, Brigham and Women's Hospital, Boston, Massachusetts [34]

Paul Farmer, MD, PhD
Kolokotrones University Professor, Harvard University; Chair, Department of Global Health and Social Medicine, Harvard Medical School; Chief, Division of Global Health Equity, Brigham and Women's Hospital; Co-Founder, Partners in Health, Boston, Massachusetts [2]

Anthony S. Fauci, MD, DSc (Hon), DM&S (Hon), DHL (Hon), DPS (Hon), DLM (Hon), DMS (Hon)
Chief, Laboratory of Immunoregulation; Director, National Institute of Allergy and Infectious Diseases, National Institutes of Health, Bethesda, Maryland [1, 188, 189, 221, 314, 326, e40]

Murray J. Favus, MD
Professor, Department of Medicine, Section of Endocrinology, Diabetes and Metabolism, Director Bone Program, University of Chicago Pritzker School of Medicine, Chicago, Illinois [287, 355]

David P. Faxon, MD
Senior Lecturer, Harvard Medical School; Vice Chair of Medicine for Strategic Planning, Department of Medicine, Brigham and Women's Hospital, Boston, Massachusetts [230, 246, e33]

David T. Felson, MD, MPH
Professor of Medicine and Epidemiology; Chair, Clinical Epidemiology Unit, Boston University School of Medicine, Boston, Massachusetts [332]

Luigi Ferrucci, MD, PhD
Director, Baltimore Longitudinal Study of Aging National Institute of Health, Baltimore, Maryland [72]

Howard L. Fields, MD, PhD
Professor of Neurology, University of California, San Francisco, San Francisco, California [11]

Gregory A. Filice, MD
Professor of Medicine, University of Minnesota; Chief, Infectious Disease Section, Veterans Affairs Medical Center, Minneapolis, Minnesota [162]

Robert Finberg, MD
Chair, Department of Medicine, University of Massachusetts Medical School, Worcester, Massachusetts [86, 132]

Joyce Fingeroth, MD
Associate Professor of Medicine, Harvard Medical School, Boston, Massachusetts [132]

Kurt Fink, MD
Instructor in Anaesthesia, Harvard Medical School; Brigham and Women's Hospital, Boston, Massachusetts [e54]

Alain Fischer, MD, PhD
University Paris Descartes, Inserm Unit 768; Immunology and Pediatric Hematology Unit, Necker Children's Hospital, Paris, France [316, e39]

Jeffrey S. Flier, MD
Caroline Shields Walker Professor of Medicine and Dean, Harvard Medical School, Boston, Massachusetts [77]

Agnes B. Fogo, MD
John L. Shapiro Professor of Pathology; Professor of Medicine and Pediatrics, Vanderbilt University Medical Center, Nashville, Tennessee [e14]

Larry C. Ford, MD
Associate Researcher, Divisions of Clinical Epidemiology and Infectious Diseases, University of Utah, Salt Lake City, Utah [31]

Jane E. Freedman, MD
Professor, Department of Medicine, University of Massachusetts Medical School, Worcester, Massachusetts [117]

Roy Freeman, MBCHB
Professor of Neurology, Harvard Medical School, Boston, Massachusetts [20]

Gyorgy Frendl, MD, PhD
Assistant Professor of Anesthesia and Critical Care, Harvard Medical School; Director of Research, Surgical Critical Care, Brigham and Women's Hospital, Boston, Massachusetts [e54]

Carl E. Freter, MD, PhD
Professor, Department of Internal Medicine, Division of Hematology/Medical Oncology, University of Missouri; Ellis Fischel Cancer Center, Columbia, Missouri [102]

Lawrence S. Friedman, MD
Professor of Medicine, Harvard Medical School; Professor of Medicine, Tufts University School of Medicine; Assistant Chief of Medicine, Massachusetts General Hospital, Boston, Massachusetts; Chair, Department of Medicine, Newton-Wellesley Hospital, Newton, Massachusetts [43]

Sonia Friedman, MD
Assistant Professor of Medicine, Harvard Medical School, Boston, Massachusetts [295]

Anne L. Fuhlbrigge, MD, MS
Assistant Professor, Harvard Medical School; Pulmonary and Critical Care Division, Brigham and Women's Hospital, Boston, Massachusetts [253]

Andre Furtado, MD
Associate Specialist at the Department of Radiology, Neuroradiology Section, University of California, San Francisco, San Francisco, California [e44]

Robert F. Gagel, MD
Professor of Medicine and Head, Division of Internal Medicine, University of Texas MD Anderson Cancer Center, Houston, Texas [351]

Nicholas B. Galifianakis, MD, MPH
Assistant Clinical Professor, Surgical Movement Disorders Center, Department of Neurology, University of California, San Francisco, San Francisco, California [e8]

John I. Gallin, MD
Director, Clinical Center, National Institutes of Health, Bethesda, Maryland [60]

Charlotte A. Gaydos, DrPh, MPH, MS
Professor of Medicine, Johns Hopkins University School of Medicine, Baltimore, Maryland [176]

J. Michael Gaziano, MD, MPH
Professor of Medicine, Harvard Medical School; Chief, Division of Aging, Brigham and Women's Hospital; Director, Massachusetts Veterans Epidemiology Center, Boston VA Healthcare System, Boston, Massachusetts [225]

Thomas A. Gaziano, MD, MSc
Assistant Professor, Harvard Medical School; Assistant Professor, Health Policy and Management, Center for Health Decision Sciences, Harvard School of Public Health; Associate Physician in Cardiovascular Medicine, Department of Cardiology, Brigham and Women's Hospital, Boston, Massachusetts [225]

Susan L. Gearhart, MD
Assistant Professor of Colorectal Surgery and Oncology, The Johns Hopkins University School of Medicine, Baltimore, Maryland [297, 298]

Robert H. Gelber, MD
Clinical Professor of Medicine and Dermatology, University of California, San Francisco, San Francisco, California [166]

Jeffrey A. Gelfand, MD
Clinical Professor of Medicine, Harvard Medical School; Physician, Massachusetts General Hospital, Boston, Massachusetts [18, 211]

Alfred L. George, Jr., MD
Professor of Medicine and Pharmacology; Chief, Division of Genetic Medicine, Vanderbilt University School of Medicine, Nashville, Tennessee [277]

Dale N. Gerding, MD
Professor of Medicine, Loyola University Chicago Stritch School of Medicine; Associate Chief of Staff for Research and Development, Edward Hines, Jr. VA Hospital, Hines, Illinois [129]

Alicia K. Gerke, MD
Associate, Division of Pulmonary and Critical Care Medicine, University of Iowa, Iowa City, Iowa [255]

Michael Geschwind, MD, PhD
Associate Professor of Neurology, Memory and Aging Center, University of California, San Francisco, School of Medicine, San Francisco, California [e8]

Marc G. Ghany, MD, MHSc
Staff Physician, Liver Diseases Branch, National Institute of Diabetes and Digestive and Kidney Diseases, National Institutes of Health, Bethesda, Maryland [301]

Michael Giladi, MD, MSc
Associate Professor of Medicine, Faculty of Medicine, Tel Aviv University, Tel Aviv, Israel [160]

Bruce C. Gilliland,† MD
Professor of Medicine and Laboratory Medicine, University of Washington School of Medicine, Seattle, Washington [337]

Roger I. Glass, MD, PhD
Director, Fogarty International Center, Bethesda, Maryland [190]

Eli Glatstein, MD
Professor and Vice Chairman, Department of Radiation Oncology, Hospital of the University of Pennsylvania, Philadelphia, Pennsylvania [223]

Peter J. Goadsby, MD, PhD, DSc, FRACP FRCP
Professor of Neurology, University of California, San Francisco, California; Honorary Consultant Neurologist, Hospital for Sick Children, London, United Kingdom [14]

Ary L. Goldberger, MD
Professor of Medicine, Harvard Medical School; Wyss Institute for Biologically Inspired Engineering, Harvard University; Beth Israel Deaconess Medical Center, Boston, Massachusetts [228, e28, e30]

David Goldblatt, PhD, MBChB, FRCP, FRCPCH
Professor of Vaccinology and Immunology; Consultant in Paediatric Immunology; Director of Clinical Research and Development; Director, NIHR Biomedical Research Centre, Institute of Child Health; University College London; Great Ormond Street Hospital for Children NHS Trust, London, United Kingdom [134]

Samuel Z. Goldhaber, MD
Professor of Medicine, Harvard Medical School; Director, Venous Thromboembolism Research Group, Cardiovascular Division, Brigham and Women's Hospital, Boston, Massachusetts [262]

Ralph Gonzales, MD, MSPH
Professor of Medicine, University of California, San Francisco, San Francisco, California [31]

Douglas S. Goodin, MD
Professor of Neurology, University of California, San Francisco School of Medicine, San Francisco, California [380]

Craig E. Gordon, MD, MS
Assistant Professor of Medicine, Boston University School of Medicine; Attending, Section of Nephrology, Boston Medical Center, Boston, Massachusetts [284]

Jeffrey I. Gordon, MD
Dr. Robert J. Glaser Distinguished University Professor; Director, Center for Genome Sciences, Washington University School of Medicine, St. Louis, Missouri [64]

Maria Luisa Gorno-Tempini, MD, PhD
Associate Professor of Neurology, Memory and Aging Center, University of California, San Francisco, San Francisco, California [e10]

Gregory A. Grabowski, MD
Professor, Departments of Pediatrics, and Molecular Genetics, Biochemistry, and Microbiology; University of Cincinnati College of Medicine, A. Graeme Mitchell Chair in Human Genetics; Director, Division of Human Genetics, Cincinnati Children's Hosptial Medical Center, Cincinnati, Ohio [361]

Alexander R. Green, MD, MPH
Assistant Professor of Medicine, Harvard Medical School; Associate Director, The Disparities Solutions Center, Massachusetts General Hospital, Boston, Massachusetts [e4]

Norton J. Greenberger, MD
Clinical Professor of Medicine, Harvard Medical School; Senior Physician, Division of Gastroenterology, Brigham and Women's Hospital, Boston, Massachusetts [311, 312, 313]

†Deceased

CONTRIBUTORS

Daryl R. Gress, MD, FAAN, FCCM
Professor of Neurocritical Care and Stroke; Professor of Neurology, University of California, San Francisco, San Francisco, California [275]

Rasim Gucalp, MD
Professor of Clinical Medicine, Albert Einstein College of Medicine; Associate Chairman for Educational Programs, Department of Oncology; Director, Hematology/Oncology Fellowship, Montefiore Medical Center, Bronx, New York [276]

Kalpana Gupta, MD, MPH
Associate Professor, Department of Medicine, Boston University School of Medicine; Chief, Section of Infectious Diseases, VA Boston Healthcare System, Boston, Massachusetts [288]

John G. Haaga, MD
Deputy Associate Director, Behavioral and Social Research Program, National Institute on Aging, National Institutes of Health, Bethesda, Maryland [70]

Chadi A. Hage, MD
Assistant Professor of Medicine, Pulmonary–Critical Care and Infectious Diseases, Roudebush VA Medical Center; Indiana University, Indianapolis, Indiana [199]

Bevra Hannahs Hahn, MD
Professor of Medicine, University of California, Los Angeles, David Geffen School of Medicine, Los Angeles, California [319]

Janet E. Hall, MD, MSc
Professor of Medicine, Harvard Medical School; Associate Physician, Massachusetts General Hospital, Boston, Massachusetts [50, 347]

Jesse B. Hall, MD, FCCP
Professor of Medicine, Anesthesia and Critical Care; Chief, Section of Pulmonary and Critical Care Medicine, University of Chicago, Chicago, Illinois [267]

Scott A. Halperin, MD
Professor of Pediatrics and Microbiology and Immunology; CIHR/Wyeth Chair in Clinical Vaccine Research; Head, Pediatric Infectious Diseases; Director, Canadian Center for Vaccinology, Dalhousie University, Halifax, Nova Scotia, Canada [148]

R. Doug Hardy, MD
Associate Professor of Internal Medicine and Pediatrics, University of Texas Southwestern Medical Center, Dallas, Texas [175]

Raymond C. Harris, MD
Ann and Roscoe R. Robinson Professor of Medicine; Chief, Division of Nephrology, Vanderbilt University School of Medicine, Nashville, Tennessee [278]

William L. Hasler, MD
Professor of Internal Medicine, Division of Gastroenterology, University of Michigan Health System, Ann Arbor, Michigan [39, 290]

Terry Hassold, PhD
Eastlick Distinguished Professor; Director, Center for Reproductive Biology, Washington State University School of Molecular Biosciences, Pullman, Washington [62]

Stephen L. Hauser, MD
Robert A. Fishman Distinguished Professor and Chairman, Department of Neurology, University of California, San Francisco, San Francisco, California [1, 366, 367, 376, 377, 380, 385, e46]

Barton F. Haynes, MD
Frederic M. Hanes Professor of Medicine and Immunology, Departments of Medicine and Immunology; Director, Duke Human Vaccine Institute, Duke University School of Medicine, Durham, North Carolina [314]

Douglas C. Heimburger, MD, MS
Professor of Medicine; Associate Director for Education and Training, Vanderbilt Institute for Global Health, Vanderbilt University School of Medicine, Nashville, Tennessee [75]

J. Claude Hemphill, III, MD, MAS
Professor of Clinical Neurology and Neurological Surgery, Department of Neurology, University of California, San Francisco; Director of Neurocritical Care, San Francisco General Hospital, San Francisco, California [275]

Patrick H. Henry, MD
Clinical Adjunct Professor of Medicine, University of Iowa, Iowa City, Iowa [59]

Katherine A. High, MD
Investigator, Howard Hughes Medical Institute; William H. Bennett Professor of Pediatrics, University of Pennsylvania School of Medicine; Director, Center for Cellular and Molecular Therapeutics, Children's Hospital of Philadelphia, Philadelphia, Pennsylvania [68, 116]

Ikuo Hirano, MD
Professor of Medicine, Division of Gastroenterology and Hepatology, Department of Medicine, Northwestern University Feinberg School of Medicine, Chicago, Illinois [38, 292]

Martin S. Hirsch, MD
Professor of Medicine, Harvard Medical School; Professor of Immunology and Infectious Diseases, Harvard School of Public Health; Physician, Massachusetts General Hospital, Cambridge, Massachusetts [182]

Helen H. Hobbs, MD
Professor of Internal Medicine and Molecular Genetics, University of Texas Southwestern Medical Center, Dallas, Texas; Investigator, Howard Hughes Medical Institute, Chevy Chase, Maryland [356]

Judith S. Hochman, MD
Harold Snyder Family Professor of Cardiology; Clinical Chief, Leon Charney Division of Cardiology; Co-Director, NYU-HHC Clinical and Translational Science Institute; Director, Cardiovascular Clinical Research Center, New York University School of Medicine, New York, New York [272]

A. Victor Hoffbrand, DM
Professor Emeritus of Haematology, University College, London; Honorary Consultant Haematologist, Royal Free Hospital, London, United Kingdom [105]

David M. Hoganson, MD
Laboratory for Tissue Engineering and Organ Fabrication Center for Regenerative Medicine, Department of Surgery, Massachusetts General Hospital, Boston, Massachusetts [69]

Charles W. Hoge, MD
Senior Scientist and Staff Psychiatrist, Center for Psychiatry and Neuroscience, Walter Reed Army Institute of Research and Water Reed Army Medical Center, Silver Spring, Maryland [e48]

Elizabeth L. Hohmann, MD
Associate Professor of Medicine and Infectious Diseases, Harvard Medical School; Massachusetts General Hospital, Boston, Massachusetts [139]

Steven M. Holland, MD
Chief, Laboratory of Clinical Infectious Diseases, National Institute of Allergy and Infectious Diseases, National Institutes of Health, Bethesda, Maryland [60, 167]

King K. Holmes, MD, PhD
Chair, Global Health; Professor of Medicine and Global Health; Adjunct Professor, Epidemiology; Director, Center for AIDS and STD; University of Washington School of Medicine; Head, Infectious Diseases Section, Harborview Medical Center, Seattle, Washington [130]

Jay H. Hoofnagle, MD
Director, Liver Diseases Research Branch, National Institute of Diabetes, Digestive and Kidney Diseases, National Institutes of Health, Bethesda, Maryland [301]

Robert Hopkin, MD
Associate Professor of Clinical Pediatrics, University of Cincinnati College of Medicine; Division of Human Genetics, Cincinnati Children's Hospital Medical Center, Cincinnati, Ohio [361]

Leora Horn, MD, MSc
Division of Hematology and Medical Oncology, Vanderbilt University School of Medicine, Nashville, Tennessee [89]

Jonathan C. Horton, MD, PhD
William F. Hoyt Professor of Neuro-ophthalmology, Professor of Ophthalmology, Neurology and Physiology, University of California, San Francisco School of Medicine, San Francisco, California [28]

Howard Hu, MD
Environmental Health Sciences, University of Michigan Schools of Public Health and Medicine, Ann Arbor, Michigan [e49]

Gary W. Hunninghake, MD
Professor, Division of Pulmonary and Critical Care Medicine, University of Iowa, Iowa City, Iowa [255]

Sharon A. Hunt, MD, FACC
Professor, Division of Cardiovascular Medicine, Stanford University, Palo Alto, California [235]

Charles G. Hurst, MD
Chief, Chemical Casualty Care Division, United States Medical Research Institute of Chemical Defense, APG-Edgewood Area, Maryland [222]

Ashraf S. Ibrahim, PhD
Associate Professor of Medicine, Geffen School of Medicine, University of California, Los Angeles (UCLA); Division of Infectious Diseases, Los Angeles Biomedical Research Institute at Harbor–UCLA Medical Center, Torrance, California [205]

David H. Ingbar, MD
Professor of Medicine, Pediatrics, and Physiology; Director, Pulmonary Allergy, Critical Care and Sleep Division, University of Minnesota School of Medicine, Minneapolis, Minnesota [272]

Alan C. Jackson, MD, FRCPC
Professor of Medicine (Neurology) and Medical Microbiology, University of Manitoba; Section Head of Neurology, Winnipeg Regional Health Authority, Winnipeg, Manitoba, Canada [195]

Lisa A. Jackson, MD, MPH
Senior Investigator, Group Health Research Institute; Research Professor, Department of Epidemiology; Adjunct Professor, Department of Medicine, University of Washington, Seattle, Washington [122]

Richard F. Jacobs, MD
Robert H. Fiser, Jr., MD Endowed Chair in Pediatrics; Professor and Chairman, Department of Pediatrics, University of Arkansas for Medical Sciences; President, Arkansas Children's Hospital Research Institute, Little Rock, Arkansas [158]

J. Larry Jameson, MD, PhD
Robert G. Dunlop Professor of Medicine; Dean, University of Pennsylvania School of Medicine; Executive Vice President of the University of Pennsylvania for the Health System, Philadelphia, Pennsylvania [1, 61, 63, 80, 100, 338, 339, 341, 346, 349, e41]

Robert T. Jensen, MD
Digestive Diseases Branch, National Institute of Diabetes; Digestive and Kidney Diseases, National Institutes of Health, Bethesda, Maryland [350]

David H. Johnson, MD, FACP
Donald W. Seldin Distinguished Chair in Internal Medicine; Professor and Chairman, Department of Internal Medicine, University of Texas Southwestern Medical School, Dallas, Texas [89]

James R. Johnson, MD
Professor of Medicine, University of Minnesota, Minneapolis, Minnesota [149]

Stuart Johnson, MD
Associate Professor of Medicine, Loyola University Chicago Stritch School of Medicine; Staff Physician, Edward Hines, Jr. VA Hospital, Hines, Illinois [129]

S. Claiborne Johnston, MD, PhD
Professor of Neurology and Epidemiology, University of California, San Francisco School of Medicine, San Francisco, California [370]

S. Andrew Josephson, MD
Associate Professor, Department of Neurology; Director, Neurohospitalist Program, University of California, San Francisco, San Francisco, California [25, e47]

Harald Jüppner, MD
Professor of Pediatrics, Endocrine Unit and Pediatric Nephrology Unit, Massachusetts General Hospital, Boston, Massachusetts [353]

Peter J. Kahrilas, MD
Gilbert H. Marquardt Professor in Medicine, Division of Gastroenterology, Department of Medicine, Northwestern University Feinberg School of Medicine, Chicago, Illinois [38, 292]

Gail Kang, MD
Assistant Clinical Professor of Neurology, Memory and Aging Center, University of California, San Francisco, San Francisco, California [e8]

Marshall M. Kaplan, MD
Professor of Medicine, Tufts University School of Medicine, Boston, Massachusetts [42, 302]

Adolf W. Karchmer, MD
Professor of Medicine, Harvard Medical School; Division of Infectious Diseases, Beth Israel Deaconess Medical Center, Boston, Massachusetts [124]

Dennis L. Kasper, MD, MA (Hon)
William Ellery Channing Professor of Medicine and Professor of Microbiology and Molecular Genetics, Harvard Medical School; Director, Channing Laboratory, Department of Medicine, Brigham and Women's Hospital, Boston, Massachusetts [1, 119, 121, 127, 146, 164]

Lloyd H. Kasper, MD
Professor of Medicine (Neurology) and Microbiology and Immunology, Dartmouth Medical School, Lebanon, New Hampshire [214]

Daniel L. Kastner, MD, PhD
Scientific Director, National Human Genome Research Institute, National Institutes of Health, Bethesda, Maryland [330]

Carol A. Kauffman, MD
Professor of Internal Medicine, University of Michigan Medical School; Chief, Infectious Diseases Section, Veterans Affairs Ann Arbor Healthcare System, Ann Arbor, Michigan [206]

Elaine T. Kaye, MD
Assistant Clinical Professor of Dermatology, Harvard Medical School, Boston, Massachusetts [17, e7]

Kenneth M. Kaye, MD
Associate Professor of Medicine, Harvard Medical School, Boston, Massachusetts [17, e7]

John A. Kessler, MD
Professor and Chair, Department of Neurology, Northwestern University Feinberg School of Medicine, Chicago, Illinois [67]

Jay S. Keystone, MD, FRCPC, MSc (CTM)
Professor of Medicine, University of Toronto, Toronto, Ontario, Canada [123]

Sundeep Khosla, MD
Professor of Medicine and Physiology, College of Medicine, Mayo Clinic, Rochester, Minnesota [46]

Elliott Kieff, MD, PhD
Harriet Ryan Albee Professor, Harvard Medical School; Chief, Infectious Diseases Division, Brigham and Women's Hospital, Boston, Massachusetts [177]

Anthony A. Killeen, MD, PhD
Associate Professor; Director of Clinical Laboratories, University of Minnesota Medical Center, Minneapolis, Minnesota [e53]

Jim Yong Kim, MD, PhD
Chair, Department of Global Health and Social Medicine, Harvard Medical School; Director, François-Xavier Bagnoud Center for Health and Human Rights, Harvard School of Public Health; Chief, Division of Global Health Equity, Brigham and Women's Hospital, Boston, Massachusetts [2]

Kami Kim, MD
Professor of Medicine (Infectious Diseases) and of Microbiology and Immunology, Albert Einstein College of Medicine, Bronx, New York [214]

Lindsay King, MD
Clinical and Research Fellow, Department of Medicine, Gastrointestinal Unit, Massachusetts General Hospital, Boston, Massachusetts [e56]

Talmadge E. King, Jr., MD
Julius R. Krevans Distinguished Professor in Internal Medicine; Chair, Department of Medicine, University of California, San Francisco, San Francisco, California [261]

Louis V. Kirchhoff, MD, MPH
Professor of Internal Medicine (Infectious Diseases) and Epidemiology, Department of Internal Medicine, The University of Iowa, Iowa City, Iowa [213]

Priya S. Kishnani, MD
Professor of Pediatrics, Duke University Medical Center, Durham, North Carolina [362]

Rob Knight, PhD
Assistant Professor, Department of Chemistry and Biochemistry, University of Colorado, Boulder, Colorado [64]

Minoru S. H. Ko, MD, PhD
Senior Investigator and Chief, Developmental Genomics and Aging Section, Laboratory of Genetics, National Institute on Aging, National Institutes of Health, Baltimore, Maryland [65]

Barbara Konkle, MD
Professor of Medicine, Hematology, University of Washington; Director, Translational Research, Puget Sound Blood Center, Seattle, Washington [58, 115]

Peter Kopp, MD
Associate Professor, Division of Endocrinology, Metabolism and Molecular Science, Northwestern University Feinberg School of Medicine, Chicago, Illinois [61]

Walter J. Koroshetz, MD
National Institute of Neurological Disorders and Stroke, National Institutes of Health, Bethesda, Maryland [382]

Thomas R. Kosten, MD
Baylor College of Medicine; Veteran's Administration Medical Center, Houston, Texas [393]

Theodore A. Kotchen, MD
Professor Emeritus, Department of Medicine; Associate Dean for Clinical Research, Medical College of Wisconsin, Milwaukee, Wisconsin [247]

Phyllis E. Kozarsky, MD
Professor of Medicine and Infectious Diseases, Emory University School of Medicine, Atlanta, Georgia [123]

Barnett S. Kramer, MD, MPH
Associate Director for Disease Prevention, Office of Disease Prevention, National Institutes of Health, Bethesda, Maryland [82]

Joel Kramer, PsyD
Clinical Professor of Neuropsychology in Neurology; Director of Neuropsychology, Memory and Aging Center, University of California, San Francisco, San Francisco, California [e10]

Stephen M. Krane, MD
Persis, Cyrus and Marlow B. Harrison Distinguished Professor of Medicine, Harvard Medical School; Massachusetts General Hospital, Boston, Massachusetts [352]

Alexander Kratz, MD, PhD, MPH
Associate Professor of Pathology and Cell Biology, Columbia University College of Physicians and Surgeons; Director, Core Laboratory, Columbia University Medical Center, New York, New York [Appendix]

John P. Kress, MD
Associate Professor of Medicine, Section of Pulmonary and Critical Care, University of Chicago, Chicago, Illinois [267]

Patricia Kritek, MD, EdM
Associate Professor, Division of Pulmonary and Critical Care Medicine, University of Washington, Seattle, Washington [34, 251, e34]

Henry M. Kronenberg, MD
Professor of Medicine, Harvard Medical School; Chief, Endocrine Unit, Massachusetts General Hospital, Boston, Massachusetts [352]

Robert F. Kushner, MD, MS
Professor of Medicine, Northwestern University Feinberg School of Medicine, Chicago, Illinois [78]

Loren Laine, MD
Professor of Medicine, University of Southern California Keck School of Medicine, Los Angeles, California [41]

Anil K. Lalwani, MD
Professor, Departments of Otolaryngology, Pediatrics, and Physiology and Neuroscience, New York University School of Medicine, New York, New York [30]

H. Clifford Lane, MD
Clinical Director; Director, Division of Clinical Research; Deputy Director, Clinical Research and Special Projects; Chief, Clinical and Molecular Retrovirology Section, Laboratory of Immunoregulation, National Institute of Allergy and Infectious Diseases, National Institutes of Health, Bethesda, Maryland [189, 221]

Carol A. Langford, MD, MHS
Director, Center for Vasculitis Care and Research, Department of Rheumatic and Immunologic Diseases, Cleveland Clinic, Cleveland, Ohio [326, 328, 336, 337, e40]

Regina C. LaRocque, MD
Assistant Professor of Medicine, Harvard Medical School; Assistant Physician, Massachusetts General Hospital, Boston, Massachusetts [128]

Wei C. Lau, MD
Associate Professor, Medical Director, Cardiovascular Center Operating Rooms; Director, Adult Cardiovascular and Thoracic Anesthesiology, University of Michigan Health System, Ann Arbor, Michigan [8]

Leslie P. Lawley, MD
Assistant Professor, Department of Dermatology, School of Medicine, Emory University, Atlanta, Georgia [52]

Thomas J. Lawley, MD
William P. Timmie Professor of Dermatology, Dean, Emory University School of Medicine, Atlanta, Georgia [51, 52, 54, e16]

Thomas H. Lee, MD, MSc
Professor of Medicine, Harvard Medical School; Network President, Partners Healthcare System, Boston, Massachusetts [12]

Jane A. Leopold, MD
Associate Professor of Medicine, Harvard Medical School; Brigham and Women's Hospital, Boston, Massachusetts [230, e33]

Nelson Leung, MD
Associate Professor of Medicine, Department of Nephrology and Hypertension, Division of Hematology, Mayo Clinic, Rochester, Minnesota [286]

Bruce D. Levy, MD
Associate Professor of Medicine, Harvard Medical School; Pulmonary and Critical Care Medicine, Brigham and Women's Hospital, Boston, Massachusetts [268]

Julia B. Lewis, MD
Professor, Department of Medicine, Division of Nephrology, Vanderbilt University Medical Center, Nashville, Tennessee [283]

Peter Libby, MD
Mallinckrodt Professor of Medicine, Harvard Medical School; Chief, Cardiovascular Medicine, Brigham and Women's Hospital, Boston, Massachusetts [224, 241, e32]

Richard W. Light, MD
Professor of Medicine, Division of Allergy, Pulmonary, and Critical Care Medicine, Vanderbilt University, Nashville, Tennessee [263]

Julie Lin, MD, MPH
Assistant Professor of Medicine, Harvard Medical School, Boston, Massachusetts [44]

Robert Lindsay, MD, PhD
Chief, Internal Medicine; Professor of Clinical Medicine, Helen Hayes Hospital, West Haverstraw, New York [354]

Marc E. Lippman, MD, MACP
Kathleen and Stanley Glaser Professor; Chairman, Department of Medicine, Deputy Director, Sylvester Comprehensive Cancer Center, University of Miami Miller School of Medicine, Miami, Florida [90]

Peter E. Lipsky, MD
Charlottesville, Virginia [318, 331]

Kathleen D. Liu, MD, PhD, MAS
Assistant Professor, Divisions of Nephrology and Critical Care Medicine, Departments of Medicine and Anesthesia, University of California, San Francisco, San Francisco, California [281]

Bernard Lo, MD
Professor of Medicine; Director, Program in Medical Ethics, University of California, San Francisco, San Francisco, California [e5]

Dan L. Longo, MD
Professor of Medicine, Harvard Medical School; Senior Physician, Brigham and Women's Hospital; Deputy Editor, New England Journal of Medicine, Boston, Massachusetts
[1, 57, 59, 66, 81, 84, 85, 100, 102, 110, 111, 188, e6, e17, e20, e21]

Nicola Longo, MD, PhD, MACP
Professor of Pediatrics; Chief, Division of Medical Genetics, Department of Pediatrics, University of Utah, Salt Lake City, Utah [364, 365]

Joseph Loscalzo, MD, PhD
Hersey Professor of the Theory and Practice of Medicine, Harvard Medical School; Chairman, Department of Medicine; Physician-in-Chief, Brigham and Women's Hospital, Boston, Massachusetts [1, 35, 36, 37, 117, 224, 226, 227, 237, 238, 243, 245, 248, 249, e13, e19]

Phillip A. Low, MD
Robert D. and Patricia E. Kern Professor of Neurology, Mayo Clinic College of Medicine, Rochester, Minnesota [375]

Daniel H. Lowenstein, MD
Dr. Robert B. and Mrs. Ellinor Aird Professor of Neurology; Director, Epilepsy Center, University of California, San Francisco, San Francisco, California [367, 369, e42]

Elyse E. Lower, MD
Medical Oncology and Hematology, University of Cincinnati; Oncology Hematology Care, Inc., Cincinnati, Ohio [329]

Franklin D. Lowy, MD
Professor of Medicine and Pathology, Columbia University College of Physicians and Surgeons, New York, New York [135]

Sheila A. Lukehart, PhD
Professor, Departments of Medicine and Global Health, University of Washington, Seattle, Washington [169, 170]

Lucio Luzzatto, MD, FRCP, FRCPath
Professor of Haematology, University of Genova, Scientific Director Istituto Toscano Tumori, Italy [106]

Lawrence C. Madoff, MD
Professor of Medicine, University of Massachusetts Medical School, Worcester, Massachusetts; Director, Division of Epidemiology and Immunization, Massachusetts Department of Public Health, Jamaica Plain, Massachusetts [119, 334, e23, e24]

Emily Nelson Maher, MD
Clinical Instructor, Department of Anesthesiology, Harvard Medical School; Brigham and Women's Hospital, Boston, Massachusetts [e57]

Adel A. F. Mahmoud, MD, PhD
Professor, Department of Molecular Biology and the Woodrow Wilson School of Public and International Affairs, Princeton University, Princeton, New Jersey [219]

Ronald V. Maier, MD
Jane and Donald D. Trunkey Professor and Vice-Chair, Surgery, University of Washington; Surgeon-in-Chief, Harborview Medical Center, Seattle, Washington [270]

Mark E. Mailliard, MD
Frederick F. Paustian Professor; Chief, Division of Gastroenterology and Hepatology, Department of Internal Medicine, University of Nebraska College of Medicine, Omaha, Nebraska [307]

Hari R. Mallidi, MD
Assistant Professor of Cardiothoracic Surgery; Director of Mechanical Circulatory Support, Stanford University Medical Center, Stanford, California [235]

Hanna Mandel, MD
Director, Pediatric Metabolic Disorders, Rambam Health Care Campus, Haifa, Israel [e18]

Brian F. Mandell, MD, PhD, MACP, FACR
Professor and Chairman of Medicine, Cleveland Clinic Lerner College of Medicine; Department of Rheumatic and Immunologic Disease, Cleveland Clinic, Cleveland, Ohio [336]

Lionel A. Mandell, MD, FRCP(C), FRCP(LOND)
Professor of Medicine, McMaster University, Hamilton, Ontario, Canada [257]

Douglas L. Mann, MD
Lewin Chair and Chief, Cardiovascular Division; Professor of Medicine, Cell Biology and Physiology, Washington University School of Medicine, St. Louis, Missouri [234]

JoAnn E. Manson, MD, DrPH
Professor of Medicine and the Michael and Lee Bell Professor of Women's Health, Harvard Medical School; Chief, Division of Preventive Medicine, Brigham and Women's Hospital, Boston, Massachusetts [348]

Eleftheria Maratos-Flier, MD
Associate Professor of Medicine, Harvard Medical School; Division of Endocrinology, Beth Israel Deaconess Medical Center, Boston, Massachusetts [77]

Francis Marchlinski, MD
Professor of Medicine; Director, Cardiac Electrophysiology, University of Pennsylvania Health System, Philadelphia, Pennsylvania [233]

Guido Marcucci, MD
Professor of Medicine; John B. and Jane T. McCoy Chair in Cancer Research; Associate Director of Translational Research, Comprehensive Cancer Center, The Ohio State University College of Medicine, Columbus, Ohio [109]

Daniel B. Mark, MD, MPH
Professor of Medicine, Duke University Medical Center; Director, Outcomes Research, Duke Clinical Research Institute, Durham, North Carolina [3]

Alexander G. Marneros, MD, PhD
Assistant Professor, Department of Dermatology, Harvard Medical School Boston, Massachusetts; Cutaneous Biology Research Center, Massachusetts General Hospital, Charlestown, Massachusetts [56]

Jeanne M. Marrazzo, MD, MPH
Associate Professor of Medicine, Division of Infectious Diseases, Harborview Medical Center, Seattle, Washington [130]

Thomas Marrie, MD
Dean, Faculty of Medicine, Dalhousie University, Halifax, Nova Scotia, Canada [174]

Gary J. Martin, MD
Raymond J. Langenbach, MD Professor of Medicine; Vice Chairman for Faculty Affairs, Department of Medicine, Northwestern University Feinberg School of Medicine, Chicago, Illinois [4]

George M. Martin, MD
Professor of Pathology Emeritus, Adjunct Professor of Genome Sciences (Retired), University of Washington, Seattle, Washington; Visiting Scholar, Molecular Biology Institute, University of California at Los Angeles, Los Angeles, California [71]

Joseph B. Martin, MD, PhD
Edward R. and Anne G. Lefler Professor, Department of Neurobiology, Harvard Medical School, Boston, Massachusetts [367]

Matthew Martinez, MD
Lehigh Valley Physician Group, Lehigh Valley Heart Specialists, Allentown, Pennsylvania [229, e29]

Susan Maslanka, PhD
Enteric Diseases Laboratory Branch, Centers for Disease Control and Prevention, Atlanta, Georgia [141]

Robert J. Mayer, MD
Stephen B. Kay Family Professor of Medicine, Harvard Medical School, Boston, Massachusetts [91]

Alexander J. McAdam, MD, PhD
Assistant Professor of Pathology, Harvard Medical School, Children's Hospital, Boston, Massachusetts [e22]

Calvin O. McCall, MD
Associate Professor, Department of Dermatology, Virginia Commonwealth University Medical Center; Chief, Dermatology Section, Hunter Holmes McGuire Veterans Affairs Medical Center, Richmond, Virginia [52]

John F. McConville, MD
Assistant Professor of Medicine, University of Chicago, Chicago, Illinois [264]

Kevin T. McVary, MD, FACS
Professor of Urology, Department of Urology, Northwestern University Feinberg School of Medicine, Chicago, Illinois [48]

Nancy K. Mello, PhD
Professor of Psychology (Neuroscience), Harvard Medical School, Boston, Massachusetts; Director, Alcohol and Drug Abuse Research Center, McLean Hospital, Belmont, Massachusetts [394]

Shlomo Melmed, MD
Senior Vice President and Dean of the Medical Faculty, Cedars-Sinai Medical Center, Los Angeles, California [339]

Jack H. Mendelson,† MD
Professor of Psychiatry (Neuroscience), Harvard Medical School, Belmont, Massachusetts [394]

Robert O. Messing, MD
Professor, Department of Neurology; Senior Associate Director, Ernest Gallo Clinic and Research Center, University of California, San Francisco, San Francisco, California [390]

M.-Marsel Mesulam, MD
Professor of Neurology, Psychiatry and Psychology, Cognitive Neurology and Alzheimer's Disease Center, Northwestern University Feinberg School of Medicine, Chicago, Illinois [26]

Susan Miesfeldt, MD
Mercy Hospital, Maine Centers for Cancer Medicine, Scarbrough, Maine [63]

Edgar L. Milford, MD
Associate Professor of Medicine, Harvard Medical School; Director, Tissue Typing Laboratory, Brigham and Women's Hospital, Boston, Massachusetts [282]

Bruce L. Miller, MD
AW and Mary Margaret Clausen Distinguished Professor of Neurology, University of California, San Francisco School of Medicine, San Francisco, California [25, 371, 383, e9, e10]

Samuel I. Miller, MD
Professor of Genome Sciences, Medicine, and Microbiology, University of Washington, Seattle, Washington [153]

Simon J. Mitchell, MB ChB, PhD
Associate Professor in Anesthesiology, Diving and Hyperbaric Medicine, Faculty of Medical and Health Sciences, University of Auckland; Consultant Anesthetist, Auckland City Hospital, Auckland, New Zealand [e52]

Thomas A. Moore, MD, FACP, FIDSA
Chairman, Department of Infectious Diseases, Ochsner Health System, New Orleans, Louisiana [208, e26]

Pat J. Morin, PhD
Senior Investigator, Laboratory of Molecular Biology and Immunology, National Institute on Aging, National Institutes of Health, Baltimore, Maryland [83]

Charles A. Morris, MD, MPH
Instructor in Medicine, Harvard Medical School; Associate Physician, Brigham and Women's Hospital, Boston, Massachusetts [e55, e57]

William J. Moss, MD, MPH
Associate Professor, Departments of Epidemiology, International Health, and Molecular Microbiology and Immunology, Johns Hopkins Bloomberg School of Public Health, Baltimore, Maryland [192]

Robert J. Motzer, MD
Professor of Medicine, Weill Cornell Medical College; Attending Physician, Genitourinary Oncology Service, Memorial Sloan-Kettering Cancer Center, New York, New York [94, 96]

David B. Mount, MD, FRCPC
Assistant Professor of Medicine, Harvard Medical School, Renal Division, VA Boston Healthcare System; Brigham and Women's Hospital, Boston, Massachusetts [45, e15]

Haralampos M. Moutsopoulos, MD, FACP, FRCP, Master ACR
Professor and Director, Department of Pathophysiology, Medical School, National University of Athens, Athens, Greece [320, 324, 327]

†Deceased

Robert S. Munford, MD
Bethesda, Maryland [271]

Nikhil C. Munshi, MD
Associate Professor of Medicine, Harvard Medical School; Associate Director, Jerome Lipper Multiple Myeloma Center, Dana Farber Cancer Institute, Boston, Massachusetts [111]

John R. Murphy, PhD
Professor of Medicine and Microbiology, Boston University School of Medicine, Boston, Massachusetts [138]

Timothy F. Murphy, MD
UB Distinguished Professor of Medicine and Microbiology, University of Buffalo, State University of New York, Buffalo, New York [145]

Barbara E. Murray, MD
J. Ralph Meadows Professor and Director, Division of Infectious Diseases, University of Texas Medical School, Houston, Texas [137]

Joseph A. Murray, MD
Professor of Medicine, Departments of Internal Medicine and Immunology, Mayo Clinic, Rochester, Minnesota [40]

Mark B. Mycyk, MD
Associate Professor, Department of Emergency Medicine, Boston University School of Medicine; Associate Professor, Department of Emergency Medicine; Rush University School of Medicine, Research Director, Division of Toxicology, Cook County Hospital, Chicago, Illinois [e50]

Robert J. Myerburg, MD
Professor, Departments of Medicine and Physiology, Division of Cardiology; AHA Chair in Cardiovascular Research, University of Miami Miller School of Medicine, Miami, Florida [273]

Hari Nadiminti, MD
Clinical Instructor, Department of Dermatology, Emory University School of Medicine, Atlanta, Georgia [87]

Edward T. Naureckas, MD
Associate Professor of Medicine, Section of Pulmonary and Critical Care Medicine, University of Chicago, Chicago, Illinois [252]

Eric G. Neilson, MD
Thomas Fearn Frist Senior Professor of Medicine and Cell and Developmental Biology, Vanderbilt University School of Medicine, Nashville, Tennessee [277, 278, 283, e14]

Gerald T. Nepom, MD, PhD
Director, Benaroya Research Institute at Virginia Mason; Director, Immune Tolerance Network; Professor, University of Washington School of Medicine, Seattle, Washington [315]

Eric J. Nestler, MD, PhD
Nash Family Professor and Chair, Department of Neuroscience; Director, Friedman Brain Institute, Mount Sinai School of Medicine, New York, New York [390]

Hartmut P. H. Neumann, MD
Head, Section Preventative Medicine, Department of Nephrology and General Medicine, Albert-Ludwigs-University of Freiburg, Germany [343]

Joseph P. Newhouse, PhD
John D. MacArthur Professor of Health Policy and Management, Department of Health Care Policy, Harvard Medical School; Department of Health Policy and Management, Harvard School of Public Health, Harvard Kennedy School; Faculty of Arts and Sciences, Harvard University, Boston, Massachusetts [e3]

Jonathan Newmark, MD
Colonel, Medical Corps, US Army; Deputy Joint Program Executive Officer, Medical Systems, Joint Program Executive Office for Chemical/Biological Defense, US Department of Defense, Falls Church, Virginia; Chemical Casualty Care Consultant to the US Army Surgeon General; Adjunct Professor of Neurology, F. Edward Hebert School of Medicine, Uniformed Services University of the Health Sciences, Bethesda, Maryland [222]

Rick A. Nishimura, MD, FACC, FACP
Judd and Mary Morris Leighton Professor of Cardiovascular Diseases; Professor of Medicine; Consultant, Division of Cardiovascular Diseases and Internal Medicine, Mayo Clinic College of Medicine, Rochester, Minnesota [229, e29]

Robert L. Norris, MD
Professor, Department of Surgery, Division of Emergency Medicine, Stanford University School of Medicine, Palo Alto, California [396]

Thomas B. Nutman, MD
Head, Helminth Immunology Section; Head, Clinical Parasitology Unit, Laboratory of Parasitic Diseases, National Institutes of Health, Bethesda, Maryland [217, 218]

Katherine L. O'Brien, MDCM, MPH, FRCPC
Associate Professor, Center for American Indian Health; Departments of International Health and Epidemiology, Johns Hopkins Bloomberg School of Public Health, Baltimore, Maryland [134]

Richard J. O'Brien, MD
Head, Product Evaluation and Demonstration, Foundation for Innovative and New Diagnostics (FIND), Geneva, Switzerland [165]

Max R. O'Donnell, MD
Assistant Professor of Medicine, Albert Einstein College of Medicine, Bronx, New York [168]

Nigel O'Farrell, MSc, MD, FRCP
Ealing Hospital, London, United Kingdom [161]

Jennifer Ogar, MS
Speech Pathologist, Memory and Aging Center, University of California, San Francisco, San Francisco, California; Acting Chief of Speech Pathology at the Department of Veterans Affairs, Martinez, California [e10]

Patrick T. O'Gara, MD
Professor of Medicine, Harvard Medical School; Director, Clinical Cardiology, Brigham and Women's Hospital, Boston, Massachusetts [227, 237, e13]

C. Warren Olanow MD, FRCPC
Department of Neurology and Neuroscience, Mount Sinai School of Medicine, New York, New York [372]

Andrew B. Onderdonk, PhD
Professor of Pathology, Harvard Medical School; Brigham and Women's Hospital, Boston, Massachusetts [e22]

Chung Owyang, MD
H. Marvin Pollard Professor of Internal Medicine; Chief, Division of Gastroenterology, University of Michigan Health System, Ann Arbor, Michigan [290, 296]

William Pao, MD, PhD
Associate Professor of Medicine, Cancer Biology, and Pathology, Division of Hematology and Medical Oncology, Vanderbilt University School of Medicine, Nashville, Tennessee [89]

Umesh D. Parashar, MBBS, MPH
Lead, Viral Gastroenteritis Epidemiology Team, Division of Viral Diseases, National Center for Immunization and Respiratory Diseases, Centers for Disease Control and Prevention, Atlanta, Georgia [190]

Shreyaskumar R. Patel, MD
Center Medical Director, Sarcoma Center; Professor of Medicine; Deputy Chairman, Department of Sarcoma Medical Oncology, MD Anderson Cancer Center, Houston, Texas [98]

David L. Paterson, MD, PhD
Professor of Medicine, University of Queensland Centre for Clinical Research; Royal Brisbane and Women's Hospital, Brisbane, Australia [150]

Gustav Paumgartner, MD
Professor Emeritus of Medicine, University of Munich, Munich, Germany [311]

David A. Pegues, MD
Hospital Epidemiologist, David Geffen School of Medicine, University of California, Los Angeles, Los Angeles, California [153]

Anton Y. Peleg, MBBS, PhD, MPH, FRACP
Infectious Diseases Physician, Senior Lecturer, and NHMRC Biomedical Fellow, Department of Infectious Diseases and Microbiology, The Alfred Hospital and Monash University, Melbourne, Victoria, Australia [150]

Florencia Pereyra, MD
Assistant Professor of Medicine, Harvard Medical School; Associate Physician, Infectious Disease Division, Brigham and Women's Hospital, Boston, Massachusetts [e23, e24]

Michael A. Pesce, PhD
Professor Emeritus of Pathology and Cell Biology, Columbia University College of Physicians and Surgeons; Columbia University Medical Center, New York, New York [Appendix]

Clarence J. Peters, MD
John Sealy Distinguished University Chair in Tropical and Emerging Virology; Professor, Department of Mirobiology and Immunology; Department of Pathology; Director for Biodefense, Center for Biodefense and Emerging Infectious Diseases, University of Texas Medical Branch, Galveston, Texas [196, 197]

Gerald B. Pier, PhD
Professor of Medicine (Microbiology and Molecular Genetics), Harvard Medical School; Microbiologist, Brigham and Women's Hospital, Boston, Massachusetts [120]

Ronald E. Polk, PharmD
Professor of Pharmacy and Medicine; Chairman, Department of Pharmacy, School of Pharmacy, Virginia Commonwealth University/ Medical College of Virginia Campus, Richmond, Virginia [133]

Richard J. Pollack, PhD
Research Associate Professor, Department of Biology, Boston University; Research Associate, Department of Immunology and Infectious Diseases, Harvard School of Public Health, Boston, Massachusetts [397]

Andrew J. Pollard, PhD, FRCPCH
Professor of Pediatric Infection and Immunity; Director of the Oxford Vaccine Group, Department of Pediatrics, University of Oxford, Oxford, United Kingdom [143]

Reuven Porat, MD
Internal Medicine Department, Tel-Aviv Sourasky Medical Centre; Sackler Faculty of Medicine, Tel-Aviv University, Tel-Aviv, Israel [16]

Daniel A. Portnoy, PhD
Professor of Biochemistry and Molecular Biology, Department of Molecular and Cell Biology, The School of Public Health, University of California, Berkeley, Berkeley, California [139]

John T. Potts, Jr., MD
Director of Research, Massachusetts General Hospital, Boston, Massachusetts [353]

Lawrie W. Powell, MD, PhD
Professor of Medicine; Director, Centre for the Advancement of Clinical Research, Royal Brisbane and Women's Hospital, Brisbane, Australia [357]

Alvin C. Powers, MD
Joe C. Davis Chair in Biomedical Science; Professor of Medicine, Molecular Physiology, and Biophysics; Director, Vanderbilt Diabetes Center; Chief, Division of Diabetes, Endocrinology, and Metabolism, Vanderbilt University School of Medicine, Nashville, Tennessee [344]

Daniel S. Pratt, MD
Assistant Professor of Medicine, Harvard Medical School; Massachusetts General Hospital, Boston, Massachusetts [42, 302]

Michael B. Prentice, MB ChB, PhD, MRCP(UK), FRCPath, FFPRCPI
Professor of Medical Microbiology, Department of Microbiology, University College Cork, Cork, Ireland [159]

Darwin J. Prockop, MD, PhD
Director and Professor, Institute for Regenerative Medicine, Texas A&M Health Science Center College of Medicine at Scott & White, Temple, Texas [363]

Stanley B. Prusiner, MD
Director, Institute for Neurodegenerative Diseases; Professor, Department of Neurology, University of California, San Francisco, San Francisco, California [383]

Howard I. Pryor, II, MD
Laboratory for Tissue Engineering and Organ Fabrication, Center for Regenerative Medicine, Department of Surgery, Massachusetts General Hospital, Boston, Massachusetts [69]

Thomas C. Quinn, MD
Professor of Medicine, Johns Hopkins University, Baltimore, Maryland; Senior Investigator, National Institute of Allergy and Infectious Diseases, National Institutes of Health, Bethesda, Maryland [176]

Gil Rabinovici, MD
Attending Neurologist, Memory and Aging Center, University of California, San Francisco, San Francisco, California [e10]

Daniel J. Rader, MD
Cooper-McClure Professor of Medicine and Pharmacology, University of Pennsylvania School of Medicine, Philadelphia, Pennsylvania [356]

Sanjay Ram, MD
Associate Professor of Medicine, Division of Infectious Diseases and Immunology, University of Massachusetts Medical School, Worcester, Massachusetts [144]

Reuben Ramphal, MD
Professor of Medicine, Molecular Genetics and Microbiology, University of Florida College of Medicine, Gainesville, Florida [152]

Kumanan Rasanathan, MBChB, MPH, FAFPHM
Technical Officer, Department of Ethics, Equity, Trade, and Human Rights, World Health Organization, Geneva, Switzerland [e1]

Neil H. Raskin, MD
Department of Neurology, University of California, San Francisco, San Francisco, San Francisco, California [14]

Anis Rassi, Jr., MD, PhD, FACC, FACP, FAHA
Scientific Director, Anis Rassi Hospital, Goiânia, Brazil [213]

James P. Rathmell, MD
Associate Professor of Anesthesia, Harvard Medical School; Chief, Division of Pain Medicine, Massachusetts General Hospital, Boston, Massachusetts [11]

Mario C. Raviglione, MD
Director, Stop TB Department, World Health Organization, Geneva, Switzerland [165]

Sharon L. Reed, MD
Professor of Pathology and Medicine; Director, Microbiology and Virology Laboratories, University of California, San Diego Medical Center, San Diego, California [e25]

Susan E. Reef, MD
Medical Epidemiologist, Centers for Disease Control and Prevention, Atlanta, Georgia [193]

Richard C. Reichman, MD
Professor of Medicine and of Microbiology and Immunology, University of Rochester School of Medicine and Dentistry, Rochester, New York [185]

John J. Reilly, Jr., MD
Executive Vice Chairman; Department of Medicine; Professor of Medicine, University of Pittsburgh, Pittsburgh, Pennsylvania [260, e34]

John T. Repke, MD
University Professor and Chairman, Department of Obstetrics and Gynecology, Pennsylvania State University College of Medicine, Obstetrician-Gynecologist-in-Chief, The Milton S. Hershey Medical Center, Hershey, Pennsylvania [7]

Victor I. Reus, MD, DFAPA, FACP
Department of Psychiatry, University of California, San Francisco School of Medicine; Langley Porter Neuropsychiatric Institute, San Francisco, San Francisco, California [391]

Joseph Rhatigan, MD
Assistant Professor of Medicine, Harvard Medical School; Assistant Professor, Harvard School of Public Health; Brigham and Women's Hospital, Boston, Massachusetts [2]

Peter A. Rice, MD
Professor of Medicine, Division of Infectious Diseases and Immunology, University of Massachusetts Medical School, Worcester, Massachusetts [144]

Stuart Rich, MD
Professor of Medicine, Department of Medicine, Section of Cardiology, University of Chicago, Chicago, Illinois [250]

Gary S. Richardson, MD
Senior Research Scientist and Staff Physician, Henry Ford Hospital, Detroit, Michigan [27]

Elizabeth Robbins, MD
Clinical Professor of Pediatrics, University of California, San Francisco, San Francisco, California [e46]

Gary L. Robertson, MD
Emeritus Professor of Medicine, Northwestern University Feinberg School of Medicine, Chicago, Illinois [340]

Russell G. Robertson, MD
Vice President for Medical Affairs, Rosalind Franklin University of Medicine and Science; Dean, Chicago Medical School, Chicago, Illinois [80]

Dan M. Roden, MD
William Stokes Professor of Experimental Therapeutics; Assistant Vice-Chancellor for Personalized Medicine, Vanderbilt University School of Medicine, Nashville, Tennessee [5]

James A. Romano, Jr., PhD, DABT
Senior Principal Life Scientist and Technical Fellow, Science Applications International Corporation, Frederick, Maryland [222]

Karen L. Roos, MD
John and Nancy Nelson Professor of Neurology and Professor of Neurological Surgery, Indiana University School of Medicine, Indianapolis, Indiana [381]

Allan H. Ropper, MD
Professor of Neurology, Harvard Medical School; Executive Vice Chair of Neurology, Raymond D. Adams Distinguished Clinician, Brigham and Women's Hospital, Boston, Massachusetts [274, 377, 378]

Roger N. Rosenberg, MD
Zale Distinguished Chair and Professor of Neurology, Department of Neurology, University of Texas Southwestern Medical Center, Dallas, Texas [373]

Myrna R. Rosenfeld, MD, PhD
Professor of Neurology and Chief, Division of Neuro-oncology, University of Pennsylvania, Philadelphia, Pennsylvania [101]

John H. Rubenstein, MD, PhD
Nina Ireland Distinguished Professor in Child Psychiatry, Center for Neurobiology and Psychiatry, Department of Psychiatry, University of California, San Francisco, San Francisco, California [390]

Michael A. Rubin, MD, PhD
Assistant Professor of Medicine, University of Utah School of Medicine, Salt Lake City, Utah [31]

Steven Rubin, MS
Acting Principal Investigator, Center for Biologics Evaluation and Research, Food and Drug Administration, Bethesda, Maryland [194]

Robert M. Russell, MD
Professor Emeritus of Medicine and Nutrition, Tufts University, Boston, Massachusetts; Office of Dietary Supplements, National Institutes of Health, Bethesda, Maryland [74]

Thomas A. Russo, MD, CM, FIDSA
Professor of Medicine and Microbiology and Immunology; Chief, Division of Infectious Diseases, University at Buffalo, State University of New York, Buffalo, New York [149, 163]

Anna Rutherford, MD, MPH
Instructor in Medicine, Harvard Medical School; Associate Physician, Division of Gastroenterology, Hepatology and Endoscopy, Brigham and Women's Hospital, Boston, Massachusetts [e56]

Edward T. Ryan, MD, DTM&H
Associate Professor of Medicine, Harvard Medical School; Associate Professor of Immunology and Infectious Diseases, Harvard School of Public Health; Director, Tropical and Geographic Medicine, Massachusetts General Hospital, Boston, Massachusetts [128, 156]

Miguel Sabria, MD
Professor of Medicine, Autonomous University of Barcelona; Chief, Infectious Diseases Section, Germans Trias I Pujl Hospital, Barcelona, Spain [147]

David J. Salant, MD
Professor of Medicine, Boston University School of Medicine; Chief, Section of Nephrology, Boston Medical Center, Boston, Massachusetts [284, 285]

Martin A. Samuels, MD, DSc(hon), FAAN, MACP, FRCP
Professor of Neurology, Harvard Medical School; Chairman, Department of Neurology, Brigham and Women's Hospital, Boston, Massachusetts [e43, e47]

Philippe Sansonetti, MD, MS
Professor, Collège de France; Institut Pasteur, Paris, France [154]

Jussi J. Saukkonen, MD
Associate Professor of Medicine, Section of Pulmonary, Allergy, and Critical Care Medicine, Boston University School of Medicine, Boston, Massachusetts [168]

Edward A. Sausville, MD, PhD
Professor, Department of Medicine, University of Maryland School of Medicine; Deputy Director and Associate Director for Clinical Research, University of Maryland Marlene and Stewart Greenebaum Cancer Center, Baltimore, Maryland [85]

Mohamed H. Sayegh, MD
Raja N. Khuri Dean, Faculty of Medicine; Professor of Medicine and Immunology; Vice President of Medical Affairs, American University of Beirut, Beirut, Lebanon; Visiting Professor of Medicine and Pediatrics, Harvard Medical School; Director, Schuster Family Transplantation Research Center, Brigham and Women's Hospital; Children's Hospital, Boston, Massachusetts [282]

David T. Scadden, MD
Gerald and Darlene Jordan Professor of Medicine, Harvard Stem Cell Institute, Harvard Medical School; Department of Stem Cell and Regenerative Biology, Massachusetts General Hospital, Boston, Massachusetts [66]

Anthony H. V. Schapira, DSc, MD, FRCP, FMedSci
University Department of Clinical Neurosciences, University College London; National Hospital for Neurology and Neurosurgery, Queen's Square, London, United Kingdom [372]

Howard I. Scher, MD
Professor of Medicine, Weill Cornell Medical College; D. Wayne Calloway Chair in Urologic Oncology; Chief, Genitourinary Oncology Service, Department of Medicine, Memorial Sloan-Kettering Cancer Center, New York, New York [94, 95]

Anne Schuchat, MD
Director, National Center for Immunization and Respiratory Diseases, Centers for Disease Control and Prevention, Atlanta, Georgia [122]

Marc A. Schuckit, MD
Distinguished Professor of Psychiatry, University of California, San Diego School of Medicine, La Jolla, California [392]

H. Ralph Schumacher, MD
Professor of Medicine, Division of Rheumatology, University of Pennsylvania, School of Medicine, Philadelphia, Pennsylvania [333]

Gordon E. Schutze, MD
Professor of Pediatrics, Section of Retrovirology; Vice President, Baylor International Pediatric AIDS Initiative at Texas Children's Hospital, Baylor College of Medicine, Houston, Texas [158]

Stuart Schwartz, PhD
Professor of Human Genetics, Medicine and Pathology, University of Chicago, Chicago, Illinois [62]

Richard M. Schwartzstein, MD
Ellen and Melvin Gordon Professor of Medicine and Medical Education; Associate Chief, Division of Pulmonary, Critical Care, and Sleep Medicine, Beth Israel Deaconess Medical Center, Harvard Medical School, Boston, Massachusetts [33]

William W. Seeley, MD
Associate Professor of Neurology, Memory and Aging Center, University of California, San Francisco, San Francisco, California [371]

Michael V. Seiden, MD, PhD
Professor of Medicine; President and CEO, Fox Chase Cancer Center, Philadelphia, Pennsylvania [97]

Julian L. Seifter, MD
Associate Professor of Medicine, Harvard Medical School; Brigham and Women's Hospital, Boston, Massachusetts [289]

David C. Seldin, MD, PhD
Chief, Section of Hematology-Oncology, Department of Medicine; Director, Amyloid Treatment and Research Program, Boston University School of Medicine; Boston Medical Center, Boston, Massachusetts [112]

Andrew P. Selwyn, MD, MBCHB
Professor of Medicine Brigham and Women's Hospital, Boston, Massachusetts [243]

Ankoor Shah, MD
Department of Medicine, Division of Rheumatology and Immunology, Duke University Medical Center, Durham, North Carolina [321]

Steven D. Shapiro, MD
Jack D. Myers Professor and Chair, Department of Medicine, University of Pittsburgh, Pittsburgh, Pennsylvania [260]

Kanade Shinkai, MD, PhD
Assistant Professor, Department of Dermatology, University of California, San Francisco, San Francisco, California [55]

William Silen, MD
Johnson and Johnson Professor Emeritus of Surgery, Harvard Medical School, Auburndale, Massachusetts [13, 299, 300]

Edwin K. Silverman, MD, PhD
Associate Professor of Medicine, Harvard Medical School; Channing Laboratory, Pulmonary and Critical Care Division, Department of Medicine, Brigham and Women's Hospital, Boston, Massachusetts [260]

Martha Skinner, MD
Professor, Department of Medicine, Boston University School of Medicine, Boston, Massachusetts [112]

Karl Skorecki, MD, FRCP(C), FASN
Annie Chutick Professor in Medicine (Nephrology); Director, Rappaport Research Institute, Technion – Israel Institute of Technology; Director, Medical and Research Development, Rambam Health Care Campus, Haifa, Israel [280, e18]

Wade S. Smith, MD, PhD
Professor of Neurology, Daryl R. Gress Endowed Chair of Neurocritical Care and Stroke; Director, University of California, San Francisco Neurovascular Service, San Francisco, San Francisco, California [275, 370]

A. George Smulian, MBBCh
Associate Professor of Medicine, University of Cincinnati College of Medicine; Chief, Infectious Disease Section, Cincinnati VA Medical Center, Cincinnati, Ohio [207]

Jeremy Sobel, MD, MPH
Medical Officer, Office of Global Health, Centers for Disease Control and Prevention, Atlanta, Georgia [141]

Kelly A. Soderberg, PhD, MPH
Director, Program Management, Duke Human Vaccine Institute, Duke University School of Medicine, Durham, North Carolina [314]

Julian Solway, MD
Walter L. Palmer Distinguished Service Professor of Medicine and Pediatrics; Associate Dean for Translational Medicine, Biological Sciences Division; Vice Chair for Research, Department of Medicine; Chair, Committee on Molecular Medicine, University of Chicago, Chicago, Illinois [252, 264]

Michael F. Sorrell, MD
Robert L. Grissom Professor of Medicine, University of Nebraska Medical Center, Omaha, Nebraska [307]

Frank E. Speizer, MD
E. H. Kass Distinguished Professor of Medicine, Channing Laboratory, Harvard Medical School; Professor of Environmental Science, Harvard School of Public Health, Boston, Massachusetts [256]

Brad Spellberg, MD
Associate Professor of Medicine, Geffen School of Medicine, University of California, Los Angeles (UCLA); Divisions of General Internal Medicine and Infectious Diseases, Los Angeles Biomedical Research Institute at Harbor–UCLA Medical Center, Torrance, California [205]

Jerry L. Spivak, MD
Professor of Medicine and Oncology, Hematology Division, Johns Hopkins University School of Medicine, Baltimore, Maryland [108]

David D. Spragg, MD
Assistant Professor of Medicine, Johns Hopkins University, Baltimore, Maryland [231, 232]

Samuel L. Stanley, Jr., MD
President, Stony Brook University, Stony Brook, New York [209]

E. William St. Clair, MD
Department of Medicine, Division of Rheumatology and Immunology, Duke University Medical Center, Durham, North Carolina [321]

Allen C. Steere, MD
Professor of Medicine, Harvard Medical School; Massachusetts General Hospital, Boston, Massachusetts [173]

Robert S. Stern, MD
Carl J. Herzog Professor of Dermatology, Harvard Medical School; Chair, Department of Dermatology, Beth Israel Deaconess Medical Center, Boston, Massachusetts [55]

Dennis L. Stevens, MD, PhD
Professor of Medicine, University of Washington School of Medicine, Seattle, Washington; Chief, Infectious Disease Section, Veterans Affairs Medical Center, Boise, Idaho [125, 142]

Lynne Warner Stevenson, MD
Professor of Medicine, Harvard Medical School; Director, Heart Failure Program, Brigham and Women's Hospital, Boston, Massachusetts [238]

Stephen E. Straus,† MD
National Institute of Allergy and Infectious Diseases, Bethesda, Maryland [e2]

Stephanie Studenski, MD, MPH
Professor of Geriatric Medicine, Department of Medicine, University of Pittsburgh School of Medicine; Staff Physician, VA Pittsburgh Geriatric Research Education and Clinical Center, Pittsburgh, Pennsylvania [72]

Lewis Sudarsky, MD
Associate Professor of Neurology, Harvard Medical School; Director of Movement Disorders, Brigham and Women's Hospital, Boston, Massachusetts [24]

Donna C. Sullivan, PhD
Professor, Department of Medicine, Division of Infectious Diseases, University of Mississippi Medical School, Jackson, Mississippi [201]

Shyam Sundar, MD
Professor of Medicine, Institute of Medical Sciences, Banaras Hindu University, Varanasi, India [212]

Paolo M. Suter, MD, MS
Professor, Clinic and Policlinic of Internal Medicine, University Hospital, Zurich, Switzerland [74]

Richard Suzman, PhD
Director, Behavioral and Social Research Program, National Institute on Aging, National Institutes of Health, Chevy Chase, Maryland [70]

Morton N. Swartz, MD
Professor of Medicine, Harvard Medical School; Chief, Jackson Firm Medical Service and Infectious Disease Unit, Massachusetts General Hospital, Boston, Massachusetts [382]

Robert A. Swerlick, MD
Alicia Leizman Stonecipher Professor and Chair of Dermatology, Emory University School of Medicine, Atlanta, Georgia [e16]

Geoffrey Tabin, MD
Professor of Ophthalmology and Visual Sciences, University of Utah School of Medicine; Director, International Ophthalmology Division, John A. Moran Eye Center; Director, Himalayan Cataract Project, Salt Lake City, Utah [e51]

Maria Carmela Tartaglia, MD, FRCPC
Clinical Instructor of Neurology, Memory and Aging Center, University of California, San Francisco, San Francisco, California [e10]

Joel D. Taurog, MD
Professor of Internal Medicine, Rheumatic Diseases Division, University of Texas Southwestern Medical Center, Dallas, Texas [325]

Stephen C. Textor, MD
Professor of Medicine, Division of Nephrology and Hypertension, Mayo Clinic, Rochester, Minnesota [286]

†Deceased

C. Louise Thwaites, MD, MBBS
Musculoskeletal Physician, Horsham, West Sussex; Oxford University Clinical Research Unit, Hospital for Tropical Diseases, Ho Chi Minh City, Vietnam [140]

Alan D. Tice, MD, FACP
Infections Limited Hawaii; John A. Burns School of Medicine, University of Hawaii, Honolulu, Hawaii [126]

Zelig A. Tochner, MD
Professor of Radiation Oncology, University of Pennsylvania School of Medicine; Medical Director, Proton Therapy Center, Philadelphia, Pennsylvania [223]

Gordon F. Tomaselli, MD
Michel Mirowski, MD Professor of Cardiology; Professor of Medicine and Cellular and Molecular Medicine; Chief, Division of Cardiology, Johns Hopkins University, Baltimore, Maryland [231, 232]

Mark Topazian, MD
Professor of Medicine, Mayo Clinic, Rochester, Minnesota [291, e36]

Barbara W. Trautner, MD, PhD
Assistant Professor, Section of Infectious Diseases, Baylor College of Medicine; The Michael E. DeBakey Veterans Affairs Medical Center, Houston VA Health Services Research and Development Center of Excellence, Houston, Texas [288]

Jeffrey M. Trent, PhD, FACMG
President and Research Director, Translational Genomics Research Institute, Phoenix, Arizona; Van Andel Research Institute, Grand Rapids, Michigan [83]

Elbert P. Trulock, MD
Rosemary and I. Jerome Flance Professor in Pulmonary Medicine, Washington University School of Medicine, St. Louis, Missouri [266]

Kenneth L. Tyler, MD
Reuler-Lewin Family Professor and Chair, Department of Neurology; Professor of Medicine and Microbiology, University of Colorado School of Medicine, Denver, Colorado; Chief of Neurology, University of Colorado Hospital, Aurora, Colorado [381]

Athanasios G. Tzioufas, MD
Professor, Department of Pathophysiology, National University of Athens School of Medicine, Athens, Greece [324]

Walter J. Urba, MD, PhD
Director of Cancer Research, Robert W. Franz Cancer Research Center, Providence Portland Medical Center, Portland, Oregon [87]

Joseph P. Vacanti, MD
John Homans Professor of Surgery, Harvard Medical School; Surgeon-in-Chief, Massachusetts General Hospital for Children; Deputy Director, Center for Regenerative Medicine, Massachusetts General Hospital, Boston, Massachusetts [69]

Jos W. M. van der Meer, MD, PhD
Professor of Medicine; Head, Department of General Internal Medicine, Radboud University, Nijmegen Medical Centre, Nijmegen, Netherlands [389]

Edouard Vannier, PhD, PharmD
Assistant Professor, Division of Geographic Medicine and Infectious Diseases, Tufts University School of Medicine; Tufts Medical Center, Boston, Massachusetts [211]

Gauri R. Varadhachary, MD
Associate Professor, Department of Gastrointestinal Medical Oncology, University of Texas MD Anderson Cancer Center, Houston, Texas [99]

John Varga, MD
John Hughes Professor of Medicine, Northwestern University Feinberg School of Medicine, Chicago, Illinois [323]

Camilo Jimenez Vasquez, MD
Assistant Professor, Department of Endocrine Neoplasia and Hormonal Disorders, Division of Internal Medicine, University of Texas MD Anderson Cancer Center, Houston, Texas [351]

Joseph M. Vinetz, MD
Professor of Medicine, Division of Infectious Diseases, Department of Medicine, University of California, San Diego, San Diego, California [171]

Indre V. Viskontas, PhD
Visiting Scholar, Memory and Aging Center, University of California, San Francisco, San Francisco, California [e9]

Panayiotis G. Vlachoyiannopoulos, MD
Associate Professor of Medicine-Immunology, Department of Pathophysiology, Medical School, National University of Athens, Athens, Greece [320]

Bert Vogelstein, MD
Professor of Oncology and Pathology; Investigator, Howard Hughes Medical Institute; Sidney Kimmel Comprehensive Cancer Center; Johns Hopkins University School of Medicine, Baltimore, Maryland [83]

Everett E. Vokes, MD
John E. Ultmann Professor and Chairman, Department of Medicine; Physician-in-Chief, University of Chicago Medical Center, Chicago, Illinois [88]

Tamara J. Vokes, MD, FACP
Professor, Department of Medicine, Section of Endocrinology, University of Chicago, Chicago, Illinois [355]

Sushrut S. Waikar, MD, MPH
Assistant Professor of Medicine, Harvard Medical School; Brigham and Women's Hospital, Boston, Massachusetts [279]

Matthew K. Waldor, MD, PhD
Edward H. Kass Professor of Medicine, Channing Laboratory, Brigham and Women's Hospital; Harvard Medical School and Howard Hughes Medical Institute, Boston, Massachusetts [156]

David H. Walker, MD
The Carmage and Martha Walls Distinguished University Chair in Tropical Diseases; Professor and Chairman, Department of Pathology; Executive Director, Center for Biodefense and Emerging Infectious Diseases, University of Texas Medical Branch, Galveston, Texas [174]

Mark F. Walker, MD
Associate Professor, Department of Neurology, Case Western Reserve University School of Medicine; Daroff-Dell'Osso Ocular Motility Laboratory, Louis Stokes Cleveland Department of Veterans Affairs Medical Center, Cleveland, Ohio [21]

B. Timothy Walsh, MD
Professor, Department of Psychiatry, College of Physicians and Surgeons, Columbia University; New York State Psychiatric Institute, New York, New York [79]

Peter D. Walzer, MD, MSc
Professor of Medicine, University of Cincinnati College of Medicine; Associate Chief of Staff for Research, Cincinnati VA Medical Center, Cincinnati, Ohio [207]

Fred Wang, MD
Professor of Medicine, Harvard Medical School; Brigham and Women's Hospital, Boston, Massachusetts [177, 183]

John W. Warren, MD
Professor of Medicine, University of Maryland School of Medicine, Baltimore, Maryland [e35]

Carl V. Washington, MD
Associate Professor of Dermatology, Winship Cancer Center, Emory University School of Medicine, Atlanta, Georgia [87]

Anthony P. Weetman, MD
University of Sheffield School of Medicine, Sheffield, United Kingdom [341]

Robert A. Weinstein, MD
The C Anderson Hedberg MD Professor of Internal Medicine, Rush Medical College; Interim Chairman, Department of Medicine, John Stroger Hospital, Chicago, Illinois [131]

Jeffrey I. Weitz, MD, FRCP(C), FACP
Professor of Medicine and Biochemistry; Executive Director, Thrombosis and Atherosclerosis Research Institute; HSFO/J. F. Mustard Chair in Cardiovascular Research, Canada Research Chair (Tier 1) in Thrombosis, McMaster University, Hamilton, Ontario, Canada [118]

Peter F. Weller, MD
Chief, Infectious Disease Division; Chief, Allergy and Inflammation Division, Beth Israel Deaconess Medical Center, Boston, Massachusetts [215-218, 220]

Patrick Y. Wen, MD
Professor of Neurology, Harvard Medical School; Dana-Farber Cancer Institute, Boston, Massachusetts [379]

Michael R. Wessels, MD
John F. Enders Professor of Pediatrics; Professor of Medicine, Harvard Medical School; Chief, Division of Infectious Diseases, Children's Hospital, Boston, Massachusetts [136]

Meir Wetzler, MD, FACP
Professor of Medicine, Roswell Park Cancer Institute, Buffalo, New York [109]

L. Joseph Wheat, MD
MiraVista Diagnostics and MiraBella Technologies, Indianapolis, Indiana [199]

A. Clinton White, Jr., MD
Director, Infectious Disease Division, Department of Internal Medicine, University of Texas Medical Branch, Galveston, Texas [220]

Nicholas J. White, MD, DSc, FRCP, F Med Sci, FRS
Professor of Tropical Medicine, Faculty of Tropical Medicine, Mahidol University, Bangkok, Thailand [210, e27]

Richard J. Whitley, MD
Distinguished Professor of Pediatrics, Loeb Eminent Scholar Chair in Pediatrics; Professor of Pediatrics, Microbiology, Medicine, and Neurosurgery, University of Alabama at Birmingham, Birmingham, Alabama [180]

John W. Winkelman, MD, PhD
Associate Professor of Psychiatry, Harvard Medical School; Medical Director, Sleep Health Centers, Brigham and Women's Hospital, Boston, Massachusetts [27]

Bruce U. Wintroub, MD
Professor and Chair, Department of Dermatology, University of California, San Francisco, San Francisco, California [55]

Andrea Wolf, MD, MPH
Instructor in Surgery, Harvard Medical School; Chief Resident in Cardiothoracic Surgery, Division of Thoracic Surgery, Brigham and Women's Hospital, Boston, Massachusetts [e55]

Allan W. Wolkoff, MD
Professor of Medicine and Anatomy and Structural Biology; Associate Chair of Medicine for Research; Chief, Division of Gastroenterology and Liver Diseases, Albert Einstein College of Medicine and Montefiore Medical Center, Bronx, New York [303]

John B. Wong, MD
Professor of Medicine, Tufts University School of Medicine; Chief, Division of Clinical Decision Making, Department of Medicine, Tufts Medical Center, Boston, Massachusetts [3]

Louis Michel Wong Kee Song, MD
Associate Professor, Division of Gastroenterology and Hepatology, Mayo Clinic, Rochester, Minnesota [291, e36]

Robert L. Wortmann, MD, FACP, MACR
Professor, Department of Medicine, Dartmouth Medical School and Dartmouth Hitchcock Medical Center, Lebanon, New Hampshire [359]

Shirley H. Wray, MB, ChB, PhD, FRCP
Professor of Neurology, Harvard Medical School; Department of Neurology, Massachusetts General Hospital, Boston, Massachusetts [e11]

Bechien U. Wu, MD
Instructor of Medicine, Harvard Medical School; Associate Physician, Division of Gastroenterology, Brigham and Women's Hospital, Boston, Massachusetts [313]

Richard Wunderink, MD
Professor of Medicine, Division of Pulmonary and Critical Care, Northwestern University Feinberg School of Medicine, Chicago, Illinois [257]

Kim B. Yancey, MD
Professor and Chair, Department of Dermatology, University of Texas Southwestern Medical Center, Dallas, Texas [51, 54]

Janet A. Yellowitz, DMD, MPH
Associate Professor; Director, Geriatric Dentistry, University of Maryland Dental School, Baltimore, Maryland [e12]

Lam Minh Yen, MD
Director, Tetanus Intensive Care Unit, Hospital for Tropical Diseases, Ho Chi Minh City, Vietnam [140]

Maria A. Yialamas, MD
Instructor, Harvard Medical School; Associate Program Director, Internal Medicine Residency, Brigham and Women's Hospital, Boston, Massachusetts [e54, e56]

Neal S. Young, MD
Chief, Hematology Branch, National Heart, Lung and Blood Institute, National Institutes of Health, Bethesda, Maryland [107]

Victor L. Yu, MD
Professor of Medicine, Department of Medicine, University of Pittsburgh Medical Center, Pittsburgh, Pennsylvania [147]

Laura A. Zimmerman, MPH
Epidemiologist, Centers for Disease Control and Prevention, Atlanta, Georgia [193]

PREFACE

Welcome to the 18th edition of *Harrison's Principles of Internal Medicine.* In the 62 years since the first edition of this textbook was published, virtually every area of medicine has evolved substantially and many new areas have emerged. In 1949, when the first edition appeared, peptic ulcer disease was thought to be caused by stress, nearly every tumor that was not resected resulted in death, rheumatic heart disease was widely prevalent, and hepatitis B and HIV infection were unknown. In the intervening years, both the infectious cause of and the cure for peptic ulcer disease were identified; advances in diagnosis and treatment made it possible to cure two-thirds of cancers; rheumatic heart disease virtually disappeared; atherosclerotic coronary artery disease waxed and then—at least in part through management of modifiable risk factors—began to wane; hepatitis B and its consequences, cirrhosis and hepatocellular carcinoma, became preventable by a vaccine; and HIV, first viewed as a uniformly fatal worldwide scourge, became a treatable chronic disease. During this same period, the amount of information required for the effective practice of medicine grew unabated, and learning options for students, residents, and practicing physicians also burgeoned to include multiple sources of information in print and electronic formats.

While retaining the founding goals of *Harrison's*, this edition has been modified extensively in light of the varied needs of the book's readers and the diverse methods and formats by which information is now acquired. The print version of the 18th edition is more reader-friendly in several respects: the book is printed in type that is easier to read than prior editions, the graphics and tables have been enhanced for ease of interpretation, and more than 300 new figures are included. This improved format requires publication of the print edition in two volumes conveniently divided by subject matter. A DVD accompanies the book and contains additional e-chapters, videos, and atlases; its image bank includes figures and photographs from the book that can be incorporated into slide presentations. All chapters have been extensively updated by experts in the field. In addition, this edition includes 25 new chapters and more than 100 new authors. The pathophysiologic approach to evaluating patients on the basis of their presentation continues to receive emphasis in an enriched section on the cardinal manifestations of disease. A new section focuses on aging, its demographics and biology, and distinctive clinical issues affecting older patients. The e-chapters have increased in number from 39 to 57 and include a new video atlas of neuro-ophthalmology, an audio-enhanced chapter on the approach to a patient with a heart murmur, a case-based teaching exercise in fluid and electrolyte imbalances and acid-base disturbances, and explorations of infectious complications of burns and bites. New videos demonstrate the neurologic examination and several commonly performed medical procedures. A new chapter focuses on neuropsychiatric problems among war veterans. E-chapters on altitude sickness and hyperbaric and diving medicine form a new section on medical effects of changes in environmental pressure.

For readers who wish to continue using *Harrison's* in a single-volume format, we are pleased to offer two new eBook versions of the 18th edition: a traditional eBook, with text and illustrations from the new edition included for reading on a portable e-reader or on a desktop, and an enhanced eBook developed especially for new tablet devices (e.g., iPad, Galaxy, Playbook, Nook) that offer high-definition resolution of multimedia content and interactive features. The *Harrison's* 18th edition enhanced eBook will contain extensive embedded video footage, including all of the new clinical procedural videos; the wonderful neurologic examination videos from Samuels and Lowenstein; examples of cardiovascular imaging and assessment; and high-resolution versions of more than 2000 color images from the book and the *Harrison's* atlases on the companion DVD. Along with other social media features, the enhanced eBook offers users the opportunity to take and share notes from lectures and their own reading. Additional resources include *Harrison's Online*, a continuously updated electronic resource that highlights and summarizes newly published articles on significant medical findings and advances. *Harrison's Self-Assessment and Board Review*, a useful study guide for board review based on information in the 18th edition, will soon be produced. *Harrison's Manual of Medicine*, a pocket version of *Harrison's Principles of Internal Medicine*, is available in both print and electronic formats.

We have many people to thank for their efforts in producing this book. First, the authors have done a superb job of producing authoritative chapters that synthesize vast amounts of scientific and clinical data to create state-of-the-art descriptions of medical disorders encompassed by internal medicine. In today's information-rich, rapidly evolving environment, they have ensured that this information is current. Helpful suggestions and critical input have been provided by a number of colleagues; particularly notable was the advice of Chung Owyang on the Gastroenterology Section. We are most grateful to our colleagues in each of our editorial offices who have kept track of the work in its various phases and facilitated communication with the authors, with the McGraw-Hill staff, and among the editors: Patricia Conrad, Emily Cowan, Patricia L. Duffey, Gregory K. Folkers, Julie B. McCoy, Elizabeth Robbins, Kristine Shontz, and Stephanie Tribuna.

The staff at McGraw-Hill has been a constant source of support and expertise. James Shanahan, Editor-in-Chief, Internal Medicine, for McGraw-Hill's Professional Publishing Division, has been a superb and insightful partner to the editors, guiding the development of the book and its related products in new formats. Kim Davis seamlessly stepped into the position of Associate Managing Editor, ensuring that the complex production of this multi-authored textbook proceeded in an efficient fashion. Paula Torres, Dominik Pucek, and Michael Crumsho oversaw the production of the new procedural and neurology videos. Phil Galea again served as Production Director on this, his final edition, and did so with a peak performance. Mary A. Murray, Director, International Rights, is retiring from McGraw Hill in 2012, after 50 years with the company. Mary joined the Blakiston Division of McGraw Hill in 1961, when Tinsley Harrison was still the editor of the book. Her first assignment was to distribute reprints of *Harrison's* chapters to the editors and contributors. For the next 23 years, Mary continued to be involved in the editorial process of *Harrison's*. In the early 1990s, she was given responsibility for licensing McGraw-Hill's medical titles; making use of her many cordial connections in global medical publishing, she licensed translations of *Harrison's* into 19 languages. We are extremely grateful to Mary for her many accomplishments in support of the book through 13 editions.

We are privileged to have compiled this 18th edition and are enthusiastic about all that it offers our readers. We learned much in the process of editing *Harrison's* and hope that you will find this edition a uniquely valuable educational resource.

THE EDITORS

PART 10

Disorders of the Cardiovascular System

SECTION 1 Introduction to Cardiovascular Disorders

SECTION 2 Diagnosis of Cardiovascular Disorders

SECTION 3 Disorders of Rhythm

SECTION 4 Disorders of the Heart

SECTION 5 Vascular Disease

CHAPTER 224

Basic Biology of the Cardiovascular System

Joseph Loscalzo
Peter Libby
Jonathan Epstein

THE BLOOD VESSEL

■ VASCULAR ULTRASTRUCTURE

Blood vessels participate in homeostasis on a moment-to-moment basis and contribute to the pathophysiology of diseases of virtually every organ system. Hence, an understanding of the fundamentals of vascular biology furnishes a foundation for understanding the normal function of all organ systems and many diseases. The smallest blood vessels—capillaries—consist of a monolayer of endothelial cells apposed to a basement membrane, adjacent to occasional smooth-muscle-like cells known as *pericytes* (Fig. 224-1*A*). Unlike larger vessels, pericytes do not invest the entire microvessel to form a continuous sheath. Veins and arteries typically have a trilaminar structure (Fig. 224-1*B–E*). The *intima* consists of a monolayer of endothelial cells continuous with those of the capillaries. The middle layer, or *tunica media*, consists of layers of smooth-muscle cells; in veins, the media can contain just a few layers of smooth-muscle cells (Fig. 224-1*B*). The outer layer, the *adventitia*, consists of looser extracellular matrix with occasional fibroblasts, mast cells, and nerve terminals. Larger arteries have their own vasculature, the *vasa vasorum*, which nourishes the outer aspects of the tunica media. The adventitia of many veins surpasses the intima in thickness.

The tone of muscular arterioles regulates blood pressure and flow through various arterial beds. These smaller arteries have a relatively thick tunica media in relation to the adventitia (Fig. 224-1*C*). Medium-size muscular arteries similarly contain a prominent tunica media (Fig. 224-1*D*); atherosclerosis commonly affects this type of muscular artery. The larger elastic arteries have a much more structured tunica media consisting of concentric bands of smooth-muscle cells, interspersed with strata of elastin-rich extracellular matrix sandwiched between layers of smooth-muscle cells (Fig. 224-1*E*). Larger arteries have a clearly demarcated internal elastic lamina that forms the barrier between the intima and the media. An external elastic lamina demarcates the media of arteries from the surrounding adventitia.

■ ORIGIN OF VASCULAR CELLS

The intima in human arteries often contains occasional resident smooth-muscle cells beneath the monolayer of vascular endothelial

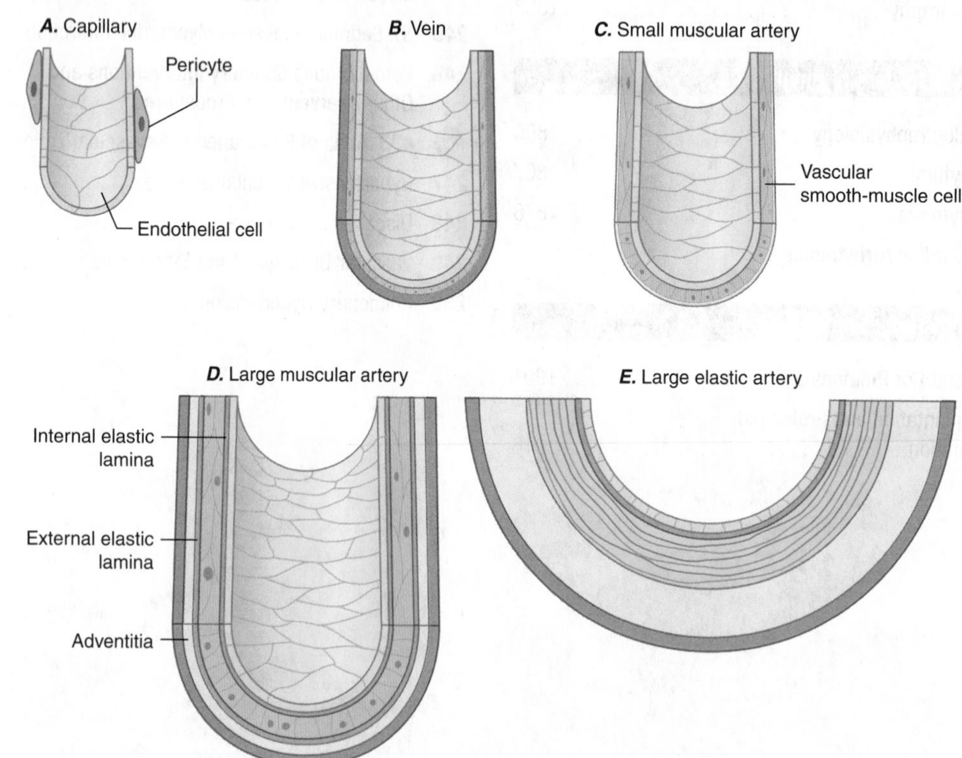

Figure 224-1 Schematics of the structures of various types of blood vessels. ***A.*** Capillaries consist of an endothelial tube in contact with a discontinuous population of pericytes. ***B.*** Veins typically have thin medias and thicker adventitias. ***C.*** A small muscular artery features a prominent tunica media. ***D.*** Larger muscular arteries have a prominent media with smooth-muscle cells embedded in a complex extracellular matrix. ***E.*** Larger elastic arteries have cylindrical layers of elastic tissue alternating with concentric rings of smooth-muscle cells.

cells. The embryonic origin of smooth-muscle cells in various types of artery differs. Some upper-body arterial smooth-muscle cells derive from the neural crest, whereas lower-body arteries generally recruit smooth-muscle cells from neighboring mesodermal structures during development. Derivatives of the proepicardial organ, which gives rise to the epicardial layer of the heart, contribute to the vascular smooth-muscle cells of the coronary arteries. Recent evidence suggests that bone marrow may give rise to both vascular endothelial cells and smooth-muscle cells, particularly under conditions of injury repair or vascular lesion formation. Indeed, the ability of bone marrow to repair an injured endothelial monolayer may contribute to maintenance of vascular health, whereas failure to do so may lead to arterial disease. The precise sources of endothelial and mesenchymal progenitor cells or their stem cell precursors remain the subject of active investigation (Chaps. 65–67).

VASCULAR CELL BIOLOGY

Endothelial cell

The key cell of the vascular intima, the endothelial cell, has manifold functions in health and disease. Most obviously, the endothelium forms the interface between tissues and the blood compartment. It therefore must regulate the entry of molecules and cells into tissues in a selective manner. The ability of endothelial cells to serve as a selectively permeable barrier fails in many vascular disorders, including atherosclerosis and hypertension. This dysregulation of permeability also occurs in pulmonary edema and other situations of "capillary leak."

The endothelium also participates in the local regulation of blood flow and vascular caliber. Endogenous substances produced by endothelial cells such as prostacyclin, endothelium-derived hyperpolarizing factor, nitric oxide (NO), and hydrogen peroxide (H_2O_2) provide tonic vasodilatory stimuli under physiologic conditions in vivo (Table 224-1). Impaired production or excess catabolism of NO impairs this endothelium-dependent vasodilator function and may contribute to excessive vasoconstriction in various pathologic situations. By contrast, endothelial cells also produce potent vasoconstrictor substances such as endothelin in a regulated fashion. Excessive production of reactive oxygen species, such as superoxide anion (O_2^-), by endothelial or smooth-muscle cells under pathologic conditions (e.g., excessive exposure to angiotensin II) can promote local oxidative stress and inactivate NO.

The endothelial monolayer contributes critically to inflammatory processes involved in normal host defenses and pathologic states. The normal endothelium resists prolonged contact with blood leukocytes; however, when activated by bacterial products such as endotoxin or proinflammatory cytokines released during infection or injury, endothelial cells express an array of leukocyte adhesion molecules that bind various classes of leukocytes. The endothelial cells appear to recruit selectively different classes of leukocytes in different pathologic conditions. The gamut of adhesion molecules and chemokines generated during acute bacterial infection tends to recruit granulocytes. In chronic inflammatory diseases such as tuberculosis and atherosclerosis, endothelial cells express adhesion molecules that favor the recruitment of mononuclear leukocytes that characteristically accumulate in these conditions.

The endothelium also dynamically regulates thrombosis and hemostasis. Nitric oxide, in addition to its vasodilatory properties, can limit platelet activation and aggregation. Like NO, prostacyclin produced by endothelial cells under normal conditions not only provides a vasodilatory stimulus but also antagonizes platelet activation and aggregation. Thrombomodulin expressed on the surface of endothelial cells binds thrombin at low concentrations and inhibits coagulation through activation of the protein C pathway, inactivating clotting factors Va and VIIIa and thus combating thrombus formation. The surface of endothelial cells contains heparan sulfate glycosaminoglycans that furnish an endogenous antithrombotic coating to the vasculature. Endothelial cells also participate actively in fibrinolysis and its regulation. They express receptors for plasminogen and plasminogen activators and produce tissue-type plasminogen activator. Through local generation of plasmin, the normal endothelial monolayer can promote the lysis of nascent thrombi.

When activated by inflammatory cytokines, bacterial endotoxin, or angiotensin II, for example, endothelial cells can produce substantial quantities of the major inhibitor of fibrinolysis, plasminogen activator inhibitor 1 (PAI-1). Thus, in pathologic circumstances, the endothelial cell may promote local thrombus accumulation rather than combat it. Inflammatory stimuli also induce the expression of the potent procoagulant tissue factor, a contributor to disseminated intravascular coagulation in sepsis.

Endothelial cells also participate in the pathophysiology of a number of immune-mediated diseases. Lysis of endothelial cells mediated by complement provides an example of immunologically mediated tissue injury. The presentation of foreign histocompatibility complex antigens by endothelial cells in solid-organ allografts can trigger immunologic rejection. In addition, immune-mediated endothelial injury may contribute in some patients with thrombotic thrombocytopenic purpura and patients with hemolytic-uremic syndrome. Thus, in addition to contributing to innate immune responses, endothelial cells participate actively in both humoral and cellular limbs of the immune response.

Endothelial cells regulate growth of the subjacent smooth-muscle cells as well. Heparan sulfate glycosaminoglycans elaborated by endothelial cells can hold smooth-muscle proliferation in check. In contrast, when exposed to various injurious stimuli, endothelial cells can elaborate growth factors and chemoattractants, such as platelet-derived growth factor, that can promote the migration and proliferation of vascular smooth-muscle cells. Dysregulated elaboration of these growth-stimulatory molecules may promote smooth-muscle accumulation in atherosclerotic lesions.

TABLE 224-1 Endothelial Functions in Health and Disease

Homeostatic Phenotype	Dysfunctional Phenotype
Vasodilation	Impaired dilation, vasoconstriction
Antithrombotic, profibrinolytic	Prothrombotic, antifibrinolytic
Anti-inflammatory	Proinflammatory
Antiproliferative	Proproliferative
Antioxidant	Prooxidant
Permselectivity	Impaired barrier function

Clinical assessment of endothelial function

Various invasive and noninvasive approaches can be used to evaluate endothelial vasodilator function in humans. Either pharmacologic agonists or increased flow stimulates the endothelium to release acutely molecular effectors that alter underlying smooth-muscle cell tone. Invasively, infusion of the cholinergic agonists acetylcholine and methacholine stimulates the release of NO from normal endothelial cells. Changes in coronary diameter can be quantitatively measured in response to an intracoronary infusion of these short-lived, rapidly acting agents. Noninvasive assessment of endothelial function in the forearm circulation typically involves occlusion of brachial artery blood flow with a blood pressure cuff, which elicits reactive hyperemia after release; the resulting flow increase normally causes endothelium-dependent vasodilation, which is measured as the change in brachial artery blood flow and diameter by ultrasound (Fig. 224-2). This approach depends on shear stress–dependent changes in endothelial release of NO after restoration of blood flow, as well as the effect of adenosine released (transiently) from ischemic tissue in the forearm.

Typically, these invasive and noninvasive approaches detect inducible vasodilatory changes in vessel diameter of ~10%. In individuals with atherosclerosis or its risk factors (especially hypertension, hypercholesterolemia, diabetes mellitus, and smoking), such studies can detect endothelial dysfunction as defined by a smaller change in diameter and, in the extreme case, a so-called paradoxical vasoconstrictor response owing to the direct effect of cholinergic agonists on vascular smooth-muscle cell tone.

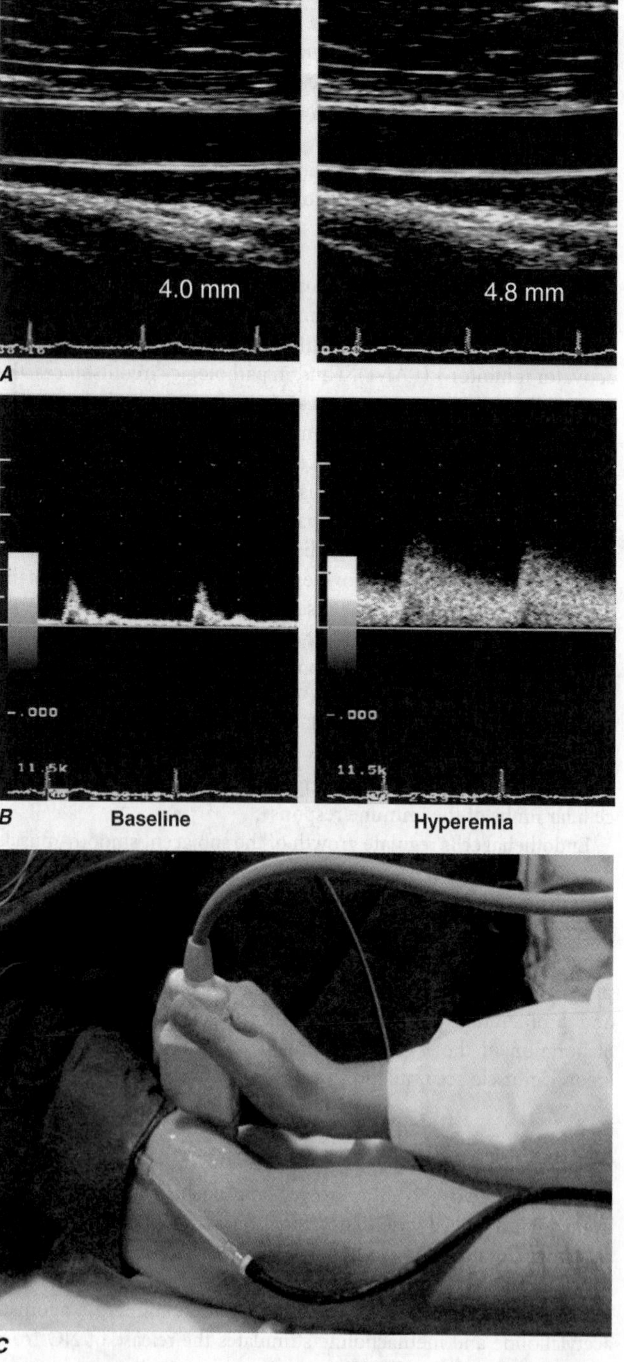

Figure 224-2 Assessment of endothelial function in vivo using blood pressure cuff-occlusion and release. Upon deflation of the cuff, changes in diameter (*A*) and blood flow (*B*) of the brachial artery are monitored with an ultrasound probe (*C*). *(Reproduced with permission of J. Vita, MD.)*

Vascular smooth-muscle cell

The vascular smooth-muscle cell, the major cell type of the media layer of blood vessels, also contributes actively to vascular pathobiology. Contraction and relaxation of smooth-muscle cells at the level of the muscular arteries controls blood pressure, and, hence, regional blood flow and the afterload experienced by the left ventricle (see below). The vasomotor tone of veins, which is governed by smooth-muscle cell tone, regulates the capacitance of the venous tree and influences the preload experienced by both ventricles. Smooth-muscle cells in the adult vessel seldom replicate. This homeostatic quiescence of smooth-muscle cells changes in conditions of arterial injury or inflammatory activation. Proliferation and migration of arterial smooth-muscle cells, which is associated with a change in phenotype characterized by lower content of contractile proteins and greater production of extracellular matrix macromolecules, can contribute to the development of arterial stenoses in atherosclerosis, arteriolar remodeling that can sustain and propagate hypertension, and the hyperplastic response of arteries injured by angioplasty or stent deployment. In the pulmonary circulation, smooth-muscle migration and proliferation contribute decisively to the pulmonary vascular disease that gradually occurs in response to sustained high-flow states such as left-to-right shunts. Such pulmonary vascular disease provides a major obstacle to the management of many patients with adult congenital heart disease. Elucidation of the signaling pathways that regulate the reversible transition of the vascular smooth-muscle cell phenotype remains an active focus of investigation. Among other mediators, microRNAs have emerged as powerful regulators of this transition, offering new targets for intervention.

The activated, phenotypically modulated smooth-muscle cells secrete the bulk of vascular extracellular matrix. Excessive production of collagen and glycosaminoglycans contributes to the remodeling and altered biology and biomechanics of arteries affected by hypertension or atherosclerosis. In larger elastic arteries, the elastin synthesized by smooth-muscle cells serves to maintain not only normal arterial structure but also hemodynamic function. The ability of the larger arteries, such as the aorta, to store the kinetic energy of systole promotes tissue perfusion during diastole. Arterial stiffness associated with aging or disease, as manifested by a widening pulse pressure, increases left ventricular afterload and portends a poor outcome.

Like endothelial cells, vascular smooth-muscle cells do not merely respond to vasomotor or inflammatory stimuli elaborated by other cell types but can themselves serve as a source of such stimuli. For example, when exposed to bacterial endotoxin or other proinflammatory stimuli, smooth-muscle cells can elaborate cytokines and other inflammatory mediators. Like endothelial cells, upon inflammatory activation, arterial smooth-muscle cells can produce prothrombotic mediators such as tissue factor, the antifibrinolytic protein PAI-1, and other molecules that modulate thrombosis and fibrinolysis. Smooth-muscle cells also elaborate autocrine growth factors that can amplify hyperplastic responses to arterial injury.

Vascular smooth-muscle cell function

Vascular smooth-muscle cells govern vessel tone. Those cells contract when stimulated by a rise in intracellular calcium concentration by calcium influx through the plasma membrane and by calcium release from intracellular stores (Fig. 224-3). In vascular

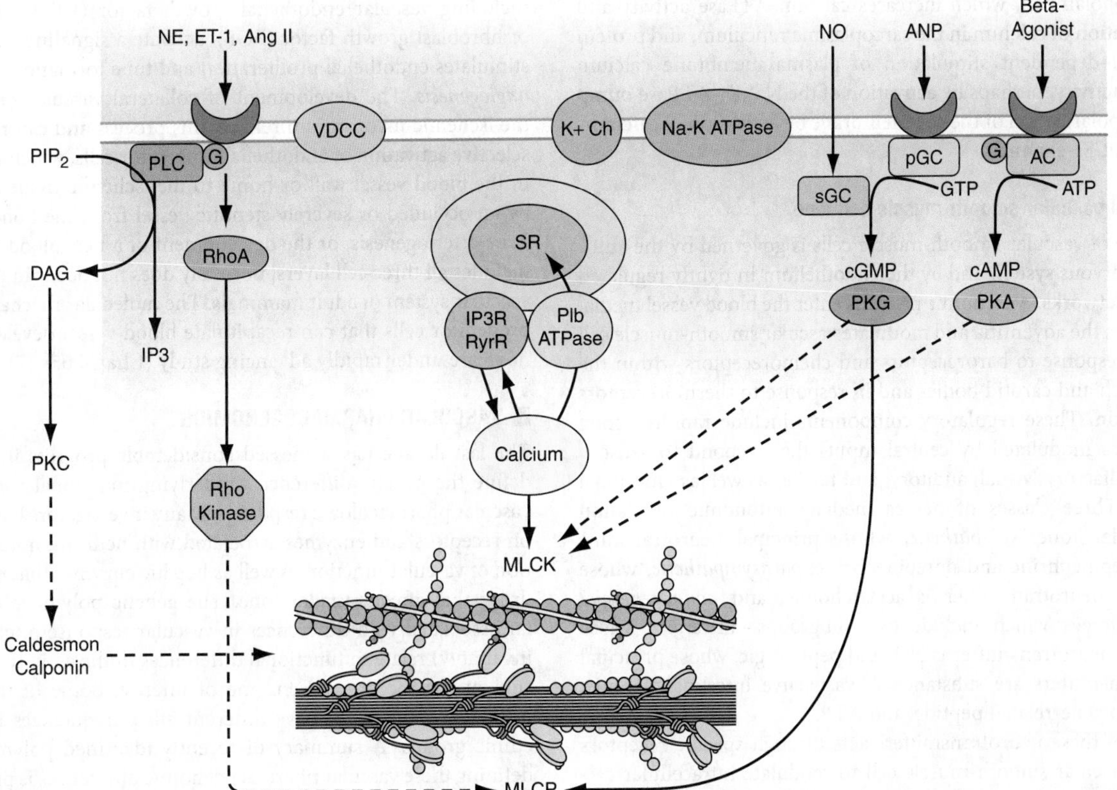

Figure 224-3 Regulation of vascular smooth-muscle cell calcium concentration and actomyosin ATPase-dependent contraction. AC, adenylyl cyclase; Ang II, angiotensin II; ANP, antrial natriuretic peptide; DAG, diacylglycerol; ET-1, endothelin-1; G, G-protein; IP_3, inositol 1,4,5-trisphosphate; MLCK, myosin light chain kinase; MLCP, myosin light chain phosphatase; NE, norepinephrine; NO, nitric oxide; pGC, particular guanylyl cyclase; PIP_2, phosphatidylinositol 4,5-bisphosphate; PKA, protein kinase A; PKC, protein kinase C; PKG, protein kinase G; PLC, phospholipase C; sGC, soluble guanylyl cyclase; SR, sarcoplasmic reticulum; VDCC, voltage-dependent calcium channel. *(Modified from B Berk, in Vascular Medicine, 3rd ed, p 23. Philadelphia, Saunders, Elsevier, 2006; with permission.)*

smooth-muscle cells, voltage-dependent L-type calcium channels open with membrane depolarization, which is regulated by energy-dependent ion pumps such as the Na^+,K^+-ATPase pump and ion channels such as the Ca^{2+}-sensitive K^+ channel. Local changes in intracellular calcium concentration, termed *calcium sparks*, result from the influx of calcium through the voltage-dependent calcium channel and are caused by the coordinated activation of a cluster of ryanodine-sensitive calcium release channels in the sarcoplasmic reticulum (see below). Calcium sparks directly augment intracellular calcium concentration and indirectly increase intracellular calcium concentration by activating chloride channels. In addition, calcium sparks reduce smooth-muscle contractility by activating large-conductance calcium-sensitive K^+ channels, hyperpolarizing the cell membrane and thereby limiting further voltage-dependent increases in intracellular calcium.

Biochemical agonists also increase intracellular calcium concentration, in this case by receptor-dependent activation of phospholipase C with hydrolysis of phosphatidylinositol 4,5-bisphosphate, resulting in generation of diacylglycerol (DAG) and inositol 1,4,5-trisphosphate (IP_3). These membrane lipid derivatives in turn activate protein kinase C and increase intracellular calcium concentration. In addition, IP_3 binds to specific receptors on the sarcoplasmic reticulum membrane to increase calcium efflux from this calcium storage pool into the cytoplasm.

Vascular smooth-muscle cell contraction is controlled principally by the phosphorylation of myosin light chain, which in the steady state depends on the balance between the actions of myosin light chain kinase and myosin light chain phosphatase. Calcium activates myosin light chain kinase through the formation of a calcium-calmodulin complex. Phosphorylation of myosin light chain by this kinase augments myosin ATPase activity and enhances contraction. Myosin light chain phosphatase dephosphorylates myosin light chain, reducing myosin ATPase activity and contractile force. Phosphorylation of the myosin-binding subunit (thr695) of myosin light chain phosphatase by Rho kinase inhibits phosphatase activity and induces calcium sensitization of the contractile apparatus. Rho kinase is itself activated by the small GTPase RhoA, which is stimulated by guanosine exchange factors and inhibited by GTPase-activating proteins.

Both cyclic AMP and cyclic GMP relax vascular smooth-muscle cells through complex mechanisms. β agonists, acting through their G-protein-coupled receptors activate adenylyl cyclase to convert ATP to cyclic AMP; NO and atrial natriuretic peptide acting directly and via a G-protein-coupled receptor, respectively, activate guanylyl cyclase to convert GTP to cyclic GMP. These agents in turn activate protein kinase A and protein kinase G, respectively, which inactivate myosin light chain kinase and decrease vascular smooth-muscle cell tone. In addition, protein kinase G can interact directly with the myosin-binding substrate subunit of myosin light chain phosphatase, increasing phosphatase activity and decreasing vascular tone. Finally, several mechanisms drive NO-dependent, protein kinase G–mediated reductions in vascular smooth-muscle cell calcium concentration, including phosphorylation-dependent inactivation of RhoA; decreased IP_3 formation; phosphorylation of the IP_3 receptor–associated cyclic GMP kinase substrate, with subsequent inhibition of IP_3 receptor function; phosphorylation of phospholamban, which increases calcium ATPase activity and sequestration of calcium in the sarcoplasmic reticulum; and protein kinase G–dependent stimulation of plasma membrane calcium ATPase activity, perhaps by activation of the Na^+,K^+-ATPase pump or hyperpolarization of the cell membrane by activation of calcium-dependent K^+ channels.

Control of vascular smooth-muscle cell tone

The tone of vascular smooth-muscle cells is governed by the autonomic nervous system and by the endothelium in tightly regulated control networks. Autonomic neurons enter the blood vessel medial layer from the adventitia and modulate vascular smooth-muscle cell tone in response to baroreceptors and chemoreceptors within the aortic arch and carotid bodies and in response to thermoreceptors in the skin. These regulatory components include rapidly acting reflex arcs modulated by central inputs that respond to sensory inputs (olfactory, visual, auditory, and tactile) as well as emotional stimuli. Three classes of nerves mediate autonomic regulation of vascular tone: *sympathetic*, whose principal neurotransmitters are epinephrine and norepinephrine; *parasympathetic*, whose principal neurotransmitter is acetylcholine; and *nonadrenergic/noncholinergic*, which include two subgroups—nitrergic, whose principal neurotransmitter is NO, and peptidergic, whose principal neurotransmitters are substance P, vasoactive intestinal peptide, calcitonin gene-related peptide, and ATP.

Each of these neurotransmitters acts through specific receptors on the vascular smooth-muscle cell to modulate intracellular calcium and, consequently, contractile tone. Norepinephrine activates α receptors, and epinephrine activates α and β receptors (adrenergic receptors); in most blood vessels, norepinephrine activates postjunctional α_1 receptors in large arteries and α_2 receptors in small arteries and arterioles, leading to vasoconstriction. Most blood vessels express β_2-adrenergic receptors on their vascular smooth-muscle cells and respond to β agonists by cyclic AMP–dependent relaxation. Acetylcholine released from parasympathetic neurons binds to muscarinic receptors (of which there are five subtypes, M_{1-5}) on vascular smooth-muscle cells to yield vasorelaxation. In addition, NO stimulates presynaptic neurons to release acetylcholine, which can stimulate the release of NO from the endothelium. Nitrergic neurons release NO produced by neuronal NO synthase, which causes vascular smooth-muscle cell relaxation via the cyclic GMP–dependent and –independent mechanisms described above. The peptidergic neurotransmitters all potently vasodilate, acting either directly or through endothelium-dependent NO release to decrease vascular smooth-muscle cell tone. For the detailed molecular physiology of the autonomic nervous system, see Chap. 375.

The endothelium modulates vascular smooth-muscle tone by the direct release of several effectors, including NO, prostacyclin, hydrogen sulfide, and endothelium-derived hyperpolarizing factor, all of which cause vasorelaxation, and endothelin, which causes vasoconstriction. The release of these endothelial effectors of vascular smooth-muscle cell tone is stimulated by mechanical (shear stress, cyclic strain, etc.) and biochemical mediators (purinergic agonists, muscarinic agonists, peptidergic agonists), with the biochemical mediators acting through endothelial receptors specific to each class. In addition to these local paracrine modulators of vascular smooth-muscle cell tone, circulating mediators can affect tone, including norepinephrine and epinephrine, vasopressin, angiotensin II, bradykinin, and the natriuretic peptides (ANP, BNP, CNP, and DNP), as discussed above.

VASCULAR REGENERATION

Growth of new blood vessels can occur in response to conditions such as chronic hypoxemia and tissue ischemia. Growth factors, including vascular endothelial growth factor (VEGF) and forms of fibroblast growth factor (FGF), activate a signaling cascade that stimulates endothelial proliferation and tube formation, defined as *angiogenesis*. The development of collateral vascular networks in the ischemic myocardium reflects this process and can result from selective activation of endothelial progenitor cells, which may reside in the blood vessel wall or home to the ischemic tissue subtended by an occluded or severely stenotic vessel from the bone marrow. True arteriogenesis, or the development of a new blood vessel that includes all three cell layers, normally does not occur in the cardiovascular system of adult mammals. The molecular mechanisms and progenitor cells that can recapitulate blood vessel development de novo are under rapidly advancing study (Chaps. 65–67).

VASCULAR PHARMACOGENOMICS

The last decade has witnessed considerable progress in efforts to define the genetic differences underlying individual variations in vascular pharmacologic responses. Many investigators have focused on receptors and enzymes associated with neurohumoral modulation of vascular function as well as hepatic enzymes that metabolize drugs that affect vascular tone. The genetic polymorphisms thus far associated with differences in vascular response often (but not invariably) relate to functional differences in the activity or expression of the receptor or enzyme of interest. Some of these polymorphisms appear to have different allele frequencies in specific ethnic groups. A summary of recently identified polymorphisms defining these vascular pharmacogenomic differences is provided in Table 224-2. For more detailed discussion, see Chap. 5.

CELLULAR BASIS OF CARDIAC CONTRACTION

CARDIAC ULTRASTRUCTURE

About three-fourths of the ventricular mass is composed of cardiomyocytes, normally 60–140 μm in length and 17–25 μm in diameter (Fig. 224-4*A*). Each cell contains multiple, rodlike cross-banded strands (myofibrils) that run the length of the cell and are composed of serially repeating structures, the sarcomeres. The cytoplasm between the myofibrils contains other cell constituents, including the single centrally located nucleus, numerous mitochondria, and the intracellular membrane system, the sarcoplasmic reticulum.

The *sarcomere*, the structural and functional unit of contraction, lies between adjacent Z lines, which are dark repeating bands that are apparent on transmission electron microscopy. The distance between Z lines varies with the degree of contraction or stretch of the muscle and ranges between 1.6 and 2.2 μm. Within the confines of the sarcomere are alternating light and dark bands, giving the myocardial fibers their striated appearance under the light microscope. At the center of the sarcomere is a dark band of constant length (1.5 μm), the A band, which is flanked by two lighter bands, the I bands, which are of variable length. The sarcomere of heart muscle, like that of skeletal muscle, consists of two sets of interdigitating myofilaments. Thicker filaments, composed principally of the protein myosin, traverse the A band; they are about 10 nm (100 Å) in diameter, with tapered ends. Thinner filaments, composed primarily of actin, course from the Z lines through the I band into the A band; they are approximately 5 nm (50 Å) in diameter and 1.0 μm in length. Thus, thick and thin filaments overlap only within the (dark) A band, whereas the (light) I band contains only thin filaments. On electron-microscopic examination, bridges may be seen to extend between the thick and thin filaments within the A band; these are myosin heads (see below) bound to actin filaments.

THE CONTRACTILE PROCESS

The sliding filament model for muscle contraction rests on the fundamental observation that both the thick and the thin filaments

TABLE 224-2 Genetic Polymorphisms in Vascular Function and Disease Risk

Gene	Polymorphic Allele	Clinical Implications
α-Adrenergic Receptors		
α_{1A}	Arg492Cys	None
α_{2B}	Glu9/G1712	Increased CHD events
α_{2C}	A2cDcl3232-325	Ethnic differences in risk of hypertension or heart failure
Angiotensin-converting enzyme (ACE)	Insertion/deletion polymorphism in intron 16	D allele or DD genotype-increased response to ACE inhibitors; inconsistent data for increased risk of atherosclerotic heart disease, and hypertension
Ang II type I receptor	1166A → C Ala-Cys	Increased response to Ang II and increased risk of pregnancy-associated hypertension
β-Adrenergic Receptors		
β_1		
	Ser49Gly	Increased HR and DCM risk
	Arg389Gly	Increased heart failure in blacks
β_2		
	Arg16Gly	Familial hypertension, increased obesity risk
	Glu27Gln	Hypertension in white type II diabetics
	Thr164Ile	Decreased agonist affinity and worse HF outcome
B2-Bradykinin receptor	Cys58Thr, Cys412Gly, Thr21Met	Increased risk of hypertension in some ethnic groups
Endothelial nitric oxide synthase (eNOS)	Nucleotide repeats in introns 4 and 13, Glu298Asp	Increased MI and venous thrombosis
	Thr785Cys	Early coronary artery disease

Abbreviations: CHD, coronary heart disease; DCM, dilated cardiomyopathy; HF, heart failure; HR, heart rate; MI, myocardial infarction.

Source: Derived from B Schaefer et al: Heart Dis 5:129, 2003.

are constant in overall length during both contraction and relaxation. With activation, the actin filaments are propelled farther into the A band. In the process, the A band remains constant in length, whereas the I band shortens and the Z lines move toward one another.

The *myosin* molecule is a complex, asymmetric fibrous protein with a molecular mass of about 500,000 Da; it has a rodlike portion that is about 150 nm (1500 Å) in length with a globular portion (head) at its end. These globular portions of myosin form the bridges between the myosin and actin molecules and are the site of ATPase activity. In forming the thick myofilament, which is composed of ~300 longitudinally stacked myosin molecules, the rodlike segments of the myosin molecules are laid down in an orderly, polarized manner, leaving the globular portions projecting outward so that they can interact with actin to generate force and shortening (Fig. 224-4*B*).

Actin has a molecular mass of about 47,000 Da. The thin filament consists of a double helix of two chains of actin molecules wound about each other on a larger molecule, tropomyosin. A group of regulatory proteins—troponins C, I, and T—are spaced at regular intervals on this filament (Fig. 224-5). In contrast to myosin, actin lacks intrinsic enzymatic activity but does combine reversibly with myosin in the presence of ATP and Ca^{2+}. The calcium ion activates the myosin ATPase, which in turn breaks down ATP, the energy source for contraction (Fig. 224-5). The activity of myosin ATPase determines the rate of forming and breaking of the actomyosin cross-bridges and ultimately the velocity of muscle contraction. In relaxed muscle, tropomyosin inhibits this interaction. *Titin* (Fig. 224-4*D*) is a large, flexible, myofibrillar protein that connects myosin to the Z line; its stretching contributes to the elasticity of the heart. Dystrophin is a long cytoskeletal protein that has an amino-terminal actin-binding domain and a carboxy-terminal domain that binds to the dystroglycan complex at adherens junctions on the cell membrane, thus tethering the sarcomere to the cell membrane at regions tightly coupled to adjacent contracting myocytes. Mutations in components of the dystrophin complex lead to muscular dystrophy and associated cardiomyopathy.

During activation of the cardiac myocyte, Ca^{2+} becomes attached to one of three components of the heterotrimer troponin C, which results in a conformational change in the regulatory protein tropomyosin; the latter, in turn, exposes the actin cross-bridge interaction sites (Fig. 224-5). Repetitive interaction between myosin heads and actin filaments is termed *cross-bridge cycling*, which results in sliding of the actin along the myosin filaments, ultimately causing muscle shortening and/or the development of tension. The splitting of ATP then dissociates the myosin cross-bridge from actin. In the presence of ATP (Fig. 224-5), linkages between actin and myosin filaments are made and broken cyclically as long as sufficient Ca^{2+} is present; these linkages cease when $[Ca^{2+}]$ falls below a critical level, and the troponin-tropomyosin complex once more prevents interactions between the myosin cross-bridges and actin filaments (Fig. 224-6).

Intracytoplasmic Ca^{2+} is a principal determinant of the inotropic state of the heart. Most agents that stimulate myocardial contractility (positive inotropic stimuli), including the digitalis glycosides and β-adrenergic agonists, increase the $[Ca^{2+}]$ in the vicinity of the myofilaments, which in turn triggers cross-bridge cycling. Increased impulse traffic in the cardiac adrenergic nerves stimulates myocardial contractility as a consequence of the release of norepinephrine from cardiac adrenergic nerve endings. Norepinephrine activates

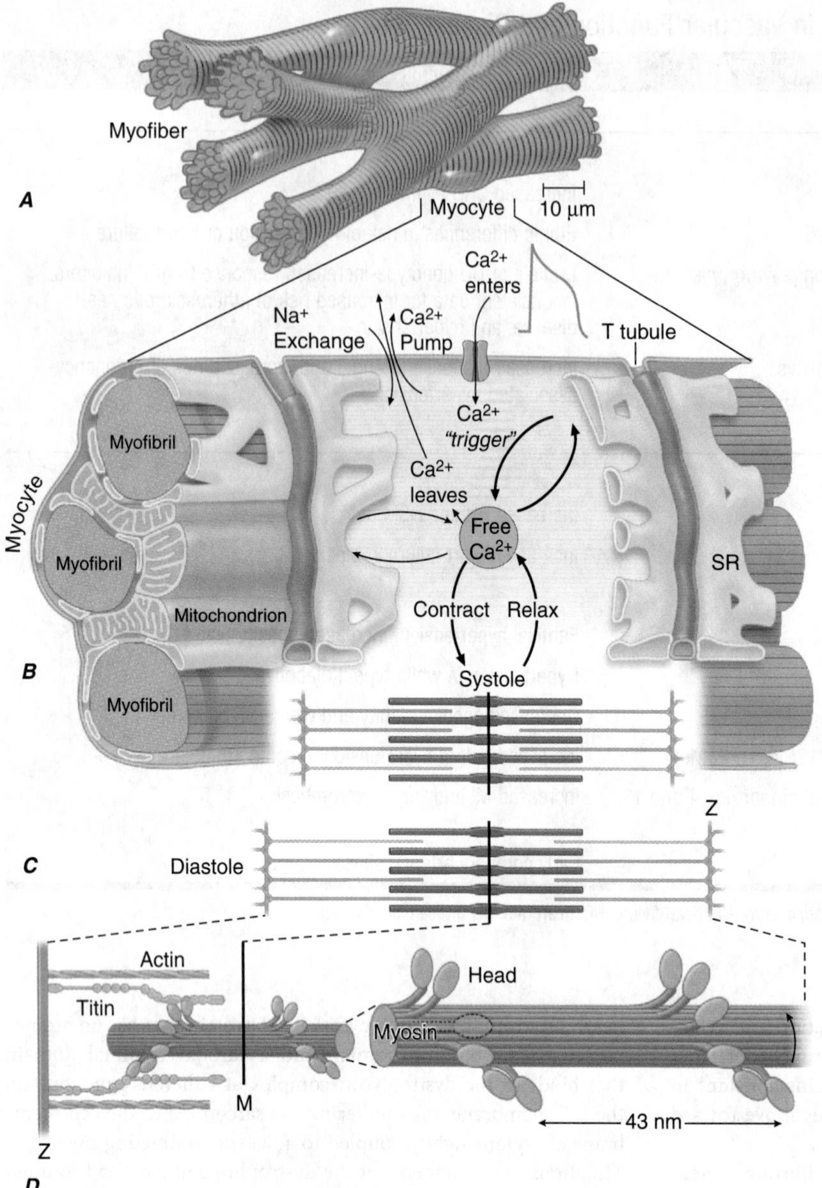

Figure 224-4 ***A*** shows the branching myocytes making up the cardiac myofibers. ***B*** illustrates the critical role played by the changing [Ca^{2+}] in the myocardial cytosol. Ca^{2+} ions are schematically shown as entering through the calcium channel that opens in response to the wave of depolarization that travels along the sarcolemma. These Ca^{2+} ions "trigger" the release of more calcium from the sarcoplasmic reticulum (SR) and thereby initiate a contraction-relaxation cycle. Eventually the small quantity of Ca^{2+} that has entered the cell leaves predominantly through an Na^+/Ca^{2+} exchanger, with a lesser role for the sarcolemmal Ca^{2+} pump. The varying actin-myosin overlap is shown for (***B***) systole, when [Ca^{2+}] is maximal, and (***C***) diastole, when [Ca^{2+}] is minimal. ***D.*** The myosin heads, attached to the thick filaments, interact with the thin actin filaments. *(From LH Opie, Heart Physiology, reprinted with permission. Copyright LH Opie, 2004.)*

myocardial β receptors and, through the G_s-stimulated guanine nucleotide-binding protein, activates the enzyme adenylyl cyclase, which leads to the formation of the intracellular second messenger cyclic AMP from ATP (Fig. 224-6). Cyclic AMP in turn activates protein kinase A (PKA), which phosphorylates the Ca^{2+} channel in the myocardial sarcolemma, thereby enhancing the influx of Ca^{2+} into the myocyte. Other functions of PKA are discussed below.

The *sarcoplasmic reticulum* (SR) (Fig. 224-7), a complex network of anastomosing intracellular channels, invests the myofibrils. Its longitudinally disposed tubules closely invest the surfaces of individual sarcomeres but have no direct continuity with the outside of the cell. However, closely related to the SR, both structurally and functionally, are the transverse tubules, or T system, formed by tubelike invaginations of the sarcolemma that extend into the myocardial fiber along the Z lines, i.e., the ends of the sarcomeres.

CARDIAC ACTIVATION

In the inactive state, the cardiac cell is electrically polarized; i.e., the interior has a negative charge relative to the outside of the cell, with a transmembrane potential of –80 to –100 mV (Chap. 231). The sarcolemma, which in the resting state is largely impermeable to Na^+, has a Na^+- and K^+-stimulating pump energized by ATP that extrudes Na^+ from the cell; this pump plays a critical role in establishing the resting potential. Thus, intracellular [K^+] is relatively high and [Na^+] is far lower; conversely, extracellular [Na^+] is high and [K^+] is low. At the same time, in the resting state, extracellular [Ca^{2+}] greatly exceeds free intracellular [Ca^{2+}].

The action potential has four phases (Fig. 231-1*B*). During the plateau of the action potential (phase 2), there is a slow inward current through L-type Ca^{2+} channels in the sarcolemma (Fig. 224-7). The depolarizing current not only extends across the surface of the cell but penetrates deeply into the cell by way of the ramifying T tubular system. The absolute quantity of Ca^{2+} that crosses the sarcolemma and the T system is relatively small and by itself appears to be insufficient to bring about full activation of the contractile apparatus. However, this Ca^{2+} current triggers the release of much larger quantities of Ca^{2+} from the SR, a process termed *Ca^{2+}-induced Ca^{2+} release*. The latter is a major determinant of intracytoplasmic [Ca^{2+}] and therefore of myocardial contractility.

Ca^{2+} is released from the SR through a Ca^{2+} release channel, a cardiac isoform of the ryanodine receptor (RyR2), which controls intracytoplasmic [Ca^{2+}] and, as in vascular smooth-muscle cells, leads to the local changes in intracellular [Ca^{2+}] called calcium sparks. A number of regulatory proteins, including *calstabin 2*, inhibit RyR2 and thereby the release of Ca^{2+} from the SR. PKA dissociates calstabin from the RyR2, enhancing Ca^{2+} release and thereby myocardial contractility. Excessive plasma catecholamine levels and cardiac sympathetic neuronal release of norepinephrine cause hyperphosphorylation of PKA, leading to calstabin 2–depleted RyR2. The latter depletes SR Ca^{2+} stores and thereby impairs cardiac contraction, leading to heart failure, and also triggers ventricular arrhythmias.

The Ca^{2+} released from the SR then diffuses toward the myofibrils, where, as already described, it combines with troponin C (Fig. 224-6). By repressing this inhibitor of contraction, Ca^{2+} activates the myofilaments to shorten. During repolarization, the activity of the Ca^{2+} pump in the SR, the SR Ca^{2+} ATPase ($SERCA_{2A}$), reaccumulates Ca^{2+} against a concentration gradient, and the Ca^{2+}

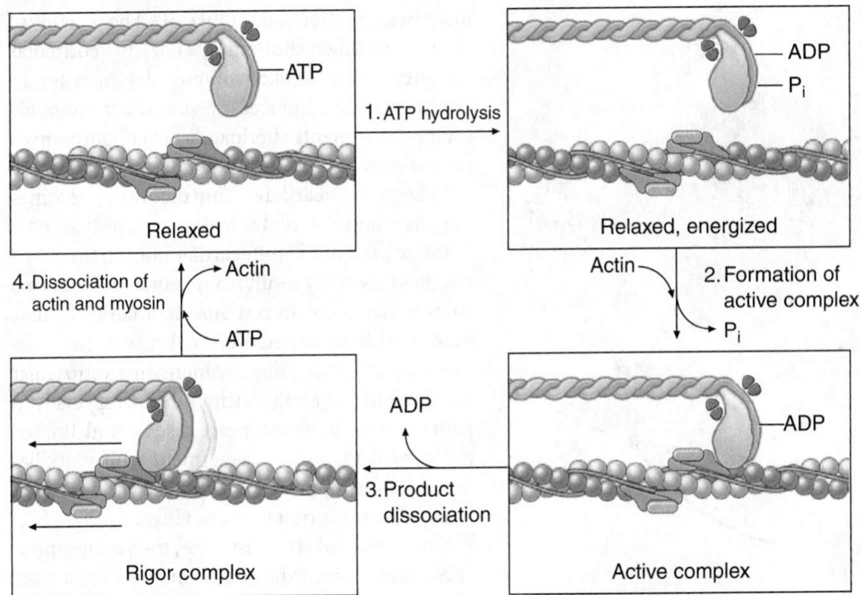

Figure 224-5 Four steps in cardiac muscle contraction and relaxation. In relaxed muscle (***upper left***), ATP bound to the myosin cross-bridge dissociates the thick and thin filaments. ***Step 1:*** Hydrolysis of myosin-bound ATP by the ATPase site on the myosin head transfers the chemical energy of the nucleotide to the activated cross-bridge (***upper right***). When cytosolic Ca^{2+} concentration is low, as in relaxed muscle, the reaction cannot proceed because tropomyosin and the troponin complex on the thin filament do not allow the active sites on actin to interact with the cross-bridges. Therefore, even though the cross-bridges are energized, they cannot interact with actin. ***Step 2:*** When Ca^{2+} binding to troponin C has exposed active sites on the thin filament, actin interacts with the myosin cross-bridges to form an active complex (***lower right***) in which the energy derived from ATP is retained in the actin-bound cross-bridge, whose orientation has not yet shifted. ***Step 3:*** The muscle contracts when ADP dissociates from the cross-bridge. This step leads to the formation of the low-energy rigor complex (***lower left***) in which the chemical energy derived from ATP hydrolysis has been expended to perform mechanical work (the "rowing" motion of the cross-bridge). ***Step 4:*** The muscle returns to its resting state, and the cycle ends when a new molecule of ATP binds to the rigor complex and dissociates the cross-bridge from the thin filament. This cycle continues until calcium is dissociated from troponin C in the thin filament, which causes the contractile proteins to return to the resting state with the cross-bridge in the energized state. ATP, adenosine triphosphate; ATPase, adenosine triphosphatase; ADP, adenosine diphosphate. *[From AM Katz: Heart failure: Cardiac function and dysfunction, in Atlas of Heart Diseases, 3rd ed, WS Colucci (ed). Philadelphia, Current Medicine, 2002. Reprinted with permission.]*

is stored in the SR by its attachment to a protein, *calsequestrin*. This reaccumulation of Ca^{2+} is an energy (ATP)-requiring process that lowers the cytoplasmic [Ca^{2+}] to a level that inhibits the actomyosin interaction responsible for contraction, and in this manner leads to myocardial relaxation. Also, there is an exchange of Ca^{2+} for Na^+ at the sarcolemma (Fig. 224-7), reducing the cytoplasmic [Ca^{2+}]. Cyclic AMP–dependent PKA phosphorylates the SR protein *phospholamban*; the latter, in turn, permits activation of the Ca^{2+} pump, thereby increasing the uptake of Ca^{2+} by the SR, accelerating the rate of relaxation and providing larger quantities of Ca^{2+} in the SR for release by subsequent depolarization, thereby stimulating contraction.

Thus, the combination of the cell membrane, transverse tubules, and SR, with their ability to transmit the action potential and release and then reaccumulate Ca^{2+}, plays a fundamental role in the rhythmic contraction and relaxation of heart muscle. Genetic or pharmacologic alterations of any component, whatever its etiology, can disturb these functions.

CONTROL OF CARDIAC PERFORMANCE AND OUTPUT

The extent of shortening of heart muscle and, therefore, the stroke volume of the ventricle in the intact heart depend on three major influences: (1) the length of the muscle at the onset of contraction, i.e., the preload; (2) the tension that the muscle is called on to develop during contraction, i.e., the afterload; and (3) the contractility of the muscle, i.e., the extent and velocity of shortening at any given preload and afterload. The major determinants of preload, afterload, and contractility are shown in Table 224-3.

The role of muscle length (preload)

The preload determines the length of the sarcomeres at the onset of contraction. The length of the sarcomeres associated with the most forceful contraction is ~2.2 μm. This length provides the optimum configuration for the interaction between the two sets of myofilaments. The length of the sarcomere also regulates the extent of activation of the contractile system, i.e., its sensitivity to Ca^{2+}. According to this concept, termed *length-dependent activation*, myofilament sensitivity to Ca^{2+} is also maximal at the optimal sarcomere length. The relation between the initial length of the muscle fibers and the developed force has prime importance for the function of heart muscle. This relationship forms the basis of Starling's law of the heart, which states that within limits, the force of ventricular contraction depends on the end-diastolic length of the cardiac muscle; in the intact heart, the latter relates closely to the ventricular end-diastolic volume.

Cardiac performance

The ventricular end-diastolic or "filling" pressure sometimes is used as a surrogate for the end-diastolic volume. In isolated heart and heart-lung preparations, the stroke volume varies directly with the end-diastolic fiber length (preload) and inversely with the arterial resistance (afterload), and as the heart fails—i.e., as its contractility declines—it delivers a progressively smaller stroke volume from a normal or even elevated end-diastolic volume. The relation between the ventricular end-diastolic pressure and the stroke work of the ventricle (the ventricular function curve) provides a useful definition of the level of contractility of the heart in the intact organism. An increase in contractility is accompanied by a shift of the ventricular function curve upward and to the left (greater stroke work at any level of ventricular end-diastolic pressure, or lower end-diastolic volume at any level of stroke work), whereas a shift downward and to the right characterizes depression of contractility (Fig. 224-8).

Ventricular afterload

In the intact heart, as in isolated cardiac muscle, the extent and velocity of shortening of ventricular muscle fibers at any level of preload and of myocardial contractility relate inversely to the afterload, i.e., the load that opposes shortening. In the intact heart, the afterload may be defined as the tension developed in the ventricular wall during ejection. Afterload is determined by the aortic pressure as well as by the volume and thickness of the ventricular cavity. Laplace's law states that the tension of the myocardial fiber is the product of the intracavitary ventricular pressure and ventricular radius divided by wall thickness. Therefore, at any particular level of

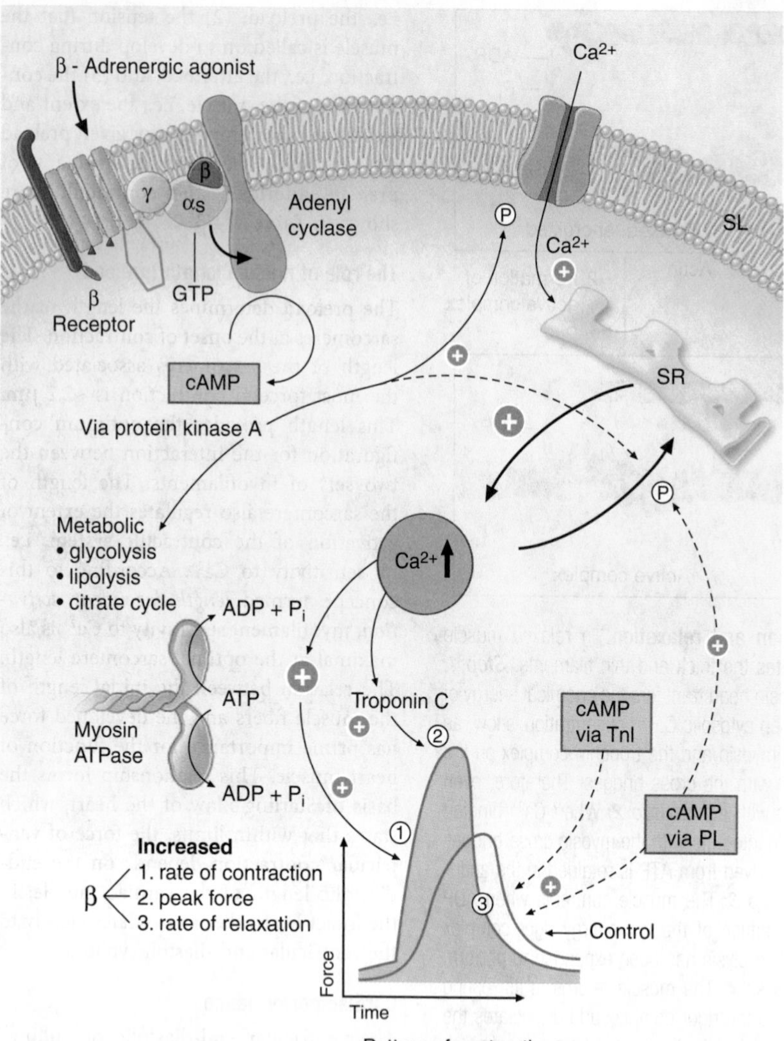

Figure 224-6 Signal systems involved in positive inotropic and lusitropic (enhanced relaxation) effects of β-adrenergic stimulation. When the β-adrenergic agonist interacts with the β receptor, a series of G protein–mediated changes leads to activation of adenylyl cyclase and the formation of cyclic adenosine monophosphate (cAMP). The latter acts via protein kinase A to stimulate metabolism (***left***) and phosphorylate the Ca^{2+} channel protein (***right***). The result is an enhanced opening probability of the Ca^{2+} channel, thereby increasing the inward movement of Ca^{2+} ions through the sarcolemma (SL) of the T tubule. These Ca^{2+} ions release more calcium from the sarcoplasmic reticulum (SR) to increase cytosolic Ca^{2+} and activate troponin C. Ca^{2+} ions also increase the rate of breakdown of adenosine triphosphate (ATP) to adenosine diphosphate (ADP) and inorganic phosphate (Pi). Enhanced myosin ATPase activity explains the increased rate of contraction, with increased activation of troponin C explaining increased peak force development. An increased rate of relaxation is explained by the fact that cAMP also activates the protein phospholamban, situated on the membrane of the SR, that controls the rate of uptake of calcium into the SR. The latter effect explains enhanced relaxation (lusitropic effect). P, phosphorylation; PL, phospholamban; TnI, troponin I. *(Modified from LH Opie, Heart Physiology, reprinted with permission. Copyright LH Opie, 2004.)*

aortic pressure, the afterload on a dilated left ventricle exceeds that on a normal-sized ventricle. Conversely, at the same aortic pressure and ventricular diastolic volume, the afterload on a hypertrophied ventricle is lower than of a normal chamber. The aortic pressure in turn depends on the peripheral vascular resistance, the physical characteristics of the arterial tree, and the volume of blood it contains at the onset of ejection.

Ventricular afterload critically regulates cardiovascular performance (Fig. 224-9). As already noted, elevations in both preload and contractility increase myocardial fiber shortening, whereas increases in afterload reduce it. The extent of myocardial fiber shortening and left ventricular size determine stroke volume. An increase in arterial pressure induced by vasoconstriction, for example, augments afterload, which opposes myocardial fiber shortening, reducing stroke volume.

When myocardial contractility becomes impaired and the ventricle dilates, afterload rises (Laplace's law) and limits cardiac output. Increased afterload also may result from neural and humoral stimuli that occur in response to a fall in cardiac output. This increased afterload may reduce cardiac output further, thereby increasing ventricular volume and initiating a vicious circle, especially in patients with ischemic heart disease and limited myocardial O_2 supply. Treatment with vasodilators has the opposite effect; when afterload is reduced, cardiac output rises (Chap. 234).

Under normal circumstances, the various influences acting on cardiac performance enumerated above interact in a complex fashion to maintain cardiac output at a level appropriate to the requirements of the metabolizing tissues (Fig. 224-9); interference with a single mechanism may not influence the cardiac output. For example, a moderate reduction of blood volume or the loss of the atrial contribution to ventricular contraction ordinarily can be sustained without a reduction in the cardiac output at rest. Under these circumstances, other factors, such as increases in the frequency of adrenergic nerve impulses to the heart, heart rate, and venous tone, will serve as compensatory mechanisms and sustain cardiac output in a normal individual.

Exercise

The integrated response to exercise illustrates the interactions among the three determinants of stroke volume: preload, afterload, and contractility (Fig. 224-8). Hyperventilation, the pumping action of the exercising muscles, and venoconstriction during exercise all augment venous return and hence ventricular filling and preload (Table 224-3). Simultaneously, the increase in the adrenergic nerve impulse traffic to the myocardium, the increased concentration of circulating catecholamines, and the tachycardia that occur during exercise combine to augment the contractility of the myocardium (Fig. 224-8, curves 1 and 2) and together elevate stroke volume and stroke work, without a change in or even a reduction of end-diastolic pressure and volume (Fig. 224-8, points A and B). Vasodilation occurs in the exercising muscles, thus tending to limit the increase in arterial pressure that otherwise would occur as cardiac output rises to levels as high as five times greater than basal levels during maximal exercise. This vasodilation ultimately allows the achievement of a greatly elevated cardiac output during exercise at an arterial pressure only moderately higher than in the resting state.

ASSESSMENT OF CARDIAC FUNCTION

Several techniques can define impaired cardiac function in clinical practice. The cardiac output and stroke volume may be depressed in the presence of heart failure, but not uncommonly, these variables are

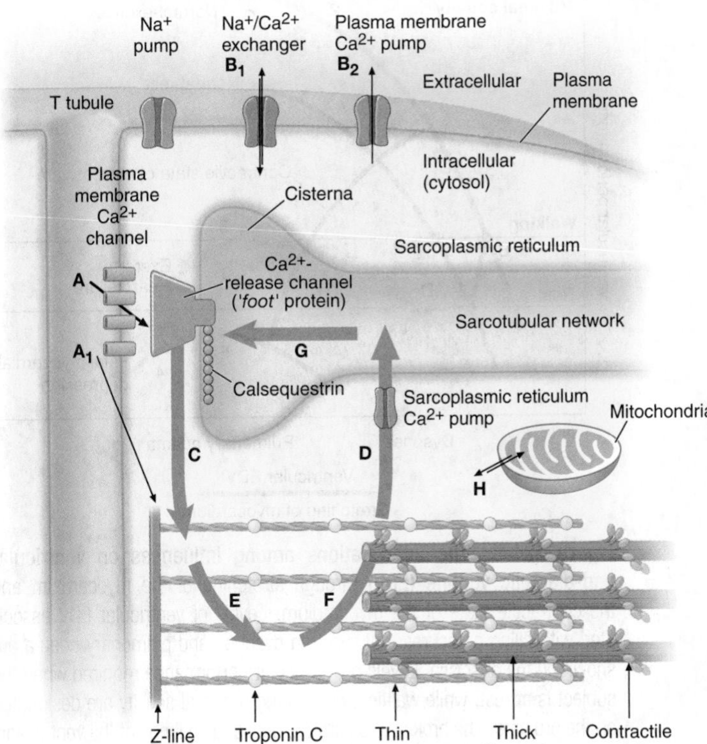

Figure 224-7 The Ca^{2+} fluxes and key structures involved in cardiac excitation-contraction coupling. The arrows denote the direction of Ca^{2+} fluxes. The thickness of each arrow indicates the magnitude of the calcium flux. Two Ca^{2+} cycles regulate excitation-contraction coupling and relaxation. The larger cycle is entirely intracellular and involves Ca^{2+} fluxes into and out of the sarcoplasmic reticulum, as well as Ca^{2+} binding to and release from troponin C. The smaller extracellular Ca^{2+} cycle occurs when this cation moves into and out of the cell. The action potential opens plasma membrane Ca^{2+} channels to allow passive entry of Ca^{2+} into the cell from the extracellular fluid (***arrow A***). Only a small portion of the Ca^{2+} that enters the cell directly activates the contractile proteins (***arrow A_1***). The extracellular cycle is completed when Ca^{2+} is actively transported back out to the extracellular fluid by way of two plasma membrane fluxes mediated by the sodium-calcium exchanger (***arrow B_1***) and the plasma membrane calcium pump (***arrow B_2***). In the intracellular Ca^{2+} cycle, passive Ca^{2+} release occurs through channels in the cisternae (***arrow C***) and initiates contraction; active Ca^{2+} uptake by the Ca^{2+} pump of the sarcotubular network (***arrow D***) relaxes the heart. Diffusion of Ca^{2+} within the sarcoplasmic reticulum (***arrow G***) returns this activator cation to the cisternae, where it is stored in a complex with calsequestrin and other calcium-binding proteins. Ca^{2+} released from the sarcoplasmic reticulum initiates systole when it binds to troponin C (***arrow E***). Lowering of cytosolic [Ca^{2+}] by the sarcoplasmic reticulum (SR) causes this ion to dissociate from troponin (***arrow F***) and relaxes the heart. Ca^{2+} also may move between mitochondria and cytoplasm (H). *(Adapted from Katz, with permission.)*

within normal limits in this condition. A somewhat more sensitive index of cardiac function is the ejection fraction, i.e., the ratio of stroke volume to end-diastolic volume (normal value = 67 ± 8%), which is frequently depressed in systolic heart failure even when the stroke volume itself is normal. Alternatively, abnormally elevated ventricular end-diastolic volume (normal value = 75 ± 20 mL/m²) or end-systolic volume (normal value = 25 ± 7 mL/m²) signifies impairment of left ventricular systolic function.

Noninvasive techniques, particularly echocardiography as well as radionuclide scintigraphy and cardiac magnetic resonance imaging (MRI) (Chap. 229), have great value in the clinical assessment of myocardial function. They provide measurements of end-diastolic and end-systolic volumes, ejection fraction, and systolic shortening rate, and they allow assessment of ventricular filling (see below) as well as regional contraction and relaxation. The latter measurements are particularly important in ischemic heart disease, as myocardial infarction causes regional myocardial damage.

A limitation of measurements of cardiac output, ejection fraction, and ventricular volumes in assessing cardiac function is that ventricular loading conditions strongly influence these variables. Thus, a depressed ejection fraction and lowered cardiac output may be observed in patients with normal ventricular function but reduced preload, as occurs in hypovolemia, or with increased afterload, as occurs in acutely elevated arterial pressure.

The end-systolic left ventricular pressure-volume relationship is a particularly useful index of ventricular performance since it does not depend on preload and afterload (Fig. 224-10). At any level of myocardial contractility, left ventricular end-systolic volume varies inversely with end-systolic pressure; as contractility declines, end-systolic volume (at any level of end-systolic pressure) rises.

■ DIASTOLIC FUNCTION

Ventricular filling is influenced by the extent and speed of myocardial relaxation, which in turn depends on the rate of uptake of Ca^{2+} by the SR; the latter may be enhanced by adrenergic activation and reduced by ischemia, which reduces the ATP available for pumping Ca^{2+} into the SR (see above). The stiffness of the ventricular wall also may impede filling. Ventricular stiffness increases with hypertrophy and conditions that infiltrate the ventricle, such as amyloid, or is caused by an extrinsic constraint (e.g., pericardial compression) (Fig. 224-11).

Ventricular filling can be assessed by continuously measuring the velocity of flow across the mitral valve, using Doppler ultrasound. Normally, the velocity of inflow is more rapid in early diastole than during atrial systole; with mild to moderately impaired relaxation, the rate of early diastolic filling declines, whereas the rate of presystolic filling rises. With further impairment of filling, the pattern is "pseudo-normalized," and early ventricular filling becomes more rapid as left atrial pressure upstream to the stiff left ventricle rises.

■ CARDIAC METABOLISM

The heart requires a continuous supply of energy (in the form of ATP) not only to perform its mechanical pumping functions, but also to regulate intracellular and transsarcolemmal ionic movements and concentration gradients. Among its pumping functions, the development of tension, the frequency of contraction, and the level of myocardial contractility are the principal determinants of the heart's substantial energy needs, making its O_2 requirements approximately 15% of that of the entire organism.

Most ATP production depends on the oxidation of substrate [glucose and free fatty acids (FFAs)]. Myocardial FFAs are derived from circulating FFAs, which result principally from lipolysis in adipose tissue, whereas the myocyte's glucose derives from plasma as well as from the cell's breakdown of its glycogen stores (glycogenolysis). These two principal sources of acetyl coenzyme A in cardiac muscle vary reciprocally. Glucose is broken down in the cytoplasm into a three-carbon product, pyruvate, which passes into the mitochondria, where it is metabolized to the two-carbon fragment,

TABLE 224-3 Determinants of Stroke Volume

I. Ventricular Preload
  A. Blood volume
  B. Distribution of blood volume
    1. Body position
    2. Intrathoracic pressure
    3. Intrapericardial pressure
    4. Venous tone
    5. Pumping action of skeletal muscles
  C. Atrial contraction

II. Ventricular Afterload
  A. Systemic vascular resistance
  B. Elasticity of arterial tree
  C. Arterial blood volume
  D. Ventricular wall tension
    1. Ventricular radius
    2. Ventricular wall thickness

III. Myocardial Contractility[a]
  A. Intramyocardial [Ca^{2+}] ↑↓
  B. Cardiac adrenergic nerve activity ↑↓[b]
  C. Circulating catecholamines ↑↓[b]
  D. Cardiac rate ↑↓[b]
  E. Exogenous inotropic agents↑
  F. Myocardial ischemia ↓
  G. Myocardial cell death (necrosis, apoptosis, autophagy) ↓
  H. Alterations of sarcomeric and cytoskeletal proteins ↓
    1. Genetic
    2. Hemodynamic overload
  I. Myocardial fibrosis ↓
  J. Chronic overexpression of neurohormones ↓
  K. Ventricular remodeling ↓
  L. Chronic and/or excessive myocardial hypertrophy ↓

[a]Arrows indicate directional effects of determinants of contractility.
[b]Contractility rises initially but later becomes depressed.

acetyl-Co-A, and undergoes oxidation. FFAs are converted to acyl-CoA in the cytoplasm and acetyl-CoA in the mitochondria. Acetyl-CoA enters the citric acid (Krebs) cycle to produce ATP by oxidative phosphorylation within the mitochondria; ATP then enters the cytoplasm from the mitochondrial compartment. Intracellular ADP, resulting from the breakdown of ATP, enhances mitochondrial ATP production.

In the fasted, resting state, circulating FFA concentrations and their myocardial uptake are high, and they furnish most of the heart's acetyl-CoA (~70%). In the fed state, with elevations of blood glucose and insulin, glucose oxidation increases and FFA oxidation subsides. Increased cardiac work, the administration of inotropic agents, hypoxia, and mild ischemia all enhance myocardial glucose uptake, glucose production resulting from glycogenolysis, and glucose metabolism to pyruvate (glycolysis). By contrast, β-adrenergic stimulation, as occurs during stress, raises the circulating levels and metabolism of FFAs in favor of glucose. Severe ischemia inhibits the cytoplasmic enzyme pyruvate dehydrogenase, and despite both glycogen and glucose breakdown, glucose is metabolized only to lactic acid (anaerobic glycolysis), which does not enter the citric

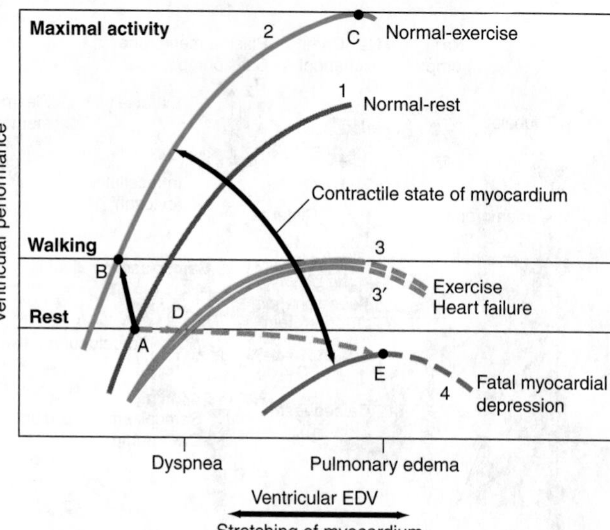

Figure 224-8 The interrelations among influences on ventricular end-diastolic volume (EDV) through stretching of the myocardium and the contractile state of the myocardium. Levels of ventricular EDV associated with filling pressures that result in dyspnea and pulmonary edema are shown on the abscissa. Levels of ventricular performance required when the subject is at rest, while walking, and during maximal activity are designated on the ordinate. The broken lines are the descending limbs of the ventricular-performance curves, which are rarely seen during life but show the level of ventricular performance if end-diastolic volume could be elevated to very high levels. For further explanation, see text. *[Modified from WS Colucci and E Braunwald: Pathophysiology of heart failure, in Braunwald's Heart Disease, 7th ed, DP Zipes et al (eds). Philadelphia: Elsevier, 2005, pp 509–538.]*

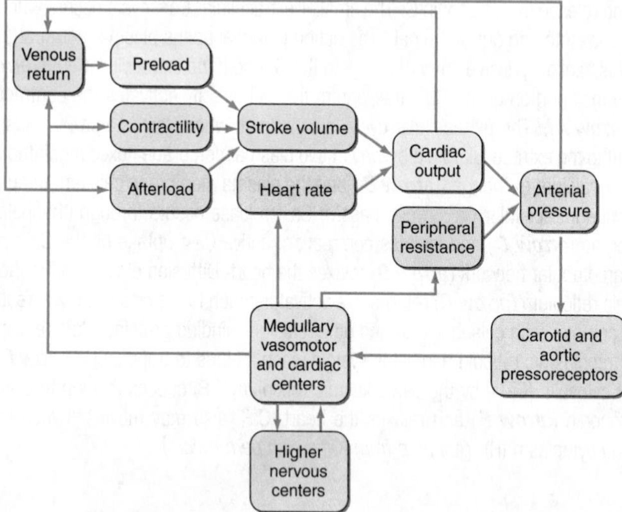

Figure 224-9 Interactions in the intact circulation of preload, contractility, and afterload in producing stroke volume. Stroke volume combined with heart rate determines cardiac output, which, when combined with peripheral vascular resistance, determines arterial pressure for tissue perfusion. The characteristics of the arterial system also contribute to afterload, an increase which reduces stroke volume. The interaction of these components with carotid and aortic arch baroreceptors provides a feedback mechanism to higher medullary and vasomotor cardiac centers and to higher levels in the central nervous system to effect a modulating influence on heart rate, peripheral vascular resistance, venous return, and contractility. *[From MR Starling: Physiology of myocardial contraction, in Atlas of Heart Failure: Cardiac Function and Dysfunction, 3rd ed, WS Colucci and E Braunwald (eds). Philadelphia: Current Medicine, 2002, pp 19–35.]*

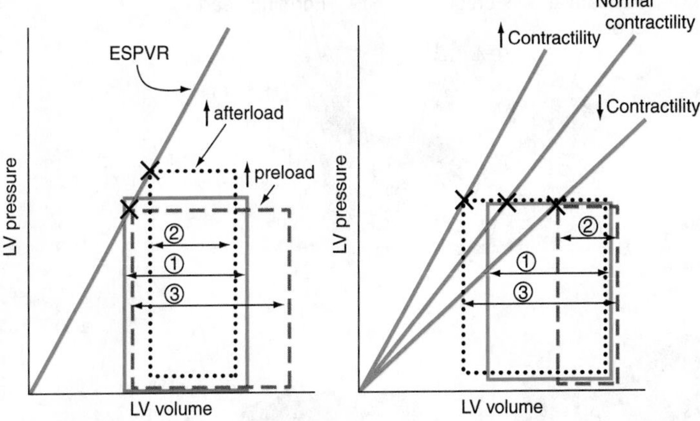

Figure 224-10 The responses of the left ventricle to increased afterload, increased preload, and increased and reduced contractility are shown in the pressure-volume plane. ***Left.*** Effects of increases in preload and afterload on the pressure-volume loop. Since there has been no change in contractility, ESPVR (the end-systolic pressure-volume relation) is unchanged. With an increase in afterload, stroke volume falls (1 → 2); with an increase in preload, stroke volume rises (1 → 3). ***Right.*** With increased myocardial contractility and constant LV end-diastolic volume, the ESPVR moves to the left of the normal line (lower end-systolic volume at any end-systolic pressure) and stroke volume rises (1 → 3). With reduced myocardial contractility, the ESPVR moves to the right; end-systolic volume is increased, and stroke volume falls (1 → 2).

acid cycle. Anaerobic glycolysis produces much less ATP than does aerobic glucose metabolism, in which glucose is metabolized to pyruvate and subsequently oxidized to CO_2. High concentrations of circulating FFAs, which can occur when adrenergic stimulation is superimposed on severe ischemia, reduce oxidative phosphorylation and also cause ATP wastage; the myocardial content of ATP

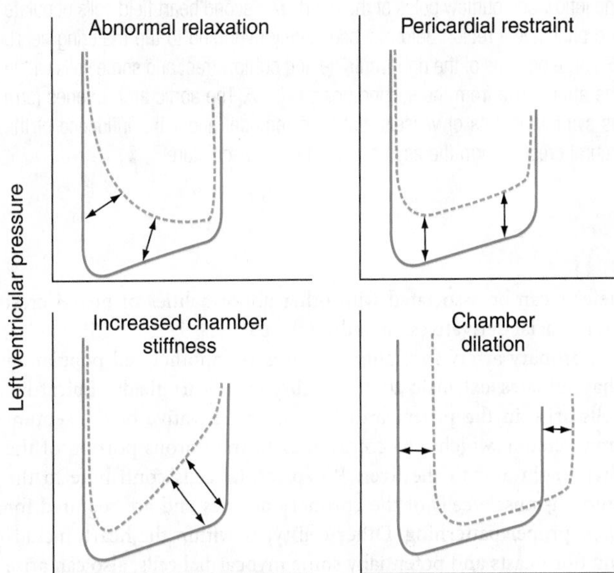

Figure 224-11 Mechanisms that cause diastolic dysfunction reflected in the pressure-volume relation. The bottom half of the pressure-volume loop is depicted. Solid lines represent normal subjects; broken lines represent patients with diastolic dysfunction. *(From JD Carroll et al: The differential effects of positive inotropic and vasodilator therapy on diastolic properties in patients with congestive cardiomyopathy. Circulation 74:815, 1986; with permission.)*

declines and impairs myocardial contraction. In addition, products of FFA breakdown can exert toxic effects on cardiac cell membranes and may be arrhythmogenic.

Myocardial energy is stored as creatine phosphate (CP), which is in equilibrium with ATP, the immediate source of energy. In states of reduced energy availability, the CP stores decline first. Cardiac hypertrophy, fibrosis, tachycardia, increased wall tension resulting from ventricular dilation, and increased intracytoplasmic [Ca^{2+}] all contribute to increased myocardial energy needs. When coupled with reduced coronary flow reserve, as occurs with obstruction of coronary arteries or abnormalities of the coronary microcirculation, an imbalance in myocardial ATP production relative to demand may occur, and the resulting ischemia can worsen or cause heart failure.

Developmental biology of the cardiovascular system

The heart is the first organ to form during embryogenesis (Fig. 224-12) and must accomplish the simultaneous challenges of circulating blood, nutrients, and oxygen to the other forming organs while continuing to grow and undergo complex morphogenetic changes. Early progenitors of the heart arise within very early crescent-shaped fields of lateral splanchnic mesoderm under the influence of multiple signals, including those derived from neural ectoderm long before neural tube closure. Early cardiac precursors express regulatory transcription factors that play reiterated roles in cardiac development, such as NKX2-5 and GATA4; these mutations are responsible for some forms of inherited congenital heart disease. Early cardiac precursors form two bilateral heart tubes, each composed of a single cell layer of endocardium surrounded by a single layer of myocardial precursors. Subsequently, a single midline heart tube is formed by the medial migration and midline fusion of these bilateral structures. The caudal, inflow region of the heart tube adopts a more rostral final position and represents the atrial anlagen, whereas the rostral, outflow portion of the tube forms the truncus arteriosus, which divides to produce the aorta and the proximal pulmonary artery. Between these extremes lie the structural precursors of the ventricles.

The linear heart tube undergoes an asymmetric looping process (the first gross evidence of left-right asymmetry in the developing embryo), which positions the portion of the heart tube destined to become the left ventricle to the left of the more rostral precursors of the right ventricle and outflow tract. Looping is coordinated with chamber specification and ballooning of various regions of the heart tube to produce the presumptive atria and ventricles.

Relatively recent work has demonstrated that significant portions of the right ventricle are formed by cells that are added to the developing heart after looping has occurred. These cells, which are derived from what is called the second heart field, derive from progenitors in the ventral pharynx and express markers that allow for their identification, including islet-1. Different embryologic origins of cells within the right and left ventricles may help explain why some forms of congenital and adult heart diseases affect these regions of the heart to varying degrees.

After looping and chamber formation, a series of septation events divide the left and right sides of the heart, separate the atria from the ventricles, and form the aorta and pulmonary artery from the truncus arteriosus. Cardiac valves form between the atria and the ventricles and between the ventricles and the outflow vessels. Early in development, the single layer of myocardial cells secretes an extracellular matrix rich in hyaluronic acid. This extracellular matrix, termed "cardiac jelly," accumulates within the endocardial cushions, precursors of the cardiac valves. Signals from overlying

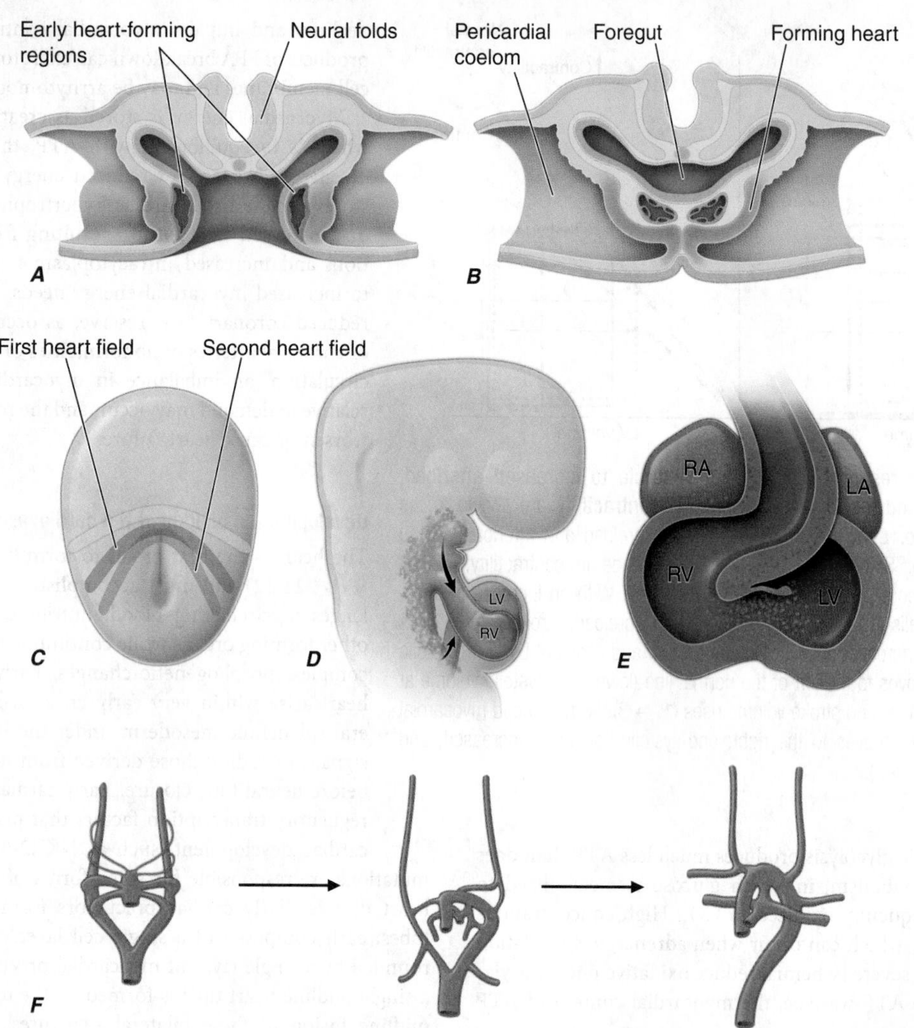

Figure 224-12 ***A.*** Schematic depiction of a transverse section through an early embryo depicts the bilateral regions where early heart tubes form. ***B.*** The bilateral heart tubes subsequently migrate to the midline and fuse to form the linear heart tube. ***C.*** At the early cardiac crescent stage of embryonic development, cardiac precursors include a primary heart field fated to form the linear heart tube and a second heart field fated to add myocardium to the inflow and outflow poles of the heart. ***D.*** Second heart field cells populate the pharyngeal region before subsequently migrating to the maturing heart. ***E.*** Large portions of the right ventricle and outflow tract and some cells within the atria derive from the second heart field. ***F.*** The aortic arch arteries form as symmetric sets of vessels that then remodel under the influence of the neural crest to form the asymmetric mature vasculature.

myocardial cells, including members of the transforming growth factor β family, trigger migration, invasion, and phenotypic changes of underlying endocardial cells, which undergo an epithelial-mesenchymal transformation and invade the cardiac jelly to cellularize the endocardial cushions. Mesenchymal components proliferate and remodel to form the mature valve leaflets.

The great vessels form as a series of bilaterally symmetric aortic arch arteries that undergo asymmetric remodeling events to form the mature vasculature. The immigration of neural crest cells that arise in the dorsal neural tube orchestrates this process. These cells are required for aortic arch remodeling and septation of the truncus arteriosus. They develop into smooth-muscle cells within the tunica media of the aortic arch, the ductus arteriosus, and the carotid arteries. Smooth-muscle cells within the descending aorta arise from a different embryologic source, the lateral plate mesoderm. Neural crest cells are sensitive to both vitamin A and folic acid, and congenital heart disease involving abnormal remodeling of the aortic arch arteries has been associated with maternal deficiencies of these vitamins. Genetic syndromes associated with aortic arch defects can be associated with other abnormalities of neural crest craniofacial derivatives, including the palate.

Coronary artery formation requires yet another cell population that initiates extrinsic to the embryonic heart fields. Epicardial cells arise in the proepicardial organ, a derivative of the septum transversum, which also contributes to the fibrous portion of the diaphragm and to the liver. Proepicardial cells contribute to the smooth-muscle cells of the coronary arteries and are required for their proper patterning. Other cell types within the heart, including fibroblasts and potentially some myocardial cells, also can arise from the proepicardium.

The cardiac conduction system, which functions both to generate and to propagate electrical impulses, develops primarily from multipotential cardiac precursors. The conduction system is composed of slow (proximal) components, such as the sinoatrial (SA) and atrioventricular (AV) nodes, as well as fast (distal) components, including the His bundle, bundle branches, and Purkinje fibers. The AV node primarily serves to delay the electrical impulse between atria and ventricles (manifesting decremental conduction), whereas the distal conduction system rapidly delivers the impulse throughout the ventricles. Significant recent attention has been focused on the embryologic origins of various components of the specialized conduction network. Precursors within the sinus venosus give rise to the SA node, whereas those within the AV canal mature into heterogeneous cell types that compose the AV node. Myocardial cells transdifferentiate into Purkinje fibers to form the distal conduction system. Fast and slow conducting cell types within the nodes and bundles are characterized by expression of distinct gap junction proteins, including connexins, and ion channels that characterize unique cell fates and electrical properties of the tissues. Developmental defects in conduction system morphogenesis and lineage determination can lead to various electrophysiologic disorders, including congenital heart block and preexcitation syndromes such as Wolff-Parkinson-White syndrome (Chap. 233).

Studies of cardiac stem and progenitor cells suggest that progressive lineage restriction results in the gradual and stepwise determination of mature cell fates within the heart, with early precursors capable of adopting endothelial, smooth-muscle, or cardiac phenotypes, and subsequent further specialization into atrial, ventricular, and specialized conduction cell types.

REGENERATING CARDIAC TISSUE

Until very recently, adult mammalian myocardial cells were viewed as fully differentiated and without regenerative potential. Evidence currently supports the existence of limited endogenous regenerative potential of mature cardiac myocytes, resident cardiac progenitors, and/or bone marrow–derived stem cells. Considerable current effort is being devoted to evaluating the utility of cells from these sources to enhance the regenerative potential of the heart. The success of such approaches would offer the exciting possibility of reconstructing an infarcted or failing ventricle (Chaps. 65 and 67).

FURTHER READINGS

Colucci WS, Braunwald E (eds): *Atlas of Heart Failure: Cardiac Function and Dysfunction*, 4th ed. Philadelphia, Current Medicine, 2004

Deanfield JE et al: Endothelial function and dysfunction: Testing and clinical relevance. Circulation 115:1285, 2007

Katz AM: *Physiology of the Heart*, 4th ed. Philadelphia, Lippincott, Williams & Wilkins, 2005

Kirby ML: *Cardiac Development*. New York, Oxford University Press, 2007

Libby P et al: The vascular endothelium and atherosclerosis, in *The Handbook of Experimental Pharmacology*, S Moncada and EA Higgs (eds). Berlin-Heidelberg, Springer-Verlag, 2006

Mahoney WM, Schwartz SM: Defining smooth muscle cells and smooth muscle cell injury. J Clin Invest 15:221, 2005

Opie LH: *Heart Physiology: From Cell to Circulation*, 4th ed. Philadelphia, Lippincott, Williams & Wilkins, 2004

———: Mechanisms of cardiac contraction and relaxation, in *Braunwald's Heart Disease*, 8th ed, P Libby et al (eds). Philadelphia, Elsevier, 2008

Wehrens XH et al: Intracellular calcium release and cardiac disease. Annu Rev Physiol 67:69, 2005

CHAPTER 225

Epidemiology of Cardiovascular Disease

Thomas A. Gaziano
J. Michael Gaziano

Cardiovascular disease (CVD) is now the most common cause of death worldwide. Before 1900, infectious diseases and malnutrition were the most common causes and CVD was responsible for less than 10% of all deaths. Today, CVD accounts for approximately 30% of deaths worldwide, including nearly 40% in high-income countries and about 28% in low- and middle-income countries.

THE EPIDEMIOLOGIC TRANSITION

The global rise in CVD is the result of an unprecedented transformation in the causes of morbidity and mortality during the twentieth and twenty-first centuries. Known as the epidemiologic transition, this shift is driven by industrialization, urbanization, and associated lifestyle changes and is taking place in every part of the world among all races, ethnic groups, and cultures. The transition is divided into four basic stages: pestilence and famine, receding pandemics, degenerative and human-made diseases, and delayed degenerative diseases. A fifth stage, characterized by an epidemic of inactivity and obesity, may be emerging in some countries (Table 225-1).

Malnutrition, infectious diseases, and high infant and child mortality rates that are offset by high fertility mark the *age of pestilence and famine*. Tuberculosis, dysentery, cholera, and influenza are often fatal, resulting in a mean life expectancy of about 30 years. Cardiovascular disease, which accounts for less than 10% of deaths, takes the form of rheumatic heart disease and cardiomyopathies due to infection and malnutrition. Approximately 10% of the world's population remains in the age of pestilence and famine.

Per capita income and life expectancy increase during the *age of receding pandemics* as the emergence of public health systems, cleaner water supplies, and improved nutrition combine to drive down deaths from infectious disease and malnutrition. Infant and childhood mortality rates also decline, but deaths due to CVD increase to between 10% and 35% of all deaths. Rheumatic valvular disease, hypertension, coronary heart disease, and stroke are the predominant forms of CVD. Almost 40% of the world's population is currently in this stage.

The *age of degenerative and human-made diseases* is distinguished by mortality from noncommunicable diseases—primarily CVD—surpassing mortality from malnutrition and infectious diseases. Caloric intake, particularly from animal fat, increases. Coronary heart disease and stroke are prevalent, and 35%–65% of all deaths can be traced to CVD. Typically, the rate of CHD deaths exceeds that of stroke by a ratio of 2:1 to 3:1. During this period, average life expectancy surpasses 50 years. Roughly 35% of the world's population falls into this category.

In the *age of delayed degenerative diseases*, CVD and cancer remain the major causes of morbidity and mortality, with CVD accounting for 40% of all deaths. However, age-adjusted CVD mortality declines, aided by preventive strategies such as smoking cessation programs and effective blood pressure control, acute

TABLE 225-1 Five Stages of the Epidemiologic Transition

Stage	Description	Deaths Related to CVD, %	Predominant CVD Type
Pestilence and famine	Predominance of malnutrition and infectious diseases as causes of death; high rates of infant and child mortality; low mean life expectancy	<10	Rheumatic heart disease, cardiomopathies caused by infection and malnutrition
Receding pandemics	Improvements in nutrition and public health lead to decrease in rates of deaths related to malnutrition and infection; precipitous decline in infant and child mortality rates	10–35	Rheumatic valvular disease, hypertension, CHD, and stroke (predominantly hemorrhagic)
Degenerative and human-made diseases	Increased fat and caloric intake and decrease in physical activity lead to emergence of hypertension and atherosclerosis; with increase in life expectancy, mortality from chronic, noncommunicable diseases exceeds mortality from malnutrition and infectious disease	35–65	CHD and stroke (ischemic and hemorrhagic)
Delayed degenerative diseases	CVD and cancer are the major causes of morbidity and mortality; better treatment and prevention efforts help avoid deaths among those with disease and delay primary events; age-adjusted CVD morality rate declines; CVD affecting older and older individuals	40–50	CHD, stroke, and congestive heart failure
Inactivity and obesity	Overweight and obesity increase at alarming rate; diabetes and hypertension increase; decline in smoking rates levels off; a minority of the population meets physical activity recommendations	Possible reversal of age-adjusted declines in mortality	CHD, stroke, and congestive heart failure, peripheral vascular disease

Abbreviations: CHD, coronary heart disease; CVD, cardiovascular disease.
Source: Adapted from AR Omran: Milbank Mem Fund Q 49:509, 1971; and SJ Olshansky, AB Ault: Milbank Q 64:355, 1986.

hospital management, and technological advances such as the availability of bypass surgery. Coronary heart disease (CHD), stroke, and congestive heart failure are the primary forms of CVD. About 15% of the world's population is now in the age of delayed degenerative diseases or is exiting this age and moving into the fifth stage of the epidemiologic transition.

In the industrialized world, physical activity continues to decline while total caloric intake increases. The resulting epidemic of overweight and obesity may signal the start of the *age of inactivity and obesity*. Rates of Type 2 diabetes mellitus, hypertension, and lipid abnormalities are on the rise, trends that are particularly evident in children. If these risk factor trends continue, age-adjusted CVD mortality rates could increase in the coming years.

THE EPIDEMIOLOGIC TRANSITION IN THE UNITED STATES

The United States, like other high-income countries, has proceeded through four stages of the epidemiologic transition. Recent trends, however, suggest that the rates of decline of some chronic and degenerative diseases have slowed. Because of the large amount of available data, the United States serves as a useful reference point for comparisons.

The age of pestilence and famine (before 1900)

The American colonies were born into pestilence and famine, with half the Pilgrims who arrived in 1620 dying of infection and malnutrition by the following spring. At the end of the 1800s, the U.S. economy was still largely agrarian, with more than 60% of the population living in rural settings. By 1900, average life expectancy had increased to about 50 years. However, tuberculosis, pneumonia, and other infectious diseases still accounted for more deaths than any other cause. CVD accounted for less than 10% of all deaths.

The age of receding pandemics (1900–1930)

By 1900, a public health infrastructure was in place: Forty states had health departments, many larger towns had major public works efforts to improve the water supply and sewage systems, municipal use of chlorine to disinfect water was widespread, pasteurization and other improvements in food handling were introduced, and the educational quality of health care personnel improved. Those changes led to dramatic declines in infectious disease mortality rates. However, the continued shift from a rural, agriculture-based economy to an urban, industrial economy had a number of consequences on risk behaviors and factors for CVD. Owing to a lack of refrigerated transport from farms to urban centers, consumption of fresh fruits and vegetables declined and consumption of meat and grains increased, resulting in diets that were higher in animal fat and processed carbohydrates. In addition, the availability of factory-rolled cigarettes made tobacco more accessible and affordable for the mass population. Age-adjusted CVD mortality rates rose from 300 per 100,000 people in 1900 to approximately 390 per 100,000 during this period, driven by rapidly rising CHD rates.

The age of degenerative and human-made diseases (1930–1965)

During this period, deaths from infectious diseases fell to fewer than 50 per 100,000 per year and life expectancy increased to almost 70 years. At the same time, the country became increasingly urbanized and industrialized, precipitating a number of important lifestyle changes. By 1955, 55% of adult men were smoking, and fat consumption accounted for approximately 40% of total calories. Lower activity levels, high-fat diets, and increased smoking pushed CVD death rates to peak levels.

The age of delayed degenerative diseases (1965–2000)

Substantial declines in age-adjusted CVD mortality rates began in the mid-1960s. In the 1970s and 1980s, age-adjusted CHD mortality rates fell approximately 2% per year and stroke rates fell 3% per year. A main characteristic of this phase is the steadily rising age at which a first CVD event occurs. Two significant advances have been credited with the decline in CVD mortality rates: new therapeutic approaches and the implementation of prevention measures. Treatments once considered advanced, such as angioplasty, bypass surgery, and implantation of defibrillators, are now considered the standard of care. Treatments for hypertension and elevated cholesterol along with the widespread use of aspirin have also contributed significantly to reducing deaths from CVD. In addition, Americans have been exposed to public health campaigns promoting lifestyle modifications effective at reducing the prevalence of smoking, hypertension, and dyslipidemia.

Is the United States entering the fifth age?

The decline in the age-adjusted CVD death rate of 3% per year through the 1970s and 1980s tapered off in the 1990s to 2%. However, CVD death rates declined by 3–5% per year during the first decade of the new millennium. In 2000, the age-adjusted CVD death rate was 341 per 100,000. By 2006, it had fallen to 263 per 100,000. Competing trends appear to be in play. On the one hand, the well-recognized increase in the prevalence of diabetes and obesity, a slowing in the rate of decline of smoking, and a leveling off in the rate of detection and treatment for hypertension are in the negative column. On the other hand, cholesterol levels continue to decline in the face of increased statin use.

CURRENT WORLDWIDE VARIATIONS

An epidemiologic transition much like that which occurred in the United States is occurring throughout the world, but unique regional features have modified aspects of the transition in various parts of the world. In terms of economic development, the world can be divided into two broad categories, (1) high-income countries and (2) low- and middle-income countries, which can be further subdivided into six distinct economic/geographic regions. Currently, 85% of the world's population lives in low- and middle-income countries, and it is those countries which are driving the rates of change in the global burden of CVD (Fig. 225-1). Three million CVD deaths occurred in high-income countries in 2001, compared with 13 million in the rest of the world.

High-income countries

Approximately 940 million people live in high-income countries, where CHD is the dominant form of CVD, with rates that tend to be twofold to fivefold higher than stroke rates. The rates of CVD in Canada, New Zealand, Australia, and Western Europe tend to be similar to those in the United States; however, among the countries of Western Europe, the absolute rates vary threefold with a clear north/south gradient. The highest CVD death rates are in the northern countries, such as Finland, Ireland, and Scotland, and the lowest rates are in the Mediterranean countries of France, Spain, and Italy. Japan is unique among the high-income countries: stroke rates increased dramatically, but CHD rates did not rise as sharply over the last century. This difference may stem in part from genetic factors, but it is more likely that the fish- and plant-based low-fat diet and resulting low cholesterol levels have played a larger role. Importantly, Japanese dietary habits are undergoing substantial changes, reflected in an increase in cholesterol levels.

Low- and middle-income countries

The World Bank groups the low- and middle-income countries (gross national income per capita less than US $9200) into six geographic regions: East Asia and the Pacific, (Eastern) Europe and Central Asia, Latin America and the Caribbean, Middle East and North Africa, South Asia, and Sub-Saharan Africa. Although communicable diseases continue to be a major cause of death, CVD has emerged as a significant health concern in low- and middle-income countries. In most, an urban/rural gradient has emerged for CHD, stroke, and hypertension, with higher rates in urban centers.

Although CVD rates are rapidly rising, there are vast differences among the regions and countries and even within individual countries (Fig. 225-2). Many factors contribute to this heterogeneity. First, the regions are in various stages of the epidemiologic transition. Second, vast differences in lifestyle and behavioral risk factors exist. Third, racial and ethnic differences may lead to altered susceptibilities to various forms of CVD. In addition, it should be noted that for most countries in these regions, accurate country-wide data on cause-specific mortality are not complete, as death certificate completion is not routine and most of those countries do not have a centralized registry for deaths.

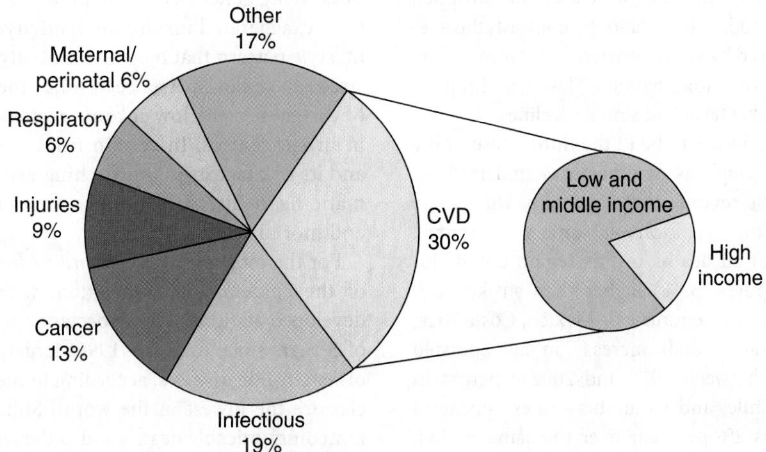

Figure 225-1 CVD data compared with other causes of death. CVD: cardiovascular disease. *(Based on data from CD Mathers et al: Deaths and Disease Burden by Cause: Global Burden of Disease Estimates for 2001 by World Bank Country Groups. Disease Control Priorities Working Paper 18. April 2004, revised January 2005.)*

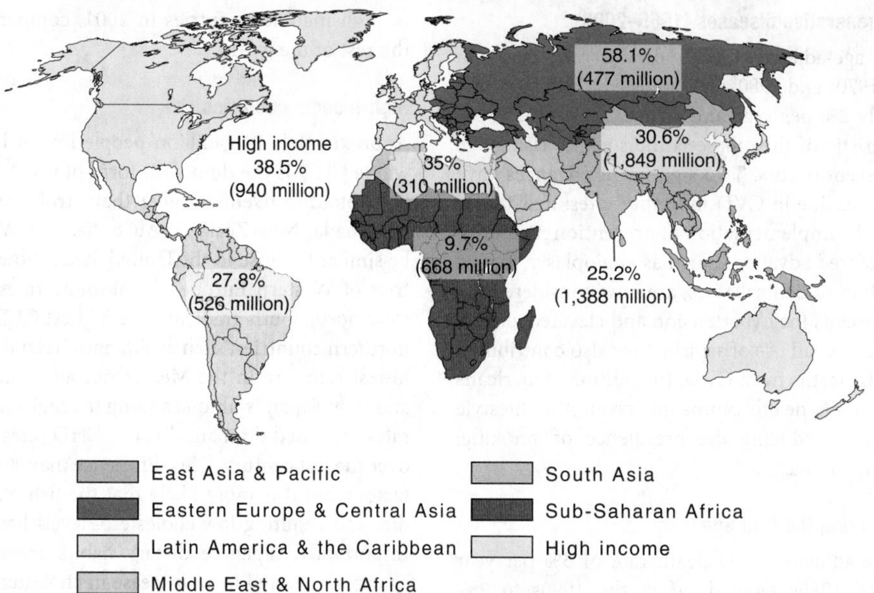

Figure 225-2 CVD death as a percentage of total deaths and total population in seven economic regions of the world defined by the World Bank *(Based on data from CD Mathers et al: Deaths and Disease Burden by Cause: Global Burden of Disease Estimates for 2001 by World Bank Country Groups. Disease Control Priorities Working Paper 18. April 2004, revised January 2005.)*

The *East Asia and Pacific* region, home to nearly 2 billion people, appears to be straddling the second and third phases of the epidemiologic transition, with China, Indonesia, and Sri Lanka's large combined population driving most of the trends. Overall, CVD is a major cause of death in China, but as in Japan, stroke (particularly hemorrhagic) causes more deaths than does CHD, in a ratio of about 3:1. However, age-adjusted CHD mortality increased 40% from 1984 to 1999, suggesting further epidemiologic transition. China also appears to have a geographic gradient like that of Western Europe, with higher CVD rates in northern China than in southern China by a factor of 6. Other countries, such as Vietnam and Cambodia, are just emerging from the pestilence and famine era.

The *Eastern Europe and Central Asia* region is firmly at the peak of the third phase, with the highest death rates (58%) due to CVD in the world, nearly double the rate of high-income countries. More troubling is that nearly 35% of deaths from CHD occur among working-age adults, which is three times the rate in the United States. In Russia, increased CVD rates have contributed to falling life expectancy, particularly for men, whose life expectancy dropped from 71.6 in 1986 to 59 years today. In Poland, by contrast, the age-adjusted mortality rate decreased by approximately 30% for men during the 1990s and slightly more among women. Slovenia, Hungary, the Czech Republic, and Slovakia have had similar declines.

In general, *Latin America* appears to be in the third phase of the epidemiologic transition, although as in other low- and middle-income regions, there is vast regional heterogeneity, with some areas in the second phase of the transition and some in the fourth. Today, approximately 28% of all deaths in this region are attributable to CVD, with CHD rates (35%) higher than stroke rates (29%). As in Eastern Europe, some countries—Mexico, Costa Rica, and Venezuela—continued an overall increase in age-adjusted CHD mortality of 3%–10% between 1970 and 2002, whereas in others—Argentina, Brazil, Chile, and Columbia—rates appear to have declined by as much as 2% per year over the same period. The *Middle East and North Africa* region appears to be entering the third phase of the epidemiologic transition, with increasing life expectancy overall and CVD death rates just below those of developed nations. CHD is responsible for 17% of all deaths, and stroke for 7%. The traditional high-fiber diet, low in fat and cholesterol, has changed rapidly. Over the last few decades, daily fat consumption has increased in most of these countries, ranging from a 13.6% increase in Sudan to a 143.3% increase in Saudi Arabia. Over 75% of Egyptians are overweight or obese, and the rate is 67% in Iraq and Jordan. Nearly 60% of Syrians of physical activity and Iraqis report that they are physically inactive (less than 10 min per day).

Most people in *South Asia* live in rural India, a country that is experiencing an alarming increase in heart disease. CVD accounted for 32% of all deaths in 2000, and an estimated 2 million deaths were expected to occur due to CHD by 2010, representing a 30% increase over the preceding decade. The transition appears to be in the Western style, with CHD as the dominant form of CVD. In 1960, CHD represented 4% of all CVD deaths in India, whereas in 1990 the proportion was >50%. This is somewhat unexpected because stroke tends to be a more dominant factor early in the epidemiologic transition. This finding may reflect inaccuracies in cause-specific mortality estimates or possibly an underlying genetic component. It has been suggested that Indians have exaggerated insulin insensitivity in response to the Western lifestyle pattern that may differentially increase rates of CHD over stroke. The South Asia region has the highest overall prevalence of diabetes in the low-income regions, with rates as high as 14% in urban centers. In certain rural areas, the prevalence of CVD and its risk factors is approaching urban rates. Nonetheless, rheumatic heart disease continues to be a major cause of morbidity and mortality.

For the most part, *sub-Saharan Africa* remains in the first phase of the epidemiologic transition, with CVD rates half those in developed nations. Life expectancy has decreased by an average of 5 years since the early 1990s largely because of HIV/AIDS and other chronic diseases, according to the World Bank; life expectancies are the lowest in the world. Still, CVD accounts for 46% of noncommunicable deaths and is the leading cause of death among adults >age 35. As more HIV/AIDS patients receive antiretroviral treatment, managing CVD risk factors such as dyslipidemia in this population requires more attention. However, hypertension continues to be the major public health concern and has resulted in

TABLE 225-2 Estimated Morbidity Related to Heart Disease: 2010-2030

Deaths	By 2010	By 2030
CVD deaths: annual number of all deaths	18.1 million	24.2 million
CVD deaths: percentage of all deaths	30.8%	32.5%
CHD deaths: percentage of all male deaths	13.1%	14.9%
CHD deaths: percentage of all female deaths	13.6%	13.1%
Stroke deaths: percentage of all male deaths	9.2%	10.4%
Stroke deaths: percentage of all female deaths	11.5%	11.8%

Abbreviations: CHD, coronary heart disease; CVD, cardiovascular disease.
Source: Adapted from J Mackay, G Mensah: *Atlas of Heart Disease and Stroke.* Geneva, World Health Organization, 2004.

stroke being the dominant form of CVD. Rheumatic heart disease is still an important cause of CVD mortality and morbidity.

GLOBAL TRENDS IN CARDIOVASCULAR DISEASE

In 1990, CVD accounted for 28% of the world's 50.4 million deaths and 9.7% of the 1.4 billion lost disability-adjusted life years (DALYs), and by 2001, CVD was responsible for 29% of all deaths and 14% of the 1.5 billion lost DALYs. By 2030, when the population is expected to reach 8.2 billion, 33% of all deaths will be the result of CVD (Table 225-2). Of these, 14.9% of deaths in men and 13.1% of deaths in women will be due to CHD. Stroke will be responsible for 10.4% of all male deaths and 11.8% of all female deaths.

In the *high-income countries*, population growth will be fueled by emigration from the low- and middle-income countries, but the populations of high-income countries will shrink as a proportion of the world's population. The modest decline in CVD death rates that began in the high-income countries in the latter third of the twentieth century will continue, but the rate of decline appears to be slowing. However, these countries are expected to see an increase in the prevalence of CVD, as well as the absolute number of deaths as the population ages.

Significant proportions of the population living in *low- and middle-income countries* have entered the third phase of the epidemiologic transition, and some are entering the fourth stage. Changing demographics play a significant role in future predictions for CVD throughout the world. For example, between 1990 and 2001, the population of Eastern Europe and Central Asia grew by 1 million people per year, whereas South Asia added 25 million people each year.

CVD rates will also have an economic impact. Even assuming no increase in CVD risk factors, most countries, but especially India and South Africa, will see a large number of people between 35 and 64 die of CVD over the next 30 years as well as an increasing level of morbidity among middle-aged people related to heart disease and stroke. In China, it is estimated that there will be 9 million deaths from CVD in 2030—up from 2.4 million in 2002—with half occurring in individuals between 35 and 64 years old.

REGIONAL TRENDS IN RISK FACTORS

As indicated earlier, the global variation in CVD rates is related to temporal and regional variations in known risk behaviors and factors. Ecological analyses of major CVD risk factors and mortality demonstrate high correlations between expected and observed mortality rates for the three main risk factors—smoking, serum cholesterol, and hypertension—and suggest that many of the regional variations are based on differences in conventional risk factors.

BEHAVIORAL RISK FACTORS

Tobacco

Every year, more than 5.5 trillion cigarettes are produced, enough to provide every person on the planet with 1,000 cigarettes. Worldwide, 1.3 billion people smoked in 2003, a number that is projected to increase to 1.6 billion by 2030. Tobacco currently causes about 5 million deaths—9% of all deaths—annually. Approximately 1.6 million are CVD-related. If current smoking patterns continue, by 2030 the global burden of disease attributable to tobacco will reach 10 million deaths annually. A unique feature of the low- and middle-income countries is easy access to smoking during the early stages of the epidemiologic transition due to the availability of relatively inexpensive tobacco products. In South Asia, the prominence of locally produced forms of tobacco other than manufactured cigarettes makes control of consumption more challenging.

Diet

Total caloric intake per capita increases as countries develop. With regard to cardiovascular disease, a key element of dietary change is an increase in intake of saturated animal fats and hydrogenated vegetable fats, which contain atherogenic trans-fatty acids, along with a decrease in intake of plant-based foods and an increase in simple carbohydrates. Fat contributes less than 20% of calories in rural China and India, less than 30% in Japan, and well above 30% in the United States. Caloric contributions from fat appear to be falling in the high-income countries. In the United States, between 1971 and 2000, the percentage of calories derived from saturated fat decreased from 13% to 11%.

Physical inactivity

The increased mechanization that accompanies the economic transition leads to a shift from physically demanding agriculture-based work to largely sedentary industry- and office-based work. In the United States, approximately one-quarter of the population does not participate in any leisure-time physical activity and only 22% report engaging in sustained physical activity for at least 30 minutes on 5 or more days per week (the current recommendation). In contrast, in countries such as China, physical activity is still integral to everyday life. Approximately 90% of the urban population walks or rides a bicycle to work, shopping, or school daily.

METABOLIC RISK FACTORS

Lipid levels

Worldwide, high cholesterol levels are estimated to cause 56% of ischemic heart disease and 18% of strokes, amounting to 4.4 million deaths annually. As countries move through the epidemiologic transition, mean population plasma cholesterol levels tend to rise. Social and individual changes that accompany urbanization clearly play a role because plasma cholesterol levels tend to be higher among urban residents than among rural residents. This shift is driven largely by greater consumption of dietary fats—primarily from animal products and processed vegetable oils—and decreased physical activity. In the high-income countries, in general, mean population cholesterol levels are falling, whereas wide variation is seen in the low- and middle-income countries.

Hypertension

Elevated blood pressure is an early indicator of the epidemiologic transition. Worldwide, approximately 62% of strokes and 49% of cases of ischemic heart disease are attributable to suboptimal (>115 mmHg systolic) blood pressure, which is believed to account for more than 7 million deaths annually. Remarkably, nearly half of this burden occurs among those with systolic blood pressure <140 mmHg, even as this level is used at the arbitrary threshold for defining hypertension in many national guidelines. Rising mean population blood pressure is apparent as populations industrialize and move from rural to urban settings. Among urban-dwelling men and women in India, for example, the prevalence of hypertension is 25.5% and 29.0%, respectively, whereas it is 14.0% and 10.8%, respectively, in rural communities. One major concern in low- and middle-income countries is the high rate of undetected, and therefore untreated, hypertension. This may explain, at least in part, the higher stroke rates in these countries in relation to CHD rates during the early stages of the transition. The high rates of hypertension, especially undiagnosed hypertension, throughout Asia probably contribute to the high prevalence of hemorrhagic stroke in the region.

Obesity

Although clearly associated with increased risk of CHD, much of the risk posed by obesity may be mediated by other CVD risk factors, including hypertension, diabetes mellitus, and lipid profile imbalances. In the mid-1980s, the World Health Organization's MONICA Project sampled 48 populations for cardiovascular risk factors. In all but one male population (China) and in most of the female populations, between 50% and 75% of adults age 35–64 years were overweight or obese. In addition, the prevalence of extreme obesity (BMI >40 kg/m^2) more than tripled, increasing from 1.3% to 4.9%. In many of the low- and middle-income countries, obesity appears to coexist with undernutrition and malnutrition. Obesity is increasing throughout the world, particularly in developing countries, where the trajectories are steeper than those experienced in the developed countries. According to the latest World Health Organization (WHO) data, this is equivalent to about 1.3 billion overweight adults in the world. A survey undertaken in 1998 found that as many as 58% of African women living in South Africa might have been overweight or obese.

Diabetes mellitus

As a consequence of, or in addition to, increasing body mass index and decreasing levels of physical activity, worldwide rates of diabetes—predominantly Type 2 diabetes—are on the rise. In 2003, 194 million adults, or 5% of the world's population, had diabetes. By 2025, this number is predicted to increase 72 percent to 333 million. By 2025, the number of people with Type 2 diabetes is projected to double in three of the six low- and middle-income regions: Middle East and North Africa, South Asia, and Sub-Saharan Africa. There appear to be clear genetic susceptibilities to diabetes mellitus in various racial and ethnic groups. For example, migration studies suggest that South Asians and Indians tend to be at higher risk than are people of European ancestry.

SUMMARY

Although CVD rates are declining in the high-income countries, they are increasing in virtually every other region of the world. The consequences of this preventable epidemic will be substantial on many levels: individual mortality and morbidity rates, family suffering, and staggering economic costs.

Three complementary strategies can be used to lessen the impact. First, the overall burden of CVD risk factors can be lowered through populationwide public health measures such as national campaigns against cigarette smoking, unhealthy diets, and physical inactivity. Second, it is important to identify higher-risk subgroups of the population that stand to benefit the most from specific, low-cost prevention interventions, including screening for and treatment of hypertension and elevated cholesterol. Simple, low-cost interventions, such as the "polypill," a regimen of aspirin, a statin, and an anithypertensive agent, also need to be explored. Third, resources should be allocated to acute as well as secondary prevention interventions. For countries with limited resources, a critical first step in developing a comprehensive plan is better assessment of cause-specific mortality and morbidity, as well as the prevalence of the major preventable risk factors.

In the meantime, the high-income countries must continue to bear the burden of research and development aimed at prevention and treatment, being mindful of the economic limitations of many countries. The concept of the epidemiologic transition provides insight into methods to alter the course of the CVD epidemic. The efficient transfer of low-cost preventive and therapeutic strategies could alter the natural course of this epidemic and thereby reduce the excess global burden of preventable CVD.

FURTHER READINGS

Gaziano T, Gaziano JM: Global burden of cardiovascular disease, in *Heart Disease: A Textbook of Cardiovascular Medicine*, 9th ed, E Braunwald (ed). Philadelphia, Elsevier Saunders, 2009

Jamison DT et al (eds): *Disease Control Priorities in Developing Countries*, 2nd ed. Washington, DC, Oxford University Press, 2006

Lawes CM et al: Global burden of blood-pressure-related disease, 2001. Lancet 371:1513, 2008

Lopez AD et al (eds): *Global Burden of Disease and Risk Factors.* Washington, DC, Oxford University Press, 2006

Shafey O et al: *The Tobacco Atlas,* 3rd ed. Atlanta: American Cancer Society, 2009

CHAPTER 226

Approach to the Patient With Possible Cardiovascular Disease

Joseph Loscalzo

THE MAGNITUDE OF THE PROBLEM

Cardiovascular diseases comprise the most prevalent serious disorders in industrialized nations and are a rapidly growing problem in developing nations (Chap. 225). Age-adjusted death rates for coronary heart disease have declined by two-thirds in the last 4 decades in the United States, reflecting the identification and reduction of risk factors as well as improved treatments and interventions for the management of coronary artery disease, arrhythmias, and heart failure. Nonetheless, cardiovascular diseases remain the most common causes of death, responsible for 35% of all deaths, almost 1 million deaths each year. Approximately one-fourth of these deaths are sudden. In addition, cardiovascular diseases are highly prevalent, diagnosed in 80 million adults, or ~35% of the adult population. The growing prevalence of obesity (Chap. 77), type 2 diabetes mellitus (Chap. 344), and metabolic syndrome (Chap. 242), which are important risk factors for atherosclerosis, now threatens to reverse the progress that has been made in the age-adjusted reduction in the mortality rate of coronary heart disease.

For many years cardiovascular disease was considered to be more common in men than in women. In fact, the percentage of all deaths secondary to cardiovascular disease is higher among women (43%) than among men (37%) (Chap. 6). In addition, although the absolute number of deaths secondary to cardiovascular disease has declined over the past decades in men, this number has actually risen in women. Inflammation, obesity, type 2 diabetes mellitus, and the metabolic syndrome appear to play more prominent roles in the development of coronary atherosclerosis in women than in men. Coronary artery disease (CAD) is more frequently associated with dysfunction of the coronary microcirculation in women than in men. Exercise electrocardiography has a lower diagnostic accuracy in the prediction of epicardial obstruction in women than in men.

CARDIAC SYMPTOMS

The symptoms caused by heart disease result most commonly from myocardial ischemia, disturbance of the contraction and/or relaxation of the myocardium, obstruction to blood flow, or an abnormal cardiac rhythm or rate. Ischemia, which is caused by an imbalance between the heart's oxygen supply and demand, is manifest most frequently as chest discomfort (Chap. 12), whereas reduction of the pumping ability of the heart commonly leads to fatigue and elevated intravascular pressure upstream of the failing ventricle. The latter results in abnormal fluid accumulation, with peripheral edema (Chap. 36) or pulmonary congestion and dyspnea (Chap. 33). Obstruction to blood flow, as occurs in valvular stenosis, can cause symptoms resembling those of myocardial failure (Chap. 234). Cardiac arrhythmias often develop suddenly, and the resulting symptoms and signs—palpitations (Chap. 37), dyspnea, hypotension, and syncope (Chap. 20)—generally occur abruptly and may disappear as rapidly as they develop.

Although dyspnea, chest discomfort, edema, and syncope are cardinal manifestations of cardiac disease, they occur in other conditions as well. Thus, dyspnea is observed in disorders as diverse as pulmonary disease, marked obesity, and anxiety (Chap. 33). Similarly, chest discomfort may result from a variety of noncardiac and cardiac causes other than myocardial ischemia (Chap. 12). Edema, an important finding in untreated or inadequately treated heart failure, also may occur with primary renal disease and in hepatic cirrhosis (Chap. 36). Syncope occurs not only with serious cardiac arrhythmias but in a number of neurologic conditions as well (Chap. 20). Whether heart disease is responsible for these symptoms frequently can be determined by carrying out a careful clinical examination (Chap. 227), supplemented by noninvasive testing using electrocardiography at rest and during exercise (Chap. 228), echocardiography, roentgenography, and other forms of myocardial imaging (Chap. 229).

Myocardial or coronary function that may be adequate at rest may be insufficient during exertion. Thus, dyspnea and/or chest discomfort that appear during activity are characteristic of patients with heart disease, whereas the opposite pattern, i.e., the appearance of these symptoms at rest and their remission during exertion, is rarely observed in such patients. It is important, therefore, to question the patient carefully about the relation of symptoms to exertion.

Many patients with cardiovascular disease may be asymptomatic both at rest and during exertion but may present with an abnormal physical finding such as a heart murmur, elevated arterial pressure, or an abnormality of the electrocardiogram (ECG) or the cardiac silhouette on the chest roentgenogram or other imaging test. It is important to assess the global risk of CAD in asymptomatic individuals, using a combination of clinical assessment and measurement of cholesterol and its fractions, as well as other biomarkers, such as C-reactive protein, in some patients (Chap. 241). Since the first clinical manifestation of CAD may be catastrophic—sudden cardiac death, acute myocardial infarction, or stroke in previous asymptomatic persons—it is mandatory to identify those at high risk of such events and institute further testing and preventive measures.

DIAGNOSIS

As outlined by the New York Heart Association (NYHA), the elements of a complete cardiac diagnosis include the systematic consideration of the following:

1. *The underlying etiology.* Is the disease congenital, hypertensive, ischemic, or inflammatory in origin?
2. *The anatomical abnormalities.* Which chambers are involved? Are they hypertrophied, dilated, or both? Which valves are affected? Are they regurgitant and/or stenotic? Is there pericardial involvement? Has there been a myocardial infarction?
3. *The physiological disturbances.* Is an arrhythmia present? Is there evidence of congestive heart failure or myocardial ischemia?
4. *Functional disability.* How strenuous is the physical activity required to elicit symptoms? The classification provided by the NYHA has been found to be useful in describing functional disability (Table 226-1).

One example may serve to illustrate the importance of establishing a complete diagnosis. In a patient who presents with exertional chest discomfort, the identification of myocardial ischemia as the etiology is of great clinical importance. However, the simple recognition of ischemia is insufficient to formulate a therapeutic strategy or prognosis until the underlying anatomical abnormalities responsible for the myocardial ischemia, e.g., coronary atherosclerosis or

TABLE 226-1 New York Heart Association Functional Classification

Class I	Class III
No limitation of physical activity	Marked limitation of physical activity
No symptoms with ordinary exertion	Less than ordinary activity causes symptoms
Class II	Asymptomatic at rest
Slight limitation of physical activity	Class IV
Ordinary activity causes symptoms	Inability to carry out any physical activity without discomfort
	Symptoms at rest

Source: Modified from The Criteria Committee of the New York Heart Association.

aortic stenosis, are identified and a judgment is made about whether other physiologic disturbances that cause an imbalance between myocardial oxygen supply and demand, such as severe anemia, thyrotoxicosis, or supraventricular tachycardia, play contributory roles. Finally, the severity of the disability should govern the extent and tempo of the workup and strongly influence the therapeutic strategy that is selected.

The establishment of a correct and complete cardiac diagnosis usually commences with the history and physical examination (Chap. 227). Indeed, the clinical examination remains the basis for the diagnosis of a wide variety of disorders. The clinical examination may then be supplemented by five types of laboratory tests: (1) ECG (Chap. 228), (2) noninvasive imaging examinations (chest roentgenogram, echocardiogram, radionuclide imaging, computed tomographic imaging, and magnetic resonance imaging (Chap. 229), (3) blood tests to assess risk [e.g., lipid determinations, C-reactive protein (Chap. 241)] or cardiac function [e.g., brain natriuretic peptide (BNP) (Chap. 234)], (4) occasionally specialized invasive examinations [i.e., cardiac catheterization and coronary arteriography (Chap. 230)], and (5) genetic tests to identify monogenic cardiac diseases [e.g., hypertrophic cardiomyopathy (Chap. 238), Marfan syndrome (Chap. 363), and abnormalities of cardiac ion channels that lead to prolongation of the QT interval and an increase in the risk of sudden death (Chap. 233)]. These tests are becoming more widely available.

FAMILY HISTORY

In eliciting the history of a patient with known or suspected cardiovascular disease, particular attention should be directed to the family history. Familial clustering is common in many forms of heart disease. Mendelian transmission of single-gene defects may occur, as in hypertrophic cardiomyopathy (Chap. 238), Marfan syndrome (Chap. 363), and sudden death associated with a prolonged QT syndrome (Chap. 233). Premature coronary disease and essential hypertension, type 2 diabetes mellitus, and hyperlipidemia (the most important risk factors for coronary artery disease) are usually polygenic disorders. Although familial transmission may be less obvious than in the monogenic disorders, it is helpful in assessing risk and prognosis in polygenic disorders. Familial clustering of cardiovascular diseases not only may occur on a genetic basis but also may be related to familial dietary or behavior patterns such as excessive ingestion of salt or calories and cigarette smoking.

ASSESSMENT OF FUNCTIONAL IMPAIRMENT

When an attempt is made to determine the severity of functional impairment in a patient with heart disease, it is helpful to ascertain the level of activity and the rate at which it is performed before symptoms develop. Thus, it is not sufficient to state that the patient complains of dyspnea. The breathlessness that occurs after running up two long flights of stairs denotes far less functional impairment than do similar symptoms that occur after taking a few steps on level ground. Also, the degree of customary physical activity at work and during recreation should be considered. The development of two-flight dyspnea in a well-conditioned marathon runner may be far more significant than the development of one-flight dyspnea in a previously sedentary person. The history should include a detailed consideration of the patient's therapeutic regimen. For example, the persistence or development of edema, breathlessness, and other manifestations of heart failure in a patient who is receiving optimal doses of diuretics and other therapies for heart failure (Chap. 234) is far graver than are similar manifestations in the absence of treatment. Similarly, the presence of angina pectoris despite treatment with optimal doses of multiple antianginal drugs (Chap. 243) is more serious than it is in a patient on no therapy. In an effort to determine the progression of symptoms, and thus the severity of the underlying illness, it may be useful to ascertain what, if any, specific tasks the patient could have carried out 6 months or 1 year earlier that he or she cannot carry out at present.

ELECTROCARDIOGRAM

(See also Chap. 228) Although an ECG usually should be recorded in patients with known or suspected heart disease, with the exception of the identification of arrhythmias, conduction abnormalities, ventricular hypertrophy, and acute myocardial infarction, it generally does not establish a specific diagnosis. The range of normal electrocardiographic findings is wide, and the tracing can be affected significantly by many noncardiac factors, such as age, body habitus, and serum electrolyte concentrations. In general, electrocardiographic changes should be interpreted in the context of other abnormal cardiovascular findings.

ASSESSMENT OF THE PATIENT WITH A HEART MURMUR

(Fig. 226-1) The cause of a heart murmur can often be readily elucidated from a systematic evaluation of its major attributes: timing, duration, intensity, quality, frequency, configuration, location, and radiation when considered in the light of the history, general physical examination, and other features of the cardiac examination, as described in Chap. 227.

The majority of heart murmurs are midsystolic and soft (grades I–II/VI). When such a murmur occurs in an asymptomatic child or young adult *without* other evidence of heart disease on clinical examination, it is usually benign and echocardiography generally is not required. By contrast, two-dimensional and Doppler echocardiography (Chap. 229) are indicated in patients with loud systolic murmurs (grades ≥III/VI), especially those that are holosystolic or late systolic, and in most patients with diastolic or continuous murmurs.

NATURAL HISTORY

Cardiovascular disorders often present acutely, as in a previously asymptomatic person who develops an acute myocardial infarction (Chap. 245), or a previously asymptomatic patient with hypertrophic cardiomyopathy (Chap. 238), or with a prolonged QT interval (Chap. 233) whose first clinical manifestation is syncope or even sudden death. However, the alert physician may recognize the patient at risk for these complications long before they occur and often can take measures to prevent their occurrence. For example, a patient with acute myocardial infarction will often have had risk factors for atherosclerosis for many years. Had these risk factors been recognized, their elimination or reduction might have delayed

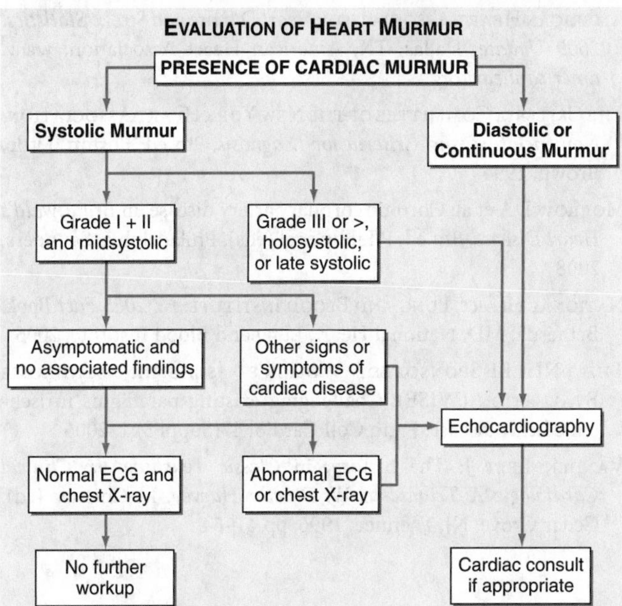

Figure 226-1 An alternative "echocardiography first" approach to the evaluation of a heart murmur that also uses the results of the electrocardiogram (ECG) and chest x-ray in asymptomatic patients with soft midsystolic murmurs and no other physical findings. This algorithm is useful for patients over age 40 years in whom the prevalence of coronary artery disease and aortic stenosis increases as the cause of systolic murmur. *[From RA O'Rourke, in Primary Cardiology, 2nd ed, E Braunwald, L Goldman (eds). Philadelphia, Saunders, 2003.]*

or even prevented the infarction. Similarly, a patient with hypertrophic cardiomyopathy may have had a heart murmur for years and a family history of this disorder. These findings could have led to an echocardiographic examination, recognition of the condition, and appropriate therapy long before the occurrence of a serious acute manifestation.

Patients with valvular heart disease or idiopathic dilated cardiomyopathy, by contrast, may have a prolonged course of gradually increasing dyspnea and other manifestations of chronic heart failure that is punctuated by episodes of acute deterioration only late in the course of the disease. Understanding the natural history of various cardiac disorders is essential for applying appropriate diagnostic and therapeutic measures to each stage of the condition, as well as for providing the patient and family with the likely prognosis.

PITFALLS IN CARDIOVASCULAR MEDICINE

Increasing subspecialization in internal medicine and the perfection of advanced diagnostic techniques in cardiology can lead to several undesirable consequences. Examples include the following:

1. Failure by the *noncardiologist* to recognize important cardiac manifestations of systemic illnesses. For example, the presence of mitral stenosis, patent foramen ovale, and/or transient atrial arrhythmia should be considered in a patient with stroke, or the presence of pulmonary hypertension and cor pulmonale should be considered in a patient with scleroderma or Raynaud's syndrome. A cardiovascular examination should be carried out to identify and estimate the severity of the cardiovascular involvement that accompanies many noncardiac disorders.
2. Failure by the *cardiologist* to recognize underlying systemic disorders in patients with heart disease. For example, hyperthyroidism should be considered in an elderly patient with atrial fibrillation and unexplained heart failure, and Lyme disease should be considered in a patient with an unexplained fluctuating atrioventricular block. A cardiovascular abnormality may provide the clue critical to the recognition of some systemic disorders. For instance, an unexplained pericardial effusion may provide an early clue to the diagnosis of tuberculosis or a neoplasm.
3. Overreliance on and overutilization of laboratory tests, particularly invasive techniques, for the evaluation of the cardiovascular system. Cardiac catheterization and coronary arteriography (Chap. 230) provide precise diagnostic information that may be crucial in developing a therapeutic plan in patients with known or suspected CAD. Although a great deal of attention has been directed to these examinations, it is important to recognize that they serve to *supplement*, not *supplant*, a careful examination carried out with clinical and noninvasive techniques. A coronary arteriogram should not be performed in lieu of a careful history in patients with chest pain suspected of having ischemic heart disease. Although coronary arteriography may establish whether the coronary arteries are obstructed and to what extent, the results of the procedure by themselves often do not provide a definitive answer to the question of whether a patient's complaint of chest discomfort is attributable to coronary atherosclerosis and whether or not revascularization is indicated.

Despite the value of invasive tests in certain circumstances, they entail some small risk to the patient, involve discomfort and substantial cost, and place a strain on medical facilities. Therefore, they should be carried out only if the results can be expected to modify the patient's management.

DISEASE PREVENTION AND MANAGEMENT

The prevention of heart disease, especially of CAD, is one of the most important tasks of primary care health givers as well as cardiologists. Prevention begins with risk assessment, followed by attention to lifestyle, such as achieving optimal weight, physical activity, smoking cessation, and then aggressive treatment of all abnormal risk factors, such as hypertension, hyperlipidemia, and diabetes mellitus (Chap. 344).

After a complete diagnosis has been established in patients with known heart disease, a number of management options are usually available. Several examples may be used to demonstrate some of the principles of cardiovascular therapeutics:

1. In the absence of evidence of heart disease, the patient should be clearly informed of this assessment and *not* be asked to return at intervals for repeated examinations. If there is no evidence of disease, such continued attention may lead to the patient's developing inappropriate concern about the possibility of heart disease.
2. If there is no evidence of cardiovascular disease but the patient has one or more risk factors for the development of ischemic heart disease (Chap. 243), a plan for their reduction should be developed and the patient should be retested at intervals to assess compliance and efficacy in risk reduction.
3. Asymptomatic or mildly symptomatic patients with valvular heart disease that is anatomically severe should be evaluated periodically, every 6 to 12 months, by clinical and noninvasive examinations. Early signs of deterioration of ventricular function may signify the need for surgical treatment before the development of disabling symptoms, irreversible myocardial damage, and excessive risk of surgical treatment (Chap. 237).
4. In patients with CAD (Chap. 243), available practice guidelines should be considered in the decision on the form of treatment (medical, percutaneous coronary intervention, or surgical revascularization). Mechanical revascularization may be employed too frequently in the United States and too infrequently in Eastern

Europe and developing nations. The mere presence of angina pectoris and/or the demonstration of critical coronary arterial narrowing at angiography should not reflexively evoke a decision to treat the patient by revascularization. Instead, these interventions should be limited to patients with CAD whose angina has not responded adequately to medical treatment or in whom revascularization has been shown to improve the natural history (e.g., acute coronary syndrome or multivessel CAD with left ventricular dysfunction).

ACKNOWLEDGMENT

Dr. Eugene Braunwald authored this chapter for the previous edition. Some of the material from the 17th edition has been carried forward.

FURTHER READINGS

Abrams J: *Synopsis of Cardiac Physical Diagnosis*, 2nd ed. Oxford, Butterworth Heinemann, 2001

American Heart Association: *Heart Disease and Stroke Statistics, 2009 Update*. Dallas, TX, American Heart Association, *www.americanheart.org*

The Criteria Committee of the New York Heart Association: *Nomenclature and Criteria for Diagnosis*, 9th ed. Boston, Little, Brown, 1994

Morrow DA et al: Chronic coronary artery disease, in *Braunwald's Heart Disease*, 8th ed, P Libby et al (eds). Philadelphia, Saunders, 2008

National Heart, Lung and Blood Institute: *FY 2005 Fact Book*. Bethesda, MD, National Heart, Lung and Blood Institute, 2006

The NHLBI-Sponsored Women's Ischemia Syndrome Evaluation (WISE): Challenging existing paradigms in ischemic heart disease. J Am Coll Cardiol 47(Suppl S):1, 2006

Vanden Belt J: The history, in *Classic Teachings in Clinical Cardiology: A Tribute to W. Proctor Harvey*, M Chizner (ed). Cedar Grove, NJ, Laennec, 1996, pp 41–54

CHAPTER 227 Physical Examination of the Cardiovascular System

Patrick T. O'Gara
Joseph Loscalzo

The approach to a patient with known or suspected cardiovascular disease begins with the time-honored traditions of a directed history and a targeted physical examination. The scope of these activities depends on the clinical context at the time of presentation, ranging from an elective ambulatory follow-up visit to a more focused emergency department encounter. There has been a gradual decline in physical examination skills over the last two decades at every level, from student to faculty specialist, a development of great concern to both clinicians and medical educators. Classic cardiac findings are recognized by only a minority of internal medicine and family practice residents. Despite popular perceptions, clinical performance does not improve predictably as a function of experience; instead, the acquisition of new examination skills may become more difficult for a busy individual practitioner. Less time is now devoted to mentored cardiovascular examinations during the training of students and residents. One widely recognized outcome of these trends is the progressive overutilization of noninvasive imaging studies to establish the presence and severity of cardiovascular disease even when the examination findings imply a low pretest probability of significant pathology. Educational techniques to improve bedside skills include repetition, patient-centered teaching conferences, and visual display feedback of auscultatory events with Doppler echocardiographic imaging.

The evidence base that links the findings from the history and physical examination to the presence, severity, and prognosis of cardiovascular disease has been established most rigorously for coronary artery disease, heart failure, and valvular heart disease. For example, observations regarding heart rate, blood pressure, signs of pulmonary congestion, and the presence of mitral regurgitation (MR) contribute importantly to bedside risk assessment in patients with acute coronary syndromes. Observations from the physical examination in this setting can inform clinical decision making before the results of cardiac biomarkers testing are known. The prognosis of patients with systolic heart failure can be predicted on the basis of the jugular venous pressure (JVP) and the presence or absence of a third heart sound (S_3). Accurate characterization of cardiac murmurs provides important insight into the natural history of many valvular and congenital heart lesions. Finally, the important role played by the physical examination in enhancing the clinician-patient relationship cannot be overestimated.

THE GENERAL PHYSICAL EXAMINATION

Any examination begins with an assessment of the general appearance of the patient, with notation of age, posture, demeanor, and overall health status. Is the patient in pain or resting quietly, dyspneic or diaphoretic? Does the patient choose to avoid certain body positions to reduce or eliminate pain, as might be the case with suspected acute pericarditis? Are there clues indicating that dyspnea may have a pulmonary cause, such as a barrel chest deformity with an increased anterior-posterior diameter, tachypnea, and pursed-lip breathing? Skin pallor, cyanosis, and jaundice can be appreciated readily and provide additional clues. A chronically ill-appearing emaciated patient may suggest the presence of long-standing heart failure or another systemic disorder, such as a malignancy. Various genetic syndromes, often with cardiovascular involvement, can also be recognized easily, such as trisomy 21, Marfan syndrome, and Holt-Oram syndrome. Height and weight should be measured routinely, and both body mass index and body surface area should be calculated. Knowledge of the waist circumference and the waist-to-hip ratio can be used to predict long-term cardiovascular risk. Mental status, level of alertness, and mood should be assessed continuously during the interview and examination.

Skin

Central cyanosis occurs with significant right-to-left shunting at the level of the heart or lungs, allowing deoxygenated blood to reach the systemic circulation. Peripheral cyanosis or acrocyanosis, in contrast, is usually related to reduced extremity blood flow due to small vessel constriction, as seen in patients with severe heart failure, shock, or peripheral vascular disease; it can be aggravated by the use of β-adrenergic blockers with unopposed α-mediated constriction. Differential cyanosis refers to isolated cyanosis affecting the lower but not the upper extremities in a patient with a large patent ductus arteriosus (PDA) and secondary pulmonary hypertension with right-to-left to shunting at the great vessel level. Hereditary telangiectasias on the lips, tongue, and mucous membranes, as part of the Osler-Weber-Rendu syndrome (hereditary hemorrhagic telangiectasia), resemble spider nevi and can be a source of right-to-left shunting when also present in the lung. Malar telangiectasias also are seen in patients with advanced mitral stenosis and scleroderma. An unusually tan or bronze discoloration of the skin may suggest hemochromatosis as the cause of the associated systolic heart failure. Jaundice, which may be visible first in the sclerae, has a broad differential diagnosis but in the appropriate setting can be consistent with advanced right heart failure and congestive hepatomegaly or late-term "cardiac cirrhosis." Cutaneous ecchymoses are seen frequently among patients taking vitamin K antagonists or antiplatelet agents such as aspirin and thienopyridines. Various lipid disorders sometimes are associated with subcutaneous xanthomas, particularly along the tendon sheaths or over the extensor surfaces of the extremities. Severe hypertriglyceridemia can be associated with eruptive xanthomatosis and lipemia retinalis. Palmar crease xanthomas are specific for type III hyperlipoproteinemia. Pseudoxanthoma elasticum, a disease associated with premature atherosclerosis, is manifested by a leathery, cobblestoned appearance of the skin in the axilla and neck creases and by angioid streaks on funduscopic examination. Extensive lentiginoses have been described in a variety of development delay–cardiovascular syndromes, including Carney syndrome, which includes multiple atrial myxomas. Cutaneous manifestations of sarcoidosis such as lupus pernio and erythema nodosum may suggest this disease as a cause of an associated dilated cardiomyopathy, especially with heart block, intraventricular conduction delay, or ventricular tachycardia.

Head and neck

Dentition and oral hygiene should be assessed in every patient both as a source of potential infection and as an index of general health. A high-arched palate is a feature of Marfan syndrome and other connective tissue disease syndromes. Bifid uvula has been described in patients with Loeys-Dietz syndrome, and orange tonsils are characteristic of Tangier disease. The ocular manifestations of hyperthyroidism have been well described. Many patients with congenital heart disease have associated hypertelorism, low-set ears, or micrognathia. Blue sclerae are a feature of osteogenesis imperfecta. An arcus senilis pattern lacks specificity as an index of coronary heart disease risk. The funduscopic examination is an often underutilized method by which to assess the microvasculature, especially among patients with established atherosclerosis, hypertension, or diabetes mellitus. A mydriatic agent may be necessary for optimal visualization. A funduscopic examination should be performed routinely in the assessment of patients with suspected endocarditis and those with a history of acute visual change. Branch retinal artery occlusion or visualization of a Hollenhorst plaque can narrow the differential diagnosis rapidly in the appropriate setting. Relapsing polychondritis may manifest as an inflamed pinna or, in its later stages, as a saddle-nose deformity because of destruction of nasal cartilage; Wegener's granulomatosis can also lead to a saddle-nose deformity.

Chest

Midline sternotomy, left posterolateral thoracotomy, or infraclavicular scars at the site of pacemaker/defibrillator generator implantation should not be overlooked and may provide the first clue regarding an underlying cardiovascular disorder in patients unable to provide a relevant history. A prominent venous collateral pattern may suggest subclavian or vena caval obstruction. If the head and neck appear dusky and slightly cyanotic and the venous pressure is grossly elevated without visible pulsations, a diagnosis of superior vena cava syndrome should be entertained. Thoracic cage abnormalities have been well described among patients with connective tissue disease syndromes. They include pectus carinatum ("pigeon chest") and pectus excavatum ("funnel chest"). Obstructive lung disease is suggested by a barrel chest deformity, especially with tachypnea, pursed-lip breathing, and use of accessory muscles. The characteristically severe kyphosis and compensatory lumbar, pelvic, and knee flexion of ankylosing spondylitis should prompt careful auscultation for a murmur of aortic regurgitation (AR). Straight back syndrome refers to the loss of the normal kyphosis of the thoracic spine and has been described in patients with mitral valve prolapse (MVP) and its variants. In some patients with cyanotic congenital heart disease, the chest wall appears to be asymmetric, with anterior displacement of the left hemithorax. The respiratory rate and pattern should be noted during spontaneous breathing, with additional attention to depth, audible wheezing, and stridor. Lung examination can reveal adventitious sounds indicative of pulmonary edema, pneumonia, or pleuritis.

Abdomen

In some patients with advanced obstructive lung disease, the point of maximal cardiac impulse may be in the epigastrium. The liver is frequently enlarged and tender in patients with chronic heart failure. Systolic pulsations over the liver signify severe tricuspid regurgitation (TR). Splenomegaly may be a feature of infective endocarditis, particularly when symptoms have persisted for weeks or months. Ascites is a nonspecific finding but may be present with advanced chronic right heart failure, constrictive pericarditis, hepatic cirrhosis, or an intraperitoneal malignancy. The finding of an elevated JVP implies a cardiovascular etiology. In nonobese patients, the aorta typically is palpated between the epigastrium and the umbilicus. The sensitivity of palpation for the detection of an abdominal aortic aneurysm (pulsatile and expansile mass) decreases as a function of body size. Because palpation alone is not sufficiently accurate to establish this diagnosis, a screening ultrasound examination is advised. The presence of an arterial bruit over the abdomen suggests high-grade atherosclerotic disease, though precise localization is difficult.

Extremities

The temperature and color of the extremities, the presence of clubbing, arachnodactyly, and pertinent nail findings can be surmised quickly during the examination. Clubbing implies the presence of central right-to-left shunting, although it has also been described in patients with endocarditis. Its appearance can range from cyanosis and softening of the root of the nail bed, to the classic loss of the normal angle between the base of the nail and the skin, to the skeletal and periosteal bony changes of hypertrophic osteoarthropathy, which is seen rarely in patients with advanced lung or liver disease. Patients with the Holt-Oram syndrome have an unopposable, "fingerized" thumb, whereas patients with Marfan syndrome may have arachnodactyly and a positive "wrist" (overlapping of the thumb and fifth finger around the wrist) or "thumb" (protrusion of the thumb beyond the ulnar aspect of the hand when the fingers are clenched over the thumb in a fist) sign. The Janeway lesions of endocarditis are nontender, slightly raised hemorrhages on the palms and soles, whereas Osler's nodes are tender, raised nodules on the pads of the fingers or toes. Splinter hemorrhages are classically identified as linear petechiae in the midposition of the nail bed and should be distinguished from the more common traumatic petechiae, which are seen closer to the distal edge.

Lower extremity or presacral edema in the setting of an elevated JVP defines volume overload and may be a feature of chronic heart failure or constrictive pericarditis. Lower extremity edema in the absence of jugular venous hypertension may be due to lymphatic or venous obstruction or, more commonly, to venous insufficiency, as further suggested by the appearance of varicosities, venous ulcers (typically medial in location), and brownish cutaneous discoloration from hemosiderin deposition (eburnation). Pitting edema can also be seen in patients who use dihydropyridine calcium channel blockers. A Homan's sign (posterior calf pain on active dorsiflexion of the foot against resistance) is neither specific nor sensitive for deep venous thrombosis. Muscular atrophy or the absence of hair along an extremity is consistent with severe arterial insufficiency or a primary neuromuscular disorder.

■ CARDIOVASCULAR EXAMINATION

Jugular venous pressure and wave form

Jugular venous pressure is the single most important bedside measurement from which to estimate the volume status. The internal jugular vein is preferred because the external jugular vein is valved and not directly in line with the superior vena cava and right atrium. Nevertheless, the external jugular vein has been used to discriminate between high and low central venous pressure (CVP) when tested among medical students, residents, and attending physicians. Precise estimation of the central venous or right atrial pressure from bedside assessment of the jugular venous waveform has proved difficult. Venous pressure traditionally has been measured as the vertical distance between the top of the jugular venous pulsation and the sternal inflection point (angle of Louis). A distance >4.5 cm at 30° elevation is considered abnormal. However, the actual distance between the mid-right atrium and the angle of Louis varies considerably as a function of both body size and the patient angle at which the assessment is made (30°, 45°, or 60°). The use of the sternal angle as a reference point leads to systematic underestimation of CVP, and this method should be used less for semiquantification than to distinguish a normal from an abnormally elevated CVP. The use of the clavicle may provide an easier reference for standardization. Venous pulsations above this level in the sitting position are clearly abnormal, as the distance between the clavicle and the right atrium is at least 10 cm. The patient should always be placed in the sitting position, with the legs dangling below the bedside, when an elevated pressure is suspected in the semisupine position. It should also be noted that bedside estimates of CVP are made in centimeters of water but must be converted to millimeters of mercury to provide correlation with accepted hemodynamic norms (1.36 cmH_2O = 1.0 mmHg).

The venous waveform sometimes can be difficult to distinguish from the carotid pulse, especially during casual inspection. Nevertheless, the venous waveform has several characteristic features, and its individual components can be appreciated in most patients (Fig. 227-1). In patients in sinus rhythm, the venous waveform is typically biphasic, whereas the carotid upstroke is monophasic.

The venous waveform is divided into several distinct peaks. The *a* wave reflects right atrial presystolic contraction and occurs just after the electrocardiographic P wave, preceding the first heart sound (S_1). A prominent *a* wave is seen in patients with reduced right ventricular compliance; a cannon *a* wave occurs with atrioventricular (AV) dissociation and right atrial contraction against a closed tricuspid valve. In a patient with a wide complex tachycardia, the appreciation of cannon *a* waves in the jugular venous waveform identifies the rhythm as ventricular in origin. The *a* wave is not present with atrial fibrillation. The *x* descent defines the fall in right atrial pressure after inscription of the *a* wave. The *c* wave interrupts this *x* descent and is followed by a further descent. The *v* wave represents atrial filling (atrial diastole) and occurs during ventricular systole. The height of the *v* wave is determined by right atrial compliance as well as the volume of blood returning to the right atrium either antegrade from the cavae or retrograde through an incompetent tricuspid valve. In patients with TR, the *v* wave is accentuated and the subsequent fall in pressure (*y* descent) is rapid. With progressive degrees of TR, the *v* wave merges with the *c* wave, and the right atrial and jugular vein waveforms become "ventricularized." The *y* descent, which follows the peak of the *v* wave, can become prolonged or blunted with obstruction to right ventricular inflow, as may occur with tricuspid stenosis (TS) or pericardial tamponade. Normally, the venous pressure should fall by at least 3 mmHg with inspiration. Kussmaul's sign is defined by either a rise or a lack of fall of the JVP with inspiration and is classically associated with constrictive pericarditis, although it has been reported in patients with restrictive cardiomyopathy, massive pulmonary embolism, right ventricular infarction, and advanced left ventricular systolic heart failure.

Venous hypertension sometimes can be elicited by performance of the abdominojugular reflex or with passive leg elevation. When these signs are positive, a volume-overloaded state with limited compliance of an overly distended or constricted venous system is present. The abdominojugular reflex is elicited with firm and consistent pressure over the upper portion of the abdomen, preferably over the right upper quadrant, for at least 10 s. A positive response is defined by a sustained rise of more than 3 cm in JVP for at least 15 s after release of the hand. Patients must be coached to refrain from breath holding or a Valsalva-like maneuver during

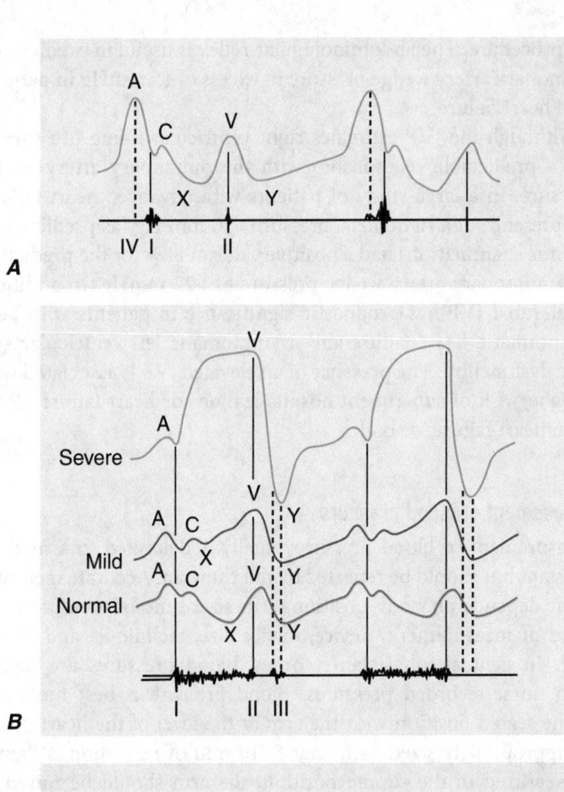

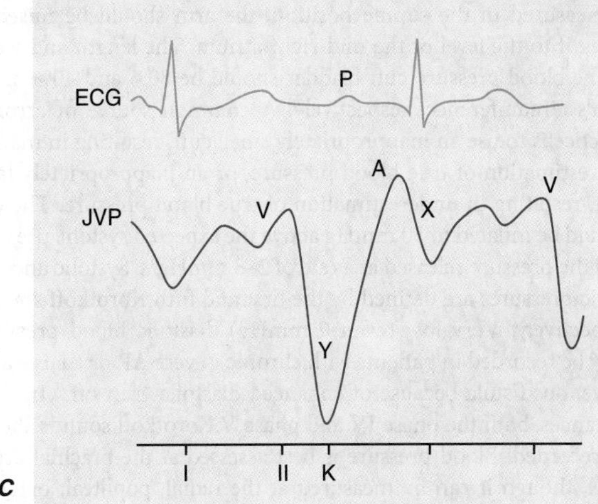

Figure 227-1 ***A.* Jugular venous pulse wave tracing** (*top*) with heart sounds (*bottom*). The A wave represents right atrial presystolic contraction and occurs just after the electrocardiographic P wave and just before the first heart sound (I). In this example, the A wave is accentuated and larger than normal due to decreased right ventricular compliance, as also suggested by the right-sided S_4 (IV). The C wave may reflect the carotid pulsation in the neck and/or an early systolic increase in right atrial pressure as the right ventricle pushes the closed tricuspid valve into the right atrium. The *x* descent follows the A wave just as atrial pressure continues to fall. The V wave represents atrial filling during ventricular systole and peaks at the second heart sound (II). The *y* descent corresponds to the fall in right atrial pressure after tricuspid valve opening. ***B.*** Jugular venous wave forms in mild (*middle*) and severe (*top*) tricuspid regurgitation, compared with normal, with phonocardiographic representation of the corresponding heart sounds below. With increasing degrees of tricuspid regurgitation, the waveform becomes "ventricularized." ***C.*** ECG (*top*), jugular venous waveform (*middle*), and heart sounds (*bottom*) in pericardial constriction. Note the prominent and rapid *y* descent, corresponding in timing to the pericardial knock (K). *(From J Abrams: Synopsis of Cardiac Physical Diagnosis, 2nd ed. Boston, Butterworth Heinemann, 2001, pp 25–35.)*

the procedure. The abdominojugular reflex is useful in predicting a pulmonary artery wedge pressure in excess of 15 mmHg in patients with heart failure.

Although the JVP estimates right ventricular filling pressure, it has a predictable relationship with the pulmonary artery wedge pressure. In a large study of patients with advanced heart failure, the presence of a right atrial pressure >10 mm Hg (as predicted on bedside examination) had a positive value of 88% for the prediction of a pulmonary artery wedge pressure of >22 mmHg. In addition, an elevated JVP has prognostic significance in patients with both symptomatic heart failure and asymptomatic left ventricular systolic dysfunction. The presence of an elevated JVP is associated with a higher risk of subsequent hospitalization for heart failure, death from heart failure, or both.

Assessment of blood pressure

Measurement of blood pressure usually is delegated to a medical assistant but should be repeated by the clinician. Accurate measurement depends on body position, arm size, time of measurement, place of measurement, device, device size, technique, and examiner. In general, physician-recorded blood pressures are higher than nurse-recorded pressures. Blood pressure is best measured in the seated position with the arm at the level of the heart, using an appropriately sized cuff, after 5–10 min of relaxation. When it is measured in the supine position, the arm should be raised to bring it to the level of the mid-right atrium. The length and width of the blood pressure cuff bladder should be 80% and 40% of the arm's circumference, respectively. A common source of error in practice is to use an inappropriately small cuff, resulting in marked overestimation of true blood pressure, or an inappropriately large cuff, resulting in underestimation of true blood pressure. The cuff should be inflated to 30 mmHg above the expected systolic pressure and the pressure released at a rate of 2–3 mmHg/s. Systolic and diastolic pressures are defined by the first and fifth Korotkoff sounds, respectively. Very low (even 0 mmHg) diastolic blood pressures may be recorded in patients with chronic, severe AR or a large arteriovenous fistula because of enhanced diastolic "run-off." In these instances, both the phase IV and phase V Korotkoff sounds should be recorded. Blood pressure is best assessed at the brachial artery level, though it can be measured at the radial, popliteal, or pedal pulse level. In general, systolic pressure increases and diastolic pressure decreases when measured in more distal arteries. Blood pressure should be measured in both arms, and the difference should be less than 10 mmHg. A blood pressure differential that exceeds this threshold may be associated with atherosclerotic or inflammatory subclavian artery disease, supravalvular aortic stenosis, aortic coarctation, or aortic dissection. Systolic leg pressures are usually as much as 20 mmHg higher than systolic arm pressures. Greater leg–arm pressure differences are seen in patients with chronic severe AR as well as patients with extensive and calcified lower extremity peripheral arterial disease. The ankle-brachial index (lower pressure in the dorsalis pedis or posterior tibial artery divided by the higher of the two brachial artery pressures) is a powerful predictor of long-term cardiovascular mortality.

The blood pressure measured in an office or hospital setting may not accurately reflect the pressure in other venues. "White coat hypertension" is defined by at least three separate clinic-based measurements >140/90 mmHg and at least two non-clinic-based measurements <140/90 mmHg in the absence of any evidence of target organ damage. Individuals with white coat hypertension may not benefit from drug therapy, although they may be more likely to develop sustained hypertension over time. Masked hypertension should be suspected when normal or even low blood pressures are recorded in patients with advanced atherosclerotic disease, especially when evidence of target organ damage is present or bruits are audible.

Orthostatic hypotension is defined by a fall in systolic pressure >20 mmHg or in diastolic pressure >10 mmHg in response to assumption of the upright posture from a supine position within 3 min. There may also be a lack of a compensatory tachycardia, an abnormal response that suggests autonomic insufficiency, as may be seen in patients with diabetes or Parkinson's disease. Orthostatic hypotension is a common cause of postural lightheadedness/syncope and should be assessed routinely in patients for whom this diagnosis might pertain. It can be exacerbated by advanced age, dehydration, certain medications, food, deconditioning, and ambient temperature.

Arterial pulse

The carotid artery pulse occurs just after the ascending aortic pulse. The aortic pulse is best appreciated in the epigastrium, just above the level of the umbilicus. Peripheral arterial pulses that should be assessed routinely include the subclavian, brachial, radial, ulnar, femoral, popliteal, dorsalis pedis, and posterior tibial. In patients in whom the diagnosis of either temporal arteritis or polymyalgia rheumatica is suspected, the temporal arteries also should be examined. Although one of the two pedal pulses may not be palpable in up to 10% of normal subjects, the pair should be symmetric. The integrity of the arcuate system of the hand is assessed by Allen's test, which is performed routinely before instrumentation of the radial artery. The pulses should be examined for their symmetry, volume, timing, contour, amplitude, and duration. If necessary, simultaneous auscultation of the heart can help identify a delay in the arrival of an arterial pulse. Simultaneous palpation of the radial and femoral pulses may reveal a femoral delay in a patient with hypertension and suspected aortic coarctation. The carotid upstrokes should never be examined simultaneously or before listening for a bruit. Light pressure should always be used to avoid precipitation of carotid hypersensitivity syndrome and syncope in a susceptible elderly individual. The arterial pulse usually becomes more rapid and spiking as a function of its distance from the heart, a phenomenon that reflects the muscular status of the more peripheral arteries and the summation of the incident and reflected waves. In general, the character and contour of the arterial pulse depend on the stroke volume, ejection velocity, vascular compliance, and systemic vascular resistance. The pulse examination can be misleading in patients with reduced cardiac output and in those with stiffened arteries from aging, chronic hypertension, or peripheral arterial disease.

The character of the pulse is best appreciated at the carotid level (Fig. 227-2). A weak and delayed pulse (*pulsus parvus et tardus*) defines severe aortic stenosis (AS). Some patients with AS may also have a slow, notched, or interrupted upstroke (anacrotic pulse) with a thrill or shudder. With chronic severe AR, by contrast, the carotid upstroke has a sharp rise and rapid fall-off (Corrigan's or water-hammer pulse). Some patients with advanced AR may have a bifid or bisferiens pulse, in which two systolic peaks can be appreciated. A bifid pulse is also described in patients with hypertrophic obstructive cardiomyopathy (HOCM), with inscription of percussion and tidal waves. A bifid pulse is easily appreciated in patients on intra-aortic balloon counterpulsation (IABP), in whom the second pulse is diastolic in timing.

Pulsus paradoxus refers to a fall in systolic pressure >10 mmHg with inspiration that is seen in patients with pericardial tamponade but also is described in those with massive pulmonary embolism, hemorrhagic shock, severe obstructive lung disease, and tension

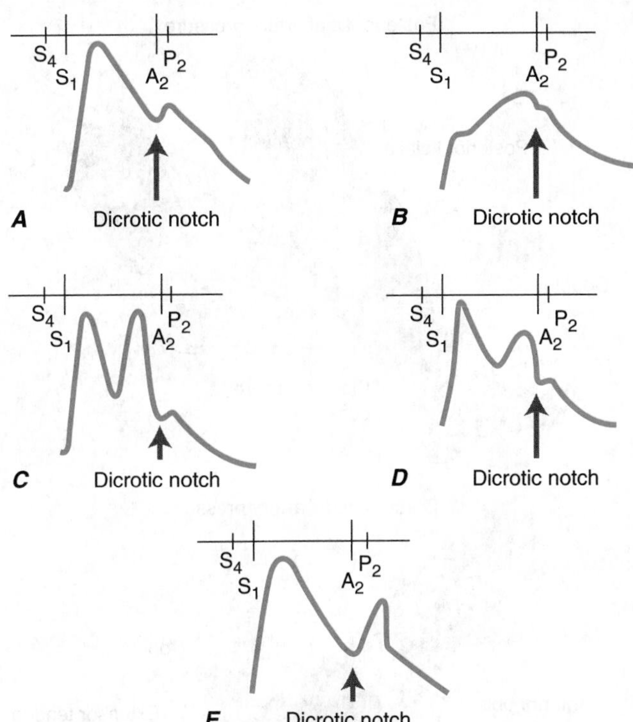

Figure 227-2 Schematic diagrams of the configurational changes in carotid pulse and their differential diagnoses. Heart sounds are also illustrated. ***A.*** Normal. S_4, fourth heart sound; S_1, first heart sound; A_2 aortic component of second heart sound; P_2 pulmonic component of second heart sound. ***B.*** Aortic stenosis. Anacrotic pulse with slow upstroke to a reduced peak. ***C.*** Bisferiens pulse with two peaks in systole. This pulse is rarely appreciated in patients with severe aortic regurgitation. ***D.*** Bisferiens pulse in hypertrophic obstructive cardiomyopathy. There is a rapid upstroke to the first peak (percussion wave) and a slower rise to the second peak (tidal wave). ***E.*** Dicrotic pulse with peaks in systole and diastole. This waveform may be seen in patients with sepsis or during intra-aortic balloon counterpulsation with inflation just after the dicrotic notch. *(From K Chatterjee, W Parmley [eds]: Cardiology: An Illustrated Text/Reference. Philadelphia, JB Lippincott, 1991).*

pneumothorax. Pulsus paradoxus is measured by noting the difference between the systolic pressure at which the Korotkoff sounds are first heard (during expiration) and the systolic pressure at which the Korotkoff sounds are heard with each heartbeat, independent of the respiratory phase. Between these two pressures, the Korotkoff sounds are heard only intermittently and during expiration. The cuff pressure must be decreased slowly to appreciate the finding. It can be difficult to measure pulsus paradoxus in patients with tachycardia, atrial fibrillation, or tachypnea. A pulsus paradoxus may be palpable at the brachial artery or femoral artery level when the pressure difference exceeds 15 mmHg. This inspiratory fall in systolic pressure is an exaggerated consequence of interventricular dependence.

Pulsus alternans, in contrast, is defined by beat-to-beat variability of pulse amplitude. It is present only when every other phase I Korotkoff sound is audible as the cuff pressure is lowered slowly, typically in a patient with a regular heart rhythm and independent of the respiratory cycle. Pulsus alternans is seen in patients with severe left ventricular systolic heart failure and is thought to be due to cyclic changes in intracellular calcium and action potential duration. Interestingly, when pulsus alternans is associated with electrocardiographic T-wave alternans, the risk for an arrhythmic event appears to be increased.

Ascending aortic aneurysms can rarely be appreciated as a pulsatile mass in the right parasternal. Appreciation of a prominent abdominal aortic pulse should prompt noninvasive imaging for better characterization. Femoral and/or popliteal artery aneurysms should be sought in patients with abdominal aortic aneurysm disease.

The level of a claudication-producing arterial obstruction can often be identified on physical examination (Fig. 227-3). For example, in a patient with calf claudication, a decrease in pulse amplitude between the common femoral and popliteal arteries will localize the obstruction to the level of the superficial femoral artery, although inflow obstruction above the level of the common femoral artery may coexist. Auscultation for carotid, subclavian, abdominal aortic, and femoral artery bruits should be routine. However, the correlation between the presence of a bruit and the degree of vascular obstruction is poor. A cervical bruit is a weak indicator of the degree of carotid artery stenosis; the absence of a bruit does not exclude the presence of significant luminal obstruction. If a bruit extends into diastole or if a thrill is present, the obstruction is generally severe. Other causes of arterial bruits include an arteriovenous fistula with enhanced flow.

The likelihood of significant lower extremity peripheral arterial disease increases with typical symptoms of claudication, cool skin, abnormalities on pulse examination, or the presence of a vascular bruit. Abnormal pulse oximetry (a >2% difference between finger and toe oxygen saturation) can be used to detect lower extremity peripheral arterial disease and is comparable in its performance characteristics to the ankle-brachial index.

Inspection and palpation of the heart

The left ventricular apex beat may be visible in the midclavicular line at the fifth intercostal space in thin-chested adults. Visible pulsations anywhere other than this expected location are abnormal. The left anterior chest wall may heave in patients with an enlarged or hyperdynamic left or right ventricle. As noted previously, a visible right upper parasternal pulsation may be suggestive of ascending aortic aneurysm disease. In thin, tall patients and patients with advanced obstructive lung disease and flattened diaphragms, the cardiac impulse may be visible in the epigastrium and should be distinguished from a pulsatile liver edge.

Palpation of the heart begins with the patient in the supine position at 30° and can be enhanced by placing the patient in the left lateral decubitus position. The normal left ventricular impulse is less than 2 cm in diameter and moves quickly away from the fingers; it is better appreciated at end expiration, with the heart closer to the anterior chest wall. Characteristics such as size, amplitude, and rate of force development should be noted.

Enlargement of the left ventricular cavity is manifested by a leftward and downward displacement of an enlarged apex beat. A sustained apex beat is a sign of pressure overload, such as that which may be present in patients with AS or chronic hypertension. A palpable presystolic impulse corresponds to the fourth heart sound (S_4) and is indicative of reduced left ventricular compliance and the forceful contribution of atrial contraction to ventricular filling. A palpable third sound (S_3), which is indicative of a rapid early filling wave in patients with heart failure, may be present even when the gallop itself is not audible. A large left ventricular aneurysm may sometimes be palpable as an ectopic impulse, discrete from the apex beat. Hypertrophic obstructive cardiomyopathy may very rarely cause a triple cadence beat at the apex with contributions from a palpable S_4 and the two components of the bisferiens systolic pulse.

Right ventricular pressure or volume overload may create a sternal lift. Signs of either TR (*cv* waves in the jugular venous pulse)

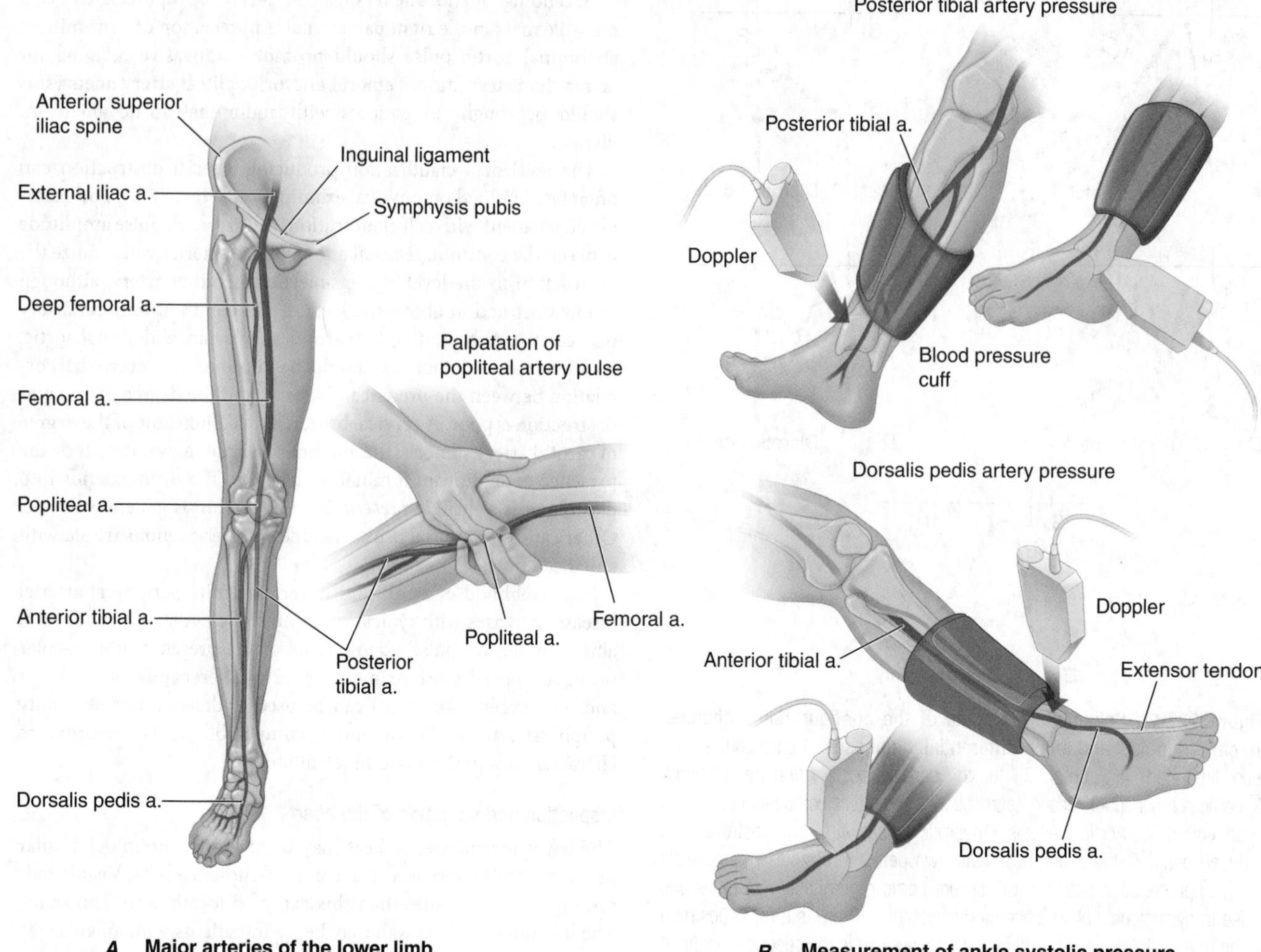

Figure 227-3 ***A.*** Anatomy of the major arteries of the leg. ***B.*** Measurement of the ankle systolic pressure. *(From NA Khan et al: JAMA 295:536, 2006.)*

and/or pulmonary arterial hypertension (a loud single or palpable P_2) would be confirmatory. The right ventricle can enlarge to the extent that left-sided events cannot be appreciated. A zone of retraction between the right and left ventricular impulses sometimes can be appreciated in patients with right ventricle pressure or volume overload when they are placed in the left lateral decubitus position. Systolic and diastolic thrills signify turbulent and high-velocity blood flow. Their locations help identify the origin of heart murmurs.

CARDIAC AUSCULTATION

Heart sounds

Ventricular systole is defined by the interval between the first (S_1) and second (S_2) heart sounds (Fig. 227-4). The first heart sound (S_1) includes mitral and tricuspid valve closure. Normal splitting can be appreciated in young patients and those with right bundle branch block, in whom tricuspid valve closure is relatively delayed. The intensity of S_1 is determined by the distance over which the anterior leaflet of the mitral valve must travel to return to its annular plane, leaflet mobility, left ventricular contractility, and the PR interval. S_1 is classically loud in the early phases of rheumatic mitral stenosis (MS) and in patients with hyperkinetic circulatory states or short PR intervals. S_1 becomes softer in the later stages of MS when the leaflets are rigid and calcified, after exposure to β-adrenergic receptor blockers, with long PR intervals, and with left ventricular contractile dysfunction. The intensity of any heart sound, however, can be reduced by any process that increases the distance between the stethoscope and the responsible cardiac event, including mechanical ventilation, obstructive lung disease, obesity, pneumothorax, and a pericardial effusion.

Aortic and pulmonic valve closure constitutes the second heart sound (S_2). With normal or physiologic splitting, the A_2–P_2 interval increases with inspiration and narrows during expiration. This physiologic interval will widen with right bundle branch block because of the further delay in pulmonic valve closure and in patients with severe MR because of the premature closure of the aortic valve. An unusually narrowly split or even a singular S_2 is a feature of pulmonary arterial hypertension. Fixed splitting of S_2, in which the A_2–P_2 interval is wide and does not change during the respiratory cycle, occurs in patients with a secundum atrial septal defect. Reversed or paradoxical splitting refers to a pathologic delay in aortic valve closure, such as that which occurs in patients with left bundle branch block, right ventricular apical pacing, severe AS, HOCM, and acute myocardial ischemia. With reversed or paradoxical splitting, the individual components of S_2 are audible at end expiration, and their interval narrows with inspiration, the opposite of what would be expected under normal physiologic conditions. P_2 is considered loud when its intensity exceeds that of A_2 at the base, when it can be palpated in the area of the proximal pulmonary artery (second left interspace), or when both components of S_2 can

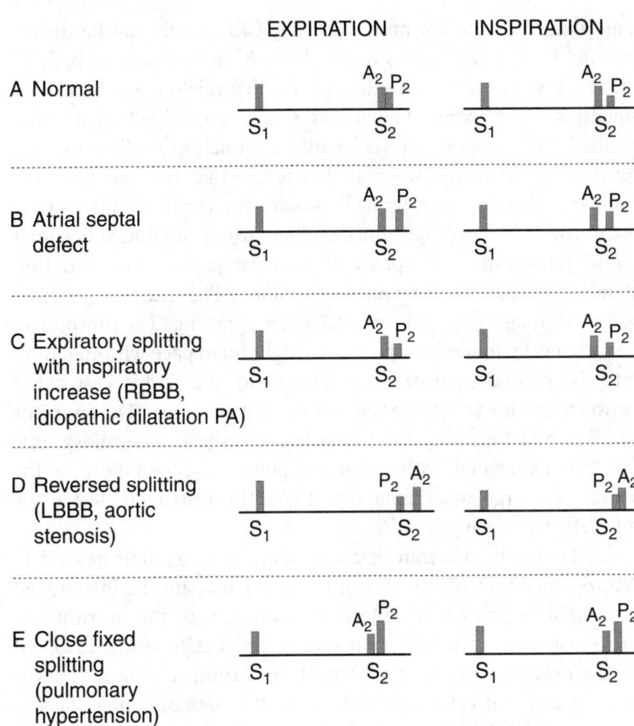

Figure 227-4 Heart sounds. ***A.*** Normal. S_1, first heart sound; S_2, second heart sound; A_2, aortic component of the second heart sound; P_2, pulmonic component of the second heart sound. ***B.*** Atrial septal defect with fixed splitting of S_2. ***C.*** Physiologic but wide splitting of S_2 with right bundle branch block. ***D.*** Reversed or paradoxical splitting of S_2 with left bundle branch block. ***E.*** Narrow splitting of S_2 with pulmonary hypertension. *(From NO Fowler: Diagnosis of Heart Disease. New York, Springer-Verlag, 1991, p 31.)*

be appreciated at the lower left sternal border or apex. The intensity of A_2 and P_2 decreases with aortic and pulmonic stenosis, respectively. In these conditions, a single S_2 may result.

Systolic sounds

An ejection sound is a high-pitched early systolic sound that corresponds in timing to the upstroke of the carotid pulse. It usually is associated with congenital bicuspid aortic or pulmonic valve disease; however, ejection sounds are also sometimes audible in patients with isolated aortic or pulmonary root dilation and normal semilunar valves. The ejection sound that accompanies bicuspid aortic valve disease becomes softer and then inaudible as the valve calcifies and becomes more rigid. The ejection sound that accompanies pulmonic stenosis (PS) moves closer to the first heart sound as the severity of the stenosis increases. In addition, the pulmonic ejection sound is the only right-sided acoustic event that decreases in intensity with inspiration. Ejection sounds are often heard more easily at the lower left sternal border than they are at the base. Nonejection sounds (clicks), which occur after the onset of the carotid upstroke, are related to mitral valve prolapse and may be single or multiple. The nonejection click may introduce a murmur. This click-murmur complex will move away from the first heart sound with maneuvers that increase ventricular preload, such as squatting. On standing, the click and murmur move closer to S_1.

Diastolic sounds

The high pitched opening snap (OS) of MS occurs after a very short interval after the second heart sound. The A_2–OS interval is inversely proportional to the height of the left atrial–left ventricular diastolic pressure gradient. The intensity of both S_1 and the OS of MS decreases with progressive calcification and rigidity of the anterior mitral leaflets. The pericardial knock (PK) is also high-pitched and occurs slightly later than the opening snap, corresponding in timing to the abrupt cessation of ventricular expansion after tricuspid valve opening and to an exaggerated *y* descent seen in the jugular venous waveform in patients with constrictive pericarditis. A tumor plop is a lower-pitched sound that rarely can be heard in patients with atrial myxoma. It may be appreciated only in certain positions and arises from the diastolic prolapse of the tumor across the mitral valve.

The third heart sound (S_3) occurs during the rapid filling phase of ventricular diastole. It can be a normal finding in children, adolescents, and young adults; however, in older patients it signifies heart failure. A left-sided S_3 is a low-pitched sound best heard over the left ventricular (LV) apex. A right-sided S_3 is usually better heard over the lower left sternal border and becomes louder with inspiration. A left-sided S_3 in patients with chronic heart failure is predictive of cardiovascular morbidity and mortality. Interestingly, an S_3 is equally prevalent among heart failure patients with and without LV systolic dysfunction.

The fourth heart sound (S_4) occurs during the atrial filling phase of ventricular diastole and indicates left ventricular presystolic expansion. An S_4 is more common among patients who derive significant benefit from the atrial contribution to ventricular filling, such as those with chronic left ventricular hypertrophy or active myocardial ischemia. An S_4 is not present with atrial fibrillation.

Cardiac murmurs

Heart murmurs result from audible vibrations that are caused by increased turbulence and are defined by their timing within the cardiac cycle. Not all murmurs are indicative of structural heart disease, and the accurate identification of a benign or functional systolic murmur often can obviate the need for additional testing in healthy subjects. The duration, frequency, configuration, and intensity of a heart murmur are dictated by the magnitude, variability, and duration of the responsible pressure difference between two cardiac chambers, the two ventricles, or the ventricles and their respective great arteries. The intensity of a heart murmur is graded on a scale of 1 to 6; a thrill is present with murmurs of grade 4 or greater intensity. Other attributes of the murmur that aid in its accurate identification include its location, radiation, and response to bedside maneuvers. Although clinicians can detect and correctly identify heart murmurs with only fair reliability, a careful and complete bedside examination usually can identify individuals with valvular heart disease for whom transthoracic echocardiography and clinical follow-up are indicated and exclude subjects for whom no further evaluation is necessary.

Systolic murmurs can be early, mid-, late, or holosystolic in timing (Fig. 227-5). Acute severe MR results in a decrescendo early systolic murmur, the characteristics of which are related to the progressive attenuation of the left ventricular to left atrial pressure gradient during systole because of the steep and rapid rise in left atrial pressure in this clinical context. Severe MR associated with posterior leaflet prolapse or flail radiates anteriorly and to the base, where it can be confused with the murmur of aortic stenosis. MR that is due to anterior leaflet involvement radiates posteriorly and to the axilla. With acute TR in patients with normal pulmonary arterty (PA) pressures, an early systolic murmur that may increase in intensity with inspiration may be heard at the left lower sternal border, with regurgitant *cv* waves visible in the jugular venous pulse.

A midsystolic murmur begins after S_1 and ends before S_2; it is typically crescendo-decrescendo in configuration. Aortic stenosis

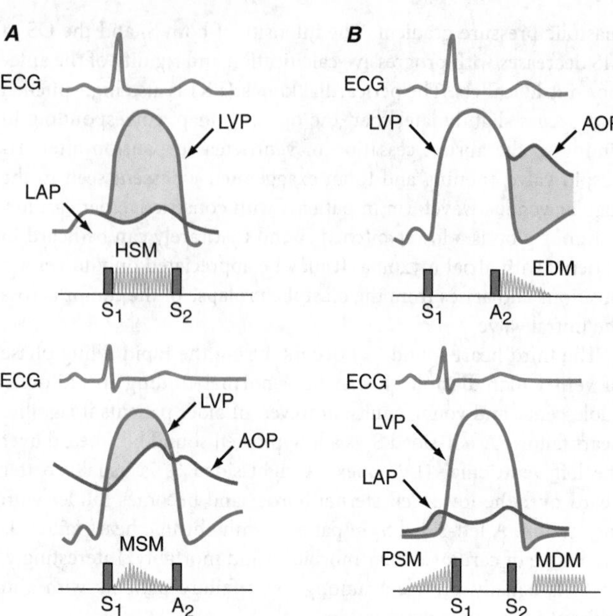

Figure 227-5 ***A.*** *Top.* Graphic representation of the systolic pressure difference (green shaded area) between left ventricle and left atrium with phonocardiographic recording of a holosystolic murmur (HSM) indicative of mitral regurgitation. ECG, electrocardiogram; LVP, left ventricular pressure; LAP, left atrial pressure; S_1, first heart sound; S_2 second heart sound. *Bottom.* Graphic representation of the systolic pressure gradient (green shaded area) between left ventricle and aorta in patient with aortic stenosis. A midsystolic murmur (MSM) with a crescendo-decrescendo configuration is recorded. AOP, aortic pressure. ***B.*** *Top.* Graphic representation of the diastolic pressure difference between the aorta and left ventricle (blue shaded area) in a patient with aortic regurgitation, resulting in a decrescendo, early diastolic murmur (EDM) beginning with A_2. *Bottom.* Graphic representation of the diastolic left atrial–left ventricular gradient (blue areas) in a patient with mitral stenosis with a mid-diastolic murmur (MDM) and late presystolic murmurs (PSM).

is the most common cause of a midsystolic murmur in an adult. It is often difficult to estimate the severity of the valve lesion on the basis of the physical examination findings, especially in older hypertensive patients with stiffened carotid arteries or patients with low cardiac output in whom the intensity of the systolic heart murmur is misleadingly soft. Examination findings consistent with severe AS would include parvus et tardus carotid upstrokes, a late-peaking grade 3 or greater midsystolic murmur, a soft A_2, a sustained LV apical impulse, and an S_4. It is sometimes difficult to distinguish aortic sclerosis from more advanced degrees of valve stenosis. The former is defined by focal thickening and calcification of the aortic valve leaflets that is not severe enough to result in obstruction. These valve changes are associated with a Doppler jet velocity across the aortic valve of 2.5 m/s or less. Patients with aortic sclerosis can have grade 2 or 3 midsystolic murmurs identical in their acoustic characteristics to the murmurs heard in patients with more advanced degrees of AS. Other causes of a midsystolic heart murmur include pulmonic valve stenosis (with or without an ejection sound), HOCM, increased pulmonary blood flow in patients with a large atrial septal defect and left-to-right shunting, and several states associated with accelerated blood flow in the absence of structural heart disease, such as fever, thyrotoxicosis, pregnancy, anemia, and normal adolescence.

The murmur of hypertrophic obstructive cardiomyopathy has features of both obstruction to left ventricular outflow and MR, as would be expected from knowledge of the pathophysiology of this condition. The systolic murmur of HOCM usually can be distinguished from other causes on the basis of its response to bedside maneuvers, including Valsalva, passive leg raising, and standing/squatting. In general, maneuvers that decrease left ventricular preload (or increase left ventricular contractility) will cause the murmur to intensify, whereas maneuvers that increase left ventricular preload or afterload will cause a decrease in the intensity of the murmur. Accordingly, the systolic murmur of HOCM becomes louder during the strain phase of the Valsalva maneuver and after standing quickly from a squatting position. The murmur becomes softer with passive leg raising and when squatting. The murmur of AS is typically loudest in the second right interspace with radiation into the carotids, whereas the murmur of HOCM is best heard between the lower left sternal border and the apex. The murmur of PS is best heard in the second left interspace. The midsystolic murmur associated with enhanced pulmonic blood flow in the setting of a large atrial septal defect (ASD) is usually loudest at the mid-left sternal border.

A late systolic murmur, heard best at the apex, indicates MVP. As previously noted, the murmur may or may not be introduced by a nonejection click. Differential radiation of the murmur, as previously described, may help identify the specific leaflet involved by the myxomatous process. The click-murmur complex behaves in a manner directionally similar to that demonstrated by the murmur of HOCM during the Valsalva and stand/squat maneuvers (Fig. 227-6). The murmur of MVP can be identified by the accompanying nonejection click.

Holosystolic murmurs are plateau in configuration and reflect a continuous and wide pressure gradient between the left ventricle and left atrium with chronic MR, the left ventricle and right ventricle with a ventricular septal defect (VSD), and the right ventricle and right atrium with TR. In contrast to acute MR, in chronic MR the left atrium is enlarged and its compliance is normal or increased to the extent that there is little if any further increase in left atrial pressure from any increase in regurgitant volume. The murmur of MR is best heard over the cardiac apex. The intensity of the murmur increases with maneuvers that increase left ventricular afterload, such as sustained hand grip. The murmur of a VSD (without significant pulmonary hypertension) is holosystolic and loudest at the mid-left sternal border, where a thrill is usually present. The murmur of TR is loudest at the lower left sternal border, increases in intensity with inspiration (Carvallo's sign), and is accompanied by visible *cv* waves in the jugular venous wave form and, on occasion, by pulsatile hepatomegaly.

Diastolic murmurs

In contrast to some systolic murmurs, diastolic heart murmurs always signify structural heart disease (Fig. 227-5). The murmur associated with acute, severe AR is relatively soft and of short duration because of the rapid rise in left ventricular diastolic pressure and the progressive diminution of the aortic-left ventricular diastolic pressure gradient. In contrast, the murmur of chronic severe AR is classically heard as a decrescendo, blowing diastolic murmur along the left sternal border in patients with primary valve pathology and sometimes along the right sternal border in patients with primary aortic root pathology. With chronic AR, the pulse pressure is wide and the arterial pulses are bounding in character. These signs of significant diastolic run-off are absent in the acute phase. The murmur of pulmonic regurgitation (PR) is also heard along the left sternal border. It is most commonly due to pulmonary hypertension and enlargement of the annulus of the pulmonic valve. S_2 is single and loud and may be palpable. There is a right ventricular/parasternal lift that is indicative of chronic right ventricular pressure overload. A

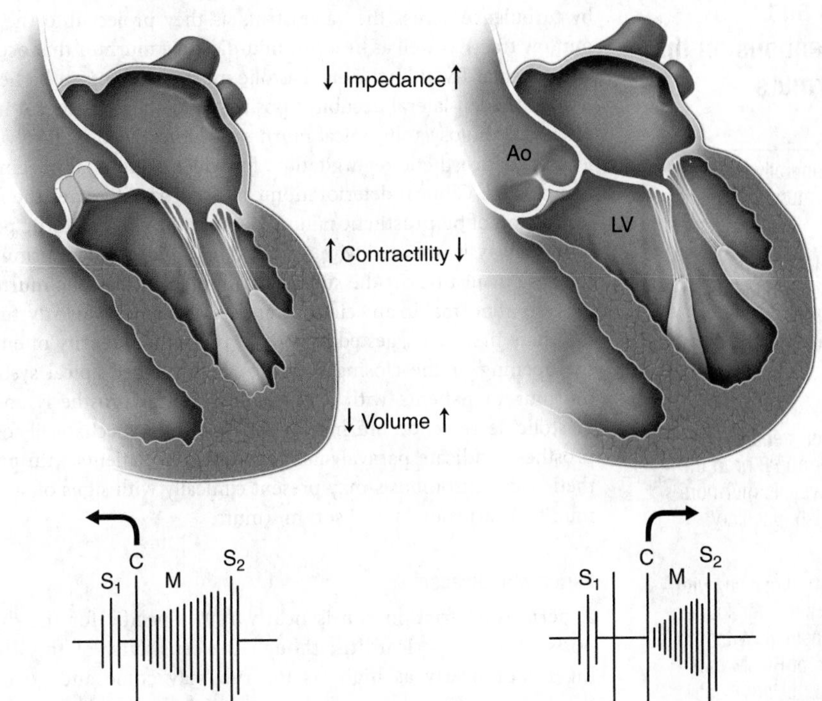

Figure 227-6. Behavior of the click (C) and murmur (M) of mitral valve prolapse with changes in loading (volume, impedance) and contractility. S_1, first heart sound; S_2, second heart sound. With standing (left side of figure), volume and impedance decrease, as a result of which the click and murmur move closer to S_1. With squatting (right), the click and murmur move away from S_1 owing to the increases in left ventricular volume and impedance (afterload). *(Adapted from RA O'Rourke, MH Crawford: Curr Prob Cardiol 1:9, 1976.)*

less impressive murmur of PR is present after repair of tetralogy of Fallot or pulmonic valve atresia. In this postoperative setting, the murmur is softer and lower-pitched and the severity of the accompanying pulmonic regurgitation can be underestimated significantly.

Mitral stenosis is the classic cause of a mid- to late diastolic murmur, which is best heard over the apex in the left lateral decubitus position and is low-pitched or rumbling and is introduced by an OS in the early stages of the rheumatic disease process. Presystolic accentuation refers to an increase in the intensity of the murmur just before the first heart sound and occurs in patients with sinus rhythm. It is absent in patients with atrial fibrillation. The auscultatory findings in patients with rheumatic tricuspid stenosis typically are obscured by left-sided events, though they are similar in nature to those described in patients with MS. "Functional" mitral or tricuspid stenosis refers to the generation of mid-diastolic murmurs that are created by increased and accelerated transvalvular diastolic flow, even in the absence of valvular obstruction, in the setting of severe MR, severe TR, or a large ASD with left-to-right shunting. The Austin Flint murmur of chronic severe AR is a low-pitched mid- to late apical diastolic murmur that sometimes can be confused with MS. The Austin Flint murmur typically decreases in intensity after exposure to vasodilators, whereas the murmur of MS may be accompanied by an opening snap and also may increase in intensity after vasodilators because of the associated increase in cardiac output. Unusual causes of a mid-diastolic murmur include atrial myxoma, complete heart block, and acute rheumatic mitral valvulitis.

Continuous murmur

A continuous murmur is predicated on a pressure gradient that persists between two cardiac chambers or blood vessels across systole and diastole. The murmurs typically begin in systole, envelop the second heart sound (S_2), and continue through some portion of diastole. They can often be difficult to distinguish from individual systolic and diastolic murmurs in patients with mixed valvular heart disease. The classic example of a continuous murmur is that associated with a patent ductus arteriosus, which usually is heard in the second or third interspace at a slight distance from the sternal border. Other causes of a continuous murmur include a ruptured sinus of Valsalva aneurysm with creation of an aortic–right atrial or right ventricular fistula, a coronary or great vessel arteriovenous fistula, and an arteriovenous fistula constructed to provide dialysis access. There are two types of benign continuous murmurs. The cervical venous hum is heard in children or adolescents in the supraclavicular fossa. It can be obliterated with firm pressure applied to the diaphragm of the stethoscope, especially when the subject turns his or her head toward the examiner. The mammary souffle of pregnancy relates to enhanced arterial blood flow through engorged breasts. The diastolic component of the murmur can be obliterated with firm pressure over the stethoscope.

Dynamic auscultation

Diagnostic accuracy can be enhanced by the performance of simple bedside maneuvers to identify heart murmurs and characterize their significance (Table 227-1). Except for the pulmonic ejection sound, right-sided events increase in intensity with inspiration and decrease with expiration; left-sided events behave oppositely (100% sensitivity, 88% specificity). As previously noted, the intensity of the murmurs associated with MR, VSD, and AR will increase in response to maneuvers that increase LV afterload, such as hand grip and vasopressors. The intensity of these murmurs will decrease after exposure to vasodilating agents. Squatting is associated with an abrupt increase in LV preload and afterload, whereas rapid standing results in a sudden decrease in preload. In patients with MVP, the click and murmur move away from the first heart sound with squatting because of the delay in onset of leaflet prolapse at higher ventricular volumes. With rapid standing, however, the click and murmur move closer to the first heart sound as prolapse occurs earlier in systole at a smaller chamber dimension. The murmur of HOCM behaves similarly, becoming softer and shorter with squatting (95% sensitivity, 85% specificity) and longer and louder on rapid standing (95% sensitivity, 84% specificity). A change in the intensity of a systolic murmur in the first beat after a premature beat or in the beat after a long cycle length in patients with atrial fibrillation suggests valvular AS rather than MR, particularly in an older patient in whom the murmur of the AS may be well transmitted to the apex (Gallavardin effect). Of note, however, the systolic murmur of HOCM also increases in intensity in the beat after a premature beat. This increase in intensity of any LV outflow murmur in the beat after a premature beat relates to the combined effects of enhanced

TABLE 227-1 Effects of Physiologic and Pharmacologic Interventions on the Intensity of Heart Murmurs and Sounds
Respiration Right-sided murmurs and sounds generally increase with inspiration, except for the PES. Left-sided murmurs and sounds are usually louder during expiration.
Valsalva maneuver Most murmurs decrease in length and intensity. Two exceptions are the systolic murmur of HOCM, which usually becomes much louder, and that of MVP, which becomes longer and often louder. After release of the Valsalva maneuver, right-sided murmurs tend to return to control intensity earlier than do left-sided murmurs.
After VPB or AF Murmurs originating at normal or stenotic semilunar valves increase in the cardiac cycle after a VPB or in the cycle after a long cycle length in AF. By contrast, systolic murmurs due to AV valve regurgitation do not change, diminish (papillary muscle dysfunction), or become shorter (MVP).
Positional changes With *standing*, most murmurs diminish, with two exceptions being the murmur of HOCM, which becomes louder, and that of MVP, which lengthens and often is intensified. With *squatting*, most murmurs become louder, but those of HOCM and MVP usually soften and may disappear. Passive leg raising usually produces the same results.
Exercise Murmurs due to blood flow across normal or obstructed valves (e.g,. PS, MS) become louder with both isotonic and submaximal isometric (hand grip) exercise. Murmurs of MR, VSD, and AR also increase with hand grip exercise. However, the murmur of HOCM often decreases with nearly maximum hand grip exercise. Left-sided S_4 and S_3 sounds are often accentuated by exercise, particularly when due to ischemic heart disease.

Abbreviations: AF, atrial fibrillation; AR, aortic regurgitation; HOCM, hypertrophic obstructive cardiomyopathy; MR, mitral regurgitation; MS, mitral stenosis; MVP, mitral valve prolapse; PES, pulmonic ejection sound; PR, pulmonic regurgitation; PS, pulmonic stenosis; TR, tricuspid regurgitation; TS, tricuspid stenosis; VPB, ventricular premature beat; VSD, ventricular septal defect.

LV filling (from the longer diastolic period) and postextrasystolic potentiation of LV contractile function. In either instance, forward flow will accelerate, causing an increase in the gradient across the LV outflow tract (dynamic or fixed) and a louder systolic murmur. In contrast, the intensity of the murmur of MR does not change in a postpremature beat, as there is relatively little change in the nearly constant LV to left atrial pressure gradient or further alteration in mitral valve flow. Bedside exercise can sometimes be performed to increase cardiac output and, secondarily, the intensity of both systolic and diastolic heart murmurs. Most left-sided heart murmurs decrease in intensity and duration during the strain phase of the Valsalva maneuver. The murmurs associated with MVP and HOCM are the two notable exceptions. The Valsalva maneuver also can be used to assess the integrity of the heart and vasculature in the setting of advanced heart failure.

Prosthetic heart valves

The first clue that prosthetic valve dysfunction may contribute to recurrent symptoms is frequently a change in the quality of the heart sounds or the appearance of a new murmur. The heart sounds with a bioprosthetic valve resemble those generated by native valves. A mitral bioprosthesis usually is associated with a grade 2 or 3 midsystolic murmur along the left sternal border (created by turbulence across the valve struts as they project into the LV outflow tract) as well as by a soft mid-diastolic murmur that occurs with normal LV filling. This diastolic murmur often can be heard only in the left lateral decubitus position and after exercise. A high pitched or holosystolic apical murmur is indicative of paravalvular leak or bioprosthetic regurgitation, for which additional imagining is indicated. Clinical deterioration can occur rapidly after the first expression of bioprosthetic failure. A tissue valve in the aortic position is always associated with a grade 2 to 3 midsystolic murmur at the base or just below the suprasternal notch. A diastolic murmur of AR is abnormal in any circumstances. Mechanical valve dysfunction may first be suggested by a decrease in the intensity of either the opening or the closing sound. A high-pitched apical systolic murmur in patients with a mechanical mitral prosthesis and a diastolic decrescendo murmur in patients with a mechanical aortic prosthesis indicate paravalvular regurgitation. Patients with prosthetic valve thrombosis may present clinically with signs of shock, muffled heart sounds, and soft murmurs.

Pericardial disease

A pericardial friction rub is nearly 100% specific for the diagnosis of acute pericarditis, though the sensitivity of this finding is not nearly as high, as the rub may come and go over the course of an acute illness or be very difficult to elicit. The rub is heard as a leathery or scratchy three-component or two-component sound, though it may be monophasic. Classically, the three components are ventricular systole, rapid early diastolic filling, and late presystolic filling after atrial contraction in patients in sinus rhythm. It is necessary to listen to the heart in several positions. Additional clues may be present from the history and 12-lead electrocardiogram. The rub typically disappears as the volume of any pericardial effusion increases. Pericardial tamponade can be diagnosed with a sensitivity of 98%, a specificity of 83%, and a positive likelihood ratio of 5.9 (95% confidence intervals 2.4 to 14) by a pulsus paradoxus that exceeds 12 mmHg in a patient with a large pericardial effusion.

The findings on physical examination are integrated with the symptoms previously elicited with a careful history to construct an appropriate differential diagnosis and proceed with indicated imaging and laboratory assessment. The physical examination is an irreplaceable component of the diagnostic algorithm and in selected patients can inform prognosis. Educational efforts to improve clinician competence eventually may result in cost saving, particularly if the indications for imaging can be influenced by the examination findings.

FURTHER READINGS

Drazner MH et al; Prognostic importance of elevated jugular venous pressure and a third heart sound in patients with heart failure. N Engl J Med 345:574, 2001

Fang JC, O'Gara PT: The history and physical examination: An evidence-based approach, in *Braunwald's Heart Disease*, 8th ed, P Libby et al (eds). Philadelphia, Saunders, 2008

Markel H: The stethoscope and the art of listening. N Engl J Med 354:551, 2006

O'Rourke RA et al: The history, physical examination, and cardiac auscultation, in *Hurst's The Heart*, 12th ed, V Fuster et al (eds). New York, McGraw-Hill, 2008

Roy CL et al: Does this patient with a pericardial effusion have cardiac tamponade? JAMA 297:1810, 2007

CHAPTER 228

Electrocardiography

Ary L. Goldberger

An electrocardiogram (ECG or EKG) is a graphic recording of electric potentials generated by the heart. The signals are detected by means of metal electrodes attached to the extremities and chest wall and then are amplified and recorded by the electrocardiograph. ECG *leads* actually display the instantaneous *differences* in potential between the electrodes.

The clinical utility of the ECG derives from its immediate availability as a noninvasive, inexpensive, and highly versatile test. In addition to its use in detecting arrhythmias, conduction disturbances, and myocardial ischemia, electrocardiography may reveal other findings related to life-threatening metabolic disturbances (e.g., hyperkalemia) or increased susceptibility to sudden cardiac death (e.g., QT prolongation syndromes).

ELECTROPHYSIOLOGY

(See also Chaps. 232 and 233) Depolarization of the heart is the initiating event for cardiac contraction. The electric currents that spread through the heart are produced by three components: cardiac pacemaker cells, specialized conduction tissue, and the heart muscle itself. The ECG, however, records only the depolarization (stimulation) and repolarization (recovery) potentials generated by the atrial and ventricular myocardium.

The depolarization stimulus for the normal heartbeat originates in the *sinoatrial* (SA) *node* (Fig. 228-1), or *sinus node*, a collection of *pacemaker cells*. These cells fire spontaneously; that is, they exhibit *automaticity*. The first phase of cardiac electrical activation is the spread of the depolarization wave through the right and left atria, followed by atrial contraction. Next, the impulse stimulates pacemaker and specialized conduction tissues in the atrioventricular (AV) nodal and His-bundle areas; together, these two regions constitute the AV junction. The bundle of His bifurcates into two main branches, the right and left bundles, which rapidly transmit depolarization wavefronts to the right and left ventricular myocardium by way of Purkinje fibers. The main left bundle bifurcates into two primary subdivisions: a left anterior fascicle and a left posterior fascicle. The depolarization wavefronts then spread through the ventricular wall, from endocardium to epicardium, triggering ventricular contraction.

Since the cardiac depolarization and repolarization waves have direction and magnitude, they can be represented by vectors. Vector analysis illustrates a central concept of electrocardiography: The ECG records the complex spatial and temporal summation of electrical potentials from multiple myocardial fibers conducted to the surface of the body. This principle accounts for inherent limitations in both ECG *sensitivity* (activity from certain cardiac regions may be canceled out or may be too weak to be recorded) and *specificity* (the same vectorial sum can result from either a selective gain or a loss of forces in opposite directions).

ECG WAVEFORMS AND INTERVALS

The ECG waveforms are labeled alphabetically, beginning with the P wave, which represents atrial depolarization (Fig. 228-2). The QRS complex represents ventricular depolarization, and the ST-T-U complex (ST segment, T wave, and U wave) represents ventricular repolarization. The J point is the junction between the end of the QRS complex and the beginning of the ST segment. Atrial repolarization is usually too low in amplitude to be detected, but it may become apparent in conditions such as acute pericarditis and atrial infarction.

The QRS-T waveforms of the surface ECG correspond in a general way with the different phases of simultaneously obtained ventricular *action potentials*, the intracellular recordings from single myocardial fibers (Chap. 232). The rapid upstroke (phase 0) of the action potential corresponds to the onset of QRS. The plateau (phase 2) corresponds to the isoelectric ST segment, and active repolarization (phase 3) corresponds to the inscription of the T wave. Factors that decrease the slope of phase 0 by impairing the influx of Na^+ (e.g., hyperkalemia and drugs such as flecainide) tend to increase QRS duration. Conditions that prolong phase 2 (amiodarone, hypocalcemia) increase the QT interval. In contrast, shortening of

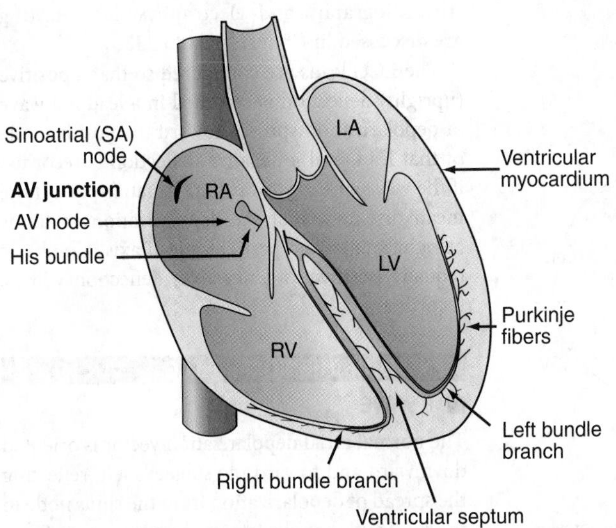

Figure 228-1 Schematic of the cardiac conduction system.

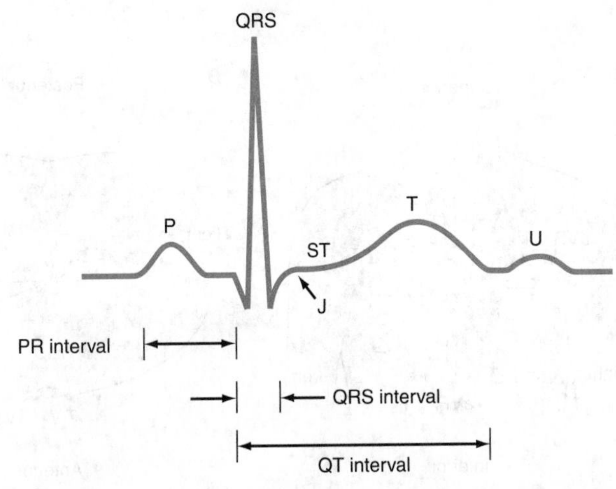

Figure 228-2 Basic ECG waveforms and intervals. Not shown is the R-R interval, the time between consecutive QRS complexes.

ventricular repolarization (phase 2), such as by digitalis administration or hypercalcemia, abbreviates the ST segment.

The electrocardiogram ordinarily is recorded on special graph paper that is divided into 1-mm^2 gridlike boxes. Since the ECG paper speed is generally 25 mm/s, the smallest (1 mm) horizontal divisions correspond to 0.04 (40 ms), with heavier lines at intervals of 0.20 s (200 ms). Vertically, the ECG graph measures the amplitude of a specific wave or deflection (1 mV = 10 mm with standard calibration; the voltage criteria for hypertrophy mentioned below are given in millimeters). There are four major ECG intervals: R-R, PR, QRS, and QT (Fig. 228-2). The heart rate (beats per minute) can be computed readily from the interbeat (R-R) interval by dividing the number of large (0.20 s) time units between consecutive R waves into 300 or the number of small (0.04 s) units into 1500. The PR interval measures the time (normally 120–200 ms) between atrial and ventricular depolarization, which includes the physiologic delay imposed by stimulation of cells in the AV junction area. The QRS interval (normally 100–110 ms or less) reflects the duration of ventricular depolarization. The QT interval includes both ventricular depolarization and repolarization times and varies inversely with the heart rate. A rate-related ("corrected") QT interval, QT_c, can be calculated as $QT/\sqrt{R\text{-}R}$ and normally is ≤0.44 s. (Some references give QT_c upper normal limits as 0.43 s in men and 0.45 s in women. Also, a number of different formulas have been proposed, without consensus, for calculating the QT_c.)

The QRS complex is subdivided into specific deflections or waves. If the initial QRS deflection in a particular lead is negative, it is termed a *Q wave*; the first positive deflection is termed an *R wave*. A negative deflection after an R wave is an *S wave*. Subsequent positive or negative waves are labeled R′ and S′, respectively. Lowercase letters (qrs) are used for waves of relatively small amplitude. An entirely negative QRS complex is termed a *QS wave*.

■ ECG LEADS

The 12 conventional ECG leads record the difference in potential between electrodes placed on the surface of the body. These leads are divided into two groups: six limb (extremity) leads and six chest (precordial) leads. The limb leads record potentials transmitted onto the *frontal plane* (Fig. 228-3*A*), and the chest leads record potentials transmitted onto the *horizontal plane* (Fig. 228-3*B*).

The spatial orientation and polarity of the six frontal plane leads is represented on the hexaxial diagram (Fig. 228-4). The six chest leads (Fig. 228-5) are unipolar recordings obtained by electrodes in the following positions: lead V_1, fourth intercostal space, just to the right of the sternum; lead V_2, fourth intercostal space, just to the left of the sternum; lead V_3, midway between V_2 and V_4; lead V_4, midclavicular line, fifth intercostal space; lead V_5, anterior axillary line, same level as V_4; and lead V_6, midaxillary line, same level as V_4 and V_5.

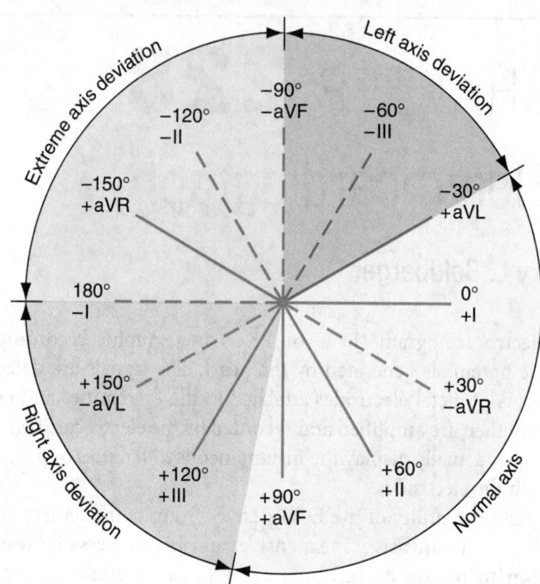

Figure 228-4 The frontal plane (limb or extremity) leads are represented on a hexaxial diagram. Each ECG lead has a specific spatial orientation and polarity. The positive pole of each lead axis (*solid line*) and the negative pole (*hatched line*) are designated by their angular position relative to the positive pole of lead I (0°). The mean electrical axis of the QRS complex is measured with respect to this display.

Together, the frontal and horizontal plane electrodes provide a three-dimensional representation of cardiac electrical activity. Each lead can be likened to a different video camera angle "looking" at the same events—atrial and ventricular depolarization and repolarization—from different spatial orientations. The conventional 12-lead ECG can be supplemented with additional leads in special circumstances. For example, right precordial leads V_3R, V_4R, etc., are useful in detecting evidence of acute right ventricular ischemia. Bedside monitors and ambulatory ECG (Holter) recordings usually employ only one or two modified leads. Intracardiac electrocardiography and electrophysiologic testing are discussed in Chaps. 232 and 233.

The ECG leads are configured so that a positive (upright) deflection is recorded in a lead if a wave of depolarization spreads toward the positive pole of that lead, and a negative deflection is recorded if the wave spreads toward the negative pole. If the mean orientation of the depolarization vector is at right angles to a particular lead axis, a biphasic (equally positive and negative) deflection will be recorded.

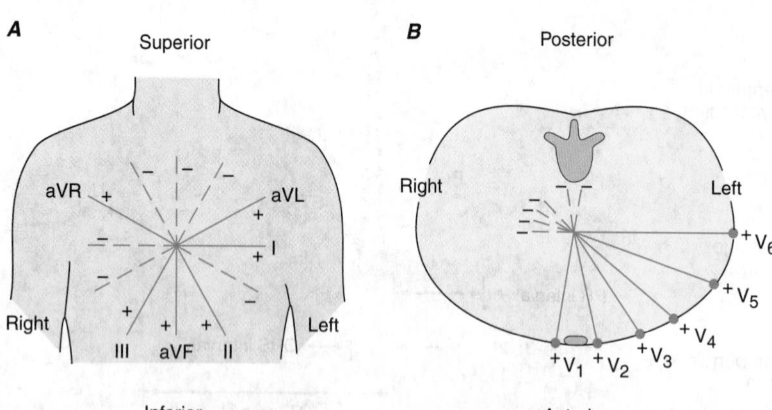

Figure 228-3 The six frontal plane (*A*) and six horizontal plane (*B*) leads provide a three-dimensional representation of cardiac electrical activity.

GENESIS OF THE NORMAL ECG

■ P WAVE

The normal atrial depolarization vector is oriented downward and toward the subject's left, reflecting the spread of depolarization from the sinus node to the right and then the left atrial myocardium. Since this vector points toward the positive pole of lead II

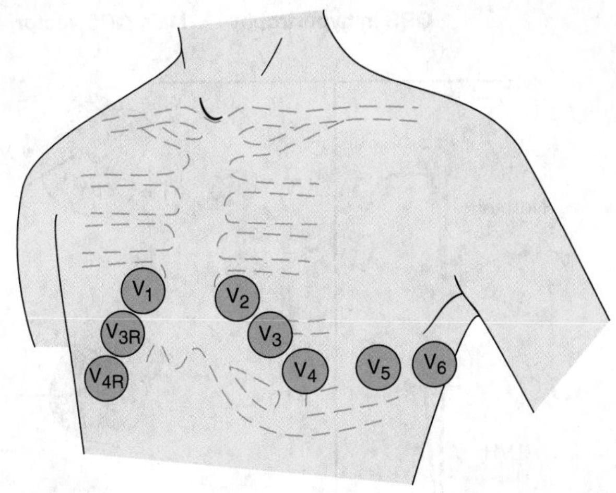

Figure 228-5 The horizontal plane (chest or precordial) leads are obtained with electrodes in the locations shown.

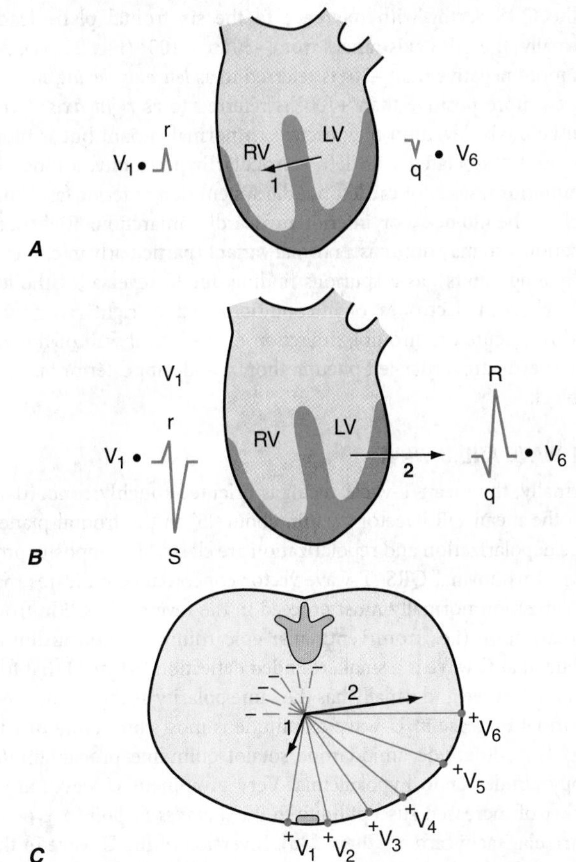

Figure 228-6 Ventricular depolarization can be divided into two major phases, each represented by a vector. ***A.*** The first phase (*arrow 1*) denotes depolarization of the ventricular septum, beginning on the left side and spreading to the right. This process is represented by a small "septal" r wave in lead V_1 and a small septal q wave in lead V_6. ***B.*** Simultaneous depolarization of the left and right ventricles (LV and RV) constitutes the second phase. Vector 2 is oriented to the left and posteriorly, reflecting the electrical predominance of the LV. *C.* Vectors (*arrows*) representing these two phases are shown in reference to the horizontal plane leads. *(After Goldberger.)*

and toward the negative pole of lead aVR, the normal P wave will be positive in lead II and negative in lead aVR. By contrast, activation of the atria from an ectopic pacemaker in the lower part of either atrium or in the AV junction region may produce retrograde P waves (negative in lead II, positive in lead aVR). The normal P wave in lead V_1 may be biphasic with a positive component reflecting right atrial depolarization, followed by a small (<1 mm²) negative component reflecting left atrial depolarization.

QRS COMPLEX

Normal ventricular depolarization proceeds as a rapid, continuous spread of activation wave fronts. This complex process can be divided into two major sequential phases, and each phase can be represented by a mean vector (Fig. 228-6). The first phase is depolarization of the interventricular septum from the left to the right and anteriorly (vector 1). The second results from the simultaneous depolarization of the right and left ventricles; it normally is dominated by the more massive left ventricle, so that vector 2 points leftward and posteriorly. Therefore, a right precordial lead (V_1) will record this biphasic depolarization process with a small positive deflection (septal r wave) followed by a larger negative deflection (S wave). A left precordial lead, e.g., V_6, will record the same sequence with a small negative deflection (septal q wave) followed by a relatively tall positive deflection (R wave). Intermediate leads show a relative increase in R-wave amplitude (normal R-wave progression) and a decrease in S-wave amplitude progressing across the chest from right to left. The precordial lead where the R and S waves are of approximately equal amplitude is referred to as the *transition zone* (usually V_3 or V_4) (Fig. 228-7).

The QRS pattern in the extremity leads may vary considerably from one normal subject to another depending on the *electrical axis* of the QRS, which describes the mean orientation

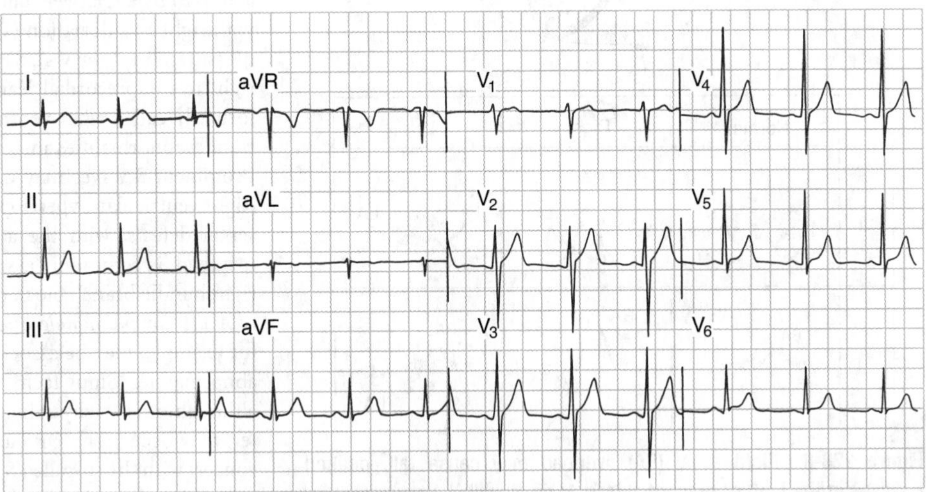

Figure 228-7 Normal electrocardiogram from a healthy subject. Sinus rhythm is present with a heart rate of 75 beats per minute. PR interval is 0.16 s; QRS interval (duration) is 0.08 s; QT interval is 0.36 s; QT_c is 0.40 s; the mean QRS axis is about +70°. The precordial leads show normal R-wave progression with the transition zone (R wave = S wave) in lead V_3.

of the QRS vector with reference to the six frontal plane leads. Normally, the QRS axis ranges from –30° to +100° (Fig. 228-4). An axis more negative than –30° is referred to as *left axis deviation*, and an axis more positive than +100° is referred to as *right axis deviation*. Left axis deviation may occur as a normal variant but is more commonly associated with left ventricular hypertrophy, a block in the anterior fascicle of the left bundle system (left anterior fascicular block or hemiblock), or inferior myocardial infarction. Right axis deviation also may occur as a normal variant (particularly in children and young adults), as a spurious finding due to reversal of the left and right arm electrodes, or in conditions such as right ventricular overload (acute or chronic), infarction of the lateral wall of the left ventricle, dextrocardia, left pneumothorax, and left posterior fascicular block.

■ T WAVE AND U WAVE

Normally, the mean T-wave vector is oriented roughly concordant with the mean QRS vector (within about 45° in the frontal plane). Since depolarization and repolarization are electrically opposite processes, this normal QRS–T-wave vector concordance indicates that repolarization normally must proceed in the reverse direction from depolarization (i.e., from ventricular epicardium to endocardium). The normal U wave is a small, rounded deflection (≤1 mm) that follows the T wave and usually has the same polarity as the T wave. An abnormal increase in U-wave amplitude is most commonly due to drugs (e.g., dofetilide, amiodarone, sotalol, quinidine, procainamide, disopyramide) or to hypokalemia. Very prominent U waves are a marker of increased susceptibility to the *torsades de pointes* type of ventricular tachycardia (Chap. 233). Inversion of the U wave in the precordial leads is abnormal and may be a subtle sign of ischemia.

MAJOR ECG ABNORMALITIES

■ CARDIAC ENLARGEMENT AND HYPERTROPHY

Right atrial overload (acute or chronic) may lead to an increase in P-wave amplitude (≥2.5 mm) (Fig. 228-8). Left atrial overload typically produces a biphasic P wave in V_1 with a broad negative component or a broad (≥120 ms), often notched P wave in one or more limb leads (Fig. 228-8). This pattern may also occur with left atrial conduction delays in the absence of actual atrial enlargement, leading to the more general designation of *left atrial abnormality*.

Right ventricular hypertrophy due to a pressure load (as from pulmonic valve stenosis or pulmonary artery hypertension) is characterized by a relatively tall R wave in lead V_1 (R ≥ S wave), usually with right axis deviation (Fig. 228-9); alternatively, there may be a qR pattern in V_1 or V_3R. ST depression and T-wave inversion in the right-to-midprecordial leads are also often present. This pattern, formerly called right ventricular "strain," is attributed to repolarization abnormalities in acutely or chronically overloaded muscle. Prominent S waves may occur in the left lateral precordial leads. Right ventricular hypertrophy due to ostium secundum–type atrial septal defects, with the accompanying right ventricular volume overload, is commonly associated with an incomplete or complete right bundle branch block pattern with a rightward QRS axis.

Acute cor pulmonale due to pulmonary embolism (Chap. 262), for example, may be associated with a normal ECG or a variety of abnormalities. Sinus tachycardia is the most common arrhythmia, although other tachyarrhythmias, such as atrial fibrillation or flutter, may occur. The QRS axis may shift to the right, sometimes in concert with the so-called $S_1Q_3T_3$ pattern (prominence of the S wave in lead I and the Q wave in lead III, with T-wave inversion in lead III). Acute right ventricular dilation also may be associated with slow R-wave progression and ST-T abnormalities in V_1 to V_4 simulating acute anterior infarction. A right ventricular conduction disturbance may appear.

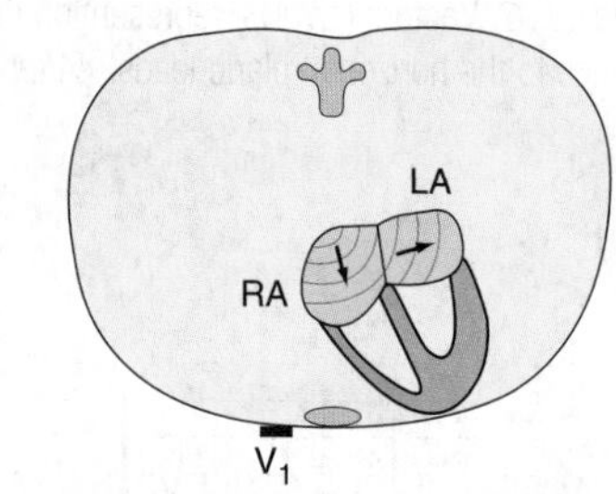

	Normal	Right	Left
II	RA LA	RA LA	RA LA
V_1	RA LA	RA LA	RA LA

Figure 228-8 Right atrial (RA) overload may cause tall, peaked P waves in the limb or precordial leads. Left atrial (LA) abnormality may cause broad, often notched P waves in the limb leads and a biphasic P wave in lead V_1 with a prominent negative component representing delayed depolarization of the LA. *(After MK Park, WG Guntheroth: How to Read Pediatric ECGs, 4th ed. St. Louis, Mosby/Elsevier, 2006.)*

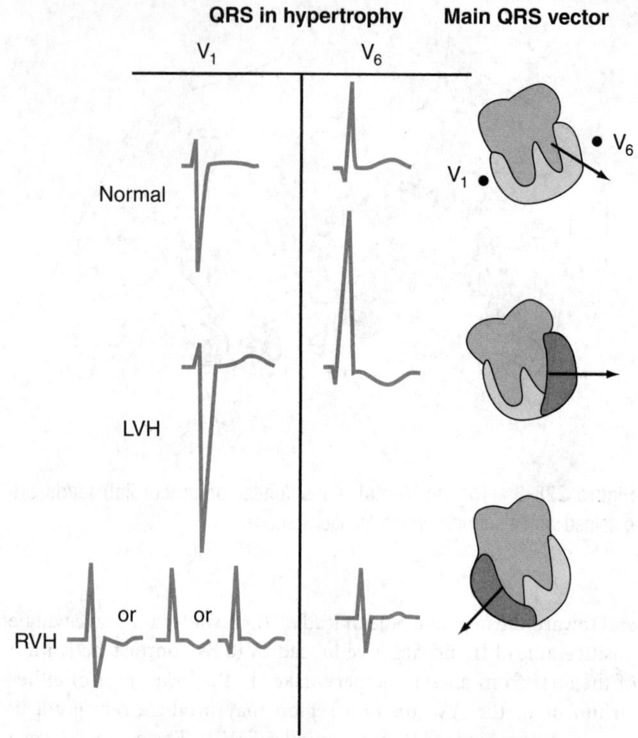

Figure 228-9 Left ventricular hypertrophy (LVH) increases the amplitude of electrical forces directed to the left and posteriorly. In addition, repolarization abnormalities may cause ST-segment depression and T-wave inversion in leads with a prominent R wave. Right ventricular hypertrophy (RVH) may shift the QRS vector to the right; this effect usually is associated with an R, RS, or qR complex in lead V_1. T-wave inversions may be present in right precordial leads.

Chronic cor pulmonale due to obstructive lung disease (Chap. 234) usually does not produce the classic ECG patterns of right ventricular hypertrophy noted above. Instead of tall right precordial R waves, chronic lung disease more typically is associated with small R waves in right-to-midprecordial leads (slow R-wave progression) due in part to downward displacement of the diaphragm and the heart. Low-voltage complexes are commonly present, owing to hyperaeration of the lungs.

A number of different voltage criteria for *left ventricular hypertrophy* (Fig. 228-9) have been proposed on the basis of the presence of tall left precordial R waves and deep right precordial S waves [e.g., SV_1 + (RV_5 or RV_6) >35 mm]. Repolarization abnormalities (ST depression with T-wave inversions, formerly called the left ventricular "strain" pattern) also may appear in leads with prominent R waves. However, prominent precordial voltages may occur as a normal variant, especially in athletic or young individuals. Left ventricular hypertrophy may increase limb lead voltage with or without increased precordial voltage (e.g., RaVL + SV_3 >20 mm in women and >28 mm in men). The presence of left atrial abnormality increases the likelihood of underlying left ventricular hypertrophy in cases with borderline voltage criteria. Left ventricular hypertrophy often progresses to incomplete or complete left bundle branch block. The sensitivity of conventional voltage criteria for left ventricular hypertrophy is decreased in obese persons and smokers. ECG evidence for left ventricular hypertrophy is a major noninvasive marker of increased risk of cardiovascular morbidity and mortality rates, including sudden cardiac death. However, because of false-positive and false-negative diagnoses, the ECG is of limited utility in diagnosing atrial or ventricular enlargement. More definitive information is provided by echocardiography (Chap. 229).

■ BUNDLE BRANCH BLOCKS

Intrinsic impairment of conduction in either the right or the left bundle system (intraventricular conduction disturbances) leads to prolongation of the QRS interval. With complete bundle branch blocks, the QRS interval is ≥120 ms in duration; with incomplete blocks, the QRS interval is between 100 and 120 ms. The QRS vector usually is oriented in the direction of the myocardial region where depolarization is delayed (Fig. 228-10). Thus, with right bundle branch block, the terminal QRS vector is oriented to the right and anteriorly (rSR′ in V_1 and qRS in V_6, typically). Left bundle branch block alters both early and later phases of ventricular depolarization. The major QRS vector is directed to the left and posteriorly. In addition, the normal early left-to-right pattern of septal activation is disrupted such that septal depolarization proceeds from right to left as well. As a result, left bundle branch block generates wide, predominantly negative (QS) complexes in lead V_1 and entirely positive (R) complexes in lead V_6. A pattern identical to that of left bundle branch block, preceded by a sharp spike, is seen in most cases of electronic right ventricular pacing because of the relative delay in left ventricular activation.

Bundle branch block may occur in a variety of conditions. In subjects without structural heart disease, right bundle branch block is seen more commonly than left bundle branch block. Right bundle branch block also occurs with heart disease, both congenital (e.g., atrial septal defect) and acquired (e.g., valvular, ischemic). Left bundle branch block is often a marker of one of four underlying conditions associated with increased risk of cardiovascular morbidity and mortality rates: coronary heart disease (frequently with impaired left ventricular function), hypertensive heart disease, aortic valve disease, and cardiomyopathy. Bundle branch blocks may be chronic or intermittent. A bundle branch block may be rate-related; for example, it often occurs when the heart rate exceeds some critical value.

Bundle branch blocks and depolarization abnormalities secondary to artificial pacemakers not only affect ventricular depolarization

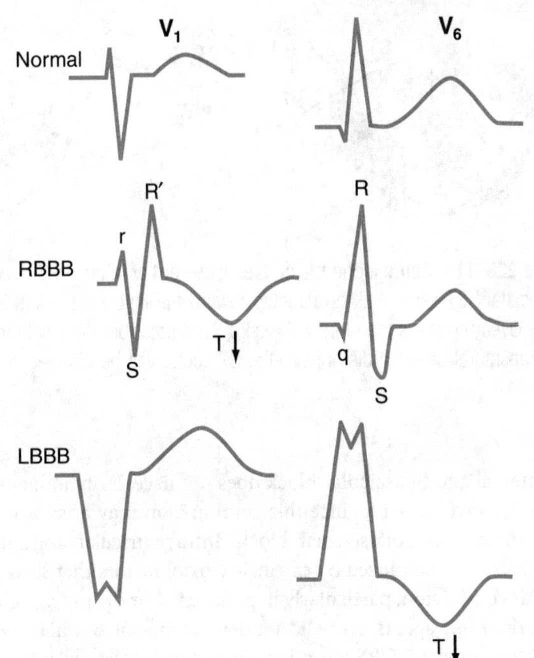

Figure 228-10 Comparison of typical QRS-T patterns in right bundle branch block (RBBB) and left bundle branch block (LBBB) with the normal pattern in leads V_1 and V_6. Note the secondary T-wave inversions (*arrows*) in leads with an rSR′ complex with RBBB and in leads with a wide R wave with LBBB.

(QRS) but also are characteristically associated with *secondary repolarization* (ST-T) abnormalities. With bundle branch blocks, the T wave is typically opposite in polarity to the last deflection of the QRS (Fig. 228-10). This discordance of the QRS–T-wave vectors is caused by the altered sequence of repolarization that occurs secondary to altered depolarization. In contrast, *primary repolarization* abnormalities are independent of QRS changes and are related instead to actual alterations in the electrical properties of the myocardial fibers themselves (e.g., in the resting membrane potential or action potential duration), not just to changes in the sequence of repolarization. Ischemia, electrolyte imbalance, and drugs such as digitalis all cause such primary ST–T-wave changes. Primary and secondary T-wave changes may coexist. For example, T-wave inversions in the right precordial leads with left bundle branch block or in the left precordial leads with right bundle branch block may be important markers of underlying ischemia or other abnormalities. A distinctive abnormality simulating right bundle branch block with ST-segment elevations in the right chest leads is seen with the Brugada pattern (Chap. 233).

Partial blocks (fascicular or "hemiblocks") in the left bundle system (left anterior or posterior fascicular blocks) generally do not prolong the QRS duration substantially but instead are associated with shifts in the frontal plane QRS axis (leftward or rightward, respectively). More complex combinations of fascicular and bundle branch blocks may occur that involve the left and right bundle system. Examples of *bifascicular block* include right bundle branch block and left posterior fascicular block, right bundle branch block with left anterior fascicular block, and complete left bundle branch block. Chronic bifascicular block in an asymptomatic individual is associated with a relatively low risk of progression to high-degree AV heart block. In contrast, new bifascicular block with acute anterior myocardial infarction carries a much greater risk of complete heart block. Alternation of right and left bundle branch block is a sign of *trifascicular disease*. However, the presence of a prolonged

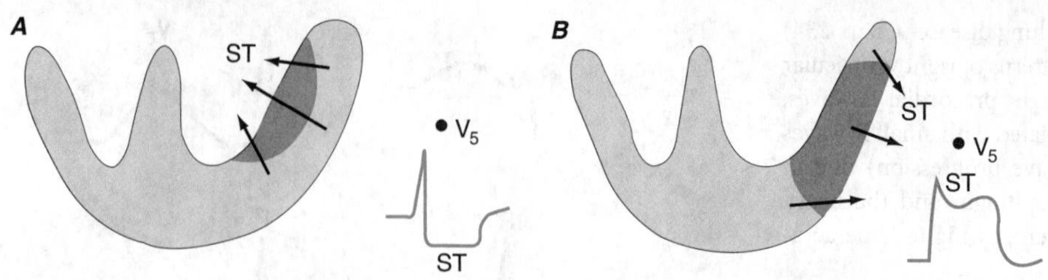

Figure 228-11 Acute ischemia causes a current of injury. With predominant subendocardial ischemia (***A***), the resultant ST vector will be directed toward the inner layer of the affected ventricle and the ventricular cavity. Overlying leads therefore will record ST depression. With ischemia involving the outer ventricular layer (***B***) (transmural or epicardial injury), the ST vector will be directed outward. Overlying leads will record ST elevation.

PR interval and bifascicular block does not necessarily indicate trifascicular involvement, since this combination may arise with AV node disease and bifascicular block. Intraventricular conduction delays also can be caused by extrinsic (toxic) factors that slow ventricular conduction, particularly hyperkalemia or drugs (e.g., class 1 antiarrhythmic agents, tricyclic antidepressants, phenothiazines).

Prolongation of QRS duration does not necessarily indicate a conduction delay but may be due to *preexcitation* of the ventricles via a bypass tract, as in Wolff-Parkinson-White (WPW) patterns (Chap. 233) and related variants. The diagnostic triad of WPW consists of a wide QRS complex associated with a relatively short PR interval and slurring of the initial part of the QRS (delta wave), with the latter effect being due to aberrant activation of ventricular myocardium. The presence of a bypass tract predisposes to reentrant supraventricular tachyarrhythmias.

MYOCARDIAL ISCHEMIA AND INFARCTION

(See also Chap. 245) The ECG is a cornerstone in the diagnosis of acute and chronic ischemic heart disease. The findings depend on several key factors: the nature of the process [reversible (i.e., ischemia) versus irreversible (i.e., infarction)], the duration (acute versus chronic), the extent (transmural versus subendocardial), and localization (anterior versus inferoposterior), as well as the presence of other underlying abnormalities (ventricular hypertrophy, conduction defects).

Ischemia exerts complex time-dependent effects on the electrical properties of myocardial cells. Severe, acute ischemia lowers the resting membrane potential and shortens the duration of the action potential. Such changes cause a voltage gradient between normal and ischemic zones. As a consequence, current flows between those regions. These currents of injury are represented on the surface ECG by deviation of the ST segment (Fig. 228-11). When the acute ischemia is *transmural*, the ST vector usually is shifted in the direction of the outer (epicardial) layers, producing ST elevations and sometimes, in the earliest stages of ischemia, tall, positive so-called hyperacute T waves over the ischemic zone. With ischemia confined primarily to the *subendocardium*, the ST vector typically shifts toward the subendocardium and ventricular cavity, so that overlying (e.g., anterior precordial) leads show ST-segment depression (with ST elevation in lead aVR). Multiple factors affect the amplitude of acute ischemic ST deviations. Profound ST elevation or depression in multiple leads usually indicates very severe ischemia. From a clinical viewpoint, the division of acute myocardial infarction into ST-segment elevation and non-ST elevation types is useful since the efficacy of acute reperfusion therapy is limited to the former group.

The ECG leads are usually more helpful in localizing regions of ST elevation than non-ST elevation ischemia. For example, acute transmural anterior (including apical and lateral) wall ischemia is reflected by ST elevations or increased T-wave positivity in one or more of the precordial leads (V_1–V_6) and leads I and aVL. Inferior wall ischemia produces changes in leads II, III, and aVF. "Posterior" wall ischemia (usually associated with lateral or inferior involvement) may be indirectly recognized by *reciprocal* ST depressions in leads V_1 to V_3 (thus constituting an ST elevation "equivalent" acute coronary syndrome). Right ventricular ischemia usually produces ST elevations in right-sided chest leads (Fig. 228-5). When ischemic ST elevations occur as the earliest sign of acute infarction, they typically are followed within a period ranging from hours to days by evolving T-wave inversions and often by Q waves occurring in the same lead distribution. Reversible transmural ischemia, for example, due to coronary vasospasm (Prinzmetal's variant angina and probably the Tako-Tsubo "stress" cardiomyopathy syndrome), may cause transient ST-segment elevations without development of Q waves, as may very early reperfusion in acute coronary syndromes. Depending on the severity and duration of ischemia, the ST elevations may resolve completely in minutes or be followed by T-wave inversions that persist for hours or even days. Patients with ischemic chest pain who present with deep T-wave inversions in multiple precordial leads (e.g., V_1–V_4) with or without cardiac enzyme elevations typically have severe obstruction in the left anterior descending coronary artery system (Fig. 228-12). In contrast, patients whose baseline ECG already shows abnormal T-wave inversions may develop T-wave normalization (pseudonormalization) during episodes of acute transmural ischemia.

With infarction, depolarization (QRS) changes often accompany repolarization (ST-T) abnormalities. Necrosis of sufficient myocardial tissue may lead to decreased R-wave amplitude or abnormal Q waves (even in the absence of transmurality) in the anterior or inferior leads (Fig. 228-13). Previously, abnormal Q waves were considered markers of transmural myocardial infarction, whereas subendocardial infarcts were thought not to produce Q waves. However, careful ECG-pathology correlative studies have indicated that transmural infarcts may occur without Q waves and that subendocardial (nontransmural) infarcts sometimes may be associated with Q waves. Therefore, infarcts are more appropriately classified as "Q-wave" or "non-Q-wave." The major acute ECG changes in syndromes of ischemic heart disease are summarized schematically

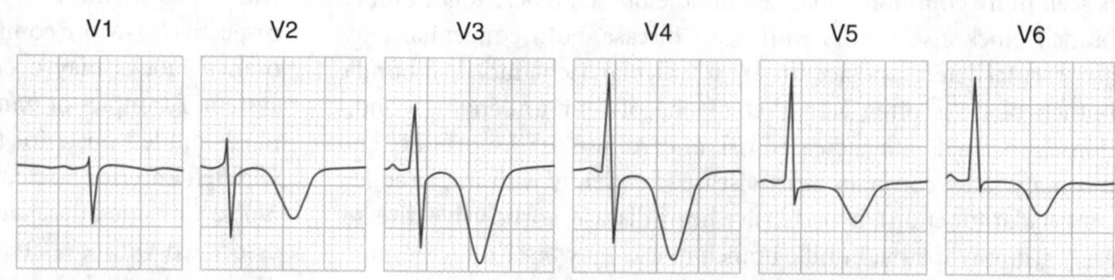

Figure 228-12 Severe anterior wall ischemia (with or without infarction) may cause prominent T-wave inversions in the precordial leads. This pattern (sometimes referred to as Wellens T waves) is usually associated with a high-grade stenosis of the left anterior descending coronary artery.

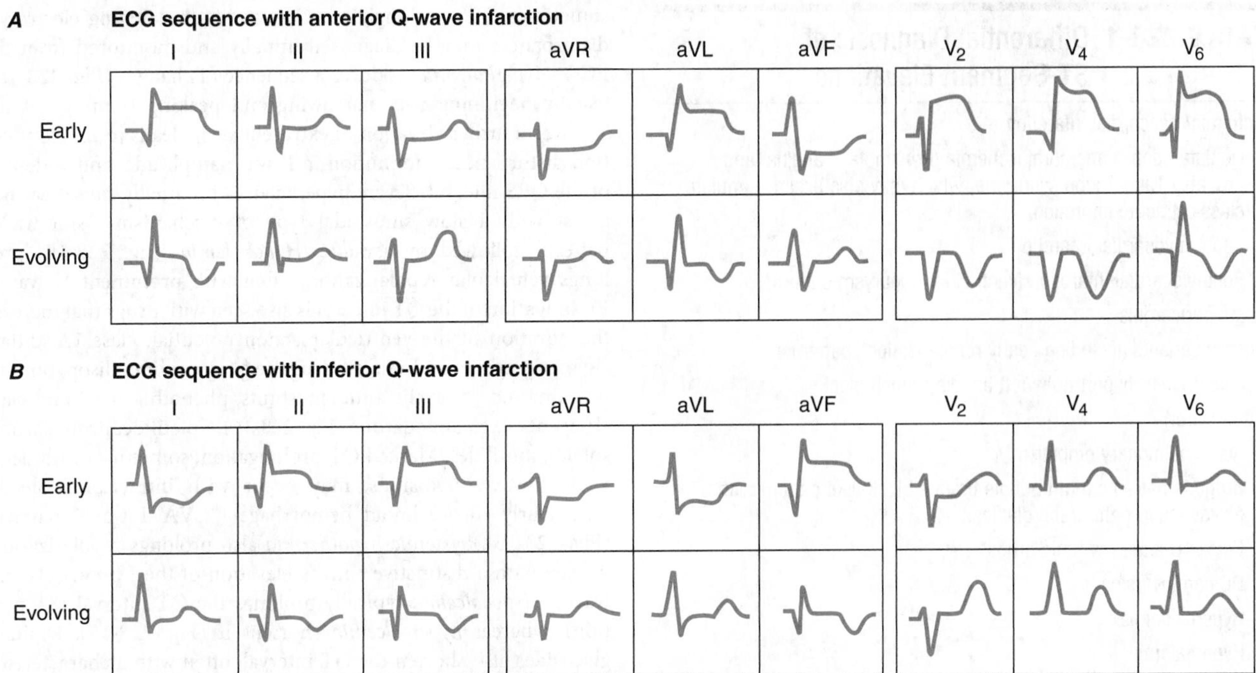

Figure 228-13 Sequence of depolarization and repolarization changes with (***A***) acute anterior and (***B***) acute inferior wall Q-wave infarctions. With anterior infarcts, ST elevation in leads I and aVL and the precordial leads may be accompanied by reciprocal ST depressions in leads II, III, and aVF. Conversely, acute inferior (or posterolateral) infarcts may be associated with reciprocal ST depressions in leads V_1 to V_3. *(After Goldberger.)*

in Fig. 228-14. Loss of depolarization forces due to posterior or lateral infarction may cause reciprocal increases in R-wave amplitude in leads V_1 and V_2 without diagnostic Q waves in any of the conventional leads. Atrial infarction may be associated with PR-segment deviations due to an atrial current of injury, changes in P-wave morphology, or atrial arrhythmias.

In the weeks and months after infarction, these ECG changes may persist or begin to resolve. Complete normalization of the ECG after Q-wave infarction is uncommon but may occur, particularly with smaller infarcts. In contrast, ST-segment elevations that persist for several weeks or more after a Q-wave infarct usually correlate with a severe underlying wall motion disorder (akinetic or dyskinetic zone), although not necessarily a frank ventricular aneurysm. ECG changes due to ischemia may occur spontaneously or may be provoked by various exercise protocols (stress electrocardiography; Chap. 243).

The ECG has important limitations in both sensitivity and specificity in the diagnosis of ischemic heart disease. Although a single normal ECG does not exclude ischemia or even acute infarction, a normal ECG *throughout* the course of an acute infarct is distinctly uncommon. Prolonged chest pain without diagnostic ECG changes therefore should always prompt a careful search for other noncoronary causes of chest pain (Chap. 12). Furthermore, the diagnostic changes of acute or evolving ischemia are often masked by the presence of left bundle branch block, electronic ventricular pacemaker patterns, and Wolff-Parkinson-White preexcitation. However, clinicians continue to overdiagnose ischemia or infarction based on the presence of ST-segment elevations or depressions; T-wave inversions; tall, positive T waves; or Q waves *not* related to ischemic heart disease (pseudoinfarct patterns). For example, ST-segment elevations simulating ischemia may occur with acute pericarditis or myocarditis, as a normal variant (including the typical "early repolarization" pattern), or in a variety of other conditions (Table 228-1). Similarly, tall, positive T waves do not invariably represent hyperacute ischemic changes but may also be caused by normal variants, hyperkalemia, cerebrovascular injury, and left ventricular volume overload due to mitral or aortic regurgitation, among other causes.

ST-segment elevations and tall, positive T waves are common findings in leads V_1 and V_2 in left bundle branch block or left ventricular hypertrophy in the absence of ischemia. The differential diagnosis of Q waves includes physiologic or positional variants, ventricular hypertrophy, acute or chronic noncoronary myocardial injury, hypertrophic cardiomyopathy, and ventricular conduction disorders. Digoxin, ventricular hypertrophy, hypokalemia, and a variety of other factors may cause ST-segment depression mimicking

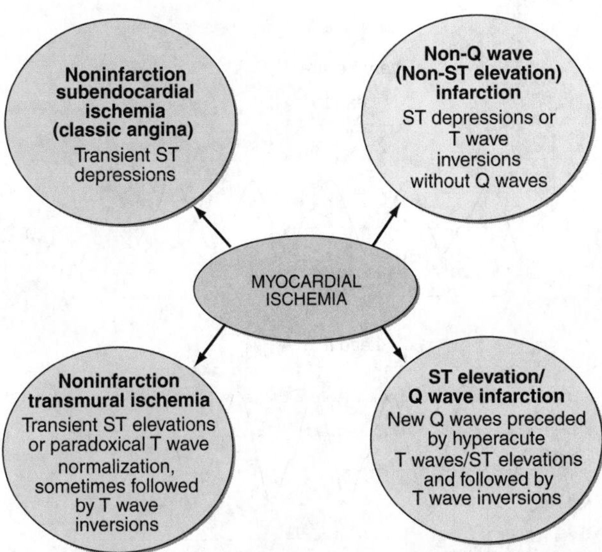

Figure 228-14 Variability of ECG patterns with acute myocardial ischemia. The ECG also may be normal or nonspecifically abnormal. Furthermore, these categorizations are not mutually exclusive. *(After Goldberger, 2006.)*

TABLE 228-1 Differential Diagnosis of ST-Segment Elevations

Ischemia/myocardial infarction
Noninfarction, transmural ischemia (Prinzmetal's angina, and probably Tako-Tsubo syndrome, which may also exactly simulate classical acute infarction)
Acute myocardial infarction
Postmyocardial infarction (ventricular aneurysm pattern)
Acute pericarditis
Normal variants (including "early repolarization" patterns)
Left ventricular hypertrophy/left bundle branch block[a]
Other (rarer)
Acute pulmonary embolism[a]
Brugada patterns (right bundle branch block–like pattern with ST elevations in right precordial leads)[a]
Class 1C antiarrhythmic drugs[a]
DC cardioversion
Hypercalcemia[a]
Hyperkalemia[a]
Hypothermia [J (Osborn) waves]
Nonischemic myocardial injury
Myocarditis
Tumor invading left ventricle
Trauma to ventricles

[a]Usually localized to V_1–V_2 or V_3.
Source: Modified from Goldberger.

subendocardial ischemia. Prominent T-wave inversion may occur with ventricular hypertrophy, cardiomyopathies, myocarditis, and cerebrovascular injury (particularly intracranial bleeds), among many other conditions.

METABOLIC FACTORS AND DRUG EFFECTS

A variety of metabolic and pharmacologic agents alter the ECG and, in particular, cause changes in repolarization (ST-T-U) and sometimes QRS prolongation. Certain life-threatening electrolyte disturbances may be diagnosed initially and monitored from the ECG. *Hyperkalemia* produces a sequence of changes (Fig. 228-15), usually beginning with narrowing and peaking (tenting) of the T waves. Further elevation of extracellular K^+ leads to AV conduction disturbances, diminution in P-wave amplitude, and widening of the QRS interval. Severe hyperkalemia eventually causes cardiac arrest with a slow sinusoidal type of mechanism ("sine-wave" pattern) followed by asystole. *Hypokalemia* (Fig. 228-16) prolongs ventricular repolarization, often with prominent U waves. Prolongation of the QT interval is also seen with drugs that increase the duration of the ventricular action potential: class 1A antiarrhythmic agents and related drugs (e.g., quinidine, disopyramide, procainamide, tricyclic antidepressants, phenothiazines) and class III agents [e.g., amiodarone (Fig. 228-16), dofetilide, dronedarone, sotalol, ibutilide]. Marked QT prolongation, sometimes with deep, wide T-wave inversions, may occur with intracranial bleeds, particularly subarachnoid hemorrhage ("CVA T-wave" pattern) (Fig. 228-16). Systemic *hypothermia* also prolongs repolarization, usually with a distinctive convex elevation of the J point (Osborn wave). *Hypocalcemia* typically prolongs the QT interval (ST portion), whereas *hypercalcemia* shortens it (Fig. 228-17). Digitalis glycosides also shorten the QT interval, often with a characteristic "scooping" of the ST–T-wave complex (*digitalis effect*).

Many other factors are associated with ECG changes, particularly alterations in ventricular repolarization. T-wave flattening, minimal T-wave inversions, or slight ST-segment depression ("nonspecific ST–T-wave changes") may occur with a variety of electrolyte and acid-base disturbances, a variety of infectious processes, central nervous system disorders, endocrine abnormalities, many drugs, ischemia, hypoxia, and virtually any type of cardiopulmonary abnormality. Although subtle ST–T-wave changes may be markers of ischemia, transient nonspecific repolarization changes may also occur after a meal or with postural (orthostatic) change, hyperventilation, or exercise in healthy individuals.

ELECTRICAL ALTERNANS

Electrical alternans—a beat-to-beat alternation in one or more components of the ECG signal—is a common type of nonlinear cardiovascular response to a variety of hemodynamic and

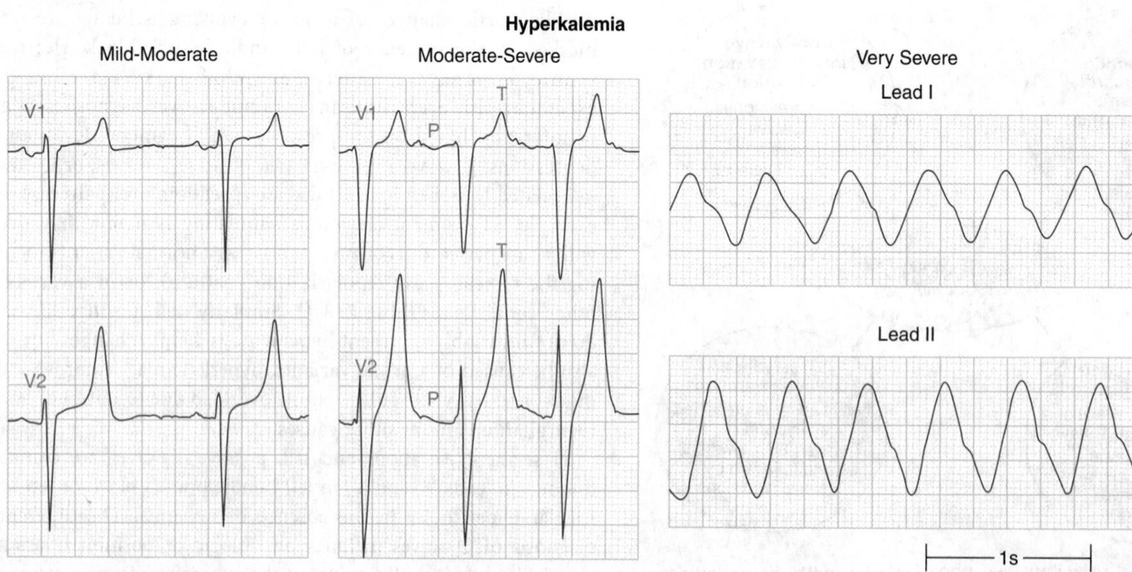

Figure 228-15 The earliest ECG change with hyperkalemia is usually peaking ("tenting") of the T waves. With further increases in the serum potassium concentration, the QRS complexes widen, the P waves decrease in amplitude and may disappear, and finally a sine-wave pattern leads to asystole unless emergency therapy is given. *(After Goldberger.)*

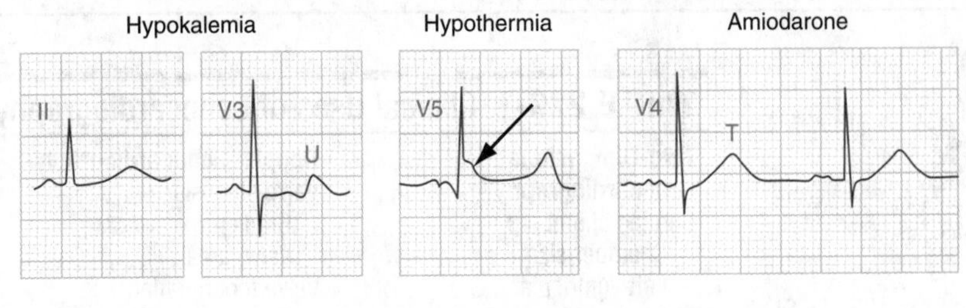

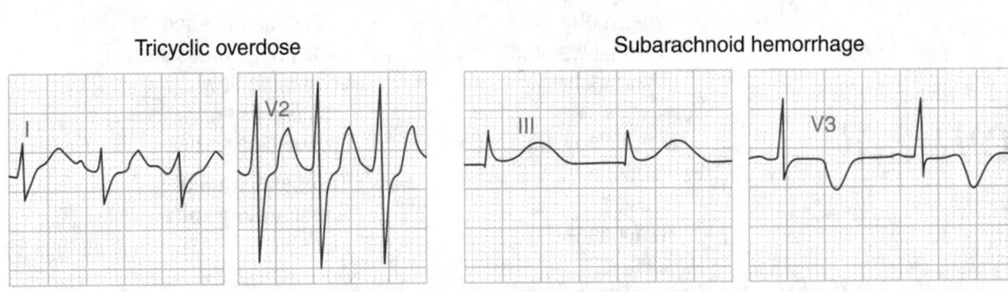

Figure 228-16 A variety of metabolic derangements, drug effects, and other factors may prolong ventricular repolarization with QT prolongation or prominent U waves. Prominent repolarization prolongation, particularly if due to hypokalemia, inherited "channelopathies," or certain pharmacologic agents, indicates increased susceptibility to *torsades des pointes*–type ventricular tachycardia (Chap. 233). Marked systemic hypothermia is associated with a distinctive convex "hump" at the J point (Osborn wave, *arrow*) due to altered ventricular action potential characteristics. Note QRS and QT prolongation along with sinus tachycardia in the case of tricyclic antidepressant overdose.

electrophysiologic perturbations. Total electrical alternans (P-QRS-T) with sinus tachycardia is a relatively specific sign of pericardial effusion, usually with cardiac tamponade. The mechanism relates to a periodic swinging motion of the heart in the effusion at a frequency exactly one-half the heart rate. Repolarization (ST-T or U wave) alternans is a sign of electrical instability and may precede ventricular tachyarrhythmias.

■ CLINICAL INTERPRETATION OF THE ECG

Accurate analysis of ECGs requires thoroughness and care. The patient's age, gender, and clinical status should always be taken into account. Many mistakes in ECG interpretation are errors of omission. Therefore, a systematic approach is essential. The following 14 points should be analyzed carefully in every ECG: (1) standardization (calibration) and technical features (including lead placement and artifacts), (2) rhythm, (3) heart rate, (4) PR interval/AV conduction, (5) QRS interval, (6) QT/QT$_c$ interval, (7) mean QRS electrical axis, (8) P waves, (9) QRS voltages, (10) precordial R-wave progression, (11) abnormal Q waves, (12) ST segments, (13) T waves, (14) U waves.

Only after analyzing all these points should the interpretation be formulated. Where appropriate, important clinical correlates or inferences should be mentioned. For example, sinus tachycardia with QRS and QT-(U) prolongation, especially in the context of changes in mental status, suggests tricyclic antidepressant overdose (Fig. 228-16). The triad of peaked T waves (hyperkalemia), a long QT due to ST-segment lengthening (hypocalcemia), and left ventricular hypertrophy (systemic hypertension) suggests chronic renal failure. Comparison with any previous ECGs is invaluable. The diagnosis and management of specific cardiac arrhythmias and conduction disturbances are discussed in Chaps. 232 and 233.

■ COMPUTERIZED ELECTROCARDIOGRAPHY

Computerized ECG systems are widely used for immediate retrieval of thousands of ECG records. Computer interpretation of ECGs still has major limitations. Incomplete or inaccurate readings are most likely with arrhythmias and complex abnormalities. Therefore, computerized interpretation (including measurements of basic ECG intervals) should not be accepted without careful clinician review.

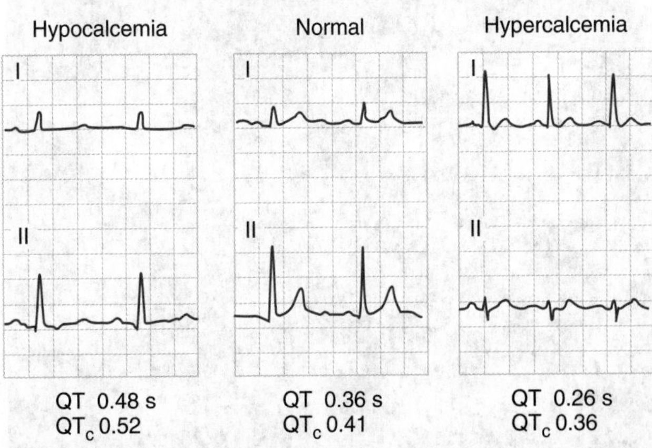

Figure 228-17 Prolongation of the Q-T interval (ST-segment portion) is typical of hypocalcemia. Hypercalcemia may cause abbreviation of the ST segment and shortening of the QT interval.

FURTHER READINGS

Goldberger AL: *Clinical Electrocardiography: A Simplified Approach*, 8th ed. St. Louis, Mosby/Elsevier, in press

Kligfield P et al: Recommendations for the standardization and interpretation of the electrocardiogram: Part I. The electrocardiogram and its standardization. J Am Coll Cardiol 49:1109, 2007

Mirvis DM, Goldberger AL: Electrocardiography, in *Braunwald's Heart Disease: A Textbook of Cardiovascular Medicine*, 9th ed, RW Bonow et al (eds). Philadelphia, Saunders, 2010

Surawicz B, Knilans TK: *Chou's Electrocardiography in Clinical Practice*, 6th ed. Philadelphia, Saunders, 2008

Wagner G et al: Recommendations for the standardization and interpretation of the electrocardiogram: Part VI. Acute myocardial ischemia. J Am Coll Cardiol 53:1003, 2009

CHAPTER 229

Noninvasive Cardiac Imaging: Echocardiography, Nuclear Cardiology, and MRI/CT Imaging

Rick A. Nishimura
Panithaya Chareonthaitawee
Matthew Martinez

Cardiovascular imaging plays an essential role in the practice of cardiology. Two-dimensional (2D) echocardiography is able to visualize the heart directly in real time using ultrasound, providing instantaneous assessment of the myocardium, cardiac chambers, valves, pericardium, and great vessels. Doppler echocardiography measures the velocity of moving red blood cells and has become a noninvasive alternative to cardiac catheterization for assessment of hemodynamics. Transesophageal echocardiography (TEE) provides a unique window for high-resolution imaging of posterior structures of the heart, particularly the left atrium, mitral valve, and aorta. Nuclear cardiology uses radioactive tracers to provide assessment of myocardial perfusion and metabolism, along with ventricular function, and is applied primarily to the evaluation of patients with ischemic heart disease. Cardiac MRI and CT can delineate cardiac structure and function with high resolution. They are particularly useful in the examination of cardiac masses, the pericardium, the great vessels, and ventricular function and perfusion. Gadolinium enhancement during cardiac MRI adds information on myocardial perfusion. Detection of coronary calcification by CT as well as direct visualization of coronary arteries by CT angiography (CTA) may be useful in selected patients with suspected coronary artery disease (CAD). This chapter provides an overview of the basic concepts of these cardiac imaging modalities as well as the clinical indications for each procedure.

ECHOCARDIOGRAPHY

■ TWO-DIMENSIONAL ECHOCARDIOGRAPHY

Basic principles

2D echocardiography uses the principle of ultrasound reflection off cardiac structures to produce images of the heart (Table 229-1). For a transthoracic echocardiogram (TTE), the imaging is performed with a handheld transducer placed directly on the chest wall. In selected patients, a TEE may be performed, in which an ultrasound transducer is mounted on the tip of an endoscope placed in the esophagus and directed toward the cardiac structures.

Current echocardiographic machines are portable and can be wheeled directly to the patient's bedside. Thus, a major advantage of echocardiography over other imaging modalities is the ability to obtain instantaneous images of the cardiac structures for immediate interpretation. Thus, echocardiography has become an ideal imaging modality for cardiac emergencies. A limitation of TTE is the inability to obtain high-quality images in all patients, especially those with a thick chest wall or severe lung disease, as ultrasound waves are poorly transmitted through lung parenchyma. Technology such as harmonic imaging and IV contrast agents (which traverse the pulmonary circulation) can be used to enhance endocardial borders in patients with poor acoustic windows.

TABLE 229-1 Clinical Uses of Echocardiography

Two-Dimensional Echocardiography	Doppler Echocardiography
Cardiac chambers	Valve stenosis
Chamber size	Gradient
Left ventricular hypertrophy	Valve area
Regional wall motion abnormalities	Valve regurgitation
Valve	Semiquantitation
Morphology and motion	Intracardiac pressures
Pericardium	Volumetric flow
Effusion	Diastolic filling
Tamponade	Intracardiac shunts
Masses	**Transesophageal Echocardiography**
Great vessels	Inadequate transthoracic images
Stress Echocardiography	Aortic disease
Two-dimensional	Infective endocarditis
Myocardial ischemia	Source of embolism
Viable myocardium	Valve prosthesis
Doppler	Intraoperative
Valve disease	

Chamber size and function

2D echocardiography is an ideal imaging modality for assessing left ventricular (LV) size and function (Fig. 229-1). A qualitative

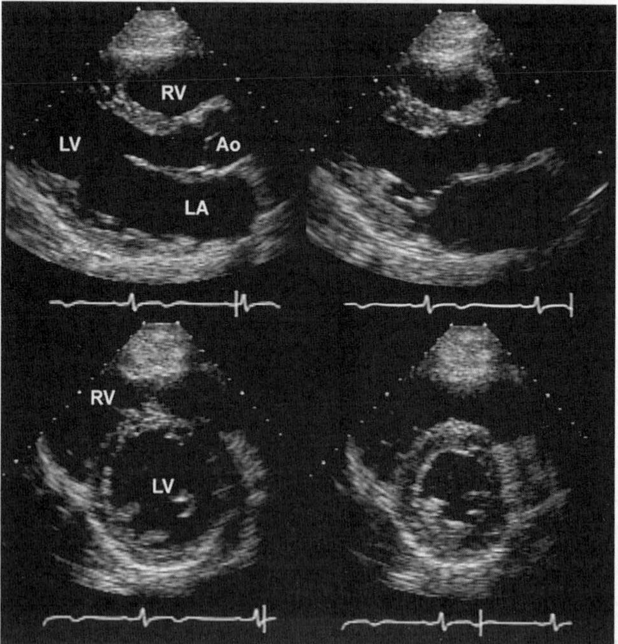

Figure 229-1 Two-dimensional echocardiographic still-frame images from a normal patient with a normal heart. Upper: Parasternal long-axis view during systole and diastole (*left*) and systole (*right*). During systole, there is thickening of the myocardium and reduction in the size of the left ventricle (LV). The valve leaflets are thin and open widely. Lower: Parasternal short-axis view during diastole (left) and systole (right) demonstrating a decrease in the left ventricular cavity size during systole as well as an increase in wall thickening. LA, left atrium; RV, right ventricle; Ao, aorta.

assessment of the ventricular cavity and systolic function can be made directly from the 2D image by experienced observers. 2D echocardiography is useful in the diagnosis of LV hypertrophy and is the imaging modality of choice for the diagnosis of hypertrophic cardiomyopathy. Other chamber sizes are assessed by visual analysis, including the left atrium and right-sided chambers.

Valve abnormalities

2D echocardiography is the "gold standard" for imaging valve morphology and motion. Leaflet thickness and mobility, valve calcification, and the appearance of subvalvular and supravalvular structures can be assessed. Valve stenosis is reliably diagnosed by the thickening and decreased mobility of the valve. 2D echocardiography is also the gold standard for the diagnosis of mitral stenosis, which produces typical tethering and diastolic doming, and the severity of the stenosis can be ascertained from a direct planimetry measurement of the mitral valve orifice. The presence and often the etiology of stenosis of the semilunar valves can be made by 2D echocardiography (Fig. 229-2), but evaluation of the severity of the stenosis requires Doppler echocardiography (see below). The diagnosis of valvular regurgitation must be made by Doppler echocardiography, but 2D echocardiography is valuable for determining the etiology of the regurgitation, as well as its effects on ventricular dimensions, shape, and function.

Pericardial disease

2D echocardiography is the imaging modality of choice for the detection of pericardial effusion, which is easily visualized as a black echolucent ovoid structure surrounding the heart (Fig. 229-3). In the hemodynamically unstable patient with pericardial tamponade, typical echo findings include a dilated inferior vena cava, right atrial collapse, and then right ventricular collapse. Echocardiographically guided pericardiocentesis has now become a standard of care.

Intracardiac masses

Intracardiac masses can be visualized on 2D echocardiography, provided that image quality is adequate. Solid masses appear as echo-dense structures, which can be located inside the cardiac chambers or infiltrating into the myocardium or pericardium. LV thrombus appears as an echo-dense structure, usually in the apical region associated with regional wall motion abnormalities. The appearance and mobility of the thrombus are predictive of embolic events. Vegetations appear as mobile linear echo densities attached to valve leaflets. Atrial myxoma can be diagnosed by the appearance of a well-circumscribed mobile mass with attachments to the atrial septum (Fig. 229-4). The high-resolution images provided by TEE may be required for further delineation of myocardial masses, especially those <1 cm in diameter.

Aortic disease

2D echocardiography can provide extremely useful information on diseases of the aorta. The proximal ascending aorta, the arch, and the distal descending aorta can usually be visualized via the

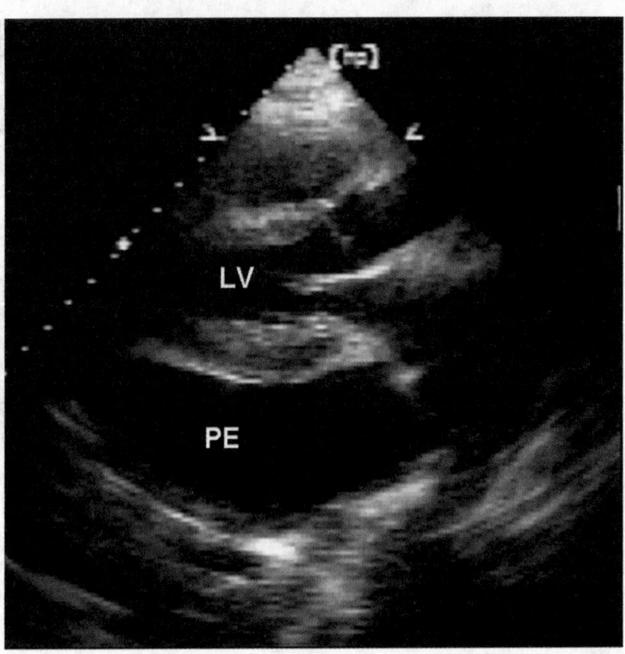

Figure 229-3 Two-dimensional echocardiographic still-frame image of a patient with a pericardial effusion. Pericardial effusion (PE) is shown as black echo-free space surrounding the heart. LV, left ventricle.

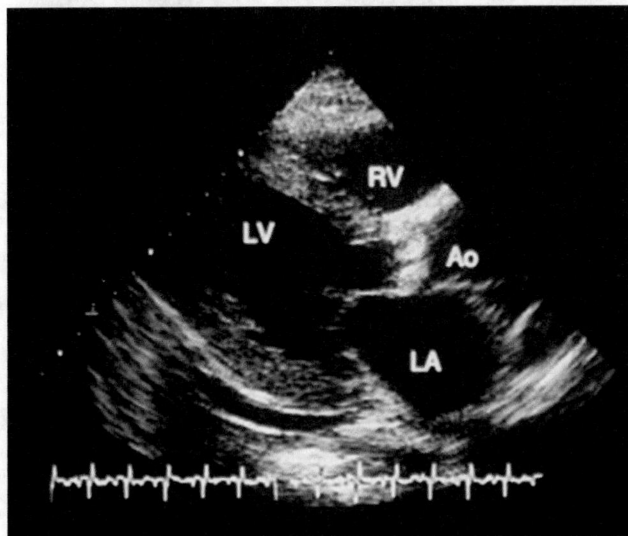

Figure 229-2 Two-dimensional echocardiographic still-frame images from a patient with aortic stenosis. Parasternal long-axis view shows a heavily calcified aortic valve. RV, right ventricle; LV, left ventricle; AO, aorta; LA, left atrium.

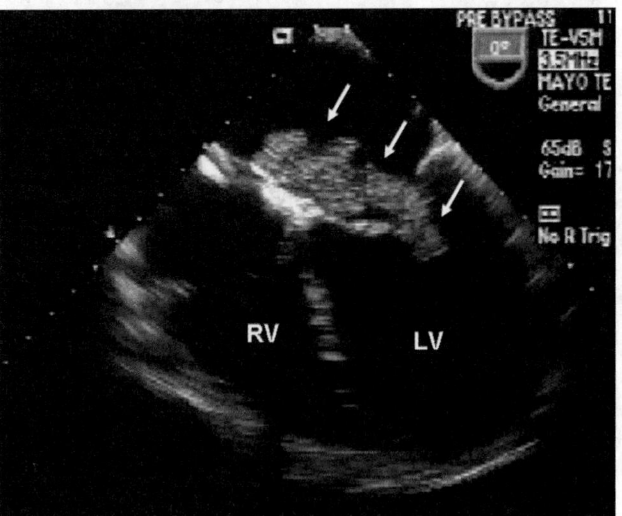

Figure 229-4 Transesophageal still-frame echocardiographic images of a patient with a left atrial myxoma. There is a large echo-dense mass in the left atrium, attached to the atrial septum. The mass moves across the mitral valve in diastole. LV, left ventricle; RV, right ventricle.

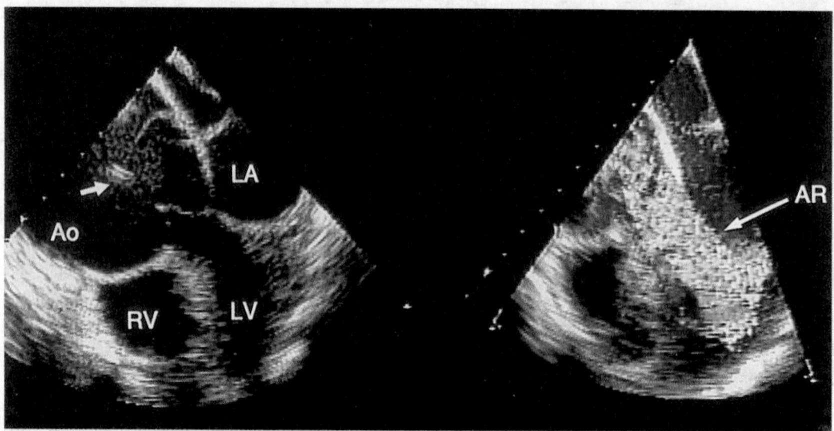

Figure 229-5 Transesophageal still-frame echocardiographic view of a patient with a dilated aorta, aortic dissection, and severe aortic regurgitation. The arrow points to the intimal flap that is seen in the dilated ascending aorta. *Left:* The long-axis apex-down view of the black-and-white two-dimensional image in diastole. *Right:* Color-flow imaging that demonstrates a large mosaic jet of aortic regurgitation. Ao, aorta; RV, right ventricle; AR, aortic regurgitation.

transthoracic approach. The definitive diagnosis of a suspected aortic dissection usually requires a TEE, which can rapidly provide high-resolution images of the proximal ascending and descending thoracic aorta (Fig. 229-5).

DOPPLER ECHOCARDIOGRAPHY

Basic principles

Doppler echocardiography uses ultrasound reflecting off moving red blood cells to measure the velocity of blood flow across valves, within cardiac chambers, and through the great vessels. Normal and abnormal blood flow patterns can be assessed noninvasively. Color-flow Doppler imaging displays the blood velocities in real time superimposed upon a 2D echocardiographic image. The different colors indicate the direction of blood flow (red toward and blue away from the transducer), with green superimposed when there is turbulent flow. Pulsed-wave Doppler measures the blood flow velocity in a specific location on the 2D echocardiographic image. Continuous-wave Doppler echocardiography can measure high velocities of blood flow directed along the line of the Doppler beam, such as occur in the presence of valve stenosis, valve regurgitation, or intracardiac shunts. These high velocities can be used to determine intracardiac pressure gradients by a modified Bernoulli equation:

$$\text{Pressure change} = 4 \text{ times } (\text{velocity})^2$$

Tissue Doppler echocardiography measures the velocity of myocardial motion. Myocardial velocities can be used to determine myocardial strain rate, which is a quantitative measure of regional myocardial contraction and relaxation.

Valve gradients

In the presence of valvular stenosis, there is an increase in the velocity of blood flow across the stenotic valve. A continuous-wave Doppler can be used to determine the pressure gradient across the valve (Fig. 229-6). A valve area can also be calculated from the Doppler velocities.

Valvular regurgitation

Valvular regurgitation is diagnosed by Doppler echocardiography when there is abnormal retrograde flow across the valve. Color-flow imaging is the Doppler method used most frequently to detect valve regurgitation by visualization of a high-velocity turbulent jet in the chamber proximal to the regurgitant valve (Fig. 229-7). The size and extent of the color-flow jet into the receiving cardiac chamber provide a semiquantitative estimate of the severity of regurgitation.

Intracardiac pressures

These can be calculated from the peak continuous-wave Doppler signal of a regurgitant lesion, which reflects the pressure gradient between two cardiac chambers. This approach is commonly applied to a tricuspid regurgitant jet, from which the systolic pressure gradient between the right atrium and right ventricle can be calculated, yielding an accurate measurement of pulmonary artery systolic pressure (Fig. 229-8).

Cardiac output

Volume flow rates (or stroke volume and cardiac output) can be reliably measured noninvasively by Doppler echocardiography. Flow is calculated as the product of the cross-sectional area of the vessel or chamber through which blood moves and the velocity of blood flow as assessed by Doppler.

Diastolic filling

Doppler echocardiography allows noninvasive evaluation of ventricular diastolic filling. The transmitral velocity curves reflect the relative pressure gradients between the left atrium and ventricle throughout diastole and are influenced by the rate of ventricular relaxation, the driving force across the valve, and the compliance of the ventricle. In the early phase of diastolic dysfunction there is primarily an impairment of LV relaxation, with reduced early transmitral flow and a compensatory increase in flow during atrial

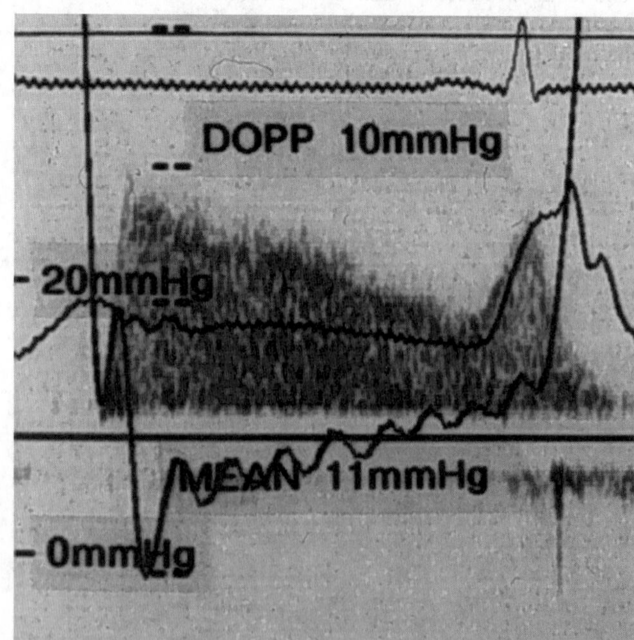

Figure 229-6 Continuous-wave Doppler of mitral valve velocities in a patient with mitral stenosis. The mean gradient calculated from Doppler (DOPP) of 10 mmHg is similar to the mean gradient of 11 mmHg from simultaneous cardiac catheterization in this patient.

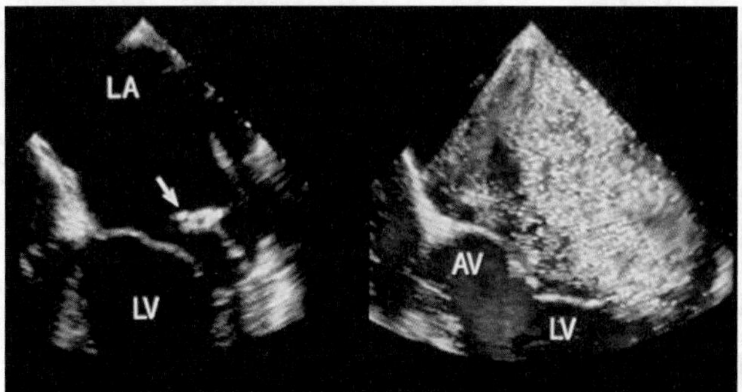

Figure 229-7 *Left:* Transesophageal echocardiographic view of a patient with severe mitral regurgitation due to a flail posterior leaflet. The arrow points to the portion of the posterior leaflet that is unsupported and moves into the left atrium during systole. *Right:* Color-flow imaging demonstrating a large mosaic jet of mitral regurgitation during systole. LA, left atrium; LV, left ventricle; AV, aortic valve.

contraction (Fig. 229-9). As disease progresses and ventricular compliance declines, left atrial pressure rises, resulting in a higher early transmitral velocity and shortening of the deceleration of flow in early diastole. Analysis of Doppler tissue velocities of annular motion and myocardial strain provides further information concerning the diastolic properties of the heart.

Congenital heart disease

2D and Doppler echocardiography have been useful in the evaluation of patients with congenital heart disease. Congenital stenotic or regurgitant valve lesions can be assessed. The detection of intracardiac shunts is possible by 2D and Doppler echocardiography. Patency of surgical shunts and conduits can also be evaluated.

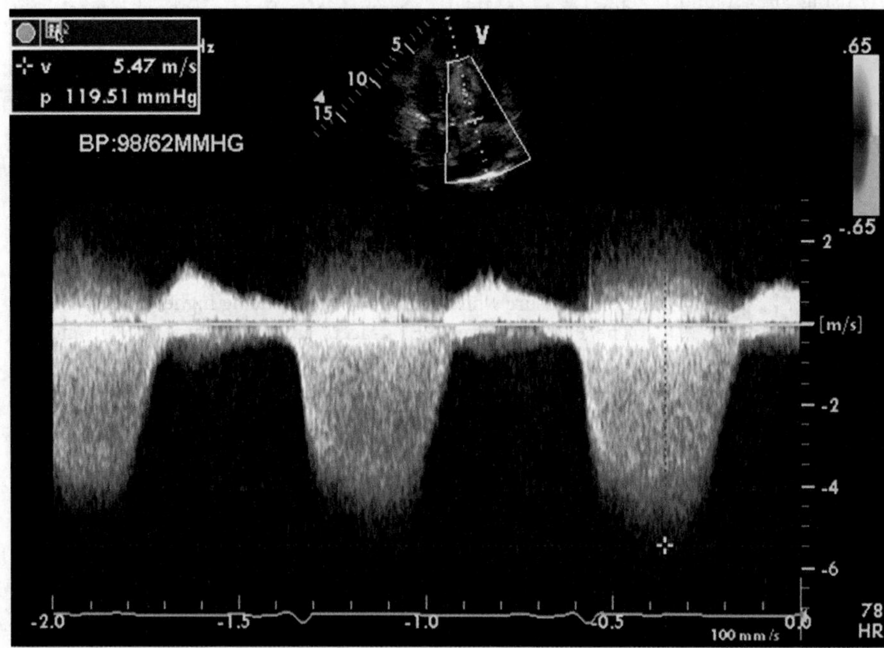

Figure 229-8 Continuous-wave Doppler of tricuspid regurgitation in a patient with pulmonary hypertension. There is an increase in the velocity to 5.4 m/s. Using the modified Bernoulli equation, the peak pressure gradient between right ventricle and right atrium during systole is 116 mmHg. Assuming a right atrial pressure of 10 mmHg, the right ventricular systolic pressure is 126 mmHg. In the absence of right ventricular outflow tract obstruction, this indicates there is severe pulmonary hypertension with a pulmonary artery systolic pressure of 126 mmHg.

STRESS ECHOCARDIOGRAPHY

2D and Doppler echocardiography are usually performed with the patient in the resting state. Further information can be obtained by reimaging during either exercise or pharmacologic stress. The primary indications for stress echocardiography are to confirm the suspicion of ischemic heart disease and determine the extent of ischemia.

A decrease in systolic contraction of an ischemic area (segment) of myocardium, termed a regional wall motion abnormality, occurs before symptoms or electrocardiographic changes (Fig. 229-10). New regional wall motion abnormalities, a decline in ejection fraction, and an increase in end-systolic volume with stress are all indicators of myocardial ischemia. Exercise stress testing is usually done with exercise protocols using either upright treadmill or bicycle exercise. In patients who are not able to exercise, pharmacologic testing can be performed by infusion of dobutamine to increase myocardial oxygen demand. Dobutamine echocardiography has also been used to assess myocardial viability in patients with poor systolic function and concomitant CAD; when used for this purpose, dobutamine is administered at lower doses than standard pharmacologic stress doses.

Doppler echocardiography can be used at rest and during exercise in patients with valvular heart disease to determine the hemodynamic response of valve gradients and pulmonary pressures (Fig. 229-11). In patients with low-output, low-gradient aortic stenosis, the response of the gradient to dobutamine stimulation is of diagnostic and therapeutic value.

TRANSESOPHAGEAL ECHOCARDIOGRAPHY

When limited information is obtained from a TTE due to poor imaging windows, TEE can be useful. Diseases of the aorta, such as aortic dissection, can be readily diagnosed by TEE. Defining the source of embolism is a common indication for TEE, as abnormalities such as atrial thrombi, patent foramen ovale, and aortic plaques can be detected. Other masses, particularly those in the atria, can be visualized. The presence of vegetations for the diagnosis of infective endocarditis and its complications can be assessed by TEE. This technique has been used before cardioversion in patients with atrial fibrillation to rule out a thrombus in the left atrium or left atrial appendage.

NUCLEAR CARDIOLOGY

BASIC PRINCIPLES OF NUCLEAR CARDIOLOGY

Nuclear (or radionuclide) imaging requires intravenous administration of radiopharmaceuticals (isotopes or tracers). Once injected, the isotope traces physiologic processes and undergoes uptake in specific organs. During this process, radiation is emitted in the form of photons, generally gamma rays, generated during radioactive decay when the nucleus of an isotope changes from one energy level to a lower one. A special camera detects these photons and creates images via a computer interface. The two most commonly used technologies in clinical nuclear cardiology are single-photon emission computed tomography (SPECT) and positron emission

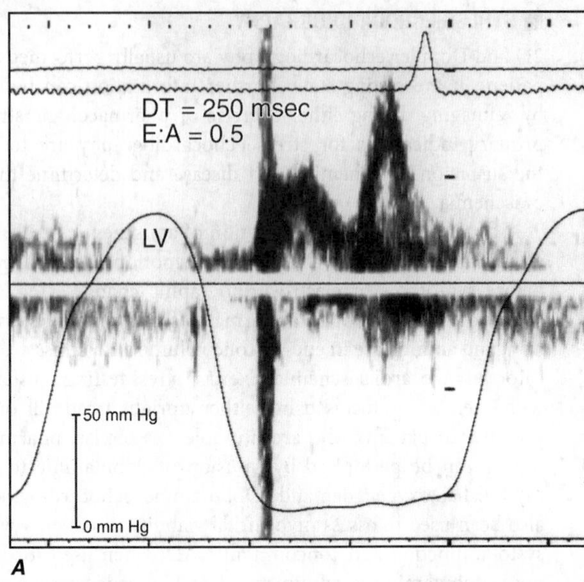

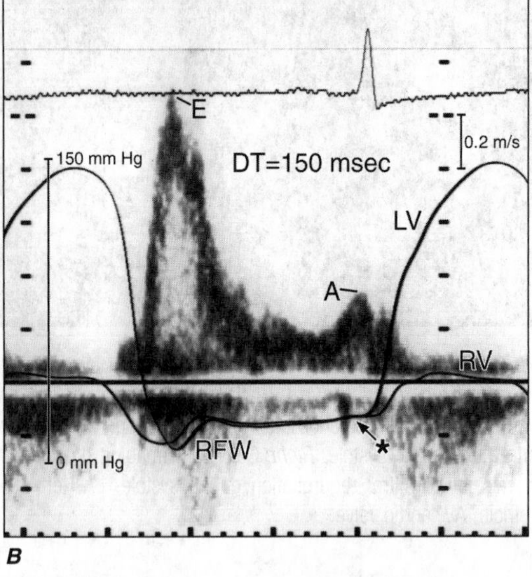

Figure 229-9 High-fidelity left ventricular (LV) pressure curves superimposed on a mitral inflow velocity curve obtained by Doppler echocardiography. The ratio of early and late diastolic flows is termed the E:A ratio. The deceleration time (DT) measures the rate of decline of early velocity and reflects the effective operative compliance of the left ventricle. *Left:* In early stages of diastolic dysfunction, there is an abnormality of relaxation. There is a decrease in the early diastolic filling and an increase with filling at atrial contraction, resulting in a low E:A ratio of 0.5, with deceleration time (DT) of 250 ms. In this instance, the LV diastolic pressure is low at 6 mmHg. *Right:* As diastolic dysfunction progresses, there is a restriction to filling, in which there is a high early diastolic velocity and low velocity at atrial contraction resulting in a high E:A ratio of 3.0, with DT of 150 ms. In this instance, the LV diastolic pressure is markedly elevated to 34 mmHg.

tomography (PET). These technologies differ in instrumentation, acquisition, resolution, and nuclides used.

CLINICAL APPLICATIONS

Assessment of myocardial perfusion and coronary artery disease

Nuclear myocardial perfusion imaging (MPI) using SPECT and more recently PET has an established role in the evaluation and management of patients with known or suspected coronary artery disease (CAD). Both SPECT and PET MRI require the injection of isotopes at rest and during stress to produce images of regional myocardial uptake proportional to regional blood flow. Normally, myocardial blood flow can be increased up to fivefold above the resting state to meet the increased myocardial oxygen demand during stress. In the presence of a fixed coronary stenosis, the inability to increase myocardial perfusion in the territory supplied by the stenosis creates a flow differential and inhomogeneous myocardial tracer uptake. In patients unable to exercise, pharmacologic agents are used to increase blood flow and create similar inhomogeneities.

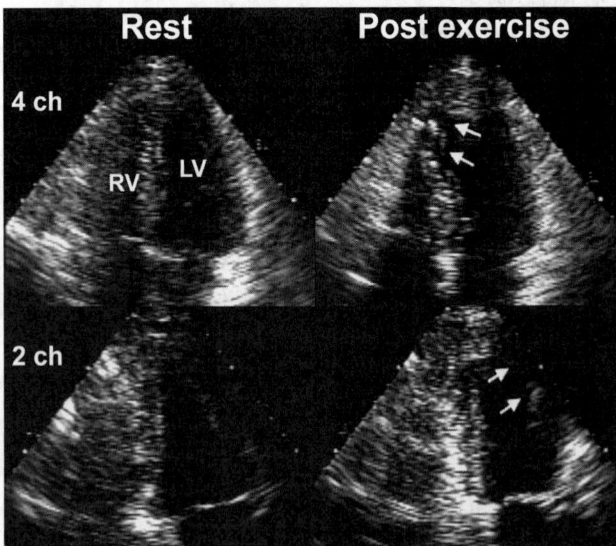

Figure 229-10 Systolic still-frame two-dimensional echocardiographic images of a patient undergoing a stress echocardiogram. During rest (*left*), there is contraction of all segments of the myocardium. During exercise (*right*), there are regional wall motion abnormalities in the anterior and anteroapical segments (*arrows*). 4ch = four-chamber view, 2ch = two-chamber views, LV = left ventricle, RV = right ventricle.

The most commonly used SPECT perfusion tracers are thallium-201 (^{201}Tl) and technetium-99m (^{99m}Tc) labeled isonitriles. ^{99m}Tc isonitriles have higher photon energies and shorter physical half-lives than ^{201}Tl, permitting injection of higher doses with less radiation exposure while concurrently producing higher-quality images. The FDA-approved PET tracers are rubidium-82 (^{82}Rb) and ^{13}N ammonia ($^{13}NH_3$) for high-dose administration and shorter imaging protocols.

Both SPECT and PET myocardial perfusion images are commonly interpreted by visual analysis, which may be supplemented with quantitative software. Normal myocardial perfusion images demonstrate uniform tracer uptake throughout the LV myocardium (Fig. 229-12). In contrast, regions with reduced myocardial blood flow demonstrate varying degrees of reduced tracer uptake (Fig. 229-13), which can be graded on a semiquantitative scale. Reduced tracer uptake in a myocardial region on both resting and stress images is called a fixed defect and is consistent with infarction. Reduced tracer uptake on the stress image with relatively preserved or improved uptake on the rest image is called a reversible defect and indicates ischemia. PET has the ability to quantify myocardial blood flow and flow reserve in absolute terms.

For the diagnosis of angiographically significant CAD, SPECT using ^{201}T1 and ^{99m}Tc isonitriles and either exercise or pharmacologic

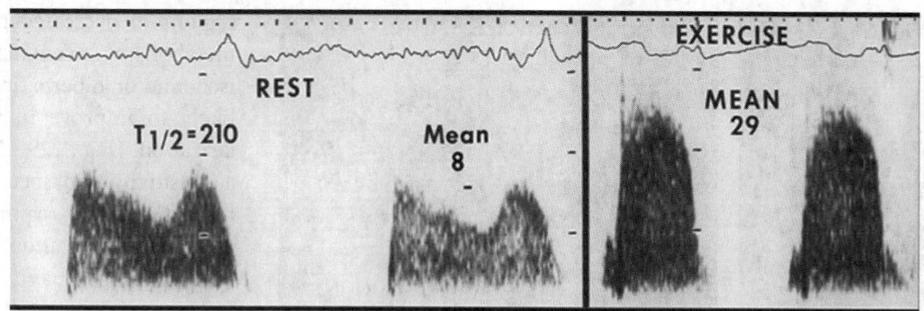

Figure 229-11 Continuous-wave Doppler echocardiogram across the mitral valve of a patient with mitral stenosis. In the resting state (*left*), there is a mean gradient of 8 mmHg. During exercise (*right*), the mean gradient rises to 29 mmHg, indicating a hemodynamically significant mitral stenosis.

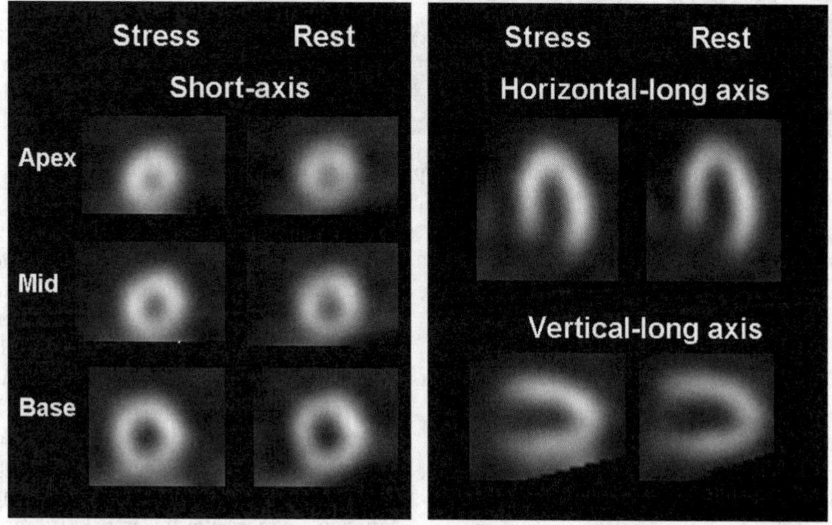

Figure 229-12 Exercise technetium-99m sestamibi images in a 65-year-old man with atypical angina. Images are shown in three standard views; stress (*left*) and rest (*right*) in each panel. There is uniform tracer uptake throughout the left ventricular myocardium at rest and peak stress in all three views.

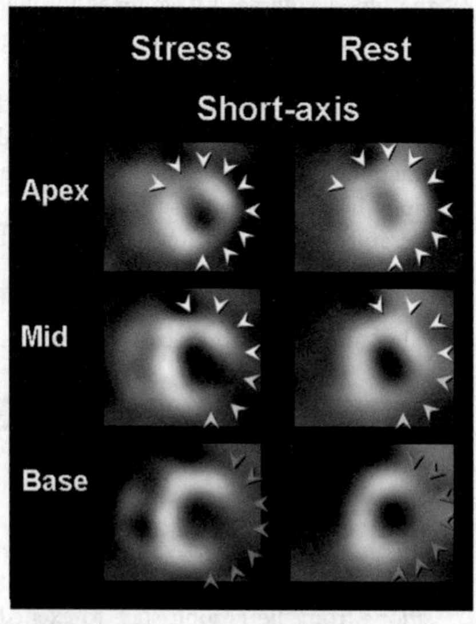

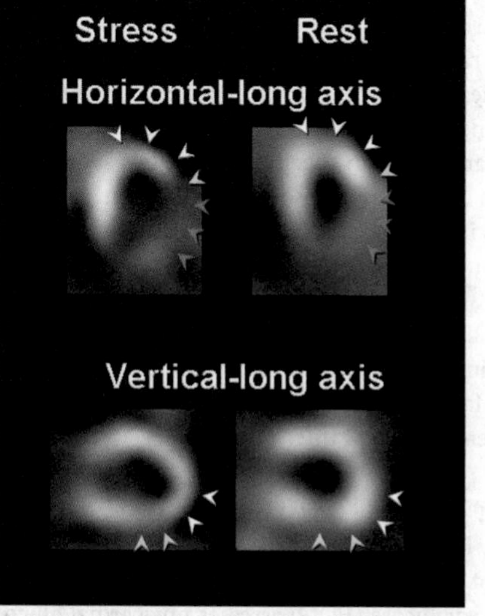

Figure 229-13 Exercise technetium-99m sestamibi and rest thallium-201 images in a 72-year-old woman with typical angina. Images are shown in three standard views, with stress (*left*) and rest (*right*) in each panel. Stress images demonstrate reduced tracer uptake in the apical, mid-anterior, mid-lateral, and mid-inferior regions (*white arrowheads*) with normal or near-normal tracer uptake in the corresponding regions on the rest images (*white arrowheads*), signifying a reversible defect consistent with ischemia. The lack of complete normalization (or reversibility) of tracer uptake on the rest images at the mid-inferior and mid-lateral region represents associated infarction in that area (*yellow arrowheads*). On both stress and rest images, the basal inferior and basal lateral regions exhibit severely reduced tracer uptake, signifying a fixed defect consistent with infarction (*red arrowheads*). Subsequent invasive coronary angiography demonstrated severe stenosis of the mid left anterior descending coronary artery and occlusion of the left circumflex coronary artery with collaterals.

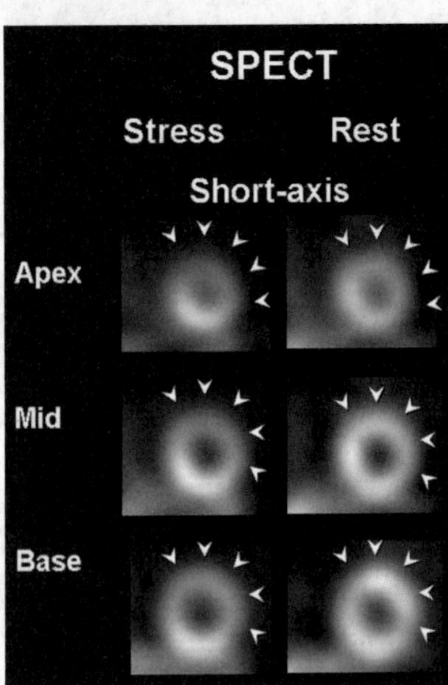

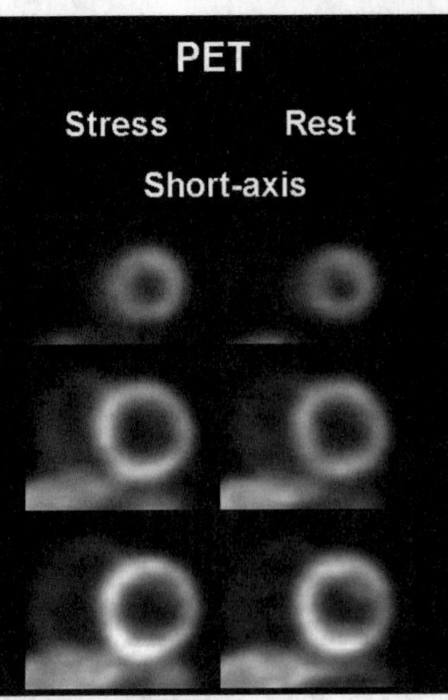

Figure 229-14 SPECT and PET images in a 67-year-old woman with atypical angina. Images are shown in short-axis views, with stress (*left*) and rest (*right*) in each panel. Shifting breast position between the rest and stress SPECT acquisitions produced an apparent reversible apical, anterior, and anterolateral attenuation artifact (*arrowheads*) resembling ischemia. With PET and its built-in attenuation correction in the same patient, the defect was not present. SPECT, single-photon emission computed tomography; PET, positron emission tomography.

stress has an average sensitivity of 87% and specificity of 73%. In comparison, PET MPI has higher accuracy (average sensitivity 90%; specificity of 89%). The robust methods for attenuation correction with PET improve the specificity, particularly in obese populations and women, while the superior resolution and higher extraction fraction of PET tracers increase the sensitivity (Fig. 229-14). PET has not been as widely used as SPECT due to decreased availability and less local experience, but PET scanners are becoming more widely available (Table 229-2).

Both SPECT and PET MPI have powerful prognostic value. In patients with normal SPECT MPI results, the annual rate of cardiac death or myocardial infarction is generally very low (<0.7%). Annual death/event rates increase with the extent and severity of imaging abnormalities and are generally about 3% in those with mild to moderate abnormalities and about 7% in those with severe abnormalities; rates are higher in specific populations such as diabetics and those with high-risk exercise treadmill results. High-risk SPECT MPI findings include severe resting or poststress LV systolic dysfunction, large or multiple stress-induced defects, or a large fixed defect with LV dilation or increased ^{201}Tl lung uptake. The incremental prognostic value of SPECT MPI has been established in many clinical settings, including populations with known CAD, prior myocardial infarction and/or revascularization, and acute chest pain in the emergency department.

Assessment of myocardial metabolism and viability

PET has traditionally been regarded as the gold standard technique for the assessment of myocardial viability. The positron-emitting tracer F-18 fluorodeoxyglucose (FDG) assesses myocardial glucose metabolism and is an indicator of myocardial viability. Because uptake is heterogeneous in normal myocardium in the fasting state, oral glucose loading or a combination of insulin and glucose infusions is used to enhance myocardial uptake. With reduced myocardial blood flow and ischemia, substrate utilization switches from fatty acids and lactate toward glucose, leading to enhanced myocardial FDG uptake. This pattern of enhanced FDG uptake in regions of decreased perfusion (termed flow/metabolism "mismatch") identifies areas of ischemic or hibernating myocardium that are likely to improve in function after revascularization (Fig. 229-15). This mismatch has a sensitivity and specificity of 92% and 63%, respectively, for regional contractile recovery after revascularization. The SPECT radiopharmaceuticals, ^{201}Tl and ^{99m}Tc isonitriles, require an intact (viable) cell membrane for uptake and also provide an assessment of myocardial viability in addition to perfusion. However, PET identifies ischemic or hibernating myocardium in 10–20% of regions otherwise classified as fibrotic (infarcted) by SPECT perfusion tracers. Patients with ischemic heart failure, who have viable myocardium identified by PET or SPECT and undergo revascularization, have a better survival than those who do not have viable myocardium or do not undergo revascularization.

Assessment of ventricular function

In addition to perfusion and metabolic information, LV systolic function and volumes are now routinely obtained with gated SPECT and PET acquisitions, as long as the heart rate is relatively constant. An automated technique determines the endocardial borders of the LV cavity, and a geometric model is used to calculate the LVEF and volumes with a high level of reproducibility. Regional wall motion can also be assessed by visual examination. The combined variables of perfusion and function are more effective in risk stratification than either alone.

Another established but less widely available nuclear technique for assessing LV function and volumes is equilibrium radionuclide angiography RNA, also known as multiple-gated blood pool acquisition (MUGA). This technique involves imaging of ^{99m}Tc-labeled albumin or red cells that are uniformly distributed throughout the blood volume. LV volumes throughout the cardiac cycle are calculated from a time-activity curve generated using regions of interest.

Innovations in hybrid imaging technology, especially PET/CT and SPECT/CT, are occurring rapidly and contribute to their emerging role in the combined assessments of anatomy and physiology in patients with suspected or known CAD. The diagnostic literature is evolving for these hybrid technologies but radiation exposure is a concern and large-scale clinical trials are still needed to validate their clinical applications, determine their prognostic value, and address their cost-effectiveness and appropriateness.

MRI AND CT IMAGING

■ MAGNETIC RESONANCE IMAGING

Basic principles

MRI is a technique based on the magnetic properties of hydrogen nuclei. In the presence of a large magnetic field, nuclear spin transitions from the ground state to excited states can be induced by an electric field, and as the nuclei relax and return to their ground state, they release energy in the form of electromagnetic radiation that is detected and processed into an image. Although the large vascular vessels can be visualized on MRI without contrast agents, gadolinium is frequently employed as a contrast agent to produce magnetic resonance angiograms (MRAs). Contrast agents also provide enhanced soft tissue contrast as well as the opportunity to

TABLE 229-2 Relative Advantages and Disadvantages of SPECT and PET

SPECT
Thallium-201
Lower radiopharmaceutical cost
Measurement of increased pulmonary uptake
Less hepatobiliary and bowel uptake
Detection of resting ischemia (hibernating myocardium)
Longer physical half-life of tracers (limiting dose administration)
Lower energy level
Technetium-99m isonitriles
Better image quality
Ventricular function assessment (gated SPECT)
Shorter imaging time
Shorter imaging protocols (patient/scheduling convenience)
Acute imaging in myocardial infarction and unstable angina
Superior quantification
PET
Robust attenuation correction
Short physical half-life of tracers
Best image quality (particularly in obese patients and women)
Shorter imaging time (particularly for rubidium-82)
Very short imaging protocols (particularly for rubidium-82)
More complex imaging protocols (particularly viability assessment)
Detection of viability
Absolute quantification
High diagnostic accuracy
Limited prognostic studies
N-13 ammonia requires on-site cyclotron
Rubidium-82 generally requires costly commercial generator
Lower radiation exposure, particularly for N-13 ammonia
High Risk Perfusion Imaging Features
Severe resting or exercise LV systolic dysfunction (EF<35%)
Stress-induced large perfusion defect (especially if anterior)
Stress-induced multiple perfusion defects of moderate size
Large, fixed perfusion defect with LV dilatation
Transient (poststress) LV dilatation
Increased lung uptake (thallium)

Abbreviatons: EF, ejection fraction; LV, left ventricle; PET, positron emission tomography; SPECT, single photon emission computed tomography.

obtain rapid angiographic images during the first pass of contrast through the vascular system.

Cardiac MRI is challenging because of the rapid motion of the heart and coronary arteries. However, both static and cine images can usually now be obtained using electrocardiographic triggering, often within short breath-holds of 10–15 s. Cine images can be acquired in any plane with excellent blood-myocardial contrast. These images can be used to quantify accurately ejection fraction, end-systolic and end-diastolic volumes, and cardiac mass with high accuracy, reliability, and reproducibility, and without the need for ionizing radiation.

Clinical utility

The multiplanar capabilities of MRI, coupled with excellent contrast and spatial resolution, provide superb images of the myocardium and great vessels. MRI is of great value in defining anatomic relationships in patients with complex congenital heart disease (Fig. 229-16) and cardiomyopathies (Fig. 229-17). Cardiac masses can be characterized and distinguished from thrombus (Fig. 229-18). In addition to defining their relationship to normal anatomic structures, MRI can determine whether a mediastinal or pulmonary mass has invaded the pericardium or heart. The entire pericardium can be visualized in multiple planes, and MRI has proved useful in characterizing pericardial effusions, pericardial thickening, and inflammation. Specialized pulse sequences can measure the velocity of blood in each pixel of the image, so that flow across valves and within blood vessels may be determined with accuracy, thereby aiding in the evaluation of valvular disease and intracardiac shunts.

MRA is a standard technique for imaging the aorta and large vessels of the chest and abdomen, with results essentially identical to conventional angiography. MRA of the coronary arteries is a much more difficult challenge, both because of the small size of these vessels and because of their rapid and complex motion during the cardiac cycle; thus, coronary MRA is not yet a reliable clinical technique.

MRI is now an accepted technology for the evaluation of patients with suspected or known coronary disease. Ventricular function and wall motion can be assessed at rest and during infusion of inotropic agents. Assessment of myocardial perfusion can be

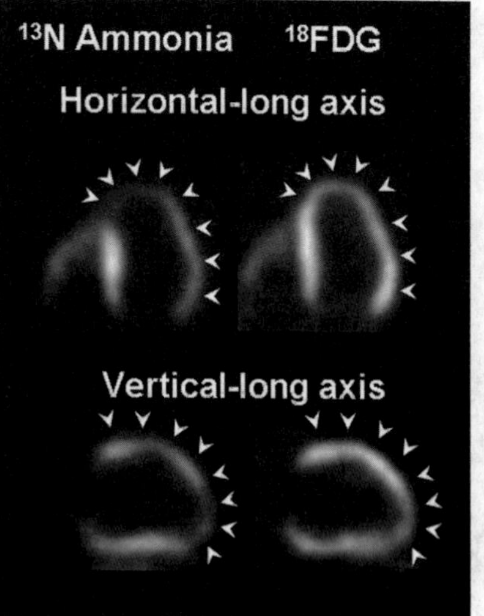

Figure 229-15 PET viability study in a 63-year-old woman with heart failure, severe LV systolic dysfunction, and severe coronary artery disease. Images are shown in three standard views, with perfusion (*left*) and glucose metabolism (*right*) in each panel. The N-13 ammonia images show a very large apical, septal, anterior, and lateral perfusion defect (*arrowheads*), but F-18 fluorodeoxyglucose (18FDG) images demonstrate relatively preserved glucose uptake in the corresponding segments (*arrowheads*). This PET perfusion-metabolism mismatch is consistent with hibernating myocardium. The patient underwent coronary artery bypass grafting surgery with improvement in left ventricular systolic function (ejection fraction increased from 26% pre- to 45% postoperatively). All regions identified as viable recovered contractile function after revascularization.

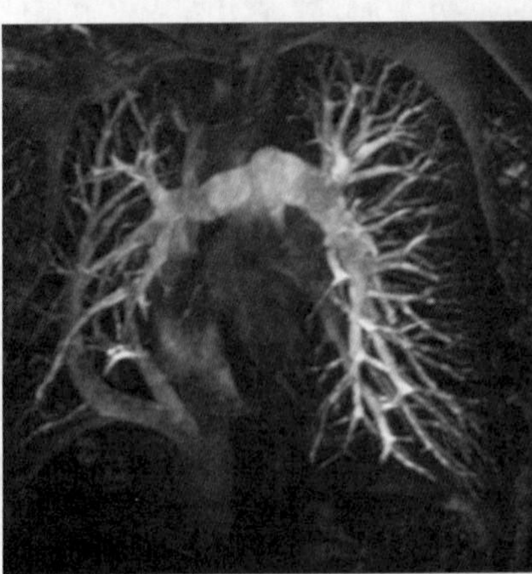
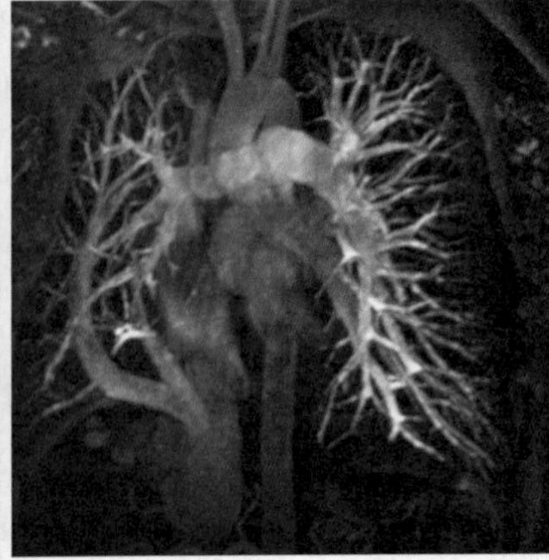

Figure 229-16 MRA scan of a patient with partial anomalous pulmonary venous drainage of the right lung into the inferior vena cava (scimitar syndrome). MRA is able to define the abnormal anatomic relationships of cardiac structures and great vessels in patients with congenital heart disease.

performed by injecting a bolus of gadolinium contrast and then continuously scanning the heart as the gadolinium passes through the cardiac chambers and into the myocardium. Relative perfusion deficits are reflected as regions of low signal intensity within the myocardium. Pharmacologic stress (typically achieved with vasodilators) can be applied during perfusion imaging to detect physiologically significant coronary artery lesions. Myocardial perfusion imaging with cardiac MRI is more sensitive than SPECT imaging for detecting subendocardial ischemia due to its enhanced spatial resolution.

Myocardial viability and infarction may be determined by imaging the heart 10–20 min after gadolinium injection, known as delayed enhancement magnetic resonance imaging. In normal myocardium, gadolinium cannot penetrate the membranes of the densely packed myocytes. Abnormal myocardial tissue accumulates excess gadolinium following intravenous injection, as ruptured myocyte membranes allow gadolinium to passively diffuse into intracellular space. In chronic infarction, the tissue concentration of gadolinium is increased due to an expansion of the intracellular space from collagenous scar (Fig. 229-18). Thus, delayed enhancement is indicative of nonviable or infarcted myocardium, the subendocardial versus transmural extent of which is accurately assessed by the high spatial resolution of MRI. The presence and pattern of gadolinium enhancement not only is useful for determining viability but also has prognostic value in the patient with an ischemic cardiomyopathy. "Myocardium at risk" following myocardial infarction can be assessed by examining the amount of myocardial edema, using T2-weighted sequences (Fig. 229-19).

Limitations of MRI

Relative contraindications to MRI include the presence of pacemakers, internal defibrillators, or cerebral aneurysm clips. A small percentage of patients are claustrophobic and unable to tolerate the examination within the relatively confined quarters of the magnet bore. Examination of clinically unstable patients and those undergoing stress testing is problematic, since close hemodynamic and electrocardiographic monitoring is difficult. Image quality in patients with significant arrhythmias is often limited. Patients with renal disease receiving gadolinium contrast may be at risk of developing nephrogenic systemic fibrosis, characterized by increased tissue deposition of collagen in the skin and development of fibrosis in skin and other organs.

■ COMPUTED TOMOGRAPHIC IMAGING

Basic principles

CT is a fast, simple, noninvasive technique that provides images of the myocardium and great vessels with excellent spatial resolution and good soft tissue contrast. The development of electron-beam

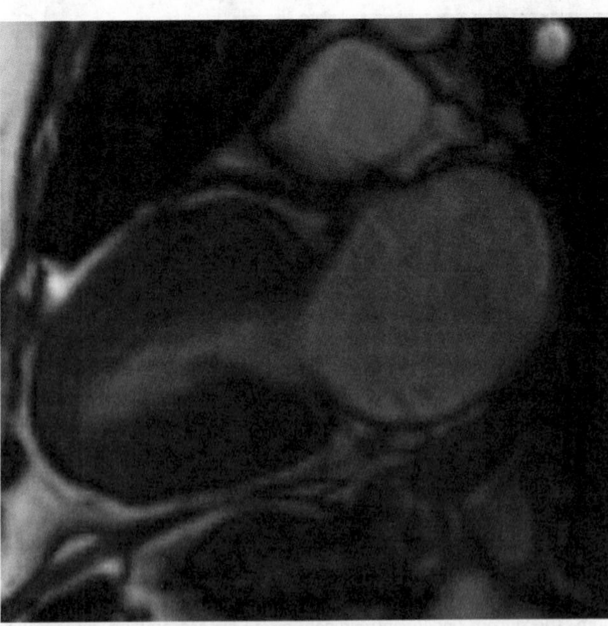

Figure 229-17 MRI scan of a patient with hypertrophic cardiomyopathy, showing the severe increase in left ventricular wall thickness. Cardiac MRI is an ideal imaging modality for diagnosing cardiomyopathies.

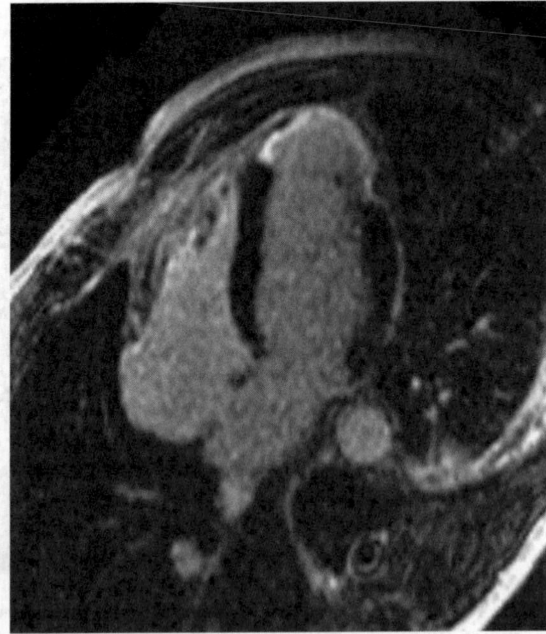

Figure 229-18 MRI scan with delayed gadolinium enhancement in a patient with a large anteroapical infarction. The gadolinium (white area) accumulated in the extracellular space in the presence of cell death from myocardial infarction.

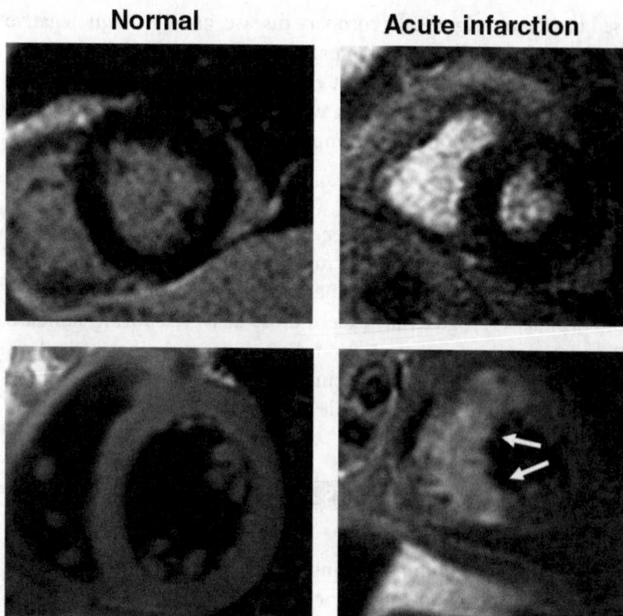

Figure 229-19 *Left*: Normal delayed enhancement and "edema"-sensitive images. *Top* (*left*): Delayed enhancement image illustrating normal black myocardium without infarction/fibrosis. *Bottom* (*left*): A triple inversion recovery sequence that is T2-weighted demonstrating normal homogenous-appearing gray myocardium. *Right:* A patient postmyocardial infarction and early revascularization without evidence of an infarction and an edematous myocardium in the septum. *Top* (*right*): Delayed enhanced with normal black myocardium without infarction or fibrosis. *Bottom* (*right*): A triple inversion recovery sequence illustrating edema in the septum without infarction. This is the area of "salvaged" myocardium.

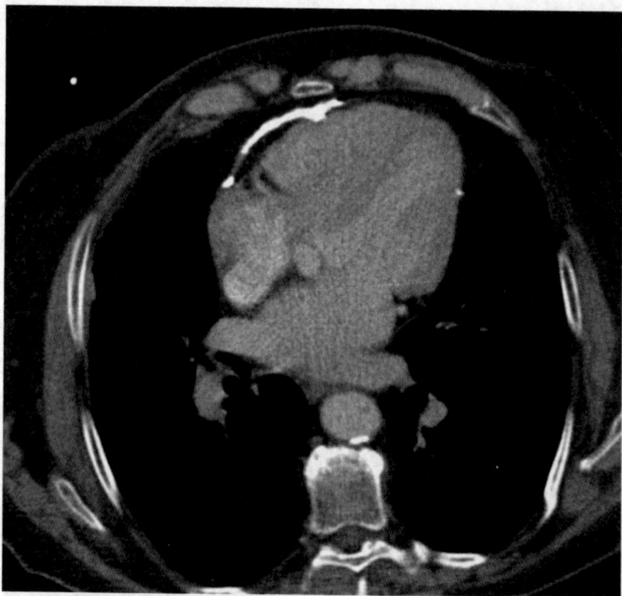

Figure 229-20 CT scan showing pericardial calcification, seen as a white linear density anterior to the myocardium.

CT and multidetector-row CT have led to improved temporal resolution and routine imaging of the beating heart. Motion-free high-spatial-resolution images are now possible with multidetector CT technology (≥64 channel) that allows imaging of the coronary arteries.

Clinical applications

Cardiac CT has important clinical applications. Pericardial calcification is easily detected by CT (Fig. 229-20). CT is useful in characterizing cardiac masses, particularly those containing fat or calcium. The ability to detect small amounts of fat with high spatial resolution makes CT an attractive technique for imaging patients with suspected arrhythmogenic right ventricular dysplasia. Cine images can be used to evaluate wall motion and to determine ejection fraction, end-diastolic and end-systolic volumes, and cardiac mass.

CT angiography (CTA) has demonstrated accuracy similar to MRA in imaging the aorta and great vessels, and CTA is the examination of choice in the evaluation of patients with suspected pulmonary embolus. CTA is an excellent imaging modality for the diagnosis of aortic dissection or penetrating ulcers. Complete visualization of the entire aorta and its branches is possible by CTA using a single contrast medial bolus injection.

Coronary calcification

Calcium in the coronary arteries occurs in atherosclerosis and is absent in the normal coronary artery (Fig. 229-21). CT is very sensitive for the detection of coronary artery calcification, and the absence of coronary calcification excludes significant epicardial coronary disease. The quantity of coronary calcification (coronary calcium score) is related to the severity of CAD and prognosis. However, the utility of CT calcification score in clinical practice in the asymptomatic patient is limited to those with a moderate risk of coronary heart disease in whom the result will change management.

Contrast-enhanced CT angiography

With the high temporal and spatial resolution of multislice spiral CT, accurate assessment of luminal narrowing in the major branches of the coronary arteries is possible in selected patients. Studies at experienced centers have shown a sensitivity and specificity of >90% for detecting coronary artery lesions as compared to cardiac catheterization. The highest accuracy has been noted in the left main and the proximal portions of the left-sided coronary arteries with decreased sensitivities in the more distal segments and in the more rapidly moving right coronary artery (Fig. 229-22).

The concept of "noninvasive coronary angiography" has generated great interest in CTA. However, as with any imaging modalities,

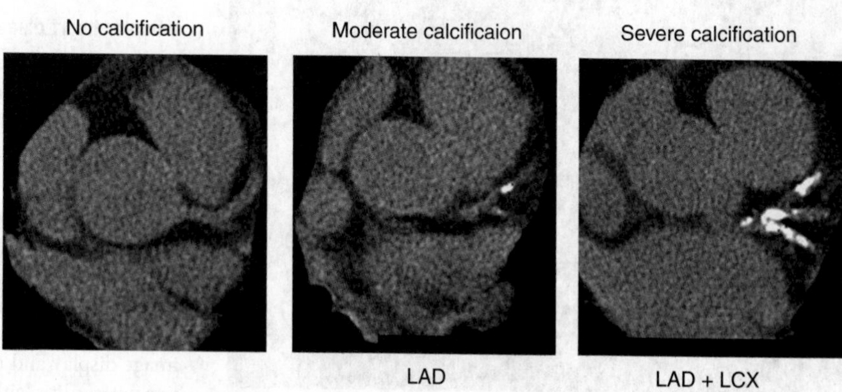

Figure 229-21 CT scans of three patients showing the ability to detect coronary calcification. *Left:* Normal coronary arteries without calcification. *Middle:* Calcification in the left anterior artery (LAD). *Right:* Severe calcification in the LAD and circumflex (CX) arteries.

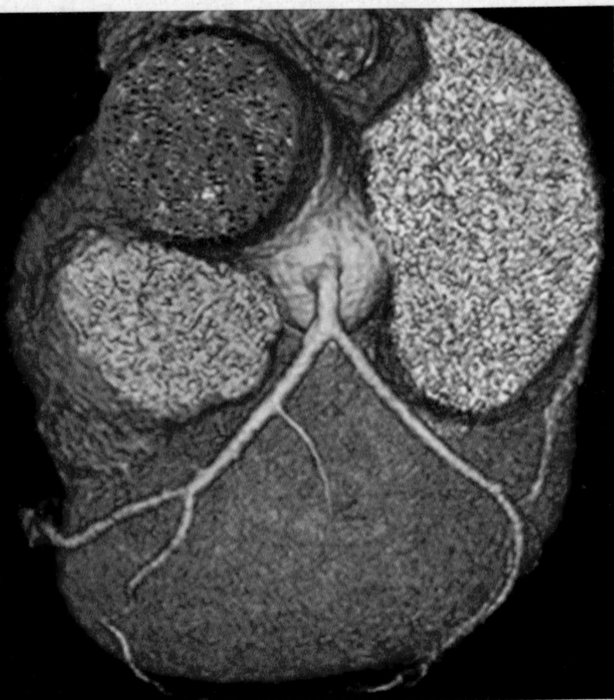

Figure 229-22 Three-dimensional volume rendered image of a contrast-enhanced CT angiogram demonstrating a normal left main coronary artery arising from the aorta and its two branches, the left anterior descending artery (*left*) and the circumflex artery (*right*).

CTA has technical limitations requiring proper patient selection and preparation. The integration of CTA into clinical practice requires knowledge of pretest diagnostic and prognostic data and the incremental information that will alter management. The well-accepted indication for coronary CTA is in the evaluation of suspected coronary artery anomalies for which CTA not only confirms the diagnosis but also shows the course of the arteries related to the great vessels (Fig. 229-23). For patients with chest pain syndromes, CTA is best

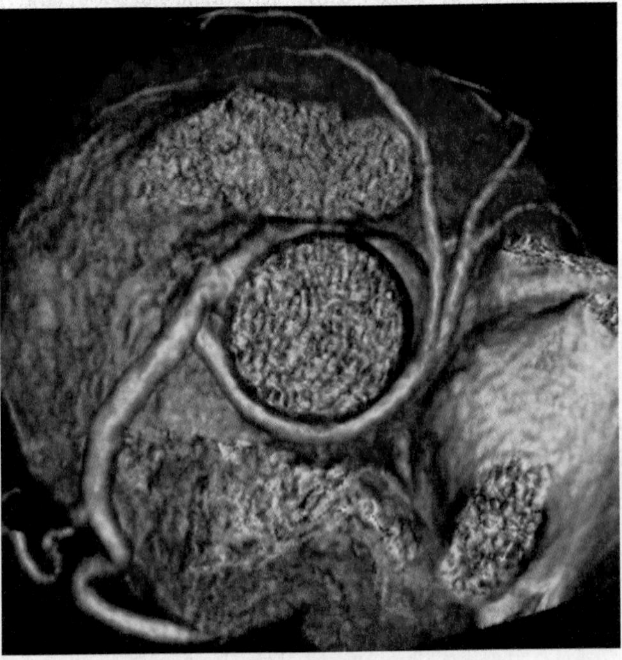

Figure 229-23 Three-dimensional volume rendered image of a contrast-enhanced CT angiogram illustrating an anomalous left coronary artery arising from the right coronary artery and traveling posterior to the aorta.

used to rule out significant coronary disease, given its high negative predictive value. Thus, it is the patient with an intermediate pretest probability of CAD who cannot exercise or has uninterpretable or equivocal results on prior testing who would be best suited for CTA. The benefit of CTA in other groups of patients is still unclear.

Limitations of CT

Limitations of CT include its dependence on ionizing radiation (in contrast to MRI) and the need for iodinated contrast. Techniques to lower radiation doses continue to evolve, as the radiation doses for coronary CTA generally exceed those delivered during standard diagnostic cardiac catheterization. Fast or irregular heart rhythms and body motion limit the accuracy of CTA. Heavy calcification and artifacts from stents preclude accurate assessment of the severity of a stenosis.

SELECTION OF IMAGING TESTS (TABLE 229-3)

■ BASIC PREMISE

The choice of the optimal imaging modality for a particular patient should be based upon the major problem being addressed, other concomitant clinical questions, as well as the local expertise and equipment available in an institution. The clinical urgency and costs of each test also need to be considered. To ensure the effective use of cardiovascular imaging tools, Appropriateness Criteria have been developed by the national societies to examine the incremental clinical benefit of imaging modalities.

■ COMMON CLINICAL QUESTIONS

Left ventricular size and function

2D echocardiography is the primary imaging modality obtained for assessment of LV cavity size, systolic function, and wall thickness. Echocardiography can also provide concomitant information on valve function, pulmonary artery pressures, and diastolic filling, which are valuable in the patient presenting with possible heart failure. The disadvantage is poor endocardial resolution in some patients and the lack of reproducible quantitative measurements.

Equilibrium radionuclide angiography can provide an accurate quantitative measurement of LV volumes and function but is not widely available and cannot be used in patients with irregular rhythms. Gated SPECT and PET measure LV systolic function and volumes as a part of myocardial perfusion and/or viability imaging but also require relatively regular rhythm. Both MRI and CT scanning provide the highest quality resolution of the endocardial border and, thus, are the most accurate of all modalities. However, they are of higher cost, lack portability, and do not provide concomitant hemodynamic information as echocardiography does.

Valvular heart disease

2D and Doppler echocardiography provide both anatomic and hemodynamic information regarding valve disease, and are the first test of choice. MRI can also visualize valve motion and determine abnormal flow velocities across valves, but there is less validation of quantitative hemodynamic measurements in comparison to echocardiography.

Pericardial disease

Echocardiography is the first imaging modality of choice in patients with suspected pericardial effusion and tamponade owing to its rapid image display and portability. For patients with suspected constrictive pericarditis, either MRI or CT scanning is the imaging modality that best delineates pericardial thickness. Hemodynamic analysis of the enhancement of ventricular interaction that occurs in pericardial constriction can be assessed by Doppler echocardiography.

TABLE 229-3 Selection of Imaging Tests

	Echo	Nuclear	CT[a]	MRI[b]
LV size/function	Initial modality of choice Low cost, portable Provides ancillary structural and hemodynamic information	Available from gated SPECT or PET imaging.	Best resolution Highest cost	Best resolution Highest cost
Valve disease	Initial modality of choice Valve motion Doppler hemodynamics			Visualize valve motion Delineate abnormal flow
Pericardial disease	Pericardial effusion Doppler hemodynamics		Pericardial thickening	Pericardial thickening
Aortic disease	TEE rapid diagnosis[c] Acute dissection		Image entire aorta Acute aneurysm Aortic dissection	Image entire aorta Aortic aneurysm Chronic dissection
Cardiac masses	TTE—large intracardiac masses TEE—smaller intracardiac masses[c]		Extracardiac masses Myocardial masses	Extracardiac masses Myocardial masses

[a]Contrast required.
[b]Relative contraindication: pacemakers, metallic objects, claustrophobic.
[c]When not seen on TTE.
Abbreviations: Echo, echocardiography; PET, positron emission tomography; SPECT, single-photon emission computed tomography; TEE, transesophageal echocardiography; TTE, transthoracic echocardiogram.

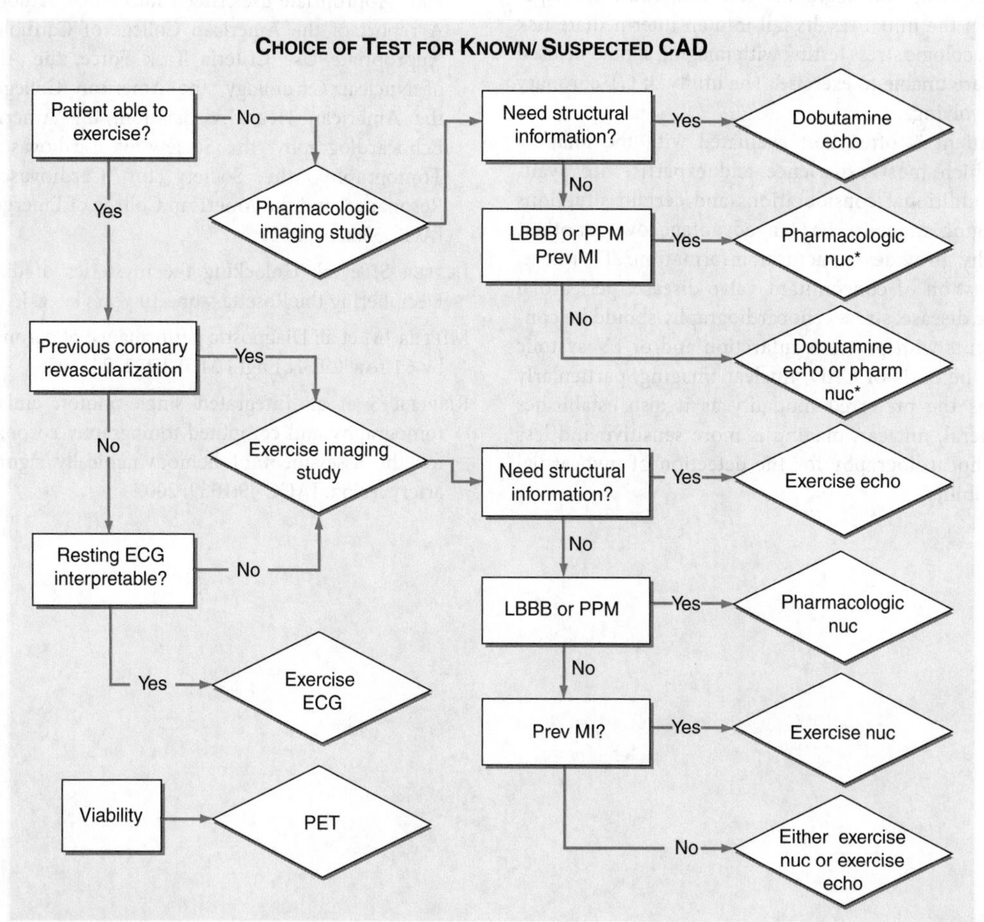

Figure 229-24 Flow diagram showing selection of initial stress test in a patient with chest pain. Patients who are able to exercise, without previous revascularization, and with an interpretable resting ECG can be tested with an exercise ECG. The appropriate imaging study for other patients depends on multiple factors (see text). LBBB, left bundle branch block; Prev MI-Reg ischemia, previous MI with a need to detect regional ischemia; Nuc, SPECT nuclear imaging study; Pharm, pharmacologic. *Consider PET if morbidly obese or female with large/dense breasts.

Aortic disease

Both CT scanning and MRI are the imaging modalities of choice for the evaluation of the stable patient with suspected aortic aneurysm or aortic dissection. In the acutely ill patient with suspected aortic dissection, either TEE or CT scanning is a reliable imaging modality.

Cardiac masses

2D TTE is the first test to rule out an intracardiac mass; masses >1.0 cm in diameter are usually well visualized. Intracardiac masses of smaller size may be visualized by TEE. CT scanning and MRI are optimal for evaluating masses extrinsic to the heart or involving the myocardium.

CHOOSING THE APPROPRIATE IMAGING TEST FOR THE EVALUATION OF KNOWN OR SUSPECTED CAD

The choice of an initial test should be based on the evaluation of the patient's resting electrocardiogram, the ability to perform exercise, the clinical features, the patient's body habitus, and the available local expertise and technology (Fig. 229-24). For the standard assessment of CAD, the exercise electrocardiographic test should be the initial consideration in patients with an interpretable electrocardiogram who are able to exercise. If there are resting electrocardiographic abnormalities, or if the patient has had prior coronary revascularization, an imaging modality (either nuclear imaging or echocardiography) should be used for initial evaluation. Imaging tests can add prognostic information to a standard exercise electrocardiographic test and, thus, are especially useful when the initial results fall into an intermediate risk category. Pharmacologic stress testing with imaging should be used in patients who are unable to exercise. The utility of CT coronary angiography is evolving.

While the patient is often best evaluated with the imaging modality for which most experience and expertise are available, there are additional considerations and certain situations where one imaging modality has an advantage over another. Echocardiography provides structural information. Therefore, if there is a question of concomitant valve disease, pericardial disease, or aortic disease, stress echocardiography should be considered. In patients with previous infarction and/or LV systolic dysfunction on the basis of CAD, nuclear imaging, particularly PET, or MRI, is the preferred modality as it also establishes viability. In general, nuclear imaging is more sensitive and less specific than echocardiography for the detection of myocardial ischemia and viability.

FURTHER READINGS

Berman DS et al: ACCF/ACR/AHA/ASNC/NASCI/SAIP/SCAI/SCCT 2009 Expert Consensus Document on Coronary CT Angiography. Circulation 119:e561, 2009

Greenland P et al: ACCF/AHA 2007 clinical expert consensus document on coronary artery calcium scoring by computed tomography in global cardiovascular risk assessment and in evaluation of patients with chest pain: A report of the American College of Cardiology Foundation Clinical Expert Consensus Task Force (ACCF/AHA Writing Committee to Update the 2000 Expert Consensus Document on Electron Beam Computed Tomography) developed in collaboration with the Society of Atherosclerosis Imaging and Prevention and the Society of Cardiovascular Computed Tomography. JACC 49:378, 2007

Hendel RC et al: ACCF/ACR/SCCT/SCMR/ASNC/NASCI/SCAI/SIR 2006 Appropriateness criteria for cardiac computed tomography and cardiac magnetic resonance imaging: A report of the American College of Cardiology Foundation Quality Strategic Directions Committee Appropriateness Criterial Working Group, American College of Radiology, Society of Cardiovascular Computed Tomography, Society for Cardiovascular Magnetic Resonance, American Society of Nuclear Cardiology, North American Society for Cardiac Imaging, Society for Cardiovascular Angiography and Interventions, and Society of Interventional Radiology. JACC 48:1475, 2006

——— et al: ACCF/ASNC/ACR/AHA/ASE/SCCT/SCMR/SNM 2009 Appropriate use criteria for cardiac radionuclide imaging: A report of the American College of Cardiology Foundation Appropriate Use Criteria Task Force, the American Society of Nuclear Cardiology, the American College of Radiology, the American Heart Association, the American Society of Echocardiography, the Society of Cardiovascular Computed Tomography, the Society for Cardiovascular Magnetic Resonance, and the American College of Emergency Physicians. JACC 53:2201, 2009

Lester SJ et al: Unlocking the mysteries of diastolic function: Deciphering the Rosetta stone 10 years later. JACC 51:679, 2008

Miller JM et al: Diagnostic performance of coronary angiography by 64-row CT. N Engl J Med 359:2324, 2008

Rispler S et al: Integrated single-photon emission computed tomography and computed tomography coronary angiography for the assessment of hemodynamically significant coronary artery lesion. JACC 49:1059, 2007

CHAPTER 230

Diagnostic Cardiac Catheterization and Coronary Angiography

Jane A. Leopold
David P. Faxon

Diagnostic cardiac catheterization and coronary angiography are considered the gold standard in the assessment of the anatomy and physiology of the heart and its associated vasculature. In 1929, Forssmann demonstrated the feasibility of cardiac catheterization in humans when he passed a urological catheter from a vein in his arm to his right atrium and documented the catheter's position in the heart by x-ray. In the 1940s, Cournand and Richards applied this technique to patients with cardiovascular disease to evaluate cardiac function.These three physicians were awarded the Nobel Prize in 1956. In 1958, Sones inadvertently performed the first selective coronary angiography when a catheter in the left ventricle slipped back across the aortic valve, engaged the right coronary artery, and power-injected 40 mL of contrast down the vessel. The resulting angiogram provided superb anatomic detail of the artery, and the patient suffered no adverse effects. Sones went on to develop selective coronary catheters, which were modified further by Judkins, who developed preformed catheters and allowed coronary artery angiography to gain widespread use as a diagnostic tool. In the United States, cardiac catheterization is the second most common operative procedure, with nearly three million procedures performed annually.

CARDIAC CATHETERIZATION

INDICATIONS, RISKS, AND PREPROCEDURE MANAGEMENT

Cardiac catheterization and coronary angiography are indicated to evaluate the extent and severity of cardiac disease in symptomatic patients and to determine if medical, surgical, or catheter-based interventions are warranted (Table 230-1). They are also used to exclude severe disease in symptomatic patients with equivocal findings on noninvasive studies and in patients with chest-pain syndromes of unclear etiology for whom a definitive diagnosis is necessary for management. Cardiac catheterization is not mandatory prior to cardiac surgery in some younger patients who have congenital or valvular heart disease that is well defined by noninvasive imaging and who do not have symptoms or risk factors that suggest concomitant coronary artery disease.

The risks associated with elective cardiac catheterization are relatively low, with a reported risk of 0.05% for myocardial infarction, 0.07% for stroke, and 0.08–0.14% for death. These risks increase substantially if the catheterization is performed emergently, during acute myocardial infarction or in hemodynamically unstable patients. Additional risks of the procedure include tachy- or brady-arrhythmias that require countershock or pharmacologic therapy, acute renal failure leading to transient or permanent dialysis, vascular complications that necessitate surgical repair, and significant access-site bleeding. Of these risks, vascular access-site bleeding is

TABLE 230-1 Indications for Cardiac Catheterization and Coronary Angiography

Coronary Artery Disease
Asymptomatic or Symptomatic
High risk for adverse outcome based on noninvasive testing
Sudden cardiac death
Sustained (>30 s) monomorphic ventricular tachycardia
Nonsustained (<30 s) polymorphic ventricular tachycardia
Symptomatic
Canadian Cardiology Society class III or IV angina on medical therapy
Unstable angina—high or intermediate risk
Chest-pain syndrome of unclear etiology and equivocal findings on noninvasive tests
Acute Myocardial Infarction
Reperfusion with primary percutaneous coronary intervention
Persistent or recurrent ischemia
Severe pulmonary edema
Cardiogenic shock or hemodynamic instability
Mechanical complications—mitral regurgitation, ventricular septal defect
Valvular Heart Disease
Suspected valve disease in symptomatic patients—dyspnea, angina, heart failure, syncope
Infective endocarditis with coronary embolization
Asymptomatic patients with aortic regurgitation and cardiac enlargement or ↓ ejection fraction
Prevalve surgery in older patients with coronary artery disease risk factors
Congestive Heart Failure
New onset with angina or suspected undiagnosed coronary artery disease
Congenital Heart Disease
Prior to surgical correction, when symptoms or noninvasive testing suggests coronary disease
Suspicion for congenital coronary anomalies
Forms of congenital heart disease associated with coronary anomalies
Pericardial Disease
Symptomatic patients with suspected cardiac tamponade or constrictive pericarditis
Cardiac Transplantation
Preoperative and postsurgical evaluation
Other Conditions
Hypertrophic cardiomyopathy with angina
Diseases of the aorta when knowledge of coronary artery involvement is necessary for management

Source: Adapted from American College of Cardiology/American Heart Association Ad Hoc Task Force on Practice Guidelines: ACC/AHA guidelines for coronary angiography. Circulation 1999;99:2345–2357.

the most common complication, occurring in 1.5–2.0% of patients, with major bleeding events associated with a worse short- and long-term outcome.

In patients who understand and accept the risks associated with cardiac catheterization, there are no absolute contraindications when the procedure is performed in anticipation of a life-saving intervention. Relative contraindications do, however, exist; these include decompensated congestive heart failure; acute renal failure; severe chronic renal insufficiency, unless dialysis is planned; bacteremia; acute stroke; active gastrointestinal bleeding; severe, uncorrected electrolyte abnormalities; a history of an anaphylactic/anaphylactoid reaction to iodinated contrast agents; and a history of allergy/bronchospasm to aspirin in patients for whom progression to a percutaneous coronary intervention is likely.

Contrast allergy and contrast-induced renal failure merit further consideration, because these adverse events may occur in otherwise healthy individuals and prophylactic measures exist to reduce risk. Allergic reactions to contrast agents occur in <5% of cases with severe anaphylactoid (clinically indistinguishable from anaphylaxis, but not mediated by an IgE mechanism) reactions occurring in 0.1%–0.2% of patients. Mild reactions manifest as nausea, vomiting, and urticaria, while severe anaphylactoid reactions lead to hypotensive shock, pulmonary edema, and cardiorespiratory arrest. Patients with a history of significant contrast allergy should be premedicated with corticosteroids and antihistamines (H_1- and H_2-blockers) and studies performed with nonionic, low-osmolar contrast agents that have a lower reported rate of allergic reactions.

Contrast-induced nephropathy, defined as an increase in creatinine >0.5 mg/dL or 25% above baseline that occurs 48–72 hours after contrast administration, occurs in ~2–7% of patients with rates of 20–30% reported in high-risk patients, including those with diabetes mellitus, congestive heart failure, chronic kidney disease, anemia, and older age. Dialysis is required in 0.3–0.7% of patients and is associated with a 5-fold increase in in-hospital mortality. For all patients, adequate intravascular volume expansion with intravenous 0.9% saline (1.0–1.5 mL/kg per hour) for 3–12 hours before and continued 6–24 hours after the procedure limits the risk of contrast-induced nephropathy. In patients with chronic kidney disease, additional pretreatment with *N*-acetylcysteine (Mucomist, 600 mg bid orally before and two days after catheterization) also decreases risk. Diabetic patients treated with metformin should stop the drug 48 hours prior to the procedure to limit the associated risk of lactic acidosis. Other strategies to decrease risk include the administration of sodium bicarbonate, although there is conflicting data regarding its efficacy; use of low- or iso-osmolar contrast agents; and limiting the volume of contrast to <100 mL per procedure.

Cardiac catheterization is performed after the patient has fasted for six hours and has received IV conscious sedation to remain awake but sedated during the procedure. All patients with suspected coronary artery disease are pretreated with 325 mg aspirin. In patients in whom the procedure is likely to progress to a percutaneous coronary intervention, a clopidogrel 600-mg loading dose followed by 75 mg daily should be started. Warfarin is held starting 48 hours prior to the catheterization to allow the international normalized ratio (INR) to fall to <2.0 and limit access-site bleeding complications. Cardiac catheterization is a sterile procedure, so antibiotic prophylaxis is not required.

■ TECHNIQUE

Cardiac catheterization and coronary angiography provide a detailed hemodynamic and anatomic assessment of the heart and coronary arteries. The selection of procedures is dependent upon the patient's symptoms and clinical condition, with some direction provided by noninvasive studies.

Vascular access

Cardiac catheterization procedures are performed using a percutaneous technique to enter the femoral artery and vein as the preferred access sites for left and right heart catheterization, respectively. A flexible sheath is inserted into the vessel over a guidewire, allowing diagnostic catheters to be introduced into the vessel and advanced toward the heart using fluoroscopic guidance. The brachial or radial artery may also be used as an arterial access site in patients with peripheral arterial disease that involves the abdominal aorta, iliac, or femoral vessels; severe iliac-artery tortuosity; morbid obesity; or preference for early postprocedure ambulation. Use of radial-artery access is gaining popularity owing to a lower rate of access-site bleeding complications. A normal Allen's test confirming dual blood supply to the hand from the radial and ulnar arteries is a prerequisite to access this site. The internal jugular vein serves as an alternate access site to the right heart when the patient has an inferior vena cava filter in place or requires prolonged hemodynamic monitoring.

Right heart catheterization

This procedure measures pressures in the right heart. Right heart catheterization is no longer a routine part of diagnostic cardiac catheterization, but it is reasonable in patients with unexplained dyspnea, valvular heart disease, pericardial disease, right and/or left ventricular dysfunction, congenital heart disease, and suspected intracardiac shunts. Right heart catheterization uses a balloon-tipped flotation catheter that is inserted into the femoral or jugular vein. Using fluoroscopic guidance, the catheter is advanced sequentially to the right atrium, right ventricle, pulmonary artery, and pulmonary wedge position (as a surrogate for left atrial pressure); in each cardiac chamber, pressure is measured and blood samples are obtained for oxygen-saturation analysis to screen for intracardiac shunts.

Left heart catheterization

This procedure measures pressures in the left heart as a determinant of left ventricular performance. With the aid of fluoroscopy, a catheter is guided to the ascending aorta and across the aortic valve into the left ventricle to provide a direct measure of left ventricular pressure. In patients with a tilting-disc prosthetic aortic valve, crossing the valve with a catheter is contraindicated and the left heart may be accessed from the right atrium using a needle-tipped catheter to puncture the atrial septum at the fossa ovalis. Once the catheter crosses from the right to the left atrium, it can be advanced across the mitral valve to the left ventricle. This technique is also used for mitral valvuloplasty. Heparin is given for prolonged procedures to limit the risk of stroke from embolism of clots that may form on the catheter.

■ HEMODYNAMICS

A comprehensive hemodynamic assessment involves obtaining pressure measurements in the right and left heart and peripheral arterial system and determining the cardiac output (Table 230-2). The shape and magnitude of the pressure waveforms provide important diagnostic information; an example of normal pressure tracings is shown in Fig. 230-1. In the absence of valvular heart disease, the atria and ventricles are "one chamber" during diastole when the tricuspid and mitral valves are open while in systole, when the pulmonary and aortic valves are open, the ventricles and their respective outflow tracts are considered "one chamber." These concepts form the basis by which hemodynamic measurements are used to assess valvular stenosis. When aortic stenosis is present, there is a systolic pressure gradient between the left ventricle and the aorta; when mitral stenosis is present, there is a diastolic

TABLE 230-2 Normal Values for Hemodynamic Measurements

Pressures (mmHg)	
Right atrium	
Mean	0–5
a wave	1–7
v wave	1–7
Right ventricle	
Peak systolic/end diastolic	17–32/1–7
Pulmonary artery	
Peak systolic/end diastolic	17–32/1–7
Mean	9–19
Pulmonary capillary wedge (mean)	4–12
Left atrium	
Mean	4–12
a wave	4–15
v wave	4–15
Left ventricle	
Peak systolic/end diastolic	90–140/5–12
Aorta	
Peak systolic/end diastolic	90–140/60–90
Mean	70–105
[Resistances (dyn-s)/cm^5]	
Systemic vascular resistance	900–1400
Pulmonary vascular resistance	40–120
Oxygen Consumption Index [(L-min)/m^2]	115–140
Arteriovenous oxygen difference (vol %)	3.5–4.8
Cardiac index [(L-min)/m^2]	2.8–4.2

pressure gradient between the pulmonary capillary wedge (left atrial) pressure and the left ventricle (Fig. 230-2). Hemodynamic measurements also discriminate between aortic stenosis and hypertrophic obstructive cardiomyopathy where the asymmetrically hypertrophied septum creates a dynamic intraventricular pressure gradient during ventricular systole. The magnitude of this obstruction is measured using an end-hole catheter positioned at the left ventricular apex that is pulled back while recording pressure; once the catheter has passed the septal obstruction and is positioned in the apex of the left ventricle, a gradient can be measured between the left ventricular apex and the aorta. Hypertrophic obstructive cardiomyopathy is confirmed by the Brockenbrough-Braunwald sign: following a premature ventricular contraction, there is an increase in the left ventricular–aorta pressure gradient with a simultaneous decrease in the aortic pulse pressure. These findings are absent in aortic stenosis.

Regurgitant valvular lesions increase volume (and pressure) in the "receiving" cardiac chamber. In severe mitral and tricuspid regurgitation, the increase in blood flow to the atria takes place during ventricular systole, leading to an increase in the *v* wave (two times greater than the mean pressure). Severe aortic regurgitation leads to a decrease in aortic diastolic pressure with a concomitant rise in left ventricular end-diastolic pressure, resulting in equalization of pressures between the two chambers at enddiastole.

Hemodynamic measurements are also used to differentiate between cardiac tamponade, constrictive pericarditis, and restrictive cardiomyopathy. In cardiac tamponade, right atrial pressure is increased with a decreased "y" descent, indicative of impaired right atrial emptying in diastole, and there is diastolic equalization of pressures in all cardiac chambers. In constrictive pericarditis, right atrial pressure is elevated with a prominent "y" descent, indicating rapid filling of the right ventricle during early diastole. A diastolic dip and plateau or "square root sign," in the ventricular waveforms due to an abrupt halt in ventricular filling during diastole; right ventricular and pulmonary artery pressures are elevated; and discordant pressure changes in the right and left ventricles with

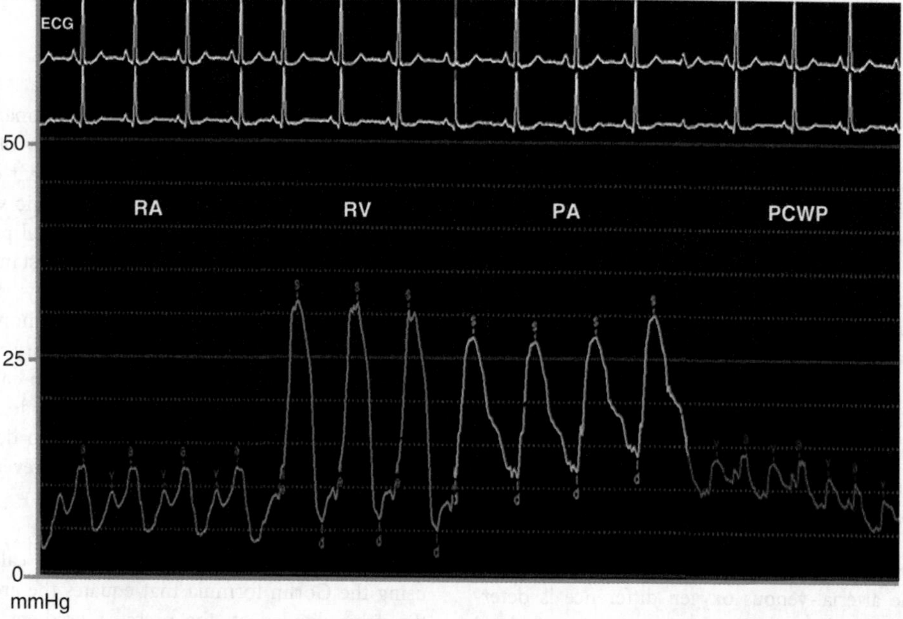

Figure 230-1 Normal hemodynamic waveforms recorded during right heart catheterization. Atrial pressure tracings have a characteristic "a" wave that reflects atrial contraction and a "*v*" wave that reflects pressure changes in the atrium during ventricular systole. Ventricular pressure tracings have a low pressure diastolic filling period and a sharp rise in pressure that occurs during ventricular systole. RA, right atrium; RV, right ventricle; PA, pulmonary artery; PCWP, pulmonary capillary wedge pressure; s, systole; d, diastole.

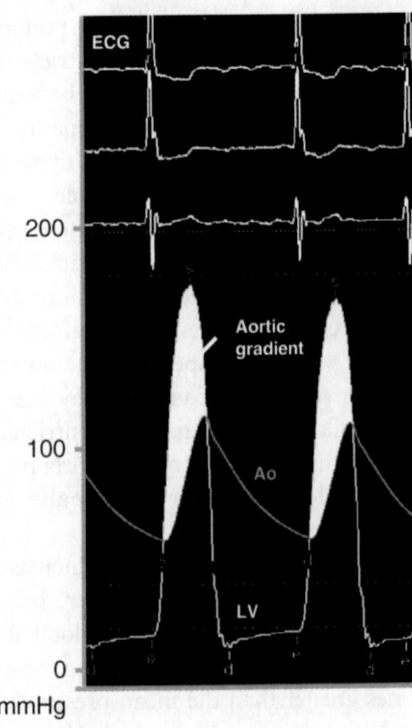

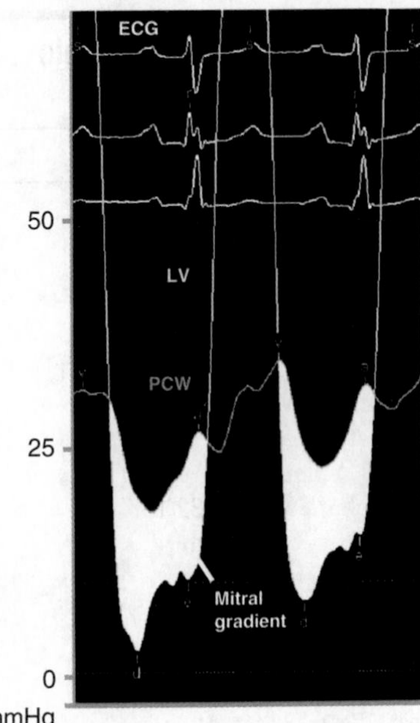

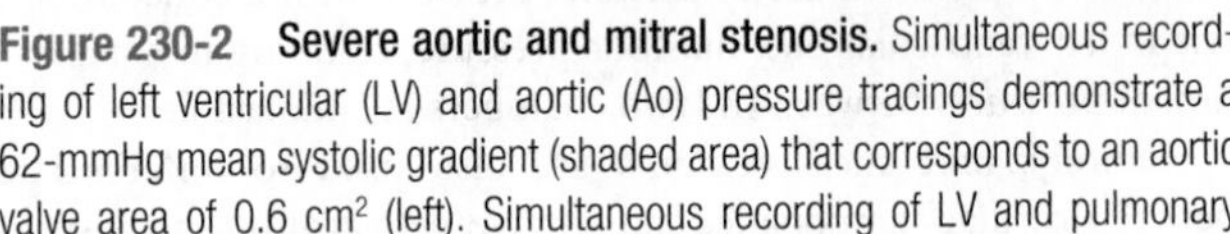

Figure 230-2 Severe aortic and mitral stenosis. Simultaneous recording of left ventricular (LV) and aortic (Ao) pressure tracings demonstrate a 62-mmHg mean systolic gradient (shaded area) that corresponds to an aortic valve area of 0.6 cm² (left). Simultaneous recording of LV and pulmonary capillary wedge (PCW) pressure tracings reveal a 14-mmHg mean diastolic gradient (shaded area) that is consistent with critical mitral stenosis (mitral valve area = 0.5 cm²). S, systole; d, diastole; e, end diastole.

inspiration (right ventricular systolic pressure increases while left ventricular systolic pressure decreases) are observed. The latter hemodynamic phenomenon is the most specific for constriction. Restrictive cardiomyopathy may be distinguished from constrictive pericarditis by a marked increase in right ventricular and pulmonary artery systolic pressures (usually >60 mmHg), a separation of the left and right ventricular diastolic pressures by >5 mmHg (at baseline or with acute volume loading), and concordant changes in left and right ventricular diastolic filling pressures with inspiration (both increase).

Cardiac output

Cardiac output is measured by the Fick method or the thermodilution technique or calculated from left ventricular angiography. Typically, the Fick method and thermodilution technique are both performed during cardiac catheterization, although the Fick method is considered more reliable in the presence of tricuspid regurgitation and in low-output states. The Fick method uses oxygen as the indicator substance and is based on the principle that the amount of a substance taken up or released by an organ (oxygen consumption) is equal to the product of its blood flow (cardiac output) and the difference in the concentration of the substance in the arterial and venous circulation (arterial-venous oxygen difference). Thus, the formula for calculating the Fick cardiac output is:

Cardiac output (L/min) = [oxygen consumption (mL/min)]/[arterial-venous oxygen difference (mL/L)]

Oxygen consumption is estimated as 125 mL oxygen/minute × body surface area, and the arterial-venous oxygen difference is determined by first calculating the oxygen carrying capacity of blood [hemoglobin (g/100 mL) × 1.36 (mL oxygen/g hemoglobin) × 10] and multiplying this product by the fractional oxygen saturation. The thermodilution method measures a substance that is injected into and adequately mixes with blood. In contemporary practice, thermodilution cardiac outputs are measured using temperature as the indicator. Measurements are made with a thermistor-tipped catheter that detects temperature deviations in the pulmonary artery after the injection of 10 mL of room-temperature normal saline into the right atrium. Cardiac output may also be calculated from the left ventriculogram by first determining left ventricular volumes in end-diastole and end-systole using the area-length method. Cardiac output is equal to the heart rate × stroke volume, which is the difference between the end-diastolic volume and the end-systolic volume.

Vascular resistance

Resistance across the systemic and pulmonary circulations is calculated by extrapolating from Ohm's law of electrical resistance and is equal to the mean pressure gradient divided by the mean flow (cardiac output). Therefore, systemic vascular resistance is [(mean aortic pressure − mean right atrial pressure)/cardiac output] multiplied by 80 to convert the resistance from Wood units to dyn-s-cm^{-5}. Similarly, the pulmonary vascular resistance is [(mean pulmonary artery − mean pulmonary capillary wedge pressure)/cardiac output] × 80. Pulmonary vascular resistance is lowered by oxygen, nitroprusside, calcium channel blockers, prostacyclin infusions, and inhaled nitric oxide; these therapies may be administered during catheterization to determine if increased pulmonary vascular resistance is fixed or reversible.

Valve area

Hemodynamic data may also be used to calculate the valve area using the Gorlin formula that equates the area to the flow across the valve divided by the pressure gradient between the cardiac chambers surrounding the valve. The formula for the assessment of valve area is: Area = [cardiac output (cm³/min)/(systolic ejection period or diastolic filling period)(heart rate)]/44.3 C × square root of the pressure gradient, where C = 1 for aortic valve and 0.85 for the mitral valve. A valve area of <1.0 cm^2 and a mean gradient of greater than 40 mmHg indicate severe aortic stenosis, while a valve area of <1.5 cm^2 and a mean gradient >5–10 mmHg is consistent with moderate-to-severe mitral stenosis; in symptomatic patients with a mitral valve area >1.5 cm^2, a mean gradient >15 mmHg, pulmonary artery pressure >60 mmHg, or a pulmonary artery wedge pressure >25 mmHg after exercise is also considered significant and may warrant intervention. The modified Hakki formula has also been used to estimate aortic valve area. This formula calculates the valve area as the cardiac output (L/min) divided by the square root of the pressure gradient. Aortic valve area calculations based on the Gorlin formula are flow-dependent and, therefore, for patients with low cardiac outputs, it is imperative to determine if a decreased valve area actually reflects a fixed stenosis or is overestimated by a low cardiac output and stroke volume that is insufficient to open the valve leaflets fully. In these instances, cautious hemodynamic manipulation using dobutamine to increase the cardiac output and recalculation of the aortic valve area may be necessary.

Intracardiac shunts

In patients with congenital heart disease, detection, localization, and quantification of the intracardiac shunt should be evaluated. A shunt should be suspected when there is unexplained arterial desaturation or increased oxygen saturation of venous blood. A "step up" or increase in oxygen content indicates the presence of a left-to-right shunt while a "step down" indicates a right-to-left shunt. The shunt is localized by detecting a difference in oxygen saturation levels of 5–7% between adjacent cardiac chambers. The severity of the shunt is determined by the ratio of pulmonary blood flow (Q_p) to the systemic blood flow (Q_s), or Q_p/Q_s = [(systemic arterial oxygen content − mixed venous oxygen content)/pulmonary vein oxygen content − pulmonary artery oxygen content]. For an atrial septal defect, a shunt ratio of 1.5 is considered significant and factored with other clinical variables to determine the need for intervention. When a congenital ventricular septal defect is present, a shunt ratio of ≥2.0 with evidence of left ventricular volume overload is a class I indication for surgical correction.

VENTRICULOGRAPHY AND AORTOGRAPHY

Ventriculography to assess left ventricular function may be performed during cardiac catheterization. A pigtail catheter is advanced retrograde across the aortic valve into the left ventricle and 30–45 mL of contrast is power-injected to visualize the left ventricular chamber during the cardiac cycle. The ventriculogram is usually performed in the right anterior oblique projection to examine wall motion and mitral valve function. Normal wall motion is observed as symmetric contraction of all segments; hypokinetic segments have decreased contraction, akinetic segments do not contract, and dyskinetic segments appear to bulge paradoxically during systole (Fig. 230-3). Ventriculography may also reveal a left ventricular aneurysm, pseudoaneurysm, or diverticulum and can be used to assess mitral valve prolapse and the severity of mitral regurgitation. The degree of mitral regurgitation is estimated by comparing the density of contrast opacification of the left atrium with that of

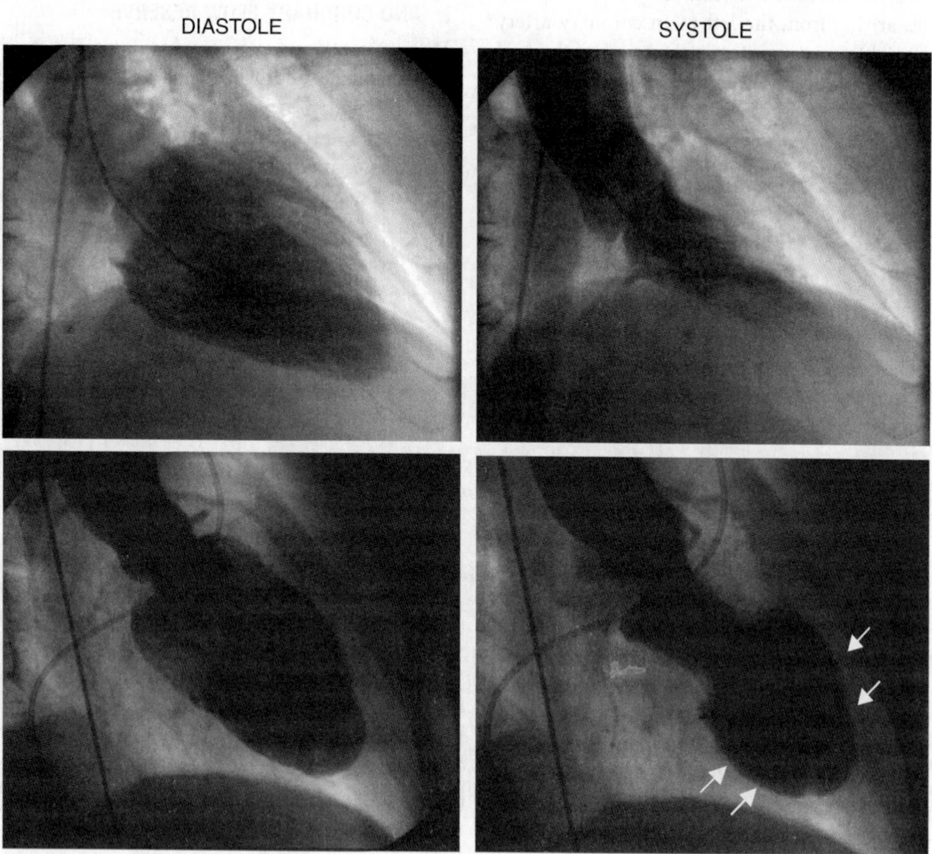

Figure 230-3 Left ventriculogram at end diastole (left) and end systole (right). In patients with normal left ventricular function, the ventriculogram reveals symmetric contraction of all walls (top). Patients with coronary artery disease may have wall motion abnormalities on ventriculography as seen in this 60-year-old male following a large anterior myocardial infarction. In systole, the anterior, apical, and inferior walls are akinetic (white arrows) (bottom).

the left ventricle. Minimal contrast reflux into the left atrium is considered 1+ mitral regurgitation while contrast density in the left atrium that is greater than that in the left ventricle with reflux of contrast into the pulmonary veins within three beats defines 4+ mitral regurgitation.

Aortography in the cardiac catheterization laboratory visualizes abnormalities of the ascending aorta, including aneurysmal dilation and involvement of the great vessels, as well as dissection with compression of the true lumen by an intimal flap that separates the true and false lumina. Aortography can also be used to identify patent saphenous vein grafts that elude selective cannulation, identify shunts that involve the aorta such as a patent ductus arteriosus, and provide a qualitative assessment of aortic regurgitation using a 1+–4+ scale similar to that used for mitral regurgitation.

CORONARY ANGIOGRAPHY

Selective coronary angiography is almost always performed during cardiac catheterization and is used to define the coronary anatomy and determine the extent of epicardial coronary artery and coronary artery bypass graft disease. Specially shaped coronary catheters are used to engage the left and right coronary ostia. Hand injection of radiopaque contrast agents create a coronary "luminogram" that is recorded on a radiographic images (cine angiography). Because the coronary arteries are three-dimensional objects that are in motion with the cardiac cycle, angiograms of the vessels using several different orthogonal projections are taken to best visualize the vessels without overlap or foreshortening.

The normal coronary anatomy is highly variable between individuals, but, in general, there are two coronary ostia and three major coronary vessels—the left anterior descending, the left circumflex, and the right coronary arteries with the left anterior descending and left circumflex arteries arising from the left main coronary artery (Fig. 230-4). When the right coronary artery is the origin of the A-V nodal branch, the posterior descending artery, and the posterior lateral vessels, the circulation is defined as right dominant; this is found in ~85% of individuals. When these branches arise from the left circumflex artery as occurs in ~5% of individuals, the circulation is defined as left dominant. The remaining ~10% of patients have a codominant circulation with vessels arising from both the right and left coronary circulation. In some patients, a ramus intermedius branch arises directly from the left main coronary artery; this finding is a normal variant. Coronary artery anomalies occur in 1–2% of patients, with separate ostia for the left anterior descending and left circumflex arteries being the most common (0.41%).

Coronary angiography visualizes coronary artery stenoses as luminal narrowings on the cine angiogram. The degree of narrowing is referred to as the percent stenosis and is determined visually by comparing the most severely diseased segment with a proximal or distal "normal segment" mg; a stenosis >50% is considered significant (Fig. 230-5). Online quantitative coronary angiography can provide a more accurate assessment of the percent stenosis and lessen the tendency to overestimate lesion severity visually. The presence of a myocardial bridge, which most commonly involves the left anterior descending artery, may be mistaken for a significant stenosis; this occurs when a portion of the vessel dips below the epicardial surface into the myocardium and is subject to compressive forces during ventricular systole. The key to differentiating a myocardial bridge from a fixed stenosis is that the "stenosed" part of the vessel returns to normal during diastole. Coronary calcification is also seen during angiography prior to the injection of contrast agents. Collateral blood vessels may be seen traversing from one vessel to the distal vasculature of a severely stenosed or totally occluded vessel. Thrombolysis in myocardial infarction (TIMI) flow grade, a measure of the relative duration of time that it takes for contrast to opacify the coronary artery fully, may provide an additional clue to the degree of lesion severity, and the presence of TIMI grade 1 or 2 flow suggests that a significant coronary artery stenosis is present.

INTRAVASCULAR ULTRASOUND, FRACTIONAL FLOW RESERVE, AND CORONARY FLOW RESERVE

During coronary angiography, intermediate stenoses (40–70%), indeterminate findings, or anatomic findings that are incongruous with the patient's symptoms may require further interrogation. In these cases, intravascular ultrasound provides a more accurate anatomic assessment of the coronary artery and the degree of coronary atherosclerosis (Fig. 230-5). Intravascular ultrasound is performed using a small flexible catheter with a 40-mHz transducer at its tip

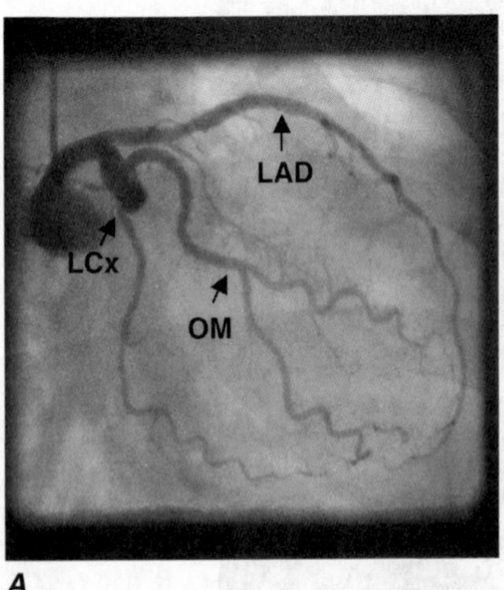

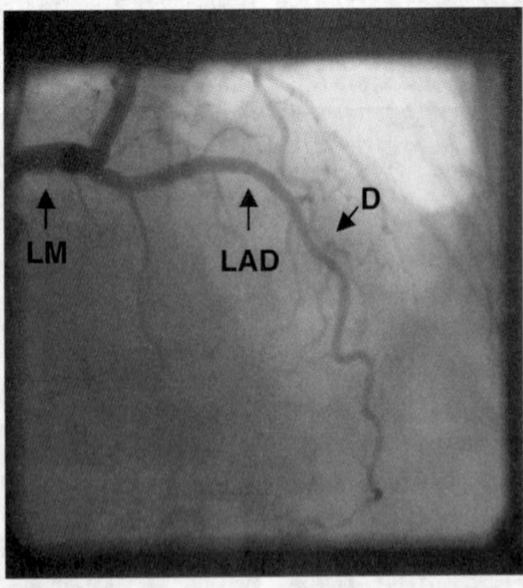

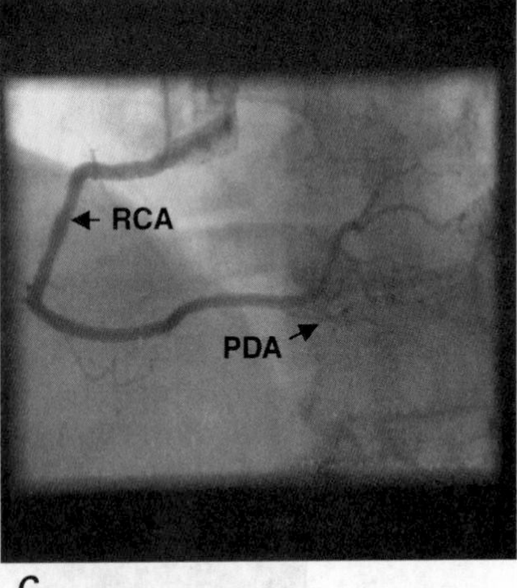

Figure 230-4 Normal coronary artery anatomy. ***A.*** Coronary angiogram showing the left circumflex (LCx) artery and its obtuse marginal (OM) branches. The left anterior descending artery (LAD) is also seen but may be foreshortened in this view. ***B.*** The LAD and its diagonal (D) branches are best seen in cranial views. In this angiogram, the left main (LM) coronary artery is also seen. ***C.*** The right coronary artery gives off the posterior descending artery (PDA) so this is a right dominant circulation.

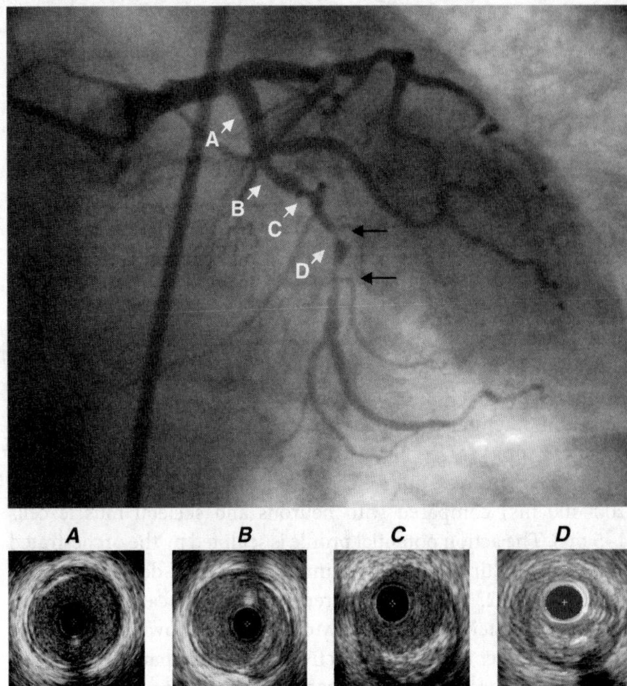

Figure 230-5 Coronary stenoses on cine angiogram and intravascular ultrasound. Significant stenoses in the coronary artery are seen as narrowings (black arrows) of the vessel. Intravascular ultrasound shows a normal segment of artery (A), areas with eccentric plaque (B, C), and near total obliteration of the lumen at the site of the significant stenosis (D). Note that the intravascular ultrasound catheter is present in the images as a black circle.

that is advanced into the coronary artery over a guidewire. Data from intravascular ultrasound studies may be used to image atherosclerotic plaque precisely, determine luminal cross-sectional area, and measure vessel size; it is also used during or following percutaneous coronary intervention to assess the stenosis and determine the adequacy of stent placement. Measurement of the fractional flow reserve provides a functional assessment of the stenosis. The fractional flow reserve is the ratio of the pressure in the coronary artery distal to the stenosis divided by the pressure in the artery proximal to the stenosis at maximal vasodilation. Fractional flow reserve is measured using a coronary pressure–sensor guidewire at rest and at maximal hyperemia following the injection of adenosine. A fractional flow reserve of <0.75 indicates a hemodynamically significant stenosis that would benefit from intervention. Measurement of coronary flow reserve is another technique to assess the functional severity of a stenosis, although this technique is used with less frequency than fractional flow reserve. The coronary flow reserve is the maximal coronary blood flow increase above resting conditions during maximal vasodilation and is a measure of both epicardial coronary artery and microvascular function. Coronary flow reserve is determined using a Doppler flow guidewire before and after the administration of adenosine to induce hyperemia. A coronary flow reserve <2:1 after maximal hyperemia is considered abnormal.

POSTPROCEDURE CARE

Once the procedure is completed, vascular access sheaths are removed. If the femoral approach is used, direct manual compression or vascular closure devices that immediately close the arteriotomy site with a staple/clip, collagen plug, or suture are used to achieve hemostasis. These devices decrease the length of bed rest (from 6 hours to 2–4 hours) and improve patient satisfaction but have not been shown definitively to be superior to manual compression with respect to access-site complications. When cardiac catheterization is performed as an elective outpatient procedure, the patient completes postprocedure bed rest in a monitored setting and is discharged home with instructions to liberalize fluids because contrast agents promote an osmotic diuresis, to avoid strenuous activity, and to observe the vascularaccess site for signs of complications. Overnight hospitalization may be required for high-risk patients with significant comorbidities, patients with complications occurring during the catheterization, or in patients who have undergone a percutaneous coronary intervention. Hypotension early after the procedure may be due to inadequate fluid replacement or retroperitoneal bleeding from the access site.

FURTHER READINGS

Baim DS (ed): *Grossman's Cardiac Catheterization, Angiography, and Intervention,* 7th ed. Baltimore, Lippincott Williams & Wilkins, 2006

Kern MJ (ed): *Hemodynamic Rounds: Interpretation of Cardiac Pathophysiology From Pressure Waveform Analysis,* 3rd ed. Hoboken, Wiley-Blackwell, 2009

Nicholls SJ et al: Intravascular ultrasound-derived measures of cornoary atherosclerotic plaque burden and clinical outcome. JACC 55:2399, 2010

Ryan TJ: The coronary angiogram and its seminal contributions to cardiovascular medicine over five decades. Circulation 106:752, 2002

Tobis J: Assessment of intermediate severity coronary lesions in the catheterization laboratory. JACC 49:839-48, 2007

CHAPTER 231 Principles of Electrophysiology

David D. Spragg
Gordon F. Tomaselli

HISTORY AND INTRODUCTION

The field of cardiac electrophysiology was ushered in with the development of the electrocardiogram (ECG) by Einthoven at the turn of the twentieth century. The recording of cellular membrane currents revealed that the body surface ECG is the timed sum of the cellular action potentials in the atria and ventricles. In the late 1960s, the development of intracavitary recording, in particular the ability to record His bundle electrograms with programmed stimulation of the heart, marked the beginning of contemporary clinical electrophysiology. Adoption of radio frequency technology to ablate cardiac tissue in the early 1990s heralded the birth of interventional cardiac electrophysiology.

The clinical problem of sudden death caused by ventricular arrhythmias, most commonly in the setting of coronary obstruction, was recognized as early as the late nineteenth century. The problem was vexing and led to the development of pharmacologic and nonpharmacologic therapies, including transthoracic defibrillators, cardiac massage, and, most recently, implantable defibrillators. Over time the limitations of antiarrhythmic drug therapy have been highlighted repeatedly in clinical trials, and now ablation and devices are first-line therapy for a number of cardiac arrhythmias.

In the last two decades, the genetic basis of a number of heritable arrhythmias has been elucidated, revealing important insights into the mechanisms not only of these rare arrhythmias but also of similar rhythm disturbances observed in more common forms of heart disease.

DESCRIPTIVE PHYSIOLOGY

The normal cardiac impulse is generated by pacemaker cells in the sinoatrial node situated at the junction of the right atrium and the superior vena cava (see Fig. 228-1). This impulse is transmitted slowly through nodal tissue to the anatomically complex atria, where it is conducted more rapidly to the atrioventricular node (AVN), inscribing the P wave of the ECG (see Fig. 228-2). There is a perceptible delay in conduction through the anatomically and functionally heterogeneous AVN. The time needed for activation of the atria and the AVN delay is represented as the PR interval of the ECG. The AVN is the only electrical connection between the atria and the ventricles in the normal heart. The electrical impulse emerges from the AVN and is transmitted to the His-Purkinje system, specifically the common bundle of His, then the left and right bundle branches, and then to the Purkinje network, facilitating activation of ventricular muscle. In normal circumstances, the ventricles are activated rapidly in a well-defined fashion that is determined by the course of the Purkinje network, and this inscribes the QRS complex (see Fig. 228-2). Recovery of electrical excitability occurs more slowly and is governed by the time of activation and duration of regional action potentials. The relative brevity of epicardial action potentials in the ventricle results in repolarization that occurs first on the epicardial surface and then proceeds to the endocardium, which inscribes a T wave normally of the same polarity as the QRS complex. The duration of activation and recovery is determined by the action potential duration represented on the body surface ECG by the QT interval (see Fig. 228-2).

Cardiac myocytes exhibit a characteristically long action potential (200–400 ms) compared with neurons and skeletal muscle cells (1–5 ms). The action potential profile is sculpted by the orchestrated activity of multiple distinctive time- and voltage-dependent ionic currents (Fig. 231-1*A*). The currents in turn are carried by transmembrane proteins that passively conduct ions down their electrochemical gradients through selective pores (ion channels), actively transport ions against their electrochemical gradient (pumps, transporters), or electrogenically exchange ionic species (exchangers).

Action potentials in the heart are regionally distinct. The regional variability in cardiac action potentials is a result of differences in the number and types of ion channel proteins expressed by different cell types in the heart. Further, unique sets of ionic currents are active in pacemaking and muscle cells, and the relative contributions of these currents may vary in the same cell type in different regions of the heart (Fig. 231-1*A*).

Ion channels are complex, multisubunit transmembrane glycoproteins that open and close in response to a number of biologic stimuli, including a change in membrane voltage, ligand binding (directly to the channel or to a G protein–coupled receptor), and mechanical deformation (Fig. 231-2). Other ion motive exchangers and transporters contribute importantly to cellular excitability in the heart. Ion pumps establish and maintain the ionic gradients across the cell membrane that serve as the driving force for current flow through ion channels. Transporters or exchangers that do not move ions in an electrically neutral manner (e.g., the sodium-calcium exchanger transports three Na^+ for one Ca^{2+}) are termed *electrogenic* and contribute directly to the action potential profile.

The most abundant superfamily of ion channels expressed in the heart is voltage gated. Several structural themes are common to all voltage-dependent ion channels. First, the architecture is modular, consisting either of four homologous subunits (e.g., K channels) or of four internally homologous domains (e.g., Na and Ca channels). Second, the proteins fold around a central pore lined by amino acids that exhibit exquisite conservation within a given channel family of like selectivity (e.g., jellyfish, eel, fruit fly, and human Na channels have very similar P segments). Third, the general strategy for activation gating (opening and closing in response to changes in membrane voltage) is highly conserved: the fourth transmembrane segment (S4), studded with positively charged residues, lies within the membrane field and moves in response to depolarization, opening the channel. Fourth, most ion channel complexes include not only the pore-forming proteins (α subunits) but also auxiliary subunits (e.g., β subunits) that modify channel function (Fig. 231-2).

Na and Ca channels are the primary carriers of depolarizing current in both the atria and the ventricles; inactivation of these currents and activation of repolarizing K currents hyperpolarize the heart cells, reestablishing the negative resting membrane potential (Fig. 231-1*B*). The *plateau phase* is a time when little current is

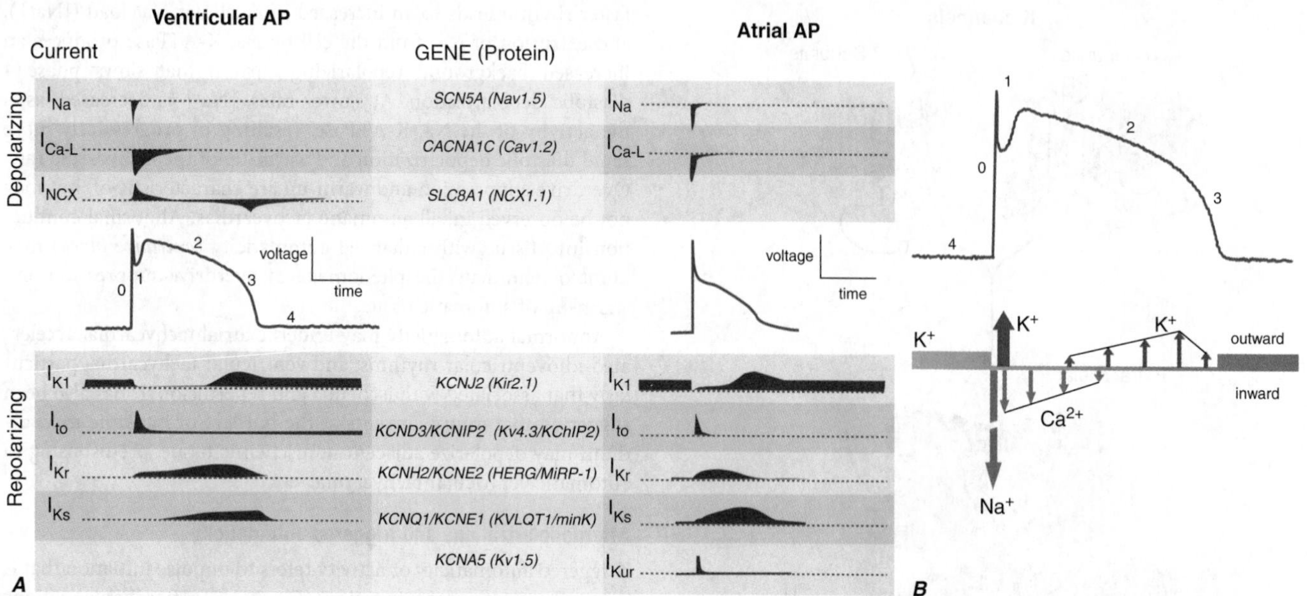

Figure 231-1 ***A.*** Cellular atrial and ventricular action potentials. Phases 0–4 are the rapid upstroke, early repolarization, plateau, late repolarization, and diastole, respectively. The ionic currents and their respective genes are shown above and below the action potentials. The currents that underlie the action potentials vary in atrial and ventricular myocytes. ***B.*** A ventricular action potential with a schematic of the ionic currents flowing during the phases of the action potential. Potassium current (I_{K1}) is the principal current during phase 4 and determines the resting membrane potential of the myocyte. Sodium current generates the upstroke of the action potential (phase 0); activation of I_{to} with inactivation of the Na current inscribes early repolarization (phase 1). The plateau (phase 2) is generated by a balance of repolarizing potassium currents and depolarizing calcium current. Inactivation of the calcium current with persistent activation of potassium currents (predominantly I_{Kr} and I_{Ks}) causes phase 3 repolarization.

flowing, and relatively minor changes in depolarizing or repolarizing currents can have profound effects on the shape and duration of the action profile. Mutations in subunits of these channel proteins produce arrhythmogenic alterations in the action potentials that cause long and short QT syndrome, idiopathic ventricular fibrillation, familial atrial fibrillation, and some forms of conduction system disease.

MECHANISMS OF CARDIAC ARRHYTHMIAS

Cardiac arrhythmias result from abnormalities of electrical impulse generation, conduction, or both. Bradyarrhythmias typically arise from disturbances in impulse formation at the level of the sinoatrial node or from disturbances in impulse propagation at any level, including exit block from the sinus node, conduction block in the AV node, and impaired conduction in the His-Purkinje system. Tachyarrhythmias can be classified according to mechanism, including enhanced automaticity (spontaneous depolarization of atrial, junctional, or ventricular pacemakers), reentry (circus propagation of a depolarizing wavefront), or triggered arrhythmias (initiated by afterdepolarizations) occurring during or immediately after cardiac repolarization, during phase 3 or 4 of the action potential. A variety of mapping and pacing maneuvers typically performed during invasive electrophysiologic testing can often determine the underlying mechanism of a tachyarrhythmia (Table 231-1).

Alterations in impulse initiation: Automaticity

Spontaneous (phase 4) diastolic depolarization underlies the property of automaticity (pacemaking) characteristic of cells in the sinoatrial (SA) and atrioventricular (AV) nodes, His-Purkinje system, coronary sinus, and pulmonary veins. Phase 4 depolarization results from the concerted action of a number of ionic currents, including K^+ currents, Ca^{2+} currents, electrogenic Na, K-ATPase, the Na-Ca exchanger, and the so-called funny, or pacemaker, current (I_f); however, the relative importance of these currents remains controversial.

The rate of phase 4 depolarization and, therefore, the firing rates of pacemaker cells are dynamically regulated. Prominent among the factors that modulate phase 4 is autonomic nervous system tone. The negative chronotropic effect of activation of the parasympathetic nervous system is a result of the release of acetylcholine that binds to muscarinic receptors, releasing G protein βγ subunits that activate a potassium current (I_{KACh}) in nodal and atrial cells. The resulting increase in K^+ conductance opposes membrane depolarization, slowing the rate of rise of phase 4 of the action potential. Conversely, augmentation of sympathetic nervous system tone increases myocardial catecholamine concentrations, which activate both α– and β–adrenergic receptors. The effect of $β_1$-adrenergic stimulation predominates in pacemaking cells, augmenting both L-type Ca current (I_{Ca-L}) and I_f, thus increasing the slope of phase 4. Enhanced sympathetic nervous system activity can dramatically increase the rate of firing of SA nodal cells, producing sinus tachycardia with rates >200 beats/min. By contrast, the increased rate of firing of Purkinje cells is more limited, rarely producing ventricular tachyarrhythmias >120 beats/min.

Normal automaticity may be affected by a number other factors associated with heart disease. Hypokalemia and ischemia may reduce the activity of Na, K-ATPase, thereby reducing the background repolarizing current and enhancing phase 4 diastolic depolarization. The end result would be an increase in the spontaneous firing rate of pacemaking cells. Modest increases in extracellular potassium may render the maximum diastolic potential more positive, thereby also increasing the firing rate of pacemaking cells. A more significant increase in $[K^+]_o$, however, renders the heart inexcitable by depolarizing the membrane potential.

Normal or enhanced automaticity of subsidiary latent pacemakers produces escape rhythms in the setting of failure of more dominant pacemakers. Suppression of a pacemaker cell by a

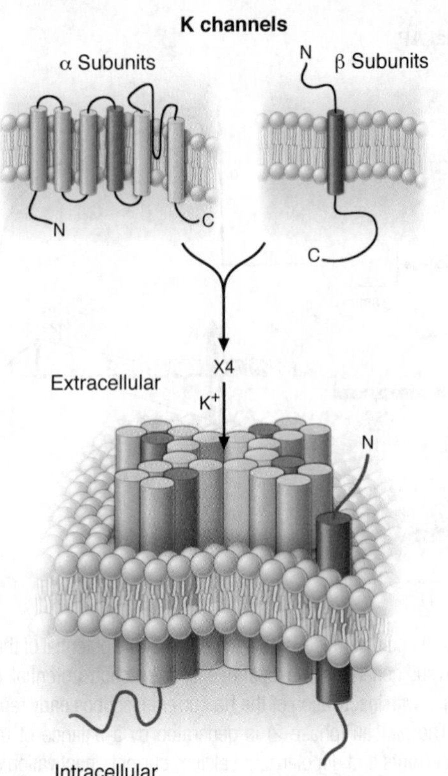

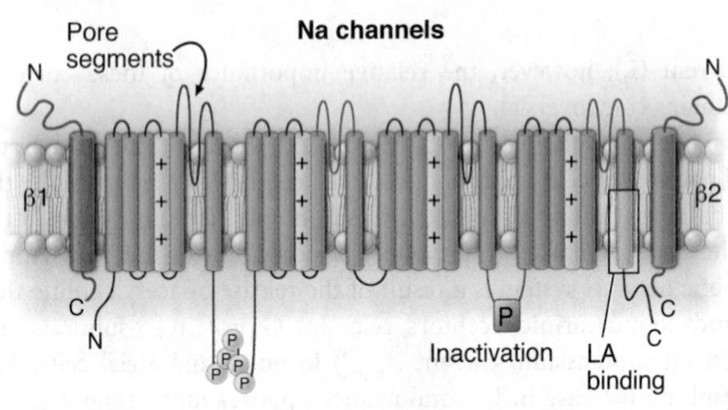

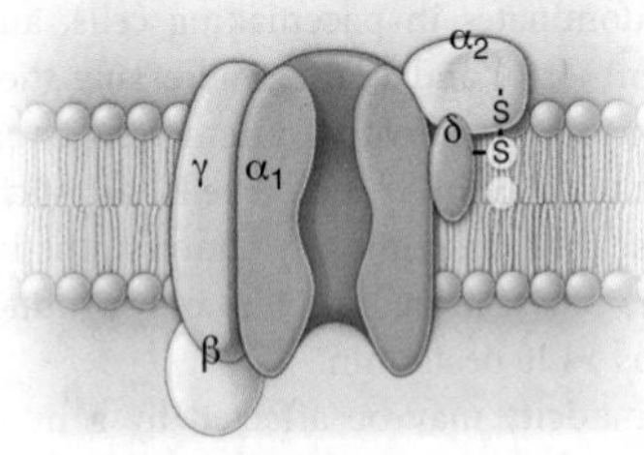

Figure 231-2 Topology and subunit composition of the voltage-dependent ion channels. Potassium channels are formed by the tetramerization of α or pore-forming subunits and one or more β subunits; only single β subunits are shown for clarity. Sodium and calcium channels are composed of α subunits with four homologous domains and one or more ancillary subunits. In all channel types the loop of protein between the fifth and sixth membrane-spanning repeat in each subunit or domain forms the ion-selective pore. In the case of the sodium channel, the channel is a target for phosphorylation, the linker between the third and fourth homologous domain is critical to inactivation, and the sixth membrane-spanning repeat in the fourth domain is important in local anesthetic antiarrhythmic drug binding.

faster rhythm leads to an increased intracellular Na^+ load ($[Na^+]_i$), and extrusion of Na^+ from the cell by Na, K-ATPase produces an increased background repolarizing current that slows phase 4 diastolic depolarization. At slower rates, $[Na^+]_i$ is decreased, as is the activity of the Na, K-ATPase, resulting in progressively more rapid diastolic depolarization and warm-up of the tachycardia rate. Overdrive suppression and warm-up are characteristic of, but may not be observed in, all automatic tachycardias. Abnormal conduction into tissue with enhanced automaticity (*entrance block*) may blunt or eliminate the phenomena of overdrive suppression and warm-up of automatic tissue.

Abnormal automaticity may underlie atrial tachycardia, accelerated idioventricular rhythms, and ventricular tachycardia, particularly that associated with ischemia and reperfusion. It has also been suggested that injury currents at the borders of ischemic myocardium may depolarize adjacent nonischemic tissue, predisposing to automatic ventricular tachycardia.

Afterdepolarizations and triggered automaticity

Triggered automaticity or activity refers to impulse initiation that is dependent on afterdepolarizations (Fig. 231-3). Afterdepolarizations are membrane voltage oscillations that occur during (early afterdepolarizations, EADs) or after (delayed afterdepolarizations, DADs) an action potential.

The cellular feature common to the induction of DADs is the presence of an increased Ca^{2+} load in the cytosol and sarcoplasmic reticulum. Digitalis glycoside toxicity, catecholamines, and ischemia all can enhance Ca^{2+} loading sufficiently to produce DADs. Accumulation of lysophospholipids in ischemic myocardium with consequent Na^+ and Ca^{2+} overload has been suggested as a mechanism for DADs and triggered automaticity. Cells from damaged areas or cells that survive a myocardial infarction may display spontaneous release of calcium from the sarcoplasmic reticulum, and this may generate "waves" of intracellular calcium elevation and arrhythmias.

EADs occur during the action potential and interrupt the orderly repolarization of the myocyte. Traditionally, EADs have been thought to arise from action potential prolongation and reactivation of depolarizing currents, but more recent experimental evidence suggests a previously unappreciated interrelationship between intracellular calcium loading and EADs. Cytosolic calcium may increase when action potentials are prolonged. This, in turn, appears to enhance L-type Ca current, further prolonging action potential duration as well as providing the inward current driving EADs. Intracellular calcium loading by action potential prolongation may also enhance the likelihood of DADs. The interrelationship among intracellular $[Ca^{2+}]$, EADs, and DADs may be one explanation for the susceptibility of hearts that are calcium loaded (e.g., in ischemia or congestive heart failure) to develop arrhythmias, particularly on exposure to action potential–prolonging drugs.

EAD-triggered arrhythmias exhibit rate dependence. In general, the amplitude of an EAD is augmented at slow rates when action potentials are longer. Indeed, a fundamental condition that underlies the development of EADs is action potential and QT prolongation. Hypokalemia, hypomagnesemia, bradycardia, and, most commonly, drugs can predispose to the generation of EADs, invariably in the context of prolonging the action potential. Antiarrhythmics with class IA and III action (see below) produce action potential and QT prolongation intended to be therapeutic but frequently causing arrhythmias. Noncardiac drugs such as phenothiazines, nonsedating antihistamines, and some antibiotics can also prolong the action potential duration and predispose to EAD-mediated triggered arrhythmias. Decreased $[K^+]_o$ paradoxically may decrease membrane potassium currents (particularly the delayed rectifier current, I_{Kr}) in

TABLE 231-1 Arrhythmia Mechanisms

Electrophysiologic Property	Molecular Components	Mechanism	Prototypic Arrhythmias
Cellular			
Impulse Initiation			
Automaticity	I_f, $I_{Ca\text{-}L}$, $I_{Ca\text{-}T}$, I_K, I_{K1}	Suppression/acceleration of phase 4	Sinus bradycardia, sinus tachycardia
Triggered automaticity	Calcium overload, I_{Ti}	DADs	Digitalis toxicity, reperfusion VT
	$I_{Ca\text{-}L}$, I_K, I_{Na}	EADs	Torsades des pointes, congenital and acquired
Excitation	I_{Na}	Suppression of phase 0	Ischemic VF
	$I_{K\text{-}ATP}$	AP shortening, inexcitability	
	$I_{Ca\text{-}L}$	Suppression	AV block
Repolarization	I_{Na}, $I_{Ca\text{-}L}$, I_K, I_{K1}, Ca^{2+} homeostasis	AP prolongation, EADs, DADs	Polymorphic VT (HF, LVH)
	$I_{Ca\text{-}L}$, K channels, Ca^{2+} homeostasis	AP shortening	Atrial fibrillation
Multicellular			
Cellular Coupling	Connexins (Cx43), I_{Na}, $I_{K\text{-}ATP}$	Decreased coupling	Ischemic VT/VF
Tissue Structure	Extracellular matrix, collagen	Excitable gap and functional reentry	Monomorphic VT, atrial fibrillation

Abbreviations: AP, action potential; AV, atrioventricular; DADs, delayed afterdepolarizations; EADs, early afterdepolarizations; HF, heart failure; LVH, left ventricular hypertrophy; VF, ventricular fibrillation; VT, ventricular tachyarrhythmia.

the ventricular myocyte, explaining why hypokalemia causes action potential prolongation and EADs. In fact, potassium infusions in patients with the congenital long QT syndrome (LQTS) and in those with drug-induced acquired QT prolongation shorten the QT interval.

EAD-mediated triggered activity probably underlies initiation of the characteristic polymorphic ventricular tachycardia, torsades des pointes, seen in patients with congenital and acquired forms of LQTS. Structural heart disease such as cardiac hypertrophy and failure may also delay ventricular repolarization (so-called electrical remodeling) and predispose to arrhythmias related to abnormalities of repolarization. The abnormalities of repolarization in hypertrophy and heart failure are often magnified by concomitant drug therapy or electrolyte disturbances.

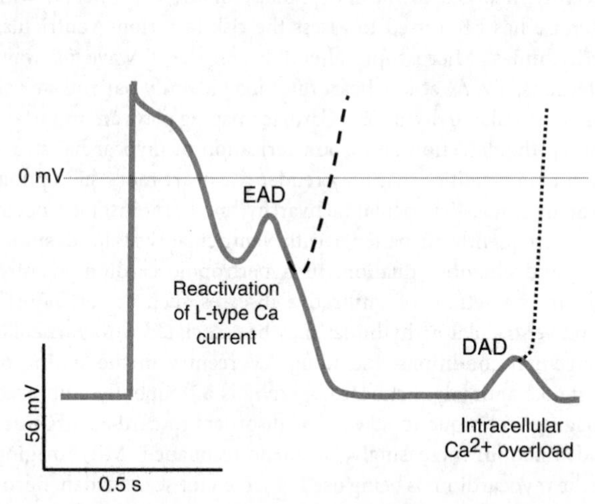

Figure 231-3 Schematic action potentials with early after depolarizations (EADs) and delayed afterdepolarizations (DADs). Afterdepolarizations are spontaneous depolarizations in cardiac myocytes. EADs occur before the end of the action potential (phases 2 and 3), interrupting repolarization. DADs occur during phase 4 of the action potential after completion of repolarization. The cellular mechanisms of EADs and DADs differ (see text).

Abnormal impulse conduction: reentry

The most common arrhythmia mechanism is reentry. Fundamentally, reentry is defined as circulation of an activation wave around an inexcitable obstacle. Thus, the requirements for reentry are two electrophysiologically dissimilar pathways for impulse propagation around an inexcitable region such that unidirectional block occurs in one of the pathways and a region of excitable tissue exists at the head of the propagating wavefront (Fig. 231-4). Structural and electrophysiologic properties of the heart may contribute to the development of the inexcitable obstacle and that of unidirectional block. The complex geometry of muscle bundles in the heart and spatial heterogeneity of cellular coupling or other active membrane properties (i.e., ionic currents) appear to be critical.

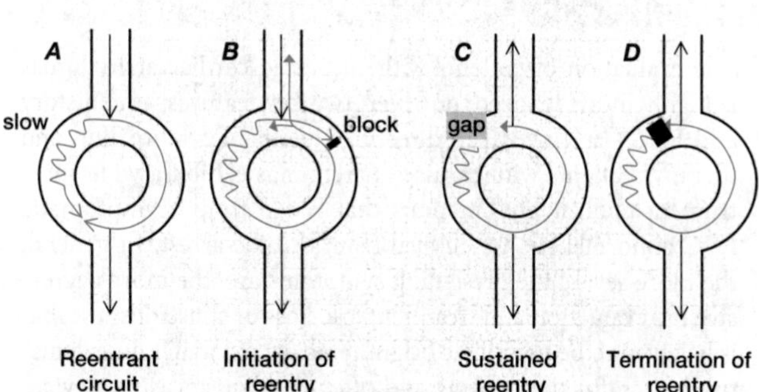

Figure 231-4 Schematic diagram of reentry. *A.* The circuit contains two limbs, one with slow conduction. ***B.*** A premature impulse blocks in the fast pathway and conducts over the slow pathway, allowing the fast pathway to recover so that the activation wave can reenter the fast pathway from the retrograde direction. ***C.*** During sustained reentry utilizing such a circuit, a gap (excitable gap) exists between the activating head of the wave and the recovering tail. ***D.*** One mechanism of termination of reentry occurs when the conduction and recovery characteristics of the circuit change and the activating head of the wave collides with the tail, extinguishing the tachycardia.

A key feature in classifying reentrant arrhythmias, particularly for therapy, is the presence and size of an excitable gap. An excitable gap exists when the tachycardia circuit is longer than the tachycardia wavelength (λ = conduction velocity × refractory period, representing the size of the circuit that can sustain reentry), allowing appropriately timed stimuli to reset propagation in the circuit. Reentrant arrhythmias may exist in the heart in the absence of an excitable gap and with a tachycardia wavelength nearly the same size as the path length. In this case, the wavefront propagates through partially refractory tissue with no anatomic obstacle and no fully excitable gap; this is referred to as *leading circle reentry*, a form of functional reentry (reentry that depends on functional properties of the tissue). Unlike excitable gap reentry, there is no fixed anatomic circuit in leading circle reentry, and it may therefore not be possible to disrupt the tachycardia with pacing or destruction of a part of the circuit. Furthermore, the circuit in leading circle reentry tends to be less stable than that in excitable gap reentrant arrhythmias, with large variations in cycle length and a predilection to termination.

Anatomically determined, excitable gap reentry can explain several clinically important tachycardias, such as AV reentry, atrial flutter, bundle branch reentry ventricular tachycardia, and ventricular tachycardia in scarred myocardium. There is strong evidence to suggest that other, less organized arrhythmias, such as atrial and ventricular fibrillation, are associated with more complex activation of the heart and are due to functional reentry.

Structural heart disease is associated with changes in conduction and refractoriness that increase the risk of reentrant arrhythmias. Chronically ischemic myocardium exhibits a downregulation of the gap junction channel protein (connexin 43) that carries intercellular ionic current. The border zones of infarcted and failing ventricular myocardium exhibit not only functional alterations of ionic currents but also remodeling of tissue and altered distribution of gap junctions. The changes in gap junction channel expression and distribution, in combination with macroscopic tissue alterations, support a role for slowed conduction in reentrant arrhythmias that complicate chronic coronary artery disease (CAD). Aged human atrial myocardium exhibits altered conduction, manifest as highly fractionated atrial electrograms, producing an ideal substrate for the reentry that may underlie the very common development of atrial fibrillation in the elderly.

APPROACH TO THE PATIENT Cardiac Arrhythmias

The evaluation of patients with suspected cardiac arrhythmias is highly individualized; however, two key features—the history and ECG—are pivotal in directing the diagnostic workup and therapy. Patients with cardiac arrhythmias exhibit a wide spectrum of clinical presentations that range from asymptomatic ECG abnormalities to survival from cardiac arrest. In general, the more severe the presenting symptoms are, the more aggressive the evaluation and treatment are. Loss of consciousness that is believed to be of cardiac origin typically mandates an exhaustive search for the etiology and often requires invasive, device-based therapy. The presence of structural heart disease and prior myocardial infarction dictates a change in the approach to the management of syncope or ventricular arrhythmias. The presence of a family history of serious ventricular arrhythmias or premature sudden death will influence the evaluation of presumed heritable arrhythmias.

The physical examination is focused on determining whether there is cardiopulmonary disease that is associated with specific cardiac arrhythmias. The absence of significant cardiopulmonary disease often, but not always, suggests benignity of the rhythm disturbance. In contrast, palpitations, syncope, or near syncope in the setting of significant heart or lung disease have more ominous implications. In addition, the physical examination may reveal the presence of a persistent arrhythmia such as atrial fibrillation.

The judicious use of noninvasive diagnostic tests is an important element in the evaluation of patients with arrhythmias, and there is no test more important than the ECG, particularly if recorded at the time of symptoms. Uncommon but diagnostically important signatures of electrophysiologic disturbances may be unearthed on the resting ECG, such as delta waves in Wolff-Parkinson-White (WPW) syndrome, prolongation or shortening of the QT interval, right precordial ST-segment abnormalities in Brugada syndrome, and epsilon waves in arrhythmogenic right ventricular dysplasia. Variants of body surface ECG recording can provide important information about arrhythmia substrates and triggers. Holter monitoring and event recording, either continuous or intermittent, record the body surface ECG over longer periods, enhancing the possibility of observing the cardiac rhythm during symptoms. Implantable long-term monitors and commercial ambulatory ECG monitoring services permit prolonged telemetric monitoring both for diagnosis and to assess the efficacy of therapy.

Long-term recordings permit the assessment of the time-varying behavior of the heart rhythm. Heart rate variability (HRV) and QT interval variability (QTV) provide noninvasive methods to assess autonomic nervous system influence on the heart. A decrease in HRV has been associated with increased sympathetic nervous system tone and increased mortality rates in patients after myocardial infarction. Signal-averaged electrocardiography (SAECG) uses signal-averaging techniques to amplify small potentials in the body surface ECG that are associated with slow conduction in the myocardium. The presence of these small potentials, referred to as *late potentials* because of their timing with respect to the QRS complex, and prolongation of the filtered (or averaged) QRS duration are indicative of slowed conduction in the ventricle and have been associated with an increased risk of ventricular arrhythmias after myocardial infarction. Exercise electrocardiography is important in determining the presence of myocardial demand ischemia; more recently, analysis of the morphology of the QT interval with exercise has been used to assess the risk of serious ventricular arrhythmias. Microscopic alterations in the T wave (T wave alternans, TWA) at low heart rates may identify patients at risk for ventricular arrhythmias. Cardiac imaging plays an important role in the detection and characterization of myocardial structural abnormalities that may render the heart more susceptible to arrhythmia. Ventricular tachyarrhythmias, for instance, occur more frequently in patients with ventricular systolic dysfunction and chamber dilation, in hypertrophic cardiomyopathy, and in the setting of infiltrative diseases such as sarcoidosis. Supraventricular arrhythmias may be associated with particular congenital conditions, including AV reentry in the setting of Ebstein's anomaly. Echocardiography is a frequently employed imaging technique to screen for disorders of cardiac structure and function. Increasingly, magnetic resonance (MR) imaging of the myocardium is being used to screen for scar burden, fibrofatty infiltration of the myocardium as seen in arrhythmogenic right ventricular cardiomyopathy, and other structural changes that affect arrhythmia susceptibility.

Head-up tilt (HUT) testing is useful in the evaluation of some patients with syncope. The physiologic response to HUT is incompletely understood; however, redistribution of blood volume and increased ventricular contractility occur consistently. Exaggerated activation of a central reflex in response to HUT produces a stereotypic response of an initial increase in heart rate, then a drop in blood pressure followed by a reduction in heart rate characteristic of neurally mediated hypotension. Other responses to HUT may be observed in patients with orthostatic hypotension and autonomic insufficiency. HUT is used most often in patients with recurrent syncope, although it may be useful in patients with single syncopal episodes with associated injury, particularly in the absence of structural heart disease. In patients with structural heart disease, HUT may be indicated in those with syncope, in whom other causes (e.g., asystole, ventricular tachyarrhythmias) have been excluded. HUT has been suggested as a useful tool in the diagnosis of and therapy for recurrent idiopathic vertigo, chronic fatigue syndrome, recurrent transient ischemic attacks, and repeated falls of unknown etiology in the elderly. Importantly, HUT is relatively contraindicated in the presence of severe CAD with proximal coronary stenoses, known severe cerebrovascular disease, severe mitral stenosis, and obstruction to left ventricular outflow (e.g., aortic stenosis). The method of HUT is variable, but the angle of tilt and the duration of upright posture are central to the diagnostic utility of the test. Pharmacologic provocation of orthostatic stress with isoproterenol, nitrates, adenosine, and edrophonium has been used to shorten the test and enhance specificity.

Electrophysiologic testing is central to the understanding and treatment of many cardiac arrhythmias. Indeed, most frequently, electrophysiologic testing is interventional, providing both diagnosis and therapy. The components of the electrophysiologic test are baseline measurements of conduction under resting and stressed (rate or pharmacologic) conditions and maneuvers, both pacing and pharmacologic, to induce arrhythmias. A number of sophisticated electrical mapping and catheter-guidance techniques have been developed to facilitate catheter-based therapeutics in the electrophysiology laboratory.

TREATMENT Cardiac Arrhythmias

ANTIARRHYTHMIC DRUG THERAPY The interaction of antiarrhythmic drugs with cardiac tissues and the resulting electrophysiologic changes are complex. An incomplete understanding of the effects of these drugs has produced serious missteps that have had adverse effects on patient outcomes and the development of newer pharmacologic agents. Currently, antiarrhythmic drugs have been relegated to an ancillary role in the treatment of most cardiac arrhythmias.

There are several explanations for the complexity of antiarrhythmic drug action: the structural similarity of target ion channels; regional differences in the levels of expression of channels and transporters, which change with disease; time and voltage dependence of drug action; and the effect of these drugs on targets other than ion channels. Because of the limitations of any scheme to classify antiarrhythmic agents, a shorthand that is useful in describing the major mechanisms of action is of some utility. Such a classification scheme was proposed in 1970 by Vaughan-Williams and later modified by Singh and Harrison. The classes of antiarrhythmic action are class I, local anesthetic effect due to blockade of Na^+ current; class II, interference with the action of catecholamines at the β-adrenergic receptor; class III, delay of repolarization due to inhibition of K^+ current or activation of depolarizing current; class IV, interference with calcium conductance (Table 231-2). The limitations of the Vaughan-Williams classification scheme include multiple actions of most drugs, overwhelming consideration of antagonism as a mechanism of action, and the fact that several agents have none of the four classes of action in the scheme.

TABLE 231-2 Antiarrhythmic Drug Actions

Drug	Class Actions				Miscellaneous Action
	I	II	III	IV	
Quinidine	++		++		α-Adrenergic blockade
Procainamide	++		++		Ganglionic blockade
Flecainide	+++		+		
Propafenone	++	+			
Sotalol		++	+++		
Dofetilide			+++		
Amiodarone	++	++	+++	+	α-Adrenergic blockade
Ibutilide			+++		Na^+ channel activator

CATHETER ABLATION The use of catheter ablation is based on the principle that there is a critical anatomic region of impulse generation or propagation that is required for the initiation and maintenance of cardiac arrhythmias. Destruction of such a critical region results in the elimination of the arrhythmia. The use of radio frequency (RF) energy in clinical medicine is nearly a century old. The first catheter ablation using a DC energy source was performed in the early 1980s by Scheinman and colleagues. By the early 1990s, RF had been adapted for use in catheter-based ablation in the heart (Fig. 231-5).

The RF frequency band (300–30,000 kHz) is used to generate energy for several biomedical applications, including coagulation and cauterization of tissues. Energy of this frequency will not stimulate skeletal muscle or the heart and heats tissue by a resistive mechanism, with the intensity of heating and tissue destruction being proportional to the delivered power. Alternative, less frequently used energy sources for catheter ablation of cardiac arrhythmias include microwaves (915 MHz or 2450 MHz), lasers, ultrasound, and freezing (cryoablation). Of these alternative ablation techniques, cryoablation is being used clinically with the most frequency, especially ablation in the region of the AV node. At temperatures just below 32°C, membrane ion transport is disrupted, producing depolarization of cells, decreased action potential amplitude and duration, and slowed conduction velocity (resulting in local conduction block)—all of which are reversible if the tissue is rewarmed in a timely fashion. Tissue cooling can be used for mapping and ablation. Cryomapping can be used to confirm the location of a desired ablation target, such as an accessory pathway in WPW syndrome, or can be used to determine the safety of ablation around the AV node by monitoring AV conduction during cooling. Another advantage of cryoablation is that once the catheter tip cools below freezing, it adheres to the tissue, increasing catheter stability independent of the rhythm or pacing.

DEVICE THERAPY Bradyarrhythmias due either to primary sinus node dysfunction or to atrioventricular conduction defects are readily treated through implantation of a permanent pacemaker. Clinical indications for pacemaker implantation often depend on the presence either of symptomatic bradycardia or

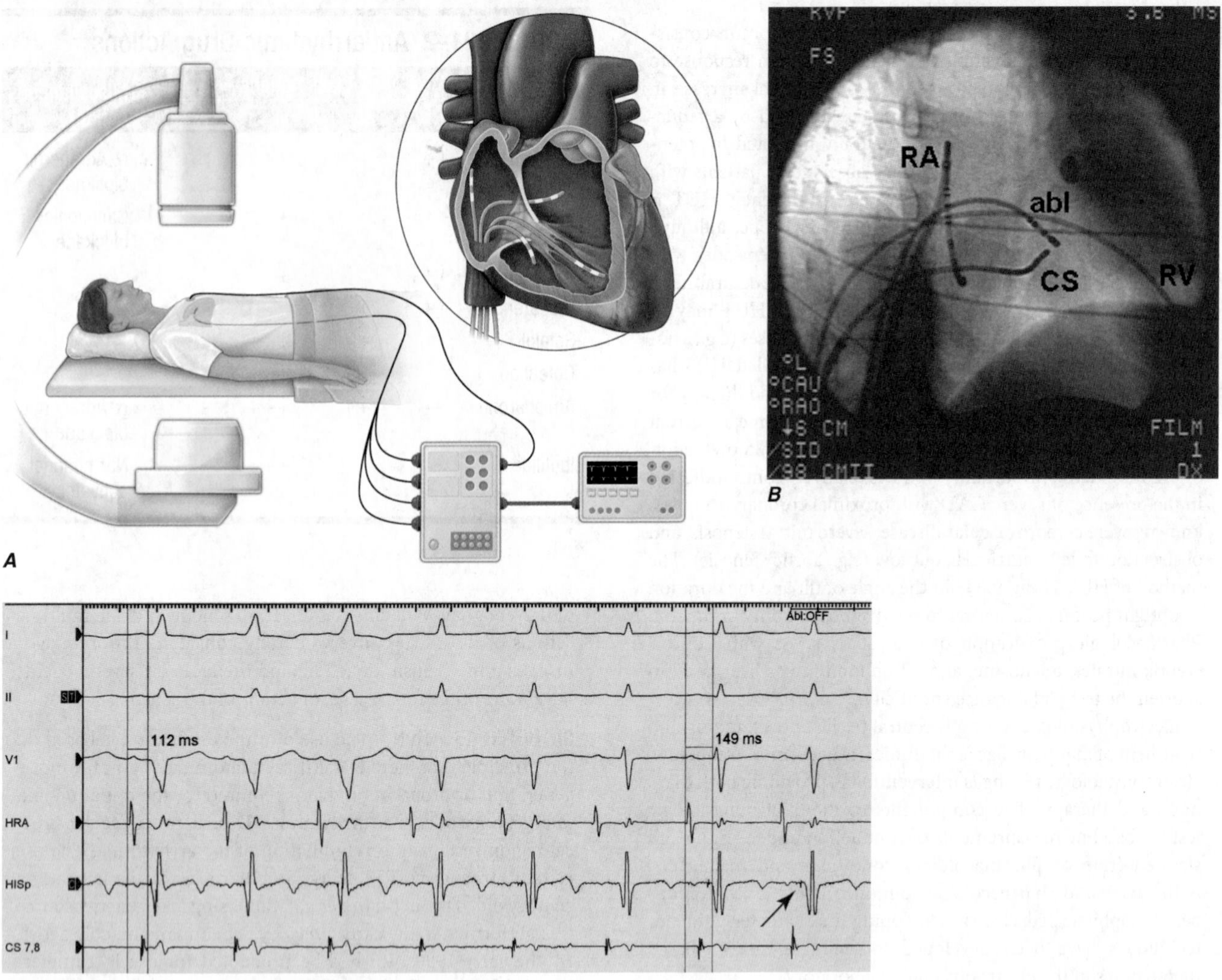

Figure 231-5 Catheter ablation of cardiac arrhythmias. ***A.*** A schematic of the catheter system and generator in a patient undergoing radiofrequency catheter ablation (RFCA); the circuit involves the catheter in the heart and a dispersive patch placed on the body surface (usually the back). The inset shows a diagram of the heart with a catheter located at the AV valve ring for ablation of an accessory pathway. ***B.*** A right anterior oblique fluoroscopic image of the catheter position for ablation of a left-sided accessory pathway. A catheter is placed in the atrial side of the mitral valve ring (abl) via a transseptal puncture. Other catheters are placed in the coronary sinus, in the right atrium (RA), and in the right ventricular (RV) apex to record local electrical activation. ***C.*** Body surface ECG recordings (I, II, V_1) and endocardial electrograms (HRA, high right atrium; HISp, proximal His bundle electrogram; CS 7,8, recordings from poles 7 and 8 of a decapolar catheter placed in the coronary sinus) during RFCA of a left-sided accessory pathway in a patient with Wolff-Parkinson-White syndrome. The QRS narrows at the fourth complex; the arrow shows the His bundle electrogram, which becomes apparent with elimination of ventricular preexcitation over the accessory pathway.

of an unreliable endogenous escape rhythm and are more fully reviewed in Chap. 232.

Ventricular tachyarrhythmias, particularly those occurring in the context of progressive structural heart diseases such as ischemic cardiomyopathy or arrhythmogenic right ventricular cardiomyopathy, may recur despite therapy with antiarrhythmic drugs or catheter ablation. In appropriate candidates, implantation of an internal cardioverter-defibrillator (ICD) may reduce mortality rates from sudden cardiac death. In a subset of patients with congestive heart failure (CHF) and ventricular mechanical dyssynchrony, ICD or pacemaker platforms can be used to provide cardiac resynchronization therapy, typically through implantation of a left ventricular pacing lead. In patients with dyssynchronous CHF, such therapy has been shown to improve both morbidity and mortality rates.

FURTHER READINGS

Akar FG, Tomaselli GF: Genetic basis of cardiac arrhythmias, in *Hurst's The Heart*, 12th ed, V Fuster et al (eds). New York, McGraw-Hill, 2007

Hille B: *Ion Channels of Excitable Membranes*, 3rd ed. Sunderland, MA, Sinauer Associates, 2001

Josephson ME: *Clinical Cardiac Electrophysiology: Techniques and Interpretations*, 4th ed. Philadelphia, Lippincott Williams & Wilkins, 2008

Saksena S, Camm AJ (eds): *Electrophysiological Disorders of the Heart*. Philadelphia, Elsevier Churchill Livingstone, 2005

Zipes DP, Jalife J (eds): *Cardiac Electrophysiology: From Cell to Bedside*, 5th ed. Philadelphia, Elsevier, 2009

CHAPTER 232

The Bradyarrhythmias

David D. Spragg
Gordon F. Tomaselli

Electrical activation of the heart normally originates in the sinoatrial (SA) node, the predominant pacemaker. Other subsidiary pacemakers in the atrioventricular (AV) node, specialized conducting system, and muscle may initiate electrical activation if the SA node is dysfunctional or suppressed. Typically, subsidiary pacemakers discharge at a slower rate and, in the absence of an appropriate increase in stroke volume, may result in tissue hypoperfusion.

Spontaneous activation and contraction of the heart are a consequence of the specialized pacemaking tissue in these anatomic locales. As described in Chap. 231, action potentials in the heart are regionally heterogeneous. The action potentials in cells isolated from nodal tissue are distinct from those recorded from atrial and ventricular myocytes (Fig. 232-1). The complement of ionic currents present in nodal cells results in a less negative resting membrane potential compared with atrial or ventricular myocytes. Electrical diastole in nodal cells is characterized by slow diastolic depolarization (phase 4), which generates an action potential as the membrane voltage reaches threshold. The action potential upstrokes (phase 0) are slow compared with atrial or ventricular myocytes, being mediated by calcium rather than sodium current. Cells with properties of SA and AV nodal tissue are electrically connected to the remainder of the myocardium by cells with an electrophysiologic phenotype between that of nodal cells and that of atrial or ventricular myocytes. Cells in the SA node exhibit the most rapid phase 4 depolarization and thus are the dominant pacemakers in a normal heart.

Bradycardia results from a failure of either impulse initiation or impulse conduction. Failure of impulse initiation may be caused by depressed automaticity resulting from a slowing or failure of phase 4 diastolic depolarization (Fig. 232-2), which may result from disease or exposure to drugs. Prominently, the autonomic nervous system modulates the rate of phase 4 diastolic depolarization and thus the firing rate of both primary (SA node) and subsidiary pacemakers. Failure of conduction of an impulse from nodal tissue to atrial or ventricular myocardium may produce bradycardia as a result of exit block. Conditions that alter the activation and connectivity of cells (e.g., fibrosis) in the heart may result in failure of impulse conduction.

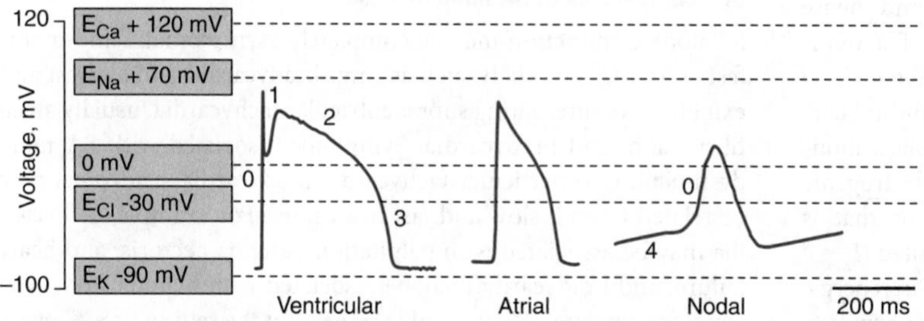

Figure 232-1 Action potential profiles recorded in cells isolated from sinoatrial or atrioventricular nodal tissue compared with those of cells from atrial or ventricular myocardium. Nodal cell action potentials exhibit more depolarized resting membrane potentials, slower phase 0 upstrokes, and phase 4 diastolic depolarization.

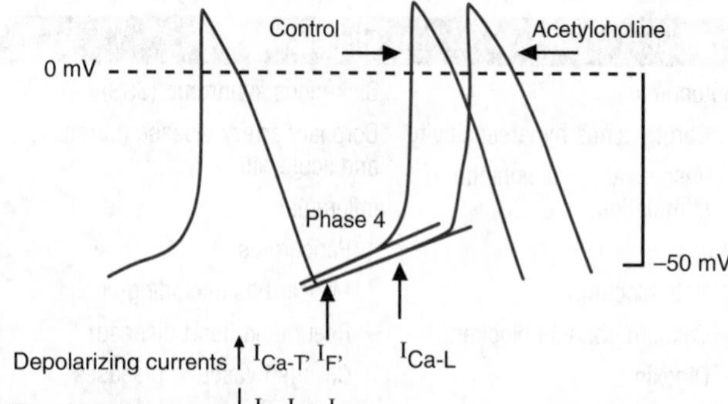

Figure 232-2 Schematics of nodal action potentials and the currents that contribute to phase 4 depolarization. Relative increases in depolarizing L- (I_{Ca-L}) and T- (I_{Ca-T}) type calcium and pacemaker currents (I_f) along with a reduction in repolarizing inward rectifier (I_{K1}) and delayed rectifier (I_K) potassium currents result in depolarization. Activation of ACh-gated (I_{KACh}) potassium current and beta blockade slow the rate of phase 4 and decrease the pacing rate. *(Modified from J Jalife et al: Basic Cardiac Electrophysiology for the Clinician, Blackwell Publishing, 1999.)*

SA node dysfunction and AV conduction block are the most common causes of pathologic bradycardia. SA node dysfunction may be difficult to distinguish from physiologic sinus bradycardia, particularly in the young. SA node dysfunction increases in frequency between the fifth and sixth decades of life and should be considered in patients with fatigue, exercise intolerance, or syncope and sinus bradycardia. Transient AV block is common in the young and probably is a result of the high vagal tone found in up to 10% of young adults. Acquired and persistent failure of AV conduction is decidedly rare in healthy adult populations, with an estimated incidence of ~200/million population per year.

Permanent pacemaking is the only reliable therapy for symptomatic bradycardia in the absence of extrinsic and reversible etiologies such as increased vagal tone, hypoxia, hypothermia, and drugs (Table 232-1). Approximately 50% of the 150,000 permanent pacemakers implanted in the United States and 20–30% of the 150,000 of those in Europe were implanted for SA node disease.

SA NODE DISEASE

Structure and physiology of the SA node

The SA node is composed of a cluster of small fusiform cells in the sulcus terminalis on the epicardial surface of the heart at the right atrial–superior vena caval junction, where they envelop the SA nodal artery. The SA node is structurally heterogeneous, but the central prototypic nodal cells have fewer distinct myofibrils than does the surrounding atrial myocardium, no intercalated disks visible on light microscopy, a poorly developed sarcoplasmic reticulum, and no T-tubules. Cells in the peripheral regions of the SA node are transitional in both structure and function. The SA nodal artery arises from the right coronary artery in 55–60% and the left circumflex artery in 40–45% of persons. The SA node is richly innervated by sympathetic and parasympathetic nerves and ganglia.

Irregular and slow propagation of impulses from the SA node can be explained by the electrophysiology of nodal cells and the structure of the SA node itself. The action potentials of SA nodal cells

TABLE 232-1 Etiologies of SA Node Dysfunction

Extrinsic	Intrinsic
Autonomic	Sick-sinus syndrome (SSS)
Carotid sinus hypersensitivity	Coronary artery disease (chronic and acute MI)
Vasovagal (cardioinhibitory) stimulation	Inflammatory
Drugs	Pericarditis
Beta blockers	Myocarditis (including viral)
Calcium channel blockers	Rheumatic heart disease
Digoxin	Collagen vascular diseases
Antiarrhythmics (class I and III)	Lyme disease
Adenosine	Senile amyloidosis
Clonidine (other sympatholytics)	Congenital heart disease
Lithium carbonate	TGA/Mustard and Fontan repairs
Cimetidine	Iatrogenic
Amitriptyline	Radiation therapy
Phenothiazines	Postsurgical
Narcotics (methadone)	Chest trauma
Pentamidine	Familial
Hypothyroidism	AD SSS, OMIM #163800 (15q24-25)
Sleep apnea	AR SSS, OMIM #608567 (3p21)
Hypoxia	SA node disease with myopia, OMIM 182190
Endotracheal suctioning (vagal maneuvers)	Kearns-Sayre syndrome, OMIM #530000
Hypothermia	Myotonic dystrophy
Increased intracranial pressure	Type 1, OMIM #160900 (19q13.2-13.3)
	Type 2, OMIM #602668 (3q13.3-q24)
	Friedreich's ataxia, OMIM #229300 (9q13, 9p23-p11)

Abbreviations: AD, autosomal dominant; AR, autosomal recessive; MI, myocardial infarction; OMIM, Online Mendelian Inheritance in Man (database); TGA, transposition of the great arteries; .

are characterized by a relatively depolarized membrane potential (Fig. 232-1) of –40 to –60 mV, slow phase 0 upstroke, and relatively rapid phase 4 diastolic depolarization compared with the action potentials recorded in cardiac muscle cells. The relative absence of inward rectifier potassium current (I_{K1}) accounts for the depolarized membrane potential; the slow upstroke of phase 0 results from the absence of available fast sodium current (I_{Na}) and is mediated by L-type calcium current (I_{Ca-L}); and phase 4 depolarization is a result of the aggregate activity of a number of ionic currents. Prominently, both L- and T-type (I_{Ca-T}) calcium currents, the pacemaker current (so-called funny current, or I_f) formed by the tetramerization of hyperpolarization-activated cyclic nucleotide-gated channels, and the electrogenic sodium-calcium exchanger provide depolarizing current that is antagonized by delayed rectifier (I_{Kr}) and acetylcholine-gated (I_{KACh}) potassium currents. I_{Ca-L}, I_{Ca-T}, and I_f are modulated by β-adrenergic stimulation and I_{KACh} by vagal stimulation, explaining the exquisite sensitivity of diastolic depolarization to autonomic nervous system activity. The slow conduction within the SA node is explained by the absence of I_{Na} and poor electrical coupling of cells in the node, resulting from sizable amounts of interstitial tissue and a low abundance of gap junctions. The poor coupling allows for graded electrophysiologic properties within the node, with the peripheral transitional cells being silenced by electrotonic coupling to atrial myocardium.

Etiology of SA nodal disease

SA nodal dysfunction has been classified as intrinsic or extrinsic. The distinction is important because extrinsic dysfunction is often reversible and generally should be corrected before pacemaker therapy is considered (Table 232-1). The most common causes of extrinsic SA node dysfunction are drugs and autonomic nervous system influences that suppress automaticity and/or compromise conduction. Other extrinsic causes include hypothyroidism, sleep apnea, and conditions likely to occur in critically ill patients such as hypothermia, hypoxia, increased intracranial pressure (Cushing's response), and endotracheal suctioning via activation of the vagus nerve.

Intrinsic sinus node dysfunction is degenerative and often is characterized pathologically by fibrous replacement of the SA node or its connections to the atrium. Acute and chronic coronary artery disease (CAD) may be associated with SA node dysfunction, although in the setting of acute myocardial infarction (MI; typically inferior), the vabnormalities are transient. Inflammatory processes may alter SA node function, ultimately producing replacement fibrosis. Pericarditis, myocarditis, and rheumatic heart disease have been associated with SA nodal disease with sinus bradycardia, sinus arrest, and exit block. Carditis associated with systemic lupus erythematosus (SLE), rheumatoid arthritis (RA), and mixed connective tissue disorders (MCTDs) may also affect SA node structure and function. Senile amyloidosis is an infiltrative disorder in patients typically in the ninth decade of life; deposition of amyloid protein in the atrial myocardium can impair SA node function. Some SA node disease is iatrogenic and results from direct injury to the SA node during cardiothoracic surgery.

Rare heritable forms of sinus node disease have been described, and several have been characterized genetically. Autosomal dominant sinus node dysfunction in conjunction with supraventricular tachycardia [(i.e., tachycardia-bradycardia variant of sick-sinus syndrome (SSS)] has been linked to mutations in the pacemaker current (I_f) subunit gene *HCN4* on chromosome 15. An autosomal recessive form of SSS with the prominent feature of atrial inexcitability and absence of P waves on the electrocardiogram (ECG) is caused by mutations in the cardiac sodium channel gene, *SCN5A*, on chromosome 3. SSS associated with myopia has been described but not genetically characterized. There are several neuromuscular diseases, including Kearns-Sayre syndrome (ophthalmoplegia, pigmentary degeneration of the retina, and cardiomyopathy) and myotonic dystrophy, that have a predilection for the conducting system and SA node.

SSS in both the young and the elderly is associated with an increase in fibrous tissue in the SA node. The onset of SSS may be hastened by coexisting disease, such as CAD, diabetes mellitus, hypertension, and valvular diseases and cardiomyopathies.

Clinical features of SA node disease

SA node dysfunction may be completely asymptomatic and manifest as an ECG anomaly such as sinus bradycardia; sinus arrest and exit block; or alternating supraventricular tachycardia, usually atrial fibrillation, and bradycardia. Symptoms associated with SA node dysfunction, in particular tachycardia-bradycardia syndrome, may be related to both slow and fast heart rates. For example, tachycardia may be associated with palpitations, angina pectoris, and heart failure, and bradycardia may be associated with hypotension, syncope, presyncope, fatigue, and weakness. In the setting of SSS, overdrive suppression of the SA node may result in prolonged pauses and syncope upon termination of the tachycardia. In many cases, symptoms associated with SA node dysfunction result from concomitant cardiovascular disease. A significant minority of patients with SSS develop signs and symptoms of heart failure that may be related to slow or fast heart rates.

One-third to one-half of patients with SA node dysfunction develop supraventricular tachycardia, usually atrial fibrillation or atrial flutter. The incidence of persistent atrial fibrillation in patients with SA node dysfunction increases with advanced age, hypertension, diabetes mellitus, left ventricular dilation, valvular heart disease, and ventricular pacing. Remarkably, some symptomatic patients may experience an improvement in symptoms with the development of atrial fibrillation, presumably from an increase in their average heart rate. Patients with the tachycardia-bradycardia variant of SSS, similar to patients with atrial fibrillation, are at risk for thromboembolism, and *those at greatest risk*, including patients ≥65 years and patients with a prior history of stroke, valvular heart disease, left ventricular dysfunction, or atrial enlargement, should be treated with anticoagulants. Up to one-quarter of patients with SA node disease will have concurrent AV conduction disease, although only a minority will require specific therapy for high-grade AV block.

The natural history of SA node dysfunction is one of varying intensity of symptoms even in patients who present with syncope. Symptoms related to SA node dysfunction may be significant, but overall mortality usually is not compromised in the absence of other significant comorbid conditions. These features of the natural history need to be taken into account in considering therapy for these patients.

Electrocardiography of SA node disease

The electrocardiographic manifestations of SA node dysfunction include sinus bradycardia, sinus pauses, sinus arrest, sinus exit block, tachycardia (in SSS), and chronotropic incompetence. It is often difficult to distinguish pathologic from physiologic sinus bradycardia. By definition, sinus bradycardia is a rhythm driven by the SA node with a rate of <60 beats/min; sinus bradycardia is very common and typically benign. Resting heart rates <60 beats/min are very common in young healthy individuals and physically conditioned subjects. A sinus rate of <40 beats/min in the awake state in the absence of physical conditioning generally is considered abnormal. Sinus pauses and sinus arrest result from failure of the SA node to discharge, producing a pause without P waves visible on the ECG (Fig. 232-3). Sinus pauses of up to 3 s are common in awake athletes, and pauses of this duration or longer may be observed in asymptomatic elderly subjects. Intermittent failure of conduction from the SA node produces sinus exit block. The severity of sinus exit block may vary in a manner similar to that of AV block (see below). Prolongation of conduction from the sinus node will not be apparent on the ECG; second-degree SA block will produce intermittent conduction from the SA node and a regularly irregular atrial rhythm.

Type I second-degree SA block results from progressive prolongation of SA node conduction with intermittent failure of the impulses originating in the sinus node to conduct to the surrounding atrial tissue. Second-degree SA block appears on the ECG as an intermittent absence of P waves (Fig. 232-4). In type II second-degree SA block, there is no change in SA node conduction before the pause. Complete or third-degree SA block results in no P waves on the ECG. Tachycardia-bradycardia syndrome is manifest as alternating sinus bradycardia and atrial tachyarrhythmias. Although atrial tachycardia, atrial flutter, and atrial fibrillation may be observed, the latter is the most common tachycardia. Chronotropic incompetence is the inability to increase the heart rate in response to exercise or other stress appropriately and is defined in greater detail below.

Diagnostic testing

SA node dysfunction is most commonly a clinical or electrocardiographic diagnosis. Sinus bradycardia or pauses on the resting ECG are rarely sufficient to diagnose SA node disease, and longer-term recording and symptom correlation generally are required. Symptoms in the absence of sinus bradyarrhythmias may be sufficient to exclude a diagnosis of SA node dysfunction.

Electrocardiographic recording plays a central role in the diagnosis and management of SA node dysfunction. Despite the limitations of the resting ECG, longer-term recording employing Holter or event monitors may permit correlation of symptoms with the cardiac rhythm. Many contemporary event monitors may be automatically triggered to record the ECG when certain programmed heart rate criteria are met. Implantable ECG monitors permit long-term recording (12–18 months) in particularly challenging patients.

Failure to increase the heart rate with exercise is referred to as *chronotropic incompetence*. This is alternatively defined as failure to reach 85% of predicted maximal heart rate at peak exercise or failure to achieve a heart rate >100 beats/min with exercise or a maximal heart rate with exercise less than two standard deviations below that of an age-matched control population. Exercise testing may be useful in discriminating chronotropic incompetence from resting bradycardia and may aid in the identification of the mechanism of exercise intolerance.

Autonomic nervous system testing is useful in diagnosing carotid sinus hypersensitivity; pauses >3 s are consistent with the diagnosis but may be present in asymptomatic elderly subjects. Determining the intrinsic heart rate (IHR) may distinguish SA node dysfunction from slow heart rates that result from high vagal tone. The normal IHR after administration of 0.2 mg/kg propranolol and 0.04 mg/kg atropine is 117.2 – (0.53 × age) in beats/min; a low IHR is indicative of SA disease.

Electrophysiologic testing may play a role in the assessment of patients with presumed SA node dysfunction and in the evaluation of syncope, particularly in the setting of structural heart disease. In this circumstance, electrophysiologic testing is used to rule out more

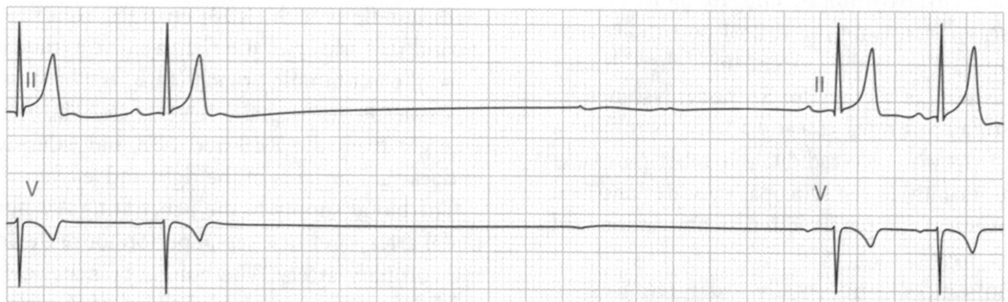

Figure 232-3 Sinus slowing and pauses on the ECG. The ECG is recorded during sleep in a young patient without heart disease. The heart rate before the pause is slow, and the PR interval is prolonged, consistent with an increase in vagal tone. The P waves have a morphology consistent with sinus rhythm. The recording is from a two-lead telemetry system in which the tracing labeled II mimics frontal lead II and V represents Modified Central Lead 1, which mimics lead V1 of the standard 12-lead ECG.

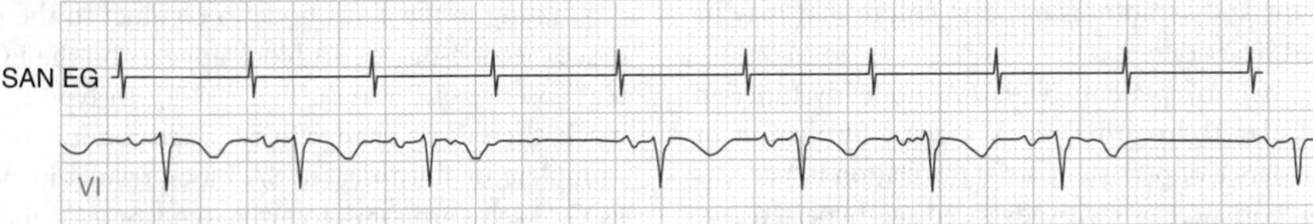

Figure 232-4 Mobitz type I SA nodal exit block. A theoretical SA node electrogram (SAN EG) is shown. Note that there is grouped beating producing a regularly irregular heart rhythm. The SA node EG rate is constant with progressive delay in exit from the node and activation of the atria, inscribing the P wave. This produces subtly decreasing P-P intervals before the pause, and the pause is less than twice the cycle length of the last sinus interval.

malignant etiologies of syncope, such as ventricular tachyarrhythmias and AV conduction block. There are several ways to assess SA node function invasively. They include the sinus node recovery time (SNRT), defined as the longest pause after cessation of overdrive pacing of the right atrium near the SA node (normal: <1500 ms or, corrected for sinus cycle length, <550 ms), and the sinoatrial conduction time (SACT), defined as one-half the difference between the intrinsic sinus cycle length and a noncompensatory pause after a premature atrial stimulus (normal <125 ms). The combination of an abnormal SNRT, an abnormal SACT, and a low IHR is a sensitive and specific indicator of intrinsic SA node disease.

TREATMENT Sinoatrial Node Dysfunction

Since SA node dysfunction is not associated with increased mortality rates, the aim of therapy is alleviation of symptoms. Exclusion of extrinsic causes of SA node dysfunction and correlation of the cardiac rhythm with symptoms is an essential part of patient management. Pacemaker implantation is the primary therapeutic intervention in patients with symptomatic SA node dysfunction. Pharmacologic considerations are important in the evaluation and management of patients with SA nodal disease. A number of drugs modulate SA node function and are extrinsic causes of dysfunction (Table 232-1). Beta blockers and calcium channel blockers increase SNRT in patients with SA node dysfunction, and antiarrhythmic drugs with class I and III action may promote SA node exit block. In general, such agents should be discontinued before decisions regarding the need for permanent pacing in patients with SA node disease are made. Chronic pharmacologic therapy for sinus bradyarrhythmias is limited. Some pharmacologic agents may improve SA node function; digitalis, for example, has been shown to shorten SNRT in patients with SA node dysfunction. Isoproterenol or atropine administered IV may increase the sinus rate acutely. Theophylline has been used both acutely and chronically to increase heart rate but has liabilities when used in patients with tachycardia-bradycardia syndrome, increasing the frequency of supraventricular tachyarrhythmias, and in patients with structural heart disease, increasing the risk of potentially serious ventricular arrhythmias. At the current time, there is only a single randomized study of therapy for SA node dysfunction. In patients with resting heart rates <50 and >30 beats/min on a Holter monitor, patients who received dual-chamber pacemakers experienced significantly fewer syncopal episodes and had symptomatic improvement compared with patients randomized to theophylline or no treatment.

In certain circumstances, sinus bradycardia requires no specific treatment or only temporary rate support. Sinus bradycardia is common in patients with acute inferior or posterior MI and can be exacerbated by vagal activation induced by pain or the use of drugs such as morphine. Ischemia of the SA nodal artery probably occurs in acute coronary syndromes more typically with involvement with the right coronary artery, and even with infarction, the effect on SA node function most often is transient.

Sinus bradycardia is a prominent feature of carotid sinus hypersensitivity and neurally mediated hypotension associated with vasovagal syncope that responds to pacemaker therapy. Carotid hypersensitivity with recurrent syncope or presyncope associated with a predominant cardioinhibitory component responds to pacemaker implantation. Several randomized trials have investigated the efficacy of permanent pacing in patients with drug-refractory vasovagal syncope, with mixed results. Although initial trials suggested that patients undergoing pacemaker implantation have fewer recurrences and a longer time to recurrence of symptoms, at least one follow-up study did not confirm these results.

The details of pacing modes and indications for pacing in SA node dysfunction are discussed below.

ATRIOVENTRICULAR CONDUCTION DISEASE

Structure and physiology of the AV node

The AV conduction axis is structurally complex, involving the atria and ventricles as well as the AV node. Unlike the SA node, the AV node is a subendocardial structure originating in the transitional zone, which is composed of aggregates of cells in the posterior-inferior right atrium. Superior, medial, and posterior transitional atrionodal bundles converge on the compact AV node. The compact AV node (~1 × 3 × 5 mm) is situated at the apex of the triangle of Koch, which is defined by the coronary sinus ostium posteriorly, the septal tricuspid valve annulus anteriorly, and the tendon of Todaro superiorly. The compact AV node continues as the penetrating AV bundle where it immediately traverses the central fibrous body and is in close proximity to the aortic, mitral, and tricuspid valve annuli; thus, it is subject to injury in the setting of valvular heart disease or its surgical treatment. The penetrating AV bundle continues through the annulus fibrosis and emerges along the ventricular septum adjacent to the membranous septum as the bundle of His. The right bundle branch (RBB) emerges from the distal AV bundle in a band that traverses the right ventricle (moderator band). In contrast, the left bundle branch (LBB) is a broad subendocardial sheet of tissue on the septal left ventricle. The Purkinje fiber network emerges from the RBB and LBB and extensively ramifies on the endocardial surfaces of the right and left ventricles, respectively.

The blood supply to the penetrating AV bundle is from the AV nodal artery and first septal perforator of the left anterior descending coronary artery. The bundle branches also have a dual blood supply from the septal perforators of the left anterior descending coronary artery and branches of the posterior descending coronary artery. The AV node is highly innervated with postganglionic sympathetic and parasympathetic nerves. The bundle of His and distal conducting system are minimally influenced by autonomic tone.

The cells that constitute the AV node complex are heterogeneous with a range of action potential profiles. In the transitional zones, the cells have an electrical phenotype between those of atrial myocytes and cells of the compact node (Fig. 232-1). Atrionodal transitional connections may exhibit *decremental conduction*, defined as slowing of conduction with increasingly rapid rates of stimulation. Fast and slow AV nodal pathways have been described, but it is controversial whether these two types of pathway are anatomically distinct or represent functional heterogeneities in different regions of the AV nodal complex. Myocytes that constitute the compact node are depolarized (resting membrane potential ~–60 mV) and exhibit action potentials with low amplitudes, slow upstrokes of phase 0 (<10 V/s), and phase 4 diastolic depolarization; high-input resistance; and relative insensitivity to external $[K^+]$. The action potential phenotype is explained by the complement of ionic currents expressed. AV nodal cells lack I_{K1} and I_{Na}; I_{Ca-L} is responsible for phase 0; and phase 4 depolarization reflects the composite activity of the depolarizing currents I_f, I_{Ca-L}, I_{Ca-T}, and I_{NCX} and the repolarizing currents I_{Kr} and I_{KACh}. Electrical coupling between cells in the AV node is tenuous due to the relatively sparse expression of gap junction channels (predominantly connexin-40) and increased extracellular volume.

The His bundle and the bundle branches are insulated from ventricular myocardium. The most rapid conduction in the heart is observed in these tissues. The action potentials exhibit very rapid upstrokes (phase 0), prolonged plateaus (phase 2), and modest automaticity (phase 4 depolarization). Gap junctions, composed largely of connexin-40, are abundant, but bundles are poorly connected transversely to ventricular myocardium.

Etiology of AV conduction disease

Conduction block from the atrium to the ventricle can occur for a variety of reasons in a number of clinical situations, and AV conduction block may be classified in a number of ways. The etiologies may be functional or structural, in part analogous to extrinsic and intrinsic causes of SA nodal dysfunction. The block may be classified by its severity from first to third degree or complete AV block or by the location of block within the AV conduction system. Table 232-2 summarizes the etiologies of AV conduction block. Those which are functional (autonomic, metabolic/endocrine, and drug-related) tend to be reversible. Most other etiologies produce structural changes, typically fibrosis, in segments of the AV conduction axis that are generally permanent. Heightened vagal tone during sleep or in well-conditioned individuals can be associated with all grades of AV block. Carotid sinus hypersensitivity, vasovagal syncope, and cough and micturition syncope may be associated with SA node slowing and AV conduction block. Transient metabolic and endocrinologic disturbances as well as a number of pharmacologic agents also may produce reversible AV conduction block.

Several infectious diseases have a predilection for the conducting system. Lyme disease may involve the heart in up to 50% of cases; 10% of patients with Lyme carditis develop AV conduction block, which is generally reversible but may require temporary pacing support. Chagas' disease, which is common in Latin America, and syphilis may produce more persistent AV conduction disturbances. Some autoimmune and infiltrative diseases may produce AV conduction block, including SLE, RA, MCTD, scleroderma, amyloidosis (primary and secondary), sarcoidosis, and hemochromatosis; rare malignancies also may impair AV conduction.

Idiopathic progressive fibrosis of the conduction system is one of the more common and degenerative causes of AV conduction block. Aging is associated with degenerative changes in the summit of the ventricular septum, central fibrous body, and aortic and mitral annuli and has been described as "sclerosis of the left cardiac skeleton." The process typically begins in the fourth decade of life and may be accelerated by atherosclerosis, hypertension, and diabetes mellitus. Accelerated forms of progressive familial heart block have been identified in families with

TABLE 232-2 Etiologies of Atrioventricular Block

Autonomic	
Carotid sinus hypersensitivity	Vasovagal
Metabolic/Endocrine	
Hyperkalemia	Hypothyroidism
Hypermagnesemia	Adrenal insufficiency
Drug-Related	
Beta blockers	Adenosine
Calcium channel blockers	Antiarrhythmics (class I and III)
Digitalis	Lithium
Infectious	
Endocarditis	Tuberculosis
Lyme disease	Diphtheria
Chagas' disease	Toxoplasmosis
Syphilis	
Heritable/Congenital	
Congenital heart disease	Facioscapulohumeral MD, OMIM #158900 (4q35)
Maternal SLE	
Kearns-Sayre syndrome, OMIM #530000	Emery-Dreifuss MD, OMIM #310300 (Xq28)
Myotonic dystrophy Type 1, OMIM #160900 (19q13.2-13.3) Type 2, OMIM #602668 (3q13.3-q24)	Progressive familial heart block, OMIM #113900 (19q13.2-q13.3, 3p21)
Inflammatory	
SLE	MCTD
Rheumatoid arthritis	Scleroderma
Infiltrative	
Amyloidosis	Hemochromatosis
Sarcoidosis	
Neoplastic/Traumatic	
Lymphoma	Radiation
Mesothelioma	Catheter ablation
Melanoma	
Degenerative	
Lev disease	Lenègre disease
Coronary Artery Disease	
Acute MI	

Abbreviations: MCTD, mixed connective tissue disease; MI, myocardial infarction; OMIM, Online Mendelian Inheritance in Man (database); SLE, systemic lupus erythematosus.

mutations in the cardiac sodium channel gene (*SCN5A*) and other loci that have been mapped to chromosomes 1 and 19.

AV conduction block has been associated with heritable neuromuscular diseases, including the nucleotide repeat disease myotonic dystrophy, the mitochondrial myopathy Kearns-Sayre syndrome (Chap. 387), and several of the monogenic muscular dystrophies. Congenital AV block may be observed in complex congenital cardiac anomalies (Chap. 236), such as transposition of the great arteries, ostium primum atrial septal defects (ASDs), ventricular septal defects (VSDs), endocardial cushion defects, and some single-ventricle defects. Congenital AV block in the setting of a structurally normal heart has been seen in children born to mothers with SLE. Iatrogenic AV block may occur during mitral or aortic valve surgery, rarely in the setting of thoracic radiation, and as a consequence of catheter ablation. AV block is a decidedly rare complication of the surgical repair of VSDs or ASDs but may complicate repairs of transposition of the great arteries.

CAD may produce transient or persistent AV block. In the setting of coronary spasm, ischemia, particularly in the right coronary artery distribution, may produce transient AV block. In acute MI, AV block transiently develops in 10–25% of patients; most commonly this is first- or second-degree AV block, but complete heart block (CHB) may also occur. Second-degree and higher-grade AV block tends to occur more often in inferior than in anterior acute MI; however, the level of block in inferior MI tends to be in the AV node with more stable, narrow escape rhythms. In contrast, acute anterior MI is associated with block in the distal AV nodal complex, His bundle, or bundle branches and results in wide complex, unstable escape rhythms and a worse prognosis with high mortality rates.

Electrocardiography and electrophysiology of AV conduction block

Atrioventricular conduction block typically is diagnosed electrocardiographically, which characterizes the severity of the conduction disturbance and allows one to draw inferences about the location of the block. AV conduction block manifests as slow conduction in its mildest forms and failure to conduct, either intermittent or persistently, in more severe varieties. First-degree AV block (PR interval >200 ms) is a slowing of conduction through the AV junction (Fig. 232-5). The site of delay is typically in the AV node but may be in the atria, bundle of His, or His-Purkinje system. A wide QRS is suggestive of delay in the distal conduction system, whereas a narrow QRS suggests delay in the AV node proper or, less commonly, in the bundle of His. In second-degree AV block there is an intermittent failure of electrical impulse conduction from atrium to ventricle. Second-degree AV block is subclassified as Mobitz type I (Wenckebach) or Mobitz type II. The periodic failure of conduction in Mobitz type I block is characterized by a progressively lengthening PR interval, shortening of the RR interval, and a pause that is less than two times the immediately preceding RR interval on the ECG. The ECG complex after the pause exhibits a shorter PR interval than that immediately preceding the pause (Fig. 232-6). This ECG pattern most often arises because of decremental conduction of electrical impulses in the AV node.

It is important to distinguish type I from type II second-degree AV nodal block because the latter has more serious prognostic implications. Type II second-degree AV block is characterized by intermittent failure of conduction of the P wave without changes in the preceding PR or RR intervals. When AV block is 2:1, it may be difficult to distinguish type I from type II block. Type II second-degree AV block typically occurs in the distal or infra-His conduction system, is often associated with intraventricular conduction delays (e.g., bundle branch block), and is more likely to proceed to higher grades of AV block than is type I second-degree AV block. Second-degree AV block (particularly type II) may be associated with a series of nonconducted P waves, referred to as *paroxysmal AV block* (Fig. 232-7), and implies significant conduction system disease and is an indication for permanent pacing. Complete failure of conduction from atrium to ventricle is referred to as complete or third-degree AV block. AV block that is intermediate between second degree and third degree is referred to as high-grade AV block and, as with CHB, implies advanced AV conduction system disease. In both cases, the block is most often distal to the AV node, and the duration of the QRS complex can be helpful in determining the level of the block. In the absence of a preexisting bundle branch block, a wide QRS escape rhythm (Fig. 232-8*B*) implies a block in the distal His or bundle branches; in contrast, a narrow QRS rhythm implies a block in the AV node or proximal His and an escape rhythm originating in the AV junction (Fig. 232-8*A*). Narrow QRS escape rhythms are typically faster and more stable than wide QRS escape rhythms and originate more proximally in the AV conduction system.

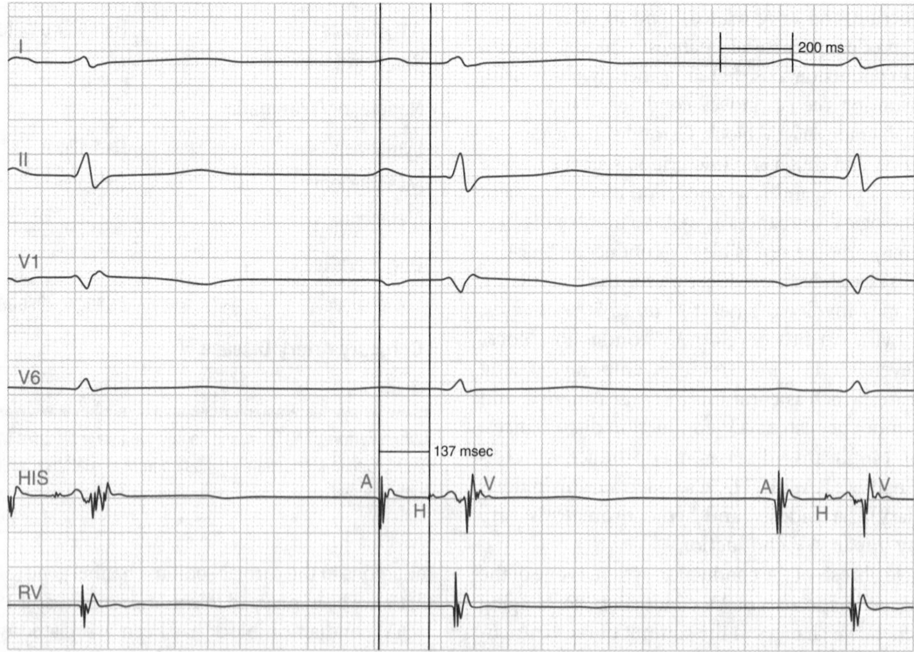

Figure 232-5 First-degree AV block with slowing of conduction in the AV node as indicated by the prolonged atrial-to-His bundle electrogram (AH) interval, in this case 157 ms. The His bundle-to-earliest ventricular activation on the surface ECG (HV) interval is normal. The normal HV interval suggests normal conduction below the AV node to the ventricle. I and V1 are surface ECG leads, HIS is the recording of the endocavitary electrogram at the His bundle position. A, H, and V are labels for the atrial, His bundle, and right ventricular electrograms, respectively.

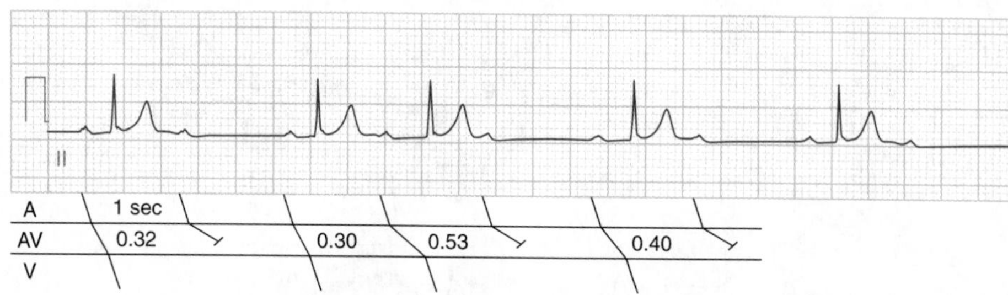

Figure 232-6 Mobitz type I second-degree AV block. The PR interval prolongs before the pause, as shown in the ladder diagram. The ECG pattern results from slowing of conduction in the AV node.

Diagnostic testing

Diagnostic testing in the evaluation of AV block is aimed at determining the level of conduction block, particularly in asymptomatic patients, since the prognosis and therapy depend on whether the block is in or below the AV node. Vagal maneuvers, carotid sinus massage, exercise, and administration of drugs such as atropine and isoproterenol may be diagnostically informative. Owing to the differences in innervation of the AV node and infranodal conduction system, vagal stimulation and carotid sinus massage slow conduction in the AV node but have less of an effect on infranodal tissue and may even improve conduction due to a reduced rate of activation of distal tissues. Conversely, atropine, isoproterenol, and exercise improve conduction through the AV node and impair infranodal conduction. In patients with congenital CHB and a narrow QRS complex, exercise typically increases heart rate; by contrast, those with acquired CHB, particularly with wide QRS, do not respond to exercise with an increase in heart rate.

Additional diagnostic evaluation, including electrophysiologic testing, may be indicated in patients with syncope and suspected high-grade AV block. This is particularly relevant if noninvasive testing does not reveal the cause of syncope or if the patient has structural heart disease with ventricular tachyarrhythmias as a cause of symptoms. Electrophysiologic testing provides more precise information regarding the location of AV conduction block and permits studies of AV conduction under conditions of pharmacologic stress and exercise. Recording of the His bundle electrogram by a catheter positioned at the superior margin of the tricuspid valve annulus provides information about conduction at all levels of the AV conduction axis. A properly recorded His bundle electrogram reveals local atrial activity, the His electrogram, and local ventricular activation; when it is monitored simultaneously with recorded body surface electrocardiographic traces, intraatrial, AV nodal, and infranodal conduction times can be assessed (Fig. 232-5). The time from the most rapid deflection of the atrial electrogram in the His bundle recording to the His electrogram (*AH interval*) represents conduction through the AV node and is normally <130 ms. The time from the His electrogram to the earliest onset of the QRS on the surface ECG (*HV interval*) represents the conduction time through the His-Purkinje system and is normally ≤55 ms.

Rate stress produced by pacing can unveil abnormal AV conduction. Mobitz I second-degree AV block at short atrial paced cycle lengths is a normal response. However, when it occurs at atrial cycle lengths >500 ms (<120 beats/min) in the absence of high vagal tone, it is abnormal. Typically, type I second-degree AV block is associated with prolongation of the AH interval, representing conduction slowing and block in the AV node. AH prolongation occasionally is due to the effect of drugs (beta blockers, calcium channel blockers, digitalis) or increased vagal tone. Atropine can be used to reverse high vagal tone; however, if AH prolongation and AV block at long pacing cycle lengths persist, intrinsic AV node disease is likely. Type II second-degree block is typically infranodal, often in the His-Purkinje system. Block below the node with prolongation of the HV interval or a His bundle electrogram with no ventricular activation (Fig. 232-9) is abnormal unless it is elicited at fast pacing rates or short coupling intervals with extra stimulation. It is often difficult to determine the type of second-degree AV block when 2:1 conduction is present; however, the finding of a His bundle electrogram after every atrial electrogram indicates that block is occurring in the distal conduction system.

Intracardiac recording at electrophysiologic study that reveals prolongation of conduction through the His-Purkinje system (i.e., long HV interval) is associated with an increased risk of progression to higher grades of block and is generally an indication for pacing. In the setting of bundle branch block, the HV interval may reveal the condition of the unblocked bundle and the prognosis for developing more advanced AV conduction block. Prolongation of the HV interval in patients with asymptomatic bundle branch block is associated with an increased risk of developing higher-grade AV block. The risk increases with greater prolongation of the HV interval such that in patients with an HV interval >100 ms, the annual incidence of complete AV block approaches 10%, indicating a need for pacing. In patients with acquired CHB, even if intermittent, there is little role for electrophysiologic testing, and pacemaker implantation is almost always indicated.

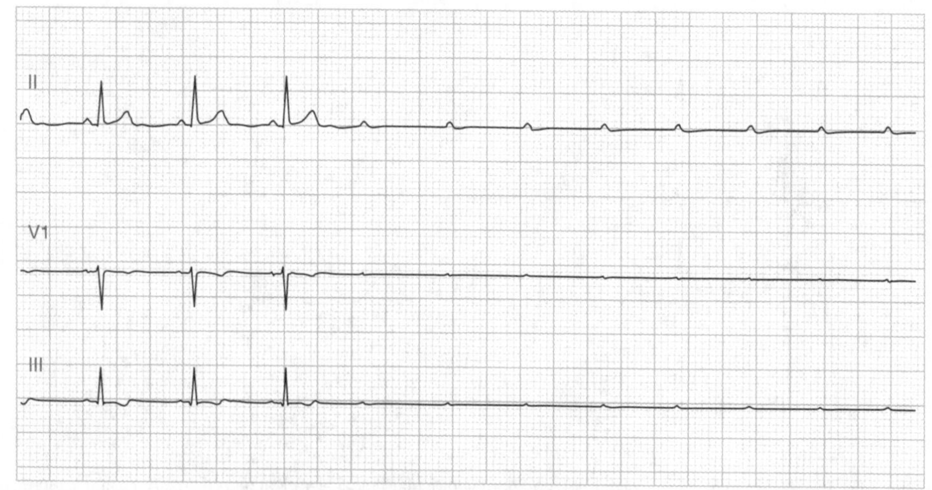

Figure 232-7 Paroxysmal AV block. Multiple nonconducted P waves after a period of sinus bradycardia with a normal PR interval. This implies significant conduction system disease, requiring permanent pacemaker implantation.

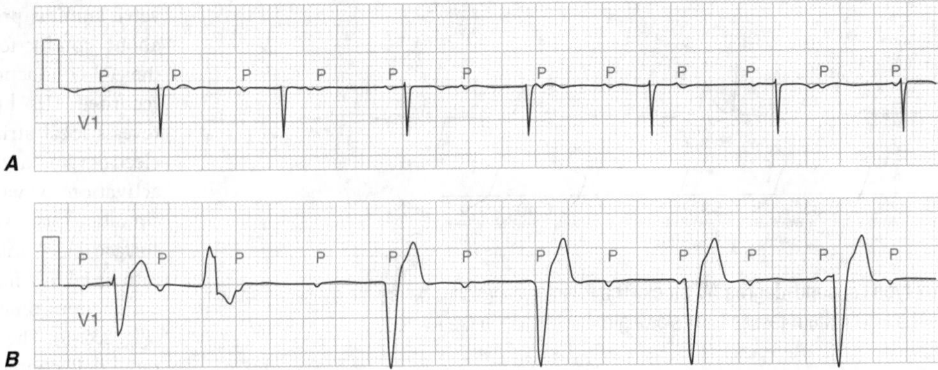

Figure 232-8 **High-grade AV block.** ***A.*** Multiple nonconducted P waves with a regular narrow complex QRS escape rhythm probably emanating from the AV junction. ***B.*** A wide complex QRS escape and a single premature ventricular contraction. In both cases there is no consistent temporal relationship between the P waves and QRS complexes.

TREATMENT Management of AV Conduction Block

Temporary or permanent artificial pacing is the most reliable treatment for patients with symptomatic AV conduction system disease. However, exclusion of reversible causes of AV block and the need for temporary heart rate support based on the hemodynamic condition of the patient are essential considerations in each patient. Correction of electrolyte derangements and ischemia, inhibition of excessive vagal tone, and withholding of drugs with AV nodal blocking properties may increase the heart rate. Adjunctive pharmacologic treatment with atropine or isoproterenol may be useful if the block is in the AV node. Since most pharmacologic treatment may take some time to initiate and become effective, temporary pacing may be necessary. The most expeditious technique is the use of transcutaneous pacing, where pacing patches are placed anteriorly over the cardiac apex (cathode) and posteriorly between the spine and the scapula or above the right nipple (anode). Acutely, transcutaneous pacing is highly effective, but its duration is limited by patient discomfort and longer-term failure to capture the ventricle owing to changes in lead impedance. If a

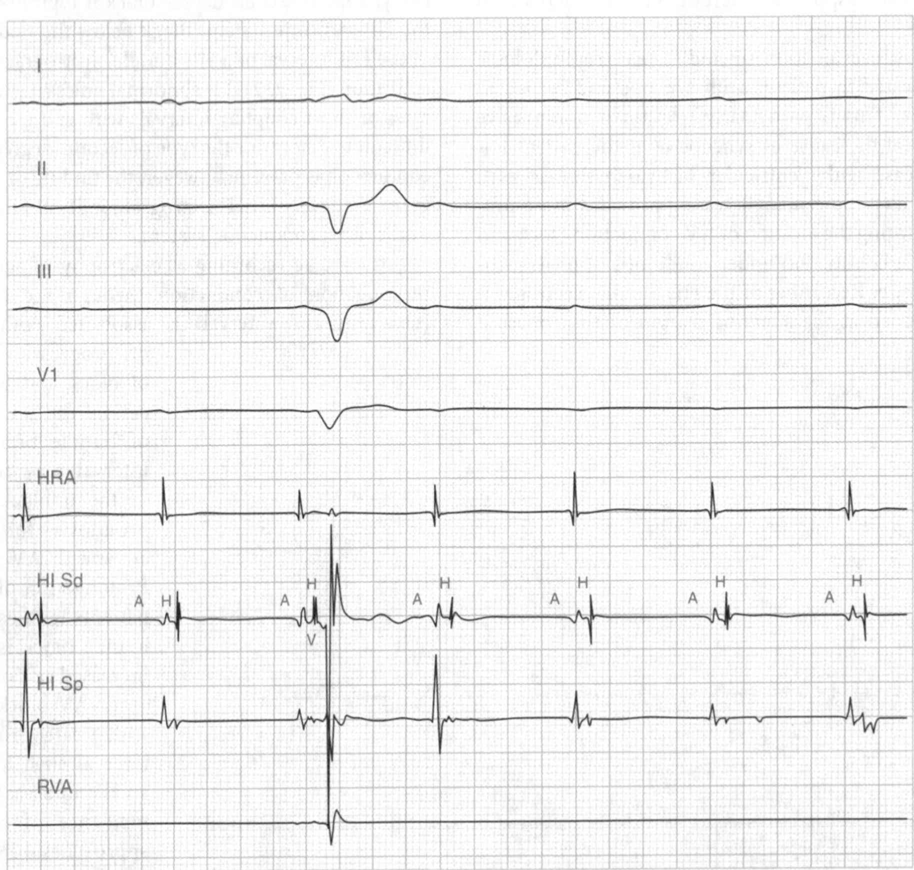

Figure 232-9 **High-grade AV block below the His.** The AH interval is normal and is not changing before the block. Atrial and His bundle electrograms are recorded consistent with block below the distal AV junction. I, II, III, and V1 are surface ECG leads. HISp, HISd, and RVA are the proximal HIS, distal HIS, and right ventricular apical electrical recordings. A, H, and V represent the atrial, His, and ventricular electrograms on the His bundle recording. *(Tracing courtesy of Dr. Joseph Marine; with permission.)*

patient requires more than a few minutes of pacemaker support, transvenous temporary pacing should be instituted. Temporary pacing leads can be placed from the jugular or subclavian venous system and advanced to the right ventricle, permitting stable temporary pacing for many days, if necessary. In most circumstances, in the absence of prompt resolution, conduction block distal to the AV node requires permanent pacemaking.

PERMANENT PACEMAKERS

Nomenclature and Complications The main therapeutic intervention in SA node dysfunction and AV conduction block is permanent pacing. Since the first implementation of permanent pacing in the 1950s, many advances in technology have resulted in miniaturization, increased longevity of pulse generators, improvement in leads, and increased functionality. To better understand pacemaker therapy for bradycardias, it is important to be familiar with the fundamentals of pacemaking. Pacemaker modes and function are named using a five-letter code. The first letter indicates the chamber(s) that is paced (O, none; A, atrium; V, ventricle; D, dual; S, single), the second is the chamber(s) in which sensing occurs (O, none; A, atrium; V, ventricle; D, dual; S, single), the third is the response to a sensed event (O, none; I, inhibition; T, triggered; D, inhibition + triggered), the fourth refers to the programmability or rate response (R, rate responsive), and the fifth refers to the existence of antitachycardia functions if present (O, none; P, antitachycardia pacing; S, shock; D, pace + shock). Almost all modern pacemakers are multiprogrammable and have the capability for rate responsiveness using one of several rate sensors: activity or motion, minute ventilation, or QT interval. The most commonly programmed modes of implanted single- and dual-chamber pacemakers are VVIR and DDDR, respectively, although multiple modes can be programmed in modern pacemakers.

Although pacemakers are highly reliable, they are subject to a number of complications related to implantation and electronic function. In adults, permanent pacemakers are most commonly implanted with access to the heart by way of the subclavian–superior vena cava venous system. Rare, but possible, acute complications of transvenous pacemaker implantation include infection, hematoma, pneumothorax, cardiac perforation, diaphragmatic/phrenic nerve stimulation, and lead dislodgment. Limitations of chronic pacemaker therapy include infection, erosion, lead failure, and abnormalities resulting from inappropriate programming or interaction with the patient's native electrical cardiac function. Rotation of the pacemaker pulse generator in its subcutaneous pocket, either intentionally or inadvertently, often referred to as "twiddler's syndrome," can wrap the leads around the generator and produce dislodgment with failure to sense or pace the heart. The small size and light weight of contemporary pacemakers make this a rare complication.

Complications stemming from chronic cardiac pacing also result from disturbances in atrioventricular synchrony and/or left ventricular mechanical synchrony. Pacing modes that interrupt or fail to restore atrioventricular synchrony may lead to a constellation of signs and symptoms, collectively referred to as pacemaker syndrome, that include neck pulsation, fatigue, palpitations, cough, confusion, exertional dyspnea, dizziness, syncope, elevation in jugular venous pressure, canon A waves, and stigmata of congestive heart failure, including edema, rales, and a third heart sound. Right ventricular apical pacing can induce dyssynchronous activation of the left ventricle, leading to compromised left ventricular (LV) systolic function, mitral valve regurgitation, and the previously mentioned stigmata of congestive heart failure. Maintenance of AV synchrony can minimize the sequelae of pacemaker syndrome. Selection of pacing modes that minimize unnecessary ventricular pacing or implantation of a device capable of right and left ventricular pacing (biventricular pacing) can help minimize the deleterious consequences of pacing-induced mechanical dyssynchrony at the ventricular level.

Pacemaker Therapy in SA Node Dysfunction Pacing in SA nodal disease is indicated to alleviate symptoms of bradycardia. Consensus guidelines published by the American Heart Association (AHA)/American College of Cardiology/Heart Rhythm Society (ACC/HRS) outline the indications for the use of pacemakers and categorize them by class based on levels of evidence. Class I conditions are those for which there is evidence or consensus of opinion that therapy is useful and effective. In class II conditions there is conflicting evidence or a divergence of opinion about the efficacy of a procedure or treatment; in class IIa conditions the weight of evidence or opinion favors treatment, and in class IIb conditions efficacy is less well established by the evidence or opinion of experts. In class III conditions, the evidence or weight of opinion indicates that the therapy is not efficacious or useful and may be harmful.

Class I indications for pacing in SA node dysfunction include documented symptomatic bradycardia, sinus node dysfunction–associated long-term drug therapy for which there is no alternative, and symptomatic chronotropic incompetence. Class IIa indications include those outlined previously in which sinus node dysfunction is suspected but not documented and for syncope of unexplained origin in the presence of major abnormalities of SA node dysfunction. Mildly symptomatic individuals with heart rates consistently <40 beats/min constitute a class IIb indication for pacing. Pacing is not indicated in patients with SA node dysfunction who do not have symptoms and in those in whom bradycardia is associated with the use of nonessential drugs (Table 232-3).

There is some controversy about the mode of pacing that should be employed in SA node disease. A number of randomized, single-blind trials of pacing mode have been performed. There are no trials that demonstrate an improvement in mortality rate with AV synchronous pacing compared with single-chamber pacing in SA node disease. In some of these studies, the incidence of atrial fibrillation and thromboembolic events was reduced with AV synchronous pacing. In trials of patients with dual-chamber pacemakers designed to compare single-chamber with dual-chamber pacing by crossover design, the need for AV synchronous pacing due to pacemaker syndrome was common. Pacing modes that preserve AV synchrony appear to be associated with a reduction in the incidence of atrial fibrillation and improved quality of life. Because of the low but finite incidence of AV conduction disease, patients with SA node dysfunction usually undergo dual-chamber pacemaker implantation.

Pacemaker Therapy in Carotid Sinus Hypersensitivity and Vasovagal Syncope Carotid sinus hypersensitivity, if accompanied by a significant cardioinhibitory component, responds well to pacing. In this circumstance, pacing is required only intermittently and single-chamber ventricular pacing is often sufficient. The mechanism of vasovagal syncope is incompletely understood but appears to involve activation of cardiac mechanoreceptors with consequent activation of neural centers that mediate vagal activation and withdrawal of sympathetic nervous system tone. Several randomized clinical trials have been performed in patients with drug-refractory vasovagal syncope, with some studies suggesting reduction in the frequency and the time to recurrent syncope in patients who were paced compared with those who were not. A recent follow-up study to one of those initial trials, however, found less convincing results, casting some doubt on the utility of pacing for vagally mediated syncope.

TABLE 232-3 Summary of Guidelines for Pacemaker Implantation in SA Node Dysfunction

Class I
1. SA node dysfunction with symptomatic bradycardia or sinus pauses
2. Symptomatic SA node dysfunction as a result of essential long-term drug therapy with no acceptable alternatives
3. Symptomatic chronotropic incompetence
4. Atrial fibrillation with bradycardia and pauses >5s
Class IIa
1. SA node dysfunction with heart rates <40 beats/min without a clear and consistent relationship between bradycardia and symptoms
2. SA node dysfunction with heart rates <40 beats/min on an essential long-term drug therapy with no acceptable alternatives, without a clear and consistent relationship between bradycardia and symptoms
3. Syncope of unknown origin when major abnormalities of SA node dysfunction are discovered or provoked by electrophysiologic testing
Class IIb
1. Mildly symptomatic patients with waking chronic heart rates <40 beats/min
Class III
1. SA node dysfunction in asymptomatic patients, even those with heart rates <40 beats/min
2. SA node dysfunction in which symptoms suggestive of bradycardia are not associated with a slow heart rate
3. SA node dysfunction with symptomatic bradycardia due to nonessential drug therapy

Source: Modified from Epstein et al, J. Am. Coll. Cardiol. 51:e1, 2008 and Gregoratos et al, J. Am. Coll. Cardiol. 40:703, 2002.

TABLE 232-4 Guideline Summary for Pacemaker Implantation in Acquired AV Block

Class I
1. Third-degree or high-grade AV block at any anatomic level associated with:
a. Symptomatic bradycardia
b. Essential drug therapy that produces symptomatic bradycardia
c. Periods of asystole >3 s or any escape rate <40 beats/min while awake
d. Postoperative AV block not expected to resolve
e. Catheter ablation of the AV junction
f. Neuromuscular diseases such as myotonic dystrophy, Kearns-Sayre syndrome, Erb dystrophy, and peroneal muscular atrophy, regardless of the presence of symptoms
2. Second-degree AV block with symptomatic bradycardia
3. Type II second-degree AV block with a wide QRS complex with or without symptoms
4. Exercise-induced second- or third-degree AV block in the absence of ischemia
5. Atrial fibrillation with bradycardia and pauses >5s
Class IIa
1. Asymptomatic third-degree AV block regardless of level
2. Asymptomatic type II second-degree AV block with a narrow QRS complex
3. Asymptomatic type II second-degree AV block with block within or below the His at electrophysiologic study
4. First- or second-degree AV block with symptoms similar to pacemaker syndrome
Class IIb
1. Marked first-degree AV block (PR interval >300 ms) in patients with LV dysfunction in whom shortening the AV delay would improve hemodynamics
2. Neuromuscular diseases such as myotonic dystrophy, Kearns-Sayre syndrome, Erb dystrophy, and peroneal muscular atrophy with any degree of AV block regardless of the presence of symptoms
Class III
1. Asymptomatic first-degree AV block
2. Asymptomatic type I second-degree AV block at the AV node level
3. AV block that is expected to resolve or is unlikely to recur (Lyme disease, drug toxicity)

Source: Modified from Epstein et al, J. Am. Coll. Cardiol. 51:e1, 2008 and Gregoratos et al, J. Am. Coll. Cardiol. 40:703, 2002.

Pacemakers in AV Conduction Disease There are no randomized trials that evaluate the efficacy of pacing in patients with AV block, as there are no reliable therapeutic alternatives for AV block and untreated high-grade AV block is potentially lethal. The consensus guidelines for pacing in acquired AV conduction block in adults provide a general outline for situations in which pacing is indicated (Table 232-4). Pacemaker implantation should be performed in any patient with symptomatic bradycardia and irreversible second- or third-degree AV block, regardless of the cause or level of block in the conducting system. Symptoms may include those directly related to bradycardia and low cardiac output or to worsening heart failure, angina, or intolerance to an essential medication. Pacing in patients with asymptomatic AV block should be individualized; situations in which pacing should be considered are patients with acquired CHB, particularly in the setting of cardiac enlargement; left ventricular dysfunction; and waking heart rates ≤40 beats/min. Patients who have asymptomatic second-degree AV block of either type should be considered for pacing if the block is demonstrated to be intra- or infra-His or is associated with a wide QRS complex. Pacing may be indicated in asymptomatic patients in special circumstances, in patients with profound first-degree AV block and left ventricular dysfunction in whom a shorter AV interval produces hemodynamic improvement, and in the setting of milder forms of AV conduction delay (first-degree AV block, intraventricular conduction delay) in patients with neuromuscular diseases that have a predilection for the conduction system, such as myotonic dystrophy and other muscular dystrophies, and Kearns-Sayre syndrome.

Pacemaker Therapy in Myocardial Infarction Atrioventricular block in acute MI is often transient, particularly in inferior infarction. The circumstances in which pacing is indicated in acute MI are persistent second- or third-degree AV block, particularly if symptomatic, and transient second- or third-degree AV block associated with bundle branch block (Table 232-5). Pacing is generally not indicated in the setting of transient AV block in the absence of intraventricular conduction delays or

TABLE 232-5 Guideline Summary for Pacemaker Implantation in AV Conduction Block in Acute Myocardial Infarction (AMI)

Class I

1. Persistent second-degree AV block in the His-Purkinje system with bilateral bundle branch block or third-degree block within or below the His after AMI
2. Transient advanced (second- or third-degree) infranodal AV block and associated bundle branch block. If the site of block is uncertain, an electrophysiologic study may be necessary
3. Persistent and symptomatic second- or third-degree AV block

Class IIb

1. Persistent second- or third-degree AV block at the AV node level

Class III

1. Transient AV block in the absence of intraventricular conduction defects
2. Transient AV block in the presence of isolated left anterior fascicular block
3. Acquired left anterior fascicular block in the absence of AV block
4. Persistent first-degree AV block in the presence of bundle branch block that is old or age-indeterminate

Source: Modified from Epstein et al, J. Am. Coll. Cardiol. 51:e1, 2008 and Gregoratos et al, J. Am. Coll. Cardiol. 40:703, 2002.

in the presence of fascicular block or first-degree AV block that develops in the setting of preexisting bundle branch block. Fascicular blocks that develop in acute MI in the absence of other forms of AV block also do not require pacing (Table 232-5 and Table 232-6).

TABLE 232-6 Indications for Pacemaker Implantation in Chronic Bifascicular and Trifascicular Block

Class I

1. Intermittent third-degree AV block
2. Type II second-degree AV block
3. Alternating bundle branch block

Class IIa

1. Syncope not demonstrated to be due to AV block when other likely causes (e.g., ventricular tachycardia) have been excluded
2. Incidental finding at electrophysiologic study of a markedly prolonged HV interval (>100 ms) in asymptomatic patients
3. Incidental finding at electrophysiologic study of pacing-induced infra-His block that is not physiologic

Class IIb

1. Neuromuscular diseases such as myotonic dystrophy, Kearns-Sayre syndrome, Erb dystrophy, and peroneal muscular atrophy with any degree of fascicular block regardless of the presence of symptoms, because there may be unpredictable progression of AV conduction disease

Class III

1. Fascicular block without AV block or symptoms
2. Fascicular block with first-degree AV block without symptoms

Source: Modified from Epstein et al, J. Am. Coll. Cardiol. 51:e1, 2008 and Gregoratos et al, J. Am. Coll. Cardiol. 40:703, 2002.

Pacemaker Therapy in Bifascicular and Trifascicular Block Distal forms of AV conduction block may require pacemaker implantation in certain clinical settings. Patients with bifascicular or trifascicular block and symptoms, particularly syncope that is not attributable to other causes, should undergo pacemaker implantation. Pacemaking is indicated in asymptomatic patients with bifascicular or trifascicular block who experience intermittent third-degree, type II second-degree AV block or alternating bundle branch block. In patients with fascicular block who are undergoing electrophysiologic study, a markedly prolonged HV interval or block below the His at long cycle lengths also may constitute an indication for permanent pacing. Patients with fascicular block and the neuromuscular diseases previously described should also undergo pacemaker implantation (Table 232-6).

Selection of Pacing Mode In general, a pacing mode that maintains AV synchrony reduces complications of pacing such as pacemaker syndrome and pacemaker-mediated tachycardia. This is particularly true in younger patients; the importance of dual-chamber pacing in the elderly, however, is not well established. Several studies have failed to demonstrate a difference in mortality rate in older patients with AV block treated with a single- (VVI) compared with a dual- (DDD) chamber pacing mode. In some of the studies that randomized pacing mode, the risk of chronic atrial fibrillation and stroke risk decreased with physiologic pacing. In patients with sinus rhythm and AV block, the very modest increase in risk with dual-chamber pacemaker implantation appears to be justified to avoid the possible complications of single-chamber pacing.

FURTHER READINGS

Bharati S et al: Sinus node dysfunction, in *Electrophysiological Disorders of the Heart*, S Saksena, AJ Camm (eds). Philadelphia, Elsevier Churchill Livingstone, 2005

Epstein AE et al: ACC/AHA/HRS 2008 Guidelines for Device-Based Therapy of Cardiac Rhythm Abnormalities: A report of the American College of Cardiology/American Heart Association Task Force on Practice Guidelines (Writing Committee to Revise the ACC/AHA/NASPE 2002 Guideline Update for Implantation of Cardiac Pacemakers and Antiarrhythmia Devices) developed in collaboration with the American Association for Thoracic Surgery and Society of Thoracic Surgeons. J Am Coll Cardiol 51:el, 2008

Goldschlager N et al: Atrioventricular block, in *Electrophysiological Disorders of the Heart*, S Saksena, AJ Camm (eds). Philadelphia, Elsevier Churchill Livingstone, 2005

———: ACC/AHA/NASPE 2008 Guidelines for device-based therapy of cardiac rhythm abnormalities. J Am Coll Cardiol 51:21, 2008

Gregoratos G et al: ACC/AHA/NASPE 2002 Guideline Update for Implantation of Cardiac Pacemakers and Antiarrhythmia Devices–summary article: A report of the American College of Cardiology/American Heart Association Task Force on Practice Guidelines (ACC/AHA/NASPE Committee to Update the 1998 Pacemaker Guidelines). J Am Coll Cardiol 40:1703, 2002

Josephson ME: *Clinical Cardiac Electrophysiology: Techniques and Interpretations*, 4th ed. Philadelphia, Lippincott Williams & Wilkins, 2008

Vijayaraman P, Ellenbogen KA: Bradyarrhythmias and pacemakers, in *Hurst's The Heart*, 12th ed, V Fuster et al (eds). New York, McGraw-Hill, 2008

CHAPTER 233 The Tachyarrhythmias

Francis Marchlinski

The term *tachyarrhythmias* typically refers to nonsustained and sustained forms of tachycardia originating from myocardial foci or reentrant circuits. The standard definition of tachycardia is a rhythm that produces a ventricular rate >100 beats per minute. This definition has some limitations in that atrial rates can exceed 100 beats per minute despite a slow ventricular rate. Furthermore, ventricular rates may exceed the baseline sinus rate and be <100 beats per minute but still represent an important "tachycardia" response, as is observed with accelerated ventricular rhythms. Premature complexes (depolarizations) are considered under the category of tachyarrhythmias because they may cause arrhythmia-related symptoms and/or serve as triggering events for more sustained forms of tachycardia.

SYMPTOMS DUE TO TACHYARRHYTHMIAS

Tachyarrhythmias classically produce symptoms of palpitations or racing of the pulse. With premature beats, skipping of the pulse or a pause may be experienced, and patients may even sense slowing of the heart rate or dizziness. A more dramatic irregularity of the pulse is experienced with chaotic rapid rhythms or tachyarrhythmias that originate in the atrium and conduct variably to the ventricles. With rapid tachyarrhythmias, hemodynamic compromise can occur, as can dizziness or syncope due to a decrease in cardiac output or breathlessness due to a marked increase in cardiac filling pressures. Occasionally, chest discomfort may be experienced that mimics symptoms of myocardial ischemia. The underlying cardiac condition typically dictates the severity of symptoms at any specific heart rate. Even patients with normal systolic left ventricular (LV) function may experience severe symptoms if diastolic compliance due to hypertrophy or valvular obstruction is present and a tachycardia develops. Hemodynamic collapse with the development of ventricular fibrillation (VF) can lead to sudden cardiac death (SCD) (Chap. 273).

DIAGNOSTIC TESTS IN EVALUATING TACHYARRHYTHMIAS

In patients who present with nonlife-threatening symptoms such as palpitations or dizziness, electrocardiographic (ECG) confirmation of an arrhythmia with the development of recurrent symptoms is essential. A 24-hour Holter monitor should be considered only for patients with daily symptoms. For intermittent symptoms that are of prolonged duration, a patient-activated event monitor can be used to obtain the ECG information without the need for continuous ECG lead attachment and recordings. A patient-activated monitor with a continuously recorded memory loop ("loop recorder") can be used to document short-lived episodes and the onset of the arrhythmia. This is the preferred monitoring technique for symptomatic patients with less frequent arrhythmia events, but it requires continuous ECG recording. A monitor that automatically triggers to record a fast rhythm can be used to detect asymptomatic arrhythmias. Patients with infrequent, severe symptoms that cannot be identified by intermittent ECG monitoring may receive an implanted loop ECG monitor that provides more extended periods of monitoring and automatic arrhythmia detection (Fig. 233-1).

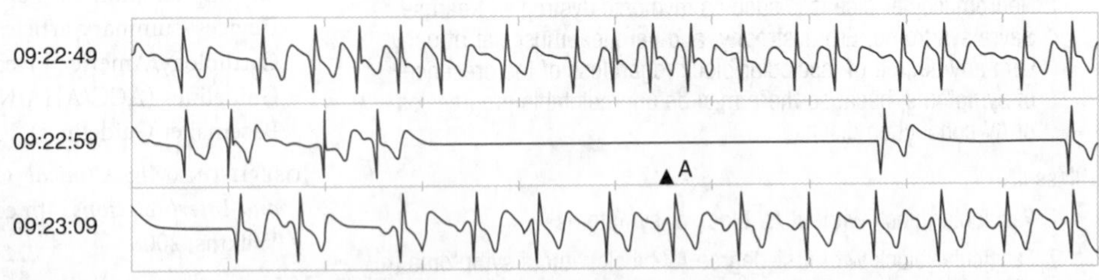

Figure 233-1 Spontaneous termination of atrial fibrillation at the time of a syncopal episode identified from implantable loop ECG recording.

In patients who present with more severe symptoms, such as syncope, outpatient monitoring may be insufficient. In patients with structural heart disease and syncope in whom there is suspicion of ventricular tachycardia (VT), hospitalization and diagnostic electrophysiologic testing are warranted, with strong consideration of an implantable cardioverter/defibrillator (ICD) device. The 12-lead ECG recorded in sinus rhythm should be assessed carefully in patients without structural heart disease for evidence of ST-segment elevation in leads V_1 and V_2 consistent with the Brugada syndrome, QT interval changes consistent with long or short QT syndromes, or a short PR interval and delta wave consistent with Wolff-Parkinson-White (WPW) syndrome. These ECG patterns identify a possible arrhythmogenic substrate that may cause intermittent life-threatening symptoms and warrant further evaluation and therapy. The individual syndromes are discussed in detail later in this chapter.

Monitoring for asymptomatic tachyarrhythmias is indicated in several specific situations. In patients with a suspected tachycardia-induced cardiomyopathy marked by chamber dilation and depression in systolic function, the demonstration of arrhythmia control is essential. Monitoring for asymptomatic ventricular premature complexes (VPCs) and nonsustained VT can be helpful in stratifying the risk of SCD in patients with depressed LV function after myocardial infarction (MI). Finally, in patients with asymptomatic atrial fibrillation (AF), anticoagulation treatment strategies depend on an accurate assessment of the presence of this arrhythmia. The duration of monitoring for asymptomatic arrhythmias may have to be extended to optimize detection capabilities.

A 12-lead ECG recording during the tachycardia can be an important diagnostic tool in identifying the mechanism and origin of a tachycardia to a degree not afforded by one- or two-lead ECG recordings. A 12-lead ECG of the tachyarrhythmia should be recorded and incorporated as a permanent part of the medical record whenever possible. For patients whose arrhythmias are provoked by exercise, an exercise test may provide an opportunity to obtain 12-lead ECG recordings of the arrhythmia and may obviate the need for more extended periods of monitoring.

Many paroxysmal supraventricular tachyarrhythmias are not associated with a significant risk of structural heart disease, and an evaluation for the presence of ischemic heart disease and cardiac function is required infrequently unless dictated by the severity or characteristics of the symptoms. However, in patients with focal or macroreentrant atrial tachycardias (ATs), atrial flutter (AFL), or AF, an evaluation of cardiac chamber size and function and of valve function is warranted. In patients with VT, an echocardiographic assessment of LV and right ventricular (RV) size and function should be the norm. Ventricular tachycardia that occurs in the setting of depressed LV function should raise the suspicion of advanced coronary artery disease (CAD). Ventricular tachycardia in the setting of isolated RV dilation should raise concern about the diagnosis of arrhythmogenic RV cardiomyopathy. Polymorphic VT in the absence of QT prolongation should always raise concern for a potentially unstable ischemic process that may need to be corrected to effect VT control.

■ MECHANISMS OF TACHYARRHYTHMIAS

Tachycardias are due to abnormalities of impulse formation and/or abnormalities of impulse propagation (Fig. 233-2).

Abnormalities in impulse formation

An increase in automaticity normally causes an increase in sinus rate and sinus tachycardia (Fig. 233-2A). Abnormal automaticity is due to an increase in the slope of phase 4 depolarization or a reduced threshold for action potential depolarization in myocardium other than the sinus node. Abnormal automaticity is thought to be responsible for most atrial premature complexes (APCs) and VPCs and some ATs. Pacing does not provoke automatic rhythms. Less commonly, abnormal impulse formation is due to triggered activity. Triggered activity is related to cellular afterdepolarizations that occur at the end of the action potential, during phase 3, and are referred to as *early afterdepolarizations;* when they occur after the action potential, during phase 4, they are referred to as *late afterdepolarizations.* Afterdepolarizations are attributable to an increase in intracellular calcium accumulation. If sufficient afterdepolarization amplitude is achieved, repeated myocardial depolarization and a tachycardic response can occur. Early afterdepolarizations may be responsible for the VPCs that trigger the polymorphic ventricular arrhythmia known as *torsades des pointes* (TDP) (p. 1890). Late afterdepolarizations are thought to be responsible for atrial, junctional, and fascicular tachyarrhythmias caused by digoxin toxicity and also appear to be the basis for catecholamine-sensitive VT originating in the outflow tract. In contrast to automatic tachycardias, those due to triggered activity (Fig. 233-2B) frequently can be provoked with pacing maneuvers.

Abnormalities in impulse propagation

Reentry is due to inhomogeneities in myocardial conduction and/or recovery properties. The presence of a unidirectional block with slow conduction to allow for retrograde recovery of the blocked myocardium allows the formation of a circuit that, if perpetuated, can sustain a tachycardia (Fig. 233-2C). These inhomogeneities are somewhat inherent but are minimized in normal myocardial activation/recovery. The inhomogeneities can be exaggerated by the presence of extra pathways, as occurs with the WPW syndrome; generalized genetically determined myocardial ion channel abnormalities, as occur with long QT syndrome (LQTS); or the interruption of normal myocardial patterns of activation due to the development of fibrosis.

Reentry appears to be the basis for most abnormal sustained supraventricular tachycardias (SVTs) and VTs. In general, reentry can be anatomically driven (fixed) based on the presence of "extra" pathways, natural anatomic barriers of conduction such as the crista terminalis, the vertical crest on the interior wall of the right atrium that separates the nontrabeculated posterior right atrium from the rest of the trabeculated right atrium located lateral to the structure, and/or extensive fibrosis created by underlying myocardial disease. This form of reentry seems to be more stable and results in a tachycardia that has a uniform (often monomorphic), repetitive appearance. Other forms of reentry appear to be more functional and are more dependent on dynamic changes in electrophysiologic properties of the myocardium. These tachycardias tend to be more unstable and may result in tachycardias that have a polymorphic appearance. Two classic examples of reentry that is primarily functional are VF due to acute myocardial ischemia and polymorphic VT in patients with a genetically determined ion channel abnormality such as the Brugada syndrome, LQTS, or catecholaminergic polymorphic VT (pp. 1894-1895).

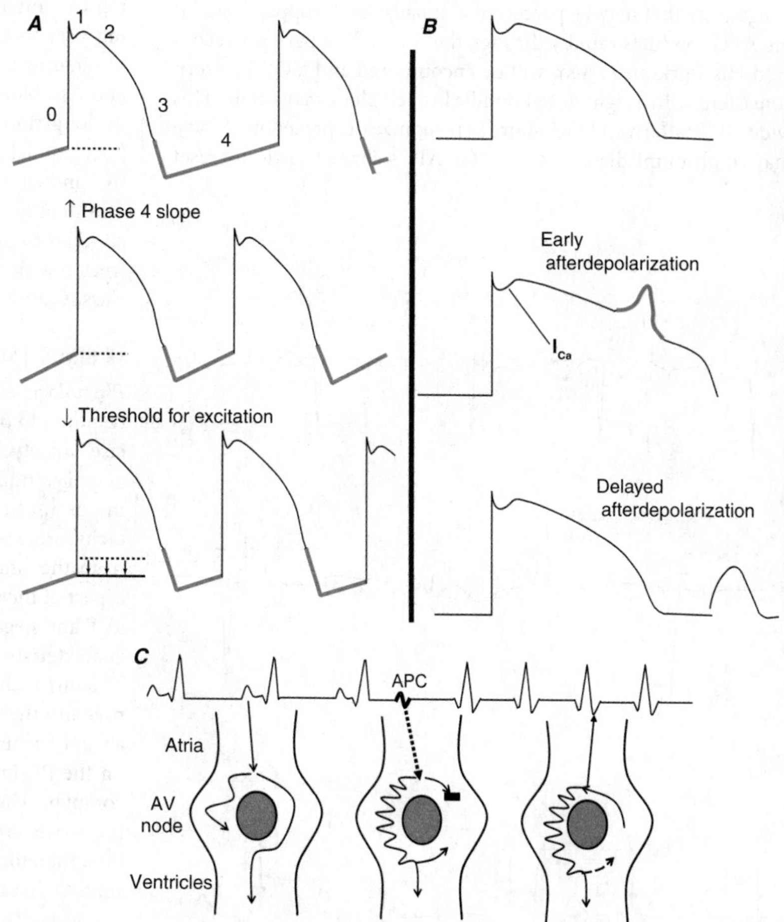

Figure 233-2 Schematic representation of the different mechanisms for arrhythmias. ***A.*** Abnormal automaticity due to an increased slope of phase 4 of the action potential or a decrease in the threshold for phase 0. ***B.*** Triggered activity due to early afterdepolarizations (EADs) during phase 3 of the action potential due to alteration of plateau currents or delayed afterdepolarizations (DADs) during phase 4 of the action potential due to intracellular calcium accumulation. ***C.*** Reentry with basic requirements of two pathways that have heterogeneous electrophysiologic properties which allows conduction to block in one pathway and propagate slowly in the other, allowing for sufficient delay so that the blocked site has time for recovery to allow for reentry or circus movement tachycardia. Shown is a typical schema for reentry in the AV node. AV, atrioventricular; APC, atrial premature complex.

SUPRAVENTRICULAR TACHYARRHYTHMIAS

ATRIAL PREMATURE COMPLEXES

Atrial premature complexes are the most common arrhythmia identified during extended ECG monitoring. The incidence of APCs frequently increases with age and with the presence of structural heart diseases. Atrial premature complexes typically are asymptomatic, although some patients experience palpitations or an irregularity of the pulse.

ECG diagnosis of APCs

The ECG diagnosis of APCs is based on the identification of a P wave that occurs before the anticipated sinus beat (Fig. 233-3*A* and *B*). The source of the APC appears to parallel the typical sites of origin for ATs. The P-wave contour typically differs from that noted during sinus rhythm, although APCs from the right atrial appendage, superior vena cava (SVC), and superior aspect of the crista terminalis in the region of the sinus node may mimic the sinus P-wave morphology. In response to an APC, the PR interval lengthens, although APCs that originate near the atrioventricular (AV) nodal region may actually have a shorter PR interval because the atrial conduction time to the junction is shortened. A very early APC may not conduct to the ventricle and can create a pulse irregularity that may be perceived as a pause or "dropped beat." If the APC conducts rapidly through the AV node, a partially recovered His-Purkinje system will be encountered and a QRS pattern consistent with a right or left bundle branch block may occur. This wide QRS pattern and the failure to recognize the preceding P wave may result in misdiagnosis of VPCs. APCs characteristically reset the sinus node. The resulting sum of the pre- and post-APC RR interval is less than two sinus PP intervals.

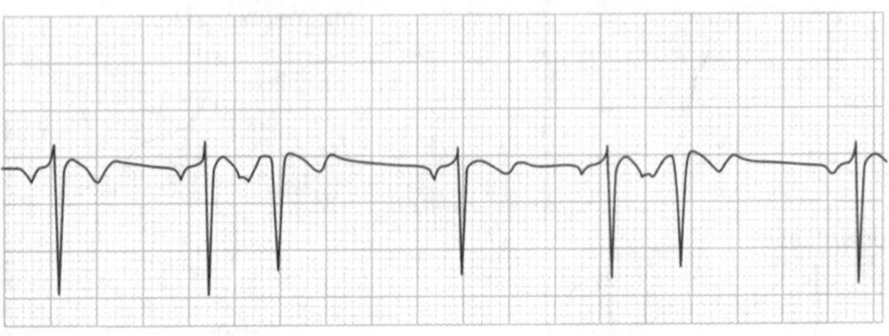
A

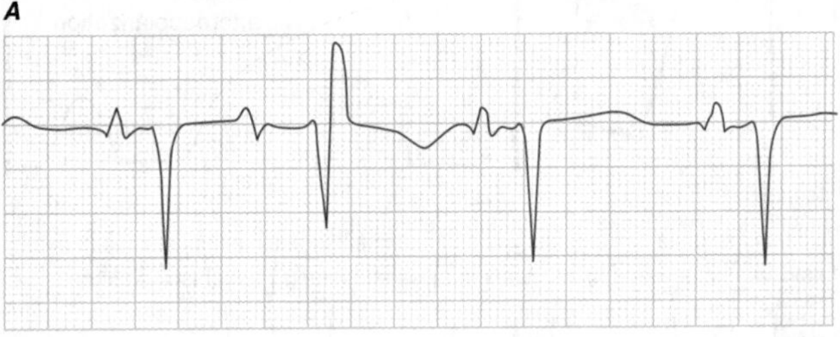
B

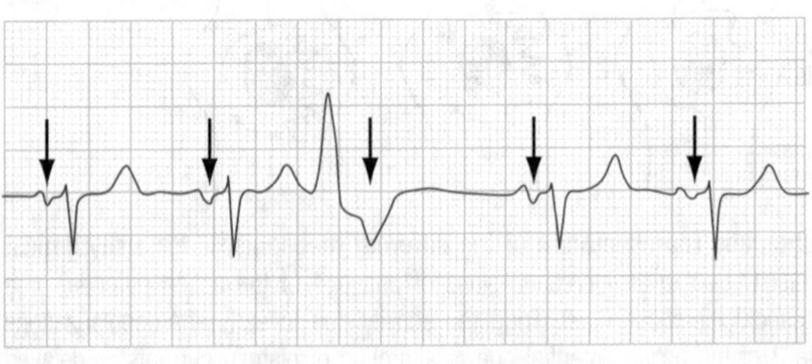
C

Figure 233-3 Atrial and ventricular premature complexes (APCs, VPCs). The APC resets the sinus node, and no compensatory pause is present ***A.*** even when conducted aberrantly in the ventricles with a bundle branch block-type QRS pattern ***B.*** VPCs tend not to reset the sinus activity (*arrows*) and will demonstrate a full compensatory pause ***C.***

TREATMENT Atrial Premature Complexes

Atrial premature complexes generally do not require intervention. For extremely symptomatic patients who do not respond to explanation and reassurance, an attempt can be made to suppress the APCs with pharmacologic agents. The repetitive focus can even be targeted for catheter ablation. Beta blockers may be tried. Of note, these agents may uncommonly exacerbate symptoms if AV block occurs with the APC and irregularity of the pulse consequently becomes more profound. The use of class IC antiarrhythmic agents may eliminate the APCs but should be avoided if structural heart disease is present.

JUNCTIONAL PREMATURE COMPLEXES

Junctional premature complexes are extremely uncommon. The complexes originate from the AV node and His bundle region and may produce retrograde atrial activation with the P wave distorting the initial or terminal portions of the QRS complex, producing pseudo Q or S waves in leads II, III, and aVF. Extrasystoles originating in the bundle of His that do not conduct to the ventricle and also block the atria can produce unexplained surface ECG PR prolongation that does not follow a typical Wenckebach periodicity (i.e., gradual PR prolongation culminating in atrial activity that fails to conduct to the ventricles). Intracardiac recordings frequently can identify a His depolarization, thus identifying the origin of the complex to the AV junction. Symptomatic patients typically may be treated with beta blockers or, if there is no structural heart disease, class IC antiarrhythmic agents.

SINUS TACHYCARDIA

Physiologic sinus tachycardia represents a normal or appropriate response to physiologic stress, such as that which occurs with exercise, anxiety, or fever. Pathologic conditions such as thyrotoxicosis, anemia, and hypotension also may produce sinus tachycardia. It is important to distinguish sinus tachycardia from other SVTs. Sinus tachycardia will produce a P-wave contour consistent with its origin from the sinus node located in the superior-lateral and posterior aspect of the right atrium. The P wave is upright in leads II, III, and aVF and negative in lead aVR. The P-wave morphology in lead V_1 characteristically has a biphasic, positive/negative contour. Onset of sinus tachycardia is gradual, and in response to carotid sinus pressure there may be some modest and transient slowing but no abrupt termination. Importantly, the diagnosis should not be based on the PR interval or the presence of a P wave before every QRS complex. The PR interval and the presence of 1:1 AV conduction properties are determined by AV nodal and His-Purkinje conduction; therefore, the PR interval can be dramatically prolonged while sinus tachycardia remains the atrial mechanism.

TREATMENT Physiologic Sinus Tachycardia

Treatment of physiologic sinus tachycardia is directed at the underlying condition causing the tachycardia response. Uncommonly, beta blockers are used to minimize the tachycardia response if it is determined to be potentially harmful, as may occur in a patient with ischemic heart disease and rate-related anginal symptoms.

Inappropriate sinus tachycardia represents an uncommon but important medical condition in which the heart rate increases either spontaneously or out of proportion to the degree of physiologic stress/exercise. Dizziness and even frank syncope often accompany the sinus tachycardia and symptoms of palpitations. The syndrome can be quite disabling. Associated symptoms of chest pain, headaches, and gastrointestinal upset are common. In many patients, the syndrome occurs after a viral illness and may resolve spontaneously over the course of 3–12 months, suggesting a postviral dysautonomia.

Excluding the diagnosis of an automatic AT that originates in the region of the sinus node can be difficult and may require invasive electrophysiologic evaluation. Frequently, patients are misdiagnosed as having an anxiety disorder with physiologic sinus tachycardia.

TREATMENT Inappropriate Sinus Tachycardia

For symptomatic patients, maintaining an increased state of hydration, salt loading, and careful titration of beta blockers to the maximum tolerated dose, administered in divided doses, frequently minimize symptoms. For severely symptomatic patients who are intolerant of or unresponsive to beta blockers, catheter ablation directed at modifying the sinus node may be effective. Because of the high recurrence rate after ablation and the frequent need for atrial pacing therapy, this intervention remains second-line treatment.

ATRIAL FIBRILLATION

(Fig. 233-4) Atrial fibrillation is the most common sustained arrhythmia. It is marked by disorganized, rapid, and irregular atrial activation. The ventricular response to the rapid atrial activation is also irregular. In an untreated patient, the ventricular rate also tends to be rapid and is entirely dependent on the conduction properties of the AV junction. Although typically the rate will vary between 120 and 160 beats per minute, in some patients it can be >200 beats per minute. In other patients, because of heightened vagal tone or intrinsic AV nodal conduction properties, the ventricular response is <100 beats per minute and occasionally even profoundly slow. The mechanism for AF initiation and maintenance, although still debated, appears to be a complex interaction between drivers responsible for the initiation and the complex anatomic atrial substrate that promotes the maintenance of multiple wavelets of (micro)reentry. The drivers appear to originate predominantly from the atrialized musculature that enters the pulmonary veins and represent either focal abnormal automaticity or triggered firing that is somewhat modulated by autonomic influences. Sustained forms of microreentry as drivers also have been documented around the orifice of pulmonary veins; nonpulmonary vein drivers also have been demonstrated. The role these drivers play in maintaining the tachycardias may be significant and may explain the success of pulmonary vein isolation procedures in eliminating more chronic or persistent forms of AF.

Although AF is common in the adult population, it is extremely unusual in children unless structural heart disease is present or there is another arrhythmia that precipitates the AF, such as paroxysmal SVT in patients with WPW syndrome. The incidence of AF increases with age such that >5% of the adult population over 70 will experience the arrhythmia. As many patients are asymptomatic with AF, it is anticipated that the overall incidence, particularly that noted in the elderly, may be more than double previously reported rates. Occasionally, AF appears to have a well-defined etiology, such as acute hyperthyroidism, an acute vagotonic episode, or acute alcohol intoxication. Acute AF is particularly common during the acute or early recovery phase of major vascular, abdominal, and thoracic surgery, in which case autonomic fluxes and/or direct mechanical irritation potentiate the arrhythmia. AF also may be triggered by other supraventricular tachycardias (p. 1888), such as AV nodal reentrant tachycardia (AVNRT), and elimination of these arrhythmias may prevent AF recurrence.

AF has clinical importance related to (1) the loss of atrial contractility, (2) the inappropriate fast ventricular response, and (3) the loss of atrial appendage contractility and emptying leading to the risk of clot formation and subsequent thromboembolic events.

Symptoms from AF vary dramatically. Many patients are asymptomatic and have no apparent hemodynamic consequences from the development of AF. Other patients experience only minor palpitations or sense irregularity of the pulse. Many patients, however, experience severe palpitations. The hemodynamic effect in patients can be quite dramatic, depending on the need for normal atrial contractility and the ventricular response. Hypotension, pulmonary congestion, and anginal symptoms may be severe in some patients. In patients with the LV diastolic dysfunction that occurs with hypertension, hypertrophic cardiomyopathy, or obstructive aortic valvular disease,

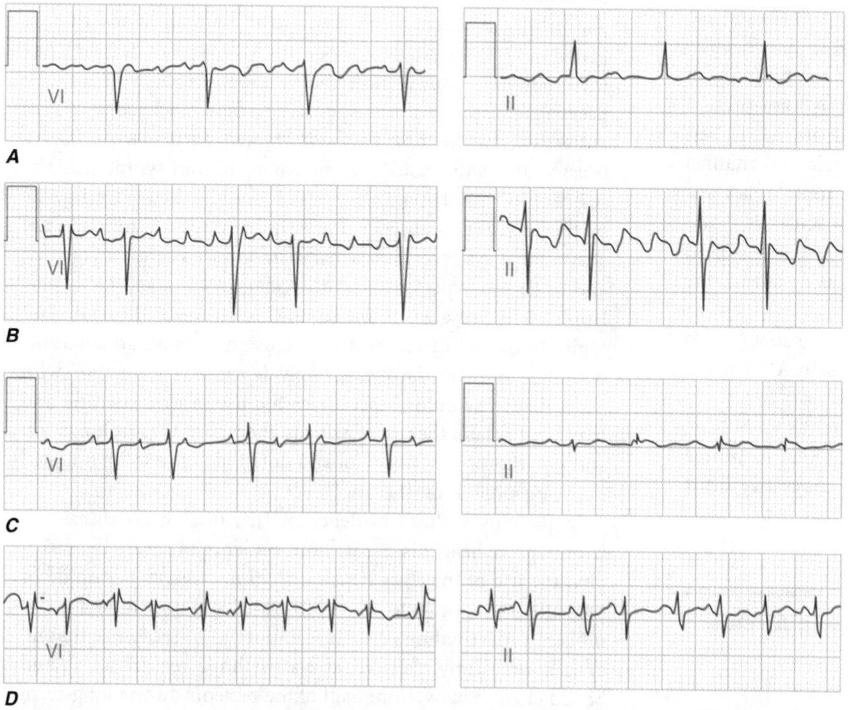

Figure 233-4 Supraventricular tachycardias with irregular ventricular rates. Atrial fibrillation ***A.*** atrial flutter ***B.*** atrial tachycardia ***C.*** and multifocal atrial tachycardia (MAT; ***D.***) are shown. The characteristics of the atrial activity with respect to the morphology and rate provide the clues to the diagnosis. The variable ventricular response to the atrial flutter and the atrial tachycardia suggest a Wenckebach-type periodicity.

symptoms may be even more dramatic, especially if the ventricular rate does not permit adequate ventricular filling. Exercise intolerance and easy fatigability are the hallmarks of poor rate control with exertion. Occasionally, the only manifestation of AF is severe dizziness or syncope associated with the pause that occurs upon termination of AF before sinus rhythm resumes (Fig. 233-1).

The ECG in AF is characterized by the lack of organized atrial activity and the irregularly irregular ventricular response. Occasionally, one needs to record from multiple ECG leads simultaneously to identify the chaotic continuous atrial activation. Lead V_1 frequently shows the appearance of organized atrial activity that mimics AFL. This occurs because the crista terminalis serves as an effective anatomic barrier to electrical conduction, and the activation of the lateral right atrium may be represented by a more uniform activation wavefront that originates over the roof of the right atrium. ECG assessment of the PP interval (<200 ms) and the chaotic P-wave morphology in the remaining ECG leads will confirm the presence of AF.

Evaluation of a patient with AF should include a search for a reversible cause of the arrhythmia, such as hyperthyroidism or anemia. An echocardiogram should be performed to determine whether there is structural heart disease. Persistent or labile hypertension should be identified and treated.

TREATMENT Atrial Fibrillation

Treatment for AF must take into account the clinical situation in which the arrhythmia is encountered, the chronicity of the AF, the status of the patient's level of anticoagulation, risk factors for stroke, the patient's symptoms, the hemodynamic impact of the AF, and the ventricular rate.

ACUTE RATE CONTROL In the absence of hemodynamic compromise that might warrant emergent cardioversion to terminate the AF, the initial goals of therapy are to (1) establish control of the ventricular rate and (2) address anticoagulation status and begin IV heparin treatment if the duration of AF is >12 h and risk factors for stroke with AF are present (Table 233-1). Ventricular rate control for acute AF is best established with beta blockers and/or the calcium channel blocking agents verapamil and diltiazem. The route of administration and dose will be dictated by the ventricular rate and clinical status. Digoxin may add to the rate-controlling benefit of the other agents but is uncommonly used as a stand-alone agent, especially in acute AF.

Anticoagulation is of particular importance in patients who have known risk factors for stroke associated with AF. Factors associated with the highest risk of stroke include a history of stroke, transient ischemic attack (TIA) or systemic embolism, and the presence of rheumatic mitral stenosis. Other identified risk factors include age >65 years, history of congestive heart failure (CHF), diabetes mellitus, hypertension, LV dysfunction, and evidence of marked left atrial enlargement (>5.0 cm). Chronic anticoagulation with warfarin targeted to achieve an international normalized ratio (INR) between 2.0 and 3.0 is recommended in patients with persistent or frequent and long-lived paroxysmal AF and risk factors. If patients have not been adequately anticoagulated and the AF is more than 24–48 h in duration, a transesophageal echocardiogram (TEE) can be performed to exclude the presence of a left atrial thrombus that might dislodge with the attempted restoration of sinus rhythm with either nonpharmacologic or pharmacologic therapy. Anticoagulation must be instituted coincident with the TEE and maintained for at least 1 month after restoration of sinus rhythm if the duration of AF has been prolonged or is unknown. Heparin is maintained routinely until the INR is 1.8 with the administration of warfarin after the TEE. For patients who do not warrant early cardioversion of AF, anticoagulation should be maintained for at least 3 weeks with the INR confirmed to be >1.8 on at least two separate occasions before attempts at cardioversion.

Termination of AF acutely may be warranted on the basis of clinical parameters and/or hemodynamic status. Confirmation of appropriate anticoagulation status as described above must be documented unless symptoms and clinical status warrant emergent intervention. Direct current transthoracic cardioversion during short-acting anesthesia is a reliable way to terminate AF. Conversion rates using a 200-J biphasic shock delivered synchronously with the QRS complex typically are >90%. Pharmacologic therapy to terminate AF is less reliable. Oral and/or IV administration of amiodarone or procainamide has only modest success. The acute IV administration of ibutilide appears to be somewhat more effective and may be used in selected patients to facilitate termination with direct current (DC) cardioversion (Tables 233-2 and 233-3).

Pharmacologic therapy to maintain sinus rhythm can be instituted once sinus rhythm has been established or in anticipation of cardioversion to attempt to maintain sinus rhythm (Table 233-3). A single episode of AF may not warrant any intervention or only a short course of beta blocker therapy. To prevent recurrent AF unresponsive to beta blockade, a trial of antiarrhythmic therapy may be warranted, particularly if the AF is associated with rapid rates and/or significant symptoms. The selection of antiarrhythmic agents should be dictated primarily by the presence or absence of CAD, depressed LV function not attributable to a reversible tachycardia-induced cardiomyopathy, and/or severe hypertension with evidence of marked LV hypertrophy. The presence of any significant structural heart disease typically narrows treatment to the use of sotalol, amiodarone, dofetilide, or dronedarone. Severely depressed LV function with heart failure symptoms precludes the use of dronedarone and may limit sotalol therapy. Owing to the risk of QT prolongation and polymorphic VT, sotalol and dofetilide have to be initiated in the hospital in most cases.

In patients without evidence of structural heart disease or hypertensive heart disease without evidence of severe hypertrophy, the use of the class IC antiarrhythmic agents flecainide or propafenone appears to be well tolerated and does not have significant proarrhythmia risk. It is important to recognize that no drug is uniformly effective, and arrhythmia recurrence should be anticipated in over one-half of the patients during long-term follow-up regardless of the type and number of agents tried. It is also important to recognize that although the maintenance of sinus rhythm has been associated with improved long-term survival, the survival outcome of patients randomized to the pharmacologic maintenance of sinus rhythm was not superior

TABLE 233-1 Risk Factors for Stroke in Atrial Fibrillation

History of stroke or transient ischemic attack	Age >75 years
	Congestive heart failure
Mitral stenosis	Left ventricular dysfunction
Hypertension	Marked left atrial enlargement (>5.0 cm)
Diabetes mellitus	Spontaneous echo contrast

TABLE 233-2 Commonly Used Antiarrhythmic Agents—Intravenous Dose Range/Primary Indication

Drug	Loading	Maintenance	Primary Indication	Class*
Adenosine	6–18 mg (rapid bolus)	N/A	Terminate reentrant SVT involving AV node	—
Amiodarone	15 mg/min for 10 min, 1 mg/min for 6 h	0.5–1 mg/min	AF, AFL, SVT, VT/VF	III
Digoxin	0.25 mg q2h until 1 mg total	0.125–0.25 mg/d	AF/AFL rate control	—
Diltiazem	0.25 mg/kg over 3–5 min (max 20 mg)	5–15 mg/h	SVT, AF/AFL rate control	IV
Esmolol	500 μg/kg over 1 min	50 μg/kg per min	AF/AFL rate control	II
Ibutilide	1 mg over 10 min if over 60 kg	N/A	Terminate AF/AFL	III
Lidocaine	1–3 mg/kg at 20–50 mg/min	1–4 mg/min	VT	IB
Metoprolol	5 mg over 3–5 min × 3 doses	1.25–5 mg q6h	SVT, AF rate control; exercise-induced VT; long QT	II
Procainamide	15 mg/kg over 60 min	1–4 mg/min	Convert/prevent AF/VT	IA
Quinidine	6–10 mg/kg at 0.3–0.5 mg/kg per min	N/A	Convert/prevent AF/VT	IA
Verapamil	5–10 mg over 3–5 min	2.5–10 mg/h	SVT, AF rate control	IV

*Classification of antiarrhythmic drugs: Class I—agents that primarily block inward sodium current; class IA agents also prolong action potential duration; class II—antisympathetic agents; class III—agents that primarily prolong action potential duration; class IV—calcium channel-blocking agents.

Abbreviations: AF, atrial fibrillation; AFL, atrial flutter; AV, atrioventricular; SVT, supraventricular tachycardia; VF, ventricular fibrillation; VT, ventricular tachycardia.

TABLE 233-3 Commonly Used Antiarrhythmic Agents: Chronic Oral Dosing/Primary Indications

Drug	Dosing Oral, mg, Maintenance	Half-Life, h	Primary Route(s) of Metabolism/Elimination	Most Common Indication	Class[a]
Acebutolol	200–400 q12h	6–7	Renal/hepatic	AF rate control/SVT Long QT/RVOT VT	II
Amiodarone	100–400 qd	40–55 d	Hepatic	AF/VT prevention	III[b]
Atenolol	25–100 per d	6–9	Renal	AF rate control/SVT Long QT/RVOT VT	II
Digoxin	0.125–0.5 qd	38–48	Renal	AF rate control	—
Diltiazem	30–60 q6h	3–4.5	Hepatic	AF rate control/SVT	IV
Disopyramide	100–300 q6–8h	4–10	Renal 50%/hepatic	AF/SVT prevention	Ia
Dofetilide	0.125–0.5 q12h	10	Renal	AF prevention	III
Dronedarone	400 q12 hr	13-19	Hepatic	AF prevention	IIIb
Flecainide	50–200 q12h	7–22	Hepatic 75%/renal	AF/SVT/VT prevention	Ic
Metoprolol	25–100 q6h	3–8	Hepatic	AF rate control/SVT Long QT/RVOT VT	II
Mexiletine	150–300 q8–12h	10–14	Hepatic	VT prevention	Ib
Moricizine	100–400 q8h	3–13	Hepatic 60%/renal	AF prevention	Ic
Nadolol	40–240 per d	10–24	Renal	Same as metoprolol	II
Procainamide	250–500 q3–6h	3–5	Hepatic/renal	AF/SVT/VT prevention	Ia
Propafenone	150–300 q8h	2–8	Hepatic	AF/SVT/VT prevention	Ic
Quinidine	300–600 q6h	6–8	Hepatic 75%/renal	AF/SVT/VT prevention	Ia
Sotalol	80–160 q12h	12	Renal	AF/VT prevention	III
Verapamil	80–120 q6–8h	4.5–12	Hepatic/renal	AF rate control/RVOT VT Idiopathic LV VT	IV

[a]Classification of antiarrhythmic drugs: Class I—agents that primarily block inward sodium current; class II—antisympathetic agents; class III—agents that primarily prolong action potential duration; class IV—calcium channel-blocking agents.

[b]Amiodarone and dronedarone both are grouped in class III, but both also have class I, II, and IV properties.

Abbreviations: AF, atrial fibrillation; LV, left ventricular; RVOT, right ventricular outflow tract; SVT, supraventricular tachycardia; VT, ventricular tachycardia.

to that of patients treated with rate control and anticoagulation in the AFFIRM and RACE trials. The AFFIRM and RACE trials compared outcome with respect to survival and thromboembolic events in patients with AF and risk factors for stroke using the two treatment strategies. It is believed that the poor outcome related to pharmacologic therapy used to maintain sinus rhythm was primarily due to the common inefficacy of such drug therapy and an increased incidence of asymptomatic AF. Many of the drugs used for rhythm control, including sotalol, amiodarone, propafenone, dronedarone, and flecainide, enhance slowing of AV nodal conduction. The absence of symptoms frequently leads to stopping anticoagulant therapy, and asymptomatic AF without anticoagulation increases stroke risk. Any consideration for stopping anticoagulation therefore must be accompanied by a prolonged period of ECG monitoring to document asymptomatic AF. It is also recommended that patients participate in monitoring by learning to take their pulse on a twice-daily basis and reliably identify its regularity if discontinuing anticoagulant therapy is contemplated seriously.

It is clear that to reduce the risk of drug-induced complications in treating AF, a thorough understanding of the drug planned to be used is critical—its dosing, metabolism, and common side effects and important drug-drug interactions. This information has been summarized in Tables 233-2, 233-3, 233-4, and 233-5 and serves as a starting point for a more complete review. In using antiarrhythmic agents that slow atrial conduction, strong consideration should be given to adding a beta blocker or a calcium channel blocker (verapamil or diltiazem) to the treatment regimen. This should help avoid a rapid ventricular response if AF is converted to "slow" AFL with the drug therapy (Fig. 233-5).

CHRONIC RATE CONTROL This is an option in patients who are asymptomatic or symptomatic due to the resulting tachycardia. Rate control is frequently difficult to achieve in patients who have paroxysmal AF. In patients with more persistent forms of AF, rate control with beta blockers, the calcium channel blockers diltiazem and verapamil, and/or digoxin frequently can be achieved. Using the drugs in combination may avoid some of the common side effects seen with high-dose monotherapy. An effort should be made to document the adequacy of rate control to reduce the risk of a tachycardia-induced cardiomyopathy. Heart rates >80 beats/min at rest or 100 beats/min with very modest physical activity are indications that rate control may be inadequate in persistent AF. Extended periods of ECG monitoring and assessment of heart rate with exercise should be considered.

In patients with symptoms resulting from inadequate rate control with pharmacologic therapy or worsening LV function

TABLE 233-4 Common Nonarrhythmic Toxicity of Most Frequently Used Antiarrhythmic Agents

Drug	Common Nonarrhythmic Toxicity
Amiodarone	Tremor, peripheral neuropathy, pulmonary inflammation, hypo- and hyperthyroidism, photosensitivity
Adenosine	Cough, flushing
Digoxin	Anorexia, nausea, vomiting, visual changes
Disopyramide	Anticholinergic effects, decreased myocardial contractility
Dofetilide	Nausea
Dronedarone	Gastointestinal intolerance, exacerbation of heart failure
Flecainide	Dizziness, nausea, headache, decreased myocardial contractility
Ibutilide	Nausea
Lidocaine	Dizziness, confusion, delirium, seizures, coma
Mexiletine	Ataxia, tremor, gait disturbances, rash, nausea
Moricizine	Mood changes, tremor, loss of mental clarity, nausea
Procainamide	Lupus erythematosus-like syndrome (more common in slow acetylators), anorexia, nausea, neutropenia
Propafenone	Taste disturbance, dyspepsia, nausea, vomiting
Quinidine	Diarrhea, nausea, vomiting, cinchonism, thrombocytopenia
Sotalol	Hypotension, bronchospasm

TABLE 233-5 Proarrhythmic Manifestations of Most Frequently Used Antiarrhythmic Agents

Drug	Common Proarrhythmic Toxicity
Amiodarone	Sinus bradycardia, AV block, increase in defibrillation threshold Rare: long QT and torsades des pointes, 1:1 ventricular conduction with atrial flutter
Adenosine	All arrhythmias potentiated by profound pauses, atrial fibrillation
Digoxin	High-grade AV block, fascicular tachycardia, accelerated junctional rhythm, atrial tachycardia
Disopyramide	Long QT and torsades des pointes, 1:1 ventricular response to atrial flutter; increased risk of some ventricular tachycardias in patients with structural heart disease
Dofetilide	Long QT and torsades des pointes
Dronedarone	Bradyarrhythmias and AV block, long QT and torsades des pointes
Flecainide	1:1 Ventricular response to atrial flutter; increased risk of some ventricular tachycardias in patients with structural heart disease; sinus bradycardia
Ibutilide	Long QT and torsades des pointes
Procainamide	Long QT and torsades des pointes, 1:1 ventricular response to atrial flutter; increased risk of some ventricular tachycardias in patients with structural heart disease
Propafenone	1:1 Ventricular response to atrial flutter; increased risk of some ventricular tachycardias in patients with structural heart disease; sinus bradycardia
Quinidine	Long QT and torsades des pointes, 1:1 ventricular response to atrial flutter; increased risk of some ventricular tachycardias in patients with structural heart disease
Sotalol	Long QT and torsades des pointes, sinus bradycardia

Abbreviation: AV, atrioventricular.

due to the persistent tachycardia, ablative therapy to attempt to eliminate atrial fibrillation, or an AV junction ablation can be performed. The AV junction ablation must be coupled with the implantation of an activity sensor pacemaker to maintain a physiologic range of heart rates. Recent evidence that RV pacing can occasionally modestly depress LV function should be taken into consideration in identifying which patients are appropriate candidates for the "ablate and pace" treatment strategy. Occasionally, biventricular pacing may be used to minimize the degree of dyssynchronization that can occur with RV apical pacing alone. Rate control treatment options must be coupled with chronic anticoagulation therapy in all cases. Trials evaluating the elimination of embolic risk by elimination or isolation of the left atrial appendage or by endovascular insertion of a left atrial appendage-occluding device may provide other treatment options that can eliminate the need for chronic anticoagulation.

CATHETER AND SURGICAL ABLATIVE THERAPY TO PREVENT RECURRENT AF Although the optimum ablation strategy has not been defined, most ablation strategies incorporate techniques that isolate the atrial muscle sleeves entering the pulmonary veins; these muscle sleeves have been identified as the source of the majority of triggers responsible for the initiation of AF. Ablation therapy is currently considered an alternative to additional pharmacologic therapy trials in patients with recurrent symptomatic AF or AF associated with poor rate control who have failed an initial attempt at rhythm control with pharmacologic management Ablative therapy appears superior to additional pharmacologic treatment aimed at rhythm control in this setting. Elimination of AF in 50–80% of patients with a catheter-based ablation procedure should be anticipated, depending on the chronicity of the AF, with additional patients becoming responsive to previously ineffective medications.

Catheter ablative therapy also holds promise in patients with more persistent forms of AF and even those with severe atrial dilation. Its confirmed efficacy suggests an important alternative to His bundle ablation and pacemaker insertion in many patients. Serious risks related to the left atrial ablation procedure, albeit low (overall 2–4%), include pulmonary vein stenosis, atrioesophageal fistula, systemic embolic events, perforation/tamponade, and phrenic nerve injury.

Surgical ablation of AF is typically performed at the time of other cardiac valve or coronary artery surgery and, less commonly, as a stand-alone procedure. The surgical Cox-Maze procedure is designed to interrupt all macroreentrant circuits that might potentially develop in the atria, thereby precluding the ability of the atria to fibrillate. In an attempt to simplify the operation, the multiple incisions of the traditional Cox-Maze procedure have been replaced with linear lines of ablation and pulmonary vein isolation using a variety of energy sources.

Severity of AF symptoms and difficulties in rate and/or rhythm control with pharmacologic therapy frequently dictate the optimum AF treatment strategy. Similar to the approach with pharmacologic rhythm control, a cautious approach to eliminating anticoagulant therapy is recommended after catheter or surgical ablation. Careful ECG monitoring for asymptomatic AF, particularly in patients with multiple risk factors for stroke, should be considered until guidelines are firmly established. If the left atrial appendage has been removed surgically, the threshold for stopping anticoagulation may be lowered. Antiarrhythmic therapy typically can be discontinued after catheter or surgical ablation of AF. However, in selected patients, satisfactory AF control may require maintenance of previously ineffective drug therapy after the ablation intervention.

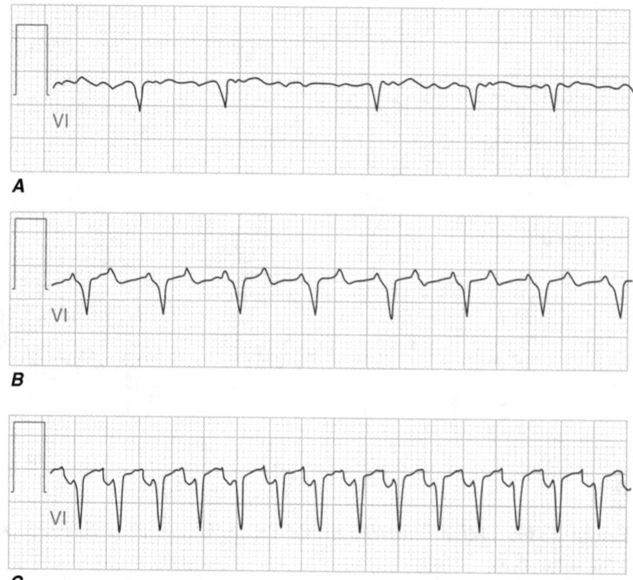

Figure 233-5 **Atrial fibrillation *A.*** transitions to "slow" atrial flutter during antiarrhythmic drug therapy. ***B.*** A rapid ventricular response with 1:1 atrioventricular conduction occurred with exercise, leading to ***C.*** symptoms of dizziness.

ATRIAL FLUTTER AND MACROREENTRANT ATRIAL TACHYCARDIAS

Macroreentrant arrhythmias involving the atrial myocardium are referred to collectively as AFL. The terms *AFL* and *macroreentrant AT* frequently are used interchangeably, with both denoting a nonfocal source of an atrial arrhythmia. The typical or most common AFL circuit rotates in a clockwise or counterclockwise direction in the right atrium around the tricuspid valve annulus. The posterior boundary of the right AFL circuit is defined by the crista terminalis, the eustachian ridge, and the inferior and superior vena cavae. Counterclockwise right AFL represents ~80% of all AFL with superiorly directed activation of the interatrial septum, which produces the saw-toothed appearance of the P waves in ECG leads II, III, and aVF. Clockwise rotation of the same right atrial circuit produces predominantly positive P waves in leads II, III, and aVF (Fig. 233-4). Macroreentrant left AFL also may develop, albeit much less commonly. This type of arrhythmia may be the sequela of surgical or catheter-based ablation procedures that create large anatomic barriers or promote slowing of conduction in the left atrium, especially around the mitral valve annulus or partially disconnected pulmonary veins. Atypical AFL or macroreentrant AT can also develop around incisions created during surgery for valvular or congenital heart disease or in and/or around large areas of atrial fibrosis.

Classic or typical right AFL has an atrial rate of 260–300 beats per minute with a ventricular response that tends to be 2:1, or typically 130–150 beats per minute. In the setting of severe atrial conduction disease and or antiarrhythmic drug therapy, the atrial rate can slow to <200 beats per minute. In this setting, a 1:1 rapid ventricular response may occur, particularly with exertion, and produce adverse hemodynamic effects (Fig. 233-5). Atypical AFL or macroreentrant AT related to prior surgical incisions and atrial fibrosis demonstrates less predictability in terms of the atrial rate and is more likely to demonstrate slower rates that overlap with those identified with focal atrial tachycardias (p. 1886).

Because lead V_1 is frequently monitored in a hospitalized patient, coarse AF may be misdiagnosed as AFL. This occurs because in both typical right AFL and coarse AF the crista terminalis in the right atrium may serve as an effective anatomic barrier. The free wall of

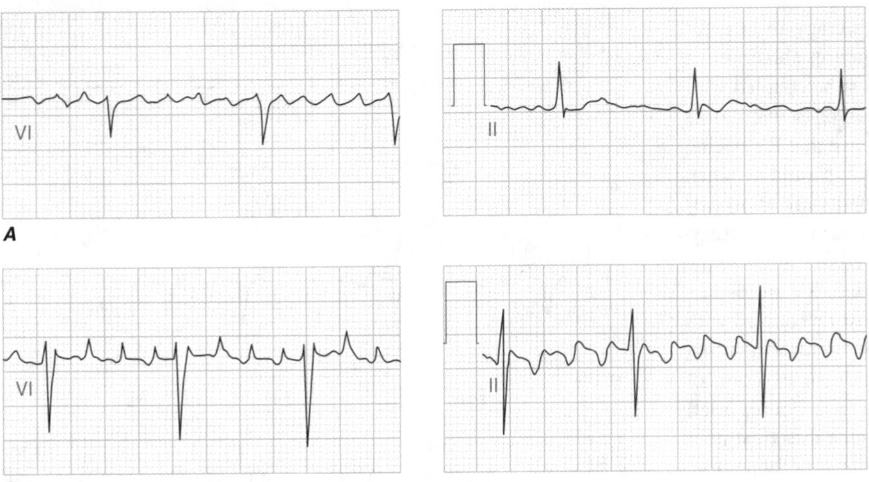

Figure 233-6 Atrial flutter/atrial fibrillation. Coarse atrial fibrillation ***A.*** contrasted with organized atrial flutter ***B.***

the right atrium, whose electrical depolarization is best reflected on the body surface by lead V_1, may demonstrate a uniform wavefront of atrial activation in both conditions. The timing of atrial activation is much more rapid in AF and always demonstrates variable atrial intervals with some intervals between defined P waves <200 ms (Fig. 233-6). A review of the other ECG leads demonstrates the disorganized atrial depolarization that is characteristic of AF. Frequently, an individual patient may alternate between AF and AFL or, less commonly, may manifest AF in one atrium and AFL in the other, making the distinction more difficult.

TREATMENT Atrial Flutter

Because of the anticipated rapid regular ventricular rate associated with AFL and the failure to respond to pharmacologic therapy directed at slowing the ventricular rate, patients frequently are treated with DC cardioversion. The organized atrial flutter activity frequently can be terminated with low-energy external cardioversion of 50–100 J. The risk of thromboembolic events associated with typical AFL is high, and anticoagulation must be managed similarly to what was described for patients with AF (p. 1882).

Asymptomatic patients with AFL may develop heart failure symptoms with tachycardia-induced severe LV dysfunction. In all patients, an effort should be made to control the ventricular rate pharmacologically or restore sinus rhythm. Rate control with calcium antagonists (diltiazem or verapamil), beta blockers, and/or digoxin may be difficult. Even higher-grade AV slowing, such as a 4:1 AV response, may be only transient and is easily overcome with activity or emotional stress. Owing to the typically faster ventricular rate, AFL tends to be poorly tolerated in comparison to AF.

In selected patients with high anesthetic risk, an attempt at pharmacologic cardioversion with procainamide, amiodarone, or ibutilide is appropriate. Antiarrhythmic drug therapy may also enhance the efficacy of DC cardioversion and the maintenance of sinus rhythm after cardioversion. Recurrence rates of AFL with pharmacologic attempts at rhythm control exceed 80% by 1 year.

Patients who manifest recurrent AFL appear to be effectively treated with catheter ablative therapy. For typical right AFL, an isthmus ablation line from the tricuspid annulus to the opening of the inferior vena cava can permanently eliminate flutter, with an anticipated success rate of >90% in most experienced centers. In patients with macroreentrant atrial tachycardia or AFL involving prior surgical incisions or catheter ablation or in areas of atrial fibrosis, detailed mapping of the arrhythmia circuit is required to design the best ablation strategy to interrupt the circuit. In selected patient with AF and typical right AFL, pharmacologic therapy may help prevent the AF but not the AFL. In this type of patient, hybrid therapy with antiarrhythmic agents coupled with a right atrial isthmus ablation may produce AF and AFL control.

MULTIFOCAL ATRIAL TACHYCARDIA

Multifocal AT (MAT) is the signature tachycardia of patients with significant pulmonary disease. The atrial rhythm is characterized by at least three distinct P-wave morphologies and often at least three different PR intervals, and the associated atrial and ventricular rates are typically between 100 and 150 beats per minute. The presence of an isoelectric baseline distinguishes this arrhythmia from AF (Fig. 233-4). The absence of any intervening sinus rhythm distinguishes MAT from normal sinus rhythm with frequent multifocal APCs, although this distinction may be moot as these processes define an electrophysiologic continuum.

TREATMENT Multifocal Atrial Tachycardia

Therapy for MAT should be directed at improving the underlying medical condition, which is typically, although not invariably, chronic obstructive or restrictive lung disease. Treatment with the calcium channel blocker verapamil also may provide some benefit. The judicious use of flecainide or propafenone may also decrease atrial arrhythmias. Patients should be screened for the presence of significant ventricular dysfunction or CAD before these agents are started. Low-dose amiodarone therapy may also control the arrhythmia and minimize the risk of pulmonary toxicity noted with the drug.

FOCAL ATRIAL TACHYCARDIAS The two general mechanisms for focal ATs can be distinguished by observations made at AT initiation and in response to adenosine. *Automatic ATs* start with a “warm-up” period over the first 3–10 complexes and, similarly, slow in rate before termination. They may respond to adenosine not only with evidence of AV block but also with gradual slowing of the atrial rhythm and termination. The initiation of automatic ATs frequently can be provoked by isoproterenol infusion. The first P wave of the tachycardia has the same morphology as the remaining waves. Some of the ATs may be triggered or provoked by burst atrial pacing but are not reliably initiated by programmed atrial stimulation.

In contrast, evidence supporting a focal reentrant AT includes the initiation of the tachycardia with programmed atrial stimulation or spontaneous premature beats. The P wave initiating the tachycardia will characteristically have a different morphology than the P wave during the sustained AT. In response to adenosine, reentrant ATs will demonstrate AV block but typically do not slow and/or terminate. Most focal ATs in the absence of

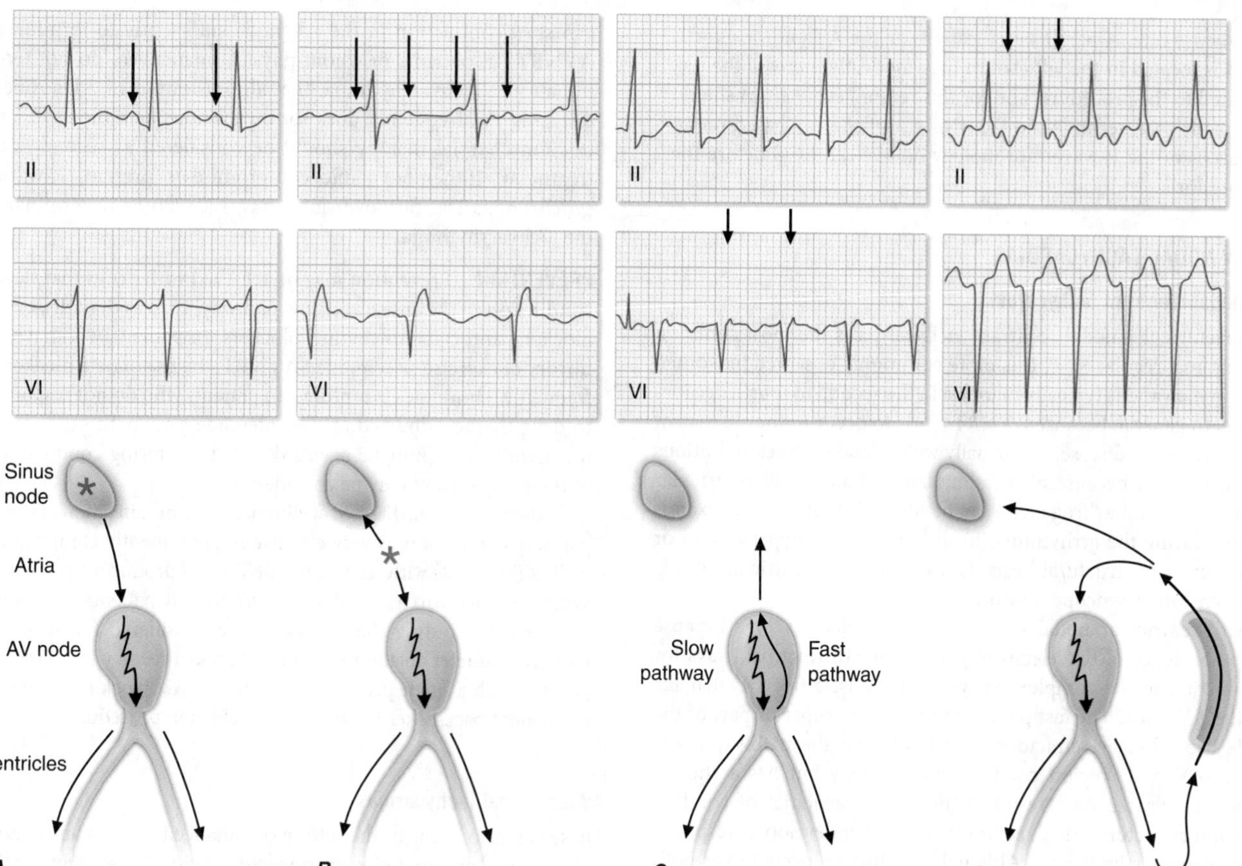

Figure 233-7 Pattern of atrial and ventricular activation and characteristic relationship of P-wave and QRS complex as recorded in leads II and V_1 during regular supraventricular tachycardias. ***A.*** Sinus tachycardia. ***B.*** Atrial tachycardia from top of the atria. ***C.*** Atrioventricular nodal reentry. ***D.*** Accessory pathway–mediated orthodromic supraventricular tachycardia.

structural heart disease originate from specific anatomic locations. These anatomic locations appear to be associated with anatomic ridges, such as the crista terminalis, the valve annuli, and the limbus of the fossa ovalis. ATs also appear to originate from the muscular sleeves associated with the cardiac thoracic veins, i.e., the SVC, the coronary sinus, and the pulmonary veins. As was indicated, repetitive firing of these foci also appears to serve as the triggering mechanism for AF in most patients.

It is important to distinguish focal ATs from reentrant tachycardias that incorporate the AV node in the circuit (Fig. 233-7). The primary distinction is related to the persistence of the AT in the presence of AV block that occurs spontaneously or is created by carotid sinus massage or the administration of adenosine (Fig. 233-4). Atrial activity drives the ventricles in AT and all changes in the PP interval accompanied by correlative changes in the RR intervals; in addition, the V–A relationship changes when the atrial rate changes. The P wave in AT is characteristically distinct from the sinus P-wave morphology, and unless there is significant AV nodal conduction delay, the PR interval is shorter than the measured RP interval when there is a 1:1 relationship between atria and ventricles (Fig. 233-7).

The P wave for ATs depends on the anatomic site of origin. In addition to attempting to create AV block to establish the diagnosis of AT, analysis of the P-wave morphology on the 12-lead ECG may help exclude AV nodal reentry, AV bypass tract–mediated reentrant tachycardias, and physiologic or inappropriate sinus tachycardia (Fig. 233-7).

The ECG distinction between focal automatic or microreentrant and macroreentrant AT or atypical AFL is not always possible. Although sustained focal ATs tend to be slower, the atrial rates frequently overlap. Focal ATs, which are more common in the absence of structural heart disease, tend to demonstrate an isolectric baseline between P waves, whereas macroreentrant ATs represent atrial activation that is continuous and an isoelectric baseline between P waves frequently is absent. In patients with a history of prior atrial surgery, one must suspect a macroreentrant mechanism. These distinctions are less important with respect to acute management but have importance related to ablation strategies and anticipated outcome (pp. 1887-1888).

TREATMENT Atrial Tachycardia

Pharmacologic treatment of AT generally is approached in a similar fashion to that of AF and AFL. AV nodal blocking agents are administered in the setting of rapid ventricular rates. Acute IV administration of procainamide or amiodarone may terminate the tachycardia. Tachycardias that do not respond to pharmacologic therapy may be terminated with electrical cardioversion. Typically, anticoagulation before treatment is not needed unless there is evidence of severe atrial dilatation, >5 cm left atrial diameter with a high risk of AF, and/or a history of coincident paroxysmal AF. Most focal ATs are readily amenable to catheter ablative therapy. In patients who fail to respond to medical therapy or who are reluctant to take chronic drug therapy, this option should be considered, with an anticipated

90% cure rate. A parahisian location for the AT and/or a focus that is located in the left atrium may modestly increase the risk related to the procedure, and for this reason, every effort should be made to determine the likely origin of the AT based on an analysis of the P-wave morphology on 12-lead ECG before the procedure.

AV NODAL TACHYCARDIAS

AV nodal reentrant tachycardia

Atrioventricular nodal reentrant tachycardia is the most common paroxysmal regular SVT. It is more commonly observed in women than in men and is typically manifest in the second to fourth decades of life. In general, because AVNRT tends to occur in the absence of structural heart disease, it is usually well tolerated. Neck pulsations are usually felt because of the simultaneous atrial and ventricular contraction, and a "frog sign" can be identified on physical examination during the arrhythmia. In the presence of hypertension or other forms of structural heart disease that limit ventricular filing, hypotension or syncope may occur.

Atrioventricular nodal reentrant tachycardia develops because of the presence of two electrophysiologically distinct pathways for conduction in the complex syncytium of muscle fibers that make up the AV node. The fast pathway in the more superior part of the node has a longer refractory period, whereas the pathway lower in the AV node region conducts more slowly but has a shorter refractory period. As a result of the inhomogeneities of conduction and refractoriness, a reentrant circuit can develop in response to premature stimulation. Although conduction occurs over both pathways during sinus rhythm, only the conduction over the fast pathway is manifest, and as a result, the PR interval is normal. APCs occurring at a critical coupling interval are blocked in the fast pathway because of the longer refractory period and are conducted slowly over the slow pathway. When sufficient conduction slowing occurs, the blocked fast pathway can recover excitability and atrial activation can occur over the fast pathway to complete the circuit. Repetitive activation down the slow and up the fast pathway results in typical AV nodal reentrant tachycardia (Fig. 233-7).

ECG Findings in AVNRT The APC initiating AVNRT is characteristically followed by a long PR interval consistent with conduction via the slow pathway. AVNRT is manifest typically as a narrow QRS complex tachycardia at rates that range from 120 to 250 beats/min. The QRS-P wave pattern associated with typical AVNRT is quite characteristic, with simultaneous activation of the atria and ventricles from the reentrant AV nodal circuit. The P wave frequently is buried inside the QRS complex and either will not be visible or will distort the initial or terminal portion of the QRS complex (Fig. 233-7). Because atrial activation originates in the region of the AV node, a negative deflection will be generated by retrograde atrial depolarization when recording ECG leads II, III, or AVF.

Occasionally, AVNRT occurs with activation in the reverse direction, conducting down the fast pathway and returning up the slow pathway. This form of AVNRT occurs much less commonly and produces a prolonged RP interval during the tachycardia with a negative P wave in leads II, III, and aVF. This atypical form of AVNRT is more easily precipitated by ventricular stimulation.

TREATMENT Atrioventricular Nodal Reentrant Tachycardia

ACUTE TREATMENT Treatment is directed at altering conduction within the AV node. Vagal stimulation, such as that which occurs with the Valsalva maneuver or carotid sinus massage, can slow conduction in the AV node sufficiently to terminate AVNRT. In patients in whom physical maneuvers do not terminate the tachyarrhythmia, the administration of adenosine, 6–12 mg IV, frequently does so. Intravenous beta blockade or calcium channel therapy should be considered as second-line treatment. If hemodynamic compromise is present, R-wave synchronous DC cardioversion using 100–200 J can terminate the tachyarrhythmia.

PREVENTION Prevention may be achieved with drugs that slow conduction in the antegrade slow pathway, such as digitalis, beta blockers, and calcium channel blockers. In patients who have a history of exercise-precipitated AVNRT, the use of beta blockers frequently eliminates symptoms. In patients who do not respond to drug therapy directed at the antegrade slow pathway, treatment with class IA or IC agents directed at altering conduction of the fast pathway may be considered.

Catheter ablation, directed at elimination or modification of slow pathway conduction, is very effective in permanently eliminating AVNRT. Patients with recurrent AVNRT that produces significant symptoms or heart rates >200 beats/min and patients reluctant to take chronic drug therapy should be considered for ablative therapy. Catheter ablation can cure AV nodal reentry in >95% of patients with a single procedure. The risk of AV block requiring a permanent pacemaker is ~1% with the ablation procedure.

AV junctional tachycardias

These can also occur in the setting of enhanced normal automaticity, abnormal automaticity, or triggered activity. These tachycardias may or may not be associated with retrograde conduction to the atria, and the P waves may appear dissociated or produce intermittent conduction and early activation of the junction. These arrhythmias may occur as a manifestation of increased adrenergic tone or drug effect in patients with sinus node dysfunction or after surgical or catheter ablation. The arrhythmia may also be a manifestation of digoxin toxicity. The most common manifestation of digoxin intoxication is the sudden regularization of the response to AF. A junctional tachycardia due to digoxin toxicity typically does not manifest retrograde conduction. Sinus activity may appear dissociated or result in intermittent capture beats with a long PR interval. If the rate is >50 beats per minute and <100 beats per minute, the term *accelerated junctional rhythm* applies. Occasionally, automatic rhythms are mimicked by AVNRT that fails to conduct to the atrium. The triggering events associated with the onset of the tachycardia may provide a clue to the appropriate diagnosis. Initiation of the tachycardia without an atrial premature beat with a gradual acceleration in rate suggests an automatic focus.

TREATMENT Atrioventricular Junctional Tachycardias

Treatment of automatic/triggered junctional tachycardias is directed at decreasing adrenergic stimulation and reversing digoxin toxicity, if present. Digoxin therapy can be withheld if toxicity is suspected, and the administration of digoxin-specific antibody fragments can rapidly reverse digoxin toxicity if the tachycardia is producing significant symptoms and rapid termination is indicated. Junctional tachycardia due to abnormal automaticity can be treated pharmacologically with beta blockers. A trial of class IA or IC drugs may also be attempted. For incessant automatic junctional tachycardia, focal catheter ablation can be performed but is associated with an increased risk of AV block.

TACHYCARDIAS ASSOCIATED WITH ACCESSORY AV PATHWAYS

Tachycardias that involve accessory pathways (APs) between atria and ventricles commonly manifest a normal QRS complex with a short or long RP interval. They must be considered in the differential diagnosis of other narrow-complex tachycardias. Importantly, most tachycardias associated with APs involve a large macroreentrant circuit that includes the ventricles (Fig. 233-7). Thus, identifying these arrhythmias as "supraventricular" is actually a misnomer, and they deserve separate consideration.

Accessory pathways are typically capable of conducting rapidly in both an antegrade and a retrograde direction. In the absence of an AP, the sinus impulse normally activates the ventricles via the AV node and His-Purkinje system, resulting in a PR interval of 120–200 ms. When an antegradely conducting AP is present, the sinus impulse bypasses the AV node and can activate the ventricles rapidly, resulting in ventricular preexcitation. The resulting PR interval is shorter than anticipated. In addition, because the initial ventricular activation is due to muscle-to-muscle conduction, as opposed to rapid spread of activation via the His-Purkinje system, the initial portion of the QRS complex is slurred, creating the characteristic "delta wave." The remaining portion of the QRS complex in sinus rhythm is created by a fusion of the ventricular activation wavefront originating from the Purkinje network and the continued spread of activation from the site of insertion of the AP (Fig. 233-8). Evidence of ventricular preexcitation includes evidence in sinus rhythm of a short PR interval and a delta wave.

The most common AP connects the left atrium to the left ventricle, followed by posterior septal, right free wall, and anterior septal APs. APs typically insert from the atrium into the adjacent ventricular myocardium. However, occasionally pathways, particularly those originating from the right atrium, can have a ventricular insertion at a site distant from the AV groove in the fascicles. These pathways conduct more slowly and are referred to as *atriofascicular accessory pathways*. Atriofascicular APs are unique in their tendency to demonstrate decremental antegrade conduction.

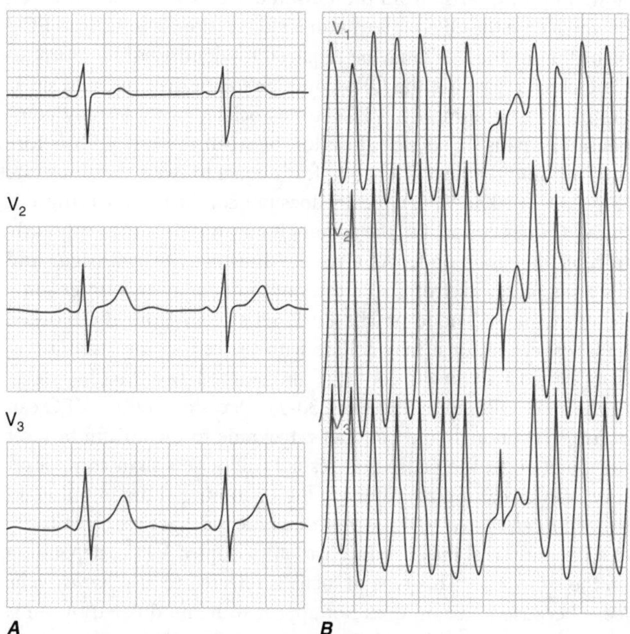

Figure 233-8 ***A.*** Sinus rhythm tracing of leads V_1–V_3 showing evidence of Wolff-Parkinson-White syndrome with short PR interval and delta wave. ***B.*** During atrial fibrillation, rapid conduction to the ventricles is observed producing a wide QRS complex tachycardia with marked irregularity of the ventricular response and morphology of the QRS complex.

Other accessory pathway connections from the AV node to the fascicles may exist. These pathways are referred to as *Mahaim fibers* and typically manifest a normal PR interval with a delta wave.

Patients with manifest preexcitation and WPW syndrome are typically subject to both macroreentrant tachycardias and a rapid response to AF (Fig. 233-8). The most common macroreentrant tachycardia associated with the WPW syndrome is referred to as *orthodromic AV reentry*. Ventricular activation occurs via the AV node and the His-Purkinje system. Conduction then returns or reenters the atria via retrograde conduction over the AP. The reentrant circuit develops because of the inhomogeneity in conduction and refractoriness in the AP and the normal AV node.

Characteristically, the AP has more rapid conduction but a longer refractory period than that of the AV node. Typical APs do not show evidence of antegrade decremental conduction. An APC can block in the AP and conduct sufficiently slowly or with decrement via the AV node to allow for retrograde recovery of activation of the AP and, in turn, of the atria (Fig. 233-7). This retrograde activation of the atria via the AP is referred to as an *echo beat*. If the pattern repeats itself, a tachycardia develops. Uncommonly, the reentrant circuit can be reversed so that the impulse reaches the ventricle via the AP and conducts retrogradely through to the atria via the His-Purkinje system and the AV node; this is referred to as *antidromic AV reentry* and/or *preexcitation macroreentry*, with the entire activation of the ventricle originating from the site of insertion of the AP. Although it is uncommon, it is important to recognize antidromic SVT. The ECG pattern during the tachycardia mimics VT originating from the site of ventricular insertion of the AP. The presence of manifest preexcitation in sinus rhythm provides a valuable clue to the diagnosis.

The second most common and potentially more serious arrhythmia associated with the WPW syndrome is rapidly conducting AF. Nearly 50% of patients with evidence of APs are predisposed to episodes of AF. In patients who have rapid antegrade conduction from the atria to the ventricles over the AP, the AP can conduct rapidly in response to AF, resulting in a faster ventricular rate than would occur normally via the AV node. The rapid ventricular rates can result in hemodynamic compromise and even precipitate VF. The QRS pattern during AF in patients with manifest preexcitation can appear quite bizarre and change on a beat-to-beat basis due to the variability in the degree of fusion from activation over the AV node (Fig. 233-8).

Concealed APs

In ~50% of patients with APs, there is no antegrade conduction over the AP; however, retrograde conduction is preserved. As a result, the AP is not manifest in sinus rhythm and is manifest only during the sustained tachycardia. The presence of a concealed AP is suggested by the timing and pattern of atrial activation during the tachycardia: the P wave typically follows ventricular activation with a short RP wave interval (Fig. 233-7). Because many APs connect the left ventricle to the left atrium, the pattern of atrial activation during the tachycardia frequently produces negative P waves in leads I and aVL. The tachycardia circuit and therefore its ECG manifestation during orthodromic tachycardia are identical both in patients with overt preexcitation in sinus rhythm and in those with concealed APs. Patients with concealed APs, although prone to episodes of AF, are not at risk for developing a rapid ventricular response to the AF.

Occasionally, APs conduct extremely slowly in a retrograde fashion, resulting in longer retrograde conduction and the development of a long RP interval during the tachycardia (*long RP tachycardia*).

Because of the presence of this dramatically slowed conduction, additional conduction slowing created by premature atrial complexes is not required for tachycardia to ensue. These patients are more prone to frequent episodes of tachycardia and can present with "incessant" tachycardias and tachycardia-induced LV cardiomyopathy. The correct diagnosis of a long RP tachycardia may be suggested by the pattern of initiation and the P-wave morphology. Frequently, however, an electrophysiologic evaluation is required to establish the diagnosis.

TREATMENT Accessory Pathway–Mediated Tachycardias

Acute treatment of AP-mediated macroreentrant orthodromic tachycardias is similar to that for AV nodal reentry and is directed at altering conduction in the AV node. Vagal stimulation with the Valsalva maneuver and carotid sinus pressure may create sufficient AV nodal slowing to terminate the AVRT. Intravenous administration of adenosine, 6–12 mg, is first-line pharmacologic therapy; IV, the calcium channel blockers verapamil and diltiazem or beta blockers may also be effective. In patients who manifest preexcitation and AF, therapy should be aimed at preventing a rapid ventricular response. In life-threatening situations, DC cardioversion should be used to terminate the AF. In nonlife-threatening situations, procainamide at a dose of 15 mg/kg administered IV over 20–30 min will slow the ventricular response and may organize and terminate AF. Ibutilide can also be used to facilitate termination of AF. During AF there may be rapid conduction over the AV node as well as the AP. Caution should be used in attempting to slow AV nodal conduction with the use of digoxin or verapamil; when administered IV, these drugs may actually result in an acute increase in rate over the AP, placing the patient at risk for development of VF. Digoxin appears to shorten the refractory period of the AP directly and thus increases the ventricular rate. Verapamil appears to shorten the refractory period indirectly by causing vasodilation and a reflex increase in sympathetic tone.

Chronic oral administration of beta blockers and/or verapamil or diltiazem may be used to prevent recurrent supraventricular reentrant tachycardias associated with APs. In patients with evidence of AF and a rapid ventricular response and in those with recurrences of SVT on AV nodal blocking drugs, strong consideration should be given to the administration of a class IA or IC antiarrhythmic drug such as quinidine, flecainide, or propafenone because these drugs slow conduction and increase refractoriness in the AP.

Patients with a history of recurrent symptomatic SVT episodes, incessant SVT, and heart rates >200 beats/min with SVT should be given strong consideration for undergoing catheter ablation. Patients who have demonstrated rapid antegrade conduction over their AP or the potential for rapid conduction should also be considered for catheter ablation. Catheter ablation therapy has been demonstrated to be successful in >95% of patients with documented WPW syndrome and appears effective regardless of age. The risk of catheter ablative therapy is low and is dictated primarily by the location of the AP. Ablation of parahisian APs is associated with a risk of heart block, and ablation in the left atrium is associated with a small but definite risk of thromboembolic phenomenon. These risks must be weighed against the potential serious complications associated with hemodynamic compromise, the risk of VF, and the severity of the patient's symptoms with AP-mediated tachycardias.

Patients who demonstrate evidence of ventricular preexcitation in the absence of any prior arrhythmia history merit special consideration. The first arrhythmia manifestation can be a rapid SVT or, albeit of low risk (<1%), a life-threatening rapid response to AF. Patients who demonstrate intermittent preexcitation during ECG monitoring or an abrupt loss of AP conduction during exercise testing are at low risk of a life-threatening rapid response to AF. All other patients should be advised of their risks and therapeutic options in advance of a documented arrhythmia event.

VENTRICULAR TACHYARRHYTHMIAS

VENTRICULAR PREMATURE COMPLEXES

The origin of premature beats in the ventricle at sites remote from the Purkinje network produces slow ventricular activation and a wide QRS complex that is typically >140 ms in duration. Ventricular premature complexes are common and increase with age and the presence of structural heart disease. VPCs can occur with a certain degree of periodicity that has become incorporated into the lexicon of electrocardiography. Ventricular premature complexes may occur in patterns of *bigeminy*, in which every sinus beat is followed by a VPC, or *trigeminy*, in which two sinus beats are followed by a VPC. VPCs may have different morphologies and are thus referred to as *multiformed.* Two successive VPCs are termed *pairs* or *couplets.* Three or more consecutive VPCs are termed *VT* when the rate is >100 beats per minute. If the repetitive VPCs terminate spontaneously and are more than three beats in duration, the arrhythmia is referred to as *nonsustained VT.*

APCs with aberrant ventricular conduction may also create a wide and early QRS complex. The premature P wave can occasionally be difficult to discern when it falls on the preceding T wave, and other clues must be used to make the diagnosis. The QRS pattern for a VPC does not appear to follow a typical right or left bundle branch block pattern as the QRS morphology is associated with aberrant atrial conduction and can be quite bizarre. On occasion, VPCs can arise from the Purkinje network of the ventricles, in which case the QRS pattern mimics aberration. The 12-lead ECG recording of the VPC may be required to identify subtle morphologic clues regarding the QRS complex to confirm its ventricular origin. Most commonly, VPCs are associated with a "fully compensatory pause" [i.e., the duration between the last QRS before the PVC and the next QRS complex is equal to twice the sinus rate (Fig. 233-3)]. The VPC typically does not conduct to the atrium. If the VPC does conduct to the atrium, it may not be sufficiently early to reset the sinus node. As a result, sinus activity will occur and the antegrade wavefront from the sinus node may encounter some delay in the AV node or His-Purkinje system from the blocked VPC wavefront, or it may collide with the retrograde atrial wavefront. Sinus activity will continue undisturbed, resulting in a delay to the next QRS complex (Fig. 233-3). Occasionally the VPC can occur early enough and conduct retrograde to the atrium to reset the sinus node; the pause that results will be less than compensatory. VPCs that fail to influence the oncoming sinus impulse are termed *interpolated VPCs.* A ventricular focus that fires repetitively at a fixed interval may produce variably coupled VPCs, depending on the sinus rate. This type of focus is referred to as a *parasystolic focus* because its firing does not appear to be modulated by sinus activity and the conducted QRS complex. The ventricular ectopy will occur at a characteristic fixed integer or multiple of these intervals. The variability in coupling relative to the underlying QRS complex and a fixed interval between complexes of ventricular origin provide the diagnostic information necessary to identify a parasystolic focus.

TREATMENT Ventricular Premature Complexes

The threshold for treatment of VPCs is high, and the treatment is directed primarily at eliminating severe symptoms associated with palpitations. VPCs of sufficient frequency can cause a reversible cardiomyopathy. Depressed LV function in the setting of ventricular bigeminy and/or frequent nonsustained VT should raise the possibility of a cardiomyopathy that is reversible with control of the ventricular arrhythmia. In the absence of structural heart disease, VPCs do not appear to have prognostic significance. In patients with structural heart disease, frequent VPCs and runs of nonsustained VT have prognostic significance and may portend an increased risk of SCD. However, no study has documented that elimination of VPCs with antiarrhythmic drug therapy reduces the risk of arrhythmic death in patients with severe structural heart disease. In fact, drug therapies that slow myocardial conduction and/or enhance dispersion of refractoriness can actually increase the risk of life-threatening arrhythmias (drug-induced QT prolongation and TDP) despite being effective at eliminating VPCs.

ACCELERATED IDIOVENTRICULAR RHYTHM (AIVR)

AIVR refers to a ventricular rhythm that is characterized by three or more complexes at a rate >40 beats per minute and <120 beats per minute. The arrhythmia mechanism causing AIVR is thought to be due to abnormal automaticity. By definition, there is an overlap between AIVR and "slow" VT; both rhythms can manifest rates between 90 and 120 beats per minute. Because AIVR tends to be a benign rhythm with different therapeutic implications, it is worthwhile to attempt to distinguish it from "slow" VT. AIVR has a characteristic gradual onset and offset and more variability in cycle length. It is typically a brief, self-limiting arrhythmia. AIVR can be seen in the absence of any structural heart disease, but it is frequently present in the setting of acute myocardial infarction (MI), cocaine intoxication, acute myocarditis, digoxin intoxication, and postoperative cardiac surgery. Sustained forms of AIVR can exist, particularly in the setting of acute MI and postoperatively. In the setting of sustained AIVR, hemodynamic compromise can occur because of the loss of AV synchrony. Patients with RV infarction associated with proximal right coronary artery occlusion are most susceptible to associated bradyarrhythmias and the hemodynamic consequences of AIVR. In these patients, acceleration of the atrial rate either by the cautious administration of atropine or by atrial pacing may be an important treatment consideration.

VENTRICULAR TACHYCARDIA

VT originates below the bundle of His at a rate >100 beats per minute; most VT patients have rates >120 beats per minute. Sustained VT at rates <120 beats per minute and even <100 beats per minute can be observed, particularly in association with the administration of antiarrhythmic agents that can slow the rate. Because of the overlap in rates with AIVR, the arrhythmia ECG characteristics and the clinical circumstance sometimes can be used to distinguish the two forms of tachycardia. Slow sustained VT is less likely to show a marked warm up in rate and the marked cycle-length oscillations seen with AIVR, and it is more likely to occur in the setting of chronic infarction or cardiomyopathy and less likely with acute infarction or myocarditis. Obviously, significant overlap may exist. Typically, slow VT will be initiated with programmed stimulation and is found to represent a large macroreentrant circuit in chronically diseased myocardium capable of supporting markedly slow conduction.

The QRS complex during VT may be uniform (monomorphic) or may vary from beat to beat (polymorphic). Polymorphic VT in

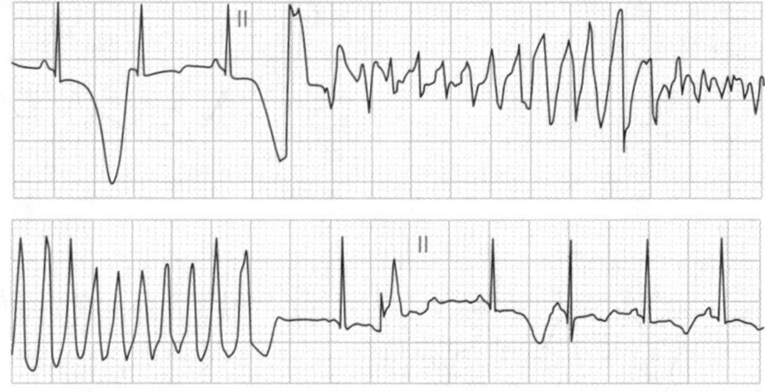

Figure 233-9 Sinus rhythm with long QT interval and the polymorphic ventricular arrhythmia torsades des pointes. Dramatic T wave alternans is present in sinus rhythm.

patients who demonstrate a long QT interval during their baseline rhythm typically is referred to as *torsades des pointes*. The polymorphic VT associated with QT prolongation dramatically oscillates around the baseline on most of the monitored ECG leads, mimicking the "turning of the points" stitching pattern (Fig. 233-9).

Monomorphic VT suggests a stable tachycardia focus in the absence of structural heart disease or a fixed anatomic abnormality that can create the substrate for a stable reentrant VT circuit when structural disease is present. Monomorphic VT tends to be a reproducible and recurrent phenomenon and may be initiated with pacing and programmed ventricular stimulation. In contrast, polymorphic VT suggests a more dynamic and/or unstable process and, by its very nature, is less reproducible. Polymorphic VT may be produced by acute ischemia, myocarditis, or dynamic changes in the QT interval and enhanced dispersion of ventricular refractoriness. Polymorphic VTs are not reliably initiated with pacing or programmed stimulation.

A time duration of 30 seconds frequently is used to distinguish sustained from nonsustained VT. Hemodynamically unstable VT that requires termination before 30 seconds or VT that is terminated by therapy from an implantable defibrillator is also typically classified as sustained. Ventricular flutter appears as a sine wave on the ECG and has a rate of >250 beats per minute. A rapid rate coupled with the sine wave nature of the arrhythmia makes it impossible to identify a discrete QRS morphology. When antiarrhythmic drugs are being administered, a sine wave appearance of the QRS complex can be observed, even at rates as low as 200 beats per minute. VF is characterized by completely disorganized ventricular activation on the surface ECG. Polymorphic ventricular arrhythmias, ventricular flutter, and VF always produce hemodynamic collapse if allowed to continue. The hemodynamic stability of a unimorphic VT depends on the presence and severity of the underlying structural heart disease, the location of the site of origin of the arrhythmia, and the heart rate.

It is important to distinguish monomorphic VT from SVT with aberrant ventricular conduction due to right or left bundle branch block.

Importantly, the sinus or baseline 12-lead ECG tracing can provide important clues that help establish the correct diagnosis of a wide complex tachycardia. The presence of an aberrant QRS pattern that matches exactly that of the wide complex rhythm strongly supports the diagnosis of SVT. A right or left bundle branch block QRS pattern that does not match the QRS and/or that is wider in duration than the QRS during the wide complex tachycardia supports the diagnosis of VT. Most patients with VT have structural heart disease and show evidence of a prior Q wave MI during sinus rhythm. Important exceptions to this rule are discussed (pp. 1894-1895). Finally, the presence of a preexcited QRS pattern on the 12-lead ECG in sinus rhythm suggests that the wide complex rhythm represents an atrial arrhythmia, such as AFL or a focal AT, with rapid

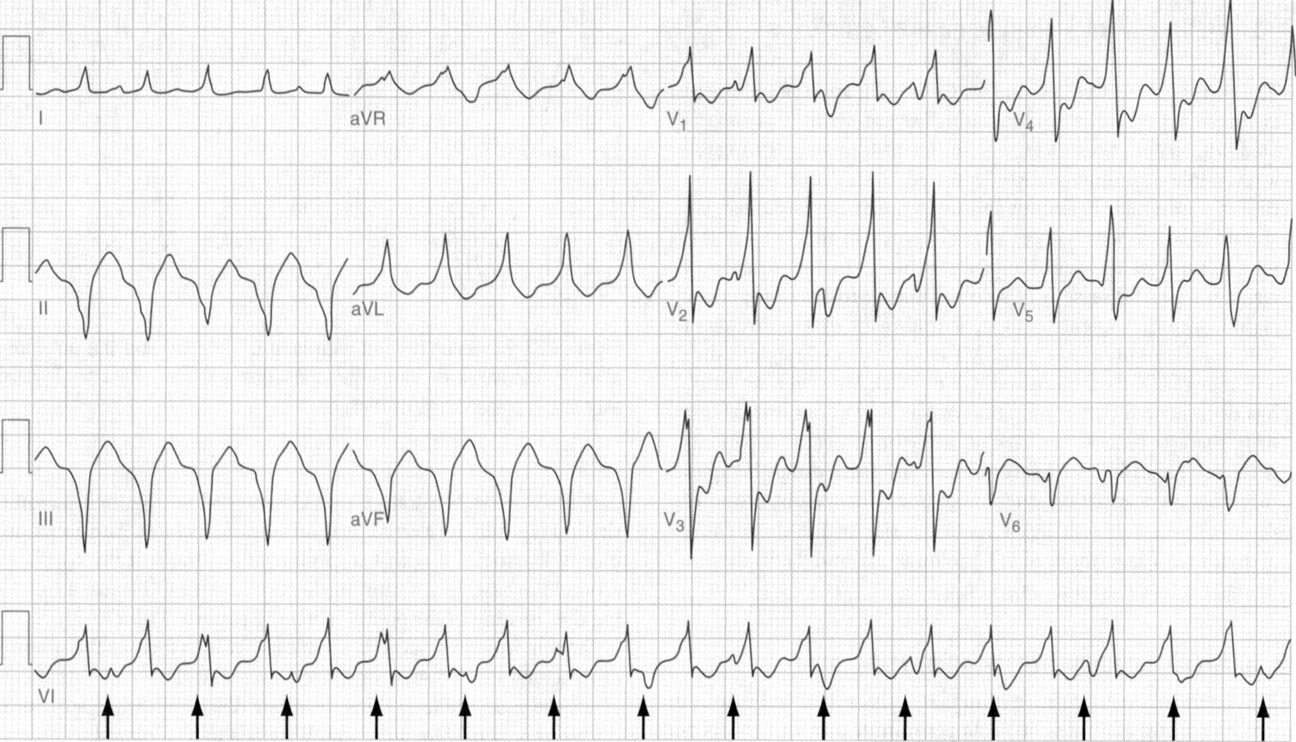

Figure 233-10 **Ventricular tachycardia.** ECG showing AV dissociation (arrows mark P waves), wide QRS >200 ms, superior frontal plane axis, slurring of the initial portion of the QRS, and large S wave in V_6—all clues to the diagnosis of ventricular tachycardia.

conduction over an AP or antidromic macroreentrant tachycardia (Fig. 233-8). If the arrhythmia is irregular with changing QRS complexes, the diagnosis of AF with ventricular preexcitation should be considered.

With the exception of some idiopathic outflow tract tachycardias, most VTs do not respond to vagal stimulation provoked by carotid sinus massage, the Valsalva maneuver, or adenosine administration. The IV administration of verapamil and/or adenosine is not recommended as a diagnostic test. Verapamil has been associated with hemodynamic collapse when administered to patients with structural heart disease and VT.

Patients with VT frequently demonstrate AV disassociation. Findings on physical examination of intermittent cannon *a* waves and variability of the first heart sound are consistent with AV dissociation. The presence of AV dissociation is characteristically marked by the presence of sinus capture or fusion beats. The presence of 1:1 ventriculoatrial conduction does not preclude a diagnosis of VT.

Additional characteristics of the 12-lead ECG during the tachycardia that suggest VT include (1) the presence of a QRS duration >140 ms in the absence of drug therapy, (2) a superior and rightward QRS frontal plane axis, (3) a bizarre QRS complex that does not mimic the characteristic QRS pattern associated with left or right bundle branch block, and (4) slurring of the initial portion of the QRS (Fig. 233-10). Table 233-6 provides a useful summary of ECG criteria that have evolved based on the described characteristics of VT.

TREATMENT Ventricular Tachycardia/Fibrillation

Sustained polymorphic VT, ventricular flutter, and VF all lead to immediate hemodynamic collapse. Emergency asynchronous defibrillation is therefore required, with at least 200-J monophasic or 100-J biphasic shock. The shock should be delivered asynchronously to avoid delays related to sensing of the QRS complex. If the arrhythmia persists, repeated shocks with the maximum energy output of the defibrillator are essential to optimize the chance of successful resuscitation. Intravenous lidocaine and/or amiodarone should be administered but should not delay repeated attempts at defibrillation.

For any monomorphic wide complex rhythm that results in hemodynamic compromise, a prompt R-wave synchronous shock is required. Conscious sedation should be provided if the hemodynamic status permits. For patients with a well-tolerated

TABLE 233-6 ECG Clues Supporting the Diagnosis of Ventricular Tachycardia

ECG Clues
AV dissociation (atrial capture, fusion beats)
QRS duration >140 ms for RBBB type V_1 morphology; V_1>160 ms for LBBB type V_1 morphology
Frontal plane axis –90° to 180°
Delayed activation during initial phase of the QRS complex
LBBB pattern—R wave in V_1, V_2>40 ms
RBBB pattern—onset of R wave to nadir of S >100 ms
Bizarre QRS pattern that does not mimic typical RBBB or LBBB QRS complex
Concordance of QRS complex in all precordial leads
RS or dominant S in V_6 for RBBB VT
Q wave in V_6 with LBBB QRS pattern
Monophasic R or biphasic qR or R/S in V_1 with RBBB pattern

Abbreviations: AV, atrioventricular; RBBB/LBBB, right/left bundle branch block.

wide complex tachycardia, the appropriate diagnosis should be established on the basis of strict ECG criteria (Table 233-6). Pharmacologic treatment to terminate monomorphic VT is not typically successful (<30%). Intravenous procainamide, lidocaine, or amiodarone can be utilized. If the arrhythmia persists, synchronous R-wave cardioversion after the administration of conscious sedation is appropriate. Selected patients with focal outflow tract tachycardias (p. 1894) who demonstrate triggered or automatic VT may respond to IV beta blocker administration. Idiopathic LV septal VT (see p. 1894) appears to respond uniquely to IV verapamil administration.

VT in patients with structural heart disease is now almost always treated with the implantation of an ICD to manage anticipated VT recurrence. The ICD can provide rapid pacing and shock therapy to treat most VTs effectively (Fig. 233-11).

Prevention of VT remains important, and >50% of patients with a history of VT and an ICD may need to be treated with adjunctive antiarrhythmic drug therapy to prevent VT recurrences or to manage atrial arrhythmias. Because of the presence of an ICD, there is more flexibility with respect to the selection of antiarrhythmic drug therapy. The use of sotalol or amiodarone represents first-line therapy for patients with a history of structural heart disease and life-threatening monomorphic or polymorphic VT not due to long QT syndrome. Importantly, sotalol has been associated with a decrease in the defibrillation threshold, which reflects the amount of energy necessary to terminate VF. Amiodarone may be better tolerated in patients with a more marginal hemodynamic status and systolic blood pressure. The risk of end-organ toxicity from amiodarone must be weighed against the ease of use and general efficacy. Antiarrhythmic drug therapy with agents such as quinidine, procainamide, and propafenone, which might not normally be used in patients with structural heart disease because of the risk of proarrhythmia, may be considered in patients with an ICD and recurrent VT.

Catheter ablative therapy for VT in patients without structural heart disease results in cure rates >90%. In patients with structural heart disease, catheter ablation that includes a strategy for eliminating unmappable/rapid VT and one that incorporates endocardial as well as epicardial mapping and ablation should be employed. In most patients, catheter ablation can reduce or eliminate the requirement for toxic drug therapy and should be considered in any patient with recurrent VT. The utilization of ablative therapy to reduce the incidence of ICD shocks for VT in patients who receive the ICD as part of primary prevention for VT is being actively investigated.

MANAGEMENT OF VT STORM Repeated VT episodes requiring external cardioversion/defibrillation or repeated appropriate ICD shock therapy are referred to as *VT storm*. Although a definition of more than two episodes in 24 h is used, most patients with VT storm will experience many more episodes. In the extreme form of VT storm, the tachycardia becomes incessant and the baseline rhythm cannot be restored for any extended period. In patients with recurrent polymorphic VT in the absence of the long QT interval, one should have a high suspicion of active ischemic disease or fulminant myocarditis. Intravenous lidocaine or amiodarone administration should be coupled with prompt assessment of the status of the coronary anatomy. Endomyocardial biopsy, if indicated by clinical circumstances, may be used to confirm the diagnosis of myocarditis, although the diagnostic yield is low. In patients who demonstrate QT prolongation and recurrent pause-dependent polymorphic VT (TDP), removal of an offending QT-prolonging drug, correction of potassium or magnesium deficiencies, and emergency pacing to prevent pauses should be considered. Intravenous beta blockade therapy should be considered for polymorphic VT storm. A targeted treatment strategy should be employed if the diagnosis of the polymorphic VT syndrome can be established. For example, quinidine or isoproterenol can be used in the treatment of Brugada syndrome (p. 40). Intraaortic balloon counterpulsation or acute coronary angioplasty may be needed to stop recurrent polymorphic VT precipitated by acute ischemia. In selected patients with a repeating VPC trigger for their polymorphic VT, the VPC can be targeted for ablation to prevent recurrent VT.

In patients with recurrent monomorphic VT, acute IV administration of lidocaine, procainamide, or amiodarone can prevent

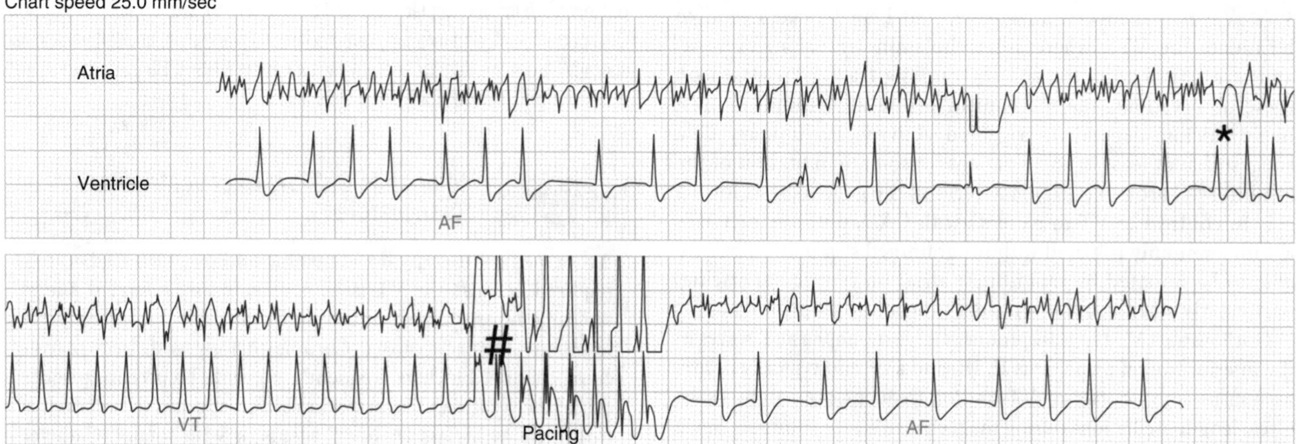

Figure 233-11 Ventricular tachycardia (VT) (*) during atrial fibrillation stopped by pacing (#) from an implantable cardioverter defibrillator (ICD) from recording stored by ICD. The atrial electrogram shows characteristic fibrillatory waves through the tracing. The ventricular electrogram shows an irregularly irregular response consistent with atrial fibrillation at the beginning of the tracing. The ventricular electrogram suddenly changes in morphology (*) and becomes regular, consistent with the diagnosis of VT. Pacing transiently accelerates the rate and interrupts the rapid VT. The patient was unaware of the life-threatening event.

recurrences. The use of such therapy is empirical, and a clinical response is not certain. Procainamide and amiodarone are more likely to slow the tachycardia and make it hemodynamically tolerated. Unfortunately, antiarrhythmic drugs, especially those that slow conduction (e.g., amiodarone, procainamide), can also facilitate recurrent VT or even result in incessant VT. VT catheter ablation can eliminate frequent recurrent or incessant VT and frequent ICD shocks. Such therapy should be deployed earlier in the course of arrhythmia events to prevent adverse consequences of recurrent VT episodes and adverse effects from antiarrhythmic drugs.

UNIQUE VT SYNDROMES

Although most ventricular arrhythmias occur in the setting of CAD with prior MI, a significant number of patients develop VT in other settings. A brief discussion of each unique VT syndrome is warranted. Information that illustrates a unique pathogenesis and enhances the ability to make the correct diagnosis and institute appropriate therapy will be highlighted.

Idiopathic outflow tract VT

VT in the absence of structural heart disease is referred to as *idiopathic VT*. There are two major varieties of these VTs. Outflow tachycardias originate in the RV and LV outflow tract regions. Approximately 80% of outflow tract VTs originate in the RV and ~20% in the LV outflow tract regions. Outflow tract VTs appear to originate from anatomic sites that form an arc that begins just above the tricuspid valve and extends along the roof of the outflow tract region to include the free wall and septal aspect of the right ventricle just beneath the pulmonic valve, the aortic valve region, and then the anterior/superior margin of the mitral valve annulus. These arrhythmias appear more commonly in women. Importantly, these ventricular arrhythmias are *rarely* associated with SCD unless manifest by very short coupled premature complexes that trigger VF. Patients manifest symptoms of palpitations with exercise, stress, and caffeine ingestion. In women, the arrhythmia is more commonly associated with hormonal triggers and can frequently be timed to the premenstrual period, gestation, and menopause. Uncommonly, the VPCs and VTs can be of sufficient frequency and duration to cause a tachycardia-induced cardiomyopathy.

The pathogenesis of outflow tract VT remains unknown, and there is no definite anatomic abnormality identified with these VTs. Vagal maneuvers, adenosine, and beta blockers tend to terminate the VTs, whereas catecholamine infusion, exercise, and stress tend to potentiate the outflow tract VTs. Based on these observations, the mechanism of the arrhythmia is most likely calcium-dependent triggered activity. Preliminary data suggest that at least in some patients, a somatic mutation of the inhibitory G protein ($G\alpha_{i2}$) may serve as the genetic basis for the VT. In contrast to VT in patients with CAD, outflow tract VTs are uncommonly initiated with programmed stimulation but are able to be initiated by rapid-burst atrial or ventricular pacing, particularly when coupled with the infusion of isoproterenol.

Outflow tract VT typically produces large monophasic R waves in the inferior frontal plane leads II, III, and aVF and typically occurs as nonsustained bursts of VT and/or frequent premature beats. Cycle length oscillations during the tachycardia are common. Since most VT originates in the RV outflow tract, the VT typically has a left bundle branch block (LBBB) pattern in lead V_1 (negative QRS vector) (Fig. 233-12). Outflow tract VTs, originating in the left ventricle, particularly those associated with an origin from the mitral valve annulus, have a right bundle branch block (RBBB) pattern in lead V_1 (positive QRS vector).

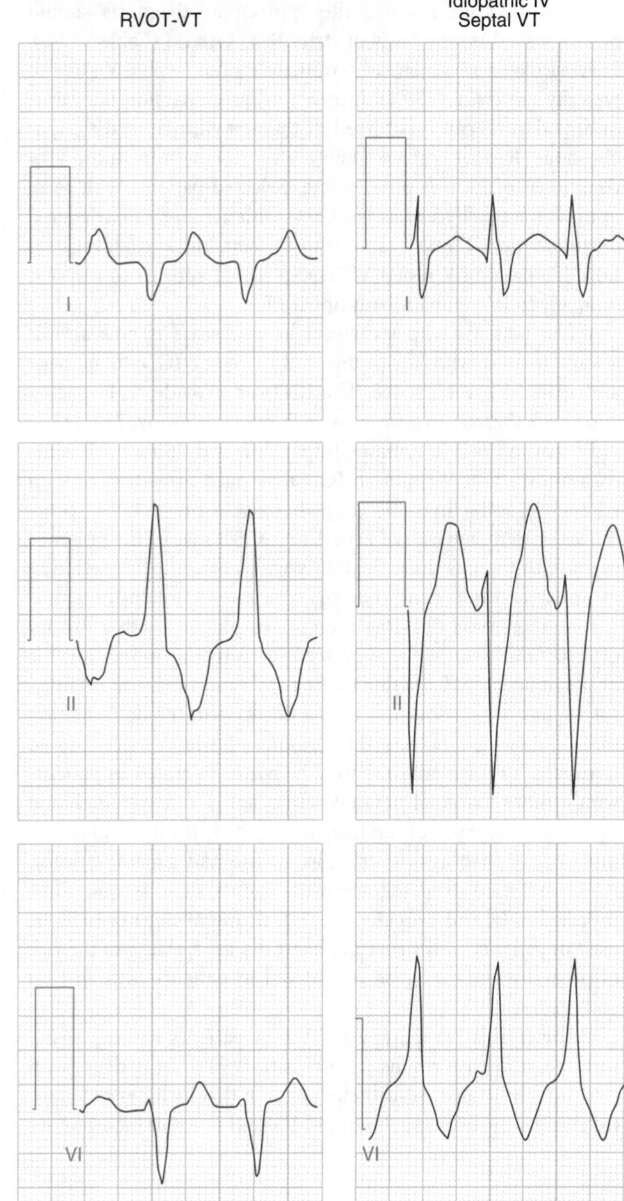

Figure 233-12 Common idiopathic ventricular tachycardia (VT) ECG patterns. Right ventricular outflow tract (RVOT) VT with typical left bundle QRS pattern in V_1 and inferiorly directed frontal plane axis, and left ventricular septal VT from the inferior septum with a narrow QRS RBBB pattern in V_1 and superior and leftward front plane QRS axis.

TREATMENT Idiopathic Outflow Tract Ventricular Tachycardia

Acute medical therapy for idiopathic outflow tract VT is rarely required because the VT is hemodynamically tolerated and is typically nonsustained. Intravenous beta blockers frequently terminate the tachycardia. Chronic therapy with beta or calcium channel blockers frequently prevents recurrent episodes of the tachycardia. The arrhythmia also appears to respond to treatment with class IA or IC agents or with sotalol. Catheter ablative therapy has been utilized successfully to eliminate the tachycardia with success rates >90%. Because of the absence of structural heart disease and the focal nature of these arrhythmias, the 12-lead ECG pattern during VT can help localize the site of origin of the arrhythmia and help facilitate catheter ablation. Efficacy of therapy is assessed with treadmill testing and/or ECG monitoring, and electrophysiologic study is performed only when the diagnosis is in question or to perform catheter ablation.

Idiopathic LV septal/fascicular VT

The second most common idiopathic VT is linked anatomically to the Purkinje system in the left ventricle. The arrhythmia mechanism appears to be macroreentry involving calcium-dependent slow response fibers that are part of the Purkinje network, although automatic tachycardias have also been observed. A 12-lead ECG morphology of the VT shows a narrow RBBB pattern and a superior leftward axis or an inferior rightward axis, depending on whether the VT originates from the posterior or anterior fascicles (Fig. 233-12). Idiopathic LV septal VT is unique in its suppression with verapamil. Beta blockers also have been used with some success as primary or effective adjunctive therapy. Catheter ablation is very effective therapy for VT resistant to drug therapy or in patients reluctant to take daily therapy, with anticipated successful elimination of VT in >90% of patients.

VT associated with LV dilated cardiomyopathy

Monomorphic and polymorphic VTs may occur in patients with nonischemic dilated cardiomyopathy (Chap. 238). Although the myopathic process may be diffuse, there appears to be a predilection for the development of fibrosis around the mitral and aortic valvular regions. Most uniform sustained VT can be mapped to these regions of fibrosis. Drug therapy is usually ineffective in preventing VT, and empirical trials of sotalol or amiodarone are usually initiated only for recurrent VT episodes after ICD implantation. VT associated with nonischemic dilated cardiomyopathy appears to be less amenable to catheter ablative therapy from the endocardium; frequently, the VT originates from epicardial areas of fibrosis and catheter access to the epicardium can be gained via a percutaneous pericardial puncture to improve the outcome of ablation techniques. In patients with a history of depressed myocardial dysfunction due to a nonischemic cardiomyopathy with an LV ejection fraction <30%, data now support the implantation of a prophylactic ICD device to reduce the risk of SCD from the first VT/VF episode effectively.

Bundle branch reentrant VT

Monomorphic VT in patients with idiopathic nonischemic cardiomyopathy or valvular cardiomyopathy is frequently due to a large macroreentrant circuit involving the various elements of the His-Purkinje network. The arrhythmia usually occurs in the presence of underlying disease of the His-Purkinje system. In sinus rhythm, an incomplete left bundle block is typically present and the time it takes to traverse the His-Purkinje network is delayed; this slow conduction serves as the substrate for reentry. Characteristically, the VT circuit rotates in an antegrade direction down the right bundle and retrograde up the left posterior or anterior fascicles and left bundle branch. As a result, bundle branch reentrant VT typically has a QRS morphology with a left bundle branch block type of pattern and a leftward superior axis (Fig. 233-13). The circuit for bundle branch (LBB) reentrant VT can occasionally rotate in the opposite direction, antegrade through the left bundle and retrograde through the right bundle, in which case a RBBB pattern during VT will be manifest.

It is important to recognize bundle branch reentrant VT because it is readily amenable to ablative therapy that targets a component of the His-Purkinje system, typically the right bundle, to block the VT circuit. Less commonly, bundle branch reentry may occur in the

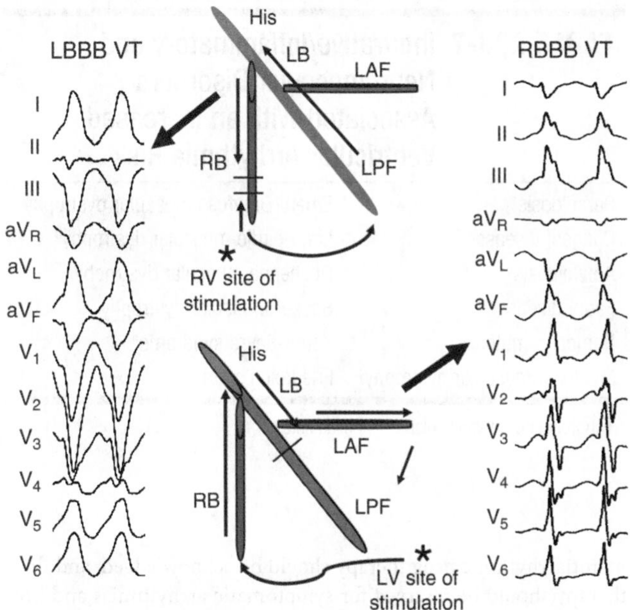

Figure 233-13 Bundle branch reentrant ventricular tachycardia (VT) showing typical QRS morphologies when VT is initiated with stimulation from the right ventricle [left bundle branch block (LBBB) VT pattern] or left ventricle [right bundle branch block (RBBB) VT pattern] and schema for circuit involving the His-Purkinje network.

absence of structural heart disease or in the setting of CAD. The use of adjunctive ICD therapy is dictated by the ability to eliminate the VT successfully and the severity of the LV dysfunction.

VT associated with hypertrophic cardiomyopathy

(See also Chap. 238) VT and VF have also been associated with hypertrophic cardiomyopathy. In patients with hypertrophic cardiomyopathy and a history of sustained VT/VF, unexplained syncope, a strong family history of SCD, LV septal thickness >30 mm, or nonsustained spontaneous VT, the risk of SCD is high and ICD implantation is usually indicated. Amiodarone, sotalol, and beta blockers have been used to control recurrent VT. Experience with ablative therapy is limited because of the infrequency with which the VT is tolerated hemodynamically. Ablation procedures that target the substrate for VT/VF and ablate areas of low voltage consistent with fibrosis, which frequently are located in apical aneurysms, appear to have promise in this setting. The WPW syndrome has been observed in patients with hypertrophic cardiomyopathy associated with *PRKAG2* mutations.

VT associated with other infiltrative cardiomyopathies and neuromuscular disorders

An increased arrhythmia risk has been identified when cardiac involvement occurs in a variety of infiltrative diseases and neuromuscular disorders (Table 233-7). Many patients manifest AV conduction disturbances and may require permanent pacemaker insertion. The decision to implant an ICD device should follow current established guidelines for patients with nonischemic cardiomyopathy, which include an LV ejection fraction < 35% or a history of unexplained syncope with significant LV dysfunction. A recent report identified AF, PR interval >240 ms, QRS 120 ms, or heart block and type 1 myotonic dystrophy as predicting a risk of sudden death. Additional study will be required to determine if patients with lesser degrees of LV dysfunction or other more diffuse myopathic disease processes also have identifiable risk and warrant primary ICD implantation. A potential proarrhythmic risk

TABLE 233-7 Infiltrative/Inflammatory and Neuromuscular Disorders Associated With an Increased Ventricular Arrhythmia Risk

Sarcoidosis[a]	Emery-Dreyfuss muscular dystrophy[a]
Chagas' disease[a]	Limb-girdle muscular dystrophy[a]
Amyloidosis[a]	Duchenne muscular dystrophy
Fabry disease	Becker muscular dystrophy
Hemochromatosis	Kearn-Sayre syndrome[a]
Myotonic muscular dystrophy[a]	Friedreich's ataxia

[a]High frequency of ventricular arrhythmias noted.

of antiarrhythmic drug therapy should be acknowledged, and drug therapy should be reserved for symptomatic arrhythmias and limited to amiodarone or sotalol if an ICD is not present.

Arrhythmogenic RV cardiomyopathy/dysplasia (ARVCM/D)

(See also Chap. 238) ARVCM/D due to a genetically determined dysplastic process or after a suspected viral myocarditis is also associated with VT/VF. The sporadic nonfamilial/nondysplastic form of RV cardiomyopathy appears to be more common; however, this may vary with ethnicity. In patients predisposed to VT, there appears to be a predominance of perivalvular fibrosis involving mostly the free wall of the right ventricle in proximity to the tricuspid and pulmonic valves. The surface ECG leads that reflect RV activation, including V_1–V_3, may show terminal notching of the QRS complex and inverted T waves in sinus rhythm. When the terminal notching is distinct and appears separated from the QRS complex, it is referred to as an *epsilon wave* (Fig. 233-14). Epsilon waves are consistent with markedly delayed ventricular activation in the region of the RV free wall near the base of the tricuspid and pulmonic valves in areas of extensive fibrosis.

In patients with ARVCM/D, echocardiography demonstrates RV enlargement with RV wall motion abnormalities and RV apical aneurysm formation. MRI may show fatty replacement of the ventricle, thinning of the RV free wall with increased fibrosis, and associated wall motion abnormalities. Because of the presence of extensive amounts of fat normally covering the epicardium in the region of the RV, caution must be used to avoid overinterpreting the MRI in trying to determine the appropriate diagnosis. Patients tend to have multiple VT morphologies. The VT will typically have a LBBB type QRS pattern in V_1 and tend to have poor R-wave progression in V_1 through V_6, consistent with an RV free-wall origin. Areas of low electrogram voltage that are identified during RV catheter endocardial sinus rhythm voltage mapping may be helpful in confirming the diagnosis. Importantly, endocardial biopsy may not identify the presence of fatty replacement or fibrosis unless directed to the basal RV free wall. The familial forms of this syndrome have been linked to a number of desmosomal protein mutations. A distinct genetic form of this syndrome, Naxos disease, consists of arrhythmogenic RV dysplasia coupled with palmar-plantar keratosis and woolly hair and is associated with a high risk of SCD in adolescents and young adults.

TREATMENT Arrhythmogenic Right Ventricular Cardiomyopathy/Dysplasia

The threshold for ICD implantation in patients with an established diagnosis of ARVCM/D is low. An ICD typically is implanted in patients deemed to have a persistent VT risk, those who have had spontaneous or inducible rapid VTs, and those who show concomitant LV cardiomyopathy. Treatment options for recurrent VT in patients with ARVCM/D include the use of the antiarrhythmic agent sotalol. Beta blockers serve as useful adjunctive therapy when coupled with other antiarrhythmic agents. Catheter ablative therapy directed at mappable sustained ventricular arrhythmias is also highly successful in controlling recurrent VT. In selected patients with multiple VT morphologies and unstable VT, linear ablation lesions directed at endocardial scars and, if required, targeting late potentials in epicardial

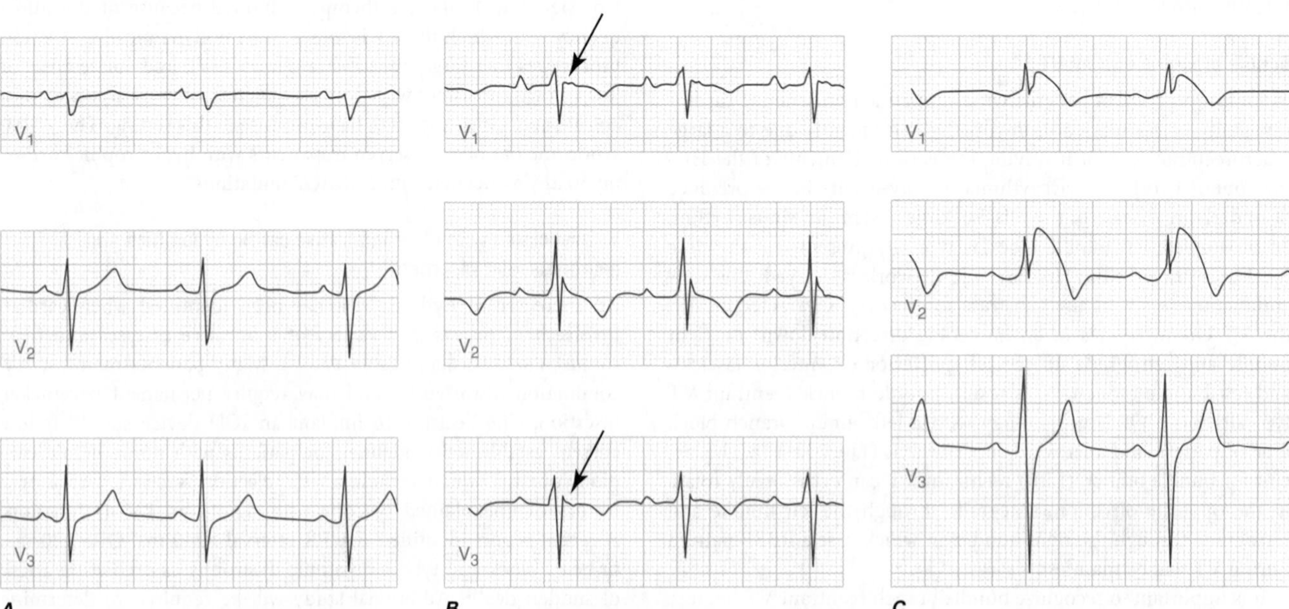

Figure 233-14 Leads V_1 to V_3 in sinus rhythm from a normal subject ***A.***, from a patient with arrhythmogenic right ventricular cardiomyopathy showing epsilon waves (*arrow*) and T-wave inversion ***B.***, and from a patient with Brugada syndrome with ST-segment elevation in V_1 and V_2 ***C.***

scars, defined by catheter-based bipolar voltage mapping, provide significant amelioration of the recurrent VT episodes.

VT after operative tetralogy of fallot repair

VT may also occur after surgical repair of tetralogy of Fallot. Patients typically develop VT many years after the surgery. VT tends to occur in patients with evidence of RV systolic dysfunction. The VT mechanism and location are typically a macroreentrant circuit around the right ventriculotomy scar to the valve annuli. Catheter ablation creating linear lesions that extend from either the pulmonic or the tricuspid annulus to the ventriculotomy scar is typically effective in preventing arrhythmia recurrences. An ICD is usually implanted in patients who manifest rapid VT, have persistent inducible VT after ablation, or have concomitant LV dysfunction.

Fascicular tachycardia caused by digoxin toxicity

Digoxin toxicity can produce increased ventricular ectopy and, when coupled with bradyarrhythmias caused by digoxin toxicity, may predispose to sustained polymorphic ventricular arrhythmias and VF. The signature VT associated with digoxin toxicity is bidirectional VT (Fig. 233-15). This unique VT is due to triggered activity associated with calcium overload resulting from the inhibition of Na^+,K^+-ATPase by digoxin. Bidirectional VT originates from the left anterior and posterior fascicles, creating a relatively narrow QRS right bundle branch (RBB) configuration with a beat-to-beat alternating right and left frontal plane QRS axis. This VT seldom is observed in the absence of digoxin toxicity. Treatment for bidirectional VT or other hemodynamically significant arrhythmias due to digoxin excess includes correction of electrolyte disorders and IV infusion of digoxin-specific Fab fragments. The antibody fragments will, over the course of 1 hour, bind digoxin and eliminate toxic effects. In the setting of normal renal function, the bound complex is secreted.

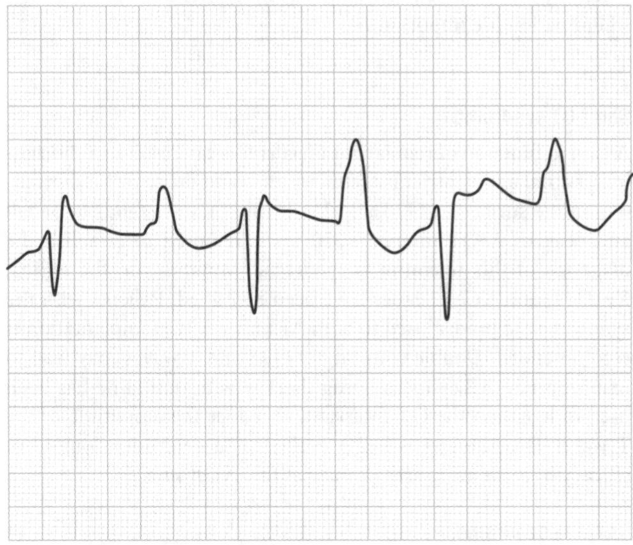

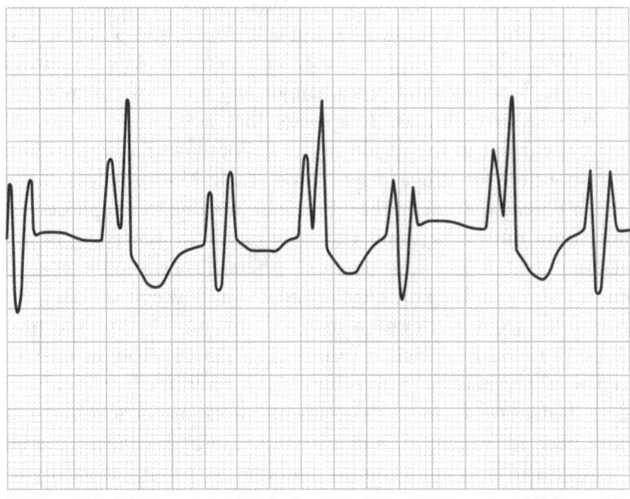

Figure 233-15 Digoxin toxic bidirectional fascicular tachycardia.

GENETICALLY DETERMINED ABNORMALITIES THAT PREDISPOSE TO POLYMORPHIC VENTRICULAR ARRHYTHMIAS

Ion channel defects that affect cardiac depolarization and repolarization may predispose to life-threatening polymorphic VT and SCD. These defects frequently produce unique ECG characteristics during sinus rhythm that facilitate the diagnosis.

Long QT syndrome

The congenital form of LQTS consists of defects in cardiac ion channels that are responsible for cardiac repolarization. Defects that enhance sodium or calcium inward currents or inhibit outward potassium currents during the plateau phase of the action potential lengthen action potential duration and, hence, the QT interval. Of the eight genetic mutations identified to date, five affect the α or β subunits of the three different potassium channels involved with repolarization (Table 233-8). Since many patients with QT prolongation do not have one of the defined mutations, it is anticipated that other genetic abnormalities affecting repolarization channel function will be identified.

The triggers for the ventricular arrhythmias are thought to be due to early afterdepolarizations potentiated by intracellular calcium accumulation from a prolonged action potential plateau. Heterogeneity of myocardial repolarization indexed by a longer

TABLE 233-8 Inherited Arrhythmia Disorders: "Channelopathies" With High Risk of Ventricular Arrhythmias

Disorder	Gene	Protein/Channel Affected
LQT1	*KCNQ1*	I_{Ks} channel α subunit
LQT2	*KCNH2* (*HERG*)	I_{Kr} channel α subunit
LQT3	*SCN5A*	I_{Na} channel α subunit
LQT4	*ANK2*	Ankyrin-B
LQT5	*KCNE1*	I_{Ks} channel β subunit
LQT6	*KCNE2*	I_{Kr} channel β subunit
LQT7	*KCNJ2*	I_{K1} channel α subunit
LQT8	*CACNA1C*	I_{Ca} channel α subunit
Jervell LN1	*KCNQ1*	I_{Ks} channel β subunit
Jervell LN2	*KCNE1*	I_{Kr} channel β subunit
Brugada syndrome	*SCN5A*	I_{Na} channel
Catecholaminergic VT	*Ry R2*	Ryanodine receptor, calsequestrin receptor
SQTS1	*KCNH2* (*HERG*)	I_{Kr} channel α subunit
SQTS2	*KCNQ1*(*KvLQT1*)	I_{Ks} channel α subunit
SQTS3	*KCNJ2*	I_{K1} channel

Abbreviations: LQT, long QT (interval); SQT, short QT (interval).

QT interval predisposes to polymorphic ventricular arrhythmias in response to the triggers (Fig. 233-9).

In most patients with LQTS, the QT interval corrected for heart rate using Bazett's formula is >460 ms in men and >480 ms in women with LQTS. Marked lengthening of the QT interval to >500 ms is clearly associated with a greater arrhythmia risk in patients with LQTS. Many affected individuals may have QT intervals that intermittently measure within a normal range or fail to shorten appropriately with exercise. Some individuals manifest the syndrome only when exposed to a drug, such as sotalol, that alters channel function.

The genotype associated with LQTS appears to influence prognosis, and identification of the genotype appears to help optimize clinical management. The first three genotypic designations of the mutations identified, LQT1, LQT2, and LQT3, appear to account for >99% of patients with clinically relevant LQTSs. Surface ECG characteristics may be helpful in distinguishing the three most common genotypes, with genetic testing being definitive.

LQT1 represents the most common genotypic abnormality. Patients with LQT1 fail to shorten or actually prolong their QT interval with exercise. The T wave in patients with LQT1 tends to be broad and constitutes the majority of the prolonged QT interval. The most common trigger for potentiating cardiac arrhythmias in patients with LQT1 is exercise, followed by emotional stress.

More than 80% of male patients have their first cardiac event by age 20, so competitive exercise should be restricted and swimming avoided for these patients. Patients tend to respond to beta blocker therapy. Patients with two LQT1 alleles have the Jervell and Lange-Nielsen syndrome, with more dramatic QT prolongation and deafness and a worse arrhythmia prognosis.

LQT2 is the second most common genotypic abnormality. The T wave tends to be notched and bifid. In LQT2 patients, the most common precipitant is emotional stress, followed by sleep or auditory stimulation. Despite the occurrence during sleep, patients typically respond to beta blocker therapy.

LQT3 is due to a mutation in the gene that encodes the cardiac sodium channel on chromosome 3. Prolongation of the action potential duration occurs because of failure to inactivate this channel. LQT3 patients have either late-onset peaked biphasic T waves or asymmetric peaked T waves. The arrhythmia events tend to be more life-threatening, and thus the prognosis for LQT3 is the poorest of all the LQTs. Male patients appear to have the worst prognosis among patients with LQT3. Most events in LQT3 patients occur during sleep, suggesting that they are at higher risk during periods of slow heart rates. Beta blockers are not recommended, and exercise is not restricted in LQT3.

TREATMENT Long QT Syndrome

The institution of ICD therapy should be strongly considered in any patient with LQTS who has demonstrated any life-threatening arrhythmia. Patients with syncope with a confirmed diagnosis based on unequivocal ECG criteria or positive genetic testing should also be given the same strong consideration. Primary prevention with prophylactic ICD implantation should be considered in male patients with LQT3 and in all patients with marked QT prolongation (>500 ms), particularly when coupled with an immediate family history of SCD. Future epidemiologic investigation may provide firmer guidelines to sort patients further on the basis of risks such as age, gender, arrhythmia history, and genetic characteristics. In all patients with documented or suspected LQTS, drugs that prolong the QT interval must be avoided. For an updated list of drugs, see *www.qtdrugs.org*.

Acquired LQTS

Patients with a genetic predisposition related to what appear to be sporadic mutations and/or single nucleotide polymorphisms can develop marked QT prolongation in response to drugs that alter repolarization currents. The QT prolongation and associated polymorphic ventricular tachycardia (TDP) are seen more frequently in women and may be a manifestation of subclinical LQTS. Drug-induced long QT and TDP frequently are potentiated by the development of hypokalemia and bradycardia. The offending drugs typically block the potassium I_{Kr} channel (Table 233-5). Since most drug effects are dose dependent, important drug-drug interactions that alter metabolism and/or alterations in elimination kinetics because of hepatic or renal dysfunction frequently contribute to the arrhythmias.

TREATMENT Acquired Long QT Syndrome

Acute therapy for acquired LQTS is directed at eliminating the offending drug therapy, reversing metabolic abnormalities by the infusion of magnesium and/or potassium, and preventing pause-dependent arrhythmias by temporary pacing or the cautious infusion of isoproterenol. Class IB antiarrhythmic agents (e.g., lidocaine) that do not cause QT prolongation may also be used, though they are frequently ineffective. Supportive therapy to allay anxiety and prevent pain with required DC shock therapy for sustained arrhythmias and efforts to facilitate drug elimination are important.

Short QT syndrome

A gain in function of repolarization currents can result in a shortening of atrial and ventricular refractoriness and marked QT shortening on the surface ECG (Table 233-8). The T wave tends to be tall and peaked. A QT interval <320 ms is required to establish the diagnosis of this uncommon syndrome. Mutations in the *HERG*, *KvLQT1*, and *KCNJ2* genes have been identified. Patients with the syndrome are predisposed to both AF and VF. ICD implantation is recommended. Double counting of QRS and T waves may lead to inappropriate ICD shocks. Drug therapy with quinidine has been used to lengthen the QT interval and reduce the amplitude of the T wave. This therapy is being evaluated to determine long-term efficacy in preventing arrhythmias in this syndrome.

Brugada syndrome

The major clinical features of Brugada syndrome include manifest, transient, or concealed ST segment elevation in V_1 to V_3 that typically can be provoked with the sodium channel-blocking drugs ajmaline, flecainide, and procainamide and a risk of polymorphic ventricular arrhythmias. It appears that a diminished inward sodium current in the region of the RV outflow tract epicardium is responsible for Brugada syndrome (Table 233-8). A loss of the action potential dome in the RV epicardium due to unopposed I_{To} potassium outward current results in dramatic shortening of the action potential. The large potential difference between the normal endocardium and rapidly depolarized RV outflow epicardium gives rise to ST-segment elevation in V_1–V_3 in sinus rhythm and predisposes to local ventricular reentry (Fig. 233-14). The majority of genetic abnormalities responsible for the syndrome have not been described; however, in ~20% of patients, mutations of *SCN5A* genes have been identified. Although identified in both genders and all races with an autosomal dominant inheritance pattern, the arrhythmia syndrome is most common in young male patients (~75%) and is thought to be responsible for the sudden and unexpected nocturnal death syndrome (SUDS) described in Southeast Asian men. The ventricular arrhythmia characteristically occurs with rest or during sleep. Fever and other sodium channel-blocking drugs have also precipitated ventricular arrhythmias.

The presence of spontaneous coved-type ST elevation in the right precordial leads and a history of syncope or aborted sudden cardiac death are predictors of an adverse outcome. Because of the overlap in *SCN5A* mutations, the association of Brugada syndrome with phenotypic LQT3 and conduction disturbances has been noted.

TREATMENT Brugada Syndrome

A drug challenge with procainamide may be important to establish the diagnosis and the probable cause of unexplained syncope when the surface ECG is equivocal (saddleback ST elevation pattern). Ajmaline and intravenous flecainide, which are not available in the United States, may have higher sensitivities for identifying the syndrome. Successful acute management of recurrent VT has been reported with isoproterenol or quinidine administration, although experience has been limited. Patients who do not benefit from beta blockers and chronic suppression with quinidine, which may lengthen epicardial action potential duration by blocking I_{TO} current, may be considered for ICD implantation. ICD treatment to manage recurrences and prevent sudden death is recommended for all patients who have had documented arrhythmia episodes and patients with syncope and positive spontaneous or provoked coved-type ECG ST-segment changes in V_1–V_3. Family members should undergo ECG screening for the presence of the abnormality. The role of programmed cardiac stimulation and the use of ICD therapy in asymptomatic patients with the Brugada-type ECG pattern remain somewhat controversial, as is provocative drug infusion and programmed stimulation in patients with borderline abnormalities and no arrhythmia symptoms. Longer-term follow-up in a larger group of these relatively low-risk patients may be required before definitive recommendations can be provided. Counseling on controversies that exist, the potential risk of fever, and inadvertent administration of tricyclic antidepressants should be considered. Genetic testing may be helpful in confirming the presence of the genetic abnormality in family members of patients who manifest the arrhythmia syndrome.

Catecholaminergic polymorphic VT

A mutation of the myocardial ryanodine release channel, which effectively creates a "leak" in calcium from the sarcoplasmic reticulum, has been identified in patients with catecholaminergic VT (Table 233-8). The accumulation of intracellular calcium potentiates delayed afterdepolarizations and triggered activity. Patients can manifest bidirectional VT, nonsustained polymorphic VT, or recurrent VF. Both an autosomal dominant familial form and sporadic forms of the disease have been described. More recently, an autosomal recessive variant associated with a mutation in the sarcoplasmic reticulum calcium-buffering protein calsequestrin has also been identified. The arrhythmias are precipitated by exercise and emotional stress (Fig. 233-16). Exercise restriction is warranted. Treatment with beta blockers and ICD implantation has been recommended. Prevention of inappropriate or easily triggered ICD shocks by proper ICD programming is essential to prevent VT storm from endogenous catecholamine release.

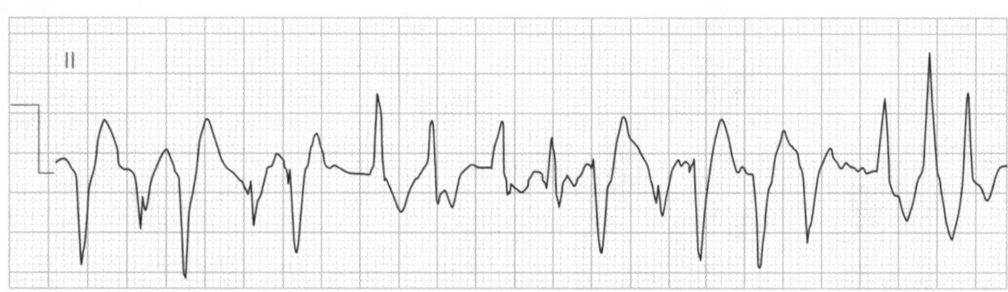

Figure 233-16 Catecholaminergic polymorphic ventricular tachycardia noted during an exercise stress test.

SPECIAL CONSIDERATION: APPROACH TO TACHYARRHYTHMIAS IN ATHLETES

The first manifestation of a tachyarrhythmia, whether benign or malignant, may occur during athletic activity. Fortunately, successful cardiopulmonary resuscitation of life-threatening ventricular arrhythmias has increased with the use of automatic external defibrillators at major sporting events and schools. Rarely, VF may be precipitated by blunt precordial blows without structural injury to the heart or chest wall (commotio cordis).

The approach to the athlete should begin with an assessment of the severity and significance of symptoms. Syncope with exertion should be assumed to be caused by a potentially lethal arrhythmia. A thorough cardiac evaluation and restricted participation in competitive sports are in order until a less life-threatening diagnosis can be established. ECG recording at the time of the symptomatic events usually can establish the diagnosis, although it may be difficult to obtain.

In patients with syncope and no ECG-documented arrhythmia, a systematic attempt to define a cardiac structural or primarily electrical abnormality with a routine ECG and a transthoracic echocardiogram is in order. Common structural abnormalities associated with fatal or life-threatening ventricular arrhythmias include hypertrophic cardiomyopathy, arrhythmogenic cardimyopathy, and acute myocarditis. Coronary anomalies should be suspected if the arrhythmia symptoms are preceded in onset by chest pain. The 12-lead ECG should be screened for the presence of preexcitation, QT prolongation, a Brugada-type ECG pattern or epsilon waves, and T-wave inversions consistent with a nonischemic RV or LV cardiomyopathy or myocarditis. Additional ECG monitoring may be required. A stress test may be appropriate to provoke arrhythmias, especially if there are recurrent symptoms. It is critical to achieve the level of exercise that precipitated the arrhythmia, which for some athletes may be a challenge for the exercise lab.

Management of an athlete with cardiac arrhythmias may be a challenge, with a tendency to discourage participation in competitive sports and institute treatment whenever there is a perception of increased risk. Guidelines for restricting athletic activity have been promulgated on the basis of expert consensus and evidence-based data and can facilitate management once a diagnosis has been established (Table 233-9). Treatment should be based on standards established for each arrhythmia syndrome. Curative catheter ablative therapy should be applied if indicated. ICD therapy, if required, is incompatible with contact sports because of the potential for blunt trauma and consequent damage to the device. Although ICDs are effective, their psychosocial impact, the potential for inappropriate shocks for sinus tachycardia, and lead-related complications must be recognized.

TABLE 233-9 Recommendations for Competitive Athletes With Selected Cardiovascular Abnormalities

Clinical Entity	Clinical Criteria	Sports Permitted
Gene carriers for arrhythmia syndromes without phenotype VT		All sports
Long QT syndrome	>0.47 s in men, >0.48 s in women	Low-intensity competitive sports
Brugada syndrome		Low-intensity competitive sports
Catecholaminergic polymorphic VT		No competitive sports
Asymptomatic Wolff-Parkinson-White syndrome	Electrophysiological study not mandatory	All sports except restriction in dangerous environments
Premature ventricular complexes		All competitive sports when no increase in PVCs or symptoms occur with exercise
Nonsustained ventricular tachycardia	No structural heart disease	All competitive sports
Nonsustained ventricular tachycardia	Structural heart disease	Only low-intensity competitive sports

Source: Adapted from ACC Bethesda Conference #36 from Pelliccia et al: J Am Coll Cardiol 52:1990–1996, 2008.

FURTHER READINGS

Antzelevitch C et al: Brugada syndrome: Report of the second consensus conference. Heart Rhythm 2:429, 2005

Cappato R et al: Updated worldwide survey on the methods, efficacy, and safety of catheter ablation for human atrial fibrillation. Circ Arrhythm Electrophysiol 3:32, 2010

Delacretaz E: Clinical practice: Supraventricular tachycardia. N Engl J Med 354:1039, 2006

Epstein AE et al: ACC/AHA/HRS 2008 Guidelines for Device-Based Therapy of Cardiac Rhythm Abnormalities: A report of the American College of Cardiology/American Heart Association Task Force on Practice Guidelines (Writing Committee to Revise the ACC/AHA/NASPE 2002 Guideline Update for Implantation of Cardiac Pacemaker and Antiarrhythmia Devices): Developed in collaboration with the American Association for Thoracic Surgery and Society of Thoracic Surgeons. Circulation 117:e350, 2008

Fuster V et al: ACC/AHA/ESC 2006 guidelines for the management of patients with atrial fibrillation. Circulation 114:e257, 2006

Groh WJ et al. Electrocardiographic abnormalities and sudden death in myotonic dystrophy type 1. N Engl J Med 358(25):2688, 2008

Josephson ME: *Clinical Cardiac Electrophysiology: Techniques and Interpretations*, 4th ed. Philadelphia, Lippincott Williams & Wilkins, 2008

Lehnart SE et al: Inherited arrhythmias: Consensus report about the diagnosis, phenotyping, molecular mechanisms, and therapeutic approaches for primary cardiomyopathies of gene mutations affecting ion channel function. Circulation 116:2325, 2007

Marchlinski FE et al: Ventricular tachycardia/ventricular fibrillation ablation in the setting of ischemic heart disease. J Cardiovasc Electrophysiol 16:59, 2005

Maron BJ, Zipes DP: Introduction: Eligibility recommendations for competitive athletes with cardiovascular abnormalities—general considerations. J Am Coll Cardiol 45:1318, 2005

Miller JM, Zipes DP: Therapy for cardiac arrhythmias, in *Braunwald's Heart Disease: A Textbook of Cardiovascular Medicine*, 7th ed. DP Zipes et al (eds). Philadelphia, Saunders, 2005, pp 712–756

Page RL: Medical management of atrial fibrillation: Future directions. Heart Rhythm 4:580, 2007

Priori SG et al: Risk stratification in the long QT syndrome. N Engl J Med 348:1866, 2003

Roden DM: Drug-induced prolongation of the QT interval. N Engl J Med 350:1013, 2004

Taylor FC et al: Systematic review of long term anticoagulation or antiplatelet treatment in patients with non-rheumatic atrial fibrillation. BMJ 322:321, 2001

Wyse DG et al: Affirm: A comparison of rate control and rhythm control in patients with atrial fibrillation. N Engl J Med 347:1825, 2002

Zipes DP et al: ACC/AHA/ESC 2006 guidelines for management of patients with ventricular arrhythmias and the prevention of sudden cardiac death. Circulation 114:e385, 2006

CHAPTER 234 Heart Failure and Cor Pulmonale

Douglas L. Mann
Murali Chakinala

HEART FAILURE

DEFINITION

Heart failure (HF) is a clinical syndrome that occurs in patients who, because of an inherited or acquired abnormality of cardiac structure and/or function, develop a constellation of clinical symptoms (dyspnea and fatigue) and signs (edema and rales) that lead to frequent hospitalizations, a poor quality of life, and a shortened life expectancy.

EPIDEMIOLOGY

HF is a burgeoning problem worldwide, with more than 20 million people affected. The overall prevalence of HF in the adult population in developed countries is 2%. HF prevalence follows an exponential pattern, rising with age, and affects 6–10% of people over age 65. Although the relative incidence of HF is lower in women than in men, women constitute at least one-half the cases of HF because of their longer life expectancy. In North America and Europe, the lifetime risk of developing HF is approximately one in five for a 40-year-old. The overall prevalence of HF is thought to be increasing, in part because current therapies for cardiac disorders, such as myocardial infarction (MI), valvular heart disease, and arrhythmias, are allowing patients to survive longer. Very little is known about the prevalence or risk of developing HF in emerging nations because of the lack of population-based studies in those countries. Although HF once was thought to arise primarily in the setting of a depressed left ventricular (LV) ejection fraction (EF), epidemiologic studies have shown that approximately one-half of patients who develop HF have a normal or preserved EF (EF ≥40–50%). Accordingly, HF patients are now broadly categorized into one of two groups: (1) HF with a depressed EF (commonly referred to as *systolic failure*) or (2) HF with a preserved EF (commonly referred to as *diastolic failure*).

ETIOLOGY

As shown in Table 234-1, any condition that leads to an alteration in LV structure or function can predispose a patient to developing HF. Although the etiology of HF in patients with a preserved EF differs from that of patients with depressed EF, there is considerable overlap between the etiologies of these two conditions. In industrialized countries, coronary artery disease (CAD) has become the predominant cause in men and women and is responsible for 60–75% of cases of HF. Hypertension contributes to the development of HF in 75% of patients, including most patients with CAD. Both CAD and hypertension interact to augment the risk of HF, as does diabetes mellitus.

TABLE 234-1 Etiologies of Heart Failure

Depressed Ejection Fraction (<40%)	
Coronary artery disease	Nonischemic dilated cardiomyopathy
Myocardial infarction[a]	Familial/genetic disorders
Myocardial ischemia[a]	Infiltrative disorders[a]
Chronic pressure overload	Toxic/drug-induced damage
Hypertension[a]	Metabolic disorder[a]
Obstructive valvular disease[a]	Viral
Chronic volume overload	Chagas' disease
Regurgitant valvular disease	Disorders of rate and rhythm
Intracardiac (left-to-right) shunting	Chronic bradyarrhythmias
Extracardiac shunting	Chronic tachyarrhythmias
Preserved Ejection Fraction (>40–50%)	
Pathologic hypertrophy	Restrictive cardiomyopathy
Primary (hypertrophic cardiomyopathies)	Infiltrative disorders (amyloidosis, sarcoidosis)
Secondary (hypertension)	Storage diseases (hemochromatosis)
Aging	Fibrosis
	Endomyocardial disorders
Pulmonary Heart Disease	
Cor pulmonale	
Pulmonary vascular disorders	
High-Output States	
Metabolic disorders	Excessive blood-flow requirements
Thyrotoxicosis	Systemic arteriovenous shunting
Nutritional disorders (beriberi)	Chronic anemia

Note: [a]Indicates conditions that can also lead to heart failure with a preserved ejection fraction.

In 20–30% of the cases of HF with a depressed EF, the exact etiologic basis is not known. These patients are referred to as having nonischemic, dilated, or idiopathic cardiomyopathy if the cause is unknown (Chap. 238). Prior viral infection or toxin exposure (e.g., alcoholic or chemotherapeutic) also may lead to a dilated cardiomyopathy. Moreover, it is becoming increasingly clear that a large number of cases of dilated cardiomyopathy are secondary to specific genetic defects, most notably those in the cytoskeleton. Most forms of familial dilated cardiomyopathy are inherited in an autosomal dominant fashion. Mutations of genes that encode cytoskeletal proteins (desmin, cardiac myosin, vinculin) and nuclear membrane proteins (laminin) have been identified thus far. Dilated cardiomyopathy also is associated with Duchenne's, Becker's, and limb-girdle muscular dystrophies. Conditions that lead to a high cardiac output (e.g., arteriovenous fistula, anemia) are seldom responsible for the development of HF in a normal heart; however, in the presence of underlying structural heart disease, these conditions can lead to overt HF.

GLOBAL CONSIDERATIONS

Rheumatic heart disease remains a major cause of HF in Africa and Asia, especially in the young. Hypertension is an important cause of HF in the African and African-American populations. Chagas' disease is still a major cause of HF in South America. Not surprisingly, anemia is a frequent concomitant factor in HF in many developing nations. As developing nations undergo socioeconomic development, the epidemiology of HF is becoming similar to that of Western Europe and North America, with CAD emerging as the single most common cause of HF. Although the contribution of diabetes mellitus to HF is not well understood, diabetes accelerates atherosclerosis and often is associated with hypertension.

PROGNOSIS

Despite many recent advances in the evaluation and management of HF, the development of symptomatic HF still carries a poor prognosis. Community-based studies indicate that 30–40% of patients die within 1 year of diagnosis and 60–70% die within 5 years, mainly from worsening HF or as a sudden event (probably because of a ventricular arrhythmia). Although it is difficult to predict prognosis in an individual, patients with symptoms at rest [New York Heart Association (NYHA) class IV] have a 30–70% annual mortality rate, whereas patients with symptoms with moderate activity (NYHA class II) have an annual mortality rate of 5–10%. Thus, functional status is an important predictor of patient outcome (Table 234-2).

TABLE 234-2 New York Heart Association Classification

Functional Capacity	Objective Assessment
Class I	Patients with cardiac disease but without resulting limitation of physical activity. Ordinary physical activity does not cause undue fatigue, palpitations, dyspnea, or anginal pain.
Class II	Patients with cardiac disease resulting in slight limitation of physical activity. They are comfortable at rest. Ordinary physical activity results in fatigue, palpitation, dyspnea, or anginal pain.
Class III	Patients with cardiac disease resulting in marked limitation of physical activity. They are comfortable at rest. Less than ordinary activity causes fatigue, palpitation, dyspnea, or anginal pain.
Class IV	Patients with cardiac disease resulting in inability to carry on any physical activity without discomfort. Symptoms of heart failure or the anginal syndrome may be present even at rest. If any physical activity is undertaken, discomfort is increased.

Source: Adapted from New York Heart Association, Inc., *Diseases of the Heart and Blood Vessels: Nomenclature and Criteria for Diagnosis,* 6th ed. Boston, Little Brown, 1964, p. 114.

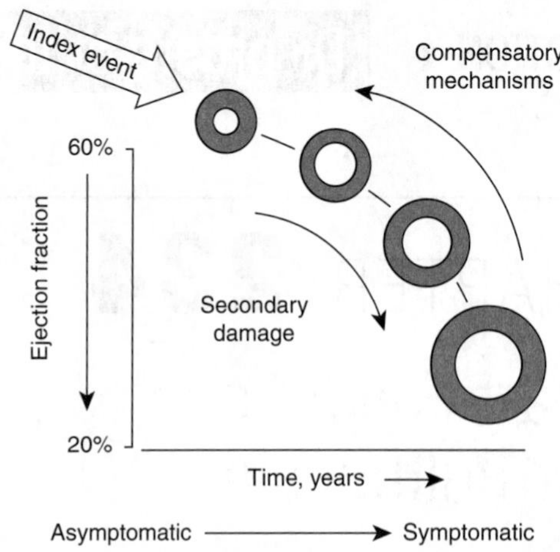

Figure 234-1 Pathogenesis of heart failure with a depressed ejection fraction. Heart failure begins after an index event produces an initial decline in the heart's pumping capacity. After this initial decline in pumping capacity, a variety of compensatory mechanisms are activated, including the adrenergic nervous system, the renin-angiotensin-aldosterone system, and the cytokine system. In the short term, these systems are able to restore cardiovascular function to a normal homeostatic range with the result that the patient remains asymptomatic. However, with time the sustained activation of these systems can lead to secondary end-organ damage within the ventricle, with worsening left ventricular remodeling and subsequent cardiac decompensation. *(From D Mann: Circulation 100:999, 1999.)*

PATHOGENESIS

Figure 234-1 provides a general conceptual framework for considering the development and progression of HF with a depressed EF. As shown, HF may be viewed as a progressive disorder that is initiated after an *index event* either damages the heart muscle, with a resultant loss of functioning cardiac myocytes, or, alternatively, disrupts the ability of the myocardium to generate force, thereby preventing the heart from contracting normally. This index event may have an abrupt onset, as in the case of a myocardial infarction (MI); it may have a gradual or insidious onset, as in the case of hemodynamic pressure or volume overloading; or it may be hereditary, as in the case of many of the genetic cardiomyopathies. Regardless of the nature of the inciting event, the feature that is common to each of these index events is that they all in some manner produce a decline in the pumping capacity of the heart. In most instances, patients remain asymptomatic or minimally symptomatic after the initial decline in pumping capacity of the heart or develop symptoms only after the dysfunction has been present for some time.

Although the precise reasons why patients with LV dysfunction may remain asymptomatic is not certain, one potential explanation is that a number of compensatory mechanisms become activated in the presence of cardiac injury and/or LV dysfunction allowing patients to sustain and modulate LV function for a period of months to years. The list of compensatory mechanisms that have been described thus far include (1) activation of the renin-angiotensin-aldosterone (RAA) and adrenergic nervous systems, which are responsible for maintaining cardiac output through increased retention of salt and water (Fig. 234-2), and (2) increased myocardial contractility. In addition, there is activation of a family of countervailing vasodilatory molecules, including the atrial and brain natriuretic peptides (ANP and BNP), prostaglandins (PGE_2 and PGI_2), and nitric oxide (NO), that offsets the excessive peripheral vascular vasoconstriction. Genetic background, sex, age, or environment may influence these compensatory mechanisms, which

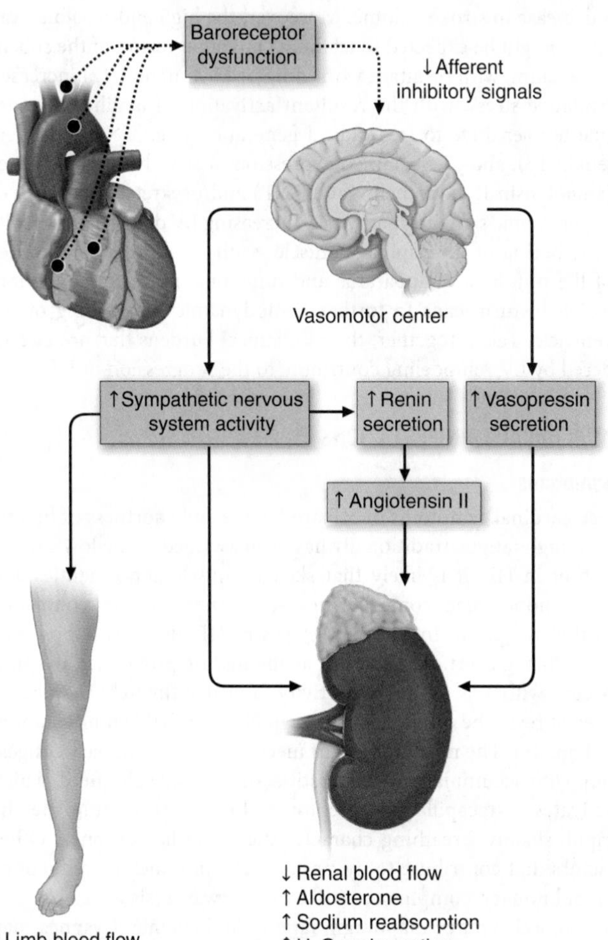

Figure 234-2 Activation of neurohormonal systems in heart failure. The decreased cardiac output in HF patients results in an "unloading" of high-pressure baroceptors (circles) in the left ventricle, carotid sinus, and aortic arch. This unloading of the peripheral baroreceptors leads to a loss of inhibitory parasympathetic tone to the central nervous system (CNS), with a resultant generalized increase in efferent sympathetic tone, and non-osmotic release of arginine vasopressin (AVP) from the pituitary. AVP [or antidiuretic hormone (ADH)] is a powerful vasoconstrictor that increases the permeability of the renal collecting ducts, leading to the reabsorption of free water. These afferent signals to the CNS also activate efferent sympathetic nervous system pathways that innervate the heart, kidney, peripheral vasculature, and skeletal muscles.

Sympathetic stimulation of the kidney leads to the release of renin, with a resultant increase in the circulating levels of angiotensin II and aldosterone. The activation of the renin-angiotensin-aldosterone system promotes salt and water retention and leads to vasoconstriction of the peripheral vasculature, myocyte hypertrophy, myocyte cell death, and myocardial fibrosis. Although these neurohormonal mechanisms facilitate short-term adaptation by maintaining blood pressure, and hence perfusion to vital organs, the same neurohormonal mechanisms are believed to contribute to end-organ changes in the heart and the circulation and to the excessive salt and water retention in advanced HF. *[Modified from A Nohria et al: Neurohormonal, renal and vascular adjustments, in Atlas of Heart Failure: Cardiac Function and Dysfunction, 4th ed, WS Colucci (ed). Philadelphia, Current Medicine Group 2002, p. 104.]*

are able to modulate LV function within a physiologic/homeostatic range so that the functional capacity of the patient is preserved or is depressed only minimally. Thus, patients may remain asymptomatic or minimally symptomatic for a period of years; however, at some point patients become overtly symptomatic, with a resultant striking increase in morbidity and mortality rates. Although the exact mechanisms that are responsible for this transition are not known, as will be discussed below, the transition to symptomatic HF is accompanied by increasing activation of neurohormonal, adrenergic, and cytokine systems that lead to a series of adaptive changes within the myocardium collectively referred to as *LV remodeling.*

In contrast to our understanding of the pathogenesis of HF with a depressed EF, our understanding of the mechanisms that contribute to the development of HF with a preserved EF is still evolving. That is, although diastolic dysfunction (see below) was thought to be the only mechanism responsible for the development of HF with a preserved EF, community-based studies suggest that additional extracardiac mechanisms may be important, such as increased vascular stiffness and impaired renal function.

BASIC MECHANISMS OF HEART FAILURE

Systolic dysfunction

LV remodeling develops in response to a series of complex events that occur at the cellular and molecular levels (Table 234-3). These changes include (1) myocyte hypertrophy, (2) alterations in the contractile properties of the myocyte, (3) progressive loss of myocytes through necrosis, apoptosis, and autophagic cell death, (4) β-adrenergic desensitization, (5) abnormal myocardial energetics and metabolism, and (6) reorganization of the extracellular matrix with dissolution of the organized structural collagen weave surrounding myocytes and subsequent replacement by an interstitial collagen matrix that does not provide structural support to the

TABLE 234-3 Overview of Left Ventricular Remodeling

Alterations in Myocyte Biology
Excitation-contraction coupling
Myosin heavy chain (fetal) gene expression
β-adrenergic desensitization
Hypertrophy
Myocytolysis
Cytoskeletal proteins
Myocardial Changes
Myocyte loss
Necrosis
Apoptosis
Autophagy
Alterations in extracellular matrix
Matrix degradation
Myocardial fibrosis
Alterations in Left Ventricular Chamber Geometry
Left ventricular (LV) dilation
Increased LV sphericity
LV wall thinning
Mitral valve incompetence

Source: Adapted from D Mann: Pathophysiology of heart failure, in *Braunwald's Heart Disease*, 8th ed, PL Libby et al (eds). Philadelphia, Elsevier, 2008, p. 550.

myocytes. The biologic stimuli for these profound changes include mechanical stretch of the myocyte, circulating neurohormones (e.g., norepinephrine, angiotensin II), inflammatory cytokines [e.g., tumor necrosis factor (TNF)], other peptides and growth factors (e.g., endothelin), and reactive oxygen species (e.g., superoxide). The sustained overexpression of these biologically active molecules is believed to contribute to the progression of HF by virtue of the deleterious effects they exert on the heart and the circulation. Indeed, this insight forms the clinical rationale for using pharmacologic agents that antagonize these systems [e.g., angiotensin-converting enzyme (ACE) inhibitors and beta blockers] in treating patients with HF.

In order to understand how the changes that occur in the failing cardiac myocyte contribute to depressed LV systolic function in HF, it is instructive first to review the biology of the cardiac muscle cell (Chap. 224). Sustained neurohormonal activation and mechanical overload result in transcriptional and posttranscriptional changes in the genes and proteins that regulate excitation-contraction coupling and cross-bridge interaction (see Figs. 224-6 and 224-7). The changes that regulate excitation-contraction include decreased function of sarcoplasmic reticulum Ca^{2+} adenosine triphosphatase (SERCA2A), resulting in decreased calcium uptake into the sarcoplamsic reticulum (SR), and hyperphosphorylation of the ryanodine receptor, leading to calcium leakage from the SR. The changes that occur in the cross-bridges include decreased expression of α-myosin heavy chain and increased expression of β-myosin heavy chain, myocytolysis, and disruption of the cytoskeletal links between the sarcomeres and the extracellular matrix. Collectively, these changes impair the ability of the myocyte to contract and therefore contribute to the depressed LV systolic function observed in patients with HF.

Diastolic dysfunction

Myocardial relaxation is an adenosine triphosphate (ATP)-dependent process that is regulated by uptake of cytoplasmic calcium into the SR by SERCA2A and extrusion of calcium by sarcolemmal pumps (see Fig. 224-7). Accordingly, reductions in ATP concentration, as occurs in ischemia, may interfere with these processes and lead to slowed myocardial relaxation. Alternatively, if LV filling is delayed because LV compliance is reduced (e.g., from hypertrophy or fibrosis), LV filling pressures will similarly remain elevated at end diastole (see Fig. 224-11). An increase in heart rate disproportionately shortens the time for diastolic filling, which may lead to elevated LV filling pressures, particularly in noncompliant ventricles. Elevated LV end-diastolic filling pressures result in increases in pulmonary capillary pressures, which can contribute to the dyspnea experienced by patients with diastolic dysfunction. In addition to impaired myocardial relaxation, increased myocardial stiffness secondary to cardiac hypertrophy and increased myocardial collagen content may contribute to diastolic failure. Importantly, diastolic dysfunction can occur alone or in combination with systolic dysfunction in patients with HF.

Left ventricular remodeling

Ventricular remodeling refers to the changes in LV mass, volume, and shape and the composition of the heart that occur after cardiac injury and/or abnormal hemodynamic loading conditions. LV remodeling may contribute independently to the progression of HF by virtue of the mechanical burdens that are engendered by the changes in the geometry of the remodeled LV. In addition to the increase in LV end-diastolic volume, LV wall thinning occurs as the left ventricle begins to dilate. The increase in wall thinning, along with the increase in afterload created by LV dilation, leads to a functional *afterload mismatch* that may contribute further to a decrease in stroke volume. Moreover, the high end-diastolic wall stress might be expected to lead to (1) hypoperfusion of the subendocardium, with resultant worsening of LV function, (2) increased oxidative stress, with the resultant activation of families of genes that are sensitive to free radical generation (e.g., TNF and interleukin 1β), and (3) sustained expression of stretch-activated genes (angiotensin II, endothelin, and TNF) and/or stretch activation of hypertrophic signaling pathways. Increasing LV dilation also results in tethering of the papillary muscles with resulting incompetence of the mitral valve apparatus and functional mitral regurgitation, which in turn leads to further hemodynamic overloading of the ventricle. Taken together, the mechanical burdens that are engendered by LV remodeling contribute to the progression of HF.

CLINICAL MANIFESTATIONS

Symptoms

The cardinal symptoms of HF are fatigue and shortness of breath. Although fatigue traditionally has been ascribed to the low cardiac output in HF, it is likely that skeletal-muscle abnormalities and other noncardiac comorbidities (e.g., anemia) also contribute to this symptom. In the early stages of HF, dyspnea is observed only during exertion; however, as the disease progresses, dyspnea occurs with less strenuous activity, and it ultimately may occur even at rest. The origin of dyspnea in HF is probably multifactorial (Chap. 33). The most important mechanism is pulmonary congestion with accumulation of interstitial or intra-alveolar fluid, which activates juxtacapillary J receptors, which in turn stimulate the rapid, shallow breathing characteristic of cardiac dyspnea. Other factors that contribute to dyspnea on exertion include reductions in pulmonary compliance, increased airway resistance, respiratory muscle and/or diaphragm fatigue, and anemia. Dyspnea may become less frequent with the onset of right ventricular (RV) failure and tricuspid regurgitation.

Orthopnea Orthopnea, which is defined as dyspnea occurring in the recumbent position, is usually a later manifestation of HF than is exertional dyspnea. It results from redistribution of fluid from the splanchnic circulation and lower extremities into the central circulation during recumbency, with a resultant increase in pulmonary capillary pressure. Nocturnal cough is a common manifestation of this process and a frequently overlooked symptom of HF. Orthopnea generally is relieved by sitting upright or sleeping with additional pillows. Although orthopnea is a relatively specific symptom of HF, it may occur in patients with abdominal obesity or ascites and patients with pulmonary disease whose lung mechanics favor an upright posture.

Paroxysmal nocturnal dyspnea (PND) This term refers to acute episodes of severe shortness of breath and coughing that generally occur at night and awaken the patient from sleep, usually 1–3 hours after the patient retires. PND may be manifest by coughing or wheezing, possibly because of increased pressure in the bronchial arteries leading to airway compression, along with interstitial pulmonary edema that leads to increased airway resistance. Whereas orthopnea may be relieved by sitting upright at the side of the bed with the legs in a dependent position, patients with PND often have persistent coughing and wheezing even after they have assumed the upright position. *Cardiac asthma* is closely related to PND, is characterized by wheezing secondary to bronchospasm, and must be differentiated from primary asthma and pulmonary causes of wheezing.

Cheyne-Stokes respiration Also referred to as periodic respiration or cyclic respiration, Cheyne-Stokes respiration is present in 40% of patients with advanced HF and usually is associated with low cardiac output. Cheyne-Stokes respiration is caused by a diminished sensitivity of the respiratory center to arterial P_{CO_2}. There is an apneic phase, during which arterial P_{O_2} falls and arterial P_{CO_2} rises. These changes in the arterial blood gas content stimulate the depressed respiratory center, resulting in hyperventilation and hypocapnia, followed by recurrence of apnea. Cheyne-Stokes respirations may be perceived by the patient or the patient's family as severe dyspnea or as a transient cessation of breathing.

Acute pulmonary edema See Chap. 272

Other symptoms

Patients with HF also may present with gastrointestinal symptoms. Anorexia, nausea, and early satiety associated with abdominal pain and fullness are common complaints and may be related to edema of the bowel wall and/or a congested liver. Congestion of the liver and stretching of its capsule may lead to right-upper-quadrant pain. Cerebral symptoms such as confusion, disorientation, and sleep and mood disturbances may be observed in patients with severe HF, particularly elderly patients with cerebral arteriosclerosis and reduced cerebral perfusion. Nocturia is common in HF and may contribute to insomnia.

PHYSICAL EXAMINATION

A careful physical examination is always warranted in the evaluation of patients with HF. The purpose of the examination is to help determine the cause of HF as well as to assess the severity of the syndrome. Obtaining additional information about the hemodynamic profile and the response to therapy and determining the prognosis are important additional goals of the physical examination.

General appearance and vital signs

In mild or moderately severe HF, the patient appears to be in no distress at rest except for feeling uncomfortable when lying flat for more than a few minutes. In more severe HF, the patient must sit upright, may have labored breathing, and may not be able to finish a sentence because of shortness of breath. Systolic blood pressure may be normal or high in early HF, but it generally is reduced in advanced HF because of severe LV dysfunction. The pulse pressure may be diminished, reflecting a reduction in stroke volume. Sinus tachycardia is a nonspecific sign caused by increased adrenergic activity. Peripheral vasoconstriction leading to cool peripheral extremities and cyanosis of the lips and nail beds is also caused by excessive adrenergic activity.

Jugular veins

(See also Chap. 227) Examination of the jugular veins provides an estimation of right atrial pressure. The jugular venous pressure is best appreciated with the patient lying recumbent, with the head tilted at 45°. The jugular venous pressure should be quantified in centimeters of water (normal ≤8 cm) by estimating the height of the venous column of blood above the sternal angle in centimeters and then adding 5 cm. In the early stages of HF, the venous pressure may be normal at rest but may become abnormally elevated with sustained (~1 min) pressure on the abdomen (positive abdominojugular reflux). Giant *v* waves indicate the presence of tricuspid regurgitation.

Pulmonary examination

Pulmonary crackles (rales or crepitations) result from the transudation of fluid from the intravascular space into the alveoli. In patients with pulmonary edema, rales may be heard widely over both lung fields and may be accompanied by expiratory wheezing (cardiac asthma). When present in patients without concomitant lung disease, rales are specific for HF. Importantly, rales are frequently absent in patients with chronic HF, even when LV filling pressures are elevated, because of increased lymphatic drainage of alveolar fluid. Pleural effusions result from the elevation of pleural capillary pressure and the resulting transudation of fluid into the pleural cavities. Since the pleural veins drain into both the systemic and the pulmonary veins, pleural effusions occur most commonly with biventricular failure. Although pleural effusions are often bilateral in HF, when they are unilateral, they occur more frequently in the right pleural space.

Cardiac examination

Examination of the heart, although essential, frequently does not provide useful information about the severity of HF. If cardiomegaly is present, the point of maximal impulse (PMI) usually is displaced below the fifth intercostal space and/or lateral to the midclavicular line, and the impulse is palpable over two interspaces. Severe LV hypertrophy leads to a sustained PMI. In some patients, a third heart sound (S_3) is audible and palpable at the apex. Patients with enlarged or hypertrophied right ventricles may have a sustained and prolonged left parasternal impulse extending throughout systole. An S_3 (or *protodiastolic gallop*) is most commonly present in patients with volume overload who have tachycardia and tachypnea, and it often signifies severe hemodynamic compromise. A fourth heart sound (S_4) is not a specific indicator of HF but is usually present in patients with diastolic dysfunction. The murmurs of mitral and tricuspid regurgitation are frequently present in patients with advanced HF.

Abdomen and extremities

Hepatomegaly is an important sign in patients with HF. When it is present, the enlarged liver is frequently tender and may pulsate during systole if tricuspid regurgitation is present. Ascites, a late sign, occurs as a consequence of increased pressure in the hepatic veins and the veins draining the peritoneum. Jaundice, also a late finding in HF, results from impairment of hepatic function secondary to hepatic congestion and hepatocellular hypoxemia and is associated with elevations of both direct and indirect bilirubin.

Peripheral edema is a cardinal manifestation of HF, but it is nonspecific and usually is absent in patients who have been treated adequately with diuretics. Peripheral edema is usually symmetric and dependent in HF and occurs predominantly in the ankles and the pretibial region in ambulatory patients. In bedridden patients, edema may be found in the sacral area (*presacral edema*) and the scrotum. Long-standing edema may be associated with indurated and pigmented skin.

Cardiac cachexia

With severe chronic HF, there may be marked weight loss and cachexia. Although the mechanism of cachexia is not entirely understood, it is probably multifactorial and includes elevation of the resting metabolic rate; anorexia, nausea, and vomiting due to congestive hepatomegaly and abdominal fullness; elevation of circulating concentrations of cytokines such as TNF; and impairment of intestinal absorption due to congestion of the intestinal veins. When present, cachexia augurs a poor overall prognosis.

DIAGNOSIS

The diagnosis of HF is relatively straightforward when the patient presents with classic signs and symptoms of HF; however, the signs and symptoms of HF are neither specific nor sensitive. Accordingly, the key to making the diagnosis is to have a high index of suspicion, particularly for high-risk patients. When these patients present with signs or symptoms of HF, additional laboratory testing should be performed.

Routine laboratory testing

Patients with new-onset HF and those with chronic HF and acute decompensation should have a complete blood count, a panel of electrolytes, blood urea nitrogen, serum creatinine, hepatic enzymes, and a urinalysis. Selected patients should have assessment for diabetes mellitus (fasting serum glucose or oral glucose tolerance test), dyslipidemia (fasting lipid panel), and thyroid abnormalities (thyroid-stimulating hormone level).

Electrocardiogram (ECG)

A routine 12-lead ECG is recommended. The major importance of the ECG is to assess cardiac rhythm and determine the presence of LV hypertrophy or a prior MI (presence or absence of Q waves) as well as to determine QRS width to ascertain whether the patient may benefit from resynchronization therapy (see below). A normal ECG virtually excludes LV systolic dysfunction.

Chest x-ray

A chest x-ray provides useful information about cardiac size and shape, as well as the state of the pulmonary vasculature, and may identify noncardiac causes of the patient's symptoms. Although patients with acute HF have evidence of pulmonary hypertension, interstitial edema, and/or pulmonary edema, the majority of patients with chronic HF do not. The absence of these findings in patients with chronic HF reflects the increased capacity of the lymphatics to remove interstitial and/or pulmonary fluid.

Assessment of LV function

Noninvasive cardiac imaging (Chap. 229) is essential for the diagnosis, evaluation, and management of HF. The most useful test is the two-dimensional (2-D) echocardiogram/Doppler, which can provide a semiquantitative assessment of LV size and function as well as the presence or absence of valvular and/or regional wall motion abnormalities (indicative of a prior MI). The presence of left atrial dilation and LV hypertrophy, together with abnormalities of LV diastolic filling provided by pulse-wave and tissue Doppler, is useful for the assessment of HF with a preserved EF. The 2-D echocardiogram/Doppler is also invaluable in assessing RV size and pulmonary pressures, which are critical in the evaluation and management of cor pulmonale (see below). Magnetic resonance imaging (MRI) also provides a comprehensive analysis of cardiac anatomy and function and is now the gold standard for assessing LV mass and volumes. MRI also is emerging as a useful and accurate imaging modality for evaluating patients with HF, both in terms of assessing LV structure and for determining the cause of HF (e.g., amyloidosis, ischemic cardiomyopathy, hemochromatosis).

The most useful index of LV function is the EF (stroke volume divided by end-diastolic volume). Because the EF is easy to measure by noninvasive testing and easy to conceptualize, it has gained wide acceptance among clinicians. Unfortunately, the EF has a number of limitations as a true measure of contractility, since it is influenced by alterations in afterload and/or preload. Nonetheless, with the exceptions indicated above, when the EF is normal (≥50%), systolic function is usually adequate, and when the EF is significantly depressed (<30–40%), contractility is usually depressed.

Biomarkers

Circulating levels of natriuretic peptides are useful adjunctive tools in the diagnosis of patients with HF. Both B-type natriuretic peptide (BNP) and N-terminal pro-BNP, which are released from the failing heart, are relatively sensitive markers for the presence of HF with depressed EF; they also are elevated in HF patients with a preserved EF, albeit to a lesser degree. However, it is important to recognize that natriuretic peptide levels increase with age and renal impairment, are more elevated in women, and can be elevated in right HF from any cause. Levels can be falsely low in obese patients and may normalize in some patients after appropriate treatment. At present, serial measurements of BNP are not recommended as a guide to HF therapy. Other biomarkers, such as troponin T and I, C-reactive protein, TNF receptors, and uric acid, may be elevated in HF and provide important prognostic information. Serial measurements of one or more biomarkers ultimately may help guide therapy in HF, but they are not currently recommended for this purpose.

Exercise testing

Treadmill or bicycle exercise testing is not routinely advocated for patients with HF, but either is useful for assessing the need for cardiac transplantation in patients with advanced HF (Chap. 235). A peak oxygen uptake (V_{o_2}) <14 mL/kg per min is associated with a relatively poor prognosis. Patients with a V_{o_2} <14 mL/kg per min have been shown, in general, to have better survival when transplanted than when treated medically.

DIFFERENTIAL DIAGNOSIS

HF resembles but should be distinguished from (1) conditions in which there is circulatory congestion secondary to abnormal salt and water retention but in which there is no disturbance of cardiac structure or function (e.g., renal failure) and (2) noncardiac causes of pulmonary edema (e.g., acute respiratory distress syndrome). In most patients who present with classic signs and symptoms of HF, the diagnosis is relatively straightforward. However, even experienced clinicians have difficulty differentiating the dyspnea that arises from cardiac and pulmonary causes (Chap. 33). In this regard, noninvasive cardiac imaging, biomarkers, pulmonary function testing, and chest x-ray may be useful. A very low BNP or N-terminal pro-BNP may be helpful in excluding a cardiac cause of dyspnea in this setting. Ankle edema may arise secondary to varicose veins, obesity, renal disease, or gravitational effects. When HF develops in patients with a preserved EF, it may be difficult to determine the relative contribution of HF to the dyspnea that occurs in chronic lung disease and/or obesity.

TREATMENT Heart Failure

HF should be viewed as a continuum that is composed of four interrelated stages. *Stage A* includes patients who are at high risk for developing HF but do not have structural heart disease or symptoms of HF (e.g., patients with diabetes mellitus or hypertension). *Stage B* includes patients who have structural heart disease but do not have symptoms of HF (e.g., patients with a previous MI and asymptomatic LV dysfunction). *Stage C* includes patients who have structural heart disease and have developed symptoms of HF (e.g., patients with a previous MI with dyspnea and fatigue). *Stage D* includes patients with refractory HF requiring special interventions (e.g., patients with refractory HF who are awaiting cardiac transplantation). In this continuum, every effort should be made to prevent HF not only by treating the preventable causes of HF (e.g., hypertension) but also by treating the patient in stages B and C with drugs that prevent disease progression (e.g., ACE inhibitors and beta blockers) and by symptomatic management of patients in stage D.

DEFINING AN APPROPRIATE THERAPEUTIC STRATEGY FOR CHRONIC HF Once patients have developed structural heart disease, their therapy depends on their NYHA functional classification (Table 234-2). Although this classification system is notoriously subjective and has large interobserver variability, it has withstood the test of time and continues to be widely applied to patients with HF. For patients who have developed LV systolic dysfunction but remain asymptomatic (class I), the goal should be to slow disease progression by blocking neurohormonal systems that lead to cardiac remodeling (see below). For patients who have developed symptoms (class II–IV), the primary goal should be to alleviate fluid retention, lessen disability, and reduce the risk of further disease progression and death. These goals generally require a strategy that combines diuretics (to control salt and water retention) with neurohormonal interventions (to minimize cardiac remodeling).

MANAGEMENT OF HF WITH DEPRESSED EJECTION FRACTION (<40%)

General Measures Clinicians should aim to screen for and treat comorbidities such as hypertension, CAD, diabetes mellitus, anemia, and sleep-disordered breathing, as these conditions tend to exacerbate HF. HF patients should be advised to stop smoking and to limit alcohol consumption to two standard drinks per day in men or one per day in women. Patients suspected of having an alcohol-induced cardiomyopathy should be urged to abstain from alcohol consumption indefinitely. Extremes of temperature and heavy physical exertion should be avoided. Certain drugs are known to make HF worse and should be avoided (Table 234-4). For example, nonsteroidal anti-inflammatory drugs, including cyclooxygenase 2 inhibitors, are not recommended in patients with chronic HF because the risk of renal failure and fluid retention is markedly increased in the presence of reduced renal function or ACE inhibitor therapy. Patients should receive immunization with influenza and pneumococcal vaccines to prevent respiratory infections. It is equally important to educate the patient and family about HF, the importance of proper diet, and the importance of compliance with the medical regimen. Supervision of outpatient care by a specially trained nurse or physician assistant and/or in specialized HF clinics has been found to be helpful, particularly in patients with advanced disease.

TABLE 234-4 Factors That May Precipitate Acute Decompensation in Patients With Chronic Heart Failure

Dietary indiscretion
Myocardial ischemia/infarction
Arrhythmias (tachycardia or bradycardia)
Discontinuation of HF therapy
Infection
Anemia
Initiation of medications that worsen HF
Calcium antagonists (verapamil, diltiazem)
Beta blockers
Nonsteroidal anti-inflammatory drugs
Antiarrhythmic agents [all class I agents, sotalol (class III)]
Anti-TNF antibodies
Alcohol consumption
Pregnancy
Worsening hypertension
Acute valvular insufficiency

Abbreviations: HF, heart failure; TNF, tumor necrosis factor.

Activity Although heavy physical labor is not recommended in HF, routine modest exercise has been shown to be beneficial in patients with NYHA class I–III HF. For euvolemic patients, regular isotonic exercise such as walking or riding a stationary-bicycle ergometer, as tolerated, should be encouraged. Exercise training results in reduced HF symptoms, increased exercise capacity, and improved quality of life.

Diet Dietary restriction of sodium (2–3 g daily) is recommended in all patients with HF and preserved or depressed EF. Further restriction (<2 g daily) may be considered in moderate to severe HF. Fluid restriction is generally unnecessary unless the patient develops hyponatremia (<130 meq/L), which may develop because of activation of the renin-angiotensin system, excessive secretion of antidiuretic hormone, or loss of salt in excess of water from diuretic use. Fluid restriction (<2 L/day) should be considered in hyponatremic patients or those whose fluid retention is difficult to control despite high doses of diuretics and sodium restriction. Vasopressin antagonists also may be useful in severe hyponatremia. Caloric supplementation is recommended for patients with advanced HF and unintentional weight loss or muscle wasting (cardiac cachexia); however, anabolic steroids are not recommended for these patients because of the potential problems with volume retention. The use of dietary supplements ("nutriceuticals") should be avoided in the management of symptomatic HF because of the lack of proven benefit and the potential for significant (adverse) interactions with proven HF therapies.

Diuretics Many of the clinical manifestations of moderate to severe HF result from excessive salt and water retention that leads to volume expansion and congestive symptoms. Diuretics (Table 234-5) are the only pharmacologic agents that can adequately control fluid retention in advanced HF, and they should be used to restore and maintain normal volume status in patients with congestive symptoms (dyspnea, orthopnea, edema) or signs of elevated filling pressures (rales, jugular venous distention, peripheral edema). Furosemide, torsemide, and bumetanide act at the loop of Henle (*loop diuretics*) by reversibly inhibiting the reabsorption of Na^+, K^+, and Cl^- in the thick ascending limb of Henle's loop; thiazides and metolazone reduce the reabsorption of Na^+ and Cl^- in the first half of the distal convoluted tubule; and potassium-sparing diuretics such as spironolactone act at the level of the collecting duct.

Although all diuretics increase sodium excretion and urinary volume, they differ in their potency and pharmacologic properties. Whereas loop diuretics increase the fractional excretion of sodium by 20–25%, thiazide diuretics increase it by only 5–10% and tend to lose their effectiveness in patients with moderate or severe renal insufficiency (creatinine >2.5 mg/dL). Hence, loop diuretics generally are required to restore normal volume status in patients with HF. Diuretics should be initiated in low doses (Table 234-5) and then carefully titrated upward to relieve signs and symptoms of fluid overload in an attempt to obtain the patient's "dry weight." This typically requires multiple dose

TABLE 234-5 Drugs for the Treatment of Chronic Heart Failure (EF <40%)

	Initiating Dose	Maximal Dose
Diuretics		
Furosemide	20–40 mg qd or bid	400 mg/d[a]
Torsemide	10–20 mg qd bid	200 mg/d[a]
Bumetanide	0.5–1 mg qd or bid	10 mg/d[a]
Hydrochlorthiazide	25 mg qd	100 mg/d[a]
Metolazone	2.5–5 mg qd or bid	20 mg/d[a]
Angiotensin-Converting Enzyme Inhibitors		
Captopril	6.25 mg tid	50 mg tid
Enalapril	2.5 mg bid	10 mg bid
Lisinopril	2.5–5 mg qd	20–35 mg qd
Ramipril	1.25–2.5 mg bid	2.5–5 mg bid
Trandolapril	0.5 mg qd	4 mg qd
Angiotensin Receptor Blockers		
Valsartan	40 mg bid	160 mg bid
Candesartan	4 mg qd	32 mg qd
Irbesartan	75 mg qd	300 mg qd[b]
Losartan	12.5 mg qd	50 mg qd
β Receptor Blockers		
Carvedilol	3.125 mg bid	25–50 mg bid
Bisoprolol	1.25 mg qd	10 mg qd
Metoprolol succinate CR	12.5–25 mg qd	Target dose 200 mg qd
Additional Therapies		
Spironolactone	12.5–25 mg qd	25–50 mg qd
Eplerenone	25 mg qd	50 mg qd
Combination of hydralazine/isosorbide dinitrate	10–25 mg/10 mg tid	75 mg/40 mg tid
Fixed dose of hydralazine/isosorbide dinitrate	37.5 mg/20 mg (one tablet) tid	75 mg/40 mg (two tablets) tid
Digoxin	0.125 mg qd	≤0.375 mg/d[b]

Notes: [a]Dose must be titrated to reduce the patient's congestive symptoms.
[b]Target dose not established.

adjustments over many days and occasionally weeks in patients with severe fluid overload. Intravenous administration of diuretics may be necessary to relieve congestion acutely and can be done safely in the outpatient setting. Once the congestion has been relieved, treatment with diuretics should be continued to prevent the recurrence of salt and water retention.

Refractoriness to diuretic therapy may represent patient nonadherence, a direct effect of chronic diuretic use on the kidney, or progression of underlying HF. The addition of thiazides or metolazone, once or twice daily, to loop diuretics may be considered in patients with persistent fluid retention despite high-dose loop diuretic therapy. Metolazone is generally more potent and much longer-acting than the thiazides in this setting as well as in patients with chronic renal insufficiency. However, chronic daily use, especially of metolazone, should be avoided if possible because of the potential for electrolyte shifts and volume depletion. Ultrafiltration and dialysis may be used in cases of refractory fluid retention that are unresponsive to high doses of diuretics and have been shown to be helpful in the short term.

Adverse Effects Diuretics have the potential to produce electrolyte and volume depletion as well as worsening azotemia. In addition, they may lead to worsening neurohormonal activation and disease progression. One of the most important adverse consequences of diuresis is alterations in potassium homeostasis (hypokalemia or hyperkalemia), which increase the risk of life-threatening arrhythmias. In general, both loop- and thiazide-type diuretics lead to hypokalemia, whereas spironolactone, eplerenone, and triamterene lead to hyperkalemia.

PREVENTING DISEASE PROGRESSION (Table 234-5) Drugs that interfere with excessive activation of the RAA system and the adrenergic nervous system can relieve the symptoms of HF with a depressed EF by stabilizing and/or reversing cardiac remodeling. In this regard, ACE inhibitors and beta blockers have emerged as the cornerstones of modern therapy for HF with a depressed EF.

ACE Inhibitors There is overwhelming evidence that ACE inhibitors should be used in symptomatic and asymptomatic patients (Figs. 234-3 and 234-4) with a depressed EF (<40%).

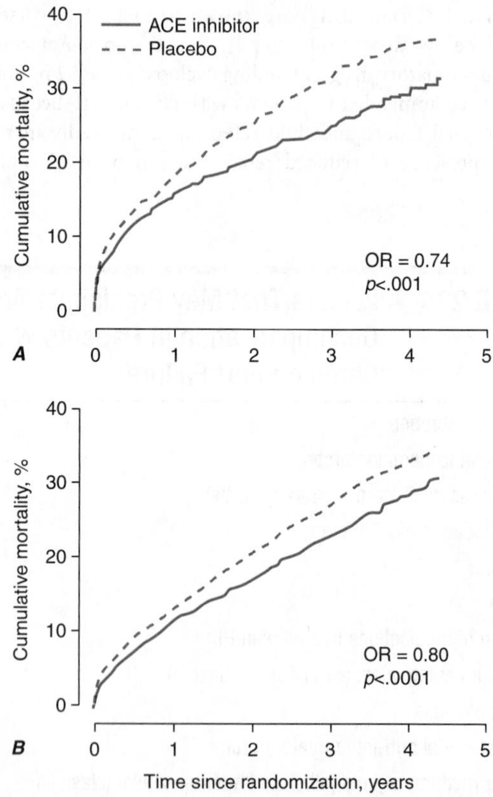

Figure 234-3 Meta-analysis of angiotensin-converting enzyme (ACE) inhibitors in heart failure patients with a depressed ejection fraction. ***A.*** The Kaplan-Meier curves for mortality for 5966 HF patients with a depressed EF treated with an ACE inhibitor after acute myocardial infarction (three trials). ***B.*** The Kaplan-Meier curves for mortality for 12,763 HF patients with a depressed EF treated with an ACE inhibitor in five clinical trials, including postinfarction trials. The benefits of ACE inhibitors were observed early and persisted long-term. *(Modified from MD Flather et al: Lancet 355:1575, 2000.)*

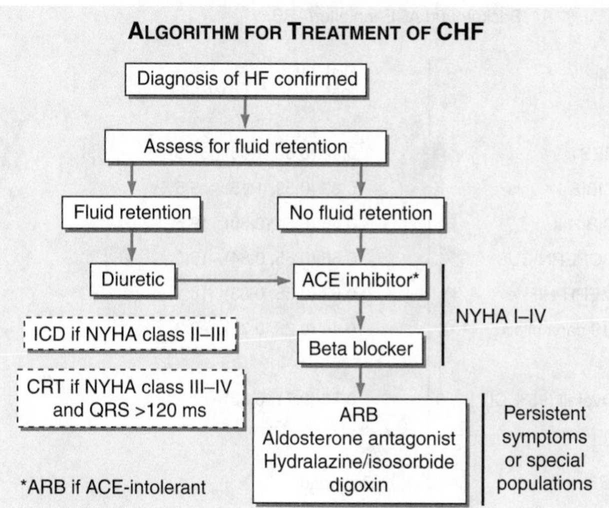

Figure 234-4 Treatment algorithm for chronic heart failure patients with a depressed ejection fraction. After the clinical diagnosis of HF is made, it is important to treat the patient's fluid retention before starting an ACE inhibitor (or an ARB if the patient is ACE-intolerant). Beta blockers should be started after the fluid retention has been treated and/or the ACE inhibitor has been uptitrated. If the patient remains symptomatic, an ARB, an aldosterone antagonist, or digoxin can be added as "triple therapy." The fixed-dose combination of hydralazine/isosorbide dinitrate should be added to an ACE inhibitor and a beta blocker in African-American patients with NYHA class II–IV HF. Device therapy should be considered in addition to pharmacologic therapy in appropriate patients. HF, heart failure; ACE, angiotensin-converting enzyme; ARB, angiotensin receptor blocker; NYHA, New York Heart Association; CRT, cardiac resynchronization therapy; ICD, implantable cardiac defibrillator.

ACE inhibitors interfere with the renin-angiotensin system by inhibiting the enzyme that is responsible for the conversion of angiotensin I to angiotensin II. However, because ACE inhibitors also inhibit kininase II, they may lead to the upregulation of bradykinin, which may further enhance the beneficial effects of angiotensin suppression. ACE inhibitors stabilize LV remodeling, improve symptoms, reduce hospitalization, and prolong life. Because fluid retention can attenuate the effects of ACE inhibitors, it is preferable to optimize the dose of diuretic before starting the ACE inhibitor. However, it may be necessary to reduce the dose of diuretic during the initiation of ACE inhibition to prevent symptomatic hypotension. ACE inhibitors should be initiated in low doses, followed by gradual increments if the lower doses have been well tolerated. The doses of ACE inhibitors should be increased until they are similar to those which have been shown to be effective in clinical trials (Table 234-5). Higher doses are more effective than lower doses in preventing hospitalization.

Adverse Effects The majority of adverse effects are related to suppression of the renin-angiotensin system. The decreases in blood pressure and mild azotemia that may occur during the initiation of therapy generally are well tolerated and do not require a decrease in the dose of the ACE inhibitor. However, if hypotension is accompanied by dizziness or if the renal dysfunction becomes severe, it may be necessary to reduce the dose of the inhibitor. Potassium retention may also become problematic if the patient is receiving potassium supplements or a potassium-sparing diuretic. Potassium retention that is not responsive to these measures may require a reduction in the dose of ACE inhibitor.

The side effects of ACE inhibitors related to kinin potentiation include a nonproductive cough (10–15% of patients) and angioedema (1% of patients). In patients who cannot tolerate ACE inhibitors because of cough or angioedema, angiotensin receptor blockers (ARBs) are the recommended first line of therapy (see below). Patients intolerant of ACE inhibitors because of hyperkalemia or renal insufficiency are likely to experience the same side effects with ARBs. In these cases, the combination of hydralazine and an oral nitrate should be considered (Table 234-5).

Angiotensin Receptor Blockers These drugs are well tolerated in patients who are intolerant of ACE inhibitors because of cough, skin rash, and angioedema. ARBs should be used in symptomatic and asymptomatic patients with an EF <40% who are ACE-intolerant for reasons other than hyperkalemia or renal insufficiency (Table 234-5). Although ACE inhibitors and ARBs inhibit the renin-angiotensin system, they do so by different mechanisms. Whereas ACE inhibitors block the enzyme responsible for converting angiotensin I to angiotensin II, ARBs block the effects of angiotensin II on the angiotensin type 1 receptor. Some clinical trials have demonstrated a therapeutic benefit from the addition of an ARB to an ACE inhibitor in patients with chronic HF. When given in concert with beta blockers, ARBs reverse the process of LV remodeling, improve patient symptoms, prevent hospitalization, and prolong life.

Adverse Effects Both ACE inhibitors and ARBs have similar effects on blood pressure, renal function, and potassium. Therefore, the problems of symptomatic hypotension, azotemia, and hyperkalemia are similar for both of these agents.

β-Adrenergic Receptor Blockers Beta-blocker therapy represents a major advance in the treatment of patients with a depressed EF (Fig. 234-5). These drugs interfere with the harmful effects of sustained activation of the adrenergic nervous system by competitively antagonizing one or more adrenergic receptors (α_1, β_1, and β_2). Although there are a number of potential benefits to blocking all three receptors, most of the deleterious effects of adrenergic activation are mediated by the β_1 receptor. When given in concert with ACE inhibitors, beta blockers reverse the process of LV remodeling, improve patient symptoms, prevent hospitalization, and prolong life. Therefore, beta blockers are indicated for patients with symptomatic or asymptomatic HF and a depressed EF <40%.

Analogous to the use of ACE inhibitors, beta blockers should be initiated in low doses (Table 234-5), followed by gradual increments in the dose if lower doses have been well tolerated. The dose of beta blocker should be increased until the doses used are similar to those which have been reported to be effective in clinical trials (Table 234-5). However, unlike ACE inhibitors, which may be titrated upward relatively rapidly, the titration of beta blockers should proceed no more rapidly than at 2-week intervals, because the initiation and/or increased dosing of these agents may lead to worsening fluid retention consequent to the withdrawal of adrenergic support to the heart and the circulation. Thus, it is important to optimize the dose of diuretic before starting therapy with beta blockers. If worsening fluid retention does occur, it is likely to do so within 3–5 days of the initiation of therapy, and it will be manifest as an increase in body weight and/or symptoms of worsening HF. The increased fluid retention usually can be managed by increasing the dose of diuretics. In some patients the dose of the beta blocker may have to be reduced.

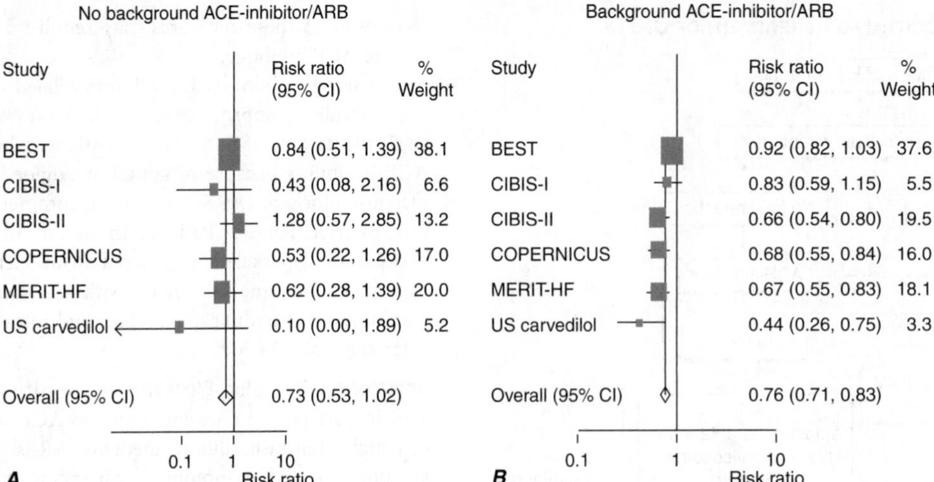

Figure 234-5 Meta-analysis of beta blockers on mortality rates in HF patients with a depressed EF. Effect of beta blockers vs. placebo in patients who were not (*A*) or who were (*B*) receiving an angiotensin-converting enzyme (ACE) inhibitor or an angiotensin receptor blocker (ARB) at baseline in six clinical trials. There was a similar impact of beta-blocker therapy on the endpoints of all-cause mortality as well as death and heart failure hospitalization in both the presence and the absence of ACE inhibitor or ARB at baseline. BEST, Beta-Blocker Evaluation of Survival Trial (bucindolol); CIBIS, Cardiac Insufficiency Bisoprolol Study (bisoprolol); COPERNICUS, Carvedilol prOsPEctive RaNdomIzed Cumulative Survival (carvedilol); MERIT-HF, Metoprolol CR/XL Randomized Intervention Trial in Heart Failure (metoprolol CR/XL). *(Modified from H Krum et al: Eur Heart J 26:2154, 2005.)*

Contrary to early reports, the aggregate results of clinical trials suggest that beta-blocker therapy is well tolerated by the great majority (≥85%) of HF patients, including patients with comorbid conditions such as diabetes mellitus, chronic obstructive lung disease, and peripheral vascular disease. Nonetheless, there is a subset of patients (10–15%) who remain intolerant to beta blockers because of worsening fluid retention or symptomatic hypotension or bradycardia.

Adverse Effects The adverse effects of beta-blocker use generally are related to the predictable complications that arise from interfering with the adrenergic nervous system. These reactions generally occur within several days of the initiation of therapy and generally are responsive to adjustments of concomitant medications, as described above. Therapy with beta blockers can lead to bradycardia and/or exacerbate heart block. Accordingly, the dose of beta blocker should be reduced if the heart rate decreases to <50 beats/min and/or second- or third-degree heart block or symptomatic hypotension develops. Beta blockers are not recommended for patients who have asthma with active bronchospasm. Beta blockers that also block the α_1 receptor can lead to vasodilatory side effects.

Aldosterone Antagonists Although classified as potassium-sparing diuretics, drugs that block the effects of aldosterone (spironolactone or eplerenone) have beneficial effects that are independent of the effects of these agents on sodium balance. Although ACE inhibition may transiently decrease aldosterone secretion, with chronic therapy there is a rapid return of aldosterone to levels similar to those before ACE inhibition. Accordingly, the administration of an aldosterone antagonist is recommended for patients with NYHA class IV or class III (previously class IV) HF who have a depressed EF (<35%) and are receiving standard therapy, including diuretics, ACE inhibitors, and beta blockers. The dose of aldosterone antagonist should be increased until the doses used are similar to those which have been shown to be effective in clinical trials (Table 234-5).

Adverse Effects The major problem with the use of aldosterone antagonists is the development of life-threatening hyperkalemia, which is more prone to occur in patients who are receiving potassium supplements or who have underlying renal insufficiency. Aldosterone antagonists are not recommended when the serum creatinine is >2.5 mg/dL (or creatinine clearance is <30 mL/min) or when the serum potassium is >5 mmol/L. Painful gynecomastia may develop in 10–15% of patients who use spironolactone, in which case eplerenone may be substituted.

SPECIAL POPULATIONS The combination of hydralazine and isosorbide dinitrate (Table 234-5) is recommended as part of standard therapy in addition to beta blockers and ACE inhibitors for African Americans with NYHA class II–IV HF. Although the exact mechanism for the effects of this combination is not known, it is believed to be secondary to the beneficial effects of NO on the peripheral circulation.

MANAGEMENT OF PATIENTS WHO REMAIN SYMPTOMATIC Additional pharmacologic therapy should be considered in patients who have persistent symptoms or progressive worsening despite optimized therapy with an ACE inhibitor and a beta blocker. Agents that may be considered as part of additional therapy include an ARB, spironolactone, the combination of hydralazine and isosorbide dinitrate, and digitalis. The optimal choice of additional drug therapy to improve the outcome further has not been firmly established. Thus, the choice of a specific agent will be influenced by clinical considerations, including renal function, serum potassium concentration, blood pressure, and race. The triple combination of an ACE inhibitor, an ARB, and an aldosterone antagonist should not be used because of the high risk of hyperkalemia.

Digoxin is recommended for patients with symptomatic LV systolic dysfunction who have concomitant atrial fibrillation, and it should be considered for patients who have signs or symptoms of HF while receiving standard therapy, including ACE inhibitors and beta blockers. Therapy with digoxin is commonly initiated and maintained at a dose of 0.125–0.25 mg daily. For the great majority of patients, the dose should be 0.125 mg daily, and the serum digoxin level should be <1 ng/mL, especially in elderly patients, patients with impaired renal function, and patients with a low lean body mass. Higher doses (and serum concentrations) appear to be less beneficial. There is no indication for using loading doses of digoxin to initiate therapy in patients with HF.

ANTICOAGULATION AND ANTIPLATELET THERAPY Patients with HF have an increased risk for arterial or venous thromboembolic events. In clinical HF trials, the rate of stroke ranges from 1.3 to 2.4% per year. Depressed LV function is believed to promote relative stasis of blood in dilated cardiac chambers with increased risk of thrombus formation. Treatment with warfarin [goal international normalized ratio (INR) 2–3] is recommended for patients with HF and chronic or paroxysmal atrial fibrillation or with a history of systemic or pulmonary emboli, including stroke or transient ischemic attack. Patients with symptomatic or asymptomatic ischemic cardiomyopathy and documented recent large anterior MI or recent MI with documented LV thrombus should be treated with warfarin (goal INR 2–3) for the initial 3 months after the MI unless there are contraindications to its use.

Aspirin is recommended in HF patients with ischemic heart disease for the prevention of MI and death. However, lower doses of aspirin (75 or 81 mg) may be preferable because of the concern of worsening of HF at higher doses.

MANAGEMENT OF CARDIAC ARRHYTHMIAS (See also Chap. 233) Atrial fibrillation occurs in 15–30% of patients with HF and is a common cause of cardiac decompensation. Most antiarrhythmic agents, with the exception of amiodarone and dofetilide, have negative inotropic effects and are proarrhythmic. Amiodarone is a class III antiarrhythmic that has few or no negative inotropic and/or proarrhythmic effects and is effective against most supraventricular arrhythmias. Amiodarone is the preferred drug for restoring and maintaining sinus rhythm, and it may improve the success of electrical cardioversion in patients with HF. Amiodarone increases the level of phenytoin and digoxin and prolongs the INR in patients taking warfarin. Therefore, it is often necessary to reduce the dose of these drugs by as much as 50% when initiating therapy with amiodarone. The risk of adverse events such as hyperthyroidism, hypothyroidism, pulmonary fibrosis, and hepatitis is relatively low, particularly when lower doses of amiodarone are used (100–200 mg/d).

Implantable cardiac defibrillators (ICDs; see below) are highly effective in treating recurrences of sustained ventricular tachycardia and/or ventricular fibrillation in HF patients with recurrent arrhythmias and/or cardiac syncope, and they may be used as stand-alone therapy or in combination with amiodarone and/or a beta blocker (Chap. 233). There is no role for treating ventricular arrhythmias with an antiarrhythmic agent without an ICD.

DEVICE THERAPY

Cardiac Resynchronization Approximately one-third of patients with a depressed EF and symptomatic HF (NYHA class III–IV) manifest a QRS duration >120 ms. This ECG finding of abnormal inter- or intraventricular conduction has been used to identify patients with dyssynchronous ventricular contraction. The mechanical consequences of ventricular dyssynchrony include suboptimal ventricular filling, a reduction in LV contractility, prolonged duration (and therefore greater severity) of mitral regurgitation, and paradoxical septal wall motion. *Biventricular pacing*, also termed *cardiac resynchronization therapy* (CRT), stimulates both ventricles nearly simultaneously, thereby improving the coordination of ventricular contraction and reducing the severity of mitral regurgitation. When CRT is added to optimal medical therapy in patients in sinus rhythm, there is a significant decrease in patient mortality rates and hospitalization and a reversal of LV remodeling, as well as improved quality of life and exercise capacity. Accordingly, CRT is recommended for patients in sinus rhythm with an EF <35% and a QRS >120 ms and those who remain symptomatic (NYHA III–IV) despite optimal medical therapy. The benefits of CRT in patients with atrial fibrillation have not been clearly established.

Implantable Cardiac Defibrillators (See also Chap. 233) The prophylactic implantation of ICDs in patients with mild to moderate HF (NYHA class II–III) has been shown to reduce the incidence of sudden cardiac death in patients with ischemic or nonischemic cardiomyopathy. Accordingly, implantation of an ICD should be considered for patients in NYHA class II–III HF with a depressed EF of <35% who are already on optimal background therapy, including an ACE inhibitor (or ARB), a beta blocker, and an aldosterone antagonist. An ICD may also be combined with a biventricular pacemaker in patients with NYHA class III–IV HF.

MANAGEMENT OF HF WITH A PRESERVED EJECTION FRACTION (>40–50%) Despite the wealth of information with respect to the evaluation and management of HF with a depressed EF, there are no proven and/or approved pharmacologic or device therapies for the management of patients with HF and a preserved EF. Therefore, it is recommended that initial treatment efforts should be focused, wherever possible, on the underlying disease process (e.g., myocardial ischemia, hypertension) associated with HF with preserved EF. Precipitating factors such as tachycardia and atrial fibrillation should be treated as quickly as possible through rate control and restoration of sinus rhythm when appropriate. Dyspnea may be treated by reducing total blood volume (dietary sodium restriction and diuretics), decreasing central blood volume (nitrates), or blunting neurohormonal activation with ACE inhibitors, ARBs, and/or beta blockers. Treatment with diuretics and nitrates should be initiated at low doses to avoid hypotension and fatigue.

ACUTE DECOMPENSATED HF

Defining an Appropriate Therapeutic Strategy The therapeutic goals for the management of acute decompensated HF (ADHF) therapy are to (1) stabilize the hemodynamic derangements that provoked the symptoms responsible for the hospitalization, (2) identify and treat the reversible factors that precipitated decompensation, and (3) reestablish an effective outpatient medical regimen that will prevent disease progression and relapse. In most instances this will require hospitalization, often in an intensive care unit (ICU) setting. Every effort should be made to identify the precipitating causes, such as infection, arrhythmias, dietary indiscretion, pulmonary embolism, infective endocarditis, occult myocardial ischemia/infarction, and environmental and/or emotional stress (Table 234-4), since removal of these precipitating events is critical to the success of treatment.

The two primary hemodynamic determinants of ADHF are elevated LV filling pressures and a depressed cardiac output. Frequently the depressed cardiac output is accompanied by an increase in systemic vascular resistance (SVR) as a result of excessive neurohormonal activation. Because these hemodynamic derangements may occur singly or together, patients with acute HF generally present with one of four basic

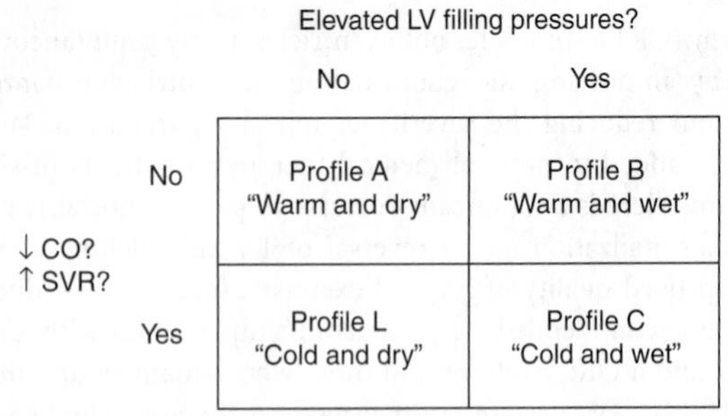

		Elevated LV filling pressures? No	Elevated LV filling pressures? Yes
↓ CO? ↑ SVR?	No	Profile A "Warm and dry"	Profile B "Warm and wet"
	Yes	Profile L "Cold and dry"	Profile C "Cold and wet"

Figure 234-6 Hemodynamic profiles in patients with acute heart failure. Most patients can be categorized into one of the four hemodynamic profiles by performing a brief bedside examination that includes examination of the neck veins, lungs, and peripheral extremities. More definitive hemodynamic information may be obtained by performing invasive hemodynamic monitoring, particularly if the patient is gravely ill or if the clinical presentation is unclear. This hemodynamic classification provides a useful guide for selecting the initial optimal therapies for the management of acute HF. LV, left ventricular; CO, cardiac output; SVR, systemic vascular resistance. *(Modified from Grady et al: Circulation 102:2443, 2000.)*

hemodynamic profiles (Fig. 234-6): normal LV filling pressure with normal perfusion (Profile A), elevated LV filling pressure with normal perfusion (Profile B), elevated LV filling pressures with decreased perfusion (Profile C), and normal or low LV filling pressure with decreased tissue perfusion (Profile L).

Accordingly, the therapeutic approach to treating patients with acute HF should be tailored to reflect the patient's hemodynamic presentation. The goal should be, whenever possible, to restore the patient to a normal hemodynamic profile (Profile A). In many instances the patient's hemodynamic presentation can be approximated from the clinical examination. For example, patients with elevated LV filling pressures may have signs of fluid retention (rales, elevated neck veins, peripheral edema) and are referred to as being "wet," whereas patients with a depressed cardiac output and an elevated SVR generally have poor tissue perfusion manifested by cool distal extremities and are referred to as being "cold." Nonetheless, it should be emphasized that patients with chronic heart failure may not have rales or evidence of peripheral edema at the time of the initial presentation with acute decompensation, and this may lead to the underrecognition of elevated filling pressures. In these patients, it may be appropriate to perform invasive hemodynamic monitoring.

Patients who are not congested and have normal tissue perfusion are referred to as being "dry" and "warm," respectively. When acute HF patients present to the hospital with Profile A, their symptoms are often due to conditions other than HF (e.g., pulmonary or hepatic disease or transient myocardial ischemia). More commonly, however, acute HF patients present with congestive symptoms ["warm and wet" (Profile B)], in which case treatment of the elevated filling pressures with diuretics and vasodilators is warranted to reduce LV filling pressures. Profile B includes most patients with acute pulmonary edema. The treatment of this life-threatening condition is described in Chap. 272.

Patients also may present with congestion and a significantly elevated SVR and reduction of cardiac output ["cold and wet" (Profile C)]. In these patients, cardiac output can be increased and LV filling pressures reduced by using intravenous vasodilators. Intravenous inotropic agents with vasodilating action [dobutamine, low-dose dopamine, milrinone (Table 234-6)] augment cardiac output by stimulating myocardial contractility as well as by functionally unloading the heart.

TABLE 234-6 Drugs for the Treatment for Acute Heart Failure

	Initiating Dose	Maximal Dose
Vasodilators		
Nitroglycerin	20 μg/min	40–400 μg/min
Nitroprusside	10 μg/min	30–350 μg/min
Nesiritide	Bolus 2 μg/kg	0.01–0.03 μg/kg per min[a]
Inotropes		
Dobutamine	1–2 μg/kg per min	2–10 μg/kg per min[b]
Milrinone	Bolus 50 μg/kg	0.1–0.75 μg/kg per min[b]
Dopamine	1–2 μg/kg per min	2–4 μg/kg per min[b]
Levosimendan	Bolus 12 μg/kg	0.1–0.2 μg/kg per min[c]
Vasoconstrictors		
Dopamine for hypotension	5 μg/kg per min	5–15 μg/kg per min
Epinephrine	0.5 μg/kg per min	50 μg/kg per min
Phenylephrine	0.3 μg/kg per min	3 μg/kg per min
Vasopressin	0.05 units/min	0.1–0.4 units/min

Notes: [a]Usually <4 μg/kg/min.

[b]Inotropes will also have vasodilatory properties.

[c]Approved outside the United States for management of acute heart failure.

Patients who present with Profile L ("cold and dry") should be carefully evaluated by right-heart catheterization for the presence of an occult elevation of LV filling pressures. If LV filling pressures are low [pulmonary capillary wedge pressure (PCWP) <12 mmHg], a cautious trial of fluid repletion may be considered. The goals of further therapy depend on the clinical situation. Therapy to reach the aforementioned goals may not be possible in some patients, particularly if they have disproportionate RV dysfunction or if they develop cardiorenal syndrome, in which renal function deteriorates during aggressive diuresis. Worsening renal dysfunction occurs in approximately 25% of patients hospitalized with HF and is associated with prolonged hospital stays and higher mortality rates after discharge.

Pharmacologic Management of Acute HF (Table 234-6)

Vasodilators After diuretics, intravenous vasodilators are the most useful medications for the management of acute HF. By stimulating guanylyl cyclase within smooth-muscle cells, nitroglycerin, nitroprusside, and nesiritide exert dilating effects on arterial resistance and venous capacitance vessels, which results in a lowering of LV filling pressure, a reduction in mitral regurgitation, and improved forward cardiac output without increasing heart rate or causing arrhythmias. Hypotension is the most common side effect of all vasodilating agents.

Intravenous *nitroglycerin* generally is begun at 20 μg/min and is increased in 20-μg increments until patient symptoms are improved or PCWP is decreased to 16 mmHg without reducing systolic blood pressure below 80 mmHg. The most common side effect of IV or oral nitrates is headache, which, if mild, can be treated with analgesics and often resolves during continued therapy. *Nitroprusside* generally is initiated at 10 μg/min and increased by 10–20 μg every 10–20 min as tolerated, with the same hemodynamic goals as described above. The rapidity of onset and offset, with a half-life of approximately 2 min, facilitates early establishment of an individual patient's optimal level of vasodilation in the ICU. The major limitation of nitroprusside is side effects from cyanide toxicity, which manifests predominantly as gastrointestinal and central nervous system manifestations and is most likely to occur in patients receiving >250 μg/min for over 48 h.

Nesiritide, the newest vasodilator, is a recombinant form of brain-type natriuretic peptide, which is an endogenous peptide secreted primarily from the LV in response to an increase in wall stress. Nesiritide is given as a bolus (2 μg/kg) followed by a fixed-dose infusion (0.01–0.03 μg/kg per min). Nesiritide effectively lowers LV filling pressures and improves symptoms during the treatment of acute HF. Headache is less common with nesiritide than with nitroglycerin. Although termed a *natriuretic peptide*, nesiritide has not been associated with major diuresis when used alone in clinical trials. It does, however, appear to potentiate the effect of concomitant diuretics such that the total required diuretic dose may be slightly lower. There have, however, been recent concerns about the adverse effects of neseritide on renal function in acute decompensated HF which may be related to the initial bolus.

Inotropic Agents Positive inotropic agents produce direct hemodynamic benefits by stimulating cardiac contractility as well as by producing peripheral vasodilation. Collectively, these hemodynamic effects result in an improvement in cardiac output and a fall in LV filling pressures.

Dobutamine, which is the most commonly used inotropic agent for the treatment of acute HF, exerts its effects by stimulating β_1 and β_2 receptors, with little effect on α_1 receptors. Dobutamine is given as a continuous infusion at an initial infusion rate of 1–2 μg/kg per min. Higher doses (>5 μg/kg per min) are frequently necessary for severe hypoperfusion; however, there is little added benefit to increasing the dose above 10 μg/kg per min. Patients maintained on chronic infusions for >72 h generally develop tachyphylaxis and require increasing doses.

Milrinone is a phosphodiesterase III inhibitor that leads to increased cyclic AMP by inhibiting its breakdown. Milrinone may act synergistically with β-adrenergic agonists to achieve a greater increase in cardiac output than is achieved with either agent alone, and it may also be more effective than dobutamine in increasing cardiac output in the presence of beta blockers. Milrinone may be administered as a bolus dose of 50 μg/kg per min, followed by a continuous infusion rate of 0.1–0.75 μg/kg per min. If the patient has a low blood pressure, many clinicians will omit the bolus dose. Because milrinone is a more effective vasodilator than dobutamine, it produces a greater reduction in LV filling pressures, albeit with a greater risk of hypotension.

Although short-term use of inotropes provides hemodynamic benefits, these agents are more prone to cause tachyarrhythmias and ischemic events than vasodilators are. Therefore, inotropes are most appropriately used in clinical settings in which vasodilators and diuretics are not helpful, such as in patients with poor systemic perfusion and/or cardiogenic shock, patients requiring short-term hemodynamic support after an MI or surgery, and patients awaiting cardiac transplantation, or as palliative care in patients with advanced HF. If patients require sustained use of intravenous inotropes, strong consideration should be given to the use of an ICD to safeguard against the proarrhythmic effects of these agents.

Vasoconstrictors Vasoconstrictors are used to support systemic blood pressure in patients with HF. Of the three agents that are commonly used (Table 234-6), dopamine is generally the first choice for therapy in situations in which modest inotropy and pressor support are required. Dopamine is an endogenous catecholamine that stimulates β_1 and α_1 receptors and dopaminergic receptors (DA_1 and DA_2) in the heart and circulation. The effects of dopamine are dose-dependent. Low doses of dopamine (<2 μg/kg per min) stimulate the DA_1 and DA_2 receptors and cause vasodilation of the splanchnic and renal vasculature. Moderate doses (2–4 μg/kg per min) stimulate the β_1 receptors and cause an increase in cardiac output with little or no change in heart rate or SVR. At higher doses (≥5 μg/kg per min) the effects of dopamine on the α_1 receptors overwhelm the dopaminergic receptors, and vasoconstriction ensues, leading to an increase in SVR, LV filling pressures, and heart rate. Significant additional inotropic and blood pressure support can be provided by epinephrine, phenylephrine, and vasopressin (Table 234-6); however, prolonged use of these agents can lead to renal and hepatic failure and can cause gangrene of the limbs. Therefore, these agents should not be administered except in true emergency situations.

Vasopressin Antagonists Vasopressin levels are often elevated in patients with HF and LV dysfunction and may contribute to the hyponatremia that develops in HF patients. Vasopressin antagonists reduce body weight and edema and normalize serum sodium in patients with hyponatremia but have not been associated with improved patient outcomes in clinical trials. Tolvaptan (oral) and conivaptan (IV) are currently approved for the treatment of hyponatremia but are not approved for the treatment of HF.

Mechanical and Surgical Interventions If pharmacologic interventions fail to stabilize a patient with refractory HF, mechanical and surgical interventions may provide effective circulatory support. These interventions include intraaortic balloon counter pulsation, percutaneous and surgically implanted LV assist devices, and cardiac transplantation (Chap. 235).

Planning for Hospital Discharge Patient education should take place during the entire hospitalization, with a specific focus on salt and fluid status and obtaining daily weights, in addition to medication schedules. Although the majority of patients hospitalized with HF can be stabilized and returned to a good level of function on an oral regimen designed to maintain stability, 30–50% of patients discharged with a diagnosis of HF are rehospitalized within 3–6 months. Although there are multiple reasons for rehospitalization, failure to meet criteria for discharge is perhaps the most common. Criteria for discharge should include at least 24 h of stable fluid status, blood pressure, and renal function on the oral regimen planned for home. Before discharge, patients should be free of dyspnea or symptomatic hypotension while at rest, washing, and walking on the ward.

COR PULMONALE

DEFINITION

Cor pulmonale, often referred to as *pulmonary heart disease*, is defined as dilation and hypertrophy of the right ventricle in response to diseases of the pulmonary vasculature and/or lung parenchyma. Historically, this definition has excluded congenital heart disease and those diseases in which the right heart fails secondary to dysfunction of the left side of the heart.

ETIOLOGY AND EPIDEMIOLOGY

Cor pulmonale develops in response to acute or chronic changes in the pulmonary vasculature and/or the lung parenchyma that are sufficient to cause pulmonary hypertension. The true prevalence of cor pulmonale is difficult to ascertain for two reasons. First, not all patients with chronic lung disease will develop cor pulmonale, and second, our ability to diagnose pulmonary hypertension and cor pulmonale by routine physical examination and laboratory testing is relatively insensitive. However, advances in 2-D echo/Doppler imaging and biomarkers (BNP) make it easier to screen for and detect cor pulmonale.

Once patients with chronic pulmonary or pulmonary vascular disease develop cor pulmonale, the prognosis worsens. Although chronic obstructive pulmonary disease (COPD) and chronic bronchitis are responsible for approximately 50% of the cases of cor pulmonale in North America (Chap. 260), any disease that affects the pulmonary vasculature (Chap. 250) or parenchyma can lead to cor pulmonale. Table 234-7 provides a list of common diseases that may lead to cor pulmonale. In contrast to COPD, the elevation in pulmonary artery pressure appears to be substantially higher in the interstitial lung diseases (Chap. 261), in which there is an inverse correlation between pulmonary artery pressure and the diffusion capacity for carbon monoxide, as well as patient survival. When cor pulmonale occurs in conjunction with obstructive sleep apnea, typically COPD or a hypoventilation syndrome [e.g., obesity hypoventilation syndrome (OHS)] is present concurrently (Chap. 265).

PATHOPHYSIOLOGY AND BASIC MECHANISMS

Although many conditions can lead to cor pulmonale, the common pathophysiologic mechanism in each case is pulmonary hypertension that is sufficient to lead to RV dilation, with or without the development of concomitant RV hypertrophy. The systemic consequences of cor pulmonale relate to alterations in cardiac output as well as salt and water homeostasis.

TABLE 234-7 Etiology of Chronic Cor Pulmonale

Diseases Leading to Hypoxemic Vasoconstriction
Chronic bronchitis
Chronic obstructive pulmonary disease
Cystic fibrosis
Chronic hypoventilation
Obesity
Neuromuscular disease
Chest wall dysfunction
Living at high altitudes
Diseases that Cause Occlusion of the Pulmonary Vascular Bed
Thromboembolic disease, acute or chronic
Pulmonary arterial hypertension
Pulmonary veno-occlusive disease
Diseases that Lead to Parenchymal Disease
Chronic bronchitis
Chronic obstructive pulmonary disease
Bronchiectasis
Cystic fibrosis
Pneumoconiosis
Sarcoidosis
Interstitial lung disease

Anatomically, the RV is a thin-walled, compliant chamber that is better suited to handle volume overload than pressure overload. Thus, the sustained pressure overload imposed by pulmonary hypertension and increased pulmonary vascular resistance eventually causes the RV to fail.

The response of the RV to pulmonary hypertension depends on the acuteness and severity of the pressure overload. Acute cor pulmonale occurs after a sudden and severe stimulus (e.g., massive pulmonary embolus), with RV dilatation and failure but no RV hypertrophy (Chap. 262). Chronic cor pulmonale, however, is associated with a more slowly evolving and progressive pulmonary hypertension that leads to initial modest RV hypertrophy and subsequent RV dilation.

Decompensation of chronic cor pulmonale can be aggravated by intermittent events that induce pulmonary vasoconstriction and RV afterload, such as hypoxemia and especially hypercarbia-induced respiratory acidosis (e.g., OHS), as well as sustained events, including COPD exacerbations, acute pulmonary emboli, and positive-pressure (mechanical) ventilation. RV failure also can be precipitated by alterations in RV volume that occur in various settings, including increased salt and fluid retention, atrial arrhythmias, polycythemia, sepsis, and a large left-to-right (extracardiac) shunt. The most common mechanisms that lead to pulmonary hypertension, including vasoconstriction, activation of the clotting cascade, and obliteration of pulmonary arterial vessels, are discussed in Chap. 250.

CLINICAL MANIFESTATIONS

Symptoms

The symptoms of chronic cor pulmonale generally are related to the underlying pulmonary disorder. Dyspnea, the most common symptom, is usually the result of the increased work of breathing secondary to changes in elastic recoil of the lung (fibrosing lung diseases), altered respiratory mechanics (e.g., overinflation with COPD), or inefficient ventilation (e.g., primary pulmonary vascular disease).Orthopnea and paroxysmal nocturnal dyspnea are rarely symptoms of isolated right HF and usually point toward concurrent left heart dysfunction. Rarely, these symptoms reflect increased work of breathing in the supine position resulting from compromised diaphragmatic excursion. Tussive or effort-related syncope may occur because of the inability of the RV to deliver blood adequately to the left side of the heart. Abdominal pain and ascites that occur with cor pulmonale are similar to the right-heart failure that ensues in chronic HF. Lower-extremity edema may occur secondary to neurohormonal activation, elevated RV filling pressures, or increased levels of carbon dioxide and hypoxemia, which can lead to peripheral vasodilation and edema formation. The symptoms of acute cor pulmonale with pulmonary embolus are reviewed in Chap. 262.

Signs

Many of the signs encountered in cor pulmonale are also present in HF patients with a depressed EF, including tachypnea, elevated jugular venous pressures, hepatomegaly, and lower-extremity edema. Patients may have prominent *v* waves in the jugular venous pulse as a result of tricuspid regurgitation. Other cardiovascular signs include an RV heave palpable along the left sternal border or in the epigastrium. The increase in intensity of the holosystolic murmur of tricuspid regurgitation with inspiration ("Carvallo's sign") may be lost eventually as RV failure worsens. Cyanosis is a late finding in cor pulmonale and is secondary to a low cardiac output with systemic vasoconstriction and ventilation-perfusion mismatches in the lung.

DIAGNOSIS

The most common cause of right-heart failure is not pulmonary parenchymal or vascular disease but left heart failure. Therefore, it is important to evaluate the patient for LV systolic and diastolic dysfunction. The ECG in severe pulmonary hypertension shows P pulmonale, right axis deviation, and RV hypertrophy. Radiographic examination of the chest may show enlargement of the main pulmonary artery, the hilar vessels, and the descending right pulmonary artery. Spirometry and lung volumes can identify obstructive and/or restrictive defects indicative of parenchymal lung diseases; arterial blood gases can demonstrate hypoxemia and/or hypercapnia. Spiral computed tomography (CT) scans of the chest are useful in diagnosing acute thromboembolic disease; however, ventilation-perfusion lung scanning remains best suited for diagnosing *chronic thromboembolic disease* (Chap. 262). A high-resolution CT scan of the chest can identify interstitial lung disease.

Two-dimensional echocardiography is useful for measuring RV thickness and chamber dimensions as well as the anatomy of the pulmonary and tricuspid valves. Location of the RV behind the sternum and its crescent shape challenge assessment of RV function by echocardiography, especially when parenchymal lung disease is present. Calculated measures of RV function [e.g., tricuspid annular plane systolic excursion (TAPSE) or the Tei Index] supplement more subjective assessments of RV function. The interventricular septum may move paradoxically during systole in the presence of pulmonary hypertension. As noted, Doppler echocardiography can be used to assess pulmonary artery pressures. MRI is also useful for assessing RV structure and function, particularly in patients who are difficult to image with 2-D echocardiography because of severe lung disease. Right-heart catheterization is useful for confirming the diagnosis of pulmonary hypertension and for excluding elevated left-heart pressures (measured as the PCWP) as a cause for right-heart failure. BNP and N-terminal BNP levels are elevated in patients with cor pulmonale secondary to RV stretch and may be dramatically elevated in acute pulmonary embolism.

TREATMENT Cor Pulmonale

The primary treatment goal of cor pulmonale is to target the underlying pulmonary disease, since this will decrease pulmonary vascular resistance and lessen RV afterload. Most pulmonary diseases that lead to chronic cor pulmonale are advanced and therefore are less amenable to treatment. General principles of treatment include decreasing work of breathing by using noninvasive mechanical ventilation and bronchodilation, as well as treating any underlying infection (Chaps. 260 and 261). Adequate oxygenation (oxygen saturation ≥90–92%) and correcting respiratory acidosis are vital for decreasing pulmonary vascular resistance and reducing demands on the RV. Patients should be transfused if they are anemic, and phlebotomy may be considered in extreme cases of polycythemia.

Diuretics are effective in RV failure, and indications are similar to those for chronic HF. One caveat of chronic diuretic use is to avoid inducing contraction alkalosis and worsening hypercapnia. Digoxin is of uncertain benefit in the treatment of cor pulmonale and may lead to arrhythmias in the setting of tissue hypoxemia and acidosis. Therefore, if digoxin is administered, it should be given at low doses and monitored carefully.

Pulmonary vasodilators can effectively improve symptoms through modest reduction of pulmonary pressures and RV afterload when isolated pulmonary arterial hypertension is present. Vasodilators are unproven in cases of pulmonary hypertension and cor pulmonale due to parenchymal lung diseases or hypoventilation syndromes. The treatment of the acute cor pulmonale that occurs with pulmonary embolus is described in Chap. 262. The treatment of pulmonary hypertension is discussed in Chap. 250.

FURTHER READINGS

Ashrafian H et al: Metabolic mechanisms in heart failure. Circulation 116:434, 2007

Bardy GH et al: Amiodarone or an implantable cardioverter-defibrillator for congestive heart failure. N Engl J Med 352:225, 2005

Chapman HA: Disorders of lung matrix remodeling. J Clin Invest 113:148, 2004

Cleland JG et al: The effect of cardiac resynchronization on morbidity and mortality in heart failure. N Engl J Med 352:1539, 2005

Friedrich EB, Bohm M: Management of end stage heart failure. Heart 93:626, 2007

Hunt SA et al: 2009 focused update incorporated into the ACC/AHA 2005 Guidelines for the Diagnosis and Management of Heart Failure in Adults: A report of the American College of Cardiology Foundation/American Heart Association Task Force on Practice Guidelines: developed in collaboration with the International Society for Heart and Lung Transplantation. Circulation 119:e391, 2009

Kessler R et al: "Natural history" of pulmonary hypertension in a series of 131 patients with chronic obstructive lung disease. Am J Respir Crit Care Med 164:219, 2001

Mann DL, Bristow MR: Mechanisms and models in heart failure: The biomechanical model and beyond. Circulation 111:2837, 2005

Mosterd A, Hoes AW: Clinical epidemiology of heart failure. Heart 93:1137, 2007

Pengo V et al: Incidence of chronic thromboembolic pulmonary hypertension after pulmonary embolism. N Engl J Med 350:2257, 2004

CHAPTER 235 Cardiac Transplantation and Prolonged Assisted Circulation

Sharon A. Hunt
Hari R. Mallidi

Advanced or end-stage heart failure is an increasingly frequent sequela, as progressively more effective palliation for the earlier stages of heart disease and prevention of sudden death associated with heart disease become more widely recognized and employed (Chap. 234). When patients with end-stage or refractory heart failure are identified, the physician is faced with the decision of advising compassionate end-of-life care or choosing to recommend extraordinary life-extending measures. For the occasional patient who is relatively young and without serious comorbidities, the latter may represent a reasonable option. Current therapeutic options are limited to cardiac transplantation (with the option of mechanical cardiac assistance as a "bridge" to transplantation) or (at least in theory) the option of permanent mechanical assistance of the circulation. In the future, it is possible that genetic modulation of ventricular function or cell-based cardiac repair will be options for such patients. Currently, both approaches are considered to be experimental.

CARDIAC TRANSPLANTATION

Surgical techniques for orthotopic transplantation of the heart were devised in the 1960s and taken into the clinical arena in 1967. The procedure did not gain widespread clinical acceptance until the introduction of "modern" and more effective immunosuppression in the early 1980s. By the 1990s, the demand for transplantable hearts met, and then exceeded, the available donor supply and leveled off at about 4,000 heart transplants annually worldwide, according to data from the Registry of the International Society for Heart and Lung Transplantation (ISHLT). Subsequently, heart transplant activity in the United States has remained stable at ~2,200/year, but worldwide activity reported to this registry has decreased somewhat. This apparent decline in numbers may be a result of the fact that reporting is legally mandated in the United States, but not elsewhere, and several countries have started their own databases.

SURGICAL TECHNIQUE

Donor and recipient hearts are excised in virtually identical operations with incisions made across the atria and atrial septum at the midatrial level (leaving the posterior walls of the atria in place) and across the great vessels just above the semilunar valves. The donor heart is generally "harvested" in an anatomically identical manner by a separate surgical team and transported from the donor hospital in a bag of iced saline solution and then is reanastomosed into the waiting recipient in the orthotopic or normal anatomic position. The only change in surgical technique since this method was first described has been a movement in recent years to move the right atrial anastamosis back to the level of the superior and inferior vena cavae to better preserve right atrial geometry and prevent atrial arrhythmias. Both methods of implantation leave the recipient with a surgically denervated heart that does not respond to any direct sympathetic or parasympathetic stimuli but does respond to circulating catecholamines. The physiologic responses of the denervated heart to the demands of exercise are atypical but quite adequate to carry on normal physical activity.

DONOR ALLOCATION SYSTEM

In the United States the allocation of donor organs is accomplished under the supervision of the United Network for Organ Sharing (UNOS), a private organization under contract to the federal government. The United States is divided geographically into eleven regions for donor heart allocation. Allocation of donor hearts within a region is decided according to a system of priority that takes into account (1) the severity of illness, (2) geographic distance from the donor, and (3) patient time on the waiting list. A physiologic limit of ~3 h of "ischemic" (out-of-body) time for hearts precludes a national sharing of hearts. This allocation system design is reissued annually and is responsive to input from a variety of constituencies, including both donor families and transplant professionals.

At the current time, highest priority according to severity of illness is assigned to patients requiring hospitalization at the transplant center for IV inotropic support with a pulmonary artery catheter in place for hemodynamic monitoring or to patients requiring mechanical circulatory support [i.e., intra-aortic balloon pump (IABP), right or left ventricular assist device (RVAD, LVAD), extracorporeal membrane oxygenation (ECMO), or mechanical ventilation]. Second highest priority is given to patients requiring ongoing inotropic support, but without a pulmonary artery catheter in place. All other patients have priority according to their time accrued on the waiting list, and matching is achieved only according to ABO blood group compatibility and gross body size compatibility, although some patients who are "pre-sensitized" and have preexisting anti-HLA antibodies (commonly multiparous women or patients previously multiply transfused) undergo prospective cross-matching with the donor. While HLA matching of donor and recipient would be ideal, the relatively small numbers of patients, as well as the time constraints involved, make such matching impractical.

INDICATIONS/CONTRAINDICATIONS

Heart failure is an increasingly common cause of death, particularly in the elderly. Most patients who reach what has recently been categorized as stage D, or refractory end-stage heart failure, are appropriately treated with compassionate end-of-life care. A subset of such patients who are younger and without significant comorbidities can be considered as candidates for heart transplantation. Exact criteria vary in different centers but generally take into consideration the patient's physiologic age and the existence of comorbidities such as peripheral or cerebrovascular disease, obesity, diabetes, cancer, or chronic infection.

RESULTS

A registry organized by the ISHLT has tracked worldwide and U.S. survival rates after heart transplantation since 1982. The most recent update reveals 83% and 76% survival 1 and 3 years posttransplant, or a posttransplant "half-life" of 10.00 years (Fig. 235-1). The quality of life in these patients is generally excellent, with well over 90% of patients in the registry returning to normal and unrestricted function following transplantation.

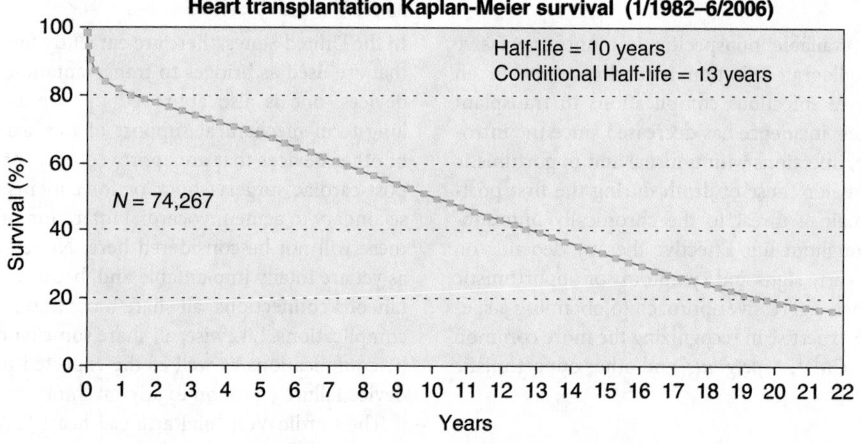

Figure 235-1 Survival was calculated using the Kaplan-Meier method, which incorporates information from all transplants for whom any follow-up has been provided. Because many patients are still alive and some patients have been lost to follow-up, the survival rates are estimates rather than exact rates because the time of death is not known for all patients. Therefore, 95% confidence limits are provided. (*From J Heart Lung Transplant 2008; 27:937–983.*)

IMMUNOSUPPRESSION

Medical regimens employed to provide suppression of the normal immune response to a solid organ allograft vary from center to center and are in a constant state of evolution, as more effective agents with improved side-effect profiles and less toxicity are introduced. All currently used regimens are nonspecific, providing general hyporeactivity to foreign antigens rather than donor-specific hyporeactivity, and also providing the attendant, and unwanted, susceptibility to infections and malignancy. Most cardiac transplant programs currently use a three-drug regimen including a calcineurin inhibitor (cyclosporine or tacrolimus), an inhibitor of T cell proliferation or differentiation (azathioprine, mycophenolate mofetil, or sirolimus), and at least a short initial course of glucocorticoids. Many programs also include an initial "induction" course of polyclonal or monoclonal anti-T cell antibodies in the perioperative period to decrease the frequency or severity of early posttransplant rejection. Most recently introduced have been monoclonal antibodies (daclizumab and basiliximab) that block the interleukin 2 receptor and may provide prevention of allograft rejection without additional global immunosuppression.

Diagnosis of cardiac allograft rejection is usually made with the use of endomyocardial biopsy, either done on a surveillance basis or in response to clinical deterioration. Biopsy surveillance is performed on a regular basis in most programs for the first year postoperatively and for the first five years in many programs. Therapy consists of augmentation of immunosuppression, the intensity and duration of which is dictated by the severity of the rejection.

LATE POSTTRANSPLANT MANAGEMENT ISSUES

Increasing numbers of heart transplant patients are surviving for years following transplantation and constitute a population of patients with a number of long-term management issues.

Allograft coronary artery disease

Despite usually having young donor hearts, cardiac allograft recipients are prone to develop coronary artery disease (CAD). This CAD is generally a diffuse, concentric, and longitudinal process that is quite different from "ordinary" atherosclerotic CAD, which is more focal and often eccentric. The underlying etiology is most likely primarily immunologic injury of the vascular endothelium, but a variety of risk factors influence its existence and progression and include nonimmunologic factors such as dyslipidemia, diabetes mellitus, and cytomegalovirus (CMV) infection. It is hoped that newer and improved immunosuppressive modalities will reduce the incidence and impact of these devastating complications, which currently account for the majority of late posttransplant deaths. Thus far, the immunosuppressive agents mycophenolate mofetil and the mammalian target of rapamycin (mTOR) inhibitors sirolimus and everolimus have been shown to be associated with short-term lesser incidence and extent of coronary intimal thickening; in anecdotal reports, institution of sirolimus was associated with some reversal of the disease. The use of statins has also been shown to be associated with a reduced incidence of this vasculopathy, and these drugs are now almost universally used in transplant recipients unless contraindicated. Palliation of the disease with percutaneous interventions is probably safe and effective in the short term, although the disease often advances relentlessly. Because of the denervated status of the organ, patients rarely experience angina pectoris, even with advanced stages of the disease.

Retransplantation is the only definitive form of therapy for advanced allograft CAD, but the scarcity of donor hearts makes the decision to pursue retransplantation a difficult one in an individual patient, as well as a difficult ethical issue.

Malignancy

The occurrence of an increased incidence of malignancy is a well-recognized sequela of any program of chronic immunosuppression, and organ transplantation is no exception. Lymphoproliferative disorders are among the most frequent posttransplant complications and, in most cases, seem to be driven by the Epstein-Barr virus. Effective therapy includes reduction of immunosuppression (a clear "double-edged sword" in the setting of a life-sustaining organ), antiviral agents, and traditional chemo- and radiotherapy. Most recently, specific antilymphocyte (CD20) therapy has shown great promise. Cutaneous malignancies (both basal cell and squamous cell carcinomas) also occur with increased frequency in transplant recipients and can pursue very aggressive courses. The role of decreasing immunosuppression for treatment of these cancers is far less clear.

Infections

The use of currently available nonspecific immunosuppressive modalities to prevent allograft rejection naturally results in an increased susceptibility to infectious complications in transplant recipients. Although their incidence has decreased since the introduction of cyclosporine, infections with unusual and opportunistic organisms remain the major cause of death during the first postoperative year and remain a threat to the chronically immunosuppressed patient throughout life. Effective therapy depends on careful surveillance for early signs and symptoms of opportunistic infection and an extremely aggressive approach to obtaining a specific diagnosis as well as expertise in recognizing the more common clinical presentations of CMV, *Aspergillus*, and other opportunistic infectious agents.

PROLONGED ASSISTED CIRCULATION

The modern era of mechanical circulatory support can be traced back to 1953, when cardiopulmonary bypass was first used in a clinical setting and ushered in the possibility of brief periods of circulatory support to permit open-heart surgery. Subsequently, a variety of extracorporeal pumps to provide circulatory support for brief periods of time have been developed. The use of a mechanical device to support the circulation for more than a few hours initially developed slowly, with the implant of a total artificial heart in 1969 in Texas by Cooley. This patient survived for 60 hours until a donor organ became available, at which point he was transplanted. Unfortunately, the patient died of pulmonary complications after transplantation. The entire field of mechanical replacement of the heart took a decade-long hiatus until the 1980s, when total artificial hearts were reintroduced with much publicity; however, they failed to produce the hoped-for treatment of end-stage heart disease. Starting in the 1970s, parallel to the development of the total artificial heart, there was intense research in the development of ventricular assist devices, which provide mechanical assistance to (rather than replacement of) the failing ventricle (currently, newer versions of the total artificial heart are in preliminary clinical trials).

Although conceived of initially as alternatives to biologic replacement of the heart, LVADs were introduced as, and are still employed primarily as, temporary "bridges" to heart transplantation in candidates who begin to fail medical therapy before a donor heart becomes available. Several devices are approved by the U.S. Food and Drug Administration (FDA) and are currently in widespread use. Those that are implantable within the body are compatible with hospital discharge and offer the patient a chance for life at home while waiting for a donor heart. However successful such "bridging" is for the individual patient, it does nothing to alleviate the scarcity of donor hearts; the ultimate goal in the field remains that of providing a reasonable alternative to biologic replacement of the heart—one that is widely and easily available and cost-effective.

CURRENT INDICATIONS AND APPLICATIONS OF VENTRICULAR ASSIST DEVICES

Currently, there are two major indications for long-term ventricular assistance. First, patients with chronic end-stage heart failure are eligible for mechanical support if they are at risk of imminent death from cardiogenic shock. Second, if patients have a left ventricular ejection fraction < 25%, peak VO_2 < 14 mL/kg/min or are dependent on inotropic therapy or support with intra-aortic balloon counterpulsation, they may be eligible for mechanical support. If they are eligible for heart transplantation, the mechanical circulatory assistance is termed "bridge to transplantation." By contrast, if the patient has a contraindication to heart transplantation, the device therapy is deemed to be "destination" left ventricular assistance therapy.

AVAILABLE DEVICES

In the United States, there are currently four FDA-approved devices that are used as bridges to transplantation in adults. Of these four devices, one is also approved for use as destination therapy or long-term mechanical support of the heart. There are a number of other devices that are approved only for short-term support for post-cardiac surgery shock or for patients with cardiogenic shock secondary to acute myocardial infarction or fulminant myocarditis; these will not be considered here. None of the long-term devices as yet are totally implantable and, because of this need for transcutaneous connections, all share a common problem with infectious complications. Likewise, all share some tendency to thromboembolic complications as well as the expected possibility of mechanical device failure common to any machine.

The CardioWest total artificial heart (TAH) (Syncardia, Tucson, AZ) is a pneumatic, biventricular, orthotopically implanted total artificial heart with an externalized driveline connecting it to its console. It consists of two spherical polyurethane chambers with polyurethane diaphragms. Inflow and outflow conduits are constructed of Dacron and contain Medtronic-Hall (Medtronic, Inc., Minneapolis, MN) valves. It is currently the only FDA-approved device for use as a bridge to transplantation in patients who have severe biventricular failure.

The Thoratec LVAD (Thoratec Corp., Pleasanton, CA) is an extracorporeal pump that takes blood from a large cannula placed in the left ventricular apex and propels it forward through an outflow cannula inserted into the ascending aorta. The pump itself sits in the paracorporeal position on the abdomen and is attached to a device console cart with wheels, allowing for limited ambulation. The extracorporeal nature of this pump allows it to be used in small adults for whom intracorporeal pumps would be too large.

The Novacor LVAD (WorldHeart, Inc., Oakland, CA) also takes blood from the left ventricular apex through a cannula and propels it into the ascending aorta through a second cannula. With this device, the pump itself is placed in a surgically created pocket in the peritoneal fascia in the abdomen. A driveline that connects to the power source is tunneled subcutaneously and usually exits in the right upper quadrant of the abdomen.

The HeartMate XVE LVAD (Thoratec Corp., Pleasanton, CA) is an intracorporeal left ventricular assist device that has an externalized driveline. The pump sits in the anterior abdominal wall with cannulae that traverse across the diaphragm. There is a drainage cannula in the left ventricular apex, and the blood is expelled from the pump into the ascending aorta via a synthetic vascular graft. This device may be used as a bridge to transplantation and patients may be discharged from the hospital with this device to await transplantation. The HeartMate XVE LVAD is now one of two FDA-approved devices for destination therapy.

The HeartMate II LVAS (Thoratec Corp., Pleasanton, CA) similarly uses a drainage cannula in the left ventricular apex to drain blood into a small chamber, where the blood is driven by an electrically powered motor that spins a rotor, accelerating blood outflow into the ascending aorta (Figure 235-2). This device is currently the only FDA-approved axial-flow pump that can be used both as a bridge to transplantation and as destination therapy. There are several other axial-flow pumps currently being investigated. These devices have fewer moving parts than previous devices and provide non-pulsatile blood flow. All current axial-flow pumps continue to require transcutaneous connections to power the electric motor. Newer, third-generation devices, which also provide non-pulsatile flow, work through a different mechanism than the axial-flow pumps and are currently being investigated. These devices are even smaller than the currently available axial-flow pumps, and their mechanism of action involves less trauma to blood cells, which may result in better durability and decreased long-term complications.

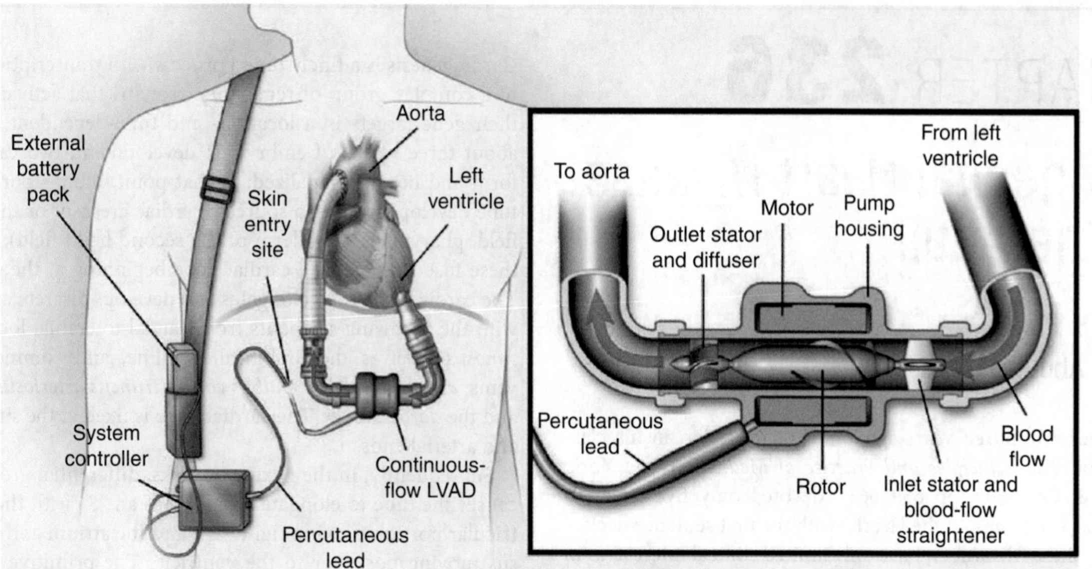

Figure 235-2 Diagram of HeartMate II left ventricular assist device. *(Reprinted with permission from Thoratec Corp., Pleasanton, CA.)*

■ RESULTS

The use of these devices in the United States is limited mainly to patients with post-cardiac surgery shock and to those who are bridged to transplantation. The results of bridging to transplantation with the available devices are quite good, with nearly 75% of younger patients receiving a transplant by 1 year and having excellent posttransplant survival rates.

Publication of the REMATCH (Randomized Evaluation of Mechanical Assistance in the Treatment of Heart Failure) trial in 2001 documented a somewhat improved survival rate in nontransplant candidates with end-stage heart disease randomized to a HeartMate XVE LVAD (albeit with a high rate of complications, especially neurologic ones) as opposed to continued medical therapy; this led to renewed interest in also using the devices as nonbiologic permanent replacement of heart function, as well as to FDA approval of one device for this indication. This outcome, in turn, led the ISHLT to initiate a Mechanical Circulatory Support database in 2002, which collects voluntary data from 60 international centers and contained data from 655 patients in its most recent publication. Only 12% of these patients had the device placed with the intention of permanent, or "destination," use, with survival rates of only 65% at 6 months and 34% at 1 year.

Several studies have evaluated the benefit of LVAD therapy as a bridge to transplantation, with the most recent data taken from a series of 133 patients who underwent implantation of a HeartMate II device. In this group of patients, 80% achieved the principal outcome (defined as survival to transplantation, recovery of heart function, or ongoing device support) at 180 days. With increased experience and improved outcomes using LVADs as a bridge to transplantation, the ability to maintain end-organ function and limit the progression of pulmonary hypertension, or even decrease pulmonary vascular resistance, makes mechanical unloading an attractive option when compared with continued inotropic support. The early bridge-to-transplantation experience demonstrated reduced posttransplantation survival when compared with medical management; however, more recent experience has shown equivalent outcomes following transplantation. This result is likely secondary to a trend toward earlier device implantation, prior to the onset of irreversible end-organ damage.

FURTHER READINGS

Garnier JL et al: Treatment of post-transplant lymphomas with anti-B-cell monoclonal antibodies. Recent Results Cancer Res 159:113, 2002

Gray NA Jr, Selzman CH: Current status of the total artificial heart. Am Heart J 152:4, 2006

Hunt SA et al: ACC/AHA 2005 guideline update for the diagnosis and management of chronic heart failure in the adult: A report of the American College of Cardiology/American Heart Association Task Force on Practice Guidelines (Writing committee to update the 2001 guidelines for the evaluation and management of heart failure). Available at *http://www.acc.org/clinical/guidelines/failure//index.pdf*

Kirklin JK et al: INTERMACS Database for Durable Devices for Circulatory Support: First Annual Report. J Heart Lung Transplant 27:1065, 2008

Mancini D et al: Use of rapamycin slows progression of cardiac transplantation vasculopathy. Circulation 108:48, 2003

Taylor DO et al: Registry of the International Society for Heart and Lung Transplantation: Twenty-sixth official adult heart transplant report—2005. J Heart Lung Transplant 228:1007, 2009

CHAPTER 236

Congenital Heart Disease in the Adult

John S. Child
Jamil Aboulhosn

A little over a hundred years ago, Sir William Osler, in his classic textbook *The Principles and Practice of Medicine* (New York, Appleton & Co, 1892, pp 659–663), devoted only five pages to "Congenital Affections of the Heart," with the first sentence declaring, that "[t]hese [disorders] have only limited clinical interest, as in a large proportion of cases the anomaly is not compatible with life, and in others nothing can be done to remedy the defect or even to relieve symptoms." Fortunately, in the intervening century, considerable progress has been made in understanding the basis for these disorders and their effective treatment.

The most common birth defects are cardiovascular in origin. These malformations are due to complex multifactorial genetic and environmental causes, but recognized chromosomal aberrations and mutations of single genes account for <10% of all cardiac malformations. Congenital heart disease (CHD) complicates ~1% of all live births in the general population—about 40,000 births/year—but occurs more frequently in the offspring (about 4–5%) of women with CHD. Owing to the remarkable surgical advances over the last 60 years, >90% of afflicted neonates and children now reach adulthood; women with CHD may now frequently successfully bear children after competent repairs. As such, the population with CHD is steadily increasing. Women with aortic disease (e.g., aortic coarctation or Marfan's syndrome) risk aortic dissection. Patients with cyanotic heart disease, pulmonary hypertension, or Marfan's syndrome with a dilated aortic root generally should not become pregnant; those with correctable lesions should be counseled about the risks of pregnancy with an uncorrected malformation versus repair and later pregnancy.

More than one million adults with operated or unoperated CHD live in the United States today and, thus, outnumber the 800,000 children with CHD. Because true surgical cures are rare, and all repairs—be they palliative or corrective—may leave residua, sequelae, or complications, most require some degree of lifetime expert surveillance. The anatomic and physiologic changes in the heart and circulation due to any specific CHD lesion are not static but, rather, progress from prenatal life to adulthood. Malformations that are benign or escape detection in childhood may become clinically significant in the adult. For example, a functionally normal congenitally bicuspid aortic valve may thicken and calcify with time, resulting in significant aortic stenosis; a well-tolerated left-to-right shunt of an atrial septal defect (ASD) may result in cardiac decompensation or pulmonary hypertension only after the fourth to fifth decade.

CARDIAC DEVELOPMENT (also see Chapter 224)

CHD is generally the result of aberrant embryonic development of a normal structure or failure of such a structure to progress beyond an early stage of embryonic or fetal development. This brief section serves to introduce the reader to normal development so that defects may be better understood; by necessity, it is not exhaustive.

Cardiogenesis is a finely tuned process with transcriptional control of a complex group of regulatory proteins that activate or inhibit their gene targets in a location- and time-dependent manner. At about three weeks of embryonic development, two cardiac cords form and become canalized; at that point, the primordial cardiac tube develops from two sources (cardiac crescent or the first heart field, pharyngeal mesoderm or the second heart field); by 21 days, these fuse into a single cardiac tube beginning at the cranial end. The cardiac tube then elongates and develops discrete constrictions with the following segments from caudal to cranial location: *sinus venosus* receives the umbilical, vitelline, and common cardinal veins: *atrium, ventricle, bulbus cordis, truncus arteriosus, aortic sac*, and the *aortic arches*. The cardiac tube is fixed at the sinus venosus and arterial ends.

Subsequently, in the next few weeks, differential growth of cells causes the tube to elongate and loop as an "S" with the bulboventricular portion moving rightward and the atrium and sinus venosus moving posterior to the ventricle. The primitive atrium and ventricle communicate via the atrioventricular canal from which the endocardial cushion develops into two parts (ventrally and dorsally). The cushions fuse and divide the atrioventricular canal into two atrioventricular inlets and also migrate to help form the ventricular septum. The primitive atrium is divided first by a *septum primum* membrane, which grows down from the superior wall to the cushions; as this fusion occurs, the mid-portion resorbs in the center forming the *ostium secundum*. Rightward of the *septum primum*, a second *septum secundum* membrane grows down from the ventral-cranial wall toward—but not reaching—the cushions, and covering most, but not all, of the *ostium secundum*, resulting in a flap of the *foramen ovale*. The primitive ventricle is partitioned by a finely tuned set of events. The interventricular septum grows up toward the cushions, and the cushions form an upper inlet septum; between the two portions is a hole called the interventricular foramen. The left and right ventricles begin to develop side by side, and the atria and their respective inlet valves align over their ventricles. Finally, these two parts of the septum fuse with the bulboventricular ridges, which, once having septated the truncus arteriosus, extend into the ventricle. The bulbocordis divides into a subaortic portion as the muscular conus resorbs, while the subpulmonary section has elongation of its muscular conus. Spiral division of the common truncus arteriosus rotates and aligns the pulmonary artery and aortic portions over their respective outflow tracts, the aortic valve moving posterior over the left ventricle (LV) outflow tract and the pulmonary valve moving anterior over the right ventricle (RV) outflow tract, with a wraparound relationship of the two great arteries.

Early on, the venous systems are bilateral and symmetric and enter two horns of the sinus venosus. Ultimately, except for the coronary sinus, most of the left-sided portions and the left sinus-venosus horn regress and the systemic venous system empties into the right horn via the inferior and superior vena cavae. The pulmonary venous system, initially connecting to the systemic venous system, develops as buds from the developing lungs fuse together in the *pulmonary venous* confluence at which point the connection to the systemic system regresses. Simultaneously, a projection from the back wall of the left atrium (the *common pulmonary vein*) grows posteriorly to merge with the confluence, which then becomes a part of the posterior left atrial wall.

The truncus arteriosus and aortic sac initially develop six paired symmetric arches, which curve posteriorly and become the paired dorsal aortae. The detailed description of the selective regression of some of the arches is not presented in this chapter. In brief summary, this process results in the development of arch 3 as the internal carotid arteries, left arch 4 as the aortic arch and right subclavian artery, and part of arch 6 as the patent ductus arteriosus. The two dorsal thoracic aortae fuse in the abdomen with persistence of the left dorsal aorta.

SPECIFIC CARDIAC DEFECTS

Tables 236-1, 236-2, and 236-3 list CHD malformations as simple, intermediate, or complex. Simple defects generally are single lesions with a shunt or a valvular malformation. Intermediate defects may have two or more simple defects. Complex defects generally have components of an intermediate defect plus more complex cardiac and vascular anatomy, often with cyanosis, and frequently with transposition complexes. The goal of these tables is to suggest when cardiology consultation or advanced CHD specialty care is needed. Patients with complex CHD (which includes most "named" surgeries that usually involve complex CHD) should virtually always be managed in conjunction with an experienced specialty adult CHD center. Patients with intermediate lesions should have an initial consultation and subsequent occasional intermittent follow-up with a cardiologist. Patients with simple lesions often may be managed by a well-informed internist or general cardiologist, although consultation with a specifically trained adult congenital cardiologist is occasionally advisable.

ATRIAL SEPTAL DEFECT

ASD is a common cardiac anomaly that may be first encountered in the adult and occurs more frequently in females. *Sinus venosus* ASD occurs high in the atrial septum near the entry of the superior vena cava into the right atrium and is associated frequently with anomalous pulmonary venous connection from the right lung to the superior vena cava or right atrium. *Ostium primum* ASDs lie adjacent to the atrioventricular valves, either of which may be deformed and regurgitant. Ostium primum ASDs are common in Down syndrome; the more complex atrioventricular septal defects with a common atrioventricular valve and a posterior defect of the basal portion of the interventricular septum are more typical of this chromosomal defect. The most common *ostium secundum* ASD involves the fossa ovalis and is midseptal in location; this should not be confused with a *patent foramen ovale*. Anatomic obliteration of the foramen ovale ordinarily follows its functional closure soon after birth, but residual "probe patency" is a common normal variant; ASD denotes a true deficiency of the atrial septum and implies functional and anatomic patency. The magnitude of the left-to-right shunt depends on the ASD size, ventricular diastolic properties, and the relative impedance in the pulmonary and systemic circulations. The left-to-right shunt causes diastolic overloading of the right ventricle and increased pulmonary blood flow. Patients with ASD are usually asymptomatic in early life, although there may be some physical underdevelopment and an increased tendency for respiratory infections; cardiorespiratory symptoms occur in many older patients. Beyond the fourth decade, a significant number of patients develop atrial arrhythmias, pulmonary arterial hypertension, bidirectional and then right-to-left shunting of blood, and right heart failure. Patients exposed to the chronic environmental hypoxemia of high altitude tend to develop pulmonary hypertension at younger ages. In older patients, left-to-right shunting across the ASD increases as progressive systemic hypertension and/or coronary artery disease (CAD) result in reduced compliance of the left ventricle.

Physical examination

Examination usually reveals a prominent RV impulse and palpable pulmonary artery pulsation. The first heart sound is normal or split, with accentuation of the tricuspid valve closure sound. Increased flow across the pulmonic valve is responsible for a midsystolic

TABLE 236-1 Simple Adult Congenital Heart Disease

Native disease
Uncomplicated congenital aortic valve disease
Mild congenital mitral valve disease (e.g., except parachute valve, cleft leaflet)
Uncomplicated small atrial septal defect
Uncomplicated small ventricular septal defect
Mild pulmonic stenosis
Repaired conditions
Previously ligated or occluded ductus arteriosus
Repaired secundum or sinus venosus atrial septal defect without residua
Repaired ventricular septal defect without residua

TABLE 236-2 Intermediate Complexity Congenital Heart Disease

Ostium primum or sinus venosus atrial septal defect
Anomalous pulmonary venous drainage, partial or total
Atrioventricular canal defects (partial or complete)
Ventricular septal defect, complicated (e.g., absent or abnormal valves or with associated obstructive lesions, aortic regurgitation)
Coarctation of the aorta
Pulmonic valve stenosis (moderate to severe)
Infundibular right ventricular outflow obstruction of significance
Pulmonary valve regurgitation (moderate to severe)
Patent ductus arteriosus (non-closed)—moderate to large
Sinus of Valsalva fistula/aneurysm
Subvalvular or supravalvular aortic stenosis

TABLE 236-3 Complex Adult Congenital Heart Disease

Cyanotic congenital heart diseases (all forms)
Eisenmenger's syndrome
Ebstein's anomaly
Tetralogy of Fallot or pulmonary atresia (all forms)
Transposition of the great arteries
Single ventricle; tricuspid or mitral atresia
Double-outlet ventricle
Truncus arteriosus
Fontan or Rastelli procedures

pulmonary outflow murmur. The second heart sound is widely split and is relatively fixed in relation to respiration. A mid-diastolic rumbling murmur, loudest at the fourth intercostal space and along the left sternal border, reflects increased flow across the tricuspid valve. In ostium primum ASD, an apical holosystolic murmur indicates associated mitral or tricuspid regurgitation or a ventricular septal defect (VSD).

These findings are altered when increased pulmonary vascular resistance causes diminution of the left-to-right shunt. Both the pulmonary outflow and tricuspid inflow murmurs decrease in intensity, the pulmonic component of the second heart sound and a systolic ejection sound are accentuated, the two components of the second heart sound may fuse, and a diastolic murmur of pulmonic regurgitation appears. Cyanosis and clubbing accompany the development of a right-to-left shunt (see "Ventricular Septal Defect" below). In adults with an ASD and atrial fibrillation, the physical findings may be confused with mitral stenosis with pulmonary hypertension because the tricuspid diastolic flow murmur and widely split second heart sound may be mistakenly thought to represent the diastolic murmur of mitral stenosis and the mitral "opening snap," respectively.

Electrocardiogram

In ostium secundum ASD, electrocardiogram (ECG) usually shows right-axis deviation and an rSr′ pattern in the right precordial leads representing enlargement of the RV outflow tract. An ectopic atrial pacemaker or first-degree heart block may occur with the sinus venous ASD. In ostium primum ASD, the RV conduction defect is accompanied by left superior axis deviation and counterclockwise rotation of the frontal plane QRS loop. Varying degrees of RV and right atrial (RA) enlargement or hypertrophy may occur with each type of defect, depending on the height of the pulmonary artery pressure. *Chest x-ray* shows an enlarged right atrium and right ventricle, and pulmonary artery and its branches; increased pulmonary vascular markings of left-to-right shunt vascularity will diminish if pulmonary vascular disease develops.

Echocardiogram

Echocardiography reveals pulmonary arterial and RV and RA dilatation with abnormal (paradoxical) ventricular septal motion in the presence of a significant right heart volume overload. The ASD may be visualized directly by two-dimensional imaging, color-flow imaging, or echocontrast. In most institutions, two-dimensional echocardiography and Doppler examination have supplanted cardiac catheterization. Transesophageal echocardiography is indicated if the transthoracic echocardiogram is ambiguous, which is often the case with sinus venosus defects, or during catheter device closure (Fig. 236-1). Cardiac catheterization is performed if inconsistencies exist in the clinical data, if significant pulmonary hypertension or associated malformations are suspected, or if CAD is a possibility.

TREATMENT Atrial Septal Defect

Operative repair, usually with a patch of pericardium or of prosthetic material or percutaneous transcatheter device closure, if the ASD is of an appropriate size and shape, should be advised for all patients with uncomplicated secundum ASD with significant left-to-right shunting, i.e., pulmonary-to-systemic flow ratios ≥2:1. Excellent results may be anticipated, at low risk, even in patients >40 years, in the absence of severe pulmonary hypertension. In ostium primum ASD, cleft mitral valves may require repair in addition to patch closure of the ASD. Closure should not be carried out in patients with small defects and trivial left-to-right shunts or in those with severe pulmonary vascular disease without a significant left-to-right shunt.

Patients with sinus venosus or ostium secundum ASDs rarely die before the fifth decade. During the fifth and sixth decades, the incidence of progressive symptoms, often leading to severe disability, increases substantially. Medical management should include prompt treatment of respiratory-tract infections; anti-arrhythmic medications for atrial fibrillation or supraventricular

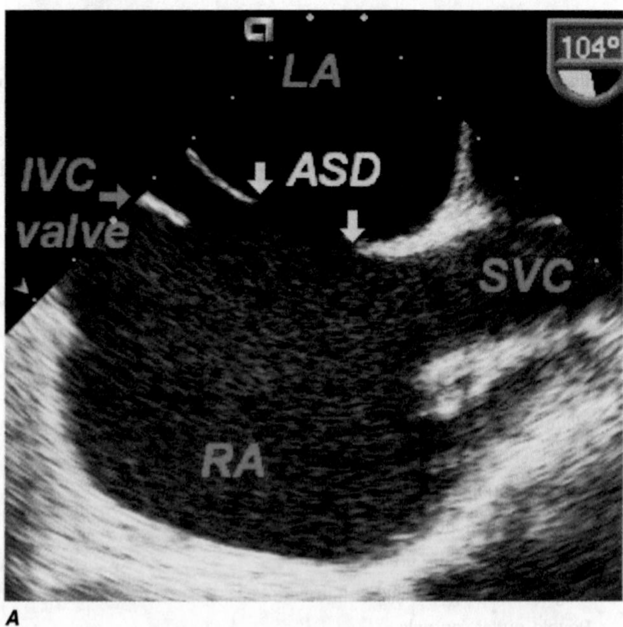

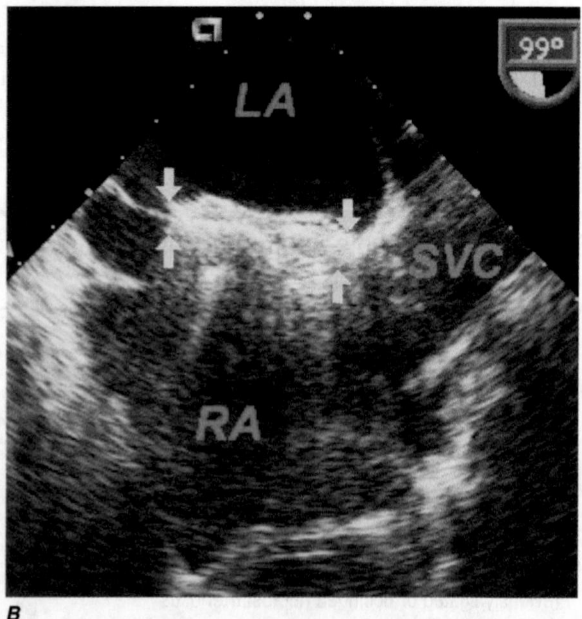

Figure 236-1 Secundum atrial septal defect. Transesophageal echocardiogram of secundum ASD and device closure. ***A.*** The atrial septal defect (ASD) between the left atrium (LA) and right atrium (RA) is shown. ***B.*** A percutaneous catheter–delivered device has occluded the defect. IVC, inferior vena cava; SVC, superior vena cava.

tachycardia; and the usual measures for hypertension, coronary disease, or heart failure (Chap. 234), if these complications occur. The risk of infective endocarditis is quite low unless the defect is complicated by valvular regurgitation or has recently been repaired with a patch or device (Chap. 124).

Ventricular septal defect

A VSD is one of the most common of all cardiac birth defects, either as isolated defects or as a component of a combination of anomalies. The VSD is usually single and situated in the membranous or midmuscular portion of the septum. The functional disturbance depends on its size and on the status of the pulmonary vascular bed. Only small- or moderate-size VSDs are seen initially in adulthood, as most patients with an isolated large VSD come to medical or surgical attention early in life.

A wide spectrum exists in the natural history of VSD, ranging from spontaneous closure to congestive cardiac failure and death in infancy. Included within this spectrum are the possible development of pulmonary vascular obstruction, RV outflow tract obstruction, aortic regurgitation, or infective endocarditis. Spontaneous closure is more common in patients born with a small VSD, which occurs in early childhood in most. The pulmonary vascular bed is often a principal determinant of the clinical manifestations and course of a given VSD and feasibility of surgical repair. Increased pulmonary arterial pressure results from increased pulmonary blood flow and/or resistance, the latter usually the result of obstructive, obliterative structural changes within the pulmonary vascular bed. It is important to quantitate and compare pulmonary-to-systemic flows and resistances in patients with severe pulmonary hypertension. The term *Eisenmenger's syndrome* is applied to patients with a large communication between the two circulations at the aortopulmonary, ventricular, or atrial levels and bidirectional or predominantly right-to-left shunts because of high resistance and obstructive pulmonary hypertension.

Patients with large VSDs and pulmonary hypertension are at greatest risk for developing pulmonary vascular obstruction. Large VSDs should be corrected surgically early in life when pulmonary vascular disease is still reversible or not yet developed. In patients with Eisenmenger syndrome, symptoms in adult life consist of exertional dyspnea, chest pain, syncope, and hemoptysis. The right-to-left shunt leads to cyanosis, clubbing, and erythrocytosis (see below). The degree to which pulmonary vascular resistance is elevated before operation is a critical factor determining prognosis. If the pulmonary vascular resistance is one-third or less of the systemic value, progression of pulmonary vascular disease after operation is unusual; however, if a moderate to severe increase in pulmonary vascular resistance exists preoperatively, either no change or a progression of pulmonary vascular disease is common postoperatively. Pregnancy is contraindicated in Eisenmenger syndrome. The mother's health is most at risk if she has a cardiovascular lesion associated with pulmonary vascular disease and pulmonary hypertension (e.g., Eisenmenger physiology or mitral stenosis) or LV outflow tract obstruction (e.g., aortic stenosis), but she is also at risk of death with any malformation that may cause heart failure or a hemodynamically important arrhythmia. The fetus is most at risk with maternal cyanosis, heart failure, or pulmonary hypertension.

RV outflow tract obstruction develops in ~5–10% of patients who present in infancy with a moderate to large left-to-right shunt. With time, as subvalvular RV outflow tract obstruction progresses, the findings in these patients whose VSD remains sizable begin to resemble more closely those of the cyanotic tetralogy of Fallot. In ~5% of patients, aortic valve regurgitation results from insufficient cusp tissue or prolapse of the cusp through the interventricular defect; the aortic regurgitation then complicates and dominates the clinical course. Two-dimensional *echocardiography* with spectral and color Doppler examination defines the number and location of defects in the ventricular septum and associated anomalies and the hemodynamic physiology of the defect(s). Hemodynamic and angiographic study may be occasionally required to assess the status of the pulmonary vascular bed and clarify details of the altered anatomy.

TREATMENT Ventricular Septal Defect

Surgery is not recommended for patients with normal pulmonary arterial pressures with small shunts (pulmonary-to-systemic flow ratios of <1.5 to 2:1). Operative correction or transcatheter closure is indicated when there is a moderate to large left-to-right shunt with a pulmonary-to-systemic flow ratio >1.5:1 or 2:1, in the absence of prohibitively high levels of pulmonary vascular resistance.

In the Eisenmenger VSD patient, pulmonary arterial vasodilators and both single-lung transplantation with intracardiac defect repair and total heart-lung transplantation show promise for improvement in symptoms (Chaps. 235 and 266). Chronic hypoxemia in cyanotic CHD results in secondary *erythrocytosis* due to increased erythropoietin production (Chap. 35). The term *polycythemia* is a misnomer; white cell counts are normal and platelet counts are normal to decreased. Compensated erythrocytosis with iron-replete equilibrium hematocrits rarely result in symptoms of hyperviscosity at hematocrits < 65% and occasionally not even with hematocrits ≥ 70%. For this reason, therapeutic phlebotomy is rarely required in compensated erythrocytosis. In contrast, patients with decompensated erythrocytosis fail to establish equilibrium with unstable, rising hematocrits and recurrent hyperviscosity symptoms. Therapeutic phlebotomy, a two-edged sword, allows temporary relief of symptoms but limits oxygen delivery, begets instability of the hematocrit, and compounds the problem by iron depletion. Iron-deficiency symptoms are usually indistinguishable from those of hyperviscosity; progressive symptoms after recurrent phlebotomy are usually due to iron depletion with hypochromic microcytosis. Iron depletion results in a larger number of smaller (microcytic) hypochromic red cells that are less capable of carrying oxygen and less deformable in the microcirculation; with more of them relative to plasma volume, viscosity is greater than for an equivalent hematocrit with fewer, larger, iron-replete, deformable cells. As such, iron-depleted erythrocytosis results in increasing symptoms due to decreased oxygen delivery to the tissues.

Hemostasis is abnormal in cyanotic CHD, due, in part, to the increased blood volume and engorged capillaries, abnormalities in platelet function, and sensitivity to aspirin or nonsteroidal anti-inflammatory agents, as well as abnormalities of the extrinsic and intrinsic coagulation system. Oral contraceptives are often contraindicated for cyanotic women because of the enhanced risk of vascular thrombosis. Adults with cyanotic CHD do not appear to be at increased risk for stroke unless there are excessive injudicious phlebotomies, inappropriate use of aspirin or anticoagulants, or the presence of atrial arrhythmias or infective endocarditis. Symptoms of hyperviscosity can be produced in any cyanotic patient with erythrocytosis if dehydration reduces plasma volume. Phlebotomy for symptoms of hyperviscosity not due to dehydration or iron deficiency is a simple outpatient removal of 500 mL of blood over 45 min with isovolumetric replacement with isotonic saline. Acute phlebotomy without volume replacement is contraindicated. Iron repletion in decompensated iron-depleted erythrocytosis reduces iron-deficiency symptoms, but must be done gradually to avoid an excessive rise in hematocrit and resulting hyperviscosity.

Patent ductus arteriosus

The ductus arteriosus is a vessel leading from the bifurcation of the pulmonary artery to the aorta just distal to the left subclavian artery. Normally, the vascular channel is open in the fetus but closes immediately after birth. The flow across the ductus is determined by the pressure and resistance relationships between the systemic and pulmonary circulations and by the cross-sectional area and length of the ductus. In most adults with this anomaly, pulmonary pressures are normal and a gradient and shunt from aorta to pulmonary artery persist throughout the cardiac cycle, resulting in a characteristic thrill and a continuous "machinery" murmur with late systolic accentuation at the upper left sternal edge. In adults who were born with a large left-to-right shunt through the ductus arteriosus, pulmonary vascular obstruction (Eisenmenger syndrome) with pulmonary hypertension, right-to-left shunting, and cyanosis have usually developed. Severe pulmonary vascular disease results in reversal of flow through the ductus; unoxygenated blood is shunted to the descending aorta; and the toes—but not the fingers—become cyanotic and clubbed, a finding termed *differential cyanosis*. The leading causes of death in adults with patent ductus are cardiac failure and infective endocarditis; occasionally severe pulmonary vascular obstruction may cause aneurysmal dilatation, calcification, and rupture of the ductus.

TREATMENT Patent Ductus Arteriosus

In the absence of severe pulmonary vascular disease and predominant left-to-right shunting of blood, the patent ductus should be surgically ligated or divided. Transcatheter closure using coils, buttons, plugs, and umbrellas has become commonplace for appropriately shaped defects. Thoracoscopic surgical approaches are considered experimental. Operation should be deferred for several months in patients treated successfully for infective endocarditis because the ductus may remain somewhat edematous and friable.

Aortic root–to-right-heart shunts

The three most common causes of aortic root–to-right-heart shunts are congenital aneurysm of an aortic sinus of Valsalva with fistula, coronary arteriovenous fistula, and anomalous origin of the left coronary artery from the pulmonary trunk. *Aneurysm of an aortic sinus of Valsalva* consists of a separation or lack of fusion between the media of the aorta and the annulus of the aortic valve. Rupture usually occurs in the third or fourth decade of life; most often, the aorticocardiac fistula is between the right coronary cusp and the right ventricle; but occasionally, when the noncoronary cusp is involved, the fistula drains into the right atrium. Abrupt rupture causes chest pain, bounding pulses, a continuous murmur accentuated in diastole, and volume overload of the heart. Diagnosis is confirmed by two-dimensional and Doppler echocardiographic studies; cardiac catheterization quantitates the left-to-right shunt, and thoracic aortography visualizes the fistula. Medical management is directed at cardiac failure, arrhythmias, or endocarditis. At operation, the aneurysm is closed and amputated, and the aortic wall is reunited with the heart, either by direct suture or with a patch or prosthesis.

Coronary arteriovenous fistula, an unusual anomaly, consists of a communication between a coronary artery and another cardiac chamber, usually the coronary sinus, right atrium, or right ventricle. The shunt is usually of small magnitude and myocardial blood flow is not usually compromised; if the shunt is large, there may be a coronary "steal" syndrome with myocardial ischemia and possible angina or ventricular arrhythmias. Potential complications include infective endocarditis; thrombus formation with occlusion or distal embolization with myocardial infarction; rupture of an aneurysmal fistula; and, rarely, pulmonary hypertension and congestive failure. A loud, superficial, continuous murmur at the lower or midsternal border usually prompts a further evaluation of asymptomatic patients. Doppler echocardiography demonstrates the site of drainage; if the site of origin is proximal, it may be detectable by two-dimensional echocardiography. Angiography (classic catheterization, CT, or magnetic resonance angiography) permits identification of the size and anatomic features of the fistulous tract, which may be closed by suture or transcatheter obliteration.

The third anomaly causing a shunt from the aortic root to the right heart is *anomalous origin of the left coronary artery from the pulmonary artery*. Myocardial infarction and fibrosis commonly lead to death within the first year, although up to 20% of patients survive to adolescence and beyond without surgical correction. The diagnosis is supported by the ECG findings of an anterolateral myocardial infarction and left ventricular hypertrophy (LVH). Operative management of adults consists of coronary artery bypass with an internal mammary artery graft or saphenous vein–coronary artery graft.

Congenital aortic stenosis

Malformations that cause obstruction to LV outflow include congenital valvular aortic stenosis, discrete subaortic stenosis, or supravalvular aortic stenosis. Bicuspid aortic valves are more common in males than in females. The congenital bicuspid aortic valve, which may initially be functionally normal, is one of the most common congenital malformations of the heart and may go undetected in early life. Because bicuspid valves may develop stenosis or regurgitation with time or be the site of infective endocarditis, the lesion may be difficult to distinguish in older adults from acquired rheumatic or degenerative calcific aortic valve disease. The dynamics of blood flow associated with a congenitally deformed, rigid aortic valve commonly lead to thickening of the cusps and, in later life, to calcification. Hemodynamically significant obstruction causes concentric hypertrophy of the LV wall. The ascending aorta is often dilated, misnamed "poststenotic" dilatation; this is due to histologic abnormalities of the aortic media similar to those in Marfan's syndrome and may result in aortic dissection. Diagnosis is made by echocardiography, which reveals the morphology of the aortic valve and aortic root and quantitates severity of stenosis or regurgitation. The clinical manifestations and hemodynamic abnormalities are discussed in Chap. 237.

TREATMENT Valvular Aortic Stenosis

Medical management includes prophylaxis against infective endocarditis and, in patients with diminished cardiac reserve, the administration of digoxin and diuretics and sodium restriction while awaiting operation. A dilated aortic root may require beta blockers. Aortic valve replacement is indicated in adults with critical obstruction, i.e., with an aortic valve area <0.45 cm^2/m^2, with symptoms secondary to LV dysfunction or myocardial ischemia, or with hemodynamic evidence of LV dysfunction. In asymptomatic children or adolescents or young adults with critical aortic stenosis without valvular calcification or these features, aortic balloon valvuloplasty is often useful (Chap. 246). If surgery is contraindicated in older patients because of a complicating medical problem such as malignancy or renal or hepatic failure, balloon valvuloplasty may provide short-term improvement. This procedure may serve as a bridge to aortic valve replacement in patients with severe heart failure.

Subaortic stenosis The *discrete* form of subaortic stenosis consists of a membranous diaphragm or fibromuscular ring encircling the LV outflow tract just beneath the base of the aortic valve. The jet impact from the subaortic stenotic jet on the underside of the aortic valve often begets progressive aortic valve fibrosis and valvular regurgitation. Echocardiography demonstrates the anatomy of the subaortic obstruction; Doppler studies show turbulence proximal to the aortic valve and can quantitate the pressure gradient and severity of aortic regurgitation. Treatment consists of complete excision of the membrane or fibromuscular ring.

Supravalvular aortic stenosis This is a localized or diffuse narrowing of the ascending aorta originating just above the level of the coronary arteries at the superior margin of the sinuses of Valsalva. In contrast to other forms of aortic stenosis, the coronary arteries are subjected to elevated systolic pressures from the left ventricle, are often dilated and tortuous, and are susceptible to premature atherosclerosis. In most patients, a genetic defect for the anomaly is located in the same chromosomal region as elastin on chromosome 7. Supravalvular aortic stenosis is the most commonly associated cardiac defect in Williams-Beuren syndrome, typically comprising the following: "elfin" facies, low nasal bridge, cheerful demeanor, mental retardation with retained language skills and love of music, supravalvular aortic stenosis, and transient hypercalcemia.

Coarctation of the aorta

Narrowing or constriction of the lumen of the aorta may occur anywhere along its length but is most common distal to the origin of the left subclavian artery near the insertion of the ligamentum arteriosum. Coarctation occurs in ~7% of patients with congenital heart disease, is more common in males than females, and is particularly frequent in patients with gonadal dysgenesis (e.g., Turner syndrome). Clinical manifestations depend on the site and extent of obstruction and the presence of associated cardiac anomalies; most commonly a bicuspid aortic valve. Circle of Willis aneurysms may occur in up to 10%, and pose a high risk of sudden rupture and death.

Most children and young adults with isolated, discrete coarctation are asymptomatic. Headache, epistaxis, cold extremities, and claudication with exercise may occur, and attention is usually directed to the cardiovascular system when a heart murmur or hypertension in the upper extremities and absence, marked diminution, or delayed pulsations in the femoral arteries are detected on physical examination. Enlarged and pulsatile collateral vessels may be palpated in the intercostal spaces anteriorly, in the axillae, or posteriorly in the interscapular area. The upper extremities and thorax may be more developed than the lower extremities. A midsystolic murmur over the left interscapular space may become continuous if the lumen is narrowed sufficiently to result in a high-velocity jet across the lesion throughout the cardiac cycle. Additional systolic and continuous murmurs over the lateral thoracic wall may reflect increased flow through dilated and tortuous collateral vessels. The ECG usually reveals LV hypertrophy. Chest x-ray may show a dilated left subclavian artery high on the left mediastinal border and a dilated ascending aorta. Indentation of the aorta at the site of coarctation and pre- and poststenotic dilatation (the "3" sign) along the left paramediastinal shadow are essentially pathognomonic. Notching of the third to ninth ribs, an important radiographic sign, is due to inferior rib erosion by dilated collateral vessels (Figs. 236-2 and 236-3). Two-dimensional echocardiography from suprasternal windows identifies the site of coarctation; Doppler quantitates the pressure gradient. Transesophageal echocardiography and MRI or three-dimensional CT allow visualization of the length and severity of the obstruction and associated collateral arteries (Figs. 236-2 and 236-3). In adults, cardiac catheterization is indicated primarily to evaluate the coronary arteries or to perform catheter-based intervention (angioplasty and stent of the coarctation).

The chief hazards of proximal aortic severe hypertension include cerebral aneurysms and hemorrhage, aortic dissection and rupture, premature coronary arteriosclerosis, and LV failure; infective endarteritis may occur on the coarctation site or endocarditis may settle on an associated bicuspid aortic valve, which is estimated to be present in up to 75% of patients.

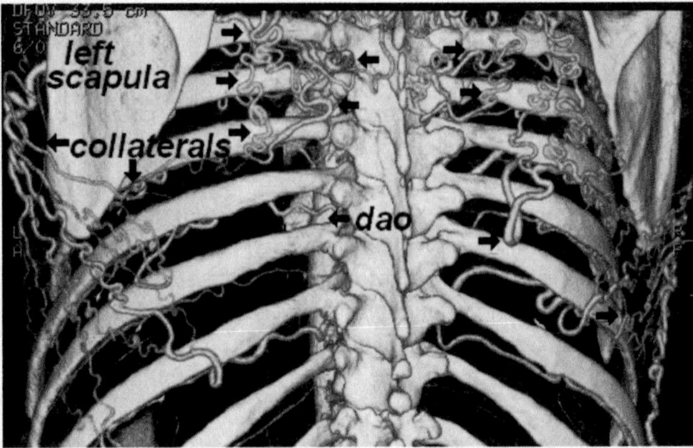

Figure 236-2 Aortic coarctation. The extensive collaterals (*left*) underneath the ribs and in the periscapular region are shown on a posterior view of a three-dimensional CT angiogram, which are responsible for rib notching on chest x-ray. dao, descending aorta.

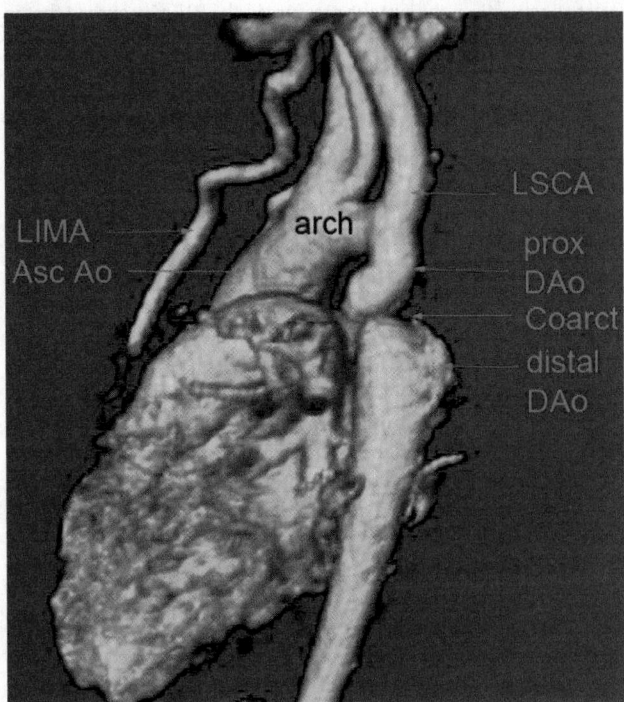

Figure 236-3 Aortic coarctation. The coarctation (Coarct) of the aorta is shown in the typical "adult" location in the descending aorta (DAo) just distal to the dilated left subclavian artery (LSCA) in this three-dimensional reconstruction of an MR angiogram. There is a post-coarct aneurysm that is in part due to intrinsic aortic medial tissue weakness. The left internal mammary artery (LIMA) is dilated. Asc Ao, ascending aorta; prox, proximal.

TREATMENT Coarctation of the Aorta

Treatment is surgical or involves percutaneous catheter balloon dilatation with stent placement; the details of selection of therapy are beyond this review. Late postoperative systemic hypertension in the absence of residual coarctation is related partly to the duration of preoperative hypertension. Follow-up of rest and exercise blood pressures is important; many have systolic hypertension only during exercise, in part due to a diffuse vasculopathy. All operated or stented coarctation patients deserve a high-quality MRI or CT procedure in follow-up.

Pulmonary stenosis with intact ventricular septum

Obstruction to RV outflow may be localized to the supravalvular, valvular, or subvalvular levels or occur at a combination of these sites. Multiple sites of narrowing of the peripheral pulmonary arteries are a feature of *rubella embryopathy* and may occur with both the familial and sporadic forms of supravalvular aortic stenosis. Valvular pulmonic stenosis (PS) is the most common form of isolated RV obstruction.

The severity of the obstructing lesion, rather than the site of narrowing, is the most important determinant of the clinical course. In the presence of a normal cardiac output, a peak systolic pressure gradient <30 mmHg indicates mild PS and >50 mmHg indicates severe PS; processes between these limits are considered to indicate moderate stenosis. Patients with mild PS are generally asymptomatic and demonstrate little or no progression in the severity of obstruction with age. In patients with more significant stenosis, the severity may increase with time. Symptoms vary with the degree of obstruction. Fatigue, dyspnea, RV failure, and syncope may limit the activity of older patients, in whom moderate or severe obstruction may prevent an augmentation of cardiac output with exercise. In patients with severe obstruction, the systolic pressure in the RV may exceed that in the LV, because the ventricular septum is intact. RV ejection is prolonged with moderate or severe stenosis, and the sound of pulmonary valve closure is delayed and soft. RV hypertrophy reduces the compliance of that chamber, and a forceful RA contraction is necessary to augment RV filling. A fourth heart sound; prominent *a* waves in the jugular venous pulse; and, occasionally, presystolic pulsations of the liver reflect vigorous atrial contraction. The clinical diagnosis is supported by a left parasternal lift and harsh systolic crescendo-decrescendo murmur and thrill at the upper left sternal border, typically preceded by a systolic ejection sound if the obstruction is due to a mobile nondysplastic pulmonary valve. The holosystolic murmur of tricuspid regurgitation may accompany severe PS, especially in the presence of congestive heart failure. Cyanosis usually reflects right-to-left shunting through a patent foramen ovale or ASD. In patients with supravalvular or peripheral pulmonary arterial stenosis, the murmur is systolic or continuous and is best heard over the area of narrowing, with radiation to the peripheral lung fields.

In mild cases, the ECG is normal, whereas moderate and severe stenoses are associated with RV hypertrophy. The chest x-ray with mild or moderate PS shows a heart of normal size with normal lung vascularity. In pulmonary valvular stenosis, dilatation of the main and left pulmonary arteries occurs in part due to the direction of the PS jet and in part due to intrinsic tissue weakness. With severe obstruction, RV hypertrophy is generally evident. The pulmonary vascularity may be reduced with severe stenosis, RV failure, and/or a right-to-left shunt at the atrial level. Two-dimensional echocardiography visualizes pulmonary-valve morphology; the outflow tract pressure gradient is quantitated by Doppler echocardiography.

TREATMENT Pulmonary Stenosis

The cardiac catheter technique of balloon valvuloplasty (Chap. 230) is usually effective. Direct surgical relief of moderate and severe obstruction may be accomplished at a low risk. Multiple stenoses of the peripheral pulmonary arteries are usually inoperable, but narrowing of a proximal branch or at the bifurcation of the main pulmonary trunk may be surgically corrected or undergo balloon dilatation and stenting.

Tetralogy of Fallot

The four components of the tetralogy of Fallot are malaligned VSD, obstruction to RV outflow, aortic override of the VSD, and RV hypertrophy due to the RV's response to aortic pressure via the large VSD (Fig. 236-4).

The severity of RV outflow obstruction determines the clinical presentation. The severity of hypoplasia of the RV outflow tract varies from mild to complete (pulmonary atresia). Pulmonary valve stenosis and supravalvular and peripheral pulmonary arterial obstruction may coexist; rarely, there is unilateral absence of a pulmonary artery (usually the left). A right-sided aortic arch and descending thoracic aorta occur in ~25%.

The relationship between the resistance of blood flow from the ventricles into the aorta and into the pulmonary artery plays a major role in determining the hemodynamic and clinical picture. When the RV outflow obstruction is severe, pulmonary blood flow is reduced markedly, and a large volume of desaturated systemic venous blood shunts right-to-left across the VSD. Severe cyanosis and erythrocytosis occur, and symptoms of systemic hypoxemia are prominent. In many infants and children, the obstruction is mild but progressive.

The ECG shows RV hypertrophy. Chest x-ray shows a normal-sized, boot-shaped heart (*coeur en sabot*) with a prominent right ventricle and a concavity in the region of the pulmonary conus. Pulmonary vascular markings are typically diminished, and the aortic arch and knob may be on the right side. Two-dimensional echocardiography demonstrates the malaligned VSD with the overriding aorta and the site and severity of PS, which may be subpulmonic (fixed or dynamic), at the pulmonary valve or in the main or branch pulmonary arteries. Classic contrast angiography may provide details regarding the RV outflow tract, pulmonary valve

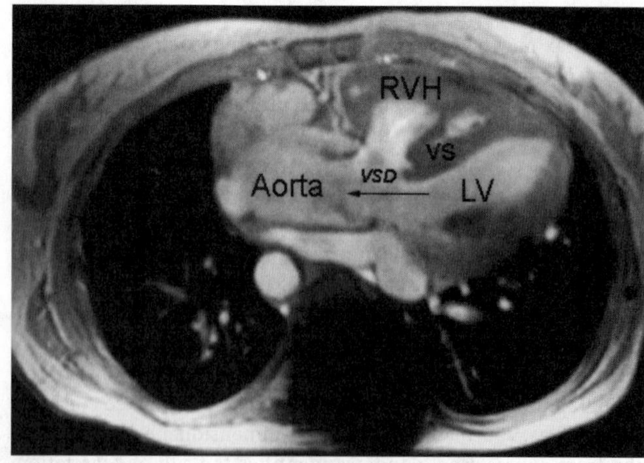

Figure 236-4 Tetralogy of Fallot. Magnetic resonance angiogram. A mid-systolic frame showing the malaligned ventricular septal defect (VSD) with the aorta overriding the ventricular septal defect. LV, left ventricle; RVH, RV hypertrophy; VS, ventricular septum.

and annulus, and caliber of the main branches of the pulmonary artery as well of possible associated aortopulmonary collaterals. Coronary arteriography identifies the anatomy and course of the coronary arteries. In experienced centers, these issues are often well demonstrated in adults by MRI (Fig. 236-4) or CT angiography with three-dimensional reconstruction.

TREATMENT Tetralogy of Fallot

For a variety of reasons, only a few adults with tetralogy of Fallot have not had some form of previous surgical intervention. Reoperation in adults is most commonly for severe pulmonary regurgitation. Long-term concerns about ventricular function persist. Ventricular and atrial arrhythmias may require medical treatment or electrophysiologic study and ablation. Interventional catheterization may be needed in selected patients (i.e., angioplasty and stenting of branch pulmonary stenosis). The aortic root has a medial tissue defect; it is commonly enlarged and associated with aortic regurgitation. Endocarditis remains a risk despite surgical repair.

Complete transposition of the great arteries

This condition is commonly called *dextro-* or *D-transposition of the great arteries.* The aorta arises rightward anteriorly from the right ventricle, and the pulmonary artery emerges leftward and posteriorly from the LV, which results in two separate parallel circulations; some communication between them must exist after birth to sustain life. Most patients have an interatrial communication, two-thirds have a patent ductus arteriosus, and about one-third have an associated VSD. Transposition is more common in males and accounts for ~10% of cyanotic heart disease. The course is determined by the degree of tissue hypoxemia, the ability of each ventricle to sustain an increased workload in the presence of reduced coronary arterial oxygenation, the nature of the associated cardiovascular anomalies, and the status of the pulmonary vascular bed. By the third decade of life, ~30% of patients will have developed decreased RV function and progressive tricuspid regurgitation, which may lead to congestive heart failure. Pulmonary vascular obstruction develops by one to two years of age in patients with an associated large VSD or large patent ductus arteriosus in the absence of obstruction to LV outflow.

TREATMENT Transposition of the Great Arteries

The balloon or blade catheter or surgical creation or enlargement of an interatrial communication in the neonate is the simplest procedure for providing increased intracardiac mixing of systemic and pulmonary venous blood. Systemic pulmonary–artery anastomosis may be indicated in the patient with severe obstruction to LV outflow and diminished pulmonary blood flow. Intracardiac repair may be accomplished by rearranging the venous returns (intra-atrial switch, i.e., Mustard or Senning operation) so that the systemic venous blood is directed to the mitral valve and, thence, to the left ventricle and pulmonary artery, while the pulmonary venous blood is diverted through the tricuspid valve and right ventricle to the aorta. The late survival after these repairs is good, but arrhythmias (e.g., atrial flutter) or conduction defects (e.g., sick sinus syndrome) occur in ~50% of such patients by 30 years after the intra-atrial switch surgery. Progressive dysfunction of the systemic subaortic right ventricle, tricuspid regurgitation, ventricular arrhythmias, or cardiac arrest and late sudden death are worrisome features. Preferably, this malformation is corrected in infancy by transposing both coronary arteries to the posterior artery and transecting, contraposing, and anastomosing the aorta and pulmonary arteries (arterial-switch operation). For those patients with a VSD in whom it is necessary to bypass a severely obstructed LV outflow tract, corrective operation employs an intracardiac ventricular baffle and extracardiac prosthetic conduit to replace the pulmonary artery (Rastelli procedure).

Single ventricle

This is a family of complex lesions with both atrioventricular valves or a common atrioventricular valve opening to a single ventricular chamber. Associated anomalies include abnormal great artery positional relationships, pulmonic valvular or subvalvular stenosis, and subaortic stenosis. Survival to adulthood depends on a relatively normal pulmonary blood flow, yet normal pulmonary resistance and good ventricular function. Modifications of the Fontan approach are generally applied to carefully selected patients with creation of a pathway(s) from the systemic veins to the pulmonary arteries.

Tricuspid atresia

This malformation is characterized by atresia of the tricuspid valve; an interatrial communication; and, frequently, hypoplasia of the right ventricle and pulmonary artery. The clinical picture is usually dominated by severe cyanosis due to obligatory admixture of systemic and pulmonary venous blood in the left ventricle. The ECG characteristically shows RA enlargement, left-axis deviation, and LV hypertrophy.

Atrial septostomy and palliative operations to increase pulmonary blood flow, often by anastomosis of a systemic artery or vein to a pulmonary artery, may allow survival to the second or third decade. A Fontan atriopulmonary or total cavopulmonary connection may then allow functional correction in those patients with normal or low pulmonary arterial resistance pressure and good LV function.

Ebstein's anomaly

Characterized by a downward displacement of the tricuspid valve into the right ventricle, due to anomalous attachment of the tricuspid leaflets, the Ebstein tricuspid valve tissue is dysplastic and results in tricuspid regurgitation. The abnormally situated tricuspid orifice produces an "atrialized" portion of the RV lying between the atrioventricular ring and the origin of the valve, which is continuous with the RA chamber. Often, the RV is hypoplastic. Although the clinical manifestations are variable, some patients come to initial attention because of either (1) progressive cyanosis from right-to-left atrial shunting, (2) symptoms due to tricuspid regurgitation and RV dysfunction, or (3) paroxysmal atrial tachyarrhythmias with or without atrioventricular bypass tracts [Wolff-Parkinson-White (WPW) syndrome]. Diagnostic findings by two-dimensional echocardiography include the abnormal positional relation between the tricuspid and mitral valves with abnormally increased apical displacement of the septal tricuspid leaflet. Tricuspid regurgitation is quantitated by Doppler examination. Surgical approaches include prosthetic replacement of the tricuspid valve when the leaflets are tethered or repair of the native valve.

Congenitally corrected transposition

The two fundamental anatomic abnormalities in this malformation are transposition of the ascending aorta and pulmonary trunk and inversion of the ventricles. This arrangement results in desaturated systemic venous blood passing from the right atrium through the mitral valve to the LV and into the pulmonary trunk, whereas oxygenated pulmonary venous blood flows from the left atrium through the tricuspid valve to the RV and into the aorta. Thus, the circulation is corrected functionally. The clinical presentation, course, and prognosis of patients with congenitally corrected transposition vary depending on the nature and severity of any complicating intracardiac anomalies and of development of dysfunction of the systemic subaortic RV. Progressive RV dysfunction and tricuspid regurgitation may also develop in one-third of patients by age 30; Ebstein-type anomalies of the left-side tricuspid atrioventricular valve are common. VSD or PS due to obstruction to outflow from the right-sided subpulmonary (anatomic left) ventricle may coexist. Complete heart block occurs at a rate of 2–10% per decade. The diagnosis of the malformation and associated lesions can be established by comprehensive two-dimensional echocardiography and Doppler examination.

Malpositions of the heart

Positional anomalies refer to conditions in which the cardiac apex is in the right side of the chest (*dextrocardia*), or at the midline (*mesocardia*), or in which there is a normal location of the heart in the left side of the chest but abnormal position of the viscera (*isolated levocardia*). Knowledge of the position of the abdominal organs and of the branching pattern of the main stem bronchi is important in categorizing these malpositions. When dextrocardia occurs without situs inversus, when the visceral situs is indeterminate, or if isolated levocardia is present, associated, often complex, multiple cardiac anomalies are usually present. In contrast, mirror-image dextrocardia is usually observed with complete situs inversus, which occurs most frequently in individuals whose hearts are otherwise normal.

SURGICALLY MODIFIED CONGENITAL HEART DISEASE

Owing to the enormous strides in cardiovascular surgical techniques that have occurred in the past 60 years, a large number of long-term survivors of corrective operations in infancy and childhood have reached adulthood. These patients are often challenging because of the diversity of anatomic, hemodynamic, and electrophysiologic residua and sequelae of cardiac operations.

The proper care of the survivor of operation for CHD requires that the clinician understand the details of the malformation before operation; pay meticulous attention to the details of the operative procedure; and recognize the postoperative residua (conditions left totally or partially uncorrected), the sequelae (conditions caused by surgery), and the complications that may have resulted from the operation. Except for ligation of an uncomplicated patent ductus arteriosus, almost every other surgical repair leaves behind or causes some abnormality of the heart and circulation that may range from trivial to serious. Intraoperative transesophageal echocardiography assists in detecting unsuspected lesions, in monitoring the repair, and in verifying a satisfactory result or directing further repair. Thus, even with results that are considered clinically to be good to excellent, continued long-term postoperative follow-up is advisable.

Cardiac operations importantly involving the atria, such as closure of ASD, repair of total or partial anomalous pulmonary venous return, or venous switch corrections of complete transposition of the great arteries (the Mustard or Senning operations), may be followed years later by sinus node or atrioventricular node dysfunction or by atrial arrhythmias (especially atrial flutter). Intraventricular surgery may also result in electrophysiologic consequences, including complete heart block necessitating pacemaker insertion to avoid sudden death. Valvular problems may arise late after initial cardiac operation. An example is the progressive stenosis of an initially nonobstructive bicuspid aortic valve in the patient who underwent aortic coarctation repair. Such aortic valves may also be the site of infective endocarditis. After repair of the ostium primum ASD, the cleft mitral valve may become progressively regurgitant. Tricuspid regurgitation may also be progressive in the postoperative patient with tetralogy of Fallot if RV outflow tract obstruction was not relieved adequately at initial surgery. In many patients with surgically modified CHD, inadequate relief of an obstructive lesion, or a residual regurgitant lesion, or a residual shunt will cause or hasten the onset of clinical signs and symptoms of myocardial dysfunction. Despite a good hemodynamic repair, many patients with a subaortic RV develop RV decompensation and signs of left heart failure. In many patients, particularly those who were cyanotic for many years before operation, a preexisting compromise in ventricular performance is due to the original underlying malformation.

A final category of postoperative problems involves the use of prosthetic valves, patches, or conduits in the operative repair. The special risks include infective endocarditis, thrombus formation, and premature degeneration and calcification of the prosthetic materials. There are many patients in whom extracardiac conduits are required to correct the circulation functionally and often to carry blood to the lungs from the right atrium or right ventricle. These conduits may develop intraluminal obstruction, and, if they include a prosthetic valve, it may show progressive calcification and thickening. Many such patients face reintervention (interventional cardiac catheterization or surgical reoperation) one or more times in their lives. Such care should be directed to centers specializing in adults with complex congenital cardiovascular malformations. The effect of pregnancy in postoperative patients depends on the outcome of the repair, including the presence and severity of residua, sequelae, or complications. Contraception is an important topic with such patients. Tubal ligation should be considered in those in whom pregnancy is strictly contraindicated.

Endocarditis prophylaxis

Two major predisposing causes of infective endocarditis are a susceptible cardiovascular substrate and a source of bacteremia. The clinical and bacteriologic profile of infective endocarditis in patients with CHD has changed with the advent of intracardiac surgery and of prosthetic devices. Prophylaxis includes both antimicrobial and hygienic measures. Meticulous dental and skin care are required. Routine antimicrobial prophylaxis is recommended for bacteremic dental procedures or instrumentation through an infected site in most patients with operated CHD, particularly if foreign material, such as a prosthetic valve, conduit, surgically constructed shunt, etc., is in place. In the case of patches, in the absence of a high-pressure patch leak, prophylaxis is usually recommended for six months until there is endothelialization. Individuals with unrepaired cyanotic heart disease are also generally recommended to receive prophylaxis (Chap. 124).

FURTHER READINGS

ABOULHOSN J, CHILD JS: Congenital Heart Disease in Adults, in *Hurst's The Heart* 12th ed, V Fuster et al (eds), New York, McGraw Medical, 2008, pp 1922–1948

———: Congenital Heart Disease in Adults, in *Hurst's The Heart Manual of Cardiology* 12th ed, V Fuster et al (eds), New York, McGraw Medical, 2009, pp 546–556

PERLOFF JK, et al: *Congenital Heart Disease in Adults* 3rd ed., Philadelphia, Saunders Elsevier, 2009, pp 1–488

WARNES CA, et al: ACC/AHA 2008 Guidelines for the Management of Adults with Congenital Heart Disease. Circulation 118:e714 2008

WEBB G et al: Congenital heart disease, in *Braunwald's Heart Disease: A Textbook of Cardiovascular Medicine*, 7th ed., D. Zipes, et al. (eds) Philadelphia, Elsevier Saunders, 2005, pp 1489–1552

CHAPTER 237

Valvular Heart Disease

Patrick O'Gara
Joseph Loscalzo

The role of the physical examination in the evaluation of patients with valvular heart disease is also considered in Chaps. e13 and 227; of electrocardiography (ECG) in Chap. 228; of echocardiography and other noninvasive imaging techniques in Chap. 229; and of cardiac catheterization and angiography in Chap. 230.

MITRAL STENOSIS

ETIOLOGY AND PATHOLOGY

Rheumatic fever is the leading cause of mitral stenosis (MS) (Table 237-1). Other less common etiologies of obstruction to left atrial outflow include congenital mitral valve stenosis, cor triatriatum, mitral annular calcification with extension onto the leaflets, systemic lupus erythematosus, rheumatoid arthritis, left atrial myxoma, and infective endocarditis with large vegetations. Pure or predominant MS occurs in approximately 40% of all patients with rheumatic heart disease and a history of rheumatic fever (Chap. 322). In other patients with rheumatic heart disease, lesser degrees of MS may accompany mitral regurgitation (MR) and aortic valve disease. With reductions in the incidence of acute rheumatic fever, particularly in temperate climates and developed countries, the incidence of MS has declined considerably over the past few decades. However, it remains a major problem in developing nations, especially in tropical and semitropical climates (see p. 1949).

In rheumatic MS, the valve leaflets are diffusely thickened by fibrous tissue and/or calcific deposits. The mitral commissures fuse, the chordae tendineae fuse and shorten, the valvular cusps become rigid, and these changes, in turn, lead to narrowing at the apex of the funnel-shaped ("fish-mouth") valve. Although the initial insult to the mitral valve is rheumatic, the later changes may be a nonspecific process resulting from trauma to the valve caused by altered flow patterns due to the initial deformity. Calcification of the stenotic mitral valve immobilizes the leaflets and narrows the orifice further. Thrombus formation and arterial embolization may arise from the calcific valve itself, but in patients with atrial fibrillation (AF), thrombi arise more frequently from the dilated left atrium (LA), particularly from within the left atrial appendage.

PATHOPHYSIOLOGY

In normal adults, the area of the mitral valve orifice is 4–6 cm^2. In the presence of significant obstruction, i.e., when the orifice area is reduced to < ~2 cm^2, blood can flow from the LA to the left ventricle (LV) only if propelled by an abnormally elevated left atrioventricular pressure gradient, the hemodynamic hallmark of MS. When the mitral valve opening is reduced to <1 cm^2, often referred to as "severe" MS, a LA pressure of ~25 mmHg is required to maintain a normal cardiac output (CO). The elevated pulmonary venous and pulmonary arterial (PA) wedge pressures reduce pulmonary compliance, contributing to exertional dyspnea. The first bouts of dyspnea are usually precipitated by clinical events that increase the rate of blood flow across the mitral orifice, resulting in further elevation of the LA pressure (see below).

To assess the severity of obstruction hemodynamically, both the transvalvular pressure gradient and the flow rate must be measured (Chap. 230). The latter depends not only on the CO but on the heart rate, as well. An increase in heart rate shortens diastole proportionately more than systole and diminishes the time available for flow across the mitral valve. Therefore, at any given level of CO, tachycardia, including that associated with rapid AF, augments the transvalvular pressure gradient and elevates further the LA pressure. Similar considerations apply to the pathophysiology of tricuspid stenosis.

The LV diastolic pressure and ejection fraction (EF) are normal in isolated MS. In MS and sinus rhythm, the elevated LA and PA wedge pressures exhibit a prominent atrial contraction pattern (*a* wave) and a gradual pressure decline after the *v* wave and mitral valve opening (*y* descent). In severe MS and whenever pulmonary vascular resistance is significantly increased, the pulmonary arterial pressure (PAP) is elevated at rest and rises further during exercise, often causing secondary elevations of right ventricular (RV) end-diastolic pressure and volume.

Cardiac output

In patients with moderate MS (mitral valve orifice 1 cm^2–1.5 cm^2), the CO is normal or almost so at rest, but rises subnormally during exertion. In patients with severe MS (valve area <1 cm^2), particularly those in whom pulmonary vascular resistance is markedly elevated, the CO is subnormal at rest and may fail to rise or may even decline during activity.

Pulmonary hypertension

The clinical and hemodynamic features of MS are influenced importantly by the level of the PAP. Pulmonary hypertension results from: (1) passive backward transmission of the elevated LA pressure; (2) pulmonary arteriolar constriction (the so-called "second stenosis"), which presumably is triggered by LA and pulmonary venous hypertension (reactive pulmonary hypertension); (3) interstitial edema in the walls of the small pulmonary vessels; and (4) at end stage, organic obliterative changes in the pulmonary vascular bed. Severe pulmonary hypertension results in RV enlargement, secondary tricuspid regurgitation (TR) and pulmonic regurgitation (PR), as well as right-sided heart failure.

SYMPTOMS

In temperate climates, the latent period between the initial attack of rheumatic carditis (in the increasingly rare circumstances in which a history of one can be elicited) and the development of symptoms due to MS is generally about two decades; most patients begin to experience disability in the fourth decade of life. Studies carried out before the development of mitral valvotomy revealed that once a patient with MS became seriously symptomatic, the disease progressed continuously to death within 2–5 years.

In patients whose mitral orifices are large enough to accommodate a normal blood flow with only mild elevations of LA pressure, marked elevations of this pressure leading to dyspnea and cough may be precipitated by sudden changes in the heart rate, volume status, or CO, as, for example, with severe exertion, excitement, fever, severe anemia, paroxysmal AF and other tachycardias, sexual intercourse, pregnancy, and thyrotoxicosis. As MS progresses, lesser degrees of stress precipitate dyspnea, the patient becomes limited in daily activities, and orthopnea and paroxysmal nocturnal dyspnea develop. The development of permanent AF often marks a turning point in the patient's course and is generally associated with acceleration of the rate at which symptoms progress.

TABLE 237-1 Major Causes of Valvular Heart Diseases

Valve Lesion	Etiologies
Mitral stenosis	Rheumatic fever
	Congenital
	Severe mitral annular calcification
	SLE, RA
Mitral regurgitation	Acute
	Endocarditis
	Papillary muscle rupture (post-MI)
	Trauma
	Chordal rupture/leaflet flail (MVP, IE)
	Chronic
	Myxomatous (MVP)
	Rheumatic fever
	Endocarditis (healed)
	Mitral annular calcification
	Congenital (cleft, AV canal)
	HOCM with SAM
	Ischemic (LV remodeling)
	Dilated cardiomyopathy
	Radiation
Aortic stenosis	Congenital (bicuspid, unicuspid)
	Degenerative calcific
	Rheumatic fever
	Radiation
Aortic regurgitation	Valvular
	Congenital (bicuspid)
	Endocarditis
	Rheumatic fever
	Myxomatous (prolapse)
	Traumatic
	Syphilis
	Ankylosing spondylitis
	Root disease
	Aortic dissection
	Cystic medial degeneration
	Marfan's syndrome
	Bicuspid aortic valve
	Nonsyndromic familial aneurysm
	Aortitis
	Hypertension
Tricuspid stenosis	Rheumatic
	Congenital
Tricuspid regurgitation	Primary
	Rheumatic
	Endocarditis
	Myxomatous (TVP)
	Carcinoid
	Radiation
	Congenital (Ebstein's)
	Trauma
	Papillary muscle injury (post-MI)
	Secondary
	RV and tricuspid annular dilatation
	Multiple causes of RV enlargement (e.g., long-standing pulmonary HTN)
	Chronic RV apical pacing
Pulmonic stenosis	Congenital
	Carcinoid
Pulmonic regurgitation	Valve disease
	Congenital
	Postvalvotomy
	Endocarditis
	Annular enlargement
	Pulmonary hypertension
	Idiopathic dilation
	Marfan's syndrome

Abbreviations: AV, atrioventricular; HOCM, hypertrophic obstructive cardiomyopathy; HTN, hypertension; IE, infective endocarditis; LV, left ventricular; MI, myocardial infarction; MVP, mitral valve prolapse; RA, rheumatoid arthritis; RV, right ventricular; SAM, systolic anterior motion of the anterior mitral valve leaflet; SLE, systemic lupus erythematosus; TVP, tricuspid valve prolapse.

Hemoptysis (Chap. 34) results from rupture of pulmonary-bronchial venous connections secondary to pulmonary venous hypertension. It occurs most frequently in patients who have elevated LA pressures without markedly elevated pulmonary vascular resistances and is rarely fatal. *Recurrent pulmonary emboli* (Chap. 262), sometimes with infarction, are an important cause of morbidity and mortality rates late in the course of MS. *Pulmonary infections,* i.e., bronchitis, bronchopneumonia, and lobar pneumonia, commonly complicate untreated MS, especially during the winter months.

Pulmonary changes

In addition to the aforementioned changes in the pulmonary vascular bed, fibrous thickening of the walls of the alveoli and pulmonary capillaries occurs commonly in MS. The vital capacity, total lung capacity, maximal breathing capacity, and oxygen uptake per unit of ventilation are reduced (Chap. 252). Pulmonary compliance falls further as pulmonary capillary pressure rises during exercise.

Thrombi and emboli

Thrombi may form in the left atria, particularly within the enlarged atrial appendages of patients with MS. Systemic embolization, the incidence of which is 10–20%, occurs more frequently in patients with AF, in patients >65 years of age, and in those with a reduced CO. However, systemic embolization may be the presenting feature in otherwise asymptomatic patients with only mild MS.

■ PHYSICAL FINDINGS

(See also Chaps. e13 and 227)

Inspection and palpation

In patients with severe MS, there may be a malar flush with pinched and blue facies. In patients with sinus rhythm and severe pulmonary hypertension or associated tricuspid stenosis (TS), the jugular venous pulse reveals prominent *a* waves due to vigorous right atrial systole. The systemic arterial pressure is usually normal or slightly low. An RV tap along the left sternal border signifies an enlarged RV. A diastolic thrill may rarely be present at the cardiac apex, with the patient in the left lateral recumbent position.

Auscultation

The first heart sound (S_1) is usually accentuated and slightly delayed. The pulmonic component of the second heart sound (P_2) also is often accentuated, and the two components of the second heart sound (S_2) are closely split. The opening snap (OS) of the mitral valve is most readily audible in expiration at, or just medial to, the cardiac apex. This sound generally follows the sound of aortic valve closure (A_2) by 0.05–0.12 s. The time interval between A_2 and OS varies inversely with the severity of the MS. The OS is followed by a low-pitched, rumbling, diastolic murmur, heard best at the apex with the patient in the left lateral recumbent position (see Fig. 227-5); it is accentuated by mild exercise (e.g., a few rapid sit-ups) carried out just before auscultation. In general, the duration of this murmur correlates with the severity of the stenosis in patients with preserved CO. In patients with sinus rhythm, the murmur often reappears or becomes louder during atrial systole (presystolic accentuation). Soft, grade I or II/VI systolic murmurs are commonly heard at the apex or along the left sternal border in patients with pure MS and do not necessarily signify the presence of MR. Hepatomegaly, ankle edema, ascites, and pleural effusion, particularly in the right pleural cavity, may occur in patients with MS and RV failure.

Associated lesions

With severe pulmonary hypertension, a pansystolic murmur produced by functional TR may be audible along the left sternal border. This murmur is usually louder during inspiration and diminishes during forced expiration (Carvallo's sign). When the CO is markedly reduced in MS, the typical auscultatory findings, including the diastolic rumbling murmur, may not be detectable (silent MS), but they may reappear as compensation is restored. The *Graham Steell murmur* of PR, a high-pitched, diastolic, decrescendo blowing murmur along the left sternal border, results from dilation of the pulmonary valve ring and occurs in patients with mitral valve disease and severe pulmonary hypertension. This murmur may be indistinguishable from the more common murmur produced by aortic regurgitation (AR), although it may increase in intensity with inspiration and is accompanied by a loud and often palpable P2.

LABORATORY EXAMINATION

ECG

In MS and sinus rhythm, the P wave usually suggests LA enlargement (see Fig. 228-8). It may become tall and peaked in lead II and upright in lead V_1 when severe pulmonary hypertension or TS complicates MS and right atrial (RA) enlargement occurs. The QRS complex is usually normal. However, with severe pulmonary hypertension, right-axis deviation and RV hypertrophy are often present.

Echocardiogram

(See also Chap. 229) Transthoracic echocardiography (TTE) with color flow and spectral Doppler imaging provides critical information, including measurements of mitral inflow velocity during early (E wave) and late (A wave in patients in sinus rhythm) diastolic filling, estimates of the transvalvular peak and mean gradients and of the mitral orifice area, the presence and severity of any associated MR, the extent of leaflet calcification and restriction, the degree of distortion of the subvalvular apparatus, and the anatomic suitability for percutaneous mitral balloon valvotomy [percutaneous mitral balloon valvuloplasty (PMBV); see below]. In addition, TTE provides an assessment of LV and RV function, chamber sizes, an estimation of the pulmonary artery pressure (PAP) based on the tricuspid regurgitant jet velocity, and an indication of the presence and severity of any associated valvular lesions. Transesophageal echocardiography (TEE) provides superior images and should be employed when TTE is inadequate for guiding management decisions. TEE is especially indicated to exclude the presence of left atrial thrombus prior to PMBV.

Chest x-ray

The earliest changes are straightening of the upper left border of the cardiac silhouette, prominence of the main pulmonary arteries, dilation of the upper lobe pulmonary veins, and posterior displacement of the esophagus by an enlarged LA. Kerley B lines are fine, dense, opaque, horizontal lines that are most prominent in the lower and mid-lung fields and that result from distention of interlobular septae and lymphatics with edema when the resting mean LA pressure exceeds approximately 20 mmHg.

DIFFERENTIAL DIAGNOSIS

Like MS, significant MR may also be associated with a prominent diastolic murmur at the apex due to increased antegrade transmitral flow, but in patients with isolated MR, this diastolic murmur commences slightly later than in patients with MS, and there is often clear-cut evidence of LV enlargement. An opening snap and increased P_2 are absent, and S_1 is soft or absent. An apical pansystolic murmur of at least grade III/VI intensity as well as an S_3 suggest significant MR. Similarly, the apical mid-diastolic murmur associated with severe AR (*Austin Flint murmur*) may be mistaken for MS but can be differentiated from it because it is not intensified in presystole and becomes softer with administration of amyl nitrite. TS, which occurs rarely in the absence of MS, may mask many of the clinical features of MS or be clinically silent; when present, the diastolic murmur of TS increases with inspiration.

Atrial septal defect (Chap. 236) may be mistaken for MS; in both conditions there is often clinical, ECG, and chest x-ray evidence of RV enlargement and accentuation of pulmonary vascularity. However, the absence of LA enlargement and of Kerley B lines and the demonstration of fixed splitting of S_2 with a grade 2 or 3 midsystolic murmur at the mid to upper left sternal border all favor atrial septal defect over MS. Atrial septal defects with large left-to-right shunts may result in functional TS because of the enhanced diastolic flow.

Left atrial myxoma (Chap. 240) may obstruct LA emptying, causing dyspnea, a diastolic murmur, and hemodynamic changes resembling those of MS. However, patients with an LA myxoma often have features suggestive of a systemic disease, such as weight loss, fever, anemia, systemic emboli, and elevated serum IgG and interleukin 6 (IL-6) concentrations. The auscultatory findings may change markedly with body position. The diagnosis can be established by the demonstration of a characteristic echo-producing mass in the LA with TTE.

CARDIAC CATHETERIZATION

Left and right heart catheterization is useful when there is a discrepancy between the clinical and TTE findings that cannot be resolved with either TEE or cardiac magnetic resonance (CMR) imaging. The growing experience with CMR for the assessment of patients with valvular heart disease may decrease the need for invasive catheterization. Catheterization is helpful in assessing associated lesions, such as aortic stenosis (AS) and AR. Catheterization and coronary angiography are not usually necessary to aid in decision-making about surgery in patients younger than 65 years of age, with typical findings of severe mitral obstruction on physical examination and TTE. In men older than 40 years of age, women older than 45 years of age, and younger patients with coronary risk factors, especially those with positive noninvasive stress tests for myocardial ischemia, coronary angiography is advisable preoperatively to identify patients with critical coronary obstructions that should be bypassed at the time of operation. Computed tomographic coronary angiography (CTCA) (Chap. 229) is now often used to screen preoperatively for the presence of coronary artery disease (CAD) in patients with valvular heart disease and low pretest likelihood of CAD. Catheterization and left ventriculography are indicated in most patients who have undergone PMBV or previous mitral valve surgery, and who have redeveloped limiting symptoms, especially if questions regarding the severity of the valve lesion(s) remain after echocardiography.

TREATMENT Mitral Stenosis

(See Fig. 237-1) Penicillin prophylaxis of group A β-hemolytic streptococcal infections (Chap. 322) for secondary prevention of rheumatic fever is important for at-risk patients with rheumatic MS (Table 237-2). Recommendations for infective endocarditis prophylaxis have recently changed. In symptomatic patients, some improvement usually occurs with restriction of sodium intake and small doses of oral diuretics. Beta blockers, nondihydropyridine calcium channel blockers (e.g., verapamil or diltiazem), and digitalis glycosides are useful in slowing the ventricular rate of patients with AF. Warfarin to an international normalized ratio (INR) of 2–3 should be administered indefinitely to patients with MS, who have AF or a history of thromboembolism. The routine use of warfarin in patients in sinus rhythm with LA enlargement (maximal dimension >5.5 cm) with or without spontaneous echo contrast is more controversial.

If AF is of relatively recent onset in a patient whose MS is not severe enough to warrant PMBV or surgical commissurotomy, reversion to sinus rhythm pharmacologically or by means of electrical countershock is indicated. Usually, cardioversion should be undertaken after the patient has had at least 3 consecutive weeks of anticoagulant treatment to a therapeutic INR. If cardioversion is indicated more urgently, then intravenous heparin should be provided and TEE performed to exclude the presence of left atrial thrombus before the procedure. Conversion to sinus rhythm is rarely successful or sustained in patients with severe MS, particularly those in whom the LA is especially enlarged or in whom AF has been present for more than 1 year.

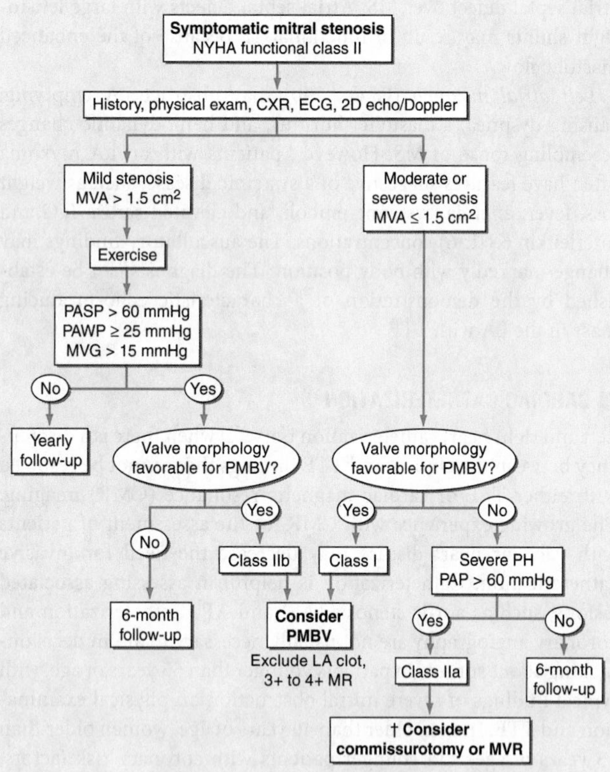

Figure 237-1 Management strategy for patients with mitral stenosis (MS) and mild symptoms. †There is controversy as to whether patients with severe MS (MVA <1 cm²) and severe pulmonary hypertension (PH) (PASP >60 mmHg) should undergo percutaneous mitral balloon valvotomy (PMBV) or mitral valve replacement (MVR) to prevent right ventricular failure. CXR, chest x-ray; ECG, electrocardiogram; echo, echocardiography; LA, left atrial; MR, mitral regurgitation; MVA, mitral valve area; MVG, mean mitral valve pressure gradient; NYHA, New York Heart Association; PASP, pulmonary artery systolic pressure; PAWP, pulmonary artery wedge pressure; 2D, 2-dimensional. *(From RO Bonow et al: J Am Coll Cardiol 48:e1, 2006; with permission.)*

TABLE 237-2 Medical Therapy of Valvular Heart Disease

Lesion	Symptom Control	Natural History
Mitral stenosis	Beta blockers, nondihydropyridine calcium channel blockers, or digoxin for rate control of AF; cardioversion for new-onset AF and HF; diuretics for HF	Warfarin for AF or thromboembolism; PCN for RF prophylaxis
Mitral regurgitation	Diuretics for HF	Warfarin for AF or thromboembolism
	Vasodilators for acute MR	Vasodilators for HTN
Aortic stenosis	Diuretics for HF	No proven therapy
Aortic regurgitation	Diuretics and vasodilators for HF	Vasodilators for HTN

Note: Antibiotic prophylaxis is recommended according to current American Heart Association guidelines. For patients with these forms of valvular heart disease, prophylaxis is indicated for a prior history of endocarditis. HF is an indication for surgical or percutaneous treatment, and the recommendations here pertain to short-term therapy prior to definitive correction of the valve lesion. For patients whose comorbidities prohibit surgery, the medical therapies listed can be continued according to available guidelines for the management of HF. See text.

Abbreviations: AF, atrial fibrillation; HF, heart failure; HTN, systemic hypertension; PCN, penicillin; RF, rheumatic fever.

Source: Adapted from NA Boon, P Bloomfield: Heart 87:395, 2002, with permission.

MITRAL VALVOTOMY Unless there is a contraindication, mitral valvotomy is indicated in symptomatic [New York Heart Association (NYHA) Functional Class II–IV] patients with isolated MS, whose effective orifice (valve area) is < ~1 cm²/m² body surface area, or <1.5 cm² in normal-sized adults. Mitral valvotomy can be carried out by two techniques: PMBV and surgical valvotomy. In PMBV (Figs. 237-2 and 237-3), a catheter is directed into the LA after transseptal puncture, and a single balloon is directed across the valve and inflated in the valvular orifice. Ideal patients have relatively pliable leaflets with little or no commissural calcium. In addition, the subvalvular structures should not be significantly scarred or thickened, and there should be no left atrial thrombus. The short- and long-term results of this procedure in appropriate patients are similar to those of surgical valvotomy, but with less morbidity and a lower periprocedural mortality rate. Event-free survival in younger (<45 years) patients with pliable valves is excellent, with rates as high as 80–90% over 3–7 years. Therefore, PMBV has become the procedure of choice for such patients when it can be performed by a skilled operator in a high-volume center.

Transthoracic echocardiography is helpful in identifying patients for the percutaneous procedure, and TEE is performed routinely to exclude left atrial thrombus at the time of the

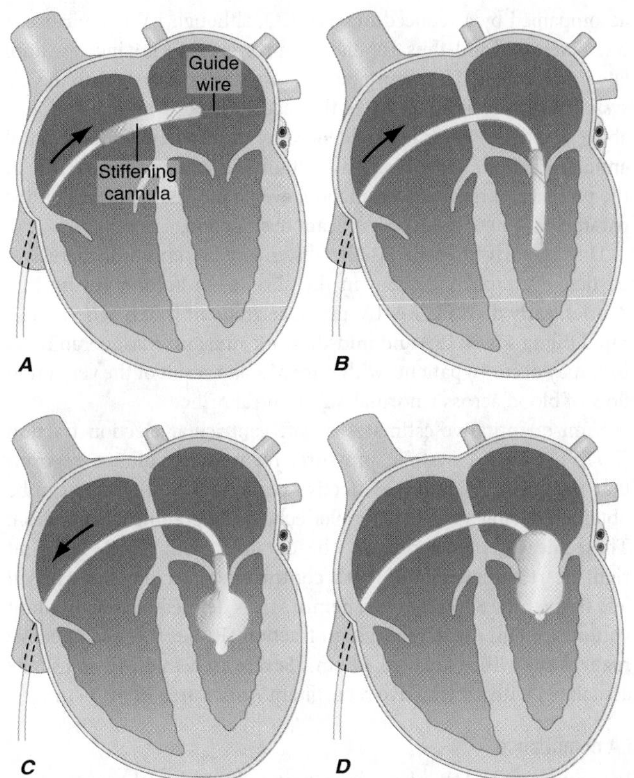

Figure 237-2 Inoue balloon technique for percutaneous mitral balloon valvotomy. ***A.*** After transseptal puncture, the deflated balloon catheter is advanced across the interatrial septum, then across the mitral valve and into the left ventricle. ***B.-D.*** The balloon is inflated stepwise within the mitral orifice.

scheduled procedure. An "echo score" has been developed to help guide decision-making. The score accounts for the degree of leaflet thickening, calcification, and mobility, and for the extent of subvalvular thickening. A lower score predicts a higher likelihood of successful PMBV.

In patients in whom PMBV is not possible or unsuccessful, or in many patients with restenosis, an "open" valvotomy using cardiopulmonary bypass is necessary. In addition to opening the valve commissures, it is important to loosen any subvalvular fusion of papillary muscles and chordae tendineae and to remove large deposits of calcium, thereby improving valvular function, as well as to remove atrial thrombi. The perioperative mortality rate is ~2%.

Successful valvotomy is defined by a 50% reduction in the mean mitral valve gradient and a doubling of the mitral valve area. Successful valvotomy, whether balloon or surgical, usually results in striking symptomatic and hemodynamic improvement and prolongs survival. However, there is no evidence that the procedure improves the prognosis of patients with slight or no functional impairment. Therefore, unless recurrent systemic embolization or severe pulmonary hypertension has occurred (PA systolic pressures >50 mmHg at rest or >60 mmHg with exercise), valvotomy is *not* recommended for patients who are entirely asymptomatic and/or who have mild stenosis (mitral valve area >1.5 cm^2). When there is little symptomatic improvement after valvotomy, it is likely that the procedure was ineffective, that it induced MR, or that associated valvular or myocardial disease was present. About half of all patients undergoing surgical mitral valvotomy require reoperation by 10 years. In the pregnant patient with MS, valvotomy should be carried out if pulmonary congestion occurs despite intensive medical treatment. PMBV is the preferred strategy in this setting and is performed with TEE and no or minimal x-ray exposure.

Mitral valve replacement (MVR) is necessary in patients with MS and significant associated MR, those in whom the valve has been severely distorted by previous transcatheter or operative manipulation, or those in whom the surgeon does not find it possible to improve valve function significantly with valvotomy. MVR is now routinely performed with preservation of the chordal attachments to optimize LV functional recovery. Perioperative mortality rates with MVR vary with age, LV function, the presence of CAD, and associated comorbidities. They average 5% overall but are lower in young patients and may be twice as high in patients >65 years of age with comorbidity rates (Table 237-3). Since there are also long-term complications of valve replacement (p. 1949), patients in whom preoperative evaluation suggests the possibility that MVR may be required should be operated on only if they have severe MS—i.e., an orifice

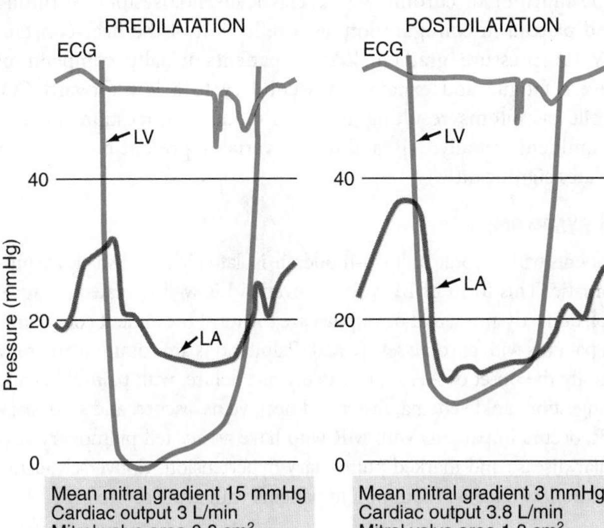

Figure 237-3 Simultaneous left atrial (LA) and left ventricular (LV) pressure before and after percutaneous mitral balloon valvuloplasty (PMBV) in a patient with severe mitral stenosis. *(Courtesy of Raymond G. McKay, MD; with permission.)*

TABLE 237-3 Mortality Rates After Valve Surgery*

Operation	Number	Unadjusted Operative Mortality (%)
AVR (isolated)	20,168	3.2
MVR (isolated)	4,616	5.0
AVR + CAB	16,678	5.0
MVR + CAB	2,479	8.8
AVR + MVR	1,239	9.0
MVP	5,617	1.8
MVP + CAB	4,932	4.8
TV surgery	6,235	9.2
PV surgery	480	6.0

*Data are for calendar year 2008, in which 912 sites reported a total of 276,308 procedures. Data are available from the Society of Thoracic Surgeons at *http://www.sts.org/documents/pdf/ndb/2ndHarvestExecutiveSummary_2009.pdf.*

Abbreviations: AVR, aortic valve replacement; CAB, coronary artery bypass; MVR, mitral valve replacement; MVP, mitral valve repair; TV surgery, tricuspid valve repair and replacement; PV surgery, pulmonic valve repair and replacement.

area ≤1 cm^2—and are in NYHA Class III, i.e., symptomatic with ordinary activity despite optimal medical therapy. The overall 10-year survival of surgical survivors is ~70%. Long-term prognosis is worse in patients >65 years of age and those with marked disability and marked depression of the CO preoperatively. Pulmonary hypertension and RV dysfunction are additional risk factors for poor outcome.

MITRAL REGURGITATION

ETIOLOGY

MR may result from an abnormality or disease process that affects any one or more of the five functional components of the mitral valve apparatus (leaflets, annulus, chordae tendineae, papillary muscles, and subjacent myocardium) (Table 237-1). Acute MR can occur in the setting of acute myocardial infarction (MI) with papillary muscle rupture (Chap. 245), following blunt chest wall trauma, or during the course of infective endocarditis. With acute MI, the posteromedial papillary muscle is involved much more frequently than the anterolateral papillary muscle because of its singular blood supply. Transient, acute MR can occur during periods of active ischemia and bouts of angina pectoris. Rupture of chordae tendineae can result in "acute-on-chronic MR" in patients with myxomatous degeneration of the valve apparatus.

Chronic MR can result from rheumatic disease, mitral valve prolapse (MVP), extensive mitral annular calcification, congenital valve defects, hypertrophic obstructive cardiomyopathy (HOCM), and dilated cardiomyopathy (Chap. 238). The rheumatic process produces rigidity, deformity, and retraction of the valve cusps and commissural fusion, as well as shortening, contraction, and fusion of the chordae tendineae. The MR associated with both MVP and HOCM is usually dynamic in nature. MR in HOCM occurs as a consequence of anterior papillary muscle displacement and systolic anterior motion of the anterior mitral valve leaflet into the narrowed LV outflow tract. Annular calcification is especially prevalent among patients with advanced renal disease and is commonly observed in women >65 years of age with hypertension and diabetes. MR may occur as a congenital anomaly (Chap. 236), most commonly as a defect of the endocardial cushions (atrioventricular cushion defects). A cleft anterior mitral valve leaflet accompanies primum atrial septal defect. Chronic MR is frequently secondary to ischemia and may occur as a consequence of ventricular remodeling, papillary muscle displacement, and leaflet tethering, or with fibrosis of a papillary muscle, in patients with healed myocardial infarction(s) and ischemic cardiomyopathy. Similar mechanisms of annular dilation and ventricular remodeling contribute to the MR that occurs among patients with nonischemic forms of dilated cardiomyopathy once the left ventricular end-diastolic dimension reaches 6 cm.

Irrespective of cause, chronic severe MR is often progressive, since enlargement of the LA places tension on the posterior mitral leaflet, pulling it away from the mitral orifice and thereby aggravating the valvular dysfunction. Similarly, LV dilation increases the regurgitation, which, in turn, enlarges the LA and LV further, causing chordal rupture and resulting in a vicious circle; hence the aphorism, "mitral regurgitation begets mitral regurgitation."

PATHOPHYSIOLOGY

The resistance to LV emptying (LV afterload) is reduced in patients with MR. As a consequence, the LV is decompressed into the LA during ejection, and with the reduction in LV size during systole, there is a rapid decline in LV tension. The initial compensation to MR is more complete LV emptying. However, LV volume increases progressively with time as the severity of the regurgitation increases and as LV contractile function deteriorates. This increase in LV volume is often accompanied by a reduced forward CO, although LV compliance is often increased and, thus, LV diastolic pressure does not increase until late in the course. The regurgitant volume varies directly with the LV systolic pressure and the size of the regurgitant orifice; as mentioned above, the latter, in turn, is influenced by the extent of LV and mitral annular dilation. Since ejection fraction (EF) rises in severe MR in the presence of normal LV function, even a modest reduction in this parameter (<60%) reflects significant dysfunction.

During early diastole, as the distended LA empties, there is a particularly rapid *y* descent in the absence of accompanying MS. A brief, early diastolic LA-LV pressure gradient [often generating a rapid filling sound (S_3) and mid-diastolic murmur masquerading as MS] may occur in patients with pure MR as a result of the very rapid flow of blood across a normal-sized mitral orifice.

Semi-quantitative estimates of left ventricular ejection fraction (LVEF), CO, PA systolic pressure, regurgitant volume, regurgitant fraction (RF), and the effective regurgitant orifice area can be obtained during a careful Doppler echocardiographic examination. These measurements can also be obtained with CMR. Left and right heart catheterization with contrast ventriculography is used less frequently. Severe, nonischemic MR is defined by a regurgitant volume ≥60 mL/beat, regurgitant fraction (RF) ≥50%, and effective regurgitant orifice area ≥0.40 cm^2. Severe ischemic MR is usually associated with an effective regurgitant orifice area of >0.3 cm^2.

LA compliance

In acute severe MR, the regurgitant volume is delivered into a normal-sized LA having normal or reduced compliance. As a result, LA pressures rise markedly for any increase in LA volume. The *v* wave in the LA pressure pulse is usually prominent, LA and pulmonary venous pressures are markedly elevated, and pulmonary edema is common. Because of the rapid rise in LA pressures during ventricular systole, the murmur of acute MR is early in timing and decrescendo in configuration ending well before S_2, as a reflection of the progressive diminution in the LV-LA pressure gradient. LV systolic function in acute MR may be normal, hyperdynamic, or reduced, depending on the clinical context.

Patients with chronic severe MR, on the other hand, develop marked LA enlargement and *increased* LA compliance with little if any increase in LA and pulmonary venous pressures for any increase in LA volume. The LA *v* wave is relatively less prominent. The murmur of chronic MR is classically holosystolic in timing and plateau in configuration, as a reflection of the near-constant LV-LA pressure gradient. These patients usually complain of severe fatigue and exhaustion secondary to a low forward CO, while symptoms resulting from pulmonary congestion are less prominent initially; AF is almost invariably present once the LA dilates significantly.

SYMPTOMS

Patients with chronic mild-to-moderate isolated MR are usually asymptomatic. This form of LV volume overload is well tolerated. Fatigue, exertional dyspnea, and orthopnea are the most prominent complaints in patients with chronic severe MR. Palpitations are common and may signify the onset of AF. Right-sided heart failure, with painful hepatic congestion, ankle edema, distended neck veins, ascites, and secondary TR, occurs in patients with MR who have associated pulmonary vascular disease and marked pulmonary hypertension. Conversely, acute pulmonary edema is common in patients with acute severe MR.

PHYSICAL FINDINGS

In patients with chronic severe MR, the arterial pressure is usually normal, although the carotid arterial pulse may show a sharp upstroke owing to the reduced forward cardiac output. A systolic thrill is often palpable at the cardiac apex, the LV is hyperdynamic with a brisk systolic impulse and a palpable rapid-filling wave (S_3), and the apex beat is often displaced laterally.

In patients with acute severe MR, the arterial pressure may be reduced with a narrow pulse pressure, the jugular venous pressure and wave forms may be normal or increased and exaggerated, the apical impulse is not displaced, and signs of pulmonary congestion are prominent.

Auscultation

S_1 is generally absent, soft, or buried in the holosystolic murmur of chronic MR. In patients with severe MR, the aortic valve may close prematurely, resulting in wide but physiologic splitting of S_2. A low-pitched S_3 occurring 0.12–0.17 s after the aortic valve closure sound, i.e., at the completion of the rapid-filling phase of the LV, is believed to be caused by the sudden tensing of the papillary muscles, chordae tendineae, and valve leaflets. It may be followed by a short, rumbling, mid-diastolic murmur, even in the absence of structural MS. A fourth heart sound is often audible in patients with *acute* severe MR who are in sinus rhythm. A presystolic murmur is not ordinarily heard with isolated MR.

A systolic murmur of at least grade III/VI intensity is the most characteristic auscultatory finding in chronic severe MR. It is usually holosystolic (see Fig. 227-5A), but as previously noted it is decrescendo and ceases in mid- to late systole in patients with acute severe MR. The systolic murmur of chronic MR is usually most prominent at the apex and radiates to the axilla. However, in patients with ruptured chordae tendineae or primary involvement of the posterior mitral leaflet with prolapse or flail, the regurgitant jet is eccentric, directed anteriorly, and strikes the LA wall adjacent to the aortic root. In this situation, the systolic murmur is transmitted to the base of the heart and, therefore, may be confused with the murmur of AS. In patients with ruptured chordae tendineae, the systolic murmur may have a cooing or "sea gull" quality, while a flail leaflet may produce a murmur with a musical quality. The systolic murmur of chronic MR not due to MVP is intensified by isometric exercise (handgrip) but is reduced during the strain phase of the Valsalva maneuver because of the associated decrease in LV preload.

LABORATORY EXAMINATION

ECG

In patients with sinus rhythm, there is evidence of LA enlargement, but RA enlargement also may be present when pulmonary hypertension is severe. Chronic severe MR is generally associated with AF. In many patients, there is no clear-cut ECG evidence of enlargement of either ventricle. In others, the signs of eccentric LV hypertrophy are present.

Echocardiogram

TTE is indicated to assess the mechanism of the MR and its hemodynamic severity. LV function can be assessed from LV end-diastolic and end-systolic volumes and EF. Observations can be made regarding leaflet structure and function, chordal integrity, LA and LV size, annular calcification, and regional and global LV systolic function. Doppler imaging should demonstrate the width or area of the color flow MR jet within the LA, the intensity of the continuous wave Doppler signal, the pulmonary venous flow contour, the early peak mitral inflow velocity, and the quantitative measures of regurgitant volume, RF, and effective regurgitant orifice area. In addition, the PA pressures can be estimated from the TR jet velocity. TTE is also indicated to follow the course of patients with chronic MR and to provide rapid assessment for any clinical change. The echocardiogram in patients with MVP is described in the next section. TEE provides greater detail than TTE (see Fig. 229-5).

Chest x-ray

The LA and LV are the dominant chambers in chronic MR. Late in the course of the disease, the LA may be massively enlarged and forms the right border of the cardiac silhouette. Pulmonary venous congestion, interstitial edema, and Kerley B lines are sometimes noted. Marked calcification of the mitral leaflets occurs commonly in patients with longstanding, combined rheumatic MR and MS. Calcification of the mitral annulus may be visualized, particularly on the lateral view of the chest. Patients with acute severe MR may have asymmetric pulmonary edema if the regurgitant jet is directed predominantly to the orifice of an upper lobe pulmonary vein.

TREATMENT Mitral Regurgitation

MEDICAL TREATMENT (See Fig. 237-4 and Table 237-2) The management of chronic severe MR depends to some degree on its cause. Warfarin should be provided once AF intervenes with a target INR of 2–3. Cardioversion should be considered depending on the clinical context and left atrial size. In contrast to the acute setting, there are no large, long-term prospective

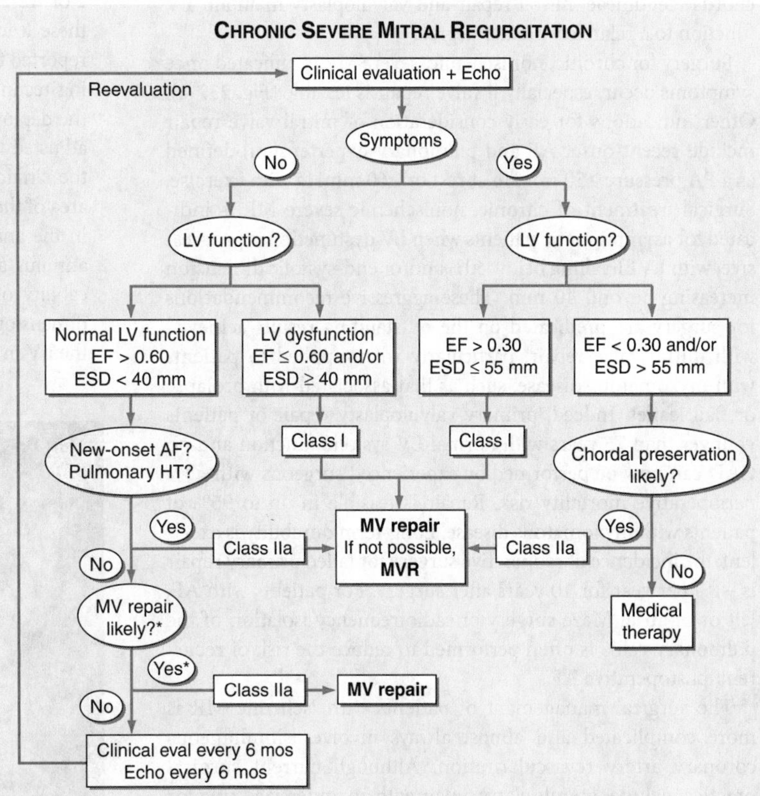

Figure 237-4 Management strategy for patients with chronic severe nonischemic mitral regurgitation. *Mitral valve (MV) repair may be performed in asymptomatic patients with normal left ventricular (LV) function if performed by an experienced surgical team and if the likelihood of successful MV repair is >90%. AF, atrial fibrillation; Echo, echocardiography; EF, ejection fraction; ESD, end-systolic dimension; eval, evaluation; HT, hypertension; MVR, mitral valve replacement. *(From RO Bonow et al: J Am Coll Cardiol 48:e1, 2006; with permission.)*

studies to substantiate the use of vasodilators for the treatment of chronic, isolated severe MR with preserved LV systolic function *in the absence of systemic hypertension.* The severity of MR in the setting of an ischemic or nonischemic dilated cardiomyopathy may diminish with aggressive, evidence-based treatment of heart failure, including the use of diuretics, beta blockers, angiotensin-converting enzyme (ACE) inhibitors, digitalis, and biventricular pacing (cardiac resynchronization therapy [CRT]). Asymptomatic patients with severe MR in sinus rhythm with normal LV size and systolic function should avoid isometric forms of exercise.

Patients with acute severe MR require urgent stabilization and preparation for surgery. Diuretics, intravenous vasodilators (particularly sodium nitroprusside), and even intraaortic balloon counterpulsation may be needed for patients with post-MI papillary muscle rupture or other forms of acute severe MR.

SURGICAL TREATMENT In the selection of patients with chronic, nonischemic, severe MR for surgical treatment, the often slowly progressive nature of the condition must be balanced against the immediate and long-term risks associated with operation. These risks are significantly lower for primary valve repair than for valve replacement (Table 237-3). Repair usually consists of valve reconstruction using a variety of valvuloplasty techniques and insertion of an annuloplasty ring. Repair spares the patient the long-term adverse consequences of valve replacement, i.e., thromboembolic and hemorrhagic complications in the case of mechanical prostheses and late valve failure necessitating repeat valve replacement in the case of bioprostheses (p. 1949). In addition, by preserving the integrity of the papillary muscles, subvalvular apparatus, and chordae tendineae, mitral repair and valvuloplasty maintain LV function to a relatively greater degree.

Surgery for chronic, nonischemic, severe MR is indicated once symptoms occur, especially if valve repair is feasible (Fig. 237-4). Other indications for early consideration of mitral valve repair include recent-onset AF and pulmonary hypertension, defined as a PA pressure ≥50 mmHg at rest or ≥60 mmHg with exercise. Surgical treatment of chronic, nonischemic severe MR is indicated for asymptomatic patients when LV dysfunction is progressive, with LVEF falling below 60% and/or end-systolic dimension increasing beyond 40 mm. These aggressive recommendations for surgery are predicated on the outstanding results achieved with mitral valve repair, particularly when applied to patients with myxomatous disease, such as that associated with prolapse or flail leaflet. Indeed, primary valvuloplasty repair of patients younger than 75 years with normal LV systolic function and no CAD can now be performed by experienced surgeons with <1% perioperative mortality risk. Repair is feasible in up to 95% of patients with myxomatous disease. Long-term durability is excellent; the incidence of reoperative surgery for failed primary repair is ~1% per year for 10 years after surgery. For patients with AF, left or bi-atrial Maze surgery or radiofrequency isolation of the pulmonary veins is often performed to reduce the risk of recurrent, postoperative AF.

The surgical management of patients with ischemic MR is more complicated and almost always involves simultaneous coronary artery revascularization. Although current surgical practice includes annuloplasty repair with an undersized ring for patients with moderate or greater degrees of MR at the time of coronary artery bypass surgery, the efficacy of this approach has not been established in prospective, randomized trials. There is also uncertainty as to whether or not valve repair or replacement is the preferred strategy, given the higher incidence of residual or recurrent MR after repair in this context compared with outcomes in patients with organic (myxomatous) disease. In patients with significantly impaired LV function (EF <30%), the risk of surgery increases, the recovery of LV performance is incomplete, and the long-term survival is reduced. However, conservative management has little to offer these patients, so operative treatment may be indicated, and the clinical and hemodynamic improvement that follows surgical treatment of patients with advanced disease is occasionally dramatic, especially when severe CAD is present and bypass grafting can be performed. The routine performance of valve repair in patients with significant MR in the setting of severe, dilated cardiomyopathy has not been shown to improve long-term survival. Patients with acute severe MR can often be stabilized temporarily with appropriate medical therapy, but surgical correction will be necessary, emergently in the case of papillary muscle rupture and within days to weeks in most other settings.

When surgical treatment is contemplated, left and right heart catheterization and left ventriculography *may* be helpful in confirming the presence of severe MR in patients in whom there is a discrepancy between the clinical and TTE findings that cannot be resolved with TEE or CMR. Coronary angiography identifies patients who require concomitant coronary revascularization.

PERCUTANEOUS MITRAL VALVE REPAIR A transcatheter approach to the treatment of either organic or functional MR may be feasible in selected patients with appropriate anatomy, although the proper role of current techniques remains under active investigation. One approach involves the deployment of a clip delivered via transeptal puncture that grasps the leading edges of the mitral leaflets in their mid-portion (anterior scallop 2–posterior scallop 2 or A2-P2, Fig. 237-5). The length and width of the gap between these leading edges have dictated patient eligibility in the trials reported to date. Preliminary results with this technically demanding technique have been favorable. A second approach involves the deployment of a device within the coronary sinus that can be adjusted to reduce its circumference, thus secondarily decreasing the circumference of the mitral annulus and the effective orifice area of the valve, much like a surgically implanted ring. Variations in the anatomic relationship of the coronary sinus to the mitral annulus and circumflex coronary artery have limited the applicability of this technique. Attempts to reduce the septal-lateral dimension of a dilated annulus using adjustable cords placed across the LV in a subvalvular location have also been investigated.

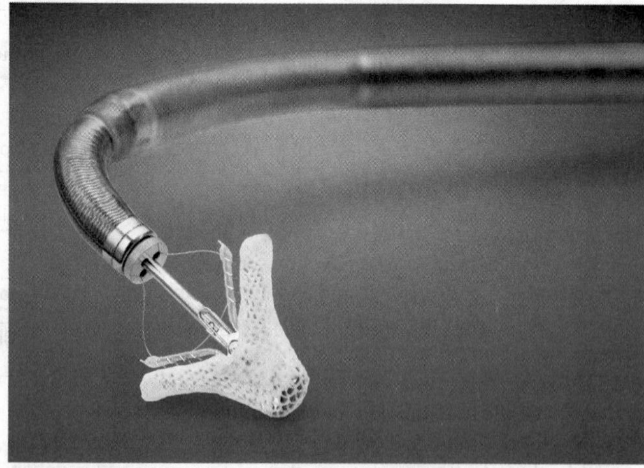

Figure 237-5 **Clip used to grasp the free edges of the anterior and posterior leaflets in their mid-sections during percutaneous repair of selected patients with mitral regurgitation.** *(Courtesy of Abbott Vascular.*

MITRAL VALVE PROLAPSE

MVP, also variously termed the *systolic click-murmur syndrome, Barlow's syndrome, floppy-valve syndrome,* and *billowing mitral leaflet syndrome,* is a relatively common but highly variable clinical syndrome resulting from diverse pathologic mechanisms of the mitral valve apparatus. Among these are excessive or redundant mitral leaflet tissue, which is commonly associated with myxomatous degeneration and greatly increased concentrations of certain glycosaminoglycans.

In most patients with MVP, the cause is unknown, but in some it appears to be a genetically determined collagen disorder. A reduction in the production of type III collagen has been incriminated, and electron microscopy has revealed fragmentation of collagen fibrils.

MVP is a frequent finding in patients with heritable disorders of connective tissue, including Marfan's syndrome (Chap. 363), osteogenesis imperfecta, and Ehlers-Danlos syndrome. MVP may be associated with thoracic skeletal deformities similar to but not as severe as those in Marfan's syndrome, such as a high-arched palate and alterations of the chest and thoracic spine, including the so-called straight back syndrome.

In most patients with MVP, myxomatous degeneration is confined to the mitral valve, although the tricuspid and aortic valves may also be affected. The posterior mitral leaflet is usually more affected than the anterior, and the mitral valve annulus is often dilated. In many patients, elongated, redundant, or ruptured chordae tendineae cause or contribute to the regurgitation.

MVP also may occur rarely as a sequel to acute rheumatic fever, in ischemic heart disease, and in various cardiomyopathies, as well as in 20% of patients with ostium secundum atrial septal defect.

MVP may lead to excessive stress on the papillary muscles, which, in turn, leads to dysfunction and ischemia of the papillary muscles and the subjacent ventricular myocardium. Rupture of chordae tendineae and progressive annular dilation and calcification contribute to valvular regurgitation, which then places more stress on the diseased mitral valve apparatus, thereby creating a vicious circle. The ECG changes (see below) and ventricular arrhythmias appear to result from regional ventricular dysfunction related to the increased stress placed on the papillary muscles.

CLINICAL FEATURES

MVP is more common in women and occurs most frequently between the ages of 15 and 30 years; the clinical course is most often benign. MVP may also be observed in older (>50 years) patients, often men, in whom MR is often more severe and requires surgical treatment. There is an increased familial incidence for some patients, suggesting an autosomal dominant form of inheritance with incomplete penetrance. MVP varies in its clinical expression, ranging from only a systolic click and murmur with mild prolapse of the posterior leaflet to severe MR due to chordal rupture and leaflet flail. The degree of myxomatous change of the leaflets can also vary widely. In many patients, the condition progresses over years or decades; in others it worsens rapidly as a result of chordal rupture or endocarditis.

Most patients are asymptomatic and remain so for their entire lives. However, in North America, MVP is now the most common cause of isolated severe MR requiring surgical treatment. Arrhythmias, most commonly ventricular premature contractions and paroxysmal supraventricular and ventricular tachycardia, as well as AF, have been reported and may cause palpitations, lightheadedness, and syncope. Sudden death is a very rare complication and occurs most often in patients with severe MR and depressed LV systolic function. There may be an excess risk of sudden death among patients with a flail leaflet. Many patients have chest pain that is difficult to evaluate; it is often substernal, prolonged, and not related to exertion, but may rarely resemble angina pectoris. Transient cerebral ischemic attacks secondary to emboli from the mitral valve due to endothelial disruption have been reported. Infective endocarditis may occur in patients with MR and/or leaflet thickening.

Auscultation

The most important finding is the mid- or late (nonejection) systolic click, which occurs 0.14 s or more after S_1 and is thought to be generated by the sudden tensing of slack, elongated chordae tendineae or by the prolapsing mitral leaflet when it reaches its maximum excursion. Systolic clicks may be multiple and may be followed by a high-pitched, late systolic crescendo-decrescendo murmur, which occasionally is "whooping" or "honking" and is heard best at the apex. The click and murmur occur earlier with standing, during the strain phase of the Valsalva maneuver, and with any intervention that decreases LV volume, exaggerating the propensity of mitral leaflet prolapse. Conversely, squatting and isometric exercises, which increase LV volume, diminish MVP; the click-murmur complex is delayed, moves away from S_1, and may even disappear. Some patients have a mid-systolic click without a murmur; others have a murmur without a click. Still others have both sounds at different times.

LABORATORY EXAMINATION

The ECG most commonly is normal but may show biphasic or inverted T waves in leads II, III, and aVF, and occasionally supraventricular or ventricular premature beats. TTE is particularly effective in identifying the abnormal position and prolapse of the mitral valve leaflets. A useful echocardiographic definition of MVP is systolic displacement (in the parasternal long axis view) of the mitral valve leaflets by at least 2 mm into the LA superior to the plane of the mitral annulus. Color flow and continuous wave Doppler imaging is helpful to evaluate the associated MR and provide semiquantitative estimates of severity. The jet lesion of MR due to MVP is most often eccentric, and assessment of RF and effective regurgitant orifice area can be difficult. TEE is indicated when more accurate information is required and is performed routinely for intraoperative guidance for valve repair. Invasive left ventriculography is rarely necessary but can also show prolapse of the posterior and sometimes of both mitral valve leaflets.

TREATMENT Mitral Valve Prolapse

Infective endocarditis prophylaxis is indicated only for patients with a prior history of endocarditis. Beta blockers sometimes relieve chest pain and control palpitations. If the patient is symptomatic from severe MR, mitral valve repair (or rarely, replacement) is indicated (Fig. 237-4). Antiplatelet agents, such as aspirin, should be given to patients with transient ischemic attacks, and if these are not effective, anticoagulants, such as warfarin, should be considered. Warfarin is also indicated once AF intervenes.

AORTIC STENOSIS

AS occurs in about one-fourth of all patients with chronic valvular heart disease; approximately 80% of adult patients with symptomatic valvular AS are male.

ETIOLOGY AND PATHOGENESIS

(Table 237-1) AS in adults is due to degenerative calcification of the aortic cusps and occurs most commonly on a substrate of congenital disease (bicuspid aortic valve [BAV]), chronic (tri-) leaflet deterioration, or previous rheumatic inflammation. A recent pathologic study of specimens removed at the time of aortic valve replacement for AS showed that 53% were bicuspid and 4% unicuspid. Contrary to previous teachings, the process of aortic valve deterioration and calcification is not a passive one, but rather one that shares many features with vascular atherosclerosis, including endothelial dysfunction, lipid accumulation, inflammatory cell activation, cytokine release, and upregulation of several signaling pathways (Fig. 237-6). Eventually, valvular myofibroblasts differentiate phenotypically into osteoblasts and actively produce bone matrix proteins that allow for the deposition of calcium hydroxyapatite crystals. Genetic polymorphisms involving the vitamin D receptor, the estrogen receptor in postmenopausal women, interleukin 10, and apolipoprotein E4 have been linked to the development of calcific AS, and a strong familial clustering of cases has been reported from western France. Several traditional atherosclerotic risk factors have also been associated with the development and progression of calcific AS, including low-density lipoprotein (LDL)-cholesterol, lipoprotein a [Lp(a)], diabetes mellitus, smoking, chronic kidney disease, and the metabolic syndrome. The presence of aortic valve sclerosis (focal thickening and calcification of the leaflets not severe enough to cause obstruction) is associated with an excess risk of cardiovascular death and MI among persons older than age 65. Approximately 30% of persons older than 65 years exhibit aortic valve sclerosis, whereas 2% exhibit frank stenosis.

Rheumatic disease of the aortic leaflets produces commissural fusion, sometimes resulting in a bicuspid-appearing valve. This condition, in turn, makes the leaflets more susceptible to trauma and ultimately leads to fibrosis, calcification, and further narrowing. By the time the obstruction to LV outflow causes serious clinical disability, the valve is usually a rigid calcified mass, and careful examination may make it difficult or even impossible to determine the etiology of the underlying process. Rheumatic AS is almost always associated with involvement of the mitral valve and with AR. Mediastinal radiation can also result in late scarring, fibrosis, and calcification of the leaflets with AS.

BICUSPID AORTIC VALVE DISEASE

A bicuspid aortic valve (BAV) is the most common congenital heart valve defect and occurs in 0.5–1.4% of the population with a 2–4:1 male to female predominance. The inheritance pattern appears to be autosomal dominant with incomplete penetrance, although some have questioned an X-linked component as suggested by the prevalence of BAV disease among patients with Turner's syndrome. The prevalence of BAV disease among first-degree relatives of an affected individual is approximately 10%. A single gene defect to explain the majority of cases has not been identified, although a mutation in the *NOTCH1* gene has been described in some families. Abnormalities in endothelial nitric oxide synthase and NKX2.5 have been implicated, as well. Aortic coarctation or medial degeneration with ascending aortic aneurysm formation occurs commonly among patients with BAV disease. Patients with BAV disease have larger aortas than patients with comparable tricuspid aortic valve disease. The aortopathy develops independent of the hemodynamic severity of the valve lesion and is a risk factor for dissection. A BAV can be a component of more complex congenital heart disease with or without other left heart obstructing lesions.

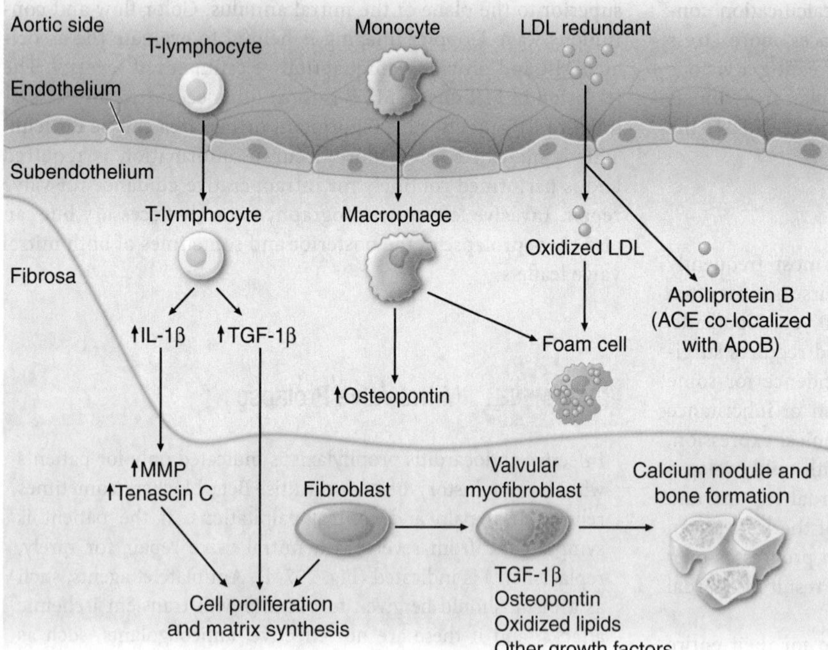

Figure 237-6 Pathogenesis of calcific aortic stenosis. Inflammatory cells infiltrate across the endothelial barrier and release cytokines that act on fibroblasts to promote cellular proliferation and matrix remodeling. LDL is oxidatively modified and taken up by macrophage scavengers to become foam cells. Angiotensin-converting enzyme colocalizes with Apo-B. A subset of myofibroblasts differentiate into an osteoblast phenotype capable of promoting bone formation. ACE, angiotensin-converting enzyme; ApoB, apolipoprotein B; LDL, low-density lipoprotein; IL, interleukin; MMP, matrix metalloproteinase; TGF, transforming growth factor. *(From RV Freeman, CM Otto: Circulation 111:3316, 2005; with permission.)*

OTHER FORMS OF OBSTRUCTION TO LEFT VENTRICULAR OUTFLOW

In addition to valvular AS, three other lesions may be responsible for obstruction to LV outflow: *hypertrophic obstructive cardiomyopathy* (Chap. 238), *discrete fibromuscular/membranous subaortic stenosis*, and *supravalvular AS* (Chap. 236). The causes of left ventricular outflow obstruction can be differentiated on the basis of the cardiac examination and Doppler echocardiographic findings.

PATHOPHYSIOLOGY

The obstruction to LV outflow produces a systolic pressure gradient between the LV and aorta. When severe obstruction is suddenly produced experimentally, the LV responds by dilation and reduction of stroke volume. However, in some patients, the obstruction may be present at birth and/or increase gradually over the course of many years, and LV contractile performance is maintained by the presence of concentric LV hypertrophy. Initially, this serves as an adaptive mechanism because it reduces toward normal the systolic stress developed by the myocardium, as predicted by the Laplace relation ($S = Pr/h$, where S = systolic wall stress, P = pressure, r = radius, and h = wall thickness). A large transaortic valve pressure gradient may exist for many years without a reduction in CO or LV dilation;

ultimately, however, excessive hypertrophy becomes maladaptive, LV systolic function declines, abnormalities of diastolic function progress, and irreversible myocardial fibrosis develops.

A mean systolic pressure gradient >40 mmHg with a normal CO or an effective aortic orifice area <~1 cm^2 (or ~<0.6 cm^2/m^2 body surface area in a normal-sized adult)—i.e., less than approximately one-third of the normal orifice area—is generally considered to represent severe obstruction to LV outflow. The elevated LV end-diastolic pressure observed in many patients with severe AS and preserved EF signifies the presence of diminished compliance of the hypertrophied LV. Although the CO at rest is within normal limits in most patients with severe AS, it usually fails to rise normally during exercise. Loss of an appropriately timed, vigorous atrial contraction, as occurs in AF or atrioventricular dissociation, may cause rapid progression of symptoms. Late in the course, contractile function deteriorates because of afterload excess, the CO and LV–aortic pressure gradient decline, and the mean LA, PA, and RV pressures rise. LV performance can be further compromised by superimposed CAD.

The hypertrophied LV causes an increase in myocardial oxygen requirements. In addition, even in the absence of obstructive CAD, coronary blood flow is impaired to the extent that ischemia can be precipitated under conditions of excess demand. Capillary density is reduced relative to wall thickness, compressive forces are increased, and the elevated LV end-diastolic pressure reduces the coronary driving pressure. The subendocardium is especially vulnerable to ischemia by this mechanism.

■ SYMPTOMS

AS is rarely of clinical importance until the valve orifice has narrowed to approximately 1 cm^2. Even severe AS may exist for many years without producing any symptoms because of the ability of the hypertrophied LV to generate the elevated intraventricular pressures required to maintain a normal stroke volume. Once symptoms occur, valve replacement is indicated.

Most patients with pure or predominant AS have gradually increasing obstruction over years, but do not become symptomatic until the sixth to eighth decades. Adult patients with BAV disease, however, develop significant valve dysfunction and symptoms one to two decades sooner. Exertional dyspnea, angina pectoris, and syncope are the three cardinal symptoms. Often, there is a history of insidious progression of fatigue and dyspnea associated with gradual curtailment of activities. *Dyspnea* results primarily from elevation of the pulmonary capillary pressure caused by elevations of LV diastolic pressures secondary to reduced left ventricular compliance and impaired relaxation. *Angina pectoris* usually develops somewhat later and reflects an imbalance between the augmented myocardial oxygen requirements and reduced oxygen availability. CAD may or may not be present, although its coexistence is common among AS patients older than age 65. *Exertional syncope* may result from a decline in arterial pressure caused by vasodilation in the exercising muscles and inadequate vasoconstriction in nonexercising muscles in the face of a fixed CO, or from a sudden fall in CO produced by an arrhythmia.

Because the CO at rest is usually well maintained until late in the course, marked fatigability, weakness, peripheral cyanosis, cachexia, and other clinical manifestations of a low CO are usually not prominent until this stage is reached. Orthopnea, paroxysmal nocturnal dyspnea, and pulmonary edema, i.e., symptoms of LV failure, also occur only in the advanced stages of the disease. Severe pulmonary hypertension leading to RV failure and systemic venous hypertension, hepatomegaly, AF, and TR are usually late findings in patients with isolated severe AS.

When AS and MS coexist, the reduction in CO induced by MS lowers the pressure gradient across the aortic valve and, thereby, masks many of the clinical findings produced by AS.

■ PHYSICAL FINDINGS

The rhythm is generally regular until late in the course; at other times, AF should suggest the possibility of associated mitral valve disease. The systemic arterial pressure is usually within normal limits. In the late stages, however, when stroke volume declines, the systolic pressure may fall and the pulse pressure narrow. The peripheral arterial pulse rises slowly to a delayed peak (*pulsus parvus et tardus*. A thrill or anacrotic "shudder" may be palpable over the carotid arteries, more commonly the left. In the elderly, the stiffening of the arterial wall may mask this important physical sign. In many patients, the *a* wave in the jugular venous pulse is accentuated. This results from the diminished distensibility of the RV cavity caused by the bulging, hypertrophied interventricular septum.

The LV impulse is usually displaced laterally. A double apical impulse (with a palpable S_4) may be recognized, particularly with the patient in the left lateral recumbent position. A systolic thrill may be present at the base of the heart to the right of the sternum when leaning forward or in the suprasternal notch.

Auscultation

An early systolic ejection sound is frequently audible in children, adolescents, and young adults with congenital BAV disease. This sound usually disappears when the valve becomes calcified and rigid. As AS increases in severity, LV systole may become prolonged so that the aortic valve closure sound no longer precedes the pulmonic valve closure sound, and the two components may become synchronous, or aortic valve closure may even follow pulmonic valve closure, causing paradoxical splitting of S_2 (Chap. 227). The sound of aortic valve closure can be heard most frequently in patients with AS who have pliable valves, and calcification diminishes the intensity of this sound. Frequently, an S_4 is audible at the apex and reflects the presence of LV hypertrophy and an elevated LV end-diastolic pressure; an S_3 generally occurs late in the course, when the LV dilates and its systolic function becomes severely compromised.

The murmur of AS is characteristically an ejection (mid) systolic murmur that commences shortly after the S_1, increases in intensity to reach a peak toward the middle of ejection, and ends just before aortic valve closure. It is characteristically low-pitched, rough and rasping in character, and loudest at the base of the heart, most commonly in the second right intercostal space. It is transmitted upward along the carotid arteries. Occasionally it is transmitted downward and to the apex, where it may be confused with the systolic murmur of MR (Gallavardin effect). In almost all patients with severe obstruction and preserved CO, the murmur is at least grade III/VI. In patients with mild degrees of obstruction or in those with severe stenosis with heart failure and low CO in whom the stroke volume and, therefore, the transvalvular flow rate are reduced, the murmur may be relatively soft and brief.

■ LABORATORY EXAMINATION

ECG

In most patients with severe AS there is LV hypertrophy. In advanced cases, ST-segment depression and T-wave inversion (LV "strain") in standard leads I and aVL and in the left precordial leads are evident. However, there is no close correlation between the ECG and the hemodynamic severity of obstruction, and the absence of ECG signs of LV hypertrophy does not exclude severe obstruction. Many patients with AS have systemic hypertension, which can also contribute to the development of hypertrophy.

Echocardiogram

The key findings on TTE are thickening, calcification, and reduced systolic opening of the valve leaflets and LV hypertrophy. Eccentric closure of the aortic valve cusps is characteristic of congenitally bicuspid valves. TEE imaging usually displays the obstructed orifice extremely well, but it is not routinely required for accurate characterization. The valve gradient and aortic valve area can be estimated by Doppler measurement of the transaortic velocity. Severe AS is defined by a valve area <1 cm^2, whereas moderate AS is defined by a valve area of 1–1.5 cm^2 and mild AS by a valve area of 1.5–2 cm^2. Aortic valve sclerosis, conversely, is accompanied by a jet velocity of less than 2.5 meters/s (peak gradient <25 mmHg). LV dilation and reduced systolic shortening reflect impairment of LV function. There is increasing experience with the use of longitudinal strain and strain rate to characterize earlier changes in LV systolic function, well before a decline in EF can be appreciated. Doppler indices of impaired diastolic function are frequently seen.

Echocardiography is useful for identifying coexisting valvular abnormalities; for differentiating valvular AS from other forms of LV outflow obstruction; and for measurement of the aortic root and proximal ascending aortic dimension. These aortic measurements are particularly important for patients with BAV disease. Dobutamine stress echocardiography is useful for the evaluation of patients with AS and severe LV systolic dysfunction (EF <0.35), in whom the severity of the AS can often be difficult to judge.

Chest x-ray

The chest x-ray may show no or little overall cardiac enlargement for many years. Hypertrophy without dilation may produce some rounding of the cardiac apex in the frontal projection and slight backward displacement in the lateral view. A dilated proximal ascending aorta may be seen along the upper right heart border in the frontal view. Aortic valve calcification may be discernible in the lateral view, but is usually readily apparent on fluoroscopic examination or by echocardiography; the absence of valvular calcification in an adult suggests that severe valvular AS is *not* present. In later stages of the disease, as the LV dilates there is increasing roentgenographic evidence of LV enlargement, pulmonary congestion, and enlargement of the LA, PA, and right heart chambers.

Catheterization

Right and left heart catheterization for invasive assessment of AS is now performed infrequently but can be useful when there is a discrepancy between the clinical and Doppler echocardiographic findings. Appropriate concerns have been raised that attempts to cross the aortic valve for measurement of left ventricular pressures are associated with a risk of cerebral embolization. Catheterization is also useful in three distinct categories of patients: (1) *patients with multivalvular disease,* in whom the role played by each valvular deformity should be defined to aid in the planning of operative treatment; (2) *young, asymptomatic patients with noncalcific congenital AS,* to define the severity of obstruction to LV outflow, since operation or percutaneous aortic balloon valvoplasty (PABV) may be indicated in these patients if severe AS is present, even in the absence of symptoms; balloon valvotomy may follow left heart catheterization in the same sitting; and (3) *patients in whom it is suspected that the obstruction to LV outflow may not be at the level of the aortic valve* but rather at the sub- or supravalvular level.

Coronary angiography is indicated to detect or exclude CAD in appropriate patients with severe AS who are being considered for surgery. The incidence of significant CAD for which bypass grafting is indicated at the time of aortic valve replacement (AVR) exceeds 50% among adult patients.

■ NATURAL HISTORY

Death in patients with severe AS occurs most commonly in the seventh and eighth decades. Based on data obtained at postmortem examination in patients before surgical treatment became widely available, the average time to death after the onset of various symptoms was as follows: angina pectoris, 3 years; syncope, 3 years; dyspnea, 2 years; congestive heart failure, 1.5–2 years. Moreover, in >80% of patients who died with AS, symptoms had existed for <4 years. Among adults dying with valvular AS, sudden death, which presumably resulted from an arrhythmia, occurred in 10–20%; however, most sudden deaths occurred in patients who had previously been symptomatic. Sudden death as the first manifestation of severe AS is very uncommon (<1% per year) in asymptomatic adult patients. Calcific AS is a progressive disease, with an annual reduction in valve area averaging 0.1 cm^2 and annual increases in the peak jet velocity and mean valve gradient averaging 0.3 meters/s and 7 mmHg, respectively (Table 237-2, Fig. 237-7).

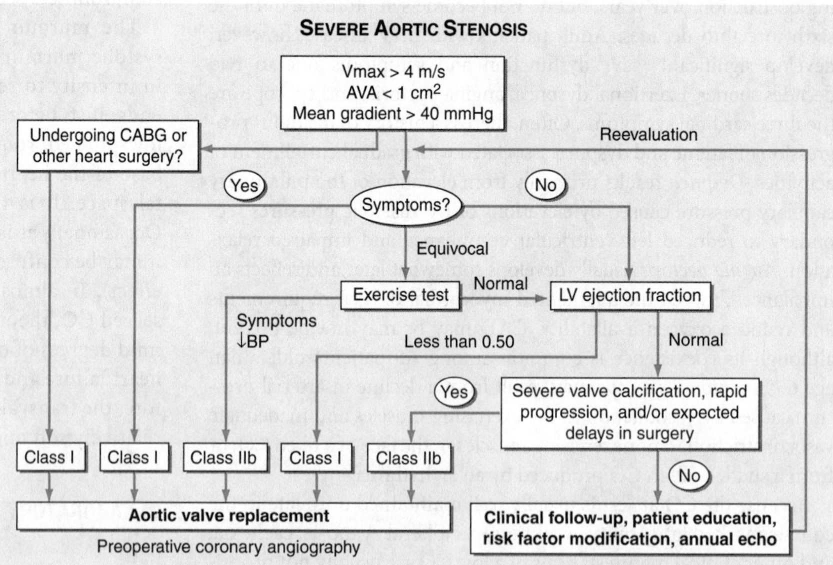

Figure 237-7 Management strategy for patients with severe aortic stenosis. Preoperative coronary angiography should be performed routinely as determined by age, symptoms, and coronary risk factors. Cardiac catheterization and angiography may also be helpful when there is a discrepancy between clinical findings and echocardiography. AVA, aortic valve area; BP, blood pressure; CABG, coronary artery bypass graft surgery; echo, echocardiography; LV, left ventricle; Vmax, maximal velocity across aortic valve by Doppler echocardiography. *(From Bonow et al. Modified from CM Otto: J Am Coll Cardiol 47:2141, 2006.)*

TREATMENT Aortic Stenosis

MEDICAL TREATMENT In patients with severe AS (valve area <1 cm^2), strenuous physical activity and competitive sports should be avoided, even in the asymptomatic stage. Care must be taken to avoid dehydration and hypovolemia to protect against a significant reduction in CO. Medications used for the treatment of hypertension or CAD, including beta blockers and ACE inhibitors, are generally safe for asymptomatic patients with preserved left ventricular systolic function. Nitroglycerin is helpful in relieving angina pectoris in patients with CAD. Retrospective studies have shown that patients with degenerative calcific AS who receive HMG-CoA reductase inhibitors ("statins") exhibit slower progression of leaflet calcification and aortic valve area reduction than those who do not. However, randomized prospective studies with either high-dose atorvastatin or combination simvastatin/ezetimibe have failed to show a measurable effect on valve-related outcomes. The use of statin medications should continue to be driven by considerations regarding primary and secondary prevention of CAD. ACE inhibitors have not been studied prospectively for AS-related outcomes. The need for endocarditis prophylaxis is restricted to AS patients with a prior history of endocarditis.

SURGICAL TREATMENT Asymptomatic patients with calcific AS and severe obstruction should be followed carefully for the development of symptoms and by serial echocardiograms for evidence of deteriorating LV function. Operation is indicated in patients with severe AS (valve area <1 cm^2 or 0.6 cm^2/m^2 body surface area) who are symptomatic, those who exhibit LV dysfunction (EF <50%), as well as those with BAV disease and an aneurysmal or expanding aortic root (maximal dimension >4.5 cm or annual increase in size >0.5 cm/year), even if they are asymptomatic. Patients with asymptomatic moderate or severe AS who are referred for CABG surgery should also have AVR. In patients without heart failure, the operative risk of AVR is approximately 3% (Table 237-3) but increases as a function of age and the need for concomitant coronary revascularization with bypass grafting. The indications for AVR in the asymptomatic patient have been the subject of intense debate over the past 5 years, as surgical outcomes in selected patients have continued to improve. Relative indications for which surgery can be considered include an abnormal response to treadmill exercise; rapid progression of AS, especially when urgent access to medical care might be compromised; very severe AS defined by a valve area <0.6 cm^2; and severe LV hypertrophy suggested by a wall thickness of >15 mm. Exercise testing can be safely performed in the asymptomatic patient, as many as one-third of whom will show signs of functional impairment.

Operation should be carried out within 3–4 months of symptom onset and certainly well before frank LV failure develops; at this late stage, the aortic valve pressure gradient declines in parallel with the CO and stroke volume (low gradient, low output AS). In such patients, the perioperative mortality risk is high (15–20%), and evidence of myocardial disease may persist even when the operation is technically successful. Long-term postoperative survival correlates with preoperative LV function. Nonetheless, in view of the even worse prognosis of such patients when they are treated medically, there is usually little choice but to advise surgical treatment, especially in patients in whom contractile reserve can be demonstrated by dobutamine echocardiography (defined by a ≥20% in stroke volume after dobutamine challenge). In patients in whom severe AS and CAD coexist, relief of the AS and revascularization may sometimes result in striking clinical and hemodynamic improvement (Table 237-3).

Because many patients with calcific AS are elderly, particular attention must be directed to the adequacy of hepatic, renal, and pulmonary function before AVR is recommended. Age alone is not a contraindication to AVR for AS. The mortality rate depends to a substantial extent on the patient's preoperative clinical and hemodynamic state. The 10-year survival rate of patients with AVR is approximately 60%. Approximately 30% of bioprosthetic valves evidence primary valve failure in 10 years, requiring re-replacement, and an approximately equal percentage of patients with mechanical prostheses develop significant hemorrhagic complications as a consequence of treatment with anticoagulants (p. 1949). Homograft AVR is usually reserved for patients with aortic valve endocarditis.

The Ross procedure involves replacement of the diseased aortic valve with the autologous pulmonic valve and implantation of a homograft in the native pulmonic position. Its use has declined considerably in the United States because of the technical complexity of the procedure and the incidence of late postoperative aortic root dilation and autograft failure with AR. There is also a low incidence of homograft stenosis.

PERCUTANEOUS BALLOON AORTIC VALVULOPLASTY This procedure is preferable to operation in many children and young adults with congenital, noncalcific AS (Chap. 236). It is not commonly used in adults with severe calcific AS because of a very high restenosis rate (80% within 1 year) and the risk of procedural complications, but on occasion it has been used successfully as a "bridge to operation" in patients with severe LV dysfunction and shock who are too ill to tolerate surgery.

PERCUTANEOUS AORTIC VALVE REPLACEMENT Transcatheter aortic valve implantation (TAVI) for treatment of AS has been performed in more than 20,000 high-risk (Society for Thoracic Surgery mortality risk >10%) adult patients worldwide using one of two available systems, a balloon-expandable valve and a self-expanding valve, both of which incorporate a pericardial prosthesis (Fig. 237-8). The aorto-iliofemoral anatomy must allow for passage of large-bore catheters; a direct, trans-LV apical approach under surgical guidance is an alternative means of delivering the valve. There are also several reports of the successful use of axillary or subclavian artery access with construction of a vascular surgical sleeve. Aortic balloon valvuloplasty is performed as a first step to create an orifice sufficient for the prosthesis. Procedural success rates now exceed 90%, and intermediate-term prosthetic function is excellent. A mild degree of paravalvular AR is common with TAVI; postprocedural heart block is observed more frequently with the self-expanding valve. Preliminary results with TAVI have been very favorable (Fig. 237-9), and it is anticipated that this technology, now clinically available in Canada and Europe, will gain regulatory approval in the United States for the treatment of patients with severe AS considered too high risk for surgical AVR. For elderly patients with symptomatic, severe AS who are deemed too high risk for surgery, TAVI has been shown in a randomized prospective trial to prolong life and improve functionality. The use of these devices for the treatment of prosthetic valve failure not due to paravalvular regurgitation ("valve-in-valve"), as an alternative to reoperative valve replacement, is also under active study.

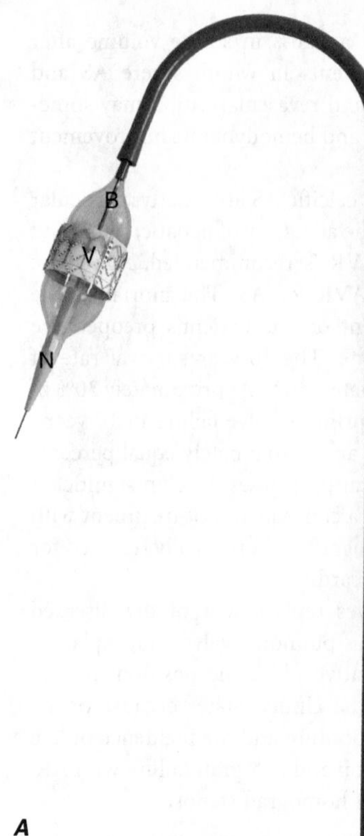

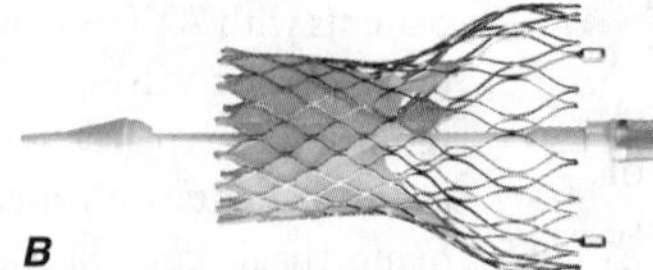

Figure 237-8 *A*. Balloon-expandable and *B* and self-expanding valves for percutaneous aortic valve replacement. B, inflated balloon; N, nose cone; V, valve. *(Part A, courtesy of Edwards Lifesciences, Irvine, CA; with permission. RetroFlex 3 is a trademark of Edwards Lifesciences Corporation. Part B, © Medtronic, Inc. 2010. Medtronic CoreValve™ Transcatheter Aortic Valve. CoreValve is a registered trademark of Medtronic, Inc.)*

AORTIC REGURGITATION

ETIOLOGY

(Table 237-1) AR may be caused by primary valve disease or by primary aortic root disease.

Primary valve disease

Rheumatic disease results in thickening, deformity, and shortening of the individual aortic valve cusps, changes that prevent their proper opening during systole and closure during diastole. A rheumatic origin is much less common in patients with isolated AR who do not have associated rheumatic mitral valve disease. Patients with congenital BAV disease may develop predominant AR, and approximately 20% of patients will require aortic valve surgery between 10 and 40 years of age. Congenital fenestrations of the aortic valve occasionally produce mild AR. Membranous subaortic stenosis often leads to thickening and scarring of the aortic valve leaflets with secondary AR. Prolapse of an aortic cusp, resulting in progressive chronic AR, occurs in approximately 15% of patients with ventricular septal defect (Chap. 236) but may also occur as an isolated phenomenon or as a consequence of myxomatous degeneration sometimes associated with mitral (p. 1937) and/or tricuspid valve involvement.

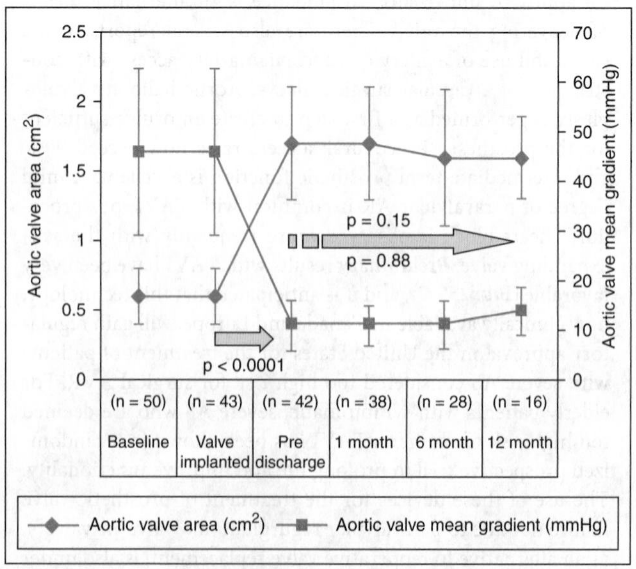

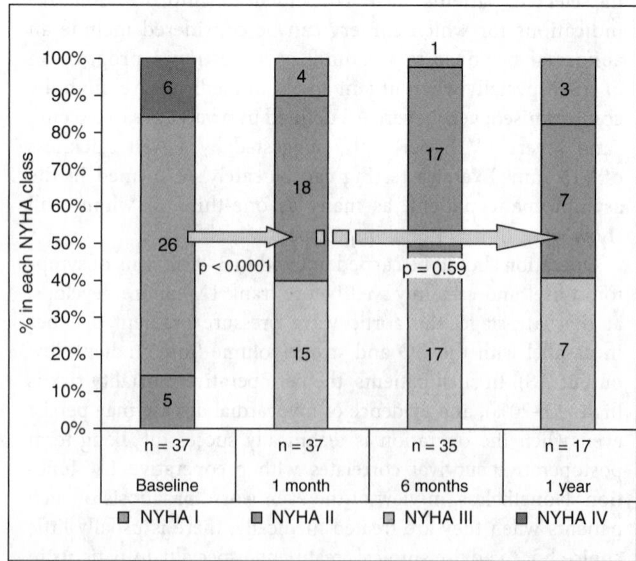

Figure 237-9 Twelve-month outcomes following percutaneous aortic valve replacement. *(Adapted from JG Webb et al: Circulation 116:755, 2007; with permission.)*

AR may result from infective endocarditis, which can develop on a valve previously affected by rheumatic disease, a congenitally deformed valve, or on a normal aortic valve, and may lead to perforation or erosion of one or more leaflets. The aortic valve leaflets may become scarred and retracted during the course of syphilis or ankylosing spondylitis and contribute further to the AR that derives primarily from the associated root disease. Although traumatic rupture or avulsion of the aortic valve is an uncommon cause of acute AR, it does represent the most frequent serious lesion in patients surviving nonpenetrating cardiac injuries. The coexistence of hemodynamically significant AS with AR usually excludes all the rarer forms of AR because it occurs almost exclusively in patients with rheumatic or congenital AR. In patients with AR due to primary valvular disease, dilation of the aortic annulus may occur secondarily and lead to worsening regurgitation.

Primary aortic root disease

AR may also be due entirely to marked aortic dilation, i.e., aortic root disease, without primary involvement of the valve leaflets; widening of the aortic annulus and separation of the aortic leaflets are responsible for the AR (Chap. 248). Cystic medial degeneration of the ascending aorta, which may or may not be associated with other manifestations of Marfan's syndrome; idiopathic dilation of the aorta; annuloaortic ectasia; osteogenesis imperfecta; and severe hypertension may all widen the aortic annulus and lead to progressive AR. Occasionally AR is caused by retrograde dissection of the aorta involving the aortic annulus. Syphilis and ankylosing spondylitis, both of which may affect aortic valves, may also be associated with cellular infiltration and scarring of the media of the thoracic aorta, leading to aortic dilation, aneurysm formation, and severe regurgitation. In syphilis of the aorta (Chap. 169), now a very rare condition, the involvement of the intima may narrow the coronary ostia, which in turn may be responsible for myocardial ischemia.

PATHOPHYSIOLOGY

The total stroke volume ejected by the LV (i.e., the sum of the effective forward stroke volume and the volume of blood that regurgitates back into the LV) is increased in patients with AR. In patients with severe AR, the volume of regurgitant flow may equal the effective forward stroke volume. In contrast to MR, in which a portion of the LV stroke volume is delivered into the low-pressure LA, in AR the entire LV stroke volume is ejected into a high-pressure zone, the aorta. An increase in the LV end-diastolic volume (increased preload) constitutes the major hemodynamic compensation for AR. The dilation and eccentric hypertrophy of the LV allow this chamber to eject a larger stroke volume without requiring any increase in the relative shortening of each myofibril. Therefore, severe AR may occur with a normal effective forward stroke volume and a normal left ventricular EF [total (forward plus regurgitant) stroke volume/end-diastolic volume], together with an elevated LV end-diastolic pressure and volume. However, through the operation of Laplace's law, LV dilation increases the LV systolic tension required to develop any given level of systolic pressure. Chronic AR is, thus, a state in which LV preload and afterload are both increased. Ultimately, these adaptive measures fail. As LV function deteriorates, the end-diastolic volume rises further and the forward stroke volume and EF decline. Deterioration of LV function often precedes the development of symptoms. Considerable thickening of the LV wall also occurs with chronic AR, and at autopsy the hearts of these patients may be among the largest encountered, sometimes weighing >1000 g.

The reverse pressure gradient from aorta to LV, which drives the AR flow, falls progressively during diastole, accounting for the decrescendo nature of the diastolic murmur. Equilibration between aortic and LV pressures may occur toward the end of diastole in patients with chronic severe AR, particularly when the heart rate is slow. In patients with acute severe AR, the LV is unprepared for the regurgitant volume load. LV compliance is normal or reduced, and LV diastolic pressures rise rapidly, occasionally to levels >40 mmHg. The LV pressure may exceed the LA pressure toward the end of diastole, and this reversed pressure gradient closes the mitral valve prematurely.

In patients with chronic severe AR, the effective forward CO usually is normal or only slightly reduced at rest, but often it fails to rise normally during exertion. An early sign of LV dysfunction is a reduction in the EF. In advanced stages there may be considerable elevation of the LA, PA wedge, PA, and RV pressures and lowering of the forward CO at rest.

Myocardial ischemia may occur in patients with AR because myocardial oxygen requirements are elevated by LV dilation, hypertrophy, and elevated LV systolic tension, and coronary blood flow may be compromised. A large fraction of coronary blood flow occurs during diastole, when arterial pressure is low, thereby reducing coronary perfusion or driving pressure. This combination of increased oxygen demand and reduced supply may cause myocardial ischemia, particularly of the subendocardium, even in the absence of concomitant CAD.

HISTORY

Approximately three-fourths of patients with pure or predominant valvular AR are men; women predominate among patients with primary valvular AR who have associated rheumatic mitral valve disease. A history compatible with infective endocarditis may sometimes be elicited from patients with rheumatic or congenital involvement of the aortic valve, and the infection often precipitates or seriously aggravates preexisting symptoms.

In patients with *acute severe AR*, as may occur in infective endocarditis, aortic dissection, or trauma, the LV cannot dilate sufficiently to maintain stroke volume, and LV diastolic pressure rises rapidly with associated marked elevations of LA and PA wedge pressures. Pulmonary edema and/or cardiogenic shock may develop rapidly.

Chronic severe AR may have a long latent period, and patients may remain relatively asymptomatic for as long as 10–15 years. However, uncomfortable awareness of the heartbeat, especially on lying down, may be an early complaint. Sinus tachycardia, during exertion or with emotion, or premature ventricular contractions may produce particularly uncomfortable palpitations as well as head pounding. These complaints may persist for many years before the development of exertional dyspnea, usually the first symptom of diminished cardiac reserve. The dyspnea is followed by orthopnea, paroxysmal nocturnal dyspnea, and excessive diaphoresis. Anginal chest pain even in the absence of CAD may occur in patients with severe AR, even in younger patients. Anginal pain may develop at rest as well as during exertion. Nocturnal angina may be a particularly troublesome symptom, and it may be accompanied by marked diaphoresis. The anginal episodes can be prolonged and often do not respond satisfactorily to sublingual nitroglycerin. Systemic fluid accumulation, including congestive hepatomegaly and ankle edema, may develop late in the course of the disease.

PHYSICAL FINDINGS

In chronic severe AR, the jarring of the entire body and the bobbing motion of the head with each systole can be appreciated, and the abrupt distention and collapse of the larger arteries are easily visible. The examination should be directed toward the detection of conditions predisposing to AR, such as bicuspid valve, endocarditis, Marfan's syndrome, and ankylosing spondylitis.

Arterial pulse

A rapidly rising "water-hammer" pulse, which collapses suddenly as arterial pressure falls rapidly during late systole and diastole

(Corrigan's pulse), and capillary pulsations, an alternate flushing and paling of the skin at the root of the nail while pressure is applied to the tip of the nail (Quincke's pulse), are characteristic of chronic severe AR. A booming "pistol-shot" sound can be heard over the femoral arteries (Traube's sign), and a to-and-fro murmur (Duroziez's sign) is audible if the femoral artery is lightly compressed with a stethoscope.

The arterial pulse pressure is widened as a result of both systolic hypertension and a lowering of the diastolic pressure. The measurement of arterial diastolic pressure with a sphygmomanometer may be complicated by the fact that systolic sounds are frequently heard with the cuff completely deflated. However, the level of cuff pressure at the time of muffling of the Korotkoff sounds (phase IV) generally corresponds fairly closely to the true intraarterial diastolic pressure. As the disease progresses and the LV end-diastolic pressure rises, the arterial diastolic pressure may actually rise as well, because the aortic diastolic pressure cannot fall below the LV end-diastolic pressure. For the same reason, acute severe AR may also be accompanied by only a slight widening of the pulse pressure. Such patients are invariably tachycardic as the heart rate increases in an attempt to preserve the CO.

Palpation

In patients with chronic severe AR, the LV impulse is heaving and displaced laterally and inferiorly. The systolic expansion and diastolic retraction of the apex are prominent. A diastolic thrill may be palpable along the left sternal border in thin-chested individuals, and a prominent systolic thrill may be palpable in the suprasternal notch and transmitted upward along the carotid arteries. This systolic thrill and the accompanying murmur do not necessarily signify the coexistence of AS. In many patients with pure AR or with combined AS and AR, the carotid arterial pulse is bisferiens, i.e., with two systolic waves separated by a trough (see Fig. 227-2*D*).

Auscultation

In patients with severe AR, the aortic valve closure sound (A_2) is usually absent. A systolic ejection sound is audible in patients with BAV disease, and occasionally an S_4 also may be heard. The murmur of chronic AR is typically a high-pitched, blowing, decrescendo diastolic murmur, heard best in the third intercostal space along the left sternal border (see Fig. 227-5*B*). In patients with mild AR, this murmur is brief, but as the severity increases, it generally becomes louder and longer, indeed holodiastolic. When the murmur is soft, it can be heard best with the diaphragm of the stethoscope and with the patient sitting up, leaning forward, and with the breath held in forced expiration. In patients in whom the AR is caused by primary valvular disease, the diastolic murmur is usually louder along the left than the right sternal border. However, when the murmur is heard best along the right sternal border, it suggests that the AR is caused by aneurysmal dilation of the aortic root. "Cooing" or musical diastolic murmurs suggest eversion of an aortic cusp vibrating in the regurgitant stream.

A mid-systolic ejection murmur is frequently audible in isolated AR. It is generally heard best at the base of the heart and is transmitted along the carotid arteries. This murmur may be quite loud without signifying aortic obstruction. A third murmur sometimes heard in patients with severe AR is the *Austin Flint murmur,* a soft, low-pitched, rumbling mid-to-late diastolic murmur. It is probably produced by the diastolic displacement of the anterior leaflet of the mitral valve by the AR stream and is not associated with hemodynamically significant mitral obstruction. The auscultatory features of AR are intensified by strenuous and sustained handgrip, which augments systemic vascular resistance.

In acute severe AR, the elevation of LV end-diastolic pressure may lead to early closure of the mitral valve, a soft S_1, a pulse pressure that is not particularly wide, and a soft, short, early diastolic murmur of AR.

LABORATORY EXAMINATION

ECG

In patients with chronic severe AR, the ECG signs of LV hypertrophy become manifest (Chap. 228). In addition, these patients frequently exhibit ST-segment depression and T-wave inversion in leads I, aVL, V_5, and V_6 ("LV strain"). Left-axis deviation and/or QRS prolongation denote diffuse myocardial disease, generally associated with patchy fibrosis, and usually signify a poor prognosis.

Echocardiogram

LV size is increased in chronic AR and systolic function is normal or even supernormal until myocardial contractility declines, as signaled by a decrease in ejection or increase in the end-systolic dimension. A rapid, high-frequency diastolic fluttering of the anterior mitral leaflet produced by the impact of the regurgitant jet is a characteristic finding. The echocardiogram is also useful in determining the cause of AR, by detecting dilation of the aortic annulus and root, aortic dissection (see Fig. 229-5), or primary leaflet pathology. With severe AR, the central jet width assessed by color flow Doppler imaging exceeds 65% of the left ventricular outflow tract, the regurgitant volume is ≥60 mL/beat, the regurgitant fraction is ≥50%, and there is diastolic flow reversal in the proximal descending thoracic aorta. The continuous wave Doppler profile shows a rapid deceleration time in patients with acute severe AR, due to the rapid increase in LV diastolic pressure. Surveillance transthoracic echocardiography forms the cornerstone of longitudinal follow-up and allows for the early detection of changes in LV size and/or function. For patients in whom echocardiography is limited by poor acoustical windows or inadequate semiquantitative assessment, gated cardiac MR imaging can be performed. This modality also allows for accurate assessment of aortic size and contour.

Chest x-ray

In chronic severe AR, the apex is displaced downward and to the left in the frontal projection. In the left anterior oblique and lateral projections, the LV is displaced posteriorly and encroaches on the spine. When AR is caused by primary disease of the aortic root, aneurysmal dilation of the aorta may be noted, and the aorta may fill the retrosternal space in the lateral view. Echocardiography, cardiac MR, and CT angiography are more sensitive than the chest x-ray for the detection of aortic root enlargement.

Cardiac catheterization and angiography

When needed, right and left heart catheterization with contrast aortography can provide confirmation of the magnitude of regurgitation and the status of LV function. Coronary angiography is performed routinely in appropriate patients prior to surgery.

TREATMENT Aortic Regurgitation

ACUTE AORTIC REGURGITATION (See Fig. 237-10) Patients with acute severe AR may respond to intravenous diuretics and vasodilators (such as sodium nitroprusside), but stabilization is usually short-lived and operation is indicated urgently. Intraaortic balloon counterpulsation is contraindicated. Beta blockers are also best avoided so as not to reduce the CO further or slow the heart rate. Surgery is the treatment of choice and is usually necessary within 24 hours of diagnosis.

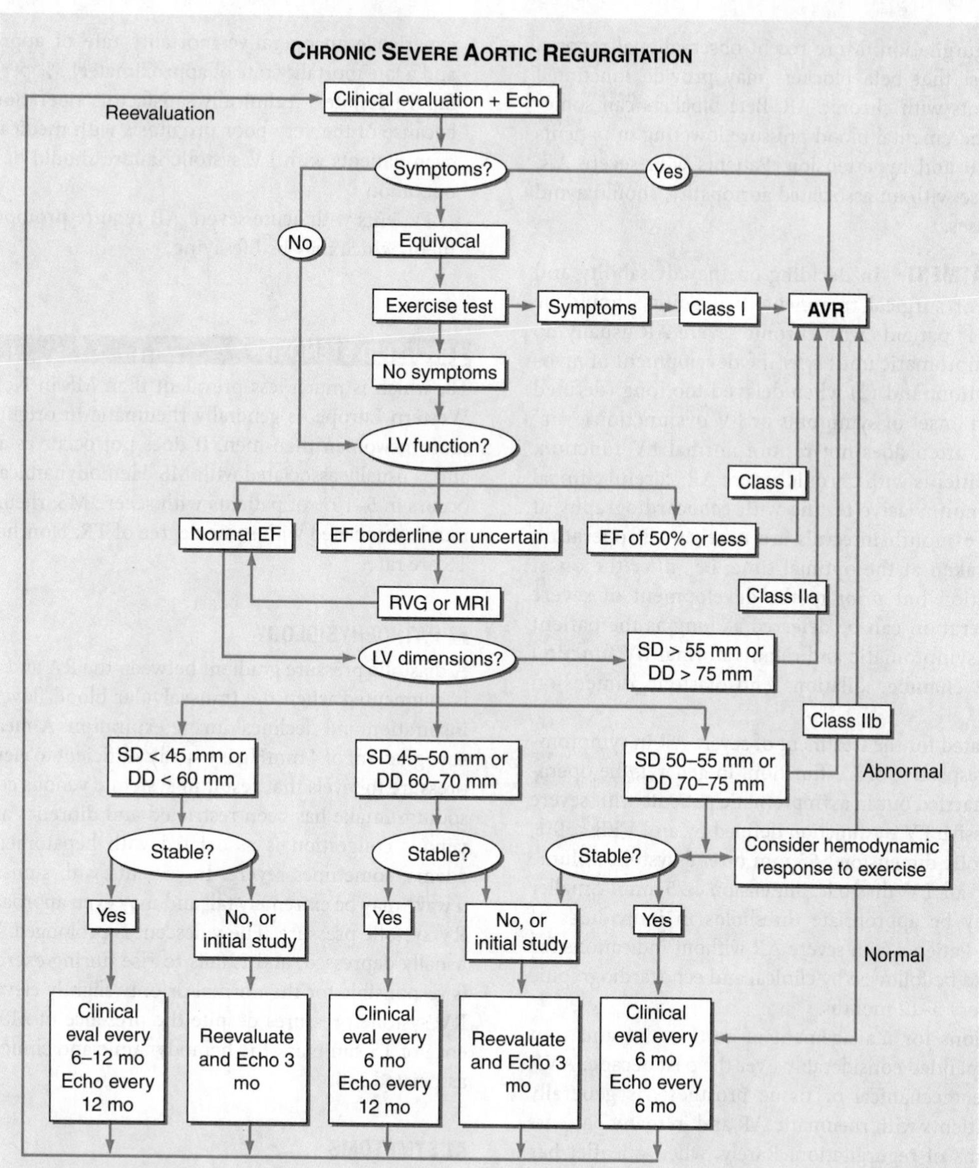

Figure 237-10 Management strategy for patients with chronic severe aortic regurgitation. Preoperative coronary angiography should be performed routinely, as determined by age, symptoms, and coronary risk factors. Cardiac catheterization and angiography may also be helpful when there is a discrepancy between clinical and echocardiographic findings. "Stable" refers to stable echocardiographic measurements. In some centers, serial follow-up may be performed with radionuclide ventriculography (RVG) or magnetic resonance imaging (MRI) rather than echocardiography (echo) to assess left ventricular (LV) volume and systolic function. AVR, aortic valve replacement; DD, end-diastolic dimension; EF, ejection fraction; eval, evaluation; SD, end-systolic dimension. *(Modified from Bonow et al.)*

CHRONIC AORTIC REGURGITATION Early symptoms of dyspnea and effort intolerance respond to treatment with diuretics; vasodilators (ACE inhibitors, dihydropyridine calcium channel blockers, or hydralazine) may be useful as well. Surgery can then be performed in a more controlled setting. The use of vasodilators to extend the compensated phase of chronic severe AR before the onset of symptoms or the development of LV dysfunction is more controversial. Expert consensus is strong regarding the need to control systolic blood pressure (goal <140 mmHg) in patients with chronic AR, and vasodilators are an excellent first choice as antihypertensive agents. It is often difficult to achieve adequate control because of the increased stroke volume that accompanies severe AR. Cardiac arrhythmias and systemic infections are poorly tolerated in patients with severe AR and must be treated promptly and vigorously. Although nitroglycerin and long-acting nitrates are not as helpful in relieving anginal pain as they are in patients with ischemic heart disease, they are worth a trial. Patients with syphilitic aortitis should receive a full course of penicillin therapy (Chap. 169). Beta blockers and the angiotensin receptor blocker, losartan, may be useful to retard the rate of aortic root enlargement in young patients with Marfan's syndrome and aortic root dilation. Early reports of the efficacy of losartan in patients with Marfan's syndrome have led to its use in other populations of patients, including those with BAV disease and aortopathy. The use of beta blockers in patients with valvular AR was previously felt to be relatively contraindicated due to concerns that the resulting slowing of the heart rate would allow more time for diastolic regurgitation. More recent observational reports, however, suggest that beta blockers may provide functional benefit in patients with chronic AR. Beta blockers can sometimes provide incremental blood pressure lowering in patients with chronic AR and hypertension. Patients with severe AR, particularly those with an associated aortopathy, should avoid isometric exercises.

SURGICAL TREATMENT In deciding on the advisability and proper timing of surgical treatment, two points should be kept in mind: (1) patients with chronic severe AR usually do not become symptomatic until *after* the development of myocardial dysfunction; and (2) when delayed too long (defined as >1 year from onset of symptoms or LV dysfunction), surgical treatment often does not restore normal LV function. Therefore, in patients with chronic severe AR, careful clinical follow-up and noninvasive testing with echocardiography at approximately 6-month intervals are necessary if operation is to be undertaken at the optimal time, i.e., *after* the onset of LV dysfunction but *prior* to the development of severe symptoms. Operation can be deferred as long as the patient both remains asymptomatic and retains normal LV function without severe chamber dilation (end-diastolic dimension >75 mm).

AVR is indicated for the treatment of severe AR in symptomatic patients irrespective of LV function. In general, the operation should be carried out in asymptomatic patients with severe AR and progressive LV dysfunction defined by an LVEF <50%, an LV end-systolic dimension >55 mm or end-systolic volume >55 mL/m^2, or an LV diastolic dimension >75 mm. Smaller dimensions may be appropriate thresholds in individuals of smaller stature. Patients with severe AR without indications for operation should be followed by clinical and echocardiographic examination every 3–12 months.

Surgical options for management of aortic valve and root disease have expanded considerably over the past decade. AVR with a suitable mechanical or tissue prosthesis is generally necessary in patients with rheumatic AR and in many patients with other forms of regurgitation. Rarely, when a leaflet has been perforated during infective endocarditis or torn from its attachments to the aortic annulus by thoracic trauma, primary surgical repair may be possible. When AR is due to aneurysmal dilation of the root, or proximal ascending aorta, rather than to primary valve involvement, it may be possible to reduce or eliminate the regurgitation by narrowing the annulus or by excising a portion of the aortic root without replacing the valve. Elective, valve-sparing aortic root reconstruction generally involves reimplantation of the valve in a contoured graft with reattachment of the coronary artery buttons into the side of the graft and is best undertaken in specialized surgical centers (Fig. 237-11). Resuspension of the native aortic valve leaflets is possible in approximately 50% of patients with acute AR in the setting of type A aortic dissection. In other conditions, however, regurgitation can be effectively eliminated only by replacing the aortic valve, the dilated or aneurysmal ascending aorta responsible for the regurgitation, and implanting a composite valve-graft conduit. This formidable procedure entails a higher risk than isolated AVR.

As in patients with other valvular abnormalities, both the operative risk and the late mortality rate are largely dependent on the stage of the disease and myocardial function at the time of operation. The overall operative mortality rate for isolated AVR is approximately 3% (Table 237-3). However, patients with marked cardiac enlargement and prolonged LV dysfunction experience an operative mortality rate of approximately 10% and a late mortality rate of approximately 5% per year due to LV failure despite a technically satisfactory operation. Nonetheless, because of the very poor prognosis with medical management, even patients with LV systolic failure should be considered for operation.

Patients with acute severe AR require prompt surgical treatment, which may be lifesaving.

TRICUSPID STENOSIS

TS, which is much less prevalent than MS in North America and Western Europe, is generally rheumatic in origin and more common in women than men. It does not occur as an isolated lesion and is usually associated with MS. Hemodynamically significant TS occurs in 5–10% of patients with severe MS; rheumatic TS is commonly associated with some degree of TR. Nonrheumatic causes of TS are rare.

PATHOPHYSIOLOGY

A diastolic pressure gradient between the RA and RV defines TS. It is augmented when the transvalvular blood flow increases during inspiration and declines during expiration. A mean diastolic pressure gradient of 4 mmHg is usually sufficient to elevate the mean RA pressure to levels that result in systemic venous congestion. Unless sodium intake has been restricted and diuretics administered, this venous congestion is associated with hepatomegaly, ascites, and edema, sometimes severe. In patients with sinus rhythm, the RA *a* wave may be extremely tall and may even approach the level of the RV systolic pressure. The *y* descent is prolonged. The CO at rest is usually depressed, and it fails to rise during exercise. The low CO is responsible for the normal or only slightly elevated LA, PA, and RV systolic pressures despite the presence of MS. Thus, the presence of TS can mask the hemodynamic and clinical features of any associated MS.

SYMPTOMS

Because the development of MS generally precedes that of TS, many patients initially have symptoms of pulmonary congestion and fatigue. Characteristically, patients with severe TS complain of relatively little dyspnea for the degree of hepatomegaly, ascites, and edema that they have. However, fatigue secondary to a low CO and discomfort due to refractory edema, ascites, and marked hepatomegaly are common in patients with TS and/or TR. In some patients, TS may be suspected for the first time when symptoms of right-sided failure persist after an adequate mitral valvotomy.

PHYSICAL FINDINGS

Because TS usually occurs in the presence of other obvious valvular disease, the diagnosis may be missed unless it is considered. Severe TS is associated with marked hepatic congestion, often resulting in cirrhosis, jaundice, serious malnutrition, anasarca, and ascites. Congestive hepatomegaly and, in cases of severe tricuspid valve disease, splenomegaly are present. The jugular veins are distended, and in patients with sinus rhythm there may be giant *a* waves. The *v* waves are less conspicuous, and because tricuspid obstruction impedes RA emptying during diastole, there is a slow *y* descent. In patients with sinus rhythm there may be prominent presystolic pulsations of the enlarged liver as well.

On auscultation, an OS of the tricuspid valve may rarely be heard approximately 0.06 s after pulmonic valve closure. The diastolic

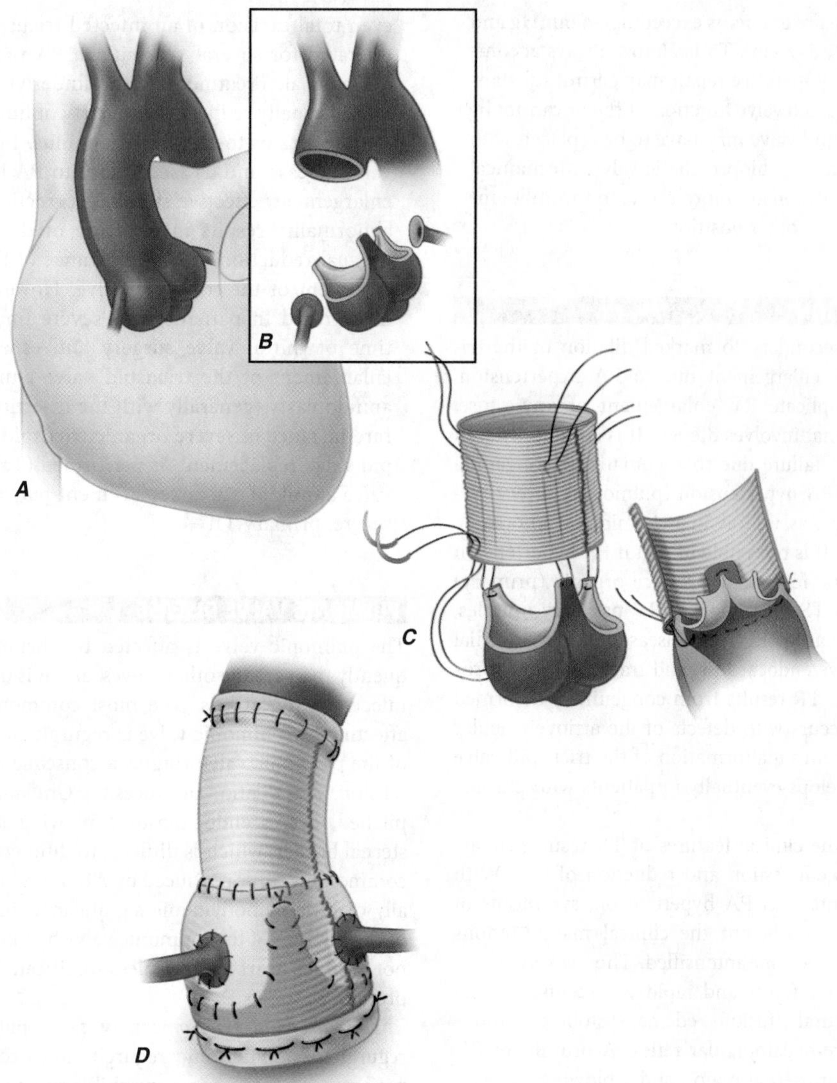

Figure 237-11 Valve-sparing aortic root reconstruction (David procedure). *(From P Steltzer et al (eds): Valvular Heart Disease: A Companion to Braunwald's Heart Disease, 3rd ed, Fig 12-27, p. 200.)*

murmur of TS has many of the qualities of the diastolic murmur of MS, and because TS almost always occurs in the presence of MS, it may be missed. However, the tricuspid murmur is generally heard best along the left lower sternal border and over the xiphoid process, and is most prominent during presystole in patients with sinus rhythm. The murmur of TS is augmented during inspiration, and it is reduced during expiration and particularly during the strain phase of the Valsalva maneuver, when tricuspid transvalvular flow is reduced.

■ LABORATORY EXAMINATION

The ECG features of RA enlargement (see Fig. 228-8) include tall, peaked P waves in lead II, as well as prominent, upright P waves in lead V_1. The *absence* of ECG evidence of right ventricular hypertrophy (RVH) in a patient with right-sided heart failure who is believed to have MS should suggest associated tricuspid valve disease. The chest x-ray in patients with combined TS and MS shows particular prominence of the RA and superior vena cava without much enlargement of the PA and with less evidence of pulmonary vascular congestion than occurs in patients with isolated MS. On echocardiographic examination, the tricuspid valve is usually thickened and domes in diastole; the transvalvular gradient can be estimated routinely by continuous wave Doppler echocardiography. TTE provides additional information regarding mitral valve structure and function, LV and RV size and function, and PA pressure.

TREATMENT Tricuspid Stenosis

Patients with TS generally exhibit marked systemic venous congestion; intensive salt restriction, bed rest, and diuretic therapy are required during the preoperative period. Such a preparatory period may diminish hepatic congestion and thereby improve hepatic function sufficiently so that the risks of operation, particularly bleeding, are diminished. Surgical relief of the TS should be carried out, preferably at the time of surgical mitral valvotomy or MVR, in patients with moderate or severe TS who have mean diastolic pressure gradients exceeding ~4 mmHg and tricuspid orifice areas <1.5–2 cm^2. TS is almost always accompanied by significant TR. Operative repair may permit substantial improvement of tricuspid valve function. If repair cannot be accomplished, the tricuspid valve may have to be replaced with a prosthesis, preferably a large bioprosthetic valve. Mechanical valves in the tricuspid position are more prone to thromboembolic complications than in other positions.

TRICUSPID REGURGITATION

Most commonly, TR is secondary to marked dilation of the tricuspid annulus from RV enlargement due to PA hypertension. Functional TR may complicate RV enlargement of any cause, including an inferior MI that involves the RV. It is commonly seen in the late stages of heart failure due to rheumatic or congenital heart disease with severe PA hypertension (pulmonary artery systolic pressure >55 mmHg), as well as in ischemic and idiopathic dilated cardiomyopathies. It is reversible in part if PA hypertension can be relieved. Rheumatic fever may produce organic (primary) TR, often associated with TS. Infarction of RV papillary muscles, tricuspid valve prolapse, carcinoid heart disease, endomyocardial fibrosis, radiation, infective endocarditis, and trauma all may produce TR. Less commonly, TR results from congenitally deformed tricuspid valves, and it occurs with defects of the atrioventricular canal, as well as with Ebstein's malformation of the tricuspid valve (Chap. 236). TR also develops eventually in patients with chronic RV apical pacing.

As is the case for TS, the clinical features of TR result primarily from systemic venous congestion and reduction of CO. With the onset of TR in patients with PA hypertension, symptoms of pulmonary congestion diminish, but the clinical manifestations of right-sided heart failure become intensified. The neck veins are distended with prominent *v* waves and rapid *y* descents, marked hepatomegaly, ascites, pleural effusions, edema, systolic pulsations of the liver, and a positive hepatojugular reflex. A prominent RV pulsation along the left parasternal region and a blowing holosystolic murmur along the lower left sternal margin, which may be intensified during inspiration and reduced during expiration or the strain of the Valsalva maneuver, are characteristic findings; AF is usually present.

The ECG may show changes characteristic of the lesion responsible for the enlargement of the RV that leads to TR, e.g., an inferior Q-wave MI or RVH. Echocardiography may be helpful by demonstrating RV dilation and prolapsing, flail, scarred, or displaced tricuspid leaflets; the diagnosis and assessment of TR can be made by color flow Doppler imaging (see Fig. 229-8). Severe TR is accompanied by hepatic vein systolic flow reversal. Continuous wave Doppler of the TR velocity profile is useful in estimating PA systolic pressure. Roentgenographic examination usually reveals enlargement of both the RA and RV.

In patients with severe TR, the CO is usually markedly reduced, and the RA pressure pulse may exhibit no *x* descent during early systole but a prominent *c-v* wave with a rapid *y* descent. The mean RA and the RV end-diastolic pressures are often elevated.

TREATMENT Tricuspid Regurgitation

Isolated TR, in the absence of PA hypertension, such as that occurring as a consequence of infective endocarditis or trauma, is usually well tolerated and does not require operation. Indeed, even total excision of an infected tricuspid valve may be well tolerated for several years if the PA pressure and resistance are normal. Treatment of the underlying cause of left heart failure usually reduces the severity of functional TR, by reducing the size of the tricuspid annulus. In patients with mitral valve disease and TR secondary to PA hypertension and RV enlargement, effective surgical correction of the mitral valve abnormality results in lowering of the PA pressures and a gradual reduction or disappearance of the TR without direct treatment of the tricuspid valve. However, recovery may be more rapid in patients with severe functional TR if, at the time of mitral valve surgery and especially when there is enlargement of the tricuspid valve annulus, tricuspid valve annuloplasty (generally with the insertion of a ring) or in the rare instance of severe organic tricuspid valve disease, tricuspid valve replacement, is performed (Table 237-3). Tricuspid valve annuloplasty or replacement may rarely be required for severe, primary TR.

PULMONIC VALVE DISEASE

The pulmonic valve is affected by rheumatic fever far less frequently than are the other valves, and it is uncommonly a nidus for infective endocarditis. The most common *acquired* abnormality affecting the pulmonic valve is regurgitation secondary to dilation of the pulmonic valve ring as a consequence of severe PA hypertension. This dilation produces the *Graham Steell murmur,* a high-pitched, decrescendo, diastolic blowing murmur along the left sternal border, which is difficult to differentiate from the far more common murmur produced by AR. Pulmonic regurgitation is usually of little hemodynamic significance; indeed, surgical removal or destruction of the pulmonic valve by infective endocarditis does not produce heart failure unless significant PA hypertension is also present.

The *carcinoid syndrome* may cause pulmonic stenosis and/or regurgitation. Pulmonic regurgitation occurs universally among patients who have undergone childhood repair of tetralogy of Fallot with reconstruction of the RV outflow tract. Congenital pulmonic stenosis is discussed in Chap. 236.

Percutaneous pulmonic valve replacement has been successfully performed in many patients with severe PR after childhood repair of tetralogy of Fallot or pulmonic valve stenosis or atresia. This procedure was introduced clinically prior to percutaneous aortic valve replacement.

MULTIPLE AND MIXED VALVULAR HEART DISEASE

Many acquired and congenital cardiac lesions may result in stenosis and/or regurgitation of one or more heart valves. For example, rheumatic fever may present with mitral (MS, MR, MS and MR), aortic (AS, AR, AS and AR), and/or tricuspid (TS, TR, TS and TR) valve involvement. The common association of secondary TR with significant mitral valve disease has been discussed previously. Aortic valve infective endocarditis may secondarily involve the mitral apparatus. Mediastinal radiation may result in aortic, mitral, and even tricuspid valve disease, most often with mixed stenosis and regurgitation. Ergotamines, and the previously used combination of fenfluramine and phentermine, may result in mixed valve lesions, as are also seen in patients with carcinoid heart disease. Patients with Marfan's syndrome may have both AR from root dilation and MR due to MVP.

The clinical assessment of patients with multiple or mixed valve disease can be challenging, With combined mitral and aortic valve disease, the hemodynamic derangements associated with the mitral lesion(s) may mask the full expression of the aortic valve disease. For example, severe mitral stenosis may decrease LV preload to the extent that the severity of AS or AR can be underappreciated. Alternatively, the development of AF during the course of MS can lead to sudden worsening in a patient whose aortic valve disease was not previously felt to be significant. In patients with mixed MS/MR or AS/AR, the regurgitant lesion usually predominates, and can be followed primarily as the trigger for surgical or transcatheter intervention as appropriate. Nevertheless, there are frequent exceptions to the rules, and careful assessment is indicated. The LV in a patient with hypertrophy in the setting of both AS and AR may not be able to dilate in response to the volume load imposed by the regurgitant lesion and, thus, show signs or lead to the development of symptoms of compromise at a relatively earlier point in the natural history. Serial echocardiography can aid in decision-making.

Similar considerations pertain to the evaluation of patients with heart valve disease and other cardiac and systemic disorders that can contribute to impaired exercise tolerance, such as hypertension, coronary artery disease, obesity, sleep apnea, and skeletal muscle deconditioning.

VALVE REPLACEMENT AND REPAIR

The results of valve replacement surgery are dependent on (1) the patient's myocardial function and general medical condition at the time of operation; (2) the technical abilities of the operative team and the quality of the postoperative care; and (3) the durability, hemodynamic characteristics, and thrombogenicity of the prosthesis. Increased perioperative mortality rate is associated with advanced age and comorbidity rate (e.g., pulmonary or renal disease, the need for nonvalvular cardiovascular surgery, diabetes mellitus) as well as with greater levels of preoperative functional disability and PA hypertension. Late complications of valve replacement include thromboemboli, bleeding due to anticoagulants, mechanical valve thrombosis, pannus ingrowth, paravalvular leak, hemolysis, structural deterioration, infective endocarditis, and prosthesis-patient mismatch (functional prosthetic valve stenosis that occurs when the prosthesis is too small relative to the patient's anatomy).

The choice between a tissue and mechanical prosthesis is essentially a trade-off between the risk of structural valve deterioration and the possible need for reoperation with a tissue valve versus the obligate need for lifelong anticoagulation and its attendant risks with a mechanical valve. The incidence of structural valve deterioration varies inversely with patient age and may be accelerated further by pregnancy or end-stage renal disease. Failure of a tissue prosthesis results in the need for reoperation in up to 30% of patients by 10 years and in 50% by 15 years. Rates of structural valve deterioration are higher for mitral than for aortic bioprostheses. This phenomenon may be due in part to the greater closing pressure to which a mitral prosthesis is exposed.

Traditionally, a mechanical prosthesis was considered preferable for a patient younger than age 65 who could take anticoagulants reliably. Bioprostheses were recommended for older patients (>65 years) who did not otherwise have an indication for anticoagulation (e.g., AF). Recent surveys of cardiac surgery in the United States, as reflected in the Society of Thoracic Surgeons database, show a clear and progressive trend favoring the implantation of bioprosthetic valves in younger (<65 years) patients. Reasons for this development include improved durability of newer generation bioprostheses, decreased risk of death or major complication at time of reoperation, the hazards of long-term anticoagulation, and patient preference to avoid anticoagulation for lifestyle reasons. Patient preference must be factored into any decision regarding the type of valve replacement. A mechanical prosthesis is reasonable for aortic or mitral valve replacement in patients younger than 65 years without a contraindication to anticoagulation. A bioprosthesis is equally reasonable for aortic or mitral valve replacement in patients younger than 65 years who elect this strategy for lifestyle reasons with full knowledge of the likely need for reoperation over time.

Bioprostheses remain the preferred valve choice for patients older than 65 years, in both the aortic and mitral position. Bioprosthetic valves are also indicated for women who expect to become pregnant, as well as for others who refuse to take anticoagulation or for whom anticoagulation may be contraindicated. Types of bioprostheses include xenografts (e.g., porcine aortic valves; cryopreserved, mounted bovine pericardial valves), homograft (allograft) aortic valves obtained from cadavers, and pulmonary autografts transplanted into the aortic position (Ross procedure). Homograft replacement may be preferred for the management of complicated aortic valve infective endocarditis.

In patients without contraindications to anticoagulants, particularly those younger than 65 years, a mechanical prosthesis is reasonable. Many surgeons now select the St. Jude prosthesis, a double-disk tilting prosthesis, for replacement of both aortic and mitral valves because of favorable hemodynamic characteristics and possible association with lower thrombogenicity. A tissue valve is preferred for tricuspid replacement.

The decision to proceed with valve replacement should be finalized only after an experienced surgeon has agreed that valve repair is either not appropriate or not feasible. As noted previously, valve repair techniques have improved considerably over the past 10–15 years, for both mitral and aortic lesions. Primary repair is often associated with a lower risk of postoperative LV functional impairment, particularly for patients with MR, and avoids the long-term risks of a prosthesis.

Antibiotic prophylaxis prior to dental procedures that involve manipulation of gingival tissue or the periapical region of teeth or perforation of the oral mucosa is indicated for patients after valve replacement or ring annuloplasty. Prosthetic valve and ventricular function should be assessed with transthoracic echocardiography 3 months after surgery and a baseline complete blood count, reticulocyte count, and serum lactate dehydrogenase (LDH) test obtained to serve as a baseline set of values should the question of hemolysis arise in the future. The intensity of anticoagulation should follow recommended guidelines.

GLOBAL BURDEN OF VALVULAR HEART DISEASE

Primary valvular heart disease ranks well below coronary heart disease, stroke, hypertension, obesity, and diabetes as major threats to the public health. Nevertheless, it is the source of significant morbidity and mortality rates. Rheumatic fever (Chap. 322) is the dominant cause of valvular heart disease in developing countries. Its prevalence has been estimated to range from as low as 1 per 100,000 school-age children in Costa Rica to as high as 150 per 100,000 in China. Rheumatic heart disease accounts for 12–65% of hospital admissions related to cardiovascular disease and 2–10% of hospital discharges in some developing countries. Prevalence and mortality rates vary among communities even within the same country as a function of crowding and the availability of medical resources and population-wide programs for detection and treatment of group A streptococcal pharyngitis. In economically deprived areas, tropical and subtropical climates (particularly on the Indian subcontinent),

Central America, and the Middle East, rheumatic valvular disease progresses more rapidly than in more-developed nations and frequently causes serious symptoms in patients younger than 20 years of age. This accelerated natural history may be due to repeated infections with more virulent strains of rheumatogenic streptococci. Approximately 16 million people live with rheumatic heart disease worldwide. As of 2000, worldwide death rates for rheumatic heart disease approximated 5.5 per 100,000 population (n = 332,000), with the highest rates reported from Southeast Asia (7.6 per 100,000).

Although there have been recent reports of isolated outbreaks of streptococcal infection in North America, valve disease in developed countries is now dominated by degenerative or inflammatory processes that lead to valve thickening, calcification, and dysfunction. The prevalence of valvular heart disease increases with age. Important left-sided valve disease may affect as many as 12–13% of adults older than the age of 75. In the United States, there were 1.5 million hospital discharges with any diagnosis of valvular heart disease in 2005, and 94,000 of these were related to surgical procedures for heart valve disease (mostly involving the aortic and mitral valves).

The incidence of infective endocarditis (Chap. 124) has increased with the aging of the population, the more widespread prevalence of vascular grafts and intracardiac devices, the emergence of more virulent multidrug-resistant microorganisms, and the growing epidemic of diabetes. Infective endocarditis has become a more frequent cause of acute valvular regurgitation. Bicuspid aortic valve disease affects as many as 0.5–1.4% of the population, and an increasing number of childhood survivors of congenital heart disease present later in life with valvular dysfunction. The global burden of valvular heart disease is expected to progress.

As is true for other health conditions, disparities in access to and quality of care for patients with valvular heart disease have been well documented. Management decisions and outcome differences based on age, gender, and race require educational efforts across all levels of providers.

FURTHER READINGS

Bonow RO et al: ACC/AHA 2006 Guidelines for the management of patients with valvular heart disease: Executive summary. Circulation 114:450, 2006

Carabello BA, Paulus WJ: Aortic stenosis. Lancet 373:956, 2009

Coats L, Bonhoeffer P: New percutaneous treatments for valve disease. Heart 93:639, 2007

Enriquez-Sarano M, Tajik AJ: Aortic regurgitation. N Engl J Med 351:1539, 2004

Feldman T, Leon MB: Prospects for percutaneous valve therapies. Circulation 116:2866, 2007

Freeman RV, Otto CM. Spectrum of calcific aortic valve disease: Pathogenesis, disease progression, and treatment strategies. Circulation 111:3316, 2005

Grube E et al: Progress and current status of percutaneous aortic valve replacement: Results of three device generations of the CoreValve Revalving system. Circ Cardiovasc Interven 1:167, 2008

Nkomo VT et al: Burden of valvular heart diseases: A population-based study. Lancet 368:1005, 2006

Otto CM, Bonow RO (eds): *Valvular Heart Disease. A Companion to Braunwald's Heart Disease*, 3rd ed. Philadelphia, Saunders Elsevier, 2009

———: Valvular heart disease, in *Braunwald's Heart Disease*, 8th ed, P Libby et al (eds). Philadelphia, Saunders, 2008

Pellikka PA et al: Outcome of 622 adults with asymptomatic, hemodynamically significant aortic stenosis during prolonged follow-up. Circulation 111:3290, 2005

Rosenhek R et al: Outcome of watchful waiting in asymptomatic severe mitral regurgitation. Circulation 113:2238, 2006

Society of Thoracic Surgeons: STS Adult Cardiovascular National Surgery Database. Period Ending 03/31/2009 Executive Summary. *http://www.sts.org/documents/pdf/ndb/2ndHarvestExecutiveSummary_2009.pdf*

———: STS national database risk calculator. *http://www.sts.org/sections/stsnationaldatabase/riskcalculator/*

Tadros TM et al: Ascending aortic dilatation associated with bicuspid aortic valve: pathophysiology, molecular biology, and clinical implications. Circulation 119:880, 2009

Webb JG et al: Percutaneous transarterial aortic valve replacement in selected high risk patients with aortic stenosis. Circulation 116:755, 2007

Wilson W et al: Prevention of infective endocarditis. Guidelines from the American Heart Association Rheumatic Fever, Endocarditis, and Kawasaki Disease Committee, Council on Cardiovascular Disease in the Young, and the Council on Clinical Cardiology, Council on Cardiovascular Surgery and Anesthesia and the Quality of Care and Outcomes Research Interdisciplinary Working Group. April 2007, *http://circ.ahajournals.org*

World Health Organization: Rheumatic fever and rheumatic heart disease. World Health Organ Tech Rep Ser 923:1, 2004

CHAPTER 238

Cardiomyopathy and Myocarditis

Lynne Warner Stevenson
Joseph Loscalzo

DEFINITION AND CLASSIFICATION

Cardiomyopathy is disease of the heart muscle. It is estimated that cardiomyopathy accounts for 5–10% of the 5–6 million patients already diagnosed with heart failure in the United States. This term is intended to exclude cardiac dysfunction that results from other structural heart disease, such as coronary artery disease, primary valve disease, or severe hypertension; however, in general usage the phrase *ischemic cardiomyopathy* is sometimes applied to describe diffuse dysfunction occurring in the presence of multivessel coronary artery disease, and *nonischemic cardiomyopathy* to describe cardiomyopathy from other causes. As of 2006, cardiomyopathies are defined as "a heterogeneous group of diseases of the myocardium associated with mechanical and/or electrical dysfunction that usually (but not invariably) exhibit inappropriate ventricular hypertrophy or dilatation and are due to a variety of causes that frequently are genetic."[1]

The traditional classification of cardiomyopathies into a triad of dilated, restrictive, and hypertrophic was based initially on autopsy specimens and later on echocardiographic findings. Dilated and hypertrophic cardiomyopathies can be distinguished on the basis of left ventricular wall thickness and cavity dimension; however, restrictive cardiomyopathy can have variably increased wall thickness and chamber dimensions that range from reduced to slightly increased, with prominent atrial enlargement. Restrictive cardiomyopathy is now defined more on the basis of abnormal diastolic function, which is also present but initially less prominent in dilated and hypertrophic cardiomyopathy. Restrictive cardiomyopathy can overlap in presentation, gross morphology, and etiology with both hypertrophic and dilated cardiomyopathies (Table 238-1).

Expanding information renders this classification triad based on phenotype increasingly inadequate to define disease or therapy. Identification of more genetic determinants of cardiomyopathy has suggested a four-way classification scheme of etiology as primary (affecting primarily the heart) and secondary to other systemic disease. The primary causes are then divided into genetic, mixed genetic and acquired, and acquired; however, in current practice the genetic information is often unavailable at the time of initial presentation, particularly in the absence of extracardiac manifestations. Many mutated genes can be associated with the same general phenotype, and one defective gene may manifest as multiple phenotypes. In addition, the bases of evidence for most therapies are still driven by clinical phenotypes. Although the proposed genetic classification does not yet guide many current clinical strategies, it will become increasingly relevant as classification of disease moves beyond individual organ pathology to more integrated systems approaches.

[1]From Maron BJ et al: Circulation 1807–1816, 2006.

GENERAL PRESENTATION

For all cardiomyopathies, the early symptoms often relate to exertional intolerance with breathlessness or fatigue, usually from inadequate cardiac reserve during exercise. These symptoms may initially go unnoticed or be attributed to other causes, commonly pulmonary. As fluid retention leads to elevation of resting filling pressures, shortness of breath may occur during routine daily activity, such as dressing, and may manifest as dyspnea or cough in the supine position. Although often considered the hallmark of congestion, peripheral edema may not appear despite severe fluid retention, particularly in younger patients. The nonspecific term *congestive heart failure* describes only the resulting syndrome of fluid retention, which is common to the three types of cardiomyopathy and also to other cardiac diseases associated with elevated filling pressures. Despite the different structural basis, all three types of cardiomyopathy can be associated with atrioventricular valve regurgitation, typical and atypical chest pain, atrial and ventricular tachyarrhythmias, and embolic events (Table 238-1). Initial evaluation begins with a detailed clinical history and examination, looking for clues to cardiac, extracardiac, and familial disease (Table 238-2). The initial evaluation, prognosis, and therapy are generally defined by the severity of cardiac and clinical dysfunction, with some distinctive features according to etiology.

GENETIC ETIOLOGIES OF CARDIOMYOPATHY

The estimated prevalence of a genetic etiology for cardiomyopathy continues to increase with increasing awareness of the importance of the family history and the availability of genetic testing. Well-recognized in hypertrophic cardiomyopathy, heritability is present in at least 30% of dilated cardiomyopathy without other clear etiology. Careful family history should elicit not only known cardiomyopathy and heart failure, but also family members who have had sudden death, often incorrectly attributed to "a massive heart attack," who have had atrial fibrillation or pacemaker implantation by middle age, or who have muscular dystrophy. The family history should be reviewed at subsequent intervals particularly regarding siblings and cousins, who may tend to manifest disease at similar ages.

Most familial cardiomyopathies are inherited in an autosomal dominant pattern, with occasional autosomal recessive and X-linked inheritance (Table 238-3). The penetrance and phenotype of a given mutation varies with other genetic, epigenetic, and environmental determinants. Some mutations are associated with primary conduction system disease as well as dilated cardiomyopathy (CDDC). With rare exceptions, such as the replacements for defective metabolic enzymes, current therapy is based on the phenotype rather than the genetic defect. However, knowledge of the genetic defect may influence prognosis and in some cases provide indication for implantable defibrillators.

Defects in sarcomeric proteins of myosin, actin, and troponin are the best characterized. While the majority of these are associated with hypertrophic cardiomyopathy, an increasing number of sarcomeric mutations have now been implicated in dilated cardiomyopathy, and some have also been associated with left ventricular noncompaction. Thus far, few mutations have been identified in excitation-contraction coupling proteins, perhaps because they are too crucial for survival to allow variation.

Many of the proteins encoded by abnormal structural genes span more than one functional area of the myocyte (Fig. 238-1). Proteins contributing to the Z-disk organize and stabilize the sarcomeres. Multiple other proteins are involved in connecting and maintaining the cytoskeleton of the myocyte. For example, desmin forms

TABLE 238-1 Presentation with Symptomatic Cardiomyopathy

	Dilated	Restrictive	Hypertrophic
Ejection fraction (normal >55%)	Usually <30% when symptoms severe	25-50%	>60%
Left ventricular diastolic dimension (normal <55 mm)	≥60 mm	<60 mm (may be decreased)	Often decreased
Left ventricular wall thickness	Decreased	Normal or increased	Markedly increased
Atrial size	Increased	Increased; may be massive	Increased; related to abnormal
Valvular regurgitation	Related to annular dilation; mitral appears earlier, during decompensation; tricuspid regurgitation in late stages	Related to endocardial involvement; frequent mitral and tricuspid regurgitation, rarely severe	Related to valve-septum interaction; mitral regurgitation
Common first symptoms	Exertional intolerance	Exertional intolerance, fluid retention early	Exertional intolerance; may have chest pain
Congestive symptoms*	Left before right, except right prominent in young adults	Right often dominates	Left-sided congestion may develop late
Arrhythmia	Ventricular tachyarrhythmia; conduction block in Chagas' disease, and some families. Atrial fibrillation.	Ventricular uncommon except in sarcoidosis conduction block in sarcoidosis and amyloidosis. Atrial fibrillation.	Ventricular tachyarrhythmias; atrial fibrillation

*Left-sided symptoms of pulmonary congestion; dyspnea on exertion, orthopnea, paroxysmal nocturnal dyspnea. Right-sided symptoms of systemic versus congestion: discomfort on bending, hepatic and abdominal distention, peripheral edema.

intermediate filaments that connect the nuclear and plasma membranes, Z-lines, and the intercalated disks between muscle cells. Desmin mutations impair the transmission of force and signaling for both cardiac and skeletal muscle, and are, thus, associated with a peripheral myopathy as well as a dilated cardiomyopathy. Most of the identified genetic defects in the Z-disk and cytoskeleton are associated with dilated cardiomyopathy.

Proteins in the sarcolemmal membrane are associated with dilated cardiomyopathy. The best known is the X-linked dystrophin, abnormalities of which cause Duchenne's and Becker's muscle dystrophy. (Interestingly, abnormal dystrophin can be acquired when the Coxsackie virus cleaves dystrophin during viral myocarditis.) This protein provides a network that supports the sarcolemma and also connects to the sarcomere. The progressive functional defect in both cardiac and skeletal muscle reflects vulnerability to mechanical stress. Dystrophin is associated at the membrane with a complex of other proteins, such as metavinculin, abnormalities of which cause dilated cardiomyopathy with autosomal dominant inheritance. Defects in the sarcolemmal channel proteins (*channelopathies*) are generally associated with primary arrhythmias, but mutations in SCN5A, distinct from those which cause the Brugada or long-QT syndromes, have been implicated in dilated cardiomyopathy.

Nuclear membrane protein defects in the myocyte can also cause skeletal myopathy in either autosomal dominant (lamin proteins) or X-linked (emerin) patterns. These are associated with a high prevalence of atrial arrhythmias and conduction system disease which, in some family members, occur without detectable cardiomyopathy.

Intercalated disks between cardiac myocytes allow mechanical and electrical coupling between cells and also connect to desmin filaments within the cell. Mutations in proteins of the desmosomal complex compromise attachment of the myocytes, which can become disconnected and die, to be replaced by fat and fibrous tissue. These areas are highly arrhythmogenic and may go on to aneurysm formation. Although it is more noticeable in the thinner right ventricle, this condition often affects both ventricles. As desmosomes are also important for elasticity of hair and skin, some defective desmosomal proteins are associated with striking "woolly hair" and thickened skin on the palm and soles.

Owing to the conservation of signaling pathways in multiple systems, we may expect to discover more extracardiac manifestations of genetic abnormalities initially considered to manifest exclusively in the heart. In contrast, the monogenic disorders of metabolism that affect the heart are already clearly recognized to affect multiple organ systems (Table 238-4). The most important currently are those defective enzymes for which specific enzyme replacement therapy can now ameliorate the course of disease, as with alpha-galactosidase-A (Fabry's disease). Abnormalities of mitochondrial DNA (maternally transmitted) impair energy production with multiple clinical manifestations, including impaired cognitive function and skeletal myopathy. The phenotypic expression is highly variable depending on the distribution of the maternal mitochondria during embryonic development. Heritable systemic diseases, such as familial amyloidosis and hemochromatosis, can affect the heart without abnormal expression of specific cardiac genes.

For any patient with suspected or proven genetic disease, family members should be considered and evaluated in a longitudinal fashion. Screening includes an echocardiogram and electrocardiogram (ECG). The indications and implications for confirmatory specific genetic testing vary depending upon the specific mutation. The profound questions raised by families about diseases shared and passed down merit serious and sensitive discussion, ideally provided by a trained genetic counselor.

DILATED CARDIOMYOPATHY

An enlarged left ventricle with decreased systolic function as measured by left ventricular ejection fraction characterizes dilated cardiomyopathy (Figs. 238-2, 238-3, 238-4). *Systolic failure* is more

TABLE 238-2 Initial Evaluation of Cardiomyopathy

Clinical Evaluation
Thorough history and physical examination to identify cardiac and noncardiac disorders[a]
Detailed family history of heart failure, cardiomyopathy, skeletal myopathy, conduction disorders and tachyarrhythmias, sudden death
History of alcohol, illicit drugs, chemotherapy or radiation therapy[a]
Assessment of ability to perform routine and desired activities[a]
Assessment of volume status, orthostatic blood pressure, body mass index[a]
Laboratory Evaluation
Electrocardiogram[a]
Chest radiograph[a]
Two-dimensional and Doppler echocardiogram[a]
Chemistry:
Serum sodium,[a] potassium,[a] calcium,[a] magnesium[a]
Fasting glucose (glycohemoglobin in DM)
Creatinine,[a] blood urea nitrogen[a]
Albumin,[a] total protein,[a] liver function tests[a]
Lipid profile
Thyroid-stimulating hormone[a]
Serum iron, transferrin saturation
Urinalysis
Creatine kinase
Hematology:
Hemoglobin/hematocrit[a]
White blood cell count with differential,[a] including eosinophils
Erythrocyte sedimentation rate
Initial Evaluation Only in Patients Selected for Possible Specific Diagnosis
Titers for infection in presence of clinical suspicion:
Acute viral (coxsackie virus, echovirus, influenza virus)
Human immunodeficiency virus,
Chagas' disease, Lyme disease, toxoplasmosis
Catheterization with coronary angiography in patients with angina who are candidates for intervention[a]
Serologies for active rheumatologic disease
Endomyocardial biopsy including sample for electron microscopy when suspecting specific diagnosis with therapeutic implications
Screening for sleep-disordered breathing

[a]Level I Recommendations from ACC/AHA Practice Guidelines for Chronic Heart Failure in the adult.

Source: From Hunt et al.

marked than the frequently accompanying diastolic dysfunction, although the latter may be functionally severe in the setting of marked volume overload. The syndrome of dilated cardiomyopathy has multiple etiologies (Table 238-5). Up to one-third of cases may be familial, as discussed below. Acquired cardiomyopathy is often attributed to a brief primary injury such as infection or toxin exposure. Some myocytes may die during the initial injury, while others survive only to have later programmed cell death, (apoptosis). As the surviving myocytes hypertrophy to accommodate the increased burden of wall stress, local and circulating factors stimulate deleterious responses that contribute to progression of disease, even in the absence of further primary injury. Dynamic remodeling of the interstitial scaffolding affects diastolic function and the amount of ventricular dilation. Mitral regurgitation commonly develops as the valvular apparatus is distorted by ventricular dilation and sometimes by focal injury to underlying myocardium and is usually substantial by the time heart failure is severe. Many cases that present "acutely" have progressed silently through these stages over months to years.

Regardless of the nature and degree of direct cell injury, the resulting functional impairment often includes some contribution from secondary responses that may be reversible. The potential reversibility of cardiomyopathy in the absence of ongoing injury remains a subject of active controversy. Almost half of all patients with truly recent onset cardiomyopathy demonstrate substantial spontaneous recovery. Some patients have dramatic improvement to near-normal ejection fractions during pharmacologic therapy, particularly notable with the β-adrenergic antagonists coupled with renin-angiotensin system inhibition. Interest in the potential for recovery of cardiomyopathy in the absence of coronary artery disease has been further stimulated by occasional "recovery" of left ventricular function in young patients after a year or more of mechanical circulatory support. The diagnosis and therapy for dilated cardiomyopathy is generally dictated by the stage of heart failure (Chap. 234), with specific aspects discussed with the relevant etiology below.

■ INFECTIVE MYOCARDITIS

Myocarditis is an inflammatory process, most commonly attributed to infectious organisms that can invade the myocardium directly, produce cardiotoxins, and trigger chronic inflammatory responses. Infective myocarditis has been reported with almost all types of infectious agents, but is most commonly associated with viral infections, the protozoan *Trypanosoma cruzi* in South America, and endomyocardial fibrosis in equatorial Africa.

Viral myocarditis in murine models begins with acute infection. After viruses enter the circulation through the respiratory or gastrointestinal tract, they can infect other organs possessing specific receptors, such as the coxsackie-adenovirus receptor on the heart. Viral invasion and replication can lead directly to myocardial injury and lysis. Viral proteases have multiple actions, of which one is to degrade the protein, dystrophin, in the myocyte membrane complex that is genetically abnormal in some muscular dystrophies. Viral antigens activate immune responses that help to contain the initial infection but may persist into later phases. Components include nonspecific cytokines, specific antibodies, and cytotoxic T-lymphocytes, which in some cases recognize myocyte proteins. There is varying evidence for a latent phase of ongoing infection with persistence of the viral genome and some viral proteins. The relative contributions of viral persistence and deleterious host immune responses to progressive dysfunction have not been clearly delineated in human disease (Fig. 238-5). The late stages are dominated by nonspecific secondary changes in gene expression, and by local and systemic neurohormonal responses, as seen for other etiologies of heart failure.

Although viral myocarditis is generally considered to be an acquired cardiomyopathy, families have been reported whose clinical disease appeared after a syndrome consistent with viral myocarditis. One possible explanation for this apparent mixed etiology is that some genetic variants of myocardial cell surface receptors bind more avidly to certain viruses, particularly coxsackie virus and adenovirus.

The typical clinical picture of myocarditis is a young adult with progressive dyspnea and weakness over a few days to weeks after a recent viral syndrome with fevers and often myalgias indicative of skeletal muscle inflammation. Some patients present with atypical or anginal-type chest pain, or with pleuritic, positional chest pain due to pericarditis with some degree of underlying myocarditis. Patients in whom ventricular tachyarrhythmias dominate the presentation may have viral myocarditis but should be evaluated for sarcoidosis or giant cell myocarditis. Patients presenting with pulmonary or systemic embolic events from intracardiac thrombi generally already have chronic, severe cardiac dysfunction.

A small number of patients present with *acute fulminant myocarditis,* with rapid progression from a severe febrile respiratory syndrome to cardiogenic shock from which multiple organ system failure, including coagulopathy, may develop. Such patients have often been discharged from the emergency department with antibiotic therapy only to return in extremis. Prompt triage is vital to provide aggressive support with high-level intravenous inotropic therapy and on occasion, mechanical circulatory support; importantly, more than half of patients with this acute presentation

TABLE 238-3 Inherited Genetic Defects Associated With Cardiomyopathy

	Gene Product	Inheritance	Cardiac Phenotype	Isolated Cardiac Phenotype	Extracardiac Manifestations
Sarcomere	*MYH7* (β myosin heavy chain)	AD	HCM, DCM, LVNC	yes	Skeletal myopathy
	MYBPC3 (myosin binding protein C)	AD	HCM, (DCM)	yes	
	TNNT2 (cardiac troponin T)	AD	HCM, DCM, LVNC	yes	
	TNNI3 (cardiac troponin I)	AD, AR	HCM, DCM, RCM	yes	
	TTN (Titin)	AD	HCM, DCM	yes	
	TPM1 (α-tropomyosin)	AD	HCM, DCM	yes	
	TNNC1 (slow troponin C)	AD	DCM	yes	
	ACTC (α-actin)	AD	HCM, DCM, (LVNC)	yes	
	MYL2 (myosin regulatory light chain)	AD	HCM	yes	Skeletal myopathy
	MYL3 (myosin essential light chain)	AD	HCM	yes	
	MYH6 (α-myosin heavy chain)	AD	HCM, (DCM)	yes	
Z-disk and Cytoskeleton	*DES* (Desmin)	AD	DCM	yes	Skeletal myopathy
	LDB3 (Cypher-ZASP)	AD	DCM, LVNC	yes	Skeletal myopathy
	MYOZ2 (Myozenin)	AD	HCM	yes	
	TCAP (Telethonin)	AD	DCM, HCM	yes	
	ANKRD1 (CARP)	AD	HCM, (DCM)	yes	
	CSRP3 (MLP)	AD	DCM, (HCM)	yes	
	OBSCN (Obscurin)	AD	HCM	yes	
	ACTN2 (α-actinin-2)	AD	DCM	yes	
	CRYAB (αB-crystallin)	AD	DCM	yes	
Nuclear Membrane	*LMNA* (Lamin A/C)	AD	CDDC	yes	Skeletal myopathy
	EMD (Emerin)	X-linked	CDDC	no	Skeletal myopathy, contractures
	TMPO (Thymopoietin)	AD	DCM	yes	
Excitation-Contraction Coupling	*PLN* (Phospholamban)	AD	DCM	yes	
	SCN5A (NAV 1.5)	AD	CDDC	yes	
	RYR2 (cardiac ryanodine receptor)	AD	ARVC	yes	

(continued)

TABLE 238-3 Inherited Genetic Defects Associated With Cardiomyopathy (*Continued*)

	Gene Product	Inheritance	Cardiac Phenotype	Isolated Cardiac Phenotype	Extracardiac Manifestations
Cellular Metabolism	*PRKAG2* (γ-subunit of AMP Kinase)	AD	HCM+	yes	
	LAMP2 (lysosomal associated membrane protein)	X-linked	HCM+	no*	Danon's disease: skeletal myopathy, cognitive impairment
	TAZ (Tafazzin)	X-linked	DCM, LVNC	no	Barth's syndrome: skeletal myopathy, cognitive impairment, neutropenia
	FXN (Frataxin)	AR	HCM	no	Friedreich's ataxia: ataxia, diabetes mellitus type 2
	ABCC9 (sulfonylurea receptor 2)	AD	DCM	yes	
	TMEM43 (transmembrane protein 43)	AD	ARVC	yes	
	GLA (α-galactosidase-A) (other systemic metabolic defects, see Table 238-4)	X-linked	HCM	yes	Fabry's disease: renal failure, angiokeratomas and painful neuropathy
Mitochondria	mitochondrial DNA	Maternal transmission	DCM, HCMc	no	MELAS, MERRF, Kearns-Sayre syndrome, ocular myopathy
Sarcolemmal Membrane	*DMD* (Dystrophin)	X-linked	DCM	no*	Duchenne's and Becker's muscular dystrophy
	DMPK (dystrophica myotonica protein kinase)	AD	DCM	no	Myotonic dystrophy type 1
	SGCD (δ-sarcoglycan)	AD	DCM	yes	
	VCL (Metavinculin)	AD	DCM	yes	
Desmosome	*DSP* (Desmoplakin)	AD, AR	ARVC	yes	Carvajal syndrome (AR)
	DSG2 (Desmoglein 2)	AD	ARVC	yes	
	DSC2 (Desmocollin 2)	AD	ARVC	yes	
	PKP2 (Plakophilin 2)	AD	ARVC	yes	
	JUP (Plakoglobin)	AD, AR	ARVC	yes	Naxos syndrome (AR)
Other	*EYA4* (Eyes Absent 4)	AD	DCM	no	Sensorineural deafness
	RBM20 (RNA binding motif 20)	AD	DCM	yes	
	PSEN1 (Presenilin-1,2)	AD	DCM	yes	Dementia

Abbreviations: AD, autosomal dominant; AR, autosomal recessive; ARVC, arrhythmogenic right ventricular cardiomyopathy; CDDC, conduction disease with dilated cardiomyopathy; DCM, dilated cardiomyopathy; HCM+, HCM with preexcitation; HCMc, HCM with conduction disease; LVNC, left ventricular noncompaction; MELAS, (mitochondrial) myopathy, encephalopathy, lactic acidosis, and strokelike episodes syndrome; MERRF, myoclonic epilepsy with ragged red fibers; RCM, restrictive cardiomyopathy.

Note: *indicates that isolated cardiac phenotype can occur in women with the x-linked defects.

Source: From Neal Lakdawala, MD, Cardiovascular Genetics, Brigham and Women's Hospital.

can survive with marked improvement within the first few weeks, often returning to near-normal systolic function.

Many patients presenting with heart failure after a viral illness actually have a long-standing cardiomyopathy that was acutely exacerbated but not caused by the new viral illness. Heart failure from any cause often worsens transiently during infection, presumably due to the myocardial depressant effects of circulating cytokines. Marked left ventricular dilation and the presence of severely elevated left-ventricular filling pressures without frank pulmonary edema suggest chronic, slowly progressive disease, which is often further supported by a history of gradual changes in exercise tolerance before the viral syndrome.

For the usual subacute presentation, the diagnosis of cardiomyopathy is confirmed by echocardiography, and further evaluation is directed to ascertain whether myocarditis is present. Troponin is often mildly elevated, and creatine kinase may be released from the cardiac injury or skeletal muscle involvement. In some cases, cardiac catheterization is performed to rule out acute ischemia. Magnetic resonance imaging is increasingly used for the diagnosis of myocarditis, which is supported by evidence of increased tissue edema and gadolinium enhancement, particularly in the mid-wall distinct from the usual coronary artery territories. Endomyocardial biopsy criteria for myocarditis require lymphocytic infiltration with evidence of myocyte necrosis (Fig. 238-6), but are met in only about

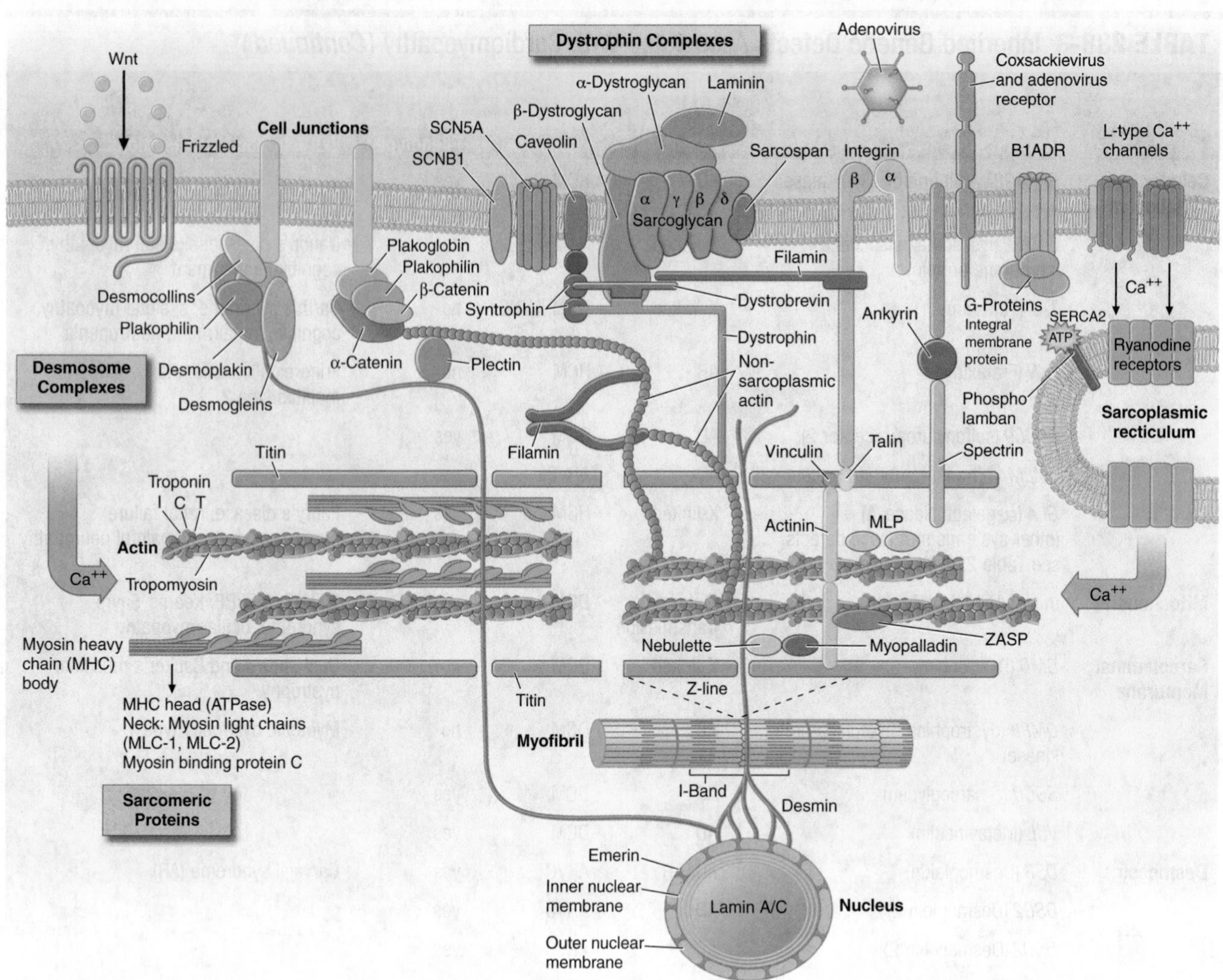

Figure 238-1 Drawing of myocyte indicating multiple sites of abnormal gene products associated with cardiomyopathy. Major functional groups include the sarcomeric proteins (actin, myosin, tropomyosin, and the associated regulatory proteins), the dystrophin complex stabilizing and connecting the cell membrane to intracellular structures, the desmosome complexes associated with cell-cell connections and stability, and multiple cytoskeletal proteins that integrate and stabilize the myocyte. ATP, adenosine triphosphate. *(Figure adapted from Jeffrey A. Towbin, MD, University of Cincinnati, with permission.)*

10–20% of classic presentations. Most biopsies in fulminant myocarditis show only marked tissue edema without a cellular infiltrate, and it is likely that many less acute cases may similarly be characterized by tissue edema and cytokine depression of myocardial function, possibly including some antibody-mediated endothelial injury, without marked cellular infiltrates. Acute and convalescent viral titers are usually sent but are more likely to be important from the public health standpoint than for the individual.

Viral myocarditis treatment is initially directed toward stabilizing the hemodynamic status and then toward adjusting neurohormonal antagonists for the treatment of heart failure as tolerated. Presentation with fulminant disease requires rapid evaluation and therapy as discussed above. For patients with subacute presentation, randomized trials have shown no benefit of immunosuppression with glucocorticoid combinations or intravenous immunoglobulin, even when the biopsy is positive for lymphocytic infiltrates; yet, immunosuppression is often used even in the absence of evidence of benefit, in part due to perceived analogy to acute cardiac transplant rejection. Animal models have shown that viral replication and myocardial injury can be worsened by immunosuppression during the early phase of infection; however, patients with persistent inflammatory myocarditis and a progressive downhill course over weeks may be treated empirically with glucocorticoids in an attempt to avoid the need for cardiac transplantation.

The true prognosis of viral myocarditis is not known, as most unrecognized cases probably resolve spontaneously, while others progress to cardiomyopathy without other obvious cause. However, among patients who have truly recent onset cardiomyopathy of less than 3–6 months' duration without other apparent etiology, almost half will have major improvement in left ventricular ejection fraction during the subsequent 6–12 months. Those patients in whom left ventricular ejection fraction and dimensions return to normal are usually considered to have residual subclinical cardiomyopathy. Neurohormonal antagonist therapy is usually continued indefinitely as tolerated, with dose adjustments to avoid side effects.

Specific viruses

In humans, viruses are often suspected but rarely confirmed as the direct cause of myocarditis. Often implicated is the picornavirus family of RNA viruses, with the enteroviruses *Coxsackie, echovirus,* and *poliovirus. Influenza,* another RNA virus, is implicated in myocarditis with varying frequency from year to year as the epitopes

TABLE 238-4 Examples of Inherited Defects in Metabolic Pathways Associated With Cardiomyopathy, Usually Restrictive or Pseudohypertrophic Phenotype

Glycogen Storage Diseases
II—Pompe's (alpha 1,4 glucosidase)
III –Forbes: de-branching enzyme (amylo 1,6 glucosidase)
Glucose Metabolism (Defective PRKAG2[a])
Fatty acid metabolism
Carnitine transport defect
Medium chain Acyl-CoA dehydrogenase
Long chain Acyl-CoA dehydrogenase
Sphingolipidoses
Fabry's disease (alpha galactosidase A)
Gaucher disease (beta-glucocerebroside)
Disorders of lysosomal function
Danon's disease—(lysosome-associated membrane protein, LAMP2)
Miscellaneous
Hemochromatosis—Fe metabolism
Familial amyloidosis—abnormal transthyretin
Barth syndrome—tafazzin defect affecting cardiolipin
Friedreich's ataxia—frataxin

[a]Gamma-2 regulatory subunit of the AMP-activated protein kinase important for glucose metabolism

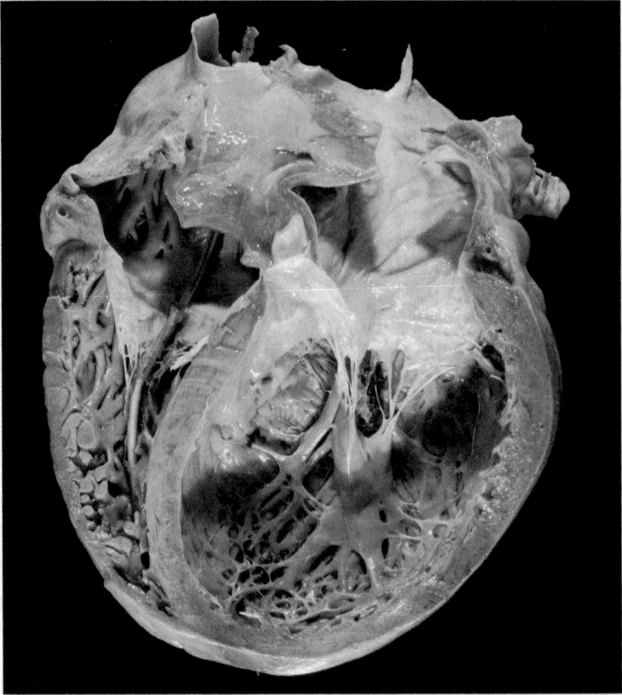

Figure 238-2 Dilated cardiomyopathy. This gross specimen of a heart removed at the time of transplantation shows massive left ventricular dilation and moderate right ventricular dilation. Although the left ventricular wall in particular appears thinned, there is significant hypertrophy of this heart, which weighs more than 800 gm (upper limit of normal = 360 g). A defibrillator lead is seen traversing the tricuspid valve into the right ventricular apex. (*Image courtesy of Robert Padera, MD, PhD, Department of Pathology, Brigham and Women's Hospital, Boston.)*

change. Of the DNA viruses, *adenovirus, variola* (smallpox) and *vaccinia* (smallpox vaccine), and the *herpesviruses (Varicella zoster, Cytomegalovirus,* and *Epstein-Barr virus)* are well-recognized as causes of myocarditis. From genetic analyses of biopsy tissue, parvovirus B19, coxsackie, adenovirus, and Epstein-Barr virus are the agents most often implicated. The role of *parvovirus B19* as a cause of myocarditis or cardiomyopathy is difficult to determine, as almost half of individuals show evidence of prior infection with this small DNA virus that causes "fifth disease" in children.

Human immunodeficiency virus (HIV) has been associated with echocardiographic abnormalities in 10–40% patients with clinical disease. Cardiomyopathy in HIV may result from cardiac involvement with other associated viruses, such as cytomegalovirus and hepatitis C. Antiviral drugs to treat chronic HIV can cause cardiomyopathy, both directly as cardiotoxins and through drug hypersensitivity. The clinical picture may be complicated by pericardial effusions and pulmonary hypertension. There is a high frequency of lymphocytic myocarditis found at autopsy, and viral particles have been demonstrated in the myocardium in some cases, consistent with direct causation.

Hepatitis C has been repeatedly implicated in cardiomyopathy, particularly in Germany and Asia. Cardiac function may improve after interferon therapy. As this cytokine itself often depresses cardiac function transiently, careful coordination of administration and ongoing clinical evaluation are critical. Involvement of the heart with hepatitis B is uncommon but can be seen when associated with systemic vasculitis (polyarteritis nodosa).

Other viral infections in which cardiac involvement is specifically implicated, beyond the depression of cardiac function during any systemic cytokine activation, include *mumps, respiratory syncytial virus,* the *arboviruses (dengue fever* and *yellow fever),* and *arenaviruses (Lassa fever).*

Parasitic myocarditis

Chagas' disease is the third most common parasitic infection in the world and the most common cause of cardiomyopathy. The protozoan *Trypanosoma cruzi* (*T. cruzi*) is usually transmitted by the bite of the reduviid bug, endemic in the rural areas of South and Central America. Transmission can also occur through blood transfusion, organ donation, from mother to fetus, and occasionally orally. While programs to eradicate the insect vector have decreased the prevalence from about 16 million to less than 10 million in South America, cases are increasingly recognized in Western developed countries. Approximately 100,000 affected individuals are currently living in the United States, most of whom contracted the disease in endemic areas.

The acute phase of Chagas' disease with parasitemia is usually unrecognized, but in fewer than 5% of cases presents clinically within a few weeks of infection, with nonspecific symptoms or occasionally with acute myocarditis and meningoencephalitis. In the absence of antiparasitic therapy, the silent stage progresses slowly over 10–30 years in almost half of patients to manifest in the cardiac and gastrointestinal systems in the chronic stages. Survival is less than 30% at 5 years after the onset of overt clinical heart failure.

Multiple pathogenetic mechanisms are implicated. The parasite itself can cause myocyte lysis and primary neuronal damage, and specific immune responses may recognize the parasites or related

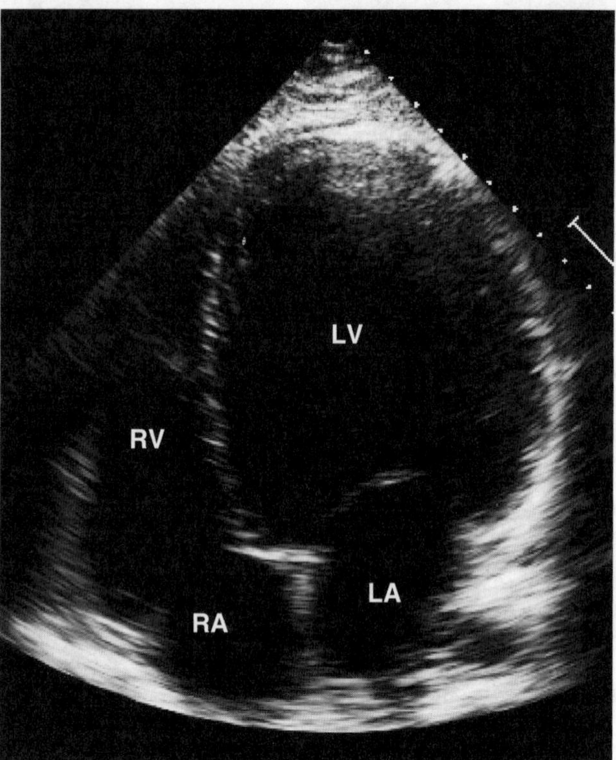

Figure 238-3 Dilated cardiomyopathy. This echocardiogram of a young man with dilated cardiomyopathy shows massive global dilation and thinning of the walls of the left ventricle (LV). The left atrium (LA) is also enlarged compared to normal. Note that the echocardiographic and pathologic images are vertically opposite, such that the LV is by convention on the top right in the echocardiographic image and bottom right in the pathologic images. *(Image courtesy of Justina Wu, MD, Brigham and Women's Hospital, Boston.)*

antigens and lead to chronic immune activation in the absence of detectable parasites. Molecular techniques have revealed persistent parasite DNA fragments in infected individuals. Further evidence for persistent infection is the eruption of parasitic skin lesions

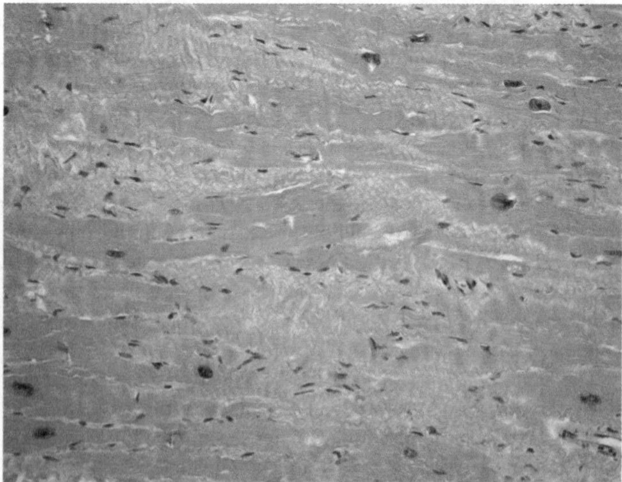

Figure 238-4 Dilated cardiomyopathy. Microscopic specimen of a dilated cardiomyopathy showing the nonspecific changes of interstitial fibrosis and myocyte hypertrophy characterized by increased myocyte size and enlarged, irregular nuclei. Hematoxylin and eosin stained section, 100× original magnification. *(Image courtesy of Robert Padera, MD, PhD, Department of Pathology, Brigham and Women's Hospital, Boston.)*

during immunosuppression after cardiac transplantation. As in postviral myocarditis, the relative roles of persistent infection and of secondary autoimmune injury have not been resolved (Fig. 238-5). An additional factor in progression of Chagas' disease is the autonomic dysfunction and microvascular damage that may contribute to cardiac and gastrointestinal disease.

Features typical of Chagas' disease are conduction system abnormalities, particularly sinus node and atrioventricular (AV) node dysfunction and right bundle branch block. Atrial fibrillation and ventricular tachyarrhythmias also occur. Small ventricular aneurysms are common, particularly at the apex. The dilated ventricles are particularly thrombogenic, giving rise to pulmonary and systemic emboli. The serologic enzyme-linked immunosorbent assay (ELISA) for the IgM has largely replaced the previous complement fixation test for diagnosis.

Treatment of the advanced stages focused on the clinical manifestations of the disease, with heart failure regimens, pacemaker-defibrillators, and anticoagulation; however, increasing emphasis is placed on antiparasitic therapy even in chronic disease. The most common effective antiparasitic therapies are benznidazole and nifurtimox, both associated with multiple severe reactions, including dermatitis, gastrointestinal distress, and neuropathy. Patients without major extracardiac disease have occasionally undergone transplantation, after which they require lifelong therapy to suppress reactivation of infection.

African trypanosomiasis infection results from the tsetse fly bite and can occur in travelers exposed during trips to Africa. The West African form is caused by *Trypanosoma brucei gambiense* and progresses silently over years. The East African form caused by *T. brucei rhodesiense* can progress rapidly through perivascular infiltration to myocarditis and heart failure, with frequent arrhythmias. The diagnosis is made by identification of trypanosomes in blood, lymph nodes, or other affected sites. Development of optimal drug regimens remains limited, and depends on the type and the stage (hemolymphatic or neurologic).

Toxoplasmosis is contracted through undercooked infected beef or pork, transmission from feline feces, organ transplantation, transfusion, or maternal-fetal transmission. Immunocompromised hosts are at greatest risk for reactivation of latent infection from cysts. The cysts have been found in up to 40% of autopsies of patients dying from HIV infection. Toxoplasmosis may present with encephalitis or chorioretinitis, and in the heart can cause myocarditis, pericardial effusion, constrictive pericarditis, and heart failure. The diagnosis may be suspected in an immunocompromised patient with myocarditis and serologic evidence of toxoplasmosis. Fortuitous sampling may reveal the cysts in the myocardium. Combination therapy can include pyrimethamine and sulfadiazine or clindamycin.

Trichinellosis is caused by *Trichinella spiralis* larva ingested with undercooked meat. Larva migrating into skeletal muscles cause myalgias, weakness, and fever. Periorbital and facial edema, and conjunctival and retinal hemorrhage may also be seen. Although the larva may occasionally invade the myocardium, clinical heart failure is rare, and when observed, attributed to the eosinophilic inflammatory response. The diagnosis is made from the specific serum antibody and is further supported by the presence of eosinophilia. Treatment includes antihelminthic drugs and glucocorticoids if inflammation is severe.

Cardiac involvement with *Echinococcus* is rare, but cysts can form and rupture in the myocardium and pericardium.

Bacterial infections

Most bacterial infections can involve the heart occasionally through direct invasion and abscess formation, but do so rarely. More commonly, contractility is depressed globally in severe infection

TABLE 238–5 Major Causes of Dilated Cardiomyopathy (With Common Examples)

Inflammatory Myocarditis	Metabolic[a]
Infective	Nutritional deficiencies: thiamine, selenium, carnitine
Viral (Coxsackie, adenovirus, HIV, hepatitis C)	Electrolyte deficiencies: calcium, phosphate, magnesium
Parasitic (*T. cruzi*—Chagas' disease, toxoplasmosis)	Endocrinopathy:
Bacterial (diphtheria)	Thyroid disease
Spirochetal (*Borellia burgdorferi*—Lyme disease)	Pheochromocytoma
Rickettsial—(Q fever)	Diabetes
Fungal (with systemic infection)	Obesity
Noninfective	Hemochromatosis
Granulomatous inflammatory disease	**Inherited Metabolic Pathway Defects (See Table 238-4)**
Sarcoidosis	**Familial[a] (See Table 238-3)**
Giant cell myocarditis	Skeletal and cardiac myopathy
Hypersensitivity myocarditis	Dystrophin-related dystrophy (Duchenne's, Becker's)
Polymyositis, dermatomyositis	Mitochondrial myopathies (e.g., Kearns-Sayre syndrome)
Collagen vascular disease	Arrhythmogenic ventricular dysplasia
Peripartum cardiomyopathy	Hemochromatosis
Transplant rejection	Associated with other systemic diseases
Toxic	Susceptibility to immune-mediated myocarditis
Alcohol	**Overlap with Restrictive Cardiomyopathy**
Catecholamines: amphetamines, cocaine	"Minimally dilated cardiomyopathy"
Chemotherapeutic agents: (anthracyclines, trastuzumab)	Hemochromatosis
Interferon	Amyloidosis
Other therapeutic agents (hydroxychloroquine, chloroquine)	Hypertrophic cardiomyopathy ("burned-out")
Drugs of misuse (emetine, anabolic steroids)	**"Idiopathic"[a]**
Heavy metals: lead, mercury	**Miscellaneous** (Shared Elements of Above Etiologies)
Occupational exposure: hydrocarbons, arsenicals	Arrhythmogenic right ventricular dysplasia (may also affect left ventricle)[a]
	Left ventricular noncompaction[a]
	Peripartum cardiomyopathy

[a]Some specific cases can be linked now to specific genetic mutation in a familial cardiomyopathy; others with similar phenotypes that appear to be acquired or idiopathic may represent genetic factors not yet identified.

and sepsis through systemic inflammatory responses. *Diphtheria* specifically affects the heart in almost one-half of cases and is the most common cause of death in patients with this infection. Once a disease of children, the prevalence of vaccines has shifted the incidence of this disease to countries where immunization is not routine and to older populations who have lost their immunity. The bacillus releases a toxin that impairs protein synthesis and may particularly affect the conduction system. The specific antitoxin should be administered as soon as possible, with higher priority than antibiotic therapy. Other systemic bacterial infections that can involve the heart include *brucellosis, chlamydophila, legionella, meningococcus, mycoplasma, psittacosis,* and *salmonellosis,* for which treatment is directed at the systemic infection.

Clostridial infections cause myocardial damage from the released toxin. Gas bubbles can be detected in the myocardium, and occasionally abscesses can form in the myocardium and pericardium. *Streptococcal infection* with β-hemolytic streptococci is most commonly associated with acute rheumatic fever, and is characterized by inflammation and fibrosis of cardiac valves and systemic connective tissue, but can also lead to a myocarditis with focal or diffuse infiltrates of mononuclear cells.

Tuberculosis can involve the myocardium directly as well as through tuberculous pericarditis, but rarely does so when the disease is treated with antibiotics. *Whipple's disease* is caused by *Tropheryma whippleii.* The usual manifestations are in the gastrointestinal tract, but pericarditis, coronary arteritis, valvular lesions, and occasionally clinical heart failure may also occur. Multidrug antituberculous regimens are effective, but the disease tends to relapse even with appropriate treatment.

Other infections

Spirochetal myocarditis has been diagnosed from myocardial biopsies containing *Borrelia burgdorferi* that causes *Lyme disease.* Lyme carditis most often presents with arthritis and conduction system

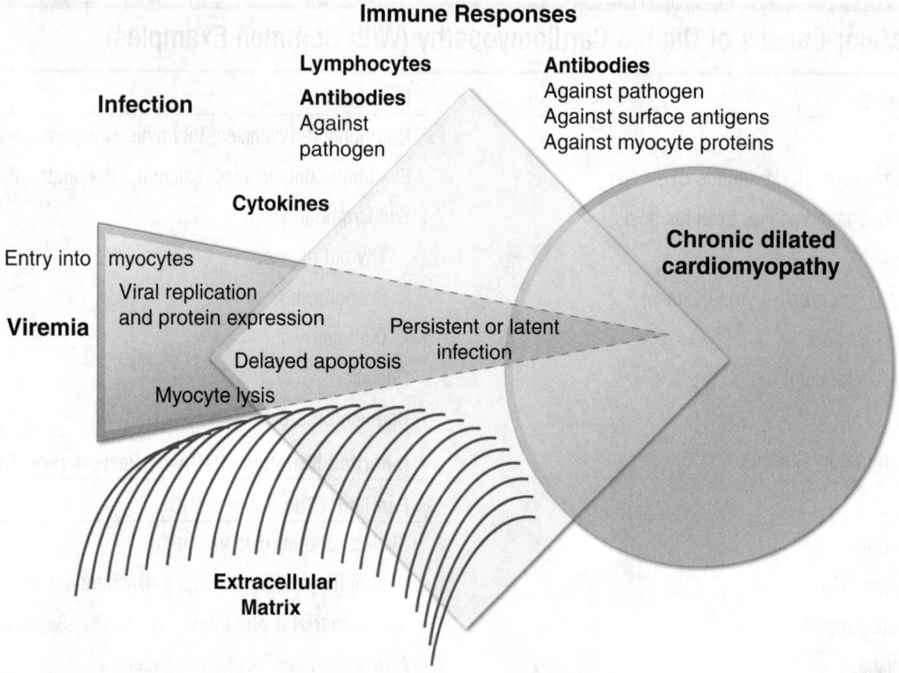

Immune Responses
Lymphocytes
Antibodies
Against pathogen
Antibodies
Against pathogen
Against surface antigens
Against myocyte proteins
Infection
Cytokines
Chronic dilated cardiomyopathy
Entry into myocytes
Viral replication and protein expression
Viremia
Persistent or latent infection
Delayed apoptosis
Myocyte lysis
Extracellular Matrix

Figure 238-5 Schematic diagram demonstrating the possible progression from infection through direct, secondary, and autoimmune responses to dilated cardiomyopathy. Most of the supporting evidence for this sequence is derived from animal models. It is not known to what degree persistent infection and/or ongoing immune responses contribute to ongoing myocardial injury in the chronic phase.

disease that resolves within 1–2 weeks of antibiotic treatment, only rarely causing clinical heart failure.

Fungal myocarditis can occur due to hematogenous or direct spread of infection from other sites, as has been described for aspergillosis, actinomycosis, blastomycosis, candidiasis, coccidioidomycosis, cryptococcosis, histoplasmosis, and mucormycosis. However, cardiac infection is rarely the dominant clinical feature of these infections.

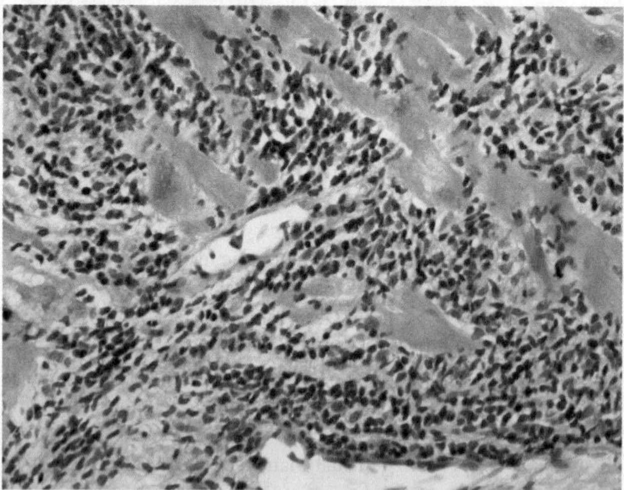

Figure 238-6 Acute myocarditis. Microscopic image of an endomyocardial biopsy showing massive infiltration with mononuclear cells and occasional eosinophils associated with clear myocyte damage. The myocyte nuclei are enlarged and reactive. Such extensive involvement of the myocardium would lead to extensive replacement fibrosis even if the inflammatory response could be suppressed. Hematoxylin and eosin stained section, 200× original magnification. *(Image courtesy of Robert Padera, MD, PhD, Department of Pathology, Brigham and Women's Hospital, Boston.)*

The **rickettsial infections,** *Q fever, Rocky Mountain spotted fever, and scrub typhus,* are frequently accompanied by ECG changes, but most clinical manifestations relate to systemic vascular involvement.

NONINFECTIVE MYOCARDITIS

Myocardial inflammation can occur without apparent preceding infection. The paradigm of noninfectious inflammation without infection is cardiac transplant rejection, from which we have learned that myocardial depression can develop and reverse quickly, that noncellular mediators such as antibodies and cytokines play a major role in addition to lymphocytes, and that myocardial antigens are exposed by prior physical injury and viral infection.

The most commonly diagnosed noninfectious inflammation is granulomatous myocarditis, including both sarcoidosis and giant cell myocarditis. Sarcoidosis, as discussed in Chap. 329, is a multisystem disease most commonly affecting the lungs, presenting in young adults with higher prevalence in African-American males. Patients with pulmonary sarcoid are at high risk for cardiac involvement, but cardiac sarcoidosis may also occur without clinical lung disease in middle-aged whites of both genders. Regional clustering of the disease supports the suspicion that the granulomatous reaction is triggered by an infectious or environmental allergen not yet identified.

The sites and density of cardiac granulomata, the time course, and the degree of extracardiac involvement are remarkably variable. Patients may present with rapid onset heart failure and ventricular tachyarrhythmias, conduction block, chest pain syndromes, or minor cardiac findings in the setting of ocular involvement, an infiltrative skin rash, or a nonspecific febrile illness. They may also present less acutely after months to years of fluctuating cardiac symptoms. When ventricular tachycardia or conduction block dominate the initial presentation of heart failure without coronary artery disease, suspicion should be high for these granulomatous myocarditides.

Depending on the time course, the ventricles may appear restrictive or dilated, at times with right ventricular predominance. Small ventricular aneurysms are common. Computed tomography of the chest often reveals pulmonary lymphadenopathy even in the absence of clinical lung disease. Metabolic imaging [positron emission tomography (PET)] of the whole chest can highlight active sarcoid lesions that are avid for glucose. Magnetic resonance imaging (MRI) of the heart can identify areas likely to be inflammatory. To rule out chronic granulomatous infections, the diagnosis usually requires pathologic confirmation. Biopsy of enlarged mediastinal nodes may provide the highest yield. The scattered granulomata of sarcoidosis can be missed on cardiac biopsy (Fig. 238-7).

Immunosuppressive treatment for sarcoidosis is initiated with high-dose glucocorticoids, which are often more effective for arrhythmias than for the heart failure. Pacemakers and implantable defibrillators are generally indicated to prevent life-threatening heart block or ventricular tachycardia, respectively. Because the inflammation often resolves into extensive fibrosis that impairs cardiac function and provides pathways for reentrant arrhythmias, the prognosis is best when the granulomata are not extensive.

Giant cell myocarditis is less common than sarcoidosis, but accounts for 10–20% of biopsy-positive cases of myocarditis. Giant cell myocarditis typically presents with rapidly progressive heart failure and tachyarrhythmias. Diffuse granulomatous lesions are surrounded by extensive inflammatory infiltrate unlikely to be missed on endomyocardial biopsy. Associated conditions are thymomas, thyroiditis, pernicious anemia, other autoimmune diseases, and occasionally recent infections. Glucocorticoid therapy is less effective than for sarcoidosis, and is sometimes combined with other immunosuppressive agents. The course is generally of rapid deterioration requiring urgent transplantation. Although the severity of presentation and myocardial histology are more fulminant than sarcoidosis, the occasional finding of giant cell myocarditis after sarcoidosis suggests that they may in some cases represent different stages of a similar disease.

Hypersensitivity myocarditis is usually an unexpected diagnosis, made when the biopsy reveals infiltration with lymphocytes and mononuclear cells with a high proportion of eosinophils. (Sometimes called eosinophilic myocarditis, this should not be confused with the hypereosinophilic syndrome in which very high circulating, often clonal populations of eosinophils cause endomyocardial fibrosis.)

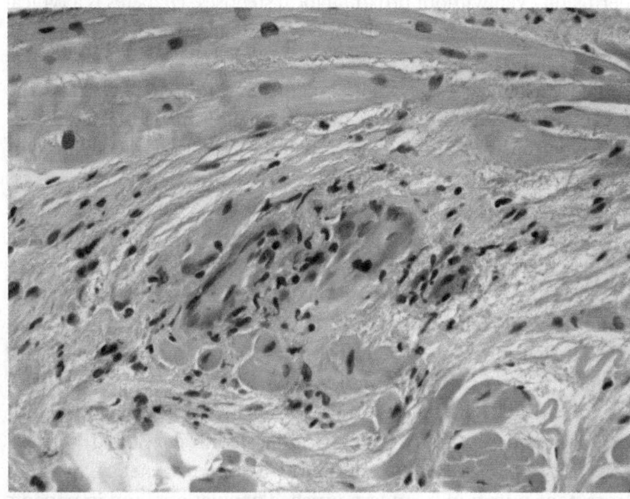

Figure 238-7 Sarcoidosis. Microscopic image of an endomyocardial biopsy showing a noncaseating granuloma and associated interstitial fibrosis typical of sarcoidosis. No microorganisms were present on special stains, and no foreign material was identified. Hematoxylin and eosin stained section, 200× original magnification. *(Image courtesy of Robert Padera, MD, PhD, Department of Pathology, Brigham and Women's Hospital, Boston.)*

Most commonly the reaction is attributed to antibiotics, particularly those taken chronically, but thiazides, anticonvulsants, indomethacin, and methyldopa have also been implicated. High-dose glucocorticoids can be curative.

Myocarditis can be associated with systemic inflammatory diseases such as polymyositis and *dermatomyositis.* While sometimes considered as an explanation for cardiac findings in patients with other inflammatory disease, such as systemic lupus erythematosus, the more common causes are pericarditis, vasculitis, pulmonary hypertension, or accelerated coronary artery disease.

Peripartum cardiomyopathy develops during the last trimester or within the first 6 months after pregnancy, with a frequency between 1:3,000 and 1:15,000 deliveries. The mechanisms remain controversial, but inflammation has been implicated. Risk factors are increased maternal age, increased parity, twin pregnancy, malnutrition, use of tocolytic therapy for premature labor, and preeclampsia or toxemia of pregnancy. As the increased circulatory demand of pregnancy can aggravate other cardiac disease that was clinically unrecognized, it is crucial to the diagnosis that there be no evidence for preexisting cardiac disorder.

Heart failure early after delivery was previously common in Nigeria, when the custom for new mothers included salt ingestion while reclining on a warm bed, which likely impaired mobilization of the excess circulating volume after delivery. In the Western world, lymphocytic myocarditis has often been found on myocardial biopsy. This inflammation has been hypothesized to reflect increased susceptibility to viral myocarditis or an autoimmune myocarditis due to cross-reactivity of anti-uterine antibodies against cardiac muscle. Another mechanism involving a prolactin cleavage fragment has been proposed based on an animal model.

■ TOXIC CARDIOMYOPATHY

Cardiotoxicity has been reported with multiple environmental and pharmacologic agents. Often these associations are seen only with very high levels of exposure or acute overdoses, respectively, in which acute electrocardiographic and hemodynamic abnormalities may reflect both direct drug effect and systemic toxicity.

Alcohol is the most common toxin implicated in chronic dilated cardiomyopathy. Excess consumption may contribute to more than 10% of cases of heart failure, including exacerbation of cases with other primary etiologies such as valvular disease or previous infarction. Toxicity is attributed both to alcohol and to its primary metabolite acetaldehyde. Polymorphisms of the genes encoding alcohol dehydrogenase and the angiotensin-converting enzyme increase the likelihood of alcoholic cardiomyopathy. Superimposed vitamin deficiencies and toxic alcohol additives are rarely implicated. The alcohol consumption necessary to produce cardiomyopathy in an otherwise normal heart has been estimated to be six drinks (about 4 ounces of pure ethanol) daily for 5–10 years, but frequent binge drinking may also be sufficient. Many patients with alcoholic cardiomyopathy are fully functional without apparent stigmata of alcoholism.

Diastolic dysfunction, mild ventricular dilation, and subclinical depression of contractility can be seen before the development of clinical heart failure. Atrial fibrillation occurs commonly. The cardiac impairment in severe alcoholic cardiomyopathy is the sum of both permanent damage and a substantial component that is reversible after cessation of alcohol consumption. Medical therapy includes neurohormonal antagonists and diuretics as needed for fluid management. Withdrawal should be supervised to avoid exacerbations of heart failure or arrhythmias, and ongoing support arranged. Even with severe disease, marked improvement can occur within 3–6 months of abstinence. Implantable defibrillators are generally deferred until an adequate period of abstinence, after which they may not be necessary if the ejection fraction has improved. With continued consumption, the prognosis is grim.

Cocaine, amphetamines, and related catecholaminergic stimulants can produce chronic cardiomyopathy as well as acute ischemia and tachyarrhythmias. Pathology reveals tiny microinfarcts consistent with small vessel ischemia. Similar findings can be seen with pheochromocytoma.

Chemotherapy agents are the most common drugs implicated in cardiomyopathy. Judicious use of these drugs requires balancing the risks of the malignancy and the risks of cardiotoxicity, as many cancers have a chronic course with prognosis no worse than heart failure.

Anthracyclines cause characteristic histologic changes of vacuolar degeneration and myofibrillar loss. Generation of reactive oxygen species involving heme compounds is currently the favored explanation for myocyte injury and fibrosis. Disruption of the large titin protein may contribute to loss of sarcomere organization. There are three different presentations of anthracycline-induced cardiomyopathy. Acute heart failure developing during administration of a single dose can be severe, but may clinically resolve in a few weeks. Early onset doxorubicin cardiotoxicity develops in about 3% of patients during or shortly after a chronic course, relating closely to total dose. It may be rapidly progressive, but may also improve to restore reasonable ventricular function. The chronic presentation differs according to whether therapy was given before or after puberty. Patients who received doxorubicin while still growing may have inadequate development of the heart to support cardiac function into the early twenties. Late after adult exposure, patients may develop the gradual onset of symptoms or an acute onset precipitated by a reversible insult, such as influenza or atrial fibrillation. Doxorubicin cardiotoxicity leads to a relatively nondilated ventricle, perhaps due to the accompanying fibrosis. Thus, the stroke volume may be severely reduced with an ejection fraction of 30–40%, which would be well tolerated in a patient with a more dilated ventricle typical of other cardiomyopathies. Therapy is that for heart failure, with careful suppression of "inappropriate" sinus tachycardia, and attention to postural hypotension that can occur in these patients. Once thought to have an inexorable downward course, some patients with doxorubicin cardiotoxicity improve under careful management to near-normal clinical function for many years.

Trastuzumab is a monoclonal antibody that interferes with cell surface receptors crucial for some tumor growth and for cardiac adaptation. The incidence of cardiotoxicity is lower than for anthracyclines but enhanced by coadministration with them. Although considered to be more often reversible, trastuzumab cardiotoxicity does not always resolve, and some patients progress to clinical heart failure and death. As with anthracycline cardiotoxicity, therapy is as usual for heart failure, but it is not clear whether or not the spontaneous rate of improvement is enhanced by neurohormonal antagonists.

Cardiotoxicity with *cyclophosphamide and ifosfamide* generally occurs acutely and with very high doses. 5-Fluorouracil, cisplatin, and some other alkylating agents can cause recurrent coronary spasm that occasionally leads to depressed contractility. Many small molecule *tyrosine kinase inhibitors* are under development for different malignancies. Although these agents are "targeted" at specific tumor receptors or pathways, the biologic conservation of signaling pathways can cause inhibitors to have "off-target" effects that include the heart and vasculature. Acute administration of *interferon-α* can cause hypotension and arrhythmias. Clinical heart failure occurring during repeated chronic administration usually resolves after discontinuation.

Other therapeutic drugs that can cause cardiotoxicity during chronic use include hydroxychloroquine, chloroquine, emetine, and antiretroviral therapies.

Toxic exposures are most commonly implicated in arrhythmias or respiratory injury acutely during accidents. Chronic exposures that can cause cardiotoxicity include hydrocarbons, fluorocarbons, arsenicals, lead, and mercury.

METABOLIC CAUSES OF DILATED CARDIOMYOPATHY

Endocrine disorders affect multiple organ systems, including the heart. *Hyperthyroidism and hypothyroidism* do not often cause clinical heart failure in an otherwise normal heart, but commonly exacerbate heart failure. The most common, current reason for thyroid abnormalities in the heart failure population is the use of amiodarone, a drug with substantial iodine content. Clinical signs of thyroid disease may be masked, so tests of thyroid function are part of the routine evaluation of cardiomyopathy. Hypothyroidism should be treated with very slow escalation of doses to avoid exacerbating tachyarrhythmias and heart failure. Hyperthyroidism should always be considered with new onset atrial fibrillation or ventricular tachycardia, or atrial fibrillation in which the rapid ventricular response is difficult to control. Hyperthyroidism and heart failure are a dangerous combination that merits very close supervision, often hospitalization, during titration of antithyroid medications, which may lead to precipitous worsening of heart failure. *Pheochromocytoma* is rare, but should be considered when a patient has heart failure and very labile blood pressure and heart rate, sometimes with episodic palpitations (Chap. 343). Most patients with pheochromocytoma have postural hypotension. In addition to α-adrenergic receptor antagonists, definitive therapy requires surgical extirpation. Very high renin states, such as those caused by renal artery stenosis, can lead to modest depression in ejection fraction with little or no ventricular dilation and markedly labile symptoms with flash pulmonary edema, related to sudden shifts in vascular tone and intravascular volume.

Controversies remain regarding whether *diabetes* and *obesity* are sufficient to cause cardiomyopathy. Most heart failure in diabetes results from epicardial coronary disease, with further increase in coronary artery risk due to accompanying hypertension and renal dysfunction. Cardiomyopathy may result in part from insulin resistance and increased advanced-glycosylation end products, which impair both systolic and diastolic function. However, much of the dysfunction can be attributed to scattered focal ischemia resulting from distal coronary artery tapering and limited microvascular perfusion even without proximal focal stenoses. Diabetes is a typical factor, along with hypertension, advanced age, and female gender, in heart failure with "preserved" ejection fraction.

The existence of a cardiomyopathy due to *obesity* is generally accepted. In addition to cardiac involvement from associated diabetes, hypertension, and vascular inflammation of the metabolic syndrome, obesity alone is associated with impaired excretion of excess volume load, which, over time, can lead to increased wall stress and secondary adaptive neurohumoral responses. The rapid clearance of natriuretic peptides by adipose tissue may contribute to fluid retention. In the absence of another obvious cause of cardiomyopathy in an obese patient with systolic dysfunction without marked ventricular dilation, effective weight reduction is often associated with major improvement in ejection fraction and clinical function.

Nutritional deficiencies can occasionally cause dilated cardiomyopathy but are not commonly implicated in developed Western countries. *Beri-beri heart disease* due to thiamine deficiency can result from poor nutrition in undernourished populations, and in patients deriving most of their calories from alcohol, and has been reported in teenagers subsisting only on highly processed foods. This disease is initially a vasodilated state with very high output heart failure that can later progress to a low output state; thiamine repletion can lead to prompt recovery of cardiovascular function. Abnormalities in *carnitine* metabolism can cause dilated or restrictive cardiomyopathies, usually in children. Deficiency of trace elements such as *selenium* can cause cardiomyopathy (Keshan's disease).

Calcium is essential for excitation-contraction coupling, serving as an inotrope when administered. Chronic deficiencies of calcium, such as can occur with hypoparathyroidism (particularly postsurgical) or intestinal dysfunction (from diarrheal syndromes and following extensive resection), can cause severe chronic heart failure that responds over days or weeks to vigorous calcium repletion. *Phosphate* is a component of high-energy compounds needed for efficient energy transfer and multiple signaling pathways. Hypophosphatemia can develop during starvation and early refeeding following a prolonged fast, and occasionally during hyperalimentation. *Magnesium* is a cofactor for thiamine-dependent reactions and for the sodium-potassium adenosine triphosphatase (ATPase), but hypomagnesemia rarely becomes sufficiently profound to cause clinical cardiomyopathy.

Hemochromatosis is variably classified as a metabolic or storage disease. It is included among the causes of restrictive cardiomyopathy, but the clinical presentation is often that of a dilated cardiomyopathy. The autosomal recessive form is related to the *HFE* gene. With up to 10% of the population heterozygous for one mutation, the clinical prevalence might be as high as 1 in 500. The lower rates observed highlight the limited penetrance of the disease, suggesting the role of additional genetic and environmental factors for clinical expression. The clinical syndrome includes cirrhosis, diabetes, and hypogonadism (Chap. 357). Hemochromatosis can also be acquired from iron overload due to hemolytic anemia and transfusions. Excess iron is deposited in the perinuclear compartment of cardiomyocytes, with resulting disruption of intracellular architecture and mitochondrial function. Diagnosis is easily made from measurement of serum iron and transferrin saturation, with a threshold of >60% for men, and >45–50% for women. Magnetic resonance imaging can help to quantitate iron stores in the liver and heart, and endomyocardial biopsy tissue can be stained for iron (Fig. 238-8). If diagnosed early, hemochromatosis can often be managed by repeated phlebotomy to remove iron. For more severe iron overload, iron chelation therapy with desferrioxamine (deferoxamine) or deferasirox can help to improve cardiac function if myocyte loss and replacement fibrosis are not too severe. Inborn disorders of metabolism occasionally present with dilated cardiomyopathy, although are most often associated with restrictive cardiomyopathy (Table 238-4).

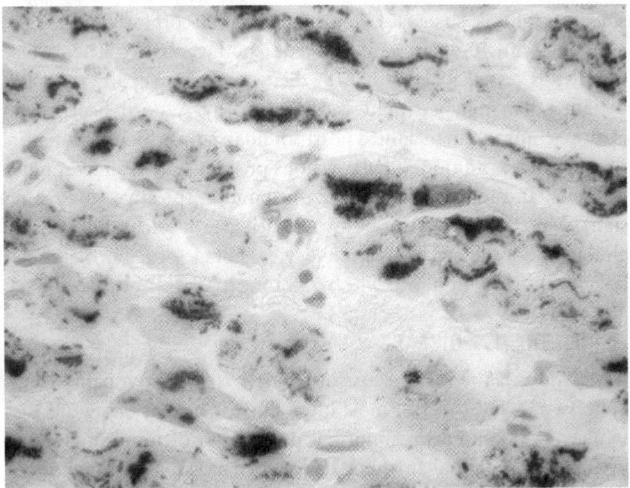

Figure 238-8 Hemochromatosis. Microscopic image of an endomyocardial biopsy showing extensive iron deposition within the cardiac myocytes with the Prussian blue stain (400× original magnification). *(Image courtesy of Robert Padera, MD, PhD, Department of Pathology, Brigham and Women's Hospital, Boston.)*

■ FAMILIAL DILATED CARDIOMYOPATHY

The recognized frequency of familial involvement in dilated cardiomyopathy has now increased to an estimated 30% (Table 238-3). The most recognizable familial syndromes are the *muscular dystrophies.* Both Duchenne's and the milder Becker's dystrophy result from abnormalities in the X-linked dystrophin gene of the sarcolemmal membrane. Skeletal myopathy is present in multiple other genetic cardiomyopathies (Table 238-3), some of which are associated with creatine kinase elevations. Mitochondrial myopathies are associated with varying degrees of skeletal involvement, biopsies of which show the characteristic "ragged red fiber" appearance. Some patients with mitochondrial myopathy have characteristic drooping eyelids. The energy deficits associated with mitochondrial abnormalities lead to multiple systemic syndromes. Other familial metabolic defects more often present as restrictive disease, but can sometimes be identified on electron microscopy of endomyocardial biopsies.

Families with a history of atrial arrhythmias, conduction system disease, and cardiomyopathy may have abnormalities of the nuclear membrane lamin proteins. While all dilated cardiomyopathies carry a risk of sudden death, a family history of cardiomyopathy with sudden death raises suspicion for a particularly arrhythmogenic mutation; affected family members may be considered for implantable defibrillators even before meeting the reduced ejection fraction threshold for primary prevention of sudden death.

A prominent family history of sudden death or ventricular tachycardia before clinical cardiomyopathy suggests genetic defects in the desmosomal proteins causing *arrhythmogenic ventricular dysplasia* (Fig. 238-9). Originally described as affecting the right ventricle [arrhythmogenic right ventricular dysplasia (ARVD)], this disorder can affect either or both ventricles. Patients often present first with ventricular tachycardia. Genetic defects in proteins of the desmosomal complex disrupt myocyte junctions and adhesions, leading to replacement of myocardium by deposits of fat. Thin ventricular walls may be recognized on echocardiography but are better visualized on MRI. The same protein also affects hair and skin, leading in some cases to a distinct syndrome of "woolly hair," and thickened palms and soles. Implantable defibrillators are usually indicated to prevent sudden death. There is variable progression to right, left, or biventricular failure.

Left ventricular noncompaction is a condition of unknown prevalence that is increasingly revealed by better imaging techniques, first by two-dimensional echocardiography and more recently by magnetic resonance imaging. The diagnostic criteria includes the presence of multiple trabeculations in the left ventricle distal to the papillary muscles, creating a "spongy" appearance of the apex; it has been associated with multiple genetic variants in the sarcomeric and other proteins such as tafazzin. The condition may be diagnosed incidentally or in patients carrying previous diagnoses of dilated, restrictive, or hypertrophic cardiomyopathy. The three cardinal clinical features are ventricular arrhythmias, embolic events, and heart failure. Treatment generally includes anticoagulation and consideration for an implantable defibrillator.

Some families inherit a susceptibility to viral-induced myocarditis. This propensity may relate to abnormalities in cell surface receptors, such as the coxsackie-adenovirus receptor, that bind viral proteins. Some may have partial homology with viral proteins such that an autoimmune response is triggered against the myocardium.

The therapy of familial dilated cardiomyopathy is dictated primarily by the stage of clinical disease and the risk for sudden death. In some cases, the familial etiology facilitates prognostic

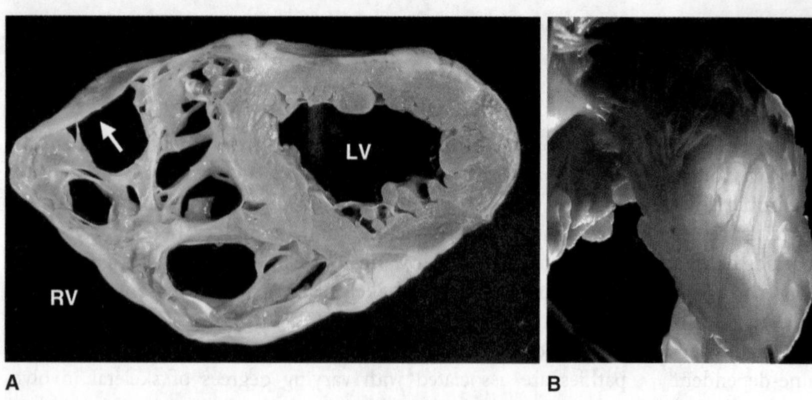

Figure 238-9 Arrhythmogenic right ventricular dysplasia. ***A.*** Cross-sectional slice of a pathology specimen removed at transplantation, showing severe dysplasia of the right ventricle (RV) with extensive fatty replacement of right ventricular myocardium. The remarkably thin right ventricular free wall is revealed by transillumination ***B.*** *(Images courtesy of Gayle Winters, MD, and Richard Mitchell, MD, PhD, Division of Pathology, Brigham and Women's Hospital, Boston.)*

decisions, particularly regarding the likelihood of recovery after a new diagnosis, which is unlikely for familial disease and frequent if the disease is acquired. The rate of progression of disease is to some extent heritable, although marked variation can be seen; however, there have been cases of remarkable clinical remission after acute presentation, likely after a reversible insult, such as infective myocarditis.

Genetic testing is less robust for dilated cardiomyopathy, for which our current understanding is similar to that for hypertrophic cardiomyopathy a decade ago. Newer molecular techniques, animal models, and databanks of cardiomyopathy patients are all contributing to the rapid expansion of the data presented in Table 238-3. However, serendipitous identification of inherited cardiomyopathy, its systemic signature, and clinical course remain crucial to continue to advance the field, one family and one gene at a time.

■ TAKO-TSUBO CARDIOMYOPATHY

The apical ballooning syndrome, or stress-induced cardiomyopathy, occurs typically in older women after sudden intense emotional or physical stress. The ventricle shows global ventricular dilation with basal contraction, forming the shape of the narrow-necked jar (*tako-tsubo*) used in Japan to trap octopi. Originally described there, it is increasingly recognized in other countries and may go unrecognized during intensive care unit (ICU) admission for noncardiac conditions. Presentations include pulmonary edema, hypotension, and chest pain with ECG changes mimicking an acute infarction. The left ventricular dysfunction extends beyond a specific coronary artery distribution and generally resolves within days to weeks, but may recur in up to 10% of patients. Animal models and ventricular biopsies suggest that this acute cardiomyopathy may result from intense sympathetic activation with heterogeneity of myocardial autonomic innervation, diffuse microvascular spasm, and/or direct catecholamine toxicity. Coronary angiography may be required to rule out acute coronary occlusion. No therapies have been proven beneficial, but reasonable strategies include nitrates for pulmonary edema, intraaortic balloon pump if needed for low output, combined alpha- and beta blockers rather than selective beta blockade if hemodynamically stable, and magnesium for arrhythmias related to QT prolongation. Anticoagulation is generally withheld due to the occasional occurrence of ventricular rupture.

■ IDIOPATHIC DILATED CARDIOMYOPATHY

Idiopathic dilated cardiomyopathy is a diagnosis of exclusion, when all other known factors have been excluded. Approximately two-thirds of dilated cardiomyopathies are still labeled as idiopathic; however, a substantial proportion of these may reflect unrecognized genetic disease. Continued reconsideration of etiology often reveals specific causes later in a patient's course.

OVERLAP BETWEEN CARDIOMYOPATHIES

The limitations of our phenotypic classification are revealed through the multiple overlaps between the etiologies and presentations of the three types. Cardiomyopathy with reduced systolic function but without severe dilation can represent early dilated cardiomyopathy, "minimally dilated cardiomyopathy," or restrictive diseases without marked increases in ventricular wall thickness. For example, sarcoidosis and hemochromatosis can present as dilated or restrictive disease. Early stages of amyloidosis sometimes appear as dilated cardiomyopathy, but can also be mistaken for hypertrophic cardiomyopathy. Progression of hypertrophic cardiomyopathy into a "burned-out" phase occurs occasionally, with decreased contractility and modest ventricular dilation. Overlaps are particularly common with the inherited metabolic disorders, which can present as any of the three major phenotypes (Fig. 238-4).

RESTRICTIVE CARDIOMYOPATHY

The least common of the triad of cardiomyopathies is restrictive cardiomyopathy, which is dominated by abnormal diastolic function, often with mildly decreased contractility and ejection fraction (usually >30–50%). Both atria are enlarged, sometimes massively. Modest left ventricular dilation can be present, usually with an end-diastolic dimension <6 cm. End-diastolic pressures are elevated in both ventricles, with preservation of cardiac output until late in the disease. Subtle exercise intolerance is usually the first symptom but is often not recognized until after clinical presentation with congestive symptoms. The restrictive diseases often present with relatively more right-sided symptoms, such as edema, abdominal discomfort, and ascites, although filling pressures are elevated in both ventricles. The cardiac impulse is less displaced than in dilated cardiomyopathy and less dynamic than in hypertrophic cardiomyopathy. A fourth heart sound is more common than a third heart sound in sinus rhythm, but atrial fibrillation is common. Jugular venous pressures often show rapid Y descents, and may increase during inspiration (positive Kussmaul's sign). Most restrictive cardiomyopathies are due to infiltration of abnormal substances between myocytes, storage of abnormal metabolic products within myocytes, or fibrotic injury (Table 238-6).

■ INFILTRATIVE DISEASE

Amyloidosis is the major cause of restrictive cardiomyopathy (Figs. 238-10, 238-11, 238-12), most often due to "primary amyloidosis" (Chap. 112) caused by abnormal production of immunoglobulin light chains. Familial amyloidosis results from an autosomal dominant mutation in transthyretin, a carrier protein for thyroxine and retinol, that is more common in African Americans than whites. Amyloidosis secondary to other chronic diseases rarely involves the heart. Senile amyloidosis with deposition of normal transthyretin or atrial natriuretic peptide usually has an indolent course and is very common beyond the seventh decade.

TABLE 238-6 Causes of Restrictive Cardiomyopathies

Infiltrative (Between Myocytes)
Amyloidosis
Primary (light chain amyloid)
Familial (abnormal transthyretin)[a]
Senile (normal transthyretin or atrial peptides)
Inherited metabolic defects[a] (see Table 238-4)
Storage (Within Myocytes)
Hemochromatosis (iron)[a]
Inherited metabolic defects[a] (see Table 238-4)
Fabry's disease
Glycogen storage disease (II, III)
Fibrotic
Radiation
Scleroderma
Endomyocardial
Possibly related fibrotic diseases
Tropical endomyocardial fibrosis
Hypereosinophilic syndrome (Löffler's endocarditis)
Carcinoid syndrome
Radiation
Drugs: e.g., serotonin, ergotamine
Overlap with Other Cardiomyopathies
Hypertrophic cardiomyopathy/"pseudohypertrophic"[a]
"Minimally dilated" cardiomyopathy
Early stage dilated cardiomyopathy
Partial recovery from dilated cardiomyopathy
Sarcoidosis
Idiopathic[a]

[a]Can be familial.

Amyloid fibrils infiltrate the myocardium, especially around the conduction system and coronary vessels. Typical clinical features are conduction block, autonomic neuropathy, renal involvement, and occasionally thickened skin lesions. Cardiac amyloid is suspected from thickened ventricular walls in conjunction with an electrocardiogram that shows low voltage. A characteristic refractile brightness in the septum on echocardiography is suggestive, but neither sensitive nor specific. Both atria are dilated, often dramatically so. The diagnosis of primary or familial can be made from biopsies of an abdominal fat pad or the rectum, but cardiac amyloidosis is most reliably identified from the myocardium (Fig. 238-12). Therapy is largely symptomatic, using diuretics as needed to treat fluid retention, which often requires high doses. Digoxin bound to the amyloid fibrils can reach toxic levels, and should therefore be used only in very low doses, if at all. There is no evidence regarding use of neurohormonal antagonists in amyloid heart disease, where the possible theoretical benefit has to be balanced against their potential side effects in light of frequent autonomic neuropathy and dependence on heart rate reserve. The risk of intracardiac thrombi may warrant chronic anticoagulation. Once heart failure develops, the median survival is 6–12 months in primary amyloidosis. Multiple myeloma is treated with chemotherapy (prednisone, melphalan, bortezomib), the extent of which is usually limited by the potential of worsening cardiac dysfunction. Colchicine can be of some benefit in inflammation-associated (AA) amyloid. Transthyretin-associated cardiac amyloid requires heart and liver transplantation, while senile cardiac amyloid is treated with conventional heart failure regimens. Immunoglobulin-associated amyloid has occasionally been treated with sequential heart transplantation and delayed bone marrow transplant, with frequent recurrence of amyloid in the transplanted heart.

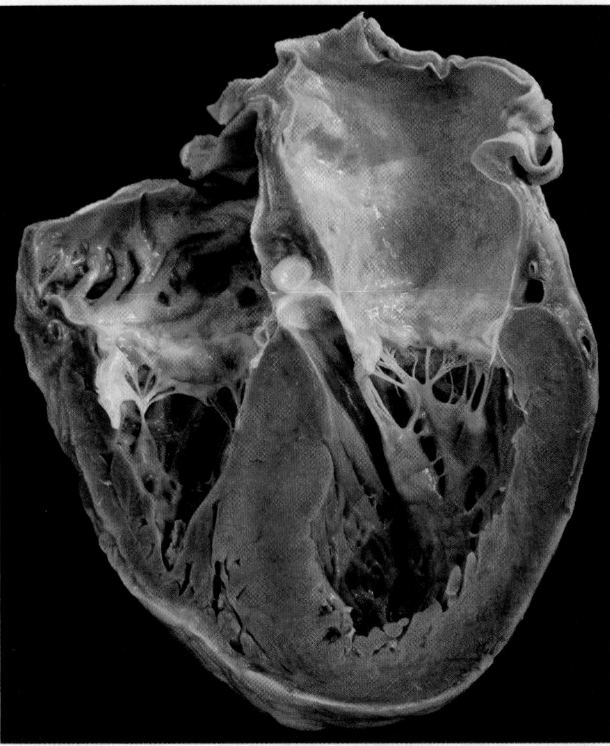

Figure 238-10 Restrictive cardiomyopathy—amyloidosis. Gross specimen of a heart with amyloidosis. The heart is firm and rubbery with a waxy cut surface. The atria are markedly dilated and the left atrial endocardium, normally smooth, has yellow-brown amyloid deposits that give texture to the surface. *(Image courtesy of Robert Padera, MD, PhD, Department of Pathology, Brigham and Women's Hospital, Boston.)*

■ DISORDERS OF METABOLIC PATHWAYS

Multiple genetic disorders of metabolic pathways can cause myocardial disease, due to infiltration of abnormal products or cells containing them between the myocytes, and storage disease, due to their accumulation within cells (Tables 238-4, 238-6). The restrictive phenotype is most common but mildly dilated cardiomyopathy may occur. Hypertrophic cardiomyopathy may be mimicked by the myocardium thickened with these abnormal products causing "pseudohypertrophy." Most of these diseases are diagnosed during childhood.

Fabry's disease results from a deficiency of the lysosomal enzyme alpha-galactosidase A caused by one of more than 160 mutations. This disorder of glycosphingolipid metabolism is an X-linked recessive disorder that may also cause clinical disease in female carriers. Glycolipid accumulation may be limited to the cardiac tissues or may also involve the skin and kidney. Electron microscopy of endomyocardial biopsy tissue shows diagnostic vesicles containing concentric lamellar figures (Fig. 238-13). Diagnosis is crucial

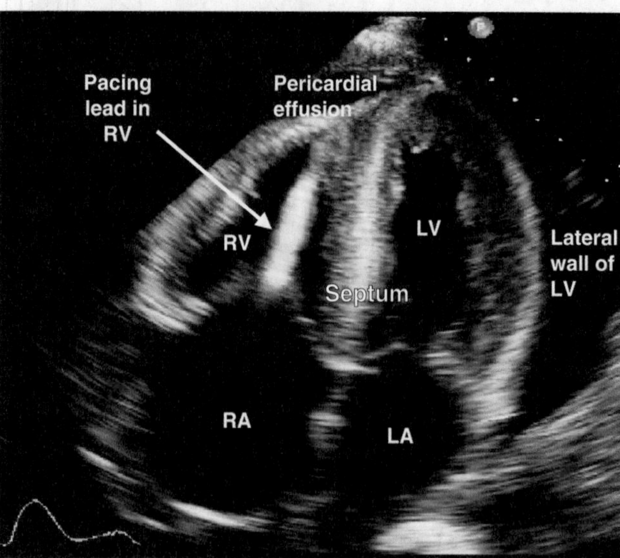

Figure 238-11 Restrictive cardiomyopathy—amyloidosis. Echocardiogram showing thickened walls of both ventricles without major chamber dilation. The atria are markedly dilated, consistent with chronically elevated ventricular filling pressures. In this example, there is a characteristic hyperrefractile "glittering" of the myocardium typical of amyloid infiltration, which is often absent (especially with more recent echocardiographic systems of better resolution). The mitral and tricuspid valves are thickened. A pacing lead is visible in the right ventricle and a pericardial effusion is evident. Note that the echocardiographic and pathologic images are vertically opposite, such that the LV is by convention on the top right in the echocardiographic image and bottom right in the pathologic images. *(Image courtesy of Justina Wu, MD, Brigham and Women's Hospital, Boston.)*

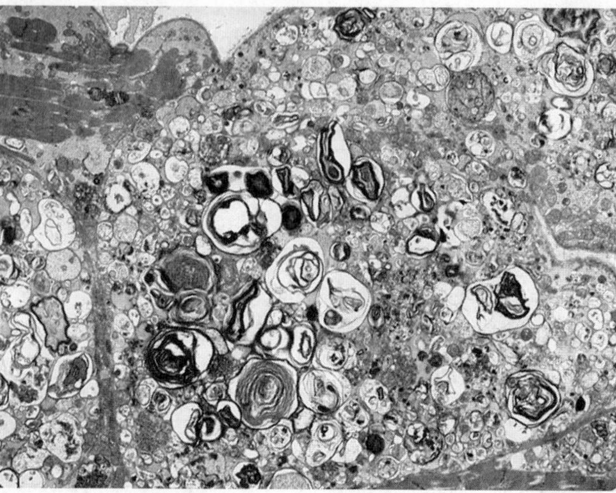

Figure 238-13 Fabry's disease. Transmission electron micrograph of a right ventricular endomyocardial biopsy specimen at high magnification showing the characteristic concentric lamellar inclusions of glycosphingolipids accumulating as a result of deficiency of the lysosomal enzyme alpha-galactosidase A. Image taken at 15,000× original magnification. *(Image courtesy of Robert Padera, MD, PhD, Department of Pathology, Brigham and Women's Hospital, Boston.)*

because enzyme replacement can reduce abnormal deposits and improve cardiac and clinical function. Enzyme replacement can also improve the course of Gaucher's disease, in which cerebroside-rich cells accumulate in multiple organs due to a deficiency of beta-glucosidase. Cerebroside-rich cells infiltrate the heart, which can also lead to a hemorrhagic pericardial effusion and valvular disease.

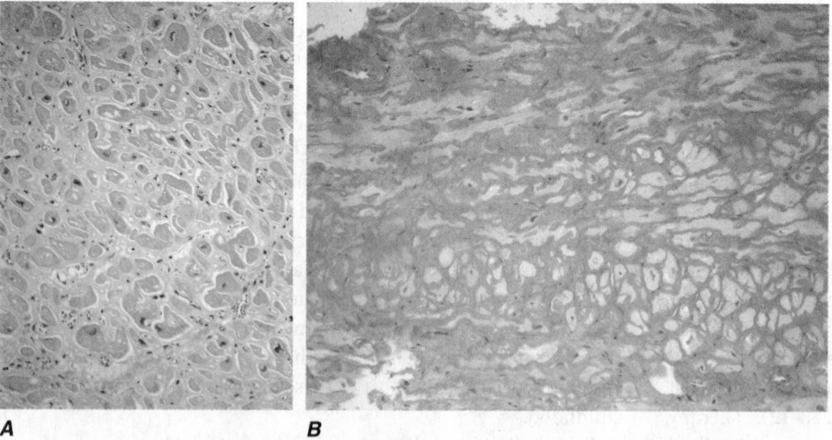

Figure 238-12 Amyloidosis—microscopic images of amyloid involving the myocardium. The left panel (hematoxylin-eosin stain) shows glassy, grey-pink amorphous material infiltrating between cardiomyocytes, which stain a darker pink. The right panel shows a sulfated blue stain that highlights the amyloid green and stains the cardiac myocytes yellow. (The Congo red stain can also be used to highlight amyloid; under polarized light, amyloid will have an apple-green birefringence when stained with Congo red). Images at 100× original magnification. *(Image courtesy of Robert Padera, MD, PhD, Department of Pathology, Brigham and Women's Hospital, Boston.)*

Glycogen storage diseases lead to accumulation of lysosomal storage products and intracellular glycogen accumulation, particularly with *glycogen storage disease type III,* due to a defective debranching enzyme. There are more than 10 types of *mucopolysaccharidoses,* in which autosomal dominant or X-linked deficiencies of lysosomal enzymes lead to the accumulation of glycosaminoglycans in the skeleton, nervous system, and heart. With characteristic facies, short stature, and frequent cognitive impairment, most individuals are diagnosed early in childhood and die before adulthood.

Carnitine is an essential cofactor in long-chain fatty acid metabolism. Multiple defects have been described that lead to carnitine deficiency, causing intracellular lipid inclusions and restrictive or dilated cardiomyopathy, often presenting in children. Fatty acid oxidation requires many metabolic steps with specific enzymes that can be deficient, with complex interactions with carnitine. Depending on the defect, cardiac and skeletal myopathy can be ameliorated with replacement of fatty acid intermediates and carnitine.

Two monogenic metabolic cardiomyopathies have recently been described as causes of increased ventricular wall thickness without an increase of muscle subunits or an increase in contractility. Mutations in the gamma-2 regulatory subunit of the adenosine monophosphate (AMP)-activated protein kinase important for glucose metabolism (PRKAG2) have been associated with a high prevalence of conduction abnormalities, such as AV block and ventricular preexcitation (Wolff-Parkinson-White syndrome). Several defects have been reported in an X-linked lysosome-associated membrane protein (LAMP2). This defect can be maternally transmitted or sporadic and has occasionally been isolated to the heart, although it often leads to a syndrome of skeletal myopathy, mental retardation, and hepatic dysfunction referred to as *Danon's disease.* Left ventricular hypertrophy appears early, often in childhood, and can progress rapidly to end-stage heart failure with low ejection fraction. Electron microscopy of these metabolic disorders shows that the myocytes are enlarged by multiple intracellular vacuoles of metabolic by-products.

FIBROTIC RESTRICTIVE CARDIOMYOPATHY

Progressive fibrosis can cause restrictive myocardial disease without dilation. Thoracic radiation, common for breast and lung cancer or mediastinal lymphoma, can produce early or late restrictive cardiomyopathy. Patients with *radiation cardiomyopathy* may present with a possible diagnosis of constrictive pericarditis, as the two conditions often coexist. Careful hemodynamic evaluation and, often, endomyocardial biopsy should be performed if considering pericardial stripping surgery, which is unlikely to be successful in the presence of underlying restrictive cardiomyopathy.

Scleroderma causes small vessel spasm and ischemia that can lead to a small, stiff heart with reduced ejection fraction without dilation. Doxorubicin causes direct myocyte injury usually leading to dilated cardiomyopathy, but the limited degree of dilation may result from increased fibrosis, which restricts remodeling.

ENDOMYOCARDIAL DISEASE

The physiologic picture of elevated filling pressures with atrial enlargement and preserved ventricular contractility with normal or reduced ventricular volumes can also result from extensive fibrosis of the endocardium, without transmural myocardial disease. For patients who have not lived in the equatorial regions, this picture is rare, and when seen is usually associated with a history of chronic hypereosinophilic syndrome (*Löffler's endocarditis*), which is more common in men than women. In this disease, persistent hypereosinophilia of >1500 eos/mm^3 for at least 6 months can cause an acute phase of eosinophilic injury in the endocardium, with systemic illness and injury to other organs. There is usually no obvious cause, but the hypereosinophilia can occasionally be explained by allergic, parasitic, or malignant disease. It is postulated to be followed by a period in which cardiac inflammation is replaced by evidence of fibrosis with superimposed thrombosis. In severe disease, the dense fibrotic layer can obliterate the ventricular apices and extend to thicken and tether the atrioventricular valve leaflets. The clinical disease may present with heart failure, embolic events, and atrial arrhythmias. While plausible, the sequence of transition has not been clearly demonstrated.

In tropical countries, up to one-quarter of heart failure may be due to *endomyocardial fibrosis,* affecting either or both ventricles. This condition shares with the previous condition the partial obliteration of the ventricular apex with fibrosis extending into the valvular inflow tract and leaflets; however, it is not clear that the etiologies are the same for all cases. Pericardial effusions frequently accompany endomyocardial fibrosis but are not common in Löffler's endocarditis. For endomyocardial fibrosis, there is no gender difference, but a higher prevalence in African American populations. While tropical endomyocardial fibrosis could represent the end-stage of previous hypereosinophilic disease triggered by endemic parasites, neither prior parasitic infection nor hypereosinophilia is usually documented. Geographic nutritional deficiencies have also been proposed as an etiology.

Medical treatment focuses on glucocorticoids and chemotherapy to suppress hypereosinophilia when present. Fluid retention may become increasingly resistant to diuretic therapy. Anticoagulation is recommended. Atrial fibrillation is associated with worse symptoms and prognosis, but may be difficult to suppress. Surgical resection of the apices and replacement of the fibrotic valves can improve symptoms, but surgical morbidity and mortality and later recurrence rates are high.

The serotonin secreted by *carcinoid* tumors can produce fibrous plaques in the endocardium and right-sided cardiac valves, occasionally affecting left-sided valves, as well. Valvular lesions may be stenotic or regurgitant. Systemic symptoms include flushing and diarrhea. Liver disease from hepatic metastases may play a role by limiting hepatic function and thereby allowing more serotonin to reach the venous circulation.

HYPERTROPHIC CARDIOMYOPATHY

Hypertrophic cardiomyopathy is characterized by marked left ventricular hypertrophy in the absence of other causes, such as hypertension or valve disease (Figs. 238-14 and 238-15). The systolic function as measured by ejection fraction is often supranormal, at times with virtual obliteration of the left ventricular cavity during systole. The hypertrophy may be asymmetric, involving the septum more than the free wall of the ventricle. Approximately one-third of symptomatic patients demonstrate a resting intraventricular gradient that impedes outflow during systole and is exacerbated by increased contractility. This was previously termed *hypertrophic obstructive cardiomyopathy* (HOCM), as distinguished from *nonobstructive hypertrophic cardiomyopathy.* Other terms that have been used include *asymmetric septal hypertrophy* (ASH) and *idiopathic hypertrophic subaortic stenosis* (IHSS). However, the accepted terminology is now hypertrophic cardiomyopathy with or without an obstructive gradient. Classically, the microscopic picture shows marked disarray of individual fibers in a characteristic whorled pattern and disarray, also at the level of the larger bundles, interspersed with fibrosis (Fig. 238-16).

The prevalence of hypertrophic cardiomyopathy is 1:500 adults. Approximately one-half of these cases occur in a recognizable auto-

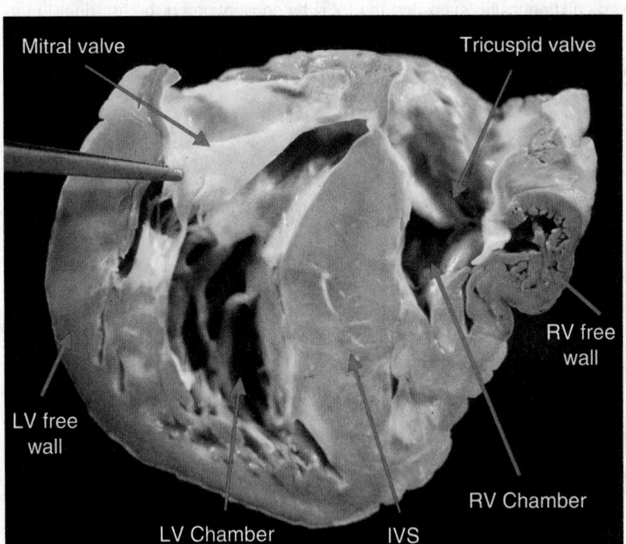

Figure 238-14 Hypertrophic cardiomyopathy. Gross specimen of a heart with hypertrophic cardiomyopathy removed at the time of transplantation, showing asymmetric septal hypertrophy (septum much thicker than left ventricular free wall) with the septum bulging into the left ventricular outflow tract causing obstruction. The forceps are retracting the anterior leaflet of the mitral valve, demonstrating the characteristic plaque of systolic anterior motion, manifest as endocardial fibrosis on the interventricular septum in a mirror-image pattern to the valve leaflet. There is patchy replacement fibrosis, and small thick walled arterioles can be appreciated grossly, especially in the interventricular septum. IVS, interventricular septum; LV, left ventricle; RV, right ventricle. *(Image courtesy of Robert Padera, MD, PhD, Department of Pathology, Brigham and Women's Hospital, Boston.)*

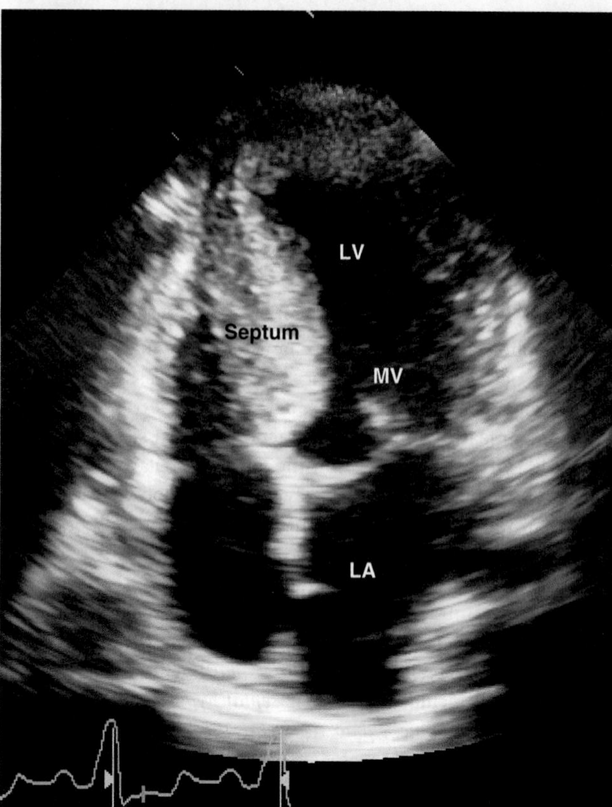

Figure 238-15 Hypertrophic cardiomyopathy. This echocardiogram of hypertrophic cardiomyopathy shows asymmetric hypertrophy of the septum compared to the lateral wall of the left ventricle (LV). The mitral valve is moving anteriorly toward the hypertrophied septum in systole. The left atrium (LA) is enlarged. Note that the echocardiographic and pathologic images are vertically opposite, such that the LV is by convention on the top right in the echocardiographic image and bottom right in the pathologic images. *(Image courtesy of Justina Wu, MD, Brigham and Women's Hospital, Boston.)*

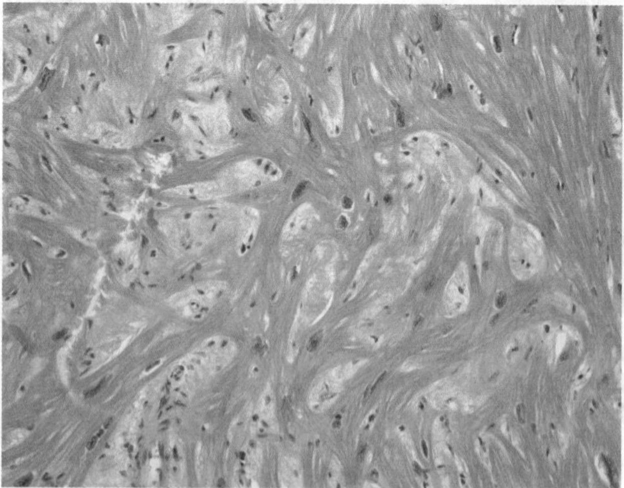

Figure 238-16 Hypertrophic cardiomyopathy. Microscopic image of hypertrophic cardiomyopathy showing the characteristic disordered myocyte architecture with swirling and branching rather than the usual parallel arrangement of myocyte fibers. Myocyte nuclei vary markedly in size and interstitial fibrosis is present. *(Image courtesy of Robert Padera, MD, PhD, Department of Pathology, Brigham and Women's Hospital, Boston.)*

somal dominant pattern, and spontaneous mutations also arise. This is the best characterized genetic cardiomyopathy, for which more than 400 individual mutations have been identified in 11 sarcomeric genes. More than 80% of the mutations are in the beta-myosin heavy chain, the cardiac myosin-binding protein C, or cardiac troponin T. Some families may demonstrate a higher incidence of early progression to end-stage heart failure or death, suggesting that their mutations are more "malignant." However, the heterogeneity of phenotypic expression within and between families confirms the influence of modifying factors from other genes and the environment.

Hypertrophic cardiomyopathy is characterized hemodynamically by diastolic dysfunction, originally attributed to the hypertrophy, fibrosis, and intraventricular gradient when present. However, studies of asymptomatic family members indicate that diastolic dysfunction is a more fundamental abnormality that can precede evidence of hypertrophy. Resting ejection fraction and cardiac output are usually normal, but peak cardiac output during exercise may be reduced due to inadequate ventricular filling at high heart rates.

DIAGNOSIS

Hypertrophic cardiomyopathy usually presents between the ages of 20 and 40 years. Dyspnea on exertion is the most common presenting symptom, reflecting elevated intracardiac filling pressures. Chest pain with either an atypical or typical exertional pattern occurs in more than half of symptomatic patients and is attributed to myocardial ischemia from high demand and abnormal intramural coronary arteries in the hypertrophied myocardium. Palpitations may result from atrial fibrillation or ventricular arrhythmias. Much less common are episodes of presyncope or syncope, often related to heavy exertion. Of grave concern is the possibility that the first manifestation of disease may be sudden death from ventricular tachycardia or fibrillation. Hypertrophic cardiomyopathy is the most common lesion found at autopsy of young athletes dying suddenly.

The physical examination typically reveals a harsh murmur heard best at the left lower sternal border, arising from both the outflow tract turbulence during ventricular ejection and the commonly associated mitral regurgitation. The gradient and the murmur may be enhanced by maneuvers that decrease ventricular volume, such as the Valsalva maneuver, or standing after squatting. They may be decreased by increasing ventricular volume or vascular resistance, such as with squatting or handgrip. A fourth heart sound is commonly heard due to decreased ventricular compliance. In patients with a significant outflow tract gradient, palpation of the carotid pulse may reveal a bifid systolic impulse, from early and delayed ejection. Patients with chronic, severe elevations in filling pressures may show signs of systemic fluid retention.

The electrocardiogram usually shows left ventricular hypertrophy, often with prominent septal Q waves that can be misdiagnosed as indicative of infarction. The diagnosis of hypertrophic cardiomyopathy is confirmed by echocardiography demonstrating left ventricular hypertrophy, which may or may not be more marked in the septum (Fig. 238-15). Intraventricular gradients to outflow can be identified by Doppler echocardiography at rest or during provocative maneuvers, such as the Valsalva maneuver. Systolic anterior motion (SAM) of the mitral valve is a classic finding on the echocardiogram. Mitral regurgitation may become severe. Cardiac catheterization can be performed to quantify the gradient, which characteristically increases after a premature ventricular contraction.

Apical hypertrophic cardiomyopathy is a variant that is uncommon in the United States; however, this variant accounts for about one-fourth of patients with hypertrophic cardiomyopathy in Japan. The electrocardiogram shows deep T-wave inversions in the precordial leads, and the echocardiogram shows a characteristic spade-like appearance with apical obliteration. It has been associated with a specific genetic defect in cardiac actin (Glu 101 Lys), but may occur with other sarcomere mutations.

The differential diagnosis of hypertrophic cardiomyopathy is limited in most patients once other cardiovascular causes for secondary hypertrophy are excluded. However, other diseases that result in thickened myocardium can appear indistinguishable on echocardiography, and are considered "pseudohypertrophic," particularly the inherited metabolic diseases (Table 238-4). The differential diagnosis between hypertrophic and restrictive cardiomyopathy may be particularly difficult when considering a diagnosis of "burned-out" hypertrophic cardiomyopathy in which systolic function has decreased. Overlap with infiltrative and restrictive myocardial diseases should be considered in the evaluation of increased left ventricular wall thickness on echocardiography, particularly when clinical features are atypical for classic hypertrophic cardiomyopathy. The metabolic defects in PRKAG2, alpha-galactosidase (Fabry's disease), and LAMP2 mutations (Tables 238-3 and 238-4) should routinely be considered during evaluation of apparent hypertrophic cardiomyopathy. With late onset without a family history of hypertrophic cardiomyopathy, amyloidosis should be carefully considered.

TREATMENT Hypertrophic Cardiomyopathy

Therapy of hypertrophic cardiomyopathy is directed to symptom management and the prevention of sudden death (Fig. 238-17); it is not known whether treatment will decrease disease progression in asymptomatic family members. Exertional dyspnea and chest pain are treated by medication to reduce heart rate and ventricular contractility with hopes of improving diastolic filling patterns. Beta-adrenergic blocking drugs and verapamil are most commonly used as initial therapy. These agents both act to decrease heart rate and increase the length of time for diastolic filling, as well as to decrease the inotropic state. If there is fluid retention, diuretic therapy will usually be necessary, but requires careful titration to avoid hypovolemia, particularly in the presence of a resting or inducible obstruction to ventricular outflow. When symptoms persist and an outflow gradient is present, addition of disopyramide is sometimes effective. Amiodarone can also improve symptoms, but is usually initiated for control of arrhythmias rather than symptoms. Anticoagulation is recommended to prevent embolic events for patients who have had atrial fibrillation.

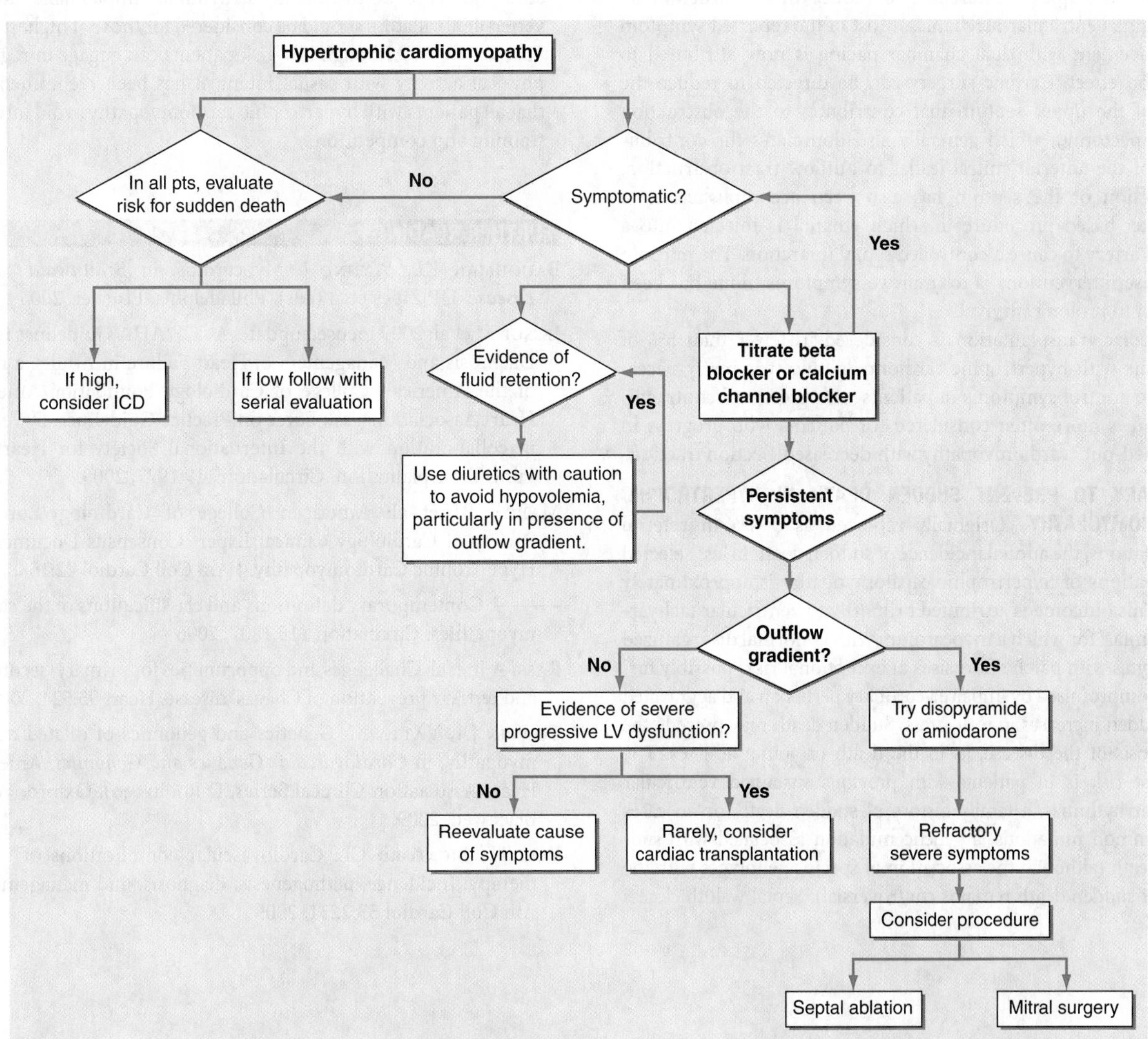

Figure 238-17 Treatment algorithm for hypertrophic cardiomyopathy depending on the presence and severity of symptoms, and the presence of an intraventricular gradient with obstruction to outflow. Note that all patients with hypertrophic cardiomyopathy should be evaluated for risk of sudden death, whether or not they require treatment for symptoms. ICD, implantable cardioverter-defibrillator; LV, left ventricular.

TABLE 238-7 Risk Factors for Sudden Death in Hypertrophic Cardiomyopathy

Major Risk Factor		Screening Technique
History of cardiac arrest or spontaneous sustained ventricular tachycardia		History
Syncope	Usually with or after exertion	History
Family history of sudden cardiac death	Or possibly with a documented gene mutation associated with high risk	Family history
Spontaneous nonsustained ventricular tachycardia	>3 beats at rate >120	Exercise or 24–48 hour ambulatory recording
LV thickness >30 mm	Present in about 10% of patients, but many sudden deaths occur with wall thickness <30 mm	Echocardiography
Abnormal blood pressure response to exercise	Systolic blood pressure fall or failure to increase at peak exercise	Maximal upright exercise testing

Abbreviation: LV, left ventricle.

Symptoms that limit routine daily life despite adjustment of medical therapies develop in fewer than 5–10% of patients, generally those with substantial obstruction to ventricular outflow. Further therapies are directed to reduce this obstruction by changing ventricular mechanics. Most of the reported symptom improvement with dual chamber pacing is now attributed to placebo effect. Cardiac surgery can be directed to reduce the size of the upper septum that contributes to the obstruction (myomectomy), which generally also dominates the contribution of the anterior mitral leaflet to outflow tract obstruction. Reduction of the septum has also been accomplished by a catheter-based procedure in which ethanol is injected into a septal artery to cause a controlled septal infarction. The purpose of these interventions is to improve symptoms; none has been shown to prolong survival.

Cardiac transplantation is considered in fewer than 5% of patients with hypertrophic cardiomyopathy. It is rarely necessary to control symptoms in patients with preserved contractility and is more often considered for patients who progress to "burned-out" cardiomyopathy with decreased ejection fraction.

THERAPY TO PREVENT SUDDEN DEATH IN HYPERTROPHIC CARDIOMYOPATHY Originally reported as 3–4% in referral populations, the annual incidence of sudden death in less selected populations of hypertrophic cardiomyopathy is approximately 1%. This outcome is attributed primarily to ventricular tachyarrhythmias, for which a myocardium with abnormal disorganized myocytes with patchy fibrosis is at exceptional risk, possibly further compromised by impaired coronary perfusion and aggravated by sudden increases in wall stress. Sudden death may precede the diagnosis of the disease, as in the death of young athletes. The highest risk is in patients with previous sustained ventricular tachyarrhythmias, a family history of sudden death, or, in cases of common mutations, a genetic mutation associated with sudden death (although the association of specific genotypes with the risk of sudden death remains controversial). Septal wall thickness >30 mm, recurrent syncope, exercise-induced hypotension, and nonsustained ventricular tachycardia are also risk factors. Areas of ventricular fibrosis detected on MRI may further identify susceptibility to life-threatening arrhythmias. Implantable cardioverter-defibrillators should be considered for those at highest risk (Table 238-7). Although low-risk patients can engage in regular physical activity with casual intent, it has been recommended that all patients with hypertrophic cardiomyopathy avoid intense training and competition.

FURTHER READINGS

Baughman KL, Wynne J: Myocarditis, in *Braunwald's Heart Disease,* DP Zipes et al (eds). Philadelphia, Elsevier, 2005

Jessup M et al: 2009 focused update: ACCF/AHA Guidelines for the Diagnosis and Management of Heart Failure in Adults: a report of the American College of Cardiology Foundation/American Heart Association Task Force on Practice Guidelines: Developed in collaboration with the International Society for Heart and Lung Transplantation. Circulation 119:1977, 2009

Maron BJ et al: American College of Cardiology/European Society of Cardiology Clinical Expert Consensus Document on Hypertrophic Cardiomyopathy. J Am Coll Cardiol 42:1688, 2003

———: Contemporary definitions and classifications of the cardiomyopathies. Circulation 113:1807, 2006

Rassi A Jr et al: Challenges and opportunities for primary, secondary, and tertiary prevention of Chagas' disease. Heart 95:524, 2009

Towbin JA, Vatta M: Genetics and genomics of dilated cardiomyopathy, in *Cardiovascular Genetics and Genomics,* American Heart Association Clinical Series, D Rodin (ed). Oxford, Wiley-Blackwell, 2009,

Yeh ET, Bickford CL: Cardiovascular complications of cancer therapy: Incidence, pathogenesis, diagnosis, and management. J Am Coll Cardiol 53:2231, 2009

CHAPTER 239
Pericardial Disease

Eugene Braunwald

NORMAL FUNCTIONS OF THE PERICARDIUM

The normal pericardium is a double-layered sac; the visceral pericardium is a serous membrane that is separated by a small quantity (15–50 mL) of fluid, an ultrafiltrate of plasma, from the fibrous parietal pericardium. The normal pericardium, by exerting a restraining force, prevents sudden dilation of the cardiac chambers, especially the right atrium and ventricle, during exercise and with hypervolemia. It also restricts the anatomic position of the heart, minimizes friction between the heart and surrounding structures, prevents displacement of the heart and kinking of the great vessels, and probably retards the spread of infections from the lungs and pleural cavities to the heart. Nevertheless, total absence of the pericardium, either congenital or after surgery, does not produce obvious clinical disease. In partial left pericardial defects, the main pulmonary artery and left atrium may bulge through the defect; very rarely, herniation and subsequent strangulation of the left atrium may cause sudden death.

ACUTE PERICARDITIS

Acute pericarditis, by far the most common pathologic process involving the pericardium, may be classified both clinically and etiologically (Table 239-1). There are four principal diagnostic features:

1. *Chest pain* is an important but not invariable symptom in various forms of acute pericarditis (Chap. 12); it is usually present in the acute infectious types and in many of the forms presumed to be related to hypersensitivity or autoimmunity. Pain is often absent in slowly developing tuberculous, postirradiation, neoplastic, and uremic pericarditis. The pain of acute pericarditis is often severe, retrosternal and left precordial, and referred to the neck, arms, or left shoulder. Often the pain is pleuritic, consequent to accompanying pleural inflammation (i.e., sharp and aggravated by inspiration and coughing), but sometimes it is a steady, constricting pain that radiates into either arm or both arms and resembles that of myocardial ischemia; therefore, confusion with acute myocardial infarction (AMI) is common. Characteristically, however, pericardial pain may be relieved by sitting up and leaning forward and is intensified by lying supine. The differentiation of AMI from acute pericarditis becomes perplexing when, with acute pericarditis, serum biomarkers of myocardial damage such as creatine kinase and troponin rise, presumably because of concomitant involvement of the epicardium in the inflammatory process (an epi-myocarditis) with resulting myocyte necrosis. However, these elevations, if they occur, are quite modest given the extensive electrocardiographic ST-segment elevation in pericarditis. This dissociation is useful in differentiating between these conditions.
2. A *pericardial friction rub* is audible in about 85% of these patients, may have up to three components per cardiac cycle, is high-pitched, and is described as rasping, scratching, or grating (Chap. 227); it can be elicited sometimes when the diaphragm of the stethoscope is applied firmly to the chest wall at the left lower sternal border. It is heard most frequently at end expiration with the patient upright and leaning forward. The rub is often inconstant, and the loud to-and-fro leathery sound may disappear within a few hours, possibly to reappear on the next day. A pericardial rub is heard throughout the respiratory cycle, whereas a pleural rub disappears when respiration is suspended.
3. The *electrocardiogram* (ECG) in acute pericarditis without massive effusion usually displays changes secondary to acute subepicardial inflammation (Fig. 239-1). It typically evolves through four stages. In stage 1, there is widespread elevation of the ST segments, often with upward concavity, involving two or three standard limb leads and V_2 to V_6, with reciprocal depressions only in aVR and sometimes V_1, as well as depression of the PR segment below the TP segment reflecting atrial involvement. Usually there are no significant changes in QRS complexes. In stage 2, after several days, the ST segments return to normal, and only then, or even later, do the T waves become inverted (stage 3). Ultimately, weeks or months after the onset of acute pericarditis, the ECG returns to normal in stage 4. In contrast, in AMI, ST elevations are convex, and reciprocal depression is usually more prominent; QRS changes occur, particularly the development of Q waves, as well as notching and loss of R-wave amplitude, and T-wave inversions are usually seen within hours *before* the ST segments have become isoelectric. Sequential ECGs are useful in distinguishing acute pericarditis from AMI. In the latter, elevated ST segments return to normal within hours (Chaps. 244 and 245).

   Early repolarization is a normal variant and may also be associated with widespread ST-segment elevation, most prominent in left precordial leads. However, in this condition the T waves are usually tall and the ST/T ratio is <0.25; importantly, this ratio is higher in acute pericarditis.
4. *Pericardial effusion* is usually associated with pain and/or the ECG changes mentioned above, as well as with an enlargement of the cardiac silhouette. Pericardial effusion is especially important clinically when it develops within a relatively short time as it may lead to cardiac tamponade (see below). Differentiation from cardiac enlargement may be difficult on physical examination, but heart sounds may be fainter with pericardial effusion. The friction rub may disappear, and the apex impulse may vanish, but sometimes it remains palpable, albeit medial to the left border of cardiac dullness. The base of the left lung may be compressed by pericardial fluid, producing *Ewart's sign*, a patch of dullness and increased fremitus (and egophony) beneath the angle of the left scapula. The chest roentgenogram may show a "water bottle" configuration of the cardiac silhouette (Fig. 239-2) but may be normal.

Diagnosis

Echocardiography (Chap. 229) is the most widely used imaging technique since it is sensitive, specific, simple, and noninvasive; may be performed at the bedside; and can identify accompanying cardiac tamponade (see below) (Fig. 239-3). The presence of pericardial fluid is recorded by two-dimensional transthoracic echocardiography as a relatively echo-free space between the posterior pericardium and left ventricular epicardium in patients with small effusions and as a space between the anterior right ventricle and the parietal pericardium just beneath the anterior chest wall in those with larger effusions. In the latter, the heart may swing freely within the pericardial sac. When severe, the extent of this motion alternates and may be associated with electrical alternans. Echocardiography allows localization and estimation of the quantity of pericardial fluid.

TABLE 239-1 Classification of Pericarditis

Clinical Classification

I. Acute pericarditis (<6 weeks)
- A. Fibrinous
- B. Effusive (serous or sanguineous)

II. Subacute pericarditis (6 weeks to 6 months)
- A. Effusive-constrictive
- B. Constrictive

III. Chronic pericarditis (>6 months)
- A. Constrictive
- B. Effusive
- C. Adhesive (nonconstrictive)

Etiologic Classification

I. Infectious pericarditis
- A. Viral (coxsackievirus A and B, echovirus, mumps, adenovirus, hepatitis, HIV)
- B. Pyogenic (pneumococcus, streptococcus, staphylococcus, *Neisseria*, *Legionella*)
- C. Tuberculous
- D. Fungal (histoplasmosis, coccidioidomycosis, *Candida*, blastomycosis)
- E. Other infections (syphilitic, protozoal, parasitic)

II. Noninfectious pericarditis
- A. Acute myocardial infarction
- B. Uremia
- C. Neoplasia
  1. Primary tumors (benign or malignant, mesothelioma)
  2. Tumors metastatic to pericardium (lung and breast cancer, lymphoma, leukemia)
- D. Myxedema
- E. Cholesterol
- F. Chylopericardium
- G. Trauma
  1. Penetrating chest wall
  2. Nonpenetrating
- H. Aortic dissection (with leakage into pericardial sac)
- I. Postirradiation
- J. Familial Mediterranean fever
- K. Familial pericarditis
  1. Mulibrey nanism[a]
- L. Acute idiopathic
- M. Whipple's disease
- N. Sarcoidosis

III. Pericarditis presumably related to hypersensitivity or autoimmunity
- A. Rheumatic fever
- B. Collagen vascular disease (systemic lupus erythematosus, rheumatoid arthritis, ankylosing spondylitis, scleroderma, acute rheumatic fever, granulomatosis with polyangiitis (Wegener's)
- C. Drug-induced (e.g., procainamide, hydralazine, phenytoin, isoniazide, minoxidil, anticoagulants, methysergide)
- D. Post-cardiac injury
  1. Postmyocardial infarction (Dressler's syndrome)
  2. Postpericardiotomy
  3. Posttraumatic

[a]An autosomal recessive syndrome characterized by growth failure, muscle hypotonia, hepatomegaly, ocular changes, enlarged cerebral ventricles, mental retardation, ventricular hypertrophy, and chronic constrictive pericarditis.

The diagnosis of pericardial fluid or thickening may be confirmed by computed tomography (CT) or magnetic resonance imaging (MRI) (Fig. 239-4). These techniques may be superior to echocardiography in detecting loculated pericardial effusions, pericardial thickening, and the presence of pericardial masses.

CARDIAC TAMPONADE

The accumulation of fluid in the pericardial space in a quantity sufficient to cause serious obstruction to the inflow of blood to the ventricles results in cardiac tamponade. This complication may be fatal if it is not recognized and treated promptly. The three most common causes of tamponade are neoplastic disease, idiopathic pericarditis, and renal failure. Tamponade may also result from bleeding into the pericardial space after cardiac operations, trauma, and treatment of patients with acute pericarditis with anticoagulants.

The three principal features of tamponade (*Beck's triad*) are hypotension, soft or absent heart sounds, and jugular venous distention with a prominent *x* descent but an absent *y* descent. There are both limitation of ventricular filling and reduction of cardiac output. The quantity of fluid necessary to produce this critical state may be as small as 200 mL when the fluid develops rapidly or >2000 mL in slowly developing effusions when the pericardium has had the opportunity to stretch and adapt to an increasing volume. Tamponade may also develop more slowly, and in these circumstances the clinical manifestations may resemble those of heart failure, including dyspnea, orthopnea, and hepatic engorgement. A high index of suspicion for cardiac tamponade is required since in many instances no obvious cause for pericardial disease is apparent, and it should be considered in any patient with otherwise unexplained enlargement of the cardiac silhouette, hypotension, and elevation of jugular venous pressure. There may be reduction in amplitude of the QRS complexes, and *electrical alternans* of the P, QRS, or T waves should raise the suspicion of cardiac tamponade.

Table 239-2 lists the features that distinguish acute cardiac tamponade from constrictive pericarditis.

Paradoxical pulse

This important clue to the presence of cardiac tamponade consists of a greater than normal (10 mmHg) inspiratory decline in systolic arterial pressure. When severe, it may be detected by palpating weakness or disappearance of the arterial pulse during inspiration, but usually sphygmomanometric measurement of systolic pressure during slow respiration is required.

Since both ventricles share a tight incompressible covering, i.e., the pericardial sac, the inspiratory enlargement of the right ventricle in cardiac tamponade compresses and reduces left ventricular volume; leftward bulging of the interventricular septum further reduces the left ventricular cavity as the right ventricle enlarges during inspiration. Thus, in cardiac tamponade the normal inspiratory augmentation of right ventricular volume causes an exaggerated reciprocal reduction in left ventricular volume. Also, respiratory distress increases the fluctuations in intrathoracic pressure, which exaggerates the mechanism just described. Right ventricular infarction (Chap. 245) may resemble cardiac tamponade with hypotension, elevated jugular venous pressure, an absent *y* descent in the jugular venous pulse, and, occasionally, pulsus paradoxus. The differences between these two conditions are shown in Table 239-2.

Paradoxical pulse occurs not only in cardiac tamponade but also in approximately one-third of patients with constrictive pericarditis (see below). This physical finding is not pathognomonic of pericardial disease because it may be observed in some cases of hypovolemic shock, acute and chronic obstructive airway disease, and pulmonary embolus.

Low-pressure tamponade refers to mild tamponade in which the intrapericardial pressure is increased from its slightly subatmospheric

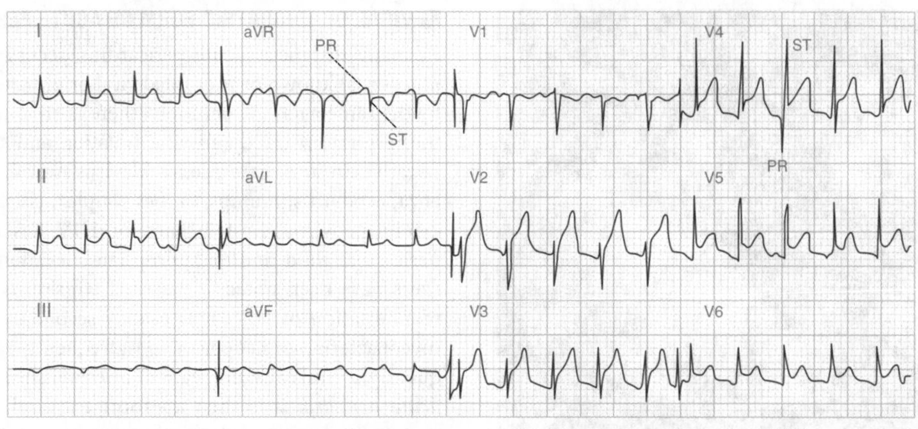

Figure 239-1 Acute pericarditis often produces diffuse ST-segment elevations (in this case in leads I, II, aVF, and V_2 to V_6) due to a ventricular current of injury. Note also the characteristic PR-segment deviation (opposite in polarity to the ST segment) due to a concomitant atrial injury current.

levels to +5 to +10 mmHg; in some instances, hypovolemia coexists. As a consequence, the central venous pressure is normal or only slightly elevated, whereas arterial pressure is unaffected and there is no paradoxical pulse. These patients are asymptomatic or complain of mild weakness and dyspnea. The diagnosis is aided by echocardiography, and both hemodynamic and clinical manifestations improve after pericardiocentesis.

Diagnosis

Since immediate treatment of cardiac tamponade may be lifesaving, prompt measures to establish the diagnosis by echocardiography should be undertaken (Fig. 239-3). When pericardial effusion causes tamponade, Doppler ultrasound shows that tricuspid and pulmonic valve flow velocities increase markedly during inspiration, whereas pulmonic vein, mitral, and aortic flow velocities diminish. Often the right ventricular cavity is reduced in diameter, and there is late diastolic inward motion (collapse) of the right ventricular free wall and the right atrium. Transesophageal echocardiography may be necessary to diagnose a loculated or hemorrhagic effusion responsible for cardiac tamponade.

TREATMENT Cardiac Tamponade

Patients with acute pericarditis should be observed frequently for the development of an effusion; if a large effusion is present, the patient should be hospitalized and pericardiocentesis carried out

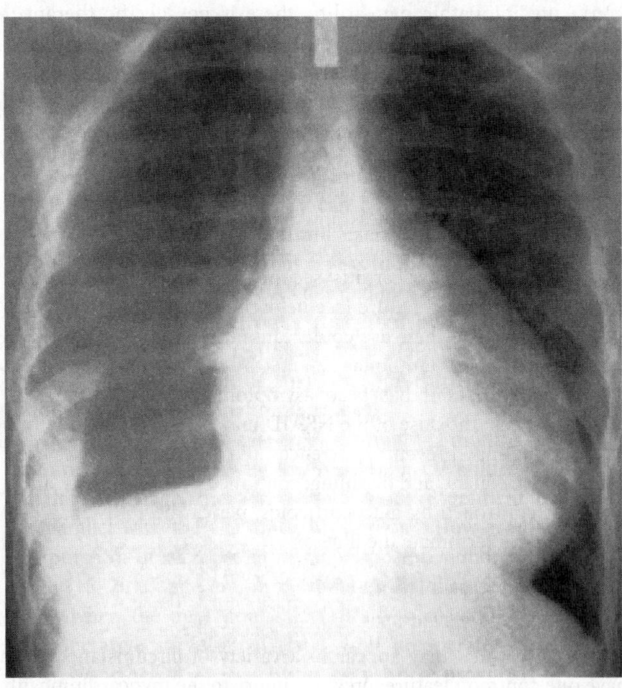

Figure 239-2 Chest radiogram from a patient with a pericardial effusion showing typical "water bottle" heart. There is also a right pleural effusion. *[From SS Kabbani, M LeWinter, in MH Crawford et al (eds): Cardiology. London, Mosby, 2001.]*

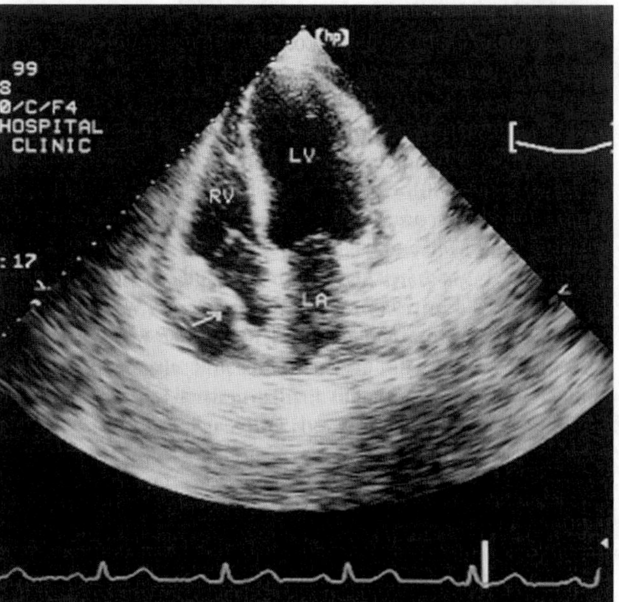

Figure 239-3 Apical four-chamber echocardiogram recorded in a patient with a moderate pericardial effusion and evidence of hemodynamic compromise. The frame is recorded in early ventricular systole, immediately after atrial contraction. Note that the right atrial wall is indented inward and its curvature is frankly reversed (*arrow*), implying elevated intrapericardial pressure above right atrial pressure. LA, left atrium; LV, left ventricle; RV, right ventricle. *[From WF Armstrong: Echocardiography, in DP Zipes et al (eds): Braunwald's Heart Disease, 7th ed. Philadelphia, Elsevier, 2005.]*

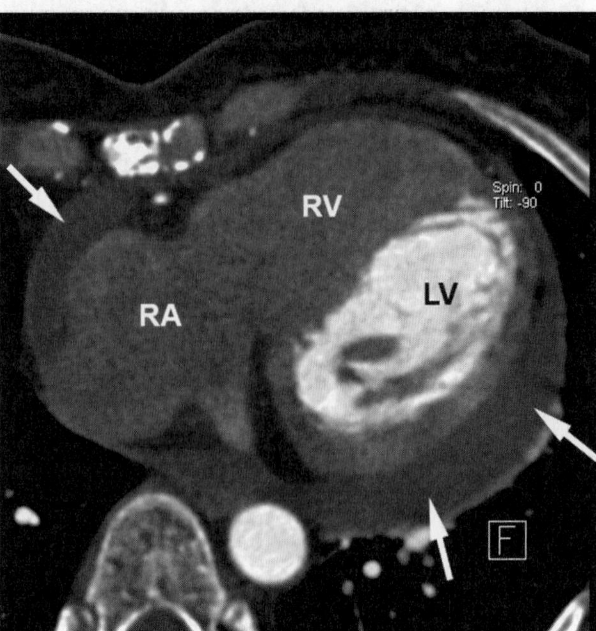

Figure 239-4 Chronic pericardial effusion in a 54-year-old female patient with Hodgkin's disease seen in contrast-enhanced 64-slice CT. The arrows point at the pericardial effusion (LV, left ventricle; RV, right ventricle; RA, right atrium). Due to the timing of the scan relative to contrast injection, only the blood in the left ventricle is contrast-enhanced, hence, the low attenuation in the right-sided chambers. *[From Achenbach S, Daniel WG: Computed Tomography of the Heart, in P Libby et al (eds): Braunwald's Heart Disease, 8th ed. Philadelphia, Elsevier, 2008.]*

or the patient should be watched closely for signs of tamponade. Arterial and venous pressures and heart rate should be monitored or followed carefully, and serial echocardiograms obtained.

PERICARDIOCENTESIS If manifestations of tamponade appear, echocardiographically or fluoroscopically guided pericardiocentesis using an apical, parasternal, or, most commonly, subxiphoid approach must be carried out at once as reduction of the elevated intrapericardial pressure may be lifesaving. Intravenous saline may be administered as the patient is being readied for the procedure, but the pericardiocentesis must not be delayed. If possible, intrapericardial pressure should be measured before fluid is withdrawn, and the pericardial cavity should be drained as completely as possible. A small, multiholed catheter advanced over the needle inserted into the pericardial cavity may be left in place to allow draining of the pericardial space if fluid reaccumulates. Surgical drainage through a limited (subxiphoid) thoracotomy may be required in recurrent tamponade, when it is necessary to remove loculated effusions, and/or when it is necessary to obtain tissue for diagnosis.

Pericardial fluid obtained from an effusion often has the physical characteristics of an exudate. Bloody fluid is most commonly due to neoplasm in the United States and tuberculosis in developing nations but may also be found in the effusion of acute rheumatic fever, post-cardiac injury, and post-myocardial infarction, as well as in the pericarditis associated with renal failure or dialysis. Transudative pericardial effusions may occur in heart failure.

The pericardial fluid should be analyzed for red and white blood cells, and cytologic studies for cancer, microscopic studies, and cultures should be obtained. The presence of DNA of *Mycobacterium tuberculosis* determined by polymerase chain reaction or an elevated adenosine deaminase activity (>30 U/L) strongly supports the diagnosis of tuberculous pericarditis (Chap. 165).

VIRAL OR IDIOPATHIC FORM OF ACUTE PERICARDITIS

In many instances, acute pericarditis occurs in association with illnesses of known or presumed viral origin and probably is caused by the same agent. Commonly, there is an antecedent infection of the respiratory tract, and viral isolation and serologic studies are negative. In some cases, coxsackievirus A or B or the virus of influenza, echovirus, mumps, herpes simplex, chickenpox, adenovirus, cytomegalovirus, Epstein-Barr, or HIV has been isolated from pericardial fluid and/or appropriate elevations in viral antibody titers have been noted. Pericardial effusion is a common cardiac manifestation of HIV; it is usually secondary to infection (often mycobacterial) or neoplasm, most frequently lymphoma. Most frequently, a viral causation cannot be established; the term *idiopathic acute pericarditis* is then appropriate. Viral or idiopathic acute pericarditis occurs at all ages but is more common in young adults and is often associated with pleural effusions and pneumonitis. The almost simultaneous development of fever and precordial pain, often 10 to 12 days after a presumed viral illness, constitutes an important feature in the differentiation of acute pericarditis from AMI, in which chest pain precedes fever. The constitutional symptoms are usually mild to moderate, and a pericardial friction rub is often audible. The disease ordinarily runs its course in a few days to 4 weeks. The ST-segment alterations in the ECG usually disappear after 1 or more weeks, but the abnormal T waves may persist for several years and be a source of confusion in persons without a clear history of pericarditis.

Pleuritis and pneumonitis frequently accompany pericarditis. Accumulation of some pericardial fluid is common, and both tamponade and constrictive pericarditis are possible complications. Recurrent (relapsing) pericarditis occurs in about one-fourth of patients with acute idiopathic pericarditis. In a smaller number, there are multiple recurrences.

TREATMENT Idiopathic Acute Pericarditis

In acute idiopathic pericarditis there is no specific therapy, but bed rest and anti-inflammatory treatment with aspirin (2–4 g/d) may be given. If this is ineffective, one of the nonsteroidal anti-inflammatory drugs (NSAIDs), such as ibuprofen (400–600 mg tid), indomethacin (25–50 mg tid), or colchicine (0.6 mg bid), is often effective. Glucocorticoids (e.g., prednisone, 40–80 mg daily) usually suppress the clinical manifestations of the acute illness and may be useful in patients in whom purulent bacterial pericarditis has been excluded and in patients with pericarditis secondary to connective tissue disorders and renal failure (see below). Anticoagulants should be avoided since their use could cause bleeding into the pericardial cavity and tamponade.

After the patient has been asymptomatic and afebrile for about a week, the dose of the NSAID may be tapered gradually. Colchicine may prevent recurrences, but when recurrences are multiple, frequent, and disabling; continued beyond 2 years; and are not controlled by glucocorticoids, pericardiectomy may be necessary to terminate the illness.

Postcardiac injury syndrome

Acute pericarditis may appear in a variety of circumstances that have one common feature: previous injury to the myocardium with blood in the pericardial cavity. The syndrome may develop after a cardiac operation (postpericardiotomy syndrome), after blunt or penetrating cardiac trauma (Chap. 240), or after perforation of the heart with a catheter. Rarely, it follows AMI.

TABLE 239-2 Features That Distinguish Cardiac Tamponade from Constrictive Pericarditis and Similar Clinical Disorders

Characteristic	Tamponade	Constrictive Pericarditis	Restrictive Cardiomyopathy	RVMI
Clinical				
Pulsus paradoxus	Common	Usually absent	Rare	Rare
Jugular veins				
Prominent *y* descent	Absent	Usually present	Rare	Rare
Prominent *x* descent	Present	Usually present	Present	Rare
Kussmaul's sign	Absent	Present	Present	Present
Third heart sound	Absent	Absent	Rare	May be present
Pericardial knock	Absent	Often present	Absent	Absent
Electrocardiogram				
Low ECG voltage	May be present	May be present	May be present	Absent
Electrical alternans	May be present	Absent	Absent	Absent
Echocardiography				
Thickened pericardium	Absent	Present	Absent	Absent
Pericardial calcification	Absent	Often present	Absent	Absent
Pericardial effusion	Present	Absent	Absent	Absent
RV size	Usually small	Usually normal	Usually normal	Enlarged
Myocardial thickness	Normal	Normal	Usually increased	Normal
Right atrial collapse and RVDC	Present	Absent	Absent	Absent
Increased early filling, ↑ mitral flow velocity	Absent	Present	Present	May be present
Exaggerated respiratory variation in flow velocity	Present	Present	Absent	Absent
CT/MRI				
Thickened/calcific pericardium	Absent	Present	Absent	Absent
Cardiac catheterization				
Equalization of diastolic pressures	Usually present	Usually present	Usually absent	Absent or present
Cardiac biopsy helpful?	No	No	Sometimes	No

Abbreviations: ECG, electrocardiograph; RV, right ventricle; RVDC, right ventricular diastolic collapse; RVMI, right ventricular myocardial infarction.

Source: From GM Brockington et al: Cardiol Clin 8:645, 1990, with permission.

The clinical picture mimics acute viral or idiopathic pericarditis. The principal symptom is the pain of acute pericarditis, which usually develops 1 to 4 weeks after the cardiac injury (1 to 3 days after AMI) but sometimes appears only after an interval of months. Recurrences are common and may occur up to 2 years or more after the injury. Pericarditis, fever with temperature up to 39°C (102.2°F), pleuritis, and pneumonitis are the outstanding features, and the bout of illness usually subsides in 1 or 2 weeks. The pericarditis may be of the fibrinous variety, or it may be a pericardial effusion, which is often serosanguineous but rarely causes tamponade. Leukocytosis, an increased sedimentation rate, and ECG changes typical of acute pericarditis may also occur.

This syndrome is probably the result of a hypersensitivity reaction to antigen that originates from injured myocardial tissue and/or pericardium. Circulating myocardial antisarcolemmal and antifibrillar autoantibodies occur frequently, but their precise role in the development of this syndrome has not been defined. Viral infection may also play an etiologic role, since antiviral antibodies are often elevated in patients who develop this syndrome after cardiac surgery.

Often no treatment is necessary aside from aspirin and analgesics. When the illness is followed by a series of disabling recurrences, therapy with an NSAID, colchicine, or a glucocorticoid is usually effective.

■ DIFFERENTIAL DIAGNOSIS

Since there is no specific test for *acute idiopathic pericarditis*, the diagnosis is one of exclusion. Consequently, all other disorders that may be associated with acute fibrinous pericarditis must be considered. A common diagnostic error is mistaking acute viral or idiopathic pericarditis for AMI and vice versa. When acute fibrinous pericarditis is associated with AMI (Chap. 245), it is characterized by fever, pain, and a friction rub in the first 4 days after the development of the infarct. ECG abnormalities (such as the appearance of Q waves, brief ST-segment elevations with reciprocal changes, and earlier T-wave changes in AMI) and the extent of the elevations of myocardial enzymes are helpful in differentiating pericarditis from AMI.

Pericarditis secondary to postcardiac injury is differentiated from acute idiopathic pericarditis chiefly by timing. If it occurs within a few days or weeks of an AMI, a chest blow, a cardiac perforation, or a cardiac operation, it may be justified to conclude that the two are probably related.

It is important to distinguish *pericarditis due to collagen vascular disease* from acute idiopathic pericarditis. Most important in the differential diagnosis is the pericarditis due to systemic lupus erythematosus (SLE; Chap. 319) or drug-induced (procainamide or hydralazine) lupus. When pericarditis occurs in the absence of any obvious underlying disorder, the diagnosis of SLE may be suggested by a rise in the titer of antinuclear antibodies. Acute pericarditis is an occasional complication of *rheumatoid arthritis, scleroderma,* and *polyarteritis nodosa,* and other evidence of these diseases is usually obvious. Asymptomatic pericardial effusion is also common in these disorders. The pericarditis of *acute rheumatic fever* is generally associated with evidence of severe pancarditis and with cardiac murmurs (Chap. 322).

Pyogenic (purulent) pericarditis is usually secondary to cardiothoracic operations, by extension of infection from the lungs or pleural cavities, from rupture of the esophagus into the pericardial sac, or from rupture of a ring abscess in a patient with infective endocarditis, or it can occur if septicemia complicates aseptic pericarditis. It is usually accompanied by fever, chills, septicemia, and evidence of infection elsewhere and generally has a poor prognosis. The diagnosis is made by examination of the pericardial fluid. Acute pericarditis may also complicate the viral, pyogenic, mycobacterial, and fungal infections that occur with HIV infection.

Pericarditis of renal failure (Chap. 280) occurs in up to one-third of patients with chronic uremia *(uremic pericarditis),* is also seen in patients undergoing chronic dialysis with normal levels of blood urea and creatinine, and is termed *dialysis-associated pericarditis.* These two forms of pericarditis may be fibrinous and are generally associated with an effusion that may be sanguineous. A pericardial friction rub is common, but pain is usually absent or mild. Treatment with an NSAID and intensification of dialysis are usually adequate. Occasionally, tamponade occurs and pericardiocentesis is required. When the pericarditis of renal failure is recurrent or persistent, a pericardial window should be created or pericardiectomy may be necessary.

Pericarditis due to *neoplastic diseases* results from extension or invasion of metastatic tumors (most commonly carcinoma of the lung and breast, malignant melanoma, lymphoma, and leukemia) to the pericardium; pain, atrial arrhythmias, and tamponade are complications that occur occasionally. Diagnosis is made by pericardial fluid cytology or pericardial biopsy. *Mediastinal irradiation* for neoplasm may cause acute pericarditis and/or chronic constrictive pericarditis. Unusual causes of acute pericarditis include syphilis, fungal infection (histoplasmosis, blastomycosis, aspergillosis, and candidiasis), and parasitic infestation (amebiasis, toxoplasmosis, echinococcosis, trichinosis).

■ CHRONIC PERICARDIAL EFFUSIONS

Chronic pericardial effusions are sometimes encountered in patients without an antecedent history of acute pericarditis. They may cause few symptoms per se, and their presence may be detected by finding an enlarged cardiac silhouette on chest roentgenogram. Tuberculosis is a common cause (Chap. 165).

Other causes

Myxedema may be responsible for chronic pericardial effusion that is sometimes massive but rarely, if ever, causes cardiac tamponade. The cardiac silhouette is markedly enlarged, and an echocardiogram distinguishes cardiomegaly from pericardial effusion. The diagnosis of myxedema can be confirmed by tests for thyroid function (Chap. 341). Myxedematous pericardial effusion responds to thyroid hormone replacement.

Neoplasms, systemic lupus erythematosus (SLE), rheumatoid arthritis, mycotic infections, radiation therapy to the chest, pyogenic infections, and chylopericardium may also cause chronic pericardial effusion and should be considered and specifically sought in such patients.

Aspiration and analysis of the pericardial fluid are often helpful in diagnosis. Pericardial fluid should be analyzed as described on p. 1974. Grossly sanguineous pericardial fluid results most commonly from a neoplasm, tuberculosis, renal failure, or slow leakage from an aortic aneurysm. Pericardiocentesis may resolve large effusions, but pericardiectomy may be required with recurrence. Intrapericardial instillation of sclerosing agents or antineoplastic agents may be used to prevent reaccumulation of fluid.

CHRONIC CONSTRICTIVE PERICARDITIS

This disorder results when the healing of an acute fibrinous or serofibrinous pericarditis or the resorption of a chronic pericardial effusion is followed by obliteration of the pericardial cavity with the formation of granulation tissue. The latter gradually contracts and forms a firm scar, which may be calcified, encasing the heart and interfering with filling of the ventricles. In developing nations where the condition is prevalent, a high percentage of cases are of tuberculous origin, but this is now an uncommon cause in North America. Chronic constrictive pericarditis may follow acute or relapsing viral or idiopathic pericarditis, trauma with organized blood clot, cardiac surgery of any type, mediastinal irradiation, purulent infection, histoplasmosis, neoplastic disease (especially breast cancer, lung cancer, and lymphoma), rheumatoid arthritis, SLE, and chronic renal failure with uremia treated by chronic dialysis. In many patients the cause of the pericardial disease is undetermined, and in them an asymptomatic or forgotten bout of viral pericarditis, acute or idiopathic, may have been the inciting event.

The basic physiologic abnormality in patients with chronic constrictive pericarditis is the inability of the ventricles to fill because of the limitations imposed by the rigid, thickened pericardium. In constrictive pericarditis, ventricular filling is unimpeded during early diastole but is reduced abruptly when the elastic limit of the pericardium is reached, whereas in cardiac tamponade, ventricular filling is impeded throughout diastole. In both conditions, ventricular end-diastolic and stroke volumes are reduced and the end-diastolic pressures in both ventricles and the mean pressures in the atria, pulmonary veins, and systemic veins are all elevated to similar levels (i.e., within 5 mmHg of one another). Despite these hemodynamic changes, myocardial function may be normal or only slightly impaired in chronic constrictive pericarditis. However, the fibrotic process may extend into the myocardium and cause myocardial scarring and atrophy, and venous congestion may then be due to the combined effects of the pericardial and myocardial lesions.

In constrictive pericarditis, the right and left atrial pressure pulses display an M-shaped contour, with prominent *x* and *y* descents. The *y* descent, which is absent or diminished in cardiac tamponade, is the most prominent deflection in constrictive pericarditis; it reflects rapid early filling of the ventricles. The *y* descent is interrupted by a rapid rise in atrial pressure during early diastole, when ventricular filling is impeded by the constricting pericardium. These characteristic changes are transmitted to the jugular veins, where they may be recognized by inspection. In constrictive pericarditis, the ventricular pressure pulses in both ventricles exhibit characteristic "square root" signs during diastole. These hemodynamic changes, although characteristic, are not pathognomonic of constrictive pericarditis and may also be observed in cardiomyopathies characterized by restriction of ventricular filling (Chap. 238) (Table 239-2).

■ CLINICAL AND LABORATORY FINDINGS

Weakness, fatigue, weight gain, increased abdominal girth, abdominal discomfort, a protuberant abdomen, and edema are common. The patient often appears chronically ill, and in advanced cases there are anasarca, skeletal muscle wasting, and cachexia. Exertional dyspnea is common, and orthopnea may occur, although it is usually not severe. Acute left ventricular failure (acute pulmonary edema) is very uncommon. The cervical veins are distended and may remain so even after intensive diuretic treatment, and venous pressure may fail to decline during inspiration (*Kussmaul's sign*). The latter is common in chronic pericarditis but may also occur in tricuspid stenosis, right ventricular infarction, and restrictive cardiomyopathy.

The pulse pressure is normal or reduced. In about one-third of cases, a paradoxical pulse can be detected. Congestive hepatomegaly is pronounced and may impair hepatic function and cause jaundice; ascites is common and is usually more prominent than dependent edema. The apical pulse is reduced and may retract in systole (*Broadbent's sign*). The heart sounds may be distant; an early third heart sound (i.e., a pericardial knock, occurring at the cardiac apex 0.09–0.12 s after aortic valve closure) is often conspicuous; it occurs with the abrupt cessation of ventricular filling. A systolic murmur of tricuspid regurgitation may be present.

The *ECG* frequently displays low voltage of the QRS complexes and diffuse flattening or inversion of the T waves. Atrial fibrillation is present in about one-third of patients. The *chest roentgenogram* shows a normal or slightly enlarged heart; pericardial calcification is most common in tuberculous pericarditis. Pericardial calcification may, however, occur in the absence of constriction.

Inasmuch as the usual physical signs of cardiac disease (murmurs, cardiac enlargement) may be inconspicuous or absent in chronic constrictive pericarditis, hepatic enlargement and dysfunction associated with jaundice and intractable ascites may lead to a mistaken diagnosis of hepatic cirrhosis. This error can be avoided if the neck veins are inspected carefully in patients with ascites and hepatomegaly. Given a clinical picture resembling hepatic cirrhosis, but with the added feature of distended neck veins, a careful search for thickening of the pericardium by imaging (see Fig. 229-6) should be carried out and may disclose this curable or remediable form of heart disease.

The transthoracic *echocardiogram* typically shows pericardial thickening, dilation of the inferior vena cava and hepatic veins, and a sharp halt in ventricular filling in early diastole, with normal ventricular systolic function and flattening of the left ventricular posterior wall. Atrial enlargement may be seen, especially in patients with long-standing constrictive physiology. There is a distinctive pattern of transvalvular flow velocity on Doppler flow-velocity echocardiography. During inspiration there is an exaggerated reduction in blood flow velocity in the pulmonary veins and across the mitral valve and a leftward shift of the ventricular septum; the opposite occurs during expiration. Diastolic flow velocity in the vena cavae into the right atrium and across the tricuspid valve increases in an exaggerated manner during inspiration and declines during expiration (Fig. 239-5). However, echocardiography cannot definitively exclude the diagnosis of constrictive pericarditis. MRI and CT

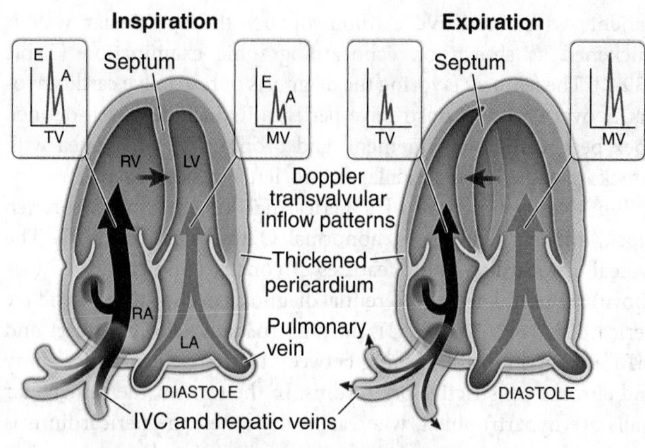

Figure 239-5 Constrictive pericarditis. Doppler schema of respirophasic changes in mitral and tricuspid inflow. Reciprocal patterns of ventricular filling are assessed on pulsed Doppler examination of mitral valve (MV) and tricuspid valve (TV) inflow.

scanning (Fig. 239-6) are more accurate than echocardiography in establishing or excluding the presence of a thickened pericardium. Pericardial thickening and even pericardial calcification, however, are not synonymous with constrictive pericarditis since they may occur without seriously impairing ventricular filling.

DIFFERENTIAL DIAGNOSIS

Like chronic constrictive pericarditis, cor pulmonale (Chap. 234) may be associated with severe systemic venous hypertension but little pulmonary congestion; the heart is usually not enlarged, and a paradoxical pulse may be present. However, in cor pulmonale, advanced parenchymal pulmonary disease is usually obvious and venous pressure *falls* during inspiration (i.e., Kussmaul's sign is negative). *Tricuspid stenosis* (Chap. 237) may also simulate chronic constrictive pericarditis; congestive hepatomegaly, splenomegaly, ascites, and venous distention may be equally prominent. However, in tricuspid stenosis, a characteristic murmur as well as the murmur of accompanying mitral stenosis is usually present.

Because constrictive pericarditis can be corrected surgically, it is important to distinguish chronic constrictive pericarditis from restrictive cardiomyopathy (Chap. 238), which has a similar physiologic abnormality (i.e., restriction of ventricular filling). In many

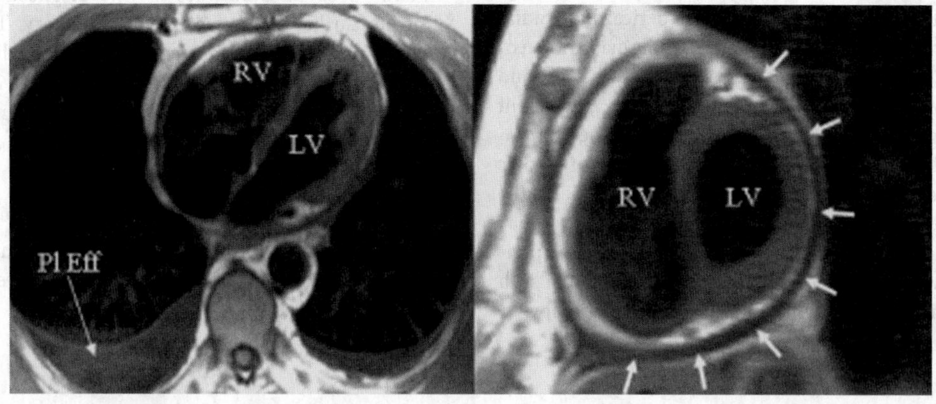

Figure 239-6 Cardiovascular magnetic resonance in a patient with constrictive pericarditis. On the right is a basal short-axis view of the ventricles showing a thickened pericardium encasing the heart (*arrows*). On the left is a transaxial view, again showing the thickened pericardium, particularly over the right heart, but also a pleural effusion (Pl Eff). LV, left ventricle; RV, right ventricle. *[From D Pennell: Cardiovascular Magnetic Resonance, in P Libby et al (eds): Braunwald's Heart Disease, 8th ed. Philadelphia, Elsevier, 2005.]*

patients with restrictive cardiomyopathy the ventricular wall is thickened as shown on echocardiographic examination (Table 239-2). The features favoring the diagnosis of restrictive cardiomyopathy over chronic constrictive pericarditis include a well-defined apex beat, cardiac enlargement, and pronounced orthopnea with attacks of acute left ventricular failure, left ventricular hypertrophy, gallop sounds (in place of a pericardial knock), bundle branch block, and, in some cases, abnormal Q waves on the ECG. The typical echocardiographic features of constrictive pericarditis (see above) are useful in the differential diagnosis in chronic constrictive pericarditis (Fig. 239-5). CT imaging (usually with contrast) and MRI are key in distinguishing between restrictive cardiomyopathy and chronic constrictive pericarditis. In the former, the ventricular walls are hypertrophied, whereas in the latter, the pericardium is thickened and sometimes calcified. When a patient has progressive, disabling, and unresponsive congestive heart failure and displays any of the features of constrictive heart disease, Doppler echocardiography to record respiratory effects on transvalvular flow and an MRI or CT scan should be obtained to detect or exclude constrictive pericarditis, since the latter is usually curable.

TREATMENT Constrictive Pericarditis

Pericardial resection is the only definitive treatment of constrictive pericarditis and should be as complete as possible. Dietary sodium restriction and diuretics are useful during preoperative preparation. Coronary arteriography should be carried out preoperatively in patients older than 50 years of age to exclude unsuspected coronary artery disease. The benefits derived from cardiac decortication are usually progressive over a period of months. The risk of this operation depends on the extent of penetration of the myocardium by the fibrotic and calcific process, the severity of myocardial atrophy, the extent of secondary impairment of hepatic and/or renal function, and the patient's general condition. Operative mortality is in the range of 5 to 10%; the patients with the most severe disease are at highest risk. Therefore, surgical treatment should, if possible, be carried out relatively early in the course.

Subacute effusive-constrictive pericarditis

This form of pericardial disease is characterized by the combination of a tense effusion in the pericardial space and constriction of the heart by thickened pericardium. It shares a number of features both with chronic pericardial effusion producing cardiac compression and with pericardial constriction. It may be caused by tuberculosis (see below), multiple attacks of acute idiopathic pericarditis, radiation, traumatic pericarditis, renal failure, scleroderma, and neoplasms. The heart is generally enlarged, and a paradoxical pulse and a prominent *x* descent (without a prominent *y* descent) are present in the atrial and jugular venous pressure pulses. After pericardiocentesis, the physiologic findings may change from those of cardiac tamponade to those of pericardial constriction. Furthermore, the intrapericardial pressure and the central venous pressure may decline, but not to normal. The diagnosis can be established by pericardiocentesis followed by pericardial biopsy. Wide excision of both the visceral and parietal pericardium is usually effective therapy.

Tuberculous pericardial disease

This chronic infection is a common cause of chronic pericardial effusion, although less so in the United States than in Africa, Asia, the Middle East, and other parts of the developing world where active tuberculosis is endemic (Chap. 165). The clinical picture is that of a chronic, systemic illness in a patient with pericardial effusion. It is important to consider this diagnosis in a patient with known tuberculosis, with HIV, and with fever, chest pain, weight loss, and enlargement of the cardiac silhouette of undetermined origin. If the etiology of chronic pericardial effusion remains obscure despite detailed analysis of the pericardial fluid (see above), a pericardial biopsy, preferably by a limited thoracotomy, should be performed. If definitive evidence is still lacking but the specimen shows granulomas with caseation, antituberculous chemotherapy (Chap. 165) is indicated.

If the biopsy specimen shows a thickened pericardium, pericardiectomy should be carried out to prevent the development of constriction. Tubercular cardiac constriction should be treated surgically while the patient is receiving antituberculous chemotherapy.

OTHER DISORDERS OF THE PERICARDIUM

Pericardial cysts appear as rounded or lobulated deformities of the cardiac silhouette, most commonly at the right cardiophrenic angle. They do not cause symptoms, and their major clinical significance lies in the possibility of confusion with a tumor, ventricular aneurysm, or massive cardiomegaly. *Tumors* involving the pericardium are most commonly secondary to malignant neoplasms originating in or invading the mediastinum, including carcinoma of the bronchus and breast, lymphoma, and melanoma. The most common *primary* malignant tumor is the mesothelioma. The usual clinical picture of malignant pericardial tumor is an insidiously developing, often bloody pericardial effusion. Surgical exploration is required to establish a definitive diagnosis and to carry out definitive or, more commonly, palliative treatment.

FURTHER READINGS

Imazio M et al: Diagnosis and management of pericardial diseases. Nat Rev Cardiol 6:743, 2009

Khandaker MH et al: Pericardial disease: Diagnosis and managemnt. Mayo Clin Proc 85:572,2010

LeWinter M: Pericardial diseases, in *Braunwald's Heart Disease*, 8th ed, P Libby et al (eds). Philadelphia, Saunders, 2008

Maisch B et al: Guidelines on the diagnosis and management of pericardial diseases executive summary: The Task Force on the Diagnosis and Management of Pericardial Diseases of the European Society of Cardiology. Eur Heart J 25:587, 2004

Mayosi BM: Contemporary trends in the epidemiology and management of cardiomyopathy and pericarditis in sub-Saharan Africa. Heart 93:1176, 2007

——— et al: Tuberculous pericarditis. Circulation 112:3608, 2005

O'Leary SM et al: Imaging the pericardium: Appearances on ECG-gated 64-detector row cardiac computed tomography. Br J Radiol 83:194,2010

CHAPTER 240

Tumors and Trauma of the Heart

Eric H. Awtry
Wilson S. Colucci

TUMORS OF THE HEART

PRIMARY TUMORS

Primary tumors of the heart are rare. Approximately three-quarters are histologically benign, and the majority of these tumors are myxomas. Malignant tumors, almost all of which are sarcomas, account for 25% of primary cardiac tumors (Table 240-1). All cardiac tumors, regardless of pathologic type, have the potential to cause life-threatening complications. Many tumors are now surgically curable; thus, early diagnosis is imperative.

Clinical presentation

Cardiac tumors may present with a wide array of cardiac and noncardiac manifestations. These manifestations depend in large part on the location and size of the tumor and are often nonspecific features of more common forms of heart disease, such as chest pain, syncope, heart failure, murmurs, arrhythmias, conduction disturbances, and pericardial effusion with or without tamponade. Additionally, embolic phenomena and constitutional symptoms may occur.

Myxoma

Myxomas are the most common type of primary cardiac tumor in all age groups, accounting for one-third to one-half of all cases at postmortem and about three-quarters of the tumors treated surgically. They occur at all ages, most commonly in the third through sixth decades, with a female predilection. Approximately 90% of myxomas are sporadic; the remainder are familial with autosomal dominant transmission. The familial variety often occurs as part of a syndrome complex (Carney complex) that includes (1) myxomas (cardiac, skin, and/or breast), (2) lentigines and/or pigmented nevi, and (3) endocrine overactivity (primary nodular adrenal cortical disease with or without Cushing's syndrome, testicular tumors, and/or pituitary adenomas with gigantism or acromegaly). Certain constellations of findings have been referred to as the *NAME* syndrome (nevi, atrial myxoma, myxoid neurofibroma, and ephelides) or the *LAMB* syndrome (lentigines, atrial myxoma, and blue nevi), although these syndromes probably represent subsets of the Carney complex. The genetic basis of this complex has not been elucidated completely; however, patients frequently have inactivating mutations in the tumor-suppressor gene *PRKAR1A*, which encodes the protein kinase A type I-α regulatory subunit.

Pathologically, myxomas are gelatinous structures that consist of myxoma cells embedded in a stroma rich in glycosaminoglycans. Most are solitary, are located in the atria (particularly the left atrium, where they usually arise from the interatrial septum in the vicinity of the fossa ovalis), and are often pedunculated on a fibrovascular stalk. In contrast to sporadic tumors, familial or syndromic tumors tend to occur in younger individuals, are often multiple, may be ventricular in location, and are more likely to recur after initial resection.

Myxomas commonly present with obstructive signs and symptoms. The most common clinical presentation mimics that of mitral valve disease: either stenosis owing to tumor prolapse into the mitral orifice or regurgitation resulting from tumor-induced valvular trauma. Ventricular myxomas may cause outflow obstruction similar to that caused by subaortic or subpulmonic stenosis. The symptoms and signs of myxoma may be sudden in onset or positional in nature, owing to the effects of gravity on tumor position. A characteristic low-pitched sound, a "tumor plop," may be appreciated on auscultation during early or mid-diastole and is thought to result from the impact of the tumor against the mitral valve or ventricular wall. Myxomas also may present with peripheral or pulmonary emboli or with constitutional signs and symptoms, including fever, weight loss, cachexia, malaise, arthralgias, rash, digital clubbing, Raynaud's phenomenon, hypergammaglobulinemia, anemia, polycythemia, leukocytosis, elevated erythrocyte sedimentation rate, thrombocytopenia, and thrombocytosis. These factors account for the frequent misdiagnosis of patients with myxomas as having endocarditis, collagen vascular disease, or a paraneoplastic syndrome.

Two-dimensional transthoracic or omniplane transesophageal echocardiography is useful in the diagnosis of cardiac myxoma and allows assessment of tumor size and determination of the site of tumor attachment, both of which are important considerations in the planning of surgical excision (Fig. 240-1). CT and MRI may provide important information regarding size, shape, composition, and surface characteristics of the tumor (Fig. 240-2).

TABLE 240-1 Relative Incidence of Primary Tumors of the Heart

Type	Number	Percent
Benign	199	58.0
Myxoma	114	33.2
Rhabdomyoma	20	5.8
Fibroma	20	5.8
Hemangioma	17	5.0
Atrioventricular nodal	10	2.9
Granular cell	4	1.2
Lipoma	2	0.6
Paraganglioma	2	0.6
Myocytic hamartoma	2	0.6
Histiocytoid cardiomyopathy	2	0.6
Inflammatory psuedotumor	2	0.6
Other benign tumors	4	1.2
Malignant	144	42.0
Sarcoma	137	39.9
Lymphoma	7	2.1

Source: Modified from A Burke, R Virmani: *Atlas of Tumor Pathology:Tumors of the Heart and Great Vessels.* Washington, DC, Armed Forces Institute of Pathology 1996, p. 231; with permission.

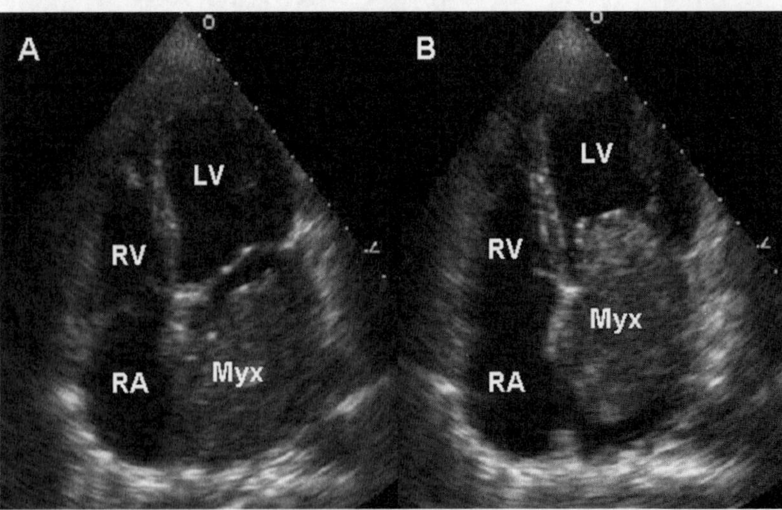

Figure 240-1 Transthoracic echocardiogram demonstrating a large atrial myxoma. The myxoma (Myx) fills the entire left atrium in systole (*panel A*) and prolapses across the mitral valve and into the left ventricle (LV) during diastole (*panel B*). RA, right atrium; RV, right ventricle. *(Courtesy of Dr. Michael Tsang; with permission.)*

Although cardiac catheterization and angiography were previously performed routinely before tumor resection, they no longer are considered mandatory when adequate noninvasive information is available and other cardiac disorders (e.g., coronary artery disease) are not considered likely. Additionally, catheterization of the chamber from which the tumor arises carries the risk of tumor embolization. Because myxomas may be familial, echocardiographic screening of first-degree relatives is appropriate, particularly if the patient is young and has multiple tumors or evidence of myxoma syndrome.

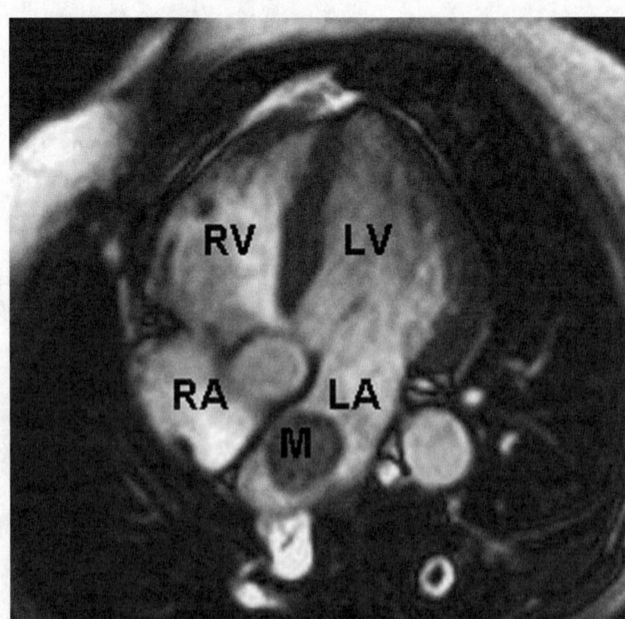

Figure 240-2 Cardiac MRI demonstrating a rounded mass (M) within the left atrium (LA). Pathologic evaluation at the time of surgery revealed it to be an atrial myxoma. LV, left ventricle; RA, right atrium; RV, right ventricle.

TREATMENT Myxoma

Surgical excision utilizing cardiopulmonary bypass is indicated regardless of tumor size and is generally curative. Myxomas recur in 12–22% of familial cases but in only 1–2% of sporadic cases. Tumor recurrence most likely is due to multifocal lesions in the former and inadequate resection in the latter.

Other benign tumors

Cardiac *lipomas*, although relatively common, are usually incidental findings at postmortem examination; however, they may grow as large as 15 cm and may present with symptoms owing to mechanical interference with cardiac function, arrhythmias, or conduction disturbances or as an abnormality of the cardiac silhouette on chest x-ray. *Papillary fibroelastomas* are the most common tumors of the cardiac valves. Although usually clinically silent, they can cause valve dysfunction and may embolize distally, resulting in transient ischemic attacks, stroke, or myocardial infarction. Therefore, these tumors should be resected even when asymptomatic. *Rhabdomyomas* and *fibromas* are the most common cardiac tumors in infants and children and usually occur in the ventricles, where they may produce mechanical obstruction to blood flow, thereby mimicking valvular stenosis, congestive heart failure (CHF), restrictive or hypertrophic cardiomyopathy, or pericardial constriction. Rhabdomyomas are probably hamartomatous growths, are multiple in 90% of cases, and are strongly associated with tuberous sclerosis. These tumors have a tendency to regress completely or partially; only tumors that cause obstruction require surgical resection. Fibromas are usually single, are often calcified, tend to grow and cause obstructive symptoms, and should be resected. *Hemangiomas* and *mesotheliomas* are generally small tumors, most often intramyocardial in location, and may cause atrioventricular (AV) conduction disturbances and even sudden death as a result of their propensity to develop in the region of the AV node. Other benign tumors arising from the heart include *teratoma, chemodectoma, neurilemoma, granular cell myoblastoma,* and *bronchogenic cysts.*

Sarcoma

Almost all primary cardiac malignancies are sarcomas, which may be of several histologic types. In general, these tumors are characterized by rapid progression that culminates in the patient's death within weeks to months from the time of presentation as a result of hemodynamic compromise, local invasion, or distant metastases. Sarcomas commonly involve the right side of the heart, are characterized by rapid growth, frequently invade the pericardial space, and may obstruct the cardiac chambers or venae cavae. Sarcomas also may occur on the left side of the heart and may be mistaken for myxomas.

TREATMENT Sarcoma

At the time of presentation these tumors have often spread too extensively to allow for surgical excision. Although there are scattered reports of palliation with surgery, radiotherapy, and/or chemotherapy, the response of cardiac sarcomas to these therapies is generally poor. The one exception appears to be cardiac lymphosarcomas, which may respond to a combination of chemo- and radiotherapy.

TUMORS METASTATIC TO THE HEART

Tumors metastatic to the heart are much more common than primary tumors, and their incidence is likely to increase as the life expectancy of patients with various forms of malignant neoplasms is extended by more effective therapy. Although cardiac metastases may occur with any tumor type, the relative incidence is especially high in malignant melanoma and, to a somewhat lesser extent, leukemia and lymphoma. In absolute terms, the most common primary originating sites of cardiac metastases are carcinoma of the breast and lung, reflecting the high incidence of those cancers. Cardiac metastases almost always occur in the setting of widespread primary disease, and most often there is either primary or metastatic disease elsewhere in the thoracic cavity. Nevertheless, cardiac metastasis occasionally may be the initial presentation of an extrathoracic tumor.

Cardiac metastases may occur via hematogenous or lymphangitic spread or by direct tumor invasion. They generally manifest as small, firm nodules; diffuse infiltration also may occur, especially with sarcomas or hematologic neoplasms. The pericardium is most often involved, followed by myocardial involvement of any chamber and, rarely, by involvement of the endocardium or cardiac valves.

Cardiac metastases are clinically apparent only ~10% of the time, are usually not the cause of the patient's presentation, and rarely are the cause of death. The vast majority occur in the setting of a previously recognized malignant neoplasm. When symptomatic, cardiac metastases may result in a variety of clinical features, including dyspnea, acute pericarditis, cardiac tamponade, ectopic tachyarrhythmias, heart block, and CHF. As with primary cardiac tumors, the clinical presentation reflects more the location and size of the tumor than its histologic type. Many of these signs and symptoms may also result from myocarditis, pericarditis, or cardiomyopathy induced by radiotherapy or chemotherapy.

Electrocardiographic (ECG) findings are nonspecific. On chest x-ray, the cardiac silhouette is most often normal but may be enlarged or exhibit a bizarre contour. Echocardiography is useful for identifying pericardial effusions and visualizing larger metastases, although CT and radionuclide imaging with gallium or thallium may define the tumor burden more clearly. Cardiac MRI offers superb image quality and plays a central role in the diagnostic evaluation of cardiac metastases and cardiac tumors in general. Pericardiocentesis may allow for a specific cytologic diagnosis in patients with malignant pericardial effusions. Angiography is rarely necessary but may delineate discrete lesions.

TREATMENT Tumors Metastatic to the Heart

Most patients with cardiac metastases have advanced malignant disease; thus, therapy is generally palliative and consists of treatment of the primary tumor. Symptomatic malignant pericardial effusions should be drained by pericardiocentesis. Concomitant instillation of a sclerosing agent (e.g., tetracycline) may delay or prevent reaccumulation of the effusion, and creation of a pericardial window allows drainage of the effusion to the pleural space.

TRAUMATIC CARDIAC INJURY

Traumatic cardiac injury may be caused by either penetrating or nonpenetrating trauma. *Penetrating injuries* most often result from gunshot or knife wounds, and the site of entry is usually obvious. *Nonpenetrating injuries* most often occur during motor vehicle accidents, either from a rapid deceleration injury or from impact of the chest against the steering wheel, and may be associated with significant cardiac injury even in the absence of external signs of thoracic trauma.

Myocardial contusions are the most common form of nonpenetrating cardiac injury and may initially be overlooked in trauma patients as the clinical focus is directed toward other, more obvious injuries. Myocardial necrosis may occur as a direct result of the blunt injury or as a result of traumatic coronary laceration or thrombosis. The contused myocardium is pathologically similar to infarcted myocardium and may be associated with atrial or ventricular arrhythmias; conduction disturbances, including bundle branch block; or ECG abnormalities resembling those of infarction or pericarditis. Thus, it is important to consider contusion as a cause of otherwise unexplained ECG changes in a trauma patient. Serum creatine kinase, myocardial bound (CK-MB) isoenzyme levels are increased in ~20% of patients who experience blunt chest trauma but may be falsely elevated in the presence of massive skeletal muscle injury. Cardiac troponin levels are more specific for identifying cardiac injury in this setting. Echocardiography is useful in detecting structural and functional sequelae of contusion, including wall motion abnormalities, pericardial effusion, valvular dysfunction, and ventricular rupture.

Rupture of the cardiac valves or their supporting structures, most commonly of the tricuspid or mitral valve, leads to acute valvular incompetence. This complication is usually heralded by the development of a loud murmur, may be associated with rapidly progressive heart failure, and can be diagnosed by either transthoracic or transesophageal echocardiography.

The most serious consequence of nonpenetrating cardiac injury is myocardial rupture, which may result in hemopericardium and tamponade (free wall rupture) or intracardiac shunting (ventricular septal rupture). Although it generally is fatal, up to 40% of patients with cardiac rupture have been reported to survive long enough to reach a specialized trauma center. Hemopericardium also may result from traumatic rupture of a pericardial vessel or a coronary artery. Additionally, a pericardial effusion may develop weeks or even months after blunt chest trauma as a manifestation of the post-cardiac injury syndrome, which resembles the post-pericardiotomy syndrome (Chap. 239).

Blunt, nonpenetrating, often innocent-appearing injuries to the chest may trigger ventricular fibrillation even in absence of overt signs of injury. This syndrome, referred to as *commotio cordis*, occurs most often in adolescents during sporting events (e.g., baseball, hockey, football, and lacrosse) and probably results from an impact to the chest wall overlying the heart during the susceptible phase of repolarization just before the peak of the T wave. Survival depends on prompt defibrillation.

Rupture of the aorta, usually just above the aortic valve or at the site of the ligamentum arteriosum, is a common consequence of nonpenetrating chest trauma and is the most common vascular deceleration injury. The clinical presentation is similar to that of aortic dissection (Chap. 248); the arterial pressure and pulse amplitude may be increased in the upper extremities and decreased in the lower extremities, and chest x-ray may reveal mediastinal widening. Occasionally, aortic rupture is contained by the aortic adventitia, resulting in a false, or *pseudo-*, aneurysm that may be discovered months or years after the initial injury.

Sudden emotional or physical trauma may precipitate a transient catecholamine-mediated cardiomyopathy referred to as *Tako-Tsubo syndrome* or the *apical ballooning syndrome* (Chap. 238).

Penetrating injuries of the heart produced by knife or bullet wounds usually result in rapid clinical deterioration and frequently in death as a result of hemopericardium/pericardial tamponade or massive hemorrhage. Nonetheless, up to half of such patients may survive long enough to reach a specialized trauma center if immediate resuscitation is performed. Prognosis in these patients relates to the mechanism of injury, their clinical condition at presentation, and the specific cardiac chamber(s) involved. Iatrogenic cardiac or coronary arterial perforation may complicate placement of central venous or intracardiac catheters, pacemaker leads, or intracoronary stents and is associated with a better prognosis than are other forms of penetrating cardiac trauma.

Traumatic rupture of a great vessel from penetrating injury is usually associated with hemothorax and, less often, hemopericardium. Local hematoma formation may compress major vessels and produce ischemic symptoms, and AV fistulas may develop, occasionally resulting in high-output CHF.

Occasionally, patients who survive penetrating cardiac injuries may subsequently present with a new cardiac murmur or CHF as a result of mitral regurgitation or an intracardiac shunt (i.e., ventricular or atrial septal defect, aortopulmonary fistula, or coronary AV fistula) that was undetected at the time of the initial injury or developed subsequently. Therefore, trauma patients should be examined carefully several weeks after the injury. If a mechanical complication is suspected, it can be confirmed by echocardiography or cardiac catheterization.

TREATMENT Traumatic Cardiac Injury

The treatment of an uncomplicated myocardial contusion is similar to the medical therapy for a myocardial infarction, except that anticoagulation is contraindicated, and should include monitoring for the development of arrhythmias and mechanical complications such as cardiac rupture (Chap. 245). Acute myocardial failure resulting from traumatic valve rupture usually requires urgent operative correction. Immediate thoracotomy should be carried out for most cases of penetrating injury or if there is evidence of cardiac tamponade and/or shock regardless of the type of trauma. Pericardiocentesis may be lifesaving in patients with tamponade but is usually only a temporizing measure while awaiting definitive surgical therapy. Pericardial hemorrhage often leads to constriction (Chap. 239), which must be treated by surgical decortication.

FURTHER READINGS

Burke A et al: Cardiac tumors: An update. Heart 94:117, 2008

Kalra MK, Abbara S: Imaging cardiac tumors. Cancer Treat Res 143:177, 2008

Mattox KL: Traumatic heart disease, in *Braunwald's Heart Disease*, 7th ed, DP Zipes et al (eds). Philadelphia, Saunders, 2005

Pretre R, Chilcott M: Blunt trauma to the heart and great vessels. N Engl J Med 336:626, 1997

Reyman K: Cardiac myxomas. N Engl J Med 333:1610, 1995

Rhee PM et al: Penetrating cardiac injuries: A population-based study. J Trauma 45:366, 1998

Sabatine M, Schoen F: Primary tumors of the heart, in *Braunwald's Heart Disease*, 7th ed, DP Zipes et al (eds). Philadelphia, Saunders, 2005

Simmers TA et al: Traumatic papillary muscle rupture. Ann Thorac Surg 72:257, 2001

Sybrandy KC et al: Diagnosing cardiac contusion: Old wisdom and new insights. Heart 89:485, 2003

Tyburski JG et al: Factors affecting prognosis with penetrating wounds of the heart. J Trauma 48:587, 2000

Vaughan CJ et al: Tumors and the heart: Molecular genetic advances. Curr Opin Cardiol 16:195, 2001

CHAPTER 241 The Pathogenesis, Prevention, and Treatment of Atherosclerosis

Peter Libby

PATHOGENESIS

Atherosclerosis remains the major cause of death and premature disability in developed societies. Moreover, current predictions estimate that by the year 2020 cardiovascular diseases, notably atherosclerosis, will become the leading global cause of total disease burden. Although many generalized or systemic risk factors predispose to its development, atherosclerosis affects various regions of the circulation preferentially and has distinct clinical manifestations that depend on the particular circulatory bed affected. Atherosclerosis of the coronary arteries commonly causes myocardial infarction (MI) (Chap. 245) and angina pectoris (Chap. 243). Atherosclerosis of the arteries supplying the central nervous system frequently provokes strokes and transient cerebral ischemia (Chap. 370). In the peripheral circulation, atherosclerosis causes intermittent claudication and gangrene and can jeopardize limb viability. Involvement of the splanchnic circulation can cause mesenteric ischemia. Atherosclerosis can affect the kidneys either directly (e.g., renal artery stenosis) or as a common site of atheroembolic disease (Chap. 248).

Even within a particular arterial bed, stenoses due to atherosclerosis tend to occur focally, typically in certain predisposed regions. In the coronary circulation, for example, the proximal left anterior descending coronary artery exhibits a particular predilection for developing atherosclerotic disease. Similarly, atherosclerosis preferentially affects the proximal portions of the renal arteries and, in the extracranial circulation to the brain, the carotid bifurcation. Indeed, atherosclerotic lesions often form at branching points of arteries which are regions of disturbed blood flow. Not all manifestations of atherosclerosis result from stenotic, occlusive disease. Ectasia and the development of aneurysmal disease, for example, frequently occur in the aorta (Chap. 248). In addition to focal, flow-limiting stenoses, nonocclusive intimal atherosclerosis also occurs diffusely in affected arteries, as shown by intravascular ultrasound and postmortem studies.

Atherogenesis in humans typically occurs over a period of many years, usually many decades. Growth of atherosclerotic plaques probably does not occur in a smooth, linear fashion but discontinuously, with periods of relative quiescence punctuated by periods of rapid evolution. After a generally prolonged "silent" period, atherosclerosis may become clinically manifest. The clinical expressions of atherosclerosis may be *chronic*, as in the development of stable, effort-induced angina pectoris or predictable and reproducible intermittent claudication. Alternatively, a dramatic *acute* clinical event such as MI, stroke, or sudden cardiac death may first herald the presence of atherosclerosis. Other individuals may never experience clinical manifestations of arterial disease despite the presence of widespread atherosclerosis demonstrated postmortem.

INITIATION OF ATHEROSCLEROSIS

An integrated view of experimental results in animals and studies of human atherosclerosis suggests that the "fatty streak" represents the initial lesion of atherosclerosis. These early lesions most often seem to arise from focal increases in the content of lipoproteins within regions of the intima. This accumulation of lipoprotein particles may not result simply from increased permeability, or "leakiness," of the overlying endothelium (Fig. 241-1). Rather, the lipoproteins may collect in the intima of arteries because they bind to constituents of the extracellular matrix, increasing the residence time of the lipid-rich particles within the arterial wall. Lipoproteins that accumulate in the extracellular space of the intima of arteries often associate with glycosaminoglycans of the arterial extracellular matrix, an interaction that may slow the egress of these lipid-rich particles from the intima. Lipoprotein particles in the extracellular space of the intima, particularly those retained by binding to matrix macromolecules, may undergo oxidative modifications. Considerable evidence supports a pathogenic role for products of oxidized lipoproteins in atherogenesis. Lipoproteins sequestered from plasma antioxidants in the extracellular space of the intima become particularly susceptible to oxidative modification, giving rise to hydroperoxides, lysophospholipids, oxysterols, and aldehydic breakdown products of fatty acids and phospholipids. Modifications of the apoprotein moieties may include breaks in the peptide backbone as well as derivatization of certain amino acid residues. Local production of hypochlorous acid by myeloperoxidase associated with inflammatory cells within the plaque yields chlorinated species such as chlorotyrosyl moieties. High-density lipoprotein (HDL) particles modified by HOCl-mediated chlorination function poorly as cholesterol acceptors, a finding that links oxidative stress with impaired reverse cholesterol transport, which is one likely mechanism of the antiatherogenic action of HDL (see below). Considerable evidence supports the presence of such oxidation products in atherosclerotic lesions. A particular member of the phospholipase family, lipoprotein-associated phospholipase A_2 (LpPL A_2), can generate proinflammatory lipids, including lysophosphatidyl choline-bearing oxidized lipid moieties from oxidized phospholipids found in oxidized low-density lipoproteins (LDLs). An inhibitor of this enzyme is in clinical development.

Leukocyte recruitment

Accumulation of leukocytes characterizes the formation of early atherosclerotic lesions (Fig. 241-1). Thus, from its very inception, atherogenesis involves elements of inflammation, a process that now provides a unifying theme in the pathogenesis of this disease. The inflammatory cell types typically found in the evolving atheroma include monocyte-derived macrophages and lymphocytes. A number of adhesion molecules or receptors for leukocytes expressed on the surface of the arterial endothelial cell probably participate in the recruitment of leukocytes to the nascent atheroma. Constituents of oxidatively modified low-density lipoprotein can augment the expression of leukocyte adhesion molecules. This example illustrates how the accumulation of lipoproteins in the arterial intima may link mechanistically with leukocyte recruitment, a key event in lesion formation.

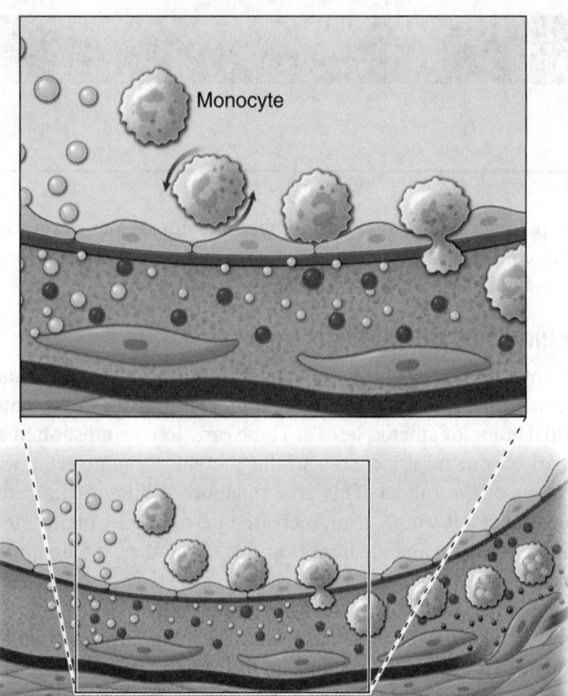

Figure 241-1 Cross-sectional view of an artery depicting steps in development of an atheroma, from left to right. The *upper panel* shows a detail of the boxed area below. The endothelial monolayer overlying the intima contacts blood. Hypercholesterolemia promotes accumulation of LDL particles (*light spheres*) in the intima. The lipoprotein particles often associate with constituents of the extracellular matrix, notably proteoglycans. Sequestration within the intima separates lipoproteins from some plasma antioxidants and favors oxidative modification. Such modified lipoprotein particles (*darker spheres*) may trigger a local inflammatory response that signals subsequent steps in lesion formation. The augmented expression of various adhesion molecules for leukocytes recruits monocytes to the site of a nascent arterial lesion.

Once adherent, some white blood cells migrate into the intima. The directed migration of leukocytes probably depends on chemoattractant factors, including modified lipoprotein particles themselves and chemoattractant cytokines (depicted by the smaller spheres), such as the chemokine macrophage chemoattractant protein-1 produced by vascular wall cells in response to modified lipoproteins. Leukocytes in the evolving fatty streak can divide and exhibit augmented expression of receptors for modified lipoproteins (scavenger receptors). These mononuclear phagocytes ingest lipids and become foam cells, represented by a cytoplasm filled with lipid droplets. As the fatty streak evolves into a more complicated atherosclerotic lesion, smooth muscle cells migrate from the media (*bottom of lower panel hairline*) through the internal elastic membrane (*solid wavy line*) and accumulate within the expanding intima, where they lay down extracellular matrix that forms the bulk of the advanced lesion (*bottom panel, right side*).

Laminar shear forces such as those encountered in most regions of normal arteries also can suppress the expression of leukocyte adhesion molecules. Sites of predilection for atherosclerotic lesions (e.g., branch points) often have disturbed flow. Ordered, pulsatile laminar shear of normal blood flow augments the production of nitric oxide by endothelial cells. This molecule, in addition to its vasodilator properties, can act at the low levels constitutively produced by arterial endothelium as a local anti-inflammatory autacoid, e.g., limiting local adhesion molecule expression. Exposure of endothelial cells to laminar shear stress increases the transcription of Krüppel-like factor 2 (KLF2) and reduces the expression of a thioredoxin-interacting protein (Txnip) that inhibits the activity of the endogenous antioxidant thioredoxin. KLF2 augments the activity of endothelial nitric oxide synthase, and reduced Txnip levels boost the function of thioredoxin. Laminar shear stress also stimulates endothelial cells to produce superoxide dismutase, an antioxidant enzyme. These examples indicate how hemodynamic forces may influence the cellular events that underlie atherosclerotic lesion initiation and potentially explain the favored localization of atherosclerotic lesions at sites that experience disturbance to laminar shear stress.

Once captured on the surface of the arterial endothelial cell by adhesion receptors, the monocytes and lymphocytes penetrate the endothelial layer and take up residence in the intima. In addition to products of modified lipoproteins, cytokines (protein mediators of inflammation) can regulate the expression of adhesion molecules involved in leukocyte recruitment. For example, interleukin 1 (IL-1) or tumor necrosis factor α (TNF-α) induce or augment the expression of leukocyte adhesion molecules on endothelial cells. Because products of lipoprotein oxidation can induce cytokine release from vascular wall cells, this pathway may provide an additional link between arterial accumulation of lipoproteins and leukocyte recruitment. Chemoattractant cytokines such as monocyte chemoattractant protein 1 appear to direct the migration of leukocytes into the arterial wall.

Foam-cell formation

Once resident within the intima, the mononuclear phagocytes mature into macrophages and become lipid-laden foam cells, a conversion that requires the uptake of lipoprotein particles by receptor-mediated endocytosis. One might suppose that the well-recognized "classic" receptor for LDL mediates this lipid uptake; however, humans or animals lacking effective LDL receptors due to genetic alterations (e.g., familial hypercholesterolemia) have abundant arterial lesions and extraarterial xanthomata rich in macrophage-derived foam cells. In addition, the exogenous cholesterol suppresses expression of the LDL receptor; thus, the level of this cell-surface receptor for LDL decreases under conditions of cholesterol excess. Candidates for alternative receptors that can mediate lipid loading of foam cells include a growing number of macrophage "scavenger" receptors, which preferentially endocytose modified lipoproteins, and other receptors for oxidized LDL or very low-density lipoprotein (VLDL). Monocyte attachment to the endothelium, migration into the intima, and maturation to form lipid-laden macrophages thus represent key steps in the formation of the fatty streak, the precursor of fully formed atherosclerotic plaques.

ATHEROMA EVOLUTION AND COMPLICATIONS

Although the fatty streak commonly precedes the development of a more advanced atherosclerotic plaque, not all fatty streaks progress to form complex atheromata. By ingesting lipids from the extracellular space, the mononuclear phagocytes bearing such scavenger receptors may remove lipoproteins from the developing lesion. Some lipid-laden macrophages may leave the artery wall, exporting lipid in the process. Lipid accumulation, and hence the propensity to form an atheroma, ensues if the amount of lipid entering the artery wall exceeds that removed by mononuclear phagocytes or other pathways.

Export by phagocytes may constitute one response to local lipid overload in the evolving lesion. Another mechanism, reverse cholesterol transport mediated by high-density lipoproteins, probably provides an independent pathway for lipid removal from atheroma. This transfer of cholesterol from the cell to the HDL particle involves specialized cell-surface molecules such as the ATP binding cassette (ABC) transporters. *ABCA1*, the gene mutated in Tangier disease, a condition characterized by very low HDL levels, transfers cholesterol from cells to nascent HDL particles and ABCG1 to mature HDL particles. "Reverse cholesterol transport" mediated by these ABC transporters allows HDL loaded with cholesterol to deliver it to hepatocytes by binding to scavenger receptor B 1 or other receptors. The liver cell can metabolize the sterol to bile acids that can be excreted. This export pathway from macrophage foam cells to peripheral cells such as hepatocytes explains part of the antiatherogenic action of HDLs. (Anti-inflammatory and antioxidant properties also may contribute to the atheroprotective effects of HDLs.) Thus, macrophages may play a vital role in the dynamic economy of lipid accumulation in the arterial wall during atherogenesis.

Some lipid-laden foam cells within the expanding intimal lesion perish. Some foam cells may die as a result of programmed cell death, or *apoptosis*. This death of mononuclear phagocytes results in the formation of the lipid-rich center, often called the *necrotic core*, in established atherosclerotic plaques. Macrophages loaded with modified lipoproteins may elaborate cytokines and growth factors that can further signal some of the cellular events in lesion complication. Whereas accumulation of lipid-laden macrophages characterizes the fatty streak, buildup of fibrous tissue formed by extracellular matrix typifies the more advanced atherosclerotic lesion. The smooth muscle cell synthesizes the bulk of the extracellular matrix of the complex atherosclerotic lesion. A number of growth factors or cytokines elaborated by mononuclear phagocytes can stimulate smooth muscle cell proliferation and production of extracellular matrix. Cytokines found in the plaque, including IL-1 and TNF-α, can induce local production of growth factors, including forms of platelet-derived growth factor (PDGF), fibroblast growth factors, and others, which may contribute to plaque evolution and complication. Other cytokines, notably interferon γ (IFN-γ) derived from activated T cells within lesions, can limit the synthesis of interstitial forms of collagen by smooth muscle cells. These examples illustrate how atherogenesis involves a complex mix of mediators that in the balance determines the characteristics of particular lesions.

The arrival of smooth muscle cells and their elaboration of extracellular matrix probably provide a critical transition, yielding a fibrofatty lesion in place of a simple accumulation of macrophage-derived foam cells. For example, PDGF elaborated by activated platelets, macrophages, and endothelial cells can stimulate the migration of smooth muscle cells normally resident in the tunica media into the intima. Such growth factors and cytokines produced locally can stimulate the proliferation of resident smooth muscle cells in the intima as well as those that have migrated from the media. Transforming growth factor β (TGF-β), among other mediators, potently stimulates interstitial collagen production by smooth muscle cells. These mediators may arise not only from neighboring vascular cells or leukocytes (a "paracrine" pathway), but also, in some instances, may arise from the same cell that responds to the factor (an "autocrine" pathway). Together, these alterations in smooth muscle cells, signaled by these mediators acting at short distances, can hasten transformation of the fatty streak into a more fibrous smooth muscle cell and extracellular matrix-rich lesion.

In addition to locally produced mediators, products of blood coagulation and thrombosis likely contribute to atheroma evolution and complication. This involvement justifies the use of the term *atherothrombosis* to convey the inextricable links between atherosclerosis and thrombosis. Fatty streak formation begins beneath a morphologically intact endothelium. In advanced fatty streaks, however, microscopic breaches in endothelial integrity may occur. Microthrombi rich in platelets can form at such sites of limited endothelial denudation, owing to exposure of the thrombogenic extracellular matrix of the underlying basement membrane. Activated platelets release numerous factors that can promote the fibrotic response, including PDGF and TGF-β. Thrombin not only generates fibrin during coagulation, but also stimulates protease-activated receptors that can signal smooth muscle migration, proliferation, and extracellular matrix production. Many arterial mural microthrombi resolve without clinical manifestation by a process of local fibrinolysis, resorption, and endothelial repair, yet can lead to lesion progression by stimulating these profibrotic functions of smooth muscle cells (Fig. 241-2*D*).

Microvessels

As atherosclerotic lesions advance, abundant plexuses of microvessels develop in connection with the artery's vasa vasorum. Newly developing microvascular networks may contribute to lesion complications in several ways. These blood vessels provide an abundant surface area for leukocyte trafficking and may serve as the portal for entry and exit of white blood cells from the established atheroma. Microvessels in the plaques may also furnish foci for intraplaque hemorrhage. Like the neovessels in the diabetic retina, microvessels in the atheroma may be friable and prone to rupture and can produce focal hemorrhage. Such a vascular leak can provoke thrombosis in situ, yielding local thrombin generation, which in turn can activate smooth muscle and endothelial cells through ligation of protease-activated receptors. Atherosclerotic plaques often contain fibrin and hemosiderin, an indication that episodes of intraplaque hemorrhage contribute to plaque complications.

Calcification As they advance, atherosclerotic plaques also accumulate *calcium*. Proteins usually found in bone also localize in atherosclerotic lesions (e.g., osteocalcin, osteopontin, and bone morphogenetic proteins). Mineralization of the atherosclerotic plaque recapitulates many aspects of bone formation, including the regulatory participation of transcription factors such as Runx2.

Plaque evolution

Although atherosclerosis research has focused much attention on proliferation of smooth muscle cells, as in the case of macrophages, smooth muscle cells also can undergo apoptosis in the atherosclerotic plaque. Indeed, complex atheromata often have a mostly fibrous character and lack the cellularity of less advanced lesions. This relative paucity of smooth muscle cells in advanced atheromata may result from the predominance of cytostatic mediators such as TGF-β and IFN-γ (which can inhibit smooth muscle cell proliferation), and also from smooth muscle cell apoptosis. Some of the same proinflammatory cytokines that activate atherogenic functions of vascular wall cells can also sensitize these cells to undergo apoptosis.

Thus, during the evolution of the atherosclerotic plaque, a complex balance between entry and egress of lipoproteins and leukocytes, cell proliferation and cell death, extracellular matrix production, and remodeling, as well as calcification and neovascularization, contribute to lesion formation. Multiple and often competing signals regulate these various cellular events. Many mediators related to atherogenic risk factors, including those derived from lipoproteins, cigarette smoking, and angiotensin II, provoke the production of proinflammatory cytokines and alter the behavior of the intrinsic vascular wall cells and infiltrating leukocytes that underlie the complex pathogenesis of these lesions. Thus, advances in vascular biology have led to increased understanding of the mechanisms that link risk factors to the pathogenesis of atherosclerosis and its complications.

■ CLINICAL SYNDROMES OF ATHEROSCLEROSIS

Atherosclerotic lesions occur ubiquitously in Western societies. Most atheromata produce no symptoms, and many never cause clinical manifestations. Numerous patients with diffuse atherosclerosis may succumb to unrelated illnesses without ever having experienced a clinically significant manifestation of atherosclerosis. What accounts for this variability in the clinical expression of atherosclerotic disease?

Arterial remodeling during atheroma formation (Fig. 241-2*A*) represents a frequently overlooked but clinically important feature of lesion evolution. During the initial phases of atheroma development, the plaque usually grows outward, in an abluminal direction. Vessels affected by atherogenesis tend to increase in diameter, a phenomenon known as *compensatory enlargement*, a type of vascular remodeling. The growing atheroma does not encroach on the arterial lumen until the burden of atherosclerotic plaque exceeds ~40% of the area encompassed by the internal elastic lamina. Thus, during much of its life history, an atheroma will not cause stenosis that can limit tissue perfusion.

Flow-limiting stenoses commonly form later in the history of the plaque. Many such plaques cause stable syndromes such as demand-induced angina pectoris or intermittent claudication in the extremities. In the coronary circulation and other circulations, even total vascular occlusion by an atheroma does not invariably lead to infarction. The hypoxic stimulus of repeated bouts of ischemia characteristically induces formation of collateral vessels in the myocardium, mitigating the consequences of an acute occlusion of an epicardial coronary artery. By contrast, many lesions that cause acute or unstable atherosclerotic syndromes, particularly in the coronary circulation, may arise from atherosclerotic plaques that do not produce a flow-limiting stenosis. Such lesions may produce only minimal luminal irregularities on traditional angiograms and often do not meet the traditional criteria for "significance" by arteriography. Thrombi arising from such nonocclusive stenoses may explain the frequency of MI as an initial manifestation of coronary artery disease (CAD) (in at least one-third of cases) in patients who report no prior history of angina pectoris, a syndrome usually caused by flow-limiting stenoses.

Plaque instability and rupture

Postmortem studies afford considerable insight into the microanatomic substrate underlying the "instability" of plaques that do not cause critical stenoses. A superficial erosion of the endothelium or a frank plaque rupture or fissure usually produces the thrombus that causes episodes of unstable angina pectoris or the occlusive and relatively persistent thrombus that causes acute MI (Fig. 241-2*B*). In the case of carotid atheromata, a deeper ulceration that provides a nidus for the formation of platelet thrombi may cause transient cerebral ischemic attacks.

Rupture of the plaque's fibrous cap (Fig. 241-2*C*) permits contact between coagulation factors in the blood and highly thrombogenic tissue factor expressed by macrophage foam cells in the plaque's lipid-rich core. If the ensuing thrombus is nonocclusive or transient, the episode of plaque disruption may not cause symptoms or may result in episodic ischemic symptoms such as rest angina. Occlusive thrombi that endure often cause acute MI, particularly in the absence of a well-developed collateral circulation that supplies the affected territory. Repetitive episodes of plaque disruption and healing provide one likely mechanism of transition of the fatty streak to a more complex fibrous lesion (Fig. 241-2D). The healing process in arteries, as in skin wounds, involves the laying down of new extracellular matrix and fibrosis.

Not all atheromata exhibit the same propensity to rupture. Pathologic studies of culprit lesions that have caused acute MI reveal several characteristic features. Plaques that have caused fatal thromboses tend to have thin fibrous caps, relatively large lipid cores, and a high content of macrophages. Morphometric studies of such culprit lesions show that at sites of plaque rupture, macrophages and T lymphocytes predominate and contain relatively few smooth muscle cells. The cells that concentrate at sites of plaque rupture bear markers of inflammatory activation. In addition, patients with active atherosclerosis and acute coronary syndromes display signs of disseminated inflammation. For example, atherosclerotic plaques

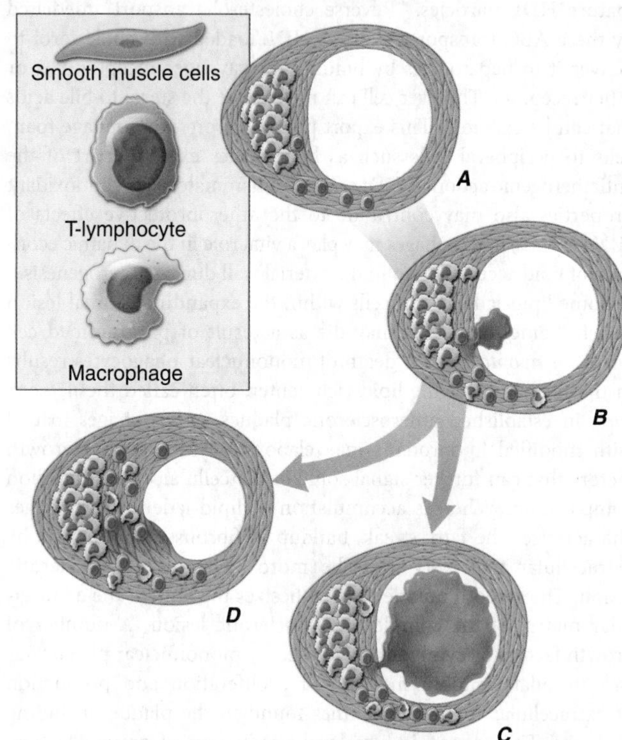

Figure 241-2 Plaque rupture, thrombosis, and healing. ***A.*** Arterial remodeling during atherogenesis. During the initial part of the life history of an atheroma, growth is often outward, preserving the caliber of the lumen. This phenomenon of "compensatory enlargement" accounts in part for the tendency of coronary arteriography to underestimate the degree of atherosclerosis. ***B.*** Rupture of the plaque's fibrous cap causes thrombosis. Physical disruption of the atherosclerotic plaque commonly causes arterial thrombosis by allowing blood coagulant factors to contact thrombogenic collagen found in the arterial extracellular matrix and tissue factor produced by macrophage-derived foam cells in the lipid core of lesions. In this manner, sites of plaque rupture form the nidus for thrombi. The normal artery wall has several fibrinolytic or antithrombotic mechanisms that tend to resist thrombosis and lyse clots that begin to form in situ. Such antithrombotic or thrombolytic molecules include thrombomodulin, tissue- and urokinase-type plasminogen activators, heparan sulfate proteoglycans, prostacyclin, and nitric oxide. ***C.*** When the clot overwhelms the endogenous fibrinolytic mechanisms, it may propagate and lead to arterial occlusion. The consequences of this occlusion depend on the degree of existing collateral vessels. In a patient with chronic multivessel occlusive coronary artery disease (CAD), collateral channels have often formed. In such circumstances, even a total arterial occlusion may not lead to myocardial infarction (MI), or it may produce an unexpectedly modest or a non-ST-segment elevation infarct because of collateral flow. In a patient with less advanced disease and without substantial stenotic lesions to provide a stimulus for collateral vessel formation, sudden plaque rupture and arterial occlusion commonly produces an ST-segment elevation infarction. These are the types of patients who may present with MI or sudden death as a first manifestation of coronary atherosclerosis. In some cases, the thrombus may lyse or organize into a mural thrombus without occluding the vessel. Such instances may be clinically silent. ***D.*** The subsequent thrombin-induced fibrosis and healing causes a fibroproliferative response that can lead to a more fibrous lesion that can produce an eccentric plaque that causes a hemodynamically significant stenosis. In this way, a nonocclusive mural thrombus, even if clinically silent or causing unstable angina rather than infarction, can provoke a healing response that can promote lesion fibrosis and luminal encroachment. Such a sequence of events may convert a "vulnerable" atheroma with a thin fibrous cap that is prone to rupture into a more "stable" fibrous plaque with a reinforced cap. Angioplasty of unstable coronary lesions may "stabilize" the lesions by a similar mechanism, producing a wound followed by healing.

and even microvascular endothelial cells at sites remote from the "culprit" lesion of an acute coronary syndrome can exhibit markers of inflammatory activation.

Inflammatory mediators regulate processes that govern the integrity of the plaque's fibrous cap and, hence, its propensity to rupture. For example, the T cell-derived cytokine IFN-γ, which is found in atherosclerotic plaques, can inhibit growth and collagen synthesis of smooth muscle cells, as noted above. Cytokines derived from activated macrophages and lesional T cells can boost production of proteolytic enzymes that can degrade the extracellular matrix of the plaque's fibrous cap. Thus, inflammatory mediators can impair the collagen synthesis required for maintenance and repair of the fibrous cap and trigger degradation of extracellular matrix macromolecules, processes that weaken the plaque's fibrous cap and enhance its susceptibility to rupture (so-called vulnerable plaques). In contrast to plaques with these features of vulnerability, those with a dense extracellular matrix and relatively thick fibrous cap without substantial tissue factor–rich lipid cores seem generally resistant to rupture and unlikely to provoke thrombosis.

Features of the biology of the atheromatous plaque, in addition to its degree of luminal encroachment, influence the clinical manifestations of this disease. This enhanced understanding of plaque biology provides insight into the diverse ways in which atherosclerosis can present clinically and the reasons why the disease may remain silent or stable for prolonged periods, punctuated by acute complications at certain times. Increased understanding of atherogenesis provides new insight into the mechanisms linking it to the risk factors discussed below, indicates the ways in which current therapies may improve outcomes, and suggests new targets for future intervention.

PREVENTION AND TREATMENT

THE CONCEPT OF ATHEROSCLEROTIC RISK FACTORS

The systematic study of risk factors for atherosclerosis emerged from a coalescence of experimental results, as well as from cross-sectional and ultimately longitudinal studies in humans. The prospective, community-based Framingham Heart Study provided rigorous support for the concept that hypercholesterolemia, hypertension, and other factors correlate with cardiovascular risk. Similar observational studies performed worldwide bolstered the concept of "risk factors" for cardiovascular disease.

From a practical viewpoint, the cardiovascular risk factors that have emerged from such studies fall into two categories: those modifiable by lifestyle and/or pharmacotherapy, and those that are immutable, such as age and sex. The weight of evidence supporting various risk factors differs. For example, hypercholesterolemia and hypertension certainly predict coronary risk, but the magnitude of the contributions of other so-called nontraditional risk factors, such as levels of homocysteine, levels of lipoprotein (a) [Lp(a)], and infection, remains controversial. Moreover, some biomarkers that predict cardiovascular risk may not participate in the causal pathway for the disease or its complications. For example, recent genetic studies suggest that C-reactive protein (CRP) does not itself mediate atherogenesis, despite its ability to predict risk. Table 241-1 lists the risk factors recognized by the current National Cholesterol Education Project Adult Treatment Panel III (ATP III). The sections below will consider some of these risk factors and approaches to their modification.

Lipid disorders

Abnormalities in plasma lipoproteins and derangements in lipid metabolism rank among the most firmly established and best understood risk factors for atherosclerosis. Chapter 356 describes the lipoprotein classes and provides a detailed discussion of lipoprotein metabolism. Current ATP III guidelines recommend

TABLE 241-1 Major Risk Factors (Exclusive of LDL Cholesterol) That Modify LDL Goals

Cigarette smoking
Hypertension (BP ≥140/90 mmHg or on antihypertensive medication)
Low HDL cholesterol* [<1.0 mmol/L (<40 mg/dL)]
Diabetes mellitus
Family history of premature CHD
CHD in male first-degree relative <55 years
CHD in female first-degree relative <65 years
Age (men ≥45 years; women ≥55 years)
Lifestyle risk factors
Obesity (BMI ≥30 kg/m²)
Physical inactivity
Atherogenic diet
Emerging risk factors
Lipoprotein(a)
Homocysteine
Prothrombotic factors
Proinflammatory factors
Impaired fasting glucose
Subclinical atherosclerosis

*HDL cholesterol ≥1.6 mmol/L (≥60 mg/dL) counts as a "negative" risk factor; its presence removes one risk factor from the total count.

Abbreviations: BMI, body mass index; BP, blood pressure; CHD, coronary heart disease; HDL, high-density lipoprotein; LDL, low-density lipoprotein.

Source: Modified from Third Report of the National Cholesterol Education Program (NCEP) Expert Panel on Detection, Evaluation, and Treatment of High Blood Cholesterol in Adults (Adult Treatment Panel III), Executive Summary. (Bethesda, MD: National Heart, Lung and Blood Institute, National Institutes of Health, 2001. NIH Publication No. 01-3670.)

lipid screening in all adults >20 years of age. The screen should include a fasting lipid profile (total cholesterol, triglycerides, LDL cholesterol, and HDL cholesterol) repeated every 5 years.

ATP III guidelines strive to match the intensity of treatment to an individual's risk. A quantitative estimate of risk places individuals in one of three treatment strata (Table 241-2). The first step in applying these guidelines involves counting an individual's risk factors (Table 241-1). Individuals with fewer than two risk factors fall into the lowest treatment intensity stratum [LDL goal <4.1 mmol/L (<160 mg/dL)]. In those with two or more risk factors, the next step involves a simple calculation that estimates the 10-year risk of developing coronary heart disease (CHD) (Table 241-2); see *http://www.nhlbi.nih.gov/guidelines/cholesterol/* for the algorithm and a downloadable risk calculator. Those with a 10-year risk ≤20% fall into the intermediate stratum [LDL goal <3.4 mmol/L (<130 mg/dL)]. Those with a calculated 10-year CHD risk of >20%, any evidence of established atherosclerosis, or diabetes (now considered a CHD risk-equivalent) fall into the most intensive treatment group [LDL goal <2.6 mmol/L (<100 mg/dL)]. Members of the ATP III panel recently suggested <1.8 mmol/L (<70 mg/dL) as a goal for very high-risk patients and an optional goal for high-risk patients based on recent clinical trial data (Table 241-2). Beyond the Framingham algorithm, there are multiple risk calculators for various

TABLE 241-2 LDL Cholesterol Goals and Cutpoints for Therapeutic Lifestyle Changes (TLC) and Drug Therapy in Different Risk Categories

	LDL Level, mmol/L (mg/dL)		
Risk Category	Goal	Initiate TLC	Consider Drug Therapy
Very high	<1.8 (<70)	≥1.8 (≥70)	≥1.8 (≥70)
ACS, or CHD w/DM, or multiple CRFs			
High	<2.6 (<100) [optional goal: <1.8 (<70)]	≥2.6 (≥100)	≥2.6 (≥100) [<2.6 (<100): consider drug Rx]
CHD or CHD risk equivalents (10-year risk >20%)			
If LDL <2.6 (<100)	<1.8 (<70)		
Moderately high	<2.6 (<100)	≥3.4 (≥130)	≥3.4 (≥130) [2.6–3.3 (100–129): consider drug Rx]
2+ risk factors (10-year risk, 10–20%)			
Moderate	<3.4 (<130)	≥3.4 (≥130)	≥4.1 (≥160)
2+ risk factors (risk <10%)			
Lower	<4.1 (<160)	≥4.1 (≥160)	≥4.9 (≥190)
0–1 risk factor			

Abbreviations: ACS, acute coronary syndrome; CHD, coronary heart disease; CRFs, coronary risk factors; DM, diabetes mellitus; LDL, low-density lipoprotein.

Source: Adapted from S Grundy et al: Circulation 110:227, 2004.

countries or regions. Risk calculators that incorporate family history of premature (CAD) and a marker of inflammation (CRP) have been validated for U.S. women and men.

The first maneuver to achieve the LDL goal involves therapeutic lifestyle changes (TLC), including specific diet and exercise recommendations established by the guidelines. According to ATP III criteria, those with LDL levels exceeding goal for their risk group by >0.8 mmol/L (>30 mg/dL) merit consideration for drug therapy. In patients with triglycerides >2.6 mmol/L (>200 mg/dL), ATP III guidelines specify a secondary goal for therapy: "non-HDL cholesterol" (simply, the HDL cholesterol level subtracted from the total cholesterol). Cutpoints for the therapeutic decision for non-HDL cholesterol are 0.8 mmol/L (30 mg/dL) more than those for LDL.

An extensive and growing body of rigorous evidence now supports the effectiveness of aggressive management of LDL. Addition of drug therapy to dietary and other nonpharmacologic measures reduces cardiovascular risk in patients with established coronary atherosclerosis and also in individuals who have not previously experienced CHD events (Fig. 241-3). As guidelines often lag the emerging clinical trial evidence base, the practitioner may elect to exercise clinical judgment in making therapeutic decisions in individual patients.

LDL-lowering therapies do not appear to exert their beneficial effect on cardiovascular events by causing a marked "regression" of stenoses. Angiographically monitored studies of lipid lowering have shown at best a modest reduction in coronary artery stenoses over the duration of study, despite abundant evidence of event reduction. These results suggest that the beneficial mechanism of lipid lowering does not require a substantial reduction in the fixed stenoses. Rather, the benefit may derive from "stabilization" of atherosclerotic lesions without decreased stenosis. Such stabilization of atherosclerotic lesions and the attendant decrease in coronary events may result from the egress of lipids or from favorably influencing aspects of the biology of atherogenesis discussed above. In addition, as sizable lesions may protrude abluminally rather than into the lumen due to complementary enlargement, shrinkage of such plaques may not be apparent on angiograms. The consistent benefit of LDL lowering by 3-hydroxy-3-methylglutaryl coenzyme A (HMG-CoA) reductase inhibitors (statins) observed in many risk groups may depend not only on their salutary effects on the lipid profile but also on direct modulation of plaque biology independent of lipid lowering.

A new class of LDL-lowering medications reduces cholesterol absorption from the proximal small bowel by targeting an enterocyte cholesterol transporter denoted Niemann-Pick C1-like 1 protein (NPC1L1). The NPC1L1 inhibitor ezetimibe provides a useful adjunct to current therapies to achieve LDL goals; however, no clinical trial evidence has yet demonstrated that ezetimibe improves CHD outcomes.

As the mechanism by which elevated LDL levels promote atherogenesis probably involves oxidative modification, several trials have tested the possibility that antioxidant vitamin therapy might reduce CHD events. Rigorous and well-controlled clinical trials have failed to demonstrate that antioxidant vitamin therapy improves CHD outcomes. Therefore, the current evidence base does *not* support the use of antioxidant vitamins for this indication.

The clinical use of effective pharmacologic strategies for lowering LDL has reduced cardiovascular events markedly, but even their optimal utilization in clinical trials prevents only a minority of these endpoints. Hence, other aspects of the lipid profile have

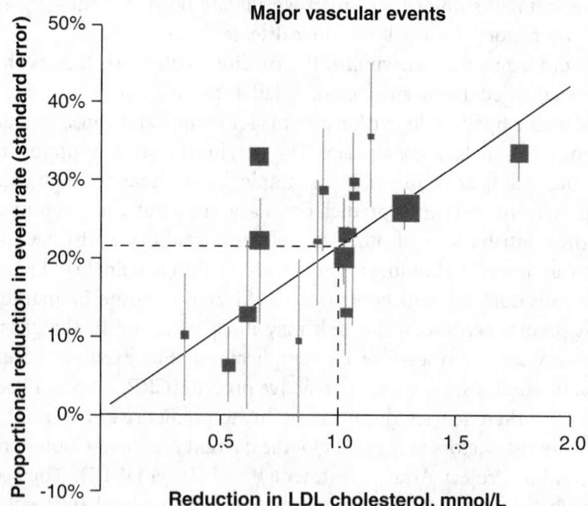

Figure 241-3 Lipid lowering reduces coronary events, as reflected on this graph showing the reduction in major cardiovascular events as a function of low-density lipoprotein level in a compendium of clinical trials with statins. *(Adapted from CTT Collaborators, Lancet 366:1267, 2005.)* The Management of Elevated Cholesterol in the Primary Prevention Group of Adult Japanese (MEGA), Treating to New Targets (TNT), and Incremental Decrease in Endpoints through Aggressive Lipid Lowering (IDEAL) studies have been added.

become tempting targets for addressing the residual burden of cardiovascular disease that persists despite aggressive LDL lowering. Indeed, in the "poststatin" era, patients with LDL levels at or below target not infrequently present with acute coronary syndromes. Low levels of HDL present a growing problem in patients with CAD as the prevalence of metabolic syndrome and diabetes increases. Blood HDL levels vary inversely with those of triglycerides, and the independent role of triglycerides as a cardiovascular risk factor remains unsettled. For these reasons, approaches to raising HDL have emerged as a prominent next hurdle in the management of dyslipidemia. Weight loss and physical activity can raise HDL. Nicotinic acid, particularly in combination with statins, can robustly raise HDL. Some clinical trial data support the effectiveness of nicotinic acid in cardiovascular risk reduction. However, flushing and pruritus remain a challenge to patient acceptance, even with improved dosage forms of nicotinic acid. A combination of nicotinic acid with an inhibitor of prostaglandin D receptor, a mediator of flushing, may limit this unwanted effect of nicotinic acid and is currently in clinical trials, but it has not received regulatory approval.

Agonists of nuclear receptors provide another potential avenue for raising HDL levels. Yet patients treated with peroxisome proliferator–activated receptors alpha and gamma (PPAR-α and -γ) agonists have not consistently shown improved cardiovascular outcomes, and at least some PPAR-agonists have been associated with worsened cardiovascular outcomes. Other agents in clinical development raise HDL levels by inhibiting cholesteryl ester transfer protein (CETP). The first of these agents to undergo large-scale clinical evaluation showed increased adverse events, leading to cessation of its development. Clinical studies currently underway will assess the effectiveness of other CETP inhibitors that lack some of the adverse off-target actions encountered with the first agent.

Hypertension

(See also Chap. 247) A wealth of epidemiologic data support a relationship between hypertension and atherosclerotic risk, and extensive clinical trial evidence has established that pharmacologic treatment of hypertension can reduce the risk of stroke, heart failure, and CHD events.

Diabetes mellitus, insulin resistance, and the metabolic syndrome

(See also Chap. 344) Most patients with diabetes mellitus die of atherosclerosis and its complications. Aging and rampant obesity underlie a current epidemic of type 2 diabetes mellitus. The abnormal lipoprotein profile associated with insulin resistance, known as *diabetic dyslipidemia*, accounts for part of the elevated cardiovascular risk in patients with type 2 diabetes. Although diabetic individuals often have LDL cholesterol levels near the average, the LDL particles tend to be smaller and denser and, therefore, more atherogenic. Other features of diabetic dyslipidemia include low HDL and elevated triglyceride levels. Hypertension also frequently accompanies obesity, insulin resistance, and dyslipidemia. Indeed, the ATP III guidelines now recognize this cluster of risk factors and provide criteria for diagnosis of the "metabolic syndrome" (Table 241-3). Despite legitimate concerns about whether clustered components confer more risk than an individual component, the metabolic syndrome concept may offer clinical utility.

Therapeutic objectives for intervention in these patients include addressing the underlying causes, including obesity and low physical activity, by initiating TLC. The ATP III guidelines provide an explicit step-by-step plan for implementing TLC, and treatment of the component risk factors should accompany TLC. Establishing that strict glycemic control reduces the risk of macrovascular

TABLE 241-3 Clinical Identification of the Metabolic Syndrome—Any Three Risk Factors

Risk Factor	Defining Level
Abdominal obesity[a]	
Men (waist circumference)[b]	>102 cm (>40 in.)
Women	>88 cm (>35 in.)
Triglycerides	>1.7 mmol/L (>150 mg/dL)
HDL cholesterol	
Men	<1 mmol/L (<40 mg/dL)
Women	<1.3 mmol/L (<50 mg/dL)
Blood pressure	≥130/≥85 mmHg
Fasting glucose	>6.1 mmol/L (>110 mg/dL)

[a]Overweight and obesity are associated with insulin resistance and the metabolic syndrome. However, the presence of abdominal obesity is more highly correlated with the metabolic risk factors than is an elevated body mass index (BMI). Therefore, the simple measure of waist circumference is recommended to identify the BMI component of the metabolic syndrome.

[b]Some male patients can develop multiple metabolic risk factors when the waist circumference is only marginally increased [e.g., 94–102 cm (37–39 in.)]. Such patients may have a strong genetic contribution to insulin resistance. They should benefit from lifestyle changes, similarly to men with categorical increases in waist circumference.

complications of diabetes has proved much more elusive than the established beneficial effects on microvascular complications such as retinopathy and renal disease. Indeed, "tight" glycemic control may increase adverse events in patients with type 2 diabetes, lending even greater importance to aggressive control of other aspects of risk in this patient population. In this regard, multiple clinical trials, including the Collaborative Atorvastatin Diabetes Study (CARDS) that addressed specifically the diabetic population, have demonstrated unequivocal benefit of HMG-CoA reductase inhibitor therapy in diabetic patients over all ranges of LDL cholesterol levels (but not those with end-stage renal disease). In view of the consistent benefit of statin treatment for diabetic populations and the thus far equivocal results with PPAR agonists, the current stance of the American Diabetic Association that statins be considered for persons with diabetes older than age 40 who have a total cholesterol level ≥135 appears amply justified. Among the oral hypoglycemic agents, metformin possesses the best evidence base for cardiovascular event reduction.

Diabetic populations appear to derive particular benefit from antihypertensive strategies that block the action of angiotensin II. Thus, the antihypertensive regimen for patients with the metabolic syndrome should include angiotensin converting-enzyme inhibitors or angiotensin receptor blockers when possible. Most of these individuals will require more than one antihypertensive agent to achieve the recently updated American Diabetes Association blood pressure goal of 130/80 mmHg.

Male sex/postmenopausal state

Decades of observational studies have verified excess coronary risk in men compared with premenopausal women. After menopause, however, coronary risk accelerates in women. At least part of the apparent protection against CHD in premenopausal women derives from their relatively higher HDL levels compared with those of men. After menopause, HDL values fall in concert with increased coronary risk. Estrogen therapy lowers LDL cholesterol and raises HDL cholesterol, changes that should decrease coronary risk.

Multiple observational and experimental studies have suggested that estrogen therapy reduces coronary risk. However, a spate of clinical trials has failed to demonstrate a net benefit of estrogen with or without progestins on CHD outcomes. In the Heart and Estrogen/Progestin Replacement Study (HERS), postmenopausal female survivors of acute MI were randomized to an estrogen/progestin combination or to placebo. This study showed no overall reduction in recurrent coronary events in the active treatment arm. Indeed, early in the 5-year course of this trial, there was a trend toward an actual increase in vascular events in the treated women. Extended follow-up of this cohort did not disclose an accrual of benefit in the treatment group. The Women's Health Initiative (WHI) study arm, using a similar estrogen plus progesterone regimen, was halted due to a small but significant hazard of cardiovascular events, stroke, and breast cancer. The estrogen without progestin arm of WHI (conducted in women without a uterus) was stopped early due to an increase in strokes, and failed to afford protection from MI or CHD death during observation over 7 years. The excess cardiovascular events in these trials may result from an increase in thromboembolism (Chap. 348). Physicians should work with women to provide information and help weigh the small but evident CHD risk of estrogen ± progestin versus the benefits for postmenopausal symptoms and osteoporosis, taking personal preferences into account. Post hoc analyses of observational studies suggest that estrogen therapy in women younger than or closer to menopause than the women enrolled in WHI might confer cardiovascular benefit. Thus, the timing in relation to menopause or the age at which estrogen therapy begins may influence its risk/benefit balance.

The lack of efficacy of estrogen therapy in cardiovascular risk reduction highlights the need for redoubled attention to known modifiable risk factors in women. The recent JUPITER trials randomized over 6000 women over age 65 without known cardiovascular disease with LDL <130 mg/dL and high-sensitivity (hs) CRP >2 mg/L to a statin or placebo. The statin-treated women had a striking reduction in cardiovascular events, as did the men. This trial, which included more women than any prior statin study, provides strong evidence supporting the efficacy of statins in women who meet those entry criteria.

Dysregulated coagulation or fibrinolysis

Thrombosis ultimately causes the gravest complications of atherosclerosis. The propensity to form thrombi and/or lyse clots once they form clearly influences the manifestations of atherosclerosis. Thrombosis provoked by atheroma rupture and subsequent healing may promote plaque growth. Certain individual characteristics can influence thrombosis or fibrinolysis and have received attention as potential coronary risk factors. For example, fibrinogen levels correlate with coronary risk and provide information about coronary risk independent of the lipoprotein profile.

The stability of an arterial thrombus depends on the balance between fibrinolytic factors such as plasmin, and inhibitors of the fibrinolytic system such as plasminogen activator inhibitor 1 (PAI-1). Individuals with diabetes mellitus or the metabolic syndrome have elevated levels of PAI-1 in plasma, and this probably contributes to the increased risk of thrombotic events. Lp(a) (Chap. 356) may modulate fibrinolysis, and individuals with elevated Lp(a) levels have increased CHD risk.

Aspirin reduces CHD events in several contexts. Chapter 243 discusses aspirin therapy in stable ischemic heart disease, Chap. 244 reviews recommendations for aspirin treatment in acute coronary syndromes, and Chap. 370 describes aspirin's role in preventing recurrent ischemic stroke. In primary prevention, pooled trial data show that low-dose aspirin treatment (81 mg/d to 325 mg on alternate days) can reduce the risk of a first MI in men. Although the recent Women's Health Study (WHS) showed that aspirin (100 mg on alternate days) reduced strokes by 17%, it did not prevent MI in women. Current American Heart Association (AHA) guidelines recommend the use of low-dose aspirin (75–160 mg/d) for women with high cardiovascular risk (≥20% 10-year risk), for men with a ≥10% 10-year risk of CHD, and for all aspirin-tolerant patients with established cardiovascular disease who lack contraindications.

Homocysteine

A large body of literature suggests a relationship between hyperhomocysteinemia and coronary events. Several mutations in the enzymes involved in homocysteine accumulation correlate with thrombosis and, in some studies, with coronary risk. Prospective studies have not shown a robust utility of hyperhomocysteinemia in CHD risk stratification. Clinical trials have not shown that intervention to lower homocysteine levels reduces CHD events. Fortification of the U.S. diet with folic acid to reduce neural tube defects has lowered homocysteine levels in the population at large. Measurement of homocysteine levels should be reserved for individuals with atherosclerosis at a young age or out of proportion to established risk factors. Physicians who advise consumption of supplements containing folic acid should consider that this treatment may mask pernicious anemia.

Inflammation

An accumulation of clinical evidence shows that markers of inflammation correlate with coronary risk. For example, plasma levels of CRP, as measured by a high-sensitivity assay (hsCRP), prospectively predict the risk of MI. CRP levels also correlate with the outcome in patients with acute coronary syndromes. In contrast to several other novel risk factors, CRP adds predictive information to that derived from established risk factors, such as those included in the Framingham score (Fig. 241-4). Recent Mendelian randomization studies do not support a causal role for CRP in cardiovascular disease. Thus, CRP serves as a validated biomarker of risk but probably not as a direct contributor to pathogenesis.

Elevations in acute-phase reactants such as fibrinogen and CRP reflect the overall inflammatory burden, not just vascular foci of inflammation. Visceral adipose tissue releases proinflammatory cytokines that drive CRP production and may represent a major extravascular stimulus to elevation of inflammatory markers in obese and overweight individuals. Indeed, CRP levels rise with body mass

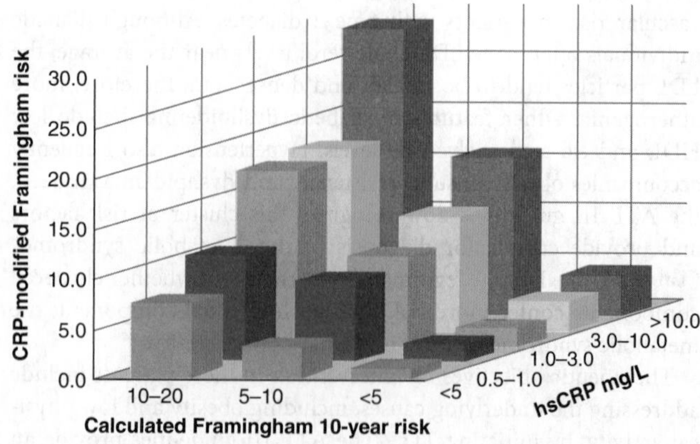

Figure 241-4 C-reactive protein (CRP) level adds to the predictive value of the Framingham score. hsCRP, high-sensitivity measurement of CRP. *(Adapted from PM Ridker et al: Circulation 109:2818, 2004.)*

Group	N	Rate
Placebo	7832	1.11
LDL ≥ 70 mg/dL, hsCRP ≥ 2 mg/L	1384	1.11
LDL < 70 mg/dL, hsCRP ≥ 2 mg/L	2921	0.62
LDL ≥ 70 mg/dL, hsCRP < 2 mg/L	726	0.54
LDL < 70 mg/dL, hsCRP < 2 mg/L	2685	0.38

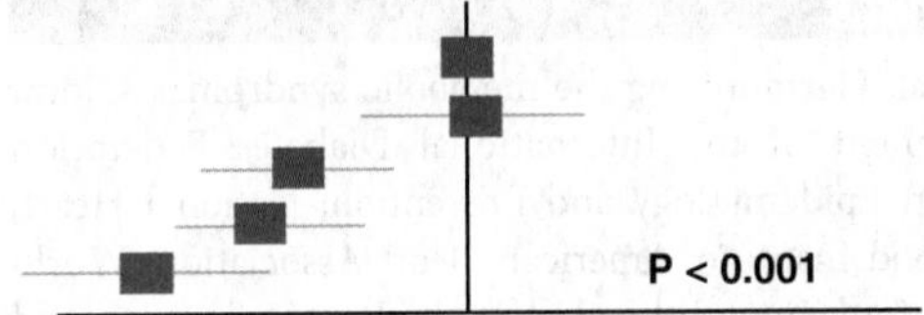

Figure 241-5 Evidence from the JUPITER study that both LDL-lowering and anti-inflammatory actions contribute to the benefit of statin therapy in primary prevention. See text for explanation. hsCRP, high-sensitivity measurement of C-reactive protein (CRP). *(Adapted from PM Ridker et al: Lancet 373:1175, 2009.)*

index (BMI), and weight reduction lowers CRP levels. Infectious agents might also furnish inflammatory stimuli related to cardiovascular risk. To date, randomized clinical trials have not supported the use of antibiotics to reduce CHD risk.

Intriguing evidence suggests that lipid-lowering therapy reduces coronary events in part by muting the inflammatory aspects of the pathogenesis of atherosclerosis. For example, in the JUPITER trial, a prespecified analysis showed that those who achieved lower levels of both LDL and CRP had better clinical outcomes than did those who only reached the lower level of either the inflammatory marker or the atherogenic lipoprotein (Fig. 241-5). Similar analyses of studies of statin treatment in patients after acute coronary syndromes showed the same pattern. The anti-inflammatory effect of statins appears independent of LDL lowering, as these two variables correlated very poorly in individual subjects in multiple clinical trials.

Lifestyle modification

The prevention of atherosclerosis presents a long-term challenge to all health care professionals and for public health policy. Both individual practitioners and organizations providing health care should strive to help patients optimize their risk factor profiles long before atherosclerotic disease becomes manifest. The current accumulation of cardiovascular risk in youth and in certain minority populations presents a particularly vexing concern from a public health perspective.

The care plan for all patients seen by internists should include measures to assess and minimize cardiovascular risk. Physicians must counsel patients about the health risks of tobacco use and provide guidance and resources regarding smoking cessation. Similarly, physicians should advise all patients about prudent dietary and physical activity habits for maintaining ideal body weight. Both National Institutes of Health (NIH) and AHA statements recommend at least 30 minutes of moderate-intensity physical activity per day. Obesity, particularly the male pattern of centripetal or visceral fat accumulation, can contribute to the elements of the metabolic syndrome (Table 241-3). Physicians should encourage their patients to take personal responsibility for behavior related to modifiable risk factors for the development of premature atherosclerotic disease. Conscientious counseling and patient education may forestall the need for pharmacologic measures intended to reduce coronary risk.

Issues in risk assessment

A growing panel of markers of coronary risk presents a perplexing array to the practitioner. Markers measured in peripheral blood include size fractions of LDL particles and concentrations of homocysteine, Lp(a), fibrinogen, CRP, PAI-1, myeloperoxidase, and lipoprotein-associated phospholipase A_2, among many others. In general, such specialized tests add little to the information available from a careful history and physical examination combined with measurement of a plasma lipoprotein profile and fasting blood glucose. The high-sensitivity CRP measurement may well prove an exception in view of its robustness in risk prediction, ease of reproducible and standardized measurement, relative stability in individuals over time, and, most important, ability to add to the risk information disclosed by standard measurements such as the components of the Framingham risk score (Fig. 241-4). The addition of information regarding a family history of premature atherosclerosis in parents (a simply obtained indicator of genetic susceptibility), together with the marker of inflammation hsCRP, permits correct reclassification of risk in individuals—especially those whose Framingham scores place them at intermediate risk. Current advisories, however, recommend the use of the hsCRP test only in individuals in this CHD event risk group (10–20%, 10-year risk).

Available data do not support the use of imaging studies to screen for subclinical disease (e.g., measurement of carotid-intima/media thickness, coronary artery calcification, and use of computed tomographic coronary angiograms). Inappropriate use of such imaging modalities may promote excessive alarm in asymptomatic individuals and prompt invasive diagnostic and therapeutic procedures of unproven value. Widespread application of such modalities for screening should await proof that clinical benefit derives from their application.

Progress in human genetics holds considerable promise for risk prediction and for individualization of cardiovascular therapy. Many reports have identified single-nucleotide polymorphisms (SNPs) in candidate genes as predictors of cardiovascular risk. To date, the validation of such genetic markers of risk and drug responsiveness in multiple populations has often proved disappointing. The advent of technology that permits relatively rapid and inexpensive genome-wide screens, in contrast to most SNP studies, has led to identification of sites of genetic variation that do reproducibly indicate heightened cardiovascular risk (e.g., chromosome 9p21). The results of genetic studies should identify new potential therapeutic targets (e.g., the enzyme mutated in autosomal dominant hypercholesterolemia, abbreviated *PCSK9*) and may lead to genetic tests that help refine cardiovascular risk assessment in the future.

■ THE CHALLENGE OF IMPLEMENTATION: CHANGING PHYSICIAN AND PATIENT BEHAVIOR

Despite declining age-adjusted rates of coronary death, cardiovascular mortality worldwide is rising due to the aging of the population, and the subsiding of communicable diseases and increased prevalence of risk factors in developing countries. Enormous challenges remain regarding translation of the current evidence base into practice. Physicians must learn how to help individuals adopt a healthy lifestyle in a culturally appropriate manner and to deploy their increasingly powerful pharmacologic tools most economically and effectively. The obstacles to implementation of current evidence-based prevention and treatment of atherosclerosis involve economics, education, physician awareness, and patient adherence to recommended regimens. Future goals in the treatment of atherosclerosis should include more widespread implementation of the current evidence-based guidelines regarding risk factor management and, when appropriate, drug therapy.

FURTHER READINGS

ALBERTI KG et al: Harmonizing the metabolic syndrome: A joint interim statement of the International Diabetes Federation Task Force on Epidemiology and Prevention; National Heart, Lung, and Blood Institute; American Heart Association; World Heart Federation; International Atherosclerosis Society; and International Association for the Study of Obesity. Circulation 120:1640, 2009

D'AGOSTINO RB et al: General cardiovascular risk profile for use in primary care: The Framingham Heart Study. Circulation 117:743, 2008

DELAHOY PJ et al: The relationship between reduction in low-density lipoprotein cholesterol by statins and reduction in risk of cardiovascular outcomes: An updated meta-analysis. Clin Ther 31:236, 2009

HAMSTEN A, ERIKSSON P: Identifying the susceptibility genes for coronary artery disease: From hyperbole through doubt to cautious optimism. J Intern Med 263:538, 2008

LIBBY P et al: Inflammation in atherosclerosis: From pathophysiology to practice. J Am Coll Cardiol 54:2129, 2009

MOSCA L et al: Evidence-based guidelines for cardiovascular disease prevention in women: 2007 update. Circulation 115:1481, 2007

RIDKER PM et al: C-reactive protein and parental history improve global cardiovascular risk prediction: The Reynolds Risk Score for men. Circulation 118:2243, 2008

SHAO B, HEINECKE JW: HDL, lipid peroxidation, and atherosclerosis. J Lipid Res 50:599, 2009

CHAPTER 242
The Metabolic Syndrome

Robert H. Eckel

The metabolic syndrome (syndrome X, insulin resistance syndrome) consists of a constellation of metabolic abnormalities that confer increased risk of cardiovascular disease (CVD) and diabetes mellitus (DM). The criteria for the metabolic syndrome have evolved since the original definition by the World Health Organization in 1998, reflecting growing clinical evidence and analysis by a variety of consensus conferences and professional organizations. The major features of the metabolic syndrome include central obesity, hypertriglyceridemia, low high-density lipoprotein (HDL) cholesterol, hyperglycemia, and hypertension (Table 242-1).

EPIDEMIOLOGY

The prevalence of metabolic syndrome varies around the world, in part reflecting the age and ethnicity of the populations studied and the diagnostic criteria applied. In general, the prevalence of metabolic syndrome increases with age. The highest recorded prevalence worldwide is in Native Americans, with nearly 60% of women ages 45–49 and 45% of men ages 45–49 meeting National Cholesterol Education Program and Adult Treatment Panel III (NCEP:ATPIII) criteria. In the United States, metabolic syndrome is less common in African-American men and more common in Mexican-American women. Based on data from the National Health and Nutrition Examination Survey (NHANES) 1999–2000, the age-adjusted prevalence of the metabolic syndrome in United States adults who did not have diabetes is 28% for men and 30% for women. In France, a cohort 30 to 60 years old has shown a <10% prevalence for each sex, although 17.5% are affected in the age range 60–64. Greater industrialization worldwide is associated with rising rates of obesity, which is anticipated to increase prevalence of

TABLE 242-1 NCEP:ATPIII 2001 and IDF Criteria for the Metabolic Syndrome

NCEP:ATPIII 2001	IDF Criteria for Central Adiposity[a]		
Three or more of the following:	**Waist circumference**		
Central obesity: Waist circumference >102 cm (M), >88 cm (F)	Men	Women	Ethnicity
Hypertriglyceridemia: Triglycerides ≥150 mg/dL or specific medication	≥94 cm	≥80 cm	Europid, Sub-Saharan African, Eastern and Middle Eastern
Low HDL cholesterol: <40 mg/dL and <50 mg/dL, respectively, or specific medication	≥90 cm	≥80 cm	South Asian, Chinese, and ethnic South and Central American
Hypertension: Blood pressure ≥130 mm systolic or ≥85 mm diastolic or specific medication	≥85 cm	≥90 cm	Japanese
Fasting plasma glucose ≥100 mg/dL or specific medication or previously diagnosed Type 2 diabetes	**Two or more of the following:**		
	Fasting triglycerides >150 mg/dL or specific medication		
	HDL cholesterol <40 mg/dL and <50 mg/dL for men and women, respectively, or specific medication		
	Blood pressure >130 mm systolic or >85 mm diastolic or previous diagnosis or specific medication		
	Fasting plasma glucose ≥100 mg/dL or previously diagnosed Type 2 diabetes		

[a]In this analysis, the following thresholds for waist circumference were used: white men, ≥94 cm; African-American men, ≥94 cm; Mexican-American men, ≥90 cm; white women, ≥80 cm; African-American women, ≥80 cm; Mexican-American women, ≥80 cm. For participants whose designation was "other race—including multiracial," thresholds that were once based on Europid cut points (≥94 cm for men and ≥80 cm for women) and once based on South Asian cut points (≥90 cm for men and ≥80 cm for women) were used. For participants who were considered "other Hispanic," the IDF thresholds for ethnic South and Central Americans were used.

Abbreviations: HDL, high-density lipoprotein; IDF, International Diabetes Foundation; NCEP:ATPIII, National Cholesterol Education Program, Adult Treatment Panel III.

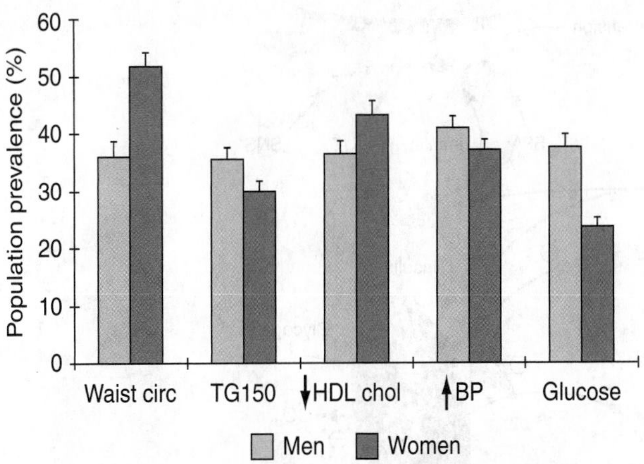

Figure 242-1 Prevalence of the metabolic syndrome components, from NHANES III. NHANES, National Health and Nutrition Examination Survey; TG, triglyceride; HDL, high-density lipoprotein; BP, blood pressure. The prevalence of elevated glucose includes individuals with known diabetes mellitus. *(Created from data in ES Ford et al: Diabetes Care 27:2444, 2004.)*

the metabolic syndrome dramatically, especially as the population ages. Moreover, the rising prevalence and severity of obesity in children is initiating features of the metabolic syndrome in a younger population.

The frequency distribution of the five components of the syndrome for the U.S. population (NHANES III) is summarized in Fig. 242-1. Increases in waist circumference predominate in women, whereas fasting triglycerides >150 mg/dL and hypertension are more likely in men.

RISK FACTORS

Overweight/obesity

Although the first description of the metabolic syndrome occurred in the early twentieth century, the worldwide overweight/obesity epidemic has been the driving force for more recent recognition of the syndrome. Central adiposity is a key feature of the syndrome, reflecting the fact that the syndrome's prevalence is driven by the strong relationship between waist circumference and increasing adiposity. However, despite the importance of obesity, patients who are normal weight may also be insulin-resistant and have the syndrome.

Sedentary lifestyle

Physical inactivity is a predictor of CVD events and related mortality rate. Many components of the metabolic syndrome are associated with a sedentary lifestyle, including increased adipose tissue (predominantly central), reduced HDL cholesterol, and a trend toward increased triglycerides, high blood pressure, and increased glucose in the genetically susceptible. Compared with individuals who watched television or videos or used the computer <1 h daily, those who carried out those behaviors for >4 h daily had a twofold increased risk of the metabolic syndrome.

Aging

The metabolic syndrome affects 44% of the U.S. population older than age 50. A greater percentage of women over age 50 have the syndrome than men. The age dependency of the syndrome's prevalence is seen in most populations around the world.

Diabetes mellitus

DM is included in both the NCEP and International Diabetes Foundation (IDF) definitions of the metabolic syndrome. It is estimated that the great majority (~75%) of patients with Type 2 diabetes or impaired glucose tolerance (IGT) have the metabolic syndrome. The presence of the metabolic syndrome in these populations relates to a higher prevalence of CVD compared with patients with Type 2 diabetes or IGT without the syndrome.

Coronary heart disease

The approximate prevalence of the metabolic syndrome in patients with coronary heart disease (CHD) is 50%, with a prevalence of 37% in patients with premature coronary artery disease (≤age 45), particularly in women. With appropriate cardiac rehabilitation and changes in lifestyle (e.g., nutrition, physical activity, weight reduction, and, in some cases, pharmacologic agents), the prevalence of the syndrome can be reduced.

Lipodystrophy

Lipodystrophic disorders in general are associated with the metabolic syndrome. Both genetic (e.g., Berardinelli-Seip congenital lipodystrophy, Dunnigan familial partial lipodystrophy) and acquired (e.g., HIV-related lipodystrophy in patients treated with highly active antiretroviral therapy) forms of lipodystrophy may give rise to severe insulin resistance and many of the components of the metabolic syndrome.

ETIOLOGY

Insulin resistance

The most accepted and unifying hypothesis to describe the pathophysiology of the metabolic syndrome is insulin resistance, which is caused by an incompletely understood defect in insulin action (Chap. 344). The onset of insulin resistance is heralded by postprandial hyperinsulinemia, followed by fasting hyperinsulinemia and, ultimately, hyperglycemia.

An early major contributor to the development of insulin resistance is an overabundance of circulating fatty acids (Fig. 242-2). Plasma albumin-bound free fatty acids (FFAs) are derived predominantly from adipose tissue triglyceride stores released by lipolytic enzymes lipase. Fatty acids are also derived from the lipolysis of triglyceride-rich lipoproteins in tissues by lipoprotein lipase (LPL). Insulin mediates both antilipolysis and the stimulation of LPL in adipose tissue. Of note, the inhibition of lipolysis in adipose tissue is the most sensitive pathway of insulin action. Thus, when insulin resistance develops, increased lipolysis produces more fatty acids, which further decrease the antilipolytic effect of insulin. Excessive fatty acids enhance substrate availability and create insulin resistance by modifying downstream signaling. Fatty acids impair insulin-mediated glucose uptake and accumulate as triglycerides in both skeletal and cardiac muscle, whereas increased glucose production and triglyceride accumulation are seen in liver.

The oxidative stress hypothesis provides a unifying theory for aging and the predisposition to the metabolic syndrome. In studies carried out in insulin-resistant subjects with obesity or Type 2 diabetes, the offspring of patients with Type 2 diabetes, and the elderly, a defect has been identified in mitochondrial oxidative phosphorylation, leading to the accumulation of triglycerides and related lipid molecules in muscle. The accumulation of lipids in muscle is associated with insulin resistance.

Increased waist circumference

Waist circumference is an important component of the most recent and frequently applied diagnostic criteria for the metabolic syndrome. However, measuring waist circumference does not reliably distinguish increases in subcutaneous adipose tissue vs. visceral

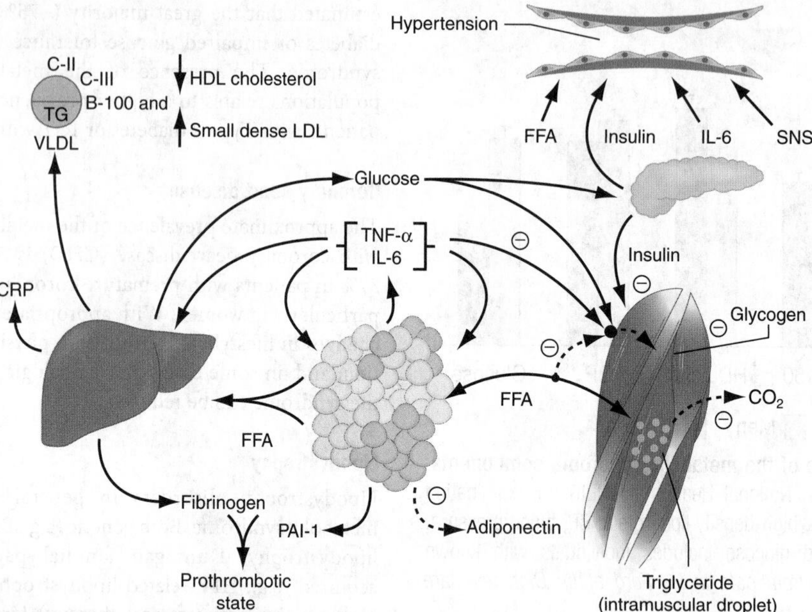

Figure 242-2 Pathophysiology of the metabolic syndrome. Free fatty acids (FFAs) are released in abundance from an expanded adipose tissue mass. In the liver, FFAs result in an increased production of glucose and triglycerides and secretion of very low density lipoproteins (VLDLs). Associated lipid/lipoprotein abnormalities include reductions in high-density lipoprotein (HDL) cholesterol and an increased density of low-density lipoproteins (LDLs). FFAs also reduce insulin sensitivity in muscle by inhibiting insulin-mediated glucose uptake. Associated defects include a reduction in glucose partitioning to glycogen and increased lipid accumulation in triglyceride (TG). Increases in circulating glucose, and to some extent FFA, increase pancreatic insulin secretion, resulting in hyperinsulinemia. Hyperinsulinemia may result in enhanced sodium reabsorption and increased sympathetic nervous system (SNS) activity and contribute to the hypertension, as might increased levels of circulating FFAs. The proinflammatory state is superimposed and contributory to the insulin resistance produced by excessive FFAs. The enhanced secretion of interleukin 6 (IL-6) and tumor necrosis factor α (TNF-α) produced by adipocytes and monocyte-derived macrophages results in more insulin resistance and lipolysis of adipose tissue triglyceride stores to circulating FFAs. IL-6 and other cytokines also enhance hepatic glucose production, VLDL production by the liver, and insulin resistance in muscle. Cytokines and FFAs also increase the hepatic production of fibrinogen and adipocyte production of plasminogen activator inhibitor 1 (PAI-1), resulting in a prothrombotic state. Higher levels of circulating cytokines also stimulate the hepatic production of C-reactive protein (CRP). Reduced production of the anti-inflammatory and insulin-sensitizing cytokine adiponectin is also associated with the metabolic syndrome. *(Reprinted from Eckel et al., with permission from Elsevier.)*

fat; this distinction requires CT or MRI. With increases in visceral adipose tissue, adipose tissue-derived FFAs are directed to the liver. In contrast, increases in abdominal subcutaneous fat release lipolysis products into the systemic circulation and avoid more direct effects on hepatic metabolism. Relative increases in visceral versus subcutaneous adipose tissue with increasing waist circumference in Asians and Asian Indians may explain the greater prevalence of the syndrome in those populations compared with African-American men in whom subcutaneous fat predominates. It is also possible that visceral fat is a marker for, but not the source of, excess postprandial FFAs in obesity.

Dyslipidemia

(See also Chap. 356) In general, FFA flux to the liver is associated with increased production of apoB-containing, triglyceride-rich very low density lipoproteins (VLDLs). The effect of insulin on this process is complex, but *hypertriglyceridemia* is an excellent marker of the insulin-resistant condition.

The other major lipoprotein disturbance in the metabolic syndrome is a *reduction in HDL cholesterol.* This reduction is a consequence of changes in HDL composition and metabolism. In the presence of hypertriglyceridemia, a decrease in the cholesterol content of HDL is a consequence of reduced cholesteryl ester content of the lipoprotein core in combination with cholesteryl ester transfer protein–mediated alterations in triglyceride, making the particle small and dense. This change in lipoprotein composition also results in increased clearance of HDL from the circulation. The relationships of these changes in HDL to insulin resistance are probably indirect, occurring in concert with the changes in triglyceride-rich lipoprotein metabolism.

In addition to HDL, low-density lipoproteins (LDLs) are modified in composition. With fasting serum triglycerides >2.0 mM (~180 mg/dL), there is almost always a predominance of small dense LDLs. Small dense LDLs are thought to be more atherogenic. They may be toxic to the endothelium, and they are able to transit through the endothelial basement membrane and adhere to glycosaminoglycans. They also have increased susceptibility to oxidation and are selectively bound to scavenger receptors on monocyte-derived macrophages. Subjects with increased small dense LDL particles and hypertriglyceridemia also have increased cholesterol content of both VLDL1 and VLDL2 subfractions. This relatively cholesterol-rich VLDL particle may contribute to the atherogenic risk in patients with metabolic syndrome.

Glucose intolerance

(See also Chap. 344) The defects in insulin action lead to impaired suppression of glucose production by the liver and kidney and reduced glucose uptake and metabolism in insulin-sensitive tissues, i.e., muscle and adipose tissue. The relationship between impaired fasting glucose (IFG) or impaired glucose tolerance (IGT) and insulin resistance is well supported by human, nonhuman primate, and rodent studies. To compensate for defects in insulin action, insulin secretion and/or clearance must be modified to sustain euglycemia. Ultimately, this compensatory mechanism fails, usually because of defects in insulin secretion, resulting in progress from IFG and/or IGT to DM.

Hypertension

The relationship between insulin resistance and hypertension is well established. Paradoxically, under normal physiologic conditions, insulin is a vasodilator with secondary effects on sodium reabsorption in the kidney. However, in the setting of insulin resistance, the vasodilatory effect of insulin is lost but the renal effect on sodium reabsorption is preserved. Sodium reabsorption is increased in whites with the metabolic syndrome but not in Africans or Asians. Insulin also increases the activity of the sympathetic nervous system, an effect that also may be preserved in the setting of the insulin resistance. Finally, insulin resistance is characterized by pathway-specific impairment in phosphatidylinositol-3-kinase signaling. In the endothelium, this may cause an imbalance between the production of nitric oxide and the secretion of endothelin 1, leading to decreased blood flow. Although these mechanisms are provocative, when insulin action is assessed by levels of fasting insulin or by the Homeostasis Model Assessment (HOMA), insulin resistance contributes only modestly to the increased prevalence of hypertension in the metabolic syndrome.

Proinflammatory cytokines

The increases in proinflammatory cytokines, including interleukin (IL)-1, IL-6, IL-18, resistin, tumor necrosis factor (TNF) α, and C-reactive protein (CRP), reflect overproduction by the expanded adipose tissue mass (Fig. 242-2). Adipose tissue-derived macrophages may be the primary source of proinflammatory cytokines locally and in the systemic circulation. It remains unclear, however, how much of the insulin resistance is caused by the paracrine vs. endocrine effects of these cytokines.

Adiponectin

Adiponectin is an anti-inflammatory cytokine produced exclusively by adipocytes. Adiponectin enhances insulin sensitivity and inhibits many steps in the inflammatory process. In the liver, adiponectin inhibits the expression of gluconeogenic enzymes and the rate of glucose production. In muscle, adiponectin increases glucose transport and enhances fatty acid oxidation, partially due to activation of adenosine monophosphate (AMP) kinase. Adiponectin is reduced in the metabolic syndrome. The relative contribution of adiponectin deficiency versus overabundance of the proinflammatory cytokines is unclear.

■ CLINICAL FEATURES

Symptoms and signs

The metabolic syndrome is typically not associated with symptoms. On physical examination, waist circumference may be expanded and blood pressure elevated. The presence of one or either of these signs should alert the clinician to search for other biochemical abnormalities that may be associated with the metabolic syndrome. Less frequently, lipoatrophy or acanthosis nigricans is found on examination. Because these physical findings typically are associated with severe insulin resistance, other components of the metabolic syndrome should be expected.

Associated diseases

Cardiovascular disease The relative risk for new-onset CVD in patients with the metabolic syndrome, in the absence of diabetes, averages between 1.5-fold and threefold. However, in an 8-year follow-up of middle-aged men and women in the Framingham Offspring Study (FOS), the population-attributable risk for patients with the metabolic syndrome to develop CVD was 34% in men and only 16% in women. In the same study, both the metabolic syndrome and diabetes predicted ischemic stroke, with greater risk for patients with the metabolic syndrome than for those with diabetes alone (19% vs. 7%), particularly in women (27% vs. 5%). Patients with metabolic syndrome are also at increased risk for peripheral vascular disease.

Type 2 diabetes Overall, the risk for Type 2 diabetes in patients with the metabolic syndrome is increased three- to fivefold. In the FOS's 8-year follow-up of middle-aged men and women, the population-attributable risk for developing Type 2 diabetes was 62% in men and 47% in women.

Other associated conditions

In addition to the features specifically associated with metabolic syndrome, insulin resistance is accompanied by other metabolic alterations. Those alterations include increases in apoB and apoC-III, uric acid, prothrombotic factors (fibrinogen, plasminogen activator inhibitor 1), serum viscosity, asymmetric dimethylarginine, homocysteine, white blood cell count, proinflammatory cytokines, CRP, microalbuminuria, nonalcoholic fatty liver disease (NAFLD) and/or nonalcoholic steatohepatitis (NASH), polycystic ovarian disease (PCOS), and obstructive sleep apnea (OSA).

Nonalcoholic fatty liver disease (See also Chap. 309) Fatty liver is relatively common. However, in NASH, both triglyceride accumulation and inflammation coexist. NASH is now present in 2–3% of the population in the United States and other Western countries. As the prevalence of overweight/obesity and the metabolic syndrome increases, NASH may become one of the more common causes of end-stage liver disease and hepatocellular carcinoma.

Hyperuricemia (See also Chap. 359) Hyperuricemia reflects defects in insulin action on the renal tubular reabsorption of uric acid, whereas the increase in asymmetric dimethylarginine, an endogenous inhibitor of nitric oxide synthase, relates to endothelial dysfunction. Microalbuminuria also may be caused by altered endothelial pathophysiology in the insulin-resistant state.

Polycystic ovary syndrome (See also Chap. 347) PCOS is highly associated with the metabolic syndrome, with a prevalence between 40 and 50%. Women with PCOS are 2–4 times more likely to have the metabolic syndrome than are women without PCOS.

Obstructive sleep apnea (See also Chap. 27) OSA is commonly associated with obesity, hypertension, increased circulating cytokines, IGT, and insulin resistance. With these associations, it is not surprising that the metabolic syndrome is frequently present. Moreover, when biomarkers of insulin resistance are compared between patients with OSA and weight-matched controls, insulin resistance is more severe in patients with OSA. Continuous positive airway pressure (CPAP) treatment in OSA patients improves insulin sensitivity.

■ DIAGNOSIS

The diagnosis of the metabolic syndrome relies on satisfying the criteria listed in Table 242-1 by using tools at the bedside and in the laboratory. The medical history should include evaluation of symptoms for OSA in all patients and PCOS in premenopausal women. Family history will help determine risk for CVD and DM. Blood pressure and waist circumference measurements provide information necessary for the diagnosis.

Laboratory tests

Fasting lipids and glucose are needed to determine if the metabolic syndrome is present. The measurement of additional biomarkers associated with insulin resistance can be individualized. Such tests might include apoB, high-sensitivity CRP, fibrinogen, uric acid, urinary microalbumin, and liver function tests. A sleep study should be performed if symptoms of OSA are present. If PCOS is suspected on the basis of clinical features and anovulation, testosterone, luteinizing hormone, and follicle-stimulating hormone should be measured.

TREATMENT The Metabolic Syndrome

LIFESTYLE (See also Chap. 78) Obesity is the driving force behind the metabolic syndrome. Thus, weight reduction is the primary approach to the disorder. With weight reduction, the improvement in insulin sensitivity is often accompanied by favorable modifications in many components of the metabolic syndrome. In general, recommendations for weight loss include a combination of caloric restriction, increased physical activity, and behavior modification. For weight reduction, caloric restriction is the most important component, whereas increases in physical activity are important for maintenance of weight loss. Some, but not all, evidence suggests that the addition of exercise to caloric restriction may promote relatively greater weight loss from the visceral depot. The tendency for weight regain after successful weight reduction underscores the need for long-lasting behavioral changes.

Diet Before prescribing a weight-loss diet, it is important to emphasize that it takes a long time for a patient to achieve an expanded fat mass; thus, the correction need not occur quickly. On the basis of ~3500 kcal = 1 lb of fat, ~500 kcal restriction daily equates to weight reduction of 1 lb per week. Diets restricted in carbohydrate typically provide a rapid initial weight loss. However, after 1 year, the amount of weight reduction is usually unchanged. Thus, adherence to the diet is more important than which diet is chosen. Moreover, there is concern about diets enriched in saturated fat, particularly for patients at risk for CVD. Therefore, a high-quality diet—i.e., enriched in fruits, vegetables, whole grains, lean poultry, and fish—should be encouraged to provide the maximum overall health benefit.

Physical Activity Before a physical activity recommendation is provided to patients with the metabolic syndrome, it is important to ensure that the increased activity does not incur risk. Some high-risk patients should undergo formal cardiovascular evaluation before initiating an exercise program. For an inactive participant, gradual increases in physical activity should be encouraged to enhance adherence and avoid injury. Although increases in physical activity can lead to modest weight reduction, 60–90 min of daily activity is required to achieve this goal. Even if an overweight or obese adult is unable to achieve this level of activity, he or she will still derive a significant health benefit from at least 30 min of moderate-intensity daily activity. The caloric value of 30 min of a variety of activities can be found at *http://www.americanheart.org/presenter.jhtml?identifier=3040364*. Of note, a variety of routine activities, such as gardening, walking, and housecleaning, require moderate caloric expenditure. Thus, physical activity need not be defined solely in terms of formal exercise such as jogging, swimming, or tennis.

Obesity (See also Chap. 78) In some patients with the metabolic syndrome, treatment options need to extend beyond lifestyle intervention. Weight-loss drugs come in two major classes: appetite suppressants and absorption inhibitors. Appetite suppressants approved by the U.S. Food and Drug Administration include phentermine (for short-term use only, 3 months) and sibutramine. Orlistat inhibits fat absorption by ~30% and is moderately effective compared to placebo (~5% weight loss). Orlistat has been shown to reduce the incidence of Type 2 diabetes, an effect that was especially evident in patients with baseline IGT.

Bariatric surgery is an option for patients with the metabolic syndrome who have a body mass index (BMI) >40 kg/m^2 or >35 kg/m^2 with comorbidities. Gastric bypass results in a dramatic weight reduction and improvement in the features of metabolic syndrome. A survival benefit has also been realized.

LDL CHOLESTEROL (See also Chap. 356) The rationale for the NCEP:ATPIII panel to develop criteria for the metabolic syndrome was to go beyond LDL cholesterol in identifying and reducing risk for CVD. The working assumption by the panel was that LDL cholesterol goals had already been achieved, and increasing evidence supports a linear reduction in CVD events with progressive lowering of LDL cholesterol. For patients with the metabolic syndrome and diabetes, LDL cholesterol should be reduced to <100 mg/dL and perhaps further in patients with a history of CVD events. For patients with the metabolic syndrome without diabetes, the Framingham risk score may predict a 10-year CVD risk that exceeds 20%. In these subjects, LDL cholesterol should also be reduced to <100 mg/dL. With a 10-year risk of <20%, however, the targeted LDL cholesterol goal is <130 mg/dL.

Diets restricted in saturated fats (<7% of calories), *trans*-fats (as few as possible), and cholesterol (<200 mg daily) should be applied aggressively. If LDL cholesterol remains above goal, pharmacologic intervention is needed. Statins (HMG-CoA reductase inhibitors), which produce a 20–60% lowering of LDL cholesterol, are generally the first choice for medication intervention. Of note, for each doubling of the statin dose, there is only ~6% additional lowering of LDL cholesterol. Side effects are rare and include an increase in hepatic transaminases and/or myopathy. The cholesterol absorption inhibitor ezetimibe is well tolerated and should be the second choice. Ezetimibe typically reduces LDL cholesterol by 15–20%. The bile acid sequestrants cholestyramine and colestipol are more effective than ezetimibe but must be used with caution in patients with the metabolic syndrome because they can increase triglycerides. In general, bile sequestrants should not be administered when fasting triglycerides are >200 mg/dL. Side effects include gastrointestinal symptoms (palatability, bloating, belching, constipation, anal irritation). Nicotinic acid has modest LDL cholesterol–lowering capabilities (<20%). Fibrates are best employed to lower LDL cholesterol when both LDL cholesterol and triglycerides are elevated. Fenofibrate may be more effective than gemfibrozil in this group.

TRIGLYCERIDES The NCEP:ATPIII has focused on non-HDL cholesterol rather than triglycerides. However, a fasting triglyceride value of <150 mg/dL is recommended. In general, the response of fasting triglycerides relates to the amount of weight reduction achieved. A weight reduction of >10% is necessary to lower fasting triglycerides.

A fibrate (gemfibrozil or fenofibrate) is the drug of choice to lower fasting triglycerides and typically achieve a 35–50% reduction. Concomitant administration with drugs metabolized by the 3A4 cytochrome P450 system (including some statins) greatly increases the risk of myopathy. In these cases, fenofibrate may be preferable to gemfibrozil. In the Veterans Affairs HDL Intervention Trial (VA-HIT), gemfibrozil was administered to men with known CHD and levels of HDL cholesterol <40 mg/dL. A coronary disease event and mortality rate benefit was experienced predominantly in men with hyperinsulinemia and/or diabetes, many of whom retrospectively were identified as having the metabolic syndrome. Of note, the amount of triglyceride lowering in the VA-HIT did not predict benefit. Although levels of LDL cholesterol did not change, a decrease in LDL particle number correlated with benefit. Although several additional clinical trials have been performed, they have not shown clear evidence that fibrates reduce CVD risk as a consequence of triglyceride lowering.

Other drugs that lower triglycerides include statins, nicotinic acid, and high doses of omega-3 fatty acids. In choosing a statin for this purpose, the dose must be high for the "less potent" statins (lovastatin, pravastatin, fluvastatin) or intermediate for the "more potent" statins (simvastatin, atorvastatin, rosuvastatin). The effect of nicotinic acid on fasting triglycerides is dose-related and less than that of fibrates (~20–40%). In patients with the metabolic syndrome and diabetes, nicotinic acid may increase fasting glucose. Omega-3 fatty acid preparations that include high doses of docosahexaenoic acid and eicosapentaenoic acid (~3.0–4.5 g daily) lower fasting triglycerides by ~40%. No interactions with fibrates or statins occur, and the main side effect is eructation with a fishy taste. This can be partially blocked by ingestion of the nutraceutical after freezing. Clinical trials of nicotinic acid or high-dose omega-3 fatty acids in patients with the metabolic syndrome have not been reported.

HDL CHOLESTEROL Beyond weight reduction, there are very few lipid-modifying compounds that increase HDL cholesterol. Statins, fibrates, and bile acid sequestrants have modest effects (5–10%), and there is no effect on HDL cholesterol with ezetimibe or omega-3 fatty acids. Nicotinic acid is the only currently available drug with predictable HDL cholesterol-raising properties. The response is dose-related and can increase HDL cholesterol ~30% above baseline. There is limited evidence at present that raising HDL has a benefit on CVD events independent of lowering LDL cholesterol, particularly in patients with the metabolic syndrome.

BLOOD PRESSURE (See also Chap. 247) The direct relationship between blood pressure and all-cause mortality rate has been well established, including patients with hypertension (>140/90) versus prehypertension (>120/80 but <140/90) versus individuals with normal blood pressure (<120/80). In patients with the metabolic syndrome without diabetes, the best choice for the first antihypertensive should usually be an angiotensin-converting enzyme (ACE) inhibitor or an angiotensin II receptor blocker, as these two classes of drugs appear to reduce the incidence of new-onset Type 2 diabetes. In all patients with hypertension, a sodium-restricted diet enriched in fruits and vegetables and low-fat dairy products should be advocated. Home monitoring of blood pressure may assist in maintaining good blood pressure control.

IMPAIRED FASTING GLUCOSE (See also Chap. 344) In patients with the metabolic syndrome and Type 2 diabetes, aggressive glycemic control may favorably modify fasting triglycerides and/or HDL cholesterol. In patients with IFG without a diagnosis of diabetes, a lifestyle intervention that includes weight reduction, dietary fat restriction, and increased physical activity has been shown to reduce the incidence of Type 2 diabetes. Metformin has also been shown to reduce the incidence of diabetes, although the effect was less than that seen with lifestyle intervention.

INSULIN RESISTANCE (See also Chap. 344) Several drug classes [biguanides, thiazolidinediones (TZDs)] increase insulin sensitivity. Because insulin resistance is the primary pathophysiologic mechanism for the metabolic syndrome, representative drugs in these classes reduce its prevalence. Both metformin and TZDs enhance insulin action in the liver and suppress endogenous glucose production. TZDs, but not metformin, also improve insulin-mediated glucose uptake in muscle and adipose tissue. Benefits of both drugs have also been seen in patients with NAFLD and PCOS, and the drugs have been shown to reduce markers of inflammation and small dense LDL.

FURTHER READINGS

Alberti KG et al: Harmonizing the metabolic syndrome: A joint interim statement of the International Diabetes Federation Task Force on Epidemiology and Prevention; National Heart, Lung, and Blood Institute; American Heart Association; World Heart Federation; International Atherosclerosis Society; and International Association for the Study of Obesity. Circulation 120:1640, 2009

Cornier MA et al: The metabolic syndrome. Endocr Rev 29:777, 2008

Eckel RH et al: The metabolic syndrome. Lancet 365:1415, 2005

Ford ES: Prevalence of the metabolic syndrome defined by the International Diabetes Federation among adults in the U.S. Diabetes Care 28:2745, 2005

Grundy SM et al: Diagnosis and management of the metabolic syndrome. An American Heart Association/National Heart, Lung, and Blood Institute scientific statement. Circulation 112:2735, 2005

———: Metabolic syndrome: Connecting and reconciling cardiovascular and diabetes worlds. J Am Coll Cardiol 47:1093, 2006

Stewart PM et al: Selective inhibitors of 11beta-hydroxysteroid dehydrogenase type 1 for patients with metabolic syndrome: Is the target liver, fat, or both? Diabetes 58:14, 2009

Valle-Gottlieb MG et al: Associations among metabolic syndrome, ischemia, inflammatory, oxidatives, and lipids biomarkers. J Clin Endocrinol Metab 95:586, 2010

Zimmet P et al: The metabolic syndrome: Progress towards one definition for an epidemic of our time. Nat Clin Pract Endocrinol Metab 4:239, 2008

CHAPTER 243

Ischemic Heart Disease

Elliott M. Antman
Andrew P. Selwyn
Joseph Loscalzo

Ischemic heart disease (IHD) is a condition in which there is an inadequate supply of blood and oxygen to a portion of the myocardium; it typically occurs when there is an imbalance between myocardial oxygen supply and demand. The most common cause of myocardial ischemia is atherosclerotic disease of an epicardial coronary artery (or arteries) sufficient to cause a regional reduction in myocardial blood flow and inadequate perfusion of the myocardium supplied by the involved coronary artery. Chapter 241 deals with the development and treatment of atherosclerosis. This chapter focuses on the chronic manifestations and treatment of ischemic heart disease. The following chapters address the acute phases of this disease.

EPIDEMIOLOGY

IHD causes more deaths and disability and incurs greater economic costs than any other illness in the developed world. IHD is the most common, serious, chronic, life-threatening illness in the United States, where 13 million persons have IHD, >6 million have angina pectoris, and >7 million have sustained a myocardial infarction. Genetic factors, a high-fat and energy-rich diet, smoking, and a sedentary lifestyle are associated with the emergence of IHD (Chap. 241). In the United States and Western Europe, it is growing among low-income groups, but primary prevention has delayed the disease to later in life in all socioeconomic groups. Despite these sobering statistics, it is worth noting that epidemiologic data show a decline in the rate of deaths due to IHD, about half of which is attributable to treatments and half to prevention by risk factor modification.

Obesity, insulin resistance, and type 2 diabetes mellitus are increasing and are powerful risk factors for IHD. With urbanization in countries with emerging economies and a growing middle class, elements of the energy-rich Western diet are being adopted. As a result, the prevalence of risk factors for and of IHD itself are both increasing rapidly in those regions such that a majority of the global burden of IHD occurs there. Population subgroups that appear to be particularly affected are men in South Asian countries, especially India and the Middle East. In light of the projection of large increases in IHD throughout the world, IHD is likely to become the most common cause of death worldwide by 2020.

PATHOPHYSIOLOGY

Central to an understanding of the pathophysiology of myocardial ischemia is the concept of myocardial supply and demand. In normal conditions, for any given level of a demand for oxygen, the myocardium will control the supply of oxygen-rich blood to prevent underperfusion of myocytes and the subsequent development of ischemia and infarction. The major determinants of myocardial oxygen demand (MVO_2) are heart rate, myocardial contractility, and myocardial wall tension (stress). An adequate supply of oxygen to the myocardium requires a satisfactory level of oxygen-carrying capacity of the blood (determined by the inspired level of oxygen, pulmonary function, and hemoglobin concentration and function) and an adequate level of coronary blood flow. Blood flows through the coronary arteries in a phasic fashion, with the majority occurring during diastole. About 75% of the total coronary resistance to flow occurs across three sets of arteries: (1) large epicardial arteries (Resistance 1 = R_1), (2) prearteriolar vessels (R_2), and (3) arteriolar and intramyocardial capillary vessels (R_3). In the absence of significant flow-limiting atherosclerotic obstructions, R_1 is trivial; the major determinant of coronary resistance is found in R_2 and R_3.

The normal coronary circulation is dominated and controlled by the heart's requirements for oxygen. This need is met by the ability of the coronary vascular bed to vary its resistance (and, therefore, blood flow) considerably while the myocardium extracts a high and relatively fixed percentage of oxygen. Normally, intramyocardial resistance vessels demonstrate an immense capacity for dilation (R_2 and R_3 decrease). For example, the changing oxygen needs of the heart with exercise and emotional stress affect coronary vascular resistance and in this manner regulate the supply of oxygen and substrate to the myocardium (*metabolic regulation*). The coronary resistance vessels also adapt to physiologic alterations in blood pressure to maintain coronary blood flow at levels appropriate to myocardial needs (*autoregulation*).

By reducing the lumen of the coronary arteries, atherosclerosis limits appropriate increases in perfusion when the demand for flow is augmented, as occurs during exertion or excitement. When the luminal reduction is severe, myocardial perfusion in the basal state is reduced. Coronary blood flow also can be limited by spasm (see Prinzmetal's angina in Chap. 244), arterial thrombi, and, rarely, coronary emboli as well as by ostial narrowing due to aortitis. Congenital abnormalities such as the origin of the left anterior descending coronary artery from the pulmonary artery may cause myocardial ischemia and infarction in infancy, but this cause is very rare in adults.

Myocardial ischemia also can occur if myocardial oxygen demands are markedly increased and particularly when coronary blood flow may be limited, as occurs in severe left ventricular hypertrophy due to aortic stenosis. The latter can present with angina that is indistinguishable from that caused by coronary atherosclerosis largely owing to subendocardial ischemia (Chap. 237). A reduction in the oxygen-carrying capacity of the blood, as in extremely severe anemia or in the presence of carboxyhemoglobin, rarely causes myocardial ischemia by itself but may lower the threshold for ischemia in patients with moderate coronary obstruction.

Not infrequently, two or more causes of ischemia coexist in a patient, such as an increase in oxygen demand due to left ventricular hypertrophy secondary to hypertension and a reduction in oxygen supply secondary to coronary atherosclerosis and anemia. Abnormal constriction or failure of normal dilation of the coronary resistance vessels also can cause ischemia. When it causes angina, this condition is referred to as *microvascular angina*.

CORONARY ATHEROSCLEROSIS

Epicardial coronary arteries are the major site of atherosclerotic disease. The major risk factors for atherosclerosis [high levels of plasma low-density lipoprotein (LDL), low plasma high-density lipoprotein (HDL), cigarette smoking, hypertension, and diabetes mellitus (Chap. 241)] disturb the normal functions of the vascular endothelium. These functions include local control of vascular tone, maintenance of an antithrombotic surface, and control of inflammatory cell adhesion and diapedesis. The loss of these defenses leads to inappropriate constriction, luminal thrombus formation, and abnormal interactions between blood cells, especially monocytes and platelets, and the activated vascular endothelium. Functional changes in the vascular milieu ultimately result in the subintimal collections of fat, smooth muscle cells, fibroblasts, and intercellular matrix that define the atherosclerotic plaque. This process develops at irregular rates in different segments of the epicardial coronary tree and leads eventually to segmental reductions in cross-sectional area, i.e., plaque formation.

There is also a predilection for atherosclerotic plaques to develop at sites of increased turbulence in coronary flow, such as at branch points in the epicardial arteries. When a stenosis reduces the diameter of an epicardial artery by 50%, there is a limitation of the ability to increase flow to meet increased myocardial demand. When the diameter is reduced by ~80%, blood flow at rest may be reduced, and further minor decreases in the stenotic orifice area can reduce coronary flow dramatically to cause myocardial ischemia at rest or with minimal stress.

Segmental atherosclerotic narrowing of epicardial coronary arteries is caused most commonly by the formation of a plaque, which is subject to rupture or erosion of the cap separating the plaque from the bloodstream. Upon exposure of the plaque contents to blood, two important and interrelated processes are set in motion: (1) platelets are activated and aggregate, and (2) the coagulation cascade is activated, leading to deposition of fibrin strands. A thrombus composed of platelet aggregates and fibrin strands traps red blood cells and can reduce coronary blood flow, leading to the clinical manifestations of myocardial ischemia.

The location of the obstruction influences the quantity of myocardium rendered ischemic and determines the severity of the clinical manifestations. Thus, critical obstructions in vessels, such as the left main coronary artery and the proximal left anterior descending coronary artery, are particularly hazardous. Chronic severe coronary narrowing and myocardial ischemia frequently are accompanied by the development of collateral vessels, especially when the narrowing develops gradually. When well developed, such vessels can by themselves provide sufficient blood flow to sustain the viability of the myocardium at rest but not during conditions of increased demand.

With progressive worsening of a stenosis in a proximal epicardial artery, the distal resistance vessels (when they function normally) dilate to reduce vascular resistance and maintain coronary blood flow. A pressure gradient develops across the proximal stenosis, and poststenotic pressure falls. When the resistance vessels are maximally dilated, myocardial blood flow becomes dependent on the pressure in the coronary artery distal to the obstruction. In these circumstances, ischemia, manifest clinically by angina or electrocardiographically by ST-segment deviation, can be precipitated by increases in myocardial oxygen demand caused by physical activity, emotional stress, and/or tachycardia. Changes in the caliber of the stenosed coronary artery due to physiologic vasomotion, loss of endothelial control of dilation (as occurs in atherosclerosis), pathologic spasm (Prinzmetal's angina), or small platelet-rich plugs also can upset the critical balance between oxygen supply and demand and thereby precipitate myocardial ischemia.

EFFECTS OF ISCHEMIA

During episodes of inadequate perfusion caused by coronary atherosclerosis, myocardial tissue oxygen tension falls and may cause transient disturbances of the mechanical, biochemical, and electrical functions of the myocardium. Coronary atherosclerosis is a focal process that usually causes nonuniform ischemia. During ischemia, regional disturbances of ventricular contractility cause segmental hypokinesia, akinesia, or, in severe cases, bulging (dyskinesia), which can reduce myocardial pump function.

The abrupt development of severe ischemia, as occurs with total or subtotal coronary occlusion, is associated with almost instantaneous failure of normal muscle relaxation and then contraction. The relatively poor perfusion of the subendocardium causes more intense ischemia of this portion of the wall (compared with the subepicardial region). Ischemia of large portions of the ventricle causes transient left ventricular failure, and if the papillary muscle apparatus is involved, mitral regurgitation can occur. When ischemia is transient, it may be associated with angina pectoris; when it is prolonged, it can lead to myocardial necrosis and scarring with or without the clinical picture of acute myocardial infarction (Chap. 245).

A wide range of abnormalities in cell metabolism, function, and structure underlie these mechanical disturbances during ischemia. The normal myocardium metabolizes fatty acids and glucose to carbon dioxide and water. With severe oxygen deprivation, fatty acids cannot be oxidized, and glucose is converted to lactate; intracellular pH is reduced, as are the myocardial stores of high-energy phosphates, i.e., ATP and creatine phosphate. Impaired cell membrane function leads to the leakage of potassium and the uptake of sodium by myocytes as well as an increase in cytosolic calcium. The severity and duration of the imbalance between myocardial oxygen supply and demand determine whether the damage is reversible (≤20 min for total occlusion in the absence of collaterals) or permanent, with subsequent myocardial necrosis (>20 min).

Ischemia also causes characteristic changes in the electrocardiogram (ECG) such as repolarization abnormalities, as evidenced by inversion of T waves and, when more severe, displacement of ST segments (Chap. 228). Transient T-wave inversion probably reflects nontransmural, intramyocardial ischemia; transient ST-segment depression often reflects patchy subendocardial ischemia; and ST-segment elevation is thought to be caused by more severe transmural ischemia. Another important consequence of myocardial ischemia is electrical instability, which may lead to isolated ventricular premature beats or even ventricular tachycardia or ventricular fibrillation (Chap. 233). Most patients who die suddenly from IHD do so as a result of ischemia-induced ventricular tachyarrhythmias (Chap. 273).

ASYMPTOMATIC VERSUS SYMPTOMATIC IHD

Postmortem studies of accident victims and military casualties in Western countries have shown that coronary atherosclerosis often begins to develop before age 20 and is widespread even among adults who were asymptomatic during life. Exercise stress tests in asymptomatic persons may show evidence of silent myocardial ischemia, i.e., exercise-induced ECG changes not accompanied by angina pectoris; coronary angiographic studies of such persons may reveal coronary artery plaques and previously unrecognized obstructions (Chap. 230). Postmortem examination of patients with such obstructions without a history of clinical manifestations of myocardial ischemia often shows macroscopic scars secondary to myocardial infarction in regions supplied by diseased coronary arteries, with or without collateral circulation. According to population studies, ~25% of patients who survive acute myocardial infarction may not come to medical attention, and these patients have the same adverse prognosis as do those who present with the classic clinical picture of acute myocardial infarction (Chap. 245). Sudden death may be unheralded and is a common presenting manifestation of IHD (Chap. 273).

Patients with IHD also can present with cardiomegaly and heart failure secondary to ischemic damage of the left ventricular myocardium that may have caused no symptoms before the development of heart failure; this condition is referred to as *ischemic cardiomyopathy*. In contrast to the asymptomatic phase of IHD, the symptomatic phase is characterized by chest discomfort due to either angina pectoris or acute myocardial infarction (Chap. 245).

Having entered the symptomatic phase, the patient may exhibit a stable or progressive course, revert to the asymptomatic stage, or die suddenly.

STABLE ANGINA PECTORIS

This episodic clinical syndrome is due to transient myocardial ischemia. Various diseases that cause myocardial ischemia as well as the numerous forms of discomfort with which it may be confused are discussed in Chap. 12. Males constitute ~70% of all patients with angina pectoris and an even greater proportion of those less than 50 years of age. It is, however, important to note that angina pectoris in women is often atypical in presentation (see below).

HISTORY

The typical patient with angina is a man >50 years or a woman >60 years of age who complains of episodes of chest discomfort, usually described as heaviness, pressure, squeezing, smothering, or choking and only rarely as frank pain. When the patient is asked to localize the sensation, he or she typically places a hand over the sternum, sometimes with a clenched fist, to indicate a squeezing, central, substernal discomfort (Levine's sign). Angina is usually crescendo-decrescendo in nature, typically lasts 2 to 5 min, and can radiate to either shoulder and to both arms (especially the ulnar surfaces of the forearm and hand). It also can arise in or radiate to the back, interscapular region, root of the neck, jaw, teeth, and epigastrium. Angina is rarely localized below the umbilicus or above the mandible. A useful finding in assessing a patient with chest discomfort is the fact that myocardial ischemic discomfort does not radiate to the trapezius muscles; that radiation pattern is more typical of pericarditis.

Although episodes of angina typically are caused by exertion (e.g., exercise, hurrying, or sexual activity) or emotion (e.g., stress, anger, fright, or frustration) and are relieved by rest, they also may occur at rest [see "Unstable Angina Pectoris," (Chap. 244)] and while the patient is recumbent (angina decubitus). The patient may be awakened at night by typical chest discomfort and dyspnea. Nocturnal angina may be due to episodic tachycardia, diminished oxygenation as the respiratory pattern changes during sleep, or expansion of the intrathoracic blood volume that occurs with recumbency; the latter causes an increase in cardiac size (end-diastolic volume), wall tension, and myocardial oxygen demand that can lead to ischemia and transient left ventricular failure.

The threshold for the development of angina pectoris may vary by time of day and emotional state. Many patients report a fixed threshold for angina, which occurs predictably at a certain level of activity, such as climbing two flights of stairs at a normal pace. In these patients, coronary stenosis and myocardial oxygen supply are fixed, and ischemia is precipitated by an increase in myocardial oxygen demand; they are said to have stable exertional angina. In other patients, the threshold for angina may vary considerably within any particular day and from day to day. In such patients, variations in myocardial oxygen supply, most likely due to changes in coronary vasomotor tone, may play an important role in defining the pattern of angina. A patient may report symptoms upon minor exertion in the morning (a short walk or shaving) yet by midday be capable of much greater effort without symptoms. Angina may also be precipitated by unfamiliar tasks, a heavy meal, exposure to cold, or a combination of these factors.

Exertional angina typically is relieved in 1 to 5 min by slowing or ceasing activities and even more rapidly by rest and sublingual nitroglycerin (see below). Indeed, the diagnosis of angina should be suspect if it does not respond to the combination of these measures. The severity of angina can be conveniently summarized by the Canadian Cardiac Society functional classification (Table 243-1). Its impact on the patient's functional capacity can be described by using the New York Heart Association functional classification (Table 243-1).

Sharp, fleeting chest pain or a prolonged, dull ache localized to the left submammary area is rarely due to myocardial ischemia. However, especially in women and diabetic patients, angina pectoris may be atypical in location and not strictly related to provoking factors. In addition, this symptom may exacerbate and remit over days, weeks, or months. Its occurrence can be seasonal, occurring more frequently in the winter in temperate climates. Anginal "equivalents" are symptoms of myocardial ischemia other than angina. They include dyspnea, nausea, fatigue, and faintness and are more common in the elderly and in diabetic patients.

TABLE 243-1 Cardiovascular Disease Classification Chart

Class	New York Heart Association Functional Classification	Canadian Cardiovascular Society Functional Classification
I	Patients have cardiac disease but *without* the resulting *limitations* of physical activity. Ordinary physical activity does not cause undue fatigue, palpitation, dyspnea, or anginal pain.	Ordinary physical activity, such as walking and climbing stairs, *does not cause angina.* Angina present with strenuous or rapid or prolonged exertion at work or recreation.
II	Patients have cardiac disease resulting in *slight limitation* of physical activity. They are comfortable at rest. Ordinary physical activity results in fatigue, palpitation, dyspnea, or anginal pain.	*Slight limitation* of ordinary activity. Walking or climbing stairs rapidly, walking uphill, walking or stair climbing after meals, in cold, or when under emotional stress or only during the few hours after awakening. Walking more than two blocks on the level and climbing more than one flight of stairs at a normal pace and in normal conditions.
III	Patients have cardiac disease resulting in *marked limitation* of physical activity. They are comfortable at rest. Less than ordinary physical activity causes fatigue, palpitation, dyspnea, or anginal pain.	*Marked limitation* of ordinary physical activity. Walking one to two blocks on the level and climbing more than one flight of stairs in normal conditions.
IV	Patients have cardiac disease resulting in *inability* to carry on any physical activity without discomfort. Symptoms of cardiac insufficiency or of the anginal syndrome may be present even at rest. If any physical activity is undertaken, discomfort is increased.	*Inability* to carry on any physical activity without discomfort—anginal syndrome *may* be present at rest.

Source: Modified from Goldman L et al: Circulation 64:1227, 1981.

Systematic questioning of a patient with suspected IHD is important to uncover the features of an unstable syndrome associated with increased risk, such as angina occurring with less exertion than in the past, occurring at rest, or awakening the patient from sleep. Since coronary atherosclerosis often is accompanied by similar lesions in other arteries, a patient with angina should be questioned and examined for peripheral arterial disease [intermittent claudication (Chap. 249)], stroke, or transient ischemic attacks (Chap. 370). It is also important to uncover a family history of premature IHD (<55 years in first-degree male relatives and <65 in female relatives) and the presence of diabetes mellitus, hyperlipidemia, hypertension, cigarette smoking, and other risk factors for coronary atherosclerosis (Chap. 241).

The history of typical angina pectoris establishes the diagnosis of IHD until proven otherwise. In patients with atypical angina (Chap. 12), the coexistence of advanced age, male sex, the postmenopausal state, and risk factors for atherosclerosis increase the likelihood of hemodynamically significant coronary disease. A particularly challenging problem is the evaluation and management of patients with persistent ischemic-type chest discomfort but no flow-limiting obstructions in their epicardial coronary arteries. This situation arises more often in women than in men. Potential etiologies include microvascular coronary disease (detectable on coronary reactivity testing in response to vasoactive agents such as intracoronary adenosine, acetylcholine, and nitroglycerin) and abnormal cardiac nociception. Treatment of microvascular coronary disease should focus on efforts to improve endothelial function, including nitrates, beta blockers, calcium antagonists, statins, and angiotensin-converting enzyme (ACE) inhibitors. Abnormal cardiac nociception is more difficult to manage and may be ameliorated in some cases by imipramine.

PHYSICAL EXAMINATION

The physical examination is often normal in patients with stable angina when they are asymptomatic. However, because of the increased likelihood of ischemic heart disease in patients with diabetes and/or peripheral arterial disease, clinicians should search for evidence of atherosclerotic disease at other sites, such as an abdominal aortic aneurysm, carotid arterial bruits, and diminished arterial pulses in the lower extremities. The physical examination also should include a search for evidence of risk factors for atherosclerosis such as xanthelasmas and xanthomas (Chap. 241). Evidence for peripheral arterial disease should be sought by evaluating the pulse contour at multiple locations and comparing the blood pressure between the arms and between the arms and the legs (ankle-brachial index). Examination of the fundi may reveal an increased light reflex and arteriovenous nicking as evidence of hypertension. There also may be signs of anemia, thyroid disease, and nicotine stains on the fingertips from cigarette smoking.

Palpation may reveal cardiac enlargement and abnormal contraction of the cardiac impulse (left ventricular dyskinesia). Auscultation can uncover arterial bruits, a third and/or fourth heart sound, and, if acute ischemia or previous infarction has impaired papillary muscle function, an apical systolic murmur due to mitral regurgitation. These auscultatory signs are best appreciated with the patient in the left lateral decubitus position. Aortic stenosis, aortic regurgitation (Chap. 237), pulmonary hypertension (Chap. 250), and hypertrophic cardiomyopathy (Chap. 238) must be excluded, since these disorders may cause angina in the absence of coronary atherosclerosis. Examination during an anginal attack is useful, since ischemia can cause transient left ventricular failure with the appearance of a third and/or fourth heart sound, a dyskinetic cardiac apex, mitral regurgitation, and even pulmonary edema. Tenderness of the chest wall, localization of the discomfort with a single fingertip on the chest, or reproduction of the pain with palpation of the chest makes it unlikely that the pain is caused by myocardial ischemia. A protuberant abdomen may indicate that the patient has the metabolic syndrome and is at increased risk for atherosclerosis.

LABORATORY EXAMINATION

Although the diagnosis of IHD can be made with a high degree of confidence from the history and physical examination, a number of simple laboratory tests can be helpful. The urine should be examined for evidence of diabetes mellitus and renal disease (including microalbuminuria) since these conditions accelerate atherosclerosis. Similarly, examination of the blood should include measurements of lipids (cholesterol—total, LDL, HDL—and triglycerides), glucose (hemoglobin A_{1C}), creatinine, hematocrit, and, if indicated based on the physical examination, thyroid function. A chest x-ray is important as it may show the consequences of IHD, i.e., cardiac enlargement, ventricular aneurysm, or signs of heart failure. These signs can support the diagnosis of IHD and are important in assessing the degree of cardiac damage. Evidence exists that an elevated level of high-sensitivity C-reactive protein (CRP) (specifically, between 0 and 3 mg/dL) is an independent risk factor for IHD and may be useful in therapeutic decision making about the initiation of hypolipidemic treatment. The major benefit of high-sensitivity CRP is in reclassifying the risk of IHD in patients in the "intermediate" risk category on the basis of traditional risk factors.

ELECTROCARDIOGRAM

A 12-lead ECG recorded at rest may be normal in patients with typical angina pectoris, but there may also be signs of an old myocardial infarction (Chap. 228). Although repolarization abnormalities, i.e., ST-segment and T-wave changes, as well as left ventricular hypertrophy and disturbances of cardiac rhythm or intraventricular conduction are suggestive of IHD, they are nonspecific, since they also can occur in pericardial, myocardial, and valvular heart disease or, in the case of the former, transiently with anxiety, changes in posture, drugs, or esophageal disease. The presence of left ventricular hypertrophy (LVH) is a significant indication of increased risk of adverse outcomes from ischemic heart disease. Of note, even though LVH and cardiac rhythm disturbances are nonspecific indicators of the development of IHD, they may be contributing factors to episodes of angina in patients in whom IHD has developed as a consequence of conventional risk factors. Dynamic ST-segment and T-wave changes that accompany episodes of angina pectoris and disappear thereafter are more specific.

STRESS TESTING

Electrocardiographic

The most widely used test for both the diagnosis of IHD and the estimation of risk and prognosis involves recording the 12-lead ECG before, during, and after exercise, usually on a treadmill (Fig. 243-1). The test consists of a standardized incremental increase in external workload (Table 243-2) while symptoms, the ECG, and arm blood pressure are monitored. Exercise duration is usually symptom-limited, and the test is discontinued upon evidence of chest discomfort, severe shortness of breath, dizziness, severe fatigue, ST-segment depression >0.2 mV (2 mm), a fall in systolic blood pressure >10 mmHg, or the development of a ventricular tachyarrhythmia. This test is used to discover any limitation in exercise performance, detect typical ECG signs of myocardial ischemia, and establish their relationship to chest discomfort. The ischemic ST-segment response generally is defined as flat or downsloping depression of the ST segment >0.1 mV below baseline (i.e., the PR segment) and lasting longer than

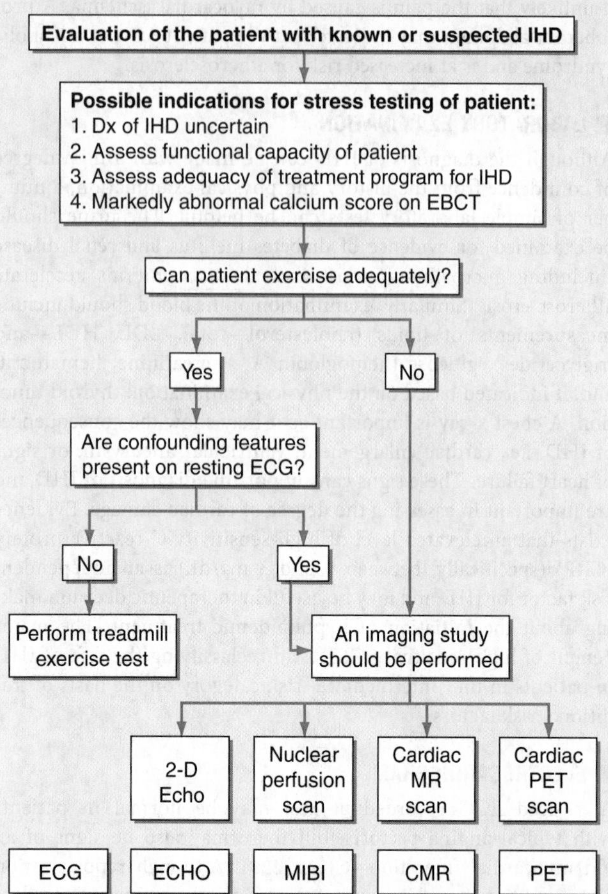

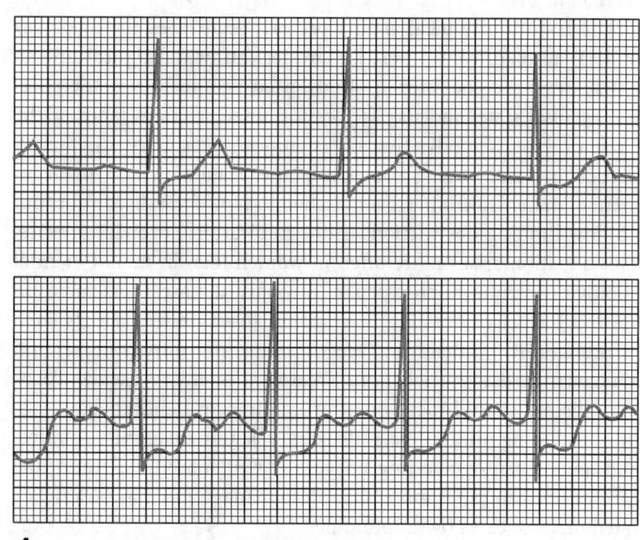

Figure 243-1 Evaluation of the patient with known or suspected ischemic heart disease. At the top of the figure is an algorithm for identifying patients who should be referred for stress testing and the decision pathway for determining whether a standard treadmill exercise with ECG monitoring alone is adequate. A specialized imaging study is necessary if the patient cannot exercise adequately (pharmacologic challenge is given) or if there are confounding features on the resting ECG (symptom-limited treadmill exercise may be used to stress the coronary circulation). At the bottom of the figure are examples of the data obtained with ECG monitoring and specialized imaging procedures. CMR, cardiac magnetic resonance; EBCT, electron beam computed tomography; ECG, electrocardiogram; ECHO, echocardiography; IHD, ischemic heart disease; MIBI, methoxyisobutyl isonitrite; MR, magnetic resonance; PET, positron emission tomography.

A. Lead V_4 at rest (*top*) and after 4½ min of exercise (*bottom*). There is 3 mm (0.3 mV) of horizontal ST-segment depression, indicating a positive test for ischemia. *[Modified from BR Chaitman, in E Braunwald et al (eds): Heart Disease, 6th ed, Philadelphia, Saunders, 2001.]*

B. 45-year-old avid jogger who began experiencing classic substernal chest pressure underwent an exercise echo study. With exercise the patient's heart rate increased from 52 to 153 bpm. The left ventricular chamber dilated with exercise, and the septal and apical portions became akinetic to dyskinetic (*red arrow*). These findings are strongly suggestive of a significant flow-limiting stenosis in the proximal left anterior descending artery, which was confirmed at coronary angiography. *[Modified from SD Solomon, in E. Braunwald et al (eds): Primary Cardiology, 2nd ed, Philadelphia, Saunders, 2003.]*

C. Stress and rest myocardial perfusion SPECT images obtained with 99m-technetium sestamibi in a patient with chest pain and dyspnea on exertion. The images demonstrate a medium-size and severe stress perfusion defect involving the inferolateral and basal inferior walls, showing nearly complete reversibility, consistent with moderate ischemia in the right coronary artery territory (*red arrows*). *(Images provided by Dr. Marcello Di Carli, Nuclear Medicine Division, Brigham and Women's Hospital, Boston, MA.)*

D. A patient with a prior myocardial infarction presented with recurrent chest discomfort. On cardiac magnetic resonance (CMR) cine imaging, a large area of anterior akinesia was noted (marked by the arrows in the top left and right images, systolic frame only). This area of akinesia was matched by a larger extent of late gadolinium-DTPA enhancements consistent with a large transmural myocardial infarction (marked by arrows in the middle left and right images). Resting (*bottom left*) and adenosine vasodilating stress (*bottom right*) first-pass perfusion images revealed reversible perfusion abnormality that extended to the inferior septum. This patient was found to have an occluded proximal left anterior descending coronary artery with extensive collateral formation. This case illustrates the utility of different modalities in a CMR examination in characterizing ischemic and infarcted myocardium. DTPA, diethylenetriamine penta-acetic acid. (*Images provided by Dr. Raymond Kwong, Cardiovascular Division, Brigham and Women's Hospital, Boston, MA.)*

E. Stress and rest myocardial perfusion PET images obtained with rubidium-82 in a patient with chest pain on exertion. The images demonstrate a large and severe stress perfusion defect involving the mid and apical anterior, anterolateral, and anteroseptal walls and the LV apex, showing complete reversibility, consistent with extensive and severe ischemia in the mid-left anterior descending coronary artery territory (*red arrows*). *(Images provided by Dr. Marcello Di Carli, Nuclear Medicine Division, Brigham and Women's Hospital, Boston, MA.)*

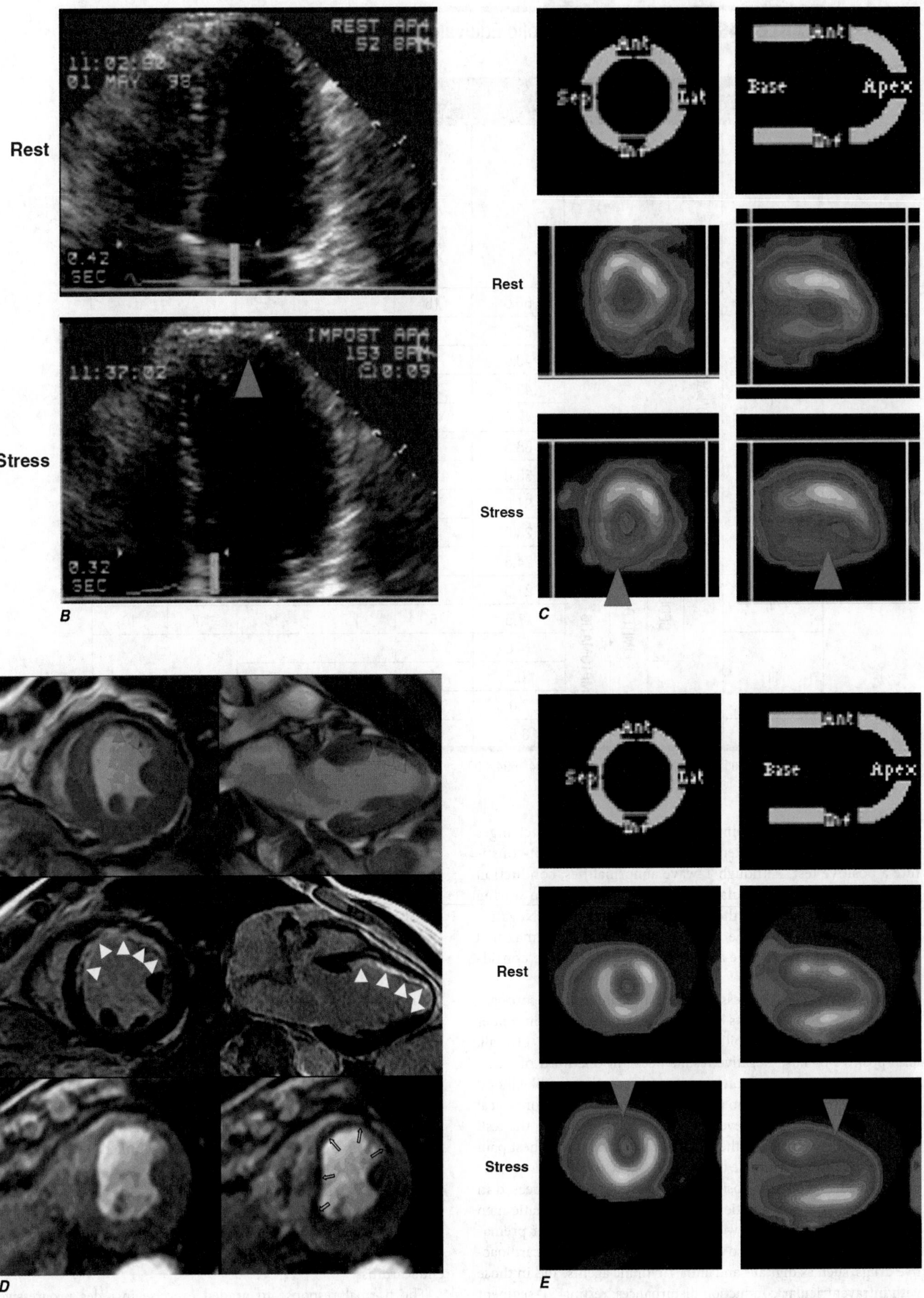

Figure 243-1 (*Continued*)

TABLE 243-2 Relation of Metabolic Equivalent Tasks (METs) to Stages in Various Testing Protocols

Functional Class	Clinical Status				O_2 Cost mL/kg/min	METS	Treadmill Protocols			
							BRUCE Modified 3 min Stage		BRUCE 3 min Stages	
							MPH	%GR	MPH	%GR
	HEALTHY, DEPENDENT ON AGE, ACTIVITY						6.0	22	6.0	22
							5.5	20	5.2	20
							5.0	18	5.0	18
NORMAL AND I					56.0	16				
					52.5	15				
					49.0	14				
					45.5	13	4.2	16	4.2	16
					42.0	12				
		SEDENTARY HEALTHY			38.5	11	3.4	14	3.4	14
					35.0	10				
					31.5	9				
					28.0	8				
			LIMITED		24.5	7	2.5	12	2.5	12
II				SYMPTOMATIC	21.0	6				
					17.5	5	1.7	10	1.7	10
III					14.0	4				
					10.5	3	1.7	5		
					7.0	2	1.7	0		
IV					3.5	1				

Source: Modified from Fletcher GF et al: Circulation 104:1694, 2001.

0.08 s (Fig. 243-1). Upsloping or junctional ST-segment changes are not considered characteristic of ischemia and do not constitute a positive test. Although T-wave abnormalities, conduction disturbances, and ventricular arrhythmias that develop during exercise should be noted, they are also not diagnostic. Negative exercise tests in which the target heart rate (85% of maximal predicted heart rate for age and sex) is not achieved are considered nondiagnostic.

In interpreting ECG stress tests, the probability that coronary artery disease (CAD) exists in the patient or population under study (i.e., pretest probability) should be considered. Overall, false-positive or false-negative results occur in one-third of cases. However, a positive result on exercise indicates that the likelihood of CAD is 98% in males who are >50 years with a history of typical angina pectoris and who develop chest discomfort during the test. The likelihood decreases if the patient has atypical or no chest pain by history and/or during the test.

The incidence of false-positive tests is significantly increased in patients with low probabilities of IHD, such as asymptomatic men <age 40 or premenopausal women with no risk factors for premature atherosclerosis. It is also increased in patients taking cardioactive drugs, such as digitalis and antiarrhythmic agents, and in those with intraventricular conduction disturbances, resting ST-segment and T-wave abnormalities, ventricular hypertrophy, or abnormal serum potassium levels. Obstructive disease limited to the circumflex coronary artery may result in a false-negative stress test since the lateral portion of the heart that this vessel supplies is not well represented on the surface 12-lead ECG. Since the overall sensitivity of exercise stress electrocardiography is only ~75%, a negative result does not exclude CAD, although it makes the likelihood of three-vessel or left main CAD extremely unlikely.

The physician should be present throughout the exercise test. It is important to measure total duration of exercise, the times to the onset of ischemic ST-segment change and chest discomfort, the external work performed (generally expressed as the stage of exercise), and the internal cardiac work performed, i.e., by the heart rate–blood pressure product. The depth of the ST-segment depression and the time needed for recovery of these ECG changes are also important. Because the risks of exercise testing are small but real—estimated at one fatality and two nonfatal complications per 10,000 tests—equipment for resuscitation should be available. Modified (heart rate–limited rather than symptom-limited) exercise tests can be performed safely in patients as early as 6 days after uncomplicated myocardial infarction (Table 243-2). Contraindications to exercise stress testing include rest angina within 48 h, unstable rhythm, severe aortic stenosis, acute myocarditis, uncontrolled heart failure, severe pulmonary hypertension, and active infective endocarditis.

The normal response to graded exercise includes progressive increases in heart rate and blood pressure. Failure of the blood pressure to increase or an actual decrease with signs of ischemia during the test is an important adverse prognostic sign, since it may reflect ischemia-induced global left ventricular dysfunction. The development of angina and/or severe (>0.2 mV) ST-segment depression at a low workload, i.e., before completion of stage II of the Bruce protocol, and/or ST-segment depression that persists >5 min after the termination of exercise increases the specificity of the test and suggests severe IHD and a high risk of future adverse events.

Cardiac imaging

(See also Chap. 229) When the resting ECG is abnormal (e.g., preexcitation syndrome, >1 mm of resting ST-segment depression, left bundle branch block, paced ventricular rhythm), information gained from an exercise test can be enhanced by stress myocardial radionuclide perfusion imaging after the intravenous administration of thallium-201 or 99m-technetium sestamibi during exercise (or with pharmacologic) stress. Contemporary data also suggest positron emission tomography (PET) imaging (with exercise or pharmacologic stress) using N-13 ammonia or rubidium-82 nuclide as another technique for assessing perfusion. Images obtained immediately after cessation of exercise to detect regional ischemia are compared with those obtained at rest to confirm reversible ischemia and regions of persistently absent uptake that signify infarction.

A sizable fraction of patients who need noninvasive stress testing to identify myocardial ischemia and increased risk of coronary events cannot exercise because of peripheral vascular or musculoskeletal disease, exertional dyspnea, or deconditioning. In these circumstances, an intravenous pharmacologic challenge is used in place of exercise. For example, dipyridamole or adenosine can be given to create a coronary "steal" by temporarily increasing flow in nondiseased segments of the coronary vasculature at the expense of diseased segments. Alternatively, a graded incremental infusion of dobutamine may be administered to increase MVO_2. A variety of imaging options are available to accompany these pharmacologic stressors (Fig. 243-1). The development of a transient perfusion defect with a tracer such as thallium-201 or 99m-technetium sestamibi is used to detect myocardial ischemia.

Echocardiography is used to assess left ventricular function in patients with chronic stable angina and patients with a history of a prior myocardial infarction, pathologic Q waves, or clinical evidence of heart failure. Two-dimensional echocardiography can assess both global and regional wall motion abnormalities of the left ventricle that are transient when due to ischemia. Stress (exercise or dobutamine) echocardiography may cause the emergence of regions of akinesis or dyskinesis that are not present at rest. Stress echocardiography, like stress myocardial perfusion imaging, is more sensitive than exercise electrocardiography in the diagnosis of IHD. Cardiac magnetic resonance (CMR) stress testing is also evolving as an alternative to radionuclide, PET, or echocardiographic stress imaging. CMR stress testing performed with dobutamine infusion can be used to assess wall motion abnormalities accompanying ischemia, as well as myocardial perfusion. CMR can be used to provide more complete ventricular evaluation using multislice MR imaging (MRI) studies.

Atherosclerotic plaques become progressively calcified over time, and coronary calcification in general increases with age. For this reason, methods for detecting coronary calcium have been developed as a measure of the presence of coronary atherosclerosis. These methods involve computed tomography (CT) applications that achieve rapid acquisition of images [electron beam (EBCT), and multidetector (MDCT) detection]. Coronary calcium detected by these imaging techniques most commonly is quantified by using the Agatston score, which is based on the area and density of calcification. Although the diagnostic accuracy of this imaging method is high (sensitivity, 90–94%; specificity, 95–97%; negative predictive value, 93–99%), its prognostic utility has not been defined. Thus, its role in CT, EBCT, and MDCT scans for the detection and management of patients with IHD has not been clarified.

CORONARY ARTERIOGRAPHY

(See also Chap. 230) This diagnostic method outlines the lumina of the coronary arteries and can be used to detect or exclude serious coronary obstruction. However, coronary arteriography provides no information about the arterial wall, and severe atherosclerosis that does not encroach on the lumen may go undetected. Of note, atherosclerotic plaques characteristically are scattered throughout the coronary tree, tend to occur more frequently at branch points, and grow progressively in the intima and media of an epicardial coronary artery at first without encroaching on the lumen, causing an outward bulging of the artery—a process referred to as remodeling (Chap. 241). Later in the course of the disease, further growth causes luminal narrowing.

Indications

Coronary arteriography is indicated in (1) patients with chronic stable angina pectoris who are severely symptomatic despite medical therapy and are being considered for revascularization, i.e., a percutaneous coronary intervention (PCI) or coronary artery bypass grafting (CABG), (2) patients with troublesome symptoms that present diagnostic difficulties in whom there is a need to confirm or rule out the diagnosis of IHD, (3) patients with known or possible angina pectoris who have survived cardiac arrest, (4) patients with angina or evidence of ischemia on noninvasive testing with clinical or laboratory evidence of ventricular dysfunction, and (5) patients judged to be at high risk of sustaining coronary events based on signs of severe ischemia on noninvasive testing, regardless of the presence or severity of symptoms (see below).

Examples of other indications for coronary arteriography include the following:

1. Patients with chest discomfort suggestive of angina pectoris but a negative or nondiagnostic stress test who require a definitive diagnosis for guiding medical management, alleviating psychological stress, career or family planning, or insurance purposes.
2. Patients who have been admitted repeatedly to the hospital for a suspected acute coronary syndrome (Chaps. 244 and 245) but in whom this diagnosis has not been established and in whom the presence or absence of CAD should be determined.
3. Patients with careers that involve the safety of others (e.g., pilots, firefighters, police) who have questionable symptoms or suspicious or positive noninvasive tests and in whom there are reasonable doubts about the state of the coronary arteries.
4. Patients with aortic stenosis or hypertrophic cardiomyopathy and angina in whom the chest pain could be due to IHD.
5. Male patients >45 years and females >55 years who are to undergo a cardiac operation such as valve replacement or repair and who may or may not have clinical evidence of myocardial ischemia.
6. Patients after myocardial infarction, especially those who are at high risk after myocardial infarction because of the recurrence of angina or the presence of heart failure, frequent ventricular premature contractions, or signs of ischemia on the stress test.
7. Patients with angina pectoris, regardless of severity, in whom noninvasive testing indicates a high risk of coronary events (poor exercise performance or severe ischemia).
8. Patients in whom coronary spasm or another nonatherosclerotic cause of myocardial ischemia (e.g., coronary artery anomaly, Kawasaki disease) is suspected.

Noninvasive alternatives to diagnostic coronary arteriography include CT angiography and cardiac MR angiography (Chap. 229).

Although these new imaging techniques can provide information about obstructive lesions in the epicardial coronary arteries, their exact role in clinical practice has not been rigorously defined. Important aspects of their use that should be noted include the substantially higher radiation exposure with CT angiography compared to conventional diagnostic arteriography and the limitations on cardiac MR imposed by cardiac movement during the cardiac cycle, especially at high heart rates.

PROGNOSIS

The principal prognostic indicators in patients known to have IHD are age, the functional state of the left ventricle, the location(s) and severity of coronary artery narrowing, and the severity or activity of myocardial ischemia. Angina pectoris of recent onset, unstable angina (Chap. 244), early postmyocardial infarction angina, angina that is unresponsive or poorly responsive to medical therapy, and angina accompanied by symptoms of congestive heart failure all indicate an increased risk for adverse coronary events. The same is true for the physical signs of heart failure, episodes of pulmonary edema, transient third heart sounds, and mitral regurgitation and for echocardiographic or radioisotopic (or roentgenographic) evidence of cardiac enlargement and reduced (<0.40) ejection fraction.

Most important, any of the following signs during noninvasive testing indicates a high risk for coronary events: inability to exercise for 6 min, i.e., stage II (Bruce protocol) of the exercise test; a strongly positive exercise test showing onset of myocardial ischemia at low workloads (≥0.1 mV ST-segment depression before completion of stage II, ≥0.2 mV ST depression at any stage, ST depression for >5 min after the cessation of exercise, a decline in systolic pressure >10 mmHg during exercise, the development of ventricular tachyarrhythmias during exercise); the development of large or multiple perfusion defects or increased lung uptake during stress radioisotope perfusion imaging; and a decrease in left ventricular ejection fraction during exercise on radionuclide ventriculography or during stress echocardiography. Conversely, patients who can complete stage III of the Bruce exercise protocol and have a normal stress perfusion scan or negative stress echocardiographic evaluation are at very low risk for future coronary events. The finding of frequent episodes of ST-segment deviation on ambulatory ECG monitoring (even in the absence of symptoms) is also an adverse prognostic finding.

On cardiac catheterization, elevations of left ventricular end-diastolic pressure and ventricular volume and reduced ejection fraction are the most important signs of left ventricular dysfunction and are associated with a poor prognosis. Patients with chest discomfort but normal left ventricular function and normal coronary arteries have an excellent prognosis. Obstructive lesions of the left main (>50% luminal diameter) or left anterior descending coronary artery proximal to the origin of the first septal artery are associated with a greater risk than are lesions of the right or left circumflex coronary artery because of the greater quantity of myocardium at risk. Atherosclerotic plaques in epicardial arteries with fissuring or filling defects indicate increased risk. These lesions go through phases of inflammatory cellular activity, degeneration, endothelial dysfunction, abnormal vasomotion, platelet aggregation, and fissuring or hemorrhage. These factors can temporarily worsen the stenosis and cause thrombosis and/or abnormal reactivity of the vessel wall, thus exacerbating the manifestations of ischemia. The recent onset of symptoms, the development of severe ischemia during stress testing (see above), and unstable angina pectoris (Chap. 244) all reflect episodes of rapid progression in coronary lesions.

With any degree of obstructive CAD, mortality is greatly increased when left ventricular function is impaired; conversely, at any level of left ventricular function, the prognosis is influenced importantly by the quantity of myocardium perfused by critically obstructed vessels. Therefore, it is essential to collect all the evidence substantiating past myocardial damage (evidence of myocardial infarction on ECG, echocardiography, radioisotope imaging, or left ventriculography), residual left ventricular function (ejection fraction and wall motion), and risk of future damage from coronary events (extent of coronary disease and severity of ischemia defined by noninvasive stress testing). The larger the quantity of established myocardial necrosis is, the less the heart is able to withstand additional damage and the poorer the prognosis is. Risk estimation must include age, presenting symptoms, all risk factors, signs of arterial disease, existing cardiac damage, and signs of impending damage (i.e., ischemia).

The greater the number and severity of risk factors for coronary atherosclerosis [advanced age (>75 years), hypertension, dyslipidemia, diabetes, morbid obesity, accompanying peripheral and/or cerebrovascular disease, previous myocardial infarction], the worse the prognosis of an angina patient. Evidence exists that elevated levels of C-reactive protein in the plasma, extensive coronary calcification on electron beam CT (see above), and increased carotid intimal thickening on ultrasound examination also indicate an increased risk of coronary events.

TREATMENT Stable Angina Pectoris

Once the diagnosis of ischemic heart disease has been made, each patient must be evaluated individually with respect to his or her level of understanding, expectations and goals, control of symptoms, and prevention of adverse clinical outcomes such as myocardial infarction and premature death. The degree of disability as well as the physical and emotional stress that precipitates angina must be recorded carefully to set treatment goals. The management plan should include the following components: (1) explanation of the problem and reassurance about the ability to formulate a treatment plan, (2) identification and treatment of aggravating conditions, (3) recommendations for adaptation of activity as needed, (4) treatment of risk factors that will decrease the occurrence of adverse coronary outcomes, (5) drug therapy for angina, and (6) consideration of revascularization.

EXPLANATION AND REASSURANCE Patients with IHD need to understand their condition and realize that a long and productive life is possible even though they have angina pectoris or have experienced and recovered from an acute myocardial infarction. Offering results of clinical trials showing improved outcomes can be of great value in encouraging patients to resume or maintain activity and return to work. A planned program of rehabilitation can encourage patients to lose weight, improve exercise tolerance, and control risk factors with more confidence.

IDENTIFICATION AND TREATMENT OF AGGRAVATING CONDITIONS A number of conditions may increase oxygen demand or decrease oxygen supply to the myocardium and may precipitate or exacerbate angina in patients with IHD. Left ventricular hypertrophy, aortic valve disease, and hypertrophic cardiomyopathy may cause or contribute to angina and should be excluded or treated. Obesity, hypertension, and hyperthyroidism should be treated aggressively to reduce the frequency and severity of anginal episodes. Decreased myocardial oxygen supply may be due to reduced oxygenation of the arterial blood (e.g., in pulmonary disease or, when carboxyhemoglobin is present, due to cigarette or cigar smoking) or decreased oxygen-carrying capacity (e.g., in anemia). Correction of these abnormalities, if present, may reduce or even eliminate angina pectoris.

ADAPTATION OF ACTIVITY Myocardial ischemia is caused by a discrepancy between the demand of the heart muscle for oxygen and the ability of the coronary circulation to meet that demand. Most patients can be helped to understand this concept and utilize it in the rational programming of activity. Many tasks that ordinarily evoke angina may be accomplished without symptoms simply by reducing the speed at which they are performed. Patients must appreciate the diurnal variation in their tolerance of certain activities and should reduce their energy requirements in the morning, immediately after meals, and in cold or inclement weather. On occasion, it may be necessary to recommend a change in employment or residence to avoid physical stress.

Physical conditioning usually improves the exercise tolerance of patients with angina and has substantial psychological benefits. A regular program of isotonic exercise that is within the limits of the individual patient's threshold for the development of angina pectoris and that does not exceed 80% of the heart rate associated with ischemia on exercise testing should be strongly encouraged. Based on the results of an exercise test, the number of metabolic equivalent tasks (METs) performed at the onset of ischemia can be estimated (Table 243-2) and a practical exercise prescription can be formulated to permit daily activities that will fall below the ischemic threshold (Table 243-3).

TREATMENT OF RISK FACTORS A *family history* of premature IHD is an important indicator of increased risk and should trigger a search for treatable risk factors such as hyperlipidemia, hypertension, and diabetes mellitus. *Obesity* impairs the treatment of other risk factors and increases the risk of adverse coronary events. In addition, obesity often is accompanied by three other risk factors: diabetes mellitus, hypertension, and hyperlipidemia. The treatment of obesity and these accompanying risk factors is an important component of any management plan. A diet low in saturated and *trans*-unsaturated fatty acids and a reduced caloric intake to achieve optimal body weight are a cornerstone in the management of chronic IHD. It is especially important to emphasize weight loss and regular exercise in patients with the metabolic syndrome or overt diabetes mellitus.

Cigarette smoking accelerates coronary atherosclerosis in both sexes and at all ages and increases the risk of thrombosis, plaque instability, myocardial infarction, and death (Chap. 241). In addition, by increasing myocardial oxygen needs and reducing oxygen supply, it aggravates angina. Smoking cessation studies

TABLE 243-3 Energy Requirements for Some Common Activities

Less Than 3 METs	3–5 METs	5–7 METs	7–9 METs	More Than 9 METs
Self-care				
Washing/shaving	Cleaning windows	Easy digging in garden	Heavy shoveling	Carrying loads upstairs (objects more than 90 lb)
Dressing	Raking	Level hand lawn mowing	Carrying objects (60–90 lb)	Climbing stairs (quickly)
Light housekeeping	Power lawn mowing	Carrying objects (30–60 lb)		Shoveling heavy snow
Desk work	Bed making/stripping			
Driving auto	Carrying objects (15–30 lb)			
Occupational				
Sitting (clerical/ assembly)	Stocking shelves (light objects	Carpentry (exterior)	Digging ditches (pick and shovel)	Heavy labor
Desk work	Light welding/carpentry	Shoveling dirt		
Standing (store clerk)		Sawing wood		
Recreational				
Golf (cart)	Dancing (social)	Tennis (singles)	Canoeing	Squash
Knitting	Golf (walking)	Snow skiing (downhill)	Mountain climbing	Ski touring
	Sailing	Light backpacking		Vigorous basketball
	Tennis (doubles)	Basketball		
		Stream fishing		
Physical conditioning				
Walking (2 mph)	Level walking (3–4 mph)	Level walking (4.5–5.0 mph)	Level jogging (5 mph)	Running more than 6 mph
Stationary bike	Level biking (6–8 mph)	Bicycling (9–10 mph)	Swimming (crawl stroke)	Bicycling (more than 13 mph)
Very light calisthenics	Light calisthenics	Swimming, breast stroke	Rowing machine	Rope jumping
			Heavy calisthenics	Walking uphill (5 mph)
			Bicycling (12 mph)	

Abbreviation: METs, metabolic equivalent tasks.

Source: Modified from WL Haskell: Rehabilitation of the coronary patient, in NK Wenger, HK Hellerstein (eds): *Design and Implementation of Cardiac Conditioning Program.* New York, Churchill Livingstone, 1978.

have demonstrated important benefits with a significant decline in the occurrence of these adverse outcomes. The physician's message must be clear and strong and supported by programs that achieve and monitor abstinence (Chap. 395). *Hypertension* (Chap. 247) is associated with an increased risk of adverse clinical events from coronary atherosclerosis as well as stroke. In addition, the left ventricular hypertrophy that results from sustained hypertension aggravates ischemia. There is evidence that long-term effective treatment of hypertension can decrease the occurrence of adverse coronary events.

Diabetes mellitus (Chap. 344) accelerates coronary and peripheral atherosclerosis and is frequently associated with dyslipidemias and increases in the risk of angina, myocardial infarction, and sudden coronary death. Aggressive control of the dyslipidemia (target LDL cholesterol <70 mg/dL) and hypertension (target BP 120/80) that are frequently found in diabetic patients is highly effective and therefore essential, as described below.

DYSLIPIDEMIA The treatment of dyslipidemia is central in aiming for long-term relief from angina, reduced need for revascularization, and reduction in myocardial infarction and death. The control of lipids can be achieved by the combination of a diet low in saturated and *trans*-unsaturated fatty acids, exercise, and weight loss. Nearly always, HMG-CoA reductase inhibitors (statins) are required and can lower LDL cholesterol (25–50%), raise HDL cholesterol (5–9%), and lower triglycerides (5–30%). A powerful treatment effect of statins on atherosclerosis, IHD, and outcomes is seen regardless of the pretreatment LDL cholesterol level. Fibrates or niacin can be used to raise HDL cholesterol and lower triglycerides (Chaps. 241 and 356). Controlled trials with lipid-regulating regimens have shown equal proportional benefit for men, women, the elderly, diabetic patients, and even smokers.

Compliance with the health-promoting behaviors listed above is generally very poor, and a conscientious physician must not underestimate the major effort required to meet this challenge. Fewer than one-half of patients in the United States discharged from the hospital with proven coronary disease receive treatment for dyslipidemia. In light of the proof that treating dyslipidemia brings major benefits, physicians need to establish treatment pathways, monitor compliance, and follow up regularly.

RISK REDUCTION IN WOMEN WITH IHD The incidence of clinical IHD in premenopausal women is very low; however, after menopause, the atherogenic risk factors increase (e.g., increased LDL, reduced HDL) and the rate of clinical coronary events accelerates to the levels observed in men. Women have not given up cigarette smoking as effectively as have men. Diabetes mellitus, which is more common in women, greatly increases the occurrence of clinical IHD and amplifies the deleterious effects of hypertension, hyperlipidemia, and smoking. Cardiac catheterization and coronary revascularization are underused in women and are performed at a later and more severe stage of the disease than in men. When cholesterol lowering, beta blockers after myocardial infarction, and coronary artery bypass grafting are applied in the appropriate patient groups, women receive the same benefits of improved outcome as do men.

DRUG THERAPY The commonly used drugs for the treatment of angina pectoris are summarized in Tables 243-4 through 243-6. Pharmacotherapy for IHD is designed to reduce the frequency of anginal episodes, myocardial infarction, and coronary death. There is a wealth of positive trial data to emphasize how important this medical management is when added to the health-promoting behaviors discussed above. To achieve maximum benefit from medical therapy for IHD, it is frequently necessary to combine agents from different classes and titrate the doses as guided by the individual profile of risk factors, symptoms, hemodynamic responses, and side effects.

NITRATES The organic nitrates are a valuable class of drugs in the management of angina pectoris (Table 243-4). Their major mechanisms of action include systemic venodilation with

TABLE 243-4 Nitroglycerin and Nitrates for Patients With Ischemic Heart Disease

Compound	Route	Dose	Duration of Effect
Nitroglycerin	Sublingual tablets	0.3–0.6 mg up to 1.5 mg	Approximately 10 min
	Spray	0.4 mg as needed	Similar to sublingual tablets
	Ointment	2% 6 × 6 in. 15 ×15 cm 7.5–40 mg	Effect up to 7 h
	Transdermal	0.2–0.8 mg/h every 12 h	8–12 h during intermittent therapy
	Oral sustained release	2.5–13 mg	4–8 h
	Intravenous	5–200 mcg/min	Tolerance may be seen in 7–8 h
Isosorbide dinitrate	Sublingual	2.5–10 mg	Up to 60 min
	Oral	5–80 mg, 2–3 times daily	Up to 8 h
	Spray	1.25 mg daily	2–3 min
	Chewable	5 mg	2–2 ½ h
	Oral slow release	40 mg 1–2 daily	Up to 8 h
	Intravenous	1.25–5.0 mg/h	Tolerance in 7–8 h
	Ointment	100 mg/24 h	Not effective
Isosorbide mononitrate	Oral	20 mg twice daily 60–240 mg once daily	12–24 h
Pentaerythritol tetranitrate	Sublingual	10 mg as needed	Not known

Source: Modified from RJ Gibbons et al.

TABLE 243-5 Properties of Beta Blockers in Clinical Use for Ischemic Heart Disease

Drugs	Selectivity	Partial Agonist Activity	Usual Dose for Angina
Acebutolol	β1	Yes	200–600 mg twice daily
Atenolol	β1	No	50–200 mg/d
Betaxolol	β1	No	10–20 mg/d
Bisoprolol	β1	No	10 mg/d
Esmolol (intravenous)[a]	β1	No	50–300 mcg/kg/min
Labetalol[b]	None	Yes	200–600 mg twice daily
Metoprolol	β1	No	50–200 mg twice daily
Nadolol	None	No	40–80 mg/day
Nebivolol	β1 (at low doses)	No	5–40 mg/day
Pindolol	None	Yes	2.5–7.5 mg 3 times daily
Propranolol	None	No	80–120 mg twice daily
Timolol	None	No	10 mg twice daily

Note: This list of beta blockers that may be used to treat patients with angina pectoris is arranged alphabetically. The agents for which there is the greatest clinical experience include atenolol, metoprolol, and propranolol. It is preferable to use a sustained-release formulation that may be taken once daily to improve the patient's compliance with the regimen.

[a]Esmolol is an ultra-short-acting beta blocker that is administered as a continuous intravenous infusion. Its rapid offset of action makes esmolol an attractive agent to use in patients with relative contraindications to beta blockade.

[b]Labetolol is a combined alpha and beta blocker.

Source: Modified from RJ Gibbons et al.

TABLE 243-6 Calcium Channel Blockers in Clinical Use for Ischemic Heart Disease

Drugs	Usual Dose	Duration of Action	Side Effects
Dihydropyridines			
Amlodipine	5–10 mg qd	Long	Headache, edema
Felodipine	5–10 mg qd	Long	Headache, edema
Isradipine	2.5–10 mg bid	Medium	Headache, fatigue
Nicardipine	20–40 mg tid	Short	Headache, dizziness, flushing, edema
Nifedipine	Immediate release:* 30–90 mg daily orally	Short	Hypotension, dizziness, flushing, nausea, constipation, edema
	Slow release: 30–180 mg orally		
Nisoldipine	20–40 mg qd	Short	Similar to nifedipine
Nondihydropyridines			
Diltiazem	Immediate release: 30–80 mg 4 times daily	Short	Hypotension, dizziness, flushing, bradycardia, edema
	Slow release: 120–320 mg qd	Long	
Verapamil	Immediate release: 80–160 mg tid	Short	Hypotension, myocardial depression, heart failure, edema, bradycardia
	Slow release: 120–480 mg qd	Long	

Note: This list of calcium channel blockers that may be used to treat patients with angina pectoris is divided into two broad classes, dihydropyridines and nondihydropyridines, and arranged alphabetically within each class. Among the dihydropyridines, the greatest clinical experience has been obtained with amlodipine and nifedipine. After the initial period of dose titration with a short-acting formulation, it is preferable to switch to a sustained-release formulation that may be taken once daily to improve patient compliance with the regimen.

*May be associated with increased risk of mortality if administered during acute myocardial infarction.

Source: Modified from RJ Gibbons et al.

concomitant reduction in left ventricular end-diastolic volume and pressure, thereby reducing myocardial wall tension and oxygen requirements; dilation of epicardial coronary vessels; and increased blood flow in collateral vessels. When metabolized, organic nitrates release nitric oxide (NO) that binds to guanylyl cyclase in vascular smooth muscle cells, leading to an increase in cyclic guanosine monophosphate, which causes relaxation of vascular smooth muscle. Nitrates also exert antithrombotic activity by NO-dependent activation of platelet guanylyl cyclase, impairment of intraplatelet calcium flux, and platelet activation.

The absorption of these agents is most rapid and complete through the mucous membranes. For this reason, nitroglycerin is most commonly administered sublingually in tablets of 0.4 or 0.6 mg. Patients with angina should be instructed to take the medication both to relieve angina and also approximately 5 min before stress that is likely to induce an episode. The value of this prophylactic use of the drug cannot be overemphasized.

Nitrates improve exercise tolerance in patients with chronic angina and relieve ischemia in patients with unstable angina as well as patients with Prinzmetal's variant angina (Chap. 244). A diary of angina and nitroglycerin use may be valuable for detecting changes in the frequency, severity, or threshold for discomfort that may signify the development of unstable angina pectoris and/or herald an impending myocardial infarction.

Long-Acting Nitrates None of the long-acting nitrates are as effective as sublingual nitroglycerin for the acute relief of angina. These organic nitrate preparations can be swallowed, chewed, or administered as a patch or paste by the transdermal route (Table 243-4). They can provide effective plasma levels for up to 24 h, but the therapeutic response is highly variable. Different preparations and/or administration during the daytime should be tried only to prevent discomfort while avoiding side effects such as headache and dizziness. Individual dose titration is important to prevent side effects. To minimize the effects of tolerance, the minimum effective dose should be used and a minimum of 8 h each day kept free of the drug to restore any useful response(s).

β-Adrenergic Blockers These drugs represent an important component of the pharmacologic treatment of angina pectoris (Table 243-5). They reduce myocardial oxygen demand by inhibiting the increases in heart rate, arterial pressure, and myocardial contractility caused by adrenergic activation. Beta blockade reduces these variables most strikingly during exercise but causes only small reductions at rest. Long-acting beta-blocking drugs or sustained-release formulations offer the advantage of once-daily dosing (Table 243-5). The therapeutic aims include relief of angina and ischemia. These drugs also can reduce mortality and reinfarction rates in patients after myocardial infarction and are moderately effective antihypertensive agents.

Relative contraindications include asthma and reversible airway obstruction in patients with chronic lung disease, atrioventricular conduction disturbances, severe bradycardia, Raynaud's phenomenon, and a history of mental depression. Side effects include fatigue, reduced exercise tolerance, nightmares, impotence, cold extremities, intermittent claudication, bradycardia (sometimes severe), impaired atrioventricular conduction, left ventricular failure, bronchial asthma, worsening claudication, and intensification of the hypoglycemia produced by oral hypoglycemic agents and insulin. Reducing the dose or even discontinuation may be necessary if these side effects develop and persist. Since sudden discontinuation can intensify ischemia, the doses should be tapered over 2 weeks. Beta blockers with relative β_1-receptor specificity such as metoprolol and atenolol may be preferable in patients with mild bronchial obstruction and insulin-requiring diabetes mellitus.

Calcium Channel Blockers Calcium channel blockers (Table 243-6) are coronary vasodilators that produce variable and dose-dependent reductions in myocardial oxygen demand, contractility, and arterial pressure. These combined pharmacologic effects are advantageous and make these agents as effective as beta blockers in the treatment of angina pectoris. They are indicated when beta blockers are contraindicated, poorly tolerated, or ineffective. Verapamil and diltiazem may produce symptomatic disturbances in cardiac conduction and bradyarrhythmias. They also exert negative inotropic actions and are more likely to aggravate left ventricular failure, particularly when used in patients with left ventricular dysfunction, especially if the patients are also receiving beta blockers. Although useful effects usually are achieved when calcium channel blockers are combined with beta blockers and nitrates, individual titration of the doses is essential with these combinations. Variant (Prinzmetal's) angina responds particularly well to calcium channel blockers (especially members of the dihydropyridine class), supplemented when necessary by nitrates (Chap. 244).

Verapamil ordinarily should not be combined with beta blockers because of the combined adverse effects on heart rate and contractility. Diltiazem can be combined with beta blockers in patients with normal ventricular function and no conduction disturbances. Amlodipine and beta blockers have complementary actions on coronary blood supply and myocardial oxygen demands. Whereas the former decreases blood pressure and dilates coronary arteries, the latter slows heart rate and decreases contractility. Amlodipine and the other second-generation dihydropyridine calcium antagonists (nicardipine, isradipine, long-acting nifedipine, and felodipine) are potent vasodilators and are useful in the simultaneous treatment of angina and hypertension. Short-acting dihydropyridines should be avoided because of the risk of precipitating infarction, particularly in the absence of concomitant beta-blocker therapy.

Choice Between Beta Blockers and Calcium Channel Blockers for Initial Therapy Since beta blockers have been shown to improve life expectancy after acute myocardial infarction (Chaps. 244 and 245) and calcium channel blockers have not, the former may also be preferable in patients with angina and a damaged left ventricle. However, calcium channel blockers are indicated in patients with the following: (1) inadequate responsiveness to the combination of beta blockers and nitrates; many of these patients do well with a combination of a beta blocker and a dihydropyridine calcium channel blocker, (2) adverse reactions to beta blockers such as depression, sexual disturbances, and fatigue, (3) angina and a history of asthma or chronic obstructive pulmonary disease, (4) sick-sinus syndrome or significant atrioventricular conduction disturbances, (5) Prinzmetal's angina, or (6) symptomatic peripheral arterial disease.

Antiplatelet Drugs Aspirin is an irreversible inhibitor of platelet cyclooxygenase and thereby interferes with platelet activation. Chronic administration of 75–325 mg orally per day has been shown to reduce coronary events in asymptomatic adult men over age 50, patients with chronic stable angina, and patients who have or have survived unstable angina and myocardial infarction. There is a dose-dependent increase in bleeding when aspirin is used chronically. It is preferable to use an enteric-coated formulation in the range of 81-162 mg/d. Administration of this drug should be considered in all patients with IHD in the absence of gastrointestinal bleeding, allergy, or dyspepsia.

Clopidogrel (300–600 mg loading and 75 mg/d) is an oral agent that blocks P2Y12 ADP receptor–mediated platelet aggregation. It provides benefits similar to those of aspirin in patients with stable chronic IHD and may be substituted for aspirin if aspirin causes the side effects listed above. Clopidogrel combined with aspirin reduces death and coronary ischemic events in patients with an acute coronary syndrome (Chap. 244) and also reduces the risk of thrombus formation in patients undergoing implantation of a stent in a coronary artery (Chap. 246). Alternative antiplatelet agents that block the P2Y12 platelet receptor such as prasugrel have been shown to be more effective than clopidogrel for prevention of ischemic events after placement of a stent for an acute coronary syndrome but are associated with an increased risk of bleeding. Although combined treatment with clopidogrel and aspirin for at least a year is recommended in patients with an acute coronary syndrome treated with implantation of a drug-eluting stent, studies have not shown any benefit from the routine addition of clopidogrel to aspirin in patients with chronic stable IHD.

OTHER THERAPIES The angiotensin-converting enzyme (ACE) inhibitors are widely used in the treatment of survivors of myocardial infarction, patients with hypertension or chronic IHD including angina pectoris, and those at high risk of vascular diseases such as diabetes. The benefits of ACE inhibitors are most evident in IHD patients at increased risk, especially if diabetes mellitus or LV dysfunction is present, and those who have not achieved adequate control of blood pressure and LDL cholesterol on beta blockers and statins. However, the routine administration of ACE inhibitors to IHD patients who have normal LV function and have achieved blood pressure and LDL goals on other therapies does not reduce the incidence of events and therefore is not cost-effective.

Despite treatment with nitrates, beta blockers, or calcium channel blockers, some patients with IHD continue to experience angina, and additional medical therapy is now available to alleviate their symptoms. Ranolazine, a piperazine derivative, may be useful for patients with chronic angina despite standard medical therapy. Its antianginal action is believed to occur via inhibition of the late inward sodium current (I_{Na}). The benefits of I_{Na} inhibition include limitation of the Na overload of ischemic myocytes and prevention of Ca^{2+} overload via the Na^+–Ca^{2+} exchanger. A dose of 500–1000 mg orally twice daily is usually well tolerated. Ranolazine is contraindicated in patients with hepatic impairment or with conditions or drugs associated with QT_c prolongation and when drugs that inhibit the CYP3A metabolic system (e.g., ketoconazole, diltiazem, verapamil, macrolide antibiotics, HIV protease inhibitors, and large quantities of grapefruit juice) are being used.

Nonsteroidal anti-inflammatory drug (NSAID) use in patients with IHD may be associated with a small but finite increased risk of MI and mortality. For this reason, they generally should be avoided in IHD patients. If they are required for symptom relief, it is advisable to coadminister aspirin and strive to use the lowest NSAID dose required for the shortest period of time.

Another class of agents open ATP-sensitive potassium channels in myocytes, leading to a reduction of free intracellular calcium ions. The major drug in this class is nicorandil, which typically is administered orally in a dose of 20 mg twice daily for prevention of angina. (Nicorandil is not available for use in the United States but is used in several other countries.)

Angina and Heart Failure Transient left ventricular failure with angina can be controlled by the use of nitrates. For patients with established congestive heart failure the increased left ventricular wall tension raises myocardial oxygen demand. Treatment of congestive heart failure with an angiotensin-converting enzyme inhibitor, a diuretic, and digoxin (Chap. 234) reduces heart size, wall tension, and myocardial oxygen demand, which helps control angina and ischemia. If the symptoms and signs of heart failure are controlled, an effort should be made to use beta blockers not only for angina but because trials in heart failure have shown significant improvement in survival. A trial of the intravenous ultra-short-acting beta blocker esmolol may be useful to establish the safety of beta blockade in selected patients. Nocturnal angina often can be relieved by the treatment of heart failure.

The combination of congestive heart failure and angina in patients with IHD usually indicates a poor prognosis and warrants serious consideration of cardiac catheterization and coronary revascularization.

CORONARY REVASCULARIZATION

Clinical trials have confirmed that with the initial diagnosis of stable IHD, it is first appropriate to initiate a thorough medical regimen as described above. Revascularization should be considered in the presence of unstable phases of the disease, intractable symptoms, severe ischemia or high-risk coronary anatomy, diabetes, and impaired LV function. *Revascularization should be employed in conjunction with but not replace the continuing need to modify risk factors and assess medical therapy.* An algorithm for integrating medical therapy and revascularization options in patients with IHD is shown in Fig. 243-2.

PERCUTANEOUS CORONARY INTERVENTION

(See also Chap. 246) Percutaneous coronary intervention (PCI) involving balloon dilatation usually accompanied by coronary stenting is widely used to achieve revascularization of the myocardium in patients with symptomatic IHD and suitable stenoses of epicardial coronary arteries. Whereas patients with stenosis of the left main coronary artery and those with three-vessel IHD (especially with diabetes and/or impaired left ventricular function) who require revascularization are best treated with CABG, PCI is widely employed in patients with symptoms and evidence of ischemia due to stenoses of one or two vessels and even in selected patients with three-vessel disease (and, perhaps, in some patients with left main disease) and may offer many advantages over surgery.

Indications and patient selection

The most common clinical indication for PCI is symptom-limiting angina pectoris, despite medical therapy, accompanied by evidence of ischemia during a stress test. PCI is more effective than medical therapy for the relief of angina. PCI improves outcomes in patients with unstable angina or when used early in the course of myocardial infarction with and without cardiogenic shock. However, in patients with stable exertional angina, clinical trials have confirmed that PCI does not reduce the occurrence of death or myocardial infarction compared to optimum medical therapy. PCI can be used to treat stenoses in native coronary arteries as well as in bypass grafts in patients who have recurrent angina after CABG.

Risks

When coronary stenoses are discrete and symmetric, two and even three vessels can be treated in sequence. However, case selection is essential to avoid a prohibitive risk of complications, which are usually due to dissection or thrombosis with vessel occlusion, uncontrolled ischemia, and ventricular failure (Chap. 246). Oral aspirin, a thienopyridine, and an antithrombin agent are given to reduce coronary thrombus formation. Left main coronary artery stenosis

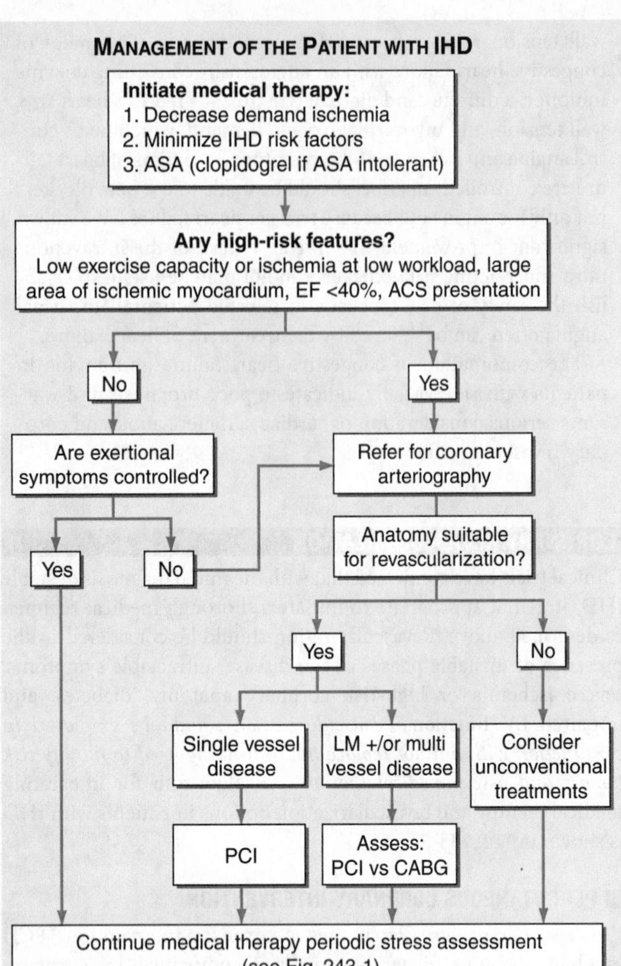

Figure 243-2 Algorithm for management of a patient with ischemic heart disease. All patients should receive the core elements of medical therapy as shown at the top of the algorithm. If high-risk features are present, as established by the clinical history, exercise test data, and imaging studies, the patient should be referred for coronary arteriography. Based on the number and location of the diseased vessels and their suitability for revascularization, the patient is treated with a percutaneous coronary intervention (PCI) or coronary artery bypass graft (CABG) surgery or should be considered for unconventional treatments. See text for further discussion. IHD, ischemic heart disease; ASA, aspirin; EF, ejection fraction; ACS, acute coronary syndrome; LM, left main.

generally is regarded as a contraindication to PCI; such patients should be treated with CABG. In selected cases such as patients with prohibitive surgical risks, PCI of an unprotected left main can be considered, but such a procedure should be performed only by a highly skilled operator; importantly, there are regional differences in the use of this approach internationally.

Efficacy

Primary success, i.e., adequate dilation (an increase in luminal diameter >20% to a residual diameter obstruction <50%) with relief of angina, is achieved in >95% of cases. Recurrent stenosis of the dilated vessels occurs in ~20% of cases within 6 months of PCI with bare metal stents, and angina will recur within 6 months in 10% of cases. Restenosis is more common in patients with diabetes mellitus, arteries with small caliber, incomplete dilation of the stenosis, long stents, occluded vessels, obstructed vein grafts, dilation of the left anterior descending coronary artery, and stenoses containing thrombi. In diseased vein grafts, procedural success has been improved by the use of capture devices or filters that prevent embolization, ischemia, and infarction.

It is usual clinical practice to administer aspirin indefinitely and a thienopyridine for 1–3 months after the implantation of a bare metal stent. Although aspirin in combination with a thienopyridine may help prevent coronary thrombosis during and shortly after PCI with stenting, there is no evidence that these medications reduce the incidence of restenosis.

The use of drug-eluting stents that locally deliver antiproliferative drugs can reduce restenosis to less than 10%. Advances in PCI, especially the availability of drug-eluting stents, have vastly extended the use of this revascularization option in patients with IHD. Of note, however, the delayed endothelial healing in the region of a drug-eluting stent also extends the period during which the patient is at risk for subacute stent thrombosis. Current recommendations are to administer aspirin indefinitely and a thienopyridine daily for at least one year after implantation of a drug-eluting stent. When a situation arises in which temporary discontinuation of antiplatelet therapy is necessary, the clinical circumstances should be reviewed with the operator who performed the PCI and a coordinated plan should be established for minimizing the risk of late stent thrombus; central to this plan is the discontinuation of antiplatelet therapy for the shortest acceptable period. The risk of stent thrombosis is dependent on stent size and length, complexity of the lesions, age, diabetes, and technique. However, compliance with dual antiplatelet therapy and individual responsiveness to platelet inhibition are very important factors as well.

Successful PCI produces effective relief of angina in >95% of cases. More than one-half of patients with symptomatic IHD who require revascularization can be treated initially by PCI. Successful PCI is less invasive and expensive than CABG and permits savings in the *initial* cost of care. Successful PCI avoids the risk of stroke associated with CABG surgery, allows earlier return to work, and allows the resumption of an active life. However, the early health-related and economic benefit of PCI is reduced over time because of the greater need for follow-up and the increased need for repeat procedures. When directly compared in patients with diabetes or three-vessel or left main coronary artery disease, CABG was superior to PCI in preventing major adverse cardiac or cerebrovascular events over a 12-month follow-up.

■ CORONARY ARTERY BYPASS GRAFTING

Anastomosis of one or both of the internal mammary arteries or a radial artery to the coronary artery distal to the obstructive lesion is the preferred procedure. For additional obstructions that cannot be bypassed by an artery, a section of a vein (usually the saphenous) is used to form a connection between the aorta and the coronary artery distal to the obstructive lesion.

Although some indications for CABG are controversial, certain areas of agreement exist:

1. The operation is relatively safe, with mortality rates <1% in patients without serious comorbid disease and normal left ventricular function and when the procedure is performed by an experienced surgical team.
2. Intraoperative and postoperative mortality rates increase with the severity of ventricular dysfunction, comorbidities, age >80 years, and lack of surgical experience. The effectiveness and risk of CABG vary widely depending on case selection and the skill and experience of the surgical team.
3. Occlusion of *venous* grafts is observed in 10 to 20% of patients during the first postoperative year and in approximately 2% per year during 5- to 7-year follow-up and 4% per year thereafter. Long-term patency rates are considerably higher for internal

mammary and radial artery implantations than for saphenous vein grafts. In patients with left anterior descending coronary artery obstruction, survival is better when coronary bypass involves the internal mammary artery rather than a saphenous vein. Graft patency and outcomes are improved by meticulous treatment of risk factors, particularly dyslipidemia.

4. Angina is abolished or greatly reduced in ~90% of patients after complete revascularization. Although this usually is associated with graft patency and restoration of blood flow, the pain may also have been alleviated as a result of infarction of the ischemic segment or a placebo effect. Within 3 years, angina recurs in about one-fourth of patients but is rarely severe.
5. Survival may be improved by operation in patients with stenosis of the left main coronary artery as well as in patients with three- or two-vessel disease with significant obstruction of the proximal left anterior descending coronary artery. The survival benefit is greater in patients with abnormal LV function (ejection fraction <50%). Survival *may* also be improved in the following patients: (a) with obstructive CAD who have survived sudden cardiac death or sustained ventricular tachycardia, (b) who have undergone previous CABG and have multiple saphenous vein graft stenoses, especially of a graft supplying the left anterior descending coronary artery, and (c) with recurrent stenosis after PCI and high-risk criteria on noninvasive testing.
6. Minimally invasive CABG through a small thoracotomy and/or off-pump surgery can reduce morbidity and shorten convalescence in suitable patients but does not appear to reduce significantly the risk of neurocognitive dysfunction postoperatively.
7. Among patients with type 2 diabetes mellitus and multivessel coronary disease, CABG surgery plus optimal medical therapy is superior to optimal medical therapy alone in preventing major cardiovascular events, a benefit mediated largely by a significant reduction in nonfatal MI. The benefits of CABG are especially evident in diabetic patients treated with an insulin-sensitizing strategy as opposed to an insulin-providing strategy.

Indications for CABG usually are based on the severity of symptoms, coronary anatomy, and ventricular function. The ideal candidate is male, is <80 years of age, has no other complicating disease, and has troublesome or disabling angina that is not adequately controlled by medical therapy or does not tolerate medical therapy. The patient wishes to lead a more active life and has severe stenoses of two or three epicardial coronary arteries with objective evidence of myocardial ischemia as a cause of the chest discomfort. Great symptomatic benefit can be anticipated in such patients. Congestive heart failure and/or left ventricular dysfunction, advanced age (>80 years), reoperation, urgent need for surgery, and the presence of diabetes mellitus are all associated with a higher perioperative mortality rate.

Left ventricular dysfunction can be due to noncontractile or hypocontractile segments that are viable but are chronically ischemic (hibernating myocardium). As a consequence of chronic reduction in myocardial blood flow, these segments downregulate their contractile function. They can be detected by using radionuclide scans of myocardial perfusion and metabolism, PET, cardiac MRI, or delayed scanning with thallium-201 or by improvement of regional functional impairment provoked by low-dose dobutamine. In such patients, revascularization improves myocardial blood flow, can return function, and can improve survival.

The choice between PCI and CABG

All the clinical characteristics of each individual patient must be used to decide on the method of revascularization (LV function, diabetes, lesion complexity, etc). A number of randomized clinical trials have compared PCI and CABG in patients with multivessel CAD who were suitable technically for both procedures. The redevelopment of angina requiring repeat coronary angiography and repeat revascularization is higher with PCI. This is a result of restenosis in the stented segment (a problem largely solved with drug-eluting stents) and the development of new stenoses in unstented portions of the coronary vasculature. It has been argued that PCI with stenting focuses on culprit lesions whereas a bypass graft to the target vessel also provides a conduit around future culprit lesions proximal to the anastomosis of the graft to the native vessel (Fig. 243-3). By contrast, stroke rates are lower with PCI.

Comparison of mortality rates in patients treated with CABG versus PCI is a complex issue. There is an early increased risk of mortality with CABG, but mortality rates appear similar in the two revascularization strategies over the long term.

Based on available evidence, it is now recommended that patients with an unacceptable level of angina despite optimal medical management be considered for coronary revascularization. Patients with single- or two-vessel disease with normal LV function and anatomically suitable lesions ordinarily are advised to undergo PCI (Chap. 246). Patients with three-vessel disease (or two-vessel disease that includes the proximal left descending coronary artery) and impaired global LV function (LV ejection fraction < 50%) or diabetes mellitus and those with left main coronary artery disease or other lesions unsuitable for catheter-based procedures should be considered for CABG as the initial method of revascularization. In light of the complexity of the decision making, it is desirable to have a multidisciplinary team, including a cardiologist and a cardiac surgeon in conjunction with the patient's primary care physician, provide input in conjunction with ascertaining the patient's preferences before committing to a particular revascularization option.

UNCONVENTIONAL TREATMENTS FOR IHD

On occasion clinicians will encounter a patient who has persistent disabling angina despite maximally tolerated medical therapy and for whom revascularization is not an option (e.g., small diffusely diseased vessels not amenable to stent implantation or acceptable targets for bypass grafting). In such situations unconventional treatments should be considered.

Enhanced external counterpulsation utilizes pneumatic cuffs on the lower extremities to provide diastolic augmentation and systolic unloading of blood pressure to decrease cardiac work and oxygen consumption while enhancing coronary blood flow. Clinical trials have shown that regular application improves angina, exercise capacity, and regional myocardial perfusion. Experimental approaches such as gene and stem cell therapies are also under active study.

ASYMPTOMATIC (SILENT) ISCHEMIA

Obstructive CAD, acute myocardial infarction, and transient myocardial ischemia are frequently asymptomatic. During continuous ambulatory ECG monitoring, the majority of ambulatory patients with typical chronic stable angina are found to have objective evidence of myocardial ischemia (ST-segment depression) during episodes of chest discomfort while they are active outside the hospital. In addition, many of these patients also have more frequent episodes of asymptomatic ischemia. Frequent episodes of ischemia (symptomatic and asymptomatic) during daily life appear to be associated with an increased likelihood of adverse coronary events (death and myocardial infarction). In addition, patients with asymptomatic ischemia after a myocardial infarction are at greater risk for a second coronary event. The widespread use of exercise ECG during

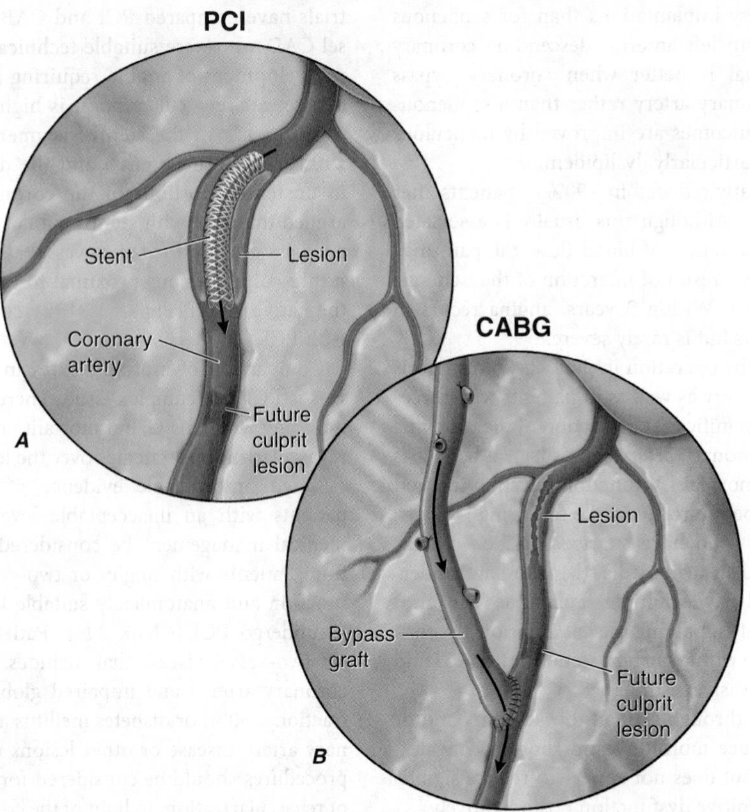

Figure 243-3 Difference in the approach to the lesion with percutaneous coronary intervention (PCI) and coronary artery bypass grafting (CABG). PCI is targeted at the "culprit" lesion or lesions, whereas CABG is directed at the epicardial vessel, including the culprit lesion or lesions and future culprits, proximal to the insertion of the vein graft, a difference that may account for the superiority of CABG, at least in the intermediate term, in patients with multivessel disease. *(Reproduced from BJ Gersh et al: N Engl J Med 352:2235, 2005.)*

routine examinations has also identified some of these previously unrecognized patients with asymptomatic CAD. Longitudinal studies have demonstrated an increased incidence of coronary events in asymptomatic patients with positive exercise tests.

TREATMENT Asymptomatic Ischemia

The management of patients with asymptomatic ischemia must be individualized. When coronary disease has been confirmed, the aggressive treatment of hypertension and dyslipidemia is essential and will decrease the risk of infarction and death. In addition, the physician should consider the following: (1) the degree of positivity of the stress test, particularly the stage of exercise at which ECG signs of ischemia appear; the magnitude and number of the ischemic zones of myocardium on imaging; and the change in LV ejection fraction that occurs on radionuclide ventriculography or echocardiography during ischemia and/or during exercise, (2) the ECG leads showing a positive response, with changes in the anterior precordial leads indicating a less favorable prognosis than changes in the inferior leads, and (3) the patient's age, occupation, and general medical condition.

Most would agree that an asymptomatic 45-year-old commercial airline pilot with significant (0.4-mV) ST-segment depression in leads V_1 to V_4 during mild exercise should undergo coronary arteriography, whereas an asymptomatic, sedentary 85-year-old retiree with 0.1-mV ST-segment depression in leads II and III during maximal activity need not. However, there is no consensus about the most appropriate approach in the large majority of patients for whom the situation is less extreme. Asymptomatic patients with silent ischemia, three-vessel CAD, and impaired LV function may be considered appropriate candidates for CABG.

The treatment of risk factors, particularly lipid lowering and blood pressure control as described above, and the use of aspirin, statins, and beta blockers after infarction have been shown to reduce events and improve outcomes in asymptomatic as well as symptomatic patients with ischemia and proven CAD. Although the incidence of asymptomatic ischemia can be reduced by treatment with beta blockers, calcium channel blockers, and long-acting nitrates, it is not clear whether this is necessary or desirable in patients who have not had a myocardial infarction.

FURTHER READINGS

Antman EM et al: Cyclooxygenase inhibition and cardiovascular risk. Circulation 112:759, 2005

Bhatt DL et al: Clopidogrel and aspirin versus aspirin alone for the prevention of atherothrombotic events. N Engl J Med 354:1706, 2006

Boden WE et al: Optimal medical therapy with or without PCI for stable coronary disease. N Engl J Med 356:1503, 2007

Chaitman BR: Ranolazine for the treatment of chronic angina and potential use in other cardiovascular conditions. Circulation 113:2462, 2006

Cleeman JI et al: Executive summary of the Third Report of the National Cholesterol Education Program (NCEP) Expert Panel on Detection, Evaluation, and Treatment of High Blood Cholesterol in Adults (Adult Treatment Panel III). JAMA 285:2486, 2001

DeFeyter PJ et al: Bypass surgery versus stenting for the treatment of multivessel disease in patients with unstable angina compared with stable angina. Circulation 105:2367, 2002

Frye RL et al: A randomized trial of therapies for type 2 diabetes and coronary artery disease. N Engl J Med 360:2503, 2009

Gibbons RJ et al: ACC/AHA 2002 guideline update for the management of patients with chronic stable angina: A report of the American College of Cardiology/American Heart Association Task Force on Practice Guidelines (Committee to Update the 1999 Guidelines for the Management of Patients with Chronic Stable Angina. J Am Coll Cardiol 41:159, 2002

Goldschmidt-Clermont PJ et al: Atherosclerosis 2005: Recent discoveries and novel hypotheses. Circulation 112:3348, 2005

Kim MC et al: Refractory angina pectoris: Mechanism and therapeutic options. J Am Coll Cardiol 39:923, 2002

Kushner FG et al: 2009 Focused Updates: ACC/AHA Guidelines for the Management of Patients With ST-Elevation Myocardial Infarction (updating the 2004 Guideline and 2007 Focused Update) and ACC/AHA/SCAI Guidelines on Percutaneous Coronary Intervention (updating the 2005 Guideline and 2007 Focused Update): A report of the American College of Cardiology Foundation/American Heart Association Task Force on Practice Guidelines. Circulation 120:2271, 2009

Lee TH et al: Noninvasive tests in patients with stable coronary artery disease. N Engl J Med 344:1840, 2001

Marasco SF et al: No improvement in neurocognitive outcomes after off-pump versus on-pump coronary revascularisation: A meta-analysis. Eur J Cardiothorac Surg 33:961, 2008

McQueen MJ et al: Lipids, lipoproteins, and apolipoproteins as risk markers of myocardial infarction in 52 countries (the INTERHEART study): A case-control study. Lancet 372:224, 2008

Mega JL et al: Cytochrome p-450 polymorphisms and response to clopidogrel. N Engl J Med 360:354, 2009

Morrow D et al: Chronic coronary artery disease, in *Braunwald's Heart Disease*, 8th ed, P Libby et al (eds). Philadelphia, Saunders, 2008

Opie LH et al: Controversies in stable coronary artery disease. Lancet 367:69, 2006

Pretre R et al: Choice of revascularization strategy for patients with coronary artery disease. JAMA 285:992, 2001

Serruys PW et al. Percutaneous coronary intervention versus coronary-artery bypass grafting for severe coronary artery disease. N Engl J Med 360:961, 2009

Van Den Brand MJBM et al: The effect of completeness of revascularization on event-free survival at one year in the ARTS trial. J Am Coll Cardiol 39:559, 2002

Weintraub WS et al: Predicting cardiovascular events with coronary calcium scoring. N Engl J Med 358:1394, 2008

CHAPTER 244

Unstable Angina and Non-ST-Segment Elevation Myocardial Infarction

Christopher P. Cannon
Eugene Braunwald

Patients with ischemic heart disease fall into two large groups: patients with chronic coronary artery disease (CAD) who most commonly present with stable angina (Chap. 243) and patients with acute coronary syndromes (ACSs). The latter group, in turn, is composed of patients with acute myocardial infarction (MI) with ST-segment elevation on their presenting electrocardiogram (ECG) (STEMI; Chap. 245) and those with unstable angina (UA) and non-ST-segment elevation MI (UA/NSTEMI; Fig. 245-1). Every year in the United States, approximately 1 million patients are admitted to hospitals with UA/NSTEMI as compared with ~300,000 patients with acute STEMI. The relative incidence of UA/NSTEMI compared to STEMI appears to be increasing. More than one-third of patients with UA/NSTEMI are women, while less than one-fourth of patients with STEMI are women.

DEFINITION

The diagnosis of UA is based largely on the clinical presentation. *Stable* angina pectoris is characterized by chest or arm discomfort that may not be described as pain but is reproducibly associated with physical exertion or stress and is relieved within 5–10 minutes by rest and/or sublingual nitroglycerin (Chaps. 12 and 343). UA is defined as angina pectoris or equivalent ischemic discomfort with at least one of three features: (1) it occurs at rest (or with minimal exertion), usually lasting >10 minutes; (2) it is severe and of new onset (i.e., within the prior 4–6 weeks); and/or (3) it occurs with a crescendo pattern (i.e., distinctly more severe, prolonged, or frequent than previously). The diagnosis of NSTEMI is established if a patient with the clinical features of UA develops evidence of myocardial necrosis, as reflected in elevated cardiac biomarkers.

PATHOPHYSIOLOGY

UA/NSTEMI is most commonly caused by a reduction in oxygen supply and/or by an increase in myocardial oxygen demand superimposed on a lesion that causes coronary arterial obstruction, usually an atherothrombotic coronary plaque. Four pathophysiologic processes that may contribute to the development of UA/NSTEMI have been identified: (1) plaque rupture or erosion with a superimposed nonocclusive thrombus, believed to be the most common cause; in such patients, NSTEMI may occur with downstream embolization of platelet aggregates and/or atherosclerotic debris; (2) dynamic obstruction [e.g., coronary spasm, as in Prinzmetal's variant angina (PVA) (p. 2020)]; (3) progressive mechanical obstruction [e.g., rapidly advancing coronary atherosclerosis or restenosis following percutaneous coronary intervention (PCI)]; and (4) UA secondary to increased myocardial oxygen demand and/or decreased supply (e.g., tachycardia, anemia). More than one of these processes may be involved.

Among patients with UA/NSTEMI studied at angiography, approximately 5% have stenosis of the left main coronary artery, 15% have three-vessel CAD, 30% have two-vessel disease, 40% have single-vessel disease, and 10% have no apparent critical epicardial coronary artery stenosis; some of the latter may have obstruction of the coronary microcirculation. The "culprit lesion" may show an eccentric stenosis with scalloped or overhanging edges and a narrow neck on angiography. Angioscopy has been reported to show "white" (platelet-rich) thrombi, as opposed to "red" (fibrin- and cell-rich) thrombi; the latter are more often seen in patients with acute STEMI. Patients with UA/NSTEMI frequently have multiple plaques at risk of disruption (vulnerable plaques).

CLINICAL PRESENTATION

History and physical examination

The clinical hallmark of UA/NSTEMI is chest pain, typically located in the substernal region or sometimes in the epigastrium, that radiates to the neck, left shoulder, and/or the left arm (Chap. 12). This discomfort is usually severe enough to be described as frank pain. Anginal "equivalents" such as dyspnea and epigastric discomfort may also occur, and these appear to be more frequent in women. The physical examination resembles that in patients with stable angina (Chap. 243) and may be unremarkable. If the patient has a large area of myocardial ischemia or a large NSTEMI, the physical findings can include diaphoresis; pale, cool skin; sinus tachycardia; a third and/or fourth heart sound; basilar rales; and, sometimes, hypotension, resembling the findings of large STEMI.

Electrocardiogram

In UA, ST-segment depression, transient ST-segment elevation, and/or T-wave inversion occur in 30 to 50% of patients. In patients with the clinical features of UA, the presence of new ST-segment deviation, even of only 0.05 mV, is an important predictor of adverse outcome. T-wave changes are sensitive for ischemia but less specific, unless they are new, deep T-wave inversions (≥0.3 mV).

Cardiac biomarkers

Patients with UA/NSTEMI who have elevated biomarkers of necrosis, such as CK-MB and troponin (a much more specific and sensitive marker of myocardial necrosis), are at increased risk for death or recurrent MI. Elevated levels of these markers distinguish patients with NSTEMI from those with UA. There is a direct relationship between the degree of troponin elevation and mortality. However, in patients *without* a clear clinical history of myocardial ischemia, minor troponin elevations have been reported and can be caused by congestive heart failure (CHF), myocarditis, or pulmonary embolism, or they may be false-positive readings. Thus, in patients with an *unclear* history, small troponin elevations may not be diagnostic of an ACS.

DIAGNOSTIC EVALUATION

(See also Chap. 12) Approximately six million persons per year in the United States present to hospital emergency departments (EDs) with a complaint of chest pain or other symptoms suggestive of ACS. A diagnosis of an ACS is established in 20 to 25% of such patients. The first step in evaluating patients with possible UA/NSTEMI is to determine the *likelihood* that CAD is the cause of the presenting symptoms. The American College of Cardiology/American Heart Association (ACC/AHA) Guidelines include, among the factors associated with a high likelihood of ACS, a prior history typical of stable angina, a history of established CAD by angiography, prior MI, CHF, new ECG changes, or elevated cardiac biomarkers.

Diagnostic pathways

Four major diagnostic tools are used in the diagnosis of UA/NSTEMI in the ED: clinical history, the ECG, cardiac markers, and stress testing (coronary imaging is an emerging option). The goals are to: (1) recognize or exclude MI (using cardiac markers), (2) evaluate for rest ischemia (using serial or continuous ECGs), and (3) evaluate for significant CAD (using provocative stress testing). Patients with a low likelihood of ischemia are usually managed with an ED-based critical pathway (which, in some institutions, is carried out in a "chest-pain unit" Fig. 244-1). Evaluation of such patients includes clinical monitoring for recurrent ischemic discomfort, serial ECGs, and cardiac markers, typically obtained at baseline and at 4–6 h and 12 h after presentation. If new elevations in cardiac markers or ECG changes are noted, the patient should be admitted to the hospital. If the patient remains pain free and the markers are negative, the patient may proceed to stress testing. CT angiography is used with increasing frequency to exclude obstructive CAD (Chap. 229).

RISK STRATIFICATION AND PROGNOSIS

Patients with documented UA/NSTEMI exhibit a wide spectrum of early (30 days) risk of death, ranging from 1 to 10%, and of new or recurrent infarction of 3–5% or recurrent ACS (5-15%). Assessment of risk can be accomplished by clinical risk scoring systems such as that developed from the Thrombolysis in Myocardial Infarction (TIMI) Trials, which includes seven independent risk factors: age ≥ 65 years, three or more risk factors for CAD, documented CAD at catheterization, development of UA/NSTEMI while on aspirin, more than two episodes of angina within the preceding 24 h, ST deviation ≥0.5 mm, and an elevated cardiac marker (Fig. 244-2). Other risk factors include diabetes mellitus, left ventricular dysfunction, renal dysfunction and elevated levels of brain natriuretic peptides and C-reactive protein. Multimarker strategies involving several biomarkers are now gaining favor, both to define more fully the pathophysiologic mechanisms underlying a given patient's presentation and to stratify the patient's risk further. Early risk assessment (especially using troponin, ST-segment changes, and/or a global risk-scoring system) is useful both in predicting the risk of recurrent cardiac events and in identifying those patients who would derive the greatest benefit from antithrombotic therapies more potent than unfractionated heparin, such as low molecular-weight heparin (LMWH) and glycoprotein IIb/IIIa inhibitors, and from an early invasive strategy. For example, in the TACTICS-TIMI 18 Trial, an early invasive strategy conferred a 40% reduction in recurrent cardiac events in patients with a positive troponin level, whereas no benefit was observed in those without detectable troponin.

TREATMENT Unstable Angina and Non-ST-Segment Elevation Myocardial Infarction

MEDICAL TREATMENT Patients with UA/NSTEMI should be placed at bed rest with continuous ECG monitoring for ST-segment deviation and cardiac arrhythmias. Ambulation is permitted if the patient shows no recurrence of ischemia (discomfort or ECG changes) and does not develop a biomarker of necrosis for 12–24 h. Medical therapy involves simultaneous anti-ischemic treatment and antithrombotic treatment.

ANTI-ISCHEMIC TREATMENT (Table 244-1) To provide relief and prevention of recurrence of chest pain, initial treatment should include bed rest, nitrates, and beta blockers.

Nitrates Nitrates should first be given sublingually or by buccal spray (0.3–0.6 mg) if the patient is experiencing ischemic pain.

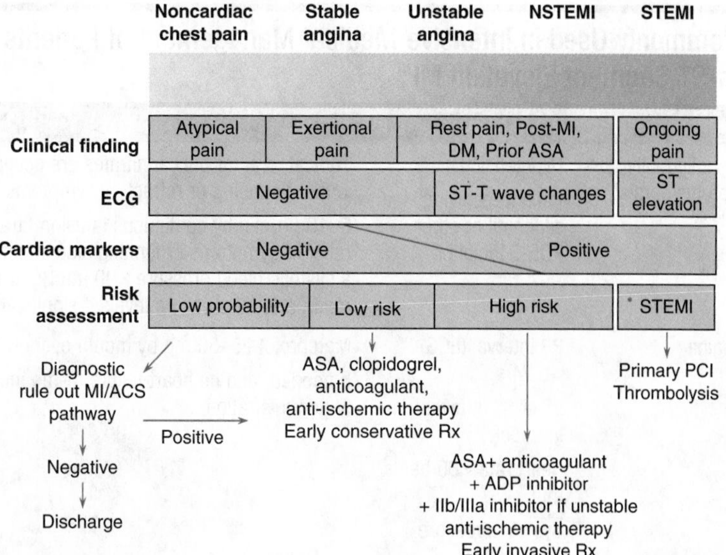

Figure 244-1 Algorithm for risk stratification and treatment of patients with suspected coronary artery disease. Using the clinical history of the type of pain and medical history, the ECG, and cardiac markers, one can identify patients who have a low likelihood of UA/NSTEMI, for whom a diagnostic "rule-out myocardial infarction (MI) or acute coronary syndrome (ACS)" is warranted. If this is negative, the patient may be discharged, but if positive, the patient is admitted and treated for UA/NSTEMI. On the other end of the spectrum, patients with acute ongoing pain and ST-segment elevation are treated with percutaneous coronary intervention (PCI) or fibrinolysis (Chap. 245). For those with UA/NSTEMI, risk stratification is used to identify patients at medium to high risk, for whom an early invasive strategy is warranted. Antithrombotic therapy should include aspirin, an anticoagulant, an ADP antagonist (clopidogrel or prasugrel), with GP IIb/IIIa inhibition considered for use during PCI. For patients at low risk, treatment with aspirin, clopidogrel, an anticoagulant such as unfractionated or low molecular–weight heparin (LMWH) or fondaparinux and anti-ischemic therapy with beta blockers and nitrates, and a conservative strategy are indicated. ASA, aspirin; DM, diabetes mellitus; ECG, electrocardiogram; MI, myocardial infarction; Rx, treatment; STEMI, ST-segment elevation myocardial infarction. *(Adapted from CP Cannon, E Braunwald, in Braunwald's Heart Disease: A Textbook of Cardiovascular Medicine, 9th ed, R Bonow et al (eds). Philadelphia, Saunders, 2011.)*

If pain persists after 3 doses given 5 min apart, intravenous nitroglycerin (5–10 μg/min using nonabsorbing tubing) is recommended. The rate of the infusion may be increased by 10 μg/min every 3–5 min until symptoms are relieved or systolic arterial pressure falls to <100 mmHg. Topical or oral nitrates (Chap. 243) can be used once the pain has resolved or they may replace intravenous nitroglycerin when the patient has been pain-free for 12–24 h. The only absolute contraindications to the use of nitrates are hypotension or the use of sildenafil or other drugs in that class within the previous 24–48 h.

Beta Adrenergic Blockers and Other Agents Beta blockers are the other mainstay of anti-ischemic treatment. Oral beta blockade targeted to a heart rate of 50–60 beats/min is recommended as first-line treatment. A caution has been raised in the new ACC/AHA guidelines for use of intravenous beta blockade in patients with any evidence of acute heart failure, where they could increase the risk of cardiogenic shock. Heart rate–slowing calcium channel blockers, e.g., verapamil or diltiazem, are recommended for patients who have persistent or recurrent symptoms after treatment with full-dose nitrates and beta blockers and in patients with contraindications to beta blockade. Additional medical therapy includes angiotensin-converting enzyme (ACE) inhibition and HMG-CoA reductase inhibitors (statins) for long-term secondary prevention. Early administration of intensive statin therapy (e.g., atorvastatin 80 mg) prior to percutaneous coronary intervention (PCI) has been shown to reduce complications, suggesting that high-dose statin therapy should be started at the time of admission.

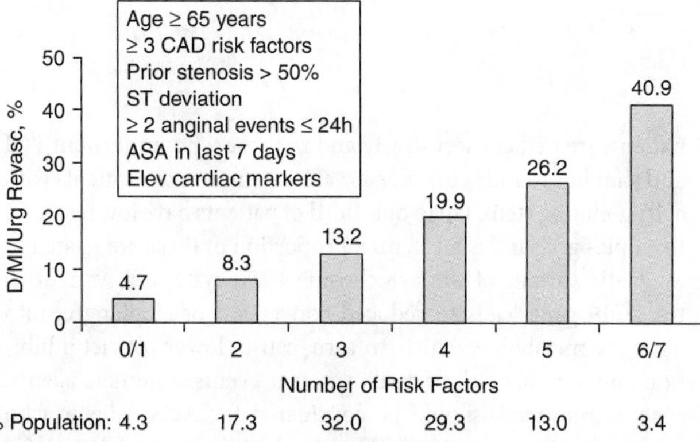

Figure 244-2 **The TIMI Risk Score for UA/NSTEMI,** a simple but comprehensive clinical risk stratification score to identify increasing risk of death, myocardial infarction, or urgent revascularization to day 14. CAD, coronary artery disease; ASA, aspirin. *(Adapted from Antman et al.)*

ANTITHROMBOTIC THERAPY (Table 244-2) This is the other main component of treatment for UA/NSTEMI. Initial treatment should begin with the platelet cyclooxygenase inhibitor aspirin (Fig. 244-3). The typical initial dose is 325 mg/d, with lower doses (75–162 mg/d) recommended for long-term therapy. The OASIS-7 trial randomized 25,087 ACS patients to receive high-dose (300–325 mg/d) vs. low-dose (75-100 mg/d) aspirin for 30 days and reported no differences in the risk of major bleeding or in efficacy over this period of time. "Aspirin resistance" has been noted in 5–10% of patients and more frequently in patients treated with lower doses of aspirin, but frequently has been related to noncompliance.

The thienopyridine, clopidogrel, an inactive prodrug that is converted into an active metabolite, which blocks the platelet $P2Y_{12}$ component or the adenosine diphosphate receptor, in

TABLE 244-1 Drugs Commonly Used in Intensive Medical Management of Patients With Unstable Angina and Non-ST Segment Elevation MI

Drug Category	Clinical Condition	When to Avoid[a]	Dosage
Nitrates	Administer sublingually, and, if symptoms persist, intravenously	Hypotension Patient receiving sildenafil or other PDE-5 inhibitor	Topical, oral, or buccal nitrates are acceptable alternatives for patients without ongoing or refractory symptoms 5–10 μg/min by continuous infusion titrated up to 75–100 μg/min until relief of symptoms or limiting side effects (headache or hypotension with a systolic blood pressure <90 mmHg or more than 30% below starting mean arterial pressure levels if significant hypertension is present)
Beta blockers[b]	Unstable angina	PR interval (ECG) >0.24 s 2° or 3° atrioventricular block Heart rate <60 beats/min Systolic pressure <90 mmHg Shock Left ventricular failure Severe reactive airway disease	Metoprolol 25–50 mg by mouth every 6 h If needed, and no heart failure, 5-mg increments by slow (over 1–2 min) IV administration
Calcium channel blockers	Patients whose symptoms are not relieved by adequate doses of nitrates and beta blockers, or in patients unable to tolerate adequate doses of one or both of these agents, or in patients with variant angina	Pulmonary edema Evidence of left ventricular dysfunction (for diltiazem or verapamil)	Dependent on specific agent
Morphine sulfate	Patients whose symptoms are not relieved after three serial sublingual nitroglycerin tablets or whose symptoms recur with adequate anti-ischemic therapy	Hypotension Respiratory depression Confusion Obtundation	2–5 mg IV dose May be repeated every 5–30 min as needed to relieve symptoms and maintain patient comfort

[a]Allergy or prior intolerance is a contraindication for all categories of drugs listed in this chart.

[b]Choice of the specific agent is not as important as ensuring that appropriate candidates receive this therapy. If there are concerns about patient intolerance owing to existing pulmonary disease, especially asthma, left ventricular dysfunction, risk of hypotension or severe bradycardia, initial selection should favor a short-acting agent, such as propranolol or metoprolol or the ultra-short-acting agent esmolol. Mild wheezing or a history of chronic obstructive pulmonary disease should prompt a trial of a short-acting agent at a reduced dose (e.g., 2.5 mg IV metoprolol, 12.5 mg oral metoprolol, or 25 μg/kg per min esmolol as initial doses) rather than complete avoidance of beta-blocker therapy.

Note: Some of the recommendations in this guide suggest the use of agents for purposes or in doses other than those specified by the U.S. Food and Drug Administration. Such recommendations are made after consideration of concerns regarding nonapproved indications. Where made, such recommendations are based on more recent clinical trials or expert consensus. IV, intravenous; ECG, electrocardiogram; 2°, second-degree; 3°, third-degree.

Source: Modified from E Braunwald et al: Circulation 90:613, 1994.

combination with aspirin, was shown in the CURE trial to confer a 20% relative reduction in cardiovascular death, MI, or stroke, compared with aspirin alone in both low- and high-risk patients, but to be associated with a moderate (absolute 1%) increase in major bleeding. Pretreatment with clopidogrel (a 300 or 600 mg loading dose, followed by 75 mg qd) is recommended prior to PCI. The OASIS-7 trial reported that one week of a higher dose of clopidogrel (600 mg loading dose and 150 mg/d for one week) did not result in an overall improvement in outcomes in ACS patients, but did so in patients receiving 325 mg of aspirin, especially those who underwent PCI.

Continued benefit of one year of treatment with the combination of clopidogrel and aspirin has been observed both in patients treated conservatively and in those who underwent PCI and should certainly continue for at least one year in patients with a drug-eluting stent. Up to one-third of patients have low response to clopidogrel, and a substantial proportion of these are related to a genetic variant of the cytochrome P450 system. A variant of the 2C19 gene leads to reduced conversion of clopidogrel into its active metabolite, which, in turn, causes lower platelet inhibition and a higher risk of cardiovascular events. Alternate agents, such as prasugrel, should be considered for ACS patients who are hyporesponsive to clopidogrel as identified by platelet and/or genetic testing, although such testing is not yet widespread.

A recently approved thienopyridine, prasugrel, has been shown to achieve a more rapid onset, and higher level of platelet

TABLE 244-2 Clinical Use of Antithrombotic Therapy

Oral Antiplatelet Therapy	
Aspirin	Initial dose of 162–325 mg nonenteric formulation followed by 75–162 mg/d of an enteric or a nonenteric formulation
Clopidogrel	Loading dose of 300-600 mg followed by 75 mg/d
Prasugrel	Pre-PCI: Loading dose 60 mg followed by 10 mg/d
Intravenous Antiplatelet Therapy	
Abciximab	0.25 mg/kg bolus followed by infusion of 0.125 μg/kg per min (maximum 10 μg/min) for 12 to 24 h
Eptifibatide	180 μg/kg bolus followed by infusion of 2.0 μg/kg per min for 72 to 96 h
Tirofiban	0.4 μg/kg per min for 30 min followed by infusion of 0.1 μg/kg per min for 48 to 96 h
Heparins*	
Unfractionated Heparin (UFH)	Bolus 60–70 U/kg (maximum 5000 U) IV followed by infusion of 12–15 U/kg per h (initial maximum 1000 U/h) titrated to a PTT 50–70 s
Enoxaparin	1 mg/kg SC every 12 h; the first dose may be preceded by a 30-mg IV bolus; renal adjustment to 1 mg/kg once daily if creatine Cl < 30 cc/min
Fondaparinux	2.5 mg SC qd
Bivalirudin	Initial bolus intravenous bolus of 0.1 mg/kg and an infusion of 0.25 mg/kg per hour. Before PCI, an additional intravenous bolus of 0.5 mg/kg was administered, and the infusion was increased to 1.75 mg/kg per hour.

*Other LMWH exist beyond those listed.

Abbreviations: IV, intravenous; SC, subcutaneously.

Source: Modified from J Anderson et al: JACO 50:e1, 2007.

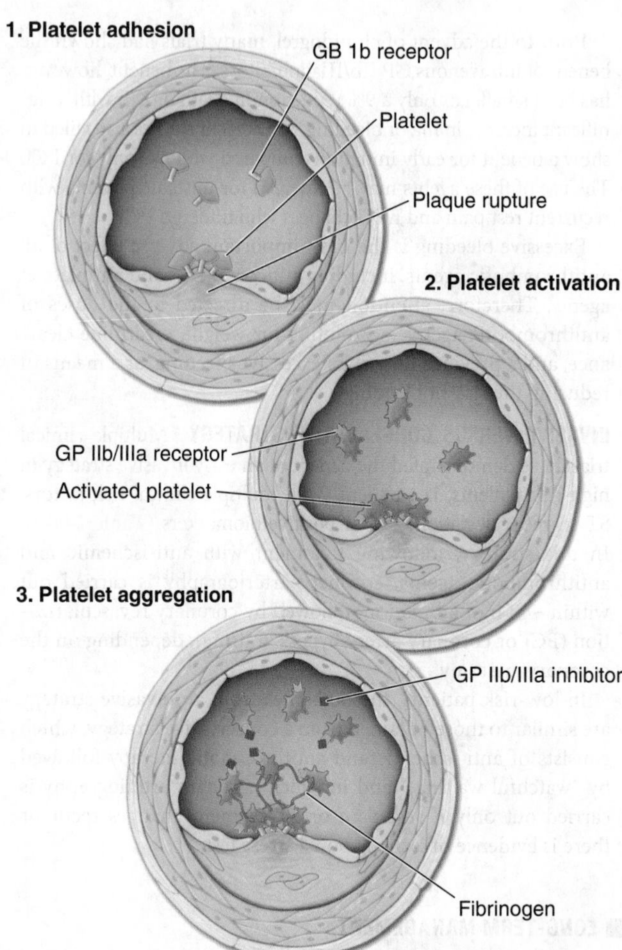

Figure 244-3 Platelets initiate thrombosis at the site of a ruptured plaque with denuded endothelium: *platelet adhesion* occurs via (1) the GP 1b receptor in conjunction with von Willebrand factor. This is followed by *platelet activation* (2), which leads to a shape change of the platelet, degranulation of the alpha and dense granules, and expression of glycoprotein IIb/IIIa receptors on the platelet surface with activation of the receptor, such that it can bind fibrinogen. The final step is *platelet aggregation* (3), in which fibrinogen (or von Willebrand factor) binds to the activated GP IIb/IIIa receptors. Aspirin (ASA) and clopidogrel act to decrease platelet activation, whereas the GP IIb/IIIa inhibitors inhibit the final step of platelet aggregation. GP, glycoprotein. [*Modified from CP Cannon, E Braunwald, in Braunwald's Heart Disease: A Textbook of Cardiovascular Medicine, 8th ed, R Bonow et al (eds). Philadelphia, Saunders, 2008.*]

inhibition than clopidogrel. It has been used in ACS patients following angiography in whom PCI is planned at a dose of 60 mg load followed by 10 mg/d for up to 15 months. The TRITON-TIMI 38 trial showed that relative to clopidogrel, prasugrel reduced the risk of cardiovascular death, MI, or stroke significantly by 19%, albeit with an increase in major bleeding. Stent thrombosis was also reduced by 52%. This agent is contraindicated in patients with prior stroke or transient ischemic attack. Ticagrelor is a novel, *reversible* ADP inhibitor that has recently been reported to reduce the risk of cardiovascular death, MI, or stroke by 16% compared with clopidogrel in a broad population of ACS patients. This agent also reduced mortality and did not increase the risk of total bleeding; it is not yet FDA approved at the time of this writing.

Four options are available for anticoagulant therapy to be added to aspirin and clopidogrel. Unfractionated heparin (UFH) is the mainstay of therapy. The low-molecular-weight heparin (LMWH), enoxaparin, has been shown in several studies to be superior to UFH in reducing recurrent cardiac events, especially in conservatively managed patients. The indirect Factor Xa inhibitor, fondaparinux, is equivalent for early efficacy compared with enoxaparin but appears to have a lower risk of major bleeding. Bivalirudin, a direct thrombin inhibitor, is similar in efficacy to either UFH or LMWH among patients treated with a GP IIb/IIIa inhibitor, but use of bivalirudin alone causes less bleeding than the combination of heparin and a GP IIb/IIIa inhibitor in patients with UA/NSTEMI undergoing catheterization and/or PCI.

Prior to the advent of clopidogrel, many trials had shown the benefit of intravenous GP IIb/IIIa inhibitors. The benefit, however, has been small, i.e., only a 9% reduction in death or MI, with a significant increase in major bleeding. Two recent studies also failed to show a benefit for early initiation compared with use only for PCI. The use of these agents may be reserved for unstable patients with recurrent rest pain and ECG changes who undergo PCI.

Excessive bleeding is the most important adverse effect of all antithrombotic agents, including anticoagulants and antiplatelet agents. Therefore, attention must be directed to the doses of antithrombotic agents, accounting for weight, creatinine clearance, and a previous history of excessive bleeding, as a means of reducing the risk of bleeding.

INVASIVE VERSUS CONSERVATIVE STRATEGY Multiple clinical trials have demonstrated the benefit of an early invasive strategy in high-risk patients, i.e., patients with multiple clinical risk factors, ST-segment deviation, and/or positive biomarkers (Table 244-3). In this strategy, following treatment with anti-ischemic and antithrombotic agents, coronary arteriography is carried out within ~48 h of admission, followed by coronary revascularization (PCI or coronary artery bypass grafting), depending on the coronary anatomy.

In low-risk patients, the outcomes from an invasive strategy are similar to those obtained from a conservative strategy, which consists of anti-ischemic and antithrombotic therapy followed by "watchful waiting," and in which coronary arteriography is carried out only if rest pain or ST-segment changes recur or there is evidence of ischemia on a stress test.

LONG-TERM MANAGEMENT

The time of hospital discharge is a "teachable moment" for the patient with UA/NSTEMI, when the physician can review and optimize the medical regimen. Risk-factor modification is key, and the caregiver should discuss with the patient the importance of smoking cessation, achieving optimal weight, daily exercise following an appropriate diet, blood-pressure control, tight control of hyperglycemia (for diabetic patients), and lipid management, as recommended for patients with chronic stable angina (Chap. 243).

TABLE 244-3 Class I Recommendations for Use of an Early Invasive Strategy*

Class I (Level of Evidence: A) Indications
Recurrent angina at rest/low-level activity despite Rx
Elevated TnT or TnI
New ST-segment depression
Rec. angina/ischemia with CHF symptoms, rales, MR
Positive stress test
EF < 0.40
Decreased BP
Sustained VT
PCI < 6 months, prior CABG
High-risk score

*Any one of the high-risk indicators.

Abbreviations: BP, blood pressure; CABG, coronary artery bypass grafting; CHF, congestive heart failure; EF, ejection fraction; MR, mitral regurgitation; PCI, percutaneous coronary intervention; Rec, recurrent; TnI, troponin I; TnT, troponin T; VT, ventricular tachycardia.

Source: J Anderson et al: JACO 50:e1, 2007.

There is evidence of benefit with long-term therapy with five classes of drugs that are directed at different components of the atherothrombotic process. Beta blockers, statins (at a high dose, e.g., atorvastatin 80 mg/d), and ACE inhibitors or angiotensin receptor blockers are recommended for long-term plaque stabilization. Antiplatelet therapy, now recommended to be the combination of aspirin and clopidogrel (or prasugrel in post PCS patients) for one year, with aspirin continued thereafter, prevents or reduces the severity of any thrombosis that would occur if a plaque were to rupture.

Observational registries have shown that patients with UA/NSTEMI at high risk, including women and the elderly as well as racial minorities, are less likely to receive evidence-based pharmacologic and interventional therapies with resultant poorer clinical outcomes and quality of life.

PRINZMETAL'S VARIANT ANGINA

In 1959 Prinzmetal et al. described a syndrome of severe ischemic pain that occurs at rest but not usually with exertion and is associated with transient ST-segment elevation. This syndrome is due to focal spasm of an epicardial coronary artery, leading to severe myocardial ischemia. The cause of the spasm is not well defined, but it may be related to hypercontractility of vascular smooth muscle due to vasoconstrictor mitogens, leukotrienes, or serotonin.

Clinical and angiographic manifestations

Patients with Prinzmetal's variant angina (PVA) are generally younger and have fewer coronary risk factors (with the exception of cigarette smoking) than patients with UA secondary to coronary atherosclerosis. Cardiac examination is usually unremarkable in the absence of ischemia. The clinical diagnosis of variant angina is made with the detection of transient ST-segment *elevation* with rest pain. Many patients also exhibit multiple episodes of asymptomatic ST-segment elevation (*silent ischemia*). Small elevations of troponin may occur in patients with prolonged attacks of variant angina.

Coronary angiography demonstrates transient coronary spasm as the diagnostic hallmark of PVA. Atherosclerotic plaques, which do not usually cause critical obstruction, in at least one proximal coronary artery occur in the majority of patients, and in them spasm usually occurs within 1 cm of the plaque. Focal spasm is most common in the right coronary artery, and it may occur at one or more sites in one artery or in multiple arteries simultaneously. Ergonovine, acetylcholine, other vasoconstrictor medications, and hyperventilation have been used to provoke focal coronary stenosis on angiography to establish the diagnosis. Hyperventilation has also been used to provoke rest angina, ST-segment elevation, and spasm on coronary arteriography.

TREATMENT Prinzmetal's Variant Angina

Nitrates and calcium channel blockers are the main agents used to treat acute episodes and to abolish recurrent episodes of PVA. Aspirin may actually increase the severity of ischemic episodes, possibly as a result of the exquisite sensitivity of coronary tone to modest changes in the synthesis of prostacyclin. The response to beta blockers is variable. Coronary revascularization may be helpful in patients who also have discrete, proximal fixed obstructive lesions.

Prognosis

Many patients with PVA pass through an acute, active phase, with frequent episodes of angina and cardiac events during the first

6 months after presentation. Long-term survival at 5 years is excellent (~90–95%). Patients with no or mild fixed coronary obstruction tend to experience a more benign course than do patients with associated severe obstructive lesions. Nonfatal MI occurs in up to 20% of patients by 5 years. Patients with PVA who develop serious arrhythmias during spontaneous episodes of pain are at a higher risk for sudden cardiac death. In most patients who survive an infarction or the initial 3- to 6-month period of frequent episodes, the condition stabilizes, and there is a tendency for symptoms and cardiac events to diminish over time.

FURTHER READINGS

Alexander KP et al: Excess dosing of antiplatelet and antithrombin agents in the treatment of non-ST-segment elevation acute coronary syndromes. JAMA 294:3108, 2005

Anderson JL et al: ACC/AHA 2007 guidelines for the management of patients with unstable angina/non-ST-elevation myocardial infarction: A report of the American College of Cardiology/American Heart Association Task Force on Practice Guidelines. Circulation 116:e148, 2007

Antman EM et al: The TIMI risk score for unstable angina/non-ST elevation MI: A method for prognostication and therapeutic decision-making. JAMA 284:835, 2000

Cannon CP, Braunwald E: Unstable angina, in *Braunwald's Heart Disease*, 9th ed, R Bonow et al (eds). Philadelphia, Saunders, 2011

Cannon CP et al: Intensive versus moderate lipid lowering with statins after acute coronary syndromes. N Engl J Med 350:1495, 2004

Giugliano RP et al: Early versus delayed, provisional eptifibatide in acute coronary syndromes. N Engl J Med 360:2176, 2009

O'Donoghue M et al: Early invasive vs. conservative treatment strategies in women and men with unstable angina and non-ST-segment elevation myocardial infarction: a meta-analysis. JAMA 300:71, 2008

Wallentin LT et al: Ticagrelor versus clopidogrel in patients with acute coronary syndromes. N Engl J Med 361:1045, 2009

Wiviott SD et al: Prasugrel versus clopidogrel in patients with acute coronary syndromes. N Engl J Med 357:2001, 2007

CHAPTER 245

ST-Segment Elevation Myocardial Infarction

Elliott M. Antman

Joseph Loscalzo

Acute myocardial infarction (AMI) is one of the most common diagnoses in hospitalized patients in industrialized countries. In the United States, approximately 650,000 patients experience a new AMI and 450,000 experience a recurrent AMI each year. The early (30-day) mortality rate from AMI is ~30%, with more than half of these deaths occurring before the stricken individual reaches the hospital. Although the mortality rate after admission for AMI has declined by ~30% over the past two decades, approximately 1 of every 25 patients who survives the initial hospitalization dies in the first year after AMI. Mortality is approximately fourfold higher in elderly patients (over age 75) as compared with younger patients.

When patients with prolonged ischemic discomfort at rest are first seen, the working clinical diagnosis is that they are suffering from an acute coronary syndrome (Fig. 245-1). The 12-lead electrocardiogram (ECG) is a pivotal diagnostic and triage tool because it is at the center of the decision pathway for management; it permits distinction of those patients presenting with ST-segment elevation from those presenting without ST-segment elevation. Serum cardiac biomarkers are obtained to distinguish unstable angina (UA) from non-ST-segment MI (NSTEMI) and to assess the magnitude of an ST-segment elevation MI (STEMI). This chapter focuses on the evaluation and management of patients with STEMI, while Chapter 244 discusses UA/NSTEMI.

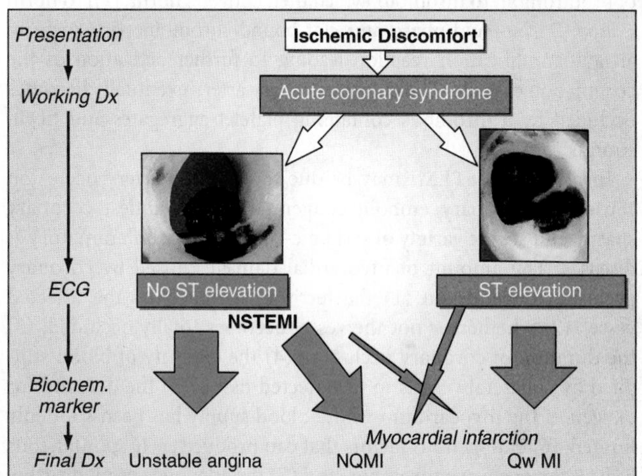

Figure 245-1 Acute coronary syndromes. Following disruption of a vulnerable plaque, patients experience ischemic discomfort resulting from a reduction of flow through the affected epicardial coronary artery. The flow reduction may be caused by a completely occlusive thrombus (***right***) or subtotally occlusive thrombus (***left***). Patients with ischemic discomfort may present with or without ST-segment elevation. Of patients with ST-segment elevation, the majority (*wide red arrow*) ultimately develop a Q wave on the ECG (QwMI), while a minority (*thin red arrow*) do not develop Q wave and, in older literature, were said to have sustained a non-Q-wave MI (NQMI). Patients who present without ST-segment elevation are suffering from either unstable angina or a non-ST-segment elevation MI (NSTEMI) (*wide green arrows*), a distinction that is ultimately made on the presence or absence of a serum cardiac marker such as CKMB or a cardiac troponin detected in the blood. The majority of patients presenting with NSTEMI do not develop a Q wave on the ECG; a minority develop a QwMI (*thin green arrow*). *(Adapted from CW Hamm et al: Lancet 358:1533, 2001, and MJ Davies: Heart 83:361, 2000; with permission from the BMJ Publishing Group.)*

PATHOPHYSIOLOGY: ROLE OF ACUTE PLAQUE RUPTURE

STEMI usually occurs when coronary blood flow decreases abruptly after a thrombotic occlusion of a coronary artery previously affected by atherosclerosis. Slowly developing, high-grade coronary artery stenoses do not typically precipitate STEMI because of the development of a rich collateral network over time. Instead, STEMI occurs when a coronary artery thrombus develops rapidly at a site of vascular injury. This injury is produced or facilitated by factors such as cigarette smoking, hypertension, and lipid accumulation. In most cases, STEMI occurs when the surface of an atherosclerotic plaque becomes disrupted (exposing its contents to the blood) and conditions (local or systemic) favor thrombogenesis. A mural thrombus forms at the site of plaque disruption, and the involved coronary artery becomes occluded. Histologic studies indicate that the coronary plaques prone to disruption are those with a rich lipid core and a thin fibrous cap (Chap. 241). After an initial platelet monolayer forms at the site of the disrupted plaque, various agonists (collagen, ADP, epinephrine, serotonin) promote platelet activation. After agonist stimulation of platelets, thromboxane A_2 (a potent local vasoconstrictor) is released, further platelet activation occurs, and potential resistance to fibrinolysis develops.

In addition to the generation of thromboxane A_2, activation of platelets by agonists promotes a conformational change in the glycoprotein IIb/IIIa receptor (Chap. 115). Once converted to its functional state, this receptor develops a high affinity for soluble adhesive proteins (i.e., integrins) such as fibrinogen. Since fibrinogen is a multivalent molecule, it can bind to two different platelets simultaneously, resulting in platelet cross-linking and aggregation.

The coagulation cascade is activated on exposure of tissue factor in damaged endothelial cells at the site of the disrupted plaque. Factors VII and X are activated, ultimately leading to the conversion of prothrombin to thrombin, which then converts fibrinogen to fibrin (Chap. 116). Fluid-phase and clot-bound thrombin participate in an autoamplification reaction leading to further activation of the coagulation cascade. The culprit coronary artery eventually becomes occluded by a thrombus containing platelet aggregates and fibrin strands.

In rare cases, STEMI may be due to coronary artery occlusion caused by coronary emboli, congenital abnormalities, coronary spasm, and a wide variety of systemic—particularly inflammatory—diseases. The amount of myocardial damage caused by coronary occlusion depends on (1) the territory supplied by the affected vessel, (2) whether or not the vessel becomes totally occluded, (3) the duration of coronary occlusion, (4) the quantity of blood supplied by collateral vessels to the affected tissue, (5) the demand for oxygen of the myocardium whose blood supply has been suddenly limited, (6) endogenous factors that can produce early spontaneous lysis of the occlusive thrombus, and (7) the adequacy of myocardial perfusion in the infarct zone when flow is restored in the occluded epicardial coronary artery.

Patients at increased risk for developing STEMI include those with multiple coronary risk factors (Chap. 241) and those with unstable angina (Chap. 244). Less common underlying medical conditions predisposing patients to STEMI include hypercoagulability, collagen vascular disease, cocaine abuse, and intracardiac thrombi or masses that can produce coronary emboli.

There have been major advances in the management of STEMI with recognition that the "chain of survival" involves a highly integrated system starting with prehospital care and extending to early hospital management so as to provide expeditious implementation of a reperfusion strategy.

CLINICAL PRESENTATION

In up to one-half of cases, a precipitating factor appears to be present before STEMI, such as vigorous physical exercise, emotional stress, or a medical or surgical illness. Although STEMI may commence at any time of the day or night, circadian variations have been reported such that clusters are seen in the morning within a few hours of awakening.

Pain is the most common presenting complaint in patients with STEMI. The pain is deep and visceral; adjectives commonly used to describe it are *heavy, squeezing*, and *crushing*, although, occasionally, it is described as stabbing or burning (Chap. 12). It is similar in character to the discomfort of angina pectoris (Chap. 243) but commonly occurs at rest, is usually more severe, and lasts longer. Typically, the pain involves the central portion of the chest and/or the epigastrium, and, on occasion, it radiates to the arms. Less common sites of radiation include the abdomen, back, lower jaw, and neck. The frequent location of the pain beneath the xiphoid and epigastrium and the patients' denial that they may be suffering a heart attack are chiefly responsible for the common mistaken impression of indigestion. The pain of STEMI may radiate as high as the occipital area but not below the umbilicus. It is often accompanied by weakness, sweating, nausea, vomiting, anxiety, and a sense of impending doom. The pain may commence when the patient is at rest, but when it begins during a period of exertion, it does not usually subside with cessation of activity, in contrast to angina pectoris.

The pain of STEMI can simulate pain from acute pericarditis (Chap. 239), pulmonary embolism (Chap. 262), acute aortic dissection (Chap. 248), costochondritis, and gastrointestinal disorders. These conditions should therefore be considered in the differential diagnosis. Radiation of discomfort to the trapezius is not seen in patients with STEMI and may be a useful distinguishing feature that suggests pericarditis is the correct diagnosis. However, *pain is not uniformly present in patients with STEMI*. The proportion of painless STEMIs is greater in patients with diabetes mellitus, and it increases with age. In the elderly, STEMI may present as sudden-onset breathlessness, which may progress to pulmonary edema. Other less common presentations, with or without pain, include sudden loss of consciousness, a confusional state, a sensation of profound weakness, the appearance of an arrhythmia, evidence of peripheral embolism, or merely an unexplained drop in arterial pressure.

PHYSICAL FINDINGS

Most patients are anxious and restless, attempting unsuccessfully to relieve the pain by moving about in bed, altering their position, and stretching. Pallor associated with perspiration and coolness of the extremities occurs commonly. The combination of substernal chest pain persisting for >30 min and diaphoresis strongly suggests STEMI. Although many patients have a normal pulse rate and blood pressure within the first hour of STEMI, about one-fourth of patients with anterior infarction have manifestations of sympathetic nervous system hyperactivity (tachycardia and/or hypertension), and up to one-half with inferior infarction show evidence of parasympathetic hyperactivity (bradycardia and/or hypotension).

The precordium is usually quiet, and the apical impulse may be difficult to palpate. In patients with anterior wall infarction, an abnormal systolic pulsation caused by dyskinetic bulging of infarcted myocardium may develop in the periapical area within the first days of the illness and then may resolve. Other physical signs of ventricular dysfunction include fourth and third heart sounds, decreased intensity of the first heart sound, and paradoxical splitting of the second heart sound (Chap. 227). A transient midsystolic or late systolic apical systolic murmur due to dysfunction of the mitral valve apparatus may be present. A pericardial friction rub is heard in many patients with transmural STEMI at some time in the course of the disease, if the patients are examined frequently. The carotid pulse is often decreased in volume, reflecting reduced stroke volume. Temperature elevations up to 38°C may be observed during the first week after STEMI. The arterial pressure is variable; in most patients with transmural infarction, systolic pressure declines by approximately 10–15 mmHg from the preinfarction state.

LABORATORY FINDINGS

Myocardial infarction (MI) progresses through the following temporal stages: (1) acute (first few hours–7 days), (2) healing (7–28 days), and (3) healed (≥29 days). When evaluating the results of diagnostic tests for STEMI, the temporal phase of the infarction must be considered. The laboratory tests of value in confirming the diagnosis may be divided into four groups: (1) ECG, (2) serum cardiac biomarkers, (3) cardiac imaging, and (4) nonspecific indices of tissue necrosis and inflammation.

■ ELECTROCARDIOGRAM

The electrocardiographic manifestations of STEMI are described in Chap. 228. During the initial stage, total occlusion of an epicardial coronary artery produces ST-segment elevation. Most patients initially presenting with ST-segment elevation ultimately evolve Q waves on the ECG. However, Q waves in the leads overlying the infarct zone may vary in magnitude and even appear only transiently, depending on the reperfusion status of the ischemic myocardium and restoration of transmembrane potentials over time. A small proportion of patients initially presenting with ST-segment elevation will not develop Q waves when the obstructing thrombus is not totally occlusive, obstruction is transient, or if a rich collateral network is present. Among patients presenting with ischemic discomfort but *without* ST-segment elevation, if a serum cardiac biomarker of necrosis (see below) is detected, the diagnosis of NSTEMI is ultimately made (Fig. 245-1). A minority of patients who present initially without ST-segment elevation may develop a Q-wave MI. Previously, it was believed that transmural MI is present if the ECG demonstrates Q waves or loss of R waves, and nontransmural MI may be present if the ECG shows only transient ST-segment and T-wave changes. However, electrocardiographic-pathologic correlations are far from perfect and terms such as *Q-wave MI*, *non-Q-wave MI*, *transmural MI*, and *nontransmural MI*, have been replaced by STEMI and NSTEMI (Fig. 245-1). Contemporary studies using MRI suggest that the development of a Q wave on the ECG is more dependent on the volume of infarcted tissue rather than the transmurality of infarction.

■ SERUM CARDIAC BIOMARKERS

Certain proteins, called serum cardiac biomarkers, are released from necrotic heart muscle after STEMI. The rate of liberation of specific proteins differs depending on their intracellular location, their molecular weight, and the local blood and lymphatic flow. Cardiac biomarkers become detectable in the peripheral blood once the capacity of the cardiac lymphatics to clear the interstitium of the infarct zone is exceeded and spillover into the venous circulation occurs. The temporal pattern of protein release is of diagnostic importance, but contemporary urgent reperfusion strategies necessitate making a decision (based largely on a combination of clinical and ECG findings) before the results of blood tests have returned from the laboratory. Rapid whole-blood bedside assays for serum cardiac markers are now available and may facilitate management decisions, particularly in patients with nondiagnostic ECGs.

Cardiac-specific troponin T (cTnT) and *cardiac-specific troponin I* (cTnI) have amino-acid sequences different from those of the skeletal muscle forms of these proteins. These differences permitted the development of quantitative assays for cTnT and cTnI with highly specific monoclonal antibodies. Since cTnT and cTnI are not normally detectable in the blood of healthy individuals but may increase after STEMI to levels >20 times higher than the upper reference limit (the highest value seen in 99% of a reference population not suffering from MI), the measurement of cTnT or cTnI is of considerable diagnostic usefulness, and they are now the preferred biochemical markers for MI (Fig. 245-2). The cardiac troponins

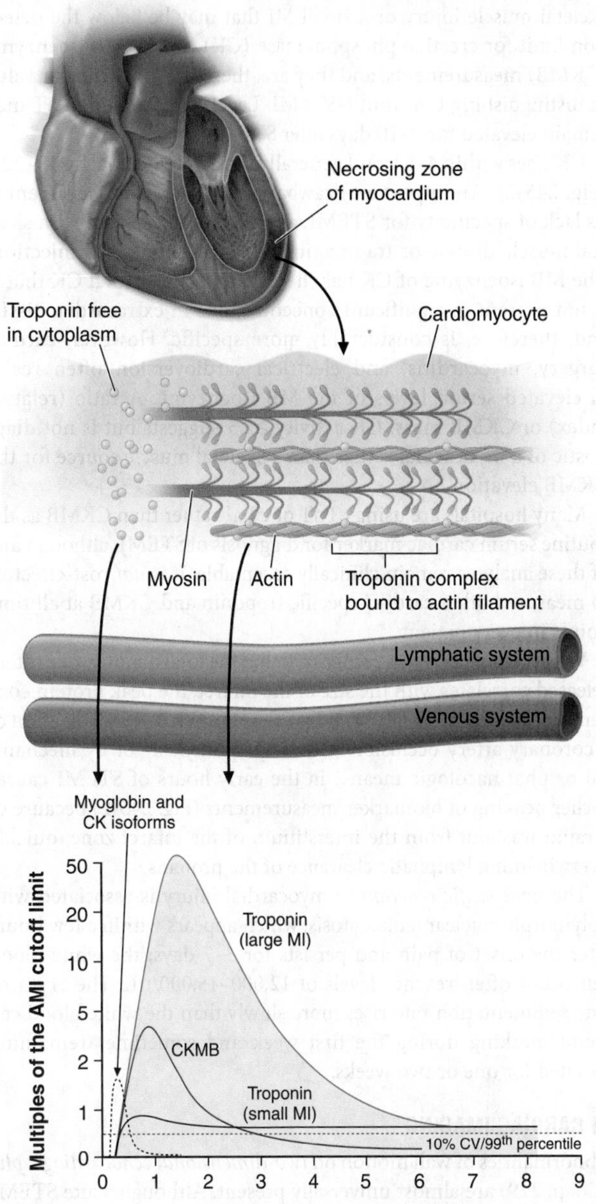

Figure 245-2 The zone of necrosing myocardium is shown at the top of the figure, followed in the middle portion of the figure by a diagram of a cardiomyocyte that is in the process of releasing biomarkers. The biomarkers that are released into the interstitium are first cleared by lymphatics followed subsequently by spillover into the venous system. After disruption of the sarcolemmal membrane of the cardiomyocyte, the cytoplasmic pool of biomarkers is released first (left-most arrow in bottom portion of figure). Markers such as myoglobin and CK isoforms are rapidly released, and blood levels rise quickly above the cutoff limit; this is then followed by a more protracted release of biomarkers from the disintegrating myofilaments that may continue for several days. Cardiac troponin levels rise to about 20 to 50 times the upper reference limit (the 99th percentile of values in a reference control group) in patients who have a "classic" acute myocardial infarction (MI) and sustain sufficient myocardial necrosis to result in abnormally elevated levels of the MB fraction of creatine kinase (CKMB). Clinicians can now diagnose episodes of microinfarction by sensitive assays that detect cardiac troponin elevations above the upper reference limit, even though CKMB levels may still be in the normal reference range (not shown). CV = coefficient of variation. *(Modified from Antman EM: Decision making with cardiac troponin tests. N Engl J Med 346:2079, 2002 and Jaffe AS, Babiun L, Apple FS: Biomarkers in acute cardiac disease: The present and the future. J Am Coll Cardiol 48:1, 2006.)*

are particularly valuable when there is clinical suspicion of either skeletal muscle injury or a small MI that may be below the detection limit for creatine phosphokinase (CK) and its MB isoenzyme (CKMB) measurements, and they are, therefore, of particular value in distinguishing UA from NSTEMI. Levels of cTnI and cTnT may remain elevated for 7–10 days after STEMI.

CK rises within 4–8 h and generally returns to normal by 48–72 h (Fig. 245-2). An important drawback of total CK measurement is its lack of specificity for STEMI, as CK may be elevated with skeletal muscle disease or trauma, including intramuscular injection. The MB isoenzyme of CK has the advantage over total CK that it is not present in significant concentrations in extracardiac tissue and, therefore, is considerably more specific. However, cardiac surgery, myocarditis, and electrical cardioversion often result in elevated serum levels of the MB isoenzyme. A ratio (relative index) of CKMB mass: CK activity ≥2.5 suggests but is not diagnostic of a myocardial rather than a skeletal muscle source for the CKMB elevation.

Many hospitals are using cTnT or cTnI rather than CKMB as the routine serum cardiac marker for diagnosis of STEMI, although any of these analytes remain clinically acceptable. It is *not* cost-effective to measure both a cardiac-specific troponin and CKMB at all time points in every patient.

While it has long been recognized that the total quantity of protein released correlates with the size of the infarct, the peak protein concentration correlates only weakly with infarct size. Recanalization of a coronary artery occlusion (either spontaneously or by mechanical or pharmacologic means) in the early hours of STEMI causes earlier peaking of biomarker measurements (Fig. 245-2) because of a rapid washout from the interstitium of the infarct zone, quickly overwhelming lymphatic clearance of the proteins.

The *nonspecific reaction* to myocardial injury is associated with polymorphonuclear leukocytosis, which appears within a few hours after the onset of pain and persists for 3–7 days; the white blood cell count often reaches levels of 12,000–15,000/μL. The erythrocyte sedimentation rate rises more slowly than the white blood cell count, peaking during the first week and sometimes remaining elevated for one or two weeks.

■ CARDIAC IMAGING

Abnormalities of wall motion on *two-dimensional echocardiography* (Chap. 229) are almost universally present. Although acute STEMI cannot be distinguished from an old myocardial scar or from acute severe ischemia by echocardiography, the ease and safety of the procedure make its use appealing as a screening tool in the Emergency Department setting. When the ECG is not diagnostic of STEMI, early detection of the presence or absence of wall motion abnormalities by echocardiography can aid in management decisions, such as whether the patient should receive reperfusion therapy [e.g., fibrinolysis or a percutaneous coronary intervention (PCI)]. Echocardiographic estimation of left ventricular (LV) function is useful prognostically; detection of reduced function serves as an indication for therapy with an inhibitor of the renin-angiotensin–aldosterone system. Echocardiography may also identify the presence of right ventricular (RV) infarction, ventricular aneurysm, pericardial effusion, and LV thrombus. In addition, Doppler echocardiography is useful in the detection and quantitation of a ventricular septal defect and mitral regurgitation, two serious complications of STEMI.

Several *radionuclide imaging techniques* (Chap. 229) are available for evaluating patients with suspected STEMI. However, these imaging modalities are used less often than echocardiography because they are more cumbersome and lack sensitivity and specificity in many clinical circumstances. Myocardial perfusion imaging with [^{201}Tl] or [^{99m}Tc]-sestamibi, which are distributed in proportion to myocardial blood flow and concentrated by viable myocardium (Chap. 243), reveal a defect ("cold spot") in most patients during the first few hours after development of a transmural infarct. Although perfusion scanning is extremely sensitive, it cannot distinguish acute infarcts from chronic scars and, thus, is not specific for the diagnosis of *acute* MI. Radionuclide ventriculography, carried out with [^{99m}Tc]-labeled red blood cells, frequently demonstrates wall motion disorders and reduction in the ventricular ejection fraction in patients with STEMI. While of value in assessing the hemodynamic consequences of infarction and in aiding in the diagnosis of RV infarction when the RV ejection fraction is depressed, this technique is nonspecific, as many cardiac abnormalities other than MI alter the radionuclide ventriculogram.

Myocardial infarction can be detected accurately with high-resolution cardiac MRI (Chap. 229) using a technique referred to as late enhancement. A standard imaging agent (gadolinium) is administered and images are obtained after a 10-min delay. Since little gadolinium enters normal myocardium, where there are tightly packed myocytes, but does percolate into the expanded intercellular region of the infarct zone, there is a bright signal in areas of infarction that appears in stark contrast to the dark areas of normal myocardium.

INITIAL MANAGEMENT

■ PREHOSPITAL CARE

The prognosis in STEMI is largely related to the occurrence of two general classes of complications: (1) electrical complications (arrhythmias) and (2) mechanical complications ("pump failure"). Most out-of-hospital deaths from STEMI are due to the sudden development of ventricular fibrillation. The vast majority of deaths due to ventricular fibrillation occur within the first 24 h of the onset of symptoms, and of these, over half occur in the first hour. Therefore, the major elements of prehospital care of patients with suspected STEMI include (1) recognition of symptoms by the patient and prompt seeking of medical attention; (2) rapid deployment of an emergency medical team capable of performing resuscitative maneuvers, including defibrillation; (3) expeditious transportation of the patient to a hospital facility that is continuously staffed by physicians and nurses skilled in managing arrhythmias and providing advanced cardiac life support; and (4) expeditious implementation of reperfusion therapy (Fig. 245-3). The greatest delay usually occurs not during transportation to the hospital but, rather, between the onset of pain and the patient's decision to call for help. This delay can best be reduced by health care professionals educating the public concerning the significance of chest discomfort and the importance of seeking early medical attention. Regular office visits with patients having a history of or who are at risk for ischemic heart disease are important "teachable moments" for clinicians to review the symptoms of STEMI and the appropriate action plan.

Increasingly, monitoring and treatment are carried out by trained personnel in the ambulance, further shortening the time between the onset of the infarction and appropriate treatment. General guidelines for initiation of fibrinolysis in the prehospital setting include the ability to transmit 12-lead ECGs to confirm the diagnosis, the presence of paramedics in the ambulance, training of paramedics in the interpretation of ECGs and management of STEMI, and online medical command and control that can authorize the initiation of treatment in the field.

MANAGEMENT IN THE EMERGENCY DEPARTMENT

In the Emergency Department, the goals for the management of patients with suspected STEMI include control of cardiac discomfort, rapid identification of patients who are candidates for urgent reperfusion therapy, triage of lower-risk patients to the appropriate

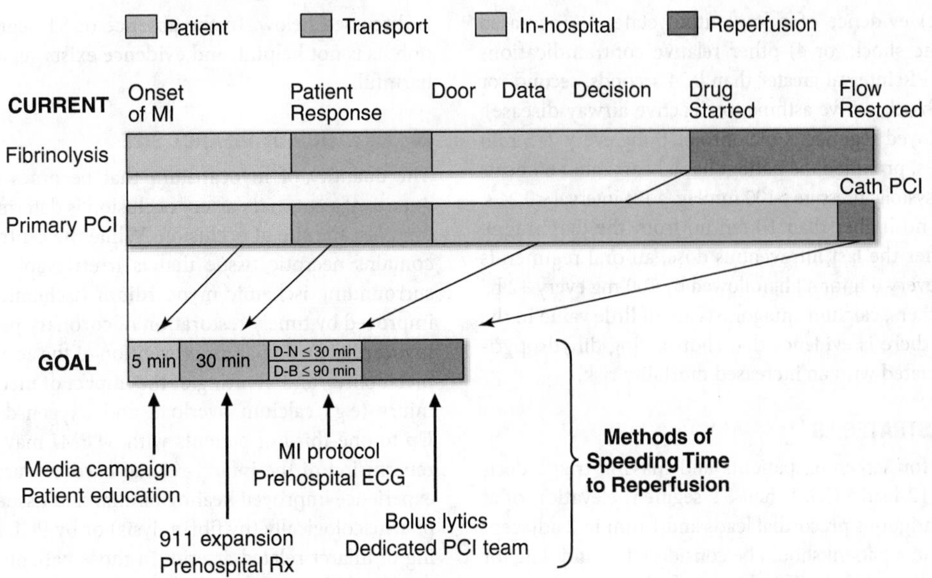

Figure 245-3 Major components of time delay between onset of symptoms from STEMI and restoration of flow in the infarct-related artery. Plotted sequentially from left to right are the times for patients to recognize symptoms and seek medical attention, transportation to the hospital, in-hospital decision making, implementation of reperfusion strategy, and restoration of flow once the reperfusion strategy has been initiated. The time to initiate fibrinolytic therapy is the "door-to-needle" (D-N) time; this is followed by the period of time required for pharmacologic restoration of flow. More time is required to move the patient to the catheterization laboratory for a percutaneous coronary interventional (PCI) procedure, referred to as the "door-to-balloon" (D-B) time, but restoration of flow in the epicardial infarct–related artery occurs promptly after PCI. At the bottom is a variety of methods for speeding the time to reperfusion along with the goals for the time intervals for the various components of the time delay. *(Adapted from CP Cannon et al: J Thromb Thrombol 1:27, 1994.)*

location in the hospital, and avoidance of inappropriate discharge of patients with STEMI. Many aspects of the treatment of STEMI are initiated in the Emergency Department and then continued during the in-hospital phase of management.

Aspirin is essential in the management of patients with suspected STEMI and is effective across the entire spectrum of acute coronary syndromes (Fig. 245-1). Rapid inhibition of cyclooxygenase-1 in platelets followed by a reduction of thromboxane A_2 levels is achieved by buccal absorption of a chewed 160–325-mg tablet in the Emergency Department. This measure should be followed by daily oral administration of aspirin in a dose of 75–162 mg.

In patients whose arterial O_2 saturation is normal, supplemental O_2 is of limited if any clinical benefit and therefore is not cost-effective. However, when hypoxemia is present, O_2 should be administered by nasal prongs or face mask (2–4 L/min) for the first 6–12 h after infarction; the patient should then be reassessed to determine if there is a continued need for such treatment.

■ CONTROL OF DISCOMFORT

Sublingual *nitroglycerin* can be given safely to most patients with STEMI. Up to three doses of 0.4 mg should be administered at about 5-min intervals. In addition to diminishing or abolishing chest discomfort, nitroglycerin may be capable of both decreasing myocardial oxygen demand (by lowering preload) and increasing myocardial oxygen supply (by dilating infarct-related coronary vessels or collateral vessels). In patients whose initially favorable response to sublingual nitroglycerin is followed by the return of chest discomfort, particularly if accompanied by other evidence of ongoing ischemia such as further ST-segment or T-wave shifts, the use of intravenous nitroglycerin should be considered. Therapy with nitrates should be avoided in patients who present with low systolic arterial pressure (<90 mmHg) or in whom there is clinical suspicion of right ventricular infarction (inferior infarction on ECG, elevated jugular venous pressure, clear lungs, and hypotension). Nitrates should not be administered to patients who have taken the phosphodiesterase-5 inhibitor sildenafil for erectile dysfunction within the preceding 24 h, because it may potentiate the hypotensive effects of nitrates. An idiosyncratic reaction to nitrates, consisting of sudden marked hypotension, sometimes occurs but can usually be reversed promptly by the rapid administration of intravenous atropine.

Morphine is a very effective analgesic for the pain associated with STEMI. However, it may reduce sympathetically mediated arteriolar and venous constriction, and the resulting venous pooling may reduce cardiac output and arterial pressure. These hemodynamic disturbances usually respond promptly to elevation of the legs, but in some patients volume expansion with intravenous saline is required. The patient may experience diaphoresis and nausea, but these events usually pass and are replaced by a feeling of well-being associated with the relief of pain. Morphine also has a vagotonic effect and may cause bradycardia or advanced degrees of heart block, particularly in patients with inferior infarction. These side effects usually respond to atropine (0.5 mg intravenously). Morphine is routinely administered by repetitive (every 5 min) intravenous injection of small doses (2–4 mg), rather than by the subcutaneous administration of a larger quantity, because absorption may be unpredictable by the latter route.

Intravenous *beta blockers* are also useful in the control of the pain of STEMI. These drugs control pain effectively in some patients, presumably by diminishing myocardial O_2 demand and hence ischemia. More important, there is evidence that intravenous beta blockers reduce the risks of reinfarction and ventricular fibrillation (see "Beta-Adrenoceptor Blockers" below). However, patient selection is important when considering beta blockers for STEMI. Oral beta-blocker therapy should be initiated in the first 24 h for patients who do not have any of the following: 1) signs of heart failure, 2) evidence of a low-output state, 3) increased risk for cardiogenic shock, or 4) other relative contraindications to beta blockade (PR interval greater than 0.24 seconds, second- or third-degree heart block, active asthma, or reactive airway disease). A commonly employed regimen is metoprolol, 5 mg every 2–5 min for a total of 3 doses, provided the patient has a heart rate >60 beats per minute (bpm), systolic pressure >100 mmHg, a PR interval <0.24 s, and rales that are no higher than 10 cm up from the diaphragm. Fifteen minutes after the last intravenous dose, an oral regimen is initiated of 50 mg every 6 h for 48 h, followed by 100 mg every 12 h.

Unlike beta blockers, calcium antagonists are of little value in the acute setting, and there is evidence that short-acting dihydropyridines may be associated with an increased mortality risk.

MANAGEMENT STRATEGIES

The primary tool for screening patients and making triage decisions is the initial 12-lead ECG. When ST-segment elevation of at least 2 mm in 2 contiguous precordial leads and 1 mm in 2 adjacent limb leads is present, a patient should be considered a candidate for *reperfusion therapy* (Fig. 245-4). The process of selecting patients for fibrinolysis versus primary PCI (angioplasty, or stenting; Chap. 246) is discussed below. In the absence of ST-segment elevation, fibrinolysis is not helpful, and evidence exists suggesting that it may be harmful.

LIMITATION OF INFARCT SIZE

The quantity of myocardium that becomes necrotic as a consequence of a coronary artery occlusion is determined by factors other than just the site of occlusion. While the central zone of the infarct contains necrotic tissue that is irretrievably lost, the fate of the surrounding ischemic myocardium (ischemic penumbra) may be improved by timely restoration of coronary perfusion, reduction of myocardial O_2 demands, prevention of the accumulation of noxious metabolites, and blunting of the impact of mediators of reperfusion injury (e.g., calcium overload and oxygen-derived free radicals). Up to one-third of patients with STEMI may achieve *spontaneous* reperfusion of the infarct-related coronary artery within 24 h and experience improved healing of infarcted tissue. Reperfusion, either pharmacologically (by fibrinolysis) or by PCI, accelerates the opening of infarct-related arteries in those patients in whom spontaneous fibrinolysis ultimately would have occurred and also greatly increases the number of patients in whom restoration of flow in the

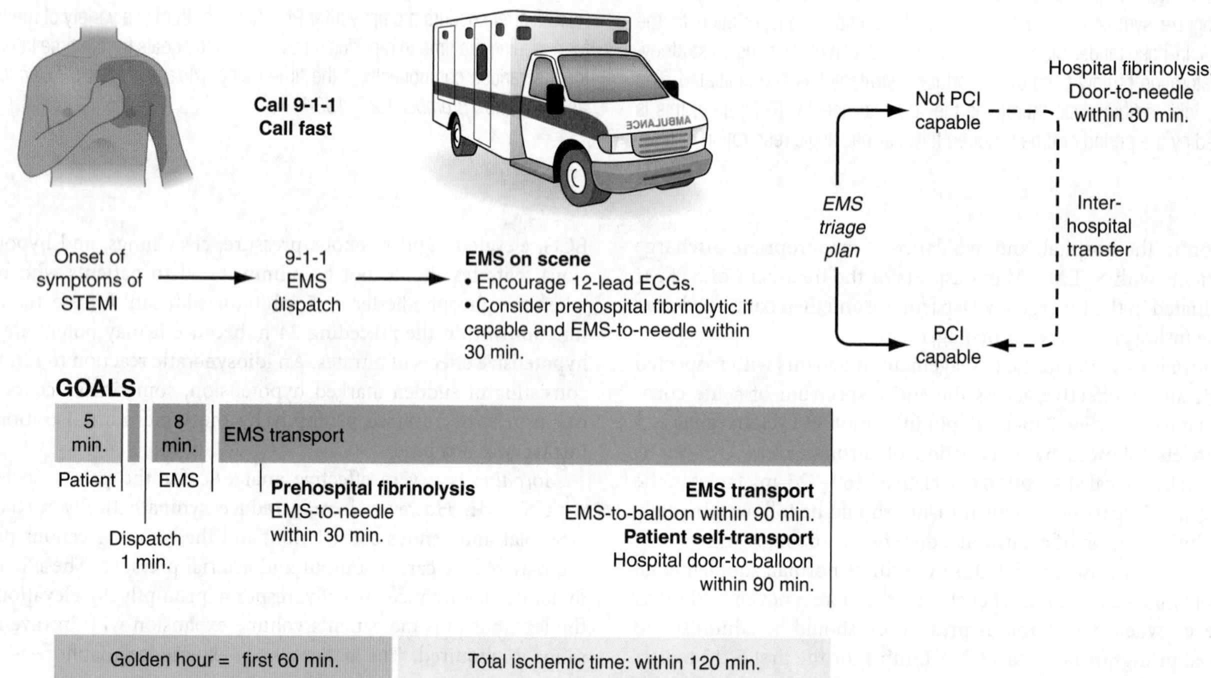

Figure 245-4 Options for transportation of patients with STEMI and initial reperfusion treatment. Patient transported by EMS after calling 911: Reperfusion in patients with STEMI can be accomplished by the pharmacologic (fibrinolysis) or catheter-based (primary PCI) approaches. Implementation of these strategies varies based on the mode of transportation of the patient and capabilities at the receiving hospital. Transport time to the hospital is variable from case to case, but the goal is to keep total ischemic time within 120 min. There are three possible scenarios: (1) If EMS has fibrinolytic capability and the patient qualifies for therapy, prehospital fibrinolysis should be started within 30 min of EMS arrival on scene. (2) If EMS is not capable of administering prehospital fibrinolysis and the patient is transported to a non-PCI-capable hospital, the hospital door-to-needle time should be within 30 min for patients in whom fibrinolysis is indicated. (3) If EMS is not capable of administering prehospital fibrinolysis and the patient is transported to a PCI-capable hospital, the hospital door-to-balloon time should be within 90 min. *Interhospital transfer*: It is also appropriate to consider emergency interhospital transfer of the patient to a PCI-capable hospital for mechanical revascularization if: (1) there is a contraindication to fibrinolysis, (2) PCI can be initiated promptly (within 90 minutes after the patient presented to the initial receiving hospital or within 60 min compared to when fibrinolysis with a fibrin-specific agent could be initiated at the initial receiving hospital), (3) fibrinolysis is administered and is unsuccessful (i.e., "rescue PCI"). Secondary nonemergency interhospital transfer can be considered for recurrent ischemia. *Patient self-transport*: Patient self-transportation is discouraged. If the patient arrives at a non-PCI-capable hospital, the door-to-needle time should be within 30 min. If the patient arrives at a PCI-capable hospital, the door-to-balloon time should be within 90 min. The treatment options and time recommended after first hospital arrival are the same. *[Adapted with permission from Antman et al: ACC/AHA guidelines for the management of patients with ST-elevation myocardial infarction: A report of the American College of Cardiology/American Heart Association Task Force on Practice Guidelines (Committee to Revise the 1999 Guidelines for the Management of Patients with Acute Myocardial Infarction).* Circulation 110:e82, 2004.*]*

infarct-related artery is accomplished. Timely restoration of flow in the epicardial infarct–related artery combined with improved perfusion of the downstream zone of infarcted myocardium results in a limitation of infarct size. Protection of the ischemic myocardium by the maintenance of an optimal balance between myocardial O_2 supply and demand through pain control, treatment of congestive heart failure (CHF), and minimization of tachycardia and hypertension extends the "window" of time for the salvage of myocardium by reperfusion strategies.

Glucocorticoids and nonsteroidal anti-inflammatory agents, with the exception of aspirin, should be avoided in patients with STEMI. They can impair infarct healing and increase the risk of myocardial rupture, and their use may result in a larger infarct scar. In addition, they can increase coronary vascular resistance, thereby potentially reducing flow to ischemic myocardium.

Primary percutaneous coronary intervention

(See also Chap. 246) PCI, usually angioplasty and/or stenting without preceding fibrinolysis, referred to as *primary PCI*, is effective in restoring perfusion in STEMI when carried out on an emergency basis in the first few hours of MI. It has the advantage of being applicable to patients who have contraindications to fibrinolytic therapy (see below) but otherwise are considered appropriate candidates for reperfusion. It appears to be more effective than fibrinolysis in opening occluded coronary arteries and, *when performed by experienced operators [≥75 PCI cases (not necessarily primary) per year] in dedicated medical centers (≥36 primary PCI cases per year)*, is associated with better short-term and long-term clinical outcomes. Compared with fibrinolysis, primary PCI is generally preferred when the diagnosis is in doubt, cardiogenic shock is present, bleeding risk is increased, or symptoms have been present for at least 2–3 h when the clot is more mature and less easily lysed by fibrinolytic drugs. However, PCI is expensive in terms of personnel and facilities, and its applicability is limited by its availability, around the clock, in only a minority of hospitals.

Fibrinolysis

If no contraindications are present (see below), fibrinolytic therapy should ideally be initiated within 30 min of presentation (i.e., door-to-needle time ≤30 min). The principal goal of fibrinolysis is prompt restoration of full coronary arterial patency. The fibrinolytic agents tissue plasminogen activator (tPA), streptokinase, tenecteplase (TNK), and reteplase (rPA) have been approved by the U.S. Food and Drug Administration for intravenous use in patients with STEMI. These drugs all act by promoting the conversion of plasminogen to plasmin, which subsequently lyses fibrin thrombi. Although considerable emphasis was first placed on a distinction between more fibrin-specific agents, such as tPA, and non-fibrin-specific agents, such as streptokinase, it is now recognized that these differences are only relative, as some degree of systemic fibrinolysis occurs with the former agents. TNK and rPA are referred to as *bolus fibrinolytics* since their administration does not require a prolonged intravenous infusion.

When assessed angiographically, flow in the culprit coronary artery is described by a simple qualitative scale called the *thrombolysis in myocardial infarction (TIMI) grading system*: grade 0 indicates complete occlusion of the infarct-related artery; grade 1 indicates some penetration of the contrast material beyond the point of obstruction but without perfusion of the distal coronary bed; grade 2 indicates perfusion of the entire infarct vessel into the distal bed, but with flow that is delayed compared with that of a normal artery; and grade 3 indicates full perfusion of the infarct vessel with normal flow. The latter is the goal of reperfusion therapy, because full perfusion of the infarct-related coronary artery yields far better results in terms of limiting infarct size, maintenance of LV function, and reduction of both short- and long-term mortality rates. Additional methods of angiographic assessment of the efficacy of fibrinolysis include counting the number of frames on the cine film required for dye to flow from the origin of the infarct-related artery to a landmark in the distal vascular bed (*TIMI frame count*) and determining the rate of entry and exit of contrast dye from the microvasculature in the myocardial infarct zone (*TIMI myocardial perfusion grade*). These methods have an even tighter correlation with outcomes after STEMI than the more commonly employed TIMI flow grade.

Fibrinolytic therapy can reduce the relative risk of in-hospital death by up to 50% when administered within the first hour of the onset of symptoms of STEMI, and much of this benefit is maintained for at least 10 years. When appropriately used, fibrinolytic therapy appears to reduce infarct size, limit LV dysfunction, and reduce the incidence of serious complications such as septal rupture, cardiogenic shock, and malignant ventricular arrhythmias. Since myocardium can be salvaged only before it has been irreversibly injured, the timing of reperfusion therapy, by fibrinolysis or a catheter-based approach, is of extreme importance in achieving maximum benefit. While the upper time limit depends on specific factors in individual patients, it is clear that every minute counts and that patients treated within 1–3 h of the onset of symptoms generally benefit most. Although reduction of the mortality rate is more modest, the therapy remains of benefit for many patients seen 3–6 h after the onset of infarction, and some benefit appears to be possible up to 12 h, especially if chest discomfort is still present and ST segments remain elevated. Compared with PCI for STEMI (primary PCI), fibrinolysis is generally the preferred reperfusion strategy for patients presenting in the first hour of symptoms, if there are logistical concerns about transportation of the patient to a suitable PCI center (experienced operator and team with a track record for a "door-to-balloon" time of <2 h), or there is an anticipated delay of at least 1 h between the time that fibrinolysis could be started versus implementation of PCI. Although patients <75 years achieve a greater relative reduction in the mortality rate with fibrinolytic therapy than do older patients, the higher *absolute* mortality rate (15–25%) in the latter results in similar absolute reductions in the mortality rates for both age groups.

tPA and the other relatively fibrin-specific plasminogen activators, rPA and TNK, are more effective than streptokinase at restoring full perfusion—i.e., TIMI grade 3 coronary flow—and have a small edge in improving survival as well. The current recommended regimen of tPA consists of a 15-mg bolus followed by 50 mg intravenously over the first 30 min, followed by 35 mg over the next 60 min. Streptokinase is administered as 1.5 million units (MU) intravenously over 1 h. rPA is administered in a double-bolus regimen consisting of a 10-MU bolus given over 2–3 min, followed by a second 10-MU bolus 30 min later. TNK is given as a single weight-based intravenous bolus of 0.53 mg/kg over 10 s. In addition to the fibrinolytic agents discussed above, pharmacologic reperfusion typically involves adjunctive antiplatelet and antithrombotic drugs, as discussed subsequently.

Alternative pharmacologic regimens for reperfusion combine an intravenous glycoprotein IIb/IIIa inhibitor with a reduced dose of a fibrinolytic agent. Compared with fibrinolytic agents that involve a prolonged infusion (e.g., tPA), such combination reperfusion regimens facilitate the rate and extent of fibrinolysis by inhibiting platelet aggregation, weakening the clot structure, and allowing penetration of the fibrinolytic agent deeper into the clot. However, combination reperfusion regimens have similar efficacy as compared with bolus fibrinolytics and are associated with an increased risk of bleeding, especially in patients >75 years. Therefore, combination reperfusion regimens are not recommended for routine use. Glycoprotein IIb/IIIa inhibitors, given alone or in combination with a reduced dose of a fibrinolytic agent as part of a preparatory regimen before planned immediate PCI (facilitated PCI), have not been shown to reduce infarct size or improve outcomes and, furthermore, are associated with increased bleeding. Facilitated PCI is, therefore, also not a strategy that is recommended for routine use.

Integrated reperfusion strategy

Evidence has emerged that suggests PCI plays an increasingly important role in the management of STEMI. Prior approaches that segregated the pharmacologic and catheter-based approaches to reperfusion have now been replaced with an integrated approach to triage and transfer of STEMI patients to receive PCI (Fig. 245-5).

Contraindications and complications

Clear contraindications to the use of fibrinolytic agents include a history of cerebrovascular hemorrhage at any time, a nonhemorrhagic stroke or other cerebrovascular event within the past year, marked hypertension (a reliably determined systolic arterial pressure >180 mmHg and/or a diastolic pressure >110 mmHg) at any time during the acute presentation, suspicion of aortic dissection, and active internal bleeding (excluding menses). While advanced age is associated with an increase in hemorrhagic complications, the benefit of fibrinolytic therapy in the elderly appears to justify its use if no other contraindications are present and the amount of myocardium in jeopardy appears to be substantial.

Relative contraindications to fibrinolytic therapy, which require assessment of the risk:benefit ratio, include current use of anticoagulants (international normalized ratio ≥2), a recent (<2 weeks) invasive or surgical procedure or prolonged (>10 min) cardiopulmonary resuscitation, known bleeding diathesis, pregnancy, a hemorrhagic ophthalmic condition (e.g., hemorrhagic diabetic retinopathy), active peptic ulcer disease, and a history of severe hypertension that is currently adequately controlled. Because of the risk of an allergic reaction, patients should not receive streptokinase if that agent had been received within the preceding five days to two years.

Allergic reactions to streptokinase occur in ~2% of patients who receive it. While a minor degree of hypotension occurs in 4–10% of patients given this agent, marked hypotension occurs, although rarely, in association with severe allergic reactions.

Hemorrhage is the most frequent and potentially the most serious complication. Because bleeding episodes that require transfusion are more common when patients require invasive procedures, unnecessary venous or arterial interventions should be avoided in patients receiving fibrinolytic agents. Hemorrhagic stroke is the

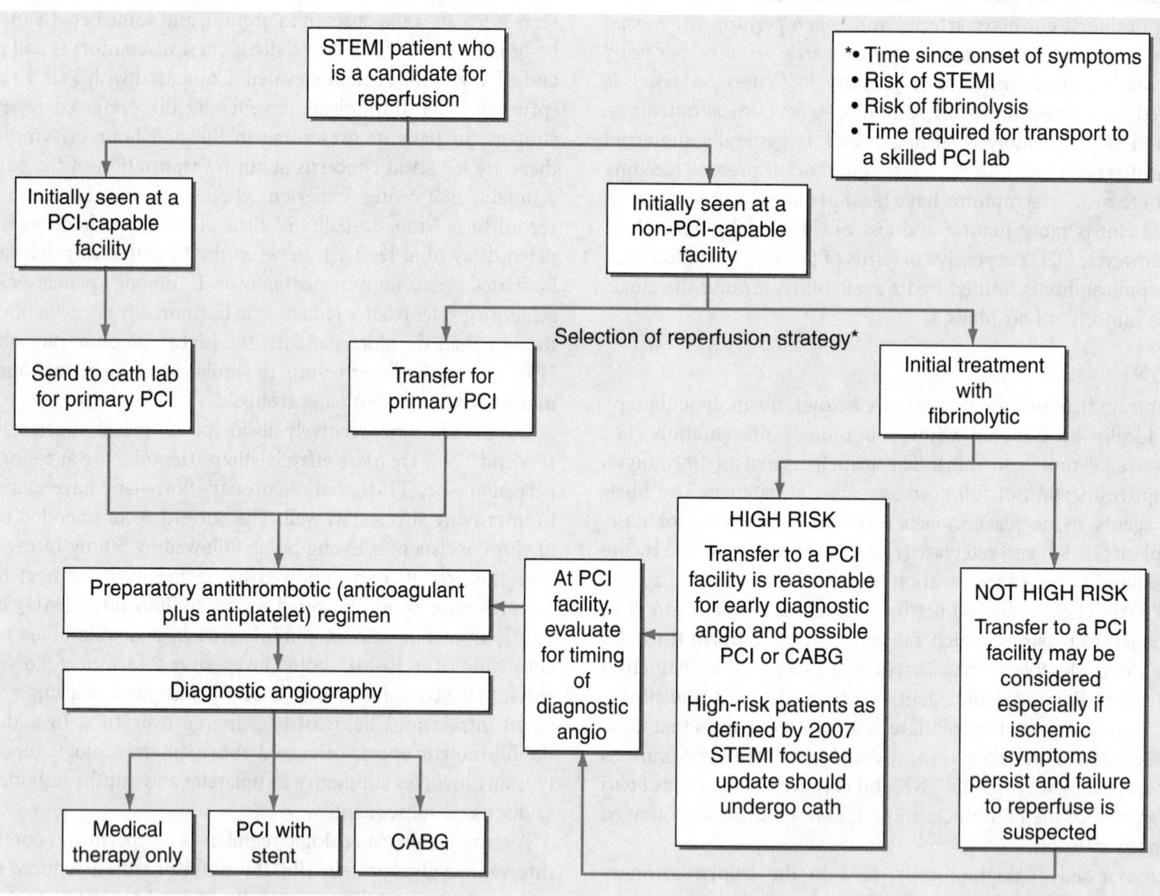

Figure 245-5 Each community and each facility in that community should have an agreed-upon plan for how STEMI patients are to be treated that includes which hospitals should receive STEMI patients from EMS units capable of obtaining diagnostic ECGs, management at the initial receiving hospital, and written criteria and agreements for expeditious transfer of patients from non-PCI-capable facilities. Patients initially seen at a PCI-capable facility (left side of diagram) should be sent promptly to the cardiac catheterization laboratory with the intent to perform primary PCI. Patients initially seen at a non-PCI-capable facility (right side of diagram) should rapidly be assessed for the optimum reperfusion therapy (see box in top right corner for assessment criteria). This may include transfer for primary PCI or initial treatment with a fibrinolytic. Following administration of a fibrinolytic, management is dictated by the patient's overall risk for death/serious complications of STEMI, and whether or not they experience recurrent ischemic symptoms or left-ventricular failure (see the two boxes at the bottom right of diagram). *[Adapted from Kushner FG et al: 2009 focused update of the ACC/AHA Guidelines for the Management of Patients with ST-Elevation Myocardial Infarction (updating the 2004 guideline and 2007 focused update): a report of the American College of Cardiology Foundation/American Heart Association Task Force on Practice Guidelines. Circulation 120:2271, 2009.]*

most serious complication and occurs in ~0.5–0.9% of patients being treated with these agents. This rate increases with advancing age, with patients >70 years experiencing roughly twice the rate of intracranial hemorrhage as those <65 years. Large-scale trials have suggested that the rate of intracranial hemorrhage with tPA or rPA is slightly higher than with streptokinase.

Cardiac catheterization and coronary angiography should be carried out after fibrinolytic therapy if there is evidence of either (1) failure of reperfusion (persistent chest pain and ST-segment elevation >90 min), in which case a *rescue PCI* should be considered; or (2) coronary artery reocclusion (re-elevation of ST segments and/or recurrent chest pain) or the development of recurrent ischemia (such as recurrent angina in the early hospital course or a positive exercise stress test before discharge), in which case an *urgent PCI* should be considered. The potential benefits of routine angiography and *elective* PCI even in asymptomatic patients following administration of fibrinolytic therapy are controversial, but such an approach may have merit given the numerous technological advances that have occurred in the catheterization laboratory and the increasing number of skilled interventionalists. Coronary artery bypass surgery should be reserved for patients whose coronary anatomy is unsuited to PCI but in whom revascularization appears to be advisable because of extensive jeopardized myocardium or recurrent ischemia.

HOSPITAL PHASE MANAGEMENT

CORONARY CARE UNITS

These units are routinely equipped with a system that permits continuous monitoring of the cardiac rhythm of each patient and hemodynamic monitoring in selected patients. Defibrillators, respirators, noninvasive transthoracic pacemakers, and facilities for introducing pacing catheters and flow-directed balloon-tipped catheters are also usually available. Equally important is the organization of a highly trained team of nurses who can recognize arrhythmias; adjust the dosage of antiarrhythmic, vasoactive, and anticoagulant drugs; and perform cardiac resuscitation, including electroshock, when necessary.

Patients should be admitted to a coronary care unit early in their illness when it is expected that they will derive benefit from the sophisticated and expensive care provided. The availability of electrocardiographic monitoring and trained personnel outside the coronary care unit has made it possible to admit lower-risk patients (e.g., those not hemodynamically compromised and without active arrhythmias) to "intermediate care units."

The duration of stay in the coronary care unit is dictated by the ongoing need for intensive care. If symptoms are controlled with oral therapy, patients may be transferred out of the coronary care unit. Also, patients who have a confirmed STEMI but who are considered to be at low risk [no prior infarction and no persistent chest discomfort, congestive heart failure (CHF), hypotension, or cardiac arrhythmias] may be safely transferred out of the coronary care unit within 24 h.

Activity

Factors that increase the work of the heart during the initial hours of infarction may increase the size of the infarct. Therefore, patients with STEMI should be kept at bed rest for the first 12 h. However, in the absence of complications, patients should be encouraged, under supervision, to resume an upright posture by dangling their feet over the side of the bed and sitting in a chair within the first 24 h. This practice is psychologically beneficial and usually results in a reduction in the pulmonary capillary wedge pressure. In the absence of hypotension and other complications, by the second or third day, patients typically are ambulating in their room with increasing duration and frequency, and they may shower or stand at the sink to bathe. By day 3 after infarction, patients should be increasing their ambulation progressively to a goal of 185 m (600 ft) at least 3 times a day.

Diet

Because of the risk of emesis and aspiration soon after STEMI, patients should receive either nothing or only clear liquids by mouth for the first 4–12 h. The typical coronary care unit diet should provide ≤30% of total calories as fat and have a cholesterol content of ≤300 mg/d. Complex carbohydrates should make up 50–55% of total calories. Portions should not be unusually large, and the menu should be enriched with foods that are high in potassium, magnesium, and fiber, but low in sodium. Diabetes mellitus and hypertriglyceridemia are managed by restriction of concentrated sweets in the diet.

Bowel management

Bed rest and the effect of the narcotics used for the relief of pain often lead to constipation. A bedside commode rather than a bedpan, a diet rich in bulk, and the routine use of a stool softener such as dioctyl sodium sulfosuccinate (200 mg/d) are recommended. If the patient remains constipated despite these measures, a laxative can be prescribed. Contrary to prior belief, it is safe to perform a gentle rectal examination on patients with STEMI.

Sedation

Many patients require sedation during hospitalization to withstand the period of enforced inactivity with tranquillity. Diazepam (5 mg), oxazepam (15–30 mg), or lorazepam (0.5–2 mg), given 3–4 times daily, is usually effective. An additional dose of any of the above medications may be given at night to ensure adequate sleep. Attention to this problem is especially important during the first few days in the coronary care unit, where the atmosphere of 24-h vigilance may interfere with the patient's sleep. However, sedation is no substitute for reassuring, quiet surroundings. Many drugs used in the coronary care unit, such as atropine, H_2 blockers, and narcotics, can produce delirium, particularly in the elderly. This effect should not be confused with agitation, and it is wise to conduct a thorough review of the patient's medications before arbitrarily prescribing additional doses of anxiolytics.

PHARMACOTHERAPY

ANTITHROMBOTIC AGENTS

The use of antiplatelet and anticoagulant therapy during the initial phase of STEMI is based on extensive laboratory and clinical evidence that thrombosis plays an important role in the pathogenesis of this condition. The primary goal of treatment with antiplatelet and anticoagulant agents is to maintain patency of the infarct-related artery, in conjunction with reperfusion strategies. A secondary goal is to reduce the patient's tendency to thrombosis and, thus, the likelihood of mural thrombus formation or deep venous thrombosis, either of which could result in pulmonary embolization. The degree to which antiplatelet and anticoagulant therapy achieves these goals partly determines how effectively it reduces the risk of mortality from STEMI.

As noted previously (see "Management in the Emergency Department" above), aspirin is the standard antiplatelet agent for patients with STEMI. The most compelling evidence for the benefits of antiplatelet therapy (mainly with aspirin) in STEMI is found in the comprehensive overview by the Antiplatelet Trialists' Collaboration. Data from nearly 20,000 patients with MI enrolled in 15 randomized trials were pooled and revealed a relative reduction of 27% in the mortality rate, from 14.2% in control patients to 10.4% in patients receiving antiplatelet agents.

Inhibitors of the P2Y12 ADP receptor prevent activation and aggregation of platelets. The addition of the P2Y12 inhibitor clopidogrel to background treatment with aspirin to STEMI patients reduces the risk of clinical events (death, reinfarction, stroke) and, in patients receiving fibrinolytic therapy, has been shown to prevent reocclusion of a successfully reperfused infarct artery. New P2Y12 ADP receptor antagonists, such as prasugrel and ticagrelor, are more effective than clopidogrel in preventing ischemic complications in STEMI patients undergoing PCI, but are associated with an increased risk of bleeding. Glycoprotein IIb/IIIa receptor inhibitors appear useful for preventing thrombotic complications in patients with STEMI undergoing PCI.

The standard anticoagulant agent used in clinical practice is unfractionated heparin (UFH). The available data suggest that when UFH is added to a regimen of aspirin and a non-fibrin-specific thrombolytic agent such as streptokinase, additional mortality benefit occurs (about 5 lives saved per 1000 patients treated). It appears that the immediate administration of intravenous UFH, in addition to a regimen of aspirin and relatively fibrin-specific fibrinolytic agents (tPA, rPA, or TNK), helps to maintain patency of the infarct-related artery. This effect is achieved at the cost of a small increased risk of bleeding. The recommended dose of UFH is an initial bolus of 60 U/kg (maximum 4000 U) followed by an initial infusion of 12 U/kg per hour (maximum 1000 U/h). The activated partial thromboplastin time during maintenance therapy should be 1.5–2 times the control value.

Alternatives to UFH for anticoagulation of patients with STEMI are the low-molecular-weight heparin (LMWH) preparations, a synthetic version of the critical pentasaccharide sequence (fondaparinux), and the direct antithrombin bivalirudin. Advantages of LMWHs include high bioavailability permitting administration subcutaneously, reliable anticoagulation without monitoring, and greater antiXa:IIa activity. Enoxaparin has been shown to reduce significantly the composite endpoints of death/nonfatal reinfarction and death/nonfatal reinfarction/urgent revascularization compared with UFH in STEMI patients who receive fibrinolysis. Treatment with enoxaparin is associated with higher rates of serious bleeding, but net clinical benefit—a composite endpoint that combines efficacy and safety—still favors enoxaparin over UFH. Interpretation of the data on fondaparinux is difficult because of the complex nature of the pivotal clinical trial evaluating it in STEMI (OASIS-6). Fondaparinux appears superior to placebo in STEMI patients not receiving reperfusion therapy, but its relative efficacy and safety compared with UFH is less certain. Owing to the risk of catheter thrombosis, fondaparinux should not be used alone at the time of coronary angiography and PCI but should be combined with another anticoagulant with antithrombin activity such as UFH or bivalirudin. Contemporary trials of bivalirudin used an open-label design to evaluate its efficacy and safety compared with UFH plus a glycoprotein IIb/IIIa inhibitor. Bivalirudin was associated with a lower rate of bleeding, largely driven by reductions in vascular access site hematomas ≥5 cm or the administration of blood transfusions.

Patients with an anterior location of the infarction, severe LV dysfunction, heart failure, a history of embolism, two-dimensional echocardiographic evidence of mural thrombus, or atrial fibrillation are at increased risk of systemic or pulmonary thromboembolism. Such individuals should receive full therapeutic levels of anticoagulant therapy (LMWH or UFH) while hospitalized, followed by at least three months of warfarin therapy.

BETA-ADRENOCEPTOR BLOCKERS

The benefits of beta blockers in patients with STEMI can be divided into those that occur immediately when the drug is given acutely and those that accrue over the long term when the drug is given for secondary prevention after an infarction. Acute intravenous beta blockade improves the myocardial O_2 supply-demand relationship, decreases pain, reduces infarct size, and decreases the incidence of serious ventricular arrhythmias. In patients who undergo fibrinolysis soon after the onset of chest pain, no incremental reduction in mortality rate is seen with beta blockers, but recurrent ischemia and reinfarction are reduced.

Thus, beta-blocker therapy after STEMI is useful for most patients [including those treated with an angiotensin-converting enzyme (ACE) inhibitor] except those in whom it is specifically contraindicated (patients with heart failure or severely compromised LV function, heart block, orthostatic hypotension, or a history of asthma) and perhaps those whose excellent long-term prognosis (defined as an expected mortality rate of <1% per year, patients <55 years, no previous MI, with normal ventricular function, no complex ventricular ectopy, and no angina) markedly diminishes any potential benefit.

INHIBITION OF THE RENIN-ANGIOTENSIN-ALDOSTERONE SYSTEM

ACE inhibitors reduce the mortality rate after STEMI, and the mortality benefits are additive to those achieved with aspirin and beta blockers. The maximum benefit is seen in high-risk patients (those who are elderly or who have an anterior infarction, a prior infarction, and/or globally depressed LV function), but evidence suggests that a short-term benefit occurs when ACE inhibitors are prescribed unselectively to all hemodynamically stable patients with STEMI (i.e., those with a systolic pressure >100 mmHg). The mechanism involves a reduction in ventricular remodeling after infarction (see "Ventricular Dysfunction" below) with a subsequent reduction in the risk of CHF. The rate of recurrent infarction may also be lower in patients treated chronically with ACE inhibitors after infarction.

Before hospital discharge, LV function should be assessed with an imaging study. ACE inhibitors should be continued indefinitely in patients who have clinically evident CHF, in patients in whom an imaging study shows a reduction in global LV function or a large regional wall motion abnormality, or in those who are hypertensive.

Angiotensin receptor blockers (ARBs) should be administered to STEMI patients who are intolerant of ACE inhibitors and who have either clinical or radiological signs of heart failure. Long-term aldosterone blockade should be prescribed for STEMI patients without significant renal dysfunction (creatinine ≥2.5 mg/dL in men and ≥2.0 mg/dL in women) or hyperkalemia (potassium ≥5.0 mEq/L) who are already receiving therapeutic doses of an ACE inhibitor, an LV ejection fraction ≤40 percent, and either symptomatic heart failure or diabetes mellitus. A multidrug regimen for inhibiting the renin-angiotensin-aldosterone system has been shown to reduce both heart failure–related and sudden cardiac death–related cardiovascular mortality after STEMI, but has not been as thoroughly explored as ACE inhibitors in STEMI patients.

OTHER AGENTS

Favorable effects on the ischemic process and ventricular remodeling (see below) previously led many physicians to routinely use *intravenous nitroglycerin* (5–10 μg/min initial dose and up to 200 μg/min as long as hemodynamic stability is maintained) for the first 24–48 h after the onset of infarction. However, the benefits of routine use of intravenous nitroglycerin are less in the contemporary era where beta-adrenoceptor blockers and ACE inhibitors are routinely prescribed for patients with STEMI.

Results of multiple trials of different calcium antagonists have failed to establish a role for these agents in the treatment of most patients with STEMI. Therefore, the routine use of calcium antagonists cannot be recommended. Strict control of blood glucose in diabetic patients with STEMI has been shown to reduce the mortality rate. Serum magnesium should be measured in all patients on admission, and any demonstrated deficits should be corrected to minimize the risk of arrhythmias.

COMPLICATIONS AND THEIR MANAGEMENT

VENTRICULAR DYSFUNCTION

After STEMI, the left ventricle undergoes a series of changes in shape, size, and thickness in both the infarcted and noninfarcted segments. This process is referred to as *ventricular remodeling* and generally precedes the development of clinically evident CHF in the months to years after infarction. Soon after STEMI, the left ventricle begins to dilate. Acutely, this results from expansion of the infarct, i.e., slippage of muscle bundles, disruption of normal myocardial cells, and tissue loss within the necrotic zone, resulting in disproportionate thinning and elongation of the infarct zone. Later, lengthening of the noninfarcted segments occurs as well. The overall chamber enlargement that occurs is related to the size and location of the infarct, with greater dilation following infarction of the anterior wall and apex of the left ventricle and causing more marked hemodynamic impairment, more frequent heart failure, and a poorer prognosis. Progressive dilation and its clinical consequences may be ameliorated by therapy with ACE inhibitors and other vasodilators (e.g., nitrates). In patients with an ejection fraction <40%, regardless of whether or not heart failure is present, ACE inhibitors or ARBs should be prescribed (see "Inhibition of the Renin-Angiotensin-Aldosterone System" above).

HEMODYNAMIC ASSESSMENT

Pump failure is now the primary cause of in-hospital death from STEMI. The extent of infarction correlates well with the degree of pump failure and with mortality, both early (within 10 days of infarction) and later. The most common clinical signs are pulmonary rales and S_3 and S_4 gallop sounds. Pulmonary congestion is also frequently seen on the chest roentgenogram. Elevated LV filling pressure and elevated pulmonary artery pressure are the characteristic hemodynamic findings, but these findings may result from a reduction of ventricular compliance (diastolic failure) and/or a reduction of stroke volume with secondary cardiac dilation (systolic failure) (Chap. 234).

A classification originally proposed by Killip divides patients into four groups: class I, no signs of pulmonary or venous congestion; class II, moderate heart failure as evidenced by rales at the lung bases, S_3 gallop, tachypnea, or signs of failure of the right side of the heart, including venous and hepatic congestion; class III, severe heart failure, pulmonary edema; and class IV, shock with systolic pressure <90 mmHg and evidence of peripheral vasoconstriction, peripheral cyanosis, mental confusion, and oliguria. When this classification was established in 1967, the expected hospital mortality rate of patients in these classes was as follows: class I, 0–5%; class II, 10–20%; class III, 35–45%; and class IV, 85–95%. With advances in management, the mortality rate in each class has fallen, perhaps by as much as one-third to one-half.

Hemodynamic evidence of abnormal global LV function appears when contraction is seriously impaired in 20–25% of the left ventricle. Infarction of ≥40% of the left ventricle usually results in cardiogenic shock (Chap. 272). Positioning of a balloon flotation (Swan-Ganz) catheter in the pulmonary artery permits monitoring of LV filling pressure; this technique is useful in patients who exhibit hypotension and/or clinical evidence of CHF. Cardiac output can also be determined with a pulmonary artery catheter. With the addition of intra-arterial pressure monitoring, systemic vascular resistance can be calculated as a guide to adjusting vasopressor and vasodilator therapy. Some patients with STEMI have markedly elevated LV filling pressures (>22 mmHg) and normal cardiac indices [2.6–3.6 L/(min/m^2)], while others have relatively low LV filling pressures (<15 mmHg) and reduced cardiac indices. The former patients usually benefit from diuresis, while the latter may respond to volume expansion.

HYPOVOLEMIA

This is an easily corrected condition that may contribute to the hypotension and vascular collapse associated with STEMI in some patients. It may be secondary to previous diuretic use, to reduced fluid intake during the early stages of the illness, and/or to vomiting associated with pain or medications. Consequently, hypovolemia should be identified and corrected in patients with STEMI and hypotension before more vigorous forms of therapy are begun. Central venous pressure reflects RV rather than LV filling pressure and is an inadequate guide for adjustment of blood volume, because LV function is almost always affected much more adversely than RV function in patients with STEMI. The optimal LV filling or pulmonary artery wedge pressure may vary considerably among patients. Each patient's ideal level (generally ~20 mmHg) is reached by cautious fluid administration during careful monitoring of oxygenation and cardiac output. Eventually, the cardiac output level plateaus, and further increases in LV filling pressure only increase congestive symptoms and decrease systemic oxygenation without raising arterial pressure.

TREATMENT Congestive Heart Failure

The management of CHF in association with STEMI is similar to that of acute heart failure secondary to other forms of heart disease (avoidance of hypoxemia, diuresis, afterload reduction, inotropic support) (Chap. 234), except that the benefits of digitalis administration to patients with STEMI are unimpressive. By contrast, diuretic agents are extremely effective, as they diminish pulmonary congestion in the presence of systolic and/or diastolic heart failure. LV filling pressure falls and orthopnea and dyspnea improve after the intravenous administration of furosemide or other loop diuretics. These drugs should be used with caution, however, as they can result in a massive diuresis with associated decreases in plasma volume, cardiac output, systemic blood pressure, and, hence, coronary perfusion. Nitrates in various forms may be used to decrease preload and congestive symptoms. Oral isosorbide dinitrate, topical nitroglycerin ointment, or intravenous nitroglycerin all have the advantage over a diuretic of lowering preload through venodilation without decreasing the total plasma volume. In addition, nitrates may improve ventricular compliance if ischemia is present, as ischemia causes an elevation of LV filling pressure. Vasodilators must be used with caution to prevent serious hypotension. As noted earlier, ACE inhibitors are an ideal class of drugs for management of ventricular dysfunction after STEMI, especially for the long term. (See "Inhibition of the Renin-Angiotensin-Aldosterone System" above.)

CARDIOGENIC SHOCK

Prompt reperfusion, efforts to reduce infarct size and treatment of ongoing ischemia and other complications of MI appear to have reduced the incidence of cardiogenic shock from 20% to about 7%. Only 10% of patients with this condition present with it on admission, while 90% develop it during hospitalization. Typically, patients who develop cardiogenic shock have severe multivessel coronary artery disease with evidence of "piecemeal" necrosis extending outward from the original infarct zone. The evaluation and management of cardiogenic shock and severe power failure after STEMI are discussed in detail in Chap. 272.

RIGHT VENTRICULAR INFARCTION

Approximately one-third of patients with inferior infarction demonstrate at least a minor degree of RV necrosis. An occasional patient with inferoposterior LV infarction also has extensive RV infarction, and rare patients present with infarction limited primarily to the RV. Clinically significant RV infarction causes signs of severe RV failure [jugular venous distention, Kussmaul's sign, hepatomegaly (Chap. 227)] with or without hypotension. ST-segment elevations of right-sided precordial ECG leads, particularly lead V_4R, are frequently present in the first 24 h in patients with RV infarction. Two-dimensional echocardiography is helpful in determining the degree of RV dysfunction. Catheterization of the right side of the heart often reveals a distinctive hemodynamic pattern resembling constrictive pericarditis (steep right atrial "y" descent and an early diastolic dip and plateau in RV waveforms) (Chap. 239). Therapy consists of volume expansion to maintain adequate RV preload and efforts to improve LV performance with attendant reduction in pulmonary capillary wedge and pulmonary arterial pressures.

ARRHYTHMIAS

(See also Chaps. 232 and 233) The incidence of arrhythmias after STEMI is higher in patients seen early after the onset of symptoms. The mechanisms responsible for infarction-related arrhythmias include autonomic nervous system imbalance, electrolyte disturbances, ischemia, and slowed conduction in zones of ischemic myocardium. An arrhythmia can usually be managed successfully if trained personnel and appropriate equipment are available when it develops. Since most deaths from arrhythmia occur during the first few hours after infarction, the effectiveness of treatment relates directly to the speed with which patients come under medical observation. The prompt management of arrhythmias constitutes a significant advance in the treatment of STEMI.

Ventricular premature beats

Infrequent, sporadic ventricular premature depolarizations occur in almost all patients with STEMI and do not require therapy. Whereas in the past, frequent, multifocal, or early diastolic ventricular extrasystoles (so-called warning arrhythmias) were routinely treated with antiarrhythmic drugs to reduce the risk of development of ventricular tachycardia and ventricular fibrillation, pharmacologic therapy is now reserved for patients with sustained ventricular arrhythmias. Prophylactic antiarrhythmic therapy (either intravenous lidocaine early or oral agents later) is contraindicated for ventricular premature beats in the absence of clinically important ventricular tachyarrhythmias, as such therapy may actually increase the mortality rate. Beta-adrenoceptor blocking agents are effective in abolishing ventricular ectopic activity in patients with STEMI and in the prevention of ventricular fibrillation. As described above (see "Beta-Adrenoceptor Blockers"), they should be used routinely in patients without contraindications. In addition, hypokalemia and hypomagnesemia are risk factors for ventricular fibrillation in patients with STEMI; to reduce the risk, the serum potassium concentration should be adjusted to approximately 4.5 mmol/L and magnesium to about 2.0 mmol/L.

Ventricular tachycardia and fibrillation

Within the first 24 h of STEMI, ventricular tachycardia and fibrillation can occur without prior warning arrhythmias. The occurrence of ventricular fibrillation can be reduced by prophylactic administration of intravenous lidocaine. However, prophylactic use of lidocaine has not been shown to reduce overall mortality from STEMI. In fact, in addition to causing possible noncardiac complications, lidocaine may predispose to an excess risk of bradycardia and asystole. For these reasons, and with earlier treatment of active ischemia, more frequent use of beta-blocking agents, and the nearly universal success of electrical cardioversion or defibrillation, routine prophylactic antiarrhythmic drug therapy *is no longer recommended.*

Sustained ventricular tachycardia that is well tolerated hemodynamically should be treated with an intravenous regimen of amiodarone (bolus of 150 mg over 10 min, followed by infusion of 1.0 mg/min for 6 h and then 0.5 mg/min) or procainamide (bolus of 15 mg/kg over 20–30 min; infusion of 1–4 mg/min); if it does not stop promptly, electroversion should be used (Chap. 233). An unsynchronized discharge of 200–300 J (monophasic wave form; approximately 50% of these energies with biphasic wave forms) is used immediately in patients with ventricular fibrillation or when ventricular tachycardia causes hemodynamic deterioration. Ventricular tachycardia or fibrillation that is refractory to electroshock may be more responsive after the patient is treated with epinephrine (1 mg intravenously or 10 mL of a 1:10,000 solution via the intracardiac route) or amiodarone (a 75–150-mg bolus).

Ventricular arrhythmias, including the unusual form of ventricular tachycardia known as torsades des pointes (Chap. 233), may occur in patients with STEMI as a consequence of other concurrent problems (such as hypoxia, hypokalemia, or other electrolyte disturbances) or of the toxic effects of an agent being administered to the patient (such as digoxin or quinidine). A search for such secondary causes should always be undertaken.

Although the in-hospital mortality rate is increased, the long-term survival is excellent in patients who survive to hospital discharge after *primary* ventricular fibrillation; i.e., ventricular fibrillation that is a primary response to acute ischemia that occurs during the first 48 h and is not associated with predisposing factors such as CHF, shock, bundle branch block, or ventricular aneurysm. This result is in sharp contrast to the poor prognosis for patients who develop ventricular fibrillation *secondary* to severe pump failure. For patients who develop ventricular tachycardia or ventricular fibrillation late in their hospital course (i.e., after the first 48 h), the mortality rate is increased both in-hospital and during long-term follow-up. Such patients should be considered for electrophysiologic study and implantation of a cardioverter/defibrillator (ICD) (Chap. 233). A more challenging issue is the prevention of sudden cardiac death from ventricular fibrillation late after STEMI in patients who have not exhibited sustained ventricular tachyarrhythmias during their index hospitalization. An algorithm for selection of patients who warrant prophylactic implantation of an ICD is shown in Fig. 245-6.

Accelerated idioventricular rhythm

Accelerated idioventricular rhythm (AIVR, "slow ventricular tachycardia"), a ventricular rhythm with a rate of 60–100 bpm, often occurs transiently during fibrinolytic therapy at the time of reperfusion. For the most part, AIVR, whether it occurs in association with fibrinolytic therapy or spontaneously, is benign and does not presage the development of classic ventricular tachycardia. Most episodes of AIVR do not require treatment if the patient is monitored carefully, as degeneration into a more serious arrhythmia is rare.

Supraventricular arrhythmias

Sinus tachycardia is the most common supraventricular arrhythmia. If it occurs secondary to another cause (such as anemia, fever, heart failure, or a metabolic derangement), the primary problem should be treated first. However, if it appears to be due to sympathetic overstimulation (e.g., as part of a hyperdynamic state), then treatment with

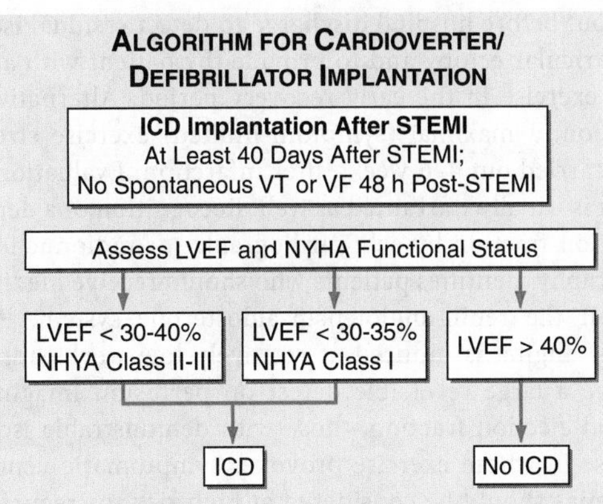

Figure 245-6 Algorithm for assessment of need for implantation of a cardioverter/defibrillator. The appropriate management is selected based upon measurement of left ventricular ejection fraction and assessment of the NYHA functional class. Patients with depressed left ventricular function at least 40 days post-STEMI are referred for insertion of an implantable cardioverter/defibrillator (ICD) if the LVEF is <30–40% and they are in NYHA class II–III or if the LVEF is <30–35% and they are in NYHA class I functional status. Patients with preserved left ventricular function (LVEF >40%) do not receive an ICD regardless of NYHA functional class. All patients are treated with medical therapy post-STEMI. *[Adapted from data contained in Zipes DP, et al: ACC/AHA/ESC 2006 guidelines for management of patients with ventricular arrhythmias and the prevention of sudden cardiac death; a report of the American College of Cardiology/American Heart Association Task Force and the European Society of Cardiology Committee for Practice Guidelines (Writing Committee to Develop Guidelines for Management of Patients with Ventricular Arrhythmias and the Prevention of Sudden Cardiac Death). J Am Coll Cardiol 48:1064, 2006.]*

a beta blocker is indicated. Other common arrhythmias in this group are atrial flutter and atrial fibrillation, which are often secondary to LV failure. Digoxin is usually the treatment of choice for supraventricular arrhythmias if heart failure is present. If heart failure is absent, beta blockers, verapamil, or diltiazem are suitable alternatives for controlling the ventricular rate, as they may also help to control ischemia. If the abnormal rhythm persists for >2 h with a ventricular rate >120 bpm, or if tachycardia induces heart failure, shock, or ischemia (as manifested by recurrent pain or ECG changes), a synchronized electroshock (100–200 J monophasic wave form) should be used.

Accelerated junctional rhythms have diverse causes but may occur in patients with inferoposterior infarction. Digitalis excess must be ruled out. In some patients with severely compromised LV function, the loss of appropriately timed atrial systole results in a marked reduction of cardiac output. Right atrial or coronary sinus pacing is indicated in such instances.

Sinus bradycardia

Treatment of sinus bradycardia is indicated if hemodynamic compromise results from the slow heart rate. Atropine is the most useful drug for increasing heart rate and should be given intravenously in doses of 0.5 mg initially. If the rate remains <50–60 bpm, additional doses of 0.2 mg, up to a total of 2.0 mg, may be given. Persistent bradycardia (<40 bpm) despite atropine may be treated with electrical pacing. Isoproterenol should be avoided.

Atrioventricular and intraventricular conduction disturbances

(See also Chap. 232) Both the in-hospital mortality rate and the post-discharge mortality rate of patients who have complete atrioventricular (AV) block in association with anterior infarction are markedly higher than those of patients who develop AV block with inferior infarction. This difference is related to the fact that heart block in inferior infarction is commonly a result of increased vagal tone and/or the release of adenosine and therefore is transient. In anterior wall infarction, however, heart block is usually related to ischemic malfunction of the conduction system, which is commonly associated with extensive myocardial necrosis.

Temporary electrical pacing provides an effective means of increasing the heart rate of patients with bradycardia due to AV block. However, acceleration of the heart rate may have only a limited impact on prognosis in patients with anterior wall infarction and complete heart block in whom the large size of the infarct is the major factor determining outcome. It should be carried out if it improves hemodynamics. Pacing does appear to be beneficial in patients with inferoposterior infarction who have complete heart block associated with heart failure, hypotension, marked bradycardia, or significant ventricular ectopic activity. A subgroup of these patients, those with RV infarction, often respond poorly to ventricular pacing because of the loss of the atrial contribution to ventricular filling. In such patients, dual-chamber AV sequential pacing may be required.

External noninvasive pacing electrodes should be positioned in a "demand" mode for patients with sinus bradycardia (rate <50 bpm) that is unresponsive to drug therapy, Mobitz II second-degree AV block, third-degree heart block, or bilateral bundle branch block (e.g., right bundle branch block plus left anterior fascicular block). Retrospective studies suggest that permanent pacing may reduce the long-term risk of sudden death due to bradyarrhythmias in the rare patient who develops combined persistent bifascicular and transient third-degree heart block during the acute phase of MI.

OTHER COMPLICATIONS

Recurrent chest discomfort

Recurrent angina develops in ~25% of patients hospitalized for STEMI. This percentage is even higher in patients who undergo successful fibrinolysis. Because recurrent or persistent ischemia often heralds extension of the original infarct or reinfarction in a new myocardial zone and is associated with a near tripling of mortality after STEMI, patients with these symptoms should be referred for prompt coronary arteriography and mechanical revascularization. Repeat administration of a fibrinolytic agent is an alternative to early mechanical revascularization.

Pericarditis

(See also Chap. 239) Pericardial friction rubs and/or pericardial pain are frequently encountered in patients with STEMI involving the epicardium. This complication can usually be managed with aspirin (650 mg 4 times daily). It is important to diagnose the chest pain of pericarditis accurately, because failure to recognize it may lead to the erroneous diagnosis of recurrent ischemic pain and/or infarct extension, with resulting inappropriate use of anticoagulants, nitrates, beta blockers, or coronary arteriography. When it occurs, complaints of pain radiating to either trapezius muscle is helpful, because such a pattern of discomfort is typical of pericarditis but rarely occurs with ischemic discomfort. Anticoagulants potentially could cause tamponade in the presence of acute pericarditis (as manifested by either pain or persistent rub) and therefore should not be used unless there is a compelling indication.

Thromboembolism

Clinically apparent thromboembolism complicates STEMI in ~10% of cases, but embolic lesions are found in 20% of patients in necropsy series, suggesting that thromboembolism is often clinically silent.

Thromboembolism is considered to be an important contributing cause of death in 25% of patients with STEMI who die after admission to the hospital. Arterial emboli originate from LV mural thrombi, while most pulmonary emboli arise in the leg veins.

Thromboembolism typically occurs in association with large infarcts (especially anterior), CHF, and a LV thrombus detected by echocardiography. The incidence of arterial embolism from a clot originating in the ventricle at the site of an infarction is small but real. Two-dimensional echocardiography reveals LV thrombi in about one-third of patients with anterior wall infarction but in few patients with inferior or posterior infarction. Arterial embolism often presents as a major complication, such as hemiparesis when the cerebral circulation is involved or hypertension if the renal circulation is compromised. When a thrombus has been clearly demonstrated by echocardiographic or other techniques or when a large area of regional wall motion abnormality is seen even in the absence of a detectable mural thrombus, systemic anticoagulation should be undertaken (in the absence of contraindications), as the incidence of embolic complications appears to be markedly lowered by such therapy. The appropriate duration of therapy is unknown, but 3–6 months is probably prudent.

Left ventricular aneurysm

The term *ventricular aneurysm* is usually used to describe *dyskinesis* or local expansile paradoxical wall motion. Normally functioning myocardial fibers must shorten more if stroke volume and cardiac output are to be maintained in patients with ventricular aneurysm; if they cannot, overall ventricular function is impaired. True aneurysms are composed of scar tissue and neither predispose to nor are associated with cardiac rupture.

The complications of LV aneurysm do not usually occur for weeks to months after STEMI; they include CHF, arterial embolism, and ventricular arrhythmias. Apical aneurysms are the most common and the most easily detected by clinical examination. The physical finding of greatest value is a double, diffuse, or displaced apical impulse. Ventricular aneurysms are readily detected by two-dimensional echocardiography, which may also reveal a mural thrombus in an aneurysm.

Rarely, myocardial rupture may be contained by a local area of pericardium, along with organizing thrombus and hematoma. Over time, this *pseudoaneurysm* enlarges, maintaining communication with the LV cavity through a narrow neck. Because a pseudoaneurysm often ruptures spontaneously, it should be surgically repaired if recognized.

POSTINFARCTION RISK STRATIFICATION AND MANAGEMENT

Many clinical and laboratory factors have been identified that are associated with an increase in cardiovascular risk after initial recovery from STEMI. Some of the most important factors include persistent ischemia (spontaneous or provoked), depressed LV ejection fraction (<40%), rales above the lung bases on physical examination or congestion on chest radiograph, and symptomatic ventricular arrhythmias. Other features associated with increased risk include a history of previous MI, age >75, diabetes mellitus, prolonged sinus tachycardia, hypotension, ST-segment changes at rest without angina ("silent ischemia"), an abnormal signal-averaged ECG, nonpatency of the infarct-related coronary artery (if angiography is undertaken), and persistent advanced heart block or a new intraventricular conduction abnormality on the ECG. Therapy must be individualized on the basis of the relative importance of the risk(s) present.

The goal of preventing reinfarction and death after recovery from STEMI has led to strategies to evaluate risk after infarction. In stable patients, submaximal exercise stress testing may be carried out before hospital discharge to detect residual ischemia and ventricular ectopy and to provide the patient with a guideline for exercise in the early recovery period. Alternatively, or in addition, a maximal (symptom-limited) exercise stress test may be carried out 4–6 weeks after infarction. Evaluation of LV function is usually warranted as well. Recognition of a depressed LV ejection fraction by echocardiography or radionuclide ventriculography identifies patients who should receive medications to inhibit the renin-angiotensin-aldosterone system. Patients in whom angina is induced at relatively low workloads, those who have a large reversible defect on perfusion imaging or a depressed ejection fraction, those with demonstrable ischemia, and those in whom exercise provokes symptomatic ventricular arrhythmias should be considered at high risk for recurrent MI or death from arrhythmia (Fig. 245-6). Cardiac catheterization with coronary angiography and/or invasive electrophysiologic evaluation is advised.

Exercise tests also aid in formulating an individualized exercise prescription, which can be much more vigorous in patients who tolerate exercise without any of the above-mentioned adverse signs. In addition, predischarge stress testing may provide an important psychological benefit, building the patient's confidence by demonstrating a reasonable exercise tolerance.

In many hospitals, a cardiac rehabilitation program with progressive exercise is initiated in the hospital and continued after discharge. Ideally, such programs should include an educational component that informs patients about their disease and its risk factors.

The usual duration of hospitalization for an uncomplicated STEMI is about 5 days. The remainder of the convalescent phase may be accomplished at home. During the first 1–2 weeks, the patient should be encouraged to increase activity by walking about the house and outdoors in good weather. Normal sexual activity may be resumed during this period. After 2 weeks, the physician must regulate the patient's activity on the basis of exercise tolerance. Most patients will be able to return to work within 2–4 weeks.

SECONDARY PREVENTION

Various secondary preventive measures are at least partly responsible for the improvement in the long-term mortality and morbidity rates after STEMI. Long-term treatment with an antiplatelet agent (usually aspirin) after STEMI is associated with a 25% reduction in the risk of recurrent infarction, stroke, or cardiovascular mortality (36 fewer events for every 1000 patients treated). An alternative antiplatelet agent that may be used for secondary prevention in patients intolerant of aspirin is clopidogrel (75 mg orally daily). ACE inhibitors or ARBs and, in appropriate patients, aldosterone antagonists should be used indefinitely by patients with clinically evident heart failure, a moderate decrease in global ejection fraction, or a large regional wall motion abnormality to prevent late ventricular remodeling and recurrent ischemic events.

The chronic routine use of oral beta-adrenoceptor blockers for at least two years after STEMI is supported by well-conducted, placebo-controlled trials.

Evidence suggests that warfarin lowers the risk of late mortality and the incidence of reinfarction after STEMI. Most physicians prescribe aspirin routinely for all patients without contraindications and add warfarin for patients at increased risk of embolism (see "Thromboembolism" above). Several studies suggest that in patients <75 years a low dose of aspirin (75–81 mg/d) in combination with warfarin administered to achieve an INR >2.0 is more effective than aspirin alone for preventing recurrent MI and embolic cerebrovascular accident. However, there is an increased risk of bleeding and a high rate of discontinuation of warfarin that has limited clinical acceptance of combination antithrombotic therapy.

There is increased risk of bleeding when warfarin is added to dual antiplatelet therapy (aspirin and clopidogrel). However, patients who have had a stent implanted and have an indication for anticoagulation should receive dual antiplatelet therapies in combination with warfarin. Such patients should also receive a proton pump inhibitor to minimize the risk of gastrointestinal bleeding and should have regular monitoring of their hemoglobin levels and stool hematest while on combination antithrombotic therapy.

Finally, risk factors for *atherosclerosis* (Chap. 224) should be discussed with the patient, and, when possible, favorably modified.

FURTHER READINGS

ANTMAN EM: ST-Elevation Myocardial Infarction: Management, in: P Libby, RO Bonow, DL Mann, DP Zipes (eds) *Braunwald's Heart Disease: A Textbook of Cardiovascular Medicine,* 8th ed, Philadelphia, Saunders Elsevier, 2008, pp 1233–1299

——: Time is muscle: Translation into practice. J Am Coll Cardiol 52:1216, 2008

BRAUNWALD E, ANTMAN EM: ST-Elevation Myocardial Infarction: Pathology, Pathophysiology, and Clinical Features in P Libby, RO Bonow, DL Mann, DP Zipes (eds) *Braunwald's Heart Disease: A Textbook of Cardiovascular Medicine,* 8th ed, Philadelphia, Saunders Elsevier, 2008, pp 1207–1232

JACOBS AK et al: Development of systems of care for ST-elevation myocardial infarction patients: executive summary. Circulation 116:217, 2007

KUSHNER FG et al: 2009 Focused Updates: ACC/AHA Guidelines for the Management of Patients With ST-Elevation Myocardial Infarction (updating the 2004 Guideline and 2007 Focused Update) and ACC/AHA/SCAI Guidelines on Percutaneous Coronary Intervention (updating the 2005 Guideline and 2007 Focused Update): A report of the American College of Cardiology Foundation/American Heart Association Task Force on Practice Guidelines. Circulation 120:2271, 2009

LLOYD-JONES D et al: Heart disease and stroke statistics—2009 update: A report from the American Heart Association Statistics Committee and Stroke Statistics Subcommittee. Circulation 119:e21, 2009

MEHRAN R et al: Bivalirudin in patients undergoing Primary angioplasty for acute myocardial infarction (HORIZONS-AMI): 1-year results of a randomised controlled trial. Lancet 374:1149, 2009

WHITE HD, CHEW DP: Acute myocardial infarction. Lancet 372:570, 2008

WIVIOTT SD et al: Prasugrel versus clopidogrel in patients with acute coronary syndromes. N Engl J Med 357:2001, 2007

CHAPTER 246

Percutaneous Coronary Interventions and Other Interventional Procedures

David P. Faxon
Deepak L. Bhatt

Percutaneous transluminal coronary angioplasty (PTCA) was first introduced by Andreas Gruentzig in 1977 as an alternative to coronary bypass surgery. The concept of percutaneous dilatation of the atherosclerotic peripheral vessels was initially demonstrated by Charles Dotter in 1964 in peripheral vessels where rigid catheters of graduated diameter were used to progressively enlarge the vessel lumen. The development of a small inelastic balloon catheter by Gruentzig allowed expansion of the technique into smaller peripheral and coronary vessels. Initial coronary experience was limited to the small percentage of patients who had single-vessel coronary disease and discrete proximal lesions due to the technical limitations of the equipment. Advances in technology and greater operator experience allowed the procedure to grow rapidly with expanded use in patients with more complex lesions and multivessel disease; by 1990 it was being performed in more than 300,000 patients annually. The addition of atherectomy devices that removed plaques aided in the growth of the procedure, but the introduction of coronary stents in 1994 was one of the major advances in the field. These devices reduced acute complications and reduced by half the significant problem of restenosis (or recurrence of the stenosis). Further reductions in restenosis were achieved by the introduction of drug-eluting stents in 2003. These stents have a polymer coating over the metal stent that is impregnated with antiproliferative agents that slowly release drugs directly into the plaque over a few months. Today, more than 1 million stents are placed in the United States per year and more than 4 million worldwide. Percutaneous coronary intervention (PCI) is the most common revascularization procedure in the United States and is performed nearly twice as often as coronary artery bypass surgery.

The field of interventional cardiology has matured to be recognized as a separate discipline in cardiology that requires specialized training. A dedicated 1-year interventional cardiology fellowship following a 3-year general cardiology fellowship and a separate board certification examination are now required to be certified in interventional cardiology. The discipline has also expanded to include interventions for structural heart disease including treatment of congenital heart disease, and valvular heart disease; it also includes interventions to treat peripheral vascular disease, including atherosclerotic and non-atherosclerotic lesions in the carotid, renal, aortic, and peripheral circulations.

TECHNIQUE

The initial procedure is performed in a similar manner as a diagnostic cardiac catheterization (Chap. 230). As is done with diagnostic catheterization, arterial access is obtained by percutaneous needle puncture into a peripheral artery. Most commonly, the arterial access site is the femoral artery, but radial artery access is gaining favor. To prevent thrombotic complications during the procedure, patients who are anticipated to need an angioplasty are given aspirin (325 mg) and clopidogrel (loading dose of 300–600 mg) before the procedure. During the procedure, anticoagulation is achieved by administration of unfractionated heparin, enoxaparin (a low-molecular-weight heparin), or bivalirudin (a direct

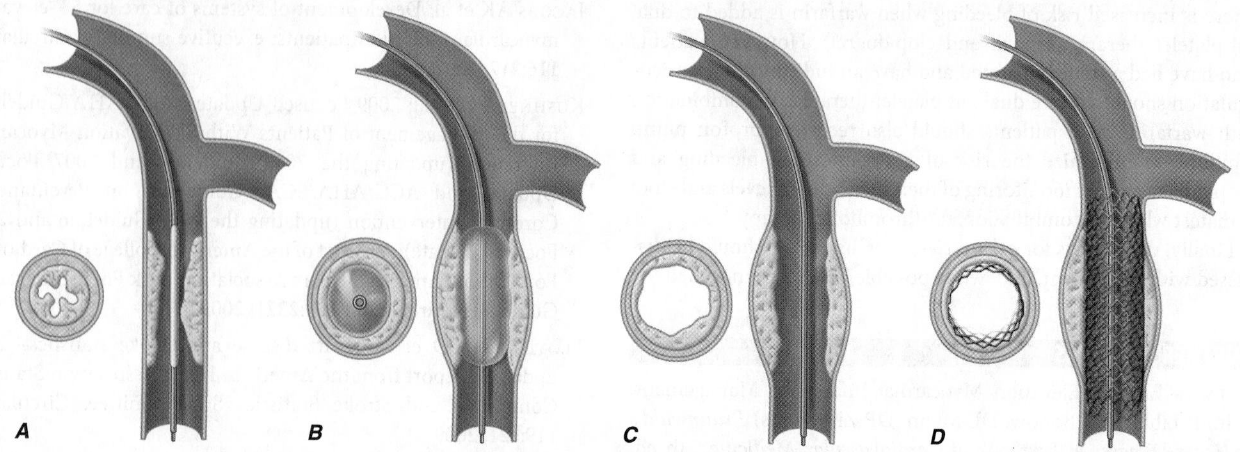

Figure 246-1 Schematic diagram of the primary mechanisms of balloon angioplasty and stenting. ***A.*** A balloon angioplasty catheter is positioned into the stenosis over a guidewire under fluoroscopic guidance. ***B.*** The balloon is inflated temporarily occluding the vessel. ***C.*** The lumen is enlarged primarily by stretching the vessel often resulting in small dissections in the neointima. ***D.*** A stent mounted on a deflated balloon is placed into the lesion and pressed against the vessel wall with balloon inflation (not shown). The balloon is deflated and removed leaving the stent permanently against the wall acting as a scaffold to hold the dissections against the wall and prevent vessel recoil. *(Adapted from EJ Topol: Textbook of Cardiovascular Medicine, 2nd ed. Philadelphia, Lippincott Williams & Wilkins, 2002.)*

thrombin inhibitor). In patients with ST-elevation myocardial infarction, high-risk acute coronary syndrome, or those with a large thrombus in the coronary artery, a glycoprotein IIb/IIIa inhibitor (abciximab, tirofiban, or eptifibatide) may also be given.

Following placement of an introducing sheath, preformed guiding catheters are used to cannulate selectively the origins of the coronary arteries. These catheters have larger internal diameters than diagnostic catheters in order to allow passage of the balloon catheter and wires. Through the guiding catheter, a flexible, steerable guidewire (diameter 0.4 mm) is negotiated down the coronary artery lumen using fluoroscopic guidance; it is then advanced through the stenosis and into the vessel beyond. This guidewire then serves as a "rail" over which angioplasty balloons, stents, or other therapeutic devices can be advanced to enlarge the narrowed segment of coronary artery. The artery is usually dilated with a balloon catheter and most often a stent is then placed with assessment of the final result by repeat angiography through the guiding catheter. The catheters and introducing sheath are removed and the artery manually held or closed using one of several arterial closure devices to achieve hemostasis. Because PCI is performed under local anesthesia and mild sedation, it requires only a short (1-day) hospitalization that decreases recovery time and hospital expense, as compared to coronary bypass surgery.

The inflated diameter of the angioplasty balloons range in size from 1.5 mm to 4.0 mm, and balloons are chosen to approximate the "normal" less diseased proximal or distal vessel without stenosis. The major advance introduced by Dr. Gruentzig was the use of inelastic balloons that do not overexpand the vessel beyond their predetermined size despite high pressures up to 10–20 atmospheres.

Angioplasty works by stretching the artery and compressing the plaque into the vessel wall, away from the lumen, enlarging the entire vessel (Figs. 246-1 and 246-2). The procedure rarely results in embolization of atherosclerotic material. Owing to inelastic elements in the plaque, the stretching of the vessel by the balloon results in small localized dissections that can protrude into the lumen and be a nidus for acute thrombus formation. If the dissections are severe, then they can obstruct the lumen or induce a thrombotic occlusion of the artery (acute closure). Stents have largely prevented this complication by holding the dissection flaps up against the vessel wall (Fig. 246-1).

Stents are currently used in more than 90% of coronary angioplasty procedures. Stents are wire meshes (usually made of stainless

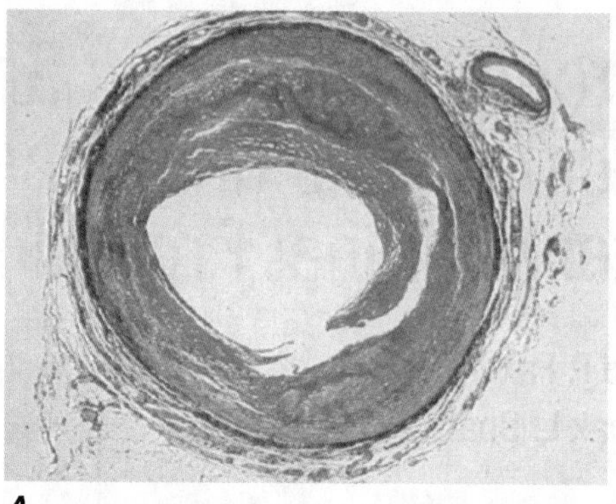

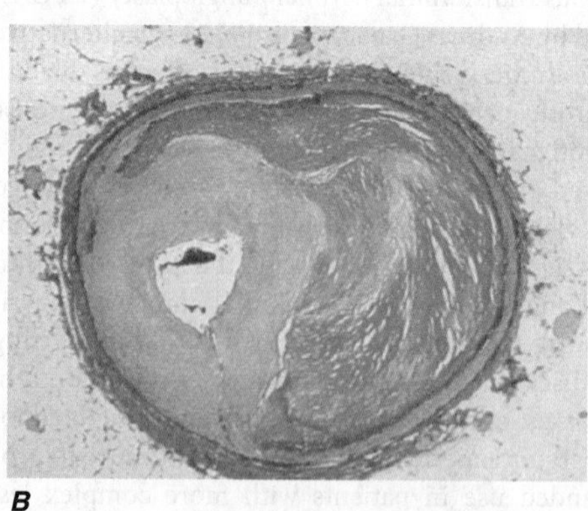

Figure 246-2 Pathology of acute effects of balloon angioplasty with intimal dissection and vessel stretching *(panel A) (From M Ueda et al: Eur Heart J 12:937, 1991; with permission)* and an example of neointimal hyperplasia and restenosis showing renarrowing of the vessel *(panel B)*. *(From CE Essed et al: Br Heart J 49:393, 1983; with permission.)*

steel) that are compressed over a deflated angioplasty balloon. When the balloon is inflated, the stent is enlarged to approximate the "normal" vessel lumen. The balloon is then deflated and removed, leaving the stent behind to provide a permanent scaffold in the artery. Owing to the design of the struts, these devices are flexible, allowing their passage through diseased and tortuous coronary vessels. Stents are rigid enough to prevent elastic recoil of the vessel and have dramatically improved the success and safety of the procedure as a result.

Drug-eluting stents were first introduced in 2003. Using a metal stent, an antiproliferative agent is attached to the stent by use of a thin polymer coating. The antiproliferative drug elutes from the stent over a 1- to 3-month period after implantation. Drug-eluting stents have been shown to reduce clinical restenosis by 50% so that in uncomplicated lesions symptomatic restenosis occurs in 5–12% of patients. Not surprisingly, this led to the rapid acceptance of these devices; currently 50–90% of all stents implanted are drug-eluting. The first-generation devices were coated with either sirolimus or paclitaxel. *Sirolimus* is an immunosuppressive agent that arrests cell proliferation in the G_1 phase. *Paclitaxel* is an inhibitor of microtubules that can arrest cell division at the M phase in high concentrations, but can have cytostatic G_1, antimigratory, and anti-inflammatory effects on smooth muscle cells at lower concentrations. Second-generation drug-eluting stents use newer agents such as everolimus, biolimus, and zotarolimus. These second-generation drug-eluting stents appear to be more effective with fewer complications than the first-generation devices. Preliminary data from long-term follow-up suggests that the second-generation drug-eluting stents have lower rates of stent thrombosis and myocardial infarction than the first-generation drug-eluting stents.

Other interventional devices include atherectomy devices, laser catheters, and thrombectomy catheters. These devices are designed to remove atherosclerotic plaque or thrombus and are used in conjunction with balloon dilatation and stent placement. Rotational atherectomy is the most commonly used adjunctive device for heavily calcified lesions and is modeled after a dentist's drill, with small round burrs of 1.5–2.5 mm at the tip of a flexible wire shaft. They are passed over the guidewire up to the stenosis and activated to rotate at 180,000 rpm in order to drill away atherosclerotic material. Because the atherosclerotic particles are <25 μm, they pass through the coronary microcirculation and rarely cause problems. The device is particularly useful in heavily calcified plaques that are resistant to balloon dilatation. Another available device is the directional atherectomy catheter. This catheter has a rigid housing at its tip that is open on one side, exposing a sliding rotating cutter. The catheter is placed in the stenosis, and a balloon on the noncutting side of the housing is inflated to push the housing up against the wall of the artery. When the cutter is rotated at 2500 rpm and advanced down the housing, it slices off atherosclerotic plaques into a distal collection chamber, allowing the plaque to be removed from the patient. Given the current advances in stents, neither rotational nor directional atherectomy is as frequently used today as in the past. Other devices include fiberoptic laser catheters that can vaporize atherosclerotic plaques. These are infrequently used today, as well. In acute myocardial infarction, specialized catheters without a balloon are used to aspirate thrombus in order to prevent embolization down the coronary vessel and to improve blood flow before angioplasty and stent placement. Data suggest that manual catheter thrombus aspiration may even reduce mortality rate in primary PCI.

PCI of degenerated saphenous vein graft lesions has been associated with a significant incidence of distal embolization of atherosclerotic material, unlike PCI of native vessel disease. A number of distal protection devices have been shown to significantly reduce embolization and myocardial infarction in this setting. Most devices work by using a collapsible wire mesh at the end of a guidewire that is expanded in the distal vessel before angioplasty. If atherosclerotic debris is dislodged, the basket captures the material, and at the end of the PCI, the basket is pulled into a delivery catheter and the debris safely removed from the patient.

SUCCESS AND COMPLICATIONS

The advances in the technology have greatly improved the success and reduced the complications of the procedure. Currently, a successful procedure (angiographic success), defined as a reduction of the stenosis to less than a 20% diameter narrowing, occurs in 95–99% of patients. The success is dependent upon the coronary anatomy, with lower success rates in patients with tortuous, small, or calcified vessels or chronic total occlusions. Chronic total occlusions have the lowest success rates and their recanalization is usually not attempted unless the occlusion is recent (within 3 months) or there are favorable anatomic features. Improvements in equipment and technique have increased the success rates of recanalization of chronic total occlusions.

Serious complications are rare but include a mortality rate of 0.1–0.3% for elective cases, a large myocardial infarction occurs in less than 3%, and stroke in less than 0.1%. Patients who are elderly (>65 years), undergoing an emergent or urgent procedure, have chronic kidney disease, present with an ST-segment elevation myocardial infarction (STEMI), or are in shock have significantly higher risk. Scoring systems can help to estimate the risk of the procedure, although no perfect scoring system has yet been developed.

Myocardial infarction during PCI can occur for multiple reasons including an acute occluding thrombus, severe coronary dissection, embolization of thrombus or atherosclerotic material, or closure of a side branch vessel at the site of angioplasty. Most myocardial infarctions are small and only detected by a rise in the creatinine phosphokinase (CPK) or troponin level after the procedure. Only those with significant enzyme elevations (more than three times the upper limit of normal) are associated with a less favorable long-term outcome. Coronary stents have largely prevented coronary dissections due to the scaffolding effect of the stent. Metallic stents are also prone to thrombotic occlusion (1–3%), either acute (<24 h) or subacute (1–30 days), which can be ameliorated by greater attention to full initial stent deployment and the use of dual antiplatelet therapy [aspirin, plus a platelet P_2Y_{12}-receptor blocker (clopidogrel or prasugrel)]. Late (30 days–1 year) and very late stent thromboses (>1 year) occur very infrequently with stents but are slightly more common with drug-eluting stents, necessitating dual antiplatelet therapy with these stents for up to 1 year or longer. Premature discontinuation of dual antiplatelet therapy particularly in the first month after implantation is associated with a significantly increased risk for stent thrombosis (three- to ninefold greater). Stent thrombosis results in death in 10–20% and a myocardial infarction in 30–70% of patients. Elective surgery that requires discontinuation of antiplatelet therapy after drug-eluting stent implantation should be postponed until after 6 months and preferably after 1 year, if at all possible.

Restenosis, or renarrowing of the dilated coronary stenosis, is the most common complication of angioplasty and occurs in 20–50% of patients with balloon angioplasty alone, 10–30% of patients with bare metal stents, and in 5–15% of patients with drug-eluting stents. The fact that stent placement provides a larger acute luminal area than balloon angioplasty alone reduces the incidence of subsequent restenosis. Drug-eluting stents further reduce restenosis through a reduction in excessive neointimal growth over the stent. If restenosis does not occur, the long-term outcome is excellent (Fig. 246-3). Clinical restenosis is recognized by recurrence of angina or symptoms within 9 months of the procedure. Most commonly, patients

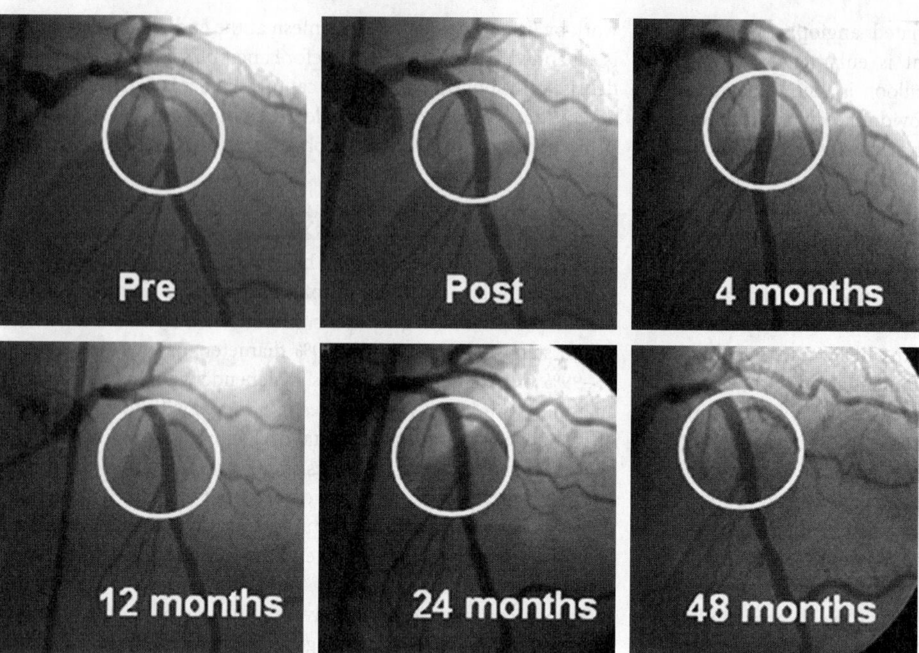

Figure 246-3 Long-term results from one of the first patients to receive a sirolimus-eluting stent from early Sao Paulo experience. *[From: GW Stone, in D Baim (ed): Cardiac Catheterization, Angiography and Intervention, 7th ed, Philadelphia, Lippincott Williams & Wilkins, 2006; with permission.]*

with clinical restenosis present with worsening angina (60–70%), but patients can present with non-ST-elevation myocardial infarction (10%) or ST-elevation myocardial infarction (5%) as well. Clinical restenosis requires confirmation of a significant stenosis at the site of the prior PCI, with repeat PCI or coronary artery bypass grafting (CABG). This is termed *target lesion revascularization* (TLR) or *target vessel revascularization* (TVR). By angiography, the incidence of restenosis is significantly higher than clinical restenosis (TLR or TVR) because many patients have mild restenosis that does not result in a recurrence of symptoms. The management of clinical restenosis is usually to repeat the PCI with balloon dilatation and, placement of a bare metal or a drug-eluting stent. Rarely, intracoronary brachytherapy using beta radiation is used. Once a patient has had restenosis, the risk of a second restenosis is further increased. The risk factors for restenosis are diabetes, long lesions, small-diameter vessels, and suboptimal initial PCI result.

The mechanism of restenosis is similar to that of wound healing, with inflammation and the migration and proliferation of smooth muscle cells that create a thick neointima (scar) that narrows the lumen at the site of dilatation (Fig. 246-2). The neointima is covered with endothelium, but it remains dysfunctional. The primary cause of restenosis in balloon angioplasty is adverse vessel remodeling with constriction of the vessel relative to the adjacent nondilated vessel. This change in remodeling can be appreciated by intravascular ultrasound but not by angiography since the latter only shows the lumen and not the entire vessel size. In addition to remodeling, excessive growth of the neointima further narrows the lumen. Stents prevent this unfavorable constrictive remodeling, and drug-eluting stents not only prevent this constriction but reduce the excessive neointimal growth as well. Common risk factors for atherosclerosis such as hyperlipidemia, hypertension, or cigarette smoking do not increase the risk of restenosis, although diabetes mellitus does.

INDICATIONS

The American College of Cardiology (ACC)/American Heart Association (AHA) guidelines extensively review the indications for PCI in patients with stable angina, unstable angina, non-ST-elevation, and ST-elevation myocardial infarction and should be referred to for a comprehensive discussion of the indications. Briefly, the two principal indications for coronary revascularization in patients with *chronic stable angina* (Chap. 243) are (1) to improve anginal symptoms in patients who remain symptomatic despite adequate medical therapy and (2) to reduce mortality rates in patients with severe coronary disease. In patients with stable angina, who are well controlled on medical therapy, older studies and the more current Clinical Outcomes Utilizing Revascularization and Aggressive Drug Evaluation (COURAGE) and Bypass Angioplasty Revascularization Investigation 2 Diabetes (BARI 2D) trials have shown that revascularization does not lead to better outcomes and can be safely delayed until symptoms worsen or evidence of severe ischemia on noninvasive testing occurs. Randomized trials done in the 1960s and 1970s showed that CABG reduced mortality rates in patients with severe three-vessel or left main coronary disease when compared with medical therapy alone regardless of the degree of symptoms. Whether PCI also confers the same degree of protection is not known as trials of PCI versus medical therapy in patients with three-vessel disease have not been conducted, but randomized trials comparing CABG and PCI have shown equal rates of death and myocardial infarction (MI) rates over 5–10 years of follow-up. Consistently these studies have also shown that PCI, despite the use of stents, is associated with a 10–30% need for repeat PCI during the first year after the procedure due largely to restenosis, although drug-eluting stents have decreased this rate. This contrasts with a need for PCI or repeat CABG in bypass patients of 2–5%.

When revascularization is indicated, the choice of PCI or CABG depends upon a number of clinical and anatomic factors (Fig. 246-4). A subgroup analysis from the Bypass Angioplasty Revascularization Investigation (BARI) randomized trial showed that patients with treated diabetes mellitus and multivessel disease fared better with CABG; however, registry experiences suggest that PCI can be done in selected diabetic patients with less-severe multivessel disease with good long-term outcome. The Synergy between Percutaneous Coronary Intervention with Taxus and Cardiac Surgery (SYNTAX) trial compared PCI with the paclitaxel drug-eluting stent to CABG in 1800 patients with three-vessel coronary disease or left main disease. The study found no difference in death or myocardial infarction at 1 year, but repeat revascularization was significantly higher in the stent-treated group (13.5 vs. 5.9%), while stroke was higher in the surgical group (2.2 vs. 0.6%). The primary endpoint of death, MI, stroke, or revascularization was significantly better with CABG due to the higher rate of revascularization in the drug-eluting stent group. Only 1 year of results are currently available and longer follow-up is needed to assess fully these two revascularization strategies in patients with severe coronary disease.

The choice of PCI versus CABG is also related to the anticipated procedural success and complications of PCI and the risks

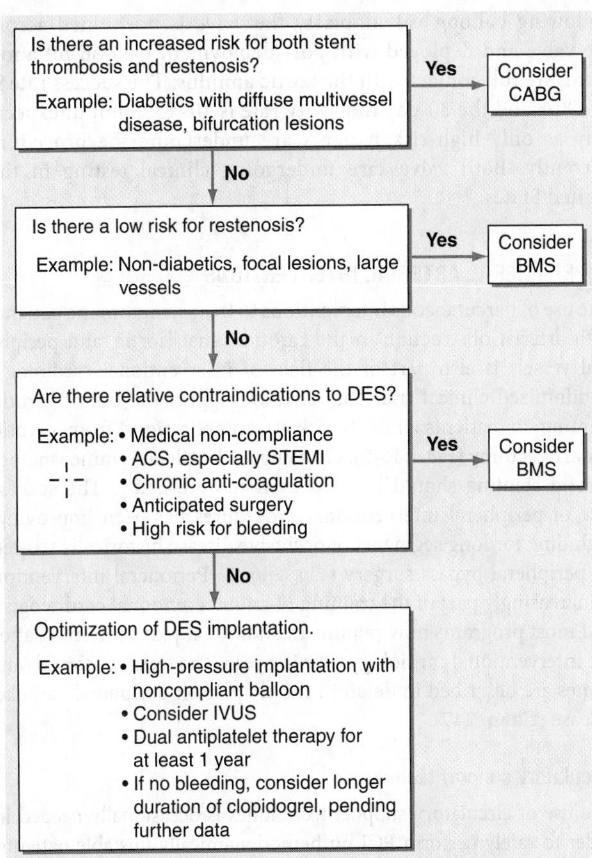

Figure 246-4 In patients requiring revascularization, several factors need to be considered in choosing between bare metal stents, drug-eluting stents, or coronary artery bypass surgery. ACS, acute coronary syndrome; BMS, bare metal stent; CABG, coronary artery bypass grafting; DES, drug-eluting stent; IVUS, intravascular ultrasound; STEMI, ST-segment elevation myocardial infarction. *(From AA Bavry, DL Bhatt: Circulation 116:696, 2007; with permission.)*

of CABG. For PCI, the characteristics of the coronary anatomy are critically important. The location of the lesion in the vessel (proximal or distal), the degree of tortuosity, and size of the vessel are considered. In addition, the lesion characteristics including the degree of the stenosis, the presence of calcium, lesion length, and presence of thrombus are assessed. The most common reason to decide not to do angioplasty is that the lesion felt to be responsible for the patient's symptoms is not treatable. This is most commonly due to the presence of a chronic total occlusion (>3 months in duration). In this setting the historical success rate has been low (30–70%) and complications are more common. A lesion classification to characterize the likelihood of success or failure of PCI has been developed by the ACC/AHA. Lesions with the highest success are called type A lesions (such as proximal noncalcified subtotal lesion) and those with the lowest success or highest complication rate are type C lesions (such as chronic total occlusions). Intermediate lesions are classified as type B1 or B2 depending on the number of unfavorable characteristics. Approximately 25–30% of patients will not be candidates for PCI due to unfavorable anatomy, whereas only 5% of CABG patients will not be candidates for surgery due to coronary anatomy. The primary reason for being considered inoperable is the presence of severe comorbidities such as advanced age, frailty, severe chronic obstructive pulmonary disease (COPD), or poor left ventricular function. Another consideration in choosing a revascularization strategy is the degree of revascularization. In patients with multivessel disease, bypass grafts can usually be placed in all vessels with significant stenosis, while PCI may be able to treat only some of the lesions due to the presence of unfavorable anatomy. The decision to do PCI versus CABG will then depend upon the importance of complete revascularization in the patient. Given the multiple factors that need to be considered in choosing the best revascularization for an individual patient with multivessel disease, it is optimal to have a discussion between the cardiac surgeon and interventional cardiologist and the physicians caring for the patient to properly weigh the choices.

Patients with acute coronary syndrome are at excess risk of short- and long-term mortality. Randomized clinical trials have shown that PCI is superior to intensive medical therapy in reducing mortality rate and myocardial infarction, with the benefit largely confined to those patients who are high risk. This includes patients with refractory ischemia, recurrent angina, positive cardiac-specific enzymes, new ST-segment depression, low ejection fraction, severe arrhythmias, or a recent PCI or CABG. PCI is preferred over surgical therapy in most high-risk patients with acute coronary syndromes unless they have severe multivessel disease or the culprit lesion responsible for the unstable presentation cannot be adequately treated. In STEMI, thrombolysis or PCI (primary PCI) are effective methods to restore coronary blood flow and salvage myocardium within the first 12 hours after onset of chest pain. Because PCI is more effective than thrombolysis, it is preferred if readily available. PCI is also performed following thrombolysis to facilitate adequate reperfusion or as a rescue procedure in those who do not achieve reperfusion from thrombolysis or in those who develop cardiogenic shock.

OTHER INTERVENTIONAL TECHNIQUES

Structural heart disease

Interventional treatment for structural heart disease (adult congenital heart disease and valvular heart disease) is a significant component of the field of interventional cardiology.

The most common adult congenital lesion to be treated with percutaneous techniques is closure of atrial septal defects (Chap. 236). The procedure is done as in a diagnostic right heart catheterization with the passage of a catheter up the femoral vein into the right atrium. With echo and fluoroscopic guidance the size and location of the defect can be accurately defined, and closure is accomplished using one of several approved devices. All devices use a left atrial and right atrial wire mesh or covered disk that are pulled together to capture the atrial septum around the defect and seal it off. The Amplatzer Septal Occluder device (AGA Medical, Minneapolis, Minnesota) is the most commonly used in the United States. The success rate in selected patients is 85–95%, and the device complications are rare and include device embolization, infection, or erosion. Closure of patent foramen ovale (PFO) is done in a similar way. PFO closure is an approved procedure in patients who have had recurrent paradoxical stroke despite adequate medical therapy including anticoagulation. The use in the treatment of migraine is under clinical investigation and is not an approved indication.

Similar devices can also be used to close patent ductus arteriosus and ventricular septal defects. Other congenital diseases that can be treated percutaneously include coarctation of the aorta, pulmonic stenosis, peripheral pulmonary stenosis, and other abnormal communications between the cardiac chambers or vessels.

The treatment of valvular heart disease is the most rapidly growing area in interventional cardiology. Until recently the only available techniques were balloon valvuoplasty for the treatment of aortic, mitral, or pulmonic stenosis (Chap. 237). Mitral valvuloplasty is the preferred treatment for symptomatic patients with rheumatic mitral stenosis who have favorable anatomy. The outcome in these patients is equal to that of surgical commissurotomy. The success is highly related to the echocardiographic appearance of the valve. The most favorable setting is commissural fusion without calcification or subchordal fusion and the absence of significant mitral regurgitation. Access is obtained from the femoral vein using a transseptal technique where a long metal catheter with a needle tip is advanced from the femoral vein through the right atrium and atrial septum at the level of the foramen ovale into the left atrium. A guidewire is advanced into the left ventricle, and a balloon-dilatation catheter is negotiated across the mitral valve and inflated to a predetermined size to enlarge the valve. The most commonly used dilatation catheter is the Inoue balloon. The technique splits the commissural fusion and commonly results in a doubling of the mitral valve area. The success of the procedure in favorable anatomy is 95% and severe complications are rare (1–2%). The most common complications are tamponade due to puncture into the pericardium and the creation of severe mitral regurgitation.

Similarly, severe aortic stenosis can be treated with balloon valvuloplasty. In this setting, the valvuloplasty balloon catheter is placed retrograde across the aortic valve from the femoral artery and briefly inflated to stretch open the valve. The success is much less favorable with an initial success rate of only 50% and a restenosis rate of 50% after 6 to 12 months. This poor success rate has limited its use to patients who are not surgical candidates or as a bridge to surgery in patients who are expected to improve sufficiently to become surgical candidates. In this setting, the mortality rate of the procedure is high (10%). Repeat aortic valvuloplasty as a treatment for aortic valve restenosis has been reported.

Percutaneous aortic valve replacement has been introduced to treat patients who are not suitable candidates for surgical aortic valve replacement. Currently, two valve models, the Edwards SAPIEN valve (Edwards Lifescience, Irvine, California) and the CoreValve ReValving system (CoreValve Inc., Irvine, California), have been approved for use in Europe. In more than 4000 cases worldwide, follow-up shows no evidence of restenosis or prosthetic valve dysfunction in the midterm. Both are placed either retrograde from the femoral artery or can be placed via the left ventricular apex following surgical exposure. The CoreValve is self-expanding, while the Edwards valve is balloon expanded. Following balloon valvuloplasty the valve is positioned across the valve and deployed with post-deployment balloon inflation to ensure full contact with the aortic annulus. The success rate is 80–90% and the 30-day mortality rate is 10–15%, not unexpectedly as only high-risk patients are undergoing the procedure currently. Both valves are undergoing clinical testing in the United States.

PERIPHERAL ARTERIAL INTERVENTIONS

The use of percutaneous interventions to treat symptomatic patients with arterial obstruction in the carotid, renal, aortic, and peripheral vessels is also part of the field of interventional cardiology. Randomized clinical trial data already support the use of carotid stenting in patients at high risk of complications from carotid endarterectomy (Fig. 246-5). Ongoing trials will determine whether carotid stenting should be used even more broadly. The success rate of peripheral interventional procedures has been improving, including for long segments of occlusive disease historically treated by peripheral bypass surgery (Fig. 246-6). Peripheral intervention is increasingly part of the training of an interventional cardiologist, and most programs now require an additional year of training after the interventional cardiology training year. The techniques and outcomes are described in detail in the chapter on peripheral vascular disease (Chap. 249).

Circulatory support techniques

The use of circulatory support techniques is occasionally needed in order to safely perform PCI on hemodynamically unstable patients. It also can be useful in helping to stabilize patients before surgical interventions. The most commonly used device is the percutaneous intraaortic balloon developed in the early 1960s. A 7-10 French 25- to 40-mL balloon catheter is placed retrograde from the femoral artery into the descending aorta between the aortic arch and the abdominal aortic bifurcation. It is connected to a helium gas inflation system that synchronizes the inflation to coincide with early diastole with deflation by mid-diastole. As a result, it increases early diastolic pressure, lowers systolic pressure, and lowers late diastolic pressure through displacement of blood from the descending aorta (counterpulsation). This results in an increase in coronary blood flow and a decrease in afterload. It is contraindicated in patients with aortic regurgitation, aortic dissection, or severe peripheral vascular disease.

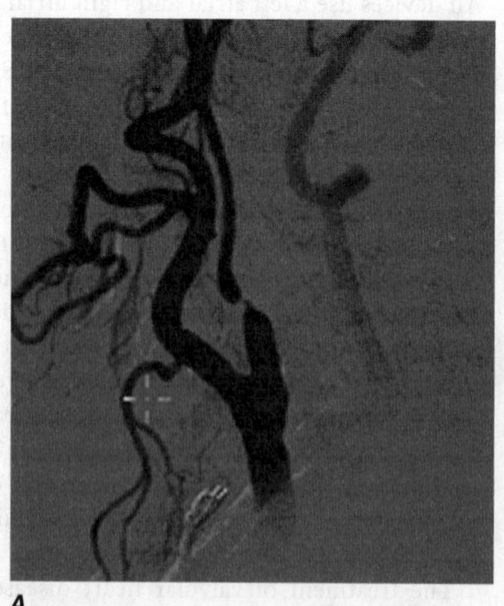
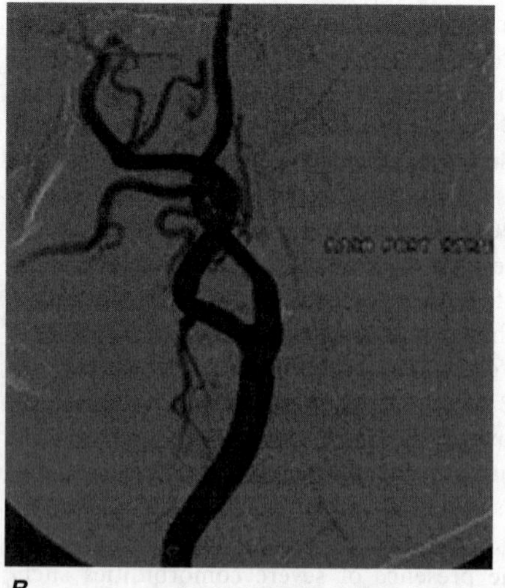

A B

Figure 246-5 An example of a high-risk patient who requires carotid revascularization, but who is not a candidate for carotid endarterectomy. Carotid artery stenting resulted in an excellent angiographic result. *(From M Belkin, DL Bhatt: Circulation 119:2302, 2009; with permission.)*

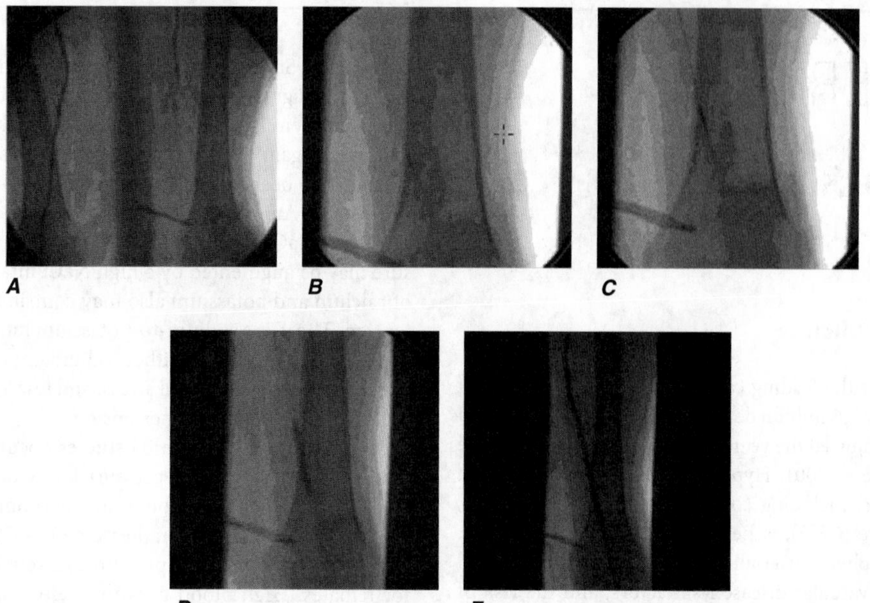

Figure 246-6 Peripheral interventional procedures have become highly effective at treating anatomic lesions previously amenable only to bypass surgery. ***A.*** Complete occlusion of the left superficial femoral artery. ***B.*** Wire and catheter advanced into subintimal space. ***C.*** Intravascular ultrasound positioned in the subintimal space to guide retrograde wire placement through the occluded vessel. ***D.*** Balloon dilation of the occlusion. ***E.*** Stent placement with excellent angiographic result. *(From A Al Mahameed, DL Bhatt: Cleve Clin J Med 73:S45, 2006; with permission.)*

The major complications are vascular and thrombotic. Intravenous heparin is given in order to reduce thrombotic complications.

Another useful tool is the Impella device (Abiomed, Danvers, Massachusetts). The catheter is placed percutaneously from the femoral artery into the left ventricle. The catheter has a small microaxial pump at its tip that can pump up to 2.5 liters per minute at a speed of 50,000 rpm from the left ventricle to the aorta. Other support devices include the hemopump and percutaneous cardiopulmonary bypass.

CONCLUSIONS

Interventional cardiology continues to expand its borders. Treatment for coronary artery disease, including complex anatomic subsets, continues to advance, encroaching on what has traditionally been treated by CABG. Technological advances such as drug-eluting stents, now already in their second generation, and manual aspiration devices are improving the results of PCI. In particular, the data for PCI preventing future ischemic events in unstable ischemic syndromes are substantial. For patients with stable coronary disease, PCI has an important role in symptom alleviation. Treatment of peripheral and cerebrovascular disease has also benefited from the application of percutaneous techniques. Structural heart disease is increasingly being treated with percutaneous options, with a high likelihood that interventional approaches will supplant open-heart surgery in a significant proportion of cases in years to come.

FURTHER READINGS

Baim DS: Percutaneous balloon angioplasty and general coronary intervention, in *Cardiac Catheterization, Angiography, and Intervention*, 7th ed, DS Baim (ed). Philadelphia, Lippincott Williams & Wilkins, 2006

BARI 2D Study Group: A randomized trial of therapies for type 2 diabetes and coronary artery disease. N Engl J Med 360:2503, 2009

Boden WE et al: Optimal medical therapy with or without PCI for stable coronary disease. N Engl J Med 356:1503, 2007

Hirsch AT et al: ACC/AHA 2005 practice guidelines for the management of patients with peripheral arterial disease (lower extremity, renal, mesenteric and abdominal aortic): Executive summary. Circulation 113:3463, 2006

King SB 3rd et al: 2007 Focused update of the ACC/AHA/SCAI 2005 guideline update for percutaneous coronary intervention: A report of the American College of Cardiology/American Heart Association Task Force on Practice Guidelines: 2007 writing group to review new evidence and update the ACC/AHA/SCAI 2005 guideline update for percutaneous coronary intervention, writing on behalf of the 2005 writing committee. Circulation 117:261, 2008

Kushner FG et al: 2009 focused updates: ACC/AHA guidelines for the management of patients with ST-elevation myocardial infarction (updating the 2004 guideline and 2007 focused update) and ACC/AHA/SCAI guidelines on percutaneous coronary intervention (updating the 2005 guideline and 2007 focused update) a report of the American College of Cardiology Foundation/American Heart Association Task Force on Practice Guidelines. J Am Coll Cardiol 54:2205, 2009)

Serruys PW et al: Percutaneous coronary intervention versus coronary artery bypass grafting for severe coronary artery disease. N Engl J Med 360:961, 2009

Smith SC et al: ACC/AHA/SCAI 2005 guideline update for percutaneous coronary intervention—summary article. A report of the American College of Cardiology/American Heart Association task force on practice guidelines (ACC/AHA/SCAI writing committee to update the 2001 guidelines for percutaneous coronary intervention). Circulation 113:156, 2006

White CJ: Catheter-based therapy for atherosclerotic renal artery stenosis. Circulation 113:1464, 2006

Yadav JS et al: Protected carotid-artery stenting versus endarterectomy in high-risk patients. N Eng J Med 351:1493, 2004

CHAPTER 247

Hypertensive Vascular Disease

Theodore A. Kotchen

Hypertension is one of the leading causes of the global burden of disease. Approximately 7.6 million deaths (13–15% of the total) and 92 million disability-adjusted life years worldwide were attributable to high blood pressure in 2001. Hypertension doubles the risk of cardiovascular diseases, including coronary heart disease (CHD), congestive heart failure (CHF), ischemic and hemorrhagic stroke, renal failure, and peripheral arterial disease. It often is associated with additional cardiovascular disease risk factors, and the risk of cardiovascular disease increases with the total burden of risk factors. Although antihypertensive therapy clearly reduces the risks of cardiovascular and renal disease, large segments of the hypertensive population are either untreated or inadequately treated.

EPIDEMIOLOGY

Blood pressure levels, the rate of age-related increases in blood pressure, and the prevalence of hypertension vary among countries and among subpopulations within a country. Hypertension is present in all populations except for a small number of individuals living in primitive, culturally isolated societies. In industrialized societies, blood pressure increases steadily during the first two decades of life. In children and adolescents, blood pressure is associated with growth and maturation. Blood pressure "tracks" over time in children and between adolescence and young adulthood. In the United States, average systolic blood pressure is higher for men than for women during early adulthood, although among older individuals the age-related rate of rise is steeper for women. Consequently, among individuals age 60 and older, systolic blood pressures of women are higher than those of men. Among adults, diastolic blood pressure also increases progressively with age until ~55 years, after which it tends to decrease. The consequence is a widening of pulse pressure (the difference between systolic and diastolic blood pressure) beyond age 60. The probability that a middle-aged or elderly individual will develop hypertension in his or her lifetime is 90%.

In the United States, based on results of the National Health and Nutrition Examination Survey (NHANES), approximately 30% (age-adjusted prevalence) of adults, or at least 65 million individuals, have hypertension (defined as any one of the following: systolic blood pressure ≥140 mmHg, diastolic blood pressure ≥90 mmHg, taking antihypertensive medications). Hypertension prevalence is 33.5% in non-Hispanic blacks, 28.9% in non-Hispanic whites, and 20.7% in Mexican Americans. The likelihood of hypertension increases with age, and among individuals age ≥60, the prevalence is 65.4%. Recent evidence suggests that the prevalence of hypertension in the United States may be increasing, possibly as a consequence of increasing obesity. The prevalence of hypertension and stroke mortality rates are higher in the southeastern United States than in other regions. In African Americans, hypertension appears earlier, is generally more severe, and results in higher rates of morbidity and mortality from stroke, left ventricular hypertrophy, CHF, and end-stage renal disease (ESRD) than in white Americans.

Both environmental and genetic factors may contribute to regional and racial variations in blood pressure and hypertension prevalence. Studies of societies undergoing "acculturation" and studies of migrants from a less to a more urbanized setting indicate a profound environmental contribution to blood pressure. Obesity and weight gain are strong, independent risk factors for hypertension. It has been estimated that 60% of hypertensives are >20% overweight. Among populations, hypertension prevalence is related to dietary NaCl intake, and the age-related increase in blood pressure may be augmented by a high NaCl intake. Low dietary intakes of calcium and potassium also may contribute to the risk of hypertension. The urine sodium-to-potassium ratio is a stronger correlate of blood pressure than is either sodium or potassium alone. Alcohol consumption, psychosocial stress, and low levels of physical activity also may contribute to hypertension.

Adoption, twin, and family studies document a significant heritable component to blood pressure levels and hypertension. Family studies controlling for a common environment indicate that blood pressure heritabilities are in the range 15–35%. In twin studies, heritability estimates of blood pressure are ~60% for males and 30–40% for females. High blood pressure before age 55 occurs 3.8 times more frequently among persons with a positive family history of hypertension.

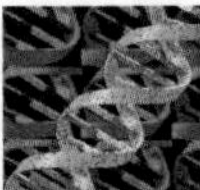

GENETIC CONSIDERATIONS

Although specific genetic variants have been identified in rare Mendelian forms of hypertension (Table 247-5), these variants are not applicable to the vast majority (>98%) of patients with essential hypertension. For most individuals, it is likely that hypertension represents a polygenic disorder in which a combination of genes acts in concert with environmental exposures to make only a modest contribution to blood pressure. Further, different subsets of genes may lead to different phenotypes associated with hypertension, e.g., obesity, dyslipidemia, insulin resistance.

Several strategies are being utilized in the search for specific hypertension-related genes. Animal models (including selectively bred rats and congenic rat strains) provide a powerful approach for evaluating genetic loci and genes associated with hypertension. Comparative mapping strategies allow for the identification of syntenic genomic regions between the rat and human genomes that may be involved in blood pressure regulation. In association studies, different alleles (or combinations of alleles at different loci) of specific candidate genes or chromosomal regions are compared in hypertensive patients and normotensive control subjects. Current evidence suggests that genes that encode components of the renin-angiotensin-aldosterone system, along with angiotensinogen and angiotensin-converting enzyme (ACE) polymorphisms, may be related to hypertension and to blood pressure sensitivity to dietary NaCl. The alpha-adducin gene is thought to be associated with increased renal tubular absorption of sodium, and variants of this gene may be associated with hypertension and salt sensitivity of blood pressure. Other genes possibly related to hypertension include genes encoding the AT_1 receptor, aldosterone synthase, and the β_2 adrenoreceptor. Genomewide association studies involve rapidly scanning markers across the entire genome to identify loci (not specific genes) associated with an observable trait (e.g., blood pressure) or a particular disease. This strategy has been facilitated by the availability of dense genotyping chips and the International HapMap. To date, the results of candidate gene studies often have not been replicated, and in contrast to several other polygenic disorders, genomewide association studies have had limited success in identifying genetic determinants of hypertension.

Preliminary evidence suggests that there may also be genetic determinants of target organ damage attributed to hypertension.

Family studies indicate significant heritability of left ventricular mass, and there is considerable individual variation in the responses of the heart to hypertension. Family studies and variations in candidate genes associated with renal damage suggest that genetic factors also may contribute to hypertensive nephropathy. Specific genetic variants have been linked to CHD and stroke.

In the future, it is possible that DNA analysis will predict individual risk for hypertension and target organ damage and will identify responders to specific classes of antihypertensive agents. However, with the exception of the rare, monogenic hypertensive diseases, the genetic variants associated with hypertension remain to be confirmed, and the intermediate steps by which these variants affect blood pressure remain to be determined.

MECHANISMS OF HYPERTENSION

To provide a framework for understanding the pathogenesis of and treatment options for hypertensive disorders, it is useful to understand factors involved in the regulation of both normal and elevated arterial pressure. Cardiac output and peripheral resistance are the two determinants of arterial pressure (Fig. 247-1). Cardiac output is determined by stroke volume and heart rate; stroke volume is related to myocardial contractility and to the size of the vascular compartment. Peripheral resistance is determined by functional and anatomic changes in small arteries (lumen diameter 100–400 μm) and arterioles.

INTRAVASCULAR VOLUME

Vascular volume is a primary determinant of arterial pressure over the long term. Sodium is predominantly an extracellular ion and is a primary determinant of the extracellular fluid volume. When NaCl intake exceeds the capacity of the kidney to excrete sodium, vascular volume initially expands and cardiac output increases. However, many vascular beds (including kidney and brain) have the capacity to autoregulate blood flow, and if constant blood flow is to be maintained in the face of increased arterial pressure, resistance within that bed must increase, since

$$\text{Blood flow} = \frac{\text{pressure across the vascular bed}}{\text{vascular resistance}}$$

The initial elevation of blood pressure in response to vascular volume expansion may be related to an increase of cardiac output; however, over time, peripheral resistance increases and cardiac output reverts toward normal. The effect of sodium on blood pressure is related to the provision of sodium with chloride; nonchloride salts of sodium have little or no effect on blood pressure. As arterial pressure increases in response to a high NaCl intake, urinary sodium excretion increases and sodium balance is maintained at the expense of an increase in arterial pressure. The mechanism for this "pressure-natriuresis" phenomenon may involve a subtle increase in the glomerular filtration rate, decreased absorbing capacity of the renal tubules, and possibly hormonal factors such as atrial natriuretic factor. In individuals with an impaired capacity to excrete sodium, greater increases in arterial pressure are required to achieve natriuresis and sodium balance.

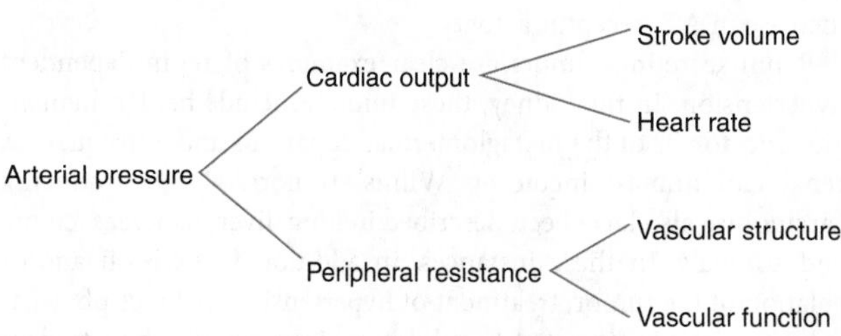

Figure 247-1 Determinants of arterial pressure.

NaCl-dependent hypertension may be a consequence of a decreased capacity of the kidney to excrete sodium, due either to intrinsic renal disease or to increased production of a salt-retaining hormone (mineralocorticoid) resulting in increased renal tubular reabsorption of sodium. Renal tubular sodium reabsorption also may be augmented by increased neural activity to the kidney. In each of these situations, a higher arterial pressure may be required to achieve sodium balance. Conversely, salt-wasting disorders are associated with low blood pressure levels. ESRD is an extreme example of volume-dependent hypertension. In ~80% of these patients, vascular volume and hypertension can be controlled with adequate dialysis; in the other 20%, the mechanism of hypertension is related to increased activity of the renin-angiotensin system and is likely to be responsive to pharmacologic blockade of renin-angiotensin.

AUTONOMIC NERVOUS SYSTEM

The autonomic nervous system maintains cardiovascular homeostasis via pressure, volume, and chemoreceptor signals. Adrenergic reflexes modulate blood pressure over the short term, and adrenergic function, in concert with hormonal and volume-related factors, contributes to the long-term regulation of arterial pressure. The three endogenous catecholamines are norepinephrine, epinephrine, and dopamine. All three play important roles in tonic and phasic cardiovascular regulation.

The activities of the adrenergic receptors are mediated by guanosine nucleotide-binding regulatory proteins (G proteins) and by intracellular concentrations of downstream second messengers. In addition to receptor affinity and density, physiologic responsiveness to catecholamines may be altered by the efficiency of receptor-effector coupling at a site "distal" to receptor binding. The receptor sites are relatively specific both for the transmitter substance and for the response that occupancy of the receptor site elicits. Norepinephrine and epinephrine are agonists for all adrenergic receptor subtypes, although with varying affinities. Based on their physiology and pharmacology, adrenergic receptors have been divided into two principal types: α and β. These types have been differentiated further into α_1, α_2, β_1, and β_2 receptors. Recent molecular cloning studies have identified several additional subtypes. α Receptors are occupied and activated more avidly by norepinephrine than by epinephrine, and the reverse is true for β receptors. α_1 Receptors are located on postsynaptic cells in smooth muscle and elicit vasoconstriction. α_2 Receptors are localized on presynaptic membranes of postganglionic nerve terminals that synthesize norepinephrine. When activated by catecholamines, α_2 receptors act as negative feedback controllers, inhibiting further norepinephrine release. In the kidney, activation of α_1-adrenergic receptors increases renal tubular reabsorption of sodium. Different classes of antihypertensive agents either inhibit α_1 receptors or act as agonists of α_2 receptors and reduce systemic sympathetic outflow. Activation of myocardial β_1 receptors stimulates the rate and strength of cardiac contraction and consequently increases cardiac output. β_1 Receptor activation also stimulates renin release from the kidney. Another class of antihypertensive agents acts by inhibiting β_1 receptors. Activation of β_2 receptors by epinephrine relaxes vascular smooth muscle and results in vasodilation.

Circulating catecholamine concentrations may affect the number of adrenoreceptors in various tissues. Downregulation of receptors may be a consequence of sustained high levels of catecholamines and provides an explanation for decreasing responsiveness, or tachyphylaxis, to catecholamines. For example, orthostatic hypotension frequently is observed in patients with pheochromocytoma, possibly due to the lack of norepinephrine-induced vasoconstriction with assumption of the upright posture. Conversely, with chronic reduction of neurotransmitter substances, adrenoreceptors may increase in number or be upregulated, resulting in increased responsiveness to the neurotransmitter. Chronic administration of agents that block adrenergic receptors may result in upregulation, and withdrawal of those agents may produce a condition of temporary hypersensitivity to sympathetic stimuli. For example, clonidine is an antihypertensive agent that is a centrally acting α_2 agonist that inhibits sympathetic outflow. Rebound hypertension may occur with the abrupt cessation of clonidine therapy, probably as a consequence of upregulation of α_1 receptors.

Several reflexes modulate blood pressure on a minute-to-minute basis. One arterial baroreflex is mediated by stretch-sensitive sensory nerve endings in the carotid sinuses and the aortic arch. The rate of firing of these baroreceptors increases with arterial pressure, and the net effect is a decrease in sympathetic outflow, resulting in decreases in arterial pressure and heart rate. This is a primary mechanism for rapid buffering of acute fluctuations of arterial pressure that may occur during postural changes, behavioral or physiologic stress, and changes in blood volume. However, the activity of the baroreflex declines or adapts to sustained increases in arterial pressure such that the baroreceptors are reset to higher pressures. Patients with autonomic neuropathy and impaired baroreflex function may have extremely labile blood pressures with difficult-to-control episodic blood pressure spikes associated with tachycardia.

In both normal-weight and obese individuals, hypertension often is associated with increased sympathetic outflow. Based on recordings of postganglionic muscle nerve activity (detected by a microelectrode inserted in a peroneal nerve in the leg), sympathetic outflow tends to be higher in hypertensive than in normotensive individuals. Sympathetic outflow is increased in obesity-related hypertension and in hypertension associated with obstructive sleep apnea. Baroreceptor activation via electrical stimulation of carotid sinus afferent nerves has been shown to lower blood pressure in patients with "resistant" hypertension. Drugs that block the sympathetic nervous system are potent antihypertensive agents, indicating that the sympathetic nervous system plays a permissive, although not necessarily a causative, role in the maintenance of increased arterial pressure.

Pheochromocytoma is the most blatant example of hypertension related to increased catecholamine production, in this instance by a tumor. Blood pressure can be reduced by surgical excision of the tumor or by pharmacologic treatment with an α_1 receptor antagonist or with an inhibitor of tyrosine hydroxylase, the rate-limiting step in catecholamine biosynthesis.

RENIN-ANGIOTENSIN-ALDOSTERONE

The renin-angiotensin-aldosterone system contributes to the regulation of arterial pressure primarily via the vasoconstrictor properties of angiotensin II and the sodium-retaining properties of aldosterone. Renin is an aspartyl protease that is synthesized as an enzymatically inactive precursor, prorenin. Most renin in the circulation is synthesized in the renal afferent renal arteriole. Prorenin may be secreted directly into the circulation or may be activated within secretory cells and released as active renin. Although human plasma contains two to five times more prorenin than renin, there is no evidence that prorenin contributes to the physiologic activity of this system. There are three primary stimuli for renin secretion: (1) decreased NaCl transport in the distal portion of the thick ascending limb of the loop of Henle that abuts the corresponding afferent arteriole (macula densa), (2) decreased pressure or stretch within the renal afferent arteriole (baroreceptor mechanism), and (3) sympathetic nervous system stimulation of renin-secreting cells via β_1 adrenoreceptors. Conversely, renin secretion is inhibited by increased NaCl transport in the thick ascending limb of the loop of Henle, by increased stretch within the renal afferent arteriole, and by

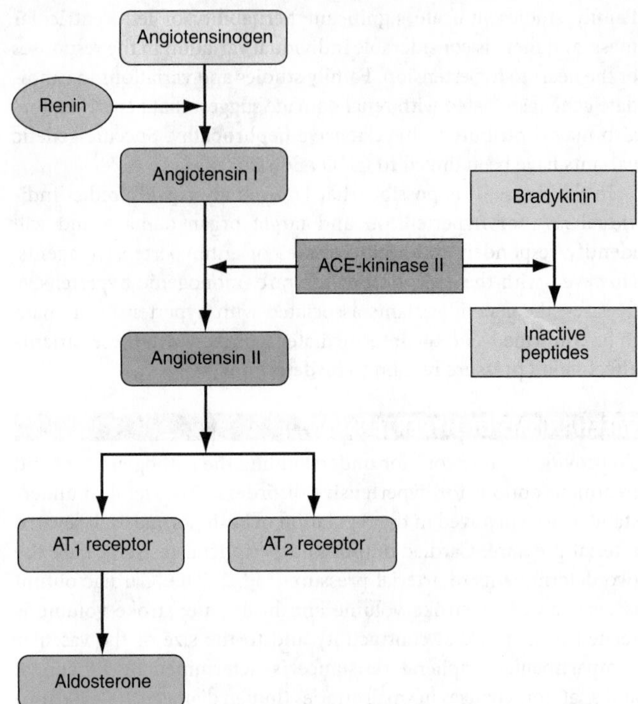

Figure 247-2 Renin-angiotensin-aldosterone axis.

β_1 receptor blockade. In addition, angiotensin II directly inhibits renin secretion due to angiotensin II type 1 receptors on juxtaglomerular cells, and renin secretion increases in response to pharmacologic blockade of either ACE or angiotensin II receptors.

Once released into the circulation, active renin cleaves a substrate, angiotensinogen, to form an inactive decapeptide, angiotensin I (Fig. 247-2). A converting enzyme, located primarily but not exclusively in the pulmonary circulation, converts angiotensin I to the active octapeptide, angiotensin II, by releasing the C-terminal histidyl-leucine dipeptide. The same converting enzyme cleaves a number of other peptides, including and thereby inactivating the vasodilator bradykinin. Acting primarily through angiotensin II type 1 (AT_1) receptors on cell membranes, angiotensin II is a potent pressor substance, the primary tropic factor for the secretion of aldosterone by the adrenal zona glomerulosa, and a potent mitogen that stimulates vascular smooth muscle cell and myocyte growth. Independent of its hemodynamic effects, angiotensin II may play a role in the pathogenesis of atherosclerosis through a direct cellular action on the vessel wall. An angiotensin II type 2 (AT_2) receptor has been characterized. It is widely distributed in the kidney and has the opposite functional effects of the AT_1 receptor. The AT_2 receptor induces vasodilation, sodium excretion, and inhibition of cell growth and matrix formation. Experimental evidence suggests that the AT_2 receptor improves vascular remodeling by stimulating smooth muscle cell apoptosis and contributes to the regulation of glomerular filtration rate. AT_1 receptor blockade induces an increase in AT_2 receptor activity.

Renin-secreting tumors are clear examples of renin-dependent hypertension. In the kidney, these tumors include benign hemangiopericytomas of the juxtaglomerular apparatus and, infrequently, renal carcinomas, including Wilms' tumors. Renin-producing carcinomas also have been described in lung, liver, pancreas, colon, and adrenals. In these instances, in addition to excision and/or ablation of the tumor, treatment of hypertension includes pharmacologic therapies targeted to inhibit angiotensin II production or action. Renovascular hypertension is another renin-mediated form of hypertension. Obstruction of the renal artery leads to decreased renal perfusion pressure, thereby stimulating renin secretion. Over time, as a consequence of secondary renal damage, this form of hypertension may become less renin dependent.

Angiotensinogen, renin, and angiotensin II are also synthesized locally in many tissues, including the brain, pituitary, aorta, arteries, heart, adrenal glands, kidneys, adipocytes, leukocytes, ovaries, testes, uterus, spleen, and skin. Angiotensin II in tissues may be formed by the enzymatic activity of renin or by other proteases, e.g., tonin, chymase, and cathepsins. In addition to regulating local blood flow, tissue angiotensin II is a mitogen that stimulates growth and contributes to modeling and repair. Excess tissue angiotensin II may contribute to atherosclerosis, cardiac hypertrophy, and renal failure and consequently may be a target for pharmacologic therapy to prevent target organ damage.

Angiotensin II is the primary tropic factor regulating the synthesis and secretion of aldosterone by the zona glomerulosa of the adrenal cortex. Aldosterone synthesis is also dependent on potassium, and aldosterone secretion may be decreased in potassium-depleted individuals. Although acute elevations of adrenocorticotropic hormone (ACTH) levels also increase aldosterone secretion, ACTH is not an important tropic factor for the chronic regulation of aldosterone.

Aldosterone is a potent mineralocorticoid that increases sodium reabsorption by amiloride-sensitive epithelial sodium channels (ENaC) on the apical surface of the principal cells of the renal cortical collecting duct (Chap. 277). Electric neutrality is maintained by exchanging sodium for potassium and hydrogen ions. Consequently, increased aldosterone secretion may result in hypokalemia and alkalosis. Because potassium depletion may inhibit aldosterone synthesis, clinically, hypokalemia should be corrected before a patient is evaluated for hyperaldosteronism.

Mineralocorticoid receptors also are expressed in the colon, salivary glands, and sweat glands. Cortisol also binds to these receptors but normally functions as a less potent mineralocorticoid than aldosterone because cortisol is converted to cortisone by the enzyme 11 β-hydroxysteroid dehydrogenase type 2. Cortisone has no affinity for the mineralocorticoid receptor. Primary aldosteronism is a compelling example of mineralocorticoid-mediated hypertension. In this disorder, adrenal aldosterone synthesis and release are independent of renin-angiotensin, and renin release is suppressed by the resulting volume expansion.

Aldosterone also has effects on nonepithelial targets. Aldosterone and/or mineralocorticoid receptor activation induces structural and functional alterations in the heart, kidney, and blood vessels, leading to myocardial fibrosis, nephrosclerosis, and vascular inflammation and remodeling, perhaps as a consequence of oxidative stress. These effects are amplified by a high salt intake. In animal models, high circulating aldosterone levels stimulate cardiac fibrosis and left ventricular hypertrophy, and spironolactone (an aldosterone antagonist) prevents aldosterone-induced myocardial fibrosis. Pathologic patterns of left ventricular geometry also have been associated with elevations of plasma aldosterone concentration in patients with essential hypertension as well as in patients with primary aldosteronism. In patients with CHF, low-dose spironolactone reduces the risk of progressive heart failure and sudden death from cardiac causes by 30%. Owing to a renal hemodynamic effect, in patients with primary aldosteronism, high circulating levels of aldosterone also may cause glomerular hyperfiltration and albuminuria. These renal effects are reversible after removal of the effects of excess aldosterone by adrenalectomy or spironolactone.

Increased activity of the renin-angiotensin-aldosterone axis is not invariably associated with hypertension. In response to a low-NaCl diet or to volume contraction, arterial pressure and volume homeostasis may be maintained by increased activity of the renin-angiotensin-aldosterone axis. Secondary aldosteronism (i.e., increased aldosterone secondary to increased renin-angiotensin), but not hypertension, also is observed in edematous states such as CHF and liver disease.

VASCULAR MECHANISMS

Vascular radius and compliance of resistance arteries are also important determinants of arterial pressure. Resistance to flow varies inversely with the fourth power of the radius, and consequently, small decreases in lumen size significantly increase resistance. In hypertensive patients, structural, mechanical, or functional changes may reduce the lumen diameter of small arteries and arterioles. Remodeling refers to geometric alterations in the vessel wall without a change in vessel volume. Hypertrophic (increased cell size, and increased deposition of intercellular matrix) or eutrophic vascular remodeling results in decreased lumen size and hence contributes to increased peripheral resistance. Apoptosis, low-grade inflammation, and vascular fibrosis also contribute to remodeling. Lumen diameter also is related to elasticity of the vessel. Vessels with a high degree of elasticity can accommodate an increase of volume with relatively little change in pressure, whereas in a semirigid vascular system, a small increment in volume induces a relatively large increment of pressure.

Hypertensive patients have stiffer arteries, and arteriosclerotic patients may have particularly high systolic blood pressures and wide pulse pressures as a consequence of decreased vascular compliance due to structural changes in the vascular wall. Recent evidence suggests that arterial stiffness has independent predictive value for cardiovascular events. Clinically, a number of devices are available to evaluate arterial stiffness or compliance, including ultrasound and magnetic resonance imaging (MRI).

Ion transport by vascular smooth muscle cells may contribute to hypertension-associated abnormalities of vascular tone and vascular growth, both of which are modulated by intracellular pH (pH_i). Three ion transport mechanisms participate in the regulation of pH_i: (1) Na^+-H^+ exchange, (2) Na^+-dependent HCO_3^--Cl^- exchange, and (3) cation-independent HCO_3^--Cl^- exchange. Based on measurements in cell types that are more accessible than vascular smooth muscle (e.g., leukocytes, erythrocytes, platelets, skeletal muscle), activity of the Na^+-H^+ exchanger is increased in hypertension, and this may result in increased vascular tone by two mechanisms. First, increased sodium entry may lead to increased vascular tone by activating Na^+-Ca^{2+} exchange and thereby increasing intracellular calcium. Second, increased pH_i enhances calcium sensitivity of the contractile apparatus, leading to an increase in contractility for a given intracellular calcium concentration. Additionally, increased Na^+-H^+ exchange may stimulate growth of vascular smooth muscle cells by enhancing sensitivity to mitogens.

Vascular endothelial function also modulates vascular tone. The vascular endothelium synthesizes and releases a spectrum of vasoactive substances, including nitric oxide, a potent vasodilator. Endothelium-dependent vasodilation is impaired in hypertensive patients. This impairment often is assessed with high-resolution ultrasonography before and after the hyperemic phase of reperfusion that follows 5 minutes of forearm ischemia. Alternatively, endothelium-dependent vasodilation may be assessed in response to an intra-arterially infused endothelium-dependent vasodilator, e.g., acetylcholine. Endothelin is a vasoconstrictor peptide produced by the endothelium, and that orally active endothelin antagonists may lower blood pressure in patients with resistant hypertension.

Currently, it is not known if the hypertension-related vascular abnormalities of ion transport and endothelial function are primary alterations or secondary consequences of elevated arterial pressure. Limited evidence suggests that vascular compliance and endothelium-dependent vasodilation may be improved by aerobic exercise, weight loss, and antihypertensive agents. It remains to be determined whether these interventions affect arterial structure and stiffness via a blood pressure–independent mechanism and whether different classes of antihypertensive agents preferentially affect vascular structure and function.

PATHOLOGIC CONSEQUENCES OF HYPERTENSION

Hypertension is an independent predisposing factor for heart failure, coronary artery disease, stroke, renal disease, and peripheral arterial disease (PAD).

HEART

Heart disease is the most common cause of death in hypertensive patients. Hypertensive heart disease is the result of structural and functional adaptations leading to left ventricular hypertrophy, CHF, abnormalities of blood flow due to atherosclerotic coronary artery disease and microvascular disease, and cardiac arrhythmias.

Both genetic and hemodynamic factors contribute to left ventricular hypertrophy. Clinically, left ventricular hypertrophy can be diagnosed by electrocardiography, although echocardiography provides a more sensitive measure of left ventricular wall thickness. Individuals with left ventricular hypertrophy are at increased risk for CHD, stroke, CHF, and sudden death. Aggressive control of hypertension can regress or reverse left ventricular hypertrophy and reduce the risk of cardiovascular disease. It is not clear whether different classes of antihypertensive agents have an added impact on reducing left ventricular mass, independent of their blood pressure–lowering effect.

CHF may be related to systolic dysfunction, diastolic dysfunction, or a combination of the two. Abnormalities of diastolic function that range from asymptomatic heart disease to overt heart failure are common in hypertensive patients. Patients with diastolic heart failure have a preserved ejection fraction, which is a measure of systolic function. Approximately one-third of patients with CHF have normal systolic function but abnormal diastolic function. Diastolic dysfunction is an early consequence of hypertension-related heart disease and is exacerbated by left ventricular hypertrophy and ischemia. Cardiac catheterization provides the most accurate assessment of diastolic function. Alternatively, diastolic function can be evaluated by several noninvasive methods, including echocardiography and radionuclide angiography.

BRAIN

Stroke is the second most frequent cause of death in the world; it accounts for 5 million deaths each year, with an additional 15 million persons having nonfatal strokes. Elevated blood pressure is the strongest risk factor for stroke. Approximately 85% of strokes are due to infarction, and the remainder are due to either intracerebral or subarachnoid hemorrhage. The incidence of stroke rises progressively with increasing blood pressure levels, particularly systolic blood pressure in individuals >65 years. Treatment of hypertension convincingly decreases the incidence of both ischemic and hemorrhagic strokes.

Hypertension also is associated with impaired cognition in an aging population, and longitudinal studies support an association between midlife hypertension and late-life cognitive decline. Hypertension-related cognitive impairment and dementia may be a consequence of a single infarct due to occlusion of a "strategic" larger vessel or multiple lacunar infarcts due to occlusive small vessel disease resulting in subcortical white matter ischemia. Several clinical trials suggest that antihypertensive therapy has a beneficial effect on cognitive function, although this remains an active area of investigation.

Cerebral blood flow remains unchanged over a wide range of arterial pressures (mean arterial pressure of 50–150 mmHg) through a process termed *autoregulation* of blood flow. In patients with the clinical syndrome of malignant hypertension, encephalopathy is related to failure of autoregulation of cerebral blood flow at the upper pressure limit, resulting in vasodilation and hyperperfusion. Signs and symptoms of hypertensive encephalopathy may include severe headache, nausea and vomiting (often of a projectile nature), focal neurologic signs, and alterations in mental status. Untreated, hypertensive encephalopathy may progress to stupor, coma, seizures, and death within hours. It is important to distinguish hypertensive encephalopathy from other neurologic syndromes that may be associated with hypertension, e.g., cerebral ischemia, hemorrhagic or thrombotic stroke, seizure disorder, mass lesions, pseudotumor cerebri, delirium tremens, meningitis, acute intermittent porphyria, traumatic or chemical injury to the brain, and uremic encephalopathy.

KIDNEY

The kidney is both a target and a cause of hypertension. Primary renal disease is the most common etiology of secondary hypertension. Mechanisms of kidney-related hypertension include a diminished capacity to excrete sodium, excessive renin secretion in relation to volume status, and sympathetic nervous system overactivity. Conversely, hypertension is a risk factor for renal injury and end-stage renal disease. The increased risk associated with high blood pressure is graded, continuous, and present throughout the distribution of blood pressure above optimal pressure. Renal risk appears to be more closely related to systolic than to diastolic blood pressure, and black men are at greater risk than white men for developing ESRD at every level of blood pressure. Proteinuria is a reliable marker of the severity of chronic kidney disease and is a predictor of its progression. Patients with high urine protein excretion (>3 g/24 h) have a more rapid rate of progression than do those with lower protein excretion rates.

Atherosclerotic, hypertension-related vascular lesions in the kidney primarily affect preglomerular arterioles, resulting in ischemic changes in the glomeruli and postglomerular structures. Glomerular injury also may be a consequence of direct damage to the glomerular capillaries due to glomerular hyperperfusion. Studies of hypertension-related renal damage, primarily in experimental animals, suggest that loss of autoregulation of renal blood flow at the afferent arteriole results in transmission of elevated pressures to an unprotected glomerulus with ensuing hyperfiltration, hypertrophy, and eventual focal segmental glomerular sclerosis. With progressive renal injury there is a loss of autoregulation of renal blood flow and glomerular filtration rate, resulting in a lower blood pressure threshold for renal damage and a steeper slope between blood pressure and renal damage. The result may be a vicious cycle of renal damage and nephron loss leading to more severe hypertension, glomerular hyperfiltration, and further renal damage. Glomerular pathology progresses to glomerulosclerosis, and eventually the renal tubules may also become ischemic and gradually atrophic. The renal lesion associated with malignant hypertension consists of fibrinoid necrosis of the afferent arterioles, sometimes extending into the glomerulus, and may result in focal necrosis of the glomerular tuft.

Clinically, macroalbuminuria (a random urine albumin/creatinine ratio >300 mg/g) or microalbuminuria (a random urine albumin/creatinine ratio 30–300 mg/g) are early markers of renal injury. These are also risk factors for renal disease progression and cardiovascular disease.

PERIPHERAL ARTERIES

In addition to contributing to the pathogenesis of hypertension, blood vessels may be a target organ for atherosclerotic disease secondary to long-standing elevated blood pressure. Hypertensive patients with arterial disease of the lower extremities are at increased risk for future cardiovascular disease. Although patients with stenotic lesions of the lower extremities may be asymptomatic, intermittent claudication is the classic symptom of PAD. This is characterized by aching pain in the calves or buttocks while walking that is relieved by rest. The ankle-brachial index is a useful approach for evaluating PAD and is defined as the ratio of noninvasively assessed ankle to brachial (arm) systolic blood pressure. An ankle-brachial index <0.90 is considered diagnostic of PAD and is associated with >50% stenosis in at least one major lower limb vessel. Several studies suggest that an ankle-brachial index <0.80 is associated with elevated blood pressure, particularly systolic blood pressure.

DEFINING HYPERTENSION

From an epidemiologic perspective, there is no obvious level of blood pressure that defines hypertension. In adults, there is a continuous, incremental risk of cardiovascular disease, stroke, and renal disease across levels of both systolic and diastolic blood pressure. The Multiple Risk Factor Intervention Trial (MRFIT), which included >350,000 male participants, demonstrated a continuous and graded influence of both systolic and diastolic blood pressure on CHD mortality, extending down to systolic blood pressures of 120 mmHg. Similarly, results of a meta-analysis involving almost 1 million participants indicate that ischemic heart disease mortality, stroke mortality, and mortality from other vascular causes are directly related to the height of the blood pressure, beginning at 115/75 mmHg, without evidence of a threshold. Cardiovascular disease risk doubles for every 20-mmHg increase in systolic and 10-mmHg increase in diastolic pressure. Among older individuals, systolic blood pressure and pulse pressure are more powerful predictors of cardiovascular disease than is diastolic blood pressure.

Clinically, hypertension may be defined as that level of blood pressure at which the institution of therapy reduces blood pressure–related morbidity and mortality. Current clinical criteria for defining hypertension generally are based on the average of two or more seated blood pressure readings during each of two or more outpatient visits. A recent classification recommends blood pressure criteria for defining normal blood pressure, prehypertension, hypertension (stages I and II), and isolated systolic hypertension, which is a common occurrence among the elderly (Table 247-1). In children and adolescents, hypertension generally is defined as systolic and/or diastolic blood pressure consistently >95th percentile for age, sex, and height. Blood pressures between the 90th and 95th percentiles are considered prehypertensive and are an indication for lifestyle interventions.

Home blood pressure and average 24-h ambulatory blood pressure measurements are generally lower than clinic blood pressures. Because ambulatory blood pressure recordings yield multiple readings throughout the day and night, they provide a more comprehensive assessment of the vascular burden of hypertension than do a limited number of office readings. Increasing evidence suggests that home blood pressures, including 24-h blood pressure recordings, more reliably predict target organ damage than do office blood pressures. Blood pressure tends to be higher in the early morning hours, soon after waking, than at other times of day. Myocardial infarction and stroke are more common in the early morning hours. Nighttime blood pressures are generally 10–20% lower than daytime blood pressures, and an attenuated nighttime blood pressure "dip" is associated with increased cardiovascular disease risk. Recommended criteria for a diagnosis of hypertension are average awake blood pressure ≥135/85 mmHg and asleep blood pressure ≥120/75 mmHg. These levels approximate a clinic blood pressure of 140/90 mmHg.

Approximately 15–20% of patients with stage 1 hypertension (as defined in Table 247-1) based on office blood pressures have average ambulatory readings <135/85 mmHg. This phenomenon, so-called white coat hypertension, also may be associated with an increased risk of target organ damage (e.g., left ventricular hypertrophy, carotid atherosclerosis, overall cardiovascular morbidity), although to a lesser extent than in individuals with elevated office and ambulatory readings. Individuals with white coat hypertension are also at increased risk for developing sustained hypertension.

CLINICAL DISORDERS OF HYPERTENSION

Depending on methods of patient ascertainment, ~80–95% of hypertensive patients are diagnosed as having "essential" hypertension (also referred to as primary or idiopathic hypertension). In the remaining 5–20% of hypertensive patients, a specific underlying disorder causing the elevation of blood pressure can be identified (Tables 247-2 and 247-3). In individuals with "secondary" hypertension, a specific mechanism for the blood pressure elevation is often more apparent.

ESSENTIAL HYPERTENSION

Essential hypertension tends to be familial and is likely to be the consequence of an interaction between environmental and genetic factors. The prevalence of essential hypertension increases with age, and individuals with relatively high blood pressures at younger ages are at increased risk for the subsequent development of hypertension. It is likely that essential hypertension represents a spectrum of disorders with different underlying pathophysiologies. In the majority of patients with established hypertension, peripheral resistance is increased and cardiac output is normal or decreased; however, in younger patients with mild or labile hypertension, cardiac output may be increased and peripheral resistance may be normal.

When plasma renin activity (PRA) is plotted against 24-h sodium excretion, ~10–15% of hypertensive patients have high PRA and

TABLE 247-1 Blood Pressure Classification

Blood Pressure Classification	Systolic, mmHg	Diastolic, mmHg
Normal	<120	*and* <80
Prehypertension	120–139	*or* 80–89
Stage 1 hypertension	140–159	*or* 90–99
Stage 2 hypertension	≥160	*or* ≥100
Isolated systolic hypertension	≥140	*and* <90

Source: Adapted from Chobanian et al.

TABLE 247-2 Systolic Hypertension With Wide Pulse Pressure

1. Decreased vascular compliance (arteriosclerosis)
2. Increased cardiac output
   a. Aortic regurgitation
   b. Thyrotoxicosis
   c. Hyperkinetic heart syndrome
   d. Fever
   e. Arteriovenous fistula
   f. Patent ductus arteriosus

TABLE 247-3 Secondary Causes of Systolic and Diastolic Hypertension

Renal	Parenchymal diseases, renal cysts (including polycystic kidney disease), renal tumors (including renin-secreting tumors), obstructive uropathy
Renovascular	Arteriosclerotic, fibromuscular dysplasia
Adrenal	Primary aldosteronism, Cushing's syndrome, 17α-hydroxylase deficiency, 11β-hydroxylase deficiency, 11-hydroxysteroid dehydrogenase deficiency (licorice), pheochromocytoma
Aortic coarctation	
Obstructive sleep apnea	
Preeclampsia/eclampsia	
Neurogenic	Psychogenic, diencephalic syndrome, familial dysautonomia, polyneuritis (acute porphyria, lead poisoning), acute increased intracranial pressure, acute spinal cord section
Miscellaneous endocrine	Hypothyroidism, hyperthyroidism, hypercalcemia, acromegaly
Medications	High-dose estrogens, adrenal steroids, decongestants, appetite suppressants, cyclosporine, tricyclic antidepressants, monamine oxidase inhibitors, erythropoietin, nonsteroidal anti-inflammatory agents, cocaine
Mendelian forms of hypertension	See Table 247-4

25% have low PRA. High-renin patients may have a vasoconstrictor form of hypertension, whereas low-renin patients may have volume-dependent hypertension. Inconsistent associations between plasma aldosterone and blood pressure have been described in patients with essential hypertension. The association between aldosterone and blood pressure is more striking in African Americans, and PRA tends to be low in hypertensive African Americans. This raises the possibility that subtle increases in aldosterone may contribute to hypertension in at least some groups of patients who do not have overt primary aldosteronism. Furthermore, spironolactone, an aldosterone antagonist, may be a particularly effective antihypertensive agent for some patients with essential hypertension, including some patients with "drug-resistant" hypertension.

OBESITY AND THE METABOLIC SYNDROME

(See also Chap. 242) There is a well-documented association between obesity (body mass index >30 kg/m^2) and hypertension. Further, cross-sectional studies indicate a direct linear correlation between body weight (or body mass index) and blood pressure. Centrally located body fat is a more important determinant of blood pressure elevation than is peripheral body fat. In longitudinal studies, a direct correlation exists between change in weight and change in blood pressure over time. Sixty percent of hypertensive adults are more than 20% overweight. It has been established that 60–70% of hypertension in adults may be directly attributable to adiposity.

Hypertension and dyslipidemia frequently occur together and in association with resistance to insulin-stimulated glucose uptake. This clustering of risk factors is often, but not invariably, associated with obesity, particularly abdominal obesity. Insulin resistance also is associated with an unfavorable imbalance in the endothelial production of mediators that regulate platelet aggregation, coagulation, fibrinolysis, and vessel tone. When these risk factors cluster, the risks for CHD, stroke, diabetes, and cardiovascular disease mortality are increased further.

Depending on the populations studied and the methodologies for defining insulin resistance, ~25–50% of nonobese, nondiabetic hypertensive persons are insulin resistant. The constellation of insulin resistance, abdominal obesity, hypertension, and dyslipidemia has been designated as the *metabolic syndrome.* As a group, first-degree relatives of patients with essential hypertension are also insulin resistant, and hyperinsulinemia (a surrogate marker of insulin resistance) may predict the eventual development of hypertension and cardiovascular disease. Although the metabolic syndrome may in part be heritable as a polygenic condition, the expression of the syndrome is modified by environmental factors, such as degree of physical activity and diet. Insulin sensitivity increases and blood pressure decreases in response to weight loss. The recognition that cardiovascular disease risk factors tend to cluster within individuals has important implications for the evaluation and treatment of hypertension. Evaluation of both hypertensive patients and individuals at risk for developing hypertension should include assessment of overall cardiovascular disease risk. Similarly, introduction of lifestyle modification strategies and drug therapies should address overall risk and not simply focus on hypertension.

RENAL PARENCHYMAL DISEASES

Virtually all disorders of the kidney may cause hypertension (Table 247-3), and renal disease is the most common cause of secondary hypertension. Hypertension is present in >80% of patients with chronic renal failure. In general, hypertension is more severe in glomerular diseases than in interstitial diseases such as chronic pyelonephritis. Conversely, hypertension may cause nephrosclerosis, and in some instances it may be difficult to determine whether hypertension or renal disease was the initial disorder. Proteinuria >1000 mg/d and an active urine sediment are indicative of primary renal disease. In either instance, the goals are to control blood pressure and retard the rate of progression of renal dysfunction.

RENOVASCULAR HYPERTENSION

Hypertension due to an occlusive lesion of a renal artery, renovascular hypertension, is a potentially curable form of hypertension. In the initial stages, the mechanism of hypertension generally is related to activation of the renin-angiotensin system. However, renin activity and other components of the renin-angiotensin system may be elevated only transiently; over time, sodium retention and recruitment of other pressure mechanisms may contribute to elevated arterial pressure. Two groups of patients are at risk for this disorder: older arteriosclerotic patients who have a plaque obstructing the renal artery, frequently at its origin, and patients with fibromuscular dysplasia. Atherosclerosis accounts for the large majority of patients with renovascular hypertension. Although fibromuscular dysplasia may occur at any age, it has a strong predilection for young white women. The prevalence in females is eightfold that in males. There are several histologic variants of fibromuscular dysplasia, including medial fibroplasia, perimedial fibroplasia, medial hyperplasia, and intimal fibroplasia. Medial fibroplasia is the most common variant and accounts for approximately two-thirds of patients. The lesions of fibromuscular dysplasia are frequently bilateral and, in contrast to atherosclerotic renovascular disease, tend to affect more distal portions of the renal artery.

In addition to the age and sex of the patient, several clues from the history and physical examination suggest a diagnosis of renovascular hypertension. The diagnosis should be considered in patients with other evidence of atherosclerotic vascular disease. Although response to antihypertensive therapy does not exclude the diagnosis, severe or refractory hypertension, recent loss of hypertension control or recent onset of moderately severe hypertension, and unexplained deterioration of renal function or deterioration of renal function associated with an ACE inhibitor should raise the possibility of renovascular hypertension. Approximately 50% of patients with renovascular hypertension have an abdominal or flank bruit, and the bruit is more likely to be hemodynamically significant if it lateralizes or extends throughout systole into diastole.

If blood pressure is adequately controlled with a simple antihypertensive regimen and renal function remains stable, there may be little impetus to pursue an evaluation for renal artery stenosis, particularly in an older patient with atherosclerotic disease and comorbid conditions. Patients with long-standing hypertension, advanced renal insufficiency, or diabetes mellitus are less likely to benefit from renal vascular repair. The most effective medical therapies include an ACE inhibitor or an angiotensin II receptor blocker; however, these agents decrease glomerular filtration rate in a stenotic kidney owing to efferent renal arteriolar dilation. In the presence of bilateral renal artery stenosis or renal artery stenosis to a solitary kidney, progressive renal insufficiency may result from the use of these agents. Importantly, the renal insufficiency is generally reversible after discontinuation of the offending drug.

If renal artery stenosis is suspected and if the clinical condition warrants an intervention such as percutaneous transluminal renal angioplasty (PTRA), placement of a vascular endoprosthesis (stent), or surgical renal revascularization, imaging studies should be the next step in the evaluation. As a screening test, renal blood flow may be evaluated with a radionuclide [^{131}I]-orthoiodohippurate (OIH) scan or glomerular filtration rate may be evaluated with a [^{99}mTc]-diethylenetriamine pentaacetic acid (DTPA) scan before and after a single dose of captopril (or another ACE inhibitor). The following are consistent with a positive study: (1) decreased relative uptake by the involved kidney, which contributes <40% of total renal function, (2) delayed uptake on the affected side, and (3) delayed washout on the affected side. In patients with normal, or nearly normal, renal function, a normal captopril renogram essentially excludes functionally significant renal artery stenosis; however, its usefulness is limited in patients with renal insufficiency (creatinine clearance <20 mL/min) or bilateral renal artery stenosis. Additional imaging studies are indicated if the scan is positive. Doppler ultrasound of the renal arteries produces reliable estimates of renal blood flow velocity and offers the opportunity to track a lesion over time. Positive studies usually are confirmed at angiography, whereas false-negative results occur frequently, particularly in obese patients. Gadolinium-contrast magnetic resonance angiography offers clear images of the proximal renal artery but may miss distal lesions. An advantage is the opportunity to image the renal arteries with an agent that is not nephrotoxic. Contrast arteriography remains the "gold standard" for evaluation and identification of renal artery lesions. Potential risks include nephrotoxicity, particularly in patients with diabetes mellitus or preexisting renal insufficiency.

Some degree of renal artery obstruction may be observed in almost 50% of patients with atherosclerotic disease, and there are several approaches for evaluating the functional significance of such a lesion to predict the effect of vascular repair on blood pressure control and renal function. Each approach has varying degrees of sensitivity and specificity, and no single test is sufficiently reliable to determine a causal relationship between a renal artery lesion and hypertension. Functionally significant lesions generally occlude more than 70% of the lumen of the affected renal artery. On angiography, the presence of collateral vessels to the ischemic kidney suggests a functionally significant lesion. A lateralizing renal vein renin ratio (ratio >1.5 of affected side/contralateral side) has a 90% predictive value for a lesion that would respond to vascular repair; however, the false-negative rate for blood pressure control is 50–60%. Measurement of the pressure gradient across a renal artery lesion does not reliably predict the response to vascular repair.

In the final analysis, a decision concerning vascular repair vs. medical therapy and the type of repair procedure should be individualized for each patient. Patients with fibromuscular disease have more favorable outcomes than do patients with atherosclerotic lesions, presumably owing to their younger age, shorter duration of hypertension, and less systemic disease. Because of its low risk-versus-benefit ratio and high success rate (improvement or cure of hypertension in 90% of patients and restenosis rate of 10%), PTRA is the initial treatment of choice for these patients. Surgical revascularization may be undertaken if PTRA is unsuccessful or if a branch lesion is present. In atherosclerotic patients, vascular repair should be considered if blood pressure cannot be controlled adequately despite optimal medical therapy or if renal function deteriorates. Surgery may be the preferred initial approach for younger atherosclerotic patients without comorbid conditions; however, for most atherosclerotic patients, depending on the location of the lesion, the initial approach may be PTRA and/or stenting. Surgical revascularization may be indicated if these approaches are unsuccessful, the vascular lesion is not amenable to PTRA or stenting, or concomitant aortic surgery is required, e.g., to repair an aneurysm. A National Institutes of Health–sponsored prospective, randomized clinical trial is in progress comparing medical therapy alone with medical therapy plus renal revascularization regarding Cardiovascular Outcomes for Renal Atherosclerotic Lesions (CORAL).

PRIMARY ALDOSTERONISM

Excess aldosterone production due to primary aldosteronism is a potentially curable form of hypertension. In patients with primary aldosteronism, increased aldosterone production is independent of the renin-angiotensin system, and the consequences are sodium retention, hypertension, hypokalemia, and low PRA. The reported prevalence of this disorder varies from <2% to ~15% of hypertensive individuals. In part, this variation is related to the intensity of screening and the criteria for establishing the diagnosis.

History and physical examination provide little information about the diagnosis. The age at the time of diagnosis is generally the third through fifth decade. Hypertension is usually mild to moderate but occasionally may be severe; primary aldosteronism should be considered in all patients with refractory hypertension. Hypertension in these patients may be associated with glucose intolerance. Most patients are asymptomatic, although, infrequently, polyuria, polydipsia, paresthesias, or muscle weakness may be present as a consequence of hypokalemic alkalosis. In a hypertensive patient with unprovoked hypokalemia (i.e., unrelated to diuretics, vomiting, or diarrhea), the prevalence of primary aldosteronism approaches 40–50%. In patients on diuretics, serum potassium <3.1 mmol/L (<3.1 meq/L) also raises the possibility of primary aldosteronism; however, serum potassium is an insensitive and nonspecific screening test. However, serum potassium is normal in ~25% of patients subsequently found to have an aldosterone-producing adenoma, and higher percentages of patients with other etiologies of primary aldosteronism are not hypokalemic. Additionally, hypokalemic hypertension may be a consequence of secondary aldosteronism, other mineralocorticoid- and glucocorticoid-induced hypertensive disorders, and pheochromocytoma.

The ratio of plasma aldosterone to plasma renin activity (PA/PRA) is a useful screening test. These measurements preferably are obtained in ambulatory patients in the morning. A ratio >30:1 in conjunction with a plasma aldosterone concentration >555 pmol/L (>20 ng/dL) reportedly has a sensitivity of 90% and a specificity of 91% for an aldosterone-producing adenoma. In a Mayo Clinic series, an aldosterone-producing adenoma subsequently was confirmed surgically in >90% of hypertensive patients with a PA/PRA ratio ≥20 and a plasma aldosterone concentration ≥415 pmol/L (≥15 ng/dL). There are, however, several caveats to interpreting the ratio. The cutoff for a "high" ratio is laboratory- and assay-dependent. Some antihypertensive agents may affect the ratio (e.g., aldosterone antagonists, angiotensin receptor antagonists, and ACE inhibitors may increase renin; aldosterone antagonists may increase aldosterone). Current recommendations are to withdraw aldosterone antagonists for at least 4 weeks before obtaining these measurements, with this caveat. The ratio has been reported to be useful as a screening test in measurements obtained with patients taking their usual antihypertensive medications. A high ratio in the absence of an elevated plasma aldosterone level is considerably less specific for primary aldosteronism since many patients with essential hypertension have low renin levels in this setting, particularly African Americans and elderly patients. In patients with renal insufficiency, the ratio may also be elevated because of decreased aldosterone clearance. In patients with an elevated PA/PRA ratio, the diagnosis of primary aldosteronism can be confirmed by demonstrating failure to suppress plasma aldosterone to <277 pmol/L (<10 ng/dL) after IV infusion of 2 L of isotonic saline over 4 h; post-saline infusion plasma aldosterone values between 138 and 277 pmol/L (5–10 ng/dL) are not determinant. Alternative confirmatory tests include failure to suppress aldosterone (based on test specific criteria) in response to an oral NaCl load, fludrocortisone, or captopril.

Several adrenal abnormalities may culminate in the syndrome of primary aldosteronism, and appropriate therapy depends on the specific etiology. Some 60–70% of patients have an aldosterone-producing adrenal adenoma. The tumor is almost always unilateral, and most often measures <3 cm in diameter. Most of the remainder of these patients have bilateral adrenocortical hyperplasia (idiopathic hyperaldosteronism). Rarely, primary aldosteronism may be caused by an adrenal carcinoma or an ectopic malignancy, e.g., ovarian arrhenoblastoma. Most aldosterone-producing carcinomas, in contrast to adrenal adenomas and hyperplasia, produce excessive amounts of other adrenal steroids in addition to aldosterone. Functional differences in hormone secretion may assist in the differential diagnosis. Aldosterone biosynthesis is more responsive to adrenocorticotropic hormone (ACTH) in patients with adenoma and more responsive to angiotensin in patients with hyperplasia. Consequently, patients with adenoma tend to have higher plasma aldosterone in the early morning that decreases during the day, reflecting the diurnal rhythm of ACTH, whereas plasma aldosterone tends to increase with upright posture in patients with hyperplasia, reflecting the normal postural response of the renin-angiotensin-aldosterone axis. However, there is some overlap in the ability of these measurements to discriminate between adenoma and hyperplasia.

Adrenal computed tomography (CT) should be carried out in all patients diagnosed with primary aldosteronism. High-resolution CT may identify tumors as small as 0.3 cm and is positive for an adrenal tumor 90% of the time. If the CT is not diagnostic, an adenoma may be detected by adrenal scintigraphy with 6 β-[I^{131}] iodomethyl-19-norcholesterol after dexamethasone suppression (0.5 mg every 6 h for 7 days); however, this technique has decreased sensitivity for adenomas <1.5 cm.

When carried out by an experienced radiologist, bilateral adrenal venous sampling for measurement of plasma aldosterone is the most accurate means of differentiating unilateral from bilateral forms of primary aldosteronism. The sensitivity and specificity of adrenal venous sampling (95% and 100%, respectively) for detecting unilateral aldosterone hypersecretion are superior to those of adrenal CT; success rates are 90–96%, and complication rates are <2.5%. One frequently used protocol involves sampling for aldosterone and cortisol levels in response to ACTH stimulation. An ipsilateral/ contralateral aldosterone ratio >4, with symmetric ACTH-stimulated cortisol levels, is indicative of unilateral aldosterone production.

Hypertension generally is responsive to surgery in patients with adenoma but not in patients with bilateral adrenal hyperplasia. Unilateral adrenalectomy, often done via a laparoscopic approach, is curative in 40–70% of patients with an adenoma. Surgery should be undertaken after blood pressure has been controlled and hypokalemia corrected. Transient hypoaldosteronism may occur up to 3 months postoperatively, resulting in hyperkalemia. Potassium should be monitored during this time, and hyperkalemia should be treated with potassium-wasting diuretics and with fludrocortisone, if needed. Patients with bilateral hyperplasia should be treated medically. The drug regimen for these patients, as well as for patients with an adenoma who are poor surgical candidates, should include an aldosterone antagonist and, if necessary, other potassium-sparing diuretics.

Glucocorticoid-remediable hyperaldosteronism is a rare, monogenic autosomal dominant disorder characterized by moderate to severe hypertension, often occurring at an early age. These patients may have a family history of hemorrhagic stroke at a young age. Hypokalemia is usually mild or absent. Normally, angiotensin II stimulates aldosterone production by the adrenal zona glomerulosa, whereas ACTH stimulates cortisol production in the zona fasciculata. Owing to a chimeric gene on chromosome 8, ACTH also regulates aldosterone secretion by the zona fasciculata in patients with glucocorticoid-remediable hyperaldosteronism. The consequence is overproduction in the zona fasciculata of both aldosterone and hybrid steroids (18-hydroxycortisol and 18-oxocortisol) due to oxidation of cortisol. The diagnosis may be established by urine excretion rates of these hybrid steroids that are 20 to 30 times normal or by direct genetic testing. Therapeutically, suppression of ACTH with low-dose glucocorticoids corrects the hyperaldosteronism, hypertension, and hypokalemia. Spironolactone is also a therapeutic option.

■ CUSHING'S SYNDROME

(See also Chap. 342) Cushing's syndrome is related to excess cortisol production due either to excess ACTH secretion (from a pituitary tumor or an ectopic tumor) or to ACTH-independent adrenal production of cortisol. Hypertension occurs in 75–80% of patients with Cushing's syndrome. The mechanism of hypertension may be related to stimulation of mineralocorticoid receptors by cortisol and increased secretion of other adrenal steroids. If clinically suspected based on phenotypic characteristics, in patients not taking exogenous glucocorticoids, laboratory screening may be carried out with measurement of 24-h excretion rates of urine free cortisol or an overnight dexamethasone-suppression test. Recent evidence suggests that late night salivary cortisol is also a sensitive and convenient screening test. Further evaluation is required to confirm the diagnosis and identify the specific etiology of Cushing's syndrome. Appropriate therapy depends on the etiology.

■ PHEOCHROMOCYTOMA

(See also Chap. 343) Catecholamine-secreting tumors are located in the adrenal medulla (pheochromocytoma) or in extra-adrenal paraganglion tissue (paraganglioma) and account for hypertension in ~0.05% of patients. If unrecognized, pheochromocytoma may result in lethal cardiovascular consequences. Clinical manifestations, including hypertension, are primarily related to increased circulating catecholamines, although some of these tumors may secrete a number of other vasoactive substances. In a small percentage of patients, epinephrine is the predominant catecholamine secreted by the tumor, and these patients may present with hypotension rather than hypertension. The initial suspicion of the diagnosis is based on symptoms and/or the association of pheochromocytoma with other disorders (Table 247-4). Approximately 20% of pheochromocytomas are familial with autosomal dominant inheritance. Inherited pheochromocytomas may be associated with multiple endocrine neoplasia (MEN) type 2A and type 2B, von Hippel-Lindau disease, and neurofibromatosis (Table 247-4). Each of these syndromes is related to specific, identifiable germ-line mutations. Additionally, mutations of succinate dehydrogenase genes are associated with paraganglioma syndromes, generally characterized by head and neck paragangliomas. Laboratory testing consists of measuring catecholamines in either urine or plasma. Genetic screening is available for evaluating patients and relatives suspected of harboring a pheochromocytoma associated with a familial syndrome. Surgical excision is the definitive treatment of pheochromocytoma and results in cure in ~90% of patients.

MISCELLANEOUS CAUSES OF HYPERTENSION

Hypertension due to *obstructive sleep apnea* is being recognized with increasing frequency (Chap. 265). Independent of obesity, hypertension occurs in >50% of individuals with obstructive sleep apnea. The severity of hypertension correlates with the severity of sleep apnea. Approximately 70% of patients with obstructive sleep apnea are obese. Hypertension related to obstructive sleep apnea also should be considered in patients with drug-resistant hypertension and patients with a history of snoring. The diagnosis can be confirmed by polysomnography. In obese patients, weight loss may alleviate or cure sleep apnea and related hypertension. Continuous positive airway pressure (CPAP) administered during sleep is an effective therapy for obstructive sleep apnea. With CPAP, patients with apparently drug-resistant hypertension may be more responsive to antihypertensive agents.

Coarctation of the aorta is the most common congenital cardiovascular cause of hypertension (Chap. 236). The incidence is 1–8 per

TABLE 247-4 Rare Mendelian Forms of Hypertension

Disease	Phenotype	Genetic Cause
Glucocorticoid-remediable hyperaldosteronism	Autosomal dominant Absent or mild hypokalemia	Chimeric 11β-hydroxylase/aldsoterone gene on chromosome 8
17α-hydroxylase deficiency	Autosomal recessive Males: pseudohermaphroditism Females: primary amenorrhea, absent secondary sexual characteristics	Random mutations of the *CYP17* gene on chromosome 10
11β-hydroxylase deficiency	Autosomal recessive Masculinization	Mutations of the *CYP11B1* gene on chromosome 8q21-q22
11β-hydroxysteroid dehydrogenase deficiency (apparent mineralocorticoid excess syndrome)	Autosomal recessive Hypokalemia, low renin, low aldosterone	Mutations in the 11β-hydroxysteroid dehydrogenase gene
Liddle's syndrome	Autosomal dominant Hypokalemia, low renin, low aldosterone	Mutation subunits of the epithelial sodium channel *SCNN1B* and *SCNN1C* genes
Pseudohypoaldosteronism type II (Gordon's syndrome)	Autosomal dominant Hyperkalemia, normal glomerular filtration rate	Linkage to chromosomes 1q31-q42 and 17p11-q21
Hypertension exacerbated in pregnancy	Autosomal dominant Severe hypertension in early pregnancy	Missense mutation with substitution of leucine for serine at codon 810 (MR_{L810})
Polycystic kidney disease	Autosomal dominant Large cystic kidneys, renal failure, liver cysts, cerebral aneurysms, valvular heart disease	Mutations in the *PKD1* gene on chromosome 16 and *PKD2* gene on chromosome 4
Pheochromocytoma	Autosomal dominant (a) Multiple endocrine neoplasia, type 2A Medullary thyroid carcinoma, hyperparathyroidism (b) Multiple endocrine neoplasia, type 2B Medullary thyroid carcinoma, mucosal neuromas, thickened corneal nerves, alimentary ganglioneuromatoses, marfanoid habitus (c) von Hippel-Lindau disease Retinal angiomas, hemangioblastomas of the cerebellum and spinal cord, renal cell carcinoma (d) Neurofibromatosis type 1 Multiple neurofibromas, café-au-lait spots	(a) Mutations in the RET protooncogene (b) Mutations in the RET protooncogene (c) Mutations in the VHL tumor-suppressor gene (d) Mutations in the NF1 tumor-suppressor gene

1000 live births. It is usually sporadic but occurs in 35% of children with Turner syndrome. Even when the anatomic lesion is surgically corrected in infancy, up to 30% of patients develop subsequent hypertension and are at risk of accelerated coronary artery disease and cerebrovascular events. Patients with less severe lesions may not be diagnosed until young adulthood. The physical findings are diagnostic and include diminished and delayed femoral pulses and a systolic pressure gradient between the right arm and the legs and, depending on the location of the coarctation, between the right and left arms. A blowing systolic murmur may be heard in the posterior left interscapular areas. The diagnosis may be confirmed by chest x-ray and transesophageal echocardiography. Therapeutic options include surgical repair and balloon angioplasty, with or without placement of an intravascular stent. Subsequently, many patients do not have a normal life expectancy but may have persistent hypertension, with death due to ischemic heart disease, cerebral hemorrhage, or aortic aneurysm.

Several additional endocrine disorders, including *thyroid diseases* and *acromegaly*, cause hypertension. Mild diastolic hypertension may be a consequence of hypothyroidism, whereas hyperthyroidism may result in systolic hypertension. *Hypercalcemia* of any etiology, the most common being primary hyperparathyroidism, may result in hypertension. Hypertension also may be related to a number of prescribed or over-the-counter *medications*.

MONOGENIC HYPERTENSION

A number of rare forms of monogenic hypertension have been identified (Table 247-4). These disorders may be recognized by their characteristic phenotypes, and in many instances the diagnosis may be confirmed by genetic analysis. Several inherited defects in adrenal steroid biosynthesis and metabolism result in mineralocorticoid-induced hypertension and hypokalemia. In patients with a 17α-hydroxylase deficiency, synthesis of sex hormones and cortisol is decreased (Fig. 247-3). Consequently, these individuals do not mature sexually; males may present with pseudohermaphroditism and females with primary amenorrhea and absent secondary sexual characteristics. Because cortisol-induced negative feedback on pituitary ACTH production is diminished, ACTH-stimulated adrenal steroid synthesis proximal to the enzymatic block is increased. Hypertension and hypokalemia are consequences of increased synthesis of mineralocorticoids proximal to the enzymatic block, particularly desoxycorticosterone. Increased steroid production and, hence, hypertension may be treated with low-dose glucocorticoids. An 11β-hydroxylase deficiency results in a salt-retaining adrenogenital syndrome that occurs in 1 in 100,000 live births. This enzymatic defect results in decreased cortisol synthesis, increased synthesis of mineralocorticoids (e.g., desoxycorticosterone), and shunting of steroid biosynthesis into the androgen pathway. In the severe form, the syndrome may present early in life, including the newborn period, with virilization and ambiguous genitalia in females and penile enlargement in males, or in older children as precocious puberty and short stature. Acne, hirsutism, and menstrual irregularities may be the presenting features when the disorder is first recognized in adolescence or early adulthood. Hypertension is less common in the late-onset forms. Patients with an 11β-hydroxysteroid dehydrogenase deficiency have an impaired capacity to metabolize cortisol to its inactive metabolite, cortisone, and hypertension is related to activation of mineralocorticoid receptors by cortisol. This defect may be inherited or acquired, due to licorice-containing glycyrrhizin acid. The same substance is present in the paste of several brands of chewing tobacco. The defect in Liddle's syndrome (Chaps. 45 and 342) results from constitutive activation of amiloride-sensitive epithelial sodium channels on the distal renal tubule, resulting in excess sodium reabsorption; the syndrome is ameliorated by amiloride. Hypertension exacerbated in pregnancy (Chap. 7) is due to activation of the mineralocorticoid receptor by progesterone.

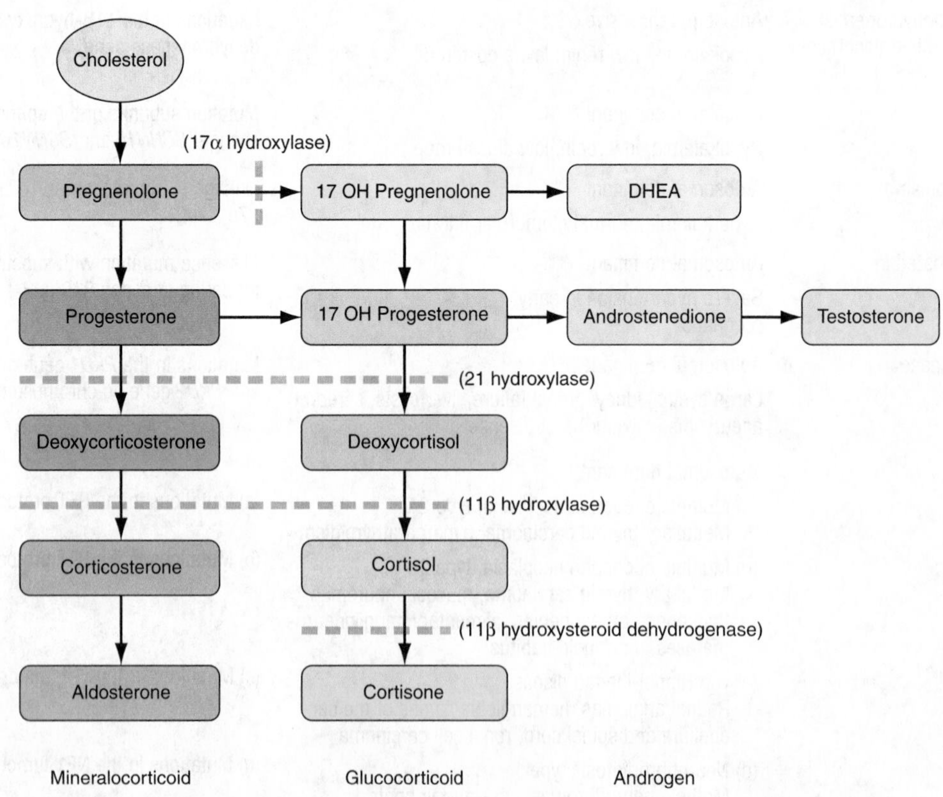

Figure 247-3 Adrenal enzymatic defects.

APPROACH TO THE PATIENT Hypertension

HISTORY The initial assessment of a hypertensive patient should include a complete history and physical examination to confirm a diagnosis of hypertension, screen for other cardiovascular disease risk factors, screen for secondary causes of hypertension, identify cardiovascular consequences of hypertension and other comorbidities, assess blood pressure–related lifestyles, and determine the potential for intervention.

Most patients with hypertension have no specific symptoms referable to their blood pressure elevation. Although popularly considered a symptom of elevated arterial pressure, headache generally occurs only in patients with severe hypertension. Characteristically, a "hypertensive headache" occurs in the morning and is localized to the occipital region. Other nonspecific symptoms that may be related to elevated blood pressure include dizziness, palpitations, easy fatigability, and impotence. When symptoms are present, they are generally related to hypertensive cardiovascular disease or to manifestations of secondary hypertension. Table 247-5 lists salient features that should be addressed in obtaining a history from a hypertensive patient.

MEASUREMENT OF BLOOD PRESSURE Reliable measurements of blood pressure depend on attention to the details of the technique and conditions of the measurement. Proper training of observers, positioning of the patient, and selection of cuff size are essential. Owing to recent regulations preventing the use of mercury because of concerns about its potential toxicity, most office measurements are made with aneroid sphygmomanometers or with oscillometric devices. These instruments should be calibrated periodically, and their accuracy confirmed. Before the blood pressure measurement is taken, the individual should be seated quietly in a chair (not the exam table) with feet on the floor for 5 min in a private, quiet setting with a comfortable room temperature. At least two measurements should be made. The center of the cuff should be at heart level, and the width of the bladder cuff should equal at least 40% of the arm circumference; the length of the cuff bladder should be enough to encircle at least 80% of the arm circumference. It is important to pay attention to cuff placement, stethoscope placement, and the rate of deflation of the cuff (2 mmHg/s). Systolic blood pressure is the first of at least two regular "tapping" Korotkoff sounds, and diastolic blood pressure is the point at which the last regular Korotkoff sound is heard. In current practice, a diagnosis of hypertension generally is based on seated, office measurements.

Currently available ambulatory monitors are fully automated, use the oscillometric technique, and typically are programmed to take readings every 15–30 min. Twenty-four-hour ambulatory blood pressure monitoring more reliably predicts cardiovascular disease risk than do office measurements. However, ambulatory monitoring is not used routinely in clinical practice and generally is reserved for patients in whom white coat hypertension is suspected. The Seventh Report of the Joint National Committee on Prevention, Detection, Evaluation, and Treatment of High Blood Pressure (JNC 7) has also recommended ambulatory monitoring for treatment resistance, symptomatic hypotension, autonomic failure, and episodic hypertension.

PHYSICAL EXAMINATION Body habitus, including weight and height, should be noted. At the initial examination, blood pressure should be measured in both arms and preferably in the supine, sitting, and standing positions to evaluate for postural hypotension. Even if the femoral pulse is normal to palpation, arterial pressure should be measured at least once in the lower extremity in patients in whom hypertension is discovered before age 30. Heart rate also should be recorded. Hypertensive individuals have an increased prevalence of atrial fibrillation. The neck should be palpated for an enlarged thyroid gland, and patients should be assessed for signs of hypo- and hyperthyroidism. Examination of blood vessels may provide clues about underlying vascular disease and should include funduscopic examination, auscultation for bruits over the carotid and femoral arteries, and palpation of femoral and pedal pulses. The retina is the only tissue in which arteries and arterioles can be examined directly. With increasing severity of hypertension and atherosclerotic disease, progressive funduscopic changes include increased arteriolar light reflex, arteriovenous crossing defects, hemorrhages and exudates, and, in patients with malignant hypertension, papilledema. Examination of the heart may reveal a loud second heart sound due to closure of the aortic valve and an S_4 gallop attributed to atrial contraction against a noncompliant left ventricle. Left ventricular hypertrophy may be detected by an enlarged, sustained, and laterally displaced apical impulse. An abdominal bruit, particularly a bruit that lateralizes and extends throughout systole into diastole, raises the possibility of renovascular hypertension. Kidneys of patients with polycystic kidney disease may be palpable in the abdomen. The physical examination also should include evaluation for signs of CHF and a neurologic examination.

LABORATORY TESTING Table 247-6 lists recommended laboratory tests in the initial evaluation of hypertensive patients.

TABLE 247-5 Patient's Relevant History

- Duration of hypertension
- Previous therapies: responses and side effects
- Family history of hypertension and cardiovascular disease
- Dietary and psychosocial history
- Other risk factors: weight change, dyslipidemia, smoking, diabetes, physical inactivity
- Evidence of secondary hypertension: history of renal disease; change in appearance; muscle weakness; spells of sweating, palpitations, tremor; erratic sleep, snoring, daytime somnolence; symptoms of hypo- or hyperthyroidism; use of agents that may increase blood pressure
- Evidence of target organ damage: history of TIA, stroke, transient blindness; angina, myocardial infarction, congestive heart failure; sexual function
- Other comorbidities

Abbreviation: TIA, transient ischemic attack.

TABLE 247-6 Basic Laboratory Tests for Initial Evaluation

System	Test
Renal	Microscopic urinalysis, albumin excretion, serum BUN and/or creatinine
Endocrine	Serum sodium, potassium, calcium, ?TSH
Metabolic	Fasting blood glucose, total cholesterol, HDL and LDL (often computed) cholesterol, triglycerides
Other	Hematocrit, electrocardiogram

Abbreviations: BUN, blood urea nitrogen; HDL, LDL, high-/low-density lipoprotein; TSH, thyroid-stimulating hormone.

Repeat measurements of renal function, serum electrolytes, fasting glucose, and lipids may be obtained after the introduction of a new antihypertensive agent and then annually or more frequently if clinically indicated. More extensive laboratory testing is appropriate for patients with apparent drug-resistant hypertension or when the clinical evaluation suggests a secondary form of hypertension.

TREATMENT Hypertension

LIFESTYLE INTERVENTIONS Implementation of lifestyles that favorably affect blood pressure has implications for both the prevention and the treatment of hypertension. Health-promoting lifestyle modifications are recommended for individuals with prehypertension and as an adjunct to drug therapy in hypertensive individuals. These interventions should address overall cardiovascular disease risk. Although the impact of lifestyle interventions on blood pressure is more pronounced in persons with hypertension, in short-term trials, weight loss and reduction of dietary NaCl have been shown to prevent the development of hypertension. In hypertensive individuals, even if these interventions do not produce a sufficient reduction in blood pressure to avoid drug therapy, the number of medications or doses required for blood pressure control may be reduced. Dietary modifications that effectively lower blood pressure are weight loss, reduced NaCl intake, increased potassium intake, moderation of alcohol consumption, and an overall healthy dietary pattern (Table 247-7).

Prevention and treatment of obesity are important for reducing blood pressure and cardiovascular disease risk. In short-term trials, even modest weight loss can lead to a reduction of blood pressure and an increase in insulin sensitivity. Average blood pressure reductions of 6.3/3.1 mmHg have been observed with a reduction in mean body weight of 9.2 kg. Regular physical activity facilitates weight loss, decreases blood pressure, and reduces the overall risk of cardiovascular disease. Blood pressure may be lowered by 30 min of moderately intense physical activity, such as brisk walking, 6–7 days a week, or by more intense, less frequent workouts.

There is individual variability in the sensitivity of blood pressure to NaCl, and this variability may have a genetic basis. Based on results of meta-analyses, lowering of blood pressure by limiting daily NaCl intake to 4.4–7.4 g (75–125 meq) results in blood pressure reductions of 3.7–4.9/0.9–2.9 mmHg in hypertensive individuals and lesser reductions in normotensive individuals. Dietary NaCl reduction also has been shown to reduce the long-term risk of cardiovascular events in adults with "prehypertension." Potassium and calcium supplementation have inconsistent, modest antihypertensive effects, and, independent of blood pressure, potassium supplementation may be associated with reduced stroke mortality. Alcohol use in persons consuming three or more drinks per day (a standard drink contains ~14 g ethanol) is associated with higher blood pressures, and a reduction of alcohol consumption is associated with a reduction of blood pressure. In patients with advanced renal disease, dietary protein restriction may have a modest effect in mitigating renal damage by reducing the intrarenal transmission of systemic arterial pressure.

The DASH (Dietary Approaches to Stop Hypertension) trial convincingly demonstrated that over an 8-week period a diet high in fruits, vegetables, and low-fat dairy products lowers blood pressure in individuals with high-normal blood pressures or mild hypertension. Reduction of daily NaCl intake to <6 g (100 meq) augmented the effect of this diet on blood pressure. Fruits and vegetables are enriched sources of potassium, magnesium, and fiber, and dairy products are an important source of calcium.

TABLE 247-7 Lifestyle Modifications to Manage Hypertension

Weight reduction	Attain and maintain BMI <25 kg/m^2
Dietary salt reduction	<6 g NaCl/d
Adapt DASH-type dietary plan	Diet rich in fruits, vegetables, and low-fat dairy products with reduced content of saturated and total fat
Moderation of alcohol consumption	For those who drink alcohol, consume ≤2 drinks/day in men and ≤1 drink/day in women
Physical activity	Regular aerobic activity, e.g., brisk walking for 30 min/d

Abbreviations: BMI, body mass index; DASH, Dietary Approaches to Stop Hypertension (trial).

PHARMACOLOGIC THERAPY Drug therapy is recommended for individuals with blood pressures ≥140/90 mmHg. The degree of benefit derived from antihypertensive agents is related to the magnitude of the blood pressure reduction. Lowering systolic blood pressure by 10–12 mmHg and diastolic blood pressure by 5–6 mmHg confers relative risk reductions of 35–40% for stroke and 12–16% for CHD within 5 years of the initiation of treatment. Risk of heart failure is reduced by >50%. Hypertension control is the single most effective intervention for slowing the rate of progression of hypertension-related chronic kidney disease.

There is considerable variation in individual responses to different classes of antihypertensive agents, and the magnitude of response to any single agent may be limited by activation of counterregulatory mechanisms that oppose the hypotensive effect of the agent. Most available agents reduce systolic blood pressure by 7–13 mmHg and diastolic blood pressure by 4–8 mmHg when corrected for placebo effect. More often than not, combinations of agents, with complementary antihypertensive mechanisms, are required to achieve goal blood pressure reductions. Selection of antihypertensive agents and combinations of agents should be individualized, taking into account age, severity of hypertension, other cardiovascular disease risk factors, comorbid conditions, and practical considerations related to cost, side effects, and frequency of dosing (Table 247-8).

Diuretics Low-dose thiazide diuretics often are used as first-line agents alone or in combination with other antihypertensive drugs. Thiazides inhibit the Na^+/Cl^- pump in the distal convoluted tubule and hence increase sodium excretion. In the long term, they also may act as vasodilators. Thiazides are safe, efficacious, inexpensive, and reduce clinical events. They provide additive blood pressure–lowering effects when combined with beta blockers, angiotensin-converting enzyme inhibitors (ACEIs), or angiotensin receptor blockers (ARBs). In contrast, addition of a diuretic to a calcium channel blocker is less effective. Usual doses of hydrochlorothiazide range from 6.25–50 mg/d. Owing to an increased incidence of metabolic side effects (hypokalemia, insulin resistance, increased cholesterol), higher doses generally are not recommended. Two potassium-sparing diuretics, amiloride and triamterene, act by inhibiting epithelial

TABLE 247-8 Examples of Oral Drugs Used in Treatment of Hypertension

Drug Class	Examples	Usual Total Daily Dose* (Dosing Frequency/Day)	Other Indications	Contraindications/Cautions
Diuretics				
Thiazides	Hydrochlorothiazide	6.25–50 mg (1–2)		Diabetes, dyslipidemia, hyperuricemia, gout, hypokalemia
	Chlorthalidone	25–50 mg (1)		
Loop diuretics	Furosemide	40–80 mg (2–3)	CHF due to systolic dysfunction, renal failure	Diabetes, dyslipidemia, hyperuricemia, gout, hypokalemia
	Ethacrynic acid	50–100 mg (2–3)		
Aldosterone antagonists	Spironolactone	25–100 mg (1–2)	CHF due to systolic dysfunction, primary aldosteronism	Renal failure, hyperkalemia
	Eplerenone	50–100 mg (1–2)		
K^+ retaining	Amiloride	5–10 mg (1–2)		Renal failure, hyperkalemia
	Triamterene	50–100 mg (1–2)		
Beta blockers				Asthma, COPD, 2nd- or 3rd-degree heart block, sick-sinus syndrome
Cardioselective	Atenolol	25–100 mg (1)	Angina, CHF due to systolic dysfunction, post-MI, sinus tachycardia, ventricular tachyarrhythmias	
	Metoprolol	25–100 mg (1–2)		
Nonselective	Propranolol	40–160 mg (2)		
	Propranolol LA	60–180 (1)		
Combined alpha/beta	Labetalol	200–800 mg (2)	?Post-MI, CHF	
	Carvedilol	12.5–50 mg (2)		
Alpha antagonists				
Selective	Prazosin	2–20 mg (2–3)	Prostatism	
	Doxazosin	1–16 mg (1)		
	Terazosin	1–10 mg (1–2)		
Nonselective	Phenoxybenzamine	20–120 mg (2–3)	Pheochromocytoma	
Sympatholytics				
Central	Clonidine	0.1–0.6 mg (2)		
	Clonidine patch	0.1–0.3 mg (1/week)		
	Methyldopa	250–1000 mg (2)		
	Reserpine	0.05–0.25 mg (1)		
	Guanfacine	0.5–2 mg (1)		
ACE inhibitors	Captopril	25–200 mg (2)	Post-MI, coronary syndromes, CHF with low ejection fraction, nephropathy	Acute renal failure, bilateral renal artery stenosis, pregnancy, hyperkalemia
	Lisinopril	10–40 mg (1)		
	Ramipril	2.5–20 mg (1–2)		
Angiotensin II antagonists	Losartan	25–100 mg (1–2)	CHF with low ejection fraction, nephropathy, ACE inhibitor cough	Renal failure, bilateral renal artery stenosis, pregnancy, hyperkalemia
	Valsartan	80–320 mg (1)		
	Candesartan	2–32 mg (1–2)		
Renin inhibitors	Aliskiren	150–300 mg (1)	Diabetic nephropathy	Pregnancy
Calcium antagonists				
Dihydropyridines	Nifedipine (long-acting)	30–60 mg (1)		
Nondihydropyridines	Verapamil (long-acting)	120–360 mg (1–2)	Post-MI, supraventricular tachycardias, angina	2nd- or 3rd-degree heart block
	Diltiazem (long-acting)	180–420 mg (1)		
Direct vasodilators	Hydralazine	25–100 mg (2)		Severe coronary artery disease
	Minoxidil	2.5–80 mg (1–2)		

*At the initiation of therapy, lower doses may be preferable for elderly patients and for select combinations of antihypertensive agents.

Abbreviations: ACE, angiotensin-converting enzyme; CHF, congestive heart failure; COPD, chronic obstructive pulmonary disease; MI, myocardial infarction.

sodium channels in the distal nephron. These agents are weak antihypertensive agents but may be used in combination with a thiazide to protect against hypokalemia. The main pharmacologic target for loop diuretics is the Na^+-K^+-$2Cl^-$ cotransporter in the thick ascending limb of the loop of Henle. Loop diuretics generally are reserved for hypertensive patients with reduced glomerular filtration rates [reflected in serum creatinine >220 μmol/L (>2.5 mg/dL)], CHF, or sodium retention and edema for some other reason, such as treatment with a potent vasodilator, e.g., minoxidil.

Blockers of the Renin-Angiotensin System ACEIs decrease the production of angiotensin II, increase bradykinin levels, and reduce sympathetic nervous system activity. ARBs provide selective blockade of AT_1 receptors, and the effect of angiotensin II on unblocked AT_2 receptors may augment their hypotensive effect. Both classes of agents are effective antihypertensive agents that may be used as monotherapy or in combination with diuretics, calcium antagonists, and alpha blocking agents. ACEIs and ARBs have been shown to improve insulin action and ameliorate the adverse effects of diuretics on glucose metabolism. Although the overall impact on the incidence of diabetes is modest, compared with amlodipine (a calcium antagonist), valsartan (an ARB) has been shown to reduce the risk of developing diabetes in high-risk hypertensive patients. ACEI/ARB combinations are less effective in lowering blood pressure than is the case when either class of these agents is used in combination with other classes of agents. In patients with vascular disease or a high risk of diabetes, combination ACEI/ARB therapy has been associated with more adverse events (e.g., cardiovascular death, myocardial infarction, stroke, and hospitalization for heart failure) without increases in benefit. However, in hypertensive patients with proteinuria, preliminary data suggest that reduction of proteinuria with ACEI/ARB combination treatment may be more effective than treatment with either agent alone.

Side effects of ACEIs and ARBs include functional renal insufficiency due to efferent renal arteriolar dilation in a kidney with a stenotic lesion of the renal artery. Additional predisposing conditions to renal insufficiency induced by these agents include dehydration, CHF, and use of nonsteroidal anti-inflammatory drugs. Dry cough occurs in ~15% of patients, and angioedema occurs in <1% of patients taking ACEIs. Angioedema occurs most commonly in individuals of Asian origin and more commonly in African Americans than in whites. Hyperkalemia due to hypoaldosteronism is an occasional side effect of both ACEIs and ARBs.

A new approach to blocking the renin-angiotensin system has been introduced into clinical practice for the treatment of hypertension: direct renin inhibitors. Blockade of the renin-angiotensin system is more complete with renin inhibitors than with ACEIs or ARBs. Aliskiren is the first of a class of oral, nonpeptide competitive inhibitors of the enzymatic activity of renin. Monotherapy with aliskiren seems to be as effective as an ACEI or ARB for lowering blood pressure, but not more effective. Further blood reductions may be achieved when aliskiren is used in combination with a thiazide diuretic, an ACEI, an ARB, or calcium antagonists. Currently, aliskiren is not considered a first-line antihypertensive agent.

Aldosterone Antagonists Spironolactone is a nonselective aldosterone antagonist that may be used alone or in combination with a thiazide diuretic. It may be a particularly effective agent in patients with low-renin essential hypertension, resistant hypertension, and primary aldosteronism. In patients with CHF, low-dose spironolactone reduces mortality and hospitalizations for heart failure when given in addition to conventional therapy with ACEIs, digoxin, and loop diuretics. Because spironolactone binds to progesterone and androgen receptors, side effects may include gynecomastia, impotence, and menstrual abnormalities. These side effects are circumvented by a newer agent, eplerenone, which is a selective aldosterone antagonist. Eplerenone has recently been approved in the United States for the treatment of hypertension.

Beta Blockers β-Adrenergic receptor blockers lower blood pressure by decreasing cardiac output, due to a reduction of heart rate and contractility. Other proposed mechanisms by which beta blockers lower blood pressure include a central nervous system effect and inhibition of renin release. Beta blockers are particularly effective in hypertensive patients with tachycardia, and their hypotensive potency is enhanced by coadministration with a diuretic. In lower doses, some beta blockers selectively inhibit cardiac β_1 receptors and have less influence on β_2 receptors on bronchial and vascular smooth muscle cells; however, there seems to be no difference in the antihypertensive potencies of cardioselective and nonselective beta blockers. Certain beta blockers have intrinsic sympathomimetic activity, and it is uncertain whether this constitutes an overall advantage or disadvantage in cardiac therapy. Beta blockers without intrinsic sympathomimetic activity decrease the rate of sudden death, overall mortality, and recurrent myocardial infarction. In patients with CHF, beta blockers have been shown to reduce the risks of hospitalization and mortality. Carvedilol and labetalol block both β receptors and peripheral α-adrenergic receptors. The potential advantages of combined β- and α-adrenergic blockade in treating hypertension remain to be determined.

α-Adrenergic Blockers Postsynaptic, selective α-adrenoreceptor antagonists lower blood pressure by decreasing peripheral vascular resistance. They are effective antihypertensive agents used either as monotherapy or in combination with other agents. However, in clinical trials of hypertensive patients, alpha blockade has not been shown to reduce cardiovascular morbidity and mortality or to provide as much protection against CHF as other classes of antihypertensive agents. These agents are also effective in treating lower urinary tract symptoms in men with prostatic hypertrophy. Nonselective α-adrenoreceptor antagonists bind to postsynaptic and presynaptic receptors and are used primarily for the management of patients with pheochromocytoma.

Sympatholytic Agents Centrally acting α_2 sympathetic agonists decrease peripheral resistance by inhibiting sympathetic outflow. They may be particularly useful in patients with autonomic neuropathy who have wide variations in blood pressure due to baroreceptor denervation. Drawbacks include somnolence, dry mouth, and rebound hypertension on withdrawal. Peripheral sympatholytics decrease peripheral resistance and venous constriction by depleting nerve terminal norepinephrine. Although they are potentially effective antihypertensive agents, their usefulness is limited by orthostatic hypotension, sexual dysfunction, and numerous drug-drug interactions.

Calcium Channel Blockers Calcium antagonists reduce vascular resistance through L-channel blockade, which reduces intracellular calcium and blunts vasoconstriction. This is a heterogeneous group of agents that includes drugs in the following three classes: phenylalkylamines (verapamil), benzothiazepines (diltiazem), and 1,4-dihydropyridines (nifedipine-like). Used alone and in combination with other agents (ACEIs, beta blockers, α_1-adrenergic blockers), calcium antagonists effectively lower blood pressure; however, it is unclear if adding a diuretic to a calcium blocker results in a further lowering of blood pressure. Side effects of flushing, headache, and edema with dihydropyridine use are related to their potencies as arteriolar dilators; edema is due to an increase in transcapillary pressure gradients, not to net salt and water retention.

Direct Vasodilators Direct vasodilators decrease peripheral resistance and concomitantly activate mechanisms that defend arterial pressure, notably the sympathetic nervous system, the renin-angiotensin-aldosterone system, and sodium retention. Usually, they are not considered first-line agents but are most effective when added to a combination that includes a diuretic and a beta blocker. Hydralazine is a potent direct vasodilator that has antioxidant and nitric oxide–enhancing actions, and minoxidil is a particularly potent agent and is used most frequently in patients with renal insufficiency who are refractory to all other drugs. Hydralazine may induce a lupus-like syndrome, and side effects of minoxidil include hypertrichosis and pericardial effusion.

COMPARISONS OF ANTIHYPERTENSIVES Based on pooling results from clinical trials, meta-analyses of the efficacy of different classes of antihypertensive agents suggest essentially equivalent blood pressure–lowering effects of the following six major classes of antihypertensive agents when used as monotherapy: thiazide diuretics, beta blockers, ACEIs, ARBs, calcium antagonists, and α_2 blockers. On average, standard doses of most antihypertensive agents reduce blood pressure by 8–10/4–7 mmHg; however, there may be subgroup differences in responsiveness. Younger patients may be more responsive to beta blockers and ACEIs, whereas patients over age 50 may be more responsive to diuretics and calcium antagonists. There is a limited relationship between plasma renin and blood pressure response. Patients with high-renin hypertension may be more responsive to ACEIs and ARBs than to other classes of agents, whereas patients with low-renin hypertension are more responsive to diuretics and calcium antagonists. Hypertensive African Americans tend to have low renin and may require higher doses of ACEIs and ARBs than whites for optimal blood pressure control, although this difference is abolished when these agents are combined with a diuretic. Beta blockers also appear to be less effective than thiazide diuretics in African Americans than in non-African Americans. Identification of genetic variants that influence blood pressure responsiveness would potentially provide a rational basis for the selection of a specific class of an antihypertensive agent in an individual patient. Early pharmacogenetic studies, utilizing either a candidate gene approach or genome-wide scans, have shown associations of gene polymorphisms with blood pressure responsiveness to specific antihypertensive drugs. However, the reported effects have generally been too small to affect clinical decisions, and associated polymorphisms remain to be confirmed in subsequent studies. Currently, in practical terms, the presence of comorbidities often influences the selection of antihypertensive agents.

A recent meta-analysis of more than 30 randomized trials of blood pressure–lowering therapy indicates that for a given reduction in blood pressure, the major drug classes seem to produce similar overall net effects on total cardiovascular events. In both nondiabetic and diabetic hypertensive patients, most trials have failed to show significant differences in cardiovascular outcomes with different drug regimens as long as equivalent decreases in blood pressure were achieved. For example, the Antihypertensive and Lipid-Lowering Treatment to prevent Heart Attack Trial (ALLHAT) demonstrated that the occurrence of coronary heart disease death and nonfatal myocardial infarction, as well as overall mortality, was virtually identical in hypertensive patients treated with either an ACEI (lisinopril), a diuretic (chlorthalidone), or a calcium antagonist (amlodipine).

However, in specific patient groups, ACEIs may have particular advantages, beyond that of blood pressure control, in reducing cardiovascular and renal outcomes. ACEIs and ARBs decrease intraglomerular pressure and proteinuria and may retard the rate of progression of renal insufficiency, not totally accounted for by their hypotensive effects, in both diabetic and nondiabetic renal diseases. Among African Americans with hypertension-related renal disease, ACEIs appear to be more effective than beta blockers or dihydropyridine calcium channel blockers in slowing, although not preventing, the decline of glomerular filtration rate. In experimental models of hypertension and diabetes, renal protection with aliskiren (a renin inhibitor) was comparable to that with ACEIs and ARBs. Independent of its blood pressure–lowering effect, aliskiren has renal protective effects in patients with hypertension, type 2 diabetes, and nephropathy. The renoprotective effect of these renin-angiotensin blockers, compared with other antihypertensive drugs, is less obvious at lower blood pressures. In most patients with hypertension and heart failure due to systolic and/or diastolic dysfunction, the use of diuretics, ACEIs or ARBs, and beta blockers is recommended to improve survival. Independent of blood pressure, in both hypertensive and normotensive individuals, ACEIs attenuate the development of left ventricular hypertrophy, improve symptomatology and risk of death from CHF, and reduce morbidity and mortality rates in post-myocardial infarction patients. Similar benefits in cardiovascular morbidity and mortality rates in patients with CHF have been observed with the use of ARBs. ACEIs provide better coronary protection than do calcium channel blockers, whereas calcium channel blockers provide more stroke protection than do either ACEIs or beta blockers. Results of a recent large, double-blind prospective clinical trial [Rationale and Design of the Avoiding Cardiovascular Events through Combination Therapy in Patients Living with Systolic Hypertension (ACCOMPLISH Trial)] indicated that combination treatment with an ACEI (benazepril) plus a calcium antagonist (amlodipine) was superior to treatment with the ACEI plus a diuretic (hydrochlorothiazide) in reducing the risk of cardiovascular events and death among high-risk patients with hypertension. However, the combination of an ACEI and a diuretic has recently been shown to produce major reductions in morbidity and mortality in the very elderly.

After a stroke, combination therapy with an ACEI and a diuretic, but not with an ARB, reduces the rate of recurrent stroke. Some of these apparent differences may reflect differences in trial design and/or patient groups.

BLOOD PRESSURE GOALS OF ANTIHYPERTENSIVE THERAPY Based on clinical trial data, the maximum protection against combined cardiovascular endpoints is achieved with pressures <135–140 mmHg for systolic blood pressure and <80–85 mmHg for diastolic blood pressure; however, treatment has not reduced cardiovascular disease risk to the level in nonhypertensive individuals. More aggressive blood pressure targets for blood pressure control (e.g., office or clinic blood pressure < 130/80 mmHg) are generally recommended for patients with diabetes, coronary heart disease, chronic kidney disease, or additional cardiovascular disease risk factors. An even lower goal blood pressure (systolic blood pressure ~120 mmHg) may be desirable for patients with proteinuria (>1 g/d) since the decline of glomerular filtration rate in these patients is particularly blood pressure–dependent. In diabetic patients, effective blood pressure control reduces the risk of cardiovascular events and death as well as the risk for microvascular disease (nephropathy, retinopathy). Risk reduction is greater in diabetic than in nondiabetic individuals. Although the optimal target blood pressure in patients with heart failure has not been established, a reasonable goal is the lowest blood pressure that is not associated with evidence of hypoperfusion.

To achieve recommended blood pressure goals, the majority of individuals with hypertension will require treatment with more than one drug. Three or more drugs frequently are needed in patients with diabetes and renal insufficiency. For most agents, reduction of blood pressure at half-standard doses is only ~20% less than at standard doses. Appropriate combinations of agents at these lower doses may have additive or almost additive effects on blood pressure with a lower incidence of side effects.

Despite theoretical concerns about decreasing cerebral, coronary, and renal blood flow by overly aggressive antihypertensive therapy, clinical trials have found no evidence for a "J-curve" phenomenon; i.e., at blood pressure reductions achieved in clinical practice, there does *not* appear to be a lower threshold for increasing cardiovascular risk. A small nonprogressive increase in the serum creatinine concentration with blood pressure reduction may occur in patients with chronic renal insufficiency. This generally reflects a hemodynamic response, not structural renal injury, indicating that intraglomerular pressure has been reduced. Blood pressure control should not be allowed to deteriorate in order to prevent a modest rise in creatinine. Even among older patients with isolated systolic hypertension, further lowering of diastolic blood pressure does not result in harm. However, relatively little information is available concerning the risk-versus-benefit ratio of antihypertensive therapy in individuals >80 years, and in this population, gradual blood pressure reduction to less aggressive target levels of control may be appropriate.

The term *resistant hypertension* refers to patients with blood pressures persistently >140/90 mmHg despite taking three or more antihypertensive agents, including a diuretic, in a reasonable combination and at full doses. Resistant or difficult-to-control hypertension is more common in patients >60 years than in younger patients. Resistant hypertension may be related to "pseudoresistance" (high office blood pressures and lower home blood pressures), nonadherence to therapy, identifiable causes of hypertension (including obesity and excessive alcohol intake), and the use of any of a number of nonprescription and prescription drugs (Table 247-3). Rarely, in older patients, pseudohypertension may be related to the inability to measure blood pressure accurately in severely sclerotic arteries. This condition is suggested if the radial pulse remains palpable despite occlusion of the brachial artery by the cuff (Osler maneuver). The actual blood pressure can be determined by direct intra-arterial measurement. Evaluation of patients with resistant hypertension might include home blood pressure monitoring to determine if office blood pressures are representative of the usual blood pressure. A more extensive evaluation for a secondary form of hypertension should be undertaken if no other explanation for hypertension resistance becomes apparent.

HYPERTENSIVE EMERGENCIES Probably due to the widespread availability of antihypertensive therapy, in the United States there has been a decline in the numbers of patients presenting with "crisis levels" of blood pressure. Most patients who present with severe hypertension are chronically hypertensive, and in the absence of acute end organ damage, precipitous lowering of blood pressure may be associated with significant morbidity and should be avoided. The key to successful management of severe hypertension is to differentiate hypertensive crises from hypertensive urgencies. The degree of target organ damage, rather than the level of blood pressure alone, determines the rapidity with which blood pressure should be lowered. Tables 247-9 and 247-10 list a number of hypertension-related emergencies and recommended therapies.

Malignant hypertension is a syndrome associated with an abrupt increase of blood pressure in a patient with underlying hypertension or related to the sudden onset of hypertension in a previously normotensive individual. The absolute level of blood pressure is not as important as its rate of rise. Pathologically, the syndrome is associated with diffuse necrotizing vasculitis, arteriolar thrombi, and fibrin deposition in arteriolar walls. Fibrinoid necrosis has been observed in arterioles of kidney, brain, retina, and other organs. Clinically, the syndrome is recognized by progressive retinopathy (arteriolar spasm, hemorrhages, exudates, and papilledema), deteriorating renal function with proteinuria, microangiopathic hemolytic anemia, and encephalopathy. In these patients, historic inquiry should include questions about the use of monamine oxidase inhibitors and recreational drugs (e.g., cocaine, amphetamines).

TABLE 247-9 Preferred Parenteral Drugs for Selected Hypertensive Emergencies

Hypertensive encephalopathy	Nitroprusside, nicardipine, labetalol
Malignant hypertension (when IV therapy is indicated)	Labetalol, nicardipine, nitroprusside, enalaprilat
Stroke	Nicardipine, labetalol, nitroprusside
Myocardial infarction/unstable angina	Nitroglycerin, nicardipine, labetalol, esmolol
Acute left ventricular failure	Nitroglycerin, enalaprilat, loop diuretics
Aortic dissection	Nitroprusside, esmolol, labetalol
Adrenergic crisis	Phentolamine, nitroprusside
Postoperative hypertension	Nitroglycerin, nitroprusside, labetalol, nicardipine
Preeclampsia/eclampsia of pregnancy	Hydralazine, labetalol, nicardipine

Source: Adapted from DG Vidt, in S Oparil, MA Weber (eds): *Hypertension*, 2nd ed. Philadelphia, Elsevier Saunders, 2005.

TABLE 247-10 Usual Intravenous Doses of Antihypertensive Agents Used in Hypertensive Emergencies*

Antihypertensive Agent	Intravenous Dose
Nitroprusside	Initial 0.3 (μg/kg)/min; usual 2–4 (μg/kg)/min; maximum 10 (μg/kg)/min for 10 min
Nicardipine	Initial 5 mg/h; titrate by 2.5 mg/h at 5–15 min intervals; max 15 mg/h
Labetalol	2 mg/min up to 300 mg *or* 20 mg over 2 min, then 40–80 mg at 10-min intervals up to 300 mg total
Enalaprilat	Usual 0.625–1.25 mg over 5 min every 6–8 h; maximum 5 mg/dose
Esmolol	Initial 80–500 μg/kg over 1 min, then 50–300 (μg/kg)/min
Phentolamine	5–15 mg bolus
Nitroglycerin	Initial 5 μg/min, then titrate by 5 μg/min at 3–5-min intervals; if no response is seen at 20 μg/min, incremental increases of 10–20 μg/min may be used
Hydralazine	10–50 mg at 30-min intervals

*Constant blood pressure monitoring is required. Start with the lowest dose. Subsequent doses and intervals of administration should be adjusted according to the blood pressure response and duration of action of the specific agent.

Although blood pressure should be lowered rapidly in patients with hypertensive encephalopathy, there are inherent risks of overly aggressive therapy. In hypertensive individuals, the upper and lower limits of autoregulation of cerebral blood flow are shifted to higher levels of arterial pressure, and rapid lowering of blood pressure to below the lower limit of autoregulation may precipitate cerebral ischemia or infarction as a consequence of decreased cerebral blood flow. Renal and coronary blood flows also may decrease with overly aggressive acute therapy. The initial goal of therapy is to reduce mean arterial blood pressure by no more than 25% within minutes to 2 h or to a blood pressure in the range of 160/100–110 mmHg. This may be accomplished with IV nitroprusside, a short-acting vasodilator with a rapid onset of action that allows for minute-to-minute control of blood pressure. Parenteral labetalol and nicardipine are also effective agents for the treatment of hypertensive encephalopathy.

In patients with malignant hypertension without encephalopathy or another catastrophic event, it is preferable to reduce blood pressure over hours or longer rather than minutes. This goal may effectively be achieved initially with frequent dosing of short-acting oral agents such as captopril, clonidine, and labetalol.

Acute, transient blood pressure elevations that last days to weeks frequently occur after thrombotic and hemorrhagic strokes. Autoregulation of cerebral blood flow is impaired in ischemic cerebral tissue, and higher arterial pressures may be required to maintain cerebral blood flow. Although specific blood pressure targets have not been defined for patients with acute cerebrovascular events, aggressive reductions of blood pressure are to be avoided. With the increasing availability of improved methods for measuring cerebral blood flow (using CT technology), studies are in progress to evaluate the effects of different classes of antihypertensive agents on both blood pressure and cerebral blood flow after an acute stroke. Currently, in the absence of other indications for acute therapy, for patients with cerebral infarction who are not candidates for thrombolytic therapy, one recommended guideline is to institute antihypertensive therapy only for patients with a systolic blood pressure >220 mmHg or a diastolic blood pressure >130 mmHg. If thrombolytic therapy is to be used, the recommended goal blood pressure is <185 mmHg systolic pressure and <110 mmHg diastolic pressure. In patients with hemorrhagic stroke, suggested guidelines for initiating antihypertensive therapy are systolic >180 mmHg or diastolic pressure >130 mmHg. The management of hypertension after subarachnoid hemorrhage is controversial. Cautious reduction of blood pressure is indicated if mean arterial pressure is >130 mmHg.

In addition to pheochromocytoma, an adrenergic crisis due to catecholamine excess may be related to cocaine or amphetamine overdose, clonidine withdrawal, acute spinal cord injuries, and an interaction of tyramine-containing compounds with monamine oxidase inhibitors. These patients may be treated with phentolamine or nitroprusside.

Treatment of hypertension in patients with acute aortic dissection is discussed in Chap. 248, and treatment of hypertension in pregnancy is discussed in Chap. 7.

FURTHER READINGS

ACCORD STUDY GROUP: Effects of intensive blood pressure control in type 2 diabetes mellitus. N Engl J Med 362:1575, 2010

ADROGUE JH, MADIAS NE: Sodium and potassium in the pathogenesis of hypertension. N Engl J Med 356:1966, 2007

ALLHAT COLLABORATIVE RESEARCH GROUP: Major outcomes in high-risk hypertensive patients randomized to angiotensin converting enzyme inhibitor or calcium channel blocker vs. diuretic: The Antihypertensive and Lipid-Lowering Treatment to Prevent Heart Attack Trial (ALLHAT). JAMA 288:2981, 2002

APPEL LJ et al: Dietary approaches to prevent and treat hypertension: A scientific statement from the American Heart Association. Hypertension 47:296, 2006

BLOOD PRESSURE LOWERING TREATMENT TRIALISTS' COLLABORATION: Effects of different blood pressure-lowering regimens on major cardiovascular events in individuals with and without diabetes mellitus. Arch Intern Med 165:1410, 2005

CASAS JP et al: Effect of inhibitors of the renin-angiotensin system and other antihypertensive drugs on renal outcomes: Systematic review and meta-analysis. Lancet 366:2026, 2005

CHOBANIAN AV et al: The Seventh Report of the Joint National Committee on Prevention, Detection, Evaluation, and Treatment of High Blood Pressure: The JNC 7 Report. JAMA 289:2560, 2003

LAW MR et al: Value of low dose combination treatment with blood pressure lowering drugs: Analysis of 354 randomised trials. Br Med J 326:1427, 2003

LAWES CMM et al: Global burden of blood pressure-related disease, 2001. Lancet 371:1513, 2008

MANCIA G: Role of outcome trials in providing information on antihypertensive treatment: Importance and limitations. Am J Hypertens 19:1, 2006

MOSER M, SETANO JF: Resistant or difficult-to-control hypertension. N Engl J Med 355:385, 2006

ONG KL et al; Prevalence, awareness, treatment, and control of hypertension among United States adults 1999–2004. Hypertension 49:69, 2007

PICKERING TG et al: Recommendations for blood pressure measurement in humans and experimental animals. Part 1: Blood pressure measurement in humans. A statement for professionals from the Subcommittee of Professional and Public Education of the American Heart Association Council on High Blood Pressure Research. Hypertension 45:142, 2005

———: Ambulatory blood-pressure monitoring. N Engl J Med 3554:2368, 2006

TEXTOR SC: Current approaches to renovascular hypertension. Med Clin North Am 93:717, 2009

WEBER MA, MATERSON BJ: Hypertension guidelines: A major reappraisal critically examines the available evidence. J Clin Hypertens (Greenwich) 12:229, 2010

CHAPTER 248
Diseases of the Aorta

Mark A. Creager
Joseph Loscalzo

The aorta is the conduit through which blood ejected from the left ventricle is delivered to the systemic arterial bed. In adults, its diameter is approximately 3 cm at the origin and in the ascending portion, 2.5 cm in the descending portion in the thorax, and 1.8–2 cm in the abdomen. The aortic wall consists of a thin intima composed of endothelium, subendothelial connective tissue, and an internal elastic lamina; a thick tunica media composed of smooth muscle cells and extracellular matrix; and an adventitia composed primarily of connective tissue enclosing the vasa vasorum and nervi vascularis. In addition to the conduit function of the aorta, its viscoelastic and compliant properties serve a buffering function. The aorta is distended during systole to allow a portion of the stroke volume and elastic energy to be stored, and it recoils during diastole so that blood continues to flow to the periphery. Because of its continuous exposure to high pulsatile pressure and shear stress, the aorta is particularly prone to injury and disease resulting from mechanical trauma. The aorta is also more prone to rupture than is any other vessel, especially with the development of aneurysmal dilation, since its wall tension, as governed by Laplace's law (i.e., proportional to the product of pressure and radius), will be increased.

CONGENITAL ANOMALIES OF THE AORTA

Congenital anomalies of the aorta usually involve the aortic arch and its branches. Symptoms such as dysphagia, stridor, and cough may occur if an anomaly causes a ring around or otherwise compresses the esophagus or trachea. Anomalies associated with symptoms include double aortic arch, origin of the right subclavian artery distal to the left subclavian artery, and right-sided aortic arch with an aberrant left subclavian artery. A Kommerell's diverticulum is an anatomic remnant of a right aortic arch. Most congenital anomalies of the aorta do not cause symptoms and are detected during catheter-based procedures. The diagnosis of suspected congenital anomalies of the aorta typically is confirmed by computed tomographic (CT) or magnetic resonance (MR) angiography. Surgery is used to treat symptomatic anomalies.

AORTIC ANEURYSM

An *aneurysm* is defined as a pathologic dilation of a segment of a blood vessel. A *true aneurysm* involves all three layers of the vessel wall and is distinguished from a *pseudoaneurysm*, in which the intimal and medial layers are disrupted and the dilated segment of the aorta is lined by adventitia only and, at times, by perivascular clot. Aneurysms also may be classified according to their gross appearance. A *fusiform aneurysm* affects the entire circumference of a segment of the vessel, resulting in a diffusely dilated artery. In contrast, a *saccular aneurysm* involves only a portion of the circumference, resulting in an outpouching of the vessel wall. Aortic aneurysms also are classified according to location, i.e., abdominal versus thoracic. Aneurysms of the descending thoracic aorta are usually contiguous with infradiaphragmatic aneurysms and are referred to as *thoracoabdominal aortic aneurysms.*

ETIOLOGY

Aortic aneurysms result from conditions that cause degradation or abnormal production of the structural components of the aortic wall: elastin and collagen. The causes of aortic aneurysms may be broadly categorized as degenerative diseases, inherited or developmental diseases, infections, vasculitis, and trauma (Table 248-1). Inflammation, proteolysis, and biomechanical wall stress contribute to the degenerative processes that characterize most aneurysms of the abdominal and descending thoracic aorta. These are mediated by B cell and T cell lymphocytes, macrophages, inflammatory cytokines, and matrix metalloproteinases that degrade elastin and

TABLE 248-1 Diseases of the Aorta: Etiology and Associated Factors

Aortic aneurysm
Degenerative/atherosclerosis
Aging
Cigarette smoking
Male gender
Family history
Cystic medial necrosis
Marfan syndrome
Loeys-Dietz syndrome
Ehlers-Danlos syndrome type IV
Familial
Bicuspid aortic valve
Chronic aortic dissection
Infective (see below)
Trauma
Acute aortic syndromes (aortic dissection, acute intramural hematoma, penetrating atherosclerotic ulcer)
Atherosclerosis
Cystic medial necrosis (see above)
Hypertension
Vasculitis (see below)
Pregnancy
Trauma
Aortic occlusion
Atherosclerosis
Thromboembolism
Aortitis
Vasculitis
Takayasu's arteritis
Giant cell arteritis
Rheumatic
HLA-B27–associated spondyloarthropathies
Behçet's syndrome
Cogan's syndrome
Idiopathic aortitis
Infective
Syphilis
Tuberculosis
Mycotic (*Salmonella*, staphylococcal, streptococcal, fungal)

collagen and alter the tensile strength and ability of the aorta to accommodate pulsatile stretch. The associated histopathology demonstrates destruction of elastin and collagen, decreased vascular smooth muscle, in-growth of new blood vessels, and inflammation. Factors associated with degenerative aortic aneurysms include aging, cigarette smoking, hypercholesterolemia, male sex, and a family history of aortic aneurysms.

The most common pathologic condition associated with degenerative aortic aneurysms is *atherosclerosis.* Many patients with aortic aneurysms have coexisting risk factors for atherosclerosis (Chap. 241), as well as atherosclerosis in other blood vessels.

Cystic medial necrosis is the histopathologic term used to describe the degeneration of collagen and elastic fibers in the tunica media of the aorta as well as the loss of medial cells that are replaced by multiple clefts of mucoid material. Cystic medial necrosis characteristically affects the proximal aorta, results in circumferential weakness and dilation, and leads to the development of fusiform aneurysms involving the ascending aorta and the sinuses of Valsalva. This condition is particularly prevalent in patients with Marfan syndrome, Loeys-Dietz syndrome, Ehlers-Danlos syndrome type IV (Chap. 363), hypertension, congenital bicuspid aortic valves, and familial thoracic aortic aneurysm syndromes; sometimes it appears as an isolated condition in patients without any other apparent disease.

Familial clusterings of aortic aneurysms occur in 20% of patients, suggesting a hereditary basis for the disease. Mutations of the gene that encodes fibrillin-1 are present in patients with Marfan syndrome. Fibrillin-1 is an important component of extracellular micofibrils, which support the architecture of elastic fibers and other connective tissue. Deficiency of fibrillin-1 in the extracellular matrix leads to excessive signaling by transforming growth factor β (TGF-β). Loeys-Dietz syndrome is caused by mutations in the genes that encode TGF-β receptors 1 (*TGFBR1*) and 2 (*TGFBR2*). Increased signaling by TGF-β and mutations of *TGFBR1* and *TGFBR2* may cause thoracic aortic aneurysms. Mutations of type III procollagen have been implicated in Ehlers-Danlos type IV syndrome. Linkage analysis has identified loci on chromosomes 5q13–14, 11q23.3–q24, and 3p24–25 in several families, although the specific alleles have not been described.

The infectious causes of aortic aneurysms include syphilis, tuberculosis, and other bacterial infections. *Syphilis* (Chap. 169) is a relatively uncommon cause of aortic aneurysm. Syphilitic periaortitis and mesoaortitis damage elastic fibers, resulting in thickening and weakening of the aortic wall. Approximately 90% of syphilitic aneurysms are located in the ascending aorta or aortic arch. *Tuberculous aneurysms* (Chap. 165) typically affect the thoracic aorta and result from direct extension of infection from hilar lymph nodes or contiguous abscesses as well as from bacterial seeding. Loss of aortic wall elasticity results from granulomatous destruction of the medial layer. A *mycotic aneurysm* is a rare condition that develops as a result of staphylococcal, streptococcal, *Salmonella*, or other bacterial or fungal infections of the aorta, usually at an atherosclerotic plaque. These aneurysms are usually saccular. Blood cultures are often positive and reveal the nature of the infective agent.

Vasculitides associated with aortic aneurysm include Takayasu's arteritis and giant cell arteritis, which may cause aneurysms of the aortic arch and descending thoracic aorta. Spondyloarthropathies such as ankylosing spondylitis, rheumatoid arthritis, psoriatic arthritis, relapsing polychondritis, and reactive arthritis (formerly known as Reiter's syndrome) are associated with dilation of the ascending aorta. Aortic aneurysms occur in patients with Behçet's syndrome (Chap. 327) and Cogan's syndrome. Aortic aneurysms also result from idiopathic aortitis. *Traumatic aneurysms* may occur after penetrating or nonpenetrating chest trauma and most commonly affect the descending thoracic aorta just beyond the site of insertion of the ligamentum arteriosum. Chronic aortic dissections are associated with weakening of the aortic wall that may lead to the development of aneurysmal dilatation.

THORACIC AORTIC ANEURYSMS

The clinical manifestations and natural history of thoracic aortic aneurysms depend on their location. Cystic medial necrosis is the most common pathology associated with ascending aortic aneurysms, whereas atherosclerosis is the condition most frequently associated with aneurysms of the aortic arch and descending thoracic aorta. The average growth rate of thoracic aneurysms is 0.1–0.2 cm per year. Thoracic aortic aneurysms associated with Marfan syndrome or aortic dissection may expand at a greater rate. The risk of rupture is related to the size of the aneurysm and the presence of symptoms, ranging approximately from 2–3% per year for thoracic aortic aneurysms <4.0 cm in diameter to 7% per year for those >6 cm in diameter. Most thoracic aortic aneurysms are asymptomatic; however, compression or erosion of adjacent tissue by aneurysms may cause symptoms such as chest pain, shortness of breath, cough, hoarseness, and dysphagia. Aneurysmal dilation of the ascending aorta may cause congestive heart failure as a consequence of aortic regurgitation, and compression of the superior vena cava may produce congestion of the head, neck, and upper extremities.

A chest x-ray may be the first test that suggests the diagnosis of a thoracic aortic aneurysm (Fig. 248-1). Findings include widening of the mediastinal shadow and displacement or compression of the trachea or left mainstem bronchus. Echocardiography, particularly transesophageal echocardiography, can be used to assess the proximal ascending aorta and descending thoracic aorta. Contrast-enhanced CT, magnetic resonance imaging (MRI), and conventional invasive aortography are sensitive and specific tests for assessment of aneurysms of the thoracic aorta and involvement of branch vessels (Fig. 248-2). In asymptomatic patients whose aneurysms are too small to justify surgery, noninvasive testing with either contrast-enhanced CT or MRI should be performed at least every 6–12 months to monitor expansion.

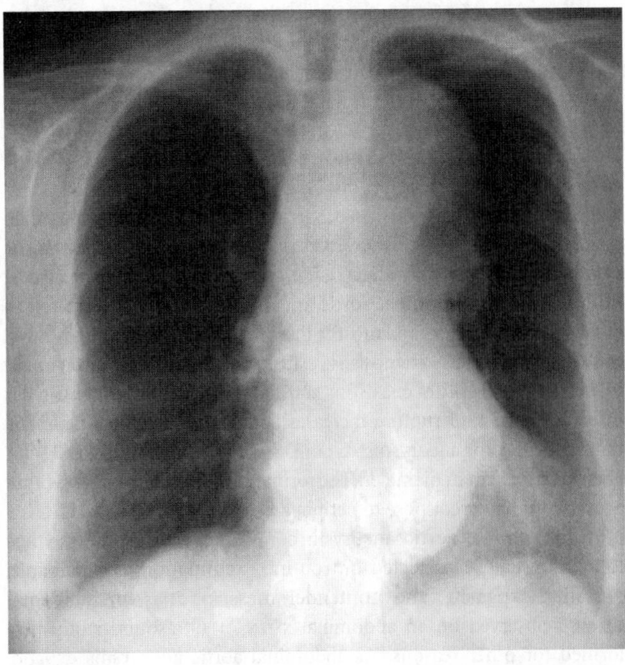

Figure 248-1 A chest x-ray of a patient with a thoracic aortic aneurysm.

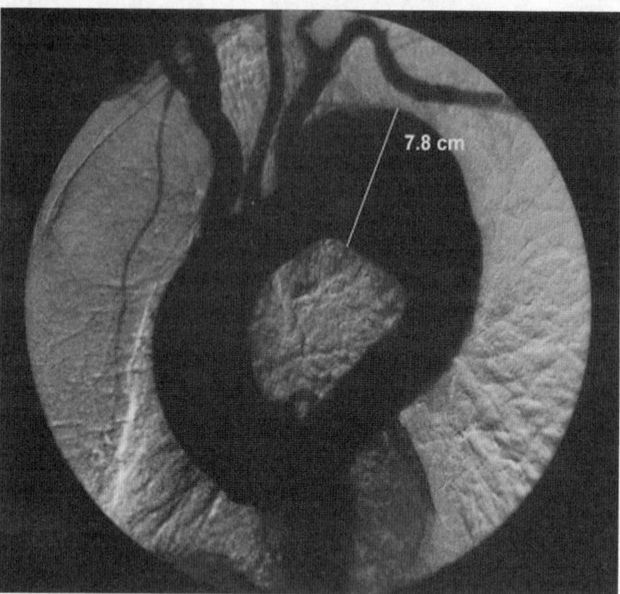

Figure 248-2 An aortogram demonstrating a large fusiform aneurysm of the descending thoracic aorta.

TREATMENT Thoracic Aortic Aneurysms

β-Adrenergic blockers currently are recommended for patients with thoracic aortic aneurysms, particularly those with Marfan syndrome, who have evidence of aortic root dilatation to reduce the rate of further expansion. Additional medical therapy should be given as necessary to control hypertension. Recent preliminary studies indicate that angiotensin receptor antagonists and angiotensin-converting enzyme inhibitors will reduce the rate of aortic dilation in patients with Marfan syndrome by blocking TGF-β signaling; clinical outcome trials of this treatment approach are in progress. Operative repair with placement of a prosthetic graft is indicated in patients with symptomatic thoracic aortic aneurysms, those in whom the ascending aortic diameter is >5.5–6 cm or the descending thoracic aortic diameter is >6.5–7 cm, and those with an aneurysm that has increased by >1 cm per year. In patients with Marfan syndrome or bicuspid aortic valve, ascending thoracic aortic aneurysms >5 cm should be considered for surgery. Endovascular repair is an alternative treatment for some patients with descending thoracic aortic aneurysms.

ABDOMINAL AORTIC ANEURYSMS

Abdominal aortic aneurysms occur more frequently in males than in females, and the incidence increases with age. Abdominal aortic aneurysms ≥4.0 cm may affect 1–2% of men older than 50 years. At least 90% of all abdominal aortic aneurysms >4.0 cm are related to atherosclerotic disease, and most of these aneurysms are below the level of the renal arteries. Prognosis is related to both the size of the aneurysm and the severity of coexisting coronary artery and cerebrovascular disease. The risk of rupture increases with the size of the aneurysm: the 5-year risk for aneurysms <5 cm is 1–2%, whereas it is 20–40% for aneurysms >5 cm in diameter. The formation of mural thrombi within aneurysms may predispose to peripheral embolization.

An abdominal aortic aneurysm commonly produces no symptoms. It usually is detected on routine examination as a palpable, pulsatile, expansile, and nontender mass, or it is an incidental finding observed on an abdominal x-ray or ultrasound study performed for other reasons. As abdominal aortic aneurysms expand, however, they may become painful. Some patients complain of strong pulsations in the abdomen; others experience pain in the chest, lower back, or scrotum. Aneurysmal pain is usually a harbinger of rupture and represents a medical emergency. More often, acute rupture occurs without any prior warning, and this complication is always life-threatening. Rarely, there is leakage of the aneurysm with severe pain and tenderness. Acute pain and hypotension occur with rupture of the aneurysm, which requires an emergency operation.

Abdominal radiography may demonstrate the calcified outline of the aneurysm; however, about 25% of aneurysms are not calcified and cannot be visualized by x-ray imaging. An abdominal ultrasound can delineate the transverse and longitudinal dimensions of an abdominal aortic aneurysm and may detect mural thrombus. Abdominal ultrasound is useful for serial documentation of aneurysm size and can be used to screen patients at risk for developing an aortic aneurysm. In one large study, ultrasound screening of men age 65–74 years was associated with a risk reduction in aneurysm-related death of 42%. For this reason, screening by ultrasonography is recommended for men age 65–75 years who have ever smoked. In addition, siblings or offspring of persons with abdominal aortic aneurysms, as well as individuals with thoracic aortic or peripheral arterial aneurysms, should be considered for screening for abdominal aortic aneurysms. CT with contrast and MRI are accurate noninvasive tests to determine the location and size of abdominal aortic aneurysms and to plan endovascular or open surgical repair (Fig. 248-3). Contrast aortography may be used for the evaluation of patients with aneurysms, but the procedure carries a small risk of complications such as bleeding, allergic reactions, and atheroembolism. Since the presence of mural thrombi may reduce the luminal size, aortography may underestimate the diameter of an aneurysm.

TREATMENT Abdominal Aortic Aneurysms

Operative repair of the aneurysm with insertion of a prosthetic graft or endovascular placement of an aortic stent graft (Fig. 248-3) is indicated for abdominal aortic aneurysms of any size that are

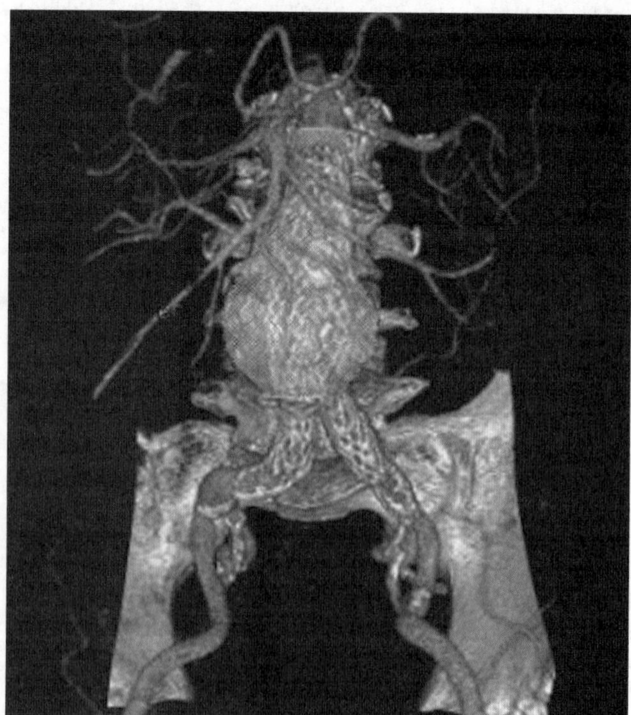

Figure 248-3 A computed tomographic angiogram (CTA) depicting a fusiform abdominal aortic aneurysm that has been treated with a bifurcated stent graft.

expanding rapidly or are associated with symptoms. For asymptomatic aneurysms, abdominal aortic aneurysm repair is indicated if the diameter is >5.5 cm. In randomized trials of patients with abdominal aortic aneurysms <5.5 cm, there was no difference in the long-term (5- to 8-year) mortality rate between those followed with ultrasound surveillance and those undergoing elective surgical repair. Thus, serial noninvasive follow-up of smaller aneurysms (<5 cm) is an alternative to immediate repair. The decision to perform an open surgical operation or endovascular repair is based in part on the vascular anatomy and comorbid conditions. Endovascular repair of abdominal aortic aneurysms has a lower short-term morbidity rate but a comparable long-term mortality rate with open surgical reconstruction. Long-term surveillance with CT or MR aortography is indicated after endovascular repair to detect leaks and possible aneurysm expansion.

In surgical candidates, careful preoperative cardiac and general medical evaluations (followed by appropriate therapy for complicating conditions) are essential. Preexisting coronary artery disease, congestive heart failure, pulmonary disease, diabetes mellitus, and advanced age add to the risk of surgery. β-Adrenergic blockers decrease perioperative cardiovascular morbidity and mortality. With careful preoperative cardiac evaluation and postoperative care, the operative mortality rate approximates 1–2%. After acute rupture, the mortality rate of emergent operation is 45–50%. Endovascular repair with stent placement is an emerging approach but at the current time is associated with a mortality rate of approximately 40%.

ACUTE AORTIC SYNDROMES

The four major acute aortic syndromes are aortic rupture (discussed above), aortic dissection, intramural hematoma, and penetrating atherosclerotic ulcer. Aortic dissection is caused by a circumferential or, less frequently, transverse tear of the intima. It often occurs along the right lateral wall of the ascending aorta where the hydraulic shear stress is high. Another common site is the descending thoracic aorta just below the ligamentum arteriosum. The initiating event is either a primary intimal tear with secondary dissection into the media or a medial hemorrhage that dissects into and disrupts the intima. The pulsatile aortic flow then dissects along the elastic lamellar plates of the aorta and creates a false lumen. The dissection usually propagates distally down the descending aorta and into its major branches, but it may propagate proximally. Distal propagation may be limited by atherosclerotic plaque. In some cases, a secondary distal intimal disruption occurs, resulting in the reentry of blood from the false to the true lumen.

There are at least two important pathologic and radiologic variants of aortic dissection: intramural hematoma without an intimal flap and penetrating atherosclerotic ulcer. Acute intramural hematoma is thought to result from rupture of the vasa vasorum with hemorrhage into the wall of the aorta. Most of these hematomas occur in the descending thoracic aorta. Acute intramural hematomas may progress to dissection and rupture. Penetrating atherosclerotic ulcers are caused by erosion of a plaque into the aortic media, are usually localized, and are not associated with extensive propagation. They are found primarily in the middle and distal portions of the descending thoracic aorta and are associated with extensive atherosclerotic disease. The ulcer can erode beyond the internal elastic lamina, leading to medial hematoma, and may progress to false aneurysm formation or rupture.

Several classification schemes have been developed for thoracic aortic dissections. DeBakey and colleagues initially classified aortic dissections as type I, in which an intimal tear occurs in the ascending aorta but involves the descending aorta as well;

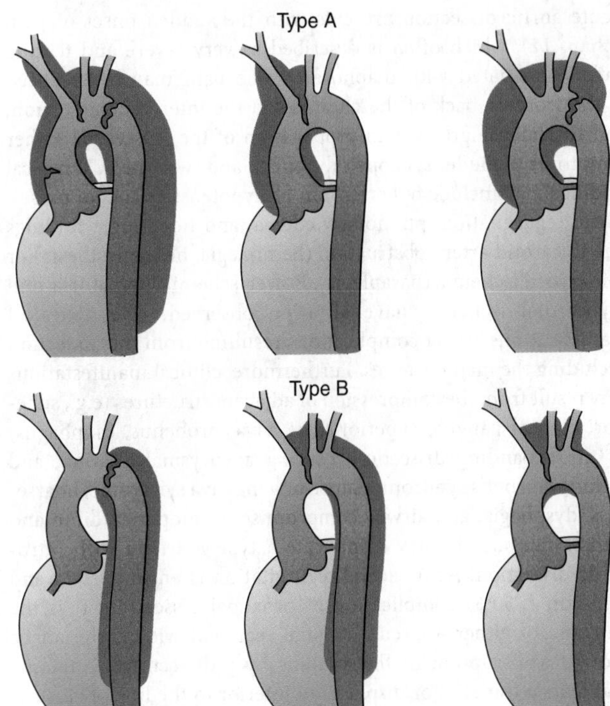

Figure 248-4 Classification of aortic dissections. Stanford classification: Type A dissections (*top panels*) involve the ascending aorta independent of site of tear and distal extension; type B dissections (*bottom panels*) involve transverse and/or descending aorta without involvement of the ascending aorta. DeBakey classification: Type I dissection involves ascending to descending aorta (*top left*); type II dissection is limited to ascending or transverse aorta, without descending aorta (*top center + top right*); type III dissection involves descending aorta only (*bottom left*). *[From DC Miller, in RM Doroghazi, EE Slater (eds): Aortic Dissection. New York, McGraw-Hill, 1983, with permission.]*

type II, in which the dissection is limited to the ascending aorta; and type III, in which the intimal tear is located in the descending aorta with distal propagation of the dissection (Fig. 248-4). Another classification (Stanford) is that of type A, in which the dissection involves the ascending aorta (proximal dissection), and type B, in which it is limited to the descending aorta (distal dissection). From a management standpoint, classification of aortic dissections and intramural hematomas into type A or B is more practical and useful, since DeBakey types I and II are managed in a similar manner.

The factors that predispose to aortic dissection include systemic hypertension, a coexisting condition in 70% of patients, and cystic medial necrosis. Aortic dissection is the major cause of morbidity and mortality in patients with Marfan syndrome (Chap. 363) and similarly may affect patients with Ehlers-Danlos syndrome. The incidence also is increased in patients with inflammatory aortitis (i.e., Takayasu's arteritis, giant cell arteritis), congenital aortic valve anomalies (e.g., bicuspid valve), coarctation of the aorta, and a history of aortic trauma. In addition, the risk of dissection is increased in otherwise normal women during the third trimester of pregnancy.

CLINICAL MANIFESTATIONS

The peak incidence of aortic dissection is in the sixth and seventh decades. Men are more affected than women by a ratio of 2:1. The presentations of aortic dissection and its variants are the consequences of intimal tear, dissecting hematoma, occlusion of involved arteries, and compression of adjacent tissues.

Acute aortic dissection presents with the sudden onset of pain (Chap. 12), which often is described as very severe and tearing and is associated with diaphoresis. The pain may be localized to the front or back of the chest, often the interscapular region, and typically migrates with propagation of the dissection. Other symptoms include syncope, dyspnea, and weakness. Physical findings may include hypertension or hypotension, loss of pulses, aortic regurgitation, pulmonary edema, and neurologic findings due to carotid artery obstruction (hemiplegia, hemianesthesia) or spinal cord ischemia (paraplegia). Bowel ischemia, hematuria, and myocardial ischemia have all been observed. These clinical manifestations reflect complications resulting from the dissection occluding the major arteries. Furthermore, clinical manifestations may result from the compression of adjacent structures (e.g., superior cervical ganglia, superior vena cava, bronchus, esophagus) by the expanding dissection, causing aneurysmal dilation, and include Horner's syndrome, superior vena cava syndrome, hoarseness, dysphagia, and airway compromise. Hemopericardium and cardiac tamponade may complicate a type A lesion with retrograde dissection. Acute aortic regurgitation is an important and common (>50%) complication of proximal dissection. It is the outcome of either a circumferential tear that widens the aortic root or a disruption of the annulus by a dissecting hematoma that tears a leaflet(s) or displaces it, inferior to the line of closure. Signs of aortic regurgitation include bounding pulses, a wide pulse pressure, a diastolic murmur often radiating along the right sternal border, and evidence of congestive heart failure. The clinical manifestations depend on the severity of the regurgitation.

In dissections involving the ascending aorta, the chest x-ray often reveals a widened superior mediastinum. A pleural effusion (usually left-sided) also may be present. This effusion is typically serosanguineous and not indicative of rupture unless accompanied by hypotension and falling hematocrit. In dissections of the descending thoracic aorta, a widened mediastinum may be observed on chest x-ray. In addition, the descending aorta may appear to be wider than the ascending portion. An electrocardiogram that shows no evidence of myocardial ischemia is helpful in distinguishing aortic dissection from myocardial infarction. Rarely, the dissection involves the right or, less commonly, left coronary ostium and causes acute myocardial infarction.

The diagnosis of aortic dissection can be established by noninvasive techniques such as echocardiography, CT, and MRI. Aortography is used less commonly because of the accuracy of these noninvasive techniques. Transthoracic echocardiography can be performed simply and rapidly and has an overall sensitivity of 60–85% for aortic dissection. For diagnosing proximal ascending aortic dissections, its sensitivity exceeds 80%; it is less useful for detecting dissection of the arch and descending thoracic aorta. Transesophageal echocardiography requires greater skill and patient cooperation but is very accurate in identifying dissections of the ascending and descending thoracic aorta but not the arch, achieving 98% sensitivity and approximately 90% specificity. Echocardiography also provides important information regarding the presence and severity of aortic regurgitation and pericardial effusion. CT and MRI are both highly accurate in identifying the intimal flap and the extent of the dissection and involvement of major arteries; each has a sensitivity and specificity >90%. They are useful in recognizing intramural hemorrhage and penetrating ulcers. MRI also can detect blood flow, which may be useful in characterizing antegrade versus retrograde dissection. The relative utility of transesophageal echocardiography, CT, and MRI depends on the availability and expertise in individual institutions as well as on the hemodynamic stability of the patient, with CT and MRI obviously less suitable for unstable patients.

TREATMENT Aortic Dissection

Medical therapy should be initiated as soon as the diagnosis is considered. The patient should be admitted to an intensive care unit for hemodynamic monitoring. Unless hypotension is present, therapy should be aimed at reducing cardiac contractility and systemic arterial pressure, and thus shear stress. For acute dissection, unless contraindicated, β-adrenergic blockers should be administered parenterally, using intravenous propranolol, metoprolol, or the short-acting esmolol to achieve a heart rate of approximately 60 beats/min. This should be accompanied by sodium nitroprusside infusion to lower systolic blood pressure to ≤120 mmHg. Labetalol (Chap. 247), a drug with both β- and α-adrenergic blocking properties, also may be used as a parenteral agent in acute therapy for dissection.

The calcium channel antagonists verapamil and diltiazem may be used intravenously if nitroprusside or β-adrenergic blockers cannot be employed. The addition of a parenteral angiotensin-converting enzyme (ACE) inhibitor such as enalaprilat to a β-adrenergic blocker also may be considered. Isolated use of a direct vasodilator such as hydralazine is contraindicated because these agents can increase hydraulic shear and may propagate the dissection.

Emergent or urgent surgical correction is the preferred treatment for acute ascending aortic dissections and intramural hematomas (type A) and for complicated type B dissections, including those characterized by propagation, compromise of major aortic branches, impending rupture, or continued pain. Surgery involves excision of the intimal flap, obliteration of the false lumen, and placement of an interposition graft. A composite valve-graft conduit is used if the aortic valve is disrupted. The overall in-hospital mortality rate after surgical treatment of patients with aortic dissection is reported to be 15–25%. The major causes of perioperative mortality and morbidity include myocardial infarction, paraplegia, renal failure, tamponade, hemorrhage, and sepsis. Endoluminal stent grafts may be considered in selected patients. Other transcatheter techniques, such as fenestration of the intimal flaps and stenting of narrowed branch vessels to increase flow to compromised organs, are used in selected patients. For uncomplicated and stable distal dissections and intramural hematomas (type B), medical therapy is the preferred treatment. The in-hospital mortality rate of medically treated patients with type B dissection is 10–20%. Long-term therapy for patients with aortic dissection and intramural hematomas (with or without surgery) consists of control of hypertension and reduction of cardiac contractility with the use of beta blockers plus other antihypertensive agents, such as ACE inhibitors or calcium antagonists. Patients with chronic type B dissection and intramural hematomas should be followed on an outpatient basis every 6–12 months with contrast-enhanced CT or MRI to detect propagation or expansion. Patients with Marfan syndrome are at high risk for postdissection complications. The long-term prognosis for patients with treated dissections is generally good with careful follow-up; the 10-year survival rate is approximately 60%.

CHRONIC ATHEROSCLEROTIC OCCLUSIVE DISEASE

Atherosclerosis may affect the thoracic and abdominal aorta. Occlusive aortic disease caused by atherosclerosis usually is confined to the distal abdominal aorta below the renal arteries. Frequently the disease extends to the iliac arteries (Chap. 249). Claudication characteristically involves the buttocks, thighs, and calves and may be associated with impotence in males (Leriche syndrome). The severity of the symptoms depends on the adequacy of collaterals. With sufficient collateral blood flow, a complete occlusion of the abdominal aorta may occur without the development of ischemic symptoms. The physical findings include the absence of femoral and other distal pulses bilaterally and the detection of an audible bruit over the abdomen (usually at or below the umbilicus) and the common femoral arteries. Atrophic skin, loss of hair, and coolness of the lower extremities usually are observed. In advanced ischemia, rubor on dependency and pallor on elevation can be seen.

The diagnosis usually is established by physical examination and noninvasive testing, including leg pressure measurements, Doppler velocity analysis, pulse volume recordings, and duplex ultrasonography. The anatomy may be defined by MRI, CT, or conventional aortography, typically performed when one is considering revascularization. Catheter-based endovascular or operative treatment is indicated in patients with lifestyle-limiting or debilitating symptoms of claudication and patients with critical limb ischemia.

■ ACUTE AORTIC OCCLUSION

Acute occlusion in the distal abdominal aorta constitutes a medical emergency because it threatens the viability of the lower extremities; it usually results from an occlusive (saddle) embolus that almost always originates from the heart. Rarely, acute occlusion may occur as the result of in situ thrombosis in a preexisting severely narrowed segment of the aorta.

The clinical picture is one of acute ischemia of the lower extremities. Severe rest pain, coolness, and pallor of the lower extremities and the absence of distal pulses bilaterally are the usual manifestations. Diagnosis should be established rapidly by MRI, CT, or aortography. Emergency thrombectomy or revascularization is indicated.

AORTITIS

Aortitis, a term referring to inflammatory disease of the aorta, may be caused by large vessel vasculitides such as Takayasu's arteritis and giant cell arteritis, rheumatic and HLA-B27–associated spondyloarthropathies, Behçet's syndrome, antineutrophil cytoplasmic antibodies (ANCA)-associated vasculitides, Cogan's syndrome, and infections such as syphilis, tuberculosis, and *Salmonella* or may be associated with retroperitoneal fibrosis. Aortitis may result in aneurysmal dilation and aortic regurgitation, occlusion of the aorta and its branch vessels, or acute aortic syndromes.

■ TAKAYASU'S ARTERITIS

This inflammatory disease often affects the ascending aorta and aortic arch, causing obstruction of the aorta and its major arteries. Takayasu's arteritis is also termed *pulseless disease* because of the frequent occlusion of the large arteries originating from the aorta. It also may involve the descending thoracic and abdominal aorta and occlude large branches such as the renal arteries. Aortic aneurysms also may occur. The pathology is a panarteritis characterized by mononuclear cells and occasionally giant cells, with marked intimal hyperplasia, medial and adventitial thickening, and, in the chronic form, fibrotic occlusion. The disease is most prevalent in young females of Asian descent but does occur in women of other geographic and ethnic origins and also in young men. During the acute stage, fever, malaise, weight loss, and other systemic symptoms may be evident. Elevations of the erythrocyte sedimentation rate and C-reactive protein are common. The chronic stages of the disease, which is intermittently active, present with symptoms related to large artery occlusion, such as upper extremity claudication, cerebral ischemia, and syncope. The process is progressive, and there is no definitive therapy. Glucocorticoids and immunosuppressive agents have been reported to be effective in some patients during the acute phase. Surgical bypass or endovascular intervention of a critically stenotic artery may be necessary.

■ GIANT CELL ARTERITIS

(See also Chap. 326) This vasculitis occurs in older individuals and affects women more often than men. Primarily large and medium-size arteries are affected. The pathology is that of focal granulomatous lesions involving the entire arterial wall; it may be associated with polymyalgia rheumatica. Obstruction of medium-size arteries (e.g., temporal and ophthalmic arteries) and major branches of the aorta and the development of aortitis and aortic regurgitation are important complications of the disease. High-dose glucocorticoid therapy may be effective when given early.

■ RHEUMATIC AORTITIS

Rheumatoid arthritis (Chap. 321), ankylosing spondylitis (Chap. 325), psoriatic arthritis (Chap. 325), reactive arthritis (formerly known as Reiter's syndrome) (Chap. 325), relapsing polychondritis, and inflammatory bowel disorders may all be associated with aortitis involving the ascending aorta. The inflammatory lesions usually involve the ascending aorta and may extend to the sinuses of Valsalva, the mitral valve leaflets, and adjacent myocardium. The clinical manifestations are aneurysm, aortic regurgitation, and involvement of the cardiac conduction system.

■ IDIOPATHIC AORTITIS

Idiopathic abdominal aortitis is characterized by adventitial and periaortic inflammation with thickening of the aortic wall. It is associated with abdominal aortic aneurysms and idiopathic retroperitoneal fibrosis. Affected individuals may present with vague constitutional symptoms, fever, and abdominal pain. Retroperitoneal fibrosis can cause ureteral obstruction and hydronephrosis. Glucocorticoids and immunosuppressive agents may reduce the inflammation.

■ INFECTIVE AORTITIS

Infective aortitis may result from direct invasion of the aortic wall by bacterial pathogens such as *Staphylococcus*, *Streptococcus*, and *Salmonella* or by fungi. These bacteria cause aortitis by infecting the aorta at sites of atherosclerotic plaque. Bacterial proteases lead to degradation of collagen, and the ensuing destruction of the aortic wall leads to the formation of a saccular aneurysm referred to as a mycotic aneurysm. Mycotic aneurysms have a predilection for the suprarenal abdominal aorta. The pathologic characteristics of the aortic wall include acute and chronic inflammation, abscesses, hemorrhage, and necrosis. Mycotic aneurysms typically affect the elderly and occur in men three times more frequently than in women. Patients may present with fever, sepsis, and chest, back, or abdominal pain; there may have been a preceding diarrheal illness. Blood cultures are positive in the majority of patients. Both CT and MRI are useful to diagnose mycotic aneurysms. Treatment includes antibiotic therapy and surgical removal of the affected part of the aorta and revascularization of the lower extremities with grafts placed in uninfected tissue.

Syphilitic aortitis is a late manifestation of luetic infection (Chap. 169) that usually affects the proximal ascending aorta, particularly the aortic root, resulting in aortic dilation and aneurysm formation. Syphilitic aortitis occasionally may involve the aortic arch or the descending aorta. The aneurysms may be saccular or fusiform and are usually asymptomatic, but compression of and erosion into adjacent structures may result in symptoms; rupture also may occur.

The initial lesion is an obliterative endarteritis of the vasa vasorum, especially in the adventitia. This is an inflammatory response to the invasion of the adventitia by the spirochetes. Destruction of the aortic media occurs as the spirochetes spread into this layer, usually via the lymphatics accompanying the vasa vasorum. Destruction of collagen and elastic tissues leads to dilation of the aorta, scar formation, and calcification. These changes account for the characteristic radiographic appearance of linear calcification of the ascending aorta.

The disease typically presents as an incidental chest radiographic finding 15–30 years after initial infection. Symptoms may result from aortic regurgitation, narrowing of coronary ostia due to syphilitic aortitis, compression of adjacent structures (e.g., esophagus), or rupture. Diagnosis is established by a positive serologic test, i.e., rapid plasmin reagin (RPR) or fluorescent treponemal antibody. Treatment includes penicillin and surgical excision and repair.

FURTHER READINGS

Blankensteijn JD et al: Two-year outcomes after conventional or endovascular repair of abdominal aortic aneurysms. N Engl J Med 352:2398, 2005

Brook BS et al: Angiotensin II blockade and aortic-root dilation in Marfan's syndrome. N Engl J Med 358:2787, 2008

Creager MA et al (eds): *Vascular Medicine: A Companion to Braunwald's Heart Disease*. Philadelphia, Saunders, 2006

Fleming C et al: Screening for abdominal aortic aneurysm: A best-evidence systematic review for the U.S. Preventive Services Task Force. Ann Intern Med 142:203, 2005

Golledge J, Eagle KA: Acute aortic dissection. Lancet 372:55, 2008

Gornik HL, Creager MA: Diseases of the aorta, in *Textbook of Cardiovascular Medicine*, 3rd ed, E Topol (ed). Philadelphia, Lippincott, Williams & Wilkins, 2007

———: Aortitis. Circulation 117:3039, 2008

Hiratzka LF et al: 2010 ACCF/AHA/AATS/ACR/ASA/SCA/SCAI/SIR/STS/SVM guidelines for the diagnosis and management of patients with Thoracic Aortic Disease: A report of the American College of Cardiology Foundation/American Heart Association Task Force on Practice Guidelines, American Association for Thoracic Surgery, American College of Radiology, American Stroke Association, Society of Cardiovascular Anesthesiologists, Society for Cardiovascular Angiography and Interventions, Society of Interventional Radiology, Society of Thoracic Surgeons, and Society for Vascular Medicine. Circulation 121:e266, 2010

Hirsch AT et al: ACC/AHA 2005 Practice Guidelines for the management of patients with peripheral arterial disease (lower extremity, renal, mesenteric, and abdominal aortic). Circulation 113:e463, 2006

Isselbacher EM: Thoracic and abdominal aortic aneurysms. Circulation 111:816, 2005

Lederle FA et al: Systematic review: Repair of unruptured abdominal aortic aneurysm. Ann Intern Med 146:735, 2007

Patel HJ, Deeb GM: Ascending and arch aorta: Pathology, natural history, and treatment. Circulation 118:188, 2008

Schermerhorn ML et al: Endovascular vs. open repair of abdominal aortic aneurysms in the Medicare population. N Engl J Med 358:464. 2008

Tsai TT et al: Acute aortic syndromes. Circulation 112:3802, 2005

CHAPTER 249

Vascular Diseases of the Extremities

Mark A. Creager

Joseph Loscalzo

ARTERIAL DISORDERS

PERIPHERAL ARTERY DISEASE

Peripheral artery disease (PAD) is defined as a clinical disorder in which there is a stenosis or occlusion in the aorta or the arteries of the limbs. Atherosclerosis is the leading cause of PAD in patients >40 years old. Other causes include thrombosis, embolism, vasculitis, fibromuscular dysplasia, entrapment, cystic adventitial disease, and trauma. The highest prevalence of atherosclerotic PAD occurs in the sixth and seventh decades of life. As in patients with atherosclerosis of the coronary and cerebral vasculature, there is an increased risk of developing PAD in cigarette smokers and in persons with diabetes mellitus, hypercholesterolemia, hypertension, or hyperhomocysteinemia.

Pathology

(See also Chap. 241) Segmental lesions that cause stenosis or occlusion are usually localized to large and medium-size vessels. The pathology of the lesions includes atherosclerotic plaques with calcium deposition, thinning of the media, patchy destruction of muscle and elastic fibers, fragmentation of the internal elastic lamina, and thrombi composed of platelets and fibrin. The primary sites of involvement are the abdominal aorta and iliac arteries (30% of symptomatic patients), the femoral and popliteal arteries (80–90% of patients), and the more distal vessels, including the tibial and peroneal arteries (40–50% of patients). Atherosclerotic lesions occur preferentially at arterial branch points, which are sites of increased turbulence, altered shear stress, and intimal injury. Involvement of the distal vasculature is most common in elderly individuals and patients with diabetes mellitus.

Clinical evaluation

Fewer than 50% of patients with PAD are symptomatic, although many have a slow or impaired gait. The most common *symptom* is intermittent claudication, which is defined as a pain, ache, cramp, numbness, or a sense of fatigue in the muscles; it occurs during exercise and is relieved by rest. The site of claudication is distal to the location of the occlusive lesion. For example, buttock, hip, and thigh discomfort occurs in patients with aortoiliac disease, whereas calf claudication develops in patients with femoral-popliteal disease. Symptoms are far more common in the lower than in the upper extremities because of the higher incidence of obstructive lesions in the former region. In patients with severe arterial occlusive disease in whom resting blood flow cannot accommodate basal nutritional needs of the tissues, critical limb ischemia may develop. Patients complain of rest pain or a feeling of cold or numbness in the foot and toes. Frequently, these symptoms occur at night when the legs are horizontal and improve when the legs are in a dependent position. With severe ischemia, rest pain may be persistent.

Important *physical findings* of PAD include decreased or absent pulses distal to the obstruction, the presence of bruits over the narrowed artery, and muscle atrophy. With more severe disease, hair loss, thickened nails, smooth and shiny skin, reduced skin temperature, and pallor or cyanosis are common physical signs. In patients with critical limb ischemia, ulcers or gangrene may occur. Elevation of the legs and repeated flexing of the calf muscles produce pallor of the soles of the feet, whereas rubor, secondary to reactive hyperemia, may develop when the legs are dependent. The time required for rubor to develop or for the veins in the foot to fill when the patient's legs are transferred from an elevated to a dependent position is related to the severity of the ischemia and the presence of collateral vessels. Patients with severe ischemia may develop peripheral edema because they keep their legs in a dependent position much of the time. Ischemic neuropathy can result in numbness and hyporeflexia.

Noninvasive testing

The history and physical examination are often sufficient to establish the diagnosis of PAD. An objective assessment of the presence and severity of disease is obtained by noninvasive techniques. Arterial pressure can be recorded noninvasively in the legs by placement of sphygmomanometric cuffs at the ankles and the use of a Doppler device to auscultate or record blood flow from the dorsalis pedis and posterior tibial arteries. Normally, systolic blood pressure in the legs and arms is similar. Indeed, ankle pressure may be slightly higher than arm pressure due to pulse-wave amplification. In the presence of hemodynamically significant stenoses, the systolic blood pressure in the leg is decreased. Thus, the ratio of the ankle and brachial artery pressures (termed the *ankle:brachial index*, or ABI) is ≥1.0 in normal individuals and <1.0 in patients with PAD; a ratio of <0.5 is consistent with severe ischemia.

Other noninvasive tests include segmental pressure measurements, segmental pulse volume recordings, duplex ultrasonography (which combines B-mode imaging and Doppler flow velocity waveform analysis examination), transcutaneous oximetry, and stress testing (usually using a treadmill). Placement of pneumatic cuffs enables assessment of systolic pressure along the legs. The presence of pressure gradients between sequential cuffs provides evidence of the presence and location of hemodynamically significant stenoses. In addition, the amplitude of the pulse volume contour becomes blunted in the presence of significant PAD. Duplex ultrasonography is used to image and detect stenotic lesions in native arteries and bypass grafts.

Treadmill testing allows the physician to assess functional limitations objectively. Decline of the ABI immediately after exercise provides further support for the diagnosis of PAD in patients with equivocal symptoms and findings on examination.

Magnetic resonance angiography (MRA), computed tomographic angiography (CTA), and conventional contrast angiography should not be used for routine diagnostic testing but are performed before potential revascularization (Fig. 249-1). Each test is useful in defining the anatomy to assist planning for catheter-based and surgical revascularization procedures.

Prognosis

The natural history of patients with PAD is influenced primarily by the extent of coexisting coronary artery and cerebrovascular disease. Approximately one-third to one-half of patients with symptomatic PAD have evidence of coronary artery disease (CAD) based on clinical presentation and electrocardiogram, and over one-half have significant CAD by coronary angiography. Patients with PAD have a 15–30% 5-year mortality rate and a two- to sixfold increased risk of death from coronary heart disease. Mortality rates are highest in those with the most severe PAD. Measurement of ABI is useful for detecting PAD and identifying persons at risk for future atherothrombotic events. The likelihood of symptomatic progression of PAD is lower than the chance of succumbing to CAD. Approximately 75–80% of nondiabetic patients who present with mild to moderate claudication remain symptomatically stable. Deterioration is likely to occur in the remainder, with approximately 1–2% of the group ultimately developing critical limb ischemia each year. Approximately 25–30% of patients with critical limb ischemia undergo amputation within 1 year. The prognosis is worse in patients who continue to smoke cigarettes or have diabetes mellitus.

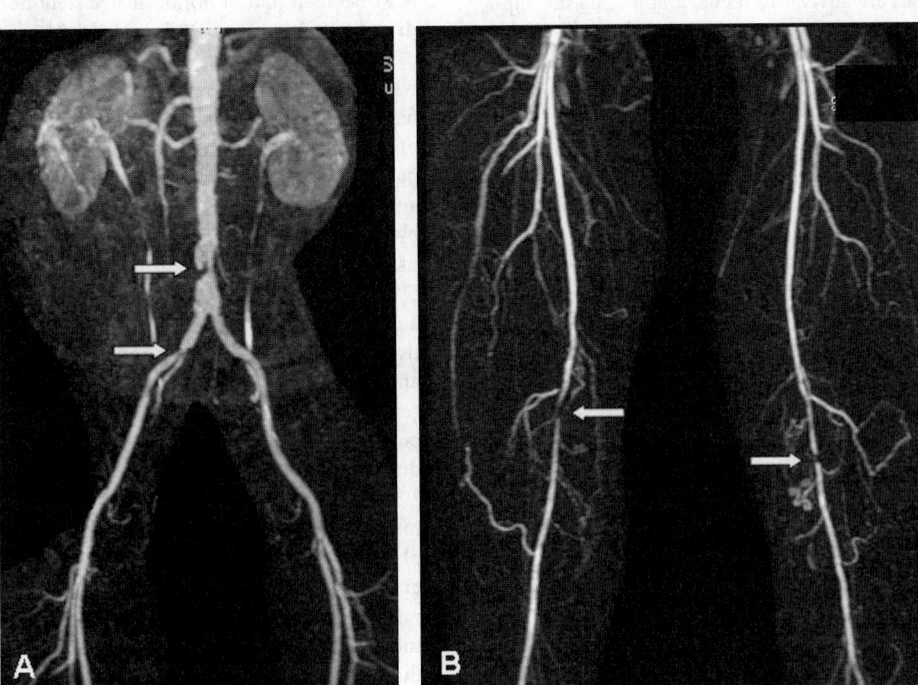

Figure 249-1 Magnetic resonance angiography of a patient with intermittent claudication, showing stenoses of the distal abdominal aorta and right iliac common iliac artery (*A*) and stenoses of the right and left superficial femoral arteries (*B*). *(Courtesy of Dr. Edwin Gravereaux, with permission.)*

TREATMENT Peripheral Artery Disease

Patients with PAD should receive therapies to reduce the risk of associated cardiovascular events, such as myocardial infarction and death, and to improve limb symptoms, prevent progression to critical limb ischemia, and preserve limb viability. Risk factor modification and antiplatelet therapy should be initiated to improve cardiovascular outcomes. The importance of discontinuing cigarette smoking cannot be overemphasized. The physician must assume a major role in this lifestyle modification. Counseling and adjunctive drug therapy with the nicotine patch, bupropion, or varenicline increase smoking cessation rates and reduce recidivism. It is important to control blood pressure in hypertensive patients. Angiotensin converting-enzyme inhibitors may reduce the risk of cardiovascular events in patients with symptomatic PAD. β-adrenergic blockers do not worsen claudication and may be used to treat hypertension, especially in patients with coexistent CAD. Treatment of hypercholesterolemia with statins is advocated to reduce the risk of myocardial infarction, stroke, and death. The National Cholesterol Education Program Adult Treatment Panel considers PAD a coronary heart disease equivalent and recommends treatment to reduce low-density lipoprotein (LDL) cholesterol to <100 mg/dL. Platelet inhibitors, including aspirin and clopidogrel, reduce the risk of adverse cardiovascular events in patients with atherosclerosis and are recommended for patients with PAD. Dual antiplatelet therapy with both aspirin and clopidogrel is not more effective than aspirin alone in reducing cardiovascular morbidity and mortality rates in patients with PAD. The anticoagulant warfarin is as effective as antiplatelet therapy in preventing adverse cardiovascular events but causes more major bleeding; therefore, it is not indicated to improve outcomes in patients with chronic PAD.

Therapies for intermittent claudication and critical limb ischemia include supportive measures, medications, nonoperative interventions, and surgery. Supportive measures include meticulous care of the feet, which should be kept clean and protected against excessive drying with moisturizing creams. Well-fitting and protective shoes are advised to reduce trauma. Elastic support hose should be avoided, as it reduces blood flow to the skin. In patients with critical limb ischemia, shock blocks under the head of the bed together with a canopy over the feet may improve perfusion pressure and ameliorate some of the rest pain.

Patients with claudication should be encouraged to exercise regularly and at progressively more strenuous levels. Supervised exercise training programs for 30- to 45-min sessions, three to five times per week for at least 12 weeks, prolong walking distance. Patients also should be advised to walk until nearly maximum claudication discomfort occurs and then rest until the symptoms resolve before resuming ambulation. Pharmacologic treatment of PAD has not been as successful as the medical treatment of CAD (Chap. 243). In particular, vasodilators as a class have not proved to be beneficial. During exercise, peripheral vasodilation occurs distal to sites of significant arterial stenoses. As a result, perfusion pressure falls, often to levels lower than that generated in the interstitial tissue by the exercising muscle. Drugs such as α-adrenergic blocking agents, calcium channel antagonists, papaverine, and other vasodilators have not been shown to be effective in patients with PAD.

Cilostazol, a phosphodiesterase inhibitor with vasodilator and antiplatelet properties, increases claudication distance by 40–60% and improves measures of quality of life. The mechanism of action accounting for its beneficial effects is not known. Pentoxifylline, a substituted xanthine derivative, increases blood flow to the microcirculation and enhances tissue oxygenation. Although several placebo-controlled studies have found that pentoxifylline increases the duration of exercise in patients with claudication, its efficacy has not been confirmed in all clinical trials. Statins appeared promising for treatment of intermittent claudication in initial clinical trials, but more studies are needed to confirm their efficacy. There is no definitive medical therapy for critical limb ischemia, although several studies have suggested that long-term parenteral administration of vasodilator prostaglandins decreases pain and facilitates healing of ulcers. Clinical trials of angiogenic growth factors are proceeding. Intramuscular gene transfer of DNA encoding vascular endothelial growth factor, fibroblast growth factor, hepatocyte growth factor, or hypoxia-inducible factor 1α, as well as administration of endothelial progenitor cells, may promote collateral blood vessel growth in patients with critical limb ischemia. Some trial results have been negative, and others encouraging. The outcome of ongoing studies will further elucidate the potential role of therapeutic angiogenesis for PAD.

REVASCULARIZATION Revascularization procedures, including catheter-based and surgical interventions, are usually indicated for patients with disabling, progressive, or severe symptoms of intermittent claudication despite medical therapy and for those with critical limb ischemia. MRA, CTA, or conventional contrast angiography should be performed to assess vascular anatomy in patients who are being considered for revascularization. Nonoperative interventions include percutaneous transluminal angiography (PTA), stent placement, and atherectomy (Chap. 246). PTA and stenting of the iliac artery are associated with higher success rates than are PTA and stenting of the femoral and popliteal arteries. Approximately 90–95% of iliac PTAs are initially successful, and the 3-year patency rate is >75%. Patency rates may be higher if a stent is placed in the iliac artery. The initial success rates for femoral-popliteal PTA and stenting are approximately 80%, with 60% 3-year patency rates. Patency rates are influenced by the severity of pretreatment stenoses; the prognosis of occlusive lesions is worse than that of nonocclusive stenotic lesions. The role of drug-eluting stents in PAD is under investigation.

Several operative procedures are available for treating patients with aortoiliac and femoral-popliteal artery disease. The preferred operative procedure depends on the location and extent of the obstruction(s) and the general medical condition of the patient. Operative procedures for aortoiliac disease include aortobifemoral bypass, axillofemoral bypass, femoro-femoral bypass, and aortoiliac endarterectomy. The most frequently used procedure is the aortobifemoral bypass using knitted Dacron grafts. Immediate graft patency approaches 99%, and 5- and 10-year graft patency in survivors is >90% and 80%, respectively. Operative complications include myocardial infarction and stroke, infection of the graft, peripheral embolization, and sexual dysfunction from interruption of autonomic nerves in the pelvis. The operative mortality rate ranges from 1–3%, mostly due to ischemic heart disease.

Operative therapy for femoral-popliteal artery disease includes in situ and reverse autogenous saphenous vein bypass grafts, placement of polytetrafluoroethylene (PTFE) or other synthetic grafts, and thromboendarterectomy. The operative mortality rate ranges from 1–3%. The long-term patency rate depends on the type of graft used, the location of the distal anastomosis, and the patency of runoff vessels beyond the anastomosis. Patency rates of femoral-popliteal saphenous vein bypass grafts approach 90% at 1 year and 70–80% at 5 years. Five-year patency rates of infrapopliteal saphenous vein bypass grafts are 60–70%. In contrast, 5-year patency rates of infrapopliteal PTFE grafts are <30%. Lumbar sympathectomy alone or as an adjunct to aortofemoral reconstruction has fallen into disfavor.

Preoperative cardiac risk assessment may identify individuals who are especially likely to experience an adverse cardiac event during the perioperative period. Patients with angina, prior myocardial infarction, ventricular ectopy, heart failure, or diabetes are among those at increased risk. Stress testing with treadmill exercise (if feasible), radionuclide myocardial perfusion imaging, or echocardiography permits further stratification of patient risk (Chap. 246). Patients with abnormal test results require close supervision and adjunctive management with anti-ischemic medications. β-adrenergic blockers and statins reduce the risk of postoperative cardiovascular complications. Coronary angiography and coronary artery revascularization compared with optimal medical therapy do not improve outcomes in most patients undergoing peripheral vascular surgery, but cardiac catheterization should be considered in patients with unstable angina and angina refractory to medical therapy as well as those suspected of having left main or three-vessel CAD.

FIBROMUSCULAR DYSPLASIA

Fibromuscular dysplasia is a hyperplastic disorder that affects medium-size and small arteries. It occurs predominantly in females and usually involves the renal and carotid arteries but can affect extremity vessels such as the iliac and subclavian arteries. The histologic classification includes intimal fibroplasia, medial dysplasia, and adventitial hyperplasia. Medial dysplasia is subdivided into medial fibroplasia, perimedial fibroplasia, and medial hyperplasia. Medial fibroplasia is the most common type and is characterized by alternating areas of thinned media and fibromuscular ridges. The internal elastic lamina usually is preserved. The iliac arteries are the limb arteries most likely to be affected by fibromuscular dysplasia. It is identified angiographically by a "string of beads" appearance caused by thickened fibromuscular ridges contiguous with thin, less-involved portions of the arterial wall. When limb vessels are involved, clinical manifestations are similar to those for atherosclerosis, including claudication and rest pain. PTA and surgical reconstruction have been beneficial in patients with debilitating symptoms or threatened limbs.

THROMBOANGIITIS OBLITERANS

Thromboangiitis obliterans (Buerger's disease) is an inflammatory occlusive vascular disorder involving small and medium-size arteries and veins in the distal upper and lower extremities. Cerebral, visceral, and coronary vessels may be affected rarely. This disorder develops most frequently in men <40 years of age. The prevalence is higher in Asians and individuals of Eastern European descent. Although the cause of thromboangiitis obliterans is not known, there is a definite relationship to cigarette smoking in patients with this disorder.

In the initial stages of thromboangiitis obliterans, polymorphonuclear leukocytes infiltrate the walls of the small and medium-size arteries and veins. The internal elastic lamina is preserved, and a cellular, inflammatory thrombus develops in the vascular lumen. As the disease progresses, mononuclear cells, fibroblasts, and giant cells replace the neutrophils. Later stages are characterized by perivascular fibrosis, organized thrombus, and recanalization.

The clinical features of thromboangiitis obliterans often include a triad of claudication of the affected extremity, Raynaud's phenomenon, and migratory superficial vein thrombophlebitis. Claudication usually is confined to the calves and feet or the forearms and hands because this disorder primarily affects distal vessels. In the presence of severe digital ischemia, trophic nail changes, painful ulcerations, and gangrene may develop at the tips of the fingers or toes. The physical examination shows normal brachial and popliteal pulses but reduced or absent radial, ulnar, and/or tibial pulses. Arteriography is helpful in making the diagnosis. Smooth, tapering segmental lesions in the distal vessels are characteristic, as are collateral vessels at sites of vascular occlusion. Proximal atherosclerotic disease is usually absent. The diagnosis can be confirmed by excisional biopsy and pathologic examination of an involved vessel.

There is no specific treatment except abstention from tobacco. The prognosis is worse in individuals who continue to smoke, but results are discouraging even in those who stop smoking. Arterial bypass of the larger vessels may be used in selected instances, as well as local debridement, depending on the symptoms and severity of ischemia. Antibiotics may be useful; anticoagulants and glucocorticoids are not helpful. If these measures fail, amputation may be required.

VASCULITIS

Other vasculitides may affect the arteries that supply the upper and lower extremities. Takayasu's arteritis and giant cell (temporal) arteritis are discussed in Chap. 326.

ACUTE ARTERIAL OCCLUSION

Acute arterial occlusion results in the sudden cessation of blood flow to an extremity. The severity of ischemia and the viability of the extremity depend on the location and extent of the occlusion and the presence and subsequent development of collateral blood vessels. There are two principal causes of acute arterial occlusion: embolism and thrombus in situ.

The most common sources of arterial emboli are the heart, aorta, and large arteries. Cardiac disorders that cause thromboembolism include atrial fibrillation, both chronic and paroxysmal; acute myocardial infarction; ventricular aneurysm; cardiomyopathy; infectious and marantic endocarditis; thrombi associated with prosthetic heart valves; and atrial myxoma. Emboli to the distal vessels may also originate from proximal sites of atherosclerosis and aneurysms of the aorta and large vessels. Less frequently, an arterial occlusion results paradoxically from a venous thrombus that has entered the systemic circulation via a patent foramen ovale or another septal defect. Arterial emboli tend to lodge at vessel bifurcations because the vessel caliber decreases at those sites; in the lower extremities, emboli lodge most frequently in the femoral artery, followed by the iliac artery, aorta, and popliteal and tibioperoneal arteries.

Acute arterial thrombosis in situ occurs most frequently in atherosclerotic vessels at the site of an atherosclerotic plaque or aneurysm and in arterial bypass grafts. Trauma to an artery may also result in the formation of an acute arterial thrombus. Arterial occlusion may complicate arterial punctures and placement of catheters; it also may result from arterial dissection if the intimal flap obstructs the artery. Less common causes include thoracic outlet compression syndrome, which causes subclavian artery occlusion, and entrapment of the popliteal artery by abnormal placement of the medial head of the gastrocnemius muscle. Polycythemia and hypercoagulable disorders (Chaps. 108 and 116) are also associated with acute arterial thrombosis.

Clinical features

The symptoms of an acute arterial occlusion depend on the location, duration, and severity of the obstruction. Often, severe pain, paresthesia, numbness, and coldness develop in the involved extremity within 1 hour. Paralysis may occur with severe and persistent ischemia. Physical findings include loss of pulses distal to the occlusion, cyanosis or pallor, mottling, decreased skin temperature, muscle stiffening, loss of sensation, weakness, and/or absent deep tendon reflexes. If acute arterial occlusion occurs in the presence of an adequate collateral circulation, as is often the case in acute graft occlusion, the symptoms and findings may be less impressive. In this situation, the patient complains about an abrupt decrease in the distance walked before claudication occurs or of modest pain and paresthesia. Pallor and coolness are evident, but sensory and motor functions generally are preserved. The diagnosis of acute arterial occlusion is usually apparent from the clinical presentation. In most circumstances, MRA, CTA, or catheter-based arteriography is used to confirm the diagnosis and demonstrate the location and extent of occlusion.

TREATMENT Acute Arterial Occlusion

Once the diagnosis is made, the patient should be anticoagulated with intravenous heparin to prevent propagation of the clot. In cases of severe ischemia of recent onset, particularly when limb viability is jeopardized, immediate intervention to ensure reperfusion is indicated. Endovascular or surgical thromboembolectomy or arterial bypass procedures are used to restore blood flow to the ischemic extremity promptly, particularly when a large proximal vessel is occluded.

Intraarterial thrombolytic therapy with recombinant tissue plasminogen activator, reteplase, or tenecteplase is often effective when acute arterial occlusion is caused by a thrombus in an atherosclerotic vessel or arterial bypass graft. Thrombolytic therapy may also be indicated when the patient's overall condition contraindicates surgical intervention or when smaller distal vessels are occluded, thus preventing surgical access. Meticulous observation for hemorrhagic complications is required during intraarterial thrombolytic therapy. Another endovascular approach to thrombus removal is percutaneous mechanical thrombectomy using devices that employ hydrodynamic forces or rotating baskets to fragment and remove the clot. These treatments may be used alone but usually are used in conjunction with pharmacologic thrombolysis. Amputation is performed when the limb is not viable, as characterized by loss of sensation, paralysis, and the absence of Doppler-detected blood flow in both arteries and veins.

If the limb is not in jeopardy, a more conservative approach that includes observation and administration of anticoagulants may be taken. Anticoagulation prevents recurrent embolism and reduces the likelihood of thrombus propagation; it can be initiated with intravenous heparin and followed by oral warfarin. Recommended doses are the same as those used for deep vein thrombosis (Chap. 262). Emboli resulting from infective endocarditis, the presence of prosthetic heart valves, or atrial myxoma often require surgical intervention to remove the cause.

ATHEROEMBOLISM

Atheroembolism constitutes a subset of acute arterial occlusion. In this condition, multiple small deposits of fibrin, platelets, and cholesterol debris embolize from proximal atherosclerotic lesions or aneurysmal sites. Large protruding aortic atheromas are a source of emboli that may lead to stroke and renal insufficiency as well as limb ischemia. Atheroembolism may occur after intraarterial procedures. Since the emboli tend to lodge in the small vessels of the muscle and skin and may not occlude the large vessels, distal pulses usually remain palpable. Patients complain of acute pain and tenderness at the site of embolization. Digital vascular occlusion may result in ischemia and the "blue toe" syndrome; digital necrosis and gangrene may develop (Fig. 249-2). Localized areas of tenderness, pallor, and livedo reticularis (see below) occur at sites of emboli. Skin or muscle biopsy may demonstrate cholesterol crystals.

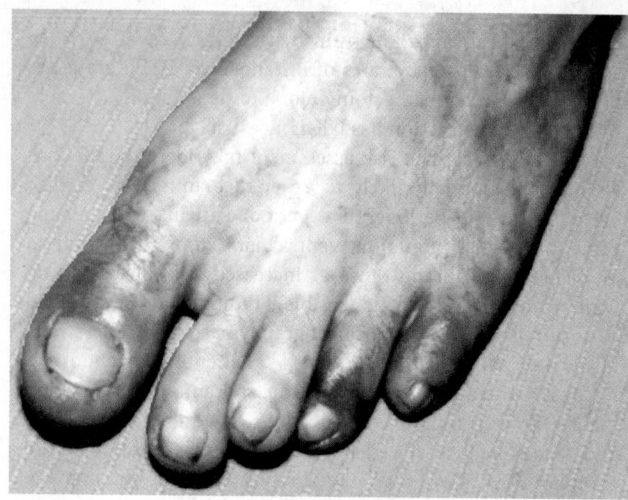

Figure 249-2 Atheroembolism causing cyanotic discoloration and impending necrosis of the toes ("blue toe" syndrome).

Ischemia resulting from atheroemboli is notoriously difficult to treat. Usually neither surgical revascularization procedures nor thrombolytic therapy is helpful because of the multiplicity, composition, and distal location of the emboli. Some evidence suggests that platelet inhibitors prevent atheroembolism. Surgical intervention to remove or bypass the atherosclerotic vessel or aneurysm that causes the recurrent atheroemboli may be necessary.

THORACIC OUTLET COMPRESSION SYNDROME

This is a symptom complex resulting from compression of the neurovascular bundle (artery, vein, or nerves) at the thoracic outlet as it courses through the neck and shoulder. Cervical ribs, abnormalities of the scalenus anticus muscle, proximity of the clavicle to the first rib, or abnormal insertion of the pectoralis minor muscle may compress the subclavian artery, subclavian vein, and brachial plexus as these structures pass from the thorax to the arm. Depending on the structures affected, thoracic outlet compression syndrome is divided into arterial, venous, and neurogenic forms. Patients with neurogenic thoracic outlet compression may develop shoulder and arm pain, weakness, and paresthesias. Patients with arterial compression may experience claudication, Raynaud's phenomenon, and even ischemic tissue loss and gangrene. Venous compression may cause thrombosis of the subclavian and axillary veins; this is often associated with effort and is referred to as *Paget-Schroetter syndrome.*

APPROACH TO THE PATIENT Thoracic Outlet Compression Syndrome

Examination of a patient with thoracic outlet compression syndrome is often normal unless provocative maneuvers are performed. Occasionally, distal pulses are decreased or absent and digital cyanosis and ischemia may be evident. Tenderness may be present in the supraclavicular fossa. In patients with axillo-subclavian venous thrombosis, the affected extremity typically is swollen. Dilated collateral veins may be apparent around the shoulder and upper arm.

Several maneuvers that support the diagnosis of thoracic outlet compression syndrome may be used to precipitate symptoms, cause a subclavian artery bruit, and diminish arm pulses. These maneuvers include the abduction and external rotation test, in which the affected arm is abducted by 90° and the shoulder is externally rotated; the scalene maneuver (extension of the neck and rotation of the head to the side of the symptoms); the costoclavicular maneuver (posterior rotation of shoulders); and the hyperabduction maneuver (raising the arm 180°). A chest x-ray will indicate the presence of cervical ribs. Duplex ultrasonography, MRA, and contrast angiography can be performed during provocative maneuvers to demonstrate thoracic outlet compression of the subclavian artery. Duplex ultrasography, magnetic resonance venography, or contrast venography can be used to diagnose axillo-subclavian vein thrombosis. Neurophysiologic tests such as the electromyogram, nerve conduction studies, and somatosensory evoked potentials may be abnormal if the brachial plexus is involved, but the diagnosis of neurogenic thoracic outlet syndrome is not necessarily excluded if these tests are normal owing to their low sensitivity.

Most patients can be managed conservatively. They should be advised to avoid the positions that cause symptoms. Many patients benefit from shoulder girdle exercises. Surgical procedures such as removal of the first rib and resection of the scalenus anticus muscle are necessary occasionally for relief of symptoms or treatment of ischemia.

POPLITEAL ARTERY ENTRAPMENT

Popliteal artery entrapment typically affects young athletic men and women when the gastrocnemius or popliteus muscle compresses the popliteal artery and causes intermittent claudication. Thrombosis, embolism, or popliteal artery aneurysm may occur. The pulse examination may be normal unless provocative maneuvers such as ankle dorsiflexion and plantar flexion are performed. The diagnosis is confirmed by duplex ultrasound, CTA, MRA, or conventional angiography. Treatment involves surgical release of the popliteal artery or vascular reconstruction.

POPLITEAL ARTERY ANEURYSM

Popliteal artery aneurysms are the most common peripheral artery aneurysms. Approximately 50% are bilateral. Patients with popliteal artery aneurysms often have aneurysms of other arteries, especially the aorta. The most common clinical presentation is limb ischemia secondary to thrombosis or embolism. Rupture occurs less frequently. Other complications include compression of the adjacent popliteal vein or peroneal nerve. Popliteal artery aneurysm can be detected by palpation and confirmed by duplex ultrasonography. Repair is indicated for symptomatic aneurysms or when the diameter exceeds 2–3 cm, owing to the risk of thrombosis, embolism, or rupture.

ARTERIOVENOUS FISTULA

Abnormal communications between an artery and a vein, bypassing the capillary bed, may be congenital or acquired. Congenital arteriovenous fistulas are a result of persistent embryonic vessels that fail to differentiate into arteries and veins; they may be associated with birthmarks, can be located in almost any organ of the body, and frequently occur in the extremities. Acquired arteriovenous fistulas either are created to provide vascular access for hemodialysis or occur as a result of a penetrating injury such as a gunshot or knife wound or as complications of arterial catheterization or surgical dissection. An uncommon cause of arteriovenous fistula is rupture of an arterial aneurysm into a vein.

The clinical features depend on the location and size of the fistula. Frequently, a pulsatile mass is palpable, and a thrill and a bruit lasting throughout systole and diastole are present over the fistula. With long-standing fistulas, clinical manifestations of chronic venous insufficiency, including peripheral edema; large, tortuous varicose veins; and stasis pigmentation become apparent because of the high venous pressure. Evidence of ischemia may occur in the distal portion of the extremity. Skin temperature is higher over the arteriovenous fistula. Large arteriovenous fistulas may result in an increased cardiac output with consequent cardiomegaly and high-output heart failure (Chap. 234).

The diagnosis is often evident from the physical examination. Compression of a large arteriovenous fistula may cause reflex slowing of the heart rate (Nicoladoni-Branham sign). Duplex ultrasonography may detect an arteriovenous fistula, especially one that affects the femoral artery and vein at the site of catheter access. Computed tomographic and conventional angiography can confirm the diagnosis and are useful in demonstrating the site and size of the arteriovenous fistula.

Management of arteriovenous fistulas may involve surgery, radiotherapy, or embolization. Congenital arteriovenous fistulas are often difficult to treat because the communications may be numerous and extensive, and new communications frequently develop after ligation of the most obvious ones. Many of these lesions are best treated conservatively using elastic support hose to reduce the consequences of venous hypertension. Occasionally, embolization with autologous material, such as fat or muscle, or with hemostatic agents, such as gelatin sponges or silicon spheres, is used to obliterate the fistula. Acquired arteriovenous fistulas are usually amenable to surgical treatment that involves division or excision of the fistula. Occasionally, autogenous or synthetic grafting is necessary to reestablish continuity of the artery and vein.

RAYNAUD'S PHENOMENON

Raynaud's phenomenon is characterized by episodic digital ischemia, manifested clinically by the sequential development of digital blanching, cyanosis, and rubor of the fingers or toes after cold exposure and subsequent rewarming. Emotional stress may also precipitate Raynaud's phenomenon. The color changes are usually well demarcated and are confined to the fingers or toes. Typically, one or more digits will appear white when the patient is exposed to a cold environment or touches a cold object. The blanching, or pallor, represents the ischemic phase of the phenomenon and results from vasospasm of digital arteries. During the ischemic phase, capillaries and venules dilate, and cyanosis results from the deoxygenated blood that is present in these vessels. A sensation of cold or numbness or paresthesia of the digits often accompanies the phases of pallor and cyanosis.

With rewarming, the digital vasospasm resolves, and blood flow into the dilated arterioles and capillaries increases dramatically. This "reactive hyperemia" imparts a bright red color to the digits. In addition to rubor and warmth, patients often experience a throbbing, painful sensation during the hyperemic phase. Although the triphasic color response is typical of Raynaud's phenomenon, some patients may develop only pallor and cyanosis; others may experience only cyanosis.

Raynaud's phenomenon is broadly separated into two categories: the idiopathic variety, termed *Raynaud's disease*, and the secondary variety, which is associated with other disease states or known causes of vasospasm (Table 249-1).

Raynaud's disease

This appellation is applied when the secondary causes of Raynaud's phenomenon have been excluded. Over 50% of patients with Raynaud's phenomenon have Raynaud's disease. Women are affected about five times more often than men, and the age of presentation is usually between 20 and 40 years. The fingers are involved more frequently than the toes. Initial episodes may involve only one or two fingertips, but subsequent attacks may involve the entire finger and may include all the fingers. The toes are affected in 40% of

TABLE 249-1 Classification of Raynaud's Phenomenon

Primary or idiopathic Raynaud's phenomenon: Raynaud's disease
Secondary Raynaud's phenomenon
Collagen vascular diseases: scleroderma, systemic lupus erythematosus, rheumatoid arthritis, dermatomyositis, polymyositis
Arterial occlusive diseases: atherosclerosis of the extremities, thromboangiitis obliterans, acute arterial occlusion, thoracic outlet syndrome
Pulmonary hypertension
Neurologic disorders: intervertebral disk disease, syringomyelia, spinal cord tumors, stroke, poliomyelitis, carpal tunnel syndrome
Blood dyscrasias: cold agglutinins, cryoglobulinemia, cryofibrinogenemia, myeloproliferative disorders, Waldenström's macroglobulinemia
Trauma: vibration injury, hammer hand syndrome, electric shock, cold injury, typing, piano playing
Drugs: ergot derivatives, methysergide, β-adrenergic receptor blockers, bleomycin, vinblastine, cisplatin

patients. Although vasospasm of the toes usually occurs in patients with symptoms in the fingers, it may happen alone. Rarely, the earlobes, the tip of the nose, and the penis are involved. Raynaud's phenomenon occurs frequently in patients who also have migraine headaches or variant angina. These associations suggest that there may be a common predisposing cause for the vasospasm.

Results of physical examination are often entirely normal; the radial, ulnar, and pedal pulses are normal. The fingers and toes may be cool between attacks and may perspire excessively. Thickening and tightening of the digital subcutaneous tissue (*sclerodactyly*) develop in 10% of patients. Angiography of the digits for diagnostic purposes is not indicated.

In general, patients with Raynaud's disease have milder forms of Raynaud's phenomenon. Fewer than 1% of these patients lose a part of a digit. After the diagnosis is made, the disease improves spontaneously in approximately 15% of patients and progresses in about 30%.

Secondary causes of Raynaud's phenomenon

Raynaud's phenomenon occurs in 80–90% of patients with systemic sclerosis (scleroderma) and is the presenting symptom in 30% (Chap. 323). It may be the only symptom of scleroderma for many years. Abnormalities of the digital vessels may contribute to the development of Raynaud's phenomenon in this disorder. Ischemic fingertip ulcers may develop and progress to gangrene and autoamputation. About 20% of patients with systemic lupus erythematosus (SLE) have Raynaud's phenomenon (Chap. 319). Occasionally, persistent digital ischemia develops and may result in ulcers or gangrene. In most severe cases, the small vessels are occluded by a proliferative endarteritis. Raynaud's phenomenon occurs in about 30% of patients with dermatomyositis or polymyositis (Chap. 388). It frequently develops in patients with rheumatoid arthritis and may be related to the intimal proliferation that occurs in the digital arteries.

Atherosclerosis of the extremities is a common cause of Raynaud's phenomenon in men >50 years. Thromboangiitis obliterans is an uncommon cause of Raynaud's phenomenon but should be considered in young men, particularly those who are cigarette smokers. The development of cold-induced pallor in these disorders may be confined to one or two digits of the involved extremity. Occasionally, Raynaud's phenomenon may follow acute occlusion of large and medium-size arteries by a thrombus or embolus. Embolization of atheroembolic debris may cause digital ischemia. The latter situation often involves one or two digits and should not be confused with Raynaud's phenomenon. In patients with thoracic outlet compression syndrome, Raynaud's phenomenon may result from diminished intravascular pressure, stimulation of sympathetic fibers in the brachial plexus, or a combination of both. Raynaud's phenomenon occurs in patients with primary pulmonary hypertension (Chap. 250); this is more than coincidental and may reflect a neurohumoral abnormality that affects both the pulmonary and digital circulations.

A variety of blood dyscrasias may be associated with Raynaud's phenomenon. Cold-induced precipitation of plasma proteins, hyperviscosity, and aggregation of red cells and platelets may occur in patients with cold agglutinins, cryoglobulinemia, or cryofibrinogenemia. Hyperviscosity syndromes that accompany myeloproliferative disorders and Waldenström macroglobulinemia should also be considered in the initial evaluation of patients with Raynaud's phenomenon.

Raynaud's phenomenon occurs often in patients whose vocations require the use of vibrating hand tools, such as chain saws or jackhammers. The frequency of Raynaud's phenomenon also seems to be increased in pianists and keyboard operators. Electric shock injury to the hands or frostbite may lead to the later development of Raynaud's phenomenon.

Several drugs have been causally implicated in Raynaud's phenomenon. They include ergot preparations, methysergide, β-adrenergic receptor antagonists, and the chemotherapeutic agents bleomycin, vinblastine, and cisplatin.

TREATMENT Raynaud's Phenomenon

Most patients with Raynaud's phenomenon experience only mild and infrequent episodes. These patients need reassurance and should be instructed to dress warmly and avoid unnecessary cold exposure. In addition to gloves and mittens, patients should protect the trunk, head, and feet with warm clothing to prevent cold-induced reflex vasoconstriction. Tobacco use is contraindicated.

Drug treatment should be reserved for severe cases. Dihydropyridine calcium channel antagonists such as nifedipine, isradipine, felodipine, and amlodipine decrease the frequency and severity of Raynaud's phenomenon. Diltiazem may be considered but is less effective. The postsynaptic α_1-adrenergic antagonist prazosin has been used with favorable responses; doxazosin and terazosin may also be effective. Topical glyceryl trinitrate may be useful in some patients. Digital sympathectomy is helpful in some patients who are unresponsive to medical therapy.

■ ACROCYANOSIS

In this condition, there is arterial vasoconstriction and secondary dilation of the capillaries and venules with resulting persistent cyanosis of the hands and, less frequently, the feet. Cyanosis may be intensified by exposure to a cold environment. Acrocyanosis may be categorized as primary or secondary to an underlying condition. In primary acrocyanosis, women are affected much more frequently than men, and the age of onset is usually <30 years. Generally, patients are asymptomatic but seek medical attention because of the discoloration. The prognosis is favorable, and pain, ulcers, and gangrene do not occur. Examination reveals normal pulses, peripheral cyanosis, and moist palms. Trophic skin changes and ulcerations do *not* occur. The disorder can be distinguished from Raynaud's phenomenon because it is persistent and not episodic, the discoloration extends proximally from the digits, and blanching does not occur. Ischemia secondary to arterial occlusive disease can usually be excluded by the presence of normal pulses. Central cyanosis and decreased arterial oxygen saturation are not present. Patients should be reassured and advised to dress warmly and avoid cold exposure. Pharmacologic intervention is not indicated.

Secondary acrocyanosis may result from hypoxemia, connective tissue diseases, atheroembolism, antiphospholipid antibodies, cold agglutinins, or cryoglobulins and is associated with anorexia nervosa and orthostatic tachycardia syndrome. Treatment should be directed at the underlying disorder.

LIVEDO RETICULARIS

In this condition, localized areas of the extremities develop a mottled or rete (netlike) appearance of reddish to blue discoloration. The mottled appearance may be more prominent after cold exposure. There are primary and secondary forms of livedo reticularis. The primary, or idiopathic, form of this disorder may be benign or associated with ulcerations. The benign form occurs more frequently in women than in men, and the most common age of onset is the third decade. Patients with the benign form are usually asymptomatic and seek attention for cosmetic reasons. These patients should be reassured and advised to avoid cold environments. No drug treatment is indicated. Primary livedo reticularis with ulceration is also called *atrophie blanche en plaque*. The ulcers are painful and may take months to heal. Secondary livedo reticularis can occur with atheroembolism (see above), SLE and other vasculitides, anticardiolipin antibodies, hyperviscosity, cryoglobulinemia, and Sneddon's syndrome (ischemic stroke and livedo reticularis). Rarely, skin ulcerations develop.

PERNIO (CHILBLAINS)

Pernio is a vasculitic disorder associated with exposure to cold; acute forms have been described. Raised erythematous lesions develop on the lower part of the legs and feet in cold weather. They are associated with pruritus and a burning sensation, and they may blister and ulcerate. Pathologic examination demonstrates angiitis characterized by intimal proliferation and perivascular infiltration of mononuclear and polymorphonuclear leukocytes. Giant cells may be present in the subcutaneous tissue. Patients should avoid exposure to cold, and ulcers should be kept clean and protected with sterile dressings. Sympatholytic drugs and dihydropyridine calcium channel antagonists may be effective in some patients.

ERYTHROMELALGIA

This disorder is characterized by burning pain and erythema of the extremities. The feet are involved more frequently than the hands, and males are affected more frequently than females. Erythromelalgia may occur at any age but is most common in middle age. It may be primary (also termed erythermalgia) or secondary. The most common causes of secondary erythromelalgia are myeloproliferative disorders such as polycythemia vera and essential thrombocytosis. Less common causes include drugs, such as calcium channel blockers, bromocriptine, and pergolide; neuropathies; connective tissue diseases such as SLE; and paraneoplastic syndromes. Patients complain of burning in the extremities that is precipitated by exposure to a warm environment and aggravated by a dependent position. The symptoms are relieved by exposing the affected area to cool air or water or by elevation. Erythromelalgia can be distinguished from ischemia secondary to peripheral arterial disorders and peripheral neuropathy because the peripheral pulses are present and the neurologic examination is normal. There is no specific treatment; aspirin may produce relief in patients with erythromelalgia secondary to myeloproliferative disease. Treatment of associated disorders in secondary erythromelalgia may be helpful.

FROSTBITE

In this condition, tissue damage results from severe environmental cold exposure or from direct contact with a very cold object. Tissue injury results from both freezing and vasoconstriction. Frostbite usually affects the distal aspects of the extremities or exposed parts of the face, such as the ears, nose, chin, and cheeks. Superficial frostbite involves the skin and subcutaneous tissue. Patients experience pain or paresthesia, and the skin appears white and waxy. After rewarming, there is cyanosis and erythema, wheal-and-flare formation, edema, and superficial blisters. Deep frostbite involves muscle, nerves, and deeper blood vessels. It may result in edema of the hand or foot, vesicles and bullae, tissue necrosis, and gangrene.

Initial treatment is rewarming, performed in an environment where reexposure to freezing conditions will not occur. Rewarming is accomplished by immersion of the affected part in a water bath at temperatures of 40°–44°C (104°–111°F). Massage, application of ice water, and extreme heat are contraindicated. The injured area should be cleansed with soap or antiseptic, and sterile dressings should be applied. Analgesics are often required during rewarming. Antibiotics are used if there is evidence of infection. The efficacy of sympathetic blocking drugs is not established. After recovery, the affected extremity may exhibit increased sensitivity to cold.

DISORDERS OF THE VEINS AND LYMPHATICS

VENOUS DISORDERS

Veins in the extremities can be broadly classified as either superficial or deep. In the lower extremity, the superficial venous system includes the greater and lesser saphenous veins and their tributaries. The deep veins of the leg accompany the major arteries. Perforating veins connect the superficial and deep systems at multiple locations. Bicuspid valves are present throughout the venous system to direct the flow of venous blood centrally.

Venous thrombosis

The presence of thrombus within a superficial or deep vein, along with the accompanying inflammatory response in the vessel wall, is termed *venous thrombosis* or *thrombophlebitis*. Initially the thrombus is composed principally of platelets and fibrin. Red cells become interspersed with fibrin, and the thrombus tends to propagate in the direction of blood flow. The inflammatory response in the vessel wall may be minimal or characterized by granulocyte infiltration, loss of endothelium, and edema.

The factors that predispose to venous thrombosis were initially described by Virchow in 1856 and include stasis, vascular damage, and hypercoagulability. Accordingly, a variety of clinical situations are associated with increased risk of venous thrombosis (Table 249-2). Venous thrombosis may occur in >50% of patients having orthopedic surgical procedures, particularly those involving the hip or knee, and in 10–40% of patients who undergo abdominal or thoracic operations. The prevalence of venous thrombosis is particularly high in patients with cancer of the pancreas, lungs, genitourinary tract, stomach, and breast. Approximately 10–20% of patients with idiopathic deep vein thrombosis have or develop clinically overt cancer; there is no consensus on whether these individuals should be subjected to intensive diagnostic workup to search for occult malignancy.

The risk of thrombosis is increased after trauma such as fractures of the spine, pelvis, femur, and tibia. Immobilization, regardless of the underlying disease, is a major predisposing cause of venous

TABLE 249-2 Conditions Associated With an Increased Risk for Development of Venous Thrombosis

Surgery
Orthopedic, thoracic, abdominal, and genitourinary procedures
Neoplasms
Pancreas, lung, ovary, testes, urinary tract, breast, stomach
Trauma
Fractures of spine, pelvis, femur, or tibia; spinal cord injuries
Immobilization
Acute myocardial infarction, congestive heart failure, stroke, postoperative convalescence
Pregnancy
Estrogen for replacement or contraception
Selective estrogen replacement modulators
Hypercoagulable states
Resistance to activated protein C; prothrombin 20210 A gene mutation deficiencies of antithrombin III, protein C, or protein S; antiphospholipid antibodies; myeloproliferative diseases; dysfibrinogenemia; disseminated intravascular coagulation
Venulitis
Thromboangiitis obliterans, Behçet's disease, homocysteinuria
Previous deep vein thrombosis

thrombosis. This may account for the relatively high incidence in patients with acute myocardial infarction or congestive heart failure. The incidence of venous thrombosis is increased during pregnancy, particularly in the third trimester, and in the first month postpartum, as well as in individuals who use oral contraceptives, postmenopausal hormone replacement therapy, or selective estrogen receptor modulators. A variety of inherited and acquired disorders that produce systemic hypercoagulability, including resistance to activated protein C (factor V Leiden); prothrombin G20210A gene mutation; antithrombin III, protein C, and protein S deficiencies; antiphospholipid syndrome; hyperhomocysteinemia; SLE; myeloproliferative diseases; dysfibrinogenemia; heparin-induced thrombocytopenia; and disseminated intravascular coagulation, are associated with venous thrombosis. Venulitis occurring in thromboangiitis obliterans, Behçet's syndrome, and homocystinuria may also cause venous thrombosis.

Deep venous thrombosis and pulmonary thromboembolism

See Chap. 262.

Superficial vein thrombosis

Thrombosis of the greater or lesser saphenous veins or their tributaries (i.e., superficial vein thrombosis) does not result in pulmonary embolism. It is associated with intravenous catheters and infusions, occurs in varicose veins, and may develop in association with deep venous thrombosis (DVT). Migrating superficial vein thrombosis is often a marker for a carcinoma and may also occur in patients with vasculitides, such as thromboangiitis obliterans. The clinical features of superficial vein thrombosis are easily distinguished from those of DVT. Patients complain of pain localized to the site of the thrombus. Examination reveals a reddened, warm, and tender cord extending along a superficial vein. The surrounding area may be red and edematous.

TREATMENT Superficial Vein Thrombosis

Treatment is primarily supportive. Initially, patients can be placed at bed rest with leg elevation and application of warm compresses. Nonsteroidal anti-inflammatory drugs may provide analgesia but may also obscure clinical evidence of thrombus propagation. If a thrombosis of the greater saphenous vein develops in the thigh and extends toward the saphenofemoral vein junction, it is reasonable to consider anticoagulant therapy to prevent extension of the thrombus into the deep system and a possible pulmonary embolism.

Varicose veins

Varicose veins are dilated, tortuous superficial veins that result from defective structure and function of the valves of the saphenous veins, intrinsic weakness of the vein wall, high intraluminal pressure, or, rarely, arteriovenous fistulas. Varicose veins can be categorized as primary or secondary. Primary varicose veins originate in the superficial system and occur two to three times as frequently in women as in men. Approximately one-half of these patients have a family history of varicose veins. Secondary varicose veins result from deep venous insufficiency and incompetent perforating veins or from deep venous occlusion that causes enlargement of superficial veins that are serving as collaterals.

Patients with venous varicosities are often concerned about the cosmetic appearance of their legs. Symptoms consist of a dull ache or pressure sensation in the legs after prolonged standing; this is relieved with leg elevation. The legs feel heavy, and mild ankle edema develops occasionally. Extensive venous varicosities may cause skin ulcerations near the ankle. Superficial venous thrombosis may be a recurring problem, and, rarely, a varicosity ruptures and bleeds. Visual inspection of the legs in the dependent position usually confirms the presence of varicose veins.

Varicose veins usually can be treated with conservative measures. Symptoms often decrease when the legs are elevated periodically, prolonged standing is avoided, and elastic support hose are worn. External compression stockings provide a counterbalance to the hydrostatic pressure in the veins. Ablative procedures, including sclerotherapy, endovenous radiofrequency or laser ablation, and surgery, may be considered to treat varicose veins in selected patients who have persistent symptoms, have recurrent superficial vein thrombosis, and/or develop skin ulceration. Ablative therapy may also be indicated for cosmetic reasons. Small, symptomatic varicose veins can be treated with sclerotherapy, in which a sclerosing solution is injected into the involved varicose vein and a compression bandage is applied. Percutaneous, endovenous delivery of radiofrequency or laser energy can be used to treat incompetent great saphenous veins. Surgical therapy usually involves ligation and stripping of the great and small saphenous veins.

Chronic venous insufficiency

Chronic venous insufficiency may result from DVT and/or valvular incompetence. After DVT, the delicate valve leaflets become thickened and contracted so that they cannot prevent retrograde flow of blood; the vein becomes rigid and thick walled. Although most veins recanalize after an episode of thrombosis, the large proximal veins may remain occluded. Secondary incompetence develops in distal valves because high pressures distend the vein and separate the leaflets. Primary deep venous valvular dysfunction may also occur without previous thrombosis. Patients with venous insufficiency often complain of a dull ache in the leg that worsens with prolonged standing and resolves with leg elevation. Examination

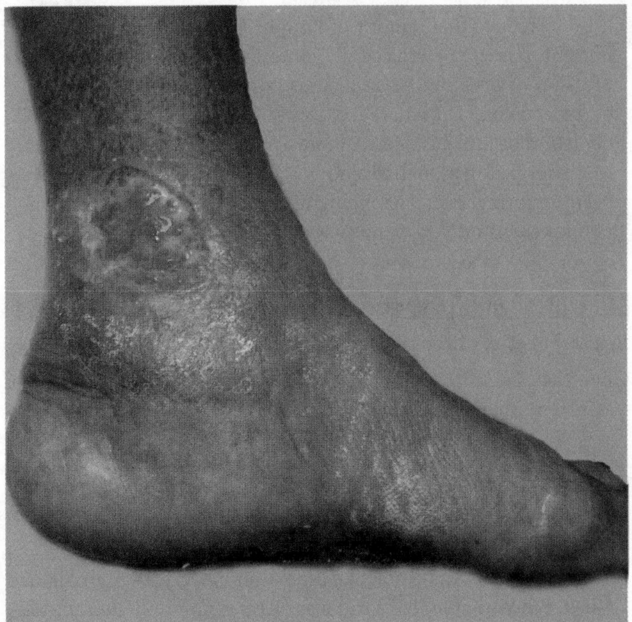

Figure 249-3 Venous insufficiency with active venous ulcer near the medial malleolus. *(Courtesy of Dr. Steven Dean, with permission.)*

demonstrates increased leg circumference, edema, and superficial varicose veins. Erythema, dermatitis, and hyperpigmentation develop along the distal aspect of the leg, and skin ulceration may occur near the medial and lateral malleoli (Fig. 249-3). Cellulitis may be a recurring problem. The CEAP (clinical, etiologic, anatomic, pathophysiologic) classification schema incorporates the range of symptoms and signs of chronic venous insufficiency to characterize its severity (Table 249-3).

Patients should be advised to avoid prolonged standing or sitting; frequent leg elevation is helpful. Graduated compression stockings should be worn during the day. These efforts should be intensified if skin ulcers develop. Ulcers should be treated with applications of wet to dry dressings or occlusive hydrocolloid dressings. Commercially available compressive dressings that consist of paste with zinc oxide, calamine, glycerin, and gelatin may be applied and should be changed weekly until healing occurs. Recurrent ulceration and severe edema may be treated by surgical interruption of incompetent communicating veins. Subfascial endoscopic perforator surgery (SEPS) is a minimally invasive technique to interrupt incompetent communicating veins. Rarely, surgical valvuloplasty and bypass of venous occlusions are employed.

TABLE 249-3 CEAP (Clinical, Etiologic, Anatomic, Pathophysiologic) Classification

C0 No visible or palpable signs of venous disease
C1 Telangiectases, reticular veins
C2 Varicose veins
C3 Edema without skin changes
C4 Skin changes, including pigmentation, eczema, lipodermatosclerosis, and *atrophie blanche*
C5 Healed venous ulcer
C6 Active venous ulcer

LYMPHATIC DISORDERS

Lymphatic capillaries are blind-ended tubes formed by a single layer of endothelial cells. The absent or widely fenestrated basement membrane of lymphatic capillaries allows access to interstitial proteins and particles. Lymphatic capillaries merge to form larger vessels that contain smooth muscle and are capable of vasomotion. Small- and medium-size lymphatic vessels empty into progressively larger channels, most of which drain into the thoracic duct. The lymphatic circulation is involved in the absorption of interstitial fluid and in the response to infection.

Lymphedema

Lymphedema may be categorized as primary or secondary (Table 249-4). The prevalence of primary lymphedema is approximately 1 per 10,000 individuals. Primary lymphedema may be secondary to agenesis, hypoplasia, or obstruction of the lymphatic vessels. It may be associated with Turner's syndrome, Klinefelter's syndrome, Noonan's syndrome, yellow nail syndrome, intestinal lymphangiectasia syndrome, and lymphangiomyomatosis. Women are affected more frequently than are men. There are three clinical subtypes: congenital lymphedema, which appears shortly after birth; lymphedema praecox, which has its onset at the time of puberty; and lymphedema tarda, which usually begins after age 35. Familial forms of congenital lymphedema (Milroy's disease) and lymphedema praecox (Meige's disease) may be inherited in an autosomal dominant manner with variable penetrance; autosomal or sex-linked recessive forms are less common.

Secondary lymphedema is an acquired condition that results from damage to or obstruction of previously normal lymphatic channels (Table 249-4). Recurrent episodes of bacterial lymphangitis, usually caused by streptococci, are a very common cause of lymphedema. The most common cause of secondary lymphedema worldwide is filariasis (Chap. 218). Tumors, such as prostate cancer and lymphoma, can also obstruct lymphatic vessels. Both surgery and radiation therapy for breast carcinoma may cause lymphedema of the upper extremity. Less common causes include tuberculosis, contact dermatitis, lymphogranuloma venereum, rheumatoid arthritis, pregnancy, and self-induced or factitious lymphedema after application of tourniquets.

Lymphedema is generally a painless condition, but patients may experience a chronic dull, heavy sensation in the leg, and most often they are concerned about the appearance of the leg. Lymphedema of the lower extremity, initially involving the foot, gradually progresses up the leg so that the entire limb becomes edematous. In the early stages, the edema is soft and pits easily with pressure. In the chronic stages, the limb has a woody texture, and the tissues become indurated and fibrotic. At this point the edema may no longer be pitting. The limb loses its normal contour, and the toes appear square. Lymphedema should be distinguished from other disorders that cause unilateral leg swelling, such as DVT and chronic venous insufficiency. In the latter condition, the edema is softer, and there is often evidence of a stasis dermatitis, hyperpigmentation,

TABLE 249-4 Causes of Lymphedema

Primary	Secondary
Congenital (includes Milroy's disease)	Recurrent lymphangitis
Lymphedema praecox [includes Nonne-Milroy-Meige (or chronic familial lymhedema of the limbs) disease]	Filariasis
	Tuberculosis
	Neoplasm
Lymphedema tarda	Surgery
	Radiation therapy

and superficial venous varicosities. Other causes of leg swelling that resemble lymphedema are pretibial myxedema and lipedema. Pretibial myxedema occurs in patients with hyperthyroidism, especially Graves' disease, and is caused by deposition of hyaluronic acid-rich protein in the dermis. Lipedema usually occurs in women and is caused by accumulation of adipose tissue in the leg from the thigh to the ankle with sparing of the feet. The evaluation of patients with lymphedema should include diagnostic studies to clarify the cause. Abdominal and pelvic ultrasound and CT can be used to detect obstructing lesions such as neoplasms. MRI may reveal edema in the epifascial compartment and identify lymph nodes and enlarged lymphatic channels. Lymphoscintigraphy and lymphangiography are rarely indicated, but either can be used to confirm the diagnosis or differentiate primary from secondary lymphedema. Lymphoscintigraphy involves the injection of radioactively labeled technetium-containing colloid into the distal subcutaneous tissue of the affected extremity. In lymphangiography, contrast material is injected into a distal lymphatic vessel that has been isolated and cannulated. In primary lymphedema, lymphatic channels are absent, hypoplastic, or ectatic. In secondary lymphedema, lymphatic channels are usually dilated, and it may be possible to determine the level of obstruction.

TREATMENT Lymphedema

Patients with lymphedema of the lower extremities must be instructed to take meticulous care of their feet to prevent recurrent lymphangitis. Skin hygiene is important, and emollients can be used to prevent drying. Prophylactic antibiotics are often helpful, and fungal infection should be treated aggressively. Patients should be encouraged to participate in physical activity; frequent leg elevation can reduce the amount of edema. Physical therapy, including massage to facilitate lymphatic drainage, may be helpful. Patients can be fitted with graduated compression hose to reduce the amount of lymphedema that develops with upright posture. Occasionally, intermittent pneumatic compression devices can be applied at home to facilitate reduction of the edema. Diuretics are contraindicated and may cause depletion of intravascular volume and metabolic abnormalities. Microsurgical lymphaticovenous anastomotic procedures have been performed to rechannel lymph flow from obstructed lymphatic vessels into the venous system.

FURTHER READINGS

Bergan J J et al: Chronic venous disease. N Engl J Med 355:488, 2006

Creager MA (ed): *Atlas of Vascular Disease*, 3rd ed. Philadelphia, Current Medicine Group, 2007

——— et al (eds): *Vascular Medicine*. Philadelphia, Saunders Elsevier, 2006

——— et al. Atherosclerotic Peripheral Vascular Disease Symposium II: Executive summary. Circulation 118:2811, 2008

Fowkes FG et al: Ankle brachial index combined with Framingham Risk Score to predict cardiovascular events and mortality: A meta-analysis. JAMA 300:197, 2008

Hirsch AT et al: ACC/AHA 2005 guidelines for the management of patients with peripheral arterial disease (lower extremity, renal, mesenteric, and abdominal aortic). J Am Coll Cardiol 47:1239, 2006

Norgren L et al: Inter-Society Consensus for the Management of Peripheral Arterial Disease (TASC II). J Vasc Surg 45:S5, 2007

Raju S, Neglen P: Clinical practice: Chronic venous insufficiency and varicose veins. N Engl J Med 360:2319, 2009

Rockson SG: Current concepts and future directions in the diagnosis and management of lymphatic vascular disease. Vasc Med 15:223, 2010

White C: Clinical practice: Intermittent claudication. N Engl J Med 356:1241, 2007

CHAPTER 250 Pulmonary Hypertension

Stuart Rich

Pulmonary hypertension, an abnormal elevation in pulmonary artery pressure, may be the result of left heart failure, pulmonary parenchymal or vascular disease, thromboembolism, or a combination of these factors. Whether the pulmonary hypertension arises from cardiac, pulmonary, or intrinsic vascular disease, it generally is a feature of advanced disease. Because the causes of pulmonary hypertension are so diverse, it is essential that the etiology underlying the pulmonary hypertension be clearly determined before beginning treatment.

PATHOPHYSIOLOGY

The right ventricle responds to an increase in pulmonary vascular resistance by increasing right ventricular (RV) systolic pressure to preserve cardiac output. In some patients, chronic changes occur in the pulmonary circulation, resulting in progressive remodeling of the vasculature, which can sustain or promote pulmonary hypertension even if the initiating factor is removed.

The ability of the RV to adapt to increased vascular resistance is influenced by several factors, including age and the rapidity of the development of pulmonary hypertension. For example, a large acute pulmonary thromboembolism can result in RV failure and shock, whereas chronic thromboembolic disease of equal severity may result in only mild exercise intolerance. Coexisting hypoxemia can impair the ability of the ventricle to compensate. Studies support the concept that RV failure occurs in pulmonary hypertension when the RV myocardium becomes ischemic as a result of excessive demands and inadequate RV coronary blood flow. The onset of RV failure, often manifest by peripheral edema, is associated with a poor outcome.

DIAGNOSIS

The most common symptom attributable to pulmonary hypertension is exertional dyspnea. Other common symptoms are fatigue, angina pectoris, syncope, near syncope, and peripheral edema.

The physical examination typically reveals increased jugular venous pressure, a reduced carotid pulse, and a palpable RV impulse. Most patients have an increased pulmonic component of the second heart sound, a right-sided fourth heart sound, and tricuspid regurgitation (Chap. 227). Peripheral cyanosis and/or edema tend to occur in later stages of the disease.

Laboratory findings

(Fig. 250-1) The chest x-ray generally shows enlarged central pulmonary arteries. The lung fields may reveal other pathology. The electrocardiogram usually shows right axis deviation and RV hypertrophy. The echocardiogram commonly demonstrates RV and right atrial enlargement, a reduction in left ventricular (LV) cavity size, and a tricuspid regurgitant jet that can be used to estimate RV systolic pressure by Doppler. Pulmonary function tests are helpful in documenting underlying obstructive airways disease, whereas high-resolution chest computed tomography (CT) is preferred to diagnose restrictive lung disease. Hypoxemia and an abnormal diffusing capacity for carbon monoxide occur with pulmonary hypertension of many causes. A perfusion lung scan is almost always abnormal in patients with thromboembolic pulmonary hypertension (Chap. 262). However, diffuse defects of a nonsegmental nature often can be seen in long-standing pulmonary hypertension in the absence of thromboemboli. Laboratory tests should include antinuclear antibody and HIV testing. Because of the high frequency of thyroid abnormalities in patients with idiopathic pulmonary hypertension, it is recommended that the thyroid-stimulating hormone level be determined periodically.

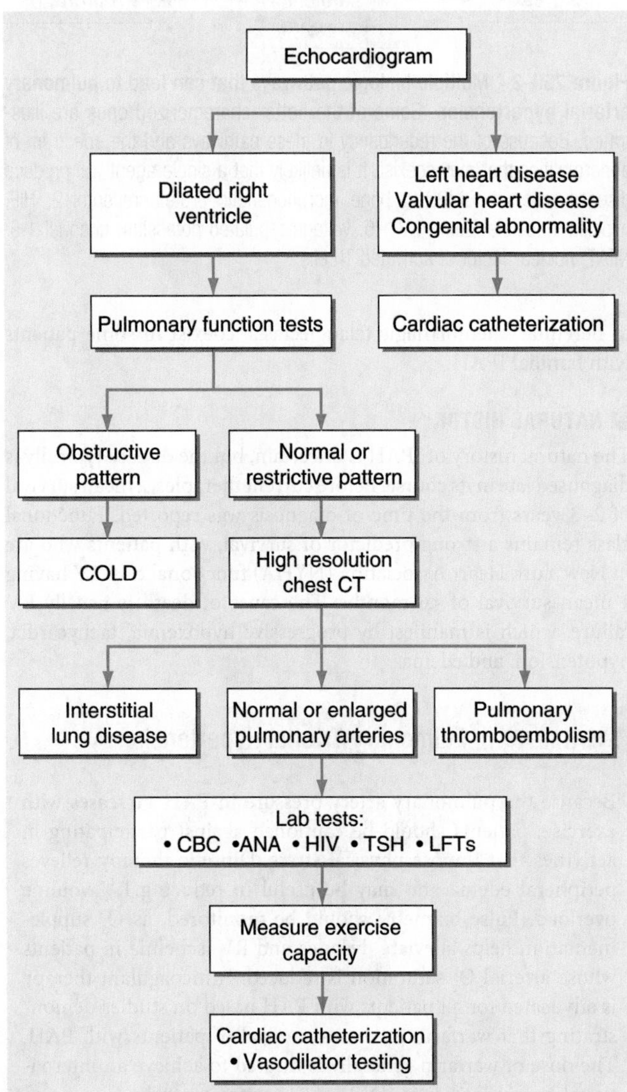

Figure 250-1 An algorithm for the workup of a patient with unexplained pulmonary hypertension. All potential etiologies and associated conditions must be investigated in a patient with clinical findings consistent with pulmonary hypertension. COLD, chronic obstructive lung disease; CBC, complete blood count; ANA, antinuclear antibodies; HIV, human immunodeficiency virus; TSH, thyroid-stimulating hormone; LFTs, liver function tests.

Cardiac catheterization

Cardiac catheterization is mandatory for accurate measurement of pulmonary artery pressure, cardiac output, and LV filling pressure as well as documentation of an underlying cardiac shunt. Care should be taken to record pressures only at end expiration. It is recommended that patients with pulmonary arterial hypertension undergo drug testing with a short-acting pulmonary vasodilator to determine the extent of pulmonary vasodilator reactivity. Inhaled nitric oxide, intravenous adenosine, and intravenous epoprostenol have comparable effects in reducing pulmonary artery pressure acutely. Nitric oxide is administered via inhalation in 10–20 parts per million. Adenosine is given in doses of 50 μg/kg per min and increased every 2 min until side effects develop. Epoprostenol is given in doses of 2 ng/kg per min and increased every 30 min until side effects develop. Patients who respond usually can be treated with calcium channel blockers and have a more favorable prognosis.

PULMONARY ARTERIAL HYPERTENSION

Pulmonary arterial hypertension (PAH) refers to a variety of diseases that include idiopathic PAH, as noted in Table 250-1. Patients with PAH have a common histopathology characterized by medial hypertrophy, eccentric and concentric intimal fibrosis, recanalized thrombi appearing as fibrous webs, and plexiform lesions.

PATHOBIOLOGY

Vasoconstriction, vascular proliferation, thrombosis, and inflammation appear to underlie the development of PAH (Fig. 250-2). Abnormalities in multiple molecular pathways and genes that regulate the pulmonary vascular endothelial and smooth muscle cells have been identified. These abnormalities include decreased expression of the voltage-regulated potassium channel, mutations in the bone morphogenetic protein-2 receptor, increased tissue factor expression, overactivation of the serotonin transporter, transcription factor activation of hypoxia-inducible factor-1 alpha, and activation of nuclear factor of activated T cells. As a result, there appears to be loss of apoptosis of the smooth muscle cells that allows their proliferation and the emergence of apoptosis-resistant endothelial cells that can obliterate the vascular lumen. In addition, thrombin deposition in the pulmonary vasculature from a procoagulant state that develops as an independent abnormality or as a result of endothelial dysfunction may amplify the vascular proliferation.

IDIOPATHIC PULMONARY ARTERIAL HYPERTENSION

Idiopathic pulmonary arterial hypertension (IPAH), formerly referred to as primary pulmonary hypertension, is uncommon, with an estimated incidence of two cases per million. There is a female predominance, with most patients presenting in the fourth and fifth decades, although the age range is from infancy to >60 years.

Familial IPAH accounts for up to 20% of cases of IPAH and is characterized by autosomal dominant inheritance and incomplete penetrance. The clinical and pathologic features of familial and sporadic IPAH are identical. Heterozygous germ-line mutations involving the gene that code the type II bone morphogenetic protein receptor (BMPR II), a member of the transforming growth factor (TGF) β superfamily, appear to account for most cases of familial IPAH. The TGF-β superfamilies include multifunctional proteins that initiate diverse cellular responses by binding to

TABLE 250-1 A Clinical Classification of Pulmonary Hypertension

Category 1. Pulmonary arterial hypertension (PAH)

Key feature: elevation in pulmonary arterial pressure (PAP) with normal pulmonary capillary wedge pressure (pcwp)

Includes:

Idiopathic (IPAH)
- Sporadic
- Familial
- Exposure to drugs or toxins
- Persistent pulmonary hypertension of the newborn
- Pulmonary capillary hemangiomatosis (PCH)

Associated with other active conditions
- Collagen vascular disease
- Congenital systemic-to-pulmonary shunts
- Portal hypertension
- HIV infection

Category 2. Pulmonary venous hypertension

Key feature: elevation in PAP with elevation in pcwp

Includes:
- Left-sided atrial or ventricular heart disease
- Left-sided valvular heart disease
- Pulmonary venous obstruction
- Pulmonary venoocclusive disease (PVOD)

Category 3. Pulmonary hypertension associated with hypoxemic lung disease

Key feature: chronic hypoxia with mild elevation of PAP

Includes:
- Chronic obstructive lung disease
- Interstitial lung disease
- Sleep-disordered breathing
- Alveolar hypoventilation disorders
- Chronic exposure to high altitude
- Developmental abnormalities

Category 4. Pulmonary hypertension due to chronic thromboembolic disease

Key feature: elevation of PA pressure with documentation of pulmonary arterial obstruction for >3 months

Includes:
- Chronic pulmonary thromboembolism
- Nonthrombotic pulmonary embolism (tumor, foreign material)

Category 5. Miscellaneous

Key feature: elevation in PAP in association with a systemic disease where a causal relationship is not clearly understood.

Includes:
- Sarcoidosis
- Chronic anemias
- Histiocytosis X
- Lymphangiomatosis
- Schistosomiasis

and activating serine/threonine kinase receptors. The low gene penetrance indicates that other risk factors or abnormalities are necessary to manifest clinical disease. Germ-line mutations in the activin-like kinase gene and endoglin gene, which have been linked

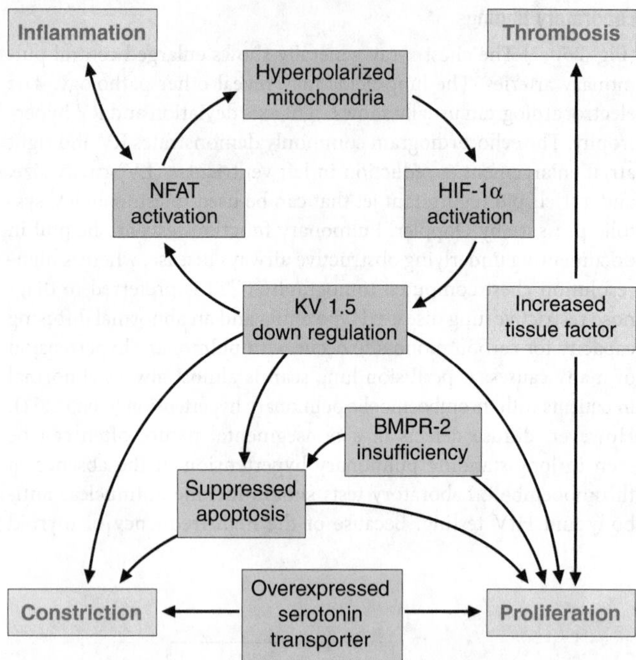

Figure 250-2 Multiple biologic pathways that can lead to pulmonary arterial hypertension. Some of the better-characterized ones are illustrated. Because of the redundancy in these pathways and the spectrum of abnormalities that may coexist, it is unlikely that a single agent will produce disease reversal. BMPR-2, bone morphogenetic protein receptor-2; HIF, hypoxia inducible factor; KV 1.5, voltage-regulated potassium channel 1.5; NFAT, nuclear factor of activated T cells.

to hereditary hemorrhagic telangiectasia, coexist in some patients with familial IPAH.

NATURAL HISTORY

The natural history of IPAH is uncertain, but the disease typically is diagnosed late in its course. Before current therapies, a mean survival of 2–3 years from the time of diagnosis was reported. Functional class remains a strong predictor of survival, with patients who are in New York Heart Association (NYHA) functional class IV having a mean survival of <6 months. The cause of death is usually RV failure, which is manifest by progressive hypoxemia, tachycardia, hypotension, and edema.

TREATMENT Pulmonary Arterial Hypertension

Because the pulmonary artery pressure in PAH increases with exercise, patients should be cautioned against participating in activities that impose physical stress. Diuretic therapy relieves peripheral edema and may be useful in reducing RV volume overload. Pulse oximetry should be monitored, as O_2 supplementation helps alleviate dyspnea and RV ischemia in patients whose arterial O_2 saturation is reduced. Anticoagulant therapy is advocated for all patients with PAH based on studies demonstrating that warfarin increases survival of patients with PAH. The dose of warfarin generally is titrated to achieve an international normalized ratio (INR) of 2–3 times control.

Several treatments are approved for PAH; they are reviewed below without making a distinction among the different types. However, the efficacy and side effects of these drugs may not be the same in all types of PAH. Other than calcium channel blockers, none of the drugs produce a significant lowering of the pulmonary arterial pressure, and their long-term effects on

TABLE 250-2 Principles of Drug Treatment of Pulmonary Arterial Hypertension

- Establish a correct diagnosis:
  Patients should undergo cardiac catheterization before initiating therapy.
- Obtain baseline assessments of the disease:
  Tests should be obtained to monitor the patient's response to therapy to know whether the treatments are effective.
- Test vasoreactivity:
  Patients should be tested at the time of diagnosis so that reactive patients are not missed.
- Reactive patients should be treated with calcium channel blockers:
  Calcium blockers in high doses are the drugs of choice.
- Nonreactive patients should be offered other therapies:
  No specific treatment has been established as first-line therapy.
- Periodic follow-up assessment of drug efficacy is essential:
  Repeat assessments should be performed within 8 weeks of initiating a new drug, as patients who do not respond initially are not likely to respond with longer exposure.
  Therapies can lose efficacy over time.
- Ineffective treatments should be replaced:
  A different treatment should be substituted rather than added.
  Patients who fail all treatments should be considered for lung transplantation.
- Benefits and risks of combination therapies are largely unknown:
  Only the addition of sildenafil to epoprostenol has been shown to be efficacious.

survival are undefined. The principles for the selection and use of the approved drug treatments are reviewed in Table 250-2.

CALCIUM CHANNEL BLOCKERS Patients who respond to short-acting vasodilators at the time of cardiac catheterization (a fall in mean pulmonary arterial pressure ≥10 mmHg and a final mean pressure <40 mmHg) should be treated with calcium channel blockers. Typically, these patients require high doses (e.g., nifedipine, 240 mg/d, or amlodipine, 20 mg/d). Patients may have dramatic reductions in pulmonary artery pressure and pulmonary vascular resistance associated with improved symptoms, regression of RV hypertrophy, and improved survival now documented to exceed 20 years. However, <20% of patients respond to calcium channel blockers in the long term. These drugs are not effective in patients who are not vasoreactive. They also have not been approved for the treatment of PAH by the U.S. Food and Drug Administration.

ENDOTHELIN RECEPTOR ANTAGONISTS The endothelin receptor antagonists *bosentan* and *ambrisentan* are approved treatments of PAH. In randomized clinical trials, both improved exercise tolerance as measured by an increase in 6-min walking distance. Therapy with bosentan is initiated at 62.5 mg bid for the first month and increased to 125 mg bid thereafter. Ambrisentan is initiated as 5 mg once daily and can be increased to 10 mg daily. Because of the high frequency of abnormal hepatic function tests associated with these drugs, primarily an increase in transaminases, it is recommended that liver function be monitored monthly throughout the duration of use. Bosentan is contraindicated in patients who are on cyclosporine or glyburide concurrently.

PHOSPHODIESTERASE-5 INHIBITORS *Sildenafil* and *tadalafil*, phosphodiesterase-5 inhibitors, are approved for the treatment of PAH. Phosphodiesterase-5 is responsible for the hydrolysis of cyclic GMP in pulmonary vascular smooth muscle, the mediator through which nitric oxide lowers pulmonary artery pressure and inhibits pulmonary vascular growth. Clinical trials have shown that both drugs improve exercise tolerance in patients with PAH. The effective dose for sildenafil is 20–80 mg tid. The effective dose for tadalafil is 40 mg once daily. The most common side effect is headache. Neither drug should be given to patients who are taking nitrovasodilators.

PROSTACYCLINS *Iloprost*, a prostacyclin analogue, is approved via inhalation for PAH. It has been shown to improve a composite measure of symptoms and exercise tolerance by 10%. Therapy can be given at either 2.5 or 5 μg per inhalation treatment via a dedicated nebulizer. The most common side effects are flushing and cough. Because of the very short half-life (<30 min) it is recommended that treatments be administered as often as every 2 h.

Epoprostenol is approved as a chronic IV treatment of PAH. Clinical trials have demonstrated an improvement in symptoms, exercise tolerance, and survival even if no acute hemodynamic response to drug challenge occurs. Drug administration requires placement of a permanent central venous catheter and infusion through an ambulatory infusion pump system. Side effects include flushing, jaw pain, and diarrhea, which are tolerated by most patients.

Treprostinil, an analogue of epoprostenol, is approved for PAH and may be given intravenously, subcutaneously, or via inhalation. Clinical trials have demonstrated an improvement in symptoms with exercise. Local pain at the infusion site with subcutaneous administration has caused most patients to switch to another therapy. Side effects are similar to those seen with epoprostenol.

The intravenous prostacyclins have the greatest efficacy as treatments for PAH and are often effective in patients who have failed all other treatments. Favorable properties include vasodilation, platelet inhibition, inhibition of vascular smooth muscle growth, and inotropic effects. It generally takes several months to titrate the dose of epoprostenol or treprostinil upward to achieve optimal clinical efficacy, which can be determined by symptoms, exercise testing, and catheterization. The optimal doses of these drugs have not been determined, but the typical doses of epoprostenol range from 25 to 40 ng/kg per min, and from 75 to 150 ng/kg per min for treprostinil. The major problem with intravenous therapy is infection related to the indwelling venous catheter, which requires close monitoring and diligence on the part of the patient. In addition, abrupt discontinuation of intravenous prostacyclins can lead to a rebound increase in pulmonary pressure.

It is recommended that every patient diagnosed with PAH be treated. Although no drug has been demonstrated to be superior as first-line therapy, many prefer to initiate treatment with an oral or inhaled form of therapy. Patients who fail to improve adequately within the first 2 months should be switched to a different therapy, as there is concern that delaying a more effective treatment may allow the disease to progress and become less responsive. The use of these drugs in combination has become popular, but the only randomized clinical trial demonstrating beneficial effects added sildenafil to patients treated with epoprostenol.

LUNG TRANSPLANTATION (See also Chap. 266) Lung transplantation is considered for patients who, while on an intravenous prostacyclin, continue to manifest right heart failure.

Acceptable results have been achieved with heart-lung, bilateral lung, and single-lung transplantation. The availability of donor organs often influences the choice of procedure.

CONDITIONS ASSOCIATED WITH PULMONARY HYPERTENSION

COLLAGEN VASCULAR DISEASE

All the collagen vascular diseases may be associated with PAH. This complication occurs commonly with the CREST syndrome (calcinosis, Raynaud's phenomenon, esophageal involvement, sclerodactyly, and telangiectasia) and in scleroderma (Chap. 323) and less frequently in systemic lupus erythematosus (Chap. 319), Sjögren's syndrome (Chap. 324), dermatomyositis, polymyositis (Chap. 326), and rheumatoid arthritis (Chap. 321). Often these patients have coexistent interstitial pulmonary fibrosis even though it may not be apparent on chest x-ray, CT, or pulmonary function tests. Consequently, they tend to have hypoxemia as an important clinical feature, along with the other classic findings of pulmonary hypertension. A fall in diffusing capacity may precede the development of pulmonary hypertension. Treatment of these patients is identical to that of patients with IPAH (see above) but is less effective. The treatment of the pulmonary hypertension, however, does not affect the natural history of the underlying collagen vascular disease.

CONGENITAL SYSTEMIC TO PULMONARY SHUNTS

It is common for large post-tricuspid cardiac shunts (e.g., ventricular septal defect, patent ductus arteriosus) to produce severe PAH (Chap. 236). Although less common, this also may occur in pretricuspid shunts (e.g., atrial septal defect, anomalous pulmonary venous drainage). In patients with uncorrected shunts, the clinical features include those associated with right-to-left shunting, such as hypoxemia and peripheral cyanosis, which worsen dramatically with exertion (Chap. 35). PAH may also occur years or even decades after surgical correction in the absence of right-to-left shunting. These patients present similarly to patients with IPAH but tend to have better long-term survival. The treatments are similar to those for IPAH.

PORTAL HYPERTENSION

Portal hypertension is associated with PAH, but the mechanism is unknown. Patients with advanced cirrhosis can have the combined features of a high-output cardiac state in association with the features of pulmonary hypertension and RV failure. Thus, a normal cardiac output may actually reflect a marked impairment of RV function. The etiology of ascites and edema can be confusing in these patients because this condition can have both cardiac and hepatic causes. Overall, these patients have a worse prognosis than do patients with IPAH. Patients with mild pulmonary hypertension who have a favorable response to epoprostenol have undergone successful liver transplantation with improvement of the pulmonary vascular disease.

ANOREXIGENS

A causal relationship has been established between exposure to several anorexigens, including aminorex and the fenfluramines, and the development of PAH. Often the pulmonary hypertension will develop years after the last exposure. Although the clinical features are identical to those of IPAH, the patients appear to be less responsive to medical treatments.

PULMONARY CAPILLARY HEMANGIOMATOSIS

Pulmonary capillary hemangiomatosis is a very rare form of pulmonary hypertension. Histologically it is characterized by the presence of infiltrating thin-walled blood vessels throughout the pulmonary interstitium and walls of the pulmonary arteries and veins. The presenting symptoms are those of IPAH but often with hypoxemia or hemoptysis as a clinical feature. The diagnosis may be suggested by findings on chest CT. The clinical course is usually one of progressive deterioration leading to death. There is no established therapy.

PULMONARY VENOUS HYPERTENSION

Pulmonary hypertension occurs as a result of increased resistance to pulmonary venous drainage. It is associated with diastolic dysfunction of the left ventricle, diseases affecting the pericardium or mitral or aortic valves, and rare entities such as cor triatriatum, left atrial myxoma, extrinsic compression of the central pulmonary veins from fibrosing mediastinitis, and pulmonary venoocclusive disease. Pulmonary venous hypertension affects the pulmonary veins and venules, producing arterialization of the external elastic lamina, medial hypertrophy, and focal eccentric intimal fibrosis. Microcirculatory lesions include capillary congestion, focal alveolar edema, and dilation of the interstitial lymphatics. Although these lesions are potentially reversible, regression may take years after the underlying cause is removed. Pulmonary venous hypertension often triggers reactive vasoconstriction in the pulmonary arterial bed and results in proliferative changes of the intima and media that can produce severe elevations in pulmonary artery pressure. Clinically it may be confusing and appear as if two separate disease processes are occurring simultaneously. The distinction is important, however, as treatments that are effective in PAH may make patients with pulmonary venous hypertension worse.

LEFT VENTRICULAR DIASTOLIC DYSFUNCTION

Pulmonary hypertension as a result of LV diastolic failure is common but often unrecognized (Chap. 234). It can occur with or without LV systolic failure. The most common risk factors are hypertensive heart disease; coronary artery disease; and impaired LV compliance related to age, diabetes, obesity, and hypoxemia. Symptoms of orthopnea and paroxysmal nocturnal dyspnea are prominent. Many patients improve considerably if LV end-diastolic pressure is lowered, but current treatments are unsatisfactory.

MITRAL VALVE DISEASE

Mitral stenosis and mitral regurgitation represent important causes of pulmonary hypertension (Chap. 237) from reactive pulmonary vasoconstriction resulting in marked elevations in pulmonary artery pressures. An echocardiogram usually shows abnormalities such as thickened mitral valve leaflets with reduced mobility or severe mitral regurgitation documented by Doppler echocardiography (Chap. 229). At cardiac catheterization, a pressure gradient between the pulmonary capillary wedge pressure and LV end-diastolic pressure is diagnostic of mitral stenosis.

In patients with mitral stenosis, corrective surgery of the mitral valve or mitral balloon valvuloplasty predictably results in a reduction in pulmonary artery pressure and pulmonary vascular resistance. Patients with mitral regurgitation, however, may not have as dramatic a response to surgery because of persistent elevations in LV end-diastolic pressure.

PULMONARY VENOOCCLUSIVE DISEASE

Pulmonary venoocclusive disease is a rare and distinct pathologic entity found in <10% of patients who present with unexplained pulmonary hypertension. Histologically it is manifest by intimal proliferation and fibrosis of the intrapulmonary veins and venules, occasionally extending to the arteriolar bed. A CT scan may reveal septal thickening, diffuse or mosaic ground-glass opacities, multiple small nodules, or areas of alveolar consolidation. Advanced pulmonary venous obstruction explains the orthopnea that can mimic LV failure, pulmonary edema noted on chest x-ray, and the increase in pulmonary capillary wedge pressure at catheterization. Effective therapy for this condition has not been established.

PULMONARY HYPERTENSION ASSOCIATED WITH LUNG DISEASE AND HYPOXEMIA

The acute hypoxic response of the pulmonary arterial smooth muscle cells involves inhibition of the potassium current, membrane depolarization, and calcium entry through L-type calcium channels. Hypoxia, acting through the small G protein RhoA, stimulates Rho kinase, which inhibits myosin vs. heavy chain in light chain phosphatase, thereby increasing phosphorylation of the light chain and augmenting contraction. Chronic hypoxia results in muscularization of the arterioles with minimal effects on the intima. When it occurs as an isolated entity, the changes produced are potentially reversible.

Although chronic hypoxia is an established cause of pulmonary hypertension, it rarely leads to an increase in the systolic pulmonary artery pressure >50 mmHg. Polycythemia in response to the hypoxemia is a characteristic finding. Hypoxia also may occur in conjunction with other causes of pulmonary hypertension associated with more extensive vascular changes. Clinically, the hypoxia has an added adverse effect. Patients with chronic hypoxia who have a marked elevation in pulmonary pressure should be evaluated for the other causes of the pulmonary hypertension.

CHRONIC OBSTRUCTIVE LUNG DISEASE

Chronic obstructive lung disease (COLD) is associated with mild pulmonary hypertension in the advanced stages (Chap. 260). The factors leading to an increase in pulmonary vascular resistance are numerous, but alveolar hypoxia is considered the predominant one. The presence of pulmonary hypertension in patients with COLD confers a worse outcome. The only effective therapy is supplemental oxygen. Clinical trials have documented that continuous oxygen therapy relieves the pulmonary vasoconstriction, reverses chronic ischemia throughout the systemic and pulmonary vascular beds, and improves survival. Long-term oxygen therapy is indicated if the resting arterial Po_2 remains <55 mmHg. Pulmonary vasodilators can worsen gas exchange and should not be used.

INTERSTITIAL LUNG DISEASE

Pulmonary hypertension is common in interstitial lung disease that results from parenchymal and vascular remodeling (Chap. 261). Coexisting hypoxemia occurs frequently and contributes to morbidity. Interstitial lung disease often is associated with the collagen vascular diseases. Many patients have pulmonary fibrosis of unknown etiology. Patients are commonly older than 50 years and report an insidious onset of progressive dyspnea and cough for months to years. It is uncommon for the mean pulmonary artery pressure to exceed 40 mmHg. The pulmonary vasodilators approved for PAH have not been shown to be helpful.

SLEEP-DISORDERED BREATHING

The incidence of pulmonary hypertension in the setting of *obstructive sleep apnea*, a common condition (Chap. 265), is <20% and is generally mild. Some patients have severe pulmonary hypertension in conjunction with sleep apnea, which may be unrelated. It is recommended that the sleep apnea and the PAH be treated as coexisting problems.

ALVEOLAR HYPOVENTILATION

Pulmonary hypertension can occur in patients with chronic hypoventilation and hypoxia secondary to thoracovertebral deformities. Symptoms are slowly progressive and are related to hypoxemia (Chap. 264). In patients with advanced disease, intermittent positive-pressure breathing and supplemental oxygen have been used successfully.

Pulmonary hypertension secondary to hypoxemia has been reported in patients with neuromuscular disease as a result of generalized weakness of the respiratory muscles and in patients with diaphragmatic paralysis, generally from trauma to the phrenic nerve. Patients with nontraumatic bilateral diaphragmatic paralysis may go unrecognized until they present with either respiratory failure or pulmonary hypertension.

PULMONARY HYPERTENSION DUE TO THROMBOEMBOLIC DISEASE

DEEP VENOUS THROMBOSIS AND PULMONARY EMBOLISM

See Chap. 262.

CHRONIC THROMBOEMBOLIC PULMONARY HYPERTENSION

Most patients treated for acute pulmonary thromboembolism with intravenous heparin and chronic oral warfarin do not develop chronic pulmonary hypertension. However, some patients have impaired fibrinolytic resolution of the thromboembolism, which leads to organization and incomplete recanalization and chronic obstruction of the pulmonary vascular bed. Because the initial pulmonary thromboembolism goes undetected or untreated, many patients are misdiagnosed as having IPAH. These patients may have underlying thrombophilic disorders, such as the lupus anticoagulant/anticardiolipin antibody syndrome, prothrombin gene mutation, or factor V Leiden (Chap. 117).

Diagnosis

The physical examination is characteristic of pulmonary hypertension but may include bruits heard over areas of the lung, representing blood flow through vessels with partial occlusion. A perfusion lung scan or contrast-enhanced spiral CT scan should reveal multiple thromboemboli. High-resolution CT scanning is necessary to document the location and proximal extent of the thromboemboli and hence the potential for operability.

TREATMENT Chronic Thromboembolic Pulmonary Hypertension

Pulmonary thromboendarterectomy is an established surgical treatment in patients whose thrombi are accessible to surgical removal. The operative mortality is <10% in experienced centers. Postoperative survivors can expect an improvement in functional class and exercise tolerance. Lifelong anticoagulation using warfarin is mandatory. Thrombolytic therapy is rarely helpful in patients with chronic thromboembolic pulmonary hypertension and may expose them to the increased risk of bleeding without potential benefit.

OTHER DISORDERS AFFECTING THE PULMONARY VASCULATURE

SARCOIDOSIS

Sarcoidosis can produce pulmonary hypertension as a result of fibrocystic lung involvement (Chap. 329) or direct cardiovascular involvement. Consequently, patients with sarcoidosis who present with progressive dyspnea and pulmonary hypertension require a thorough evaluation. There is a subset of patients with sarcoidosis and severe pulmonary hypertension who exhibit a favorable response to epoprostenol therapy.

SICKLE CELL DISEASE

Cardiovascular system abnormalities are prominent in the clinical spectrum of sickle cell disease, including pulmonary hypertension. The etiology is multifactorial, including hemolysis, hypoxemia, thromboembolism, chronic high cardiac output, and chronic liver disease. The presence of pulmonary hypertension in patients with sickle cell disease is associated with higher mortality. Intensification of sickle cell disease–specific therapy appears to reduce the morbidity. Clinical trials assessing drugs to treat pulmonary hypertension are ongoing, but the efficacy of those drugs is unknown.

SCHISTOSOMIASIS

Although extremely rare in North America, schistosomiasis is one of the most common causes of pulmonary hypertension worldwide (Chap. 219). The development of pulmonary hypertension occurs in the setting of hepatosplenic disease and portal hypertension. Studies suggest that inflammation from the infection triggers the pulmonary vascular changes that occur. The diagnosis is confirmed by finding the parasite ova in the urine or stools of patients with symptoms, which can be difficult. The efficacy of therapies directed toward pulmonary hypertension in these patients is unknown.

HIV INFECTION

The mechanism by which HIV infection produces pulmonary hypertension is unknown (Chap. 189). Although the incidence is estimated at 1 per 200 cases, the marked rise in the prevalence of HIV infection worldwide could have a significant impact on the frequency with which these entities are seen in combination. The evaluation and treatments are identical to those for IPAH. Treatment of the HIV infection does not appear to affect the severity or natural history of the underlying pulmonary hypertension.

FURTHER READINGS

CONDLIFFE R: Connective tissue disease-associated pulmonary arterial hypertension in the modern treatment era. Am J Respir Crit Care Med 179:151, 2009

DILLER GP, GATZOULIS MA: Pulmonary vascular disease in adults with congenital heart disease. Circulation 115:1039, 2007

MACCHIA A et al: Systematic review of trials using vasodilators in pulmonary arterial hypertension: Why a new approach is needed. Am Heart J 159:245, 2010

MCLAUGHLIN VV et al: ACCF/AHA Expert consensus document on pulmonary hypertension. J Am Coll Cardiol 53;1573, 2009

RABINOVITCH M: Molecular pathogenesis of pulmonary arterial hypertension. J Clin Invest 118:2372, 2008

RICH S, MCLAUGHLIN VV: Pulmonary hypertension, in *Braunwald's Heart Disease: A Textbook of Cardiovascular Medicine*, 8th ed, P Libby et al (eds). Philadelphia, Elsevier Saunders, 2008

PART 11

Disorders of the Respiratory System

SECTION 1 Diagnosis of Respiratory Disorders

SECTION 2 Diseases of the Respiratory System

CHAPTER 251

Approach to the Patient With Disease of the Respiratory System

Patricia Kritek
Augustine Choi

The majority of diseases of the respiratory system fall into one of three major categories: (1) obstructive lung diseases; (2) restrictive disorders; and (3) abnormalities of the vasculature. Obstructive lung diseases are most common and primarily include disorders of the airways such as asthma, chronic obstructive pulmonary disease (COPD), bronchiectasis, and bronchiolitis. Diseases resulting in restrictive pathophysiology include parenchymal lung diseases, abnormalities of the chest wall and pleura, as well as neuromuscular disease. Disorders of the pulmonary vasculature are not always recognized and include pulmonary embolism, pulmonary hypertension, and pulmonary venoocclusive disease. Although many specific diseases fall into these major categories, both infective and neoplastic processes can affect the respiratory system and may result in myriad pathologic findings, including obstruction, restriction, and pulmonary vascular disease (see Table 251-1).

The majority of respiratory diseases present with abnormal gas exchange. Disorders can also be grouped into the categories of gas exchange abnormalities, including hypoxemic, hypercarbic, or combined impairment. Importantly, many diseases of the lung do not manifest gas exchange abnormalities.

As with the evaluation of most patients, the approach to a patient with disease of the respiratory system begins with a thorough history. A focused physical examination is helpful in further categorizing the specific pathophysiology. Many patients will subsequently undergo pulmonary function testing, chest imaging, blood and sputum analysis, a variety of serologic or microbiologic studies, and diagnostic procedures, such as bronchoscopy. This step-wise approach is discussed in detail below.

TABLE 251-1 Categories of Respiratory Disease

Category	Examples
Obstructive lung disease	Asthma
	COPD
	Bronchiectasis
	Bronchiolitis
Restrictive pathophysiology—parenchymal disease	Idiopathic pulmonary fibrosis (IPF)
	Asbestosis
	Desquamative interstitial pneumonitis (DIP)
	Sarcoidosis
Restrictive pathophysiology—neuromuscular weakness	Amyotrophic lateral sclerosis (ALS)
	Guillain-Barré syndrome
Restrictive pathophysiology—chest wall/pleural disease	Kyphoscoliosis
	Ankylosing spondylitis
	Chronic pleural effusions
Pulmonary vascular disease	Pulmonary embolism
	Pulmonary arterial hypertension (PAH)
Malignancy	Bronchogenic carcinoma (non-small-cell and small cell)
	Metastatic disease
Infectious diseases	Pneumonia
	Bronchitis
	Tracheitis

Abbreviation: COPD, chronic obstructive pulmonary disease.

HISTORY

■ DYSPNEA AND COUGH

The cardinal symptoms of respiratory disease are dyspnea and cough (Chaps. 33 and 34). Dyspnea can result from many causes, some of which are not predominantly caused by lung pathology. The words a patient uses to describe breathlessness or shortness of breath can suggest certain etiologies of the dyspnea. Patients with obstructive lung disease often complain of "chest tightness" or "inability to get a deep breath," whereas patients with congestive heart failure more commonly report "air hunger" or a sense of suffocation.

The tempo of onset and duration of a patient's dyspnea are helpful in determining the etiology. Acute shortness of breath is usually associated with sudden physiological changes, such as laryngeal edema, bronchospasm, myocardial infarction, pulmonary embolism, or pneumothorax. Patients with underlying lung disease commonly have progressive shortness of breath or episodic dyspnea. Patients with COPD and idiopathic pulmonary fibrosis (IPF) have a gradual progression of dyspnea on exertion, punctuated by acute exacerbations of shortness of breath. In contrast, most asthmatics have normal breathing the majority of the time and have recurrent episodes of dyspnea usually associated with specific triggers, such as an upper respiratory tract infection or exposure to allergens.

Specific questioning should focus on factors that incite the dyspnea, as well as any intervention that helps resolve the patient's shortness of breath. Of the obstructive lung diseases, asthma is most likely to have specific triggers related to sudden onset of dyspnea, although this can also be true of COPD. Many patients with lung disease report dyspnea on exertion. It is useful to determine the degree of activity that results in shortness of breath as it gives the clinician a gauge of the patient's degree of disability. Many patients adapt their level of activity to accommodate progressive limitation. For this reason it is important, particularly in older patients, to delineate the activities in which they engage and how they have changed over time. Dyspnea on exertion is often an early symptom of underlying lung or heart disease and warrants a thorough evaluation.

Cough is the other common presenting symptom that generally indicates disease of the respiratory system. The clinician should inquire about the duration of the cough, whether or not it associated with sputum production, and any specific triggers that induce it. Acute cough productive of phlegm is often a symptom of infection of the respiratory system, including processes affecting the upper airway (e.g., sinusitis, tracheitis) as well as the lower airways (e.g., bronchitis, bronchiectasis) and lung parenchyma (e.g., pneumonia). Both the quantity and quality of the sputum, including whether it is blood-streaked or frankly bloody, should be determined. Hemoptysis warrants an evaluation as delineated in Chap. 34.

Chronic cough (defined as persisting for more than 8 weeks) is commonly associated with obstructive lung diseases, particularly asthma and chronic bronchitis, as well as "nonrespiratory" diseases, such as gastroesophageal reflux (GERD) and postnasal drip. Diffuse parenchymal lung diseases, including idiopathic pulmonary fibrosis, frequently present with a persistent, nonproductive cough. As with dyspnea, all causes of cough are not respiratory in origin, and assessment should consider a broad differential, including cardiac and gastrointestinal diseases as well as psychogenic causes.

ADDITIONAL SYMPTOMS

Patients with respiratory disease may complain of wheezing, which is suggestive of airways disease, particularly asthma. Hemoptysis, which must be distinguished from epistaxis or hematemesis, can be a symptom of a variety of lung diseases, including infections of the respiratory tract, bronchogenic carcinoma, and pulmonary embolism. Chest pain or discomfort is also often thought to be respiratory in origin. As the lung parenchyma is not innervated with pain fibers, pain in the chest from respiratory disorders usually results from either diseases of the parietal pleura (e.g., pneumothorax) or pulmonary vascular diseases (e.g., pulmonary hypertension). As many diseases of the lung can result in strain on the right side of the heart, patients may also present with symptoms of cor pulmonale, including abdominal bloating or distention, and pedal edema (Chap. 234).

ADDITIONAL HISTORY

A thorough social history is an essential component of the evaluation of patients with respiratory disease. All patients should be asked about current or previous cigarette smoking as this exposure is associated with many diseases of the respiratory system, most notably COPD and bronchogenic lung cancer but also a variety of diffuse parenchymal lung diseases [e.g., desquamative interstitial pneumonitis (DIP) and pulmonary Langerhans cell histiocytosis]. For most disorders, the duration and intensity of exposure to cigarette smoke increases the risk of disease. There is growing evidence that "second-hand smoke" is also a risk factor for respiratory tract pathology; for this reason, patients should be asked about parents, spouses, or housemates who smoke. It is becoming less common for patients to be exposed to cigarette smoke on the job, but for older patients, an occupational history should include the potential for heavy cigarette smoke exposure (e.g., flight attendants working prior to prohibition of smoking on airplanes).

Possible inhalational exposures should be explored, including those at the work place (e.g., asbestos, wood smoke) and those associated with leisure (e.g., pigeon excrement from pet birds, paint fumes) (Chap. 256). Travel predisposes to certain infections of the respiratory tract, most notably the risk of tuberculosis. Potential exposure to fungi found in specific geographic regions or climates (e.g., *Histoplasma capsulatum*) should be explored.

Associated symptoms of fever and chills should raise the suspicion of infective etiologies, both pulmonary and systemic. Some systemic diseases, commonly rheumatologic or autoimmune, present with respiratory tract manifestations. Review of systems should include evaluation for symptoms that suggest undiagnosed rheumatologic disease. These may include joint pain or swelling, rashes, dry eyes, dry mouth, or constitutional symptoms. Additionally, carcinomas from a variety of primary sources commonly metastasize to the lung and cause respiratory symptoms. Finally, therapy for other conditions, including both radiation and medications, can result in diseases of the chest.

PHYSICAL EXAMINATION

The clinician's suspicion for respiratory disease often begins with a patient's vital signs. The respiratory rate is often informative, whether elevated (tachypnea) or depressed (hypopnea). In addition, pulse oximetry should be measured as many patients with respiratory disease will have hypoxemia, either at rest or with exertion.

Simple observation of the patient is informative. Patients with respiratory disease may be in distress, often using accessory muscles of respiration to breathe. Severe kyphoscoliosis can result in restrictive pathophysiology. Inability to complete a sentence in conversation is generally a sign of severe impairment and should result in an expedited evaluation of the patient.

AUSCULTATION

The majority of the manifestations of respiratory disease present with abnormalities of the chest examination. Wheezes suggest airway obstruction and are most commonly a manifestation of asthma. Peribronchial edema in the setting of congestive heart failure, often referred to as "cardiac asthma," can also result in diffuse wheezes as can any other process that causes narrowing of small airways. For this reason, clinicians must take care not to attribute all wheezing to asthma.

Rhonchi are a manifestation of obstruction of medium-sized airways, most often with secretions. In the acute setting, this may be a sign of viral or bacterial bronchitis. Chronic rhonchi suggest bronchiectasis or COPD. Bronchiectasis, or permanent dilation and irregularity of the bronchi, often causes what is referred to as a "musical chest" with a combination of rhonchi, pops, and squeaks. Stridor or a low-pitched, focal inspiratory wheeze usually heard over the neck, is a manifestation of upper airway obstruction and should result in an expedited evaluation of the patient as it can precede complete upper airway obstruction and respiratory failure.

Crackles, or rales, are commonly a sign of alveolar disease. A variety of processes that fill the alveoli with fluid result in crackles. Pneumonia, or infection of the lower respiratory tract and air spaces, may cause crackles. Pulmonary edema, of cardiogenic or noncardiogenic cause, is associated with crackles, generally more prominent at the bases. Interestingly, diseases that result in fibrosis of the interstitium (e.g., IPF) also result in crackles often sounding like Velcro being ripped apart. Although some clinicians make a distinction between "wet" and "dry" crackles, this has not been shown to be a reliable way to differentiate among etiologies of respiratory disease.

One way to help distinguish between crackles associated with alveolar fluid and those associated with interstitial fibrosis is to assess for egophony. Egophony is the auscultation of the sound "AH" instead of "EEE" when a patient phonates "EEE." This change in note is due to abnormal sound transmission through consolidated lung and will be present in pneumonia but not in IPF. Similarly, areas of alveolar filling have increased whispered pectoriloquy as well as transmission of larger airway sounds (i.e., bronchial breath sounds in a lung zone where vesicular breath sounds are expected).

The lack of breath sounds or diminished breath sounds can also help determine the etiology of respiratory disease. Patients with emphysema often have a quiet chest with diffusely decreased breath sounds. A pneumothorax or pleural effusion may present with an area of absent breath sounds, although this is not always the case.

REMAINDER OF CHEST EXAMINATION

In addition to auscultation, percussion of the chest helps distinguish among pathologic processes of the respiratory system. Diseases of the pleural space are often suggested by differences in percussion note. An area of dullness may suggest a pleural effusion, whereas hyperresonance, particularly at the apex, can indicate air in the pleural space (i.e., pneumothorax).

Tactile fremitus will be increased in areas of lung consolidation, such as pneumonia, and decreased with pleural effusion. Decreased diaphragmatic excursion can suggest neuromuscular weakness manifesting as respiratory disease or hyperinflation associated with COPD.

Careful attention should also be paid to the cardiac examination with particular emphasis on signs of right heart failure as it is associated with chronic hypoxemic lung disease and pulmonary vascular disease. The clinician should feel for a right ventricular heave and listen for a prominent P2 component of the second heart sound, as well as a right-sided S4.

OTHER SYSTEMS

Pedal edema, if symmetric, may suggest cor pulmonale, and if asymmetric may be due to deep venous thrombosis and associated pulmonary embolism. Jugular venous distention may also be a sign of volume overload associated with right heart failure. Pulsus paradoxus is an ominous sign in a patient with obstructive lung disease as it is associated with significant negative intrathoracic (pleural) pressures required for ventilation, and impending respiratory failure.

As stated earlier, rheumatologic disease may manifest primarily as lung disease. Owing to this association, particular attention should be paid to joint and skin examination. Clubbing can be found in many lung diseases, including cystic fibrosis, IPF, and lung cancer, although it can also be associated with inflammatory bowel disease or as a congenital finding of no clinical importance. Patients with COPD do not usually have clubbing; thus, this sign should warrant an investigation for second process, most commonly an unrecognized bronchogenic carcinoma, in these patients. Cyanosis is seen in hypoxemic respiratory disorders that result in more than 5 g/dL deoxygenated hemoglobin.

DIAGNOSTIC EVALUATION

The sequence of studies is dictated by the clinician's differential diagnosis determined by the history and physical examination. Acute respiratory symptoms are often evaluated with multiple tests obtained at the same time in order to diagnose any life threatening diseases rapidly (e.g., pulmonary embolism or multilobar pneumonia). In contrast, chronic dyspnea and cough can be evaluated in a more protracted, step-wise fashion.

PULMONARY FUNCTION TESTING

(See also Chap. 253) The initial pulmonary function test obtained is spirometry. This study is used to assess for obstructive pathophysiology as seen in asthma, COPD, and bronchiectasis. A diminished forced expiratory volume in 1 second (FEV_1)/forced vital capacity (FVC) (often defined as less than 70% of predicted value) is diagnostic of obstruction. History as well as further testing can help distinguish among different obstructive diseases. COPD is almost exclusively seen in cigarette smokers. Asthmatics often show an acute response to inhaled bronchodilators (e.g., albuterol). In addition to the measurements of FEV_1 and FVC, the clinician should examine the flow-volume loop. A plateau of the inspiratory or expiratory curves suggests large airway obstruction in extrathoracic and intrathoracic locations, respectively.

Normal spirometry or spirometry with symmetric decreases in FEV_1 and FVC warrants further testing, including lung volume measurement and the diffusion capacity of the lung for carbon monoxide (D_LCO). A total lung capacity (TLC) less than 80% of the predicted value for a patient's age, race, gender, and height defines restrictive pathophysiology. Restriction can result from parenchymal disease, neuromuscular weakness, or chest wall or pleural diseases. Restriction with impaired gas exchange, as indicated by a decreased D_LCO, suggests parenchymal lung disease. Additional testing, such as maximal expiratory pressure (MEP) and maximal inspiratory pressure (MIP), can help diagnose neuromuscular weakness. Normal spirometry, normal lung volumes, and a low D_LCO should prompt further evaluation for pulmonary vascular disease.

Arterial blood gas testing is often also helpful in assessing respiratory disease. Hypoxemia, while usually apparent with pulse oximetry, can be further evaluated with the measurement of arterial PO_2 and the calculation of an alveolar gas and arterial blood oxygen tension difference [(A-a)DO_2]. It should also be noted that at times, most often due to abnormal hemoglobins or non-oxygen hemoglobin-ligand complexes, pulse oximetry can be misleading (such as observed with carboxyhemoglobin). Diseases that cause ventilation-perfusion mismatch or shunt physiology will have an increased (A-a)DO_2 at rest. Arterial blood gas testing also allows for the measurement of arterial PCO_2. Most commonly, acute or chronic obstructive lung disease presents with hypercarbia; however, many diseases of the respiratory system can cause hypercarbia if the resulting increase in work of breathing is greater than that which allows a patient to sustain an adequate minute ventilation.

CHEST IMAGING

(See Chap. e34) Most patients with disease of the respiratory system will undergo imaging of the chest as part of initial evaluation. Clinicians should generally begin with a plain chest radiograph, preferably posterior-anterior (PA) and lateral films. Several findings, including opacities of the parenchyma, blunting of the costophrenic angles, mass lesions, and volume loss, can be very helpful in determining an etiology. It should be noted that many diseases of the respiratory system, particularly those of the airways and pulmonary vasculature, are associated with a normal chest radiograph.

Subsequent computed tomography of the chest (CT scan) is often obtained. The CT scan allows better delineation of parenchymal processes, pleural disease, masses or nodules, and large airways. If administered with contrast, the pulmonary vasculature can be assessed with particular utility for determination of pulmonary emboli. Intravenous contrast also allows lymph nodes to be delineated in greater detail.

FURTHER STUDIES

Depending on the clinician's suspicion, a variety of other studies may be obtained. Concern for large airway lesions may warrant bronchoscopy. This procedure may also be used to sample the alveolar space with bronchoalveolar lavage (BAL) or to obtain nonsurgical lung biopsies. Blood testing may include assessment for hypercoagulable states in the setting of pulmonary vascular disease, serologic testing for infectious or rheumatologic disease, or assessment of inflammatory markers or leukocyte counts (e.g., eosinophils). Sputum evaluation for malignant cells or microorganisms may be appropriate. An echocardiogram to assess right- and left-sided heart function is often obtained. Finally, at times, a surgical lung biopsy is needed to diagnose certain diseases of the respiratory system. All of these studies will be guided by the preceding history, physical examination, pulmonary function testing, and chest imaging.

FURTHER READINGS

IRWIN RS et al: Diagnosis and management of cough executive summary: ACCP evidence-based clinical practice guidelines. Chest 129:1S, 2006

MANNING HL, SCHWARTZSTEIN RM: Pathophysiology of dyspnea. N Engl J Med 333:1547, 1995

SCHWARTZSTEIN RM, PARKER MJ: *Respiratory Physiology: A Clinical Approach.* Philadelphia, Lippincott, 2006

WEINBERGER SE et al: *Principles of Pulmonary Medicine*, 5th ed. Philadelphia, Saunders, 2008

CHAPTER 252

Disturbances of Respiratory Function

Edward T. Naureckas
Julian Solway

INTRODUCTION

The primary function of the respiratory system is to oxygenate blood and eliminate carbon dioxide, which requires that blood come into virtual contact with fresh air to facilitate diffusion of respiratory gases between blood and gas. This process occurs in the lung alveoli, where blood flowing through alveolar wall capillaries is separated from alveolar gas by an extremely thin membrane of flattened endothelial and epithelial cells, across which respiratory gases diffuse and equilibrate. Blood flow through the lung is unidirectional via a continuous vascular path, along which venous blood absorbs oxygen from and loses CO_2 to inspired gas. The path for airflow, in contrast, reaches a dead end at the alveolar walls; as such, the alveolar space must be ventilated tidally, with inflow of fresh gas and outflow of alveolar gas alternating periodically at the respiratory rate (RR). To achieve an enormous alveolar surface area (typically 70 m^2) for blood-gas diffusion within the modest volume of a thoracic cavity (typically 7 L), nature has distributed both blood flow and ventilation among millions of tiny alveoli through multigenerational branching of both pulmonary arteries and bronchial airways. As a consequence of variations in tube lengths and calibers along these pathways, and of the effects of gravity, tidal pressure fluctuations, and anatomic constraints from the chest wall, there is variation among alveoli in their relative ventilations and perfusions. Not surprisingly, for the lung to be most efficient in exchanging gas, the fresh gas ventilation of a given alveolus must be matched to its perfusion.

For the respiratory system to succeed in oxygenating blood and eliminating carbon dioxide, it must be able to ventilate the lung tidally to freshen alveolar gas; it must provide for perfusion of the individual alveolus in a manner proportional to its ventilation; and it must allow for adequate diffusion of respiratory gases between alveolar gas and capillary blood. Furthermore, it must be able to accommodate severalfold increases in the demand for oxygen uptake or CO_2 elimination imposed by metabolic needs or acid-base derangement. Given these multiple requirements for normal operation, it is not surprising that many diseases disturb respiratory function. Here, we consider in greater detail the physiologic determinants of lung ventilation and perfusion, and how their matching distributions and rapid gas diffusion allow for normal gas exchange. We also discuss how common diseases derange these normal functions, and thereby impair gas exchange—or at least raise the work of the respiratory muscles or heart to maintain adequate respiratory function.

VENTILATION

It is useful to think about the respiratory system as having three independently functioning components—the lung including its airways, the neuromuscular system, and the chest wall; the latter includes everything that is not lung or active neuromuscular system. As such, the mass of the respiratory muscles is part of the chest wall, while the force they generate is part of the neuromuscular system; the abdomen (especially an obese abdomen) and the heart (especially an enlarged heart) are, for these purposes, part of the chest wall. Each of these three components has mechanical properties that relate to its enclosed volume, or in the case of the neuromuscular system, the respiratory system volume at which it is operating, and to the rate of change of its volume (i.e., flow).

■ VOLUME-RELATED MECHANICAL PROPERTIES—STATICS

Figure 252-1 shows the volume-related properties of each component of the respiratory system. Due both to surface tension at the air-liquid interface between alveolar wall lining fluid and alveolar gas and to elastic recoil of the lung tissue itself, the lung requires a positive transmural pressure difference between alveolar gas and its pleural surface to stay inflated; this difference is called the elastic recoil pressure of the lung, and it increases with lung volume. Importantly, the lung becomes rather stiff at high lung volumes, so that relatively small volume changes are accompanied by large changes in transpulmonary pressure; in contrast, the lung is compliant at lower lung volumes, including

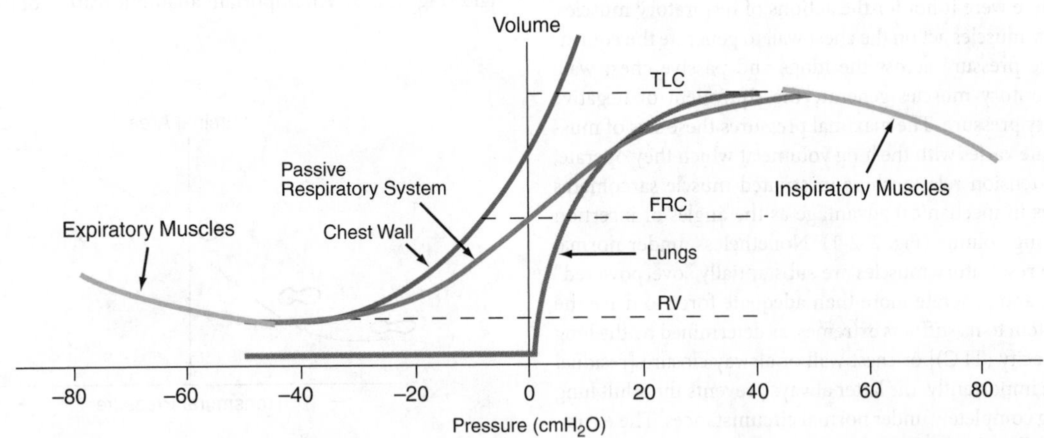

Figure 252-1 Pressure-volume curves of the isolated lung, isolated chest wall, combined respiratory system, inspiratory muscles, and expiratory muscles. FRC, functional residual capacity; RV, residual volume; TLC, total lung capacity.

those at which tidal breathing normally occurs. Note that at zero inflation pressure, even normal lungs retain some air in the alveoli. This occurs because the small peripheral airways of the lung are tethered open by radially outward pull from inflated lung parenchyma attached to adventitia; as the lung deflates during exhalation, those small airways are pulled open progressively less, and eventually they close, trapping some gas in the alveoli. This effect can be exaggerated with age and especially with obstructive airways diseases, resulting in gas trapping at quite large lung volumes.

The elastic behavior of the passive chest wall (i.e., in the absence of neuromuscular activation) differs markedly from that of the lung. Whereas the lung tends toward full deflation with no distending (transmural) pressure, the chest wall encloses a large volume when pleural pressure equals body surface (atmospheric) pressure. Furthermore, the chest wall is compliant at high enclosed volumes, readily expanding even further in response to increases in transmural pressure. The chest wall also remains compliant at small negative transmural pressures (i.e., when pleural pressure falls slightly below atmospheric pressure), but as the volume enclosed by the chest wall becomes quite small in response to large negative transmural pressures, the passive chest wall becomes stiff due to squeezing together of ribs and intercostal muscles, diaphragm stretch, displacement of abdominal contents, and straining of ligaments and bony articulations. Under normal circumstances, the lung and the passive chest wall enclose essentially the same volume, the only difference between these being the volumes of the pleural fluid and of the lung parenchyma (both quite small). As such, and because the lung and chest wall function in mechanical series, the pressure required to displace the passive respiratory system (lungs + chest wall) at any volume is simply the sum of the elastic recoil pressure of the lungs and the transmural pressure across the chest wall. When plotted against respiratory system volume, this relationship assumes a sigmoid shape, exhibiting stiffness at high lung volumes (imparted by the lung), stiffness at low lung volumes (imparted by the chest wall, or sometimes by airway closure), and compliance in the middle range of lung volumes. There is also a passive resting point of the respiratory system, attained when alveolar gas pressure equals body surface pressure (i.e., the transrespiratory system pressure is zero). At this volume [called *functional residual capacity* (FRC)], the outward recoil of the chest wall is balanced exactly by the inward recoil of the lung. As these recoils are transmitted through the pleural fluid, the latter is pulled both outward and inward simultaneously at FRC, and, thus, its pressure falls below atmospheric pressure (typically, –5 cmH_2O).

The normal passive respiratory system would equilibrate at FRC and remain there were it not for the actions of respiratory muscles. The inspiratory muscles act on the chest wall to generate the equivalent of positive pressure across the lungs and passive chest wall, while the expiratory muscles generate the equivalent of negative transrespiratory pressure. The maximal pressures these sets of muscles can generate varies with the lung volume at which they operate, due to length-tension relationships in striated muscle sarcomeres and to changes in mechanical advantage as the angles of insertion change with lung volume (Fig. 252-1). Nonetheless, under normal conditions the respiratory muscles are substantially "overpowered" for their roles, and generate more than adequate force to drive the respiratory system to its stiffness extremes, as determined by the lung [total lung capacity (TLC)] or chest wall or airway closure [residual volume (RV)]; importantly, the latter always prevents the adult lung from emptying completely under normal circumstances. The excursion between full and minimal lung inflation is called vital capacity (VC; Fig. 252-2), and is readily seen to be the difference between volumes at two unrelated stiffness extremes—one determined by the lung (TLC) and the other determined by the chest wall or airways (RV). Thus, although VC is easy to measure (see below), it tells one little about the intrinsic properties of the respiratory system. It is much more useful, as we shall see, for the clinician to know TLC and RV individually.

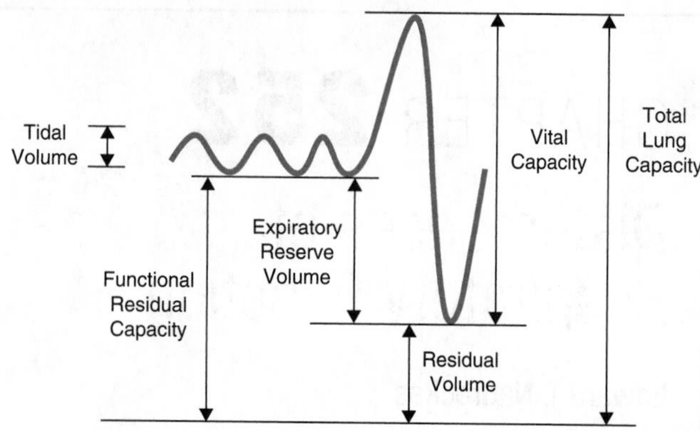

Figure 252-2 Spirogram demonstrating a slow vital capacity maneuver and various lung volumes.

■ FLOW-RELATED MECHANICAL PROPERTIES—DYNAMICS

The passive chest wall and active neuromuscular system do exhibit mechanical behaviors related to the rate of change of volume, but these become quantitatively important only at markedly supraphysiologic breathing frequencies (e.g., during high-frequency mechanical ventilation), and, thus, we shall not address these here. In contrast, the dynamic airflow properties of the lung substantially determine the ability to ventilate and contribute importantly to the work of breathing, and are often deranged by disease. Understanding these properties is, therefore, well worthwhile.

As with flow of any fluid (gas or liquid) in any tube, maintenance of airflow within the pulmonary airways requires a pressure gradient that falls along the direction of flow, the magnitude of which is determined by the flow rate and the frictional resistance to flow. During quiet tidal breathing, the pressure gradients driving inspiratory or expiratory flow are small owing to the very low frictional resistance of normal pulmonary airways (normally <2 cmH_2O/L per second). However, during rapid exhalation another phenomenon reduces flow below that which would have been expected were frictional resistance the only impediment to flow. This phenomenon is called dynamic airflow limitation, and it occurs because the bronchial airways through which air is exhaled are collapsible rather than rigid (Fig. 252-3). An important anatomic feature of the pulmonary

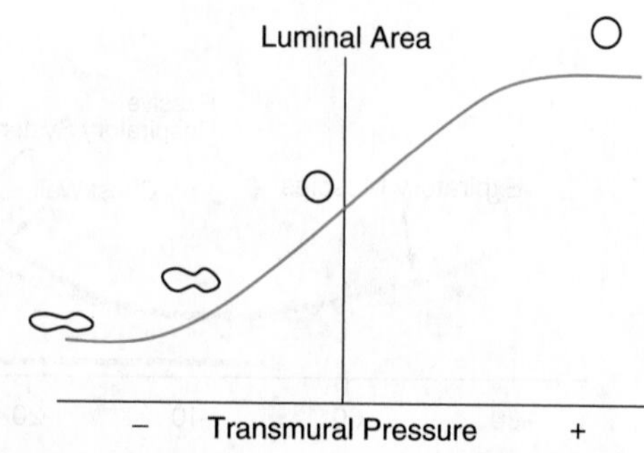

Figure 252-3 Luminal area versus transmural pressure relationship. Transmural pressure represents the pressure difference across the airway wall from inside to outside.

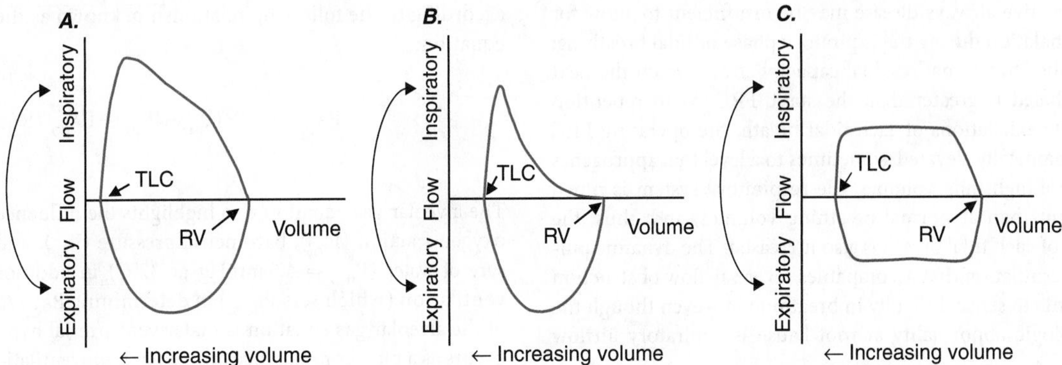

Figure 252-4 Flow-volume loops. ***A.*** Normal. ***B.*** Airflow obstruction. ***C.*** Fixed central airway obstruction. RV, residual volume; TLC, total lung capacity.

airways is its treelike branching structure. While the individual airways in each successive generation, from most proximal (trachea) to most distal (respiratory bronchioles), are smaller than those of the parent generation, their number increases exponentially such that the summed cross-sectional area of the airways becomes very large toward the lung periphery. Because flow (volume/time) is constant along the airway tree, the velocity of airflow (flow/summed cross-sectional area) is much greater in the central airways than in the peripheral airways. During exhalation, gas leaving the alveoli must therefore gain velocity as it proceeds toward the mouth. The energy required for this "convective" acceleration is drawn from the component of gas energy manifested as its local pressure, thereby reducing intraluminal gas pressure (the Bernoulli effect), reducing airway transmural pressure, reducing airway size (Fig. 252-3), and reducing flow. If one tries to exhale more forcefully, the local velocity increases further and reduces airway size further, resulting in no net increase in flow. Under these circumstances, flow has reached its maximum possible value, or its flow limit. Lungs normally exhibit such dynamic airflow limitation. The maximum value of flow is related to the gas density, airway cross-section and distensibility, the elastic recoil pressure of the lung, and the frictional pressure loss to the flow-limiting airway site. Under normal conditions, maximal expiratory flow falls with lung volume (Fig. 252-4), due primarily to the dependence of lung recoil pressure on lung volume (Fig. 252-1). In pulmonary fibrosis, lung recoil pressure is increased at any lung volume, and, thus, the maximum expiratory flow is relatively elevated when considered in relation to lung volume. Conversely, in emphysema, lung recoil pressure is reduced, which is a principal mechanism by which maximal expiratory flows fall. Diseases that narrow the airway lumen at any transmural pressure, such as asthma or chronic bronchitis, or which cause excessive airway collapsibility, like tracheomalacia, also reduce maximal expiratory flow.

The Bernoulli effect also acts during inspiration, but the more negative pleural pressures during inspiration lower the pressure outside of airways, thereby increasing transmural pressure and promoting airway expansion. Thus, inspiratory airflow limitation seldom occurs due to diffuse pulmonary airway disease. Conversely, extrathoracic airway narrowing (as due to a tracheal adenoma or post-tracheostomy stricture) can lead to inspiratory airflow limitation (Fig. 252-4).

The phenomenon of flow limitation and the importance of airway size and distensibility and of upstream pressure (lung elastic recoil pressure for forced exhalation) can easily be appreciated by sniffing through one's nose with low, medium, or substantial effort. If one keeps the nostrils relaxed, increasing from low to medium inspiratory effort raises inspiratory flow through the nose somewhat, but inhaling even harder will likely not increase inspiratory nasal airflow more but, rather, will just collapse the nares, a manifestation of dynamic airflow limitation. One can increase inspiratory nasal airflow, however, by flaring one's nostrils using the alae nasi muscles. This increases nostril area (reducing velocity for a given flow through the nares) and stiffens the nostril walls (reducing their narrowing in response to negative transmural pressure). Springlike nasal strips sometimes used by football players have the same effect. In patients with obstructive sleep apnea (OSA), a narrowed and excessively compliant pharyngeal airway also collapses in response to negative transmural pressure generated by the Bernoulli effect and by inspiratory frictional pressure loss in the nose (which is why an upper respiratory infection often worsens OSA). Increasing the upstream driving pressure from which these phenomena lower intrapharyngeal gas pressure with positive nasal airway pressure keeps pharyngeal transmural pressure positive, preventing inspiratory airflow limitation. Inspiratory airflow limitation in the nose or in the pharynx of patients with OSA closely parallels expiratory flow limitation in the lung.

■ WORK OF BREATHING

In health, the elastic (volume change–related) and dynamic (flow-related) loads that must be overcome to ventilate the lungs at rest are small, and the work required of the respiratory muscles is minimal. However, the work of breathing can increase considerably, due either to requirement for substantially increased ventilation, an abnormally increased mechanical load, or both. As discussed below, the rate of ventilation is primarily set by the need to eliminate carbon dioxide, and, thus, ventilation increases during exercise (sometimes more than 20-fold) and during metabolic acidosis as a compensatory response. Naturally, the work rate required to overcome the elasticity of the respiratory system increases with both the depth and frequency of tidal breaths, while the work required to overcome the dynamic load increases with total ventilation. A modest increase of ventilation is most efficiently achieved by increasing tidal volume but not respiratory rate, which is the normal ventilatory response to lower level exercise. At high levels of exercise, deep breathing persists, but respiratory rate also increases. The pattern chosen by the respiratory controller minimizes the work of breathing.

Work of breathing also increases when disease reduces the compliance of the respiratory system or increases the resistance to airflow. The former occurs commonly in diseases of the lung parenchyma (interstitial processes or fibrosis, alveolar filling diseases such as pulmonary edema or pneumonia, or substantial lung resection), and the latter occurs in obstructive airways diseases such as asthma, chronic bronchitis, emphysema, and cystic fibrosis. Furthermore, severe airflow obstruction can functionally reduce the compliance of the respiratory system by leading to dynamic hyperinflation. In this scenario, expiratory flows slowed by the obstructive airways disease may be insufficient to allow for complete exhalation during the expiratory phase of tidal breathing; as a result, the "functional residual capacity" from which the next breath is inhaled is greater than the static FRC. With repetition of incomplete exhalations of each tidal breath, the operating FRC becomes dynamically elevated, sometimes to a level that approaches TLC. At these high lung volumes, the respiratory system is much less compliant than at normal breathing volumes, and, thus, the elastic work of each tidal breath is also increased. The dynamic pulmonary hyperinflation that accompanies severe airflow obstruction causes patients to sense difficulty in breathing in—even though the pathophysiologic abnormality at root cause is expiratory airflow obstruction.

■ ADEQUACY OF VENTILATION

As noted above, the respiratory control system that sets the rate of ventilation responds to chemical signals, including arterial carbon dioxide and oxygen tensions and blood pH, and to volitional needs, such as the need to inhale deeply before playing a long phrase on the trumpet. Disturbances in ventilation are discussed in Chap. 264. Here, we focus on the relationship between ventilation of the lung and carbon dioxide elimination.

At the end of each tidal exhalation, the conducting airways are filled with alveolar gas that had not reached the mouth when expiratory flow stopped. During the ensuing inhalation, fresh gas immediately enters the airway tree at the mouth, but the gas first entering the alveoli at the start of inhalation is that same alveolar gas in the conducting airways that had just left the alveoli. As such, fresh gas does not enter the alveoli until the volume of the conducting airways has been inspired. This volume is called the anatomic dead space. Quiet breathing with tidal volumes smaller than the anatomic dead space introduces no fresh gas into the alveoli at all; only that part of the inspired tidal volume (V_T) that is greater than the dead space (V_D) introduces fresh gas into the alveoli. Importantly, the dead space can be further increased functionally if some of the inspired tidal volume is delivered to a part of the lung that receives no pulmonary blood flow, and, thus, cannot contribute to gas exchange, as can occur in the portion of the lung distal to a large pulmonary embolus. As such, exhaled minute ventilation ($\dot{V}_E = V_T \times RR$) includes a component of dead space ventilation ($\dot{V}_D = V_D \times RR$) and a component of fresh gas alveolar ventilation ($\dot{V}_A = [V_T - V_D] \times RR$). Carbon dioxide elimination from the alveoli is equal to $\dot{V}_A$ times the difference in CO_2 fraction between inspired air (essentially zero) and alveolar gas (typically ~5.6%, after correcting for humidification of inspired air, corresponding to 40 mmHg). In the steady state, the alveolar fraction of CO_2 is equal to the metabolic CO_2 production divided by the alveolar ventilation. Because, as discussed below, alveolar and arterial CO_2 tensions are equal, and because the respiratory controller normally strives to maintain arterial P_{CO_2} (Pa_{CO_2}) at ~40 mmHg, the adequacy of alveolar ventilation is reflected in Pa_{CO_2}. If Pa_{CO_2} falls much below 40 mmHg, alveolar hyperventilation is present, and if Pa_{CO_2} exceeds 40 mmHg, then alveolar hypoventilation is present. Ventilatory failure is characterized by extreme alveolar hypoventilation.

As a consequence of oxygen uptake of alveolar gas into capillary blood, alveolar oxygen tension falls below that of inspired gas. The rate of oxygen uptake (determined by the body's metabolic oxygen consumption) is related to the average rate of metabolic carbon dioxide production and their ratio, called the "respiratory quotient" ($R = \dot{V}_{CO_2}/\dot{V}_{O_2}$), depends largely on the fuel being metabolized. For a typical American diet, R is usually around 0.85, and more oxygen is absorbed than CO_2 is excreted. Together, these phenomena allow the estimation of alveolar oxygen tension, according to the following relationship, known as the alveolar gas equation:

$$PA_{O_2} = FI_{O_2} \times (P_{bar} - P_{H_2O}) - PA_{CO_2}/R$$

The alveolar gas equation also highlights the influences of inspired oxygen fraction (FI_{O_2}), barometric pressure (P_{bar}), and vapor pressure of water (P_{H_2O} = 47 mmHg at 37°C) in addition to alveolar ventilation (which sets PA_{CO_2}) in determining PA_{O_2}. An implication of the alveolar gas equation is that severe arterial hypoxemia rarely occurs as a pure consequence of alveolar hypoventilation at sea level while breathing air. The potential for alveolar hypoventilation to induce severe hypoxemia with otherwise normal lungs increases as Pbar falls with increasing altitude.

GAS EXCHANGE

■ DIFFUSION

For oxygen to be delivered to the peripheral tissues, it must pass from alveolar gas into alveolar capillary blood by diffusing through alveolar membrane. The aggregate alveolar membrane is highly optimized for this process, with a very large surface area and minimal thickness. Diffusion through the alveolar membrane is so efficient in the human lung that in most circumstances its hemoglobin becomes fully oxygen saturated by the time a red blood cell has traveled just one-third the length of the alveolar capillary. As such, uptake of alveolar oxygen is ordinarily limited by the amount of blood transiting the alveolar capillaries rather than how rapidly oxygen can diffuse across the membrane; thus, oxygen uptake from the lung is said to be "perfusion limited." Carbon dioxide also equilibrates rapidly across the alveolar membrane. Thus, the oxygen and CO_2 tensions in capillary blood leaving a normal alveolus are essentially equal to those in alveolar gas. In only rare circumstances is oxygen uptake from normal lungs diffusion-limited, which can occur at high altitude and/or by high-performance athletes exerting maximum effort. Diffusion limitation can also occur in interstitial lung disease if substantially thickened alveolar walls remain perfused.

■ VENTILATION-PERFUSION HETEROGENEITY

As noted above, for gas exchange to be most efficient, the ventilation to each individual alveolus should be matched to the perfusion to its accompanying capillaries for each of millions of alveoli. Due to the differential effects of gravity on lung mechanics and blood flow throughout the lung, and due to differences of airway and vascular architecture among various respiratory paths, there is minor ventilation/perfusion heterogeneity even in the normal lung; however, $\dot{V}/\dot{Q}$ heterogeneity can be particularly marked in disease. Two extreme examples are (1) ventilation of unperfused lung distal to a pulmonary embolus, in which ventilation of the physiologic dead space is "wasted" in the sense that it does not contribute to gas exchange; and (2) perfusion of nonventilated lung, a condition known as a "shunt." The latter allows venous blood to pass through the lung unaltered; when mixed with fully oxygenated blood leaving other well-ventilated lung units, shunted venous blood disproportionately lowers the mixed arterial Pa_{O_2}, due to the nonlinear oxygen content versus the P_{O_2} relationship of hemoglobin (Fig. 252-5). Furthermore, the resulting arterial hypoxemia is refractory to supplemental inspired oxygen. This is because raising inspired FI_{O_2} has no effect on alveolar gas tensions in nonventilated alveoli, and while raising inspired FI_{O_2} does increase PA_{O_2} in ventilated alveoli, the oxygen content of

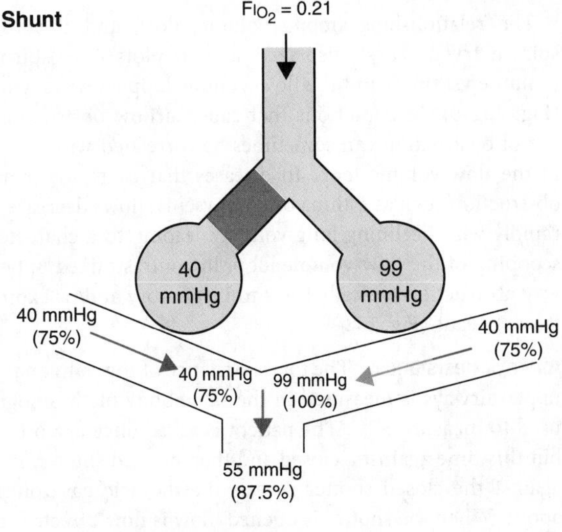

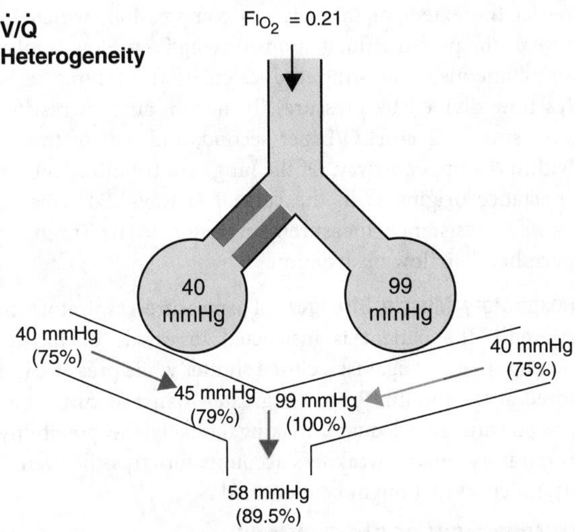

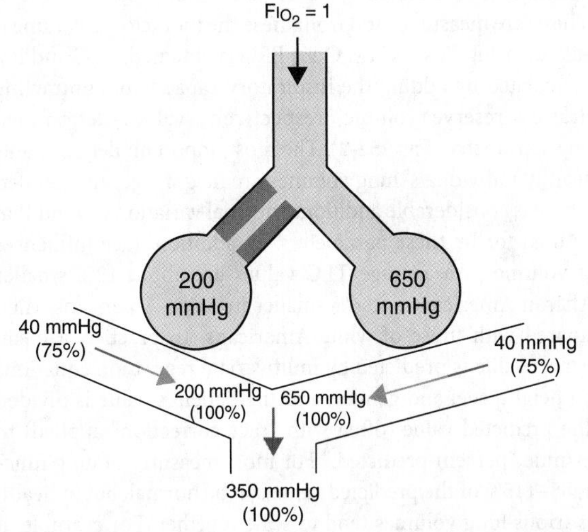

Figure 252-5 Influence of air vs oxygen breathing on mixed arterial oxygenation in shunt and ventilation/perfusion heterogeneity. Partial pressure of oxygen (mmHg) and oxygen saturations are shown for mixed venous blood, end capillary blood for normal versus affected alveoli, and for mixed arterial blood.

blood exiting ventilated units increases only slightly as hemoglobin will already have been nearly fully saturated and the solubility of oxygen in plasma is quite small.

More commonly occurring than the two extreme examples given above is a widening of the distribution of ventilation/perfusion ratios; such $\dot{V}/\dot{Q}$ heterogeneity is a common consequence of lung disease. In this circumstance, perfusion of relatively underventilated alveoli results in the incomplete oxygenation of exiting blood. When mixed with well-oxygenated blood leaving higher $\dot{V}/\dot{Q}$ regions, this partially preoxygenated blood disproportionately lowers arterial Pa_{O_2}, although to a lower extent than does a similar perfusion fraction of blood leaving regions of pure shunt. In addition, in contrast to shunt regions, inhalation of supplemental oxygen does raise the PA_{O_2} even in relatively underventilated low $\dot{V}/\dot{Q}$ regions, and so the arterial hypoxemia induced by $\dot{V}/\dot{Q}$ heterogeneity is typically responsive to oxygen therapy (Fig. 252-5).

In sum, arterial hypoxemia can be caused by substantial reduction of inspired oxygen tension, by severe alveolar hypoventilation, or by perfusion of relatively underventilated (low $\dot{V}/\dot{Q}$) or completely unventilated (shunt) lung regions, and, in unusual circumstances, by limitation of gas diffusion.

APPROACH TO THE PATIENT Disturbances of Respiratory Function

There are many diseases that injure the respiratory system, but there are relatively few ways in which it responds to that injury. For this reason, the pattern of physiologic abnormalities may or may not provide sufficient information to discriminate among conditions. The following studies are commonly used to characterize a patient's respiratory function and often lead to a better understanding of the underlying disorder.

MEASUREMENT OF VENTILATORY FUNCTION

Lung Volumes Figure 252-2 demonstrates a spirometry tracing in which the volume of air entering or exiting the lung is plotted over time. In a slow vital capacity maneuver, the subject inhales from FRC, fully inflating the lungs to TLC, and then the patient exhales slowly to RV; VC is the difference between TLC and RV, and represents the maximum excursion of the respiratory system. Spirometry discloses relative volume changes during these maneuvers, but cannot reveal the absolute volumes at which they occur. To determine absolute lung volumes, two approaches are commonly used—inert gas dilution and body plethysmography. In the former, a known amount of a nonabsorbable inert gas (usually helium or neon) is inhaled in a single large breath or is rebreathed from a closed circuit; the inert gas is diluted by the gas resident in the lung at the time of inhalation, and its final concentration reveals the volume of resident gas contributing to the dilution. A drawback of this method is that regions of the lung that ventilate poorly (e.g., due to airflow obstruction) may not receive much inspired inert gas and so do not contribute to its dilution. As such, inert gas dilution often underestimates true lung volumes.

In the second approach, FRC is determined by measuring the compressibility of gas within the chest, which is proportional to the volume of gas being compressed. The patient sits in a body plethysmograph, a chamber usually made of transparent plastic to minimize claustrophobia, and at the end of a normal tidal breath (i.e., when lung volume is FRC) is instructed to pant against a closed shutter, thus, periodically compressing air within the lung slightly. Pressure fluctuations at the mouth and volume fluctuations within the body box (equal but opposite to those of the chest) are measured, and from these the thoracic gas volume is calculated using Boyle's law. Once FRC is obtained, TLC and RV are calculated by adding the inspiratory capacity or subtracting expiratory reserve volume, respectively, values determined during spirometry (Fig. 252-2). The most important determinants of healthy individuals' lung volumes are height, age, and gender, but there is considerable additional normal variation beyond that accounted for by these parameters. In addition, race influences lung volumes; on average TLC values are about 12% smaller in African Americans and 6% smaller in Asian Americans when compared with those of white Americans. In practice, a mean "normal" value is predicted by multivariate regression equations using height, age, and gender, and the patient's value is divided by the predicted value (often with "race correction" applied) to determine "percent predicted." For most measures of lung function, 85–115% of the predicted value can be normal, but in health the various lung volumes tend to scale together. For example, if one is "normal big" with TLC 110% of the predicted value, then all other lung volumes and spirometry values will also approximate 110% of their respective predicted values. This pattern is particularly helpful in evaluating airflow, as discussed below.

Air Flow As noted above, spirometry plays a key role in lung volume determination. But even more often, spirometry is used to measure air flow, which reflects the dynamic properties of the lung. During a forced vital capacity maneuver, the patient inhales to TLC and then exhales rapidly and forcefully to RV; this ensures that flow limitation has been achieved, so that the precise effort made has little influence on actual flow. The total amount of air exhaled is the forced vital capacity (FVC) and the amount of air exhaled in the first second is the forced expiratory volume in one second (FEV_1); note that FEV_1 is a flow rate, as it reveals volume change per time. As with lung volumes, an individual's maximal expiratory flows should be compared to predicted values based on height, age, and gender. While the FEV_1/FVC ratio is typically reduced in airflow obstruction, airflow obstruction can also reduce FVC by raising RV. If this occurs, the FEV_1/FVC ratio may be "artifactually normal," erroneously suggesting that airflow obstruction is absent. To circumvent this problem, it is useful to compare FEV_1 as a fraction of its predicted value with TLC as a fraction of its predicted value. In health, these are usually similar. In contrast, even an FEV_1 value that is 95% of its predicted value may actually be relatively low if TLC is 110% of its respective prediction. In this case, airflow obstruction might be present, despite the "normal" value for FEV_1.

The relationships among volume, flow, and time during spirometry are best displayed in two plots—the spirogram (volume vs. time) and the flow-volume loop (flow vs. volume) (Fig. 252-4). In conditions that cause airflow obstruction, the site of obstruction can sometimes be correlated with the shape of the flow-volume loop. In diseases that cause lower airway obstruction such as asthma or emphysema, flows decrease more rapidly with declining lung volumes leading to a characteristic scooping of the flow-volume loop. In contrast, fixed upper airway obstruction typically leads to inspiratory and/or expiratory flow plateaus (Fig. 252-4).

Airways Resistance The total resistance of the pulmonary and upper airways is measured in the same body plethysmography used to measure FRC. The patient is asked once again to pant, but this time against a closed and then opened shutter. Panting against the closed shutter reveals the thoracic gas volume as above. When the shutter is opened, flow is now directed to and from the body box, so that volume fluctuations in the box reveal the extent of thoracic gas compression, which in turn reveals the pressure fluctuations driving flow. Flow is measured simultaneously, allowing the calculation of lung resistance (as flow divided by pressure). In health, airways resistance is very small, <2 cmH_2O/L per second, and half of this resides within the upper airway. Of the lung's contribution, most of the resistance originates in the central airways. For this reason, airways resistance measurement tends to be insensitive to peripheral airflow obstruction.

Respiratory Muscle Strength To measure respiratory muscle strength, the patient is instructed to exhale or inhale with maximum effort against a closed shutter while pressure is monitored at the mouth. Pressures greater than ±60 cmH_2O at FRC are considered adequate, making unlikely the possibility that respiratory muscle weakness accounts for any other ventilatory dysfunction that might be identified.

MEASUREMENT OF GAS EXCHANGE

Diffusing Capacity This test uses a small (and safe) amount of carbon monoxide to measure gas exchange across the alveolar membrane during a 10-second breath hold. Carbon monoxide in exhaled breath is analyzed to determine the quantity of CO absorbed by crossing the alveolar membrane and combining with hemoglobin in red blood cells. This "single-breath diffusing capacity" [diffusion capacity of the lung for carbon monoxide (DL_{CO})] value increases with the surface area available for diffusion and the amount of hemoglobin within the capillaries, and varies inversely with alveolar membrane thickness. Thus, DL_{CO} decreases in diseases that thicken or destroy alveolar membranes (e.g., pulmonary fibrosis, emphysema), curtail the pulmonary vasculature (e.g., pulmonary hypertension), or reduce alveolar capillary hemoglobin (e.g., anemia). Single-breath diffusing capacity may be elevated in acute congestive heart failure, asthma, polycythemia, and pulmonary hemorrhage.

Arterial Blood Gases The effectiveness of gas exchange can be assessed by measuring the partial pressures of oxygen and carbon dioxide in a sample of blood obtained by arterial puncture. The oxygen content of blood (Ca_{O_2}) depends upon arterial saturation (%O_2Sat), which is set by Pa_{O_2}, pH, and Pa_{CO_2} according to the oxyhemoglobin dissociation curve; Ca_{O_2} can also be measured by oximetry (see below):

$$Ca_{O_2}\ (mL/dL) = 1.34\ (mL/dL/g) \times [hemoglobin](g) \times \%O_2Sat + 0.003\ (mL/dL/mmHg) \times Pa_{O_2}\ (mmHg)$$

Pulse Oximetry Continuous monitoring of arterial blood gases requires either repeated arterial punctures or an indwelling arterial catheter, and so may be difficult in many circumstances. Instead, the oxygen saturation fraction of hemoglobin can be measured continuously using pulse oximetry, a tool that measures the absorbance by hemoglobin of several wavelengths of light transmitted across a finger, toe, or ear by a noninvasive probe. However, since oxygen content varies relatively little with Pa_{O_2} at saturations above 90%, it is difficult to know the precise Pa_{O_2} using this device. In addition, as noted above, Pa_{CO_2} is needed to fully assess the mechanism of hypoxemia, a value that is not revealed by pulse oximetry.

CLINICAL CORRELATIONS: TYPICAL EXAMPLES

This chapter has highlighted the physiologic processes underlying respiratory system function and the techniques used by clinicians to assess them. Figure 252-6 lists abnormalities in pulmonary function testing typically found in a number of common respiratory disorders and highlights the simultaneous occurrence of multiple physiologic abnormalities. Importantly, some of these respiratory disorders can coexist, which results in more complex superposition of these abnormalities.

VENTILATORY RESTRICTION DUE TO INCREASED ELASTIC RECOIL—EXAMPLE: IDIOPATHIC PULMONARY FIBROSIS

Idiopathic pulmonary fibrosis raises lung recoil at all lung volumes, thereby lowering TLC, FRC, and RV, as well as FVC. Maximal expiratory flows are also reduced compared with normal values, but are relatively elevated when considered in relation to lung volumes. The latter occurs both because the increased lung recoil drives greater maximal flow at any lung volume and because airway diameters are relatively increased due to greater radially outward traction exerted on bronchi by the stiff lung parenchyma. Airway resistance is also normal, for the same reason. Pulmonary capillaries are destroyed by the fibrotic process resulting in marked reduction in diffusing capacity. Oxygenation is often severely reduced due to persistent perfusion of alveolar units that are relatively underventilated due to fibrosis of nearby (and mechanically linked) lung. The flow-volume loop looks like a miniature version of a normal loop but is shifted toward lower absolute lung volumes and displays maximum expiratory flows that are increased for any given volume when compared to the normal tracing.

VENTILATORY RESTRICTION DUE TO CHEST WALL ABNORMALITY—EXAMPLE: MODERATE OBESITY

As the size of the average American continues to increase, this pattern may become the most commonly seen of pulmonary function abnormalities. In moderate obesity, the outward recoil of the chest wall is blunted due to the weight of chest wall fat and to the space occupied by intraabdominal fat. As such, preserved inward recoil of the lung now overbalances the reduced outward recoil of the chest wall, and FRC falls. Because respiratory muscle strength and lung recoil remain normal, TLC is typically unchanged (although TLC may fall in massive obesity) and RV is normal (but may be reduced in massive obesity). Mild hypoxemia may be present, due to perfusion of alveolar units that are poorly ventilated because of airway closure that occurs in dependent portions of the lung while breathing near the reduced FRC. Flows remain normal, as does DL_{CO}, unless obstructive sleep apnea (which often accompanies obesity) and associated chronic intermittent hypoxemia have induced pulmonary arterial hypertension, in which case DL_{CO} may be low.

VENTILATORY RESTRICTION DUE TO REDUCED MUSCLE STRENGTH—EXAMPLE: MYASTHENIA GRAVIS

FRC remains normal, as both lung recoil and passive chest wall recoil are normal. However, TLC is low and RV is elevated, as respiratory muscle strength is insufficient to push the passive respiratory

	Restriction due to increased lung elastic recoil (pulmonary fibrosis)	Restriction due to chest wall abnormality (moderate obesity)	Restriction due to respiratory muscle weakness (myasthenia gravis)	Obstruction due to airway narrowing (acute asthma)	Obstruction due to decreased elastic recoil (severe emphysema)
TLC	60%	95%	75%	100%	130%
FRC	60%	65%	100%	104%	220%
RV	60%	100%	120%	120%	310%
FVC	60%	92%	60%	90%	60%
FEV_1	75%	92%	60%	35% pre-b.d. 75% post-b.d.	35% pre-b.d. 38% post-b.d.
R_{aw}	1.0	1.0	1.0	2.5	1.5
DL_{CO}	60%	95%	80%	120%	40%

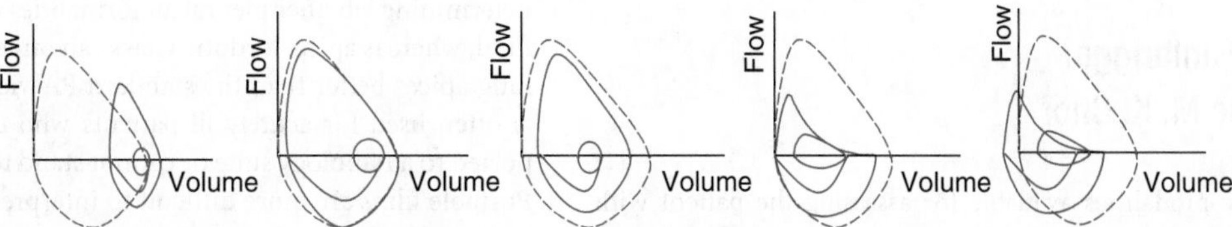

Figure 252-6 Commonly seen abnormalities of pulmonary function (see text). Pulmonary function values are expressed as percent of normal predicted values, except for R_{aw}, which is expressed as $cmH_2O/L/s$ (normal <2 $cmH_2O/L/s$). The figures at the bottom of each column show typical configuration of flow-volume loops in each condition, including the flow-volume relationship during tidal breathing. b.d., bronchodilator; DL_{CO}, diffusion capacity of lung for carbon monoxide; FEV_1, forced expiratory volume in one second; FRC, functional residual capacity; FVC, forced vital capacity; R_{aw}, airways resistance; RV, residual volume; TLC, total lung capacity.

system fully toward either volume extreme. Caught between the low TLC and the elevated RV, FVC and FEV_1 are reduced as "innocent bystanders." As airway size and the lung vasculature are unaffected, both airways resistance (R_{aw}) and DL_{CO} are normal. Oxygenation is normal unless weakness becomes so severe that the patient has insufficient strength to reopen collapsed alveoli during sighs, with resulting atelectasis.

AIRFLOW OBSTRUCTION DUE TO DECREASED AIRWAY DIAMETER—EXAMPLE: ACUTE ASTHMA

During an episode of acute asthma, luminal narrowing due to smooth muscle constriction and inflammation and thickening within the small- and medium-sized bronchi raise frictional resistance and reduce airflow. Scooping of the flow-volume loop is caused by reduction of airflow, especially at lower lung volumes. Often, airflow obstruction can be reversed by inhalation of β_2-adrenergic agonists acutely or by treatment with inhaled steroids chronically. Total lung capacity (TLC) usually remains normal (although elevated TLC is sometimes seen in long-standing asthma), but FRC may be dynamically elevated. RV is often increased due to exaggerated airway closure at low lung volumes, and this elevation of RV reduces FVC. Because central airways are narrowed, airways resistance is usually elevated. Mild arterial hypoxemia is often present due to perfusion of relatively underventilated alveoli distal to obstructed airways (and is responsive to oxygen supplementation), but DL_{CO} is normal or mildly elevated.

AIRFLOW OBSTRUCTION DUE TO DECREASED ELASTIC RECOIL—EXAMPLE: SEVERE EMPHYSEMA

Loss of lung elastic recoil in severe emphysema results in pulmonary hyperinflation, of which elevated TLC is the hallmark. FRC is more severely elevated due both to loss of lung elastic recoil and to dynamic hyperinflation (the same phenomenon as autoP-EEP, which is the unintended positive end-expiratory pressure). Residual volume is very severely elevated due to airway closure and because exhalation toward RV may take so long that RV cannot be reached before the patient must inhale again. Both FVC and FEV_1 are markedly decreased, the former due to the severe elevation of RV, and the latter because loss of lung elastic recoil reduces the pressure driving maximal expiratory flow and also reduces tethering open of small intrapulmonary airways. The flow-volume loop demonstrates marked scooping of the flow-volume loop, with an initial transient spike of flow attributable largely to expulsion of air from collapsing central airways at the onset of forced exhalation. Otherwise, the central airways remain relatively unaffected, so R_{aw} is normal in "pure" emphysema. Loss of alveolar surface and capillaries in the alveolar walls reduces DL_{CO}, but because poorly ventilated emphysematous acini are also poorly perfused (due to loss of their capillaries), arterial hypoxemia is usually not seen at rest until emphysema becomes very severe. However, during exercise, Pa_{O_2} may fall precipitously if extensive destruction of the pulmonary vasculature prevents a sufficient increase in cardiac output and mixed venous oxygen content falls substantially. Under these circumstances, any venous admixture through low $\dot{V}/\dot{Q}$ units has a particularly marked effect in lowering mixed arterial oxygen tension.

ACKNOWLEDGEMENT

The authors wish to acknowledge the contribution of Dr. Steven E. Weinberger and Irene M. Rosen to this chapter in previous edits and the helpful contributions of Drs. Mary Strek and Jeff Jacobson.

FURTHER READINGS

Hyatt RE et al: *Interpretation of Pulmonary Function Testing*, 3rd ed. Philadelphia, Lippincott Williams & Wilkins, 2009

MacIntyre N: Standardization of the single-breath determination of carbon monoxide uptake in the lung. Eur Respir J 26:720, 2005

Miller MR et al: Standardization of spirometry. Eur Respir J 26:319, 2005

Wanger J: Standardization of measurements of lung volumes. Eur Respir J 26:511, 2005

Weinberger SE: *Principles of Pulmonary Medicine*, 4th ed. Philadelphia, Saunders, 2004

CHAPTER 253

Diagnostic Procedures in Respiratory Disease

Anne L. Fuhlbrigge
Augustine M. K. Choi

The diagnostic modalities available for assessing the patient with suspected or known respiratory system disease include imaging studies and techniques for acquiring biologic specimens, some of which involve direct visualization of part of the respiratory system. Methods to characterize the functional changes developing as a result of disease, including pulmonary function tests and measurements of gas exchange, are discussed in Chap. 252.

IMAGING STUDIES

ROUTINE RADIOGRAPHY

Routine chest radiography, generally including both posteroanterior (PA) and lateral views, is an integral part of the diagnostic evaluation of diseases involving the pulmonary parenchyma, the pleura, and, to a lesser extent, the airways and the mediastinum (see Chaps. 251 and e34). Lateral decubitus views are often useful for determining whether pleural abnormalities represent freely flowing fluid, whereas apical lordotic views can often visualize disease at the lung apices better than the standard PA view. Portable equipment is often used for acutely ill patients who either cannot be transported to a radiology suite or cannot stand for PA and lateral views. Portable films are more difficult to interpret owing to several limitations: (1) the single antero posterior (AP) projection obtained; (2) variability in over- and underexposure of film; (3) a shorter focal spot-film distance leading to lack of edge sharpness, and loss of fine detail; and (4) magnification of the cardiac silhouette and other anterior structures by the AP projection. Common radiographic patterns and their clinical correlates are reviewed in Chap. e34.

Advances in computer technology and the availability of reusable radiation detectors have allowed the development of digital or computed radiography. The images obtained in this format can be subjected to significant postprocessing analysis to improve diagnostic information. In addition, the benefit of immediate availability of the images, the ability to store images electronically, and the facility of transfer within or between health care systems have led many hospital systems to convert to digital systems.

COMPUTED TOMOGRAPHY

Computed tomography (CT) offers several advantages over routine chest radiography (Figs. 253-1*A*, *B* and 253-2*A*, *B*; see also Figs. 261-3, 261-4, and 268-4). First, the use of cross-sectional images allows distinction between densities that would be superimposed on plain radiographs. Second, CT is far better than routine radiographic studies at characterizing tissue density, distinguishing subtle density differences between adjacent structures, and providing accurate size assessment of lesions.

CT is particularly valuable in assessing hilar and mediastinal disease (which is often poorly characterized by plain radiography), in identifying and characterizing disease adjacent to the chest wall or spine (including pleural disease), and in identifying areas of fat density or calcification in pulmonary nodules (Fig. 253-2). Its utility in the assessment of mediastinal disease has made CT an important tool in the staging of lung cancer (Chap. 89), as an assessment of tumor involvement of mediastinal lymph nodes is critical to proper staging. With the additional use of contrast material, CT also makes it possible to distinguish vascular from nonvascular structures, which is particularly important in distinguishing lymph nodes and masses from vascular structures primarily in the mediastinum, and vascular disorders such as pulmonary embolism.

In high-resolution CT (HRCT), the thickness of individual cross-sectional images is ~1–2 mm, rather than the usual 7–10 mm in conventional CT. The visible detail on HRCT scans allows better recognition of subtle parenchymal and airway disease, thickened interlobular septa, ground-glass opacification, small nodules, and the abnormally thickened or dilated airways seen in bronchiectasis. Using HRCT, characteristic patterns are recognized for many interstitial lung diseases such as lymphangitic carcinoma, idiopathic pulmonary fibrosis, sarcoidosis, and eosinophilic granuloma. However, there is debate about, the settings in which the presence of a characteristic pattern on HRCT eliminates the need for obtaining lung tissue to make a diagnosis.

HELICAL CT SCANNING

Recent advances in computer processing have allowed the development of helical CT scanning. Helical CT technology results in faster scans with improved contrast enhancement and thinner collimation. The image is obtained during a single breath-holding maneuver that allows less motion artifact. In addition, helical CT scanning allows the collection of continuous data over a larger volume of lung than is possible with conventional CT. Data from the imaging procedure can be reconstructed as images in planes other than the traditional cross-sectional (axial) view, including coronal, or sagittal planes (Fig. 253-3*A*). Finally, sophisticated volumetric "3D" representations of structures can be produced (Fig. 253-3*B*) including the ability to perform a *virtual bronchoscopy,* mimicking direct visualization through a bronchoscope (Fig. 253-4).

MULTIDETECTOR CT (MDCT)

Refinements in detector technology have allowed production of scanners with additional detectors along the scanning axis (*z*-axis). These scanners, called *multidetector CT* (MDCT) scanners, can obtain multiple slices in a single rotation that are thinner and can be acquired in a shorter period of time. This results in enhanced resolution and increased image reconstruction ability. As the technology has progressed, higher numbers (2, 4, 6, 8, 10, 16, 32, 40 and currently up to 64) of detectors are used to produce

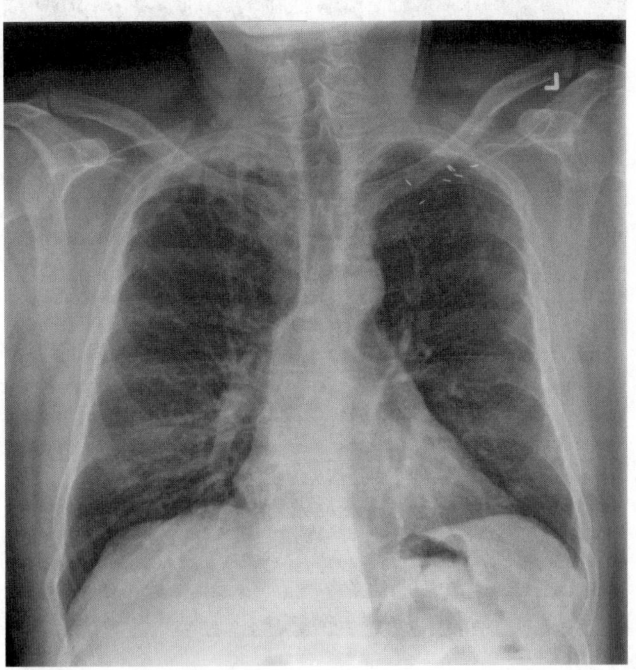

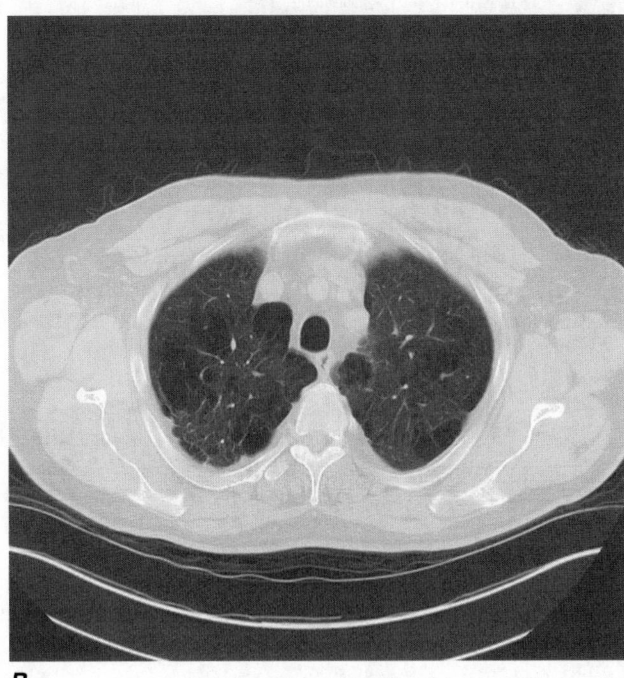

Figure 253-1 Chest x-ray (A) and CT scan (B) from a patient with emphysema. The extent and distribution of emphysema are not well appreciated on plain film but clearly evident on CT scan obtained.

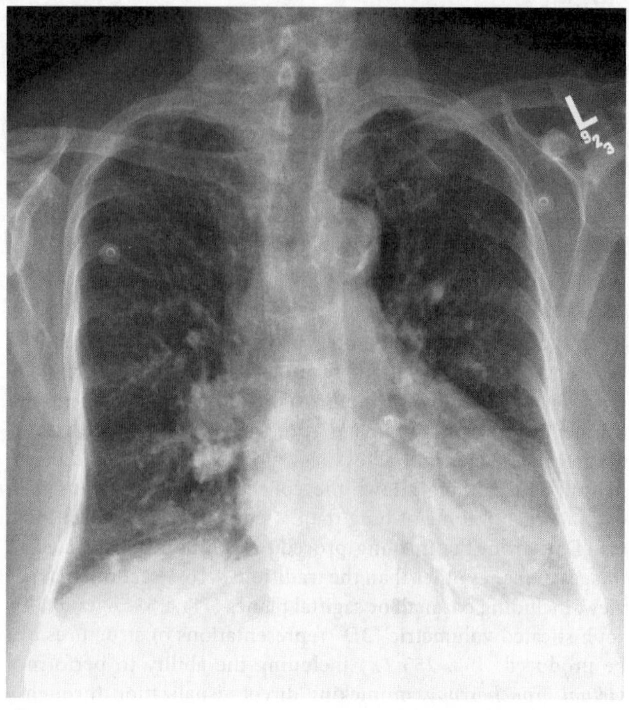

A

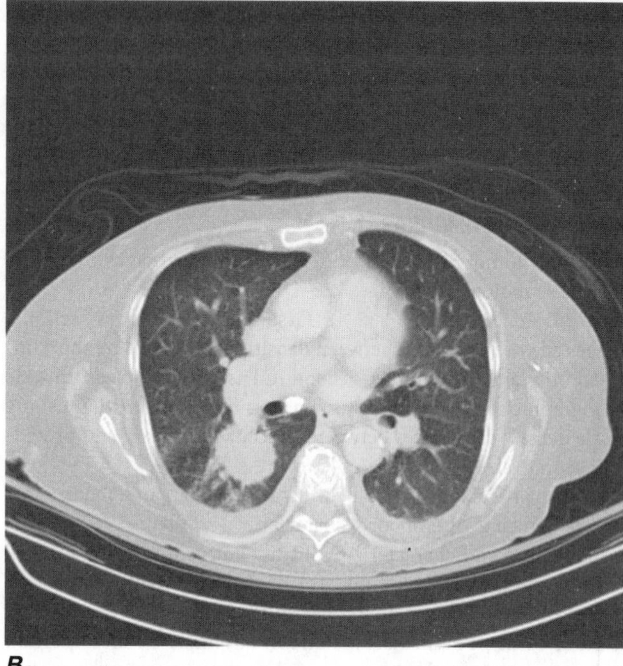

B

Figure 253-2 Chest x-ray (*A*) and CT scan (*B*) demonstrating a right lower-lobe mass. The mass is not well appreciated on the plain film because of the hilar structures and known calcified adenopathy. CT is superior to plain radiography for the detection of abnormal mediastinal densities and the distinction of masses from adjacent vascular structures.

clearer final images. The development of MDCT allows for even shorter breath holds, which are beneficial for all patients but especially children, the elderly, and the critically ill. However, it should be noted that despite the advantages of MDCT, there is an increase in radiation dose compared to single-detector CT to consider. With MDCT, the additional detectors along the *z*-axis result in improved use of the contrast bolus. In addition, the shorter breath holds secondary to faster scanning times and

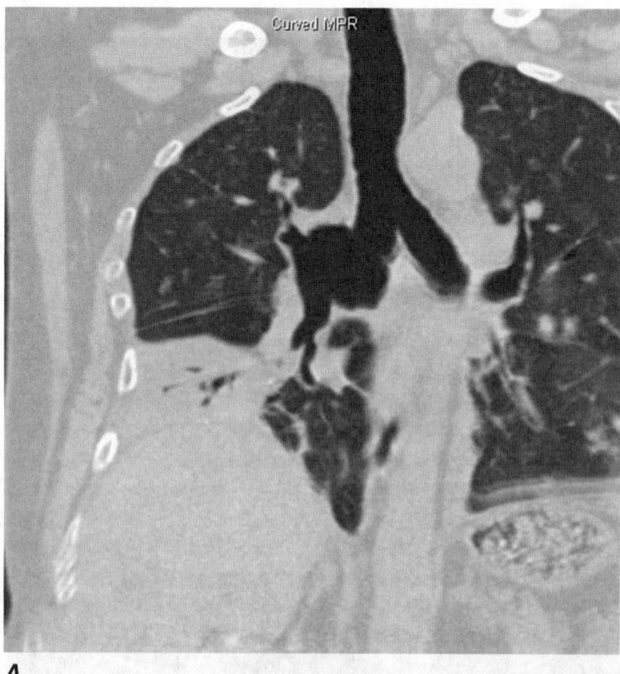

A

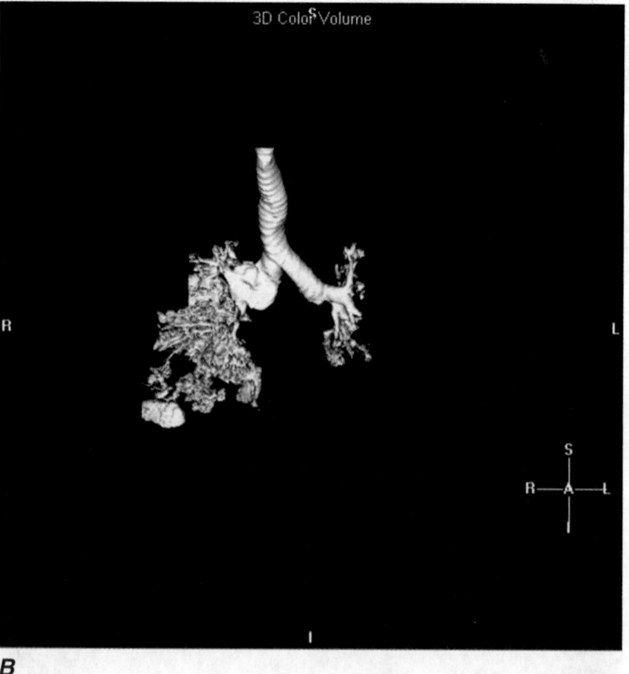

B

Figure 253-3 Spiral CT with reconstruction of images in planes other than axial view. Spiral CT in a lung transplant patient with a dehiscence and subsequent aneurysm of the anastomosis. CT images were reconstructed in the sagittal view (***A***) and using digital subtraction to view images of the airways only (***B***), which demonstrate the exact location and extent of the abnormality.

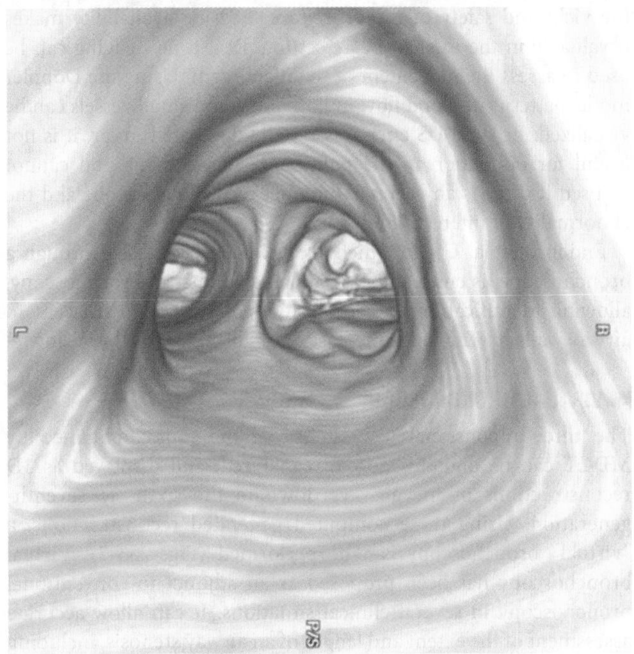

Figure 253-4 MRA image of the vasculature of a patient after lung transplant. The image demonstrates the detailed view of the vasculature that can be obtained using digital subtraction techniques. Images from a patient after lung transplant show the venous and arterial anastomosis on the right; a slight narrowing is seen at the site of the anastomosis, which is considered within normal limits and not suggestive of obstruction.

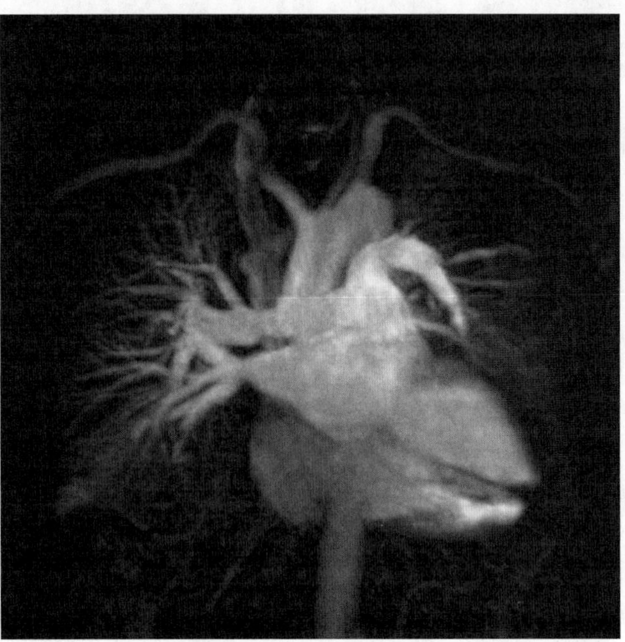

Figure 253-5 Virtual bronchoscopic image of the trachea. The view projected is one that would be obtained from the trachea looking down to the carina. The left and right main stem airways are seen bifurcating from the carina.

increased resolution have all led to improved imaging of the pulmonary vasculature and the ability to detect segmental and subsegmental emboli. In contrast to pulmonary angiography, CT pulmonary angiography (CTPA) also allows simultaneous detection of parenchymal abnormalities that may be contributing to a patient's clinical presentation. Secondary to these advantages and increasing availability, CTPA has rapidly become the test of choice for many clinicians in the evaluation of pulmonary embolism; it is considered equal to pulmonary angiography in terms of accuracy, and with less associated risks.

MAGNETIC RESONANCE IMAGING

The role of magnetic resonance (MR) imaging in the evaluation of respiratory system disease is less well-defined than that of CT. Magnetic resonance provides poorer spatial resolution and less detail of the pulmonary parenchyma, and for these reasons is currently not considered a substitute for CT in imaging the thorax. However, the use of hyperpolarized gas in conjunction with MR has led to the investigational use of MR for imaging the lungs, particularly in obstructive lung disease. Of note, MR examinations are difficult to obtain among several subgroups of patients. Patients who cannot lie still or who cannot lie on their backs may have MR images that are of poor quality; some tests require patients to hold their breaths for 15 to 25 seconds at a time in order to get good MR images. MR is generally avoided in unstable and/or ventilated patients and those with severe trauma because of the hazards of the MR environment and the difficulties in monitoring patients within the MR room. The presence of metallic foreign bodies, pacemakers, and intracranial aneurysm clips also preclude use of MR.

An advantage of MR is the use of nonionizing electromagnetic radiation. Additionally, MR is well suited to distinguish vascular from nonvascular structures without the need for contrast. Blood vessels appear as hollow tubular structures because flowing blood does not produce a signal on MR imaging. Therefore, MR can be useful in demonstrating pulmonary emboli, defining aortic lesions such as aneurysms or dissection, or other vascular abnormalities (Fig. 253-5) if radiation and IV contrast medium cannot be used. Gadolinium can be used as an intravascular contrast agent for MR angiography (MRA); however, synchronization of data acquisition with the peak arterial bolus is one of the major challenges of MRA; the flow of contrast medium from the peripheral injection site to the vessel of interest is affected by a number of factors including heart rate, stroke volume, and the presence of proximal stenotic lesions.

NUCLEAR MEDICINE TECHNIQUES

Nuclear imaging depends on the selective uptake of various compounds by organs of the body. In thoracic imaging, these compounds are concentrated by one of three mechanisms: blood pool or compartmentalization (e.g., within the heart), physiologic incorporation (e.g., bone or thyroid) and capillary blockage (e.g., lung scan). Radioactive isotopes can be administered by either the IV or inhaled routes or both. When injected intravenously, albumin macroaggregates labeled with [^{99m}Tc] become lodged in pulmonary capillaries; the distribution of the trapped radioisotope follows the distribution of blood flow. When inhaled, radiolabeled xenon gas can be used to demonstrate the distribution of ventilation. Using these techniques, ventilation-perfusion lung scanning was a commonly used technique for the evaluation of pulmonary embolism. Pulmonary thromboembolism produces one or more regions of ventilation-perfusion mismatch [i.e., regions in which there is a defect in perfusion that follows the distribution of a vessel and that is not accompanied by a corresponding defect in ventilation (Chap. 262)]. However, with advances in CT scanning, scintigraphic imaging has been largely replaced by CT angiography in patients with suspected pulmonary embolism.

Another common use of ventilation-perfusion scans is in patients with impaired lung function, who are being considered for lung resection. Because many patients with bronchogenic carcinoma have coexisting chronic obstructive pulmonary disease (COPD), the question arises as to whether or not a patient can tolerate lung resection. The distribution of the isotope(s) can be used to assess the regional distribution of blood flow and ventilation, allowing the physician to estimate the level of postoperative lung function.

POSITRON EMISSION TOMOGRAPHIC SCANNING

Positron emission tomographic (PET) scanning is commonly used to identify malignant lesions in the lung, based on their increased uptake and metabolism of glucose. The technique involves injection of a radiolabeled glucose analogue, [^{18}F]-fluoro-2-deoxyglucose (FDG), which is taken up by metabolically active malignant cells. However, FDG is trapped within the cell following phosphorylation, and the unstable [^{18}F] decays by emission of positrons, which can be detected by a specialized PET camera or by a gamma camera that has been adapted for imaging of positron-emitting nuclides. This technique has been used in the evaluation of solitary pulmonary nodules and in staging lung cancer through the detection or exclusion of mediastinal lymph node involvement and identification of extrathoracic disease. The limited anatomical definition of radionuclide imaging has been improved by the development of hybrid imaging that allows the superimposition of nuclear medicine and CT images, a technique known as functional–anatomical mapping. Today, most PET scans are performed using instruments with combined PET and CT scanners. The hybrid PET/CT scans provide images that help pinpoint the abnormal metabolic activity to anatomical structures seen on CT. The combined scans provide more accurate diagnoses than the two scans performed separately. FDG–PET can differentiate benign from malignant lesions as small as 1 cm. However, false-negative findings can occur in lesions with low metabolic activity such as carcinoid tumors and bronchioloalveolar cell carcinomas, or in lesions <1 cm in which the required threshold of metabolically active malignant cells is not present for PET diagnosis. False-positive results can be seen due to FDG uptake in inflammatory conditions such as pneumonia and granulomatous diseases.

PULMONARY ANGIOGRAPHY

The pulmonary arterial system can be visualized by pulmonary angiography, in which radiopaque contrast medium is injected through a catheter placed in the pulmonary artery. When performed in cases of pulmonary embolism, pulmonary angiography demonstrates the consequences of an intravascular thrombus—either a defect in the lumen of a vessel (a filling defect) or an abrupt termination (cutoff) of the vessel. Other, less common indications for pulmonary angiography include visualization of a suspected pulmonary arteriovenous malformation and assessment of pulmonary arterial invasion by a neoplasm. The risks associated with modern arteriography are extremely small, generally of greatest concern in patients with severe pulmonary hypertension. With advances in CT scanning, MDCT angiography (MDCTA) is replacing conventional angiography for the diagnosis of pulmonary embolism.

ULTRASOUND

Diagnostic ultrasound (US) produces images using echoes or reflection of the ultrasound beam from interfaces between tissues with differing acoustic properties. US is nonionizing and safe to perform on pregnant patients and children. It is helpful in the detection and localization of pleural abnormalities, and a quick and effective way of guiding percutaneous needle biopsy of peripheral lung, pleural, or chest wall lesions. US is also helpful in identifying septations within loculated collections and can facilitate placement of a needle for sampling of pleural liquid (i.e., for thoracentesis), improving the yield and safety of the procedure. Bedside availability makes it valuable in the intensive care setting. Real-time imaging can be used to assess the movement of the diaphragm. Using the Doppler mode, patterns of blood flow in both large and small vessels can be visualized. Because US energy is rapidly dissipated in air, it is not useful for evaluation of the pulmonary parenchyma and cannot be used if there is any aerated lung between the US probe and the abnormality of interest.

Endobronchial US, in which the US probe is passed through a bronchoscope, is emerging as a valuable adjunct to bronchoscopy, allowing identification and localization of pathology adjacent to airway walls or within the mediastinum, discussed further below.

VIRTUAL BRONCHOSCOPY

The three-dimensional (3D) image of the thorax obtained by MDCT can be digitally stored, reanalyzed, and displayed as 3D reconstructions of the airways down to the sixth- to seventh-generation. Using these computed generated reconstructions, a "virtual" bronchoscopy can be performed (Fig. 253-5). Virtual bronchoscopy has been proposed as an adjunct to conventional bronchoscopy in several clinical situations: It can allow accurate assessment of the extent and length of an airway stenosis, including the airway distal to the narrowing; it can provide useful information about the relationship of the airway abnormality to adjacent mediastinal structures; and it allows preprocedure planning for therapeutic bronchoscopy to help ensure the appropriate equipment is available for the procedure. Virtual bronchoscopy can also be used to perform noninvasive follow-up of patients with treated airway lesions. Navigational systems using virtual bronchoscopy have been developed to allow pathfinding to guide the bronchoscopist to a peripheral region within the lung, allowing peripheral lung lesions to be sampled more efficiently. Finally, with the advent of endobronchial lung volume reduction surgery in the management of pulmonary emphysema, virtual bronchoscopy may be able to help target the area of peripheral lung for endobronchial valve procedures. The extent of emphysema in each segmental region together with other anatomic details may help in choosing the most appropriate subsegments. However, software packages for the generation of virtual bronchoscopic images are relatively early in development and their utilization and potential impact on patient care are still unknown. In addition to allowing virtual bronchoscopy, advances in computing capabilities and digital imaging allow the bronchoscopic images obtained through a real bronchoscopic examination to be stored as digital images and reviewed after completion of the procedure.

MEDICAL TECHNIQUES FOR OBTAINING BIOLOGIC SPECIMENS

COLLECTION OF SPUTUM

Sputum can be collected either by spontaneous expectoration or after inhalation of an irritating aerosol such as hypertonic saline. The latter method, called *sputum induction,* is commonly used to obtain sputum for diagnostic studies, either because sputum is not spontaneously being produced or because of an expected higher yield of certain types of findings. Knowledge of the appearance and quality of the sputum specimen obtained is especially important when one is interested in Gram's method and culture. Because sputum consists mainly of secretions from the tracheobronchial tree rather than the upper airway, the finding of alveolar macrophages and other inflammatory cells is consistent with a lower respiratory tract origin of the sample, whereas the presence of squamous epithelial cells in a "sputum" sample indicates contamination by secretions from the upper airways.

In addition to processing for routine bacterial pathogens by Gram's method and culture, sputum can be processed for a variety of other pathogens, including staining and culture for mycobacteria or fungi, culture for viruses, and staining for *Pneumocystis jiroveci*. In the specific case of sputum obtained for evaluation of *P. jiroveci* pneumonia in a patient infected with HIV, for example, sputum should be collected by induction rather than spontaneous expectoration, and an immunofluorescent stain should be used to detect the organisms. Cytologic staining of sputum for malignant cells, using the traditional Papanicolaou method, allows noninvasive evaluation for suspected lung cancer. Traditional stains and cultures are now also being supplemented in some cases by immunologic techniques and by molecular biologic methods, including the use of polymerase chain reaction amplification and DNA probes.

PERCUTANEOUS NEEDLE ASPIRATION (TRANSTHORACIC)

A needle can be inserted through the chest wall into a pulmonary lesion to aspirate material for analysis by cytologic or microbiologic techniques. Aspiration can be performed to obtain a diagnosis or to decompress and/or drain a fluid collection. The procedure is usually carried out under CT or ultrasound guidance to assist positioning of the needle and assure localization in the lesion. The low potential risk of this procedure (intrapulmonary bleeding or creation of a pneumothorax with collapse of the underlying lung) in experienced hands is usually acceptable owing to the information obtained. However, a limitation of the technique is sampling error due to the small size of the tissue sample. Thus, findings other than a specific cytologic or microbiologic diagnosis are of limited clinical value.

THORACENTESIS

Sampling of pleural liquid by thoracentesis is commonly performed for diagnostic purposes or, in the case of a large effusion, for palliation of dyspnea. Diagnostic sampling, either by blind needle aspiration or after localization by US, allows the collection of liquid for microbiologic and cytologic studies. Analysis of the fluid obtained for its cellular composition and chemical constituents, including glucose, protein, and lactate dehydrogenase, allows the effusion to be classified as either exudative or transudative (Chap. 263).

BRONCHOSCOPY

Bronchoscopy is the process of direct visualization of the tracheobronchial tree. Although bronchoscopy is now performed almost exclusively with flexible fiberoptic instruments, rigid bronchoscopy, generally performed in an operating room on a patient under general anesthesia, still has a role in selected circumstances, primarily because of a larger suction channel and the fact that the patient can be ventilated through the bronchoscope channel. These situations include the retrieval of a foreign body and the suctioning of a massive hemorrhage, for which the small suction channel of the bronchoscope may be insufficient.

FLEXIBLE FIBEROPTIC BRONCHOSCOPY

This outpatient procedure is usually performed in an awake but sedated patient (conscious sedation). The bronchoscope is passed through either the mouth or the nose, between the vocal cords, and into the trachea. The ability to flex the scope makes it possible to visualize virtually all airways to the level of subsegmental bronchi. The bronchoscopist is able to identify endobronchial pathology, including tumors, granulomas, bronchitis, foreign bodies, and sites of bleeding. Samples from airway lesions can be taken by several methods, including washing, brushing, and biopsy. Washing involves instillation of sterile saline through a channel of the bronchoscope and onto the surface of a lesion. A portion of the liquid is collected by suctioning through the bronchoscope, and the recovered material can be analyzed for cells (cytology) or organisms (by standard stains and cultures). Brushing or biopsy of the surface of the lesion, using a small brush or biopsy forceps at the end of a long cable inserted through a channel of the bronchoscope, allows recovery of cellular material or tissue for analysis by standard cytologic and histopathologic methods.

The bronchoscope can be used to sample material not only from the regions that can be directly visualized (i.e., the airways) but also from the more distal pulmonary parenchyma. With the bronchoscope wedged into a subsegmental airway, aliquots of sterile saline can be instilled through the scope, allowing sampling of cells and organisms even from alveolar spaces. This procedure, called *bronchoalveolar lavage*, has been particularly useful for the recovery of organisms such as *P. jiroveci* in patients with HIV infection.

Brushing and biopsy of the distal lung parenchyma can also be performed with the same instruments that are used for endobronchial sampling. These instruments can be passed through the scope into small airways, where they penetrate the airway wall, allowing biopsy of peribronchial alveolar tissue. This procedure, called *transbronchial biopsy*, is used when there is either relatively diffuse disease or a localized lesion of adequate size. With the aid of fluoroscopic imaging, the bronchoscopist is able to determine not only whether and when the instrument is in the area of abnormality, but also the proximity of the instrument to the pleural surface. If the forceps are too close to the pleural surface, there is a risk of violating the visceral pleura and creating a pneumothorax; the other potential complication of transbronchial biopsy is pulmonary hemorrhage. The incidence of these complications is less than several percent.

TRANSBRONCHIAL NEEDLE ASPIRATION (TBNA)

Another procedure involves use of a hollow-bore needle passed through the bronchoscope for sampling of tissue adjacent to the trachea or a large bronchus. The needle is passed through the airway wall (transbronchial), and cellular material can be aspirated from mass lesions or enlarged lymph nodes, generally in a search for malignant cells. Other promising new techniques that are not yet widely available include fluorescence bronchoscopy (to detect early endobronchial malignancy) and endobronchial ultrasound (to better identify and localize peribronchial and mediastinal pathology). Mediastinoscopy has been considered the gold standard for mediastinal staging; however, TBNA allows sampling from the lungs and surrounding lymph nodes without the need for surgery or general anesthesia.

ENDOBRONCHIAL ULTRASOUND (EBUS)–TRANSBRONCHIAL NEEDLE ASPIRATION (TBNA)

Further advances in needle aspiration techniques have been accomplished with the development of endobronchial ultrasound (EBUS). The technology uses an ultrasonic bronchoscope fitted with a probe that allows for needle aspiration of mediastinal and hilar lymph nodes guided by real-time US images. This procedure offers access to more difficult-to-reach areas and smaller lymph nodes in the staging of malignancies. EBUS–TBNA has the potential to access the same paratracheal and subcarinal lymph node stations as mediastinoscopy, but also extends out to the hilar lymph nodes (levels 10 and 11).The usefulness of EBUS for clinical indications other than lung cancer is unclear, although studies on sarcoidosis point to the effectiveness of endobronchial ultrasonography in diagnosing this disease.

INTERVENTIONAL PULMONOLOGY (IP)

Interventional pulmonology was initially developed to focus on procedures to help palliate patients with advanced thoracic malignancies. However, the availability of advanced bronchoscopic and pleuroscopic techniques is enabling interventional pulmonologists to provide alternatives to surgery for patients with a wide variety of thoracic disorders and problems. IP can be defined as "the art and science of medicine as related to the performance of diagnostic and invasive therapeutic procedures that which require additional training and expertise beyond that which required in a standard pulmonary medicine training program."

A central role for an IP physician is the acquisition of tissue for diagnosing mass lesions within the thorax. Several techniques already discussed are part of the day-to-day procedural armamentarium used by an IP physician. TBNA to obtain cytologic, histologic, or microbiologic sampling of lesions within the airway wall, the lung parenchyma, and mediastinum. TBNA is frequently performed in combination with EBUS to improve diagnostic yield. Transthoracic needle aspiration and biopsy (TTNA/B) refers to the percutaneous sampling of lesions involving the chest wall, lung parenchyma, and mediastinum for cytologic, histopathologic, or microbiologic examinations.

AUTOFLUORESCENCE BRONCHOSCOPY

Autofluorescence bronchoscopy (AFB) uses bronchoscopes with an additional light source that allows an experienced operator (interventional pulmonologist or surgeon) to distinguish between normal and abnormal tissue. This technique can be used as a screening tool in high-risk individuals to inspect the tracheobronchial tree in order to identify premalignant lesions (airway dysplasia) and carcinoma in situ.

MEDICAL THORACOSCOPY

Medical thoracoscopy (or pleuroscopy) focuses on the diagnosis of pleural-based problems. The procedure is performed with a conventional rigid or a semirigid pleuroscope (similar in design to a bronchoscope and enabling the operator to inspect the pleural surface, sample and/or drain pleural fluid, or perform targeted biopsies of the parietal pleura). Medical thoracoscopy can be performed in the endoscopy suite or operating room with the patient under conscious sedation and local anesthesia. In contrast, video-assisted thoracoscopic surgery (VATS) requires general anesthesia and is only performed in the OR. A common diagnostic indication for medical thoracoscopy is the evaluation of a pleural effusion or biopsy of presumed parietal pleural carcinomatosis. It can also be used to place a chest tube under visual guidance, or perform chemical or talc pleurodesis, a therapeutic intervention to prevent a recurrent pleural effusion (usually malignant) or recurrent pneumothorax.

THERAPEUTIC BRONCHOSCOPY

The bronchoscope may provide the opportunity for treatment as well as diagnosis. A central role of the IP physican is the performance of therapeutic bronchoscopy. For example, an aspirated foreign body may be retrieved with an instrument passed through the bronchoscope (either flexible or rigid), and bleeding may be controlled with a balloon catheter similarly introduced. Newer interventional techniques performed through a bronchoscope include methods for achieving and maintaining patency of airways that are partially or completely occluded, especially by tumors. These techniques include laser therapy, cryotherapy, argon plasma coagulation, electrocautery, balloon bronchoplasty and dilation, and stent placement. Many IP physicians are also trained in performing percutaneous tracheotomy.

SURGICAL TECHNIQUES FOR OBTAINING BIOLOGIC SPECIMENS

Evaluation and diagnosis of disorders of the chest commonly involve collaboration between pulmonologists and thoracic surgeons. While procedures such as mediastinoscopy, VATS, and thoracotomy are performed by thoracic surgeons, there is overlap in many minimally invasive techniques that can be performed by a pulmonologist or a thoracic surgeon.

MEDIASTINOSCOPY AND MEDIASTINOTOMY

Proper staging of lung cancer is of paramount concern when determining a treatment regimen. Although CT and PET scanning are useful for determining the size and nature of mediastinal lymph nodes as part of the staging of lung cancer, tissue biopsy and histopathologic examination are often critical for the diagnosis of mediastinal masses or enlarged mediastinal lymph nodes. The two major surgical procedures used to obtain specimens from masses or nodes in the mediastinum are mediastinoscopy (via a suprasternal approach) and mediastinotomy (via a parasternal approach). Both procedures are performed under general anesthesia by a qualified surgeon. In the case of suprasternal mediastinoscopy, a rigid mediastinoscope is inserted at the suprasternal notch and passed into the mediastinum along a pathway just anterior to the trachea. Tissue can be obtained with biopsy forceps passed through the scope, sampling masses or nodes that are in a paratracheal or pretracheal position (levels 2R, 2L, 3, 4R, 4L). Aortopulmonary lymph nodes (levels 5, 6) are not accessible by this route and thus are commonly sampled by parasternal mediastinotomy (the Chamberlain procedure). This approach involves a parasternal incision and dissection directly down to a mass or node that requires biopsy.

As an alternative to surgery, a bronchoscope can be used to perform TBNA (discussed above) to obtain tissue from the mediastinum, and, when combined with EBUS, can allow access to the same lymph node stations associated with mediastinoscopy, but also extend access out to the hilar lymph nodes (levels 10, 11). Finally, endoscopic ultrasound (EUS)–fine-needle aspiration (FNA) is a second procedure that complements EBUS–FNA in the staging of lung cancer. EUS–FNA is performed via the esophagus and is ideally suited for sampling lymph nodes in the posterior mediastinum (levels 7, 8, 9). Because US imaging cannot penetrate air filled spaces, the area directly anterior to the trachea cannot accurately be assessed and is a "blind spot" for EUS–FNA. However, EBUS–FNA can visualize the anterior lymph nodes and can complement EUS–FNA. The combination of EUS–FNA and EBUS–FNA is a technique that is becoming an alternative to surgery for staging the mediastinum in thoracic malignancies.

VIDEO-ASSISTED THORACIC SURGERY

Advances in video technology have allowed the development of thoracoscopy, or VATS, for the diagnosis and management of pleural as well as parenchymal lung disease. This procedure is performed in the operating room using single-lung ventilation with double-lumen endotracheal intubation and involves the passage of a rigid scope with a distal lens through a trocar inserted into the pleura. A high-quality image is shown on a monitor screen, allowing the operator to manipulate instruments passed into the pleural space through separate small intercostal incisions. With these instruments the operator can biopsy lesions of the pleura under direct visualization. In addition, this procedure is now used commonly to biopsy peripheral lung tissue or to remove peripheral nodules for both diagnostic and therapeutic purposes. This much less invasive procedure has largely supplanted the traditional "open lung biopsy" performed via thoracotomy. The decision to use a VATS technique versus performing an open thoracotomy is made by the thoracic surgeon and is based on whether a patient can tolerate the single-lung ventilation that is required to allow adequate visualization of the lung. With further advances in instrumentation and experience, VATS can be used to perform procedures previously requiring thoracotomy, including stapled lung biopsy, resection of pulmonary nodules, lobectomy, pneumonectomy, pericardial window, or other standard thoracic surgical procedures; but allows them to be performed in a minimally invasive manner.

THORACOTOMY

Although frequently replaced by VATS, thoracotomy remains an option for the diagnostic sampling of lung tissue. It provides the largest amount of material, and it can be used to biopsy and/or excise lesions that are too deep or too close to vital structures for removal by VATS. The choice between VATS and thoracotomy needs to be made on a case-by-case basis.

ACKNOWLEDGMENT

We wish to acknowledge Dr. Scott Manaker and Dr. Steven Weinberger for their contributions to prior versions of this chapter.

FURTHER READINGS

Brown MA, Semelka RC: *MRI: Basic Principles and Applications,* 3rd ed. Hoboken, Wiley-Liss, 2003

Detterbeck FC. Evolution and science, progress and change. Thorax 62:654, 2007

———, et al: Seeking a home for a PET. Defining the appropriate place for positron emission tomography imaging in the diagnosis of pulmonary nodules or masses. Parts 1 and 2. Chest 125:2294, 2300, 2004

De Wever W et al: Multidetector CT-generated virtual bronchoscopy: An illustrated review of the potential clinical indications. Eur Respir J 23:776, 2004

———: Virtual bronchoscopy: Accuracy and usefulness—an overview. Semin Ultrasound CT MR 26:364, 2005

Kalra MK, Saini S: A practical approach to MDCT, in *MDCT: A Practical Approach,* S Saini et al (eds). Milan, Springer, 2006

Kavanagh JJ et al: Pulmonary embolism imaging with MDCT, in *MDCT: A Practical Approach*, S Saini et al (eds). Milan, Springer, 2006

Lee P, Colt HG: State of the art: Pleuroscopy. J Thorac Oncol 2:663, 2007

Medford ARL et al: Mediastinal staging procedures in lung cancer: EBUS, TBNA and mediastinoscopy. Curr Opin Pulmon Med 15:334, 2009

Moghissi K et al: Current indications and future perspective of fluorescence bronchoscopy: A review study. Photodiagn Photodyn Ther 5:238, 2008

Muller NL, Silva CIS: Normal chest radiograph, in *Imaging of the Chest*, vol. 1, NL Muller, CIS Silva (eds). Philadelphia, Saunders/Elsevier, 2008

Patel S, Kazerooni EA: Helical CT for the evaluation of acute pulmonary embolism. AJR Am J Roentgenol 185:135, 2005

Varela-Lema L et al: Effectiveness and safety of endobronchial ultrasound–transbronchial needle aspiration: A systematic review. Eur Respir J 33:1156, 2009

Wahidi MM et al: State of the art interventional pulmonology. Chest 131:261, 2007

Wallace MB et al. Minimally invasive endoscopic staging of suspected lung cancer. JAMA 299:540, 2008

Weinberger SE (ed): *Principles of Pulmonary Medicine,* 4th ed. Philadelphia, Saunders, 2004

CHAPTER 254 Asthma

Peter J. Barnes

Asthma is a syndrome characterized by airflow obstruction that varies markedly, both spontaneously and with treatment. Asthmatics harbor a special type of inflammation in the airways that makes them more responsive than nonasthmatics to a wide range of triggers, leading to excessive narrowing with consequent reduced airflow and symptomatic wheezing and dyspnea. Narrowing of the airways is usually reversible, but in some patients with chronic asthma there may be an element of irreversible airflow obstruction. The increasing global prevalence of asthma, the large burden it now imposes on patients, and the high health care costs have led to extensive research into its mechanisms and treatment.

PREVALENCE

Asthma is one of the most common chronic diseases globally and currently affects approximately 300 million people worldwide. The prevalence of asthma has risen in affluent countries over the last 30 years but now appears to have stabilized, with approximately 10–12% of adults and 15% of children affected by the disease. In developing countries where the prevalence of asthma had been much lower, there is a rising prevalence, which is associated with increased urbanization. The prevalence of atopy and other allergic diseases has also increased over the same time, suggesting that the reasons for the increase are likely to be systemic rather than confined to the lungs. This epidemiologic observation suggests that there is a maximum number of individuals in the community, who are likely to be affected by asthma, most likely by genetic predisposition. Most patients with asthma in affluent countries are atopic, with allergic sensitization to the house dust mite *Dermatophagoides pteronyssinus* and other environmental allergens.

Because asthma is both common and frequently complicated by the effects of smoking on the lungs, it is difficult to be certain about the natural history of the disease in adults. Asthma can present at any age, with a peak age of 3 years. In childhood, twice as many males as females are asthmatic, but by adulthood the sex ratio has equalized. The commonly held belief that children "grow out of their asthma" is justified to some extent. Long-term studies that have followed children until they reach the age of 40 years suggest that many with asthma become asymptomatic during adolescence but that asthma returns in some during adult life, particularly in those with persistent symptoms and severe asthma. Adults with asthma, including those with onset during adulthood, rarely become permanently asymptomatic. The severity of asthma does not vary significantly within a given patient; those with mild asthma rarely progress to more severe disease, whereas those with severe asthma usually have severe disease at the onset.

Deaths from asthma are uncommon, and in many affluent countries have been steadily declining over the last decade. A rise in asthma mortality seen in several countries during the 1960s was associated with increased use of short-acting β_2-adrenergic agonists (as rescue therapy), but there is now compelling evidence that the more widespread use of inhaled corticosteroids (ICS) in patients with persistent asthma is responsible for the decrease in mortality in recent years. Major risk factors for asthma deaths are poorly controlled disease with frequent use of bronchodilator inhalers, lack of corticosteroid therapy, and previous admissions to hospital with near-fatal asthma.

It has proved difficult to agree on a definition of asthma, but there is good agreement on the description of the clinical syndrome and disease pathology. Until the etiologic mechanisms of the disease are better understood, it will be difficult to provide an accurate definition.

ETIOLOGY

Asthma is a heterogeneous disease with interplay between genetic and environmental factors. Several risk factors have been implicated (Table 254-1).

ATOPY

Atopy is the major risk factor for asthma, and nonatopic individuals have a very low risk of developing asthma. Patients with asthma commonly suffer from other atopic diseases, particularly allergic rhinitis, which may be found in over 80% of asthmatic patients, and atopic dermatitis (eczema). Atopy may be found in 40–50% of the population in affluent countries, with only a proportion of atopic individuals becoming asthmatic. This observation suggests that some other environmental or genetic factor(s) predispose to the development of asthma in atopic individuals. The allergens that lead to sensitization are usually proteins that have protease activity, and the most common allergens are derived from house dust mites, cat and dog fur, cockroaches (in inner cities), grass and tree pollens, and rodents (in laboratory workers). Atopy is due to the genetically determined production of specific IgE antibody, with many patients showing a family history of allergic diseases.

TABLE 254-1 Risk Factors and Triggers Involved in Asthma

Endogenous Factors	Environmental Factors
Genetic predisposition	Indoor allergens
Atopy	Outdoor allergens
Airway hyperresponsiveness	Occupational sensitizers
Gender	Passive smoking
Ethnicity?	Respiratory infections
Obesity?	
Early viral infections?	
Triggers	
Allergens	
Upper respiratory tract viral infections	
Exercise and hyperventilation	
Cold air	
Sulfur dioxide and irritant gases	
Drugs (β-blockers, aspirin)	
Stress	
Irritants (household sprays, paint fumes)	

INTRINSIC ASTHMA

A minority of asthmatic patients (approximately 10%) have negative skin tests to common inhalant allergens and normal serum concentrations of IgE. These patients, with nonatopic or intrinsic asthma, usually show later onset of disease (adult-onset asthma), commonly have concomitant nasal polyps, and may be aspirin-sensitive. They usually have more severe, persistent asthma. Little is understood about mechanism, but the immunopathology in bronchial biopsies and sputum appears to be identical to that found in atopic asthma. There is recent evidence for increased local production of IgE in the airways, suggesting that there may be common IgE-mediated mechanisms; staphylococcal enterotoxins, which serve as "superantigens," have been implicated.

INFECTIONS

Although viral infections are common as triggers of asthma exacerbations, it is uncertain whether they play a role in etiology. There is some association between respiratory syncytial virus infection in infancy and the development of asthma, but the specific pathogenesis is difficult to elucidate, as this infection is very common in children. More recently, atypical bacteria such as *Mycoplasma* and *Chlamydophila,* have been implicated in the mechanism of severe asthma, but thus far, the evidence is not very convincing of a true association.

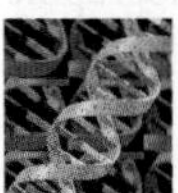

GENETIC CONSIDERATIONS

The familial association of asthma and a high degree of concordance for asthma in identical twins indicate a genetic predisposition to the disease; however, whether or not the genes predisposing to asthma are similar or in addition to those predisposing to atopy is not yet clear. It now seems likely that different genes may also contribute to asthma specifically, and there is increasing evidence that the severity of asthma is also genetically determined. Genetic screens with classical linkage analysis and single-nucleotide polymorphisms of various candidate genes indicate that asthma is polygenic, with each gene identified having a small effect that is often not replicated in different populations. This observation suggests that the interaction of many genes is important, and these may differ in different populations. The most consistent findings have been associations with polymorphisms of genes on chromosome 5q, including the T helper 2 (T_H2) cells interleukin (IL)-4, IL-5, IL-9, and IL-13, which are associated with atopy. There is increasing evidence for a complex interaction between genetic polymorphisms and environmental factors that will require very large population studies to unravel. Novel genes that have been associated with asthma, including *ADAM-33*, *DPP-10*, and *GPRA*, have also been identified by positional cloning, but their function in disease pathogenesis is not yet clear. Recent genome-wide association studies have identified further novel genes, although, again, their functional role is not yet clear. Genetic polymorphisms may also be important in determining the response to asthma therapy. For example, the Arg-Gly-16 variant in the β_2-receptor has been associated with reduced response to β_2-agonists, and repeats of an Sp1 recognition sequence in the promoter region of 5-lipoxygenase may affect the response to antileukotrienes. However, these effects are small and inconsistent and do not yet have any implications for asthma therapy.

ENVIRONMENTAL FACTORS

It is likely that environmental factors in early life determine which atopic individuals become asthmatic. The increasing prevalence of asthma, particularly in developing countries, over the last few decades also indicates the importance of environmental mechanisms interacting with a genetic predisposition.

Hygiene hypothesis

The observation that allergic sensitization and asthma were less common in children with older siblings first suggested that lower levels of infection may be a factor in affluent societies that increase the risks of asthma. This "hygiene hypothesis" proposes that lack of infections in early childhood preserves the T_H2 cell bias at birth, whereas exposure to infections and endotoxin results in a shift toward a predominant protective T_H1 immune response. Children brought up on farms who are exposed to a high level of endotoxin are less likely to develop allergic sensitization than children raised on dairy farms. Intestinal parasite infection may also be associated with a reduced risk of asthma. While there is considerable epidemiologic support for the hygiene hypothesis, it cannot account for the parallel increase in T_H1-driven diseases such as diabetes mellitus over the same period.

Diet

The role of dietary factors is controversial. Observational studies have shown that diets low in antioxidants such as vitamin C and vitamin A, magnesium, selenium, and omega-3 polyunsaturated fats (fish oil) or high in sodium and omega-6 polyunsaturates are associated with an increased risk of asthma. Vitamin D deficiency may also predispose to the development of asthma. However, interventional studies with supplementary diets have not supported an important role for these dietary factors. Obesity is also an independent risk factor for asthma, particularly in women, but the mechanisms are thus far unknown.

Air pollution

Air pollutants such as sulfur dioxide, ozone, and diesel particulates, may trigger asthma symptoms, but the role of different air pollutants in the etiology of the disease is much less certain. Most evidence argues against an important role for air pollution as asthma is no more prevalent in cities with a high ambient level of traffic pollution than in rural areas with low levels of pollution. Asthma had a much lower prevalence in East Germany compared to West Germany despite a much higher level of air pollution, but since reunification these differences have decreased as eastern Germany has become more affluent. Indoor air pollution may be more important with exposure to nitrogen oxides from cooking stoves and exposure to passive cigarette smoke. There is some evidence that maternal smoking is a risk factor for asthma, but it is difficult to dissociate this association from an increased risk of respiratory infections.

Allergens

Inhaled allergens are common triggers of asthma symptoms and have also been implicated in allergic sensitization. Exposure to house dust mites in early childhood is a risk factor for allergic sensitization and asthma, but rigorous allergen avoidance has not shown any evidence for a reduced risk of developing asthma. The increase in house dust mites in centrally heated poorly ventilated homes with fitted carpets has been implicated in the increasing prevalence of asthma in affluent countries. Domestic pets, particularly cats, have also been associated with allergic sensitization, but early exposure to cats in the home may be protective through the induction of tolerance.

Occupational exposure

Occupational asthma is relatively common and may affect up to 10% of young adults. Over 200 sensitizing agents have been identified. Chemicals such as toluene diisocyanate and trimellitic anhydride, may lead to sensitization independent of atopy. Individuals may also be exposed to allergens in the workplace such as small animal allergens in laboratory workers and fungal amylase in wheat flour in bakers. Occupational asthma may be suspected when symptoms improve during weekends and holidays.

■ OTHER FACTORS

Several other factors have been implicated in the etiology of asthma, including lower maternal age, duration of breast-feeding, prematurity and low birthweight, and inactivity, but are unlikely to contribute to the recent global increase in asthma prevalence. There is also an association with acetaminophen (paracetamol) consumption in childhood, which remains unexplained.

PATHOGENESIS

Asthma is associated with a specific chronic inflammation of the mucosa of the lower airways. One of the main aims of treatment is to reduce this inflammation.

■ PATHOLOGY

The pathology of asthma has been revealed through examining the lungs at autopsy of patients who have died of asthma and from bronchial biopsies in patients with usually mild asthma. The airway mucosa is infiltrated with activated eosinophils and T lymphocytes, and there is activation of mucosal mast cells. The degree of inflammation is poorly related to disease severity and may be found in atopic patients without asthma symptoms. The inflammation is reduced by treatment with ICS. A characteristic finding is thickening of the basement membrane due to subepithelial collagen deposition. This feature is also found in patients with eosinophilic bronchitis presenting as cough who do not have asthma and is, therefore, likely to be a marker of eosinophilic inflammation in the airway as eosinophils release fibrogenic factors. The epithelium is often shed or friable, with reduced attachments to the airway wall and increased numbers of epithelial cells in the lumen. The airway wall itself may be thickened and edematous, particularly in fatal asthma. Another common finding in fatal asthma is occlusion of the airway lumen by a mucous plug, which is comprised of mucous glycoproteins secreted from goblet cells and plasma proteins from leaky bronchial vessels (Fig. 254-1). There is also vasodilation and increased numbers of blood vessels (angiogenesis). Direct observation by bronchoscopy indicates that the airways may be narrowed, erythematous, and edematous. The pathology of asthma is remarkably uniform in different types of asthma, including atopic, nonatopic, occupational, aspirin-sensitive, and pediatric asthma. These pathologic changes are found in all airways, but do not extend to the lung parenchyma; peripheral airway inflammation is found particularly in patients with severe asthma. The involvement of airways may be patchy and this is consistent with bronchographic findings of uneven narrowing of the airways.

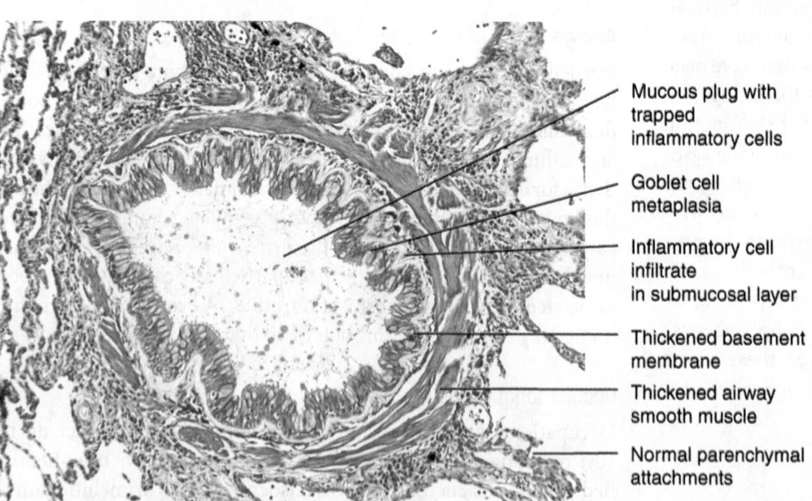

Figure 254-1 Histopathology of a small airway in fatal asthma. The lumen is occluded with a mucous plug, there is goblet cell metaplasia, and the airway wall is thickened, with an increase in basement membrane thickness and airway smooth muscle. *(Courtesy of Dr. J. Hogg, University of British Colombia.)*

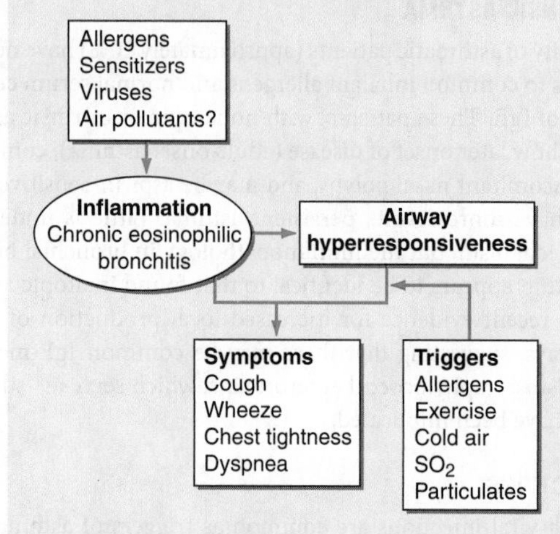

Figure 254-2 Inflammation in the airways of asthmatic patients leads to airway hyperresponsiveness and symptoms. So_2, sulfur dioxide.

■ INFLAMMATION

There is inflammation in the respiratory mucosa from the trachea to terminal bronchioles, but with a predominance in the bronchi (cartilaginous airways). Considerable research has identified the major cellular components of inflammation, but it is still uncertain how inflammatory cells interact and how inflammation translates into the symptoms of asthma (Fig. 254-2). There is good evidence that the specific pattern of airway inflammation in asthma is associated with airway hyperresponsiveness (AHR), the physiologic abnormality of asthma, which is correlated with variable airflow obstruction. The pattern of inflammation in asthma is characteristic of allergic diseases, with similar inflammatory cells seen in the nasal mucosa in rhinitis. However, an indistinguishable pattern of inflammation is found in intrinsic asthma, and this may reflect local rather than systemic IgE production. Although most attention has focused on the acute inflammatory changes seen in asthma, this is a chronic condition, with inflammation persisting over many years in most patients. The mechanisms involved in persistence of inflammation in asthma are still poorly understood. Superimposed on this chronic inflammatory state are acute inflammatory episodes, which correspond to exacerbations of asthma. Many inflammatory cells are known to be involved in asthma with no key cell that is predominant (Fig. 254-3).

Mast cells

Mast cells are important in initiating the acute bronchoconstrictor responses to allergens and several other indirectly acting stimuli such as exercise and hyperventilation (via osmolality or thermal changes), as well as fog. Activated mast cells are found at the airway surface in asthma patients and also in the airway smooth-muscle layer, whereas this is not seen in normal subjects or patients with eosinophilic bronchitis. Mast

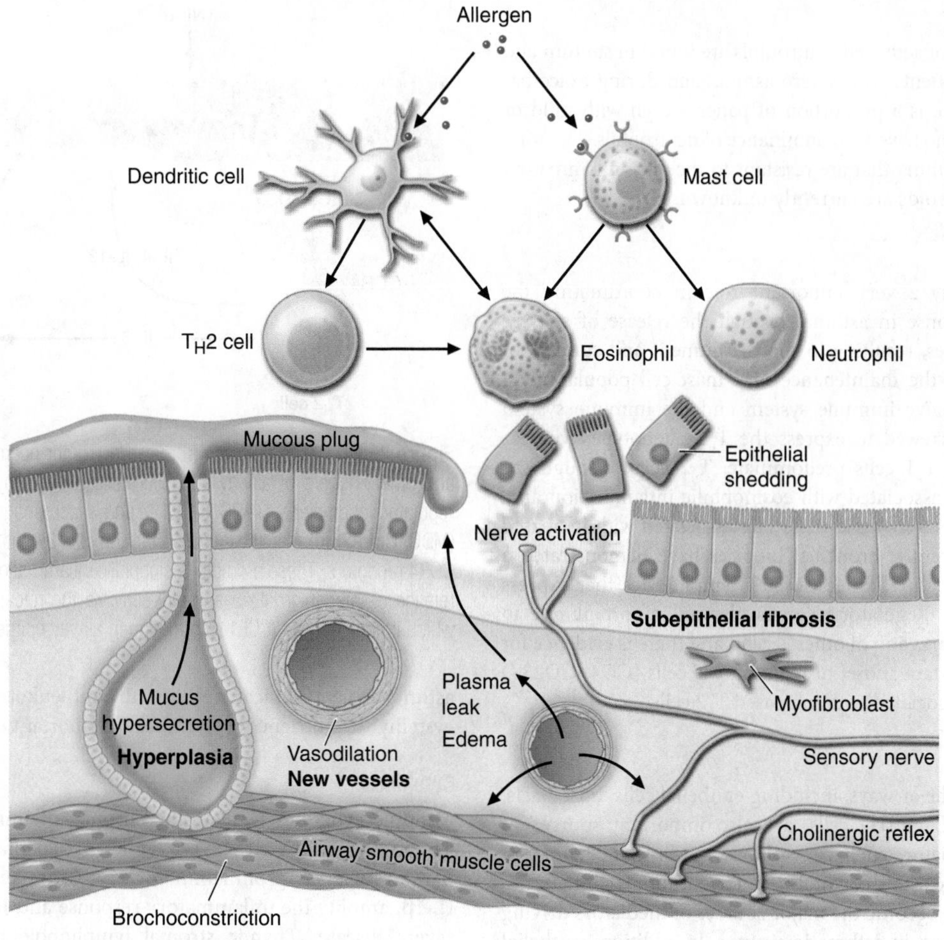

Figure 254-3 The pathophysiology of asthma is complex with participation of several interacting inflammatory cells, which result in acute and chronic inflammatory effects on the airway.

cells are activated by allergens through an IgE-dependent mechanism, and binding of specific IgE to mast cells renders them more sensitive to activation. The importance of IgE in the pathophysiology of asthma has been highlighted by clinical studies with humanized anti-IgE antibodies, which inhibit IgE-mediated effects, reduce asthma symptoms, and reduce exacerbations. There are, however, uncertainties about the role of mast cells in more chronic allergic inflammatory events. Mast cells release several bronchoconstrictor mediators, including histamine, prostaglandin D_2, and cysteinyl-leukotrienes, but also several cytokines, chemokines, growth factors, and neurotrophins.

Macrophages and dendritic cells

Macrophages, which are derived from blood monocytes, may traffic into the airways in asthma and may be activated by allergens via low-affinity IgE receptors ($Fc_{\varepsilon}RII$). Macrophages have the capacity to initiate a type of inflammatory response via the release of a certain pattern of cytokines, but these cells also release anti-inflammatory mediators (e.g., IL-10) and, thus, their roles in asthma are uncertain. Dendritic cells are specialized macrophage-like cells in the airway epithelium, which are the major antigen-presenting cells. Dendritic cells take up allergens, process them to peptides, and migrate to local lymph nodes where they present the allergenic peptides to uncommitted T-lymphocytes to program the production of allergen-specific T cells. Immature dendritic cells in the respiratory tract promote T_H2 cell differentiation and require cytokines such as IL-12 and tumor necrosis factor α (TNF-α), to promote the normally preponderant T_H1 response. The cytokine thymic stromal lymphopoietin (TSLP) released from epithelial cells in asthmatic patients instructs dendritic cells to release chemokines that attract T_H2 cells into the airways.

Eosinophils

Eosinophil infiltration is a characteristic feature of asthmatic airways. Allergen inhalation results in a marked increase in activated eosinophils in the airways at the time of the late reaction. Eosinophils are linked to the development of AHR through the release of basic proteins and oxygen-derived free radicals. Eosinophil recruitment involves adhesion of eosinophils to vascular endothelial cells in the airway circulation due to interaction between adhesion molecules, migration into the submucosa under the direction of chemokines, and their subsequent activation and prolonged survival. Blocking antibodies to IL-5 causes a profound and prolonged reduction in circulating and sputum eosinophils, but is not associated with reduced AHR or asthma symptoms, although in selected patients with steroid-resistant airway eosinophils, there is a reduction in exacerbations. Eosinophilic inflammation is also found in patients with chronic cough (eosinophilic bronchitis) who do not have AHR or clinical features of asthma. Increasing evidence suggests that eosinophils may be important in release of growth factors involved in airway remodeling, in exacerbations but not in AHR.

Neutrophils

Increased numbers of activated neutrophils are found in sputum and airways of some patients with severe asthma and during exacerbations, although there is a proportion of patients even with mild or moderate asthma who have a predominance of neutrophils. The roles of neutrophils in asthma that are resistant to the anti-inflammatory effects of corticosteroids are currently unknown.

T lymphocytes

T lymphocytes play a very important role in coordinating the inflammatory response in asthma through the release of specific patterns of cytokines, resulting in the recruitment and survival of eosinophils and in the maintenance of a mast cell population in the airways. The naïve immune system and the immune system of asthmatics are skewed to express the T_H2 phenotype, whereas in normal airways T_H1 cells predominate. T_H2 cells, through the release of IL-5, are associated with eosinophilic inflammation and, through the release of IL-4 and IL-13, are associated with increased IgE formation. Recently, bronchial biopsies have demonstrated a preponderance of natural killer $CD4^+$ T lymphocytes that express high levels of IL-4. Regulatory T cells play an important role in determining the expression of other T cells, and there is evidence for a reduction in a certain subset of regulatory T cells (CD4+CD25+) in asthma that is associated with increased T_H2 cells.

Structural cells

Structural cells of the airways, including epithelial cells, fibroblasts, and airway smooth-muscle cells, are also important sources of inflammatory mediators such as cytokines and lipid mediators, in asthma. Indeed, because structural cells far outnumber inflammatory cells, they may become the major sources of mediators driving chronic inflammation in asthmatic airways. In addition, epithelial cells may have key roles in translating inhaled environmental signals into an airway inflammatory response, and are probably major target cells for ICS.

INFLAMMATORY MEDIATORS

Many different mediators have been implicated in asthma, and they may have a variety of effects on the airways that could account for the pathologic features of asthma (Fig. 254-4). Mediators such as histamine, prostaglandin D_2, and cysteinyl-leukotrienes contract airway smooth muscle, increase microvascular leakage, increase airway mucus secretion, and attract other inflammatory cells. Because each mediator has many effects, the role of individual mediators in the pathophysiology of asthma is not yet clear. Although the multiplicity of mediators makes it unlikely that preventing the synthesis or action of a single mediator will have a major impact in clinical

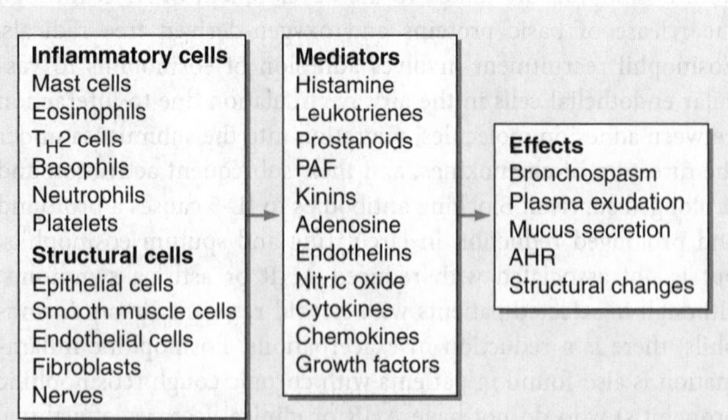

Figure 254-4 Many cells and mediators are involved in asthma and lead to several effects on the airways.

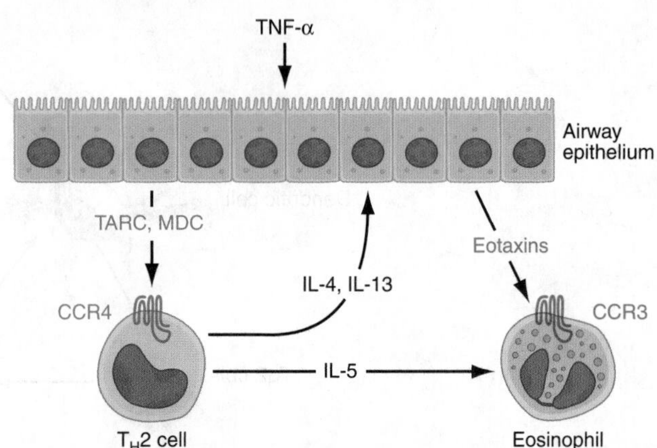

Figure 254-5 Chemokines in asthma. Tumor necrosis factor α (TNF-α) and other triggers of airway epithelial cells release thymus and activation-regulated chemokine (TARC, CCL17) and macrophage-derived chemokine (MDC, CCL22) from epithelial cells that attract T_H2 cells via activation of their CCR4 receptors. These promote eosinophilic inflammation directly through the release of interleukin (IL)-5 and indirectly via the release of IL-4 and IL-13, which induce eotaxin (CCL11) formation in airway epithelial cells.

asthma, recent clinical studies with antileukotrienes suggest that cysteinyl-leukotrienes have clinically important effects.

Cytokines

Multiple cytokines regulate the chronic inflammation of asthma. The TH2 cytokines IL-4, IL-5, and IL-13 mediate allergic inflammation, whereas proinflammatory cytokines such as TNF-α and IL-1β, amplify the inflammatory response and play a role in more severe disease. Thymic stromal lymphopoietin is an upstream cytokine released from epithelial cells of asthmatics that orchestrates the release of chemokines that selectively attract T_H2 cells. Some cytokines such as IL-10 and IL-12 are anti-inflammatory and may be deficient in asthma.

Chemokines

Chemokines are involved in attracting inflammatory cells from the bronchial circulation into the airways. Eotaxin (CCL11) is selectively attractant to eosinophils via CCR3 and is expressed by epithelial cells of asthmatics, whereas CCL17 (TARC) and CCL22 (MDC) from epithelial cells attract T_H2 cells via CCR4 (Fig. 254-5).

Oxidative stress

There is increased oxidative stress in asthma as activated inflammatory cells such as macrophages and eosinophils that produce reactive oxygen species. Evidence for increased oxidative stress in asthma is provided by the increased concentrations of 8-isoprostane (a product of oxidized arachidonic acid) in exhaled breath condensates and increased ethane (a product of lipid peroxidation) in the expired air of asthmatic patients. Increased oxidative stress is related to disease severity, may amplify the inflammatory response, and may reduce responsiveness to corticosteroids.

Nitric oxide

Nitric oxide (NO) is produced by several cells in the airway by NO synthases, particularly airway epithelial cells and macrophages. The level of NO in the expired air of patients with asthma is higher than normal and is related to the eosinophilic inflammation. Increased NO may contribute to the bronchial vasodilation observed in asthma. Exhaled NO is increasingly used in the diagnosis and monitoring of asthmatic inflammation, although it is not yet used routinely in clinical practice.

Transcription factors

Proinflammatory transcription factors such as nuclear factor-κB (NF-κB) and activator protein-1, are activated in asthmatic airways and orchestrate the expression of multiple inflammatory genes. More specific transcription factors that are involved include nuclear factor of activated T cells and GATA-3, which regulate the expression of T_H2 cytokines in T cells.

■ EFFECTS OF INFLAMMATION

The chronic inflammatory response has several effects on the target cells of the airways, resulting in the characteristic pathophysiologic changes associated with asthma. Asthma may be regarded as a disease with continuous inflammation and repair proceeding simultaneously. Important advances continue to be made in our understanding of these changes, but, despite these new insights, the relationship between chronic inflammatory processes and asthma symptoms is often not clear.

Airway epithelium

Airway epithelial shedding may be important in contributing to AHR and may explain how several mechanisms, such as ozone exposure, virus infections, chemical sensitizers, and allergen exposure, can lead to its development, as all of these stimuli may lead to epithelial disruption. Epithelial damage may contribute to AHR in a number of ways, including loss of its barrier function to allow penetration of allergens; loss of enzymes (such as neutral endopeptidase) that degrade certain peptide inflammatory mediators; loss of a relaxant factor (so called epithelial-derived relaxant factor); and exposure of sensory nerves, which may lead to reflex neural effects on the airway.

Fibrosis

In all asthmatic patients, the basement membrane is apparently thickened due to subepithelial fibrosis with deposition of types III and V collagen below the true basement membrane and is associated with eosinophil infiltration, presumably through the release of profibrotic mediators such as transforming growth factor-β. Mechanical manipulations can alter the phenotype of airway epithelial cells in a profibrotic fashion. In more severe patients, there is also fibrosis within the airway wall, which may contribute to irreversible narrowing of the airways.

Airway smooth muscle

There is still debate about the role of abnormalities in airway smooth muscle in asthmatic airways. In vitro airway smooth muscle from asthmatic patients usually shows no increased responsiveness to constrictors. Reduced responsiveness to β-agonists has also been reported in postmortem or surgically removed bronchi from asthmatics, although the number of β-receptors is not reduced, suggesting that β-receptors have been uncoupled. These abnormalities of airway smooth-muscle may be secondary to the chronic inflammatory process. Inflammatory mediators may modulate the ion channels that serve to regulate the resting membrane potential of airway smooth-muscle cells, thus altering the level of excitability of these cells. In asthmatic airways there is also a characteristic hypertrophy and hyperplasia of airway smooth muscle, which is presumably the result of stimulation of airway smooth-muscle cells by various growth factors such as platelet-derived growth factor (PDGF) or endothelin-1 released from inflammatory or epithelial cells.

Vascular responses

There is increased airway mucosal blood flow in asthma. The bronchial circulation may play an important role in regulating airway caliber, since an increase in the vascular volume may contribute to airway narrowing. Increased airway blood flow may be important in removing inflammatory mediators from the airway, and may play a role in the development of exercise-induced asthma. There is an increase in the number of blood vessels in asthmatic airways as a result of angiogenesis in response to growth factors, particularly vascular-endothelial growth factor. Microvascular leakage from postcapillary venules in response to inflammatory mediators is observed in asthma, resulting in airway edema and plasma exudation into the airway lumen.

Mucus hypersecretion

Increased mucus secretion contributes to the viscid mucous plugs that occlude asthmatic airways, particularly in fatal asthma. There is evidence for hyperplasia of submucosal glands that are confined to large airways and of increased numbers of epithelial goblet cells. IL-4 and IL-13 induce mucus hypersecretion in experimental models of asthma.

Neural effects

Various defects in autonomic neural control may contribute to AHR in asthma, but these are likely to be secondary to the disease, rather than primary defects. Cholinergic pathways, through the release of acetylcholine acting on muscarinic receptors, cause bronchoconstriction and may be activated reflexly in asthma. Inflammatory mediators may activate sensory nerves, resulting in reflex cholinergic bronchoconstriction or release of inflammatory neuropeptides. Inflammatory products may also sensitize sensory nerve endings in the airway epithelium such that the nerves become hyperalgesic. Neurotrophins, which may be released from various cell types in airways, including epithelial cells and mast cells, may cause proliferation and sensitization of airway sensory nerves. Airway nerves may also release neurotransmitters, such as substance P, which have inflammatory effects.

■ AIRWAY REMODELING

Several changes in the structure of the airway are characteristically found in asthma, and these may lead to irreversible narrowing of the airways. Population studies have shown a greater decline in lung function over time than in normal subjects; however, most patients with asthma preserve normal or near-normal lung function throughout life if appropriately treated. This observation suggests that the accelerated decline in lung function occurs in a smaller proportion of asthmatics, and these are usually patients with more severe disease. There is some evidence that the early use of ICS may reduce the decline in lung function. The characteristic structural changes are increased airway smooth muscle, fibrosis, angiogenesis, and mucus hyperplasia.

ASTHMA TRIGGERS

Several stimuli trigger airway narrowing, wheezing, and dyspnea in asthmatic patients. While the previous view held that these should be avoided, it is now seen as evidence for poor control and an indicator of the need to increase controller (preventive) therapy.

■ ALLERGENS

Inhaled allergens activate mast cells with bound IgE directly leading to the immediate release of bronchoconstrictor mediators, resulting in the early response that is reversed by bronchodilators. Often, experimental allergen challenge is followed by a late response when there is airway edema and an acute inflammatory response with increased eosinophils and neutrophils that are not very reversible with bronchodilators. The most common allergens to trigger asthma are *Dermatophagoides* species, and environmental exposure leads to low-grade chronic symptoms that are perennial. Other perennial allergens are derived from cats and other domestic pets, as well as cockroaches. Other allergens, including grass pollen, ragweed, tree pollen, and fungal spores, are seasonal. Pollens usually cause allergic rhinitis rather than asthma, but in thunderstorms the pollen grains are disrupted and the particles that may be released can trigger severe asthma exacerbations (thunderstorm asthma).

VIRUS INFECTIONS

Upper respiratory tract virus infections such as rhinovirus, respiratory syncytial virus, and coronavirus are the most common triggers of acute severe exacerbations and may invade epithelial cells of the lower as well as the upper airways. The mechanism whereby these viruses cause exacerbations is poorly understood, but there is an increase in airway inflammation with increased numbers of eosinophils and neutrophils. There is evidence for reduced production of type I interferons by epithelial cells from asthmatic patients, resulting in increased susceptibility to these viral infections and a greater inflammatory response.

PHARMACOLOGIC AGENTS

Several drugs may trigger asthma. Beta-adrenergic blockers commonly acutely worsen asthma, and their use may be fatal. The mechanisms are not clear but are likely mediated through increased cholinergic bronchoconstriction. All beta blockers need to be avoided and even selective β_2 blocker or topical application (e.g., timolol eye drops) may be dangerous. Angiotensin-converting enzyme inhibitors are theoretically detrimental as they inhibit breakdown of kinins, which are bronchoconstrictors; however, they rarely worsen asthma, and the characteristic cough is no more frequent in asthmatics than in nonasthmatics. Aspirin may worsen asthma in some patients (aspirin-sensitive asthma is discussed below under "Special Considerations").

EXERCISE

Exercise is a common trigger of asthma, particularly in children. The mechanism is linked to hyperventilation, which results in increased osmolality in airway lining fluid and triggers mast cell mediator release, resulting in bronchoconstriction. Exercise-induced asthma (EIA) typically begins after exercise has ended, and recovers spontaneously within about 30 minutes. EIA is worse in cold, dry climates than in hot, humid conditions. It is, therefore, more common in sports such as cross-country running in cold weather, overland skiing, and ice hockey than in swimming. It may be prevented by prior administration of β_2-agonists and antileukotrienes, but is best prevented by regular treatment with ICS, which reduce the population of surface mast cells required for this response.

PHYSICAL FACTORS

Cold air and hyperventilation may trigger asthma through the same mechanisms as exercise. Laughter may also be a trigger. Many patients report worsening of asthma in hot weather and when the weather changes. Some asthmatics become worse when exposed to strong smells or perfumes, but the mechanism of this response is uncertain.

FOOD

There is little evidence that allergic reactions to food lead to increased asthma symptoms, despite the belief of many patients that their symptoms are triggered by particular food constituents. Exclusion diets are usually unsuccessful at reducing the frequency of episodes. Some foods such as shellfish and nuts may induce anaphylactic reactions that may include wheezing. Patients with aspirin-induced asthma may benefit from a salicylate-free diet, but these are difficult to maintain. Certain food additives may trigger asthma. Metabisulfite, which is used as a food preservative, may trigger asthma through the release of sulfur dioxide gas in the stomach. Tartrazine, a yellow food-coloring agent, was believed to be a trigger for asthma, but there is little convincing evidence for this.

AIR POLLUTION

Increased ambient levels of sulfur dioxide, ozone, and nitrogen oxides are associated with increased asthma symptoms.

OCCUPATIONAL FACTORS

Several substances found in the workplace may act as sensitizing agents, as discussed above, but may also act as triggers of asthma symptoms. Occupational asthma is characteristically associated with symptoms at work with relief on weekends and holidays. If removed from exposure within the first 6 months of symptoms, there is usually complete recovery. More persistent symptoms lead to irreversible airway changes, and, thus, early detection and avoidance are important.

HORMONAL FACTORS

Some women show premenstrual worsening of asthma, which can occasionally be very severe. The mechanisms are not completely understood, but are related to a fall in progesterone and in severe cases may be improved by treatment with high doses of progesterone or gonadotropin-releasing factors. Thyrotoxicosis and hypothyroidism can both worsen asthma, although the mechanisms are uncertain.

GASTROESOPHAGEAL REFLUX

Gastroesophageal reflux is common in asthmatic patients as it is increased by bronchodilators. Although acid reflux might trigger reflex bronchoconstriction, it rarely causes asthma symptoms, and antireflux therapy fails to reduce asthma symptoms in most patients.

STRESS

Many asthmatics report worsening of symptoms with stress. There is no doubt that psychological factors can induce bronchoconstriction through cholinergic reflex pathways. Paradoxically, very severe stress such as bereavement usually does not worsen, and may even improve, asthma symptoms.

PATHOPHYSIOLOGY

Limitation of airflow is due mainly to bronchoconstriction, but airway edema, vascular congestion, and luminal occlusion with exudate may also contribute. This results in a reduction in forced expiratory volume in 1 second (FEV_1), FEV_1/forced vital capacity (FVC) ratio, and peak expiratory flow (PEF), as well as an increase in airway resistance. Early closure of peripheral airway results in lung hyperinflation, (air trapping) and increased residual volume, particularly during acute exacerbations and in severe persistent asthma. In more severe asthma, reduced ventilation and increased pulmonary blood flow result in mismatching of ventilation and perfusion and in bronchial hyperemia. Ventilatory failure is very uncommon, even in patients with severe asthma, and arterial P_{CO_2} tends to be low due to increased ventilation.

AIRWAY HYPERRESPONSIVENESS

AHR is the characteristic physiologic abnormality of asthma and describes the excessive bronchoconstrictor response to multiple inhaled triggers that would have no effect on normal airways. The increase in AHR is linked to the frequency of asthma symptoms, and, thus, an important aim of therapy is to reduce AHR. Increased bronchoconstrictor responsiveness is seen with *direct* bronchoconstrictors such as histamine and methacholine, which contract airway smooth muscle, but is characteristically also seen with many *indirect* stimuli, which release bronchoconstrictors from mast cells or activate sensory nerves. Most of the triggers for asthma symptoms appear to act indirectly, including allergens, exercise, hyperventilation, fog (via mast cell activation), irritant dusts, and sulfur dioxide (via a cholinergic reflex).

CLINICAL FEATURES AND DIAGNOSIS

The characteristic symptoms of asthma are wheezing, dyspnea, and coughing, which are variable, both spontaneously and with therapy. Symptoms may be worse at night and patients typically awake in the early morning hours. Patients may report difficulty in filling their lungs with air. There is increased mucus production in some patients, with typically tenacious mucus that is difficult to expectorate. There may be increased ventilation and use of accessory muscles of ventilation. Prodromal symptoms may precede an attack, with itching under the chin, discomfort between the scapulae, or inexplicable fear (impending doom).

Typical physical signs are inspiratory, and to a greater extent expiratory, rhonchi throughout the chest, and there may be hyperinflation. Some patients, particularly children, may present with a predominant nonproductive cough (cough-variant asthma). There may be no abnormal physical findings when asthma is under control.

DIAGNOSIS

The diagnosis of asthma is usually apparent from the symptoms of variable and intermittent airways obstruction, but is usually confirmed by objective measurements of lung function.

Lung function tests

Simple spirometry confirms airflow limitation with a reduced FEV_1, FEV_1/FVC ratio, and PEF. Reversibility is demonstrated by a >12% and 200-mL increase in FEV_1 15 minutes after an inhaled short-acting β_2-agonist or in some patients by a 2 to 4 week trial of oral corticosteroids (OCS) (prednisone or prednisolone 30–40 mg daily). Measurements of PEF twice daily may confirm the diurnal variations in airflow obstruction. Flow-volume loops show reduced peak flow and reduced maximum expiratory flow. Further lung function tests are rarely necessary, but whole body plethysmography shows increased airway resistance and may show increased total lung capacity and residual volume. Gas diffusion is usually normal, but there may be a small increase in gas transfer in some patients.

Airway responsiveness

The increased AHR is normally measured by methacholine or histamine challenge with calculation of the provocative concentration that reduces FEV_1 by 20% (PC_{20}). This is rarely useful in clinical practice, but can be used in the differential diagnosis of chronic cough and when the diagnosis is in doubt in the setting of normal pulmonary function tests. Occasionally exercise testing is done to demonstrate the postexercise bronchoconstriction if there is a predominant history of EIA. Allergen challenge is rarely necessary and should only be undertaken by a specialist if specific occupational agents are to be identified.

Hematologic tests

Blood tests are not usually helpful. Total serum IgE and specific IgE to inhaled allergens [radioallergosorbent test (RAST)] may be measured in some patients.

Imaging

Chest roentgenography is usually normal but in more severe patients may show hyperinflated lungs. In exacerbations, there may be evidence of a pneumothorax. Lung shadowing usually indicates pneumonia or eosinophilic infiltrates in patients with bronchopulmonary aspergillosis. High-resolution CT may show areas of bronchiectasis in patients with severe asthma, and there may be thickening of the bronchial walls, but these changes are not diagnostic of asthma.

Skin tests

Skin prick tests to common inhalant allergens are positive in allergic asthma and negative in intrinsic asthma, but are not helpful in diagnosis. Positive skin responses may be useful in persuading patients to undertake allergen avoidance measures.

Exhaled nitric oxide

Exhaled NO is now being used as a noninvasive test to measure eosinophilic airway inflammation. The typically elevated levels in asthma are reduced by ICS, so this may be a test of compliance with therapy. It may also be useful in demonstrating insufficient anti-inflammatory therapy.

DIFFERENTIAL DIAGNOSIS

It is usually not difficult to differentiate asthma from other conditions that cause wheezing and dyspnea. Upper airway obstruction by a tumor or laryngeal edema can mimic severe asthma, but patients typically present with stridor localized to large airways. The diagnosis is confirmed by a flow-volume loop that shows a reduction in inspiratory as well as expiratory flow, and bronchoscopy to demonstrate the site of upper airway narrowing. Persistent wheezing in a specific area of the chest may indicate endobronchial obstruction with a foreign body. Left ventricular failure may mimic the wheezing of asthma but basilar crackles are present in contrast to asthma.

Eosinophilic pneumonias and systemic vasculitis, including Churg-Strauss syndrome and polyarteritis nodosa, may be associated with wheezing. Chronic obstructive pulmonary disease (COPD) is usually easy to differentiate from asthma as symptoms show less variability, never completely remit, and show much less (or no) reversibility to bronchodilators. Approximately 10% of COPD patients have features of asthma, with increased sputum eosinophils and a response to oral corticosteroids; these patients probably have both diseases concomitantly.

TREATMENT Asthma

The treatment of asthma is straightforward and the majority of patients are now managed by internists and family doctors with effective and safe therapies. There are several aims of therapy (Table 254-2). Most emphasis has been placed on drug therapy, but several nonpharmacologic approaches have also been used. The main drugs for asthma can be divided into bronchodilators, which give rapid relief of symptoms mainly through relaxation of airway smooth muscle, and controllers, which inhibit the underlying inflammatory process.

BRONCHODILATOR THERAPIES Bronchodilators act primarily on airway smooth muscle to reverse the bronchoconstriction of asthma. This gives rapid relief of symptoms but has little or no effect on the underlying inflammatory process. Thus, bronchodilators are not sufficient to control asthma in patients with

TABLE 254-2 Aims of Asthma Therapy

- Minimal (ideally no) chronic symptoms, including nocturnal
- Minimal (infrequent) exacerbations
- No emergency visits
- Minimal (ideally no) use of a required β_2-agonist
- No limitations on activities, including exercise
- Peak expiratory flow circadian variation <20%
- (Near) normal PEF
- Minimal (or no) adverse effects from medicine

Abbreviation: PEF, peak expiratory flow.

persistent symptoms. There are three classes of bronchodilators in current use: β_2-adrenergic agonists, anticholinergics, and theophylline; of these, β_2-agonists are by far the most effective.

β_2-Agonists β_2-Agonists activate β_2-adrenergic receptors, which are widely expressed in the airways. β_2-Receptors are coupled through a stimulatory G protein to adenylyl cyclase, resulting in increased intracellular cyclic adenosine monophosphate (AMP), which relaxes smooth muscle cells and inhibits certain inflammatory cells, particularly mast cells.

Mode of Action The primary action of β_2-agonists is to relax airway smooth-muscle cells of all airways, where they act as functional antagonists, reversing and preventing contraction of airway smooth-muscle cells by all known bronchoconstrictors. This generalized action is likely to account for their great efficacy as bronchodilators in asthma. There are also additional nonbronchodilator effects that may be clinically useful, including inhibition of mast cell mediator release, reduction in plasma exudation, and inhibition of sensory nerve activation (Table 254-3). Inflammatory cells express small numbers of β_2-receptors, but these are rapidly downregulated with β_2-agonist activation so that, in contrast to corticosteroids, there are no effects on inflammatory cells in the airways and there is no reduction in AHR.

Clinical Use β_2-Agonists are usually given by inhalation to reduce side effects. Short-acting β_2-agonists (SABAs) such as albuterol and terbutaline have a duration of action of 3–6 hours. They have a rapid onset of bronchodilation and are, therefore, used as needed for symptom relief. Increased use of SABAs indicates that asthma is not controlled. They are also useful in preventing EIA if taken prior to exercise. SABAs are used in high doses by nebulizer or via a metered-dose inhaler with a spacer. Long-acting β_2-agonists (LABAs) include salmeterol and formoterol, both of which have a duration of action over 12 hours and are given twice daily by inhalation. LABAs have replaced the regular use of SABAs, but LABAs should not be given in the absence of ICS therapy as they do not control the underlying inflammation. They do, however, improve asthma control and reduce exacerbations when added to ICS, which allows asthma to be controlled at lower doses of corticosteroids. This observation has led to the widespread use of fixed combination inhalers that contain a corticosteroid and a LABA, which have proved to be highly effective in the control of asthma.

TABLE 254-3 Effects of β-Adrenergic Agonists on Airways

- Relaxation of airway smooth muscle (proximal and distal airways)
- Inhibition of mast cell mediator release
- Inhibition of plasma exudation and airway edema
- Increased mucociliary clearance
- Increased mucus secretion
- Decreased cough
- No effect on chronic inflammation

Side Effects Adverse effects are not usually a problem with β_2-agonists when given by inhalation. The most common side effects are muscle tremor and palpitations, which are seen more commonly in elderly patients. There is a small fall in plasma potassium due to increased uptake by skeletal muscle cells, but this effect does not usually cause any clinical problem.

Tolerance Tolerance is a potential problem with any agonist given chronically, but while there is down-regulation of β_2-receptors, this does not reduce the bronchodilator response as there is a large receptor reserve in airway smooth-muscle cells. By contrast, mast cells become rapidly tolerant, but their tolerance may be prevented by concomitant administration of ICS.

Safety The safety of β_2-agonists has been an important issue. There is an association between asthma mortality and the amount of SABA used, but careful analysis demonstrates that the increased use of rescue SABAs reflects poor asthma control, which is a risk factor for asthma death. The slight excess in mortality that has been associated with the use of LABAs is related to the lack of use of concomitant ICS, as the LABA therapy fails to suppress the underlying inflammation. This highlights the importance of always using an ICS when LABAs are given, which is most conveniently achieved by using a combination inhaler.

Anticholinergics Muscarinic receptor antagonists such as ipratropium bromide, prevent cholinergic nerve-induced bronchoconstriction and mucus secretion. They are much less effective than β_2-agonists in asthma therapy as they inhibit only the cholinergic reflex component of bronchoconstriction, whereas β_2-agonists prevent all bronchoconstrictor mechanisms. Anticholinergics are, therefore, only used as an additional bronchodilator in patients with asthma that is not controlled by other inhaled medications. High doses may be given by nebulizer in treating acute severe asthma but should only be given following β_2-agonists, as they have a slower onset of bronchodilation.

Side effects are not usually a problem as there is little or no systemic absorption. The most common side effect is dry mouth; in elderly patients, urinary retention and glaucoma may also be observed.

Theophylline Theophylline was widely prescribed as an oral bronchodilator several years ago, especially as it was inexpensive. It has now fallen out of favor as side effects are common and inhaled β_2-agonists are much more effective as bronchodilators. The bronchodilator effect is due to inhibition of phosphodiesterases in airway smooth-muscle cells, which increases cyclic AMP, but doses required for bronchodilation commonly cause side effects that are mediated mainly by phosphodiesterase inhibition. There is increasing evidence that theophylline at lower doses has anti-inflammatory effects, and these are likely to be mediated through different molecular mechanisms. There is evidence that theophylline activates the key nuclear enzyme histone deacetylase-2, which is a critical mechanism for switching off activated inflammatory genes.

Clinical Use Oral theophylline is usually given as a slow-release preparation once or twice daily as this gives more stable plasma concentrations than normal theophylline tablets. It may be used as an additional bronchodilator in patients with severe asthma when plasma concentrations of 10–20 mg/L are required, although these concentrations are often associated with side effects. Low doses of theophylline, giving plasma concentrations of 5–10 mg/L, have additive effects to ICS and are particularly useful in patients with severe asthma. Indeed, withdrawal of theophylline from these patients may result in marked deterioration in asthma control. At low doses, the drug is well tolerated. IV aminophylline (a soluble salt of theophylline) was used for the treatment of severe asthma but has now been largely replaced by high doses of inhaled SABAs, which are more effective and have fewer side effects. Aminophylline is occasionally used (via slow IV infusion) in patients with severe exacerbations that are refractory to SABAs.

Side Effects Oral theophylline is well absorbed and is largely inactivated in the liver. Side effects are related to plasma concentrations; measurement of plasma theophylline may be useful in determining the correct dose. The most common side effects are nausea, vomiting, and headaches and are due to phosphodiesterase inhibition. Diuresis and palpitations may also occur, and at high concentrations cardiac arrhythmias, epileptic seizures, and death may occur due to adenosine A_1-receptor antagonism. Theophylline side effects are related to plasma concentration and are rarely observed at plasma concentrations below 10 mg/L. Theophylline is metabolized by CYP450 in the liver, and, thus, plasma concentrations may be elevated by drugs that block CYP450 such as erythromycin and allopurinol. Other drugs may also reduce clearance by other mechanisms leading to increased plasma concentrations (Table 254-4).

CONTROLLER THERAPIES

Inhaled Corticosteroids ICS are by far the most effective controllers for asthma, and their early use has revolutionized asthma therapy.

TABLE 254-4 Factors Affecting Clearance of Theophylline

Increased Clearance
• Enzyme induction (rifampicin, phenobarbitone, ethanol)
• Smoking (tobacco, marijuana)
• High-protein, low-carbohydrate diet
• Barbecued meat
• Childhood
Decreased Clearance
• Enzyme inhibition (cimetidine, erythromycin, ciprofloxacin, allopurinol, zileuton, zafirlukast)
• Congestive heart failure
• Liver disease
• Pneumonia
• Viral infection and vaccination
• High carbohydrate diet
• Old age

Mode of Action ICS are the most effective anti-inflammatory agents used in asthma therapy, reducing inflammatory cell numbers and their activation in the airways. ICS reduce eosinophils in the airways and sputum, and numbers of activated T lymphocytes and surface mast cells in the airway mucosa. These effects may account for the reduction in AHR that is seen with chronic ICS therapy.

The molecular mechanism of action of corticosteroids involves several effects on the inflammatory process. The major effect of corticosteroids is to switch off the transcription of multiple activated genes that encode inflammatory proteins such as cytokines, chemokines, adhesion molecules, and inflammatory enzymes. This effect involves several mechanisms, including inhibition of the transcription factors NF-κB and activator protein (AP)-1, but an important mechanism is recruitment of histone deacetylase-2 to the inflammatory gene complex, which reverses the histone acetylation associated with increased gene transcription. Corticosteroids also activate anti-inflammatory genes such as mitogen-activated protein (MAP) kinase phosphatase-1, and increase the expression of β_2-receptors. Most of the metabolic and endocrine side effects of corticosteroids are also mediated through transcriptional activation.

Clinical Use ICS are by far the most effective controllers in the management of asthma and are beneficial in treating asthma of any severity and age. ICS are usually given twice daily, but some may be effective once daily in mildly symptomatic patients. ICS rapidly improve the symptoms of asthma, and lung function improves over several days. They are effective in preventing asthma symptoms, such as EIA and nocturnal exacerbations, but also prevent severe exacerbations. ICS reduce AHR, but maximal improvement may take several months of therapy. Early treatment with ICS appears to prevent irreversible changes in airway function that occur with chronic asthma. Withdrawal of ICS results in slow deterioration of asthma control, indicating that they suppress inflammation and symptoms, but do not cure the underlying condition. ICS are now given as first-line therapy for patients with persistent asthma, but if they do not control symptoms at low doses, it is usual to add a LABA as the next step.

Side Effects Local side effects include hoarseness (dysphonia) and oral candidiasis, which may be reduced with the use of a large-volume spacer device. There has been concern about systemic side effects from lung absorption, but many studies have demonstrated that ICS have minimal systemic effects (Fig. 254-6). At the highest recommended doses, there may be some suppression of plasma and urinary cortisol concentrations, but there is no convincing evidence that long-term treatment leads to impaired growth in children or to osteoporosis in adults. Indeed effective control of asthma with ICS reduces the number of courses of OCS that are needed and, thus, reduces systemic exposure to ICS.

Systemic Corticosteroids Corticosteroids are used intravenously (hydrocortisone or methylprednisolone) for the treatment of acute severe asthma, although several studies now show that OCS are as effective and easier to administer. A course of OCS (usually prednisone or prednisolone 30–45 mg once daily for 5–10 days) is used to treat acute exacerbations of asthma; no tapering of the dose is needed. Approximately 1% of asthma patients may require maintenance treatment with OCS; the lowest dose necessary to maintain control needs to be determined. Systemic side effects, including truncal obesity, bruising, osteoporosis, diabetes, hypertension, gastric

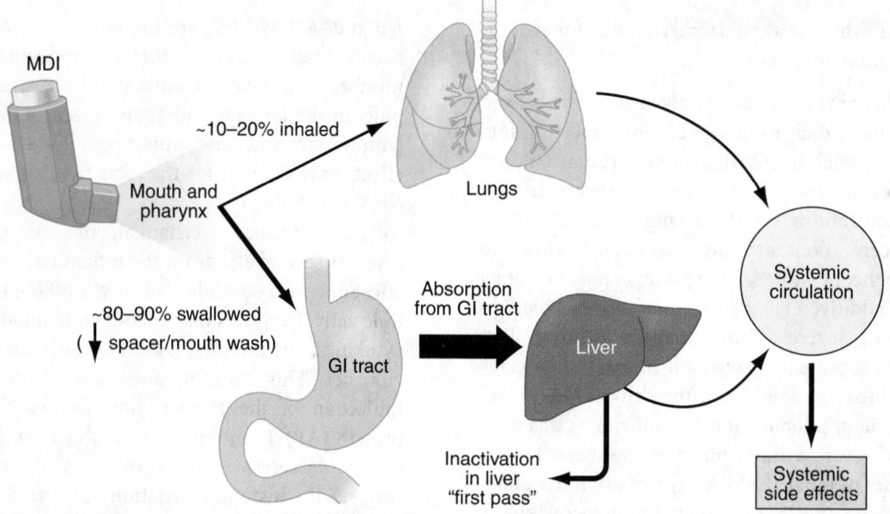

Figure 254-6 Pharmacokinetics of inhaled corticosteroids.

ulceration, proximal myopathy, depression, and cataracts, may be a major problem, and steroid-sparing therapies may be considered if side effects are a significant problem. If patients require maintenance treatment with OCS, it is important to monitor bone density so that preventive treatment with bisphosphonates or estrogen in postmenopausal women may be initiated if bone density is low. Intramuscular triamcinolone acetonide is a depot preparation that is occasionally used in noncompliant patients, but proximal myopathy is a major problem with this therapy.

Antileukotrienes Cysteinyl-leukotrienes are potent bronchoconstrictors, cause microvascular leakage, and increase eosinophilic inflammation through the activation of cys-LT_1-receptors. These inflammatory mediators are produced predominantly by mast cells and, to a lesser extent, eosinophils in asthma. Antileukotrienes such as montelukast and zafirlukast, block cys-LT_1-receptors and provide modest clinical benefit in asthma. They are less effective than ICS in controlling asthma and have less effect on airway inflammation, but are useful as an add-on therapy in some patients not controlled with low doses of ICS, although they are less effective than LABAs. They are given orally once or twice daily and are well tolerated. Some patients show a better response than others to antileukotrienes, but this has not been convincingly linked to any genomic differences in the leukotriene pathway.

Cromones Cromolyn sodium and nedocromil sodium are asthma controller drugs that appear to inhibit mast cell and sensory nerve activation and are, therefore, effective in blocking trigger-induced asthma such as EIA and allergen- and sulfur dioxide–induced symptoms. Cromones have relatively little benefit in the long-term control of asthma due to their short duration of action (at least four times daily by inhalation). They are very safe and were popular in the treatment of childhood asthma, although now low doses of ICS are preferred as they are more effective and have a proven safety profile.

Steroid-Sparing Therapies Various immunomodulatory treatments have been used to reduce the requirement for OCS in patients with severe asthma, who have serious side effects with this therapy. Methotrexate, cyclosporin A, azathioprine, gold, and IV gamma globulin have all been used as steroid-sparing therapies, but none of these treatments has any long-term benefit and each is associated with a relatively high risk of side effects.

Anti-IgE Omalizumab is a blocking antibody that neutralizes circulating IgE without binding to cell-bound IgE and, thus, inhibits IgE-mediated reactions. This treatment has been shown to reduce the number of exacerbations in patients with severe asthma and may improve asthma control. However, the treatment is very expensive and is only suitable for highly selected patients who are not controlled on maximal doses of inhaler therapy and have a circulating IgE within a specified range. Patients should be given a 3 to 4-month trial of therapy to show objective benefit. Omalizumab is usually given as a subcutaneous injection every 2–4 weeks and appears not to have significant side effects, although anaphylaxis is very occasionally seen.

Immunotherapy Specific immunotherapy using injected extracts of pollens or house dust mites has not been very effective in controlling asthma and may cause anaphylaxis. Side effects may be reduced by sublingual dosing. It is not recommended in most asthma treatment guidelines because of lack of evidence of clinical efficacy.

Alternative Therapies Nonpharmacologic treatments, including hypnosis, acupuncture, chiropraxis, breathing control, yoga, and speleotherapy, may be popular with some patients. However, placebo-controlled studies have shown that each of these treatments lacks efficacy and cannot be recommended. However, they are not detrimental and may be used as long as conventional pharmacologic therapy is continued.

Future Therapies It has proved very difficult to discover novel pharmaceutical therapies, particularly as current therapy with corticosteroids and β_2-agonists is so effective in the majority of patients. There is, however, a need for the development of new therapies for patients with refractory asthma who have side effects with systemic corticosteroids. Antagonists of specific mediators have little or no benefit in asthma, apart from antileukotrienes, which have rather weak effects, presumably reflecting the fact that multiple mediators are involved. Blocking antibodies against IL-5 may reduce exacerbations in highly selected patients who have sputum eosinophils despite high doses of corticosteroids, whereas anti-TNF-α antibodies are not effective in severe asthma. Novel anti-inflammatory treatments that are in

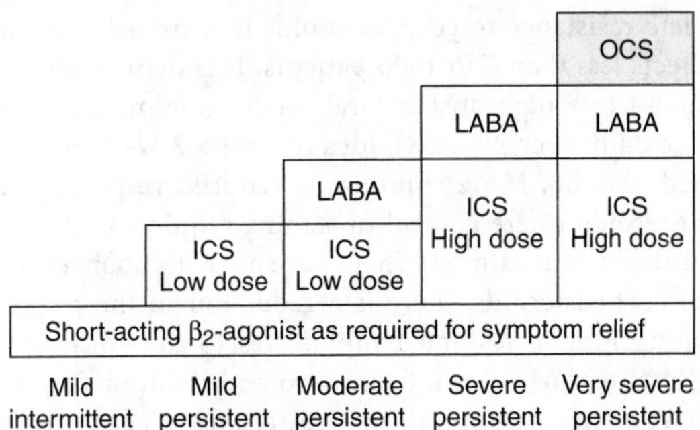

Figure 254-7 Stepwise approach to asthma therapy according to the severity of asthma and ability to control symptoms. ICS, inhaled corticosteroids; LABA, long-acting β_2-agonist; OCS, oral corticosteroid.

clinical development include inhibitors of phosphodiesterase-4, NF-κB and p38 MAP kinase. However, these drugs, which act on signal transduction pathways common to many cells, are likely to have troublesome side effects, necessitating their delivery by inhalation. Safer and more effective immunotherapy using T-cell peptide fragments of allergens or DNA vaccination are also being investigated. Bacterial products, such as CpG oligonucleotides that stimulate T_H1 immunity or regulatory T cells, are also currently under evaluation.

MANAGEMENT OF CHRONIC ASTHMA There are several aims of chronic therapy in asthma (Table 254-2). It is important to establish the diagnosis objectively using spirometry or PEF measurements at home. Triggers that worsen asthma control, such as allergens or occupational agents, should be avoided, whereas triggers, such as exercise and fog, which result in transient symptoms, provide an indication that more controller therapy is needed.

Stepwise Therapy For patients with mild, intermittent asthma, a short-acting β_2-agonist is all that is required (Fig. 254-7). However, use of a reliever medication more than three times a week indicates the need for regular controller therapy. The treatment of choice for all patients is an ICS given twice daily. It is usual to start with an intermediate dose [e.g., 200 (μg) bid of (beclomethasone dipropionate) BDP] or equivalent and to decrease the dose if symptoms are controlled after three months. If symptoms are not controlled, a LABA should be added, which is most conveniently given by switching to a combination inhaler. The dose of controller should be adjusted accordingly, as judged by the need for a rescue inhaler. Low doses of theophylline or an antileukotriene may also be considered as an add-on therapy, but these are less effective than LABAs. In patients with severe asthma, low-dose oral theophylline is also helpful, and when there is irreversible airway narrowing, the long-acting anticholinergic tiotropium bromide may be tried. If asthma is not controlled despite the maximal recommended dose of inhaled therapy, it is important to check compliance and inhaler technique. In these patients, maintenance treatment with an OCS may be needed and the lowest dose that maintains control should be used. Occasionally omalizumab may be tried in steroid-dependent asthmatics who are not well controlled. Once asthma is controlled, it is important to slowly decrease therapy in order to find the optimal dose to control symptoms.

Education Patients with asthma need to understand how to use their medications and the difference between reliever and controller therapies. Education may improve compliance, particularly with ICS. All patients should be taught how to use their inhalers correctly. In particular, they need to understand how to recognize worsening of asthma and how to step up therapy. Written action plans have been shown to reduce hospital admissions and morbidity rates in adults and children, and are recommended particularly in patients with unstable disease who have frequent exacerbations.

ACUTE SEVERE ASTHMA

Exacerbations of asthma are feared by patients and may be life threatening. One of the main aims of controller therapy is to prevent exacerbations; in this respect, ICS and combination inhalers are very effective.

CLINICAL FEATURES

Patients are aware of increasing chest tightness, wheezing, and dyspnea that are often not or poorly relieved by their usual reliever inhaler. In severe exacerbations patients may be so breathless that they are unable to complete sentences and may become cyanotic. Examination usually shows increased ventilation, hyperinflation, and tachycardia. Pulsus paradoxus may be present, but this is rarely a useful clinical sign. There is a marked fall in spirometric values and PEF. Arterial blood gases on air show hypoxemia and P_{CO_2} is usually low due to hyperventilation. A normal or rising P_{CO_2} is an indication of impending respiratory failure and requires immediate monitoring and therapy. A chest roentgenogram is not usually informative, but may show pneumonia or pneumothorax.

TREATMENT Acute Severe Asthma

A high concentration of oxygen should be given by face mask to achieve oxygen saturation of >90%. The mainstay of treatment are high doses of SABAs given either by nebulizer or via a metered-dose inhaler with a spacer. In severely ill patients with impending respiratory failure, IV β_2-agonists may be given. An inhaled anticholinergic may be added if there is not a satisfactory response to β_2-agonists alone, as there are additive effects. In patients who are refractory to inhaled therapies, a slow infusion of aminophylline may be effective, but it is important to monitor blood levels, especially if patients have already been treated with oral theophylline. Magnesium sulfate given intravenously or by nebulizer has also been shown to be effective when added to inhaled β_2-agonists, and is relatively well tolerated but is not routinely recommended. Prophylactic intubation may be indicated for impending respiratory failure, when the P_{CO_2} is normal or rises. For patients with respiratory failure, it is necessary to intubate and institute ventilation. These patients may benefit from an anesthetic such as halothane if they have not responded to conventional bronchodilators. Sedatives should never be given as they may depress ventilation. Antibiotics should not be used routinely unless there are signs of pneumonia.

REFRACTORY ASTHMA

Although most patients with asthma are easily controlled with appropriate medication, a small proportion of patients (approximately 5% of asthmatics) are difficult to control despite maximal inhaled therapy. Some of these patients will require maintenance treatment with OCS. In managing these patients, it is important to investigate and correct any mechanisms that may be aggravating asthma. There are two major patterns of difficult asthma: some patients have persistent symptoms and poor lung function, despite appropriate therapy, whereas others may have normal or near normal lung function but intermittent, severe (sometimes life-threatening) exacerbations.

MECHANISMS

The most common reason for poor control of asthma is noncompliance with medication, particularly ICS. Compliance with ICS may be low because patients do not feel any immediate clinical benefit or may be concerned about side effects. Compliance with ICS is difficult to monitor as there are no useful plasma measurements that can be made. Compliance may be improved by giving the ICS as a combination with a LABA that gives symptom relief. Compliance with OCS may be measured by suppression of plasma cortisol and the expected concentration of prednisone/prednisolone in the plasma. There are several factors that may make asthma more difficult to control, including exposure to high, ambient levels of allergens or unidentified occupational agents. Severe rhinosinusitis may make asthma more difficult to control; upper airway disease should be vigorously treated. Gastroesophageal reflux is common among asthmatics due to bronchodilator therapy, but there is little evidence that it is a significant factor in worsening asthma, and treatment of the reflux is not usually effective at improving asthma symptoms. Some patients may have chronic infection with *Mycoplasma pneumoniae* or *Chlamydophila pneumoniae* and benefit from treatment with a macrolide antibiotic. Drugs such as beta-adrenergic blockers, aspirin, and other cyclooxygenase (COX) inhibitors may worsen asthma. Some women develop severe premenstrual worsening of asthma, which is unresponsive to corticosteroids and requires treatment with progesterone or gonadotropin-releasing factors. Few systemic diseases make asthma more difficult to control, but hyper- and hypothyroidism may increase asthma symptoms and should be investigated if suspected.

Relatively little is known about the pathology of refractory asthma, as biopsy studies are more difficult in these patients. Some patients show the typical eosinophilic pattern of inflammation, whereas others have a predominantly neutrophilic pattern. There may be an increase in T_H1 cells and CD8 lymphocytes compared to mild asthma and increased expression of TNF-α. Structural changes in the airway, including fibrosis, angiogenesis, and airway smooth-muscle thickening, are more commonly seen in these patients.

DIFFERENTIAL DIAGNOSIS

Some patients who apparently have difficult-to-control asthma have vocal cord dysfunction, resulting in wheezing or stridor. This symptom is thought to be an attention-seeking hysterical conversion syndrome and may lead to escalating doses of asthma therapy with some patients taking high doses of oral corticosteroids. It may be recognized by the characteristic discrepancy between tests of forced expiration, such as FEV_1 and PEF, and relatively normal airway resistance. Direct inspection by laryngoscopy may confirm adduction of the vocal cords at the time of symptoms. This condition is usually difficult to manage, but it is important that patients be weaned off OCS and ICS. Speech therapy is sometimes beneficial. Some patients with COPD may be diagnosed as asthmatic and may show the characteristic poor response to corticosteroids and bronchodilators, but this situation is complicated by the fact that some patients with COPD also have concomitant asthma.

CORTICOSTEROID-RESISTANT ASTHMA

A few patients with asthma show a poor response to corticosteroid therapy and may have various molecular abnormalities that impair the anti-inflammatory action of corticosteroids. Complete resistance to corticosteroids is extremely uncommon and affects less than 1 in 1000 patients. It is defined by a failure to respond to a high dose of oral prednisone/prednisolone (40 mg once daily over 2 weeks), ideally with a 2-week run-in with matched placebo. More common is reduced responsiveness to corticosteroids where control of asthma requires OCS (corticosteroid-dependent asthma). In all patients with poor responsiveness to corticosteroids, there is a reduction in the response of circulating monocytes and lymphocytes to the anti-inflammatory effects of corticosteroids in vitro and reduced skin blanching in response to topical corticosteroids. There are several mechanisms that have been described, including an excess of the transcription factor AP-1, an increase in the alternatively spliced form of the glucocorticoid receptor (GR)-β, an abnormal pattern of histone acetylation in response to corticosteroids, a defect in IL-10 production, and a reduction in histone deacetylase activity (as in COPD). These observations suggest that there are likely to be heterogeneous mechanisms for corticosteroid resistance; whether these mechanisms are genetically determined has yet to be decided.

BRITTLE ASTHMA

Some patients show chaotic variations in lung function despite taking appropriate therapy. Some show a persistent pattern of variability and may require oral corticosteroids or, at times, continuous infusion of β_2-agonists (type I brittle asthma), whereas others have generally normal or near-normal lung function but precipitous, unpredictable falls in lung function that may result in death (type 2 brittle asthma). These latter patients are difficult to manage as they do not respond well to corticosteroids, and the worsening of asthma does not reverse well with inhaled bronchodilators. The most effective therapy is subcutaneous epinephrine, which suggests that the worsening is likely to be a localized airway anaphylactic reaction with edema. In some of these patients, there may be allergy to specific foods. These patients should be taught to self-administer epinephrine and should carry a medical warning accordingly.

TREATMENT Refractory Asthma

Refractory asthma is difficult to control, by definition. It is important to check compliance and the correct use of inhalers and to identify and eliminate any underlying triggers. Low doses of theophylline may be helpful in some patients, and theophylline withdrawal has been found to worsen in many patients. Most of these patients will require maintenance treatment with oral corticosteroids, and the minimal dose that achieves satisfactory control should be determined by careful dose titration. Steroid-sparing therapies are rarely effective. In some patients with allergic asthma, omalizumab is effective, particularly when there are frequent exacerbations. Anti-TNF therapy is not effective in severe asthma and should not be used. A few patients may benefit from infusions of β_2-agonists. New therapies are needed for these patients, who currently consume a disproportionate amount of health care spending.

SPECIAL CONSIDERATIONS

Although asthma is usually straightforward to manage, there are some situations that may require additional investigation and different therapy.

■ ASPIRIN-SENSITIVE ASTHMA

A small proportion (1–5%) of asthmatics become worse with aspirin and other COX inhibitors, although this is much more commonly seen in severe cases and in those patients with frequent hospital admission. Aspirin-sensitive asthma is a well defined subtype of asthma that is usually preceded by perennial rhinitis and nasal polyps in nonatopic patients with a late onset of the disease. Aspirin, even in small doses, characteristically provokes rhinorrhea, conjunctival irritation, facial flushing, and wheezing. There is a genetic predisposition to increased production of cysteinyl-leukotrienes with functional polymorphism of *cys*-leukotriene C synthase. Asthma is triggered by COX inhibitors, but is persistent even in their absence. All nonselective COX inhibitors should be avoided, but selective COX2 inhibitors are safe to use when an anti-inflammatory analgesic is needed. Aspirin-sensitive asthma responds to usual therapy with ICS. Although antileukotrienes should be effective in these patients, they are no more effective than in allergic asthma. Occasionally, aspirin desensitization is necessary, but this should only be undertaken in specialized centers.

■ ASTHMA IN THE ELDERLY

Asthma may start at any age, including in elderly patients. The principles of management are the same as in other asthmatics, but side effects of therapy may be a problem, including muscle tremor with β_2-agonists and more systemic side effects with ICS. Comorbidities are more frequent in this age group, and interactions with drugs such as β_2-blockers, COX inhibitors, and agents that may affect theophylline metabolism need to be considered. COPD is more likely in elderly patients and may coexist with asthma. A trial of OCS may be very useful in documenting the steroid responsiveness of asthma.

■ PREGNANCY

Approximately one-third of asthmatic patients who are pregnant improve during the course of a pregnancy, one-third deteriorate, and one-third are unchanged. It is important to maintain good control of asthma as poor control may have adverse effects on fetal development. Compliance may be a problem as there is often concern about the effects of antiasthma medications on fetal development. The drugs that have been used for many years in asthma therapy have now been shown to be safe and without teratogenic potential. These drugs include short-acting β_2-agonists, ICS, and theophylline; there is less safety information about newer classes of drugs such as LABAs, antileukotrienes, and anti-IgE. If an OCS is needed, it is better to use prednisone rather than prednisolone as it cannot be converted to the active prednisolone by the fetal liver, thus protecting the fetus from systemic effects of the corticosteroid. There is no contraindication to breast-feeding when patients are using these drugs.

■ CIGARETTE SMOKING

Approximately 20% of asthmatics smoke, which may adversely affect asthma in several ways. Smoking asthmatics have more severe disease, more frequent hospital admissions, a faster decline in lung function, and a higher risk of death from asthma than nonsmoking asthmatics. There is evidence that smoking interferes with the anti-inflammatory actions of corticosteroids, necessitating higher doses for asthma control. Smoking cessation improves lung function and reduces the steroid resistance, and, thus, vigorous smoking cessation strategies should be used. Some patients report a temporary worsening of asthma when they first stop smoking, which could be due to the loss of the bronchodilating effect of NO in cigarette smoke.

■ SURGERY

If asthma is well controlled, there is no contraindication to general anesthesia and intubation. Patients who are treated with OCS will have adrenal suppression and should be treated with an increased dose of OCS immediately prior to surgery. Patients with FEV_1 <80% of their normal levels should also be given a boost of OCS prior to surgery. High-maintenance doses of corticosteroids may be a contraindication to surgery because of increased risks of infection and delayed wound healing.

■ BRONCHOPULMONARY ASPERGILLOSIS

Bronchopulmonary aspergillosis (BPA) is uncommon and results from an allergic pulmonary reaction to inhaled spores of *Aspergillus fumigatus* and, occasionally, other *Aspergillus* species. A skin prick test to *A. fumigatus* is always positive, whereas serum *Aspergillus* precipitins are low or undetectable. Characteristically, there are fleeting eosinophilic infiltrates in the lungs, particularly in the upper lobes. Airways become blocked with mucoid plugs rich in eosinophils, and patients may cough up brown plugs and have hemoptysis. BPA may result in bronchiectasis, particularly affecting central airways, if not suppressed by corticosteroids. Asthma is controlled in the usual way by ICS, but it is necessary to give a course of OCS if any sign of worsening or pulmonary shadowing is found. Treatment with the oral antifungal itraconazole is beneficial in preventing exacerbations.

FURTHER READINGS

Barnes PJ: How corticosteroids control inflammation. Br J Pharmacol 148:245, 2006.

———: Cytokine networks in asthma and chronic obstructive pulmonary disease. J Clin Invest 118:3546, 2008

———: Immunology of asthma and chronic obstructive pulmonary disease. Nat Immunol Rev 8:183, 2008

——— et al: *Asthma and COPD*, 2nd ed. Amsterdam, Elsevier, 2009

Bateman ED et al: Global strategy for asthma management and prevention: GINA executive summary. Eur Respir J 31:143, 2008

Eder W et al: The asthma epidemic. N Engl J Med 355:2226, 2006

Fanta CH: Asthma. N Engl J Med 360:1002, 2009

Farooque SP, Lee TH: Aspirin-sensitive respiratory disease. Annu Rev Physiol 71:465, 2009

Hamid Q, Tulic M: Immunobiology of asthma. Annu Rev Physiol 71:489, 2009

———: New therapies for asthma: Is there any progress? Trends Pharmacol Sci 31:355, 2010

Lazarus SC: Emergency treatment of asthma. N Engl J Med 363:755, 2010

Wenzel SE, Busse WW: Severe asthma: Lessons from the Severe Asthma Research Program. J Allergy Clin Immunol 119:14, 2007

CHAPTER 255

Hypersensitivity Pneumonitis and Pulmonary Infiltrates With Eosinophilia

Alicia K. Gerke
Gary W. Hunninghake

HYPERSENSITIVITY PNEUMONITIS

First described in 1874, hypersensitivity pneumonitis (HP), or extrinsic allergic alveolitis, is an inflammatory disorder of the lung involving alveolar walls and terminal airways that is induced by repeated inhalation of a variety of organic agents in a susceptible host. The expression of HP depends on factors related to the host susceptibility and the inciting agent. The frequency of HP varies with the environmental exposure and the specific antigen involved, which often depends on season, geographic location, or presence of certain industries.

ETIOLOGY

Agents implicated as causes of HP are diverse and include those listed in Table 255-1. The common name of each disease often reflects the occupational or avocational risk associated with that disease. In the United States, the most common types of HP are farmer's lung, bird fancier's lung, and chemical worker's lung. In *farmer's lung*, inhalation of proteins, such as thermophilic bacteria and fungal spores that are present in moldy bedding and feed, are most commonly responsible for the development of HP. These antigens are probably also responsible for the etiology of *mushroom worker's disease* (moldy composted growth medium), bagassosis (moldy sugar cane), and water-related exposure (molds in air conditioners or humidifiers). *Hot tub lung* refers to a hypersensitivity reaction to *Mycobacterium avium complex*, which is present in hot tubs or whirlpools and is differentiated from actual infection. *Bird fancier's lung* (and the related disorders of duck fever, turkey handler's lung, and dove pillow's lung) is a response to inhalation of proteins from feathers and droppings. *Chemical worker's lung* is an example of how simple chemicals, such as isocyanates, may also cause immune-mediated diseases. Interestingly, cigarette smoking has been associated with decreased incidence of HP; however, smoking may lead to a more progressive or severe course of HP once the disease is present.

PATHOGENESIS

The finding that precipitating antibodies against extracts of moldy hay were demonstrable in most patients with farmer's lung led to the early conclusion that HP was an immune complex–mediated reaction. Subsequent investigations of HP in human beings and animal models provided evidence for the importance of cell-mediated hypersensitivity. The very early (acute) reaction is characterized by an increase in polymorphonuclear leukocytes in the alveoli and small airways. This early lesion is followed by an influx of mononuclear cells into the lung and the formation of granulomas that appear to be the result of a classic delayed (T cell–mediated) hypersensitivity reaction to repeated inhalation of antigen and adjuvant-active materials. Studies in animal models suggest that the disease is a T_H1-mediated immune response to antigen, with interferon γ, interleukin (IL)-12, and possibly IL-18 contributing to disease expression. Most likely, multiple cytokines [including also IL-1β, transforming growth factor β (TGF-β), tumor necrosis factor α (TNF-α) and others] interact to promote HP; their source includes both alveolar macrophages and T lymphocytes in the lung. Data support a genetic predisposition to the development of HP; certain polymorphisms of the TNF-α promoter region and major histocompatibility complex reportedly confer an enhanced susceptibility to pigeon breeder's disease.

After inhalation of an antigenic particle, the attraction and accumulation of inflammatory cells in the lung may be due to one or more of the following mechanisms: induction of the adhesion molecules L-selectin and E-selectin, elaboration by dendritic cells of CC chemokine 1 (DC-CK-1/CCL18), or increased expression of CXCR3/CXCL10 by $CD4^+$ and $CD8^+$ lymphocytes. Increased levels of Fas protein and FasL in the lung (which would be expected to suppress inflammation by induction of T cell apoptosis) is counterbalanced by increased expression of the inducible antiapoptotic gene *Bcl-xL*, resulting in a lower overall level of pulmonary lymphocyte apoptosis in HP patients.

Bronchoalveolar lavage (BAL) in patients with HP consistently demonstrates an increase in T lymphocytes in lavage fluid (a finding that is also observed in patients with other granulomatous lung disorders). Patients with recent or continual exposure to antigen may have an increase in polymorphonuclear leukocytes in lavage fluid, which has been associated with lung fibrosis. A role for oxidant injury has been proposed in HP. Several markers of oxidative stress are reported to be increased during exacerbation of HP and are reduced by treatment with glucocorticoids.

CLINICAL PRESENTATION

The clinical picture is that of an interstitial pneumonitis, which varies from patient to patient and seems related to the frequency and intensity of exposure to the causative antigen and, perhaps, other host factors. The presentation can be acute, subacute, or chronic. In the *acute* form, symptoms such as cough, fever, chills, malaise, and dyspnea may occur 6 to 8 h after exposure to the antigen and usually clear within a few days if there is no further exposure to antigen; it often closely resembles an influenza-like illness. The *subacute* form often appears insidiously over a period of weeks marked by cough and dyspnea and may progress to cyanosis and severe dyspnea, requiring hospitalization. In some patients, a subacute form of the disease may persist after an acute presentation of the disorder, especially if there is continued exposure to antigen. In most patients with the acute or subacute form of HP, the symptoms, signs, and other manifestations of HP disappear within days, weeks, or months if the causative agent is no longer inhaled. Transformation to a chronic form of the disease may occur, but the frequency of such progression is uncertain.

Continuous low-level antigen exposure or repeated episodes can also lead to chronic disease with more subtle symptoms, accounting for delayed or uncertain diagnosis over a long period of time. This may occur without a prior history of acute or subacute manifestations. The *chronic* form of HP may be clinically indistinguishable from pulmonary fibrosis in its later stages. Symptoms include cough, weight loss, malaise, and gradual increase in dyspnea. Physical examination may reveal inspiratory crackles and digital clubbing. Imaging shows interstitial fibrosis or emphysema. Progressive worsening may result in dependence on supplemental oxygen, pulmonary hypertension, or respiratory failure. Pulmonary fibrosis is the clinical manifestation of HP with the greatest predictive value for mortality. Fibrosis appears most prominent in hypersensitivity pneumonitis associated with birds, while emphysema is often more common in farmer's lung.

TABLE 255-1 Selected Examples of Hypersensitivity Pneumonitis (HP)

Disease	Antigen	Source of Antigen
Bagassosis	Thermophilic actinomycetes[a]	"Moldy" bagasse (sugar cane)
Bird fancier's, breeder's, or handler's lung[b]	Parakeet, pigeon, chicken, turkey proteins	Avian droppings or feathers
Cephalosporium HP	Contaminated basement (sewage)	*Cephalosporium*
Cheese washer's lung	*Penicillium casei*	Moldy cheese
Chemical worker's lung[b]	Isocyanates	Polyurethane foam, varnishes, lacquer
Coffee worker's lung	Coffee bean dust	Coffee beans
Compost lung	*Aspergillus*	Compost
Detergent worker's disease	*Bacillus subtilis* enzymes (subtilisins)	Detergent
Familial HP	*Bacillus subtilis*	Contaminated wood dust in walls
Farmer's lung[b]	Thermophilic actinomycetes[a]	"Moldy" hay, grain, silage
Fish food lung	Unknown	Fish food
Fish meal worker's lung	Fish meal dust	Fish meal
Furrier's lung	Animal fur dust	Animal pelts
Hot tub lung	*Cladosporium* spp., *Mycobacterium avium* complex	Mold on ceiling; contaminated water
Humidifier or air conditioner lung (ventilation pneumonitis)	*Aureobasidium pullulans, Candida albicans,* Thermophilic actinomycetes,[a] *Mycobacterium* spp., other microorganisms	Contaminated water in humidification or forced-air air conditioning systems
Japanese summer-type HP	*Trichosporon cutaneum, T. asahii,* and *T. mucoides*	House dust, bird droppings
Laboratory worker's HP	Male rat urine	Laboratory rat
Lycoperdonosis	*Lycoperdon* puffballs	Puffball spores
Malt worker's lung	*Aspergillus fumigatus* or *A. clavatus*	Moldy barley
Maple bark disease	*Cryptostroma corticale*	Maple bark
Metalworking fluid lung	*Mycobacterium* spp., *Pseudomonas* spp.	Contaminated metalworking fluid
Miller's lung	*Sitophilus granarius* (wheat weevil)	Infested wheat flour
Miscellaneous medication	Amiodarone, bleomycin, efavirenz, gemcitabine, hydralazine, hydroxyurea, isoniazid, methotrexate, paclitaxel, penicillin, procarbazine, propranolol, riluzole, sirolimus, sulfasalazine	Medication
Mushroom worker's lung	Thermophilic actinomycetes,[a] *Hypsizygus marmoreus, Bunashimeji,* and other exotic mushrooms	Mushroom compost; mushrooms
Pituitary snuff taker's lung	Animal proteins	Heterologous pituitary snuff
Potato riddler's lung	Thermophilic actinomycetes,[a] *Aspergillus*	"Moldy" hay around potatoes
Sauna taker's lung	*Aureobasidium* spp., other	Contaminated sauna water
Sausage worker's lung	*Penicillium nalgiovense*	Dry sausage mold
Sequoiosis	*Aureobasidium, Graphium* spp.	Redwood sawdust
Streptomyces albus HP	*Streptomyces albus*	Contaminated fertilizer
Suberosis	*Penicillium glabrum* and *Chrysonilia sitophila*	Cork dust
Tap water lung	*Mycobacteria* spp.	Contaminated tap water
Thatched roof disease	*Saccharomonospora viridis*	Dried grasses and leaves
Tobacco worker's disease	*Aspergillus* spp.	Mold on tobacco
Winegrower's lung	*Botrytis cinerea*	Mold on grapes
Wood trimmer's disease	*Rhizopus* spp., *Mucor* spp.	Contaminated wood trimmings
Woodman's disease	*Penicillium* spp.	Oak and maple trees
Woodworker's lung	Wood dust, *Alternaria*	Oak, cedar, pine, and mahogany dusts

[a]Thermophilic actinomycetes species include *Micropolyspora faeni, Thermoactinomyces vulgaris, T. saccharri, T. viridis,* and *T. candidus.*

[b]Most common causes of hypersensitivity pneumonitis in the United States.

■ DIAGNOSIS

All forms of the disease may be associated with elevations in erythrocyte sedimentation rate, C-reactive protein, rheumatoid factor, lactate dehydrogenase, or serum immunoglobulins. Following acute exposure to an antigen, neutrophilia and lymphopenia are frequently present. Eosinophilia is not a feature. Examination for *serum precipitins* against suspected antigens, such as those listed in Table 255-1, is an important part of the diagnostic workup and should be performed on any patient with interstitial lung disease, especially if a suggestive exposure history is elicited. The occurrence of precipitins indicates sufficient exposure to the causative agent for generation of an immunologic response and is one of the major diagnostic criteria; however, the diagnosis of HP is not established solely by the presence of precipitins, as they are found in sera of many individuals exposed to appropriate antigens who demonstrate no other evidence of HP. False-negative results may occur because of unreliable testing techniques or an inappropriate choice of antigens. Extraction of antigens from the suspected source may at times be helpful.

Chest x-ray shows no specific or distinctive changes in HP. It can be normal even in symptomatic patients. The acute or subacute phases may be associated with poorly defined, patchy, or diffuse infiltrates; with discrete, nodular infiltrates; or with air-space consolidation. In the chronic phase, the chest x-ray usually shows a diffuse reticulonodular infiltrate. Honeycombing may eventually develop as the condition progresses. Apical sparing is common, suggesting that disease severity correlates with inhaled antigen load, but no particular distribution or pattern is classic for HP. Abnormalities rarely seen in HP include pleural effusion or thickening and significant hilar adenopathy.

High-resolution chest CT has become the procedure of choice for imaging of HP. Although pathognomonic features have not been identified, acute HP may appear with diffuse "ground-glass" infiltrates, a reticulonodular pattern, or confluent alveolar opacification. In subacute disease, centrilobular nodules and "ground-glass" changes predominate, and expiratory views may demonstrate air trapping or mosaic perfusion (Fig. 255-1). This pattern is more common in individuals whose exposure to antigen continues rather than in those in whom removal from antigen exposure has occurred. In chronic HP, diffuse changes include patchy emphysema and interstitial fibrosis; subpleural linear opacities and honeycombing are also common. The findings are often similar (but not identical) to idiopathic pulmonary fibrosis.

Pulmonary function studies in all forms of HP may show a restrictive or an obstructive pattern with loss of lung volumes, impaired diffusing capacity, and decreased compliance. Resting or exercise-induced hypoxemia may be seen. Bronchospasm and bronchial hyperreactivity are sometimes found in acute HP. With antigen avoidance, the pulmonary function abnormalities are usually reversible in acute and subacute disease.

BAL is used in some centers to aid in diagnostic evaluation. A marked lymphocytic alveolitis on BAL is almost universal, although not pathognomonic. Lymphocytes are typically activated and show a decreased helper/suppressor ratio, although this ratio can be variable depending on dose and duration of exposure. Alveolar neutrophilia is also prominent acutely, but tends to fade in the absence of recurrent exposure. Bronchoalveolar mastocytosis may correlate with disease activity.

Lung biopsy, obtained through flexible bronchoscopy, open-lung procedures, or thoracoscopy, may be diagnostic. Although the histopathology is distinctive, it may not be pathognomonic of HP (Fig. 255-2). When the biopsy is taken during the active phase of disease, typical findings include an interstitial alveolar infiltrate consisting of plasma cells, lymphocytes, and occasional eosinophils and neutrophils, usually accompanied by loose, noncaseating peribronchial granulomas. Some degree of bronchiolitis is found in about one-half the cases. Rarely, bronchiolitis obliterans with organizing pneumonia (BOOP) (Chap. 261) may be present. In subacute disease, the triad of mononuclear bronchiolitis; interstitial infiltrates of lymphocytes and plasma cells; and single, nonnecrotizing, randomly scattered parenchymal granulomas without mural vascular involvement is consistent with HP. Interstitial fibrosis may be present, but most often is mild in earlier stages of the disease. Chronic HP has variable pathology and may resemble nonspecific interstitial pneumonia, organizing pneumonia, or usual interstitial pneumonia; granulomas may or may not be present. Centrilobular fibrosis, peribronchial inflammation with fibrosis, bridging fibrosis, and emphysema are common.

A *prediction rule* for the clinical diagnosis of HP has been developed by the International HP Study Group. Six significant predictors of HP (exposure to a known antigen, positive predictive antibodies

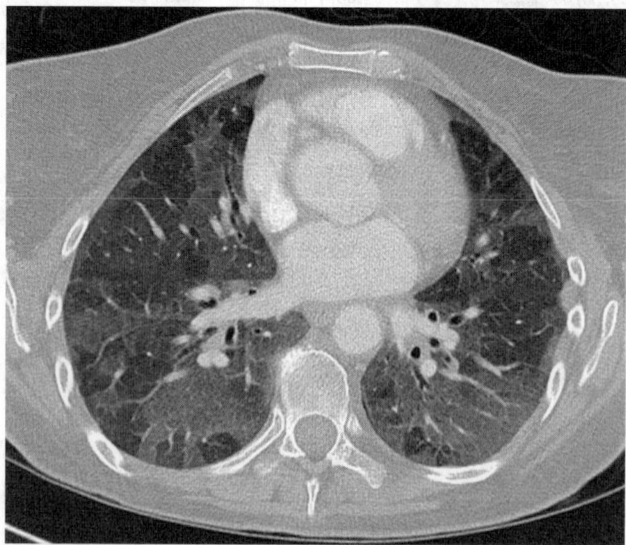

Figure 255-1 Chest CT scan of a patient with subacute hypersensitivity pneumonitis in which scattered regions of ground-glass infiltrates in a mosaic pattern consistent with air trapping are seen bilaterally. This patient had *bird fancier's lung. (Courtesy of TJ Gross; with permission.)*

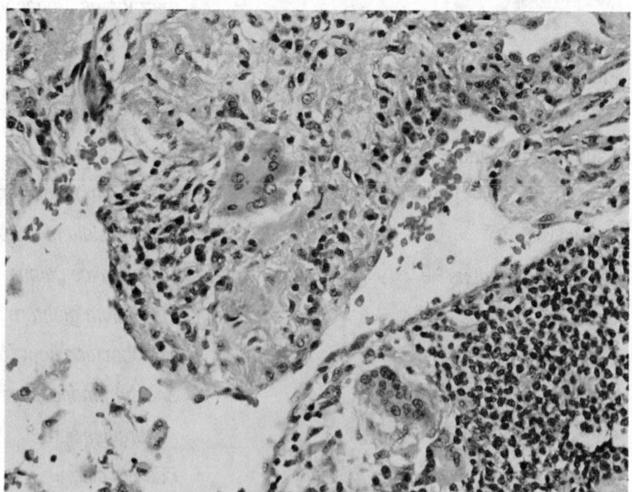

Figure 255-2 Open-lung biopsy from a patient with subacute hypersensitivity pneumonitis demonstrating a loose, nonnecrotizing granuloma made up of histiocytes and multinucleated giant cells. Peribronchial inflammatory infiltrate made up of lymphocytes and plasma cells is also seen. *(Courtesy of TJ Gross; with permission.)*

to the antigen, recurrent episodes of symptoms, inspiratory crackles, symptoms developing 4–8 h after exposure, and weight loss) were retrospectively developed then validated in a separate cohort. This diagnostic paradigm has a high predictive value in the diagnosis of HP, without the need for invasive testing. In cases where only a subset of the criteria is fulfilled, the diagnosis is less certain. It is clear, however, that the diagnosis of HP is established by (1) consistent symptoms, physical findings, pulmonary function tests, and radiographic tests; (2) a history of exposure to a recognized antigen; and (3) ideally, identification of an antibody to that antigen. Symptoms upon re-exposure to the suspected antigen also support the diagnosis. In some circumstances, BAL and/or lung biopsy may be needed. The most important tool in diagnosing HP continues to be a high index of suspicion.

DIFFERENTIAL DIAGNOSIS

Chronic HP may often be difficult to distinguish from a number of other interstitial lung disorders (Chap. 261). A negative history for use of relevant drugs and no evidence of a systemic disorder usually exclude the presence of drug-induced lung disease or a collagen vascular disorder. BAL often shows predominance of neutrophils in idiopathic pulmonary fibrosis and a predominance of CD4+ lymphocytes in sarcoidosis. Hilar/paratracheal lymphadenopathy or evidence of multisystem involvement also favors the diagnosis of sarcoidosis. In some patients, a lung biopsy may be required to differentiate chronic HP from other interstitial diseases. The lung disease associated with acute or subacute HP may clinically resemble other disorders that present with systemic symptoms and recurrent pulmonary infiltrates, including the allergic bronchopulmonary mycoses and other eosinophilic pneumonias. Eosinophilic pneumonia is often associated with asthma and is typified by peripheral eosinophilia; neither of these is a feature of HP. Allergic bronchopulmonary aspergillosis (ABPA) is the most common example of the allergic bronchopulmonary mycoses and is sometimes confused with HP because of the presence of precipitating antibodies to *Aspergillus fumigatus*. ABPA is associated with allergic (atopic) asthma. Acute HP may be confused with *organic dust toxic syndrome* (ODTS), a condition that is more common than HP. ODTS follows heavy exposure to organic dusts and is characterized by transient fever and muscle aches, with or without dyspnea and cough. Serum precipitins are absent, and the chest x-ray is usually normal. This distinction is important, as ODTS is a self-limited disorder without significant long-term sequelae, whereas continued antigen exposure in HP can result in permanent disability. Massive exposure to moldy silage may result in a syndrome termed *pulmonary mycotoxicosis*, with fever, chills, and cough and the presence of pulmonary infiltrates within a few hours of exposure. No previous sensitization is required, and precipitins are absent to *Aspergillus*, the suspected causative agent.

TREATMENT Hypersensitivity Pneumonitis

Because effective treatment depends largely on avoiding the antigen, identification of the causative agent and its source is essential. This is usually possible if the physician takes a detailed environmental and occupational history or, if necessary, visits the patient's environment. The simplest way to avoid the incriminated agent is to remove the patient from the environment or remove the source of the agent from the patient's environment. This recommendation cannot be taken lightly when it completely changes the lifestyle or livelihood of the patient. In many cases, the source of exposure (birds, humidifiers, molds, etc.) can be removed. Pollen masks, personal dust respirators, airstream helmets, and ventilated helmets with a supply of fresh air are increasingly efficient means of purifying inhaled air. If symptoms recur or physiologic abnormalities progress in spite of these measures, more effective measures to avoid antigen exposure must be pursued. The chronic form of HP typically results from low-grade or recurrent exposure over many months to years, and the lung disease may already be partially or completely irreversible. These patients are usually advised to avoid all possible contact with the offending agent.

Patients with the *acute,* recurrent form of HP usually recover without need for glucocorticoids. *Subacute* HP may be associated with severe symptoms and marked physiologic impairment and may continue to progress for several days despite hospitalization. Urgent establishment of the diagnosis and prompt institution of glucocorticoid treatment are indicated in such patients. Prednisone at a dosage of 1 mg/kg per d or its equivalent is continued for 7 to 14 days and then tapered over the ensuing 2 to 6 weeks at a rate that depends on the patient's clinical status. Patients with *chronic* HP may gradually recover without therapy following environmental control. In many patients, however, a trial of prednisone may be useful to obtain maximal reversibility of the lung disease. Following initial prednisone therapy (1 mg/kg per d for 2 to 4 weeks), the drug is tapered to the lowest dosage that will maintain the functional status of the patient. Many patients will not require or benefit from long-term therapy if there is no further exposure to antigen. Although a short course of corticosteroids has been shown to accelerate recovery from the acute stage, glucocorticoid therapy does not appear to have an effect on long-term prognosis of farmer's lung. Improvement of lung function may continue over a few months to years.

PULMONARY INFILTRATES WITH EOSINOPHILIA

Pulmonary infiltrates with eosinophilia (PIE, eosinophilic pneumonias) include distinct individual syndromes characterized by eosinophilic pulmonary infiltrates and, commonly, peripheral blood eosinophilia. Since Loeffler's initial description of a transient, benign syndrome of migratory pulmonary infiltrates and peripheral blood eosinophilia of unknown cause, this group of disorders has been enlarged to include several diseases of both known and unknown etiology (Table 255-2). These diseases may be considered as immunologically mediated lung diseases, but are not to be confused with HP, in which eosinophilia is *not* a feature. In differentiating the etiologies of this heterogeneous group of lung disorders, an extensive history and full examination of all organ systems are essential.

When an eosinophilic pneumonia is associated with bronchial asthma, it is important to determine if the patient has atopic asthma

TABLE 255-2 Pulmonary Infiltrates With Eosinophilia

Etiology Known
Allergic bronchopulmonary mycoses
Parasitic infestations
Drug reactions
Eosinophilia-myalgia syndrome
Idiopathic
Loeffler's syndrome
Acute eosinophilic pneumonia
Chronic eosinophilic pneumonia
Allergic granulomatosis of Churg and Strauss
Hypereosinophilic syndrome

TABLE 255-3 Diagnostic Features of Allergic Bronchopulmonary Aspergillosis (ABPA)

Main Diagnostic Criteria
Bronchial asthma
Pulmonary infiltrates
Peripheral eosinophilia (>1000/μL)
Immediate wheal-and-flare response to *Aspergillus fumigatus*
Serum precipitins to *A. fumigatus*
Elevated serum IgE
Central bronchiectasis
Other Diagnostic Features
History of brownish plugs in sputum
Culture of *A. fumigatus* from sputum
Elevated IgE (and IgG) class antibodies specific for *A. fumigatus*

and has wheal-and-flare skin reactivity to *Aspergillus* or other relevant fungal antigens. If so, other criteria should be sought for the diagnosis of ABPA (Table 255-3) or other, rarer examples of allergic bronchopulmonary mycosis such as those caused by *Penicillium, Candida, Curvularia,* or *Helminthosporium* spp. *A. fumigatus* is the most common cause of ABPA. The chest roentgenogram in ABPA may show transient, recurrent infiltrates or may suggest the presence of proximal bronchiectasis. High-resolution chest CT is a sensitive, noninvasive technique for the recognition of proximal bronchiectasis. The bronchial asthma of ABPA likely involves an IgE-mediated hypersensitivity, whereas the bronchiectasis associated with this disorder is thought to result from a deposition of immune complexes in proximal airways. Adequate treatment usually requires the long-term use of systemic glucocorticoids. Another eosinophilic process associated with asthma is Churg-Strauss syndrome, or allergic angiitis granulomatosis, which presents with necrotizing eosinophilic vasculitis and eosinophilic infiltration of multiple organs, including the lung.

A travel history or evidence of recent immigration should prompt the consideration of parasite-associated disorders. *Tropical eosinophilia* is usually caused by filarial infection; however, eosinophilic pneumonias also occur with other parasites such as *Ascaris* spp., *Ancyclostoma* spp., *Toxocara* spp., and *Strongyloides stercoralis.* Tropical eosinophilia due to *Wuchereria bancrofti* or *W. malayi* occurs most commonly in southern Asia, Africa, and South America and is treated successfully with diethylcarbamazine. In the United States, *Strongyloides* is endemic to the Southeastern and Appalachian regions. Even in cases of known foreign travel, identification of the causative agent is not always possible, as exemplified by 18 cases (2 fatal) of acute eosinophilic pneumonia reported amongst U.S. military personnel deployed in Iraq.

In the United States, *drug-induced eosinophilic pneumonias* are the most common cause of eosinophilic pulmonary infiltrates. These are exemplified by acute reactions to nitrofurantoin, which may begin 2 h to 10 days after nitrofurantoin is started, with symptoms of dry cough, fever, chills, and dyspnea; an eosinophilic pleural effusion accompanying patchy or diffuse pulmonary infiltrates may also occur. Other drugs associated with eosinophilic pneumonias include sulfonamides, penicillin, chlorpropamide, thiazides, tricyclic antidepressants, hydralazine, gold salts, isoniazid, indomethacin, and others. One report has identified anti-TNF-α monoclonal antibody therapy as a cause of eosinophilic pneumonitis. Treatment consists of withdrawal of the incriminated drugs or toxins and the use of glucocorticoids, if necessary.

The group of primary (idiopathic) eosinophilic pneumonias consists of diseases of varying severity. *Loeffler's syndrome* was originally reported as a benign, acute eosinophilic pneumonia of unknown cause characterized by migrating pulmonary infiltrates and minimal clinical manifestations. In some patients, these clinical characteristics prove to be secondary to parasites or drugs. *Acute eosinophilic pneumonia* is an idiopathic acute febrile illness of <7 days' duration with severe hypoxemia, pulmonary infiltrates, pleural effusions, and no history of asthma. BAL fluid reveals greater than 25% eosinophils (normally less than 2% in nonsmokers); however, the peripheral eosinophilia tends to develop later in the course and may not be apparent on initial presentation. *Chronic eosinophilic pneumonia* presents with significant systemic symptoms including fever, chills, night sweats, cough, anorexia, and weight loss of several weeks' to months' duration. The chest x-ray classically shows peripheral infiltrates, and pulmonary function testing reveals obstruction. Peripheral blood and BAL eosinophilia is more pronounced than in the acute form. Some patients also have bronchial asthma of the intrinsic or nonallergic type. For both acute and chronic disease, dramatic clearing of symptoms and chest x-ray is often noted after initiation of glucocorticoid therapy In contrast to acute eosinophilic pneumonia, chronic eosinophilic pneumonia tends to recur and may require repeated treatment.

The *hypereosinophilic syndrome* is characterized by presence of >1500 eosinophils per microliter of peripheral blood for 6 months or longer; lack of evidence for parasitic, allergic, or other known causes of eosinophilia; and signs or symptoms of multisystem organ dysfunction. Consistent features are blood and bone marrow eosinophilia with tissue infiltration by relatively mature eosinophils. The heart may be involved with tricuspid valve abnormalities or endomyocardial fibrosis and a restrictive, biventricular cardiomyopathy (Chap. 238). Other organs affected typically include the lungs, liver, spleen, skin, and nervous system. Therapy of the disorder consists of glucocorticoids and/or hydroxyurea, plus therapy as needed for cardiac dysfunction, which is frequently responsible for much of the morbidity and mortality in this syndrome. Pulmonary eosinophilia has also been associated with T cell lymphoma and has been reported following *lung* and *bone marrow transplantation.*

GLOBAL PICTURE OF HYPERSENSITIVITY PNEUMONITIS AND PULMONARY INFILTRATES WITH EOSINOPHILIA

HP is more prevalent outside of the United States than within, and the range of antigen responses is somewhat different. Internationally, bird breeder's lung is the most common form of HP. Rather than being associated with avocational exposures, bird-raising practices, highlighted by the emerging threat of avian influenza, lead to substantial exposure to workers involved in poultry husbandry and processing. This increases antigen exposure enormously, in comparison to U.S. workers, and enhances the risk of HP. Importantly, it is the most common cause of pediatric HP and has been reported in individuals as young as 4 years, presenting as a chronic cough.

Farmer's lung, one of the earliest reported causes of HP, appears to be waning worldwide. This is likely in response to changing agricultural practices; increased use of masks and impermeable barriers in hay storage has reduced the exposure and proliferation of thermophilic bacteria, and thus HP.

The international manifestations of HP resemble those of the U.S. disease. Many industrialized nations have increasingly reported HP due to mycobacteria and pseudomonads in contaminated metal-working fluids. The prevalence of these environmental contaminants greatly depends on workplace hygiene practices. Some forms of HP are almost exclusively geographically limited, such as summer-type hypersensitivity pneumonitis in Japan from exposure to *Trichosporon cutaneum* associated with birds. Likewise, cork worker's pneumonitis (suberosis), caused by exposure to contaminated corks, is almost exclusively seen in Spain and southern Europe because of the regional cork industry. However, one of the causative antigens (*Chrysonilia sitophila*) is also reported to be an antigen in lung diseases associated with logging in Canada. In Spain, esparto, a member of the grass family, is used as a fiber for the weaving of mats, baskets, and ropes; it is also incorporated into traditional plaster construction. In both of its uses, it has been associated with HP (most likely due to contamination with *A. fumigatus*), again geographically limited because of the utility of the product, though not of the underlying fungal antigen. Exposure to exotic mushrooms is greater in Asia than in the United States, and this has recently been linked to cases of HP.

Pulmonary infiltrates with eosinophilia are also a greater international than U.S. health burden. In this case, parasitic infestation is far more common than drug-induced lung disease, but the manifestations are similar.

ACKNOWLEDGMENTS

We acknowledge the contribution of Dr. Joel N. Kline to this chapter in the previous edition.

FURTHER READINGS

Allen JN: Drug-induced eosinophilic lung disease. Clin Chest Med 25:77, 2004

Cooray JH, Ismail MM: Re-examination of the diagnostic criteria of tropical pulmonary eosinophilia. Respir Med 93:655, 1999

Cormier Y et al: High-resolution computed tomographic characteristics in acute farmer's lung and in its follow-up. Eur Resp J 16:56, 2000

Fink JN et al: Needs and opportunities for research in hypersensitivity pneumonitis. Am J Respir Crit Care Med 171:792, 2005

Lacasse Y et al: Clinical diagnosis of hypersensitivity pneumonitis. Am J Respir Crit Care Med 168:962, 2003

Miyazaki Y et al: Clinical predictors and histologic appearance of acute exacerbations in chronic hypersensitivity pneumonitis. Chest 134(6):1265, 2008

Selman M et al: Hypersensitivity pneumonitis caused by fungi. Proc Am Thorac Soc 7:229, 2010

Shorr AF et al: Acute eosinophilic pneumonia among U.S. military personnel deployed in or near Iraq. JAMA 292:2997, 2004

Silva CI et al: Hypersensitivity pneumonitis: Spectrum of high-resolution CT and pathologic findings. Am J Roentgenol 188:334, 2007

Zacharisen MC et al: The long-term outcome in acute, subacute, and chronic forms of pigeon breeder's disease hypersensitivity pneumonitis. Ann Allergy Asthma Immunol 88:175, 2002

CHAPTER 256

Occupational and Environmental Lung Disease

John R. Balmes

Frank E. Speizer

Occupational and environmental lung diseases are difficult to distinguish from those of nonenvironmental origin. Virtually all major categories of pulmonary disease can be caused by environmental agents, and environmentally related disease usually presents clinically in a manner indistinguishable from that of disease not caused by such agents. In addition, the etiology of many diseases may be multifactorial; occupational and environmental factors may interact with other factors (such as smoking and genetic risk). It is often only after a careful exposure history is taken that the underlying workplace or general environmental exposure is uncovered.

Why is knowledge of occupational or environmental etiology so important? Patient management and prognosis are affected significantly by such knowledge. For example, patients with occupational asthma or hypersensitivity pneumonitis often cannot be managed adequately without cessation of exposure to the offending agent. Establishment of cause may have significant legal and financial implications for a patient who no longer can work in his or her usual job. Other exposed people may be identified as having the disease or prevented from getting it. In addition, new associations between exposure and disease may be identified (e.g., nylon flock worker's lung disease and diacetyl-induced bronchiolitis obliterans).

Although the exact proportion of lung disease due to occupational and environmental factors is unknown, a large number of individuals are at risk. For example, 15–20% of the burden of adult asthma and chronic obstructive pulmonary disease (COPD) has been estimated to be due to occupational factors.

HISTORY AND PHYSICAL EXAMINATION

The patient's history is of paramount importance in assessing any potential occupational or environmental exposure. Inquiry into specific work practices should include questions about the specific contaminants involved, the presence of visible dusts, chemical odors, the size and ventilation of workspaces, the use of respiratory protective equipment, and whether co-workers have similar complaints. The temporal association of exposure at work and symptoms may provide clues to occupation-related disease. In addition, the patient must be questioned about alternative sources of exposure to potentially toxic agents, including hobbies, home characteristics, exposure to secondhand smoke, and proximity to traffic or industrial facilities. Short-term and long-term exposures to potential toxic agents in the distant past also must be considered.

Workers in the United States have the right to know about potential hazards in their workplaces under federal Occupational Safety and Health Administration (OSHA) regulations. Employers must provide specific information about potential hazardous agents in products being used through Material Safety Data Sheets as well as training in personal protective equipment and environmental control procedures. Reminders posted in the workplace may warn workers about hazardous substances. However, the introduction of new processes and/or new chemical compounds may change exposure significantly, and often only the employee on the production line is aware of the change. For the physician caring for a patient with a suspected work-related illness, a visit to the work site can be very instructive. Alternatively, an affected worker can request an inspection by OSHA.

The physical examination of patients with environmentally related lung diseases may help determine the nature and severity of the pulmonary condition but usually does not contribute information that points to a specific etiology.

PULMONARY FUNCTION TESTS AND CHEST IMAGING

Exposures to inorganic and organic dusts can cause interstitial lung disease that presents with a restrictive pattern and a decreased diffusing capacity (Chap. 252). Similarly, exposures to a number of organic dusts or chemical agents may result in occupational asthma or COPD that is characterized by airway obstruction. Measurement of change in forced expiratory volume (FEV_1) before and after a working shift can be used to detect an acute bronchoconstrictive response. For example, an acute decrement of FEV_1 over the first work shift of the week is a characteristic feature of cotton textile workers with byssinosis (an obstructive airway disorder with features of both asthma and chronic bronchitis).

The chest radiograph is useful in detecting and monitoring the pulmonary response to mineral dusts, certain metals, and organic dusts capable of inducing hypersensitivity pneumonitis. The International Labour Organisation (ILO) International Classification of Radiographs of Pneumoconioses classifies chest radiographs by the nature and size of opacities seen and the extent of involvement of the parenchyma. In general, small rounded opacities are seen in silicosis or coal worker's pneumoconiosis and small linear opacities are seen in asbestosis. The profusion of such opacities is rated by using a 12-point scheme. Although useful for epidemiologic studies and screening large numbers of workers, the ILO system can be problematic when applied to an individual worker's chest radiograph. With dusts causing rounded opacities, the degree of involvement on the chest radiograph may be extensive, whereas pulmonary function may be only minimally impaired. In contrast, in pneumoconiosis causing linear, irregular opacities like those seen in asbestosis, the radiograph may lead to underestimation of the severity of the impairment until relatively late in the disease. For patients with a history of asbestos exposure, conventional computed tomography (CT) is more sensitive for the detection of pleural thickening and high-resolution CT (HRCT) improves the detection of asbestosis.

Other procedures that may be of use in identifying the role of environmental exposures in causing lung disease include evaluation of heavy metal concentrations in urine (cadmium in battery plant workers), skin prick testing or specific IgE antibody titers for evidence of immediate hypersensitivity to agents capable of inducing occupational asthma (flour antigens in bakers), specific IgG precipitating antibody titers for agents capable of causing hypersensitivity pneumonitis (pigeon antigen in bird handlers), and assays for specific cell-mediated immune responses (beryllium lymphocyte proliferation testing in nuclear workers or tuberculin skin testing in health care workers). Sometimes a bronchoscopy to obtain transbronchial biopsies of lung tissue may be required for histologic diagnosis (chronic beryllium disease). Rarely, video-assisted thoracoscopic surgery to obtain a larger sample of lung tissue may be required to determine the specific diagnosis of environmentally induced lung disease (hypersensitivity pneumonitis or giant cell interstitial pneumonitis due to cobalt exposure).

EXPOSURE ASSESSMENT

If reliable environmental sampling data are available, that information should be used in assessing a patient's exposure. Since many of the chronic diseases result from exposure over many years, current environmental measurements should be combined with work histories to arrive at estimates of past exposure.

In situations in which individual exposure to specific agents—either in a work setting or via ambient air pollutants—has been determined, the chemical and physical characteristics of those agents affect both the inhaled dose and the site of deposition in the respiratory tract. Water-soluble gases such as ammonia and sulfur dioxide are absorbed in the lining fluid of the upper and proximal airways and thus tend to produce irritative and bronchoconstrictive responses. In contrast, nitrogen dioxide and phosgene, which are less soluble, may penetrate to the bronchioles and alveoli in sufficient quantities to produce acute chemical pneumonitis that can be life-threatening.

Particle size of air contaminants must also be considered. Because of their settling velocities in air, particles >10–15 μm in diameter do not penetrate beyond the nose and throat. Particles <10 μm in size are deposited below the larynx. These particles are divided into three size fractions on the basis of their size characteristics and sources. Particles ~2.5–10 μm (coarse-mode fraction) contain crustal elements such as silica, aluminum, and iron. These particles mostly deposit relatively high in the tracheobronchial tree. Although the total mass of an ambient sample is dominated by these larger respirable particles, the number of particles, and therefore the surface area on which potential toxic agents can deposit and be carried to the lower airways, is dominated by particles <2.5 μm (fine-mode fraction). These fine particles are created primarily by the burning of fossil fuels or high-temperature industrial processes resulting in condensation products from gases, fumes, or vapors. The smallest particles, those <0.1 μm in size, represent the ultrafine fraction and make up the largest number of particles; they tend to remain in the airstream and deposit in the lung only on a random basis as they come into contact with the alveolar walls. If they do deposit, however, particles of this size range may penetrate into the circulation and be carried to extrapulmonary sites. New technologies create particles of this size ("nanoparticles") for use in many commercial applications. Besides the size characteristics of particles and the solubility of gases, the actual chemical composition, mechanical properties, and immunogenicity or infectivity of inhaled material determine in large part the nature of the diseases found among exposed persons.

OCCUPATIONAL EXPOSURES AND PULMONARY DISEASE

Table 256-1 provides broad categories of exposure in the workplace and diseases associated with chronic exposure in those industries.

ASBESTOS-RELATED DISEASES

Asbestos is a generic term for several different mineral silicates, including chrysolite, amosite, anthophyllite, and crocidolite. In addition to workers involved in the production of asbestos products (mining, milling, and manufacturing), many workers in the shipbuilding and construction trades, including pipe fitters and boilermakers, were occupationally exposed because asbestos was widely used during the twentieth century for its thermal and electrical insulation properties. Asbestos also was used in the manufacture of fire-resistant textiles, in cement and floor tiles, and in friction materials such as brake and clutch linings.

Exposure to asbestos is not limited to persons who directly handle the material. Cases of asbestos-related diseases have been encountered in individuals with only bystander exposure, such as painters and electricians who worked alongside insulation workers in a shipyard. Community exposure resulted from the use of asbestos-containing mine and mill tailings as landfill, road surface, and playground material (e.g., Libby, MT, the site of a vermiculite mine in which the ore was contaminated with asbestos). Finally, exposure can occur from the disturbance of naturally occurring asbestos (e.g., from increasing residential development in the foothills of the Sierra Mountains in California).

Asbestos has largely been replaced in the developed world with synthetic mineral fibers such as fiberglass and refractory ceramic fibers, but it continues to be used increasingly in the developing world. Despite current OSHA regulations mandating adequate training for any worker potentially exposed to asbestos, exposure continues among inadequately trained and protected demolition

TABLE 256-1 Categories of Occupational Exposure and Associated Respiratory Conditions

Occupational Exposures	Nature of Respiratory Responses	Comment
Inorganic Dusts		
Asbestos: mining, processing, construction, ship repair	Fibrosis (asbestosis), pleural disease, cancer, mesothelioma	Virtually all new mining and construction with asbestos done in developing countries
Silica: mining, stone cutting, sandblasting, quarrying	Fibrosis (silicosis), progressive massive fibrosis (PMF), cancer, tuberculosis, chronic obstructive pulmonary disease (COPD)	Improved protection in United States, persistent risk in developing countries
Coal dust: mining	Fibrosis (coal worker's pneumoconiosis), PMF, COPD	Risk persists in certain areas of United States, increasing in countries where new mines open
Beryllium: processing alloys for high-tech industries	Acute pneumonitis (rare), chronic granulomatous disease, lung cancer (highly suspect)	Risk in high-tech industries persists
Other metals: aluminum, chromium, cobalt, nickel, titanium, tungsten carbide, or "hard metal" (contains cobalt)	Wide variety of conditions from acute pneumonitis to lung cancer and asthma	New diseases appear with new process development
Organic Dusts		
Cotton dust: milling, processing	Byssinosis (an asthma-like syndrome), chronic bronchitis, COPD	Increasing risk in developing countries with drop in United States as jobs shift overseas
Grain dust: elevator agents, dock workers, milling, bakers	Asthma, chronic bronchitis, COPD	Risk shifting more to migrant labor pool
Other agricultural dusts: fungal spores, vegetable products, insect fragments, animal dander, bird and rodent feces, endotoxins, microorganisms, pollens	Hypersensitivity pneumonitis (farmer's lung), asthma, chronic bronchitis	Important in migrant labor pool but also resulting from in-home exposures
Toxic chemicals: wide variety of industries, see Table 256-2	Asthma, chronic bronchitis, COPD, hypersensitivity pneumonitis, pneumoconiosis, and cancer	Reduced risk with recognized hazards; increasing risk for developing countries where controlled labor practices are less stringent
Other respiratory environmental agents: uranium and radon daughters, secondhand tobacco smoke, polycyclic hydrocarbons, biomass smoke, diesel exhaust, welding fumes, wood finishing	Occupational exposures estimated to contribute to up to 10% of all lung cancers; chronic bronchitis, COPD, and fibrosis	In-home exposures important; in developing countries biomass smoke is a major risk factor for COPD among women

workers. The major health effects from exposure to asbestos are pleural and pulmonary fibrosis, cancers of the respiratory tract, and pleural and peritoneal mesothelioma.

Asbestosis is a diffuse interstitial fibrosing disease of the lung that is directly related to the intensity and duration of exposure. The disease resembles other forms of diffuse interstitial fibrosis (Chap. 261). Usually, moderate to severe exposure has taken place for at least 10 years before the disease becomes manifest, and it may occur after exposure to any of the asbestiform fiber types. The mechanisms by which asbestos fibers induce lung fibrosis are not completely understood but are known to involve oxidative injury due to the generation of reactive oxygen species by the transition metals on the surface of the fibers as well as from cells engaged in phagocytosis.

The chest radiograph can be used to detect the pulmonary manifestations of asbestos exposure. Past exposure is specifically indicated by pleural plaques, which are characterized by either thickening or calcification along the parietal pleura, particularly along the lower lung fields, the diaphragm, and the cardiac border. Without additional manifestations, pleural plaques imply only exposure, not pulmonary impairment. Benign pleural effusions also may occur. The fluid is typically a serous or bloody exudate. The effusion may be slowly progressive or may resolve spontaneously. Irregular or linear opacities, evidence of asbestosis that usually are first noted in the lower lung fields and spreading into the middle and upper lung fields, occur as the disease progresses. An indistinct heart border or a "ground-glass" appearance in the lung fields is seen in some cases. In cases in which the x-ray changes are less obvious, HRCT may show distinct changes of subpleural curvilinear lines 5–10 mm in length that appear to be parallel to the pleural surface (Fig. 256-1).

Pulmonary function testing in asbestosis reveals a restrictive pattern with a decrease in both lung volumes and diffusing capacity. There may also be evidence of mild airflow obstruction (due to peribronchiolar fibrosis).

No specific therapy is available for the management of patients with asbestosis. The supportive care is the same as that given to any patient with diffuse interstitial fibrosis of any cause. In general, newly diagnosed cases will have resulted from exposures that occurred many years before.

Lung cancer (Chap. 89) is the most common cancer associated with asbestos exposure. The excess frequency of lung cancer (all histologic types) in asbestos workers is associated with a minimum latency of 15–19 years between first exposure and development of the disease. Persons with more exposure are at greater risk of disease. In addition, there is a significant interactive effect of smoking and asbestos exposure that results in greater risk than what would be expected from the additive effect of each factor.

Mesotheliomas (Chap. 263), both pleural and peritoneal, are also associated with asbestos exposure. In contrast to lung cancers, these tumors do not appear to be associated with smoking. Relatively short-term asbestos exposures of ≤1–2 years or less, occurring up to 40 years in the past, have been associated with the development of mesotheliomas (an observation that emphasizes the importance of obtaining a complete environmental exposure history). Although the risk of mesothelioma is much less than that of lung cancer among asbestos-exposed workers, over 2000 cases were reported in the United States per year at the start of the twenty-first century.

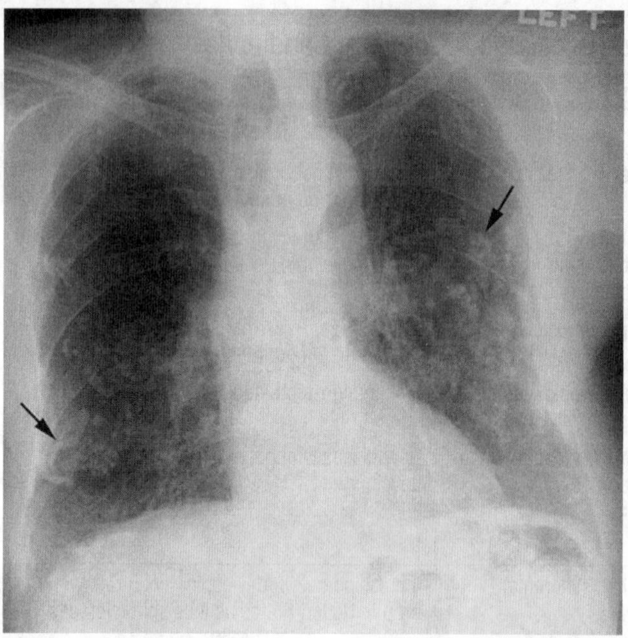

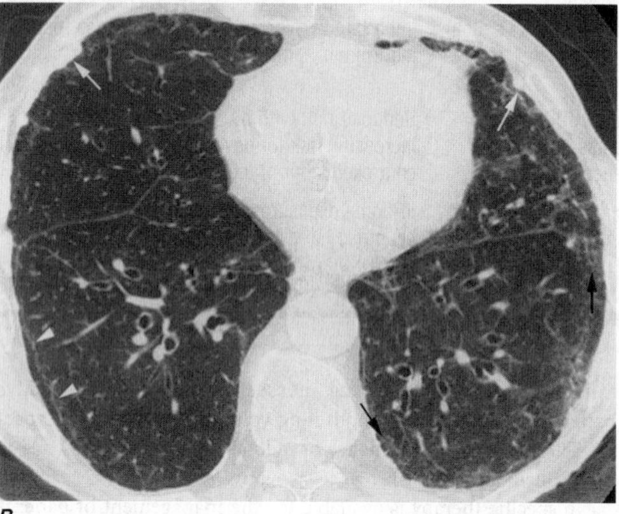

Figure 256-1 Asbestosis: ***A.*** Frontal chest radiograph shows bilateral calcified pleural plaques consistent with asbestos-related pleural disease. Poorly defined linear and reticular abnormalities are seen in the lower lobes bilaterally. ***B.*** Axial high-resolution computed tomography of the thorax obtained through the lung bases shows bilateral, subpleural reticulation (*black arrows*), representing fibrotic lung disease due to asbestosis. Subpleural lines are also present (*arrowheads*), characteristic of, though not specific for, asbestosis. Calcified pleural plaques representing asbestos-related pleural disease (*white arrows*) are also evident.

Although ~50% of mesotheliomas metastasize, the tumor generally is locally invasive, and death usually results from local extension. Most patients present with effusions that may obscure the underlying pleural tumor. In contrast to the findings in effusion due to other causes, because of the restriction placed on the chest wall, no shift of mediastinal structures toward the opposite side of the chest will be seen. The major diagnostic problem is differentiation from peripherally spreading pulmonary adenocarcinoma or adenocarcinoma that has metastasized to pleura from an extrathoracic primary site. Although cytologic examination of pleural fluid may suggest the diagnosis, biopsy of pleural tissue, generally with video-assisted thoracic surgery, and special immunohistochemical staining usually are required. There is no effective therapy.

Since epidemiologic studies have shown that >80% of mesotheliomas may be associated with asbestos exposure, documented mesothelioma in a patient with occupational or environmental exposure to asbestos may be compensable.

SILICOSIS

In spite of being one of the oldest known occupational pulmonary hazards, *free silica* (SiO_2), or crystalline quartz, is still a major cause of disease. The major occupational exposures include mining; stonecutting; employment in abrasive industries such as stone, clay, glass, and cement manufacturing; foundry work; packing of silica flour; and quarrying, particularly of granite. Most often, pulmonary fibrosis due to silica exposure (silicosis) occurs in a dose-response fashion after many years of exposure.

Workers heavily exposed through sandblasting in confined spaces, tunneling through rock with a high quartz content (15–25%), or the manufacture of abrasive soaps may develop acute silicosis with as little as 10 months of exposure. The clinical and pathologic features of acute silicosis are similar to those of pulmonary alveolar proteinosis (Chap. 261). The chest radiograph may show profuse miliary infiltration or consolidation, and there is a characteristic HRCT pattern known as "crazy paving" (Fig. 256-2). The disease may be quite severe and progressive despite the discontinuation of exposure. Whole-lung lavage may provide symptomatic relief and slow the progression.

With long-term, less intense exposure, small rounded opacities in the upper lobes may appear on the chest radiograph after 15–20 years of exposure (*simple silicosis*). Calcification of hilar nodes may occur in as many as 20% of cases and produces a characteristic "eggshell" pattern. Silicotic nodules may be identified more readily by HRCT (Fig. 256-3). The nodular fibrosis may be progressive in the absence of further exposure, with coalescence and formation of nonsegmental conglomerates of irregular masses >1 cm in diameter (*complicated silicosis*). These masses can become quite large, and when this occurs, the term *progressive massive fibrosis* (PMF) is applied. Significant functional impairment with both restrictive and obstructive components may be associated with this form of silicosis.

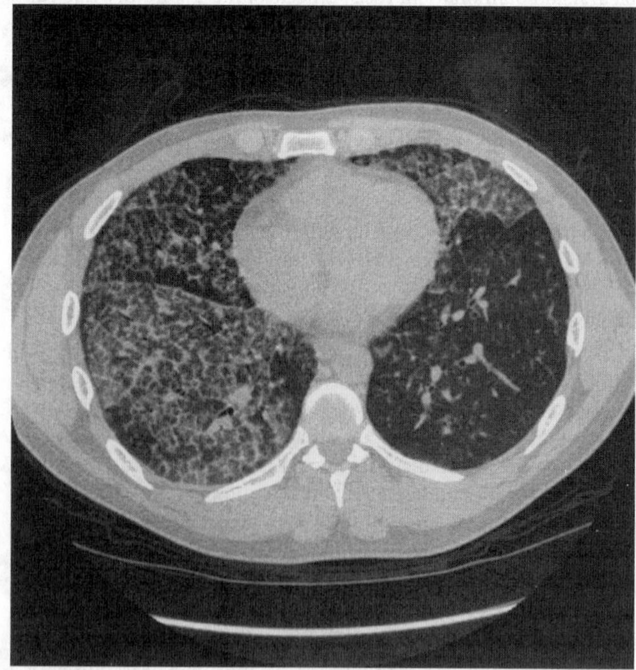

Figure 256-2 Acute silicosis. This high-resolution computed tomography scan shows multiple small nodules consistent with silicosis but also diffuse ground-glass densities with thickened intralobular and interlobular septa producing polygonal shapes. This has been referred to as "crazy paving."

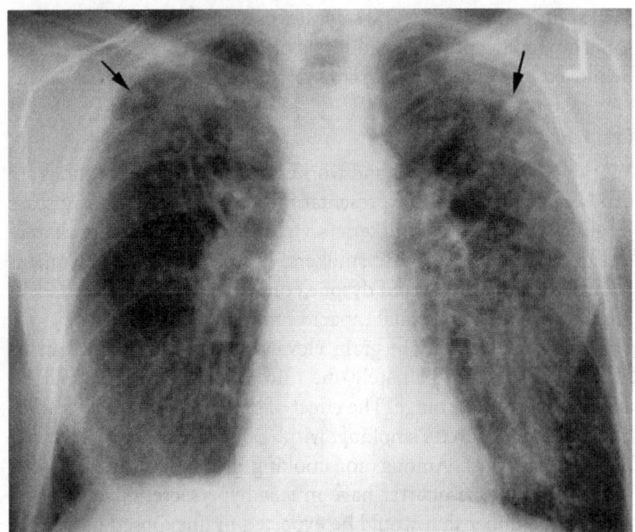

A

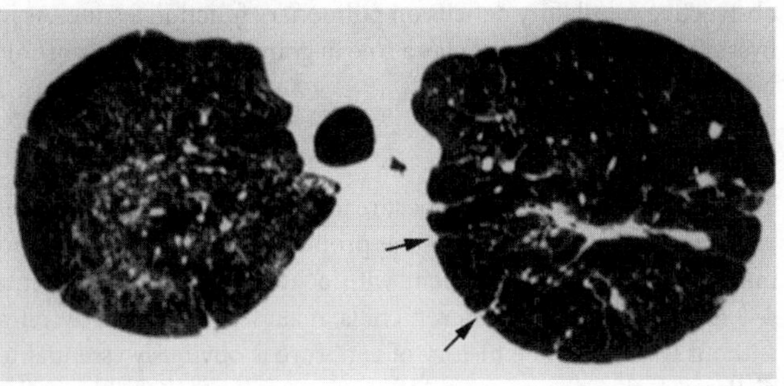

B

Figure 256-3 Chronic silicosis. ***A.*** Frontal chest radiograph in a patient with silicosis shows variably sized, poorly defined nodules (*arrows*) predominating in the upper lobes, ***B.*** Axial thoracic computed tomography image through the lung apices shows numerous small nodules, more pronounced in the right upper lobe. A number of the nodules are subpleural in location (*arrows*).

Because silica is cytotoxic to alveolar macrophages, patients with silicosis are at greater risk of acquiring lung infections that involve these cells as a primary defense (*Mycobacterium tuberculosis*, atypical mycobacteria and fungi). Because of the increased risk of active tuberculosis, the recommended treatment of latent tuberculosis in these patients is longer. Another potential clinical complication of silicosis is autoimmune connective tissue disorders such as rheumatoid arthritis and scleroderma. In addition, there are sufficient epidemiologic data that the International Agency for Research on Cancer lists silica as a probable lung carcinogen.

Other, less hazardous silicates include fuller's earth, kaolin, mica, diatomaceous earths, silica gel, soapstone, carbonate dusts, and cement dusts. The production of fibrosis in workers exposed to these agents is believed to be related either to the free silica content of these dusts or, for substances that contain no free silica, to the potentially large dust loads to which these workers may be exposed.

Other silicates, including *talc dusts*, may be contaminated with asbestos and/or free silica. Fibrosis and/or pleural or lung cancer have been associated with chronic exposure to commercial talc.

COAL WORKER'S PNEUMOCONIOSIS (CWP)

Occupational exposure to *coal dust* can lead to CWP, which has enormous social, economic, and medical significance in every nation in which coal mining is an important industry. Simple radiographically identified CWP is seen in ~10% of all coal miners and in as many as 50% of anthracite miners with more than 20 years' work on the coal face. The prevalence of disease is lower in workers in bituminous coal mines.

With prolonged exposure to coal dust (i.e., 15–20 years), small, rounded opacities similar to those of silicosis may develop. As in silicosis, the presence of these nodules (*simple CWP*) usually is not associated with pulmonary impairment. Much of the symptomatology associated with simple CWP appears to be due to the effects of coal dust on the development of chronic bronchitis and COPD (Chap. 260). The effects of coal dust are additive to those of cigarette smoking.

Complicated CWP is manifested by the appearance on the chest radiograph of nodules ranging from 1 cm in diameter to the size of an entire lobe, generally confined to the upper half of the lungs. As in silicosis, this condition can progress to PMF that is accompanied by severe lung function deficits and associated with premature mortality. Despite improvements in technology to protect coal miners, cases of PMF still occur in the United States at a disturbing rate.

Caplan's syndrome (Chap. 321), first described in coal miners but subsequently found in patients with silicosis, includes seropositive rheumatoid arthritis with characteristic pneumoconiotic nodules. Silica has immunoadjuvant properties and is often present in anthracitic coal dust.

CHRONIC BERYLLIUM DISEASE

Beryllium is a lightweight metal with tensile strength that has good electrical conductivity and is valuable in the control of nuclear reactions through its ability to quench neutrons. Although beryllium may produce an acute pneumonitis, it is far more commonly associated with a chronic granulomatous inflammatory disease that is similar to sarcoidosis (Chap. 329). Unless one inquires specifically about occupational exposures to beryllium in the manufacture of alloys, ceramics, or high-technology electronics in a patient with sarcoidosis, one may miss entirely the etiologic relationship to the occupational exposure. What distinguishes chronic beryllium disease (CBD) from sarcoidosis is evidence of a specific cell-mediated immune response (i.e., delayed hypersensitivity) to beryllium.

The test that usually provides this evidence is the beryllium lymphocyte proliferation test (BeLPT). The BeLPT compares the in vitro proliferation of lymphocytes from blood or bronchoalveolar lavage in the presence of beryllium salts with that of unstimulated cells. Proliferation is usually measured by lymphocyte uptake of radiolabeled thymidine.

Chest imaging findings are similar to those of sarcoidosis (nodules along septal lines) except that hilar adenopathy is somewhat less common. As with sarcoidosis, pulmonary function test results may show restrictive and/or obstructive ventilatory deficits and decreased diffusing capacity. With early disease, both chest imaging studies and pulmonary function tests may be normal. Fiberoptic bronchoscopy with transbronchial lung biopsy usually is required to make the diagnosis of CBD. In a beryllium-sensitized individual, the presence of noncaseating granulomas or monocytic infiltration in lung tissue establishes the diagnosis. Accumulation of beryllium-specific CD4+ T cells occurs in the granulomatous inflammation seen on lung biopsy. CBD is one of the best studied examples of gene-environment interaction. Susceptibility to CBD is highly associated with human leukocyte antigen DP (HLA-DP) alleles that have a glutamic acid in position 69 of the β chain.

Other metals, including aluminum and titanium dioxide, have been rarely associated with a sarcoid-like reaction in lung tissue. Exposure to dust containing tungsten carbide, also known as "hard metal," may produce giant cell interstitial pneumonitis. Cobalt is a constituent of tungsten carbide and is the likely etiologic agent of both the interstitial pneumonitis and the occupational asthma that may occur. The most common exposures to tungsten carbide occur in tool and dye, saw blade, and drill bit manufacture. Diamond polishing may also involve exposure to cobalt dust. The same Glu69 polymorphism of the

HLA-DP β chain that confers increased risk of CBD also appears to increase the risk of cobalt-induced giant cell interstitial pneumonitis.

In patients with interstitial lung disease, one should always inquire about exposure to metal fumes and/or dusts. Especially when sarcoidosis appears to be the diagnosis, one should always consider possible CBD.

OTHER INORGANIC DUSTS

Most of the inorganic dusts discussed thus far are associated with the production of either dust macules or interstitial fibrotic changes in the lung. Other inorganic and organic dusts (see categories in Table 256-1), along with some of the dusts previously discussed, are associated with chronic mucus hypersecretion (chronic bronchitis), with or without reduction of expiratory flow rates. Cigarette smoking is the major cause of these conditions, and any effort to attribute some component of the disease to occupational and environmental exposures must take cigarette smoking into account. Most studies suggest an additive effect of dust exposure and smoking. The pattern of the irritant dust effect is similar to that of cigarette smoking, suggesting that small airway inflammation may be the initial site of pathologic response in those cases and continued exposure may lead to chronic bronchitis and COPD.

ORGANIC DUSTS

Some of the specific diseases associated with organic dusts are discussed in detail in the chapters on asthma (Chap. 254) and hypersensitivity pneumonitis (Chap. 255). Many of these diseases are named for the specific setting in which they are found, e.g., farmer's lung, malt worker's disease, and mushroom worker's disease. Often the temporal relation of symptoms to exposure furnishes the best evidence for the diagnosis. Three occupational exposures are singled out for discussion here because they affect the largest proportions of workers.

Cotton dust (byssinosis)

Workers occupationally exposed to cotton dust (but also to flax, hemp, or jute dust) in the production of yarns for textiles and rope making are at risk for an asthma-like syndrome known as byssinosis. Exposure occurs throughout the manufacturing process but is most pronounced in the portions of the factory involved with the treatment of the cotton before spinning, i.e., blowing, mixing, and carding (straightening of fibers). The risk of byssinosis is associated with both cotton dust and endotoxin levels in the workplace environment.

Byssinosis is characterized clinically as occasional (early-stage) and then regular (late-stage) chest tightness toward the end of the first day of the workweek ("Monday chest tightness"). In epidemiologic studies, depending on the level of exposure via the carding room air, up to 80% of employees may show a significant drop in FEV_1 over the course of a Monday shift.

Initially the symptoms do not recur on subsequent days of the week. However, in 10–25% of workers, the disease may be progressive, with chest tightness recurring or persisting throughout the workweek. After >10 years of exposure, workers with recurrent symptoms are more likely to have an obstructive pattern on pulmonary function testing. The highest grades of impairment generally are seen in smokers.

Reduction of dust exposure is of primary importance to the management of byssinosis. Dust levels can be controlled by the use of exhaust hoods, general increases in ventilation, and wetting procedures, but respiratory protective equipment appears to be required during certain operations to prevent workers from being exposed to levels of cotton dust that exceed the current OSHA-permissible exposure level. Regular surveillance of pulmonary function in cotton dust–exposed workers using spirometry before and after the workshift is required by OSHA. All workers with persistent symptoms or significantly reduced levels of pulmonary function should be moved to areas of lower risk of exposure.

Grain dust

Worldwide, many farmers and workers in grain storage facilities are exposed to grain dust. The presentation of obstructive airway disease in grain dust–exposed workers is virtually identical to the characteristic findings in cigarette smokers, i.e., persistent cough, mucus hypersecretion, wheeze and dyspnea on exertion, and reduced FEV_1 and FEV_1/FVC (forced vital capacity) ratio (Chap. 252).

Dust concentrations in grain elevators vary greatly but can be >10,000 μg/m^3; approximately one-third of the particles, by weight, are in the respirable range. The effect of grain dust exposure is additive to that of cigarette smoking, with ~50% of workers who smoke having symptoms. Among nonsmoking grain elevator operators, approximately one-quarter have mucus hypersecretion, about five times the number that would be expected in unexposed nonsmokers. Smoking grain dust–exposed workers are more likely to have obstructive ventilatory deficits on pulmonary function testing. As in byssinosis, endotoxin may play a role in grain dust–induced chronic bronchitis and COPD.

Farmer's lung

This condition results from exposure to moldy hay containing spores of thermophilic actinomycetes that produce a hypersensitivity pneumonitis (Chap. 255). A patient with acute farmer's lung presents 4–8 h after exposure with fever, chills, malaise, cough, and dyspnea without wheezing. The history of exposure is obviously essential to distinguish this disease from influenza or pneumonia with similar symptoms. In the chronic form of the disease, the history of repeated attacks after similar exposure is important in differentiating this syndrome from other causes of patchy fibrosis (e.g., sarcoidosis).

A wide variety of other organic dusts are associated with the occurrence of hypersensitivity pneumonitis (Chap. 255). For patients who present with hypersensitivity pneumonitis, specific and careful inquiry about occupations, hobbies, and other home environmental exposures is necessary to uncover the source of the etiologic agent.

TOXIC CHEMICALS

Exposure to toxic chemicals affecting the lung generally involves gases and vapors. A common accident is one in which the victim is trapped in a confined space where the chemicals have accumulated to toxic levels. In addition to the specific toxic effects of the chemical, the victim often sustains considerable anoxia, which can play a dominant role in determining whether the individual survives.

Table 256-2 lists a variety of toxic agents that can produce acute and sometimes life-threatening reactions in the lung. All these agents in sufficient concentrations have been demonstrated, at least in animal studies, to affect the lower airways and disrupt alveolar architecture, either acutely or as a result of chronic exposure. Some of these agents may be generated acutely in the environment (see below).

Firefighters and fire victims are at risk of *smoke inhalation*, an important cause of acute cardiorespiratory failure. Smoke inhalation kills more fire victims than does thermal injury. Carbon monoxide poisoning with resulting significant hypoxemia can be life-threatening (Chap. e50). Synthetic materials (plastic, polyurethanes), when burned, may release a variety of other toxic agents (such as cyanide and hydrochloric acid), and this must be considered in evaluating smoke inhalation victims. Exposed victims may have some degree of lower respiratory tract inflammation and/or pulmonary edema.

Exposure to certain highly reactive, low-molecular-weight agents used in the manufacture of synthetic polymers, paints, and coatings (*diisocyanates* in polyurethanes, *aromatic amines* and *acid anhydrides* in epoxies) are associated with a high risk of occupational asthma. Although this occupational asthma manifests clinically as if sensitization has occurred, an IgE antibody–mediated mechanism is not necessarily involved. Hypersensitivity pneumonitis–like reactions also have been described in diisocyanate and acid anhydride–exposed workers.

Fluoropolymers such as Teflon, which at normal temperatures produce no reaction, become volatilized upon heating. The inhaled agents cause a characteristic syndrome of fever, chills, malaise, and occasionally mild wheezing, leading to the diagnosis of *polymer fume fever*. A similar self-limited, influenza-like syndrome—*metal fume fever*—results from acute exposure to fumes or smoke containing zinc oxide. The syndrome may begin several hours after work and resolves within 24 h, only to return on repeated exposure. Welding of galvanized steel is the most common exposure leading to metal fume fever.

Two other agents have been recently associated with potentially severe interstitial lung disease. Occupational exposure to nylon flock has been shown to induce a lymphocytic bronchiolitis, and workers exposed to diacetyl used to provide "butter" flavor in the manufacture of microwave popcorn and other foods have developed bronchiolitis obliterans (Chap. 261).

World Trade Center disaster

A consequence of the attack on the World Trade Center (WTC) on September 11, 2001, was relatively heavy exposure of a large number of firefighters and other rescue workers to the dust generated by the

TABLE 256-2 Selected Common Toxic Chemical Agents That Affect the Lung

Agent(s)	Selected Exposures	Acute Effects from High or Accidental Exposure	Chronic Effects from Relatively Low Exposure
Acid anhydrides	Manufacture of resin esters, polyester resins, thermoactivated adhesives	Nasal irritation, cough	Asthma, chronic bronchitis, hypersensitivity pneumonitis
Acid fumes: H_2SO_4, HNO_3	Manufacture of fertilizers, chlorinated organic compounds, dyes, explosives, rubber products, metal etching, plastics	Mucous membrane irritation, followed by chemical pneumonitis 2–3 days later	Bronchitis and suggestion of mildly reduced pulmonary function in children with lifelong residential exposure to high levels
Acrolein and other aldehydes	By-product of burning plastics, woods, tobacco smoke	Mucous membrane irritant, decrease in lung function	Upper respiratory tract irritation
Ammonia	Refrigeration; petroleum refining; manufacture of fertilizers, explosives, plastics, and other chemicals	Same as for acid fumes, but bronchiectasis also has been reported	Upper respiratory tract irritation, chronic bronchitis
Cadmium fumes	Smelting, soldering, battery production	Mucous membrane irritant, acute respiratory distress syndrome (ARDS)	Chronic obstructive pulmonary disease (COPD)
Formaldehyde	Manufacture of resins, leathers, rubber, metals, and woods; laboratory workers, embalmers; emission from urethane foam insulation	Same as for acid fumes	Nasopharyngeal cancer
Halides and acid salts (Cl, Br, F)	Bleaching in pulp, paper, textile industry; manufacture of chemical compounds; synthetic rubber, plastics, disinfectant, rocket fuel, gasoline	Mucous membrane irritation, pulmonary edema; possible reduced FVC 1–2 yrs after exposure	Upper respiratory tract irritation, epistaxis, tracheobronchitis
Hydrogen sulfide	By-product of many industrial processes, oil, other petroleum processes and storage	Increase in respiratory rate followed by respiratory arrest, lactic acidosis, pulmonary edema, death	Conjunctival irritation, chronic bronchitis, recurrent pneumonitis
Isocyanates (TDI, HDI, MDI)	Production of polyurethane foams, plastics, adhesives, surface coatings	Mucous membrane irritation, dyspnea, cough, wheeze, pulmonary edema	Upper respiratory tract irritation, cough, asthma, hypersensitivity pneumonitis, reduced lung function
Nitrogen dioxide	Silage, metal etching, explosives, rocket fuels, welding, by-product of burning fossil fuels	Cough, dyspnea, pulmonary edema may be delayed 4–12 h; possible result from acute exposure: bronchiolitis obliterans in 2–6 wks	Emphysema in animals, ?chronic bronchitis, associated with reduced lung function in children with lifelong residential exposure
Ozone	Arc welding, flour bleaching, deodorizing, emissions from copying equipment, photochemical air pollutant	Mucous membrane irritant, pulmonary hemorrhage and edema, reduced pulmonary function transiently in children and adults, and increased hospitalization with exposure to summer haze	Excess cardiopulmonary mortality rates
Phosgene	Organic compound, metallurgy, volatilization of chlorine-containing compounds	Delayed onset of bronchiolitis and pulmonary edema	Chronic bronchitis
Sulfur dioxide	Manufacture of sulfuric acid, bleaches, coating of nonferrous metals, food processing, refrigerant, burning of fossil fuels, wood pulp industry	Mucous membrane irritant, epistaxis, bronchospasm (especially in people with asthma)	Chronic bronchitis

collapse of the buildings. Environmental monitoring and chemical characterization of WTC dust has revealed a wide variety of potentially toxic constituents, although much of the dust was pulverized cement. Possibly because of the high alkalinity of WTC dust, significant cough, wheeze, and phlegm production occurred among firefighters and cleanup crews. New cough and wheeze syndromes also occurred among local residents. Initial longitudinal follow-up of New York firefighters suggests that heavier exposure to WTC dust is associated with accelerated decline of lung function. Ongoing follow-up will provide data on whether massive exposure to this irritant dust has led to the development of chronic respiratory disease.

■ OCCUPATIONAL RESPIRATORY CARCINOGENS

Exposures at work have been estimated to contribute to 10% of all lung cancer cases. In addition to asbestos, other agents either proven or suspected to be respiratory carcinogens include acrylonitrile, arsenic compounds, beryllium, bis(chloromethyl) ether, chromium (hexavalent), formaldehyde (nasal), isopropanol (nasal sinuses), mustard gas, nickel carbonyl (nickel smelting), polyaromatic hydrocarbons (coke oven emissions and diesel exhaust), secondhand tobacco smoke, silica (both mining and processing), talc (possible asbestos contamination in both mining and milling), vinyl chloride (sarcomas), wood (nasal cancer only), and uranium. Workers at risk of radiation-related lung cancer include not only those involved in mining or processing uranium but also those exposed in underground mining operations of other ores where radon daughters may be emitted from rock formations.

■ ASSESSMENT OF DISABILITY

Patients who have lung disease may not be able to continue to work in their usual jobs because of respiratory symptoms. *Disability* is the term used to describe the decreased ability to work due to the effects of a medical condition. Physicians are generally able to assess physiologic dysfunction, or *impairment*, but the rating of disability for compensation of loss of income also involves nonmedical factors such as the education and employability of the individual. The disability rating scheme differs with the compensation-granting agency. For example, the U.S. Social Security Administration requires that an individual be unable to do any work (i.e., *total* disability) before he or she will receive income replacement payments. Many state workers' compensation systems allow for payments for *partial* disability. In the Social Security scheme no determination of cause is done, whereas work-relatedness must be established in workers' compensation systems.

For respiratory impairment rating, resting pulmonary function tests (spirometry and diffusing capacity) are used as the initial assessment tool, with cardiopulmonary exercise testing (to assess maximal oxygen consumption) used if the results of the resting tests do not correlate with the patient's symptoms. Methacholine challenge (to assess airway reactivity) can also be useful in patients with asthma who have normal spirometry when evaluated. Some compensation agencies (e.g., Social Security) have proscribed disability classification schemes based on pulmonary function test results. When no specific scheme is proscribed, the *Guidelines of the American Medical Association* should be used.

Evaluating relation to work exposure requires a detailed work history, as previously discussed in this chapter. Occasionally, as with some cases of suspected occupational asthma, challenge to the putative agent in the work environment with repeated pulmonary function measures may be required.

GENERAL ENVIRONMENTAL EXPOSURES

■ OUTDOOR AIR POLLUTION

In 1971, the U.S. government established national air quality standards for several pollutants believed to be responsible for excess cardiorespiratory diseases. Primary standards regulated by the U.S. Environmental Protection Agency (EPA) designed to protect the public health with an adequate margin of safety exist for sulfur dioxide, particulates matter, nitrogen dioxide, ozone, lead, and carbon monoxide. Standards for each of these pollutants are updated regularly through an extensive review process conducted by the EPA. (For details on current standards, go to *http://www.epa.gov/air/criteria.html*.)

Pollutants are generated from both stationary sources (power plants and industrial complexes) and mobile sources (automobiles), and none of the regulated pollutants occurs in isolation. Furthermore, pollutants may be changed by chemical reactions after being emitted. For example, sulfur dioxide and particulate matter emissions from a coal-fired power plant may react in air to produce acid sulfates and aerosols, which can be transported long distances in the atmosphere. Oxidizing substances such as oxides of nitrogen and volatile organic compounds from automobile exhaust may react with sunlight to produce ozone. Although originally thought to be confined to Los Angeles, photochemically derived pollution ("smog") is now known to be a problem throughout the United States and in many other countries. Both acute and chronic effects of these exposures have been documented in large population studies.

The symptoms and diseases associated with air pollution are the same as conditions commonly associated with cigarette smoking. In addition, decreased growth of lung function and asthma have been associated with chronic exposure to only modestly elevated levels of traffic-related gases and respirable particles. Multiple population-based time-series studies within cities have demonstrated excess health care utilization for asthma and other cardiopulmonary conditions and mortality rates. Cohort studies comparing cities that have relatively high levels of particulate exposures with less polluted communities suggest excess morbidity and mortality rates from cardiopulmonary conditions in long-term residents of the former. The strong epidemiologic evidence that fine particulate matter is a risk factor for cardiovascular morbidity and mortality has prompted toxicologic investigations into the underlying mechanisms. The inhalation of fine particles from combustion sources probably generates oxidative stress followed by local injury and inflammation in the lungs that in turn lead to autonomic and systemic inflammatory responses that can induce endothelial dysfunction and/or injury. Recent research findings on the health effects of air pollutants have led to stricter U.S. ambient air quality standards for ozone, oxides of nitrogen, and particulate matter as well as greater emphasis on publicizing pollution alerts to encourage individuals with significant cardiopulmonary impairment to stay indoors during high-pollution episodes.

■ INDOOR EXPOSURES

Secondhand tobacco smoke (Chap. 395), radon gas, wood smoke, and other biologic agents generated indoors must be considered. Several studies have shown that the respirable particulate load in any household is directly proportional to the number of cigarette smokers living in that home. Increases in prevalence of respiratory illnesses, especially asthma, and reduced levels of pulmonary function measured with simple spirometry have been found in the children of smoking parents in a number of studies. Recent meta-analyses for lung cancer and cardiopulmonary diseases, combining data from multiple secondhand tobacco smoke epidemiologic studies, suggest an ~25% increase in relative risk for each condition, even after adjustment for major potential confounders.

Exposure to *radon gas* in homes is a risk factor for lung cancer. The main radon product (radon 222) is a gas that results from the decay series of uranium 238, with the immediate precursor being radium 226. The amount of radium in earth materials determines how much radon gas will be emitted. Outdoors, the concentrations are trivial. Indoors, levels are dependent on the sources, the ventilation rate of the space, and the size of the space into which the gas is emitted. Levels associated with excess lung cancer risk may be present in as many as 10% of the houses in the United States. When smokers reside in the home, the problem is potentially greater, since the molecular size of radon particles allows them to attach readily to smoke particles that are inhaled. Fortunately, technology is available for assessing and reducing the level of exposure.

Other indoor exposures of concern are bioaerosols that contain antigenic material (fungi, cockroaches, dust mites, and pet danders) associated with an increased risk of atopy and asthma. Indoor chemical agents include strong cleaning agents (bleach, ammonia), formaldehyde, perfumes, pesticides, and oxides of nitrogen from gas appliances. Nonspecific responses associated with "tight-building syndrome," perhaps better termed "building-associated illness," in which no particular agent has been implicated, have included a wide variety of complaints, among them respiratory symptoms that are relieved only by avoiding exposure in the building in question. The degree to which "smells" and other sensory stimuli are involved in the triggering of potentially incapacitating psychological or physical responses has yet to be determined, and the long-term consequences of such environmental exposures are unknown.

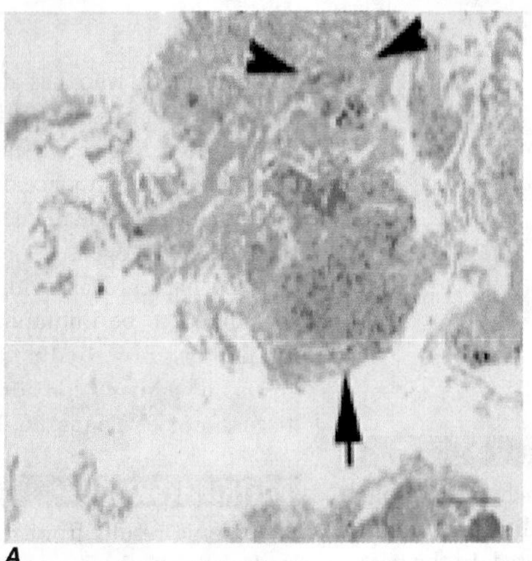

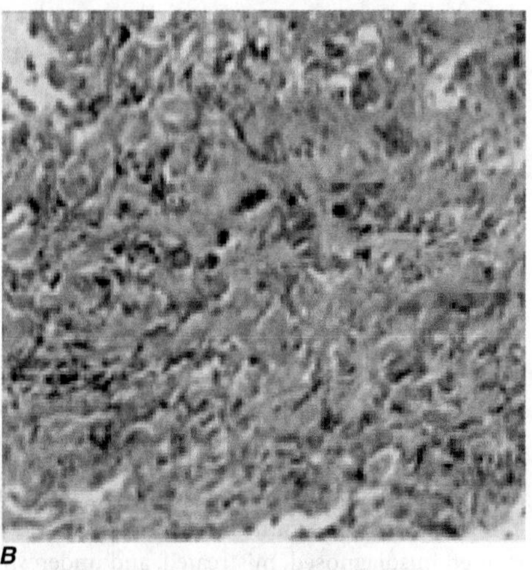

Figure 256-4 Histopathologic features of biomass smoke–induced interstitial lung disease. ***A.*** Anthracitic pigment is seen accumulating along alveolar septae (*arrowheads*) and within a pigmented dust macule (*single arrow*). ***B.*** A high-power photomicrograph contains a mixture of fibroblasts and carbon-laden macrophages.

PORTAL OF ENTRY

The lung is a primary point of entry into the body for a number of toxic agents that affect other organ systems. For example, the lung is a route of entry for benzene (bone marrow), carbon disulfide (cardiovascular and nervous systems), cadmium (kidney), and metallic mercury (kidney, central nervous system). Thus, in any disease state of obscure origin, it is important to consider the possibility of inhaled environmental agents. Such consideration can sometimes furnish the clue needed to identify a specific external cause for a disorder that might otherwise be labeled "idiopathic."

Global considerations

Indoor exposure to *biomass smoke* (wood, dung, crop residues, charcoal) is estimated to be responsible for ~3% of worldwide disability-adjusted life-years (DALYs) lost, due to acute lower respiratory infections in children and COPD and lung cancer in women. This burden of disease places indoor exposure to biomass smoke as the second leading environmental hazard for poor health, just behind unsafe water, sanitation, and hygiene, and is 3.5 times larger than the burden attributed to outdoor air pollution.

More than one-half of the world's population uses biomass fuel for cooking, heating, or baking. This occurs predominantly in the rural areas of developing countries. Because many families burn biomass fuels in open stoves, which are highly inefficient, and inside homes with poor ventilation, women and young children are exposed on a daily basis to high levels of smoke. In these homes, 24-h mean levels of fine particulate matter, a component of biomass smoke, have been reported to be 2–30 times higher than the National Ambient Air Quality Standards set by the U.S. EPA.

Epidemiologic studies have consistently shown associations between exposure to biomass smoke and both chronic bronchitis and COPD, with odds ratios ranging between 3 and 10 and increasing with longer exposures. In addition to the common occupational exposure to biomass smoke of women in developing countries, men from such countries may be occupationally exposed. Because of increased migration to the United States from developing countries, clinicians need to be aware of the chronic respiratory effects of exposure to biomass smoke, which can include interstitial lung disease (Fig. 256-4). Evidence is beginning to emerge that improved stoves with chimneys can reduce biomass smoke–induced respiratory illness in both children and women.

FURTHER READINGS

Aldrich TK et al: Lung function in rescue workers at the World Trade Center after 7 years. N Engl J Med 362:1263, 2010

Balmes JR: When smoke gets in your lungs. Proc Am Thorac Soc 7:98, 2010

Chen TM et al: Outdoor air pollution: Overview and historical perspective. Am J Med Sci 333:230, 2007

Cummings KJ et al: A reconsideration of acute beryllium disease. Environ Health Perspect 117:1250, 2009

Currie GP et al: An overview of how asbestos exposure affects the lung. BMJ 339:b3209, 2009

Jerrett M et al: Long-term ozone exposure and mortality. N Engl J Med 360:1085, 2009

Rees D, Murray J: Silica, silicosis and tuberculosis. Int J Tuberc Lung Dis 11:474, 2007

Romieu I et al: Improved biomass stove intervention in rural Mexico: Impact on the respiratory health of women. Am J Respir Crit Care Med 180:649, 2009

Samuel G, Maier LA: Immunology of chronic beryllium disease. Curr Opin Allergy Clin Immunol 8:126, 2008

Suganuma N et al: Reliability of the proposed international classification of high-resolution computed tomography for occupational and environmental respiratory diseases. J Occup Health 51:210, 2009

Torén K, Blanc PD: Asthma caused by occupational exposures is common—a systematic analysis of estimates of the population-attributable fraction. BMC Pulm Med 9:7, 2009

CHAPTER 257

Pneumonia

Lionel A. Mandell
Richard Wunderink

DEFINITION

Pneumonia is an infection of the pulmonary parenchyma. Despite being the cause of significant morbidity and mortality, pneumonia is often misdiagnosed, mistreated, and underestimated. In the past, pneumonia was typically classified as community-acquired (CAP), hospital-acquired (HAP), or ventilator-associated (VAP). Over the past two decades, however, some persons presenting as outpatients with onset of pneumonia have been found to be infected with the multidrug-resistant (MDR) pathogens previously associated with HAP. Factors responsible for this phenomenon include the development and widespread use of potent oral antibiotics, earlier transfer of patients out of acute-care hospitals to their homes or various lower-acuity facilities, increased use of outpatient IV antibiotic therapy, general aging of the population, and more extensive immunomodulatory therapies. The potential involvement of these MDR pathogens has led to a new category of pneumonia—termed *health care–associated pneumonia* (HCAP)—distinct from CAP. Conditions associated with HCAP and the likely pathogens are listed in Table 257-1.

Although the new classification system has been helpful in designing empirical antibiotic strategies, it is not without disadvantages. Not all MDR pathogens are associated with all risk factors (Table 257-1). Moreover, HCAP is a distillation of multiple risk factors, and each patient must be considered individually. For example, the risk of infection with MDR pathogens for a nursing home resident who has dementia but can independently dress, ambulate, and eat is quite different from the risk for a patient who is in a chronic vegetative state with a tracheostomy and a percutaneous feeding tube in place. In addition, risk factors for MDR infection do not preclude the development of pneumonia caused by the usual CAP pathogens.

This chapter deals with pneumonia in patients who are not considered to be immunocompromised. Pneumonia in severely immunocompromised patients, some of whom overlap with the groups of patients considered in this chapter, warrants separate discussion (see Chaps. 86, 132, and 189).

TABLE 257-1 Clinical Conditions Associated With and Likely Pathogens in Health Care–Associated Pneumonia

	Pathogen			
Condition	MRSA	*Pseudomonas aeruginosa*	*Acinetobacter* spp.	MDR Enterobacteriaceae
Hospitalization for ≥48 h	X	X	X	X
Hospitalization for ≥2 days in prior 3 months	X	X	X	X
Nursing home or extended-care-facility residence	X	X	X	X
Antibiotic therapy in preceding 3 months		X		X
Chronic dialysis	X			
Home infusion therapy	X			
Home wound care	X			
Family member with MDR infection	X			X

Abbreviations: MDR, multidrug-resistant; MRSA, methicillin-resistant *Staphylococcus aureus*.

PATHOPHYSIOLOGY

Pneumonia results from the proliferation of microbial pathogens at the alveolar level and the host's response to those pathogens. Microorganisms gain access to the lower respiratory tract in several ways. The most common is by aspiration from the oropharynx. Small-volume aspiration occurs frequently during sleep (especially in the elderly) and in patients with decreased levels of consciousness. Many pathogens are inhaled as contaminated droplets. Rarely, pneumonia occurs via hematogenous spread (e.g., from tricuspid endocarditis) or by contiguous extension from an infected pleural or mediastinal space.

Mechanical factors are critically important in host defense. The hairs and turbinates of the nares capture larger inhaled particles before they reach the lower respiratory tract. The branching architecture of the tracheobronchial tree traps particles on the airway lining, where mucociliary clearance and local antibacterial factors either clear or kill the potential pathogen. The gag reflex and the cough mechanism offer critical protection from aspiration. In addition, the normal flora adhering to mucosal cells of the oropharynx, whose components are remarkably constant, prevents pathogenic bacteria from binding and thereby decreases the risk of pneumonia caused by these more virulent bacteria.

When these barriers are overcome or when the microorganisms are small enough to be inhaled to the alveolar level, resident alveolar macrophages are extremely efficient at clearing and killing pathogens. Macrophages are assisted by local proteins (e.g., surfactant proteins A and D) that have intrinsic opsonizing properties or antibacterial or antiviral activity. Once engulfed by the macrophage, the pathogens—even if they are not killed—are eliminated via either the mucociliary elevator or the lymphatics and no longer represent an infectious challenge. Only when the capacity of the alveolar macrophages to ingest or kill the microorganisms is exceeded does clinical pneumonia become manifest. In that situation, the alveolar macrophages initiate the inflammatory response to bolster lower respiratory tract defenses. The host inflammatory response, rather than the proliferation of microorganisms, triggers the clinical syndrome of pneumonia. The release of inflammatory mediators, such as interleukin (IL)-1 and tumor necrosis factor (TNF), results in fever. Chemokines, such as IL-8 and granulocyte colony-stimulating factor, stimulate the release of neutrophils and their attraction to the lung, producing both peripheral leukocytosis and increased purulent secretions. Inflammatory mediators released by macrophages and the newly recruited neutrophils create an alveolar capillary leak equivalent to that seen in the acute respiratory distress syndrome (ARDS), although in pneumonia this leak is localized (at least initially). Even erythrocytes can cross the alveolar-capillary membrane, with consequent hemoptysis. The capillary leak results in a radiographic infiltrate and rales detectable on auscultation, and hypoxemia results from alveolar filling. Moreover, some bacterial pathogens appear to interfere with the hypoxemic vasoconstriction that would normally occur with fluid-filled alveoli, and this interference can result in severe hypoxemia. Increased respiratory drive in the systemic inflammatory response syndrome (SIRS; Chap. 271) leads to respiratory alkalosis. Decreased compliance due to capillary leak, hypoxemia, increased respiratory drive, increased secretions, and occasionally infection-related bronchospasm all lead to dyspnea. If severe enough, the changes in lung mechanics secondary to reductions in lung volume and compliance and the intrapulmonary shunting of blood may cause the patient's death.

PATHOLOGY

Classic pneumonia evolves through a series of pathologic changes. The initial phase is one of *edema,* with the presence of a proteinaceous exudate—and often of bacteria—in the alveoli. This phase is rarely evident in clinical or autopsy specimens because it is so rapidly followed by a *red hepatization* phase. The presence of erythrocytes in the cellular intraalveolar exudate gives this second stage its name, but neutrophil influx is more important from the standpoint of host defense. Bacteria are occasionally seen in pathologic specimens collected during this phase. In the third phase, *gray hepatization,* no new erythrocytes are extravasating, and those already present have been lysed and degraded. The neutrophil is the predominant cell, fibrin deposition is abundant, and bacteria have disappeared. This phase corresponds with successful containment of the infection and improvement in gas exchange. In the final phase, *resolution,* the macrophage reappears as the dominant cell type in the alveolar space, and the debris of neutrophils, bacteria, and fibrin has been cleared, as has the inflammatory response.

This pattern has been described best for lobar pneumococcal pneumonia and may not apply to pneumonias of all etiologies, especially viral or *Pneumocystis* pneumonia. In VAP, respiratory bronchiolitis may precede the development of a radiologically apparent infiltrate. Because of the microaspiration mechanism, a bronchopneumonia pattern is most common in nosocomial pneumonias, whereas a lobar pattern is more common in bacterial CAP. Despite the radiographic appearance, viral and *Pneumocystis* pneumonias represent alveolar rather than interstitial processes.

COMMUNITY-ACQUIRED PNEUMONIA

■ ETIOLOGY

The extensive list of potential etiologic agents in CAP includes bacteria, fungi, viruses, and protozoa. Newly identified pathogens include hantaviruses, metapneumoviruses, the coronavirus responsible for severe acute respiratory syndrome (SARS), and community-acquired strains of methicillin-resistant *Staphylococcus aureus* (MRSA). Most cases of CAP, however, are caused by relatively few pathogens (Table 257-2). Although *Streptococcus pneumoniae* is most common, other organisms must also be considered in light of the patient's risk factors and severity of illness. In most cases, it is most useful to think of the potential causes as either "typical" bacterial pathogens or "atypical" organisms. The former category includes *S. pneumoniae, Haemophilus influenzae,* and (in selected patients) *S. aureus* and gram-negative bacilli such as *Klebsiella pneumoniae* and *Pseudomonas aeruginosa.* The "atypical" organisms include *Mycoplasma pneumoniae* and *Chlamydia pneumoniae* (in outpatients) and *Legionella* spp. (in inpatients) as well as respiratory viruses such as influenza viruses, adenoviruses, and respiratory syncytial viruses. Data suggest that a virus may be responsible for up to 18% of cases of CAP that require admission to the hospital. The atypical organisms cannot be cultured on standard media, nor can they be seen on Gram's stain. The frequency and importance of atypical pathogens have significant implications for therapy. These organisms are intrinsically resistant to all β-lactam agents and must be treated with a macrolide, a fluoroquinolone, or a tetracycline. In the ~10–15% of CAP cases that are polymicrobial, the etiology often includes a combination of typical and atypical pathogens.

TABLE 257-2 Microbial Causes of Community-Acquired Pneumonia, by Site of Care

	Hospitalized Patients	
Outpatients	Non-ICU	ICU
Streptococcus pneumoniae	*S. pneumoniae*	*S. pneumoniae*
Mycoplasma pneumoniae	*M. pneumoniae*	*Staphylococcus aureus*
Haemophilus influenzae	*Chlamydia pneumoniae*	*Legionella* spp.
C. pneumoniae		Gram-negative bacilli
Respiratory viruses[a]	*H. influenzae*	*H. influenzae*
	Legionella spp.	
	Respiratory viruses[a]	

[a]Influenza A and B viruses, adenoviruses, respiratory syncytial viruses, parainfluenza viruses.

Note: Pathogens are listed in descending order of frequency. ICU, intensive care unit.

Anaerobes play a significant role only when an episode of aspiration has occurred days to weeks before presentation for pneumonia. The combination of an unprotected airway (e.g., in patients with alcohol or drug overdose or a seizure disorder) and significant gingivitis constitutes the major risk factor. Anaerobic pneumonias are often complicated by abscess formation and significant empyemas or parapneumonic effusions.

S. aureus pneumonia is well known to complicate influenza infection. However, MRSA has been reported as the primary etiologic agent of CAP. While this entity is still relatively uncommon, clinicians must be aware of its potentially serious consequences such as necrotizing pneumonia. Two important developments have led to this problem: the spread of MRSA from the hospital setting to the community and the emergence of genetically distinct strains of MRSA in the community. The former circumstance is more likely to result in HCAP, whereas the novel community-acquired MRSA (CA-MRSA) strains have infected healthy individuals who have had no association with health care.

Unfortunately, despite a careful history and physical examination as well as routine radiographic studies, the causative pathogen in a case of CAP is difficult to predict with any degree of certainty; in more than one-half of cases, a specific etiology is never determined. Nevertheless, epidemiologic and risk factors may suggest the involvement of certain pathogens (Table 257-3).

TABLE 257-3 Epidemiologic Factors Suggesting Possible Causes of Community-Acquired Pneumonia

Factor	Possible Pathogen(s)
Alcoholism	*Streptococcus pneumoniae,* oral anaerobes, *Klebsiella pneumoniae, Acinetobacter* spp., *Mycobacterium tuberculosis*
COPD and/or smoking	*Haemophilus influenzae, Pseudomonas aeruginosa, Legionella* spp., *S. pneumoniae, Moraxella catarrhalis, Chlamydia pneumoniae*
Structural lung disease (e.g., bronchiectasis)	*P. aeruginosa, Burkholderia cepacia, Staphylococcus aureus*
Dementia, stroke, decreased level of consciousness	Oral anaerobes, gram-negative enteric bacteria
Lung abscess	CA-MRSA, oral anaerobes, endemic fungi, *M. tuberculosis,* atypical mycobacteria
Travel to Ohio or St. Lawrence river valleys	*Histoplasma capsulatum*
Travel to southwestern United States	Hantavirus, *Coccidioides* spp.
Travel to Southeast Asia	*Burkholderia pseudomallei,* avian influenza virus
Stay in hotel or on cruise ship in previous 2 weeks	*Legionella* spp.
Local influenza activity	Influenza virus, *S. pneumoniae, S. aureus*
Exposure to bats or birds	*H. capsulatum*
Exposure to birds	*Chlamydia psittaci*
Exposure to rabbits	*Francisella tularensis*
Exposure to sheep, goats, parturient cats	*Coxiella burnetii*

Abbreviations: CA-MRSA, community-acquired methicillin-resistant *Staphylococcus aureus;* COPD, chronic obstructive pulmonary disease.

■ EPIDEMIOLOGY

In the United States, ~80% of the 4 million CAP cases that occur annually are treated on an outpatient basis, and ~20% are treated in the hospital. CAP results in more than 600,000 hospitalizations, 64 million days of restricted activity, and 45,000 deaths annually. The overall yearly cost associated with CAP is estimated at $9–10 billion. The incidence rates are highest at the extremes of age. The overall annual rate in the United States is 12 cases per 1000 persons, but the figure increases to 12–18 per 1000 among children <4 years of age and to 20 per 1000 among persons >60 years of age.

The risk factors for CAP in general and for pneumococcal pneumonia in particular have implications for treatment regimens. Risk factors for CAP include alcoholism, asthma, immunosuppression, institutionalization, and an age of ≥70 years versus 60–69 years. Risk factors for pneumococcal pneumonia include dementia, seizure disorders, heart failure, cerebrovascular disease, alcoholism, tobacco smoking, chronic obstructive pulmonary disease (COPD), and HIV infection. CA-MRSA pneumonia is more likely in patients with skin colonization or infection with CA-MRSA. Enterobacteriaceae tend to infect patients who have recently been hospitalized and/or received antibiotic therapy or who have comorbidities such as alcoholism, heart failure, or renal failure. *P. aeruginosa* is a particular problem in patients with severe structural lung disease, such as bronchiectasis, cystic fibrosis, or severe COPD. Risk factors for *Legionella* infection include diabetes, hematologic malignancy, cancer, severe renal disease, HIV infection, smoking, male gender, and a recent hotel stay or ship cruise. (Many of these risk factors would now reclassify as HCAP some cases that were previously designated CAP.)

■ CLINICAL MANIFESTATIONS

CAP can vary from indolent to fulminant in presentation and from mild to fatal in severity. The various signs and symptoms that depend on the progression and severity of the infection include both constitutional findings and manifestations limited to the lung and associated structures. In light of the pathobiology of the disease, many of the findings are to be expected.

The patient is frequently febrile with tachycardia or may have a history of chills and/or sweats. Cough may be either nonproductive or productive of mucoid, purulent, or blood-tinged sputum. Depending on severity, the patient may be able to speak in full sentences or may be very short of breath. If the pleura is involved, the patient may experience pleuritic chest pain. Up to 20% of patients may have gastrointestinal symptoms such as nausea, vomiting, and/or diarrhea. Other symptoms may include fatigue, headache, myalgias, and arthralgias.

Findings on physical examination vary with the degree of pulmonary consolidation and the presence or absence of a significant pleural effusion. An increased respiratory rate and use of accessory muscles of respiration are common. Palpation may reveal increased or decreased tactile fremitus, and the percussion note can vary from dull to flat, reflecting underlying consolidated lung and pleural fluid, respectively. Crackles, bronchial breath sounds, and possibly a pleural friction rub may be heard on auscultation. The clinical presentation may not be so obvious in the elderly, who may initially display new-onset or worsening confusion and few other manifestations. Severely ill patients may have septic shock and evidence of organ failure.

■ DIAGNOSIS

When confronted with possible CAP, the physician must ask two questions: Is this pneumonia, and, if so, what is the likely etiology? The former question is typically answered by clinical and radiographic methods, whereas the latter requires the aid of laboratory techniques.

Clinical diagnosis

The differential diagnosis includes both infectious and noninfectious entities such as acute bronchitis, acute exacerbations of chronic bronchitis, heart failure, pulmonary embolism, and radiation pneumonitis. The importance of a careful history cannot be overemphasized. For example, known cardiac disease may suggest worsening pulmonary edema, while underlying carcinoma may suggest lung injury secondary to irradiation. Epidemiologic clues, such as recent travel to areas with known endemic pathogens (e.g., the U.S. southwest), may alert the physician to specific possibilities (Table 257-3).

Unfortunately, the sensitivity and specificity of the findings on physical examination are less than ideal, averaging 58% and 67%, respectively. Therefore, chest radiography is often necessary to differentiate CAP from other conditions. Radiographic findings may include risk factors for increased severity (e.g., cavitation or multilobar involvement). Occasionally, radiographic results suggest an etiologic diagnosis. For example, pneumatoceles suggest infection with *S. aureus,* and an upper-lobe cavitating lesion suggests tuberculosis. CT is rarely necessary but may be of value in a patient with suspected postobstructive pneumonia caused by a tumor or foreign body. For outpatients, the clinical and radiologic assessments are usually all that is done before treatment for CAP is started since most laboratory results are not available soon enough to influence initial management significantly. In certain cases, the availability of rapid point-of-care outpatient diagnostic tests can be very important (e.g., rapid diagnosis of influenza virus infection can prompt specific anti-influenza drug treatment and secondary prevention).

Etiologic diagnosis

The etiology of pneumonia usually cannot be determined solely on the basis of clinical presentation; instead, the physician must rely upon the laboratory for support. Except for the 2% of CAP patients who are admitted to the intensive care unit (ICU), no data exist to show that treatment directed at a specific pathogen is statistically superior to empirical therapy. The benefit of establishing a microbial etiology can therefore be questioned, particularly in light of the cost of diagnostic testing. However, a number of reasons can be advanced for attempting an etiologic diagnosis. Identification of an unexpected pathogen allows narrowing of the initial empirical regimen that decreases antibiotic selection pressure, lessening the risk of resistance. Pathogens with important public safety implications such as *Mycobacterium tuberculosis* and influenza virus, may be found in some cases. Finally, without culture and susceptibility data, trends in resistance cannot be followed accurately, and appropriate empirical therapeutic regimens are harder to devise.

Gram's stain and culture of sputum The main purpose of the sputum Gram's stain is to ensure that a sample is suitable for culture. However, Gram's staining may also identify certain pathogens (e.g., *S. pneumoniae, S. aureus,* and gram-negative bacteria) by their characteristic appearance. To be adequate for culture, a sputum sample must have >25 neutrophils and <10 squamous epithelial cells per low-power field. The sensitivity and specificity of the sputum Gram's stain and culture are highly variable. Even in cases of proven bacteremic pneumococcal pneumonia, the yield of positive cultures from sputum samples is ≤50%.

Some patients, particularly elderly individuals, may not be able to produce an appropriate expectorated sputum sample. Others may already have started a course of antibiotics that can interfere with culture results at the time a sample is obtained. Inability to produce sputum can be a consequence of dehydration, and the correction of this condition may result in increased sputum production and a more obvious infiltrate on chest radiography. For patients admitted to the ICU and intubated, a deep-suction aspirate or bronchoalveolar lavage sample (obtained either via bronchoscopy or non-bronchoscopically) has a high yield on culture when sent to the microbiology laboratory as soon as possible. Since the etiologies in severe CAP are somewhat different from those in milder disease (Table 257-2), the greatest benefit of staining and culturing respiratory secretions is to alert the physician of unsuspected and/or resistant pathogens and to permit appropriate modification of therapy. Other stains and cultures (e.g., specific stains for *M. tuberculosis* or fungi) may be useful as well.

Blood cultures The yield from blood cultures, even when samples are collected before antibiotic therapy, is disappointingly low. Only ~5–14% of cultures of blood from patients hospitalized with CAP are positive, and the most frequently isolated pathogen is *S. pneumoniae.* Since recommended empirical regimens all provide pneumococcal coverage, a blood culture positive for this pathogen has little, if any, effect on clinical outcome. However, susceptibility data may allow narrowing of antibiotic therapy in appropriate cases. Because of the low yield and the lack of significant impact on outcome, blood cultures are no longer considered *de rigueur* for all hospitalized CAP patients. Certain high-risk patients—including those with neutropenia secondary to pneumonia, asplenia, or complement deficiencies; chronic liver disease; or severe CAP—should have blood cultured.

Antigen tests Two commercially available tests detect pneumococcal and certain *Legionella* antigens in urine. The test for *L. pneumophila* detects only serogroup 1, but this serogroup accounts for most community-acquired cases of Legionnaires' disease. The sensitivity and specificity of the *Legionella* urine antigen test are as high as 90% and 99%, respectively. The pneumococcal urine antigen test is also quite sensitive and specific (80% and >90%, respectively). Although false-positive results can be obtained with samples from pneumococcus-colonized children, the test is generally reliable. Both tests can detect antigen even after the initiation of appropriate antibiotic therapy. Other antigen tests include a rapid test for influenza virus and direct fluorescent antibody tests for influenza virus and respiratory syncytial virus; the latter tests are only poorly sensitive.

Polymerase chain reaction Polymerase chain reaction (PCR) tests, which amplify a microorganism's DNA or RNA, are available for a number of pathogens, including *L. pneumophila* and mycobacteria. In addition, a multiplex PCR can detect the nucleic acid of *Legionella* spp., *M. pneumoniae,* and *C. pneumoniae.* However, the use of these PCR assays is generally limited to research studies. In patients with pneumococcal pneumonia, an increased bacterial load documented by PCR is associated with an increased risk of septic shock, need for mechanical ventilation, and death. Such a test could conceivably help identify patients suitable for ICU admission.

Serology A fourfold rise in specific IgM antibody titer between acute- and convalescent-phase serum samples is generally considered diagnostic of infection with the pathogen in question. In the past, serologic tests were used to help identify atypical pathogens as well as selected unusual organisms such as *Coxiella burnetii.* Recently, however, they have fallen out of favor because of the time required to obtain a final result for the convalescent-phase sample.

TREATMENT Community-Acquired Pneumonia

SITE OF CARE The cost of inpatient management exceeds that of outpatient treatment by a factor of 20, and hospitalization accounts for most CAP-related expenditures. Thus the decision to admit a patient with CAP to the hospital has considerable implications. Certain patients clearly can be managed at home, and others clearly require treatment in the hospital, but the choice is sometimes difficult. Tools that objectively assess the risk of adverse outcomes, including severe illness and death, can minimize unnecessary hospital admissions. There are currently two sets of criteria: the Pneumonia Severity Index (PSI), a prognostic model used to identify patients at low risk of dying; and the CURB-65 criteria, a severity-of-illness score.

To determine the PSI, points are given for 20 variables, including age, coexisting illness, and abnormal physical and laboratory findings. On the basis of the resulting score, patients are assigned to one of five classes with the following mortality rates: class 1, 0.1%; class 2, 0.6%; class 3, 2.8%; class 4, 8.2%; and class 5, 29.2%. Clinical trials demonstrate that routine use of the PSI results in lower admission rates for class 1 and class 2 patients. Patients in classes 4 and 5 should be admitted to the hospital, while those in class 3 should ideally be admitted to an observation unit until a further decision can be made.

The CURB-65 criteria include five variables: confusion (C); urea >7 mmol/L (U); respiratory rate ≥30/min (R); blood pressure, systolic ≤90 mmHg or diastolic ≤60 mmHg (B); and age ≥65 years (65). Patients with a score of 0, among whom the 30-day mortality rate is 1.5%, can be treated outside the hospital. With a score of 2, the 30-day mortality rate is 9.2%, and patients should be admitted to the hospital. Among patients with scores of ≥3, mortality rates are 22% overall; these patients may require admission to an ICU.

It is not clear which assessment tool is superior. The PSI is less practical in a busy emergency room setting because of the need to assess 20 variables. While the CURB-65 criteria are easily remembered, they have not been studied as extensively. Whichever system is used, these objective criteria must always be tempered by careful consideration of factors relevant to individual patients, including the ability to comply reliably with an oral antibiotic regimen and the resources available to the patient outside the hospital. In fact, neither the PSI nor CURB-65 is ideal for determining the need for ICU care. The severity criteria proposed by the Infectious Diseases Society of America (IDSA) and the American Thoracic Society (ATS) in their guidelines for the management of CAP are better suited to this purpose.

ANTIBIOTIC RESISTANCE Antimicrobial resistance is a significant problem that threatens to diminish our therapeutic armamentarium. Misuse of antibiotics results in increased antibiotic selection pressure that can affect resistance locally or even globally by clonal dissemination. For CAP, the main resistance issues currently involve *S. pneumoniae* and CA-MRSA.

S. pneumoniae In general, pneumococcal resistance is acquired (1) by direct DNA incorporation and remodeling resulting from contact with closely related oral commensal bacteria, (2) by the process of natural transformation, or (3) by mutation of certain genes.

The cutoff for penicillin susceptibility in pneumonia has recently been raised from a minimal inhibitory concentration (MIC) of ≤0.6 μg/mL to an MIC of ≤2 μg/mL. Cutoffs for intermediate resistance have been raised to 4 μg/mL (from 0.1–1 μg/mL) and ≥8 μg/mL (from ≥2 μg/mL), respectively. These changes in susceptibility thresholds have resulted in a dramatic decrease in the proportion of pneumococcal isolates considered nonsusceptible. For meningitis, MIC thresholds remain at the former levels. Fortunately, resistance to penicillin appeared to plateau even before the change in MIC thresholds. Pneumococcal resistance to β-lactam drugs is due solely to low-affinity penicillin-binding proteins. Risk factors for penicillin-resistant pneumococcal infection include recent antimicrobial therapy, an age of <2 years or >65 years, attendance at day-care centers, recent hospitalization, and HIV infection.

In contrast to penicillin resistance, resistance to macrolides is increasing through several mechanisms. *Target-site modification* is caused by ribosomal methylation in 23S rRNA encoded by the *ermB* gene, resulting in resistance to macrolides, lincosamides, and streptogramin B–type antibiotics. This MLSB phenotype is associated with high-level resistance, with typical MICs of ≥64 μg/mL. The *efflux mechanism* encoded by the *mef* gene (*M phenotype*) is usually associated with low-level resistance (MICs, 1–32 μg/mL). These two mechanisms account for ~45% and ~65%, respectively, of resistant pneumococcal isolates in the United States. High-level resistance to macrolides is more common in Europe, whereas lower-level resistance seems to predominate in North America. Although clinical failures with macrolides have been reported, many experts think that these drugs still have a role to play in the management of pneumococcal pneumonia in North America.

Pneumococcal resistance to fluoroquinolones (e.g., ciprofloxacin and levofloxacin) has been reported. Changes can occur in one or both target sites (topoisomerases II and IV); changes in these two sites usually result from mutations in the *gyrA* and *parC* genes, respectively. The increasing number of pneumococcal isolates that, although still testing susceptible to fluoroquinolones, already have a mutation in one target site is of concern. Such organisms may be more likely to undergo a second step mutation that will render them fully resistant to fluoroquinolones. In addition, an efflux pump may play a role in pneumococcal resistance to fluoroquinolones.

Isolates resistant to drugs from three or more antimicrobial classes with different mechanisms of action are considered MDR. The propensity for an association of pneumococcal resistance to penicillin with reduced susceptibility to other drugs such as macrolides, tetracyclines, and trimethoprim-sulfamethoxazole, is also of concern. In the United States, 58.9% of penicillin-resistant pneumococcal isolates from blood are also resistant to macrolides.

The most important risk factor for antibiotic-resistant pneumococcal infection is use of a specific antibiotic within the previous 3 months. Therefore, a patient's history of prior antibiotic treatment is a critical factor in avoiding the use of an inappropriate antibiotic.

CA-MRSA CAP due to MRSA may be caused by infection with the classic hospital-acquired strains or with the more recently identified, genotypically and phenotypically distinct community-acquired strains. Most infections with the former strains have been acquired either directly or indirectly by contact with the health care environment and would now be classified as HCAP. In some hospitals, CA-MRSA strains are displacing the classic hospital-acquired strains—a trend suggesting that the newer strains may be more robust.

Methicillin resistance in *S. aureus* is determined by the *mecA* gene, which encodes for resistance to all β-lactam drugs. At least five *staphylococcal chromosomal cassette mec* (*SCCmec*) types have been described. The typical hospital-acquired strain usually has type II or III, whereas CA-MRSA has a type IV SCC*mec* element. CA-MRSA isolates tend to be less resistant than the older hospital-acquired strains and are often susceptible to trimethoprim-sulfamethoxazole, clindamycin, and tetracycline in addition to vancomycin and linezolid. However, CA-MRSA strains may also carry genes for superantigens, such as enterotoxins B and C and Panton-Valentine leukocidin, a membrane-tropic toxin that can create cytolytic pores in polymorphonuclear neutrophils, monocytes, and macrophages.

Gram-Negative Bacilli A detailed discussion of resistance among gram-negative bacilli is beyond the scope of this chapter (see Chap. 149). Fluoroquinolone resistance among isolates of *Escherichia coli* from the community appears to be increasing. *Enterobacter* spp. are typically resistant to cephalosporins; the drugs of choice for use against these bacteria are usually fluoroquinolones or carbapenems. Similarly, when infections due to bacteria producing extended-spectrum β-lactamases are documented or suspected, a fluoroquinolone or a carbapenem should be used; these MDR strains are more likely to be involved in HCAP.

INITIAL ANTIBIOTIC MANAGEMENT Since the physician rarely knows the etiology of CAP at the outset of treatment, initial therapy is usually empirical and is designed to cover the most likely pathogens (Table 257-4). In all cases, antibiotic treatment

TABLE 257-4 Empirical Antibiotic Treatment of Community-Acquired Pneumonia

Outpatients
Previously healthy and no antibiotics in past 3 months
• A macrolide [clarithromycin (500 mg PO bid) or azithromycin (500 mg PO once, then 250 mg qd)] *or*
• Doxycycline (100 mg PO bid)
Comorbidities or antibiotics in past 3 months: select an alternative from a different class
• A respiratory fluoroquinolone [moxifloxacin (400 mg PO qd), gemifloxacin (320 mg PO qd), levofloxacin (750 mg PO qd)] *or*
• A β-lactam [preferred: high-dose amoxicillin (1 g tid) or amoxicillin/clavulanate (2 g bid); alternatives: ceftriaxone (1–2 g IV qd), cefpodoxime (200 mg PO bid), cefuroxime (500 mg PO bid)] *plus* a macrolide[a]
In regions with a high rate of "high-level" pneumococcal macrolide resistance,[b] consider alternatives listed above for patients with comorbidities.
Inpatients, Non-ICU
• A respiratory fluoroquinolone [moxifloxacin (400 mg PO or IV qd), gemifloxacin (320 mg PO qd), levofloxacin (750 mg PO or IV qd)]
• A β-lactam[c] [cefotaxime (1–2 g IV q8h), ceftriaxone (1–2 g IV qd), ampicillin (1–2 g IV q4–6h), ertapenem (1 g IV qd in selected patients)] *plus* a macrolide[d] [oral clarithromycin or azithromycin (as listed above for previously healthy patients) or IV azithromycin (1 g once, then 500 mg qd)]
Inpatients, ICU
• A β-lactam[e] [cefotaxime (1–2 g IV q8h), ceftriaxone (2 g IV qd), ampicillin-sulbactam (2 g IV q8h)] *plus*
• Azithromycin or a fluoroquinolone (as listed above for inpatients, non-ICU)
Special Concerns
If *Pseudomonas* is a consideration
• An antipneumococcal, antipseudomonal β-lactam [piperacillin/tazobactam (4.5 g IV q6h), cefepime (1–2 g IV q12h), imipenem (500 mg IV q6h), meropenem (1 g IV q8h)] *plus* either ciprofloxacin (400 mg IV q12h) or levofloxacin (750 mg IV qd)
• The above β-lactams *plus* an aminoglycoside [amikacin (15 mg/kg qd) or tobramycin (1.7 mg/kg qd) and azithromycin]
• The above β-lactams[f] *plus* an aminoglycoside *plus* an antipneumococcal fluoroquinolone
If CA-MRSA is a consideration
• Add linezolid (600 mg IV q12h) or vancomycin (1 g IV q12h).

[a]Doxycycline (100 mg PO bid) is an alternative to the macrolide.
[b]MICs of >16 μg/mL in 25% of isolates.
[c]A respiratory fluoroquinolone should be used for penicillin-allergic patients.
[d]Doxycycline (100 mg IV q12h) is an alternative to the macrolide.
[e]For penicillin-allergic patients, use a respiratory fluoroquinolone and aztreonam (2 g IV q8h).
[f]For penicillin-allergic patients, substitute aztreonam.
Abbreviations: CA-MRSA, community-acquired methicillin-resistant *Staphylococcus aureus;* ICU, intensive care unit.

should be initiated as expeditiously as possible. The CAP treatment guidelines in the United States (summarized in Table 257-4) represent joint statements from the IDSA and the ATS; the Canadian guidelines come from the Canadian Infectious Disease Society and the Canadian Thoracic Society. In these guidelines, coverage is always provided for the pneumococcus and the atypical pathogens. In contrast, guidelines from some European countries do not always include atypical coverage based on local epidemiologic data. The U.S.–Canadian approach is supported by retrospective data from several studies of administrative databases including thousands of patients. Atypical pathogen coverage provided by the addition of a macrolide to a cephalosporin or by the use of a fluoroquinolone alone has been consistently associated with a significant reduction in mortality rates compared with those for β-lactam coverage alone.

Therapy with a macrolide or a fluoroquinolone within the previous 3 months is associated with an increased likelihood of infection with a resistant strain of *S. pneumoniae.* For this reason, a fluoroquinolone-based regimen should be used for patients recently given a macrolide, and vice versa (Table 257-4).

Once the etiologic agent(s) and susceptibilities are known, therapy may be altered to target the specific pathogen(s). However, this decision is not always straightforward. If blood cultures yield *S. pneumoniae* sensitive to penicillin after 2 days of treatment with a macrolide plus a β-lactam or with a fluoroquinolone alone, should therapy be switched to penicillin alone? The concern here is that a β-lactam alone would not be effective in the potential 15% of cases with atypical co-infection. No standard approach exists. In all cases, the individual patient and the various risk factors must be considered.

Management of bacteremic pneumococcal pneumonia is also controversial. Data from nonrandomized studies suggest that combination therapy (especially with a macrolide and a β-lactam) is associated with a lower mortality rate than monotherapy, particularly in severely ill patients. The exact reason is unknown, but possible explanations include an additive or synergistic antibacterial effect, antimicrobial tolerance, atypical co-infection, or the immunomodulatory effects of the macrolides.

For patients with CAP who are admitted to the ICU, the risk of infection with *P. aeruginosa* or CA-MRSA is increased, and coverage should be considered when a patient has risk factors or a Gram's stain suggestive of these pathogens (Table 257-4). If CA-MRSA infection is suspected, either linezolid or vancomycin should be added to the initial empirical regimen. There is concern about vancomycin's loss of potency against MRSA; in addition, vancomycin does not reach significant concentrations in epithelial lining fluid, whereas concentrations of linezolid at this site exceed the MIC for MRSA during the entire dosing interval.

Although hospitalized patients have traditionally received initial therapy by the IV route, some drugs—particularly the fluoroquinolones—are very well absorbed and can be given orally from the outset to select patients. For patients initially treated IV, a switch to oral treatment is appropriate as long as the patient can ingest and absorb the drugs, is hemodynamically stable, and is showing clinical improvement.

The duration of treatment for CAP has generated considerable interest. Patients were previously treated for 10–14 days, but studies with fluoroquinolones and telithromycin suggest that a 5-day course is sufficient for otherwise uncomplicated CAP. Even a single dose of ceftriaxone has been associated with a significant cure rate. A longer course is required for patients with bacteremia, metastatic infection, or infection with a virulent pathogen such as *P. aeruginosa* or CA-MRSA.

GENERAL CONSIDERATIONS In addition to appropriate antimicrobial therapy, certain general considerations apply in dealing with CAP, HCAP, or HAP/VAP. Adequate hydration, oxygen therapy for hypoxemia, and assisted ventilation when necessary are critical to the success of therapy. Patients with severe CAP who remain hypotensive despite fluid resuscitation may have adrenal insufficiency and may respond to glucocorticoid treatment. Immunomodulatory therapy in the form of drotrecogin alfa (activated) should be considered for CAP patients with persistent septic shock and APACHE II scores of ≥25, particularly if the infection is caused by *S. pneumoniae.* The value of other forms of adjunctive therapy, including glucocorticoids, statins, and angiotensin-converting enzyme inhibitors, remains unproven in the management of CAP.

Failure to Improve Patients who are slow to respond to therapy should be reevaluated at about day 3 (sooner if their condition is worsening rather than simply not improving), and a number of possible scenarios should be considered. A number of noninfectious conditions can mimic pneumonia, including pulmonary edema, pulmonary embolism, lung carcinoma, radiation and hypersensitivity pneumonitis, and connective tissue disease involving the lungs. If the patient has CAP and treatment is aimed at the correct pathogen, the lack of response may be explained in a number of ways. The pathogen may be resistant to the drug selected, or a sequestered focus (e.g., a lung abscess or empyema) may be blocking access of the antibiotic(s) to the pathogen. The patient may be getting either the wrong drug or the correct drug at the wrong dose or frequency of administration. It is also possible that CAP is the correct diagnosis but that an unsuspected pathogen (e.g., CA-MRSA, *M. tuberculosis,* or a fungus) is the cause. Nosocomial superinfections—both pulmonary and extrapulmonary—are possible explanations for failure to improve or worsening. In all cases of delayed response or deteriorating condition, the patient must be carefully reassessed and appropriate studies initiated. These studies may include such diverse procedures as CT and bronchoscopy.

Complications As in other severe infections, common complications of severe CAP include respiratory failure, shock and multiorgan failure, coagulopathy, and exacerbation of comorbid illnesses. Three particularly noteworthy conditions are metastatic infection, lung abscess, and complicated pleural effusion. Metastatic infection (e.g., brain abscess or endocarditis), although unusual, deserves immediate attention by the physician, with a detailed workup and proper treatment. Lung abscess may occur in association with aspiration or with infection caused by a single CAP pathogen such as CA-MRSA, *P. aeruginosa,* or (rarely) *S. pneumoniae.* Aspiration pneumonia is typically a mixed polymicrobial infection involving both aerobes and anaerobes. In either scenario, drainage should be established, and antibiotics that cover the known or suspected pathogens should be administered. A significant pleural effusion should be tapped for both diagnostic and therapeutic purposes. If the fluid has a pH of <7, a glucose level of <2.2 mmol/L, and a lactate dehydrogenase concentration of >1000 U/L or if bacteria are seen or cultured, then the fluid should be drained; a chest tube is usually required.

Follow-Up Fever and leukocytosis usually resolve within 2–4 days in otherwise healthy patients with CAP, but physical findings may persist longer. Chest radiographic abnormalities are slowest to resolve and may require 4–12 weeks to clear, with the speed of clearance depending on the patient's age and underlying lung disease. Patients may be discharged from the hospital once their clinical conditions are stable, with no active medical problems requiring hospital care. The site of residence after discharge (nursing home, home with family, home alone) is an important consideration, particularly for elderly patients. For a patient whose condition is improving and who (if hospitalized) has been discharged, a follow-up radiograph can be done ~4–6 weeks later. If relapse or recurrence is documented, particularly in the same lung segment, the possibility of an underlying neoplasm must be considered.

PROGNOSIS

The prognosis of CAP depends on the patient's age, comorbidities, and site of treatment (inpatient or outpatient). Young patients without comorbidity do well and usually recover fully after ~2 weeks. Older patients and those with comorbid conditions can take several weeks longer to recover fully. The overall mortality rate for the outpatient group is <1%. For patients requiring hospitalization, the overall mortality rate is estimated at 10%, with ~50% of deaths directly attributable to pneumonia.

PREVENTION

The main preventive measure is vaccination. The recommendations of the Advisory Committee on Immunization Practices should be followed for influenza and pneumococcal vaccines. In the event of an influenza outbreak, unprotected patients at risk from complications should be vaccinated immediately and given chemoprophylaxis with either oseltamivir or zanamivir for 2 weeks—i.e., until vaccine-induced antibody levels are sufficiently high. Because of an increased risk of pneumococcal infection, even among patients without obstructive lung disease, smokers should be strongly encouraged to stop smoking.

An available 7-valent pneumococcal conjugate vaccine produces T cell–dependent antigens that result in long-term immunologic memory. Administration of this vaccine to children has led to an overall decrease in the prevalence of antimicrobial-resistant pneumococci and in the incidence of invasive pneumococcal disease among both children and adults. However, vaccination can be followed by the replacement of vaccine serotypes with nonvaccine serotypes (e.g., 19A and 35B).

HEALTH CARE–ASSOCIATED PNEUMONIA

HCAP represents a transition between classic CAP and typical HAP. The definition of HCAP is still in some degree of flux because of a lack of large-scale studies. Several of the studies that are available have been limited to patients with culture-positive pneumonia. In these studies, the incidence of MDR pathogens in HCAP was as high as or higher than in HAP/VAP. MRSA in particular was more common in HCAP than in traditional HAP/VAP. Conversely, prospective studies in nontertiary-care centers have found a low incidence of MDR pathogens in HCAP.

The patients at greatest risk for HCAP are not well defined. Patients from nursing homes are not always at elevated risk for infection with MDR pathogens. Careful evaluation of nursing home residents with pneumonia suggests that their risk of MDR infection is low if they have not recently received antibiotics and are independent in most activities of daily living. Conversely, nursing home patients are at increased risk of infection with influenza virus and other atypical pneumonia pathogens. Undue concern about MDR pathogens occasionally results in a failure to cover atypical pathogens in treating nursing home patients. In addition, patients receiving home infusion therapy or undergoing chronic dialysis are probably at particular risk for MRSA pneumonia but may not be at greater risk for infection with *Pseudomonas* or *Acinetobacter* than are other patients who develop CAP.

In general, the management of HCAP due to MDR pathogens is similar to that of MDR HAP/VAP. This topic will therefore be covered in subsequent sections on HAP and VAP. The prognosis of HCAP is intermediate between that of CAP and VAP and is closer to that of HAP.

VENTILATOR-ASSOCIATED PNEUMONIA

Most research on VAP has focused on illness in the hospital setting. However, the information and principles based on this research can be applied to non-ICU HAP and HCAP as well. The greatest difference between VAP and HCAP/HAP is the return to dependence on expectorated sputum for a microbiologic diagnosis of VAP (as for that of CAP), which is further complicated by frequent colonization by pathogens in patients with HAP or HCAP.

Etiology

Potential etiologic agents of VAP include both MDR and non-MDR bacterial pathogens (Table 257-5). The non-MDR group is nearly identical to the pathogens found in severe CAP (Table 257-2); it is not surprising that such pathogens predominate if VAP develops in the first 5–7 days of the hospital stay. However, if patients have other risk factors for HCAP, MDR pathogens are a consideration, even early in the hospital course. The relative frequency of individual MDR pathogens can vary significantly from hospital to hospital and even between different critical care units within the same institution. Most hospitals have problems with *P. aeruginosa* and MRSA, but other MDR pathogens are often institution-specific. Less commonly, fungal and viral pathogens cause VAP, usually affecting severely immunocompromised patients. Rarely, community-associated viruses cause mini-epidemics, usually when introduced by ill health care workers.

Epidemiology

Pneumonia is a common complication among patients requiring mechanical ventilation. Prevalence estimates vary between 6 and 52 cases per 100 patients, depending on the population studied. On any given day in the ICU, an average of 10% of patients will have pneumonia—VAP in the overwhelming majority of cases. The frequency of diagnosis is not static but changes with the duration of mechanical ventilation, with the highest hazard ratio in the first 5 days and a plateau in additional cases (1% per day) after ~2 weeks. However, the cumulative rate among patients who remain ventilated for as long as 30 days is as high as 70%. These rates often do not reflect the recurrence of VAP in the same patient. Once a ventilated patient is transferred to a chronic-care facility or to home, the incidence of pneumonia drops significantly, especially in the absence of other risk factors for pneumonia. However, in chronic ventilator units, purulent tracheobronchitis becomes a significant issue, often interfering with efforts to wean patients off mechanical ventilation.

Three factors are critical in the pathogenesis of VAP: colonization of the oropharynx with pathogenic microorganisms, aspiration of these organisms from the oropharynx into the lower respiratory tract, and compromise of the normal host defense mechanisms. Most risk factors and their corresponding prevention strategies pertain to one of these three factors (Table 257-6).

TABLE 257-5 Microbiologic Causes of Ventilator-Associated Pneumonia

Non-MDR Pathogens	MDR Pathogens
Streptococcus pneumoniae	*Pseudomonas aeruginosa*
Other *Streptococcus* spp.	MRSA
Haemophilus influenzae	*Acinetobacter* spp.
MSSA	Antibiotic-resistant Enterobacteriaceae
Antibiotic-sensitive Enterobacteriaceae	*Enterobacter* spp.
Escherichia coli	ESBL-positive strains
Klebsiella pneumoniae	*Klebsiella* spp.
Proteus spp.	*Legionella pneumophila*
Enterobacter spp.	*Burkholderia cepacia*
Serratia marcescens	*Aspergillus* spp.

Abbreviations: ESBL, extended-spectrum β-lactamase; MDR, multidrug-resistant; MRSA, methicillin-resistant *Staphylococcus aureus;* MSSA, methicillin-sensitive *S. aureus.*

TABLE 257-6 Pathogenic Mechanisms and Corresponding Prevention Strategies for Ventilator-Associated Pneumonia

Pathogenic Mechanism	Prevention Strategy
Oropharyngeal colonization with pathogenic bacteria	
Elimination of normal flora	Avoidance of prolonged antibiotic courses
Large-volume oropharyngeal aspiration around time of intubation	Short course of prophylactic antibiotics for comatose patients[a]
Gastroesophageal reflux	Postpyloric enteral feeding[b]; avoidance of high gastric residuals, prokinetic agents
Bacterial overgrowth of stomach	Prophylactic agents that raise gastric pH[b]; selective decontamination of digestive tract with nonabsorbable antibiotics[b]
Cross-infection from other colonized patients	Hand washing, especially with alcohol-based hand rub; intensive infection control education[a]; isolation; proper cleaning of reusable equipment
Large-volume aspiration	Endotracheal intubation; avoidance of sedation; decompression of small-bowel obstruction
Microaspiration around endotracheal tube	
Endotracheal intubation	Noninvasive ventilation[a]
Prolonged duration of ventilation	Daily awakening from sedation,[a] weaning protocols[a]
Abnormal swallowing function	Early percutaneous tracheostomy[a]
Secretions pooled above endotracheal tube	Head of bed elevated[a]; continuous aspiration of subglottic secretions with specialized endotracheal tube[a]; avoidance of reintubation; minimization of sedation and patient transport
Altered lower respiratory host defenses	Tight glycemic control[b]; lowering of hemoglobin transfusion threshold; specialized enteral feeding formula

[a]Strategies demonstrated to be effective in at least one randomized controlled trial.
[b]Strategies with negative randomized trials or conflicting results.

The most obvious risk factor is the endotracheal tube, which bypasses the normal mechanical factors preventing aspiration. While the presence of an endotracheal tube may prevent large-volume aspiration, microaspiration is actually exacerbated by secretions pooling above the cuff. The endotracheal tube and the concomitant need for suctioning can damage the tracheal mucosa, thereby facilitating tracheal colonization. In addition, pathogenic bacteria can form a glycocalyx biofilm on the tube's surface that protects them from both antibiotics and host defenses. The bacteria can also be dislodged during suctioning and can reinoculate the trachea, or tiny fragments of glycocalyx can embolize to distal airways, carrying bacteria with them.

In a high percentage of critically ill patients, the normal oropharyngeal flora is replaced by pathogenic microorganisms. The most important risk factors are antibiotic selection pressure, cross-infection from other infected/colonized patients or contaminated equipment, and malnutrition. Of these factors, antibiotic exposure poses the greatest risk by far. Pathogens such as *P. aeruginosa* almost never cause infection in patients without prior exposure to antibiotics. The recent emphasis on hand hygiene has lowered the cross-infection rate.

How the lower respiratory tract defenses become overwhelmed remains poorly understood. Almost all intubated patients experience microaspiration and are at least transiently colonized with pathogenic bacteria. However, only around one-third of colonized patients develop VAP. Colony counts increase to high levels, sometimes days before the development of clinical pneumonia; these increases suggest that the final step in VAP development, independent of aspiration and oropharyngeal colonization, is the overwhelming of host defenses. Severely ill patients with sepsis and trauma appear to enter a state of immunoparalysis several days after admission to the ICU—a time that corresponds to the greatest risk of developing VAP. The mechanism of this immunosuppression is not clear, although several factors have been suggested. Hyperglycemia affects neutrophil function, and trials suggest that keeping the blood sugar close to normal with exogenous insulin may have beneficial effects, including a decreased risk of infection. More frequent transfusions also adversely affect the immune response.

Clinical manifestations

The clinical manifestations are generally the same in VAP as in all other forms of pneumonia: fever, leukocytosis, increase in respiratory secretions, and pulmonary consolidation on physical examination, along with a new or changing radiographic infiltrate. The frequency of abnormal chest radiographs before the onset of pneumonia in intubated patients and the limitations of portable radiographic technique make interpretation of radiographs more difficult than in patients who are not intubated. Other clinical features may include tachypnea, tachycardia, worsening oxygenation, and increased minute ventilation.

Diagnosis

No single set of criteria is reliably diagnostic of pneumonia in a ventilated patient. The inability to identify such patients compromises efforts to prevent and treat VAP and even calls into question estimates of the impact of VAP on mortality rates.

Application of clinical criteria consistently results in overdiagnosis of VAP, largely because of three common findings in at-risk patients: (1) tracheal colonization with pathogenic bacteria in patients with endotracheal tubes, (2) multiple alternative causes of radiographic infiltrates in mechanically ventilated patients, and (3) the high frequency of other sources of fever in critically ill patients. The differential diagnosis of VAP includes a number of entities such as atypical pulmonary edema, pulmonary contusion, alveolar hemorrhage, hypersensitivity pneumonitis, ARDS, and pulmonary embolism. Clinical findings in ventilated patients with fever and/or leukocytosis may have alternative causes, including antibiotic-associated diarrhea, sinusitis, urinary tract infection, pancreatitis, and drug fever. Conditions mimicking pneumonia are often documented in patients in whom VAP has been ruled out by accurate diagnostic techniques. Most of these alternative diagnoses do not require antibiotic treatment; require antibiotics different from those used to treat VAP; or require some additional intervention, such as surgical drainage or catheter removal, for optimal management.

This diagnostic dilemma has led to debate and controversy. The major question is whether a quantitative-culture approach as a means of eliminating false-positive clinical diagnoses is superior to the clinical approach enhanced by principles learned from quantitative-culture studies. The most recent IDSA/ATS guidelines for HCAP suggest that either approach is clinically valid.

Quantitative-culture approach The essence of the quantitative-culture approach is to discriminate between colonization and true infection by determining the bacterial burden. The more distal in the respiratory tree the diagnostic sampling, the more specific the results and therefore the lower the threshold of growth necessary to diagnose pneumonia and exclude colonization. For example, a quantitative endotracheal aspirate yields proximate samples, and the diagnostic threshold is 10^6 cfu/mL. The protected specimen brush method, in contrast, obtains distal samples and has a threshold of 10^3 cfu/mL. Conversely, sensitivity declines as more distal secretions are obtained, especially when they are collected blindly (i.e., by a technique other than bronchoscopy). Additional tests that may increase the diagnostic yield include Gram's stain, differential cell counts, staining for intracellular organisms, and detection of local protein levels elevated in response to infection.

Several studies have compared patient cohorts managed by the various quantitative-culture methods. While these studies documented issues of relative sensitivity and specificity, outcomes were not significantly different for the various groups of patients. The IDSA/ATS guidelines suggest that all these methods are appropriate and that the choice depends on availability and local expertise.

The Achilles heel of the quantitative approach is the effect of antibiotic therapy. With sensitive microorganisms, a single antibiotic dose can reduce colony counts below the diagnostic threshold. Recent changes in antibiotic therapy are the most significant. After 3 days, the operating characteristics of the tests are almost the same as if no antibiotic therapy has been given. Conversely, colony counts above the diagnostic threshold during antibiotic therapy suggest that the current antibiotics are ineffective. Even the normal host response may be sufficient to reduce quantitative-culture counts below the diagnostic threshold if sampling is delayed. In short, expertise in quantitative-culture techniques is critical, with a specimen obtained as soon as pneumonia is suspected and before antibiotic therapy is initiated or changed.

In a study comparing the quantitative with the clinical approach, use of bronchoscopic quantitative cultures resulted in significantly less antibiotic use at 14 days after study entry and lower rates of mortality and severity-adjusted mortality at 28 days. In addition, more alternative sites of infection were found in patients randomized to the quantitative-culture strategy. A critical aspect of this study was that antibiotic treatment was initiated only in patients whose gram-stained respiratory sample was positive or who displayed signs of hemodynamic instability. Fewer than one-half as many patients were treated for pneumonia in the bronchoscopy group, and only one-third as many microorganisms were cultured.

TABLE 257-7 Clinical Pulmonary Infection Score (CPIS)

Criterion	Score
Fever (°C)	
≥38.5 but ≤38.9	1
>39 or <36	2
Leukocytosis	
<4000 or >11,000/μL	1
Bands >50%	1 (additional)
Oxygenation (mmHg)	
Pa_{O_2}/FI_{O_2} <250 and no ARDS	2
Chest radiograph	
Localized infiltrate	2
Patchy or diffuse infiltrate	1
Progression of infiltrate (no ARDS or CHF)	2
Tracheal aspirate	
Moderate or heavy growth	1
Same morphology on Gram's stain	1 (additional)
Maximal score[a]	12

[a]At the time of the original diagnosis, the progression of the infiltrate is not known and tracheal aspirate culture results are often unavailable; thus, the maximal score is initially 8–10.

Abbreviations: ARDS, acute respiratory distress syndrome; CHF, congestive heart failure.

Other studies that did not demonstrate a similar beneficial impact of quantitative culture on outcomes did not tightly link antibiotic treatment to the results of quantitative culture and other tests.

Clinical approach The lack of specificity of a clinical diagnosis of VAP has led to efforts to improve the diagnostic criteria. The Clinical Pulmonary Infection Score (CPIS) was developed by weighting of the various clinical criteria usually used for the diagnosis of VAP (Table 257-7). Use of the CPIS allows the selection of low-risk patients who may need only short-course antibiotic therapy or no treatment at all. Moreover, studies have demonstrated that the absence of bacteria in gram-stained endotracheal aspirates makes pneumonia an unlikely cause of fever or pulmonary infiltrates. These findings, coupled with a heightened awareness of the alternative diagnoses possible in patients with suspected VAP, can prevent inappropriate treatment for this disease. Furthermore, data show that the absence of an MDR pathogen in tracheal aspirate cultures eliminates the need for MDR coverage when empirical antibiotic therapy is narrowed. Since the most likely explanations for the mortality benefit of bronchoscopic quantitative cultures are decreased antibiotic selection pressure (which reduces the risk of subsequent infection with MDR pathogens) and identification of alternative sources of infection, a clinical diagnostic approach that incorporates such principles may result in similar outcomes.

TREATMENT Ventilator-Associated Pneumonia

Many studies have demonstrated higher mortality rates with inappropriate than with appropriate empirical antibiotic therapy. The key to appropriate antibiotic management of VAP is an appreciation of the patterns of resistance of the most likely pathogens in any given patient.

ANTIBIOTIC RESISTANCE If it were not for the risk of infection with MDR pathogens (Table 257-1), VAP could be treated with the same antibiotics used for severe CAP. However, antibiotic selection pressure leads to the frequent involvement of MDR pathogens by selecting either for drug-resistant isolates of common pathogens (MRSA and extended-spectrum β-lactamase–positive Enterobacteriaceae) or for intrinsically resistant pathogens (*P. aeruginosa* and *Acinetobacter* spp.). Frequent use of β-lactam drugs, especially cephalosporins, appears to be the major risk factor for infection with MRSA and extended spectrum β-lactamase–positive strains.

P. aeruginosa has demonstrated the ability to develop resistance to all routinely used antibiotics. Unfortunately, even if initially sensitive, *P. aeruginosa* isolates have also shown a propensity to develop resistance during treatment. Either derepression of resistance genes or selection of resistant clones within the large bacterial inoculum associated with most pneumonias may be the cause. *Acinetobacter* spp., *Stenotrophomonas maltophilia*, and *Burkholderia cepacia* are intrinsically resistant to many of the empirical antibiotic regimens employed (see below). VAP caused by these pathogens emerges during treatment of other infections, and resistance is always evident at initial diagnosis.

EMPIRICAL THERAPY Recommended options for empirical therapy are listed in Table 257-8. Treatment should be started once diagnostic specimens have been obtained. The major factor in the selection of agents is the presence of risk factors for MDR pathogens. Choices among the various options listed depend on local patterns of resistance and the patient's prior antibiotic exposure.

The majority of patients *without* risk factors for MDR infection can be treated with a single agent. The major difference

TABLE 257-8 Empirical Antibiotic Treatment of Health Care–Associated Pneumonia

Patients without Risk Factors for MDR Pathogens

Ceftriaxone (2 g IV q24h) *or*

Moxifloxacin (400 mg IV q24h), ciprofloxacin (400 mg IV q8h), or levofloxacin (750 mg IV q24h) *or*

Ampicillin/sulbactam (3 g IV q6h) *or*

Ertapenem (1 g IV q24h)

Patients with Risk Factors for MDR Pathogens

1. A β-lactam:
   Ceftazidime (2 g IV q8h) or cefepime (2 g IV q8–12h) *or*
   Piperacillin/tazobactam (4.5 g IV q6h), imipenem (500 mg IV q6h or 1 g IV q8h), or meropenem (1 g IV q8h) ***plus***
2. A second agent active against gram-negative bacterial pathogens:
   Gentamicin or tobramycin (7 mg/kg IV q24h) or amikacin (20 mg/kg IV q24h) *or*
   Ciprofloxacin (400 mg IV q8h) or levofloxacin (750 mg IV q24h) ***plus***
3. An agent active against gram-positive bacterial pathogens:
   Linezolid (600 mg IV q12h) *or*
   Vancomycin (15 mg/kg, up to 1 g IV, q12h)

Abbreviation: MDR, multidrug-resistant.

from CAP is the markedly lower incidence of atypical pathogens in VAP; the exception is *Legionella,* which can be a nosocomial pathogen, especially with breakdowns in the treatment of potable water in the hospital.

The standard recommendation for patients *with* risk factors for MDR infection is for three antibiotics: two directed at *P. aeruginosa* and one at MRSA. The choice of a β-lactam agent provides the greatest variability in coverage, yet the use of the broadest-spectrum agent—a carbapenem, even in an antibiotic combination—still represents inappropriate initial therapy in 10–15% of cases.

SPECIFIC TREATMENT Once an etiologic diagnosis is made, broad-spectrum empirical therapy can be modified to address the known pathogen specifically. For patients with MDR risk factors, antibiotic regimens can be reduced to a single agent in more than one-half of cases and to a two-drug combination in more than one-quarter of cases. Only a minority of cases require a complete course with three drugs. A negative tracheal-aspirate culture or growth below the threshold for quantitative cultures, especially if the sample was obtained before any antibiotic change, strongly suggests that antibiotics should be discontinued. Identification of other confirmed or suspected sites of infection may require ongoing antibiotic therapy, but the spectrum of pathogens (and the corresponding antibiotic choices) may be different from those for VAP. If the CPIS decreases over the first 3 days, antibiotics should be stopped after 8 days. An 8-day course of therapy is just as effective as a 2-week course and is associated with less frequent emergence of antibiotic-resistant strains.

The major controversy regarding specific therapy for VAP concerns the need for ongoing combination treatment of *Pseudomonas* infection. No randomized controlled trials have demonstrated a benefit of combination therapy with a β-lactam and an aminoglycoside, nor have subgroup analyses in other trials found a survival benefit with such a regimen. The unacceptably high rates of clinical failure and death for VAP caused by *P. aeruginosa* despite combination therapy (see "Failure to Improve," below) indicate that better regimens are needed—including, perhaps, aerosolized antibiotics.

VAP caused by MRSA is associated with a 40% clinical failure rate when treated with standard-dose vancomycin. One proposed solution is the use of high-dose individualized treatment, although the risk of renal toxicity increases with this strategy. In addition, the MIC of vancomycin has been increasing, and a high percentage of clinical failures occur when the MIC is in the upper range of sensitivity (i.e., 1.5–2 μg/mL). Linezolid appears to be more efficacious than the standard dose of vancomycin and may be the preferred agent in patients with renal insufficiency and in those infected with high-MIC isolates of MRSA.

FAILURE TO IMPROVE Treatment failure is not uncommon in VAP, especially in that caused by MDR pathogens. In addition to the 40% failure rate for MRSA infection treated with vancomycin, VAP due to *Pseudomonas* has a 50% failure rate, no matter what the regimen. The causes of clinical failure vary with the pathogen(s) and the antibiotic(s). Inappropriate therapy can usually be minimized by use of the recommended triple-drug regimen (Table 257-8). However, the emergence of β-lactam resistance during therapy is an important problem, especially in infection with *Pseudomonas* and *Enterobacter* spp. Recurrent VAP caused by the same pathogen is possible because the biofilm on endotracheal tubes allows reintroduction of the microorganism. However, studies of VAP caused by *Pseudomonas* show that approximately one-half of recurrent cases are caused by a new strain. Inadequate local levels of vancomycin are the likely cause of treatment failure in VAP due to MRSA.

Treatment failure is very difficult to diagnose. Pneumonia due to a new superinfection, the presence of extrapulmonary infection, and drug toxicity must be considered in the differential diagnosis of treatment failure. Serial CPIS appears to track the clinical response accurately, while repeat quantitative cultures may clarify the microbiologic response. A persistently elevated or rising CPIS value by day 3 of therapy is likely to indicate failure. The most sensitive component of the CPIS is improvement in oxygenation.

COMPLICATIONS Apart from death, the major complication of VAP is prolongation of mechanical ventilation, with corresponding increases in length of stay in the ICU and in the hospital. In most studies, an additional week of mechanical ventilation because of VAP is common. The additional expense of this complication often warrants costly and aggressive efforts at prevention.

In rare cases, some types of necrotizing pneumonia (e.g., that due to *P. aeruginosa*) result in significant pulmonary hemorrhage. More commonly, necrotizing infections result in the long-term complications of bronchiectasis and parenchymal scarring leading to recurrent pneumonias. The long-term complications of pneumonia are underappreciated. Pneumonia results in a catabolic state in a patient already nutritionally at risk. The muscle loss and general debilitation from an episode of VAP often require prolonged rehabilitation and, in the elderly, commonly result in an inability to return to independent function and the need for nursing home placement.

FOLLOW-UP Clinical improvement, if it occurs, is usually evident within 48–72 h of the initiation of antimicrobial treatment. Because findings on chest radiography often worsen initially during treatment, they are less helpful than clinical criteria as an indicator of clinical response in severe pneumonia. Seriously ill patients with pneumonia often undergo follow-up chest radiography daily, at least until they are being weaned off mechanical ventilation. Once a patient has been extubated and is in stable condition, follow-up radiographs may not be necessary for a few weeks.

Prognosis

VAP is associated with significant mortality. Crude mortality rates of 50–70% have been reported, but the real issue is attributable mortality. Many patients with VAP have underlying diseases that would result in death even if VAP did not occur. Attributable mortality exceeded 25% in one matched cohort study. Patients who develop VAP are at least twice as likely to die as those who do not. Some of the variability in VAP mortality rates is clearly related to the type of patient and ICU studied. VAP in trauma patients is not associated with attributable mortality, possibly because many of the patients were otherwise healthy before being injured. However, the causative pathogen also plays a major role. Generally, MDR pathogens are associated with significantly greater attributable mortality than non-MDR pathogens. Pneumonia caused by some pathogens (e.g., *S. maltophilia*) is simply a marker for a patient whose immune system is so compromised that death is almost inevitable.

Prevention

(Table 257-6) Because of the significance of the endotracheal tube as a risk factor for VAP, the most important preventive intervention is to avoid endotracheal intubation or at least to minimize its duration. Successful use of noninvasive ventilation via a nasal or full-face mask avoids many of the problems associated with endotracheal tubes. Strategies that minimize the duration of ventilation through daily holding of sedation and formal weaning protocols have also been highly effective in preventing VAP.

Unfortunately, a tradeoff in risks is sometimes required. Aggressive attempts to extubate early may result in reintubation(s) and increase aspiration, posing a risk of VAP. Heavy continuous sedation increases the risk, but self-extubation because of too little sedation is also a risk. The tradeoffs also apply to antibiotic therapy. Short-course antibiotic prophylaxis can decrease the risk of VAP in comatose patients requiring intubation, and data suggest that antibiotics decrease VAP rates in general. However, the major benefit appears to be a decrease in the incidence of early-onset VAP, which is usually caused by the less pathogenic non-MDR microorganisms. Conversely, prolonged courses of antibiotics consistently increase the risk of VAP caused by the more lethal MDR pathogens. Despite its virulence and associated mortality, VAP caused by *Pseudomonas* is rare among patients who have not recently received antibiotics.

Minimizing the amount of microaspiration around the endotracheal tube cuff is also a strategy for avoidance of VAP. Simply elevating the head of the bed (at least 30° above horizontal but preferably 45°) decreases VAP rates. Specially modified endotracheal tubes that allow removal of the secretions pooled above the cuff may also prevent VAP. The risk-to-benefit ratio of transporting the patient outside the ICU for diagnostic tests or procedures should be carefully considered, since VAP rates are increased among transported patients.

Emphasis on the avoidance of agents that raise gastric pH and on oropharyngeal decontamination has been diminished by the equivocal and conflicting results of more recent clinical trials. The role in the pathogenesis of VAP that is played by the overgrowth of bacterial components of the bowel flora in the stomach has also been downplayed. MRSA and the nonfermenters *P. aeruginosa* and *Acinetobacter* spp. are not normally part of the bowel flora but reside primarily in the nose and on the skin, respectively. Therefore, an emphasis on controlling overgrowth of the bowel flora may be relevant only in certain populations, such as liver transplant recipients and patients who have undergone other major intraabdominal procedures or who have bowel obstruction.

In outbreaks of VAP due to specific pathogens, the possibility of a breakdown in infection control measures (particularly contamination of reusable equipment) should be investigated. Even high rates of pathogens that are already common in a particular ICU may be a result of cross-infection. Education and reminders of the need for consistent hand washing and other infection control practices can minimize this risk.

HOSPITAL-ACQUIRED PNEUMONIA

While significantly less well studied than VAP, HAP in nonintubated patients—both inside and outside the ICU—is similar to VAP. The main differences are in the higher frequency of non-MDR pathogens and the better underlying host immunity in nonintubated patients. The lower frequency of MDR pathogens allows monotherapy in a larger proportion of cases of HAP than of VAP.

The only pathogens that may be more common in the non-VAP population are anaerobes. The greater risk of macroaspiration by nonintubated patients and the lower oxygen tensions in the lower respiratory tract of these patients increase the likelihood of a role for anaerobes. While more common in patients with HAP, anaerobes are usually only contributors to polymicrobial pneumonias except in patients with large-volume aspiration or in the setting of bowel obstruction/ileus. As in the management of CAP, specific therapy targeting anaerobes probably is not indicated (unless gross aspiration is a concern) since many of the recommended antibiotics are active against anaerobes.

Diagnosis is even more difficult for HAP in the nonintubated patient than for VAP. Lower respiratory tract samples appropriate for culture are considerably more difficult to obtain from nonintubated patients. Many of the underlying diseases that predispose a patient to HAP are also associated with an inability to cough adequately. Since blood cultures are infrequently positive (<15% of cases), the majority of patients with HAP do not have culture data on which antibiotic modifications can be based. Therefore, de-escalation of therapy is less likely in patients with risk factors for MDR pathogens. Despite these difficulties, the better host defenses in non-ICU patients result in lower mortality rates than are documented for VAP. In addition, the risk of antibiotic failure is lower in HAP.

FURTHER READINGS

American Thoracic Society/Infectious Diseases Society of America: Guidelines for the management of adults with hospital-acquired, ventilator-associated, and healthcare-associated pneumonia. Am J Respir Crit Care Med 171:388, 2005

Chastre J, Fagon JY: Ventilator-associated pneumonia. Am J Respir Crit Care Med 165:867, 2002

Fagon JY et al: Invasive and noninvasive strategies for management of suspected ventilator-associated pneumonia. A randomized trial. Ann Intern Med 132:621, 2000

Fine MJ et al: A prediction rule to identify low-risk patients with community-acquired pneumonia. N Engl J Med 336:243, 1997

Lim WS et al: Defining community acquired pneumonia severity on presentation to hospital: An international derivation and validation study. Thorax 58:377, 2003

Mandell LA et al: Infectious Diseases Society of America/American Thoracic Society consensus guidelines on the management of community-acquired pneumonia. Clin Infect Dis 44(Suppl 2): S27, 2007

Singh N et al: Short-course empiric antibiotic therapy for patients with pulmonary infiltrates in the intensive care unit. A proposed solution for indiscriminate antibiotic prescription. Am J Respir Crit Care Med 162:505, 2000

Vanderkooi OG et al: Predicting antimicrobial resistance in invasive pneumococcal infections. Clin Infect Dis 40:1288, 2005

PART 11 Disorders of the Respiratory System

CHAPTER 258 Bronchiectasis and Lung Abscess

Rebecca M. Baron
John G. Bartlett

BRONCHIECTASIS

Bronchiectasis refers to an irreversible airway dilation that involves the lung in either a focal or a diffuse manner and that classically has been categorized as cylindrical or tubular (the most common form), varicose, or cystic.

ETIOLOGY

Bronchiectasis can arise from infectious or noninfectious causes (Table 258-1). Clues to the underlying etiology are often provided by the pattern of lung involvement. *Focal bronchiectasis* refers to bronchiectatic changes in a localized area of the lung and can be a consequence of obstruction of the airway—either extrinsic (e.g., due to compression by adjacent lymphadenopathy or parenchymal tumor mass) or intrinsic (e.g., due to an airway tumor or aspirated foreign body, a scarred/stenotic airway, or bronchial atresia from congenital underdevelopment of the airway). *Diffuse bronchiectasis* is characterized by widespread bronchiectatic changes throughout the lung and often arises from an underlying systemic or infectious disease process.

More pronounced involvement of the upper lung fields is most common in cystic fibrosis (CF) and is also observed in postradiation fibrosis, corresponding to the lung region encompassed by the radiation port. Bronchiectasis with predominant involvement of the lower lung fields usually has its source in chronic recurrent aspiration (e.g., due to esophageal motility disorders like those in scleroderma), end-stage fibrotic lung disease (e.g., traction bronchiectasis from idiopathic pulmonary fibrosis), or recurrent immunodeficiency-associated infections (e.g., hypogammaglobulinemia). Bronchiectasis resulting from infection by nontuberculous mycobacteria [NTM; most commonly the *Mycobacterium avium-intracellulare* complex (MAC)] often preferentially affects the midlung fields. Congenital causes of bronchiectasis with predominant midlung field involvement include the dyskinetic/immotile cilia syndrome. Finally, predominant involvement of the central airways is reported in association with allergic bronchopulmonary aspergillosis (ABPA), in which an immune-mediated reaction to *Aspergillus* damages the bronchial wall. Congenital causes of central airway–predominant bronchiectasis resulting from cartilage deficiency include tracheobronchomegaly (Mounier-Kuhn syndrome) and Williams-Campbell syndrome.

In many cases, the etiology of bronchiectasis is not determined. In case series, as many as 25–50% of patients referred for bronchiectasis have idiopathic disease.

EPIDEMIOLOGY

The epidemiology of bronchiectasis varies greatly with the underlying etiology. For example, patients born with CF often develop significant clinical bronchiectasis in late adolescence or early adulthood, although atypical presentations of CF in adults in their thirties and forties are also possible. In contrast, bronchiectasis resulting from MAC infection

TABLE 258-1 Major Etiologies of Bronchiectasis and Proposed Workup

Pattern of Lung Involvement by Bronchiectasis	Etiology by Categories (with Specific Examples)	Workup
Focal	Obstruction (e.g., aspirated foreign body, tumor mass)	Chest imaging (chest x-ray and/or chest CT); bronchoscopy
Diffuse	Infection (e.g., bacterial, nontuberculous mycobacterial)	Gram's stain/culture; stains/cultures for acid-fast bacilli and fungi. If no pathogen is identified, consider bronchoscopy with bronchoalveolar lavage (BAL)
	Immunodeficiency (e.g., hypogammaglobulinemia, HIV infection, bronchiolitis obliterans after lung transplantation)	Complete blood count with differential; immunoglobulin measurement; HIV testing
	Genetic causes (e.g., cystic fibrosis, Kartagener's syndrome, α_1 antitrypsin deficiency)	Measurement of chloride levels in sweat (for cystic fibrosis), α_1 antitrypsin levels; nasal or respiratory tract brush/biopsy (for dyskinetic/immotile cilia syndrome); genetic testing
	Autoimmune or rheumatologic causes (e.g., rheumatoid arthritis, Sjögren's syndrome, inflammatory bowel disease); immune-mediated disease (e.g., allergic bronchopulmonary aspergillosis)	Clinical examination with careful joint exam, serologic testing (e.g., for rheumatoid factor). Consider workup for allergic bronchopulmonary aspergillosis, especially in patients with refractory asthma[a]
	Recurrent aspiration	Test of swallowing function and general neuromuscular strength
	Miscellaneous (e.g., yellow nail syndrome; traction bronchiectasis from postradiation fibrosis or idiopathic pulmonary fibrosis)	Guided by clinical condition
	Idiopathic	Exclusion of other causes

[a]Skin testing for *Aspergillus* reactivity; measurement of serum precipitins for *Aspergillus*, serum IgE levels, serum eosinophils, etc.

classically affects nonsmoking women older than age 50 years. In general, the incidence of bronchiectasis increases with age. Bronchiectasis is more common among women than among men.

In areas where tuberculosis is prevalent, bronchiectasis more frequently occurs as a sequela of granulomatous infection. Focal bronchiectasis can arise from extrinsic compression of the airway by enlarged granulomatous lymph nodes and/or from development of intrinsic obstruction as a result of erosion of a calcified lymph node through the airway wall (e.g., broncholithiasis). Especially in reactivated tuberculosis, parenchymal destruction from infection can result in areas of more diffuse bronchiectasis. Apart from cases associated with tuberculosis, an increased incidence of non-CF bronchiectasis with an unclear underlying mechanism has been reported as a significant problem in developing nations. It has been suggested that the high incidence of malnutrition in certain areas may predispose to immune dysfunction and development of bronchiectasis.

PATHOGENESIS AND PATHOLOGY

The most widely cited mechanism of infectious bronchiectasis is the "vicious cycle hypothesis," in which susceptibility to infection and poor mucociliary clearance result in microbial colonization of the bronchial tree. Some organisms, such as *Pseudomonas aeruginosa*, exhibit a particular propensity for colonizing damaged airways and evading host defense mechanisms. Impaired mucociliary clearance can result from inherited conditions such as CF or dyskinetic cilia syndrome, and it has been proposed that a single severe infection (e.g., pneumonia caused by *Bordetella pertussis* or *Mycoplasma pneumoniae*) can result in significant airway damage and poor secretion clearance. The presence of the microbes incites continued chronic inflammation, with consequent damage to the airway wall, continued impairment of secretion and microbial clearance, and ongoing propagation of the infectious/inflammatory cycle. Moreover, it has been proposed that mediators released directly from bacteria can interfere with mucociliary clearance.

Classic studies of the pathology of bronchiectasis from the 1950s demonstrated significant small-airway wall inflammation and larger-airway wall destruction as well as dilation, with loss of elastin, smooth muscle, and cartilage. It has been proposed that inflammatory cells in the small airways release proteases and other mediators, such as reactive oxygen species and proinflammatory cytokines, that damage the larger-airway walls. Furthermore, the ongoing inflammatory process in the smaller airways results in airflow obstruction. It is believed that antiproteases, such as α_1 antitrypsin, play an important role in neutralizing the damaging effects of neutrophil elastase and in enhancing bacterial killing. In addition to emphysema, bronchiectasis has been observed in patients with α_1 antitrypsin deficiency.

Proposed mechanisms for noninfectious bronchiectasis include immune-mediated reactions that damage the bronchial wall (e.g., those associated with systemic autoimmune conditions such as Sjögren's syndrome and rheumatoid arthritis). *Traction bronchiectasis* refers to dilated airways arising from parenchymal distortion as a result of lung fibrosis (e.g., postradiation fibrosis or idiopathic pulmonary fibrosis).

CLINICAL MANIFESTATIONS

The most common clinical presentation is a persistent productive cough with ongoing production of thick, tenacious sputum. Physical findings often include crackles and wheezing on lung auscultation, and some patients with bronchiectasis exhibit clubbing of the digits. Mild to moderate airflow obstruction is often detected on pulmonary function tests, overlapping with that seen at presentation with other conditions, such as chronic obstructive pulmonary disease (COPD). Acute exacerbations of bronchiectasis are usually characterized by changes in the nature of sputum production, with increased volume and purulence. However, typical signs and symptoms of lung infection, such as fever and new infiltrates, may not be present.

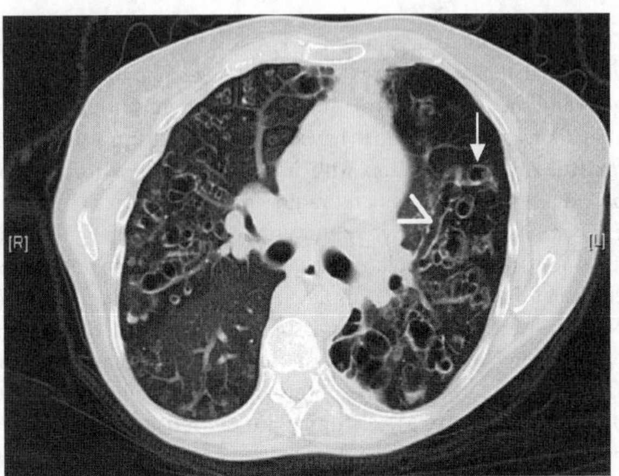

Figure 258-1 Representative chest CT image of severe bronchiectasis. This patient's CT demonstrates many severely dilated airways, seen both longitudinally (arrowhead) and in cross-section (arrow).

DIAGNOSIS

The diagnosis is usually based on presentation with a persistent chronic cough and sputum production accompanied by consistent radiographic features. While chest radiographs lack sensitivity, the presence of "tram tracks" indicating dilated airways is consistent with bronchiectasis. Chest CT is more specific for bronchiectasis and is the imaging modality of choice for confirming the diagnosis. CT findings include airway dilation (detected as parallel "tram tracks" or as the "signet-ring sign"—a cross-sectional area of the airway with a diameter at least 1.5 times that of the adjacent vessel), lack of bronchial tapering (including the presence of tubular structures within 1 cm from the pleural surface), bronchial wall thickening in dilated airways, inspissated secretions (e.g., the "tree-in-bud" pattern), or cysts emanating from the bronchial wall (especially pronounced in cystic bronchiectasis; Fig. 258-1).

APPROACH TO THE PATIENT Bronchiectasis

The evaluation of a patient with bronchiectasis entails elicitation of a clinical history, chest imaging, and a workup to determine the underlying etiology. Evaluation of focal bronchiectasis almost always requires bronchoscopy to exclude airway obstruction by an underlying mass or foreign body. A workup for diffuse bronchiectasis includes analysis for the major etiologies (Table 258-1). Pulmonary function testing is an important component of a functional assessment of the patient.

TREATMENT Bronchiectasis

Treatment of infectious bronchiectasis is directed at the control of active infection and improvements in secretion clearance and bronchial hygiene so as to decrease the microbial load within the airways and minimize the risk of repeated infections.

ANTIBIOTIC TREATMENT Antibiotics targeting the causative or presumptive pathogen (with *Haemophilus influenzae* and *P. aeruginosa* isolated commonly) should be administered in acute exacerbations, usually for a minimum of 7–10 days.

Decisions about treatment of NTM infection can be difficult, given that these organisms can be colonizers as well as pathogens and the prolonged treatment course often is not well tolerated. Consensus guidelines have advised that diagnostic criteria for true clinical infection with NTM should be considered in patients with symptoms and radiographic findings of lung disease who have at least two sputum samples positive on culture; at least one bronchoalveolar lavage (BAL) fluid sample positive on culture; a biopsy sample displaying histopathologic features of NTM infection (e.g., granuloma or a positive stain for acid-fast bacilli) along with one positive sputum culture; or a pleural fluid sample (or a sample from another sterile extrapulmonary site) positive on culture. MAC strains are the most common NTM pathogens, and the recommended regimen for HIV-negative patients includes a macrolide combined with rifampin and ethambutol. Consensus guidelines also recommend macrolide susceptibility testing for clinically significant MAC isolates.

BRONCHIAL HYGIENE The numerous approaches employed to enhance secretion clearance in bronchiectasis include hydration and mucolytic administration, aerosolization of bronchodilators and hyperosmolar agents (e.g., hypertonic saline), and chest physiotherapy (e.g., postural drainage, traditional mechanical chest percussion via hand clapping to the chest, or use of devices such as an oscillatory positive expiratory pressure flutter valve or a high-frequency chest wall oscillation vest). The mucolytic dornase (DNase) is recommended routinely in CF-related bronchiectasis but not in non-CF bronchiectasis, given concerns about lack of efficacy and potential harm in the non-CF population.

ANTI-INFLAMMATORY THERAPY It has been proposed that control of the inflammatory response may be of benefit in bronchiectasis, and relatively small-scale trials have yielded evidence of alleviated dyspnea, decreased need for inhaled β-agonists, and reduced sputum production with inhaled glucocorticoids. However, no significant differences in lung function or bronchiectasis exacerbation rates have been observed. Risks of immunosuppression and adrenal suppression must be carefully considered with use of anti-inflammatory therapy in infectious bronchiectasis. Nevertheless, administration of oral/systemic glucocorticoids may be important in treating bronchiectasis due to certain etiologies, such as ABPA, or noninfectious bronchiectasis due to underlying conditions, especially that in which an autoimmune condition is believed to be active (e.g., rheumatoid arthritis or Sjögren's syndrome). Patients with ABPA may also benefit from a prolonged course of treatment with the oral antifungal agent itraconazole.

REFRACTORY CASES In select cases, surgery can be considered, with resection of a focal area of suppuration. In advanced cases, lung transplantation can be considered.

COMPLICATIONS

In more severe cases of infectious bronchiectasis, recurrent infections and repeated courses of antibiotics can lead to microbial resistance to antibiotics. In certain cases, combinations of antibiotics that have their own independent toxicity profiles may be necessary to treat resistant organisms.

Recurrent infections can result in injury to superficial mucosal vessels, with bleeding and, in severe cases, life-threatening hemoptysis. Management of massive hemoptysis usually requires intubation to stabilize the patient, identifying the source of bleeding, and protecting the nonbleeding lung. Control of bleeding often necessitates bronchial artery embolization and, in severe cases, surgery.

PROGNOSIS

Outcomes of bronchiectasis vary widely with the underlying etiology and may also be influenced by the frequency of exacerbations and (in infectious cases) the specific pathogens involved. In one study, the decline of lung function in patients with non-CF bronchiectasis was similar to that in patients with COPD, with the forced expiratory volume in 1 s (FEV_1) declining by 50–55 mL per year as opposed to 20–30 mL per year for healthy controls.

PREVENTION

Reversal of an underlying immunodeficient state (e.g., by administration of gamma globulin for immunoglobulin-deficient patients) and vaccination of patients with chronic respiratory conditions (e.g., influenza and pneumococcal vaccines) can decrease the risk of recurrent infections. Patients who smoke should be counseled about smoking cessation.

After resolution of an acute infection in patients with recurrences (e.g., ≥3 episodes per year), the use of suppressive antibiotics to minimize the microbial load and reduce the frequency of exacerbations has been proposed, although there is less consensus with regard to this approach in non-CF-associated bronchiectasis than there is in patients with CF-related bronchiectasis. Possible suppressive treatments include (1) administration of an oral antibiotic (e.g., ciprofloxacin) daily for 1–2 weeks per month; (2) use of a rotating schedule of oral antibiotics (to minimize the risk of development of drug resistance); (3) administration of a macrolide antibiotic daily or three times per week (with mechanisms of possible benefit related to non-antimicrobial properties, such as anti-inflammatory effects and reduction of gram-negative bacillary biofilms); (4) inhalation of aerosolized antibiotics [e.g., tobramycin inhalation solution (TOBI)] by select patients on a rotating schedule (e.g., 30 days on, 30 days off) with the goal of decreasing the microbial load without encountering the side effects of systemic drug administration; and (5) intermittent administration of IV antibiotics (e.g., "clean-outs") for patients with more severe bronchiectasis and/or resistant pathogens.

In addition, ongoing, consistent attention to bronchial hygiene can promote secretion clearance and decrease the microbial load in the airways.

LUNG ABSCESS

The term *lung abscess* refers to a microbial infection of the lung that results in necrosis of the pulmonary parenchyma. *Necrotizing pneumonia* or *lung gangrene* refers to multiple small pulmonary abscesses in contiguous areas of the lung, usually resulting from a more virulent infection.

CLASSIFICATION

Lung abscesses are classified by clinical and pathologic features including the tempo of progression, the presence or absence of an associated underlying lesion, and the microbial pathogen responsible. Duration defines the infection as *acute* versus *chronic*, with the dividing line usually at 4–6 weeks. Abscesses occurring in the presence of underlying pulmonary lesions, including tumors or systemic conditions (e.g., HIV infection), are referred to as *secondary*; those that occur in the absence of underlying pulmonary lesions are considered *primary*. The term *nonspecific lung abscess* refers to cases in which no likely pathogen is recovered from expectorated sputum; most such cases are presumed to be due to anaerobic bacteria. *Putrid lung abscess* is a term applied to anaerobic bacterial lung abscesses, which are characterized by distinctive foul-smelling breath, sputum, or empyema fluid.

ETIOLOGY

The likely etiologic agent, appropriate diagnostic testing, and appropriate treatment are frequently indicated by the characteristics of the

TABLE 258-2 Microbial Pathogens Causing Cavitary Lung Infection

Aspiration-Prone Host
Anaerobic bacteria plus microaerophilic and/or anaerobic streptococci, *Gemella* spp.
Embolic (endovascular) lesions: usually *Staphylococcus aureus, Pseudomonas aeruginosa, Fusobacterium necrophorum*[a]
Endemic fungi: *Histoplasma, Blastomyces, Coccidioides* spp.
Mycobacteria: *M. tuberculosis, M. kansasii, M. avium*
Immunocompromised Host
M. tuberculosis, Nocardia asteroides, Rhodococcus equi, Legionella spp., *P. aeruginosa*, Enterobacteriaceae (especially *Klebsiella pneumoniae*), *Aspergillus* spp., *Cryptococcus* spp.
Previously Healthy Host
Bacteria: *S. aureus*,[b] *S. milleri, K. pneumoniae*, group A *Streptococcus*; *Gemella, Legionella*, and *Actinomyces* spp.
Parasites: *Entamoeba histolytica, Paragonimus westermani, Strongyloides stercoralis*

[a]Lemierre's disease.
[b]Often in a young patient with influenza.

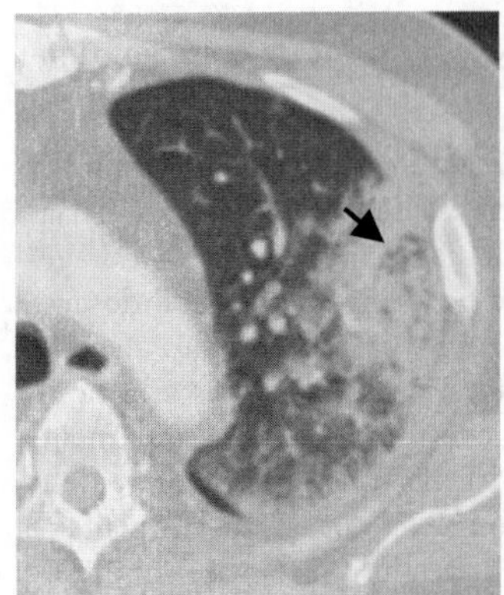

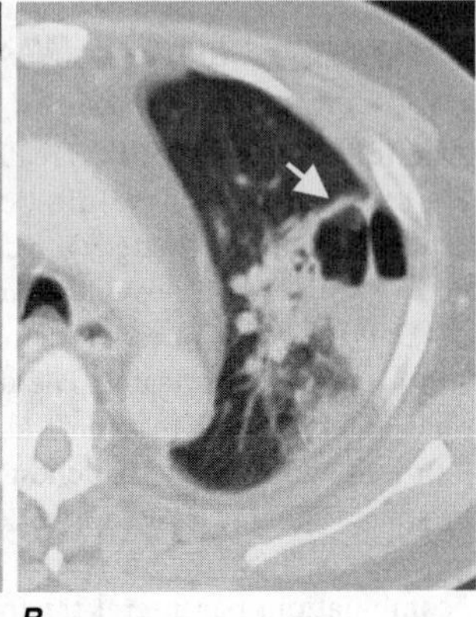

Figure 258-2 Representative chest CT demonstrating development of lung abscesses. This patient was immunocompromised due to underlying lymphoma and developed severe *Pseudomonas aeruginosa* pneumonia, as represented by a left lung infiltrate with concern for central regions of necrosis (**panel A,** black arrow). Two weeks later, areas of cavitation with air fluid levels were visible in this region and were consistent with the development of lung abscesses (**panel B,** white arrow). *(Images provided by Dr. Ritu Gill, Division of Chest Radiology, Brigham and Women's Hospital, Boston.)*

host and the disease process. A variety of microbial pathogens cause lung abscess (Table 258-2). Most nonspecific lung abscesses are presumed to be due to anaerobic bacteria. Mycobacteria, especially *M. tuberculosis*, are a very important cause of pulmonary infections and abscess formation. Fungi and some parasites also cause lung abscess. An acute lung abscess developing in a young, previously healthy patient, especially in conjunction with influenza, is likely to involve *Staphylococcus aureus*; this pathogen generally is seen easily on sputum Gram's stain and culture, and presumptive treatment for methicillin-resistant *S. aureus* is urgent. In an immunocompromised host, suspected pathogens include enteric gram-negative bacilli—especially *Klebsiella pneumoniae* but also agents that are found almost exclusively in patients with defective cell-mediated immunity, such as *Nocardia asteroides* and *Rhodococcus equi.* Lung abscess acquired in other countries may involve *Burkholderia pseudomallei* or *Paragonimus westermani.*

Multiple pulmonary lesions that are not caused by microbes may resemble lung abscess. These include the lesions of pulmonary infarction, bronchiectasis, necrotizing carcinoma, pulmonary sequestration, vasculitides [e.g., periarteritis nodosa, granulomatosis with polyangiitis (Wegener's), Goodpasture syndrome], and cysts or bullae with fluid collections. In some cases, multiple lung abscesses result from septic emboli, most commonly in association with tricuspid valve endocarditis.

CLINICAL FEATURES

The classic presentation of nonspecific lung abscess is an indolent infection that evolves over several days or weeks, usually in a host who has a predisposition to aspiration. A common feature is periodontal infection with pyorrhea or gingivitis. Anaerobes and aerobic or microaerophilic streptococci that colonize the upper airways are implicated in these lesions. The usual symptoms are fatigue, cough, sputum production, and fever. Chills are uncommon. Many patients have evidence of chronic disease, such as weight loss and anemia. Some patients have putrid-smelling sputum indicative of the presence of anaerobes; the foul odor is presumably due to the organisms' production of short-chain fatty acids, such as butyric or succinic acid. Some patients have pleurisy due to pleural involvement by contiguous spread or by a bronchopleural fistula. The pleurisy may be severe and may be the symptom that prompts medical evaluation. Sequential x-rays or CT scans show the evolution of this lesion from pneumonitis to cavitation, a process that generally requires 7–14 days in experimental animals (Fig. 258-2).

DIAGNOSIS

Lung abscess can usually be detected with standard imaging, including chest x-ray and CT (Fig. 258-2). The latter is clearly preferred for precise definition of the lesion and its location and possibly for detection of underlying lesions. Lymphadenopathy is not associated with bacterial lung abscess; thus this finding suggests an alternative diagnosis.

Microbiologic studies include stains and cultures of expectorated sputum to detect aerobic bacterial pathogens. However, clinical correlations are very important because sputum cultures (especially those that do not satisfy standard cytologic criteria) are unreliable. In appropriate settings, it is important to consider cultures for fungi and mycobacteria. Anaerobic bacteria, the most common causes of primary lung abscess, are not detected in expectorated sputum cultures, and in any case the specimen is subject to anaerobic contamination as it traverses the upper airways. Alternative specimens that may be useful include pleural fluid obtained by thoracentesis in patients who have empyema and quantitative bronchoalveolar lavage (BAL) specimens if they are processed promptly and appropriately for anaerobic bacteria. Many reports describe the use of transtracheal aspiration to bypass the upper airways and obtain a specimen for meaningful anaerobic culture. This procedure, which was used extensively in the 1970s, has largely been abandoned out of concern about adverse consequences and because of a general decline in the pursuit of an etiologic agent in pulmonary infections. Another invasive method for bypassing contamination by the flora of the upper airways is transthoracic needle aspiration under CT guidance; the popularity of this procedure has increased in recent years. In most cases, the etiology of anaerobic lung abscess is clear: the host is prone to aspiration and has an abscess in a dependent pulmonary segment, with no other likely cause. As stated above, putrid breath, sputum, or empyema fluid indicates anaerobic infection.

TREATMENT Lung Abscess

ANTIBIOTIC SELECTION Treatment depends on the presumed or established etiology. Infections caused by anaerobic bacteria should usually be treated with clindamycin; the initial IV dosage of 600 mg four times daily can be changed to an oral dosage of 300 mg four times daily once the patient becomes afebrile and improves clinically. The duration of therapy is arbitrary, but many experts recommend continuation of oral treatment until imaging shows that chest lesions have cleared or have left a small, stable scar. A shorter course may be effective. An alternative to clindamycin is any β-lactam/β-lactamase inhibitor combination; parenteral treatment may be followed by orally administered amoxicillin/clavulanate. Carbapenems are also effective against anaerobic bacteria as well as streptococci, but the published data with these drugs in the treatment of anaerobic pulmonary infections are sparse. Penicillin was previously regarded as a preferred drug for these infections, but many oral anaerobes produce β-lactamases, and clindamycin proved superior to penicillin G in a randomized clinical trial. Metronidazole is highly active against virtually all anaerobes but not against aerobic microaerophilic streptococci, which play an important role in mixed infections. In therapeutic trials, metronidazole has done poorly unless combined with a β-lactam or another agent active against aerobic and microaerophilic streptococci.

Persistence of fever beyond 5–7 days or progression of the infiltrate suggests failure of therapy and a need to exclude factors such as obstruction, complicating empyema, and involvement of antibiotic-resistant bacteria. Many patients with uncomplicated lung abscesses and all those with atypical presentations or unresponsive abscesses should undergo bronchoscopy and/or CT to detect a possible associated anatomic lesion, such as a tumor, or a foreign body. Quantitative bacteriologic studies using a protected brush catheter or BAL are much less reliable when done after antibiotic therapy. Postural drainage was previously popular for patients with lung abscess, but aggressive attempts to implement this strategy may result in spillage to other pulmonary segments, leading to airway obstruction and clinical deterioration.

Lung abscess due to *S. aureus* is usually treated with vancomycin at a dosage that targets a trough serum level of 15–20 μg/mL. The main alternative is linezolid. Daptomycin should not be used for pulmonary infections. Lung abscesses caused by aerobic gram-negative bacteria need to be treated according to the results of antibiotic sensitivity tests. Most common among the pathogens involved are *K. pneumoniae* (especially the K1 strain in Taiwan) and *P. aeruginosa* in patients with severe chronic lung disease or compromised immune defenses. Pseudomonal lung abscesses usually require prolonged courses of parenteral antibiotics. Carbapenems or β-lactams are frequently combined with aminoglycosides; oral fluoroquinolones are often effective initially, but resistance is common with prolonged use. Aerosolized colistin and aminoglycosides are sometimes used to augment other therapy, but the efficacy of this approach is variable.

Surgery for lung abscesses was developed at the time penicillin became available in the late 1940s. The relative roles of penicillin and resectional surgery were hotly debated at that time, but by the late 1950s penicillin was favored. Initially the standard choice for most lung abscesses, penicillin was subsequently supplanted by the options summarized above. Recent large-scale reviews indicate that, in general, surgery is now reserved for ~10–12% of patients. The major indications for surgery are failure to respond to medical management, suspected neoplasm, and hemorrhage. Failure to respond to antibiotics is usually due to an obstructed bronchus and an extremely large abscess (>6 cm in diameter) or to infection involving relatively resistant bacteria, such as *P. aeruginosa*. The usual procedure is lobectomy. An alternative intervention that is becoming popular is percutaneous drainage under CT guidance. Aspirate samples for assay of possible pathogens should be carefully collected.

RESPONSE TO THERAPY Patients with lung abscess usually show clinical improvement, with decreased fever, within 3–5 days of initiation of antibiotic treatment. Defervescence can be expected within 5–10 days. Patients with fevers persisting for 7–14 days should undergo bronchoscopy or other diagnostic tests to better define anatomic changes and microbiologic findings. Cultures of expectorated sputum are not likely to be helpful at this juncture except for detecting pathogens such as mycobacteria and fungi. The response to therapy apparent on serial chest radiographs is delayed in comparison with the clinical course. In fact, infiltrates usually progress during the first 3 days of treatment in approximately one-half of patients. Pleural involvement is relatively common and may develop in dramatic fashion. The most common causes of failures of medical management include a failure to drain pleural collections, an inappropriate choice of antimicrobial therapy, an obstructed bronchus that prevents drainage, a "giant" abscess, a resistant pathogen, or refractory lesions due to immunocompromise.

FURTHER READINGS

BRONCHIECTASIS

Barbato A et al: Primary ciliary dyskinesia: A consensus statement on diagnostic and treatment approaches in children. Eur Respir J 34:1264, 2009

Cantin L et al: Bronchiectasis. AJR Am J Roentgenol 193:W158, 2009

Griffith DE et al: An official ATS/IDSA statement: Diagnosis, treatment, and prevention of nontuberculous mycobacterial diseases. Am J Respir Crit Care Med 175:367, 2007

Kapur N et al: Inhaled steroids for bronchiectasis. Cochrane Database Syst Rev Jan 21(1):CD000996, 2009

Martinez-Garcia MA et al: Factors associated with lung function decline in adult patients with stable non-cystic fibrosis bronchiectasis. Chest 132:1565, 2007

Parr DG et al: Prevalence and impact of bronchiectasis in alpha1-antitrypsin deficiency. Am J Respir Crit Care Med 176:1215, 2007

Seitz AE et al: Trends and burdens of bronchiectasis-associated hospitalizations in the United States, 1993–2006. Chest 138:944, 2010

Shoemark A et al: Aetiology in adult patients with bronchiectasis. Respir Med 101:1163, 2007

Stevens DA et al: A randomized trial of itraconazole in allergic bronchopulmonary aspergillosis. N Engl J Med 342:756, 2000

Weycker D et al: Prevalence and economic burden of bronchiectasis (obstructive airways disease). Clin Pulm Med 12:205, 2005

LUNG ABSCESS

Allewelt M et al: Ampicillin + sulbactam vs clindamycin +/− cephalosporin for the treatment of aspiration pneumonia and primary lung abscess. Clin Microbiol Infect 10:163, 2004

Bartlett JG: The role of anaerobic bacteria in lung abscess. Clin Infect Dis 40:923, 2005

——: Anaerobic bacterial infections of the lung and pleural space. Clin Infect Dis 16:S248, 1993

Fernández-Sabé N et al: Efficacy and safety of sequential amoxicillin-clavulanate in the treatment of anaerobic lung infections. Eur J Clin Microbiol Infect Dis 22:185, 2003

Francis JS et al: Severe community-onset pneumonia in healthy adults caused by methicillin-resistant *Staphylococcus aureus* carrying Panton-Valentine leukocidin genes. Clin Infect Dis 40:100, 2005

Moreira Jda S et al: Lung abscess: Analysis of 252 consecutive cases diagnosed between 1968 and 2004. J Bras Pneumol 32:136, 2006

Shinzato T, Saito A: The *Streptococcus milleri* group as a cause of pulmonary infections. Clin Infect Dis 21(Suppl 3):S238, 1995

Takayanagi N et al: Etiology and outcome of community-acquired lung abscess. Respiration 80:98, 2010

Vardakas KZ et al: Comparison of community-acquired pneumonia due to methicillin-resistant and methicillin-susceptible *Staphylococcus aureus* producing the Panton-Valentine leukocidin. Int J Tuberc Lung Dis 13:1476, 2009

Wang JL et al: Changing bacteriology of adult community-acquired lung abscess in Taiwan: *Klebsiella pneumoniae* vs. anaerobes. Clin Infect Dis 40:915, 2005

CHAPTER 259
Cystic Fibrosis

Richard C. Boucher

Cystic fibrosis (CF) is a monogenic disorder that presents as a multisystem disease. The first signs and symptoms typically occur in childhood, but about 5% of patients in the United States are diagnosed as adults. Due to improvements in therapy, >46% of patients are now adults (≥18 years old) and 16.4% are past the age of 30. The median survival is >37.4 years for patients with CF; thus, CF is no longer only a pediatric disease, and internists must be prepared to recognize and treat its many complications. CF is characterized by chronic bacterial infection of the airways that leads to bronchiectasis and bronchiolectasis, exocrine pancreatic insufficiency and intestinal dysfunction, abnormal sweat gland function, and urogenital dysfunction.

PATHOGENESIS

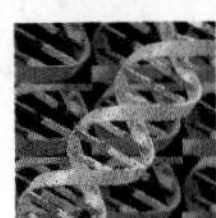

GENETIC CONSIDERATIONS

CF is an autosomal recessive disease resulting from mutations in the *CFTR* gene located on chromosome 7. The mutations in the *CFTR* gene fall into five major classes, as depicted in Fig. 259-1. Classes I–III mutations are considered "severe," as indexed by pancreatic insufficiency and high sweat NaCl values (see below). Class IV and V mutations can be "mild," i.e., associated with pancreatic sufficiency and intermediate/normal sweat NaCl values.

The prevalence of CF varies with the ethnic origin of a population. CF is detected in approximately 1 in 3000 live births in the Caucasian population of North America and northern Europe, 1 in 17,000 live births of African Americans, and 1 in 90,000 live births of the Asian population of Hawaii. The most common mutation in the *CFTR* gene (~70% of CF chromosomes) is a 3-bp deletion (a class II mutation) that results in an absence of phenylalanine at amino acid position 508 (ΔF_{508}) of the CF gene protein product, known as cystic fibrosis transmembrane conductance regulator (CFTR). The large number (>1500) of relatively uncommon (<2% each) mutations identified in the *CFTR* gene makes genetic testing challenging.

CFTR PROTEIN

The CFTR protein is a single polypeptide chain, containing 1480 amino acids, that functions both as a cyclic AMP–regulated Cl^- channel and a regulator of other ion channels. The fully processed form of CFTR localizes to the plasma membrane in normal epithelia. Biochemical studies indicate that the ΔF_{508} mutation leads to improper maturation and intracellular degradation of the mutant CFTR protein. Thus, absence of CFTR in the plasma membrane is central to the molecular pathophysiology of the ΔF_{508} mutation and other classes I–II mutations. Classes III–IV

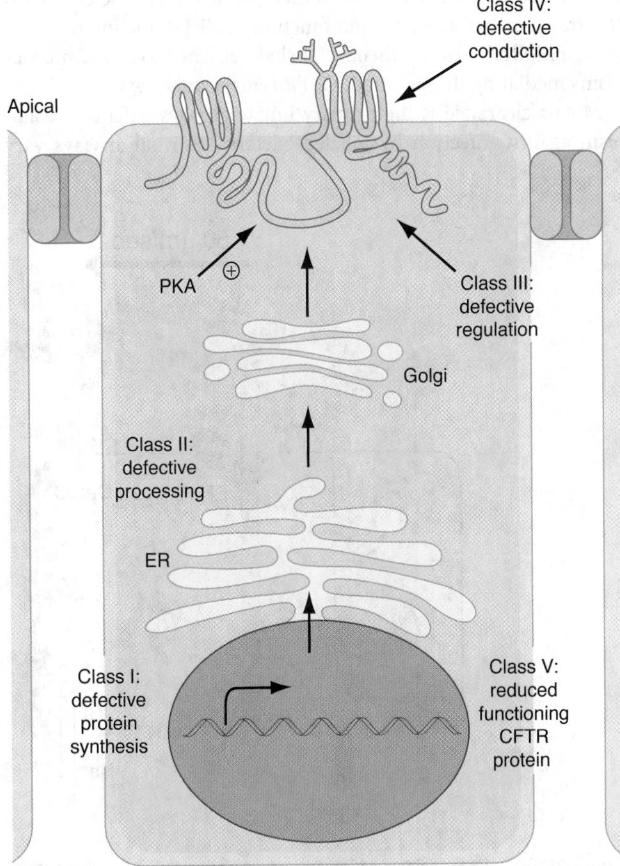

Figure 259-1 Schema describing classes of genetic mutations in CFTR gene and effects on CFTR protein/function. Note the ΔF_{508} mutation is a class II mutation and, like class I mutations, would be predicted to produce no mature CFTR protein in the apical membrane. CFTR, cystic fibrosis transmembrane conductance regulator.

mutations produce CFTR proteins that are fully processed but are nonfunctional or only partially functional in the plasma membrane. Class V mutations include splicing mutations that produce small amounts of functional CFTR.

EPITHELIAL DYSFUNCTION

The epithelia affected by CF exhibit different functions in their native state, i.e., some are volume-absorbing (airways and distal intestinal epithelia), and some are salt- but not volume-absorbing (sweat duct), whereas others are volume-secretory (proximal intestine and pancreas). Given this diversity of native activities, it is not surprising that CF produces organ-specific effects on electrolyte and water transport. However, the unifying concept is that all affected tissues express abnormal ion transport function.

ORGAN-SPECIFIC PATHOPHYSIOLOGY

Lung

The diagnostic biophysical hallmark of CF airway epithelia is the raised transepithelial electric potential difference (PD), which reflects both the rate of active ion transport and epithelial resistance to ion flow. CF airway epithelia exhibit abnormalities in both active Cl^- secretion and Na^+ absorption (Fig. 259-2). The Cl^- secretory defect reflects the absence of cyclic AMP–dependent kinase and protein kinase C–regulated Cl^- transport mediated by CFTR itself. An important observation is that there is also a molecularly distinct Ca^{2+}-activated Cl^- channel (CaCC, TMEM16a) expressed in the apical membrane. This channel can substitute for CFTR with regard to Cl^- secretion and is a potential therapeutic target. The abnormal Na^+ transport reflects a second function of CFTR, its function as a tonic inhibitor of the epithelial Na^+ channel. The molecular mechanisms mediating this action of CFTR remain unknown.

Mucus clearance is the primary innate airways defense mechanism against infection by inhaled bacteria. Normal airways vary the rates of active Na^+ absorption and Cl^- secretion to adjust the volume of liquid (water), i.e., "hydration," on airway surfaces for efficient mucus clearance. The central hypothesis of CF airways pathophysiology is that the faulty regulation of Na^+ absorption and inability to secrete Cl^- via CFTR reduce the volume of liquid on airway surfaces; i.e., they are "dehydrated." Dehydration of both the mucus and the periciliary liquid layers produces adhesion of mucus to the airway surface, which leads to a failure to clear mucus from the airways both by ciliary and cough-dependent mechanisms. The absence of a strict correspondence between gene-mutation class and severity of lung disease suggests important roles for modifier genes and gene-environmental interactions.

The infection that characterizes CF airways involves the mucus layer rather than epithelial or airway wall invasion. The predisposition of CF airways to chronic infection by *Staphylococcus aureus* and *Pseudomonas aeruginosa* is consistent with failure to clear mucus. Recently, it has been demonstrated that the O_2 tension is very low in CF mucus, and adaptations to hypoxemia are important determinants of the physiology of bacteria in the CF lung. Indeed, both mucus stasis and mucus hypoxemia contribute to (1) the propensity for *Pseudomonas* to grow in biofilm colonies within CF airway mucus and (2) the presence of strict anaerobes in CF lungs.

Gastrointestinal tract

The gastrointestinal effects of CF are diverse. In the exocrine pancreas, the absence of the CFTR Cl^- channel in the apical membrane of pancreatic ductal epithelia limits the function of an apical membrane Cl^--HCO_3^- exchanger to secrete bicarbonate and Na^+ (by a passive process) into the duct. The failure to secrete Na^+ HCO_3^- and water leads to retention of enzymes in the pancreas and destruction of virtually all pancreatic tissue. Because of the lack of Cl^- and water secretion, the CF intestinal epithelium fails to flush secreted mucins and other macromolecules from intestinal crypts. The diminished

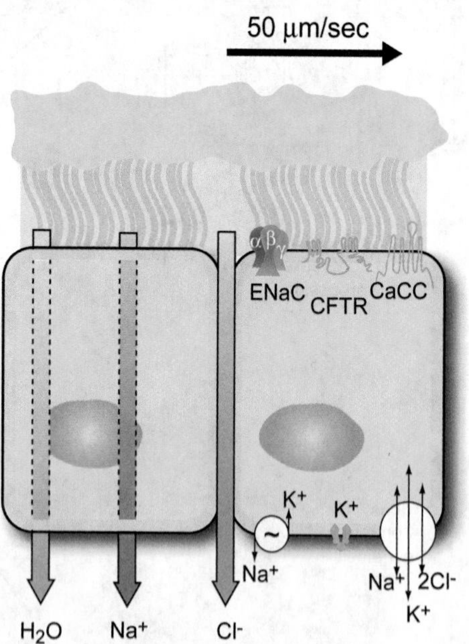

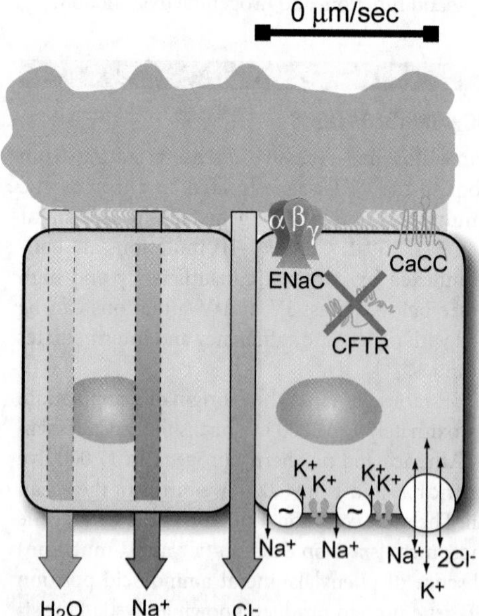

Figure 259-2 Comparison of ion transport properties of normal (top) and CF (bottom) airway epithelia. The vectors describe routes and magnitudes of Na^+ and Cl^- transport that is accompanied by osmotically driven water flow. The normal basal pattern for ion transport is absorption of Na^+ from the lumen via an amiloride-sensitive epithelial Na^+ channel (ENaC) composed of α, β, and γ ENaC subunits. This process is accelerated in CF. The capacity to initiate cyclic AMP–mediated Cl^- secretion is diminished in CF airway epithelia due to abnormal maturation/dysfunction of the CFTR Cl^- channel. The accelerated Na^+ absorption in CF reflects the absence of CFTR inhibitory effects on Na^+ channels. A Ca^{2+}-activated Cl^- channel, likely a product of the TMEM16a gene, is expressed in normal and CF apical membranes and can be activated by extracellular ATP. Horizontal arrows depict velocity of mucociliary clearance (µm/sec).

CFTR-mediated liquid secretion may be exacerbated by excessive absorption of liquid, reflecting abnormalities of CFTR-mediated regulation of Na^+ absorption (both mediated by Na^+ channels and possibly other Na^+ transporters, e.g., Na^+-H^+ exchangers). Both dysfunctions lead to dehydrated intraluminal contents and intestinal obstruction. In the hepatobiliary system, defective hepatic ductal salt (Cl^-) and water secretion causes thickened biliary secretions, focal biliary cirrhosis, and bile-duct proliferation in approximately 25–30% of patients with CF. The inability of the CF gallbladder epithelium to secrete salt and water can lead to both chronic cholecystitis and cholelithiasis.

Sweat gland

CF patients secrete nearly normal volumes of sweat in the sweat acinus, but are not able to absorb NaCl from the sweat duct due to the inability to absorb Cl^- via CFTR across ductal epithelial cells. This sweat gland dysfunction is typically measured by measuring Cl^- concentrations in sweat collected after iontophoresis of cholinergic agonists.

CLINICAL FEATURES

Most patients with CF present with signs and symptoms of the disease in childhood. Approximately 20% of patients present within the first 24 h of life with gastrointestinal obstruction, termed *meconium ileus*. Other common presentations within the first year or two of life include respiratory tract symptoms, most prominently cough and/or recurrent pulmonary infiltrates, and failure to thrive. A significant proportion of patients (~5%), however, are diagnosed after age 18.

RESPIRATORY TRACT

Upper respiratory tract disease is almost universal in patients with CF. Chronic sinusitis is common in childhood, and the incidence of nasal polyps, which often requires treatment with topical steroids and/or surgery, approaches 25%.

In the lower respiratory tract, the first symptom of CF is cough. With time, the cough becomes persistent and produces viscous, purulent, often greenish-colored sputum. There are protracted periods of clinical stability interrupted by "pulmonary exacerbations," often triggered by viral infections, and defined by increased cough, weight loss, low-grade fever, increased sputum volume, and decrements in pulmonary function. Over the course of years, the exacerbation frequency increases and the recovery of lost lung function becomes incomplete, leading to respiratory failure.

CF patients exhibit a characteristic sputum microbiology. *Haemophilus influenzae* and *S. aureus* are often the first organisms recovered from lung secretions in newly diagnosed CF patients. *P. aeruginosa*, often mucoid and antibiotic-resistant, is typically cultured from lower respiratory tract secretions thereafter. *Burkholderia cepacia* is also recovered from CF sputum and is pathogenic. Patient-to-patient spread of certain strains of these organisms mandates strict infection control in the hospital. Other gram-negative rods recovered from CF sputum include *Alcaligenes xylosoxidans*, *B. gladioli*; and, occasionally, *Proteus*, *Escherichia coli*, and *Klebsiella*. Up to 50% of CF patients have *Aspergillus fumigatus* in their sputum, and up to 10% of these patients exhibit the syndrome of allergic bronchopulmonary aspergillosis. *Mycobacterium tuberculosis* is rare in patients with CF. However, 10–20% of adult patients with CF have sputum cultures positive for nontuberculous mycobacteria, and in some patients, these microorganisms are associated with disease.

The first lung-function abnormalities in CF children, increased ratios of residual volume to total lung capacity, suggest that small-airways disease is the first functional lung abnormality in CF. As disease progresses, both reversible and irreversible changes in forced vital capacity (FVC) and forced expiratory volume in 1 s (FEV_1) develop. The reversible component reflects the accumulation of intraluminal secretions and/or airway reactivity, which occurs in 40–60% of patients with CF. The irreversible component reflects chronic destruction of the airway wall and bronchiolitis.

The earliest chest x-ray change in CF lungs is hyperinflation, reflecting small-airways obstruction. Later, signs of luminal mucus impaction, bronchial cuffing, and finally bronchiectasis, e.g., ring shadows, are noted. For reasons that remain speculative, the right upper lobe displays the earliest and most severe changes.

CF pulmonary disease is associated with many intermittent complications. Pneumothorax is common (>10% of patients). The production of small amounts of blood in sputum is common in CF patients with advanced pulmonary disease. Massive hemoptysis is life-threatening. With advanced lung disease, clubbing of digits appears in virtually all patients with CF. As late events, respiratory failure and cor pulmonale are prominent features of CF.

GASTROINTESTINAL TRACT

Meconium ileus in infants presents with abdominal distention, failure to pass stool, and emesis. The abdominal flat plate can be diagnostic, with small intestinal air-fluid levels, a granular appearance representing meconium, and a small colon. In children and young adults, a syndrome termed *distal intestinal obstruction syndrome* (DIOS) occurs, which presents with right lower quadrant pain, loss of appetite, occasionally emesis, and often a palpable mass. DIOS can be confused with appendicitis, whose frequency is not increased in CF patients.

Exocrine pancreatic insufficiency occurs in >90% of patients with CF. Insufficient pancreatic enzyme secretion yields protein and fat malabsorption, with frequent, bulky, foul-smelling stools. Signs and symptoms of malabsorption of fat-soluble vitamins, including vitamins E and K, are also noted. Pancreatic beta cells are spared early, but function decreases with age. This effect, plus inflammation-induced insulin resistance, causes hyperglycemia and a requirement for insulin in >29% of older patients with CF (>35 years).

GENITOURINARY SYSTEM

Late onset of puberty is common in both males and females with CF. More than 95% of male patients with CF are azoospermic, reflecting obliteration of the vas deferens due to defective liquid secretion. Some 20% of CF women are infertile due to effects of chronic lung disease on the menstrual cycle and thick, tenacious cervical mucus that blocks sperm migration. Most pregnancies produce viable infants, and CF women breast-feed infants normally.

DIAGNOSIS

The diagnosis of CF rests on the combination of clinical criteria and abnormal CFTR function as documented by sweat tests, nasal PD measurements, and *CFTR* mutation analysis. Elevated sweat Cl^- values are nearly pathognomonic for CF. The sweat concentration values for Cl^- (and Na^+) vary with age, but, typically, a Cl^- concentration of >70 meq/L in adults discriminates between CF and other lung diseases. DNA analysis of the most common mutations identify CF mutations in >90% of affected patients. The nasal PD measurement can document CFTR dysfunction if the sweat Cl^- test is normal or borderline and two CF mutations are not identified. DNA analysis is performed routinely in patients with CF, because pancreatic genotype-phenotype relationships have been identified and mutation class–specific treatments are being developed.

Between 1 and 2% of patients with the clinical syndrome of CF have normal sweat Cl^- values. In most of these patients, the nasal transepithelial PD is raised into the diagnostic range for CF, and sweat acini do not secrete in response to injected β-adrenergic agonists. A single mutation of the *CFTR* gene, 3849 + 10 kb C→T, is associated with most CF patients with normal sweat Cl^- values.

TREATMENT Cystic Fibrosis

The major objectives of therapy for CF are to promote clearance of secretions and control infection in the lung, provide adequate nutrition, and prevent intestinal obstruction. Ultimately, therapies that restore the processing of misfolded mutant *CFTR* or gene therapy may be the treatments of choice.

LUNG DISEASE More than 95% of CF patients die of complications from lung infection. Theoretically, promoting clearance of adherent mucus should both treat and prevent progression of CF lung disease, whereas antibiotics principally reduce the bacterial burden in the CF lung.

The time-honored techniques for clearing pulmonary secretions are exercise, flutter valves, and chest percussion. Regular use of these maneuvers is effective in preserving lung function. Inhaled hypertonic saline (7%) has demonstrated efficacy in restoring mucus clearance and pulmonary function in short-term studies and in reducing acute exacerbations in a long-term (one-year) study. Hypertonic saline is safe but produces bronchoconstriction in some patients, which can be prevented with coadministered bronchodilators. Inhaled hypertonic saline is becoming a standard of care for all CF patients.

Pharmacologic agents for increasing mucus clearance are in use and in development. An important adjunct to secretion clearance can be recombinant human DNAse, which degrades DNA in CF sputum, increases airflow during short-term administration, and increases the time between pulmonary exacerbations. Most patients receive a therapeutic trial of DNAse for several months to test for efficacy. Clinical trials of experimental drugs aimed at restoring salt and water content of secretions are under way, but these drugs are not yet available for clinical use.

Antibiotics are used to treat lung infection, and their selection is guided by sputum culture results. However, because routine hospital microbiologic cultures are performed under conditions that do not mimic conditions in the CF lung, (e.g., hypoxemia) clinical efficacy often does not correlate with sensitivity testing. Because of increased total-body clearance and volume of distribution of antibiotics in CF patients, the required doses are higher for patients with CF.

Early intervention with antibiotics in infants with infection may eradicate *P. aeruginosa* for extended periods. In older patients with established infection, suppression of bacterial growth is the therapeutic goal. Azithromycin (250 mg/d or 500 mg three times weekly) is often used chronically, although it is unclear whether its actions are antimicrobial or anti-inflammatory. Inhaled aminoglycosides, (e.g., tobramycin 300 mg bid) are also used. "Mild exacerbations," as defined by increased cough and mucus production, are treated with additional oral antibiotics. Oral agents used to treat *Staphylococcus* include a semisynthetic penicillin or a cephalosporin. Oral ciprofloxacin may reduce pseudomonal bacterial counts and control symptoms, but its clinical utility is limited by emergence of resistant organisms. Accordingly, it is often used with an inhaled antibiotic, either tobramycin or colistin (75 mg bid). More severe exacerbations require intravenous antibiotics. Intravenous therapy is given both in hospital and outpatient settings. Usually, two drugs with different mechanisms of action (e.g., a cephalosporin and an aminoglycoside) are used to treat *P. aeruginosa* to minimize emergence of resistant organisms. Drug dosage should be monitored so that levels for gentamicin or tobramycin peak at ranges of ~10 μg/mL and exhibit troughs of <2 μg/mL. Antibiotics directed at *Staphylococcus* and/or *H. influenzae* are added, depending on culture results.

Inhaled β-adrenergic agonists can be useful to control airways constriction, but long-term benefit has not been shown. Oral glucocorticoids may reduce airway inflammation, but their long-term use is limited by adverse side effects; however, they may be useful for treating allergic bronchopulmonary aspergillosis.

The chronic damage to airway walls reflects in part the destructive activities of proteolytic enzymes generated, in part, by inflammatory cells. Specific antiprotease therapies are not available. However, a subset of adolescents with CF may benefit from long-term, high-dose nonsteroidal (ibuprofen) therapy.

Pulmonary complications often require acute interventions. Atelectasis requires treatment with inhaled hypertonic saline, chest physiotherapy, and antibiotics. Pneumothoraxes involving ≤10% of the lung can be observed, but chest tubes are required to expand a collapsed, diseased lung. Small-volume hemoptysis typically requires treatment of lung infection and assessment of coagulation and vitamin K status. For massive hemoptysis, bronchial artery embolization should be performed. The most ominous complications of CF are respiratory failure and cor pulmonale. The most effective conventional therapy for these conditions is vigorous medical management of the lung disease and O_2 supplementation. Ultimately, the only effective treatment for respiratory failure in CF is lung transplantation (Chap. 266). The 2-year survival for lung transplantation exceeds 60%, and transplant-patient deaths result principally from obliterative bronchiolitis.

GASTROINTESTINAL DISEASE Maintenance of adequate nutrition is critical for the health of the CF patient. Most (>90%) CF patients require pancreatic enzyme replacement. Capsules generally contain between 4000 and 20,000 units of lipase. The dose of enzymes (typically no more than 2500 units/kg per meal, to avoid risk of fibrosing colonopathy) is adjusted on the basis of weight, abdominal symptomatology, and stool character. Replacement of fat-soluble vitamins, particularly vitamins E and K, is usually required. Hyperglycemia most often becomes manifest in the adult and typically requires insulin treatment.

For treatment of acute distal intestinal obstruction, megalodiatrizoate or other hypertonic radiocontrast materials delivered by enema to the terminal ileum are used. For control of symptoms, adjustment of pancreatic enzymes and solutions containing osmotically active agents, (e.g., propyleneglycol) is recommended. Persistent symptoms may indicate a gastrointestinal malignancy, which is increased in incidence in patients with CF.

Cholestatic liver disease occurs in about 8% of CF patients. Treatment with urodeoxycholic acid is often initiated, but has not been shown to influence the course of hepatic disease. End-stage liver disease occurs in about 5% of CF patients and is treated by transplantation.

OTHER ORGAN COMPLICATIONS Dehydration due to heat-induced salt loss occurs more readily in CF patients. CF patients also have an increased incidence of osteoarthropathy, renal stones, and osteoporosis, particularly following transplant.

PSYCHOSOCIAL FACTORS CF imposes a tremendous burden on patients, and depression is common. Health insurance, career options, family planning, and life expectancy become major issues. Thus, assisting patients with the psychosocial adjustments required by CF is critical.

FURTHER READINGS

BOUCHER RC: Airway surface dehydration in cystic fibrosis: pathogenesis and therapy. Ann Rev Med 58:157, 2007

BOYLE MP: Cystic fibrosis: Year in review. Curr Opin Pulm Med 16:583, 2010

DAVIES JC et al: Cystic fibrosis. Br Med J 335:1255, 2007

DAVIS PB: Cystic fibrosis since 1938. Am J Respir Crit Care Med 173:475, 2006

ELIZUR A et al: Airway inflammation in cystic fibrosis. Chest 133:489, 2008

ELKINS MR et al: A controlled trial of long-term inhaled hypertonic saline in patients with cystic fibrosis. N Engl J Med 354:229, 2006

FERKOL T et al: Cystic fibrosis pulmonary exacerbations. J Pediatr 148:259, 2006

FLUME PA, STENBIT A: Making the diagnosis of cystic fibrosis. Am J Med Sci 335:51, 2008

GUGGINO WB, STANTON BA: New insights into cystic fibrosis: molecular switches that regulate CFTR. Nat Rev Mol Cell Biol 7:426, 2006

CHAPTER 260

Chronic Obstructive Pulmonary Disease

John J. Reilly, Jr.
Edwin K. Silverman
Steven D. Shapiro

Chronic obstructive pulmonary disease (COPD) is defined as a disease state characterized by airflow limitation that is not fully reversible (*http://www.goldcopd.com/*). COPD includes *emphysema*, an anatomically defined condition characterized by destruction and enlargement of the lung alveoli; *chronic bronchitis*, a clinically defined condition with chronic cough and phlegm; and *small airways disease*, a condition in which small bronchioles are narrowed. COPD is present only if chronic airflow obstruction occurs; chronic bronchitis *without* chronic airflow obstruction is *not* included within COPD.

COPD is the fourth leading cause of death and affects >10 million persons in the United States. COPD is also a disease of increasing public health importance around the world. Estimates suggest that COPD will rise from the sixth to the third most common cause of death worldwide by 2020.

RISK FACTORS

CIGARETTE SMOKING

By 1964, the Advisory Committee to the Surgeon General of the United States had concluded that cigarette smoking was a major risk factor for mortality from chronic bronchitis and emphysema. Subsequent longitudinal studies have shown accelerated decline in the volume of air exhaled within the first second of the forced expiratory maneuver (FEV_1) in a dose-response relationship to the intensity of cigarette smoking, which is typically expressed as pack-years (average number of packs of cigarettes smoked per day multiplied by the total number of years of smoking). This dose-response relationship between reduced pulmonary function and cigarette smoking intensity accounts for the higher prevalence rates for COPD with increasing age. The historically higher rate of smoking among males is the likely explanation for the higher prevalence of COPD among males; however, the prevalence of COPD among females is increasing as the gender gap in smoking rates has diminished in the past 50 years.

Although the causal relationship between cigarette smoking and the development of COPD has been absolutely proved, there is considerable variability in the response to smoking. Although pack-years of cigarette smoking is the most highly significant predictor of FEV_1 (Fig. 260-1), only 15% of the variability in FEV_1 is explained by pack-years. This finding suggests that additional environmental and/or genetic factors contribute to the impact of smoking on the development of airflow obstruction.

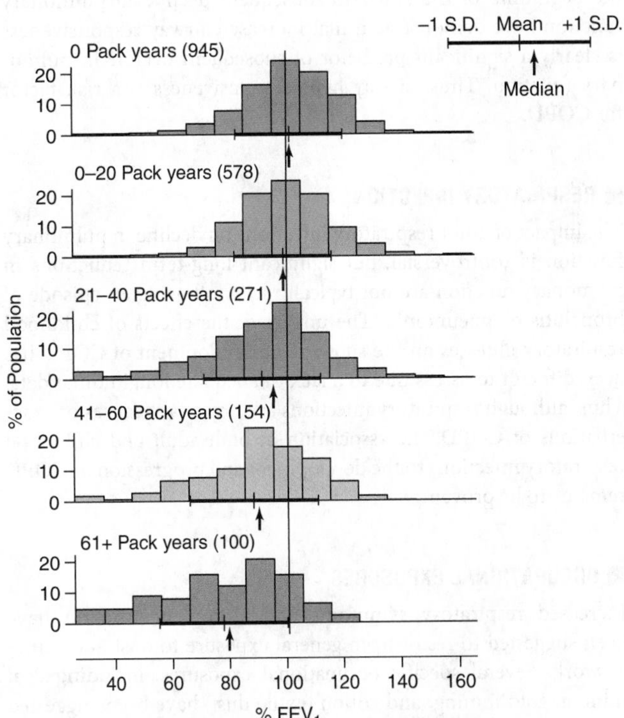

Figure 260-1 Distributions of forced expiratory volume in 1 s (FEV_1) values in a general population sample, stratified by pack-years of smoking. Means, medians, and ±1 standard deviation of percent predicted FEV_1 are shown for each smoking group. Although a dose-response relationship between smoking intensity and FEV_1 was found, marked variability in pulmonary function was observed among subjects with similar smoking histories. *(From B Burrows et al: Am Rev Respir Dis 115:95, 1977; with permission.)*

Although cigar and pipe smoking may also be associated with the development of COPD, the evidence supporting such associations is less compelling, likely related to the lower dose of inhaled tobacco by-products during cigar and pipe smoking.

AIRWAY RESPONSIVENESS AND COPD

A tendency for increased bronchoconstriction in response to a variety of exogenous stimuli, including methacholine and histamine, is one of the defining features of asthma (Chap. 254). However, many patients with COPD also share this feature of airway hyperresponsiveness. The considerable overlap between persons with asthma and those with COPD in airway responsiveness, airflow obstruction, and pulmonary symptoms led to the formulation of the Dutch hypothesis. This suggests that asthma, chronic bronchitis, and emphysema are variations of the same basic disease, which is modulated by environmental and genetic factors to produce these pathologically distinct entities. The alternative British hypothesis contends that asthma and COPD are fundamentally different diseases: Asthma is viewed as largely an allergic phenomenon, while COPD results from smoking-related inflammation and damage. Determination of the validity of the Dutch hypothesis vs. the British hypothesis awaits identification of the genetic predisposing factors for asthma and/or COPD, as well as the interactions between these postulated genetic factors and environmental risk factors. Of note, several genes related to the proteinase-antiproteinase hypothesis have been implicated as genetic determinants for both COPD and asthma, including *ADAM33* and macrophage elastase (*MMP12*) as described below.

Longitudinal studies that compared airway responsiveness at the beginning of the study to subsequent decline in pulmonary function have demonstrated that increased airway responsiveness is clearly a significant predictor of subsequent decline in pulmonary function. Thus, airway hyperresponsiveness is a risk factor for COPD.

RESPIRATORY INFECTIONS

The impact of adult respiratory infections on decline in pulmonary function is controversial, but significant long-term reductions in pulmonary function are not typically seen following an episode of bronchitis or pneumonia. The impact of the effects of childhood respiratory illnesses on the subsequent development of COPD has been difficult to assess due to a lack of adequate longitudinal data. Thus, although respiratory infections are important causes of exacerbations of COPD, the association of both adult and childhood respiratory infections to the development and progression of COPD remains to be proven.

OCCUPATIONAL EXPOSURES

Increased respiratory symptoms and airflow obstruction have been suggested to result from general exposure to dust and fumes at work. Several specific occupational exposures, including coal mining, gold mining, and cotton textile dust, have been suggested as risk factors for chronic airflow obstruction. Although nonsmokers in these occupations developed some reductions in FEV_1, the importance of dust exposure as a risk factor for COPD, independent of cigarette smoking, is not certain for most of these exposures. However, a recent study found that coal mine dust exposure was a significant risk factor for emphysema in both smokers and nonsmokers. In most cases, the magnitude of these occupational exposures on COPD risk is likely substantially less important than the effect of cigarette smoking.

AMBIENT AIR POLLUTION

Some investigators have reported increased respiratory symptoms in those living in urban compared to rural areas, which may relate to increased pollution in the urban settings. However, the relationship of air pollution to chronic airflow obstruction remains unproved. Prolonged exposure to smoke produced by biomass combustion—a common mode of cooking in some countries—also appears to be a significant risk factor for COPD among women in those countries. However, in most populations, ambient air pollution is a much less important risk factor for COPD than cigarette smoking.

PASSIVE, OR SECOND-HAND, SMOKING EXPOSURE

Exposure of children to maternal smoking results in significantly reduced lung growth. In utero tobacco smoke exposure also contributes to significant reductions in postnatal pulmonary function. Although passive smoke exposure has been associated with reductions in pulmonary function, the importance of this risk factor in the development of the severe pulmonary function reductions in COPD remains uncertain.

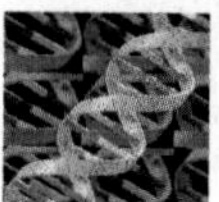

GENETIC CONSIDERATIONS

Although cigarette smoking is the major environmental risk factor for the development of COPD, the development of airflow obstruction in smokers is highly variable. Severe α_1 antitrypsin (α_1AT) deficiency is a proven genetic risk factor for COPD; there is increasing evidence that other genetic determinants also exist.

α_1 Antitrypsin deficiency

Many variants of the protease inhibitor (PI or SERPINA1) locus that encodes α_1AT have been described. The common M allele is associated with normal α_1AT levels. The S allele, associated with slightly reduced α_1AT levels, and the Z allele, associated with markedly reduced α_1AT levels, also occur with frequencies >1% in most white populations. Rare individuals inherit null alleles, which lead to the absence of any α_1AT production through a heterogeneous collection of mutations. Individuals with two Z alleles or one Z and one null allele are referred to as Pi^Z, which is the most common form of severe α_1AT deficiency.

Although only 1–2% of COPD patients are found to have severe α_1AT deficiency as a contributing cause of COPD, these patients demonstrate that genetic factors can have a profound influence on the susceptibility for developing COPD. Pi^Z individuals often develop early-onset COPD, but the ascertainment bias in the published series of Pi^Z individuals—which have usually included many Pi^Z subjects who were tested for α_1AT deficiency because they had COPD—means that the fraction of Pi^Z individuals who will develop COPD and the age-of-onset distribution for the development of COPD in Pi^Z subjects remain unknown. Approximately 1 in 3000 individuals in the United States inherits severe α_1AT deficiency, but only a small minority of these individuals has been recognized. The clinical laboratory test used most frequently to screen for α_1AT deficiency is measurement of the immunologic level of α_1AT in serum (see "Laboratory Findings").

A significant percentage of the variability in pulmonary function among Pi^Z individuals is explained by cigarette smoking; cigarette smokers with severe α_1AT deficiency are more likely to develop COPD at early ages. However, the development of COPD in Pi^Z subjects, even among current or ex-smokers, is not absolute. Among Pi^Z nonsmokers, impressive variability has been noted in the development of airflow obstruction. Asthma and male gender also appear to increase the risk of COPD in Pi^Z subjects. Other genetic and/or environmental factors likely contribute to this variability.

Specific treatment in the form of α_1AT augmentation therapy is available for severe α_1AT deficiency as a weekly IV infusion (see "Treatment," below).

The risk of lung disease in heterozygous Pi^{MZ} individuals, who have intermediate serum levels of α_1AT (~60% of Pi^{MM} levels), is controversial. Although previous general population surveys have not typically shown increased rates of airflow obstruction in Pi^{MZ} compared to Pi^{MM} individuals, case-control studies that compared COPD patients to control subjects have usually found an excess of Pi^{MZ} genotypes in the COPD patient group. Several recent large population studies have suggested that Pi^{MZ} subjects are at slightly increased risk for the development of airflow obstruction, but it remains unclear if all Pi^{MZ} subjects are at slightly increased risk for COPD or if a subset of Pi^{MZ} subjects are at substantially increased risk for COPD due to other genetic or environmental factors.

Other genetic risk factors

Studies of pulmonary function measurements performed in general population samples have suggested that genetic factors other than PI type influence variation in pulmonary function. Familial aggregation of airflow obstruction within families of COPD patients has also been demonstrated.

Association studies have compared the distribution of variants in candidate genes hypothesized to be involved in the development of COPD in COPD patients and control subjects. However, the results have been quite inconsistent, often due to underpowered studies. However, a recent association study comprising 8300 patients and 7 separate cohorts found that a minor allele SNP of *MMP12* (rs2276109) associated with decreased MMP-12 expression has a positive effect on lung function in children with asthma and in adult smokers. Recent genome-wide association studies have identified several COPD loci, including a region near the hedgehog interacting protein (*HHIP*) gene on chromosome 4 and a cluster of genes on chromosome 15 (including components of the nicotinic acetylcholine receptor) that likely contain COPD susceptibility determinants, but the specific genetic determinants in those regions have yet to be definitively identified.

NATURAL HISTORY

The effects of cigarette smoking on pulmonary function appear to depend on the intensity of smoking exposure, the timing of smoking exposure during growth, and the baseline lung function of the individual; other environmental factors may have similar effects. Most individuals follow a steady trajectory of increasing pulmonary function with growth during childhood and adolescence, followed by a gradual decline with aging. Individuals appear to track in their quartile of pulmonary function based upon environmental and genetic factors that put them on different tracks. The risk of eventual mortality from COPD is closely associated with reduced levels of FEV_1. A graphic depiction of the natural history of COPD is shown as a function of the influences on tracking curves of FEV_1 in Fig. 260-2. Death or disability from COPD can result from a normal rate of decline after a reduced growth phase (curve *C*), an early initiation of pulmonary function decline after normal growth (curve *B*), or an accelerated decline after normal growth (curve *D*). The rate of decline in pulmonary function can be modified by changing environmental exposures (i.e., quitting smoking), with smoking cessation at an earlier age providing a more beneficial effect than smoking cessation after marked reductions in pulmonary function have already developed. Genetic factors likely contribute to the level of pulmonary function achieved during growth and to the rate of decline in response to smoking and potentially to other environmental factors as well.

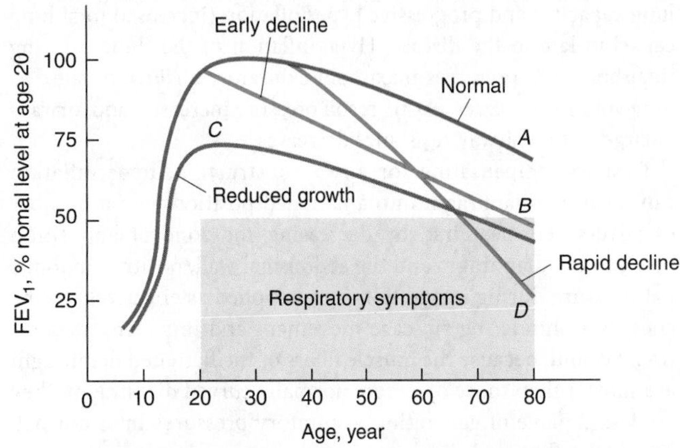

Figure 260-2 Hypothetical tracking curves of FEV_1 for individuals throughout their life spans. The normal pattern of growth and decline with age is shown by curve *A*. Significantly reduced FEV_1 (<65% of predicted value at age 20) can develop from a normal rate of decline after a reduced pulmonary function growth phase (curve *C*), early initiation of pulmonary function decline after normal growth (curve *B*), or accelerated decline after normal growth (curve *D*). *(From B Rijcken: Doctoral dissertation, p 133, University of Groningen, 1991; with permission.)*

PATHOPHYSIOLOGY

Persistent reduction in forced expiratory flow rates is the most typical finding in COPD. Increases in the residual volume and the residual volume/total lung capacity ratio, nonuniform distribution of ventilation, and ventilation-perfusion mismatching also occur.

AIRFLOW OBSTRUCTION

Airflow limitation, also known as airflow obstruction, is typically determined by spirometry, which involves forced expiratory maneuvers after the subject has inhaled to total lung capacity. Key parameters obtained from spirometry include FEV_1 and the total volume of air exhaled during the entire spirometric maneuver [forced vital capacity (FVC)]. Patients with airflow obstruction related to COPD have a chronically reduced ratio of FEV_1/FVC. In contrast to asthma, the reduced FEV_1 in COPD seldom shows large responses to inhaled bronchodilators, although improvements up to 15% are common. Asthma patients can also develop chronic (not fully reversible) airflow obstruction.

Airflow during forced exhalation is the result of the balance between the elastic recoil of the lungs promoting flow and the resistance of the airways limiting flow. In normal lungs, as well as in lungs affected by COPD, maximal expiratory flow diminishes as the lungs empty because the lung parenchyma provides progressively less elastic recoil and because the cross-sectional area of the airways falls, raising the resistance to airflow. The decrease in flow coincident with decreased lung volume is readily apparent on the expiratory limb of a flow-volume curve. In the early stages of COPD, the abnormality in airflow is only evident at lung volumes at or below the functional residual capacity (closer to residual volume), appearing as a scooped-out lower part of the descending limb of the flow-volume curve. In more advanced disease the entire curve has decreased expiratory flow compared to normal.

HYPERINFLATION

Lung volumes are also routinely assessed in pulmonary function testing. In COPD there is often "air trapping" (increased residual volume and increased ratio of residual volume to total lung capacity) and progressive hyperinflation (increased total lung capacity) late in the disease. Hyperinflation of the thorax during tidal breathing preserves maximum expiratory airflow, because as lung volume increases, elastic recoil pressure increases, and airways enlarge so that airway resistance decreases.

Despite compensating for airway obstruction, hyperinflation can push the diaphragm into a flattened position with a number of adverse effects. First, by decreasing the zone of apposition between the diaphragm and the abdominal wall, positive abdominal pressure during inspiration is not applied as effectively to the chest wall, hindering rib cage movement and impairing inspiration. Second, because the muscle fibers of the flattened diaphragm are shorter than those of a more normally curved diaphragm, they are less capable of generating inspiratory pressures than normal. Third, the flattened diaphragm (with increased radius of curvature, r) must generate greater tension (t) to develop the transpulmonary pressure (p) required to produce tidal breathing. This follows from Laplace's law, $p = 2t/r$. Also, because the thoracic cage is distended beyond its normal resting volume, during tidal breathing the inspiratory muscles must do work to overcome the resistance of the thoracic cage to further inflation instead of gaining the normal assistance from the chest wall recoiling outward toward its resting volume.

■ GAS EXCHANGE

Although there is considerable variability in the relationships between the FEV_1 and other physiologic abnormalities in COPD, certain generalizations may be made. The Pa_{O_2} usually remains near normal until the FEV_1 is decreased to ~50% of predicted, and even much lower FEV_1 values can be associated with a normal Pa_{O_2}, at least at rest. An elevation of arterial level of carbon dioxide (Pa_{CO_2}) is not expected until the FEV_1 is <25% of predicted and even then may not occur. Pulmonary hypertension severe enough to cause cor pulmonale and right ventricular failure due to COPD typically occurs in individuals who have marked decreases in FEV_1 (<25% of predicted) and chronic hypoxemia (Pa_{O_2} <55 mmHg); however, recent evidence suggests that some patients will develop significant pulmonary hypertension independent of COPD severity (Chap. 250).

Nonuniform ventilation and ventilation-perfusion mismatching are characteristic of COPD, reflecting the heterogeneous nature of the disease process within the airways and lung parenchyma. Physiologic studies are consistent with multiple parenchymal compartments having different rates of ventilation due to regional differences in compliance and airway resistance. Ventilation-perfusion mismatching accounts for essentially all of the reduction in Pa_{O_2} that occurs in COPD; shunting is minimal. This finding explains the effectiveness of modest elevations of inspired oxygen in treating hypoxemia due to COPD and therefore the need to consider problems other than COPD when hypoxemia is difficult to correct with modest levels of supplemental oxygen in the patient with COPD.

PATHOLOGY

Cigarette smoke exposure may affect the large airways, small airways (≤2 mm diameter), and alveoli. Changes in large airways cause cough and sputum, while changes in small airways and alveoli are responsible for physiologic alterations. Emphysema and small airway pathology are both present in most persons with COPD; however, they do not appear to be mechanistically related to each other, and their relative contributions to obstruction vary from one person to another.

■ LARGE AIRWAY

Cigarette smoking often results in mucous gland enlargement and goblet cell hyperplasia leading to cough and mucus production that define chronic bronchitis, but these abnormalities are not related to airflow limitation. Goblet cells not only increase in number but in extent through the bronchial tree. Bronchi also undergo squamous metaplasia, predisposing to carcinogenesis and disrupting mucociliary clearance. Although not as prominent as in asthma, patients may have smooth-muscle hypertrophy and bronchial hyperreactivity leading to airflow limitation. Neutrophil influx has been associated with purulent sputum of upper respiratory tract infections. Independent of its proteolytic activity, neutrophil elastase is among the most potent secretagogues identified.

■ SMALL AIRWAYS

The major site of increased resistance in most individuals with COPD is in airways ≤2 mm diameter. Characteristic cellular changes include goblet cell metaplasia, with these mucus-secreting cells replacing surfactant-secreting Clara cells. Infiltration of mononuclear phagocytes is also prominent. Smooth-muscle hypertrophy may also be present. These abnormalities may cause luminal narrowing by fibrosis, excess mucus, edema, and cellular infiltration. Reduced surfactant may increase surface tension at the air-tissue interface, predisposing to airway narrowing or collapse. Respiratory bronchiolitis with mononuclear inflammatory cells collecting in distal airway tissues may cause proteolytic destruction of elastic fibers in the respiratory bronchioles and alveolar ducts where the fibers are concentrated as rings around alveolar entrances.

Because small airway patency is maintained by the surrounding lung parenchyma that provides radial traction on bronchioles at points of attachment to alveolar septa, loss of bronchiolar attachments as a result of extracellular matrix destruction may cause airway distortion and narrowing in COPD.

■ LUNG PARENCHYMA

Emphysema is characterized by destruction of gas-exchanging air spaces, i.e., the respiratory bronchioles, alveolar ducts, and alveoli. Their walls become perforated and later obliterated with coalescence of small distinct air spaces into abnormal and much larger air spaces. Macrophages accumulate in respiratory bronchioles of essentially all young smokers. Bronchoalveolar lavage fluid from such individuals contains roughly five times as many macrophages as lavage from nonsmokers. In smokers' lavage fluid, macrophages comprise >95% of the total cell count, and neutrophils, nearly absent in nonsmokers' lavage, account for 1–2% of the cells. T lymphocytes, particularly CD8+ cells, are also increased in the alveolar space of smokers.

Emphysema is classified into distinct pathologic types, the most important being centriacinar and panacinar. *Centriacinar emphysema*, the type most frequently associated with cigarette smoking, is characterized by enlarged air spaces found (initially) in association with respiratory bronchioles. Centriacinar emphysema is usually most prominent in the upper lobes and superior segments of lower lobes and is often quite focal. *Panacinar emphysema* refers to abnormally large air spaces evenly distributed within and across acinar units. Panacinar emphysema is usually observed in patients with α_1AT deficiency, which has a predilection for the lower lobes. Distinctions between centriacinar and panacinar emphysema are interesting and may ultimately be shown to have different mechanisms of pathogenesis. However, garden-variety smoking-related emphysema is usually mixed, particularly in advanced cases, and these pathologic classifications are not helpful in the care of patients with COPD.

PATHOGENESIS

Airflow limitation, the major physiologic change in COPD, can result from both small airway obstruction and emphysema, as

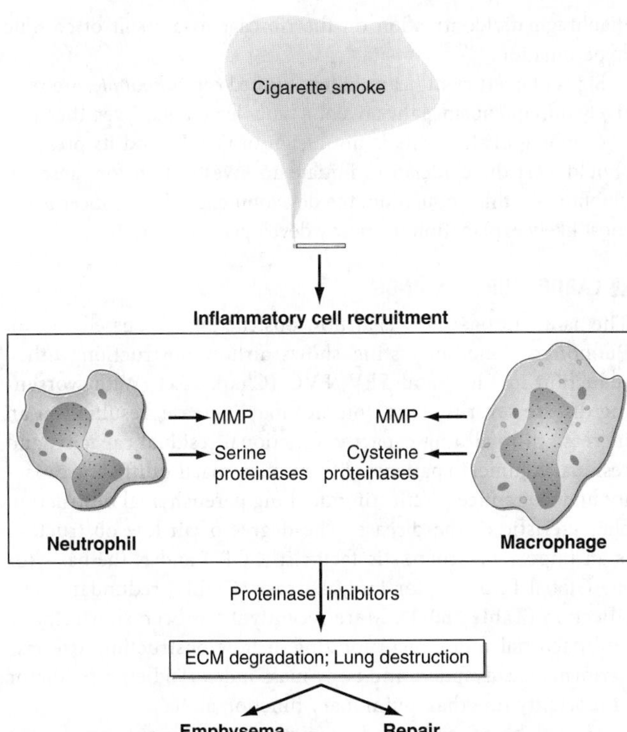

Figure 260-3 Pathogenesis of emphysema. Upon long-term exposure to cigarette smoke, inflammatory cells are recruited to the lung; they release proteinases in excess of inhibitors, and if repair is abnormal, this leads to air space destruction and enlargement or emphysema. ECM, extracellular matrix; MMP, matrix metalloproteinase.

discussed above. Pathologic findings that can contribute to small airway obstruction are described above, but their relative importance is unknown. Fibrosis surrounding the small airways appears to be a significant contributor. Mechanisms leading to collagen accumulation around the airways in the face of increased collagenase activity remain an enigma. Although seemingly counterintuitive, there are several potential mechanisms whereby a proteinase can predispose to fibrosis, including proteolytic activation of transforming growth factor β (TGF-β). Largely due to greater similarity of animal air spaces than airways to humans, we know much more about mechanisms involved in emphysema than small airway obstruction.

The dominant paradigm of the pathogenesis of emphysema comprises four interrelated events (Fig. 260-3): (1) Chronic exposure to cigarette smoke may lead to inflammatory cell recruitment within the terminal air spaces of the lung. (2) These inflammatory cells release elastolytic proteinases that damage the extracellular matrix of the lung. (3) Structural cell death results from oxidant stress and loss of matrix-cell attachment. (4) Ineffective repair of elastin and other extracellular matrix components result in air space enlargement that defines pulmonary emphysema.

THE ELASTASE:ANTIELASTASE HYPOTHESIS

Elastin, the principal component of elastic fibers, is a highly stable component of the extracellular matrix that is critical to the integrity of the lung. The elastase:antielastase hypothesis proposed in the mid-1960s states that the balance of elastin-degrading enzymes and their inhibitors determines the susceptibility of the lung to destruction resulting in air space enlargement. This hypothesis was based on the clinical observation that patients with genetic deficiency in α_1AT, the inhibitor of the serine proteinase neutrophil elastase, were at increased risk of emphysema, and that instillation of elastases, including neutrophil elastase, to experimental animals results in emphysema. The elastase:antielastase hypothesis remains a prevailing mechanism for the development of emphysema. However, a complex network of immune and inflammatory cells and additional proteinases that contribute to emphysema have subsequently been identified.

INFLAMMATION AND EXTRACELLULAR MATRIX PROTEOLYSIS

Macrophages patrol the lower air space under normal conditions. Upon exposure to oxidants from cigarette smoke, macrophages become activated, producing proteinases and chemokines that attract other inflammatory cells. One mechanism of macrophage activation occurs via oxidant-induced inactivation of histone deacetylase-2, shifting the balance toward acetylated or loose chromatin, exposing nuclear factor κB sites and resulting in transcription of matrix metalloproteinases, proinflammatory cytokines such as interleukin 8 (IL-8), and tumor necrosis factor α (TNF-α); this leads to neutrophil recruitment. CD8+ T cells are also recruited in response to cigarette smoke and release interferon inducible protein-10 (IP-10, CXCL-7) that in turn leads to macrophage production of macrophage elastase [matrix metalloproteinase-12 (MMP-12)]. Matrix metalloproteinases and serine proteinases, most notably neutrophil elastase, work together by degrading the inhibitor of the other, leading to lung destruction. Proteolytic cleavage products of elastin also serve as a macrophage chemokine, fueling this destructive positive feedback loop.

Autoimmune mechanisms have recently been identified in COPD and may promote the progression of disease. Increased B cells and lymphoid follicles are present in patients, particularly those with advanced disease. Antibodies have been found against elastin fragments, as well; IgG autoantibodies with avidity for pulmonary epithelium and the potential to mediate cytotoxicity have been detected.

Concomitant cigarette smoke–induced loss of cilia in the airway epithelium and impaired macrophage phagocytosis predispose to bacterial infection with neutrophilia. In end-stage lung disease, long after smoking cessation there remains an exuberant inflammatory response, suggesting that mechanisms of cigarette smoke–induced inflammation that initiate the disease differ from mechanisms that sustain inflammation after smoking cessation.

Cell death

Air space enlargement with loss of alveolar units obviously requires disappearance of both extracellular matrix and cells. Cell death can occur from increased oxidant stress both directly from cigarette smoke and from inflammation. Animal models have used endothelial and epithelial cell death as a means to generate transient air space enlargement. Uptake of apoptotic cells by macrophages results in production of growth factors and dampens inflammation, promoting lung repair. Cigarette smoke impairs macrophage uptake of apoptotic cells, limiting repair.

Ineffective repair

The ability of the adult lung to repair damaged alveoli appears limited. It is unlikely that the process of septation that is responsible for alveologenesis during lung development can be reinitiated. The capacity of stem cells to repopulate the lung is under active investigation. It appears difficult for an adult human to completely restore an appropriate extracellular matrix, particularly functional elastic fibers.

CLINICAL PRESENTATION

HISTORY

The three most common symptoms in COPD are cough, sputum production, and exertional dyspnea. Many patients have such symptoms for months or years before seeking medical attention. Although the development of airflow obstruction is a gradual process, many patients date the onset of their disease to an acute illness or exacerbation. A careful history, however, usually reveals the presence of symptoms prior to the acute exacerbation. The development of exertional dyspnea, often described as increased effort to breathe, heaviness, air hunger, or gasping, can be insidious. It is best elicited by a careful history focused on typical physical activities and how the patient's ability to perform them has changed. Activities involving significant arm work, particularly at or above shoulder level, are particularly difficult for patients with COPD. Conversely, activities that allow the patient to brace the arms and use accessory muscles of respiration are better tolerated. Examples of such activities include pushing a shopping cart, walking on a treadmill, or pushing a wheelchair. As COPD advances, the principal feature is worsening dyspnea on exertion with increasing intrusion on the ability to perform vocational or avocational activities. In the most advanced stages, patients are breathless doing simple activities of daily living.

Accompanying worsening airflow obstruction is an increased frequency of exacerbations (described below). Patients may also develop resting hypoxemia and require institution of supplemental oxygen.

PHYSICAL FINDINGS

In the early stages of COPD, patients usually have an entirely normal physical examination. Current smokers may have signs of active smoking, including an odor of smoke or nicotine staining of fingernails. In patients with more severe disease, the physical examination is notable for a prolonged expiratory phase and may include expiratory wheezing. In addition, signs of hyperinflation include a barrel chest and enlarged lung volumes with poor diaphragmatic excursion as assessed by percussion. Patients with severe airflow obstruction may also exhibit use of accessory muscles of respiration, sitting in the characteristic "tripod" position to facilitate the actions of the sternocleidomastoid, scalene, and intercostal muscles. Patients may develop cyanosis, visible in the lips and nail beds.

Although traditional teaching is that patients with predominant emphysema, termed "pink puffers," are thin and noncyanotic at rest and have prominent use of accessory muscles, and patients with chronic bronchitis are more likely to be heavy and cyanotic ("blue bloaters"), current evidence demonstrates that most patients have elements of both bronchitis and emphysema and that the physical examination does not reliably differentiate the two entities.

Advanced disease may be accompanied by systemic wasting, with significant weight loss, bitemporal wasting, and diffuse loss of subcutaneous adipose tissue. This syndrome has been associated with both inadequate oral intake and elevated levels of inflammatory cytokines (TNF-α). Such wasting is an independent poor prognostic factor in COPD. Some patients with advanced disease have paradoxical inward movement of the rib cage with inspiration (Hoover's sign), the result of alteration of the vector of diaphragmatic contraction on the rib cage as a result of chronic hyperinflation.

Signs of overt right heart failure, termed *cor pulmonale,* are relatively infrequent since the advent of supplemental oxygen therapy.

Clubbing of the digits is not a sign of COPD, and its presence should alert the clinician to initiate an investigation for causes of clubbing. In this population, the development of lung cancer is the most likely explanation for newly developed clubbing.

LABORATORY FINDINGS

The hallmark of COPD is airflow obstruction (discussed above). Pulmonary function testing shows airflow obstruction with a reduction in FEV_1 and FEV_1/FVC (Chap. 252). With worsening disease severity, lung volumes may increase, resulting in an increase in total lung capacity, functional residual capacity, and residual volume. In patients with emphysema, the diffusing capacity may be reduced, reflecting the lung parenchymal destruction characteristic of the disease. The degree of airflow obstruction is an important prognostic factor in COPD and is the basis for the Global Initiative for Lung Disease (GOLD) redundant classification (Table 260-1). More recently it has been shown that a multifactorial index incorporating airflow obstruction, exercise performance, dyspnea, and body mass index is a better predictor of mortality rate than pulmonary function alone.

Arterial blood gases and oximetry may demonstrate resting or exertional hypoxemia. Arterial blood gases provide additional information about alveolar ventilation and acid-base status by measuring arterial P_{CO_2} and pH. The change in pH with P_{CO_2} is 0.08 units/10 mmHg acutely and 0.03 units/10 mmHg in the chronic state. Knowledge of the arterial pH therefore allows the classification of ventilatory failure, defined as P_{CO_2} >45 mmHg, into acute or chronic conditions. The arterial blood gas is an important component of the evaluation of patients presenting with symptoms of an exacerbation. An elevated hematocrit suggests the presence of chronic hypoxemia, as does the presence of signs of right ventricular hypertrophy.

Radiographic studies may assist in the classification of the type of COPD. Obvious bullae, paucity of parenchymal markings, or hyperlucency suggests the presence of emphysema.

TABLE 260-1 GOLD Criteria for COPD Severity

GOLD Stage	Severity	Symptoms	Spirometry
0	At Risk	Chronic cough, sputum production	Normal
I	Mild	With or without chronic cough or sputum production	FEV_1/FVC <0.7 and FEV_1 ≥80% predicted
IIA	Moderate	With or without chronic cough or sputum production	FEV_1/FVC <0.7 and 50% ≤FEV_1 <80% predicted
III	Severe	With or without chronic cough or sputum production	FEV_1/FVC <0.7 and 30% ≤FEV_1 <50% predicted
IV	Very Severe	With or without chronic cough or sputum production	FEV_1/FVC <0.7 and FEV_1 <30% predicted or FEV_1 <50% predicted with respiratory failure or signs of right heart failure

Abbreviation: GOLD, Global Initiative for Lung Disease.
Source: From RA Pauwels et al.

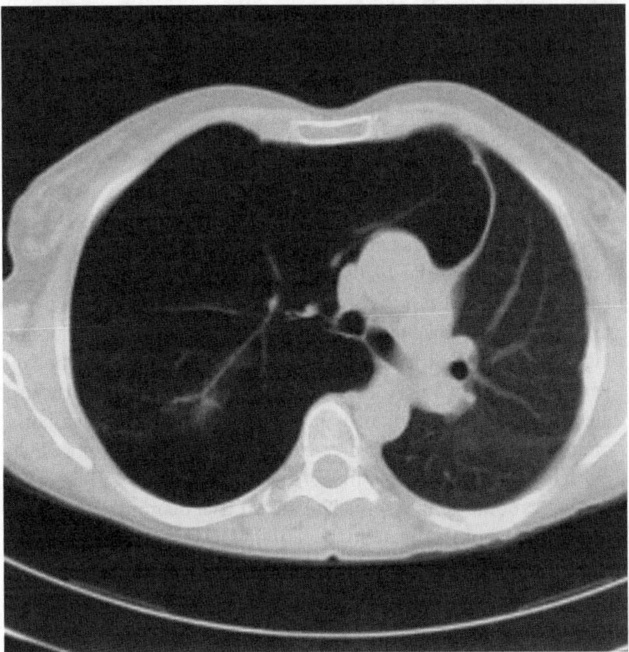

Figure 260-4 Chest CT scan of a patient with COPD who underwent a left single-lung transplant. Note the reduced parenchymal markings in the right lung (*left side of figure*) as compared to the left lung, representing emphysematous destruction of the lung, and mediastinal shift to the left, indicative of hyperinflation.

Increased lung volumes and flattening of the diaphragm suggest hyperinflation but do not provide information about chronicity of the changes. Computed tomography (CT) scan is the current definitive test for establishing the presence or absence of emphysema in living subjects (Fig. 260-4). From a practical perspective, the CT scan does little to influence therapy of COPD except in those individuals considering surgical therapy for their disease (described below).

Recent guidelines have suggested testing for α_1AT deficiency in all subjects with COPD or asthma with chronic airflow obstruction. Measurement of the serum α_1AT level is a reasonable initial test. For subjects with low α_1AT levels, the definitive diagnosis of α_1AT deficiency requires protease inhibitor (PI) type determination. This is typically performed by isoelectric focusing of serum, which reflects the genotype at the PI locus for the common alleles and many of the rare PI alleles as well. Molecular genotyping of DNA can be performed for the common PI alleles (M, S, and Z).

TREATMENT Chronic Obstructive Pulmonary Disease

STABLE PHASE COPD Only three interventions—smoking cessation, oxygen therapy in chronically hypoxemic patients, and lung volume reduction surgery in selected patients with emphysema—have been demonstrated to influence the natural history of patients with COPD. There is currently suggestive, but not definitive, evidence that the use of inhaled glucocorticoids may alter mortality rate (but not lung function). All other current therapies are directed at improving symptoms and decreasing the frequency and severity of exacerbations. The institution of these therapies should involve an assessment of symptoms, potential risks, costs, and benefits of therapy. This should be followed by an assessment of response to therapy, and a decision should be made whether or not to continue treatment.

PHARMACOTHERAPY

Smoking Cessation (See also Chap. 395) It has been shown that middle-aged smokers who were able to successfully stop smoking experienced a significant improvement in the rate of decline in pulmonary function, returning to annual changes similar to that of nonsmoking patients. Thus, all patients with COPD should be strongly urged to quit and educated about the benefits of quitting. An emerging body of evidence demonstrates that combining pharmacotherapy with traditional supportive approaches considerably enhances the chances of successful smoking cessation. There are three principal pharmacologic approaches to the problem: bupropion, originally developed as an antidepressant medication; nicotine replacement therapy available as gum, transdermal patch, inhaler, and nasal spray; and varenicline, a nicotinic acid receptor agonist/antagonist. Current recommendations from the U.S. Surgeon General are that all adult, nonpregnant smokers considering quitting be offered pharmacotherapy, in the absence of any contraindication to treatment.

Bronchodilators In general, bronchodilators are used for symptomatic benefit in patients with COPD. The inhaled route is preferred for medication delivery as the incidence of side effects is lower than that seen with the use of parenteral medication delivery.

Anticholinergic Agents Ipratropium bromide improves symptoms and produces acute improvement in FEV_1. Tiotropium, a long-acting anticholinergic, has been shown to improve symptoms and reduce exacerbations. Studies of both ipratropium and tiotropium have failed to demonstrate that either influences the rate of decline in FEV_1. In a large randomized clinical trial, there was a trend toward reduced mortality rate in the tiotropium-treated patients that approached, but did not reach, statistical significance. Side effects are minor, and a trial of inhaled anticholinergics is recommended in symptomatic patients with COPD.

Beta Agonists These provide symptomatic benefit. The main side effects are tremor and tachycardia. Long-acting inhaled β agonists, such as salmeterol, have benefits comparable to ipratropium bromide. Their use is more convenient than short-acting agents. The addition of a β agonist to inhaled anticholinergic therapy has been demonstrated to provide incremental benefit. A recent report in asthma suggests that those patients, particularly African Americans, using a long-acting β agonist without concomitant inhaled corticosteroids have an increased risk of deaths from respiratory causes. The applicability of these data to patients with COPD is unclear.

Inhaled Glucocorticoids Although a recent trial demonstrated an apparent benefit from the regular use of inhaled glucocorticoids on the rate of decline of lung function, a number of other well-designed randomized trials have not. Patients studied included those with mild to severe airflow obstruction and current and ex-smokers. Patients with significant acute response to inhaled β agonists were excluded from many of these trials, which may impact the generalizability of the findings. Their use has been associated with increased rates of oropharyngeal candidiasis and an increased rate of loss of bone density. Available data suggest that inhaled glucocorticoids reduce exacerbation frequency by ~25%. The impact of inhaled corticosteroids on mortality rates in COPD is controversial. A meta-analysis and several retrospective studies suggest a mortality benefit, but in a recently published randomized trial, differences in mortality rate approached, but did not reach, conventional criteria for statistical significance. A trial of inhaled glucocorticoids should be considered in patients with frequent exacerbations, defined as two or more per year, and in patients who demonstrate a significant amount of acute reversibility in response to inhaled bronchodilators.

Oral Glucocorticoids The chronic use of oral glucocorticoids for treatment of COPD is not recommended because of an unfavorable benefit/risk ratio. The chronic use of oral glucocorticoids is associated with significant side effects, including osteoporosis, weight gain, cataracts, glucose intolerance, and increased risk of infection. A recent study demonstrated that patients tapered off chronic low-dose prednisone (~10 mg/d) did not experience any adverse effect on the frequency of exacerbations, health-related quality of life, or lung function. On average, patients lost ~4.5 kg (~10 lb) when steroids were withdrawn.

Theophylline Theophylline produces modest improvements in expiratory flow rates and vital capacity and a slight improvement in arterial oxygen and carbon dioxide levels in patients with moderate to severe COPD. Nausea is a common side effect; tachycardia and tremor have also been reported. Monitoring of blood theophylline levels is typically required to minimize toxicity.

Oxygen Supplemental O_2 is the only pharmacologic therapy demonstrated to unequivocally decrease mortality rates in patients with COPD. For patients with resting hypoxemia (resting O_2 saturation ≤88% or <90% with signs of pulmonary hypertension or right heart failure), the use of O_2 has been demonstrated to have a significant impact on mortality rate. Patients meeting these criteria should be on continual oxygen supplementation, as the mortality benefit is proportional to the number of hours/day oxygen is used. Various delivery systems are available, including portable systems that patients may carry to allow mobility outside the home.

Supplemental O_2 is commonly prescribed for patients with exertional hypoxemia or nocturnal hypoxemia. Although the rationale for supplemental O_2 in these settings is physiologically sound, the benefits of such therapy are not well substantiated.

Other Agents *N*-acetyl cysteine has been used in patients with COPD for both its mucolytic and antioxidant properties. A prospective trial failed to find any benefit with respect to decline in lung function or prevention of exacerbations. Specific treatment in the form of IV α_1AT augmentation therapy is available for individuals with severe α_1AT deficiency. Despite sterilization procedures for these blood-derived products and the absence of reported cases of viral infection from therapy, some physicians recommend hepatitis B vaccination prior to starting augmentation therapy. Although biochemical efficacy of α_1AT augmentation therapy has been shown, a randomized controlled trial of α_1AT augmentation therapy has not definitively established the efficacy of augmentation therapy in reducing decline of pulmonary function. Eligibility for α_1AT augmentation therapy requires a serum α_1AT level <11 μM (approximately 50 mg/dL). Typically, Pi^Z individuals will qualify, although other rare types associated with severe deficiency (e.g., null-null) are also eligible. Since only a fraction of individuals with severe α_1AT deficiency will develop COPD, α_1AT augmentation therapy is not recommended for severely α_1AT-deficient persons with normal pulmonary function and a normal chest CT scan.

NONPHARMACOLOGIC THERAPIES

General Medical Care Patients with COPD should receive the influenza vaccine annually. Polyvalent pneumococcal vaccine is also recommended, although proof of efficacy in this patient population is not definitive.

Pulmonary Rehabilitation This refers to a treatment program that incorporates education and cardiovascular conditioning. In COPD, pulmonary rehabilitation has been demonstrated to improve health-related quality of life, dyspnea, and exercise capacity. It has also been shown to reduce rates of hospitalization over a 6- to 12-month period.

Lung Volume Reduction Surgery (LVRS) Surgery to reduce the volume of lung in patients with emphysema was first introduced with minimal success in the 1950s and was reintroduced in the 1990s. Patients are excluded if they have significant pleural disease, a pulmonary artery systolic pressure >45 mmHg, extreme deconditioning, congestive heart failure, or other severe comorbid conditions. Patients with an FEV_1 <20% of predicted and either diffusely distributed emphysema on CT scan or diffusing capacity of lung for carbon monoxide (DL_{CO}) <20% of predicted have an increased mortality rate after the procedure and thus are not candidates for LVRS.

The National Emphysema Treatment trial demonstrated that LVRS offers both a mortality benefit and a symptomatic benefit in certain patients with emphysema. The anatomic distribution of emphysema and postrehabilitation exercise capacity are important prognostic characteristics. Patients with upper lobe–predominant emphysema and a low postrehabilitation exercise capacity are most likely to benefit from LVRS.

Lung Transplantation (See also Chap. 266) COPD is currently the second leading indication for lung transplantation (Fig. 260-4). Current recommendations are that candidates for lung transplantation should be <65 years; have severe disability despite maximal medical therapy; and be free of comorbid conditions such as liver, renal, or cardiac disease. In contrast to LVRS, the anatomic distribution of emphysema and the presence of pulmonary hypertension are not contraindications to lung transplantation. Unresolved issues concerning lung transplantation and COPD include whether single- or double-lung transplant is the preferred procedure.

EXACERBATIONS OF COPD Exacerbations are a prominent feature of the natural history of COPD. Exacerbations are episodes of increased dyspnea and cough and change in the amount and character of sputum. They may or may not be accompanied by other signs of illness, including fever, myalgias, and sore throat. Self-reported health-related quality of life correlates with frequency of exacerbations more closely than it does with the degree of airflow obstruction. Economic analyses have shown that >70% of COPD-related health care expenditures go to emergency department visits and hospital care; this translates to >$10 billion annually in the United States. The frequency of exacerbations increases as airflow obstruction increases; patients with moderate to severe airflow obstruction [GOLD stages III, IV (Table 260-1)] on average have one to three episodes per year. However, some individuals with very severe airflow obstruction do not have frequent exacerbations; the history of prior exacerbations is a strong predictor of future exacerbations.

The approach to the patient experiencing an exacerbation includes an assessment of the severity of the patient's illness, both acute and chronic components; an attempt to identify the precipitant of the exacerbation; and the institution of therapy.

Precipitating Causes and Strategies to Reduce Frequency of Exacerbations A variety of stimuli may result in the final common pathway of airway inflammation and increased symptoms that are characteristic of COPD exacerbations. Bacterial infections play a role in many, but by no means all, episodes. Viral respiratory infections are present in approximately one-third of COPD exacerbations. In a significant minority of instances (20–35%), no specific precipitant can be identified.

Despite the frequent implication of bacterial infection, chronic suppressive or "rotating" antibiotics are not beneficial in patients with COPD. This is in contrast to their efficacy in patients with bronchiectasis due to cystic fibrosis, in whom suppressive antibiotics have been shown to reduce frequency of hospital admissions.

The role of pharmacotherapy in reducing exacerbation frequency is less well studied. Chronic oral glucocorticoids are not recommended for this purpose. Inhaled glucocorticoids reduce the frequency of exacerbations by 25–30% in most analyses. The use of inhaled glucocorticoids should be considered in patients with frequent exacerbations or those who have an asthmatic component, i.e., significant reversibility on pulmonary function testing or marked symptomatic improvement after inhaled bronchodilators. Similar magnitudes of reduction have been reported for anticholinergic and long-acting beta-agonist therapy. The influenza vaccine has been shown to reduce exacerbation rates in patients with COPD.

Patient Assessment An attempt should be made to establish the severity of the exacerbation as well as the severity of preexisting COPD. The more severe either of these two components, the more likely that the patient will require hospital admission. The history should include quantification of the degree of dyspnea by asking about breathlessness during activities of daily living and typical activities for the patient. The patient should be asked about fever; change in character of sputum; any ill contacts; and associated symptoms such as nausea, vomiting, diarrhea, myalgias, and chills. Inquiring about the frequency and severity of prior exacerbations can provide important information.

The physical examination should incorporate an assessment of the degree of distress of the patient. Specific attention should be focused on tachycardia, tachypnea, use of accessory muscles, signs of perioral or peripheral cyanosis, the ability to speak in complete sentences, and the patient's mental status. The chest examination should establish the presence or absence of focal findings, degree of air movement, presence or absence of wheezing, asymmetry in the chest examination (suggesting large airway obstruction or pneumothorax mimicking an exacerbation), and the presence or absence of paradoxical motion of the abdominal wall.

Patients with severe underlying COPD, who are in moderate or severe distress or those with focal findings should have a chest x-ray. Approximately 25% of x-rays in this clinical situation will be abnormal, with the most frequent findings being pneumonia and congestive heart failure. Patients with advanced COPD, those with a history of hypercarbia, those with mental status changes (confusion, sleepiness), or those in significant distress should have an arterial blood-gas measurement. The presence of hypercarbia, defined as a P_{CO_2} >45 mmHg, has important implications for treatment (discussed below). In contrast to its utility in the management of exacerbations of asthma, measurement of pulmonary function has not been demonstrated to be helpful in the diagnosis or management of exacerbations of COPD.

There are no definitive guidelines concerning the need for inpatient treatment of exacerbations. Patients with respiratory acidosis and hypercarbia, significant hypoxemia, or severe underlying disease or those whose living situation is not conducive to careful observation and the delivery of prescribed treatment should be admitted to the hospital.

ACUTE EXACERBATIONS

Bronchodilators Typically, patients are treated with an inhaled β agonist, often with the addition of an anticholinergic agent. These may be administered separately or together, and the frequency of administration depends on the severity of the exacerbation. Patients are often treated initially with nebulized therapy, as such treatment is often easier to administer in older patients or to those in respiratory distress. It has been shown, however, that conversion to metered-dose inhalers is effective when accompanied by education and training of patients and staff. This approach has significant economic benefits and also allows an easier transition to outpatient care. The addition of methylxanthines (such as theophylline) to this regimen can be considered, although convincing proof of its efficacy is lacking. If added, serum levels should be monitored in an attempt to minimize toxicity.

Antibiotics Patients with COPD are frequently colonized with potential respiratory pathogens, and it is often difficult to identify conclusively a specific species of bacteria responsible for a particular clinical event. Bacteria frequently implicated in COPD exacerbations include *Streptococcus pneumoniae, Haemophilus influenzae,* and *Moraxella catarrhalis.* In addition, *Mycoplasma pneumoniae* or *Chlamydia pneumoniae* are found in 5–10% of exacerbations. The choice of antibiotic should be based on local patterns of antibiotic susceptibility of the above pathogens as well as the patient's clinical condition. Most practitioners treat patients with moderate or severe exacerbations with antibiotics, even in the absence of data implicating a specific pathogen.

Glucocorticoids Among patients admitted to the hospital, the use of glucocorticoids has been demonstrated to reduce the length of stay, hasten recovery, and reduce the chance of subsequent exacerbation or relapse for a period of up to 6 months. One study demonstrated that 2 weeks of glucocorticoid therapy produced benefit indistinguishable from 8 weeks of therapy. The GOLD guidelines recommend 30–40 mg of oral prednisolone or its equivalent for a period of 10–14 days. Hyperglycemia, particularly in patients with preexisting diagnosis of diabetes, is the most frequently reported acute complication of glucocorticoid treatment.

Oxygen Supplemental O_2 should be supplied to keep arterial saturations ≥90%. Hypoxemic respiratory drive plays a small role in patients with COPD. Studies have demonstrated that in patients with both acute and chronic hypercarbia, the administration of supplemental O_2 does not reduce minute ventilation. It does, in some patients, result in modest increases in arterial P_{CO_2}, chiefly by altering ventilation-perfusion relationships within the lung. This should not deter practitioners from providing the oxygen needed to correct hypoxemia.

Mechanical Ventilatory Support The initiation of noninvasive positive-pressure ventilation (NIPPV) in patients with respiratory failure, defined as Pa_{CO_2} >45 mmHg, results in a significant reduction in mortality rate, need for intubation, complications of therapy, and hospital length of stay. Contraindications to NIPPV include cardiovascular instability, impaired mental status or inability to cooperate, copious secretions or the inability to clear secretions, craniofacial abnormalities or trauma precluding effective fitting of mask, extreme obesity, or significant burns.

Invasive (conventional) mechanical ventilation via an endotracheal tube is indicated for patients with severe respiratory distress despite initial therapy, life-threatening hypoxemia, severe hypercarbia and/or acidosis, markedly impaired mental status, respiratory arrest, hemodynamic instability, or other complications. The goal of mechanical ventilation is to correct the aforementioned conditions. Factors to consider during mechanical ventilatory support include the need to provide sufficient expiratory time in patients with severe airflow obstruction and the presence of auto-PEEP (positive end-expiratory pressure), which can result in patients having to generate significant respiratory effort to trigger a breath during a demand mode of ventilation. The mortality rate of patients requiring mechanical ventilatory support is 17–30% for that particular hospitalization. For patients age >65 admitted to the intensive care unit for treatment, the mortality rate doubles over the next year to 60%, regardless of whether mechanical ventilation was required.

FURTHER READINGS

American Thoracic Society/European Respiratory Society Task Force: Standards for the diagnosis and management of patients with COPD [Internet]. Version 1.2. New York: American Thoracic Society; 2004 [updated September 8, 2005]. Available from *http://www-test.thoracic.org/copd/*

Fiore MC et al: *Treating Tobacco Use and Dependence,* Clinical Practice Guideline. Rockville, MD: U.S. Department of Health and Human Services. Public Health Service, June 2000

Hunninghake GM et al: MMP12, lung function, and COPD in high-risk populations. N Engl J Med 361:2599, 2009

Ito K et al: Decreased histone deacetylase activity in chronic obstructive pulmonary disease. N Engl J Med 352:1967, 2005

Mannino DM, Buist AS: Global burden of COPD: Risk factors, prevalence, and future trends. Lancet 370:765, 2007

Rabe KF et al: Global strategy for the diagnosis, management and prevention of chronic obstructive pulmonary disease: GOLD executive summary. Am J Respir Crit Care Med 176:532, 2007

——et al: Update in chronic obstructive pulmonary disease 2006. Am J Respir Crit Care Med 175:1222, 2007

Sin DD et al: Inhaled corticosteroids and mortality in chronic obstructive pulmonary disease. Thorax 60:992, 2005

Wise RA, Tashkin DP: Optimizing treatment of chronic obstructive pulmonary disease: An assessment of current therapies. Am J Med 120:S4, 2007

CHAPTER 261
Interstitial Lung Diseases

Talmadge E. King, Jr.

Patients with interstitial lung diseases (ILDs) come to medical attention mainly because of the onset of progressive exertional dyspnea or a persistent nonproductive cough. Hemoptysis, wheezing, and chest pain may be present. Often, the identification of interstitial opacities on chest x-ray focuses the diagnostic approach on one of the ILDs.

ILDs represent a large number of conditions that involve the parenchyma of the lung—the alveoli, the alveolar epithelium, the capillary endothelium, and the spaces between those structures—as well as the perivascular and lymphatic tissues. The disorders in this heterogeneous group are classified together because of similar clinical, roentgenographic, physiologic, or pathologic manifestations. These disorders often are associated with considerable rates of morbidity and mortality, and there is little consensus regarding the best management of most of them.

ILDs have been difficult to classify because >200 known individual diseases are characterized by diffuse parenchymal lung involvement, either as the primary condition or as a significant part of a multiorgan process, as may occur in the connective tissue diseases (CTDs). One useful approach to classification is to separate the ILDs into two groups based on the major underlying histopathology: (1) those associated with predominant inflammation and fibrosis and (2) those with a predominantly granulomatous reaction in interstitial or vascular areas (Table 261-1). Each of these groups can be subdivided further according to whether the cause is known or unknown. For each ILD there may be an acute phase, and there is usually a chronic one as well. Rarely, some are recurrent, with intervals of subclinical disease.

Sarcoidosis (Chap. 329), idiopathic pulmonary fibrosis (IPF), and pulmonary fibrosis associated with CTDs (Chaps. 319–326) are the most common ILDs of unknown etiology. Among the ILDs of known cause, the largest group includes occupational and environmental exposures, especially the inhalation of inorganic dusts, organic dusts, and various fumes or gases (Chaps. 255 and 256) (Table 261-2). A clinical diagnosis is possible for many forms of ILD, especially if an occupational and environmental history is pursued aggressively. High-resolution computed tomography (HRCT) scanning improves the diagnostic accuracy and may eliminate the need for tissue examination in many cases, especially in IPF. For other forms, tissue examination, usually obtained by thoracoscopic lung biopsy, is critical to confirmation of the diagnosis.

PATHOGENESIS

The ILDs are nonmalignant disorders and are not caused by identified infectious agents. The precise pathway(s) leading from injury to fibrosis is not known. Although there are multiple initiating agent(s) of injury, the immunopathogenic responses of lung tissue are limited, and the mechanisms of repair have common features (Fig. 261-1).

As mentioned above, the two major histopathologic patterns are a granulomatous pattern and a pattern in which inflammation and fibrosis predominate.

Granulomatous lung disease

This process is characterized by an accumulation of T lymphocytes, macrophages, and epithelioid cells organized into discrete structures (granulomas) in the lung parenchyma. The granulomatous lesions can progress to fibrosis. Many patients with granulomatous lung disease remain free of severe impairment of lung function or, when symptomatic, improve after treatment. The main differential diagnosis is between sarcoidosis (Chap. 329) and hypersensitivity pneumonitis (Chap. 255).

Inflammation and fibrosis

The initial insult is an injury to the epithelial surface that causes inflammation in the air spaces and alveolar walls (Fig. 261-2). If the disease becomes chronic, inflammation spreads to adjacent portions of the interstitium and vasculature and eventually causes interstitial fibrosis. Important histopathologic patterns found in the ILDs include usual interstitial pneumonia (UIP), nonspecific interstitial pneumonia, respiratory bronchiolitis/desquamative interstitial pneumonia, organizing pneumonia, diffuse alveolar damage (acute or organizing), and lymphocytic interstitial pneumonia. The development of irreversible scarring (fibrosis) of alveolar walls, airways, or vasculature is the most feared outcome in all of these conditions because it is often progressive and leads to significant derangement of ventilatory function and gas exchange.

TABLE 261-1 Major Categories of Alveolar and Interstitial Inflammatory Lung Disease

Lung Response: Alveolitis, Interstitial Inflammation, and Fibrosis	
Known Cause	
Asbestos	Residual of acute respiratory distress syndrome
Fumes, gases	Smoking-related
Drugs (antibiotics, amiodarone, gold) and chemotherapy drugs	Desquamative interstitial pneumonia
Radiation	Respiratory bronchiolitis–associated interstitial lung disease
Aspiration pneumonia	Langerhans cell granulomatosis (eosinophilic granuloma of the lung)
Unknown Cause	
Idiopathic interstitial pneumonias	Pulmonary alveolar proteinosis
Idiopathic pulmonary fibrosis (usual interstitial pneumonia)	Lymphocytic infiltrative disorders (lymphocytic interstitial pneumonitis associated with connective tissue disease)
Acute interstitial pneumonia (diffuse alveolar damage)	Eosinophilic pneumonias
Cryptogenic organizing pneumonia (bronchiolitis obliterans with organizing pneumonia)	Lymphangioleiomyomatosis
Nonspecific interstitial pneumonia	Amyloidosis
Connective tissue diseases	Inherited diseases
Systemic lupus erythematosus, rheumatoid arthritis, ankylosing spondylitis, systemic sclerosis, Sjögren's syndrome, polymyositis-dermatomyositis	Tuberous sclerosis, neurofibromatosis, Niemann-Pick disease, Gaucher's disease, Hermansky-Pudlak syndrome
Pulmonary hemorrhage syndromes	Gastrointestinal or liver diseases (Crohn's disease, primary biliary cirrhosis, chronic active hepatitis, ulcerative colitis)
Goodpasture's syndrome, idiopathic pulmonary hemosiderosis, isolated pulmonary capillaritis	Graft-versus-host disease (bone marrow transplantation; solid organ transplantation)
Lung Response: Granulomatous	
Known Cause	
Hypersensitivity pneumonitis (organic dusts)	Inorganic dusts: beryllium, silica
Unknown Cause	
Sarcoidosis	Bronchocentric granulomatosis
Granulomatous vasculitides	Lymphomatoid granulomatosis
Granulomatosis with polyangiitis (Wegener's), allergic granulomatosis of Churg-Strauss	

HISTORY

Duration of illness

Acute presentation (days to weeks), although unusual, occurs with allergy (drugs, fungi, helminths), acute interstitial pneumonia (AIP), eosinophilic pneumonia, and hypersensitivity pneumonitis. These conditions may be confused with atypical pneumonias because of diffuse alveolar opacities on chest x-ray. *Subacute presentation* (weeks to months) may occur in all ILDs but is seen especially in sarcoidosis, drug-induced ILDs, the alveolar hemorrhage syndromes, cryptogenic organizing pneumonia (COP), and the acute immunologic pneumonia that complicates systemic lupus erythematosus (SLE) or polymyositis. In most ILDs the symptoms and signs form a *chronic presentation* (months to years). Examples include IPF, sarcoidosis, pulmonary Langerhans cell histiocytosis (PLCH) (also known as Langerhans cell granulomatosis, eosinophilic granuloma, or histiocytosis X), pneumoconioses, and CTDs. *Episodic presentations* are unusual and include eosinophilic pneumonia, hypersensitivity pneumonitis, COP, vasculitides, pulmonary hemorrhage, and Churg-Strauss syndrome.

Age

Most patients with sarcoidosis, ILD associated with CTD, lymphangioleiomyomatosis (LAM), PLCH, and inherited forms of ILD (familial IPF, Gaucher's disease, Hermansky-Pudlak syndrome) present between the ages of 20 and 40 years. Most patients with IPF are older than 60 years.

Gender

LAM and pulmonary involvement in tuberous sclerosis occur exclusively in premenopausal women. In addition, ILD in Hermansky-Pudlak syndrome and in the CTDs is more common in women; an exception is ILD in rheumatoid arthritis (RA), which is more common in men. IPF is more common in men. Because of occupational exposures, pneumoconioses also occur more frequently in men.

Family history

Familial lung fibrosis has been associated with mutations in three genes: the surfactant protein C gene, the surfactant protein A2 gene, and the ATP-binding cassette transporter A3 gene. Familial lung fibrosis is characterized by several patterns of interstitial pneumonia, including nonspecific interstitial pneumonia, desquamative interstitial pneumonia, and UIP. Older age, male sex, and a history of cigarette smoking have been identified as risk factors for familial lung fibrosis. Family associations (with an autosomal dominant pattern) have been identified in tuberous sclerosis and neurofibromatosis. Familial clustering has been identified increasingly in sarcoidosis. The genes responsible for several rare ILDs have been identified,

TABLE 261-2 Estimated Relative Frequency of the Interstitial Lung Diseases

Diagnosis	Relative Frequency, %
Idiopathic interstitial pneumonias	40
Idiopathic pulmonary fibrosis	55
Nonspecific interstitial pneumonia	25
Respiratory bronchiolitis—ILD and desquamative interstitial pneumonia	15
Cryptogenic organizing pneumonia	3
Acute interstitial pneumonia	<1
Occupational and environmental	26
Sarcoidosis	10
Connective tissue diseases	9
Drug and radiation	1
Pulmonary hemorrhage syndromes	<1
Other	13

Source: From DB Coultas, R Hubbard, in JP Lynch III (ed): *Lung Biology in Health and Disease*. New York, Marcel Dekker, 2004; S Garantziotis et al: J Clin Invest 114:319, 2004.

i.e., alveolar microlithiasis, Gaucher's disease, Hermansky-Pudlak syndrome, and Niemann-Pick disease, along with the genes for surfactant homeostasis in pulmonary alveolar proteinosis and for control of cell growth and differentiation in LAM.

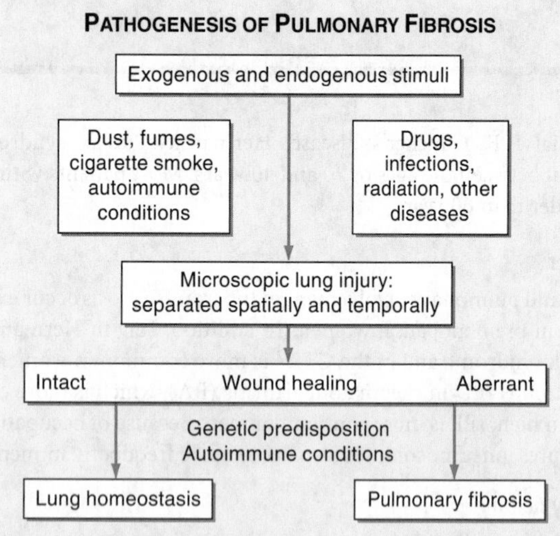

Figure 261-1 Proposed mechanism for the pathogenesis of pulmonary fibrosis. The lung is naturally exposed to repetitive injury from a variety of exogenous and endogenous stimuli. Several local and systemic factors (e.g., fibroblasts, circulating fibrocytes, chemokines, growth factors, and clotting factors) contribute to tissue healing and functional recovery. Dysregulation of this intricate network through genetic predisposition, autoimmune conditions, or superimposed diseases can lead to aberrant wound healing, with the result of pulmonary fibrosis. Alternatively, excessive injury to the lung may overwhelm even intact reparative mechanisms and lead to pulmonary fibrosis. *(From S Garantziotis et al: J Clin Invest 114:319, 2004.)*

Smoking history

Two-thirds to 75% of patients with IPF and familial lung fibrosis have a history of smoking. Patients with PLCH, respiratory bronchiolitis/desquamative interstitial pneumonia (DIP), Goodpasture's syndrome, respiratory bronchiolitis, and pulmonary alveolar proteinosis are usually current or former smokers.

Occupational and environmental history

A strict chronologic listing of the patient's lifelong employment must be sought, including specific duties and known exposures. In hypersensitivity pneumonitis (see Fig. 255-1), respiratory symptoms, fever, chills, and an abnormal chest roentgenogram are often temporally related to a hobby (pigeon breeder's disease) or to the workplace (farmer's lung) (Chap. 255). Symptoms may diminish or disappear after the patient leaves the site of exposure for several days; similarly, symptoms may reappear when the patient returns to the exposure site.

Other important past history

Parasitic infections may cause pulmonary eosinophilia, and therefore a travel history should be taken in patients with known or suspected ILD. History of risk factors for HIV infection should be elicited because several processes may occur at the time of initial presentation or during the clinical course, e.g., HIV infection, organizing pneumonia, AIP, lymphocytic interstitial pneumonitis, and diffuse alveolar hemorrhage.

Respiratory symptoms and signs

Dyspnea is a common and prominent complaint in patients with ILD, especially the idiopathic interstitial pneumonias, hypersensitivity pneumonitis, COP, sarcoidosis, eosinophilic pneumonias, and PLCH. Some patients, especially patients with sarcoidosis, silicosis, PLCH, hypersensitivity pneumonitis, lipoid pneumonia, or lymphangitis carcinomatosis, may have extensive parenchymal lung disease on chest x-ray without significant dyspnea, especially early in the course of the illness. Wheezing is an uncommon manifestation of ILD but has been described in patients with chronic eosinophilic pneumonia, Churg-Strauss syndrome, respiratory bronchiolitis, and sarcoidosis. Clinically significant chest pain is uncommon in most ILDs. However, substernal discomfort is common in sarcoidosis. Sudden worsening of dyspnea, especially if associated with acute chest pain, may indicate a spontaneous pneumothorax, which occurs in PLCH, tuberous sclerosis, LAM, and neurofibromatosis. Frank hemoptysis and blood-streaked sputum are rarely presenting manifestations of ILD but can be seen in the diffuse alveolar hemorrhage (DAH) syndromes, LAM, tuberous sclerosis, and the granulomatous vasculitides. Fatigue and weight loss are common in all ILDs.

PHYSICAL EXAMINATION

The findings are usually not specific. Most commonly, physical examination reveals tachypnea and bibasilar end-inspiratory dry crackles, which are common in most forms of ILD associated with inflammation but are less likely to be heard in the granulomatous lung diseases. Crackles may be present in the absence of radiographic abnormalities on the chest radiograph. Scattered late inspiratory high-pitched rhonchi—so-called inspiratory squeaks—are heard in patients with bronchiolitis. The cardiac examination is usually normal except in the middle or late stages of the disease, when findings of pulmonary hypertension and cor pulmonale may become evident (Chap. 250). Cyanosis and clubbing of the digits occur in some patients with advanced disease.

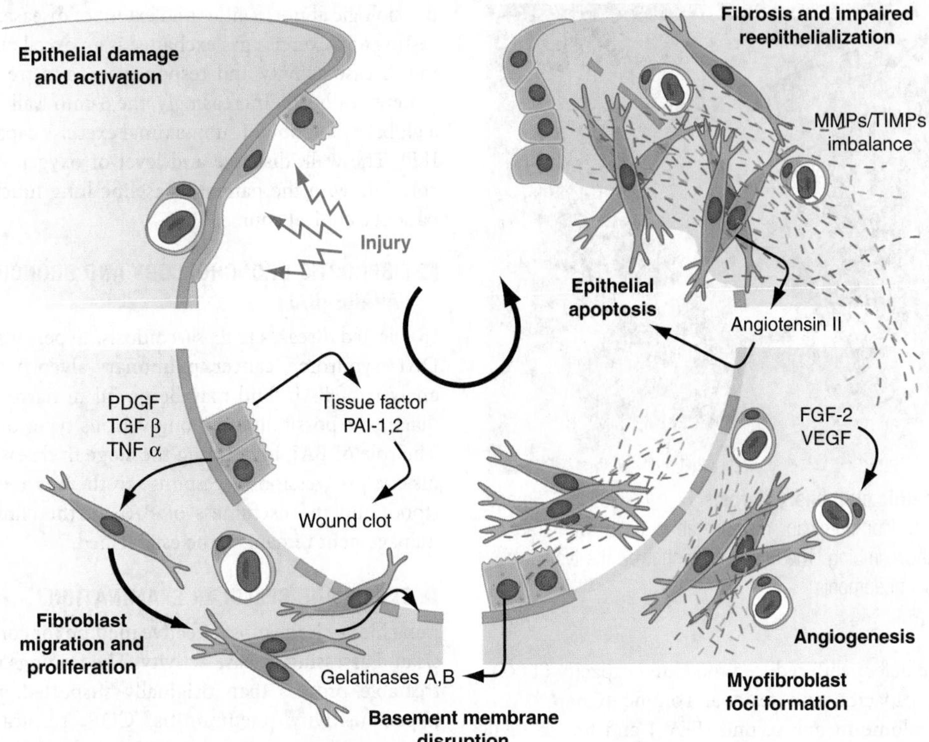

Figure 261-2 Cellular basis for the pathogenesis of interstitial lung disease. Multiple microinjuries damage and activate alveolar epithelial cells (*top left*), which in turn induce an antifibrinolytic environment in the alveolar spaces, enhancing wound clot formation. Alveolar epithelial cells secrete growth factors and induce migration and proliferation of fibroblasts and differentiation into myofibroblasts (*bottom left*). Subepithelial myofibroblasts and alveolar epithelial cells produce gelatinases that may increase basement membrane disruption and allow fibroblast–myofibroblast migration (*bottom right*). Angiogenic factors induce neovascularization. Both intraalveolar and interstitial myofibroblasts secrete extracellular matrix proteins, mainly collagens. An imbalance between interstitial collagenases and tissue inhibitors of metalloproteinases provokes the progressive deposit of extracellular matrix (*top right*). Signals responsible for myofibroblast apoptosis seem to be absent or delayed in usual interstitial pneumonia, increasing cell survival. Myofibroblasts produce angiotensinogen that, as angiotensin II, provokes alveolar epithelial cell death, further impairing reepithelialization. Abbreviations: FGF-2, fibroblast growth factor 2; MMPs, metalloproteinases; PAI-1, PAI-2, plasminogen activator inhibitor 1, 2; PDGF, platelet-derived growth factor; TGF-β, transforming growth factor β; TIMPs, tissue inhibitors of metalloproteinases; TNF-α, tumor necrosis factor α; VEGF, vascular endothelial growth factor. *(From M Selman et al: Ann Intern Med 134:136, 2001, with permission.)*

■ LABORATORY

Antinuclear antibodies and anti-immunoglobulin antibodies (rheumatoid factors) are identified in some patients, even in the absence of a defined CTD. A raised lactate dehydrogenase (LDH) level is a nonspecific finding common to ILDs. Elevation of the serum level of angiotensin-converting enzyme is common in sarcoidosis. Serum precipitins confirm exposure when hypersensitivity pneumonitis is suspected, although they are not diagnostic of the process. Antineutrophil cytoplasmic or anti-basement membrane antibodies are useful if vasculitis is suspected. The electrocardiogram is usually normal unless pulmonary hypertension is present; then it demonstrates right-axis deviation, right ventricular hypertrophy, or right atrial enlargement or hypertrophy. Echocardiography also reveals right ventricular dilation and/or hypertrophy in the presence of pulmonary hypertension.

■ CHEST IMAGING STUDIES

Chest x-ray

ILD may be first suspected on the basis of an abnormal chest radiograph, which most commonly reveals a bibasilar reticular pattern. A nodular or mixed pattern of alveolar filling and increased reticular markings also may be present. A subgroup of ILDs exhibit nodular opacities with a predilection for the upper lung zones [sarcoidosis, PLCH, chronic hypersensitivity pneumonitis, silicosis, beryliosis, RA (necrobiotic nodular form), ankylosing spondylitis]. The chest x-ray correlates poorly with the clinical or histopathologic stage of the disease. The radiographic finding of honeycombing correlates with pathologic findings of small cystic spaces and progressive fibrosis; when present, it portends a poor prognosis. In most cases, the chest radiograph is nonspecific and usually does not allow a specific diagnosis.

Computed tomography

High-resolution computed tomography is superior to the plain chest x-ray for early detection and confirmation of suspected ILD (Fig. 261-3). In addition, HRCT allows better assessment of the extent and distribution of disease, and it is especially useful in the investigation of patients with a normal chest radiograph. Coexisting disease is often best recognized on HRCT scanning, e.g., mediastinal adenopathy, carcinoma, or emphysema. In the appropriate clinical setting HRCT may be sufficiently characteristic to preclude the need for lung biopsy in IPF, sarcoidosis, hypersensitivity pneumonitis, asbestosis, lymphangitic carcinoma, and PLCH. When a lung biopsy is required, HRCT scanning is useful for determining the most appropriate area from which biopsy samples should be taken.

■ PULMONARY FUNCTION TESTING

Spirometry and lung volumes

Measurement of lung function is important in assessing the extent of pulmonary involvement in patients with ILD. Most forms of ILD

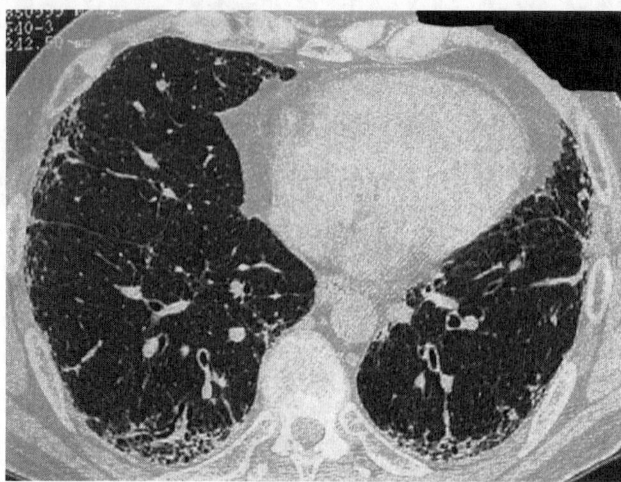

Figure 261-3 Idiopathic pulmonary fibrosis. High-resolution CT image shows bibasal, peripheral predominant reticular abnormality with traction bronchiectasis and honeycombing. The lung biopsy showed the typical features of usual interstitial pneumonia.

produce a restrictive defect with reduced total lung capacity (TLC), functional residual capacity, and residual volume (Chap. 252). Forced expiratory volume in one second (FEV_1) and forced vital capacity (FVC) are reduced, but these changes are related to the decreased TLC. The FEV_1/FVC ratio is usually normal or increased. Lung volumes decrease as lung stiffness worsens with disease progression. A few disorders produce interstitial opacities on chest x-ray and obstructive airflow limitation on lung function testing (uncommon in sarcoidosis and hypersensitivity pneumonitis but common in tuberous sclerosis and LAM). Pulmonary function studies have been proved to have prognostic value in patients with idiopathic interstitial pneumonias, particularly IPF and nonspecific interstitial pneumonia (NSIP).

Diffusing capacity

A reduction in the diffusing capacity of the lung for carbon monoxide (DL_{CO}) is a common but nonspecific finding in most ILDs. This decrease is due in part to effacement of the alveolar capillary units but, more important, to mismatching of ventilation and perfusion ($\dot{V}/\dot{Q}$). Lung regions with reduced compliance due to either fibrosis or cellular infiltration may be poorly ventilated but may still maintain adequate blood flow, and the ventilation-perfusion mismatch in these regions acts like true venous admixture. The severity of the reduction in DL_{CO} does not correlate with disease stage.

Arterial blood gas

The resting arterial blood gas may be normal or reveal hypoxemia (secondary to a mismatching of ventilation to perfusion) and respiratory alkalosis. A normal arterial O_2 tension (or saturation by oximetry) at rest does not rule out significant hypoxemia during exercise or sleep. Carbon dioxide (CO_2) retention is rare and is usually a manifestation of end-stage disease.

CARDIOPULMONARY EXERCISE TESTING

Because hypoxemia at rest is not always present and because severe exercise-induced hypoxemia may go undetected, it is useful to perform exercise testing with measurement of arterial blood gases to detect abnormalities of gas exchange. Arterial oxygen desaturation, a failure to decrease dead space appropriately with exercise [i.e., a high V_D/V_T (dead space/tidal volume) ratio (Chap. 252)], and an excessive increase in respiratory rate with a lower than expected recruitment of tidal volume provide useful information about physiologic abnormalities and extent of disease. Serial assessment of resting and exercise gas exchange is an excellent method for following disease activity and responsiveness to treatment, especially in patients with IPF. Increasingly, the 6-min walk test is used to obtain a global evaluation of submaximal exercise capacity in patients with ILD. The walk distance and level of oxygen desaturation tend to correlate with the patient's baseline lung function and mirror the patient's clinical course.

FIBEROPTIC BRONCHOSCOPY AND BRONCHOALVEOLAR LAVAGE (BAL)

In selected diseases (e.g., sarcoidosis, hypersensitivity pneumonitis, DAH syndrome, cancer, pulmonary alveolar proteinosis), cellular analysis of BAL fluid may be useful in narrowing the differential diagnostic possibilities among various types of ILD (Table 261-3). The role of BAL in defining the stage of disease and assessment of disease progression or response to therapy remains poorly understood, and the usefulness of BAL in the clinical assessment and management remains to be established.

TISSUE AND CELLULAR EXAMINATION

Lung biopsy is the most effective method for confirming the diagnosis and assessing disease activity. The findings may identify a more treatable process than originally suspected, particularly chronic hypersensitivity pneumonitis, COP, respiratory bronchiolitis–associated ILD, or sarcoidosis. Biopsy should be obtained before the initiation of treatment. A definitive diagnosis avoids confusion and anxiety later in the clinical course if the patient does not respond to therapy or experiences serious side effects from it.

Fiberoptic bronchoscopy with multiple transbronchial lung biopsies (four to eight biopsy samples) is often the initial procedure of choice, especially when sarcoidosis, lymphangitic carcinomatosis, eosinophilic pneumonia, Goodpasture's syndrome, or infection is suspected. If a specific diagnosis is not made by transbronchial biopsy, surgical lung biopsy by video-assisted thoracic surgery or open thoracotomy is indicated. Adequate-sized biopsies from multiple sites, usually from two lobes, should be obtained. Relative contraindications to lung biopsy include serious cardiovascular disease, honeycombing and other roentgenographic evidence of diffuse end-stage disease, severe pulmonary dysfunction, and other major operative risks, especially in the elderly.

TREATMENT Interstitial Lung Disease

Although the course of ILD is variable, progression is common and often insidious. All treatable possibilities should be carefully considered. Since therapy does not reverse fibrosis, the major goals of treatment are permanent removal of the offending agent, when known, and early identification and aggressive suppression of the acute and chronic inflammatory process, thereby reducing further lung damage. Hypoxemia (Pa_{O_2} <55 mmHg) at rest and/or with exercise should be managed with supplemental oxygen. Management of cor pulmonale may be required as the disease progresses (Chaps. 234 and 250). Pulmonary rehabilitation has been shown to improve the quality of life in patients with ILD.

DRUG THERAPY Glucocorticoids are the mainstay of therapy for suppression of the alveolitis present in ILD, but the success rate is low. There have been no placebo-controlled trials of glucocorticoids in ILD, and so there is no direct evidence that steroids improve survival in many of the diseases for which they are commonly used. Glucocorticoid therapy is recommended for symptomatic ILD patients with eosinophilic pneumonias, COP, CTD, sarcoidosis, hypersensitivity pneumonitis, acute

TABLE 261-3 Diagnostic Value of Bronchoalveolar Lavage in Interstitial Lung Disease

Condition	Bronchoalveolar Lavage Finding
Sarcoidosis	Lymphocytosis; CD4:CD8 ratio >3.5 most specific of diagnosis
Hypersensitivity pneumonitis	Marked lymphocytosis (>50%)
Organizing pneumonia	Foamy macrophages; mixed pattern of increased cells characteristic; decreased CD4:CD8 ratio
Eosinophilic lung disease	Eosinophils >25%
Diffuse alveolar bleeding	Hemosiderin-laden macrophages, red blood cells
Diffuse alveolar damage, drug toxicity	Atypical hyperplastic type II pneumocytes
Opportunistic infections	*Pneumocystis carinii*, fungi, cytomegalovirus-transformed cells
Lymphangitic carcinomatosis, alveolar cell carcinoma, pulmonary lymphoma	Malignant cells
Alveolar proteinosis	Milky effluent, foamy macrophages and lipoproteinaceous intraalveolar material (periodic acid–Schiff stain–positive)
Lipoid pneumonia	Fat globules in macrophages
Pulmonary Langerhans cell histiocytosis	Increased CD1+ Langerhans cells, electron microscopy demonstrating Birbeck granule in lavaged macrophage (expensive and difficult to perform)
Asbestos-related pulmonary disease	Dust particles, ferruginous bodies
Berylliosis	Positive lymphocyte transformation test to beryllium
Silicosis	Dust particles by polarized light microscopy
Lipoidosis	Accumulation of specific lipopigment in alveolar macrophages

inorganic dust exposures, acute radiation pneumonitis, DAH, and drug-induced ILD. In organic dust disease, glucocorticoids are recommended for both the acute and chronic stages.

The optimal dose and proper length of therapy with glucocorticoids in the treatment of most ILDs are not known. A common starting dose is prednisone, 0.5–1 mg/kg in a once-daily oral dose (based on the patient's lean body weight). This dose is continued for 4–12 weeks, at which time the patient is reevaluated. If the patient is stable or improved, the dose is tapered to 0.25–0.5 mg/kg and is maintained at this level for an additional 4–12 weeks, depending on the course. Rapid tapering or a shortened course of glucocorticoid treatment can result in recurrence. If the patient's condition continues to decline on glucocorticoids, a second agent (see below) often is added and the prednisone dose is lowered to or maintained at 0.25 mg/kg per d.

Cyclophosphamide and azathioprine (1–2 mg/kg lean body weight per day), with or without glucocorticoids, have been tried with variable success in IPF, vasculitis, progressive systemic sclerosis, and other ILDs. An objective response usually requires at least 8–12 weeks to occur. In situations in which these drugs have failed or could not be tolerated, other agents, including methotrexate, colchicine, penicillamine, and cyclosporine, have been tried. However, their role in the treatment of ILDs remains to be determined.

Many cases of ILD are chronic and irreversible despite the therapy discussed above, and lung transplantation may then be considered (Chap. 266).

INDIVIDUAL FORMS OF ILD

IDIOPATHIC PULMONARY FIBROSIS

IPF is the most common form of idiopathic interstitial pneumonia. Separating IPF from other forms of lung fibrosis is an important step in the evaluation of all patients presenting with ILD. IPF has a distinctly poor response to therapy and a bad prognosis.

Clinical manifestations

Exertional dyspnea, a nonproductive cough, and inspiratory crackles with or without digital clubbing may be present on physical examination. HRCT lung scans typically show patchy, predominantly basilar, subpleural reticular opacities, often associated with traction bronchiectasis and honeycombing (Fig. 261-3). Atypical findings that should suggest an alternative diagnosis include extensive ground-glass abnormality, nodular opacities, upper or midzone predominance, and prominent hilar or mediastinal lymphadenopathy. Pulmonary function tests often reveal a restrictive pattern, a reduced DL_{CO}, and arterial hypoxemia that is exaggerated or elicited by exercise.

Histologic findings

Confirmation of the presence of the UIP pattern on histologic examination is essential to confirm this diagnosis. Transbronchial biopsies are not helpful in making the diagnosis of UIP, and surgical biopsy usually is required. The histologic hallmark and chief diagnostic criterion of UIP is a heterogeneous appearance at low magnification with alternating areas of normal lung, interstitial inflammation, foci of proliferating fibroblasts, dense collagen fibrosis, and honeycomb changes. These histologic changes affect the peripheral, subpleural parenchyma most severely. The interstitial inflammation is usually patchy and consists of a lymphoplasmacytic infiltrate in the alveolar septa, associated with hyperplasia of type 2 pneumocytes. The fibrotic zones are composed mainly of dense collagen, although scattered foci of proliferating fibroblasts are a consistent finding. The extent of fibroblastic proliferation is predictive of disease progression. Areas of honeycomb change are composed of cystic fibrotic air spaces that frequently are lined by bronchiolar epithelium and filled with mucin. Smooth-muscle hyperplasia is commonly seen in areas of fibrosis and honeycomb change. A fibrotic pattern with some features similar to UIP may be found in the chronic stage of several specific disorders, such as pneumoconioses (e.g., asbestosis), radiation injury, certain drug-induced lung diseases (e.g., nitrofurantoin), chronic aspiration, sarcoidosis, chronic hypersensitivity pneumonitis, organized chronic eosinophilic pneumonia, and PLCH. Commonly, other histopathologic features are present in these situations, thus allowing separation of these lesions from the UIP-like pattern. Consequently, the term *usual interstitial pneumonia* is used for patients in whom the lesion is idiopathic and not associated with another condition.

TREATMENT Management Issues in Patients with IPF

Untreated patients with IPF show continued progression of their disease and have a high mortality rate. There is no effective therapy for IPF. Chronic microaspiration secondary to gastroesophageal reflux may play a role in the pathogenesis and natural history of IPF. Patients with IPF and coexisting emphysema [combined pulmonary fibrosis and emphysema (CPFE)] are more likely to require long-term oxygen therapy and develop pulmonary hypertension and may have a more dismal outcome than those without emphysema.

Patients with IPF may have acute deterioration secondary to infections, pulmonary embolism, or pneumothorax. Heart failure and ischemic heart disease are common problems in patients with IPF, accounting for nearly one-third of deaths. These patients also commonly experience an accelerated phase of rapid clinical decline that is associated with a poor prognosis (so-called acute exacerbations of IPF). These acute exacerbations are defined by worsening of dyspnea within a few days to 4 weeks; newly developing diffuse ground-glass abnormality and/or consolidation superimposed on a background reticular or honeycomb pattern consistent with the UIP pattern; worsening hypoxemia; and absence of infectious pneumonia, heart failure, and sepsis. The rate of these acute exacerbations ranges from 10–57%, apparently depending on the length of follow-up. During these episodes, the histopathologic pattern of diffuse alveolar damage is often found on the background of UIP. No therapy has been found to be effective in the management of acute exacerbations of IPF. Often mechanical ventilation is required, but it is usually not successful, with a hospital mortality rate of up to three-fourths of patients. In those who survive, a recurrence of acute exacerbation is common and usually results in death at those times.

Lung transplantation should be considered for patients who experience progressive deterioration despite optimal medical management and who meet the established criteria (Chap. 266).

NONSPECIFIC INTERSTITIAL PNEUMONIA

This condition defines a subgroup of the idiopathic interstitial pneumonias that can be distinguished clinically and pathologically from UIP, DIP, AIP, and idiopathic BOOP. Importantly, many cases with this histopathologic pattern occur in the context of an underlying disorder, such as a connective tissue disease, drug-induced ILD, or chronic hypersensitivity pneumonitis.

Patients with idiopathic NSIP have clinical, serologic, radiographic, and pathologic characteristics highly suggestive of autoimmune disease and meet the criteria for undifferentiated connective tissue disease. Idiopathic NSIP is a subacute restrictive process with a presentation similar to that of IPF but usually at a younger age, most commonly in women who have never smoked. It is often associated with a febrile illness. HRCT shows bilateral, subpleural ground-glass opacities, often associated with lower lobe volume loss (Fig. 261-4). Patchy areas of airspace consolidation and reticular abnormalities may be present, but honeycombing is unusual. The key histopathologic feature of NSIP is the uniformity

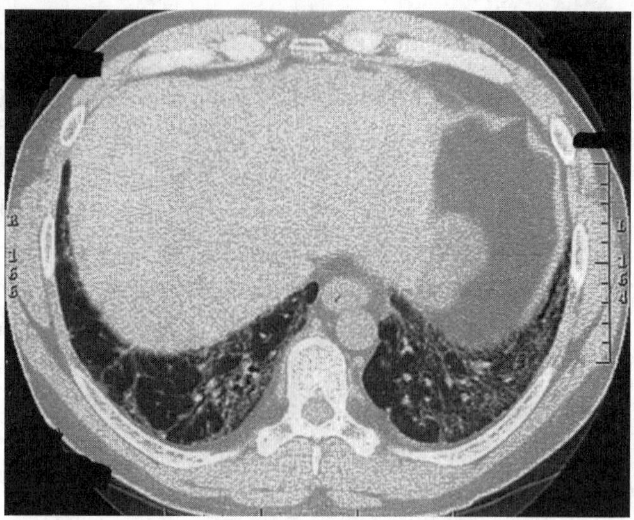

Figure 261-4 Nonspecific interstitial pneumonia. High-resolution CT through the lower lung shows volume loss with extensive ground-glass abnormality, reticular abnormality, and traction bronchiectasis. There is sparing on the lung immediately adjacent to the pleura. Histology showed a combination of inflammation and mild fibrosis.

of interstitial involvement across the biopsy section, and this may be predominantly cellular or fibrosing. There is less temporal and spatial heterogeneity than in UIP, and little or no honeycombing is found. The cellular variant is rare. Unlike patients with IPF (UIP), the majority of patients with NSIP have a good prognosis (5-year mortality rate estimated at <15%), with most showing improvement after treatment with glucocorticoids, often used in combination with azathioprine.

ACUTE INTERSTITIAL PNEUMONIA (HAMMAN-RICH SYNDROME)

AIP is a rare, fulminant form of lung injury characterized histologically by diffuse alveolar damage on lung biopsy. Most patients are older than 40 years. AIP is similar in presentation to the acute respiratory distress syndrome (ARDS) (Chap. 268) and probably corresponds to the subset of cases of idiopathic ARDS. The onset is usually abrupt in a previously healthy individual. A prodromal illness, usually lasting 7–14 days before presentation, is common. Fever, cough, and dyspnea are common manifestations at presentation. Diffuse, bilateral, air-space opacification is present on the chest radiograph. HRCT scans show bilateral, patchy, symmetric areas of ground-glass attenuation. Bilateral areas of air-space consolidation also may be present. A predominantly subpleural distribution may be seen. The diagnosis of AIP requires the presence of a clinical syndrome of idiopathic ARDS and pathologic confirmation of organizing diffuse alveolar damage. Therefore, lung biopsy is required to confirm the diagnosis. Most patients have moderate to severe hypoxemia and develop respiratory failure. Mechanical ventilation is often required. The mortality rate is high (>60%), with most patients dying within 6 months of presentation. Recurrences have been reported. However, those who recover often have substantial improvement in lung function. The main treatment is supportive. It is not clear that glucocorticoid therapy is effective.

CRYPTOGENIC ORGANIZING PNEUMONIA

COP is a clinicopathologic syndrome of unknown etiology. The onset is usually in the fifth and sixth decades. The presentation may be of a flulike illness with cough, fever, malaise, fatigue, and weight loss. Inspiratory crackles are frequently present on examination. Pulmonary function is usually impaired, with a restrictive defect and arterial hypoxemia being most common. The roentgenographic manifestations are distinctive, revealing bilateral, patchy, or diffuse alveolar opacities in the presence of normal lung volume. Recurrent and migratory pulmonary opacities are common. HRCT shows areas of air-space consolidation, ground-glass opacities, small nodular opacities, and bronchial wall thickening and dilation. These changes occur more frequently in the periphery of the lung and in the lower lung zone. Lung biopsy shows granulation tissue within small airways, alveolar ducts, and airspaces, with chronic inflammation in the surrounding alveoli. Glucocorticoid therapy induces clinical recovery in two-thirds of patients. A few patients have rapidly progressive courses with fatal outcomes despite glucocorticoids.

Foci of organizing pneumonia is a nonspecific reaction to lung injury found adjacent to other pathologic processes or as a component of other primary pulmonary disorders [e.g., cryptococcosis, granulomatosis with polyangiitis (Wegener's), lymphoma, hypersensitivity pneumonitis, and eosinophilic pneumonia]. Consequently, the clinician must carefully reevaluate any patient found to have this histopathologic lesion to rule out these possibilities.

ILD ASSOCIATED WITH CIGARETTE SMOKING

Desquamative interstitial pneumonia

DIP is a rare but distinct clinical and pathologic entity found almost exclusively in cigarette smokers. The histologic hallmark is the extensive accumulation of macrophages in intraalveolar spaces with minimal interstitial fibrosis. The peak incidence is in the fourth and fifth decades. Most patients present with dyspnea and cough. Lung function testing shows a restrictive pattern with reduced DL_{CO} and arterial hypoxemia. The chest x-ray and HRCT scans usually show diffuse hazy opacities. Clinical recognition of DIP is important because the process is associated with a better prognosis (10-year survival rate is ~70%) in response to smoking cessation. There are no clear data showing that systemic glucocorticoids are effective in DIP.

Respiratory bronchiolitis–associated ILD

Respiratory bronchiolitis–associated ILD (RB-ILD) is considered to be a subset of DIP and is characterized by the accumulation of macrophages in peribronchial alveoli. The clinical presentation is similar to that of DIP. Crackles are often heard on chest examination and occur throughout inspiration; sometimes they continue into expiration. The process is best seen on HRCT lung scanning, which shows bronchial wall thickening, centrilobular nodules, ground-glass opacity, and emphysema with air trapping. RB-ILD appears to resolve in most patients after smoking cessation alone.

Pulmonary Langerhans cell histiocytosis

This is a rare, smoking-related, diffuse lung disease that primarily affects men between the ages of 20 and 40 years. The clinical presentation varies from an asymptomatic state to a rapidly progressive condition. The most common clinical manifestations at presentation are cough, dyspnea, chest pain, weight loss, and fever. Pneumothorax occurs in ~25% of patients. Hemoptysis and diabetes insipidus are rare manifestations. The radiographic features vary with the stage of the disease. The combination of ill-defined or stellate nodules (2–10 mm in diameter), reticular or nodular opacities, bizarre-shaped upper zone cysts, preservation of lung volume, and sparing of the costophrenic angles are characteristics of PLCH. HRCT that reveals a combination of nodules and thin-walled cysts is virtually diagnostic of PLCH. The most common pulmonary function abnormality is a markedly reduced DL_{CO}, although varying degrees of restrictive disease, airflow limitation, and diminished exercise capacity may occur. The characteristic histopathologic finding in PLCH is the presence of nodular sclerosing lesions that contain Langerhans cells accompanied by mixed cellular infiltrates. The nodular lesions are poorly defined and are distributed in a bronchiolocentric fashion with intervening normal lung parenchyma. As the disease advances, fibrosis progresses to involve adjacent lung tissue, leading to pericicatricial air space enlargement, which accounts for the concomitant cystic changes. Discontinuance of smoking is the key treatment, resulting in clinical improvement in one-third of patients. Most patients with PLCH experience persistent or progressive disease. Death due to respiratory failure occurs in ~10% of patients.

ILD ASSOCIATED WITH CONNECTIVE TISSUE DISORDERS

Clinical findings suggestive of a CTD (musculoskeletal pain, weakness, fatigue, fever, joint pain or swelling, photosensitivity, Raynaud's phenomenon, pleuritis, dry eyes, dry mouth) should be sought in any patient with ILD. The CTDs may be difficult to rule out since the pulmonary manifestations occasionally precede the more typical systemic manifestations by months or years. The most common form of pulmonary involvement is the nonspecific interstitial pneumonia histopathologic pattern. However, determining the precise nature of lung involvement in most of the CTDs is difficult due to the high incidence of lung involvement caused by disease-associated complications of esophageal dysfunction (predisposing to aspiration and secondary infections), respiratory muscle weakness (atelectasis and secondary infections), complications of therapy (opportunistic infections), and associated malignancies.

Progressive systemic sclerosis (PSS)

(See also Chap. 323) Clinical evidence of ILD is present in about one-half of patients with PSS, and pathologic evidence in three-quarters. Pulmonary function tests show a restrictive pattern and impaired diffusing capacity, often before any clinical or radiographic evidence of lung disease appears. Pulmonary vascular disease alone or in association with pulmonary fibrosis, pleuritis, or recurrent aspiration pneumonitis is strikingly resistant to current modes of therapy.

Rheumatoid arthritis

(See also Chap. 321) ILD associated with RA is more common in men. Pulmonary manifestations of RA include pleurisy with or without effusion, ILD in up to 20% of cases, necrobiotic nodules (nonpneumoconiotic intrapulmonary rheumatoid nodules) with or without cavities, Caplan's syndrome (rheumatoid pneumoconiosis), pulmonary hypertension secondary to rheumatoid pulmonary vasculitis, organized pneumonia, and upper airway obstruction due to crico-arytenoid arthritis.

Systemic lupus erythematosus

(See also Chap. 319) Lung disease is a common complication in SLE. Pleuritis with or without effusion is the most common pulmonary manifestation. Other lung manifestations include the following: atelectasis, diaphragmatic dysfunction with loss of lung volumes, pulmonary vascular disease, pulmonary hemorrhage, uremic pulmonary edema, infectious pneumonia, and organized pneumonia. Acute lupus pneumonitis characterized by pulmonary capillaritis leading to alveolar hemorrhage is uncommon. Chronic, progressive ILD is uncommon. It is important to exclude pulmonary infection. Although pleuropulmonary involvement may not be evident clinically, pulmonary function testing, particularly DL_{CO}, reveals abnormalities in many patients with SLE.

Polymyositis and dermatomyositis (PM/DM)

(See also Chap. 388) ILD occurs in ~10% of patients with PM/DM. Diffuse reticular or nodular opacities with or without an alveolar component occur radiographically, with a predilection for the lung bases. ILD occurs more commonly in the subgroup of patients with an anti-Jo-1 antibody that is directed to histidyl tRNA synthetase. Weakness of respiratory muscles contributing to aspiration pneumonia may be present. A rapidly progressive illness characterized by diffuse alveolar damage may cause respiratory failure.

Sjögren's syndrome

(See also Chap. 324) General dryness and lack of airway secretion cause the major problems of hoarseness, cough, and bronchitis. Lymphocytic interstitial pneumonitis, lymphoma, pseudolymphoma, bronchiolitis, and bronchiolitis obliterans are associated with this condition. Lung biopsy is frequently required to establish a precise pulmonary diagnosis. Glucocorticoids have been used in the management of ILD associated with Sjögren's syndrome with some degree of clinical success.

DRUG-INDUCED ILD

Many classes of drugs have the potential to induce diffuse ILD, which is manifest most commonly as exertional dyspnea and nonproductive cough. A detailed history of the medications taken by the patient is needed to identify drug-induced disease, including over-the-counter medications, oily nose drops, and petroleum products (mineral oil). In most cases, the pathogenesis is unknown, although a combination of direct toxic effects of the drug (or its metabolite) and indirect inflammatory and immunologic events are likely. The onset of the illness may be abrupt and fulminant, or it may be insidious, extending over weeks to months. The drug may have been taken for several years before a reaction develops (e.g., amiodarone), or the lung disease may occur weeks to years after the drug has been discontinued (e.g., carmustine). The extent and severity of disease are usually dose-related. Treatment consists of discontinuation of any possible offending drug and supportive care.

EOSINOPHILIC PNEUMONIA

(See Chap. 255)

PULMONARY ALVEOLAR PROTEINOSIS (PAP)

Although not strictly an ILD, PAP resembles and is therefore considered with these conditions. It has been proposed that a defect in macrophage function, more specifically an impaired ability to process surfactant, may play a role in the pathogenesis of PAP. This diffuse disease is characterized by the accumulation of an amorphous, periodic acid–Schiff-positive lipoproteinaceous material in the distal air spaces. There is little or no lung inflammation, and the underlying lung architecture is preserved. PAP is an autoimmune disease with a neutralizing antibody of immunoglobulin G isotype against granulocyte-macrophage colony-stimulating factor (GM-CSF). These findings suggest that neutralization of GM-CSF bioactivity by the antibody causes dysfunction of alveolar macrophages, which results in reduced surfactant clearance. There are three distinct classes of PAP: acquired (>90% of all cases), congenital, and secondary. *Congenital PAP* is transmitted in an autosomal recessive manner and is caused by homozygosity for a frameshift mutation (121ins2) in the *SP-B* gene, which leads to an unstable SP-B mRNA, reduced protein levels, and *secondary disturbances of SP-C processing. Secondary PAP* is rare among adults and is caused by lysinuric protein intolerance, acute silicosis and other inhalational syndromes, immunodeficiency disorders, and malignancies (almost exclusively of hematopoietic origin) and hematopoietic disorders.

The typical age of presentation is 30–50 years, and males predominate. The clinical presentation is usually insidious and is manifested by progressive exertional dyspnea, fatigue, weight loss, and low-grade fever. A nonproductive cough is common, but occasionally expectoration of "chunky" gelatinous material may occur. Polycythemia, hypergammaglobulinemia, and increased LDH levels are common. Markedly elevated serum levels of lung surfactant proteins A and D have been found in PAP. In the absence of any known secondary cause of PAP, an elevated serum anti-GM-CSF titer is highly sensitive and specific for the diagnosis of acquired PAP. BAL fluid levels of anti-GM-CSF antibodies correlate better with the severity of PAP than do serum titers. Radiographically, bilateral symmetric alveolar opacities located centrally in middle and lower lung zones result in a "bat-wing" distribution. HRCT shows a ground-glass opacification and thickened intralobular structures and interlobular septa. Whole-lung lavage(s) through a double-lumen endotracheal tube provides relief to many patients with dyspnea or progressive hypoxemia and also may provide long-term benefit.

PULMONARY LYMPHANGIOLEIOMYOMATOSIS

Pulmonary LAM is a rare condition that afflicts premenopausal women and should be suspected in young women with "emphysema," recurrent pneumothorax, or chylous pleural effusion. It is often misdiagnosed as asthma or chronic obstructive pulmonary disease. Pathologically, LAM is characterized by the proliferation of atypical pulmonary interstitial smooth muscle and cyst formation. The immature-appearing smooth-muscle cells react with monoclonal antibody HMB45, which recognizes a 100-kDa glycoprotein (gp100) originally found in human melanoma cells. Whites are affected much more commonly than are members of other racial groups. The disease accelerates during pregnancy and abates after oophorectomy. Common complaints at presentation are dyspnea, cough, and chest pain. Hemoptysis may be life threatening. Spontaneous pneumothorax occurs in 50% of patients; it may be bilateral and necessitate pleurodesis. Meningioma and renal angiomyolipomas (hamartomas), characteristic findings in the genetic disorder tuberous sclerosis, are also common in patients with LAM. Chylothorax, chyloperitoneum (chylous ascites), chyluria, and chylopericardium are other complications. Pulmonary function testing usually reveals an obstructive or mixed obstructive-restrictive pattern, and gas exchange is often abnormal. HRCT shows thin-walled cysts surrounded by normal lung without zonal predominance. Progression is common, with a median survival of 8–10 years from diagnosis. No therapy is of proven benefit in LAM. Progesterone (10 mg/d), luteinizing hormone–releasing hormone analogues, and sirolimus have been used. Oophorectomy is no longer recommended, and estrogen-containing drugs should be discontinued. Lung transplantation offers the only hope for cure despite reports of recurrent disease in the transplanted lung.

SYNDROMES OF ILD WITH DIFFUSE ALVEOLAR HEMORRHAGE

Injury to arterioles, venules, and the alveolar septal (alveolar wall or interstitial) capillaries can result in hemoptysis secondary to disruption of the alveolar-capillary basement membrane. This results in bleeding into the alveolar spaces, which characterizes DAH. Pulmonary capillaritis, characterized by a neutrophilic infiltration of the alveolar septae, may lead to necrosis of these structures, loss of capillary structural integrity, and the pouring of red blood cells into the alveolar space. Fibrinoid necrosis of the interstitium and red blood cells within the interstitial space are sometimes seen. Bland pulmonary hemorrhage (i.e., DAH without inflammation of the alveolar structures) also may occur.

The clinical onset is often abrupt, with cough, fever, and dyspnea. Severe respiratory distress requiring ventilatory support may be evident at initial presentation. Although hemoptysis is expected, it can be absent at the time of presentation in one-third of the cases. For patients without hemoptysis, new alveolar opacities, a falling hemoglobin level, and hemorrhagic BAL fluid point to the diagnosis. The chest radiograph is nonspecific and most commonly shows new patchy or diffuse alveolar opacities. Recurrent episodes of DAH may lead to pulmonary fibrosis, resulting in interstitial opacities on the chest radiograph. An elevated white blood cell count and falling hematocrit are common. Evidence for impaired renal function caused by focal segmental necrotizing glomerulonephritis, usually with crescent formation, also may be present.

Varying degrees of hypoxemia may occur and are often severe enough to require ventilatory support. DL_{CO} may be increased, resulting from the increased hemoglobin within the alveoli compartment. Evaluation of either lung or renal tissue by immunofluorescent techniques indicates an absence of immune complexes (pauci-immune) in granulomatosis with polyangiitis (Wegener's), microscopic polyangiitis pauci-immune glomerulonephritis, and isolated pulmonary capillaritis. A granular pattern is found in the CTDs, particularly SLE, and a characteristic linear deposition is found in Goodpasture's syndrome. Granular deposition of IgA-containing immune complexes is present in Henoch-Schönlein purpura.

The mainstay of therapy for the DAH associated with systemic vasculitis, CTD, Goodpasture's syndrome, and isolated pulmonary capillaritis is IV methylprednisolone, 0.5–2 g daily in divided doses for up to 5 days, followed by a gradual tapering, and then maintenance on an oral preparation. Prompt initiation of therapy is important, particularly in the face of renal insufficiency, since early initiation of therapy has the best chance of preserving renal function. The decision to start other immunosuppressive therapy (cyclophosphamide or azathioprine) acutely depends on the severity of illness.

Goodpasture's syndrome

Pulmonary hemorrhage and glomerulonephritis are features in most patients with this disease. Autoantibodies to renal glomerular and lung alveolar basement membranes are present. This syndrome can present and recur as DAH without an associated glomerulonephritis. In such cases, circulating anti-basement membrane antibody is often absent, and the only way to establish the diagnosis is by demonstrating linear immunofluorescence in lung tissue. The underlying histology may be bland hemorrhage or DAH associated with capillaritis. Plasmapheresis has been recommended as adjunctive treatment.

INHERITED DISORDERS ASSOCIATED WITH ILD

Pulmonary opacities and respiratory symptoms typical of ILD can develop in related family members and in several inherited diseases. These diseases include the phakomatoses, tuberous sclerosis and neurofibromatosis (Chap. 379), and the lysosomal storage diseases, Niemann-Pick disease and Gaucher disease (Chap. 361). The Hermansky-Pudlak syndrome is an autosomal recessive disorder in which granulomatous colitis and ILD may occur. It is characterized by oculocutaneous albinism, bleeding diathesis secondary to platelet dysfunction, and the accumulation of a chromolipid, lipofuscin material in cells of the reticuloendothelial system. A fibrotic pattern is found on lung biopsy, but the alveolar macrophages may contain cytoplasmic ceroid-like inclusions.

ILD WITH A GRANULOMATOUS RESPONSE IN LUNG TISSUE OR VASCULAR STRUCTURES

Inhalation of organic dusts, which cause hypersensitivity pneumonitis, or of inorganic dust, such as silica, which elicits a granulomatous inflammatory reaction leading to ILD, produces diseases of known etiology (Table 261-1) that are discussed in Chaps. 255 and 256. Sarcoidosis (Chap. 329) is prominent among granulomatous diseases of unknown cause in which ILD is an important feature.

Granulomatous vasculitides

(See also Chap. 326) The granulomatous vasculitides are characterized by pulmonary angiitis (i.e., inflammation and necrosis of blood vessels) with associated granuloma formation (i.e., infiltrates of lymphocytes, plasma cells, epithelioid cells, or histiocytes, with or without the presence of multinucleated giant cells, sometimes with tissue necrosis). The lungs are almost always involved, although any organ system may be affected. Granulomatosis with polyangiitis (Wegener's) and allergic angiitis and granulomatosis (Churg-Strauss syndrome) primarily affect the lung but are associated with a systemic vasculitis as well. The granulomatous vasculitides generally limited to the lung include necrotizing sarcoid granulomatosis and benign lymphocytic angiitis and granulomatosis. Granulomatous infection and pulmonary angiitis due to irritating embolic material (e.g., talc) are important known causes of pulmonary vasculitis.

LYMPHOCYTIC INFILTRATIVE DISORDERS

This group of disorders features lymphocyte and plasma cell infiltration of the lung parenchyma. The disorders either are benign or can behave as low-grade lymphomas. Included are angioimmunoblastic lymphadenopathy with dysproteinemia, a rare lymphoproliferative disorder characterized by diffuse lymphadenopathy, fever, hepatosplenomegaly, and hemolytic anemia, with ILD in some cases.

Lymphocytic interstitial pneumonitis

This rare form of ILD occurs in adults, some of whom have an autoimmune disease or dysproteinemia. It has been reported in patients with Sjögren's syndrome and HIV infection.

Lymphomatoid granulomatosis

This multisystem disorder of unknown etiology is an angiocentric malignant (T cell) lymphoma characterized by a polymorphic lymphoid infiltrate, an angiitis, and granulomatosis. Although it may affect virtually any organ, it is most frequently characterized by pulmonary, skin, and central nervous system involvement.

BRONCHOCENTRIC GRANULOMATOSIS

Rather than a specific clinical entity, bronchocentric granulomatosis (BG) is a descriptive histologic term that is applied to an uncommon and nonspecific pathologic response to a variety of airway injuries. There is evidence that BG is caused by a hypersensitivity reaction to *Aspergillus* or other fungi in patients with asthma. About one-half of the patients described have had chronic asthma with severe wheezing and peripheral blood eosinophilia. In patients with asthma, BG probably represents one pathologic manifestation of allergic bronchopulmonary aspergillosis or another allergic mycosis. In patients without asthma, BG has been associated with RA and a variety of infections, including tuberculosis, echinococcosis, histoplasmosis, coccidioidomycosis, and nocardiosis. The chest roentgenogram reveals irregularly shaped nodular or mass lesions with ill-defined margins, which are usually unilateral and solitary, with upper lobe predominance. Glucocorticoids are the treatment of choice, often with an excellent outcome, although recurrences may occur as therapy is tapered or stopped.

GLOBAL CONSIDERATIONS

Limited epidemiologic data exist describing the prevalence or incidence of ILD in the general population. With a few exceptions, e.g., sarcoidosis and certain occupational and environmental exposures, there appear to be no significant differences in the prevalence or incidence of ILD among various populations. For sarcoidosis, there are important environmental, racial, and genetic differences (Chap. 329).

FURTHER READINGS

American Thoracic Society/European Respiratory Society: Idiopathic pulmonary fibrosis: Diagnosis and treatment: International consensus statement. Am J Respir Crit Care Med 161:646, 2000

———: International multidisciplinary consensus classification of the idiopathic interstitial pneumonias. Am J Respir Crit Care Med 165:277, 2002

Collard HR et al: Acute exacerbations of idiopathic pulmonary fibrosis. Am J Respir Crit Care Med 176:636, 2007

El-Zammar OA, Katzenstein AL: Pathological diagnosis of granulomatous lung disease: A review. Histopathology 50:289, 2007

Kinder BW et al: Idiopathic nonspecific interstitial pneumonia: Lung manifestation of undifferentiated connective tissue disease? Am J Respir Crit Care Med176:691, 2007

King TE Jr: Clinical advances in the diagnosis and therapy of the interstitial lung diseases. Am J Respir Crit Care Med 172:268, 2005

Klingsberg RC et al: Current clinical trials for the treatment of idiopathic pulmonary fibrosis. Respirology 15:19, 2010

Kottmann RM et al: Determinants of initiation and progression of idiopathic pulmonary fibrosis. Respirology 14:917, 2009

Raghu G et al: An Official TS/ERS/JRS/ALAT Statement: Idiopathic Pulmonary Fibrosis: Evidence-based Guidelines for Diagnosis and Management. Am J Respir Crit Care Med 183:788, 2011

Selman M et al: Idiopathic pulmonary fibrosis: Prevailing and evolving hypotheses about its pathogenesis and implications for therapy. Ann Intern Med 134:136, 2001

Seymour JF, Presneill JJ: Pulmonary alveolar proteinosis: Progress in the first 44 years. Am J Respir Crit Care Med 166:215, 2002

Travis WD et al: Idiopathic nonspecific interstitial pneumonia: Report of an American Thoracic Society project. Am J Respir Crit Care Med 177:1338, 2008

Wells AU et al: Interstitial lung disease guideline. Thorax 63:v1, 2008

CHAPTER 262 Deep Venous Thrombosis and Pulmonary Thromboembolism

Samuel Z. Goldhaber

EPIDEMIOLOGY

Venous thromboembolism (VTE), which encompasses deep venous thrombosis (DVT) and pulmonary embolism (PE), is one of the three major cardiovascular causes of death, along with myocardial infarction and stroke. VTE can cause death from PE or, among survivors, chronic thromboembolic pulmonary hypertension and postphlebitic syndrome. The U.S. Surgeon General has declared that PE is the most common preventable cause of death among hospitalized patients. Medicare has labeled PE and DVT occurring after total hip or knee replacement as unacceptable "never events" and no longer reimburses hospitals for the incremental expenses associated with treating this postoperative complication. New nonprofit organizations have begun educating health care professionals and the public on the medical consequences of VTE, along with risk factors and warning signs.

Between 100,000 and 300,000 VTE-related deaths occur annually in the United States. Mortality rates and length of hospital stay are decreasing as charges for hospital care increase. Approximately three of four symptomatic VTE events occur in the community, and the remainder are hospital acquired. Approximately 14 million (M) hospitalized patients are at moderate to high risk for VTE in the United States annually: 6 M major surgery patients and 8 M medical patients with comorbidities such as heart failure, cancer, and stroke. The prophylaxis paradigm has changed from voluntary to mandatory compliance with guidelines to prevent VTE among hospitalized patients. With an estimated 370,000 PE-related deaths annually in Europe, the projected direct cost for VTE-associated care exceeds 3 billion euros per year. In Japan, as the lifestyle becomes more westernized, the rate of VTE appears to be increasing.

The long-term effects of nonfatal VTE lower the quality of life. Chronic thromboembolic pulmonary hypertension is often disabling and causes breathlessness. A late effect of DVT is *postphlebitic syndrome*, which eventually occurs in more than one-half of DVT patients. Postphlebitic syndrome (also known as *postthrombotic syndrome* or *chronic venous insufficiency*) is a delayed complication of DVT that causes the venous valves of the leg to become incompetent and exude interstitial fluid. Patients complain of chronic ankle or calf swelling and leg aching, especially after prolonged standing. In its most severe form, postphlebitic syndrome causes skin ulceration, especially in the medial malleolus of the leg. There is no effective medical therapy for this condition.

Prothrombotic states

Thrombophilia contributes to the risk of venous thrombosis. The two most common autosomal dominant genetic mutations are factor V Leiden, which causes resistance to activated protein C (which inactivates clotting factors V and VIII), and the prothrombin gene mutation, which increases the plasma prothrombin concentration (Chaps. 58 and 117). Antithrombin, protein C, and protein S are naturally occurring coagulation inhibitors. Deficiencies of these inhibitors are associated with VTE but are rare. Hyperhomocysteinemia can increase the risk of VTE, but lowering the homocysteine level with folate, vitamin B_6, or vitamin B_{12} does not reduce the incidence of VTE. Antiphospholipid antibody syndrome is the most common acquired cause of thrombophilia and is associated with venous or arterial thrombosis. Other common predisposing factors include cancer, systemic arterial hypertension, chronic obstructive pulmonary disease, long-haul air travel, air pollution, obesity, cigarette smoking, eating large amounts of red meat, oral contraceptives, pregnancy, postmenopausal hormone replacement, surgery, and trauma.

PATHOPHYSIOLOGY

Embolization

When venous thrombi are dislodged from their site of formation, they embolize to the pulmonary arterial circulation or, paradoxically, to the arterial circulation through a patent foramen ovale or atrial septal defect. About one-half of patients with pelvic vein thrombosis or proximal leg DVT develop PE, which is often asymptomatic. Isolated calf vein thrombi pose a much lower risk of PE but are the most common source of paradoxical embolism. These tiny thrombi can traverse a patent foramen ovale or atrial septal defect, unlike larger, more proximal leg thrombi. With increased use of chronic indwelling central venous catheters for hyperalimentation and chemotherapy, as well as more frequent insertion of permanent pacemakers and internal cardiac defibrillators, upper extremity venous thrombosis is becoming a more common problem. These thrombi rarely embolize and cause PE.

Physiology

The most common gas exchange abnormalities are hypoxemia (decreased arterial P_{O_2}) and an increased alveolar-arterial O_2 tension gradient, which represents the inefficiency of O_2 transfer across the lungs. Anatomic dead space increases because breathed gas does not enter gas exchange units of the lung. Physiologic dead space increases because ventilation to gas exchange units exceeds venous blood flow through the pulmonary capillaries.

Other pathophysiologic abnormalities include the following:

1. *Increased pulmonary vascular resistance* due to vascular obstruction or platelet secretion of vasoconstricting neurohumoral agents such as serotonin. Release of vasoactive mediators can produce ventilation-perfusion mismatching at sites remote from the embolus, thereby accounting for a potential discordance between a small PE and a large alveolar-arterial O_2 gradient.
2. *Impaired gas exchange* due to increased alveolar dead space from vascular obstruction, hypoxemia from alveolar hypoventilation relative to perfusion in the nonobstructed lung, right-to-left shunting, and impaired carbon monoxide transfer due to loss of gas exchange surface.
3. *Alveolar hyperventilation* due to reflex stimulation of irritant receptors.
4. *Increased airway resistance* due to constriction of airways distal to the bronchi.
5. *Decreased pulmonary compliance* due to lung edema, lung hemorrhage, or loss of surfactant.

Right-ventricular (RV) dysfunction

Progressive right heart failure is the usual cause of death from PE. As pulmonary vascular resistance increases, RV wall tension rises and causes further RV dilation and dysfunction. RV contraction continues even after the left ventricle (LV) starts relaxing at end-systole. Consequently, the interventricular septum bulges into and compresses an intrinsically normal left ventricle. Diastolic LV impairment develops, attributable to septal displacement, and results in reduced LV distensibility and impaired LV filling during diastole. Increased RV wall tension also compresses the right coronary artery, diminishes subendocardial perfusion, limits myocardial oxygen supply, and may precipitate myocardial ischemia and RV infarction. Underfilling of the LV may lead to a fall in left-ventricular cardiac output and systemic arterial pressure, thereby provoking myocardial ischemia due to compromised coronary artery perfusion. Eventually, circulatory collapse and death may ensue.

DIAGNOSIS

Clinical evaluation

VTE mimics other illnesses, and PE is known as "the Great Masquerader," making diagnosis difficult. Occult PE is especially hard to detect when it occurs concomitantly with overt heart failure or pneumonia. In such circumstances, clinical improvement often fails to occur despite standard medical treatment of the

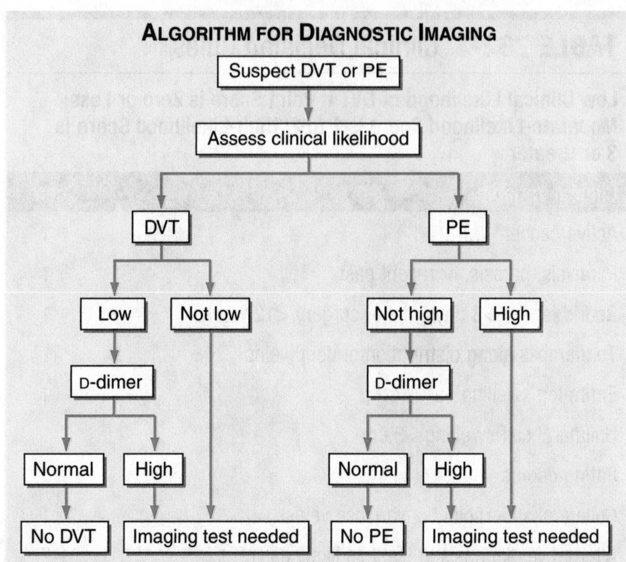

Figure 262-1 How to decide whether diagnostic imaging is needed. For assessment of clinical likelihood, see Table 262-1.

concomitant illness. This scenario is a clinical clue to the possible coexistence of PE.

For patients who have DVT, the most common history is a cramp in the lower calf that persists for several days and becomes more uncomfortable as time progresses. For patients who have PE, the most common history is unexplained breathlessness.

In evaluating patients with possible VTE, the initial task is to decide on the clinical likelihood of the disorder. Patients with a low likelihood of DVT or a low-to-moderate likelihood of PE can undergo initial diagnostic evaluation with D-dimer testing alone (see "Blood tests") without obligatory imaging tests (Fig. 262-1). If the D-dimer is abnormally elevated, imaging tests are the next step.

Point score methods are useful for estimating the clinical likelihood of DVT and PE (Table 262-1).

Clinical syndromes

The differential diagnosis is critical because not all leg pain is due to DVT and not all dyspnea is due to PE (Table 262-2). Sudden, severe calf discomfort suggests a ruptured Baker's cyst. Fever and chills usually herald cellulitis rather than DVT, though DVT may be present concomitantly. Physical findings, if present at all, may consist only of mild palpation discomfort in the lower calf. Massive DVT is much easier to recognize. The patient presents with marked thigh swelling and tenderness during palpation of the common femoral vein. In extreme cases, patients are unable to walk or may require a cane, crutches, or a walker.

If the leg is diffusely edematous, DVT is unlikely. More probable is an acute exacerbation of venous insufficiency due to postphlebitic syndrome. Upper extremity venous thrombosis may present with asymmetry in the supraclavicular fossa or in the circumference of the upper arms. A prominent superficial venous pattern may be evident on the anterior chest wall.

Patients with *massive PE* present with systemic arterial hypotension and usually have anatomically widespread thromboembolism. Those with *moderate to large PE* have RV hypokinesis on echocardiography but normal systemic arterial pressure. Patients with *small to moderate PE* have both normal right heart function and normal systemic arterial pressure. They have an excellent prognosis with adequate anticoagulation.

TABLE 262-1 Clinical Decision Rules

Low Clinical Likelihood of DVT if Point Score Is Zero or Less; Moderate-Likelihood Score Is 1 to 2; High-Likelihood Score Is 3 or Greater

Clinical Variable	Score
Active cancer	1
Paralysis, paresis, or recent cast	1
Bedridden for >3 days; major surgery <12 weeks	1
Tenderness along distribution of deep veins	1
Entire leg swelling	1
Unilateral calf swelling >3 cm	1
Pitting edema	1
Collateral superficial nonvaricose veins	1
Alternative diagnosis at least as likely as DVT	−2

High Clinical Likelihood of PE if Point Score Exceeds 4

Clinical Variable	Score
Signs and symptoms of DVT	3.0
Alternative diagnosis less likely than PE	3.0
Heart rate >100/min	1.5
Immobilization >3 days; surgery within 4 weeks	1.5
Prior PE or DVT	1.5
Hemoptysis	1.0
Cancer	1.0

The presence of *pulmonary infarction* usually indicates a small PE but one that is exquisitely painful because it lodges peripherally, near the innervation of pleural nerves. Pleuritic chest pain is more common with small, peripheral emboli. However, larger, more central PEs can occur concomitantly with peripheral pulmonary infarction.

Nonthrombotic PE may be easily overlooked. Possible etiologies include fat embolism after pelvic or long bone fracture, tumor embolism, bone marrow, and air embolism. Cement embolism and bony fragment embolism can occur after total hip or knee replacement. Intravenous drug users may inject themselves with a wide array of substances that can embolize such as hair, talc, and cotton. *Amniotic fluid embolism* occurs when fetal membranes leak or tear at the placental margin. Pulmonary edema in this syndrome probably is due to alveolar capillary leakage.

Dyspnea is the most common symptom of PE, and tachypnea is the most common sign. Dyspnea, syncope, hypotension, or cyanosis indicates a massive PE, whereas pleuritic pain, cough, or hemoptysis often suggests a small embolism situated distally near the pleura. On physical examination, young and previously healthy individuals may appear anxious but otherwise seem well, even with an anatomically large PE. They may have dyspnea only with moderate exertion. They often lack "classic" signs such as tachycardia, low-grade fever, neck vein distention, and an accentuated pulmonic component of the second heart sound. Sometimes paradoxical bradycardia occurs.

TABLE 262-2 Differential Diagnosis

DVT
Ruptured Baker's cyst
Cellulitis
Postphlebitic syndrome/venous insufficiency
PE
Pneumonia, asthma, chronic obstructive pulmonary disease
Congestive heart failure
Pericarditis
Pleurisy: "viral syndrome," costochondritis, musculoskeletal discomfort
Rib fracture, pneumothorax
Acute coronary syndrome
Anxiety

Nonimaging diagnostic modalities

Nonimaging tests are best utilized in combination with clinical likelihood assessment of DVT or PE (Fig. 262-1).

Blood tests The quantitative *plasma* D*-dimer enzyme-linked immunosorbent assay (ELISA)* rises in the presence of DVT or PE because of the breakdown of fibrin by plasmin. Elevation of D-dimer indicates endogenous although often clinically ineffective thrombolysis. The sensitivity of the D-dimer is >80% for DVT (including isolated calf DVT) and >95% for PE. The D-dimer is less sensitive for DVT than for PE because the DVT thrombus size is smaller. The D-dimer is a useful "rule out" test. More than 95% of patients with a normal (<500 ng/mL) D-dimer do not have PE. The D-dimer assay is not specific. Levels increase in patients with myocardial infarction, pneumonia, sepsis, cancer, and the postoperative state and those in the second or third trimester of pregnancy. Therefore, D-dimer rarely has a useful role among hospitalized patients, because levels are frequently elevated due to systemic illness.

Contrary to classic teaching, *arterial blood gases* lack diagnostic utility for PE, even though both P_{O_2} and P_{CO_2} often decrease. Among patients suspected of having PE, neither the room air arterial P_{O_2} nor calculation of the alveolar-arterial O_2 gradient can reliably differentiate or triage patients who actually have PE at angiography.

Elevated cardiac biomarkers Serum troponin and plasma heart-type fatty acid–binding protein levels increase because of RV microinfarction. Myocardial stretch results in elevation of brain natriuretic peptide or NT-pro-brain natriuretic peptide. Elevated cardiac biomarkers predict an increase in major complications and mortality from PE.

Electrocardiogram The most frequently cited abnormality, in addition to sinus tachycardia, is the S1Q3T3 sign: an S wave in lead I, a Q wave in lead III, and an inverted T wave in lead III (Chap. 228). This finding is relatively specific but insensitive. Perhaps the most common abnormality is T-wave inversion in leads V_1 to V_4.

Noninvasive imaging modalities

Venous ultrasonography Ultrasonography of the deep venous system (Table 262-3) relies on loss of vein compressibility as the primary criterion for DVT. When a normal vein is imaged in cross-section, it readily collapses with gentle manual pressure from the ultrasound transducer. This creates the illusion of a "wink." With acute DVT, the vein loses its compressibility because of passive distention by acute thrombus. The diagnosis of acute DVT is even more secure when thrombus is directly visualized. It appears homogeneous and has low echogenicity (Fig. 262-2). The vein itself often appears mildly dilated, and collateral channels may be absent.

TABLE 262-3 Ultrasonography of the Deep Leg Veins

Criteria for Establishing the Diagnosis of Acute DVT
Lack of vein compressibility (principal criterion)
Vein does not "wink" when gently compressed in cross-section
Failure to appose walls of vein due to passive distention
Direct Visualization of Thrombus
Homogeneous
Low echogenicity
Abnormal Doppler Flow Dynamics
Normal response: calf compression augments Doppler flow signal and confirms vein patency proximal and distal to Doppler
Abnormal response: flow blunted rather than augmented with calf compression

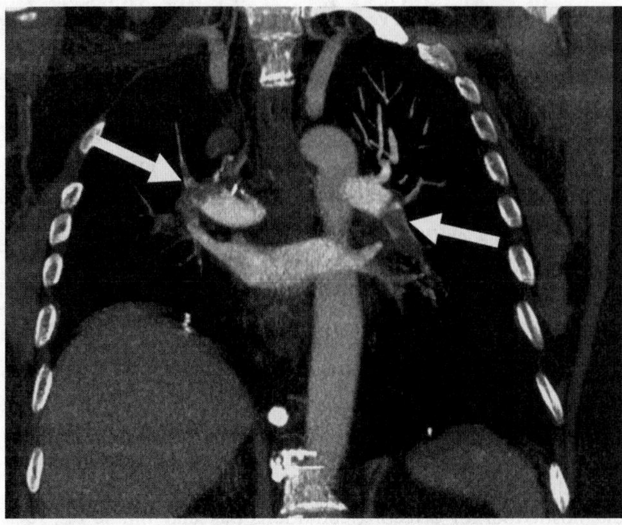

Figure 262-3 **Large bilateral proximal PE** on a coronal chest CT image in a 54-year-old man with lung cancer and brain metastases. He had developed sudden onset of chest heaviness and shortness of breath while at home. There are filling defects in the main and segmental pulmonary arteries bilaterally (*white arrows*). Only the left upper lobe segmental artery is free of thrombus.

Venous flow dynamics can be examined with Doppler imaging. Normally, manual calf compression causes augmentation of the Doppler flow pattern. Loss of normal respiratory variation is caused by an obstructing DVT or by any obstructive process within the pelvis. Because DVT and PE are so closely related and are both treated with anticoagulation (see "Treatment Deep Venous Thrombosis") confirmed DVT is usually an adequate surrogate for PE. In contrast, a normal venous ultrasound does not exclude PE. About one-half of patients with PE have no imaging evidence of DVT, probably because the clot already has embolized to the lung or is in the pelvic veins, where ultrasonography is usually inadequate. In patients without DVT, the ultrasound examination may identify other reasons for leg discomfort, such as a Baker's cyst (also known as a popliteal or synovial cyst) or a hematoma. For patients with a technically poor or nondiagnostic venous ultrasound, one should consider alternative imaging modalities for DVT, such as computed tomography (CT) and magnetic resonance imaging.

Chest roentgenography A normal or nearly normal chest x-ray often occurs in PE. Well-established abnormalities include focal oligemia (Westermark's sign), a peripheral wedged-shaped density

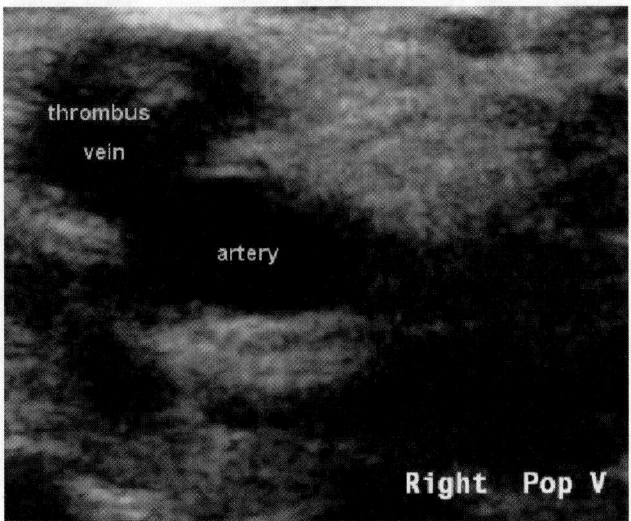

Figure 262-2 **Acute popliteal DVT on venous ultrasound** in a 56-year-old man receiving chemotherapy for lung cancer.

above the diaphragm (Hampton's hump), and an enlarged right descending pulmonary artery (Palla's sign).

Chest CT Computed tomography of the chest with intravenous contrast is the principal imaging test for the diagnosis of PE (Fig. 262-3). Multidetector-row spiral CT acquires all chest images with ≤1 mm of resolution during a short breath hold. This generation of CT scanners can image small peripheral emboli. Sixth-order branches can be visualized with resolution superior to that of conventional invasive contrast pulmonary angiography. The CT scan also obtains excellent images of the RV and LV and can be used for risk stratification along with its use as a diagnostic tool. In patients with PE, RV enlargement on chest CT indicates an increased likelihood of death within the next 30 days compared with PE patients who have normal RV size on chest CT. When imaging is continued below the chest to the knee, pelvic and proximal leg DVT also can be diagnosed by CT scanning. In patients without PE, the lung parenchymal images may establish alternative diagnoses not apparent on chest x-ray that explain the presenting symptoms and signs such as pneumonia, emphysema, pulmonary fibrosis, pulmonary mass, and aortic pathology. Sometimes asymptomatic early-stage lung cancer is diagnosed incidentally.

Lung scanning Lung scanning has become a second-line diagnostic test for PE, used mostly for patients who cannot tolerate intravenous contrast. Small particulate aggregates of albumin labeled with a gamma-emitting radionuclide are injected intravenously and are trapped in the pulmonary capillary bed. The perfusion scan defect indicates absent or decreased blood flow, possibly due to PE. Ventilation scans, obtained with a radiolabeled inhaled gas such as xenon or krypton, improve the specificity of the perfusion scan. Abnormal ventilation scans indicate abnormal nonventilated lung, thereby providing possible explanations for perfusion defects other than acute PE, such as asthma and chronic obstructive pulmonary disease. A high-probability scan for PE is defined as one that indicates two or more segmental perfusion defects in the presence of normal ventilation.

The diagnosis of PE is very unlikely in patients with normal and nearly normal scans but is about 90% certain in patients with high-probability scans. Unfortunately, most patients have nondiagnostic scans, and fewer than one-half of patients with angiographically confirmed PE have a high probability scan. As many as 40% of patients with high clinical suspicion for PE and "low-probability" scans do, in fact, have PE at angiography.

Magnetic resonance (MR) (contrast-enhanced) When ultrasound is equivocal, MR venography with gadolinium contrast is an excellent imaging modality to diagnose DVT. MR imaging should be considered for suspected VTE patients with renal insufficiency or contrast dye allergy. MR pulmonary angiography may detect large proximal PE but is not reliable for smaller segmental and subsegmental PE.

Echocardiography Echocardiography is *not* a reliable diagnostic imaging tool for acute PE because most patients with PE have normal echocardiograms. However, echocardiography is a very useful diagnostic tool for detecting conditions that may mimic PE, such as acute myocardial infarction, pericardial tamponade, and aortic dissection.

Transthoracic echocardiography rarely images thrombus directly. The best-known indirect sign of PE on transthoracic echocardiography is McConnell's sign: hypokinesis of the RV free wall with normal motion of the RV apex.

One should consider transesophageal echocardiography when CT scanning facilities are not available or when a patient has renal failure or severe contrast allergy that precludes administration of contrast despite premedication with high-dose steroids. This imaging modality can identify saddle, right main, or left main PE.

Invasive diagnostic modalities

Pulmonary angiography Chest CT with contrast (see above) has virtually replaced invasive pulmonary angiography as a diagnostic test. Invasive catheter-based diagnostic testing is reserved for patients with technically unsatisfactory chest CTs and those in whom an interventional procedure such as catheter-directed thrombolysis or embolectomy is planned. A definitive diagnosis of PE depends on visualization of an intraluminal filling defect in more than one projection. Secondary signs of PE include abrupt occlusion ("cut-off") of vessels, segmental oligemia or avascularity, a prolonged arterial phase with slow filling, and tortuous, tapering peripheral vessels.

Contrast phlebography Venous ultrasonography has virtually replaced contrast phlebography as the diagnostic test for suspected DVT.

Integrated diagnostic approach

An integrated diagnostic approach (Fig. 262-1) streamlines the workup of suspected DVT and PE (Fig. 262-4).

TREATMENT Deep Venous Thrombosis

PRIMARY THERAPY VERSUS SECONDARY PREVENTION *Primary therapy* consists of clot dissolution with thrombolysis or removal of PE by embolectomy. Anticoagulation with heparin and warfarin or placement of an inferior vena caval filter constitutes *secondary prevention* of recurrent PE rather than primary therapy.

RISK STRATIFICATION Rapid and accurate risk stratification is critical in determining the optimal treatment strategy. The presence of hemodynamic instability, RV dysfunction, RV enlargement, or elevation of the troponin level due to RV microinfarction can identify high-risk patients. RV hypokinesis on echocardiography, RV enlargement on chest CT, and troponin elevation predict an increased mortality rate from PE.

Primary therapy should be reserved for patients at high risk of an adverse clinical outcome. When RV function remains normal in a hemodynamically stable patient, a good clinical outcome is highly likely with anticoagulation alone (Fig. 262-5).

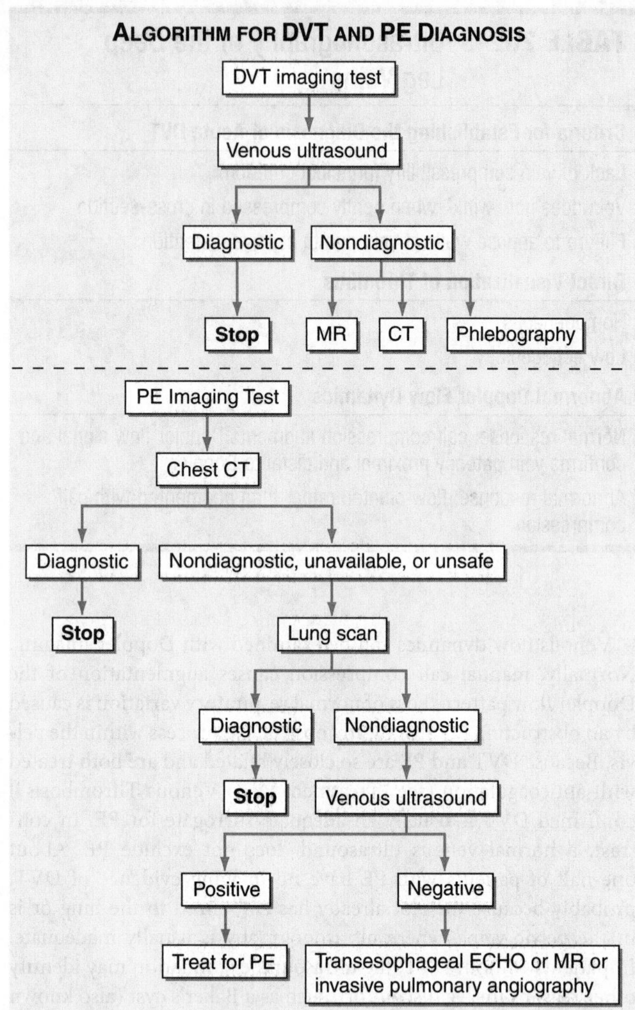

Figure 262-4 Imaging tests to diagnose DVT and PE.

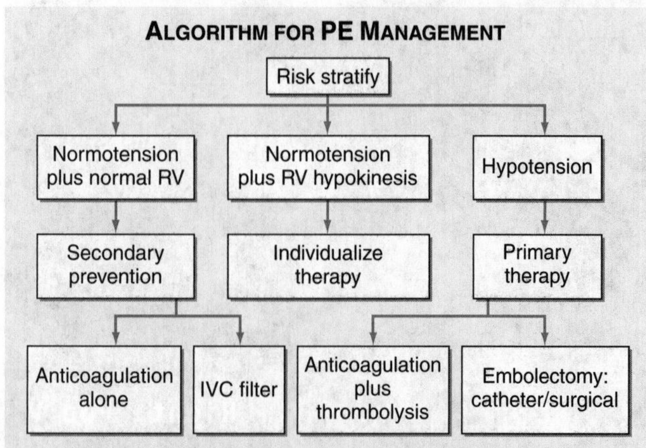

Figure 262-5 Acute management of pulmonary thromboembolism. RV, right ventricular; IVC, inferior vena cava.

TREATMENT Massive Pulmonary Embolism

ANTICOAGULATION Anticoagulation is the foundation for successful treatment of DVT and PE (Table 262-4). Immediately effective anticoagulation is initiated with a parenteral drug: unfractionated heparin (UFH), low-molecular-weight heparin (LMWH), or fondaparinux. One should use a direct thrombin inhibitor—argatroban, lepirudin, or bivalirudin—in patients with proven or suspected heparin-induced thrombocytopenia. Parenteral agents are continued as a transition or "bridge" to stable, long-term anticoagulation with a vitamin K antagonist (exclusively warfarin in the United States). Warfarin requires 5–7 days to achieve a therapeutic effect. During that period, one should overlap the parenteral and oral agents. After 5–7 days of anticoagulation, residual thrombus begins to endothelialize in the vein or pulmonary artery. However, anticoagulants do *not* directly dissolve thrombus that already exists.

Unfractionated Heparin Unfractionated heparin anticoagulates by binding to and accelerating the activity of antithrombin, thus preventing additional thrombus formation and permitting endogenous fibrinolytic mechanisms to lyse clot that already has formed. UFH is dosed to achieve a target activated partial thromboplastin time (aPTT) that is 2–3 times the upper limit of the laboratory normal. This is usually equivalent to an aPTT of 60–80 s. For UFH, a typical intravenous bolus is 5000–10,000 units followed by a continuous infusion of 1000–1500 U/h. Nomograms based on a patient's weight may assist in adjusting the dose of heparin. The most popular nomogram utilizes an initial bolus of 80 U/kg, followed by an initial infusion rate of 18/kg per h.

The major advantage of UFH is its short half-life. This is especially useful if the patient may undergo an invasive procedure such as embolectomy. The major disadvantage of UFH is that achieving the target aPTT is empirical and may require repeated blood sampling and heparin dose adjustment every 4–6 hours. Furthermore, patients are at risk of developing heparin-induced thrombocytopenia.

Low-Molecular-Weight Heparins These fragments of UFH exhibit less binding to plasma proteins and endothelial cells and consequently have greater bioavailability, a more predictable dose response, and a longer half-life than does UFH. No monitoring or dose adjustment is needed unless the patient is markedly obese or has chronic kidney disease.

TABLE 262-4 Anticoagulation of VTE

Immediate Parenteral Anticoagulation
Unfractionated heparin, bolus and continuous infusion, to achieve aPTT two to three times the upper limit of the laboratory normal, *or*
Enoxaparin 1 mg/kg twice daily with normal renal function, *or*
Dalteparin 200 U/kg once daily or 100 U/kg twice daily, with normal renal function, *or*
Tinzaparin 175 U/kg once daily with normal renal function, *or*
Fondaparinux weight-based once daily; adjust for impaired renal function
Warfarin Anticoagulation
Usual start dose is 5 mg
Titrate to INR, target 2.0–3.0
Continue parenteral anticoagulation for a minimum of 5 days and until two sequential INR values, at least 1 day apart, achieve the target INR range.

There are two commonly used LMWH preparations in the United States: enoxaparin and dalteparin. *Enoxaparin* is approved as a bridge to warfarin for VTE. *Dalteparin* is also approved as monotherapy without warfarin for symptomatic VTE patients with cancer in a dose of 200 U/kg once daily for 30 days, followed by 150 U/kg once daily for months 2–6. These weight-adjusted LMWH doses must be reduced in patients with chronic kidney disease because the kidneys metabolize LMWH.

Fondaparinux Fondaparinux, an anti-Xa pentasaccharide, is administered as a once-daily subcutaneous injection in a prefilled syringe to treat DVT and PE as a "bridge" to warfarin. No laboratory monitoring is required. Patients weighing <50 kg receive 5 mg, patients weighing 50–100 kg receive 7.5 mg, and patients weighing >100 kg receive 10 mg. Fondaparinux is synthesized in a laboratory and, unlike LMWH or UFH, is not derived from animal products. It does not cause heparin-induced thrombocytopenia. The dose must be adjusted downward for patients with renal dysfunction because the kidneys metabolize the drug.

Warfarin This vitamin K antagonist prevents carboxylation activation of coagulation factors II, VII, IX, and X. The full effect of warfarin requires at least 5 days even if the prothrombin time, used for monitoring, becomes elevated more rapidly. If warfarin is initiated as monotherapy during an acute thrombotic illness, a paradoxical exacerbation of hypercoagulability can increase the likelihood of thrombosis rather than prevent it. Overlapping UFH, LMWH, or fondaparinux with warfarin for at least 5 days can counteract the early procoagulant effect of unopposed warfarin.

Warfarin Dosing In an average-size adult, warfarin usually is initiated in a dose of 5 mg. Doses of 7.5 or 10 mg can be used in obese or large-framed young patients who are otherwise healthy. Patients who are malnourished or who have received prolonged courses of antibiotics are probably deficient in vitamin K and should receive smaller initial doses of warfarin, such as 2.5 mg. The prothrombin time is standardized by calculating the international normalized ratio (INR), which assesses the anticoagulant effect of warfarin (Chap. 58). The target INR is usually 2.5, with a range of 2.0–3.0.

The warfarin dose is titrated to achieve the target INR. Proper dosing is difficult because hundreds of drug-drug and drug-food interactions affect warfarin metabolism. Variables such as increasing age and comorbidities such as systemic illness reduce the required warfarin dose. Pharmacogenomics may provide more precise initial dosing of warfarin, especially for patients who require unusually large or small doses. *CYP2C9* variant alleles impair the hydroxylation of S-warfarin, thereby lowering the dose requirement. Variants in the gene encoding the vitamin K epoxide reductase complex 1 (*VKORC1*) can predict whether patients require low, moderate, or high warfarin doses. Nevertheless, more than half of warfarin dosing variability is caused by clinical factors such as age, sex, weight, concomitant drugs, and comorbid illnesses.

Nomograms have been developed (*www.warfarindosing.org*) to help clinicians initiate warfarin dosing based on clinical information and, if available, pharmacogenetic data. However, most practitioners utilize empirical dosing with an "educated guess." Centralized anticoagulation clinics have improved the efficacy and safety of warfarin dosing. Patients maintain a therapeutic INR more often if they self-monitor their INR with a home point-of-care fingerstick machine rather than obtaining a coagulation laboratory INR. The patient subgroup with the best results self-adjusts warfarin doses as well as self-tests INRs.

Novel Anticoagulants Novel oral anticoagulants are administered in a fixed dose, establish effective anticoagulation within hours of administration, require no laboratory coagulation monitoring, and have few of the drug-drug or drug-food interactions that make warfarin so difficult to dose. Rivaroxaban, a factor Xa inhibitor, and dabigatran, a direct thrombin inhibitor, are approved in Canada and Europe for prevention of VTE after total hip and total knee replacement. In a large-scale trial of acute VTE treatment, dabigatran was as effective as warfarin and had less nonmajor bleeding. Because of these drugs' rapid onset of action and relatively short half-life compared with warfarin, "bridging" with a parenteral anticoagulant is not required.

Complications of Anticoagulants The most serious adverse effect of anticoagulation is hemorrhage. For life-threatening or intracranial hemorrhage due to heparin or LMWH, protamine sulfate can be administered. There is no specific antidote for bleeding caused by fondaparinux or direct thrombin inhibitors.

Major bleeding from warfarin is best managed with prothrombin complex concentrate. With non-life threatening bleeding in a patient who can tolerate large volume, fresh-frozen plasma can be used. Recombinant human coagulation factor VIIa (rFVIIa), FDA-approved for bleeding in hemophiliacs, is an off-label option to manage catastrophic bleeding from warfarin. For minor bleeding or to manage an excessively high INR in the absence of bleeding, oral vitamin K may be administered.

Heparin-induced thrombocytopenia (HIT) and osteopenia are far less common with LMWH than with UFH. Thrombosis due to HIT should be managed with a direct thrombin inhibitor: argatroban for patients with renal insufficiency and lepirudin for patients with hepatic failure. In the setting of percutaneous coronary intervention, one should administer bivalirudin.

During pregnancy, warfarin should be avoided if possible because of warfarin embryopathy, which is most common with exposure during the sixth through twelfth week of gestation. However, women can take warfarin postpartum and breast-feed safely. Warfarin can also be administered safely during the second trimester.

Duration of Hospital Stay Acute DVT patients with good family and social support, permanent residence, telephone service, and no hearing or language impairment often can be managed as outpatients. They, a family member, or a visiting nurse must administer a parenteral anticoagulant. Warfarin dosing can be titrated to the INR and adjusted on an outpatient basis.

Acute PE patients, who traditionally have required hospital stays of 5–7 days for intravenous heparin as a "bridge" to warfarin, can be considered for abbreviated hospitalization if they have a reliable support system at home and an excellent prognosis. Criteria include clinical stability, absence of chest pain or shortness of breath, normal RV size and function, and normal levels of cardiac biomarkers.

Duration of Anticoagulation Patients with PE after surgery, trauma, or estrogen exposure (from oral contraceptives, pregnancy, or postmenopausal therapy) ordinarily have a low rate of recurrence after 3–6 months of anticoagulation. For DVT isolated to an upper extremity or calf that has been provoked by surgery, trauma, estrogen, or an indwelling central venous catheter or pacemaker, 3 months of anticoagulation suffices. For provoked proximal leg DVT or PE, 3 to 6 months of anticoagulation is sufficient. For patients with cancer and VTE, the consensus is to prescribe 3–6 months of LMWH as monotherapy without warfarin and to continue anticoagulation indefinitely unless the patient is rendered cancer-free. However, there is uncertainty whether subsequent anticoagulation should continue with LMWH or whether the patient should be placed on warfarin.

Among patients with idiopathic, unprovoked VTE, the recurrence rate is high after cessation of anticoagulation. VTE that occurs during long-haul air travel is considered unprovoked. It appears that unprovoked VTE is often a chronic illness, with latent periods between flares of recurrent episodes. American College of Chest Physicians (ACCP) guidelines recommend considering anticoagulation for an indefinite duration with a target INR between 2 and 3 for patients with idiopathic VTE. An alternative approach after the first 6 months of anticoagulation is to reduce the intensity of anticoagulation and to lower the target INR range to between 1.5 and 2.

Counterintuitively, the presence of genetic mutations such as heterozygous factor V Leiden and prothrombin gene mutation do not appear to increase the risk of recurrent VTE. However, patients with moderate or high levels of anticardiolipin antibodies probably warrant indefinite-duration anticoagulation even if the initial VTE was provoked by trauma or surgery.

INFERIOR VENA CAVAL (IVC) FILTERS The two principal indications for insertion of an IVC filter are (1) active bleeding that precludes anticoagulation and (2) recurrent venous thrombosis despite intensive anticoagulation. Prevention of recurrent PE in patients with right heart failure who are not candidates for fibrinolysis and prophylaxis of extremely high-risk patients are "softer" indications for filter placement. The filter itself may fail by permitting the passage of small- to medium-size clots. Large thrombi may embolize to the pulmonary arteries via collateral veins that develop. A more common complication is caval thrombosis with marked bilateral leg swelling.

Paradoxically, by providing a nidus for clot formation, filters double the DVT rate over the ensuing 2 years after placement. Retrievable filters can now be placed for patients with an anticipated temporary bleeding disorder or for patients at temporary high risk of PE, such as individuals undergoing bariatric surgery who have a prior history of perioperative PE. The filters can be retrieved up to several months after insertion unless thrombus forms and is trapped within the filter. The retrievable filter becomes permanent if it remains in place or if, for technical reasons such as rapid endothelialization, it cannot be removed.

MAINTAINING ADEQUATE CIRCULATION For patients with massive PE and hypotension, one should administer 500 mL of normal saline. Additional fluid should be infused with extreme caution because excessive fluid administration exacerbates RV wall stress, causes more profound RV ischemia, and worsens LV compliance and filling by causing further interventricular septal shift toward the LV. Dopamine and dobutamine are first-line inotropic agents for treatment of PE-related shock. There should be a low threshold for initiating these pressors. Often, a "trial-and-error" approach works best; one should consider norepinephrine, vasopressin, or phenylephrine.

FIBRINOLYSIS Successful fibrinolytic therapy rapidly reverses right heart failure and may result in a lower rate of death and recurrent PE by (1) dissolving much of the anatomically obstructing pulmonary arterial thrombus, (2) preventing the continued release of serotonin and other neurohumoral factors that exacerbate pulmonary hypertension, and (3) lysing much of the source of the thrombus in the pelvic or deep leg veins, thereby decreasing the likelihood of recurrent PE.

The preferred fibrinolytic regimen is 100 mg of recombinant tissue plasminogen activator (tPA) administered as a continuous peripheral intravenous infusion over 2 hours. Patients appear to respond to fibrinolysis for up to 14 days after the PE has occurred.

Contraindications to fibrinolysis include intracranial disease, recent surgery, and trauma. The overall major bleeding rate is about 10%, including a 1–3% risk of intracranial hemorrhage. Careful screening of patients for contraindications to fibrinolytic therapy (Chap. 245) is the best way to minimize bleeding risk.

TABLE 262-5 Prevention of Venous Thromboembolism

Condition	Prophylaxis Strategy
High-risk general surgery	Mini-UFH *or* LMWH
Thoracic surgery	Mini-UFH + IPC
Cancer surgery, including gynecologic cancer surgery	LMWH, consider 1 month of prophylaxis
Total hip replacement, total knee replacement, hip fracture surgery	LMWH, fondaparinux (a pentasaccharide) 2.5 mg SC, once daily, *or* (except for total knee replacement) warfarin (target INR 2.5); rivaroxaban or dalteparin in countries where it is approved
Neurosurgery	IPC
Neurosurgery for brain tumor	Mini-UFH *or* LMWH, + IPC + predischarge venous ultrasonography
Benign gynecologic surgery	Mini-UFH
Medically ill patients	Mini-UFH *or* LMWH
Anticoagulation contraindicated	IPC
Long-haul air travel	Consider LMWH for very high-risk patients

Note: Mini-UFH, mini-dose unfractionated heparin, 5000 units subcutaneously twice (less effective) or three times daily (more effective); LMWH, low-molecular-weight heparin, typically in the United States enoxaparin, 40 mg once daily, or dalteparin, 2500 or 5000 units once daily; IPC, intermittent pneumatic compression devices.

The only FDA-approved indication for PE fibrinolysis is massive PE. For patients with preserved systolic blood pressure and submassive PE with moderate or severe RV dysfunction, ACCP guidelines for fibrinolysis recommend individual patient risk assessment of the thrombotic burden versus the bleeding risk.

PULMONARY EMBOLECTOMY The risk of intracranial hemorrhage with fibrinolysis has prompted a renaissance of surgical embolectomy. More prompt referral before the onset of irreversible cardiogenic shock and multisystem organ failure and improved surgical technique have resulted in a high survival rate. A possible alternative to open surgical embolectomy is catheter embolectomy. New-generation catheters are under development.

PULMONARY THROMBOENDARTERECTOMY Chronic thromboembolic pulmonary hypertension occurs in 2–4% of acute PE patients. Therefore, PE patients who have initial pulmonary hypertension (usually diagnosed with Doppler echocardiography) should be followed up at about 6 weeks with a repeat echocardiogram to determine whether pulmonary arterial pressure has normalized. Patients impaired by dyspnea due to chronic thromboembolic pulmonary hypertension should be considered for pulmonary thromboendarterectomy, which, if successful, can markedly reduce, and at times even cure, pulmonary hypertension (Chap. 250). The operation requires median sternotomy, cardiopulmonary bypass, deep hypothermia, and periods of hypothermic circulatory arrest. The mortality rate at experienced centers is approximately 5%.

EMOTIONAL SUPPORT Patients with VTE may feel overwhelmed when they learn that they are susceptible to recurrent PE or DVT. They worry about the health of their families and the genetic implications of their illness. Those who are advised to discontinue warfarin after 3–6 months of therapy may feel especially vulnerable. At Brigham and Woman's Hospital a physican-nurse-facilitated PE support group has been maintained for patients and has met monthly for more than 15 years.

PREVENTION OF POSTPHLEBITIC SYNDROME Daily use of below-knee 30- to 40-mmHg vascular compression stockings will halve the rate of developing postphlebitic syndrome. These stockings should be prescribed as soon as DVT is diagnosed and should be fitted carefully to maximize their benefit. When patients are in bed, the stockings need not be worn.

PREVENTION OF VTE

Prophylaxis (Table 262-5) is of paramount importance because VTE is difficult to detect and poses a profound medical and economic burden. Computerized reminder systems can increase the use of preventive measures and at Brigham and Women's Hospital have reduced the symptomatic VTE rate by more than 40%. Patients who have undergone total hip or knee replacement or cancer surgery will benefit from extended pharmacologic prophylaxis for a total of 4–5 weeks.

FURTHER READINGS

Ageno W et al: Cardiovascular risk factors and venous thromboembolism: A meta-analysis. Circulation 117:93, 2008

Dalen JE: Should patients with venous thromboembolism be screened for thrombophilia? Am J Med 121:458, 2008

Dennis M et al: Effectiveness of thigh-length graduated compression stockings to reduce the risk of deep vein thrombosis after stroke (CLOTS trial 1): A multicentre, randomised controlled trial. Lancet 373:1958, 2009

Dentali F et al: Meta-analysis: Anticoagulant prophylaxis to prevent symptomatic venous thromboembolism in hospitalized medical patients. Ann Intern Med 146:278, 2007

Geerts WH et al: Prevention of venous thromboembolism: American College of Chest Physicians Evidence-Based Clinical Practice Guidelines (8th ed). Chest 133:381S, 2008

Glynn RJ et al: A randomized trial of rosuvastatin in the prevention of venous thromboembolism. N Engl J Med 360:1851, 2009

Kucher N, Goldhaber SZ: Management of massive pulmonary embolism. Circulation 112:e28, 2005

Park B et al: Recent trends in clinical outcomes and resource utilization for pulmonary embolism in the United States: Findings from the nationwide inpatient sample. Chest 136: 983, 2009

Piazza G, Goldhaber SZ: The acutely decompensated right ventricle. Chest 128:1836, 2005

Prandoni P et al: Residual thrombosis on ultrasonography to guide the duration of anticoagulation in patients with deep venous thrombosis: A randomized trial. Ann Intern Med 150:577, 2009

Spencer FA et al: Venous thromboembolism in the outpatient setting. Arch Intern Med 167:1471, 2007

Todd JL, Tapson VF: Thrombolytic therapy for acute pulmonary embolism: A critical appraisal. Chest 135:1321, 2009

Torbicki A et al: Guidelines on the diagnosis and management of acute pulmonary embolism: The Task Force for the Diagnosis and Management of Acute Pulmonary Embolism of the European Society of Cardiology (ESC). Eur Heart J 29:2276, 2008

Van Belle A et al: Effectiveness of managing suspected pulmonary embolism using an algorithm combining clinical probability, D-dimer testing, and computed tomography. JAMA 295:172, 2006

CHAPTER 263
Disorders of the Pleura and Mediastinum

Richard W. Light

DISORDERS OF THE PLEURA

PLEURAL EFFUSION

The pleural space lies between the lung and the chest wall and normally contains a very thin layer of fluid, which serves as a coupling system. A pleural effusion is present when there is an excess quantity of fluid in the pleural space.

Etiology

Pleural fluid accumulates when pleural fluid formation exceeds pleural fluid absorption. Normally, fluid enters the pleural space from the capillaries in the parietal pleura and is removed via the lymphatics in the parietal pleura. Fluid also can enter the pleural space from the interstitial spaces of the lung via the visceral pleura or from the peritoneal cavity via small holes in the diaphragm. The lymphatics have the capacity to absorb 20 times more fluid than is formed normally. Accordingly, a pleural effusion may develop when there is excess pleural fluid formation (from the interstitial spaces of the lung, the parietal pleura, or the peritoneal cavity) or when there is decreased fluid removal by the lymphatics.

Diagnostic approach

When a patient is found to have a pleural effusion, an effort should be made to determine the cause (Fig. 263-1). The first step is to determine whether the effusion is a transudate or an exudate. A *transudative pleural effusion* occurs when *systemic factors* that influence the formation and absorption of pleural fluid are altered. The leading causes of transudative pleural effusions in the United States are left-ventricular failure and cirrhosis. An *exudative pleural effusion* occurs when *local factors* that influence the formation and absorption of pleural fluid are altered. The leading causes of exudative pleural effusions are bacterial pneumonia, malignancy, viral infection, and pulmonary embolism. The primary reason for making this differentiation is that additional diagnostic procedures are indicated with exudative effusions to define the cause of the local disease.

Transudative and exudative pleural effusions are distinguished by measuring the lactate dehydrogenase (LDH) and protein levels in the pleural fluid. Exudative pleural effusions meet at least one of the following criteria, whereas transudative pleural effusions meet none:

1. Pleural fluid protein/serum protein >0.5
2. Pleural fluid LDH/serum LDH >0.6
3. Pleural fluid LDH more than two-thirds normal upper limit for serum

These criteria misidentify ~25% of transudates as exudates. If one or more of the exudative criteria are met and the patient is clinically thought to have a condition producing a transudative effusion, the difference between the protein levels in the serum and the pleural fluid should be measured. If this gradient is >31 g/L (3.1 g/dL), the exudative categorization by these criteria can be ignored because almost all such patients have a transudative pleural effusion.

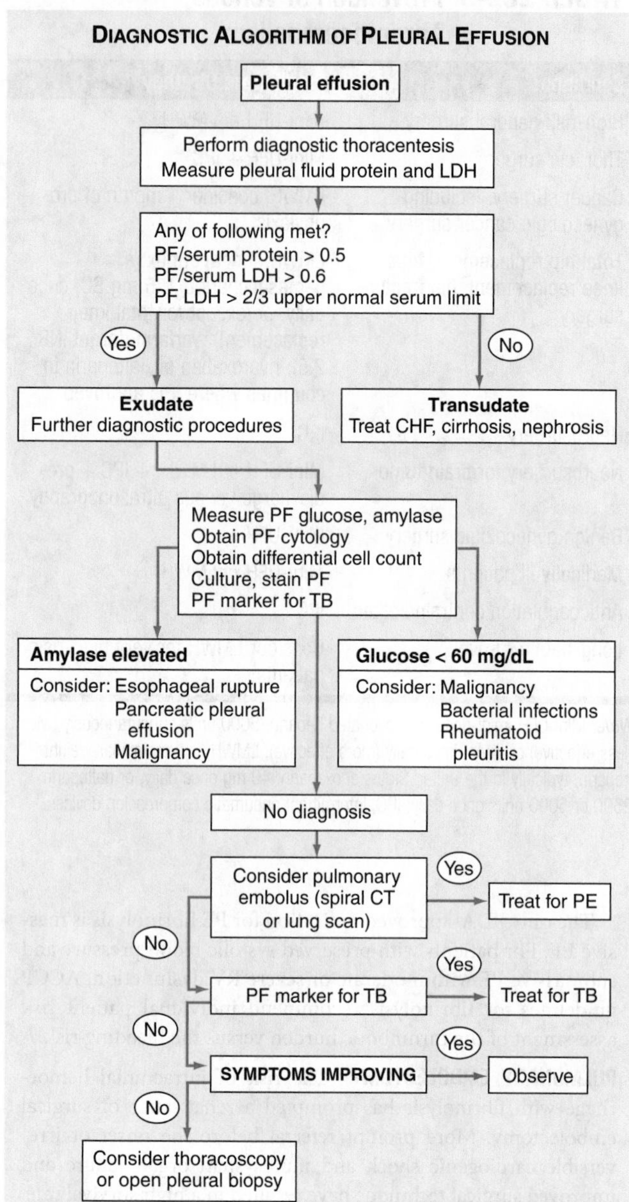

Figure 263-1 Approach to the diagnosis of pleural effusions. CHF, congestive heart failure; CT, computed tomography; LDH, lactate dehydrogenase; PE, pulmonary embolism; TB, tuberculosis; PF, pleural fluid.

If a patient has an exudative pleural effusion, the following tests on the pleural fluid should be obtained: description of the appearance of the fluid, glucose level, differential cell count, microbiologic studies, and cytology.

Effusion due to heart failure

The most common cause of pleural effusion is left-ventricular failure. The effusion occurs because the increased amounts of fluid in the lung interstitial spaces exit in part across the visceral pleura; this overwhelms the capacity of the lymphatics in the parietal pleura to remove fluid. In patients with heart failure, a diagnostic thoracentesis should be performed if the effusions are not bilateral and comparable in size, if the patient is febrile, or if the patient has pleuritic chest pain to verify that the patient has a transudative effusion. Otherwise the patient's heart failure is treated. If the effusion persists despite therapy, a diagnostic thoracentesis should be performed. A pleural fluid N-terminal pro-brain natriuretic peptide (NT-proBNP) >1500 pg/mL is virtually diagnostic of an effusion secondary to congestive heart failure.

Hepatic hydrothorax

Pleural effusions occur in ~5% of patients with cirrhosis and ascites. The predominant mechanism is the direct movement of peritoneal fluid through small openings in the diaphragm into the pleural space. The effusion is usually right-sided and frequently is large enough to produce severe dyspnea.

Parapneumonic effusion

Parapneumonic effusions are associated with bacterial pneumonia, lung abscess, or bronchiectasis and are probably the most common cause of exudative pleural effusion in the United States. *Empyema* refers to a grossly purulent effusion.

Patients with aerobic bacterial pneumonia and pleural effusion present with an acute febrile illness consisting of chest pain, sputum production, and leukocytosis. Patients with anaerobic infections present with a subacute illness with weight loss, a brisk leukocytosis, mild anemia, and a history of some factor that predisposes them to aspiration.

The possibility of a parapneumonic effusion should be considered whenever a patient with bacterial pneumonia is initially evaluated. The presence of free pleural fluid can be demonstrated with a lateral decubitus radiograph, computed tomography (CT) of the chest, or ultrasound. If the free fluid separates the lung from the chest wall by >10 mm, a therapeutic thoracentesis should be performed. Factors indicating the likely need for a procedure more invasive than a thoracentesis (in increasing order of importance) include the following:

1. Loculated pleural fluid
2. Pleural fluid pH <7.20
3. Pleural fluid glucose <3.3 mmol/L (<60 mg/dL)
4. Positive Gram stain or culture of the pleural fluid
5. Presence of gross pus in the pleural space

If the fluid recurs after the initial therapeutic thoracentesis and if any of these characteristics are present, a repeat thoracentesis should be performed. If the fluid cannot be completely removed with the therapeutic thoracentesis, consideration should be given to inserting a chest tube and instilling a fibrinolytic agent (e.g., tissue plasminogen activator, 10 mg) or performing a thoracoscopy with the breakdown of adhesions. Decortication should be considered when these measures are ineffective.

Effusion secondary to malignancy

Malignant pleural effusions secondary to metastatic disease are the second most common type of exudative pleural effusion. The three tumors that cause ~75% of all malignant pleural effusions are lung carcinoma, breast carcinoma, and lymphoma. Most patients complain of dyspnea, which is frequently out of proportion to the size of the effusion. The pleural fluid is an exudate, and its glucose level may be reduced if the tumor burden in the pleural space is high.

The diagnosis usually is made via cytology of the pleural fluid. If the initial cytologic examination is negative, thoracoscopy is the best next procedure if malignancy is strongly suspected. At the time of thoracoscopy, a procedure such as pleural abrasion should be performed to effect a pleurodesis. An alternative to thoracoscopy is CT- or ultrasound-guided needle biopsy of pleural thickening or nodules. Patients with a malignant pleural effusion are treated symptomatically for the most part, since the presence of the effusion indicates disseminated disease and most malignancies associated with pleural effusion are not curable with chemotherapy. The only symptom that can be attributed to the effusion itself is dyspnea. If the patient's lifestyle is compromised by dyspnea and if the dyspnea is relieved with a therapeutic thoracentesis, one of the following procedures should be considered: (1) insertion of a small indwelling catheter or (2) tube thoracostomy with the instillation of a sclerosing agent such as doxycycline, 500 mg.

Mesothelioma

Malignant mesotheliomas are primary tumors that arise from the mesothelial cells that line the pleural cavities; most are related to asbestos exposure. Patients with mesothelioma present with chest pain and shortness of breath. The chest radiograph reveals a pleural effusion, generalized pleural thickening, and a shrunken hemithorax. Thoracoscopy or open pleural biopsy is usually necessary to establish the diagnosis. Chest pain should be treated with opiates, and shortness of breath with oxygen and/or opiates.

Effusion secondary to pulmonary embolization

The diagnosis most commonly overlooked in the differential diagnosis of a patient with an undiagnosed pleural effusion is pulmonary embolism. Dyspnea is the most common symptom. The pleural fluid is almost always an exudate. The diagnosis is established by spiral CT scan or pulmonary arteriography (Chap. 262). Treatment of a patient with a pleural effusion secondary to pulmonary embolism is the same as it is for any patient with pulmonary emboli. If the pleural effusion increases in size after anticoagulation, the patient probably has recurrent emboli or another complication, such as a hemothorax or a pleural infection.

Tuberculous pleuritis

(See also Chap. 165) In many parts of the world, the most common cause of an exudative pleural effusion is tuberculosis (TB), but tuberculous effusions are relatively uncommon in the United States. Tuberculous pleural effusions usually are associated with primary TB and are thought to be due primarily to a hypersensitivity reaction to tuberculous protein in the pleural space. Patients with tuberculous pleuritis present with fever, weight loss, dyspnea, and/or pleuritic chest pain. The pleural fluid is an exudate with predominantly small lymphocytes. The diagnosis is established by demonstrating high levels of TB markers in the pleural fluid (adenosine deaminase >40 IU/L or interferon γ >140 pg/mL). Alternatively, the diagnosis can be established by culture of the pleural fluid, needle biopsy of the pleura, or thoracoscopy. The recommended treatments of pleural and pulmonary TB are identical (Chap. 165).

Effusion secondary to viral infection

Viral infections are probably responsible for a sizable percentage of undiagnosed exudative pleural effusions. In many series, no diagnosis is established for ~20% of exudative effusions, and these effusions resolve spontaneously with no long-term residua. The importance of these effusions is that one should not be too aggressive in trying to establish a diagnosis for the undiagnosed effusion, particularly if the patient is improving clinically.

Chylothorax

A chylothorax occurs when the thoracic duct is disrupted and chyle accumulates in the pleural space. The most common cause of chylothorax is trauma (most frequently thoracic surgery), but it also may result from tumors in the mediastinum. Patients with chylothorax present with dyspnea, and a large pleural effusion is present on the chest radiograph. Thoracentesis reveals milky fluid, and biochemical analysis reveals a triglyceride level that exceeds 1.2 mmol/L (110 mg/dL). Patients with chylothorax and no obvious trauma should have a lymphangiogram and a mediastinal CT scan to assess the mediastinum for lymph nodes. The treatment of choice for most chylothoraxes is insertion of a chest tube plus the administration of octreotide. If these modalities fail, a pleuroperitoneal shunt should be placed unless the patient has chylous ascites. An alternative treatment is ligation of the thoracic duct. Patients with chylothoraxes should not undergo prolonged tube thoracostomy with chest tube drainage because this will lead to malnutrition and immunologic incompetence.

Hemothorax

When a diagnostic thoracentesis reveals bloody pleural fluid, a hematocrit should be obtained on the pleural fluid. If the hematocrit is more than one-half of that in the peripheral blood, the patient is considered to have a hemothorax. Most hemothoraxes are the result of trauma; other causes include rupture of a blood vessel or tumor. Most patients with hemothorax should be treated with tube thoracostomy, which allows continuous quantification of bleeding. If the bleeding emanates from a laceration of the pleura, apposition of the two pleural surfaces is likely to stop the bleeding. If the pleural hemorrhage exceeds 200 mL/h, consideration should be given to thoracoscopy or thoracotomy.

Miscellaneous causes of pleural effusion

There are many other causes of pleural effusion (Table 263-1). Key features of some of these conditions are as follows: If the pleural fluid amylase level is elevated, the diagnosis of esophageal rupture or pancreatic disease is likely. If the patient is febrile, has predominantly polymorphonuclear cells in the pleural fluid, and has no pulmonary parenchymal abnormalities, an intraabdominal abscess should be considered.

The diagnosis of an asbestos pleural effusion is one of exclusion. Benign ovarian tumors can produce ascites and a pleural effusion (Meigs' syndrome), as can the ovarian hyperstimulation syndrome. Several drugs can cause pleural effusion; the associated fluid is usually eosinophilic. Pleural effusions commonly occur after coronary

TABLE 263-1 Differential Diagnoses of Pleural Effusions

Transudative Pleural Effusions	
1. Congestive heart failure	5. Peritoneal dialysis
2. Cirrhosis	6. Superior vena cava obstruction
3. Pulmonary embolization	7. Myxedema
4. Nephrotic syndrome	8. Urinothorax
Exudative Pleural Effusions	
1. Neoplastic diseases	6. Post-coronary artery bypass surgery
a. Metastatic disease	7. Asbestos exposure
b. Mesothelioma	8. Sarcoidosis
2. Infectious diseases	9. Uremia
a. Bacterial infections	10. Meigs' syndrome
b. Tuberculosis	11. Yellow nail syndrome
c. Fungal infections	12. Drug-induced pleural disease
d. Viral infections	a. Nitrofurantoin
e. Parasitic infections	b. Dantrolene
3. Pulmonary embolization	c. Methysergide
4. Gastrointestinal disease	d. Bromocriptine
a. Esophageal perforation	e. Procarbazine
b. Pancreatic disease	f. Amiodarone
c. Intraabdominal abscesses	g. Dasatinib
d. Diaphragmatic hernia	13. Trapped lung
e. After abdominal surgery	14. Radiation therapy
f. Endoscopic variceal sclerotherapy	15. Post-cardiac injury syndrome
g. After liver transplant	16. Hemothorax
5. Collagen vascular diseases	17. Iatrogenic injury
a. Rheumatoid pleuritis	18. Ovarian hyperstimulation syndrome
b. Systemic lupus erythematosus	19. Pericardial disease
c. Drug-induced lupus	20. Chylothorax
d. Immunoblastic lymphadenopathy	
e. Sjögren's syndrome	
f. Granulomatosis with polyangiitis (Wegener's)	
g. Churg-Strauss syndrome	

artery bypass surgery. Effusions occurring within the first weeks are typically left-sided and bloody, with large numbers of eosinophils, and respond to one or two therapeutic thoracenteses. Effusions occurring after the first few weeks are typically left-sided and clear yellow, with predominantly small lymphocytes, and tend to recur. Other medical manipulations that induce pleural effusions include abdominal surgery; radiation therapy; liver, lung, or heart transplantation; and the intravascular insertion of central lines.

PNEUMOTHORAX

Pneumothorax is the presence of gas in the pleural space. A *spontaneous pneumothorax* is one that occurs without antecedent trauma to the thorax. A *primary spontaneous pneumothorax* occurs in the absence of underlying lung disease, whereas a *secondary pneumothorax* occurs in its presence. A *traumatic pneumothorax* results from penetrating or nonpenetrating chest injuries. A *tension pneumothorax* is a pneumothorax in which the pressure in the pleural space is positive throughout the respiratory cycle.

Primary spontaneous pneumothorax

Primary spontaneous pneumothoraxes are usually due to rupture of apical pleural blebs, small cystic spaces that lie within or immediately under the visceral pleura. Primary spontaneous pneumothoraxes occur almost exclusively in smokers; this suggests that these patients have subclinical lung disease. Approximately one-half of patients with an initial primary spontaneous pneumothorax will have a recurrence. The initial recommended treatment for primary spontaneous pneumothorax is simple aspiration. If the lung does not expand with aspiration or if the patient has a recurrent pneumothorax, thoracoscopy with stapling of blebs and pleural abrasion is indicated. Thoracoscopy or thoracotomy with pleural abrasion is almost 100% successful in preventing recurrences.

Secondary pneumothorax

Most secondary pneumothoraxes are due to chronic obstructive pulmonary disease, but pneumothoraxes have been reported with virtually every lung disease. Pneumothorax in patients with lung disease is more life-threatening than it is in normal individuals because of the lack of pulmonary reserve in these patients. Nearly all patients with secondary pneumothorax should be treated with tube thoracostomy. Most should also be treated with thoracoscopy or thoracotomy with the stapling of blebs and pleural abrasion. If the patient is not a good operative candidate or refuses surgery, pleurodesis should be attempted by the intrapleural injection of a sclerosing agent such as doxycycline.

Traumatic pneumothorax

Traumatic pneumothoraxes can result from both penetrating and nonpenetrating chest trauma. Traumatic pneumothoraxes should be treated with tube thoracostomy unless they are very small. If a hemopneumothorax is present, one chest tube should be placed in the superior part of the hemithorax to evacuate the air and another should be placed in the inferior part of the hemithorax to remove the blood. Iatrogenic pneumothorax is a type of traumatic pneumothorax that is becoming more common. The leading causes are transthoracic needle aspiration, thoracentesis, and the insertion of central intravenous catheters. Most can be managed with supplemental oxygen or aspiration, but if these measures are unsuccessful, a tube thoracostomy should be performed.

Tension pneumothorax

This condition usually occurs during mechanical ventilation or resuscitative efforts. The positive pleural pressure is life-threatening both because ventilation is severely compromised and because the positive pressure is transmitted to the mediastinum, resulting in decreased venous return to the heart and reduced cardiac output.

Difficulty in ventilation during resuscitation or high peak inspiratory pressures during mechanical ventilation strongly suggest the diagnosis. The diagnosis is made by physical examination showing an enlarged hemithorax with no breath sounds, hyperresonance to percussion, and shift of the mediastinum to the contralateral side. Tension pneumothorax must be treated as a medical emergency. If the tension in the pleural space is not relieved, the patient is likely to die from inadequate cardiac output or marked hypoxemia. A large-bore needle should be inserted into the pleural space through the second anterior intercostal space. If large amounts of gas escape from the needle after insertion, the diagnosis is confirmed. The needle should be left in place until a thoracostomy tube can be inserted.

DISORDERS OF THE MEDIASTINUM

The mediastinum is the region between the pleural sacs. It is separated into three compartments. The *anterior mediastinum* extends from the sternum anteriorly to the pericardium and brachiocephalic vessels posteriorly. It contains the thymus gland, the anterior mediastinal lymph nodes, and the internal mammary arteries and veins. The *middle mediastinum* lies between the anterior and posterior mediastina and contains the heart; the ascending and transverse arches of the aorta; the venae cavae; the brachiocephalic arteries and veins; the phrenic nerves; the trachea, the main bronchi, and their contiguous lymph nodes; and the pulmonary arteries and veins. The *posterior mediastinum* is bounded by the pericardium and trachea anteriorly and the vertebral column posteriorly. It contains the descending thoracic aorta, the esophagus, the thoracic duct, the azygos and hemiazygos veins, and the posterior group of mediastinal lymph nodes.

MEDIASTINAL MASSES

The first step in evaluating a mediastinal mass is to place it in one of the three mediastinal compartments, since each has different characteristic lesions. The most common lesions in the anterior mediastinum are thymomas, lymphomas, teratomatous neoplasms, and thyroid masses. The most common masses in the middle mediastinum are vascular masses, lymph node enlargement from metastases or granulomatous disease, and pleuropericardial and bronchogenic cysts. In the posterior mediastinum, neurogenic tumors, meningoceles, meningomyeloceles, gastroenteric cysts, and esophageal diverticula are commonly found.

CT scanning is the most valuable imaging technique for evaluating mediastinal masses and is the only imaging technique that should be done in most instances. Barium studies of the gastrointestinal tract are indicated in many patients with posterior mediastinal lesions, since hernias, diverticula, and achalasia are readily diagnosed in this manner. An ^{131}I scan can efficiently establish the diagnosis of intrathoracic goiter.

A definite diagnosis can be obtained with mediastinoscopy or anterior mediastinotomy in many patients with masses in the anterior or middle mediastinal compartments. A diagnosis can be established without thoracotomy via percutaneous fine-needle aspiration biopsy or endoscopic transesophageal or endobronchial ultrasound-guided biopsy of mediastinal masses in most cases. Alternative ways to establish the diagnosis are video-assisted thoracoscopy, mediastinoscopy, and mediastinotomy. In many cases the diagnosis can be established and the mediastinal mass removed with video-assisted thoracoscopy.

ACUTE MEDIASTINITIS

Most cases of acute mediastinitis either are due to esophageal perforation or occur after median sternotomy for cardiac surgery. Patients with esophageal rupture are acutely ill with chest pain and dyspnea due to the mediastinal infection. The esophageal rupture can occur spontaneously or as a complication of esophagoscopy or the insertion of a Blakemore tube. Appropriate treatment consists of exploration of the mediastinum with primary repair of the esophageal tear and drainage of the pleural space and the mediastinum.

The incidence of mediastinitis after median sternotomy is 0.4–5.0%. Patients most commonly present with wound drainage. Other presentations include sepsis and a widened mediastinum. The diagnosis usually is established with mediastinal needle aspiration. Treatment includes immediate drainage, debridement, and parenteral antibiotic therapy, but the mortality rate still exceeds 20%.

CHRONIC MEDIASTINITIS

The spectrum of chronic mediastinitis ranges from granulomatous inflammation of the lymph nodes in the mediastinum to fibrosing mediastinitis. Most cases are due to histoplasmosis or TB, but sarcoidosis, silicosis, and other fungal diseases are at times causative. Patients with granulomatous mediastinitis are usually asymptomatic. Those with fibrosing mediastinitis usually have signs of compression of a mediastinal structure such as the superior vena cava or large airways, phrenic or recurrent laryngeal nerve paralysis, or obstruction of the pulmonary artery or proximal pulmonary veins. Other than antituberculous therapy for tuberculous mediastinitis, no medical or surgical therapy has been demonstrated to be effective for mediastinal fibrosis.

PNEUMOMEDIASTINUM

In this condition, there is gas in the interstices of the mediastinum. The three main causes are (1) alveolar rupture with dissection of air into the mediastinum, (2) perforation or rupture of the esophagus, trachea, or main bronchi, and (3) dissection of air from the neck or the abdomen into the mediastinum. Typically, there is severe substernal chest pain with or without radiation into the neck and arms. The physical examination usually reveals subcutaneous emphysema in the suprasternal notch and *Hamman's sign*, which is a crunching or clicking noise synchronous with the heartbeat and is best heard in the left lateral decubitus position. The diagnosis is confirmed with the chest radiograph. Usually no treatment is required, but the mediastinal air will be absorbed faster if the patient inspires high concentrations of oxygen. If mediastinal structures are compressed, the compression can be relieved with needle aspiration.

FURTHER READINGS

Gilbert S et al: Endobronchial ultrasound as a diagnostic tool in patients with mediastinal lymphadenopathy. Ann Thorac Surg 88:896, 2009

Light RW: Pleural effusion. N Engl J Med 346:1971, 2002

———: *Pleural Diseases*, 5th ed. Philadelphia, Lippincott Williams & Wilkins, 2006

Porcel JM et al: Biomarkers of heart failure in pleural fluid. Chest 163:671, 2009.

———: Pleural fluid tests to identify complicated parapneumonic effusions. Curr Opin Pulm Med 16:357, 2010

Warren WH et al: Identification of clinical factors predicting Pleurx catheter removal in patients treated for malignant pleural effusion. Eur J Cardiothorac Surg 33:89, 2008

CHAPTER 264

Disorders of Ventilation

John F. McConville

Julian Solway

DEFINITION AND PHYSIOLOGY

In health the arterial level of carbon dioxide (Pa_{CO_2}) is maintained between 37 and 43 mmHg at sea level. All disorders of ventilation result in abnormal measurements of Pa_{CO_2}. This chapter reviews chronic ventilatory disorders that are reflected in abnormal Pa_{CO_2}.

The continuous production of CO_2 by cellular metabolism necessitates its efficient elimination by the respiratory system. The relationship between CO_2 production and Pa_{CO_2} is described by the equation, $Pa_{CO_2} = (k)(\dot{V}_{CO_2})/\dot{V}A$, where $\dot{V}_{CO_2}$ represents the carbon dioxide production, k is a constant and $\dot{V}A$ is fresh gas alveolar ventilation (Chap. 252). $\dot{V}A$ can be calculated as minute ventilation x(1-Vd/Vt), where the dead space fraction Vd/Vt represents the portion of a tidal breath that remains within the conducting airways at the conclusion of inspiration and does not, therefore, contribute to alveolar ventilation. As such, all disturbances of Pa_{CO_2} must reflect altered CO_2 production, minute ventilation, or dead space fraction.

Diseases that alter $\dot{V}_{CO_2}$ are often acute (sepsis, burns, or pyrexia, for example), and their contribution to ventilatory abnormalities and/or respiratory failure is reviewed elsewhere. Chronic ventilatory disorders typically involve inappropriate levels of minute ventilation or increased dead space fraction. Characterization of these disorders requires a review of the normal respiratory cycle.

The spontaneous cycle of inspiration and expiration is automatically generated in the brainstem. Two groups of neurons located within the medulla are particularly important: the dorsal respiratory group (DRG) and the ventral respiratory column (VRC). These neurons have widespread projections, including the descending projections into the contralateral spinal cord, where they perform many functions. They initiate activity in the phrenic nerve/diaphragm, project to the upper airway muscle groups and spinal respiratory neurons, and innervate the intercostal and abdominal muscles that participate in normal respiration. The DRG acts as the initial integration site for many of the afferent nerves relaying information about the partial pressure of arterial oxygen (Pa_{O_2}), Pa_{CO_2}, pH, and blood pressure from the carotid and aortic chemoreceptors and baroreceptors to the central nervous system (CNS). In addition, the vagus nerve relays information from stretch receptors and juxtapulmonary-capillary receptors in the lung parenchyma and chest wall to the DRG. The respiratory rhythm is generated within the VRC, as well as the more rostrally located parafacial respiratory group (pFRG), which is particularly important for the generation of active expiration. One particularly important area within the VRC is the so-called pre-Bötzinger complex. This area is responsible for the generation of various forms of inspiratory activity, and lesioning of the pre-Bötzinger complex leads to the complete cessation of breathing. The neural output of these medullary respiratory networks can be voluntarily suppressed or augmented by input from higher brain centers and the autonomic nervous system. During normal sleep there is an attenuated response to hypercapnia and hypoxemia resulting in mild nocturnal hypoventilation that corrects upon awakening.

Once neural input has been delivered to the respiratory pump muscles, normal gas exchange requires an adequate amount of respiratory muscle strength to overcome the elastic and resistive loads of the respiratory system (Fig. 264-1*A*, Chap. 252). In health, the strength of the respiratory muscles readily accomplishes this, and normal respiration continues indefinitely. Reduction in respiratory drive or neuromuscular competence or substantial increase in respiratory load can diminish minute ventilation, resulting in hypercapnia (Fig. 264-1*B*). Alternatively, if normal respiratory muscle strength is coupled with excessive respiratory drive, then alveolar hyperventilation ensues and leads to hypocapnia (Fig. 264-1*C*).

HYPOVENTILATION

CLINICAL FEATURES

Diseases that reduce minute ventilation or increase dead space fall into four major categories: parenchymal lung and chest wall disease, sleep disordered breathing, neuromuscular disease, and respiratory drive disorders (Fig. 264-1*B*). The clinical manifestations of hypoventilation syndromes are nonspecific (Table 264-1) and vary depending on the severity of hypoventilation, the rate at which hypercapnia develops, the degree of compensation for respiratory acidosis, and the underlying disorder. Patients with parenchymal lung or chest wall disease typically present with shortness of breath and diminished exercise tolerance. Episodes of increased dyspnea and sputum production are hallmarks of obstructive lung diseases, such as chronic obstructive pulmonary disease (COPD), whereas progressive dyspnea and cough are common in interstitial lung diseases. Excessive daytime somnolence, poor quality sleep, and snoring are common among patients with sleep-disordered breathing. Sleep disturbance and orthopnea are also described in neuromuscular disorders. As neuromuscular weakness progresses, the respiratory muscles, including the diaphragm, are placed at a mechanical disadvantage in the supine position due to the upward movement of the abdominal contents. New-onset orthopnea is frequently a sign of reduced respiratory muscle force generation. More commonly, however, extremity weakness or bulbar symptoms develop prior to sleep disturbance in neuromuscular diseases, such as amyotrophic lateral sclerosis (ALS) or muscular dystrophy. Patients with respiratory drive disorders do not have symptoms distinguishable from other causes of chronic hypoventilation.

The clinical course of patients with chronic hypoventilation from neuromuscular or chest wall disease follows a characteristic sequence: An asymptomatic stage where daytime Pa_{O_2} and Pa_{CO_2} are normal, followed by nocturnal hypoventilation, initially during rapid eye movement (REM) sleep and later in non-REM sleep. Finally, if vital capacity drops further, daytime hypercapnia develops. Symptoms can develop at any point along this time course and often depend on the pace of respiratory muscle functional decline. Regardless of cause, the hallmark of all alveolar hypoventilation syndromes is an increase in alveolar P_{CO_2} (PA_{CO_2}) and, therefore, in Pa_{CO_2}. The resulting respiratory acidosis eventually leads to a compensatory increase in plasma bicarbonate concentration. The increase in PA_{CO_2} results in an obligatory decrease in PA_{O_2}, often resulting in hypoxemia. If severe, the hypoxemia manifests clinically as cyanosis and can stimulate erythropoiesis, thereby inducing secondary erythrocytosis. The combination of chronic hypoxemia and hypercapnia may also induce pulmonary vasoconstriction, leading eventually to pulmonary hypertension, right-ventricular hypertrophy, and right heart failure.

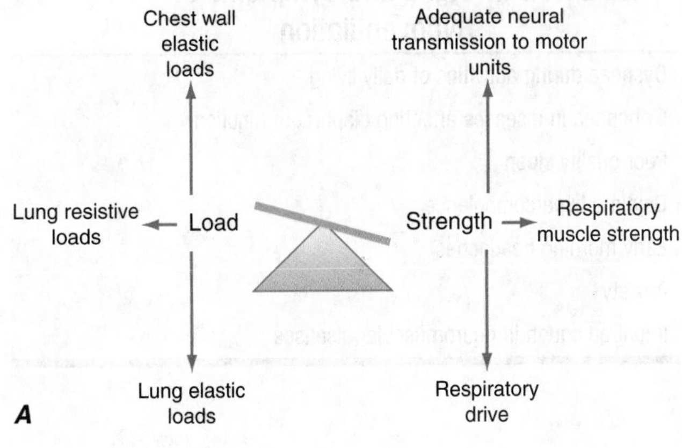

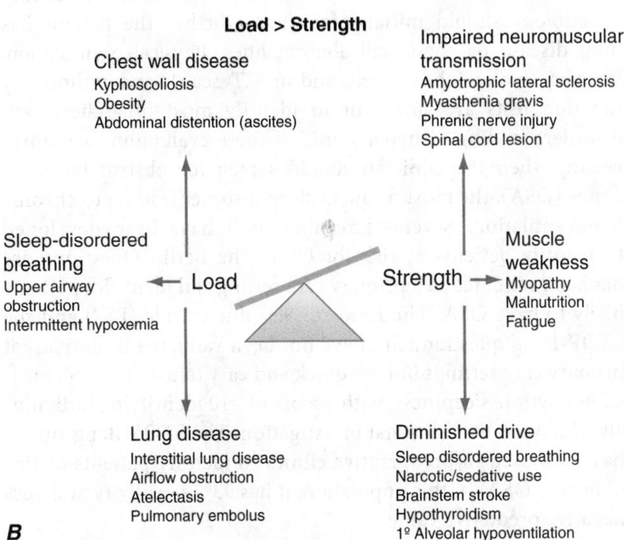

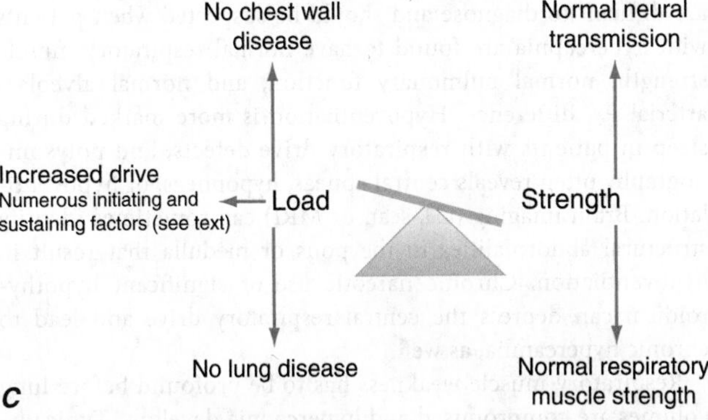

Figure 264-1 Examples of balance between respiratory system strength and load. *A.* Excess respiratory muscle strength in health. *B.* Load greater than strength. *C.* Increased drive with acceptable strength.

DIAGNOSIS

Elevated plasma bicarbonate in the absence of volume depletion is suggestive of hypoventilation. An arterial blood gas demonstrating elevated Pa_{CO_2} with a normal pH confirms chronic

TABLE 264-1 Signs and Symptoms of Hypoventilation

Dyspnea during activities of daily living
Orthopnea in diseases affecting diaphragm function
Poor quality sleep
Daytime hypersomnolence
Early morning headaches
Anxiety
Impaired cough in neuromuscular diseases

alveolar hypoventilation. The subsequent evaluation to identify an etiology should initially focus on whether the patient has lung disease or chest wall abnormalities. Physical examination, imaging studies (chest x-ray and/or CT scan), and pulmonary function tests are sufficient to identify most lung/chest wall disorders leading to hypercapnia. If these evaluations are unrevealing, then the clinician should screen for obstructive sleep apnea (OSA), the most frequent sleep disorder leading to chronic hypoventilation. Several screening tools have been developed to identify patients at risk for OSA. The Berlin Questionnaire has been validated in a primary care setting and identifies patients likely to have OSA. The Epworth Sleepiness Scale (ESS) and the STOP-Bang questionnaire have not been validated in outpatient primary care settings but are quick and easy to use. The ESS measures daytime sleepiness, with a score of ≥10 identifying individuals who warrant additional investigation. The STOP-Bang survey has been used in preoperative clinics to identify patients at risk of having OSA. In this population, it has 93% sensitivity and 90% negative predictive value.

If the ventilatory apparatus (lung, airways, chest wall) is not responsible for chronic hypercapnia, then the focus should shift to respiratory drive and neuromuscular disorders. There is an attenuated increase in minute ventilation in response to elevated CO_2 and/or low O_2 in respiratory drive disorders. These diseases are difficult to diagnose and should be suspected when patients with hypercapnia are found to have normal respiratory muscle strength, normal pulmonary function, and normal alveolar-arterial P_{O_2} difference. Hypoventilation is more marked during sleep in patients with respiratory drive defects, and polysomnography often reveals central apneas, hypopneas, or hypoventilation. Brain imaging (CT scan or MRI) can sometimes identify structural abnormalities in the pons or medulla that result in hypoventilation. Chronic narcotic use or significant hypothyroidism can depress the central respiratory drive and lead to chronic hypercapnia, as well.

Respiratory muscle weakness has to be profound before lung volumes are compromised and hypercapnia develops. Typically, physical examination reveals decreased strength in major muscle groups prior to the development of hypercapnia. Measurement of maximum inspiratory and expiratory pressures or forced vital capacity (FVC) can be used to monitor for respiratory muscle involvement in diseases with progressive muscle weakness. These patients also have increased risk for sleep-disordered breathing, including hypopneas, central and obstructive apneas, and hypoxemia. Nighttime oximetry and polysomnography are helpful in better characterizing sleep disturbances in this patient population.

TREATMENT Hypoventilation

Nocturnal noninvasive positive-pressure ventilation (NIPPV) has been used successfully in the treatment of hypoventilation and apneas, both central and obstructive, in patients with neuromuscular and chest wall disorders. Nocturnal NIPPV has been shown to improve daytime hypercapnia, prolong survival, and improve health-related quality of life when daytime hypercapnia is documented. ALS guidelines recommend nocturnal NIPPV if symptoms of hypoventilation exist AND one of the following criteria is present: Pa_{CO_2} ≥45 mmHg; nocturnal oximetry demonstrates oxygen saturation ≤88% for 5 consecutive minutes; maximal inspiratory pressure <60 cm H_2O; and FVC <50% predicted. However, at present there is inconclusive evidence to support preemptive nocturnal NIPPV use in all patients with neuromuscular and chest wall disorders who demonstrate nocturnal, but not daytime, hypercapnia. Nevertheless, at some point the institution of full-time ventilatory support with either pressure or volume-preset modes is required in progressive neuromuscular disorders. There is less evidence to direct the timing of this decision, but ventilatory failure requiring mechanical ventilation and chest infections related to ineffective cough are frequent triggers for the institution of full-time ventilatory support.

Treatment of chronic hypoventilation from lung or neuromuscular diseases should be directed at the underlying disorder. Pharmacologic agents that stimulate respiration, such as medroxyprogesterone and acetazolamide, have been poorly studied in chronic hypoventilation and should not replace treatment of the underlying disease process. Regardless of the cause, excessive metabolic alkalosis should be corrected, as plasma bicarbonate levels elevated out of proportion to the degree of chronic respiratory acidosis can result in additional hypoventilation. When indicated, administration of supplemental oxygen is effective in attenuating hypoxemia, polycythemia, and pulmonary hypertension.

Phrenic nerve or diaphragm pacing is a potential therapy for patients with hypoventilation from high cervical spinal cord lesions or respiratory drive disorders. Prior to surgical implantation, patients should have nerve conduction studies to ensure normal bilateral phrenic nerve function. Small case series suggest that effective diaphragmatic pacing can improve quality of life in these patients.

HYPOVENTILATION SYNDROMES

OBESITY HYPOVENTILATION SYNDROME

The diagnosis of obesity hypoventilation syndrome (OHS) requires: body mass index (BMI) ≥30 kg/m^2, sleep-disordered breathing and chronic daytime alveolar hypoventilation, defined as Pa_{CO2} ≥45 mmHg, and Pa_{O_2} < 70 mmHg in the absence of other known causes of hypercapnia. In almost 90% of cases, the sleep-disordered breathing is in the form of OSA. Several international studies in different populations confirm that the overall prevalence of obstructive sleep apnea syndrome, defined by an apnea hypopnea index ≥5 AND daytime sleepiness, is approximately 3–4% in middle-aged men and 2% in middle-aged women. Thus, the population at risk for the development of OHS continues to rise as the worldwide obesity epidemic persists. Although no population-based prevalence studies of OHS have been performed, some estimates suggest there may be as many as 500,000 individuals with OHS in the United States.

Several studies suggest that severe obesity (BMI >40 kg/m^2) and severe OSA apnea-hypopnea index [(AHI) >30 events per hour] are risk factors for the development of OHS. The pathogenesis of hypoventilation in these patients is multifactorial and incompletely understood. Defects in central respiratory drive have been demonstrated in OHS patients but often improve with treatment. This suggests central defects may not be the primary disturbance that leads to chronic hypercapnia. The treatment of OHS is similar to that for OSA: weight reduction and continuous positive airway pressure (CPAP) therapy during sleep. CPAP improves daytime hypercapnia and hypoxemia in the majority of patients with OHS. There is not conclusive evidence to suggest that bilevel positive airway pressure (BiPAP) is superior to CPAP. Bilevel positive airway pressure should be reserved for patients not able to tolerate high levels of CPAP support or patients that remain hypoxemic despite resolution of obstructive respiratory events.

CENTRAL HYPOVENTILATION SYNDROME

This syndrome can present later in life or in the neonatal period where it is often called Ondine's curse or congenital central hypoventilation syndrome (CCHS). Abnormalities in the gene encoding PHOX2b, a transcription factor with a role in neuronal development, have been implicated in the pathogenesis of congenital central hypoventilation syndrome. Regardless of the age of onset, these patients have absent respiratory response to hypoxia or hypercapnia, mildly elevated Pa_{CO_2} while awake, and markedly elevated Pa_{CO_2} during non-REM sleep. Interestingly, these patients are able to augment their ventilation and "normalize" Pa_{CO_2} during exercise. These patients typically require NIPPV or mechanical ventilation as therapy and should be considered for phrenic nerve or diaphragmatic pacing at centers with experience performing these procedures.

HYPERVENTILATION

CLINICAL FEATURES

Hyperventilation is defined as ventilation in excess of metabolic requirements (CO_2 production) leading to a reduction in Pa_{CO_2}. The physiology of patients with chronic hyperventilation is poorly understood, and there is no typical clinical presentation. Symptoms can include dyspnea, paresthesias, tetany, headache, dizziness, visual disturbances, and atypical chest pain. Because symptoms can be so diverse, patients with chronic hyperventilation present to a variety of health care providers, including internists, neurologists, psychologists, psychiatrists, and pulmonologists.

It is helpful to think of hyperventilation as having initiating and sustaining factors. Some investigators believe that an initial event leads to increased alveolar ventilation and a drop in Pa_{CO_2} to ~20 mmHg. The ensuing onset of chest pain, breathlessness, paresthesia, or altered consciousness can be alarming. The resultant increase in minute volume to relieve these acute symptoms only serves to exacerbate symptoms that are often misattributed by the patient and health care workers to cardiopulmonary disorders. An unrevealing evaluation for causes of these symptoms often results in patients being anxious and fearful of additional attacks. It is important to note that *anxiety disorders and panic attacks are NOT synonymous with hyperventilation.* Anxiety can be both an initiating and sustaining factor in the pathogenesis of chronic hyperventilation, but these are not necessary for the development of chronic hypocapnia.

DIAGNOSIS

Respiratory symptoms associated with acute hyperventilation can be the initial manifestation of systemic illnesses such as diabetic ketoacidosis. Causes of acute hyperventilation need to be excluded before a diagnosis of chronic hyperventilation is considered. Arterial blood gas sampling that demonstrates a compensated respiratory alkalosis with a near-normal pH, low Pa_{CO_2} and low calculated bicarbonate are necessary to confirm chronic hyperventilation. Other causes of respiratory alkalosis, such as mild asthma, need to be diagnosed and treated before chronic hyperventilation can be considered. A high index of suspicion is required as increased minute ventilation can be difficult to detect on physical examination. Once chronic hyperventilation is established, a sustained 10% increase in alveolar ventilation is enough to perpetuate hypocapnia. This increase can be accomplished with subtle changes in the respiratory pattern, such as occasional sigh breaths or yawning two to three times per minute.

TREATMENT Hyperventilation

There are few well-controlled treatment studies of chronic hyperventilation because of its diverse features and the lack of a universally accepted diagnostic process. Clinicians often spend considerable time identifying initiating factors, excluding alternative diagnoses and discussing the patient's concerns and fears. In some patients, reassurance and frank discussion about hyperventilation can be liberating. Identifying and eliminating habits that perpetuate hypocapnia, such as frequent yawning or sigh breathing, can be helpful. Some evidence suggests that breathing exercises and diaphragmatic retraining may be beneficial for some patients. The evidence for using medications to treat hyperventilation is scant. Beta-blockers may be helpful in patients with sympathetically mediated symptoms, such as palpitations and tremors.

ACKNOWLEDGMENT

We would like to acknowledge Eliot A. Phillipson for earlier versions of this chapter and Jan-Marino Ramirez for his careful critique and helpful suggestions.

FURTHER READINGS

Chung F et al: STOP Questionnaire: A tool to screen patients for obstructive sleep apnea. Anesthesiology 108:812, 2008

Douglas IS et al: Acute-on-chronic respiratory failure, in *Principles of Critical Care*, 3rd ed, JB Hall et al (eds). McGraw-Hill, 2005

Gardner WN: The pathophysiology of hyperventilation disorders. Chest 109:516, 1996

Laffey JG, Kavanagh BP: Hypocapnia. N Engl J Med 347:43, 2002

Littleton SW, Mokhlesi B: The Pickwickian syndrome-obesity hypoventilation syndrome. Clin Chest Med 30:467, 2009

Simonds AK: Recent advances in respiratory care for neuromuscular disease. Chest 130:1879, 2006

CHAPTER 265

Sleep Apnea

Neil J. Douglas

OBSTRUCTIVE SLEEP APNEA

Obstructive sleep apnea/hypopnea syndrome (OSAHS) is one of the most important medical conditions identified in the last 50 years. It is a major cause of morbidity, a significant cause of mortality, and the most common medical cause of daytime sleepiness. Central sleep apnea is a rare clinical problem. Other sleep disorders are discussed in Chap. 27.

DEFINITION

OSAHS is defined as the coexistence of unexplained excessive daytime sleepiness with at least five obstructed breathing events (apnea or hypopnea) per hour of sleep (Table 265-1). This event threshold may have to be increased in the elderly. *Apneas* are defined in adults as breathing pauses lasting ≥10 s and hypopneas as events ≥10 s in which there is continued breathing but ventilation is reduced by at least 50% from the previous baseline during sleep. As a syndrome, OSAHS is the association of a clinical picture with specific abnormalities on testing; asymptomatic individuals with abnormal breathing during sleep should not be labeled as having OSAHS.

MECHANISM OF OBSTRUCTION

Apneas and hypopneas are caused by the airway being sucked closed on inspiration during sleep. This occurs as the upper-airway dilating muscles—like all striated muscles—relax during sleep. In patients with OSAHS, the dilating muscles fail to oppose negative pressure within the airway during inspiration. The primary defect is not in the upper-airway muscles, which function normally in OSAHS patients when awake. These patients have narrow upper airways already during wakefulness, but when they are awake, their airway dilating muscles have increased activity, which ensures airway patency. However, during sleep, muscle tone falls and the airway narrows; snoring may commence before the airway occludes, and apnea results. Apneas and hypopneas terminate when the subject arouses, i.e., wakens briefly, from sleep. This arousal is sometimes too subtle to be seen on the electroencephalogram but may be detected by cardiac acceleration, blood pressure elevation, or increase in sympathetic tone. The arousal results in return of upper-airway dilating muscle tone, and thus airway patency is resumed.

Factors predisposing to OSAHS by narrowing the pharynx include obesity—in Western populations around 50% of OSAHS patients have a body mass index (BMI) >30 kg/m^2—and shortening of the mandible and/or maxilla. This change in jaw shape may be subtle and can be familial. Hypothyroidism and acromegaly predispose to OSAHS by narrowing the upper airway with tissue infiltration. Other predisposing factors for OSAHS include male sex and middle age (40–65 years), myotonic dystrophy, Ehlers-Danlos syndrome, and, perhaps, smoking.

EPIDEMIOLOGY

OSAHS occurs in around 1–4% of middle-aged males and is about half as common in women. The syndrome also occurs in childhood—usually associated with tonsil or adenoid enlargement—and in the elderly, although the frequency is slightly lower in old age. Irregular breathing during sleep *without* daytime sleepiness is much more common, occurring in perhaps a quarter of the middle-aged male population. As these individuals are asymptomatic, they do not have OSAHS, but there is increasing epidemiologic evidence of an association of irregular breathing during sleep with increased vascular risk even in the nonsleepy.

CLINICAL FEATURES

Randomized controlled treatment trials have shown that OSAHS causes daytime sleepiness; impaired vigilance, cognitive performance and driving; depression; disturbed sleep; and hypertension. Daytime sleepiness may range from mild to irresistible and can be indistinguishable from that in narcolepsy (Chap. 27). The sleepiness may cause inability to work effectively, damage interpersonal

TABLE 265-1 Clinical Indicators in the Sleepy Patient

	OSAHS	Narcolepsy	IHS
Age of onset (years)	35–60	10–30	10–30
Cataplexy	No	Yes	No
Night sleep			
Duration	Normal	Normal	Long
Awakenings	Occasional	Frequent	Rare
Snoring	Yes, loud	Occasional	Occasional
Morning drunkenness	Occasional	Occasional	Common
Daytime naps			
Frequency	Usually few	Many	Few
Time of day	Afternoon/evening	Afternoon/evening	Morning
Duration	<1 h	<1 h	>1 h

Note: Features suggesting obstructive sleep apnea/hypopnea syndrome (OSAHS), narcolepsy, or idiopathic hypersomnolence (IHS).

relationships, and prevent socializing. The somnolence is dangerous, with a three- to sixfold risk of road accidents. Experiments with normal subjects repeatedly aroused from sleep indicate that the sleepiness results, at least in part, from the repetitive sleep disruption associated with the breathing abnormality. Other symptoms include difficulty concentrating, unrefreshing nocturnal sleep, nocturnal choking, nocturia, and decreased libido. Partners report nightly loud snoring in all postures, which may be punctuated by the silence of apneas.

Cardiovascular and cerebrovascular events

OSAHS raises 24-h mean blood pressure. The increase is greater in those with recurrent nocturnal hypoxemia, is at least 4–5 mmHg, and may be as great as 10 mmHg in those with >20% arterial oxygen desaturations per hour of sleep. This rise probably results from a combination of surges in blood pressure accompanying each arousal at apnea/hypopnea termination and from the associated 24-h increases in sympathetic tone.

Epidemiologic data in normal populations indicate that this rise in blood pressure would increase the risk of myocardial infarction by around 20% and that of stroke by about 40%. Although there are no long-term randomized controlled trials to indicate whether this is true in OSAHS patients—such studies would be unethical—observational studies suggest an increase in cardiovascular and stroke risk in patients with untreated OSAHS. Furthermore, epidemiologic studies suggest increased vascular risk in normal subjects with raised apneas and hypopneas during sleep. Patients with recent stroke have a high frequency of apneas and hypopneas during sleep. These seem largely to be a consequence, not a cause, of the stroke and to decline over the weeks after the vascular event. There is no evidence that treating the apneas and hypopneas improves stroke outcome.

Diabetes mellitus

The association of OSAHS with diabetes mellitus is not due only to the fact that obesity is common in both conditions. Increased apneas and hypopneas during sleep are associated with insulin resistance independent of obesity. In addition, uncontrolled trials suggest OSAHS can aggravate diabetes and that treating OSAHS in patients who also have diabetes decreases their insulin requirements.

Liver

Hepatic dysfunction also has been associated with irregular breathing during sleep. Non-alcohol-drinking subjects with apneas and hypopneas during sleep were found to have raised liver enzymes and more steatosis and fibrosis on liver biopsy, independent of body weight.

Anesthetic risk

Patients with OSAHS are at increased risk perioperatively as their upper airways may obstruct during the recovery period or as a consequence of sedation. Patients whom anesthesiologists have difficulty intubating are much more likely to have irregular breathing during sleep. Anesthesiologists should thus take preoperative sleep histories and take the appropriate precautions with patients who might have OSAHS.

Differential diagnosis

(See also Chap. 27) Causes of sleepiness that may need to be distinguished include (Table 265-1) the following:

- *Insufficient sleep:* this usually can be diagnosed by history.
- *Shift work:* a major cause of sleepiness, especially in those >40 years old.
- *Psychological/psychiatric causes:* depression is a major cause of sleepiness.
- *Drugs:* both stimulant and sedative drugs can produce sleepiness.
- *Narcolepsy:* around 50 times less common than OSAHS, narcolepsy is usually evident from childhood or the teens and is associated with cataplexy.
- *Idiopathic hypersomnolence:* this is an ill-defined condition typified by long sleep duration and sleepiness.
- *Phase alteration syndromes:* both the phase delay and the less common phase advancement syndromes are characterized by sleepiness at the appropriate time of day.

Who to refer for diagnosis

Anyone whose troublesome sleepiness is not readily explained and rectified by considering the differential diagnosis above should be referred to a sleep specialist. The guideline the author uses for patients with troublesome sleepiness includes those with an Epworth Sleepiness Score >11 (Table 265-2) and also those whose sleepiness during work or driving poses problems. The Epworth Score is not a perfect measure for detecting sleepiness, as many whose lives are troubled by frequently fighting sleepiness but who never doze will correctly give themselves a low Epworth Score. The patient and his or her partner often give divergent scores for the patient's sleepiness, and in such cases the higher of the two scores should be used.

Diagnosis

OSAHS requires lifelong treatment, and the diagnosis has to be made or excluded with certainty. This will hinge on obtaining a

TABLE 265-2 Epworth Sleepiness Score

How often are you likely to doze off or fall asleep in the following situations, in contrast to feeling just tired? This refers to your usual way of life in recent times. Even if you have not done some of these things recently, try to work out how they would have affected you. Use the following scale to choose the *most appropriate number* for each situation:

0 = would *never* doze

1 = *slight* chance of dozing

2 = *moderate* chance of dozing

3 = *high* chance of dozing

Situation	Score
Sitting and reading	....
Watching TV	....
Sitting, inactive in a public place (e.g., a theater or a meeting)	....
As a passenger in a car for an hour without a break	....
Lying down to rest in the afternoon when circumstances permit	....
Sitting and talking to someone	....
Sitting quietly after lunch without alcohol	....
In a car, while stopped for a few minutes in traffic	....
TOTAL	....

Source: From MW Johns: Sleep 14:540, 1991.

good sleep history from the patient and partner, with both completing sleep questionnaires, including the Epworth Sleepiness Score (Table 265-2). Physical examination must include assessment of obesity, jaw structure, the upper airway, blood pressure, and possible predisposing causes, including hypothyroidism and acromegaly (see above).

In those with appropriate clinical features, the diagnostic test must demonstrate recurrent breathing pauses during sleep. This may be full polysomnography with recording of multiple respiratory and neurophysiologic signals during sleep (Chap. 27). Increasingly, especially outside the United States, most diagnostic tests are "limited studies"—recording respiratory and oxygenation patterns overnight without neurophysiologic recording. Such approaches in expert hands produce good patient outcomes and are cost-effective. It is sensible to use such limited sleep studies as the first-line diagnostic test and then allow positively diagnosed patients to proceed to treatment. A reasonable approach at present is for patients with troublesome sleepiness but negative limited studies to have polysomnography to exclude or confirm OSAHS.

TREATMENT Obstructive Sleep Apnea

WHOM TO TREAT There is evidence from robust randomized controlled trials (RCTs) that treatment improves symptoms, sleepiness, driving, cognition, mood, quality of life, and blood pressure in patients who have an Epworth Score >11, troublesome sleepiness while driving or working, and >15 apneas + hypopneas per hour of sleep. For those with similar degrees of sleepiness and 5–15 events per hour of sleep, RCTs indicate improvements in symptoms, including subjective sleepiness, with less strong evidence indicating gains in cognition and quality of life. There is no evidence of blood pressure improvements in this group. There is no robust evidence that treating nonsleepy subjects improves their symptoms, function, or blood pressure, and so treatment cannot be advocated for this large group, although this may change with further RCTs or less obtrusive therapy.

HOW TO TREAT All patients diagnosed with OSAHS should have the condition and its significance explained to them and their partners. This should be accompanied by written and/or Web-based information and a discussion of the implications of the local driving regulations. Rectifiable predispositions should be discussed; this often includes weight loss and alcohol reduction both to reduce weight and because alcohol acutely decreases upper-airway dilating muscle tone, thus predisposing to obstructed breathing. Sedative drugs, which also impair airway tone, should be carefully withdrawn.

Continuous Positive Airway Pressure (CPAP) CPAP therapy works by blowing the airway open during sleep, usually with pressures of 5–20 mmHg. CPAP has been shown in randomized placebo-controlled trials to improve breathing during sleep, sleep quality, sleepiness, blood pressure, vigilance, cognition, and driving ability as well as mood and quality of life in patients with OSAHS. However, this is obtrusive therapy, and care must be taken to explain the need for the treatment to patients and their partners and to intensively support patients on CPAP with telephone or Web support and regular follow-up. Initiation should include finding the most comfortable mask from the ranges of several manufacturers and trying the system for at least 30 min during the day to prepare for the overnight trial. An overnight monitored trial of CPAP is used to identify the pressure required to keep the patient's airway patent. The development of pressure-varying CPAP machines has made an in-lab CPAP night trial unnecessary, but treatment must be initiated in a supportive environment. Thereafter, patients can be treated with fixed-pressure CPAP machines set at the determined pressure or with a self-adjusting intelligent CPAP device. The main side effect of CPAP is airway drying, which can be countered by using an integral heated humidifier. CPAP use is imperfect, but around 94% of patients with severe OSAHS are still using their therapy after 5 years on objective monitoring.

Mandibular Repositioning Splint (MRS) Also called oral devices, MRSs work by holding the lower jaw and the tongue forward, thereby widening the pharyngeal airway. MRSs have been shown in RCTs to improve OSAHS patients' breathing during sleep, daytime somnolence, and blood pressure. As there are many devices with differing designs with unknown relative efficacy, these results cannot be generalized to all MRSs. Self-reports of the use of devices long-term suggest high dropout rates.

Surgery Four forms of surgery have a role in OSAHS, although it must be remembered that these patients have a raised perioperative risk. Bariatric surgery can be curative in the morbidly obese. Tonsillectomy can be highly effective in children but rarely in adults. Tracheostomy is curative but rarely used because of the associated morbidity rate but should not be overlooked in severe cases. Jaw advancement surgery—particularly maxillomandibular osteotomy—is effective in those with retrognathia (posterior displacement of the mandible) and should be considered particularly in young and thin patients. There is no robust evidence that pharyngeal surgery, including uvulopalatopharyngoplasty (whether by scalpel, laser, or thermal techniques) helps OSAHS patients.

Drugs Unfortunately, no drugs are clinically useful in the prevention or reduction of apneas and hypopneas. A marginal improvement in sleepiness in patients who remain sleepy despite CPAP can be produced by modafinil, but the clinical value is debatable and the financial cost is significant.

CHOICE OF TREATMENT CPAP and MRS are the two most widely used and best evidence-based therapies. Direct comparisons in RCTs indicate better outcomes with CPAP in terms of apneas and hypopneas, nocturnal oxygenation, symptoms, quality of life, mood, and vigilance. Adherence to CPAP is generally better than that to an MRS, and there is evidence that CPAP improves driving, whereas there are no such data on MRSs. Thus, CPAP is the current treatment of choice. However, MRSs are evidence-based second-line therapy in those who fail CPAP. In younger, thinner patients, maxillomandibular advancement should be considered.

HEALTH RESOURCES Untreated OSAHS patients are heavy users of health care and dangerous drivers; they also work beneath their potential. Treatment of OSAHS with CPAP is cost-effective in terms of reducing the health care costs of associated illness and associated accidents.

CENTRAL SLEEP APNEA

Central sleep apneas (CSAs) are respiratory pauses caused by lack of respiratory effort. They occur occasionally in normal subjects, particularly at sleep onset and in rapid eye movement (REM) sleep, and are transiently increased after ascent to altitude. Recurrent CSA is most commonly found in the presence of cardiac failure or neurologic disease, especially stroke. Spontaneous central sleep syndrome is rare and can be classified on the basis of the arterial P_{CO_2}.

Hypercapnic CSA occurs in conjunction with diminished ventilatory drive in Ondine's curse (central alveolar hypoventilation). Patients with normocapnic spontaneous CSA have a normal or low arterial P_{CO_2} when awake, with brisk ventilatory responses to hypercapnia. This combination results in unstable ventilatory control, with subjects breathing close to or below their apneic threshold for P_{CO_2} during sleep; this apneic tendency is compounded by cycles of arousal-induced hyperventilation, inducing further hypocapnia.

CLINICAL FEATURES

Patients may present with sleep maintenance insomnia, which is relatively unusual in OSAHS. Daytime sleepiness may occur.

INVESTIGATION

Many apneas previously labeled central because of absent thoracoabdominal movement are actually obstructive, identification of movement being particularly difficult in the very obese. CSA can be identified with certainty only if either esophageal pressure or respiratory muscle electromyography is recorded and shown to be absent during the events.

TREATMENT Central Sleep Apnea

Patients with underlying cardiac failure should have their failure treated appropriately. CPAP may improve outcome but is difficult to initiate and has not been shown to improve survival. Patients with spontaneous normocapnic CSA may be treated with acetazolamide. In a minority of patients, CPAP is effective, perhaps because in some patients with OSAHS, pharyngeal collapse initiates reflex inhibition of respiration, and this is prevented by CPAP. Oxygen and nocturnal nasal positive-pressure ventilation also may be tried.

FURTHER READINGS

Bradley TD et al: Obstructive sleep apnoea and its cardiovascular consequences. Lancet 373:82, 2009

Eckert DJ et al: Central sleep apnea: Pathophysiology and treatment. Chest 131:595, 2007

Engleman HM et al: Randomized crossover trial of two treatments for sleep apnea/hypopnea syndrome: Continuous positive airway pressure and mandibular repositioning splint. Am J Respir Crit Care Med 165:855, 2002

Marin JM et al: Long-term cardiovascular outcomes in men with obstructive sleep apnoea-hypopnoea with or without treatment with continuous positive airway pressure: An observational study. Lancet 365:1046, 2005

Pack AL et al: Risk factors for excessive sleepiness in older adults. Ann Neurol 59:893, 2006

Somers VK et al: Sleep apnea and vascular disease. Circulation 118:1080, 2008

Sundaram S et al: Surgery for obstructive sleep apnoea in adults. Cochrane Database Syst Rev 2008, CD001004

Whitelaw WA et al: Clinical usefulness of home oximetry compared with polysomnography for assessment of sleep apnea. Am J Respir Crit Care Med 171:188, 2005

Yaggi HK et al: Obstructive sleep apnea as a risk factor for stroke and death. N Engl J Med 353:2034, 2005

Young T et al: Sleep disordered breathing and mortality: Eighteen-year follow-up of the Wisconsin sleep cohort. Sleep 31:1071, 2008

CHAPTER 266

Lung Transplantation

Elbert P. Trulock

Lung transplantation is a therapeutic consideration for many patients with nonmalignant end-stage lung disease, and it prolongs survival and improves quality of life in appropriately selected recipients. Since 1985 more than 25,000 procedures have been recorded worldwide, and ~2200 transplants have been reported annually in recent years.

INDICATIONS

The indications span the gamut of lung diseases. The most common indications in the last few years have been chronic obstructive pulmonary disease (COPD), ~30%; idiopathic pulmonary fibrosis (IPF), ~30%; cystic fibrosis (CF), ~15%; α_1-antitrypsin deficiency emphysema, ~3%; and idiopathic pulmonary arterial hypertension (IPAH), ~2%. Other diseases have accounted for the balance of primary indications, and retransplantation has accounted for ~4% of procedures.

RECIPIENT SELECTION

Transplantation should be considered when other therapeutic options have been exhausted and when the patient's prognosis is expected to improve as a result of the procedure. Survival rates after transplantation can be compared with predictive indices for the patient's disease, but each patient's clinical course must be integrated into the assessment, too. Moreover, quality of life is a primary motive for transplantation for many patients, and the prospect of improved quality-adjusted survival is often attractive even if the survival advantage itself may be marginal.

Disease-specific consensus guidelines for referring patients for evaluation and for proceeding with transplantation are summarized in Table 266-1 and are linked to clinical, physiologic, radiographic, and pathologic features that influence the prognosis of the respective diseases. Candidates for lung transplantation are also thoroughly screened for comorbidities that might affect the outcome adversely. Conditions such as systemic hypertension, diabetes mellitus, gastroesophageal reflux, and osteoporosis are not unusual, but if uncomplicated and adequately managed, they do not disqualify patients from transplantation. The upper age limit is ~65–70 years at most centers.

Standard exclusions include HIV infection, chronic active hepatitis B or C infection, uncontrolled or untreatable pulmonary or extrapulmonary infection, uncured malignancy, active cigarette smoking, drug or alcohol dependency, irreversible physical deconditioning, chronic nonadherence with medical care, significant disease of another vital organ (e.g., heart, liver, or kidney), and psychiatric or psychosocial situations that could substantially interfere with posttransplantation management. Other problems that may compromise the outcome constitute relative contraindications. Some typical issues are ventilator-dependent respiratory failure, previous thoracic surgical procedures, obesity, and coronary artery

TABLE 266-1 Disease-Specific Guidelines for Referral and Transplantation

Chronic Obstructive Pulmonary Disease
Referral
BODE index >5
Transplantation
BODE index 7–10
or
any of the following criteria:
Hospitalization for exacerbation, with Pa_{CO_2} >50 mmHg
Pulmonary hypertension or cor pulmonale despite oxygen therapy
FEV_1<20% with either DL_{CO} <20% or diffuse emphysema
Cystic Fibrosis/Bronchiectasis
Referral
FEV_1<30% or rapidly declining FEV_1
Hospitalization in ICU for exacerbation
Increasing frequency of exacerbations
Refractory or recurrent pneumothorax
Recurrent hemoptysis not controlled by bronchial artery embolization
Transplantation
Oxygen-dependent respiratory failure
Hypercapnia
Pulmonary hypertension
Idiopathic Pulmonary Fibrosis
Referral
Pathologic or radiographic evidence of UIP regardless of vital capacity
Transplantation
Pathologic or radiographic evidence of UIP
and
any of the following criteria
DL_{CO} <39%
Decrement in FVC ≥10% during 6 months of follow-up
Decrease in Sp_{O_2} below 88% during a 6-min walk test
Honeycombing on HRCT (fibrosis score >2)
Idiopathic Pulmonary Arterial Hypertension
Referral
NYHA functional class III or IV regardless of therapy
Rapidly progressive disease
Transplantation
Failing therapy with intravenous epoprostenol (or equivalent drug)
Persistent NYHA functional class III or IV on maximal medical therapy
Low (<350 m) or declining 6-min walk test
Cardiac index <2 L/min/m^2
Right atrial pressure >15 mmHg

Abbreviations: BODE, body-mass index (B), airflow obstruction (O), dyspnea (D), exercise capacity (E); FVC, forced vital capacity; FEV_1, forced expiratory volume in 1 s; DL_{CO}, diffusing capacity for carbon monoxide; Pa_{CO_2}, partial pressure of carbon dioxide in arterial blood; Sp_{O_2}, arterial oxygen saturation by pulse oximetry; ICU, intensive care unit; UIP, usual interstitial pneumonitis; HRCT, high-resolution computed tomography; NYHA, New York Heart Association.

Source: Summarized from Orens et al. For BODE index, BR Celli et al: N Engl J Med 350:1005, 2004.

disease. Chronic infection with antibiotic-resistant *Pseudomonas* species, *Burkholderia* species, *Aspergillus* species, or nontuberculous mycobacteria is a unique concern in some patients with CF. The potential impact of these and other factors has to be judged in clinical context to determine an individual candidate's suitability for transplantation.

■ WAITING LIST AND ORGAN ALLOCATION

Organ allocation policies are influenced by medical, ethical, geographic, and political factors, with systems varying from country to country. Regardless of the system, potential recipients are placed on a waiting list and must be matched for blood group compatibility and, with some latitude, for lung size with an acceptable donor. Most lungs are procured from deceased donors after brain death, but only ~15–17% of brain-death organ donors yield either one or two lungs suitable for transplantation. Lungs from donors after cardiac death have been utilized to a limited extent.

A priority algorithm for allocating donor lungs was implemented in the United States in 2005. A lung allocation score that is based on the patient's risk of death on the waiting list and likelihood of survival after transplantation determines priority. The score can range from zero to 100, and precedence for transplantation is ranked from highest to lowest scores. Both the lung disease and its severity affect a patient's score; parameters in the score must be updated biannually but can be submitted for calculation of a new score whenever the patient's condition changes. The median score for all candidates on the waiting list is usually ~34–35, but the distribution of scores tends to be higher among patients with IPF and CF than among patients with COPD and IPAH. Under this priority system, the median waiting time for transplantation has fallen to <6 months, and the annual number of deaths on the waiting list has dropped by ~50%. The main indication for transplantation has also shifted from COPD to IPF. Overall survival rates in the first two years after transplantation have not changed substantially under this system; however, recipients with lung allocation scores >60 have had lower survival rates in the first two years compared with recipients with lower scores.

■ TRANSPLANT PROCEDURE

Bilateral transplantation is mandatory for CF and other forms of bronchiectasis because the risk of spillover infection from a remaining native lung precludes single-lung transplantation. Heart-lung transplantation is obligatory for Eisenmenger syndrome with complex anomalies that cannot be readily repaired in conjunction with lung transplantation and for concomitant end-stage lung and heart disease. However, cardiac replacement is not necessary for cor pulmonale because right ventricular function will recover when pulmonary vascular afterload is normalized by lung transplantation.

Either bilateral or single-lung transplantation is an option for other diseases unless there is a special consideration, but bilateral transplantation has been utilized increasingly for most indications. Recently, ~65% of procedures in the United States have been bilateral, and in the international registry, ~55% of transplants for COPD, ~50% for IPF, and ~90% for IPAH have been bilateral.

Living donor lobar transplantation has a limited role in adult lung transplantation. It has been performed predominantly in teenagers or young adults with CF, and it usually has been reserved for patients who were unlikely to survive the wait for a deceased organ donor.

■ POSTTRANSPLANTATION MANAGEMENT

Induction therapy with an antilymphocyte globulin or an interleukin 2 receptor antagonist is utilized by ~50% of centers, and a three-drug maintenance immunosuppressive regimen that includes a calcineurin inhibitor (cyclosporine or tacrolimus), a purine synthesis antagonist (azathioprine or a mycophenolic acid precursor), and prednisone is traditional. Subsequently, other drugs, such as sirolimus, may be substituted into the regimen for various reasons. Prophylaxis for *Pneumocystis jiroveci* pneumonia is standard, and prophylaxis against cytomegalovirus (CMV) infection and fungal infection is part of many protocols. The dose of cyclosporine, tacrolimus, and sirolimus is adjusted by blood-level monitoring. All these agents are metabolized by the hepatic cytochrome P450 system, and interactions with medications that affect this pathway can significantly alter the clearance and blood level of these drugs.

Routine management focuses on monitoring the allograft, regulating immunosuppressive therapy, and detecting problems or complications expeditiously. Regular contact with a nurse coordinator, physician follow-up, chest radiographs, blood tests, and spirometry are customary, and periodic surveillance bronchoscopies are employed in some programs. If recovery is uncomplicated, lung function rapidly improves and then stabilizes by 3–6 months after transplantation. Subsequently, the variation in spirometric measurements is small, and a sustained decline of ≥10–15% signals a potentially significant problem.

OUTCOMES

Survival

Major registries publish survival (Table 266-2) and other outcomes annually (*www.ishlt.org; www.ustransplant.org*). In the international registry, survival half-life for the main indications is in the range of 4–6 years; however, age and transplant procedure have a significant impact on outcome. For recipients 18–59 years of age, the survival half-life is 5–6 years, but it decreases to 4 years for those 60–65 years old and to 3 years for those >65 years old. Survival over 10 years has been significantly better after bilateral transplantation than after unilateral transplantation for COPD, α_1-antitrypsin deficiency emphysema, IPF, and IPAH.

The main sources of perioperative mortality include technical complications of the operation, primary graft dysfunction, and infections. Acute rejection and CMV infection are common problems in the first year, but neither is usually fatal. Beyond the first year, chronic rejection and non-CMV infections cause the majority of deaths.

Function

Regardless of the disease, successful transplantation impressively restores cardiopulmonary function. After bilateral transplantation, pulmonary function tests are typically normal; after unilateral transplantation, a mild abnormality characteristic of the remaining diseased lung is still apparent. Formal exercise testing usually demonstrates some impairment in maximum work rate and maximum oxygen uptake, but few recipients report any limitation to activities of daily living.

Quality of life

Both overall and health-related quality of life are enhanced. With multidimensional profiles, improvements extend across most domains and are sustained longitudinally unless chronic rejection or another complication develops. Other problems that detract from quality of life include renal dysfunction and drug side effects.

Cost

The cost of transplantation depends on the health care system, other health care policies, and economic factors that vary from country to country. In the United States in 2008 the average billed charge per transplant for the period 30 days before transplantation through 180 days after the transplant admission was $450,400 for single-lung transplantation and $657,800 for bilateral lung transplantation. For bilateral transplantation, the total cost included the following charges: all care during 30 days before transplantation, $20,700; donor organ procurement, $96,500; hospital transplant admission, $344,700; physician fees during transplant admission, $59,300; all inpatient and outpatient care during 180 days after transplant admission, $113,800; and all outpatient drugs, including immunosuppressants, from discharge for the transplant to 180 days after transplant admission, $22,800.

TABLE 266-2 Recipient Survival, by Pretransplantation Diagnosis (1990–2006)

Diagnosis	*n*	Survival Rate, %				
		3 Months	1 Year	3 Years	5 Years	10 Years
Chronic obstructive pulmonary disease						
Bilateral	2444	93	85	69	57	31
Single	5316	90	81	63	47	19
α_1-Antitrypsin deficiency emphysema						
Bilateral	956	88	79	67	58	36
Single	969	87	77	61	51	28
Cystic fibrosis	3275	90	82	66	56	39
Idiopathic pulmonary fibrosis						
Bilateral	1290	81	72	59	48	28
Single	2641	85	73	56	43	19
Idiopathic pulmonary arterial hypertension						
Bilateral	710	75	69	59	51	33
Single	260	71	61	51	41	24
Sarcoidosis	506	83	70	56	51	31

Source: Data from *www.ishlt.org/registries/slides.asp?slides=heartLungRegistry.*

TABLE 266-3 Major Potential Complications of Lung Transplantation and Immunosuppression

Category	Complication
Allograft	Primary graft dysfunction; anastomotic dehiscence or stenosis; ischemic airway injury with bronchostenosis or bronchomalacia; rejection; infection; recurrence of primary disease (sarcoidosis, lymphangioleiomyomatosis, giant cell interstitial pneumonitis, diffuse panbronchiolitis, pulmonary alveolar proteinosis, Langerhans cell histiocytosis)
Thoracic	Phrenic nerve injury—diaphragmatic dysfunction; recurrent laryngeal nerve injury—vocal cord dysfunction; cervical ganglia injury—Horner's syndrome; pneumothorax; pleural effusion; chylothorax; empyema
Cardiovascular	Intraoperative or perioperative air embolism; postoperative pericarditis; perioperative myocardial injury/infarction; venous thromboembolism; supraventricular dysrhythmias; systemic hypertension
Gastrointestinal	Esophagitis [especially *Candida*, herpes, or cytomegalovirus (CMV)]; gastroparesis; gastroesophageal reflux; diarrhea (*Clostridium difficile*; medications, especially mycophenolate mofetil and sirolimus); colitis (*C. difficile*; CMV)
Hepatobiliary	Hepatitis (especially CMV or medications); acalculous cholecystitis
Renal	Calcineurin inhibitor nephropathy; hemolytic-uremic syndrome (thrombotic microangiopathy)
Neurologic	Tremors; seizures; reversible posterior leukoencephalopathy; headaches
Musculoskeletal	Steroid myopathy; rhabdomyolysis (cyclosporine + HMG-CoA reductase inhibitor treatment); osteoporosis; avascular necrosis
Metabolic	Obesity; diabetes mellitus; hyperlipidemia; idiopathic hyperammonemia
Hematologic	Anemia; leukopenia; thrombocytopenia; thrombotic microangiopathy
Oncologic	Lymphoproliferative disease and lymphoma; skin cancers; other malignancies

Complications

Lung transplantation can be complicated by a variety of problems (Table 266-3). Aside from predicaments that are unique to transplantation, side effects and toxicities of the immunosuppressive medications can cause new medical problems or aggravate preexisting conditions.

Graft dysfunction

Primary graft dysfunction (PGD) is an acute lung injury that is a manifestation of multiple potential insults to the donor organ inherent in the transplantation process. The principal clinical features are diffuse pulmonary infiltrates and hypoxemia within 72 h of transplantation; however, the presentation can be mimicked by pulmonary venous obstruction, hyperacute rejection, pulmonary edema, and pneumonia.

The severity is variable, and a standardized grading system has been established. Up to 50% of recipients may have some degree of PGD, and ~10–20% have severe PGD. The treatment follows the conventional, supportive paradigm for acute lung injury. Inhaled nitric oxide and extracorporeal membrane oxygenation have been used in severe cases; retransplantation also has been performed, but retransplantation in the first 30 days has a poor survival rate (~30% at 1 year). Most recipients with mild PGD recover, but the mortality rate for severe PGD has been ~40–60%. PGD also is associated with longer postoperative ventilator support, longer intensive care unit and hospital stays, higher costs, and excess morbidity rates and severe PGD is probably a risk factor for the later development of chronic rejection.

Airway complications

The bronchial blood supply to the donor lung is disrupted during procurement. Bronchial revascularization during transplantation is technically feasible in some cases, but it is not widely practiced. Consequently, after implantation the donor bronchus is dependent on retrograde bronchial blood flow from the pulmonary circulation and is vulnerable to ischemia.

The spectrum of airway problems includes anastomotic necrosis and dehiscence, occlusive granulation tissue, anastomotic or bronchial stenosis, and bronchomalacia. The incidence has been in the range of 7–18%, but the associated mortality rate has been low. These problems usually can be managed bronchoscopically with techniques such as simple endoscopic debridement, laser photoresection, balloon dilatation, and bronchial stenting.

Rejection

Rejection is the main limitation to better medium- and long-term survival. It is an immunologic response to alloantigen recognition, and both cell-mediated and antibody-mediated (humoral) cascades can play a role. Cellular rejection is effected by T lymphocyte interactions with donor alloantigens, mainly in the major histocompatibility complex (MHC), whereas humoral rejection is driven by antibodies to donor MHC alloantigens or possibly to non-MHC antigens on epithelial or endothelial cells.

Rejection often is categorized as acute or chronic without mention of the mechanism. Acute rejection is cell-mediated, and its incidence is highest in the first 6–12 months after transplantation. In contrast, chronic rejection generally emerges later, and both alloimmune and nonalloimmune fibroproliferative reactions may contribute to its pathogenesis.

Acute cellular rejection

With current immunosuppressive regimens, ~25–40% of recipients have acute rejection in the first year. Acute cellular rejection (ACR) can be clinically silent, or it can be manifested by nonspecific symptoms or signs that may include cough, low-grade fever, dyspnea, hypoxemia, inspiratory crackles, interstitial infiltrates, and declining lung function; however, clinical impression is not reliable. The diagnosis is confirmed by transbronchial biopsies showing the characteristic lymphocytic infiltrates around arterioles or bronchioles, and a standardized pathologic scheme is used to grade the biopsies.

Minimal ACR on a surveillance biopsy in a clinically stable recipient often is left untreated, but higher grades generally are treated regardless of the clinical situation. Treatment usually includes a short course of high-dose steroid therapy and adjustment of the maintenance immunosuppressive regimen. Most episodes respond to this approach; however, more intensive therapy is sometimes necessary for persistent or recurrent episodes.

Chronic rejection

This complication is the main impediment to better long-term survival rates, and it is the source of substantial morbidity rates because of its impact on lung function and quality of life. Clinically, it is characterized physiologically by airflow limitation and pathologically by bronchiolitis obliterans; the process is denoted bronchiolitis obliterans syndrome (BOS). Transbronchial biopsies are relatively insensitive for detecting bronchiolitis obliterans, and pathologic confirmation is not required for diagnosis. Thus, after other causes of graft dysfunction have been excluded, the diagnosis of BOS is based primarily on a sustained decrement (≥20%) in forced expiratory volume in 1s (FEV_1), although smaller declines in FEV_1 (≥10%) or in forced expiratory flow $FEF_{25-75\%}$ may presage BOS. Spirometric criteria for diagnosis and staging of BOS have been standardized.

The prevalence of BOS approaches 50% by 5 years after transplantation. Antecedent ACR is the main risk factor, but PGD, CMV pneumonitis, other community-acquired respiratory viral infections, and gastroesophageal reflux have been implicated as well. BOS can present acutely and imitate infectious bronchitis, or it can manifest as an insidious decline in lung function. The chest radiograph is typically unchanged; computed tomography may reveal mosaic perfusion, air trapping, ground-glass opacities, or bronchiolectasis. Bronchoscopy is indicated to eliminate other processes, but transbronchial biopsies identify bronchiolitis obliterans in a minority of cases.

BOS usually is treated with augmented immunosuppression, but there is no consensus about therapy. Strategies include changes in the maintenance drug regimen, including the addition of azithromycin, antilymphocyte globulin, photopheresis, and total lymphoid irradiation. Although therapy may stabilize lung function, the overall results of treatment have been disappointing; median survival after onset has been ~3–4 years. Retransplantation is a consideration if clinical circumstances and other comorbidities are not prohibitive, but survival has been inferior to that with primary transplantation.

Humoral rejection

The role of antibody-mediated rejection is still evolving. Hyperacute rejection is caused by preformed human leukocyte (HLA) antibodies in the recipient, but it is minimized by pretransplantation antibody screening coupled with virtual or direct cross-matching with any potential donor. Donor-specific HLA antibodies develop after transplantation in up to 50% of recipients, and their presence has been associated with an increased risk of both ACR and BOS and with poorer overall survival. However, the mechanisms by which these antibodies could contribute to ACR or BOS or could otherwise be detrimental have not been unraveled. Formal criteria for antibody-mediated rejection have been defined for renal transplantation, but few cases in lung transplantation fulfill them. Nonetheless, episodes of acute lung allograft dysfunction occasionally have been attributed directly to antibody-mediated injury. If treatment is indicated, therapies that may deplete antibodies include plasmapheresis, intravenous immune globulin, and rituximab.

Infection

The lung allograft is especially susceptible to infection, which has been one of the leading causes of death. In addition to a blunted immune response from the immunosuppressive drugs, other normal defenses are compromised: the cough reflex is diminished, and mucociliary clearance is impaired in the transplanted lung. The spectrum of infections includes both opportunistic and nonopportunistic pathogens.

Bacterial bronchitis or pneumonia can occur at any time, but it is very common in the perioperative period. Later, bronchitis occurs frequently in recipients with BOS, and *Pseudomonas aeruginosa* or methicillin-resistant *Staphylococcus aureus* is often the culprit.

CMV is the most common viral infection. Although gastroenteritis, colitis, and hepatitis can occur, CMV viremia and CMV pneumonia are the main illnesses. Most episodes occur in the first 6 months, and treatment with ganciclovir is effective unless resistance develops. Other community-acquired viruses such as influenza, parainfluenza, and respiratory syncytial virus also contribute to respiratory complications. The most problematic fungal infections are caused by *Aspergillus* species. The spectrum encompasses simple pulmonary colonization, tracheobronchitis, invasive pulmonary aspergillosis, and disseminated aspergillosis, and the clinical scenario dictates treatment.

Other complications

Other potential complications are listed in Table 266-3. Many of them are related to side effects or toxicities of the immunosuppressive drugs. Management of these general medical problems is guided by standard practices, but the complex milieu of transplantation requires close collaboration and good communication among health care providers.

FURTHER READINGS

Belperio JA et al: Chronic lung allograft rejection: Mechanisms and therapy. Proc Am Thorac Soc 6:108, 2009

Bhorade SM, Stern E: Immunosuppression for lung transplantation. Proc Am Thorac Soc 6:47, 2009

Boasquevisque CHR et al: Surgical techniques: Lung transplant and lung volume reduction. Proc Am Thorac Soc 6:66, 2009

Chan KM et al: Nonmedical therapy for chronic obstructive pulmonary disease. Proc Am Thorac Soc 6:137, 2009

Christie JD et al: The Registry of the International Society for Heart and Lung Transplantation: Twenty-sixth Official Adult Lung and Heart-Lung Transplantation Report-2009. J Heart Lung Transplant 28:1031, 2009

Kreider M, Kotloff RM: Selection of candidates for lung transplantation. Proc Am Thorac Soc 6:20, 2009

Lee JC, Christie JD: Primary graft dysfunction. Proc Am Thorac Soc 6: 39, 2009

Lyu DM, Zamora MR: Medical complications of lung transplantation. Proc Am Thorac Soc 6:101, 2009

Martinu T et al: Acute rejection and humoral sensitization in lung transplant recipients. Proc Am Thorac Soc 6:54, 2009

Orens JB, Garrity ER Jr: General overview of lung transplantation and review of organ allocation. Proc Am Thorac Soc 6:13, 2009

——— et al: International guidelines for the selection of lung transplant candidates: 2006 update—a consensus report from the pulmonary scientific council of the International Society for Heart and Lung Transplantation. J Heart Lung Transplant 25:745, 2006

REMUND KF et al: Infections relevant to lung transplantation. Proc Am Thorac Soc 6:94, 2009

SANTACRUZ JF, MEHTA AC: Airway complications and management after lung transplantation: Ischemia, dehiscence, and stenosis. Proc Am Thorac Soc 6:79, 2009

SWEET SC: Pediatric lung transplantation. Proc Am Thorac Soc 6:122, 2009

VAN RAEMDONCK D et al: Lung donor selection and management. Proc Am Thorac Soc 6:28, 2009

YUSEN RD: Technology and outcomes assessment in lung transplantation. Proc Am Thorac Soc 6:128, 2009

PART 12

Critical Care Medicine

SECTION 1 Respiratory Critical Care

SECTION 2 Shock and Cardiac Arrest

SECTION 3 Neurologic Critical Care

SECTION 4 Oncologic Emergencies

CHAPTER 267 Approach to the Patient With Critical Illness

John P. Kress
Jesse B. Hall

The care of critically ill patients requires a thorough understanding of pathophysiology and is centered initially on resuscitation of patients at extremes of physiologic deterioration. This resuscitation is often fast-paced and occurs early without a detailed awareness of the patients' chronic medical problems. While physiologic stabilization is taking place, intensivists attempt to gather important background medical information to supplement the real-time assessment of the patients' current physiologic conditions. Numerous tools are available to assist intensivists in the accurate assessment of pathophysiology and management to incipient organ failure, offering a window of opportunity for diagnosing and treating underlying disease(s) in a stabilized patient. Indeed, the use of invasive interventions such as mechanical ventilation and renal replacement therapy is commonplace in the intensive care unit. An appreciation of the risks and benefits of such aggressive and often invasive interventions is vital to assure an optimal patient outcome. Nonetheless, intensivists must recognize when patients' chances for recovery are remote or impossible and counsel and comfort dying patients and their significant others. Critical care physicians often must redirect the goals of care from resuscitation and cure to comfort when the resolution of an underlying illness is not possible.

ASSESSMENT OF SEVERITY OF ILLNESS

Categorization of a patient's illness into grades of severity occurs frequently in the intensive care unit (ICU). Numerous severity-of-illness (SOI) scoring systems have been developed and validated over the last two decades. Although these scoring systems have been validated as tools to assess populations of critically ill patients, their utility in predicting individual patient outcomes is not clear.

SOI scoring systems are important for defining populations of critically ill patients. This allows effective comparison of groups of patients enrolled in clinical trials. To be assured that a purported benefit of a therapy is real, investigators must be assured that different groups involved in a clinical trial have similar illness severities. SOI scores are also useful in guiding hospital administrative policies. Allocation of resources such as nursing and ancillary care can be directed by such scoring systems. SOI scoring systems also can assist in the assessment of quality of ICU care over time. Scoring system validations are based on the premise that increasing age, the presence of chronic medical illnesses, and increasingly severe derangements from normal physiology are associated with increased mortality rates. All currently existing SOI scoring systems are derived from patients who already have been admitted to the ICU. There are no established scoring systems available that purport to direct clinicians' decision-making regarding criteria for admission to an ICU.

Currently, the most commonly utilized scoring systems are the APACHE (acute physiology and chronic health evaluation) system and the SAPS (simplified acute physiology score) system. These systems were designed to predict outcomes in critical illness and use common variables that include age; vital signs; assessments of respiratory, renal, and neurologic function; and an evaluation of chronic medical illnesses.

APACHE II SCORING SYSTEM

The APACHE II system is the most commonly used SOI scoring system in North America. Age, type of ICU admission (after elective surgery vs. nonsurgical or after emergency surgery), a chronic health problem score, and 12 physiologic variables (the most severely abnormal of each in the first 24 h of ICU admission) are used to derive a score. The predicted hospital mortality is derived from a formula that takes into account the APACHE II score, the need for emergency surgery, and a weighted, disease-specific diagnostic category (Table 267-1). The relationship between APACHE II score and mortality is illustrated in Fig. 267-1. Updated versions of the APACHE scoring system (APACHE III and APACHE IV) have been published. APACHE III is derived from a larger database than APACHE II and utilizes a daily clinical update protocol to provide daily modification of predicted mortality. APACHE IV uses a modified statistical model of logistic regression; it is the most recently released version of this scoring system.

THE SAPS SCORING SYSTEM

The SAPS II score, used more frequently in Europe, was derived in a manner similar to the APACHE scores. This score is not disease-specific but, rather, incorporates three underlying disease variables (AIDS, metastatic cancer, and hematologic malignancy).

Severity of illness scoring systems cannot be used to predict survival in individual patients. Accordingly, the use of these scoring systems to direct therapy and clinical decision-making cannot be recommended at present. Instead, these tools should be used as important data to complement clinical bedside decision-making.

SHOCK

(See also Chap. 270)

INITIAL EVALUATION

Shock is a common condition necessitating admission to the ICU or occurring in the course of critical care. Shock is defined by the presence of multisystem end organ hypoperfusion. Clinical indicators include reduced mean arterial pressure (MAP), tachycardia, tachypnea, cool skin and extremities, acute altered mental status, and oliguria. Hypotension is usually, though not always, present. The end result of multiorgan hypoperfusion is tissue hypoxia, often clinically manifested by lactic acidosis. Since the MAP is the product of cardiac output and systemic vascular resistance (SVR), reductions in blood pressure can be caused by decreased cardiac output and/or decreased SVR. Accordingly, the initial evaluation of a hypotensive patient should include an assessment of the adequacy of cardiac output; this should be part of the earliest assessment of the patient by the

TABLE 267-1 Calculation of Acute Physiology and Chronic Health Evaluation II (APACHE II)[a]

Acute Physiology Score

Score	4	3	2	1	0	1	2	3	4
Rectal temperature, °C	≥41	39.0–40.9		38.5–38.9	36.0–38.4	34.0–35.9	32.0–33.9	30.0–31.9	≤29.9
Mean blood pressure, mmHg	≥160	130–159	110–129		70–109		50–69		≤49
Heart rate	≥180	140–179	110–139		70–109		55–69	40–54	≤39
Respiratory rate	≥50	35–49		25–34	12–24	10–11	6–9		≤5
Arterial pH	≥7.70	7.60–7.69		7.50–7.59	7.33–7.49		7.25–7.32	7.15–7.24	<7.15
Oxygenation									
If FI_{O_2} > 0.5, use (A – a) D_{O_2}	≥500	350–499	200–349		<200				
If FI_{O_2} ≤ 0.5, use Pa_{O_2}					>70	61–70		55–60	<55
Serum sodium, meq/L	≥180	160–179	155–159	150–154	130–149		120–129	111–119	≤110
Serum potassium, meq/L	≥7.0	6.0–6.9		5.5–5.9	3.5–5.4	3.0–3.4	2.5–2.9		<2.5
Serum creatinine, mg/dL	≥3.5	2.0–3.4	1.5–1.9		0.6–1.4		<0.6		
Hematocrit	≥60		50–59.9	46–49.9	30–45.9		20–29.9		<20
WBC count, 10^3/mL	≥40		20–39.9	15–19.9	3–14.9		1–2.9		<1

Glasgow Coma Score[b,c]

Eye Opening	Verbal (Nonintubated)	Verbal (Intubated)	Motor Activity
4—Spontaneous	5—Oriented and talks	5—Seems able to talk	6—Verbal command
3—Verbal stimuli	4—Disoriented and talks	3—Questionable ability to talk	5—Localizes to pain
2—Painful stimuli	3—Inappropriate words	1—Generally unresponsive	4—Withdraws to pain
1—No response	2—Incomprehensible sounds		3—Decorticate
	1—No response		2—Decerebrate
			1—No response

Points Assigned to Age and Chronic Disease as Part of the APACHE II Score

Age, Years	Score
<45	0
45–54	2
55–64	3
65–74	5
≥75	6

Chronic Health (History of Chronic Conditions)[d]	Score
None	0
If patient is admitted after elective surgery	2
If patient is admitted after emergency surgery or for reason other than after elective surgery	5

[a] APACHE II score is the sum of the acute physiology score (vital signs, oxygenation, laboratory values), Glasgow coma score, age, and chronic health points. Worst values during first 24 h in the ICU should be used.

[b] Glasgow coma score (GCS) = eye-opening score + verbal (intubated or nonintubated) score + motor score.

[c] For GCS component of acute physiology score, subtract GCS from 15 to obtain points assigned.

[d] Chronic health conditions: liver, cirrhosis with portal hypertension or encephalopathy; cardiovascular, class IV angina (at rest or with minimal self-care activities); pulmonary, chronic hypoxemia or hypercapnia, polycythemia, ventilator dependent; kidney, chronic peritoneal or hemodialysis; immune, immunocompromised host.

Note: (A – a) D_{O_2}, alveolar-arterial oxygen difference; WBC, white blood (cell) count.

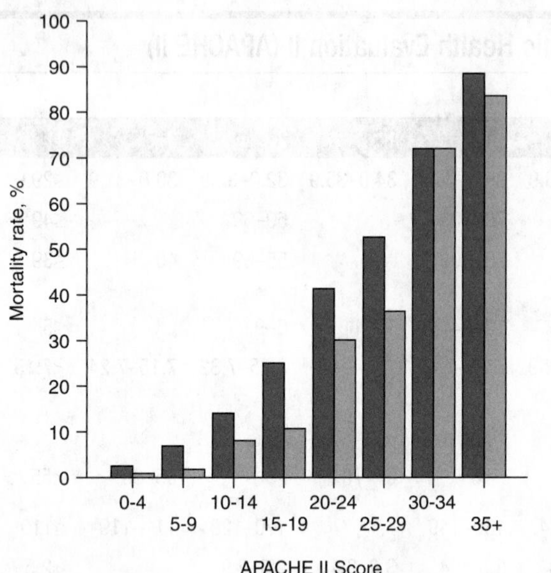

Figure 267-1 APACHE II survival curve. Blue, nonoperative; green, postoperative.

clinician at the bedside once shock is contemplated (Fig. 267-2). Clinical evidence of *diminished* cardiac output includes a narrow pulse pressure—a marker that correlates with stroke volume—and cool extremities with delayed capillary refill. Signs of *increased* cardiac output include a widened pulse pressure (particularly with a reduced diastolic pressure), warm extremities with bounding pulses, and rapid capillary refill. If a hypotensive patient has clinical signs of increased cardiac output, one can infer that the reduced blood pressure is a result of decreased SVR.

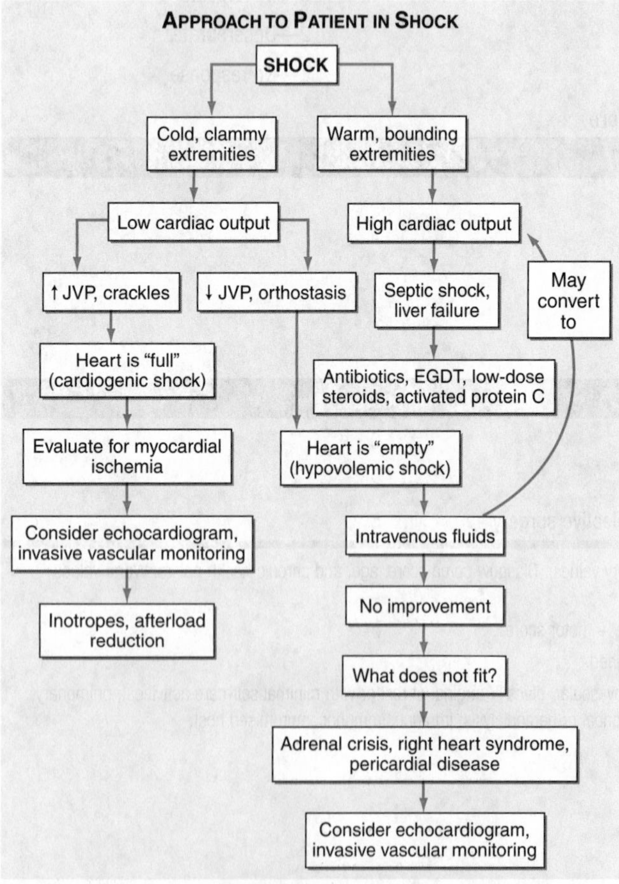

Figure 267-2 Approach to patient in shock. EGDT, early goal-directed therapy; JVP, jugular venous pulse.

In hypotensive patients with signs of a reduced cardiac output, an assessment of intravascular and cardiac volume status is appropriate. A hypotensive patient with decreased intravascular volume status may have a history suggesting hemorrhage or other volume losses (e.g., vomiting, diarrhea, polyuria). The jugular venous pressure (JVP) may be reduced in such a patient, although the change in right atrial pressure as a function of spontaneous respiration is a better predictor of fluid responsiveness (Fig. 267-3). Patients with fluid-responsive (i.e., hypovolemic) shock also may manifest large changes in pulse pressure as a function of respiration during positive-pressure mechanical ventilation (Fig. 267-4). A hypotensive patient with increased intravascular volume status and cardiac dysfunction may have S_3 and/or S_4 gallops on examination, increased JVP, extremity edema, and crackles on lung auscultation. The chest x-ray may show cardiomegaly, widening of the vascular pedicle, Kerley B lines, and pulmonary edema. Chest pain and electrocardiographic changes consistent with ischemia may be noted (Chap. 272).

In hypotensive patients with clinical evidence of increased cardiac output, a search for causes of decreased SVR is appropriate. The most common cause of high cardiac output hypotension is sepsis (Chap. 271). Other causes of high cardiac output hypotension include liver failure, severe pancreatitis, burns and other trauma that elicit the systemic inflammatory response syndrome (SIRS), anaphylaxis, thyrotoxicosis, and peripheral arteriovenous shunts.

In summary, the most common categories of shock are hypovolemic, cardiogenic, and high cardiac output with decreased SVR (high-output hypotension). Certainly these categories may overlap and occur simultaneously (e.g., hypovolemic and septic shock).

The initial assessment of a patient in shock as outlined above should take only a few minutes. It is important that aggressive, early resuscitation is instituted based on the initial assessment, particularly since early resuscitation of septic and cardiogenic shock may improve survival (see below). If the initial bedside assessment yields equivocal or confounding data, more objective assessments such as echocardiography and/or invasive vascular monitoring may be useful. The goal of early resuscitation is to reestablish adequate tissue perfusion to prevent or minimize end organ injury.

MECHANICAL VENTILATORY SUPPORT

(See also Chap. 269) During the initial resuscitation of patients in shock, principles of advanced cardiac life support should be followed. Since patients in shock may be obtunded and unable to protect the airway, an early assessment of the patient's airway is mandatory during resuscitation from shock. Early intubation and mechanical ventilation often are required. Reasons for the institution of endotracheal intubation and mechanical ventilation include acute hypoxemic respiratory failure and ventilatory failure, which frequently accompany shock. Acute hypoxemic respiratory failure may occur in patients with cardiogenic shock and pulmonary edema (Chap. 272) as well as in those in septic shock with pneumonia or acute respiratory distress syndrome (ARDS) (Chaps. 268 and 271). Ventilatory failure often occurs as a result of an increased load on the respiratory system. This load may present in the form of acute metabolic acidosis (often lactic acidosis) or decreased compliance of the lungs ("stiff" lungs) as a result of pulmonary edema. Inadequate perfusion to respiratory muscles in the setting of shock may be another reason for early intubation and mechanical ventilation. Normally, the respiratory muscles receive a very small percentage of the cardiac output. However, in patients who are in shock with respiratory distress for the reasons listed above, the percentage

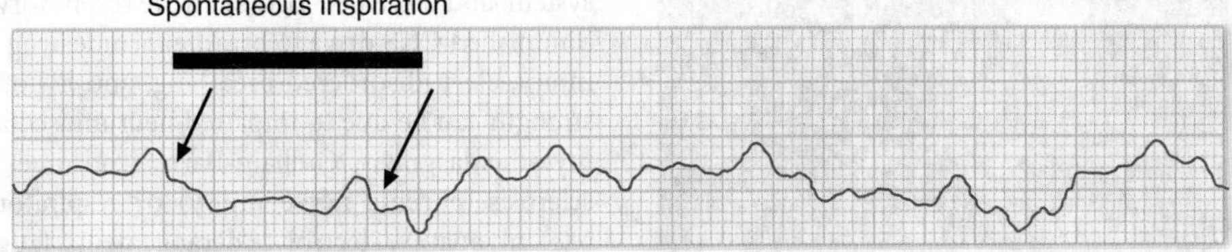

Figure 267-3 Right atrial pressure change during spontaneous respiration in a patient with shock who will increase cardiac output in response to intravenous fluid administration. The right atrial pressure decreases from 7 mmHg to 4 mmHg. The horizontal bar marks the time of spontaneous inspiration.

of cardiac output dedicated to respiratory muscles may increase tenfold or more. Lactic acid production from inefficient respiratory muscle activity presents an additional ventilatory load.

Mechanical ventilation may relieve the patient of the work of breathing and allow redistribution of a limited cardiac output to other vital organs, often with an improvement in lactic acidosis. Patients demonstrate signs of respiratory distress with a number of clinical signs, including inability to speak full sentences, accessory use of respiratory muscles, paradoxical abdominal muscle activity, extreme tachypnea (>40 breaths/min), and decreasing respiratory rate despite an increasing drive to breathe. When patients with shock are treated with mechanical ventilation, a major goal of ventilator settings is to assume all or the majority of work of breathing, facilitating a state of minimal respiratory muscle work. With the institution of mechanical ventilation for shock, further declines in MAP are frequently seen. The reasons for this include impeded venous return with positive-pressure ventilation, reduced endogenous catecholamine secretion once the stress associated with respiratory failure abates, and the actions of drugs used to facilitate endotracheal intubation (e.g., barbiturates, benzodiazepines, opiates), all of which may result in hypotension. Accordingly, hypotension should be anticipated after endotracheal intubation and positive-pressure ventilation. Many of these patients have a component of hypovolemia, which may respond to IV volume administration. Fig. 267-2 summarizes the diagnosis and treatment of different types of shock. For further discussion of individual forms of shock, see Chaps. 270, 271, and 272.

RESPIRATORY FAILURE

Respiratory failure is one of the most common reasons patients are admitted to the ICU. In some ICUs, ≥75% of patients require mechanical ventilation during their stay. Respiratory failure can be categorized mechanistically, based on pathophysiologic derangements in respiratory function. Accordingly, four different types of respiratory failure can be described, based on these pathophysiologic derangements.

Type I, acute hypoxemic respiratory failure

This occurs when alveolar flooding and subsequent intrapulmonary shunt physiology occur. Alveolar flooding may be a consequence of pulmonary edema, pneumonia, or alveolar hemorrhage. Pulmonary edema can be further categorized as occurring due to elevated pulmonary microvascular pressures as seen in heart failure and intravascular volume overload or ARDS ("low-pressure pulmonary edema"; Chap. 268) and represents an extreme degree of lung injury. This syndrome is defined by diffuse bilateral airspace edema seen on chest radiography, the absence of left atrial hypertension, and profound shunt physiology (Fig. 267-5) in a clinical setting in which this syndrome is known to occur, including sepsis, gastric aspiration, pneumonia, near-drowning, multiple blood transfusions, and pancreatitis. The mortality rate of patients with ARDS was traditionally very high (50–70%), although recent changes in ventilator management strategy have led to reports of mortality rates closer to 30% (see below).

For many years, physicians have suspected that mechanical ventilation of patients with acute lung injury and ARDS may propagate lung injury. Cyclical collapse and reopening of alveoli may be partly responsible for this. As seen in Fig. 267-6, the pressure-volume relationship of the lung in ARDS is not linear. Alveoli may collapse at very low lung volumes. Animal studies have suggested that stretching and overdistention of injured alveoli during mechanical ventilation can further injure the lung. Concern over this alveolar overdistention, termed *ventilator-induced "volutrauma,"* led to a multicenter, randomized, prospective trial to compare traditional ventilator strategies for acute lung injury and ARDS (large tidal volume—12 mL/kg ideal body weight) to a low tidal volume (6 mL/kg ideal body weight). This study showed a dramatic reduction in mortality rate in the low tidal volume group (large tidal volume—39.8% mortality rate versus low tidal volume—31% mortality rate) and confirmed that ventilator management could affect outcomes in these patients. In addition, a "fluid conservative" management strategy [maintaining a relatively low central venous pressure (CVP) or

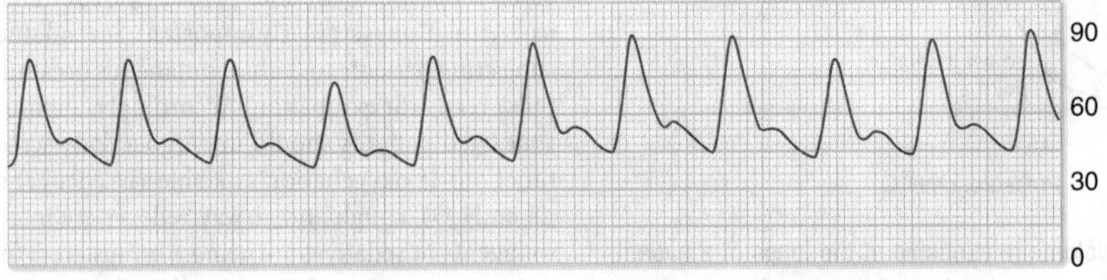

Figure 267-4 Pulse pressure change during mechanical ventilation in a patient with shock who will increase cardiac output in response to intravenous fluid administration. The pulse pressure (systolic minus diastolic blood pressure) changes during mechanical ventilation in a patient with septic shock.

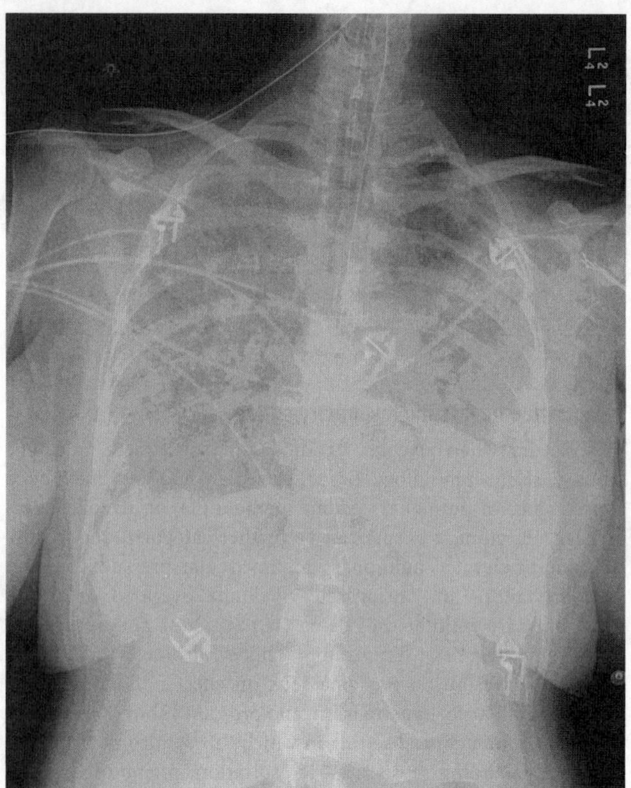

Figure 267-5 Chest radiograph of a patient with ARDS. ARDS, acute respiratory distress syndrome.

pulmonary capillary wedge pressure (PCWP)] is associated with the need for fewer days of mechanical ventilation compared with a "fluid liberal" management strategy (maintaining a relatively high CVP or PCWP) in acute lung injury and ARDS.

Type II respiratory failure

This type of respiratory failure occurs as a result of alveolar hypoventilation and results in the inability to eliminate carbon dioxide effectively. Mechanisms by which this occurs are categorized by impaired central nervous system (CNS) drive to breathe, impaired strength with failure of neuromuscular function in the respiratory system, and increased load(s) on the respiratory system. Reasons for diminished CNS drive to breathe include drug overdose, brainstem injury, sleep-disordered breathing, and hypothyroidism. Reduced strength can be due to impaired neuromuscular transmission (e.g., myasthenia gravis, Guillain-Barré syndrome, amyotrophic lateral sclerosis, phrenic nerve injury) or respiratory muscle weakness (e.g., myopathy, electrolyte derangements, fatigue).

The overall load on the respiratory system can be subclassified into increased resistive loads (e.g., bronchospasm), loads due to reduced lung compliance [e.g., alveolar edema, atelectasis, intrinsic positive end-expiratory pressure (autoPEEP)—see below], loads due to reduced chest wall compliance (e.g., pneumothorax, pleural effusion, abdominal distention), and loads due to increased minute ventilation requirements (e.g., pulmonary embolus with increased dead space fraction, sepsis).

The mainstays of therapy for type II respiratory failure are treatments directed at reversing the underlying cause(s) of ventilatory failure. Noninvasive positive-pressure ventilation using a mechanical ventilator with a tight-fitting face or nasal mask that avoids endotracheal intubation often can stabilize these patients. This approach has been shown to be beneficial in treating patients with exacerbations of chronic obstructive pulmonary disease. Noninvasive ventilation has been tested less extensively in other types of type II respiratory failure but may be attempted nonetheless in the absence of contraindications (hemodynamic instability, inability to protect airway, respiratory arrest).

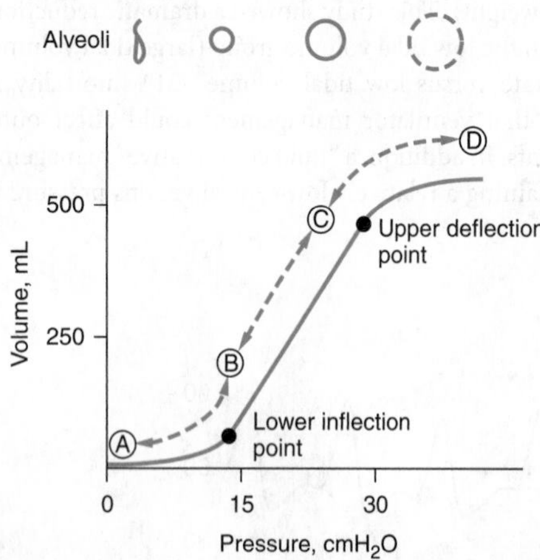

Figure 267-6 Pressure-volume relationship of the lungs of a patient with ARDS. At the lower inflection point, collapsed alveoli begin to open, and the lung compliance changes. At the upper deflection point, alveoli become overdistended. The shape and size of alveoli are illustrated at the top. ARDS, acute respiratory distress syndrome.

Type III respiratory failure

This form of respiratory failure occurs as a result of lung atelectasis. Because atelectasis occurs so commonly in the perioperative period, this is also called perioperative respiratory failure. After general anesthesia, decreases in functional residual capacity lead to collapse of dependent lung units. Such atelectasis can be treated by frequent changes in position, chest physiotherapy, upright positioning, and aggressive control of incisional and/or abdominal pain. Noninvasive positive-pressure ventilation may also be used to reverse regional atelectasis.

Type IV respiratory failure

This form results from hypoperfusion of respiratory muscles in patients in shock. Normally, respiratory muscles consume <5% of the total cardiac output and O_2 delivery. Patients in shock often experience respiratory distress due to pulmonary edema (e.g., patients in cardiogenic shock), lactic acidosis, and anemia. In this setting, up to 40% of the cardiac output may be distributed to the respiratory muscles. Intubation and mechanical ventilation can allow redistribution of the cardiac output away from the respiratory muscles and back to vital organs while the shock is treated.

CARE OF THE MECHANICALLY VENTILATED PATIENT

(See also Chap. 269) Whereas a thorough understanding of the pathophysiology of respiratory failure is essential to optimize patient care, recognition of a patient's readiness to be liberated from mechanical ventilation is similarly important. Several studies have shown that subjecting patients to daily spontaneous breathing trials can identify those ready for extubation. Accordingly, all intubated, mechanically ventilated patients should undergo a daily screening of respiratory function. If oxygenation is stable (i.e., Pa_{O_2}/Fi_{O_2} >200 and PEEP ≤5 cmH_2O), cough and airway reflexes are intact, and no vasopressor agents or sedatives are being administered, the patient has passed the screening test and should undergo a spontaneous breathing trial. This trial consists of a period of breathing through the endotracheal tube without ventilator support [both continuous positive airway pressure (CPAP) of 5 cmH_2O and an open T-piece breathing system can be used] for 30–120 min. The spontaneous breathing trial is declared a failure and stopped if *any* of the following occur: (1) respiratory rate >35/min for >5 min, (2) O_2 saturation <90%, (3) heart rate >140/min or a 20% increase or decrease from baseline, (4) systolic blood pressure <90 mmHg or >180 mmHg, (5) increased anxiety or diaphoresis. If, at the end of the spontaneous breathing trial, the ratio of the respiratory rate and tidal volume in liters (f/V_T) is <105, the patient can be extubated. Such protocol-driven approaches to patient care can have an important impact on the duration of mechanical ventilation and length of stay in the ICU. In spite of such a careful approach to liberation from mechanical ventilation, up to 10% of patients will develop respiratory distress after extubation and may require resumption of mechanical ventilation. Many of these patients will require reintubation. The use of noninvasive ventilation in patients who fail extubation may be associated with worse outcomes compared with immediate reintubation.

Mechanically ventilated patients frequently require sedatives and analgesics. Most patients undergoing mechanical ventilation experience pain, which can be elicited by the presence of the endotracheal tube and endotracheal suctioning. Accordingly, early attention to pain control is extremely important. Opiates are the mainstay of therapy for pain control in mechanically ventilated patients. After adequate pain control has been assured, additional indications for sedation for mechanically ventilated patients include anxiolysis; treatment of subjective dyspnea; psychosis; facilitation of nursing care; reduction of autonomic hyperactivity, which may precipitate myocardial ischemia; and reduction of total O_2 consumption (V_{O_2}).

Neuromuscular blocking agents are occasionally needed to facilitate mechanical ventilation in patients with profound dyssynchrony with the ventilator despite optimal sedation. The use of neuromuscular blocking agents may result in prolonged weakness—a myopathy known as the *postparalytic syndrome*. For this reason, these agents typically are used as a last resort when aggressive sedation fails to achieve patient-ventilator synchrony. Because neuromuscular blocking agents result in pharmacologic paralysis without altering mental status, sedative-induced amnesia is mandatory when these agents are administered.

Amnesia can be achieved reliably with benzodiazepines such as lorazepam and midazolam as well as the IV anesthetic agent propofol. Outside the setting of pharmacologic paralysis, there are few data supporting the idea that amnesia is mandatory in all patients who require intubation and mechanical ventilation. Since many of these patients have impaired hepatic and renal function, sedatives and opiates may accumulate in critically ill patients when they are given for prolonged periods. A protocol-driven approach to sedation of mechanically ventilated patients with daily interruption of sedative infusions paired with daily spontaneous breathing trials has been shown to prevent excessive drug accumulation and shorten the duration of mechanical ventilation and length of stay in the ICU.

MULTIORGAN SYSTEM FAILURE

The syndrome of multiorgan system failure is a common problem associated with critical illness. This syndrome is defined by the simultaneous presence of physiologic dysfunction and/or failure of two or more organs. Typically, this occurs in the setting of severe sepsis, shock of any kind, severe inflammatory conditions such as pancreatitis, and trauma. The fact that multiorgan system failure occurs commonly in the ICU is a testament to our current ability to stabilize and support single-organ failure. The ability to support single-organ failure aggressively (e.g., mechanical ventilation for respiratory failure, renal replacement therapy for acute renal failure) has affected rates of early mortality in critical illness greatly. As a result, it is uncommon for critically ill patients to die in the initial stages of resuscitation. Instead, many patients succumb to critical illness later in the ICU stay, after the initial presenting problem has been stabilized.

Although there is debate regarding specific definitions of organ failure, several general principles governing the syndrome of multiorgan system failure apply. First, organ failure, no matter how defined, must persist beyond 24 h. Second, mortality risk increases as patients accrue additional failing. Third, prognosis is worsened by increased duration of organ failure. These observations remain true across various critical care settings (e.g., medical versus surgical). SIRS is a common basis for multiorgan system failure. Although infection is a common cause of SIRS, "sterile" triggers such as pancreatitis, trauma, and burns often are invoked to explain multiorgan system failure.

MONITORING IN THE ICU

Because respiratory and circulatory failure occurs commonly in critically ill patients, monitoring of the respiratory and cardiovascular systems is undertaken frequently in the ICU. Evaluation of respiratory gas exchange is routine in critical illness. The "gold standard" remains arterial blood-gas analysis, in which pH, partial pressures of O_2 and CO_2, and O_2 saturation are measured directly. With arterial blood-gas analysis, the two main functions of the lung—oxygenation of arterial blood and elimination of CO_2—can be assessed directly. Importantly, the blood pH, which has a profound effect on the drive to breathe, can be assessed only by sampling arterial blood. Though sampling of arterial blood is generally safe, it may be painful and cannot provide continuous information for clinicians routinely. In light of these limitations, noninvasive monitoring of respiratory function is often employed in the critical care setting.

PULSE OXIMETRY

This is the most commonly utilized noninvasive monitor of respiratory function. This technique takes advantage of differences in the absorptive properties of oxygenated and deoxygenated hemoglobin. At wavelengths of 660 nm, oxyhemoglobin reflects light more effectively than does deoxyhemoglobin, whereas the reverse is true in the infrared spectrum (940 nm). A pulse oximeter passes both wavelengths of light through a perfused digit such as a finger, and the relative intensity of light transmission at these two wavelengths is recorded. This allows the derivation of the relative percentage of oxyhemoglobin. Since arterial pulsations produce phasic changes in the intensity of transmitted light, the pulse oximeter is designed to detect only light of alternating intensity. This allows distinction of arterial and venous blood O_2 saturations.

Respiratory system mechanics

These can be measured in patients during mechanical ventilation (Chap. 269). When volume-controlled modes of mechanical ventilation are used, accompanying airway pressures can be easily measured, assuming the patient is passive. The peak airway pressure is determined by two variables: airway resistance and respiratory system compliance. At the end of inspiration, inspiratory flow can be stopped transiently. This end-inspiratory pause (*plateau pressure*) is a static measurement, affected only by respiratory system compliance, not airway resistance. Therefore, during volume-controlled ventilation, the difference between the peak (airway resistance + respiratory system compliance) and plateau (respiratory system compliance only) airway pressures provides a quantitative assessment of airway resistance. Accordingly, during volume-controlled ventilation, patients with increases in airway resistance typically have increased peak airway pressures as well as abnormally high gradients between peak and plateau airway pressures (typically >15 cmH_2O). The compliance of the respiratory system is defined by the change in pressure of the respiratory system per unit change in volume.

The respiratory system can be divided further into two components: the lungs and the chest wall. Normally, respiratory system compliance is ~100 mL per cmH_2O. Pathophysiologic processes such as pleural effusions, pneumothorax, and increased abdominal girth from ascites all reduce chest wall compliance. Lung compliance may be reduced by pneumonia, pulmonary edema from any cause, or autoPEEP. Accordingly, patients with abnormalities in compliance of the respiratory system (lungs and/or chest wall) typically have elevated peak *and* plateau airway pressures but a normal gradient between peak and plateau airway pressures. AutoPEEP occurs when there is insufficient time for emptying of alveoli before the next inspiratory cycle. Since the alveoli have not decompressed completely, alveolar pressure remains positive at end exhalation (functional residual capacity). This phenomenon results most commonly from critical narrowing of distal airways in disease processes such as asthma and chronic obstructive pulmonary disease. AutoPEEP with resulting alveolar overdistention may result in diminished lung compliance, reflected by abnormally increased plateau airway pressures. Modern mechanical ventilators allow breath-to-breath display of pressure and flow, which may allow detection of problems such as patient-ventilator dyssynchrony, airflow obstruction, and autoPEEP (Fig. 267-7).

CIRCULATORY STATUS

Oxygen delivery (Q_{O_2}) is a function of cardiac output and the content of O_2 in the arterial blood (Ca_{O_2}). The Ca_{O_2} is determined by the hemoglobin concentration, the arterial hemoglobin saturation, and dissolved O_2 not bound to hemoglobin. For normal adults:

$$Q_{O_2} = 50 \text{ dL/min} \times [1.39 \times 15 \text{ g/dL (hemoglobin concentration)} \times 1.0 \text{ (hemoglobin \% saturation)} + 0.0031 \times 100 \text{ } (Pa_{O_2})]$$
$$= 50 \text{ dL/min (cardiac output)} \times 21.16 \text{ mL } O_2 \text{ per dL blood } (Ca_{O_2})$$
$$= 1058 \text{ mL } O_2 \text{ per min}$$

It is apparent that the vast majority of O_2 delivered to tissues is bound to hemoglobin and that the dissolved O_2 (Pa_{O_2}) contributes

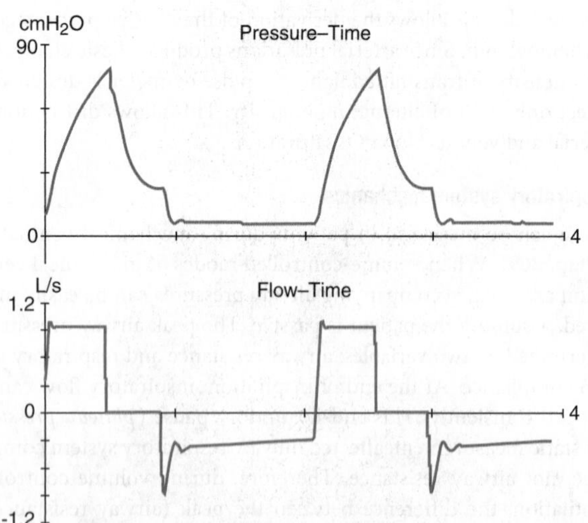

Figure 267-7 Increased airway resistance with autoPEEP. The top waveform (airway pressure vs. time) shows a large difference between the peak airway pressure (80 cmH_2O) and the plateau airway pressure (20 cmH_2O). The bottom waveform (flow vs. time) demonstrates airflow throughout expiration (reflected by the flow tracing on the negative portion of the abscissa) that persists up to the next inspiratory effort.

very little to O_2 content in arterial blood or O_2 delivery. Normally, the content of O_2 in mixed venous blood ($C\bar{v}_{O_2}$) is 15.76 mL O_2 per dL blood, since the mixed venous blood is 75% saturated. Therefore, the normal tissue extraction ratio for O_2 is $Ca_{O_2} - C\bar{v}_{O_2}/Ca_{O_2}$ ([21.16–15.76]/21.16) or ~25%. A pulmonary artery catheter allows measurements of O_2 delivery and O_2 extraction ratio.

The mixed venous O_2 saturation allows assessment of global tissue perfusion. A reduced mixed venous O_2 saturation may be caused by inadequate cardiac output, reduced hemoglobin concentration, and/or reduced arterial O_2 saturation. An abnormally high O_2 consumption (V_{O_2}) may also lead to a reduced mixed venous O_2 saturation if O_2 delivery is not concomitantly increased. Abnormally increased V_{O_2} by peripheral tissues may be caused by a multitude of problems, such as fever, agitation, shivering, and thyrotoxicosis.

The pulmonary artery catheter originally was designed as a tool to guide therapy in acute myocardial infarction but is currently used in the ICU for evaluation and treatment of a variety of other conditions, such as ARDS, septic shock, congestive heart failure, and acute renal failure. This device has never been validated as a tool associated with reduction in morbidity and mortality rates. Indeed, despite numerous prospective studies, there has been no report of mortality or morbidity rate benefit associated with the use of the pulmonary artery catheter in any setting. Accordingly, it appears that the routine use of pulmonary artery catheterization is not indicated as a monitor to characterize the circulatory status in most critically ill patients.

Recent data suggest that static measurements of circulatory parameters (e.g., CVP, PCWP) do not provide reliable information on the circulatory status of critically ill patients. In contrast, dynamic assessments measuring the impact of breathing on the circulation are more reliable predictors of responsiveness to IV fluid administration. A decrease in CVP of >1 mmHg during inspiration in a spontaneously breathing patient has been shown to predict an increase in cardiac output after IV fluid administration. Similarly, a changing pulse pressure during mechanical ventilation has been shown to predict an increase in cardiac output after IV fluid administration in patients with septic shock.

PREVENTION OF COMPLICATIONS OF CRITICAL ILLNESS

Sepsis in the critical care unit

(See also Chap. 271) Sepsis is a significant problem in the care of critically ill patients. It is the leading cause of death in noncoronary ICUs in the United States, with case rates expected to increase as the population ages with a greater percentage of people vulnerable to infection.

Many therapeutic interventions in the ICU are invasive and predispose patients to infectious complications. These interventions include endotracheal intubation, indwelling vascular catheters, nasally placed enteral feeding tubes, transurethral bladder catheters, and other catheters placed into sterile body cavities (e.g., tube thoracostomy, percutaneous intraabdominal drainage catheters). The longer such devices remain in place, the more prone to these infections patients become. For example, ventilator-associated pneumonia (VAP) correlates strongly with the duration of intubation and mechanical ventilation. Therefore, an important aspect of preventive care is the timely removal of invasive devices as soon as they are no longer needed. Multidrug-resistant organisms are commonplace in the ICU.

An important aspect of critical care is infection control in the ICU. Simple measures such as frequent hand washing are effective but underutilized strategies. Protective isolation of patients with colonization or infection by drug-resistant organisms is another frequently used strategy in the critical care setting. A recent study utilizing silver-coated endotracheal tubes reported a significant reduction in VAP incidence. Studies evaluating multifaceted, evidence-based strategies to decrease catheter-related bloodstream infections have shown improved outcomes from using measures such as hand washing, full-barrier precautions during insertion, chlorhexidine skin preparation, avoidance of the femoral site, and timely catheter removal.

Deep venous thromboses (DVTs)

All ICU patients are at high risk for this complication because of their predilection for being immobile. Therefore, all should receive some form of prophylaxis against DVT. The most commonly employed forms of prophylaxis are subcutaneous low-dose heparin injections and sequential compression devices for the lower extremities. Observational studies report an alarming incidence of the occurrence of DVTs despite the use of these standard prophylactic regimens. Heparin prophylaxis may result in heparin-induced thrombocytopenia (HIT), another relatively common nosocomial complication in critically ill patients.

Low-molecular-weight heparins such as enoxaparin are more effective than unfractionated heparin for DVT prophylaxis in high-risk patients, such as those undergoing orthopedic surgery, and they have a lower incidence of HIT. Fondaparinux, a selective factor Xa inhibitor, is even more effective than enoxaparin in high-risk orthopedic patients.

Stress ulcers

Prophylaxis against stress ulcers is frequently administered in most ICUs; typically, histamine-2 antagonists are given. Currently available data suggest that high-risk patients, such as those with coagulopathy, shock, or respiratory failure requiring mechanical ventilation, benefit from such prophylactic treatment.

Nutrition and glycemic control

These are important issues in critically ill patients that may be associated with respiratory failure, impaired wound healing, and dysfunctional immune response. Early enteral feeding is reasonable, though no data are available to suggest that this improves patient outcome per se. Certainly, enteral feeding, if possible, is preferred over parenteral nutrition, which is associated with numerous complications, including hyperglycemia, fatty liver, cholestasis, and sepsis. In addition, enteral feeding may prevent bacterial translocation across the gut mucosa. Tight glucose control is another area of controversy in critical care. Although one study showed a significant mortality benefit when glucose levels were aggressively normalized in a large group of surgical ICU patients, more recent data suggest that tight glucose control in a large population of both medical and surgical ICU patients resulted in increased rates of mortality.

ICU-acquired weakness

This occurs frequently in patients who survive critical illness. It is particularly common in those with SIRS and/or sepsis. Neuropathies and myopathies both have been described, most commonly after ~1 week in the ICU. The mechanisms behind ICU-acquired weakness syndromes are poorly understood. Intensive insulin therapy may reduce polyneuropathy of critical illness. A recent study of very early physical and occupational therapy in mechanically ventilated critically ill patients reported significant improvements in functional independence at hospital discharge, as well as reduced duration of mechanical ventilation and delirium.

Anemia

This is a common problem in critically ill patients. Studies have shown that the vast majority of ICU patients are anemic. Furthermore, most have anemia of chronic inflammation. Phlebotomy contributes significantly to anemia in ICU patients. Studies have demonstrated that erythropoietin levels are inappropriately reduced in most ICU patients and that exogenous erythropoietin administration may reduce transfusion requirements in the ICU. The hemoglobin level that merits transfusion in critically ill patients has been a long-standing area of controversy. A large, multicenter study involving patients in many different ICU settings challenged the conventional notion that a hemoglobin level of 100 g/L (10 g/dL) is needed in critically ill patients. Red blood cell transfusion is associated with impairment of immune function and increased risk of infections as well as acute lung injury and volume overload, all of which may explain the findings in this study. A conservative transfusion strategy should be the rule in managing critically ill patients who are not actively hemorrhaging.

Acute renal failure

(See also Chap. 279) This occurs in a significant percentage of critically ill patients. The most common underlying etiology is acute tubular necrosis, usually precipitated by hypoperfusion and/or nephrotoxic agents. Currently, there are no pharmacologic agents available for prevention of renal injury in critical illness. A recent study showed convincingly that low-dose dopamine is *not* effective in protecting the kidneys from acute injury.

NEUROLOGIC DYSFUNCTION IN CRITICALLY ILL PATIENTS

Delirium

(See also Chaps. 25 and 274) This state is defined by (1) an acute onset of changes or fluctuations in the course of mental status, (2) inattention, (3) disorganized thinking, and (4) an altered level of consciousness (i.e., other than alert). Delirium is reported to occur in over 80% of mechanically ventilated ICU patients and can be detected by the Confusion Assessment Method (CAM)-ICU. This assessment asks patients to answer simple questions and perform simple tasks and can be completed by the bedside nurse in ~2 min. The differential diagnosis of delirium in ICU patients is broad and includes infectious etiologies (including sepsis), medications (particularly sedatives and analgesics), drug withdrawal, metabolic/electrolyte derangements, intracranial pathology (e.g., stroke, intracranial hemorrhage), seizures, hypoxia, hypertensive crisis, shock, and vitamin deficiencies (particularly thiamine). Patients with ICU delirium have increases in hospital length of stay, time on mechanical ventilation, cognitive impairment at hospital discharge, and 6-month mortality rate. Interventions to reduce ICU delirium have been described recently. The use of the novel sedative dexmedetomidine was associated with reduced ICU delirium compared with midazolam. In addition, as mentioned above in the section "ICU-Acquired Weakness," very early physical and occupational therapy in mechanically ventilated patients also has been demonstrated to reduce delirium.

Anoxic cerebral injury

(See also Chap. 275) This condition is common after cardiac arrest and often results in severe and permanent brain injury in patients whose cardiac arrest is resuscitated. Active cooling of patients after cardiac arrest has been shown to improve neurologic outcomes. Therefore, patients who present to the ICU after circulatory arrest from ventricular fibrillation or pulseless ventricular tachycardia should be actively cooled with cooling blankets and ice packs if necessary to achieve a core body temperature of 32–34°C.

Stroke

(See also Chap. 370) This is a common cause of neurologic critical illness. Hypertension must be managed carefully, since abrupt reductions in blood pressure may be associated with further brain ischemia and injury. Acute ischemic stroke treated with tissue plasminogen activator (tPA) has an improved neurologic outcome when treatment is given within 3 h of onset of symptoms. The mortality rate is not improved when tPA is compared with placebo, despite the improved neurologic outcome. Cerebral hemorrhage is significantly higher in patients given tPA. A treatment benefit is not seen when tPA therapy is given beyond 3 h. Heparin has not been shown to demonstrate improved outcomes convincingly in patients with acute ischemic stroke.

Subarachnoid hemorrhage

(See also Chap. 370) This may occur secondary to aneurysm rupture and is often complicated by cerebral vasospasm, rebleeding, and hydrocephalus. Vasospasm can be detected by either transcranial Doppler assessment or cerebral angiography; it is typically treated with the calcium channel blocker nimodipine, aggressive IV fluid administration, and therapy aimed at increasing blood pressure, typically with vasoactive drugs such as phenylephrine. The IV fluids and vasoactive drugs (hypertensive hypervolemic therapy) are used to overcome the cerebral vasospasm. Early surgical clipping of aneurysms is advocated by most authorities to prevent complications related to rebleeding. Hydrocephalus, typically heralded by a decreased level of consciousness, may require ventriculostomy drainage.

Status epilepticus

(See also Chap. 369) Recurrent or relentless seizure activity is a medical emergency. Cessation of seizure activity is required to prevent irreversible neurologic injury. Lorazepam is the most effective benzodiazepine for treating status epilepticus and is the treatment of choice for controlling seizures acutely. Phenytoin or fosphenytoin should be given concomitantly since lorazepam has a short half-life. Other drugs, such as gabapentin, carbamazepine, and phenobarbital, should be reserved for patients with contraindications to phenytoin (e.g., allergy or pregnancy) or ongoing seizures despite phenytoin.

Brain death

(See also Chap. 275) Though critically ill patients usually die from irreversible cessation of circulatory and respiratory function, a diagnosis of death also may be established by irreversible cessation of all functions of the entire brain, including the brainstem, even if circulatory and respiratory function remains intact on artificial life support. Patients must demonstrate absence of cerebral function (unresponsive to all external stimuli) and brainstem functions [e.g., unreactive pupils, absent ocular movement to head turning or ice water irrigation of ear canals, positive apnea test (no drive to breathe)]. Absence of brain function must have an established cause and be permanent without possibility of recovery (e.g., must confirm the absence of sedative effect, hypothermia, hypoxemia, neuromuscular paralysis, or severe hypotension). If there is uncertainty about the cause of coma, studies of cerebral blood flow and electroencephalography should be performed.

WITHHOLDING AND WITHDRAWING CARE

(See also Chap. 9) Withholding and withdrawing of care occurs commonly in the ICU setting. The Task Force on Ethics of the Society of Critical Care Medicine reported that it is ethically sound to withhold or withdraw care if a patient or surrogate makes such a request or if the goals of therapy are not achievable according to the physician. Since all medical treatments are justified by their expected benefits, the loss of such an expectation justifies the act of withdrawing or withholding such treatment. Thus, the act of withdrawing care is fundamentally similar to the act of withholding care. An underlying stipulation derived from this report is that an informed patient should have his or her wishes respected with regard to life-sustaining therapy. Implicit in this stipulation is the need to ensure that patients are thoroughly and accurately informed regarding the plausibility and expected results of various therapies.

The act of informing patients and/or surrogate decision makers is the responsibility of the physician and other health care providers. If a patient or surrogate desires therapy deemed futile by the treating physician, the physician is not obligated ethically to provide such treatment. Rather, arrangements may be made to transfer the patient's care to another care provider. Whether the decision to withdraw life support should be initiated by the physician or left to surrogate decision makers is not clear. A recent study reported that slightly more than half of surrogate decision makers preferred to receive such a recommendation, whereas the rest did not. Critical care providers should meet regularly with patients and/or surrogates to discuss prognosis when the withholding or withdrawal of care is being considered. After a consensus among caregivers has been reached regarding withholding or withdrawal of care, this should be relayed to the patient and/or surrogate decision maker. If a decision to withhold or withdraw life-sustaining care for a patient has been reached, aggressive attention to analgesia and anxiolysis is needed. Opiates and benzodiazepines are typically used to achieve these goals.

FURTHER READINGS

Abraham E et al: Drotrecogin alfa (activated) for adults with severe sepsis and a low risk of death. N Engl J Med 353:1332, 2005

The Acute Respiratory Distress Syndrome Network: Ventilation with lower tidal volumes as compared with traditional tidal volumes for acute lung injury and the acute respiratory distress syndrome. N Engl J Med 342:1301, 2000

Cook DJ et al: Deep venous thrombosis in medical-surgical critically ill patients: Prevalence, incidence, and risk factors. Crit Care Med 33:1565, 2005

Esteban A et al: Noninvasive positive-pressure ventilation for respiratory failure after extubation. N Engl J Med 350:2452, 2004

Girard T et al: Efficacy and safety of a paired sedation and ventilator weaning protocol for mechanically ventilated patients in intensive care (Awakening and Breathing Controlled trial): A randomised controlled trial. Lancet 371:126, 2008

The Hypothermia after Cardiac Arrest Study Group: Mild therapeutic hypothermia to improve the neurologic outcome after cardiac arrest. N Engl J Med 346:549, 2002

The National Heart, Lung, and Blood Institute Acute Respiratory Distress Syndrome (ARDS) Clinical Trials Network: Comparison of two fluid-management strategies in acute lung injury. N Engl J Med 354:2564, 2006

The Nice-Sugar Study Investigators: Intensive versus glucose control in critically ill patients. N Engl J Med 360:1283, 2009

Pronovost P et al: An intervention to decrease catheter-related bloodstream infections in the ICU. N Engl J Med 355:2725, 2006

Schweikert WD et al: Early physical and occupational therapy in mechanically ventilated, critically ill patients: A randomised controlled trial. Lancet 373:1874, 2009

Shah MR et al: Impact of the pulmonary artery catheter in critically ill patients: Meta-analysis of randomized clinical trials. JAMA 294:1664, 2005

Task Force on Ethics of the Society of Critical Care Medicine: Consensus report on the ethics of forgoing life-sustaining treatments in the critically ill. Crit Care Med 18:1424, 1990

CHAPTER 268

Acute Respiratory Distress Syndrome

Bruce D. Levy
Augustine M. K. Choi

Acute respiratory distress syndrome (ARDS) is a clinical syndrome of severe dyspnea of rapid onset, hypoxemia, and diffuse pulmonary infiltrates leading to respiratory failure. ARDS is caused by diffuse lung injury from many underlying medical and surgical disorders. The lung injury may be direct, as occurs in toxic inhalation, or indirect, as occurs in sepsis (Table 268-1). The clinical features of ARDS are listed in Table 268-2. Acute lung injury (ALI) is a less severe disorder but has the potential to evolve into ARDS (Table 268-2). The arterial (a) P_{O_2} (in mmHg)/F_{IO_2} (inspiratory O_2 fraction) <200 mmHg is characteristic of ARDS, while a Pa_{O_2}/F_{IO_2} between 200 and 300 identifies patients with ALI who are likely to benefit from aggressive therapy.

The annual incidences of ALI and ARDS are estimated to be up to 80/100,000 and 60/100,000, respectively. Approximately 10% of all intensive care unit (ICU) admissions suffer from acute respiratory failure, with ~20% of these patients meeting criteria for ALI or ARDS.

■ ETIOLOGY

While many medical and surgical illnesses have been associated with the development of ALI and ARDS, most cases (>80%) are caused by a relatively small number of clinical disorders, namely, severe sepsis syndrome and/or bacterial pneumonia (~40–50%), trauma, multiple transfusions, aspiration of gastric contents, and drug overdose. Among patients with trauma, pulmonary contusion, multiple bone fractures, and chest wall trauma/flail chest are the most frequently reported surgical conditions in ARDS, whereas head trauma, near-drowning, toxic inhalation, and burns are rare causes. The risks of developing ARDS are increased in patients suffering from more than one predisposing medical or surgical condition (e.g., the risk for ARDS increases from 25% in patients with severe trauma to 56% in patients with trauma and sepsis).

TABLE 268-1 Clinical Disorders Commonly Associated With ARDS

Direct Lung Injury	Indirect Lung Injury
Pneumonia	Sepsis
Aspiration of gastric contents	Severe trauma
Pulmonary contusion	Multiple bone fractures
Near-drowning	Flail chest
Toxic inhalation injury	Head trauma
	Burns
	Multiple transfusions
	Drug overdose
	Pancreatitis
	Postcardiopulmonary bypass

TABLE 268-2 Diagnostic Criteria for ALI and ARDS

Oxygenation	Onset	Chest Radiograph	Absence of Left Atrial Hypertension
ALI: Pa_{O_2}/F_{IO_2} ≤ 300 mmHg ARDS: Pa_{O_2}/F_{IO_2} ≤ 200 mmHg	Acute	Bilateral alveolar or interstitial infiltrates	PCWP ≤ 18 mmHg *or* no clinical evidence of increased left atrial pressure

Abbreviations: ALI, acute lung injury; ARDS, acute respiratory distress syndrome; F_{IO_2}, inspired O_2 percentage; Pa_{O_2}, arterial partial pressure of O_2; PCWP, pulmonary capillary wedge pressure.

Several other clinical variables have been associated with the development of ARDS. These include older age, chronic alcohol abuse, metabolic acidosis, and severity of critical illness. Trauma patients with an acute physiology and chronic health evaluation (APACHE) II score ≥16 (Chap. 267) have a 2.5-fold increase in the risk of developing ARDS, and those with a score >20 have an incidence of ARDS that is more than threefold greater than those with APACHE II scores ≤9.

■ CLINICAL COURSE AND PATHOPHYSIOLOGY

The natural history of ARDS is marked by three phases—exudative, proliferative, and fibrotic—each with characteristic clinical and pathologic features (Fig. 268-1).

Exudative phase

(Figure. 268-2) In this phase, alveolar capillary endothelial cells and type I pneumocytes (alveolar epithelial cells) are injured, leading to the los-s of the normally tight alveolar barrier to fluid and macromolecules. Edema fluid that is rich in protein accumulates in the interstitial and alveolar spaces. Significant concentrations of cytokines (e.g., interleukin 1, interleukin 8, and tumor necrosis factor α) and lipid mediators (e.g., leukotriene B_4) are present in the lung in this acute phase. In response to proinflammatory mediators, leukocytes (especially neutrophils) traffic into the pulmonary interstitium and alveoli. In addition, condensed

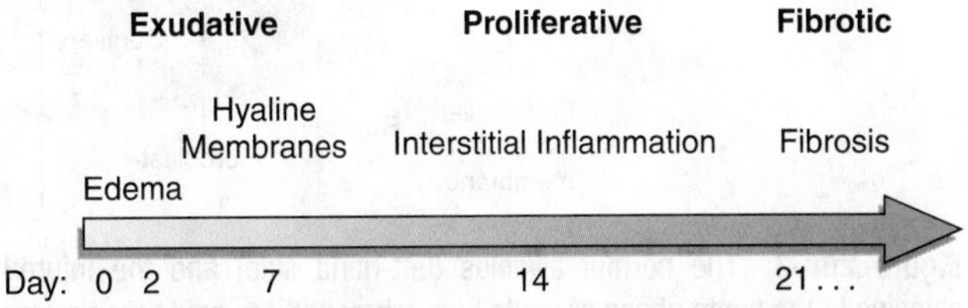

Figure 268-1 Diagram illustrating the time course for the development and resolution of ARDS. The exudative phase is notable for early alveolar edema and neutrophil-rich leukocytic infiltration of the lungs with subsequent formation of hyaline membranes from diffuse alveolar damage. Within 7 days, a proliferative phase ensues with prominent interstitial inflammation and early fibrotic changes. Approximately 3 weeks after the initial pulmonary injury, most patients recover. However, some patients enter the fibrotic phase, with substantial fibrosis and bullae formation.

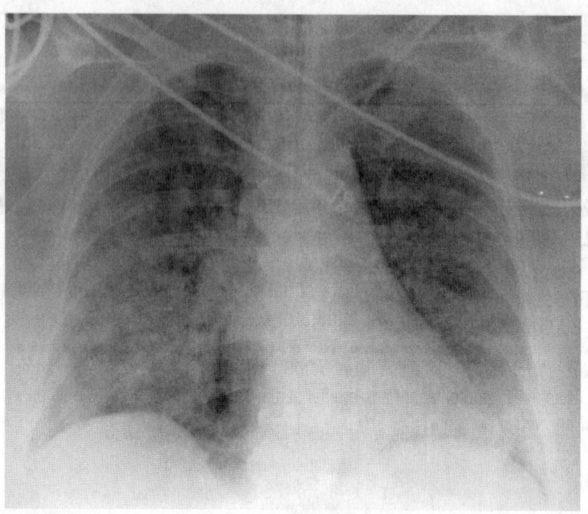

Figure 268-2 A representative anteroposterior (AP) chest x-ray in the exudative phase of ARDS that shows diffuse interstitial and alveolar infiltrates, that can be difficult to distinguish from left ventricular failure.

plasma proteins aggregate in the air spaces with cellular debris and dysfunctional pulmonary surfactant to form hyaline membrane whorls. Pulmonary vascular injury also occurs early in ARDS, with vascular obliteration by microthrombi and fibrocellular proliferation (Fig. 268-3).

Alveolar edema predominantly involves *dependent* portions of the lung, leading to diminished aeration and atelectasis. Collapse of large sections of dependent lung markedly decreases lung compliance. Consequently, intrapulmonary shunting and hypoxemia develop and the work of breathing rises, leading to dyspnea. The pathophysiologic alterations in alveolar spaces are exacerbated by microvascular occlusion that leads to reductions in pulmonary arterial blood flow to ventilated portions of the lung, increasing the dead space, and to pulmonary hypertension. Thus, in addition to severe hypoxemia, hypercapnia secondary to an increase in pulmonary dead space is also prominent in early ARDS.

The exudative phase encompasses the first 7 days of illness after exposure to a precipitating ARDS risk factor, with the patient experiencing the onset of respiratory symptoms. Although usually present within 12–36 hours after the initial insult, symptoms can be delayed by 5–7 days. Dyspnea develops with a sensation of rapid

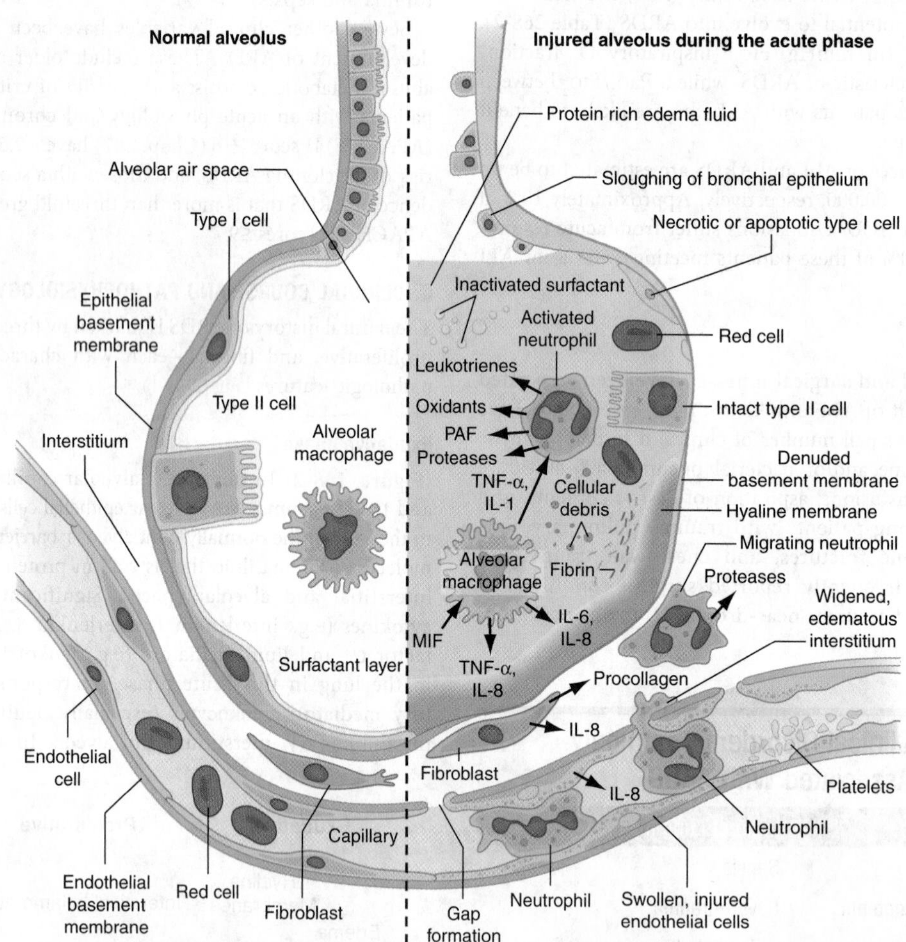

Figure 268-3 The normal alveolus (left-hand side) and the injured alveolus in the acute phase of acute lung injury and the acute respiratory distress syndrome (right-hand side). In the acute phase of the syndrome (right-hand side), there is sloughing of both the bronchial and alveolar epithelial cells, with the formation of protein-rich hyaline membranes on the denuded basement membrane. Neutrophils are shown adhering to the injured capillary endothelium and marginating through the interstitium into the air space, which is filled with protein-rich edema fluid. In the air space, an alveolar macrophage is secreting cytokines, interleukins 1, 6, 8, and 10 (IL-1, -6, -8, and -10) and tumor necrosis factor α (TNF-α), that act locally to stimulate chemotaxis and activate neutrophils. Macrophages also secrete other cytokines, including IL-1, -6, and -10. IL-1 can also stimulate the production of extracellular matrix by fibroblasts. Neutrophils can release oxidants, proteases, leukotrienes, and other proinflammatory molecules, such as platelet-activating factor (PAF). A number of antiinflammatory mediators are also present in the alveolar milieu, including IL-1–receptor antagonist, soluble TNF-α receptor, autoantibodies against IL-8, and cytokines such as IL-10 and -11 (not shown). The influx of protein-rich edema fluid into the alveolus has led to the inactivation of surfactant. MIF, macrophage inhibitory factor. (*From Ware and Matthay, with permission.*)

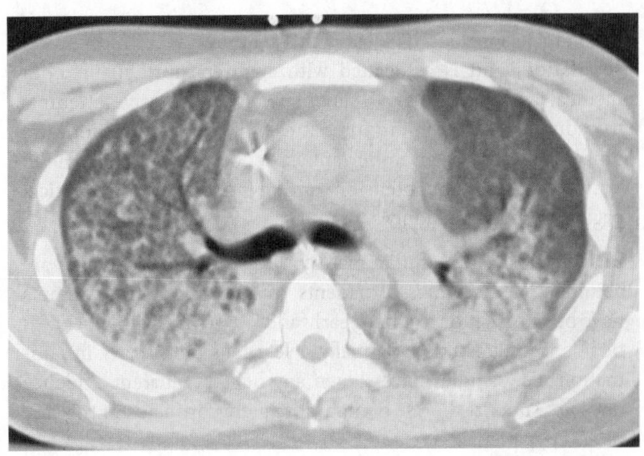

Figure 268-4 A representative computed tomographic scan of the chest during the exudative phase of ARDS in which *dependent* alveolar edema and atelectasis predominate.

shallow breathing and an inability to get enough air. Tachypnea and increased work of breathing frequently result in respiratory fatigue and ultimately in respiratory failure. Laboratory values are generally nonspecific and primarily indicative of underlying clinical disorders. The chest radiograph usually reveals alveolar and interstitial opacities involving at least three-quarters of the lung fields (Fig. 268-2). While characteristic for ARDS or ALI, these radiographic findings are not specific and can be indistinguishable from cardiogenic pulmonary edema (Chap. 272). Unlike the latter, however, the chest x-ray in ARDS rarely shows cardiomegaly, pleural effusions, or pulmonary vascular redistribution. Chest computed tomographic (CT) scanning in ARDS reveals extensive heterogeneity of lung involvement (Fig. 268-4).

Because the early features of ARDS and ALI are nonspecific, alternative diagnoses must be considered. In the differential diagnosis of ARDS, the most common disorders are cardiogenic pulmonary edema, diffuse pneumonia, and alveolar hemorrhage. Less frequent diagnoses to consider include acute interstitial lung diseases [e.g., acute interstitial pneumonitis (Chap. 261)], acute immunologic injury [e.g., hypersensitivity pneumonitis (Chap. 255)], toxin injury (e.g., radiation pneumonitis), and neurogenic pulmonary edema.

Proliferative phase

This phase of ARDS usually lasts from day 7 to day 21. Most patients recover rapidly and are liberated from mechanical ventilation during this phase. Despite this improvement, many still experience dyspnea, tachypnea, and hypoxemia. Some patients develop progressive lung injury and early changes of pulmonary fibrosis during the proliferative phase. Histologically, the first signs of resolution are often evident in this phase with the initiation of lung repair, organization of alveolar exudates, and a shift from a neutrophil- to a lymphocyte-predominant pulmonary infiltrate. As part of the reparative process, there is a proliferation of type II pneumocytes along alveolar basement membranes. These specialized epithelial cells synthesize new pulmonary surfactant and differentiate into type I pneumocytes. The presence of alveolar type III procollagen peptide, a marker of pulmonary fibrosis, is associated with a protracted clinical course and increased mortality from ARDS.

Fibrotic phase

While many patients with ARDS recover lung function 3–4 weeks after the initial pulmonary injury, some will enter a fibrotic phase that may require long-term support on mechanical ventilators and/or supplemental oxygen. Histologically, the alveolar edema and inflammatory exudates of earlier phases are now converted to extensive alveolar duct and interstitial fibrosis. Acinar architecture is markedly disrupted, leading to emphysema-like changes with large bullae. Intimal fibroproliferation in the pulmonary microcirculation leads to progressive vascular occlusion and pulmonary hypertension. The physiologic consequences include an increased risk of pneumothorax, reductions in lung compliance, and increased pulmonary dead space. Patients in this late phase experience a substantial burden of excess morbidity. Lung biopsy evidence for pulmonary fibrosis in any phase of ARDS is associated with increased mortality.

TREATMENT Acute Respiratory Distress Syndrome

GENERAL PRINCIPLES Recent reductions in ARDS/ALI mortality are largely the result of general advances in the care of critically ill patients (Chap. 267). Thus, caring for these patients requires close attention to (1) the recognition and treatment of the underlying medical and surgical disorders (e.g., sepsis, aspiration, trauma); (2) minimizing procedures and their complications; (3) prophylaxis against venous thromboembolism, gastrointestinal bleeding, aspiration, excessive sedation, and central venous catheter infections; (4) prompt recognition of nosocomial infections; and (5) provision of adequate nutrition.

MANAGEMENT OF MECHANICAL VENTILATION (See also Chap. 269) Patients meeting clinical criteria for ARDS frequently fatigue from increased work of breathing and progressive hypoxemia, requiring mechanical ventilation for support.

Ventilator-Induced Lung Injury Despite its life-saving potential, mechanical ventilation can aggravate lung injury. Experimental models have demonstrated that ventilator-induced lung injury appears to require two processes: repeated alveolar overdistention and recurrent alveolar collapse. Clearly evident by chest CT (Fig. 268-4), ARDS is a heterogeneous disorder, principally involving dependent portions of the lung with relative sparing of other regions. Because of their differing compliance, attempts to fully inflate the consolidated lung may lead to overdistention and injury to the more "normal" areas of the lung. Ventilator-induced injury can be demonstrated in experimental models of ALI, with high tidal volume (V_T) ventilation resulting in additional, synergistic alveolar damage. These findings led to the hypothesis that ventilating patients suffering from ALI or ARDS with lower V_Ts would protect against ventilator-induced lung injury and improve clinical outcomes.

A large-scale, randomized controlled trial sponsored by the National Institutes of Health and conducted by the ARDS Network compared low V_T (6 mL/kg predicted body weight) ventilation to conventional V_T (12 mL/kg predicted body weight) ventilation. Mortality was significantly lower in the low V_T patients (31%) compared to the conventional V_T patients (40%). This improvement in survival represents the most substantial benefit in ARDS mortality demonstrated for *any* therapeutic intervention in ARDS to date.

Prevention of Alveolar Collapse In ARDS, the presence of alveolar and interstitial fluid and the loss of surfactant can lead to a marked reduction of lung compliance. Without an increase in end-expiratory pressure, significant alveolar collapse can occur at end-expiration, impairing oxygenation. In most clinical settings, positive end-expiratory pressure (PEEP) is empirically set to minimize FIO_2 and maximize PaO_2. On most modern mechanical ventilators, it is possible to construct a static pressure–volume curve for the respiratory system. The lower inflection point on the curve represents alveolar opening (or "recruitment"). The pressure at this point, usually 12–15 mmHg in ARDS, is a theoretical "optimal PEEP" for alveolar recruitment. Titration of the PEEP to the lower inflection point on the static pressure–volume curve has been hypothesized to keep the lung open, improving oxygenation and protecting against lung injury. Three large randomized trials have investigated the utility of PEEP-based strategies to keep the lung open. In all three trials, improvement in lung function was evident but there were no significant differences in overall mortality. Until more data become available on the clinical utility of high PEEP, it is advisable to set PEEP to minimize F_{IO_2} and optimize Pa_{O_2} (Chap. 269). Measurement of esophageal pressures to estimate transpulmonary pressure may help identify an optimal PEEP in some patients.

Oxygenation can also be improved by increasing mean airway pressure with "inverse ratio ventilation." In this technique, the inspiratory (*I*) time is lengthened so that it is longer than the expiratory (*E*) time (*I*:*E* > 1:1). With diminished time to exhale, dynamic hyperinflation leads to increased end-expiratory pressure, similar to ventilator-prescribed PEEP. This mode of ventilation has the advantage of improving oxygenation with lower peak pressures than conventional ventilation. Although inverse ratio ventilation can improve oxygenation and help reduce F_{IO_2} to ≤0.60 to avoid possible oxygen toxicity, no mortality benefit in ARDS has been demonstrated. Recruitment maneuvers that transiently increase PEEP to "recruit" atelectatic lung can also increase oxygenation, but a mortality benefit has not been established.

In several randomized trials, mechanical ventilation in the prone position improved arterial oxygenation, but its effect on survival and other important clinical outcomes remains uncertain. Moreover, unless the critical-care team is experienced in "proning," repositioning critically ill patients can be hazardous, leading to accidental endotracheal extubation, loss of central venous catheters, and orthopedic injury. Until validation of its efficacy, prone-position ventilation should be reserved for only the most critically ill ARDS patients.

Other Strategies in Mechanical Ventilation Several additional mechanical ventilation strategies that utilize specialized equipment have been tested in ARDS patients, most with mixed or disappointing results in adults. These include high-frequency ventilation (HFV) [i.e., ventilating at extremely high respiratory rates (5–20 cycles per second) and low V_Ts (1–2 mL/kg)]. Partial liquid ventilation (PLV) with perfluorocarbon, an inert, high-density liquid that easily solubilizes oxygen and carbon dioxide, has revealed promising preliminary data on pulmonary function in patients with ARDS but also without survival benefit. Lung-replacement therapy with extracorporeal membrane oxygenation (ECMO), which provides a clear survival benefit in neonatal respiratory distress syndrome, may also have utility in select adult patients with ARDS.

Data in support of the efficacy of "adjunctive" ventilator therapies (e.g., high PEEP, inverse ratio ventilation, recruitment maneuvers, prone positioning, HFV, ECMO, and PLV) remain incomplete, so these modalities are not routinely used.

FLUID MANAGEMENT (See also Chap. 267) Increased pulmonary vascular permeability leading to interstitial and alveolar edema rich in protein is a central feature of ARDS. In addition, impaired vascular integrity augments the normal increase in extravascular lung water that occurs with increasing left atrial pressure. Maintaining a normal or low left atrial filling pressure minimizes pulmonary edema and prevents further decrements in arterial oxygenation and lung compliance, improves pulmonary mechanics, shortens ICU stay and the duration of mechanical ventilation, and is associated with a lower mortality in both medical and surgical ICU patients. Thus, aggressive attempts to reduce left atrial filling pressures with fluid restriction and diuretics should be an important aspect of ARDS management, limited only by hypotension and hypoperfusion of critical organs such as the kidneys.

GLUCOCORTICOIDS Inflammatory mediators and leukocytes are abundant in the lungs of patients with ARDS. Many attempts have been made to treat both early and late ARDS with glucocorticoids to reduce this potentially deleterious pulmonary inflammation. Few studies have shown any benefit. Current evidence does *not* support the use of high-dose glucocorticoids in the care of ARDS patients.

OTHER THERAPIES Clinical trials of surfactant replacement and multiple other medical therapies have proved disappointing. Inhaled nitric oxide (NO) can transiently improve oxygenation but does not improve survival or decrease time on mechanical ventilation. Therefore, the use of NO is *not* currently recommended in ARDS.

RECOMMENDATIONS Many clinical trials have been undertaken to improve the outcome of patients with ARDS; most have been unsuccessful in modifying the natural history. The large number and uncertain clinical efficacy of ARDS therapies can make it difficult for clinicians to select a rational treatment plan, and these patients' critical illnesses can tempt physicians to try unproven and potentially harmful therapies. While results of large clinical trials must be judiciously administered to *individual* patients, evidence-based recommendations are summarized in Table 268-3, and an algorithm for the initial therapeutic goals and limits in ARDS management is provided in Fig. 268-5.

TABLE 268-3 Evidence-Based Recommendations for ARDS Therapies

Treatment	Recommendation*
Mechanical ventilation:	
Low tidal volume	A
Minimize left atrial filling pressures	B
High-PEEP or "open lung"	C
Prone position	C
Recruitment maneuvers	C
ECMO	C
High-frequency ventilation	D
Glucocorticoids	D
Surfactant replacement, inhaled nitric oxide, and other anti-inflammatory therapy (e.g., ketoconazole, PGE_1, NSAIDs)	D

*A, recommended therapy based on strong clinical evidence from randomized clinical trials; B, recommended therapy based on supportive but limited clinical data; C, indeterminate evidence: recommended only as alternative therapy; D, not recommended based on clinical evidence against efficacy of therapy.

Abbreviations: ARDS, acute respiratory distress syndrome; ECMO, extracorporeal membrane oxygenation; NSAIDs, nonsteroidal anti-inflammatory drugs; PEEP, positive end-expiratory pressure; PGE_1, prostaglandin E_1.

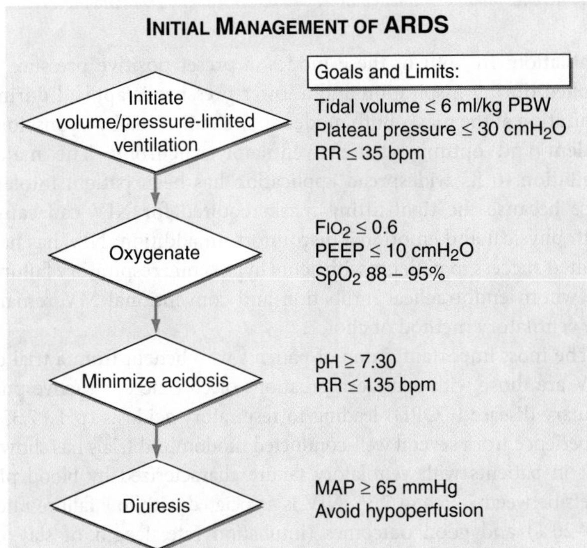

Figure 268-5 Algorithm for the initial management of ARDS. Clinical trials have provided evidence-based therapeutic goals for a stepwise approach to the early mechanical ventilation, oxygenation, and correction of acidosis and diuresis of critically ill patients with ARDS.

PROGNOSIS

Mortality

Recent mortality estimates for ARDS range from 26 to 44%. There is substantial variability, but a trend toward improved ARDS outcomes appears evident. Of interest, mortality in ARDS is largely attributable to nonpulmonary causes, with sepsis and nonpulmonary organ failure accounting for >80% of deaths. Thus, improvement in survival is likely secondary to advances in the care of septic/infected patients and those with multiple organ failure (Chap. 267).

Several risk factors for mortality to help estimate prognosis have been identified. Similar to the risk factors for developing ARDS, the major risk factors for ARDS mortality are also nonpulmonary. Advanced age is an important risk factor. Patients >75 years of age have a substantially increased mortality (~60%) compared to those <45 (~20%). Also, patients >60 years of age with ARDS and sepsis have a threefold higher mortality compared to those <60. Preexisting organ dysfunction from chronic medical illness is an important additional risk factor for increased mortality. In particular, chronic liver disease, cirrhosis, chronic alcohol abuse, chronic immunosuppression, sepsis, chronic renal disease, any nonpulmonary organ failure, and increased APACHE III scores (Chap. 267) have also been linked to increased ARDS mortality. Several factors related to the presenting clinical disorders also increase the risk for ARDS mortality. Patients with ARDS from direct lung injury (including pneumonia, pulmonary contusion, and aspiration; Table 268-1) have nearly twice the mortality of those with indirect causes of lung injury, while surgical and trauma patients with ARDS, especially those without direct lung injury, have a better survival rate than other ARDS patients.

Surprisingly, there is little value in predicting ARDS mortality from the Pao_2/Fio_2 ratio and any of the following measures of the severity of lung injury: the level of PEEP used in mechanical ventilation, the respiratory compliance, the extent of alveolar infiltrates on chest radiography, and the lung injury score (a composite of all these variables). However, recent data indicate that an early (within 24 hours of presentation) elevation in dead space and the oxygenation index may predict increased mortality from ARDS.

Functional recovery in ARDS survivors

While it is common for patients with ARDS to experience prolonged respiratory failure and remain dependent on mechanical ventilation for survival, it is a testament to the resolving powers of the lung that the majority of patients recover nearly normal lung function. Patients usually recover their maximum lung function within 6 months. One year after endotracheal extubation, more than one-third of ARDS survivors have normal spirometry values and diffusion capacity. Most of the remaining patients have only mild abnormalities in their pulmonary function. Unlike the risk for mortality, recovery of lung function is strongly associated with the extent of lung injury in early ARDS. Low static respiratory compliance, high levels of required PEEP, longer durations of mechanical ventilation, and high lung injury scores are all associated with worse recovery of pulmonary function. When caring for ARDS survivors, it is important to be aware of the potential for a substantial burden of emotional and respiratory symptoms. There are significant rates of depression and posttraumatic stress disorder in ARDS survivors.

ACKNOWLEDGMENT

The authors acknowledge the contribution to this chapter by the previous author, Dr. Steven D. Shapiro.

FURTHER READINGS

Fan E et al: Ventilatory management of acute lung injury and acute respiratory distress syndrome. JAMA 294:2889, 2005

Tomashefski JF Jr.: Pulmonary pathology of acute respiratory distress syndrome. Clin Chest Med 21:435, 2000

Ware LB, Matthay MA: The acute respiratory distress syndrome. N Engl J Med 342:1334, 2000

Wheeler AP, Bernard GR: Acute lung injury and the acute respiratory distress syndrome: A clinical review. Lancet 369:1553, 2007

WEB SITES

ARDS Support Center for patient-oriented education: *www.ards.org*

ARDS Network clinical trials information: *www.ardsnet.org*

ARDS Foundation: *www.ardsusa.org*

CHAPTER 269
Mechanical Ventilatory Support

Bartolome R. Celli

MECHANICAL VENTILATORY SUPPORT

Mechanical ventilation is a therapeutic method that is used to assist or replace spontaneous breathing. The primary indication for initiation of mechanical ventilation is respiratory failure, of which there are two basic types: *hypoxemic* respiratory failure, which is present when arterial O_2 saturation (Sao_2) <90% occurs despite an increased inspired O_2 fraction, and *hypercarbic* respiratory failure, which is characterized by arterial PCO_2 values >50 mmHg. When it is chronic, neither of the two types is obligatorily treated with mechanical ventilation, but when acute, mechanical ventilation may be lifesaving.

INDICATIONS

The most common reasons for instituting mechanical ventilation are acute respiratory failure with hypoxemia (acute respiratory distress syndrome, heart failure with pulmonary edema, pneumonia, sepsis, complications of surgery and trauma), which accounts for ~65% of all ventilated cases, followed by causes of hypercarbic ventilatory failure such as coma (15%), exacerbations of chronic obstructive pulmonary disease (13%), and neuromuscular diseases (5%). The primary objectives of mechanical ventilation are to decrease the work of breathing, thus avoiding respiratory muscle fatigue, and to reverse life-threatening hypoxemia and progressive respiratory acidosis.

In some cases, mechanical ventilation is used as an adjunct to other forms of therapy, such as its use in reducing cerebral blood flow in patients with increased intracranial pressure. Mechanical ventilation also is used frequently in conjunction with endotracheal intubation to prevent aspiration of gastric contents in otherwise unstable patients during gastric lavage for suspected drug overdose or during gastrointestinal endoscopy. In critically ill patients, intubation and mechanical ventilation may be indicated before essential diagnostic or therapeutic studies if it appears that respiratory failure may occur during those maneuvers.

TYPES OF MECHANICAL VENTILATION

In its broadest sense, there are two distinct methods for ventilating patients: noninvasive ventilation (NIV) and invasive ventilation or conventional mechanical ventilation (MV).

Noninvasive ventilation

Noninvasive ventilation has been gaining more acceptance because it is effective in certain conditions, such as acute or chronic respiratory failure, and is associated with fewer complications, namely, pneumonia and tracheolaryngeal trauma. Noninvasive ventilation usually is provided by using a tight-fitting face mask or nasal mask similar to the masks traditionally used for treatment of sleep apnea. Noninvasive ventilation has proved highly effective in patients with respiratory failure from acute exacerbations of chronic obstructive pulmonary disease and is most frequently implemented by using bilevel positive airway pressure ventilation or pressure support ventilation. In both of these modes, a preset positive pressure is applied during inspiration and a lower pressure is applied during expiration at the mask. Both modes are well tolerated by a conscious patient and optimize patient-ventilator synchrony. The major limitation to its widespread application has been patient intolerance because the tight-fitting mask required for NIV can cause both physical and emotional discomfort. In addition, NIV has had limited success in patients with acute hypoxemic respiratory failure, for whom endotracheal intubation and conventional MV remain the ventilatory method of choice.

The most important group of patients who benefit from a trial of NIV are those with acute exacerbations of chronic obstructive pulmonary disease (COPD) leading to respiratory acidosis (pH <7.35). Experience from several well-conducted randomized trials has shown that in patients with ventilatory failure characterized by blood pH levels between 7.25 and 7.35, NIV is associated with low failure rates (15–20%) and good outcomes (intubation rate, length of stay in intensive care, and in some series mortality rates). In more severely ill patients with pH <7.25, the rate of NIV failure is inversely related to the severity of respiratory acidosis, with greater failure as the pH decreases. In patients with milder acidosis (pH >7.35), NIV is not better than conventional therapy that includes controlled oxygen delivery and pharmacotherapy for exacerbations of COPD (systemic corticosteroids, bronchodilators, and, if needed, antibiotics).

Despite its benign outcomes, NIV is not useful in the majority of cases of respiratory failure and is contraindicated in patients with the conditions listed in Table 269-1. Experience shows that NIV can delay lifesaving ventilatory support in those cases and actually results in aspiration or hypoventilation. Once NIV is initiated, patients should be monitored; a reduction in respiratory frequency and a decrease in the use of accessory muscles (scalene, sternomastoid, and intercostals) are good clinical indicators of adequate therapeutic benefit. Arterial blood gases should be obtained at least within hours of the initiation of therapy to ensure that NIV is having the desired effect and that it is safe to continue its application. Lack of benefit within that time frame should alert one to the possible need for conventional MV.

Conventional mechanical ventilation

Conventional mechanical ventilation is implemented once a cuffed tube is inserted into the trachea to allow conditioned gas (warmed, oxygenated, and humidified) to be delivered to the airways and lungs at pressures above atmospheric pressure. Great care has to be taken during the act of intubation to avoid brain-damaging hypoxia. In some patients, intubation can be achieved without added sedation. In most patients, the administration of mild sedation

TABLE 269-1 Contraindications for Noninvasive Ventilation

Cardiac or respiratory arrest
Severe encephalopathy
Severe gastrointestinal bleed
Hemodynamic instability
Unstable angina and myocardial infarction
Facial surgery or trauma
Upper airway obstruction
High-risk aspiration and/or inability to protect airways
Inability to clear secretions

may help facilitate the procedure. Opiates and benzodiazepines are good choices but can have a deleterious effect on hemodynamics in patients with depressed cardiac function or low systemic vascular resistance. Morphine can promote histamine release from tissue mast cells and may worsen bronchospasm in patients with asthma; fentanyl, sufentanil, and alfentanil are acceptable alternatives. Ketamine may increase systemic arterial pressure and has been associated with hallucinatory responses; it should be used with caution in patients with hypertensive crisis or a history of psychiatric disorders. Newer agents such as etomidate and propofol have been used for both induction and maintenance of anesthesia in ventilated patients. They are shorter-acting, and etomidate has fewer adverse hemodynamic effects, but both agents are significantly more expensive than older agents. Great care must be taken to avoid the use of neuromuscular paralysis during intubation; in particular, the use of agents whose mechanism of action includes depolarization at the neuromuscular junction, such as succinylcholine chloride, should be avoided in patients with renal failure, tumor lysis syndrome, crush injuries, medical conditions associated with elevated serum potassium levels, and muscular dystrophy syndromes.

PRINCIPLES OF MECHANICAL VENTILATION

Once the patient has been intubated, the basic principles of applying MV are *to optimize oxygenation while avoiding overstretch and collapse/rerecruitment ventilator-induced lung injury (VILI)*. This concept, which is illustrated in Fig. 269-1, has gained acceptance because of important empirical and experimental evidence linking high airway pressures and volumes and overstretching the lung with collapse/rerecruitment with poor outcomes. Although normalization of pH through elimination of CO_2 is desirable, the risk of lung damage associated with the large volume and high pressures needed to achieve this goal has led to the acceptance of permissive hypercapnia. This approach has been found to be well tolerated when care is taken to avoid excess acidosis by pH buffering.

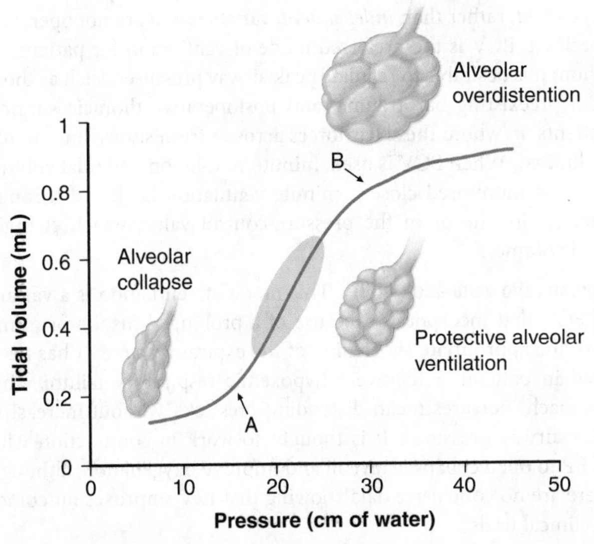

Figure 269-1 Hypothetical pressure-volume curve of the lung in a patient on MV. Alveoli tend to close if the distending pressure falls below the lower inflection point (A), whereas they overstretch if the pressure within them is higher than that of the upper inflection point (B). Collapse and opening of ventilated alveoli are associated with poor outcomes in patients with acute respiratory failure. Protective ventilation (*hatched lines*), using lower tidal volume (6 mL/kg of ideal body weight) and maintaining positive end-expiratory pressure to prevent overstretching and collapse/opening of alveoli, has resulted in improved survival in patients on MV.

MODES OF VENTILATION

Mode refers to the manner in which ventilator breaths are triggered, cycled, and limited. The *trigger,* either an inspiratory effort or a time-based signal, defines what the ventilator senses to initiate an assisted breath. *Cycle* refers to the factors that determine the end of inspiration. For example, in volume-cycled ventilation, inspiration ends when a specific tidal volume is delivered. Other types of cycling include pressure cycling and time cycling. The *limiting factors* are operator-specified values, such as airway pressure, that are monitored by transducers internal to the ventilator circuit throughout the respiratory cycle; if the specified values are exceeded, inspiratory flow is terminated, and the ventilator circuit is vented to atmospheric pressure or the specified pressure at the end of expiration [positive end-expiratory pressure (PEEP)]. Most patients are ventilated with assist control ventilation, intermittent mandatory ventilation, or pressure-support ventilation, with the latter two modes often used simultaneously (Table 269-2).

Assist control ventilation (ACMV)

This is the most widely used mode of ventilation. In this mode, an inspiratory cycle is initiated either by the patient's inspiratory effort or, if none is detected within a specified time window, by a timer signal within the ventilator. Every breath delivered, whether patient- or timer-triggered, consists of the operator-specified tidal volume. Ventilatory rate is determined either by the patient or by the operator-specified backup rate, whichever is of higher frequency. ACMV commonly is used for initiation of mechanical ventilation because it ensures a backup minute ventilation in the absence of an intact respiratory drive and allows for synchronization of the ventilator cycle with the patient's inspiratory effort.

Problems can arise when ACMV is used in patients with tachypnea due to nonrespiratory or nonmetabolic factors, such as anxiety, pain, and airway irritation. Respiratory alkalemia may develop and trigger myoclonus or seizures. Dynamic hyperinflation leading to increased intrathoracic pressures (so-called auto-PEEP) may occur if the patient's respiratory mechanics are such that inadequate time is available for complete exhalation between inspiratory cycles. Auto-PEEP can limit venous return, decrease cardiac output, and increase airway pressures, predisposing to barotrauma.

Intermittent mandatory ventilation (IMV)

With this mode, the operator sets the number of mandatory breaths of fixed volume to be delivered by the ventilator; between those breaths, the patient can breathe spontaneously. In the most frequently used synchronized mode (SIMV), mandatory breaths are delivered in synchrony with the patient's inspiratory efforts at a frequency determined by the operator. If the patient fails to initiate a breath, the ventilator delivers a fixed-tidal-volume breath and resets the internal timer for the next inspiratory cycle. SIMV differs from ACMV in that only the preset number of breaths is ventilator-assisted.

SIMV allows patients with an intact respiratory drive to exercise inspiratory muscles between assisted breaths, making it useful for both supporting and weaning intubated patients. SIMV may be difficult to use in patients with tachypnea because they may attempt to exhale during the ventilator-programmed inspiratory cycle. When this occurs, the airway pressure may exceed the inspiratory pressure limit, the ventilator-assisted breath will be aborted, and minute volume may drop below that programmed by the operator. In this setting, if the tachypnea is in response to respiratory or metabolic acidosis, a change in ACMV will increase minute ventilation and help normalize the pH while the underlying process is further evaluated and treated.

TABLE 269-2 Characteristics of the Most Commonly Used Forms of Mechanical Ventilation

Ventilatory Mode	Variables Set by User (Independent)	Variables Monitored by User (Dependent)	Trigger Cycle Limit	Advantages	Disadvantages
ACMV (assist control ventilation)	Tidal volume Ventilator rate F_{IO_2} PEEP level Pressure limit	Peak, mean, and plateau airway pressures VE ABG I/E ratio	Patient effort Timer Pressure limit	Patient control Guaranteed ventilation	Potential to hyperventilate, Barotrauma and volume trauma Every effective breath generates a ventilator volume
IMV (intermittent mandatory ventilation)	Tidal volume Mandatory Ventilator Rate F_{IO_2} PEEP level Pressure limit Between breaths patients can breathe spontaneously	Peak, mean, and plateau airway pressures VE ABG I/E ratio	Patient effort Timer Pressure limit	Patient control Comfort from spontaneous breaths Guaranteed ventilation	Potential dysynchrony May result in hypoventilation
PSV (pressure support ventilation)	Inspiratory pressure level F_{IO_2} PEEP Pressure limit	Tidal volume Respiratory rate VE ABG	Pressure limit Inspiratory flow	Patient control Comfort Assures synchrony	No timer backup May result in hypoventilation
NIV (noninvasive ventilation)	Inspiratory and expiratory pressure level F_{IO_2}	Tidal volume Respiratory rate VE ABG	Pressure limit Inspiratory flow	Patient control	Mask interface may cause discomfort and facial bruising Leaks are common Hypoventilation

Abbreviations: ABG, arterial blood gases; F_{IO_2}, fraction of inspired oxygen; PEEP, positive end-expiratory pressure; I/E, inspiratory to expiratory time ratio; VE, minute ventilation.

Pressure-support ventilation (PSV)

This form of ventilation is patient-triggered, flow-cycled, and pressure-limited. It provides graded assistance and differs from the other two modes in that the operator sets the pressure level (rather than the volume) to augment every spontaneous respiratory effort. The level of pressure is adjusted by observing the patient's respiratory frequency. During PSV, the inspiration is terminated when inspiratory airflow falls below a certain level; in most ventilators, this flow rate cannot be adjusted by the operator. When PSV is used, patients receive ventilator assistance only when the ventilator detects an inspiratory effort. PSV frequently is used in combination with SIMV to ensure volume-cycled backup for patients whose respiratory drive is depressed. PSV frequently is well tolerated by most patients who are being weaned; PSV parameters can be set to provide full or nearly full ventilatory support and can be withdrawn to load the respiratory muscles gradually.

There are other modes of ventilation, and each has its own acronym, making it very difficult to understand for those unfamiliar with the terms. All these modes are modifications of the manner and duration in which pressure is applied to the airway and lungs and of the interaction between the mechanical assistance provided by the ventilator and the patient's respiratory effort. Although their use in acute respiratory failure is limited, the following have been used with varying levels of enthusiasm and adoption.

Pressure-control ventilation (PCV) This form of ventilation is time-triggered, time-cycled, and pressure-limited. During the inspiratory phase, a specified pressure is imposed at the airway opening throughout inspiration. Since the inspiratory airway pressure is specified by the operator, tidal volume and inspiratory flow rate are *dependent*, rather than *independent*, variables and are not operator-specified. PCV is the preferred mode of ventilation for patients in whom it is desirable to regulate peak airway pressures, such as those with preexisting barotrauma, and postoperative thoracic surgical patients, in whom the shear forces across a fresh suture line should be limited. When PCV is used, minute ventilation and tidal volume must be monitored closely; minute ventilation is altered through changes in rate or in the pressure-control value, which changes tidal volume.

Inverse ratio ventilation (IRV) This mode of ventilation is a variant of PCV that incorporates the use of a prolonged inspiratory time with the appropriate shortening of the expiratory time. It has been used in patients with severe hypoxemic respiratory failure. This approach increases mean distending pressures without increasing peak airway pressures. It is thought to work in conjunction with PEEP to open collapsed alveoli and improve oxygenation, although there are no conclusive data showing that IRV improves outcomes in clinical trials.

Continuous positive airway pressure (CPAP) This is not a true support mode of ventilation because all ventilation occurs through the patient's spontaneous efforts. The ventilator provides fresh gas to the breathing circuit with each inspiration and sets the circuit to a constant, operator-specified pressure. CPAP is used to assess extubation potential in patients who have been effectively weaned and require little ventilator support and patients with intact respiratory system function who require an endotracheal tube for airway protection.

NONCONVENTIONAL VENTILATORY STRATEGIES

Several nonconventional ventilator strategies have been evaluated for their ability to improve oxygenation and reduce mortality rates in patients with advanced hypoxemic respiratory failure. These strategies include high-frequency oscillatory ventilation (HFOV), airway pressure release ventilation (APRV), extracorporeal membrane oxygenation (BCMO), and partial liquid ventilation (PLV) using perfluorocarbons. Although case reports and small uncontrolled cohort studies have shown benefit, randomized controlled trials have failed to demonstrate consistent improvements in outcome with any of these strategies. Currently, these approaches should be considered "salvage" techniques and considered for patients with hypoxemia refractory to conventional therapy. Prone positioning of patients with refractory hypoxemia has been explored because in theory it would tend to improve ventilation-perfusion matching. Although this is conceptually appealing and simple to implement, several randomized trial in patients with acute lung injury did not demonstrate a survival advantage with prone positioning despite demonstration of a transient physiologic benefit. The administration of nitric oxide (NO) gas, which has bronchodilator and pulmonary vasodilator effects when delivered through the airways and has been shown to improve arterial oxygenation in many patients with advanced hypoxemic respiratory failure, also failed to improve outcomes in patients with advanced hypoxemic respiratory failure.

Newer, promising strategies are intended to improve patient-ventilator synchrony, a major practical problem during MV. Currently, the more advanced new ventilators allow patients to trigger the ventilator with their own effort while also incorporating flow algorithms that allow termination of cycles once certain preset criteria are reached; this approach has greatly improved patient-ventilator synchrony and comfort. More recently, new modes of ventilation that synchronize not only the timing but also the levels of assistance to match the patient's effort have been developed. Proportional assist ventilation (PAV) and neurally adjusted ventilatory assist ventilation (NAV) are two modes that are designed to deliver assisted breaths through algorithms incorporating not only pressure, volume, and time but also overall respiratory resistance and compliance in the case of PAV and neural activation of the diaphragm in the case of NAV. Although these modes result in better patient-ventilator synchrony, their practical use in the everyday management of patients on MV needs further study.

PROTECTIVE VENTILATORY STRATEGY

Whichever mode of MV is used, in acute respiratory failure the evidence from several important controlled trials indicates that the use of a protective ventilation approach guided by the principles outlined below and summarized in Fig. 269-1 is safe and offers the best chance of a good outcome:

1. Set a target tidal volume close to 6 mL/kg of ideal body weight.
2. Prevent plateau pressure (static pressure in the airway at the end of inspiration) over 30 cmH_2O.
3. Use the lowest possible fraction of inspired oxygen (F_{IO_2}) to keep Sa_{O_2} ≥90%.
4. Adjust the PEEP to maintain alveolar patency while preventing overdistention and closure/reopening.

With the application of these techniques, the mortality rate among patients with acute hypoxemic respiratory failure has decreased to ~30% from close to 50% a decade ago.

PATIENT MANAGEMENT

Once the patient has been stabilized with respect to gas exchange, definitive therapy for the underlying process responsible for respiratory failure is initiated. Subsequent modifications in ventilator therapy must be provided in parallel with changes in the patient's clinical status. As improvement in respiratory function is noted, the first priority is to reduce the level of mechanical ventilator support. Patients on full ventilator support should be monitored frequently with the goal of switching to a mode that allows for weaning as soon as possible. Protocols and guidelines that can be applied by paramedical personnel when physicians are not readily available have proved to be of value in shortening ventilator and intensive care unit (ICU) time, with very good outcomes. Patients whose condition continues to deteriorate after ventilator support is initiated may require increased O_2, PEEP, or one of the alternative modes of ventilation.

GENERAL SUPPORT DURING VENTILATION

Patients started on mechanical ventilation usually require sedation and analgesia to maintain an acceptable level of comfort. Often, this consists of a combination of a benzodiazepine and an opiate administered intravenously. Medications commonly used for this purpose include lorazepam, midazolam, diazepam, morphine, and fentanyl. The use of oversedation must be avoided in the ICU. Indeed, recent trials evaluating the effect of daily interruption of sedation in patients with improved ventilatory status show that this results in shorter time on the ventilator and shorter ICU stay.

Immobilized patients in the ICU who are on mechanical ventilator support are at increased risk for deep venous thrombosis and decubitus ulcers. To prevent venous thrombosis, prophylaxis in the form of subcutaneous heparin and/or pneumatic compression boots is prescribed frequently. Fractionated low-molecular-weight heparin appears to be equally effective for this purpose. To help prevent decubitus ulcers, frequent changes in body position and the use of soft mattress overlays and air mattresses are employed. Prophylaxis against diffuse gastrointestinal mucosal injury is indicated for patients on MV. Histamine-receptor antagonists (H_2-receptor antagonists), antacids, and cytoprotective agents such as Carafate (sucralfate) have all been used for this purpose and appear to be effective. Nutrition support by enteral feeding through either a nasogastric or an orogastric tube should be initiated and maintained whenever possible. Delayed gastric emptying is common in critically ill patients on sedative medications but often responds to promotility agents such as metoclopramide. Parenteral nutrition is an alternative to enteral nutrition in patients with severe gastrointestinal pathology who need prolonged MV.

COMPLICATIONS OF MECHANICAL VENTILATION

Endotracheal intubation and mechanical ventilation have direct and indirect effects on the lung and upper airways, the cardiovascular system, and the gastrointestinal system. Pulmonary complications include barotrauma, nosocomial pneumonia, oxygen toxicity, tracheal stenosis, and deconditioning of respiratory muscles. Barotrauma and volutrauma overdistend and disrupt lung tissue; may be clinically manifest by interstitial emphysema, pneumomediastinum, subcutaneous emphysema, or pneumothorax; and can result in the liberation of cytokines from overdistended tissues, further promoting tissue injury. Clinically significant pneumothorax requires tube thoracostomy. Intubated patients are at high risk for ventilator-associated pneumonia (VAP) as a result of aspiration from the upper airways through small leaks around the endotracheal tube cuff; the most common organisms responsible for this condition are *Pseudomonas aeruginosa*, enteric gram-negative rods, and *Staphylococcus aureus*. Because this condition is associated with high mortality rates, early initiation of empirical antibiotics directed against likely pathogens is recommended. *Hypotension* resulting from elevated intrathoracic pressures with decreased venous return is almost always responsive to intravascular volume repletion. In patients who are judged to have respiratory failure on the basis of alveolar edema but in whom the cardiac or pulmonary origin of the edema is unclear, hemodynamic monitoring with a pulmonary arterial catheter may be of value in helping to clarify the cause of the edema.

Gastrointestinal effects of positive-pressure ventilation include stress ulceration and mild to moderate cholestasis.

WEANING FROM MECHANICAL VENTILATION

It is important to consider discontinuation of mechanical ventilation once the underlying respiratory disease begins to reverse. Although the predictive capacities of multiple clinical and physiologic variables have been explored, the consensus from a weaning task force includes the following recommendations: (1) lung injury is stable/resolving, (2) gas exchange is adequate with low PEEP/FIO_2 (<8 cmH_2O and FIO <0.5), (3) hemodynamic variables are stable (patient off vasopressors), and (4) patient is capable of initiating spontaneous breaths. This "screen" should be done at least daily. If the patient is deemed capable of beginning weaning, the recommendation of the task force is to perform a spontaneous breathing trial (SBT) because several randomized trials support the value of this approach (Fig. 269-2). The SBT involves an integrated patient assessment during spontaneous breathing with little or no ventilator support. The SBT is usually implemented with a T-piece using 1–5 cmH_2O CPAP or a T-piece with 5–7 cmH_2O or PSV from the ventilator to offset the resistance from the endotracheal tube. Once it is determined that the patient can breath spontaneously, a decision must be made about the removal of the artificial airway; this should be done only when it is concluded that the patient has the ability to protect the airway, is able to cough and clear secretions, and is alert enough to follow commands. In addition, other factors must be taken into account, such as the possible difficulty in replacing the tube if that is anticipated. If upper airway difficulty is suspected, an evaluation using a "cuff leak" test (assessing the presence of air movement around a deflated endotracheal tube cuff) is supported by some internists. Despite the application of all of these methods, ~10–15% of extubated patients require reintubation. Several studies suggest that NIV can be used to avert reintubation; this has been particularly useful in patients with ventilatory failure secondary to COPD exacerbation. In this group, earlier extubation with the use of prophylactic NIV has shown good results. The use of NIV to facilitate weaning in other causes of respiratory failure is not currently indicated.

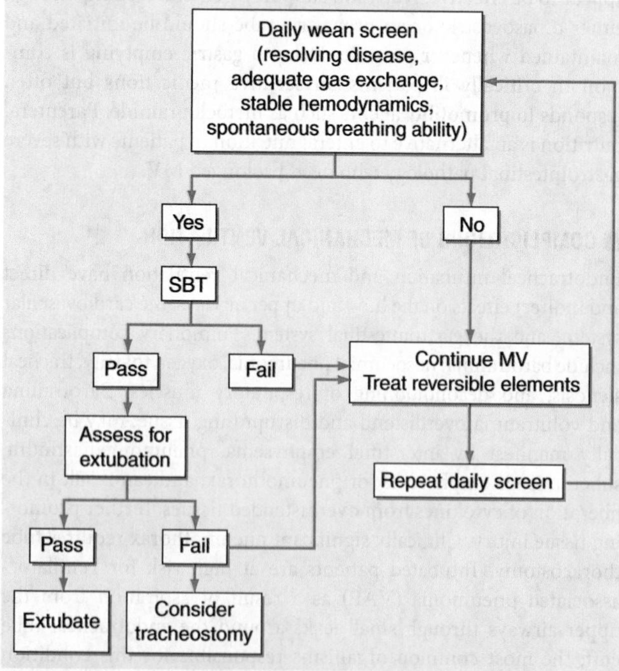

Figure 269-2 Flow chart to guide daily approach to managing patients considered for weaning. If the patient fails attempts at extubation, a tracheostomy should be considered.

Prolonged mechanical ventilation and tracheostomy

From 5 to 13% of patients on MV will go on to require prolonged MV (>21 days). In these patients, critical care personnel have to make a decision about whether and when to perform a tracheostomy. This decision is individually based on the risk and benefits of tracheostomy and prolonged intubation and the patient's preferences and expected clinical outcomes. A tracheostomy is thought to be more comfortable, require less sedation, and provide a more secure airway, and it seems to reduce weaning time. However, tracheostomy carries the risk of complications, which occur in 5–40% of the procedures and include bleeding, cardiopulmonary arrest, hypoxia due to airway loss, structural damage, postoperative pneumothorax, pneumomediastinum, and wound infection. In patients with long-term tracheostomy, tracheal stenosis, granulation, and the erosion of the innominate artery are complex complications. It is generally agreed that if a patient is in need of MV for more than 10–14 days, a tracheostomy is indicated and should be planned under optimal conditions. Whether it is completed at the bedside or as an operative procedure depends on the local resources and experience. Some 5–10% of patients are deemed unable to wean in the ICU. These patients may benefit from transfer to special units where a multidisciplinary approach, including nutrition optimization, physical therapy with rehabilitation, and slower weaning methods, including SIMV with PSV, results in up to 30% successful weaning. Unfortunately, close to 2% of ventilated patients may ultimately remain unable to wean and become dependent on ventilatory support to maintain life. Most of these patients remain in chronic care institutions, although some who have strong social, economical, and family support may achieve a fulfilling life with home mechanical ventilation.

ACKNOWLEDGMENT

Portions of this chapter were retained from the work of the previous author, Edward Ingenito, MD.

FURTHER READINGS

THE ACUTE RESPIRATORY DISTRESS SYNDROME NETWORK: Ventilation with lower tidal volumes as compared with traditional tidal volumes for acute lung injury and the acute respiratory distress syndrome. N Engl J Med 342:1301, 2000

BOLES JM et al: Weaning from mechanical ventilation. Eur Respir J 29:1033, 2007

ESTEBAN A et al: Non-invasive ventilation for respiratory failure after extubation. N Engl J Med 350:2452, 2004

MACINTYRE N (ed): *Controversies in Mechanical Ventilation*. Clinics in Chest Medicine. Philadelphia, Elsevier Saunders, 2008

MERCAT A et al: Positive and end-expiratory pressure setting in adults with acute lung injury and acute respiratory distress syndrome: A randomized controlled trial. JAMA 299:646, 2008

SCALISE PI, VOTTO J: Weaning from long term mechanical ventilation. Chron Respir Dis 2:99, 2005

CHAPTER 270 Approach to the Patient With Shock

Ronald V. Maier

Shock is the clinical syndrome that results from inadequate tissue perfusion. Irrespective of cause, the hypoperfusion-induced imbalance between the delivery of and requirements for oxygen and substrate leads to cellular dysfunction. The cellular injury created by the inadequate delivery of oxygen and substrates also induces the production and release of damage-associated molecular patterns (DAMPs or "danger signals") and inflammatory mediators that further compromise perfusion through functional and structural changes within the microvasculature. This leads to a vicious cycle in which impaired perfusion is responsible for cellular injury that causes maldistribution of blood flow, further compromising cellular perfusion; the latter ultimately causes multiple organ failure (MOF) and, if the process is not interrupted, leads to death. The clinical manifestations of shock are also the result, in part, of autonomic neuroendocrine responses to hypoperfusion as well as the breakdown in organ function induced by severe cellular dysfunction (Fig. 270-1).

When very severe and/or persistent, inadequate oxygen delivery leads to irreversible cell injury; only rapid restoration of oxygen delivery can reverse the progression of the shock state. The fundamental approach to management, therefore, is to recognize overt and impending shock in a timely fashion and to intervene emergently to restore perfusion. This often requires the expansion or reexpansion of intravascular blood volume. Control of any inciting pathologic process (e.g., continued hemorrhage, impairment of cardiac function, or infection), must occur simultaneously.

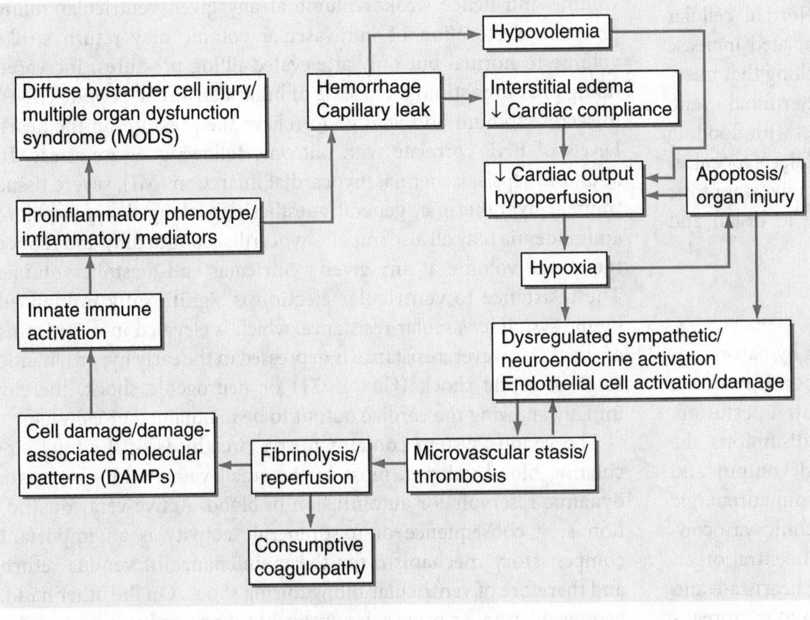

Figure 270-1 Shock-induced vicious cycle.

Clinical shock is usually accompanied by hypotension (i.e., a mean arterial pressure (MAP) <60 mmHg in previously normotensive persons). Multiple classification schemes have been developed in an attempt to synthesize the seemingly dissimilar processes leading to shock. Strict adherence to a classification scheme may be difficult from a clinical standpoint because of the frequent combination of two or more causes of shock in any individual patient, but the classification shown in Table 270-1 provides a useful reference point from which to discuss and further delineate the underlying processes.

TABLE 270-1 Classification of Shock

Hypovolemic	Septic
Traumatic	Hyperdynamic (early)
Cardiogenic	Hypodynamic (late)
Intrinsic	Neurogenic
Compressive	Hypoadrenal

PATHOGENESIS AND ORGAN RESPONSE

MICROCIRCULATION

Normally when cardiac output falls, systemic vascular resistance rises to maintain a level of systemic pressure that is adequate for perfusion of the heart and brain at the expense of other tissues such as muscle, skin, and especially the gastrointestinal (GI) tract. Systemic vascular resistance is determined primarily by the luminal diameter of arterioles. The metabolic rates of the heart and brain are high, and their stores of energy substrate are low. These organs are critically dependent on a continuous supply of oxygen and nutrients, and neither tolerates severe ischemia for more than brief periods (minutes). Autoregulation (i.e., the maintenance of blood flow over a wide range of perfusion pressures), is critical in sustaining cerebral and coronary perfusion despite significant hypotension. However, when MAP drops to ≤60 mmHg, blood flow to these organs falls, and their function deteriorates.

Arteriolar vascular smooth muscle has both α- and β-adrenergic receptors. The α_1 receptors mediate vasoconstriction, while the β_2 receptors mediate vasodilation. Efferent sympathetic fibers release norepinephrine, which acts primarily on α_1 receptors as one of the most fundamental compensatory responses to reduced perfusion pressure. Other constrictor substances that are increased in most forms of shock include angiotensin II, vasopressin, endothelin 1, and thromboxane A_2. Both norepinephrine and epinephrine are released by the adrenal medulla, and the concentrations of these catecholamines in the bloodstream rise. Circulating vasodilators in shock include prostacyclin [prostaglandin (PG) I_2], nitric oxide (NO), and, importantly, products of local metabolism such as adenosine that match flow to the tissue's metabolic needs. The balance between these various vasoconstrictors and vasodilators influences acting upon the microcirculation determines local perfusion.

Transport to cells depends on microcirculatory flow; capillary permeability; the diffusion of oxygen, carbon dioxide, nutrients, and products of metabolism through the interstitium; and the exchange of these products across cell membranes. Impairment of the microcirculation that is central to the pathophysiologic responses in the late stages of all forms of shock, results in the derangement of cellular metabolism that is ultimately responsible for organ failure.

The endogenous response to mild or moderate hypovolemia is an attempt at restitution of intravascular volume through alterations in hydrostatic pressure and osmolarity. Constriction of arterioles leads to reductions in both the capillary hydrostatic pressure and the number of capillary beds perfused, thereby limiting the capillary surface area across which filtration occurs. When filtration is reduced while intravascular oncotic pressure remains constant or rises, there is net reabsorption of fluid into the vascular bed, in accord with Starling's law of capillary interstitial liquid exchange. Metabolic changes (including hyperglycemia and elevations in the products of glycolysis, lipolysis, and proteolysis) raise extracellular osmolarity, leading to an osmotic gradient that increases interstitial and intravascular volume at the expense of intracellular volume.

CELLULAR RESPONSES

Interstitial transport of nutrients is impaired in shock, leading to a decline in intracellular high-energy phosphate stores. Mitochondrial dysfunction and uncoupling of oxidative phosphorylation are the most likely causes for decreased amounts of adenosine triphosphate (ATP). As a consequence, there is an accumulation of hydrogen ions, lactate, and other products of anaerobic metabolism. As shock progresses, these vasodilator metabolites override vasomotor tone, causing further hypotension and hypoperfusion. Dysfunction of cell membranes is thought to represent a common end-stage pathophysiologic pathway in the various forms of shock. Normal cellular transmembrane potential falls, and there is an associated increase in intracellular sodium and water, leading to cell swelling that interferes further with microvascular perfusion. In a preterminal event, homeostasis of calcium via membrane channels is lost with flooding of calcium intracellularly and a concomitant extracellular hypocalcemia. There is also evidence for a widespread but selective apoptotic (programmed cell-death) loss of cells, contributing to organ and immune failure.

NEUROENDOCRINE RESPONSE

Hypovolemia, hypotension, and hypoxia are sensed by baroreceptors and chemoreceptors that contribute to an autonomic response that attempts to restore blood volume, maintain central perfusion, and mobilize metabolic substrates. Hypotension disinhibits the vasomotor center, resulting in increased adrenergic output and reduced vagal activity. Release of norepinephrine from adrenergic neurons induces significant peripheral and splanchnic vasoconstriction, a major contributor to the maintenance of central organ perfusion, while reduced vagal activity increases the heart rate and cardiac output. Loss of vagal activity is also recognized to upregulate the innate immunity inflammatory response. The effects of circulating epinephrine released by the adrenal medulla in shock are largely metabolic, causing increased glycogenolysis and gluconeogenesis and reduced pancreatic insulin release. However, epinephrine also inhibits production and release of inflammatory mediators through stimulation of β-adrenergic receptors on innate immune cells.

Severe pain or other stresses cause the hypothalamic release of adrenocorticotropic hormone (ACTH). This stimulates cortisol secretion that contributes to decreased peripheral uptake of glucose and amino acids, enhances lipolysis, and increases gluconeogenesis. Increased pancreatic secretion of glucagon during stress accelerates hepatic gluconeogenesis and further elevates blood glucose concentration. These hormonal actions act synergistically to increase blood glucose for both selective tissue metabolism and the maintenance of blood volume. Many critically ill patients have recently been shown to exhibit low plasma cortisol levels and an impaired response to ACTH stimulation, which is linked to a decrease in survival. The importance of the cortisol response to stress is illustrated by the profound circulatory collapse that occurs in patients with adrenal cortical insufficiency (Chap. 342).

Renin release is increased in response to adrenergic discharge and reduced perfusion of the juxtaglomerular apparatus in the kidney. Renin induces the formation of angiotensin I that is then converted to angiotensin II, an extremely potent vasoconstrictor and stimulator of aldosterone release by the adrenal cortex and of vasopressin by the posterior pituitary. Aldosterone contributes to the maintenance of intravascular volume by enhancing renal tubular reabsorption of sodium, resulting in the excretion of a low-volume, concentrated, sodium-free urine. Vasopressin has a direct action on vascular smooth muscle, contributing to vasoconstriction, and acts on the distal renal tubules to enhance water reabsorption.

CARDIOVASCULAR RESPONSE

Three variables—ventricular filling (preload), the resistance to ventricular ejection (afterload), and myocardial contractility—are paramount in controlling stroke volume (Chap. 224). Cardiac output, the major determinant of tissue perfusion, is the product of stroke volume and heart rate. Hypovolemia leads to decreased ventricular preload that in turn reduces the stroke volume. An increase in heart rate is a useful but limited compensatory mechanism to maintain cardiac output. A shock-induced reduction in myocardial compliance is frequent, reducing ventricular end-diastolic volume and hence stroke volume at any given ventricular filling pressure. Restoration of intravascular volume may return stroke volume to normal but only at elevated filling pressures. Increased filling pressures stimulate release of brain natriuretic peptide (BNP) to secrete sodium and volume to relieve the pressure on the heart. Levels of BNP correlate with outcome following severe stress. In addition, sepsis, ischemia, myocardial infarction (MI), severe tissue trauma, hypothermia, general anesthesia, prolonged hypotension, and acidemia may all also impair myocardial contractility and reduce the stroke volume at any given ventricular end-diastolic volume. The resistance to ventricular ejection is significantly influenced by the systemic vascular resistance, which is elevated in most forms of shock. However, resistance is depressed in the early hyperdynamic stage of septic shock (Chap. 271) or neurogenic shock, thereby initially allowing the cardiac output to be maintained or elevated.

The venous system contains nearly two-thirds of the total circulating blood volume, most in the small veins, and serves as a dynamic reservoir for autoinfusion of blood. Active venoconstriction as a consequence of α-adrenergic activity is an important compensatory mechanism for the maintenance of venous return and therefore of ventricular filling during shock. On the other hand, venous dilation, as occurs in neurogenic shock, reduces ventricular filling and hence stroke volume and potentially cardiac output.

■ PULMONARY RESPONSE

The response of the pulmonary vascular bed to shock parallels that of the systemic vascular bed, and the relative increase in pulmonary vascular resistance, particularly in septic shock, may exceed that of the systemic vascular resistance, leading to right heart failure. Shock-induced tachypnea reduces tidal volume and increases both dead space and minute ventilation. Relative hypoxia and the subsequent tachypnea induce a respiratory alkalosis. Recumbency and involuntary restriction of ventilation secondary to pain reduce functional residual capacity and may lead to atelectasis. Shock and, in particular, resuscitation-induced oxidant radical generation, is recognized as a major cause of acute lung injury and subsequent acute respiratory distress syndrome (ARDS; Chap. 268). These disorders are characterized by noncardiogenic pulmonary edema secondary to diffuse pulmonary capillary endothelial and alveolar epithelial injury, hypoxemia, and bilateral diffuse pulmonary infiltrates. Hypoxemia results from perfusion of underventilated and nonventilated alveoli. Loss of surfactant and lung volume in combination with increased interstitial and alveolar edema reduces lung compliance. The work of breathing and the oxygen requirements of respiratory muscles increase.

■ RENAL RESPONSE

Acute kidney injury (Chap. 279), a serious complication of shock and hypoperfusion, occurs less frequently than heretofore because of early aggressive volume repletion. Acute tubular necrosis is now more frequently seen as a result of the interactions of shock, sepsis, the administration of nephrotoxic agents (such as aminoglycosides and angiographic contrast media), and rhabdomyolysis; the latter may be particularly severe in skeletal muscle trauma. The physiologic response of the kidney to hypoperfusion is to conserve salt and water. In addition to decreased renal blood flow, increased afferent arteriolar resistance accounts for diminished glomerular filtration rate (GFR) that together with increased aldosterone and vasopressin is responsible for reduced urine formation. Toxic injury causes necrosis of tubular epithelium and tubular obstruction by cellular debris with back leak of filtrate. The depletion of renal ATP stores that occurs with prolonged renal hypoperfusion contributes to subsequent impairment of renal function.

■ METABOLIC DERANGEMENTS

During shock, there is disruption of the normal cycles of carbohydrate, lipid, and protein metabolism. Through the citric acid cycle, alanine in conjunction with lactate, which is converted from pyruvate in the periphery in the presence of oxygen deprivation enhances the hepatic production of glucose. With reduced availability of oxygen, the breakdown of glucose to pyruvate, and ultimately lactate, represents an inefficient cycling of substrate with minimal net energy production. An elevated plasma lactate/pyruvate ratio is preferable to lactate alone as a measure of anaerobic metabolism and reflects inadequate tissue perfusion. Decreased clearance of exogenous triglycerides coupled with increased hepatic lipogenesis causes a significant rise in serum triglyceride concentrations. There is increased protein catabolism as energy substrate, a negative nitrogen balance, and, if the process is prolonged, severe muscle wasting.

■ INFLAMMATORY RESPONSES

Activation of an extensive network of proinflammatory mediator systems by the innate immune system plays a significant role in the progression of shock and contributes importantly to the development of multiple organ injury, dysfunction (MOD), and failure (MOF) (Fig. 270-2). In those surviving the acute insult, there is a prolonged endogenous counterregulatory response to "turn off" or balance the excessive proinflammatory response. If balance is restored, the patient does well. If the response is excessive, adaptive immunity is

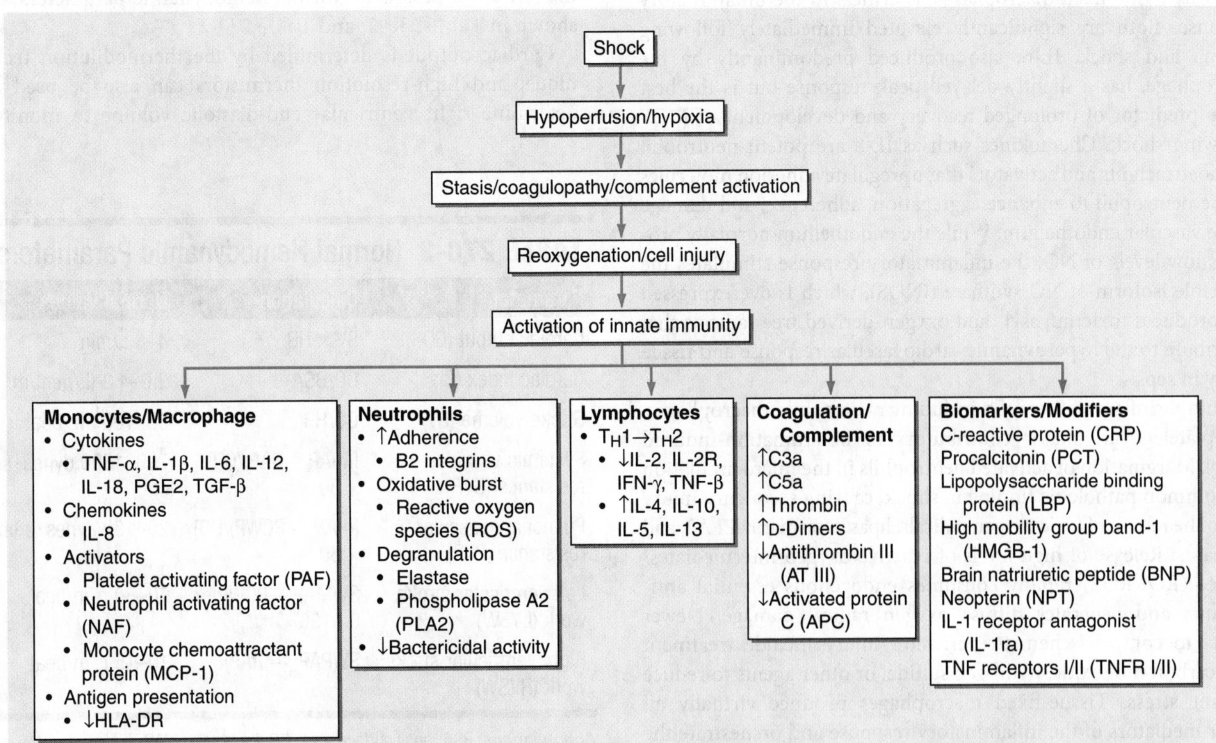

Figure 270-2 **A schematic of the host immunoinflammatory response to shock.**

suppressed and the patient is highly susceptible to secondary nosocomial infections, which may then drive the inflammatory response and lead to delayed MOF.

Multiple humoral mediators are activated during shock and tissue injury. The complement cascade, activated through both the classic and alternate pathways, generates the anaphylatoxins C3a and C5a (Chap. 314). Direct complement fixation to injured tissues can progress to the C5-C9 attack complex, causing further cell damage. Activation of the coagulation cascade (Chap. 116) causes microvascular thrombosis, with subsequent fibrinolysis leading to repeated episodes of ischemia and reperfusion. Components of the coagulation system (e.g., thrombin), are potent proinflammatory mediators that cause expression of adhesion molecules on endothelial cells and activation of neutrophils, leading to microvascular injury. Coagulation also activates the kallikrein-kininogen cascade, contributing to hypotension.

Eicosanoids are vasoactive and immunomodulatory products of arachidonic acid metabolism that include cyclooxygenase-derived prostaglandins (PGs) and thromboxane A_2, as well as lipoxygenase-derived leukotrienes and lipoxins. Thromboxane A_2 is a potent vasoconstrictor that contributes to the pulmonary hypertension and acute tubular necrosis of shock. PGI_2 and PGE_2 are potent vasodilators that enhance capillary permeability and edema formation. The cysteinyl leukotrienes LTC_4 and LTD_4 are pivotal mediators of the vascular sequelae of anaphylaxis, as well as of shock states resulting from sepsis or tissue injury. LTB_4 is a potent neutrophil chemoattractant and secretagogue that stimulates the formation of reactive oxygen species. Platelet-activating factor, an ether-linked, arachidonyl-containing phospholipid mediator, causes pulmonary vasoconstriction, bronchoconstriction, systemic vasodilation, increased capillary permeability, and the priming of macrophages and neutrophils to produce enhanced levels of inflammatory mediators.

Tumor necrosis factor α (TNF-α), produced by activated macrophages, reproduces many components of the shock state, including hypotension, lactic acidosis, and respiratory failure. Interleukin 1β (IL-1β), originally defined as "endogenous pyrogen" and produced by tissue-fixed macrophages, is critical to the inflammatory response. Both are significantly elevated immediately following trauma and shock. IL-6, also produced predominantly by the macrophage, has a slightly delayed peak response but is the best single predictor of prolonged recovery and development of MOF following shock. Chemokines such as IL-8 are potent neutrophil chemoattractants and activators that upregulate adhesion molecules on the neutrophil to enhance aggregation, adherence, and damage to the vascular endothelium. While the endothelium normally produces low levels of NO, the inflammatory response stimulates the inducible isoform of NO synthase (iNOS), which is overexpressed and produces toxic nitrosyl- and oxygen-derived free radicals that contribute to the hyperdynamic cardiovascular response and tissue injury in sepsis.

Multiple inflammatory cells, including neutrophils, macrophages, and platelets, are major contributors to inflammation-induced injury. Margination of activated neutrophils in the microcirculation is a common pathologic finding in shock, causing secondary injury due to the release of toxic oxygen radicals, lipases, primarily PLA2, and proteases. Release of high levels of reactive oxygen intermediates/species (ROI/ROS) rapidly consumes endogenous essential antioxidants and generates diffuse oxygen radical damage. Newer efforts to control ischemia/reperfusion injury include treatment with carbon monoxide, hydrogen sulfide, or other agents to reduce oxidant stress. Tissue-fixed macrophages produce virtually all major mediators of the inflammatory response and orchestrate the progression and duration of the inflammatory response. A major source of activation of the monocyte/macrophage is through the highly conserved membrane toll-like receptors (TLRs) that recognize DAMPs such as HMGB-1, and pathogen-associated molecular patterns (PAMPs) such as endotoxins released following tissue injury, and by pathogenic microbial organisms, respectively. Toll-like receptors also appear important for the chronic inflammation seen in Crohn's disease, ulcerative colitis, and transplant rejection. The variability in individual responses is a genetic predisposition that, in part, is due to single nucleotide polymorphisms (SNPs) in genetic sequences affecting the function and production of various inflammatory mediators.

TREATMENT Shock

MONITORING Patients in shock require care in an ICU. Careful and continuous assessment of the physiologic status is necessary. Arterial pressure through an indwelling line, pulse, and respiratory rate should be monitored continuously; a Foley catheter should be inserted to follow urine flow; and mental status should be assessed frequently. Sedated patients should be allowed to awaken ("drug holiday") daily to assess their neurologic status and to shorten duration of ventilator support.

There is ongoing debate as to the indications for using the flow-directed pulmonary artery catheter (PAC, Swan-Ganz catheter). Most patients in the ICU can be safely managed without the use of a PAC. However, in shock with significant ongoing blood loss, fluid shifts, and underlying cardiac dysfunction, a PAC may be useful. The PAC is placed percutaneously via the subclavian or jugular vein through the central venous circulation and right heart into the pulmonary artery. There are ports both proximal in the right atrium and distal in the pulmonary artery to provide access for infusions and for cardiac output measurements. Right atrial and pulmonary artery pressures (PAPs) are measured, and the pulmonary capillary wedge pressure (PCWP) serves as an approximation of the left atrial pressure. Normal hemodynamic parameters are shown in Table 230-2 and Table 270-2.

Cardiac output is determined by the thermodilution technique, and high-resolution thermistors can also be used to determine right ventricular end-diastolic volume to monitor

TABLE 270-2 Normal Hemodynamic Parameters

Parameter	Calculation	Normal Values
Cardiac output (CO)	SV × HR	4–8 L/min
Cardiac index (CI)	CO/BSA	2.6–4.2 (L/min)/m^2
Stroke volume (SV)	CO/HR	50–100 mL/beat
Systemic vascular resistance (SVR)	[(MAP – RAP)/CO] × 80	700–1600 dynes · s/cm^5
Pulmonary vascular resistance (PVR)	[(PAP_m – PCWP)/CO] × 80	20–130 dynes · s/cm^5
Left ventricular stroke work (LVSW)	SV(MAP – PCWP) × 0.0136	60–80 g-m/beat
Right ventricular stroke work (RVSW)	SV(PAP_m – RAP)	10–15 g-m/beat

Abbreviations: BSA, body surface area; HR, heart rate; MAP, mean arterial pressure; PAP_m, pulmonary artery pressure—mean; PCWP, pulmonary capillary wedge pressure; RAP, right atrial pressure.

further the response of the right heart to fluid resuscitation. A PAC with an oximeter port offers the additional advantage of on-line monitoring of the mixed venous oxygen saturation, an important index of overall tissue perfusion. Systemic and pulmonary vascular resistances are calculated as the ratio of the pressure drop across these vascular beds to the cardiac output (Chap. 230). Determinations of oxygen content in arterial and venous blood, together with cardiac output and hemoglobin concentration, allow calculation of oxygen delivery, oxygen consumption, and oxygen-extraction ratio (Table 270-3). The hemodynamic patterns associated with the various forms of shock are shown in Table 270-4.

In resuscitation from shock, it is critical to restore tissue perfusion and optimize oxygen delivery, hemodynamics, and cardiac function rapidly. A reasonable goal of therapy is to achieve a normal mixed venous oxygen-saturation and arterio-venous oxygen-extraction ratio. To enhance oxygen delivery, red cell mass, arterial oxygen saturation, and cardiac output may be augmented singly or simultaneously. An increase in oxygen delivery not accompanied by an increase in oxygen consumption implies that oxygen availability is adequate and that oxygen consumption is not flow dependent. Conversely, an elevation of oxygen consumption with increased delivery implies that the oxygen supply was inadequate. However, cautious interpretation is required due to the link among increased oxygen delivery, cardiac work, and oxygen consumption. A reduction in systemic vascular resistance accompanying an increase in cardiac output indicates that compensatory vasoconstriction is reversing due to improved tissue perfusion. The determination of stepwise expansion of blood volume on cardiac performance allows identification of the optimum preload (Starling's law). An algorithm for the resuscitation of the patient in shock is shown in Fig. 270-3.

TABLE 270-3 Oxygen Transport Calculations

Parameter	Calculation	Normal Values
Oxygen-carrying capacity of hemoglobin		1.39 mL/g
Plasma O_2 concentration		$P_{O_2} \times 0.0031$
Arterial O_2 concentration (Ca_{O_2})	$1.39\ Sa_{O_2} + 0.0031\ Pa_{O_2}$	20 vol%
Venous O_2 concentration (Cv_{O_2})	$1.39\ Sv_{O_2} + 0.0031\ Pv_{O_2}$	15.5 vol%
Arteriovenous O_2 difference ($Ca_{O_2} - Cv_{O_2}$)	$1.39\ (Sa_{O_2} - Sv_{O_2}) +$ $0.0031\ (Pa_{O_2} - Pv_{O_2})$	3.5 vol%
Oxygen delivery (D_{O_2})	$Ca_{O_2} \times$ CO (L/min) $\times$ 10 (dL/L) $1.39\ Sa_{O_2} \times CO \times 10$	800–1600 mL/min
Oxygen uptake (V_{O_2})	$(Ca_{O_2} - Cv_{O_2}) \times CO \times 10$ $1.39\ (Sa_{O_2} - Sv_{O_2}) \times CO \times 10$	150–400 mL/min
Oxygen delivery index ($D_{O_2}I$)	D_{O_2}/BSA	520–720 (mL/min)/m^2
Oxygen uptake index ($V_{O_2}I$)	V_{O_2}/BSA	115–165 (mL/min)/m^2
Oxygen extraction ratio (O_2ER)	$[1 - (V_{O_2}/D_{O_2})] \times 100$	22–32%

Abbreviations: BSA, body surface area; CO, cardiac output; P_{O_2}, partial pressure of oxygen; Pa_{O_2}, partial pressure of O_2 in arterial blood; Pv_{O_2}, partial pressure of O_2 in venous blood; Sa_{O_2}, saturation of hemoglobin with O_2 in arterial blood; Sv_{O_2}, saturation of hemoglobin with O_2 in venous blood.

TABLE 270-4 Physiologic Characteristics of the Various Forms of Shock

Type of Shock	CVP and PCWP	Cardiac Output	Systemic Vascular Resistance	Venous O_2 Saturation
Hypovolemic	↓	↓	↑	↓
Cardiogenic	↑	↓	↑	↓
Septic				
Hyperdynamic	↓↑	↑	↓	↑
Hypodynamic	↓↑	↓	↑	↑↓
Traumatic	↓	↓↑	↑↓	↓
Neurogenic	↓	↓	↓	↓
Hypoadrenal	↓↑	↓	=↓	↓

Abbreviations: CVP, central venous pressure; PCWP, pulmonary capillary wedge pressure.

SPECIFIC FORMS OF SHOCK

HYPOVOLEMIC SHOCK

This most common form of shock results either from the loss of red blood cell mass and plasma from hemorrhage or from the loss of plasma volume alone due to extravascular fluid sequestration or GI, urinary, and insensible losses. The signs and symptoms of nonhemorrhagic hypovolemic shock are the same as those of hemorrhagic shock, although they may have a more insidious onset. The normal physiologic response to hypovolemia is to maintain perfusion of the brain and heart while attempting to restore an effective circulating blood volume. There is an increase in sympathetic activity, hyperventilation, collapse of venous capacitance vessels, release of stress hormones, and an attempt to replace the loss of intravascular volume through the recruitment of interstitial and intracellular fluid and by reduction of urine output.

Mild hypovolemia (≤20% of the blood volume) generates mild tachycardia but relatively few external signs, especially in a supine young patient (Table 270-5). With moderate hypovolemia (~20–40% of the blood volume), the patient becomes increasingly anxious and tachycardic; although normal blood pressure may be maintained in the supine position, there may be significant postural hypotension and tachycardia. If hypovolemia is severe (≥40% of the blood volume), the classic signs of shock appear; the blood pressure declines and becomes unstable even in the supine position, and the patient develops marked tachycardia, oliguria, and agitation or confusion. Perfusion of the central nervous system is well maintained until shock becomes severe. Hence, mental obtundation is an ominous clinical sign. The transition from mild to severe hypovolemic shock can be insidious or extremely rapid. If severe shock is not reversed rapidly, especially in elderly patients and those with comorbid illnesses, death is imminent. A very narrow time frame separates the derangements found in severe shock that can be reversed with aggressive resuscitation from those of progressive decompensation and irreversible cell injury.

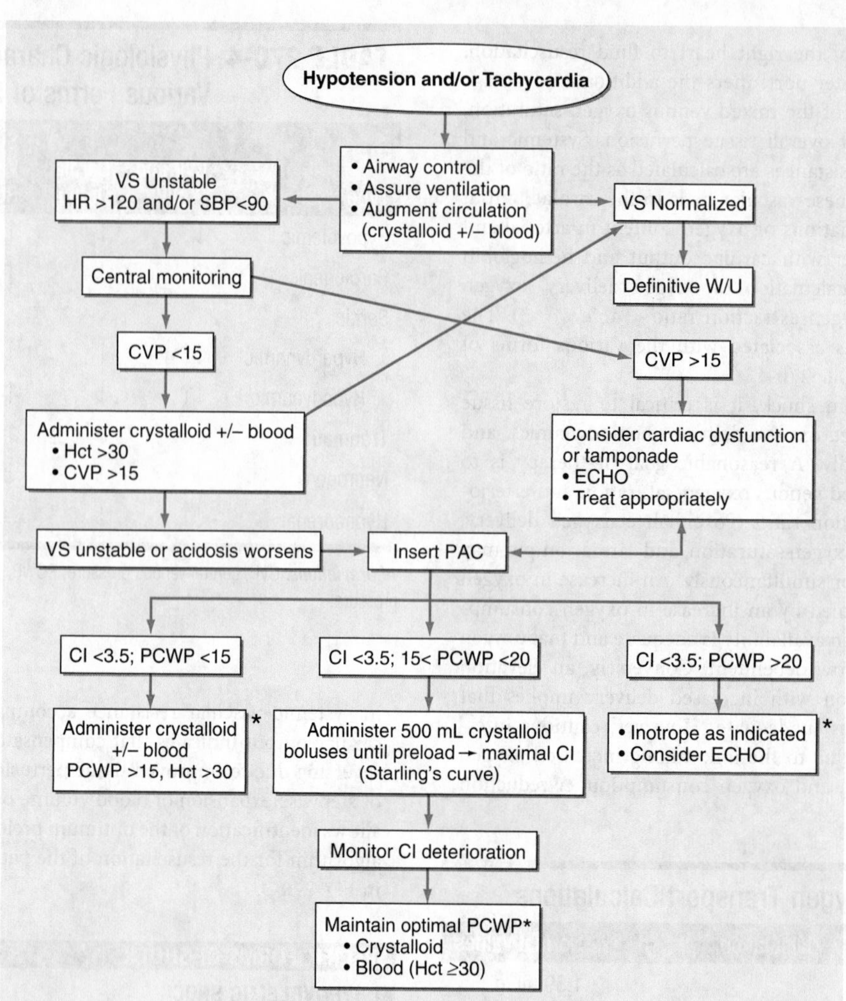

Figure 270-3 An algorithm for the resuscitation of the patient in shock. *Monitor SV_{O_2}, SVRI, and RVEDVI as additional markers of correction for perfusion and hypovolemia. Consider age-adjusted CI. SV_{O_2}, saturation of hemoglobin with O_2 in venous blood; SVRI, systemic vascular resistance index; RVEDVI, right-ventricular end-diastolic volume index. CI, cardiac index in (L/min) per m^2; CVP, central venous pressure; ECHO, echocardiogram; Hct, hematocrit; HR, heart rate; PAC, pulmonary artery catheter; PCWP, pulmonary capillary wedge pressure in mmHg; SBP, systolic blood pressure; VS, vital signs; W/U, work up.

Diagnosis

Hypovolemic shock is readily diagnosed when there are signs of hemodynamic instability and the source of volume loss is obvious. The diagnosis is more difficult when the source of blood loss is occult, as into the GI tract, or when plasma volume alone is depleted. Even after acute hemorrhage, hemoglobin and hematocrit values do not change until compensatory fluid shifts have occurred or exogenous fluid is administered. Thus, an initial normal hematocrit does not disprove the presence of significant blood loss. Plasma losses cause hemoconcentration, and free water loss leads to hypernatremia. These findings should suggest the presence of hypovolemia.

It is essential to distinguish between hypovolemic and cardiogenic shock (Chap. 272) because, while both may respond to volume initially, definitive therapy differs significantly. Both forms are associated with a reduced cardiac output and a compensatory sympathetic mediated response characterized by tachycardia and elevated systemic vascular resistance. However, the findings in cardiogenic shock of jugular venous distention, rales, and an S_3 gallop distinguish it from hypovolemic shock and signify that ongoing volume expansion is undesirable and may cause further organ dysfunction.

TABLE 270-5 Hypovolemic Shock

Mild (<20% Blood Volume)	Moderate (20–40% Blood Volume)	Severe (>40% Blood Volume)
Cool extremities	Same, plus:	Same, plus:
Increased capillary refill time	Tachycardia	Hemodynamic instability
Diaphoresis	Tachypnea	Marked tachycardia
Collapsed veins	Oliguria	Hypotension
Anxiety	Postural changes	Mental status deterioration (coma)

TREATMENT Hypovolemic Shock

Initial resuscitation requires rapid reexpansion of the circulating intravascular blood volume along with interventions to control ongoing losses. In accordance with Starling's law (Chap. 224), stroke volume and cardiac output rise with the increase in preload. After resuscitation, the compliance of the ventricles may remain reduced due to increased interstitial fluid in the myocardium. Therefore, elevated filling pressures are frequently required to maintain adequate ventricular performance.

Volume resuscitation is initiated with the rapid infusion of either isotonic saline (although care must be taken to avoid hyperchloremic acidosis from loss of bicarbonate buffering capacity and replacement with excess chloride) or a balanced salt solution such as Ringer's lactate (being cognizant of the presence of potassium and potential renal dysfunction) through large-bore intravenous lines. Data, particularly on severe traumatic brain injury (TBI), regarding benefits of small volumes of hypertonic saline that more rapidly restore blood pressure are variable, but tend to show improved survival thought to be linked to immunomodulation. No distinct benefit from the use of colloid has been demonstrated, and in trauma patients it is associated with a higher mortality, particularly in patients with TBI. The infusion of 2–3 L of salt solution over 20–30 min should restore normal hemodynamic parameters. Continued hemodynamic instability implies that shock has not been reversed and/or there are significant ongoing blood or other volume losses. Continuing acute blood loss, with hemoglobin concentrations declining to ≤100 g/L (10 g/dL), should initiate blood transfusion, preferably as fully cross-matched recently banked (<14 days old) blood. Resuscitated patients are often coagulopathic due to deficient clotting factors in crystalloids and banked packed red blood cells (PRBCs). Early administration of component therapy during massive transfusion [fresh-frozen plasma (FFP) and platelets] approaching a 1:1 ratio of PRBC/FFP appears to improve survival. In extreme emergencies, type-specific or O-negative packed red cells may be transfused. Following severe and/or prolonged hypovolemia, inotropic support with norepinephrine, vasopressin, or dopamine may be required to maintain adequate ventricular performance *but only after* blood volume has been restored. Increases in peripheral vasoconstriction with inadequate resuscitation leads to tissue loss and organ failure. Once hemorrhage is controlled and the patient has stabilized, blood transfusions should not be continued unless the hemoglobin is <~7g/dL. Studies have demonstrated an increased survival in patients treated with this restrictive blood transfusion protocol.

Successful resuscitation also requires support of respiratory function. Supplemental oxygen should always be provided, and endotracheal intubation may be necessary to maintain arterial oxygenation. Following resuscitation from isolated hemorrhagic shock, end-organ damage is frequently less than following septic or traumatic shock. This may be due to the absence of massive activation of the inflammatory innate immune response and consequent nonspecific organ injury and failure.

TRAUMATIC SHOCK

Shock following trauma is, in large measure, due to hemorrhage. However, even when hemorrhage has been controlled, patients can continue to suffer loss of plasma volume into the interstitium of injured tissues. These fluid losses are compounded by injury-induced inflammatory responses that which contribute to the secondary microcirculatory injury. Proinflammatory mediators are induced by DAMPs released from injured tissue and are recognized by the highly conserved membrane receptors of the TLR family (see "Inflammatory Responses" above). These receptors on cells of the innate immune system, particularly the circulating monocyte, tissue-fixed macrophage, and dendritic cell, are potent activators of an excessive proinflammatory phenotype in response to cellular injury. This causes secondary tissue injury and maldistribution of blood flow, intensifying tissue ischemia and leading to multiple organ system failure. In addition, direct structural injury to the heart, chest, or head can also contribute to shock. For example, pericardial tamponade or tension pneumothorax impairs ventricular filling, while myocardial contusion depresses myocardial contractility.

TREATMENT Traumatic Shock

Inability of the patient to maintain a systolic blood pressure ≥90 mmHg after trauma-induced hypovolemia is associated with a mortality rate up to ~50%. To prevent this decompensation of homeostatic mechanisms, therapy must be promptly administered.

The initial management of the seriously injured patient requires attention to the "ABCs" of resuscitation: assurance of an *airway* (A), adequate ventilation (*breathing*, B), and establishment of an adequate blood volume to support the *circulation* (C). Control of ongoing hemorrhage requires immediate attention. Early stabilization of fractures, debridement of devitalized or contaminated tissues, and evacuation of hematomata all reduce the subsequent inflammatory response to the initial insult and minimize damaged-tissue release of DAMPs and subsequent diffuse organ injury. Supplementation of depleted endogenous antioxidants also reduces subsequent organ failure and mortality.

CARDIOGENIC SHOCK

See Chap. 272.

COMPRESSIVE CARDIOGENIC SHOCK

With extrinsic compression, the heart and surrounding structures are less compliant, and therefore normal filling pressures generate inadequate diastolic filling and stroke volume. Blood or fluid within the poorly distensible pericardial sac may cause tamponade (Chap. 239). Any cause of increased intrathoracic pressure such as tension pneumothorax, herniation of abdominal viscera through a diaphragmatic hernia, or excessive positive-pressure ventilation to support pulmonary function, can also cause compressive cardiogenic shock while simultaneously impeding venous return and preload. Although initially responsive to increased filling pressures produced by volume expansion, as compression increases, cardiogenic shock recurs. The window of opportunity gained by volume loading may be very brief until irreversible shock recurs. Diagnosis and intervention must occur urgently.

The diagnosis of compressive cardiogenic shock is most frequently based on clinical findings, the chest radiograph, and an echocardiogram. The diagnosis of compressive cardiac shock may be more difficult to establish in the setting of trauma when hypovolemia and cardiac compression are present simultaneously. The classic findings of pericardial tamponade include the triad of hypotension, neck vein distention, and muffled heart sounds (Chap. 239). Pulsus paradoxus (i.e., an inspiratory reduction in systolic pressure >10 mmHg), may also be noted. The diagnosis is confirmed by echocardiography, and treatment consists of immediate pericardiocentesis or open subxiphoid pericardial window. A tension pneumothorax produces ipsilateral decreased breath sounds, tracheal deviation away from the affected thorax, and jugular venous distention. Radiographic findings include increased intrathoracic volume, depression of the diaphragm of the affected hemithorax, and shifting of the mediastinum to the contralateral side. Chest decompression must be carried out immediately, and, ideally, should occur based on clinical findings rather than awaiting a chest radiograph. Release of air and restoration of normal cardiovascular dynamics are both diagnostic and therapeutic.

SEPTIC SHOCK

See Chap. 271.

NEUROGENIC SHOCK

Interruption of sympathetic vasomotor input after a high cervical spinal cord injury, inadvertent cephalad migration of spinal anesthesia, or devastating head injury may result in neurogenic shock. In addition to arteriolar dilation, venodilation causes pooling in the venous system, which decreases venous return and cardiac output. The extremities are often warm, in contrast to the usual sympathetic vasoconstriction-induced coolness in hypovolemic or cardiogenic shock. Treatment involves a simultaneous approach to the relative hypovolemia and to the loss of vasomotor tone. Excessive volumes of fluid may be required to restore normal hemodynamics if given alone. Once hemorrhage has been ruled out, norepinephrine or a pure α-adrenergic agent (phenylephrine) may be necessary to augment vascular resistance and maintain an adequate mean arterial pressure.

HYPOADRENAL SHOCK

(See also Chap. 342) The normal host response to the stress of illness, operation, or trauma requires that the adrenal glands hypersecrete cortisol in excess of that normally required. Hypoadrenal shock occurs in settings in which unrecognized adrenal insufficiency complicates the host response to the stress induced by acute illness or major surgery. Adrenocortical insufficiency may occur as a consequence of the chronic administration of high doses of exogenous glucocorticoids. In addition, recent studies have shown that critical illness, including trauma and sepsis, may also induce a relative hypoadrenal state. Other, less common causes include adrenal insufficiency secondary to idiopathic atrophy, use of etomidate for intubation, tuberculosis, metastatic disease, bilateral hemorrhage, and amyloidosis. The shock produced by adrenal insufficiency is characterized by loss of homeostasis with reductions in systemic vascular resistance, hypovolemia, and reduced cardiac output. The diagnosis of adrenal insufficiency may be established by means of an ACTH stimulation test but is inconsistent.

TREATMENT Hypoadrenal Shock

In the persistently hemodynamically unstable patient, dexamethasone sodium phosphate, 4 mg, should be given intravenously. This agent is preferred if empiric therapy is required because, unlike hydrocortisone, it does not interfere with the ACTH stimulation test. If the diagnosis of absolute or relative adrenal insufficiency is established as shown by nonresponse to corticotropin stimulation (cortisol ≤9 μg/dL change poststimulation), the patient has a reduced risk of death if treated with hydrocortisone, 100 mg every 6–8 h, and tapered as the patient achieves hemodynamic stability. Simultaneous volume resuscitation and pressor support are required. The need for simultaneous mineralocoid is unclear.

ADJUNCTIVE THERAPIES

The sympathomimetic amines dobutamine, dopamine, and norepinephrine are widely used in the treatment of all forms of shock. Dobutamine is inotropic with simultaneous afterload reduction, thus minimizing cardiac-oxygen consumption increases as cardiac output increases. Dopamine is an inotropic and chronotropic agent that also supports vascular resistance in those whose blood pressure will not tolerate peripheral vascular dilation. Norepinephrine primarily supports blood pressure through vasoconstriction and increases myocardial oxygen consumption while placing marginally perfused tissues such as extremities and splanchnic organs, at risk for ischemia or necrosis, but it is also inotropic without chronotropy. Arginine-vasopressin (antidiuretic hormone) is being used increasingly to increase afterload and may better protect vital organ blood flow and prevent pathologic vasodilation.

REWARMING

Hypothermia is a frequent adverse consequence of massive volume resuscitation (Chap. 19). The infusion of large volumes of refrigerated blood products and room temperature crystalloid solutions can rapidly drop core temperatures if fluid is not run through warming devices. Hypothermia may depress cardiac contractility and thereby further impair cardiac output and oxygen delivery/utilization. Hypothermia, particularly temperatures <35°C (<95°F), directly impairs the coagulation pathway, sometimes causing a significant coagulopathy. Rapid rewarming to >35°C (>95°F) significantly decreases the requirement for blood products and produces an improvement in cardiac function. The most effective method for rewarming is endovascular countercurrent warmers through femoral vein cannulation. This process does not require a pump and can rewarm from 30° to 35°C (86° to 95°F) in 30–60 minutes.

FURTHER READINGS

ARDS Clinical Trials Network: Pulmonary-artery versus central venous catheter to guide treatment of acute lung injury. N Engl J Med 354:2213, 2006

Egi M et al: Selecting a vasopressor drug for vasoplegic shock after adult cardiac surgery: A systematic literature review. Ann Thor Surg 83:715, 2007

Englehart MS et al: Measurement of acid-base resuscitation endpoints: Lactate, base deficit, bicarbonate or what? Curr Opin Crit Care 12:569, 2006

Gonzales EA et al: Fresh frozen plasma should be given earlier to patients receiving massive transfusion. J Trauma 62:112, 2007

Hebert PC et al: Clinical consequence of anemia and red cell transfusion in the critically ill. Crit Care Clin 20:225, 2004

Jones AE et al: Goal-directed hemodynamic optimization in the post-cardiac arrest syndrome: A systematic review. Resuscitation 77:26, 2008

Matsuda N et al: Systemic inflammatory response syndrome (SIRS): Molecular pathophysiology and gene therapy. J Pharmacol Sci 101:189, 2006

Rivers EP et al: The influence of early hemodynamic optimization on biomarker patterns of severe sepsis and septic shock. Crit Care Med 35:2016, 2007

The Safe Study Investigators: Saline or albumin for fluid resuscitation in patients with traumatic brain injury. N Engl J Med 537:874, 2007

Sprung CL et al: Hydrocortisone therapy for patients with septic shock. N Engl J Med 358:111, 2008

CHAPTER 271

Severe Sepsis and Septic Shock

Robert S. Munford

DEFINITIONS

(See Table 271-1) Animals mount both local and systemic responses to microbes that traverse their epithelial barriers and enter underlying tissues. Fever or hypothermia, leukocytosis or leukopenia, tachypnea, and tachycardia are the cardinal signs of the systemic response, that is often called the *systemic inflammatory response syndrome* (SIRS). SIRS may have an infectious or a noninfectious etiology. If infection is suspected or proven, a patient with SIRS is said to have *sepsis*. When sepsis is associated with dysfunction of organs distant from the site of infection, the patient has *severe sepsis*. Severe sepsis may be accompanied by hypotension or evidence of hypoperfusion. When hypotension cannot be corrected by infusing fluids, the diagnosis is *septic shock*. These definitions were developed by consensus conference committees in 1992 and 2001 and have been widely used; there is evidence that the different stages may form a continuum.

ETIOLOGY

Sepsis can be a response to any class of microorganism. Microbial invasion of the bloodstream is not essential, since local inflammation can also elicit distant organ dysfunction and hypotension. In fact, blood cultures yield bacteria or fungi in only ~20–40% of cases of severe sepsis and 40–70% of cases of septic shock. Individual gram-negative or gram-positive bacteria account for ~70% of these isolates; the remainder are fungi or a mixture of microorganisms (Table 271-2). In patients whose blood cultures are negative, the etiologic agent is often established by culture or microscopic examination of infected material from a local site; specific identification of microbial DNA or RNA in blood or tissue samples is also used. In some case series, a majority of patients with a clinical picture of severe sepsis or septic shock have had negative microbiologic data.

EPIDEMIOLOGY

Severe sepsis is a contributing factor in >200,000 deaths per year in the United States. The incidence of severe sepsis and septic shock

TABLE 271-1 Definitions Used to Describe the Condition of Septic Patients

Bacteremia	Presence of bacteria in blood, as evidenced by positive blood cultures
Septicemia	Presence of microbes or their toxins in blood
Systemic inflammatory response syndrome (SIRS)	Two or more of the following conditions: (1) fever (oral temperature >38°C) or hypothermia (<36°C); (2) tachypnea (>24 breaths/min); (3) tachycardia (heart rate >90 beats/min); (4) leukocytosis (>12,000/μL), leukopenia (<4,000/μL), or >10% bands; may have a noninfectious etiology
Sepsis	SIRS that has a proven or suspected microbial etiology
Severe sepsis (similar to "sepsis syndrome")	Sepsis with one or more signs of organ dysfunction—for example: 1. *Cardiovascular:* Arterial systolic blood pressure ≤90 mmHg or mean arterial pressure ≤70 mmHg that responds to administration of intravenous fluid 2. *Renal:* Urine output <0.5 mL/kg per hour for 1 h despite adequate fluid resuscitation 3. *Respiratory:* Pa_{O_2}/FI_{O_2} ≤250 or, if the lung is the only dysfunctional organ, ≤200 4. *Hematologic:* Platelet count <80,000/μL or 50% decrease in platelet count from highest value recorded over previous 3 days 5. *Unexplained metabolic acidosis:* A pH ≤7.30 or a base deficit ≥5.0 mEq/L and a plasma lactate level >1.5 times upper limit of normal for reporting lab 6. *Adequate fluid resuscitation:* Pulmonary artery wedge pressure ≥12 mmHg or central venous pressure ≥8 mmHg
Septic shock	Sepsis with hypotension (arterial blood pressure <90 mmHg systolic, or 40 mmHg less than patient's normal blood pressure) for at least 1 h despite adequate fluid resuscitation; *or* Need for vasopressors to maintain systolic blood pressure ≥90 mmHg *or* mean arterial pressure ≥70 mmHg
Refractory septic shock	Septic shock that lasts for >1 h and does not respond to fluid or pressor administration
Multiple-organ dysfunction syndrome (MODS)	Dysfunction of more than one organ, requiring intervention to maintain homeostasis
Predisposition–infection–response–organ dysfunction (PIRO)	A grading system that stratifies patients according to four key aspects of illness; attempts to define subgroups of patients, reducing heterogeneity in clinical trials
Critical illness– related corticosteroid insufficiency (CIRCI)	Inadequate corticosteroid activity for the patient's severity of illness; should be suspected when hypotension is not relieved by fluid administration

Source: Adapted from the American College of Chest Physicians/Society of Critical Care Medicine Consensus Conference Committee.

TABLE 271-2 Microorganisms Involved in Episodes of Severe Sepsis at Eight Academic Medical Centers

Microorganisms	Episodes with Bloodstream Infection, % (*n* = 436)	Episodes with Documented Infection but No Bloodstream Infection, % (*n* = 430)	Total Episodes, % (*n* = 866)
Gram-negative bacteria[a]	35	44	40
Gram-positive bacteria[b]	40	24	31
Fungi	7	5	6
Polymicrobial	11	21	16
Classic pathogens[c]	<5	<5	<5

[a]Enterobacteriaceae, pseudomonads, *Haemophilus* spp., other gram-negative bacteria.
[b]*Staphylococcus aureus*, coagulase-negative staphylococci, enterococci, *Streptococcus pneumoniae*, other streptococci, other gram-positive bacteria.
[c]Such as *Neisseria meningitidis*, *S. pneumoniae*, *Haemophilus influenzae*, and *Streptococcus pyogenes*.
Source: Adapted from Sands et al., 1997.

has increased over the past 30 years, and the annual number of cases is now >700,000 (~3 per 1000 population). Approximately two-thirds of the cases occur in patients with significant underlying illness. Sepsis-related incidence and mortality rates increase with age and preexisting comorbidity. The rising incidence of severe sepsis in the United States is attributable to the aging of the population, the increasing longevity of patients with chronic diseases, and the relatively high frequency with which sepsis develops in patients with AIDS. The widespread use of immunosuppressive drugs, indwelling catheters, and mechanical devices also plays a role.

Invasive bacterial infections are prominent causes of death around the world, particularly among young children. In sub-Saharan Africa, for example, careful screening for positive blood cultures found that community-acquired bacteremia accounted for at least one-fourth of deaths of children >1 year of age. Nontyphoidal *Salmonella* species, *Streptococcus pneumoniae*, *Haemophilus influenzae*, and *Escherichia coli* were the most commonly isolated bacteria. Bacteremic children often had HIV infection or were severely malnourished.

PATHOPHYSIOLOGY

Most cases of severe sepsis are triggered by bacteria or fungi that do not ordinarily cause systemic disease in immunocompetent hosts (Table 271-2). To survive within the human body, these microbes often exploit deficiencies in host defenses, indwelling catheters or other foreign matter, or obstructed fluid drainage conduits. Microbial pathogens, in contrast, can circumvent innate defenses because they (1) lack molecules that can be recognized by host receptors (see below) or (2) elaborate toxins or other virulence factors. In both cases, the body can mount a vigorous inflammatory reaction that results in severe sepsis yet fails to kill the invaders. The septic response may also be induced by microbial exotoxins that act as superantigens (e.g., toxic shock syndrome toxin 1; Chap. 135) as well as by many pathogenic viruses.

Host mechanisms for sensing microbes

Animals have exquisitely sensitive mechanisms for recognizing and responding to certain highly conserved microbial molecules. Recognition of the lipid A moiety of lipopolysaccharide (LPS, also called *endotoxin*; Chap. 120) is the best-studied example. A host protein (LPS-binding protein) binds lipid A and transfers the LPS to CD14 on the surfaces of monocytes, macrophages, and neutrophils. LPS then is passed to MD-2, that is bound to toll-like receptor (TLR) 4 to form a molecular complex that transduces the LPS recognition signal to the interior of the cell. This signal rapidly triggers the production and release of mediators, such as tumor necrosis factor (TNF; see below), that amplify the LPS signal and transmit it to other cells and tissues. Bacterial peptidoglycan and lipopeptides elicit responses in animals that are generally similar to those induced by LPS; whereas these molecules also may be transferred by CD14, they interact with different TLRs. Having numerous TLR-based receptor complexes (11 different TLRs have been identified so far in humans) allows animals to recognize many conserved microbial molecules; others include lipopeptides (TLR2/1, TLR2/6), flagellin (TLR5), undermethylated DNA sequences (TLR9), and double-stranded RNA (TLR3, TLR7). The ability of some TLRs to serve as receptors for host ligands (e.g., hyaluronans, heparan sulfate, saturated fatty acids) raises the possibility that they also play a role in producing noninfectious sepsis-like states. Other host pattern-recognition proteins that are important for sensing microbial invasion include the intracellular NOD1 and NOD2 proteins, which recognize discrete fragments of bacterial peptidoglycan; early complement components (principally in the alternative pathway); and mannose-binding lectin and C-reactive protein, which activate the classic complement pathway.

A host's ability to recognize certain microbial molecules may influence both the potency of its own defenses and the pathogenesis of severe sepsis. For example, MD-2–TLR4 best senses LPS that has a hexaacyl lipid A moiety (i.e., one with six fatty acyl chains). Most of the commensal aerobic and facultatively anaerobic gram-negative bacteria that trigger severe sepsis and shock (including *E. coli*, *Klebsiella*, and *Enterobacter*) make this lipid A structure. When they invade human hosts, often through breaks in an epithelial barrier, they are typically confined to the subepithelial tissue by a localized inflammatory response. Bacteremia, if it occurs, is intermittent and low-grade, as these bacteria are efficiently cleared from the bloodstream by TLR4-expressing Kupffer cells and splenic macrophages. These mucosal commensals seem to induce severe sepsis most often by triggering severe local tissue inflammation rather than by circulating within the bloodstream. One exception is *Neisseria meningitidis*. Its hexaacyl LPS seems to be shielded from host recognition by its polysaccharide capsule. This protection may allow meningococci to transit undetected from the nasopharyngeal mucosa into the bloodstream, where they can infect vascular endothelial cells and release large amounts of endotoxin. Host recognition of lipid A may nonetheless influence pathogenesis, as meningococci that produce pentaacyl LPS were isolated from the blood of patients with less severe coagulopathy than was found in patients whose isolates produced hexaacyl lipid A. In contrast, gram-negative bacteria that make lipid A with fewer than six acyl chains (*Yersinia pestis*, *Francisella tularensis*, *Vibrio vulnificus*, *Pseudomonas aeruginosa*, and *Burkholderia pseudomallei*, among others) are poorly recognized by MD-2–TLR4. When these bacteria enter the body, they may initially induce relatively little inflammation. When they do trigger severe sepsis, it is often after they have multiplied to high density in tissues and blood. The importance of LPS recognition in disease pathogenesis has been shown by engineering a virulent strain of *Y. pestis*, which makes tetraacyl LPS at 37°C, to produce hexaacyl LPS; unlike its virulent parent, the mutant strain stimulates local inflammation and is rapidly cleared from tissues. For at least one large class of microbes—gram-negative aerobic bacteria—the pathogenesis of sepsis thus depends, at least in part, upon whether the bacterium's major signal molecule, LPS, can be sensed by the host.

Local and systemic host responses to invading microbes

Recognition of microbial molecules by tissue phagocytes triggers the production and/or release of numerous host molecules (cytokines, chemokines, prostanoids, leukotrienes, and others) that increase blood flow to the infected tissue, enhance the permeability of local blood vessels, recruit neutrophils to the site of infection, and elicit pain. These reactions are familiar elements of local inflammation, the body's frontline innate immune mechanism for eliminating microbial invaders. Systemic responses are activated by neural and/or humoral communication with the hypothalamus and brainstem; these responses enhance local defenses by increasing blood flow to the infected area, augmenting the number of circulating neutrophils, and elevating blood levels of numerous molecules (such as the microbial recognition proteins discussed above) that have anti-infective functions.

Cytokines and other mediators Cytokines can exert endocrine, paracrine, and autocrine effects (Chap. 314). TNF-α stimulates leukocytes and vascular endothelial cells to release other cytokines (as well as additional TNF-α), to express cell-surface molecules that enhance neutrophil-endothelial adhesion at sites of infection, and to increase prostaglandin and leukotriene production. Whereas blood levels of TNF-α are not elevated in individuals with localized infections, they increase in most patients with severe sepsis or septic shock. Moreover, IV infusion of TNF-α can elicit the characteristic abnormalities of SIRS. In animals, larger doses of TNF-α induce shock and death.

Although TNF-α is a central mediator, it is only one of many proinflammatory molecules that contribute to innate host defense. Chemokines, most prominently interleukin (IL)-8 and IL-17, attract circulating neutrophils to the infection site. IL-1β exhibits many of the same activities as TNF-α. TNF-α, IL-1β, interferon (IFN) γ, IL-12, IL-17, and other proinflammatory cytokines probably interact synergistically with one another and with additional mediators. The nonlinearity and multiplicity of these interactions have made it difficult to interpret the roles played by individual mediators in both tissues and blood.

Coagulation factors Intravascular thrombosis, a hallmark of the local inflammatory response, may help wall off invading microbes and prevent infection and inflammation from spreading to other tissues. IL-6 and other mediators promote intravascular coagulation initially by inducing blood monocytes and vascular endothelial cells to express tissue factor (Chap. 58). When tissue factor is expressed on cell surfaces, it binds to factor VIIa to form an active complex that can convert factors X and IX to their enzymatically active forms. The result is activation of both extrinsic and intrinsic clotting pathways, culminating in the generation of fibrin. Clotting is also favored by impaired function of the protein C–protein S inhibitory pathway and depletion of antithrombin and proteins C and S, while fibrinolysis is prevented by increased plasma levels of plasminogen activator inhibitor 1. Thus, there may be a striking propensity toward intravascular fibrin deposition, thrombosis, and bleeding; this propensity has been most apparent in patients with intravascular endothelial infections such as meningococcemia (Chap. 143). Evidence points to tissue factor–expressing microparticles derived from leukocytes as a potential trigger for intravascular coagulation. Contact-system activation occurs during sepsis but contributes more to the development of hypotension than to disseminated intravascular coagulation (DIC).

Control mechanisms Elaborate control mechanisms operate within both local sites of inflammation and the systemic compartment.

Local control mechanisms Host recognition of invading microbes within subepithelial tissues typically ignites immune responses that rapidly kill the invader and then subside to allow tissue recovery. The anti-inflammatory forces that put out the fire and clean up the battleground include molecules that neutralize or inactivate microbial signals. Among these molecules are intracellular factors (e.g., suppressor of cytokine signaling 3 and IL-1 receptor–associated kinase 3) that diminish the production of proinflammatory mediators by neutrophils and macrophages; anti-inflammatory cytokines (IL-10, IL-4); and molecules derived from essential polyunsaturated fatty acids (lipoxins, resolvins, and protectins) that promote tissue restoration. Enzymatic inactivation of microbial signal molecules (e.g., LPS) may be required to restore homeostasis; a leukocyte enzyme, acyloxyacyl hydrolase, has been shown to prevent prolonged inflammation by inactivating LPS in mice.

Systemic control mechanisms The signaling apparatus that links microbial recognition to cellular responses in tissues is less active in the blood. For example, whereas LPS-binding protein plays a role in recognizing the presence of LPS, in plasma it also prevents LPS signaling by transferring LPS molecules into plasma lipoprotein particles that sequester the lipid A moiety so that it cannot interact with cells. At the high concentrations found in blood, LPS-binding protein also inhibits monocyte responses to LPS, and the soluble (circulating) form of CD14 strips off LPS that has bound to monocyte surfaces.

Systemic responses to infection also diminish cellular responses to microbial molecules. Circulating levels of anti-inflammatory cytokines (e.g., IL-10) increase even in patients with mild infections. Glucocorticoids inhibit cytokine synthesis by monocytes in vitro; the increase in blood cortisol levels early in the systemic response presumably plays a similarly inhibitory role. Epinephrine inhibits the TNF-α response to endotoxin infusion in humans while augmenting and accelerating the release of IL-10; prostaglandin E_2 has a similar "reprogramming" effect on the responses of circulating monocytes to LPS and other bacterial agonists. Cortisol, epinephrine, IL-10, and C-reactive protein reduce the ability of neutrophils to attach to vascular endothelium, favoring their demargination and thus contributing to leukocytosis while preventing neutrophil-endothelial adhesion in uninflamed organs. The available evidence thus suggests that the body's systemic responses to injury and infection normally prevent inflammation within organs distant from a site of infection. There is also evidence that these responses may be immunosuppressive.

The acute-phase response increases the blood concentrations of numerous molecules that have anti-inflammatory actions. Blood levels of IL-1 receptor antagonist often greatly exceed those of circulating IL-1β, for example, and this excess may inhibit the binding of IL-1β to its receptors. High levels of soluble TNF receptors neutralize TNF-α that enters the circulation. Other acute-phase proteins are protease inhibitors or antioxidants; these may neutralize potentially harmful molecules released from neutrophils and other inflammatory cells. Increased hepatic production of hepcidin promotes the sequestration of iron in hepatocytes, intestinal epithelial cells, and erythrocytes; this effect reduces iron acquisition by invading microbes while contributing to the normocytic, normochromic anemia associated with inflammation.

It can thus be concluded that both local and systemic responses to infectious agents benefit the host in important ways. Most of these responses and the molecules responsible for them have been highly conserved during animal evolution and therefore may be adaptive. Elucidating how they contribute to lethality—i.e., become maladaptive—remains a major challenge for sepsis research.

Organ dysfunction and shock

As the body's responses to infection intensify, the mixture of circulating cytokines and other molecules becomes very complex: elevated blood levels of more than 50 molecules have been found in patients with septic shock. Although high concentrations of both pro- and anti-inflammatory molecules are found, the net mediator balance in the plasma of these extremely sick patients seems to be anti-inflammatory. For example, blood leukocytes from patients with severe sepsis are often hyporesponsive to agonists such as LPS. In patients with severe sepsis, persistence of leukocyte hyporesponsiveness has been associated with an increased risk of dying. Apoptotic death of B cells, follicular dendritic cells, and CD4+ T lymphocytes also may contribute significantly to the immunosuppressive state.

Endothelial injury Many investigators have favored widespread vascular endothelial injury as the major mechanism for multiorgan dysfunction. In keeping with this idea, one study found high numbers of vascular endothelial cells in the peripheral blood of septic patients. Leukocyte-derived mediators and platelet-leukocyte-fibrin thrombi may contribute to vascular injury, but the vascular endothelium also seems to play an active role. Stimuli such as TNF-α induce vascular endothelial cells to produce and release cytokines, procoagulant molecules, platelet-activating factor, nitric oxide, and other mediators. In addition, regulated cell-adhesion molecules promote the adherence of neutrophils to endothelial cells. While these responses can attract phagocytes to infected sites and activate their antimicrobial arsenals, endothelial cell activation can also promote increased vascular permeability, microvascular thrombosis, DIC, and hypotension.

Tissue oxygenation may decrease as the number of functional capillaries is reduced by luminal obstruction due to swollen endothelial cells, decreased deformability of circulating erythrocytes, leukocyte-platelet-fibrin thrombi, or compression by edema fluid. On the other hand, studies using orthogonal polarization spectral imaging of the microcirculation in the tongue found that sepsis-associated derangements in capillary flow could be reversed by applying acetylcholine to the surface of the tongue or by giving nitroprusside intravenously; these observations suggest a neuroendocrine basis for the loss of capillary filling. Oxygen utilization by tissues may also be impaired by a state of "hibernation" in which ATP production is diminished as oxidative phosphorylation decreases; nitric oxide may be responsible for inducing this response.

Remarkably, poorly functioning "septic" organs usually appear normal at autopsy. There is typically very little necrosis or thrombosis, and apoptosis is largely confined to lymphoid organs and the gastrointestinal tract. Moreover, organ function usually returns to normal if patients recover. These points suggest that organ dysfunction during severe sepsis has a basis that is principally biochemical, not structural.

Septic shock The hallmark of septic shock is a decrease in peripheral vascular resistance that occurs despite increased levels of vasopressor catecholamines. Before this vasodilatory phase, many patients experience a period during which oxygen delivery to tissues is compromised by myocardial depression, hypovolemia, and other factors. During this "hypodynamic" period, the blood lactate concentration is elevated and central venous oxygen saturation is low. Fluid administration is usually followed by the hyperdynamic, vasodilatory phase during which cardiac output is normal (or even high) and oxygen consumption declines despite adequate oxygen delivery. The blood lactate level may be normal or increased, and normalization of central venous oxygen saturation may reflect either improved oxygen delivery or left-to-right shunting.

Prominent hypotensive molecules include nitric oxide, β-endorphin, bradykinin, platelet-activating factor, and prostacyclin. Agents that inhibit the synthesis or action of each of these mediators can prevent or reverse endotoxic shock in animals. However, in clinical trials, neither a platelet-activating factor receptor antagonist nor a bradykinin antagonist improved survival rates among patients with septic shock, and a nitric oxide synthase inhibitor, L-N^G-methylarginine HCl, actually increased the mortality rate. Remarkably, recent findings indicate that exogenous nitrite can protect mice from challenge with TNF or LPS. Nitrite provides a storage pool from which nitric oxide can be generated in hypoxic and/or acidic conditions. These findings should renew interest in the possibility of exploiting nitric oxide metabolism to improve survival rates among septic patients.

Severe sepsis: A single pathogenesis?

In some cases, circulating bacteria and their products almost certainly elicit multiorgan dysfunction and hypotension by directly stimulating inflammatory responses within the vasculature. In patients with fulminant meningococcemia, for example, mortality rates have correlated directly with blood levels of endotoxin and bacterial DNA and with the occurrence of DIC (Chap. 143). In most patients infected with other gram-negative bacteria, in contrast, circulating bacteria or bacterial molecules may reflect uncontrolled infection at a local tissue site and have little or no direct impact on distant organs; in these patients, inflammatory mediators or neural signals arising from the local site seem to be the key triggers for severe sepsis and septic shock. In a large series of patients with positive blood cultures, the risk of developing severe sepsis was strongly related to the site of primary infection: bacteremia arising from a pulmonary or abdominal source was eightfold more likely to be associated with severe sepsis than was bacteremic urinary tract infection, even after the investigators controlled for age, the kind of bacteria isolated from the blood, and other factors. A third pathogenesis may be represented by severe sepsis due to superantigen-producing *Staphylococcus aureus* or *Streptococcus pyogenes*; the T cell activation induced by these toxins produces a cytokine profile that differs substantially from that elicited by gram-negative bacterial infection. Further evidence for different pathogenetic pathways has come from observations that the pattern of mRNA expression in peripheral-blood leukocytes from children with sepsis is different for gram-positive, gram-negative, and viral pathogens.

The pathogenesis of severe sepsis thus may differ according to the infecting microbe, the ability of the host's innate defense mechanisms to sense it, the site of the primary infection, the presence or absence of immune defects, and the prior physiologic status of the host. Genetic factors are probably important as well, yet despite much study only a few allelic polymorphisms (e.g., in the IL-1β gene) have been associated with sepsis severity in more than one or two analyses. Further studies in this area are needed.

CLINICAL MANIFESTATIONS

The manifestations of the septic response are superimposed on the symptoms and signs of the patient's underlying illness and primary infection. The rate at which severe sepsis develops may differ from patient to patient, and there are striking individual variations in presentation. For example, some patients with sepsis are normo- or hypothermic; the absence of fever is most common in neonates, in elderly patients, and in persons with uremia or alcoholism.

Hyperventilation is often an early sign of the septic response. Disorientation, confusion, and other manifestations of encephalopathy may also develop early on, particularly in the elderly and in individuals with preexisting neurologic impairment. Focal neurologic signs are uncommon, although preexisting focal deficits may become more prominent.

Hypotension and DIC predispose to acrocyanosis and ischemic necrosis of peripheral tissues, most commonly the digits. Cellulitis, pustules, bullae, or hemorrhagic lesions may develop when hematogenous bacteria or fungi seed the skin or underlying soft tissue. Bacterial toxins may also be distributed hematogenously and elicit diffuse cutaneous reactions. On occasion, skin lesions may suggest specific pathogens. When sepsis is accompanied by cutaneous petechiae or purpura, infection with *N. meningitidis* (or, less commonly, *H. influenzae*) should be suspected (Fig. e7-42); in a patient who has been bitten by a tick while in an endemic area, petechial lesions also suggest Rocky Mountain spotted fever (Fig. 174-1). A cutaneous lesion seen almost exclusively in neutropenic patients is ecthyma gangrenosum, usually caused by *P. aeruginosa*. It is a bullous lesion, surrounded by edema, that undergoes central hemorrhage and necrosis (Fig. 152-1). Histopathologic examination shows bacteria in and around the wall of a small vessel, with little or no neutrophilic response. Hemorrhagic or bullous lesions in a septic patient who has recently eaten raw oysters suggest *V. vulnificus* bacteremia, while such lesions in a patient who has recently suffered a dog bite may indicate bloodstream infection due to *Capnocytophaga canimorsus* or *C. cynodegmi*. Generalized erythroderma in a septic patient suggests the toxic shock syndrome due to *S. aureus* or *S. pyogenes*.

Gastrointestinal manifestations such as nausea, vomiting, diarrhea, and ileus may suggest acute gastroenteritis. Stress ulceration can lead to upper gastrointestinal bleeding. Cholestatic jaundice, with elevated levels of serum bilirubin (mostly conjugated) and alkaline phosphatase, may precede other signs of sepsis. Hepatocellular or canalicular dysfunction appears to underlie most cases, and the results of hepatic function tests return to normal with resolution of the infection. Prolonged or severe hypotension may induce acute hepatic injury or ischemic bowel necrosis.

Many tissues may be unable to extract oxygen normally from the blood, so that anaerobic metabolism occurs despite near-normal mixed venous oxygen saturation. Blood lactate levels rise early because of increased glycolysis as well as impaired clearance of the resulting lactate and pyruvate by the liver and kidneys. The blood glucose concentration often increases, particularly in patients with diabetes, although impaired gluconeogenesis and excessive insulin release on occasion produce hypoglycemia. The cytokine-driven acute-phase response inhibits the synthesis of transthyretin while enhancing the production of C-reactive protein, fibrinogen, and complement components. Protein catabolism is often markedly accelerated. Serum albumin levels decline as a result of decreased hepatic synthesis and the movement of albumin into interstitial spaces.

■ MAJOR COMPLICATIONS

Cardiopulmonary complications

Ventilation-perfusion mismatching produces a fall in arterial P_{O2} early in the course. Increasing alveolar epithelial injury and capillary permeability result in increased pulmonary water content, which decreases pulmonary compliance and interferes with oxygen exchange. In the absence of pneumonia or heart failure, progressive diffuse pulmonary infiltrates and arterial hypoxemia (Pa_{O2}/FI_{O2}, <300) indicate the development of acute lung injury; more severe hypoxemia (Pa_{O2}/FI_{O2}, <200) denotes the acute respiratory distress syndrome (ARDS). Acute lung injury or ARDS develops in ~50% of patients with severe sepsis or septic shock. Respiratory muscle fatigue can exacerbate hypoxemia and hypercapnia. An elevated pulmonary capillary wedge pressure (>18 mmHg) suggests fluid volume overload or cardiac failure rather than ARDS. Pneumonia caused by viruses or by *Pneumocystis* may be clinically indistinguishable from ARDS.

Sepsis-induced hypotension (see "Septic Shock," above) usually results initially from a generalized maldistribution of blood flow and blood volume and from hypovolemia that is due, at least in part, to diffuse capillary leakage of intravascular fluid. Other factors that may decrease effective intravascular volume include dehydration from antecedent disease or insensible fluid losses, vomiting or diarrhea, and polyuria. During early septic shock, systemic vascular resistance is usually elevated and cardiac output may be low. After fluid repletion, in contrast, cardiac output typically increases and systemic vascular resistance falls. Indeed, normal or increased cardiac output and decreased systemic vascular resistance distinguish septic shock from cardiogenic, extracardiac obstructive, and hypovolemic shock; other processes that can produce this combination include anaphylaxis, beriberi, cirrhosis, and overdoses of nitroprusside or narcotics.

Depression of myocardial function, manifested as increased end-diastolic and systolic ventricular volumes with a decreased ejection fraction, develops within 24 h in most patients with severe sepsis. Cardiac output is maintained despite the low ejection fraction because ventricular dilatation permits a normal stroke volume. In survivors, myocardial function returns to normal over several days. Although myocardial dysfunction may contribute to hypotension, refractory hypotension is usually due to low systemic vascular resistance, and death results from refractory shock or the failure of multiple organs rather than from cardiac dysfunction per se.

Adrenal insufficiency

The diagnosis of adrenal insufficiency may be very difficult in critically ill patients. Whereas a plasma cortisol level of ≤15 μg/mL (≤10 μg/mL if the serum albumin concentration is <2.5 mg/dL) indicates adrenal insufficiency (inadequate production of cortisol), many experts now feel that the ACTH (CoSyntropin®) stimulation test is not useful for detecting less profound degrees of corticosteroid deficiency in patients who are critically ill. The concept of critical illness–related corticosteroid insufficiency (CIRCI; Table 271-1) was proposed to encompass the different mechanisms that may produce corticosteroid activity that is inadequate for the severity of a patient's illness. Although CIRCI may result from structural damage to the adrenal gland, it is more commonly due to reversible dysfunction of the hypothalamic-pituitary axis or to tissue corticosteroid resistance resulting from abnormalities of the glucocorticoid receptor or increased conversion of cortisol to cortisone. The major clinical manifestation of CIRCI is hypotension that is refractory to fluid replacement and requires pressor therapy. Some classic features of adrenal insufficiency, such as hyponatremia and hyperkalemia, are usually absent; others, such as eosinophilia and modest hypoglycemia, may sometimes be found. Specific etiologies include fulminant *N. meningitidis* bacteremia, disseminated tuberculosis, AIDS (with cytomegalovirus, *Mycobacterium avium-intracellulare*, or *Histoplasma capsulatum* disease), or the prior use of drugs that diminish glucocorticoid production, such as glucocorticoids, megestrol, etomidate, or ketoconazole.

Renal complications

Oliguria, azotemia, proteinuria, and nonspecific urinary casts are frequently found. Many patients are inappropriately polyuric; hyperglycemia may exacerbate this tendency. Most renal failure is due to acute tubular necrosis induced by hypotension or capillary injury, although some patients also have glomerulonephritis, renal cortical necrosis, or interstitial nephritis. Drug-induced renal damage may complicate therapy, particularly when hypotensive patients are given aminoglycoside antibiotics.

Coagulopathy

Although thrombocytopenia occurs in 10–30% of patients, the underlying mechanisms are not understood. Platelet counts are usually very low (<50,000/μL) in patients with DIC; these low counts may reflect diffuse endothelial injury or microvascular thrombosis, yet thrombi have only infrequently been found upon biopsy of septic organs.

Neurologic complications

When the septic illness lasts for weeks or months, "critical illness" polyneuropathy may prevent weaning from ventilatory support and produce distal motor weakness. Electrophysiologic studies are diagnostic. Guillain-Barré syndrome, metabolic disturbances, and toxin activity must be ruled out.

■ IMMUNOSUPPRESSION

Patients with severe sepsis are often profoundly immunosuppressed. Manifestations include loss of delayed-type hypersensitivity reactions to common antigens, failure to control the primary infection, and increased risk for secondary infections (e.g., by opportunists such as *Stenotrophomonas maltophilia, Acinetobacter calcoaceticus-baumannii*, and *Candida albicans*). Approximately one-third of patients experience reactivation of herpes simplex virus, varicella-zoster virus, or cytomegalovirus infections; the latter are thought to contribute to adverse outcomes in some instances.

■ LABORATORY FINDINGS

Abnormalities that occur early in the septic response may include leukocytosis with a left shift, thrombocytopenia, hyperbilirubinemia, and proteinuria. Leukopenia may develop. The neutrophils may contain toxic granulations, Döhle bodies, or cytoplasmic vacuoles. As the septic response becomes more severe, thrombocytopenia worsens (often with prolongation of the thrombin time, decreased fibrinogen, and the presence of D-dimers, suggesting DIC), azotemia and hyperbilirubinemia become more prominent, and levels of aminotransferases rise. Active hemolysis suggests clostridial bacteremia, malaria, a drug reaction, or DIC; in the case of DIC, microangiopathic changes may be seen on a blood smear.

During early sepsis, hyperventilation induces respiratory alkalosis. With respiratory muscle fatigue and the accumulation of lactate, metabolic acidosis (with increased anion gap) typically supervenes. Evaluation of arterial blood gases reveals hypoxemia that is initially correctable with supplemental oxygen but whose later refractoriness to 100% oxygen inhalation indicates right-to-left shunting. The chest radiograph may be normal or may show evidence of underlying pneumonia, volume overload, or the diffuse infiltrates of ARDS. The electrocardiogram may show only sinus tachycardia or nonspecific ST–T-wave abnormalities.

Most diabetic patients with sepsis develop hyperglycemia. Severe infection may precipitate diabetic ketoacidosis that may exacerbate hypotension (Chap. 344). Hypoglycemia occurs rarely. The serum albumin level declines as sepsis continues. Hypocalcemia is rare.

■ DIAGNOSIS

There is no specific diagnostic test for the septic response. Diagnostically sensitive findings in a patient with suspected or proven infection include fever or hypothermia, tachypnea, tachycardia, and leukocytosis or leukopenia (Table 271-1); acutely altered mental status, thrombocytopenia, an elevated blood lactate level, or hypotension also should suggest the diagnosis. The septic response can be quite variable, however. In one study, 36% of patients with severe sepsis had a normal temperature, 40% had a normal respiratory rate, 10% had a normal pulse rate, and 33% had normal white blood cell counts. Moreover, the systemic responses of uninfected patients with other conditions may be similar to those characteristic of sepsis. Noninfectious etiologies of SIRS (Table 271-1) include pancreatitis, burns, trauma, adrenal insufficiency, pulmonary embolism, dissecting or ruptured aortic aneurysm, myocardial infarction, occult hemorrhage, cardiac tamponade, postcardiopulmonary bypass syndrome, anaphylaxis, tumor-associated lactic acidosis, and drug overdose.

Definitive etiologic diagnosis requires isolation of the microorganism from blood or a local site of infection. At least two blood samples should be obtained (from two different venipuncture sites) for culture; in a patient with an indwelling catheter, one sample should be collected from each lumen of the catheter and another via venipuncture. In many cases, blood cultures are negative; this result can reflect prior antibiotic administration, the presence of slow-growing or fastidious organisms, or the absence of microbial invasion of the bloodstream. In these cases, Gram's staining and culture of material from the primary site of infection or from infected cutaneous lesions may help establish the microbial etiology. Identification of microbial DNA in peripheral-blood or tissue samples by polymerase chain reaction may also be definitive. The skin and mucosae should be examined carefully and repeatedly for lesions that might yield diagnostic information. With overwhelming bacteremia (e.g., pneumococcal sepsis in splenectomized individuals; fulminant meningococcemia; or infection with *V. vulnificus, B. pseudomallei*, or *Y. pestis*), microorganisms are sometimes visible on buffy coat smears of peripheral blood.

TREATMENT Severe Sepsis and Septic Shock

Patients in whom sepsis is suspected must be managed expeditiously. This task is best accomplished by personnel who are experienced in the care of the critically ill. Successful management requires urgent measures to treat the infection, to provide hemodynamic and respiratory support, and to eliminate the offending microorganisms. These measures should be initiated within 1 h of the patient's presentation with severe sepsis or septic shock. Rapid assessment and diagnosis are therefore essential.

ANTIMICROBIAL AGENTS Antimicrobial chemotherapy should be started as soon as samples of blood and other relevant sites have been obtained for culture. A large retrospective review of patients who developed septic shock found that the interval between the onset of hypotension and the administration of appropriate antimicrobial chemotherapy was the major determinant of outcome; a delay of as little as 1 h was associated with lower survival rates. Use of inappropriate antibiotics, defined on the basis of local microbial susceptibilities and published guidelines for empirical therapy (see below), was associated with fivefold lower survival rates, even among patients with negative cultures.

It is therefore very important to promptly initiate empirical antimicrobial therapy that is effective against both gram-positive and gram-negative bacteria (Table 271-3). Maximal recommended doses of antimicrobial drugs should be given intravenously, with adjustment for impaired renal function when necessary. Available information about patterns of antimicrobial susceptibility among bacterial isolates from the community, the hospital, and the patient should be taken into account. When culture results become available, the regimen can often be simplified, as a single antimicrobial agent is usually adequate for the treatment of a known pathogen. Meta-analyses have concluded that, with one exception, combination antimicrobial therapy is not superior to monotherapy for treating gram-negative bacteremia; the exception is that aminoglycoside monotherapy for *P. aeruginosa* bacteremia is less effective than the combination of an aminoglycoside with an antipseudomonal β-lactam agent. Empirical antifungal therapy should be strongly

TABLE 271-3 Initial Antimicrobial Therapy for Severe Sepsis With No Obvious Source in Adults With Normal Renal Function

Clinical Condition	Antimicrobial Regimens (Intravenous Therapy)
Immunocompetent adult	The many acceptable regimens include (1) piperacillin-tazobactam (3.375 g q4–6h); (2) imipenem-cilastatin (0.5 g q6h) or meropenem (1 g q8h); or (3) cefepime (2 g q12h). If the patient is allergic to β-lactam agents, use ciprofloxacin (400 mg q12h) or levofloxacin (500–750 mg q12h) plus clindamycin (600 mg q8h). Vancomycin (15 mg/kg q12h) should be added to each of the above regimens.
Neutropenia (<500 neutrophils/μL)	Regimens include (1) imipenem-cilastatin (0.5 g q6h) or meropenem (1 g q8h) or cefepime (2 g q8h); (2) piperacillin-tazobactam (3.375 g q4h) plus tobramycin (5–7 mg/kg q24h). Vancomycin (15 mg/kg q12h) should be added if the patient has an indwelling vascular catheter, has received quinolone prophylaxis, or has received intensive chemotherapy that produces mucosal damage; if staphylococci are suspected; if the institution has a high incidence of MRSA infections; or if there is a high prevalence of MRSA isolates in the community. Empirical antifungal therapy with an echinocandin (for caspofungin: a 70-mg loading dose, then 50 mg daily) or a lipid formulation of amphotericin B should be added if the patient is hypotensive or has been receiving broad-spectrum antibacterial drugs.
Splenectomy	Cefotaxime (2 g q6–8h) or ceftriaxone (2 g q12h) should be used. If the local prevalence of cephalosporin-resistant pneumococci is high, add vancomycin. If the patient is allergic to β-lactam drugs, vancomycin (15 mg/kg q12h) plus either moxifloxacin (400 mg q24h) or levofloxacin (750 mg q24h) or aztreonam (2 g q8h) should be used.
IV drug user	Vancomycin (15 mg/kg q12h)
AIDS	Cefepime (2 g q8h) or piperacillin-tazobactam (3.375 g q4h) plus tobramycin (5–7 mg/kg q24h) should be used. If the patient is allergic to β-lactam drugs, ciprofloxacin (400 mg q12h) or levofloxacin (750 mg q12h) plus vancomycin (15 mg/kg q12h) plus tobramycin should be used.

Abbreviation: MRSA, methicillin-resistant *Staphylococcus aureus.*

Source: Adapted in part from WT Hughes et al: Clin Infect Dis 25:551, 1997; and DN Gilbert et al: The Sanford Guide to Antimicrobial Therapy, 2009.

considered if the septic patient is already receiving broad-spectrum antibiotics or parenteral nutrition, has been neutropenic for ≥5 days, has had a long-term central venous catheter, or has been hospitalized in an intensive care unit for a prolonged period. The chosen antimicrobial regimen should be reconsidered daily in order to provide maximal efficacy with minimal resistance, toxicity, and cost.

Most patients require antimicrobial therapy for at least 1 week. The duration of treatment is typically influenced by factors such as the site of tissue infection, the adequacy of surgical drainage, the patient's underlying disease, and the antimicrobial susceptibility of the microbial isolate(s). The absence of an identified microbial pathogen is not necessarily an indication for discontinuing antimicrobial therapy, since "appropriate" antimicrobial regimens seem to be beneficial in both culture-negative and culture-positive cases.

REMOVAL OF THE SOURCE OF INFECTION Removal or drainage of a focal source of infection is essential. In one series, a focus of ongoing infection was found in ~80% of surgical intensive care patients who died of severe sepsis or septic shock. Sites of occult infection should be sought carefully, particularly in the lungs, abdomen, and urinary tract. Indwelling IV or arterial catheters should be removed and the tip rolled over a blood agar plate for quantitative culture; after antibiotic therapy has been initiated, a new catheter should be inserted at a different site. Foley and drainage catheters should be replaced. The possibility of paranasal sinusitis (often caused by gram-negative bacteria) should be considered if the patient has undergone nasal intubation. Even in patients without abnormalities on chest radiographs, CT of the chest may identify unsuspected parenchymal, mediastinal, or pleural disease. In the neutropenic patient, cutaneous sites of tenderness and erythema, particularly in the perianal region, must be carefully sought. In patients with sacral or ischial decubitus ulcers, it is important to exclude pelvic or other soft tissue pus collections with CT or MRI. In patients with severe sepsis arising from the urinary tract, sonography or CT should be used to rule out ureteral obstruction, perinephric abscess, and renal abscess. Sonographic or CT imaging of the upper abdomen may disclose evidence of cholecystitis, bile duct dilatation, and pus collections in the liver, subphrenic space, or spleen.

HEMODYNAMIC, RESPIRATORY, AND METABOLIC SUPPORT The primary goals are to restore adequate oxygen and substrate delivery to the tissues as quickly as possible and to improve tissue oxygen utilization and cellular metabolism. Adequate organ perfusion is thus essential. Circulatory adequacy is assessed by measurement of arterial blood pressure and monitoring of parameters such as mentation, urine output, and skin perfusion. Indirect indices of oxygen delivery and consumption, such as central venous oxygen saturation, may also be useful. Initial management of hypotension should include the administration of IV fluids, typically beginning with 1–2 L of normal saline over 1–2 h. To avoid pulmonary edema, the central venous pressure should be maintained at 8–12 cmH_2O. The urine output rate should be kept at >0.5 mL/kg per hour by continuing fluid administration; a diuretic such as furosemide may be used if needed. In about one-third of patients, hypotension and organ hypoperfusion respond to fluid resuscitation; a reasonable goal is to maintain a mean arterial blood pressure of >65 mmHg (systolic pressure >90 mmHg). If these guidelines cannot be met by volume infusion, vasopressor therapy is indicated (Chap. 272). Titrated doses of norepinephrine or dopamine should be administered through a central catheter. If myocardial dysfunction produces elevated cardiac filling pressures and low cardiac output, inotropic therapy with dobutamine is recommended.

In patients with septic shock, plasma vasopressin levels increase transiently but then decrease dramatically. Early studies found that vasopressin infusion can reverse septic shock in some patients, reducing or eliminating the need for catecholamine pressors. More recently, a randomized clinical trial that compared vasopressin plus norepinephrine with norepinephrine alone in 776 patients with pressor-dependent septic shock found no difference between treatment groups in the primary study outcome, 28-day mortality. Although vasopressin may have benefited patients who required less norepinephrine, its role in the treatment of septic shock seems to be a minor one overall.

CIRCI should be strongly considered in patients who develop hypotension that does not respond to fluid replacement therapy. Hydrocortisone (50 mg IV every 6 h) should be given; if clinical improvement occurs over 24–48 h, most experts would continue hydrocortisone therapy for 5–7 days before slowly tapering and discontinuing it. Meta-analyses of recent clinical trials have concluded that hydrocortisone therapy hastens recovery from septic shock without increasing long-term survival.

Ventilator therapy is indicated for progressive hypoxemia, hypercapnia, neurologic deterioration, or respiratory muscle failure. Sustained tachypnea (respiratory rate, >30 breaths/min) is frequently a harbinger of impending respiratory collapse; mechanical ventilation is often initiated to ensure adequate oxygenation, to divert blood from the muscles of respiration, to prevent aspiration of oropharyngeal contents, and to reduce the cardiac afterload. The results of recent studies favor the use of low tidal volumes (6 mL/kg of ideal body weight, or as low as 4 mL/kg if the plateau pressure exceeds 30 cmH_2O). Patients undergoing mechanical ventilation require careful sedation, with daily interruptions; elevation of the head of the bed helps to prevent nosocomial pneumonia. Stress-ulcer prophylaxis with a histamine H_2-receptor antagonist may decrease the risk of gastrointestinal hemorrhage in ventilated patients.

Erythrocyte transfusion is generally recommended when the blood hemoglobin level decreases to ≤7 g/dL, with a target level of 9 g/dL in adults. Erythropoietin is not used to treat sepsis-related anemia. Bicarbonate is sometimes administered for severe metabolic acidosis (arterial pH <7.2), but there is little evidence that it improves either hemodynamics or the response to vasopressor hormones. DIC, if complicated by major bleeding, should be treated with transfusion of fresh-frozen plasma and platelets. Successful treatment of the underlying infection is essential to reverse both acidosis and DIC. Patients who are hypercatabolic and have acute renal failure may benefit greatly from intermittent hemodialysis or continuous veno-venous hemofiltration.

GENERAL SUPPORT In patients with prolonged severe sepsis (i.e., lasting more than 2 or 3 days), nutritional supplementation may reduce the impact of protein hypercatabolism; the available evidence, which is not strong, favors the enteral delivery route. Prophylactic heparinization to prevent deep venous thrombosis is indicated for patients who do not have active bleeding or coagulopathy; when heparin is contraindicated, compression stockings or an intermittent compression device should be used. Recovery is also assisted by prevention of skin breakdown, nosocomial infections, and stress ulcers.

The role of tight control of the blood glucose concentration in recovery from critical illness has been addressed in numerous controlled trials. Meta-analyses of these trials have concluded that use of insulin to lower blood glucose levels to 100–120 mg/dL is potentially harmful and does not improve survival rates. Most experts now recommend using insulin only if it is needed to maintain the blood glucose concentration below ~150 mg/dL. Patients receiving intravenous insulin must be monitored frequently (every 1–2 h) for hypoglycemia.

OTHER MEASURES Despite aggressive management, many patients with severe sepsis or septic shock die. Numerous interventions have been tested for their ability to improve survival rates among patients with severe sepsis. The list includes endotoxin-neutralizing proteins, inhibitors of cyclooxygenase or nitric oxide synthase, anticoagulants, polyclonal immunoglobulins, glucocorticoids, a phospholipid emulsion, and antagonists to TNF-α, IL-1, platelet-activating factor, and bradykinin. Unfortunately, none of these agents has improved rates of survival among patients with severe sepsis/septic shock in more than one large-scale, randomized, placebo-controlled clinical trial. Many factors have contributed to this lack of reproducibility, including (1) heterogeneity in the patient populations studied, the primary infection sites, the preexisting illnesses, and the inciting microbes; and (2) the nature of the "standard" therapy also used. A dramatic example of this problem was seen in a trial of tissue factor pathway inhibitor (Fig. 271-1). Whereas the drug appeared to improve survival rates after 722 patients had been studied ($p = .006$), it did not do so in the next 1032 patients, and the overall result was negative. This inconsistency argues that the results of a clinical trial may not apply to individual patients, even within a carefully selected patient population. It also suggests that, at a minimum, a sepsis intervention should show a significant survival benefit in more than one placebo-controlled, randomized clinical trial before it is accepted as routine clinical practice. In one prominent attempt to reduce patient heterogeneity in clinical trials, experts have called for changes that would restrict these trials to patients who have similar underlying diseases (e.g., major trauma) and inciting infections (e.g., pneumonia). The goal of the predisposition–infection–response–organ dysfunction (PIRO) grading system for classification of septic patients (Table 271-1) is similar. Other investigators have used

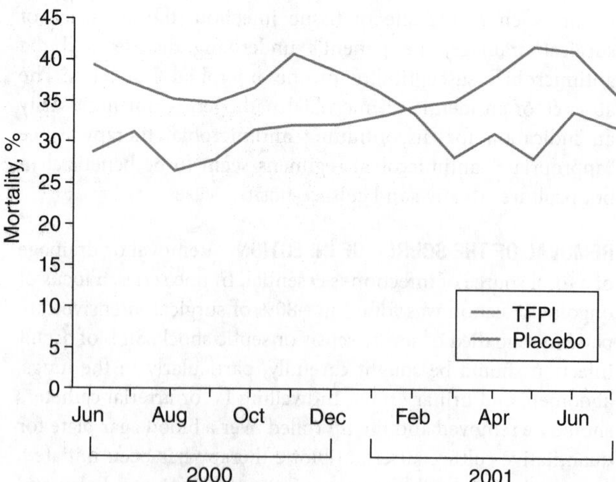

Figure 271-1 Mortality rates among patients who received tissue factor pathway inhibitor (TFPI) or placebo, shown as the running average over the course of the clinical trial. The drug seemed highly efficacious at the interim analysis in December 2000, but this trend reversed later in the trial. Demonstrating that therapeutic agents for sepsis have consistent, reproducible efficacy has been extremely difficult, even within well-defined patient populations. *(Reprinted with permission from Abraham et al.)*

specific biomarkers, such as IL-6 levels in blood or the expression of HLA-DR on peripheral-blood monocytes, to identify the patients most likely to benefit from certain interventions. Multivariate risk stratification based on easily measurable clinical variables should be used with each of these approaches.

Recombinant activated protein C (aPC) was the first drug to be approved by the U.S. Food and Drug Administration for the treatment of patients with severe sepsis or septic shock. Approval was based on the results of a single randomized controlled trial in which the drug was given within 24 h of the patient's first sepsis-related organ dysfunction; the 28-day survival rate was significantly higher among aPC recipients who were very sick (APACHE II score, ≥25) before infusion of the protein than among placebo-treated controls. Subsequent trials failed to show a benefit of aPC treatment in patients who were less sick (APACHE II score, <25) or in children. A second trial of aPC in high-risk patients is now under way in Europe. Given the drug's known toxicity (increased risk of severe bleeding) and uncertain performance in clinical practice, many experts are awaiting the results of the European trial before recommending further use of aPC. Other agents in ongoing or planned clinical trials include intravenous immunoglobulin, a small-molecule endotoxin antagonist (eritoran), and granulocyte-macrophage colony-stimulating factor that was recently reported to restore monocyte immunocompetence in patients with sepsis-associated immunosuppression.

A careful retrospective analysis found that the apparent efficacy of all sepsis therapeutics studied to date has been greatest among the patients at greatest risk of dying before treatment; conversely, use of many of these drugs has been associated with increased mortality rates among patients who are less ill. The authors proposed that neutralizing one of many different mediators may help patients who are very sick, whereas disrupting the mediator balance may be harmful to patients whose adaptive defense mechanisms are working well. This analysis suggests that if more aggressive early resuscitation improves survival rates among sicker patients, it will become more difficult to obtain additional benefit from other therapies; that is, if an intervention improves patients' risk status, moving them into a "less severe illness" category, it will be harder to show that adding another agent to the therapeutic regimen is beneficial.

THE SURVIVING SEPSIS CAMPAIGN An international consortium has advocated "bundling" multiple therapeutic maneuvers into a unified algorithmic approach that will become the standard of care for severe sepsis. In theory, such a strategy could improve care by mandating measures that seem to bring maximal benefit, such as the rapid administration of appropriate antimicrobial therapy; on the other hand, this approach would deemphasize physicians' experience and judgment and minimize the consideration of potentially important differences between patients. Bundling multiple therapies into a single package also obscures the efficacy and toxicity of the individual measures. Caution should be engendered by the fact that two of the key elements of the initial algorithm have now been withdrawn for lack of evidence, while a third remains unproven and controversial.

PROGNOSIS

Approximately 20–35% of patients with severe sepsis and 40–60% of patients with septic shock die within 30 days. Others die within the ensuing 6 months. Late deaths often result from poorly controlled infection, immunosuppression, complications of intensive care, failure of multiple organs, or the patient's underlying disease. Case-fatality rates are similar for culture-positive and culture-negative severe sepsis. Prognostic stratification systems such as APACHE II indicate that factoring in the patient's age, underlying condition, and various physiologic variables can yield estimates of the risk of dying of severe sepsis. Age and prior health status are probably the most important risk factors (Fig. 271-2). In patients with no known preexisting morbidity, the case-fatality rate remains below 10% until the fourth decade of life, after which it gradually increases to exceed 35% in the very elderly. Death is significantly more likely in severely septic patients with preexisting illness, especially during the third to fifth decades. Septic shock is also a strong predictor of short- and long-term mortality.

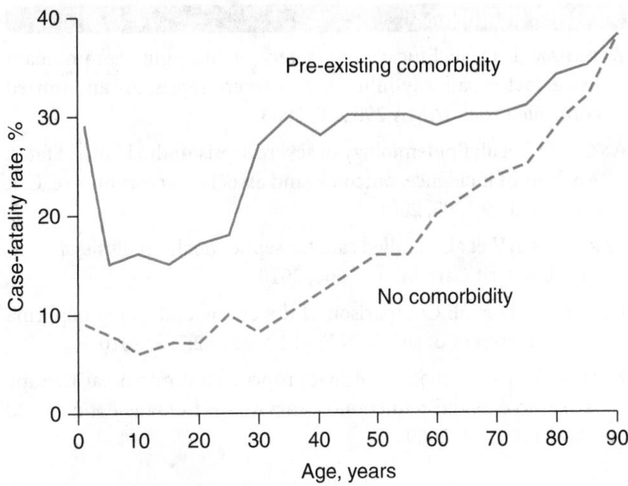

Figure 271-2 Influence of age and prior health status on outcome from severe sepsis. With modern therapy, fewer than 10% of previously healthy young individuals (below 35 years of age) die with severe sepsis; the case-fatality rate then increases slowly through middle and old age. The most commonly identified etiologic agents in patients who die are *Staphylococcus aureus, Streptococcus pyogenes, S. pneumoniae,* and *Neisseria meningitidis.* Individuals with preexisting comorbidities are at greater risk of dying of severe sepsis at any age. The etiologic agents in these cases are likely to be *S. aureus, Pseudomonas aeruginosa,* various Enterobacteriaceae, enterococci, or fungi. *(Adapted from Angus et al., 2001.)*

PREVENTION

Prevention offers the best opportunity to reduce morbidity and mortality from severe sepsis. In developed countries, most episodes of severe sepsis and septic shock are complications of nosocomial infections. These cases might be prevented by reducing the number of invasive procedures undertaken, by limiting the use (and duration of use) of indwelling vascular and bladder catheters, by reducing the incidence and duration of profound neutropenia (<500 neutrophils/μL), and by more aggressively treating localized nosocomial infections. Indiscriminate use of antimicrobial agents and glucocorticoids should be avoided, and optimal infection-control measures (Chap. 131) should be used. Studies indicate that 50–70% of patients who develop nosocomial severe sepsis or septic shock have experienced a less severe stage of the septic response (e.g., SIRS, sepsis) on at least one previous day in the hospital. Research is needed to identify patients at increased risk and to develop adjunctive agents that can modulate the septic response before organ dysfunction or hypotension occurs.

FURTHER READINGS

Abraham E et al: Efficacy and safety of tifacogin (recombinant tissue factor pathway inhibitor) in severe sepsis: A randomized controlled trial. JAMA 290:238, 2003

Angus DC et al: Epidemiology of severe sepsis in the United States: Analysis of incidence, outcome, and associated costs of care. Crit Care Med 29:1303, 2001

Barochia AV et al: Bundled care for septic shock: Analysis of clinical trials. Crit Care Med 38:668, 2010

DeBacker D et al: Comparison of dopamine and norepinephrine in the treatment of shock. N Engl J Med 362:779, 2010

Kumar A et al: Initiation of inappropriate antimicrobial therapy results in a 5-fold reduction of survival in human septic shock. Chest 136:1237, 2009

Marik PE: Critical illness-related corticosteroid insufficiency. Chest 135:181, 2009

Munford RS: Sensing gram-negative bacterial lipopolysaccharides: A human disease determinant? Infect Immun 76:454, 2008

Sands KE et al: Epidemiology of sepsis syndrome in 8 academic medical centers. JAMA 278:234, 1997

Toussaint S, Gerlach H: Activated protein C for sepsis. N Engl J Med 361:2646, 2009

Vincent J-L et al: Evolving concepts in sepsis definitions. Crit Care Clin 25:665, 2009

CHAPTER 272

Cardiogenic Shock and Pulmonary Edema

Judith S. Hochman

David H. Ingbar

Cardiogenic shock and pulmonary edema are life-threatening conditions that should be treated as medical emergencies. The most common etiology for both is severe left ventricular (LV) dysfunction that leads to pulmonary congestion and/or systemic hypoperfusion (Fig. 272-1). The pathophysiology of pulmonary edema and shock is discussed in Chaps. 33 and 270, respectively.

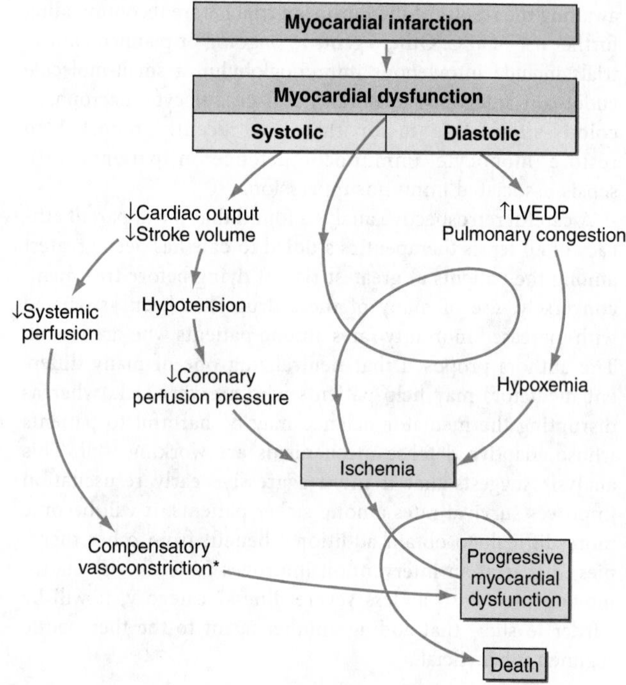

Figure 272-1 Pathophysiology of cardiogenic shock. Systolic and diastolic myocardial dysfunction results in a reduction in cardiac output and often pulmonary congestion. Systemic and coronary hypoperfusion occur, resulting in progressive ischemia. Although a number of compensatory mechanisms are activated in an attempt to support the circulation, these compensatory mechanisms may become maladaptive and produce a worsening of hemodynamics. *Release of inflammatory cytokines after myocardial infarction may lead to inducible nitric oxide expression, excess nitric oxide, and inappropriate vasodilation. This causes further reduction in systemic and coronary perfusion. A vicious spiral of progressive myocardial dysfunction occurs that ultimately results in death if it is not interrupted. LVEDP, left ventricular end-diastolic pressure. *(From SM Hollenberg et al: Ann Intern Med 131:47, 1999.)*

CARDIOGENIC SHOCK

Cardiogenic shock (CS) is characterized by systemic hypoperfusion due to severe depression of the cardiac index [<2.2 (L/min)/m^2] and sustained systolic arterial hypotension (<90 mmHg) despite an elevated filling pressure [pulmonary capillary wedge pressure (PCWP) >18 mmHg]. It is associated with in-hospital mortality rates >50%. The major causes of CS are listed in Table 272-1. Circulatory failure based on cardiac dysfunction may be caused by primary myocardial failure, most commonly secondary to acute myocardial infarction (MI) (Chap. 245), and less frequently by cardiomyopathy or myocarditis (Chap. 238), cardiac tamponade (Chap. 239), or critical valvular heart disease (Chap. 237).

Incidence

CS is the leading cause of death of patients hospitalized with MI. Early reperfusion therapy for acute MI decreases the incidence of CS. The rate of CS complicating acute MI was 20% in the 1960s, stayed at ~8% for >20 years, but decreased to 5–7% in the first decade of this millennium. Shock typically is associated with ST elevation MI (STEMI) and is less common with non-ST elevation MI (Chap. 245).

LV failure accounts for ~80% of cases of CS complicating acute MI. Acute severe mitral regurgitation (MR), ventricular septal rupture (VSR), predominant right ventricular (RV) failure, and free wall rupture or tamponade account for the remainder.

Pathophysiology

CS is characterized by a vicious circle in which depression of myocardial contractility, usually due to ischemia, results in reduced cardiac output and arterial pressure (BP), which result in hypoperfusion of the myocardium and further ischemia and depression of cardiac

TABLE 272-1 Etiologies of Cardiogenic Shock (CS)[a] and Cardiogenic Pulmonary Edema

Etiologies of Cardiogenic Shock or Pulmonary Edema
Acute myocardial infarction/ischemia
LV failure
VSR
Papillary muscle/chordal rupture—severe MR
Ventricular free wall rupture with subacute tamponade
Other conditions complicating large MIs
Hemorrhage
Infection
Excess negative inotropic or vasodilator medications
Prior valvular heart disease
Hyperglycemia/ketoacidosis
Post-cardiac arrest
Post-cardiotomy
Refractory sustained tachyarrhythmias
Acute fulminant myocarditis
End-stage cardiomyopathy
Left ventricular apical ballooning
Takotsubo's cardiomyopathy
Hypertrophic cardiomyopathy with severe outflow obstruction
Aortic dissection with aortic insufficiency or tamponade
Pulmonary embolus
Severe valvular heart disease
Critical aortic or mitral stenosis
Acute severe aortic or MR
Toxic-metabolic
Beta-blocker or calcium channel antagonist overdose
Other Etiologies of Cardiogenic Shock[b]
RV failure due to:
Acute myocardial infarction
Acute coronary pulmonale
Refractory sustained bradyarrhythmias
Pericardial tamponade
Toxic/metabolic
Severe acidosis, severe hypoxemia

[a]The etiologies of CS are listed. Most of these can cause pulmonary edema instead of shock or pulmonary edema with CS.
[b]These cause CS but not pulmonary edema.
Abbreviations: LV, left ventricular; VSR, ventricular septal rupture; MR, mitral regurgitation; MI, myocardial infarction; RV, right ventricular.

output (Fig. 272-1). Systolic myocardial dysfunction reduces stroke volume and, together with diastolic dysfunction, leads to elevated LV end-diastolic pressure and PCWP as well as to pulmonary congestion. Reduced coronary perfusion leads to worsening ischemia and progressive myocardial dysfunction and a rapid downward spiral, which, if uninterrupted, is often fatal. A systemic inflammatory response syndrome may accompany large infarctions and shock. Inflammatory cytokines, inducible nitric oxide synthase, and excess nitric oxide and peroxynitrite may contribute to the genesis of CS as they do to that of other forms of shock (Chap. 270). Lactic acidosis from poor tissue perfusion and hypoxemia from pulmonary edema may result from pump failure and then contribute to the vicious circle by worsening myocardial ischemia and hypotension. Severe acidosis (pH <7.25) reduces the efficacy of endogenous and exogenously administered catecholamines. Refractory sustained ventricular or atrial tachyarrhythmias can cause or exacerbate CS.

Patient profile

In patients with acute MI, older age, female sex, prior MI, diabetes, and anterior MI location are all associated with an increased risk of CS. Shock associated with a first inferior MI should prompt a search for a mechanical cause. Reinfarction soon after MI increases the risk of CS. Two-thirds of patients with CS have flow-limiting stenoses in all three major coronary arteries, and 20% have stenosis of the left main coronary artery. CS may rarely occur in the absence of significant stenosis, as seen in LV apical ballooning/Takotsubo's cardiomyopathy.

Timing

Shock is present on admission in only one-quarter of patients who develop CS complicating MI; one-quarter develop it rapidly thereafter, within 6 h of MI onset. Another quarter develop shock later on the first day. Subsequent onset of CS may be due to reinfarction, marked infarct expansion, or a mechanical complication.

Diagnosis

Due to the unstable condition of these patients, supportive therapy must be initiated simultaneously with diagnostic evaluation (Fig. 272-2). A focused history and physical examination should be performed, blood specimens sent to the laboratory, and an electrocardiogram (ECG) and chest x-ray obtained.

Echocardiography is an invaluable diagnostic tool in patients suspected of CS.

Clinical findings Most patients have continuing chest pain and dyspnea and appear pale, apprehensive, and diaphoretic. Mentation may be altered, with somnolence, confusion, and agitation. The pulse is typically weak and rapid, often in the range of 90–110 beats/min, or severe bradycardia due to high-grade heart block may be present. Systolic blood pressure is reduced (<90 mmHg) with a narrow pulse pressure (<30 mmHg), but occasionally BP may be maintained by very high systemic vascular resistance. Tachypnea, Cheyne-Stokes respirations, and jugular venous distention may be present. The precordium is typically quiet, with a weak apical pulse. S_1 is usually soft, and an S_3 gallop may be audible. Acute, severe MR and VSR usually are associated with characteristic systolic murmurs (Chap. 245). Rales are audible in most patients with LV failure causing CS. Oliguria (urine output <30 mL/h) is common.

Laboratory findings The white blood cell count is typically elevated with a left shift. In the absence of prior renal insufficiency, renal function is initially normal, but blood urea nitrogen and creatinine rise progressively. Hepatic transaminases may be markedly elevated due to liver hypoperfusion. Poor tissue perfusion may result in an anion-gap acidosis and elevation of the lactic acid level. Before support with supplemental O_2, arterial blood gases usually demonstrate hypoxemia and metabolic acidosis, which may be compensated by respiratory alkalosis. Cardiac markers, creatine phosphokinase and its MB fraction, and troponins I and T are markedly elevated.

Electrocardiogram In CS due to acute MI with LV failure, Q waves and/or >2-mm ST elevation in multiple leads or left bundle branch block are usually present. More than one-half of all infarcts associated with shock are anterior. Global ischemia due to severe left main

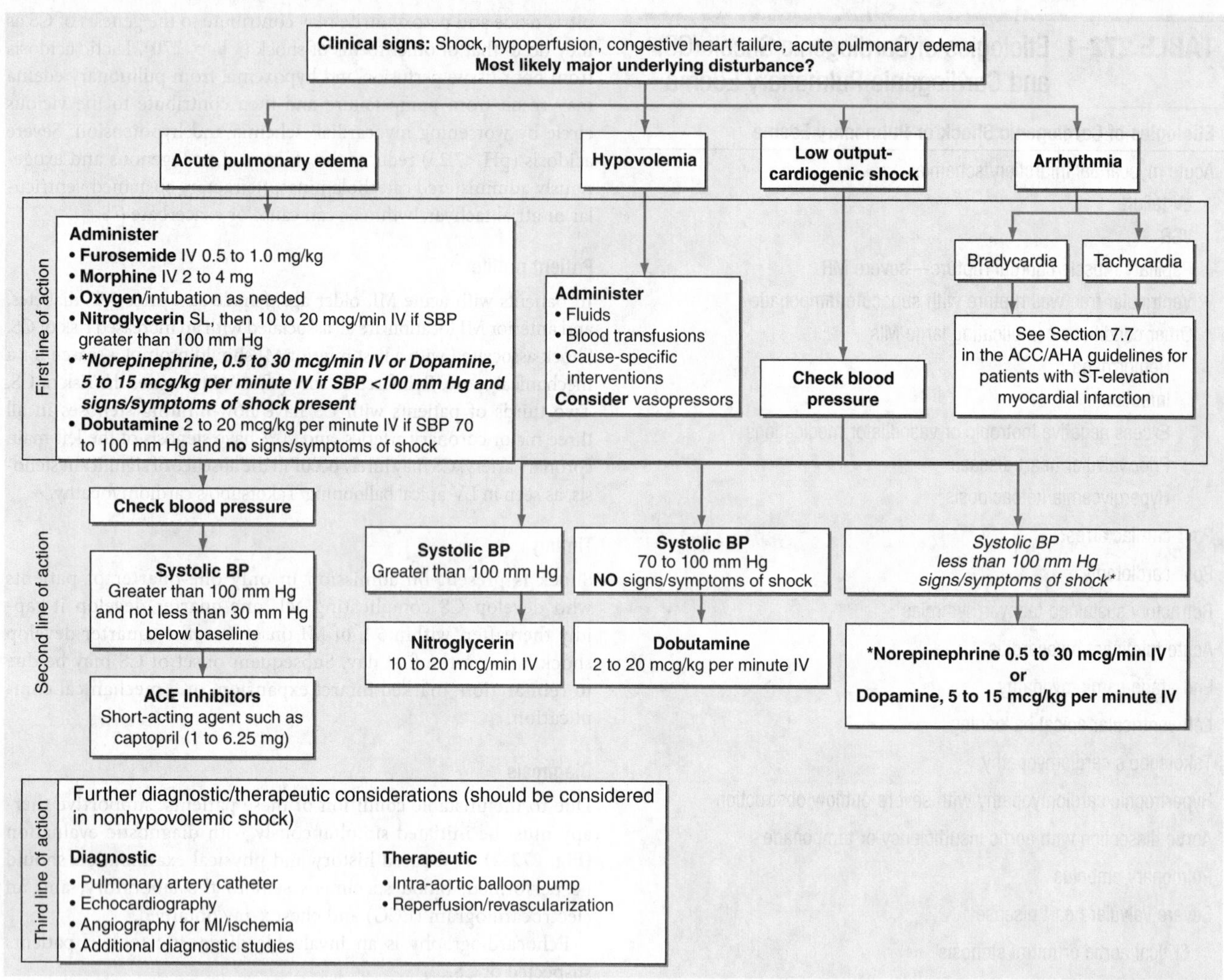

Figure 272-2 The emergency management of patients with cardiogenic shock, acute pulmonary edema, or both is outlined. *Furosemide: <0.5 mg/kg for new-onset acute pulmonary edema without hypervolemia; 1 mg/kg for acute on chronic volume overload, renal insufficiency. †For management of bradycardia and tachycardia, see Chaps. 232 and 233. *Indicates modification from published guidelines. ACE, angiotensin-converting enzyme; BP, blood pressure; MI, myocardial infarction. *(Modified from Guidelines 2000 for Cardiopulmonary Resuscitation and Emergency Cardiovascular Care. Part 7:The era of reperfusion: Section 1: Acute coronary syndromes (acute myocardial infarction). The American Heart Association in collaboration with the International Liaison Committee on Resuscitation. Circulation 102:I172, 2000.)*

stenosis usually is accompanied by severe (e.g., >3 mm) ST depressions in multiple leads.

Chest roentgenogram The chest x-ray typically shows pulmonary vascular congestion and often pulmonary edema, but these findings may be absent in up to a third of patients. The heart size is usually normal when CS results from a first MI but is enlarged when it occurs in a patient with a previous MI.

Echocardiogram A two-dimensional echocardiogram with color-flow Doppler (Chap. 229) should be obtained promptly in patients with suspected CS to help define its etiology. Doppler mapping demonstrates a left-to-right shunt in patients with VSR and the severity of MR when the latter is present. Proximal aortic dissection with aortic regurgitation or tamponade may be visualized, or evidence for pulmonary embolism may be obtained (Chap. 262).

Pulmonary artery catheterization There is controversy regarding the use of pulmonary artery (Swan-Ganz) catheters in patients with established or suspected CS (Chaps. 230 and 267). Their use is generally recommended for measurement of filling pressures and cardiac output to confirm the diagnosis and optimize the use of IV fluids, inotropic agents, and vasopressors in persistent shock (Table 272-2). Blood samples for O_2 saturation measurement should be obtained from the right atrium, right ventricle, and pulmonary artery to rule out a left-to-right shunt. Mixed venous O_2 saturations are low and arteriovenous (AV) O_2 differences are elevated, reflecting low cardiac index and high fractional O_2 extraction. However, when a systemic inflammatory response syndrome accompanies CS, AV O_2 differences may not be elevated (Chap. 270). The PCWP is elevated. However, use of sympathomimetic amines may return these measurements and the systemic BP to normal. Systemic vascular resistance may be low, normal, or elevated in CS. Equalization of right- and left-sided filling pressures (right atrial and PCWP) suggests cardiac tamponade as the cause of CS (Chap. 239).

Left heart catheterization and coronary angiography Measurement of LV pressure and definition of the coronary anatomy provide useful information and are indicated in most patients with CS complicating MI. Cardiac catheterization should be performed

TABLE 272-2 Hemodynamic Patterns[a]

	RA, mmHg	RVS, mmHg	RVD, mmHg	PAS, mmHg	PAD, mmHg	PCW, mmHg	CI, (L/min)/m^2	SVR, (dyn · s)/cm^5
Normal values	<6	<25	0–12	<25	0–12	<6–12	≥2.5	(800–1600)
MI without pulmonary edema[b]	—	—	—	—	—	~13 (5–18)	~2.7 (2.2–4.3)	—
Pulmonary edema	↔↑	↔↑	↔↑	↑	↑	↑	↔↓	↑
Cardiogenic shock								
LV failure	↔↑	↔↑	↔↑	↔↑	↑	↑	↓	↔↑
RV failure[c]	↑	↓↔↑[d]	↑	↓↔↑[d]	↔↓↑[d]	↓↔↑[d]	↓	↑
Cardiac tamponade	↑	↔↑	↑	↔↑	↔↑	↔↑	↓	↑
Acute mitral regurgitation	↔↑	↑	↔↑	↑	↑	↑	↔↓	↔↑
Ventricular septal rupture	↑	↔↑	↑	↔↑	↔↑	↔↑	↑PBF ↓SBF	↔↑
Hypovolemic shock	↓	↔↓	↔↓	↓	↓	↓	↓	↑
Septic shock	↓	↔↓	↔↓	↓	↓	↓	↑	↓

[a]There is significant patient-to-patient variation. Pressure may be normalized if cardiac output is low.

[b]Forrester et al classified nonreperfused MI patients into four hemodynamic subsets. (From Forrester JS et al: N Engl J Med 295:1356, 1976.) PCWP and CI in clinically stable subset 1 patients are shown. Values in parentheses represent range.

[c]"Isolated" or predominant RV failure.

[d]PCW and PA pressures may rise in RV failure after volume loading due to RV dilation, right-to-left shift of the interventricular septum, resulting in impaired LV filling. When biventricular failure is present, the patterns are similar to those shown for LV failure.

Abbreviations: CI, cardiac index; MI, myocardial infarction; P/SBF, pulmonary/systemic blood flow; PAS/D, pulmonary artery systolic/diastolic; PCW, pulmonary capillary wedge; RA, right atrium; RVS/D, right ventricular systolic/diastolic; SVR, systemic vascular resistance.

Source: Table prepared with the assistance of Krishnan Ramanathan, MD.

when there is a plan and capability for immediate coronary intervention (see below) or when a definitive diagnosis has not been made by other tests.

TREATMENT Acute Myocardial Infarction

GENERAL MEASURES (Fig. 272-2) In addition to the usual treatment of acute MI (Chap. 245), initial therapy is aimed at maintaining adequate systemic and coronary perfusion by raising systemic BP with vasopressors and adjusting volume status to a level that ensures optimum LV filling pressure. There is interpatient variability, but the values that generally are associated with adequate perfusion are systolic BP ~90 mmHg or mean BP >60 mmHg and PCWP >20 mmHg. Hypoxemia and acidosis must be corrected; most patients require ventilatory support with either endotracheal intubation or noninvasive ventilation to correct these abnormalities and reduce the work of breathing (see "Pulmonary Edema," below). Negative inotropic agents should be discontinued, and the doses of renally cleared medications adjusted. Hyperglycemia should be controlled with insulin. Bradyarrhythmias may require transvenous pacing. Recurrent ventricular tachycardia or rapid atrial fibrillation may require immediate treatment (Chap. 233).

VASOPRESSORS Various IV drugs may be used to augment BP and cardiac output in patients with CS. All have important disadvantages, and none has been shown to change the outcome in patients with established shock. *Norepinephrine* is a potent vasoconstrictor and inotropic stimulant that is useful for patients with CS. As first line of therapy norepinephrine was associated with fewer adverse events, including arrhythmias, compared to a dopamine randomized trial of patients with several eteologies of circulatory shock. Although it did not significantly improve survival compared to dopamine, its relative safety suggests that norepinephrine is reasonable as initial vasopressor therapy. Norepinephrine should be started at a dose of 2 to 4 μg/min and titrated upward as necessary. If systemic perfusion or systolic pressure cannot be maintained at >90 mmHg with a dose of 15 μg/min, it is unlikely that a further increase will be beneficial.

Dopamine has varying hemodynamic effects based on the dose; at low doses (≤ 2 μg/kg per min), it dilates the renal vascular bed, although its outcome benefits at this low dose have not been demonstrated conclusively; at moderate doses (2–10 μg/kg per min), it has positive chronotropic and inotropic effects as a consequence of β-adrenergic receptor stimulation. At higher doses, a vasoconstrictor effect results from α-receptor stimulation. It is started at an infusion rate of 2–5 μg/kg per min, and the dose is increased every 2–5 min to a maximum of 20–50 μg/kg per min. *Dobutamine* is a synthetic sympathomimetic amine with positive inotropic action and minimal positive chronotropic activity at low doses (2.5 μg/kg per min) but moderate chronotropic activity at higher doses. Although the usual dose is up to 10 μg/kg per min, its vasodilating activity precludes its use when a vasoconstrictor effect is required.

AORTIC COUNTERPULSATION In CS, mechanical assistance with an intraaortic balloon pumping (IABP) system capable of augmenting both arterial diastolic pressure and cardiac output is helpful in rapidly stabilizing patients. A sausage-shaped balloon is introduced percutaneously into the aorta via the femoral artery; the balloon is automatically inflated during early diastole, augmenting coronary blood flow. The balloon collapses in early systole, reducing the afterload against which the LV ejects. IABP improves hemodynamic status temporarily in most patients. In contrast to vasopressors and inotropic agents, myocardial O_2 consumption is reduced, ameliorating ischemia. IABP is useful as a stabilizing measure in patients with CS before and during cardiac catheterization and percutaneous coronary intervention (PCI) or before urgent surgery. IABP is contraindicated if aortic regurgitation is present or aortic dissection is suspected. Ventricular assist devices may be considered for eligible young patients with refractory shock as a bridge to cardiac transplantation (Chap. 235).

REPERFUSION-REVASCULARIZATION The rapid establishment of blood flow in the infarct-related artery is essential in the management of CS and forms the centerpiece of management. The randomized SHOCK Trial demonstrated that 132 lives were saved per 1000 patients treated with early revascularization with PCI or coronary artery bypass graft (CABG) compared with initial medical therapy including IABP with fibrinolytics followed by delayed revascularization. The benefit is seen across the risk strata and is sustained up to 11 years after an MI. Early revascularization with PCI or CABG is a class I recommendation for patients age <75 years with ST elevation or left bundle branch block MI who develop CS within 36 h of MI and who can be revascularized within 18 h of the development of CS. When mechanical revascularization is not possible, IABP and fibrinolytic therapy are recommended. Older patients who are suitable candidates for aggressive care also should be offered early revascularization.

Prognosis

Within this high-risk condition, there is a wide range of expected death rates based on age, severity of hemodynamic abnormalities, severity of the clinical manifestations of hypoperfusion, and the performance of early revascularization.

■ SHOCK SECONDARY TO RIGHT VENTRICULAR INFARCTION

Although transient hypotension is common in patients with RV infarction and inferior MI (Chap. 245), persistent CS due to RV failure accounts for only 3% of CS complicating MI. The salient features of RV shock are absence of pulmonary congestion, high right atrial pressure (which may be seen only after volume loading), RV dilation and dysfunction, only mildly or moderately depressed LV function, and predominance of single-vessel proximal right coronary artery occlusion. Management includes IV fluid administration to optimize right atrial pressure (10–15 mmHg); avoidance of excess fluids, which cause a shift of the interventricular septum into the LV; sympathomimetic amines; IABP; and the early reestablishment of infarct-artery flow.

■ MITRAL REGURGITATION

(See also Chap. 245) Acute severe MR due to papillary muscle dysfunction and/or rupture may complicate MI and result in CS and/or pulmonary edema. This complication most often occurs on the first day, with a second peak several days later. The diagnosis is confirmed by echo-Doppler. Rapid stabilization with IABP is recommended, with administration of dobutamine as needed to raise cardiac output. Reducing the load against which the LV pumps (afterload) reduces the volume of regurgitant flow of blood into the left atrium. Mitral valve surgery is the definitive therapy and should be performed early in the course in suitable candidates.

■ VENTRICULAR SEPTAL RUPTURE

(See also Chap. 245) Echo-Doppler demonstrates shunting of blood from the left to the right ventricle and may visualize the opening in the interventricular septum. Timing and management are similar to those for MR with IABP support and surgical correction for suitable candidates.

■ FREE WALL RUPTURE

Myocardial rupture is a dramatic complication of STEMI that is most likely to occur during the first week after the onset of symptoms; its frequency increases with the age of the patient. The clinical presentation typically is a sudden loss of pulse, blood pressure, and consciousness but sinus rhythm on ECG (pulseless electrical activity) due to cardiac tamponade (Chap. 239). Free wall rupture may also result in CS due to subacute tamponade when the pericardium temporarily seals the rupture sites. Definitive surgical repair is required.

■ ACUTE FULMINANT MYOCARDITIS

(See also Chap. 238) Myocarditis can mimic acute MI with ST deviation or bundle branch block on the ECG and marked elevation of cardiac markers. Acute myocarditis causes CS in a small proportion of cases. These patients are typically younger than those with CS due to acute MI and often do not have typical ischemic chest pain. Echocardiography usually shows global LV dysfunction. Initial management is the same as for CS complicating acute MI (Fig. 272-2) but does not involve coronary revascularization.

PULMONARY EDEMA

The etiologies and pathophysiology of pulmonary edema are discussed in Chap. 33.

Diagnosis

Acute pulmonary edema usually presents with the rapid onset of dyspnea at rest, tachypnea, tachycardia, and severe hypoxemia. Rales and wheezing due to airway compression from peribronchial cuffing may be audible. Hypertension is usually present due to release of endogenous catecholamines.

It is often difficult to distinguish between cardiogenic and noncardiogenic causes of acute pulmonary edema. *Echocardiography* may identify systolic and diastolic ventricular dysfunction and valvular lesions. Pulmonary edema associated with electrocardiographic ST elevation and evolving Q waves is usually diagnostic of acute MI and should prompt immediate institution of MI protocols and coronary artery reperfusion therapy (Chap. 245). Brain natriuretic peptide levels, when substantially elevated, support heart failure as the etiology of acute dyspnea with pulmonary edema (Chap. 234).

The use of a *Swan-Ganz catheter* permits measurement of PCWP and helps differentiate high-pressure (cardiogenic) from normal-pressure (noncardiogenic) causes of pulmonary edema. Pulmonary artery catheterization is indicated when the etiology of the pulmonary edema is uncertain, when it is refractory to therapy, or when it is accompanied by hypotension. Data derived from use of a catheter often alter the treatment plan, but the impact on mortality rates has not been demonstrated.

TREATMENT Pulmonary Edema

The treatment of pulmonary edema depends on the specific etiology. In light of the acute, life-threatening nature of the condition, a number of measures must be applied immediately to support the circulation, gas exchange, and lung mechanics. In addition, conditions that frequently complicate pulmonary edema, such as infection, acidemia, anemia, and renal failure, must be corrected.

SUPPORT OF OXYGENATION AND VENTILATION Patients with acute cardiogenic pulmonary edema generally have an identifiable cause of acute LV failure—such as arrhythmia, ischemia/infarction, or myocardial decompensation (Chap. 234)—that can be rapidly treated, with improvement in gas exchange. In contrast, noncardiogenic edema usually resolves much less quickly, and most patients require mechanical ventilation.

Oxygen Therapy Support of oxygenation is essential to ensure adequate O_2 delivery to peripheral tissues, including the heart.

Positive-Pressure Ventilation Pulmonary edema increases the work of breathing and the O_2 requirements of this work, imposing a significant physiologic stress on the heart. When oxygenation or ventilation is not adequate in spite of supplemental O_2, positive-pressure ventilation by face or nasal mask or by endotracheal intubation should be initiated. Noninvasive ventilation (Chap. 269) can rest the respiratory muscles, improve oxygenation and cardiac function, and reduce the need for intubation. In refractory cases, mechanical ventilation can relieve the work of breathing more completely than can noninvasive ventilation. Mechanical ventilation with positive end-expiratory pressure can have multiple beneficial effects on pulmonary edema: (1) decreases both preload and afterload, thereby improving cardiac function, (2) redistributes lung water from the intraalveolar to the extraalveolar space, where the fluid interferes less with gas exchange, and (3) increases lung volume to avoid atelectasis.

REDUCTION OF PRELOAD In most forms of pulmonary edema, the quantity of extravascular lung water is determined by both the PCWP and the intravascular volume status.

Diuretics The "loop diuretics" furosemide, bumetanide, and torsemide are effective in most forms of pulmonary edema, even in the presence of hypoalbuminemia, hyponatremia, or hypochloremia. Furosemide is also a venodilator that reduces preload rapidly, before any diuresis, and is the diuretic of choice. The initial dose of furosemide should be ≤0.5 mg/kg, but a higher dose (1 mg/kg) is required in patients with renal insufficiency, chronic diuretic use, or hypervolemia or after failure of a lower dose.

Nitrates Nitroglycerin and isosorbide dinitrate act predominantly as venodilators but have coronary vasodilating properties as well. They are rapid in onset and effective when administered by a variety of routes. Sublingual nitroglycerin (0.4 mg × 3 every 5 min) is first-line therapy for acute cardiogenic pulmonary edema. If pulmonary edema persists in the absence of hypotension, sublingual may be followed by IV nitroglycerin, commencing at 5–10 μg/min. IV nitroprusside (0.1–5 μg/kg per min) is a potent venous and arterial vasodilator. It is useful for patients with pulmonary edema and hypertension but is not recommended in states of reduced coronary artery perfusion. It requires close monitoring and titration using an arterial catheter for continuous BP measurement.

Morphine Given in 2- to 4-mg IV boluses, morphine is a transient venodilator that reduces preload while relieving dyspnea and anxiety. These effects can diminish stress, catecholamine levels, tachycardia, and ventricular afterload in patients with pulmonary edema and systemic hypertension.

Angiotensin-Converting Enzyme (ACE) Inhibitors ACE inhibitors reduce both afterload and preload and are recommended for hypertensive patients. A low dose of a short-acting agent may be initiated and followed by increasing oral doses. In acute MI with heart failure, ACE inhibitors reduce short- and long-term mortality rates.

Other Preload-Reducing Agents IV recombinant brain natriuretic peptide (nesiritide) is a potent vasodilator with diuretic properties and is effective in the treatment of cardiogenic pulmonary edema. It should be reserved for refractory patients and is not recommended in the setting of ischemia or MI.

Physical Methods Reduction of venous return reduces preload. Patients without hypotension should be maintained in the sitting position with the legs dangling along the side of the bed.

Inotropic and Inodilator Drugs The sympathomimetic amines dopamine and dobutamine (see above) are potent inotropic agents. The bipyridine phosphodiesterase-3 inhibitors (inodilators), such as milrinone (50 μg/kg followed by 0.25–0.75 μg/kg per min), stimulate myocardial contractility while promoting peripheral and pulmonary vasodilation. Such agents are indicated in patients with cardiogenic pulmonary edema and severe LV dysfunction.

Digitalis Glycosides Once a mainstay of treatment because of their positive inotropic action (Chap. 234), digitalis glycosides are rarely used at present. However, they may be useful for control of ventricular rate in patients with rapid atrial fibrillation or flutter and LV dysfunction, since they do not have the negative inotropic effects of other drugs that inhibit atrioventricular nodal conduction.

Intraaortic Counterpulsation IABP may help relieve cardiogenic pulmonary edema. It is indicated as a stabilizing measure when acute severe mitral regurgitation or ventricular septal rupture causes refractory pulmonary edema, especially in preparation for surgical repair. IABP or LV-assist devices (Chap. 235) are useful as bridging therapy to cardiac transplantation in patients with refractory pulmonary edema secondary to myocarditis or cardiomyopathy.

Treatment of Tachyarrhythmias and Atrial-Ventricular Resynchronization (See also Chap. 233) Sinus tachycardia or atrial fibrillation can result from elevated left atrial pressure and sympathetic stimulation. Tachycardia itself can limit LV filling time and raise left atrial pressure further. Although relief of pulmonary congestion will slow the sinus rate or ventricular response in atrial fibrillation, a primary tachyarrhythmia may require cardioversion. In patients with reduced LV function and without atrial contraction or with lack of synchronized atrioventricular contraction, placement of an atrioventricular sequential pacemaker should be considered (Chap. 232).

Stimulation of Alveolar Fluid Clearance Recent mechanistic studies on alveolar epithelial ion transport have defined a variety of ways to upregulate the clearance of solute and water from the alveolar space. In patients with acute lung injury (noncardiogenic pulmonary edema), IV β-adrenergic agonist treatment decreases extravascular lung water, but the outcome benefit is uncertain.

SPECIAL CONSIDERATIONS

The risk of iatrogenic cardiogenic shock In the treatment of pulmonary edema vasodilators lower BP, and, particularly when used in combination, their use may lead to hypotension, coronary artery hypoperfusion, and shock (Fig. 272-1). In general, patients with a *hypertensive* response to pulmonary edema tolerate and benefit from these medications. In normotensive patients, low doses of single agents should be instituted sequentially, as needed.

Acute Coronary Syndromes (See also Chap. 245) Acute STEMI complicated by pulmonary edema is associated with in-hospital mortality rates of 20–40%. After immediate stabilization, coronary artery blood flow must be reestablished rapidly. When available, primary PCI is preferable; alternatively, a fibrinolytic agent should be administered. Early coronary angiography and revascularization by PCI or CABG also are indicated for patients with non-ST elevation acute coronary syndrome. IABP use may be required to stabilize patients for coronary angiography if hypotension develops or for refractory pulmonary edema in patients with LV failure who are candidates for revascularization.

Unusual Types of Edema Specific etiologies of pulmonary edema may require particular therapy. Reexpansion pulmonary edema can develop after removal of air or fluid that has been in the pleural space for some time. These patients may develop hypotension or oliguria resulting from rapid fluid shifts into the lung. Diuretics and preload reduction are contraindicated, and intravascular volume repletion often is needed while supporting oxygenation and gas exchange.

High-altitude pulmonary edema often can be prevented by use of dexamethasone, calcium channel-blocking drugs, or long-acting inhaled β_2-adrenergic agonists. Treatment includes descent from altitude, bed rest, oxygen, and, if feasible, inhaled nitric oxide; nifedipine may also be effective.

For pulmonary edema resulting from upper airway obstruction, recognition of the obstructing cause is key, since treatment then is to relieve or bypass the obstruction.

FURTHER READINGS

Antman EM: Treatment of ST elevation myocardial infarction, in *Braunwald's Heart Disease*, 8th ed, P Libby et al (eds). Philadelphia, Saunders, 2008

——— et al: ACC/AHA Guidelines for the management of patients with acute myocardial infarction: A report of the American College of Cardiology/American Heart Association task force on practice guidelines (Committee on Management of Acute Myocardial Infarction). J Am Coll Cardiol 44:671, 2004

Goldberg RJ, et al: Thirty-year trends (1975 to 2005) in the magnitude of, management of, and hospital death rates associated with cardiogenic shock in patients with acute myocardial infarction: A population-based perspective. Circulation 119:1211, 2009

Hochman JS, Ohman EM: *Cardiogenic Shock*, American Heart Association Clinical Series, E Antman (ed). New York, Wiley-Blackwell, 2008

——— et al: Early revascularization and long-term survival in cardiogenic shock complicating acute myocardial infarction. JAMA 295:2511, 2006

Matthay MA, Ingbar DH (eds): *Pulmonary Edema. Lung Biology in Health and Disease*, vol 116. New York, Marcel Dekker, 1998

Okuda M: A multidisciplinary overview of cardiogenic shock. Shock 25:557, 2006

Reynolds HR, Hochman JS: Cardiogenic shock: Current concepts and improving outcomes. Circulation 117:686, 2008

Ware LB, Matthay MA: Clinical practice: Acute pulmonary edema. N Engl J Med 353:2788, 2005

CHAPTER 273

Cardiovascular Collapse, Cardiac Arrest, and Sudden Cardiac Death

Robert J. Myerburg
Agustin Castellanos

OVERVIEW AND DEFINITIONS

Sudden cardiac death (SCD) is defined *as natural death due to cardiac causes* in a person who may or may not have previously recognized heart disease but in whom the time and mode of death are *unexpected*. In the context of time, "sudden" is defined for most clinical and epidemiologic purposes as *1 h or less* between a change in clinical status heralding the onset of the terminal clinical event and the cardiac arrest itself. An exception is unwitnessed deaths, in which pathologists may expand the definition of time to 24 h after the victim was last seen to be alive and stable.

The overwhelming majority of natural deaths are caused by cardiac disorders. However, it is common for underlying heart diseases—often far advanced—to go unrecognized before the fatal event. As a result, up to two-thirds of all SCDs occur as the first clinical expression of previously undiagnosed disease or in patients with known heart disease, the extent of which suggests low risk. The magnitude of sudden *cardiac* death as a public health problem is highlighted by the estimate that ~50% of all cardiac deaths are sudden and unexpected, accounting for a total SCD burden estimated to range from <200,000 to >450,000 deaths each year in the United States. SCD is a direct consequence of cardiac arrest, which may be reversible if addressed promptly. Since resuscitation techniques and emergency rescue systems are available to respond to victims of out-of-hospital cardiac arrest, which was uniformly fatal in the past, understanding the SCD problem has practical clinical importance.

Because of community-based interventions, victims may remain biologically alive for days or even weeks after a cardiac arrest that has resulted in irreversible central nervous system damage. Confusion in terms can be avoided by adhering strictly to definitions of cardiovascular collapse, cardiac arrest, and death (Table 273-1). Although cardiac arrest is often potentially reversible by appropriate and timely interventions, death is biologically, legally, and literally an absolute and irreversible event. Death may be delayed in a survivor of cardiac arrest, but "survival after sudden death" is an irrational term. When biologic death of a cardiac arrest victim is delayed because of interventions, the relevant pathophysiologic event remains the sudden and unexpected cardiac arrest that leads ultimately to death, even though delayed by interventions. The language used should reflect the fact that the index event was a cardiac arrest and that death was due to its delayed consequences. Accordingly, for statistical purposes, deaths that occur during hospitalization or within 30 days after resuscitated cardiac arrest are counted as sudden deaths.

TABLE 273-1 Distinction Between Cardiovascular Collapse, Cardiac Arrest, and Death

Term	Definition	Qualifiers	Mechanisms
Cardiovascular collapse	Sudden loss of effective blood flow due to cardiac and/or peripheral vascular factors that may reverse spontaneously (e.g., neurocardiogenic syncope, vasovagal syncope) or require interventions (e.g., cardiac arrest)	Nonspecific term: includes cardiac arrest and its consequences and transient events that characteristically revert spontaneously	Same as "Cardiac Arrest," plus vasodepressor syncope or other causes of transient loss of blood flow
Cardiac arrest	Abrupt cessation of cardiac mechanical function, which may be reversible by a prompt intervention but will lead to death in its absence	Rare spontaneous reversions; likelihood of successful intervention relates to mechanism of arrest, clinical setting, and prompt return of circulation	Ventricular fibrillation, ventricular tachycardia, asystole, bradycardia, pulseless electrical activity, mechanical factors
Sudden cardiac death	Sudden, irreversible cessation of all biological functions	None	

Source: Modified from Myerburg and Castellanos, 2008, with permission of publisher.

CLINICAL DEFINITION OF FORMS OF CARDIOVASCULAR COLLAPSE

Cardiovascular collapse is a general term connoting loss of sufficient cerebral blood flow to maintain consciousness due to acute dysfunction of the heart and/or peripheral vasculature. It may be caused by vasodepressor syncope (vasovagal syncope, postural hypotension with syncope, neurocardiogenic syncope; Chap. 20), a transient severe bradycardia, or cardiac arrest. The latter is distinguished from the transient forms of cardiovascular collapse in that it usually requires an intervention to restore spontaneous blood flow. In contrast, vasodepressor syncope and other primary bradyarrhythmic syncopal events are transient and non-life-threatening, with spontaneous return of consciousness.

The most common electrical mechanism for cardiac arrest is ventricular fibrillation (VF), which is responsible for 50–80% of cardiac arrests. Severe persistent bradyarrhythmias, asystole, and pulseless electrical activity [PEA: organized electrical activity, unusually slow, without mechanical response, formerly called electromechanical dissociation (EMD)] cause another 20–30%. Pulseless sustained ventricular tachycardia (a rapid arrhythmia distinct from PEA) is a less common mechanism. Acute low cardiac output states, having a precipitous onset, also may present clinically as a cardiac arrest. These hemodynamic causes include massive acute pulmonary emboli, internal blood loss from a ruptured aortic aneurysm, intense anaphylaxis, and cardiac rupture with tamponade after myocardial infarction (MI). Sudden deaths due to these causes are not included in the SCD category.

ETIOLOGY, INITIATING EVENTS, AND CLINICAL EPIDEMIOLOGY

Clinical, epidemiologic, and pathologic studies have provided information on the underlying *structural abnormalities* in victims of SCD and identified subgroups at high risk for SCD. In addition, studies of clinical physiology have begun to identify *transient functional factors* that may convert a long-standing underlying structural abnormality from a stable to an unstable state, leading to the onset of cardiac arrest (Table 273-2).

Cardiac disorders constitute the most common causes of sudden *natural* death. After an initial peak incidence of sudden death between birth and 6 months of age [the sudden infant death syndrome (SIDS)], the incidence of sudden death declines sharply and remains low through childhood and adolescence. Among adolescents and young adults, the incidence of SCD is approximately 1 per 100,000 population per year. The incidence begins to increase in adults over age 30 years, reaching a second peak in the age range 45–75 years, when it approximates 1–2 per 1000 per year among the unselected adult population. Increasing age within this range is associated with increasing risk for sudden *cardiac* death (Fig. 273-1A). From 1 to 13 years of age, only one of five sudden *natural* deaths is due to cardiac causes. Between 14 and 21 years of age, the proportion increases to 30%, and it rises to 88% in the middle-aged and elderly.

Young and middle-aged men and women have different susceptibilities to SCD, but the sex differences decrease with advancing age. The difference in risk for SCD parallels the differences in age-related risks for other manifestations of coronary heart disease (CHD) between men and women. As the gender gap for manifestations of CHD closes in the sixth to eighth decades of life, the excess risk of SCD in males progressively narrows. Despite the lower incidence among younger women, coronary risk factors such as cigarette smoking, diabetes, hyperlipidemia, and hypertension are highly influential, and SCD remains an important clinical and epidemiologic problem. The incidence of SCD among the African-American population appears to be higher than it is among the white population; the reasons remain uncertain.

Genetic factors contribute to the risk of acquiring CHD and its expression as acute coronary syndromes, including SCD. In addition, however, there are data suggesting a familial predisposition to SCD as a specific form of expression of CHD. A parental history of SCD as an initial coronary event increases the probability of a similar expression in the offspring. In a number of less common syndromes, such as hypertrophic cardiomyopathy, congenital long QT interval syndromes, right ventricular dysplasia, and the syndrome of right bundle branch block and nonischemic ST-segment elevations (Brugada syndrome), there is a specific inherited risk of ventricular arrhythmias and SCD (Chap. 233).

The structural causes of and functional factors contributing to the SCD syndrome are listed in Table 273-2. Worldwide, and especially in Western cultures, coronary atherosclerotic heart disease is the most common structural abnormality associated with SCD in middle-aged and older adults. Up to 80% of all SCDs in the United States are due to the consequences of coronary atherosclerosis. The nonischemic cardiomyopathies (dilated and hypertrophic, collectively; Chap. 231) account for another 10–15% of SCDs, and all the remaining diverse etiologies cause only 5–10% of all SCDs. The inherited arrhythmia syndromes (see above and Table 273-2) are proportionally more common causes in adolescents and young adults. For some of these syndromes, such as hypertrophic cardiomyopathy (Chap. 238), the risk of SCD increases significantly after the onset of puberty.

Transient ischemia in a previously scarred or hypertrophied heart, hemodynamic and fluid and electrolyte disturbances, fluctuations in autonomic nervous system activity, and transient

TABLE 273-2 Cardiac Arrest and Sudden Cardiac Death

Structural Associations and Causes
I. Coronary heart disease
A. Coronary artery abnormalities
1. Chronic atherosclerotic lesions
2. Acute (active) lesions (plaque fissuring, platelet aggregation, acute thrombosis)
3. Anomalous coronary artery anatomy
B. Myocardial Infarction
1. Healed
2. Acute
II. Myocardial hypertrophy
A. Secondary
B. Hypertrophic cardiomyopathy
1. Obstructive
2. Nonobstructive
III. Dilated cardiomyopathy—primary muscle disease
IV. Inflammatory and infiltrative disorders.
A. Myocarditis
B. Noninfectious inflammatory diseases
C. Infiltrative diseases
V. Valvular heart disease
VI. Electrophysiologic abnormalities, structural
A. Anomalous pathways in Wolff-Parkinson-White syndrome
B. Conducting system disease
VII. Inherited disorders associated with electrophysiological abnormalities (congenital long QT syndromes, right ventricular dysplasia, Brugada syndrome, catecholaminergic polymorphic ventricular tachycardia, etc.)
Functional Contributing Factors
I. Alterations of coronary blood flow
A. Transient ischemia
B. Reperfusion after ischemia
II. Low cardiac output states
A. Heart failure
1. Chronic
2. Acute decompensation
B. Shock
III. Systemic metabolic abnormalities
A. Electrolyte imbalance (e.g., hypokalemia)
B. Hypoxemia, acidosis
IV. Neurologic disturbances
A. Autonomic fluctuations: central, neural, humoral
B. Receptor function
V. Toxic responses
A. Proarrhythmic drug effects
B. Cardiac toxins (e.g., cocaine, digitalis intoxication)
C. Drug interactions

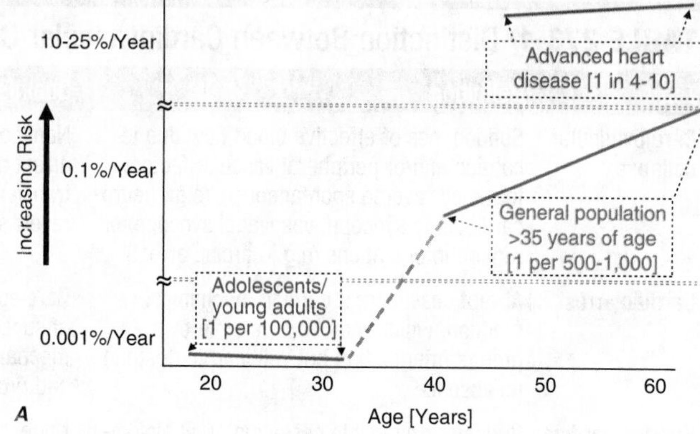

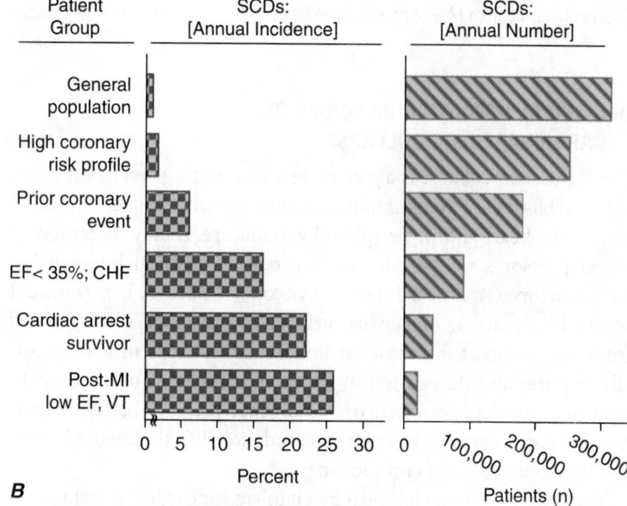

Figure 273-1 *Panel A* **demonstrates age-related risk for SCD.** For the general population age 35 years and older, SCD risk is 0.1–0.2 percent per year (1 per 500–1000 population). Among the general population of adolescents and adults younger than age 30 years, the overall risk of SCD is 1 per 100,000 population, or 0.001% per year. The risk of SCD increases dramatically beyond age 35 years. The greatest rate of increase is between 40 and 65 years (vertical axis is discontinuous). Among patients older than 30 years of age, with advanced structural heart disease and markers of high risk for cardiac arrest, the event rate may exceed 25% per year, and age-related risk attenuates. *(Modified from Myerburg and Castellanos 2008, with permission of publisher.)* ***Panel B*** **demonstrates the incidence of SCD in population subgroups** and the relation of total number of events per year to incidence figures. Approximations of subgroup incidence figures and the related population pool from which they are derived are presented. Approximately 50% of all cardiac deaths are sudden and unexpected. The incidence triangle on the left ("Percent/Year") indicates the approximate percentage of sudden and nonsudden deaths in each of the population subgroups indicated, ranging from the lowest percentage in unselected adult populations (0.1–2% per year) to the highest percentage in patients with VT or VF during convalescence after an MI (approximately 50% per year). The triangle on the right indicates the total number of events per year in each of these groups to reflect incidence in context with the size of the population subgroups. The highest risk categories identify the smallest number of total annual events, and the lowest incidence category accounts for the largest number of events per year. EF, ejection fraction; VT, ventricular tachycardia; VF, ventricular fibrillation; MI, myocardial infarction. *(After RJ Myerburg et al: Circulation 85:2, 1992.)*

electrophysiologic changes caused by drugs or other chemicals (e.g., proarrhythmia) have all been implicated as mechanisms responsible for the transition from electrophysiologic stability to instability. In addition, reperfusion of ischemic myocardium may cause transient electrophysiologic instability and arrhythmias.

■ PATHOLOGY

Data from postmortem examinations of SCD victims parallel the clinical observations on the prevalence of CHD as the major structural etiologic factor. More than 80% of SCD victims have pathologic findings of CHD. The pathologic description often includes a combination of long-standing, extensive atherosclerosis of the epicardial coronary arteries and unstable coronary artery lesions, which include various permutations of eroded, fissured, or ruptured plaques; platelet aggregates; hemorrhage; and/or thrombosis. As many as 70–75% of males who die suddenly have preexisting healed MIs, whereas only 20–30% have recent acute MIs, despite the prevalence of unstable plaques and thrombi. The latter suggests transient ischemia as the mechanism of onset. Regional or global left ventricular (LV) hypertrophy often coexists with prior MIs.

PREDICTION AND PREVENTION OF CARDIAC ARREST AND SUDDEN CARDIAC DEATH

SCD accounts for approximately one-half the total number of cardiovascular deaths. As shown in Fig. 273-1*B*, the very high risk subgroups provide more focused populations ("percent per year") for predicting cardiac arrest or SCD, but the representation of such subgroups within the overall population burden of SCD, indicated by the absolute number of events ("events per year"), is relatively small. The requirements for achieving a major population impact are effective prevention of underlying diseases and/or new epidemiologic probes that will allow better resolution of specific high-risk subgroups within the large general populations.

Strategies for predicting and preventing SCD are classified as primary and secondary. *Primary prevention*, as defined in various implantable defibrillator trials, refers to the attempt to identify individual patients at specific risk for SCD and institute preventive strategies. *Secondary prevention* refers to measures taken to prevent recurrent cardiac arrest or death in individuals who have survived a previous cardiac arrest. A third category consists of interventions intended to abort sudden cardiac arrests, thus avoiding their progression to death. This focuses primarily on out-of-hospital response strategies.

The primary prevention strategies currently used depend on the magnitude of risk among the various population subgroups. Because the annual incidence of SCD among the unselected adult population is limited to 1–2 per 1000 population per year (Fig. 273-1) and >30% of all SCDs due to coronary artery disease occur as the first clinical manifestation of the disease (Fig. 273-2*A*), the only currently practical strategies are profiling for risk of developing CHD and risk factor control (Fig. 273-2*B*). The most powerful long-term risk factors include age, cigarette smoking, elevated serum cholesterol, diabetes mellitus, elevated blood pressure, LV hypertrophy, and nonspecific electrocardiographic abnormalities. Markers of inflammation (e.g., levels of C-reactive protein) that may predict plaque destabilization have been added to risk classifications. The presence of multiple risk factors progressively increases incidence, but not sufficiently or specifically enough to warrant therapies targeted to potentially fatal arrhythmias (Fig. 273-1*A*). However, recent studies offer the hope that genetic markers for specific risk may become available. These studies suggest that a family history of SCD associated with acute coronary syndromes predicts a higher likelihood of cardiac arrest as the initial manifestation of coronary artery disease in first-degree family members.

After coronary artery disease has been identified in a patient, additional strategies for risk profiling become available (Fig. 273-2*B*), but the majority of SCDs occur among the large unselected groups rather than in the specific high-risk subgroups that become evident among populations with established disease (compare events per year with percent per year in Fig. 273-1*B*). After a major cardiovascular event, such as acute coronary syndromes, recent onset of heart failure, and survival after out-of-hospital cardiac arrest, the highest risk of death occurs during the initial 6–18 months after the event and then plateaus toward the baseline risk associated with the extent of underlying disease. However, many of the early deaths are nonsudden, diluting the potential benefit of strategies targeted specifically to SCD. Thus, although post-MI beta-blocker therapy has an identifiable benefit for both early SCD and nonsudden mortality risk, a total mortality benefit for ICD therapy early after MI has not been observed.

Among patients in the acute, convalescent, and chronic phases of myocardial infarction (Chap. 245), subgroups at high absolute risk of SCD can be identified. During the acute phase, the potential risk of cardiac arrest from onset through the first 48 h may be as high as 15%, emphasizing the importance for patients to respond promptly to the onset of symptoms. Those who survive acute-phase VF, however, are not at continuing risk for recurrent cardiac arrest indexed to that event. During the convalescent phase after MI (3 days to ~6 weeks), an episode of sustained ventricular tachycardia (VT) or VF, which is usually associated with a large infarct, predicts a natural history mortality risk of >25% at 12 months. At least one-half of the deaths are sudden. Aggressive intervention techniques may reduce this incidence.

After passage into the chronic phase of MI, the longer-term risk for total mortality and SCD mortality is predicted by a number of factors (Fig. 273-2*B*). The most important for both SCD and nonsudden death is the extent of myocardial damage sustained as a result of the acute MI. This is measured by the magnitude of reduction of the ejection fraction (EF) and/or the occurrence of heart failure. Various studies have demonstrated that ventricular arrhythmias identified by ambulatory monitoring contribute significantly to this risk, especially in patients with an EF <40%. In addition, inducibility of VT or VF during electrophysiologic testing of patients who have ambient ventricular arrhythmias [premature ventricular contractions (PVCs) and nonsustained VT] and an EF <35 or 40% is a strong predictor of SCD risk. Patients in this subgroup are now considered candidates for implantable cardioverter defibrillators (ICDs) (see below). Risk falls off sharply with EFs >40% after MI and the absence of ambient arrhythmias and conversely is high with EFs <30% even without the ambient arrhythmia markers.

The cardiomyopathies (dilated and hypertrophic, Chap. 238) are the second most common category of diseases associated with risk of SCD, after CHD (Table 273-2). Some risk factors have been identified, largely related to extent of disease, documented ventricular arrhythmias, and symptoms of arrhythmias (e.g., syncope). The less common causes of SCD include valvular heart disease (primarily aortic) and inflammatory and infiltrative disorders of the myocardium. The latter include viral myocarditis, sarcoidosis, and amyloidosis.

Among adolescents and young adults, rare inherited disorders such as hypertrophic cardiomyopathy, the long QT interval syndromes, right ventricular dysplasia, and the Brugada syndrome have received attention as important causes of SCD because of advances in genetics and the ability to identify some of those at risk before a fatal event. The subgroup of young competitive athletes has received special attention. The incidence of SCD among athletes appears to be higher than it is for the general adolescent and young adult population, perhaps up to 1 in 75,000. Hypertrophic

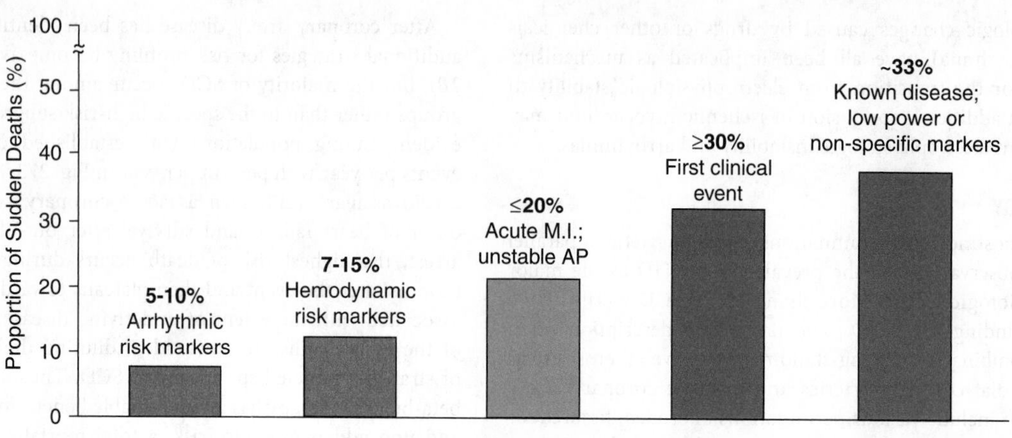

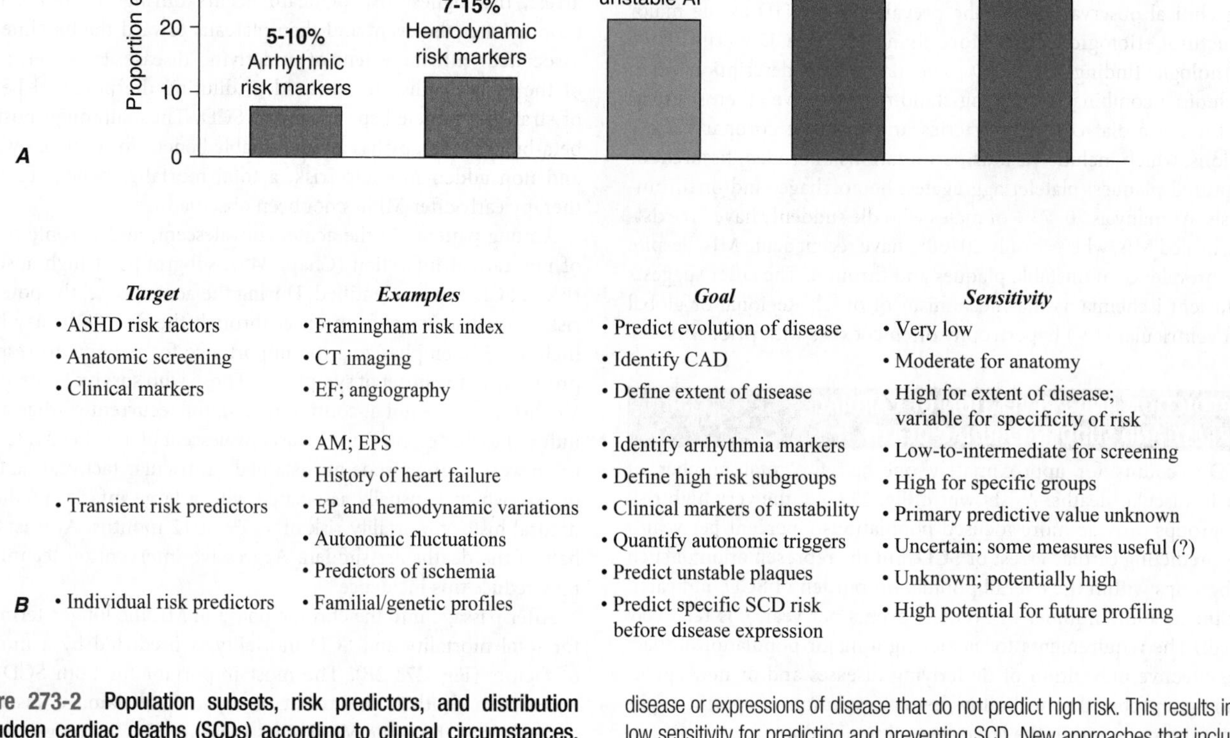

B

Target	*Examples*	*Goal*	*Sensitivity*
• ASHD risk factors	• Framingham risk index	• Predict evolution of disease	• Very low
• Anatomic screening	• CT imaging	• Identify CAD	• Moderate for anatomy
• Clinical markers	• EF; angiography	• Define extent of disease	• High for extent of disease; variable for specificity of risk
	• AM; EPS	• Identify arrhythmia markers	• Low-to-intermediate for screening
	• History of heart failure	• Define high risk subgroups	• High for specific groups
• Transient risk predictors	• EP and hemodynamic variations	• Clinical markers of instability	• Primary predictive value unknown
	• Autonomic fluctuations	• Quantify autonomic triggers	• Uncertain; some measures useful (?)
	• Predictors of ischemia	• Predict unstable plaques	• Unknown; potentially high
• Individual risk predictors	• Familial/genetic profiles	• Predict specific SCD risk before disease expression	• High potential for future profiling

Figure 273-2 Population subsets, risk predictors, and distribution of sudden cardiac deaths (SCDs) according to clinical circumstances. ***A.*** The population subset with high-risk arrhythmia markers in conjunction with low ejection fraction is a group at high risk of SCD but accounts for <10% of the total SCD burden attributable to coronary artery disease. In contrast, nearly two-thirds of all SCD victims present with SCD as the first and only manifestation of underlying disease or have known disease but are considered relatively low risk because of the absence of high-risk markers. ***B.*** Risk profile for prediction and prevention of SCD is difficult. The highest absolute numbers of events occur among the general population who may have risk factors for coronary heart disease or expressions of disease that do not predict high risk. This results in a low sensitivity for predicting and preventing SCD. New approaches that include epidemiologic modeling of transient risk factors and methods of predicting individual patient risk offer hope for greater sensitivity in the future. AP, angina pectoris; ASHD, arteriosclerotic heart disease; CAD, coronary artery disease; EPS, electrophysiologic study; HRV, heart rate variability. *(Modified from Myerburg RJ: J Cardiovasc Electrophysiol 2001; 12:369–381, reproduced with permission of the publisher.)*

cardiomyopathy (Chap. 238) is the most common cause in the United States, compared with Italy, where more comprehensive screening programs remove potential victims from the population of athletes.

Secondary prevention strategies should be applied to surviving victims of a cardiac arrest that was not associated with an acute MI or a transient risk of SCD (e.g., drug exposures, correctable electrolyte imbalances). Multivessel coronary artery disease and dilated cardiomyopathy, especially with markedly reduced left ventricular EF predict a 1- to 2-year risk of recurrence of an SCD or cardiac arrest of up to 30% in the absence of specific interventions (see below). The presence of life-threatening arrhythmias with long QT syndromes or right ventricular dysplasia are also associated with increased risks.

CLINICAL CHARACTERISTICS OF CARDIAC ARREST

PRODROME, ONSET, ARREST, DEATH

SCD may be presaged by days to months of increasing angina, dyspnea, palpitations, easy fatigability, and other nonspecific complaints. However, these *prodromal symptoms* are generally predictive of any major cardiac event; they are not specific for predicting SCD.

The *onset of the clinical transition,* leading to cardiac arrest, is defined as an acute change in cardiovascular status preceding cardiac arrest by up to 1 h. When the onset is instantaneous or abrupt, the probability that the arrest is cardiac in origin is >95%. Continuous electrocardiographic (ECG) recordings fortuitously obtained at the onset of a cardiac arrest commonly demonstrate changes in cardiac electrical activity during the minutes or hours before the event. There is a tendency for the heart rate to increase and for advanced grades of PVCs to evolve. Most cardiac arrests that are caused by VF begin with a run of nonsustained or sustained VT, which then degenerates into VF.

The probability of achieving successful resuscitation from cardiac arrest is related to the interval from onset of loss of circulation to institution of resuscitative efforts, the setting in which the event occurs, the mechanism (VF, VT, PEA, asystole), and the clinical status of the patient before the cardiac arrest. Return of circulation and survival rates as a result of defibrillation decrease almost linearly from the first minute to 10 min. After 5 min, survival rates are no better than 25–30% in out-of-hospital settings. Those settings in which it is possible to institute prompt cardiopulmonary resuscitation (CPR) followed by prompt defibrillation provide a better chance of a successful outcome. However, the outcome in intensive care units and other in-hospital environments is heavily influenced by the patient's preceding clinical status. The immediate outcome is good for cardiac arrest occurring in the intensive care unit in the presence of an acute cardiac event or transient metabolic disturbance, but survival among patients with far-advanced chronic cardiac disease or advanced noncardiac diseases (e.g., renal failure, pneumonia, sepsis, diabetes, cancer) is low and not much better in the in-hospital than in the out-of-hospital setting. Survival from unexpected cardiac arrest in unmonitored areas in a hospital is not much better than that it is for witnessed out-of-hospital arrests. Since implementation of community response systems, survival from out-of-hospital cardiac arrest has improved although it still remains low, under most circumstances. Survival probabilities in public sites exceed those in the home environment.

The success rate for initial resuscitation and survival to hospital discharge after an out-of-hospital cardiac arrest depends heavily on the mechanism of the event. When the mechanism is pulseless VT, the outcome is best; VF is the next most successful; and asystole and PEA generate dismal outcome statistics. Advanced age also adversely influences the chances of successful resuscitation.

Progression to biologic death is a function of the mechanism of cardiac arrest and the length of the delay before interventions. VF or asystole without CPR within the first 4–6 min has a poor outcome even if defibrillation is successful because of superimposed brain damage; there are few survivors among patients who had no life support activities for the first 8 min after onset. Outcome statistics are improved by lay bystander intervention (basic life support—see below) before definitive interventions (advanced life support) especially when followed by early successful defibrillation. In regard to the latter, evaluations of deployment of automatic external defibrillators (AEDs) in communities (e.g., police vehicles, large buildings, airports, and stadiums) are beginning to generate encouraging data. Increased deployment is to be encouraged.

Death during the hospitalization after a successfully resuscitated cardiac arrest relates closely to the severity of central nervous system injury. Anoxic encephalopathy and infections subsequent to prolonged respirator dependence account for 60% of the deaths. Another 30% occur as a consequence of low cardiac output states that fail to respond to interventions. Recurrent arrhythmias are the least common cause of death, accounting for only 10% of in-hospital deaths.

In the setting of acute MI (Chap. 245), it is important to distinguish between primary and secondary cardiac arrests. *Primary cardiac arrests* are those which occur in the absence of hemodynamic instability, and *secondary cardiac arrests* are those which occur in patients in whom abnormal hemodynamics dominate the clinical picture before cardiac arrest. The success rate for immediate resuscitation in primary cardiac arrest during acute MI in a monitored setting should exceed 90%. In contrast, as many as 70% of patients with secondary cardiac arrest succumb immediately or during the same hospitalization.

TREATMENT Cardiac Arrest

An individual who collapses suddenly is managed in five stages: (1) initial evaluation and basic life support if arrest is confirmed, (2) public access defibrillation (when available), (3) advanced life support, (4) postresuscitation care, and (5) long-term management. The initial response, including confirmation of loss of circulation, followed by basic life support and public access defibrillation, can be carried out by physicians, nurses, paramedical personnel, and trained laypersons. There is a requirement for increasingly specialized skills as the patient moves through the stages of advanced life support, postresuscitation care, and long-term management.

INITIAL EVALUATION AND BASIC LIFE SUPPORT Confirmation that a sudden collapse is indeed due to a cardiac arrest includes prompt observations of the state of consciousness, respiratory movements, skin color, and the presence or absence of pulses in the carotid or femoral arteries. For lay responders, the pulse check is no longer recommended. As soon as a cardiac arrest is suspected, confirmed, or even considered to be impending, calling an emergency rescue system (e.g., 911) is the immediate priority. With the development of AEDs that are easily used by nonconventional emergency responders, an additional layer for response has evolved (see below).

Agonal respiratory movements may persist for a short time after the onset of cardiac arrest, but it is important to observe for severe stridor with a persistent pulse as a clue to aspiration of a foreign body or food. If this is suspected, a Heimlich maneuver (see below) may dislodge the obstructing body. A precordial blow, or "thump," delivered firmly with a clenched fist to the junction of the middle and lower thirds of the sternum may occasionally revert VT or VF, but there is concern about converting VT to VF. Therefore, it is recommended to use precordial thumps as a life support technique only when monitoring and defibrillation are available. This conservative application of the technique remains controversial.

The third action during the initial response is to clear the airway. The head is tilted back and the chin lifted so that the oropharynx can be explored to clear the airway. Dentures or foreign bodies are removed, and the Heimlich maneuver is performed if there is reason to suspect that a foreign body is lodged in the oropharynx. If respiratory arrest precipitating cardiac arrest is suspected, a second precordial thump is delivered after the airway is cleared.

Basic life support, more popularly known as CPR, is intended to maintain organ perfusion until definitive interventions can be instituted. The elements of CPR are the maintenance of ventilation of the lungs and compression of the chest. Mouth-to-mouth respiration may be used if no specific rescue equipment is immediately available (e.g., plastic oropharyngeal airways, esophageal obturators, masked Ambu bag). Conventional ventilation techniques during single-responder CPR require that the lungs be inflated twice in succession after every 30 chest compressions. Recent data suggest that interrupting chest compressions to perform mouth-to-mouth respiration may be less effective than a continuous chest compression strategy.

Chest compression is based on the assumption that cardiac compression allows the heart to maintain a pump function by sequential filling and emptying of its chambers, with competent valves maintaining forward direction of flow. The palm of one hand is placed over the lower sternum, with the heel of the other resting on the dorsum of the lower hand. The sternum is depressed, with the arms remaining straight, at a rate of approximately 100 per minute. Sufficient force is applied to depress the sternum 4–5 cm, and relaxation is abrupt.

AUTOMATED EXTERNAL DEFIBRILLATION (AED) AEDs that are easily used by nonconventional responders, such as nonparamedic firefighters, police officers, ambulance drivers, trained security guards, and minimally trained or untrained laypersons, have been developed. This advance has inserted another level of response into the cardiac arrest paradigm. A number of studies have demonstrated that AED use by nonconventional responders in strategic response systems and public access lay responders can improve cardiac arrest survival rates. This strategy is based on shortening the time to the first defibrillation attempt while awaiting the arrival of advanced life support.

ADVANCED CARDIAC LIFE SUPPORT (ACLS) ACLS is intended to achieve adequate ventilation, control cardiac arrhythmias, stabilize blood pressure and cardiac output, and restore organ perfusion. The activities carried out to achieve these goals include (1) defibrillation/cardioversion and/or pacing, (2) intubation with an endotracheal tube, and (3) insertion of an intravenous line. The speed with which defibrillation/cardioversion is achieved is an important element in successful resuscitation, both for restoration of spontaneous circulation and for protection of the central nervous system. Immediate defibrillation should precede intubation and insertion of an intravenous line; CPR should be carried out while the defibrillator is being charged. As soon as a diagnosis of VF or VT is established, a shock of at least 300 J should be delivered when one is using a monophasic waveform device or 120–150 J with a biphasic waveform. Additional shocks are escalated to a maximum of 360 J monophasic (200 J biphasic) if the initial shock does not successfully revert VT or VF. However, it is now recommended that five cycles of CPR be carried out before repeated shocks, if the first shock fails to restore an organized rhythm, or 60–90 s of CPR before the first shock if 5 min has elapsed between the onset of cardiac arrest and ability to deliver a shock (see 2005 update of guidelines for cardiopulmonary resuscitation and emergency cardiac care at *http://circ.ahajournals.org/content/vol112/24_suppl.toc.*

Epinephrine, 1 mg intravenously, is given after failed defibrillation, and attempts to defibrillate are repeated. The dose of epinephrine may be repeated after intervals of 3–5 min (Fig. 273-3A). Vasopressin (a single 40-unit dose given IV) has been suggested as an alternative to epinephrine.

If the patient is less than fully conscious upon reversion or if two or three attempts fail, prompt intubation, ventilation, and arterial blood gas analysis should be carried out. Ventilation with O_2 (room air if O_2 is not immediately available) may promptly reverse hypoxemia and acidosis. A patient who is persistently acidotic after successful defibrillation and intubation should be given 1 meq/kg $NaHCO_3$ initially and an additional 50% of the dose repeated every 10–15 min. However, it should not be used routinely.

After initial unsuccessful defibrillation attempts or with persistent/recurrent electrical instability, antiarrhythmic therapy should be instituted. Intravenous amiodarone has emerged as the initial treatment of choice (150 mg over 10 min, followed by 1 mg/min for up to 6 h and 0.5 mg/min thereafter) (Fig. 273-3A). For cardiac arrest due to VF in the early phase of an acute coronary syndrome, a bolus of 1 mg/kg of lidocaine may be given intravenously as an alternative, and the dose may be repeated in 2 min. It also may be tried in patients in whom amiodarone is unsuccessful. Intravenous procainamide (loading infusion of 100 mg/5 min to a total dose of 500–800 mg, followed by continuous infusion at 2–5 mg/min) is now rarely used in this setting but may be tried for persisting, hemodynamically stable arrhythmias. Intravenous calcium gluconate is no longer considered safe or necessary for routine administration. It is used only in patients in whom acute hyperkalemia is known to be the triggering event for resistant VF, in the presence of known hypocalcemia, or in patients who have received toxic doses of calcium channel antagonists.

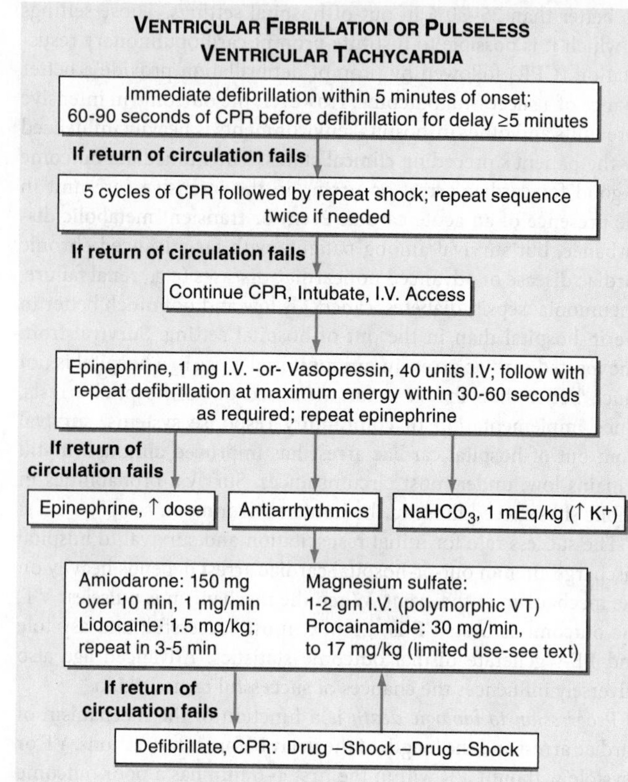

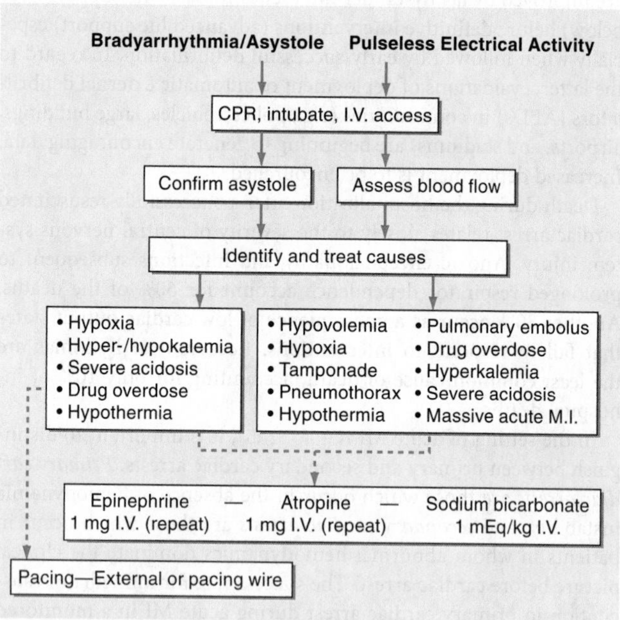

Figure 273-3 ***A.* The algorithm of ventricular fibrillation** or pulseless ventricular tachycardia begins with defibrillation attempts. If that fails, it is followed by epinephrine and then antiarrhythmic drugs. See text for details. ***B.* The algorithms for bradyarrhythmia/asystole** (*left*) or pulseless electrical activity (*right*) are dominated first by continued life support and a search for reversible causes. Subsequent therapy is nonspecific and is accompanied by a low success rate. See text for details. CPR, cardiopulmonary resuscitation; MI, myocardial infarction.

Cardiac arrest due to bradyarrhythmias or asystole (B/A cardiac arrest) is managed differently (Fig. 273-3B). The patient is promptly intubated, CPR is continued, and an attempt is made to control hypoxemia and acidosis. Epinephrine and/or atropine are given intravenously or by an intracardiac route. External pacing devices are used to attempt to establish a regular rhythm. The success rate may be good when B/A arrest is due to acute inferior wall myocardial infarction or to correctable airway obstruction or drug-induced respiratory depression or with prompt resuscitation efforts. For acute airway obstruction, prompt removal of foreign bodies by the Heimlich maneuver or, in hospitalized patients, by intubation and suctioning of obstructing secretions in the airway is often successful. The prognosis is generally very poor in other causes of this form of cardiac arrest, such as end-stage cardiac or noncardiac diseases. Treatment of PEA is similar to that for bradyarrhythmias, but its outcome is also dismal.

POSTRESUSCITATION CARE This phase of management is determined by the clinical setting of the cardiac arrest. *Primary VF* in acute MI (not accompanied by low-output states) (Chap. 245) is generally very responsive to life support techniques and easily controlled after the initial event. In the in-hospital setting, respirator support is usually not necessary or is needed for only a short time, and hemodynamics stabilize promptly after defibrillation or cardioversion. In *secondary VF* in acute MI (those events in which hemodynamic abnormalities predispose to the potentially fatal arrhythmia), resuscitative efforts are less often successful, and in patients who are successfully resuscitated, the recurrence rate is high. The clinical picture and outcome are dominated by hemodynamic instability and the ability to control hemodynamic dysfunction. Bradyarrhythmias, asystole, and PEA are commonly secondary events in hemodynamically unstable patients. The in-hospital phase of care of an out-of-hospital cardiac arrest survivor is dictated by specific clinical circumstances. The most difficult is the presence of anoxic encephalopathy, which is a strong predictor of in-hospital death. A recent addition to the management of this condition is induced hypothermia to reduce metabolic demands and cerebral edema.

The outcome after in-hospital cardiac arrest associated with noncardiac diseases is poor, and in the few successfully resuscitated patients, the postresuscitation course is dominated by the nature of the underlying disease. Patients with end-stage cancer, renal failure, acute central nervous system disease, and uncontrolled infections, as a group, have a survival rate of <10% after in-hospital cardiac arrest. Some major exceptions are patients with transient airway obstruction, electrolyte disturbances, proarrhythmic effects of drugs, and severe metabolic abnormalities, most of whom may have a good chance of survival if they can be resuscitated promptly and stabilized while the transient abnormalities are being corrected.

LONG-TERM MANAGEMENT AFTER SURVIVAL OF OUT-OF-HOSPITAL CARDIAC ARREST Patients who survive cardiac arrest without irreversible damage to the central nervous system and who achieve hemodynamic stability should have diagnostic testing to define appropriate therapeutic interventions for their long-term management. This aggressive approach is driven by the fact that survival after out-of-hospital cardiac arrest is followed by a 10–25% mortality rate during the first 2 years after the event, and there are data suggesting that significant survival benefits can be achieved by prescription of an implantable cardioverter-defibrillator (ICD).

Among patients in whom an acute ST elevation MI, or transient and reversible myocardial ischemia, is identified as the specific mechanism triggering an out-of-hospital cardiac arrest, the management is dictated in part by the transient nature of life-threatening arrhythmia risk during the acute coronary syndrome (ACS) and in part by the extent of permanent myocardial damage that results. Cardiac arrest during the acute ischemic phase is not an ICD indication, but survivors of cardiac arrest not associated with an ACS do benefit. In addition, patients who survive MI with an ejection fraction less than 30–35% appear to benefit from ICDs.

For patients with cardiac arrest determined to be due to a treatable transient ischemic mechanism, particularly with higher EFs, catheter interventional, surgical, and/or pharmacologic anti-ischemic therapy is generally accepted for long-term management.

Survivors of cardiac arrest due to other categories of disease, such as the hypertrophic or dilated cardiomyopathies and the various rare inherited disorders (e.g., right ventricular dysplasia, long QT syndrome, Brugada syndrome, catecholaminergic polymorphic VT, and so-called idiopathic VF), are all considered ICD candidates.

PREVENTION OF SCD IN HIGH-RISK INDIVIDUALS WITHOUT PRIOR CARDIAC ARREST

Post-MI patients with EFs <35% and other markers of risk such as ambient ventricular arrhythmias, inducible ventricular tachyarrhythmias in the electrophysiology laboratory, and a history of heart failure are considered candidates for ICDs 30 days or more after the MI. Total mortality benefits in the range of a 20–35% reduction over 2–5 years have been observed in a series of clinical trials. One study suggested that an EF <30% was a sufficient marker of risk to indicate ICD benefit, and another demonstrated benefit for patients with Functional Class 2 or 3 heart failure and ejection fractions ≤35%, regardless of etiology (ischemic or nonischemic) or the presence of ambient or induced arrhythmias (see Chaps. 233 and 234). There appears to be a gradient of increasing ICD benefit with EFs ranging lower than the threshold indications. However, patients with very low EFs (e.g., <20%) may receive less benefit.

Decision making for primary prevention in disorders other than coronary artery disease and dilated cardiomyopathy is generally driven by observational data and judgment based on clinical observations. Controlled clinical trials providing evidence-based indicators for ICDs are lacking for these smaller population subgroups. In general, for the rare disorders listed above, indicators of arrhythmic risk such as syncope, documented ventricular tachyarrhythmias, aborted cardiac arrest or a family history of premature SCD in some conditions, and a number of other clinical or ECG markers may be used as indicators for ICDs.

FURTHER READINGS

Huikuri H et al: Sudden death due to cardiac arrhythmias. N Engl J Med 345:1473, 2001

International Liaison Committee on Resuscitation: 2005 International Consensus on Cardiopulmonary Resuscitation and Emergency Cardiovascular Care Science with Treatment Recommendations. Circulation 112(Suppl III):III-1–III-136, 2005, *http://circ.ahajournals.org/content/vol112/24_suppl/*

Kokolis S et al: Ventricular arrhythmias and sudden cardiac death. Prog Cardiovasc Dis 48:426, 2006

Marenco JP et al: Improving survival from sudden cardiac arrest: The role of the automated external defibrillator. JAMA 285:1193, 2001

Maron BJ, Pelliccia A: The heart of trained athletes: Cardiac remodeling and the risks of sports, including sudden death. Circulation 114:1633, 2006

Myerburg RJ, Castellanos A: Cardiac arrest and sudden cardiac death, in *Braunwald's Heart Disease*, 8th ed, P Libby et al (eds). Philadelphia, Saunders, 2008

——— et al: Indications for implantable cardioverter-defibrillators based on evidence and judgment. J Am Coll Cardiol 54:747, 2009

Noseworthy PA, Newton-Cheh C: Genetic determinants of sudden cardiac death. Circulation 118:1854, 2008

Wik L et al: Delaying defibrillation to give basic cardiopulmonary resuscitation to patients with out-of-hospital ventricular fibrillation: A randomized trial. JAMA 289:1389, 2003

CHAPTER 274
Coma

Allan H. Ropper

Coma is among the most common and striking problems in general medicine. It accounts for a substantial portion of admissions to emergency wards and occurs on all hospital services. Coma demands immediate attention and requires an organized approach.

There is a continuum of states of reduced alertness, the most severe form being *coma*, defined as a deep sleeplike state from which the patient cannot be aroused. *Stupor* refers to a higher degree of arousability in which the patient can be transiently awakened only by vigorous stimuli, accompanied by motor behavior that leads to avoidance of uncomfortable or aggravating stimuli. *Drowsiness*, which is familiar to all persons, simulates light sleep and is characterized by easy arousal and the persistence of alertness for brief periods. Drowsiness and stupor are usually accompanied by some degree of confusion (Chap. 25). A precise narrative description of the level of arousal and of the type of responses evoked by various stimuli as observed at the bedside is preferable to ambiguous terms such as *lethargy*, *semicoma*, or *obtundation*.

Several other conditions that render patients unresponsive and thereby simulate coma are considered separately because of their special significance. The *vegetative state* signifies an awake but nonresponsive state in a patient who has emerged from coma. In the vegetative state, the eyelids may open, giving the appearance of wakefulness. Respiratory and autonomic functions are retained. Yawning, coughing, swallowing, as well as limb and head movements persist and the patient may follow visually presented objects, but there are few, if any, meaningful responses to the external and internal environment—in essence, an "awake coma." The term *vegetative* is unfortunate as it is subject to misinterpretation. There are always accompanying signs that indicate extensive damage in both cerebral hemispheres, e.g., decerebrate or decorticate limb posturing and absent responses to visual stimuli (see below). In the closely related but less severe *minimally conscious state*, the patient has rudimentary vocal or motor behaviors, often spontaneous, but some in response to touch, visual stimuli, or command. Cardiac arrest with cerebral hypoperfusion and head injuries are the most common causes of the vegetative and minimally conscious states (Chaps. 273 and 275). The prognosis for regaining mental faculties once the vegetative state has supervened for several months is very poor, and after a year, almost nil, hence the term *persistent vegetative state*. Most reports of dramatic recovery, when investigated carefully, are found to yield to the usual rules for prognosis but there have been rare instances in which recovery has occurred to a severely disabled condition and, in rare childhood cases, to an even better state. The possibility of incorrectly attributing meaningful behavior to patients in the vegetative and minimally conscious states has created inordinate problems and anguish for families. On the other hand, the question of whether these patients lack any capability for cognition has been reopened by functional imaging studies demonstrating, in a small proportion of posttraumatic cases, cerebral activation in response to external stimuli.

Apart from the above conditions, several syndromes that affect alertness are prone to be misinterpreted as stupor or coma. *Akinetic mutism* refers to a partially or fully awake state in which the patient is able to form impressions and think, as demonstrated by later recounting of events, but remains virtually immobile and mute. The condition results from damage in the regions of the medial thalamic nuclei or the frontal lobes (particularly lesions situated deeply or on the orbitofrontal surfaces) or from extreme hydrocephalus. The term *abulia* describes a milder form of akinetic mutism characterized by mental and physical slowness and diminished ability to initiate activity. It is also usually the result of damage to the frontal lobes and its connections (Chap. 26). *Catatonia* is a curious hypomobile and mute syndrome that occurs as part of a major psychosis, usually schizophrenia or major depression. Catatonic patients make few voluntary or responsive movements, although they blink, swallow, and may not appear distressed. There are nonetheless signs that the patient is responsive, although it may take ingenuity on the part of the examiner to demonstrate them. For example, eyelid elevation is actively resisted, blinking occurs in response to a visual threat, and the eyes move concomitantly with head rotation, all of which are inconsistent with the presence of a brain lesion causing unresponsiveness. It is characteristic but not invariable in catatonia for the limbs to retain the postures in which they have been placed by the examiner ("waxy flexibility," or catalepsy). With recovery, patients often have some memory of events that occurred during their catatonic stupor. Catatonia is superficially similar to akinetic mutism, but clinical evidence of cerebral damage such as Babinski signs and hypertonicity of the limbs is lacking. The special problem of coma in brain death is discussed below.

The *locked-in state* describes yet another type of pseudocoma in which an awake patient has no means of producing speech or volitional movement but retains voluntary vertical eye movements and lid elevation, thus allowing the patient to signal with a clear mind. The pupils are normally reactive. Such individuals have written entire treatises using Morse code. The usual cause is an infarction or hemorrhage of the ventral pons that transects all descending motor (corticospinal and corticobulbar) pathways. A similar awake but de-efferented state occurs as a result of total paralysis of the musculature in severe cases of Guillain-Barré syndrome (Chap. 385), critical illness neuropathy (Chap. 275), and pharmacologic neuromuscular blockade.

THE ANATOMY AND PHYSIOLOGY OF COMA

Almost all instances of diminished alertness can be traced to widespread abnormalities of the cerebral hemispheres or to reduced activity of a special thalamocortical alerting system termed the *reticular activating system* (RAS). The proper functioning of this system, its ascending projections to the cortex, and the cortex itself are required to maintain alertness and coherence of thought. It follows that the principal causes of coma are (1) lesions that damage the RAS in the upper midbrain or its projections; (2) destruction of large portions of both cerebral hemispheres; and (3) suppression of reticulocerebral function by drugs, toxins, or metabolic derangements such as hypoglycemia, anoxia, uremia, and hepatic failure.

The proximity of the RAS to midbrain structures that control pupillary function and eye movements permits clinical localization of the cause of coma in many cases. Pupillary enlargement with loss of light reaction and loss of vertical and adduction movements of the eyes suggests that the lesion is in the upper brainstem. Conversely, preservation of pupillary light reactivity and of eye movements absolves the upper brainstem and indicates that widespread structural lesions or metabolic suppression of the cerebral hemispheres is responsible for coma.

Coma due to cerebral mass lesions and herniations

The cranial cavity is separated into compartments by infoldings of the dura. The two cerebral hemispheres are separated by the falx, and the anterior and posterior fossae by the tentorium. Herniation refers to displacement of brain tissue into a compartment that it normally does not occupy. Coma and many of its associated signs can be attributed to these tissue shifts, and certain clinical features are characteristic of specific herniations (Fig. 274-1). They are in essence "false localizing" signs since they derive from compression of brain structures at a distance from the mass.

The most common herniations are those in which a part of the brain is displaced from the supratentorial to the infratentorial compartment through the tentorial opening; this is referred to as *transtentorial* herniation. *Uncal transtentorial* herniation refers to impaction of the anterior medial temporal gyrus (the uncus) into the tentorial opening just anterior to and adjacent to the midbrain (Fig. 274-1A). The uncus compresses the third nerve as it traverses the subarachnoid space, causing enlargement of the ipsilateral pupil (putatively because the fibers subserving parasympathetic pupillary function are located peripherally in the nerve). The coma that follows is due to compression of the midbrain against the opposite tentorial edge by the displaced parahippocampal gyrus (Fig. 274-2). Lateral displacement of the midbrain may compress the opposite cerebral peduncle, producing a Babinski's sign and hemiparesis contralateral to the original hemiparesis (the Kernohan-Woltman sign). Herniation may also compress the anterior and posterior cerebral arteries as they pass over the tentorial reflections, with resultant brain infarction. The distortions may also entrap portions of the ventricular system, resulting in hydrocephalus.

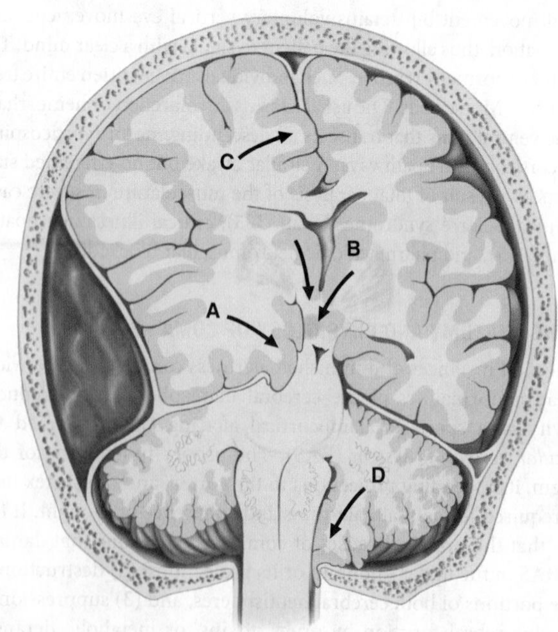

Figure 274-1 Types of cerebral herniation. (*A*) uncal; (*B*) central; (*C*) transfalcial; (*D*) foraminal.

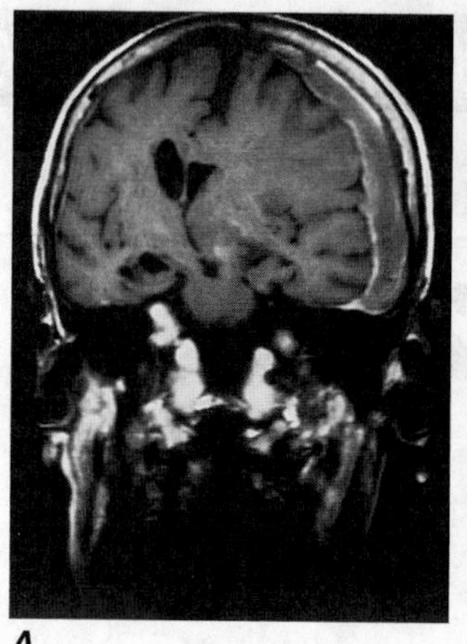

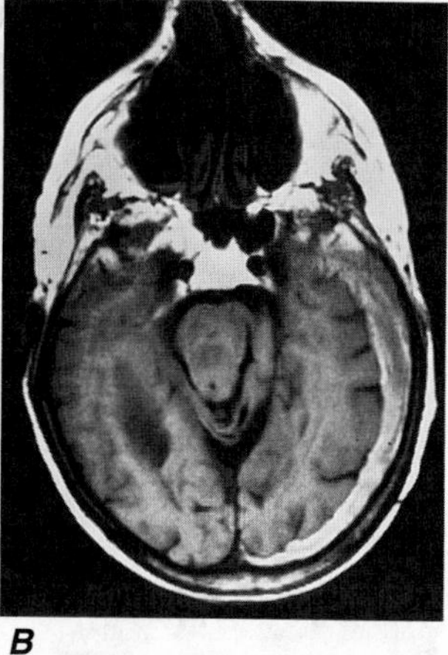

Figure 274-2 Coronal (*A*) and axial (*B*) magnetic resonance images from a stuporous patient with a left third nerve palsy as a result of a large left-sided subdural hematoma (seen as a gray-white rim). The upper midbrain and lower thalamic regions are compressed and displaced horizontally away from the mass, and there is transtentorial herniation of the medial temporal lobe structures, including the uncus anteriorly. The lateral ventricle opposite to the hematoma has become enlarged as a result of compression of the third ventricle.

Central transtentorial herniation denotes a symmetric downward movement of the thalamic medial structures through the tentorial opening with compression of the upper midbrain (Fig. 274-1B). Miotic pupils and drowsiness are the heralding signs. Both temporal and central transtentorial herniations have been considered causes of progressive compression of the brainstem, with initial damage to the midbrain, then the pons, and finally the medulla. The result is a sequence of neurologic signs that corresponds to each affected level. Other forms of herniation are *transfalcial herniation* (displacement of the cingulate gyrus under the falx and across the midline, Fig. 274-1C), and *foraminal herniation* (downward forcing of the cerebellar tonsils into the foramen magnum, Fig. 274-1D), which causes compression of the medulla, respiratory arrest, and death.

A direct relationship between the various configurations of transtentorial herniation and coma is not always found. Drowsiness and stupor can occur with moderate horizontal displacement of the diencephalon (thalamus), before transtentorial herniation is evident. This lateral shift may be quantified on axial images of CT and MRI scans (Fig. 274-2). In cases of *acutely appearing masses*, horizontal displacement of the pineal calcification of 3–5 mm is generally associated with drowsiness, 6–8 mm with stupor, and >9 mm with coma. Intrusion of the medial temporal lobe into the tentorial opening is also apparent on MRI and CT scans as obliteration of the cisterna that surround the upper brainstem.

Coma due to metabolic disorders

Many systemic metabolic abnormalities cause coma by interrupting the delivery of energy substrates (e.g., hypoxia, ischemia, hypoglycemia) or by altering neuronal excitability (drug and alcohol intoxication, anesthesia, and epilepsy). The same metabolic abnormalities that produce coma may, in milder forms, induce an acute confusional state. Thus, in metabolic encephalopathies, clouded consciousness and coma are in a continuum.

Cerebral neurons are fully dependent on cerebral blood flow (CBF) and the delivery of oxygen and glucose. CBF is ~75 mL per 100g/min in gray matter and 30 mL per 100 g/min in white matter (mean ~55 mL per 100 g/min); oxygen consumption is 3.5 mL per 100 g/min, and glucose utilization is 5 mg per 100 g/min. Brain stores of glucose provide energy for ~2 minutes after blood flow is interrupted, and oxygen stores last 8–10 seconds after the cessation of blood flow. Simultaneous hypoxia and ischemia exhaust glucose more rapidly. The electroencephalogram (EEG) rhythm in these circumstances becomes diffusely slowed, typical of metabolic encephalopathies, and as conditions of substrate delivery worsen, eventually brain electrical activity ceases.

Unlike hypoxia-ischemia, which causes neuronal destruction, most metabolic disorders such as hypoglycemia, hyponatremia, hyperosmolarity, hypercapnia, hypercalcemia, and hepatic and renal failure cause only minor neuropathologic changes. The causes of the reversible effects of these conditions on the brain are not understood but may result from impaired energy supplies, changes in ion fluxes across neuronal membranes, and neurotransmitter abnormalities. For example, the high ammonia concentration of hepatic coma interferes with cerebral energy metabolism and with the Na^+, K^+-ATPase pump, increases the number and size of astrocytes, and causes increased concentrations of potentially toxic products of ammonia metabolism; it may also affect neurotransmitters, including the production of putative "false" neurotransmitters that are active at receptor sites. Apart from hyperammonemia, which of these mechanisms is of critical importance is not clear. The mechanism of the encephalopathy of renal failure is also not known. Unlike ammonia, urea does not produce central nervous system (CNS) toxicity and a multifactorial causation has been proposed for the encephalopathy, including increased permeability of the blood-brain barrier to toxic substances such as organic acids and an increase in brain calcium and cerebrospinal fluid (CSF) phosphate content.

Coma and seizures are common accompaniments of large shifts in sodium and water balance in the brain. These changes in osmolarity arise from systemic medical disorders, including diabetic ketoacidosis, the nonketotic hyperosmolar state, and hyponatremia from any cause (e.g., water intoxication, excessive secretion of antidiuretic hormone, or atrial natriuretic peptides). Sodium levels <125 mmol/L induce confusion, and <115 mmol/L are associated with coma and convulsions. In hyperosmolar coma, the serum osmolarity is generally >350 mosmol/L. Hypercapnia depresses the level of consciousness in proportion to the rise in carbon dioxide (CO_2) tension in the blood. *In all of these metabolic encephalopathies, the degree of neurologic change depends to a large extent on the rapidity with which the serum changes occur.* The pathophysiology of other metabolic encephalopathies such as hypercalcemia, hypothyroidism, vitamin B_{12} deficiency, and hypothermia are incompletely understood but must also reflect derangements of CNS biochemistry, membrane function, and neurotransmitters.

Epileptic coma

Generalized electrical discharges of the cortex (*seizures*) are associated with coma, even in the absence of epileptic motor activity (*convulsions*). The self-limited coma that follows a seizure, the *postictal state*, may be due to exhaustion of energy reserves or effects of locally toxic molecules that are the by-product of seizures. The postictal state produces a pattern of continuous, generalized slowing of the background EEG activity similar to that of other metabolic encephalopathies.

Toxic (including drug-induced) coma

This common class of encephalopathy is in large measure reversible and leaves no residual damage provided there has not been cardiorespiratory failure. Many drugs and toxins are capable of depressing nervous system function. Some produce coma by affecting both the brainstem nuclei, including the RAS, and the cerebral cortex. The combination of cortical and brainstem signs, which occurs in certain drug overdoses, may lead to an incorrect diagnosis of structural brainstem disease. Overdose of medications that have atropinic actions produces signs such as dilated pupils, tachycardia, and dry skin; opiate overdose produces pinpoint pupils <1 mm in diameter.

Coma due to widespread damage to the cerebral hemispheres

This category, comprising a number of unrelated disorders, results from widespread structural cerebral damage, thereby simulating a metabolic disorder of the cortex. Hypoxia-ischemia is perhaps the best known and one in which it is not possible initially to distinguish the acute reversible effects of hypoperfusion and oxygen deprivation of the brain from the subsequent effects of neuronal damage. Similar bihemispheral damage is produced by disorders that occlude small blood vessels throughout the brain; examples include cerebral malaria, thrombotic thrombocytopenic purpura, and hyperviscosity. Diffuse white matter damage from cranial trauma or inflammatory demyelinating diseases causes a similar syndrome of coma.

APPROACH TO THE PATIENT: Coma

Acute respiratory and cardiovascular problems should be attended to prior to neurologic assessment. In most instances, a complete medical evaluation, except for vital signs, funduscopy, and examination for nuchal rigidity, may be deferred until the neurologic evaluation has established the severity and nature of coma. The approach to the patient with coma from cranial trauma is discussed in Chap. 378.

HISTORY In many cases, the cause of coma is immediately evident (e.g., trauma, cardiac arrest, or reported drug ingestion). In the remainder, certain points are especially useful: (1) the circumstances and rapidity with which neurologic symptoms developed; (2) the antecedent symptoms (confusion, weakness, headache, fever, seizures, dizziness, double vision, or vomiting); (3) the use of medications, illicit drugs, or alcohol; and (4) chronic liver, kidney, lung, heart, or other medical disease. Direct interrogation of family, observers, and ambulance technicians on the scene, in person or by telephone, is an important part of the evaluation.

GENERAL PHYSICAL EXAMINATION Fever suggests a systemic infection, bacterial meningitis, encephalitis, heat stroke, neuroleptic malignant syndrome, malignant hyperthermia due to anesthetics or anticholinergic drug intoxication; only rarely is it attributable to a lesion that has disturbed hypothalamic temperature-regulating centers ("*central fever*"). A slight elevation in temperature may follow vigorous convulsions. Hypothermia is observed with exposure; alcoholic, barbiturate, sedative, or phenothiazine intoxication; hypoglycemia; peripheral circulatory failure; or extreme hypothyroidism. Hypothermia itself causes coma only when the temperature is <31°C (87.8°F). Tachypnea may indicate systemic acidosis or pneumonia or rarely infiltration of the brain with lymphoma. Aberrant respiratory patterns that reflect brainstem disorders are discussed below. Marked hypertension suggests hypertensive encephalopathy, but it may also be secondary to a rapid rise in intracranial pressure (ICP) (the Cushing response) most often after cerebral hemorrhage or head injury. Hypotension is characteristic of coma from alcohol or barbiturate intoxication, internal hemorrhage, myocardial infarction, sepsis, profound hypothyroidism, or Addisonian crisis.

The funduscopic examination can detect subarachnoid hemorrhage (subhyaloid hemorrhages), hypertensive encephalopathy (exudates, hemorrhages, vessel-crossing changes, papilledema), and increased ICP (papilledema). Cutaneous petechiae suggest thrombotic thrombocytopenic purpura, meningococcemia, or a bleeding diathesis associated with an intracerebral hemorrhage. Cyanosis, reddish or anemic skin coloration are other indications of an underlying systemic disease responsible for the coma.

NEUROLOGIC EXAMINATION The patient should first be observed without intervention by the examiner. Tossing about in the bed, reaching up toward the face, crossing legs, yawning, swallowing, coughing, or moaning reflect a drowsy state that is close to normal awakeness. Lack of restless movements on one side or an outturned leg suggests a hemiplegia. Intermittent twitching movements of a foot, finger, or facial muscle may be the only sign of seizures. Multifocal myoclonus almost always indicates a metabolic disorder, particularly uremia, anoxia, drug intoxication (especially with lithium or haloperidol), or a prion disease (Chap. 383). In a drowsy and confused patient, bilateral *asterixis* is a certain sign of metabolic encephalopathy or drug intoxication.

Decorticate rigidity and *decerebrate rigidity*, or "posturing," describe stereotyped arm and leg movements occurring spontaneously or elicited by sensory stimulation. Flexion of the elbows and wrists and supination of the arm (decortication) suggests bilateral damage rostral to the midbrain, whereas extension of the elbows and wrists with pronation (decerebration) indicates damage to motor tracts in the midbrain or caudal diencephalon. The less frequent combination of arm extension with leg flexion or flaccid legs is associated with lesions in the pons. These concepts have been adapted from animal work and cannot be applied with precision to coma in humans. In fact, acute and widespread disorders of any type, regardless of location, frequently cause limb extension, and almost all extensor posturing becomes predominantly flexor as time passes.

LEVEL OF AROUSAL A sequence of increasingly intense stimuli is used to determine the threshold for arousal and the motor response of each side of the body. The results of testing may vary from minute to minute, and serial examinations are most useful. Tickling the nostrils with a cotton wisp is a moderate stimulus to arousal—all but deeply stuporous and comatose patients will move the head away and arouse to some degree. An even greater degree of responsiveness is present if the patient uses his hand to remove an offending stimulus. Pressure on the knuckles or bony prominences and pinprick stimulation are humane forms of noxious stimuli; pinching the skin causes unsightly ecchymoses and is generally not necessary but may be useful in eliciting abduction withdrawal movements of the limbs. Posturing in response to noxious stimuli indicates severe damage to the corticospinal system, whereas abduction-avoidance movement of a limb is usually purposeful and denotes an intact corticospinal system. Posturing may also be unilateral and coexists with purposeful limb movements, reflecting incomplete damage to the motor system.

BRAINSTEM REFLEXES Assessment of brainstem function is essential to localization of the lesion in coma (Fig. 274-3). The brainstem reflexes that are conveniently examined are pupillary size and reaction to light, spontaneous and elicited eye movements, corneal responses, and the respiratory pattern. As a rule, coma is due to bilateral hemispheral disease when these brainstem activities are preserved, particularly the pupillary reactions and eye movements. However, the presence of abnormal brainstem signs does not always indicate that the primary lesion is in the brainstem because hemispheral masses can cause secondary brainstem pathology by transtentorial herniation.

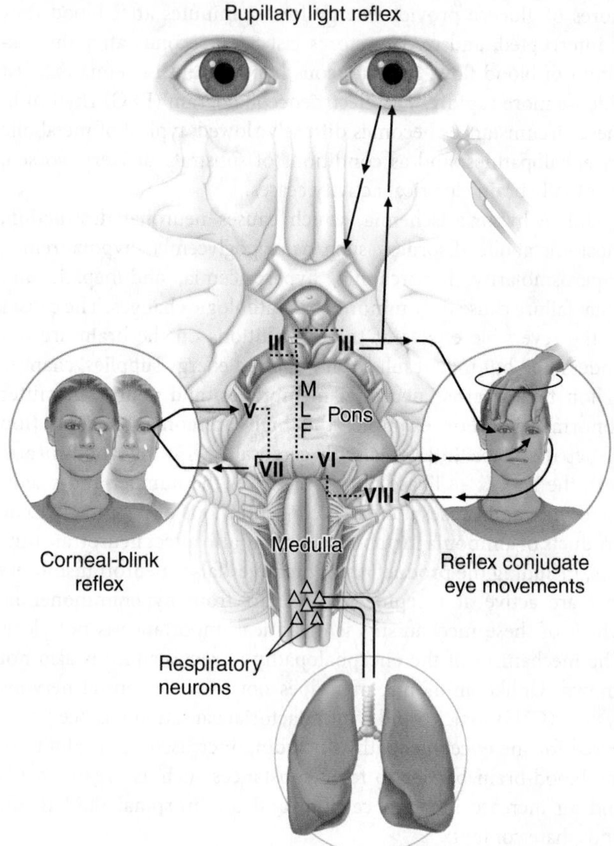

Figure 274-3 Examination of brainstem reflexes in coma. Midbrain and third nerve function are tested by pupillary reaction to light, pontine function by spontaneous and reflex eye movements and corneal responses, and medullary function by respiratory and pharyngeal responses. Reflex conjugate, horizontal eye movements are dependent on the medial longitudinal fasciculus (MLF) interconnecting the sixth and contralateral third nerve nuclei. Head rotation (oculocephalic reflex) or caloric stimulation of the labyrinths (oculovestibular reflex) elicits contraversive eye movements (for details see text).

Pupillary Signs Pupillary reactions are examined with a bright, diffuse light (not an ophthalmoscope). Reactive and round pupils of midsize (2.5–5 mm) essentially exclude midbrain damage, either primary or secondary to compression. A response to light may be difficult to appreciate in pupils <2 mm in diameter, and bright room lighting mutes pupillary reactivity. One enlarged and poorly reactive pupil (>6 mm) signifies compression or stretching of the third nerve from the effects of a cerebral mass above. Enlargement of the pupil contralateral to a hemispheral mass may occur but is infrequent. An oval and slightly eccentric pupil is a transitional sign that accompanies early midbrain–third nerve compression. The most extreme pupillary sign, bilaterally dilated and unreactive pupils, indicates severe midbrain damage, usually from compression by a supratentorial mass. Ingestion of drugs with anticholinergic activity, the use of mydriatic eye drops, and direct ocular trauma are among the causes of misleading pupillary enlargement.

Unilateral miosis in coma has been attributed to dysfunction of sympathetic efferents originating in the posterior hypothalamus and descending in the tegmentum of the brainstem to the cervical cord. It is therefore of limited localizing value but is an occasional finding in patients with a large cerebral hemorrhage that affects the thalamus. Reactive and bilaterally small (1–2.5 mm) but not pinpoint pupils are seen in metabolic encephalopathies or in deep bilateral hemispheral lesions such as hydrocephalus or thalamic hemorrhage. Even smaller reactive pupils (<1 mm) characterize narcotic or barbiturate overdoses but also occur with extensive pontine hemorrhage. The response to naloxone and the presence of reflex eye movements (see below) assist in distinguishing these.

Ocular Movements The eyes are first observed by elevating the lids and noting the resting position and spontaneous movements of the globes. Lid tone, tested by lifting the eyelids and noting their resistance to opening and the speed of closure, is progressively reduced as unresponsiveness progresses. Horizontal divergence of the eyes at rest is normal in drowsiness. As coma deepens, the ocular axes may become parallel again.

Spontaneous eye movements in coma often take the form of conjugate horizontal roving. This finding alone exonerates damage in the midbrain and pons and has the same significance as normal reflex eye movements (see below). Conjugate horizontal ocular deviation to one side indicates damage to the pons on the opposite side or alternatively, to the frontal lobe on the same side. This phenomenon is summarized by the following maxim: *The eyes look toward a hemispheral lesion and away from a brainstem lesion.* Seizures also drive the eyes to one side but usually with superimposed clonic movements of the globes. The eyes may occasionally turn paradoxically away from the side of a deep hemispheral lesion ("wrong-way eyes"). The eyes turn down and inward with thalamic and upper midbrain lesions, typically thalamic hemorrhage. "Ocular bobbing" describes brisk downward and slow upward movements of the eyes associated with loss of horizontal eye movements and is diagnostic of bilateral pontine damage, usually from thrombosis of the basilar artery. "Ocular dipping" is a slower, arrhythmic downward movement followed by a faster upward movement in patients with normal reflex horizontal gaze; it indicates diffuse cortical anoxic damage.

The oculocephalic reflexes, elicited by moving the head from side to side or vertically and observing eye movements in the direction opposite to the head movement, depend on the integrity of the ocular motor nuclei and their interconnecting tracts that extend from the midbrain to the pons and medulla (Fig. 274-3). The movements, called somewhat inappropriately "doll's eyes" (which refers more accurately to the reflex elevation of the eyelids with flexion of the neck), are normally suppressed in the awake patient. The ability to elicit them therefore indicates both reduced cortical influence on the brainstem and intact brainstem pathways, indicating that coma is caused by a lesion or dysfunction in the cerebral hemispheres. The opposite, an absence of reflex eye movements, usually signifies damage within the brainstem but can result infrequently from overdoses of certain drugs. Normal pupillary size and light reaction distinguishes most drug-induced comas from structural brainstem damage.

Thermal, or "caloric," stimulation of the vestibular apparatus (oculovestibular response) provides a more intense stimulus for the oculocephalic reflex but provides essentially the same information. The test is performed by irrigating the external auditory canal with cool water in order to induce convection currents in the labyrinths. After a brief latency, the result is tonic deviation of both eyes to the side of cool-water irrigation and nystagmus in the opposite direction. (The acronym "COWS" has been used to remind generations of medical students of the direction of nystagmus—"*c*old water *o*pposite, *w*arm water *s*ame.") The loss of induced conjugate ocular movements indicates brainstem damage. The presence of corrective nystagmus indicates that the frontal lobes are functioning and connected to the brainstem; thus functional or hysterical coma is likely.

By touching the cornea with a wisp of cotton, a response consisting of brief bilateral lid closure is normally observed. The corneal reflex depends on the integrity of pontine pathways between the fifth (afferent) and both seventh (efferent) cranial nerves; in conjunction with reflex eye movements, it is a useful test of pontine function. CNS-depressant drugs diminish or eliminate the corneal responses soon after reflex eye movements are paralyzed but before the pupils become unreactive to light. The corneal (and pharyngeal) response may be lost for a time on the side of an acute hemiplegia.

Respiratory Patterns These are of less localizing value in comparison to other brainstem signs. Shallow, slow, but regular breathing suggests metabolic or drug depression. Cheyne-Stokes respiration in its classic cyclic form, ending with a brief apneic period, signifies bihemispheral damage or metabolic suppression and commonly accompanies light coma. Rapid, deep (Kussmaul) breathing usually implies metabolic acidosis but may also occur with pontomesencephalic lesions. Tachypnea occurs with lymphoma of the CNS. Agonal gasps are the result of lower brainstem (medullary) damage and are recognized as the terminal respiratory pattern of severe brain damage. A number of other cyclic breathing variations have been described but are of lesser significance.

LABORATORY STUDIES AND IMAGING

The studies that are most useful in the diagnosis of coma are: chemical-toxicologic analysis of blood and urine, cranial CT or MRI, EEG, and CSF examination. Arterial blood gas analysis is helpful in patients with lung disease and acid-base disorders. The metabolic aberrations commonly encountered in clinical practice require measurement of electrolytes, glucose, calcium, osmolarity, and renal (blood urea nitrogen) and hepatic (NH_3) function. Toxicologic analysis is necessary in any case of acute coma where the diagnosis is not immediately clear. However, the presence of exogenous drugs or toxins, especially alcohol, does not exclude the possibility that other factors, particularly head trauma, are also contributing to the clinical state. An ethanol level of 43 mmol/L (0.2 g/dL) in nonhabituated patients generally causes impaired mental activity; a level of >65 mmol/L (0.3 g/dL) is associated with stupor. The development of tolerance may allow the chronic alcoholic to remain awake at levels >87 mmol/L (0.4 g/dL).

The availability of CT and MRI has focused attention on causes of coma that are detectable by imaging (e.g., hemorrhage, tumor, or hydrocephalus). Resorting primarily to this approach, although at times expedient, is imprudent because most cases of coma (and confusion) are metabolic or toxic in origin. Furthermore, the notion that a normal CT scan excludes anatomic lesion as the cause of coma is erroneous. Bilateral hemisphere infarction, acute brainstem infarction, encephalitis, meningitis, mechanical shearing of axons as a result of closed head trauma, sagittal sinus thrombosis, and subdural hematoma isodense to adjacent brain are some of the disorders that may not be detected. Nevertheless, if the source of coma remains unknown, a scan should be obtained.

The EEG (Chap. e45) is useful in metabolic or drug-induced states but is rarely diagnostic, except when coma is due to clinically unrecognized seizure, to herpesvirus encephalitis, or to prion (Creutzfeldt-Jakob) disease. The amount of background slowing of the EEG is a reflection of the severity of an encephalopathy. Predominant high-voltage slowing (δ or triphasic waves) in the frontal regions is typical of metabolic coma, as from hepatic failure, and widespread fast (β) activity implicates sedative drugs (e.g., diazepines, barbiturates). A special pattern of "alpha coma," defined by widespread, variable 8- to 12-Hz activity, superficially resembles the normal α rhythm of waking but, unlike normal α activity, is not altered by environmental stimuli. Alpha coma results from pontine or diffuse cortical damage and is associated with a poor prognosis. Normal α activity on the EEG, which is suppressed by stimulating the patient, also alerts the clinician to the locked-in syndrome or to hysteria or catatonia. The most important use of EEG recordings in coma is to reveal clinically inapparent epileptic discharges.

Lumbar puncture is performed less frequently than in the past for coma diagnosis because neuroimaging effectively excludes intracerebral and extensive subarachnoid hemorrhage. However, examination of the CSF remains indispensable in the diagnosis of meningitis and encephalitis. For patients with an altered level of consciousness, it is generally recommended that an imaging study be performed prior to lumbar puncture to exclude a large intracranial mass lesion. Blood culture and antibiotic administration usually precede the imaging study if meningitis is suspected (Chap. e46).

■ DIFFERENTIAL DIAGNOSIS OF COMA

(Table 274-1) The causes of coma can be divided into three broad categories: those without focal neurologic signs (e.g., metabolic and toxic encephalopathies); meningitis syndromes, characterized by fever or stiff neck and an excess of cells in the spinal fluid (e.g., bacterial meningitis, subarachnoid hemorrhage); and conditions associated with prominent focal signs (e.g., stroke, cerebral hemorrhage). In most instances, coma is part of an obvious medical problem, such as drug ingestion, hypoxia, stroke, trauma, or liver or kidney failure. Conditions that cause sudden coma include drug ingestion, cerebral hemorrhage, trauma, cardiac arrest, epilepsy, or basilar artery embolism. Coma that appears subacutely is usually related to a preexisting medical or neurologic problem or, less often, to secondary brain swelling of a mass such as tumor or cerebral infarction.

When cerebrovascular disease is the cause of coma, diagnosis can be difficult (Chap. 370). The most common diseases are (1) basal ganglia and thalamic hemorrhage (acute but not instantaneous onset, vomiting, headache, hemiplegia, and characteristic eye signs); (2) pontine hemorrhage (sudden onset, pinpoint pupils, loss of reflex eye movements and corneal responses, ocular bobbing, posturing, hyperventilation, and excessive sweating); (3) cerebellar hemorrhage (occipital headache, vomiting, gaze paresis, and inability to stand); (4) basilar artery thrombosis (neurologic prodrome or warning spells, diplopia, dysarthria, vomiting, eye movement and corneal response abnormalities, and asymmetric limb paresis); and (5) subarachnoid hemorrhage (precipitous coma after headache and vomiting). The most common stroke, infarction in the territory of the middle cerebral artery, does not generally cause coma, but edema surrounding large infarctions may expand during the first few days and act as a mass.

The syndrome of acute hydrocephalus accompanies many intracranial diseases, particularly subarachnoid hemorrhage. It is characterized by headache and sometimes vomiting that may progress quickly to coma with extensor posturing of the limbs, bilateral Babinski signs, small unreactive pupils, and impaired oculocephalic movements in the vertical direction.

If the history and examination do not indicate the cause of coma, then information obtained from CT or MRI is needed. The majority of medical causes of coma can be established without a neuroimaging study. Sometimes imaging results can be misleading such as when small subdural hematomas or old strokes are found, but the patient's coma is due to intoxication.

TABLE 274-1 Differential Diagnosis of Coma

1. Diseases that cause no focal or lateralizing neurologic signs, usually with normal brainstem functions; CT scan and cellular content of the CSF are normal
   a. Intoxications: alcohol, sedative drugs, opiates, etc.
   b. Metabolic disturbances: anoxia, hyponatremia, hypernatremia, hypercalcemia, diabetic acidosis, nonketotic hyperosmolar hyperglycemia, hypoglycemia, uremia, hepatic coma, hypercarbia, addisonian crisis, hypo- and hyperthyroid states, profound nutritional deficiency
   c. Severe systemic infections: pneumonia, septicemia, typhoid fever, malaria, Waterhouse-Friderichsen syndrome
   d. Shock from any cause
   e. Postseizure states, status epilepticus, subclinical epilepsy
   f. Hypertensive encephalopathy, eclampsia
   g. Severe hyperthermia, hypothermia
   h. Concussion
   i. Acute hydrocephalus
2. Diseases that cause meningeal irritation with or without fever, and with an excess of WBCs or RBCs in the CSF, usually without focal or lateralizing cerebral or brainstem signs; CT or MRI shows no mass lesion
   a. Subarachnoid hemorrhage from ruptured aneurysm, arteriovenous malformation, trauma
   b. Acute bacterial meningitis
   c. Viral encephalitis
   d. Miscellaneous: fat embolism, cholesterol embolism, carcinomatous and lymphomatous meningitis, etc.
3. Diseases that cause focal brainstem or lateralizing cerebral signs, with or without changes in the CSF; CT and MRI are abnormal
   a. Hemispheral hemorrhage (basal ganglionic, thalamic) or infarction (large middle cerebral artery territory) with secondary brainstem compression
   b. Brainstem infarction due to basilar artery thrombosis or embolism
   c. Brain abscess, subdural empyema
   d. Epidural and subdural hemorrhage, brain contusion
   e. Brain tumor with surrounding edema
   f. Cerebellar and pontine hemorrhage and infarction
   g. Widespread traumatic brain injury
   h. Metabolic coma (see above) with preexisting focal damage
   i. Miscellaneous: Cortical vein thrombosis, herpes simplex encephalitis, multiple cerebral emboli due to bacterial endocarditis, acute hemorrhagic leukoencephalitis, acute disseminated (postinfectious) encephalomyelitis, thrombotic thrombocytopenic purpura, cerebral vasculitis, gliomatosis cerebri, pituitary apoplexy, intravascular lymphoma, etc.

Abbreviations: CSF, cerebrospinal fluid; RBCs, red blood cells; WBCs, white blood cells.

■ BRAIN DEATH

This is a state of cessation of cerebral function with preservation of cardiac activity and maintenance of somatic function by artificial means. It is the only type of brain damage recognized as equivalent to death. Several sets of criteria have been advanced for the diagnosis of brain death and it is essential to adhere to those standards endorsed by the local medical community. Ideal criteria are simple, can be assessed at the bedside, and allow no chance of diagnostic error. They contain three essential elements: (1) widespread cortical destruction that is reflected by deep coma and unresponsiveness to all forms of stimulation; (2) global brainstem damage demonstrated by absent pupillary light reaction and by the loss of oculovestibular and corneal reflexes; and (3) destruction of the medulla, manifested by complete apnea. The heart rate is invariant and unresponsive to atropine. Diabetes insipidus is often present but may only develop hours or days after the other clinical signs of brain death. The pupils are usually midsized but may be enlarged; they should not, however, be small. Loss of deep tendon reflexes is not required because the spinal cord remains functional. Babinski signs are generally absent and the toe response is often flexor.

Demonstration that apnea is due to irreversible medullary damage requires that the Pco_2 be high enough to stimulate respiration during a test of spontaneous breathing. *Apnea testing* can be done safely by the use of diffusion oxygenation prior to removing the ventilator. This is accomplished by preoxygenation with 100% oxygen, which is then sustained during the test by oxygen administered through a tracheal cannula. co_2 tension increases ~0.3–0.4 kPa/min (2–3 mmHg/min) during apnea. At the end of a period of observation, typically several minutes, arterial Pco_2 should be at least >6.6–8.0 kPa (50–60 mmHg) for the test to be valid. Apnea is confirmed if no respiratory effort has been observed in the presence of a sufficiently elevated Pco_2. Other techniques, including the administration of co_2 to accelerate the test, are used in special circumstances. The test is usually stopped if there is serious cardiovascular instability.

An isoelectric EEG may be used as a confirmatory test for total cerebral damage. Radionuclide brain scanning, cerebral angiography, or transcranial Doppler measurements may also be included to demonstrate the absence of CBF but they have not been extensively correlated with pathologic changes.

The possibility of profound drug-induced or hypothermic depression of the nervous system should be excluded, and some period of observation, usually 6–24 hours, is desirable, during which the clinical signs of brain death are sustained. It is advisable to delay clinical testing for at least 24 hours if a cardiac arrest has caused brain death or if the inciting disease is not known.

Although it is largely accepted in Western society that the respirator can be disconnected from a brain-dead patient, problems frequently arise because of poor communication and inadequate preparation of the family by the physician. Reasonable medical practice, ideally with the agreement of the family, allows the removal of support or transfer out of an intensive care unit of patients who are not brain dead but whose neurologic conditions are nonetheless hopeless.

TREATMENT Coma

The immediate goal in a comatose patient is prevention of further nervous system damage. Hypotension, hypoglycemia, hypercalcemia, hypoxia, hypercapnia, and hyperthermia should be corrected rapidly. An oropharyngeal airway is adequate to keep the pharynx open in a drowsy patient who is breathing normally. Tracheal intubation is indicated if there is apnea, upper airway obstruction, hypoventilation, or emesis, or if the patient is liable to aspirate because of coma. Mechanical ventilation is required if there is hypoventilation or a need to induce hypocapnia in order to lower ICP. IV access is established, and naloxone and dextrose are administered if narcotic overdose or hypoglycemia are possibilities; thiamine is given along with glucose to avoid provoking Wernicke's disease in malnourished patients. In cases of suspected basilar thrombosis with brainstem ischemia, IV heparin or a thrombolytic agent is often utilized, after cerebral hemorrhage has been excluded by a neuroimaging study. Physostigmine may awaken patients with anticholinergic-type drug overdose but should be used only with careful monitoring; many physicians believe that it should only be used to treat anticholinergic overdose–associated cardiac arrhythmias. The use of benzodiazepine antagonists offers some prospect of improvement after overdose of soporific drugs and has transient benefit in hepatic encephalopathy.

Administration of hypotonic solutions should be monitored carefully in any serious acute brain illness because of the potential for exacerbating brain swelling. Cervical spine injuries must not be overlooked, particularly before attempting intubation or evaluation of oculocephalic responses. Fever and meningismus indicate an urgent need for examination of the CSF to diagnose meningitis. If the lumbar puncture in a case of suspected meningitis is delayed, an antibiotic such as a third-generation cephalosporin may be administered, preferably after obtaining blood cultures. The management of raised ICP is discussed in Chap. 275.

PROGNOSIS

One hopes to avoid the anguishing outcome of a patient who is left severely disabled or vegetative. The uniformly poor outcome of the persistent vegetative state has already been mentioned. Children and young adults may have ominous early clinical findings such as abnormal brainstem reflexes and yet recover; temporization in offering a prognosis in this group of patients is wise. Metabolic comas have a far better prognosis than traumatic ones. All systems for estimating prognosis in adults should be taken as approximations, and medical judgments must be tempered by factors such as age, underlying systemic disease, and general medical condition. In an attempt to collect prognostic information from large numbers of patients with head injury, the Glasgow Coma Scale was devised; empirically, it has predictive value in cases of brain trauma (Table 378-2). For anoxic and metabolic coma, clinical signs such as the pupillary and motor responses after 1 day, 3 days, and 1 week have been shown to have predictive value (Fig. 275-4). Other studies suggest that the absence of corneal responses may have the most discriminative value. The absence of the cortical waves of the somatosensory evoked potentials has also proved a strong indicator of poor outcome in coma from any cause.

There have been recent advances using functional imaging that demonstrate some preserved cognitive abilities of vegetative and minimally conscious patients. In one series, about 10% of such patients could be trained to activate the frontal or temporal lobes in response to requests by an examiner to imagine certain visuospatial tasks. In one case, a rudimentary form of one-way communication could be established. There are also reports in a limited number of patients of improvement in cognitive function with the implantation of thalamic-stimulating electrodes. It is prudent to avoid generalizations from these experiments.

FURTHER READINGS

Booth CM et al: Is this patient dead, vegetative, or severely impaired? JAMA 291:870, 2004

Monti MM et al: Willful modulation of brain activity in disorders of consciousness. N Engl J Med 362:579, 2010

Posner JB et al: *Plum and Posner's Diagnosis of Stupor and Coma*, 4th ed. New York, Oxford University Press, 2007

Ropper AH et al: *Neurological and Neurosurgical Intensive Care*, 4th ed. New York, Lippincott Williams & Wilkins, 2004

Wijdicks EF et al: Neuropathology of brain death in the modern transplant era. Neurology 70:1234, 2008

Young GB: Clinical Practice. Neurologic prognosis after cardiac arrest. N Engl J Med 361:605, 2009

——— Wijdicks EF: Disorders of Consciousness, in *Handbook of Clinical Neurology*, v 90, 3rd series, MJ Aminoff et al (eds). Edinburg, Elsevier, 2008

CHAPTER 275

Neurologic Critical Care, Including Hypoxic-Ischemic Encephalopathy, and Subarachnoid Hemorrhage

J. Claude Hemphill, III
Wade S. Smith
Daryl R. Gress

Life-threatening neurologic illness may be caused by a primary disorder affecting any region of the neuraxis or may occur as a consequence of a systemic disorder such as hepatic failure, multisystem organ failure, or cardiac arrest (Table 275-1). Neurologic critical care focuses on preservation of neurologic tissue and prevention of secondary brain injury caused by ischemia, edema, and elevated intracranial pressure (ICP). Management of other organ systems proceeds concurrently and may need to be modified in order to maintain the overall focus on neurologic issues.

PATHOPHYSIOLOGY

Brain edema

Swelling, or edema, of brain tissue occurs with many types of brain injury. The two principal types of edema are vasogenic and cytotoxic. *Vasogenic edema* refers to the influx of fluid and solutes into the brain through an incompetent blood-brain barrier (BBB). In the normal cerebral vasculature, endothelial tight junctions associated with astrocytes create an impermeable barrier (the BBB), through which access into the brain interstitium is dependent upon specific transport mechanisms. The BBB may be compromised in ischemia, trauma, infection, and metabolic derangements. Typically, vasogenic edema develops rapidly following injury. *Cytotoxic edema* refers to cellular swelling and occurs in a variety of settings, including brain ischemia and trauma. Early astrocytic swelling is a hallmark of ischemia. Brain edema that is clinically significant usually represents a combination of vasogenic and cellular components. Edema can lead to increased ICP as well as tissue shifts and brain displacement from focal processes (Chap. 274). These tissue shifts can cause injury by mechanical distention and compression in addition to the ischemia of impaired perfusion consequent to the elevated ICP.

Ischemic cascade and cellular injury

When delivery of substrates, principally oxygen and glucose, is inadequate to sustain cellular function, a series of interrelated biochemical reactions known as the *ischemic cascade* is initiated (see Fig. 370-2). The release of excitatory amino acids, especially glutamate, leads to influx of calcium and sodium ions, which disrupt cellular homeostasis. An increased intracellular calcium concentration may activate proteases and lipases, which then lead to lipid peroxidation and free radical–mediated cell membrane injury. Cytotoxic edema ensues, and ultimately necrotic cell death and tissue infarction occur. This pathway to irreversible cell death

TABLE 275-1 Neurologic Disorders in Critical Illness

Localization Along Neuroaxis	Syndrome
Central Nervous System	
Brain: Cerebral hemispheres	Global encephalopathy
	Delirium
	Sepsis
	Organ failure—hepatic, renal
	Medication related—sedatives, hypnotics, analgesics, H_2 blockers, antihypertensives
	Drug overdose
	Electrolyte disturbance—hyponatremia, hypoglycemia
	Hypotension/hypoperfusion
	Hypoxia
	Meningitis
	Subarachnoid hemorrhage
	Wernicke's disease
	Seizure—postictal or nonconvulsive status
	Hypertensive encephalopathy
	Hypothyroidism—myxedema
	Focal deficits
	Ischemic stroke
	Tumor
	Abscess, subdural empyema
	Subdural/epidural hematoma
Brainstem	Mass effect and compression
	Ischemic stroke, intraparenchymal hemorrhage
	Hypoxia
Spinal cord	Mass effect and compression
	Disk herniation
	Epidural hematoma
	Ischemia—hypotension/embolic
	Epidural abscess
	Trauma, central cord syndrome
Peripheral Nervous System	
Peripheral nerve	
Axonal	Critical illness polyneuropathy
	Possible neuromuscular blocking agent complication
	Metabolic disturbances, uremia, hyperglycemia
	Medication effects—chemotherapeutic, antiretroviral
Demyelinating	Guillain-Barré syndrome
	Chronic inflammatory demyelinating polyneuropathy
Neuromuscular junction	Prolonged effect of neuromuscular blockade
	Medication effects—aminoglycosides
	Myasthenia gravis, Lambert-Eaton syndrome
Muscle	Critical illness myopathy
	Septic myopathy
	Cachectic myopathy—with or without disuse atrophy
	Electrolyte disturbances—hypokalemia/hyperkalemia, hypophosphatemia
	Acute quadriplegic myopathy

is common to ischemic stroke, global cerebral ischemia, and traumatic brain injury. *Penumbra* refers to areas of ischemic brain tissue that have not yet undergone irreversible infarction, implying that these regions are potentially salvageable if ischemia can be reversed. Factors that may exacerbate ischemic brain injury include systemic hypotension and hypoxia, which further reduce substrate delivery to vulnerable brain tissue, and fever, seizures, and hyperglycemia, which can increase cellular metabolism, outstripping compensatory processes. Clinically, these events are known as *secondary brain insults* because they lead to exacerbation of the primary brain injury. Prevention, identification, and treatment of secondary brain insults are fundamental goals of management.

An alternative pathway of cellular injury is *apoptosis*. This process implies programmed cell death, which may occur in the setting of ischemic stroke, global cerebral ischemia, traumatic brain injury, and possibly intracerebral hemorrhage. Apoptotic cell death can be distinguished histologically from the necrotic cell death of ischemia and is mediated through a different set of biochemical pathways. At present, interventions for prevention and treatment of apoptotic cell death remain less well defined than those for ischemia. Excitotoxicity and mechanisms of cell death are discussed in more detail in Chap. 366.

Cerebral perfusion and autoregulation

Brain tissue requires constant perfusion in order to ensure adequate delivery of substrate. The hemodynamic response of the brain has the capacity to preserve perfusion across a wide range of systemic blood pressures. Cerebral perfusion pressure (CPP), defined as the mean systemic arterial pressure (MAP) minus the ICP, provides the driving force for circulation across the capillary beds of the brain. *Autoregulation* refers to the physiologic response whereby cerebral blood flow (CBF) is regulated via alterations in cerebrovascular resistance in order to maintain perfusion over wide physiologic changes such as neuronal activation or changes in hemodynamic function. If systemic blood pressure drops, cerebral perfusion is preserved through vasodilation of arterioles in the brain; likewise, arteriolar vasoconstriction occurs at high systemic pressures to prevent hyperperfusion, resulting in fairly constant perfusion across a wide range of systemic blood pressures (Fig. 275-1). At the extreme limits of MAP or CPP (high or low), flow becomes directly related to perfusion pressure. These autoregulatory changes occur in the microcirculation and are mediated by vessels below the resolution of those seen on angiography. CBF is also strongly influenced by pH and Pa_{CO_2}. CBF increases with hypercapnia and acidosis and decreases with hypocapnia and alkalosis. This forms the basis for the use of hyperventilation to lower ICP, and this effect on ICP is mediated through a decrease in intracranial blood volume. Cerebral autoregulation is a complex process critical to the normal homeostatic functioning of the brain, and this process may be disordered focally and unpredictably in disease states such as traumatic brain injury and severe focal cerebral ischemia.

Cerebrospinal fluid and intracranial pressure

The cranial contents consist essentially of brain, cerebrospinal fluid (CSF), and blood. CSF is produced principally in the choroid plexus of each lateral ventricle, exits the brain via the foramens of Luschka and Magendi, and flows over the cortex to be absorbed into the venous system along the superior sagittal sinus. Approximately 150 mL of CSF are contained within the ventricles and surrounding the brain and spinal cord; the cerebral blood volume is also ~150 mL. The bony skull offers excellent protection for the brain but allows little tolerance for additional volume. Significant increases in volume eventually result in increased ICP. Obstruction of CSF outflow, edema of cerebral tissue, or increases in volume from tumor or hematoma may increase ICP. Elevated ICP diminishes cerebral perfusion and can lead to tissue ischemia. Ischemia in turn may lead to vasodilation via autoregulatory mechanisms designed to restore cerebral perfusion. However, vasodilation also increases cerebral blood volume, which in turn then increases ICP, lowers CPP, and provokes further ischemia (Fig. 275-2). This vicious cycle is commonly seen in traumatic brain injury, massive intracerebral hemorrhage, and large hemispheric infarcts with significant tissue shifts.

APPROACH TO THE PATIENT Severe CNS Dysfunction

Critically ill patients with severe central nervous system dysfunction require rapid evaluation and intervention in order to limit primary and secondary brain injury. Initial neurologic evaluation should be performed concurrent with stabilization of basic respiratory, cardiac, and hemodynamic parameters. Significant barriers may exist to neurologic assessment in the

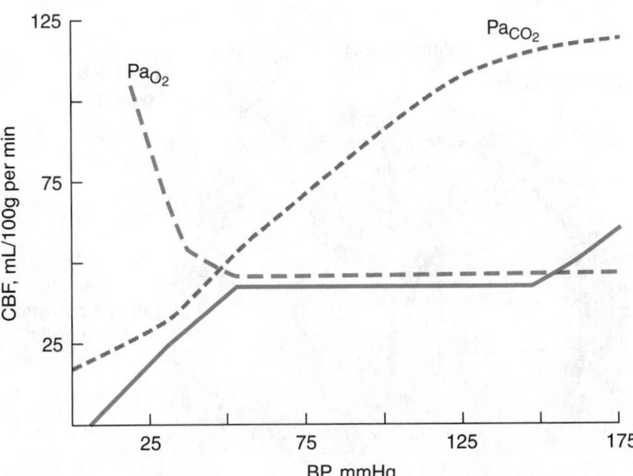

Figure 275-1 Autoregulation of cerebral blood flow (*solid line*). Cerebral perfusion is constant over a wide range of systemic blood pressure. Perfusion is increased in the setting of hypoxia or hypercarbia. BP, blood pressure; CBF, cerebral blood flow. *(Reprinted with permission from HM Shapiro: Anesthesiology 43:447, 1975. Copyright 1975, Lippincott Company.)*

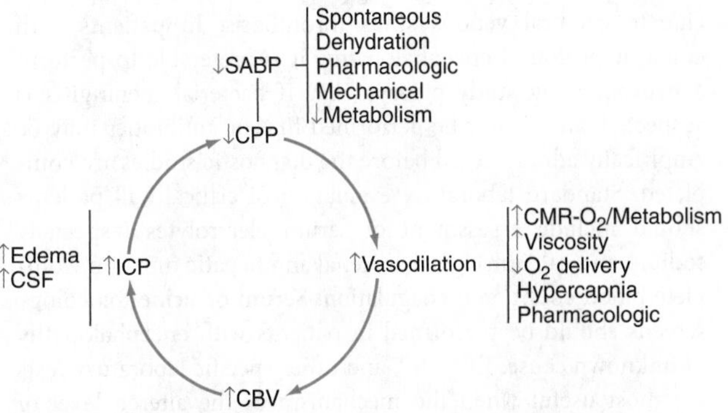

Figure 275-2 Ischemia and vasodilatation. Reduced cerebral perfusion pressure (CPP) leads to increased ischemia, vasodilation, increased intracranial pressure (ICP), and further reductions in CPP, a cycle leading to further neurologic injury. CBV, cerebral blood volume; CMR, cerebral metabolic rate; CSF, cerebrospinal fluid; SABP, systolic arterial blood pressure. *(Adapted from MJ Rosner et al: J Neurosurg 83:949, 1995; with permission.)*

critical care unit, including endotracheal intubation and the use of sedative or paralytic agents to facilitate procedures.

An impaired level of consciousness is common in critically ill patients. The essential first task in assessment is to determine whether the cause of dysfunction is related to a diffuse, usually metabolic, process or whether a focal, usually structural, process is implicated. Examples of diffuse processes include metabolic encephalopathies related to organ failure, drug overdose, or hypoxia-ischemia. Focal processes include ischemic and hemorrhagic stroke and traumatic brain injury, especially with intracranial hematomas. Since these two categories of disorders have fundamentally different causes, treatments, and prognoses, the initial focus is on making this distinction rapidly and accurately. The approach to the comatose patient is discussed in Chap. 274; etiologies are listed in Table 274-1.

Minor focal deficits may be present on the neurologic examination in patients with metabolic encephalopathies. However, the finding of prominent focal signs such as pupillary asymmetry, hemiparesis, gaze palsy, or paraplegia should suggest the possibility of a structural lesion. All patients with a decreased level of consciousness associated with focal findings should undergo an urgent neuroimaging procedure, as should all patients with coma of unknown etiology. CT scanning is usually the most appropriate initial study because it can be performed quickly in critically ill patients and demonstrates hemorrhage, hydrocephalus, and intracranial tissue shifts well. MRI may provide more specific information in some situations, such as acute ischemic stroke (diffusion-weighted imaging, DWI) and cerebral venous sinus thrombosis (magnetic resonance venography, MRV). Any suggestion of trauma from the history or examination should alert the examiner to the possibility of cervical spine injury and prompt an imaging evaluation using plain x-rays, CT, or MRI.

Other diagnostic studies are best utilized in specific circumstances, usually when neuroimaging studies fail to reveal a structural lesion and the etiology of the altered mental state remains uncertain. Electroencephalography (EEG) can be important in the evaluation of critically ill patients with severe brain dysfunction. The EEG of metabolic encephalopathy typically reveals generalized slowing. One of the most important uses of EEG is to help exclude inapparent seizures, especially nonconvulsive status epilepticus. Untreated continuous or frequently recurrent seizures may cause neuronal injury, making the diagnosis and treatment of seizures crucial in this patient group. Lumbar puncture (LP) may be necessary to exclude infectious processes, and an elevated opening pressure may be an important clue to cerebral venous sinus thrombosis. In patients with coma or profound encephalopathy, it is preferable to perform a neuroimaging study prior to LP. If bacterial meningitis is suspected, an LP may be performed first or antibiotics may be empirically administered before the diagnostic studies are completed. Standard laboratory evaluation of critically ill patients should include assessment of serum electrolytes (especially sodium and calcium), glucose, renal and hepatic function, complete blood count, and coagulation. Serum or urine toxicology screens should be performed in patients with encephalopathy of unknown cause. EEG, LP, and other specific laboratory tests are most useful when the mechanism of the altered level of consciousness is uncertain; they are not routinely performed in clear-cut cases of stroke or traumatic brain injury.

Monitoring of ICP can be an important tool in selected patients. In general, patients who should be considered for ICP monitoring are those with primary neurologic disorders, such as stroke or traumatic brain injury, who are at significant risk for secondary brain injury due to elevated ICP and decreased CPP. Included are patients with the following: severe traumatic brain injury [Glasgow Coma Scale (GCS) score ≤ 8 (Table 378-2)]; large tissue shifts from supratentorial ischemic or hemorrhagic stroke; or hydrocephalus from subarachnoid hemorrhage (SAH), intraventricular hemorrhage, or posterior fossa stroke. An additional disorder in which ICP monitoring can add important information is fulminant hepatic failure, in which elevated ICP may be treated with barbiturates or, eventually, liver transplantation. In general, ventriculostomy is preferable to ICP monitoring devices that are placed in the brain parenchyma, because ventriculostomy allows CSF drainage as a method of treating elevated ICP. However, parenchymal ICP monitoring is most appropriate for patients with diffuse edema and small ventricles (which may make ventriculostomy placement more difficult) or any degree of coagulopathy (in which ventriculostomy carries a higher risk of hemorrhagic complications) (Fig 275-3).

Treatment of Elevated ICP Elevated ICP may occur in a wide range of disorders, including head trauma, intracerebral hemorrhage, SAH with hydrocephalus, and fulminant hepatic failure. Because CSF and blood volume can be redistributed initially, by the time elevated ICP occurs, intracranial compliance is severely impaired. At this point, any small increase in the volume of CSF, intravascular blood, edema, or a mass lesion may result in a significant increase in ICP and a decrease in cerebral perfusion. This is a fundamental mechanism of secondary ischemic brain injury and constitutes an emergency that requires immediate attention. In general, ICP should be maintained at <20 mmHg and CPP should be maintained at ≥60 mmHg.

Interventions to lower ICP are ideally based on the underlying mechanism responsible for the elevated ICP (Table 275-2). For example, in hydrocephalus from SAH, the principal cause of elevated ICP is impairment of CSF drainage. In this setting, ventricular drainage of CSF is likely to be sufficient and most appropriate. In head trauma and stroke, cytotoxic edema may be most responsible, and the use of osmotic agents such as mannitol or hypertonic saline becomes an appropriate early step. As

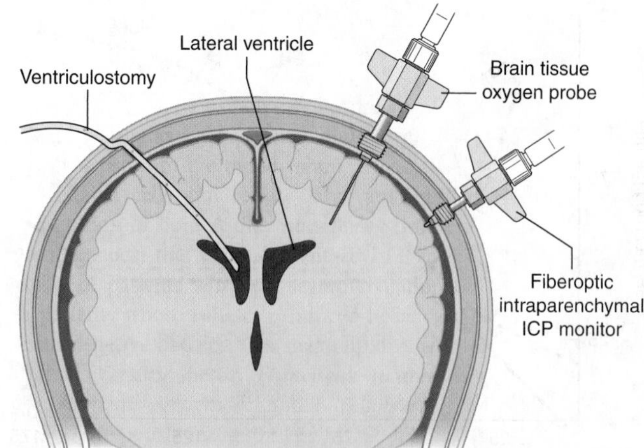

Figure 275-3 Intracranial pressure and brain tissue oxygen monitoring. A ventriculostomy allows for drainage of cerebrospinal fluid to treat elevated intracranial pressure (ICP). Fiberoptic ICP and brain tissue oxygen monitors are usually secured using a screwlike skull bolt. Cerebral blood flow and microdialysis probes (not shown) may be placed in a manner similar to the brain tissue oxygen probe.

TABLE 275-2 Stepwise Approach to Treatment of Elevated Intracranial Pressure*

Insert ICP monitor—ventriculostomy versus parenchymal device
General goals: maintain ICP <20 mmHg and CPP ≥60 mmHg
For ICP >20–25 mmHg for >5 min:

1. Drain CSF via ventriculostomy (if in place)
2. Elevate head of the bed; midline head position
3. Osmotherapy—mannitol 25–100 g q4h as needed (maintain serum osmolality <320 mosmol) or hypertonic saline (30 mL, 23.4% NaCl bolus)
4. Glucocorticoids—dexamethasone 4 mg q6h for vasogenic edema from tumor, abscess (avoid glucocorticoids in head trauma, ischemic and hemorrhagic stroke)
5. Sedation (e.g., morphine, propofol, or midazolam); add neuromuscular paralysis if necessary (patient will require endotracheal intubation and mechanical ventilation at this point, if not before)
6. Hyperventilation—to $PaCO_2$ 30–35 mmHg
7. Pressor therapy—phenylephrine, dopamine, or norepinephrine to maintain adequate MAP to ensure CPP ≥ 60 mmHg (maintain euvolemia to minimize deleterious systemic effects of pressors)
8. Consider second-tier therapies for refractory elevated ICP
   a. High-dose barbiturate therapy ("pentobarb coma")
   b. Aggressive hyperventilation to $PaCO_2$ <30 mmHg
   c. Hypothermia
   d. Hemicraniectomy

*Throughout ICP treatment algorithm, consider repeat head CT to identify mass lesions amenable to surgical evacuation.

Abbreviations: CPP, cerebral perfusion pressure; CSF, cerebrospinal fluid; MAP, mean arterial pressure; $PaCO_2$, arterial partial pressure of carbon dioxide.

described above, elevated ICP may cause tissue ischemia, and, if cerebral autoregulation is intact, the resulting vasodilation can lead to a cycle of worsening ischemia. Paradoxically, administration of vasopressor agents to increase mean arterial pressure may actually lower ICP by improving perfusion, thereby allowing autoregulatory vasoconstriction as ischemia is relieved and ultimately decreasing intracranial blood volume.

Early signs of elevated ICP include drowsiness and a diminished level of consciousness. Neuroimaging studies may reveal evidence of edema and mass effect. Hypotonic IV fluids should be avoided, and elevation of the head of the bed is recommended. Patients must be carefully observed for risk of aspiration and compromise of the airway as the level of alertness declines. Coma and unilateral pupillary changes are late signs and require immediate intervention. Emergent treatment of elevated ICP is most quickly achieved by intubation and hyperventilation, which causes vasoconstriction and reduces cerebral blood volume. In order to avoid provoking or worsening cerebral ischemia, hyperventilation is best used for short periods of time until a more definitive treatment can be instituted. Furthermore, the effects of hyperventilation on ICP are short-lived, often lasting only for several hours because of the buffering capacity of the cerebral interstitium, and rebound elevations of ICP may accompany abrupt discontinuation of hyperventilation. As the level of consciousness declines to coma, the ability to follow the neurologic status of the patient by examination deteriorates and measurement of ICP assumes greater importance. If a ventriculostomy device is in place, direct drainage of CSF to reduce ICP is possible. Finally, high-dose barbiturates, decompressive hemicraniectomy, or hypothermia are sometimes used for refractory elevations of ICP, although these have significant side effects and have not been proven to improve outcome.

Secondary Brain Insults Patients with primary brain injuries, whether due to trauma or stroke, are at risk for ongoing secondary ischemic brain injury. Because secondary brain injury can be a major determinant of a poor outcome, strategies for minimizing secondary brain insults are an integral part of the critical care of all patients. While elevated ICP may lead to secondary ischemia, most secondary brain injury is mediated through other clinical events that exacerbate the ischemic cascade already initiated by the primary brain injury. Episodes of secondary brain insults are usually not associated with apparent neurologic worsening. Rather, they lead to cumulative injury limiting eventual recovery, which manifests as higher mortality rate or worsened long-term functional outcome. Thus, close monitoring of vital signs is important, as is early intervention to prevent secondary ischemia. Avoiding hypotension and hypoxia is critical, as significant hypotensive events (systolic blood pressure < 90 mmHg) as short as 10 min in duration have been shown to adversely influence outcome after traumatic brain injury. Even in patients with stroke or head trauma who do not require ICP monitoring, close attention to adequate cerebral perfusion is warranted. Hypoxia (pulse oximetry saturation < 90%), particularly in combination with hypotension, also leads to secondary brain injury. Likewise, fever and hyperglycemia both worsen experimental ischemia and have been associated with worsened clinical outcome after stroke and head trauma. Aggressive control of fever with a goal of normothermia is warranted but may be difficult to achieve with antipyretic medications and cooling blankets. The value of newer surface or intravascular temperature control devices for the management of refractory fever is under investigation. The use of IV insulin infusion is encouraged for control of hyperglycemia as this allows better regulation of serum glucose levels than SC insulin. A reasonable goal is to maintain the serum glucose level at <7.8 mmol/L (<140 mg/dL), although episodes of hypoglycemia appear equally detrimental and the optimal targets remain uncertain. New cerebral monitoring tools that allow continuous evaluation of brain tissue oxygen tension, CBF, and metabolism (via microdialysis) may further improve the management of secondary brain injury.

CRITICAL CARE DISORDERS OF THE CENTRAL NERVOUS SYSTEM

HYPOXIC-ISCHEMIC ENCEPHALOPATHY

This occurs from lack of delivery of oxygen to the brain because of hypotension or respiratory failure. Causes include myocardial infarction, cardiac arrest, shock, asphyxiation, paralysis of respiration, and carbon monoxide or cyanide poisoning. In some circumstances, hypoxia may predominate. Carbon monoxide and cyanide poisoning are termed *histotoxic hypoxia* since they cause a direct impairment of the respiratory chain.

Clinical manifestations

Mild degrees of pure hypoxia, such as occur at high altitudes, cause impaired judgment, inattentiveness, motor incoordination, and, at times, euphoria. However, with hypoxia-ischemia, such as occurs with circulatory arrest, consciousness is lost within seconds. If circulation is restored within 3–5 min, full recovery may occur, but if hypoxia-ischemia lasts beyond 3–5 min, some degree of permanent cerebral damage usually results. Except in extreme cases, it may be difficult to judge the precise degree of hypoxia-ischemia, and some patients make a relatively full recovery after even 8–10 min of global cerebral ischemia. The distinction between pure hypoxia and hypoxia-ischemia is important, since a Pa_{O_2} as low as 20 mmHg (2.7 kPa) can be well tolerated if it develops gradually and normal blood pressure is maintained, but short durations of very low or absent cerebral circulation may result in permanent impairment.

Clinical examination at different time points after a hypoxic-ischemic insult (especially cardiac arrest) is useful in assessing prognosis for long-term neurologic outcome. The prognosis is better for patients with intact brainstem function, as indicated by normal pupillary light responses and intact oculocephalic (doll's eyes), oculovestibular (caloric), and corneal reflexes (Fig. 275-4). Absence of these reflexes and the presence of persistently dilated pupils that do not react to light are grave prognostic signs. A uniformly dismal prognosis from hypoxic-ischemic coma is conveyed by an absent pupillary light reflex or extensor or absent motor response to pain on day 3 following the injury. Electrophysiologically, the bilateral absence of the N20 component of the somatosensory evoked potential (SSEP) in the first several days also conveys a poor prognosis. A very elevated serum level (>33 μg/L) of the biochemical marker neuron-specific enolase (NSE) is indicative of brain damage after resuscitation from cardiac arrest and predicts a poor outcome. However, at present, SSEPs and NSE levels may be difficult to obtain in a timely fashion, with SSEP testing requiring substantial expertise in interpretation and NSE measurements not yet standardized. Whether administration of mild hypothermia after cardiac arrest (see "Treatment") will alter the usefulness of these clinical and electrophysiologic predictors is unknown. Long-term consequences of hypoxic-ischemic encephalopathy include persistent coma or a vegetative state (Chap. 274), dementia, visual agnosia (Chap. 26), parkinsonism, choreoathetosis, cerebellar ataxia, myoclonus, seizures, and an amnestic state, which may be a consequence of selective damage to the hippocampus.

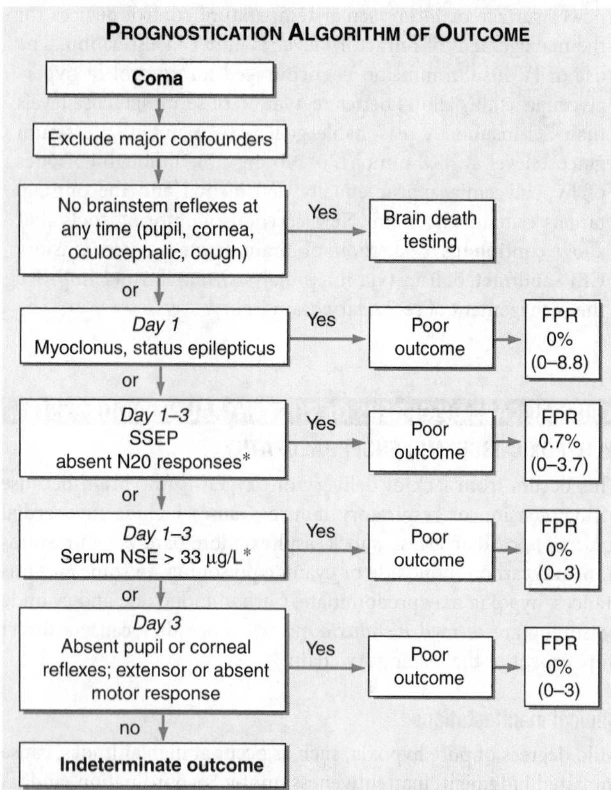

Figure 275-4 Prognostication of outcome in comatose survivors of cardiopulmonary resuscitation. Numbers in parentheses are 95% confidence intervals. Confounders could include use of sedatives or neuromuscular blocking agents, hypothermia therapy, organ failure, or shock. Tests denoted with an asterisk (*) may not be available in a timely and standardized manner. SSEP, somatosensory evoked potentials; NSE, neuron-specific enolase; FPR, false-positive rate (Chap. 3). *(From Wijdicks et al, with permission.)*

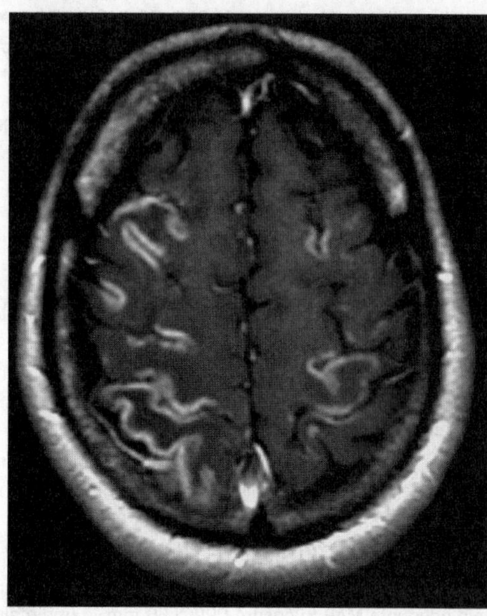

Figure 275-5 Cortical laminar necrosis in hypoxic-ischemic encephalopathy. T1-weighted postcontrast MRI shows cortical enhancement in a watershed distribution consistent with laminar necrosis.

Pathology

Principal histologic findings are extensive multifocal or diffuse laminar cortical necrosis (Fig. 275-5), with almost invariable involvement of the hippocampus. The hippocampal CA1 neurons are vulnerable to even brief episodes of hypoxia-ischemia, perhaps explaining why selective persistent memory deficits may occur after brief cardiac arrest. Scattered small areas of infarction or neuronal loss may be present in the basal ganglia, hypothalamus, or brainstem. In some cases, extensive bilateral thalamic scarring may affect pathways that mediate arousal, and this pathology may be responsible for the persistent vegetative state. A specific form of hypoxic-ischemic encephalopathy, so-called watershed infarcts, occurs at the distal territories between the major cerebral arteries and can cause cognitive deficits, including visual agnosia, and weakness that is greater in proximal than in distal muscle groups.

Diagnosis

Diagnosis is based upon the history of a hypoxic-ischemic event such as cardiac arrest. Blood pressure <70 mmHg systolic or Pa_{O_2} <40 mmHg is usually necessary, although both absolute levels as well as duration of exposure are important determinants of cellular injury. Carbon monoxide intoxication can be confirmed by measurement of carboxyhemoglobin and is suggested by a cherry red color of the skin, although the latter is an inconsistent clinical finding.

TREATMENT Hypoxic-Ischemic Encephalopathy

Treatment should be directed at restoration of normal cardiorespiratory function. This includes securing a clear airway, ensuring adequate oxygenation and ventilation, and restoring cerebral perfusion, whether by cardiopulmonary resuscitation, fluid, pressors, or cardiac pacing. Hypothermia may target the neuronal cell injury cascade and has substantial neuroprotective properties in experimental models of brain injury. In two trials, mild hypothermia (33°C) improved functional outcome in patients who remained comatose after resuscitation from a cardiac arrest. Treatment was initiated within minutes of cardiac resuscitation and continued for 12 h in one study and 24 h in the other. Potential complications of hypothermia include coagulopathy and an increased risk of infection. Based upon these studies, the International Liaison Committee on Resuscitation issued the following advisory statement in 2003: "Unconscious adult patients with spontaneous circulation after out-of-hospital cardiac arrest should be cooled to 32°–34°C for 12–24 h when the initial rhythm was ventricular fibrillation."

Severe carbon monoxide intoxication may be treated with hyperbaric oxygen. Anticonvulsants may be needed to control seizures, although these are not usually given prophylactically. Posthypoxic myoclonus may respond to oral administration of clonazepam at doses of 1.5–10 mg daily or valproate at doses of 300–1200 mg daily in divided doses. Myoclonic status epilepticus within 24 h after a primary circulatory arrest generally portends a very poor prognosis, even if seizures are controlled.

Carbon monoxide and cyanide intoxication can also cause a delayed encephalopathy. Little clinical impairment is evident when the patient first regains consciousness, but a parkinsonian syndrome characterized by akinesia and rigidity without tremor may develop. Symptoms can worsen over months, accompanied by increasing evidence of damage in the basal ganglia as seen on both CT and MRI.

METABOLIC ENCEPHALOPATHIES

Altered mental states, variously described as confusion, delirium, disorientation, and encephalopathy, are present in many patients with severe illness in an intensive care unit (ICU). Older patients are particularly vulnerable to delirium, a confusional state characterized by disordered perception, frequent hallucinations, delusions, and sleep disturbance. This is often attributed to medication effects, sleep deprivation, pain, and anxiety. The presence of delirium is associated with worsened outcome in critically ill patients, even in those without an identifiable central nervous system pathology such as stroke or brain trauma. In these patients, the cause of delirium is often multifactorial, resulting from organ dysfunction, sepsis, and especially the use of medications given to treat pain, agitation, or anxiety. Critically ill patients are often treated with a variety of sedative and analgesic medications, including opiates, benzodiazepines, neuroleptics, and sedative-anesthetic medications, such as propofol. Recent studies suggest that in critically ill patients requiring sedation, the use of the centrally acting α_2 agonist dexmedetomidine reduces delirium and shortens the duration of mechanical ventilation compared to the use of benzodiazepines such as lorazepam or midazolam. The presence of family members in the ICU may also help to calm and orient agitated patients, and in severe cases, low doses of neuroleptics (e.g., haloperidol 0.5–1 mg) can be useful. Current strategies focus on limiting the use of sedative medications when this can be done safely.

In the ICU setting, several metabolic causes of an altered level of consciousness predominate. Hypercarbic encephalopathy can present with headache, confusion, stupor, or coma. Hypoventilation syndrome occurs most frequently in patients with a history of chronic CO_2 retention who are receiving oxygen therapy for emphysema or chronic pulmonary disease (Chap. 264). The elevated Pa_{CO_2} leading to CO_2 narcosis may have a direct anesthetic effect, and cerebral vasodilation from increased Pa_{CO_2} can lead to increased ICP. Hepatic encephalopathy is suggested by asterixis and can occur in chronic liver failure or acute fulminant hepatic failure. Both hyperglycemia and hypoglycemia can cause encephalopathy, as can hypernatremia and hyponatremia. Confusion, impairment of eye movements, and gait ataxia are the hallmarks of acute Wernicke's disease (see below).

SEPSIS-ASSOCIATED ENCEPHALOPATHY

Pathogenesis

In patients with sepsis, the systemic response to infectious agents leads to the release of circulating inflammatory mediators that appear to contribute to encephalopathy. Critical illness, in association with the systemic inflammatory response syndrome (SIRS), can lead to multisystem organ failure. This syndrome can occur in the setting of apparent sepsis, severe burns, or trauma, even without clear identification of an infectious agent. Many patients with critical illness, sepsis, or SIRS develop encephalopathy without obvious explanation. This condition is broadly termed *sepsis-associated encephalopathy*. While the specific mediators leading to neurologic dysfunction remain uncertain, it is clear that the encephalopathy is not simply the result of metabolic derangements of multiorgan failure. The cytokines tumor necrosis factor, interleukin (IL)-1, IL-2, and IL-6 are thought to play a role in this syndrome.

Diagnosis

Sepsis-associated encephalopathy presents clinically as a diffuse dysfunction of the brain without prominent focal findings. Confusion, disorientation, agitation, and fluctuations in level of alertness are typical. In more profound cases, especially with hemodynamic compromise, the decrease in level of alertness can be more prominent, at times resulting in coma. Hyperreflexia and frontal release signs such as a grasp or snout reflex (Chap. 26) can be seen. Abnormal movements such as myoclonus, tremor, or asterixis can occur. Sepsis-associated encephalopathy is quite common, occurring in the majority of patients with sepsis and multisystem organ failure. Diagnosis is often difficult because of the multiple potential causes of neurologic dysfunction in critically ill patients and requires exclusion of structural, metabolic, toxic, and infectious (e.g., meningitis or encephalitis) causes. The mortality rate of patients with sepsis-associated encephalopathy severe enough to produce coma approaches 50%, although this principally reflects the severity of the underlying critical illness and is not a direct result of the encephalopathy. Patients dying from severe sepsis or septic shock may have elevated levels of the serum brain injury biomarker S-100β and neuropathologic findings of neuronal apoptosis and cerebral ischemic injury. However, successful treatment of the underlying critical illness almost always results in complete resolution of the encephalopathy, with profound long-term cognitive disability being uncommon.

CENTRAL PONTINE MYELINOLYSIS

This disorder typically presents in a devastating fashion as quadriplegia and pseudobulbar palsy. Predisposing factors include severe underlying medical illness or nutritional deficiency; most cases are associated with rapid correction of hyponatremia or with hyperosmolar states. The pathology consists of demyelination without inflammation in the base of the pons, with relative sparing of axons and nerve cells. MRI is useful in establishing the diagnosis (Fig. 275-6) and may also identify partial forms that present as confusion, dysarthria, and/or disturbances of conjugate gaze without quadriplegia. Occasional cases present with lesions outside of the brainstem. Therapeutic guidelines for the restoration of severe hyponatremia should aim for gradual correction, i.e., by ≤10 mmol/L (10 meq/L) within 24 h and 20 mmol/L (20 meq/L) within 48 h.

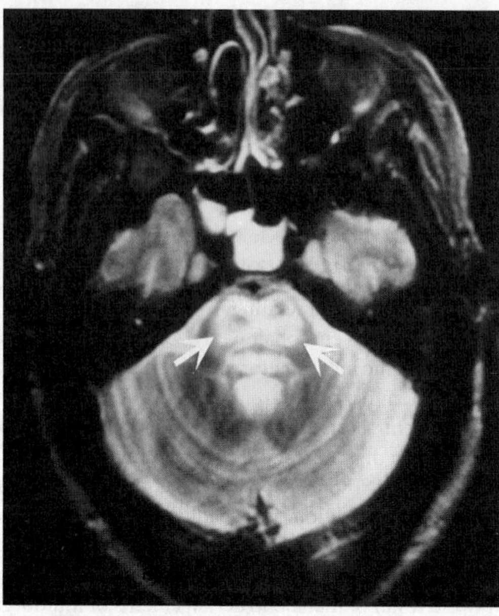

Figure 275-6 Central pontine myelinolysis. Axial T2-weighted MR scan through the pons reveals a symmetric area of abnormal high signal intensity within the basis pontis (*arrows*).

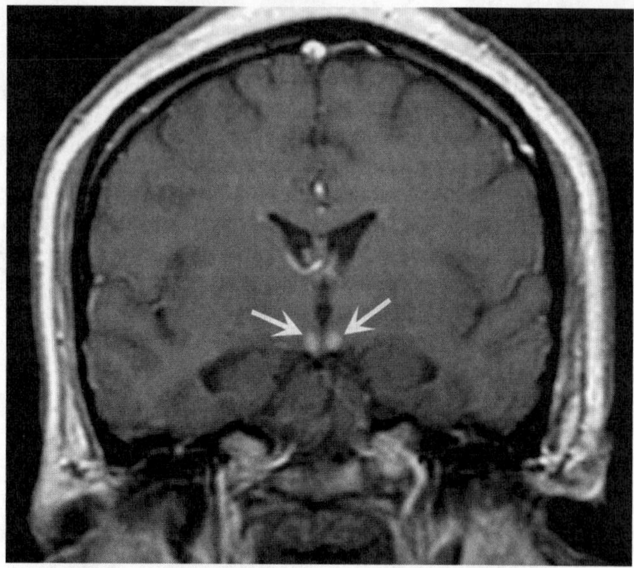

Figure 275-7 Wernicke's disease. Coronal T1-weighted postcontrast MRI reveals abnormal enhancement of the mammillary bodies (*arrows*), typical of acute Wernicke's encephalopathy.

WERNICKE'S DISEASE

Wernicke's disease is a common and preventable disorder due to a deficiency of thiamine (Chap. 74). In the United States, alcoholics account for most cases, but patients with malnutrition due to hyperemesis, starvation, renal dialysis, cancer, AIDS, or rarely gastric surgery are also at risk. The characteristic clinical triad is that of ophthalmoplegia, ataxia, and global confusion. However, only one-third of patients with acute Wernicke's disease present with the classic clinical triad. Most patients are profoundly disoriented, indifferent, and inattentive, although rarely they have an agitated delirium related to ethanol withdrawal. If the disease is not treated, stupor, coma, and death may ensue. Ocular motor abnormalities include horizontal nystagmus on lateral gaze, lateral rectus palsy (usually bilateral), conjugate gaze palsies, and rarely ptosis. Gait ataxia probably results from a combination of polyneuropathy, cerebellar involvement, and vestibular paresis. The pupils are usually spared, but they may become miotic with advanced disease.

Wernicke's disease is usually associated with other manifestations of nutritional disease, such as polyneuropathy. Rarely, amblyopia or myelopathy occurs. Tachycardia and postural hypotension may be related to impaired function of the autonomic nervous system or to the coexistence of cardiovascular beriberi. Patients who recover show improvement in ocular palsies within hours after the administration of thiamine, but horizontal nystagmus may persist. Ataxia improves more slowly than the ocular motor abnormalities. Approximately half recover incompletely and are left with a slow, shuffling, wide-based gait and an inability to tandem walk. Apathy, drowsiness, and confusion improve more gradually. As these symptoms recede, an amnestic state with impairment in recent memory and learning may become more apparent (*Korsakoff's psychosis*). Korsakoff's psychosis is frequently persistent; the residual mental state is characterized by gaps in memory, confabulation, and disordered temporal sequencing.

Pathology

Periventricular lesions surround the third ventricle, aqueduct, and fourth ventricle, with petechial hemorrhages in occasional acute cases and atrophy of the mamillary bodies in most chronic cases. There is frequently endothelial proliferation, demyelination, and some neuronal loss. These changes may be detected by MRI scanning (Fig. 275-7). The amnestic defect is related to lesions in the dorsal medial nuclei of the thalamus.

Pathogenesis

Thiamine is a cofactor of several enzymes, including transketolase, pyruvate dehydrogenase, and α-ketoglutarate dehydrogenase. Thiamine deficiency produces a diffuse decrease in cerebral glucose utilization and results in mitochondrial damage. Glutamate accumulates owing to impairment of α-ketoglutarate dehydrogenase activity and, in combination with the energy deficiency, may result in excitotoxic cell damage.

TREATMENT Wernicke's Disease

Wernicke's disease is a medical emergency and requires immediate administration of thiamine, in a dose of 100 mg either IV or IM. The dose should be given daily until the patient resumes a normal diet and should be begun prior to treatment with IV glucose solutions. Glucose infusions may precipitate Wernicke's disease in a previously unaffected patient or cause a rapid worsening of an early form of the disease. For this reason, thiamine should be administered to all alcoholic patients requiring parenteral glucose.

CRITICAL CARE DISORDERS OF THE PERIPHERAL NERVOUS SYSTEM

Critical illness with disorders of the peripheral nervous system (PNS) arises in two contexts: (1) primary neurologic diseases that require critical care interventions such as intubation and mechanical ventilation, and (2) secondary PNS manifestations of systemic critical illness, often involving multisystem organ failure. The former include acute polyneuropathies such as Guillain-Barré syndrome (Chap. 385), neuromuscular junction disorders including myasthenia gravis (Chap. 386) and botulism (Chap. 141), and primary muscle disorders such as polymyositis (Chap. 388). The latter result either from the systemic disease itself or as a consequence of interventions.

General principles of respiratory evaluation in patients with PNS involvement, regardless of cause, include assessment of pulmonary mechanics, such as maximal inspiratory force (MIF) and vital capacity (VC), and evaluation of strength of bulbar muscles. Regardless of the cause of weakness, endotracheal intubation should be considered when the MIF falls to <–25 cmH_2O or the VC is <1 L. Also, patients with severe palatal weakness may require endotracheal intubation in order to prevent acute upper airway obstruction or recurrent aspiration. Arterial blood gases and oxygen saturation from pulse oximetry are used to follow patients with potential respiratory compromise from PNS dysfunction. However, intubation and mechanical ventilation should be undertaken based on clinical assessment rather than waiting until oxygen saturation drops or CO_2 retention develops from hypoventilation. Noninvasive mechanical ventilation may be considered initially in lieu of endotracheal intubation but is generally insufficient in patients with severe bulbar weakness or ventilatory failure with hypercarbia. Principles of mechanical ventilation are discussed in Chap. 269.

NEUROPATHY

While encephalopathy may be the most obvious neurologic dysfunction in critically ill patients, dysfunction of the PNS is also quite common. It is typically present in patients with prolonged critical illnesses lasting several weeks and involving sepsis; clinical suspicion is aroused when there is failure to wean from mechanical ventilation despite improvement of the underlying sepsis and critical illness. *Critical illness polyneuropathy* refers to the most common PNS complication related to critical illness; it is seen in the setting of prolonged critical illness, sepsis, and multisystem organ failure. Neurologic findings include diffuse weakness, decreased reflexes, and distal sensory loss. Electrophysiologic studies demonstrate a diffuse, symmetric, distal axonal sensorimotor neuropathy, and pathologic studies have confirmed axonal degeneration. The precise mechanism of critical illness polyneuropathy remains unclear, but circulating factors such as cytokines, which are associated with sepsis and SIRS, are thought to play a role. It has been reported that up to 70% of patients with the sepsis syndrome have some degree of neuropathy, although far fewer have a clinical syndrome profound enough to cause severe respiratory muscle weakness requiring prolonged mechanical ventilation or resulting in failure to wean. Aggressive glycemic control with insulin infusions appears to decrease the risk of critical illness polyneuropathy. Treatment is otherwise supportive, with specific intervention directed at treating the underlying illness. While spontaneous recovery is usually seen, the time course may extend over weeks to months and necessitate long-term ventilatory support and care even after the underlying critical illness has resolved.

DISORDERS OF NEUROMUSCULAR TRANSMISSION

A defect in neuromuscular transmission may be a source of weakness in critically ill patients. Myasthenia gravis may be a consideration; however, persistent weakness secondary to impaired neuromuscular junction transmission is almost always due to administration of drugs. A number of medications impair neuromuscular transmission; these include antibiotics, especially aminoglycosides, and beta-blocking agents. In the ICU, the nondepolarizing neuromuscular blocking agents (nd-NMBAs), also known as muscle relaxants, are most commonly responsible. Included in this group of drugs are such agents as pancuronium, vecuronium, rocuronium, and atracurium. They are often used to facilitate mechanical ventilation or other critical care procedures, but with prolonged use persistent neuromuscular blockade may result in weakness even after discontinuation of these agents hours or days earlier. Risk factors for this prolonged action of neuromuscular blocking agents include female sex, metabolic acidosis, and renal failure.

Prolonged neuromuscular blockade does not appear to produce permanent damage to the PNS. Once the offending medications are discontinued, full strength is restored, although this may take days. In general, the lowest dose of neuromuscular blocking agent should be used to achieve the desired result and, when these agents are used in the ICU, a peripheral nerve stimulator should be used to monitor neuromuscular junction function.

MYOPATHY

Critically ill patients, especially those with sepsis, frequently develop muscle wasting, often in the face of seemingly adequate nutritional support. The assumption has been that this represents a catabolic myopathy brought about as a result of multiple factors, including elevated cortisol and catecholamine release and other circulating factors induced by the SIRS. In this syndrome, known as *cachectic myopathy*, serum creatine kinase levels and electromyography (EMG) are normal. Muscle biopsy shows type II fiber atrophy. Panfascicular muscle fiber necrosis may also occur in the setting of profound sepsis. This so-called *septic myopathy* is characterized clinically by weakness progressing to a profound level over just a few days. There may be associated elevations in serum creatine kinase and urine myoglobin. Both EMG and muscle biopsy may be normal initially but eventually show abnormal spontaneous activity and panfascicular necrosis with an accompanying inflammatory reaction. Both of these myopathic syndromes may be considered under the broader heading of *critical illness myopathy*.

Acute quadriplegic myopathy describes a clinical syndrome of severe weakness seen in the setting of glucocorticoid and nd-NMBA use. The most frequent scenario in which this is encountered is the asthmatic patient who requires high-dose glucocorticoids and nd-NMBA to facilitate mechanical ventilation. This muscle disorder is not due to prolonged action of nd-NMBAs at the neuromuscular junction but, rather, is an actual myopathy with muscle damage; it has occasionally been described with high-dose glucocorticoid use alone. Clinically this syndrome is most often recognized when a patient fails to wean from mechanical ventilation despite resolution of the primary pulmonary process. Pathologically, there may be vacuolar changes in both type I and type II muscle fibers with evidence of regeneration. Acute quadriplegic myopathy has a good prognosis. If patients survive their underlying critical illness, the myopathy invariably improves and most patients return to normal. However, because this syndrome is a result of true muscle damage, not just prolonged blockade at the neuromuscular junction, this process may take weeks or months, and tracheotomy with prolonged ventilatory support may be necessary. Some patients do have residual long-term weakness, with atrophy and fatigue limiting ambulation. At present, it is unclear how to prevent this myopathic complication, except by avoiding use of nd-NMBAs, a strategy not always possible. Monitoring with a peripheral nerve stimulator can help to avoid the overuse of these agents. However, this is more likely to prevent the complication of prolonged neuromuscular junction blockade than it is to prevent this myopathy.

SUBARACHNOID HEMORRHAGE

Subarachnoid hemorrhage (SAH) renders the brain critically ill from both primary and secondary brain insults. Excluding head trauma, the most common cause of SAH is rupture of a saccular aneurysm. Other causes include bleeding from a vascular malformation (arteriovenous malformation or dural arterial-venous fistula) and extension into the subarachnoid space from a primary intracerebral hemorrhage. Some idiopathic SAHs are localized to the perimesencephalic cisterns and are benign; they probably have a venous or capillary source, and angiography is unrevealing.

Saccular ("berry") aneurysm

Autopsy and angiography studies have found that about 2% of adults harbor intracranial aneurysms, for a prevalence of 4 million persons in the United States; the aneurysm will rupture, producing SAH, in 25,000–30,000 cases per year. For patients who arrive alive at hospital, the mortality rate over the next month is about 45%. Of those who survive, more than half are left with major neurologic deficits as a result of the initial hemorrhage, cerebral vasospasm with infarction, or hydrocephalus. If the patient survives but the aneurysm is not obliterated, the rate of rebleeding is about 20% in the first 2 weeks, 30% in the first month, and about 3% per year afterwards. Given these alarming figures, the major therapeutic emphasis is on preventing the predictable early complications of the SAH.

Unruptured, asymptomatic aneurysms are much less dangerous than a recently ruptured aneurysm. The annual risk of rupture for aneurysms <10 mm in size is ~0.1%, and for aneurysms ≥10 mm in size is ~0.5–1%; the surgical morbidity rate far exceeds these percentages. Because of the longer length of exposure to risk of rupture, younger patients with aneurysms >10 mm in size may benefit from prophylactic treatment. As with the treatment of asymptomatic carotid stenosis, this risk-benefit strongly depends on the complication rate of treatment.

Giant aneurysms, those >2.5 cm in diameter, occur at the same sites (see below) as small aneurysms and account for 5% of cases. The three most common locations are the terminal internal carotid artery, middle cerebral artery (MCA) bifurcation, and top of the basilar artery. Their risk of rupture is ~6% in the first year after identification and may remain high indefinitely. They often cause symptoms by compressing the adjacent brain or cranial nerves.

Mycotic aneurysms are usually located distal to the first bifurcation of major arteries of the circle of Willis. Most result from infected emboli due to bacterial endocarditis causing septic degeneration of arteries and subsequent dilation and rupture. Whether these lesions should be sought and repaired prior to rupture or left to heal spontaneously is controversial.

Pathophysiology Saccular aneurysms occur at the bifurcations of the large- to medium-sized intracranial arteries; rupture is into the subarachnoid space in the basal cisterns and often into the parenchyma of the adjacent brain. Approximately 85% of aneurysms occur in the anterior circulation, mostly on the circle of Willis. About 20% of patients have multiple aneurysms, many at mirror sites bilaterally. As an aneurysm develops, it typically forms a neck with a dome. The length of the neck and the size of the dome vary greatly and are important factors in planning neurosurgical obliteration or endovascular embolization. The arterial internal elastic lamina disappears at the base of the neck. The media thins, and connective tissue replaces smooth-muscle cells. At the site of rupture (most often the dome) the wall thins, and the tear that allows bleeding is often ≤0.5 mm long. Aneurysm size and site are important in predicting risk of rupture. Those >7 mm in diameter and those at the top of the basilar artery and at the origin of the posterior communicating artery are at greater risk of rupture.

Clinical manifestations Most unruptured intracranial aneurysms are completely asymptomatic. Symptoms are usually due to rupture and resultant SAH, although some unruptured aneurysms present with mass effect on cranial nerves or brain parenchyma. At the moment of aneurysmal rupture with major SAH, the ICP suddenly rises. This may account for the sudden transient loss of consciousness that occurs in nearly half of patients. Sudden loss of consciousness may be preceded by a brief moment of excruciating headache, but most patients first complain of headache upon regaining consciousness. In 10% of cases, aneurysmal bleeding is severe enough to cause loss of consciousness for several days. In ~45% of cases, severe headache associated with exertion is the presenting complaint. The patient often calls the headache "the worst headache of my life"; however, the most important characteristic is sudden onset. Occasionally, these ruptures may present as headache of only moderate intensity or as a change in the patient's usual headache pattern. The headache is usually generalized, often with neck stiffness, and vomiting is common.

Although sudden headache in the absence of focal neurologic symptoms is the hallmark of aneurysmal rupture, focal neurologic deficits may occur. Anterior communicating artery or MCA bifurcation aneurysms may rupture into the adjacent brain or subdural space and form a hematoma large enough to produce mass effect. The deficits that result can include hemiparesis, aphasia, and abulia.

Occasionally, prodromal symptoms suggest the location of a progressively enlarging unruptured aneurysm. A third cranial nerve palsy, particularly when associated with pupillary dilation, loss of ipsilateral (but retained contralateral) light reflex, and focal pain above or behind the eye, may occur with an expanding aneurysm at the junction of the posterior communicating artery and the internal carotid artery. A sixth nerve palsy may indicate an aneurysm in the cavernous sinus, and visual field defects can occur with an expanding supraclinoid carotid or anterior cerebral artery aneurysm. Occipital and posterior cervical pain may signal a posterior inferior cerebellar artery or anterior inferior cerebellar artery aneurysm (Chap. 370). Pain in or behind the eye and in the low temple can occur with an expanding MCA aneurysm. Thunderclap headache is a variant of migraine that simulates an SAH. Before concluding that a patient with sudden, severe headache has thunderclap migraine, a definitive workup for aneurysm or other intracranial pathology is required.

Aneurysms can undergo small ruptures and leaks of blood into the subarachnoid space, so-called *sentinel bleeds*. Sudden unexplained headache at any location should raise suspicion of SAH and be investigated, because a major hemorrhage may be imminent.

The initial clinical manifestations of SAH can be graded using the Hunt-Hess or World Federation of Neurosurgical Societies classification schemes (Table 275-3). For ruptured aneurysms, prognosis for good outcomes falls as the grade increases. For example, it is

TABLE 275-3 Grading Scales for Subarachnoid Hemorrhage

Grade	Hunt-Hess Scale	World Federation of Neurosurgical Societies (WFNS) Scale
1	Mild headache, normal mental status, no cranial nerve or motor findings	GCS[a] score 15, no motor deficits
2	Severe headache, normal mental status, may have cranial nerve deficit	GCS score 13–14, no motor deficits
3	Somnolent, confused, may have cranial nerve or mild motor deficit	GCS score 13–14, with motor deficits
4	Stupor, moderate to severe motor deficit, may have intermittent reflex posturing	GCS score 7–12, with or without motor deficits
5	Coma, reflex posturing or flaccid	GCS score 3–6, with or without motor deficits

[a]Glasgow Coma Scale: See Table 378-2.

unusual for a Hunt-Hess grade 1 patient to die if the aneurysm is treated, but the mortality rate for grade 4 and 5 patients may be as high as 80%.

Delayed neurologic deficits There are four major causes of delayed neurologic deficits: rerupture, hydrocephalus, vasospasm, and hyponatremia.

1. *Rerupture.* The incidence of rerupture of an untreated aneurysm in the first month following SAH is ~30%, with the peak in the first 7 days. Rerupture is associated with a 60% mortality rate and poor outcome. Early treatment eliminates this risk.
2. *Hydrocephalus.* Acute hydrocephalus can cause stupor and coma and can be mitigated by placement of an external ventricular drain. More often, subacute hydrocephalus may develop over a few days or weeks and causes progressive drowsiness or slowed mentation (abulia) with incontinence. Hydrocephalus is differentiated from cerebral vasospasm with a CT scan, CT angiogram, transcranial Doppler (TCD) ultrasound, or conventional x-ray angiography. Hydrocephalus may clear spontaneously or require temporary ventricular drainage. Chronic hydrocephalus may develop weeks to months after SAH and manifest as gait difficulty, incontinence, or impaired mentation. Subtle signs may be a lack of initiative in conversation or a failure to recover independence.
3. *Vasospasm.* Narrowing of the arteries at the base of the brain following SAH causes symptomatic ischemia and infarction in ~30% of patients and is the major cause of delayed morbidity and death. Signs of ischemia appear 4–14 days after the hemorrhage, most often at 7 days. The severity and distribution of vasospasm determine whether infarction will occur.

   Delayed vasospasm is believed to result from direct effects of clotted blood and its breakdown products on the arteries within the subarachnoid space. In general, the more blood that surrounds the arteries, the greater the chance of symptomatic vasospasm. Spasm of major arteries produces symptoms referable to the appropriate vascular territory (Chap. 370). All of these focal symptoms may present abruptly, fluctuate, or develop over a few days. In most cases, focal spasm is preceded by a decline in mental status.

   Vasospasm can be detected reliably with conventional x-ray angiography, but this invasive procedure is expensive and carries the risk of stroke and other complications. TCD ultrasound is based on the principle that the velocity of blood flow within an artery will rise as the lumen diameter is narrowed. By directing the probe along the MCA and proximal anterior cerebral artery (ACA), carotid terminus, and vertebral and basilar arteries on a daily or every-other-day basis, vasospasm can be reliably detected and treatments initiated to prevent cerebral ischemia (see below). CT angiography is another method that can detect vasospasm.

   Severe cerebral edema in patients with infarction from vasospasm may increase the ICP enough to reduce cerebral perfusion pressure. Treatment may include mannitol, hyperventilation, and hemicraniectomy; moderate hypothermia may have a role as well.
4. *Hyponatremia.* Hyponatremia may be profound and can develop quickly in the first 2 weeks following SAH. There is both natriuresis and volume depletion with SAH, so that patients become both hyponatremic and hypovolemic. Both atrial natriuretic peptide and brain natriuretic peptide have a role in producing this "cerebral salt-wasting syndrome." Typically, it clears over the course of 1–2 weeks and, in the setting of SAH, should not be treated with free-water restriction as this may increase the risk of stroke (see below).

Laboratory evaluation and imaging (Fig. 275-8) The hallmark of aneurysmal rupture is blood in the CSF. More than 95% of cases

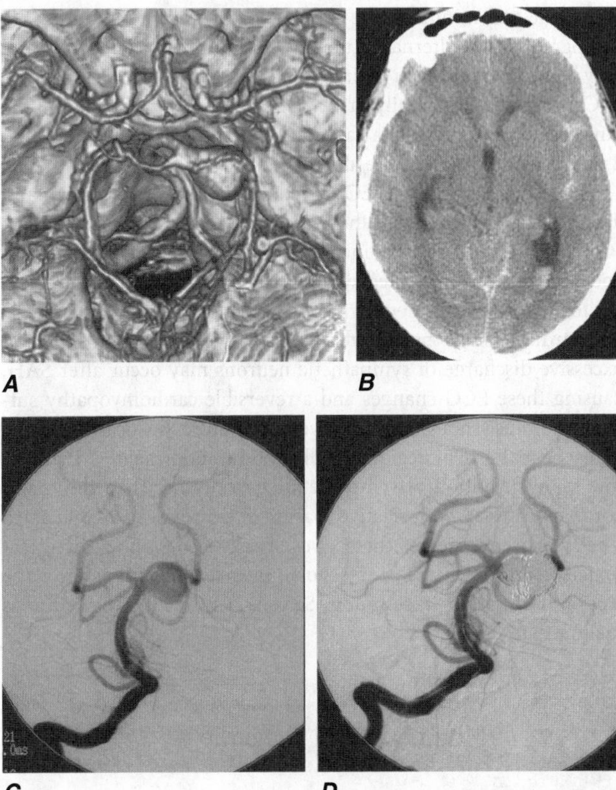

Figure 275-8 Subarachnoid hemorrhage. ***A.*** CT angiography revealing an aneurysm of the left superior cerebellar artery. ***B.*** Noncontrast CT scan at the level of the third ventricle revealing subarachnoid blood (*bright*) in the left sylvian fissure and within the left lateral ventricle. ***C.*** Conventional anteroposterior x-ray angiogram of the right vertebral and basilar artery showing the large aneurysm. ***D.*** Conventional angiogram following coil embolization of the aneurysm, whereby the aneurysm body is filled with platinum coils delivered through a microcatheter navigated from the femoral artery into the aneurysm neck.

have enough blood to be visualized on a high-quality noncontrast CT scan obtained within 72 h. If the scan fails to establish the diagnosis of SAH and no mass lesion or obstructive hydrocephalus is found, a lumbar puncture should be performed to establish the presence of subarachnoid blood. Lysis of the red blood cells and subsequent conversion of hemoglobin to bilirubin stains the spinal fluid yellow within 6–12 h. This xanthochromic spinal fluid peaks in intensity at 48 h and lasts for 1–4 weeks, depending on the amount of subarachnoid blood.

The extent and location of subarachnoid blood on noncontrast CT scan help locate the underlying aneurysm, identify the cause of any neurologic deficit, and predict delayed vasospasm. A high incidence of symptomatic vasospasm in the MCA and ACA has been found when early CT scans show subarachnoid clots >5 × 3 mm in the basal cisterns or layers of blood >1 mm thick in the cerebral fissures. CT scans less reliably predict vasospasm in the vertebral, basilar, or posterior cerebral arteries.

Lumbar puncture prior to an imaging procedure is indicated only if a CT scan is not available at the time of the suspected SAH. Once the diagnosis of hemorrhage from a ruptured saccular aneurysm is suspected, four-vessel conventional x-ray angiography (both carotids and both vertebrals) is generally performed to localize and define the anatomic details of the aneurysm and to determine if other unruptured aneurysms exist (Fig. 275-8C). At some centers, the ruptured aneurysm can be treated using endovascular techniques at the time of the initial angiogram as a way to expedite treatment and minimize the number of invasive procedures. CT angiography is an alternative method for locating the aneurysm and may be sufficient to plan definitive therapy.

Close monitoring (daily or twice daily) of electrolytes is important because hyponatremia can occur precipitously during the first 2 weeks following SAH (see above).

The electrocardiogram (ECG) frequently shows ST-segment and T-wave changes similar to those associated with cardiac ischemia. Prolonged QRS complex, increased QT interval, and prominent "peaked" or deeply inverted symmetric T waves are usually secondary to the intracranial hemorrhage. There is evidence that structural myocardial lesions produced by circulating catecholamines and excessive discharge of sympathetic neurons may occur after SAH, causing these ECG changes and a reversible cardiomyopathy sufficient to cause shock or congestive heart failure. Echocardiography reveals a pattern of regional wall motion abnormalities that follow the distribution of sympathetic nerves rather than the major coronary arteries, with relative sparing of the ventricular wall apex. The sympathetic nerves themselves appear to be injured by direct toxicity from the excessive catecholamine release. An asymptomatic troponin elevation is common. Serious ventricular dysrhythmias are unusual.

TREATMENT Subarachnoid Hemorrhage

Early aneurysm repair prevents rerupture and allows the safe application of techniques to improve blood flow (e.g., induced hypertension and hypervolemia) should symptomatic vasospasm develop. An aneurysm can be "clipped" by a neurosurgeon or "coiled" by an endovascular surgeon. Surgical repair involves placing a metal clip across the aneurysm neck, thereby immediately eliminating the risk of rebleeding. This approach requires craniotomy and brain retraction, which is associated with neurologic morbidity. Endovascular techniques involve placing platinum coils, or other embolic material, within the aneurysm via a catheter that is passed from the femoral artery. The aneurysm is packed tightly to enhance thrombosis and over time is walled off from the circulation (Fig. 275-8*D*). The only prospective randomized trial of surgery versus endovascular treatment for ruptured aneurysm, the International Subarachnoid Aneurysm Trial (ISAT), was terminated early when 24% of patients treated with endovascular therapy were dead or dependent at 1 year compared to 31% treated with surgery, a significant 23% relative reduction. After 5 years, risk of death was lower in the coiling group, although the proportion of survivors who were independent was the same in both groups. Risk of rebleeding was low, but more common in the coiling group. Also, because some aneurysms have a morphology that is not amenable to endovascular treatment, surgery remains an important treatment option. Centers that combine both endovascular and neurosurgical expertise likely offer the best outcomes for patients, and there are reliable data showing that centers that specialize in aneurysm treatment have improved mortality rates.

The medical management of SAH focuses on protecting the airway, managing blood pressure before and after aneurysm treatment, preventing rebleeding prior to treatment, managing vasospasm, treating hydrocephalus, treating hyponatremia, and preventing pulmonary embolus.

Intracranial hypertension following aneurysmal rupture occurs secondary to subarachnoid blood, parenchymal hematoma, acute hydrocephalus, or loss of vascular autoregulation. Patients who are stuporous should undergo emergent ventriculostomy to measure ICP and to treat high ICP in order to prevent cerebral ischemia. Medical therapies designed to combat raised ICP (e.g., mild hyperventilation, mannitol, and sedation) can also be used as needed. High ICP refractory to treatment is a poor prognostic sign.

Prior to definitive treatment of the ruptured aneurysm, care is required to maintain adequate cerebral perfusion pressure while avoiding excessive elevation of arterial pressure. If the patient is alert, it is reasonable to lower the blood pressure to normal using nicardipine, labetolol, or esmolol. If the patient has a depressed level of consciousness, ICP should be measured and the cerebral perfusion pressure targeted to 60–70 mmHg. If headache or neck pain is severe, mild sedation and analgesia are prescribed. Extreme sedation is avoided because it can obscure changes in neurologic status. Adequate hydration is necessary to avoid a decrease in blood volume predisposing to brain ischemia.

Seizures are uncommon at the onset of aneurysmal rupture. The quivering, jerking, and extensor posturing that often accompany loss of consciousness with SAH are probably related to the sharp rise in ICP rather than seizure. However, anticonvulsants are sometimes given as prophylactic therapy since a seizure could theoretically promote rebleeding.

Glucocorticoids may help reduce the head and neck ache caused by the irritative effect of the subarachnoid blood. There is no good evidence that they reduce cerebral edema, are neuroprotective, or reduce vascular injury, and their routine use therefore is not recommended.

Antifibrinolytic agents are not routinely prescribed but may be considered in patients in whom aneurysm treatment cannot proceed immediately. They are associated with a reduced incidence of aneurysmal rerupture but may also increase the risk of delayed cerebral infarction and deep-vein thrombosis (DVT).

Vasospasm remains the leading cause of morbidity and mortality following aneurysmal SAH. Treatment with the calcium channel antagonist nimodipine (60 mg PO every 4 h) improves outcome, perhaps by preventing ischemic injury rather than reducing the risk of vasospasm. Nimodipine can cause significant hypotension in some patients, which may worsen cerebral ischemia in patients with vasospasm. Symptomatic cerebral vasospasm can also be treated by increasing the cerebral perfusion pressure by raising mean arterial pressure through plasma volume expansion and the judicious use of IV vasopressor agents, usually phenylephrine or norepinephrine. Raised perfusion pressure has been associated with clinical improvement in many patients, but high arterial pressure may promote rebleeding in unprotected aneurysms. Treatment with induced hypertension and hypervolemia generally requires monitoring of arterial and central venous pressures; it is best to infuse pressors through a central venous line as well. Volume expansion helps prevent hypotension, augments cardiac output, and reduces blood viscosity by reducing the hematocrit. This method is called "triple-H" (hypertension, hemodilution, and hypervolemic) therapy.

If symptomatic vasospasm persists despite optimal medical therapy, intraarterial vasodilators and percutaneous transluminal angioplasty are considered. Vasodilatation by direct angioplasty appears to be permanent, allowing triple-H therapy to be tapered sooner. The pharmacologic vasodilators (verapamil and nicardipine) do not last more than about 24 h, and therefore multiple treatments may be required until the subarachnoid blood is reabsorbed. Although intraarterial papaverine is an effective vasodilator, there is evidence that papaverine may be neurotoxic, so its use should generally be avoided.

Acute hydrocephalus can cause stupor or coma. It may clear spontaneously or require temporary ventricular drainage. When chronic hydrocephalus develops, ventricular shunting is the treatment of choice.

Free-water restriction is contraindicated in patients with SAH at risk for vasospasm because hypovolemia and hypotension may occur and precipitate cerebral ischemia. Many patients continue to experience a decline in serum sodium despite receiving parenteral fluids containing normal saline. Frequently, supplemental oral salt coupled with normal saline will mitigate hyponatremia, but often patients also require hypertonic saline. Care must be taken not to correct serum sodium too quickly in patients with marked hyponatremia of several days' duration, as central pontine myelinolysis may occur.

All patients should have pneumatic compression stockings applied to prevent pulmonary embolism. Unfractionated heparin administered subcutaneously for DVT prophylaxis can be initiated immediately following endovascular treatment and within days following craniotomy and surgical clipping and is a useful adjunct to pneumatic compression stockings. Treatment of pulmonary embolus depends on whether the aneurysm has been treated and whether or not the patient has had a craniotomy. Systemic anticoagulation with heparin is contraindicated in patients with ruptured and untreated aneurysms. It is a relative contraindication following craniotomy for several days, and it may delay thrombosis of a coiled aneurysm. Following craniotomy, use of inferior vena cava filters is preferred to prevent further pulmonary emboli, while systemic anticoagulation with heparin is preferred following successful endovascular treatment.

FURTHER READINGS

Latronico N et al: Neuromuscular sequelae of critical illness. Curr Opin Crit Care 11:381, 2005

Liou AK et al: To die or not to die for neurons in ischemia, traumatic brain injury and epilepsy: A review on the stress-activated signaling pathways and apoptotic pathways. Prog Neurobiol 69:103, 2003

Molyneux A et al: Risk of recurrent subarachnoid haemorrhage, death, or dependence and standardised mortality ratios after clipping or coiling of an intracranial aneurysm in the International Subarachnoid Aneurysm Trial (ISAT): Long-term follow-up. Lancet Neurol 8:427, 2009

Morandi A et al: Delirium in the intensive care unit. Int Rev Psych 21:43, 2009

Nolan JP et al: Therapeutic hypothermia after cardiac arrest: An advisory statement by the Advanced Life Support Task Force of the International Liaison Committee on Resuscitation. Circulation 108:118, 2003

Posner JB et al: *Plum and Posner's Diagnosis of Stupor and Coma*, 4th ed. New York, Oxford University Press, 2007

Rossetti AO et al: Prognostication after cardiac arrest and hypothermia: A prospective study. Ann Neurol 67:301, 2010

Wijdicks EFM et al: Practice parameter: Prediction of outcome in comatose survivors after cardiopulmonary resuscitation (an evidence-based review). Neurology 67:203, 2006

CHAPTER 276
Oncologic Emergencies

Rasim Gucalp
Janice Dutcher

Emergencies in patients with cancer may be classified into three groups: pressure or obstruction caused by a space-occupying lesion, metabolic or hormonal problems (paraneoplastic syndromes, Chap. 100), and treatment-related complications.

STRUCTURAL-OBSTRUCTIVE ONCOLOGIC EMERGENCIES

SUPERIOR VENA CAVA SYNDROME

Superior vena cava syndrome (SVCS) is the clinical manifestation of superior vena cava (SVC) obstruction, with severe reduction in venous return from the head, neck, and upper extremities. Malignant tumors, such as lung cancer, lymphoma, and metastatic tumors, are responsible for the majority of SVCS cases. With the expanding use of intravascular devices (e.g., permanent central venous access catheters, pacemaker/defibrillator leads), the prevalence of benign causes of SVCS is increasing now, accounting for at least 40% of cases. Lung cancer, particularly of small cell and squamous cell histologies, accounts for approximately 85% of all cases of malignant origin. In young adults, malignant lymphoma is a leading cause of SVCS. Hodgkin's lymphoma involves the mediastinum more commonly than other lymphomas but rarely causes SVCS. When SVCS is noted in a young man with a mediastinal mass, the differential diagnosis is lymphoma vs primary mediastinal germ cell tumor. Metastatic cancers to the mediastinum, such as testicular and breast carcinomas, account for a small proportion of cases. Other causes include benign tumors, aortic aneurysm, thyromegaly, thrombosis, and fibrosing mediastinitis from prior irradiation, histoplasmosis, or Behçet's syndrome. SVCS as the initial manifestation of Behçet's syndrome may be due to inflammation of the SVC associated with thrombosis.

Patients with SVCS usually present with neck and facial swelling (especially around the eyes), dyspnea, and cough. Other symptoms include hoarseness, tongue swelling, headaches, nasal congestion, epistaxis, hemoptysis, dysphagia, pain, dizziness, syncope, and lethargy. Bending forward or lying down may aggravate the symptoms. The characteristic physical findings are dilated neck veins; an increased number of collateral veins covering the anterior chest wall; cyanosis; and edema of the face, arms, and chest. More severe cases include proptosis, glossal and laryngeal edema, and obtundation. The clinical picture is milder if the obstruction is located above the azygos vein. Symptoms are usually progressive, but in some cases they may improve as collateral circulation develops.

Signs and symptoms of cerebral and/or laryngeal edema, though rare, are associated with a poorer prognosis and require urgent evaluation. Seizures are more likely related to brain metastases than to cerebral edema from venous occlusion. Patients with small cell lung cancer and SVCS have a higher incidence of brain metastases than those without SVCS.

Cardiorespiratory symptoms at rest, particularly with positional changes, suggest significant airway and vascular obstruction and limited physiologic reserve. Cardiac arrest or respiratory failure can occur, particularly in patients receiving sedatives or undergoing general anesthesia.

Rarely, esophageal varices may develop. These are "downhill" varices based on the direction of blood flow from cephalad to caudad (in contrast to "uphill" varices associated with caudad to cephalad flow from portal hypertension). If the obstruction to the SVC is proximal to the azygous vein, varices develop in the upper one-third of the esophagus. If the obstruction involves or is distal to the azygous vein, varices occur in the entire length of the esophagus. Variceal bleeding may be a late complication of chronic SVCS.

The diagnosis of SVCS is a clinical one. The most significant chest radiographic finding is widening of the superior mediastinum, most commonly on the right side. Pleural effusion occurs in only 25% of patients, often on the right side. The majority of these effusions are exudative and occasionally chylous. However, a normal chest radiograph is still compatible with the diagnosis if other characteristic findings are present. CT provides the most reliable view of the mediastinal anatomy. The diagnosis of SVCS requires diminished or absent opacification of central venous structures with prominent collateral venous circulation. MRI has no advantages over CT. Invasive procedures, including bronchoscopy, percutaneous needle biopsy, mediastinoscopy, and even thoracotomy, can be performed by a skilled clinician without any major risk of bleeding. For patients with a known cancer, a detailed workup usually is not necessary, and appropriate treatment may be started after obtaining a CT scan of the thorax. For those with no history of malignancy, a detailed evaluation is essential to rule out benign causes and determine a specific diagnosis to direct the appropriate therapy.

TREATMENT Superior Vena Cava Syndrome

The one potentially life-threatening complication of a superior mediastinal mass is tracheal obstruction. Upper airway obstruction demands emergent therapy. Diuretics with a low-salt diet, head elevation, and oxygen may produce temporary symptomatic relief. Glucocorticoids may be useful at shrinking lymphoma masses; they are of no benefit in patients with lung cancer.

Radiation therapy is the primary treatment for SVCS caused by non-small cell lung cancer and other metastatic solid tumors. Chemotherapy is effective when the underlying cancer is small cell carcinoma of the lung, lymphoma, or germ cell tumor. SVCS recurs in 10–30% of patients; it may be palliated with the use of intravascular self-expanding stents (Fig. 276-1). Early stenting may be necessary in patients with severe symptoms; however, the prompt increase in venous return after stenting may precipitate heart failure and pulmonary edema. Surgery may provide immediate relief for patients in whom a benign process is the cause.

Clinical improvement occurs in most patients, although this improvement may be due to the development of adequate collateral circulation. The mortality associated with SVCS does not relate to caval obstruction but rather to the underlying cause.

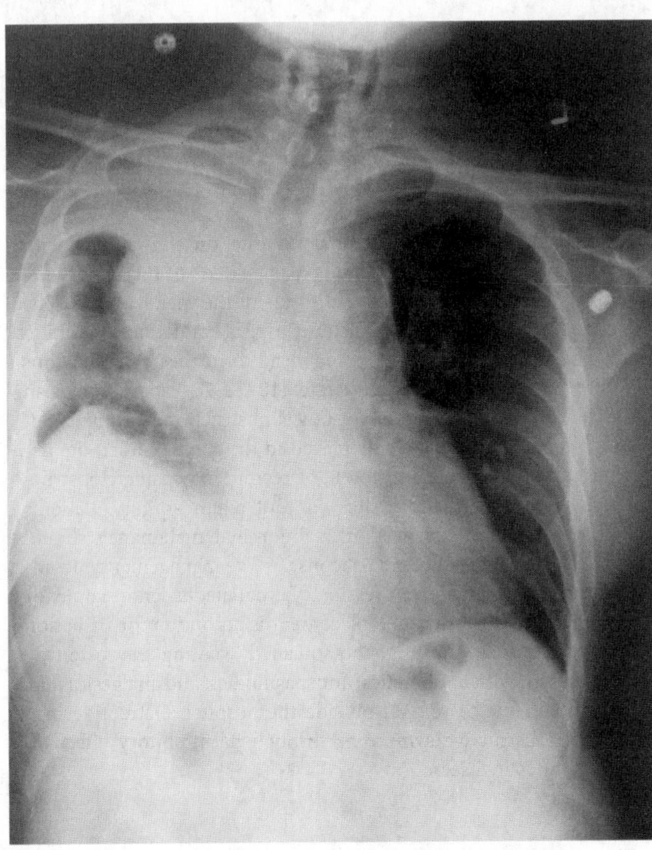

A

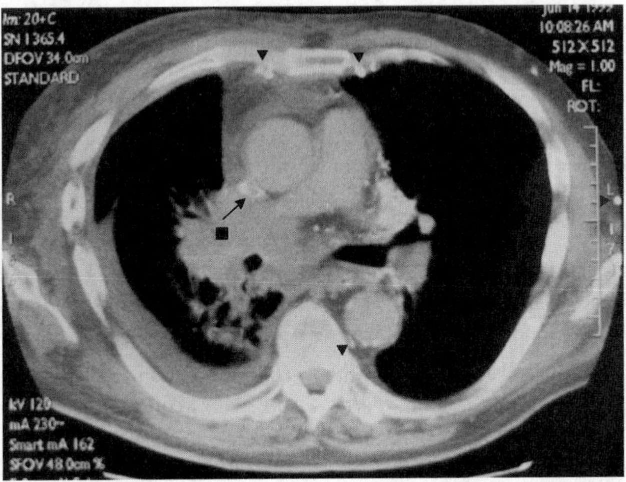

B

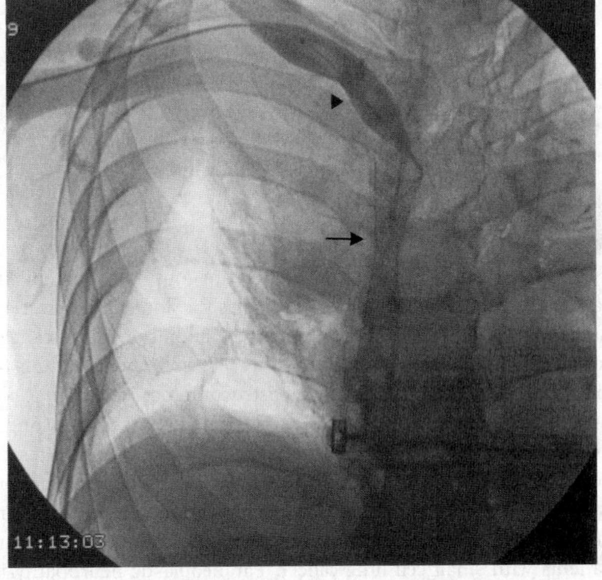

C

Figure 276-1 Superior vena cava syndrome. *A.* Chest radiographs of a 59-year-old man with recurrent SVCS caused by non-small cell lung cancer showing right paratracheal mass with right pleural effusion. ***B.*** CT of same patient demonstrating obstruction of SVC with thrombosis (*arrow*) by the lung cancer (*square*) and collaterals (*arrowheads*). ***C.*** Balloon angioplasty (*arrowhead*) with Wallstent (*arrow*) in same patient.

SVCS AND CENTRAL VENOUS CATHETERS IN ADULTS The use of long-term central venous catheters has become common practice in patients with cancer. Major vessel thrombosis may occur. In these cases, catheter removal should be combined with anticoagulation to prevent embolization. SVCS in this setting, if detected early, can be treated by fibrinolytic therapy without sacrificing the catheter. The routine use of low-dose warfarin or low-molecular-weight heparin to prevent thrombosis related to permanent central venous access catheters in cancer patients is not recommended.

■ PERICARDIAL EFFUSION/TAMPONADE

Malignant pericardial disease is found at autopsy in 5–10% of patients with cancer, most frequently with lung cancer, breast cancer, leukemias, and lymphomas. Cardiac tamponade as the initial presentation of extrathoracic malignancy is rare. The origin is not malignancy in about 50% of cancer patients with symptomatic pericardial disease, but it can be related to irradiation, drug-induced pericarditis, hypothyroidism, idiopathic pericarditis, infection, or autoimmune diseases. Two types of radiation pericarditis occur: an acute inflammatory, effusive pericarditis occurring within months of irradiation, which usually resolves spontaneously, and a chronic effusive pericarditis that may appear up to 20 years after radiation therapy and is accompanied by a thickened pericardium.

Most patients with pericardial metastasis are asymptomatic. However, the common symptoms are dyspnea, cough, chest pain, orthopnea, and weakness. Pleural effusion, sinus tachycardia, jugular venous distention, hepatomegaly, peripheral edema, and cyanosis are the most frequent physical findings. Relatively specific diagnostic findings, such as paradoxical pulse, diminished heart sounds, pulsus alternans (pulse waves alternating between those of greater and lesser amplitude with successive beats), and friction rub are less common than with nonmalignant pericardial disease. Chest radiographs and ECG reveal abnormalities in 90% of patients, but half of these abnormalities are nonspecific. Echocardiography is the most helpful diagnostic test. Pericardial fluid may be serous, serosanguineous, or hemorrhagic, and cytologic examination of pericardial fluid is diagnostic in most patients. Cancer patients with pericardial effusion containing malignant cells on cytology have a very poor survival, about 7 weeks.

TREATMENT Pericardial Effusion/Tamponade

Pericardiocentesis with or without the introduction of sclerosing agents, the creation of a pericardial window, complete pericardial stripping, cardiac irradiation, or systemic chemotherapy are effective treatments. Acute pericardial tamponade with life-threatening hemodynamic instability requires immediate drainage of fluid. This can be quickly achieved by pericardiocentesis. The recurrence rate after percutaneous catheter drainage is about 20%. Sclerotherapy (pericardial instillation of bleomycin, mitomycin C, or tetracycline) may decrease recurrences. Alternatively, subxiphoid pericardiotomy can be performed in 45 min under local anesthesia. Thoracoscopic pericardial fenestration can be employed for benign causes; however, 60% of malignant pericardial effusions recur after this procedure.

INTESTINAL OBSTRUCTION

Intestinal obstruction and reobstruction are common problems in patients with advanced cancer, particularly colorectal or ovarian carcinoma. However, other cancers, such as lung or breast cancer and melanoma, can metastasize within the abdomen, leading to intestinal obstruction. Typically, obstruction occurs at multiple sites in peritoneal carcinomatosis. Melanoma has a predilection to involve the small bowel; this involvement may be isolated and resection may result in prolonged survival. Intestinal pseudoobstruction is caused by infiltration of the mesentery or bowel muscle by tumor, involvement of the celiac plexus, or paraneoplastic neuropathy in patients with small cell lung cancer. Paraneoplastic neuropathy is associated with IgG antibodies reactive to neurons of the myenteric and submucosal plexuses of the jejunum and stomach. Ovarian cancer can lead to authentic luminal obstruction or to pseudoobstruction that results when circumferential invasion of a bowel segment arrests the forward progression of peristaltic contractions.

The onset of obstruction is usually insidious. Pain is the most common symptom and is usually colicky in nature. Pain can also be due to abdominal distention, tumor masses, or hepatomegaly. Vomiting can be intermittent or continuous. Patients with complete obstruction usually have constipation. Physical examination may reveal abdominal distention with tympany, ascites, visible peristalsis, high-pitched bowel sounds, and tumor masses. Erect plain abdominal films may reveal multiple air-fluid levels and dilation of the small or large bowel. Acute cecal dilation to >12–14 cm is considered a surgical emergency because of the high likelihood of rupture. CT scan is useful in differentiating benign from malignant causes of obstruction in patients who have undergone surgery for malignancy. Malignant obstruction is suggested by a mass at the site of obstruction or prior surgery, adenopathy, or an abrupt transition zone and irregular bowel thickening at the obstruction site. Benign obstruction is more likely when CT shows mesenteric vascular changes, a large volume of ascites, or a smooth transition zone and smooth bowel thickening at the obstruction site. The prognosis for the patient with cancer who develops intestinal obstruction is poor; median survival is 3–4 months. About 25–30% of patients are found to have intestinal obstruction due to causes other than cancer. Adhesions from previous operations are a common benign cause. Ileus induced by vinca alkaloids, narcotics, or other drugs is another reversible cause.

TREATMENT Intestinal Obstruction

The management of intestinal obstruction in patients with advanced malignancy depends on the extent of the underlying malignancy and the functional status of the major organs. The initial management should include surgical evaluation. Operation is not always successful and may lead to further complications with a substantial mortality rate (10–20%). Laparoscopy can diagnose and treat malignant bowel obstruction in some cases. Self-expanding metal stents placed in the gastric outlet, duodenum, proximal jejunum, colon, or rectum may palliate obstructive symptoms at those sites without major surgery. Patients known to have advanced intraabdominal malignancy should receive a prolonged course of conservative management, including nasogastric decompression. Percutaneous endoscopic or surgical gastrostomy tube placement is an option for palliation of nausea and vomiting, the so-called "venting gastrostomy." Treatment with antiemetics, antispasmodics, and analgesics may allow patients to remain outside the hospital. Octreotide may relieve obstructive symptoms through its inhibitory effect on gastrointestinal secretion.

URINARY OBSTRUCTION

Urinary obstruction may occur in patients with prostatic or gynecologic malignancies, particularly cervical carcinoma; metastatic disease from other primary sites such as carcinomas of the breast, stomach, lung, colon, and pancreas; or lymphomas. Radiation therapy to pelvic tumors may cause fibrosis and subsequent ureteral obstruction. Bladder outlet obstruction is usually due to prostate and cervical cancers and may lead to bilateral hydronephrosis and renal failure.

Flank pain is the most common symptom. Persistent urinary tract infection, persistent proteinuria, or hematuria in patients with cancer should raise suspicion of ureteral obstruction. Total anuria and/or anuria alternating with polyuria may occur. A slow, continuous rise in the serum creatinine level necessitates immediate evaluation. Renal ultrasound is the safest and cheapest way to identify hydronephrosis. The function of an obstructed kidney can be evaluated by a nuclear scan. CT scan can reveal the point of obstruction and identify a retroperitoneal mass or adenopathy.

TREATMENT Urinary Obstruction

Obstruction associated with flank pain, sepsis, or fistula formation is an indication for immediate palliative urinary diversion. Internal ureteral stents can be placed under local anesthesia. Percutaneous nephrostomy offers an alternative approach for drainage. In the case of bladder outlet obstruction due to malignancy, a suprapubic cystostomy can be used for urinary drainage.

MALIGNANT BILIARY OBSTRUCTION

This common clinical problem can be caused by a primary carcinoma arising in the pancreas, ampulla of Vater, bile duct, or liver or by metastatic disease to the periductal lymph nodes or liver parenchyma. The most common metastatic tumors causing biliary obstruction are gastric, colon, breast, and lung cancers. Jaundice, light-colored stools, dark urine, pruritus, and weight loss due to malabsorption are usual symptoms. Pain and secondary infection are uncommon in malignant biliary obstruction. Ultrasound, CT scan, or percutaneous transhepatic or endoscopic retrograde cholangiography will identify the site and nature of the biliary obstruction.

TREATMENT Malignant Biliary Obstruction

Palliative intervention is indicated only in patients with disabling pruritus resistant to medical treatment, severe malabsorption, or infection. Stenting under radiographic control, surgical bypass, or radiation therapy with or without chemotherapy may alleviate the obstruction. The choice of therapy should be based on the site of obstruction (proximal vs distal), the type of tumor (sensitive to radiotherapy, chemotherapy, or neither), and the general condition of the patient. In the absence of pruritus, biliary obstruction may be a largely asymptomatic cause of death.

SPINAL CORD COMPRESSION

Malignant spinal cord compression (MSCC) is defined as compression of the spinal cord and/or cauda equina by an extradural tumor mass. The minimum radiologic evidence for cord compression is indentation of the theca at the level of clinical features. Spinal cord compression occurs in 5–10% of patients with cancer. Epidural tumor is the first manifestation of malignancy in about 10% of patients. The underlying cancer is usually identified during the initial evaluation; lung cancer is the most common cause of MSCC.

Metastatic tumor involves the vertebral column more often than any other part of the bony skeleton. Lung, breast, and prostate cancer are the most frequent offenders. Multiple myeloma also has a high incidence of spine involvement. Lymphomas, melanoma, renal cell cancer, and genitourinary cancers also cause cord compression. The thoracic spine is the most common site (70%), followed by the lumbosacral spine (20%) and the cervical spine (10%). Involvement of multiple sites is most frequent in patients with breast and prostate carcinoma. Cord injury develops when metastases to the vertebral body or pedicle enlarge and compress the underlying dura. Another cause of cord compression is direct extension of a paravertebral lesion through the intervertebral foramen. These cases usually involve a lymphoma, myeloma, or pediatric neoplasm. Parenchymal spinal cord metastasis due to hematogenous spread is rare. Intramedullary metastases can be seen in lung cancer, multiple myeloma, renal cell cancer, and breast cancer and are frequently associated with brain metastases and leptomeningeal disease.

Expanding extradural tumors induce injury through several mechanisms. Obstruction of the epidural venous plexus leads to edema. Local production of inflammatory cytokines enhances blood flow and edema formation. Compression compromises blood flow leading to ischemia. Production of vascular endothelial growth factor is associated with spinal cord hypoxia and has been implicated as a potential cause of damage after spinal cord injury.

The most common initial symptom in patients with spinal cord compression is localized back pain and tenderness due to involvement of vertebrae by tumor. Pain is usually present for days or months before other neurologic findings appear. It is exacerbated by movement and by coughing or sneezing. It can be differentiated from the pain of disk disease by the fact that it worsens when the patient is supine. Radicular pain is less common than localized back pain and usually develops later. Radicular pain in the cervical or lumbosacral areas may be unilateral or bilateral. Radicular pain from the thoracic roots is often bilateral and is described by patients as a feeling of tight, band-like constriction around the thorax and abdomen. Typical cervical radicular pain radiates down the arm; in the lumbar region, the radiation is down the legs. *Lhermitte's sign*, a tingling or electric sensation down the back and upper and lower limbs upon flexing or extending the neck, may be an early sign of cord compression. Loss of bowel or bladder control may be the presenting symptom but usually occurs late in the course. Occasionally patients present with ataxia of gait without motor and sensory involvement due to involvement of the spinocerebellar tract.

On physical examination, pain induced by straight leg raising, neck flexion, or vertebral percussion may help to determine the level of cord compression. Patients develop numbness and paresthesias in the extremities or trunk. Loss of sensibility to pinprick is as common as loss of sensibility to vibration or position. The upper limit of the zone of sensory loss is often one or two vertebrae below the site of compression. Motor findings include weakness, spasticity, and abnormal muscle stretching. An extensor plantar reflex reflects significant compression. Deep tendon reflexes may be brisk. Motor and sensory loss usually precedes sphincter disturbance. Patients with autonomic dysfunction may present with decreased anal tonus, decreased perineal sensibility, and a distended bladder. The absence of the anal wink reflex or the bulbocavernosus reflex confirms cord involvement. In doubtful cases, evaluation of postvoiding urinary residual volume can be helpful. A residual volume of >150 mL suggests bladder dysfunction. Autonomic dysfunction is an unfavorable prognostic factor. Patients with progressive neurologic symptoms should have frequent neurologic examinations and rapid therapeutic intervention. Other illnesses that may mimic cord compression include osteoporotic vertebral collapse, disk disease, pyogenic abscess or vertebral tuberculosis, radiation myelopathy, neoplastic leptomeningitis, benign tumors, epidural hematoma, and spinal lipomatosis.

Cauda equina syndrome is characterized by low back pain; diminished sensation over the buttocks, posterior-superior thighs, and perineal area in a saddle distribution; rectal and bladder dysfunction; sexual impotence; absent bulbocavernous, patellar, and Achilles' reflexes; and variable amount of lower-extremity weakness. This reflects compression of nerve roots as they form the cauda equina after leaving the spinal cord.

Patients with cancer who develop back pain should be evaluated for spinal cord compression as quickly as possible (Fig. 276-2). Treatment is more often successful in patients who are ambulatory and still have sphincter control at the time treatment is initiated. Patients should have a neurologic examination and plain films of the spine. Those whose physical examination suggests cord compression should receive dexamethasone (6 mg intravenously every 6 h), starting immediately.

Erosion of the pedicles (the "winking owl" sign) is the earliest radiologic finding of vertebral tumor. Other radiographic changes include increased intrapedicular distance, vertebral destruction, lytic or sclerotic lesions, scalloped vertebral bodies, and vertebral body collapse. Vertebral collapse is not a reliable indicator of the presence of tumor; about 20% of cases of vertebral collapse, particularly those in older patients and postmenopausal women, are due not to cancer but to osteoporosis. Also, a normal appearance on plain films of the spine does not exclude the diagnosis of cancer. The role of bone scans in the detection of cord compression is not clear; this method is sensitive but less specific than spinal radiography.

The full-length image of the cord provided by MRI is the imaging procedure of choice. Multiple epidural metastases are noted in 25% of patients with cord compression, and their presence influences treatment plans. On T1-weighted images, good contrast is noted between the cord, cerebrospinal fluid, and extradural lesions.

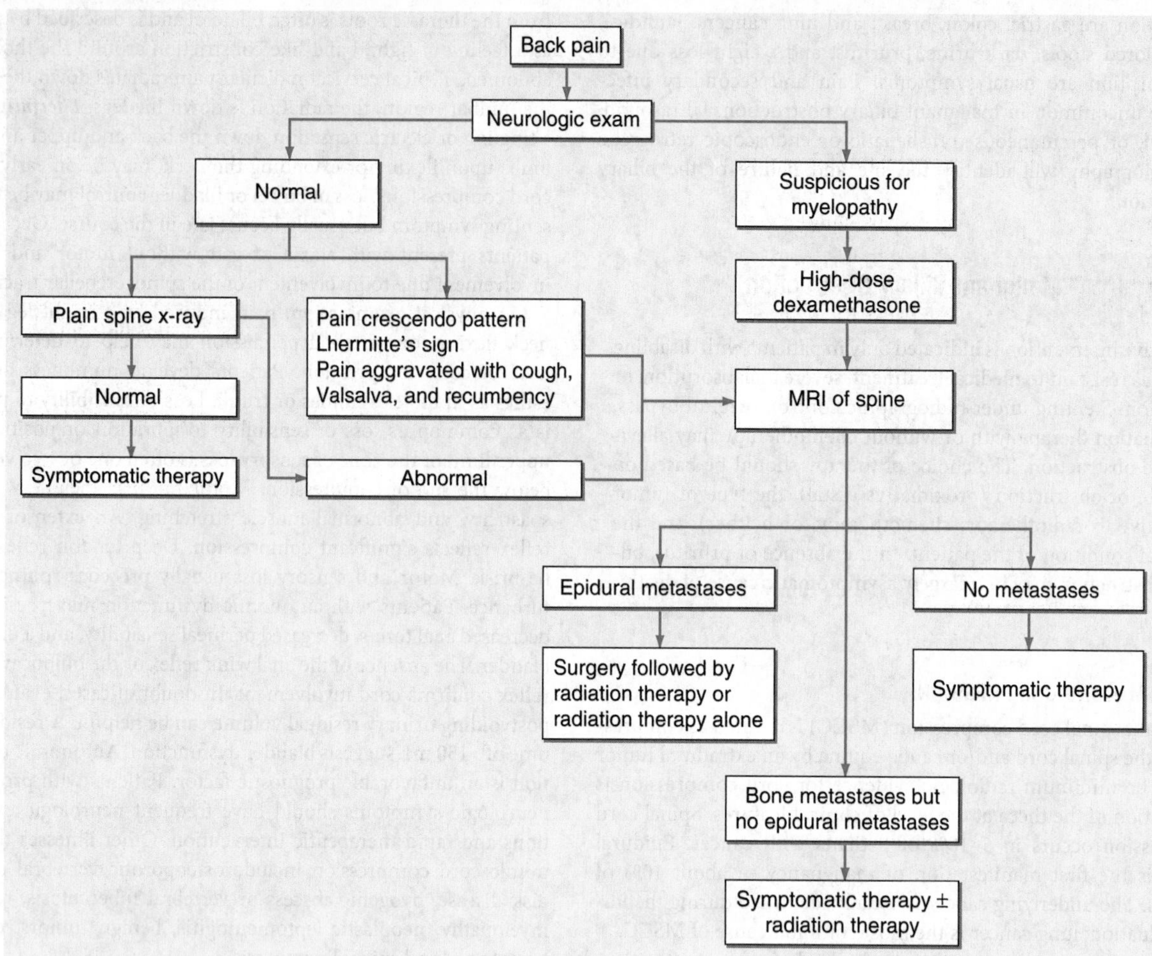

Figure 276-2 Management of cancer patients with back pain.

Owing to its sensitivity in demonstrating the replacement of bone marrow by tumor, MRI can show which parts of a vertebra are involved by tumor. MRI also visualizes intraspinal extradural masses compressing the cord. T2-weighted images are most useful for the demonstration of intramedullary pathology. Gadolinium-enhanced MRI can help to delineate intramedullary disease. MRI is as good as or better than myelography plus postmyelogram CT scan in detecting metastatic epidural disease with cord compression. Myelography should be reserved for patients who have poor MR images or who cannot undergo MRI promptly. CT scan in conjunction with myelography enhances the detection of small areas of spinal destruction.

In patients with cord compression and an unknown primary tumor, a simple workup including chest radiography, mammography, measurement of prostate-specific antigen, and abdominal CT usually reveals the underlying malignancy.

TREATMENT Spinal Cord Compression

The treatment of patients with spinal cord compression is aimed at relief of pain and restoration/preservation of neurologic function (Fig. 276-2).

Radiation therapy plus glucocorticoids is generally the initial treatment of choice for most patients with spinal cord compression. Up to 75% of patients treated when still ambulatory remain ambulatory, but only 10% of patients with paraplegia recover walking capacity. Indications for surgical intervention include unknown etiology, failure of radiation therapy, a radioresistant tumor type (e.g., melanoma or renal cell cancer), pathologic fracture dislocation, and rapidly evolving neurologic symptoms. Laminectomy is done for tissue diagnosis and for the removal of posteriorly localized epidural deposits in the absence of vertebral body disease. Because most cases of epidural spinal cord compression are due to anterior or anterolateral extradural disease, resection of the anterior vertebral body along with the tumor, followed by spinal stabilization, has achieved good results. A randomized trial showed that patients who underwent an operation followed by radiotherapy (within 14 days) retained the ability to walk significantly longer than those treated with radiotherapy alone. Surgically treated patients also maintained continence and neurologic function significantly longer than patients in the radiation group. The length of survival was not significantly different in the two groups, although there was a trend toward longer survival in the surgery group. The study drew some criticism for the poorer than expected results in the patients who did not go to surgery. However, patients should be evaluated for surgery if they are expected to survive longer than 3 months. Conventional radiotherapy has a role after surgery. Chemotherapy may have a role in patients with chemosensitive tumors who have had prior radiotherapy to the same region and who are not candidates for surgery. Most patients with prostate cancer who develop cord compression have already had hormonal therapy; however, for those who have not, androgen deprivation is combined with surgery and radiotherapy.

Patients with metastatic vertebral tumors may benefit from percutaneous vertebroplasty or kyphoplasty, the injection of acrylic cement into a collapsed vertebra to stabilize the fracture. Pain palliation is common, and local antitumor effects have been noted. Cement leakage may cause symptoms in about 10% of patients. Bisphosphonates may be helpful in prevention of SCC in patients with bony involvement.

The histology of the tumor is an important determinant of both recovery and survival. Rapid onset and progression of signs and symptoms are poor prognostic features.

INCREASED INTRACRANIAL PRESSURE

About 25% of patients with cancer die with intracranial metastases. The cancers that most often metastasize to the brain are lung and breast cancers and melanoma. Brain metastases often occur in the presence of systemic disease, and they frequently cause major symptoms, disability, and early death. The initial presentation of brain metastases from a previously unknown primary cancer is common. Lung cancer is most commonly the primary malignancy. Chest CT scans and brain MRI as the initial diagnostic studies can identify a biopsy site in most patients.

The signs and symptoms of a metastatic brain tumor are similar to those of other intracranial expanding lesions: headache, nausea, vomiting, behavioral changes, seizures, and focal, progressive neurologic changes. Occasionally the onset is abrupt, resembling a stroke, with the sudden appearance of headache, nausea, vomiting, and neurologic deficits. This picture is usually due to hemorrhage into the metastasis. Melanoma, germ cell tumors, and renal cell cancers have a particularly high incidence of intracranial bleeding. The tumor mass and surrounding edema may cause obstruction of the circulation of cerebrospinal fluid, with resulting hydrocephalus. Patients with increased intracranial pressure may have papilledema with visual disturbances and neck stiffness. As the mass enlarges, brain tissue may be displaced through the fixed cranial openings, producing various herniation syndromes.

CT scan and MRI are equally effective in the diagnosis of brain metastases. CT scan with contrast should be used as a screening procedure. The CT scan shows brain metastases as multiple enhancing lesions of various sizes with surrounding areas of low-density edema. If a single lesion or no metastases are visualized by contrast-enhanced CT, MRI of the brain should be performed. Gadolinium-enhanced MRI is more sensitive than CT at revealing meningeal involvement and small lesions, particularly in the brainstem or cerebellum.

Intracranial hypertension secondary to tretinoin therapy has been reported.

TREATMENT Increased Intracranial Pressure

Dexamethasone is the best initial treatment for all symptomatic patients with brain metastases. If signs and symptoms of brain herniation (particularly headache, drowsiness, and papilledema) are present, the patient should be intubated and hyperventilated to maintain Pco_2 between 25 and 30 mmHg and should receive infusions of mannitol (1–1.5 g/kg) every 6 h. Other measures include head elevation, fluid restriction, and hypertonic saline with diuretics. Patients with multiple lesions should receive whole-brain radiation. Patients with a single brain metastasis and with controlled extracranial disease may be treated with surgical excision followed by whole-brain radiation therapy, especially if they are younger than 60 years. Radioresistant tumors should be resected if possible. Stereotactic radiosurgery is an effective treatment for inaccessible or recurrent lesions. With a gamma knife or linear accelerator, multiple small, well-collimated beams of ionizing radiation destroy lesions seen on MRI. Some patients with increased intracranial pressure associated with hydrocephalus may benefit from shunt placement. If neurologic deterioration is not reversed with medical therapy, ventriculotomy to remove cerebrospinal fluid (CSF) or craniotomy to remove tumors or hematomas may be necessary.

NEOPLASTIC MENINGITIS

Tumor involving the leptomeninges is a complication of both primary central nervous system (CNS) tumors and tumors that metastasize to the CNS. The incidence is estimated at 3–8% of patients with cancer. Melanoma, breast and lung cancer, lymphoma (including AIDS-associated), and acute leukemia are the most common causes. Synchronous intraparenchymal brain metastases are evident in 11–31% of patients with neoplastic meningitis.

Patients typically present with multifocal neurologic signs and symptoms, including headache, gait abnormality, mental changes, nausea, vomiting, seizures, back or radicular pain, and limb weakness. Signs include cranial nerve palsies, extremity weakness, paresthesia, and decreased deep tendon reflexes.

Diagnosis is made by demonstrating malignant cells in the CSF; however, up to 40% of patients may have false-negative CSF cytology. An elevated CSF protein level is nearly always present (except in HTLV-1–associated adult T cell leukemia). Patients with neurologic signs and symptoms consistent with neoplastic meningitis who have a negative CSF cytology but an elevated CSF protein level should have the spinal tap repeated at least three times for cytologic examination before the diagnosis is rejected. MRI findings suggestive of neoplastic meningitis include leptomeningeal, subependymal, dural, or cranial nerve enhancement; superficial cerebral lesions; and communicating hydrocephalus. Spinal cord imaging by MRI is a necessary component of the evaluation of nonleukemia neoplastic meningitis as ~20% of patients have cord abnormalities, including intradural enhancing nodules that are diagnostic for leptomeningeal involvement. Cauda equina lesions are common, but lesions may be seen anywhere in the spinal canal. Radiolabeled CSF flow studies are abnormal in up to 70% of patients with neoplastic meningitis; ventricular outlet obstruction, abnormal flow in the spinal canal, or impaired flow over the cerebral convexities may affect distribution of intrathecal chemotherapy resulting in decreased efficacy or increased toxicity. Radiation therapy may correct CSF flow abnormalities before use of intrathecal chemotherapy. Neoplastic meningitis can also lead to intracranial hypertension and hydrocephalus. Placement of a ventriculoperitoneal shunt may effectively palliate symptoms in these patients.

The development of neoplastic meningitis usually occurs in the setting of uncontrolled cancer outside the CNS; thus, prognosis is poor (median survival 10–12 weeks). However, treatment of the neoplastic meningitis may successfully alleviate symptoms and control the CNS spread.

TREATMENT Neoplastic Meningitis

Intrathecal chemotherapy, usually methotrexate, cytarabine, or thiotepa, is delivered by lumbar puncture or by an intraventricular reservoir (Ommaya) three times a week until the CSF is free of malignant cells. Injections are given twice a week for a month and then weekly for a month. An extended-release preparation of cytarabine (Depocyte) has a longer half-life and is more effective than other formulations. Among solid tumors, breast cancer responds best to therapy. Patients with neoplastic meningitis from either acute leukemia or lymphoma may be cured of their CNS disease if the systemic disease can be eliminated.

SEIZURES

Seizures occurring in a patient with cancer can be caused by the tumor itself, by metabolic disturbances, by radiation injury, by cerebral infarctions, by chemotherapy-related encephalopathies, or by CNS infections. Metastatic disease to the CNS is the most common cause of seizures in patients with cancer. However, seizures occur more frequently in primary brain tumors than in metastatic brain lesions. Seizures are a presenting symptom of CNS metastasis in 6–29% of cases. Approximately 10% of patients with CNS metastasis eventually develop seizures. Tumors that affect the frontal, temporal, and parietal lobes are more commonly associated with seizures than are occipital lesions. The presence of frontal lesions correlates with early seizures, and the presence of hemispheric symptoms increases the risk for late seizures. Both early and late seizures are uncommon in patients with posterior fossa and sellar lesions. Seizures are common in patients with CNS metastases from melanoma and low-grade primary brain tumors. Very rarely, cytotoxic drugs such as etoposide, busulfan, and chlorambucil cause seizures. Another cause of seizures related to drug therapy is reversible posterior leukoencephalopathy syndrome (RPLS). RPLS is associated with administration of cisplatin, 5-fluorouracil, bleomycin, vinblastine, vincristine, etoposide, paclitaxel, ifosfamide, cyclophosphamide, doxorubicin, cytarabine, methotrexate, oxaliplatin, cyclosporine, tacrolimus, and bevacizumab. RPLS is characterized by headache, altered consciousness, generalized seizures, visual disturbances, hypertension, and posterior cerebral white matter vasogenic edema on CT/MRI. Seizures may begin focally but are typically generalized.

TREATMENT Seizures

Patients in whom seizures due to CNS metastases have been demonstrated should receive anticonvulsive treatment with phenytoin. Prophylactic anticonvulsant therapy is not recommended unless the patient is at high risk for late seizures (melanoma primary, hemorrhagic metastases, treatment with radiosurgery). Serum phenytoin levels should be monitored closely and the dosage adjusted according to serum levels. Phenytoin induces the hepatic metabolism of dexamethasone, reducing its half-life, while dexamethasone may decrease phenytoin levels. Most antiseizure medications induce CYP450, which alters the metabolism of antitumor agents, including irinotecan, taxanes, and etoposide as well as molecular targeted agents, including imatinib, gefitinib, erlotinib, and tipifarnib. Levetiracetam and topiramate are anticonvulsant agents not metabolized by the hepatic cytochrome P450 system and do not alter the metabolism of antitumor agents.

PULMONARY AND INTRACEREBRAL LEUKOSTASIS

Hyperleukocytosis and the leukostasis syndrome associated with it is a potentially fatal complication of acute leukemia (particularly myeloid leukemia) that can occur when the peripheral blast cell count is >100,000/mL. The frequency of hyperleukocytosis is 5–13% in acute myelid leukemia (AML) and 10–30% in acute lymphoid leukemia; however, leukostasis is rare in lymphoid leukemia. At such high blast cell counts, blood viscosity is increased, blood flow is slowed by aggregates of tumor cells, and the primitive myeloid leukemic cells are capable of invading through the endothelium and causing hemorrhage. Brain and lung are most commonly affected. Patients with brain leukostasis may experience stupor, headache, dizziness, tinnitus, visual disturbances, ataxia, confusion, coma, or sudden death. Administration of 600 cGy of whole-brain irradiation can protect against this complication and can be followed by rapid institution of antileukemic therapy. Hydroxyurea, 3-5 grams, can rapidly reduce a high blast cell count while the accurate diagnostic workup is in progress. Pulmonary leukostasis may present as respiratory distress, hypoxemia, and progress to respiratory failure. Chest radiographs may be normal but usually show interstitial or alveolar infiltrates. Arterial blood gas results should be interpreted cautiously. Rapid consumption of plasma oxygen by the markedly increased number of white blood cells can cause spuriously low arterial oxygen tension. Pulse oximetry is the most accurate way of assessing oxygenation in patients with hyperleukocytosis. Leukapheresis may be helpful in decreasing circulating blast counts. Treatment of the leukemia can result in pulmonary hemorrhage from lysis of blasts in the lung, called *leukemic cell lysis pneumopathy*. Intravascular volume depletion and unnecessary blood transfusions may increase blood viscosity and worsen the leukostasis syndrome. Leukostasis is very rarely a feature of the high white cell counts associated with chronic lymphoid or chronic myeloid leukemia.

When acute promyelocytic leukemia is treated with differentiating agents like tretinoin and arsenic trioxide, cerebral or pulmonary leukostasis may occur as tumor cells differentiate into mature neutrophils. This complication can be largely avoided by using cytotoxic chemotherapy together with the differentiating agents.

HEMOPTYSIS

Hemoptysis may be caused by nonmalignant conditions, but lung cancer accounts for a large proportion of cases. Up to 20% of patients with lung cancer have hemoptysis some time in their course. Endobronchial metastases from carcinoid tumors, breast cancer, colon cancer, kidney cancer, and melanoma may also cause hemoptysis. The volume of bleeding is often difficult to gauge. Massive hemoptysis is defined as >200–600 mL of blood produced in 24 h. However, any hemoptysis should be considered massive if it threatens life. When respiratory difficulty occurs, hemoptysis should be treated emergently. The first priorities are to maintain the airway, optimize oxygenation, and stabilize the hemodynamic status. *Often patients can tell where the bleeding is occurring.* They should be placed bleeding side down and given supplemental oxygen. If large-volume bleeding continues or the airway is compromised, the patient should be intubated and undergo emergency bronchoscopy. If the site of bleeding is detected, either the patient undergoes a definitive surgical procedure or the lesion is treated with a neodymium:yttrium-aluminum-garnet (Nd:YAG) laser. The surgical option is preferred. Bronchial artery embolization may control brisk bleeding in 75–90% of patients, permitting the definitive surgical procedure to be done more safely. Embolization without definitive surgery is associated with rebleeding in 20–50% of patients. Recurrent hemoptysis usually responds to a second embolization procedure. A postembolization syndrome characterized by pleuritic pain, fever, dysphagia, and leukocytosis may occur; it lasts 5–7 days and resolves with symptomatic treatment. Bronchial or esophageal wall necrosis, myocardial infarction, and spinal cord infarction are rare complications.

Pulmonary hemorrhage with or without hemoptysis in hematologic malignancies is often associated with fungal infections, particularly *Aspergillus* sp. After granulocytopenia resolves, the lung infiltrates in aspergillosis may cavitate and cause massive hemoptysis. Thrombocytopenia and coagulation defects should be corrected, if possible. Surgical evaluation is recommended in patients with aspergillosis-related cavitary lesions.

Bevacizumab, an antibody to vascular endothelial growth factor (VEGF) that inhibits angiogenesis, has been associated with life-threatening hemoptysis in patients with non-small cell lung cancer, particularly squamous cell histology. Non-small cell lung cancer patients with cavitary lesions have higher risk for pulmonary hemorrhage.

AIRWAY OBSTRUCTION

Airway obstruction refers to a blockage at the level of the mainstem bronchi or above. It may result either from intraluminal tumor growth or from extrinsic compression of the airway. The most common cause of malignant upper airway obstruction is invasion from an adjacent primary tumor, most commonly lung cancer, followed by esophageal, thyroid, and mediastinal malignancies. Extrathoracic primary tumors such as renal, colon, or breast cancer can cause airway obstruction through endobronchial and/or mediastinal lymph node metastases. Patients may present with dyspnea, hemoptysis, stridor, wheezing, intractable cough, postobstructive pneumonia, or hoarseness. Chest radiographs usually demonstrate obstructing lesions. CT scans reveal the extent of tumor. Cool, humidified oxygen, glucocorticoids, and ventilation with a mixture of helium and oxygen (Heliox) may provide temporary relief. If the obstruction is proximal to the larynx, a tracheostomy may be lifesaving. For more distal obstructions, particularly intrinsic lesions incompletely obstructing the airway, bronchoscopy with laser treatment, photodynamic therapy, or stenting can produce immediate relief in most patients (Fig. 276-3). However, radiation therapy (either external-beam irradiation or brachytherapy) given together with glucocorticoids may also open the airway. Symptomatic extrinsic compression may be palliated by stenting. Patients with primary airway tumors such as squamous cell carcinoma, carcinoid tumor, adenocystic carcinoma, or non-small cell lung cancer should have surgery.

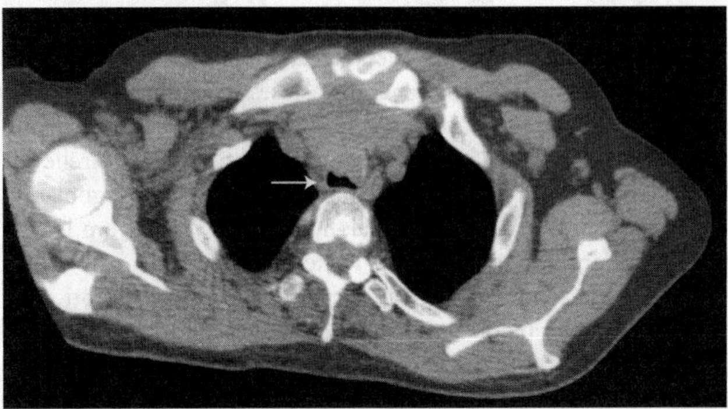
A

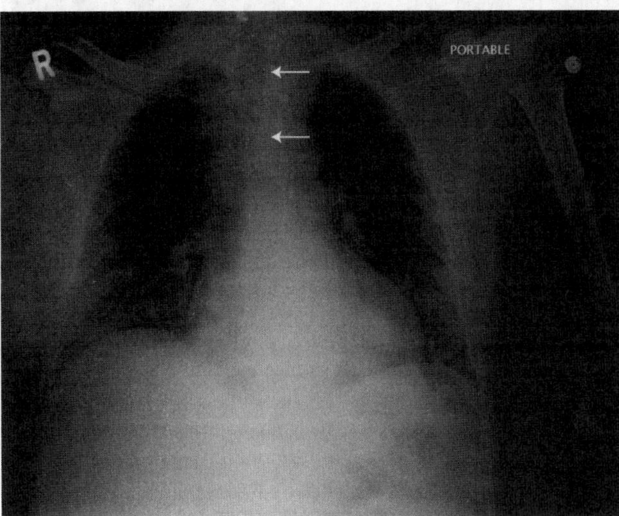

B

Figure 276-3 Airway obstruction. ***A.*** CT scan of a 62-year-old man with tracheal obstruction caused by renal carcinoma showing paratracheal mass (*A*) with tracheal invasion/obstruction (*arrow*). ***B.*** Chest x-ray of same patient after stent (*arrows*) placement.

METABOLIC EMERGENCIES

HYPERCALCEMIA

Hypercalcemia is the most common paraneoplastic syndrome. Its pathogenesis and management are discussed fully in Chaps. 100 and 353.

SYNDROME OF INAPPROPRIATE SECRETION OF ANTIDIURETIC HORMONE (SIADH)

Hyponatremia is a common electrolyte abnormality in cancer patients, and SIADH is the most common cause among patients with cancer. SIADH is discussed fully in Chaps. 100 and 339.

LACTIC ACIDOSIS

Lactic acidosis is a rare and potentially fatal metabolic complication of cancer. The body produces about 1500 mmols of lactic acid per day, most of which is metabolized by the liver. Normally, this lactate is generated by the skin (25%), muscle (25%), red cells (20%), brain (20%), and gut (10%). Lactic acidosis may occur as a consequence of increased production or decreased hepatic metabolism. Normal venous levels of lactate are 0.5–2.2 mmol/L (4.5–19.8 mg/dL). Lactic acidosis associated with sepsis and circulatory failure is a common preterminal event in many malignancies. Lactic acidosis in the absence of hypoxemia may occur in patients with leukemia, lymphoma, or solid tumors. Extensive involvement of the liver by tumor is often present. In most cases, decreased metabolism and increased production by the tumor both contribute to lactate accumulation. Tumor cell overexpression of certain glycolytic enzymes and mitochondrial dysfunction can contribute to its increased lactate production. HIV-infected patients have an increased risk of aggressive lymphoma; lactic acidosis that occurs in such patients may be related either to the rapid growth of the tumor or from toxicity of nucleoside reverse transcriptase inhibitors. Symptoms of lactic acidosis include tachypnea, tachycardia, change of mental status, and hepatomegaly. The serum level of lactic acid may reach 10–20 mmol/L (90–180 mg/dL). Treatment is aimed at the underlying disease. *The danger from lactic acidosis is from the acidosis, not the lactate.* Sodium bicarbonate should be added if acidosis is very severe or if hydrogen ion production is very rapid and uncontrolled. The prognosis is poor.

HYPOGLYCEMIA

Persistent hypoglycemia is occasionally associated with tumors other than pancreatic islet cell tumors. Usually these tumors are large; tumors of mesenchymal origin, hepatomas, or adrenocortical tumors may cause hypoglycemia. Mesenchymal tumors are usually located in the retroperitoneum or thorax. Obtundation, confusion, and behavioral aberrations occur in the postabsorptive period and may precede the diagnosis of the tumor. These tumors often secrete incompletely processed insulin-like growth factor II (IGF-II), a hormone capable of activating insulin receptors and causing hypoglycemia. Tumors secreting incompletely processed big IGF-II are characterized by an increased IGF-II to IGF-I ratio, suppressed insulin and C-peptide level, and inappropriately low growth hormone and β-hydroxybutyrate concentrations. Rarely, hypoglycemia is due to insulin secretion by a non-islet cell carcinoma. The development of hepatic dysfunction from liver metastases and increased glucose consumption by the tumor can contribute to hypoglycemia. If the tumor cannot be resected, hypoglycemia symptoms may be relieved by the administration of glucose, glucocorticoids, or glucagon.

Hypoglycemia can be artifactual; hyperleukocytosis from leukemia, myeloproliferative diseases, leukemoid reactions, or colony-stimulating factor treatment can increase glucose consumption in the test tube after blood is drawn, leading to pseudohypoglycemia.

ADRENAL INSUFFICIENCY

In patients with cancer, adrenal insufficiency may go unrecognized because the symptoms, such as nausea, vomiting, anorexia, and orthostatic hypotension, are nonspecific and may be mistakenly attributed to progressive cancer or to therapy. Primary adrenal insufficiency may develop owing to replacement of both glands by metastases (lung, breast, colon, or kidney cancer; lymphoma), to removal of both glands, or to hemorrhagic necrosis in association with sepsis or anticoagulation. Impaired adrenal steroid synthesis occurs in patients being treated for cancer with mitotane, ketoconazole, or aminoglutethimide or undergoing rapid reduction in glucocorticoid therapy. Rarely, metastatic replacement causes primary adrenal insufficiency as the first manifestation of an occult malignancy. Metastasis to the pituitary or hypothalamus is found at autopsy in up to 5% of patients with cancer, but associated secondary adrenal insufficiency is rare. Megestrol acetate, used to manage cancer and HIV-related cachexia, may suppress plasma levels of cortisol and adrenocorticotropic hormone (ACTH). Patients taking megestrol may develop adrenal insufficiency, and even those whose adrenal dysfunction is not symptomatic may have inadequate adrenal reserve if they become seriously ill. Paradoxically, some patients may develop Cushing's syndrome and/or hyperglycemia because of the glucocorticoid-like activity of megestrol acetate. Cranial irradiation for childhood brain tumors may affect the hypothalamus-pituitary-adrenal axis, resulting in secondary adrenal insufficiency.

Acute adrenal insufficiency is potentially lethal. Treatment of suspected adrenal crisis is initiated after the sampling of serum cortisol and ACTH levels (Chap. 342).

TREATMENT-RELATED EMERGENCIES

TUMOR LYSIS SYNDROME

Tumor lysis syndrome (TLS) is characterized by hyperuricemia, hyperkalemia, hyperphosphatemia, and hypocalcemia and is caused by the destruction of a large number of rapidly proliferating neoplastic cells. Acidosis may also develop. Acute renal failure occurs frequently.

TLS is most often associated with the treatment of Burkitt's lymphoma, acute lymphoblastic leukemia, and other rapidly proliferating lymphomas, but it also may be seen with chronic leukemias and, rarely, with solid tumors. This syndrome has been seen in patients with chronic lymphocytic leukemia after treatment with nucleosides like fludarabine. TLS has been observed with administration of glucocorticoids, hormonal agents such as letrozole and tamoxifen, and monoclonal antibodies such as rituximab and gemtuzumab. TLS usually occurs during or shortly (1–5 days) after chemotherapy. Rarely, spontaneous necrosis of malignancies causes TLS.

Hyperuricemia may be present at the time of chemotherapy. Effective treatment kills malignant cells and leads to increased serum uric acid levels from the turnover of nucleic acids. Owing to the acidic local environment, uric acid can precipitate in the tubules, medulla, and collecting ducts of the kidney, leading to renal failure. Lactic acidosis and dehydration may contribute to the precipitation of uric acid in the renal tubules. The finding of uric acid crystals in the urine is strong evidence for uric acid nephropathy. The ratio of urinary uric acid to urinary creatinine is >1 in patients with acute hyperuricemic nephropathy and <1 in patients with renal failure due to other causes.

Hyperphosphatemia, which can be caused by the release of intracellular phosphate pools by tumor lysis, produces a reciprocal depression in serum calcium, which causes severe neuromuscular irritability and tetany. Deposition of calcium phosphate in the kidney and hyperphosphatemia may cause renal failure. Potassium is the principal intracellular cation, and massive destruction of malignant cells may lead to hyperkalemia. Hyperkalemia in patients with renal failure may rapidly become life-threatening by causing ventricular arrhythmias and sudden death.

The likelihood that TLS will occur in patients with Burkitt's lymphoma is related to the tumor burden and renal function. Hyperuricemia and high serum levels of lactate dehydrogenase (LDH >1500 U/L), both of which correlate with total tumor burden, also correlate with the risk of TLS. In patients at risk for TLS, pretreatment evaluations should include a complete blood count, serum chemistry evaluation, and urine analysis. High leukocyte and platelet counts may artificially elevate potassium levels ("pseudohyperkalemia") due to lysis of these cells after the blood is drawn. In these cases, plasma potassium instead of serum potassium should be followed. In pseudohyperkalemia, no electrocardiographic abnormalities are present. In patients with abnormal baseline renal function, the kidneys and retroperitoneal area should be evaluated by sonography and/or CT to rule out obstructive uropathy. Urine output should be watched closely.

TREATMENT Tumor Lysis Syndrome

Recognition of risk and prevention are the most important steps in the management of this syndrome (Fig. 276-4). The standard preventive approach consists of allopurinol, urinary alkalinization, and aggressive hydration. Intravenous allopurinol may be given in patients who cannot tolerate oral therapy. In some cases, uric acid levels cannot be lowered sufficiently with the standard preventive approach. Rasburicase (recombinant urate oxidase) can be effective in these instances. Urate oxidase is missing from primates and catalyzes the conversion of poorly soluble uric acid to readily soluble allantoin. Rasburicase acts rapidly, decreasing uric acid levels within hours; however, it may cause hypersensitivity reactions such as bronchospasm, hypoxemia, and hypotension. Rasburicase should also be administered to high-risk patients for TLS prophylaxis. Rasburicase is contraindicated in patients with glucose-6-phosphate dehydrogenase deficiency who are unable to break down hydrogen peroxide, an end product of the urate oxidase reaction. Despite aggressive prophylaxis, TLS and/or oliguric or anuric renal failure may occur. Care should be taken to prevent worsening of symptomatic hypocalcemia by induction of alkalosis during bicarbonate infusion. Administration of sodium bicarbonate may also lead to urinary precipitation of calcium phosphate, which is less soluble at alkaline pH. Dialysis is often necessary and should be considered early in the course. Hemodialysis is preferred. Hemofiltration offers a gradual, continuous method of removing cellular by-products and fluid. The prognosis is excellent, and renal function recovers after the uric acid level is lowered to ≤10 mg/dL.

HUMAN ANTIBODY INFUSION REACTIONS

The initial infusion of human or humanized antibodies (e.g., rituximab, gemtuzumab, trastuzumab) is associated with fever, chills,

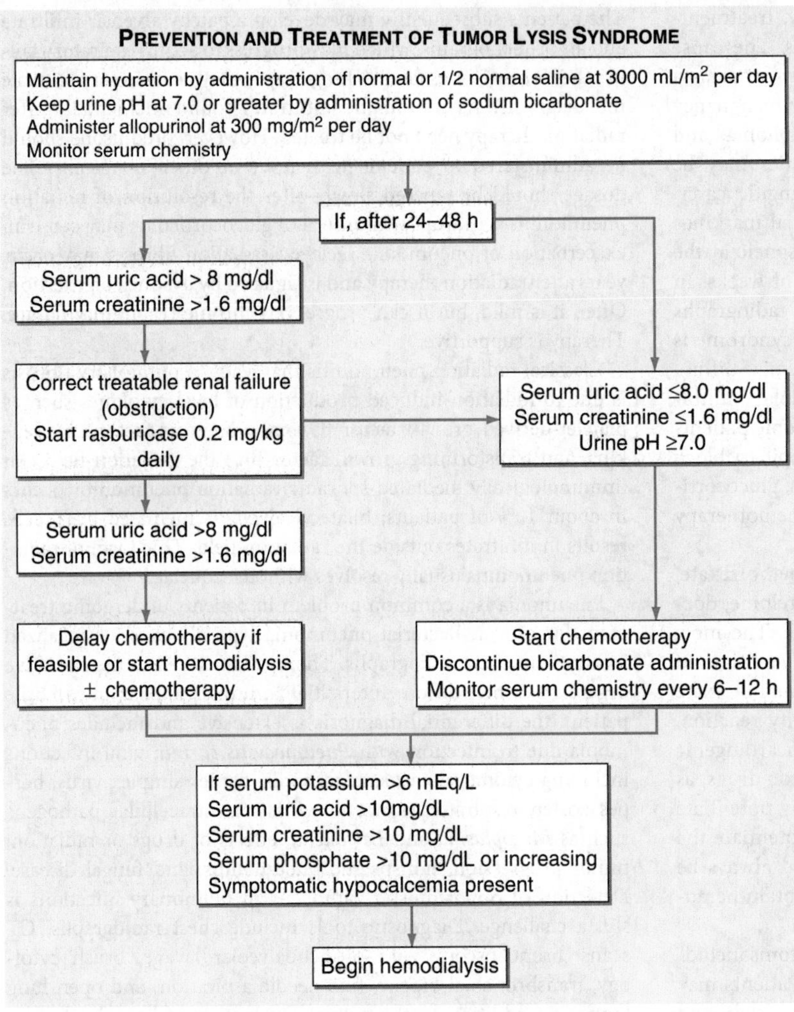
PREVENTION AND TREATMENT OF TUMOR LYSIS SYNDROME
Maintain hydration by administration of normal or 1/2 normal saline at 3000 mL/m2 per day
Keep urine pH at 7.0 or greater by administration of sodium bicarbonate
Administer allopurinol at 300 mg/m2 per day
Monitor serum chemistry
If, after 24–48 h
Serum uric acid > 8 mg/dl
Serum creatinine >1.6 mg/dl
Correct treatable renal failure (obstruction)
Start rasburicase 0.2 mg/kg daily
Serum uric acid ≤8.0 mg/dl
Serum creatinine ≤1.6 mg/dl
Urine pH ≥7.0
Serum uric acid >8 mg/dl
Serum creatinine >1.6 mg/dl
Delay chemotherapy if feasible or start hemodialysis ± chemotherapy
Start chemotherapy
Discontinue bicarbonate administration
Monitor serum chemistry every 6–12 h
If serum potassium >6 mEq/L
Serum uric acid >10mg/dL
Serum creatinine >10 mg/dL
Serum phosphate >10 mg/dL or increasing
Symptomatic hypocalcemia present
Begin hemodialysis

Figure 276-4 Management of patients at high risk for the tumor lysis syndrome.

nausea, asthenia, and headache in up to half of treated patients. Bronchospasm and hypotension occur in 1% of patients. Severe manifestations including pulmonary infiltrates, acute respiratory distress syndrome, and cardiogenic shock occur rarely. Laboratory manifestations include elevated hepatic aminotransferase levels, thrombocytopenia, and prolongation of prothrombin time. The pathogenesis is thought to be activation of immune effector processes (cells and complement) and release of inflammatory cytokines, such as tumor necrosis factor α and interleukin 6 (cytokine release syndrome). Severe reactions from rituximab have occurred with high numbers (more than 50 × 10^9 lymphocytes) of circulating cells bearing the target antigen (CD 20) and have been associated with a rapid fall in circulating tumor cells, mild electrolyte evidence of TLS, and very rarely, with death. In addition, increased liver enzymes, D-dimer, LDH, and prolongation of the prothrombin time may occur. Diphenhydramine, hydrocortisone, and acetaminophen can often prevent or suppress the infusion-related symptoms. If they occur, the infusion is stopped and restarted at half the initial infusion rate after the symptoms have abated. Severe "cytokine release syndrome" may require intensive support for acute respiratory distress syndrome (ARDS) and resistant hypotension.

HEMOLYTIC-UREMIC SYNDROME

Hemolytic-uremic syndrome (HUS) and, less commonly, thrombotic thrombocytopenic purpura (TTP) (Chap. 286) may rarely occur after treatment with antineoplastic drugs including mitomycin, cisplatin, bleomycin, and gemcitabine. It occurs most often in patients with gastric, lung, colorectal, pancreatic, and breast carcinoma. In one series, 35% of patients were without evident cancer at the time this syndrome appeared. Secondary HUS/TTP has also been reported as a rare but sometimes fatal complication of bone marrow transplantation.

HUS usually has its onset 4–8 weeks after the last dose of chemotherapy, but it is not rare to detect it several months later. HUS is characterized by microangiopathic hemolytic anemia, thrombocytopenia, and renal failure. Dyspnea, weakness, fatigue, oliguria, and purpura are also common initial symptoms and findings. Systemic hypertension and pulmonary edema frequently occur. Severe hypertension, pulmonary edema, and rapid worsening of hemolysis and renal function may occur after a blood or blood product transfusion. Cardiac findings include atrial arrhythmias, pericardial friction rub, and pericardial effusion. Raynaud's phenomenon is part of the syndrome in patients treated with bleomycin.

Laboratory findings include severe to moderate anemia associated with red blood cell fragmentation and numerous schistocytes on peripheral smear. Reticulocytosis, decreased plasma haptoglobin, and an LDH level document hemolysis. The serum bilirubin level is usually normal or slightly elevated. The Coombs' test is negative. The white cell count is usually normal, and thrombocytopenia (<100,000/μL) is almost always present. Most patients have a normal coagulation profile, although some have mild elevations in thrombin time and in levels of fibrin degradation products. The serum creatinine level is elevated at presentation and shows a pattern of subacute worsening within weeks of the initial azotemia. The urinalysis reveals hematuria, proteinuria, and granular or hyaline casts; and circulating immune complexes may be present.

The basic pathologic lesion appears to be deposition of fibrin in the walls of capillaries and arterioles, and these deposits are similar to those seen in HUS due to other causes. These microvascular abnormalities involve mainly the kidneys and rarely occur in other organs. The pathogenesis of chemotherapy-related HUS is unknown. Other forms of HUS/TTP are related to a decrease in processing of von Willebrand factor by a protease called ADAMTS13.

The case fatality rate is high; most patients die within a few months. There is no consensus on the optimal treatment for chemotherapy-induced HUS. Treatment modalities for HUS/TTP including immunocomplex removal (plasmapheresis, immunoadsorption, or exchange transfusion), antiplatelet/anticoagulant therapies, immunosuppressive therapies, and plasma exchange employed varying degrees of success. Rituximab is successfully used in patients with chemotherapy-induced HUS as well as in ADAMTS13-deficient TTP.

NEUTROPENIA AND INFECTION

These remain the most common serious complications of cancer therapy. They are covered in detail in Chap. 86.

PULMONARY INFILTRATES

Patients with cancer may present with dyspnea associated with diffuse interstitial infiltrates on chest radiographs. Such infiltrates may be due to progression of the underlying malignancy, treatment-related toxicities, infection, and/or unrelated diseases. The cause may be multifactorial; however, most commonly they occur as a consequence of treatment. Infiltration of the lung by malignancy has been described in patients with leukemia, lymphoma, and breast and other solid cancers. Pulmonary lymphatics may be involved diffusely by neoplasm (pulmonary lymphangitic carcinomatosis), resulting in a diffuse increase in interstitial markings on chest radiographs. The patient is often mildly dyspneic at the onset, but pulmonary failure develops over a period of weeks. In some patients, dyspnea precedes changes on the chest radiographs and is accompanied by a nonproductive cough. This syndrome is characteristic of solid tumors. In patients with leukemia, diffuse microscopic neoplastic peribronchial and peribronchiolar infiltration is frequent but may be asymptomatic. However, some patients present with diffuse interstitial infiltrates, an alveolar capillary block syndrome, and respiratory distress. In these situations, glucocorticoids can provide symptomatic relief, but specific chemotherapy should always be started promptly.

Several cytotoxic agents, such as bleomycin, methotrexate, busulfan, nitrosoureas, gemcitabine, mitomycin, vinorelbine, docetaxel, and ifosfamide may cause pulmonary damage. The most frequent presentations are interstitial pneumonitis, alveolitis, and pulmonary fibrosis. Some cytotoxic agents, including methotrexate and procarbazine, may cause an acute hypersensitivity reaction. Cytosine arabinoside has been associated with noncardiogenic pulmonary edema. Administration of multiple cytotoxic drugs, as well as radiotherapy and preexisting lung disease, may potentiate the pulmonary toxicity. Supplemental oxygen may potentiate the effects of drugs and radiation injury. Patients should always be managed with the lowest FIO_2 that is sufficient to maintain hemoglobin saturation.

The onset of symptoms may be insidious, with symptoms including dyspnea, nonproductive cough, and tachycardia. Patients may have bibasilar crepitant rales, end-inspiratory crackles, fever, and cyanosis. The chest radiograph generally shows an interstitial and sometimes an intraalveolar pattern that is strongest at the lung bases and may be symmetric. A small effusion may occur. Hypoxemia with decreased carbon monoxide diffusing capacity is always present. Glucocorticoids may be helpful in patients in whom pulmonary toxicity is related to radiation therapy or to chemotherapy. Treatment is otherwise supportive.

Molecular targeted agents, imatinib, erlotinib, and gefitinib are potent inhibitors of tyrosine kinases. These drugs may cause interstitial lung disease. In the case of gefitinib, preexisting fibrosis, poor performance status, and prior thoracic irradiation are independent risk factors; this complication has a high fatality rate. In Japan, incidence of interstitial lung disease associated with gefitinib was about 4.5% compared to 0.5% in the United States. Temsirolimus, a derivative of rapamycin, is an agent that blocks the effects of mTOR, an enzyme that has an important role in regulating the synthesis of proteins that control cell division. It may cause ground-glass opacities in the lung with or without diffuse interstitial disease and lung parenchymal consolidation.

Radiation pneumonitis and/or fibrosis is a relatively frequent side effect of thoracic radiation therapy. It may be acute or chronic. Radiation-induced lung toxicity is a function of the irradiated lung volume, dose per fraction, and radiation dose. The larger the irradiated lung field, the higher the risk for radiation pneumonitis. The use of concurrent chemoradiation increases pulmonary toxicity. Radiation pneumonitis usually develops from 2 to 6 months after completion of radiotherapy. The clinical syndrome, which varies in severity, consists of dyspnea, cough with scanty sputum, low-grade fever, and an initial hazy infiltrate on chest radiographs. The infiltrate and tissue damage usually are confined to the radiation field. The patients subsequently may develop a patchy alveolar infiltrate and air bronchograms, which may progress to acute respiratory failure that is sometimes fatal. A lung biopsy may be necessary to make the diagnosis. Asymptomatic infiltrates found incidentally after radiation therapy need not be treated. However, prednisone should be administered to patients with fever or other symptoms. The dosage should be tapered slowly after the resolution of radiation pneumonitis, as abrupt withdrawal of glucocorticoids may cause an exacerbation of pneumonia. Delayed radiation fibrosis may occur years after radiation therapy and is signaled by dyspnea on exertion. Often it is mild, but it can progress to chronic respiratory failure. Therapy is supportive.

Classical radiation pneumonitis that leads to pulmonary fibrosis is due to radiation-induced production of local cytokines such as platelet-derived growth factor β, tumor necrosis factor, interleukins, and transforming growth factor β in the radiation field. An immunologically mediated sporadic radiation pneumonitis occurs in about 10% of patients; bilateral alveolitis mediated by T cells results in infiltrates outside the radiation field. This form of radiation pneumonitis usually resolves without sequelae.

Pneumonia is a common problem in patients undergoing treatment for cancer. Bacterial pneumonia typically causes a localized infiltrate on chest radiographs. Therapy is tailored to the causative organism. When diffuse interstitial infiltrates appear in a febrile patient, the differential diagnosis is extensive and includes pneumonia due to infection with *Pneumocystis carinii*; viral infections including cytomegalovirus, adenovirus, herpes simplex virus, herpes zoster, respiratory syncytial virus, or intracellular pathogens such as *Mycoplasma* and *Legionella*; effects of drugs or radiation; tumor progression; nonspecific pneumonitis; and fungal disease. Detection of opportunistic pathogens in pulmonary infections is still a challenge. Diagnostic tools include chest radiographs, CT scans, bronchoscopy with bronchoalveolar lavage, brush cytology, transbronchial biopsy, fine-needle aspiration, and open lung biopsy. In addition to the culture, evaluation of bronchoalveolar lavage fluid for *P. carinii* by polymerase chain reaction (PCR) and serum galactomannan test improve the diagnostic yield. Patients with cancer who are neutropenic and have fever and local infiltrates on chest radiograph should be treated initially with broad-spectrum antibiotics. A new or persistent focal infiltrate not responding to broad-spectrum antibiotics argues for initiation of empiric antifungal therapy. When diffuse bilateral infiltrates develop in patients with febrile neutropenia, broad-spectrum antibiotics plus trimethoprim-sulfamethoxazole, with or without erythromycin, should be initiated. Addition of an antiviral agent is necessary in some settings, such as patients undergoing allogeneic hematopoietic stem cell transplantation. If the patient does not improve in 4 days, open lung biopsy is the procedure of choice. Bronchoscopy with bronchoalveolar lavage may be used in patients who are poor candidates for surgery.

In patients with pulmonary infiltrates who are afebrile, heart failure and multiple pulmonary emboli are in the differential diagnosis.

NEUTROPENIC ENTEROCOLITIS

Neutropenic enterocolitis (typhlitis) is the inflammation and necrosis of the cecum and surrounding tissues that may complicate the treatment of acute leukemia. Nevertheless, it may involve any segment of the gastrointestinal tract including small intestine, appendix, and colon. This complication has also been seen in patients with other forms of cancer treated with taxanes and in patients receiving high-dose chemotherapy (Fig. 276-5). The patient develops right lower quadrant abdominal pain, often with rebound tenderness and a tense, distended abdomen, in a setting of fever and neutropenia. Watery diarrhea (often containing sloughed mucosa) and bacteremia are common, and bleeding

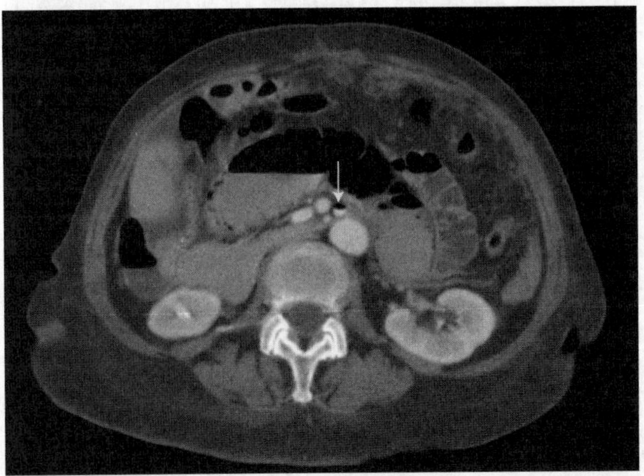

A

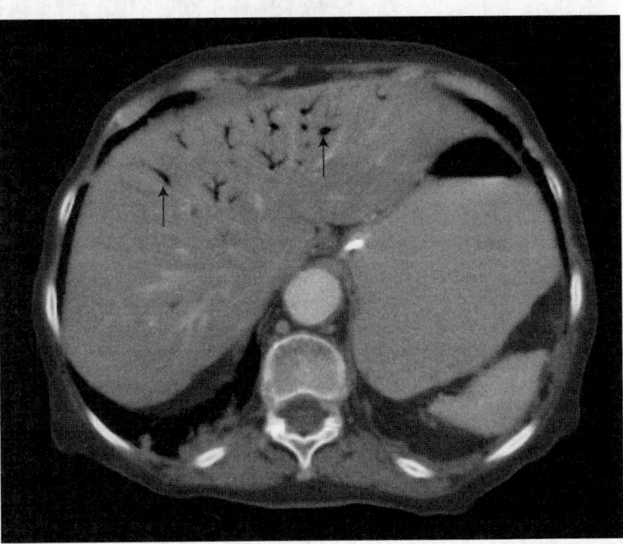

B

Figure 276-5 Abdominal CT scans of a 72-year-old woman with neutropenic enterocolitis secondary to chemotherapy. ***A.*** Air in inferior mesenteric vein (*arrow*) and bowel wall with pneumatosis intestinalis. ***B.*** CT scans of upper abdomen demonstrating air in portal vein (*arrows*).

may occur. Plain abdominal films are generally of little value in the diagnosis; CT scan may show marked bowel wall thickening, particularly in the cecum, with bowel wall edema, mesenteric stranding, and ascites. Patients with bowel wall thickness >10 mm on ultrasonogram have higher mortality rates. However, bowel wall thickening is significantly more prominent in patients with *Clostridium difficile* colitis. Pneumatosis intestinalis is a more specific finding, seen only in those with neutropenic enterocolitis and ischemia. The combined involvement of the small and large bowel suggests a diagnosis of neutropenic enterocolitis. Rapid institution of broad-spectrum antibiotics and nasogastric suction may reverse the process. Surgical intervention is reserved for severe cases of neutropenic enterocolitis with evidence of perforation, peritonitis, gangrenous bowel, or gastrointestinal hemorrhage despite correction of any coagulopathy.

C. difficile colitis is increasing in incidence. Newer strains of *C. difficile* produce about 20 times more of toxins A and B compared to previously studied strains. *C. difficile* risk is also increased with chemotherapy. Antibiotic coverage for *C. difficile* should be added if pseudomembranous colitis cannot be excluded.

HEMORRHAGIC CYSTITIS

Hemorrhagic cystitis can develop in patients receiving cyclophosphamide or ifosfamide. Both drugs are metabolized to acrolein, which is a strong chemical irritant that is excreted in the urine. Prolonged contact or high concentrations may lead to bladder irritation and hemorrhage. Symptoms include gross hematuria, frequency, dysuria, burning, urgency, incontinence, and nocturia. The best management is prevention. Maintaining a high rate of urine flow minimizes exposure. In addition, 2-mercaptoethanesulfonate (mesna) detoxifies the metabolites and can be coadministered with the instigating drugs. Mesna usually is given three times on the day of ifosfamide administration in doses that are each 20% of the total ifosfamide dose. If hemorrhagic cystitis develops, the maintenance of a high urine flow may be sufficient supportive care. If conservative management is not effective, irrigation of the bladder with a 0.37–0.74% formalin solution for 10 min stops the bleeding in most cases. *N*-acetylcysteine may also be an effective irrigant. Prostaglandin (carboprost) can inhibit the process. In extreme cases, ligation of the hypogastric arteries, urinary diversion, or cystectomy may be necessary.

Hemorrhagic cystitis also occurs in patients who undergo bone marrow transplantation (BMT). In the BMT setting, early-onset hemorrhagic cystitis is related to drugs in the treatment regimen (e.g., cyclophosphamide), and late-onset hemorrhagic cystitis is usually due to the polyoma virus BKV or adenovirus type 11. BKV load in urine alone or in combination with acute graft-versus-host disease correlate with development of hemorrhagic cystitis. Viral causes are usually detected by PCR-based diagnostic tests. Treatment of viral hemorrhagic cystitis is largely supportive, with reduction in doses of immunosuppressive agents, if possible. No antiviral therapy is approved, though cidofovir is reported to be effective in small series.

HYPERSENSITIVITY REACTIONS TO ANTINEOPLASTIC DRUGS

Many antineoplastic drugs may cause hypersensitivity reaction (HSR). These reactions are unpredictable and potentially life-threatening. Most reactions occur during or within hours of parenteral drug administration. Taxanes, platinum compounds, asparaginase, etoposide, and biologic agents, including rituximab, bevacizumab, trastuzumab, gemtuzumab, cetuximab, and alemtuzumab, are more commonly associated with acute HSR than are other agents. Acute hypersensitivity reactions to some drugs, such as taxanes, occur during the first or second dose administered. HSR from platinum compounds occurs after prolonged exposure. Skin testing may identify patients with high risk for HSR after carboplatin exposure. Premedication with histamine H_1 and H_2 receptor antagonists and glucocorticoids reduce the incidence of hypersensitivity reaction to taxanes, particularly paclitaxel. Despite premedication, HSR may still occur. In these cases, re-treatment may be attempted with care, but use of alternative agents may be required.

FURTHER READINGS

Albanell J, Baselga J: Systemic therapy emergencies. Semin Oncol 27:347, 2000

Coiffier B, Riouffol C: Management of tumor lysis syndrome in adults. Expert Rev Anticancer Ther 7:233, 2007

Davis MP et al: Modern management of cancer-related intestinal obstruction. Curr Oncol Rep 2:343, 2000

Gleissner B et al: Neoplastic meningitis. Lancet Neurol 5:443, 2006

Loblaw DA et al: Systematic review of the diagnosis and management of malignant extradural spinal cord compression: The Cancer Care Ontario Practice Guidelines Initiative's neuro-oncology disease site group. J Clin Oncol 23:2028, 2005

Maggi E et al: Acute infusion reactions induced by monoclonal antibody therapy. Expert Rev Clin Immunol 7:55, 2011

Ripamonti C et al: Respiratory problems in advanced cancer. Support Care Cancer 10:204, 2002

Samphao S et al: Oncological emergencies: Clinical importance and principles of management. Eur J Cancer Care (Engl) 19:707, 2010

Wan JF, Bezjak A: Superior vena cava syndrome. Emerg Med Clin North Am 27:243, 2009

Wright FC et al: Predictors of survival in patients with non-curative stage IV cancer and malignant bowel obstruction. J Surg Oncol 101:425, 2010

Zanotti KM et al: Prevention and management of antineoplastic-induced hypersensitivity reactions; Drug Saf 24:767, 2001

PART 13

Disorders of the Kidney and Urinary Tract

CHAPTER 277 Cellular and Molecular Biology of the Kidney

Alfred L. George, Jr.
Eric G. Neilson

The kidney is one of the most highly differentiated organs in the body. At the conclusion of embryologic development, nearly 30 different cell types form a multitude of filtering capillaries and segmented nephrons enveloped by a dynamic interstitium. This cellular diversity modulates a variety of complex physiologic processes. Endocrine functions, the regulation of blood pressure and intraglomerular hemodynamics, solute and water transport, acid-base balance, and removal of drug metabolites are all accomplished by intricate mechanisms of renal response. This breadth of physiology hinges on the clever ingenuity of nephron architecture that evolved as complex organisms came out of water to live on land.

EMBRYOLOGIC DEVELOPMENT

Kidneys develop from intermediate mesoderm under the timed or sequential control of a growing number of genes, described in Fig. 277-1. The transcription of these genes is guided by morphogenic cues that invite two ureteric buds to each penetrate bilateral metanephric blastema, where they induce primary mesenchymal cells to form early nephrons. This induction involves a number of complex signaling pathways mediated by Pax2, Six2, WT-1, Wnt9b, c-Met, fibroblast growth factor, transforming growth factor β, glial cell-derived neurotrophic factor, hepatocyte growth factor, and epidermal growth factor. The two ureteric buds emerge from posterior nephric ducts and mature into separate collecting systems that eventually form a renal pelvis and ureter. Induced mesenchyme undergoes mesenchymal epithelial transitions to form comma-shaped bodies at the proximal end of each ureteric bud leading to the formation of S-shaped nephrons that cleft and enjoin with penetrating endothelial cells derived from sprouting angioblasts. Under the influence of vascular endothelial growth factor A (VEGF-A), these penetrating cells form capillaries with surrounding mesangial cells that differentiate into a glomerular filter for plasma water and solute. The ureteric buds branch, and each branch produces a new set of nephrons. The number of branching events ultimately determines the total number of nephrons in each kidney. There are approximately 900,000 glomeruli in each kidney in normal birth weight adults and as few as 225,000 in low birth weight adults—producing the latter in numerous comorbid risks.

Glomeruli evolve as complex capillary filters with fenestrated endothelia under the guiding influence of VEGF-A and angiopoietin-1 secreted by adjacently developing podocytes. Epithelial podocytes facing the urinary space envelop the exterior basement membrane supporting these emerging endothelial capillaries. Podocytes are partially polarized and periodically fall off into the urinary space by epithelial-mesenchymal transition, and to a lesser extent apoptosis, only to be replenished by migrating parietal epithelia from Bowman's capsule. Failing replenishment results in heavy proteinuria. Podocytes attach to the basement membrane by special foot processes and share a slit-pore membrane with their neighbor. The slit-pore membrane forms a filter for plasma water and solute by the synthetic interaction of nephrin, annexin-4, CD2AP, FAT, ZO-1, P-cadherin, podocin, TRPC6, PLCE1, and neph 1–3 proteins. Mutations in many of these proteins also result in heavy proteinuria. The glomerular capillaries are embedded in a mesangial matrix shrouded by parietal and proximal tubular epithelia forming Bowman's capsule. Mesangial cells have an embryonic lineage consistent with arteriolar or juxtaglomerular cells and contain contractile actin-myosin fibers. These mesangial cells make contact with glomerular capillary loops, and their local matrix holds them in condensed arrangement.

Between nephrons lies the renal interstitium. This region forms a functional space surrounding glomeruli and their downstream tubules, which are home to resident and trafficking cells such as fibroblasts, dendritic cells, occasional lymphocytes, and lipid-laden macrophages. The cortical and medullary capillaries, which siphon off solute and water following tubular reclamation of glomerular filtrate, are also part of the interstitial fabric as well as a web of

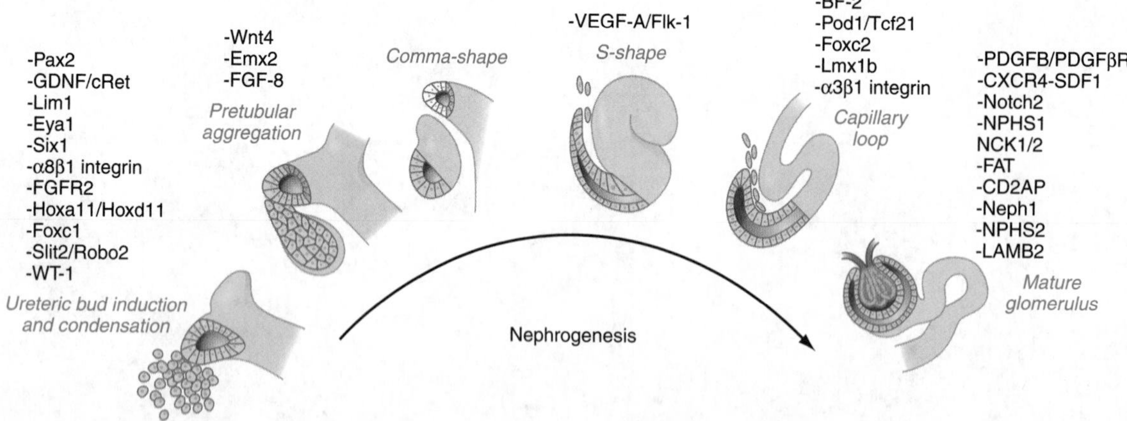

Figure 277-1 Genes controlling renal nephrogenesis. A growing number of genes have been identified at various stages of glomerulotubular development in the mammalian kidney. The genes listed have been tested in various genetically modified mice, and their location corresponds to the classical stages of kidney development postulated by Saxen in 1987. GDNF, giant cell line-derived neutrophilic factor; FGFR2, fibroblast growth factor receptor 2; WT-1, Wilms' tumor gene 1; FGF-8, fibroblast growth factor 8; VEGF–A/Flk-1, vascular endothelial growth factor–A/fetal liver kinase-1; PDGFβ, platelet-derived growth factor β; PDGFβR, PDGFβ receptor; SDF-1, stromal-derived factor 1; NPHS1, nephrin; NCK1/2, NCK-adaptor protein; CD2AP, CD2-associated protein; NPHS2, podocin; LAMB2, laminin beta-2.

connective tissue that supports the kidney's emblematic architecture of folding tubules. The relational precision of these structures determines the unique physiology of the kidney.

Each nephron is partitioned during embryologic development into a proximal tubule, descending and ascending limbs of the loop of Henle, distal tubule, and the collecting duct. These classic tubular segments build from subsegments lined by highly unique epithelia serving regional physiology. All nephrons have the same structural components, but there are two types whose structure depend on their location within the kidney. The majority of nephrons are cortical, with glomeruli located in the mid-to-outer cortex. Fewer nephrons are juxtamedullary, with glomeruli at the boundary of the cortex and outer medulla. Cortical nephrons have short loops of Henle, whereas juxtamedullary nephrons have long loops of Henle. There are critical differences in blood supply as well. The peritubular capillaries surrounding cortical nephrons are shared among adjacent nephrons. By contrast, juxtamedullary nephrons depend on individual capillaries called *vasa recta*. Cortical nephrons perform most of the glomerular filtration because there are more of them and because their afferent arterioles are larger than their respective efferent arterioles. The juxtamedullary nephrons, with longer loops of Henle, create a hyperosmolar gradient for concentrating urine. How developmental instructions specify the differentiation of all these unique epithelia among various tubular segments is still unknown.

DETERMINANTS AND REGULATION OF GLOMERULAR FILTRATION

Renal blood flow normally drains approximately 20% of the cardiac output, or 1000 mL/min. Blood reaches each nephron through the afferent arteriole leading into a glomerular capillary where large amounts of fluid and solutes are filtered to form the tubular fluid. The distal ends of the glomerular capillaries coalesce to form an efferent arteriole leading to the first segment of a second capillary network (cortical peritubular capillaries or medullary vasa recta) surrounding the tubules (Fig. 277-2A). Thus, nephrons have two capillary beds arranged in a series separated by the efferent arteriole that regulates the hydrostatic pressure in both capillary beds. The distal capillaries empty into small venous branches that coalesce into larger veins to eventually form the renal vein.

The hydrostatic pressure gradient across the glomerular capillary wall is the primary driving force for glomerular filtration. Oncotic pressure within the capillary lumen, determined by the concentration of unfiltered plasma proteins, partially offsets the hydrostatic pressure gradient and opposes filtration. As the oncotic pressure rises along the length of the glomerular capillary, the driving force for filtration falls to zero on reaching the efferent arteriole. Approximately 20% of the renal plasma flow is filtered into Bowman's space, and the ratio of glomerular filtration rate (GFR) to renal plasma flow determines the filtration fraction. Several factors, mostly hemodynamic, contribute to the regulation of filtration under physiologic conditions.

Although glomerular filtration is affected by renal artery pressure, this relationship is not linear across the range of physiologic blood pressures due to autoregulation of GFR. Autoregulation of glomerular filtration is the result of three major factors that modulate either afferent or efferent arteriolar tone: these include an autonomous vasoreactive (myogenic) reflex in the afferent arteriole, *tubuloglomerular feedback*, and angiotensin II–mediated vasoconstriction of the efferent arteriole. The myogenic reflex is a first line of defense against fluctuations in renal blood flow. Acute changes in renal perfusion pressure evoke reflex constriction or dilatation of the afferent arteriole in response to increased or decreased pressure, respectively. This phenomenon helps protect the glomerular capillary from sudden changes in systolic pressure.

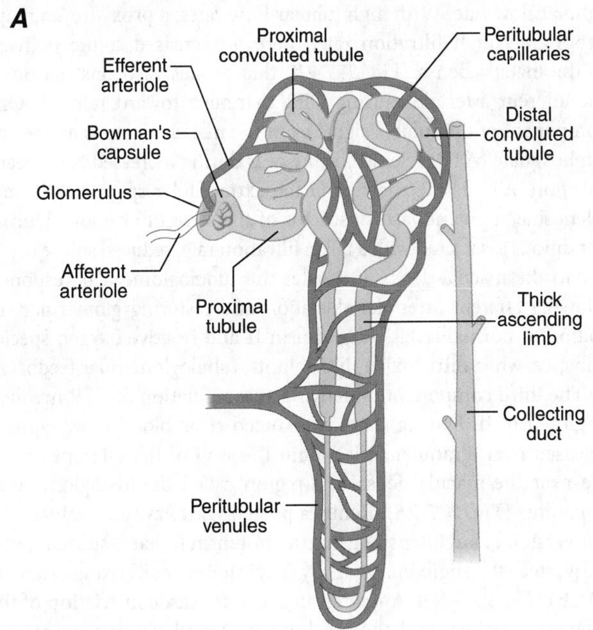

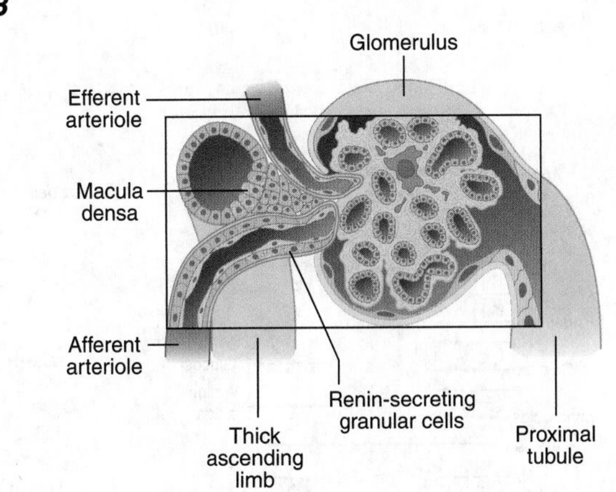

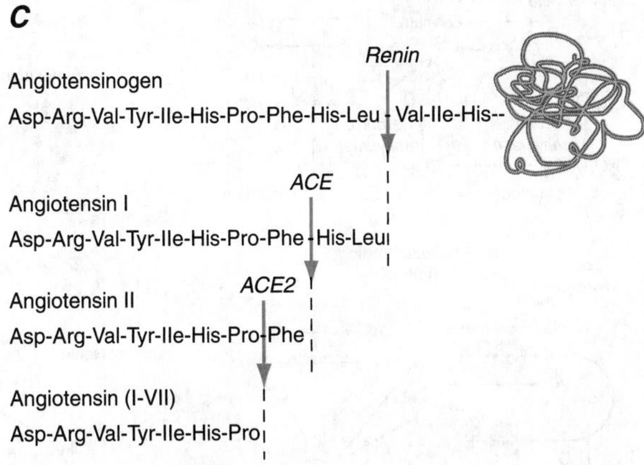

Figure 277-2 Renal microcirculation and the renin-angiotensin system. ***A.*** Diagram illustrating relationships of the nephron with glomerular and peritubular capillaries. ***B.*** Expanded view of the glomerulus with its juxtaglomerular apparatus including the macula densa and adjacent afferent arteriole. ***C.*** Proteolytic processing steps in the generation of angiotensins.

Tubuloglomerular feedback changes the rate of filtration and tubular flow by reflex vasoconstriction or dilatation of the afferent arteriole. Tubuloglomerular feedback is mediated by specialized cells in the thick ascending limb of the loop of Henle called the *macula densa* that act as sensors of solute concentration and tubular flow rate. With high tubular flow rates, a proxy for an inappropriately high filtration rate, there is increased solute delivery to the macula densa (Fig. 277-2B) that evokes vasoconstriction of the afferent arteriole causing GFR to return toward normal. One component of the soluble signal from the macula densa is adenosine triphosphate (ATP) released by the cells during increased NaCl reabsorption. ATP is metabolized in the extracellular space to generate adenosine, a potent vasoconstrictor of the afferent arteriole. During conditions associated with a fall in filtration rate, reduced solute delivery to the macula densa attenuates the tubuloglomerular response, allowing afferent arteriolar dilatation and restoring glomerular filtration to normal levels. Angiotensin II and reactive oxygen species enhance, while nitric oxide (NO) blunts, tubuloglomerular feedback.

The third component underlying autoregulation of GFR involves angiotensin II. During states of reduced renal blood flow, renin is released from granular cells within the wall of the afferent arteriole near the macula densa in a region called the juxtaglomerular apparatus (Fig. 277-2B). Renin, a proteolytic enzyme, catalyzes the conversion of angiotensinogen to angiotensin I, that is subsequently converted to angiotensin II by angiotensin-converting enzyme (ACE) (Fig. 277-2C). Angiotensin II evokes vasoconstriction of the efferent arteriole, and the resulting increased glomerular hydrostatic pressure elevates filtration to normal levels.

MECHANISMS OF RENAL TUBULAR TRANSPORT

The renal tubules are composed of highly differentiated epithelia that vary dramatically in morphology and function along the nephron (Fig. 277-3). The cells lining the various tubular segments form monolayers connected to one another by a specialized region of the adjacent lateral membranes called the *tight junction*. Tight junctions form an occlusive barrier that separates the lumen of the tubule from the interstitial spaces surrounding the tubule and also apportions the cell membrane into discrete domains: the apical membrane facing the tubular lumen and the basolateral membrane facing the interstitium. This regionalization allows cells to allocate membrane proteins and lipids asymmetrically. Owing to this feature, renal epithelial cells are said to be *polarized*. The asymmetric assignment of membrane proteins, especially proteins mediating transport processes, provides the machinery for directional movement of fluid and solutes by the nephron.

EPITHELIAL SOLUTE TRANSPORT

There are two types of epithelial transport. Movement of fluid and solutes sequentially across the apical and basolateral cell membranes (or vice versa) mediated by transporters, channels, or pumps is called *cellular transport*. By contrast, movement of fluid and solutes

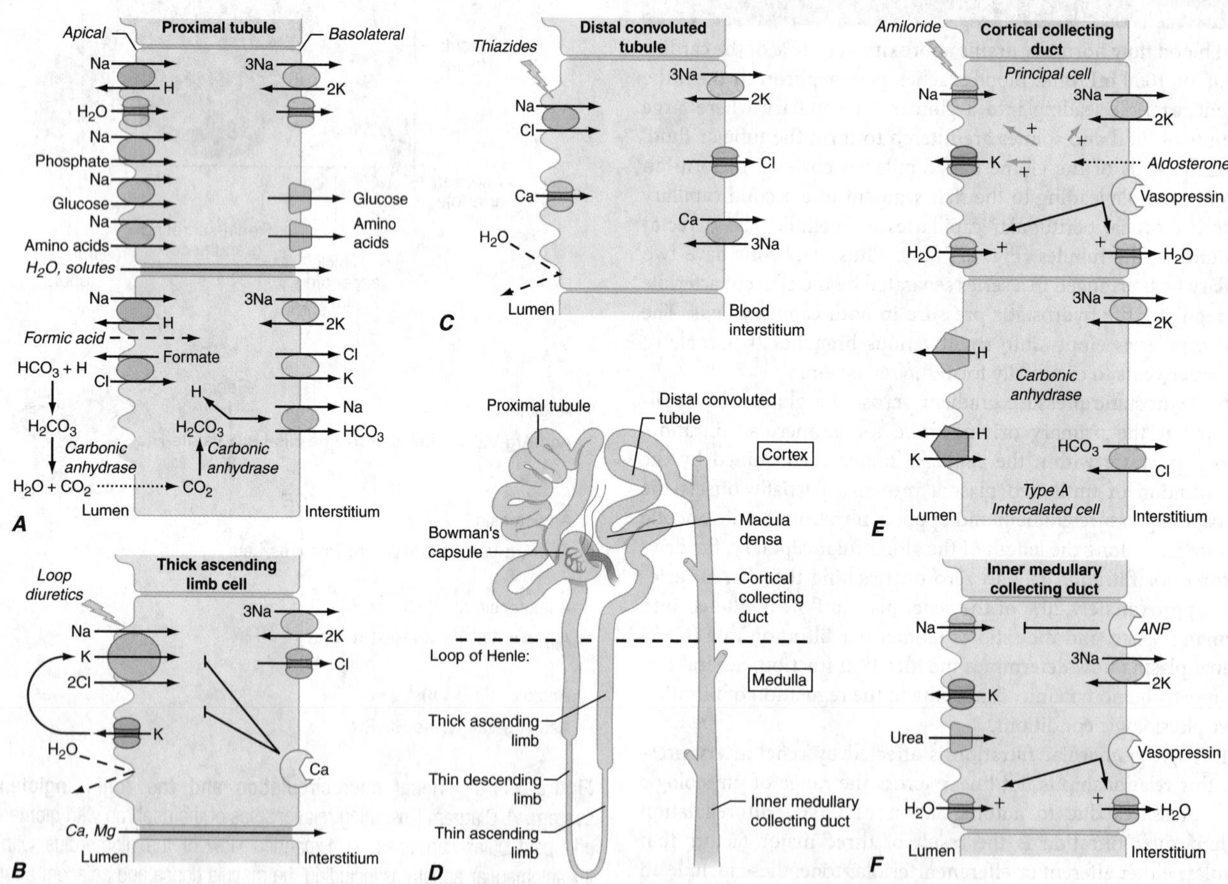

Figure 277-3 Transport activities of the major nephron segments. Representative cells from five major tubular segments are illustrated with the lumen side (apical membrane) facing left and interstitial side (basolateral membrane) facing right. ***A.*** Proximal tubular cells. ***B.*** Typical cell in the thick ascending limb of the loop of Henle. ***C.*** Distal convoluted tubular cell. ***D.*** Overview of entire nephron. ***E.*** Cortical collecting duct cells. ***F.*** Typical cell in the inner medullary collecting duct. The major membrane transporters, channels, and pumps are drawn with arrows indicating the direction of solute or water movement. For some events, the stoichiometry of transport is indicated by numerals preceding the solute. Targets for major diuretic agents are labeled. The actions of hormones are illustrated by arrows with plus signs for stimulatory effects and lines with perpendicular ends for inhibitory events. Dotted lines indicate free diffusion across cell membranes. The dashed line indicates water impermeability of cell membranes in the thick ascending limb and distal convoluted tubule.

through the narrow passageway between adjacent cells is called *paracellular transport.* Paracellular transport occurs through tight junctions, indicating that they are not completely "tight." Indeed, some epithelial cell layers allow rather robust paracellular transport to occur (*leaky epithelia*), whereas other epithelia have more effective tight junctions (*tight epithelia*). In addition, because the ability of ions to flow through the paracellular pathway determines the electrical resistance across the epithelial monolayer, leaky and tight epithelia are also referred to as low or high-resistance epithelia, respectively. The proximal tubule contains leaky epithelia, whereas distal nephron segments such as the collecting duct, contain tight epithelia. Leaky epithelia are most well suited for bulk fluid reabsorption, whereas tight epithelia allow for more refined control and regulation of transport.

MEMBRANE TRANSPORT

Cell membranes are composed of hydrophobic lipids that repel water and aqueous solutes. The movement of solutes and water across cell membranes is made possible by discrete classes of integral membrane proteins, including channels, pumps, and transporters. These different mechanisms mediate specific types of transport activities, including *active transport* (pumps), *passive transport* (channels), *facilitated diffusion* (transporters), and *secondary active transport* (cotransporters). Active transport requires metabolic energy generated by the hydrolysis of ATP. Active transport pumps are ion-translocating ATPases, including the ubiquitous Na^+/K^+-ATPase, the H^+-ATPases, and Ca^{2+}-ATPases. Active transport creates asymmetric ion concentrations across a cell membrane and can move ions against a chemical gradient. The potential energy stored in a concentration gradient of an ion such as Na^+ can be utilized to drive transport through other mechanisms (secondary active transport). Pumps are often *electrogenic*, meaning they can create an asymmetric distribution of electrostatic charges across the membrane and establish a voltage or membrane potential. The movement of solutes through a membrane protein by simple diffusion is called passive transport. This activity is mediated by channels created by selectively permeable membrane proteins, and it allows solute or water to move across a membrane driven by favorable *concentration gradients* or *electrochemical potential.* Examples in the kidney include water channels (aquaporins), K^+ channels, epithelial Na^+ channels, and Cl^- channels. Facilitated diffusion is a specialized type of passive transport mediated by simple transporters called *carriers* or *uniporters*. For example, hexose transporters such as GLUT2 mediate glucose transport by tubular cells. These transporters are driven by the concentration gradient for glucose that is highest in extracellular fluids and lowest in the cytoplasm due to rapid metabolism. Many other transporters operate by translocating two or more ions/solutes in concert either in the same direction (*symporters* or *cotransporters*) or in opposite directions (*antiporters* or *exchangers*) across the cell membrane. The movement of two or more ions/solutes may produce no net change in the balance of electrostatic charges across the membrane (*electroneutral*), or a transport event may alter the balance of charges (*electrogenic*). Several inherited disorders of renal tubular solute and water transport occur as a consequence of mutations in genes encoding a variety of channels, transporter proteins, and their regulators (Table 277-1).

SEGMENTAL NEPHRON FUNCTIONS

Each anatomic segment of the nephron has unique characteristics and specialized functions enabling selective transport of solutes and water (Fig. 277-3). Through sequential events of reabsorption and secretion along the nephron, tubular fluid is progressively conditioned into urine. Knowledge of the major tubular mechanisms responsible for solute and water transport is critical for understanding hormonal regulation of kidney function and the pharmacologic manipulation of renal excretion.

PROXIMAL TUBULE

The proximal tubule is responsible for reabsorbing ~60% of filtered NaCl and water, as well as ~90% of filtered bicarbonate and most critical nutrients such as glucose and amino acids. The proximal tubule utilizes both cellular and paracellular transport mechanisms. The apical membrane of proximal tubular cells has an expanded surface area available for reabsorptive work created by a dense array of microvilli called the *brush border*, and leaky tight junctions enable high-capacity fluid reabsorption.

Solute and water pass through these tight junctions to enter the lateral intercellular space where absorption by the peritubular capillaries occurs. Bulk fluid reabsorption by the proximal tubule is driven by high oncotic pressure and low hydrostatic pressure within the peritubular capillaries. Physiologic adjustments in GFR made by changing efferent arteriolar tone cause proportional changes in reabsorption, a phenomenon known as *glomerulotubular balance.* For example, vasoconstriction of the efferent arteriole by angiotensin II will increase glomerular capillary hydrostatic pressure but lower pressure in the peritubular capillaries. At the same time, increased GFR and filtration fraction raise oncotic pressure near the end of the glomerular capillary. These changes, a lowered hydrostatic and increased oncotic pressure, increase the driving force for fluid absorption by the peritubular capillaries.

Cellular transport of most solutes by the proximal tubule is coupled to the Na^+ concentration gradient established by the activity of a basolateral Na^+/K^+-ATPase (Fig. 277-3A). This active transport mechanism maintains a steep Na^+ gradient by keeping intracellular Na^+ concentrations low. Solute reabsorption is coupled to the Na^+ gradient by Na^+-dependent transporters such as Na^+-glucose and Na^+-phosphate cotransporters. In addition to the paracellular route, water reabsorption also occurs through the cellular pathway enabled by constitutively active water channels (aquaporin-1) present on both apical and basolateral membranes. Small, local *osmotic gradients* close to plasma membranes generated by cellular Na^+ reabsorption are likely responsible for driving directional water movement across proximal tubule cells, but reabsorption along the proximal tubule does not produce a net change in tubular fluid osmolality.

Proximal tubular cells reclaim bicarbonate by a mechanism dependent on carbonic anhydrases. Filtered bicarbonate is first titrated by protons delivered to the lumen by Na^+/H^+ exchange. The resulting carbonic acid (H_2CO_3) is metabolized by brush border carbonic anhydrase to water and carbon dioxide. Dissolved carbon dioxide then diffuses into the cell, where it is enzymatically hydrated by cytoplasmic carbonic anhydrase to re-form carbonic acid. Finally, intracellular carbonic acid dissociates into free protons and bicarbonate anions, and bicarbonate exits the cell through a basolateral Na^+/HCO_3^- cotransporter. This process is saturable, resulting in urinary bicarbonate excretion when plasma levels exceed the physiologically normal range (24–26 meq/L). Carbonic anhydrase inhibitors such as acetazolamide, a class of weak diuretic agents, block proximal tubule reabsorption of bicarbonate and are useful for alkalinizing the urine.

Chloride is poorly reabsorbed throughout the first segment of the proximal tubule, and a rise in Cl^- concentration counterbalances the removal of bicarbonate anion from tubular fluid. In later proximal tubular segments, cellular Cl^- reabsorption is initiated by apical exchange of cellular formate for higher luminal concentrations of Cl^-. Once in the lumen, formate anions are titrated by H^+ (provided by Na^+/H^+ exchange) to generate neutral formic acid, which can diffuse passively across the apical membrane back into the cell where it dissociates a proton and is recycled. Basolateral Cl^- exit is mediated by a K^+/Cl^- cotransporter.

Reabsorption of glucose is nearly complete by the end of the proximal tubule. Cellular transport of glucose is mediated by apical

TABLE 277-1 Inherited Disorders Affecting Renal Tubular Ion and Solute Transport

Disease or Syndrome	Gene	OMIM[a]
Disorders Involving the Proximal Tubule		
Proximal renal tubular acidosis	Sodium bicarbonate cotransporter (*SLC4A4*, 4q21)	604278
Fanconi-Bickel syndrome	Glucose transporter, GLUT2 (*SLC2A2*, 3q26.2)	227810
Isolated renal glycosuria	Sodium glucose cotransporter (*SLC5A2*, 16p11.2)	233100
Cystinuria		
Type I	Cystine, dibasic and neutral amino acid transporter (*SLC3A1*, 2p16.3)	220100
Nontype I	Amino acid transporter, light subunit (*SLC7A9*, 19q13.1)	600918
Lysinuric protein intolerance	Amino acid transporter (*SLC7A7*, 4q11.2)	222700
Hartnup disorder	Neutral amino acid transporter (*SLC6A19*, 5p15.33)	34500
Hereditary hypophosphatemic rickets with hypercalcemia	Sodium phosphate cotransporter (*SLC34A3*, 9q34)	241530
Renal hypouricemia		
Type 1	Urate-anion exchanger (*SLC22A12*, 11q13)	220150
Type 2	Urate transporter, GLUT9 (*SLC2A9*, 4p16.1)	612076
Dent's disease	Chloride channel, ClC-5 (*CLCN5*, Xp11.22)	300009
X-linked recessive nephrolithiasis with renal failure	Chloride channel, ClC-5 (*CLCN5*, Xp11.22)	310468
X-linked recessive hypophosphatemic rickets	Chloride channel, ClC-5 (*CLCN5*, Xp11.22)	307800
Disorders Involving the Loop of Henle		
Bartter's syndrome		
Type 1	Sodium, potassium chloride cotransporter (*SLC12A1*, 15q21.1)	241200
Type 2	Potassium channel, ROMK (*KCNJ1*, 11q24)	601678
Type 3	Chloride channel, ClC-Kb (*CLCNKB*, 1p36)	602023
with sensorineural deafness	Chloride channel accessory subunit, Barttin (*BSND*, 1p31)	602522
Autosomal dominant hypocalcemia with Bartter-like syndrome	Calcium-sensing receptor (*CASR*, 3q13.33))	601199
Familial hypocalciuric hypercalcemia	Calcium-sensing receptor (*CASR*, 3q13.33)	145980
Primary hypomagnesemia	Claudin-16 or paracellin-1 (*CLDN16* or *PCLN1*, 3q27)	248250
Isolated renal magnesium loss	Sodium potassium ATPase, γ_1-subunit (*ATP1G1*, 11q23)	154020
Disorders Involving the Distal Tubule and Collecting Duct		
Gitelman's syndrome	Sodium chloride cotransporter (*SLC12A3*, 16q13)	263800
Primary hypomagnesemia with secondary hypocalcemia	Melastatin-related transient receptor potential cation channel 6 (*TRPM6*, 9q22)	602014
Pseudoaldosteronism (Liddle's syndrome)	Epithelial sodium channel β and γ subunits (*SCNN1B*, *SCNN1G*, 16p12.1)	177200
Recessive pseudohypoaldosteronism Type 1	Epithelial sodium channel, α, β, and γ subunits (*SCNN1A*, 12p13; *SCNN1B*, *SCNN1G*, 16pp12.1)	264350
Pseudohypoaldosteronism Type 2 (Gordon's hyperkalemia-hypertension syndrome)	Kinases WNK-1, WNK-4 (*WNK1*, 12p13; *WNK4*, 17q21.31)	145260
X-linked nephrogenic diabetes insipidus	Vasopressin V2 receptor (AVPR2, Xq28)	304800
Nephrogenic diabetes insipidus (autosomal)	Water channel, aquaporin-2 (*AQP2*, 12q13)	125800
Distal renal tubular acidosis		
autosomal dominant	Anion exchanger-1 (*SLC4A1*, 17q21.31)	179800
autosomal recessive	Anion exchanger-1 (*SLC4A1*, 17q21.31)	602722
with neural deafness	Proton ATPase, β1 subunit (*ATP6V1B1*, 2p13.3)	192132
with normal hearing	Proton ATPase, 116-kD subunit (*ATP6V0A4*, 7q34)	602722

[a]Online Mendelian Inheritance in Man database (*http://www.ncbi.nlm.nih.gov/Omim*).

Na$^+$-glucose cotransport coupled with basolateral, facilitated diffusion by a glucose transporter. This process is also saturable, leading to glycosuria when plasma levels exceed 180–200 mg/dL, as seen in untreated diabetes mellitus.

The proximal tubule possesses specific transporters capable of secreting a variety of organic acids (carboxylate anions) and bases (mostly primary amine cations). Organic anions transported by these systems include urate, ketoacid anions, and several protein-bound drugs not filtered at the glomerulus (penicillins, cephalosporins, and salicylates). Probenecid inhibits renal organic anion secretion and can be clinically useful for raising plasma concentrations of certain drugs like penicillin and oseltamivir. Organic cations secreted by the proximal tubule include various biogenic amine neurotransmitters (dopamine, acetylcholine, epinephrine, norepinephrine, and histamine) and creatinine. The ATP-dependent transporter P-glycoprotein is highly expressed in brush border membranes and secretes several medically important drugs, including cyclosporine, digoxin, tacrolimus, and various cancer chemotherapeutic agents. Certain drugs like cimetidine and trimethoprim compete with endogenous compounds for transport by the organic cation pathways. While these drugs elevate serum creatinine levels, there is no change in the actual GFR.

The proximal tubule, through distinct classes of Na$^+$-dependent and Na$^+$-independent transport systems, reabsorbs amino acids efficiently. These transporters are specific for different groups of amino acids. For example, cystine, lysine, arginine, and ornithine are transported by a system comprising two proteins encoded by the *SLC3A1* and *SLC7A9* genes. Mutations in either *SLC3A1* or *SLC7A9* impair reabsorption of these amino acids and cause the disease cystinuria. Peptide hormones such as insulin and growth hormone, β_2-microglobulin, albumin, and other small proteins, are taken up by the proximal tubule through a process of absorptive endocytosis and are degraded in acidified endocytic lysosomes. Acidification of these vesicles depends on a vacuolar H$^+$-ATPase and Cl$^-$ channel. Impaired acidification of endocytic vesicles because of mutations in a Cl$^-$ channel gene (*CLCN5*) causes low molecular weight proteinuria in Dent's disease. Renal ammoniagenesis from glutamine in the proximal tubule provides a major tubular fluid buffer to ensure excretion of secreted H$^+$ ion as NH_4^+ by the collecting duct. Cellular K$^+$ levels inversely modulate ammoniagenesis, and in the setting of high serum K$^+$ from hypoaldosteronism, reduced ammoniagenesis facilitates the appearance of Type IV renal tubular acidosis.

LOOP OF HENLE

The loop of Henle consists of three major segments: descending thin limb, ascending thin limb, and ascending thick limb. These divisions are based on cellular morphology and anatomic location, but also correlate with specialization of function. Approximately 15–25% of filtered NaCl is reabsorbed in the loop of Henle, mainly by the thick ascending limb. The loop of Henle has an important role in urinary concentration by contributing to the generation of a hypertonic medullary interstitium in a process called *countercurrent multiplication*. The loop of Henle is the site of action for the most potent class of diuretic agents (loop diuretics) and also contributes to reabsorption of calcium and magnesium ions.

The descending thin limb is highly water permeable owing to dense expression of constitutively active aquaporin-1 water channels. By contrast, water permeability is negligible in the ascending limb. In the thick ascending limb, there is a high level of secondary active salt transport enabled by the Na$^+$/K$^+$/2Cl$^-$ cotransporter on the apical membrane in series with basolateral Cl$^-$ channels and Na$^+$/K$^+$-ATPase (Fig. 277-3*B*). The Na$^+$/K$^+$/2Cl$^-$ cotransporter is the primary target for loop diuretics. Tubular fluid K$^+$ is the limiting substrate for this cotransporter (tubular concentration of K$^+$ is similar to plasma, about 4 meq/L), but transporter activity is maintained by K$^+$ recycling through an apical potassium channel. An inherited disorder of the thick ascending limb, Bartter's syndrome, also results in a salt-wasting renal disease associated with hypokalemia and metabolic alkalosis; loss-of-function mutations in one of five distinct genes encoding components of the Na$^+$/K$^+$/2Cl$^-$ cotransporter (*NKCC2*), apical K$^+$ channel (*KCNJ1*), or basolateral Cl$^-$ channel (*CLCNKB, BSND*), or calcium-sensing receptor (*CASR*) can cause Bartter's syndrome.

Potassium recycling also contributes to a positive electrostatic charge in the lumen relative to the interstitium that promotes divalent cation (Mg^{2+} and Ca^{2+}) reabsorption through a paracellular pathway. A Ca^{2+}-sensing, G-protein–coupled receptor (CaSR) on basolateral membranes regulates NaCl reabsorption in the thick ascending limb through dual signaling mechanisms utilizing either cyclic AMP or eicosanoids. This receptor enables a steep relationship between plasma Ca^{2+} levels and renal Ca^{2+} excretion. Loss-of-function mutations in CaSR cause familial hypercalcemic hypocalciuria because of a blunted response of the thick ascending limb to extracellular Ca^{2+}. Mutations in *CLDN16* encoding paracellin-1, a transmembrane protein located within the tight junction complex, leads to familial hypomagnesemia with hypercalcuria and nephrocalcinosis, suggesting that the ion conductance of the paracellular pathway in the thick limb is regulated.

The loop of Henle contributes to urine-concentrating ability by establishing a *hypertonic medullary interstitium* that promotes water reabsorption by the downstream inner medullary collecting duct. *Countercurrent multiplication* produces a hypertonic medullary interstitium using two countercurrent systems: the loop of Henle (opposing descending and ascending limbs) and the vasa recta (medullary peritubular capillaries enveloping the loop). The countercurrent flow in these two systems helps maintain the hypertonic environment of the inner medulla, but NaCl reabsorption by the thick ascending limb is the primary initiating event. Reabsorption of NaCl without water dilutes the tubular fluid and adds new osmoles to medullary interstitial fluid. Because the descending thin limb is highly water permeable, osmotic equilibrium occurs between the descending limb tubular fluid and the interstitial space, leading to progressive solute trapping in the inner medulla. Maximum medullary interstitial osmolality also requires partial recycling of urea from the collecting duct.

DISTAL CONVOLUTED TUBULE

The distal convoluted tubule reabsorbs ~5% of the filtered NaCl. This segment is composed of a tight epithelium with little water permeability. The major NaCl-transporting pathway utilizes an apical membrane, electroneutral thiazide-sensitive Na$^+$/Cl$^-$ cotransporter in tandem with basolateral Na$^+$/K$^+$-ATPase and Cl$^-$ channels (Fig. 277-3C). Apical Ca^{2+}-selective channels (TRPV5) and basolateral Na$^+$/Ca^{2+} exchange mediate calcium reabsorption in the distal convoluted tubule. Ca^{2+} reabsorption is inversely related to Na$^+$ reabsorption and is stimulated by parathyroid hormone. Blocking apical Na$^+$/Cl$^-$ cotransport will reduce intracellular Na$^+$, favoring increased basolateral Na$^+$/Ca^{2+} exchange and passive apical Ca^{2+} entry. Loss-of-function mutations of *SLC12A3* encoding the apical Na$^+$/Cl$^-$ cotransporter cause Gitelman's syndrome, a salt-wasting disorder associated with hypokalemic alkalosis and hypocalciuria. Mutations in genes encoding WNK kinases, WNK-1 and WNK-4, cause pseudohypoaldosteronism type II or Gordon's syndrome characterized by familial hypertension with hyperkalemia. WNK kinases influence the activity of several tubular ion transporters. Mutations in this disorder lead to overactivity of the apical Na$^+$/Cl$^-$ cotransporter in the distal convoluted tubule as the primary stimulus for increased salt reabsorption, extracellular volume expansion, and hypertension. Hyperkalemia may be caused by diminished activity of apical K$^+$ channels in the collecting duct, a primary route for K^+ secretion. Mutations in *TRPM6* encoding Mg^{2+} permeable ion channels also cause familial hypomagnesemia with hypocalcemia. A molecular complex of TRPM6 and TRPM7 proteins is critical for Mg^{2+} reabsorption in the distal convoluted tubule.

COLLECTING DUCT

The collecting duct modulates the final composition of urine. The two major divisions, the cortical collecting duct and inner medullary collecting duct, contribute to reabsorbing ~4–5% of filtered Na^+ and are important for hormonal regulation of salt and water balance. The cortical collecting duct contains *high-resistance epithelia* with two cell types. Principal cells are the main water, Na^+-reabsorbing, and K^+-secreting cells, and the site of action of aldosterone, K^+-sparing diuretics, and mineralocorticoid receptor antagonists such as spironolactone. The other cells are type A and B intercalated cells. Type A intercalated cells mediate acid secretion and bicarbonate reabsorption also under the influence of aldosterone. Type B intercalated cells mediate bicarbonate secretion and acid reabsorption.

Virtually all transport is mediated through the cellular pathway for both principal cells and intercalated cells. In principal cells, passive apical Na^+ entry occurs through the amiloride-sensitive, epithelial Na^+ channel (ENaC) with basolateral exit via the Na^+/K^+-ATPase (Fig. 277-3*E*). This Na^+ reabsorptive process is tightly regulated by aldosterone and is physiologically activated by a variety of proteolytic enzymes that cleave extracellular domains of ENaC; plasmin in the tubular fluid of nephrotic patients, for example, activates ENaC, leading to sodium retention. Aldosterone enters the cell across the basolateral membrane, binds to a cytoplasmic mineralocorticoid receptor, and then translocates into the nucleus, where it modulates gene transcription, resulting in increased Na^+ reabsorption and K^+ secretion. Activating mutations in ENaC increase Na^+ reclamation and produce hypokalemia, hypertension, and metabolic alkalosis (Liddle's syndrome). The potassium-sparing diuretics amiloride and triamterene block ENaC, causing reduced Na^+ reabsorption.

Principal cells secrete K^+ through an apical membrane potassium channel. Several forces govern the secretion of K^+. Most importantly, the high intracellular K^+ concentration generated by Na^+/K^+-ATPase creates a favorable concentration gradient for K^+ secretion into tubular fluid. With reabsorption of Na^+ without an accompanying anion, the tubular lumen becomes negative relative to the cell interior, creating a favorable electrical gradient for secretion of potassium. When Na^+ reabsorption is blocked, the electrical component of the driving force for K^+ secretion is blunted and this explains lack of excess urinary K^+ loss during treatment with potassium-sparing diuretics. K^+ secretion is also promoted by aldosterone actions that increase regional Na^+ transport favoring more electronegativity and by increasing the number and activity of potassium channels. Fast tubular fluid flow rates that occur during volume expansion or diuretics acting "upstream" of the cortical collecting duct also increase K^+ secretion, as does the presence of relatively nonreabsorbable anions (including bicarbonate and semisynthetic penicillins) that contribute to the lumen-negative potential. Off-target effects of certain antibiotics such as trimethoprim and pentamidine, block ENaCs and predispose to hyperkalemia, especially when renal K^+ handling is impaired for other reasons. Principal cells, as described below, also participate in water reabsorption by increased water permeability in response to vasopressin.

Intercalated cells do not participate in Na^+ reabsorption but instead mediate acid-base secretion. These cells perform two types of transport: active H^+ transport mediated by H^+-ATPase (proton pump), and Cl^-/HCO_3^- exchange. Intercalated cells arrange the two transport mechanisms on opposite membranes to enable either acid or base secretion. Type A intercalated cells have an apical proton pump that mediates acid secretion and a basolateral Cl^-/HCO_3^- anion exchanger for bicarbonate reabsorption (Fig. 277-3*E*); aldosterone increases the number of H^+-ATPase pumps, sometimes contributing to the development of metabolic alkalosis. By contrast, type B intercalated cells have the anion exchanger on the apical membrane to mediate bicarbonate secretion while the proton pump resides on the basolateral membrane to enable acid reabsorption. Under conditions of acidemia, the kidney preferentially uses type A intercalated cells to secrete the excess H^+ and generate more HCO_3^-. The opposite is true in states of bicarbonate excess with alkalemia where the type B intercalated cells predominate. An extracellular protein called *hensin* mediates this adaptation.

Inner medullary collecting duct cells share many similarities with principal cells of the cortical collecting duct. They have apical Na^+ and K^+ channels that mediate Na^+ reabsorption and K^+ secretion, respectively (Fig. 277-3*F*). Inner medullary collecting duct cells also have vasopressin-regulated water channels (aquaporin-2 on the apical membrane, aquaporin-3 and -4 on the basolateral membrane). The antidiuretic hormone vasopressin binds to the V2 receptor on the basolateral membrane and triggers an intracellular signaling cascade through G-protein–mediated activation of adenylyl cyclase, resulting in an increase in the cellular levels of cyclic AMP. This signaling cascade stimulates the insertion of water channels into the apical membrane of the inner medullary collecting duct cells to promote increased water permeability. This increase in permeability enables water reabsorption and production of concentrated urine. In the absence of vasopressin, inner medullary collecting duct cells are water impermeable, and urine remains dilute.

Sodium reabsorption by inner medullary collecting duct cells is also inhibited by the natriuretic peptides called *atrial natriuretic peptide* or *renal natriuretic peptide* (urodilatin); the same gene encodes both peptides but uses different posttranslational processing of a common preprohormone to generate different proteins. Atrial natriuretic peptides are secreted by atrial myocytes in response to volume expansion, whereas urodilatin is secreted by renal tubular epithelia. Natriuretic peptides interact with either apical (urodilatin) or basolateral (atrial natriuretic peptides) receptors on inner medullary collecting duct cells to stimulate guanylyl cyclase and increase levels of cytoplasmic cGMP. This effect in turn reduces the activity of the apical Na^+ channel in these cells and attenuates net Na^+ reabsorption, producing natriuresis.

The inner medullary collecting duct transports urea out of the lumen, returning urea to the interstitium, where it contributes to the hypertonicity of the medullary interstitium. Urea is recycled by diffusing from the interstitium into the descending and ascending limbs of the loop of Henle.

HORMONAL REGULATION OF SODIUM AND WATER BALANCE

The balance of solute and water in the body is determined by the amounts ingested, distributed to various fluid compartments, and excreted by skin, bowel, and kidneys. *Tonicity*, the osmolar state determining the volume behavior of cells in a solution, is regulated by water balance (Fig. 277-4*A*), and *extracellular blood volume* is regulated by Na^+ balance (Fig. 277-4*B*). The kidney is a critical modulator of both physiologic processes.

WATER BALANCE

Tonicity depends on the variable concentration of *effective osmoles* inside and outside the cell causing water to move in either direction across its membrane. Classic effective osmoles, like Na^+, K^+, and their anions, are solutes trapped on either side of a cell membrane, where they collectively partition and obligate water to move and find equilibrium in proportion to retained solute; Na^+/K^+-ATPase keeps most K^+ inside cells and most Na^+ outside. Normal tonicity (~280 mosmol/L) is rigorously defended by osmoregulatory mechanisms

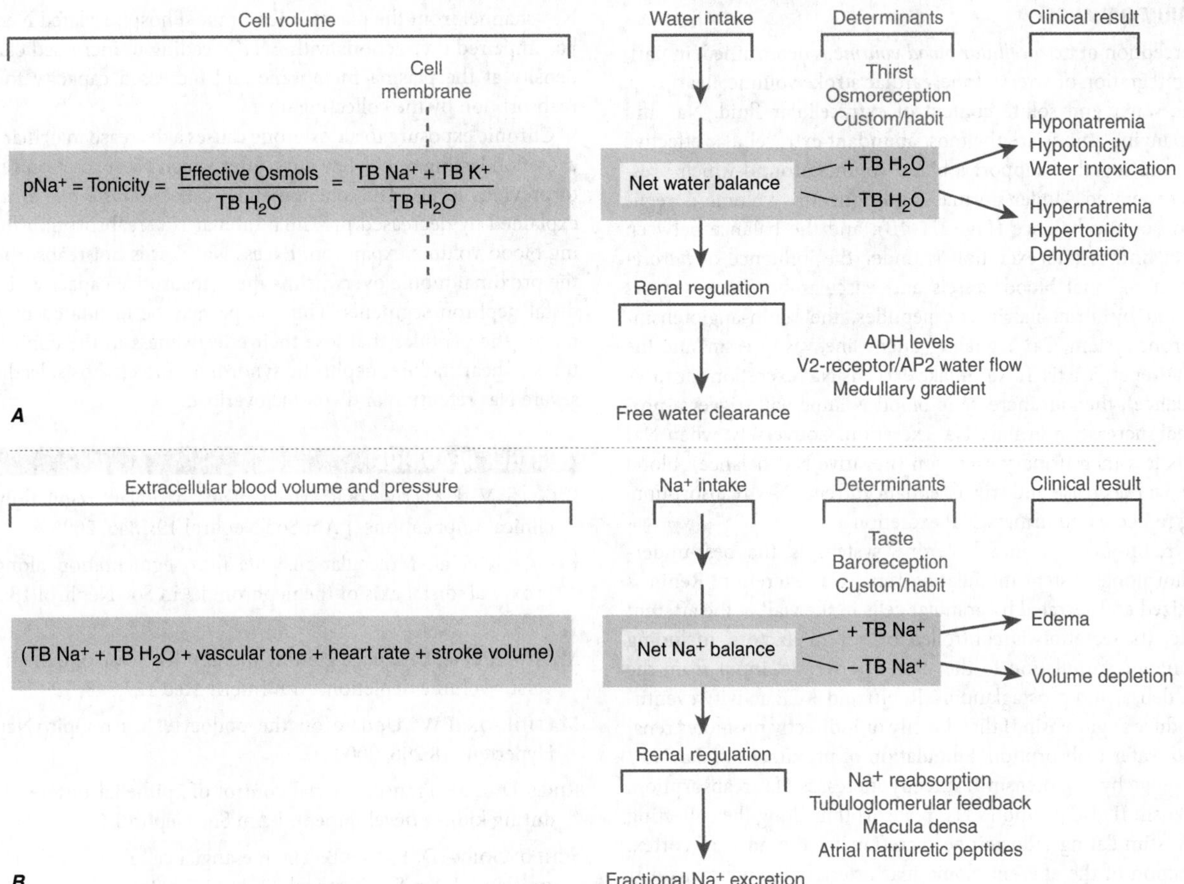

Figure 277-4 Determinants of sodium and water balance. ***A.*** Plasma Na^+ concentration is a surrogate marker for plasma tonicity, the volume behavior of cells in a solution. Tonicity is determined by the number of effective osmols in the body divided by the total body H_2O (TB H_2O), which translates simply into the total body Na (TB Na^+) and anions outside the cell separated from the total body K (TB K^+) inside the cell by the cell membrane. Net water balance is determined by the integrated functions of thirst, osmoreception, Na reabsorption, vasopressin release, and the strength of the medullary gradient in the kidney, keeping tonicity within a narrow range of osmolality around 280 mosmol/L. When water metabolism is disturbed and total body water increases, hyponatremia, hypotonicity, and water intoxication occur; when total body water decreases, hypernatremia, hypertonicity, and dehydration occur. ***B.*** Extracellular blood volume and pressure are an integrated function of total body Na^+ (TB Na^+), total body H_2O (TB H_2O), vascular tone, heart rate, and stroke volume that modulates volume and pressure in the vascular tree of the body. This extracellular blood volume is determined by net Na balance under the control of taste, baroreception, habit, Na^+ reabsorption, macula densa/tubuloglomerular feedback, and natriuretic peptides. When Na^+ metabolism is disturbed and total body Na^+ increases, edema occurs; when total body Na^+ is decreased, volume depletion occurs. ADH, antidiuretic hormone; AQP2, aquaporin-2.

that control water balance to protect tissues from inadvertent *dehydration* (cell shrinkage) or *water intoxication* (cell swelling), both of which are deleterious to cell function (Fig. 277-4*A*).

The mechanisms that control osmoregulation are distinct from those governing extracellular volume, although there is some shared physiology in both processes. While cellular concentrations of K^+ have a determinant role in any level of tonicity, the routine surrogate marker for assessing clinical tonicity is the concentration of serum Na^+. Any reduction in total body water, which raises the Na^+ concentration, triggers a brisk sense of thirst and conservation of water by decreasing renal water excretion mediated by release of vasopressin from the posterior pituitary. Conversely, a decrease in plasma Na^+ concentration triggers an increase in renal water excretion by suppressing the secretion of vasopressin. While all cells expressing mechanosensitive TRPV1, 2, or 4 channels, among potentially other sensors, respond to changes in tonicity by altering their volume and Ca^{2+} concentration, only $TRPV^+$ neuronal cells connected to the organum vasculosum of the lamina terminalis are *osmoreceptive.* Only these cells, because of their neural connectivity and adjacency to a minimal blood-brain barrier, modulate the downstream release of vasopressin by the posterior lobe of the pituitary gland. Secretion is stimulated primarily by changing tonicity and secondarily by other nonosmotic signals such as variable blood volume, stress, pain, nausea, and some drugs. The release of vasopressin by the posterior pituitary increases linearly as plasma tonicity rises above normal, although this varies, depending on the perception of extracellular volume (one form of cross-talk between mechanisms that adjudicate blood volume and osmoregulation). Changing the intake or excretion of water provides a means for adjusting plasma tonicity; thus, osmoregulation governs water balance.

The kidneys play a vital role in maintaining water balance through the regulation of renal water excretion. The ability to concentrate urine to an osmolality exceeding that of plasma enables water conservation, while the ability to produce urine more dilute than plasma promotes excretion of excess water. For water to enter or exit a cell, the cell membrane must express aquaporins. In the kidney, aquaporin 1 is constitutively active in all water-permeable segments of the proximal and distal tubules, while vasopressin-regulated aquaporins 2, 3, and 4 in the inner medullary collecting duct promote rapid water permeability. Net water reabsorption is ultimately driven by the osmotic gradient between dilute tubular fluid and a hypertonic medullary interstitium.

SODIUM BALANCE

The perception of *extracellular blood volume* is determined, in part, by the integration of arterial tone, cardiac stroke volume, heart rate, and the water and solute content of extracellular fluid. Na^+ and accompanying anions are the most abundant extracellular effective osmols and together support a blood volume around which pressure is generated. Under normal conditions, this volume is regulated by sodium balance (Fig. 277-4*B*), and the balance between daily Na^+ intake and excretion is under the influence of *baroreceptors* in regional blood vessels and vascular hormone sensors modulated by atrial natriuretic peptides, the renin-angiotensin-aldosterone system, Ca^{2+} signaling, adenosine, vasopressin, and the neural adrenergic axis. If Na^+ intake exceeds Na^+ excretion (positive Na^+ balance), then an increase in blood volume will trigger a proportional increase in urinary Na^+ excretion. Conversely, when Na^+ intake is less than urinary excretion (negative Na^+ balance), blood volume will decrease and trigger enhanced renal Na^+ reabsorption, leading to decreased urinary Na^+ excretion.

The renin-angiotensin-aldosterone system is the best-understood hormonal system modulating renal Na^+ excretion. Renin is synthesized and secreted by granular cells in the wall of the afferent arteriole. Its secretion is controlled by several factors, including β_1-adrenergic stimulation to the afferent arteriole, input from the macula densa, and prostaglandins. Renin and ACE activity eventually produce angiotensin II that directly or indirectly promotes renal Na^+ and water reabsorption. Stimulation of proximal tubular Na^+/H^+ exchange by angiotensin II directly increases Na^+ reabsorption. Angiotensin II also promotes Na^+ reabsorption along the collecting duct by stimulating aldosterone secretion by the adrenal cortex. Constriction of the efferent glomerular arteriole by angiotensin II indirectly increases the filtration fraction and raises peritubular capillary oncotic pressure to promote tubular Na^+ reabsorption. Finally, angiotensin II inhibits renin secretion through a negative feedback loop. Alternative metabolism of angiotensin by ACE2 generates the vasodilatory peptide angiotensin 1-7 that acts through Mas receptors to counterbalance several actions of angiotensin II on blood pressure and renal function (Fig. 277-2*C*).

Aldosterone is synthesized and secreted by granulosa cells in the adrenal cortex. It binds to cytoplasmic mineralocorticoid receptors in the collecting duct principal cells that increase activity of ENaC, apical membrane K^+ channel, and basolateral Na^+/K^+-ATPase. These effects are mediated in part by aldosterone-stimulated transcription of the gene encoding serum/glucocorticoid-induced kinase 1 (SGK1). The activity of ENaC is increased by SGK1-mediated phosphorylation of Nedd4-2, a protein that promotes recycling of the Na^+ channel from the plasma membrane. Phosphorylated Nedd4-2 has impaired interactions with ENaC, leading to increased channel density at the plasma membrane and increased capacity for Na^+ reabsorption by the collecting duct.

Chronic exposure to aldosterone causes a decrease in urinary Na^+ excretion lasting only a few days, after which Na^+ excretion returns to previous levels. This phenomenon, called *aldosterone escape*, is explained by decreased proximal tubular Na^+ reabsorption following blood volume expansion. Excess Na^+ that is not reabsorbed by the proximal tubule overwhelms the reabsorptive capacity of more distal nephron segments. This escape may be facilitated by atrial natriuretic peptides that lose their effectiveness in the clinical settings of heart failure, nephrotic syndrome, and cirrhosis, leading to severe Na^+ retention and volume overload.

FURTHER READINGS

Bhalla V, Hallows KR: Mechanisms of ENaC regulation and clinical implications. J Am Soc Nephrol 19:1845, 2008

Kopan R et al: Molecular insights into segmentation along the proximal–distal axis of the nephron. J Am Soc Nephrol 18:2014, 2007

Mange K et al: Language guiding therapy: The case of dehydration versus volume depletion. Ann Intern Med 127:848, 1997

Mathieson PW: Update on the podocyte. Curr Opin Nephrol Hypertens 18:206, 2009

Ribes D et al: Transcriptional control of epithelial differentiation during kidney development. J Am Soc Nephrol 14:S9, 2003

Schlöndorff D, Banas B: The mesangial cell revisited: No cell is an island. J Am Soc Nephrol 20: 1179, 2009

Schrier RT: Decreased effective blood volume in edematous disorders: What does this mean? J Am Soc Nephrol 18:2028, 2007

Schrier RW, Ecder T: Gibbs memorial lecture: Unifying hypothesis of body fluid volume regulation. Mt Sinai J Med 68:350, 2001

Vaughan MR, Quaggin SE: How do mesangial and endothelial cells form the glomerular tuft? J Am Soc Nephrol 19:24, 2008

Verbalis JG: How does the brain sense osmolality? J Am Soc Nephrol 18:3056, 2007

Wang WH, Giebisch G: Regulation of potassium (K) handling in the renal collecting duct. Pflugers Arch 458:157, 2009

Wiseman AC, Linas S: Disorders of potassium and acid-base balance. Am J Kidney Dis 45:941, 2005

CHAPTER 278

Adaption of the Kidney to Renal Injury

Raymond C. Harris
Eric G. Neilson

The size of a kidney and the total number of nephrons formed late in embryologic development depend on the degree to which the ureteric bud undergoes branching morphogenesis. Humans have between 225,000 and 900,000 nephrons in each kidney, a number that mathematically hinges on whether ureteric branching goes to completion or is terminated prematurely by one or two cycles. Although the signaling mechanisms regulating cycle number are incompletely understood, these final rounds of branching likely determine how well the kidney will adapt to the physiologic demands of blood pressure and body size, various environmental stresses, or unwanted inflammation leading to chronic renal failure.

One of the intriguing generalities regarding chronic renal failure is that residual nephrons hyperfunction to compensate for the loss of those nephrons succumbing to primary disease. This compensation depends on adaptive changes produced by renal hypertrophy and adjustments in *tubuloglomerular feedback* and *glomerulotubular balance*, as advanced in the *intact nephron hypothesis* by Neal Bricker in 1969. Some physiologic adaptations to nephron loss also produce unintended clinical consequences explained by Bricker's *trade-off hypothesis* in 1972, and eventually some adaptations accelerate the deterioration of residual nephrons, as described by Barry Brenner in his *hyperfiltration hypothesis* in 1982. These three important notions regarding chronic renal failure form a conceptual basis for understanding common pathophysiology leading to uremia.

COMMON MECHANISMS OF PROGRESSIVE RENAL DISEASE

When the initial complement of nephrons is reduced by a sentinel event, such as unilateral nephrectomy, the remaining kidney adapts by enlarging and increasing its glomerular filtration rate. If the kidneys were initially normal, the filtration rate usually returns to 80% of normal for two kidneys. The remaining kidney grows by *compensatory renal hypertrophy* with very little cellular proliferation. This unique event is accomplished by increasing the size of each cell along the nephron, which is accommodated by the elasticity or growth of interstitial spaces under the renal capsule. The mechanism of this *compensatory renal hypertrophy* is only partially understood; studies suggest roles for angiotensin II transactivation of heparin-binding epithelial growth factor, PI3K, and p27^{kip1}, a cell cycle protein that prevents tubular cells exposed to angiotensin II from proliferating, and the mammalian target of rapamycin (mTOR), which mediates new protein synthesis.

Hyperfiltration during pregnancy or in humans born with one kidney or who lose one to trauma or transplantation generally produces no ill consequences. By contrast, experimental animals that undergo resection of 80% of their renal mass, or humans who have persistent injury that destroys a comparable amount of renal tissue, progress to end-stage disease (Fig. 278-1). Clearly, there is a critical amount of primary nephron loss that produces maladaptive deterioration in remaining nephrons. This maladaptive response is referred to clinically as *renal progression*, and the pathologic correlate of renal progression is the relentless advance of tubular atrophy and tissue fibrosis. The mechanism for this maladaptive response is the focus of intense investigation. A unified theory of *renal progression* is just starting to emerge, and most importantly, this progression follows a final common pathway regardless of whether renal injury begins in glomeruli or within the tubulointerstitium.

There are six mechanisms that hypothetically unify this final common pathway. If injury begins in glomeruli, these sequential steps build on each other: (1) persistent glomerular injury produces local hypertension in capillary tufts, increases their single-nephron glomerular filtration rate and engenders protein leak into the tubular fluid; (2) significant glomerular proteinuria, accompanied by increases in the local production of angiotensin II, facilitates a downstream cytokine bath that induces the accumulation of interstitial mononuclear cells; (3) the initial appearance of interstitial neutrophils is quickly replaced by a gathering of macrophages and T lymphocytes, which form a nephritogenic immune response producing interstitial nephritis; (4) some tubular epithelia respond to this inflammation by disaggregating from their basement membrane and adjacent sister cells to undergo *epithelial-mesenchymal transitions* forming new interstitial fibroblasts; and finally (5) surviving fibroblasts lay down a collagenous matrix that disrupts adjacent capillaries and tubular nephrons, eventually leaving an acellular scar. The details of these complex events are outlined below (Fig. 278-2).

Significant ablation of renal mass results in *hyperfiltration* characterized by an increase in the rate of *single-nephron glomerular filtration*. The remaining nephrons lose their ability to autoregulate, and systemic hypertension is transmitted to the glomerulus. Both the *hyperfiltration* and *intraglomerular* hypertension stimulate the eventual appearance of glomerulosclerosis. Angiotensin II acts as an essential mediator of increased *intraglomerular* capillary pressure by selectively increasing efferent arteriolar vasoconstriction relative

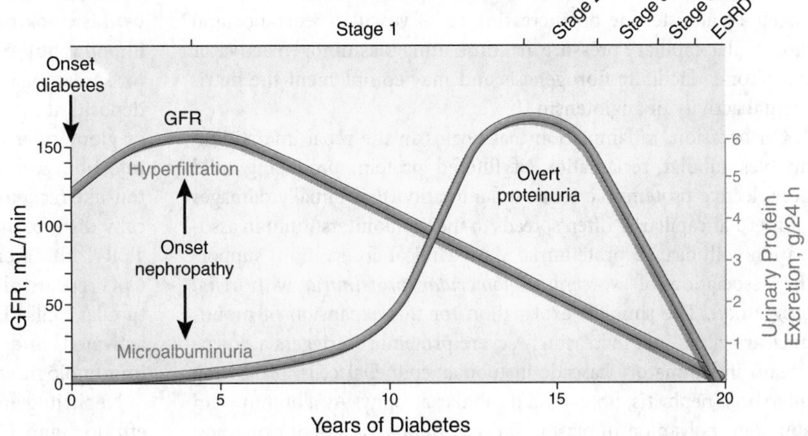

Figure 278-1 Progression of chronic renal injury. Although various types of renal injury have their own unique rates of progression, one of the best understood is that associated with type I diabetic nephropathy. Notice the early increase in glomerular filtration rate, followed by inexorable decline associated with increasing proteinuria. Also indicated is the National Kidney Foundation K/DOQI classification of the stages of chronic kidney disease.

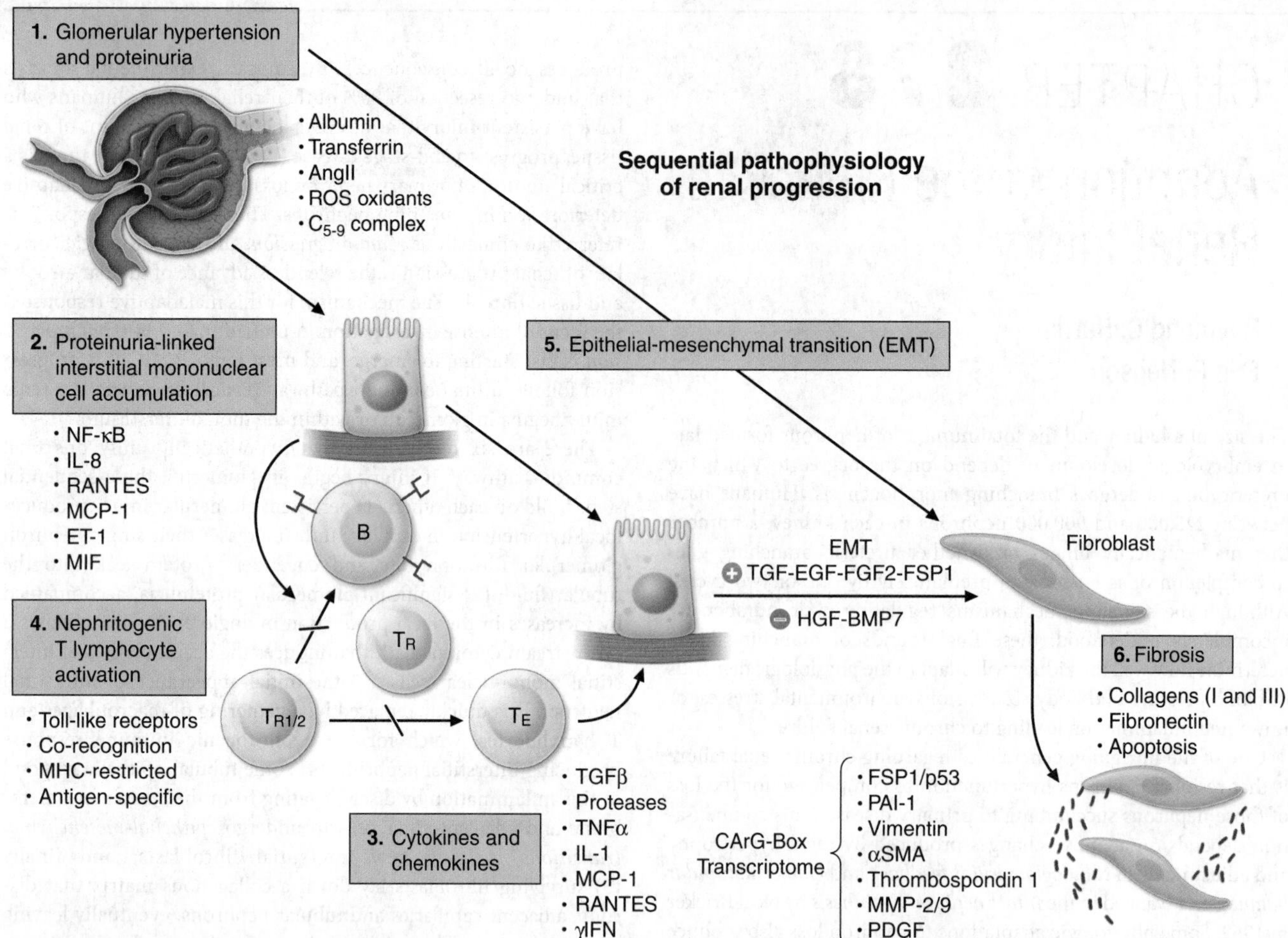

Figure 278-2 Mechanisms of renal progression. The general mechanisms of renal progression advance sequentially through six stages that include hyperfiltration, proteinuria, cytokine bath, mononuclear cell infiltration, epithelial-mesenchymal transition, and fibrosis. *(Modified from Harris and Neilson.)*

to afferent arteriolar tone. Angiotensin II impairs glomerular size selectivity, induces protein ultrafiltration, and increases intracellular Ca^{2+} in podocytes, which alters podocyte function. Diverse vasoconstrictor mechanisms, including blockade of nitric oxide synthase and activation of angiotensin II and thromboxane receptors, can also induce oxidative stress in surrounding renal tissue. Finally, the effects of aldosterone on increasing renal vascular resistance and glomerular capillary pressure, or stimulating plasminogen activator inhibitor-1, facilitate fibrogenesis and may complement the detrimental activity of angiotensin II.

On occasion, inflammation that begins in the renal interstitium disables tubular reclamation of filtered protein, producing mild nonselective proteinuria. Renal inflammation that initially damages glomerular capillaries often spreads to the tubulointerstitium in association with heavier proteinuria. Many clinical observations support the association of worsening *glomerular proteinuria* with *renal progression*. The simplest explanation for this expansion of mononuclear cells is that increasingly severe proteinuria triggers a downstream inflammatory cascade in tubular epithelial cells, producing interstitial nephritis, fibrosis, and tubular atrophy. As albumin is an abundant polyanion in plasma and can bind a variety of cytokines, chemokines, and lipid mediators, it is likely these small albumin-carried molecules initiate the tubular inflammation brought on by proteinuria. Furthermore, glomerular injury either adds activated mediators to the proteinuric filtrate or alters the balance of cytokine inhibitors and activators such that attainment of a critical level of activated cytokines eventually damages downstream tubular nephron.

Tubular epithelia bathed in these complex mixtures of proteinuric cytokines respond by increasing their secretion of chemokines and relocating NF-κB to the nucleus to induce the proinflammatory release of transforming growth factor β (TGF-β), platelet-derived growth factor–BB (PDGF-BB), and fibroblast growth factor 2 (FGF-2). Inflammatory cells are drawn into the renal interstitium by this cytokine milieu. This interstitial spreading reduces the likelihood that the kidney will survive. The immunologic mechanisms for spreading include loss of tolerance to parenchymal self, immune deposits that share cross-reactive epitopes in either compartment or glomerular injury that reveals a new interstitial epitope. Drugs, infection, and metabolic defects also induce autoimmunity through toll-like receptors (TLRs) that bind to ligands with an immunologically distinct molecular pattern. Bacterial and viral ligands activate TLRs but interestingly so do Tamm-Horsfall protein, bacterial CpG repeats, and RNA that is released nonspecifically from injured tubular cells. Dendritic cells and macrophages are subsequently activated, and circulating T cells engage in the formal cellular immunologic response.

Nephritogenic interstitial T cells are a mix of $CD4^+$ helper, $CD17^+$ effector, and $CD8^+$ cytotoxic lymphocytes. Presumptive evidence of antigen-driven T cells found by examining the DNA sequence of T cell receptors suggests a polyclonal expansion responding to multiple epitopes. Some experimental interstitial lesions are histologically analogous to a cutaneous delayed-type hypersensitivity reaction, and more intense reactions sometimes induce granuloma formation. The cytotoxic activity of antigen-reactive

T cells probably accounts for tubular cell destruction and atrophy. Cytotoxic T cells synthesize proteins with serine esterase activity as well as pore-forming proteins, which can effect membrane damage much like the activated membrane attack complex of the complement cascade. Such enzymatic activity provides a structural explanation for target cell lysis.

One long-term consequence of tubular epithelia and adjacent endothelia exposed to cytokines is the profibrotic activation of *epithelial/endothelial-mesenchymal transition* (EMT). Persistent cytokine activity during renal inflammation and disruption of underlying basement membranes by local proteases initiates the process of transition. Rather than collapsing into the tubular lumens and dying, some epithelia become fibroblasts while translocating back into the interstitial space behind deteriorating tubules through holes in the ruptured basement membrane; the contribution of endothelial cells from interstitial vessels may be equally important. Wnt proteins, integrin-linked kinases, insulin-like growth factors, EGF, FGF-2, and TGF-β are among the classic modulators of EMT. Fibroblasts that deposit collagen during fibrogenesis also replicate locally at sites of persistent inflammation. Estimates indicate that more than half of the total fibroblasts found in fibrotic renal tissues are products of the proliferation of newly transitioned or preexisting fibroblasts. Fibroblasts are stimulated to multiply by activation of cognate cell-surface receptors for PDGF and TGF-β.

Tubulointerstitial scars are composed principally of fibronectin, collagen types I and III, and tenascin, but other glycoproteins such as thrombospondin, SPARC, osteopontin, and proteoglycan may be also important. Although tubular epithelia can synthesize collagens I and III and are modulated by a variety of growth factors, these epithelia disappear through transition and tubular atrophy, leaving fibroblasts as the major contributor to matrix production. After fibroblasts acquire a synthetic phenotype, expand their population, and locally migrate around areas of inflammation, they begin to deposit fibronectin, which provides a scaffold for interstitial collagens. When fibroblasts outdistance their survival factors, they die from apoptosis, leaving an acellular scar.

RESPONSE TO REDUCTION IN NUMBERS OF FUNCTIONING NEPHRONS

As mentioned above, the response to the loss of many functioning nephrons produces an increase in renal blood flow with glomerular *hyperfiltration*, which is the result of increased vasoconstriction in postglomerular efferent arterioles relative to preglomerular afferent arterioles, increasing the *intraglomerular* capillary pressure and filtration fraction. Persistent intraglomerular hypertension is associated with progressive nephron destruction. Although the hormonal and metabolic factors mediating *hyperfiltration* are not fully understood, a number of vasoconstrictive and vasodilatory substances have been implicated, chief among them being angiotensin II. Angiotensin II incrementally vasoconstricts the efferent arteriole, and studies in animals and humans demonstrate that interruption of the renin-angiotensin system with either angiotensin-converting inhibitors or angiotensin II receptor blockers will decrease *intraglomerular* capillary pressure, decrease proteinuria, and slow the rate of nephron destruction. The vasoconstrictive agent endothelin has also been implicated in *hyperfiltration*, and increases in afferent vasodilatation have been attributed, at least in part, to local prostaglandins and release of endothelium-derived nitric oxide. Finally, hyperfiltration may be mediated in part by a resetting of the kidney's intrinsic autoregulatory mechanism of glomerular filtration by a *tubuloglomerular feedback system*. This feedback originates from the macula densa and modulates renal blood flow and glomerular filtration (see Chap. 277).

Even with the loss of functioning nephrons, there is some continued maintenance of *glomerulotubular balance*, by which the residual tubules adapt to increases in *single nephron glomerular filtration* with appropriate alterations in reabsorption or excretion of filtered water and solutes in order to maintain homeostasis. *Glomerulotubular balance* results both from tubular hypertrophy and from regulatory adjustments in tubular oncotic pressure or solute transport along the proximal tubule. Some studies indicate these alterations in tubule size and function may themselves be maladaptive, and as a trade-off, predispose to further tubule injury.

TUBULAR FUNCTION IN CHRONIC RENAL FAILURE

SODIUM

Na^+ ions are reclaimed along many parts of the nephron by various transport mechanisms (see Chapter 278). This transport function and its contribution to maintaining extracellular blood volume usually remains near normal until limitations from advanced renal disease inadequately excrete dietary Na^+ intake. Prior to this point and throughout renal progression, increasing the fractional excretion of Na^+ in final urine at progressively reduced rates of glomerular filtration provides a mechanism of early adaptation. Na^+ excretion increases predominantly by decreasing Na^+ reabsorption in the loop of Henle and distal nephron. An increase in the osmotic obligation of residual nephrons increases tubular water and lowers the concentration of Na^+ in tubular fluid, reducing efficient Na^+ reclamation; increased excretion of inorganic and organic anions also obligates more Na^+ excretion. In addition, hormonal influences, notably increased expression of atrial natriuretic peptides that increase distal Na^+ excretion, play an important role in maintaining net Na^+ excretion. Although many details of these adjustments are only understood conceptually, it is an example of a trade-off by which initial adjustments following the loss of functioning nephrons leads to compensatory responses that maintain homeostasis. Eventually, with advancing nephron loss, the atrial natriuretic peptides lose their effectiveness and Na^+ retention results in intravascular volume expansion, edema, and worsening hypertension.

URINARY DILUTION AND CONCENTRATION

Patients with progressive renal injury gradually lose the capacity either to dilute or concentrate their urine, and urine osmolality becomes relatively fixed about 350 mOsm/L (specific gravity ~1.010). Although the absolute ability of a single nephron to excrete water free of solute may not be impaired, the reduced number of functioning nephrons obligates increased fractional solute excretion by residual nephrons, and this greater obligation impairs the ability to dilute tubular fluid maximally. Similarly, urinary concentrating ability falls as more water is needed to hydrate an increasing solute load. Tubulointerstitial damage also creates insensitivity to the antidiuretic effects of vasopressin along the collecting duct or loss of the medullary gradient that eventually disturbs control of variation in urine osmolality. Patients with moderate degrees of chronic renal failure often complain of *nocturia* as a manifestation of this fixed urine osmolality, and they are prone to extracellular volume depletion if they do not keep up with the persistent loss of Na^+ or to hypotonicity if they drink too much water.

POTASSIUM

Renal excretion is the major pathway for reducing excess total body K^+. Normally, the kidney excretes 90% of dietary K^+, while 10% is excreted in the stool with a trivial amount lost to sweat. Although the colon possesses some capacity to increase K^+ excretion—up to 30% of ingested K^+ may be excreted in the stool of patients with worsening renal failure, the majority of the K^+ load continues to be excreted by the kidneys due to elevation in levels of serum K^+ that increase filtered load. Aldosterone also regulates collecting duct Na^+ reabsorption and K^+ secretion. Aldosterone is released from the

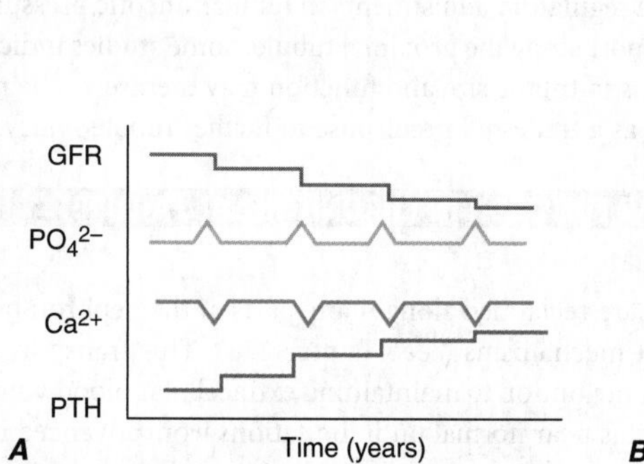

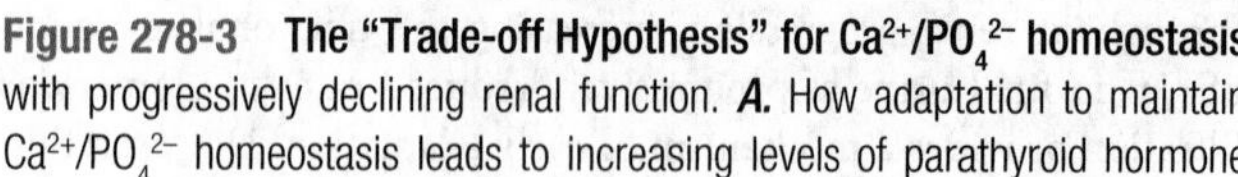

Figure 278-3 The "Trade-off Hypothesis" for Ca^{2+}/PO_4^{2-} homeostasis with progressively declining renal function. ***A.*** How adaptation to maintain Ca^{2+}/PO_4^{2-} homeostasis leads to increasing levels of parathyroid hormone *("classic" presentation from Slatopolsky et al.: Kidney Int 4:141, 1973).* ***B.*** current understanding of the underlying mechanisms for this Ca^{2+}/PO_4^{2-} trade-off.

adrenal cortex not only in response to the renin-angiotensin system but also in direct response to elevated levels of serum K^+ and, for a while, a compensatory increase in the capacity of the collecting duct to secrete K^+ keeps up with *renal progression.* As serum K^+ levels rise with renal failure, circulating levels of aldosterone also increase over what is required to maintain normal levels of blood volume.

■ ACID-BASE REGULATION

The kidneys excrete 1 meq/kg/day of noncarbonic H^+ ion on a normal diet. To do this, all of the filtered HCO_3^{2-} needs to be reabsorbed proximally so that H^+ pumps in the intercalated cells of the collecting duct can secrete H^+ ions that are subsequently trapped by urinary buffers, particularly phosphates and ammonia (see Chap. 277). While remaining nephrons increase their solute load with loss of renal mass, the ability to maintain total body H^+ excretion is often impaired by the gradual loss of H^+ pumps or with reductions in ammoniagenesis leading to development of a non-delta acidosis. Although hypertrophy of the proximal tubules initially increases their ability to reabsorb filtered HCO_3^{2-} and increases ammoniagenesis, with progressive loss of nephrons this compensation is eventually overwhelmed. In addition, with advancing renal failure, ammoniagenesis is further inhibited by elevation in levels of serum K^+, producing type IV renal tubular acidosis. Once the glomerular filtration rate falls below 25 mL/min, noncarbonic organic acids accumulate, producing a delta metabolic acidosis. Hyperkalemia can also inhibit tubular HCO_3^{2-} reabsorption, as can extracellular volume expansion and elevated levels of parathyroid hormone. Eventually, as the kidneys fail, the level of serum HCO_3^{2-} falls severely, reflecting the exhaustion of all body buffer systems, including bone.

■ CALCIUM AND PHOSPHATE

The kidney and gut play an important role in the regulation of serum levels of Ca^{2+} and PO_4^{2-}. With decreasing renal function and the appearance of tubulointerstitial nephritis, the expression of 1α-hydroxylase by the proximal tubule is reduced, lowering levels of calcitriol and Ca^{2+} absorption by the gut. Loss of nephron mass with progressive renal failure also gradually reduces the excretion of PO_4^{2-} and Ca^{2+}, and elevations in serum PO_4^{2-} further lower serum levels of Ca^{2+}, causing sustained secretion of parathyroid hormone. Unregulated increases in levels of parathyroid hormone cause Ca^{2+} mobilization from bone, Ca^{2+}/PO_4^{2-} precipitation in vascular tissues, abnormal bone remodeling, decreases in tubular bicarbonate reabsorption, and increases in renal PO_4^{2-} excretion. While elevated serum levels of parathyroid hormone initially maintain serum PO_4^{2-} near normal, with progressive nephron destruction, the capacity for renal PO_4^{2-} excretion is overwhelmed, the serum PO_4^{2-} elevates, and bone is progressively demineralized from secondary hyperparathyroidism. These adaptations evoke another classic functional trade-off (Fig. 278-3).

MODIFIERS INFLUENCING THE PROGRESSION OF RENAL DISEASE

Well-described risk factors for the progressive loss of renal function include systemic hypertension, diabetes, and activation of the renin-angiotensin-aldosterone system (Table 278-1). Poor glucose control will aggravate *renal progression* in both diabetic and non-diabetic renal disease. Angiotensin II produces *intraglomerular* hypertension and stimulates fibrogenesis. Aldosterone also serves as an independent fibrogenic mediator of progressive nephron loss apart from its role in modulating Na^+ and K^+ homeostasis. Genetic factors also play a role. There is recent, exciting evidence that risk alleles for *APOL1* underlies the increased susceptibility of African Americans to development of progressive kidney injury.

Lifestyle choices also affect the progression of renal disease. Cigarette smoking either predisposes or accelerates the progression of nephron loss. Whether the effect of cigarettes is related to systemic hemodynamic alterations or specific damage to the renal microvasculature and/or tubules is unclear. Increases in fetuin-A, decreases in adiponectin, and increases in lipid oxidation associated with obesity also accelerate cardiovascular disease and progressive renal damage. Recent epidemiologic studies also confirm an association between high

TABLE 278-1 Potential Modifiers of Renal Disease Progression

Hypertension	Hyperlipidemia
Renin-angiotensin system activation	Abnormal calcium/phosphorus homeostasis
Angiotensin II	Cigarette smoking
Aldosterone	Intrinsic paucity in nephron number
Diabetes	Prematurity/low birth weight
Obesity	Genetic predisposition
Excessive dietary protein	Genetic factors

protein diets and progression of renal disease. Progressive nephron loss in experimental animals, and possibly in humans, is slowed by adherence to a low protein diet. Although a large multicenter trial, the Modification of Diet in Renal Disease, did not provide conclusive evidence that dietary protein restriction could retard progression to renal failure in humans, secondary analyses and a number of meta-analyses suggest a renoprotective effect from supervised low-protein diets in the range of 0.6–0.75 g/kg/day. Repair of chronic low serum bicarbonate levels during renal progression increases kidney survival. Abnormal Ca^{2+} and PO_4^{2-} metabolism in chronic kidney disease also plays a role in renal progression, and administration of calcitriol or its analogues can attenuate progression in a variety of models of chronic kidney disease.

An intrinsic paucity in the number of functioning nephrons predisposes to the development of renal disease. A reduced number of nephrons leads to permanent hypertension, either through direct renal damage or *hyperfiltration* producing glomerulosclerosis, or by primary induction of systemic hypertension that further exacerbates glomerular barotrauma. Younger individuals with hypertension who die suddenly as a result of trauma have 47% fewer glomeruli per kidney than age-matched controls.

A consequence of low birth weight is a relative deficit in the number of total nephrons, and low birth weight associates in adulthood with more hypertension and renal failure, among other abnormalities. In this regard, in addition or instead of a genetic predisposition to development of a specific disease or condition such as low birth weight, different epigenetic phenomena may produce varying clinical phenotypes from a single genotype depending upon maternal exposure to different environmental stimuli during gestation, a phenomena known as *developmental plasticity*. A specific clinical phenotype can also be selected in response to an adverse environmental exposure during critical periods of intrauterine development, also known as *fetal programming*. In the United States, there is at least a twofold increased incidence of low birth weight among blacks compared with whites, much but not all of which can be attributed to maternal age, health, or socioeconomic status.

As in other conditions producing nephron loss, the glomeruli of low-birth-weight individuals enlarge and associate with early *hyperfiltration* to maintain normal levels of renal function. With time, the resulting *intraglomerular* hypertension initiates a progressive decline in residual hyperfunctioning nephrons, ultimately accelerating renal failure. In African Americans, as well as other populations at increased risk for kidney failure, such as Pima Indians and Australian aborigines, large glomeruli are seen at early stages of kidney disease. An association between low birth weight and the development of albuminuria and nephropathy is reported for both diabetic and nondiabetic renal disease.

FURTHER READINGS

Brenner BM: Remission of renal disease: Recounting the challenge, acquiring the goal. J Clin Invest 110:1753, 2002

de Brito-Ashurst I et al: Bicarbonate supplementation slows progression of CKD and improves nutritional status. J Am Soc Nephrol 20: 2075, 2009

Genovese G et al: Association of trypanolytic ApoL1 variants with kidney disease in African Americans. Science 329:841, 2010

Harris RC, Neilson EG: Towards a unified theory of renal progression. Annu Rev Med 57:365, 2006

Ix JH, Sharma K: Mechanisms linking obesity, chronic kidney disease, and fatty liver disease: The roles of fetuin-A, adiponectin, and AMPK. J Am Soc Nephrol 21:406, 2010

Kao WH et al: MYH9 is associated with nondiabetic end-stage renal disease in African Americans. Nat Genet 40:1185, 2008

Luyckx VA, Brenner BM: The clinical importance of nephron mass. J Am Soc Nephrol 21:898, 2010

Peti-Peterdi J, Harris RC: Macula densa sensing and signaling mechanisms of renin release. J Am Soc Nephrol 21:1093, 2010

Slatopolsky E, Bricker NS: The role of phosphorus restriction in the prevention of secondary hyperparathyroidism in chronic renal disease. Kidney Int 4:141, 1973

——— et al: Calcium, phosphorus and vitamin D disorders in uremia. Contr Nephrol 149:261, 2005

Zandi-Nejad K et al: Adult hypertension and kidney disease: The role of fetal programming. Hypertension 47:502, 2006

CHAPTER 279

Acute Kidney Injury

Sushrut S. Waikar

Joseph V. Bonventre

Acute kidney injury (AKI), previously known as acute renal failure, is characterized by the sudden impairment of kidney function resulting in the retention of nitrogenous and other waste products normally cleared by the kidneys. AKI is not a single disease but, rather, a designation for a heterogeneous group of conditions that share common diagnostic features: specifically, an increase in the blood urea nitrogen (BUN) concentration and/or an increase in the plasma or serum creatinine (SCr) concentration, often associated with a reduction in urine volume. AKI can range in severity from asymptomatic and transient changes in laboratory parameters of glomerular filtration rate (GFR), to overwhelming and rapidly fatal derangements in effective circulating volume regulation and electrolyte and acid-base composition of the plasma.

Changing the name of a syndrome as well known as "acute renal failure" does not occur frequently. We will summarize some of the reasons why the name was changed to "acute kidney injury." The term *failure* reflects only part of the spectrum of damage to the kidney that occurs clinically. In most cases of damage, the reduction in kidney function is modest. Nevertheless, this modest change has been documented to be associated with negative effects on outcome, albeit not nearly as ominous as seen with large decreases in kidney function associated with frank kidney failure that often requires acute dialysis therapies. Furthermore, the term *renal* is not well understood in the general population and this makes communication with patients and family more challenging; hence "kidney" has replaced "renal."

EPIDEMIOLOGY

AKI complicates 5–7% of acute care hospital admissions and up to 30% of admissions to the intensive care unit. AKI is also a major medical complication in the developing world, particularly in the setting of diarrheal illnesses, infectious diseases like malaria and leptospirosis, and natural disasters such as earthquakes. The incidence of AKI has grown by more than fourfold in the United States since 1988 and is estimated to have a yearly incidence of 500 per 100,000 population, higher than the yearly incidence of stroke. AKI is associated with a markedly increased risk of death in hospitalized individuals, particularly in those admitted to the ICU where in-hospital mortality rates may exceed 50%.

AKI in the developing world

The epidemiology of AKI differs tremendously between developed and developing countries, owing to differences in demographics, economics, geography, and comorbid disease burden. While certain features of AKI are common to both—particularly since urban centers of some developing countries increasingly resemble those in the developed world—many etiologies for AKI are region-specific such as envenomations from snakes, spiders, caterpillars, and bees; infectious causes such as malaria and leptospirosis; and crush injuries and resultant rhabdomyolysis from earthquakes.

ETIOLOGY AND PATHOPHYSIOLOGY

The causes of AKI have traditionally been divided into three broad categories: prerenal azotemia, intrinsic renal parenchymal disease, and postrenal obstruction (Fig. 279-1).

PRERENAL AZOTEMIA

Prerenal azotemia (from "azo," meaning nitrogen, and "-emia") is the most common form of AKI. It is the designation for a rise in SCr or BUN concentration due to inadequate renal plasma flow and intraglomerular hydrostatic pressure to support normal glomerular filtration. The most common clinical conditions associated with prerenal azotemia are hypovolemia, decreased cardiac output, and medications that interfere with renal autoregulatory responses such as nonsteroidal anti-inflammatory drugs (NSAIDs) and inhibitors of angiotensin II (Fig. 279-2). Prerenal azotemia may coexist with other forms of intrinsic AKI. Prolonged periods of prerenal azotemia may lead to ischemic injury, often termed acute tubular necrosis, or ATN. By definition, prerenal azotemia involves no parenchymal damage to the kidney and is rapidly reversible once intraglomerular hemodynamics are restored.

Normal GFR is maintained in part by the relative resistances of the afferent and efferent renal arterioles, which determine the glomerular plasma flow and the transcapillary hydraulic pressure gradient that drive glomerular ultrafiltration. Mild degrees of hypovolemia and reductions in cardiac output elicit compensatory renal physiologic changes. Because renal blood flow accounts for 20% of the cardiac output, renal vasoconstriction and salt and water reabsorption occur as a homeostatic response to decreased effective circulating volume or cardiac output in order to maintain blood pressure and increase intravascular volume to sustain perfusion to the cerebral and coronary vessels. Mediators of this response include angiotensin II, norepinephrine, and vasopressin (also termed antidiuretic hormone). Glomerular filtration can be maintained despite reduced renal blood flow by angiotensin II–mediated renal efferent vasoconstriction, which maintains glomerular capillary hydrostatic pressure closer to normal and thereby prevents marked reductions in GFR if renal blood flow reduction is not excessive.

In addition, a myogenic reflex within the afferent arteriole leads to dilation in the setting of low perfusion pressure, thereby maintaining glomerular perfusion. Intrarenal biosynthesis of vasodilator prostaglandins (prostacyclin, prostaglandin E2), kallikrein and kinins, and possibly nitric oxide (NO) also increase in response to low renal perfusion pressure. Autoregulation is also accomplished by tubuloglomerular feedback, in which decreases in solute delivery to the macula densa (specialized cells within the proximal tubule) elicit dilation of the juxtaposed afferent arteriole in order to maintain glomerular perfusion, a mechanism mediated, in part, by NO. There is a limit, however, to the ability of these counterregulatory mechanisms to maintain GFR in the face of systemic hypotension. Even in healthy adults, renal autoregulation usually fails once the systolic blood pressure falls below 80 mmHg.

A number of factors determine the robustness of the autoregulatory response and, thereby, the risk of prerenal azotemia. Atherosclerosis, long-standing hypertension, and older age can lead to hyalinosis and myointimal hyperplasia, causing structural narrowing of the intrarenal arterioles and impaired capacity for renal afferent vasodilation. In chronic kidney disease, renal afferent vasodilation may be operating at maximal capacity in order to maximize GFR in response to reduced functional renal mass. Drugs can affect the compensatory changes evoked to maintain GFR.

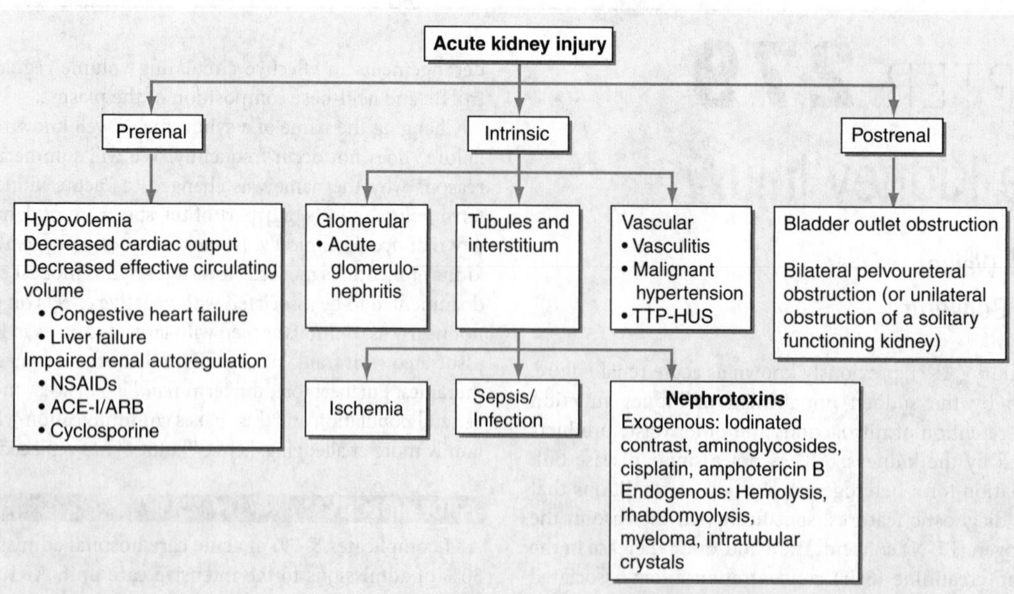

Figure 279-1 Classification of the major causes of acute kidney injury. ACE-1, angiotensin-converting enzyme 1; ARB, angiotensin receptor blocker; NSAIDs, nonsteroidal anti-inflammatory drugs; TTP-HUS, thrombotic thrombocytopenic purpura-hemolytic uremic syndrome.

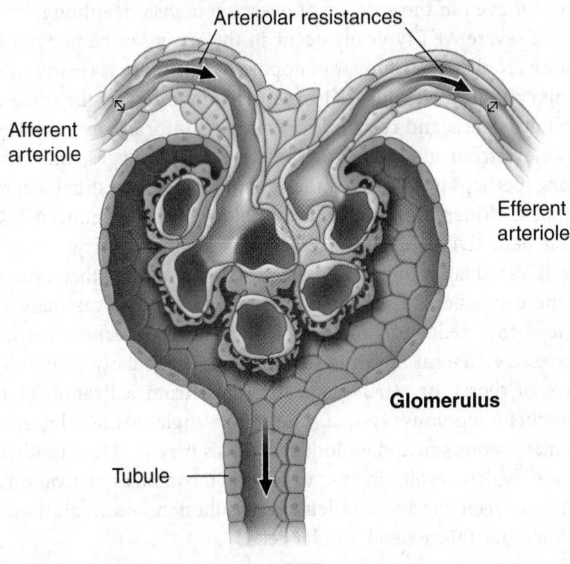

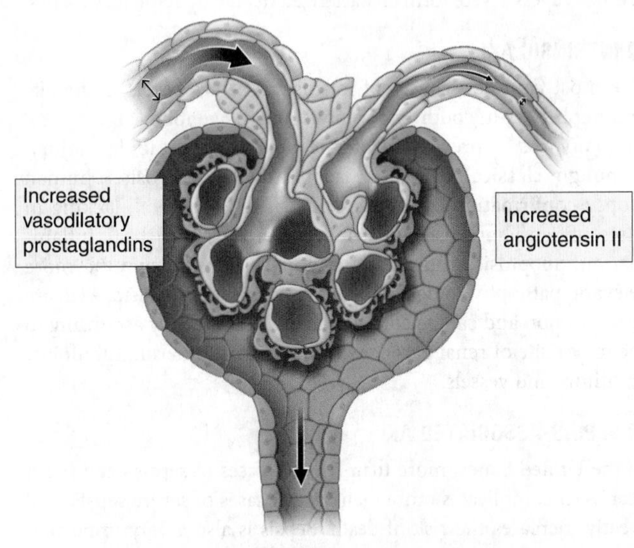

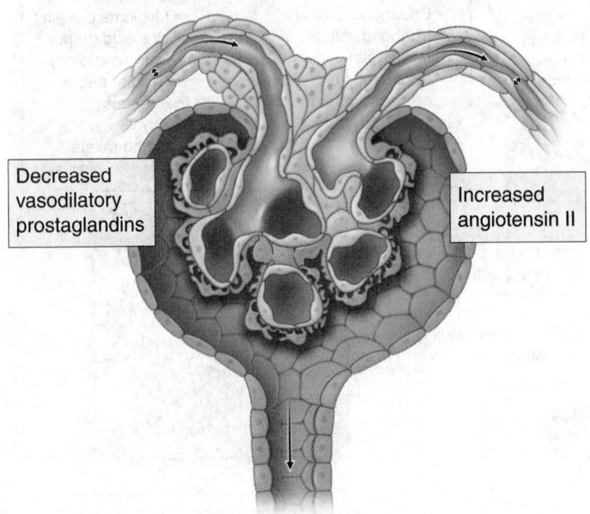

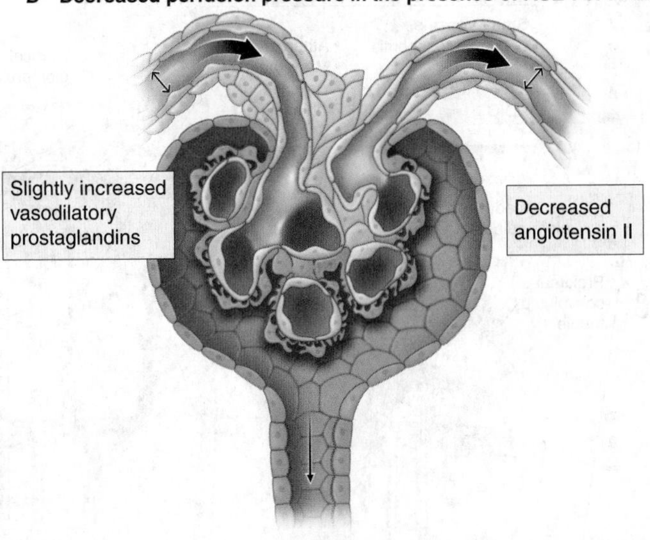

Figure 279-2 Intrarenal Mechanisms for Autoregulation of the Glomerular Filtration Rate (GFR) under Decreased Perfusion Pressure and Reduction of the GFR by Drugs. Panel A shows normal conditions and a normal GFR. Panel B shows reduced perfusion pressure within the autoregulatory range. Normal glomerular capillary pressure is maintained by afferent vasodilatation and efferent vasoconstriction. Panel C shows reduced perfusion pressure with a nonsteroidal anti-inflammatory drug (NSAID). Loss of vasodilatory prostaglandins increases afferent resistance; this causes the glomerular capillary pressure to drop below normal values and the GFR to decrease. Panel D shows reduced perfusion pressure with an angiotensin-converting enzyme (ACE-I) inhibitor or an angiotensin receptor blocker (ARB). Loss of angiotensin II action reduces efferent resistance; this causes the glomerular capillary pressure to drop below normal values and the GFR to decrease. *(From N Engl J Med 2007;357:797-805; with permission.)*

NSAIDs inhibit renal prostaglandin production, limiting renal afferent vasodilation. ACE inhibitors and angiotensin receptor blockers (ARBs) limit renal efferent vasoconstriction; this effect is particularly pronounced in patients with bilateral renal artery stenosis or unilateral renal artery stenosis (in the case of a solitary functioning kidney) because renal efferent vasoconstriction is needed to maintain GFR due to low renal perfusion. The combined use of nonsteroidal anti-inflammatory agents with ACE inhibitors or ARBs poses a particularly high risk for developing prerenal azotemia.

Many individuals with advanced cirrhosis exhibit a unique hemodynamic profile that resembles prerenal azotemia despite total body volume overload. Systemic vascular resistance is markedly reduced due to primary arterial vasodilation in the splanchnic circulation, resulting ultimately in activation of vasoconstrictor responses similar to those seen in hypovolemia. AKI is a common complication in this setting, and it can be triggered by volume depletion and spontaneous bacterial peritonitis. A particularly poor prognosis is seen in the case of type 1 hepatorenal syndrome, in which AKI without an alternate cause (e.g., infection, shock, nephrotoxic drugs) persists despite volume administration and withholding of diuretics. Type 2 hepatorenal syndrome is a less severe form characterized mainly by refractory ascites.

INTRINSIC AKI

The most common causes of intrinsic AKI are sepsis, ischemia, and nephrotoxins, both endogenous and exogenous (Fig. 279-3). In many cases, prerenal azotemia advances to tubular injury. Although classically termed "acute tubular necrosis," human biopsy confirmation of tubular necrosis is, in general, lacking in cases of sepsis and ischemia; indeed, processes such as inflammation, apoptosis, and altered regional perfusion may be more relevant pathophysiologically. Other causes of intrinsic AKI are less common and can be conceptualized anatomically according to the major site of renal parenchymal damage: glomeruli, tubulointerstitium, and vessels.

SEPSIS-ASSOCIATED AKI

In the United States, more than 700,000 cases of sepsis occur each year. AKI complicates more than 50% of cases of severe sepsis, and greatly increases the risk of death. Sepsis is also a very important cause of AKI in the developing world. Decreases in GFR with sepsis can occur even in the absence of overt hypotension, although most cases of severe AKI typically occur in the setting of hemodynamic collapse requiring vasopressor support. While there is clearly tubular injury associated with AKI in sepsis as manifest by the presence of tubular debris and casts in the urine, postmortem examinations of kidneys from individuals with severe sepsis suggest that other factors, perhaps related to inflammation and interstitial edema, must be considered in the pathophysiology of sepsis-induced AKI.

The hemodynamic effects of sepsis—arising from generalized arterial vasodilation, mediated in part by cytokines that upregulate the expression of inducible NO synthase in the vasculature—can lead to a reduction in GFR. The operative mechanisms may be excessive efferent arteriole vasodilation, particularly early in the course of sepsis, or renal vasoconstriction from activation of the sympathetic nervous system, the renin-angiotensin-aldosterone system, vasopressin, and endothelin. Sepsis may lead to endothelial damage, which results in microvascular thrombosis, activation of reactive oxygen species, and leukocyte adhesion and migration, all of which may injure renal tubular cells.

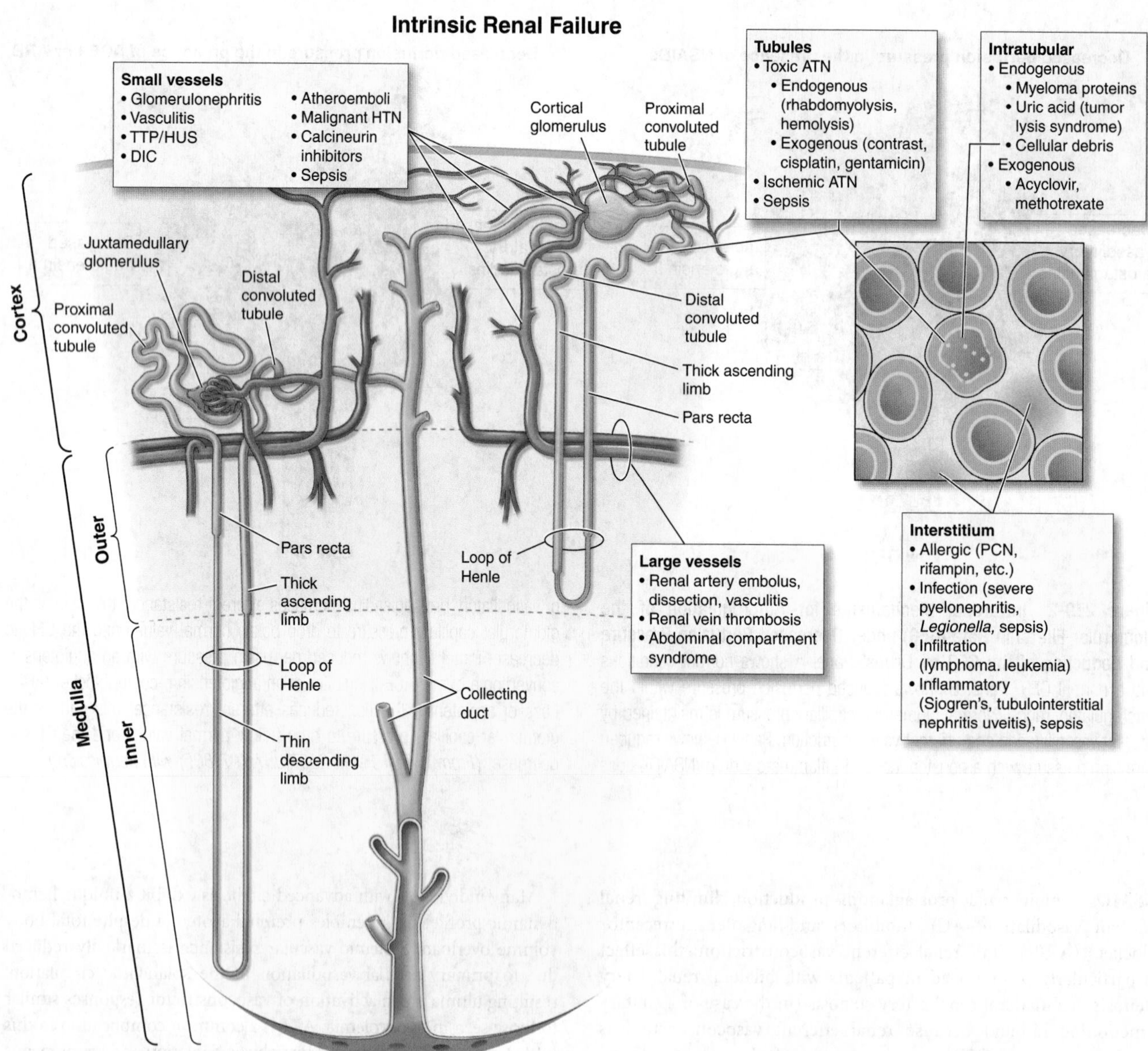

Figure 279-3 Major causes of intrinsic acute kidney injury. ATN, acute tubular necrosis; DIC, disseminated intravascular coagulation; HTN, hypertensive nephropathy; MTX, methotrexate; PCN, penicillin; TTP/HUS, thrombotic thrombocytopenic purpura/hemolytic uremic syndrome; TINU, tubulointerstitial nephritis-uveitis.

■ ISCHEMIA-ASSOCIATED AKI

Healthy kidneys receive 20% of the cardiac output and account for 10% of resting oxygen consumption, despite constituting only 0.5% of the human body mass. The kidneys are also the site of one of the most hypoxic regions in the body, the renal medulla. The outer medulla is particularly vulnerable to ischemic damage because of the architecture of the blood vessels that supply oxygen and nutrients to the tubules. Enhanced leukocyte-endothelial interactions in the small vessels lead to inflammation and reduced local blood flow to the metabolically very active S3 segment of the proximal tubule, which depends on oxidative metabolism for survival. Ischemia alone in a normal kidney is usually not sufficient to cause severe AKI, as evidenced by the relatively low risk of severe AKI even after total interruption of renal blood flow during suprarenal aortic clamping or cardiac arrest. Clinically, AKI more commonly develops when ischemia occurs in the context of limited renal reserve (e.g., chronic kidney disease or older age) or coexisting insults such as sepsis, vasoactive or nephrotoxic drugs, rhabdomyolysis, and the systemic inflammatory states associated with burns and pancreatitis. Prerenal azotemia and ischemia-associated AKI represent a continuum of the manifestations of renal hypoperfusion. Persistent preglomerular vasoconstriction may be a common underlying cause of the reduction in GFR seen in AKI; implicated factors for vasoconstriction include activation of tubuloglomerular feedback from enhanced delivery of solute to the macula densa following proximal tubule injury, increased basal vascular tone and reactivity to vasoconstrictive agents, and decreased vasodilator responsiveness. Other contributors to low GFR include backleak of filtrate across ischemic and denuded tubular epithelium and mechanical obstruction of tubules from necrotic debris (Fig. 279-4).

Postoperative AKI

Ischemia-associated AKI is a serious complication in the postoperative period, especially after major operations involving significant blood loss and intraoperative hypotension. The procedures most commonly associated with AKI are cardiac surgery with cardiopulmonary bypass (particularly for combined valve and bypass procedures), vascular procedures with aortic cross clamping, and intraperitoneal procedures. Severe AKI requiring dialysis occurs in approximately 1% of cardiac and vascular surgery procedures. The risk of severe AKI has been less well studied for major intraperitoneal procedures, but appears to be of comparable magnitude. Common risk factors for postoperative AKI include underlying chronic kidney disease, older age, diabetes mellitus, congestive heart failure, and emergency procedures. The pathophysiology of AKI following cardiac surgery is multifactorial. Major AKI risk factors are common in the population undergoing cardiac surgery. The use of nephrotoxic agents including iodinated contrast for cardiac imaging prior to surgery may increase the risk of AKI. Cardiopulmonary bypass is a unique hemodynamic state characterized by nonpulsatile flow and exposure of the circulation to extracorporeal circuits. Longer duration of cardiopulmonary bypass is a risk factor for AKI. In addition to ischemic injury from sustained hypoperfusion, cardiopulmonary bypass may cause AKI through a number of mechanisms including extracorporeal circuit activation of leukocytes and inflammatory processes, hemolysis with resultant pigment nephropathy (see below), and aortic injury with resultant atheroemboli. AKI from atheroembolic disease, which can also occur following percutaneous catheterization of the aorta, or spontaneously, is due to cholesterol crystal embolization resulting in partial or total occlusion of multiple small arteries within the kidney. Over time, a foreign body reaction can result in intimal proliferation, giant cell formation, and further narrowing of the vascular lumen, accounting for the generally subacute (over a period of weeks rather than days) decline in renal function.

Burns and acute pancreatitis

Extensive fluid losses into the extravascular compartments of the body frequently accompany severe burns and acute pancreatitis. AKI is an ominous complication of burns, affecting 25% of individuals with more than 10% total body surface area involvement. In addition to severe hypovolemia resulting in decreased cardiac output and increased neurohormonal activation, burns and acute pancreatitis both lead to dysregulated inflammation and an increased risk of sepsis and acute lung injury, all of which may facilitate the development and progression of AKI. Individuals undergoing massive fluid resuscitation for trauma, burns, and acute pancreatitis can also develop the abdominal compartment syndrome, where markedly elevated intraabdominal pressures, usually higher than 20 mmHg, lead to renal vein compression and reduced GFR.

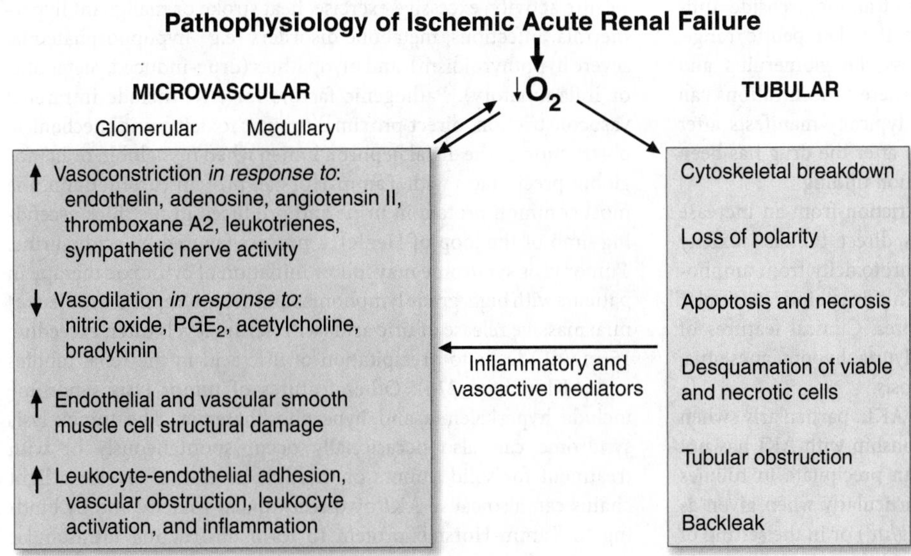

Figure 279-4 Interacting microvascular and tubular events contributing to the pathophysiology of ischemic acute kidney injury. PGE_2, prostaglandin E_2. *(From J Am Soc Nephrol 14:2199, 2003.)*

Diseases of the microvasculature leading to ischemia

Microvascular causes of AKI include the thrombotic microangiopathies [antiphospholipid antibody syndrome, radiation nephritis, malignant nephrosclerosis, and thrombotic thrombocytopenic purpura/hemolytic uremic syndrome (TTP-HUS)], scleroderma, and atheroembolic disease. Large vessel diseases associated with AKI include renal artery dissection, thromboembolism, thrombosis, and renal vein compression or thrombosis.

■ NEPHROTOXIN-ASSOCIATED AKI

The kidney has very high susceptibility to nephrotoxicity due to extremely high blood perfusion and concentration of circulating substances along the nephron where water is reabsorbed and in the medullary interstitium; this results in high-concentration exposure of toxins to tubular, interstitial, and endothelial cells. Nephrotoxic injury occurs in response to a number of pharmacologic compounds with diverse structures, endogenous substances, and environmental exposures. All structures of the kidney are vulnerable to toxic injury, including the tubules, interstitium, vasculature, and collecting system. As with other forms of AKI, risk factors for nephrotoxicity include older age, chronic kidney disease (CKD), and prerenal azotemia. Hypoalbuminemia may increase the risk of some forms of nephrotoxin-associated AKI due to increased free circulating drug concentrations.

Contrast agents

Iodinated contrast agents used for cardiovascular and CT imaging are a leading cause of AKI. The risk of AKI, or "contrast nephropathy," is negligible in those with normal renal function but increases markedly in the setting of chronic kidney disease, particularly diabetic nephropathy. The most common clinical course of contrast nephropathy is characterized by a rise in SCr beginning 24–48 hours following exposure, peaking within 3–5 days, and resolving within 1 week. More severe, dialysis-requiring AKI is uncommon except in the setting of significant preexisting chronic kidney disease, often in association with congestive heart failure or other coexisting causes for ischemia-associated AKI. Patients with multiple myeloma and renal disease are particularly susceptible. Low fractional excretion of sodium and relatively benign urinary sediment without features of tubular necrosis (see below) are common findings. Contrast nephropathy is thought to occur from a combination of factors, including (1) hypoxia in the renal outer medulla due to perturbations in renal microcirculation and occlusion of small vessels; (2) cytotoxic damage to the tubules directly or via the generation of oxygen free radicals, especially since the concentration of the agent within the tubule is markedly increased; and (3) transient tubule obstruction with precipitated contrast material. Other diagnostic agents implicated as a cause of AKI are high-dose gadolinium used for MRI and oral sodium phosphate solutions used as bowel purgatives.

Antibiotics

Several antimicrobial agents are commonly associated with AKI. *Aminoglycosides and amphotericin B* both cause tubular necrosis. Nonoliguric AKI (i.e., without a significant reduction in urine volume) accompanies 10–30% of courses of aminoglycoside antibiotics, even when plasma levels are in the therapeutic range. Aminoglycosides are freely filtered across the glomerulus and then accumulate within the renal cortex, where concentrations can greatly exceed those of the plasma. AKI typically manifests after 5–7 days of therapy and can present even after the drug has been discontinued. Hypomagnesemia is a common finding.

Amphotericin B causes renal vasoconstriction from an increase in tubuloglomerular feedback as well as direct tubular toxicity mediated by reactive oxygen species. Nephrotoxicity from amphotericin B is dose and duration dependent. This drug binds to tubular membrane cholesterol and introduces pores. Clinical features of amphotericin B nephrotoxicity include polyuria, hypomagnesemia, hypocalcemia, and nongap metabolic acidosis.

Vancomycin may be associated with AKI, particularly when trough levels are high, but a causal relationship with AKI has not been definitively established. *Acyclovir* can precipitate in tubules and cause AKI by tubular obstruction, particularly when given as an intravenous bolus at high doses (500 mg/m^2) or in the setting of hypovolemia. *Foscarnet, pentamidine*, and *cidofovir* (less commonly prescribed antimicrobials) are also frequently associated with AKI due to tubular toxicity. AKI secondary to acute interstitial nephritis can occur as a consequence of a number of antibiotics, including *penicillins, cephalosporins, quinolones, sulfonamides*, and *rifampin*.

Chemotherapeutic agents

Cisplatin and *carboplatin* are accumulated by proximal tubular cells and cause necrosis and apoptosis. Intensive hydration regimens have reduced the incidence of cisplatin nephrotoxicity, but it remains a dose-limiting toxicity. *Ifosfamide* may cause hemorrhagic cystitis and tubular toxicity, manifested as Type II renal tubular acidosis (Fanconi's syndrome), polyuria, hypokalemia, and a modest decline in GFR. Antiangiogenesis agents such as *bevacizumab*, can cause proteinuria and hypertension via injury to the glomerular microvasculature (thrombotic microangiopathy). Other antineoplastic agents such as mitomycin C and gemcitabine may cause thrombotic microangiopathy with resultant AKI.

Toxic ingestions

Ethylene glycol, present in automobile antifreeze, is metabolized to oxalic acid, glycolaldehyde, and glyoxylate, which may cause AKI through direct tubular injury. Diethylene glycol is an industrial agent that has been the cause of outbreaks of severe AKI around the world due to adulteration of pharmaceutical preparations. The metabolite 2-hydroxyethoxyacetic acid (HEAA) is thought to be responsible for tubular injury. Melamine contamination of foodstuffs has led to nephrolithiasis and AKI, either through intratubular obstruction or possibly direct tubular toxicity. Aristolochic acid was found to be the cause of "Chinese herb nephropathy" and "Balkan nephropathy" due to contamination of medicinal herbs or farming. The list of environmental toxins is likely to grow and contribute to a better understanding of previously catalogued "idiopathic" chronic tubular interstitial disease, a common diagnosis in both the developed and developing world.

Endogenous toxins

AKI may be caused by a number of endogenous compounds, including myoglobin, hemoglobin, uric acid, and myeloma light chains. Myoglobin can be released by injured muscle cells, and hemoglobin can be released during massive hemolysis leading to pigment nephropathy. Rhabdomyolysis may result from traumatic crush injuries, muscle ischemia during vascular or orthopedic surgery, compression during coma or immobilization, prolonged seizure activity, excessive exercise, heat stroke or malignant hyperthermia, infections, metabolic disorders (e.g., hypophosphatemia, severe hypothyroidism), and myopathies (drug-induced, metabolic, or inflammatory). Pathogenic factors for AKI include intrarenal vasoconstriction, direct proximal tubular toxicity, and mechanical obstruction of the distal nephron lumen when myoglobin or hemoglobin precipitates with Tamm-Horsfall protein (uromodulin, the most common protein in urine and produced in the thick ascending limb of the loop of Henle), a process favored by acidic urine. Tumor lysis syndrome may follow initiation of cytotoxic therapy in patients with high-grade lymphomas and acute lymphoblastic leukemia; massive release of uric acid (with serum levels often exceeding 15 mg/dL) leads to precipitation of uric acid in the renal tubules and AKI (Chap. 276). Other features of tumor lysis syndrome include hyperkalemia and hyperphosphatemia. The tumor lysis syndrome can also occasionally occur spontaneously or with treatment for solid tumors or multiple myeloma. Myeloma light chains can also cause AKI by direct tubular toxicity and by binding to Tamm-Horsfall protein to form obstructing intratubular casts. Hypercalcemia, which can also be seen in multiple myeloma, may cause AKI by intense renal vasoconstriction and volume depletion.

Allergic acute tubulointerstitial disease and other causes of intrinsic AKI

While many of the ischemic and toxic causes of AKI previously described result in tubulointerstitial disease, many drugs are also associated with the development of an allergic response characterized by an inflammatory infiltrate and often peripheral and urinary eosinophilia. AKI may be caused by severe infections and infiltrative diseases. Diseases of the glomeruli or vasculature can lead to AKI by compromising blood flow within the renal circulation. Glomerulonephritis or vasculitis are relatively uncommon but potentially severe causes of AKI that may necessitate timely treatment with immunosuppressive agents or therapeutic plasma exchange.

■ POSTRENAL ACUTE KIDNEY INJURY

(See also Chap. 289) Postrenal AKI occurs when the normally unidirectional flow of urine is acutely blocked either partially or totally, leading to increased retrograde hydrostatic pressure and interference with glomerular filtration. Obstruction to urinary flow may be caused by functional or structural derangements anywhere from the renal pelvis to the tip of the urethra (Fig. 279-5). Normal urinary flow rate does not rule out the presence of partial obstruction, since the GFR is normally two orders of magnitude higher than the urinary flow rate. For AKI to occur in healthy individuals, obstruction must affect both kidneys unless only one kidney is functional, in which case unilateral obstruction can cause AKI. Unilateral obstruction may cause AKI in the setting of significant underlying CKD or in rare cases from reflex vasospasm of the contralateral kidney. Bladder neck obstruction is a common cause of postrenal AKI and can be due to prostate disease (benign prostatic hypertrophy or prostate cancer), neurogenic bladder, or therapy with anticholinergic drugs. Obstructed Foley catheters can cause postrenal AKI if not recognized and relieved. Other causes of lower tract obstruction are blood clots, calculi, and urethral strictures. Ureteric obstruction can occur from intraluminal obstruction (e.g., calculi, blood clots, sloughed renal papillae), infiltration of the ureteric wall (e.g., neoplasia), or external compression (e.g., retroperitoneal fibrosis, neoplasia, abscess, or inadvertent surgical damage). The pathophysiology of postrenal AKI involves hemodynamic alterations triggered by an abrupt increase in intratubular pressures. An initial period of hyperemia from afferent arteriolar dilation is followed by intrarenal vasoconstriction from the generation of angiotensin II, thromboxane A2, and vasopressin, and a reduction in NO production. Reduced GFR is due to underperfusion of glomeruli and, possibly, changes in the glomerular ultrafiltration coefficient.

DIAGNOSTIC EVALUATION (TABLE 279-1)

The presence of AKI is usually inferred by an elevation in the SCr concentration. AKI is currently defined by a rise of at least 0.3 mg/dL or 50% higher than baseline within a 24–48-hours period or a reduction in urine output to 0.5 mL/kg per hour for longer than 6 hours. It is important to recognize that given this definition, some patients with AKI will not have tubular or glomerular damage (e.g., prerenal azotemia). The distinction between AKI and chronic kidney disease is important for proper diagnosis and treatment. The distinction is straightforward when a recent baseline SCr concentration is available, but more difficult in the many instances in which the baseline is unknown. In such cases, clues suggestive of chronic kidney disease can come from radiologic studies (e.g., small, shrunken kidneys with cortical thinning on renal ultrasound, or evidence of renal osteodystrophy) or laboratory tests such as normocytic anemia or secondary hyperparathyroidism with hyperphosphatemia and hypocalcemia, consistent with CKD. No set of tests, however, can rule out AKI superimposed on CKD since AKI is a frequent complication in patients with CKD, further complicating the distinction. Serial blood tests showing continued substantial rise of SCr is clear evidence of AKI. Once the diagnosis of AKI is established, its cause needs to be determined.

■ HISTORY AND PHYSICAL EXAMINATION

The clinical context, careful history taking, and physical examination often narrow the differential diagnosis for the cause of AKI. Prerenal azotemia should be suspected in the setting of vomiting,

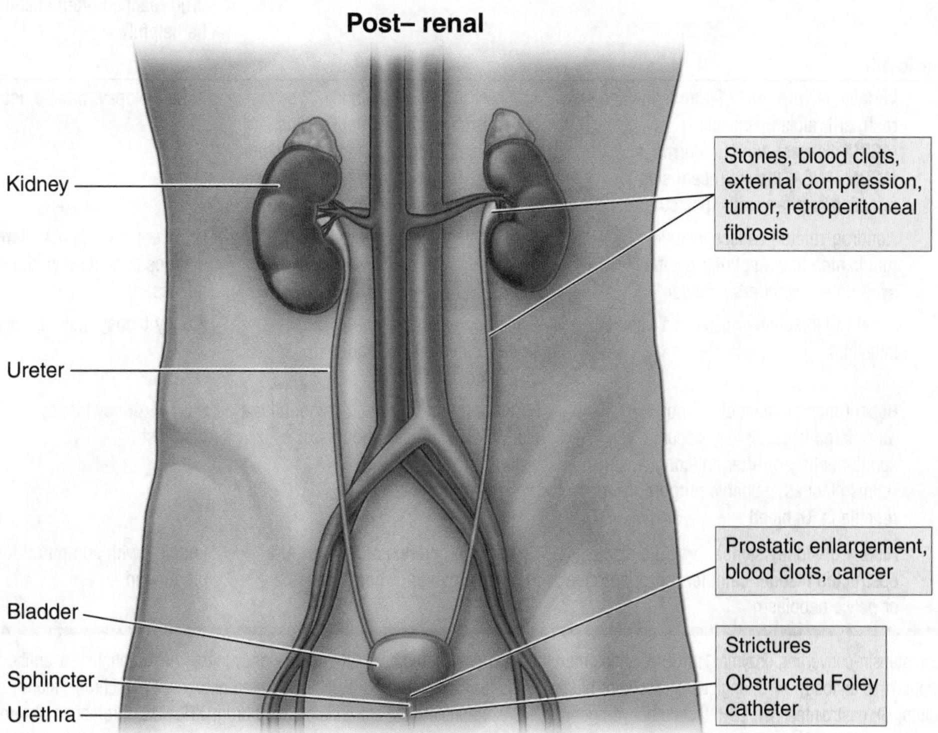

Figure 279-5 Anatomic sites and causes of obstruction leading to postrenal acute kidney injury.

TABLE 279-1 Major Causes, Clinical Features, and Diagnostic Studies for Acute Kidney Injury

Etiology	Clinical Features	Laboratory Features	Comments
Prerenal azotemia	History of poor fluid intake or fluid loss (hemorrhage, diarrhea, vomiting, sequestration into extravascular space); NSAID/ACE-I/ARB; heart failure; evidence of volume depletion (tachycardia, absolute or postural hypotension, low jugular venous pressure, dry mucous membranes), decreased effective circulatory volume (cirrhosis, heart failure)	BUN/creatinine ratio above 20, FeNa <1%, hyaline casts in urine sediment, urine specific gravity >1.018, urine osmolality >500 mOsm/kg	Low FeNa, high specific gravity and osmolality may not be seen in the setting of CKD, diuretic use; BUN elevation out of proportion to creatinine may alternatively indicate upper GI bleed or increased catabolism. Response to restoration of hemodynamics is most diagnostic.
Sepsis-associated AKI	Sepsis, sepsis syndrome, or septic shock. Overt hypotension not always seen in mild to moderate AKI	Positive culture from normally sterile body fluid; urine sediment often contains granular casts, renal tubular epithelial cell casts	FeNa may be low (<1%), particularly early in the course, but is usually >1% and osmolality <500 mOsm/kg
Ischemia-associated AKI	Systemic hypotension, often superimposed upon sepsis and/or reasons for limited renal reserve such as older age, CKD	Urine sediment often contains granular casts, renal tubular epithelial cell casts. FeNa typically >1%.	
Nephrotoxin-Associated AKI: Endogenous			
Rhabdomyolysis	Traumatic crush injuries, seizures, immobilization	Elevated myoglobin, creatine kinase; urinalysis heme positive with few red blood cells	FeNa may be low (<1%)
Hemolysis	Recent blood transfusion with transfusion reaction	Anemia, elevated LDH, low haptoglobin	FeNa may be low (<1%); evaluation for transfusion reaction
Tumor lysis	Recent chemotherapy	Hyperphosphatemia, hypocalcemia, hyperuricemia	
Multiple myeloma	Age >60 years, constitutional symptoms, bone pain	Monoclonal spike in urine or serum electrophoresis; low anion gap	Bone marrow or renal biopsy can be diagnostic
Contrast nephropathy	Exposure to iodinated contrast	Characteristic course is rise in SCr within 1–2 d, peak within 3–5 d, recovery within 7 d	FeNa may be low (<1%)
Nephrotoxin-Associated AKI: Exogenous			
Tubular injury	Aminoglycoside antibiotics, cisplatin, tenofovir, zoledronate	Urine sediment often contains granular casts, renal tubular epithelial cell casts. FeNa typically >1%.	
Interstitial nephritis	Recent medication exposure; can have fever, rash arthralgias	Eosinophilia, sterile pyuria; often nonoliguric	Urine eosinophils have limited diagnostic accuracy; systemic signs of drug reaction often absent; kidney biopsy may be helpful
Other Causes of Intrinsic AKI			
Glomerulonephritis/ vasculitis	Variable (Chap. 283) features include skin rash, arthralgias, sinusitis (AGBM disease), lung hemorrhage (AGBM, ANCA, lupus), recent skin infection or pharyngitis (poststreptococcal)	ANA, ANCA, AGBM antibody, hepatitis serologies, cryoglobulins, blood culture, decreased complement levels, ASO titer (abnormalities of these tests depending on etiology)	Kidney biopsy may be necessary
Interstitial nephritis	Nondrug-related causes include tubulointerstitial nephritis-uveitis (TINU) syndrome, *Legionella* infection	Eosinophilia, sterile pyuria; often nonoliguric	Urine eosinophils have limited diagnostic accuracy; kidney biopsy may be necessary
TTP/HUS	Recent GI infection or use of calcineurin inhibitors	Schistocytes on peripheral blood smear, elevated LDH, anemia, thrombocytopenia	Kidney biopsy may be necessary
Atheroembolic disease	Recent manipulation of the aorta or other large vessels; may occur spontaneously or after anticoagulation; retinal plaques, palpable purpura, livedo reticularis, GI bleed	Hypocomplementemia, eosinophiluria (variable), variable amounts of proteinuria	Skin or kidney biopsy can be diagnostic
Postrenal AKI	History of kidney stones, prostate disease, obstructed bladder catheter, retroperitoneal or pelvic neoplasm	No specific findings other than AKI; may have pyuria or hematuria	Imaging with computed tomography or ultrasound

Abbreviations: ACE-1, angiotensin-converting enzyme-1; AGBM, antiglomerular basement membrane; AKI, acute kidney injury; ANA, antinuclear antibody; ANCA, antineutrophilic cytoplasmic antibody; ARB, angiotensin receptor blocker; ASO, antistreptolysin O; BUN, blood urea nitrogen; CKD, chronic kidney disease; FeNa, fractional excretion of sodium; GI, gastrointestinal; LDH, lactate dehydrogenase; NSAID, nonsteroidal anti-inflammatory drug. TTP/HUS, thrombotic thrombocytopenic purpura/hemolytic uremic syndrome.

diarrhea, glycosuria causing polyuria, and several medications including diuretics, NSAIDs, ACE inhibitors, and ARBs. Physical signs of orthostatic hypotension, tachycardia, reduced jugular venous pressure, decreased skin turgor, and dry mucous membranes are often present in prerenal azotemia. A history of prostatic disease, nephrolithiasis, or pelvic or paraaortic malignancy would suggest the possibility of postrenal AKI. Whether or not symptoms are present early during obstruction of the urinary tract depends on the location of obstruction. Colicky flank pain radiating to the groin suggests acute ureteric obstruction. Nocturia and urinary frequency or hesitancy can be seen in prostatic disease. Abdominal fullness and suprapubic pain can accompany massive bladder enlargement. Definitive diagnosis of obstruction requires radiologic investigations.

A careful review of all medications is imperative in the evaluation of an individual with AKI. Not only are medications frequently a cause of AKI but doses of administered medications must be adjusted for estimated GFR. Idiosyncratic reactions to a wide variety of medications can lead to allergic interstitial nephritis, which may be accompanied by fever, arthralgias, and a pruritic erythematous rash. The absence of systemic features of hypersensitivity, however, does not exclude the diagnosis of interstitial nephritis.

AKI accompanied by palpable purpura, pulmonary hemorrhage, or sinusitis raises the possibility of systemic vasculitis with glomerulonephritis. Atheroembolic disease can be associated with livedo reticularis and other signs of emboli to the legs. A tense abdomen should prompt consideration of acute abdominal compartment syndrome, which requires measurement of bladder pressure. Signs of limb ischemia may be clues to the diagnosis of rhabdomyolysis.

URINE FINDINGS

Complete anuria early in the course of AKI is uncommon except in the following situations: complete urinary tract obstruction, renal artery occlusion, overwhelming septic shock, severe ischemia (often with cortical necrosis), or severe proliferative glomerulonephritis or vasculitis. A reduction in urine output (oliguria, defined as <400 mL/24 h) usually denotes more significant AKI (i.e., lower GFR) than when urine output is preserved. Oliguria is associated with worse clinical outcomes. Preserved urine output can be seen in nephrogenic diabetes insipidus characteristic of longstanding urinary tract obstruction, tubulointerstitial disease, or nephrotoxicity from cisplatin or aminoglycosides, among other causes. Red or brown urine may be seen with or without gross hematuria; if the color persists in the supernatant after centrifugation, then pigment nephropathy from rhabdomyolysis or hemolysis should be suspected.

The urinalysis and urine sediment examination are invaluable tools, but they require clinical correlation because of generally limited sensitivity and specificity (Fig. 279-6) (Chap. e14). In the absence of preexisting proteinuria from CKD, AKI from ischemia or nephrotoxins leads to mild proteinuria (<1 g/d). Greater proteinuria in AKI suggests damage to the glomerular ultrafiltration barrier or excretion of myeloma light chains; the latter are not detected with conventional urine dipsticks (which detect albumin) and require the sulfosalicylic acid test or immunoelectrophoresis. Atheroemboli can cause a variable degree of proteinuria. Extremely heavy proteinuria ("nephrotic range," >3.5 g/d) can occasionally be seen in glomerulonephritis, vasculitis, or interstitial nephritis (particularly from NSAIDs). AKI can also complicate cases of minimal change disease, a cause of the nephrotic syndrome (Chap. 277). If the dipstick is positive for hemoglobin but few red blood cells are evident in the urine sediment, then rhabdomyolysis or hemolysis should be suspected.

Prerenal azotemia may present with hyaline casts or an unremarkable urine sediment exam. Postrenal AKI may also lead to an unremarkable sediment, but hematuria and pyuria may be seen depending on the cause of obstruction. AKI from ATN due to ischemic injury, sepsis, or certain nephrotoxins has characteristic urine sediment findings: pigmented "muddy brown" granular casts and tubular epithelial cell casts. These findings may be absent in more than 20% of cases, however. Glomerulonephritis may lead to dysmorphic red blood cells or red blood cell casts. Interstitial nephritis may lead to white blood cell casts. The urine sediment findings overlap somewhat in glomerulonephritis and interstitial nephritis, and a diagnosis is not always possible on the basis of the

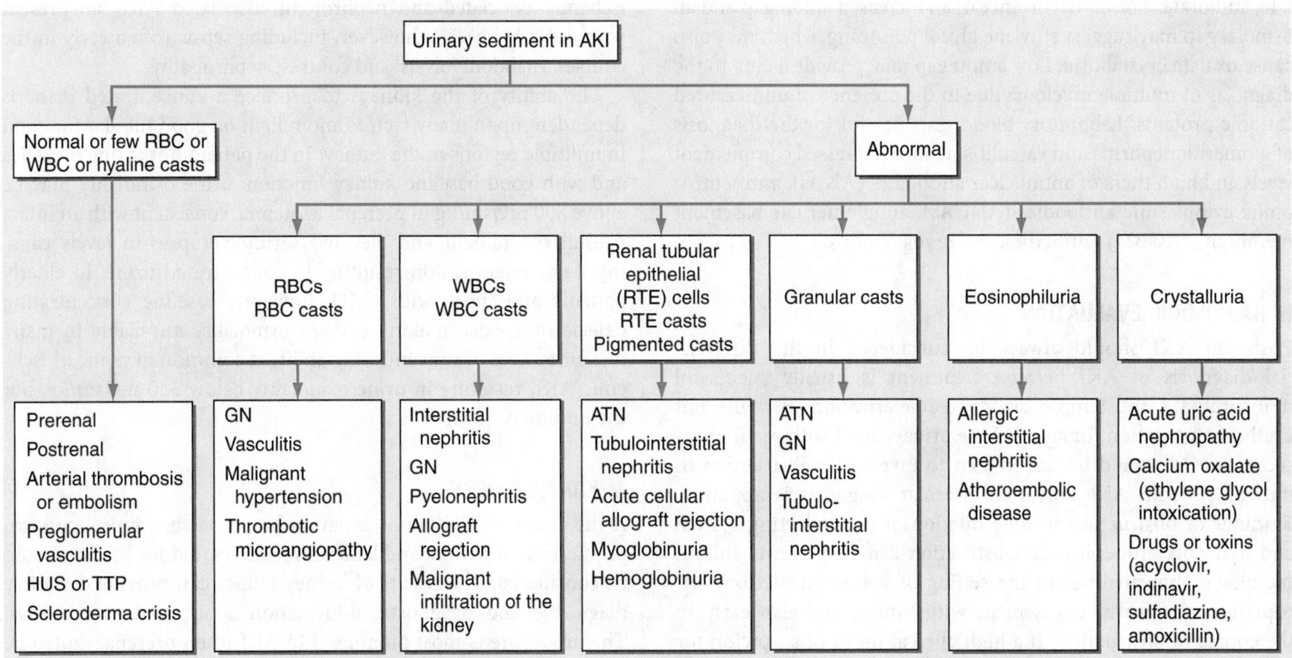

Figure 279-6 Interpretation of urinary sediment findings in acute kidney injury. GN, glomerulonephritis; RTE, renal tubular epithelial. *[Adapted from L Yang, JV Bonventre: Diagnosis and clinical evaluation of acute kidney injury. In Comprehensive Nephrology, 4th ed. J Floege et al (eds). Philadelphia, Elsevier, 2010.]*

urine sediment alone. Urine eosinophils have a limited role in differential diagnosis; they can be seen in interstitial nephritis, pyelonephritis, cystitis, atheroembolic disease, or glomerulonephritis. Crystalluria may be important diagnostically. The finding of oxalate crystals in AKI should prompt an evaluation for ethylene glycol toxicity. Abundant uric acid crystals may be seen in the tumor lysis syndrome.

BLOOD LABORATORY FINDINGS

Certain forms of AKI are associated with characteristic patterns in the rise and fall of SCr. Prerenal azotemia typically leads to modest rises in SCr that return to baseline with improvement in hemodynamic status. Contrast nephropathy leads to a rise in SCr within 24–48 hours, peak within 3–5 days, and resolution within 5–7 days. In comparison, atheroembolic disease usually manifests with more subacute rises in SCr, although severe AKI with rapid increases in SCr can occur in this setting. With many of the epithelial cell toxins such as aminoglycoside antibiotics and cisplatin, the rise in SCr is characteristically delayed for 4–5 days to 2 weeks after initial exposure.

A complete blood count may provide diagnostic clues. Anemia is common in AKI and is usually multifactorial in origin. It is not related to an effect of AKI solely on production of red blood cells since this effect in isolation takes longer to manifest. Severe anemia in the absence of bleeding may reflect hemolysis, multiple myeloma, or thrombotic microangiopathy (e.g., HUS or TTP). Other laboratory findings of thrombotic microangiopathy include thrombocytopenia, schistocytes on peripheral blood smear, elevated lactate dehydrogenase level, and low haptoglobin content. Peripheral eosinophilia can accompany interstitial nephritis, atheroembolic disease, polyarteritis nodosa, and Churg-Strauss vasculitis.

AKI often leads to hyperkalemia, hyperphosphatemia, and hypocalcemia. Marked hyperphosphatemia with accompanying hypocalcemia, however, suggests rhabdomyolysis or the tumor lysis syndrome. Creatinine phosphokinase levels and serum uric acid are elevated in rhabdomyolysis, while tumor lysis syndrome shows normal or marginally elevated creatine kinase and markedly elevated serum uric acid. The anion gap may be increased with any cause of uremia due to retention of anions such as phosphate, hippurate, sulfate, and urate. The co-occurrence of an increased anion gap and an osmolal gap may suggest ethylene glycol poisoning, which may also cause oxalate crystalluria. Low anion gap may provide a clue to the diagnosis of multiple myeloma due to the presence of unmeasured cationic proteins. Laboratory blood tests helpful for the diagnosis of glomerulonephritis and vasculitis include depressed complement levels and high titers of antinuclear antibodies (ANAs), antineutrophilic cytoplasmic antibodies (ANCAs), antiglomerular basement membrane (AGBM) antibodies, and cryoglobulins.

RADIOLOGIC EVALUATION

Postrenal AKI should always be considered in the differential diagnosis of AKI because treatment is usually successful if instituted early. Simple bladder catheterization can rule out urethral obstruction. Imaging of the urinary tract with renal ultrasound or CT should be undertaken to investigate obstruction in individuals with AKI unless an alternate diagnosis is apparent. Findings of obstruction include dilation of the collecting system and hydroureteronephrosis. Obstruction can be present without radiologic abnormalities in the setting of volume depletion, retroperitoneal fibrosis, encasement with tumor, and also early in the course of obstruction. If a high clinical index of suspicion for obstruction persists despite normal imaging, antegrade or retrograde pyelography should be performed. Imaging may also provide additional helpful information about kidney size and echogenicity to assist in the distinction between acute versus CKD. Large kidneys observed in these studies suggest the possibility of diabetic nephropathy, HIV-associated nephropathy, infiltrative diseases, or occasionally acute interstitial nephritis. Vascular imaging may be useful if venous or arterial obstruction is suspected, but the risks of contrast administration should be kept in mind. MRI with gadolinium-based contrast agents should be avoided if possible in severe AKI due to the possibility of inducing nephrogenic system fibrosis, a rare but serious complication seen most commonly in patients with end-stage renal disease.

RENAL FAILURE INDICES

Several indices have been used to help differentiate prerenal azotemia from intrinsic AKI when the tubules are malfunctioning. The low tubular flow rate and increased recycling of urea seen in prerenal azotemia may cause a disproportionate elevation of the BUN compared to creatinine. Other causes of disproportionate BUN elevation need to be kept in mind, however, including upper gastrointestinal bleeding, hyperalimentation, increased tissue catabolism, and glucocorticoid use.

The fractional excretion of sodium (FeNa) is the fraction of the filtered sodium load that is reabsorbed by the tubules and is a measure of both the kidney's ability to reabsorb sodium as well as endogenously and exogenously administered factors that affect tubular reabsorption. As such, it depends on sodium intake, effective intravascular volume, GFR, and intact tubular reabsorptive mechanisms. With prerenal azotemia, the FeNa may be below 1%, suggesting avid tubular sodium reabsorption. In patients with CKD, a FeNa significantly above 1% can still be present despite a prerenal state. The FeNa may also be above 1% despite hypovolemia due to treatment with diuretics. Low FeNa is often seen in glomerulonephritis (and other disorders), and, hence, should not be taken as prima facie evidence of prerenal azotemia. Low FeNa is therefore suggestive but not synonymous with effective intravascular volume depletion, and should not be used as the sole guide for volume management. The response of urine output to crystalloid or colloid fluid administration may be both diagnostic and therapeutic in prerenal azotemia. In ischemic AKI, the FeNa is frequently above 1% because of tubular injury and resultant inability to reabsorb sodium. Several causes of ischemia-associated and nephrotoxin-associated AKI can present with FeNa below 1%, however, including sepsis (often early in the course), rhabdomyolysis, and contrast nephropathy.

The ability of the kidneys to produce a concentrated urine is dependent upon many factors and reliant on good tubular function in multiple regions of the kidney. In the patient not taking diuretics and with good baseline kidney function, urine osmolality may be above 500 mOsm/kg in prerenal azotemia, consistent with an intact medullary gradient and elevated serum vasopressin levels causing water reabsorption resulting in concentrated urine. In elderly patients and those with CKD, however, baseline concentrating defects may exist, making urinary osmolality unreliable in many instances. Loss of concentrating ability is common in septic or ischemic AKI, resulting in urine osmolality below 350 mOsm/kg, but the finding is not specific.

KIDNEY BIOPSY

If the cause of AKI is not apparent based on the clinical context, physical examination, and laboratory studies, kidney biopsy should be considered. The results of kidney biopsy can provide definitive diagnostic and prognostic information about acute and CKDs. The procedure is most often used in AKI when prerenal azotemia, postrenal AKI, and ischemic or nephrotoxic AKI have been deemed unlikely, and other possible diagnoses are being considered such as glomerulonephritis, vasculitis, interstitial nephritis, myeloma kidney, HUS and TTP, and allograft dysfunction. Kidney biopsy is associated with a risk of bleeding, which can be severe and organ or life threatening in patients with thrombocytopenia or coagulopathy.

NOVEL BIOMARKERS

BUN and creatinine are functional biomarkers of glomerular filtration rather than tissue injury biomarkers and, therefore, may be suboptimal for the diagnosis of actual parenchymal kidney damage. BUN and creatinine are also relatively slow to rise after kidney injury. Several novel kidney injury biomarkers have been investigated and show great promise for the early and accurate diagnosis of AKI. *Kidney injury molecule-1 (KIM-1)* is a type 1 transmembrane protein that is abundantly expressed in proximal tubular cells injured by ischemia or nephrotoxins such as cisplatin. KIM-1 is not expressed in appreciable quantities in the absence of tubular injury or in extrarenal tissues. KIM-1's functional role may be to confer phagocytic properties to tubular cells, enabling them to clear debris from the tubular lumen after kidney injury. KIM-1 can be detected shortly after ischemic or nephrotoxic injury in the urine and, therefore, may be an easily tested biomarker in the clinical setting. *Neutrophil gelatinase associated lipocalin* (*NGAL*, also known as lipocalin-2 or siderocalin) is another leading novel biomarker of AKI. NGAL was first discovered as a protein in granules of human neutrophils. NGAL can bind to iron siderophore complexes and may have tissue-protective effects in the proximal tubule. NGAL is highly upregulated after inflammation and kidney injury and can be detected in the plasma and urine within 2 hours of cardiopulmonary bypass–associated AKI. Other injury markers that are being studied in an attempt to increase the early recognition of injury and predict the outcome in AKI are listed in Table 279-2.

COMPLICATIONS

The kidney plays a central role in homeostatic control of volume status, blood pressure, plasma electrolyte composition, and acid-base balance, and for excretion of nitrogenous and other waste products. Complications associated with AKI are, therefore, protean, and depend on the severity of AKI and other associated conditions. Mild to moderate AKI may be entirely asymptomatic, particularly early in the course.

UREMIA

Buildup of nitrogenous waste products, manifested as an elevated BUN concentration, is a hallmark of AKI. BUN itself poses little direct toxicity at levels below 100 mg/dL. At higher concentrations, mental status changes and bleeding complications can arise. Other toxins normally cleared by the kidney may be responsible for the symptom complex known as uremia. Few of the many possible uremic toxins have been definitively identified. The correlation of BUN and SCr concentrations with uremic symptoms is extremely variable, due in part to differences in urea and creatinine generation rates across individuals.

HYPERVOLEMIA AND HYPOVOLEMIA

Expansion of extracellular fluid volume is a major complication of oliguric and anuric AKI, due to impaired salt and water excretion. The result can be weight gain, dependent edema, increased jugular venous pressure, and pulmonary edema; the latter can be life threatening. Pulmonary edema can also occur from volume overload and hemorrhage in pulmonary renal syndromes. AKI may also induce or exacerbate acute lung injury characterized by increased vascular permeability and inflammatory cell infiltration in lung parenchyma. Recovery from AKI can sometimes be accompanied by polyuria, which, if untreated, can lead to significant volume depletion. The polyuric phase of recovery may be due to an osmotic diuresis from retained urea and other waste products as well as delayed recovery of tubular reabsorptive functions.

HYPONATREMIA

Administration of excessive hypotonic crystalloid or isotonic dextrose solutions can result in hypoosmolality and hyponatremia, which, if severe, can cause neurologic abnormalities, including seizures.

HYPERKALEMIA

Abnormalities in plasma electrolyte composition can be mild or life threatening. Frequently the most concerning complication of AKI is hyperkalemia. Marked hyperkalemia is particularly common in rhabdomyolysis, hemolysis, and tumor lysis syndrome due to release of intracellular potassium from damaged cells. Potassium affects the cellular membrane potential of cardiac and neuromuscular tissues. Muscle weakness may be a symptom of hyperkalemia. The more serious complication of hyperkalemia is due to effects on cardiac conduction, leading to potentially fatal arrhythmias.

ACIDOSIS

Metabolic acidosis, usually accompanied by an elevation in the anion gap, is common in AKI, and can further complicate acid-base and potassium balance in individuals with other causes of acidosis, including sepsis, diabetic ketoacidosis, or respiratory acidosis.

HYPERPHOSPHATEMIA AND HYPOCALCEMIA

AKI can lead to hyperphosphatemia, particularly in highly catabolic patients or those with AKI from rhabdomyolysis, hemolysis, and tumor lysis syndrome. Metastatic deposition of calcium phosphate can lead to hypocalcemia. AKI-associated hypocalcemia may also arise from derangements in the vitamin D–parathyroid axis. Hypocalcemia is often asymptomatic but can lead to perioral paresthesias, muscle cramps, seizures, carpopedal spasms, and prolongation of the QT interval on electrocardiography. Calcium levels should be corrected for the degree of hypoalbuminemia, if present, or ionized calcium levels should be followed. Mild, asymptomatic hypocalcemia does not require treatment.

BLEEDING

Hematologic complications of AKI include anemia and bleeding, both of which are exacerbated by coexisting disease processes such as sepsis, liver disease, and disseminated intravascular coagulation. Direct hematologic effects from AKI-related uremia include decreased erythropoiesis and platelet dysfunction.

INFECTIONS

Infections are a common precipitant of AKI and also a dreaded complication of AKI. Impaired host immunity has been described in end-stage renal disease and may be operative in severe AKI.

CARDIAC COMPLICATIONS

The major cardiac complications of AKI are arrhythmias, pericarditis, and pericardial effusion.

MALNUTRITION

AKI is often a severely hypercatabolic state, and, therefore, malnutrition is a major complication.

TABLE 279-2 Biomarkers of Acute Kidney Injury

Biomarker	Comments	Detection	Species
Alanine aminopeptidase (AAP)	1. Proximal tubule brush border enzyme 2. Instability may limit clinical utility	Colorimetry	Rat, dog, human
Alkaline phosphatase (AP)	1. Proximal tubule brush border enzyme. Human intestinal alkaline phosphatase is specific for proximal tubular S3 segment; human tissue nonspecific alkaline phosphatase is specific for S1 and S2 segments 2. Levels may not correlate with extent of functional injury 3. Instability may limit clinical utility	Colorimetry	Rat, human
α-Glutathione-*S*-transferase (α-GST)	1. Proximal tubule cytosolic enzyme 2. Requires stabilization buffer for specimen storage and processing 3. Upregulated in AKI and renal cell carcinoma	ELISA	Mouse, rat, human
γ-Glutamyl transpeptidase (γGT)	1. Proximal tubule brush border enzyme 2. Instability requires samples to be analyzed quickly after collection, limiting clinical utility	Colorimetry	Rat, human
N-Acetyl-β-(D) glucosaminidase (NAG)	1. Proximal tubule lysosomal enzyme 2. More stable than other urinary enzymes 3. Extensive preclinical and clinical data in a variety of conditions (nephrotoxicant exposure, cardiopulmonary bypass, delayed renal allograft function, etc.) 4. Endogenous urea may inhibit activity	Colorimetry	Mouse, rat, human
β_2-Microglobulin	1. Light chain of the MHC I molecule expressed on the cell surface of all nucleated cells 2. Monomeric form is filtered by the glomerulus and reabsorbed by the proximal tubule cells 3. Early marker of tubular dysfunction in a variety of conditions 4. Instability in acidic urine limits clinical utility	ELISA Nephelometry	Mouse, rat, human
α_1-Microglobulin	1. Synthesized by the liver 2. Filtered by the glomerulus and reabsorbed by proximal tubule cells 3. Early marker of tubular dysfunction; high levels may predict poorer outcome 4. Stable across physiologic urinary pH	ELISA Nephelometry	Mouse, rat, human
Retinol-binding protein	1. Synthesized by liver, involved in vitamin A transport 2. Filtered by glomerulus and reabsorbed by proximal tubule cells 3. Early marker of tubular dysfunction 4. Increased stability in acidic urine when compared to β_2-microglobulin	ELISA Nephelometry	Mouse, rat, human
Cystatin C	1. Important extracellular inhibitor of cysteine proteases 2. Filtered by the glomerulus and reabsorbed by proximal tubule cells 3. Elevated urinary levels reflect tubular dysfunction; high levels may predict poorer outcome	ELISA Nephelometry	Mouse, rat, human
Microalbumin	1. Established marker for monitoring progression of chronic kidney disease 2. Elevated urinary levels may be indicative of proximal tubular damage 3. Lack of specificity for AKI may limit its utility	ELISA Immunoturbidimetry	Mouse, rat, dog, monkey, human
Kidney injury molecule-1 (KIM-1)	1. Type-1 cell membrane glycoprotein upregulated in dedifferentiated proximal tubule epithelial cells 2. Ectodomain is shed and can be quantitated in urine following AKI in preclinical and clinical studies 3. Elevated urinary levels are highly sensitive and specific for AKI 4. Upregulated following various models of preclinical and clinical AKI, fibrosis, renal cell carcinoma, and polycystic kidney disease	ELISA, Luminex®-based assay	Zebrafish, mouse, rat, dog, monkey, human
Clusterin	1. Expressed on dedifferentiated proximal tubular epithelial cells 2. Elevated kidney and urinary levels are very sensitive for AKI in preclinical models 3. Upregulated in various rodent models of AKI, fibrosis, renal cell carcinoma, and polycystic kidney disease 4. No clinical study demonstrating its use	ELISA	Mouse, rat, dog, monkey, human

(continued)

TABLE 279-2 Biomarkers of Acute Kidney Injury (*Continued*)

Biomarker	Comments	Detection	Species
Neutrophil gelatinase associated lipocalin (NGAL)	1. Initially identified bound to gelatinase in specific granules of the neutrophils, but also may be induced in epithelial cells in the setting of inflammation or malignancy 2. Expression upregulated in kidney proximal tubule cells and urine following ischemic or cisplatin induced renal injury 3. Found to be an early indicator of AKI following cardiopulmonary bypass 4. Specificity for AKI in setting of sepsis and pyuria need to be further established	ELISA Luminex®-based assay	Mouse, rat, human
Interleukin-18 (IL-18)	1. Cytokine with broad immunomodulatory properties, particularly in setting of ischemic injury 2. Constitutively expressed in distal tubules; strong immunoreactivity in proximal tubules with transplant rejection 3. Elevated urinary levels found to be early marker of AKI and independent predictor of mortality in critically ill patients	ELISA Luminex®-based assay	Mouse, rat, human
Cysteine-rich protein (CYR-61)	1. Induced in proximal straight tubules of kidney and secreted in the urine within 3–6 h following ischemic kidney injury 2. Urinary levels decrease rapidly in spite of progression of injury indicating stability issue 3. No clinical study demonstrating its use 4. No quantitative method established	Western blot	Mouse, rat, human
Osteopontin	1. Upregulated in various rodent models of AKI 2. The induction correlates with inflammation and tubulointerstitial fibrosis 3. No clinical study demonstrating its use	ELISA	Mouse, rat, monkey, human
Liver fatty acid–binding protein (L-FABP)	1. Expressed in proximal tubule epithelial cells 2. Current evidence suggests clinical utility as a biomarker in CKD and diabetic nephropathy 3. Additional studies necessary to determine utility in setting of preclinical and clinical AKI	ELISA	Mouse, rat, human
Sodium/hydrogen exchanger isoform (NHE3)	1. Most abundant sodium transporter in the renal tubule 2. Urinary levels found to discriminate between prerenal azotemia and AKI in ICU patients 3. Samples require considerable processing, limiting assay throughput	Immunoblotting	Mouse, rat, human
Exosomal fetuin-A	1. Acute phase protein synthesized in the liver and secreted into the circulation 2. Levels in proximal tubule cell cytoplasm correspond to degree of injury 3. Urinary levels found to be much higher in ICU patients with AKI compared to ICU patients without AKI and healthy volunteers 4. Samples require considerable processing, limiting assay throughput 5. Additional studies necessary to determine utility in setting of preclinical and clinical AKI	Immunoblotting	Rat, human

Abbreviations: AKI, acute kidney injury; ELISA, enzyme-linked immunosorbent assay; ICU, intensive care unit; RCC, renal cell carcinoma.

TREATMENT Acute Kidney Injury

PREVENTION AND TREATMENT The management of individuals with and at risk for AKI varies according to the underlying cause (Table 279-3). Common to all are several principles. Optimization of hemodynamics, correction of fluid and electrolyte imbalances, discontinuation of nephrotoxic medications, and dose adjustment of administered medications are all critical. Common causes of AKI such as sepsis and ischemic ATN, do not yet have specific therapies once injury is established, but meticulous clinical attention is needed to support the patient until (if) AKI resolves. The kidney possesses remarkable capacity to repair itself after even severe, dialysis-requiring AKI. However, some patients with AKI do not recover fully and may remain dialysis dependent.

Prerenal Azotemia Prevention and treatment of prerenal azotemia requires optimization of renal perfusion. The composition of replacement fluids should be targeted to the type of fluid lost. Severe acute blood loss should be treated with packed red blood cells. Isotonic crystalloid and/or colloid should be used for less severe acute hemorrhage or plasma loss in the case of burns and pancreatitis. Crystalloid solutions are less expensive and probably equally efficacious as colloid solutions. Crystalloid has been reported to be preferable to albumin in the setting of traumatic brain injury. Isotonic crystalloid (e.g., 0.9% saline) or colloid should be used for volume resuscitation in severe hypovolemia, whereas hypotonic crystalloids (e.g., 0.45% saline) suffice for less severe hypovolemia. Excessive chloride administration from 0.9% saline may lead to hyperchloremic metabolic acidosis. Use of bicarbonate-containing solutions (e.g., dextrose water with 150 mEq sodium bicarbonate) should be used if metabolic acidosis is a concern.

Optimization of cardiac function in the cardiorenal syndrome (i.e., renal hypoperfusion from poor cardiac output) may require use of inotropic agents, preload- and afterload-reducing agents, antiarrhythmic drugs, and mechanical aids such as an intraaortic balloon pump. Invasive hemodynamic monitoring to guide therapy may be necessary.

Cirrhosis and Hepatorenal Syndrome Fluid management in individuals with cirrhosis, ascites, and AKI is challenging because of the frequent difficulty in ascertaining intravascular volume status. Administration of intravenous fluids as a volume challenge may be required diagnostically as well as therapeutically. Excessive volume administration may, however, result in worsening ascites and pulmonary compromise in the setting of hepatorenal syndrome or AKI due to superimposed spontaneous bacterial peritonitis. Peritonitis should be ruled out by culture of ascitic fluid. Albumin may prevent AKI in those treated with antibiotics for spontaneous bacterial peritonitis. The definitive treatment of the hepatorenal syndrome is orthotopic liver transplantation. Bridge therapies that have shown promise include terlipressin (a vasopressin analog), combination therapy with octreotide (a somatostatin analog) and midodrine (an α1-adrenergic agonist), and norepinephrine, all in combination with intravenous albumin (25–50 mg per day, maximum 100 g/d).

Intrinsic AKI Several agents have been tested and have failed to show benefit in the treatment of ischemic acute tubular injury. These include atrial natriuretic peptide, low-dose dopamine, endothelin antagonists, loop diuretics, calcium channel blockers, α-adrenergic receptor blockers, prostaglandin analogs, antioxidants, antibodies against leukocyte adhesion molecules, and insulin-like growth factor and many others. Most studies have enrolled patients with severe and well-established AKI, and treatment may have been initiated too late. Novel kidney injury biomarkers may provide an opportunity to test agents earlier in the course of AKI.

AKI due to acute glomerulonephritis or vasculitis may respond to immunosuppressive agents and/or plasmapheresis (Chap. 277). Allergic interstitial nephritis due to medications requires discontinuation of the offending agent. Glucocorticoids have been used, but not tested in randomized trials, in cases where AKI persists or worsens despite discontinuation of the suspected medication. AKI due to scleroderma (scleroderma renal crisis) should be treated with ACE inhibitors.

Early and aggressive volume repletion is mandatory in patients with rhabdomyolysis, who may require 10 L of fluid per day. Alkaline fluids (e.g., 75 mmol sodium bicarbonate added to 0.45% saline) may be beneficial in preventing tubular injury and cast formation, but carry the risk of worsening hypocalcemia. Diuretics may be used if fluid repletion is adequate but unsuccessful in achieving urinary flow rates of 200–300 mL/h. There is no specific therapy for established AKI in rhabdomyolysis, other than dialysis in severe cases or general supportive care to maintain fluid and electrolyte balance and tissue perfusion. Careful attention must be focused on calcium and phosphate status because of precipitation in damaged tissue and released when the tissue heals.

Postrenal AKI Prompt recognition and relief of urinary tract obstruction can forestall the development of permanent structural damage induced by urinary stasis. The site of obstruction defines the treatment approach. Transurethral or suprapubic bladder catheterization may be all that is needed initially for

TABLE 279-3 Management of Ischemia- and Nephrotoxin-Associated AKI

General Issues

1. Optimization of systemic and renal hemodynamics through volume resuscitation and judicious use of vasopressors
2. Elimination of nephrotoxic agents (e.g., ACE inhibitors, ARBs, NSAIDs, aminoglycosides) if possible
3. Initiation of renal replacement therapy when indicated

Specific Issues

1. Nephrotoxin-specific
   a. Rhabdomyolysis: consider forced alkaline diuresis
   b. Tumor lysis syndrome: allopurinol or rasburicase
2. Volume overload
   a. Salt and water restriction
   b. Diuretics
   c. Ultrafiltration
3. Hyponatremia
   a. Restriction of enteral free water intake, minimization of hypotonic intravenous solutions including those containing dextrose
4. Hyperkalemia
   a. Restriction of dietary potassium intake
   b. Discontinuation of potassium-sparing diuretics, ACE inhibitors, ARBs, NSAIDs
   c. Loop diuretics to promote urinary potassium loss
   d. Potassium binding ion-exchange resin (sodium polystyrene sulfonate)
   e. Insulin (10 units regular) and glucose (50 mL of 50% dextrose) to promote entry of potassium intracellularly
   f. Inhaled beta-agonist therapy to promote entry of potassium intracellularly
   g. Calcium gluconate or calcium chloride (1 g) to stabilize the myocardium
5. Metabolic acidosis
   a. Sodium bicarbonate (if pH <7.2 to keep serum bicarbonate >15 mmol/L)
   b. Administration of other bases e.g., THAM
   c. Renal replacement therapy
6. Hyperphosphatemia
   a. Restriction of dietary phosphate intake
   b. Phosphate binding agents (calcium acetate, sevelamer hydrochloride, aluminum hydroxide—taken with meals)
7. Hypocalcemia
   a. Calcium carbonate or calcium gluconate if symptomatic
8. Hypermagnesemia
   a. Discontinue Mg^{2+} containing antacids
9. Hyperuricemia
   a. Acute treatment is usually not required except in the setting of tumor lysis syndrome (see above)
10. Nutrition
    a. Sufficient protein and calorie intake to avoid negative nitrogen balance
11. Drug dosing
    a. Careful attention to dosages and frequency of administration of drugs, adjustment for degree of renal failure

Abbreviations: ACE, angiotensin-converting enzyme; ARBs, angiotensin receptor blocker; NSAIDs, nonsteroidal anti-inflammatory drug; TRAM, tris (hydroxymethyl) aminomethane.

urethral strictures or functional bladder impairment. Ureteric obstruction may be treated by percutaneous nephrostomy tube placement or ureteral stent placement. Relief of obstruction is usually followed by an appropriate diuresis for several days. In rare cases, severe polyuria persists due to tubular dysfunction and may require continued administration of intravenous fluids and electrolytes for a period of time.

SUPPORTIVE MEASURES

Volume Management Hypervolemia in oliguric or anuric AKI may be life threatening due to acute pulmonary edema, especially since many patients have coexisting pulmonary disease, and AKI likely increases pulmonary vascular permeability. Fluid and sodium should be restricted, and diuretics may be used to increase the urinary flow rate. There is no evidence that increasing urine output itself improves the natural history of AKI, but diuretics may help to avoid the need for dialysis in some cases. In severe cases of volume overload, furosemide may be given as a bolus (200 mg) followed by an intravenous drip (10–40 mg/h), with or without a thiazide diuretic. Diuretic therapy should be stopped if there is no response. Dopamine in low doses may transiently increase salt and water excretion by the kidney in prerenal states, but clinical trials have failed to show any benefit in patients with intrinsic AKI. Because of the risk of arrhythmias and potential bowel ischemia, it has been argued that the risks of dopamine may outweigh the benefits in the treatment or prevention of AKI.

Electrolyte and acid-base abnormalities The treatment of dysnatremias and hyperkalemia is described in Chap. 45. Metabolic acidosis is not treated unless severe (pH <7.20 and serum bicarbonate <15 mmol/L). Acidosis can be treated with oral or intravenous sodium bicarbonate (Chap. 47), but overcorrection should be avoided because of the possibility of metabolic alkalosis, hypocalcemia, hypokalemia, and volume overload. Hyperphosphatemia is common in AKI and can usually be treated by limiting intestinal absorption of phosphate using phosphate binders (calcium carbonate, calcium acetate, sevelamer, or aluminum hydroxide). Hypocalcemia does not usually require therapy unless symptoms are present.

Malnutrition Protein energy wasting is common in AKI, particularly in the setting of multisystem organ failure. Inadequate nutrition may lead to starvation ketoacidosis and protein catabolism. Excessive nutrition may increase the generation of nitrogenous waste and lead to worsening azotemia. Total parenteral nutrition requires large volumes of fluid administration and may complicate efforts at volume control.

Anemia The anemia seen in AKI is usually multifactorial and is not improved by erythropoiesis stimulating agents, due to their delayed onset of action and the presence of bone marrow resistance in critically ill patients. Uremic bleeding may respond to desmopressin or estrogens, but may require dialysis in the case of longstanding or severe uremia. Gastrointestinal prophylaxis with proton pump inhibitors or histamine (H_2) receptor blockers is required. Venous thromboembolism prophylaxis is important and should be tailored to the clinical setting; low-molecular-weight heparins and factor Xa inhibitors have unpredictable pharmacokinetics in severe AKI and should be avoided.

Dialysis Indications and Modalities (See also Chap. 281) Dialysis is indicated when medical management fails to control volume overload, hyperkalemia, acidosis, in some toxic ingestions, and when there are severe complications of uremia (asterixis, pericardial rub or effusion, encephalopathy, uremic bleeding). The timing of dialysis is still a matter of debate. Late initiation of dialysis carries the risk of avoidable volume, electrolyte, and metabolic complications of AKI. On the other hand, initiating dialysis too early may unnecessarily expose individuals to intravenous lines and invasive procedures, with the attendant risks of infection, bleeding, procedural complications, and hypotension. The initiation of dialysis should not await the development of a life-threatening complication of renal failure. Many nephrologists initiate dialysis for AKI empirically when the BUN exceeds 100 mg/dL in patients without clinical signs of recovery of kidney function.

The available modes for renal replacement therapy in AKI require either access to the peritoneal cavity (for peritoneal dialysis) or the large blood vessels (for hemodialysis, hemofiltration, and other hybrid procedures). Small solutes are removed across a semipermeable membrane down their concentration gradient ("diffusive" clearance) and/or along with the movement of plasma water ("convective" clearance). The choice of modality is often dictated by the immediate availability of technology and the expertise of medical staff. Peritoneal dialysis is performed through a temporary intraperitoneal catheter. It is rarely used in the United States for AKI in adults but has enjoyed widespread use internationally, particularly when hemodialysis technology is not available. Dialysate solution is instilled into and removed from the peritoneal cavity at regular intervals in order to achieve diffusive and convective clearance of solutes across the peritoneal membrane; ultrafiltration of water is achieved by the presence of an osmotic gradient across the peritoneal membrane, typically due to high concentrations of dextrose in the dialysate. Being a continuous procedure, it is often better tolerated than intermittent procedures like hemodialysis in hypotensive patients. Peritoneal dialysis may not be sufficient for hypercatabolic patients due to inherent limitations in dialysis efficacy.

Hemodialysis can be employed intermittently or continuously, and can be done through convective clearance, diffusive clearance, or a combination of the two. Vascular access is through the femoral, internal jugular, or subclavian veins. Hemodialysis is an intermittent procedure that removes solutes through diffusive and convective clearance. Hemodialysis is performed 3–4 h per d, three to four times per week, and is the most common form of renal replacement therapy for AKI. One of the major complications of hemodialysis is hypotension, particularly in the critically ill.

Continuous intravascular procedures were developed in the early 1980s to treat hemodynamically unstable patients without inducing the rapid shifts of volume, osmolarity, and electrolytes characteristic of intermittent hemodialysis. Continuous renal replacement therapy (CRRT) can be performed by convective clearance [continuous venovenous hemofiltration (CVVH)], in which large volumes of plasma water (and accompanying solutes) are forced across the semipermeable membrane by means of hydrostatic pressure; the plasma water is then replaced by a physiologic crystalloid solution. CRRT can also be performed by diffusive clearance [continuous venovenous hemodialysis (CVVHD)], a technology similar to hemodialysis except at lower blood flow and dialysate flow rates. A hybrid therapy combines both diffusive and convective clearance [continuous venovenous hemodiafiltration (CVVHDF)]. To achieve some of the advantages of CRRT without the need for 24-h staffing of the procedure, a newer form of therapy has been introduced, termed slow low-efficiency dialysis (SLED) or extended daily dialysis (EDD). In this therapy, blood flow and dialysate flow are higher than in CVVHD, but the treatment time is reduced to 12 h.

The optimal dose of dialysis for AKI is not clear. Daily intermittent hemodialysis and high-dose CRRT do not confer a demonstrable survival or renal recovery advantage, but care should be taken to avoid undertreatment. Studies have failed to show that continuous therapies are superior to intermittent therapies. If available, CRRT is often preferred in patients with severe hemodynamic instability, cerebral edema, or significant volume overload.

OUTCOME AND PROGNOSIS

The development of AKI is associated with a significantly increased risk of in-hospital and long-term mortality, longer length of stay, and increased costs. Prerenal azotemia, with the exception of the cardiorenal and hepatorenal syndromes, and postrenal azotemia carry a better prognosis than most cases of intrinsic AKI. The kidneys may recover even after severe, dialysis-requiring AKI. Survivors of an episode of AKI requiring temporary dialysis, however, are at extremely high risk for progressive CKD, and up to 10% may develop end-stage renal disease. Postdischarge care under the supervision of a nephrologist for aggressive secondary prevention of kidney disease is prudent. Patients with AKI are more likely to die prematurely after they leave the hospital even if their kidney function has recovered.

FURTHER READINGS

Bonventre JV: Pathophysiology of AKI: Injury and normal and abnormal repair. Contrib Nephrol 165:9, 2010

——— et al: Next-generation biomarkers for detecting kidney toxicity. Nat Biotechnol 28:436, 2010

Chertow GM et al: Acute kidney injury, mortality, length of stay, and costs in hospitalized patients. J Am Soc Nephrol 16:3365, 2005

Coca SG et al: Biomarkers for the diagnosis and risk stratification of acute kidney injury: A systematic review. Kidney Int 73:1008, 2008

Devarajan P: Update on mechanisms of ischemic acute kidney injury. J Am Soc Nephrol 17:1503, 2006

Waikar SS, Bonventre JV: Creatinine kinetics and the definition of acute kidney injury. J Am Soc Nephrol 20:672, 2009

Wald R: Chronic dialysis and death among survivors of acute kidney injury requiring dialysis. JAMA 302:1532, 2009.

CHAPTER 280 Chronic Kidney Disease

Joanne M. Bargman
Karl Skorecki

Chronic kidney disease (CKD) encompasses a spectrum of different pathophysiologic processes associated with abnormal kidney function and a progressive decline in glomerular filtration rate (GFR). Table 280-1 provides a widely accepted classification, based on guidelines of the National Kidney Foundation [Kidney Dialysis Outcomes Quality Initiative (KDOQI)], in which stages of CKD are defined according to the estimated GFR.

TABLE 280-1 Classification of Chronic Kidney Disease (CKD)

Stage	GFR, mL/min per 1.73 m^2
0	>90[a]
1	≥90[b]
2	60–89
3	30–59
4	15–29
5	<15

[a]With risk factors for CKD (see text).
[b]With demonstrated kidney damage (e.g., persistent proteinuria, abnormal urine sediment, abnormal blood and urine chemistry, abnormal imaging studies).
Abbreviation: GFR, glomerular filtration rate.
Source: Modified from National Kidney Foundation. K/DOQI Clinical Practice Guidelines for Chronic Kidney Disease: Evaluation, classification and stratification. Am J Kidney Dis 39:suppl 1, 2002.

The term *chronic renal failure* applies to the process of continuing significant irreversible reduction in nephron number and typically corresponds to CKD stages 3–5. The pathophysiologic processes and adaptations associated with chronic renal failure will be the focus of this chapter. The dispiriting term *end-stage renal disease* represents a stage of CKD where the accumulation of toxins, fluid, and electrolytes normally excreted by the kidneys results in the *uremic syndrome*. This syndrome leads to death unless the toxins are removed by renal replacement therapy, using dialysis or kidney transplantation. These latter interventions are discussed in Chaps. 281 and 282. *End-stage renal disease* will be supplanted in this chapter by the term *stage 5 CKD*.

PATHOPHYSIOLOGY OF CHRONIC KIDNEY DISEASE

The pathophysiology of CKD involves two broad sets of mechanisms of damage: (1) initiating mechanisms specific to the underlying etiology (e.g., genetically determined abnormalities in kidney development or integrity, immune complex deposition and inflammation in certain types of glomerulonephritis, or toxin exposure in certain diseases of the renal tubules and interstitium) and (2) a set of progressive mechanisms, involving hyperfiltration and hypertrophy of the remaining viable nephrons, that are a common consequence following long-term reduction of renal mass, irrespective of underlying etiology (Chap. 278). The responses to reduction in nephron number are mediated by vasoactive hormones, cytokines, and growth factors. Eventually, these short-term adaptations of hypertrophy and hyperfiltration become maladaptive as the increased pressure and flow predisposes to distortion of glomerular architecture, associated with sclerosis and dropout of the remaining nephrons (Fig. 280-1). Increased intrarenal activity of the renin-angiotensin axis appears to contribute both to the initial adaptive hyperfiltration and to the subsequent maladaptive hypertrophy and sclerosis, the latter, in part, owing to the stimulation of transforming growth factor β (TGF-β). This process explains why a reduction in renal mass from an isolated insult may lead to a progressive decline in renal function over many years (Fig. 280-2).

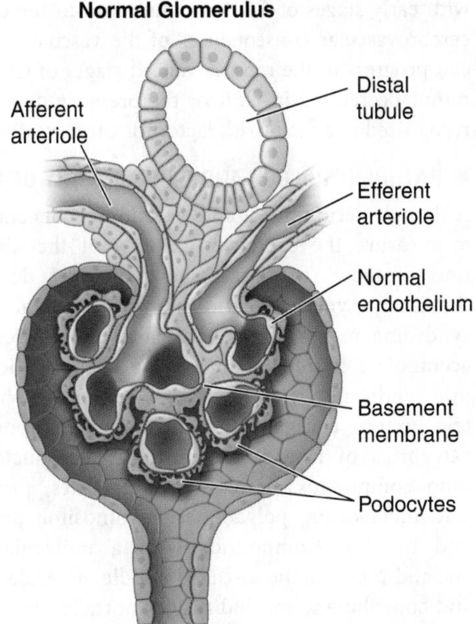

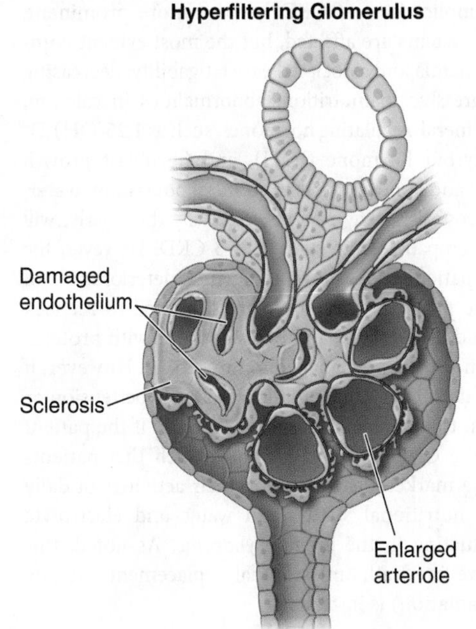

Figure 280-1 Left: Schema of the normal glomerular architecture. Right: Secondary glomerular changes associated with a reduction in nephron number, including enlargement of capillary lumens and focal adhesions, which are thought to occur consequent to compensatory hyperfiltration and hypertrophy in the remaining nephrons. *(Modified from JR Ingelfinger: N Engl J Med 348:99, 2003.)*

IDENTIFICATION OF RISK FACTORS AND STAGING OF CKD

It is important to identify factors that increase the risk for CKD, even in individuals with normal GFR. Risk factors include hypertension, diabetes mellitus, autoimmune disease, older age, African ancestry, a family history of renal disease, a previous episode of acute kidney injury, and the presence of proteinuria, abnormal urinary sediment, or structural abnormalities of the urinary tract.

Recent research in the genetics of predisposition to common complex diseases (Chap. 61) has revealed DNA sequence variants at a number of genetic loci that are associated with common forms of CKD. A striking example is the finding of allelic versions of the *APOL1* gene, of West African population ancestry, which contributes to the several-fold higher frequency of certain common etiologies of CKD (e.g., focal segmental glomerulosclerosis) observed among African and Hispanic Americans. The prevalence in West African populations seems to have an evolutionary basis, since these same variants offer protection from tropical pathogens.

In order to stage CKD, it is necessary to estimate the GFR. Two equations commonly used to estimate GFR are shown in Table 280-2 and incorporate the measured plasma creatinine concentration, age, sex, and ethnic origin. Many laboratories now report an estimated GFR, or "eGFR," using one of these equations.

The normal annual mean decline in GFR with age from the peak GFR (~120 mL/min per 1.73 m^2) attained during the third decade of life is ~1 mL/min per year per 1.73 m^2, reaching a mean value of 70 mL/min per 1.73 m^2 at age 70. The mean GFR is lower in women than in men. For example, a woman in her 80s with a normal serum creatinine may have a GFR of just 50 mL/min per 1.73 m^2. Thus, even a mild elevation in serum creatinine concentration [e.g., 130 μmol/L (1.5 mg/dL)] often signifies a substantial reduction in GFR in most individuals.

Measurement of albuminuria is also helpful for monitoring nephron injury and the response to therapy in many forms of CKD, especially chronic glomerular diseases. While an accurate 24-h urine collection is the criterion standard for measurement of albuminuria, the measurement of protein-to-creatinine ratio in a spot first-morning urine sample is often more practical to obtain and correlates well, but not perfectly, with 24-h urine collections.

TABLE 280-2 Recommended Equations for Estimation of Glomerular Filtration Rate (GFR) Using Serum Creatinine Concentration (P_{Cr}), Age, Sex, Race, and Body Weight

1. Equation from the Modification of Diet in Renal Disease study*
   Estimated GFR (mL/min per 1.73 m^2) = $1.86 \times (P_{Cr})^{-1.154} \times (\text{age})^{-0.203}$
   Multiply by 0.742 for women
   Multiply by 1.21 for African Americans
2. Cockcroft-Gault equation
   Estimated creatinine clearance (mL/min)
   $$= \frac{(140-\text{age}) \times \text{body weight (kg)}}{72 \times P_{Cr}\ (\text{mg/dL})}$$
   Multiply by 0.85 for women

*Equation is *available* in hand-held calculators and in tabular form.
Source: Adapted from AS Levey et al: Am J Kidney Dis 39: S1, 2002, with permission.

Persistence in the urine of >17 mg of albumin per gram of creatinine in adult males and 25 mg albumin per gram of creatinine in adult females usually signifies chronic renal damage. *Microalbuminuria* refers to the excretion of amounts of albumin too small to detect by urinary dipstick or conventional measures of urine protein. It is a good screening test for early detection of renal disease, and may be a marker for the presence of microvascular disease in general. If a patient has a large amount of excreted albumin, there is no reason to test for microalbuminuria.

Stages 1 and 2 CKD are usually not associated with any symptoms arising from the decrement in GFR. However, there may be symptoms from the underlying renal disease itself, such as edema in patients with nephrotic syndrome or signs of hypertension secondary to the renal parenchymal disease in patients with polycystic kidney disease, some forms of glomerulonephritis, and many other parenchymal and vascular renal diseases, even with well-preserved GFR. If the decline in GFR progresses to stages 3 and 4, clinical and laboratory complications of CKD become more prominent. Virtually all organ systems are affected, but the most evident complications include anemia and associated easy fatigability; decreasing appetite with progressive malnutrition; abnormalities in calcium, phosphorus, and mineral-regulating hormones, such as $1,25(OH)_2D_3$ (calcitriol), parathyroid hormone (PTH), and fibroblast growth factor 23 (FGF-23); and abnormalities in sodium, potassium, water, and acid-base homeostasis. Many patients, especially the elderly, will have eGFR values compatible with stage 2 or 3 CKD. However, the majority of these patients will show no further deterioration of renal function. The primary care physician is advised to recheck kidney function, and if it is stable and not associated with proteinuria, the patient can usually be managed in this setting. However, if there is evidence of decline of GFR and uncontrolled hypertension or proteinuria, referral to a nephrologist is appropriate. If the patient progresses to stage 5 CKD, toxins accumulate such that patients usually experience a marked disturbance in their activities of daily living, well-being, nutritional status, and water and electrolyte homeostasis, eventuating in the *uremic syndrome.* As noted, this state will culminate in death unless renal replacement therapy (dialysis or transplantation) is instituted.

ETIOLOGY AND EPIDEMIOLOGY

It has been estimated from population survey data that at least 6% of the adult population in the United States has CKD at stages 1 and 2. An unknown subset of this group will progress to more advanced stages of CKD. An additional 4.5% of the U.S. population is estimated to have stages 3 and 4 CKD. Table 280-3 lists the five most frequent categories of causes of CKD, cumulatively accounting for greater than 90% of the CKD disease burden worldwide. The relative contribution of each category varies among different geographic regions. The most frequent cause of CKD in North America and Europe is diabetic nephropathy, most often secondary to type 2 diabetes mellitus. Patients with newly diagnosed CKD often also present with hypertension. When no overt evidence for a primary glomerular or tubulointerstitial kidney disease process is present, CKD is often attributed to hypertension. However, it is now appreciated that such individuals can be considered in two categories. The first includes patients with a silent primary glomerulopathy, such as focal segmental glomerulosclerosis, without the overt nephrotic or nephritic manifestations of glomerular disease (Chap. 283). The second includes patients in whom progressive nephrosclerosis and hypertension is the renal correlate of a systemic vascular disease, often also involving large- and small-vessel cardiac and cerebral pathology. This latter combination is especially common in the elderly, in whom chronic renal ischemia as a cause of CKD may be underdiagnosed. The increasing incidence of CKD in the elderly has been ascribed, in part, to decreased mortality rate from the cardiac and cerebral complications of atherosclerotic vascular disease, enabling a greater segment of the population to manifest the renal component of generalized vascular disease. Nevertheless, it should be appreciated that the vast majority of such patients with early stages of CKD will succumb to the cardiovascular and cerebrovascular consequences of the vascular disease before they can progress to the most advanced stages of CKD. Indeed, even a minor decrement in GFR or the presence of albuminuria is now recognized as a major risk factor for cardiovascular disease.

TABLE 280-3 Leading Categories of Etiologies of CKD*

- Diabetic glomerular disease
- Glomerulonephritis
- Hypertensive nephropathy
  - Primary glomerulopathy with hypertension
  - Vascular and ischemic renal disease
- Autosomal dominant polycystic kidney disease
- Other cystic and tubulointerstitial nephropathy

*Relative contribution of each category varies with geographic region.

PATHOPHYSIOLOGY AND BIOCHEMISTRY OF UREMIA

Although serum urea and creatinine concentrations are used to measure the excretory capacity of the kidneys, accumulation of these two molecules themselves do not account for the many symptoms and signs that characterize the uremic syndrome in advanced renal failure. Hundreds of toxins that accumulate in renal failure have been implicated in the uremic syndrome. These include water-soluble, hydrophobic, protein-bound, charged, and uncharged compounds. Additional categories of nitrogenous excretory products include guanidino compounds, urates and hippurates, products of nucleic acid metabolism, polyamines, myoinositol, phenols, benzoates, and indoles. Compounds with a molecular mass between 500 and 1500 Da, the so-called middle molecules, are also retained and contribute to morbidity and mortality. It is thus evident that the serum concentrations of urea and creatinine should be viewed as being readily measured, but incomplete, surrogate markers for these compounds, and monitoring the levels of urea and creatinine in the patient with impaired kidney function represents a vast oversimplification of the uremic state.

The uremic syndrome and the disease state associated with advanced renal impairment involve more than renal excretory failure. A host of metabolic and endocrine functions normally performed by the kidneys is also impaired or suppressed, and this results in anemia, malnutrition, and abnormal metabolism of carbohydrates, fats, and proteins. Furthermore, plasma levels of many hormones, including PTH, FGF-23, insulin, glucagon, steroid hormones including vitamin D and sex hormones, and prolactin, change with renal failure as a result of urinary retention, decreased degradation, or abnormal regulation. Finally, progressive renal impairment is associated with worsening systemic inflammation. Elevated levels of C-reactive protein are detected along with other acute-phase reactants, while levels of so-called negative acute-phase reactants, such as albumin and fetuin, decline with progressive renal impairment, even in nonproteinuric kidney disease. Thus, the inflammation associated with renal impairment is important in the malnutrition-inflammation-atherosclerosis/calcification syndrome, which contributes in turn to the acceleration of vascular disease and comorbidity rate associated with advanced kidney disease.

In summary, the pathophysiology of the uremic syndrome can be divided into manifestations in three spheres of dysfunction: (1) those consequent to the accumulation of toxins that normally undergo renal excretion, including products of protein metabolism; (2) those consequent to the loss of other renal functions, such as fluid and electrolyte homeostasis and hormone regulation; and (3) progressive systemic inflammation and its vascular and nutritional consequences.

CLINICAL AND LABORATORY MANIFESTATIONS OF CHRONIC KIDNEY DISEASE AND UREMIA

Uremia leads to disturbances in the function of virtually every organ system. Chronic dialysis can reduce the incidence and severity of many of these disturbances, so that the overt and florid manifestations of uremia have largely disappeared in the modern health setting. However, as indicated in Table 280-4, even optimal dialysis therapy is not completely effective as renal replacement therapy, because some disturbances resulting from impaired renal function fail to respond to dialysis.

TABLE 280-4 Clinical Abnormalities in Uremia[a]

Fluid and electrolyte disturbances	Neuromuscular disturbances	Dermatologic disturbances
Volume expansion (I)	Fatigue (I)[b]	Pallor (I)[b]
Hyponatremia (I)	Sleep disorders (P)	Hyperpigmentation (I, P, or D)
Hyperkalemia (I)	Headache (P)	Pruritus (P)
Hyperphosphatemia (I)	Impaired mentation (I)[b]	Ecchymoses (I)
Endocrine-metabolic disturbances	Lethargy (I)[b]	Nephrogenic fibrosing dermopathy (D)
Secondary hyperparathyroidism (I or P)	Asterixis (I)	Uremic frost (I)
Adynamic bone (D)	Muscular irritability	**Gastrointestinal disturbances**
Vitamin D–deficient osteomalacia (I)	Peripheral neuropathy (I or P)	Anorexia (I)
Carbohydrate resistance (I)	Restless legs syndrome (I or P)	Nausea and vomiting (I)
Hyperuricemia (I or P)	Myoclonus (I)	Gastroenteritis (I)
Hypertriglyceridemia (I or P)	Seizures (I or P)	Peptic ulcer (I or P)
Increased Lp(a) level (P)	Coma (I)	Gastrointestinal bleeding (I, P, or D)
Decreased high-density lipoprotein level (P)	Muscle cramps (P or D)	Idiopathic ascites (D)
Protein-energy malnutrition (I or P)	Dialysis disequilibrium syndrome (D)	Peritonitis (D)
Impaired growth and development (P)	Myopathy (P or D)	**Hematologic and immunologic disturbances**
Infertility and sexual dysfunction (P)	**Cardiovascular and pulmonary disturbances**	Anemia (I)[b]
Amenorrhea (I/P)	Arterial hypertension (I or P)	Lymphocytopenia (P)
β_2-Microglobulin–associated amyloidosis (P or D)	Congestive heart failure or pulmonary edema (I)	Bleeding diathesis (I or D)[b]
	Pericarditis (I)	Increased susceptibility to infection (I or P)
	Hypertrophic or dilated cardiomyopathy (I, P, or D)	Leukopenia (D)
	Uremic lung (I)	Thrombocytopenia (D)
	Accelerated atherosclerosis (P or D)	
	Hypotension and arrhythmias (D)	
	Vascular calcification (P or D)	

[a]Virtually all abnormalities in this table are completely reversed in time by successful renal transplantation. The response of these abnormalities to hemodialysis or peritoneal dialysis therapy is more variable. (I) denotes an abnormality that usually improves with an optimal program of dialysis and related therapy; (P) denotes an abnormality that tends to persist or even progress, despite an optimal program; (D) denotes an abnormality that develops only after initiation of dialysis therapy.
[b]Improves with dialysis and erythropoietin therapy.
Abbreviation: Lp(a), lipoprotein A.

FLUID, ELECTROLYTE, AND ACID-BASE DISORDERS

Sodium and water homeostasis

In most patients with stable CKD, the total-body content of sodium and water is modestly increased, although this may not be apparent on clinical examination. Normal renal function guarantees that the tubular reabsorption of filtered sodium and water is adjusted so that urinary excretion matches intake. Many forms of renal disease (e.g., glomerulonephritis) disrupt this glomerulotubular balance such that dietary intake of sodium exceeds its urinary excretion, leading to sodium retention and attendant extracellular fluid volume (ECFV) expansion. This expansion may contribute to hypertension, which itself can accelerate the nephron injury. As long as water intake does not exceed the capacity for water clearance, the ECFV expansion will be isotonic and the patient will have a normal plasma sodium concentration and effective osmolality (Chap. 278). Hyponatremia is not commonly seen in CKD patients but, when present, can respond to water restriction. If the patient has evidence of ECFV expansion (peripheral edema, sometimes hypertension poorly responsive to therapy), he or she should be counseled regarding salt restriction. Thiazide diuretics have limited utility in stages 3–5 CKD, such that administration of loop diuretics, including furosemide, bumetanide, or torsemide, may also be needed. Resistance to loop diuretics in renal failure often mandates use of higher doses than those used in patients with near-normal kidney function. The combination of loop diuretics with metolazone, which inhibits the sodium chloride co-transporter of the distal convoluted tubule, can help effect renal salt excretion. Ongoing diuretic resistance with intractable edema and hypertension in advanced CKD may serve as an indication to initiate dialysis.

In addition to problems with salt and water excretion, some patients with CKD may instead have impaired renal conservation of sodium and water. When an extrarenal cause for fluid loss, such as gastrointestinal (GI) loss, is present, these patients may be prone to ECFV depletion because of the inability of the failing kidney to reclaim filtered sodium adequately. Furthermore, depletion of ECFV, whether due to GI losses or overzealous diuretic therapy, can further compromise kidney function through underperfusion, or a "prerenal" basis, leading to acute-on-chronic kidney failure. In this setting, cautious volume repletion with normal saline may return the ECFV to normal and restore renal function to baseline without having to intervene with dialysis.

Potassium homeostasis

In CKD, the decline in GFR is not necessarily accompanied by a parallel decline in urinary potassium excretion, which is predominantly mediated by aldosterone-dependent secretory events in distal nephron segments. Another defense against potassium retention in these patients is augmented potassium excretion in the GI tract. Notwithstanding these two homeostatic responses, hyperkalemia may be precipitated in certain settings. These include increased dietary potassium intake, protein catabolism, hemolysis, hemorrhage, transfusion of stored red blood cells, and metabolic acidosis. In addition, a host of medications can inhibit renal potassium excretion. The most important medications in this respect include the angiotensin-converting enzyme (ACE) inhibitors, angiotensin receptor blockers (ARBs), and spironolactone and other potassium-sparing diuretics such as amiloride, eplerenone, and triamterene.

Certain causes of CKD can be associated with earlier and more severe disruption of potassium-secretory mechanisms in the distal nephron, out of proportion to the decline in GFR. These include conditions associated with hyporeninemic hypoaldosteronism, such as diabetes, and renal diseases that preferentially affect the distal nephron, such as obstructive uropathy and sickle cell nephropathy.

Hypokalemia is not common in CKD and usually reflects markedly reduced dietary potassium intake, especially in association with excessive diuretic therapy or concurrent GI losses. Hypokalemia can also occur as a result of primary renal potassium wasting in association with other solute transport abnormalities, such as Fanconi's syndrome, renal tubular acidosis, or other forms of hereditary or acquired tubulointerstitial disease. However, even with these conditions, as the GFR declines, the tendency to hypokalemia diminishes and hyperkalemia may supervene. Therefore, the use of potassium supplements and potassium-sparing diuretics should be constantly reevaluated as GFR declines.

Metabolic acidosis

Metabolic acidosis is a common disturbance in advanced CKD. The majority of patients can still acidify the urine, but they produce less ammonia and, therefore, cannot excrete the normal quantity of protons in combination with this urinary buffer. Hyperkalemia, if present, further depresses ammonia production. The combination of hyperkalemia and hyperchloremic metabolic acidosis is often present, even at earlier stages of CKD (stages 1–3), in patients with diabetic nephropathy or in those with predominant tubulointerstitial disease or obstructive uropathy; this is a non-anion-gap metabolic acidosis. Treatment of hyperkalemia may increase renal ammonia production, improve renal generation of bicarbonate, and improve the metabolic acidosis.

With worsening renal function, the total urinary net daily acid excretion is usually limited to 30–40 mmol, and the anions of retained organic acids can then lead to an anion-gap metabolic acidosis. Thus, the non-anion-gap metabolic acidosis that can be seen in earlier stages of CKD may be complicated by the addition of an anion-gap metabolic acidosis as CKD progresses. In most patients, the metabolic acidosis is mild; the pH is rarely <7.35 and can usually be corrected with oral sodium bicarbonate supplementation. Animal and human studies have suggested that even modest degrees of metabolic acidosis may be associated with the development of protein catabolism. Alkali supplementation may attenuate the catabolic state and possibly slow CKD progression and accordingly is recommended when the serum bicarbonate concentration falls below 20–23 mmol/L. The concomitant sodium load mandates careful attention to volume status and the potential need for diuretic agents.

TREATMENT Fluid, Electrolyte, and Acid-Base Disorders

Adjustments in the dietary intake of salt and use of loop diuretics, occasionally in combination with metolazone, may be needed to maintain euvolemia. In contrast, overzealous salt restriction or diuretic use can lead to ECFV depletion and precipitate a further decline in GFR. The rare patient with salt-losing nephropathy may require a sodium-rich diet or salt supplementation. Water restriction is indicated only if there is a problem with hyponatremia. Otherwise, patients with CKD and an intact thirst mechanism may be instructed to drink fluids in a quantity that keeps them just ahead of their thirst. Intractable ECFV expansion, despite dietary salt restriction and diuretic therapy, may be an indication to start renal replacement therapy. Hyperkalemia often responds to dietary restriction of potassium, avoidance of potassium supplements (including occult sources, such as dietary salt substitutes) as well as potassium-retaining medications (especially ACE inhibitors or ARBs), or the use of kaliuretic diuretics. Kaliuretic diuretics promote urinary potassium excretion, while potassium-binding resins, such as calcium resonium or sodium polystyrene, can promote potassium loss through the GI tract and may reduce the incidence of hyperkalemia in CKD patients. Intractable hyperkalemia is an indication (although uncommon) to consider institution of dialysis in a CKD patient. The renal tubular acidosis and subsequent anion-gap metabolic acidosis in progressive CKD will respond to alkali supplementation, typically with sodium bicarbonate. Recent studies suggest that this replacement should be considered when the serum bicarbonate concentration falls below 20–23 mmol/L to avoid the protein catabolic state seen with even mild degrees of metabolic acidosis and to slow the progression of CKD.

DISORDERS OF CALCIUM AND PHOSPHATE METABOLISM

The principal complications of abnormalities of calcium and phosphate metabolism in CKD occur in the skeleton and the vascular bed, with occasional severe involvement of extraosseous soft tissues. It is likely that disorders of bone turnover and disorders of vascular and soft tissue calcification are related to each other (Fig. 280-2).

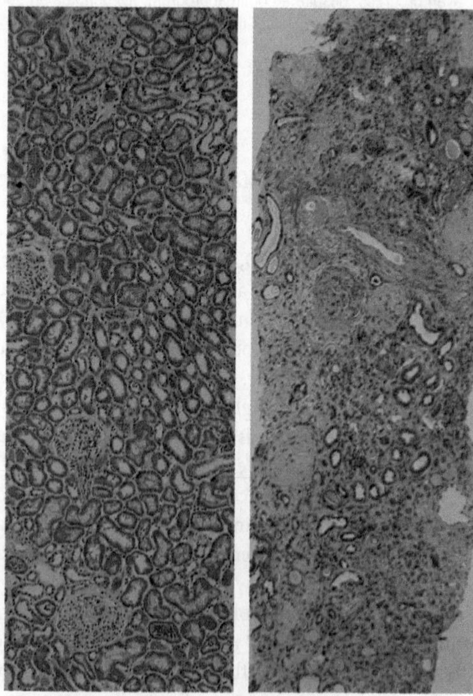

Figure 280-2 Left: Low-power photomicrograph of a normal kidney showing normal glomeruli and healthy tubulointerstitium without fibrosis. **Right:** Low-power photomicrograph of chronic kidney disease with sclerosis of many glomeruli and severe tubulointerstitial fibrosis *(Masson trichrome, × 40 magnification. Slides courtesy of the late Dr. Andrew Herzenberg.)*

Bone manifestations of CKD

The major disorders of bone disease can be classified into those associated with high bone turnover with increased PTH levels (including osteitis fibrosa cystica, the classic lesion of secondary hyperparathyroidism) and low bone turnover with low or normal PTH levels (adynamic bone disease and osteomalacia).

The pathophysiology of secondary hyperparathyroidism and the consequent high-turnover bone disease is related to abnormal mineral metabolism through the following events: (1) declining GFR leads to reduced excretion of phosphate and, thus, phosphate retention; (2) the retained phosphate stimulates increased synthesis of PTH and growth of parathyroid gland mass; and (3) decreased levels of ionized calcium, resulting from diminished calcitriol production by the failing kidney as well as phosphate retention, also stimulate PTH production. Low calcitriol levels contribute to hyperparathyroidism, both by leading to hypocalcemia and also by a direct effect on PTH gene transcription. These changes start to occur when the GFR falls below 60 mL/min.

Fibroblast growth factor 23 (FGF-23) is part of a family of phosphatonins that promotes renal phosphate excretion. Recent studies have shown that levels of this hormone, secreted by osteocytes, increases early in the course of CKD. It may defend normal serum phosphorus in at least three ways: (1) increased renal phosphate excretion; (2) stimulation of PTH, which also increases renal phosphate excretion; and (3) suppression of the formation of $1,25(OH)_2D_3$, leading to diminished phosphorus absorption from the gastrointestinal tract. Interestingly, high levels of FGF-23 are also an independent risk factor for left ventricular hypertrophy and mortality in dialysis patients. Moreover, elevated levels of FGF-23 may indicate the need for therapeutic intervention (e.g., phosphate restriction), even when serum phosphate levels are within the normal range.

Hyperparathyroidism stimulates bone turnover and leads to *osteitis fibrosa cystica*. Bone histology shows abnormal osteoid, bone and bone marrow fibrosis, and in advanced stages, the formation of bone cysts, sometimes with hemorrhagic elements so that they appear brown in color, hence the term *brown tumor*. Clinical manifestations of severe hyperparathyroidism include bone pain and fragility, brown tumors, compression syndromes, tumors, and erythropoietin resistance in part related to the bone marrow fibrosis. Furthermore, PTH itself is considered a uremic toxin, and high levels are associated with muscle weakness, fibrosis of cardiac muscle, and nonspecific constitutional symptoms.

Low-turnover bone disease can be grouped into two categories—adynamic bone disease and osteomalacia. In the latter condition, there is accumulation of unmineralized bone matrix that may be caused by a number of processes, including vitamin D deficiency, metabolic acidosis, and in the past aluminum deposition. Adynamic bone disease is increasing in prevalence, especially among diabetics and the elderly. It is characterized by reduced bone volume and mineralization and may result from excessive suppression of PTH production, chronic inflammation, or both. Suppression of PTH can result from the use of vitamin D preparations or from excessive calcium exposure in the form of calcium-containing phosphate binders or high-calcium dialysis solutions. Complications of adynamic bone disease include an increased incidence of fracture and bone pain and an association with increased vascular and cardiac calcification.

Calcium, phosphorus, and the cardiovascular system

Recent epidemiologic evidence has shown a strong association between hyperphosphatemia and increased cardiovascular mortality rate in patients with stage 5 CKD and even in patients with earlier stages of CKD. Hyperphosphatemia and hypercalcemia are associated with increased vascular calcification, but it is unclear whether the excessive mortality rate is mediated by this mechanism. Studies using CT and electron-beam CT scanning show that CKD patients have calcification of the media in coronary arteries and even heart valves that appear to be orders of magnitude greater than that in patients without renal disease. The magnitude of the calcification is proportional to age and hyperphosphatemia and is also associated with low PTH levels and low bone turnover. It is possible that in patients with advanced kidney disease, ingested calcium cannot be deposited in bones with low turnover and, therefore, is deposited at extraosseous sites, such as the vascular bed and soft tissues. It is interesting in this regard that there is also an association between osteoporosis and vascular calcification in the general population. Finally, there is recent evidence indicating that hyperphosphatemia can induce a change in gene expression in vascular cells to an osteoblast-like profile, leading to vascular calcification and even ossification.

Other complications of abnormal mineral metabolism

Calciphylaxis (calcific uremic arteriolopathy) is a devastating condition seen almost exclusively in patients with advanced CKD. It is heralded by livedo reticularis and advances to patches of ischemic necrosis, especially on the legs, thighs, abdomen, and breasts (Fig. 280-3). Pathologically, there is evidence of vascular occlusion in association with extensive vascular and soft tissue calcification. It appears that this condition is increasing in incidence. Originally it was ascribed to severe abnormalities in calcium and phosphorus control in dialysis patients, usually associated with advanced hyperparathyroidism. However, more recently, calciphylaxis has been seen with increasing frequency in the absence of severe hyperparathyroidism. Other etiologies have been suggested, including the increased use of oral calcium as a phosphate binder. Warfarin is commonly used in hemodialysis patients, and one of the effects of warfarin therapy is to decrease the vitamin K–dependent regeneration of matrix GLA protein. This latter protein is important in preventing vascular calcification. Thus, warfarin treatment is considered a risk factor for calciphylaxis, and if a patient develops this syndrome, this medication should be discontinued and replaced with alternative forms of anticoagulation.

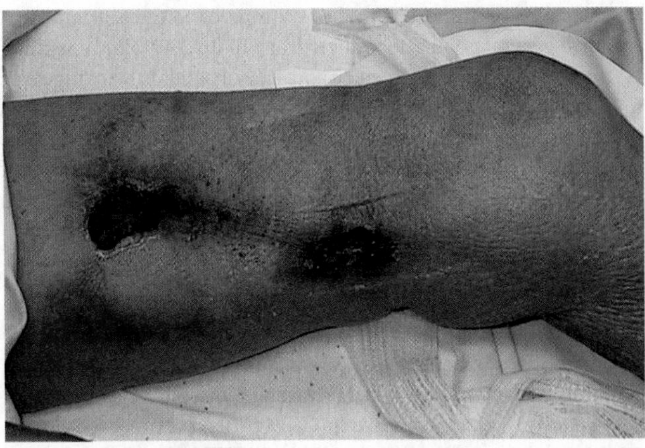

Figure 280-3 Calciphylaxis. This peritoneal dialysis patient was on chronic warfarin therapy for prophylactic anticoagulation for a mechanical heart valve. She slept with the dialysis catheter pressed between her legs. A small abrasion was followed by progressive skin necrosis along the catheter tract on her inner thighs. Despite treatment with hyperbaric oxygen, intravenous thiosulfate, and discontinuation of warfarin, she succumbed to systemic complications of the necrotic process.

TREATMENT Disorders of Calcium and Phosphate Metabolism

The optimal management of secondary hyperparathyroidism and osteitis fibrosa is prevention. Once the parathyroid gland mass is very large, it is difficult to control the disease. Careful attention should be paid to the plasma phosphate concentration in CKD patients, who should be counseled on a low-phosphate diet as well as the appropriate use of phosphate-binding agents. These are agents that are taken with meals and complex the dietary phosphate to limit its GI absorption. Examples of phosphate binders are calcium acetate and calcium carbonate. A major side effect of calcium-based phosphate binders is total-body calcium accumulation and hypercalcemia, especially in patients with low-turnover bone disease. Sevelamer and lanthanum are non-calcium-containing polymers that also function as phosphate binders; they do not predispose CKD patients to hypercalcemia and may attenuate calcium deposition in the vascular bed.

Calcitriol exerts a direct suppressive effect on PTH secretion and also indirectly suppresses PTH secretion by raising the concentration of ionized calcium. However, calcitriol therapy may result in hypercalcemia and/or hyperphosphatemia through increased GI absorption of these minerals. Certain analogues of calcitriol are available (e.g., paricalcitol) that suppress PTH secretion with less attendant hypercalcemia.

Recognition of the role of the extracellular calcium-sensing receptor has led to the development of calcimimetic agents that enhance the sensitivity of the parathyroid cell to the suppressive effect of calcium. This class of drug, which includes cinacalcet, produces a dose-dependent reduction in PTH and plasma calcium concentration in some patients.

Current KDOQI guidelines recommend a target PTH level between 150 and 300 pg/mL, recognizing that very low PTH levels are associated with adynamic bone disease and possible consequences of fracture and ectopic calcification.

CARDIOVASCULAR ABNORMALITIES

Cardiovascular disease is the leading cause of morbidity and mortality in patients at every stage of CKD. The incremental risk of cardiovascular disease in those with CKD compared to the age- and sex-matched general population ranges from 10- to 200-fold, depending on the stage of CKD. Between 30 and 45% of patients reaching stage 5 CKD already have advanced cardiovascular complications. As a result, most patients with CKD succumb to cardiovascular disease (Fig. 280-4) before ever reaching stage 5 CKD. Thus, the focus of patient care in earlier CKD stages should be directed to prevention of cardiovascular complications.

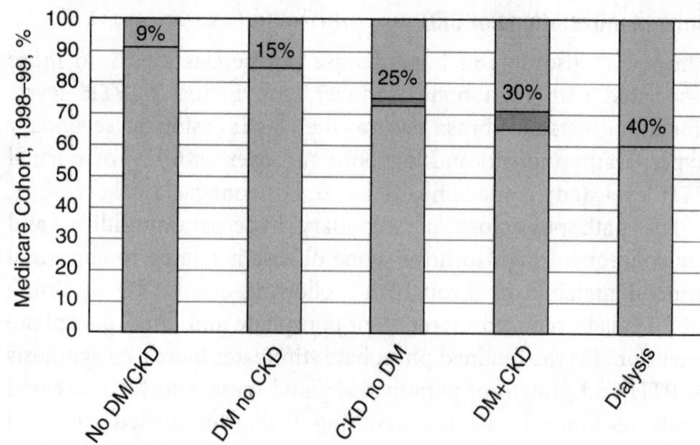

Figure 280-4 U.S. Renal Data System showing increased likelihood of dying rather than starting dialysis or reaching stage 5 chronic kidney disease (CKD). 1, Death; 2, ESRD/D; 3, event-free. DM; diabetes mellitus. *(Adapted from RN Foley et al: J Am Soc Nephrol 16:489-95, 2005.)*

Ischemic vascular disease

The presence of any stage of CKD is a major risk factor for ischemic cardiovascular disease, including occlusive coronary, cerebrovascular, and peripheral vascular disease. The increased prevalence of vascular disease in CKD patients derives from both traditional ("classic") and nontraditional (CKD-related) risk factors. Traditional risk factors include hypertension, hypervolemia, dyslipidemia, sympathetic overactivity, and hyperhomocysteinemia. The CKD-related risk factors comprise anemia, hyperphosphatemia, hyperparathyroidism, sleep apnea, and generalized inflammation. The inflammatory state associated with a reduction in kidney function is reflected in increased circulating acute-phase reactants, such as inflammatory cytokines and C-reactive protein, with a corresponding fall in the "negative acute-phase reactants," such as serum albumin and fetuin. The inflammatory state appears to accelerate vascular occlusive disease, and low levels of fetuin may permit more rapid vascular calcification, especially in the face of hyperphosphatemia. Other abnormalities seen in CKD may augment myocardial ischemia, including left ventricular hypertrophy and microvascular disease. Coronary reserve, defined as the increase in coronary blood flow in response to greater demand, is also attenuated. There is diminished availability of nitric oxide because of increased concentration of asymmetric dimethyl-1-arginine and increased scavenging by reactive oxygen species. In addition, hemodialysis, with its attendant episodes of hypotension and hypovolemia, may further aggravate coronary ischemia. Interestingly, however, the largest increment in cardiovascular mortality rate in dialysis patients is not necessarily directly associated with documented acute myocardial infarction but, instead, presents with congestive heart failure and all of its manifestations, including sudden death.

Cardiac troponin levels are frequently elevated in CKD without evidence of acute ischemia. The elevation complicates the diagnosis of acute myocardial infarction in this population. Serial measurements may be needed, and if the level is unchanged, it is possible that there is no acute myocardial ischemia. On the other hand, an increase upon subsequent testing suggests cardiac injury. Therefore, the trend in levels over the hours after presentation may be more informative than a single, elevated level. Interestingly, consistently elevated levels are an independent prognostic factor for adverse cardiovascular events in this population.

Heart failure

Abnormal cardiac function secondary to myocardial ischemia, left ventricular hypertrophy, and frank cardiomyopathy, in combination with the salt and water retention that can be seen with CKD, often results in heart failure or even episodes of pulmonary edema. Heart failure can be a consequence of diastolic or systolic dysfunction, or both. A form of "low-pressure" pulmonary edema can also occur in advanced CKD, manifesting as shortness of breath and a "bat wing" distribution of alveolar edema fluid on the chest x-ray. This finding can occur even in the absence of ECFV overload and is associated with normal or mildly elevated pulmonary capillary wedge pressure. This process has been ascribed to increased permeability of alveolar capillary membranes as a manifestation of the uremic state, and it responds to dialysis. Other CKD-related risk factors, including anemia and sleep apnea, may contribute to the risk of heart failure.

Hypertension and left ventricular hypertrophy

Hypertension is one of the most common complications of CKD. It usually develops early during the course of CKD and is associated with adverse outcomes, including the development of ventricular hypertrophy and a more rapid loss of renal function. Many studies have shown a relationship between the level of blood pressure and the rate of progression of diabetic and non-diabetic kidney disease. Left ventricular hypertrophy and dilated cardiomyopathy are among the strongest risk factors for cardiovascular morbidity and mortality in patients with CKD and are thought to be related primarily, but not exclusively, to prolonged hypertension and ECFV overload. In addition, anemia and the placement of an arteriovenous fistula for hemodialysis can generate a high cardiac output state and consequent heart failure.

The absence of hypertension may signify the presence of a salt-wasting form of renal disease, the effect of antihypertensive therapy, or volume depletion or may signify poor left ventricular function. Indeed, in epidemiologic studies of dialysis patients, low blood pressure actually carries a worse prognosis than does high blood pressure. This mechanism, in part, accounts for the "reverse causation" seen in dialysis patients, wherein the presence of traditional risk factors, such as hypertension, hyperlipidemia, and obesity, appear to portend a better prognosis. Importantly, these observations derive from cross-sectional studies of late-stage CKD patients and should not be interpreted to discourage appropriate management of these risk factors in CKD patients, especially at early stages. In contrast to the general population, it is possible that in late-stage CKD, low blood pressure, reduced body mass index, and hypolipidemia indicate the presence of an advanced malnutrition-inflammation state, with poor prognosis.

The use of exogenous erythropoiesis-stimulating agents can increase blood pressure and the requirement for antihypertensive drugs. Chronic ECFV overload is also a contributor to hypertension, and improvement in blood pressure can often be seen with the use of dietary sodium restriction, diuretics, and fluid removal with dialysis. Nevertheless, because of activation of the renin-angiotensin-aldosterone axis and other disturbances in the balance of vasoconstrictors and vasodilators, some patients remain hypertensive despite careful attention to ECFV status.

TREATMENT Cardiovascular Abnormalities

MANAGEMENT OF HYPERTENSION There are two overall goals of therapy for hypertension in these patients: to slow the progression of the kidney disease itself, and to prevent the extrarenal complications of high blood pressure, such as cardiovascular disease and stroke. In all patients with CKD, blood pressure should be controlled to levels recommended by national guideline panels. In CKD patients with diabetes or proteinuria >1 g per 24 h, blood pressure should be reduced to 125/75, if achievable without prohibitive adverse effects. Salt restriction should be the first line of therapy. When volume management alone is not sufficient, the choice of antihypertensive agent is similar to that in the general population. The ACE inhibitors and ARBs slow the rate of decline of kidney function, but occasionally can precipitate an episode of acute kidney injury, especially when used in patients with ischemic renovascular disease. The use of ACE inhibitors and ARBs may also be complicated by the development of hyperkalemia. Often the concomitant use of a kaliuretic diuretic, such as metolazone, can improve potassium excretion in addition to improving blood pressure control. Potassium-sparing diuretics should be used with caution or avoided altogether in most patients. Indeed, increased usage of spironolactone for the management of heart failure has resulted in an increase in serious hyperkalemic events in patients with reduced kidney function.

MANAGEMENT OF CARDIOVASCULAR DISEASE There are many strategies available to treat the traditional and nontraditional risk factors in CKD patients. While these have been proved effective in the general population, there is little evidence for their benefit in patients with advanced CKD, especially those on dialysis. Certainly hypertension, elevated serum levels of homocysteine, and dyslipidemia promote atherosclerotic disease and are treatable complications of CKD. Renal disease complicated by nephrotic syndrome is associated with a very atherogenic lipid profile and hypercoagulability, which increases the risk of occlusive vascular disease. Since diabetes mellitus and hypertension are the two most frequent causes of advanced CKD, it is not surprising that cardiovascular disease is the most frequent cause of death in dialysis patients. The role of "inflammation" may be quantitatively more important in patients with kidney disease, and the treatment of more traditional risk factors may result in only modest success. However, modulation of traditional risk factors may be the only weapon in the therapeutic armamentarium for these patients until the nature of inflammation in CKD and its treatment are better understood.

Lifestyle changes, including regular exercise, should be advocated but are not often implemented. Hyperlipidemia in patients with CKD should be managed according to national guidelines. If dietary measures are not sufficient, preferred lipid-lowering medications, such as statins, should be used. Again, the use of these agents has not been of proven benefit for patients with advanced CKD.

Pericardial disease

Chest pain with respiratory accentuation, accompanied by a friction rub, is diagnostic of pericarditis. Classic electrocardiographic abnormalities include PR-interval depression and diffuse ST-segment elevation. Pericarditis can be accompanied by pericardial effusion that is seen on echocardiography and can rarely lead to tamponade. However, the pericardial effusion can be asymptomatic, and pericarditis can be seen without significant effusion.

Pericarditis is observed in advanced uremia, and with the advent of timely initiation of dialysis, is not as common as it once was. It is now more often observed in underdialyzed, nonadherent patients than in those starting dialysis.

TREATMENT Pericardial Disease

Uremic pericarditis is an absolute indication for the urgent initiation of dialysis or for intensification of the dialysis prescription in those already receiving dialysis. Because of the propensity to hemorrhage in pericardial fluid, hemodialysis should be performed without heparin. A pericardial drainage procedure should be considered in patients with recurrent pericardial effusion, especially with echocardiographic signs of impending tamponade. Nonuremic causes of pericarditis and effusion include viral, malignant, tuberculous, and autoimmune etiologies. It may also be seen after myocardial infarction and as a complication of treatment with the antihypertensive drug minoxidil.

TABLE 280-5 Causes of Anemia in CKD

Relative deficiency of erythropoietin
Diminished red blood cell survival
Bleeding diathesis
Iron deficiency
Hyperparathyroidism/bone marrow fibrosis
"Chronic inflammation"
Folate or vitamin B_{12} deficiency
Hemoglobinopathy
Comorbid conditions: hypo/hyperthyroidism, pregnancy, HIV-associated disease, autoimmune disease, immunosuppressive drugs

HEMATOLOGIC ABNORMALITIES

Anemia

A normocytic, normochromic anemia is observed as early as stage 3 CKD and is almost universal by stage 4. The primary cause in patients with CKD is insufficient production of erythropoietin (EPO) by the diseased kidneys. Additional factors include iron deficiency, acute and chronic inflammation with impaired iron utilization ("anemia of chronic disease"), severe hyperparathyroidism with consequent bone marrow fibrosis, and shortened red cell survival in the uremic environment. In addition, comorbid conditions such as hemoglobinopathy can worsen the anemia (Table 280-5).

The anemia of CKD is associated with a number of adverse pathophysiologic consequences, including decreased tissue oxygen delivery and utilization, increased cardiac output, ventricular dilation, and ventricular hypertrophy. Clinical manifestations include fatigue and diminished exercise tolerance, angina, heart failure, decreased cognition and mental acuity, and impaired host defense against infection. In addition, anemia may play a role in growth retardation in children with CKD. While many studies in CKD patients have found that anemia and resistance to exogenous EPO are associated with a poor prognosis, the relative contribution to a poor outcome of the low hematocrit itself, versus inflammation as a cause of the anemia, remains unclear.

TREATMENT Anemia

The availability of recombinant human EPO and modified EPO products, such as darbepoetin-alpha, has been one of the most significant advances in the care of renal patients since the introduction of dialysis and renal transplantation. The routine use of these products has obviated the need for regular blood transfusions in severely anemic CKD patients, thus dramatically reducing the incidence of transfusion-associated infections and iron overload. Frequent blood transfusions in dialysis patients also leads to the development of allo-antibodies that could sensitize the patient to donor kidney antigens and make renal transplantation more problematic.

Adequate bone marrow iron stores should be available before treatment with EPO is initiated. Iron supplementation is usually essential to ensure an optimal response to EPO in patients with CKD because the demand for iron by the marrow frequently exceeds the amount of iron that is immediately available for erythropoiesis (measured by percent transferrin saturation), as well as the amount in iron stores (measured by serum ferritin). For the CKD patient not yet on dialysis or the patient treated with peritoneal dialysis, oral iron supplementation should be attempted. If there is GI intolerance, the patient may have to undergo IV iron infusion. For patients on hemodialysis, IV iron can be administered during dialysis. In addition to iron, an adequate supply of other major substrates and cofactors for red cell production must be ensured, including vitamin B_{12} and folate. Anemia resistant to recommended doses of EPO in the face of adequate iron stores may be due to some combination of the following: acute or chronic inflammation, inadequate dialysis, severe hyperparathyroidism, chronic blood loss or hemolysis, chronic infection, or malignancy. Patients with a hemoglobinopathy, such as sickle cell disease or thalassemia, will usually not respond normally to exogenous EPO; however, an increase in hemoglobin concentration is still seen in many of these patients. Blood transfusions increase the risk of hepatitis, iron overload, and transplant sensitization; they should be avoided unless the anemia fails to respond to EPO and the patient is symptomatic.

At least three randomized, controlled trials of erythropoietin-stimulating agents in CKD have failed to show an improvement in cardiovascular outcomes with this therapy. Indeed, there has been an indication that the use of EPO in CKD may be associated with an increased risk of stroke in those with type 2 diabetes, an increase in thromboembolic events, and perhaps a faster progression to the need for dialysis. Therefore, any benefit in terms of improvement of anemic symptoms needs to be balanced against the potential cardiovascular risk of EPO therapy in CKD. While further studies are needed, it is quite clear that complete normalization of the hemoglobin concentration has not been demonstrated to be of incremental benefit to CKD patients. Current practice is to target a hemoglobin concentration of 100–115 g/L.

Abnormal hemostasis

Patients with later stages of CKD may have a prolonged bleeding time, decreased activity of platelet factor III, abnormal platelet aggregation and adhesiveness, and impaired prothrombin consumption. Clinical manifestations include an increased tendency to bleeding and bruising, prolonged bleeding from surgical incisions, menorrhagia, and spontaneous GI bleeding. Interestingly, CKD patients also have a greater susceptibility to thromboembolism, especially if they have renal disease that includes nephrotic-range proteinuria. The latter condition results in hypoalbuminemia and renal loss of anticoagulant factors, which can lead to a thrombophilic state.

TREATMENT Abnormal Hemostasis

Abnormal bleeding time and coagulopathy in patients with renal failure may be reversed temporarily with desmopressin (DDAVP), cryoprecipitate, IV conjugated estrogens, blood transfusions, and EPO therapy. Optimal dialysis will usually correct a prolonged bleeding time.

Given the coexistence of bleeding disorders and a propensity to thrombosis that is unique in the CKD patient, decisions about anticoagulation that have a favorable risk-benefit profile in the general population may not be applicable to the patient with advanced CKD. One example is warfarin anticoagulation for atrial fibrillation: the decision to anticoagulate should be made on an individual basis in the CKD patient, as there appears to be a greater risk of bleeding complications.

Certain anticoagulants, such as fractionated low-molecular-weight heparin, may need to be avoided or dose adjusted in these patients, with monitoring of factor Xa activity where available. It is often more prudent to use conventional high-molecular-weight heparin, titrated to the measured partial thromboplastin time, in hospitalized patients requiring an alternative to warfarin anticoagulation.

NEUROMUSCULAR ABNORMALITIES

Central nervous system (CNS), peripheral, and autonomic neuropathy as well as abnormalities in muscle structure and function are all well-recognized complications of CKD. Retained nitrogenous metabolites and middle molecules, including PTH, contribute to the pathophysiology of neuromuscular abnormalities. Subtle clinical manifestations of uremic neuromuscular disease usually become evident at stage 3 CKD. Early manifestations of CNS complications include mild disturbances in memory and concentration and sleep disturbance. Neuromuscular irritability, including hiccups, cramps, and fasciculations or twitching of muscles, becomes evident at later stages. In advanced untreated kidney failure, asterixis, myoclonus, seizures, and coma can be seen.

Peripheral neuropathy usually becomes clinically evident after the patient reaches stage 4 CKD, although electrophysiologic and histologic evidence occurs earlier. Initially, sensory nerves are involved more than motor, lower extremities more than upper, and distal parts of the extremities more than proximal. The "restless leg syndrome" is characterized by ill-defined sensations of sometimes debilitating discomfort in the legs and feet relieved by frequent leg movement. If dialysis is not instituted soon after onset of sensory abnormalities, motor involvement follows, including muscle weakness. Evidence of peripheral neuropathy without another cause (e.g., diabetes mellitus) is a firm indication for starting renal replacement therapy. Many of the complications described above will resolve with dialysis, although subtle nonspecific abnormalities may persist. Successful renal transplantation may reverse residual neurologic changes.

GASTROINTESTINAL AND NUTRITIONAL ABNORMALITIES

Uremic fetor, a urine-like odor on the breath, derives from the breakdown of urea to ammonia in saliva and is often associated with an unpleasant metallic taste (dysgeusia). Gastritis, peptic disease, and mucosal ulcerations at any level of the GI tract occur in uremic patients and can lead to abdominal pain, nausea, vomiting, and GI bleeding. These patients are also prone to constipation, which can be worsened by the administration of calcium and iron supplements. The retention of uremic toxins also leads to anorexia, nausea, and vomiting.

Protein restriction may be useful to decrease nausea and vomiting; however, it may put the patient at risk for malnutrition and should be carried out, if possible, in consultation with a registered dietitian specializing in the management of CKD patients. Protein-energy malnutrition, a consequence of low protein and caloric intake, is common in advanced CKD and is often an indication for initiation of renal replacement therapy. In addition to diminished intake, these patients are resistant to the anabolic actions of insulin and other hormones and growth factors. Metabolic acidosis and the activation of inflammatory cytokines can promote protein catabolism. Assessment for protein-energy malnutrition should begin at stage 3 CKD. A number of indices are useful in this assessment and include dietary history, including food diary and subjective global assessment; edema-free body weight; and measurement of urinary protein nitrogen appearance. Dual-energy x-ray absorptiometry is now widely used to estimate lean body mass versus ECFV. Adjunctive tools include clinical signs, such as skin-fold thickness, mid-arm muscle circumference, and additional laboratory tests such as serum pre-albumin and cholesterol levels. Nutritional guidelines for patients with CKD are summarized in the "Treatment" section below.

ENDOCRINE-METABOLIC DISTURBANCES

Glucose metabolism is impaired in CKD, as evidenced by a slowing of the rate at which blood glucose levels decline after a glucose load. However, fasting blood glucose is usually normal or only slightly elevated, and the mild glucose intolerance does not require specific therapy. Because the kidney contributes to insulin removal from the circulation, plasma levels of insulin are slightly to moderately elevated in most uremic patients, both in the fasting and postprandial states. Because of this diminished renal degradation of insulin, patients on insulin therapy may need progressive reduction in dose as their renal function worsens. Many hypoglycemic agents require dose reduction in renal failure, and some, such as metformin, are contraindicated when the GFR is less than half of normal.

In women with CKD, estrogen levels are low, and menstrual abnormalities and inability to carry pregnancies to term are common. When the GFR has declined to ~40 mL/min, pregnancy is associated with a high rate of spontaneous abortion, with only ~20% of pregnancies leading to live births, and pregnancy may hasten the progression of the kidney disease itself. Women with CKD who are contemplating pregnancy should consult first with a nephrologist in conjunction with an obstetrician specializing in high-risk pregnancy. Men with CKD have reduced plasma testosterone levels, and sexual dysfunction and oligospermia may supervene. Sexual maturation may be delayed or impaired in adolescent children with CKD, even among those treated with dialysis. Many of these abnormalities improve or reverse with intensive dialysis or most importantly with successful renal transplantation.

DERMATOLOGIC ABNORMALITIES

Abnormalities of the skin are prevalent in progressive CKD. Pruritus is quite common and one of the most vexing manifestations of the uremic state. In advanced CKD, even on dialysis, patients may become more pigmented, and this is felt to reflect the deposition of retained pigmented metabolites, or *urochromes*. Although many of the cutaneous abnormalities improve with dialysis, pruritus is often tenacious. The first lines of management are to rule out unrelated skin disorders, such as scabies, and to treat hyperphosphatemia, which can cause itch. EPO therapy was initially reported to improve uremic pruritus, although that is not always the case. Local moisturizers, mild topical glucocorticoids, oral antihistamines, and ultraviolet radiation have been reported to be helpful.

A skin condition unique to CKD patients called *nephrogenic fibrosing dermopathy* consists of progressive subcutaneous induration, especially on the arms and legs. The condition is similar to scleromyxedema and is seen in patients with CKD who have been exposed to the magnetic resonance contrast agent gadolinium. Current recommendations are that patients with CKD stage 2 (GFR 30–59 mL/min) should minimize exposure to gadolinium, and those with CKD stages 3–5 (GFR < 30 mL/min) should avoid the use of gadolinium agents unless it is medically necessary. Concomitant liver disease appears to be a risk factor. However, no patient should be denied an imaging investigation that is critical to clinical management, and under such circumstances, rapid removal of gadolinium by hemodialysis (even in patients not yet receiving renal replacement therapy) shortly after the imaging procedure may mitigate this sometimes devastating complication

EVALUATION AND MANAGEMENT OF PATIENTS WITH CKD

INITIAL APPROACH

History and physical examination

Symptoms and overt signs of kidney disease are often subtle or absent until renal failure supervenes. Thus, the diagnosis of kidney disease often surprises patients and may be a cause of skepticism and denial. Particular aspects of the history that are germane to renal disease include a history of hypertension (which can cause CKD or more commonly be a consequence of CKD), diabetes mellitus, abnormal urinalyses, and problems with pregnancy such as preeclampsia or early pregnancy loss. A careful drug history should be elicited: patients may not volunteer use of analgesics, for example. Other drugs to consider include nonsteroidal anti-inflammatory agents, gold, penicillamine, antimicrobials, chemotherapeutic agents, antiretroviral agents, proton pump inhibitors, phosphate-containing bowel cathartics, and lithium, as well as prior exposure to medical imaging radiocontrast agents. In evaluating the uremic syndrome, questions about appetite, weight loss, nausea, hiccups, peripheral edema, muscle cramps, pruritus, and restless legs are especially helpful. A careful family history of kidney disease, together with assessment of manifestations in other organ systems such as auditory, visual, integumentary and others, may lead to the diagnosis of a heritable form of CKD (e.g., Alport or Fabry syndrome, cystinuria, among others) or shared environmental exposure to nephrotoxic agents (e.g., heavy metals, aristolochic acid). It should be noted that clustering of CKD, sometimes of different etiologies, is often observed within families.

The physical examination should focus on blood pressure and target organ damage from hypertension. Thus, funduscopy and precordial examination (left ventricular heave, a fourth heart sound) should be carried out. Funduscopy is important in the diabetic patient, as it may show evidence of diabetic retinopathy, which is associated with nephropathy. Other physical examination manifestations of CKD include edema and sensory polyneuropathy. The finding of asterixis or a pericardial friction rub not attributable to other causes usually signifies the presence of the uremic syndrome.

Laboratory investigation

Laboratory studies should focus on a search for clues to an underlying causative or aggravating disease process and on the degree of renal damage and its consequences. Serum and urine protein electrophoresis, looking for multiple myeloma, should be obtained in all patients >35 years with unexplained CKD, especially if there is associated anemia and elevated, or even inappropriately normal, serum calcium concentration in the face of renal insufficiency. In the presence of glomerulonephritis, autoimmune diseases such as lupus and underlying infectious etiologies such as hepatitis B and C and HIV should be assessed. Serial measurements of renal function should be obtained to determine the pace of renal deterioration and ensure that the disease is truly chronic rather than acute or subacute and hence potentially reversible. Serum concentrations of calcium, phosphorus, vitamin D, and PTH should be measured to evaluate metabolic bone disease. Hemoglobin concentration, iron, B_{12}, and folate should also be evaluated. A 24-h urine collection may be helpful, as protein excretion >300 mg may be an indication for therapy with ACE inhibitors or ARBs.

Imaging studies

The most useful imaging study is a renal ultrasound, which can verify the presence of two kidneys, determine if they are symmetric, provide an estimate of kidney size, and rule out renal masses and evidence of obstruction. Since it takes time for kidneys to shrink as a result of chronic disease, the finding of bilaterally small kidneys supports the diagnosis of CKD of long-standing duration, with an irreversible component of scarring. If the kidney size is normal, it is possible that the renal disease is acute or subacute. The exceptions are diabetic nephropathy (where kidney size is increased at the onset of diabetic nephropathy before CKD with loss of GFR supervenes), amyloidosis, and HIV nephropathy, where kidney size may be normal in the face of CKD. Polycystic kidney disease that has reached some degree of renal failure will almost always present with enlarged kidneys with multiple cysts (Chap. 284). A discrepancy >1 cm in kidney length suggests either a unilateral developmental abnormality or disease process or renovascular disease with arterial insufficiency affecting one kidney more than the other. The diagnosis of renovascular disease can be undertaken with different techniques, including Doppler sonography, nuclear medicine studies, or CT or MRI studies. If there is a suspicion of reflux nephropathy (recurrent childhood urinary tract infection, asymmetric renal size with scars on the renal poles), a voiding cystogram may be indicated. However, in most cases by the time the patient has CKD, the reflux has resolved, and even if still present, repair does not improve renal function. Radiographic contrast imaging studies are not particularly helpful in the investigation of CKD. Intravenous or intraarterial dye should be avoided where possible in the CKD patient, especially with diabetic nephropathy, because of the risk of radiographic contrast dye–induced renal failure. When unavoidable, appropriate precautionary measures include avoidance of hypovolemia at the time of contrast exposure, minimization of the dye load, and choice of radiographic contrast preparations with the least nephrotoxic potential. Additional measures thought to attenuate contrast-induced worsening of renal function include judicious administration of sodium bicarbonate–containing solutions and *N*-acetyl-cysteine.

Renal biopsy

In the patient with bilaterally small kidneys, renal biopsy is not advised because (1) it is technically difficult and has a greater likelihood of causing bleeding and other adverse consequences, (2) there is usually so much scarring that the underlying disease may not be apparent, and (3) the window of opportunity to render disease-specific therapy has passed. Other contraindications to renal biopsy include uncontrolled hypertension, active urinary tract infection, bleeding diathesis (including ongoing anticoagulation), and severe obesity. Ultrasound-guided percutaneous biopsy is the favored approach, but a surgical or laparoscopic approach can be considered, especially in the patient with a single kidney where direct visualization and control of bleeding are crucial. In the CKD patient in whom a kidney biopsy is indicated (e.g., suspicion of a concomitant or superimposed active process such as interstitial nephritis or in the face of accelerated loss of GFR), the bleeding time should be measured, and, if increased, desmopressin should be administered immediately prior to the procedure.

A brief run of hemodialysis (without heparin) may also be considered prior to renal biopsy to normalize the bleeding time.

ESTABLISHING THE DIAGNOSIS AND ETIOLOGY OF CKD

The most important initial diagnostic step in the evaluation of a patient presenting with elevated serum creatinine is to distinguish newly diagnosed CKD from acute or subacute renal failure because the latter two conditions may respond to therapy specific to the disease. Previous measurements of serum creatinine concentration are particularly helpful in this regard. Normal values from recent months or even years suggest that the current extent of renal dysfunction could be more acute, and hence reversible, than might otherwise be appreciated. In contrast, elevated serum creatinine concentration in the past suggests that the renal disease represents the progression of a chronic process. Even if there is evidence of chronicity, there is the possibility of a superimposed acute process (e.g., ECFV depletion, urinary infection or obstruction, or nephrotoxin exposure) supervening on the chronic condition. If the history suggests multiple systemic manifestations of recent onset (e.g., fever, polyarthritis, and rash), it should be assumed that renal insufficiency is part of the acute process.

Some of the laboratory tests and imaging studies outlined above can be helpful. Evidence of metabolic bone disease with hyperphosphatemia, hypocalcemia, and elevated PTH and bone alkaline phosphatase levels suggests chronicity. Normochromic, normocytic anemia suggests that the process has been ongoing for some time.

The finding of bilaterally reduced kidney size (<8.5 cm in all but the smallest adults) favors CKD.

While renal biopsy can usually be performed in early CKD (stages 1–3), it is not always indicated. For example, in a patient with a history of type 1 diabetes mellitus for 15–20 years with retinopathy, nephrotic-range proteinuria, and absence of hematuria, the diagnosis of diabetic nephropathy is very likely and biopsy is usually not necessary. However, if there were some other finding not typical of diabetic nephropathy, such as hematuria or white blood cell casts, or absence of diabetic retinopathy, some other disease may be present and a biopsy may be indicated. Ischemic nephropathy is usually diagnosed clinically by the presence of long-standing hypertension, evidence of ischemic disease elsewhere (e.g., cardiac or peripheral vascular disease), and the finding of nonnephrotic proteinuria in the absence of urinary blood or red cell casts. It is important to consider progressive ischemic nephropathy because a small subset of these patients may respond to revascularization procedures, although this remains controversial.

In the absence of a clinical diagnosis, renal biopsy may be the only recourse to establish an etiology in early-stage CKD. However, as noted above, once the CKD is advanced and the kidneys are small and scarred, there is little utility and significant risk in attempting to arrive at a specific diagnosis.

TREATMENT Chronic Kidney Disease

Treatments aimed at specific causes of CKD are discussed elsewhere. Among others, these include optimized glucose control in diabetes mellitus, immunomodulatory agents for glomerulonephritis, and emerging specific therapies to retard cytogenesis in polycystic kidney disease. The optimal timing of both specific and nonspecific therapy is usually well before there has been a measurable decline in GFR and certainly before CKD is established (Table 280-6). It is helpful to sequentially measure and plot the rate of decline of GFR in all patients. Any acceleration in the rate of decline should prompt a search for superimposed acute or subacute processes that may be reversible. These include ECFV depletion, uncontrolled hypertension, urinary tract infection, new obstructive uropathy, exposure to nephrotoxic agents [such as nonsteroidal anti-inflammatory drugs (NSAIDs) or radiographic dye], and reactivation or flare of the original disease, such as lupus or vasculitis.

SLOWING THE PROGRESSION OF CKD There is variation in the rate of decline of GFR among patients with CKD. However, the following interventions should be considered in an effort to stabilize or slow the decline of renal function.

Reducing Intraglomerular Hypertension and Proteinuria Increased intraglomerular filtration pressures and glomerular hypertrophy develop as a response to loss of nephron number from different kidney diseases. This response is maladaptive, as it promotes the ongoing decline of kidney function even if the inciting process has been treated or spontaneously resolved. Control of systemic and glomerular hypertension is important in slowing the progression of CKD. Therefore, in addition to reduction of cardiovascular disease risk, antihypertensive therapy in patients with CKD also aims to slow the progression of nephron injury by reducing intraglomerular hypertension. Elevated blood pressure increases proteinuria by increasing its flux across the glomerular capillaries. Conversely, the renoprotective effect of antihypertensive medications is gauged through the consequent reduction of proteinuria. Thus, the more effective a given treatment is in lowering protein excretion, the greater the subsequent impact on protection from decline in GFR. This observation is the basis for the treatment guideline establishing 125/75 mmHg as the target blood pressure in proteinuric CKD patients.

ACE inhibitors and ARBs inhibit the angiotensin-induced vasoconstriction of the efferent arterioles of the glomerular microcirculation. This inhibition leads to a reduction in both intraglomerular filtration pressure and proteinuria. Several controlled studies have shown that these drugs are effective in slowing the progression of renal failure in patients with advanced stages of both diabetic and nondiabetic CKD. This slowing in progression of CKD is strongly associated with the proteinuria-lowering effect. In the absence of an anti-proteinuric response with either agent alone, combined treatment with both ACE inhibitors and ARBs has been considered. The combination is associated with a greater reduction in proteinuria compared to either agent alone. Insofar as reduction in proteinuria is a surrogate for improved renal outcome, the combination would appear to be advantageous. However, a recent randomized, controlled study found a greater incidence of acute renal failure and adverse cardiac events from such combination therapy. It is uncertain, therefore, whether the ACE plus ARB therapy can be advised routinely. Adverse effects from these agents include cough and angioedema with ACE inhibitors, anaphylaxis, and hyperkalemia with either class. A progressive increase in serum creatinine concentration with these agents may suggest the presence of renovascular disease within the large or small arteries. Development of these side effects may mandate the use of second-line antihypertensive agents instead of the ACE inhibitors or ARBs. Among the calcium channel blockers, diltiazem and verapamil may exhibit superior antiproteinuric and renoprotective effects compared to the dihydropyridines. At least two different categories of response can be considered: one in which progression is strongly associated with systemic and intraglomerular hypertension and proteinuria (e.g., diabetic nephropathy, glomerular diseases) and in which ACE inhibitors and ARBs are likely to be the first choice; and another in which proteinuria is mild or absent initially (e.g., adult polycystic kidney disease and other tubulointerstitial diseases), where the contribution of intraglomerular hypertension is less prominent, and other antihypertensive agents can be useful for control of systemic hypertension.

TABLE 280-6 Clinical Action Plan

Stage	Description	GFR, mL/min per 1.73 m^2	Action*
1	Kidney damage with normal or ↑ GFR	≥90	Diagnosis and treatment, treatment of comorbid conditions, slowing progression, CVD risk reduction
2	Kidney damage with mild ↓ GFR	60–89	Estimating progression
3	Moderate ↓ GFR	30–59	Evaluating and treating complications
4	Severe ↓ GFR	15–29	Preparation for kidney replacement therapy
5	Kidney failure	<15 (or dialysis)	Kidney replacement (if uremia present)

*Includes actions from preceding stages.

Abbreviations: CVD, cardiovascular disease; GFR, glomerular filtration rate.

Source: National Kidney Foundation: Am J Kidney Dis 39:S1, 2002.

SLOWING PROGRESSION OF DIABETIC RENAL DISEASE (See also Chap. 344) Diabetic nephropathy is now the leading cause of CKD requiring renal replacement therapy in many parts of the world, and its prevalence is increasing disproportionately in the developing world. Furthermore, the prognosis of diabetic patients on dialysis is poor, with survival comparable to many forms of cancer. Accordingly, it is mandatory to develop strategies whose aim is to prevent or slow the progression of diabetic nephropathy in these patients.

Control of Blood Glucose Excellent glycemic control reduces the risk of kidney disease and its progression in both type 1 and type 2 diabetes mellitus. It is recommended that plasma values for preprandial glucose be kept in the 5.0–7.2 mmol/L (90–130 mg/dL) range and hemoglobin A_{1C} should be < 7%. As the GFR decreases with progressive nephropathy, the use and dose of oral hypoglycemics needs to be reevaluated. For example, chlorpropamide may be associated with prolonged hypoglycemia in patients with decreased renal function; metformin can cause lactic acidosis in the patient with renal impairment and should be discontinued when the GFR is reduced; and the thiazolidinediones (e.g., rosiglitazone, pioglitazone, and others), may increase renal salt and water absorption and aggravate volume-overload states, and contribute to adverse cardiovascular events. Finally, as renal function declines, renal degradation of administered insulin will also decline, so that less insulin may be required for glycemic control.

Control of Blood Pressure and Proteinuria Hypertension is found in the majority of type 2 diabetic patients at diagnosis. This finding correlates with the presence of albuminuria and is a strong predictor of cardiovascular events and nephropathy. Microalbuminuria, the finding of albumin in the urine not detectable by the urine dipstick, precedes the decline in GFR and heralds renal and cardiovascular complications. Testing for microalbumin is recommended in all diabetic patients, at least annually. If the patient already has established proteinuria, then testing for microalbumin is not necessary. Antihypertensive treatment reduces albuminuria and diminishes its progression even in normotensive diabetic patients. In addition to treatment of hypertension in general, the use of ACE inhibitors and ARBs in particular is associated with additional renoprotection. These salutary effects are mediated by reducing intraglomerular pressure and inhibition of angiotensin-driven sclerosing pathways, in part through inhibition of TGF-β-mediated pathways. Recent studies have highlighted the benefit of renin-angiotensin axis blockade on the development of retinopathy in diabetic patients, but do not necessarily show a clear-cut renal benefit of intervention at the very earliest stages, prior to onset of overt proteinuria. In any case, as noted above, the combination of ACE inhibitors with ARBs is not recommended.

Protein Restriction While protein restriction has been advocated to reduce symptoms associated with uremia, it may also slow the rate of renal decline at earlier stages of renal disease. This concept is based on clinical and experimental evidence that protein-mediated hyperfiltration contributes to ongoing decline in renal function in many different forms of renal disease. A number of studies have shown that protein restriction may be effective in slowing the progression of CKD, especially proteinuric and diabetic renal diseases. However, the Modification of Diet in Renal Disease study was unable to demonstrate a robust benefit in delaying progression to advanced stages of CKD with dietary restriction of protein intake. Nonetheless, restriction of dietary protein intake has been recommended for CKD patients. KDOQI clinical practice guidelines include a daily protein intake of between 0.60 and 0.75 g/kg per day, depending upon patient adherence, comorbid disease, presence of proteinuria, and nutritional status. It is further advised that at least 50% of the protein intake be of high biologic value. As patients approach stage 5 CKD, spontaneous protein intake tends to decrease, and patients may enter a state of protein-energy malnutrition. In these circumstances, a protein intake of up to 0.90 g/kg per day might be recommended, again with an emphasis on proteins of high biologic value.

Sufficient energy intake is important to prevent protein-calorie malnutrition, and 35 kcal/kg is recommended. Monitoring of parameters of nutritional status must accompany the dietary intervention, using the parameters outlined above in the section on GI and nutritional abnormalities

MANAGING OTHER COMPLICATIONS OF CHRONIC KIDNEY DISEASE

Medication Dose Adjustment Although the loading dose of most drugs is not affected by CKD because no renal elimination is used in the calculation, the maintenance doses of many drugs will need to be adjusted. For those agents in which >70% excretion is by a nonrenal route, such as hepatic elimination, dose adjustment may not be needed. Some drugs that should be avoided include metformin, meperidine, and oral hypoglycemics that are eliminated by the kidney. NSAIDs should be avoided because of the risk of further worsening of kidney function. Many antibiotics, antihypertensives, and antiarrhythmics may require a reduction in dosage or change in the dose interval. Several online web-based databases for dose adjustment of medications according to stage of CKD or estimated GFR are available (e.g., *http://www.globalrph.com/renaldosing2.htm*). Nephrotoxic medical imaging radiocontrast agents and gadolinium should be avoided or used according to strict guidelines when medically necessary as described above.

Preparation for Renal Replacement Therapy (See also Chap. 282) Temporary relief of symptoms and signs of impending uremia, such as anorexia, nausea, vomiting, lassitude, and pruritus, may sometimes be achieved with protein restriction. However, this carries a significant risk of protein-energy malnutrition, and thus plans for more long-term management should be in place.

Maintenance dialysis and kidney transplantation has extended the lives of hundreds of thousands of patients with CKD worldwide. Clear indications for initiation of renal replacement therapy for patients with CKD include uremic pericarditis, encephalopathy, intractable muscle cramping, anorexia, and nausea not attributable to reversible causes such as peptic ulcer disease, evidence of malnutrition, and fluid and electrolyte abnormalities, principally hyperkalemia or ECF volume overload, that are refractory to other measures.

Recommendations for the optimal time for initiation of renal replacement therapy have been established by the National Kidney Foundation in their KDOQI Guidelines and are based on recent evidence demonstrating that delaying initiation of renal replacement therapy until patients are malnourished or have severe uremic complications leads to a worse prognosis on dialysis or with transplantation. Because of the interindividual variability in the severity of uremic symptoms and renal function, it is ill-advised to assign an arbitrary urea nitrogen or creatinine level to the need to start dialysis. Moreover, patients may become accustomed to chronic uremia and deny symptoms, only to find that they feel better with dialysis and realize in retrospect how poorly they were feeling before its initiation.

Previous studies suggested that starting dialysis before the onset of severe symptoms and signs of uremia were associated with prolongation of survival. This led to the concept of "healthy" start and is congruent with the philosophy that it is better to keep patients feeling well all along rather than allowing them to become ill with uremia before trying to return them to better health with dialysis or transplantation. Although recent studies have not confirmed a clear association of early-start dialysis with improved patient survival, there is still merit in this approach. On a practical level, advanced preparation may help to avoid problems with the dialysis process itself (e.g., a poorly functioning fistula for hemodialysis or malfunctioning peritoneal dialysis catheter) and thus preempt the morbidity associated with resorting to the insertion of temporary hemodialysis access with its attendant risks of sepsis, bleeding, and thrombosis.

Patient Education Social, psychological, and physical preparation for the transition to renal replacement therapy and the choice of the optimal initial modality are best accomplished with a gradual approach involving a multidisciplinary team. Along with conservative measures discussed in the sections above, it is important to prepare patients with an intensive educational program, explaining the likelihood and timing of initiation of renal replacement therapy and the various forms of therapy available. The more knowledgeable that patients are about hemodialysis (both in-center and home-based), peritoneal dialysis, and kidney transplantation, the easier and more appropriate will be their decisions. Patients who are provided with educational programs are more likely to choose home-based dialysis therapy. This approach is of societal benefit because home-based therapy is less expensive and is associated with improved quality of life. The educational programs should be commenced no later than stage 4 CKD so that the patient has sufficient time and cognitive function to learn the important concepts, to make informed choices, and implement preparatory measures for renal replacement therapy.

Exploration of social service support is also important. In those who may perform home dialysis or undergo preemptive renal transplantation, early education of family members for selection and preparation of a home dialysis helper, or a biologically or emotionally related potential living kidney donor, should occur long before the onset of symptomatic renal failure.

Kidney transplantation (Chap. 282) offers the best potential for complete rehabilitation, because dialysis replaces only a small fraction of the kidneys' filtration function and none of the other renal functions, including endocrine and anti-inflammatory effects. Generally, kidney transplantation follows a period of dialysis treatment, although preemptive kidney transplantation (usually from a living donor) can be carried out if it is certain that the renal failure is irreversible.

IMPLICATIONS FOR GLOBAL HEALTH

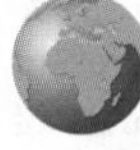

In distinction to the natural decline and successful eradication of many devastating infectious diseases, there is rapid growth in the prevalence of metabolic and vascular disease in developing countries. Diabetes mellitus is becoming increasingly prevalent in these countries, perhaps due in part to change in dietary habits, diminished physical activity, and weight gain. Therefore, it follows that there will be a proportionate increase in vascular and renal disease. Healthcare agencies must plan for improved screening for early detection, prevention, and treatment plans in these nations and must start considering options for improved availability of renal replacement therapies.

FURTHER READINGS

Abboud H, Heinrich WL: Clinical practice: Stage IV chronic kidney disease. N Engl J Med 362:56, 2010

Eknoyan G et al: The burden of kidney disease: Improving global outcomes. Kidney Int 66:1310, 2004

Go A et al: Chronic kidney disease and the risks of death, cardiovascular events, and hospitalization. N Engl J Med 351:1296, 2004

Golestaneh L et al: Uremic memory: The role of acute kidney injury in long-term outcomes. Kidney Int 76:813, 2009

Ketteler M et al: Calcification and cardiovascular health: New insights into an old phenomenon. Hypertension 47:1027, 2006

Kottgen A: Genome-wide association studies in nephrology. Am J Kidney Dis 56:743, 2010

Kronenberg F: Emerging risk factors and markers of chronic kidney disease progression. Nat Rev Nephrol 5:677, 2009

Levey AS et al: CKD: Common, harmful and treatable—World Kidney Day 2007. Am J Kidney Dis 2:401, 2007

Meyer TW et al: Uremia. N Engl J Med 357:1316, 2007

National Kidney Foundation: Kidney Disease Outcomes Quality Initiative Clinical Practice Guidelines for Nutrition in Chronic Renal Failure. Am J Kidney Dis 35 (suppl 2): S1, 2000

———: K/DOQI Clinical Practice Guidelines for Chronic Kidney Disease: Evaluation, classification and stratification. Am J Kidney Dis 39 (suppl 1), 2000

Sarnak M et al: Kidney disease as a risk factor for development of cardiovascular disease: A statement from the American Heart Association Councils on Kidney in Cardiovascular Disease, High Blood Pressure Research, Clinical Cardiology, and Epidemiology and Prevention. Circulation 108:2154, 2003

Strong K et al: Preventing chronic disease: How many lives can we save? Lancet 366:1578, 2005

Taal MW et al: Predicting initiation and progression of chronic kidney disease: Developing renal risk scores. Kidney Int 70:1694, 2006

Tonelli: M et al: Using proteinuria and estimated glomerular filtration rate to classify risk in patients with chronic kidney disease: A cohort study. Ann Intern Med 154:12, 2011

CHAPTER 281 Dialysis in the Treatment of Renal Failure

Kathleen D. Liu
Glenn M. Chertow

Dialysis may be required for the treatment of either acute or chronic kidney disease. The use of continuous renal replacement therapies (CRRTs) and slow low-efficiency dialysis (SLED) is specific to the management of acute renal failure and is discussed in Chap. 279. These modalities are performed continuously (CRRT) or over 6–12 hours per session (SLED), in contrast to the 3–4 hours of an intermittent hemodialysis session. Advantages and disadvantages of CRRT and SLED are discussed in Chap. 279.

Peritoneal dialysis is rarely used in developed countries for the treatment of acute renal failure because of the increased risk of infection and (as will be discussed in more detail below) less efficient clearance per unit of time. The focus of the majority of this chapter will be on the use of peritoneal and hemodialysis for end-stage renal disease (ESRD).

With the widespread availability of dialysis, the lives of hundreds of thousands of patients with ESRD have been prolonged. In the United States alone, there are now approximately 530,000 patients with ESRD, the vast majority of whom require dialysis. The incidence rate for ESRD is 350 cases per million population per year. The incidence of ESRD is disproportionately higher in African Americans (approximately 1000 per million population per year) as compared with white Americans (275 per million population per year). In the United States, the leading cause of ESRD is diabetes mellitus, currently accounting for nearly 55% of newly diagnosed cases of ESRD. Approximately one-third (33%) of patients have ESRD that has been attributed to hypertension, although it is unclear whether in these cases hypertension is the cause or a consequence of vascular disease or other unknown causes of kidney failure. Other prevalent causes of ESRD include glomerulonephritis, polycystic kidney disease, and obstructive uropathy.

Globally, mortality rates for patients with ESRD are lowest in Europe and Japan but very high in the developing world because of the limited availability of dialysis. In the United States, the mortality rate of patients on dialysis is approximately 18–20% per year, with a 5-year survival rate of approximately 30–35%. Deaths are due mainly to cardiovascular diseases and infections (approximately 50 and 15% of deaths, respectively). Older age, male sex, nonblack race, diabetes mellitus, malnutrition, and underlying heart disease are important predictors of death.

TREATMENT OPTIONS FOR ESRD PATIENTS

Commonly accepted criteria for initiating patients on maintenance dialysis include the presence of uremic symptoms, the presence of hyperkalemia unresponsive to conservative measures, persistent extracellular volume expansion despite diuretic therapy, acidosis refractory to medical therapy, a bleeding diathesis, and a creatinine clearance or estimated glomerular filtration rate (GFR) below 10 mL/min per 1.73 m^2 (see Chap. 280 for estimating equations). Timely referral to a nephrologist for advanced planning and creation of a dialysis access, education about ESRD treatment options, and management of the complications of advanced chronic kidney disease (CKD), including hypertension, anemia, acidosis, and secondary hyperparathyroidism, is advisable. Recent data have suggested that a sizable fraction of ESRD cases result following episodes of acute renal failure, particularly among persons with underlying CKD.

In ESRD, treatment options include hemodialysis (in center or at home); peritoneal dialysis, as either continuous ambulatory peritoneal dialysis (CAPD) or continuous cyclic peritoneal dialysis (CCPD); or transplantation (Chap. 282). Although there are significant geographic variations and differences in practice patterns, hemodialysis remains the most common therapeutic modality for ESRD (>90% of patients) in the United States. In contrast to hemodialysis, peritoneal dialysis is continuous, but much less efficient, in terms of solute clearance. While no large-scale clinical trials have been completed comparing outcomes among patients randomized to either hemodialysis or peritoneal dialysis, outcomes associated with both therapies are similar in most reports, and the decision of which modality to select is often based on personal preferences and quality-of-life considerations.

HEMODIALYSIS

Hemodialysis relies on the principles of solute diffusion across a semipermeable membrane. Movement of metabolic waste products takes place down a concentration gradient from the circulation into the dialysate. The rate of diffusive transport increases in response to several factors, including the magnitude of the concentration gradient, the membrane surface area, and the mass transfer coefficient of the membrane. The latter is a function of the porosity and thickness of the membrane, the size of the solute molecule, and the conditions of flow on the two sides of the membrane. According to laws of diffusion, the larger the molecule, the slower its rate of transfer across the membrane. A small molecule, such as urea (60 Da), undergoes substantial clearance, whereas a larger molecule, such as creatinine (113 Da), is cleared less efficiently. In addition to diffusive clearance, movement of waste products from the circulation into the dialysate may occur as a result of ultrafiltration. Convective clearance occurs because of solvent drag, with solutes being swept along with water across the semipermeable dialysis membrane.

THE DIALYZER

There are three essential components to hemodialysis: the dialyzer, the composition and delivery of the dialysate, and the blood delivery system (Fig. 281-1). The dialyzer is a plastic chamber with the ability to perfuse blood and dialysate compartments simultaneously at very high flow rates. The surface area of modern dialysis membranes in adult patients is usually in the range of 1.5–2.0 m^2. The hollow-fiber dialyzer is the most common in use in the United States. These dialyzers are composed of bundles of capillary tubes through which blood circulates while dialysate travels on the outside of the fiber bundle.

Recent advances have led to the development of many different types of membrane material. Broadly, there are four categories of dialysis membranes: cellulose, substituted cellulose, cellulosynthetic, and synthetic. Over the past three decades, there has been a gradual switch from cellulose-derived to synthetic membranes, because the latter are more "biocompatible." *Bioincompatibility* is generally defined as the ability of the membrane to activate the complement cascade. Cellulosic membranes are bioincompatible because of the presence of free hydroxyl groups on the membrane surface. In contrast, with the substituted cellulose membranes (e.g., cellulose acetate) or the cellulosynthetic membranes, the hydroxyl groups are chemically bound to either acetate or tertiary amino groups, resulting in limited complement activation. Synthetic membranes, such as polysulfone, polymethylmethacrylate, and polyacrylonitrile

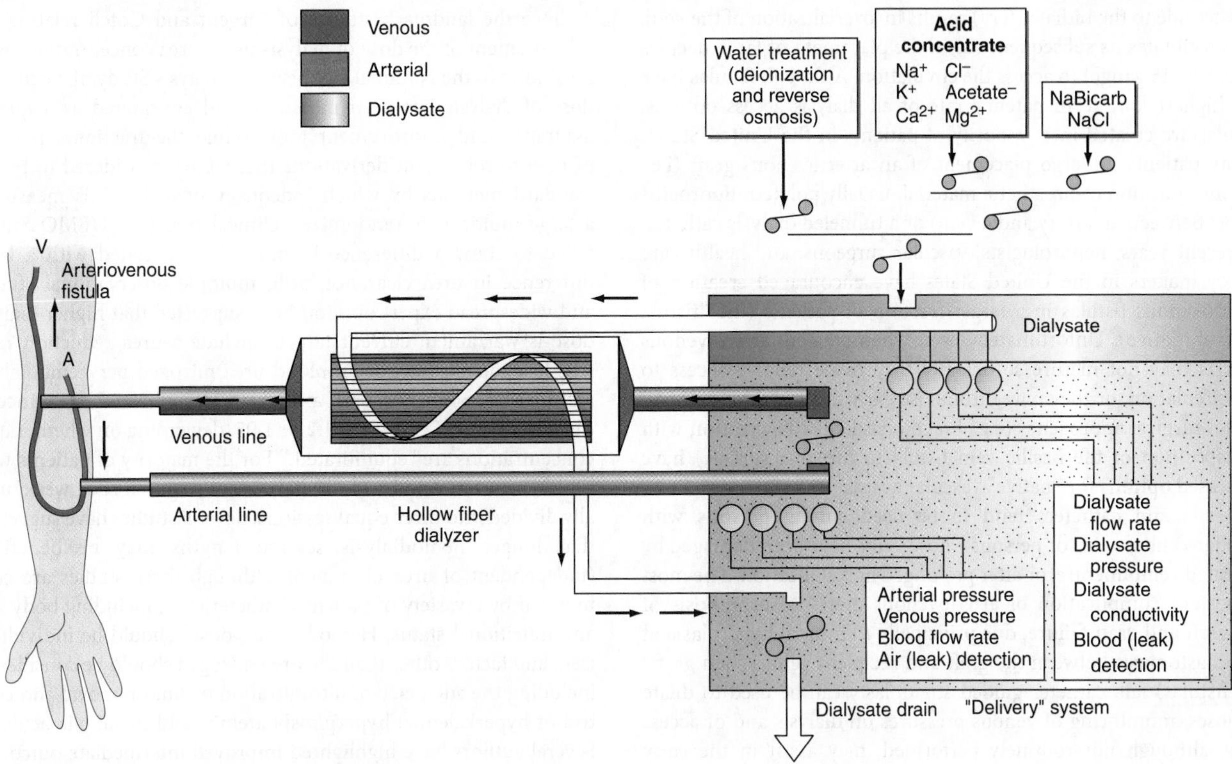

Figure 281-1 Schema for hemodialysis.

membranes, are even more biocompatible because of the absence of these hydroxyl groups. The majority of dialyzers now manufactured in the United States are derived from polysulfone or newer derivatives (polyarylethersulfone).

Reprocessing and reuse of hemodialyzers are often employed for patients on maintenance hemodialysis in the United States. However, as the manufacturing costs for disposable dialyzers have declined, more and more outpatient dialysis facilities are no longer reprocessing dialyzers. In most centers employing reuse, only the dialyzer unit is reprocessed and reused, whereas in the developing world blood lines are also frequently reused. The reprocessing procedure can be either manual or automated. It consists of the sequential rinsing of the blood and dialysate compartments with water, a chemical cleansing step with reverse ultrafiltration from the dialysate to the blood compartment, the testing of the patency of the dialyzer, and, finally, disinfection of the dialyzer. Formaldehyde, peracetic acid–hydrogen peroxide, glutaraldehyde, and bleach have all been used as reprocessing agents.

DIALYSATE

The potassium concentration of dialysate may be varied from 0 to 4 mmol/L depending on the predialysis serum potassium concentration. The usual dialysate calcium concentration in U.S. hemodialysis centers is 1.25 mmol/L (2.5 meq/L), although modification may be required in selected settings (e.g., higher dialysate calcium concentrations may be used in patients with hypocalcemia associated with secondary hyperparathyroidism or following parathyroidectomy). The usual dialysate sodium concentration is 140 mmol/L. Lower dialysate sodium concentrations are associated with a higher frequency of hypotension, cramping, nausea, vomiting, fatigue, and dizziness in some patients, although may attenuate thirst. In patients who frequently develop hypotension during their dialysis run, "sodium modeling" to counterbalance urea-related osmolar gradients is often employed. With sodium modeling, the dialysate sodium concentration is gradually lowered from the range of 145–155 mmol/L to isotonic concentrations (140 mmol/L) near the end of the dialysis treatment, typically declining either in steps or in a linear or exponential fashion. Higher dialysate sodium concentrations and sodium modeling may predispose patients to positive sodium balance; thus, these strategies to ameliorate intradialytic hypotension may be undesirable in hypertensive patients or in patients with large interdialytic weight gains. Because patients are exposed to approximately 120 L of water during each dialysis treatment, water used for the dialysate is subjected to filtration, softening, deionization, and, ultimately, reverse osmosis. During the reverse osmosis process, water is forced through a semipermeable membrane at very high pressure to remove microbiologic contaminants and >90% of dissolved ions.

BLOOD DELIVERY SYSTEM

The blood delivery system is composed of the extracorporeal circuit in the dialysis machine and the dialysis access. The dialysis machine consists of a blood pump, dialysis solution delivery system, and various safety monitors. The blood pump moves blood from the access site, through the dialyzer, and back to the patient. The blood flow rate may range from 250–500 mL/min, depending largely on the type and integrity of the vascular access. Negative hydrostatic pressure on the dialysate side can be manipulated to achieve desirable fluid removal or *ultrafiltration.* Dialysis membranes have different ultrafiltration coefficients (i.e., mL removed/min per mmHg) so that along with hydrostatic changes, fluid removal can be varied. The dialysis solution delivery system dilutes the concentrated dialysate with water and monitors the temperature, conductivity, and flow of dialysate.

DIALYSIS ACCESS

The fistula, graft, or catheter through which blood is obtained for hemodialysis is often referred to as a *dialysis access.* A native fistula created by the anastomosis of an artery to a vein (e.g., the Brescia-Cimino fistula, in which the cephalic vein is anastomosed end-to-side to the radial artery) results in arterialization of the vein. This facilitates its subsequent use in the placement of large needles (typically 15 gauge) to access the circulation. Although fistulas have the highest long-term patency rate of all dialysis access options, fistulas are created in a minority of patients in the United States. Many patients undergo placement of an arteriovenous graft (i.e., the interposition of prosthetic material, usually polytetrafluoroethylene, between an artery and a vein) or a tunneled dialysis catheter. In recent years, nephrologists, vascular surgeons, and health care policy makers in the United States have encouraged creation of arteriovenous fistulas in a larger fraction of patients (the "fistula first" initiative). Unfortunately, even when created, arteriovenous fistulas may not mature sufficiently to provide reliable access to the circulation, or they may thrombose early in their development. Novel surgical approaches (e.g., brachiobasilic fistula creation with transposition of the basilic vein fistula to the arm surface) have increased options for "native" vascular access.

Grafts and catheters tend to be used among persons with smaller-caliber veins or persons whose veins have been damaged by repeated venipuncture, or after prolonged hospitalization. The most important complication of arteriovenous grafts is thrombosis of the graft and graft failure, due principally to intimal hyperplasia at the anastomosis between the graft and recipient vein. When grafts (or fistulas) fail, catheter-guided angioplasty can be used to dilate stenoses; monitoring of venous pressures on dialysis and of access flow, although not routinely performed, may assist in the early recognition of impending vascular access failure. In addition to an increased rate of access failure, grafts and (in particular) catheters are associated with much higher rates of infection than fistulas.

Intravenous large-bore catheters are often used in patients with acute and chronic kidney disease. For persons on maintenance hemodialysis, tunneled catheters (either two separate catheters or a single catheter with two lumens) are often used when arteriovenous fistulas and grafts have failed or are not feasible due to anatomic considerations. These catheters are tunneled under the skin; the tunnel reduces bacterial translocation from the skin, resulting in a lower infection rate than with nontunneled temporary catheters. Most tunneled catheters are placed in the internal jugular veins; the external jugular, femoral, and subclavian veins may also be used.

Nephrologists, interventional radiologists, and vascular surgeons generally prefer to avoid placement of catheters into the subclavian veins; while flow rates are usually excellent, subclavian stenosis is a frequent complication and, if present, will likely prohibit permanent vascular access (i.e., a fistula or graft) in the ipsilateral extremity. Infection rates may be higher with femoral catheters. For patients with multiple vascular access complications and no other options for permanent vascular access, tunneled catheters may be the last "lifeline" for hemodialysis. Translumbar or transhepatic approaches into the inferior vena cava may be required if the superior vena cava or other central veins draining the upper extremities are stenosed or thrombosed.

GOALS OF DIALYSIS

The hemodialysis procedure is targeted at removing both low- and high-molecular-weight solutes. The procedure consists of pumping heparinized blood through the dialyzer at a flow rate of 300–500 mL/min, while dialysate flows in an opposite *counter-current* direction at 500–800 mL/min. The efficiency of dialysis is determined by blood and dialysate flow through the dialyzer as well as dialyzer characteristics (i.e., its efficiency in removing solute). The *dose* of dialysis, which is currently defined as a derivation of the fractional urea clearance during a single dialysis treatment, is further governed by patient size, residual kidney function, dietary protein intake, the degree of anabolism or catabolism, and the presence of comorbid conditions.

Since the landmark studies of Sargent and Gotch relating the measurement of the dose of dialysis using urea concentrations with morbidity in the National Cooperative Dialysis Study, the *delivered* dose of dialysis has been measured and considered as a quality assurance and improvement tool. While the fractional removal of urea nitrogen and derivations thereof are considered to be the standard methods by which "adequacy of dialysis" is measured, a large multicenter randomized clinical trial (the HEMO Study) failed to show a difference in mortality associated with a large difference in urea clearance. Still, multiple observational studies and widespread expert opinion have suggested that higher dialysis dose is warranted; current targets include a urea reduction ratio (the fractional reduction in blood urea nitrogen per hemodialysis session) of >65–70% and a body water–indexed clearance × time product (KT/V) above 1.2 or 1.05, depending on whether urea concentrations are "equilibrated." For the majority of patients with ESRD, between 9 and 12 h of dialysis are required each week, usually divided into three equal sessions. Several studies have suggested that longer hemodialysis session lengths may be beneficial (independent of urea clearance), although these studies are confounded by a variety of patient characteristics, including body size and nutritional status. Hemodialysis "dose" should be individualized, and factors other than the urea nitrogen should be considered, including the adequacy of ultrafiltration or fluid removal and control of hyperkalemia, hyperphosphatemia, and metabolic acidosis. Several authors have highlighted improved intermediate outcomes associated with more frequent hemodialysis (i.e., more than three times a week), although these studies are also confounded by multiple factors. A randomized clinical trial is currently under way to test whether more frequent dialysis results in differences in a variety of physiologic and functional markers.

COMPLICATIONS DURING HEMODIALYSIS

Hypotension is the most common acute complication of hemodialysis, particularly among patients with diabetes mellitus. Numerous factors appear to increase the risk of hypotension, including excessive ultrafiltration with inadequate compensatory vascular filling, impaired vasoactive or autonomic responses, osmolar shifts, overzealous use of antihypertensive agents, and reduced cardiac reserve. Patients with arteriovenous fistulas and grafts may develop high output cardiac failure due to shunting of blood through the dialysis access; on rare occasions, this may necessitate ligation of the fistula or graft. Because of the vasodilatory and cardiodepressive effects of acetate, its use as the buffer in dialysate was once a common cause of hypotension. Since the introduction of bicarbonate-containing dialysate, dialysis-associated hypotension has become less common. The management of hypotension during dialysis consists of discontinuing ultrafiltration, the administration of 100–250 mL of isotonic saline or 10 mL of 23% saturated hypertonic saline, or administration of salt-poor albumin. Hypotension during dialysis can frequently be prevented by careful evaluation of the dry weight and by ultrafiltration modeling, such that more fluid is removed at the beginning rather than the end of the dialysis procedure. Additional maneuvers include the performance of sequential ultrafiltration followed by dialysis, cooling of the dialysate during dialysis treatment; and avoiding heavy meals during dialysis. Midodrine, a selective α_1 adrenergic pressor agent, has been advocated by some practitioners, although there is insufficient evidence of its safety and efficacy to support its routine use.

Muscle cramps during dialysis are also a common complication of the procedure. The etiology of dialysis-associated cramps remains obscure. Changes in muscle perfusion because of excessively aggressive volume removal, particularly below the estimated dry weight, and the use of low-sodium–containing dialysate, have been proposed as precipitants of dialysis-associated cramps. Strategies that may be used to prevent cramps include reducing volume removal during dialysis, ultrafiltration profiling, and the use of higher concentrations of sodium in the dialysate or sodium modeling (see above).

Anaphylactoid reactions to the dialyzer, particularly on its first use, have been reported most frequently with the bioincompatible cellulosic-containing membranes. With the gradual phasing out of cuprophane membranes in the United States, dialyzer reactions have become uncommon. Dialyzer reactions can be divided into two types, A and B. Type A reactions are attributed to an IgE-mediated intermediate hypersensitivity reaction to ethylene oxide used in the sterilization of new dialyzers. This reaction typically occurs soon after the initiation of a treatment (within the first few minutes) and can progress to full-blown anaphylaxis if the therapy is not promptly discontinued. Treatment with steroids or epinephrine may be needed if symptoms are severe. The type B reaction consists of a symptom complex of nonspecific chest and back pain, which appears to result from complement activation and cytokine release. These symptoms typically occur several minutes into the dialysis run and typically resolve over time with continued dialysis.

Cardiovascular disease constitutes the major cause of death in patients with ESRD. Cardiovascular mortality and event rates are higher in dialysis patients than in patients posttransplantation, although rates are extraordinarily high in both populations. The underlying cause of cardiovascular disease is unclear but may be related to shared risk factors (e.g., diabetes mellitus, hypertension, atherosclerotic and arteriosclerotic vascular disease), chronic inflammation, massive changes in extracellular volume (especially with high interdialytic weight gains), inadequate treatment of hypertension, dyslipidemia, anemia, dystrophic vascular calcification, hyperhomocysteinemia, and, perhaps, alterations in cardiovascular dynamics during the dialysis treatment. Few studies have targeted cardiovascular risk reduction in ESRD patients; none have demonstrated consistent benefit. Two clinical trials of statin agents in ESRD demonstrated significant reductions in low-density lipoprotein (LDL) cholesterol concentrations but no significant reductions in death or cardiovascular events [Die Deutsche Diabetes Dialyse Studie (4D) and AURORA studies]. Nevertheless, most experts recommend conventional cardioprotective strategies (e.g., lipid-lowering agents, aspirin, β-adrenergic antagonists) in dialysis patients based on the patients' cardiovascular risk profile, which appears to be increased by more than an order of magnitude relative to persons unaffected by kidney disease.

PERITONEAL DIALYSIS

In peritoneal dialysis, 1.5–3 L of a dextrose-containing solution is infused into the peritoneal cavity and allowed to dwell for a set period of time, usually 2–4 h. As with hemodialysis, toxic materials are removed through a combination of convective clearance generated through ultrafiltration and diffusive clearance down a concentration gradient. The clearance of solutes and water during a peritoneal dialysis exchange depends on the balance between the movement of solute and water into the peritoneal cavity versus absorption from the peritoneal cavity. The rate of diffusion diminishes with time and eventually stops when equilibration between plasma and dialysate is reached. Absorption of solutes and water from the peritoneal cavity occurs across the peritoneal membrane into the peritoneal capillary circulation and via peritoneal lymphatics into the lymphatic circulation. The rate of peritoneal solute transport varies from patient to patient and may be altered by the presence of infection (peritonitis), drugs, and physical factors such as position and exercise.

FORMS OF PERITONEAL DIALYSIS

Peritoneal dialysis may be carried out as CAPD, CCPD, or a combination of both. In CAPD, dialysis solution is manually infused into the peritoneal cavity during the day and exchanged three to five times daily. A nighttime dwell is frequently instilled at bedtime and remains in the peritoneal cavity through the night. The drainage of spent dialysate is performed manually with the assistance of gravity to move fluid out of the abdomen. In CCPD, exchanges are performed in an automated fashion, usually at night; the patient is connected to an automated cycler that performs a series of exchange cycles while the patient sleeps. The number of exchange cycles required to optimize peritoneal solute clearance varies by the peritoneal membrane characteristics; as with hemodialysis, experts suggest careful tracking of solute clearances to ensure dialysis "adequacy."

Peritoneal dialysis solutions are available in volumes typically ranging from 1.5 to 3 L. Lactate is the preferred buffer in peritoneal dialysis solutions. The most common additives to peritoneal dialysis solutions are heparin to prevent obstruction of the dialysis catheter lumen with fibrin and antibiotics during an episode of acute peritonitis. Insulin may also be added in patients with diabetes mellitus.

ACCESS TO THE PERITONEAL CAVITY

Access to the peritoneal cavity is obtained through a peritoneal catheter. Catheters used for maintenance peritoneal dialysis are flexible, being made of silicone rubber with numerous side holes at the distal end. These catheters usually have two Dacron cuffs to promote fibroblast proliferation, granulation, and invasion of the cuff. The scarring that occurs around the cuffs anchors the catheter and seals it from bacteria tracking from the skin surface into the peritoneal cavity; it also prevents the external leakage of fluid from the peritoneal cavity. The cuffs are placed in the preperitoneal plane and ~2 cm from the skin surface.

The *peritoneal equilibrium test* is a formal evaluation of peritoneal membrane characteristics that measures the transfer rates of creatinine and glucose across the peritoneal membrane. Patients are classified as low, low–average, high–average, and high transporters. Patients with rapid equilibration (i.e., high transporters) tend to absorb more glucose and lose efficiency of ultrafiltration with long daytime dwells. High transporters also tend to lose larger quantities of albumin and other proteins across the peritoneal membrane. In general, patients with rapid transporting characteristics require more frequent, shorter dwell time exchanges, nearly always obligating use of a cycler for feasibility. Slower (low and low–average) transporters tend to do well with fewer exchanges. The efficiency of solute clearance also depends on the volume of dialysate infused. Larger volumes allow for greater solute clearance, particularly with CAPD in patients with low and low–average transport characteristics. Interestingly, solute clearance also increases with physical activity, presumably related to more efficient flow dynamics within the peritoneal cavity.

As with hemodialysis, the optimal dose of peritoneal dialysis is unknown. Several observational studies have suggested that higher rates of urea and creatinine clearance (the latter generally measured in L/week) are associated with lower mortality rates and fewer uremic complications. However, a randomized clinical trial [Adequacy of Peritoneal Dialysis in Mexico (ADEMEX)] failed to show a significant reduction in mortality or complications with a relatively large increment in urea clearance. In general, patients on peritoneal dialysis do well when they retain residual kidney function. The rates of technique failure increase with years on dialysis and have been correlated with loss of residual function to a greater extent than loss of peritoneal membrane capacity. Recently, a nonabsorbable carbohydrate (icodextrin) has been introduced as an alternative osmotic agent. Studies have demonstrated more efficient ultrafiltration with icodextrin than with dextrose-containing solutions. Icodextrin is typically used as the "last fill" for patients on CCPD or for the longest dwell in patients on CAPD. For some patients in whom CCPD does not provide sufficient solute clearance, a hybrid approach can be adopted where one or more daytime exchanges are added to the CCPD regimen. While this approach can enhance solute clearance and prolong a patient's capacity to remain on peritoneal dialysis, the burden of the hybrid approach can be overwhelming to some.

COMPLICATIONS DURING PERITONEAL DIALYSIS

The major complications of peritoneal dialysis are peritonitis, catheter-associated nonperitonitis infections, weight gain and other metabolic disturbances, and residual uremia (especially among patients with no residual kidney function).

Peritonitis typically develops when there has been a break in sterile technique during one or more of the exchange procedures. Peritonitis is usually defined by an elevated peritoneal fluid leukocyte count (100/mm^3, of which at least 50% are polymorphonuclear neutrophils); these cutoffs are lower than in spontaneous bacterial peritonitis because of the presence of dextrose in peritoneal dialysis solutions and rapid bacterial proliferation in this environment without antibiotic therapy. The clinical presentation typically consists of pain and cloudy dialysate, often with fever and other constitutional symptoms. The most common culprit organisms are gram-positive cocci, including *Staphylococcus,* reflecting the origin from the skin. Gram-negative rod infections are less common; fungal and mycobacterial infections can be seen in selected patients, particularly after antibacterial therapy. Most cases of peritonitis can be managed either with intraperitoneal or oral antibiotics, depending on the organism; many patients with peritonitis do not require hospitalization. In cases where peritonitis is due to hydrophilic gram negative rods (e.g., *Pseudomonas* sp.) or yeast, antimicrobial therapy is usually not sufficient, and catheter removal is required to ensure complete eradication of infection. Nonperitonitis catheter-associated infections (often termed *tunnel infections*) vary widely in severity. Some cases can be managed with local antibiotic or silver nitrate administration, while others are severe enough to require parenteral antibiotic therapy and catheter removal.

Peritoneal dialysis is associated with a variety of metabolic complications. As noted above, albumin and other proteins can be lost across the peritoneal membrane in concert with the loss of metabolic wastes. The hypoproteinemia induced by peritoneal dialysis obligates a higher dietary protein intake in order to maintain nitrogen balance. Hyperglycemia and weight gain are also common complications of peritoneal dialysis. Several hundred calories in the form of dextrose are absorbed each day, depending on the concentration employed. Peritoneal dialysis patients, particularly those with type II diabetes mellitus, are then prone to other complications of insulin resistance, including hypertriglyceridemia. On the positive side, the continuous nature of peritoneal dialysis usually allows for a more liberal diet, due to continuous removal of potassium and phosphorus—two major dietary components whose accumulation can be hazardous in ESRD.

GLOBAL PERSPECTIVE

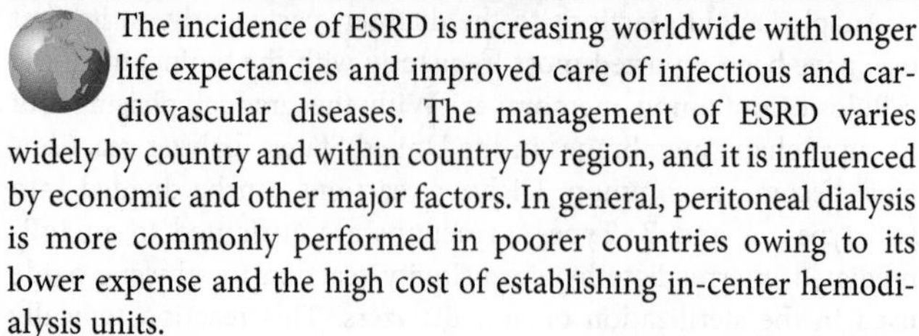

The incidence of ESRD is increasing worldwide with longer life expectancies and improved care of infectious and cardiovascular diseases. The management of ESRD varies widely by country and within country by region, and it is influenced by economic and other major factors. In general, peritoneal dialysis is more commonly performed in poorer countries owing to its lower expense and the high cost of establishing in-center hemodialysis units.

ACKNOWLEDGMENT

We are grateful to Dr. Ajay Singh and Dr. Barry Brenner, authors of "Dialysis in the Treatment of Renal Failure" in the 16th edition of Harrison's, for contributions to this chapter.

FURTHER READINGS

BURKART JM et al: Peritoneal dialysis, in *Brenner and Rector's The Kidney,* 7th ed, BM Brenner (ed). Philadelphia, Saunders, 2004

EKNOYAN G et al: Effect of dialysis dose and membrane flux in maintenance hemodialysis. N Engl J Med 346:2010, 2002

FELLSTROM BC et al: Rosuvastatin and cardiovascular events in patients undergoing hemodialysis. N Engl J Med 360:1395, 2009

FORNI LG, HILTON PJ: Current concepts: Continuous hemofiltration in the treatment of acute renal failure. N Engl J Med 336:1303, 1997

HIMMELFARB J, KLIGER AS: End-stage renal disease measures of quality. Annu Rev Med 58:387, 2007

NATIONAL KIDNEY FOUNDATION: Kidney Disease Quality Initiative Clinical Practice Guidelines: Hemodialysis and peritoneal dialysis adequacy, 2001. Available online: *http://www.kidney.org/professionals/kdoqi/guidelines.cfm*

PANIAGUA R et al: Effects of increased peritoneal clearances on mortality rates in peritoneal dialysis: ADEMEX, a prospective, randomized, controlled trial. J Am Soc Nephrol 13:1307, 2002

RAYNER HC et al: Vascular access results from the Dialysis Outcomes and Practice Patterns Study (DOPPS): Performance against Kidney Disease Outcomes Quality Initiative (K/DOQI) Clinical Practice Guidelines. Am J Kidney Dis 44:S22, 2004

U.S. RENAL DATA SYSTEM: USRDS 2009 Annual Data Report: Atlas of End-Stage Renal Disease in the United States. Bethesda, National Institutes of Health, National Institute of Diabetes and Digestive and Kidney Disease, 2009

WANNER C et al: Atorvastatin in patients with type 2 diabetes mellitus undergoing hemodialysis. N Engl J Med 353: 238, 2005

CHAPTER 282

Transplantation in the Treatment of Renal Failure

Anil Chandraker
Edgar L. Milford
Mohamed H. Sayegh

Transplantation of the human kidney is the treatment of choice for advanced chronic renal failure. Worldwide, tens of thousands of these procedures have been performed. When azathioprine and prednisone initially were used as immunosuppressive drugs in the 1960s, the results with properly matched familial donors were superior to those with organs from deceased donors: 75–90% compared with 50–60% graft survival rates at 1 year. During the 1970s and 1980s, the success rate at the 1-year mark for deceased-donor transplants rose progressively. Currently, deceased-donor grafts have an 89% 1-year survival and living-donor grafts have a 95% 1-year survival. Although there has been improvement in long-term survival, it has not been as impressive as the short-term survival, and currently the "average" ($t_{1/2}$) life expectancy of a living-donor graft is around 20 years and that of a deceased-donor graft is close to 14 years.

Mortality rates after transplantation are highest in the first year and are age-related: 2% for ages 18–34 years, 3% for ages 35–49 years, and 6.8% for ages ≥50–60 years. These rates compare favorably with those in the chronic dialysis population even after risk adjustments for age, diabetes, and cardiovascular status. Occasionally, acute irreversible rejection may occur after many months of good function, especially if the patient neglects to take the prescribed immunosuppressive drugs. Most grafts, however, succumb at varying rates to a chronic process consisting of interstitial fibrosis, tubular atrophy, vasculopathy, and glomerulopathy, the pathogenesis of which is incompletely understood. Overall, transplantation returns most patients to an improved lifestyle and an improved life expectancy compared with patients on dialysis. There are at least 100,000 patients with functioning kidney transplants in the United States, and when one adds in the numbers of kidney transplants in centers around the world, the total activity is doubled.

RECENT ACTIVITY AND RESULTS

In 2008 there were more than 10,500 deceased-donor kidney transplants and 6000 living-donor transplants in the United States, with the ratio of deceased to living donors being stable over the last few years. The backlog of patients with end-stage renal disease (ESRD) has been increasing every year, and it always lags behind the number of available donors. As the number of patients with end-stage kidney disease increases, the demand for kidney transplants continues to increase. In 2008, 33,051 new registrants were added to the waiting list and under 17,000 patients were transplanted. This imbalance is set to worsen over the coming years with the predicted increased rates of obesity and diabetes worldwide. In an attempt to increase utilization of deceased-donor kidneys and reduce discard rates of organs, criteria for the use of so-called expanded criteria donor (ECD) kidneys and kidneys from donors after cardiac death (DCD) have been developed (Table 282-1). ECD kidneys are usually used for older patients who are expected to fare less well on dialysis.

TABLE 282-1 Definition of an Expanded Criteria Donor (ECD) and a Non-Heart-Beating Donor [Donation After Cardiac Death (DCD)]

Expanded Criteria Donor (ECD)
Deceased donor >60 years
Deceased donor >50 years and hypertension and creatinine >1.5 mg/dL
Deceased donor >50 years and hypertension and death caused by cerebrovascular accident (CVA)
Deceased donor >50 years and death caused by CVA and creatinine >1.5 mg/dL
Donation after Cardiac Death[a] (DCD)
I Brought in dead
II Unsuccessful resuscitation
III Awaiting cardiac arrest
IV Cardiac arrest after brainstem death
V Cardiac arrest in a hospital patient

[a]Kidneys can be used for transplantation from categories II–V but are commonly only used from categories III and IV. The survival of these kidneys has not been shown to be inferior to that of deceased-donor kidneys.

Note: Kidneys can be bought ECD and DCD. ECD kidneys have been shown to have a poorer survival, and there is a separate shorter waiting list for ECD kidneys. They are generally utilized for patients for whom the benefits of being transplanted earlier outweigh the associated risks of using an ECD kidney.

The overall results of transplantation are presented in Table 282-2 as the survival of grafts and of patients. At the 1-year mark, graft survival is higher for living-donor recipients, most likely because those grafts are not subject to as much ischemic injury. The more powerful drugs now in use for immunosuppression have almost equalized the risk of graft rejection in all patients for the first year. At 5 and 10 years, however, there has been a steeper decline in survival of those with deceased-donor kidneys.

RECIPIENT SELECTION

There are few absolute contraindications to renal transplantation. The transplant procedure is relatively noninvasive, as the organ is placed in the inguinal fossa without entering the peritoneal cavity. Recipients without perioperative complications often can be discharged from the hospital in excellent condition within 5 days of the operation.

Virtually all patients with ESRD who receive a transplant have a higher life expectancy than do risk-matched patients who remain on dialysis. Even though diabetic patients and older candidates have a higher mortality rate than other transplant recipients, their survival is improved with transplantation compared with remaining on dialysis. This global benefit of transplantation as a treatment modality poses substantial ethical issues for policy makers, as the number of deceased kidneys available is far from sufficient to meet the current needs of the candidates. The current standard of care is that the candidate should have a life expectancy of >5 years to be put on a deceased organ wait list. Even for living donation, the candidate should have >5 years of life expectancy. This standard has been established because the benefits of kidney transplantation

TABLE 282-2 Mean Rates of Graft and Patient Survival for Kidneys Transplanted in the United States from 1992 to 2002[a]

	1-Year Follow-Up		5-Year Follow-Up		10-Year Follow-Up	
	Grafts, %	Patients, %	Grafts, %	Patients, %	Grafts, %	Patients, %
Deceased donor	89	95	67	81	41	61
Living donor	95	98	80	90	56	76

[a]All patients transplanted are included, and the follow-up unadjusted survival data from the 1-, 5-, and 10-year periods are presented to show the attrition rates over time within the two types of organ donors.

Source: Data from Summary Tables, 2004 and 2005 Annual Reports, Scientific Registry of Transplant Recipients.

over dialysis are realized only after a perioperative period in which the mortality rate is higher in transplanted patients than in dialysis patients with comparable risk profiles.

All candidates must have a thorough risk-versus-benefit evaluation before being approved for transplantation. In particular, an aggressive approach to diagnosis of correctable coronary artery disease, presence of latent or indolent infection (HIV, hepatitis B or C, tuberculosis), and neoplasm should be a routine part of the candidate workup. Most transplant centers consider overt AIDS and active hepatitis absolute contraindications to transplantation because of the high risk of opportunistic infection. Some centers are now transplanting individuals with hepatitis and even HIV infection under strict protocols to determine whether the risks and benefits favor transplantation over dialysis.

Among the few absolute "immunologic" contraindications to transplantation is the presence of a potentially harmful antibody against the donor kidney at the time of the anticipated transplant. Harmful antibodies that can cause very early graft loss include natural antibodies against the ABO blood group antigens and antibodies against human leukocyte antigen (HLA) class I (A, B, C) or class II (DR) antigens. These antibodies are routinely excluded by proper screening of the candidate's ABO compatibility, HLA typing of donor and recipient, and direct cross-matching of candidate serum with lymphocytes of the donor.

DONOR SELECTION

Donors can be deceased or volunteer living donors. The latter are usually family members selected to have at least partial compatibility for HLA antigens. Living volunteer donors should be normal on physical examination and of the same major ABO blood group, because crossing major blood group barriers prejudices survival of the allograft. It is possible, however, to transplant a kidney of a type O donor into an A, B, or AB recipient. Selective renal arteriography should be performed on donors to rule out the presence of multiple or abnormal renal arteries because the surgical procedure is difficult and the ischemic time of the transplanted kidney is long when there are vascular abnormalities. Transplant surgeons are now using a laparoscopic method to isolate and remove the living donor's kidney. This operation has the advantage of less evident surgical scars, and, because there is less tissue trauma, the laparoscopic donors have a substantially shorter hospital stay and less discomfort than those who have the traditional surgery. Deceased donors should be free of malignant neoplastic disease, hepatitis, and HIV because of possible transmission to the recipient. Increased risk of graft failure exists when the donor is elderly or has renal failure and when the kidney has a prolonged period of ischemia and storage.

In the United States, there is a coordinated national system of regulations, allocation support, and outcomes analysis for kidney transplantation called the Organ Procurement Transplant Network. It is now possible to remove deceased-donor kidneys and maintain them for up to 48 h on cold pulsatile perfusion or simple flushing and cooling. This approach permits adequate time for typing, cross-matching, transportation, and selection problems to be solved.

TISSUE TYPING AND CLINICAL IMMUNOGENETICS

Matching for antigens of the HLA major histocompatibility gene complex (Chap. 315) is an important criterion for selection of donors for renal allografts. Each mammalian species has a single chromosomal region that encodes the strong, or major, transplantation antigens, and this region on the human sixth chromosome is called *HLA*. HLA antigens have been classically defined by serologic techniques, but methods to define specific nucleotide sequences in genomic DNA are increasingly being used. Other "minor" antigens may play crucial roles, in addition to the ABH(O) blood groups and endothelial antigens that are not shared with lymphocytes. The Rh system is not expressed on graft tissue. Evidence for designation of HLA as the genetic region that encodes major transplantation antigens comes from the success rate in living related donor renal and bone marrow transplantation, with superior results in HLA-identical sibling pairs. Nevertheless, 5% of HLA-identical renal allografts are rejected, often within the first weeks after transplantation. These failures represent states of prior sensitization to non-HLA antigens. Non-HLA minor antigens are relatively weak when initially encountered and are, therefore, suppressible by conventional immunosuppressive therapy. Once priming has occurred, however, secondary responses are much more refractory to treatment.

LIVING DONORS

When first-degree relatives are donors, graft survival rates at 1 year are 5–7% greater than those for deceased-donor grafts. The 5-year survival rates still favor a partially matched (3/6 HLA mismatched) family donor over a randomly selected cadaver donor (Table 282-3). In addition, living donors provide the advantage of immediate availability. For both living and deceased donors, the 5-year outcomes are poor if there is a complete (6/6) HLA mismatch.

The survival rate of living unrelated renal allografts is as high as that of perfectly HLA-matched cadaver renal transplants and comparable to that of kidneys from living relatives. This outcome is probably a consequence of both short cold ischemia time and the extra care taken to document that the condition and renal function of the donor are optimal before proceeding with a living unrelated donation. It is illegal in the United States to purchase organs for transplantation.

Concern has been expressed about the potential risk to a volunteer kidney donor of premature renal failure after several years of increased blood flow and hyperfiltration per nephron in the

TABLE 282-3 Effect of HLA-A, -B, -DR Mismatching on Kidney Graft Survival

Degree of Donor Mismatch	1-Year Survival, %	5-Year Survival, %
Cadaver donor (all)	89.2	61.3
0/6-HLA mismatch	91.3	68.2
3/6-HLA mismatch	90.1	60.8
6/6-HLA mismatch	85.2	55.3
Living related donor (all)	94.7	76.0
0/6-HLA mismatch	96.7	87.0
3/6-HLA mismatch	94.3	73.2
6/6-HLA mismatch	92.7	57.7

Note: 0-mismatched related donor transplants are virtually all from HLA-identical siblings, whereas 3/6-mismatched transplants can be one haplotype mismatched (1-A, 1-B, and 1-DR antigen) from a parent, child, or sibling; 6/6-HLA-mismatched living related kidneys are derived from siblings or relatives outside the nuclear family.

remaining kidney. There are a few reports of the development of hypertension, proteinuria, and even lesions of focal segmental sclerosis in donors over long-term follow-up. Difficulties in donors followed for ≥20 years are unusual, however, and it may be that having a single kidney becomes significant only when another condition, such as hypertension, is superimposed. It is also desirable to consider the risk of development of type 1 diabetes mellitus in a family member who is a potential donor to a diabetic renal failure patient. Anti-insulin and anti-islet cell antibodies should be measured, and glucose tolerance tests should be performed in such donors to exclude a prediabetic state.

PRESENSITIZATION

A positive cytotoxic cross-match of recipient serum with donor T lymphocytes representing anti-HLA class I is usually predictive of an acute vasculitic event termed *hyperacute rejection.* Patients with anti-HLA antibodies can be transplanted safely if careful cross-matching of donor blood lymphocytes with recipient serum is performed. The known sources of such sensitization are blood transfusion, a prior transplant, and pregnancy. Patients sustained by dialysis often show fluctuating antibody titers and specificity patterns. At the time of assignment of a cadaveric kidney, cross-matches are performed with at least a current serum. Previously analyzed antibody specificities and additional cross-matches are performed accordingly. The minimal purpose for the cross-match is avoidance of hyperacute rejection mediated by recipient antibodies to donor HLA class I antigens. More sensitive tests, such as the use of flow cytometry, can be useful for avoidance of accelerated, and often untreatable, early graft rejection in patients receiving second or third transplants. Donor T lymphocytes, which express only class I antigens, are used as targets for detection of anti–class I (HLA-A and -B) antibodies.

Preformed anti–class II (HLA-DR) antibodies against the donor carry a higher risk of graft loss as well, particularly in recipients who have suffered early loss of a prior kidney transplant. B lymphocytes expressing both class I and class II antigens are used in these assays. Non-HLA antigens restricted in expression to endothelium and sometimes monocytes have been described, but clinical relevance is not well established. A series of minor histocompatibility antigens do not elicit antibodies, and sensitization to these antigens is detectable only by cytotoxic T cells, an assay too cumbersome for routine use. Desensitization before transplantation by reducing the level of antidonor antibodies via plasmapheresis of blood and administration of pooled immunoglobulin or both has been useful in reducing the hazard of hyperacute rejection.

IMMUNOLOGY OF REJECTION

Both cellular and humoral (antibody-mediated) effector mechanisms can play roles in kidney transplant rejection. Antibodies can also initiate a form of antibody-dependent but cell-mediated cytotoxicity by recipient cells that bear receptors for the Fc portion of immunoglobulin.

Cellular rejection is mediated by lymphocytes that respond to HLA antigens expressed within the organ. The CD4+ lymphocyte responds to class II (HLA-DR) incompatibility by proliferating and releasing proinflammatory cytokines that augment the proliferative response of both CD4+ and CD8+ cells. CD8+ cytotoxic lymphocyte precursors respond primarily to class I (HLA-A, -B) antigens and mature into cytotoxic effector cells. The cytotoxic effector ("killer") T cells cause organ damage through direct contact and lysis of donor target cells. The natural role of HLA antigen molecules is to present processed peptide fragments of antigen to T lymphocytes, the fragments residing in a "groove" of the HLA molecule distal to the cell surface. T cells can be directly stimulated by intact nonself HLA molecules expressed on donor parenchymal cells and residual donor leukocytes residing in the kidney interstitium. In addition, donor HLA molecules can be processed by a variety of donor or recipient cells capable of antigen presentation of peptides and then presented to T cells in the same manner as most other antigens. The former mode of stimulation is sometimes called *direct presentation,* and the latter mode *indirect presentation* (Fig. 282-1). There is evidence that non-HLA antigens can also play a role in renal transplant rejection episodes. Recipients who receive a kidney from an HLA-identical sibling can have rejection episodes and require maintenance immunosuppression, whereas identical twin transplants require no immunosuppression. There are documented non-HLA antigens, such as an endothelial-specific antigen system with limited polymorphism and a tubular antigen, that can be targets of humoral or cellular rejection responses, respectively.

IMMUNOSUPPRESSIVE TREATMENT

Immunosuppressive therapy, as currently available, generally suppresses all immune responses, including those to bacteria, fungi, and even malignant tumors. In the 1950s, when clinical renal transplantation began, sublethal total-body irradiation was employed. We have now reached the point where sophisticated pharmacologic immunosuppression is available, but it still has the hazard of promoting infection and malignancy. In general, all clinically useful drugs are more selective to primary than to memory immune responses. Agents to suppress the immune response are discussed in the following paragraphs, and those currently in clinical use are listed in Table 282-4.

DRUGS

Azathioprine, an analogue of mercaptopurine, was for two decades the keystone to immunosuppressive therapy in humans but has given way to more effective agents. This agent can inhibit synthesis of DNA, RNA, or both. Therapy with azathioprine in doses of 1.5–2 mg/kg per d is generally added to cyclosporine as a means of decreasing the requirements for the latter. Reduction in the dose is required because of leukopenia and occasionally thrombocytopenia. Excessive amounts of azathioprine may also cause jaundice, anemia, and alopecia. If it is essential to administer allopurinol concurrently, the azathioprine dose must be reduced. As inhibition of xanthine oxidase delays degradation, this combination is best avoided.

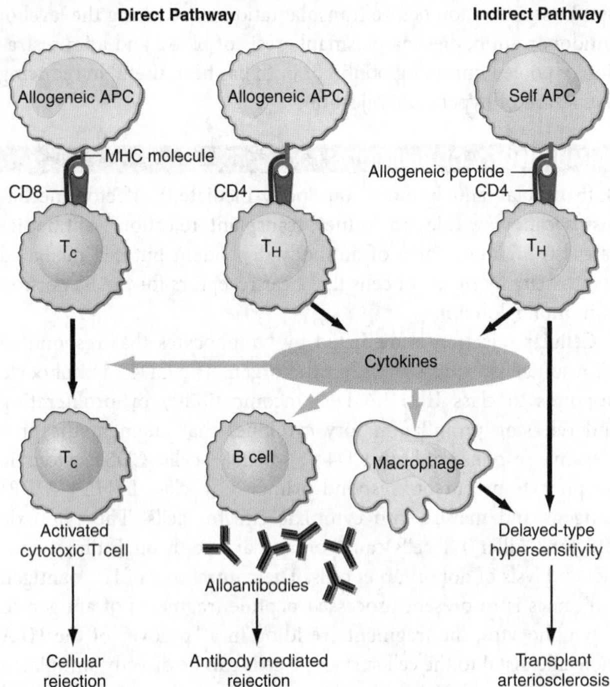

Figure 282-1 Recognition pathways for major histocompatibility complex (MHC) antigens. Graft rejection is initiated by CD4 helper T lymphocytes (T_H) having antigen receptors that bind to specific complexes of peptides and MHC class II molecules on antigen-presenting cells (APC). In transplantation, in contrast to other immunologic responses, there are two sets of T cell clones involved in rejection. In the direct pathway the class II MHC of donor allogeneic APCs is recognized by CD4 T_H cells that bind to the intact MHC molecule, and class I MHC allogeneic cells are recognized by CD8 T cells. The latter generally proliferate into cytotoxic cells (T_C). In the indirect pathway, the incompatible MHC molecules are processed into peptides that are presented by the self-APCs of the recipient. The indirect, but not the direct, pathway is the normal physiologic process in T cell recognition of foreign antigens. Once T_H cells are activated, they proliferate and, by secretion of cytokines and direct contact, exert strong helper effects on macrophages, T_C, and B cells. *(From MH Sayegh, LH Turka, N Engl J Med, 338:1813, 1998.*

Mycophenolate mofetil or mycophenolate sodium, both of which are metabolized to mycophenolic acid, is now used in place of azathioprine in most centers. It has a similar mode of action and a mild degree of gastrointestinal toxicity but produces minimal bone marrow suppression. Its advantage is its increased potency in preventing or reversing rejection. Patients with hyperuricemia can be given allopurinol without adjustment of the mycophenolic acid dose. The usual dose is 2–3 g/d in divided doses.

Glucocorticoids are important adjuncts to immunosuppressive therapy. Among all the agents employed, prednisone has effects that are easiest to assess, and in large doses it is usually effective for the reversal of rejection. In general, 200–300 mg prednisone is given immediately before or at the time of transplantation, and the dose is reduced to 30 mg within a week. The side effects of the glucocorticoids, particularly impairment of wound healing and predisposition to infection, make it desirable to taper the dose as rapidly as possible in the immediate postoperative period. Many centers now have protocols for early discontinuance or avoidance of steroids because of long-term adverse effects on bone, skin, and glucose metabolism. For treatment of acute rejection, methylprednisolone, 0.5–1 g IV, is administered immediately upon diagnosis of beginning rejection and continued once daily for 3 days. When the drug is effective, the results are usually apparent within 96 h. Such "pulse" doses are not effective in chronic rejection. Most patients whose renal function is stable after 6 months or a year do not require large doses of prednisone; maintenance doses of 10–15 mg/d are the rule. Many patients tolerate an alternate-day course of steroids without an increased risk of rejection. A major effect of steroids is on the monocyte-macrophage system, preventing the release of interleukin (IL) 6 and IL-1.

Cyclosporine is a fungal peptide with potent immunosuppressive activity. It acts on the calcineurin pathway to block transcription of mRNA for IL-2 and other proinflammatory cytokines, thereby inhibiting T cell proliferation. Although it works alone, cyclosporine is more effective in conjunction with glucocorticoids and mycophenolate. Clinical results with tens of thousands of renal transplants have been impressive. Among its toxic effects (nephrotoxicity, hepatotoxicity, hirsutism, tremor, gingival hyperplasia, diabetes), only nephrotoxicity presents a serious management problem and is further discussed below.

TABLE 282-4 Maintenance Immunosuppressive Drugs

Agent	Pharmacology	Mechanisms	Side Effects
Glucocorticoids	Increased bioavailability with hypoalbuminemia and liver disease; prednisone/prednisolone generally used	Binds cytosolic receptors and heat shock proteins. Blocks transcription of IL-1,-2,-3,-6, TNF-α, and IFN-γ	Hypertension, glucose intolerance, dyslipidemia, osteoporosis
Cyclosporine (CsA)	Lipid-soluble polypeptide, variable absorption, microemulsion more predictable	Trimolecular complex with cyclophilin and calcineurin → block in cytokine (e.g., IL-2) production; however, stimulates TGF-β production	Nephrotoxicity, hypertension, dyslipidemia, glucose intolerance, hirsutism/hyperplasia of gums
Tacrolimus (FK506)	Macrolide, well absorbed	Trimolecular complex with FKBP-12 and calcineurin → block in cytokine (e.g., IL-2) production; may stimulate TGF-β production	Similar to CsA, but hirsutism/hyperplasia of gums unusual, and diabetes more likely
Azathioprine	Mercaptopurine analogue	Hepatic metabolites inhibit purine synthesis	Marrow suppression (WBC > RBC > platelets)
Mycophenolate mofetil (MMF)	Metabolized to mycophenolic acid	Inhibits purine synthesis via inosine monophosphate dehydrogenase	Diarrhea/cramps; dose-related liver and marrow suppression is uncommon
Sirolimus	Macrolide, poor oral bioavailability	Complexes with FKBP-12 and then blocks p70 S6 kinase in the IL-2 receptor pathway for proliferation	Hyperlipidemia, thrombocytopenia

Abbreviations: FKBP-12, FK506 binding protein 12; IFN, interferon; IL, interleukin; RBC, red blood cells; TGF, transforming growth factor; TNF, tumor necrosis factor; WBC, white blood cells.

Tacrolimus (previously called FK506) is a fungal macrolide that has the same mode of action as cyclosporine as well as a similar side-effect profile; it does not, however, produce hirsutism or gingival hyperplasia. De novo diabetes mellitus is more common with tacrolimus. The drug was first used in liver transplantation and may substitute for cyclosporine entirely or be tried as an alternative in renal patients whose rejections are poorly controlled by cyclosporine.

Sirolimus (previously called rapamycin) is another fungal macrolide but has a different mode of action; i.e., it inhibits T cell growth factor signaling pathways, preventing the response to IL-2 and other cytokines. Sirolimus can be used in conjunction with cyclosporine or tacrolimus, or with mycophenolic acid, to avoid calcineurin inhibitors. Its use with tacrolimus alone shows promise as a steroid-sparing regimen, especially in patients who would benefit from pancreatic islet cell transplantation, where steroids have an adverse effect on islet survival.

ANTIBODIES TO LYMPHOCYTES

When serum from animals made immune to host lymphocytes is injected into the recipient, a marked suppression of cellular immunity to the tissue graft results. The action on cell-mediated immunity is greater than the action on humoral immunity. A globulin fraction of serum [antilymphocyte globulin (ALG)] is the agent generally employed. For use in humans, peripheral human lymphocytes, thymocytes, or lymphocytes from spleens or thoracic duct fistulas have been injected into horses, rabbits, or goats to produce antilymphocyte serum, from which the globulin fraction is then separated. A rabbit antithymocyte globulin (thymoglobulin) is the agent most commonly in use currently. Monoclonal antibodies against defined lymphocyte subsets offer a more precise and standardized form of therapy. OKT3 is directed to the CD3 molecules that form a portion of the T cell antigen-receptor complex and is thus expressed on all mature T cells.

Another approach to more selective therapy is to target the 55-kDa alpha chain of the IL-2 receptor, which is expressed only on T cells that have been recently activated. Two such antibodies to the IL-2 receptor, in which either a chimeric protein has been made between mouse Fab with human Fc (basiliximab) or the antibody has been "humanized" by splicing the combining sites of the mouse into a molecule that is 90% human IgG (daclizumab), are in use for prophylaxis of acute rejection in the immediate posttransplant period. They are effective at decreasing the acute rejection rate and have few adverse side effects.

More recently, two new strategies have involved administration of engineered biologic agents: a depleting T cell antibody (alemtuzumab) as induction therapy to minimize maintenance immunosuppression and a fusion protein (Belatacept) to block B7 T cell costimulatory signals. The latter has shown promise in phase 2 trials and is currently being tested in phase 3 trials in kidney transplantation. Both of these new biologics as well as antilymphocyte globulin are increasingly being used as "induction" therapy at the time of transplantation to minimize or eliminate the use of either steroids or calcineurin inhibitors because of their perceived toxicities. The next step in the evolution of this therapeutic strategy, which has already been achieved in the short term in small numbers of immunologically well-matched patients, is the elimination of all maintenance immunosuppression therapy altogether.

CLINICAL COURSE AND MANAGEMENT OF THE RECIPIENT

Adequate hemodialysis should be performed within 48 h of surgery, and care should be taken that the serum potassium level is not markedly elevated so that intraoperative cardiac arrhythmias can be averted. The diuresis that commonly occurs postoperatively must be carefully monitored. In some instances, it may be massive, reflecting the inability of ischemic tubules to regulate sodium and water excretion; with large diureses, massive potassium losses may occur. Most chronically uremic patients have some excess of extracellular fluid, and it is useful to maintain an expanded fluid volume in the immediate postoperative period. Acute tubular necrosis (ATN) may cause immediate oliguria or may follow an initial short period of graft function. ATN is most likely when cadaveric donors have been underperfused or if the interval between cessation of blood flow and organ harvest (warm ischemic time) is more than a few minutes. Recovery usually occurs within 3 weeks, although periods as long as 6 weeks have been reported. Superimposition of rejection on ATN is common, and the differential diagnosis may be difficult without a graft biopsy. Cyclosporine therapy prolongs ATN, and some patients do not diurese until the dose is reduced drastically. Many centers avoid starting cyclosporine for the first several days, using ALG or a monoclonal antibody along with mycophenolic acid and prednisone until renal function is established. Figure 282-2 illustrates an algorithm followed by many transplant centers for early posttransplant management of recipients at high or low risk of early renal dysfunction.

THE REJECTION EPISODE

Early diagnosis of rejection allows prompt institution of therapy to preserve renal function and prevent irreversible damage. Clinical evidence of rejection is rarely characterized by fever, swelling, and tenderness over the allograft. Rejection may present only with a rise in serum creatinine, with or without a reduction in urine volume. The focus should be on ruling out other causes of functional deterioration.

Doppler ultrasonography or magnetic resonance angiography may be useful in ascertaining changes in the renal vasculature and in renal blood flow, even in the absence of changes in urinary flow. Thrombosis of the renal vein occurs rarely; it may be reversible if it is caused by technical factors and intervention is prompt. Diagnostic ultrasound is the procedure of choice to rule out urinary obstruction or to confirm the presence of perirenal collections of urine, blood, or lymph. When renal function has been good initially, a rise in the serum creatinine level is the most sensitive and reliable indicator of possible rejection and may be the only sign.

Calcineurin inhibitors (cyclosporine and tacrolimus) may cause deterioration in renal function in a manner similar to a rejection episode. In fact, rejection processes tend to be more indolent with these inhibitors, and the only way to make a diagnosis may be by renal biopsy. Calcineurin inhibitors have an afferent arteriolar constrictor effect on the kidney and may produce permanent vascular and interstitial injury after sustained high-dose therapy. The addition of angiotensin-converting enzyme (ACE) inhibitors or nonsteroidal anti-inflammatory drugs is likely to raise serum creatinine levels. The former are generally safe to use after the early months, whereas the latter are best avoided in all renal transplant patients. There is no universally accepted lesion that makes a diagnosis of calcineurin inhibitor toxicity, although interstitial fibrosis, isometric tubular vacuolization, and thickening of arteriolar walls have been noted by some. Basically, if the biopsy does not reveal moderate and active cellular rejection activity, the serum creatinine most likely will respond to a reduction in dose. Blood levels of drug can be useful if they are very high or very low but do not correlate precisely with renal function, although serial changes in a patient can be useful. If rejection activity is present in the biopsy, appropriate therapy is indicated. The first rejection episode is usually treated with IV administration of methylprednisolone, 500–1000 mg daily for 3 days. Failure to respond is an indication for antibody therapy, usually with OKT3 or antithymocyte globulin.

Biopsy may be necessary to confirm the presence of rejection; when evidence of antibody-mediated injury is present with endothelial injury and deposition of complement component C4d is detected by fluorescence labeling, one can usually detect the

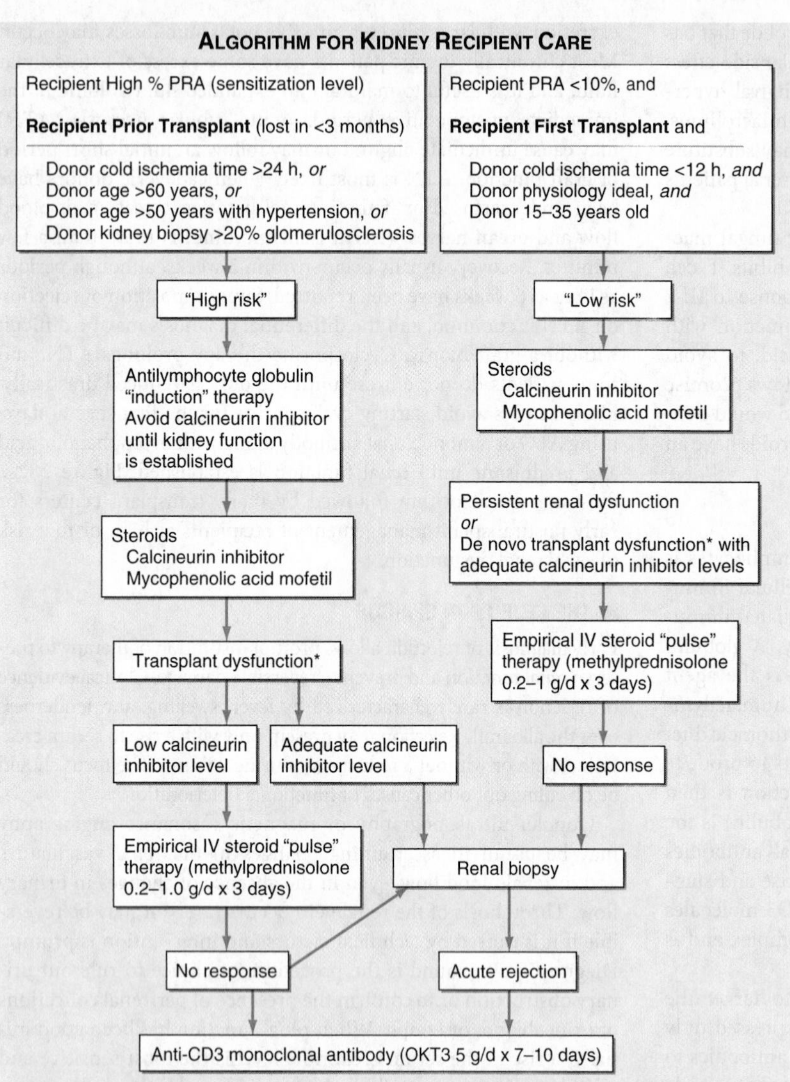

Figure 282-2 A typical algorithm for early posttransplant care of a kidney recipient. If any of the recipient or donor "high-risk" factors exist, more aggressive management is called for. Low-risk patients can be treated with a standard immunosuppressive regimen. Patients at higher risk of rejection or early ischemic and nephrotoxic transplant dysfunction are often induced with an antilymphocyte globulin to provide more potent early immunosuppression or to spare calcineurin nephrotoxicity. *When there is early transplant dysfunction, prerenal, obstructive, and vascular causes must be ruled out by ultrasonographic examination. The panel reactive antibody (PRA) is a quantitation of how much antibody is present in a candidate against a panel of cells representing the distribution of antigens in the donor pool. APC, antigen-presenting cell; MHC, major histocompatibility complex.

antibody in recipient blood. The prognosis is poor, and aggressive use of plasmapheresis, immunoglobulin infusions, or anti-CD20 monoclonal antibody (rituximab) that targets B lymphocytes is indicated.

MANAGEMENT PROBLEMS

The usual clinical manifestations of infection in the posttransplant period are blunted by immunosuppressive therapy. The major toxic effect of azathioprine is bone marrow suppression, which is less likely with mycophenolic acid, whereas calcineurin inhibitors have no marrow effects. All drugs predispose to unusual opportunistic infections, however. The typical times after transplantation when the most common opportunistic infections occur are shown in Table 282-5. The signs and symptoms of infection may be masked or distorted. Fever without obvious cause is common, and only after days or weeks may it become apparent that it has a viral or fungal origin. Bacterial infections are most common during the first month after transplantation. The importance of blood cultures in such patients cannot be overemphasized because systemic infection without obvious foci is common, although wound infections with or without urinary fistulas are the most common. Particularly ominous are rapidly occurring pulmonary lesions, which may result in death within 5 days of onset. When these lesions become apparent, immunosuppressive agents should be discontinued, except for maintenance doses of prednisone.

Aggressive diagnostic procedures, including transbronchial and open-lung biopsy, are frequently indicated. In the case of *Pneumocystis carinii* (Chap. 207) infection, trimethoprim-sulfamethoxazole (TMP-SMX) is the treatment of choice; amphotericin B has been used effectively in systemic fungal infections. Prophylaxis against *P. carinii* with daily or alternate-day low-dose TMP-SMX is very effective. Involvement of the oropharynx with *Candida* (Chap. 203) may be treated with local nystatin. Tissue-invasive fungal infections require treatment with systemic agents such as fluconazole. Small doses (a total of 300 mg) of amphotericin given over a period of 2 weeks may be effective in fungal infections refractory to fluconazole. Macrolide antibiotics, especially ketoconazole and erythromycin, and some calcium channel blockers (diltiazem, verapamil) compete with calcineurin inhibitors for P450 catabolism and cause elevated levels of these immunosuppressive drugs. Analeptics, such as phenytoin and carbamazepine, will increase catabolism to result in low levels. *Aspergillus* (Chap. 204), *Nocardia* (Chap. 162), and especially cytomegalovirus (CMV) (Chap. 182) infections also occur.

CMV is a common and dangerous DNA virus in transplant recipients. It does not generally appear until the end of the first posttransplant month. Active CMV infection is sometimes associated, or occasionally confused, with rejection episodes. Patients at highest risk for severe CMV disease are those without anti-CMV antibodies who receive a graft from a CMV antibody–positive donor (15% mortality). Valganciclovir is a cost-effective and bioavailable oral form of ganciclovir that has been proved effective in both prophylaxis and treatment of CMV disease. Early diagnosis in a febrile patient with clinical suspicion of CMV disease can be made by determining CMV viral load in the blood. A rise in IgM antibodies to CMV is also diagnostic. Culture of CMV from blood may be less sensitive. Tissue invasion of CMV is common in the gastrointestinal tract and lungs. CMV retinopathy occurs late in the course, if untreated. Treatment of active CMV disease with valganciclovir is always indicated. In many patients immune to CMV, viral activation can occur with major immunosuppressive regimens.

The polyoma group (BK, JC, SV40) is another class of DNA viruses that can become dormant in kidneys and can be activated by immunosuppression. When reactivation occurs with BK, there is a 50% chance of progressive fibrosis and loss of the graft within 1 year by the activated virus. Risk of infection is associated with the overall degree of immunosuppression rather than the individual immunosuppressive drugs used. Renal biopsy is necessary for the diagnosis. There have been promising results with leflunomide,

TABLE 282-5 The Most Common Opportunistic Infections in Renal Transplant Recipients

Peritransplant (<1 month)	Late (>6 months)
Wound infections	*Aspergillus*
Herpesvirus	*Nocardia*
Oral candidiasis	BK virus (polyoma)
Urinary tract infection	Herpes zoster
Early (1–6 months)	Hepatitis B
Pneumocystis carinii	Hepatitis C
Cytomegalovirus	
Legionella	
Listeria	
Hepatitis B	
Hepatitis C	

cidofovir, and quinolone anitibiotics (which are effective against polyoma helicase), but it is most important to reduce the immunosuppressive load.

The complications of glucocorticoid therapy are well known and include gastrointestinal bleeding, impairment of wound healing, osteoporosis, diabetes mellitus, cataract formation, and hemorrhagic pancreatitis. The treatment of unexplained jaundice in transplant patients should include cessation or reduction of immunosuppressive drugs if hepatitis or drug toxicity is suspected. Therapy in such circumstances often does not result in rejection of a graft, at least for several weeks. Acyclovir is effective in therapy for herpes simplex virus infections.

CHRONIC LESIONS OF THE TRANSPLANTED KIDNEY

Although 1-year transplant survival is excellent, most recipients experience progressive decline in kidney function over time thereafter. Chronic renal transplant dysfunction can be caused by recurrent disease, hypertension, cyclosporine or tacrolimus nephrotoxicity, chronic immunologic rejection, secondary focal glomerulosclerosis, or a combination of these pathophysiologies. Chronic vascular changes with intimal proliferation and medial hypertrophy are commonly found. Control of systemic and intrarenal hypertension with ACE inhibitors is thought to have a beneficial influence on the rate of progression of chronic renal transplant dysfunction. Renal biopsy can distinguish subacute cellular rejection from recurrent disease or secondary focal sclerosis.

MALIGNANCY

The incidence of tumors in patients on immunosuppressive therapy is 5–6%, or approximately 100 times greater than that in the general population in the same age range. The most common lesions are cancer of the skin and lips and carcinoma in situ of the cervix, as well as lymphomas such as non-Hodgkin's lymphoma. The risks are increased in proportion to the total immunosuppressive load administered and the time elapsed since transplantation. Surveillance for skin and cervical cancers is necessary.

OTHER COMPLICATIONS

Hypercalcemia after transplantation may indicate failure of hyperplastic parathyroid glands to regress. Aseptic necrosis of the head of the femur is probably due to preexisting hyperparathyroidism, with aggravation by glucocorticoid treatment. With improved management of calcium and phosphorus metabolism during chronic dialysis, the incidence of parathyroid-related complications has fallen dramatically. Persistent hyperparathyroid activity may require subtotal parathyroidectomy.

Hypertension may be caused by (1) native kidney disease, (2) rejection activity in the transplant, (3) renal artery stenosis if an end-to-end anastomosis was constructed with an iliac artery branch, and (4) renal calcineurin inhibitor toxicity. This toxicity may improve with reduction in dose. Whereas ACE inhibitors may be useful, calcium channel blockers are more frequently used initially. Amelioration of hypertension to the range of 120–130/70–80 mmHg should be the goal in all patients.

Although most transplant patients have robust production of erythropoietin and normalization of hemoglobin, *anemia* is commonly seen in the posttransplant period. Often the anemia is attributable to bone marrow–suppressant immunosuppressive medications such as azathioprine, mycophenolic acid, and sirolimus. Gastrointestinal bleeding is a common side effect of high-dose and long-term steroid administration. Many transplant patients have creatinine clearances of 30–50 mL/min and can be considered in the same way as other patients with chronic renal insufficiency for anemia management, including supplemental erythropoietin.

Chronic hepatitis, particularly when due to hepatitis B virus, can be a progressive, fatal disease over a decade or so. Patients who are persistently hepatitis B surface antigen–positive are at higher risk, according to some studies, but the presence of hepatitis C virus is also a concern when one embarks on a course of immunosuppression in a transplant recipient.

Both chronic dialysis and renal transplant patients have a higher incidence of death from myocardial infarction and stroke than does the population at large, and this is particularly true in diabetic patients. Contributing factors are the use of glucocorticoids and sirolimus, as well as hypertension. Recipients of renal transplants have a high prevalence of coronary artery and peripheral vascular diseases. The percentage of deaths from these causes has been slowly rising as the numbers of transplanted diabetic patients and the average age of all recipients increase. More than 50% of renal recipient mortality is attributable to cardiovascular disease. In addition to strict control of blood pressure and blood lipid levels, close monitoring of patients for indications of further medical or surgical intervention is an important part of management.

FURTHER READINGS

Chandraker A et al: Transplantation immunobiology, in *Brenner and Rector's The Kidney*, 8th ed, B Brenner (ed). Philadelphia, Saunders, 2008, pp 2101–2126

Denton MD et al: Immunosuppressive strategies in renal transplantation. Lancet 353:1083, 1999

Kawai T et al: HLA-mismatched renal transplantation without maintenance immunosuppression. N Engl J Med 358:353, 2008

Li XC et al: Costimulatory pathways in transplantation: Challenges and new developments. Immunol Rev 229:271, 2009

Mahoney RJ et al: B-cell crossmatching and kidney allograft outcome in 9031 United States transplant recipients. Hum Immunol 63:324, 2002

Pescovitz MD, Govani M: Sirolimus and mycophenolate mofetil for calcineurin-free immunosuppression in renal transplant recipients. Am J Kidney Dis 38:S16, 2001

Sayegh MH, Carpenter CB: Transplantation 50 years later—progress, challenges and promises. N Engl J Med 351:2761, 2004

Vicenti F, Kirk AD: What's next in the pipeline. Am J Transplant 8:1972, 2008

Vo AA et al: Rituximab and intravenous immune globulin for desensitization during renal transplantation. N Engl J Med 359:242, 2008

CHAPTER 283 Glomerular Diseases

Julia B. Lewis
Eric G. Neilson

Two human kidneys harbor nearly 1.8 million glomerular capillary tufts. Each glomerular tuft resides within Bowman's space. The capsule circumscribing this space is lined by parietal epithelial cells that transition into tubular epithelia forming the proximal nephron or migrate into the tuft to replenish podocytes. The glomerular capillary tuft derives from an afferent arteriole that forms a branching capillary bed embedded in mesangial matrix (Fig. 283-1). This capillary network funnels into an efferent arteriole, which passes filtered blood into cortical peritubular capillaries or medullary vasa recta that supply and exchange with a folded tubular architecture. Hence the glomerular capillary tuft, fed and drained by arterioles, represents an arteriolar portal system. Fenestrated endothelial cells resting on a glomerular basement membrane (GBM) line glomerular capillaries. Delicate foot processes extending from epithelial podocytes shroud the outer surface of these capillaries, and podocytes interconnect to each other by slit-pore membranes forming a selective filtration barrier.

The glomerular capillaries filter 120–180 L/d of plasma water containing various solutes for reclamation or discharge by downstream tubules. Most large proteins and all cells are excluded from filtration by a physicochemical barrier governed by pore size and negative electrostatic charge. The mechanics of filtration and reclamation are quite complicated for many solutes (Chap. 271). For example, in the case of serum albumin, the glomerulus is an imperfect barrier. Although albumin has a negative charge, which would tend to repel the negatively charged GBM, it only has a physical radius of 3.6 nm, while pores in the GBM and slit-pore membranes have a radius of 4 nm. Consequently, variable amounts of albumin inevitably cross the filtration barrier to be reclaimed by megalin and cubilin receptors along the proximal tubule. Remarkably, humans with normal nephrons do not excrete more than 8–10 mg of albumin in daily voided urine, approximately 20–60% of total excreted protein. This amount of albumin, and other proteins, can rise to gram quantities following glomerular injury.

The breadth of diseases affecting the glomerulus is expansive because the glomerular capillaries can be injured in a variety of ways, producing many different lesions and several unique changes

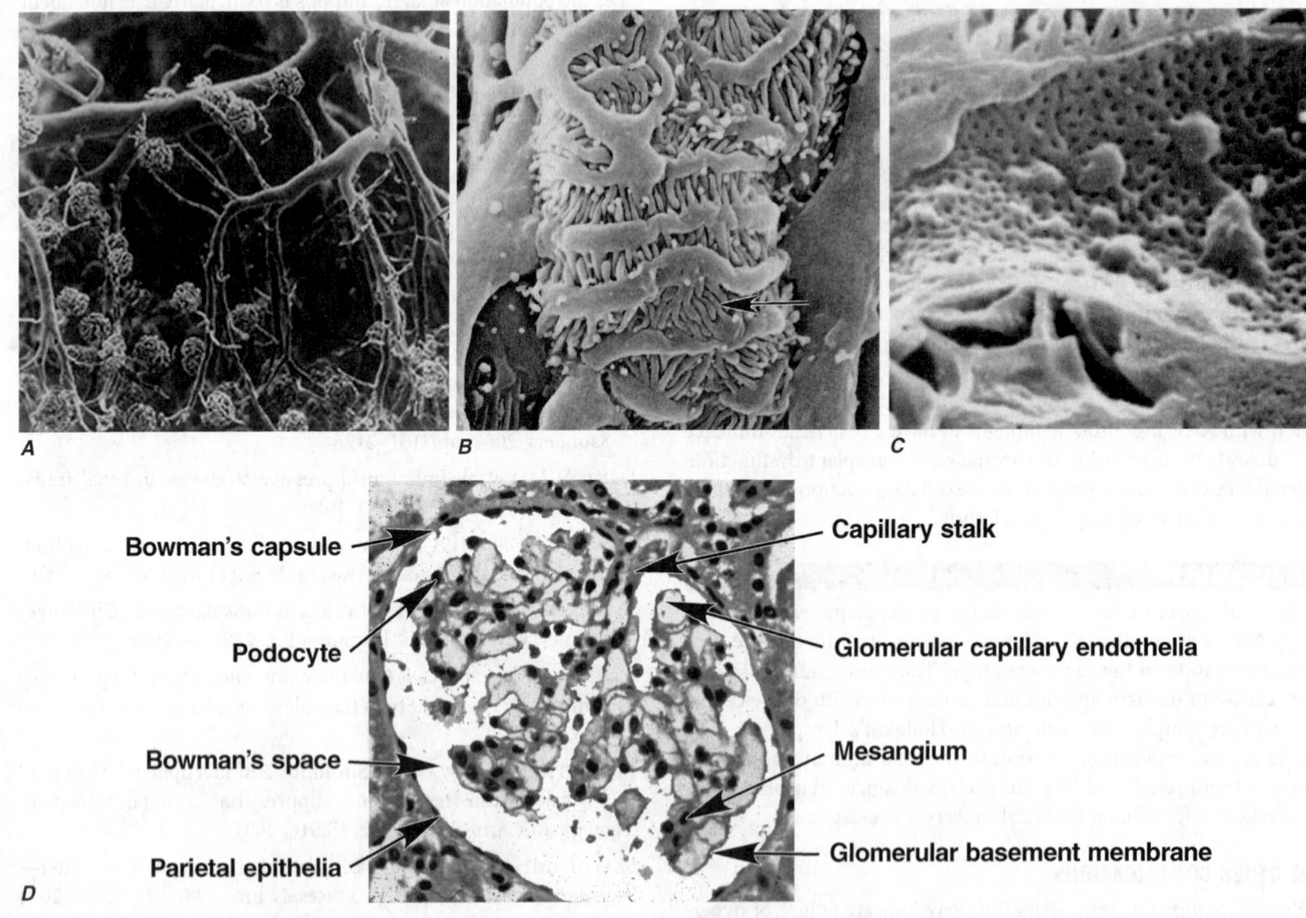

Figure 283-1 Glomerular architecture. ***A.*** The glomerular capillaries form from a branching network of renal arteries, arterioles, leading to an afferent arteriole, glomerular capillary bed (tuft), and a draining efferent arteriole. *(From VH Gattone II et al: Hypertension 5:8, 1983.)* ***B.*** Scanning electron micrograph of podocytes that line the outer surface of the glomerular capillaries (*arrow* shows foot process). ***C.*** Scanning electron micrograph of the fenestrated endothelia lining the glomerular capillary. ***D.*** The various normal regions of the glomerulus on light microscopy *(A–C, courtesy of Dr. Vincent Gattone, Indiana University; with permission).*

to urinalysis. Some order to this vast subject is brought by grouping all of these diseases into a smaller number of clinical syndromes.

PATHOGENESIS OF GLOMERULAR DISEASE

There are many forms of glomerular disease with pathogenesis variably linked to the presence of genetic mutations, infection, toxin exposure, autoimmunity, atherosclerosis, hypertension, emboli, thrombosis, or diabetes mellitus. Even after careful study, however, the cause often remains unknown, and the lesion is called *idiopathic.* Specific or unique features of pathogenesis are mentioned with the description of each of the glomerular diseases later in this chapter.

Some glomerular diseases result from genetic mutations producing familial disease or a founder effect: congenital nephrotic syndrome from mutations in *NPHS1* (nephrin) and *NPHS2* (podocin) affect the slit-pore membrane at birth, and *TRPC6* cation channel mutations produce *focal segmental glomerulosclerosis (FSGS)* in adulthood; polymorphisms in the gene encoding apolipoprotein L1, *APOL1* are a major risk for nearly 70% of African Americans with nondiabetic end-stage renal disease (ESRD), particularly FSGS; mutations in complement factor H associate with *membranoproliferative glomerulonephritis (MPGN)* or *atypical hemolytic uremic syndrome (aHUS),* type II partial lipodystrophy from mutations in genes encoding lamin A/C, or PPARγ cause a metabolic syndrome associated with MPGN, which is sometimes accompanied by dense deposits and C3 nephritic factor; Alport's syndrome, from mutations in the genes encoding for the α3, α4, or α5 chains of type IV collagen, produces *split-basement membranes* with *glomerulosclerosis;* and lysosomal storage diseases, such as α-galactosidase A deficiency causing Fabry's disease and *N*-acetylneuraminic acid hydrolase deficiency causing nephrosialidosis, produce FSGS.

Systemic hypertension and atherosclerosis can produce pressure stress, ischemia, or lipid oxidants that lead to *chronic glomerulosclerosis. Malignant hypertension* can quickly complicate glomerulosclerosis with fibrinoid necrosis of arterioles and glomeruli, thrombotic microangiopathy, and acute renal failure. *Diabetic nephropathy* is an acquired sclerotic injury associated with thickening of the GBM secondary to the long-standing effects of hyperglycemia, advanced glycosylation end products, and reactive oxygen species.

Inflammation of the glomerular capillaries is called *glomerulonephritis.* Most glomerular or mesangial antigens involved in *immune-mediated glomerulonephritis* are unknown (Fig. 283-2). Glomerular epithelial or mesangial cells may shed or express epitopes that mimic other immunogenic proteins made elsewhere in the body. Bacteria, fungi, and viruses can directly infect the kidney producing their own antigens. Autoimmune diseases like idiopathic *membranous glomerulonephritis (MGN)* or MPGN are confined to the kidney, while systemic inflammatory diseases like *lupus nephritis* or *granulomatosis with polyangiitis (Wegener's)* spread to the kidney, causing secondary glomerular injury. *Antiglomerular basement membrane disease* producing Goodpasture's syndrome primarily injures both the lung and kidney because of the narrow distribution of the α3 NC1 domain of type IV collagen that is the target antigen.

Local activation of Toll-like receptors on glomerular cells, deposition of immune complexes, or complement injury to glomerular structures induces mononuclear cell infiltration, which subsequently leads to an adaptive immune response attracted to the kidney by local release of chemokines. Neutrophils, macrophages, and T cells are drawn by chemokines into the glomerular tuft, where they react with antigens and epitopes on or near somatic cells or their structures, producing more cytokines and proteases that damage the mesangium, capillaries, and/or the GBM. While the adaptive immune response is similar to that of other tissues, early T cell activation plays an important role in the mechanism of glomerulonephritis. Antigens presented by class II major histocompatibility complex (MHC) molecules on macrophages and dendritic cells in conjunction with associative recognition molecules engage the CD4/8 T cell repertoire.

Mononuclear cells by themselves can injure the kidney, but autoimmune events that damage glomeruli classically produce a humoral immune response. *Poststreptococcal glomerulonephritis, lupus nephritis,* and idiopathic *membranous nephritis* typically are associated with immune deposits along the GBM, while anti-GBM antibodies produce the linear binding of anti-GBM disease. Preformed circulating immune complexes can precipitate along the subendothelial side of the GBM, while other immune deposits form in situ on the subepithelial side. These latter deposits accumulate when circulating autoantibodies find their antigen trapped along the subepithelial edge of the GBM. Immune deposits in the glomerular mesangium may result from the deposition of preformed circulating complexes or in situ antigen-antibody interactions. Immune deposits stimulate the release of local proteases and activate the complement cascade, producing C_{5-9} attack complexes. In addition, local oxidants damage glomerular structures, producing proteinuria and effacement of the podocytes. Overlapping etiologies or pathophysiologic mechanisms can produce similar glomerular lesions, suggesting that downstream molecular and cellular responses often converge toward common patterns of injury.

PROGRESSION OF GLOMERULAR DISEASE

Persistent glomerulonephritis that worsens renal function is always accompanied by interstitial nephritis, renal fibrosis, and tubular atrophy (Fig. e14-27). What is not so obvious, however, is that renal failure in glomerulonephritis best correlates histologically with the appearance of tubulointerstitial nephritis rather than with the type of inciting glomerular injury.

Loss of renal function due to interstitial damage is explained hypothetically by several mechanisms. The simplest explanation is that urine flow is impeded by tubular obstruction as a result of interstitial inflammation and fibrosis. Thus, obstruction of the tubules with debris or by extrinsic compression results in aglomerular nephrons. A second mechanism suggests that interstitial changes, including interstitial edema or fibrosis, alter tubular and vascular architecture and thereby compromise the normal tubular transport of solutes and water from tubular lumen to vascular space. This failure increases the solute and water content of the tubule fluid, resulting in isosthenuria and polyuria. Adaptive mechanisms related to tubuloglomerular feedback also fail, resulting in a reduction of renin output from the juxtaglomerular apparatus trapped by interstitial inflammation. Consequently, the local vasoconstrictive influence of angiotensin II on the glomerular arterioles decreases, and filtration drops owing to a generalized decrease in arteriolar tone. A third mechanism involves changes in vascular resistance due to damage of peritubular capillaries. The cross-sectional volume of these capillaries is decreased by interstitial inflammation, edema, or fibrosis. These structural alterations in vascular resistance affect renal function through two mechanisms. First, tubular cells are very metabolically active, and, as a result, decreased perfusion leads to ischemic injury. Second, impairment of glomerular arteriolar outflow leads to increased intraglomerular hypertension in less-involved glomeruli; this selective intraglomerular hypertension aggravates and extends *mesangial sclerosis* and *glomerulosclerosis* to less-involved glomeruli. Regardless of the exact mechanism, early *acute tubulointerstitial nephritis* (Fig. e14-27) suggests potentially recoverable renal function, while the development of *chronic interstitial fibrosis* prognosticates permanent loss (Fig. e14-30).

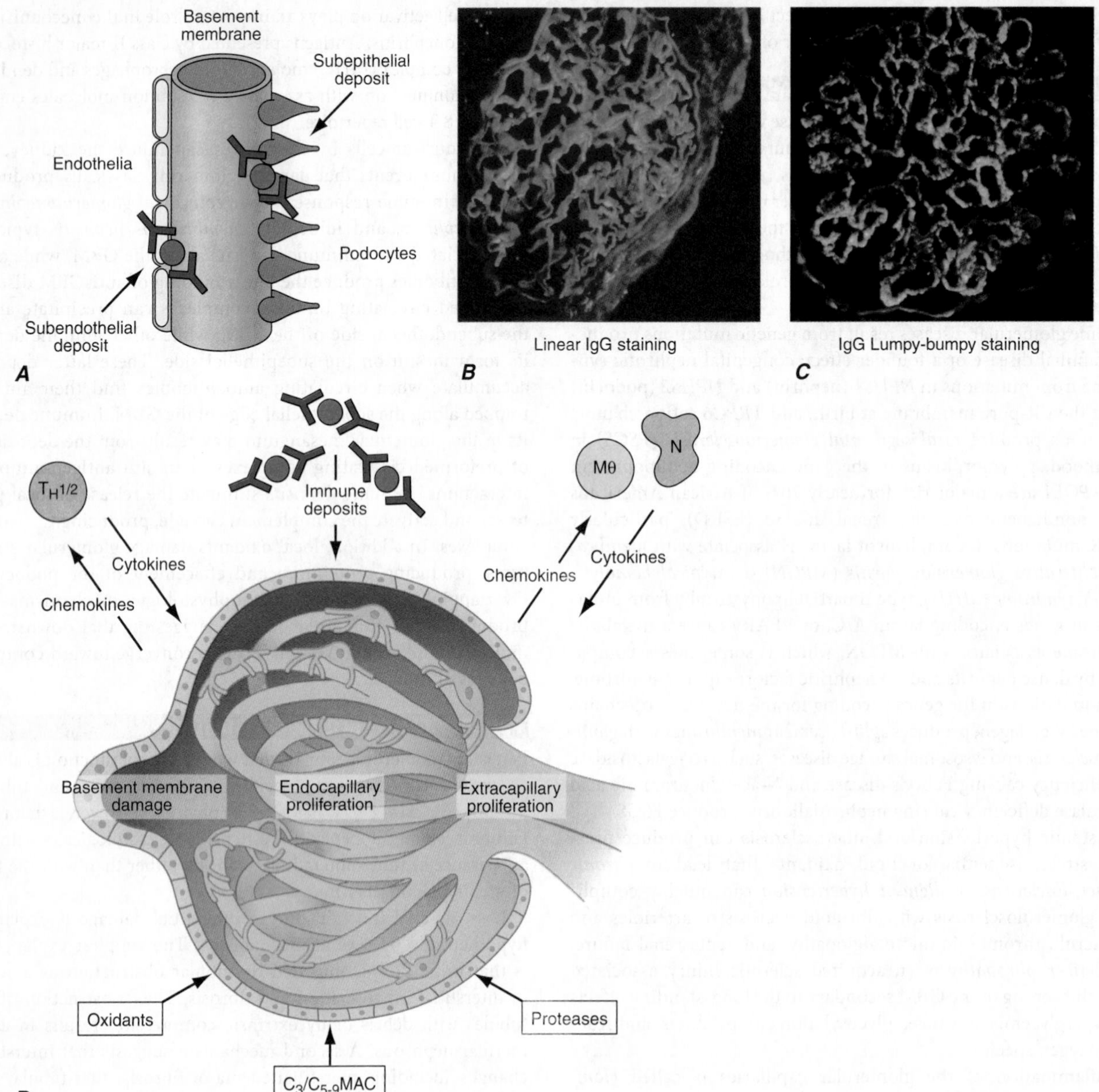

Figure 283-2 The glomerulus is injured by a variety of mechanisms. ***A.*** Preformed immune deposits can precipitate from the circulation and collect along the glomerular basement membrane (GBM) in the subendothelial space or can form in situ along the subepithelial space. ***B.*** Immunofluorescent staining of glomeruli with labeled anti-IgG demonstrating linear staining from a patient with anti-GBM disease or immune deposits from a patient with membranous glomerulonephritis. ***C.*** The mechanisms of glomerular injury have a complicated pathogenesis. Immune deposits and complement deposition classically draw macrophages and neutrophils into the glomerulus. T lymphocytes may follow to participate in the injury pattern as well. ***D.*** Amplification mediators as locally derived oxidants and proteases expand this inflammation, and, depending on the location of the target antigen and the genetic polymorphisms of the host, basement membranes are damaged with either endocapillary or extracapillary proliferation.

Persistent damage to glomerular capillaries spreads to the tubulointerstitium in association with proteinuria. There is an untested hypothesis that efferent arterioles leading from inflamed glomeruli carry forward inflammatory mediators, which induces downstream interstitial nephritis, resulting in fibrosis. Glomerular filtrate from injured glomerular capillaries adherent to Bowman's capsule may also be misdirected to the periglomerular interstitium. Most nephrologists believe, however, that proteinuric glomerular filtrate forming tubular fluid is the primary route to downstream tubulointerstitial injury, although none of these hypotheses are mutually exclusive.

The simplest explanation for the effect of proteinuria on the development of interstitial nephritis is that increasingly severe proteinuria, carrying activated cytokines and lipoproteins producing reactive oxygen species, triggers a downstream inflammatory cascade in and around epithelial cells lining the tubular nephron. These effects induce T lymphocyte and macrophage infiltrates in the interstitial spaces along with fibrosis and tubular atrophy.

Tubules disaggregate following direct damage to their basement membranes, leading to epithelial-mesenchymal transitions forming more interstitial fibroblasts at the site of injury. Transforming growth factor β (TGF-β), fibroblast growth factor 2 (FGF-2), hypoxemia-inducible factor 1α (HIF-1α), and platelet-derived growth factor (PDGF) are particularly active in this transition. With persistent nephritis, fibroblasts multiply and lay down tenascin and a fibronectin scaffold for the polymerization of new interstitial collagen types I/III. These events form scar tissue through a process called fibrogenesis. In experimental studies, bone morphogenetic protein 7 and hepatocyte growth factor can reverse early fibrogenesis and preserve tubular architecture. When fibroblasts outdistance their survival factors, apoptoses occurs, and the permanent renal scar becomes acellular, leading to irreversible renal failure.

APPROACH TO THE PATIENT Glomerular Disease

HEMATURIA, PROTEINURIA, AND PYURIA Patients with glomerular disease usually have some hematuria with varying degrees of proteinuria. Hematuria is typically asymptomatic. As few as three to five red blood cells in the spun sediment from first-voided morning urine is suspicious. The diagnosis of glomerular injury can be delayed because patients will not realize they have *microscopic hematuria,* and only rarely with the exception of IgA nephropathy and sickle cell disease is *gross hematuria* present. When working up microscopic hematuria, perhaps accompanied by minimal proteinuria (<500 mg/24 h), it is important to exclude anatomic lesions, such as malignancy of the urinary tract, particularly in older men. Microscopic hematuria may also appear with the onset of benign prostatic hypertrophy, interstitial nephritis, papillary necrosis, hypercalciuria, renal stones, cystic kidney diseases, or renal vascular injury. However, when red blood cell casts (Fig. e14-34) or dysmorphic red blood cells are found in the sediment, glomerulonephritis is likely.

Sustained proteinuria >1–2 g/24 h is also commonly associated with glomerular disease. Patients often will not know they have proteinuria unless they become edematous or notice foaming urine on voiding. *Sustained proteinuria* has to be distinguished from lesser amounts of so-called *benign proteinuria* in the normal population (Table 283-1). This latter class of proteinuria is nonsustained, generally <1 g/24 h, and is sometimes called *functional* or *transient proteinuria.* Fever, exercise, obesity, sleep apnea, emotional stress, and congestive heart failure can explain transient proteinuria. Proteinuria only seen with upright posture is called *orthostatic proteinuria* and has a benign prognosis. Isolated proteinuria sustained over multiple clinic visits is found in diabetic nephropathy, *nil lesion, mesangioproliferative glomerulonephritis,* and FSGS. Proteinuria in most adults with glomerular disease is *nonselective,* containing albumin and a mixture of other serum proteins, while in children with nil lesion from *minimal change disease,* the proteinuria is *selective* and composed largely of albumin.

Some patients with inflammatory glomerular disease, such as acute poststreptococcal glomerulonephritis or MPGN, have *pyuria* characterized by the presence of considerable numbers of leukocytes. This latter finding has to be distinguished from urine infected with bacteria.

CLINICAL SYNDROMES Various forms of glomerular injury can also be parsed into several distinct syndromes on clinical grounds (Table 283-2). These syndromes, however, are not always mutually exclusive. There is an *acute nephritic syndrome* producing 1–2 g/24 h of proteinuria, hematuria with red blood cell casts, pyuria, hypertension, fluid retention, and a rise in serum creatinine associated with a reduction in glomerular filtration. If glomerular inflammation develops slowly, the serum creatinine will rise gradually over many weeks, but if the serum creatinine rises quickly, particularly over a few days, acute nephritis is sometimes called *rapidly progressive glomerulonephritis* (RPGN); the histopathologic term *crescentic glomerulonephritis* is the pathologic equivalent of the clinical presentation of RPGN. When patients with RPGN present with lung hemorrhage from Goodpasture's syndrome, antineutrophil cytoplasmic antibodies (ANCA)-associated small-vessel vasculitis, lupus erythematosus, or cryoglobulinemia, they are often diagnosed as having a *pulmonary-renal syndrome. Nephrotic syndrome* describes the onset of heavy proteinuria (>3.0 g/24 h), hypertension, hypercholesterolemia, hypoalbuminemia, edema/anasarca, and microscopic hematuria; if only large amounts of proteinuria are present without clinical manifestations, the condition is sometimes called *nephrotic-range proteinuria.* The glomerular filtration rate (GFR) in these patients may initially be normal or, rarely, higher than normal, but with persistent hyperfiltration and continued nephron loss, it typically declines over months to years. Patients with a *basement membrane syndrome* either have genetically abnormal basement membranes (Alport's syndrome) or an autoimmune response to basement membrane collagen IV (Goodpasture's syndrome) associated with microscopic hematuria, mild to heavy proteinuria, and hypertension with variable elevations in serum creatinine. *Glomerular-vascular syndrome* describes patients with vascular injury producing hematuria and moderate proteinuria. Affected individuals can have vasculitis, thrombotic microangiopathy, antiphospholipid syndrome, or, more commonly, a systemic disease such as atherosclerosis, cholesterol emboli, hypertension, sickle cell anemia, and autoimmunity. *Infectious disease-associated syndrome* is most important if one has an international perspective. Save for subacute bacterial endocarditis in the Western Hemisphere, malaria and schistosomiasis may be the most common causes of glomerulonephritis throughout the world, closely followed by HIV and chronic hepatitis B and C. These infectious diseases produce a variety of inflammatory reactions in glomerular capillaries, ranging from nephrotic syndrome to acute nephritic injury, and urinalyses that demonstrate a combination of hematuria and proteinuria.

These six general categories of syndromes are usually determined at the bedside with the help of a history and physical examination, blood chemistries, renal ultrasound, and urinalysis. These initial studies help frame further diagnostic workup that typically involves some testing of the serum for the presence of various proteins (HIV and hepatitis B and C antigens), antibodies [anti-GBM, antiphospholipid, antistreptolysin O (ASO), anti-DNAse, antihyaluronidase, ANCA, anti-DNA, cryoglobulins, anti-HIV, and anti-hepatitis B and C antibodies] or depletion of complement components (C_3 and C_4). The bedside history and physical examination can also help determine whether the glomerulonephritis is isolated to the kidney (*primary glomerulonephritis*) or is part of a systemic disease (*secondary glomerulonephritis*).

TABLE 283-1 Urine Assays for Albuminuria/Proteinuria

	24-Hour Albumin[a] (mg/24 h)	Albumin[a]/ Creatinine Ratio (mg/g)	Dipstick Proteinuria	24-Hour Urine Protein[b] (mg/24 h)
Normal	8–10	<30	–	<150
Microalbuminuria	30–300	30–300	–/Trace/1+	–
Proteinuria	>300	>300	Trace–3+	>150

[a]Albumin detected by radioimmunoassay.
[b]Albumin represents 30–70% of the total protein excreted in the urine.

TABLE 283-2 Patterns of Clinical Glomerulonephritis

Glomerular Syndromes	Proteinuria	Hematuria	Vascular Injury
Acute Nephritic Syndromes			
Poststreptococcal glomerulonephritis[a]	+/++	++/+++	–
Subacute bacterial endocarditis[a]	+/++	++	–
Lupus nephritis[a]	+/++	++/+++	–
Antiglomerular basement membrane disease[a]	++	++/+++	–
IgA nephropathy[a]	+/++	++/+++[c]	–
ANCA small-vessel vasculitis[a]			
Granulomatosis with polyangiitis (Wegener's)	+/++	++/+++	++++
Microscopic polyangiitis	+/++	++/+++	++++
Churg-Strauss syndrome	+/++	++/+++	++++
Henoch-Schönlein purpura[a]	+/++	++/+++	++++
Cryoglobulinemia[a]	+/++	++/+++	++++
Membranoproliferative glomerulonephritis[a]	++	++/+++	–
Mesangioproliferative glomerulonephritis	+	+/++	–
Pulmonary-Renal Syndromes			
Goodpasture's syndrome[a]	++	++/+++	–
ANCA small-vessel vasculitis[a]			
Granulomatosis with polyangiitis (Wegener's)	+/++	++/+++	++++
Microscopic polyangiitis	+/++	++/+++	++++
Churg-Strauss syndrome	+/++	++/+++	++++
Henoch-Schönlein purpura[a]	+/++	++/+++	++++
Cryoglobulinemia[a]	+/++	++/+++	++++
Nephrotic Syndromes			
Minimal change disease	++++	–	–
Focal segmental glomerulosclerosis	+++/++++	+	–
Membranous glomerulonephritis	++++	+	–
Diabetic nephropathy	++/++++	–/+	–
AL and AA amyloidosis	+++/++++	+	+/++
Light-chain deposition disease	+++	+	–
Fibrillary-immunotactoid disease	+++/++++	+	+
Fabry's disease	+	+	–
Basement Membrane Syndromes			
Anti-GBM disease[a]	++	++/+++	–
Alport's syndrome	++	++	–
Thin basement membrane disease	+	++	–
Nail-patella syndrome	++/+++	++	–
Glomerular Vascular Syndromes			
Atherosclerotic nephropathy	+	+	+++
Hypertensive nephropathy[b]	+/++	+/++	++
Cholesterol emboli	+/++	++	+++
Sickle cell disease	+/++	++[c]	+++
Thrombotic microangiopathies	++	++	+++
Antiphospholipid syndrome	++	++	+++

(continued)

TABLE 283-2 Patterns of Clinical Glomerulonephritis (*Continued*)

Glomerular Syndromes	Proteinuria	Hematuria	Vascular Injury
ANCA small-vessel vasculitis[a]			
Granulomatosis with polyangiitis (Wegener's)	+/++	++/+++	++++
Microscopic polyangiitis	+/++	++/+++	++++
Churg-Strauss syndrome	+++	++/+++	++++
Henoch-Schönlein purpura[a]	+/++	++/+++	++++
Cryoglobulinemia[a]	+/++	++/+++	++++
AL and AA amyloidosis	+++/++++	+	+/++
Infectious Disease–Associated Syndromes			
Poststreptococcal glomerulonephritis[a]	+/++	++/+++	–
Subacute bacterial endocarditis[a]	+/++	++	–
HIV	+++	+/++	–
Hepatitis B and C	+++	+/++	–
Syphilis	+++	+	–
Leprosy	+++	+	–
Malaria	+++	+/++	–
Schistosomiasis	+++	+/++	–

[a]Can present as rapidly progressive glomerulonephritis (RPGN); sometimes called crescentic glomerulonephritis.
[b]Can present as a malignant hypertensive crisis producing an aggressive fibrinoid necrosis in arterioles and small arteries with microangiopathic hemolytic anemia.
[c]Can present with gross hematuria.
Abbreviations: AA, amyloid A; AL, amyloid L; ANCA, antineutrophil cytoplasmic antibodies; GBM, glomerular basement membrane.

When confronted with an abnormal urinalysis and elevated serum creatinine, with or without edema or congestive heart failure, one must consider whether the glomerulonephritis is *acute* or *chronic.* This assessment is best made by careful history (last known urinalysis or serum creatinine during pregnancy or insurance physical, evidence of infection, or use of medication or recreational drugs); the size of the kidneys on renal ultrasound examination; and how the patient feels at presentation. Chronic glomerular disease often presents with decreased kidney size. Patients who quickly develop renal failure are fatigued and weak; feel miserable; often have uremic symptoms associated with nausea, vomiting, fluid retention, and somnolence. Primary glomerulonephritis presenting with renal failure that has progressed slowly, however, can be remarkably asymptomatic, as are patients with acute glomerulonephritis without much loss in renal function. Once this initial information is collected, selected patients who are clinically stable, have adequate blood clotting parameters, and are willing and able to receive treatment are encouraged to have a renal biopsy. Biopsies can be done safely with an ultrasound-guided biopsy gun.

RENAL PATHOLOGY

A renal biopsy in the setting of glomerulonephritis quickly identifies the type of glomerular injury and often suggests a course of treatment. The biopsy is processed for light microscopy using stains for *hematoxylin and eosin (H&E)* to assess cellularity and architecture, *periodic acid–Schiff (PAS)* to stain carbohydrate moieties in the membranes of the glomerular tuft and tubules, *Jones-methenamine silver* to enhance basement membrane structure, *Congo red* for amyloid deposits, and *Masson's trichrome* to identify collagen deposition and assess the degree of glomerulosclerosis and interstitial fibrosis. Biopsies are also processed for direct immunofluorescence using conjugated antibodies against IgG, IgM, and IgA to detect the presence of "lumpy-bumpy" immune deposits or "linear" IgG or IgA antibodies bound to GBM, antibodies against trapped complement proteins (C_3 and C_4), or specific antibodies against a relevant antigen. High-resolution electron microscopy can clarify the principal location of immune deposits and the status of the basement membrane.

Each region of a renal biopsy is assessed separately. By light microscopy, glomeruli (at least 10 and ideally 20) are reviewed individually for discrete lesions; <50% involvement is considered *focal,* and >50% is *diffuse.* Injury in each glomerular tuft can be *segmental,* involving a portion of the tuft, or *global,* involving most of the glomerulus. Glomeruli having *proliferative* characteristics show increased cellularity. When cells in the capillary tuft proliferate, it is called *endocapillary,* and when cellular proliferation extends into Bowman's space, it is called *extracapillary. Synechiae* are formed when epithelial podocytes attach to Bowman's capsule in the setting of glomerular injury; *crescents,* which in some cases may be the extension of synechiae, develop when fibrocellular/fibrin collections fill all or part of Bowman's space; and *sclerotic* glomeruli show acellular, amorphous accumulations of proteinaceous material throughout the tuft with loss of functional capillaries and normal mesangium. Since *age-related glomerulosclerosis* is common in adults, one can estimate the background percentage of sclerosis by dividing the patient's age in half and subtracting 10. Immunofluorescent and electron microscopy can detect the presence and location of *subepithelial, subendothelial,* or *mesangial* immune deposits, or *reduplication* or *splitting* of the basement membrane. In the other regions of the biopsy, the vasculature surrounding glomeruli and tubules can show *angiopathy, vasculitis,* the presence of *fibrils*, or *thrombi*. The tubules can be assessed for adjacency to one another; separation can be the result of edema, tubular dropout, or collagen deposition resulting from interstitial fibrosis. Interstitial fibrosis is an ominous sign of irreversibility and progression to renal failure.

ACUTE NEPHRITIC SYNDROMES

Acute nephritic syndromes classically present with hypertension, hematuria, red blood cell casts, pyuria, and mild to moderate proteinuria. Extensive inflammatory damage to glomeruli causes a fall in GFR and eventually produces uremic symptoms with salt and water retention, leading to edema and hypertension.

POSTSTREPTOCOCCAL GLOMERULONEPHRITIS

Poststreptococcal glomerulonephritis is prototypical for *acute endocapillary proliferative glomerulonephritis.* The incidence of poststreptococcal glomerulonephritis has dramatically decreased in developed countries and in these locations is typically sporadic; epidemics are less common. Acute poststreptococcal glomerulonephritis in underdeveloped countries usually affects children between the ages of 2 and 14 years, but in developed countries is more typical in the elderly, especially in association with debilitating conditions. It is more common in males, and the familial or cohabitant incidence is as high as 40%. Skin and throat infections with particular M types of streptococci (nephritogenic strains) antedate glomerular disease; M types 47, 49, 55, 2, 60, and 57 are seen following impetigo and M types 1, 2, 4, 3, 25, 49, and 12 with pharyngitis. Poststreptococcal glomerulonephritis due to impetigo develops 2–6 weeks after skin infection and 1–3 weeks after streptococcal pharyngitis.

The renal biopsy in poststreptococcal glomerulonephritis demonstrates hypercellularity of mesangial and endothelial cells, glomerular infiltrates of polymorphonuclear leukocytes, granular subendothelial immune deposits of IgG, IgM, C_3, C_4, and C_{5-9}, and subepithelial deposits (which appear as "humps") (Fig. e14-6). (See Glomerular Schematic 1.) Poststreptococcal glomerulonephritis is an immune-mediated disease involving putative streptococcal antigens, circulating immune complexes, and activation of complement in association with cell-mediated injury. Many candidate antigens have been proposed over the years; candidates from nephritogenic streptococci of interest at the moment are: a cationic cysteine proteinase known as streptococcal pyrogenic exotoxin B (SPEB) that is generated by proteolysis of a zymogen precursor (zSPEB) and, NAPlr, the nephritis-associated plasmin receptor. These two antigens have biochemical affinity for plasmin, bind as complexes facilitated by this relationship, and both activate the alternate complement pathway. The nephritogenic antigen, SPEB, has been demonstrated inside the subepithelial "humps" on biopsy.

The classic presentation is an acute nephritic picture with hematuria, pyuria, red blood cell casts, edema, hypertension, and oliguric renal failure, which may be severe enough to appear as RPGN. Systemic symptoms of headache, malaise, anorexia, and flank pain (due to swelling of the renal capsule) are reported in as many as 50% of cases. Five percent of children and 20% of adults have proteinuria in the nephrotic range. In the first week of symptoms, 90% of patients will have a depressed CH_{50} and decreased levels of C_3 with normal levels of C_4. Positive rheumatoid factor (30–40%), cryoglobulins and circulating immune complexes (60–70%), and ANCA against myeloperoxidase (10%) are also reported. Positive cultures for streptococcal infection are inconsistently present (10–70%), but increased titers of ASO (30%), anti-DNAse, (70%), or antihyaluronidase antibodies (40%) can help confirm the diagnosis. Consequently, the diagnosis of poststreptococcal glomerulonephritis rarely requires a renal biopsy. A subclinical disease is reported in some series to be four to five times as common as clinical nephritis, and these latter cases are characterized by asymptomatic microscopic hematuria with low serum C_3 complement levels.

Treatment is supportive, with control of hypertension, edema, and dialysis as needed. Antibiotic treatment for streptococcal infection should be given to all patients and their cohabitants. There is no role for immunosuppressive therapy, even in the setting of crescents. Recurrent poststreptococcal glomerulonephritis is rare despite repeated streptococcal infections. Early death is rare in children but does occur in the elderly. Overall, the prognosis is good, with permanent renal failure being very uncommon, less than 1% in children. Complete resolution of the hematuria and proteinuria in the majority of children occurs within 3–6 weeks of the onset of nephritis but 3–10% of children may have persistent microscopic hematuria, non-nephrotic proteinuria, or hypertension. The prognosis in elderly patients is worse with a high incidence of azotemia (up to 60%), nephrotic-range proteinuria, and end-stage renal disease.

Glomerular schematic 1

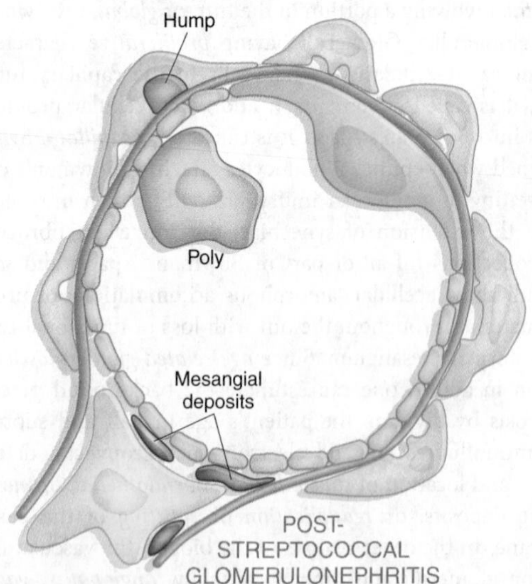

SUBACUTE BACTERIAL ENDOCARDITIS

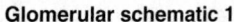

Endocarditis-associated glomerulonephritis is typically a complication of subacute bacterial endocarditis, particularly in patients who remain untreated for a long time, have negative blood cultures, or have right-sided endocarditis. Glomerulonephritis is unusual in acute bacterial endocarditis because it takes 10–14 days to develop immune complex–mediated injury, by which time the patient has been treated, often with emergent surgery. Grossly, the kidneys in subacute bacterial endocarditis have subcapsular hemorrhages with a "flea-bitten" appearance, and microscopy on renal biopsy reveals focal proliferation around foci of necrosis associated with abundant mesangial, subendothelial, and subepithelial immune deposits of IgG, IgM, and C_3. Patients who present with a clinical picture of RPGN have crescents. Embolic infarcts or septic abscesses may also be present. The pathogenesis hinges on the renal deposition of circulating immune complexes in the kidney with complement activation. Patients present with gross or microscopic hematuria, pyuria, and mild proteinuria or, less commonly, RPGN with rapid loss of renal function. A normocytic anemia, elevated erythrocyte sedimentation rate, hypocomplementemia, high titers of rheumatoid factor, type III cryoglobulins, and circulating immune complexes are often present. Levels of serum creatinine may be elevated at diagnosis, but with modern therapy there is little progression to chronic renal failure. Primary treatment is eradication of the infection with 4–6 weeks of antibiotics, and if accomplished expeditiously, the prognosis for renal recovery is good. ANCA-associated vasculitis sometimes accompanies or is confused with subacute bacterial endocarditis (SBE) and should be ruled out, as the treatment is different.

As variants of persistent bacterial infection in blood, glomerulonephritis can occur in patients with ventriculoatrial and ventriculoperitoneal shunts; pulmonary, intraabdominal, pelvic, or cutaneous infections; and infected vascular prostheses. The clinical presentation of these conditions is variable and includes proteinuria, microscopic hematuria, and acute renal failure. Blood cultures are usually positive and serum complement levels low, and there may be elevated levels of C-reactive proteins, rheumatoid factor, antinuclear antibodies, and cryoglobulins. Renal lesions include membranoproliferative glomerulonephritis (MPGN), diffuse proliferative glomerulonephritis (DPGN), or mesangioproliferative glomerulonephritis, sometimes leading to RPGN. Treatment focuses on eradicating the infection, with most patients treated as if they have endocarditis.

LUPUS NEPHRITIS

Lupus nephritis is a common and serious complication of systemic lupus erythematosus (SLE) and most severe in African-American female adolescents. Thirty to fifty percent of patients will have clinical manifestations of renal disease at the time of diagnosis, and 60% of adults and 80% of children develop renal abnormalities at some point in the course of their disease. Lupus nephritis results from the deposition of circulating immune complexes, which activate the complement cascade leading to complement-mediated damage, leukocyte infiltration, activation of procoagulant factors, and release of various cytokines. In situ immune complex formation following glomerular binding of nuclear antigens, particularly necrotic nucleosomes, also plays a role in renal injury. The presence of antiphospholipid antibodies may also trigger a thrombotic microangiopathy in a minority of patients.

The clinical manifestations, course of disease, and treatment of lupus nephritis are closely linked to renal pathology. The most common clinical sign of renal disease is proteinuria, but hematuria, hypertension, varying degrees of renal failure, and active urine sediment with red blood cell casts can all be present. Although significant renal pathology can be found on biopsy even in the absence of major abnormalities in the urinalysis, most nephrologists do not biopsy patients until the urinalysis is convincingly abnormal. The extrarenal manifestations of lupus are important in establishing a firm diagnosis of systemic lupus because, while serologic abnormalities are common in lupus nephritis, they are not diagnostic. Anti-dsDNA antibodies that fix complement correlate best with the presence of renal disease. Hypocomplementemia is common in patients with acute lupus nephritis (70–90%) and declining complement levels may herald a flare. Although urinary biomarkers of lupus nephritis are being identified to assist in predicting renal flares, renal biopsy is the only reliable method of identifying the morphologic variants of lupus nephritis.

The World Health Organization (WHO) workshop in 1974 first outlined several distinct patterns of lupus-related glomerular injury; these were modified in 1982. In 2004 the International Society of Nephrology in conjunction with the Renal Pathology Society again updated the classification. This latest version of lesions seen on biopsy (Table 283-3) best defines clinicopathologic correlations, provides valuable prognostic information, and forms the basis for modern treatment recommendations. Class I nephritis describes normal glomerular histology by any technique or normal light microscopy with minimal mesangial deposits on immunofluorescent or electron microscopy. Class II designates mesangial immune complexes with *mesangial proliferation.* Both class I and II lesions are typically associated with minimal renal manifestation and normal renal function; nephrotic syndrome is rare. Patients with lesions limited to the renal mesangium have an excellent prognosis and generally do not need therapy for their lupus nephritis.

TABLE 283-3 Classification for Lupus Nephritis

Class I	Minimal mesangial	Normal histology with mesangial deposits
Class II	Mesangial proliferation	Mesangial hypercellularity with expansion of the mesangial matrix
Class III	Focal nephritis	Focal endocapillary ± extracapillary proliferation with focal subendothelial immune deposits and mild mesangial expansion
Class IV	Diffuse nephritis	Diffuse endocapillary ± extracapillary proliferation with diffuse subendothelial immune deposits and mesangial alterations
Class V	Membranous nephritis	Thickened basement membranes with diffuse subepithelial immune deposits; may occur with class III or IV lesions and is sometimes called mixed membranous and proliferative nephritis
Class VI	Sclerotic nephritis	Global sclerosis of nearly all glomerular capillaries

Note: Revised in 2004 by the International Society of Nephrology-Renal Pathology Society Study Group.

The subject of lupus nephritis is presented under acute nephritic syndromes because of the aggressive and important proliferative lesions seen in class III–V renal disease. Class III describes *focal lesions with proliferation or scarring,* often involving only a segment of the glomerulus (Fig. e14-12). Class III lesions have the most varied course. Hypertension, an active urinary sediment, and proteinuria are common with nephrotic-range proteinuria in 25–33% of patients. Elevated serum creatinine is present in 25% of patients. Patients with mild proliferation involving a small percentage of glomeruli respond well to therapy with steroids alone, and fewer than 5% progress to renal failure over 5 years. Patients with more severe proliferation involving a greater percentage of glomeruli have a far worse prognosis and lower remission rates. Treatment of those patients is the same as that for class IV lesions. Most nephrologists believe that class III lesions are simply an early presentation of class IV disease. Others believe severe class III disease is a discrete lesion also requiring aggressive therapy. Class IV describes *global, diffuse proliferative lesions* involving the vast majority of glomeruli. Patients with class IV lesions commonly have high anti-DNA antibody titers, low serum complement, hematuria, red blood cell casts, proteinuria, hypertension, and decreased renal function; 50% of patients have nephrotic-range proteinuria. Patients with crescents on biopsy often have a rapidly progressive decline in renal function (Fig. e14-12). Without treatment, this aggressive lesion has the worst renal prognosis. However, if a remission—defined as a return to near-normal renal function and proteinuria ≤330 mg/dL per day—is achieved with treatment, renal outcomes are excellent. Current evidence suggests that inducing a remission with administration of high-dose steroids and either cyclophosphamide or mycophenolate mofetil for 2–6 months, followed by maintenance therapy with lower doses of steroids and mycophenolate mofetil, best balances the likelihood of successful remission with the side effects of therapy. There is no consensus on use of high-dose intravenous methylprednisolone versus oral prednisone, monthly intravenous cyclophosphamide versus daily oral cyclophosphamide, or other immunosuppressants such as cyclosporine, tacrolimus, rituximab, or azathioprine. Nephrologists tend to avoid prolonged use of cyclophosphamide in patients of childbearing age without first banking eggs or sperm.

The class V lesion describes subepithelial immune deposits producing a *membranous pattern;* a subcategory of class V lesions is associated with proliferative lesions and is sometimes called *mixed membranous and proliferative disease* (Fig. e14-11); this category of injury is treated like class IV glomerulonephritis. Sixty percent of patients present with nephrotic syndrome or lesser amounts of proteinuria. Patients with lupus nephritis class V, like patients with *idiopathic membranous nephropathy,* are predisposed to renal-vein thrombosis and other thrombotic complications. A minority of patients with class V will present with hypertension and renal dysfunction. There are conflicting data on the clinical course, prognosis, and appropriate therapy for patients with class V disease, which may reflect the heterogeneity of this group of patients. Patients with severe nephrotic syndrome, elevated serum creatinine, and a progressive course will probably benefit from therapy with steroids in combination with other immunosuppressive agents. Therapy with inhibitors of the renin-angiotensin system also may attenuate the proteinuria. Antiphospholipid antibodies present in lupus may result in glomerular microthromboses and complicate the course in up to 20% of lupus nephritis patients. The renal prognosis is worse even with anticoagulant therapy.

Patients with any of the above lesions also can transform to another lesion; hence patients often require reevaluation, including repeat renal biopsy. Lupus patients with class VI lesions have greater than 90% *sclerotic glomeruli* and end-stage renal disease with interstitial fibrosis. As a group, approximately 20% of patients with lupus nephritis will reach end-stage disease, requiring dialysis or transplantation. Systemic lupus tends to become quiescent once there is renal failure, perhaps due to the immunosuppressant effects of uremia. Renal transplantation in renal failure from lupus, usually performed after approximately 6 months of inactive disease, results in allograft survival rates comparable to patients transplanted for other reasons.

ANTIGLOMERULAR BASEMENT MEMBRANE DISEASE

Patients who develop autoantibodies directed against glomerular basement antigens frequently develop a glomerulonephritis termed *antiglomerular basement membrane (anti-GBM) disease.* When they present with lung hemorrhage and glomerulonephritis, they have a pulmonary-renal syndrome called *Goodpasture's syndrome.* The target epitopes for this autoimmune disease lie in the quaternary structure of $\alpha3$ NC1 domain of collagen IV. MHC-restricted T cells initiate the autoantibody response because humans are not tolerant to the epitopes created by this quaternary structure. The epitopes are normally sequestered in the collagen IV hexamer and can be exposed by infection, smoking, oxidants, or solvents. Goodpasture's syndrome appears in two age groups: in young men in their late 20s and in men and women in their 60–70s. Disease in the younger age group is usually explosive, with hemoptysis, a sudden fall in hemoglobin, fever, dyspnea, and hematuria. Hemoptysis is largely confined to smokers, and those who present with lung hemorrhage as a group do better than older populations who have prolonged, asymptomatic renal injury; presentation with oliguria is often associated with a particularly bad outcome. The performance of an urgent kidney biopsy is important in suspected cases of Goodpasture's syndrome to confirm the diagnosis and assess prognosis. Renal biopsies typically show *focal* or *segmental necrosis* that later, with aggressive destruction of the capillaries by cellular proliferation, leads to crescent formation in Bowman's space (Fig. e14-14). As these lesions progress, there is concomitant interstitial nephritis with fibrosis and tubular atrophy.

The presence of anti-GBM antibodies and complement is recognized on biopsy by linear immunofluorescent staining for IgG (rarely IgA). In testing serum for anti-GBM antibodies, it is particularly important that the $\alpha3$ NC1 domain of collagen IV alone be used as the target. This is because nonnephritic antibodies against the $\alpha1$ NC1 domain are seen in paraneoplastic syndromes and cannot be discerned from assays that use whole basement membrane fragments as the binding target. Between 10 and 15% of sera from patients with Goodpasture's syndrome also contain ANCA antibodies against myeloperoxidase. This subset of patients has a vasculitis-associated variant, which has a surprisingly good prognosis with treatment. Prognosis at presentation is worse if there are >50% crescents on renal biopsy with advanced fibrosis, if serum creatinine is >5–6 mg/dL, if oliguria is present, or if there is a need for acute dialysis. Although frequently attempted, most of these latter patients will not respond to plasmapheresis and steroids. Patients with advanced renal failure who present with hemoptysis should still be treated for their lung hemorrhage, as it responds to plasmapheresis and can be lifesaving. Treated patients with less severe disease typically respond to 8–10 treatments of plasmapheresis accompanied by oral prednisone and cyclophosphamide in the first 2 weeks. Kidney transplantation is possible, but because there is risk of recurrence, experience suggests that patients should wait for 6 months and until serum antibodies are undetectable.

IgA NEPHROPATHY

Berger first described the glomerulonephritis now termed *IgA nephropathy.* It is classically characterized by episodic hematuria associated with the deposition of IgA in the mesangium. IgA nephropathy is one of the most common forms of glomerulonephritis worldwide. There is a male preponderance, a peak incidence in the second and third decades of life, and rare familial clustering. There are geographic differences in the prevalence of IgA nephropathy, with 30% prevalence along the Asian and Pacific Rim and 20% in southern Europe, compared to a much lower prevalence in northern Europe and North America. It was initially hypothesized that variation in detection, in part, accounted for regional differences. With clinical care in nephrology becoming more uniform, this variation in prevalence more likely reflects true differences among racial and ethnic groups.

IgA nephropathy is predominantly a sporadic disease but susceptibility to it has been shown uncommonly to have a genetic component depending on geography and the existence of "founder effects." Familial forms of IgA nephropathy are more common in northern Italy and eastern Kentucky. No single causal gene has been identified. Clinical and laboratory evidence suggests close similarities between Henoch-Schönlein purpura and IgA nephropathy. Henoch-Schönlein purpura is distinguished clinically from IgA nephropathy by prominent systemic symptoms, a younger age (<20 years old), preceding infection, and abdominal complaints. Deposits of IgA are also found in the glomerular mesangium in a variety of systemic diseases, including chronic liver disease, Crohn's disease, gastrointestinal adenocarcinoma, chronic bronchiectasis, idiopathic interstitial pneumonia, dermatitis herpetiformis, mycosis fungoides, leprosy, ankylosing spondylitis, relapsing polychondritis, and Sjögren's syndrome. IgA deposition in these entities is not usually associated with clinically significant glomerular inflammation or renal dysfunction and thus is not called IgA nephropathy.

Glomerular schematic 2

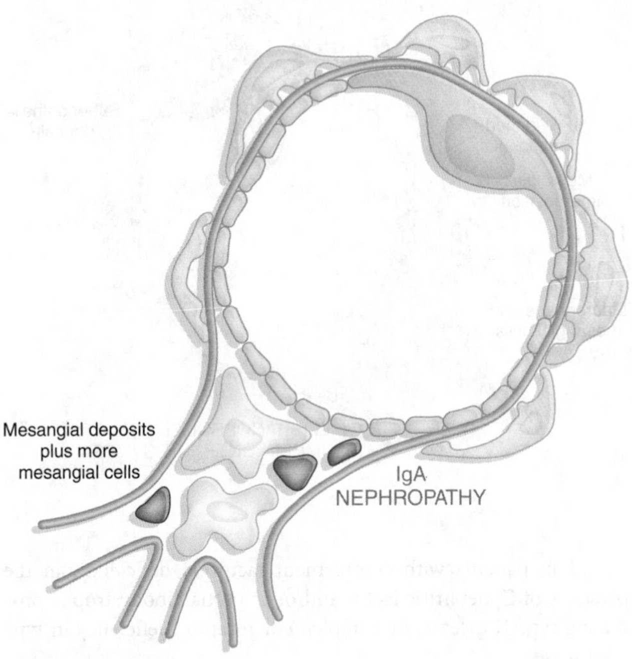

IgA nephropathy is an immune complex–mediated glomerulonephritis defined by the presence of diffuse mesangial IgA deposits often associated with mesangial hypercellularity. (See Glomerular Schematic 2.) IgM, IgG, C_3, or immunoglobulin light chains may be codistributed with IgA. IgA deposited in the mesangium is typically polymeric and of the IgA1 subclass, the pathogenic significance of which is not clear. Abnormalities have been described in IgA production by plasma cells, particularly secretory IgA; in IgA clearance, predominately by the liver; in mesangial IgA clearance and receptors for IgA; and in growth factor and cytokine-mediated events. Currently, however, abnormalities in the *O*-glycosylation of the hinge region of IgA seem to best account for the pathogenesis of sporadic IgA nephropathy. Despite the presence of elevated serum IgA levels in 20–50% of patients, IgA deposition in skin biopsies in 15–55% of patients, or elevated levels of secretory IgA and IgA-fibronectin complexes, a renal biopsy is necessary to confirm the diagnosis. Although the immunofluorescent pattern of IgA on renal biopsy defines IgA nephropathy in the proper clinical context, a variety of histologic lesions may be seen on light microscopy (Fig. e14-8), including DPGN; *segmental sclerosis;* and, rarely, *segmental necrosis with cellular crescent formation,* which typically presents as RPGN.

The two most common presentations of IgA nephropathy are recurrent episodes of macroscopic hematuria during or immediately following an upper respiratory infection often accompanied by proteinuria or persistent asymptomatic microscopic hematuria. Nephrotic syndrome, however, is uncommon. Proteinuria can also first appear late in the course of the disease. Rarely patients present with acute renal failure and a rapidly progressive clinical picture. IgA nephropathy is a benign disease for the majority of patients, and 5–30% of patients may go into a complete remission, with others having hematuria but well preserved renal function. In the minority of patients who have progressive disease, progression is slow, with renal failure seen in only 25–30% of patients with IgA nephropathy over 20–25 years. This risk varies considerably among populations. Cumulatively, risk factors for the loss of renal function identified thus far account for less than 50% of the variation in observed outcome but include the presence of hypertension or proteinuria, the absence of episodes of macroscopic hematuria, male age, older age of onset, and extensive glomerulosclerosis or interstitial fibrosis on renal biopsy. Several analyses in large populations of patients found persistent proteinuria for 6 months or longer to have the greatest predictive power for adverse renal outcomes.

There is no agreement on optimal treatment. Both large studies that include patients with multiple glomerular diseases and small studies of patients with IgA nephropathy support the use of angiotensin-converting enzyme (ACE) inhibitors in patients with proteinuria or declining renal function. Tonsillectomy, steroid therapy, and fish oil have all been suggested in small studies to benefit select patients with IgA nephropathy. When presenting as RPGN, patients typically receive steroids, cytotoxic agents, and plasmapheresis.

ANCA SMALL-VESSEL VASCULITIS

A group of patients with small-vessel vasculitis (arterioles, capillaries, and venules; rarely small arteries) and glomerulonephritis have serum ANCA; the antibodies are of two types, anti-proteinase 3 (PR3) or anti-myeloperoxidase (MPO) (Chap. 326); Lamp-2 antibodies have also been reported experimentally as potentially pathogenic. ANCA are produced with the help of T cells and activate leukocytes and monocytes, which together damage the walls of small vessels. Endothelial injury also attracts more leukocytes and extends the inflammation. Granulomatosis with polyangiitis (Wegener's), microscopic polyangiitis, and Churg-Strauss syndrome belong to this group because they are ANCA-positive and have a *pauci-immune glomerulonephritis* with few immune complexes in small vessels and glomerular capillaries. Patients with any of these three diseases can have any combination of the above serum antibodies, but anti-PR3 antibodies are more common in granulomatosis with polyangiitis (Wegener's) and anti-MPO antibodies are more common in microscopic polyangiitis or Churg-Strauss. While each of these diseases have some unique clinical features, most features do not predict relapse or progression, and as a group they are generally treated in the same way. Since mortality is high without treatment, virtually all patients receive urgent treatment. Induction therapy usually includes some combination of plasmapheresis, methylprednisolone, and cyclophosphamide. The benefit of plasmapheresis in this setting is uncertain. Monthly "pulse" IV cyclophosphamide to induce remission of ANCA-associated vasculitis is as effective as daily oral cyclophosphamide and results in reduced cumulative adverse events but may be associated with increased relapses. Steroids are tapered soon after acute inflammation subsides, and patients are maintained on cyclophosphamide or azathioprine for up to a year to minimize the risk of relapse.

Granulomatosis with polyangiitis (Wegener's)

Patients with this disease classically present with fever, purulent rhinorrhea, nasal ulcers, sinus pain, polyarthralgias/arthritis, cough, hemoptysis, shortness of breath, microscopic hematuria, and 0.5–1 g/24 h of proteinuria; occasionally there may be cutaneous purpura and mononeuritis multiplex. Presentation without renal involvement is termed *limited granulomatosis with polyangiitis (Wegener's)*, although some of these patients will show signs of renal injury later. Chest x-ray often reveals nodules and persistent infiltrates, sometimes with cavities. Biopsy of involved tissue will show a small-vessel vasculitis and adjacent noncaseating granulomas. Renal biopsies during active disease demonstrate *segmental necrotizing glomerulonephritis* without immune deposits (Fig. e14-13). The cause of granulomatosis with polyangiitis (Wegener's) is unknown. In case-controlled studies there is greater risk associated with exposure to silica dust. The disease is also more common in patients with α_1-antitrypsin deficiency, which is an inhibitor of PR3. Relapse after achieving remission is more common in patients with granulomatosis with polyangiitis (Wegener's) than the other ANCA-associated vasculitis, necessitating diligent follow-up care.

Microscopic polyangiitis

Clinically, these patients look somewhat similar to those with granulomatosis with polyangiitis (Wegener's), except they rarely have significant lung disease or destructive sinusitis. The distinction is made on biopsy, where the vasculitis in microscopic polyangiitis is without granulomas. Some patients will also have injury limited to the capillaries and venules.

Churg-Strauss syndrome

When small-vessel vasculitis is associated with peripheral eosinophilia, cutaneous purpura, mononeuritis, asthma, and allergic rhinitis, a diagnosis of Churg-Strauss syndrome is considered. Hypergammaglobulinemia, elevated levels of serum IgE, or the presence of rheumatoid factor sometimes accompanies the allergic state. Lung inflammation, including fleeting cough and pulmonary infiltrates, often precedes the systemic manifestations of disease by years; lung manifestations are rarely absent. A third of patients may have exudative pleural effusions associated with eosinophils. Small-vessel vasculitis and *focal segmental necrotizing glomerulonephritis* can be seen on renal biopsy, usually absent eosinophils or granulomas. The cause of Churg-Strauss syndrome is autoimmune, but the inciting factors are unknown. Interestingly, some asthma patients treated with leukotriene receptor antagonists will develop this vasculitis.

MEMBRANOPROLIFERATIVE GLOMERULONEPHRITIS

MPGN is sometimes called *mesangiocapillary glomerulonephritis* or *lobar glomerulonephritis*. It is an immune-mediated glomerulonephritis characterized by thickening of the GBM with mesangioproliferative changes; 70% of patients have hypocomplementemia. MPGN is rare in African Americans, and idiopathic disease usually presents in childhood or young adulthood. MPGN is subdivided pathologically into type I, type II, and type III disease. *Type I MPGN* is commonly associated with persistent hepatitis C infections, autoimmune diseases like lupus or cryoglobulinemia, or neoplastic diseases (Table 283-4). *Types II and III MPGN* are usually idiopathic,

TABLE 283-4 Membranoproliferative Glomerulonephritis

Type I Disease (Most Common)
Idiopathic
Subacute bacterial endocarditis
Systemic lupus erythematosus
Hepatitis C ± cryoglobulinemia
Mixed cryoglobulinemia
Hepatitis B
Cancer: Lung, breast, and ovary (germinal)
Type II Disease (Dense Deposit Disease)
Idiopathic
C_3 nephritic factor–associated
Partial lipodystrophy
Type III Disease
Idiopathic
Complement receptor deficiency

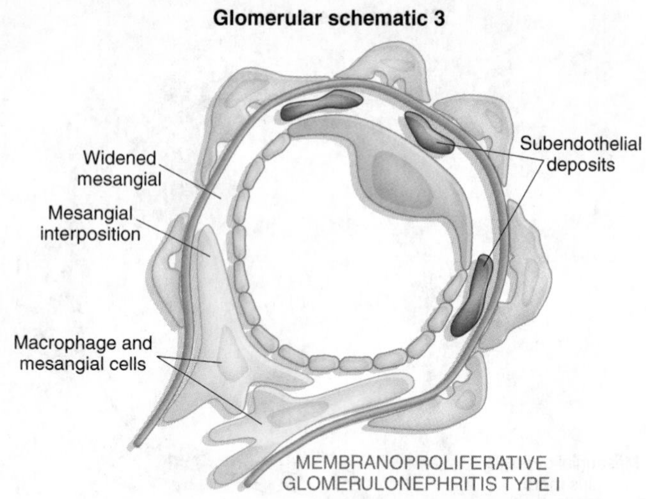

except in patients with complement factor H deficiency, in the presence of C_3 nephritic factor and/or in partial lipodystrophy producing type II disease, or complement receptor deficiency in type III disease.

Type I MPGN, the most proliferative of the three types, shows mesangial proliferation with lobular segmentation on renal biopsy and mesangial interposition between the capillary basement membrane and endothelial cells, producing a double contour sometimes called *tram-tracking* (Fig. e14-9). (See Glomerular Schematic 3.) Subendothelial deposits with low serum levels of C_3 are typical, although 50% of patients have normal levels of C_3 and occasional intramesangial deposits. Low serum C_3 and a dense thickening of the GBM containing ribbons of dense deposits and C_3 characterize type II MPGN, sometimes called *dense deposit disease* (Fig. e14-10). Classically, the glomerular tuft has a lobular appearance; intramesangial deposits are rarely present and subendothelial deposits are generally absent. Proliferation in type III MPGN is less common than the other two types and is often focal; mesangial interposition is rare, and subepithelial deposits can occur along widened segments of the GBM that appear laminated and disrupted.

Type I MPGN is secondary to glomerular deposition of circulating immune complexes or their in situ formation. Types II and III MPGN may be related to "nephritic factors," which are autoantibodies that stabilize C_3 convertase and allow it to activate serum C_3. Patients with MPGN present with proteinuria, hematuria, and pyuria (30%), systemic symptoms of fatigue and malaise that are most common in children with type I disease, or an acute nephritic picture with RPGN and a speedy deterioration in renal function in up to 25% of patients. Low serum C_3 levels are common. Fifty percent of patients with MPGN develop end-stage disease 10 years after diagnosis, and 90% have renal insufficiency after 20 years. Nephrotic syndrome, hypertension, and renal insufficiency all predict poor outcome. In the presence of proteinuria, treatment with inhibitors of the renin-angiotensin system is prudent. Evidence for treatment with dipyridamole, Coumadin (warfarin), or cyclophosphamide is not strongly established. There is some evidence supporting the efficacy of treatment of *primary MPGN* with steroids, particularly in children, as well as reports of efficacy with plasma exchange and other immunosuppressive drugs. In *secondary MPGN*, treating the associated infection, autoimmune disease, or neoplasms is of demonstrated benefit. In particular, pegylated interferon and ribavirin are useful in reducing viral load. Although all primary renal diseases can recur over time in transplanted renal allografts, patients with MPGN are well known to be at risk for not only a histologic recurrence but also a clinically significant recurrence with loss of graft function.

MESANGIOPROLIFERATIVE GLOMERULONEPHRITIS

Mesangioproliferative glomerulonephritis is characterized by expansion of the mesangium, sometimes associated with mesangial hypercellularity; thin, single contoured capillary walls; and mesangial immune deposits. Clinically, it can present with varying degrees of proteinuria and, commonly, hematuria. Mesangioproliferative disease may be seen in IgA nephropathy, *Plasmodium falciparum* malaria, resolving postinfectious glomerulonephritis, and class II nephritis from lupus, all of which can have a similar histologic appearance. With these secondary entities excluded, the diagnosis of *primary mesangioproliferative glomerulonephritis* is made in less than 15% of renal biopsies. As an immune-mediated renal lesion with deposits of IgM, C1q, and C_3, the clinical course is variable. Patients with isolated hematuria may have a very benign course, and those with heavy proteinuria occasionally progress to renal failure. There is little agreement on treatment, but some clinical reports suggest benefit from use of inhibitors of the renin-angiotensin system, steroid therapy, and even cytotoxic agents.

NEPHROTIC SYNDROME

Nephrotic syndrome classically presents with heavy proteinuria, minimal hematuria, hypoalbuminemia, hypercholesterolemia, edema, and hypertension. If left undiagnosed or untreated, some of these syndromes will progressively damage enough glomeruli to cause a fall in GFR, producing renal failure.

Therapies for various causes of nephrotic syndrome are noted under individual disease headings below. In general, all patients with hypercholesterolemia secondary to nephrotic syndrome should be treated with lipid-lowering agents because they are at increased risk for cardiovascular disease. Edema secondary to salt and water retention can be controlled with the judicious use of diuretics, avoiding intravascular volume depletion. Venous complications secondary to the hypercoagulable state associated with nephrotic syndrome can be treated with anticoagulants. The losses of various serum binding proteins, such as thyroid-binding globulin, lead to alterations in functional tests. Lastly, proteinuria itself is hypothesized to be nephrotoxic, and treatment of proteinuria with inhibitors of the renin-angiotensin system can lower urinary protein excretion.

MINIMAL CHANGE DISEASE

Minimal change disease (MCD), sometimes known as *nil lesion,* causes 70–90% of nephrotic syndrome in childhood but only 10–15% of nephrotic syndrome in adults. Minimal change disease usually presents as a primary renal disease but can be associated with several other conditions, including Hodgkin's disease, allergies, or use of nonsteroidal anti-inflammatory agents; significant interstitial nephritis often accompanies cases associated with nonsteroidal use. Minimal change disease on renal biopsy shows no obvious glomerular lesion by light microscopy and is negative for deposits by immunofluorescent microscopy, or occasionally shows small amounts of IgM in the mesangium (Fig. e14-1). (See Glomerular Schematic 4.) Electron microscopy, however, consistently demonstrates an effacement of the foot process supporting the epithelial podocytes with weakening of slit-pore membranes. The pathophysiology of this lesion is uncertain. Most agree there is a circulating cytokine, perhaps related to a T cell response that alters capillary charge and podocyte integrity. The evidence for cytokine-related immune injury is circumstantial and is suggested by the presence of preceding allergies, altered cell-mediated immunity

Glomerular schematic 4

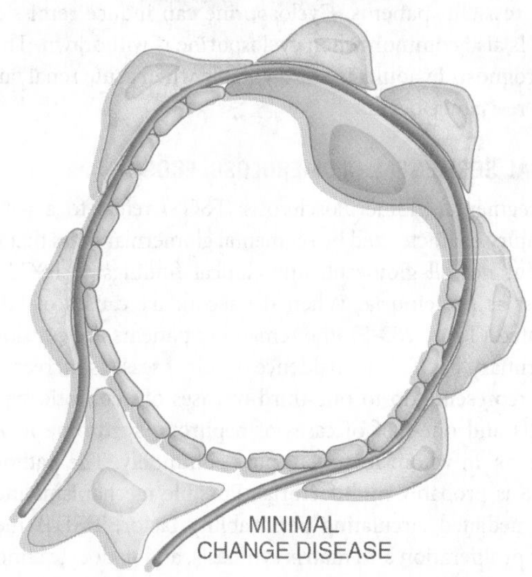

during viral infections, and the high frequency of remissions with steroids.

Minimal change disease presents clinically with the abrupt onset of edema and nephrotic syndrome accompanied by acellular urinary sediment. Average urine protein excretion reported in 24 hours is 10 grams with severe hypoalbuminemia. Less common clinical features include hypertension (30% in children, 50% in adults), microscopic hematuria (20% in children, 33% in adults), atopy or allergic symptoms (40% in children, 30% in adults), and decreased renal function (<5% in children, 30% in adults). The appearance of acute renal failure in adults is often seen more commonly in patients with low serum albumin and intrarenal edema (nephrosarca) that is responsive to intravenous albumin and diuretics. This presentation must be distinguished from acute renal failure secondary to hypovolemia. Acute tubular necrosis and interstitial inflammation is also reported. In children, the abnormal urine principally contains albumin with minimal amounts of higher-molecular-weight proteins, and is sometimes called *selective proteinuria.* Although up to 30% of children have a spontaneous remission, all children today are treated with steroids; only children who are nonresponders are biopsied in this setting. Primary responders are patients who have a complete remission (<0.2 mg/24 h of proteinuria) after a single course of prednisone; steroid-dependent patients relapse as their steroid dose is tapered. Frequent relapsers have two or more relapses in the 6 months following taper, and steroid-resistant patients fail to respond to steroid therapy. Adults are not considered steroid-resistant until after 4 months of therapy. Ninety to 95% of children will develop a complete remission after 8 weeks of steroid therapy, and 80–85% of adults will achieve complete remission, but only after a longer course of 20–24 weeks. Patients with steroid resistance may have FSGS on repeat biopsy. Some hypothesize that if the first renal biopsy does not have a sample of deeper corticomedullary glomeruli, then the correct early diagnosis of FSGS may be missed.

Relapses occur in 70–75% of children after the first remission, and early relapse predicts multiple subsequent relapses. The frequency of relapses decreases after puberty, although there is an increased risk of relapse following the rapid tapering of steroids in all groups. Relapses are less common in adults but are more resistant to subsequent therapy. Prednisone is first-line therapy, either given daily or on alternate days. Other immunosuppressive drugs, such as cyclophosphamide, chlorambucil, and mycophenolate mofetil, are saved for frequent relapsers, steroid-dependent, or steroid-resistant patients. Cyclosporine can induce remission, but relapse is also common when cyclosporine is withdrawn. The long-term prognosis in adults is less favorable when acute renal failure or steroid resistance occurs.

FOCAL SEGMENTAL GLOMERULOSCLEROSIS

Focal segmental glomerulosclerosis (FSGS) refers to a pattern of renal injury characterized by segmental glomerular scars that involve some but not all glomeruli; the clinical findings of FSGS largely manifest as proteinuria. When the secondary causes of FSGS are eliminated (Table 283-5), the remaining patients are considered to have primary FSGS. The incidence of this disease is increasing, and it now represents up to one-third of cases of nephrotic syndrome in adults and one-half of cases of nephrotic syndrome in African Americans, in whom it is seen more commonly. The pathogenesis of FSGS is probably multifactorial. Possible mechanisms include a T cell–mediated circulating permeability factor, TGF-β–mediated cellular proliferation and matrix synthesis, and podocyte abnormalities associated with genetic mutations. Risk polymorphisms at the *APOL1* locus encoding apolipoprotein L1 expressed in podocytes substantially explain the increased burden of FSGS among African Americans with or without HIV-associated disease.

The pathologic changes of FSGS are most prominent in glomeruli located at the corticomedullary junction (Fig. e14-2), so if the renal biopsy specimen is from superficial tissue, the lesions can be missed, which sometimes leads to a misdiagnosis of MCD. In addition to focal and segmental scarring, other variants have been

TABLE 283-5 Focal Segmental Glomerulosclerosis

Primary focal segmental glomerulosclerosis
Secondary focal segmental glomerulosclerosis
Viruses: HIV/Hepatitis B/Parvovirus
Hypertensive nephropathy
Reflux nephropathy
Cholesterol emboli
Drugs: Heroin/analgesics/pamidronate
Oligomeganephronia
Renal dysgenesis
Alport's syndrome
Sickle cell disease
Lymphoma
Radiation nephritis
Familial podocytopathies
NPHS1 mutation/nephrin
NPHS2 mutation/podocin
TRPC6 mutation/cation channel
ACTN4 mutation/actinin
α-Galactosidase A deficiency/Fabry's disease
N-acetylneuraminic acid hydrolase deficiency/nephrosialidosis

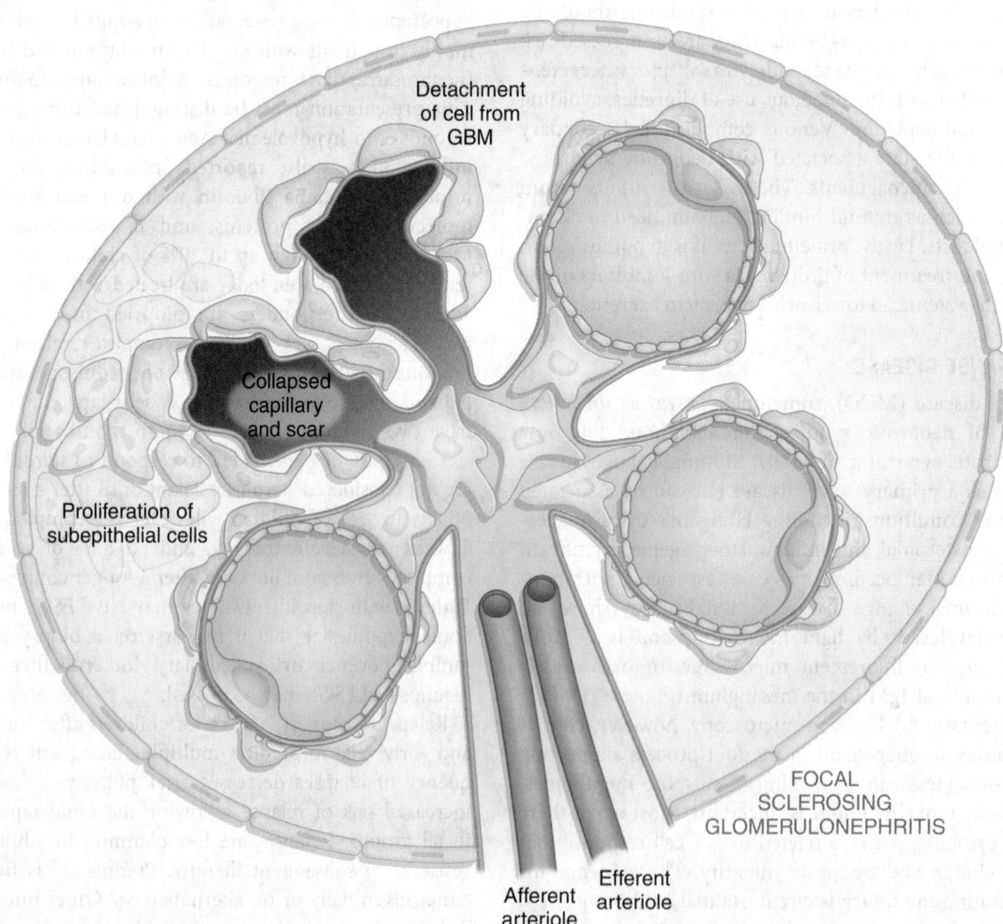

described, including cellular lesions with *endocapillary hypercellularity* and heavy proteinuria; *collapsing glomerulopathy* (Fig. e14-3) with segmental or global glomerular collapse and a rapid decline in renal function; a hilar stalk lesion (Fig. e14-4) or the *glomerular tip lesion* (Fig. e14-5), which may have a better prognosis. (See Glomerular Schematic 5.)

FSGS can present with hematuria, hypertension, any level of proteinuria or renal insufficiency. Nephrotic-range proteinuria, African-American race, and renal insufficiency are associated with a poor outcome, with 50% of patients reaching renal failure in 6–8 years. FSGS rarely remits spontaneously, but treatment-induced remission of proteinuria significantly improves prognosis. Treatment of patients with *primary FSGS* should include inhibitors of the renin-angiotensin system. Based on retrospective studies, patients with nephrotic-range proteinuria can be treated with steroids but respond far less often and after a longer course of therapy than patients with MCD. Proteinuria remits in only 20–45% of patients receiving a course of steroids over 6–9 months. Limited evidence suggests the use of cyclosporine in steroid-responsive patients helps ensure remissions. Relapse frequently occurs after cessation of cyclosporine therapy, and cyclosporine itself can lead to a deterioration of renal function due to its nephrotoxic effects. A role for other agents that suppress the immune system has not been established. Primary FSGS recurs in 25–40% of patients given allografts at end-stage disease, leading to graft loss in half of those cases. The treatment of *secondary FSGS* typically involves treating the underlying cause and controlling proteinuria. There is no role for steroids or other immunosuppressive agents in secondary FSGS.

MEMBRANOUS GLOMERULONEPHRITIS

Membranous glomerulonephritis (MGN), or *membranous nephropathy* as it is sometimes called, accounts for approximately 30% of cases of nephrotic syndrome in adults, with a peak incidence between the ages of 30 and 50 years and a male to female ratio of 2:1. It is rare in childhood and the most common cause of nephrotic syndrome in the elderly. In 25–30% of cases, MGN is associated with a malignancy (solid tumors of the breast, lung, colon), infection (hepatitis B, malaria, schistosomiasis), or rheumatologic disorders like lupus or rarely rheumatoid arthritis (Table 283-6).

Uniform thickening of the basement membrane along the peripheral capillary loops is seen by light microscopy on renal biopsy (Fig. e14-7); this thickening needs to be distinguished from that seen in diabetes and amyloidosis. (See Glomerular Schematic 6.)

TABLE 283-6 Membranous Glomerulonephritis

Primary/idiopathic membranous glomerulonephritis

Secondary membranous glomerulonephritis

- Infection: Hepatitis B and C, syphilis, malaria, schistosomiasis, leprosy, filariasis
- Cancer: Breast, colon, lung, stomach, kidney, esophagus, neuroblastoma
- Drugs: gold, mercury, penicillamine, nonsteroidal anti-inflammatory agents, probenecid
- Autoimmune diseases: systemic lupus erythematosus, rheumatoid arthritis, primary biliary cirrhosis, dermatitis herpetiformis, bullous pemphigoid, myasthenia gravis, Sjögren's syndrome, Hashimoto's thyroiditis
- Other systemic diseases: Fanconi's syndrome, sickle cell anemia, diabetes, Crohn's disease, sarcoidosis, Guillain-Barré syndrome, Weber-Christian disease, angiofollicular lymph node hyperplasia

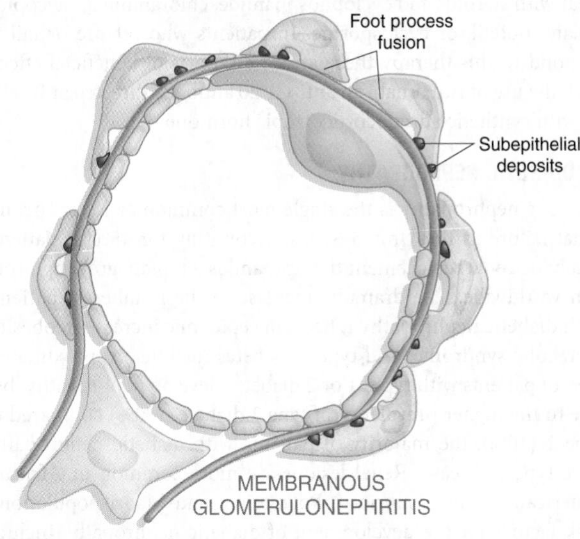

Immunofluorescence demonstrates diffuse granular deposits of IgG and C_3, and electron microscopy typically reveals electron-dense subepithelial deposits. While different stages (I–V) of progressive membranous lesions have been described, some published analyses indicate the degree of tubular atrophy or interstitial fibrosis is more predictive of progression than is the stage of glomerular disease. The presence of subendothelial deposits or the presence of tubuloreticular inclusions strongly points to a diagnosis of membranous lupus nephritis, which may precede the extrarenal manifestations of lupus. Work in Heyman nephritis, an animal model of MGN, suggests that glomerular lesions result from in situ formation of immune complexes with megalin receptor–associated protein as the putative antigen. This antigen is not found in human podocytes, but human antibodies have been described against neutral endopeptidase expressed by podocytes, hepatitis antigens B/C, *Helicobacter pylori* antigens, and tumor antigens. In a newer study, autoantibodies against the M-type phospholipase A_2 receptor (PLA_2R) circulate and bind to a conformational epitope present in the receptor on human podocytes, producing in situ deposits characteristic of idiopathic membranous nephropathy. Other renal diseases and secondary membranous nephropathy do not appear to involve such autoantibodies. Eighty percent of patients with MGN present with nephrotic syndrome and nonselective proteinuria. Microscopic hematuria is seen in up to 50% of patients but is seen less commonly than in IgA nephropathy or FSGS. Spontaneous remissions occur in 20–33% of patients and often occur late in the course after years of nephrotic syndrome, which make treatment decisions difficult. One-third of patients continue to have relapsing nephrotic syndrome but maintain normal renal function, and approximately another third of patients develop renal failure or die from the complications of nephrotic syndrome. Male gender, older age, hypertension, and the persistence of proteinuria are associated with worse prognosis. Although thrombotic complications are a feature of all nephrotic syndromes, MGN has the highest reported incidences of renal vein thrombosis, pulmonary embolism, and deep vein thrombosis. Prophylactic anticoagulation is controversial but has been recommended for patients with severe or prolonged proteinuria in the absence of risk factors for bleeding.

In addition to the treatment of edema, dyslipidemia, and hypertension, inhibition of the renin-angiotensin system is recommended. Therapy with immunosuppressive drugs is also recommended for patients with primary MGN and persistent proteinuria (>3.0 g/24 h). The choice of immunosuppressive drugs for therapy is controversial, but current recommendations based on small clinical studies are to treat with steroids and cyclophosphamide, chlorambucil, mycophenolate mofetil, or cyclosporine. In patients who relapse or fail to respond to this therapy there are case reports of beneficial effects with the use of rituximab, an anti-CD20 antibody directed at B cells, or with synthetic adrenocorticotropic hormone.

DIABETIC NEPHROPATHY

Diabetic nephropathy is the single most common cause of chronic renal failure in the United States, accounting for 45% of patients receiving renal replacement therapy, and is a rapidly growing problem worldwide. The dramatic increase in the number of patients with diabetic nephropathy reflects the epidemic increase in obesity, metabolic syndrome, and type 2 diabetes mellitus. Approximately 40% of patients with types 1 or 2 diabetes develop nephropathy, but due to the higher prevalence of type 2 diabetes (90%) compared to type 1 (10%), the majority of patients with diabetic nephropathy have type 2 disease. Renal lesions are more common in African-American, Native American, Polynesian, and Maori populations. Risk factors for the development of diabetic nephropathy include hyperglycemia, hypertension, dyslipidemia, smoking, a family history of diabetic nephropathy, and gene polymorphisms affecting the activity of the renin-angiotensin-aldosterone axis.

Within 1–2 years after the onset of clinical diabetes, morphologic changes appear in the kidney. Thickening of the GBM is a sensitive indicator for the presence of diabetes but correlates poorly with the presence or absence of clinically significant nephropathy. The composition of the GBM is altered notably with a loss of heparan sulfate moieties that form the negatively charged filtration barrier. This change results in increased filtration of serum proteins into the urine, predominately negatively charged albumin. The expansion of the mesangium due to the accumulation of extracellular matrix correlates with the clinical manifestations of diabetic nephropathy (see stages in Fig. e14-20). This expansion in mesangial matrix is associated with the development of *mesangial sclerosis.* Some patients also develop eosinophilic, PAS$^+$ nodules called *nodular glomerulosclerosis* or *Kimmelstiel-Wilson nodules.* Immunofluorescence microscopy often reveals the nonspecific deposition of IgG (at times in a linear pattern) or complement staining without immune deposits on electron microscopy. Prominent vascular changes are frequently seen with hyaline and hypertensive arteriosclerosis. This is associated with varying degrees of chronic glomerulosclerosis and tubulointerstitial changes. Renal biopsies from patients with types 1 and 2 diabetes are largely indistinguishable.

These pathologic changes are the result of a number of postulated factors. Multiple lines of evidence support an important role for increases in glomerular capillary pressure (intraglomerular hypertension) in alterations in renal structure and function. Direct effects of hyperglycemia on the actin cytoskeleton of renal mesangial and vascular smooth-muscle cells as well as diabetes-associated changes in circulating factors such as atrial natriuretic factor, angiotensin II, and insulin-like growth factor (IGF) may account for this. Sustained glomerular hypertension increases matrix production, alterations in the GBM with disruption in the filtration barrier (and hence proteinuria), and glomerulosclerosis. A number of factors have also been identified that alter matrix production, including the accumulation of advanced glycosylation end products, circulating factors including growth hormone, IGF-I, angiotensin II, connective tissue growth factor, TGF-β, and dyslipidemia.

The natural history of diabetic nephropathy in patients with types 1 and 2 diabetes is similar. However, since the onset of Type 1 diabetes is readily identifiable and the onset of type 2 diabetes is not, a patient newly diagnosed with type 2 diabetes may have renal disease for many years before nephropathy is discovered and presents as *advanced diabetic nephropathy.* At the onset of diabetes, renal hypertrophy and glomerular hyperfiltration are present. The degree of glomerular hyperfiltration correlates with the subsequent risk of clinically significant nephropathy. In the approximately 40% of patients with diabetes who develop diabetic nephropathy, the earliest manifestation is an increase in albuminuria detected by sensitive radioimmunoassay (Table 283-1). Albuminuria in the range of 30–300 mg/24 h is called *microalbuminuria.* In patients with types 1 or 2 diabetes, microalbuminuria appears 5–10 years after the onset of diabetes. It is currently recommended to test patients with type 1 disease for microalbuminuria 5 years after diagnosis of diabetes and yearly thereafter, and, because the time of onset of type 2 diabetes is often unknown, to test type 2 patients at the time of diagnosis of diabetes and yearly thereafter.

Patients with small rises in albuminuria increase their levels of urinary albumin excretion, typically reaching dipstick positive levels of proteinuria (>300 mg albuminuria) 5–10 years after the onset of early albuminuria. Microalbuminuria is a potent risk factor for cardiovascular events and death in patients with type 2 diabetes. Many patients with type 2 diabetes and microalbuminuria succumb to cardiovascular events before they progress to proteinuria or renal failure. Proteinuria in frank diabetic nephropathy can be variable, ranging from 500 mg to 25 g/24 h, and is often associated with nephrotic syndrome. More than 90% of patients with type 1 diabetes and nephropathy have diabetic retinopathy, so the absence of retinopathy in type 1 patients with proteinuria should prompt consideration of a diagnosis other than diabetic nephropathy; only 60% of patients with type 2 diabetes with nephropathy have diabetic retinopathy. There is a highly significant correlation between the presence of retinopathy and the presence of Kimmelstiel-Wilson nodules (Fig. e14-20). Also, characteristically, patients with advanced diabetic nephropathy have normal to enlarged kidneys, in contrast to other glomerular diseases where kidney size is usually decreased. Using the above epidemiologic and clinical data, and in the absence of other clinical or serologic data suggesting another disease, diabetic nephropathy is usually diagnosed without a renal biopsy. After the onset of proteinuria, renal function inexorably declines, with 50% of patients reaching renal failure over another 5–10 years; thus, from the earliest stages of microalbuminuria, it usually takes 10–20 years to reach end-stage renal disease. Hypertension may predict which patients develop diabetic nephropathy, as the presence of hypertension accelerates the rate of decline in renal function. Once renal failure appears, however, survival on dialysis is far shorter for patients with diabetes compared to other dialysis patients. Survival is best for patients with type 1 diabetes who receive a transplant from a living related donor.

Good evidence supports the benefits of blood sugar and blood pressure control as well as inhibition of the renin-angiotensin system in retarding the progression of diabetic nephropathy. In patients with type 1 diabetes, intensive control of blood sugar clearly prevents the development or progression of diabetic nephropathy. The evidence for benefit of intensive blood glucose control in patients with type 2 diabetes is less certain, with current studies reporting conflicting results. Some, but not all, trials have reported increased mortality rate associated with intensive blood glucose control and the safety of $HgbA_1C$ goals less than 7% in patients with type 2 diabetes is currently unclear.

Controlling systemic blood pressure decreases renal and cardiovascular adverse events in this high-risk population. The vast majority of patients with diabetic nephropathy require three or more antihypertensive drugs to achieve this goal. Drugs that inhibit the renin-angiotensin system, independent of their effects on systemic blood pressure, have been shown in numerous large clinical trials to slow the progression of diabetic nephropathy at early (microalbuminuria) and late (proteinuria with reduced glomerular filtration) stages, independent of any effect they may have on systemic blood pressure. Since angiotensin II increases efferent arteriolar resistance and, hence, glomerular capillary pressure, one key mechanism for the efficacy of ACE inhibitors or angiotensin receptor blockers (ARBs) is reducing glomerular hypertension. Patients with type 1 diabetes for 5 years, who develop albuminuria or declining renal function should be treated with ACE inhibitors. Patients with type 2 diabetes and microalbuminuria or proteinuria may be treated with ACE inhibitors or ARBs. Less compelling evidence supports therapy with a combination of two drugs (ACE inhibitors, ARBs, renin inhibitors, or aldosterone antagonists) that suppress several components of the renin-angiotensin system.

GLOMERULAR DEPOSITION DISEASES

Plasma cell dyscrasias producing excess light chain immunoglobulin sometimes lead to the formation of glomerular and tubular deposits that cause heavy proteinuria and renal failure; the same is true for the accumulation of serum amyloid A protein fragments seen in several inflammatory diseases. This broad group of proteinuric patients has *glomerular deposition disease.*

Light chain deposition disease

The biochemical characteristics of nephrotoxic light chains produced in patients with light chain malignancies often confer a specific pattern of renal injury; that of either *cast nephropathy* (Fig. e14-17), which causes renal failure but not heavy proteinuria or amyloidosis, or light chain deposition disease (Fig. e14-16), which produces nephrotic syndrome with renal failure. These latter patients produce kappa light chains that do not have the biochemical features necessary to form amyloid fibrils. Instead, they self-aggregate and form granular deposits along the glomerular capillary and mesangium, tubular basement membrane, and Bowman's capsule. When predominant in glomeruli, nephrotic syndrome develops, and about 70% of patients progress to dialysis. Light-chain deposits are not fibrillar and do not stain with Congo red, but they are easily detected with anti–light chain antibody using immunofluorescence or as granular deposits on electron microscopy. A combination of the light chain rearrangement, self-aggregating properties at neutral pH, and abnormal metabolism probably contribute to the deposition. Treatment for light chain deposition disease is treatment of the primary disease. As so many patients with light chain deposition disease progress to renal failure, the overall prognosis is grim.

Renal amyloidosis

Most *renal amyloidosis* is either the result of primary fibrillar deposits of immunoglobulin light chains known as amyloid L (AL), or secondary to fibrillar deposits of serum amyloid A (AA) protein fragments (Chap. 112). Even though both occur for different reasons, their clinicopathophysiology is quite similar and will be discussed together. Amyloid infiltrates the liver, heart, peripheral nerves, carpal tunnel, upper pharynx, and kidney, producing restrictive cardiomyopathy, hepatomegaly, macroglossia, and heavy proteinuria sometimes associated with renal vein thrombosis. In systemic AL amyloidosis, also called *primary amyloidosis,* light chains produced in excess by clonal plasma cell dyscrasias are made into fragments by macrophages so they can self-aggregate at acid pH. A disproportionate number of these light chains (75%) are of the *lambda* class. About 10% of these patients have overt myeloma with lytic bone lesions and infiltration of the bone marrow with >30% plasma cells; nephrotic syndrome is common, and about 20% of patients progress to dialysis. AA amyloidosis is sometimes called *secondary amyloidosis* and also presents as nephrotic syndrome. It is due to deposition of β-pleated sheets of serum amyloid A protein, an acute phase reactant whose physiologic functions include cholesterol transport, immune cell attraction, and metalloproteases activation. Forty percent of patients with AA amyloid have rheumatoid arthritis, and another 10% have ankylosing spondylitis or psoriatic arthritis; the rest derive from other lesser causes. Less common in Western countries but more common in Mediterranean regions, particularly in Sephardic and Iraqi Jews, is familial Mediterranean fever (FMF). FMF is caused by a mutation in the gene encoding pyrin, while Muckle-Wells syndrome, a related disorder, results from a mutation in cryopyrin; both proteins are important in the apoptosis of leukocytes early in inflammation; such proteins with pyrin domains are part of a new pathway called the *inflammasome.* Receptor mutations in tumor necrosis factor receptor 1 (TNFR1)-associated periodic syndrome also produce chronic inflammation and secondary amyloidosis. Fragments of serum amyloid A protein increase and self-aggregate by attaching to receptors for advanced glycation end products in the extracellular environment; nephrotic syndrome is common, and about 40–60% of patients progress to dialysis. AA and AL amyloid fibrils are detectable with Congo red or in more detail with electron microscopy (Fig. e14-15). Currently developed serum free light chain nephelometry assays are useful in the early diagnosis and follow-up of disease progression. Biopsy of involved liver or kidney is diagnostic 90% of the time when the pretest probability is high; abdominal fat pad aspirates are positive about 70% of the time, but apparently less so when looking for AA amyloid. Amyloid deposits are distributed along blood vessels and in the mesangial regions of the kidney. The treatment for primary amyloidosis is not particularly effective; melphalan and autologous hematopoietic stem cell transplantation can delay the course of disease in about 30% of patients. Secondary amyloidosis is also relentless unless the primary disease can be controlled. Some new drugs in development that disrupt the formation of fibrils may be available in the future.

Fibrillary-immunotactoid glomerulopathy

Fibrillary-immunotactoid glomerulopathy is a rare (<1.0% of renal biopsies) morphologically defined disease characterized by glomerular accumulation of nonbranching randomly arranged fibrils. Some classify amyloid and nonamyloid fibril-associated renal disease all as fibrillary glomerulopathies with immunotactoid glomerulopathy reserved for nonamyloid fibrillary disease not associated with a systemic illness. Others define fibrillary glomerulonephritis as a nonamyloid fibrillary disease with fibrils 12–24 nm and immunotactoid glomerulonephritis with fibrils >30 nm. In either case, fibrillar/microtubular deposits of oligoclonal or oligotypic immunoglobulins and complement appear in the mesangium and along the glomerular capillary wall. Congo red stains are negative. The cause of this "nonamyloid" glomerulopathy is mostly idiopathic; reports of immunotactoid glomerulonephritis describe an occasional association with chronic lymphocytic leukemia or B cell lymphoma. Both disorders appear in adults in the fourth decade with moderate to heavy proteinuria, hematuria, and a wide variety of histologic lesions, including DPGN, MPGN, MGN, or mesangioproliferative glomerulonephritis. Nearly half of patients develop renal failure over a few years. There is no consensus on treatment of this uncommon disorder. The disease has been reported to recur following renal transplantation in a minority of cases.

FABRY'S DISEASE

Fabry's disease is an X-linked inborn error of globotriaosylceramide metabolism secondary to deficient lysosomal α-galactosidase A activity, resulting in excessive intracellular storage of globotriaosylceramide. Affected organs include the vascular endothelium, heart, brain, and kidneys. Classically, Fabry's disease presents in childhood in males with acroparesthesias, angiokeratoma, and hypohidrosis. Over time male patients develop cardiomyopathy,

Glomerular schematic 7

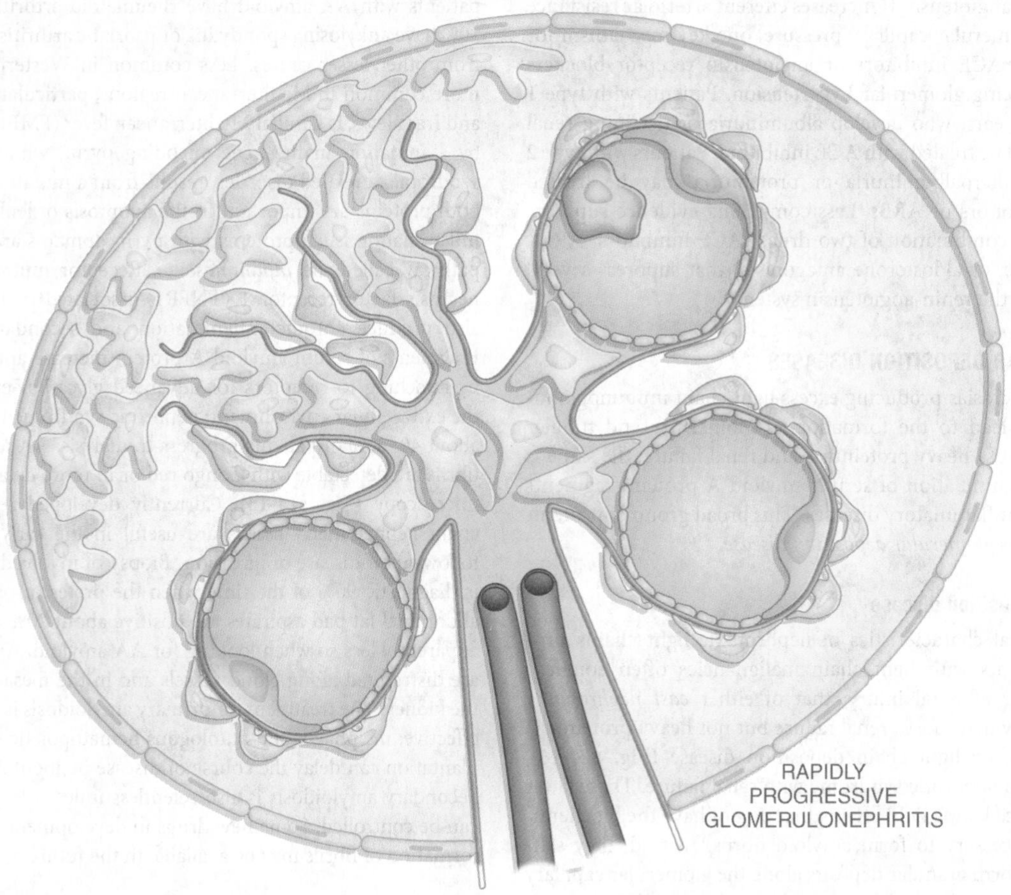

cerebrovascular disease, and renal injury, with an average age of death around 50 years of age. Hemizygotes with hypomorphic mutations sometimes present in the fourth to sixth decade with single-organ involvement. Rarely, dominant-negative α-galactosidase A mutations or female heterozygotes with unfavorable X inactivation present with mild single-organ involvement. Rare females develop severe manifestations including renal failure but do so later in life than males. Renal biopsy reveals enlarged glomerular visceral epithelial cells packed with small clear vacuoles containing globotriaosylceramide; vacuoles may also be found in parietal and tubular epithelia (Fig. e14-18). These vacuoles of electron-dense materials in parallel arrays (zebra bodies) are easily seen on electron microscopy. Ultimately, renal biopsies reveal FSGS. The nephropathy of Fabry's disease typically presents in the third decade as mild to moderate proteinuria, sometimes with microscopic hematuria or nephrotic syndrome. Urinalysis may reveal oval fat bodies and birefringent glycolipid globules under polarized light (Maltese cross). Renal biopsy is necessary for definitive diagnosis. Progression to renal failure occurs by the fourth or fifth decade. Treatment with inhibitors of the renin-angiotensin system is recommended. Treatment with recombinant α-galactosidase A clears microvascular endothelial deposits of globotriaosylceramide from the kidneys, heart, and skin. The degree of organ involvement at the time when enzyme replacement is initiated is crucial. In patients with advanced organ involvement, progression of disease occurs despite enzyme replacement therapy. Variable responses to enzyme therapy may be due to the occurrence of neutralizing antibodies or differences in uptake of the enzyme. Graft and patient survival following renal transplantation in patients with Fabry's are similar to other causes of end-stage renal disease.

PULMONARY-RENAL SYNDROMES

Several diseases can present with catastrophic hemoptysis and glomerulonephritis associated with varying degrees of renal failure. The usual causes include Goodpasture's syndrome, granulomatosis with polyangiitis (Wegener's), microscopic polyangiitis, Churg-Strauss vasculitis, and, rarely, Henoch-Schönlein purpura or cryoglobulinemia. Each of these diseases can also present without hemoptysis and are discussed in detail in "Acute Nephritic Syndromes," above. (See Glomerular Schematic 7.) Pulmonary bleeding in this setting is life-threatening and often results in airway intubation, and acute renal failure requires dialysis. Diagnosis is difficult initially because biopsies and serologic testing take time. Treatment with plasmapheresis and methylprednisolone is often empirical and temporizing until results of testing are available.

BASEMENT MEMBRANE SYNDROMES

All kidney epithelia, including podocytes, rest on basement membranes assembled into a planar surface through the interweaving of collagen IV with laminins, nidogen, and sulfated proteoglycans. Structural abnormalities in GBM associated with hematuria are characteristic of several familial disorders related to the expression of collagen IV genes. The extended family of collagen IV contains six chains, which are expressed in different tissues at different stages of embryonic development. All epithelial basement membranes early in human development are composed of interconnected triple-helical protomers rich in α1.α1.α2(IV) collagen. Some specialized tissues undergo a developmental switch replacing α1.α1.α2(IV) protomers with an α3.α4.α5(IV) collagen network; this switch occurs in the kidney (glomerular and tubular basement membrane), lung, testis, cochlea, and eye, while an α5.α5.α6(IV) network appears in skin, smooth muscle, and esophagus and along Bowman's capsule in the kidney. This switch probably occurs because the α3.α4.α5(IV) network is more resistant to proteases and ensures the structural longevity of critical tissues. When basement membranes are the target of glomerular disease, they produce moderate proteinuria, some hematuria, and progressive renal failure.

ANTI-GBM DISEASE

Autoimmune disease where antibodies are directed against the α3 NC1 domain of collagen IV produces an *anti-GBM disease* often associated with RPGN and/or a pulmonary-renal syndrome called *Goodpasture's syndrome*. Discussion of this disease is covered in "Acute Nephritic Syndromes," above.

ALPORT'S SYNDROME

Classically, patients with Alport's syndrome develop hematuria, thinning and splitting of the GBMs, mild proteinuria (<1–2 g/24 h), which appears late in the course, followed by chronic glomerulosclerosis leading to renal failure in association with sensorineural deafness. Some patients develop lenticonus of the anterior lens capsule, "dot and fleck" retinopathy, and rarely, mental retardation or leiomyomatosis. Approximately 85% of patients with Alport's syndrome have an X-linked inheritance of mutations in the α5(IV) collagen chain on chromosome Xq22–24. Female carriers have variable penetrance depending on the type of mutation or the degree of mosaicism created by X inactivation. Fifteen percent of patients have autosomal recessive disease of the α3(IV) or α4(IV) chains on chromosome 2q35–37. Rarely, some kindred have an autosomal dominant inheritance of dominant-negative mutations in α3(IV) or α4(IV) chains.

Pedigrees with the X-linked syndrome are quite variable in their rate and frequency of tissue damage leading to organ failure. Seventy percent of patients have the juvenile form with nonsense or missense mutations, reading frame shifts, or large deletions and generally develop renal failure and sensorineural deafness by age 30. Patients with splice variants, exon skipping, or missense mutations of α-helical glycines generally deteriorate after the age of 30 (adult form) with mild or late deafness. Early severe deafness, lenticonus, or proteinuria suggests a poorer prognosis. Usually females from X-linked pedigrees have only microhematuria, but up to 25% of carrier females have been reported to have more severe renal manifestations. Pedigrees with the autosomal recessive form of the disease have severe early disease in both females and males with asymptomatic parents.

Clinical evaluation should include a careful eye examination and hearing tests. However, the absence of extrarenal symptoms does not rule out the diagnosis. Since α5(IV) collagen is expressed in the skin, some X-linked Alport patients can be diagnosed with a skin biopsy revealing the lack of the α5(IV) collagen chain on immunofluorescent analysis. Other patients with suspected disease require a renal biopsy. Alport's patients early in their disease typically have thin basement membranes on renal biopsy (Fig. e14-19), which thicken over time into multilamellations surrounding lucent areas that often contain granules of varying density—the so-called split basement membrane. In any Alport kidney there are areas of thinning mixed with splitting of the GBM. Tubules drop out, glomeruli scar, and the kidney eventually succumbs to interstitial fibrosis. Primary treatment is control of systemic hypertension and use of ACE inhibitors to slow renal progression. Although patients who receive renal allografts usually develop anti-GBM antibodies directed toward the collagen epitopes absent in their native kidney, overt Goodpasture's syndrome is rare and graft survival is good.

THIN BASEMENT MEMBRANE DISEASE

Thin basement membrane disease (TBMD) characterized by persistent or recurrent hematuria is not typically associated with proteinuria, hypertension, or loss of renal function or extrarenal disease. Although not all cases are familial (perhaps a founder effect), it usually presents in childhood in multiple family members and is also called *benign familial hematuria*. Cases of TBMD have genetic defects in type IV collagen but in contrast to Alport behave as an autosomal dominant disorder that in ~40% of families segregates with the *COL(IV) α3/COL(IV) α4* loci. Mutations in these loci can result in a spectrum of disease ranging from TBMD to autosomal dominant or recessive Alport's. The GBM shows diffuse thinning compared to normal values for the patient's age in otherwise normal biopsies (Fig. e14-19). The vast majority of patients have a benign course.

NAIL-PATELLA SYNDROME

Patients with nail-patella syndrome develop iliac horns on the pelvis and dysplasia of the dorsal limbs involving the patella, elbows, and nails, variably associated with neural-sensory hearing impairment, glaucoma, and abnormalities of the GBM and podocytes, leading to hematuria, proteinuria, and FSGS. The syndrome is autosomal dominant, with haploinsufficiency for the *LIM* homeodomain transcription factor LMX1B; pedigrees are extremely variable in the penetrance for all features of the disease. LMX1B regulates the expression of genes encoding α3 and α4 chains of collagen IV, interstitial type III collagen, podocin, and CD2AP that help form the slit-pore membranes connecting podocytes. Mutations in the LIM domain region of *LMX1B* associate with glomerulopathy, and renal failure appears in as many as 30% of patients. Proteinuria or isolated hematuria is discovered throughout life, but usually by the third decade, and is inexplicably more common in females. On renal biopsy there is lucent damage to the lamina densa of the GBM, an increase in collagen III fibrils along glomerular capillaries and in the mesangium, and damage to the slit-pore membrane, producing heavy proteinuria not unlike that seen in congenital nephrotic syndrome. Patients with renal failure do well with transplantation.

GLOMERULAR-VASCULAR SYNDROMES

A variety of diseases result in classic vascular injury to the glomerular capillaries. Most of these processes also damage blood vessels elsewhere in the body. The group of diseases discussed here lead to vasculitis, renal endothelial injury, thrombosis, ischemia, and/or lipid-based occlusions.

ATHEROSCLEROTIC NEPHROPATHY

Aging in the developed world is commonly associated with the occlusion of coronary and systemic blood vessels. The reasons for this include obesity, insulin resistance, smoking, hypertension, and diets rich in lipids that deposit in the arterial and arteriolar circulation, producing local inflammation and fibrosis of small blood vessels. When the renal arterial circulation is involved, the glomerular microcirculation is damaged, leading to *chronic nephrosclerosis*. Patients with GFRs <60 mL/min have more cardiovascular events and hospitalizations than those with higher filtration rates. Several aggressive lipid disorders can accelerate this process, but most of the time atherosclerotic progression to chronic nephrosclerosis is associated with poorly controlled hypertension. Approximately 10% of glomeruli are normally sclerotic by age 40, rising to 20% by age 60 and 30% by age 80. Serum lipid profiles in humans are greatly affected by *apolipoprotein E* polymorphisms; the E4 allele is accompanied by increases in serum cholesterol and is more closely associated with atherogenic profiles in patients with renal failure. Mutations in E2 alleles, particularly in Japanese patients, produce a specific renal abnormality called *lipoprotein glomerulopathy* associated with glomerular lipoprotein thrombi and capillary dilation.

HYPERTENSIVE NEPHROSCLEROSIS

Uncontrolled systemic hypertension causes permanent damage to the kidneys in about 6% of patients with elevated blood pressure. As many as 27% of patients with end-stage kidney disease have hypertension as a primary cause. Although there is not a clear correlation between the extent or duration of hypertension and the risk of end-organ damage, *hypertensive nephrosclerosis* is fivefold more frequent in African Americans than whites. Risk alleles associated with *APOL1*, a functional gene for apolipoprotein L1 expressed in podocytes substantially explains the increased burden of end-stage renal disease among African Americans. Associated risk factors for progression to end-stage kidney disease include age, sex, race, smoking, hypercholesterolemia, duration of hypertension, low birth weight, and preexisting renal injury. Kidney biopsies in patients with hypertension, microhematuria, and moderate proteinuria demonstrate arteriolosclerosis, chronic nephrosclerosis, and interstitial fibrosis in the absence of immune deposits (Fig. e14-21). Today, based on a careful history, physical examination, urinalysis, and some serologic testing, the diagnosis of chronic nephrosclerosis is usually inferred without a biopsy. Treating hypertension is the best way to avoid progressive renal failure; most guidelines recommend lowering blood pressure to <130/80 mmHg if there is preexisting diabetes or kidney disease. In the presence of kidney disease, most patients begin therapy with two drugs, classically a thiazide diuretic and an ACE inhibitor; most will require three drugs. There is strong evidence in African Americans with hypertensive nephrosclerosis that therapy initiated with an ACE inhibitor can slow the rate of decline in renal function independent of effects on systemic blood pressure. Malignant acceleration of hypertension complicates the course of chronic nephrosclerosis, particularly in the setting of scleroderma or cocaine use (Fig. e14-24). The hemodynamic stress of malignant hypertension leads to fibrinoid necrosis of small blood vessels, thrombotic microangiography, a nephritic urinalysis, and acute renal failure. In the setting of renal failure, chest pain, or papilledema, the condition is treated as a hypertensive emergency. Slightly lowering the blood pressure often produces an immediate reduction in GFR that improves as the vascular injury attenuates and autoregulation of blood vessel tone is restored.

CHOLESTEROL EMBOLI

Aging patients with clinical complications from atherosclerosis sometimes shower cholesterol crystals into the circulation—either spontaneously or, more commonly, following an endovascular procedure with manipulation of the aorta—or with use of systemic anticoagulation. Spontaneous emboli may shower acutely or shower subacutely and somewhat more silently. Irregular emboli trapped in the microcirculation produce ischemic damage that induces an inflammatory reaction. Depending on the location of the atherosclerotic plaques releasing these cholesterol fragments, one may see cerebral transient ischemic attacks; livedo reticularis in the lower extremities; Hollenhorst plaques in the retina with visual field cuts; necrosis of the toes; and acute glomerular capillary injury leading to *focal segmental glomerulosclerosis* sometimes associated with hematuria, mild proteinuria, and loss of renal function, which typically progresses over a few years. Occasional patients have fever, eosinophilia, or eosinophiluria. A skin biopsy of an involved area may be diagnostic. Since tissue fixation dissolves the cholesterol, one typically sees only residual, biconvex clefts in involved vessels (Fig. e14-22). There is no therapy to reverse embolic occlusions, and steroids do not help. Controlling blood pressure and lipids and cessation of smoking are usually recommended for prevention.

SICKLE CELL DISEASE

Although individuals with SA-hemoglobin are usually asymptomatic, most will gradually develop hyposthenuria due to subclinical infarction of the renal medulla, thus predisposing them to volume depletion; interestingly, there is an unexpectedly high prevalence of sickle trait among dialysis patients who are African American. Patients with homozygous SS-sickle cell disease develop chronic vasoocclusive disease in many organs. Polymers of deoxygenated SS-hemoglobin distort the shape of red blood cells. These cells attach to endothelia and obstruct small blood vessels, producing frequent, random, and painful sickle cell crises over time. Vessel occlusions in the kidney produce glomerular hypertension, FSGS, interstitial nephritis, and renal infarction associated with hyposthenuria, microscopic hematuria, and even gross hematuria; some patients also present with MPGN. By the second or third decade of life, persistent vasoocclusive disease in the kidney leads to varying degrees of renal failure, and some patients end up on dialysis. Treatment is directed to reducing the frequency of painful crises and administering ACE inhibitors in the hope of delaying a progressive decline in renal function. In sickle cell patients undergoing renal transplantation, renal graft survival is comparable to African Americans in the general transplant population.

THROMBOTIC MICROANGIOPATHIES

Thrombotic thrombocytopenic purpura (TTP) and *hemolytic-uremic syndrome* (HUS) represent a spectrum of thrombotic microangiopathies. Thrombotic thrombocytopenic purpura and hemolytic-uremic syndrome share the general features of idiopathic thrombocytopenic purpura, hemolytic anemia, fever, renal failure, and neurologic disturbances. When patients, particularly children, have more evidence of renal injury, their condition tends to be called HUS. In adults with neurologic disease, it is considered to be TTP. In adults there is often a mixture of both, which is why they are often called TTP/HUS. On examination of kidney tissue there is evidence of *glomerular capillary endotheliosis* associated with platelet thrombi, damage to the capillary wall, and formation of fibrin material in and around glomeruli (Fig. e14-23). These tissue findings are similar to what is seen in preeclampsia/HELLP (*h*emolysis, *e*levated *l*iver enzymes, and *l*ow *p*latelet count syndrome), malignant hypertension, and the antiphospholipid syndrome. Thrombotic thrombocytopenic purpura/hemolytic-uremic syndrome is also seen in pregnancy; with the use of oral contraceptives or quinine; in renal transplant patients given OKT3 for rejection; in patients taking the calcineurin inhibitors, cyclosporine and tacrolimus, or in patients taking the antiplatelet agents, ticlopidine and clopidogrel; or following HIV infection.

Although there is no agreement on how much they share a final common pathophysiology, two general groups of patients are recognized: childhood HUS associated with enterohemorrhagic diarrhea and TTP/HUS in adults. Childhood HUS is caused by a toxin released by *Escherichia coli* 0157:H7 and occasionally by *Shigella dysenteriae.* This shiga toxin (verotoxin) directly injures endothelia, enterocytes, and renal cells, causing apoptosis, platelet clumping, and intravascular hemolysis by binding to the glycolipid receptors (Gb3). These receptors are more abundant along endothelia in children compared to adults. Shiga toxin also inhibits the endothelial production of ADAMTS13. In familial cases of adult TTP/HUS, there is a genetic deficiency of the ADAMTS13 metalloprotease that cleaves large multimers of von Willebrand's factor. Absent ADAMTS13, these large multimers cause platelet clumping and intravascular hemolysis. An antibody to ADAMTS13 is found in many sporadic cases of adult TTP/HUS, but not all; many patients also have antibodies to the thrombospondin receptor on selected endothelial cells in small vessels or increased levels of plasminogen-activator inhibitor 1 (PAI-1). Some children with complement protein deficiencies express atypical HUS (aHUS), which can be treated with liver transplant. The treatment of adult TTP/HUS is daily plasmapheresis, which can be lifesaving. Plasmapheresis is given until the platelet count rises, but in relapsing patients it normally is continued well after the platelet count improves, and in resistant patients twice-daily exchange may be helpful. Most patients respond within 2 weeks of daily plasmapheresis. Since TTP/HUS often has an autoimmune basis, there is an anecdotal role in relapsing patients for using splenectomy, steroids, immunosuppressive drugs, or rituximab, an anti-CD20 antibody. Patients with childhood HUS from infectious diarrhea are not given antibiotics, as antibiotics are thought to accelerate the release of the toxin and the diarrhea is usually self-limited. No intervention appears superior to supportive therapy in children with postdiarrheal HUS.

ANTIPHOSPHOLIPID ANTIBODY SYNDROME (SEE CHAP. 320)

INFECTIOUS DISEASE–ASSOCIATED SYNDROMES

A number of infectious diseases will injure the glomerular capillaries as part of a systemic reaction producing an immune response or from direct infection of renal tissue. Evidence of this immune response is collected by glomeruli in the form of immune deposits that damage the kidney, producing moderate proteinuria and hematuria. Some of these infectious diseases represent the most common causes of glomerulonephritis in many parts of the world.

POST-STREPTOCOCCAL GLOMERULONEPHRITIS

This form of glomerulonephritis is one of the classic complications of streptococcal infection. The discussion of this disease can be found in the section on *acute nephritic syndromes.*

SUBACUTE BACTERIAL ENDOCARDITIS

Renal injury from persistent bacteremia absent the continued presence of a foreign body, regardless of cause, is treated presumptively as if the patient has endocarditis. The discussion of this disease can be found in the section on *acute nephritic syndromes.*

HUMAN IMMUNODEFICIENCY VIRUS

Renal disease is an important complication of HIV disease. The risk of development of end-stage renal disease is much higher in HIV-infected African Americans than in HIV-infected whites. About 50% of HIV-infected patients with kidney disease have HIV-associated nephropathy (HIVAN) on biopsy. The lesion in HIVAN is FSGS, characteristically revealing a collapsing glomerulopathy (Fig. e14-3) with visceral epithelial cell swelling, microcystic dilatation of renal tubules, and tubuloreticular inclusion. Renal epithelial cells express replicating HIV virus, but host immune responses also play a role in the pathogenesis. MPGN and DPGN have also been reported but more commonly in HIV-infected whites and in patients coinfected with hepatitis B or C. HIV-associated TTP has also been reported. Other renal lesions include DPGN, IgA nephropathy, and MCD. Renal biopsy may be indicated to distinguish between these lesions.

HIV patients with FSGS typically present with nephrotic-range proteinuria and hypoalbuminemia, but unlike patients with other etiologies for nephrotic syndrome, they do not commonly have hypertension, edema, or hyperlipidemia. Renal ultrasound also reveals large, echogenic kidneys despite the finding that renal function in some patients declines rapidly. Treatment with inhibitors of the renin-angiotensin system decreases the proteinuria. Effective antiretroviral therapy benefits both the patient and the kidney and improves survival of HIV-infected patient with chronic kidney disease (CKD) or end-stage renal disease. In HIV-infected patients not yet on therapy, the presence of HIVAN is an indication to initiate therapy. Following the introduction of antiretroviral therapy, survival on dialysis for the HIV-infected patient has improved dramatically and is equivalent in patients treated with hemodialysis or peritoneal dialysis. Renal transplants in HIV-infected patients without detectable viral loads or histories of opportunistic infections have a better survival benefit over dialysis. Following transplantation, patient and graft survival are similar to the general transplant population despite frequent rejections.

HEPATITIS B AND C

Typically infected patients present with microscopic hematuria, nonnephrotic or nephrotic-range proteinuria, and hypertension. There is a close association between hepatitis B infection and polyarteritis nodosa with vasculitis appearing generally in the first 6 months following infection. Renal manifestations include renal artery aneurysms, renal infarction, and ischemic scars. Alternatively, the hepatitis B carrier state can produce a MGN that is more common in children than adults, or MPGN that is more common in adults than in children. Renal histology is indistinguishable from idiopathic MGN or type I MPGN. Viral antigens are found in the renal deposits. There are no good treatment guidelines, but interferon α-2b and lamivudine have been used to some effect in small studies. Children have a good prognosis, with 60–65% achieving spontaneous remission within 4 years. In contrast, 30% of adults have renal insufficiency and 10% have renal failure 5 years after diagnosis.

Up to 30% of patients with chronic hepatitis C infection have some renal manifestations. Patients often present with type II mixed cryoglobulinemia, nephrotic syndrome, microscopic hematuria, abnormal liver function tests, depressed C3 levels, anti–hepatitis C virus (HCV) antibodies, and viral RNA in the blood. The renal lesions most commonly seen, in order of decreasing frequency, are *cryoglobulinemic glomerulonephritis, MGN,* and *type I MPGN.* Treatment with pegylated interferon and ribavirin is typical to reduce the viral load.

OTHER VIRUSES

Other viral infections are occasionally associated with glomerular lesions, but cause and effect are not well established. These viral infections and their respective glomerular lesions include: cytomegalovirus producing MPGN; influenza and anti-GBM disease; measles-associated endocapillary proliferative glomerulonephritis, with measles antigen in the capillary loops and mesangium; parvovirus causing mild proliferative or mesangioproliferative glomerulonephritis or FSGS; mumps and mesangioproliferative glomerulonephritis; Epstein-Barr virus producing MPGN, diffuse proliferative nephritis, or IgA nephropathy; dengue hemorrhagic fever causing endocapillary proliferative glomerulonephritis; and coxsackievirus producing *focal glomerulonephritis* or DPGN.

SYPHILIS

Secondary syphilis, with rash and constitutional symptoms, develops weeks to months after the chancre first appears and occasionally presents with the nephrotic syndrome from MGN caused by subepithelial immune deposits containing treponemal antigens. Other lesions have also rarely been described including interstitial syphilitic nephritis. The diagnosis is confirmed with nontreponemal and treponemal tests for *Treponema pallidum.* The renal lesion responds to treatment with penicillin or an alternative drug, if allergic. Additional testing for other sexually transmitted diseases is an important part of disease management.

LEPROSY

Despite aggressive eradication programs, approximately 400,000 new cases of leprosy appear annually worldwide. The diagnosis is best made in patients with multiple skin lesions accompanied by sensory loss in affected areas, using skin smears showing paucibacillary or multibacillary infection (WHO criteria). Leprosy is caused by infection with *Mycobacterium leprae* and can be classified by Ridley-Jopling criteria into various types: tuberculoid, borderline tuberculoid, mid-borderline and borderline lepromatous, and lepromatous. Renal involvement in leprosy is related to the quantity of bacilli in the body, and the kidney is one of the target organs during splanchnic localization. In some series, all cases with borderline lepromatous and lepromatous types of leprosy have various forms of renal involvement including FSGS, mesangioproliferative glomerulonephritis, or renal amyloidosis; much less common are the renal lesions of DPGN and MPGN. Treatment with dapsone, rifampicin, and clofazimine can eradicate the infection in nearly all patients.

MALARIA

There are 300–500 million incident cases of malaria each year worldwide, and the kidney is commonly involved. Glomerulonephritis is due to immune complexes containing malarial antigens that are implanted in the glomerulus. In malaria from *P. falciparum,* mild proteinuria is associated with subendothelial deposits, mesangial deposits, and mesangioproliferative glomerulonephritis that usually resolve with treatment. In quartan malaria from infection with *P. malariae,* children are more commonly affected and renal involvement is more severe. Transient proteinuria and microscopic hematuria can resolve with treatment of the infection. However, resistant nephrotic syndrome with progression to renal failure over 3–5 years does happen, as <50% of patients respond to steroid therapy. Affected patients with nephrotic syndrome have thickening of the glomerular capillary walls, with subendothelial deposits of IgG, IgM, and C_3 associated with a sparse membranoproliferative lesion. The rare mesangioproliferative glomerulonephritis reported with *P. vivax* or *P. ovale* typically has a benign course.

SCHISTOSOMIASIS

Schistosomiasis affects more than 300 million people worldwide and primarily involves the urinary and gastrointestinal tracts. Glomerular involvement varies with the specific strain of schistosomiasis; *Schistosoma mansoni* is most commonly associated with clinical renal disease, and the glomerular lesions can be classified: Class I is a *mesangioproliferative glomerulonephritis;* class II is an *extracapillary proliferative glomerulonephritis;* class III is a *membranoproliferative glomerulonephritis;* class IV is a *focal segmental glomerulonephritis;* and class V lesions have *amyloidosis.* Classes I–II often remit with treatment of the infection, but classes III and IV lesions are associated with IgA immune deposits and progress despite antiparasitic and/or immunosuppressive therapy.

OTHER PARASITES

Renal involvement with toxoplasmosis infections is rare. When it occurs, patients present with nephrotic syndrome and have a histologic picture of MPGN. Fifty percent of patients with leishmaniasis will have mild to moderate proteinuria and microscopic hematuria, but renal insufficiency is rare. Acute DPGN, MGN, and mesangioproliferative glomerulonephritis have all been observed on biopsy. Filariasis and trichinosis are caused by nematodes and are sometimes associated with glomerular injury presenting with proteinuria, hematuria, and a variety of histologic lesions that typically resolve with eradication of the infection.

FURTHER READINGS

Beck LH Jr, Salant DJ: Glomerular and tubulointerstitial diseases. Prim Care 35:265, 2008

Berthoux FC et al: Natural history of primary IgA nephropathy. Semin Nephrol 28:4, 2008

Bomback AS, Appel GB: Updates on the treatment of lupus nephritis. J Am Soc Nephrol 21:2028, 2010

Falk RJ, Jennette JC: ANCA disease: Where is this field heading? J Am Soc Nephrol 21:745, 2010

Freedman BI, Sedor Jr: Hypertension-associated kidney disease: perhaps no more. J Am Soc Nephrol 19: 2047, 2008

Hudson BG et al: Alport and Goodpasture syndromes and the type IV collagen family. N Engl J Med 348:2543, 2003

Peti-Peterdi J, Sipos A: A high-powered view of the filtration barrier. J Am Soc Nephrol 21:1835, 2010

Rodriguez-Iturbe B, Musser JM: The current state of poststreptococcal glomerulonephritis. J Am Soc Nephrol 19: 1855, 2008

Smith RJH et al: New approaches to the treatment of dense deposit disease. J Am Soc Nephrol 18: 2447, 2007

Tervaert TW et al: Pathologic classification of diabetic nephropathy. J Am Soc Nephrol 21:556, 2010

Tryggvason K et al: Hereditary proteinuria syndromes and mechanisms of proteinuria. N Engl J Med 354:1387, 2006

CHAPTER 284

Polycystic Kidney Disease and Other Inherited Tubular Disorders

David J. Salant
Craig E. Gordon

INTRODUCTION

The polycystic kidney diseases are among the most common life-threatening inherited diseases worldwide and frequently cause kidney failure. Autosomal dominant polycystic kidney disease (ADPKD) is seen predominantly in adults (Fig. 284-1), whereas autosomal recessive polycystic kidney disease (ARPKD) is mainly a disease of childhood. Renal cysts also are seen in several other hereditary kidney diseases (Table 284-1), some of which may have defects in a common signaling pathway with ADPKD and ARPKD. Other inherited tubular diseases manifest primarily with alterations in fluid, electrolyte, acid-base, and mineral balance (Table 284-2).

■ AUTOSOMAL DOMINANT POLYCYSTIC KIDNEY DISEASE

Etiology and pathogenesis

ADPKD is a systemic disorder resulting from mutations in either the *PKD-1* or the *PKD-2* gene. The *PKD-1*-encoded protein, polycystin-1, is a large receptor-like molecule, whereas the *PKD-2* gene product, polycystin-2, has features of a calcium channel protein. Both are transmembrane proteins that are present throughout all segments of the nephron. They have been localized to the luminal surface of tubular cells in primary cilia, where they appear to serve as flow sensors; on the basal surface in focal adhesion complexes; and on the lateral surface in adherens junctions. The proteins are thought to function independently, or as a complex, to regulate fetal and adult epithelial cell gene transcription, apoptosis, differentiation, and cell-matrix interactions. Disruption of these processes leads to epithelial dedifferentiation, unregulated proliferation and apoptosis, altered cell polarity, disorganization of surrounding extracellular matrix, excessive fluid secretion, and abnormal expression of several genes, including some that encode growth factors. Vasopressin-mediated elevation of cyclic AMP levels in cyst epithelia plays a major role in cystogenesis by stimulating cell proliferation and fluid secretion into the cyst lumen through apical chloride and aquaporin channels. Cyst formation begins in utero from any point along the nephron, although <5% of total nephrons are thought to be involved. As the cysts accumulate fluid, they enlarge, separate entirely from the nephron, compress the neighboring renal parenchyma, and progressively compromise renal function.

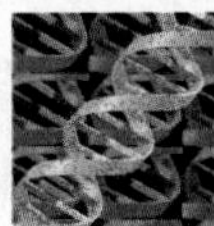

GENETIC CONSIDERATIONS

ADPKD occurs in 1:400–1:1000 individuals worldwide and accounts for ~4% of end-stage renal disease (ESRD) in the United States. ADPKD is equally prevalent in all ethnic and racial groups. Over 90% of cases are inherited as an autosomal dominant trait, with the remainder probably representing spontaneous mutations. Mutations in the *PKD-1* gene on chromosome 16 (ADPKD-1) account for 85% of cases, and mutations in the *PKD-2* gene on chromosome 4 (ADPKD-2) account for the remainder. A few families appear to have a defect at a site that is different from either of these loci. Direct mutation analysis of isolated cysts suggests that there is loss of heterozygosity, whereby a somatic mutation in the normal allele of a small number of tubular epithelial cells leads to unregulated clonal proliferation of the cells that ultimately form the cyst lining.

Clinical features

Phenotypic heterogeneity is a hallmark of ADPKD, as evidenced by family members who have the same mutation but have a different clinical course. Affected individuals are often asymptomatic into the fourth or fifth decade. Presenting symptoms and signs include abdominal discomfort, hematuria, urinary tract infection, incidental discovery of hypertension, abdominal masses, elevated serum creatinine, and cystic kidneys on imaging studies (Fig. 284-1*A* and *B*). Frequently, the diagnosis is made before the onset of symptoms, when asymptomatic members in affected families request screening. In most patients, renal function declines progressively over the course of 10–20 years from the time of diagnosis, but not everyone with ADPKD develops ESRD; it occurs in about 60% of these patients by age 70. Those with ADPKD-2 tend to have later onset and slower progression. Hypertension is common and often precedes renal dysfunction, perhaps mediated by increased activity of the renin-angiotensin system. There is only mild proteinuria, and impaired urinary concentrating ability manifests early as polyuria and nocturia. Risk factors for progressive kidney disease include younger age at diagnosis, black race, male sex, presence of polycystin-1

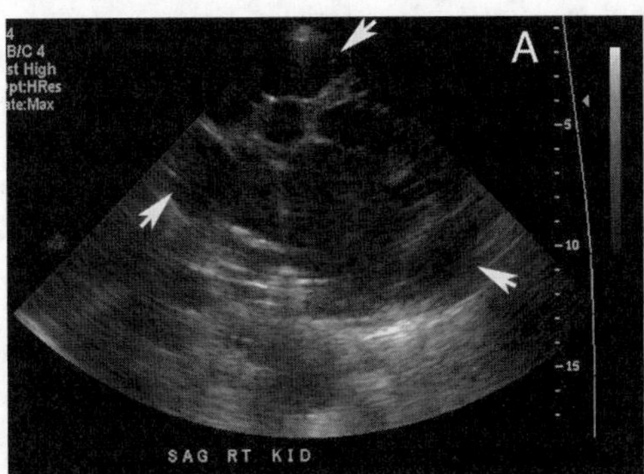

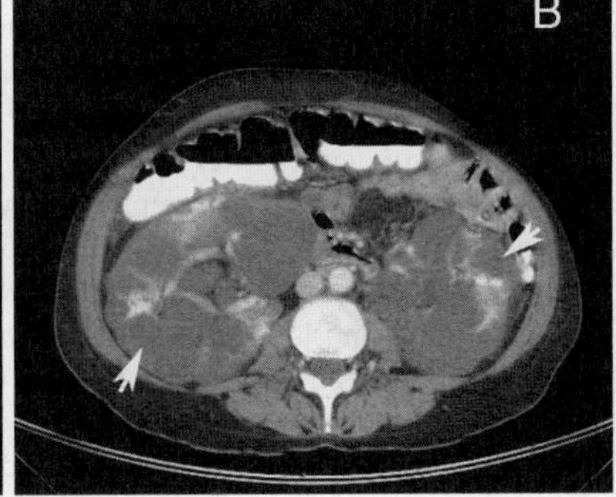

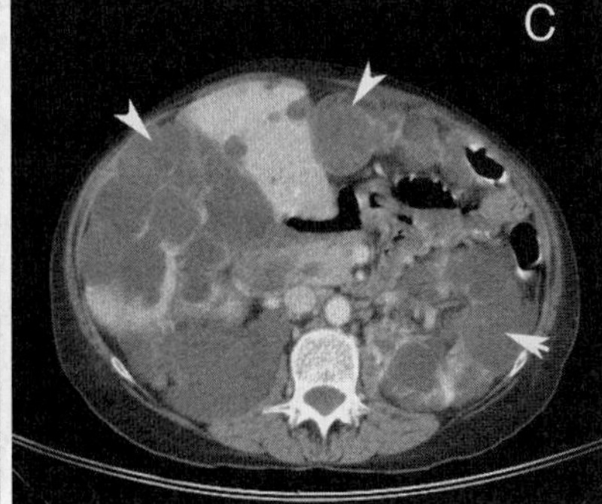

Figure 284-1 Renal ultrasonogram and contrast-enhanced abdominal CT scan in a 56-year-old woman with autosomal dominant polycystic kidney disease. ***A.*** Sonogram of the right kidney showing numerous cysts of varying sizes (*arrows*). ***B.*** Abdominal CT scan demonstrating bilaterally enlarged kidneys with large cysts (*arrows*). ***C.*** Multiple liver cysts (*arrowheads*) and renal cysts (*arrow*) are seen in an upper abdominal image.

TABLE 284-1 Inherited Cystic Kidney Diseases

Disease (OMIM)	Mode of Inheritance	Locus	Gene	Protein	Renal Abnormalities	Extrarenal Abnormalities
Autosomal dominant polycystic kidney disease (601313, 173910)	AD	16p13	*PKD1*	Polycystin-1	Cortical and medullary cysts	Cerebral aneurysms; liver cysts, other[a]
	AD	4q21	*PKD2*	Polycystin-2	Cortical and medullary cysts	Cerebral aneurysms; liver cysts, other[a]
Autosomal recessive polycystic kidney disease (263200)	AR	6p21	*PKHD1*	Fibrocystin (polyductin)	Distal tubule and collecting duct cysts	Hepatic fibrosis; Caroli's disease
Nephronophthisis I (juvenile/adolescent, 256100)[b]	AR	2q13	*NPHP1*	Nephrocystin	Small fibrotic kidneys; medullary cysts	Retinitis pigmentosa
Nephronophthisis II (infantile, 602088)[b]	AR	9q31	*NPHP2 (INVS)*	Inversin	Large kidneys; widespread cysts	Situs inversus
Nephronophthisis III (juvenile/adolescent, 604387)[b]	AR	3q22	*NPHP3*	Nephrocystin-3	Small fibrotic kidneys; medullary cysts	Retinitis pigmentosa; hepatic fibrosis
Medullary cystic kidney disease (174000, 603860)	AD	1q21	*MCKD1*	Unknown	Small fibrotic kidneys; medullary cysts	None
	AD	16p12	*MCKD2 (UMOD)*	Uromodulin (Tamm-Horsfall protein)	Small fibrotic kidneys; medullary cysts	Hyperuricemia and gout
Tuberous sclerosis (191100)	AD	9q34	*TSC1*	Hamartin	Renal cysts; angiomyolipomas; renal cell carcinoma	Facial angiofibromas; CNS hamartomas
	AD	16p13	*TSC2*	Tuberin	Renal cysts; angiomyolipomas; renal cell carcinoma	Facial angiofibromas; CNS hamartomas
Von Hippel-Lindau disease (608537)	AD	3p26-p25	*VHL*	pVHL	Renal cysts; renal cell carcinoma	Retinal angiomas; CNS hemangioblastomas; pheochromocytomas

[a]See text for details.

[b]The three variants of nephronophthisis listed in the table are the most prevalent of the currently described 11 forms of nephronophthisis. Each variant has similar renal abnormalities but varying extrarenal phenotypes.

Abbreviations: AD, autosomal dominant; AR, autosomal recessive; OMIM, online Mendelian inheritance in man.

mutation, and hypertension. There is a close correlation between the rate of kidney expansion, as measured by magnetic resonance imaging (MRI) scanning, and the rate of decline in kidney function. Dull, persistent flank and abdominal pain and early satiety are common due to the mass effect of the enlarged kidneys or liver. Cyst rupture or hemorrhage into a cyst may produce acute flank pain or symptoms and signs of localized peritonitis. Gross hematuria may result from cyst rupture into the collecting system or from uric acid or calcium oxalate kidney stones. Nephrolithiasis occurs in about 20% of patients. Urinary tract infection, including acute pyelonephritis, occurs with increased frequency in ADPKD. Infection in a kidney cyst is a particularly serious complication. It is most often due to Gram-negative bacteria and presents with flank pain, fever, and chills. Blood cultures are frequently positive, but urine culture may be negative because infected kidney cysts do not communicate directly with the collecting system. Distinguishing between infection and cyst hemorrhage is often challenging, and the diagnosis relies mainly on clinical and bacteriologic findings. Radiologic and nuclear imaging studies are generally not helpful.

Numerous extrarenal manifestations of ADPKD highlight the systemic nature of the disease. Patients with ADPKD have a twofold to fourfold increased risk of subarachnoid or cerebral hemorrhage from a ruptured intracranial aneurysm compared with the general population. Saccular aneurysms of the anterior cerebral circulation may be detected in up to 10% of asymptomatic patients on magnetic resonance angiography (MRA) screening, but most are small, have a low risk of spontaneous rupture, and do not merit the risk of intervention. In general, hemorrhage tends to occur before age 50 years, in patients with a family history of intracranial hemorrhage, and in those who have survived a previous bleed, have aneurysms >10 mm, and have uncontrolled hypertension. Other vascular abnormalities include aortic root and annulus dilation. Cardiac valvular abnormalities occur in 25% of patients, most commonly mitral valve prolapse and aortic regurgitation. Although most valvular lesions are asymptomatic, some may progress over time and warrant valve replacement. The incidence of hepatic cysts is 83% by MRI in patients age 15–46 years. Most patients are asymptomatic with normal liver function tests, but hepatic cysts may bleed, become infected, rupture, and cause pain. Although the frequency of liver cysts is equal between the sexes, women are more likely to have massive cysts (Fig. 284-1*C*). Colonic diverticulae are common, with a higher incidence of perforation in patients with ADPKD. Abdominal wall and inguinal hernias also occur with a higher frequency than in the general population.

Diagnosis and screening

Most often, the diagnosis of ADPKD is made from a positive family history and imaging studies showing large kidneys with multiple

TABLE 284-2 Inherited Tubular Disorders

Disease (OMIM)	Mode of Inheritance	Locus	Gene	Protein	Renal Abnormalities	Extrarenal Abnormalities
Bartter's syndrome						
Type 1 (601678)	AR	15q15	*SLC12A1*	NKCC2	Salt wasting; hypokalemia	
Type 2 (241200)	AR	11q24	*KCNJ1*	ROMK	Salt wasting; hypokalemia	
Type 3 (607364)	AR	1p36	*ClCNKb*	CLC-Kb	Salt wasting; hypokalemia	
Type 4 (602023)	AR	1p31	*BSND*	Barttin	Salt wasting; hypokalemia	Sensorineural deafness
Type 5 (601199)	AD	3q13	*CASR*	CASR	Salt wasting; hypokalemia	
Gitelman's syndrome (263800)	AR	16q13	*SLC12A3*	NCCT	Salt wasting; hypokalemia; hypomagnesemia	
Pseudohypoaldosteronism type I (264350, 177735)	AR	16p13 16p13 12p13	*SCNN1B* *SCNN1G* *SCNN1A*	α, β, or γ subunit of ENaC	Hyperkalemia; salt wasting	Increased lung secretions and lung infections
	AD	4q31	*NR3C2*	Mineralocorticoid receptor (type I)	Hyperkalemia; salt wasting	
Familial hypomagnesemia with hypercalciuria and nephrocalcinosis (FHHNC) (248250, 248190)	AR	3q27 1p34	*CLDN16* *CLDN19*	Claudin 16 Claudin 19	Hypomagnesemia; nephrocalcinosis	Ocular abnormalities (claudin 19 defect only)
Hypomagnesemia with secondary hypocalcemia (HSH) (602014)	AR	9q22	*TRPM6*	TRPM6	Hypomagnesemia; hypocalcemia	
Autosomal dominant hypomagnesemia (154020)	AD	11q23	*FXYD2*	γ subunit of basolateral Na/K-ATPase of DCT	Hypomagnesemia; hypocalciuria	
Autosomal dominant hypoparathyroidism (601199)	AD	3q13	*CASR*	CASR	Hypocalcemia; hypercalciuria; hypomagnesemia	
Isolated autosomal recessive hypomagnesemia (611718)	AR	4q25	*EGF*	EGF	Hypomagnesemia	
Liddle's syndrome (177200)	AD	16p13	*SCNN1B* *SCNN1G*	β and γ subunits of ENaC	Hypertension; hypokalemia; alkalosis	
Pseudohypoaldosteronism type II (Gordon's syndrome, 145260)	AD	12p13 17q21	*WNK1* *WNK4*	WNK 1 WNK 4	Hypertension; hyperkalemia	
Nephrogenic DI type 1 (304800)	XL	Xq28	*AVPR2*	AVPR2	Renal concentrating defect	
Nephrogenic DI type 2 (125800)	AR, AD	12q13	*AQP2*	AQP2	Renal concentrating defect	
Nephrogenic syndrome of inappropriate antidiuresis (300539)	XL	Xq28	*AVPR2*	AVPR2	Hyponatremia	
Distal renal tubular acidosis (267300, 602722, 259730, 179800)	AR	2cenq13 7q33	*ATP6V1B1* *ATP6VOA4*	H^+-ATPase (B1) H^+-ATPase (α4)	Hyperchloremic metabolic acidosis; nephrocalcinosis	Sensorineural deafness (B1 defect only); growth retardation
	AR	8q22	*CA2*	CA2	Proximal and distal RTA	Osteopetrosis, short stature, mental retardation
	AD	17q21	*SLC4A1*	AE1	Distal RTA	
Proximal renal tubular acidosis (604278)	AR	4q21	*SLC4A4*	NBC-1	Moderate hyperchloremic metabolic acidosis	Glaucoma; band keratopathy
Cystinuria (220100)	AR	2p16 19q13	*SLC3A1* *SLC7A9*	$rBATb^{o,+}AT1$	Cystine stones; dibasic aminoaciduria	
Hartnup disease (234500)	AR	5p15	*SLC6A19*	B^oAT1	Neutral aminoaciduria	Dermatitis, ataxia; dementia
Dent's disease (300009)	XL	Xp11	*CLCN5*	CLC-5	Fanconi syndrome; nephrocalcinosis	Osteomalacia; rickets

(*continued*)

TABLE 284-2 Inherited Tubular Disorders (*Continued*)

Disease (OMIM)	Mode of Inheritance	Locus	Gene	Protein	Renal Abnormalities	Extrarenal Abnormalities
Cystinosis (219800)	AR	17p13	*CTNS*	Cystinosin	Fanconi syndrome; progressive kidney failure	Ocular, muscular, liver, gonadal, and thyroid involvement
Renal glucosuria (233100)	AR	16p11	*SLC5A2*	SGLT2	Glucosuria	
Hereditary hypophosphatemic rickets with hypercalciuria (HHRH, 241530)	AR	9q34	*SLC34A3*	Sodium-phosphate co-transporter	Hypophoshatemia; hypercalciuria	Rickets
Vitamin D–dependent rickets type I (VDDR I, 264700)	AR	12q14.1	*CYP27B1*	25-vitamin D_3-1-α-hydroxylase	Hypocalcemia	Rickets

Abbreviations: AD, autosomal dominant; AE1, anion exchanger 1; AR, autosomal recessive; AT1, amino acid transporter; AVPR2, arginine vasopressin receptor 2; CA2, carbonic anhydrase II; CASR, calcium-sensing receptor; CLC-5, chloride channel 5; CLC-Kb, chloride channel Kb; DI, diabetes insipidus; ENaC, amiloride-sensitive epithelial sodium channel; NBC, sodium-bicarbonate co-transporter; NCCT, thiazide-senstitive Na-Cl co-transporter; NKCC2, Na-K-2Cl co-transporter; OMIM, online Mendelian inheritance in man; rBAT, renal basic amino acid transport glycoprotein; ROMK, renal outer medullary potassium channel; SGLT2, sodium/glucose co-transporter.TRPM6, transient receptor potential cation channel, subfamily M, member 6; WNK, with no lysine (K); XL, X-linked;

bilateral cysts and possibly liver cysts (Fig. 284-1). Criteria for the diagnosis of ADPKD by ultrasonography in asymptomatic individuals account for the later onset of ADPKD-2 and assume that the genotype of the individual and family being tested is unknown. The presence of three or more cysts in one or both kidneys is required to diagnose ADPKD in patients age 15–39 years with a specificity and positive predictive value of 100%; sensitivity varies from 82 to 96% for persons age 15–29 and 30–39 years, respectively. The presence of two or more cysts in each kidney is associated with a sensitivity and specificity of 90% and 100%, respectively, in patients age 40–59 years. In subjects older than 60 years, the presence of four or more cysts in each kidney is required to diagnose ADPKD because of the increased frequency of benign simple cysts, whereas fewer than two renal cysts in at-risk individuals age ≥40 years is sufficient to exclude the disease. Computed tomography (CT) scan and T2-weighted MRI are more sensitive for detecting presymptomatic disease in young patients. Genetic linkage analysis and mutational screening for *ADPKD-1* and *ADPKD-2* is available for equivocal cases, especially when a young adult from an affected family is being considered as a potential kidney donor. Genetic counseling is essential for those being screened. Screening for asymptomatic intracranial aneurysms should be restricted to patients with a personal or family history of intracranial hemorrhage and those in high-risk occupations. Intervention should be limited to aneurysms larger than 10 mm.

TREATMENT Autosomal Dominant Polycystic Kidney Disease

No treatment has been proved to prevent cyst growth or the decline in kidney function. Hypertension control with a target blood pressure of 130/80 mmHg or less is recommended according to Joint National Committee (JNC) VII guidelines. A multidrug approach that includes agents to inhibit the renin-angiotensin system is frequently required. Studies are investigating the role of angiotensin-converting enzyme (ACE) inhibitors and angiotensin receptor blockers (ARBs) in slowing growth of kidney volume and loss of glomerular filtration rate (GFR). Lipid-soluble antimicrobials such as trimethoprim-sulfamethoxazole and fluoroquinolones that have good cyst penetration are the preferred therapy for infected kidney and liver cysts. Pain management occasionally requires cyst drainage by percutaneous aspiration, sclerotherapy with alcohol, or, rarely, surgical drainage. Patients with ADPKD appear to have a survival advantage on either peritoneal or hemodialysis compared with patients with other causes of ESRD. Those undergoing kidney transplantation may require bilateral nephrectomy if the kidneys are massively enlarged or have been the site of infected cysts. Posttransplantation survival rates are similar to those of patients with other causes of kidney failure, but these patients remain at risk for the extrarenal complications of ADPKD. Studies in animal models of inherited cystic diseases have identified promising therapeutic strategies, including vasopressin V2 receptor antagonists that suppress cyst growth by lowering intracellular cAMP, and inhibitors of cell dedifferentiation and proliferation that target the epidermal growth factor receptor tyrosine kinase and the mammalian target of rapamycin (mTOR). Clinical trials of these agents are ongoing.

AUTOSOMAL RECESSIVE POLYCYSTIC KIDNEY DISEASE

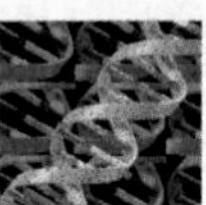

GENETIC CONSIDERATIONS

ARPKD is primarily a disease of infants and children. The incidence is 1:20,000 births. The kidneys are enlarged, with small cysts, <5 mm, limited to the collecting tubules. The ARPKD gene on chromosome 6p21, *PKHD1*, encodes several alternatively spliced transcripts (Table 284-1). The largest transcript produces a multidomain transmembrane protein termed *fibrocystin (polyductin)* that is found in the cortical and medullary collecting ducts and the thick ascending limb of Henle's loop in the kidney as well as in biliary and pancreatic duct epithelia. Like the polycystins, fibrocystin has receptor-like features and may be involved in cell-cell and cell-matrix interactions. Fibrocystin, the polycystins, and several proteins involved in animal models of PKD are located in association with primary cilia on the tubular epithelial cell apical surface; this suggests that they may cooperate in a mechanosensory pathway. A large number of different mutations have been identified throughout *PKHD1* and are unique to individual families. Most patients are compound heterozygotes. Those with two truncating mutations frequently die shortly after birth, whereas those who survive beyond the neonatal period generally have at least one missense mutation. Mutations in *PKHD1* have also been identified in about 30% of children with congenital hepatic fibrosis (Caroli's syndrome) without evident kidney involvement.

Clinical features

The clinical presentation of ARPKD is highly variable. Up to 50% of affected neonates die of pulmonary hypoplasia, the result of oligohydramnios from severe intrauterine kidney disease. About 80% of those who survive the neonatal period are still alive after 10 years; however, one-third will have developed ESRD. Enlarged kidneys may be detected soon after birth as bilateral abdominal masses. Impaired urinary concentrating ability and metabolic acidosis ensue as tubular function deteriorates. Hypertension often occurs in the first few years of life. Kidney function deteriorates progressively from childhood into early adult life. Longer-term survivors frequently develop complications of portal hypertension from periportal fibrosis.

Diagnosis

Ultrasonography reveals large, echogenic kidneys. The diagnosis can be made in utero after 24 weeks of gestation in severe cases, but cysts generally become visible only after birth. The absence of renal cysts in either parent on ultrasonography helps distinguish ARPKD from ADPKD in older patients. The wide range of different mutations and the large size of the gene complicate molecular diagnosis, although prenatal diagnosis is possible by gene linkage to the *PKHD1* locus in families with a previous confirmed ARPKD birth.

TREATMENT Autosomal Recessive Polycystic Kidney Disease

There is no specific therapy for ARPKD. Improvements in neonatal intensive care, blood pressure management, dialysis, and kidney transplantation have led to survival into adulthood. Complications of hepatic fibrosis may necessitate liver transplantation. Future therapies may target aberrant cell signaling mechanisms, as in ADPKD.

NEPHRONOPHTHISIS

Genetics and pathogenesis

Nephronophthisis (NPHP) is the most common genetic cause of ESRD in childhood and adolescence. Eleven distinct genetic mutations with autosomal recessive inheritance have been identified to date and produce different renal and extrarenal manifestations of NPHP (Table 284-1). Although their precise functions are unclear, the defective protein products, named nephrocystins and inversin, localize to the primary cilium and associated basal body of renal epithelial cells, similar to the polycystins and fibrocystin. NPHP is classified into infantile, juvenile, and adolescent forms based on the age of ESRD onset. In juvenile NPHP, the most common form, the kidneys are shrunken and histology shows tubular atrophy, thickening of tubular basement membranes, diffuse interstitial fibrosis, and microscopic medullary cysts. In the infantile form, the kidneys are large with histology similar to that of the juvenile form except that medullary cysts are more prominent and develop earlier.

Clinical features

In juvenile NPHP symptoms typically appear after 1 year of age. Impaired tubular function causes salt wasting and defective urinary concentration and acidification. Patients may present with polyuria, polydipsia, volume depletion, or systemic acidosis. Hypertension is usually absent due to salt wasting. Progressive kidney failure and volume depletion lead to growth retardation. On average, ESRD occurs by age 3 in the infantile form, age 13 in the juvenile form, and age 19 in the adolescent form. Up to 15% of patients with juvenile NPHP have extrarenal manifestations (Table 284-1), most commonly retinitis pigmentosa (Senior-Loken syndrome). Other abnormalities include blindness from amaurosis, oculomotor apraxia, cerebellar ataxia (Joubert syndrome), polydactyly, mental retardation, hepatic fibrosis, and ventricular septal defect. Situs inversus is seen in some cases of infantile NPHP, consistent with mutation in *INVS (NPHP2)*, a gene critical for left-right patterning in the embryo.

Diagnosis

The diagnosis of NPHP should be considered in patients with a family history of kidney disease, early-onset progressive renal failure, and a bland urine sediment with minimal proteinuria. Ultrasonography reveals small hyperechoic kidneys in juvenile NPHP and large kidneys with cysts in the infantile form.

TREATMENT Nephronophthisis

There is no specific therapy to prevent loss of kidney function in NPHP. Salt and water replacement are required for patients with salt wasting and polyuria. Therapy should include sodium bicarbonate or citrate for acidosis, management of chronic kidney disease, and timely institution of dialysis and kidney transplantation. NPHP does not recur in transplanted kidneys.

MEDULLARY CYSTIC KIDNEY DISEASE

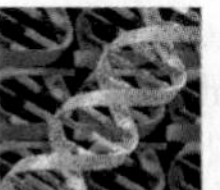

GENETIC CONSIDERATIONS

The medullary cystic kidney diseases (MCKDs) generally present in young adults. Two genetic loci have been defined, both with autosomal dominant transmission (Table 284-1). The locus for MCKD1 has been mapped to chromosome 1q21. Mutations in the uromodulin gene (*UMOD*) that encodes the Tamm-Horsfall mucoprotein on chromosome 16p12 have been identified in MCKD2.

Clinical features

As with NPHP, patients with MCKD have atrophic kidneys with diffuse interstitial fibrosis, cysts restricted to the renal medulla, salt wasting, and polyuria. Disease onset is later than in NPHP. Consequently, there is no growth retardation, salt wasting is milder, and ESRD occurs later, usually between ages 20 and 70. There are no extrarenal manifestations in MCKD1, but most patients with MCKD2 have severe hyperuricemia and precocious onset of gout.

Diagnosis

MCKD should be considered in young adults with a family history suggesting dominant inheritance of kidney disease who present with progressive renal failure, bland urinalysis with little or no proteinuria, and small dense kidneys with medullary cysts on radiographic imaging. The presence of hyperuricemia and gout is a further clue to the diagnosis of MCKD2, which can be confirmed by mutation analysis of *UMOD*.

TREATMENT Medullary Cystic Kidney Disease

There is no specific therapy for MCKD. Allopurinol is indicated for patients with gout and is reasonable for those with asymptomatic hyperuricemia, although there is no evidence that it prevents progressive renal failure in MCKD2. Dialysis and transplantation outcomes appear to be favorable. The disease does not recur in transplanted kidneys.

■ TUBEROUS SCLEROSIS

Tuberous sclerosis (TS) is an autosomal dominant disorder that affects 1 in 6000 people. It results from mutations in either the *TSC1* gene encoding hamartin or the *TSC2* gene encoding tuberin (Table 284-1). Hamartin and tubulin form a complex that is thought to negatively regulate cell growth and proliferation through inhibition of mTOR. The presence of either mutation produces uncontrolled proliferation in numerous tissues, including the kidneys, skin, central nervous system, and heart. The kidneys are affected in 80% of patients. Renal TS occurs in three forms: renal angiomyolipomas, renal cysts, and renal cell carcinoma. Angiomyolipomas are the most common renal abnormality. They occur bilaterally, are often multiple, and are usually asymptomatic; however, they may cause spontaneous bleeding, flank pain, hematuria, and life-threatening retroperitoneal hemorrhage. Large lesions, >4 cm, are more likely to be symptomatic and may require transcatheter arterial embolization or surgical excision. Cysts are usually asymptomatic and are not evident on imaging studies until adulthood. Rarely, cysts may be large and numerous, sometimes leading to ESRD and producing a clinical scenario that can be confused with ADPKD, especially if there are few other systemic manifestations of TS. Multicentric renal cell carcinomas occur with increased frequency in TS. Patients with TS should be screened for renal involvement at initial diagnosis with ultrasonography or CT. Those with cysts or angiomyolipomas require regular imaging to monitor for the development of renal cell carcinoma.

■ VON HIPPEL-LINDAU DISEASE

Von Hippel-Lindau disease (VHL) is a rare autosomal dominant disease characterized by abnormal angiogenesis with benign and malignant tumors that affect multiple tissues. The disease is inherited as a mutation in one allele of the *VHL* tumor-suppressor gene. Somatic mutation of the normal allele leads to retinal angiomas, central nervous system (CNS) hemangioblastomas, pheochromocytomas and multicentric clear cell cysts, hemangiomas, and adenomas of the kidney. The kidneys are affected in three-quarters of patients, and half these patients develop clear cell carcinomas in the renal cysts. It is noteworthy that *VHL* mutations also account for 60% of spontaneous clear cell carcinomas of the kidney. The mean age of diagnosis of renal cell carcinoma in VHL disease is 44 years, and 70% of patients who survive to age 60 develop renal cell carcinoma. The high risk of renal cell carcinoma mandates periodic surveillance (usually yearly in adults) by CT or MRI. Routine screening and awareness of the natural history of lesions has enabled renal-sparing approaches to disease management. Tumors <3 cm in size require careful monitoring for growth, whereas partial nephrectomy is indicated in those >3 cm in the absence of metastasis. Nonsurgical renal-sparing strategies, including percutaneous radio frequency ablation and selective arterial embolization, have shown promise in short-term trials.

■ MEDULLARY SPONGE KIDNEY

Pathology and clinical features

Medullary sponge kidney (MSK) is a relatively common benign condition of unknown cause characterized by ectasia of the papillary collecting ducts of one or both kidneys. Urinary stasis in the dilated ducts, hypocitraturia, and occasionally incomplete distal renal tubular acidosis (dRTA) contribute to the formation of small calcium-containing calculi. Most cases are asymptomatic or are discovered during investigation of hematuria. Symptomatic patients typically present as young adults with renal colic and nephrolithiasis or recurrent urinary tract infections; however, MSK also may affect children. Most cases are sporadic, although MSK has been found rarely in association with other congenital anomalies of the urinary tract and with congenital hepatic ductal ectasia (Caroli's disease).

Diagnosis

MSK is characteristically seen as hyperdense papillae with clusters of small stones on renal ultrasonography or abdominal x-ray (Fig. 284-2). The classical "paintbrush-like" features of MSK, representing the ectatic collecting ducts, are best seen on intravenous urography. However, this procedure has been supplanted by contrast-enhanced, high-resolution helical CT with digital reconstruction (Fig. 284-2).

TREATMENT Medullary Sponge Kidney

No treatment is necessary in asymptomatic individuals, aside from maintaining high fluid intake to reduce the risk of nephrolithiasis. Recurrent stone formation should prompt a metabolic evaluation and treatment as in any stone former (Chap. 287). In patients with hypocitraturia and incomplete dRTA, treatment with potassium citrate helps prevent new stone formation. Urinary tract infections should be treated promptly.

HEREDITARY DISORDERS OF SODIUM, POTASSIUM, AND MAGNESIUM HANDLING WITHOUT HYPERTENSION

Inherited forms of hypochloremic metabolic alkalosis and hypokalemia without hypertension are due to genetic mutations of various ion transporters and channels of the thick ascending limb of Henle's loop (TAL) and distal convoluted tubule (DCT) (Table 284-2 and Fig. 284-3). In 1962 Bartter described two patients with a syndrome of metabolic alkalosis, hypovolemia, and failure to thrive associated with juxtaglomerular apparatus hyperplasia, hyperaldosteronism, and normal blood pressure. Subsequently, Gitelman identified a similar but milder syndrome accompanied by hypomagnesemia from urinary magnesium wasting and presenting in later childhood and adolescence. These disorders are now known to occur sporadically or result from genetically heterogeneous loss-of-function autosomal recessive mutations that cause salt-losing tubulopathy.

■ BARTTER'S SYNDROME AND GITELMAN'S SYNDROME

Genetics and pathogenesis

Bartter's syndrome may result from mutations affecting any of five ion transport proteins in the TAL. The proteins affected include the apical loop diuretic–sensitive sodium-potassium-chloride co-transporter NKCC2 (type 1), the apical potassium channel ROMK (type 2), and the basolateral chloride channel ClC-Kb (type 3). Bartter's type 4 results from mutations in barttin, an essential subunit of ClC-Ka and ClC-Kb that enables transport of the chloride channels to the cell surface. Barttin is also expressed in the inner ear; this accounts for the deafness invariably associated with Bartter's type 4. A Bartter-like phenotype (type 5) with associated hypocalcemia has been described in patients with autosomal dominant gain-of-function mutations in the extracellular calcium-sensing receptor (CaSR). Unregulated activation of this G protein–coupled receptor inhibits sodium reabsorption in the TAL. The TAL transporters function in an integrated manner to maintain both the electrical potential difference and the sodium gradient between the lumen and the cell (Fig. 284-3). Loss of the lumen-positive electrical transport potential that normally drives the paracellular reabsorption of sodium, calcium, and magnesium causes NaCl wasting, hypercalciuria, and mild hypomagnesemia. As expected, the clinical syndrome mimics the effects of chronic ingestion of a loop diuretic.

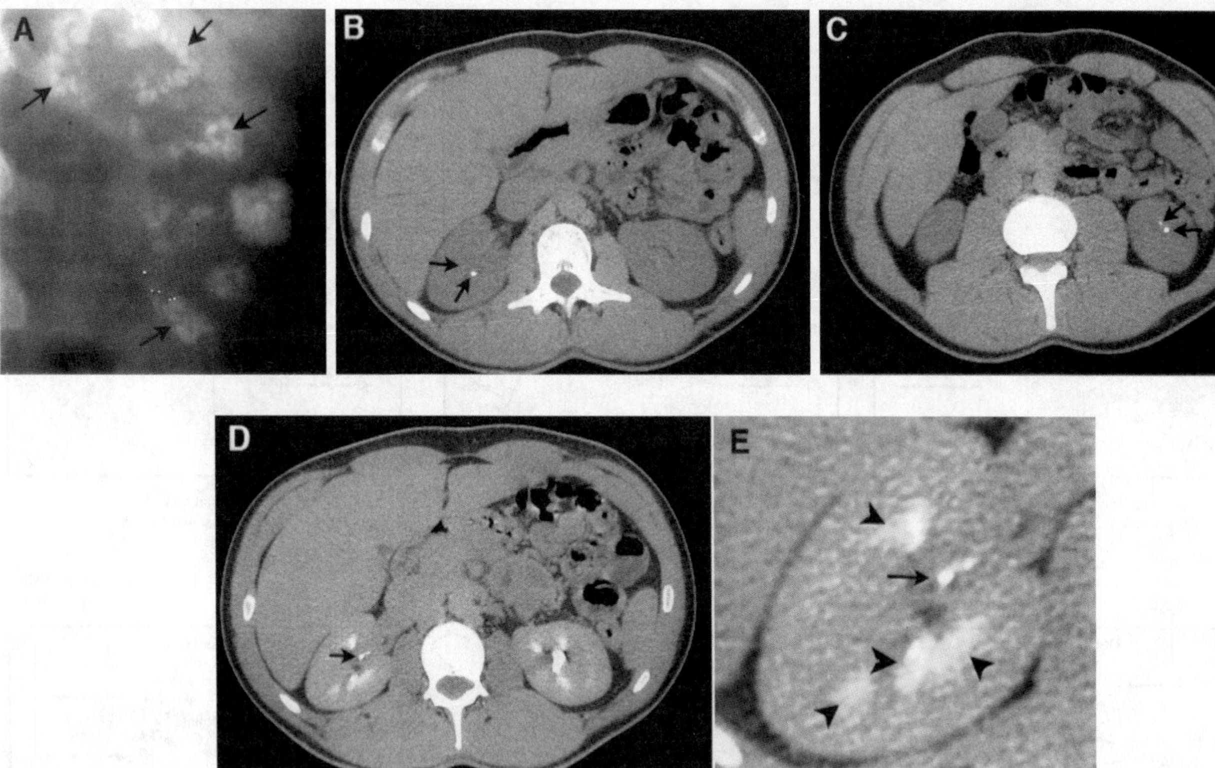

Figure 284-2 Radiographs of medullary sponge kidney disease. ***A.*** Plain x-ray film of a patient with a history of recurrent nephrolithiasis showing clusters of stones in the papillae (arrows). ***B–E.*** CT scan of an 18-year-old male patient investigated for persistent microscopic hematuria. ***B*** and ***C.*** CT without contrast showing a few small stones in the papillae (*arrows*). ***D*** and ***E.*** Contrast-enhanced CT of the same region shown in *B.* In addition to the stone (*arrow*), a blush of contrast is seen filling the ectatic collecting ducts (*arrowheads*).

Gitelman's syndrome is due to mutations in the thiazide-sensitive Na-Cl co-transporter, NCCT, in the DCT. Defects in NCCT in Gitelman's syndrome impair sodium and chloride reabsorption in the DCT (Fig. 284-3) and thus resemble the effects of thiazide diuretics. It remains unclear how this defect leads to severe magnesium wasting.

In both Bartter's and Gitelman's syndromes, hypovolemia from impaired sodium and chloride reabsorption in either the TAL or the DCT activates the renin-angiotensin-aldosterone system (RAAS). The consequent hyperaldosteronism, together with increased distal flow and sodium delivery, stimulates increased sodium reabsorption in the collecting tubules via the epithelial sodium channel (ENaC). This promotes increased potassium and hydrogen ion secretion, causing hypokalemia and metabolic alkalosis. Additionally, in Bartter's syndrome, RAAS activation causes increased levels of cyclooxygenase 2 (COX-2) and marked overproduction of renal prostaglandins (PGE_2), and this exacerbates the polyuria and electrolyte abnormalities.

Clinical features

Bartter's syndrome Bartter's syndrome is a rare disease that most often presents in the neonatal period or early childhood with polyuria, polydipsia, salt craving, and growth retardation. Blood pressure is normal or low. Metabolic abnormalities include hypokalemia, hypochloremic metabolic alkalosis, decreased urinary concentrating and diluting ability, hypercalciuria with nephrocalcinosis, mild hypomagnesemia, and increased urinary prostaglandin excretion. Hyperprostaglandin E syndrome is a particularly severe form of Bartter's syndrome in which neonates present with pronounced volume depletion and failure to thrive, as well as fever, vomiting, and diarrhea from PGE_2 overproduction. In the antenatal period, fetal polyuria may cause maternal polyhydramnios and premature labor. Sensorineural deafness occurs in patients with barttin gene mutations (type 4). Patients with severe Bartter's syndrome who survive early childhood may develop chronic kidney disease from nephrocalcinosis or from tubular atrophy and interstitial fibrosis from severe persistent hypokalemia. Patients with Bartter's syndrome type 3 have a phenotype intermediate between those of Bartter's and Gitelman's syndromes, consistent with mutation of the ClC-Kb chloride channel in both the TAL and the DCT with preservation of the ClC-Ka chloride channel in the TAL. This disease occurs predominantly in African-American patients and resembles most closely the classic syndrome described by Bartter. Onset is generally later in childhood, patients have mild or no nephrocalcinosis, and prostaglandin excretion is normal.

Gitelman's syndrome Gitelman's syndrome is more common than Bartter's syndrome and has a generally milder clinical course with a later age of presentation. It is characterized by prominent neuromuscular symptoms and signs, including fatigue, weakness, carpopedal spasm, cramps, and tetany.

Diagnosis

Hypokalemia and hypochloremic metabolic alkalosis without hypertension are more often due to surreptitious vomiting or diuretic abuse than to Bartter's or Gitelman's syndrome. In contrast to Bartter's and Gitelman's syndromes, urinary chloride levels are very low in patients with surreptitious vomiting. Diuretic abuse can be diagnosed by screening the urine for the offending agents. Gitelman's syndrome is distinguished from most forms of Bartter's syndrome by the presence of severe hypomagnesemia and hypocalciuria.

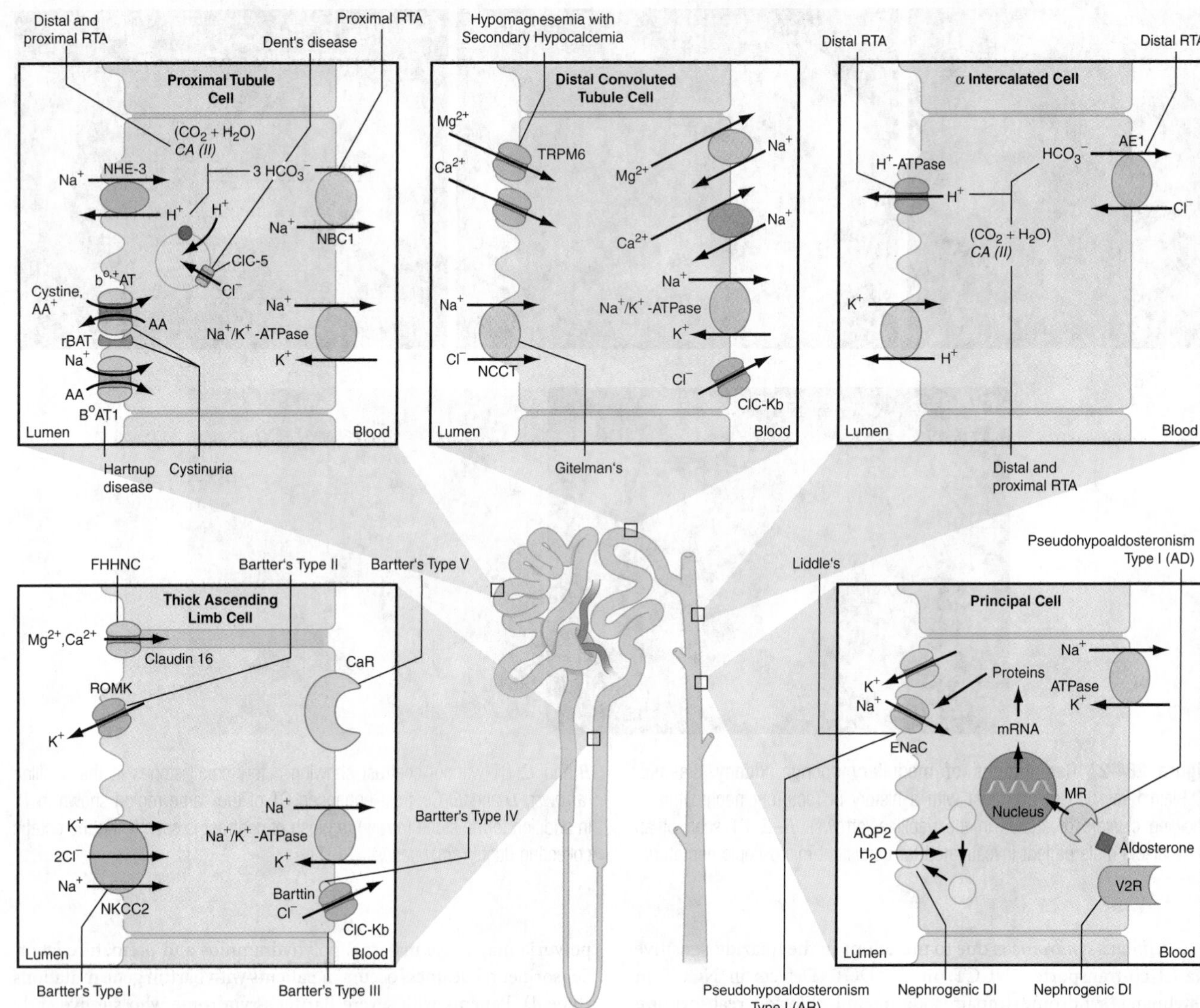

Figure 284-3 Schematic representation of channels, transporters, and enzymes associated with hereditary renal tubular disorders. AD, autosomal dominant; AR, autosomal recessive; DI, diabetes insipidus; NKCC2, Na-K-2Cl co-transporter; ROMK, renal outer medullary potassium channel; AQP2, aquaporin-2; CLC-Kb, chloride channel Kb; CaR, calcium-sensing receptor; NCCT, thiazide-senstitive Na-Cl co-transporter; ENaC, amiloride-sensitive epithelial sodium channel; TRPM6, transient receptor potential cation channel, subfamily M, member 6; WNK, with no lysine (K); V2R, arginine vasopressin receptor 2; MR, mineralocorticoid receptor; RTA, renal tubular acidosis; CA (II), carbonic anhydrase II; AE1, anion exchanger 1; NBC1; sodium-bicarbonate co-transporter; rBAT, renal basic amino acid transport glycoprotein; AT1, amino acid transporter; CLC-5, chloride channel 5; AA, amino acids.

TREATMENT Bartter's Syndrome and Gitelman's Syndrome

Both conditions require lifelong therapy with potassium and magnesium supplements and liberal salt intake. High doses of spironolactone or amiloride treat the hypokalemia, alkalosis, and magnesium wasting. Nonsteroidal anti-inflammatory drugs (NSAIDs) reduce the polyuria and salt wasting in Bartter's syndrome but are ineffective in Gitelman's syndrome. They may be lifesaving in hyperprostaglandin E syndrome and can be given in the form of a COX-2 inhibitor to avoid the gastrointestinal side effects of long-term high-dose NSAIDs. In Gitelman's syndrome, magnesium repletion is essential to correct the hypokalemia and control muscle weakness, tetany, and metabolic alkalosis; however, it may prove difficult in patients wasting large amounts of magnesium.

PSEUDOHYPOALDOSTERONISM TYPE 1

Patients with type 1 pseudohypoaldosteronism present with severe renal salt wasting and hyperkalemia. Although these findings resemble mineralocorticoid deficiency, plasma renin activity and aldosterone levels are elevated. Defective salt handling is the result of autosomal recessive loss-of-function mutations of the α, β, or γ subunit of the ENaC or autosomal dominant mutations of one allele of the mineralocorticoid receptor (Table 284-2 and Fig. 284-3). The autosomal recessive form is a multisystem disorder with a severe phenotype, often manifesting in the neonatal period with renal salt wasting, vomiting, hyponatremia, hyperkalemia, acidosis, and failure to thrive. Impaired channel activity in the skin and lungs can produce excess sodium and chloride loss in sweat, excess fluid in the airways, and a propensity for lower respiratory tract infections that mimic cystic fibrosis. In contrast, the autosomal dominant form has a more benign course that is limited mainly to renal salt wasting and hyperkalemia. Aggressive salt replacement and management of hyperkalemia can lead to survival into adulthood, and symptoms may become less severe with time, especially in the dominant form. In the latter, high-dose fludrocortisone or carbenoxolone provides additional benefit by increasing mineralocorticoid activity and partly restoring the functional defect in the mutant receptor.

MAGNESIUM WASTING DISORDERS

In addition to Gitelman's syndrome, several hereditary disorders cause urinary magnesium wasting (Table 284-2 and Fig. 284-3). These disorders include autosomal recessive familial hypomagnesemia with hypercalciuria and nephrocalcinosis (FHHNC), autosomal recessive hypomagnesemia with secondary hypocalcemia (HSH), autosomal dominant hypomagnesemia, autosomal dominant hypoparathyroidism, and isolated autosomal recessive hypomagnesemia (Chap. 353). Common clinical features are the early onset of spasms, tetany, and seizures as well as associated or secondary disturbances in calcium homeostasis.

Familial hypomagnesemia with hypercalciuria and nephrocalcinosis

FHHNC is the first example of a disorder attributable to a defective protein involved in paracellular ion transport. *CLDCN16* encodes claudin 16 (previously known as paracellin-1), a member of the claudin family of proteins that are involved in tight junction formation. Claudin 16 is expressed in the TAL of Henle's loop and the DCT. Claudin 16 is thought to be an essential component of the paracellular pathway for Mg, and Ca to a lesser extent, reabsorption in the TAL. Clinical manifestations begin in infancy and include hypomagnesemia that is refractory to oral supplementation, hypercalciuria, and nephrocalcinosis. Recurrent urinary tract infections and nephrolithiasis have also been observed. Patients with mutations of claudin 19 have a similar phenotype but also manifest ocular defects, including corneal calcifications and chorioretinitis.

Hypomagnesemia with secondary hypocalcemia

Hypomagnesemia in HSH results from a defect in the TRPM6 channel, a member of the transient receptor potential (TRP) family of cation transport channels. TRPM6 is expressed in intestinal epithelia and the DCT and is thought to mediate transepithelial magnesium transport. Symptoms are attributable to hypomagnesemia with secondary impairment of parathyroid function and hypocalcemia. Seizures and muscle spasms occur in infancy, and restoration of magnesium and calcium levels requires high doses of oral magnesium supplementation.

Other hereditary hypomagnesemic disorders

Mutations of the sodium-potassium-ATPase γ subunit can cause an autosomal dominant hypomagnesemia. Activating mutations of the CaSR in autosomal dominant hypoparathyroidism primarily manifest as hypocalcemia, but hypomagnesemia has been reported in 50% of these patients. Mutations in epidermal growth factor (EGF) result in isolated autosomal recessive hypomagnesemia due to impaired activation of the EGF receptor and consequent failure to activate TRPM6.

HEREDITARY TUBULAR DISORDERS CAUSING HYPERTENSION DUE TO SALT RETENTION

LIDDLE'S SYNDROME

Liddle's syndrome mimics a state of aldosterone excess by the presence of early and severe hypertension, often accompanied by hypokalemia and metabolic alkalosis, but plasma aldosterone and renin levels are low. This disorder is due to unregulated sodium reabsorption by an overactive ENaC in the cortical collecting duct (Fig. 284-3). Deletional mutations of the intracellular domain of the β or γ subunit of ENaC (Table 284-2) prevent binding of the ubiquitin ligase Nedd4-2 that normally targets the channel for proteasomal degradation. This results in an inability to downregulate the number of channels despite a high intracellular sodium concentration. Increased potassium and hydrogen ion secretion follow the lumen-negative electrical potential that results from chloride-independent sodium reabsorption. Amiloride or triamterene blocks ENaC and, combined with salt restriction, provides effective therapy for the hypertension and hypokalemia.

PSEUDOHYPOALDOSTERONISM TYPE II (FAMILIAL HYPERKALEMIC HYPERTENSION; GORDON'S SYNDROME)

Pseudohypoaldosteronism type II is a rare autosomal dominant disease that manifests in adolescence or early adulthood with thiazide-responsive low-renin hypertension, hyperkalemia, and metabolic acidosis with normal renal function. Mutations have been identified in the WNK kinases 1 and 4 that lead to increased activity of the thiazide-sensitive sodium chloride channel, NCCT. This causes hypertension from enhanced salt reabsorption in the DCT and impaired distal secretion of potassium and hydrogen ion, all of which can be corrected with thiazide diuretics.

INHERITED DISORDERS OF WATER HANDLING

HEREDITARY NEPHROGENIC DIABETES INSIPIDUS

Hereditary nephrogenic diabetes insipidus (NDI) is a rare monogenic disease that usually presents in infancy with severe vasopressin-resistant polyuria, dehydration, failure to thrive, and dilute urine despite the presence of hypernatremia.

Genetics and pathogenesis

Vasopressin [antidiuretic hormone (ADH)]-stimulated water reabsorption in the collecting duct is mediated by the type 2 vasopressin receptor (V2R) on the basal surface of principal cells. Activation of the adenylyl cyclase–cAMP pathway phosphorylates vesicle-associated aquaporin-2 (AQP2) water channels and stimulates their insertion into the apical plasma membrane. Water enters the cells from the tubular lumen through AQP2 and exits along an osmotic gradient into the hypertonic medulla and vasa rectae via basal AQP3/4 channels (Fig. 284-3). X-linked mutations of *AVPR2,* the gene that encodes V2R, account for about 90% of cases of hereditary NDI, such that the expression of the receptor on the cell surface is impaired. The remaining cases are due to various autosomal recessive or dominant mutations of *AQP2* that cause the water channels to be retained within the cytosol (Table 284-2). The effect of these mutations is an inability to concentrate the urine and conserve water despite high plasma levels of vasopressin. Penetrance is variable in heterozygous female carriers of X-linked NDI, and some have a moderate concentrating defect that may be exacerbated in pregnancy due to placental vasopressinase.

Clinical features

Whereas NDI in adults is most often acquired from lithium therapy, hypercalcemia, and partial chronic urinary obstruction, hereditary NDI typically presents in infancy. Unlike other polyuric syndromes such as Bartter's and Gitelman's syndromes, conservation of electrolytes is normal, and hypernatremia is entirely from the loss of water. Recurrent episodes of dehydration and hypernatremia can lead to seizures and mental retardation. Although renal function is otherwise normal, chronically high urine flow causes dilation of the ureters and bladder and may cause bladder dysfunction and obstructive uropathy.

Diagnosis

The diagnosis in infants and children with hereditary NDI is usually apparent from the family history and clinical presentation. The diagnosis can be confirmed by the presence of high plasma levels of vasopressin in the face of polyuria and hypotonic urine. This may be especially useful in adults with partial NDI to distinguish the polyuric state from central diabetes insipidus or psychogenic polydipsia (Chap. 340). Genetic screening for mutations in *AVPR2* and *AQP2* is available in research centers and can be performed to identify affected infants from families at risk of NDI to begin treatment and avoid dehydration and its consequences.

TREATMENT Hereditary Nephrogenic Diabetes Insipidus

Early diagnosis and treatment with abundant water intake have enabled many patients to live to adulthood with normal mental and physical development. Exogenous vasopressin is ineffective, and because these patients can excrete up to 20 L of urine per day, maintaining adequate water intake is challenging. Thiazide diuretics and salt restriction can reduce urine output by inducing a state of mild volume contraction, thereby promoting increased proximal reabsorption of isotonic fluid and inhibiting the delivery of free water to the collecting duct. A combination thiazide-amiloride formulation will avoid thiazide-induced hypokalemia, and indomethacin may further reduce urine output by inhibiting prostaglandin synthesis.

NEPHROGENIC SYNDROME OF INAPPROPRIATE ANTIDIURESIS

Activating mutations of the V2R result in hyponatremia, inappropriately elevated urinary osmolality, and undetectable arginine vasopressin (AVP) levels in affected males. This syndrome results from missense mutations of *AVPR2* on the X chromosome, which cause constitutive activation of V2R and inappropriate water reabsorption. Heterozygous female carriers may be at risk of hyponatremia when exposed to large volumes of hypotonic fluids.

INHERITED RENAL TUBULAR ACIDOSIS

Non-anion-gap (hyperchloremic) metabolic acidosis from proximal tubular bicarbonate wasting or impaired distal net acid excretion may be a primary (sporadic or inherited) tubular disorder or may be acquired secondary to a variety of conditions (Chap. 47). There are three forms of renal tubular acidosis (RTA). Types 1 and 2 may be acquired or primary, whereas the most common form, type 4 RTA, usually is acquired in association with moderate renal dysfunction and is characterized by hyperkalemia.

TYPE 1 (DISTAL) RTA

Clinical features and diagnosis

In distal RTA the kidneys are unable to acidify the urine to pH <5.5 in the presence of systemic metabolic acidosis or after acid loading as a result of impaired hydrogen ion secretion or bicarbonate reabsorption in the distal nephron. Other features include hypokalemia, hypocitraturia, hypercalciuria, nephrocalcinosis, and/or nephrolithiasis. Chronic untreated acidosis may cause rickets or osteomalacia. Inheritance of primary dRTA includes autosomal dominant and autosomal recessive forms with a broad spectrum of clinical expression. Autosomal recessive dRTA most often presents in infancy with severe acidosis, failure to thrive, impaired growth, and impaired kidney function from nephrocalcinosis. Many patients with autosomal dominant dRTA, and some with recessive disease, are asymptomatic, and RTA is discovered incidentally in adolescence or adulthood during evaluation for kidney stones. In the absence of systemic acidosis, the diagnosis of incomplete dRTA is suggested by hypocitraturia and hypercalciuria and can be confirmed by failure of the urine to acidify to pH <5.5 after acid loading.

Genetics and pathophysiology

Primary dRTA may be hereditary or sporadic with autosomal recessive and autosomal dominant forms. Several kindreds with autosomal recessive dRTA have been identified in Southeast Asia and in areas of the world where parental consanguinity is high. The cellular basis for dRTA lies in dysfunction at the level of the α type intercalated cell of the cortical collecting duct (Fig. 284-3). Mutations affecting subunits of the H^+-ATPase proton pump on the luminal surface impair hydrogen ion secretion and account for most forms of autosomal recessive dRTA and are often associated with early-onset sensorineural hearing loss (Table 284-2). Autosomal dominant dRTA results from mutations involving the chloride-bicarbonate exchanger, AE1, on the basolateral membrane. Anion exchange by the mutant AE1 is normal, but aberrant targeting of AE1 from the basal to the apical plasma membrane is believed to cause bicarbonate loss into the urine instead of reabsorption. Bi-allelic mutations of AE1 may impair transport activity and account for some cases of recessive disease (Table 284-2). A syndrome of osteopetrosis, short stature, and mental retardation, so-called marble-brain disease with dRTA, is due to mutations in carbonic anhydrase II. Urinary potassium wasting and defective urinary concentration are characteristic of dRTA. Calcium is released from bone in the process of buffering of acid and results in hypercalciuria. Enhanced proximal citrate absorption accounts for hypocitraturia and, together with hypercalciuria, predisposes to nephrocalcinosis and formation of calcium phosphate stones.

TREATMENT Type 1 (Distal) RTA

Early initiation of alkali replacement at doses equivalent to 1–3 mmol/kg per day of bicarbonate in divided doses will usually correct the acidosis, hypokalemia, and hypocitraturia, maintaining growth and preventing bone disease in early-onset dRTA. Citrate is generally tolerated better than sodium bicarbonate and can be given as the potassium or sodium salt, depending on the severity of hypokalemia. In patients who present later with kidney stones, large fluid intake and sufficient alkali to restore normal acid-base balance correct the hypocitraturia and reduce hypercalciuria, thereby inhibiting the formation of new stones.

TYPE 2 (PROXIMAL) RTA

Proximal RTA (pRTA) is the result of impaired bicarbonate reabsorption in the proximal tubule, where the bulk of filtered bicarbonate is recovered (Fig. 284-3). It is most often secondary to various autoimmune, drug-induced, infiltrative, or other tubulopathies (Chap. 47) or results from tubular injury from inherited diseases in which endogenous metabolites accumulate and produce tubular injury. Such inherited disorders include Wilson's disease, cystinosis, tyrosinemia, galactosemia, hereditary fructose intolerance, glycogen storage disease type I, and Lowe's syndrome. In this situation pRTA is only one of several abnormalities that constitute Fanconi syndrome. Other features are hyperphosphaturia, hyperuricosuria, hypercalciuria, nonselective aminoaciduria, and glycosuria. In addition to hyperchloremic acidosis, rickets and osteomalacia are the predominant effects of Fanconi syndrome.

A rare infantile form of primary pRTA with isolated proximal tubular bicarbonate wasting is due to homozygous mutations of the proximal tubule basolateral sodium-bicarbonate co-transporter NBC1 (Table 284-2). This co-transporter is the main mechanism by which bicarbonate moves from the proximal tubule cell back into the blood. Other manifestations include short stature and mental retardation. An ocular phenotype that includes bilateral glaucoma, cataracts, and band keratopathy reflects a role of NBC1 in maintaining normal fluid balance in the eye and clarity of the lens.

TREATMENT Type 2 (Proximal) RTA

It is difficult to restore normal acid-base balance in patients with pRTA despite large amounts of alkali. This is the case because they continue to waste bicarbonate (fractional excretion >15%) until the serum level falls below a threshold, usually about 15–17 mmol/L, at which time bicarbonate is completely reabsorbed distally and the urine is maximally acidified with pH <5.5. When the serum bicarbonate concentration is raised above the threshold with alkali therapy, bicarbonate wasting recurs and causes hypokalemia as potassium is secreted to maintain luminal electroneutrality. Thus, treatment of pRTA requires 5–15 mmol/kg per day of bicarbonate together with supplemental potassium.

OTHER MONOGENIC DISORDERS OF PROXIMAL TUBULAR FUNCTION (FIG. 284-3)

CYSTINURIA

Cystinuria is an autosomal recessive disorder of cystine and dibasic amino acid (ornithine, arginine, and lysine) transport in the proximal tubule and intestinal epithelial cells. With a prevalence of about 1 in 10,000, it represents one of the more common heritable diseases. Impaired tubular absorption leads to high concentrations of cystine, which is insoluble in the acid environment of the renal tubules. Clinical severity varies from asymptomatic cystine crystalluria in heterozygous carriers to the frequent passage of gravel and cystine stones, ureteral obstruction, recurrent urinary infections, formation of staghorn calculi, and progressive kidney failure in homozygotes. The median onset of nephrolithiasis is 12 years. The disease is due to mutations in one of two genes, *SLC3A1* and *SLC7A9* (Table 284-2). *SLC3A1* encodes rBAT, a high-affinity, sodium-independent transporter for dibasic amino acids. The protein product of *SLC7A9*, $b^{0,+}AT$, is a catalytic subunit that associates with rBAT to form the active transporter. Diagnosis of cystinuria is established by a positive family history, the finding of hexagonal cystine crystals on urinalysis, and 24-h urinary cystine excretion that exceeds 400 mg (normal less than 30 mg/d).

TREATMENT Cystinuria

The mainstay of treatment is hydration to achieve a urine output of 2.5 L/d or more to reduce urine cystine concentration to <300 mg/L, together with urine alkalinization to pH 7.0–7.5 with potassium citrate, and sodium restriction. Cystine is an oxidized dimer that is formed by linking two cysteine residues via a disulfide bond between the -SH groups. Thus, in intractable cases, thiol derivatives such as penicillamine, tiopronin, and captopril may be added as chelation therapy to dissociate the cystine molecule into more soluble disulfide compounds. Various stone removal and urinary drainage procedures are often required.

HARTNUP DISEASE

Hartnup disease is an autosomal recessive condition caused by a defect in intestinal and renal transport of neutral amino acids. The major clinical manifestations are cerebellar ataxia and a pellagra-like skin rash. Other than aminoaciduria, the kidneys are unaffected. The defective gene, *SLC6A19*, encodes a sodium-dependent and chloride-independent neutral amino acid transporter (B^0AT1), which is expressed predominately in the small intestine and proximal tubule of the kidney (Table 284-2). Amino acids such as tryptophan that are retained in the intestinal lumen are converted to indole compounds that are toxic to the CNS. Abnormal tryptophan metabolism also leads to a niacin deficiency that accounts for the skin manifestations. Symptoms are aggravated by a protein-deficient diet and are alleviated with a high-protein diet and nicotinamide supplements.

DENT'S DISEASE

Dent's disease and X-linked recessive nephrolithiasis are unusual forms of Fanconi syndrome due to X-linked mutations of the gene encoding CLC-5, a voltage-gated chloride channel (Table 284-2). The disorders are characterized by childhood onset of low-molecular-weight proteinuria, hypercalciuria, nephrocalcinosis, and nephrolithiasis. Rickets or osteomalacia occurs in 25% of patients, and progressive renal failure from interstitial fibrosis, tubular atrophy, and glomerulosclerosis commonly develops in adulthood. CLC-5 serves to maintain the electrical gradient and acid environment established in proximal tubular cell endosomes by proton-ATPase, which is necessary for the degradation of low-molecular-weight proteins normally filtered by the glomerulus. Defects in CLC-5 appear to disrupt this process and lead to tubular cell dysfunction.

TREATMENT Dent's Disease

Treatment is directed at controlling hypercalciuria by dietary salt restriction and thiazide diuretics, which favor calcium reabsorption. Restriction of dietary calcium is not recommended.

CYSTINOSIS

Cystinosis is a rare multisystem autosomal recessive disease caused by mutations of cystinosin, a hydrogen ion–driven transporter responsible for exporting cystine from lysosomes. Accumulation of insoluble cystine leads to crystal formation in proximal tubular cells and other organs. Cystinosis occurs in infantile (nephropathic), adolescent, and adult forms. The nephropathic form is the most common, with clinical signs developing between 3 and 6 months of age, including Fanconi syndrome, salt and water wasting, growth retardation, rickets, vomiting, constipation, and unexplained fever. End-stage renal disease occurs by age 10 in the infantile form of the disease but after age 15 in the intermediate form. Extrarenal manifestations result from cystine accumulation in organs and include photophobia and blindness, muscular weakness from carnitine deficiency, hepatomegaly, hypothyroidism, delayed pubertal development, and late-onset neurologic disease. The adult form of cystinosis is largely asymptomatic except for photophobia. The diagnosis is made by measuring elevated cystine content of peripheral blood leukocytes.

TREATMENT Cystinosis

Treatment includes replacement of fluid and electrolyte losses related to Fanconi syndrome and polyuria. L-Carnitine supplementation is recommended to achieve normal plasma carnitine levels. Cysteamine provides a direct treatment of the disease that converts cystine to cysteine, which can exit the lysosome. Cysteamine should be started promptly upon the diagnosis of cystinosis as it preserves kidney function, prevents hypothyroidism, and improves growth. Kidney transplantation is the treatment of choice for ESRD as cystinosis does not recur in transplanted kidneys, but the extrarenal manifestations persist and may progress.

RENAL GLUCOSURIA

Isolated glucosuria in the presence of a normal blood glucose concentration is due to mutations in *SLC5A2*, the gene that encodes the high-capacity sodium-glucose co-transporter SGLT2 in the proximal renal tubule (Table 284-2). Subjects with this disorder are usually asymptomatic and do not have other features of proximal tubular dysfunction. Depending on the severity of the defect, the tubular maximum for glucose reabsorption may fall well within normal blood glucose levels and lead to >50 g/d of glucosuria. Such patients may have polyuria from osmotic diuresis.

RENAL PHOSPHATE WASTING

Renal phosphate wasting resulting in hypophosphatemia and rickets or osteomalacia may be part of a generalized disorder of proximal tubular function, as in Fanconi syndrome, or an isolated phenomenon. Isolated phosphaturia is most often due to the inhibition of renal tubular phosphate reabsorption by one or another phosphaturic hormone, with FGF-23 playing a major role (Chap. 352). An exception is hereditary hypophosphatemic rickets with hypercalciuria (HHRH), an autosomal recessive disorder due to mutations in *SLC34A3*, the gene encoding the proximal tubule sodium-phosphate co-transporter, NPT-2c (Table 284-2). Defective phosphate reabsorption causes renal phosphate wasting and stunted growth from rickets. The low serum phosphorus levels stimulate 1-hydroxylation of vitamin D, which increases intestinal calcium absorption, suppresses parathyroid hormone (PTH) secretion, and results in hypercalciuria. High levels of 1,25-dihydroxyvitamin D help distinguish HHRH from hormonal causes of hyperphosphaturia (Chap. 352). Treatment is directed at phosphate repletion.

VITAMIN D–DEPENDENT RICKETS

Vitamin D–dependent rickets exists in two forms that manifest with hypocalcemia, hypophosphatemia, elevated PTH levels, and the skeletal abnormalities of rickets and osteomalacia. Tetany may be present in severe cases. Vitamin D–dependent rickets type I is an autosomal recessive disease that results from mutations in *CYP27B1*, the gene that encodes $25(OH)D_3$-1α-hydroxylase, an enzyme in the proximal tubule that catalyzes the hydroxylation and activation of $25(OH)D_3$ into $1,25(OH)_2D_3$ (Table 284-2). It can be treated with physiologic replacement doses of $1,25(OH)_2D_3$. In contrast, autosomal recessive vitamin D–dependent rickets type II is due to end organ resistance to $1,25(OH)_2D_3$ as a result of mutations in the vitamin D receptor (Chap. 353).

FURTHER READINGS

Camargo SM et al: Aminoacidurias: Clinical and molecular aspects. Kidney Int 73:918, 2008

Crino PB et al: The tuberous sclerosis complex. N Engl J Med 355:1345, 2006

Devonald MA, Karet FE: Renal epithelial traffic jams and one-way streets. J Am Soc Nephrol 15:1370, 2004

Grantham JJ: Autosomal dominant polycystic kidney disease. N Engl J Med 359:1477, 2008

Guay-Woodford L: Other cystic kidney diseases, in *Comprehensive Clinical Nephrology*, 2nd ed, RJ Johnson, J Feehally (eds). New York, Saunders, 2003

Hart TC et al: Mutations of the UMOD gene are responsible for medullary cystic kidney disease 2 and familial juvenile hyperuricaemic nephropathy. J Med Genet 39:882, 2002

Hildebrandt F et al: Nephronophthisis: Disease mechanisms of a ciliopathy. J Am Soc Nephrol 11:1937, 2000; 20:23, 2009

Jeck N et al: Salt handling in the distal nephron: Lessons learned from inherited human disorders. Am J Physiol Regul Integr Comp Physiol 288:R782, 2005

Knoers NVAM: Inherited forms of renal hypomagnesemia: An update. Pediatr Nephrol 24:697, 2009

Laing CM et al: Renal tubular acidosis: Developments in our understanding of the molecular basis. Int J Biochem Cell Biol 37:1151, 2005

Sands JM, Bichet DG: Nephrogenic diabetes insipidus. Ann Intern Med 144:186, 2006

Saunier S et al: Nephronophthisis. Curr Opin Genet Dev 15:324, 2005

Siroky BJ: Renal involvement in tuberous sclerosis complex and von Hippel-Lindau disease: Shared disease mechanisms? Nat Clin Pract Nephrol 5:143, 2009

Torres VE, Harris PC: Mechanisms of disease: Autosomal dominant and recessive polycystic kidney diseases. Nat Clin Pract Nephrol 2:40, 2006

CHAPTER 285

Tubulointerstitial Diseases of the Kidney

Laurence H. Beck
David J. Salant

Inflammation or fibrosis of the renal interstitium and atrophy of the tubular compartment are common consequences of diseases that target the glomeruli or vasculature. Distinct from these secondary phenomena, however, are a group of disorders that primarily affect the tubules and interstitium, with relative sparing of the glomeruli and renal vessels. Such disorders are conveniently divided into acute and chronic tubulointerstitial nephritis (TIN) (Table 285-1).

Acute TIN most often presents with acute renal failure (Chap. 279). The acute nature of this group of disorders may be caused by aggressive inflammatory infiltrates that lead to tissue edema, tubular cell injury, and compromised tubular flow, or by frank obstruction of the tubules with casts, cellular debris, or crystals. There is sometimes flank pain due to distention of the renal capsule. Urinary sediment is often active with leukocytes and cellular casts, but depends on the exact nature of the disorder in question.

The clinical features of chronic TIN are more indolent and may manifest with disorders of tubular function, including polyuria from impaired concentrating ability (nephrogenic diabetes insipidus), defective proximal tubular reabsorption leading to features of Fanconi syndrome [glycosuria, phosphaturia, aminoaciduria, hypokalemia- and type II renal tubular acidosis (RTA) from bicarbonaturia], or non-anion-gap metabolic acidosis and hyperkalemia (type IV RTA) due to impaired ammoniagenesis, as well as progressive azotemia [rising creatinine and blood urea nitrogen (BUN)]. There is often modest proteinuria (rarely >2 g/d) attributable to decreased tubular reabsorption of filtered proteins; however, nephrotic-range albuminuria may occur in some conditions due to the development of secondary focal segmental glomerulosclerosis (FSGS). Renal ultrasonography may reveal changes of "medical renal disease," such as increased echogenicity of the renal parenchyma with loss of corticomedullary differentiation, prominence of the renal pyramids, and cortical scarring in some conditions. The predominant pathology in chronic TIN is interstitial fibrosis with patchy mononuclear cell infiltration and widespread tubular atrophy, luminal dilation, and thickening of tubular basement membranes. Because of the nonspecific nature of the histopathology, biopsy specimens rarely provide a specific diagnosis. Thus, diagnosis relies on careful analysis of history, drug or toxin exposure, associated symptoms, and imaging studies.

ACUTE INTERSTITIAL NEPHRITIS

In 1897 Councilman reported on eight cases of acute interstitial nephritis (AIN) in the Medical and Surgical Reports of the Boston City Hospital; three as a postinfectious complication of scarlet fever and two from diphtheria. Later, he described the lesion as "an acute inflammation of the kidney characterized by cellular and fluid exudation in the interstitial tissue, accompanied by, but not dependant on, degeneration of the epithelium; the exudation is not purulent in character, and the lesions may be both diffuse and focal." Today

TABLE 285-1 Classification of the Causes of Tubulointerstitial Diseases of the Kidney

Acute Tubulointerstitial Disorders
Acute Interstitial Nephritis
Therapeutic agents
• Antibiotics (β-lactams, sulfonamides, quinolones, vancomycin, erythromycin, minocycline, rifampin, ethambutol, acyclovir)
• Nonsteroidal anti-inflammatory drugs, COX-2 inhibitors
• Diuretics (rarely thiazides, loop diuretics, triamterene)
• Anticonvulsants (phenytoin, valproate, carbamazepine, phenobarbital)
• Miscellaneous (proton pump inhibitors, H_2 blockers, captopril, mesalazine, indinavir, allopurinol)
Infection
• Bacteria (*Streptococcus, Staphylococcus, Legionella, Salmonella, Brucella, Yersinia, Corynebacterium diphtheriae*)
• Viruses (EBV, CMV, hantavirus, polyomavirus, HIV)
• Miscellaneous (*Leptospira, Rickettsia, Mycoplasma*)
Autoimmune
• Tubulointerstitial nephritis with uveitis (TINU)
• Sjögren's syndrome
• Systemic lupus erythematosus
• Granulomatous interstitial nephritis
• IgG4-related systemic disease
• Idiopathic autoimmune interstitial nephritis
Acute obstructive disorders
• Light chain cast nephropathy ("myeloma kidney")
• Acute phosphate nephropathy
• Acute urate nephropathy
Chronic Tubulointerstitial Disorders
• Vesicoureteral reflux/reflux nephropathy
• Sickle cell disease
• Chronic exposure to toxins or therapeutic agents
• Analgesics, especially those containing phenacetin
• Lithium
• Heavy metals (lead, cadmium)
• Aristolochic acid (Chinese herbal and Balkan endemic nephropathies)
• Calcineurin inhibitors (cyclosporine, tacrolimus)
Metabolic Disturbances
• Hypercalcemia and/or nephrocalcinosis
• Hyperuricemia
• Prolonged hypokalemia
• Hyperoxaluria
• Cystinosis (see Chap. 284)
Cystic and Hereditary Disorders (see Chap. 284)
• Polycystic kidney disease
• Nephronophthisis
• Adult medullary cystic disease
• Medullary sponge kidney
Miscellaneous
• Aging
• Chronic glomerulonephritis
• Chronic urinary tract obstruction
• Ischemia and vascular disease
• Radiation nephritis (rare)

Abbreviations: CMV, cytomegalovirus; COX, cyclooxygenase; EBV, Epstein-Barr virus.

AIN is far more often encountered as an allergic reaction to a drug (Table 285-1). Immune-mediated AIN may also occur as part of a known autoimmune syndrome, but in some cases there is no identifiable cause despite features suggestive of an immunological etiology (Table 285-1).

ALLERGIC INTERSTITIAL NEPHRITIS

Although biopsy-proven AIN accounts for no more than ~15% of cases of unexplained acute renal failure, this is likely a substantial underestimate of the true incidence. This is because potentially offending medications are more often identified and empirically discontinued in a patient noted to have a rising serum creatinine, without the benefit of a renal biopsy to establish the diagnosis of AIN.

Clinical features

The classic presentation of AIN, namely, fever, rash, peripheral eosinophilia, and oliguric renal failure occurring after 7–10 days of treatment with methicillin or another β-lactam antibiotic is the exception rather than the rule. More often, patients are found incidentally to have a rising serum creatinine or present with symptoms attributable to acute renal failure (Chap. 279). Atypical reactions can occur; most notably nonsteroidal anti-inflammatory drug (NSAID)-induced AIN, in which fever, rash and eosinophilia are rare, but acute renal failure with heavy proteinuria is common. A particularly severe and rapid-onset AIN may occur upon reintroduction of rifampin after a drug-free period. More insidious reactions to the agents listed in Table 285-1 may lead to progressive tubulointerstitial damage. Examples include proton pump inhibitors and, rarely, sulfonamide and 5-aminosalicylate (mesalazine and sulfasalazine) derivatives and antiretrovirals.

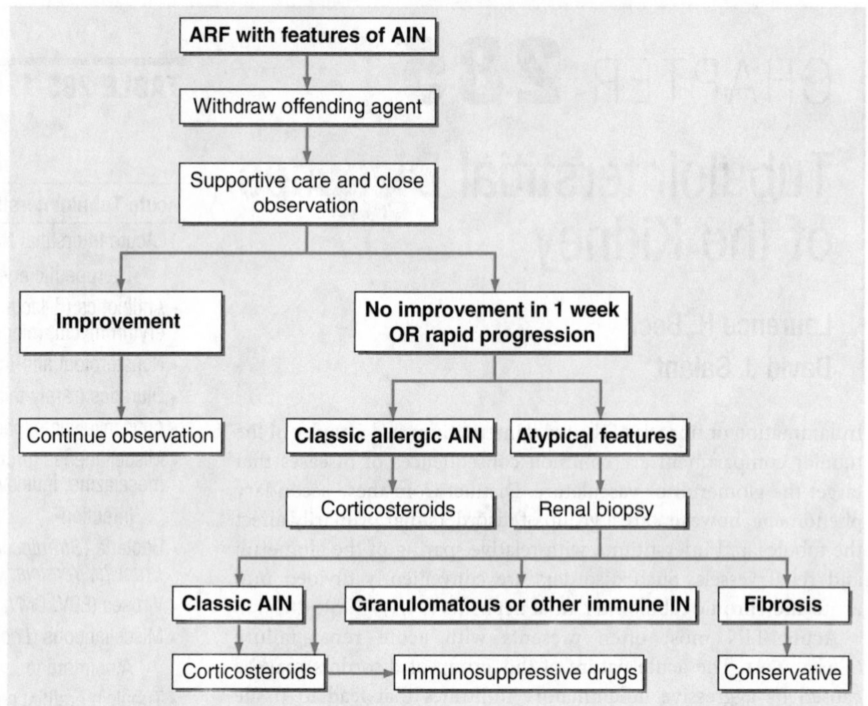

Figure 285-1 Algorithm for the treatment of allergic and other immune-mediated acute interstitial nephritis (AIN). ARF, acute renal failure. See text for immunosuppressive drugs used for refractory or relapsing AIN. *(Modified from S Reddy, DJ Salant: Ren Fail 20:829, 1998.)*

Diagnosis

Finding otherwise unexplained renal failure with or without oliguria and exposure to a potentially offending agent usually points to the diagnosis. Peripheral blood eosinophilia adds supporting evidence but is present in only a minority of patients. Urinalysis reveals pyuria with white blood cell casts and hematuria. Urinary eosinophils are neither sensitive nor specific for AIN; therefore, testing is not recommended. Renal biopsy is generally not required for diagnosis but reveals extensive interstitial and tubular infiltration of leukocytes, including eosinophils.

TREATMENT Allergic Interstitial Nephritis

Discontinuation of the offending agent often leads to reversal of the renal injury. However, depending on the duration of exposure and degree of tubular atrophy and interstitial fibrosis that has occurred, the renal damage may not be completely reversible. Glucocorticoid therapy may accelerate renal recovery, but does not appear to impact long-term renal survival. It is best reserved for those cases with severe renal failure in which dialysis is imminent or if renal function continues to deteriorate despite stopping the offending drug (Fig. 285-1 and Table 285-2).

SJÖGREN'S SYNDROME

Sjögren's syndrome is a systemic autoimmune disorder that primarily targets the exocrine glands, especially the lacrimal and salivary glands, and thus results in symptoms, such as dry eyes and mouth, that constitute the "sicca syndrome" (Chap. 324). Tubulointerstitial nephritis with a predominant lymphocytic infiltrate is the most

TABLE 285-2 Indications for Corticosteroids and Immunosuppressives in Interstitial Nephritis

Absolute Indications
• Sjögren's syndrome
• Sarcoidosis
• SLE interstitial nephritis
• Adults with TINU
• Idiopathic and other granulomatous interstitial nephritis
Relative Indications
• Drug-induced or idiopathic AIN with:
Rapid progression of renal failure
Diffuse infiltrates on biopsy
Impending need for dialysis
Delayed recovery
• Children with TINU
• Postinfectious AIN with delayed recovery (?)

Abbreviations: AIN, acute interstitial nephritis; SLE, systemic lupus erythematosus; TINU, tubulointerstitial nephritis with uveitis.
Source: Modified from S Reddy, DJ Salant: Ren Fail 20:829, 1998.

common renal manifestation of Sjögren's syndrome and can be associated with distal RTA, nephrogenic diabetes insipidus, and moderate renal failure. Diagnosis is strongly supported by positive serologic testing for anti-Ro (SS-A) and anti-La (SS-B) antibodies. A large proportion of patients with Sjögren's syndrome also have polyclonal hypergammaglobulinemia. Treatment is initially with glucocorticoids, although patients may require maintenance therapy with azathioprine or mycophenolate mofetil to prevent relapse (Fig. 285-1 and Table 285-2).

■ TUBULOINTERSTITIAL NEPHRITIS WITH UVEITIS (TINU)

TINU is a systemic autoimmune disease of unknown etiology. It accounts for fewer than 5% of all cases of AIN, affects females three times more often than males, and has a median age of onset of 15 years. Its hallmark feature, in addition to a lymphocyte-predominant interstitial nephritis (Fig. 285-2), is a painful anterior uveitis, often bilateral and accompanied by blurred vision and photophobia. Diagnosis is often confounded by the fact that the ocular symptoms precede or accompany the renal disease in only one-third of cases. Additional extrarenal features include fever, anorexia, weight loss, abdominal pain, and arthralgia. The presence of such symptoms as well as elevated creatinine, sterile pyuria, mild proteinuria, features of the Fanconi syndrome, and elevated erythrocyte sedimentation rate should raise suspicion for this disorder. Serologies suggestive of the more common autoimmune diseases are usually negative, and TINU is often a diagnosis of exclusion after other causes of uveitis and renal disease, such as Sjögren's syndrome, Behçet's disease, sarcoidosis, and systemic lupus erythematosus, have been considered. Clinical symptoms are typically self-limited in children, but are more apt to follow a relapsing course in adults. The renal and ocular manifestations generally respond well to oral glucocorticoids, although maintenance therapy with agents such as methotrexate, azathioprine, or mycophenolate may be necessary to prevent relapses (Fig. 285-1 and Table 285-2).

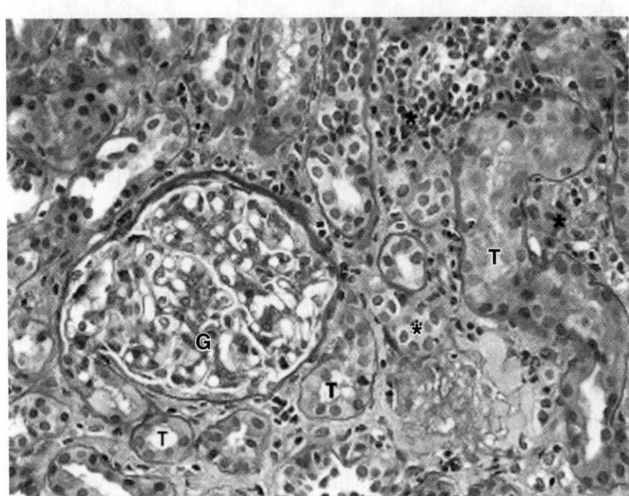

Figure 285-2 Acute interstitial nephritis (AIN) in a patient who presented with acute iritis, low-grade fever, erythrocyte sedimentation rate of 103, pyuria and cellular casts on urinalysis, and a newly elevated serum creatinine of 2.4 mg/dL. Both the iritis and AIN improved after intravenous methylprednisolone. This PAS-stained renal biopsy shows a mononuclear cell interstitial infiltrate (asterisks) and edema separating the tubules (T) and a normal glomerulus (G). Some of the tubules contain cellular debris and infiltrating inflammatory cells. The findings in this biopsy are indistinguishable from those that would be seen in a case of drug-induced AIN. PAS, Periodic acid–Schiff.

■ SYSTEMIC LUPUS ERYTHEMATOSUS

An interstitial mononuclear cell inflammatory reaction often accompanies the glomerular lesion in most cases of class III or IV lupus nephritis (Chap. 283), and deposits of immune complexes can be identified in tubule basement membranes in about 50%. Occasionally, however, the tubulointerstitial inflammation predominates and may manifest with azotemia and type IV RTA rather than features of glomerulonephritis.

■ GRANULOMATOUS INTERSTITIAL NEPHRITIS

Some patients may present with features of AIN but follow a protracted and relapsing course. Renal biopsy in such patients reveals a more chronic inflammatory infiltrate with granulomas and multinucleated giant cells. Most often, no associated disease or cause is found; however, some of these cases may have or subsequently develop the pulmonary, cutaneous, or other systemic manifestations of *sarcoidosis* such as hypercalcemia. Most patients experience some improvement in renal function if treated early with glucocorticoids before the development of significant interstitial fibrosis and tubular atrophy (Table 285-2). Other immunosuppressive agents may be required for those who relapse frequently upon steroid withdrawal (Fig. 285-1). Tuberculosis should be ruled out before starting treatment because this too is a rare cause of granulomatous interstitial nephritis.

■ IgG4-RELATED SYSTEMIC DISEASE

A form of AIN characterized by a dense inflammatory infiltrate containing IgG4-expressing plasma cells can occur as a part of a recently described syndrome known as IgG4-related systemic disease. Autoimmune pancreatitis, sclerosing cholangitis, retroperitoneal fibrosis, and a chronic sclerosing sialadenitis (mimicking Sjögren's syndrome) may variably be present as well. Fibrotic lesions that form pseudotumors in the affected organs soon replace the initial inflammatory infiltrates and often lead to biopsy or excision for fear of true malignancy. Although the involvement of IgG4 in the pathogenesis is not understood, glucocorticoids have been successfully used as first-line treatment in this group of disorders, once they are correctly diagnosed.

■ IDIOPATHIC AIN

Some patients present with typical clinical and histologic features of AIN but have no evidence of drug exposure or clinical or serologic features of an autoimmune disease. The presence in some cases of autoantibodies to a tubular antigen, similar to that identified in rats with an induced form of interstitial nephritis, suggests that an autoimmune response may be involved. Like TINU and granulomatous interstitial nephritis, idiopathic AIN is responsive to glucocorticoid therapy but may follow a relapsing course requiring maintenance treatment with another immunosuppressive agent (Fig. 285-1 and Table 285-2).

■ INFECTION-ASSOCIATED AIN

AIN may also occur as a local inflammatory reaction to microbial infection (Table 285-1) and should be distinguished from acute bacterial pyelonephritis (Chap. 288). Acute bacterial pyelonephritis does not generally cause acute renal failure unless it affects both kidneys or causes septic shock. Presently, infection-associated AIN is most often seen in immunocompromised patients, particularly renal transplant recipients with reactivation of polyomavirus BK (Chaps. 132 and 282).

■ CRYSTAL DEPOSITION DISORDERS AND OBSTRUCTIVE TUBULOPATHIES

Acute renal failure may occur when crystals of various types are deposited in tubular cells and interstitium or when they obstruct tubules. Oliguric acute renal failure, often accompanied by flank pain from tubular obstruction, may occur in patients treated with sulfadiazine for toxoplasmosis, indinavir for HIV, and intravenous acyclovir for severe herpesvirus infections. Urinalysis reveals "sheaf of wheat" sulfonamide crystals, individual or parallel clusters of needle-shaped indinavir crystals, or red-green birefringement needle-shaped crystals of acyclovir. This adverse effect is generally precipitated by hypovolemia and is reversible with saline volume repletion and drug withdrawal. Distinct from the obstructive disease, a frank AIN from indinavir crystal deposition has also been reported.

Acute tubular obstruction is also the cause of oliguric renal failure in patients with *acute urate nephropathy.* It typically results from severe hyperuricemia from tumor lysis syndrome in patients with lympho- or myeloproliferative disorders treated with cytotoxic agents, but also may occur spontaneously before the treatment has been initiated (Chap. 276). Uric acid crystallization in the tubules and collecting system leads to partial or complete obstruction of the collecting ducts, renal pelvis, or ureter. A dense precipitate of birefringent uric acid crystals is found in the urine, usually in association with microscopic or gross hematuria. Prophylactic allopurinol reduces the risk of uric acid nephropathy but is of no benefit once tumor lysis has occurred. Once oliguria has developed, attempts to increase tubular flow and solubility of uric acid with alkaline diuresis may be of some benefit; however, emergent treatment with hemodialysis or rasburicase, a recombinant urate oxidase, is usually required to rapidly lower uric acid levels and restore renal function.

Calcium oxalate crystal deposition in tubular cells and interstitium may lead to permanent renal dysfunction in patients who survive ethylene glycol intoxication, in patients with enteric hyperoxaluria from ileal resection or small-bowel bypass surgery, and in patients with hereditary hyperoxaluria (Chap. 287). *Acute phosphate nephropathy* is an uncommon but serious complication of oral Phospho-soda used as a laxative or for bowel preparation for colonoscopy. It is the result of calcium phosphate crystal deposition in tubules and interstitium and occurs especially in subjects with underlying renal impairment and hypovolemia. Consequently, Phospho-soda should be avoided in patients with chronic kidney disease.

LIGHT CHAIN CAST NEPHROPATHY

Patients with multiple myeloma may develop acute renal failure in the setting of hypovolemia, infection, or hypercalcemia or after exposure to NSAIDs or radiographic contrast media. The diagnosis of light chain cast nephropathy (LCCN)—commonly known as *myeloma kidney*—should be considered in patients who fail to recover when the precipitating factor is corrected or in any elderly patient with otherwise unexplained acute renal failure.

In this disorder, filtered monoclonal immunoglobulin light chains (Bence-Jones proteins) form intratubular aggregates with secreted Tamm-Horsfall protein in the distal tubule. Casts, in addition to obstructing the tubular flow in affected nephrons, incite a giant cell or foreign body reaction and can lead to tubular rupture, resulting in interstitial fibrosis (Fig. 285-3). Although LCCN generally occurs in patients with known multiple myeloma and a large plasma cell burden, the disorder should also be considered as a possible diagnosis in patients who have known monoclonal gammopathy even in the absence of frank myeloma. Filtered monoclonal light chains may also cause less pronounced renal manifestations in the absence of obstruction, due to direct toxicity to proximal tubular cells and intracellular crystal formation. This may result in isolated tubular disorders such as RTA or the full Fanconi syndrome.

Diagnosis

Clinical clues to the diagnosis include anemia, bone pain, hypercalcemia, and an abnormally narrow anion gap due to hypoalbuminemia and hypergammaglobulinemia. Urinary dipsticks detect albumin but not immunoglobulin light chains; however, laboratory detection of increased amounts of protein in a spot urine specimen and a negative dipstick result are highly suggestive that the urine contains Bence-Jones protein. Serum and urine should both be sent for protein electrophoresis and for immunofixation for the detection and identification of a potential monoclonal band. A sensitive method is now clinically available to detect urine and serum free light chains.

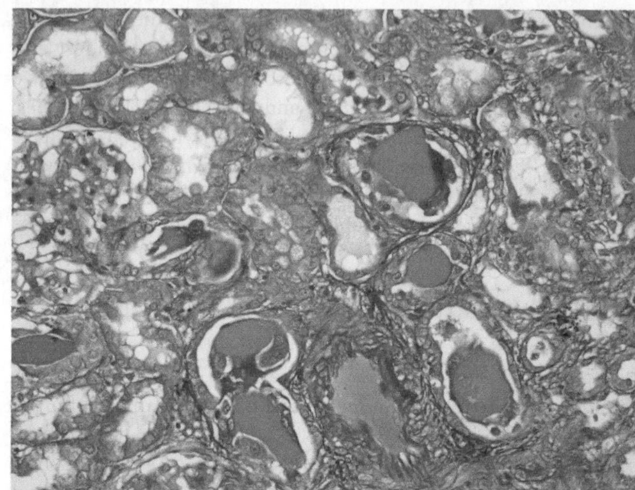

Figure 285-3 Histologic appearance of myeloma cast nephropathy. A hematoxylin-eosin-stained kidney biopsy shows many atrophic tubules filled with eosinophilic casts (consisting of Bence-Jones protein), which are surrounded by giant cell reactions. *(Courtesy of Dr. Michael N. Koss, University of Southern California Keck School of Medicine; with permission.)*

TREATMENT Light Chain Cast Nephropathy

The goals of treatment are to correct precipitating factors such as hypovolemia and hypercalcemia, discontinue potential nephrotoxic agents, and treat the underlying plasma cell dyscrasia (Chap. 111); plasmapheresis to remove light chains is of questionable value for LCCN.

LYMPHOMATOUS INFILTRATION OF THE KIDNEY

Interstitial infiltration by malignant B lymphocytes is a common autopsy finding in patients dying of chronic lymphocytic leukemia and non-Hodgkin's lymphoma; however, this is usually an incidental finding. Rarely, such infiltrates may cause massive enlargement of the kidneys and oliguric acute renal failure. Although high-dose glucocorticoids and subsequent chemotherapy often results in recovery of renal function, the prognosis in such cases is generally poor.

CHRONIC TUBULOINTERSTITIAL DISEASES

Improved occupational and public health measures, together with the banning of over-the-counter phenacetin-containing analgesics, has led to a dramatic decline in the incidence of chronic interstitial nephritis (CIN) from heavy metal—particularly lead and cadmium—exposure and analgesic nephropathy in North America. Today, CIN is most often the result of renal ischemia or secondary to a primary glomerular disease (Chap. 283). Other important forms of CIN are the result of developmental anomalies or inherited diseases such as reflux nephropathy or sickle cell nephropathy and may not be recognized until adolescence or adulthood. Whereas it is impossible to reverse damage that has already occurred, further deterioration may be prevented or at least slowed in such cases by treating glomerular hypertension, a common denominator in the development of secondary FSGS and progressive loss of functioning nephrons. Therefore, awareness and early detection of patients at risk may prevent them from developing end-stage renal disease (ESRD).

VESICOURETERAL REFLUX AND REFLUX NEPHROPATHY

Reflux nephropathy is the consequence of vesicoureteral reflux (VUR) or other urologic anomalies in early childhood. It was previously called *chronic pyelonephritis* because it was believed to result from recurrent urinary tract infections (UTIs) in childhood. VUR stems from abnormal retrograde urine flow from the bladder into one or both ureters and kidneys because of mislocated and incompetent ureterovesical valves (Fig. 285-4). Although high-pressure sterile reflux may impair normal growth of the kidneys, when coupled with recurrent UTIs in early childhood, the result is

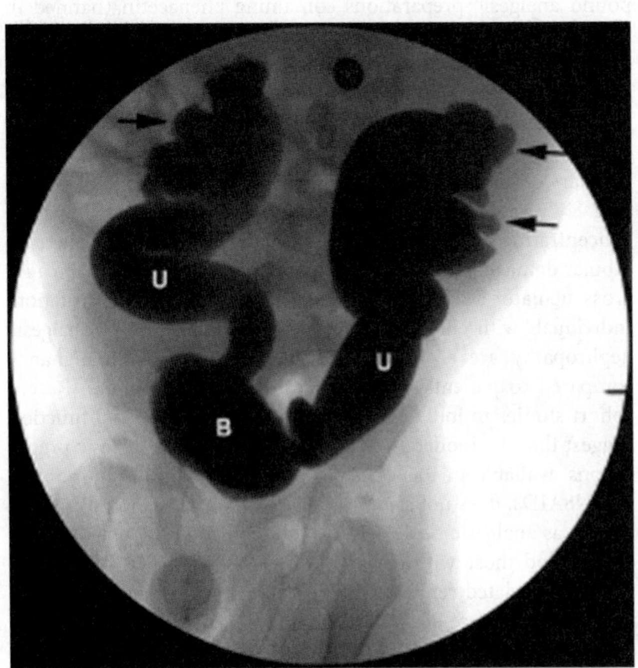

A

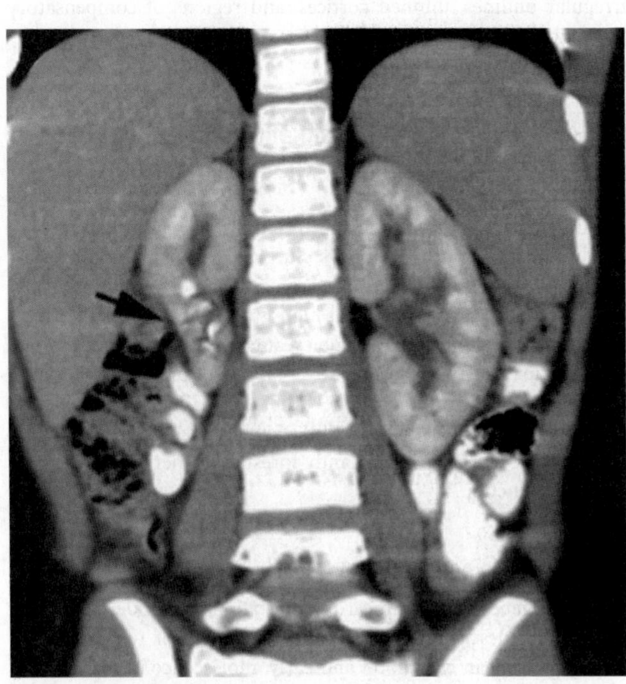

B

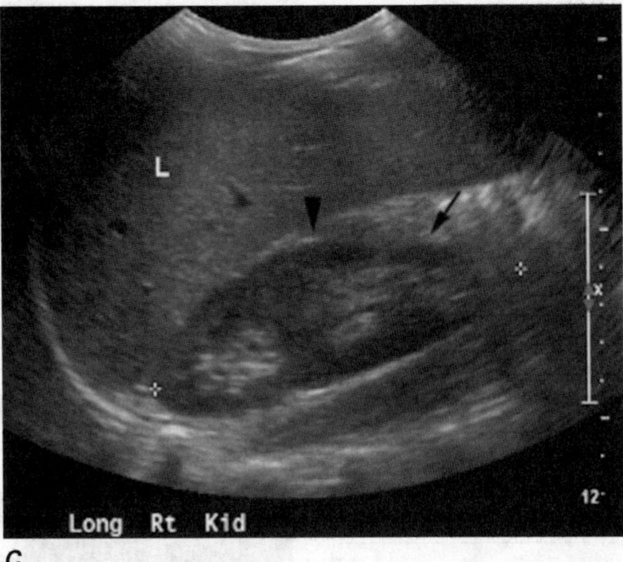

C

Figure 285-4 Radiographs of vesicoureteral reflux (VUR) and reflux nephropathy. ***A***. Voiding cystourethrogram in a 7-month-old baby with bilateral high-grade VUR evidenced by clubbed calyces (arrows) and dilated tortuous ureters (U) entering the bladder (B). ***B***. Abdominal CT scan (coronal plane reconstruction) in a child showing severe scarring of the lower portion of the right kidney (arrow). ***C***. Sonogram of the right kidney showing loss of parenchyma at the lower pole due to scarring (arrow) and hypertrophy of the mid-region (arrowhead). *(Courtesy of Dr. George Gross, University of Maryland Medical Center; with permission.)*

patchy interstitial scarring and tubular atrophy. Loss of functioning nephrons leads to hypertrophy of the remnant glomeruli and eventual secondary FSGS. Reflux nephropathy often goes unnoticed until early adulthood when chronic kidney disease is detected during routine evaluation or during pregnancy. Affected adults are frequently asymptomatic, but may give a history of prolonged bed-wetting or recurrent UTIs during childhood, and exhibit variable renal insufficiency, hypertension, mild to moderate proteinuria, and unremarkable urine sediment. When both kidneys are affected, the disease often progresses inexorably over several years to end-stage kidney disease, despite the absence of ongoing urinary infections or reflux. A single affected kidney may go undetected, except for the presence of hypertension. Renal ultrasound in adults characteristically shows asymmetric small kidneys with irregular outlines, thinned cortices, and regions of compensatory hypertrophy (Fig. 285-4).

TREATMENT Vesicoureteral Reflux and Reflux Nephropathy

Maintenance of a sterile urine in childhood has been shown to limit scarring of the kidneys. Surgical reimplantation of the ureters into the bladder to restore competency is indicated in young children with persistent high-grade reflux but is ineffective and is not indicated in adolescents or adults after scarring has occurred. Aggressive control of blood pressure with an angiotensin-converting enzyme inhibitor (ACEI) or angiotensin receptor blocker (ARB) and other agents is effective in reducing proteinuria and may significantly forestall further deterioration of renal function.

SICKLE CELL NEPHROPATHY

The pathogenesis and clinical manifestations of sickle cell nephropathy are described in Chap. 286. Evidence of tubular injury may be evident in childhood and early adolescence in the form of polyuria due to decreased concentrating ability or type IV renal tubular acidosis years before there is significant nephron loss and proteinuria from secondary FSGS. Early recognition of these subtle renal abnormalities or development of microalbuminuria in a child with sickle cell disease may warrant consultation with a nephrologist and/or therapy with low-dose ACEIs. Papillary necrosis may result from ischemia due to sickling of red cells in the relatively hypoxemic and hypertonic medullary vasculature and present with gross hematuria and ureteric obstruction by sloughed ischemic papillae (Table 285-3).

TUBULOINTERSTITIAL ABNORMALITIES ASSOCIATED WITH GLOMERULONEPHRITIS

Primary glomerulopathies are often associated with damage to tubules and interstitium. This may occasionally be due to the same pathologic process affecting the glomerulus and tubulointerstitium, as is the case with immune-complex deposition in lupus nephritis. More often, however, chronic tubulointerstitial changes occur as a secondary consequence of prolonged glomerular dysfunction. Potential mechanisms by which glomerular disease might cause tubulointerstitial injury include proteinuria-mediated damage to the epithelial cells, activation of tubular cells by cytokines and complement, or reduced peritubular blood flow leading to downstream tubulointerstitial ischemia, especially in the case of glomeruli that are globally obsolescent due to severe glomerulonephritis. It is often difficult to discern the initial cause of injury by renal biopsy in a patient who presents with advanced renal disease in this setting.

TABLE 285-3 Major Causes of Papillary Necrosis

Analgesic nephropathy
Sickle cell nephropathy
Diabetes with urinary tract infection
Prolonged NSAID use (rare)

Abbreviation: NSAID, nonsteroidal anti-inflammatory.

ANALGESIC NEPHROPATHY

Analgesic nephropathy results from the long-term use of compound analgesic preparations containing phenacetin (banned in the United States since 1983), aspirin, and caffeine. In its classic form, analgesic nephropathy is characterized by renal insufficiency, papillary necrosis (Table 285-3) attributable to the presumed concentration of the drug to toxic levels in the inner medulla, and a radiographic constellation of small, scarred kidneys with papillary calcifications best appreciated by computed tomography (Fig. 285-5). Patients may also have polyuria due to impaired concentrating ability and non-anion-gap metabolic acidosis from tubular damage. Shedding of a sloughed necrotic papilla can cause gross hematuria and ureteric colic due to ureteral obstruction. Individuals with end-stage kidney disease as a result of analgesic nephropathy are at increased risk of a urothelial malignancy compared to patients with other causes of renal failure. Recent cohort studies in individuals with normal baseline renal function suggest that the moderate chronic use of current analgesic preparations available in the United States, including acetaminophen and NSAIDs, does not seem to cause the constellation of findings known as analgesic nephropathy, although volume-depleted individuals and those with chronic kidney disease are at higher risk of NSAID-related renal toxicity. Nonetheless, it is recommended that heavy users of acetaminophen and NSAIDs be screened for evidence of renal disease.

CHINESE HERBAL NEPHROPATHY AND BALKAN NEPHROPATHY

Nontraditional (alternative or herbal) medications can also lead to progressive tubulointerstitial disease. In Chinese herbal nephropathy, first described in young women taking Chinese herbal preparations as part of a weight-loss regimen, one of the offending agents

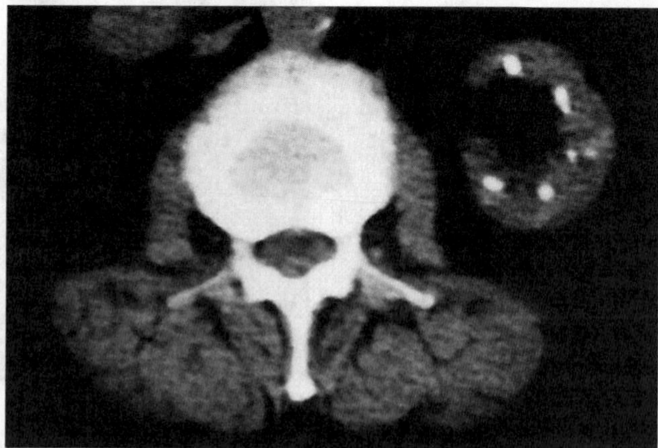

Figure 285-5 Radiologic appearance of analgesic nephropathy. A non-contrast CT scan shows an atrophic left kidney with papillary calcifications in a garland pattern. *(Reprinted by permission from Macmillan Publishers, Ltd., MM Elseviers et al., Kidney International 48:1316, 1995.)*

has been identified as aristolochic acid, a botanical product and known rodent carcinogen from the plant *Aristolochia*. This chemical, after prolonged exposure, produces renal interstitial fibrosis with a relative paucity of cellular infiltrates. The urine sediment is bland, with rare leukocytes and only mild proteinuria. Anemia may be disproportionately severe relative to the level of renal dysfunction. Like analgesic nephropathy, Chinese herbal nephropathy has been associated with a long-term increased risk of bladder and ureteral malignancies. There is recent evidence that Balkan endemic nephropathy, a chronic tubulointerstitial nephritis found primarily in towns along the tributaries of the Danube River, may also be linked to aristolochic acid as a result of contamination of local grain preparations. Although other environmental factors for Balkan endemic nephropathy, such as the mycotoxin ochratoxin A or water-soluble hydrocarbons leached from the coal deposits in the area, have been proposed as causative agents, current evidence appears to be strongest for aristolochic acid. It has been proposed that Chinese herbal nephropathy and Balkan endemic nephropathy be collectively known as aristolochic acid nephropathy.

LITHIUM-ASSOCIATED NEPHROPATHY

The use of lithium salts for the treatment of manic-depressive illness may have several renal sequelae, the most common of which is nephrogenic diabetes insipidus manifesting as polyuria and polydipsia. Lithium accumulates in principal cells of the collecting duct by entering through the epithelial sodium channel (ENaC), where it inhibits glycogen synthase kinase 3β and downregulates vasopressin-regulated aquaporin water channels. Less frequently, chronic tubulointerstitial nephritis develops after prolonged (greater than 10–20 years) lithium use and is most likely to occur in patients that have experienced repeated episodes of toxic lithium levels. Findings on renal biopsy include interstitial fibrosis and tubular atrophy that are out of proportion to the degree of glomerulosclerosis or vascular disease, a sparse lymphocytic infiltrate, and small cysts or dilation of the distal tubule and collecting duct that are highly characteristic of this disorder. The degree of interstitial fibrosis correlates both with duration and cumulative dose of lithium. Individuals with lithium-associated nephropathy are typically asymptomatic, with minimal proteinuria, few urinary leukocytes, and normal blood pressure. Some patients develop more severe proteinuria due to secondary FSGS, which may contribute to further loss of renal function.

TREATMENT Lithium-Associated Nephropathy

Renal function should be followed regularly in patients taking lithium, and caution should be exercised in patients with underlying renal disease. The use of amiloride to inhibit lithium entry via ENaC has been effective to prevent and treat lithium-induced nephrogenic diabetes insipidus, but it is not clear if it will prevent lithium-induced CIN. Once lithium-associated nephropathy is detected, the discontinuation of lithium in attempt to forestall further renal deterioration can be problematic, as lithium is an effective mood stabilizer that is often incompletely substituted by other agents. Furthermore, despite discontinuation of lithium, chronic renal disease in such patients is often irreversible and can slowly progress to end-stage kidney disease. The most prudent approach is to monitor lithium levels frequently and adjust dosing to avoid toxic levels (preferably <1 meq/L). This is especially important as lithium is cleared less effectively as renal function declines. In those cases that develop significant proteinuria, ACEI or ARB treatment should be initiated.

CALCIURIN-INHIBITOR NEPHROTOXICITY

The calcineurin inhibitor (CNI) immunosuppressive agents cyclosporine and tacrolimus can cause both acute and chronic renal injury. Acute forms can result from vascular causes such as vasoconstriction or the development of thrombotic microangiopathy, or can be due to a toxic tubulopathy. Chronic CNI-induced renal injury is typically seen in solid organ (including heart-lung and liver) transplant recipients and manifests with a slow but irreversible reduction of glomerular filtration rate, with mild proteinuria and arterial hypertension. Hyperkalemia is a relatively common complication and is caused, in part, by tubular resistance to aldosterone. The histologic changes in renal tissue include patchy interstitial fibrosis and tubular atrophy, often in a "striped" pattern. In addition, the intrarenal vasculature often demonstrates hyalinosis, and focal glomerulosclerosis can be present as well. Similar changes may occur in patients receiving CNIs for autoimmune diseases, although the doses are generally lower than those used for organ transplantation. Dose reduction or CNI avoidance appears to mitigate the chronic tubulointerstitial changes, but may increase the risk of rejection and graft loss.

HEAVY METAL (LEAD) NEPHROPATHY

Heavy metals, such as lead or cadmium, can lead to a chronic tubulointerstitial process after prolonged exposure. The disease entity is no longer commonly diagnosed, because such heavy metal exposure has been greatly reduced due to the known health risks from lead and the consequent removal of lead from most commercial products and fuels. Nonetheless, occupational exposure is possible in workers involved in the manufacture or destruction of batteries, removal of lead paint, or manufacture of alloys and electrical equipment (cadmium) in countries where industrial regulation is less stringent. In addition, ingestion of moonshine whiskey distilled in lead-tainted containers has been one of the more frequent sources of lead exposure.

Early signs of chronic lead intoxication are attributable to proximal tubule dysfunction, particularly hyperuricemia as a result of diminished urate secretion. The triad of "saturnine gout," hypertension, and renal insufficiency should prompt a practitioner to ask specifically about lead exposure. Unfortunately, evaluating lead burden is not as straightforward as ordering a blood test; the preferred methods involve measuring urinary lead after infusion of a chelating agent or by radiographic fluoroscopy of bone. Several recent studies have shown an association between chronic low-level lead exposure and decreased renal function, although either of these two factors may have been the primary event. In those patients who have CIN of unclear origin and an elevated total body lead burden, repeated treatments of lead chelation therapy have been shown to slow the decline in renal function.

METABOLIC DISORDERS

Disorders leading to excessively high or low levels of certain electrolytes and products of metabolism can also lead to chronic kidney disease if untreated.

CHRONIC URIC ACID NEPHROPATHY

The constellation of pathologic findings that represent *gouty nephropathy* are very uncommon nowadays and are more of historical interest than clinical importance, as gout is typically well managed with allopurinol and other agents. However, there is emerging evidence that hyperuricemia is an independent risk factor for the development of chronic kidney disease, perhaps through endothelial damage. The complex interactions of hyperuricemia, hypertension, and renal failure are still incompletely understood.

Presently, gouty nephropathy is most likely to be encountered in patients with severe tophaceous gout and prolonged hyperuricemia from a hereditary disorder of purine metabolism (Chap. 359). Histologically, the distinctive feature of gouty nephropathy is the presence of crystalline deposits of uric acid and monosodium urate salts in the kidney parenchyma. These deposits not only cause intrarenal obstruction but also incite an inflammatory response, leading to lymphocytic infiltration, foreign-body giant cell reaction, and eventual fibrosis, especially in the medullary and papillary regions of the kidney. Since patients with gout frequently suffer from hypertension and hyperlipidemia, degenerative changes of the renal arterioles may constitute a striking feature of the histologic abnormality, out of proportion to the other morphologic defects. Clinically, gouty nephropathy is an insidious cause of chronic kidney disease. Early in its course, glomerular filtration rate may be near normal, often despite morphologic changes in medullary and cortical interstitium, proteinuria, and diminished urinary concentrating ability. Treatment with allopurinol and urine alkalinization is generally effective in preventing uric acid nephrolithiasis and the consequences of recurrent kidney stones; however, gouty nephropathy may be intractable to such measures. Furthermore, the use of allopurinol in asymptomatic hyperuricemia has not been consistently shown to improve renal function.

HYPERCALCEMIC NEPHROPATHY

(See also Chap. 353) Chronic hypercalcemia, as occurs in primary hyperparathyroidism, sarcoidosis, multiple myeloma, vitamin D intoxication, or metastatic bone disease, can cause tubulointerstitial disease and progressive renal failure. The earliest lesion is a focal degenerative change in renal epithelia, primarily in collecting ducts, distal tubules, and loops of Henle. Tubular cell necrosis leads to nephron obstruction and stasis of intrarenal urine, favoring local precipitation of calcium salts and infection. Dilation and atrophy of tubules eventually occurs, as does interstitial fibrosis, mononuclear leukocyte infiltration, and interstitial calcium deposition (nephrocalcinosis). Calcium deposition may also occur in glomeruli and the walls of renal arterioles.

Clinically, the most striking defect is an inability to maximally concentrate the urine, due to reduced collecting duct responsiveness to AVP and defective transport of sodium and chloride in the loop of Henle. Reductions in both glomerular filtration rate and renal blood flow can occur, both in acute and in prolonged hypercalcemia. Eventually, uncontrolled hypercalcemia leads to severe tubulointerstitial damage and overt renal failure. Abdominal x-rays may demonstrate nephrocalcinosis as well as nephrolithiasis, the latter due to the hypercalciuria that often accompanies hypercalcemia.

Treatment consists of reducing the serum calcium concentration toward normal and correcting the primary abnormality of calcium metabolism (Chap. 353). Renal dysfunction of acute hypercalcemia may be completely reversible. Gradual progressive renal insufficiency related to chronic hypercalcemia, however, may not improve even with correction of the calcium disorder.

HYPOKALEMIC NEPHROPATHY

Patients with prolonged and severe hypokalemia from chronic laxative or diuretic abuse, surreptitious vomiting, or primary aldosteronism may develop a reversible tubular lesion characterized by vacuolar degeneration of proximal and distal tubular cells. Eventually, tubular atrophy and cystic dilation accompanied by interstitial fibrosis may ensue, leading to irreversible chronic kidney disease. Timely correction of the hypokalemia will prevent further progression, but persistent hypokalemia can cause ESRD.

GLOBAL PERSPECTIVE

The causes of acute and chronic interstitial nephritis vary widely across the globe. Analgesic nephropathy continues to be seen in countries where phenacetin-containing compound analgesic preparations are readily available. Adulterants in unregulated herbal and traditional medicaments pose a threat of toxic interstitial nephritis, as exemplified by aristolochic acid contamination of herbal slimming preparations. Contamination of food sources with toxins, such as the recent outbreak of nephrolithiasis and acute renal failure from melamine contamination of infant milk formula, poses a continuing risk. Likewise, Balkan endemic nephropathy appears likely to be the result of aristolochic acid contamination of grain preparations. While industrial exposure to lead and cadmium has largely disappeared as a cause of chronic interstitial nephritis in developed nations, it remains a risk for nephrotoxicity in countries where such exposure is less well controlled. Conversely, the widespread use of proton pump inhibitors for gastroesophageal reflux disease (GERD) and Phospho-soda prior to screening colonoscopy has introduced a new spectrum of drug-induced kidney diseases to wealthier nations.

ACKNOWLEDGMENT

We are grateful to Drs. Alan Yu and Barry Brenner, authors of "Tubulointerstitial Diseases of the Kidney" in the 17th edition of Harrison's, for contributions to this chapter.

FURTHER READINGS

Appel GB: The treatment of acute interstitial nephritis: More data at last. Kidney Int 73:905, 2008

Batuman V: Proximal tubular injury in myeloma. Contrib Nephrol 153:87, 2007

Beck LH Jr, Salant DJ: Glomerular and tubulointerstitial diseases. Prim Care 35:265, 2008

Becker GJ, Kincaid-Smith P: Reflux nephropathy: The glomerular lesion and progression of renal failure. Pediatr Nephrol 7:365, 1993

Brewster UC, Perazella MA: Proton pump inhibitors and the kidney: Critical review. Clin Nephrol 68:65, 2007

De Broe ME, Elseviers MM: Over-the-counter analgesic use. J Am Soc Nephrol 20:2098, 2009

Geevasinga N et al: Proton pump inhibitors and acute interstitial nephritis. Clin Gastroenterol Hepatol 4:597, 2006

Grunfeld JP, Rossier BC: Lithium nephrotoxicity revisited. Nat Rev Nephrol 5:270, 2009

Henrich WL et al: Non-contrast-enhanced computerized tomography and analgesic-related kidney disease: Report of the National Analgesic Nephropathy Study. J Am Soc Nephrol 17:1472, 2006

Isnard Bagnis C et al: Herbs and the kidney. Am J Kidney Dis 44:1, 2004

CHAPTER 286
Vascular Injury to the Kidney

Stephen C. Textor
Nelson Leung

The renal vasculature is unusually complex with rich arteriolar flow to the cortex in excess of metabolic requirements, consistent with its primary function as a filtering organ. After delivering blood to cortical glomeruli, the postglomerular circulation supplies deeper medullary segments that support energy-dependent solute transport at multiple levels of the renal tubule. These postglomerular vessels carry less blood, and high oxygen consumption leaves the deeper medullary regions at the margin of hypoxemia. Vascular disorders that commonly threaten the blood supply of the kidney include large vessel atherosclerosis, fibromuscular diseases, and embolic, inflammatory, and primary hematologic disorders that produce microvascular injury.

ATHEROSCLEROSIS AND KIDNEY CIRCULATION

■ MICROVASCULAR DISEASE

The glomerular capillary endothelium shares susceptibility to oxidative stress, pressure injury, and inflammation with other vascular territories. Rates of urinary albumin excretion (UAE) are predictive of systemic atherosclerotic disease events. Increased UAE may develop years before cardiovascular events. UAE and the risk of cardiovascular events are both reduced with pharmacologic therapy such as statins. Experimental studies demonstrate functional changes and rarefaction of renal microvessels under conditions of accelerated atherosclerosis and/or compromise of proximal perfusion pressures with large vessel disease (Fig. 286-1).

■ MACROVASCULAR DISEASE

Large-vessel renal artery occlusive disease can result from extrinsic compression of the vessel, fibromuscular dysplasias, or most commonly, from atherosclerotic disease. Any disorder that reduces perfusion pressure to the kidney can activate mechanisms that tend to restore renal pressures at the expense of developing systemic hypertension. Because restoration of perfusion pressures can reverse these pathways, renal artery stenosis is considered a specifically treatable "secondary" cause of hypertension.

Renal artery stenosis is common and often has only minor hemodynamic effects. Fibromuscular dysplasia (FMD) is reported in 3–5% of normal subjects presenting as potential kidney donors without hypertension. It may present clinically with hypertension in younger individuals (between age 15 and 50), most often women. FMD does not often threaten kidney function, but sometimes produces total occlusion and can be associated with renal artery aneurysms. Atherosclerotic renal artery stenosis (ARAS) is common in the general population (6.8% of a community-based sample above age 65), a prevalence that increases with age and for patients with other vascular conditions such as coronary artery disease (18–23%) and/or peripheral aortic or lower extremity disease (more than 30%). If untreated, ARAS progresses in nearly 50% of cases over a 5-year period, sometimes to total occlusion. Intensive treatment of arterial blood pressure and statin therapy appear to slow these rates and improve clinical outcomes.

Critical levels of stenosis lead to a reduction in perfusion pressure that activates the renin-angiotensin system, reduces sodium excretion, and activates sympathetic adrenergic pathways. These events lead to systemic hypertension characterized by angiotensin dependence in the early stages, widely varying pressures, loss of circadian blood pressure (BP) rhythms, and accelerated target organ injury, including left ventricular hypertrophy and renal fibrosis. Renovascular hypertension can be treated with agents that block the renin-angiotensin system and other drugs that modify these pressor pathways. It can also be treated with restoration of renal blood flow by either endovascular or surgical revascularization. In most cases, patients require continued antihypertensive drug therapy because revascularization alone rarely lowers BP to normal.

ARAS and systemic hypertension tend to affect both the post-stenotic and contralateral kidneys, reducing overall glomerular filtration rate (GFR) in ARAS. When kidney function is threatened by large vessel disease primarily, it has been labeled *ischemic nephropathy*. Unlike FMD, ARAS develops in patients with other risk factors for atherosclerosis and is commonly superimposed upon preexisting small vessel disease in the kidney resulting from hypertension, aging, and diabetes. Nearly 85% of patients considered for renal revascularization have stage 3–5 chronic kidney

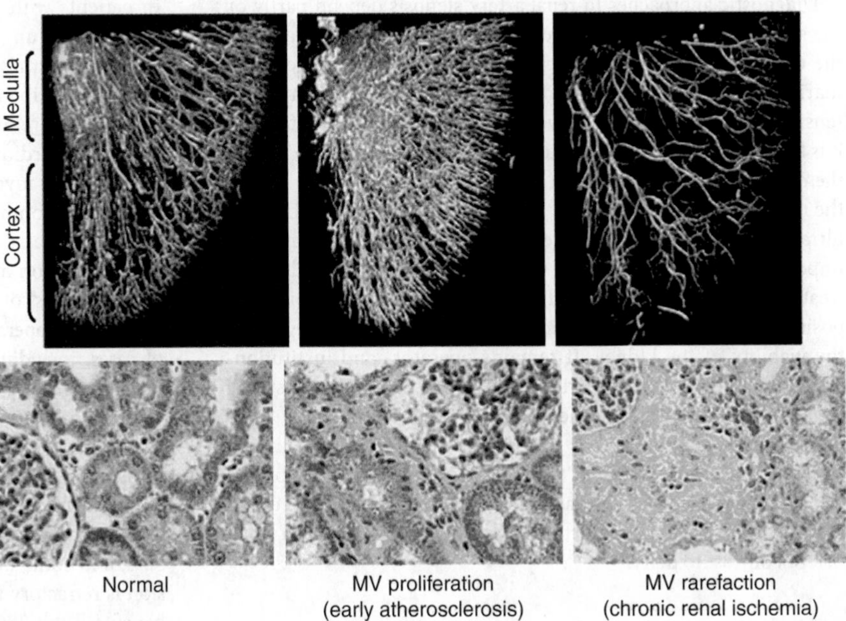

Figure 286-1 Examples of micro-CT images from vessels defined by radiopaque casts injected into the renal vasculature. These illustrate the complex, dense cortical capillary network supplying the kidney cortex that can either proliferate or succumb to rarefaction under the influence of atherosclerosis and/or occlusive disease. Changes in blood supply are followed by tubulointerstitial fibrosis and loss of kidney function. MV, microvascular *(From LO Lerman, AR Chade: Curr Opin Nephrol Hyper 18:160, 2009, with permission.)*

TABLE 286-1 Summary of Imaging Modalities for Evaluating the Kidney Vasculature

Perfusion Studies to Assess Differential Renal Blood Flow			
Captopril renography with technetium ^{99m}Tc mertiatide (^{99m}Tc MAG3)	Captopril-mediated fall in filtration pressure amplifies differences in renal perfusion	Normal study excludes renovascular hypertension	Multiple limitations in patients with advanced atherosclerosis or creatinine >2.0 mg/dL (177 μmol/L)
Nuclear imaging with technetium mertiatide or technetium-labeled pentetic acid (DTPA) to estimate fractional flow to each kidney	Estimates fractional flow to each kidney	Allows calculation of single-kidney glomerular filtration rate	Results may be influenced by other conditions, e.g., obstructive uropathy
Vascular Studies to Evaluate the Renal Arteries			
Duplex ultrasonography	Shows the renal arteries and measures flow velocity as a means of assessing the severity of stenosis	Inexpensive; widely available	Heavily dependent on operator's experience; less useful than invasive angiography for the diagnosis of fibromuscular dysplasia and abnormalities in accessory renal arteries
Magnetic resonance angiography	Shows the renal arteries and perirenal aorta	Not nephrotoxic, but concerns for gadolinium toxicity exclude use in GFR <30 mL/min/1.73 m^2; provides excellent images	Expensive; gadolinium excluded in renal failure, unable to visualize stented vessels
Computed tomographic angiography	Shows the renal arteries and perirenal aorta	Provides excellent images; stents do not cause artifacts	Expensive, moderate volume of contrast required, potentially nephrotoxic
Intra-arterial angiography	Shows location and severity of vascular lesion	Considered "gold standard" for diagnosis of large vessel disease, usually performed simultaneous with planned intervention	Expensive, associated hazard of atheroemboli, contrast toxicity, procedure-related complications, e.g., dissection

Abbrevations: DTPA, diethylenetriamine pentaacetic acid (pentetic acid); GFR, glomerular filtration rate.

disease (CKD) with GFR below 60 mL/min per 1.73 m^2. The presence of ARAS is a strong predictor of morbidity- and mortality-related cardiovascular events, independent of whether renal revascularization is undertaken.

Diagnostic approaches to renal artery stenosis depend partly on the specific issues to be addressed. Noninvasive characterization of the renal vasculature may be achieved by several techniques summarized in (Table 286-1). Although activation of the renin-angiotensin system is a key step in developing renovascular hypertension, it is transient. Levels of renin activity are therefore subject to timing, the effects of drugs and sodium intake, and do not reliably predict the response to vascular therapy. Renal artery velocities by Doppler ultrasound above 200 cm/s generally predict hemodynamically important lesions (above 60% vessel lumen occlusion), although treatment trials require velocity above 300 cm/s to avoid false positives. The renal resistive index has predictive value regarding the viability of the kidney. It remains operator- and institution-dependent, however. Captopril-enhanced renography has a strong negative predictive value when entirely normal. Magnetic resonance angiography (MRA) is now less often used, as gadolinium contrast has been associated with nephrogenic systemic fibrosis. Contrast-enhanced CT with vascular reconstruction provides excellent vascular images and functional assessment, but carries a small risk of contrast toxicity.

TREATMENT Renal Artery Stenosis

While restoring renal blood flow and perfusion seems intuitively beneficial for high-grade occlusive lesions, revascularization procedures also pose hazards and expense. Patients with FMD are commonly younger females with otherwise normal vessels and a long life expectancy. These patients often respond well to percutaneous renal artery angioplasty. If blood pressure can be controlled to goal levels and kidney function remains stable in patients with ARAS, it may be argued that medical therapy with follow-up for disease progression is equally effective. Prospective trials up to now fail to identify compelling benefits for interventional procedures regarding short-term results of blood pressure and renal function, although long-term studies regarding cardiovascular outcomes such as stroke, congestive heart failure, myocardial infarction, and end-stage renal failure are not yet complete. Medical therapy should include blockade of the renin-angiotensin system, attainment of goal blood pressures, cessation of tobacco, statins, and aspirin.

Techniques of renal revascularization are improving. With experienced operators, major complications develop in about 9% of cases, including renal artery dissection, capsular perforation, hemorrhage, and occasional atheroembolic disease. Although not common, atheroembolic disease can be catastrophic and accelerate both hypertension and kidney failure, exactly the events that revascularization is intended to prevent. Although renal blood flow usually can be restored by endovascular stenting, recovery of renal function is limited to about 25% of cases, with no change in 50%, and some deterioration evident in others. When hypertension is refractory to effective therapy, revascularization offers real benefits. Table 286-2 summarizes currently accepted guidelines for considering renal revascularization.

ATHEROEMBOLIC RENAL DISEASE

Emboli to the kidneys arise most frequently as a result of cholesterol crystals breaking free of atherosclerotic vascular plaque and lodging in downstream microvessels. Most clinical atheroembolic events

TABLE 286-2 Clinical Factors Favoring Medical Therapy and Revascularization or Surveillance for Renal Artery Stenosis

Factors Favoring Medical Therapy and Revascularization for Renal Artery Stenosis
• Progressive decline in GFR during treatment of systemic hypertension
• Failure to achieve adequate blood pressure control with optimal medical therapy (medical failure)
• Rapid or recurrent decline in the GFR in association with a reduction in systemic pressure
• Decline in the GFR during therapy with ACE inhibitors or ARBs
• Recurrent congestive heart failure in a patient in whom the adequacy of left ventricular function does not explain a cause
Factors Favoring Medical Therapy and Surveillance of Renal Artery Disease
• Controlled blood pressure with stable renal function (e.g., stable renal insufficiency)
• Stable renal artery stenosis without progression on surveillance studies (e.g., serial duplex ultrasound)
• Very advanced age and/or limited life expectancy
• Extensive comorbidity that make revascularization too risky
• High risk for or previous experience with atheroembolic disease
• Other concomitant renal parenchymal diseases that cause progressive renal dysfunction (e.g., interstitial nephritis, diabetic nephropathy)

Abbreviations: ACE, angiotensin-converting enzyme; ARBs, angiotensin receptor blockers; GFR, glomerular filtration rate.

follow angiographic procedures, often of the coronary vessels. It has been argued that nearly all vascular interventional procedures lead to plaque fracture and release of microemboli, but clinical manifestations develop only in a fraction of these. The incidence of clinical atheroemboli has been increasing with more vascular procedures and longer life spans. Atheroembolic renal disease is suspected in more than 3% of end-stage renal disease (ESRD) in elderly subjects and is likely underdiagnosed. It is more frequent in males with history of diabetes, hypertension, and ischemic cardiac disease. Atheroemboli in the kidney are strongly associated with aortic aneurysmal disease and renal artery stenosis. Most clinical cases can be associated with precipitating events, such as angiography, vascular surgery, anticoagulation with heparin, thrombolytic therapy, or trauma. Clinical manifestations of this syndrome commonly develop between 1 and 14 days after an inciting event and may continue to develop for weeks thereafter. Systemic embolic disease manifestations, such as fever, abdominal pain, and weight loss are present in less than half of patients, although cutaneous manifestations including livedo reticularis and localized toe gangrene may be more common. Worsening hypertension and deteriorating kidney function are common, sometimes reaching a malignant phase. Progressive renal failure can occur and require dialytic support. These cases often develop after a stuttering onset over many weeks and have an ominous prognosis. Mortality rate after 1 year reaches 38%, and although some may eventually recover sufficiently to no longer require dialysis, many do not.

Beyond the clinical manifestations above, laboratory findings include rising creatinine, eosinophilia (60–80%), elevated sedimentation rate, and hypocomplementemia (15%). Establishing this diagnosis can be difficult and is often by exclusion. Definitive diagnosis depends upon kidney biopsy demonstrating microvessel occlusion with cholesterol crystals that leave a "cleft" in the vessel. Biopsies obtained from patients undergoing surgical revascularization of the kidney indicate that silent cholesterol emboli are frequently present before any further manipulation is performed.

No effective therapy is available for atheroembolic disease once it has developed. Withdrawal of anticoagulation is recommended. Late recovery of kidney function after supportive measures sometimes occurs, and statin therapy may improve outcome. The role of embolic protection devices in the renal circulation is unclear, but a few prospective trials have failed to demonstrate major benefits. These devices are limited to distal protection during the endovascular procedure and offer no protection from embolic debris after removal.

THROMBOEMBOLIC RENAL DISEASE

Thrombotic occlusion of renal vessels or branch arteries can lead to declining renal function and hypertension. It is difficult to diagnose and is often overlooked, especially in elderly patients. Thrombosis can develop as a result of local vessel abnormalities, such as local dissection, trauma, or inflammatory vasculitis. While hypercoagulability conditions sometimes present as renal artery thrombosis, this is rare. It can also derive from distant embolic events, e.g., the left atrium in patients with atrial fibrillation or from fat emboli originating from traumatized tissue, most commonly large bone fractures. Cardiac sources include vegetations from subacute bacterial endocarditis. Systemic emboli to the kidneys may also arise from the venous circulation if right-to-left shunting occurs, e.g., through a patent foramen ovale.

Clinical manifestations vary depending upon the rapidity of onset and extent of occlusion. Acute arterial thrombosis may produce flank pain, fever, leukocytosis, nausea, and vomiting. If kidney infarction results, enzymes such as lactate dehydrogenase (LDH) rise to extreme levels. If both kidneys are affected, renal function will decline precipitously with a drop in urine output. If a single kidney is involved, renal functional changes may be minor. Hypertension related to sudden release of renin from ischemic tissue can develop rapidly, so long as some viable tissue in the "peri-infarct" border zone remains. If the infarct zone demarcates precisely, the rise in blood pressure and renin activity may resolve. Diagnosis of renal infarction may be established by vascular imaging with MR, CT angiography, or arteriography (Figs. 286-2*A* and *B*).

■ MANAGEMENT OF ARTERIAL THROMBOSIS OF THE KIDNEY

Options for interventions of newly detected arterial occlusion include surgical reconstruction, anticoagulation, thrombolytic therapy, endovascular procedures, and supportive care, particularly antihypertensive drug therapy. Application of these methods depends upon the patient's overall condition, the precipitating factors (e.g., local trauma or systemic illness), the magnitude of renal tissue and function at risk, and the likelihood of recurrent events in the future. For unilateral disease, e.g., arterial dissection with thrombosis, supportive care with anticoagulation may suffice. Acute, bilateral occlusion is potentially catastrophic, producing anuric renal failure. Depending upon the precipitating event, surgical or thrombolytic therapies can sometimes restore kidney viability.

MICROVASCULAR INJURY AND HYPERTENSION

■ ARTERIOLONEPHROSCLEROSIS

"Malignant" hypertension

Although BP rises with age, it has long been recognized that some individuals develop rapidly progressive BP elevations with target organ injury including retinal hemorrhages, encephalopathy, and declining kidney function. Placebo arms during the controlled trials of hypertension therapy identified progression to severe levels in

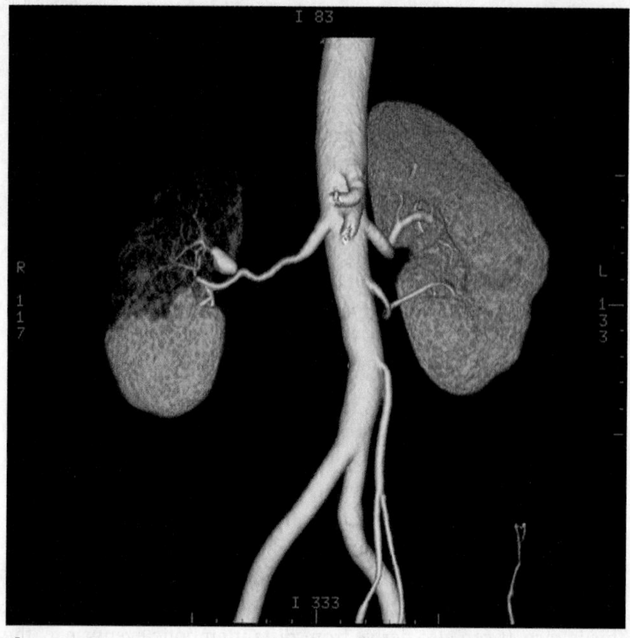

A

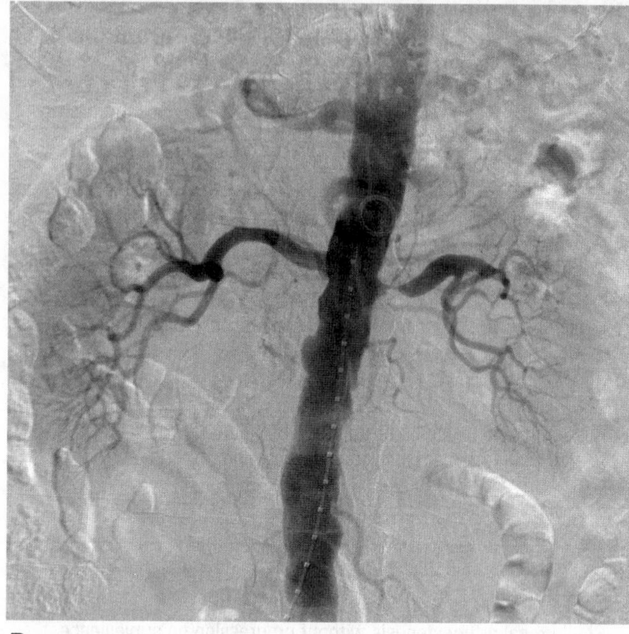

B

Figure 286-2 ***A.*** **CT angiogram illustrating loss of circulation to the upper pole of the right kidney in a patient with fibromuscular disease and a renal artery aneurysm.** Activation of the renin-angiotensin system produced rapidly developing hypertension. ***B.*** Angiogram illustrating high-grade renal artery stenosis affecting the left kidney. This lesion is often part of widespread atherosclerosis and sometimes is an extension of aortic plaque. This lesion develops in older individuals with preexisting atherosclerotic risk factors.

20% of subjects over 5 years. If untreated, patients with target organ injury including papilledema and declining kidney function suffered mortality rates in excess of 50% over 6–12 months, hence the designation "malignant." Postmortem studies of such patients identified vascular lesions, designated "fibrinoid necrosis," with breakdown of the vessel wall, deposition of eosinophilic material including fibrin, and a perivascular cellular infiltrate. A separate lesion was identified in the larger interlobular arteries in many patients with hyperplastic proliferation of the vascular wall cellular elements, deposition of collagen, and separation of layers, designated the "onionskin" lesion. For many of these patients, fibrinoid necrosis led to obliteration of glomeruli and loss of tubular structures. Progressive kidney failure ensued and without dialysis support led to early mortality in untreated malignant-phase hypertension. These vascular changes could develop with pressure-related injury from a variety of hypertensive pathways, including but not limited to activation of the renin-angiotensin system, and severe vasospasm associated with catecholamine release. Occasionally endothelial injury is sufficient to induce microangiopathic hemolysis as discussed below.

Antihypertensive therapy is the mainstay of therapy for malignant hypertension. With effective BP reduction, manifestations of vascular injury including microangiopathic hemolysis and renal dysfunction can improve over time. Whereas mortality in series reported before the era of drug therapy suggested that 1-year mortality rates exceeded 90%, current survival over 5 years exceeds 50%.

Malignant hypertension is less common in Western countries, although it persists in parts of the world where medical care and antihypertensive drug therapy are less available. It most commonly develops in patients with treated hypertension that neglect to take medications, or who may use vasospastic drugs, such as cocaine. Renal abnormalities typically include rising serum creatinine, occasionally hematuria and proteinuria. Biochemical findings may include evidence of hemolysis (anemia, schistocytes, and reticulocytosis) and changes associated with kidney failure. African-American males are more likely to develop rapidly progressive hypertension and kidney failure than are whites in the United States. Genetic polymorphisms (MYH9) that are common in the African-American population and predispose to subtle focal sclerosing glomerular disease may be responsible, with hypertension developing secondary to renal disease in this instance.

"Hypertensive nephrosclerosis"

Based on experience with malignant hypertension and epidemiologic evidence linking BP with long-term risks of kidney failure, it has long been assumed that lesser degrees of hypertension induce less severe, but prevalent changes in kidney vessels and loss of kidney function. As a result, a large portion of patients reaching ESRD without a specific etiologic diagnosis are assigned the designation "hypertensive nephrosclerosis." Pathologic examination commonly identifies afferent arteriolar thickening with deposition of homogeneous eosinophilic material (*hyaline arteriolosclerosis*) associated with narrowing of vascular lumina. Clinical manifestations include retinal vessel changes associated with hypertension (arteriolar narrowing, crossing changes), left ventricular hypertrophy, and elevated blood pressure. The role of these vascular changes in kidney function is unclear. Postmortem and biopsy samples from normotensive kidney donors demonstrate similar vessel changes associated with aging, dyslipidemia, and glucose intolerance. While BP reduction does slow progression of proteinuric kidney diseases and is warranted to reduce the excessive cardiovascular risks associated with CKD, antihypertensive therapy does not alter the course of kidney dysfunction identified specifically as hypertensive nephrosclerosis.

THROMBOTIC MICROANGIOPATHY

Thrombotic microangiopathy (TMA) refers to injured endothelial cells that are thickened, swollen, or detached mainly from arterioles and capillaries. Platelet and hyaline thrombi causing partial or complete occlusion are integral to the histopathology. TMA is the histologic result of microangiopathic hemolytic anemia (MAHA), which consumes platelets and erythrocytes and is characterized by thrombocytopenia and schistocytes. In the kidney, TMA is characterized by swelling of the endocapillary cells (endotheliosis), fibrin thrombi, platelet plugs, arterial intimal fibrosis, and membranoproliferative changes. In severe cases, the fibrin thrombi may extend into the arteriolar vascular pole producing glomerular collapse and sometimes cortical necrosis. Secondary focal segmental glomerulosclerosis may be seen in individuals who recover from acute TMA. Diseases that present with this lesion include thrombotic thrombocytopenia (TTP), hemolytic-uremia syndrome (HUS), malignant hypertension, scleroderma renal crisis, antiphospholipid syndrome, preeclampsia/HELLP (*h*emolysis, *e*levated *l*iver enzymes, *l*ow *p*latelet count) syndrome, HIV infection, and radiation nephropathy.

HEMOLYTIC-UREMIC SYNDROME (HUS)/THROMBOTIC THROMBOCYTOPENIC PURPURA (TTP)

HUS and TTP are the prototypes of MAHA. Whether they represent a spectrum of the same disease or two distinct entities continues to be debated. Histologically, the diseases are inseparable, but they differ regarding epidemiology and pathophysiology. Typical HUS usually affects children (most under the age of 5) and is preceded by hemorrhagic diarrhea. Typical TTP affects individuals in their thirties and forties. Neurologic symptoms are more common in TTP and have significant morbidity and mortality rates if not treated with plasma exchange, while plasma exchange is ineffective in most HUS. The argument is strengthened with the discovery of a disintegrin and metalloproteinase with a thrombospondin type 1 motif member 13 (ADAMTS13), a von Willebrand factor (vWF) cleaving protease that is either absent or inactive in TTP but not in HUS. However, neurologic symptoms can occur in HUS, and low ADAMTS13 activity has been identified in HUS cases. Furthermore, plasma infusion/exchange is effective in some HUS. As a result, the distinction between the two is blurred, and they are often identified simply as HUS/TTP.

HEMOLYTIC-UREMIC SYNDROME

There are at least four variants of HUS. The most common is D+ HUS referring to its association with bacterial gastroenteritis. This typically affects young children (<5 years), but adults are also susceptible. More than 80% of cases are preceded within a week by diarrhea, often bloody. Gastrointestinal symptoms include abdominal pain, cramping, and vomiting. Fever is typically absent. Neurologic symptoms are common and may include lethargy, encephalopathy, seizures, and even cerebral infarction. The pathogenic agent linked to D+ HUS is the shiga toxin, also referred to as *verotoxin*. This toxin is produced by certain strains of *Escherichia coli* and *Shigella dysenteriae*. In the United States and Europe, the most common shiga-toxigenic *E. coli* (STEC) strain is the 0157:H7. Other strains such as 0157/H$^-$, 0111:H$^-$, 026:H11/H$^-$, and 0145:H28 can also produce shiga toxin. Once shiga toxin enters the circulation, it binds to neutrophils and preferentially localizes in the kidney, where it causes damage to the endothelial cells. This results in platelet aggregation, which initiates the microangiopathic process. Another bacterium associated with HUS is *Streptococcus pneumoniae*. This bacterium produces a neuraminidase that cleaves the *N*-acetyl neuraminic acid moieties that cover the Thomsen-Friedenreich antigen on platelets and endothelial cells. Exposure of this normally cryptic antigen to preformed IgM results in severe MAHA.

Another variant produces atypical HUS (aHUS), caused by congenital complement dysregulation rather than a toxin. These patients have low C3 levels, a characteristic of alternative pathway activation. The most common cause is a deficiency of factor H, which has been linked to families with aHUS. Factor H competes with factor B to prevent the formation of C3b,Bb and acts as a cofactor for factor I, which proteolytically degrades C3b. More than 70 mutations of the factor H gene have been identified. Most are missense mutations that produce normal levels of factor H with abnormalities mainly in the C-terminus region, which affect its binding to C3b. Other mutations result in low or complete absence of the protein. Deficiencies in other complement regulatory proteins such as factor I, factor B, membrane cofactor protein or MCP (CD46), C3, complement factor H–related protein 1 (CFHR1), CFHR3, and CFHR5 have also been described. Finally, an autoimmune variant of HUS has been discovered. Deficient for CHFR protein and factor H autoantibody–positive (DEAP), HUS occurs when an autoantibody is formed against factor H. DEAP-HUS is often associated with a deletion of an 84-kb fragment of the chromosome that encodes for CFHR1 and CFHR3. The autoantibody blocks the binding of factor H to C3b and surface-bound C3 convertase.

THROMBOTIC THROMBOCYTOPENIC PURPURA

Traditionally TTP is characterized by the pentad (hemolytic anemia, thrombocytopenia, neurologic symptoms, fever, and renal failure). Classic TTP is differentiated from HUS by neurologic involvement. However, in practice, differentiation between TTP and HUS is unreliable due to overlap in clinical manifestations. TTP has been linked with the absence or marked decreased activity in the metalloprotease ADAMTS13 specific for vWF, although this is not universally present. Even complete absence of ADAMTS13 alone does not produce TTP. Most often, an additional trigger (such as infection, surgery, pancreatitis, or pregnancy) initiates clinical TTP.

Data from the Oklahoma TTP/HUS Registry reveal an incidence rate of 11.3 per 10^6 patients. The median age of the patients was 40 years. Higher frequency was noted among blacks, with an incidence more than nine times higher than non-blacks. Women have nearly three times the incidence, similar to the demographics for systemic lupus erythematosus. If untreated, TTP has a mortality rate exceeding 90%. Even with modern therapy, 20% of the patients die within the first month from complications of microvascular thrombosis.

Several subtypes of TTP have been described. The classic form is acquired or idiopathic TTP, which usually follows an infection, malignancy, or an intense inflammatory reaction such as pancreatitis. This variant typically occurs with deficiency of ADAMTS13 or its activity and is the result of an autoantibody. The autoantibody (IgG or IgM) can either increase clearance of ADAMTS13 or inhibit its activity. A hereditary form with congenital deficiency of ADAMTS13 is seen in patients with Upshaw-Schulman characterized by MAHA and thrombocytopenia. TTP in these patients can start within the first weeks of life, but in others, may not start until several years of age. Environmental and genetic factors are thought to influence the development of TTP. Plasma transfusion is effective as a prevention and treatment during the TTP episodes.

Drug-induced TTP/TMA is a recognized complication of chemotherapeutic agents, immunosuppressive agents, antiplatelet agents, and quinine. Two mechanisms are responsible for drug-induced TMA. With chemotherapeutic agents (mitomycin C, gemcitabine, etc.) and immunosuppressive agents (cyclosporine, tacrolimus, and sirolimus), endothelial damage is the main cause of the MAHA. This process is usually dose-dependent. Alternatively, drugs can induce autoantibodies that produce TMA. Suppression of ADAMTS13 activity and formation of an autoantibody has been detected in patients exposed to ticlopidine. Quinine appears to induce autoantibodies against granulocytes, lymphocytes, endothelial cells, and platelet glycoprotein IbB/IX or IIb/IIIa complexes but not to ADAMTS13. Quinine-associated TTP is more common in women. Autoantibody-associated TTP can occur after a single dose in patients who had previous exposure to the drug. Most patients developing TTP from clopidogrel do not have either autoantibodies or decreased

ADAMTS13 activity. Drugs that inhibit vascular endothelial growth factor (VEGF) sometimes produce TMA. The mechanism is not fully understood.

Treatment of HUS/TTP should be based on the pathophysiologic pathways that are identified. Autoantibody-mediated TTP and DEAP HUS should be treated with plasma exchange or plasmapheresis. In addition to removing the autoantibodies, plasma exchange replaces ADAMTS13. Twice-daily plasma exchanges, vincristine, and rituximab occasionally have been found to be effective in refractory cases. Plasma infusion is usually sufficient for congenital TTP such as Upshaw-Schulman syndrome. Plasma exchange should be considered if larger volumes of plasma are necessary. TTP secondary to drug-induced autoantibodies responds well to plasma exchange, while drugs that cause endothelial damage may not. D+ HUS should be treated with supportive measures. Plasma exchange has not been found to be effective. Antimotility agents and antibiotics increase the incidence of HUS and should be avoided. Conversely, plasma infusion/exchange may be beneficial in aHUS by repleting complement regulatory proteins. Antibiotics and washed red cells should be given in neuraminidase-associated HUS. Plasma and whole blood should be avoided since they contain IgM, which would exacerbate the MAHA. The coexistence of factor H and ADAMTS13 deficiency can exacerbate TTP and make it less responsive to plasma infusion, illustrating the complexity of managing these disorders.

TRANSPLANTATION-ASSOCIATED THROMBOTIC MICROANGIOPATHY (TA-TMA)

TA-TMA can develop after hematopoietic stem cell transplantation (HSCT) with an incidence of 8.2%. Etiologic factors include conditioning regimens, immunosuppression, infections, and graft-versus-host disease. Other risk factors include female sex, age, and human leukocyte antigen (HLA)-mismatched donor grafts. TA-TMA usually occurs within the first 100 days after HSCT. Table 286-3 lists definitions of TA-TMA currently used for clinical trials. A firm diagnosis may be difficult because thrombocytopenia, anemia, and renal insufficiency are common in the posttransplant period. TA-TMA carries a high mortality rate (75% within 3 months). Plasma exchange is beneficial in less than 50% of patients, most of whom have more than 5% ADAMTS13 activity. Calciuria inhibitors should be discontinued, and substitution with daclizumab [antibody to the interleukin 2 (IL-2) receptor] is recommended. Treatment with rituximab and defibrotide may also be helpful.

TABLE 286-3 Criteria for Establishing Microangiopathic Kidney Injury Associated With Hematopoietic Stem Cell Transplantation

International Working Group	Blood and Marrow Transplant Clinical Trials Network Toxicity Committee
>4% schistocytes in the blood	RBC fragmentation and at least 2 schistocytes per high-power field
De novo, prolonged, or progressive thrombocytopenia	Concurrent increase in LDH above baseline
A sudden and persistent increase in LDH	Negative direct and indirect Coombs test
Decrease in hemoglobin or increased RBC transfusion requirement	Concurrent renal and/or neurologic dysfunction without other explanations
Decrease in haptoglobin concentration	

Note: These features underscore the need to identify pathways of hemolysis and thrombocytopenia that accompany deterioration of kidney function.
Abbreviations: LDH, lactate dehydrogenase; RBC, red blood cell.

HIV-RELATED TMA

TMA is mainly a complication encountered before widespread use of highly active retroviral therapy for HIV. It is seen in patients with advanced AIDS and low CD4 count, although it occasionally can be the first manifestation of HIV infection. The presence of MAHA thrombocytopenia and renal failure are suggestive, but renal biopsy is required to establish the diagnosis since HIV is associated with several other renal diseases. The median platelet count is 77,000/μL with a range of 10,000 to 160,000/μL, which may prohibit a renal biopsy in some patients. Cytomegalovirus (CMV) coinfection may also be a risk factor. The mechanism of injury is unclear, but HIV may induce apoptosis in endothelial cells. Plasma exchange is effective and is recommended in conjunction with antiviral therapy.

RADIATION NEPHROPATHY

Radiation can produce microangiopathic injury after either local or total body irradiation. The kidney is one of the most radiosensitive organs, and injury can result with as little as 4–5 Gy exposure. It is characterized by renal insufficiency, proteinuria, and hypertension usually presenting 6 months or longer after radiation exposure. Renal biopsy reveals classic TMA in the kidney with damage to glomerular, tubular, and vascular cells. Systemic evidence for MAHA is rare. Because of its high incidence after allogeneic HSCT, it is often referred to as bone marrow transplant (BMT) nephropathy. No specific therapy is available, although some evidence supports treatment with renin-angiotensin system blockade.

SCLERODERMA (PROGRESSIVE SYSTEMIC SCLEROSIS)

Scleroderma commonly affects the kidney, with 52% of subjects with widespread scleroderma having renal involvement sometime during the follow-up period. Of these, 19% were due to scleroderma renal crisis (SRC). Other renal manifestations in scleroderma include transient (prerenal) or medication-related forms of acute kidney injury [e.g., D-penicillamine, nonsteroidal anti-inflammatory drugs (NSAIDs), or cyclosporine]. SRC occurs in patients with diffuse systemic sclerosis (12 vs. 2% in limited systemic sclerosis). SRC is the most severe manifestation, characterized by accelerated hypertension, a rapid decline in renal function, nephrotic proteinuria, and hematuria. Retinopathy and encephalopathy may accompany the hypertension. Salt and water retention with microvascular injury can lead to pulmonary edema. Other manifestations include myocarditis, pericarditis, and arrhythmias, which denote an especially poor prognosis. Although MAHA is present in over half of the patients, coagulopathy is rare.

The renal lesion in SRC is characterized by arcuate artery intimal and medial proliferation with luminal narrowing. This lesion is described as *onionskinning* and can be accompanied by glomerular collapse due to reduced blood flow. Histologically it is indistinguishable from malignant hypertension. Fibrinoid necrosis and thrombosis are common. Before the availability of angiotensin-converting enzyme (ACE) inhibitors, the mortality rate for SRC at 1 month was greater than 90%. Introduction of renin-angiotensin system blockade has lowered the mortality rate to 30% at 3 years. Nearly two-thirds of patients with SRC require dialysis support. Half of those needing dialysis as a result of SRC will recover renal function (median time = 1 year). Glomerulonephritis and vasculitis associated with antineutrophil cytoplasmic antibodies (ANCAs) and systemic lupus erythematosus have been described in patients with scleroderma. An association has been found with antinuclear antibodies' (ANAs) speckled pattern and anti-RNA polymerase antibodies (I and III). Anti-U3-RNP may identify young patients at risk for SRC. Anticentromere antibody (ACA), however, is a negative predictor of SRC. Because of the overlap between SRC and other autoimmune disorders, a renal biopsy is recommended for patients with atypical renal involvement, especially if hypertension is absent.

Treatment with ACE inhibition is the first-line therapy unless contraindicated. The goal of therapy is to reduce systolic blood pressure by 20 mmHg and diastolic by 10 mmHg every 24 hours until blood pressure is normalized. Additional antihypertensive therapy may be added once the ACE inhibition is maximized. Both ACE inhibitors and angiotensin II receptor antagonists are effective, although published data show that treatment is superior with ACE inhibitors. ACE inhibition alone does not prevent SRC, although it reduces the role of hypertension. Intravenous iloprost has been used in Europe for blood pressure management and improvement of renal perfusion. Kidney transplantation is not recommended for 2 years after the start of dialysis, since delayed recovery may occur.

ANTIPHOSPHOLIPID SYNDROME (APS)

Antiphospholipid syndrome (Chap. 320) can be either primary or secondary to systemic lupus erythematosus. It is characterized by systemic thrombosis (arterial and venous) and fetal morbidity mediated by antiphospholipid antibodies (aPLs). The aPLs are mainly anticardiolipin (aCL) antibodies, which can be IgG, IgM, or IgA, lupus anticoagulant (LA), and anti-β-2 glycoprotein I antibodies (antiβ2GPI). Patients with both aCL and antiβ2GPI appear to have the highest risk of thrombosis. The vascular compartment within the kidney is the main site of renal involvement. Arteriosclerosis is commonly present in the arcuate and intralobular arteries. In the intralobular arteries, fibrous intimal hyperplasia characterized by intimal thickening secondary to intense myofibroblastic intimal cellular proliferation with extracellular matrix deposition is frequently seen along with onionskinning. Arterial and arteriolar fibrous and fibrocellular occlusions are present in over two-thirds of the biopsies. Cortical necrosis and focal cortical atrophy may result from vascular occlusion. TMA is commonly present in the renal biopsies, although signs of MAHA and platelet consumption are usually absent. TMA is especially common in the catastrophic variant of APS. In patients with secondary antiphospholipid syndrome (APS), other glomerulopathies may be present including membranous nephropathy, minimal change disease, focal segmental glomerulosclerosis, and pauci-immune crescentic glomerulonephritis.

Large vessels can be involved in APS and may form the proximal nidus near the ostium for thrombosis of the renal artery. Renal vein thrombosis can occur and should be suspected in patients with lupus anticoagulant LA who develop nephrotic range proteinuria. Progression to end-stage renal disease can occur, and thrombosis may form in the vascular access and the renal allografts. Hypertension is common. Treatment entails lifelong anticoagulation. Glucocorticoids may be beneficial in accelerated hypertension. Immunosuppression and plasma exchange may be helpful for catastrophic episodes of APS, but themselves do not reduce recurrent thrombosis.

HELLP SYNDROME

HELLP (*h*emolysis, *el*evated *l*iver enzymes, *l*ow *p*latelets) syndrome is a dangerous complication of pregnancy. Occurring in 0.5–0.9% of all pregnancies and 10–20% of cases with severe preeclampsia, it has a mortality rate that ranges between 7.4 and 34%. Most commonly occurring in the third trimester, 10% of cases occur before week 27 and 30% postpartum. Although most consider HELLP to be a severe form of preeclampsia, nearly 20% are not preceded by preeclampsia. HELLP patients have increased inflammatory markers [C-reactive protein (CRP), IL-1Ra, and IL-6] as compared to preeclampsia alone.

Renal failure occurs in half of patients with HELLP, although the etiology is not well understood. Limited data suggest renal failure is the result of a combination of preeclampsia and acute tubular necrosis from HELLP. Renal histologic findings are those of TMA with endothelial cell swelling and occlusion of the capillary lumens, but luminal thrombi are typically absent. However, thrombi become more common in severe eclampsia and HELLP. Although renal failure is common, the organ that defines this syndrome is the liver. Subcapsular hepatic hematomas sometimes produce spontaneous rupture of the liver and can be a life-threatening complication. Neurologic complications such as strokes, cerebral infarcts, cerebral and brainstem hemorrhage, and cerebral edema are other major potentially life-threatening complications. Nonfatal complications include placental abruption, permanent vision loss due to Purtscher-like (hemorrhagic and vasoocclusive vasculopathy) retinopathy, pulmonary edema, bleeding, and fetal demise.

The HELLP syndrome shares many features with other forms of MAHA. Distinguishing the specific disorders is complicated by the fact that both aHUS and TTP flares can be triggered by pregnancy. Patients with antiphospholipid syndrome have a higher risk of HELLP. A history of episodes of MAHA before pregnancy is helpful. Serum levels of ADAMTS13 activity is reduced (30–60%) in HELLP but not to the levels seen in TTP (<5%). Some authors suggest using LDH to AST ratio for diagnosis. Patients with HELLP and preeclampsia have an LDH to AST ratio of 13 to 1 versus 29 to 1 in patients without preeclampsia. Other markers such as antithrombin III (decreased in HELLP but not in TTP) and D-dimer (elevated in HELLP but not in TTP) may aid in the diagnosis. HELLP syndrome resolves spontaneously in most cases after delivery, although a portion of HELLP occurs postpartum. Glucocorticoids may decrease inflammatory markers, although two randomized, controlled trials failed to confirm beneficial effects. Plasma exchange should be considered if the hemolysis is refractory to glucocorticoids and/or delivery, especially if TTP had not been ruled out.

SICKLE CELL NEPHROPATHY

Renal complications in sickle cell disease (SCD) result from occlusion of the vasa recta in the renal medulla. The low partial pressure of oxygen and high osmolarity predispose to hemoglobin S polymerization and erythrocyte sickling. Sequelae include hyposthenuria, hematuria, and papillary necrosis. The kidney responds by increasing blood flow and GFR mediated by prostaglandins. This dependence on prostaglandins may explain why patients with SCD experience greater reduction of GFR by NSAIDs than others. The glomeruli are typically enlarged. Intracapillary fragmentation and phagocytosis of sickled erythrocytes are thought to be responsible for the membranoproliferative glomerulonephritis-like lesion, and focal segmental glomerulosclerosis is sometimes seen. Proteinuria is present in 20–30% of the patients, and nephrotic range proteinuria is associated with renal failure. ACE inhibitors reduce proteinuria, although data are lacking on prevention of renal failure. Patients with SCD are also more prone to acute renal failure. The cause is thought to reflect microvascular occlusion associated with nontraumatic rhabdomyolysis, high fever, infection, and generalized sickling. Chronic kidney disease is present in 12–20% of patients. Despite the frequency of renal disease, hypertension is uncommon in patients with SCD.

RENAL VEIN THROMBOSIS

Renal vein thrombosis (RVT) can either present with flank pain, tenderness, hematuria, rapid decline in renal function, and proteinuria or it can be silent. Occasionally, RVT is identified during workup for pulmonary embolism. The left renal vein is more commonly involved and two-thirds of cases are bilateral. Etiologies can be divided into three broad categories: endothelial damage, venous stasis, and hypercoagulable states. Homocystinuria, endovascular intervention, and surgery can produce vascular endothelial damage. Dehydration, which is more common in males, is a common cause of stasis in the pediatric population. Stasis also can result from compression and kinking of the renal veins from retroperitoneal processes such as retroperitoneal fibrosis and abdominal neoplasms. Thrombosis can occur throughout the renal circulation with antiphospholipid antibody syndrome. RVT can also be secondary to nephrotic syndrome, particularly membranous nephropathy. Other hypercoagulable states associated with RVT include proteins C and S, antithrombin deficiency, factor V Leiden, disseminated malignancy, and oral contraceptives.

Diagnostic screening can be performed with Doppler ultrasound, which is more sensitive than ultrasound alone. The most sensitive test is CT angiography, which is nearly 100% sensitive. MR angiography is another option but is more expensive and requires sedation in pediatric patients. Treatment for RVT is anticoagulation and therapy for the underlying cause. Endovascular thrombolysis may be considered in severe cases. Occasionally nephrectomy may be undertaken for life-threatening complications. Vena caval filters are often used to prevent migration of the thrombi.

FURTHER READINGS

de Mast Q, Beutler JJ: The prevalence of atherosclerotic renal artery stenosis in risk groups: A systematic literature review. J Hypertens 27:1333, 2009

Denton CP: Renal manifestations of systemic sclerosis—clinical features and outcome assessment. Rheumatology 47(Suppl 5): v54, 2008

Garovic V, Textor SC: Renovascular hypertension and ischemic nephropathy. Circulation 112:1362, 2005

George JN: The thrombotic thrombocytopenic purpura and hemolytic uremic syndromes: Overview of pathogenesis (Experience of the Oklahoma TTP-HUS Registry, 1989–2007). Kidney Int Suppl 112:S8, 2009

Nochy D et al: The intrarenal vascular lesions associated with primary antiphospholipid syndrome. J Am Soc Nephrol 10:507, 1999

Penn H, Denton CP: Diagnosis, management and prevention of scleroderma renal disease. Curr Opin Rheumatol 20:692, 2008

Slovut DP, Olin JW: Current concepts: Fibromuscular dysplasia. N Engl J Med 350:1862, 2004

CHAPTER 287

Nephrolithiasis

John R. Asplin
Fredric L. Coe
Murray J. Favus

Kidney stones are one of the most common urologic problems. In the United States, ~13% of men and 7% of women will develop a kidney stone during their lifetimes, and the prevalence is increasing throughout the industrialized world.

■ TYPES OF STONES

Calcium salts, uric acid, cystine, and struvite are the constituents of most kidney stones in the western hemisphere (Chap. e14). Calcium oxalate and calcium phosphate stones make up 75–85% of the total (Table 287-1) and those constituents may be admixed in the same stone. Calcium phosphate in stones is usually hydroxyapatite [$Ca_5(PO_4)_3OH$] or, less commonly, brushite ($CaHPO_4H_2O$), although the incidence of brushite stones is increasing.

Calcium stones are more common in men; the average age of onset is the third to fourth decade. Approximately 50% of people who form a single calcium stone form another within the next 10 years, and some form multiple recurrent stones. The average rate of new stone formation in recurrent stone formers is about one stone every 3 years. *Uric acid stones* account for 5–10% of kidney stones and are also more common in men. Five percent of stones are *struvite*, whereas *cystine stones* are uncommon, accounting for ~1% of cases in most series of nephrolithiasis.

■ MANIFESTATIONS OF STONES

As stones grow on the surfaces of the renal papillae or within the collecting system, they do not necessarily produce symptoms. Asymptomatic stones may be discovered during the course of radiographic studies undertaken for unrelated reasons. Stones are a common cause of isolated hematuria. Stones become symptomatic when they enter the ureter or occlude the ureteropelvic junction, causing pain and obstruction.

Stone passage

A stone can traverse the ureter without symptoms, but passage usually produces pain and bleeding. The pain begins gradually, usually in the flank, but increases over the next 20–60 min to become so severe that narcotics may be needed for its control. The pain may remain in the flank or spread downward and anteriorly toward the ipsilateral loin, testis, or vulva. A stone in the portion of the ureter within the bladder wall causes frequency, urgency, and dysuria that may be confused with urinary tract infection. The vast majority of ureteral stones <0.5 cm in diameter pass spontaneously.

Helical computed tomography (CT) scanning without radiocontrast enhancement is now the standard radiologic procedure for diagnosis of nephrolithiasis. The advantages of CT include detection of uric acid stones in addition to the traditional radiopaque stones, no exposure to the risk of radiocontrast agents, and possible diagnosis of other causes of abdominal pain in a patient suspected of having renal colic from stones. Ultrasound is not as sensitive as CT in detecting renal or ureteral stones. Standard abdominal x-rays may be used to monitor patients for formation and growth of kidney stones, as they are less expensive

TABLE 287-1 Major Causes of Renal Stones

Stone Type and Causes	Percent of all Stones[a]	Percent Occurrence of Specific Causes[a]	Ratio of Males to Females	Etiology	Diagnosis	Treatment
Calcium stones	75–85		2:1 to 3:1			
Idiopathic hypercalciuria		50–55	2:1	? Hereditary	Normocalcemia, unexplained hypercalciuria[b]	Low-sodium, low-protein diet; thiazide diuretics
Hyperuricosuria		20	4:1	Diet	Urine uric acid >750 mg per 24 h (women), >800 mg per 24 h (men)	Allopurinol or low-purine diet
Primary hyperparathyroidism		3–5	3:10	Neoplasia	Hypercalcemia with nonsuppressed parathyroid hormone	Surgery
Distal renal tubular acidosis		Rare	1:1	Hereditary or acquired	Hyperchloremic acidosis, minimum urine pH >5.5	Alkali replacement
Dietary hyperoxaluria		10–30	1:1	High-oxalate diet or low-calcium diet	Urine oxalate >40 mg per 24 h	Low-oxalate, normal-calcium diet
Enteric hyperoxaluria		~1–2	1:1	Bowel surgery	Urine oxalate >75 mg per 24 h	Low-oxalate diet and oral calcium pills
Primary hyperoxaluria		Rare	1:1	Hereditary	Urine oxalate and glycolic or l-glyceric acid increased	Fluids, pyridoxine, citrate and neutral phosphate
Hypocitraturia		20–40	1:1 to 2:1	? Hereditary, diet	Urine citrate <320 mg per 24 h	Alkali supplements
Idiopathic stone disease		20	2:1	Unknown	None of the above present	Oral phosphate, fluids
Uric acid stones	5–10					
Metabolic syndrome		~30	1:1	Diet	Glucose intolerance, obesity, hyperlipidemia	Alkali and allopurinol if daily urine uric acid >1000 mg
Gout		~30	3:1 to 4:1	Hereditary	Clinical diagnosis	Alkali and allopurinol
Idiopathic		~30	1:1	? Hereditary	Uric acid stones, no gout	Alkali and allopurinol if daily urine uric acid >1000 mg
Dehydration		?	1:1	Intestinal, habit	History, intestinal fluid loss	Alkali, fluids, reversal of cause
Lesch-Nyhan syndrome		Rare	Males only	Hereditary	Reduced hypoxanthine-guanine phosphoribosyltransferase level	Allopurinol
Cystine stones	1		1:1	Hereditary	Stone type; elevated cystine excretion	Massive fluids, alkali, D-penicillamine if needed
Struvite stones	5		1:3	Infection	Stone type	Antimicrobial agents and judicious surgery

[a]Values are percentages of patients who form a particular type of stone and who display each specific cause of stones.

[b]Urine calcium >300 mg/24 h (men), 250 mg/24 h (women), or 4 mg/kg per 24 h either sex. Hyperthyroidism, Cushing's syndrome, sarcoidosis, malignant tumors, immobilization, vitamin D intoxication, rapidly progressive bone disease, and Paget's disease all cause hypercalciuria and must be excluded in diagnosis of idiopathic hypercalciuria.

and provide less radiation exposure than CT scans. Calcium, cystine, and struvite stones are all radiopaque on standard x-rays, whereas uric acid stones are radiolucent.

Other syndromes

Staghorn calculi Struvite, cystine, and uric acid stones often grow too large to enter the ureter. They gradually fill the renal pelvis and may extend outward through the infundibula to the calyces themselves. Very large staghorn stones can have surprisingly few symptoms and may lead to the eventual loss of kidney function.

Nephrocalcinosis Calcium stones grow on the papillae. Most break loose and cause colic, but they may remain in place so that multiple papillary calcifications are found by x-ray, a condition termed *nephrocalcinosis*. Papillary nephrocalcinosis is common in hereditary distal renal tubular acidosis (RTA) and in other types of severe hypercalciuria. In medullary sponge kidney disease (Chap. 284), calcification may occur in dilated distal collecting ducts.

Infection

Although urinary tract infection is not a direct consequence of stone disease, it can occur after instrumentation and surgery of the urinary tract, which are used frequently in the treatment of stone disease. Stone disease and urinary tract infection can enhance their respective seriousness and interfere with treatment. Obstruction of an infected kidney by a stone may lead to sepsis and extensive damage of renal tissue, since it converts the urinary tract proximal to the obstruction into a closed space that can become an abscess. Stones may harbor bacteria in the stone matrix, leading to recurrent urinary tract infection, and infection due to bacteria that have the enzyme urease can cause stones composed of struvite.

Activity of stone disease

In active disease, new stones are forming or preformed stones are growing. Sequential radiographs are needed to document the growth or appearance of new stones and ensure that passed stones are actually newly formed, not preexistent.

PATHOGENESIS OF STONES

Urinary stones usually arise because of the breakdown of a delicate balance between solubility and precipitation of salts. The kidneys must conserve water, but they must excrete materials that have low solubility. These two opposing requirements must be balanced during adaptation to diet, climate, and activity. The problem is mitigated to some extent by the fact that urine contains substances such as pyrophosphate, citrate, and glycoproteins that inhibit crystallization. These protective mechanisms are less than perfect. When urine becomes supersaturated with insoluble materials, because excretion rates are excessive and/or because water conservation is extreme, crystals form and may grow and aggregate to form a stone.

Supersaturation

A solution in equilibrium with a solid phase is said to be saturated with respect to that substance. If the concentration of a substance in a solution is above the saturation point, the solution is said to be supersaturated and can support the growth of crystals, and if supersaturation is excessive, new crystals can begin to develop spontaneously. Excessive supersaturation is common in stone formation.

Calcium, oxalate, and phosphate form many soluble complexes among themselves and with other substances in urine, such as citrate. As a result, their free ion activities are below their chemical concentrations. Reduction in ligands such as citrate can increase ion activity and therefore supersaturation. Urine supersaturation can be increased by dehydration or by overexcretion of calcium, oxalate, phosphate, cystine, or uric acid. Urine pH is also important; phosphate and uric acid are acids that dissociate readily over the physiologic range of urine pH. Alkaline urine contains more dibasic phosphate, favoring deposits of brushite and apatite. Below a urine pH of 5.5, uric acid crystals predominate, whereas phosphate crystals are rare. The solubility of calcium oxalate is not influenced by changes in urine pH. Measurements of supersaturation in a 24-h urine sample probably underestimate the risk of precipitation. Transient dehydration, variation of urine pH, and postprandial bursts of overexcretion may cause spikes in supersaturation.

Crystallization

When urine supersaturation is excessive, crystals begin to nucleate. Once formed, crystal nuclei will grow in size if urine is supersaturated with respect to that crystal phase. Multiple crystals can then aggregate to form a kidney stone. For a kidney stone to form, crystals must be retained in the renal pelvis long enough to grow and aggregate to a clinically significant size. Recent studies have shown that common calcium oxalate kidney stones form as overgrowths on apatite plaques in the renal papillae. These plaques, called Randall's plaques, provide an excellent surface for heterogeneous nucleation of calcium oxalate salts. The Randall's plaques begin in the deep medulla in the basement membrane of the thin limb of the loop of Henle and then spread through the interstitium to the basement membrane of the papillary urothelium. If the urothelium becomes damaged, the plaque is exposed to the urine, and calcium oxalate crystals form on the plaque, accumulating a clinically significant mass to form a stone. Calcium phosphate stone formers, particularly formers of brushite, do not follow this pattern. Inner medullary collecting ducts are plugged with apatite crystals, and stones form as extension of those plugs. Unlike in calcium oxalate stone formers, renal papillae are often fibrotic and deformed.

EVALUATION AND TREATMENT OF PATIENTS WITH NEPHROLITHIASIS

Most patients with nephrolithiasis have remediable metabolic disorders that cause stones and can be detected by chemical analyses of serum and urine. Adults with recurrent kidney stones and children with even a single kidney stone should be evaluated. A practical outpatient evaluation consists of two 24-h urine collections, with a corresponding blood sample; measurements of serum and urine calcium, uric acid, electrolytes, and creatinine, along with urine pH, volume, oxalate, and citrate should be made. Since stone risks vary with diet, activity, and environment, at least one urine collection should be made on a weekend when the patient is at home and another on a workday. When possible, the composition of kidney stones should be determined because treatment depends on stone type (Table 287-1). No matter what disorders are found, every patient should be counseled to avoid dehydration and drink copious amounts of water. The efficacy of high fluid intake was confirmed in a prospective study of first-time stone formers. Increasing urine volume to 2.5 L per day resulted in a 50% reduction of stone recurrence compared with the control group.

TREATMENT Nephrolithiasis

The management of stones already present in the kidneys or urinary tract requires a combined medical and surgical approach. The specific treatment depends on the location of the stone, the extent of obstruction, the nature of the stone, the function of the affected and unaffected kidneys, the presence or absence of urinary tract infection, the progress of stone passage, and the risks of operation or anesthesia in light of the clinical state of the patient. Medical therapy can enhance passage of ureteral stones. Oral α_1-adrenergic blockers relax ureteral muscle and have been shown to reduce time to stone passage and the need for surgical removal of small stones. Severe obstruction, infection, intractable pain, and serious bleeding are indications for removal of a stone.

Advances in urologic technology have rendered open surgery for stones a rare event. There are now three alternatives for stone removal. *Extracorporeal lithotripsy* causes the in situ fragmentation of stones in the kidney, renal pelvis, or ureter by exposing them to shock waves. After multiple shock waves, most stones are reduced to powder that moves through the ureter into the bladder. *Percutaneous nephrolithotomy* requires the passage of a nephroscope into the renal pelvis through a small incision in the flank. Stones are then disrupted by a small ultrasound transducer or holmium laser. The third method is *ureteroscopy* with stone disruption using a holmium laser. Ureteroscopy generally is used for stones in the ureter, but some surgeons are now using ureteroscopy for stones in the renal pelvis as well.

Calcium stones

Idiopathic Hypercalciuria This condition is the most common metabolic abnormality found in patients with nephrolithiasis (Table 287-1). It is familial and is probably a polygenic trait, although there are some rare monogenic causes of hypercalciuria and kidney stones such as Dent's disease, which is an X-linked disorder characterized by hypercalciuria, nephrocalcinosis, and progressive kidney failure. Idiopathic hypercalciuria is diagnosed by the presence of hypercalciuria without hypercalcemia and the absence of other systemic disorders known to affect mineral metabolism. Vitamin D overactivity through either high calcitriol levels or excess vitamin D receptor is a likely explanation for the hypercalciuria in many patients. Recent studies have shown that a polymorphism (Arg990Gly) of the calcium-sensing receptor, which leads to activation of the receptor, is more common in hypercalciuric subjects and probably contributes to higher urine calcium excretion. Hypercalciuria contributes to stone formation by raising urine saturation with respect to calcium oxalate and calcium phosphate.

TREATMENT Hypercalciuria

For many years the standard therapy for hypercalciuria was dietary calcium restriction. However, studies have shown that low-calcium diets increase the risk of incident stone formation, perhaps by reducing the amount of calcium in the intestine to bind oxalate, thereby increasing urine oxalate levels. A 5-year prospective trial compared the efficacy of a low-calcium diet to a low-protein, low-sodium, normal-calcium diet in preventing stone recurrence in male calcium stone formers. The group on the low-calcium diet had a significantly greater rate of stone relapse. In addition, hypercalciuric stone formers have reduced bone mineral density and an increased risk of fracture compared with the non-stone-forming population. Low calcium intake probably contributes to the low bone mineral density. In sum, low-calcium diets are of unknown efficacy in preventing stone formation and carry a long-term risk of bone disease, making low-sodium and low-protein diets a superior treatment option. If diet therapy is not sufficient to prevent stones, thiazide diuretics may be used. Thiazide diuretics lower urine calcium and are effective in preventing the formation of stones. Three 3-year randomized trials have shown a 50% decrease in stone formation in the thiazide-treated groups compared with the placebo-treated controls. The drug effect requires slight contraction of the extracellular fluid volume, and high dietary NaCl intake reduces its therapeutic effect. Thiazide-induced hypokalemia should be treated aggressively since hypokalemia will reduce urine citrate, an important inhibitor of calcium crystallization.

Hyperuricosuria About 20% of calcium oxalate stone formers are hyperuricosuric, primarily because of an excessive intake of purine from meat and fish. The mechanism of stone formation probably involves salting out calcium oxalate by urate. A low-purine diet is desirable but difficult for many patients to achieve. The alternative is allopurinol, which has been shown to be effective in a randomized, controlled trial.

Primary hyperparathyroidism (See also Chap. 353) The diagnosis of this condition is established by documenting that hypercalcemia that cannot be otherwise explained is accompanied by inappropriately elevated serum concentrations of parathyroid hormone. Hypercalciuria, which usually is present, raises the urine supersaturation of calcium phosphate and/or calcium oxalate (Table 287-1). Calcium oxalate stones form on interstitial apatite plaque, whereas calcium phosphate stones form on apatite crystals, obstructing collecting ducts. In patients who have hyperparathyroidism, the Arg990Gly polymorphism of the calcium-sensing receptor leads to higher urine calcium excretion and an increased risk of nephrolithiasis. Prompt diagnosis of hyperparathyroidism is important because parathyroidectomy should be carried out before recurrent stones or renal damage occurs.

Distal renal tubular acidosis (See also Chap. 284) The defect in this condition seems to reside in the distal nephron, which cannot establish a normal pH gradient between urine and blood, leading to hyperchloremic acidosis. The diagnosis is suggested by a minimum urine pH >5.5 in the presence of systemic acidosis. Hypercalciuria, an alkaline urine, and a low urine citrate level increase urine saturation with respect to calcium phosphate. Calcium phosphate stones form, nephrocalcinosis is common, and osteomalacia or rickets may occur. Apatite deposits form in inner medullary collecting ducts and cause extensive medullary tubular interstitial nephropathy, which can lead to reduced kidney function. Renal tubular acidosis may be genetic, secondary to a systemic disease, or caused by a medication. Topiramate, a drug commonly used for seizures and migraines, inhibits the enzyme carbonic anhydrase and may cause calcium nephrolithiasis.

Treatment with supplemental alkali reduces hypercalciuria and limits the production of new stones. The preferred form of alkali is potassium citrate, which is given at a dose of 0.5–2.0 meq/kg body weight in two to three divided doses per day. In incomplete distal renal tubular acidosis, systemic acidosis is absent, but urine pH cannot be lowered below 5.5 after an exogenous acid load. Incomplete RTA may develop in some patients who form calcium oxalate stones because of idiopathic hypercalciuria; the importance of RTA in producing stones in this situation is uncertain, and thiazide treatment is a reasonable alternative. Alkali also can be used in incomplete RTA. In treating patients with alkali, it is prudent to monitor changes in urine citrate and pH. If urine pH increases without an increase in citrate, calcium phosphate supersaturation will increase and stone disease may worsen.

Hyperoxaluria Oxalate is a metabolic end product in humans. Urine oxalate comes from diet and endogenous metabolic production, with ~40–50% originating from dietary sources. The upper limit of normal for oxalate excretion is generally considered to be 40–50 mg per day. Mild hyperoxaluria (50–80 mg/d) usually is caused by excessive intake of high-oxalate foods such as spinach, nuts, and chocolate. In addition, low-calcium diets may promote hyperoxaluria as there is less calcium available to bind oxalate in the intestine. Enteric hyperoxaluria is a consequence of small-bowel disease, resulting in fat malabsorption. Oxalate excretion is often >100 mg per day. Enteric hyperoxaluria may be caused by jejunoileal bypass for obesity, pancreatic insufficiency, or extensive small-intestine involvement from Crohn's disease. With fat malabsorption, calcium in the bowel lumen is bound by fatty acids instead of oxalate, which is left free for absorption in the colon. Delivery of unabsorbed fatty acids and bile salts to the colon injures the colonic mucosa and enhances oxalate absorption. Recent studies have shown that modern bariatric surgery for obesity that involves bypassing intestinal segments, such as Roux-en-Y gastric bypass and biliopancreatic diversions, may lead to hyperoxaluria that can cause kidney failure as well as kidney stones. The mechanism of hyperoxaluria has not been well studied.

Primary hyperoxaluria is a rare autosomal recessive disease that causes severe hyperoxaluria. Patients usually present with recurrent calcium oxalate stones during childhood. Primary hyperoxaluria type 1 is due to a deficiency in the peroxisomal enzyme alanine:glyoxylate aminotransferase. Type 2 is due to a deficiency of D-glyceric dehydrogenase. Severe hyperoxaluria from any cause can lead to stone formation and produce tubulointerstitial nephropathy (Chap. 285).

TREATMENT Hyperoxaluria

Patients with mild to moderate hyperoxaluria should be treated with a diet low in oxalate and with a normal intake of calcium and magnesium to reduce oxalate absorption. Enteric hyperoxaluria can be treated with a low-fat, low-oxalate diet and calcium supplements, given with meals, to bind oxalate in the gut lumen. The oxalate-binding resin cholestyramine provides an additional form of therapy. Treatment for primary hyperoxaluria includes a high fluid intake, neutral phosphate, potassium citrate, and pyridoxine (25–200 mg/d). Even with aggressive therapy, irreversible renal failure may occur. Liver transplantation to correct the enzyme defect, combined with kidney transplantation, has been successfully utilized in patients with primary hyperoxaluria.

Hypocitraturia Urine citrate prevents calcium stone formation by creating a soluble complex with calcium, effectively reducing free urine calcium. Hypocitraturia is found in 20–40% of stone formers either as a single disorder or in combination with other metabolic abnormalities. It can be secondary to systemic disorders such as RTA, chronic diarrheal illness, and hypokalemia, or it may be a primary disorder, in which case it is called *idiopathic hypocitraturia.*

TREATMENT Hypocitraturia

Treatment is with alkali, which increases urine citrate excretion; generally, bicarbonate or citrate salts are used. Potassium salts are preferred as sodium loading increases urinary excretion of calcium, reducing the effectiveness of treatment. Two randomized, placebo-controlled trials have demonstrated the effectiveness of citrate supplements in calcium oxalate stone formers. Lemonade and other citrate-rich beverages have been used to treat hypocitraturia, although the increase in urine citrate is not as great as is seen with pharmacologic dosing of citrate salts.

Idiopathic calcium lithiasis Some patients have no metabolic cause for stones despite a thorough metabolic evaluation (Table 287-1). The best treatment appears to be high fluid intake so that the urine specific gravity remains at ≤1.005 throughout the day and night. Thiazide diuretics and citrate therapy may help reduce crystallization of calcium salts, but there have been no prospective trials in this patient population. Oral phosphate at a dose of 2 g phosphorus daily may lower urine calcium and increase urine pyrophosphate, thereby reducing the rate of recurrence. Orthophosphate causes mild nausea and diarrhea, but tolerance may improve with continued intake.

Uric acid stones

Persistently acidic urine is the major risk factor for uric acid stone formation. When urine pH is low, the protonated form of uric acid predominates and is soluble in urine at concentrations of 100 mg/L. Concentrations above this level represent supersaturation that causes crystals and stones to form. Common causes of acidic urine and uric acid stones include metabolic syndrome, chronic diarrheal states, gout, and idiopathic uric acid lithiasis. As the prevalence of obesity increases, metabolic syndrome is becoming an increasingly important cause of uric acid stone formation, as insulin resistance leads to a decrease in ammoniagenesis, requiring that the metabolic acid load be excreted as titratable acid. Hyperuricosuria, when present, increases supersaturation, but urine of low pH can be supersaturated with uric acid even though the daily excretion rate is normal. Myeloproliferative syndromes, chemotherapy for malignant tumors, and Lesch-Nyhan syndrome cause such massive production of uric acid and consequent hyperuricosuria that stones and uric acid sludge form even at a normal urine pH. Obstruction of the renal tubules by uric acid crystals can cause acute renal failure.

TREATMENT Uric Acid Lithiasis

The two goals of treatment are to raise urine pH and lower excessive urine uric acid excretion to <1 g/d. Supplemental alkali, 1–3 meq/kg of body weight per day, should be given in three or four divided doses, one of which should be given at bedtime. The goal of treatment should be a urine pH between 6 and 6.5 in a 24-h urine collection. Increasing urine pH above 6.5 will not provide additional benefit in preventing uric acid crystallization but increases the risk of calcium phosphate stone formation. The form of the alkali may be important. Potassium citrate may reduce the risk of calcium salts crystallizing when urine pH is increased, whereas sodium alkali salts may increase the risk. A low-purine diet should be instituted in uric acid stone formers with hyperuricosuria. Patients who continue to form uric acid stones despite treatment with fluids, alkali, and a low-purine diet should have allopurinol added to their regimen.

Cystinuria and cystine stones

(See also Chap. 364) In this inherited disorder, proximal tubular and jejunal transport of the dibasic amino acids cystine, lysine, arginine, and ornithine is defective, and excessive amounts are lost in the urine. Clinical disease is due solely to the insolubility of cystine. Cystine crystals plug terminal collecting ducts, and stones may grow as an extension of those plugs. Damage to the papillae and medulla from crystal obstruction is the probable reason why kidney function is reduced in cystinuria compared with routine stone disease.

Pathogenesis Cystinuria occurs because of defective transport of dibasic amino acids by the brush borders of renal tubule and intestinal epithelial cells. Disease-causing mutations have been identified in both the heavy and light chains of a heteromeric amino acid transporter found in the proximal tubule of the kidney. Cystinuria is classified into two main types, based on the urinary excretion of cystine in obligate heterozygotes. In type I cystinuria, heterozygotes have normal urine cystine excretion; thus, type I has an autosomal recessive pattern of inheritance. A gene on chromosome 2 that has been designated *SLC3A1* encodes the heavy chain of the transporter and has been found to be abnormal in type I. In non-type I cystinuria, heterozygotes have moderately elevated urine cystine excretion, with homozygotes having a much higher urine cystine excretion. Non-type I is inherited as a dominant trait with incomplete penetrance. Non-type I is due to mutations in the *SLC7A9* gene on chromosome 19, which encodes the light chain of the heteromeric transporter. In rare cases, mutations of the *SLC7A9* gene can lead to a type I phenotype.

Diagnosis Cystine stones are formed only by patients with cystinuria, but 10% of stones in cystinuric patients do not contain cystine;

therefore, every stone former should be screened for the disease. The sediment from a first morning urine specimen in many patients with homozygous cystinuria reveals typical hexagonal, platelike cystine crystals. Cystinuria can also be detected by using the urine sodium nitroprusside test. Because the test is sensitive, it is positive for cystinuria in many asymptomatic heterozygotes. A positive nitroprusside test or the finding of cystine crystals in the urine sediment should be evaluated by measurement of daily cystine excretion. Cystine stones seldom form in adults unless urine excretion is at least 300 mg/d.

TREATMENT Cystinuria and Cystine Stones

High fluid intake, even at night, is the cornerstone of therapy. Daily urine volume should exceed 3 L. Raising urine pH with alkali is helpful provided that the urine pH exceeds 7.5. A low-salt diet (100 mmol/d) can reduce cystine excretion up to 40%. Because side effects are common, drugs such as penicillamine and tiopronin, which form mixed soluble disulfide cysteine-drug complexes, should be used only when fluid loading, salt reduction, and alkali therapy are ineffective. Low-methionine diets have not proved to be practical for clinical use, but patients should avoid protein gluttony.

Struvite stones

These stones are a result of urinary infection with bacteria, usually *Proteus* species, which possess urease, an enzyme that degrades urea to NH_3 and CO_2. The NH_3 hydrolyzes to NH_4^+ and raises urine pH to 8 or 9. The NH_4^+ precipitates PO_4^{3-} and Mg^{2+} to form $MgNH_4PO_4$ (struvite). Struvite does not form in urine in the absence of infection, because NH_4^+ concentration is low in urine that is alkaline in response to physiologic stimuli. Chronic *Proteus* infection can occur because of impaired urinary drainage, urologic instrumentation or surgery, and especially with chronic antibiotic treatment, which can favor the dominance of *Proteus* in the urinary tract. The presence of struvite crystals in urine, rectangular prisms that resemble coffin lids, indicates infection with urease-producing organisms.

TREATMENT Struvite Stones

Complete removal of the stone with subsequent sterilization of the urinary tract is the treatment of choice for patients who can tolerate the procedures. Percutaneous nephrolithotomy is the preferred surgical approach for most patients. At times, extracorporeal lithotripsy may be used in combination with a percutaneous approach. Open surgery is rarely required. Irrigation of the renal pelvis and calyces with hemiacidrin, a solution that dissolves struvite, can reduce recurrence after surgery. Stone-free rates of 50–90% have been reported after surgical intervention. Antimicrobial treatment is best reserved for dealing with acute infection and for maintenance of a sterile urine after surgery. Urine cultures and culture of stone fragments removed at surgery should guide the choice of antibiotic. For patients who are not candidates for surgical removal of a stone, acetohydroxamic acid, an inhibitor of urease, can be used. Unfortunately, acetohydroxamic acid has many side effects, such as headache, tremor, and thrombophlebitis, that limit its use.

FURTHER READINGS

Al-Ansari A et al: Efficacy of tamsulosin in the management of lower ureteral stones: A randomized double-blind placebo-controlled study of 100 patients. Urology 75:4, 2010

Asplin JR: Evaluation of the kidney stone patient. Semin Nephrol 28:99, 2008

Cameron MA, Sakhaee K: Uric acid nephrolithiasis. Urol Clin North Am 34:335, 2007

Miller NL et al: A formal test of the hypothesis that idiopathic calcium oxalate stones grow on Randall's plaque. BJU Int 103:966, 2009

Patel BN et al: Prevalence of hyperoxaluria after bariatric surgery. J Urol 181:161, 2009

Vezzoli G et al: R990G polymorphism of calcium-sensing receptor does produce a gain-of-function and predispose to primary hypercalciuria. Kidney Int 71:1155, 2007

CHAPTER 288

Urinary Tract Infections, Pyelonephritis, and Prostatitis

Kalpana Gupta
Barbara W. Trautner

Urinary tract infection (UTI) is a common and painful human illness that, fortunately, is rapidly responsive to modern antibiotic therapy. In the preantibiotic era, UTI caused significant morbidity. Hippocrates, writing about a disease that appears to have been acute cystitis, said that the illness could last for a year before either resolving or worsening to involve the kidneys. When chemotherapeutic agents used to treat UTI were introduced in the early twentieth century, they were relatively ineffective, and persistence of infection after 3 weeks of therapy was common. Nitrofurantoin, which became available in the 1950s, was the first tolerable and effective agent for the treatment of UTI.

Since the most common manifestation of UTI is acute cystitis and since acute cystitis is far more prevalent among women than among men, most clinical research on UTI has involved women. Many studies have enrolled women from college campuses or large health maintenance organizations in the United States. Therefore, when reviewing the literature and recommendations concerning UTI, clinicians must consider whether the findings are applicable to their patient populations.

DEFINITIONS

UTI may be asymptomatic (subclinical infection) or symptomatic (disease). Thus, the term *UTI* encompasses a variety of clinical entities, including asymptomatic bacteriuria (ABU), cystitis, prostatitis, and pyelonephritis. The distinction between symptomatic UTI and ABU has major clinical implications. Both UTI and ABU connote the presence of bacteria in the urinary tract, usually accompanied by white blood cells and inflammatory cytokines in the urine. However, ABU occurs in the absence of symptoms attributable to the bacteria in the urinary tract and does not usually require treatment, while UTI has more typically been assumed to imply symptomatic disease that warrants antimicrobial therapy. Much of the literature concerning UTI, particularly catheter-associated infection, does not differentiate between UTI and ABU. In this chapter, the term *UTI* denotes symptomatic disease; *cystitis*, symptomatic infection of the bladder; and *pyelonephritis*, symptomatic infection of the kidneys. *Uncomplicated UTI* refers to acute cystitis or pyelonephritis in nonpregnant outpatient women without anatomic abnormalities or instrumentation of the urinary tract; *complicated UTI* is a catch-all term that encompasses all other types of UTI. *Recurrent UTI* is not necessarily complicated; individual episodes can be uncomplicated and treated as such. *Catheter-associated bacteriuria* can be either symptomatic (CAUTI) or asymptomatic.

EPIDEMIOLOGY AND RISK FACTORS

Except among infants and the elderly, UTI occurs far more commonly in females than in males. During the neonatal period, the incidence of UTI is slightly higher among males than among females because male infants more commonly have congenital urinary tract anomalies. After 50 years of age, obstruction from prostatic hypertrophy becomes common in men, and the incidence of UTI is almost as high among men as among women. Between 1 year and ~50 years of age, UTI and recurrent UTI are predominantly diseases of females. The prevalence of ABU is ~5% among women between ages 20 and 40 and may be as high as 40–50% among elderly women and men.

As many as 50–80% of women in the general population acquire at least one UTI during their lifetime—uncomplicated cystitis in most cases. Recent use of a diaphragm with spermicide, frequent sexual intercourse, and a history of UTI are independent risk factors for acute cystitis. Cystitis is temporally related to recent sexual intercourse, with a sixtyfold increase in the relative odds of acute cystitis in the 48 h after intercourse. In healthy postmenopausal women, sexual activity, diabetes mellitus, and incontinence are risk factors for UTI.

Many factors predisposing women to cystitis also increase the risk of pyelonephritis. Factors independently associated with pyelonephritis in young healthy women include frequent sexual intercourse, a new sexual partner, a UTI in the previous 12 months, a maternal history of UTI, diabetes, and incontinence. The common risk factors for cystitis and pyelonephritis are not surprising given that pyelonephritis typically arises through the ascent of bacteria from the bladder to the upper urinary tract. However, pyelonephritis can occur without clear antecedent cystitis.

About 20–30% of women who have had one episode of UTI will have recurrent episodes. Early recurrence (within 2 weeks) is usually regarded as relapse rather than reinfection and may indicate the need to evaluate the patient for a sequestered focus. Intracellular pods of infecting organisms within the bladder epithelium have been demonstrated in animal models of UTI, but the importance of this phenomenon in humans is not yet clear. The rate of recurrence ranges from 0.3 to 7.6 infections per patient per year, with an average of 2.6 infections per year. It is not uncommon for multiple recurrences to follow an initial infection, resulting in clustering of episodes. Clustering may be related temporally to the presence of a new risk factor or to the sloughing of the protective outer bladder epithelial layer in response to bacterial attachment during acute cystitis. The likelihood of a recurrence decreases with increasing time since the last infection. A case-control study of predominantly white premenopausal women with recurrent UTI identified frequent sexual intercourse, use of spermicide, a new sexual partner, a first UTI before 15 years of age, and a maternal history of UTI as independent risk factors for recurrent UTI. The only consistently documented behavioral risk factors for recurrent UTI include frequent sexual intercourse and spermicide use. In postmenopausal women, anatomic factors affecting bladder emptying, such as cystoceles, urinary incontinence, and residual urine, are most strongly associated with recurrent UTI.

In pregnant women, ABU has clinical consequences, and both screening for and treatment of this condition are indicated. Specifically, ABU during pregnancy is associated with preterm birth and perinatal mortality for the fetus and with pyelonephritis for the mother. A Cochrane meta-analysis found that treatment of ABU in pregnant women decreased the risk of pyelonephritis by 75%.

The majority of men with UTI have a functional or anatomic abnormality of the urinary tract, most commonly urinary obstruction secondary to prostatic hypertrophy. That said, not all men with UTI have detectable urinary abnormalities; this point is particularly relevant for men ≤45 years of age. Lack of circumcision is also associated with an increased risk of UTI, because *Escherichia coli* is more likely to colonize the glans and prepuce and subsequently migrate into the urinary tract.

Women—but not men—with diabetes have a two- to threefold higher rate of ABU and UTI than women without diabetes. Increased duration of diabetes and the use of insulin rather than oral medication are also associated with a higher risk of UTI among women with diabetes. Poor bladder function, obstruction in urinary flow, and incomplete voiding are additional factors commonly found in patients with diabetes that increase the risk of UTI. Impaired cytokine secretion may contribute to ABU in diabetic women.

ETIOLOGY

The uropathogens causing UTI vary by clinical syndrome but are usually enteric gram-negative rods that have migrated to the urinary tract. The susceptibility patterns of these organisms vary by clinical syndrome and by geography. In acute uncomplicated cystitis in the United States, the etiologic agents are highly predictable: *E. coli* accounts for 75–90% of isolates; *Staphylococcus saprophyticus* for 5–15% (with particularly frequent isolation from younger women); and *Klebsiella* species, *Proteus* species, *Enterococcus* species, *Citrobacter* species, and other organisms for 5–10%. Similar etiologic agents are found in Europe and Brazil. The spectrum of agents causing uncomplicated pyelonephritis is similar, with *E. coli* predominating. In complicated UTI (e.g., CAUTI), *E. coli* remains the predominant organism, but other aerobic gram-negative rods, such as *Klebsiella* species, *Proteus* species, *Citrobacter* species, *Acinetobacter* species, *Morganella* species, and *Pseudomonas aeruginosa*, also are frequently isolated. Gram-positive bacteria (e.g., enterococci and *Staphylococcus aureus*), and yeasts are also important pathogens in complicated UTI. Data on etiology and resistance are generally obtained from laboratory surveys and should be understood in the context that organism identification is performed only in cases in which urine is sent for culture—i.e., typically when complicated UTI or pyelonephritis is suspected. The available data demonstrate a worldwide increase in the resistance of *E. coli* to antibiotics commonly used to treat UTI. North American and European surveys of *E. coli* isolates from women with acute cystitis have documented rates of resistance to trimethoprim-sulfamethoxazole (TMP-SMX) greater than 20% and rates of resistance to ciprofloxacin between 5% and 10% in some regions. Since resistance rates vary by local geographic region, with individual patient characteristics, and over time, it is important to use current and local data when choosing a treatment regimen.

PATHOGENESIS

The urinary tract can be viewed as an anatomic unit united by a continuous column of urine extending from the urethra to the kidneys. In the majority of UTIs, bacteria establish infection by ascending from the urethra to the bladder. Continuing ascent up the ureter to the kidney is the pathway for most renal parenchymal infections. However, introduction of bacteria into the bladder does not inevitably lead to sustained and symptomatic infection. The interplay of host, pathogen, and environmental factors determines whether tissue invasion and symptomatic infection will ensue (Fig. 288-1). For example, bacteria often enter the bladder after sexual intercourse, but normal voiding and innate host defense mechanisms in the bladder eliminate these organisms. Any foreign body in the urinary tract, such as a urinary catheter or stone, provides an inert surface for bacterial colonization. Abnormal micturition and/or significant residual urine volume promotes true infection. In the simplest of terms, anything that increases the likelihood of bacteria entering the bladder and staying there increases the risk of UTI.

Bacteria can also gain access to the urinary tract through the bloodstream. However, hematogenous spread accounts for <2% of documented UTIs and usually results from bacteremia caused by relatively virulent organisms, such as *Salmonella* and *S. aureus*. Indeed, the isolation of either of these pathogens from a patient without a catheter or other instrumentation warrants a search for a bloodstream source. Hematogenous infections may produce focal abscesses or areas of pyelonephritis within a kidney and result in positive urine cultures. The pathogenesis of candiduria is distinct in that the hematogenous route is common. The presence of *Candida* in the urine of a noninstrumented immunocompetent patient implies either genital contamination or potentially widespread visceral dissemination.

Environmental factors

Vaginal ecology In women, vaginal ecology is an important environmental factor affecting the risk of UTI. Colonization of the vaginal introitus and perirurethral area with organisms from the intestinal flora (usually *E. coli*) is the critical initial step in the pathogenesis of UTI. Sexual intercourse is associated with an increased risk of vaginal colonization with *E. coli* and thereby increases the risk of UTI. Nonoxynol-9 in spermicide is toxic to the normal vaginal microflora and thus is likewise associated with an increased risk of *E. coli* vaginal colonization and bacteriuria. In postmenopausal women, the previously predominant vaginal lactobacilli are replaced with gram-negative colonization. The use of topical estrogens to prevent UTI in postmenopausal women is controversial; given the side effects of systemic hormone replacement, oral estrogens should not be used to prevent UTI.

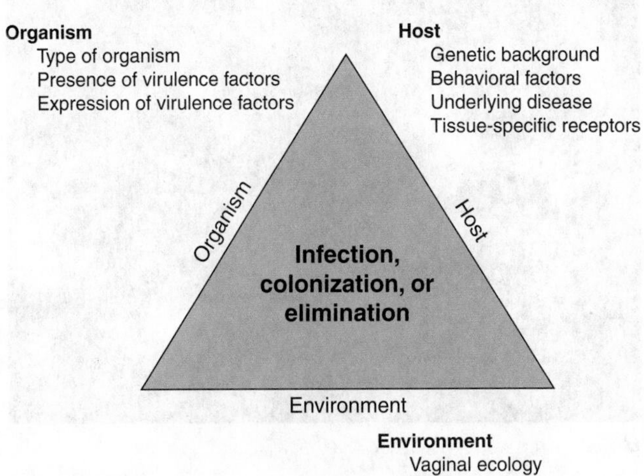

Figure 288-1 Pathogenesis of urinary tract infection. The relationship between specific host, pathogen, and environmental factors determines the clinical outcome.

Anatomic and functional abnormalities Any condition that permits urinary stasis or obstruction predisposes the individual to UTI. Foreign bodies such as stones or urinary catheters provide an inert surface for bacterial colonization and formation of a persistent biofilm. Thus, vesicoureteral reflux, ureteral obstruction secondary to prostatic hypertrophy, neurogenic bladder, and urinary diversion surgery create an environment favorable to UTI. In persons with such conditions, *E. coli* strains lacking typical urinary virulence factors are often the cause of infection. Inhibition of ureteral peristalsis and decreased ureteral tone leading to vesicoureteral reflux are important in the pathogenesis of pyelonephritis in pregnant women. Anatomic factors—specifically, the distance of the urethra from the anus—are considered to be the primary reason why UTI is predominantly an illness of young women rather than of young men.

Host factors

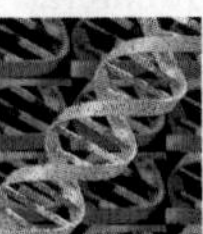

The genetic background of the host influences the individual's susceptibility to recurrent UTI, at least among women. A familial disposition to UTI and to pyelonephritis is well documented. Women with recurrent UTI are more likely to have had their first UTI before age 15 years and to have a maternal history of UTI. A component of the underlying pathogenesis of this familial predisposition to recurrent UTI may be persistent vaginal colonization with *E. coli*, even during asymptomatic periods. Vaginal and periurethral mucosal cells from women with recurrent UTI bind threefold more uropathogenic bacteria than do mucosal cells from women without recurrent infection. Epithelial cells from susceptible women may possess specific types or greater numbers of receptors to which *E. coli* can bind, thereby facilitating colonization and invasion. Mutations in host response genes (e.g., those coding for Toll-like receptors and the interleukin 8 receptor) have also been linked to recurrent UTI and pyelonephritis. Polymorphisms in the interleukin 8–specific receptor gene *CXCR1* are associated with increased susceptibility to pyelonephritis. Lower-level expression of *CXCR1* on the surface of neutrophils impairs neutrophil-dependent host defense against bacterial invasion of the renal parenchyma.

Microbial factors

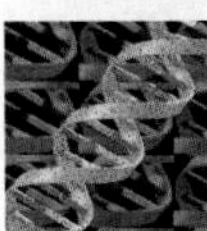

An anatomically normal urinary tract presents a stronger barrier to infection than a compromised urinary tract. Thus, strains of *E. coli* that cause invasive symptomatic infection of the urinary tract in otherwise normal hosts often possess and express genetic virulence factors, including surface adhesins that mediate binding to specific receptors on the surface of uroepithelial cells. The best-studied adhesins are the P fimbriae, hairlike protein structures that interact with a specific receptor on renal epithelial cells. (The letter *P* denotes the ability of these fimbriae to bind to blood group antigen P, which contains a D-galactose-D-galactose residue.) P fimbriae are important in the pathogenesis of pyelonephritis and subsequent bloodstream invasion from the kidney.

Another adhesin is the type 1 pilus (fimbria), which all *E. coli* strains possess but not all *E. coli* strains express. Type 1 pili are thought to play a key role in initiating *E. coli* bladder infection; they mediate binding to uroplakins on the luminal surface of bladder uroepithelial cells. The binding of type 1 fimbriae of *E. coli* to receptors on uroepithelial cells initiates a complex series of signaling events that leads to apoptosis and exfoliation of uroepithelial cells, with the attached *E. coli* organisms carried away in the urine.

APPROACH TO THE PATIENT Clinical Manifestations

The most important issue to be addressed when a UTI is suspected is the characterization of the clinical syndrome as ABU, uncomplicated cystitis, pyelonephritis, prostatitis, or complicated UTI. This information will shape the diagnostic and therapeutic approach.

Asymptomatic Bacteriuria A diagnosis of ABU can be considered only when the patient does not have local or systemic symptoms referable to the urinary tract. The clinical presentation is usually that of a patient who undergoes a screening urine culture for a reason unrelated to the genitourinary tract and is incidentally found to have bacteriuria. The presence of systemic signs or symptoms such as fever, altered mental status, and leukocytosis in the setting of a positive urine culture does not merit a diagnosis of symptomatic UTI unless other potential etiologies have been considered.

Cystitis The typical symptoms of cystitis are dysuria, urinary frequency, and urgency. Nocturia, hesitancy, suprapubic discomfort, and gross hematuria are often noted as well. Unilateral back or flank pain is generally an indication that the upper urinary tract is involved. Fever is also an indication of invasive infection of either the kidney or the prostate.

Pyelonephritis Mild pyelonephritis can present as low-grade fever with or without lower-back or costovertebral-angle pain, whereas severe pyelonephritis can manifest as high fever, rigors, nausea, vomiting, and flank and/or loin pain. Symptoms are generally acute in onset, and symptoms of cystitis may not be present. Fever is the main feature distinguishing cystitis and pyelonephritis. The fever of pyelonephritis typically exhibits a high, spiking "picket-fence" pattern and resolves over 72 h of therapy. Bacteremia develops in 20–30% of cases of pyelonephritis. Patients with diabetes may present with obstructive uropathy associated with acute papillary necrosis when the sloughed papillae obstruct the ureter. Papillary necrosis may also be evident in some cases of pyelonephritis complicated by obstruction, sickle cell disease, analgesic nephropathy, or combinations of these conditions. In the rare cases of bilateral papillary necrosis, a rapid rise in the serum creatinine level may be the first indication of the condition. *Emphysematous* pyelonephritis is a particularly severe form of the disease that is associated with the production of gas in renal and perinephric tissues and occurs almost exclusively in diabetic patients (Fig. 288-2). *Xanthogranulomatous* pyelonephritis occurs when chronic urinary obstruction (often by staghorn calculi), together with chronic infection, leads to suppurative destruction of renal tissue (Fig. 288-3). On pathologic examination, the residual

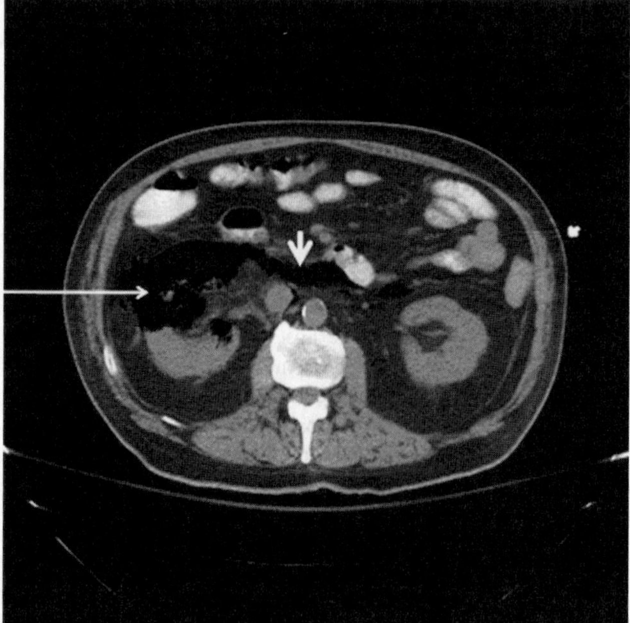

Figure 288-2 Emphysematous pyelonephritis. Infection of the right kidney of a diabetic man by *Escherichia coli*, a gas-forming, facultative anaerobic uropathogen, has led to destruction of the renal parenchyma (*arrow*) and tracking of gas through the retroperitoneal space (*arrowhead*).

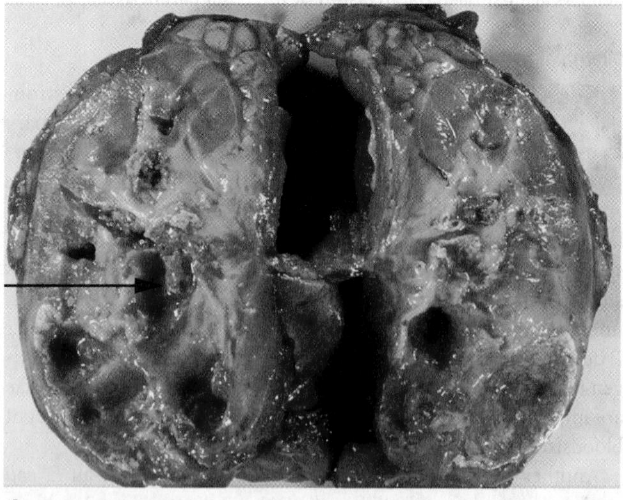

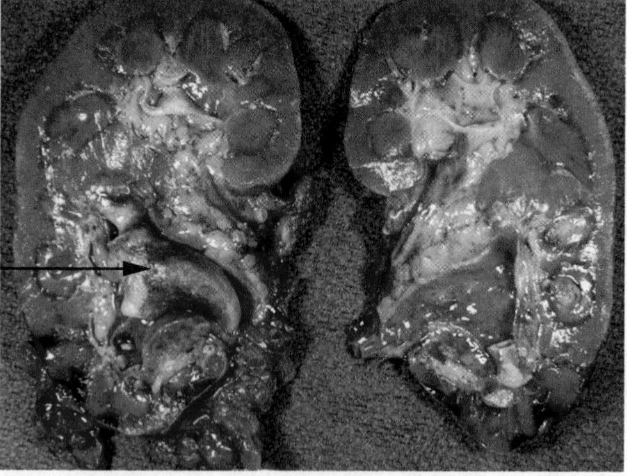

Figure 288-3 Xanthogranulomatous pyelonephritis. ***A.*** This photograph shows extensive destruction of renal parenchyma due to long-standing suppurative inflammation. The precipitating factor was obstruction by a staghorn calculus, which has been removed, leaving a depression (*arrow*). The mass effect of xanthogranulomatous pyelonephritis can mimic renal malignancy. ***B.*** A large staghorn calculus (*arrow*) is seen obstructing the renal pelvis and calyceal system. The lower pole of the kidney shows areas of hemorrhage and necrosis with collapse of cortical areas. *(Both images: Courtesy of Dharam M. Ramnani, MD, Virginia Urology Pathology Laboratory, Richmond, VA.)*

renal tissue frequently has a yellow coloration with infiltration by lipid-laden macrophages. Pyelonephritis can also be complicated by intraparenchymal abscess formation; this situation should be suspected when a patient has continued fever and/or bacteremia despite antibacterial therapy.

Prostatitis Prostatitis includes both infectious and noninfectious abnormalities of the prostate gland. Infections can be acute or chronic, are almost always bacterial in nature, and are far less common than the noninfectious entity of chronic pelvic pain syndrome (formerly known as chronic prostatitis). Acute bacterial prostatitis presents as dysuria, frequency, and pain in the prostatic, pelvic, or perineal area. Fever and chills are usually present, and symptoms of bladder outlet obstruction are common. Chronic bacterial prostatitis presents more insidiously as recurrent episodes of cystitis, sometimes with associated pelvic and perineal pain. Men who present with recurrent cystitis should be evaluated for a prostatic focus.

Complicated UTI Complicated UTI presents as a symptomatic episode of cystitis or pyelonephritis in a man or woman with an anatomic predisposition to infection, with a foreign body in the urinary tract, or with factors predisposing to a delayed response to therapy.

DIAGNOSTIC TOOLS

History

The diagnosis of any the UTI syndromes or ABU begins with a detailed history (Fig. 288-4). The history given by the patient has a high predictive value in uncomplicated cystitis. A meta-analysis evaluating the probability of acute UTI on the basis of history and physical findings concluded that, in women presenting with at least one symptom of UTI (dysuria, frequency, hematuria, or back pain) and without complicating factors, the probability of acute cystitis or pyelonephritis is 50%. The even higher rates of accuracy of self-diagnosis among women with recurrent UTI probably account for the success of patient-initiated treatment of recurrent cystitis. If vaginal discharge and complicating factors are absent and risk factors for UTI are present, then the probability of UTI is close to 90%, and no laboratory evaluation is needed. Similarly, a combination of dysuria and urinary frequency in the absence of vaginal discharge increases the probability of UTI to 96%. Further laboratory evaluation with dipstick testing or urine culture is not necessary in such patients before the initiation of definitive therapy.

When the patient's history is applied as a diagnostic tool, it is important to recall that the studies included in the meta-analysis cited above did not enroll children, adolescents, pregnant women, men, or patients with complicated UTI. One significant concern is that sexually transmitted disease—that caused by *Chlamydia trachomatis* in particular—may be inappropriately treated as UTI. This concern is particularly relevant for female patients under the age of 25. The differential diagnosis to be considered when women present with dysuria includes cervicitis (*C. trachomatis*, *Neisseria gonorrhoeae*), vaginitis (*Candida albicans*, *Trichomonas vaginalis*), herpetic urethritis, interstitial cystitis, and noninfectious vaginal or vulvar irritation. Women with more than one sexual partner and inconsistent use of condoms are at high risk for both UTI and sexually transmitted disease, and symptoms alone do not always distinguish between these conditions.

The urine dipstick test, urinalysis, and urine culture

Useful diagnostic tools include the urine dipstick test and urinalysis, both of which provide point-of-care information, and the urine culture, which can retrospectively confirm a prior diagnosis. Understanding the parameters of the dipstick test is important in interpreting its results. Only members of the family Enterobacteriaceae convert nitrate to nitrite, and enough nitrite must accumulate in the urine to reach the threshold of detection. If a woman with acute cystitis is forcing fluids and voiding frequently, the dipstick test for nitrite is less likely to be positive, even when *E. coli* is present. The leukocyte esterase test detects this enzyme in the host's polymorphonuclear leukocytes in the urine, whether the cells are intact or lysed. Many reviews have attempted to describe the diagnostic accuracy of dipstick testing. The bottom line for clinicians is that a urine dipstick test can confirm the diagnosis of uncomplicated cystitis in a patient with a reasonably high pretest probability of this disease. Either nitrite or leukocyte esterase positivity can be interpreted as a positive result. Blood in the urine may also suggest a diagnosis of UTI. A dipstick test negative for both nitrite and leukocyte esterase in the same type of patient should prompt consideration of other explanations for the patient's symptoms and collection of urine for culture. A negative dipstick test is not sufficiently sensitive to rule out bacteriuria in pregnant women, in whom it is important to detect all episodes of bacteriuria. Performance characteristics of the dipstick test differ in men (highly specific) and in noncatheterized nursing home residents (highly sensitive).

Urine microscopy reveals pyuria in nearly all cases of cystitis and hematuria in ~30% of cases. In current practice, most hospital laboratories use an automated system rather than manual examination for urine microscopy. A machine aspirates a sample of the urine and then classifies the particles in the urine by size, shape, contrast, light scatter, volume, and other properties. These automated systems can be overwhelmed by high numbers of dysmorphic red blood cells, white blood cells, or crystals; in general, counts of bacteria are less accurate than are counts of red and white blood cells. Our clinical recommendation is that the patient's symptoms and presentation should outweigh an incongruent result on automated urinalysis.

The detection of bacteria in a urine culture is the diagnostic "gold standard" for UTI; unfortunately, however, culture results do not become available until 24 h after the patient's presentation. Identifying specific organism(s) can require an additional 24 h. Studies of women with symptoms of cystitis have found that a colony count threshold of $>10^2$ bacteria/mL is more sensitive (95%) and specific (85%) than a threshold of 10^5/mL for the diagnosis of acute cystitis in women. In men, the minimal level indicating infection appears to be 10^3/mL. Urine specimens frequently become contaminated with the normal microbial flora of the distal urethra, vagina, or skin. These contaminants can grow to high numbers if the collected urine is allowed to stand at room temperature. In most instances, a culture that yields mixed bacterial species is contaminated except in settings of long-term catheterization, chronic urinary retention, or the presence of a fistula between the urinary tract and the gastrointestinal or genital tract.

DIAGNOSIS

The approach to diagnosis is influenced by which of the clinical UTI syndromes is suspected (Fig. 288-4).

Uncomplicated cystitis in women

Uncomplicated cystitis in women can be treated on the basis of history alone. However, if the symptoms are not specific or if a reliable history cannot be obtained, then a urine dipstick test should be performed. A positive nitrite or leukocyte esterase result in a woman with one symptom of UTI increases the probability of UTI from 50% to ~80%, and empirical treatment can be considered without further testing. In this setting, a negative dipstick result does not rule out UTI, and a urine culture, close clinical follow-up, and possibly a pelvic examination are recommended. These recommendations are made with the caveat that factors associated with complicated UTI, such as pregnancy, are not present.

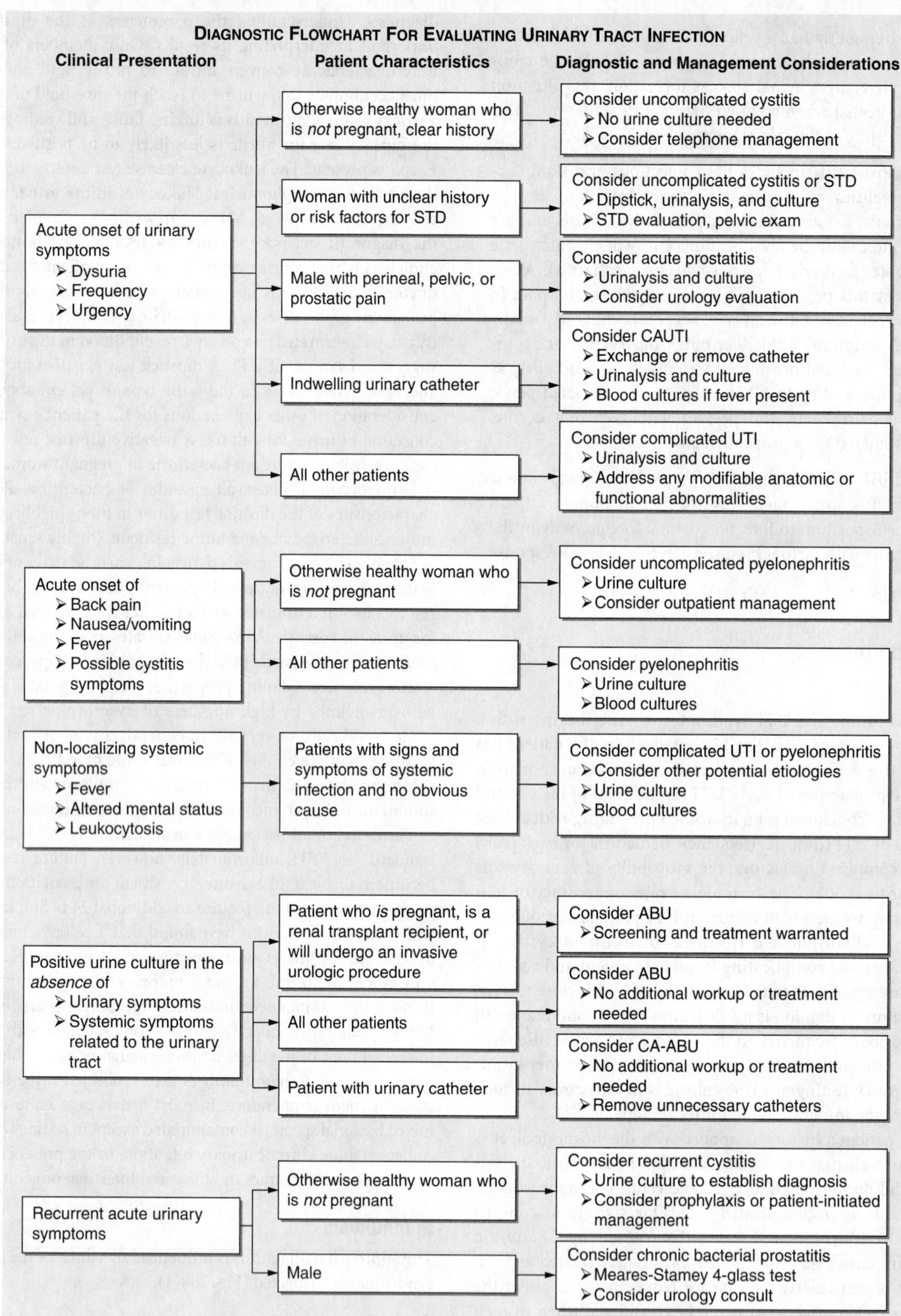

Figure 288-4 Diagnostic approach to urinary tract infection. STD, sexually transmitted disease; CAUTI, catheter-associated UTI; ABU, asymptomatic bacteriuria; CA-ABU, catheter-associated ABU.

Cystitis in men

The signs and symptoms of cystitis in men are similar to those in women, but this disease differs in several important ways in the male population. Collection of urine for culture is strongly recommended when a man has symptoms of UTI, as the documentation of bacteriuria can differentiate the less common syndromes of acute and chronic bacterial prostatitis from the very common entity of chronic pelvic pain syndrome, which is not associated with bacteriuria and thus is not usually responsive to antibacterial therapy. If the diagnosis is unclear, localization cultures using the two- or four-glass Meares-Stamey test (urine collection after prostate massage) should be undertaken to differentiate between bacterial and nonbacterial prostatic syndromes, and the patient should be referred to a urologist. Men with febrile UTI often have an elevated serum level of prostate-specific antigen as well as an enlarged prostate and enlarged seminal vesicles on ultrasound—findings indicative of prostate involvement. In 85 men with febrile UTI, symptoms of urinary retention, early recurrence of UTI, hematuria at follow-up, and voiding difficulties were predictive of surgically correctable disorders. Men with none of these symptoms had normal upper and lower urinary tracts on urologic workup.

Asymptomatic bacteriuria

The diagnosis of ABU involves both microbiologic and clinical criteria. The microbiologic criterion is usually ≥10^5 bacterial cfu/mL except in catheter-associated disease, in which case ≥10^2 cfu/mL is the cutoff. The clinical criterion is that the person has no signs or symptoms referable to UTI.

TREATMENT Urinary Tract Infections

Antimicrobial therapy is warranted for any symptomatic UTI. The choice of antimicrobial agent and the dose and duration of therapy depend on the site of infection and the presence or absence of complicating conditions. Each category of UTI warrants a different approach based on the particular clinical syndrome.

UNCOMPLICATED CYSTITIS IN WOMEN Since the species and antimicrobial susceptibilities of the bacteria that cause acute uncomplicated cystitis are highly predictable, many episodes of uncomplicated cystitis can be managed over the telephone (Fig. 288-4). Most patients with other UTI syndromes require further diagnostic evaluation. Although the risk of serious complications with telephone management appears to be low, studies of telephone management algorithms generally have involved otherwise healthy white women who are at low risk for complications of UTI.

In 1999, TMP-SMX was recommended as the first-line agent for treatment of uncomplicated UTI in the published guidelines of the Infectious Diseases Society of America. Antibiotic resistance among uropathogens causing uncomplicated cystitis has since increased, appreciation of the importance of collateral damage (as defined below) has increased, and newer agents have been studied. Unfortunately, there is no longer a single best agent for acute uncomplicated cystitis.

Collateral damage refers to the adverse ecologic effects of antimicrobial therapy, including killing of the normal flora and selection of drug-resistant organisms. Outbreaks of *Clostridium difficile* infection offer an example of collateral damage in the hospital environment. The implication of collateral damage in this context is that a drug that is highly efficacious for the treatment of UTI is not necessarily the optimal first-line agent if it also has pronounced secondary effects on the normal flora or is likely to change resistance patterns. Drugs used for UTI that have a minimal effect on fecal flora include pivmecillinam, fosfomycin, and nitrofurantoin. In contrast, trimethoprim, TMP-SMX, quinolones, and ampicillin affect the fecal flora more significantly; these drugs are notably the agents for which rising resistance levels have been documented.

Several effective therapeutic regimens are available for acute uncomplicated cystitis in women (Table 288-1). Well-studied first-line agents include TMP-SMX and nitrofurantoin. Second-line agents include fluoroquinolone and β-lactam compounds. Single-dose fosfomycin treatment for acute cystitis is widely used in Europe but has produced mixed results in randomized trials. Pivmecillinam is not currently available in the United States or Canada but is a popular agent in some European countries. The pros and cons of other therapies are discussed briefly below.

TABLE 288-1 Treatment Strategies for Acute Uncomplicated Cystitis

Drug and Dose	Estimated Clinical Efficacy (%)	Estimated Bacterial Efficacy (%)	Common Side Effects
Nitrofurantoin, 100 mg bid × 5–7 d	84–95	86–92	Nausea, headache
TMP-SMX, 1 DS tablet bid × 3 d	90–100	91–100	Rash, urticaria, nausea, vomiting, hematologic abnormalities
Fosfomycin, 3-g single-dose sachet	70–91	78–83	Diarrhea, nausea, headache
Pivmecillinam, 400 mg bid × 3–7 d	55–82	74–84	Nausea, vomiting, diarrhea
Fluoroquinolones, dose varies by agent; 3-d regimen	85–95	81–98	Nausea, vomiting, diarrhea, headache, drowsiness, insomnia
β-Lactams, dose varies by agent; 5- to 7-d regimen	79–98	74–98	Diarrhea, nausea, vomiting, rash, urticaria

Note: Efficacy rates are averages or ranges calculated from the data and studies included in the 2010 Infectious Diseases Society of America/European Society of Clinical Microbiology and Infectious Diseases Guideline for Treatment of Uncomplicated UTI. TMP-SMX, trimethoprim-sulfamethoxazole; DS, double-strength.

Traditionally, TMP-SMX has been recommended as first-line treatment for acute cystitis, and it remains appropriate to consider the use of this drug in regions with resistance rates not exceeding 20%. TMP-SMX resistance has clinical significance: in TMP-SMX-treated patients with resistant isolates, the time to symptom resolution is longer and rates of both clinical and microbiologic failure are higher. Individual host factors associated with an elevated risk of UTI caused by a strain of *E. coli* resistant to TMP-SMX include recent use of TMP-SMX or another antimicrobial agent and recent travel to an area with high rates of TMP-SMX resistance. The optimal setting for empirical use of TMP-SMX is uncomplicated UTI in a female patient who has an established relationship with the practitioner and who can thus seek further care if her symptoms do not respond promptly.

Resistance to nitrofurantoin remains low despite >60 years of use. Since this drug affects bacterial metabolism in multiple pathways, several mutational steps are required for the development of resistance. Nitrofurantoin remains highly active against *E. coli* and most non–*E. coli* isolates. *Proteus*, *Pseudomonas*, *Serratia*, *Enterobacter*, and yeasts are all intrinsically resistant to this drug. Although nitrofurantoin has traditionally been prescribed as a 7-day regimen, similar microbiologic and clinical efficacies are noted with a 5-day course of nitrofurantoin or a 3-day course of TMP-SMX for treatment of women with acute cystitis; 3-day courses of nitrofurantoin are not recommended for acute cystitis. Nitrofurantoin does not reach significant levels in tissue and cannot be used to treat pyelonephritis.

Most fluoroquinolones are highly effective for short-course therapy for cystitis; the exception is moxifloxacin, which does not achieve adequate urinary levels. The fluoroquinolones commonly used for UTI include ofloxacin, ciprofloxacin, and levofloxacin. The main concern about fluoroquinolone use for acute cystitis is the propagation of fluoroquinolone resistance, not only among uropathogens but also among other organisms causing more serious and difficult-to-treat infections at other sites. Fluoroquinolone use is also a factor driving the emergence of *C. difficile* outbreaks in hospital settings. Most experts now call for restricting fluoroquinolones to specific instances of uncomplicated cystitis in which other antimicrobial agents are not suitable. Quinolone use in the elderly has been associated with an increased risk of Achilles tendon rupture.

Except for pivmecillinam, β-lactam agents generally have not performed as well as TMP-SMX or fluoroquinolones in acute cystitis. Rates of pathogen eradication are lower and relapse rates are higher with β-lactam drugs. The generally accepted explanation is that β-lactams fail to eradicate uropathogens from the vaginal reservoir. A proposed role for intracellular biofilm communities is intriguing. Many strains of *E. coli* that are resistant to TMP-SMX are also resistant to amoxicillin and cephalexin; thus, these drugs should be used only for patients infected with susceptible strains.

Urinary analgesics are appropriate in certain situations to speed resolution of bladder discomfort. The urinary tract analgesic phenazopyridine is widely used but can cause significant nausea. Combination analgesics containing urinary antiseptics (methenamine, methylene blue), a urine-acidifying agent (sodium phosphate), and an antispasmodic agent (hyoscyamine) are also available.

PYELONEPHRITIS Since patients with pyelonephritis have tissue-invasive disease, the treatment regimen chosen should have a very high likelihood of eradicating the causative organism and should reach therapeutic blood levels quickly. High rates of TMP-SMX-resistant *E. coli* in patients with pyelonephritis have made fluoroquinolones the first-line therapy for acute uncomplicated pyelonephritis. Whether the fluoroquinolones are given orally or parenterally depends on the patient's tolerance for oral intake. A randomized clinical trial demonstrated that a 7-day course of therapy with oral ciprofloxacin (500 mg twice daily, with or without an initial IV 400-mg dose) was highly effective for the initial management of pyelonephritis in the outpatient setting. Oral TMP-SMX (one double-strength tablet twice daily for 14 days) is also effective for treatment of acute uncomplicated pyelonephritis if the uropathogen is known to be susceptible. If the pathogen's susceptibility is not known and TMP-SMX is used, an initial IV 1-g dose of ceftriaxone is recommended. Oral β-lactam agents are less effective than the fluoroquinolones and should be used with caution and close follow-up. Options for parenteral therapy for uncomplicated pyelonephritis include fluoroquinolones, an aminoglycoside with or without ampicillin, an extended-spectrum cephalosporin with or without an aminoglycoside, or a carbapenem. Combinations of a β-lactam and a β-lactamase inhibitor (e.g., ampicillin-sulbactam, ticarcillin-clavulanate, and piperacillin-tazobactam) or imipenem-cilastatin can be used in patients with more complicated histories, previous episodes of pyelonephritis, or recent urinary tract manipulations; in general, the treatment of such patients should be guided by urine culture results. Once the patient has responded clinically, oral therapy should be substituted for parenteral therapy.

UTI IN PREGNANT WOMEN Nitrofurantoin, ampicillin, and the cephalosporins are considered relatively safe in early pregnancy. One retrospective case-control study suggesting an association between nitrofurantoin and birth defects awaits confirmation. Sulfonamides should clearly be avoided both in the first trimester (because of possible teratogenic effects) and near term (because of a possible role in the development of kernicterus). Fluoroquinolones are avoided because of possible adverse effects on fetal cartilage development. Ampicillin and the cephalosporins have been used extensively in pregnancy and are the drugs of choice for the treatment of asymptomatic or symptomatic UTI in this group of patients. For pregnant women with overt pyelonephritis, parenteral β-lactam therapy with or without aminoglycosides is the standard of care.

UTI IN MEN Since the prostate is involved in the majority of cases of febrile UTI in men, the goal in these patients is to eradicate the prostatic infection as well as the bladder infection. In men with apparently uncomplicated UTI, a 7- to 14-day course of a fluoroquinolone or TMP-SMX is recommended. If acute bacterial prostatitis is suspected, antimicrobial therapy should be initiated after urine and blood are obtained for cultures. Therapy can be tailored to urine culture results and should be continued for 2–4 weeks. For documented chronic bacterial prostatitis, a 4- to 6-week course of antibiotics is often necessary. Recurrences, which are not uncommon in chronic prostatitis, often warrant a 12-week course of treatment.

COMPLICATED UTI Complicated UTI (other than that discussed above) occurs in a heterogeneous group of patients with a wide variety of structural and functional abnormalities of the urinary tract and kidneys. The range of species and their susceptibility to antimicrobial agents are likewise heterogeneous. As a consequence, therapy for complicated UTI must be individualized and guided by urine culture results. Frequently, a patient with complicated UTI will have prior urine culture data that can be used to guide empirical therapy while current culture results are awaited. Xanthogranulomatous pyelonephritis is treated with nephrectomy. Percutaneous drainage can be used as the initial therapy in emphysematous pyelonephritis and can be followed by elective nephrectomy as needed. Papillary necrosis with obstruction requires intervention to relieve the obstruction and to preserve renal function.

ASYMPTOMATIC BACTERIURIA Treatment of ABU does not decrease the frequency of symptomatic infections or complications except in pregnant women, persons undergoing urologic surgery, and perhaps neutropenic patients and renal transplant recipients. Treatment of ABU in pregnant women and patients undergoing urologic procedures should be directed by urine culture results. In all other populations, screening for and treatment of ABU are discouraged. The majority of cases of catheter-associated bacteriuria are asymptomatic and do not warrant antimicrobial therapy.

CATHETER-ASSOCIATED UTI Multiple institutions have released guidelines for the treatment of CAUTI, which is defined by bacteriuria and symptoms in a catheterized patient. The signs and symptoms either are localized to the urinary tract or can include otherwise unexplained systemic manifestations, such as fever. The accepted threshold for bacteriuria varies from $\geq 10^3$ cfu/mL to $\geq 10^5$ cfu/mL.

The formation of biofilm—a living layer of uropathogens—on the urinary catheter is central to the pathogenesis of CAUTI and affects both therapeutic and preventive strategies. Organisms in a biofilm are relatively resistant to killing by antibiotics, and eradication of a catheter-associated biofilm is difficult without removal of the device itself. Furthermore, because catheters provide a conduit for bacteria to enter the bladder, bacteriuria is inevitable with long-term catheter use.

The typical signs and symptoms of UTI, including pain, urgency, dysuria, fever, peripheral leukocytosis, and pyuria, have less predictive value for the diagnosis of infection in catheterized patients.

Furthermore, the presence of bacteria in the urine of a patient who is febrile and catheterized does not necessarily predict CAUTI, and other explanations for the fever should be considered.

The etiology of CAUTI is diverse, and urine culture results are essential to guide treatment. Fairly good evidence supports the practice of catheter change during treatment for CAUTI. The goal is to remove biofilm-associated organisms that could serve as a nidus for reinfection. Pathology studies reveal that many patients with long-term catheters have occult pyelonephritis. A randomized trial in persons with spinal cord injury who were practicing intermittent catheterization found that relapse was more common after 3 days of therapy than after 14 days. In general, a 7- to 14-day course of antibiotics is recommended, but further studies on the optimal duration of therapy are needed.

In the setting of long-term catheter use, systemic antibiotics, bladder-acidifying agents, antimicrobial bladder washes, topical disinfectants, and antimicrobial drainage-bag solutions have all been ineffective at preventing the onset of bacteriuria and have been associated with the emergence of resistant organisms. The best strategy for prevention of CAUTI is to avoid insertion of unnecessary catheters and to remove catheters once they are no longer necessary. Evidence is insufficient to recommend suprapubic catheters and condom catheters as alternatives to indwelling urinary catheters as a means to prevent CAUTI. However, intermittent catheterization may be preferable to long-term indwelling urethral catheterization in certain populations (e.g., spinal cord–injured persons) to prevent both infectious and anatomic complications. Antimicrobial catheters impregnated with silver or nitrofurazone have not been shown to provide significant clinical benefit in terms of reducing rates of symptomatic UTI.

CANDIDURIA The appearance of *Candida* in the urine is an increasingly common complication of indwelling catheterization, particularly for patients in the intensive care unit, those taking broad-spectrum antimicrobial drugs, and those with underlying diabetes mellitus. *C. albicans* is still the most common isolate, although *C. glabrata* and other non-*albicans* species are also isolated frequently. The clinical presentation varies from an asymptomatic laboratory finding to pyelonephritis and even sepsis. In asymptomatic patients, removal of the urethral catheter results in resolution of candiduria in more than one-third of cases. Treatment is recommended for patients who have symptomatic cystitis or pyelonephritis and for those who are at high risk for disseminated disease. High-risk patients include those with neutropenia, those who are undergoing urologic manipulation, and low-birth-weight infants. Fluconazole (200–400 mg/d for 14 days) achieves high levels in urine and is the first-line regimen for *Candida* infections of the urinary tract. The newer azoles and echinocandins are characterized by only low-level urinary excretion and thus are not recommended, although cases of successful eradication of candiduria with some of these agents have been reported. For *Candida* isolates with high levels of resistance to fluconazole, oral flucytosine and/or parenteral amphotericin B are options. Bladder irrigation with amphotericin B generally is not recommended.

PREVENTION OF RECURRENT UTI IN WOMEN

Recurrence of uncomplicated cystitis in reproductive-age women is common, and a preventive strategy is indicated if recurrent UTIs are interfering with a patient's lifestyle. The threshold of two or more symptomatic episodes per year is not absolute; decisions about interventions should take the patient's preferences into account.

Three prophylactic strategies are available: continuous, postcoital, or patient-initiated therapy. Continuous prophylaxis and postcoital prophylaxis usually entail low doses of TMP-SMX, a fluoroquinolone, or nitrofurantoin. These regimens are all highly effective during the period of active antibiotic intake. Typically, a prophylactic regimen is prescribed for 6 months and then discontinued, at which point the rate of recurrent UTI often returns to baseline. If bothersome infections recur, the prophylactic program can be reinstituted for a longer period.

Patient-initiated therapy involves supplying the patient with materials for urine culture and self-medication with a course of antibiotics at the first symptoms of infection. The urine culture is refrigerated and delivered to the physician's office for confirmation of the diagnosis. When an established and reliable patient-provider relationship exists, the urine culture can be omitted as long as the symptomatic episodes respond completely to short-course therapy and are not followed by relapse.

PROGNOSIS

Cystitis is a risk factor for recurrent cystitis and pyelonephritis. ABU is common among elderly and catheterized patients but does not in itself increase the risk of death. The relationships among recurrent UTI, chronic pyelonephritis, and renal insufficiency have been widely studied. In the absence of anatomic abnormalities, recurrent infection in children and adults does not lead to chronic pyelonephritis or to renal failure. Moreover, infection does not play a primary role in chronic interstitial nephritis; the primary etiologic factors in this condition are analgesic abuse, obstruction, reflux, and toxin exposure. In the presence of underlying renal abnormalities (particularly obstructing stones), infection as a secondary factor can accelerate renal parenchymal damage. In spinal cord–injured patients, use of a long-term indwelling bladder catheter is a well-documented risk factor for bladder cancer. Chronic bacteriuria resulting in chronic inflammation is one possible explanation for this observation.

FURTHER READINGS

Bent S et al: Does this woman have acute uncomplicated urinary tract infection? JAMA 287:2701, 2002

Fihn SD: Clinical practice. Acute uncomplicated urinary tract infection in women. N Engl J Med 349:259, 2003

Gupta K et al: International clinical practice guidelines for the treatment of acute uncomplicated cystitis and pyelonephritis in women: A 2010 update by the Infectious Diseases Society of America and the European Society for Microbiology and Infectious Diseases. Clin Infect Dis 52:e103, 2011

Gupta K et al: Patient-initiated treatment of uncomplicated recurrent urinary tract infections in young women. Ann Intern Med 135:9, 2001

Hooton TM et al: Diagnosis, prevention, and treatment of catheter-associated urinary tract infection in adults: 2009 international clinical practice guidelines from the Infectious Diseases Society of America. Clin Infect Dis 50:625, 2010

Johnson JR et al: Systematic review: Antimicrobial urinary catheters to prevent catheter-associated urinary tract infection in hospitalized patients. Ann Intern Med 144:116, 2006

Le BV, Schaeffer AJ: Genitourinary pain syndromes, prostatitis, and lower urinary tract symptoms. Urol Clin North Am 36:527, 2009

Nicolle LE et al: Infectious Diseases Society of America guidelines for the diagnosis and treatment of asymptomatic bacteriuria in adults. Clin Infect Dis 40:643, 2005

Saint S et al: The effectiveness of a clinical practice guideline for the management of presumed uncomplicated urinary tract infection in women. Am J Med 106:636, 1999

Trautner BW: Management of catheter-associated urinary tract infection. Curr Opin Infect Dis 23:76, 2010

CHAPTER 289
Urinary Tract Obstruction

Julian L. Seifter

Obstruction to the flow of urine, with attendant stasis and elevation in urinary tract pressure, impairs renal and urinary conduit functions and is a common cause of acute and chronic kidney disease (obstructive nephropathy). With early relief of obstruction, the defects in function usually disappear completely. However, chronic obstruction may produce permanent loss of renal mass (renal atrophy) and excretory capability, as well as enhanced susceptibility to local infection and stone formation. Early diagnosis and prompt therapy are, therefore, essential to minimize the otherwise devastating effects of obstruction on kidney structure and function.

ETIOLOGY

Obstruction to urine flow can result from *intrinsic* or *extrinsic mechanical blockade* as well as from *functional defects* not associated with fixed occlusion of the urinary drainage system. Mechanical obstruction can occur at any level of the urinary tract, from the renal calyces to the external urethral meatus. Normal points of narrowing, such as the ureteropelvic and ureterovesical junctions, bladder neck, and urethral meatus, are common sites of obstruction. When obstruction is above the level of the bladder, unilateral dilatation of the ureter (*hydroureter*) and renal pyelocalyceal system (*hydronephrosis*) occur; lesions at or below the level of the bladder cause bilateral involvement.

Common forms of obstruction are listed in Table 289-1. Childhood causes include *congenital malformations*, such as narrowing of the ureteropelvic junction and abnormal insertion of the ureter into the bladder, the most common cause. Vesicoureteral reflux in the absence of urinary tract infection or bladder neck obstruction often resolves with age. Reinsertion of the ureter into the bladder is indicated if reflux is severe and unlikely to improve spontaneously, if renal function deteriorates, or if urinary tract infections recur despite chronic antimicrobial therapy. Vesicoureteral reflux may cause prenatal hydronephrosis and, if severe, can lead to recurrent urinary infections and renal scarring in childhood. Posterior urethral valves are the most common cause of bilateral hydronephrosis in boys. In adults, urinary tract obstruction (UTO) is due mainly to *acquired defects*. Pelvic tumors, calculi, and urethral stricture predominate. Ligation of, or injury to, the ureter during pelvic or colonic surgery can lead to hydronephrosis which, if unilateral, may remain undetected. Obstructive uropathy may also result from extrinsic neoplastic (carcinoma of cervix or colon) or inflammatory disorders. Lymphomas and pelvic or colonic neoplasms with retroperitoneal involvement are causes of ureteral obstruction.

Functional impairment of urine flow usually results from disorders that involve both the ureter and bladder. Causes include neurogenic bladder, often with adynamic ureter, and vesicoureteral reflux. Reflux in children may result in severe unilateral or bilateral hydroureter and hydronephrosis. Urinary retention may be the consequence of alpha-adrenergic and anticholinergic agents, as well as opiates. Hydronephrosis in pregnancy is due to relaxational effects of progesterone on smooth muscle of the renal pelvis, as well as ureteral compression by the enlarged uterus.

CLINICAL FEATURES AND PATHOPHYSIOLOGY

The pathophysiology and clinical features of UTO are summarized in Table 289-2. *Pain*, the symptom that most commonly leads to medical attention, is due to distention of the collecting system or renal capsule. Pain severity is influenced more by the rate at which distention develops than by the degree of distention. Acute supravesical obstruction, as from a stone lodged in a ureter (see Chap. 287), is associated with excruciating pain, known as *renal colic*. This pain often radiates to the lower abdomen, testes, or labia. By contrast,

TABLE 289-1 Common Mechanical Causes of Urinary Tract Obstruction

Ureter	Bladder Outlet	Urethra
Congenital		
Ureteropelvic junction narrowing or obstruction	Bladder neck obstruction	Posterior urethral valves
Ureterovesical junction narrowing or obstruction and reflux	Ureterocele	Anterior urethral valves
Ureterocele		Stricture
Retrocaval ureter		Meatal stenosis
		Phimosis
Acquired Intrinsic Defects		
Calculi	Benign prostatic hyperplasia	Stricture
Inflammation	Cancer of prostate	Tumor
Infection	Cancer of bladder	Calculi
Trauma	Calculi	Trauma
Sloughed papillae	Diabetic neuropathy	Phimosis
Tumor	Spinal cord disease	
Blood clots	Anticholinergic drugs and α-adrenergic antagonists	
Acquired Extrinsic Defects		
Pregnant uterus	Carcinoma of cervix, colon	Trauma
Retroperitoneal fibrosis	Trauma	
Aortic aneurysm		
Uterine leiomyomata		
Carcinoma of uterus, prostate, bladder, colon, rectum		
Lymphoma		
Pelvic inflammatory disease, endometriosis		
Accidental surgical ligation		

TABLE 289-2 Pathophysiology of Bilateral Ureteral Obstruction

Hemodynamic Effects	Tubule Effects	Clinical Features
Acute		
↑Renal blood flow	↑Ureteral and tubule pressures	Pain (capsule distention)
↓GFR	↑Reabsorption of Na^+, urea, water	Azotemia
↓Medullary blood flow		Oliguria or anuria
↑Vasodilator prostaglandins, nitric oxide		
Chronic		
↓ Renal blood flow	↓Medullary osmolarity	Azotemia
↓↓GFR	↓Concentrating ability	Hypertension
↑Vasoconstrictor prostaglandins	Structural damage; parenchymal atrophy	AVP-insensitive polyuria
		Natriuresis
↑Renin-angiotensin production	↓Transport functions for Na^+, K^+, H^+	Hyperkalemic, hyperchloremic acidosis
Release of Obstruction		
Slow ↑ in GFR (variable)	↓Tubule pressure	Postobstructive diuresis
	↑Solute load per nephron (urea, NaCl)	Potential for volume depletion and electrolyte imbalance due to losses of Na^+, K^+, PO_4^{2-}, Mg^{2+}, and water
	Natriuretic factors present	

Abbreviations: AVP, arginine vasopressin; GFR, glomerular filtration rate.

more insidious causes of obstruction, such as chronic narrowing of the ureteropelvic junction, may produce little or no pain and yet result in total destruction of the affected kidney. Flank pain that occurs only with micturition is pathognomonic of vesicoureteral reflux. Hesitancy and straining to initiate the urinary stream, postvoid dribbling, urinary frequency, and incontinence are common with obstruction at or below the level of the bladder.

Obstruction of urine flow results in an increase in hydrostatic pressures proximal to the site of obstruction. It is this buildup of pressure that leads to the accompanying pain, the distention of the collecting system in the kidney, and elevated intratubular pressures that initiate tubular dysfunction. As the increased hydrostatic pressure is expressed in the urinary space of the glomeruli, further filtration decreases or stops completely.

Azotemia develops when overall excretory function is impaired, often in the setting of bladder outlet obstruction, bilateral renal pelvic or ureteric obstruction, or unilateral disease in a patient with a solitary functioning kidney. Complete bilateral obstruction should be suspected when acute renal failure is accompanied by anuria. Any patient with renal failure otherwise unexplained, or with a history of nephrolithiasis, hematuria, diabetes mellitus, prostatic enlargement, pelvic surgery, trauma, or tumor should be evaluated for UTO.

In the acute setting, partial, bilateral obstruction may mimic prerenal azotemia with concentrated urine and sodium retention. However, with more prolonged obstruction, symptoms of *polyuria* and *nocturia* commonly accompany partial UTO and result from diminished renal concentrating ability. Impairment of transcellular salt reabsorption in the proximal tubule, medullary thick ascending limb of Henle, and collecting duct cells is due to down-regulation of transport proteins including the Na^+, K^+ adenosine triphosphatase (ATPase), NaK_2Cl cotransporter (NKCC) in the thick ascending limb, and the epithelial Na^+ channel (ENaC) in collecting duct cells. Consequences include failure to produce urine free of salt (natriuresis), and loss of medullary hypertonicity producing a urinary concentrating defect. In addition to direct effects on renal transport mechanisms, increased PGE2 (due to induction of COX-2), angiotensin-II (with its down-regulation of Na^+ transporters), and atrial natriuretic peptide (ANP) (due to volume expansion in the azotemic patient) contribute to the decreased salt reabsorption along the nephron.

Dysregulation of aquaporin-2 water channels in the collecting duct contributes to the polyuria. The defect usually does not improve with administration of vasopressin and is therefore a form of acquired nephrogenic diabetes insipidus.

Wide fluctuations in urine output in a patient with azotemia should always raise the possibility of intermittent or partial UTO. If fluid intake is inadequate, severe dehydration and hypernatremia may develop. However, as with other causes of poor renal function, excesses of salt and water intake may result in edema and hyponatremia.

Partial bilateral UTO often results in *acquired distal renal tubular acidosis, hyperkalemia,* and *renal salt wasting.* The H^+-ATPase, situated on the apical membrane of the intercalated cells of the collecting duct, is critical for distal H^+ secretion. The trafficking of intracellular H^+ pumps from the cytoplasm to the cell membrane is disrupted in UTO. The decreased function of the ENaC, in the apical membrane of neighboring collecting duct principal cells, contributes to decreased Na^+ reabsorption (salt-wasting), decreased electronegativity of the tubule lumen, and therefore decreased K^+ secretion via K^+ channels (hyperkalemia) and H^+ secretion via the H^+-ATPases [distal renal tubular acidosis (RTA)]. Proximal tubule ammoniagenesis, important to the elimination of H^+ as $NH4^+$, is impaired. These defects in tubule function are often accompanied by renal tubulointerstitial damage. Azotemia with hyperkalemia and metabolic acidosis should prompt consideration of UTO.

The renal interstitium becomes edematous and infiltrated with mononuclear inflammatory cells early in UTO. Later, interstitial fibrosis and atrophy of the papillae and medulla occur and precede these processes in the cortex. The increase in angiotensin-II noted in UTO contributes to the inflammatory response and fibroblast accumulation through mechanisms involving profibrotic cytokines. With time, this process leads to chronic kidney damage.

UTO must always be considered in patients with urinary tract infections or urolithiasis. Urinary stasis encourages the growth of organisms. Urea-splitting bacteria are associated with magnesium ammonium phosphate (struvite) calculi. *Hypertension* is frequent in acute and subacute unilateral obstruction and is usually a consequence of increased release of renin by the involved kidney. Chronic kidney disease from bilateral UTO, often associated with extracellular volume expansion, may result in significant hypertension. *Erythrocytosis,* an infrequent complication of obstructive uropathy, is secondary to increased erythropoietin production.

DIAGNOSIS

A history of difficulty in voiding, pain, infection, or change in urinary volume is common. Evidence for distention of the kidney or urinary bladder can often be obtained by palpation and percussion of the abdomen. A careful rectal and genital examination may reveal enlargement or nodularity of the prostate, abnormal rectal sphincter tone, or a rectal or pelvic mass.

Urinalysis may reveal hematuria, pyuria, and bacteriuria. The urine sediment is often normal, even when obstruction leads to marked azotemia and extensive structural damage. An abdominal scout film may detect nephrocalcinosis or a radiopaque stone. As indicated in Fig. 289-1, if UTO is suspected, a bladder catheter should be inserted. Abdominal ultrasonography should be performed to evaluate renal and bladder size, as well as pyelocalyceal contour. Ultrasonography is approximately 90% specific and sensitive for detection of hydronephrosis. False-positive results are associated with diuresis, renal cysts, or the presence of an extrarenal pelvis, a normal congenital variant. Congenital ureteropelvic junction (UPJ) obstruction may be mistaken for renal cystic disease. Hydronephrosis may be absent on ultrasound when obstruction is less than 48 hours in duration or associated with volume contraction, staghorn calculi, retroperitoneal fibrosis, or infiltrative renal disease. Duplex Doppler ultrasonography may detect an increased resistive index in urinary obstruction.

Recent advances in technology have led to alternatives to the once standard intravenous urogram in the further evaluation of UTO. The high-resolution multidetector row CT scan in particular has advantages of visualizing the retroperitoneum, as well as identifying both intrinsic and extrinsic sites of obstruction. Noncontrast CT scans improve visualization of the urinary tract in the patient with renal impairment and are safer for patients at risk for contrast nephropathy. MR urography is a promising technique but at this time not superior to the CT scan and carries the risk of certain gadolinium agents in patients with renal insufficiency, i.e., nephrogenic systemic fibrosis. The intravenous urogram may define the site of obstruction and demonstrate dilatation of the calyces, renal pelvis, and ureter above the obstruction. The ureter may be tortuous in chronic obstruction. Radionuclide scans are able to give differential renal function but give less anatomic detail than CT or intravenous urography (IVU).

To facilitate visualization of a suspected lesion in a ureter or renal pelvis, *retrograde* or *antegrade urography* should be attempted. These procedures do not carry risk of contrast-induced acute renal failure in patients with renal insufficiency. The retrograde approach involves catheterization of the involved ureter under cystoscopic control, while the antegrade technique necessitates percutaneous placement of a catheter into the renal pelvis. While the antegrade approach may provide immediate decompression of a unilateral obstructing lesion, many urologists initially attempt the retrograde approach unless the catheterization is unsuccessful.

Voiding cystourethrography is of value in the diagnosis of vesicoureteral reflux and bladder neck and urethral obstructions. Postvoiding films reveal residual urine. Endoscopic visualization by the urologist often permits precise identification of lesions involving the urethra, prostate, bladder, and ureteral orifices.

TREATMENT Urinary Tract Obstruction

UTO complicated by infection requires immediate relief of obstruction to prevent development of generalized sepsis and progressive renal damage. Sepsis necessitates prompt urologic intervention. Drainage may be achieved by nephrostomy, ureterostomy, or ureteral, urethral, or suprapubic catheterization. Prolonged antibiotic treatment may be necessary. Chronic or recurrent infections in a poorly functioning obstructed kidney may necessitate nephrectomy. When infection is not present, surgery is often delayed until acid-base, fluid, and electrolyte status is restored. Nevertheless, the site of obstruction should be ascertained as soon as feasible. Elective relief of obstruction is usually recommended in patients with urinary retention, recurrent urinary tract infections, persistent pain, or progressive loss of renal function. Benign prostatic hypertrophy may be treated medically with alpha adrenergic blockers and 5α-reductase inhibitors. Functional obstruction secondary to neurogenic bladder may be decreased with the combination of frequent voiding and cholinergic drugs.

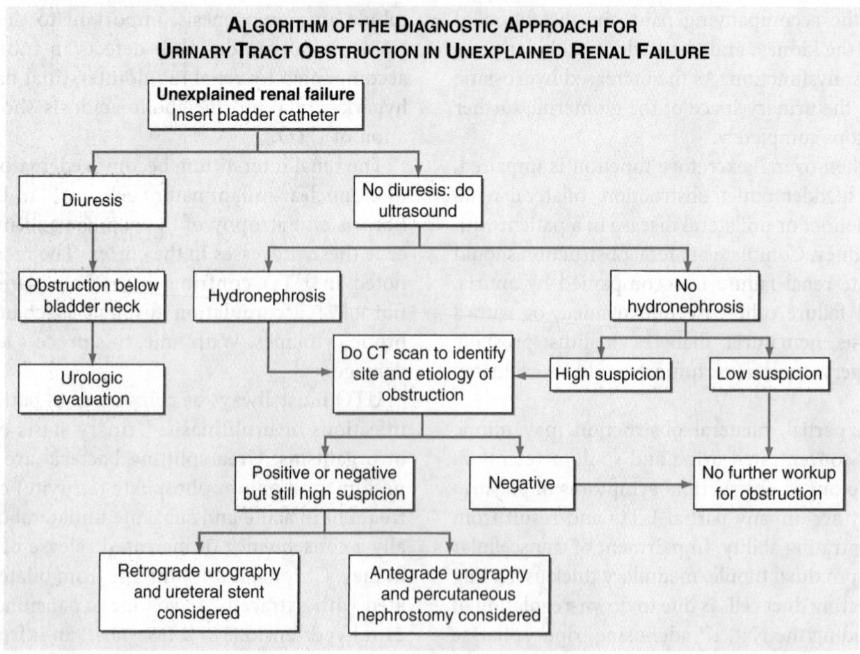

Figure 289-1 Diagnostic approach for urinary tract obstruction in unexplained renal failure. CT, computed tomography.

PROGNOSIS

With relief of obstruction, the prognosis regarding return of renal function depends largely on whether irreversible renal damage has occurred. When obstruction is not relieved, the course will depend mainly on whether the obstruction is complete or incomplete and bilateral or unilateral, as well as whether or not urinary tract infection is also present. Complete obstruction with infection can lead to total destruction of the kidney within days. Partial return of glomerular filtration rate may follow relief of complete obstruction of 1 and 2 weeks' duration, but after 8 weeks of obstruction, recovery is unlikely. In the absence of definitive evidence of irreversibility, every effort should be made to decompress the obstruction in the hope of restoring renal function at least partially. A renal radionuclide scan, performed after a prolonged period of decompression, may be used to predict the reversibility of renal dysfunction.

POSTOBSTRUCTIVE DIURESIS

Relief of bilateral, but not unilateral, complete obstruction commonly results in polyuria, which may be massive. The urine is usually hypotonic and may contain large amounts of sodium chloride, potassium, phosphate, and magnesium. The natriuresis is due in part to the excretion of retained urea (osmotic diuresis), natriuretic factors accumulated during uremia and depressed salt and water reabsorption when urine flow is reestablished. In the majority of patients this diuresis results in the *appropriate* excretion of the excesses of retained salt and water. When extracellular volume and composition return to normal, the diuresis usually abates spontaneously. Occasionally, iatrogenic expansion of extracellular volume is responsible for, or sustains, the diuresis observed in the postobstructive period. Replacement with intravenous fluids in amounts less than urinary losses usually avoids this complication. More aggressive fluid management is required in the setting of hypovolemia, hypotension, or disturbances in serum electrolyte concentrations.

The loss of electrolyte-free water with urea may result in hypernatremia. Serum and urine sodium and osmolal concentrations should guide the use of appropriate intravenous replacement. Often replacement with 0.45% saline is required. Relief of obstruction may be followed by urinary salt and water losses severe enough to provoke profound dehydration and vascular collapse. In these patients, decreased tubule reabsorptive capacity is probably responsible for the marked diuresis. Appropriate therapy in such patients includes intravenous administration of salt-containing solutions to replace sodium and volume deficits.

FURTHER READINGS

Campbell SC, Walsh PC: Pathophysiology of urinary tract obstruction, in *Campbell-Walsh Urology,* vol 2, 9th ed, J Wein (ed). Philadelphia, Saunders, 2007, pp 1195–1226

Frokiaer J, Zeidel ML: Urinary tract obstruction, in *Brenner and Rector's The Kidney,* 8th ed, BM Brenner (ed). Philadelphia, Saunders, 2007, pp 1239–1259

Klahr S: Urinary tract obstruction, in *Diseases of the Kidney,* 7th ed, RW Schrier, CW Gottschalk (eds). Boston, Little, Brown, 2001, pp 751–787

Williams B et al: Pathophysiology and treatment of ureteropelvic junction obstruction. Curr Urol Rep 8:111, 2007

PART 14

Disorders of the Gastrointestinal System

SECTION 1 Disorders of the Alimentary Tract

SECTION 2 Liver and Biliary Tract Disease

SECTION 3 Disorders of the Pancreas

CHAPTER 290

Approach to the Patient With Gastrointestinal Disease

William L. Hasler
Chung Owyang

ANATOMIC CONSIDERATIONS

The gastrointestinal (GI) tract extends from the mouth to the anus and is composed of several organs with distinct functions. Specialized independently controlled thickened sphincters that assist in gut compartmentalization separate the organs. The gut wall is organized into well-defined layers that contribute to functional activities in each region. The mucosa is a barrier to luminal contents or as a site for transfer of fluids or nutrients. Gut smooth muscle mediates propulsion from one region to the next. Many GI organs possess a serosal layer that provides a supportive foundation but that also permits external input.

Interactions with other organ systems serve the needs both of the gut and the body. Pancreaticobiliary conduits deliver bile and enzymes into the duodenum. A rich vascular supply is modulated by GI tract activity. Lymphatic channels assist in gut immune activities. Intrinsic gut wall nerves provide the basic controls for propulsion and fluid regulation. Extrinsic neural input provides volitional or involuntary control to degrees that are specific for each gut region.

FUNCTIONS OF THE GASTROINTESTINAL TRACT

The GI tract serves two main functions—assimilating nutrients and eliminating waste. The gut anatomy is organized to serve these functions. In the mouth, food is processed, mixed with salivary amylase, and delivered to the gut lumen. The esophagus propels the bolus into the stomach; the lower esophageal sphincter prevents oral reflux of gastric contents. The esophageal mucosa has a protective squamous histology, which does not permit significant diffusion or absorption. Propulsive esophageal activities are exclusively aboral and coordinate with relaxation of the upper and lower esophageal sphincters on swallowing.

The stomach furthers food preparation by triturating and mixing the bolus with pepsin and acid. Gastric acid also sterilizes the upper gut. The proximal stomach serves a storage function by relaxing to accommodate the meal. The distal stomach exhibits phasic contractions that propel solid food residue against the pylorus, where it is repeatedly propelled proximally for further mixing before it is emptied into the duodenum. Finally, the stomach secretes intrinsic factor for vitamin B_{12} absorption.

The small intestine serves most of the nutrient absorptive function of the gut. The intestinal mucosa exhibits villus architecture to provide maximal surface area for absorption and is endowed with specialized enzymes and transporters. Triturated food from the stomach mixes with pancreatic juice and bile in the duodenum to facilitate digestion. Pancreatic juice contains the main enzymes for carbohydrate, protein, and fat digestion as well as bicarbonate to optimize the pH for activation of these enzymes. Bile secreted by the liver and stored in the gallbladder is essential for intestinal lipid digestion. The proximal intestine is optimized for rapid absorption of nutrient breakdown products and most minerals, while the ileum is better suited for absorption of vitamin B_{12} and bile acids. The small intestine also aids in waste elimination. Bile contains by-products of erythrocyte degradation, toxins, metabolized and unmetabolized medications, and cholesterol. Motor function of the small intestine delivers indigestible food residue and sloughed enterocytes into the colon for further processing. The small intestine terminates in the ileocecal junction, a sphincteric structure that prevents coloileal reflux and maintains small-intestinal sterility.

The colon prepares the waste material for controlled evacuation. The colonic mucosa dehydrates the stool, decreasing daily fecal volumes from 1000–1500 mL delivered from the ileum to 100–200 mL expelled from the rectum. The colonic lumen possesses a dense bacterial colonization that ferments undigested carbohydrates and short-chain fatty acids. Whereas transit times in the esophagus are on the order of seconds and times in the stomach and small intestine range from minutes to a few hours, propagation through the colon takes more than one day in most individuals. Colonic motor patterns exhibit a to-and-fro character that facilitates slow fecal desiccation. The proximal colon serves to mix and absorb fluid, while the distal colon exhibits peristaltic contractions and mass actions that function to expel the stool. The colon terminates in the anus, a structure with volitional and involuntary controls to permit retention of the fecal bolus until it can be released in a socially convenient setting.

EXTRINSIC MODULATION OF GUT FUNCTION

GI function is modified by influences outside of the gut. Unlike other organ systems, the gut is in continuity with the outside environment. Thus, protective mechanisms are vigilant against deleterious effects of foods, medications, toxins, and infectious organisms. Mucosal immune mechanisms include chronic lymphocyte and plasma cell populations in the epithelial layer and lamina propria backed up by lymph node chains to prevent noxious agents from entering the circulation. All substances absorbed into the bloodstream are filtered through the liver via the portal venous circulation. In the liver, many drugs and toxins are detoxified by a variety of mechanisms. Although intrinsic nerves control most basic gut activities, extrinsic neural input modulates many functions. Two activities under voluntary control are swallowing and defecation. Many normal GI reflexes involve extrinsic vagus or splanchnic nerve pathways. The brain gut axis further alters function in regions not under volitional regulation. As an example, stress has potent effects on gut motor, secretory, and sensory functions.

OVERVIEW OF GASTROINTESTINAL DISEASES

GI diseases develop as a result of abnormalities within or outside of the gut and range in severity from those that produce mild symptoms and no long-term morbidity to those with intractable symptoms or adverse outcomes. Diseases may be localized to one organ or exhibit diffuse involvement at many sites.

■ CLASSIFICATION OF GI DISEASES

GI diseases are manifestations of alterations in nutrient assimilation or waste evacuation or in the activities supporting these main functions.

Impaired digestion and absorption

Diseases of the stomach, intestine, biliary tree, and pancreas can disrupt digestion and absorption. The most common intestinal maldigestion syndrome, lactase deficiency, produces gas and diarrhea after dairy products and has no adverse outcomes. Other intestinal enzyme deficiencies produce similar symptoms after ingestion of other simple sugars. Conversely, celiac disease, bacterial overgrowth, infectious enteritis, Crohn's ileitis, and radiation damage, which affect digestion and/or absorption more diffusely, produce anemia, dehydration, electrolyte disorders, or malnutrition. Gastric hypersecretory conditions such as Zollinger-Ellison syndrome damage the intestinal mucosa, impair pancreatic enzyme activation, and accelerate transit due to excess gastric acid. Biliary obstruction from stricture or neoplasm impairs fat digestion. Impaired pancreatic enzyme release in chronic pancreatitis or pancreatic cancer decreases intraluminal digestion and can lead to malnutrition.

Altered secretion

Selected GI diseases result from dysregulation of gut secretion. Gastric acid hypersecretion occurs in Zollinger-Ellison syndrome, G cell hyperplasia, retained antrum syndrome, and some individuals with duodenal ulcers. Conversely, patients with atrophic gastritis or pernicious anemia release little or no gastric acid. Inflammatory and infectious small-intestinal and colonic diseases produce fluid loss through impaired absorption or enhanced secretion. Common intestinal and colonic hypersecretory conditions cause diarrhea and include acute bacterial or viral infection, chronic *Giardia* or cryptosporidia infections, small-intestinal bacterial overgrowth, bile salt diarrhea, microscopic colitis, diabetic diarrhea, and abuse of certain laxatives. Less common causes include large colonic villus adenomas and endocrine neoplasias with tumor overproduction of secretagogue transmitters like vasoactive intestinal polypeptide.

Altered gut transit

Impaired gut transit may be secondary to mechanical obstruction. Esophageal occlusion often results from acid-induced stricture or neoplasm. Gastric outlet obstruction develops from peptic ulcer disease or gastric cancer. Small-intestinal obstruction most commonly results from adhesions but may also occur with Crohn's disease, radiation- or drug-induced strictures, and less likely malignancy. The most common cause of colonic obstruction is colon cancer, although inflammatory strictures develop in patients with inflammatory bowel disease, after certain infections such as diverticulitis, or with some drugs.

Retardation of propulsion also develops from disordered motor function. Achalasia is characterized by impaired esophageal body peristalsis and incomplete lower esophageal sphincter relaxation. Gastroparesis is the symptomatic delay in gastric emptying of meals due to impaired gastric motility. Intestinal pseudoobstruction causes marked delays in small-bowel transit due to enteric nerve or intestinal smooth-muscle injury. Slow-transit constipation is produced by diffusely impaired colonic propulsion. Constipation also is produced by outlet abnormalities such as rectal prolapse, intussusception, or dyssynergia—a failure of anal or puborectalis relaxation upon attempted defecation.

Disorders of rapid propulsion are less common than those with delayed transit. Rapid gastric emptying occurs in postvagotomy dumping syndrome, with gastric hypersecretion, and in some cases of functional dyspepsia and cyclic vomiting syndrome. Exaggerated intestinal or colonic motor patterns may be responsible for diarrhea in irritable bowel syndrome. Accelerated transit with hyperdefecation is noted in hyperthyroidism.

Immune dysregulation

Many inflammatory GI conditions are consequences of altered gut immune function. The mucosal inflammation of celiac disease results from dietary ingestion of gluten-containing grains. Some patients with food allergy also exhibit altered immune populations. Eosinophilic esophagitis and eosinophilic gastroenteritis are inflammatory disorders with prominent mucosal eosinophils. Ulcerative colitis and Crohn's disease are disorders of uncertain etiology that produce mucosal injury primarily in the lower gut. The microscopic colitides, lymphocytic and collagenous colitis, exhibit colonic subepithelial infiltrates without visible mucosal damage. Bacterial, viral, and protozoal organisms may produce ileitis or colitis in selected patient populations.

Impaired gut blood flow

Different GI regions are at variable risk for ischemic damage from impaired blood flow. Rare cases of gastroparesis result from blockage of the celiac and superior mesenteric arteries. More commonly encountered are intestinal and colonic ischemia that are consequences of arterial embolus, arterial thrombosis, venous thrombosis, or hypoperfusion from dehydration, sepsis, hemorrhage, or reduced cardiac output. These may produce mucosal injury, hemorrhage, or even perforation. Some cases of radiation enterocolitis exhibit reduced mucosal blood flow.

Neoplastic degeneration

All GI regions are susceptible to malignant degeneration to varying degrees. In the United States, colorectal cancer is most common and usually presents after age 50 years. Worldwide, gastric cancer is prevalent especially in certain Asian regions. Esophageal cancer develops with chronic acid reflux or after an extensive alcohol or tobacco use history. Small-intestinal neoplasms are rare and occur with underlying inflammatory disease. Anal cancers arise after prior anal infection or inflammation. Pancreatic and biliary cancers elicit severe pain, weight loss, and jaundice and have poor prognoses. Hepatocellular carcinoma usually arises in the setting of chronic viral hepatitis or cirrhosis secondary to other causes. Most GI cancers exhibit carcinomatous histology; however, lymphomas and other cell types also are observed.

Disorders without obvious organic abnormalities

The most common GI disorders show no abnormalities on biochemical or structural testing and include irritable bowel syndrome, functional dyspepsia, functional chest pain, and functional heartburn. These disorders exhibit altered gut motor function; however, the pathogenic relevance of these abnormalities is uncertain. Exaggerated visceral sensory responses to noxious stimulation may cause discomfort in these disorders. Symptoms in other patients result from altered processing of visceral pain sensations in the central nervous system. Functional bowel patients with severe symptoms may exhibit significant emotional disturbances on psychometric testing. Subtle immunologic defects may contribute to functional symptoms as well.

Genetic influences

Although many GI diseases result from environmental factors, others exhibit hereditary components. Family members of inflammatory bowel disease patients show a genetic predisposition to disease development themselves. Colonic and esophageal malignancies arise in certain inherited disorders. Rare genetic dysmotility syndromes are described. Familial clustering is even observed in the functional bowel disorders, although this may be secondary learned familial illness behavior rather than a true hereditary factor.

SYMPTOMS OF GASTROINTESTINAL DISEASE

The most common GI symptoms are abdominal pain, heartburn, nausea and vomiting, altered bowel habits, GI bleeding, and jaundice (Table 290-1). Others are dysphagia, anorexia, weight loss, fatigue, and extraintestinal symptoms.

Abdominal pain

Abdominal pain results from GI disease and extraintestinal conditions involving the genitourinary tract, abdominal wall, thorax, or spine. Visceral pain generally is midline in location and vague in character, while parietal pain is localized and precisely described. Common inflammatory diseases with pain include peptic ulcer, appendicitis, diverticulitis, inflammatory bowel disease, and infectious enterocolitis. Other intraabdominal causes of pain include gallstone disease and pancreatitis. Noninflammatory visceral sources include mesenteric ischemia and neoplasia. The most common causes of abdominal pain are irritable bowel syndrome and functional dyspepsia.

Heartburn

Heartburn, a burning substernal sensation, is reported intermittently by at least 40% of the population. Classically, heartburn is felt to result from excess gastroesophageal reflux of acid. However, some cases exhibit normal esophageal acid exposure and may result from reflux of nonacidic material or heightened sensitivity of esophageal mucosal nerves.

Nausea and vomiting

Nausea and vomiting are caused by GI diseases, medications, toxins, acute and chronic infection, endocrine disorders, labyrinthine conditions, and central nervous system disease. The best-characterized GI etiologies relate to mechanical obstruction of the upper gut; however, disorders of propulsion including gastroparesis and intestinal pseudoobstruction also elicit prominent symptoms. Nausea and vomiting also are commonly reported by patients with irritable bowel syndrome and functional disorders of the upper gut (including chronic idiopathic nausea and functional vomiting).

Altered bowel habits

Altered bowel habits are common complaints of patients with GI disease. Constipation is reported as infrequent defecation, straining with defecation, passage of hard stools, or a sense of incomplete fecal evacuation. Causes of constipation include obstruction, motor disorders of the colon, medications, and endocrine diseases such as hypothyroidism and hyperparathyroidism. Diarrhea is reported as frequent defecation, passage of loose or watery stools, fecal urgency, or a similar sense of incomplete evacuation. The differential diagnosis of diarrhea is broad and includes infections, inflammatory causes, malabsorption, and medications. Irritable bowel syndrome produces constipation, diarrhea, or an alternating bowel pattern. Fecal mucus is common in irritable bowel syndrome, while pus characterizes inflammatory disease. Steatorrhea develops with malabsorption.

GI bleeding

Hemorrhage may develop from any gut organ. Most commonly, upper GI bleeding presents with melena or hematemesis, whereas lower GI bleeding produces passage of bright red or maroon stools. However, briskly bleeding upper sites can elicit voluminous red rectal bleeding, while slowly bleeding ascending colon sites may produce melena. Chronic slow GI bleeding may present with iron deficiency anemia. The most common upper GI causes of bleeding are ulcer disease, gastroduodenitis, and esophagitis. Other etiologies include portal hypertensive causes, malignancy, tears across the gastroesophageal junction, and vascular lesions. The most prevalent lower GI sources of hemorrhage include hemorrhoids, anal fissures, diverticula, ischemic colitis, and arteriovenous malformations. Other causes include neoplasm, inflammatory bowel disease, infectious colitis, drug-induced colitis, and other vascular lesions.

Jaundice

Jaundice results from prehepatic, intrahepatic, or posthepatic disease. Posthepatic causes of jaundice include biliary diseases such as choledocholithiasis, acute cholangitis, primary sclerosing cholangitis, other strictures, and neoplasm and pancreatic disorders, such as acute and chronic pancreatitis, stricture, and malignancy.

TABLE 290-1 Common Causes of Common GI Symptoms

Abdominal Pain	Nausea and Vomiting	Diarrhea	GI Bleeding	Obstructive Jaundice
Appendicitis	Medications	Infection	Ulcer disease	Bile duct stones
Gallstone disease	GI obstruction	Poorly absorbed sugars	Esophagitis	Cholangiocarcinoma
Pancreatitis	Motor disorders	Inflammatory bowel disease	Varices	Cholangitis
Diverticulitis	Functional bowel disorder	Microscopic colitis	Vascular lesions	Sclerosing cholangitis
Ulcer disease	Enteric infection	Functional bowel disorder	Neoplasm	Ampullary stenosis
Esophagitis	Pregnancy	Celiac disease	Diverticula	Ampullary carcinoma
GI obstruction	Endocrine disease	Pancreatic insufficiency	Hemorrhoids	Pancreatitis
Inflammatory bowel disease	Motion sickness	Hyperthyroidism	Fissures	Pancreatic tumor
Functional bowel disorder	Central nervous system disease	Ischemia	Inflammatory bowel disease	
Vascular disease		Endocrine tumor	Infectious colitis	
Gynecologic causes				
Renal stone				

Other symptoms

Other symptoms are manifestations of GI disease. Dysphagia, odynophagia, and unexplained chest pain suggest esophageal disease. A globus sensation is reported with esophagopharyngeal conditions, but also occurs with functional GI disorders. Weight loss, anorexia, and fatigue are nonspecific symptoms of neoplastic, inflammatory, gut motility, pancreatic, small-bowel mucosal, and psychiatric conditions. Fever is reported with inflammatory illness, but malignancies also evoke febrile responses. GI disorders also produce extraintestinal symptoms. Inflammatory bowel disease is associated with hepatobiliary dysfunction, skin and eye lesions, and arthritis. Celiac disease may present with dermatitis herpetiformis. Jaundice can produce pruritus. Conversely, systemic diseases can have GI consequences. Systemic lupus may cause gut ischemia, presenting with pain or bleeding. Overwhelming stress or severe burns may lead to gastric ulcer formation.

EVALUATION OF THE PATIENT WITH GASTROINTESTINAL DISEASE

Evaluation of the patient with GI disease begins with a careful history and examination. Subsequent investigation with a variety of tools designed to test gut structure or function are indicated in selected cases. Some patients exhibit normal findings on diagnostic testing. In these individuals, validated symptom profiles are employed to confidently diagnose a functional bowel disorder.

HISTORY

The history of the patient with suspected GI disease has several components. Symptom timing suggests specific etiologies. Symptoms of short duration commonly result from acute infection, toxin exposure, or abrupt inflammation or ischemia. Long-standing symptoms point to underlying chronic inflammatory or neoplastic conditions or functional bowel disorders. Symptoms from mechanical obstruction, ischemia, inflammatory bowel disease, and functional bowel disorders are worsened by meals. Conversely, ulcer symptoms may be relieved by eating or antacids. Symptom patterns and duration may suggest underlying etiologies. Ulcer pain occurs at intermittent intervals lasting weeks to months, while biliary colic has a sudden onset and lasts up to several hours. Pain from acute inflammation as with acute pancreatitis is severe and persists for days to weeks. Meals elicit diarrhea in some cases of inflammatory bowel disease and irritable bowel syndrome. Defecation relieves discomfort in inflammatory bowel disease and irritable bowel syndrome. Functional bowel disorders are exacerbated by stress. Sudden awakening from sound sleep suggests organic rather than functional disease. Diarrhea from malabsorption usually improves with fasting, while secretory diarrhea persists without oral intake.

Symptom relation to other factors narrows the list of diagnostic possibilities. Obstructive symptoms with prior abdominal surgery raise concern for adhesions, whereas loose stools after gastrectomy or gallbladder excision suggest dumping syndrome or postcholecystectomy diarrhea. Symptom onset after travel prompts a search for enteric infection. Medications may produce pain, altered bowel habits, or GI bleeding. Lower GI bleeding likely results from neoplasms, diverticula, or vascular lesions in an older person and from anorectal abnormalities or inflammatory bowel disease in a younger individual. Celiac disease is prevalent in people of northern European descent, while inflammatory bowel disease is more common in certain Jewish populations. A sexual history may raise concern for sexually transmitted diseases or immunodeficiency.

For more than two decades, working groups have been convened to devise symptom criteria to improve the confident diagnosis of functional bowel disorders and to minimize the numbers of unnecessary diagnostic tests performed. The most widely accepted symptom-based criteria are the Rome criteria. When tested against findings of structural investigations, the Rome criteria exhibit diagnostic specificities exceeding 90% for many of the functional bowel disorders.

PHYSICAL EXAMINATION

The physical exam complements information from the history. Abnormal vital signs provide diagnostic clues and determine the need for acute intervention. Fever suggests inflammation or neoplasm. Orthostasis is found with significant blood loss, dehydration, sepsis, or autonomic neuropathy. Skin, eye, or joint findings may point to specific diagnoses. Neck exam with swallowing assessment evaluates dysphagia. Cardiopulmonary disease may present with abdominal pain or nausea, thus lung and cardiac exams are important. Pelvic examination tests for a gynecologic source of abdominal pain. Rectal exam may detect blood, indicating gut mucosal injury or neoplasm or a palpable inflammatory mass in appendicitis. Metabolic conditions and gut motor disorders have associated peripheral neuropathy.

Inspection of the abdomen may reveal distention from obstruction, tumor, or ascites or vascular abnormalities with liver disease. Ecchymoses develop with severe pancreatitis. Auscultation can detect bruits or friction rubs from vascular disease or hepatic tumors. Loss of bowel sounds signifies ileus, while high-pitched, hyperactive sounds characterize intestinal obstruction. Percussion assesses liver size and can detect shifting dullness from ascites. Palpation assesses for hepatosplenomegaly as well as neoplastic or inflammatory masses. Abdominal exam is helpful in evaluating unexplained pain. Intestinal ischemia elicits severe pain but little tenderness. Patients with visceral pain may exhibit generalized discomfort, while those with parietal pain or peritonitis have directed pain, often with involuntary guarding, rigidity, or rebound. Patients with musculoskeletal abdominal wall pain may note tenderness exacerbated by Valsalva or straight-leg lift maneuvers.

TOOLS FOR PATIENT EVALUATION

Laboratory, radiographic, and functional tests can assist in diagnosis of suspected GI disease. The GI tract also is amenable to internal evaluation with upper and lower endoscopy and to examination of luminal contents. Histopathologic exams of GI tissues complement these tests.

Laboratory

Selected laboratory tests facilitate the diagnosis of GI disease. Iron-deficiency anemia suggests mucosal blood loss, while vitamin B_{12} deficiency results from small-intestinal, gastric, or pancreatic disease. Either also can result from inadequate oral intake. Leukocytosis and increased sedimentation rates and C-reactive proteins are found in inflammatory conditions, while leukopenia is seen in viremic illness. Severe vomiting or diarrhea elicits electrolyte disturbances, acid-base abnormalities, and elevated blood urea nitrogen. Pancreaticobiliary or liver disease is suggested by elevated pancreatic or liver chemistries. Thyroid chemistries, cortisol, and calcium levels are obtained to exclude endocrinologic causes of GI symptoms. Pregnancy testing is considered for women with unexplained nausea. Serologic tests can screen for celiac disease, inflammatory bowel disease, rheumatologic diseases like lupus or scleroderma, and paraneoplastic dysmotility syndromes. Hormone levels are obtained for suspected endocrine neoplasia. Intraabdominal malignancies produce other tumor markers including the carcinoembryonic antigen CA 19-9 and α-fetoprotein. Blood testing also monitors medication therapy in some diseases, as with thiopurine metabolite levels in inflammatory bowel disease. Other body fluids are sampled under certain circumstances. Ascitic fluid is analyzed for infection, malignancy, or findings of portal hypertension. Cerebrospinal fluid is obtained for suspected central nervous system causes of vomiting. Urine samples screen for carcinoid, porphyria, and heavy metal intoxication.

Luminal contents

Luminal contents can be examined for diagnostic clues. Stool samples are cultured for bacterial pathogens, examined for leukocytes and parasites, or tested for *Giardia* antigen. Duodenal aspirates can be examined for parasites or cultured for bacterial overgrowth. Fecal fat is quantified in possible malabsorption. Stool electrolytes can be measured in diarrheal conditions. Laxative screens are done when laxative abuse is suspected. Gastric acid is quantified to rule out Zollinger-Ellison syndrome. Esophageal pH testing is done for refractory symptoms of acid reflux, whereas impedance techniques assess for nonacidic reflux. Pancreatic juice is analyzed for enzyme or bicarbonate content to exclude pancreatic exocrine insufficiency.

Endoscopy

The gut is accessible with endoscopy, which can provide the diagnosis of the causes of bleeding, pain, nausea and vomiting, weight loss, altered bowel function, and fever. Table 290-2 lists the most common indications for the major endoscopic procedures. Upper endoscopy evaluates the esophagus, stomach, and duodenum, while colonoscopy assesses the colon and distal ileum. Upper endoscopy is advocated as the initial structural test performed in patients with suspected ulcer disease, esophagitis, neoplasm, malabsorption, and Barrett's metaplasia because of its ability to directly visualize as well as biopsy the abnormality. Colonoscopy is the procedure of choice for colon cancer screening and surveillance as well as diagnosis of colitis secondary to infection, ischemia, radiation, and inflammatory bowel disease. Sigmoidoscopy examines the colon up to the splenic flexure and is currently used to exclude distal colonic inflammation or obstruction in young patients not at significant risk for colon cancer. For elusive GI bleeding secondary to arteriovenous malformations or superficial ulcers, small-intestinal examination is performed with push enteroscopy, capsule endoscopy, or double-balloon enteroscopy. Capsule endoscopy also can visualize small-intestinal Crohn's disease in individuals with negative barium radiography. Endoscopic retrograde cholangiopancreaticography (ERCP) provides diagnoses of pancreatic and biliary disease. Endoscopic ultrasound is useful for evaluating extent of disease in GI malignancy as well as exclusion of choledocholithiasis, evaluation of pancreatitis, drainage of pancreatic pseudocysts, and assessment of anal continuity.

Radiography/nuclear medicine

Radiographic tests evaluate diseases of the gut and extraluminal structures. Oral or rectal contrast agents like barium provide mucosal definition from the esophagus to the rectum. Contrast radiography also assesses gut transit and pelvic floor dysfunction. Barium swallow is the initial procedure for evaluation of dysphagia to exclude subtle rings or strictures and assess for achalasia, whereas small-bowel contrast radiology reliably diagnoses intestinal tumors and Crohn's ileitis. Contrast enemas are performed when colonoscopy is unsuccessful or contraindicated. Ultrasound and computed tomography (CT) evaluate regions not accessible by endoscopy or contrast studies, including the liver, pancreas, gallbladder, kidneys, and retroperitoneum. These tests are useful for diagnosis of mass lesions, fluid collections, organ enlargement, and in the case of ultrasound gallstones. CT and magnetic resonance (MR) colonography are being evaluated as alternatives to colonoscopy for colon cancer screening. MR imaging assesses the pancreaticobiliary ducts to

TABLE 290-2 Common Indications for Endoscopy

Upper Endoscopy	Colonoscopy	Endoscopic Retrograde Cholangiopancreatography	Endoscopic Ultrasound	Capsule Endoscopy	Double Balloon Endoscopy
Dyspepsia despite treatment	Cancer screening	Jaundice	Staging of malignancy	Obscure GI bleeding	Ablation of small-intestinal bleeding sources
Dyspepsia with signs of organic disease	Lower GI bleeding	Postbiliary surgery complaints	Characterize and biopsy submucosal mass	Suspected Crohn's disease of the small intestine	Biopsy of suspicious small-intestinal masses/ulcers
Refractory vomiting	Anemia	Cholangitis	Bile duct stones		
Dysphagia	Diarrhea	Gallstone pancreatitis	Chronic pancreatitis		
Upper GI bleeding	Polypectomy	Pancreatic/biliary/ampullary tumor	Drain pseudocyst		
Anemia	Obstruction	Unexplained pancreatitis	Large gastric folds		
Weight loss	Biopsy radiologic abnormality	Pancreatitis with unrelenting pain	Anal continuity		
Malabsorption	Cancer surveillance: family history prior polyp/cancer, colitis	Fistulas			
Biopsy radiologic abnormality	Palliate neoplasm	Biopsy radiologic abnormality			
Polypectomy	Remove foreign body	Pancreaticobiliary drainage			
Place gastrostomy	Place stent across stenosis	Sample bile			
Barrett's surveillance		Sphincter of Oddi manometry			
Palliate neoplasm					
Sample duodenal tissue/fluid					
Remove foreign body					
Endoscopic mucosal resection or ablation of dysplastic Barrett's mucosa					
Place stent across stenosis					

exclude neoplasm, stones, and sclerosing cholangitis, and the liver to characterize benign and malignant tumors. Specialized CT or MR enterography can assess intensity of inflammatory bowel disease. Angiography excludes mesenteric ischemia and determines spread of malignancy. Angiographic techniques also access the biliary tree in obstructive jaundice. CT and MR techniques can be used to screen for mesenteric occlusion, thereby limiting exposure to angiographic dyes. Positron emission tomography can facilitate distinguishing malignant from benign disease in several organ systems.

Scintigraphy both evaluates structural abnormalities and quantifies luminal transit. Radionuclide bleeding scans localize bleeding sites in patients with brisk hemorrhage so that therapy with endoscopy, angiography, or surgery may be directed. Radiolabeled leukocyte scans can search for intraabdominal abscesses not visualized on CT. Biliary scintigraphy is complementary to ultrasound in the assessment of cholecystitis. Scintigraphy to quantify esophageal and gastric emptying are well established, while techniques to measure small intestinal or colonic transit are less widely used.

Histopathology

Gut mucosal biopsies obtained at endoscopy evaluate for inflammatory, infectious, and neoplastic disease. Deep rectal biopsies assist with diagnosis of Hirschsprung's disease or amyloid. Liver biopsy is indicated in cases with abnormal liver chemistries, unexplained jaundice, following liver transplant to exclude rejection, and to characterize the degree of inflammation in patients with chronic viral hepatitis prior to initiating antiviral therapy. Biopsies obtained during CT or ultrasound can evaluate for other intraabdominal conditions not accessible by endoscopy.

Functional testing

Tests of gut function provide important data when structural testing is nondiagnostic. In addition to gastric acid and pancreatic function testing, functional testing of motor activity is provided by manometric techniques. Esophageal manometry is useful for suspected achalasia, whereas small-intestinal manometry tests for pseudoobstruction. A wireless motility capsule is now available to measure transit and contractile activity in the stomach, small intestine, and colon in a single test. Anorectal manometry with balloon expulsion testing is employed for unexplained incontinence or constipation from outlet dysfunction. Anorectal manometry and electromyography also assess anal function in fecal incontinence. Biliary manometry tests for sphincter of Oddi dysfunction with unexplained biliary pain. Measurement of breath hydrogen while fasting and after oral mono- or oligosaccharide challenge can screen for carbohydrate intolerance and small-intestinal bacterial overgrowth.

TREATMENT Gastrointestinal Disease

Management options for the patient with GI disease depend on the cause of symptoms. Available treatments include modifications in dietary intake, medications, interventional endoscopy or radiology techniques, surgery, and therapies directed to external influences.

NUTRITIONAL MANIPULATION Dietary modifications for GI disease include treatments that only reduce symptoms, therapies that correct pathologic defects, and measures that replace normal food intake with enteral or parenteral formulations. Changes that improve symptoms but do not reverse an organic abnormality include lactose restriction for lactase deficiency, liquid meals in gastroparesis, carbohydrate restrictions with dumping syndrome, and high-fiber diets in irritable bowel syndrome. The gluten-free diet for celiac disease exemplifies a modification that serves as primary therapy to reduce mucosal inflammation. Enteral medium-chain triglycerides replace normal fats with short-gut syndrome or severe ileal disease. Perfusion of liquid meals through a gastrostomy is performed in those who cannot swallow safely. Enteral feeding through a jejunostomy is considered for gastric dysmotility syndromes that preclude feeding into the stomach. Intravenous hyperalimentation is employed for individuals with generalized gut malfunction who cannot tolerate or who cannot be sustained with enteral nutrition.

PHARMACOTHERAPY Several medications are available to treat GI diseases. Considerable health care resources are expended on over-the-counter remedies. Many prescription drug classes are offered as short-term or continuous therapy of GI illness. A plethora of alternative treatments have gained popularity in GI conditions for which traditional therapies provide incomplete relief.

Over-the-Counter Agents Over-the-counter agents are reserved for mild GI symptoms. Antacids and histamine H_2 antagonists decrease symptoms in gastroesophageal reflux and dyspepsia, whereas antiflatulents and adsorbents reduce gaseous symptoms. More potent acid inhibitors such as proton pump inhibitors are now available over the counter for treatment of chronic gastroesophageal reflux disease (GERD). Fiber supplements, stool softeners, enemas, and laxatives are used for constipation. Laxatives are categorized as stimulants, osmotic agents (including isotonic preparations containing polyethylene glycol), and poorly absorbed sugars. Nonprescription antidiarrheal agents include bismuth subsalicylate, kaolin-pectin combinations, and loperamide. Supplemental enzymes include lactase pills for lactose intolerance and bacterial α-galactosidase to treat excess gas. In general, use of a nonprescription preparation for more than a short time for chronic persistent symptoms should be supervised by a health care provider.

Prescription Drugs Prescription drugs for GI diseases are a major focus of attention from pharmaceutical companies. Potent acid suppressants including drugs that inhibit the proton pump are advocated for acid reflux when over-the-counter preparations are inadequate. Cytoprotective agents rarely are used for upper gut ulcers. Prokinetic drugs stimulate GI propulsion in gastroparesis and pseudoobstruction. Prosecretory drugs are prescribed for constipation refractory to other agents. Prescription antidiarrheals include opiate drugs, anticholinergic antispasmodics, tricyclics, bile acid binders, and serotonin antagonists. Antispasmodics and antidepressants also are useful for functional abdominal pain, whereas narcotics are used for pain control in organic conditions such as disseminated malignancy and chronic pancreatitis. Antiemetics in several classes reduce nausea and vomiting. Potent pancreatic enzymes decrease malabsorption and pain from pancreatic disease. Antisecretory drugs such as the somatostatin analogue octreotide treat hypersecretory states. Antibiotics treat ulcer disease secondary to *Helicobacter pylori*, infectious diarrhea, diverticulitis, intestinal bacterial overgrowth, and Crohn's disease. Some cases of irritable bowel syndrome (especially those with diarrhea) respond to nonabsorbable antibiotic therapy. Anti-inflammatory and immunosuppressive drugs are used in ulcerative colitis, Crohn's disease, microscopic colitis, refractory celiac disease, and gut vasculitis. Chemotherapy with or without radiotherapy is offered for GI malignancies. Most GI carcinomas respond poorly to such therapy, whereas lymphomas may be cured with such intervention.

Alternative Therapies Alternative treatments are marketed to treat selected GI symptoms. Ginger, acupressure, and acustimulation have been advocated for nausea, while pyridoxine has been investigated for nausea of first-trimester pregnancy. Probiotics containing active bacterial cultures are used as adjuncts in some cases of infectious diarrhea and irritable bowel syndrome. Probiotics that selectively nourish benign luminal bacteria may ultimately show benefit in functional disorders as well. Low-potency pancreatic enzyme preparations are sold as general digestive aids but have little evidence to support their efficacy.

ENTERIC THERAPIES/INTERVENTIONAL ENDOSCOPY AND RADIOLOGY Simple luminal interventions are commonly performed for GI diseases. Nasogastric tube suction decompresses the upper gut in ileus or mechanical obstruction. Nasogastric lavage of saline or water in the patient with upper GI hemorrhage determines the rate of bleeding and helps evacuate blood prior to endoscopy. Enteral feedings can be initiated through a nasogastric or nasoenteric tube. Enemas relieve fecal impaction or assist in gas evacuation in acute colonic pseudoobstruction. A rectal tube can be left in place to vent the distal colon in colonic pseudoobstruction and other colonic distention disorders.

In addition to its diagnostic role, endoscopy has therapeutic capabilities in certain settings. Cautery techniques can stop hemorrhage from ulcers, vascular malformations, and tumors. Injection with vasoconstrictor substances or sclerosants is used for bleeding ulcers, vascular malformations, varices, and hemorrhoids. Endoscopic encirclement of varices and hemorrhoids with constricting bands stops hemorrhage from these sites, while endoscopically placed clips can occlude arterial bleeding sites. Endoscopy can remove polyps or debulk lumen-narrowing malignancies. Endoscopic mucosal resection and radio frequency techniques can remove or ablate some cases of Barrett's esophagus with dysplasia. Endoscopic sphincterotomy of the ampulla of Vater relieves symptoms of choledocholithiasis. Obstructions of the gut lumen and pancreaticobiliary tree are relieved by endoscopic dilatation or placement of plastic or expandable metal stents. In cases of acute colonic pseudoobstruction, colonoscopy is employed to withdraw luminal gas. Finally, endoscopy is commonly used to insert feeding tubes.

Radiologic measures also are useful in GI disease. Angiographic embolization or vasoconstriction decreases bleeding from sites not amenable to endoscopic intervention. Dilatation or stenting with fluoroscopic guidance relieves luminal strictures. Contrast enemas can reduce volvulus and evacuate air in acute colonic pseudoobstruction. CT and ultrasound help drain abdominal fluid collections, in many cases obviating the need for surgery. Percutaneous transhepatic cholangiography relieves biliary obstruction when ERCP is contraindicated. Lithotripsy can fragment gallstones in patients who are not candidates for surgery. In some instances, radiologic approaches offer advantages over endoscopy for gastroenterostomy placement. Finally, central venous catheters for parenteral nutrition may be placed using radiographic techniques.

SURGERY Surgery is performed to cure disease, control symptoms without cure, maintain nutrition, or palliate unresectable neoplasm. Medication-unresponsive ulcerative colitis, diverticulitis, cholecystitis, appendicitis, and intraabdominal abscess are curable with surgery, while only symptom control without cure is possible with Crohn's disease. Surgery is mandated for ulcer complications such as bleeding, obstruction, or perforation and intestinal obstructions that persist after conservative care. Fundoplication of the gastroesophageal junction is performed for severe ulcerative esophagitis and drug-refractory symptomatic acid reflux. Achalasia responds to operations to relieve lower esophageal sphincter pressure. Operations for motor disorders have been introduced including implanted electrical stimulators for gastroparesis and electrical devices and artificial sphincters for fecal incontinence. Surgery may be needed to place a jejunostomy for long-term enteral feedings. The threshold for performing surgery depends on the clinical setting. In all cases, the benefits of operation must be weighed against the potential for postoperative complications.

THERAPY DIRECTED TO EXTERNAL INFLUENCES In some conditions, GI symptoms respond to treatments directed outside the gut. Psychological therapies including psychotherapy, behavior modification, hypnosis, and biofeedback have shown efficacy in functional bowel disorders. Patients with significant psychological dysfunction and those with little response to treatments targeting the gut are likely to benefit from this form of therapy.

FURTHER READINGS

Kahrilas PJ et al: American Gastroenterological Association Institute technical review on the management of gastroesophageal reflux disease. Gastroenterology 135:1392, 2008

Lichtenstein GR et al: American Gastroenterological Association Institute technical review on corticosteroids, immunomodulators, and infliximab in inflammatory bowel disease. Gastroenterology 130:940, 2006

Longstreth GF et al: Functional bowel disorders. Gastroenterology 130:1480, 2006

Rex DK et al: American College of Gastroenterology guidelines for colorectal cancer screening 2008. Am J Gastroenterol 104:739, 2009

Yamada T (ed): *Textbook of Gastroenterology*, 5th ed. Hoboken, NJ, Wiley-Blackwell, 2008

CHAPTER 291

Gastrointestinal Endoscopy

Louis Michel Wong Kee Song
Mark Topazian

Gastrointestinal endoscopy has been attempted for over 200 years, but the introduction of semirigid gastroscopes in the middle of the twentieth century marked the dawn of the modern endoscopic era. Since then, rapid advances in endoscopic technology have led to dramatic changes in the diagnosis and treatment of many digestive diseases. Innovative endoscopic devices and new endoscopic treatment modalities continue to expand the use of endoscopy in patient care.

Flexible endoscopes provide either an optical image (transmitted over fiberoptic bundles) or an electronic video image (generated by a charge-coupled device in the tip of the endoscope). Operator controls permit deflection of the endoscope tip; fiberoptic bundles bring light to the tip of the endoscope; and working channels allow washing, suctioning, and the passage of instruments. Progressive changes in the diameter and stiffness of endoscopes have improved the ease and patient tolerance of endoscopy.

ENDOSCOPIC PROCEDURES

UPPER ENDOSCOPY

Upper endoscopy, also referred to as esophagogastroduodenoscopy (EGD), is performed by passing a flexible endoscope through the mouth into the esophagus, stomach, bulb, and second duodenum. The procedure is the best method of examining the upper gastrointestinal mucosa. While the upper gastrointestinal radiographic series has similar accuracy for diagnosis of duodenal ulcer (Fig. 291-1), EGD is superior for detection of gastric ulcers (Fig. 291-2) and flat mucosal lesions such as Barrett's esophagus (Fig. 291-3), and it permits directed biopsy and endoscopic therapy. Intravenous conscious sedation is given to most patients in the United States to ease the anxiety and discomfort of the procedure, although in many countries EGD is routinely performed with topical pharyngeal anesthesia only. Patient tolerance of unsedated EGD is improved by the use of an ultrathin, 5-mm diameter endoscope that can be passed transorally or transnasally.

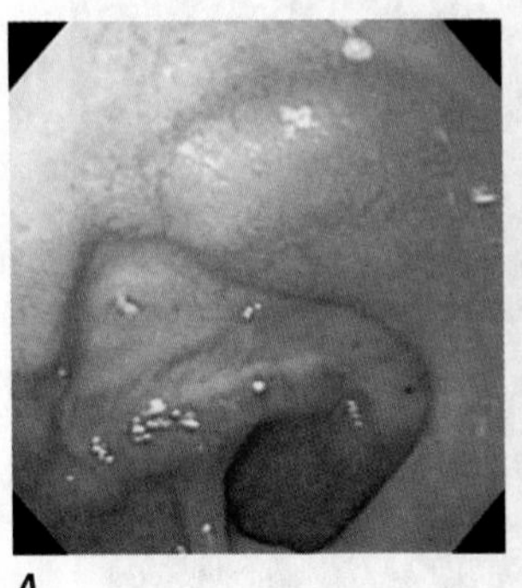
A

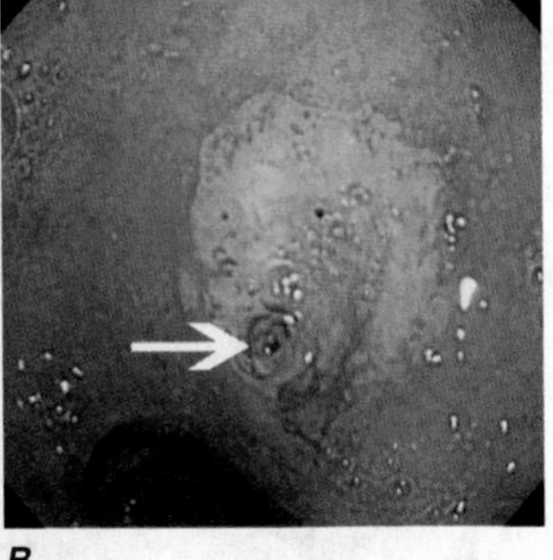
B

Figure 291-1 Duodenal ulcers. ***A.*** Ulcer with a clean base. ***B.*** Ulcer with a visible vessel (*arrow*) in a patient with recent hemorrhage.

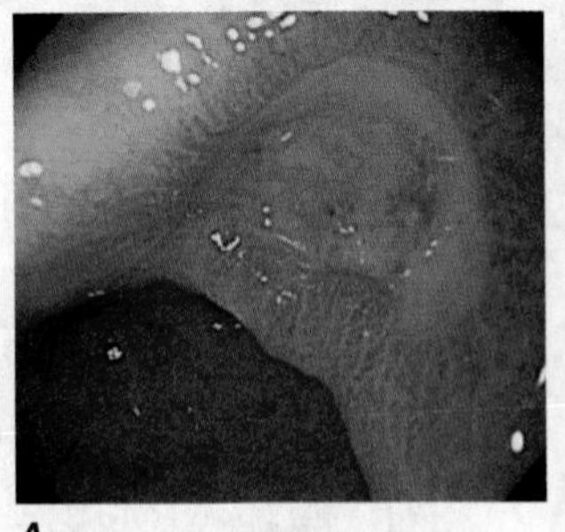
A

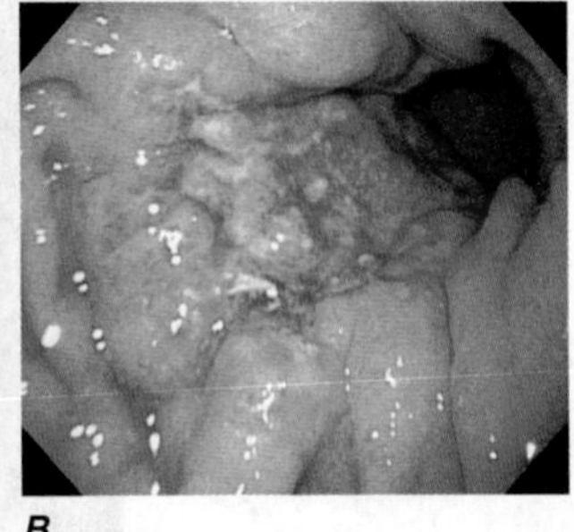
B

Figure 291-2 Gastric ulcers. ***A.*** Benign gastric ulcer. ***B.*** Malignant gastric ulcer involving greater curvature of stomach.

COLONOSCOPY

Colonoscopy is performed by passing a flexible colonoscope through the anal canal into the rectum and colon. The cecum is reached in >95% of cases, and the terminal ileum can often be examined. Colonoscopy is the gold standard for diagnosis of colonic mucosal disease. Colonoscopy has greater sensitivity than barium enema for colitis (Fig. 291-4), polyps (Fig. 291-5), and cancer (Fig. 291-6). CT colonography is an emerging technology that rivals colonoscopy's accuracy for detection of polyps and cancer. Conscious sedation is usually given before colonoscopy in the United States, although a willing patient and a skilled examiner can complete the procedure without sedation in many cases.

FLEXIBLE SIGMOIDOSCOPY

Flexible sigmoidoscopy is similar to colonoscopy but visualizes only the rectum and a variable portion of the left colon, typically to 60 cm from the anal verge. This procedure causes abdominal cramping, but it is brief and is usually performed without sedation. Flexible sigmoidoscopy is primarily used for evaluation of diarrhea and rectal outlet bleeding.

SMALL-BOWEL ENDOSCOPY

Three techniques are currently used to evaluate the small intestine, most often in patients presenting with presumed small-bowel bleeding. For *capsule endoscopy* the patient swallows a disposable capsule that contains a complementary metal oxide silicon (CMOS) chip camera. Color still images (Fig. 291-7) are transmitted wirelessly to an external receiver at several frames per second until the capsule's battery is exhausted or it is passed into the toilet. Although capsule endoscopy enables visualization of the jejunal and ileal mucosa beyond the reach of a conventional endoscope, it remains solely a diagnostic procedure at present.

Push enteroscopy is performed with a long endoscope similar in design to an upper endoscope. The enteroscope is pushed down the small bowel, sometimes with the help of a stiffening overtube that extends from the mouth to the small intestine. The proximal to mid-jejunum is usually reached, and the endoscope's instrument channel allows for biopsies or endoscopic therapy.

Deeper insertion into the small bowel can be accomplished by *single-* or *double-balloon enteroscopy* or *spiral enteroscopy* (Fig. 291-8). These instruments enable pleating of the small intestine onto an overtube (Video e36-1). With balloon-assisted enteroscopy, the entire small bowel can be visualized in some patients when both the oral and anal routes of insertion are used. Biopsies and endoscopic therapy can be performed throughout the visualized small bowel (Fig. 291-9).

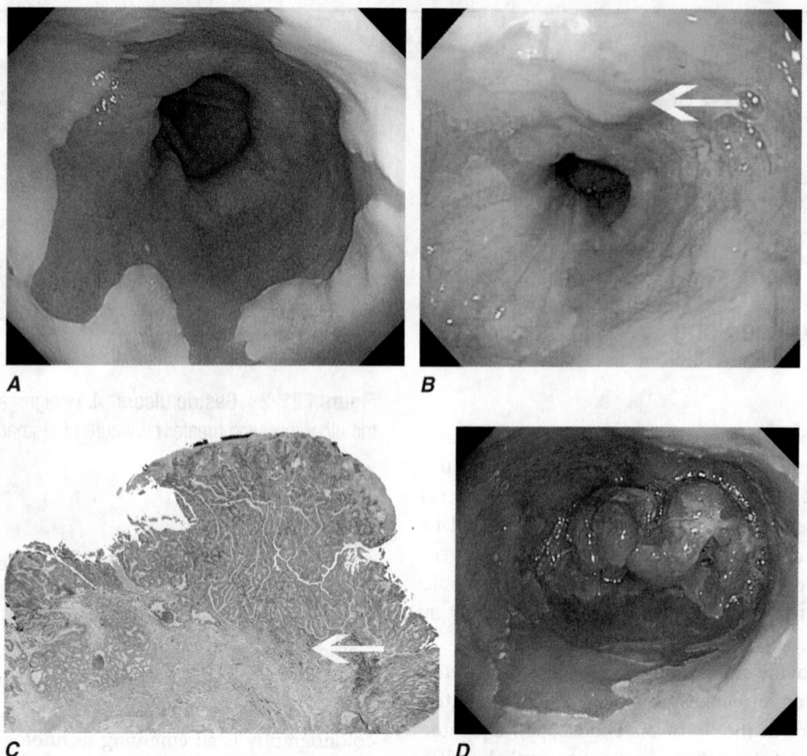

Figure 291-3 Barrett's esophagus. ***A.*** Pink tongues of Barrett's mucosa extending proximally from the gastroesophageal junction. ***B.*** Barrett's esophagus with a suspicious nodule (*arrow*) identified during endoscopic surveillance. ***C.*** Histologic finding of intramucosal adenocarcinoma in the endoscopically resected nodule. Tumor extends into the esophageal submucosa (*arrow*). ***D.*** Barrett's esophagus with locally advanced adenocarcinoma.

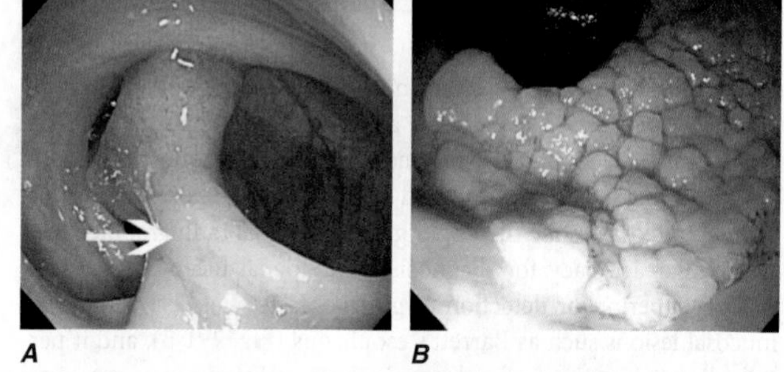

Figure 291-5 Colonic polyps. ***A.*** Pedunculated colon polyp on a thick stalk covered with normal mucosa (*arrow*). ***B.*** Sessile rectal polyp.

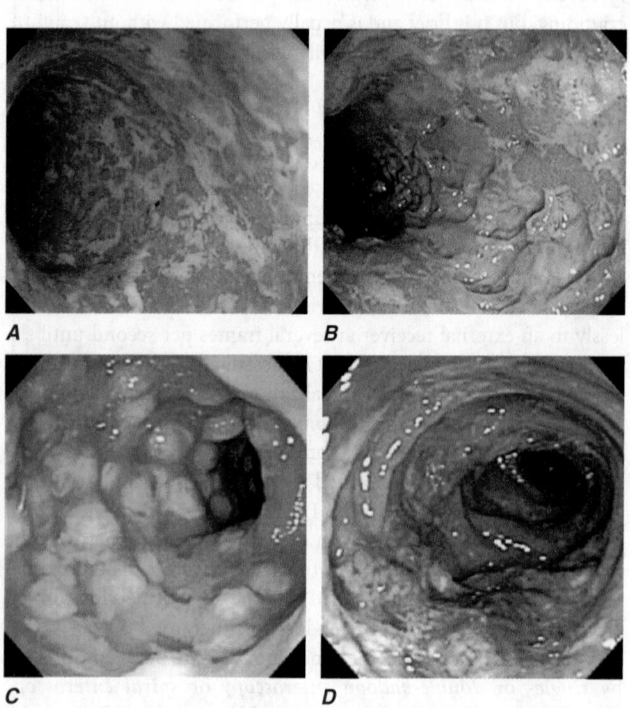

Figure 291-4 Causes of colitis. ***A.*** Chronic ulcerative colitis with diffuse ulcerations and exudates. ***B.*** Severe Crohn's colitis with deep ulcers. ***C.*** Pseudomembranous colitis with yellow, adherent pseudomembranes. ***D.*** Ischemic colitis with patchy mucosal edema, subepithelial hemorrhage, and cyanosis.

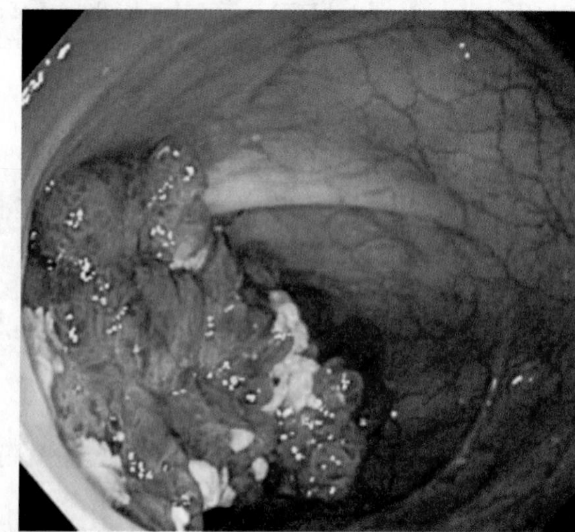

Figure 291-6 Colon adenocarcinoma growing into the lumen.

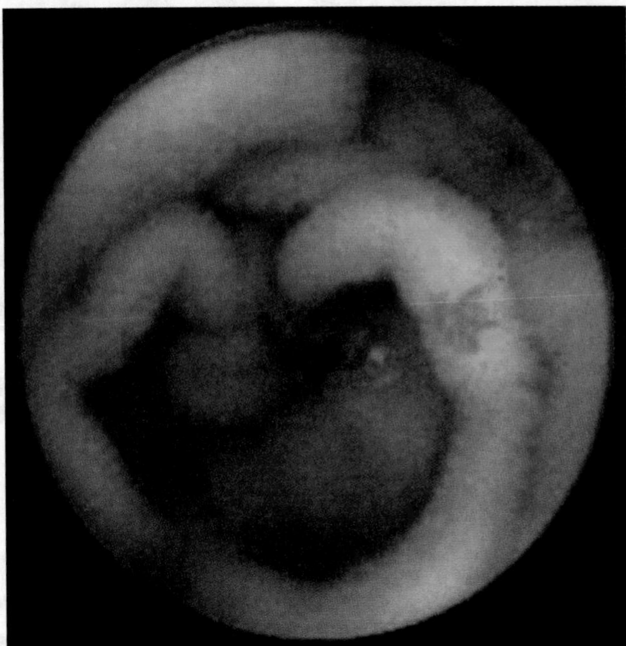

Figure 291-7 Capsule endoscopy image of jejunal vascular ectasia.

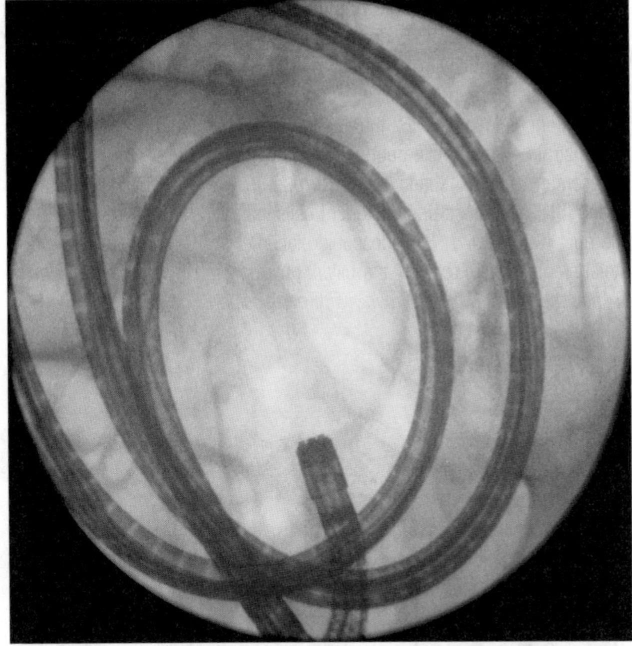

Figure 291-8 Radiograph of a double-balloon enteroscope in the small intestine.

ENDOSCOPIC RETROGRADE CHOLANGIOPANCREATOGRAPHY (ERCP)

During ERCP, a side-viewing endoscope is passed through the mouth to the duodenum, the ampulla of Vater is identified and cannulated with a thin plastic catheter, and radiographic contrast material is injected into the bile duct and pancreatic duct under fluoroscopic guidance (Fig. 291-10). When indicated, the sphincter of Oddi can be opened using the technique of endoscopic sphincterotomy (Fig. 291-11). Stones can be retrieved from the ducts, biopsies can be performed, strictures can be dilated and/or stented (Fig. 291-12), and ductal leaks can be stented (Fig. 291-13). ERCP is often performed for therapy but remains important in diagnosis, especially for ductal strictures and bile duct stones.

ENDOSCOPIC ULTRASOUND (EUS)

EUS utilizes high-frequency ultrasound transducers incorporated into the tip of a flexible endoscope. Ultrasound images are obtained of the gut wall and adjacent organs, vessels, and lymph nodes. By sacrificing depth of ultrasound penetration and bringing the ultrasound transducer close to the area of interest via endoscopy, high-resolution images are obtained. EUS provides the most accurate preoperative local staging of esophageal, pancreatic, and rectal malignancies (Fig. 291-14), although it does not detect most distant metastases. EUS is also useful for diagnosis of bile duct stones, gallbladder disease, submucosal gastrointestinal lesions, and chronic pancreatitis. Fine-needle aspirates and core biopsies of masses and lymph nodes in the posterior mediastinum, abdomen, pancreas, retroperitoneum, and pelvis can be obtained under EUS guidance (Fig. 291-15).

NATURAL ORIFICE TRANSLUMINAL ENDOSCOPIC SURGERY (NOTES)

NOTES is an evolving collection of endoscopic methods that entail passage of an endoscope or its accessories through the wall of the gastrointestinal tract (e.g., stomach) to perform diagnostic or therapeutic interventions. Some NOTES procedures, such as percutaneous endoscopic gastrostomy (PEG) or endoscopic necrosectomy of pancreatic necrosis, are established clinical procedures (Video e36-2); others, such as endoscopic appendectomy, cholecystectomy, and tubal ligation, are in development, and their ultimate clinical application is presently unclear. NOTES is currently an area of intense innovation and endoscopic research.

RISKS OF ENDOSCOPY

Medications used during conscious sedation may cause respiratory depression or allergic reactions. All endoscopic procedures carry some risk of bleeding and gastrointestinal perforation. These risks are quite low with diagnostic upper endoscopy and colonoscopy (<1:1000 procedures), although the risk is as high as 2:100 when

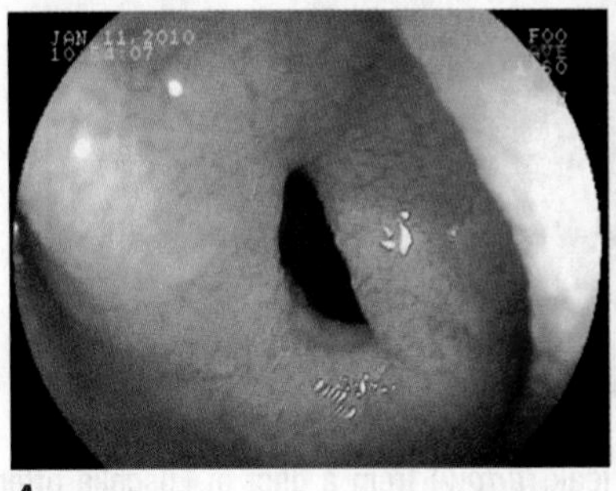

A

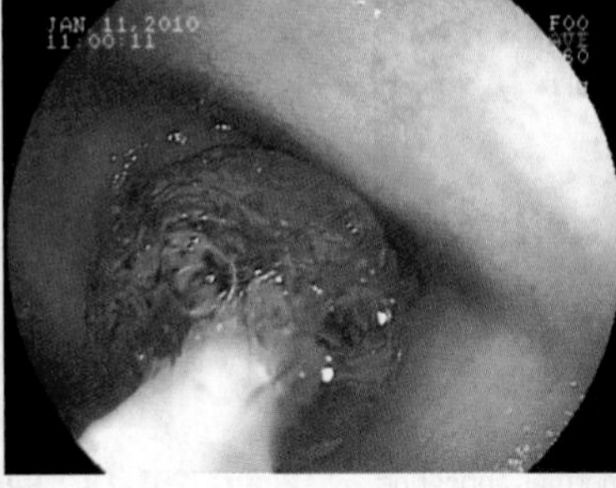

B

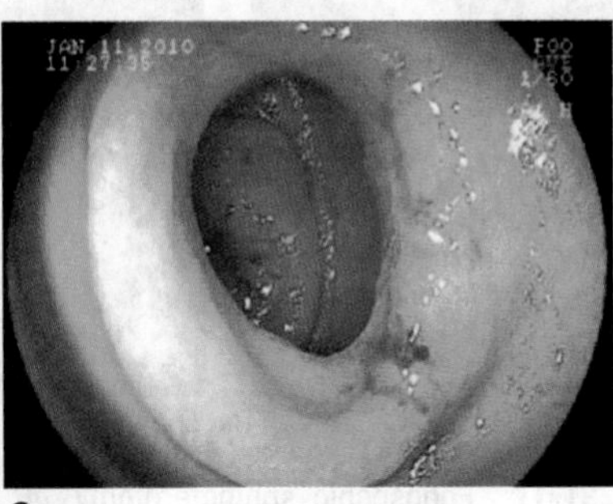

C

Figure 291-9 Nonsteroidal anti-inflammatory (NSAID)-induced proximal ileal stricture diagnosed by double-balloon endoscopy. ***A.*** Ileal stricture causing obstructive symptoms. ***B.*** Balloon dilatation of the ileal stricture. ***C.*** Appearance of stricture after dilatation.

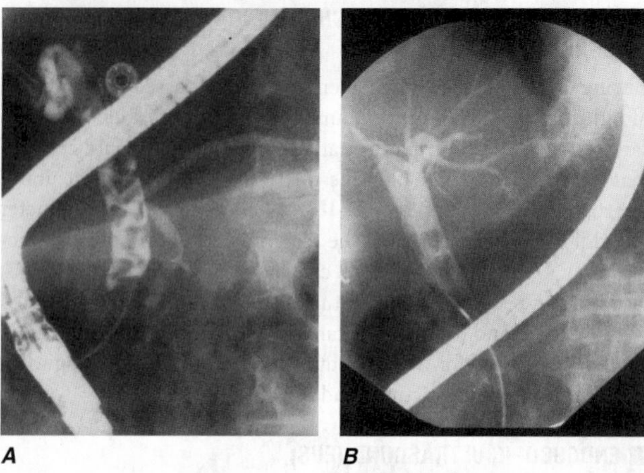

Figure 291-10 Endoscopic retrograde cholangiopancreatography (ERCP) for bile duct stones with cholangitis. ***A.*** Faceted bile duct stones are demonstrated in the common bile duct. ***B.*** After endoscopic sphincterotomy, the stones are extracted with a Dormia basket. A small abscess communicates with the left hepatic duct.

therapeutic procedures such as polypectomy, control of hemorrhage, or stricture dilatation are performed. Bleeding and perforation are rare with flexible sigmoidoscopy. The risks for diagnostic EUS (without needle aspiration) are similar to the risks for diagnostic upper endoscopy.

Infectious complications are unusual with most endoscopic procedures. Some procedures carry a higher incidence of postprocedure bacteremia, and prophylactic antibiotics may be indicated (Table 291-1).

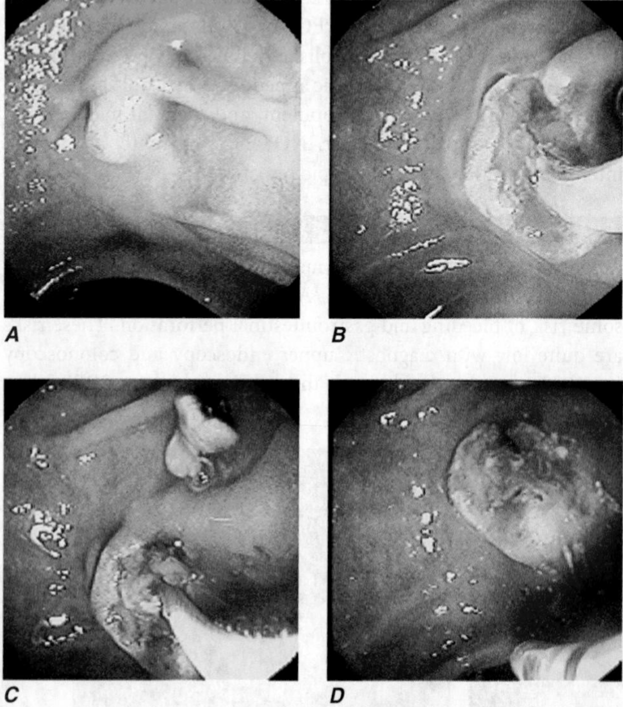

Figure 291-11 Endoscopic sphincterotomy. ***A.*** A normal-appearing ampulla of Vater. ***B.*** Sphincterotomy is performed with electrocautery. ***C.*** Bile duct stones are extracted with a balloon catheter. ***D.*** Final appearance of the sphincterotomy.

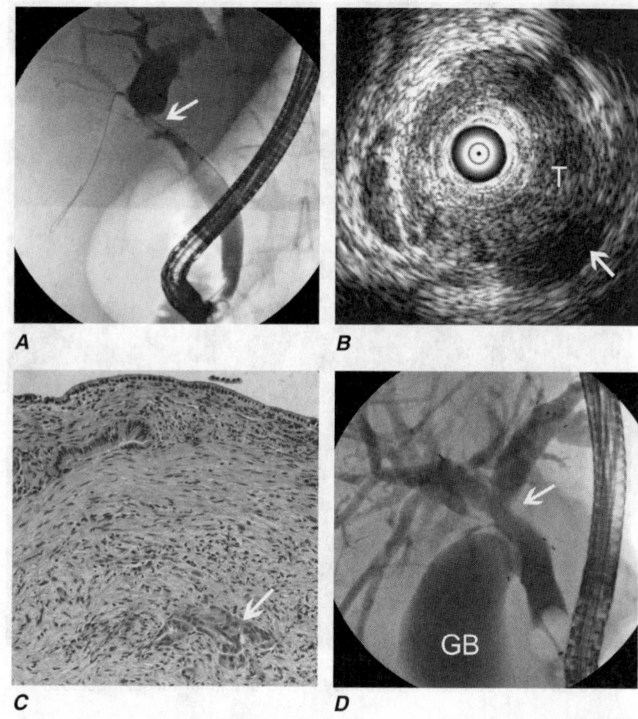

Figure 291-12 Endoscopic diagnosis, staging, and palliation of hilar cholangiocarcinoma. ***A.*** Endoscopic retrograde cholangiopancreatography (ERCP) in a patient with obstructive jaundice demonstrates a malignant-appearing stricture of the biliary confluence extending into the left and right intrahepatic ducts. ***B.*** Intraductal ultrasound of the biliary stricture demonstrates marked bile duct wall thickening due to tumor (T) with partial encasement of the hepatic artery (*arrow*). ***C.*** Intraductal biopsy obtained during ERCP demonstrates malignant cells infiltrating the submucosa of the bile duct wall (*arrow*). ***D.*** Endoscopic placement of bilateral self-expanding metal stents (arrow) relieves the biliary obstruction. GB, gallbladder. (*Image C courtesy of Dr. Thomas Smyrk; with permission.)*

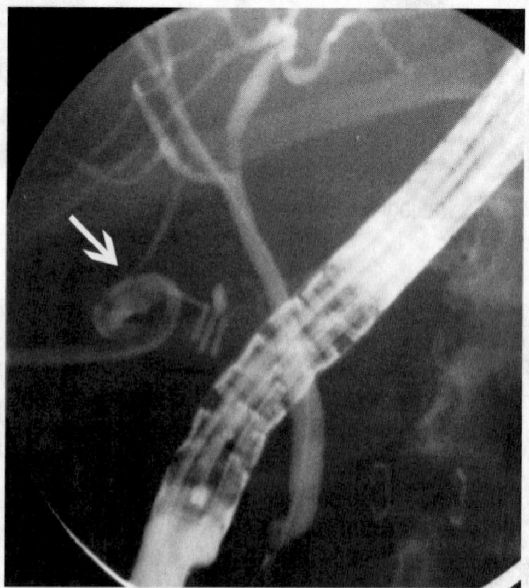

Figure 291-13 Bile leak (*arrow*) from a duct of Luschka after laparoscopic cholecystectomy. Contrast leaks from a small right intrahepatic duct into the gallbladder fossa, then flows into the pigtail of a percutaneous drainage catheter.

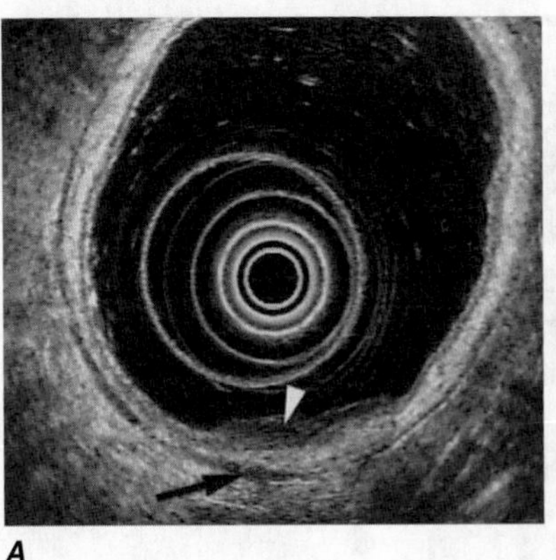

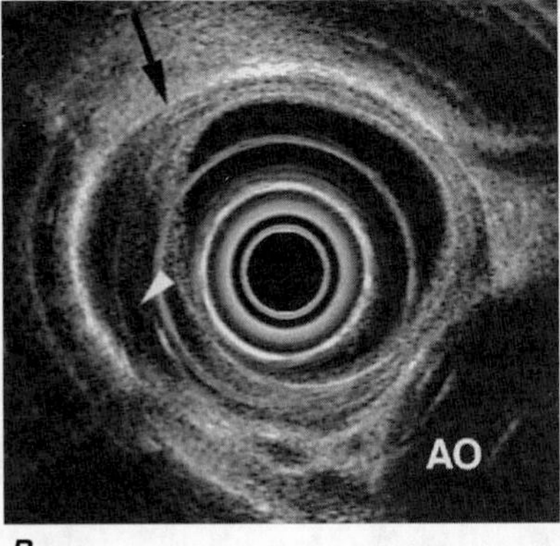

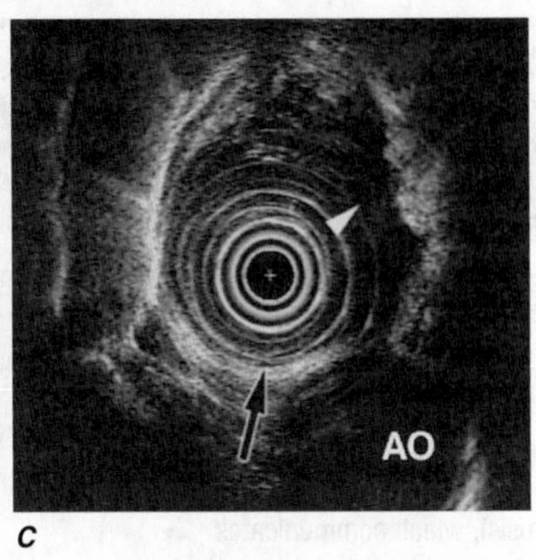

Figure 291-14 Local staging of gastrointestinal cancers with endoscopic ultrasound. In each example the white arrowhead marks the primary tumor and the black arrow indicates the muscularis propria (mp) of the intestinal wall. ***A.*** T1 gastric cancer. The tumor does not invade the mp. ***B.*** T2 esophageal cancer. The tumor invades the mp. ***C.*** T3 esophageal cancer. The tumor extends through the mp into the surrounding tissue, and focally abuts the aorta. AO, aorta.

ERCP carries additional risks. Pancreatitis occurs in about 5% of patients undergoing ERCP and in up to 25% of patients with sphincter of Oddi dysfunction. Young anicteric patients with normal ducts are at increased risk. Post-ERCP pancreatitis is usually mild and self-limited but may rarely result in prolonged hospitalization, surgery, diabetes, or death. Bleeding occurs in 1% of endoscopic sphincterotomies. Ascending cholangitis, pseudocyst infection, retroperitoneal perforation, and abscess may occur as a result of ERCP.

Percutaneous gastrostomy tube placement during EGD is associated with a 10–15% incidence of complications, most often wound infections. Fasciitis, pneumonia, bleeding, buried bumper syndrome, and colonic injury may result from gastrostomy tube placement.

URGENT ENDOSCOPY

ACUTE GASTROINTESTINAL HEMORRHAGE

Endoscopy is an important diagnostic and therapeutic technique for patients with acute gastrointestinal hemorrhage. Although gastrointestinal bleeding stops spontaneously in most cases, some patients will have persistent or recurrent hemorrhage that may be life-threatening. Clinical predictors of rebleeding help identify patients most likely to benefit from urgent endoscopy and endoscopic, angiographic, or surgical hemostasis.

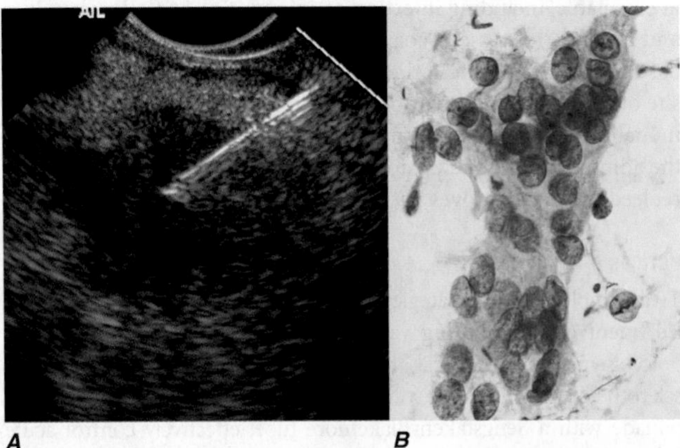

Figure 291-15 Endoscopic ultrasound (EUS)-guided fine-needle aspiration (FNA). ***A.*** Ultrasound image of a 22-gauge needle passed through the duodenal wall and positioned in a hypoechoic pancreatic head mass. ***B.*** Micrograph of aspirated malignant cells. *(Image B courtesy of Dr. Michael R. Henry; with permission.)*

Initial evaluation

The initial evaluation of the bleeding patient focuses on the magnitude of hemorrhage as reflected by the postural vital signs, the frequency of hematemesis or melena, and (in some cases) findings on nasogastric lavage. Decreases in hematocrit and hemoglobin lag behind the clinical course and are not reliable gauges of the magnitude of acute bleeding. This initial evaluation, completed well before the bleeding source is confidently identified, guides immediate supportive care of the patient and helps determine the timing of endoscopy. The severity of the initial hemorrhage is the most important indication for urgent endoscopy, since a large initial bleed increases the likelihood of ongoing or recurrent bleeding. Patients with resting hypotension, repeated hematemesis, bloody nasogastric aspirate that does not clear with large volume lavage, or orthostatic change in vital signs, or those requiring blood transfusions, should be considered for urgent endoscopy. In addition, patients with cirrhosis, coagulopathy, respiratory or renal failure, and those over 70 years of age are more likely to have significant rebleeding.

Bedside evaluation also suggests an upper or lower gastrointestinal source of bleeding in most patients. Over 90% of patients with melena are bleeding proximal to the ligament of Treitz, and about 90% of patients with hematochezia are bleeding from the colon. Melena can result from bleeding in the small bowel or right colon, especially in older patients with slow colonic transit. Conversely, some patients with massive hematochezia may be bleeding from an upper gastrointestinal source, such as a gastric Dieulafoy's lesion or duodenal ulcer, with rapid intestinal transit. Early upper endoscopy should be considered in such patients.

Endoscopy should be performed after the patient has been resuscitated with intravenous fluids and transfusions as necessary. Marked coagulopathy or thrombocytopenia is usually treated before endoscopy, since correction of these abnormalities may lead to resolution of bleeding, and techniques for endoscopic hemostasis are limited in such patients. Metabolic derangements should also be addressed. Tracheal intubation for airway protection should be considered before upper endoscopy in patients with repeated recent hematemesis and suspected variceal hemorrhage.

Most patients with impressive hematochezia can undergo colonoscopy after a rapid colonic purge with a polyethylene glycol solution; the preparation fluid may be administered via a nasogastric tube. Colonoscopy has a higher diagnostic yield than radionuclide bleeding scans or angiography in lower gastrointestinal bleeding, and endoscopic therapy can be applied in some cases. In a minority of cases, endoscopic assessment is hindered by poor visualization

TABLE 291-1 Antibiotic Prophylaxis for Endoscopic Procedures

Patient Condition	Procedure Contemplated	Goal of Prophylaxis	Periprocedural Antibiotic Prophylaxis
All cardiac conditions	Any endoscopic procedure	Prevention of infective endocarditis	Not indicated
Bile-duct obstruction in the absence of cholangitis	ERCP with complete drainage	Prevention of cholangitis	Not recommended
Bile-duct obstruction in absence of cholangitis	ERCP with anticipated incomplete drainage (e.g., PSC, hilar strictures)	Prevention of cholangitis	Recommended; continue antibiotics after the procedure
Sterile pancreatic fluid collection (e.g., pseudocyst, necrosis), which communicates with pancreatic duct	ERCP	Prevention of cyst infection	Recommended
Sterile pancreatic fluid collection	Transmural drainage	Prevention of cyst infection	Recommended
Solid lesion along upper GI tract	EUS-FNA	Prevention of local infection	Not recommended[a]
Solid lesion along lower GI tract	EUS-FNA	Prevention of local infection	Insufficient data to make firm recommendation[b]
Cystic lesions along GI tract (including mediastinum)	EUS-FNA	Prevention of cyst infection	Recommended
All patients	Percutaneous endoscopic feeding tube placement	Prevention of peristomal infection	Recommended
Cirrhosis with acute GI bleeding	Required for all patients, regardless of endoscopic procedures	Prevention of infectious complications and reduction of mortality	Upon admission[c]
Synthetic vascular graft and other nonvalvular cardiovascular devices	Any endoscopic procedure	Prevention of graft and device infection	Not recommended[d]
Prosthetic joints	Any endoscopic procedure	Prevention of septic arthritis	Not recommended[e]

[a]Low rates of bacteremia and local infection.

[b]Endoscopists may choose on a case by case basis.

[c]Risk for bacterial infection associated with cirrhosis and GI bleeding is well established.

[d]No reported cases of infection associated with endoscopy.

[e]Very low risk of infection.

Abbreviations: ERCP, endoscopic retrograde cholangiopancreatography; EUS-FNA, endoscopic ultrasound–fine-needle aspiration; PSC, primary sclerosing cholangitis.

Source: Adapted from S Banerjee et al: Gastrointest Endosc 67:719, 2008; with permission from Elsevier.

due to persistent vigorous bleeding with recurrent hemodynamic instability, and other techniques (such as angiography or emergent subtotal colectomy) must be employed. In such patients, massive bleeding originating from an upper gastrointestinal source should also be considered and excluded by upper endoscopy. The anal and rectal mucosa should be visualized endoscopically early in the course of massive rectal bleeding, as bleeding lesions in or close to the anal canal may be identified that are amenable to endoscopic or surgical transanal hemostatic techniques.

Peptic ulcer

The endoscopic appearance of peptic ulcers provides useful prognostic information and guides the need for endoscopic therapy in patients with acute hemorrhage (Fig. 291-16). A clean-based ulcer is associated with a low, 3–5% risk of rebleeding; patients with melena and a clean-based ulcer are often discharged home from the emergency room or endoscopy suite if they are young, reliable, and otherwise healthy. Flat pigmented spots and adherent clots covering the ulcer base have a 10 and 20% risk of rebleeding, respectively. Endoscopic therapy is often considered for an ulcer with an adherent clot. When a platelet plug is seen protruding from a vessel wall in the base of an ulcer (so-called sentinel clot or visible vessel), the risk of rebleeding from the ulcer is 40%. This finding generally leads to endoscopic therapy to decrease the rebleeding rate. Occasionally, active spurting from an ulcer is seen with >90% risk of ongoing bleeding without therapy.

Endoscopic therapy of ulcers with high-risk stigmata typically lowers the rebleeding rate to 5–10%. Several hemostatic techniques are available, including injection of epinephrine or a sclerosant into and around the vessel, "coaptive coagulation" of the vessel in the base of the ulcer using a thermal probe that is pressed against the site of bleeding, placement of hemoclips, or a combination of these modalities (Video e36-3). In conjunction with endoscopic therapy, the administration of a proton pump inhibitor decreases the risk of rebleeding and improves patient outcome.

Varices

Two complementary strategies guide therapy of bleeding varices: local treatment of the bleeding varices and treatment of the underlying portal hypertension. Local therapies, including endoscopic variceal sclerotherapy, endoscopic variceal band ligation, and balloon tamponade with a Sengstaken-Blakemore tube, effectively control acute hemorrhage in most patients, although therapies that decrease portal pressure (pharmacologic treatment, surgical shunts, or radiologically placed intrahepatic portosystemic shunts) also play an important role.

Endoscopic variceal ligation (EVL) is indicated for the prevention of a first bleed from large esophageal varices (Fig. 291-17), particularly in patients in whom beta blockers are contraindicated

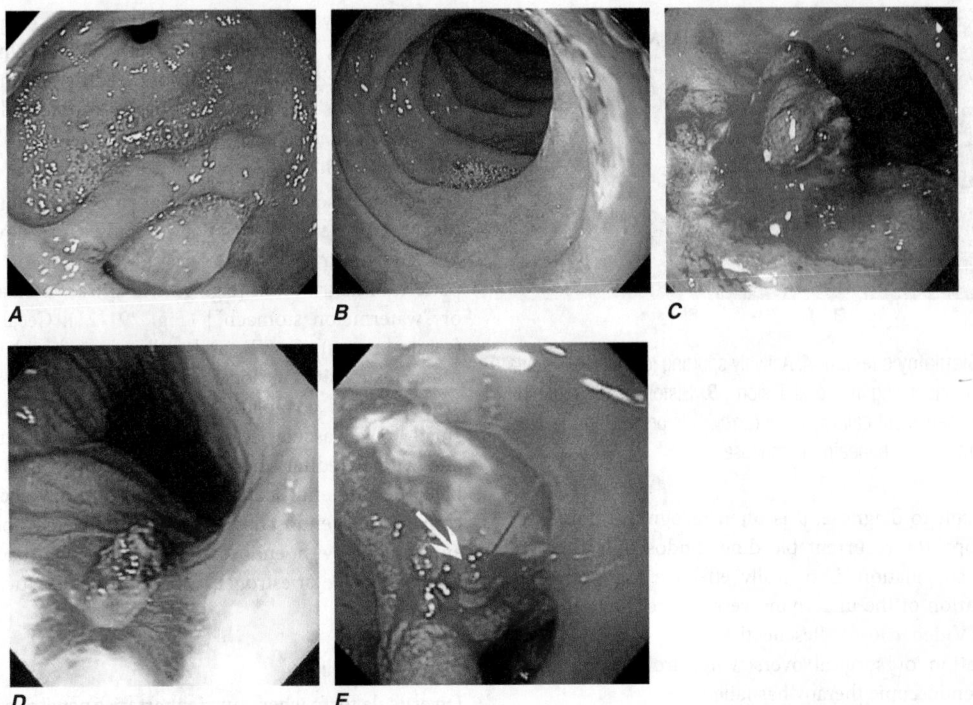

Figure 291-16 Stigmata of hemorrhage in peptic ulcers. ***A.*** Gastric antral ulcer with a clean base. ***B.*** Duodenal ulcer with flat pigmented spots. ***C.*** Duodenal ulcer with a dense adherent clot. ***D.*** Gastric ulcer with a pigmented protuberance/visible vessel. ***E.*** Duodenal ulcer with active spurting (*arrow*).

or not tolerated (primary prophylaxis). EVL is also the preferred endoscopic therapy for control of active esophageal variceal bleeding and for subsequent eradication of esophageal varices (secondary prophylaxis). During EVL, a varix is suctioned into a cap fitted on the end of the endoscope, and a rubber band is released from the cap, ligating the varix (Video e36-4). EVL controls acute hemorrhage in up to 90% of patients. Complications of EVL, such as post-banding ulcer bleeding and esophageal stenosis, are uncommon. Endoscopic variceal sclerotherapy (EVS) involves the injection of a sclerosing, thrombogenic solution into or next to the esophageal varices. EVS also controls acute hemorrhage in most patients but has a higher complication rate than EVL. These techniques are used when varices are actively bleeding during endoscopy or (more commonly) when varices are the only identifiable cause of acute hemorrhage. Bleeding from large gastric fundic varices (Fig. 291-18) is best treated with endoscopic cyanoacrylate ("glue") injection (Video e36-5), since EVL or EVS of these varices are associated with a high rebleeding rate. Complications of cyanoacrylate injection include infection and glue embolization to other organs, such as the lungs, brain, and spleen.

After treatment of the acute hemorrhage, an elective course of endoscopic therapy can be undertaken with the goal of eradicating esophageal varices and preventing rebleeding months to years later. However, this chronic therapy is less successful, preventing long-term rebleeding in ~50% of patients. Pharmacologic therapies that decrease portal pressure have similar efficacy, and the two modalities may be combined.

Dieulafoy's lesion

This lesion, also called *persistent caliber artery*, is a large-caliber arteriole that runs immediately beneath the gastrointestinal mucosa and bleeds through a pinpoint mucosal erosion (Fig. 291-19). Dieulafoy's lesion is seen most commonly on the lesser curvature of the proximal stomach, causes impressive arterial hemorrhage,

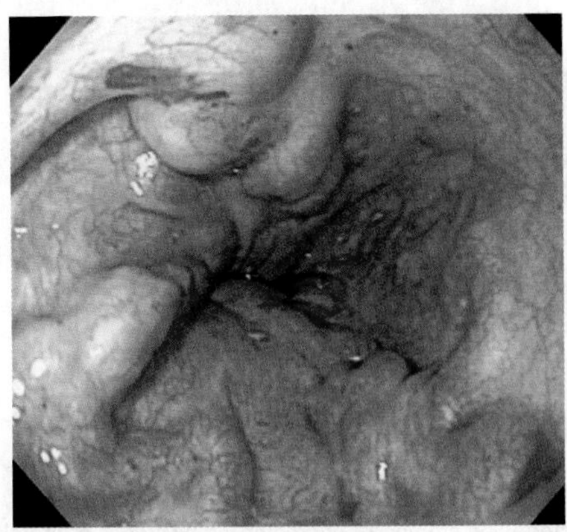

Figure 291-17 Esophageal varices.

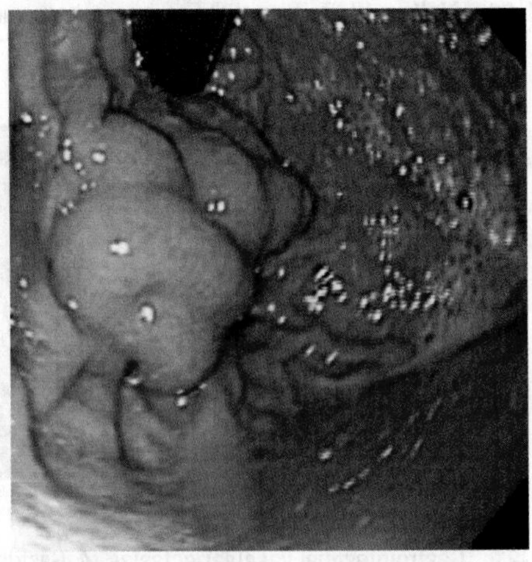

Figure 291-18 Gastric fundic varices.

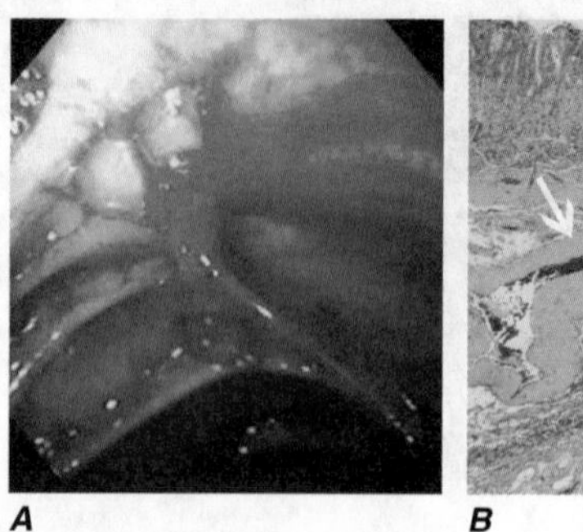

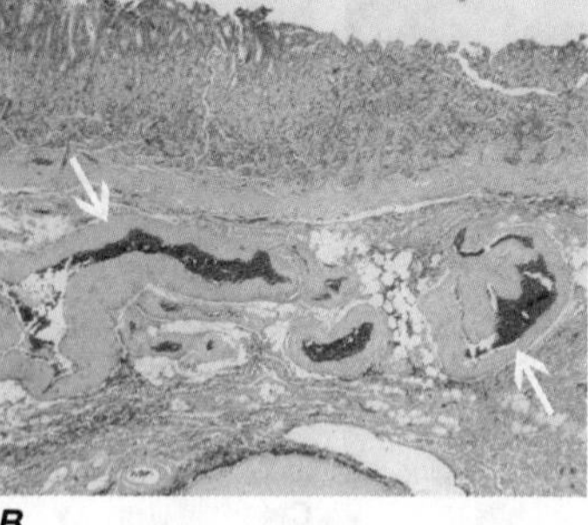

Figure 291-19 Dieulafoy's lesion. ***A.*** Actively spurting jejunal Dieulafoy's lesion. There is no underlying mucosal lesion. ***B.*** Histology of a gastric Dieulafoy's lesion. A persistent caliber artery (*arrows*) is present in the gastric submucosa, immediately beneath the mucosa.

and may be difficult to diagnose; it is often recognized only after repeated endoscopy for recurrent bleeding. Endoscopic therapy, such as thermal coagulation, is typically effective for control of bleeding and ablation of the underlying vessel once the lesion has been identified (Video e36-6). Rescue therapies, such as angiographic embolization or surgical oversewing, are considered in situations where endoscopic therapy has failed.

Mallory-Weiss tear

A Mallory-Weiss tear is a linear mucosal rent near or across the gastroesophageal junction that is often associated with retching or vomiting (Fig. 291-20). When the tear disrupts a submucosal arteriole, brisk hemorrhage may result. Endoscopy is the best method of diagnosis, and an actively bleeding tear can be treated endoscopically with epinephrine injection, coaptive coagulation, band ligation, or hemoclips (Video e36-7). Unlike peptic ulcer, a Mallory-Weiss tear with a nonbleeding sentinel clot in its base rarely rebleeds and thus does not necessitate endoscopic therapy.

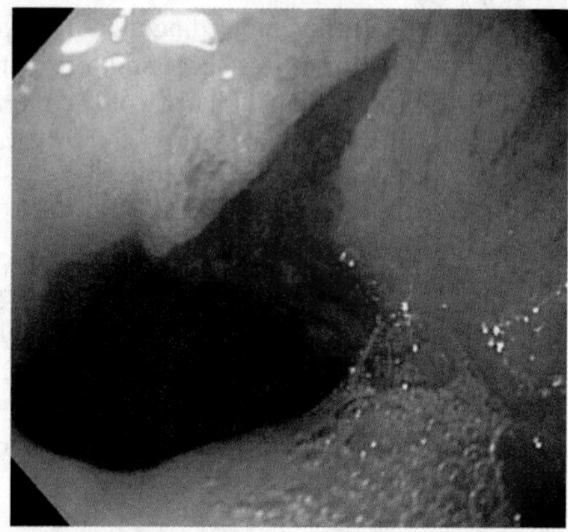

Figure 291-20 Mallory-Weiss tear at the gastroesophageal junction.

Vascular ectasias

Vascular ectasias are flat mucosal vascular anomalies that are best diagnosed by endoscopy. They usually cause slow intestinal blood loss and occur either in a sporadic fashion or in a well-defined pattern of distribution [e.g., gastric antral vascular ectasia (GAVE) or "watermelon stomach"] (Fig. 291-21). Cecal vascular ectasias (senile lesions), GAVE, and radiation-induced rectal ectasias are often responsive to local endoscopic ablative therapy, such as argon plasma coagulation (Video e36-8). Patients with diffuse small-bowel vascular ectasias (associated with chronic renal failure and with hereditary hemorrhagic telangiectasia) may continue to bleed despite endoscopic treatment of easily accessible lesions by conventional endoscopy. These patients may benefit from deep enteroscopy with endoscopic therapy, pharmacologic treatment with octreotide or estrogen/progesterone therapy, or intraoperative enteroscopy.

Colonic diverticula

Diverticula form where nutrient arteries penetrate the muscular wall of the colon en route to the colonic mucosa (Fig. 291-22). The artery found in the base of a diverticulum may bleed, causing painless and impressive hematochezia. Colonoscopy is indicated in patients with hematochezia and suspected diverticular hemorrhage, since other causes of bleeding (such as vascular ectasias, colitis, and colon cancer) must be excluded. In addition, an actively bleeding diverticulum may be seen and treated during colonoscopy (Video e36-9).

GASTROINTESTINAL OBSTRUCTION AND PSEUDOOBSTRUCTION

Endoscopy is useful for evaluation and treatment of some forms of gastrointestinal obstruction. An important exception is small bowel obstruction due to surgical adhesions, which is generally not diagnosed or treated endoscopically. Esophageal, gastroduodenal, and colonic obstruction or pseudoobstruction can all be diagnosed and often managed endoscopically.

Acute esophageal obstruction

Esophageal obstruction by impacted food (Fig. 291-23) or an ingested foreign body is a potentially life-threatening event and represents an endoscopic emergency. Left untreated, the patient may develop esophageal ulceration, ischemia, and perforation. Patients with persistent esophageal obstruction often have hypersalivation and are usually unable to swallow water; endoscopy is generally

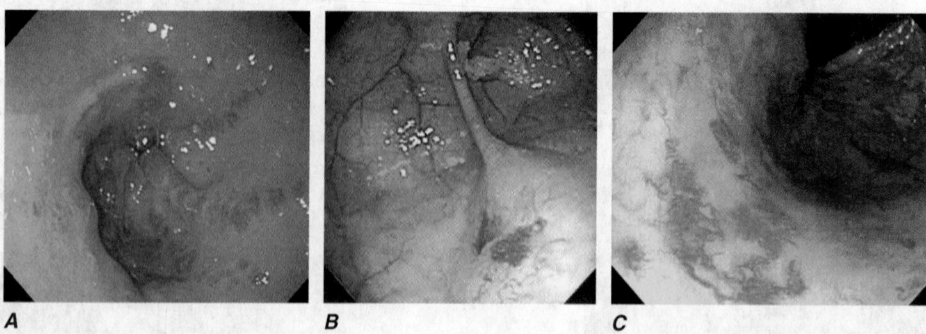

Figure 291-21 Gastrointestinal vascular ectasias. ***A.*** Gastric antral vascular ectasia ("watermelon stomach") characterized by stripes of prominent flat or raised vascular ectasias. ***B.*** Cecal vascular ectasias. ***C.*** Radiation-induced vascular ectasias of the rectum in a patient previously treated for prostate cancer.

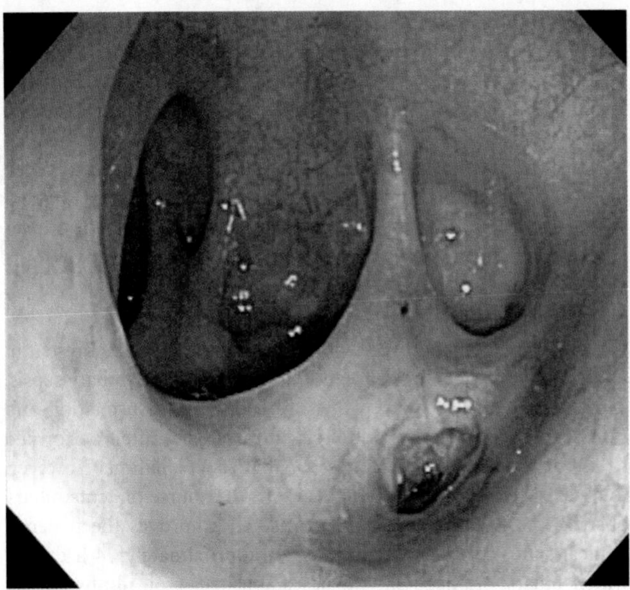

Figure 291-22 Colonic diverticula.

the best initial test in such patients, since endoscopic removal of the obstructing material is usually possible, and the presence of an underlying esophageal pathology can often be determined. Radiographs of the chest and neck should be considered before endoscopy in patients with fever, obstruction for ≥24 h, or ingestion of a sharp object such as a fishbone. Radiographic contrast studies interfere with subsequent endoscopy and are not advisable in most patients with a clinical picture of esophageal obstruction. Occasionally, sublingual nifedipine or nitrates, or intravenous glucagon, may resolve an esophageal food impaction, but in most patients an underlying web, ring, or stricture is present and endoscopic removal of the obstructing food bolus is necessary.

Gastric outlet obstruction

Obstruction of the gastric outlet is commonly caused by gastric, duodenal, or pancreatic malignancy, or chronic peptic ulceration with stenosis of the pylorus. Patients vomit partially digested food many hours after eating. Gastric decompression with a nasogastric tube and subsequent lavage for removal of retained material is the

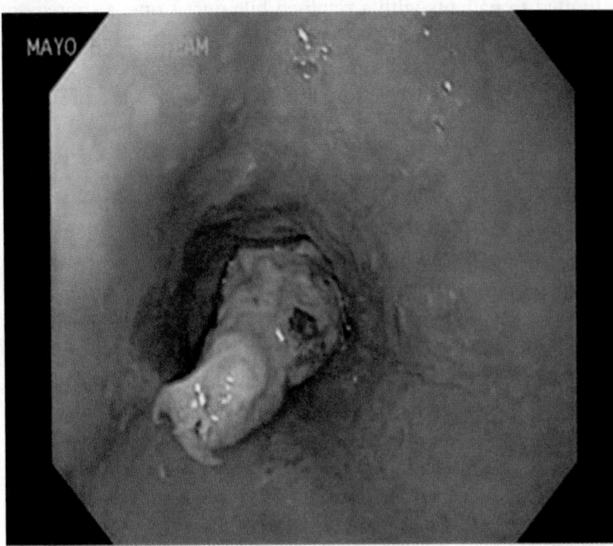

Figure 291-23 Esophageal food (meat) impaction.

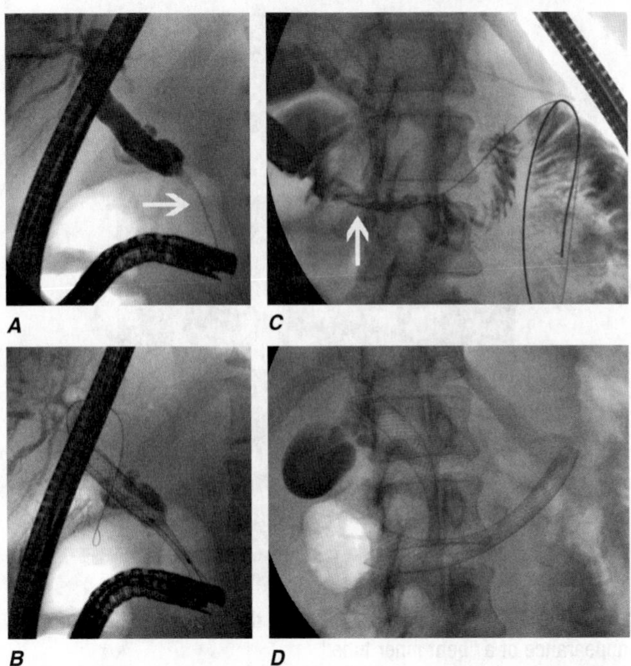

Figure 291-24 Biliary and duodenal self-expanding metal stents (SEMS) for obstruction caused by pancreatic cancer. ***A.*** Endoscopic retrograde cholangiopancreatography (ERCP) demonstrates a distal bile duct stricture (*arrow*). ***B.*** A biliary SEMS is placed. ***C.*** Contrast injection demonstrates a duodenal stricture (*arrow*). ***D.*** Biliary and duodenal SEMS in place.

first step in treatment. The diagnosis can then be confirmed with a saline load test, if desired. Endoscopy is useful for diagnosis and treatment. Patients with benign pyloric stenosis may be treated with endoscopic balloon dilatation of the pylorus, and a course of endoscopic dilatation results in long-term relief of symptoms in about 50% of patients. Malignant gastric outlet obstruction can be relieved with endoscopically placed expandable stents (Fig. 291-24) in patients with inoperable malignancy.

Colonic obstruction and pseudoobstruction

These both present with abdominal distention and discomfort; tympany; and a dilated, air-filled colon on plain abdominal radiography. The radiographic appearance can be characteristic of a particular condition, such as sigmoid volvulus (Fig. 291-25). Both structural obstruction and pseudoobstruction may lead to colonic perforation if untreated. Acute colonic pseudoobstruction is a form of colonic ileus that is usually attributable to electrolyte disorders, narcotic and anticholinergic medications, immobility (as after surgery), and retroperitoneal hemorrhage or mass. Multiple causative factors are often present. Colonoscopy, water-soluble contrast enema, or CT may be used to look for an obstructing lesion and differentiate obstruction from pseudoobstruction. One of these diagnostic studies should be strongly considered if the patient does not have clear risk factors for pseudoobstruction, if radiographs do not show air in the rectum, or if the patient fails to improve when underlying causes of pseudoobstruction have been addressed. The risk of cecal perforation in pseudoobstruction rises when the cecal diameter exceeds 12 cm, and decompression of the colon may be achieved using intravenous neostigmine or via colonoscopic decompression (Fig. 291-26). Most patients should receive a trial of conservative therapy (with correction of electrolyte disorders, removal of offending medications, and increased mobilization) before undergoing an invasive decompressive procedure for colonic pseudoobstruction.

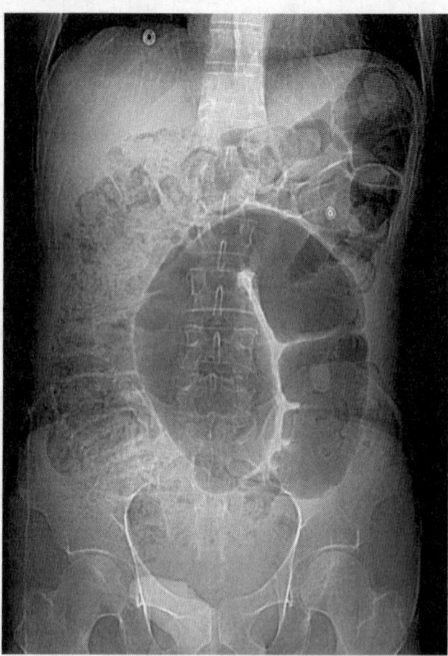

Figure 291-25 Sigmoid volvulus with the characteristic radiologic appearance of a "bent inner tube."

Colonic obstruction is an indication for urgent intervention. Emergent diverting colostomy may be performed with a subsequent second operation after bowel preparation to treat the underlying cause of obstruction. Colonoscopic placement of an expandable stent is an alternative that can relieve malignant obstruction without emergency surgery and permit bowel preparation for an elective one-stage operation (Fig. 291-27).

ACUTE BILIARY OBSTRUCTION

The steady, severe pain that occurs when a gallstone acutely obstructs the common bile duct often brings patients to a hospital. The diagnosis of a ductal stone is suspected when the patient is jaundiced or when serum liver tests or pancreatic enzyme levels are elevated; it is confirmed by direct cholangiography (performed endoscopically, percutaneously, or during surgery). ERCP is currently the primary means of diagnosing and treating common bile duct stones in most hospitals in the United States (Figs. 291-10 and 291-11).

Bile duct imaging

While transabdominal ultrasound diagnoses only a minority of bile duct stones, magnetic resonance cholangiopancreatography (MRCP) and EUS are >90% accurate and have an important role in diagnosis. Examples of these modalities are shown in Fig. 291-28.

If the suspicion for a bile duct stone is high and urgent treatment is required (as in a patient with obstructive jaundice and biliary sepsis), ERCP is the procedure of choice, since it remains the gold standard for diagnosis and allows for immediate treatment (Video e36-10). If a persistent bile duct stone is unlikely (as in a patient with gallstone pancreatitis), ERCP may be supplanted by less invasive imaging techniques, such as EUS or MRCP.

Ascending cholangitis

Charcot's triad of jaundice, abdominal pain, and fever is present in about 70% of patients with ascending cholangitis and biliary sepsis. These patients are managed initially with fluid resuscitation and intravenous antibiotics. Abdominal ultrasound is often performed to assess for gallbladder stones and bile duct dilation. However, the bile duct may not be dilated early in the course of acute biliary obstruction. Medical management usually improves the patient's clinical status, providing a window of approximately 24 h during which biliary drainage should be established, typically by ERCP. Undue delay can result in recrudescence of overt sepsis and increased morbidity and mortality rates. In addition to Charcot's triad, the additional presence of shock and confusion (Reynolds's pentad) is associated with high mortality rate and should prompt an urgent intervention to restore biliary drainage.

Gallstone pancreatitis

Gallstones may cause acute pancreatitis as they pass through the ampulla of Vater. The occurrence of gallstone pancreatitis usually implies passage of a stone into the duodenum, and only about 20% of patients harbor a persistent stone in the ampulla or the common bile duct. Retained stones are more common in patients with jaundice, rising serum liver tests following hospitalization, severe pancreatitis, or superimposed ascending cholangitis.

Urgent ERCP decreases the morbidity rate of gallstone pancreatitis in a subset of patients with retained bile duct stones. It is unclear whether the benefit of ERCP is mainly attributable to treatment and prevention of ascending cholangitis or to relief of pancreatic duct obstruction. ERCP is warranted early in the course of gallstone pancreatitis if ascending cholangitis is suspected, especially in a jaundiced patient. Urgent ERCP also appears to benefit patients predicted to have severe pancreatitis using a clinical index of severity such as the Glasgow or Ranson score. Since the benefit of ERCP is limited to patients with a retained bile duct stone, a strategy of initial MRCP or EUS for diagnosis decreases the utilization of ERCP in gallstone pancreatitis and improves clinical outcomes by limiting the occurrence of ERCP-related complications.

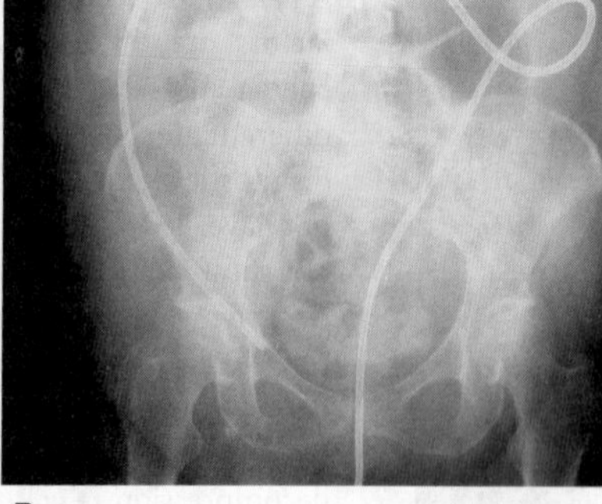

Figure 291-26 Acute colonic pseudoobstruction. ***A.*** Acute colonic dilatation occurring in a patient soon after knee surgery. ***B.*** Colonoscopic placement of decompression tube with marked improvement in colonic dilatation.

ELECTIVE ENDOSCOPY

DYSPEPSIA

Dyspepsia is a chronic or recurrent burning discomfort or pain in the upper abdomen that may be caused by diverse processes such as gastroesophageal reflux, peptic ulcer disease, and "nonulcer dyspepsia," a heterogeneous category that includes disorders of motility, sensation, and somatization. Gastric and esophageal malignancies are less common causes of dyspepsia. Careful history-taking allows accurate differential diagnosis of dyspepsia in only about half of patients. In the remainder, endoscopy can be a useful diagnostic tool, especially in

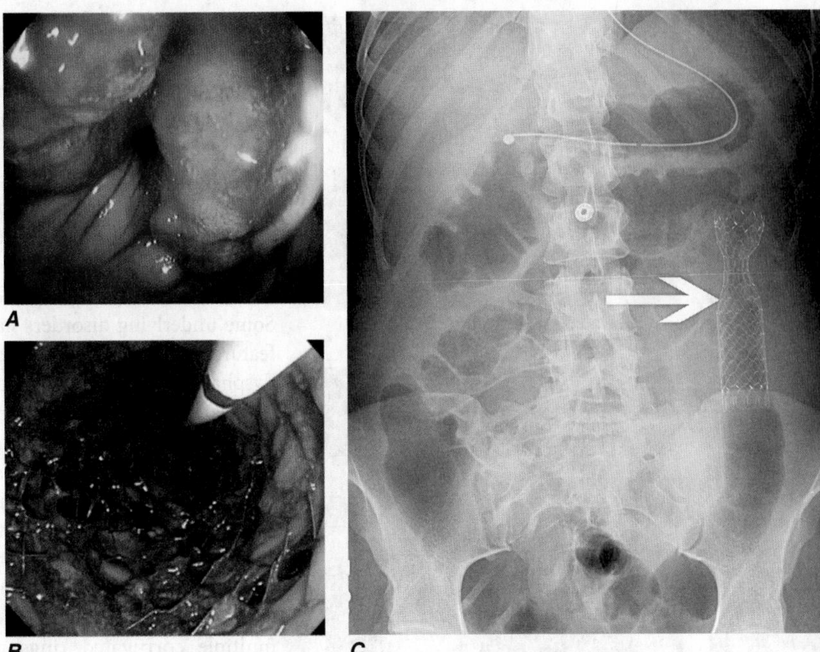

Figure 291-27 Obstructing colonic carcinoma. ***A.*** Colonic adenocarcinoma causing marked luminal narrowing of the descending colon. ***B.*** Endoscopic placement of a self-expanding metal stent. ***C.*** Radiograph of expanded stent across the obstructing tumor with a residual waist (*arrow*). *(Image A courtesy of Dr. Glenn Alexander; with permission.)*

patients whose symptoms are not resolved by an empirical trial of symptomatic treatment. Endoscopy should be performed at the outset in patients with dyspepsia and alarm features, such as weight loss or iron deficiency anemia.

GASTROESOPHAGEAL REFLUX DISEASE (GERD)

When classic symptoms of gastroesophageal reflux are present, such as water brash and substernal heartburn, presumptive diagnosis and empirical treatment are often sufficient. Endoscopy is a sensitive test for diagnosis of esophagitis (Fig. 291-29), but will miss nonerosive reflux disease (NERD) since some patients have symptomatic reflux without esophagitis. The most sensitive test for diagnosis of GERD is 24-h ambulatory pH monitoring. Endoscopy is indicated in patients with reflux symptoms refractory to antisecretory therapy; in those with alarm symptoms such as dysphagia, weight loss, or gastrointestinal bleeding; and in those with recurrent dyspepsia after treatment that is not clearly due to reflux on clinical grounds alone. Endoscopy may be considered in patients with long-standing (≥10 years) GERD with frequent symptoms, as they have a sixfold increased risk of harboring Barrett's esophagus compared to a patient with <1 year of reflux symptoms. Patients with Barrett's esophagus (Fig. 291-3) generally undergo a surveillance program of periodic endoscopy with biopsies to detect dysplasia or early carcinoma.

Barrett's esophagus

Barrett's esophagus is specialized columnar metaplasia that replaces the normal squamous mucosa of the distal esophagus in some persons with GERD. Barrett's epithelium is a major risk factor for

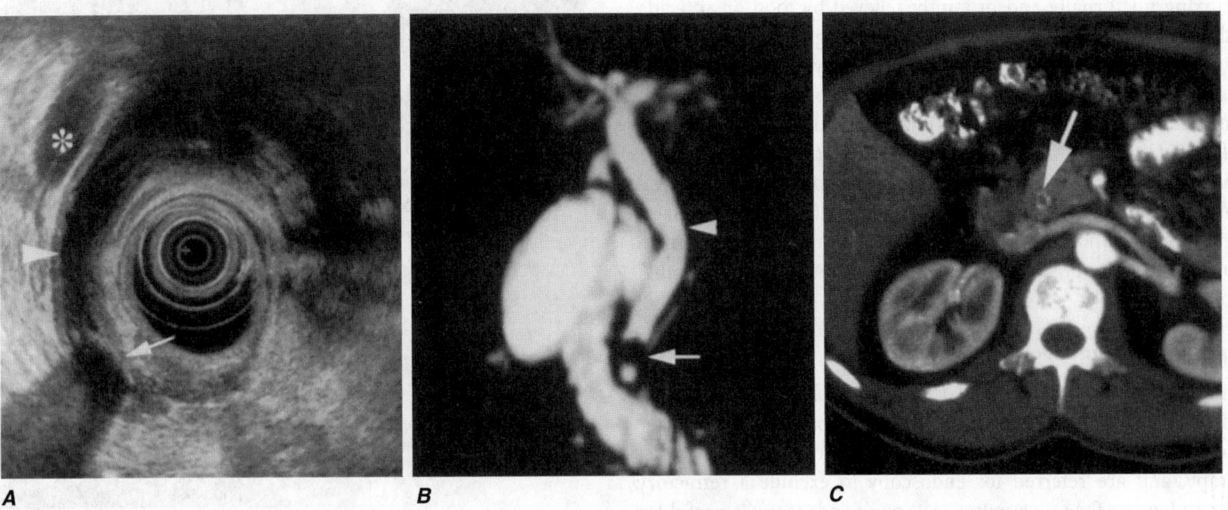

Figure 291-28 Methods of bile duct imaging. Arrows mark bile duct stones. Arrowheads indicate the common bile duct, and the asterisk marks the portal vein. ***A.*** Endoscopic ultrasound (EUS). ***B.*** Magnetic resonance cholangiopancreatography (MRCP). ***C.*** Helical computed tomography (CT).

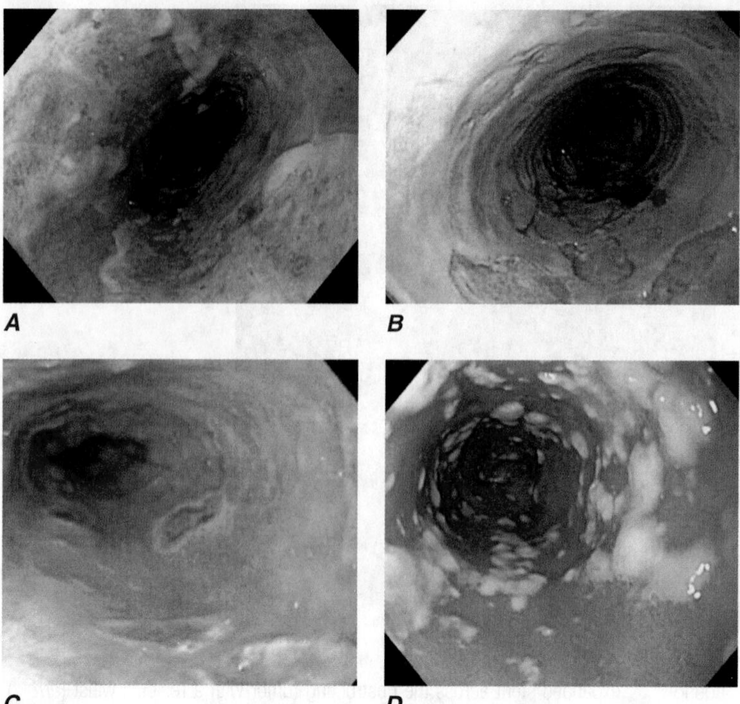

Figure 291-29 Causes of esophagitis. ***A.*** Severe reflux esophagitis with mucosal ulceration and friability. ***B.*** Cytomegalovirus esophagitis. ***C.*** Herpes simplex virus esophagitis with target-type shallow ulcerations. ***D.*** Candida esophagitis with white plaques adherent to the esophageal mucosa.

adenocarcinoma of the esophagus and is readily detected endoscopically, due to proximal displacement of the squamocolumnar junction (Fig. 291-3). A screening EGD for Barrett's esophagus may be considered in patients with a chronic history (>10 year) of GERD symptoms. Endoscopic biopsy is the gold standard for confirmation of Barrett's esophagus, and for dysplasia or cancer arising in Barrett's mucosa. Endoscopic therapies such as endoscopic mucosal resection (EMR) (Video e36-11), endoscopic submucosal dissection (ESD), photodynamic therapy (PDT), and radiofrequency ablation (RFA) are effective modalities for treatment of high-grade dysplasia and intramucosal cancer in Barrett's esophagus.

■ PEPTIC ULCER

Peptic ulcer classically causes epigastric gnawing or burning, often occurring nocturnally and promptly relieved by food or antacids. Although endoscopy is the most sensitive diagnostic test for peptic ulcer, it is not a cost-effective strategy in young patients with ulcer-like dyspeptic symptoms unless endoscopy is available at low cost. Patients with suspected peptic ulcer should be evaluated for *Helicobacter pylori* infection. Serology (past or present infection), urea breath testing (current infection), and stool tests are noninvasive and less costly than endoscopy with biopsy. Patients with alarm symptoms and those with persistent symptoms despite treatment should undergo endoscopy to exclude gastric malignancy and other etiologies.

■ NONULCER DYSPEPSIA

Nonulcer dyspepsia may be associated with bloating and, unlike peptic ulcer, tends not to remit and recur. Most patients describe marginal relief on acid-reducing, prokinetic, or anti-*Helicobacter* therapy, and are referred for endoscopy to exclude a refractory ulcer and assess for other causes. Although endoscopy is useful for excluding other diagnoses, its impact on the treatment of patients with nonulcer dyspepsia is limited.

■ DYSPHAGIA

About 50% of patients presenting with difficulty swallowing have a mechanical obstruction; the remainder has a motility disorder, such as achalasia or diffuse esophageal spasm. Careful history-taking often points to a presumptive diagnosis and leads to the appropriate use of diagnostic tests. Esophageal strictures (Fig. 291-30) typically cause progressive dysphagia, first for solids, then for liquids; motility disorders often cause intermittent dysphagia for both solids and liquids. Some underlying disorders have characteristic historic features: Schatzki's ring (Fig. 291-31) causes episodic dysphagia for solids, typically at the beginning of a meal; oropharyngeal motor disorders typically present with difficulty initiating deglutition (*transfer dysphagia*) and nasal reflux or coughing with swallowing; and achalasia may cause nocturnal regurgitation of undigested food.

When mechanical obstruction is suspected, endoscopy is a useful initial diagnostic test, since it permits immediate biopsy and/or dilatation of strictures, masses, or rings. The presence of linear furrows and multiple corrugated rings throughout a narrowed esophagus (*feline esophagus*) should raise suspicion for eosinophilic esophagitis, an increasingly recognized cause for recurrent dysphagia and food impaction (Fig. 291-32). Blind or forceful passage of an endoscope may lead to perforation in a patient with stenosis of the cervical esophagus or a Zenker's diverticulum, but gentle passage of an endoscope under direct visual guidance is reasonably safe. Endoscopy can miss a subtle stricture or ring in some patients.

When transfer dysphagia is evident or an esophageal motility disorder is suspected, esophageal radiography and/or a video-swallow study are the best initial diagnostic tests. The oropharyngeal swallowing mechanism, esophageal peristalsis, and the lower esophageal sphincter can all be assessed. In some disorders, subsequent esophageal manometry may also be important for diagnosis.

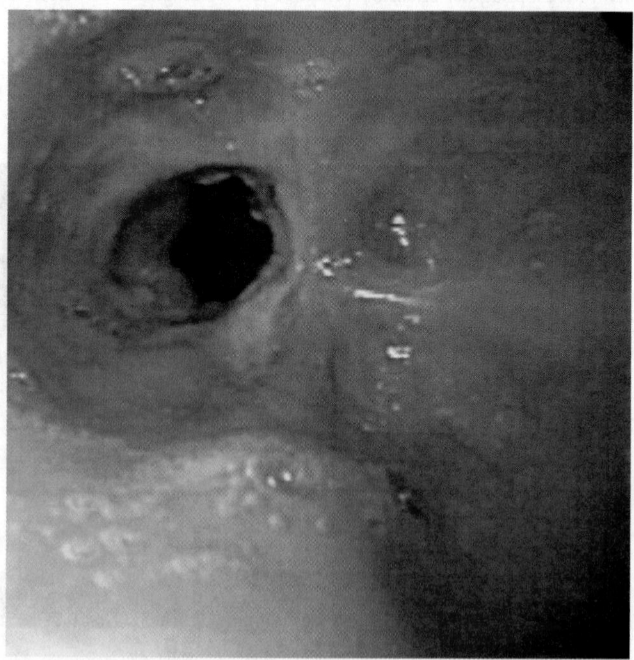

Figure 291-30 Peptic esophageal stricture associated with ulceration and scarring of the distal esophagus.

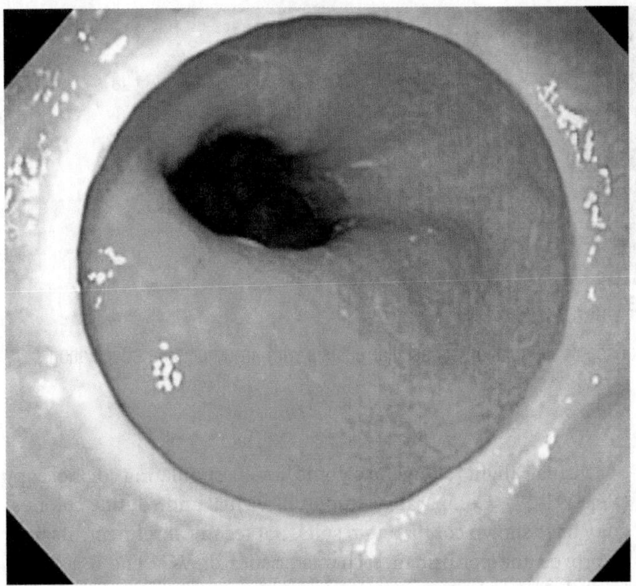

Figure 291-31 **Schatzki's ring at the** gastroesophageal junction.

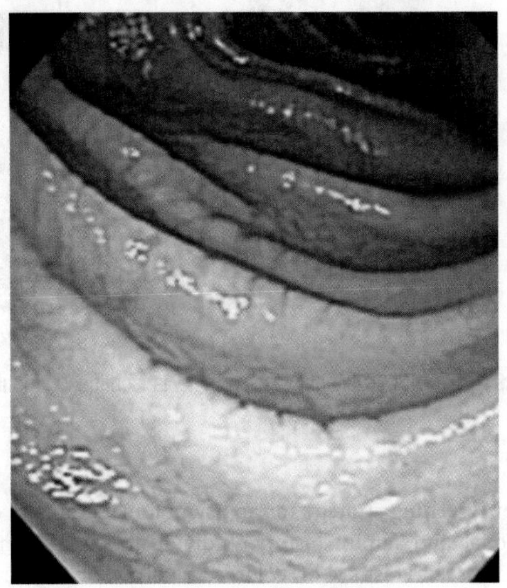

Figure 291-33 Scalloped duodenal folds in a patient with celiac sprue.

■ ANEMIA AND OCCULT BLOOD IN THE STOOL

Iron-deficiency anemia may be attributed to poor iron absorption (as in celiac sprue) or, more commonly, chronic blood loss. Intestinal bleeding should be strongly suspected in men and postmenopausal women with iron-deficiency anemia, and colonoscopy is indicated in such patients, even in the absence of detectable occult blood in the stool. Approximately 30% will have large colonic polyps, 10% will have colorectal cancer, and a few additional patients will have colonic vascular lesions. When a convincing source of blood loss is not found in the colon, upper gastrointestinal endoscopy should be considered; if no lesion is found, duodenal biopsies should be obtained to exclude sprue (Fig. 291-33). Small bowel evaluation with capsule endoscopy or deep enteroscopy may be appropriate if both EGD and colonoscopy are unrevealing (Fig. 291-34).

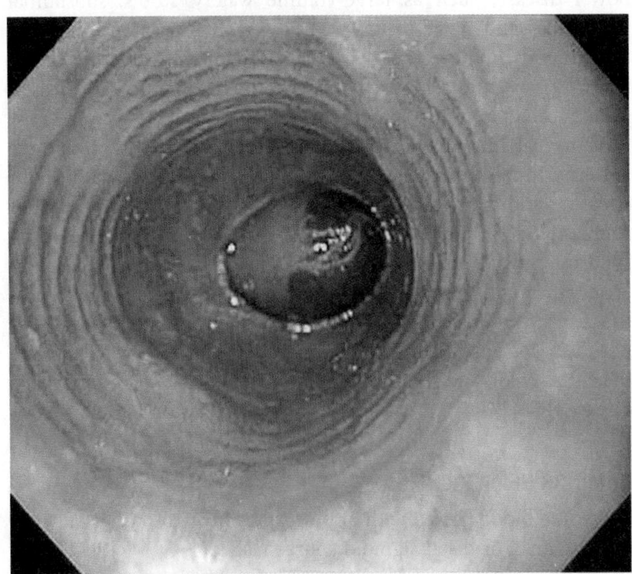

Figure 291-32 **Eosinophilic esophagitis with multiple circular rings of the esophagus creating a corrugated appearance, and an impacted grape at the narrowed esophagogastric junction.** The diagnosis requires biopsy with histologic finding of >15–20 eosinophils/high power field.

Tests for occult blood in the stool detect hemoglobin or the heme moiety and are most sensitive for colonic blood loss, although they will also detect larger amounts of upper gastrointestinal bleeding. Patients over age 50 with occult blood in normal-appearing stool should undergo colonoscopy to diagnose or exclude colorectal neoplasia. The diagnostic yield is lower than in iron-deficiency anemia. Whether upper endoscopy is also indicated depends on the patient's symptoms.

The small intestine may be the source of chronic intestinal bleeding, especially if colonoscopy and upper endoscopy are not diagnostic. The utility of small bowel evaluation varies with the clinical setting and is most important in patients in whom bleeding causes chronic or recurrent anemia. In contrast to the low diagnostic yield of small bowel radiography, positive findings on capsule endoscopy are seen in 50–70% of patients with suspected small-intestinal bleeding. The most common finding is mucosal vascular ectasias. Deep enteroscopy may follow capsule endoscopy for biopsy of lesions or to provide specific therapy, such as argon plasma coagulation of vascular ectasias (Fig. 291-35, Video e36-8).

■ COLORECTAL CANCER SCREENING

The majority of colon cancers develop from preexisting colonic adenomas, and colorectal cancer can be largely prevented by the detection and removal of adenomatous polyps (Video e36-12). The

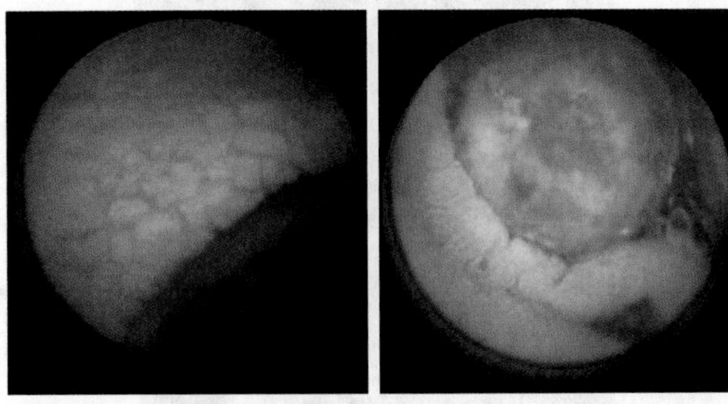

Figure 291-34 **Capsule endoscopy images of a mildly scalloped jejunal fold (left) and an ileal tumor (right) in a patient with celiac sprue.** *(Images courtesy of Dr. Elizabeth Rajan; with permission.)*

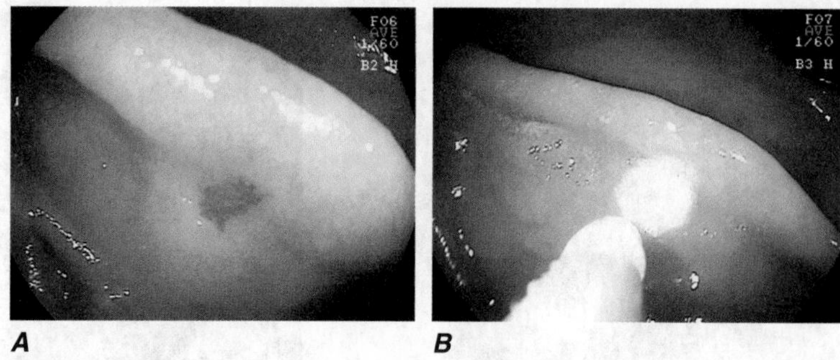

Figure 291-35 ***A.*** Mid-jejunal vascular ectasia identified by double-balloon endoscopy. ***B.*** Ablation of vascular ectasia with argon plasma coagulation.

choice of screening strategy for an asymptomatic person depends on personal and family history. Individuals with inflammatory bowel disease, a history of colorectal polyps or cancer, family members with adenomatous polyps or cancer, or certain familial cancer syndromes (Fig. 291-36) are at increased risk for colorectal cancer. An individual without these factors is generally considered at average risk.

Screening strategies are summarized in Table 291-2. While stool tests for occult blood have been shown to decrease mortality rate from colorectal cancer, they do not detect some cancers and many polyps, and direct visualization of the colon is a more effective screening strategy. Either sigmoidoscopy or colonoscopy may be used for cancer screening in asymptomatic average-risk individuals. The use of sigmoidoscopy was based on the historical finding that the majority of colorectal cancers occurred in the rectum and left colon, and that patients with right-sided colon cancers had left-sided polyps. Over the past several decades, however, the distribution of colon cancers has changed, with proportionally fewer rectal and left-sided cancers than in the past. Large studies of colonoscopy for screening of average-risk individuals show that cancers are roughly equally distributed between left and right colon and half of patients with right-sided lesions have no polyps in the left colon. Visualization of the entire colon thus appears to be the optimal strategy for colorectal cancer screening and prevention.

Virtual colonoscopy (VC) is a radiologic technique that images the colon with CT following rectal insufflation of the colonic lumen. Computer rendering of CT images generates an electronic display of a virtual "flight" along the colonic lumen, simulating colonoscopy (Fig. 291-37). Comparative studies of virtual and routine colonoscopy have shown conflicting results, but technical refinements have improved the performance characteristics of VC. The use of VC for colorectal cancer screening may become more widespread in the future, particularly at institutions with demonstrated skill with this technique. Findings detected during virtual colonoscopy often require subsequent conventional colonoscopy for confirmation and treatment.

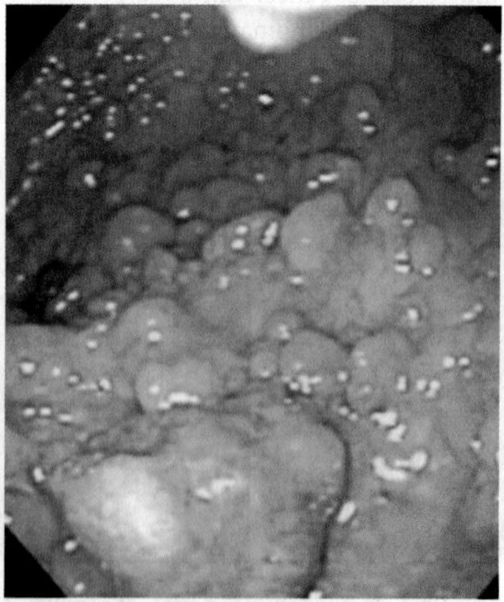

Figure 291-36 Innumerable colon polyps of various sizes in a patient with familial adenomatous polyposis syndrome.

■ DIARRHEA

Most cases of diarrhea are acute, self-limited, and due to infections or medication. Chronic diarrhea (lasting >6 weeks) is more often due to a primary inflammatory, malabsorptive, or motility disorder; is less likely to resolve spontaneously; and generally requires diagnostic evaluation. Patients with chronic diarrhea or severe, unexplained acute diarrhea often undergo endoscopy if stool tests for pathogens are unrevealing. The choice of endoscopic testing depends on the clinical setting.

Patients with colonic symptoms and findings such as bloody diarrhea, tenesmus, fever, or leukocytes in stool generally undergo sigmoidoscopy or colonoscopy to assess for colitis (Fig. 291-4). Sigmoidoscopy is an appropriate initial test in most patients. Conversely, patients with symptoms and findings suggesting small-bowel disease, such as large-volume watery stools, substantial weight loss, and malabsorption of iron, calcium, or fat may undergo upper endoscopy with duodenal aspirates for assessment of bacterial overgrowth and biopsies for assessment of mucosal diseases, such as celiac sprue.

Many patients with chronic diarrhea do not fit either of these patterns. In the setting of a long-standing history of alternating constipation and diarrhea dating to early adulthood, without findings such as blood in the stool or anemia, a diagnosis of irritable bowel syndrome may be made without direct visualization of the bowel. Steatorrhea and upper abdominal pain may prompt evaluation of the pancreas rather than the gut. Patients whose chronic diarrhea is not easily categorized often undergo initial colonoscopy to examine the entire colon and terminal ileum for inflammatory or neoplastic disease (Fig. 291-38).

■ MINOR HEMATOCHEZIA

Bright red blood passed with or on formed brown stool usually has a rectal, anal, or distal sigmoid source (Fig. 291-39). Patients with even trivial amounts of hematochezia should be investigated with flexible sigmoidoscopy and anoscopy to exclude polyps or cancers in the distal colon. Patients reporting red blood on the toilet tissue only, without blood in the toilet or on the stool, are generally bleeding from a lesion in the anal canal. Careful external inspection,

TABLE 291-2 Colorectal Cancer Screening Strategies

	Choices/Recommendations	Comments
Average-Risk Patients		
Asymptomatic individuals ≥50 years of age (≥45 years of age for African Americans)	Colonoscopy every 10 years*	Preferred cancer prevention strategy
	Annual fecal immunochemical test (FIT) for occult bleeding, fecal DNA testing every 3 years	Cancer detection strategy; fails to detect many polyps and some cancers
	CT colonography every 5 years	Evolving technology (see text)
	Flexible sigmoidoscopy every 5 years	Fails to detect proximal colon polyps and cancers
	Double-contrast barium enema every 5 years	Less sensitive than colonoscopy or CT colonography, misses some rectosigmoid polyps and cancers
Personal History of Polyps or Colorectal Cancer		
1 or 2 small (<1 cm) adenomas with low-grade dysplasia	Repeat colonoscopy in 5 years	Assuming complete polyp resection
3 to 9 adenomas, or any adenoma ≥1 cm or containing high-grade dysplasia or villus features	Repeat colonoscopy in 3 years; subsequent colonoscopy based on findings	Assuming complete polyp resection
≥10 adenomas	Colonoscopy in <3 years based on clinical judgment	Consider evaluation for FAP or HNPCC; see recommendations below
Piecemeal removal of a sessile polyp	Exam in 2 to 6 months to verify complete removal	
Small (<1 cm) hyperplastic polyps of sigmoid and rectum	Colonoscopy in 10 years	
>2 serrated polyps, or any serrated or hyperplastic polyp ≥1 cm	Repeat colonoscopy in 3 years	
Incompletely removed serrated polyp ≥1 cm	Exam in 2 to 6 months to verify complete removal	
Colon cancer	Evaluate entire colon around the time of resection, then repeat colonoscopy in 3 years	
Inflammatory Bowel Disease		
Long-standing (>8 years) ulcerative colitis or Crohn's colitis, or left-sided ulcerative colitis of >15 years' duration	Colonoscopy with biopsies every 1 to 3 years	
Family History of Polyps or Colorectal Cancer		
First-degree relatives with only small tubular adenomas	Same as average risk	
Single first-degree relative with CRC or advanced adenoma at age ≥60 years	Same as average risk	
Single first-degree relative with CRC or advanced adenoma at age <60 years, OR two first-degree relatives with CRC or advanced adenomas at any age	Colonoscopy every 5 years beginning at age 40 years or 10 years younger than age at diagnosis of the youngest affected relative	
FAP	Sigmoidoscopy or colonoscopy annually, beginning at age 10–12 years	Consider genetic counseling and testing
HNPCC	Colonoscopy every 2 years beginning at age 20–25 years until age 40, then annually thereafter	Consider histologic evaluation for microsatellite instability in tumor specimens of patients who meet Bethesda criteria; consider genetic counseling and testing

*Assumes good colonic preparation and complete exam to cecum.

Abbreviations: CRC, colorectal cancer; FAP, familial adenomatous polyposis; HNPCC, hereditary nonpolyposis colorectal cancer.

Source: Adapted from Winawer SJ et al: Gastroenterology 130:1872, 2006 and Levin B et al: CA Cancer J Clin 58:130, 2008.

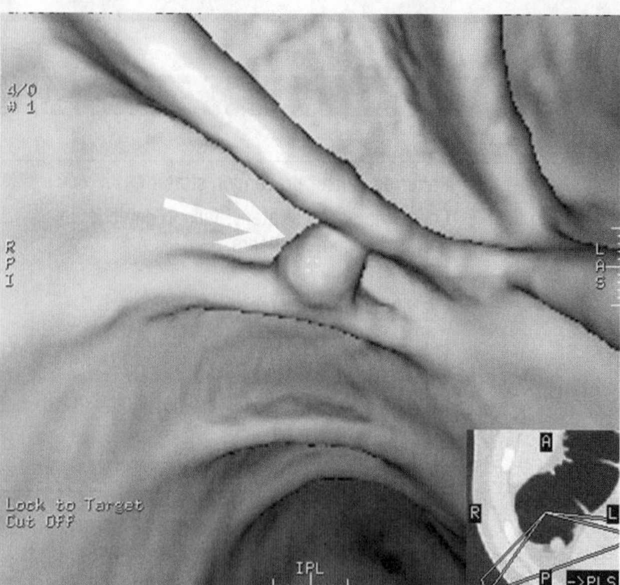

Figure 291-37 **Virtual colonoscopy image of a colon polyp** (*arrow*). *(Image courtesy of Dr. Jeff Fidler; with permission.)*

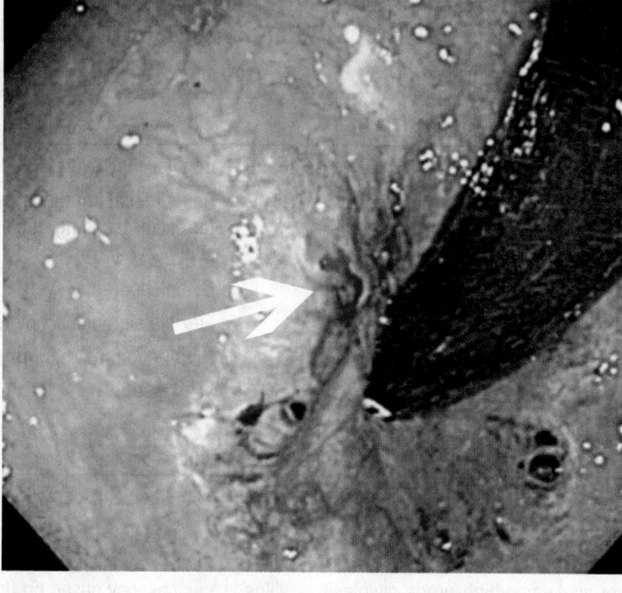

Figure 291-39 Internal hemorrhoids with bleeding (*arrow*) as seen on a retroflexed view of the rectum.

digital examination, and proctoscopy with anoscopy are sufficient for diagnosis in most cases.

PANCREATITIS

About 20% of patients with pancreatitis have no identified cause after routine clinical investigation (including a review of medication and alcohol use, measurement of serum triglyceride and calcium levels, abdominal ultrasonography, and CT). Endoscopic assessment leads to a specific diagnosis in the majority of such patients, often altering clinical management. Endoscopic investigation is particularly appropriate if the patient has had more than one episode of pancreatitis.

Microlithiasis, or the presence of microscopic crystals in bile, is a leading cause of previously unexplained acute pancreatitis and is sometimes seen during abdominal ultrasonography as layering sludge or flecks of floating, echogenic material in the gallbladder. Gallbladder bile can be obtained for microscopic analysis by administering a cholecystokinin analogue during endoscopy, causing contraction of the gallbladder. Bile is suctioned from the duodenum as it drains from the papilla, and the darkest fraction is examined for cholesterol crystals or bilirubinate granules. The combination of EUS of the gallbladder and bile microscopy is probably the most sensitive means of diagnosing microlithiasis.

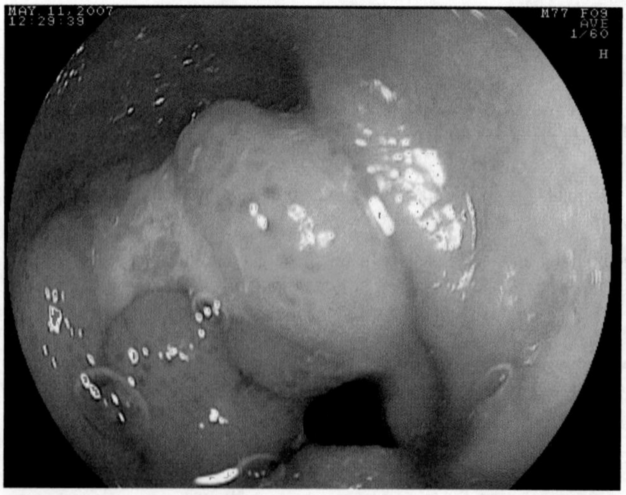

Previously undetected chronic pancreatitis, pancreatic malignancy, or pancreas divisum may be diagnosed by either ERCP or EUS. Sphincter of Oddi dysfunction or stenosis is a potential cause for pancreatitis and can be diagnosed by manometric studies performed during ERCP. Autoimmune pancreatitis may require EUS-guided pancreatic biopsy for histologic diagnosis.

Severe pancreatitis often results in pancreatic fluid collections. Both pseudocysts and areas of organized pancreatic necrosis can be drained into the stomach or duodenum endoscopically, using transpapillary and transmural endoscopic techniques. Pancreatic necrosis can be treated by direct endoscopic necrosectomy (Video e36-2).

Figure 291-38 **Ulcerated ileal carcinoid tumor.**

CANCER STAGING

Local staging of esophageal, gastric, pancreatic, bile duct, and rectal cancers can be obtained with EUS (Fig. 291-14). EUS with fine-needle aspiration (Fig. 291-15) currently provides the most accurate preoperative assessment of local tumor and nodal staging, but it does not detect most distant metastases. Details of the local tumor stage can guide treatment decisions including resectability and need for neoadjuvant therapy. EUS with transesophageal needle biopsy may also be used to assess the presence of non-small cell lung cancer in mediastinal nodes.

OPEN-ACCESS ENDOSCOPY

Direct scheduling of endoscopic procedures by primary care physicians without preceding gastroenterology consultation, or *open-access endoscopy,* is common. When the indications for endoscopy are clear-cut and appropriate, the procedural risks are low, and the patient understands what to expect, open-access endoscopy streamlines patient care and decreases costs.

Patients referred for open-access endoscopy should have a recent history, physical examination, and medication review. A copy of such an evaluation should be available when the patient comes to the endoscopy suite. Patients with unstable cardiovascular or respiratory conditions should not be referred directly for open-access endoscopy. Patients with particular conditions and undergoing certain procedures should be prescribed prophylactic antibiotics prior to endoscopy (Table 291-1). In addition, patients taking anticoagulants and/or antiplatelet drugs may require adjustment of these agents before endoscopy based on the procedure risk for bleeding and condition risk for a thromboembolic event (Figs. 291-40 and 291-41). Common indications for open-access EGD include dyspepsia resistant to a trial of appropriate therapy; dysphagia; gastrointestinal bleeding; and persistent anorexia or early satiety. Open-access colonoscopy is often requested in men or postmenopausal women with iron-deficiency anemia, in patients over age 50 with occult blood in the stool, in patients with a previous history of colorectal adenomatous polyps or cancer, and for colorectal cancer screening. Flexible sigmoidoscopy is commonly performed as an open-access procedure.

When patients are referred for open-access colonoscopy, the primary care provider may need to choose a colonic preparation. Commonly used oral preparations include polyethylene glycol lavage solution, with or without citric acid. A "split-dose" regimen improves the quality of colonic preparation. Sodium phosphate purgatives may cause fluid and electrolyte abnormalities and renal toxicity, especially in patients with renal failure or congestive heart failure and those over 70 years of age.

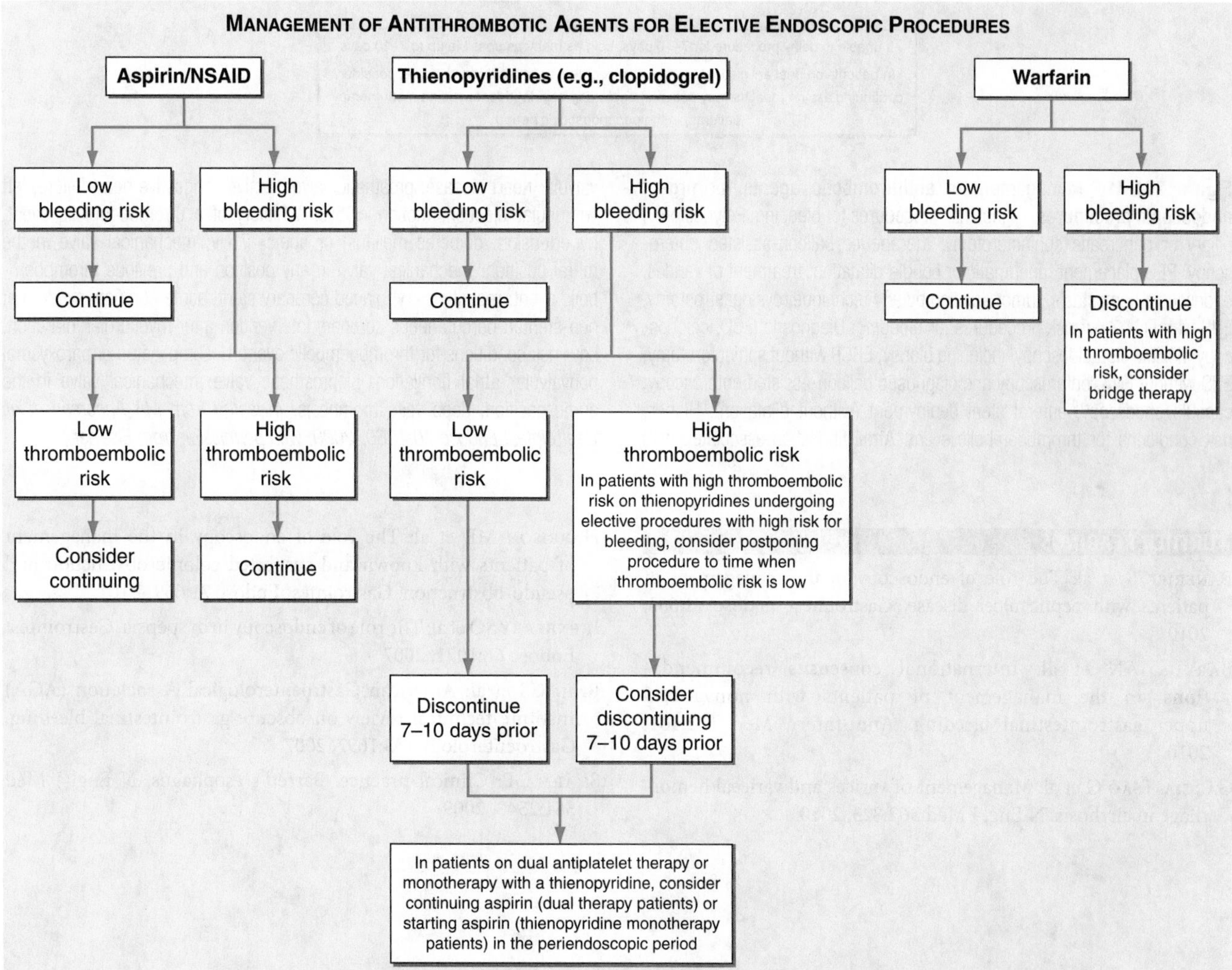

Figure 291-40 Management of antithrombotic agents for elective endoscopic procedures. Higher-risk procedures for bleeding: Polypectomy, biliary or pancreatic sphincterotomy, therapeutic balloon-assisted enteroscopy, PEG placement, pneumatic or bougie dilatation, treatment of varices, endoscopic hemostasis, tumor ablation by any technique, cystogastrostomy, EUS with FNA. Low-risk procedures for bleeding: Diagnostic (EGD, colonoscopy, flexible sigmoidoscopy) including biopsy, ERCP without sphincterotomy, EUS without FNA, enteroscopy and diagnostic balloon-assisted enteroscopy, capsule endoscopy, enteral stent deployment (without dilatation). Higher-risk conditions for thromboembolic event: Atrial fibrillation associated with valvular heart disease, prosthetic valves, active congestive heart failure, left ventricular ejection fraction <35%, a history of a thromboembolic event, hypertension, diabetes mellitus, or age >75 y; mechanical valve in the mitral position; mechanical valve in any position and previous thromboembolic event; recently (<1 y) placed coronary stent; acute coronary syndrome; non-stented percutaneous coronary intervention after myocardial infarction. Low-risk conditions for thromboembolic event: Uncomplicated or paroxysmal nonvalvular atrial fibrillation; bioprosthetic valve; mechanical valve in the aortic position; deep vein thrombosis. *(Adapted from MA Anderson et al: Gastrointest Endosc 70:1060, 2009; with permission from Elsevier.)*

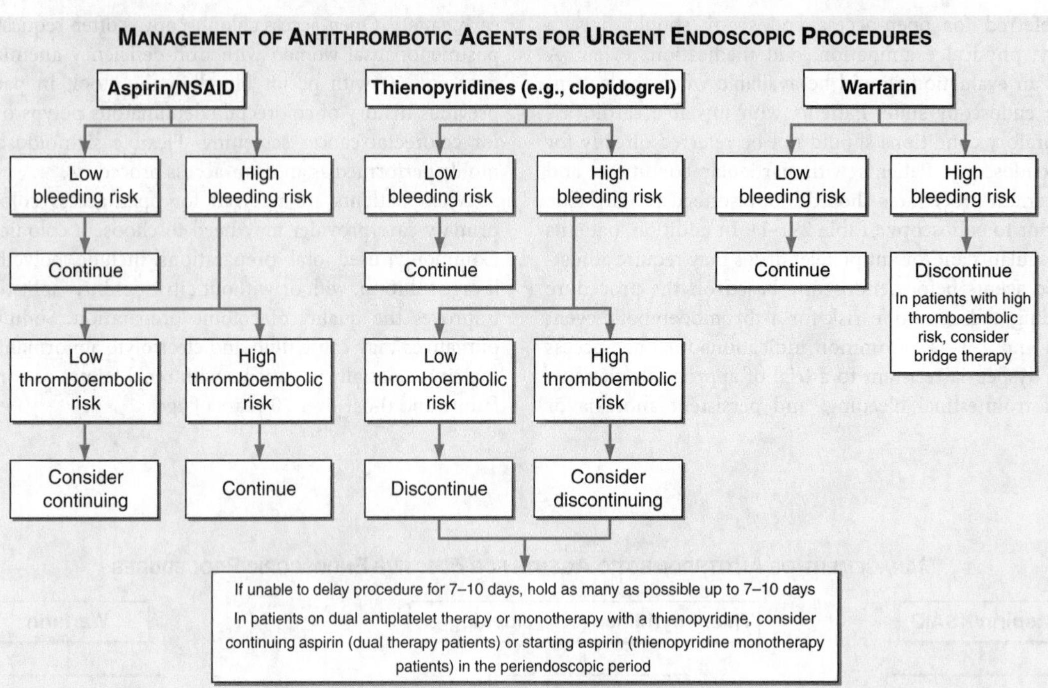

Figure 291-41 Management of antithrombotic agents for urgent endoscopic procedures. Higher-risk procedures for bleeding: Polypectomy, biliary or pancreatic sphincterotomy, therapeutic balloon-assisted enteroscopy, PEG placement, pneumatic or bougie dilatation, treatment of varices, endoscopic hemostasis, tumor ablation by any technique, cystogastrostomy, EUS with FNA. Low-risk procedures for bleeding: Diagnostic (EGD, colonoscopy, flexible sigmoidoscopy) including biopsy, ERCP without sphincterotomy, EUS without FNA, enteroscopy and diagnostic balloon-assisted enteroscopy, capsule endoscopy, enteral stent deployment (without dilatation). Higher-risk conditions for thromboembolic event: Atrail fibrillation associated with valvular heart disease, prosthetic valves, active congestive heart failure, left ventricular ejection fraction <35%, a history of a thromboembolic event, hypertension, diabetes mellitus, or age > 75 y; mechanical valve in the mitral position; mechanical valve in any position and previous thromboembolic event; recently (>1y) placed coronary stent; acute coronary syndrome; non-stented percutaneous coronary intervention after myocardial infarction. Low-risk conditions for thromboembolic event: Uncomplicated or paroxysmal nonvalvular atrial fibrillation; bioprosthetic valve; mechanical valve in the aortic position, deep vein thrombosis. *(Adapted from MA Anderson et al: Gastrointest Endosc 70:1060, 2009; with permission from Elsevier.)*

FURTHER READINGS

Banerjee S et al: The role of endoscopy in the management of patients with peptic ulcer disease. Gastrointest Endosc 71:663, 2010

Barkun AN et al: International consensus recommendations on the management of patients with nonvariceal upper gastrointestinal bleeding. Ann Intern Med 152:101, 2010

Garcia-Tsao G et al: Management of varices and variceal hemorrhage in cirrhosis. N Engl J Med 362:823, 2010

Harrison ME et al: The role of endoscopy in the management of patients with known and suspected colonic obstruction and pseudo-obstruction. Gastrointest Endosc 71:669, 2010

Ikenberry SO et al: The role of endoscopy in dyspepsia. Gastrointest Endosc 66:1071, 2007

Raju GS et al: American Gastroenterological Association (AGA) Institute technical review on obscure gastrointestinal bleeding. Gastroenterology 133:1697, 2007

Sharma P: Clinical practice. Barrett's esophagus. N Engl J Med 361:2548, 2009

CHAPTER 292

Diseases of the Esophagus

Peter J. Kahrilas
Ikuo Hirano

ESOPHAGEAL STRUCTURE AND FUNCTION

The esophagus is a hollow muscular tube coursing through the posterior mediastinum joining the hypopharynx to the stomach with a sphincter at each end. It functions to transport food and fluid between these ends, otherwise remaining empty. The physiology of swallowing, esophageal motility, and oral and pharyngeal dysphagia are described in Chap. 38. Esophageal diseases can be manifested by impaired function or pain. Key functional impairments are swallowing disorders and excessive gastroesophageal reflux. Pain, sometimes indistinguishable from cardiac chest pain, can result from inflammation, infection, dysmotility, or neoplasm.

SYMPTOMS OF ESOPHAGEAL DISEASE

The clinical history remains central to the evaluation of esophageal symptoms. A thoughtfully obtained history will often expedite management. Important details include weight gain or loss, gastrointestinal bleeding, dietary habits including the timing of meals, smoking, and alcohol consumption. The major esophageal symptoms are heartburn, regurgitation, chest pain, dysphagia, odynophagia, and globus sensation.

Heartburn (pyrosis), the most common esophageal symptom, is characterized by a discomfort or burning sensation behind the sternum that arises from the epigastrium and may radiate toward the neck. Heartburn is an intermittent symptom, most commonly experienced after eating, during exercise, and while lying recumbent. The discomfort is relieved with drinking water or antacid but can occur frequently and interfere with normal activities including sleep. The association between heartburn and gastroesophageal reflux disease (GERD) is so strong that empirical therapy for GERD has become accepted management. However, the term "heartburn" is often misused and/or referred to with other terms such as "indigestion" or "repeating," making it important to clarify the intended meaning.

Regurgitation is the effortless return of food or fluid into the pharynx without nausea or retching. Patients report a sour or burning fluid in the throat or mouth that may also contain undigested food particles. Bending, belching, or maneuvers that increase intraabdominal pressure can provoke regurgitation. A clinician needs to discriminate among regurgitation, vomiting, and rumination. *Vomiting* is preceded by nausea and accompanied by retching. *Rumination* is a behavior in which recently swallowed food is regurgitated and then reswallowed repetitively for up to an hour. Although there is some linkage between rumination and mental deficiency, the behavior is also exhibited by unimpaired individuals who sometimes even find it pleasurable.

Chest pain is a common esophageal symptom with characteristics similar to cardiac pain, sometimes making this distinction difficult. Esophageal pain is usually experienced as a pressure type sensation in the mid chest, radiating to the mid back, arms, or jaws. The similarity to cardiac pain is likely because the two organs share a nerve plexus and the nerve endings in the esophageal wall have poor discriminative ability among stimuli. Esophageal distention or even chemostimulation (e.g., with acid) will often be perceived as chest pain. Gastroesophageal reflux is the most common cause of esophageal chest pain.

Esophageal *dysphagia* (see also Chap. 38) is often described as a feeling of food "sticking" or even lodging in the chest. Important distinctions are between uniquely solid food dysphagia as opposed to liquid and solid, episodic versus constant dysphagia, and progressive versus static dysphagia. If the dysphagia is for liquids as well as solid food, it suggests a motility disorder such as achalasia. Conversely, uniquely solid food dysphagia is suggestive of a stricture, ring, or tumor. Of note, a patient's localization of food hang-up in the esophagus is notoriously imprecise. Approximately 30% of distal esophageal obstructions are perceived as cervical dysphagia. In such instances, the absence of concomitant symptoms generally associated with oropharyngeal dysphagia such as aspiration, nasopharyngeal regurgitation, cough, drooling, or obvious neuromuscular compromise should suggest an esophageal etiology.

Odynophagia is pain either caused by or exacerbated by swallowing. Odynophagia is more common with pill or infectious esophagitis than with reflux esophagitis and should prompt a search for these entities. When odynophagia does occur in GERD, it is likely related to an esophageal ulcer or deep erosion.

Globus sensation, alternatively labeled "globus hystericus," is the perception of a lump or fullness in the throat that is felt irrespective of swallowing. Although such patients are frequently referred for an evaluation of dysphagia, globus sensation is often relieved by the act of swallowing. As implied by its alternative name (globus hystericus), globus sensation often occurs in the setting of anxiety or obsessive-compulsive disorders. Clinical experience teaches that it is often attributable to GERD.

Water brash is excessive salivation resulting from a vagal reflex triggered by acidification of the esophageal mucosa. This is not a common symptom. Afflicted individuals will describe the unpleasant sensation of the mouth rapidly filling with salty thin fluid, often in the setting of concomitant heartburn.

DIAGNOSTIC STUDIES

ENDOSCOPY

Endoscopy, also known as esophagogastroduodenoscopy (EGD) is the best test for the evaluation of the proximal gastrointestinal tract. Modern instruments produce high-quality color images of the esophageal, gastric, and duodenal lumen. Endoscopes also have an instrumentation channel through which biopsy forceps, sclerotherapy catheters, balloon dilators, or cautery devices can be utilized. The key advantages of endoscopy over barium radiography are: (1) increased sensitivity for the detection of mucosal lesions, (2) vastly increased sensitivity for the detection of abnormalities mainly identifiable by an abnormal color such as Barrett's metaplasia, (3) the ability to obtain biopsy specimens for histologic examination of suspected abnormalities, and (4) the ability to dilate strictures during the examination. The main disadvantage of endoscopy is that it usually necessitates the use of conscious sedation with medicines such as midazolam (Versed), meperidine (Demerol), or fentanyl.

RADIOGRAPHY

Contrast radiography of the esophagus, stomach, and duodenum can demonstrate barium reflux, hiatal hernia, mucosal granularity, erosions, ulcerations, and strictures. The sensitivity of radiography compared with endoscopy for detecting esophagitis reportedly ranges from 22–95%, with higher grades of esophagitis (i.e., ulceration or stricture) exhibiting greater detection rates. Conversely, the sensitivity of barium radiography for detecting esophageal strictures is greater than that of endoscopy, especially when the study is done in conjunction with barium-soaked bread or a 13-mm barium tablet. Barium studies also provide an assessment of esophageal function and morphology that may be undetected on endoscopy. Hypopharyngeal pathology and disorders of the cricopharyngeal muscle are better appreciated on radiographic examination, particularly with videofluoroscopic recording. The major shortcoming of barium radiography is that it rarely obviates the need for endoscopy. Either a positive or a negative study is usually followed by an endoscopic evaluation either to clarify findings in the case of a positive examination or to add a level of certainty in the case of a negative one.

ENDOSCOPIC ULTRASOUND

Endoscopic ultrasound (EUS) instruments combine an endoscope with an ultrasound transducer to create a transmural image of the tissue surrounding the endoscope tip. The key advantage of EUS over alternative radiologic imaging techniques is much greater resolution attributable to the proximity of the ultrasound transducer to the area being examined. Available devices can provide either radial imaging (360-degree, cross-sectional) or a curved linear image that can guide fine-needle aspiration of imaged structures such as lymph nodes or tumors. Major esophageal applications of EUS are to stage esophageal cancer, to evaluate dysplasia in Barrett's esophagus, and to assess submucosal tumors.

ESOPHAGEAL MANOMETRY

Esophageal manometry, or motility testing, entails positioning a pressure sensing catheter within the esophagus and then observing the contractility following test swallows. The upper and lower esophageal sphincters appear as zones of high pressure that relax on swallowing while the intersphincteric esophagus exhibits peristaltic contractions. Manometry is used to diagnose motility disorders (achalasia, diffuse esophageal spasm) and to assess peristaltic integrity prior to the surgery for reflux disease. Technological advances have rebranded esophageal manometry as high-resolution esophageal pressure topography (Fig. 292-1). Manometry can also be combined with intraluminal impedance monitoring. Impedance recordings utilize a catheter with a series of paired electrodes. Esophageal luminal contents in contact with the electrodes decrease (liquid) or increase (air) the impedance signal allowing detection of anterograde or retrograde transit of esophageal bolus transit.

REFLUX TESTING

GERD is often diagnosed in the absence of endoscopic esophagitis, which would otherwise define the disease. This occurs in the settings of partially treated disease, an abnormally sensitive esophageal mucosa, or without obvious explanation. In such instances, reflux testing can demonstrate excessive esophageal exposure to refluxed gastric juice, the physiologic abnormality of GERD. This can be done by ambulatory 24- to 48-hour esophageal pH recording using either a wireless pH-sensitive transmitter that is anchored to the esophageal mucosa or with a transnasally positioned wire electrode with the tip stationed in the distal esophagus. Either way, the outcome is expressed as the percentage of the day that the pH was less than 4 (indicative of recent acid reflux), with values exceeding 5% indicative of GERD. Reflux testing is useful with atypical symptoms or an inexplicably poor response to therapy. Intraluminal impedance monitoring can be added to pH monitoring to detect reflux events irrespective of whether or not they are acidic, potentially increasing the sensitivity of the study.

STRUCTURAL DISORDERS

HIATAL HERNIA

Hiatus hernia is a herniation of viscera, most commonly the stomach, into the mediastinum through the esophageal hiatus of the diaphragm. Four types of hiatus hernia are distinguished with type I, or sliding hiatal hernia comprising at least 95% of the overall total. A sliding hiatal hernia is one in which the gastroesophageal junction and gastric cardia slide upward as a result of weakening of the phrenoesophageal ligament attaching the gastroesophageal junction to the diaphragm at the hiatus. True to its name, sliding hernias enlarge with increased intraabdominal pressure, swallowing, and respiration. The incidence of sliding hernias increases with age and conceptually, results from wear and tear: increased intraabdominal pressure from abdominal obesity, pregnancy, etc., and hereditary factors predisposing to the condition. The main significance of sliding hernias is the propensity of affected individuals to have GERD.

Types II, III, and IV hiatal hernias are all subtypes of paraesophageal hernia in which the herniation into the mediastinum includes a visceral structure other than the gastric cardia. With type II and III paraesophageal hernias, the gastric fundus also herniates with the distinction being that in type II, the gastroesophageal junction remains fixed at the hiatus, while type III is a mixed sliding/paraesophageal hernia. With type IV hiatal hernias, viscera other than the stomach

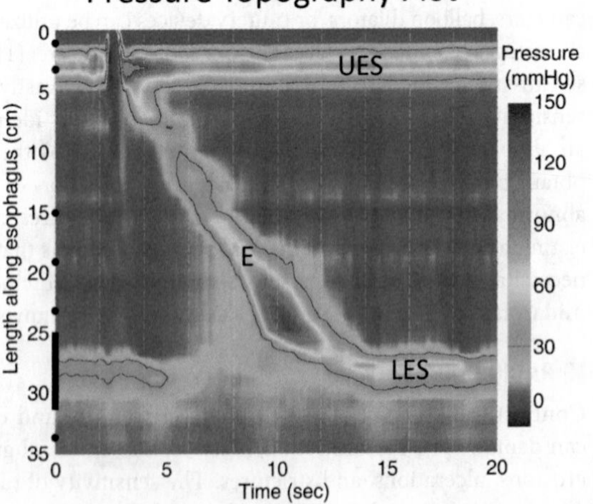

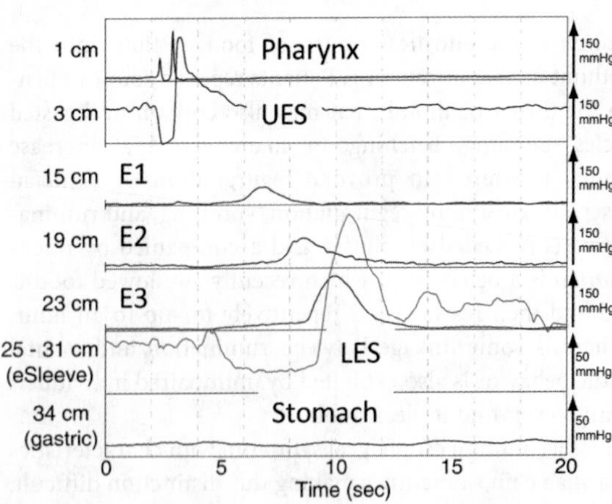

Figure 292-1 **High-resolution esophageal pressure topography *(right)* and conventional manometry *(left)* of a normal swallow.** LES, lower esophageal sphincter; E, esophageal body; UES, upper esophageal sphincter.

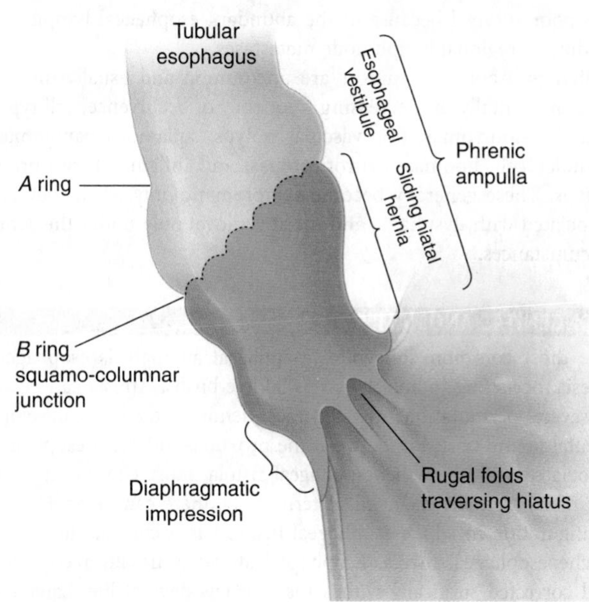

Figure 292-2 Radiographic anatomy of the gastroesophageal junction.

herniate into the mediastinum, most commonly the colon. With type II and III paraesophageal hernias, the stomach inverts as it herniates and large paraesophageal hernias can lead to an upside down stomach, gastric volvulus, and even strangulation of the stomach. Because of this risk, surgical repair is often advocated for large paraesophageal hernias.

RINGS AND WEBS

A lower esophageal mucosal ring, also called a *B ring*, is a thin membranous narrowing at the squamocolumnar mucosal junction (Fig. 292-2). Its origin is unknown but B rings are demonstrable in about 15% of people and are usually asymptomatic. When the lumen diameter is less than 13 mm, distal rings are usually associated with episodic solid food dysphagia and are called *Schatzki rings*. Patients typically present older than 40 years, consistent with an acquired rather than congenital origin. Schatzki ring is one of the most common causes of intermittent food impaction, also known as "steakhouse syndrome" as meat is a typical instigator. Symptomatic rings are easily treated by dilatation.

Web-like constrictions higher in the esophagus can be of congenital or inflammatory origin. Asymptomatic cervical esophageal webs are demonstrated in about 10% of people and typically originate along the anterior aspect of the esophagus. When circumferential, they can cause intermittent dysphagia to solids similar to Schatzki rings and are similarly treated with dilatation. The combination of symptomatic proximal esophageal webs and iron-deficiency anemia in middle-aged women constitutes Plummer-Vinson syndrome.

DIVERTICULA

Esophageal diverticula are categorized by location with the most common being epiphrenic, hypopharyngeal (Zenker's), and mid esophageal. Epiphrenic and Zenker's diverticula are false diverticula involving herniation of the mucosa and submucosa through the muscular layer of the esophagus. These lesions result from increased intraluminal pressure associated with distal obstruction. In the case of Zenker's, the obstruction is a stenotic cricopharyngeus muscle (upper esophageal sphincter) and the hypopharyngeal herniation most commonly occurs in an area of natural weakness known as *Killian's triangle* (Fig. 292-3). Small Zenker's diverticula are usually asymptomatic but when they enlarge sufficiently to retain food and saliva they can be associated with dysphagia, halitosis, and aspiration. Treatment is by surgical diverticulectomy and cricopharyngeal myotomy or a marsupialization procedure in which an endoscopic stapling device is used to divide the cricopharyngeus.

Epiphrenic diverticula are usually associated with achalasia or a distal esophageal stricture. Mid-esophageal diverticula may be caused by traction from adjacent inflammation (classically tuberculosis) in which case they are true diverticula involving all layers of the esophageal wall, or by pulsion associated with esophageal motor disorders. Mid-esophageal and epiphrenic diverticula are usually asymptomatic until they enlarge sufficiently to retain food and cause dysphagia and regurgitation. Symptoms attributable to the diverticula tend to correlate more with the underlying esophageal disorder than the size of the diverticula. Large diverticula can be removed surgically, usually in conjunction with a myotomy if the underlying cause is achalasia. Diffuse intramural esophageal

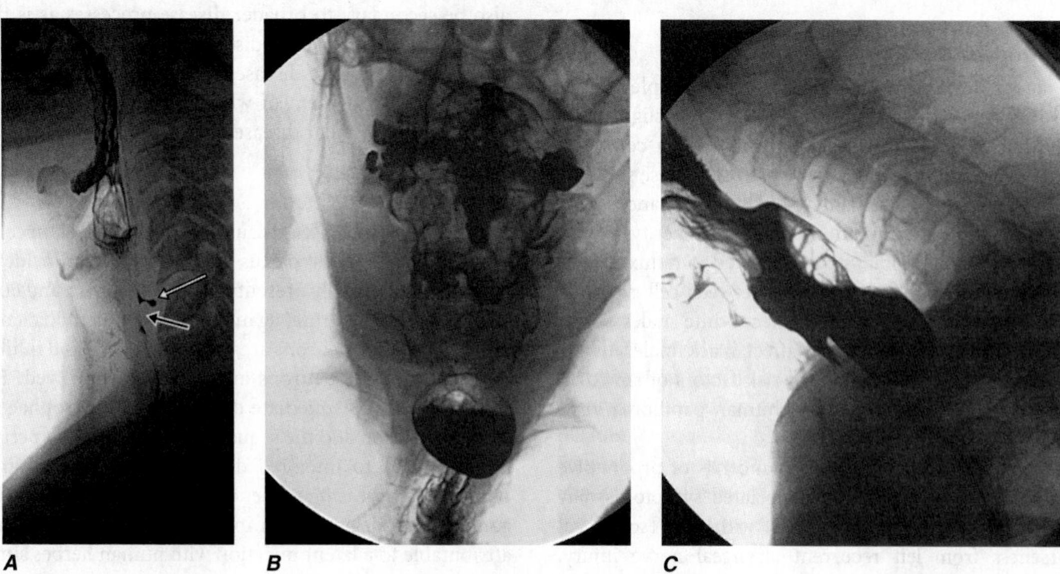

Figure 292-3 Examples of small (*left*) and large (*middle, right*) Zenker's diverticulum arising from Killian's triangle in the distal hypopharynx. Smaller diverticula are evident only during the swallow, whereas larger ones retain food and fluid.

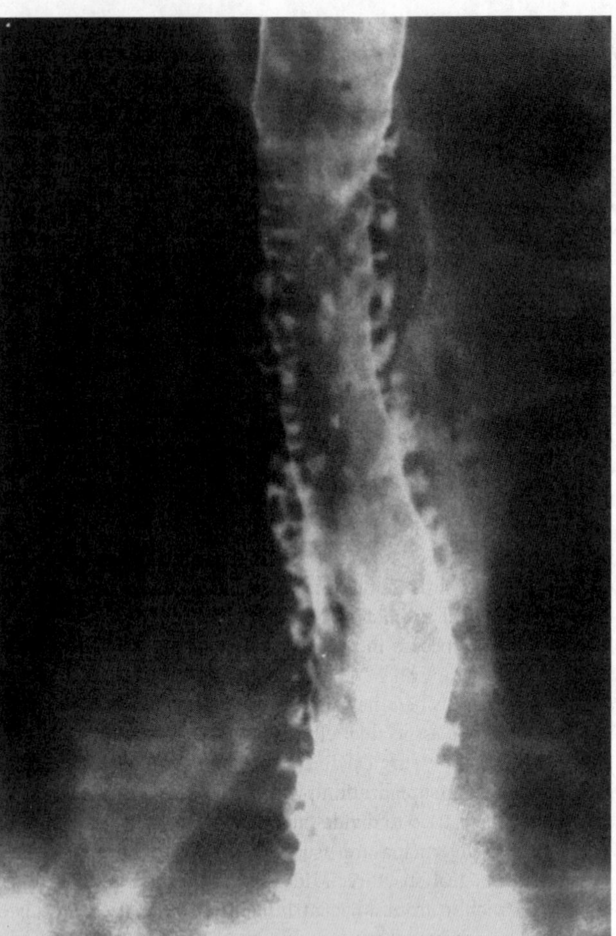

Figure 292-4 Intramural esophageal pseudodiverticulosis associated with chronic obstruction. Invaginations of contrast into the esophageal wall outline deep esophageal glands.

diverticulosis is a rare entity that results from dilatation of the excretory ducts of submucosal esophageal glands (Fig. 292-4). Esophageal candidiasis and proximal esophageal strictures are commonly found in association with this disorder.

TUMORS

Esophageal cancer occurs in about 4.5:100,000 people in the United States with the associated mortality being only slightly less at 4.4:100,000. It is about 10 times less common than colorectal cancer but kills about one-quarter as many patients. These statistics emphasize both the rarity and lethality of esophageal cancer. One notable trend is the shift of dominant esophageal cancer type from squamous cell to adenocarcinoma, strongly linked to reflux disease and Barrett's metaplasia. Other distinctions between cell types are the predilection for adenocarcinoma to affect white males in the distal esophagus and squamous cell to affect black males in the more proximal esophagus with the added risk factors of smoking, alcohol consumption, caustic injury, and human papilloma virus infection (Chap. 91).

The typical presentation of esophageal cancer is of progressive solid food dysphagia and weight loss. Associated symptoms may include odynophagia, iron deficiency, and, with mid-esophageal tumors, hoarseness from left recurrent laryngeal nerve injury. Generally, these are indications of locally invasive or even metastatic disease manifest by tracheoesophageal fistulas, and vocal cord paralysis. Even when detected as a small lesion, esophageal cancer has poor survival because of the abundant esophageal lymphatics leading to regional lymph node metastases.

Benign esophageal tumors are uncommon and usually discovered incidentally. In decreasing frequency of occurrence, cell types include leiomyomas, fibrovascular polyps, squamous papillomas, granular cell, lipomas, neurofibromas, and inflammatory fibroid polyps. These generally become symptomatic only when they are associated with dysphagia and merit removal only under the same circumstances.

CONGENITAL ANOMALIES

The most common congenital esophageal anomaly is esophageal atresia, occurring in about 1 in 5,000 live births. Atresia can occur in several permutations, the common denominator being developmental failure of fusion between the proximal and distal esophagus associated with a tracheoesophageal fistula, most commonly with the distal segment excluded. Alternatively, there can be an H-type configuration in which esophageal fusion has occurred, but with a tracheoesophageal fistula. Esophageal atresia is usually recognized and corrected surgically within the first few days of life. Later life complications include dysphagia from anastomotic strictures or absent peristalsis and reflux, which can be severe. Less common developmental anomalies include congenital esophageal stenosis, webs, and duplications.

Dysphagia can also result from congenital abnormalities that cause extrinsic compression of the esophagus. In dysphagia lusoria, the esophagus is compressed by an aberrant right subclavian artery arising from the descending aorta and passing behind the esophagus. Alternatively vascular rings may surround and constrict the esophagus.

Heterotopic gastric mucosa, also known as an esophageal inlet patch, is a focus of gastric type epithelium in the proximal cervical esophagus; the estimated prevalence is 4.5%. The inlet patch is thought to result from incomplete replacement of embryonic columnar epithelium with squamous epithelium. The majority of patches are asymptomatic, but acid production can occur as most contain fundic type gastric epithelium with parietal cells.

ESOPHAGEAL MOTALITY DISORDERS

Esophageal motility disorders are diseases attributable to esophageal neuromuscular dysfunction commonly associated with dysphagia, chest pain, or heartburn. The major entities are achalasia, diffuse esophageal spasm (DES), and GERD. Motility disorders can also be secondary to broader disease processes as is the case with pseudoachalasia, Chagas' disease, and scleroderma. Not included in this discussion are diseases affecting the pharynx and proximal esophagus, impairment of which is almost always part of a more global neuromuscular disease process.

ACHALASIA

Achalasia is a rare disease caused by loss of ganglion cells within the esophageal myenteric plexus with a population incidence of about 1:100,000 and usually presenting between age 25 and 60. With long-standing disease, virtual aganglionosis is noted. Excitatory (cholinergic) ganglionic neurons are variably affected and inhibitory (nitric oxide) ganglionic neurons are necessarily involved. Functionally, inhibitory neurons mediate deglutitive lower esophageal sphincter (LES) relaxation and the sequential propagation of peristalsis. Their absence leads to impaired deglutitive LES relaxation and absent peristalsis. Increasing evidence suggests that the ultimate cause of ganglion cell degeneration in achalasia is an autoimmune process attributable to a latent infection with human herpes simplex virus 1 combined with genetic susceptibility.

Long-standing achalasia is characterized by progressive dilatation and sigmoid deformity of the esophagus with hypertrophy of the

LES. Clinical manifestations may include dysphagia, regurgitation, chest pain, and weight loss. Most patients report solid and liquid food dysphagia. Regurgitation occurs when food, fluid, and secretions are retained in the dilated esophagus. Patients with advanced achalasia are at risk for bronchitis, pneumonia, or lung abscess from chronic regurgitation and aspiration. Chest pain is frequent early in the course of achalasia, thought to result from esophageal spasm. Patients describe a squeezing, pressure-like retrosternal pain, sometimes radiating to the neck, arms, jaw, and back. Paradoxically, some patients complain of heartburn that may be a chest pain equivalent. Treatment of achalasia is less effective in relieving chest pain than it is in relieving dysphagia or regurgitation.

The differential diagnosis of achalasia includes DES, Chagas' disease, and pseudoachalasia. Chagas' disease is endemic in areas of central Brazil, Venezuela, and northern Argentina, spread by the bite of the reduvid (kissing) bug that transmits the protozoan, *Trypanosoma cruzi*. The chronic phase of the disease develops years after infection and results from destruction of autonomic ganglion cells throughout the body, including the heart, gut, urinary tract, and respiratory tract. Tumor infiltration, most commonly seen with carcinoma in the gastric fundus or distal esophagus can mimic idiopathic achalasia. The resultant "pseudoachalasia" accounts for up to 5% of suspected cases and is more likely with advanced age, abrupt onset of symptoms (<1 year), and weight loss. Hence, endoscopy should be part of the evaluation of achalasia. When the clinical suspicion for pseudoachalasia is high and endoscopy nondiagnostic, CT scanning or endoscopic ultrasonography may be of value. Rarely, pseudoachalasia can result from a paraneoplastic syndrome with circulating antineuronal antibodies.

Achalasia is diagnosed by barium swallow x-ray and/or esophageal manometry; endoscopy has a relatively minor role other than to exclude pseudoachalasia. The barium swallow x-ray appearance is of a dilated esophagus with poor emptying, an air-fluid level, and tapering at the LES giving it a beak-like appearance (Fig. 292-5). Occasionally, an epiphrenic diverticulum is observed. In long-standing achalasia, the esophagus may assume a sigmoid configuration. The diagnostic criteria for achalasia with esophageal manometry are impaired LES relaxation and absent peristalsis. High-resolution manometry has somewhat advanced this diagnosis; three subtypes of achalasia are differentiated based on the pattern of pressurization in the nonperistaltic esophagus (Fig. 292-6). Because manometry identifies early disease before esophageal dilatation and food retention, it is the most sensitive diagnostic test.

There is no known way of preventing or reversing achalasia. Therapy is directed at reducing LES pressure so that gravity and

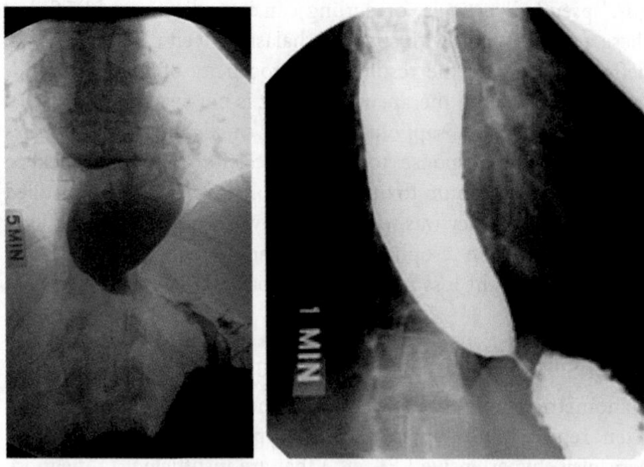

Figure 292-5 Achalasia with esophageal dilatation, tapering at the gastroesophageal junction and an air-fluid level within the esophagus. The example on the left shows sigmoid deformity with very advanced disease.

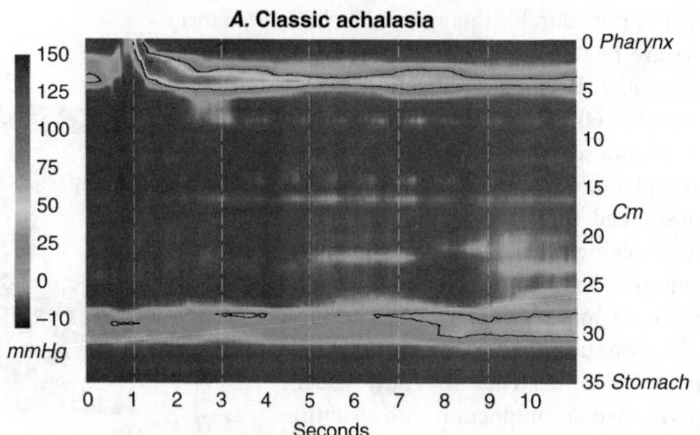

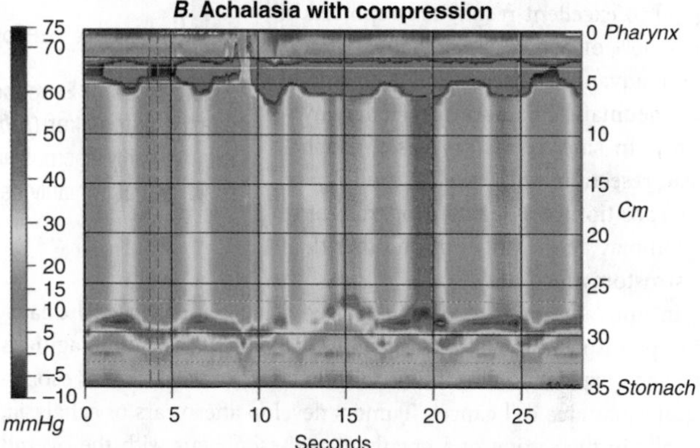

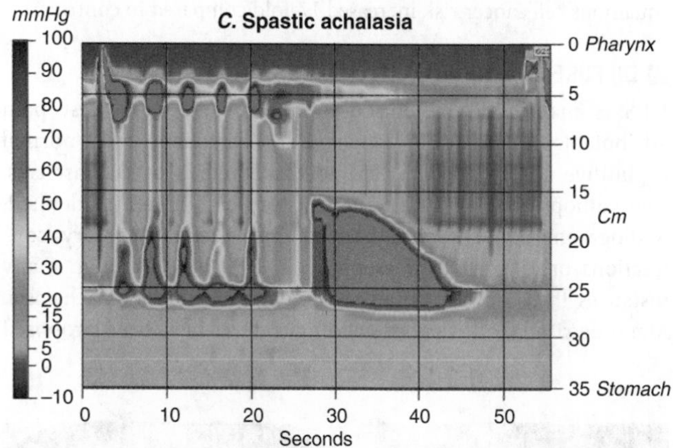

Figure 292-6 Three subtypes of achalasia: classic (*Panel A*), with esophageal compression (*Panel B*), and spastic achalasia (*Panel C*) imaged with pressure topography. All are characterized by impaired lower esophageal sphincter (LES) relaxation and absent peristalsis. However, classic achalasia has minimal pressurization of the esophageal body while substantial fluid pressurization is observed in achalasia with esophageal compression and spastic esophageal contractions are observed with spastic achalasia.

esophageal pressurization promote esophageal emptying. Peristalsis rarely, if ever, returns. LES pressure can be reduced by pharmacologicals therapy, forceful dilatation, or surgical myotomy. No large, controlled trials of the therapeutic alternatives exist and the optimal approach is debated. Pharmacologicals therapies are relatively ineffective but are often used as temporizing therapies. Nitrates or calcium channel blockers are administered before eating, advising caution because of their effects on blood pressure. Botulinum toxin, injected into the LES under endoscopic guidance, inhibits acetylcholine release from nerve endings and improves dysphagia in about 66% of cases for at least 6 months. Sildenafil, or alternative phosphodiesterase inhibitors, effectively decrease LES pressure, but practicalities limit their clinical use in achalasia.

The only durable therapies for achalasia are pneumatic dilatation and Heller myotomy. Pneumatic dilatation, with a reported efficacy ranging from 32–98%, is an endoscopic technique using a noncompliant, cylindrical balloon dilator positioned across the LES and inflated to a diameter of 3–4 cm. The major complication is perforation with a reported incidence of 1–5%. The most common surgical procedure for achalasia is laparoscopic Heller myotomy, usually performed in conjunction with an antireflux procedure (partial fundoplication); good to excellent results are reported in 62–100% of cases. Occasionally, patients with advanced disease fail to respond to pneumatic dilatation or Heller myotomy. In such refractory cases, esophageal resection with gastric pull-up or interposition of a segment of transverse colon may be the only option other than gastrostomy feeding.

Figure 292-8 Esophageal pressure topography of the two major variants of esophageal spasm: spastic nutcracker (*left*) and diffuse esophageal spasm (*right*). Spastic nutcracker is defined by the extraordinarily vigorous and repetitive contractions with normal peristaltic onset. Diffuse esophageal spasm is similar but primarily defined by a rapid propagation at the onset of the contraction.

In untreated or inadequately treated achalasia, esophageal dilatation predisposes to stasis esophagitis. Prolonged stasis esophagitis is the likely explanation for the association between achalasia and esophageal squamous cell cancer. Tumors develop after years of achalasia, usually in the setting of a greatly dilated esophagus with the overall squamous cell cancer risk increased 17-fold compared to controls.

DIFFUSE ESOPHAGEAL SPASM (DES)

DES is manifested by episodes of dysphagia and chest pain attributable to abnormal esophageal contractions with normal deglutitive LES relaxation. Beyond that, there is little consensus. The pathophysiology and natural history of DES are ill defined. Radiographically, DES has been characterized by tertiary contractions or a "corkscrew esophagus" (Fig. 292-7), but in many instances these abnormalities are actually indicative of achalasia. Manometrically, a variety of defining features have been proposed including uncoordinated ("spastic") activity in the distal esophagus, spontaneous and repetitive contractions, or high amplitude and prolonged contractions. Greatest consensus exists with the concept that simultaneous contractions define DES. All of these definitions lead to patients with a variety of disorders being diagnosed as DES. In fact, high-resolution manometry suggests that DES, when defined in a restrictive fashion (Fig. 292-8), is actually much less common than achalasia and suspected cases are often incorrectly categorized achalasia.

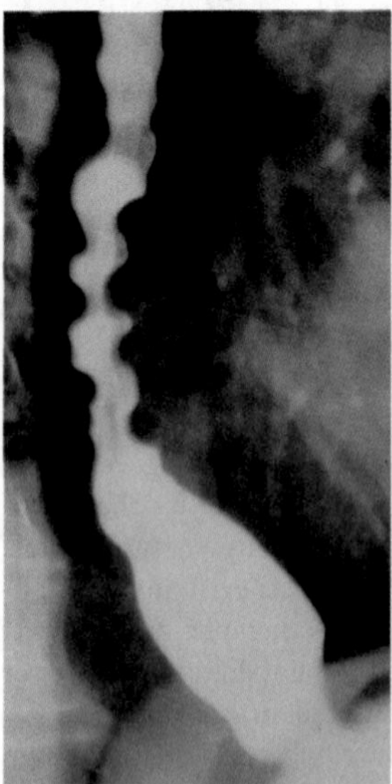

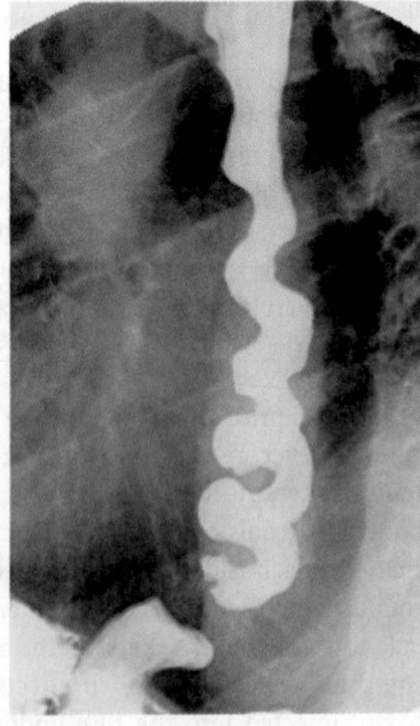

Figure 292-7 Diffuse esophageal spasm. The characteristic "corkscrew" esophagus results from spastic contraction of the circular muscle in the esophageal wall; more precisely, this is actually a helical array of muscle. These findings are also seen with spastic achalasia.

Esophageal chest pain closely mimics angina pectoris. Features suggesting esophageal pain include pain that is nonexertional, prolonged, interrupts sleep, is meal-related, is relieved with antacids, and is accompanied by heartburn, dysphagia, or regurgitation. However, all of these features exhibit overlap with cardiac pain, which still must be the primary consideration. Furthermore, even within the spectrum of esophageal diseases, both chest pain and dysphagia are also characteristic of peptic or infectious esophagitis. Only after these more common entities have been excluded by evaluation and/or treatment should a diagnosis of DES be pursued.

Although the defining criteria are currently disputed, DES is diagnosed by manometry. Endoscopy is useful to identify alternative structural and inflammatory lesions that may cause chest pain. Radiographically, a "corkscrew esophagus," "rosary bead esophagus," pseudodiverticula, or curling can be indicative of DES, but these are also found with spastic achalasia. Given these vagaries of defining DES, and the resultant heterogeneity of patients identified for inclusion in therapeutic trials, it is not surprising that trial results have been disappointing. Only small, uncontrolled trials exist, reporting response to nitrates, calcium channel blockers, hydralazine, botulinum toxin, and anxiolytics. The only controlled trial showing efficacy was with an anxiolytic. Surgical therapy (long myotomy or even esophagectomy) should be considered only with severe weight loss or unbearable pain. These indications are extremely rare.

NONSPECIFIC MANOMETRIC FINDINGS

Manometric studies done to evaluate chest pain and/or dysphagia often report minor abnormalities (hypertensive or hypotensive peristalsis, hypertensive LES, etc.) that are insufficient to diagnose either achalasia or DES. These findings are of unclear significance. Reflux and psychiatric diagnoses, particularly anxiety and depression, are common among such individuals. A lower visceral pain threshold and symptoms of irritable bowel syndrome are noted in more than half of such patients. Consequently, therapy for these individuals should either target the most common esophageal disorder, GERD, or more global conditions such as depression or somatization neurosis that are found to be coexistent.

GASTROESOPHAGEAL REFLUX DISEASE (GERD)

The current conception of GERD is to encompass a family of conditions with the commonality that they are caused by the gastroesophageal reflux resulting in either troublesome symptoms or an array of potential esophageal and extraesophageal manifestations. It is estimated that 15% of adults in the United States are affected by GERD, although such estimates are based only on self-reported chronic heartburn. With respect to the esophagus, the spectrum of injury includes esophagitis, stricture, Barrett's esophagus, and adenocarcinoma (Fig. 292-9). Of particular concern is the rising incidence of esophageal adenocarcinoma, an epidemiologic trend that parallels the increasing incidence of GERD. There were about 8,000 incident cases of esophageal adenocarcinoma in the United States in 2010 (half of all esophageal cancers); it is estimated that this disease burden has increased two- to sixfold in the last 20 years.

PATHOPHYSIOLOGY

The best defined subset of GERD patients, albeit a minority overall, have esophagitis. Esophagitis occurs when refluxed gastric acid and pepsin cause necrosis of the esophageal mucosa causing erosions and ulcers. Note that some degree of gastroesophageal reflux is normal, physiologically intertwined with the mechanism of belching (transient LES relaxation), but esophagitis results from excessive reflux, often accompanied by impaired clearance of the refluxed gastric juice. Restricting reflux to that which is physiologically intended depends on the anatomic and physiologic integrity of the esophagogastric junction, a complex sphincter comprised of both the LES and the surrounding crural diaphragm. Three dominant mechanisms of esophagogastric junction incompetence are recognized: (1) transient LES relaxations (a vagovagal reflex in which LES relaxation is elicited by gastric distention), (2) LES hypotension, or (3) anatomic distortion of the esophagogastric junction inclusive of hiatus hernia. Of note, the third factor, esophagogastric junction anatomic disruption, is both significant unto itself and also because it interacts with the first two mechanisms. Transient LES relaxations account for at least 90% of reflux in normal subjects or GERD patients without hiatus hernia, but patients with hiatus hernia have a more heterogeneous mechanistic profile. Factors tending to exacerbate reflux regardless of mechanism are abdominal obesity, pregnancy, gastric hypersecretory states, delayed gastric emptying, disruption of esophageal peristalsis, and gluttony.

After acid reflux, peristalsis returns the refluxed fluid to the stomach and acid clearance is completed by titration of the residual acid by bicarbonate contained in swallowed saliva. Consequently, two causes of prolonged acid clearance are impaired peristalsis and reduced salivation. Impaired peristaltic emptying can be attributable to disrupted peristalsis or superimposed reflux associated with a hiatal hernia. With superimposed reflux, fluid retained within a sliding hiatal hernia refluxes back into the esophagus during swallow-related LES relaxation, a phenomenon that does not normally occur.

Inherent in the pathophysiologic model of GERD is that gastric juice is harmful to the esophageal epithelium. However, gastric acid hypersecretion is usually not a dominant factor in the development of esophagitis. An obvious exception is with Zollinger-Ellison syndrome, which is associated with severe esophagitis in about 50% of patients. Another caveat is with chronic *H. pylori* gastritis, which may have a protective effect by inducing atrophic gastritis with concomitant hypoacidity. Pepsin, bile, and pancreatic enzymes within gastric secretions can also injure the esophageal epithelium, but their noxious properties are either lessened in an acidic environment or dependent on acidity for activation. Bile warrants attention because it persists in refluxate despite acid-suppressing medications. Bile can transverse the cell membrane, imparting severe cellular injury in a weakly acidic environment, and has also been invoked as a cofactor in the pathogenesis of Barrett's metaplasia and adenocarcinoma. Hence, the causticity of gastric refluxate extends beyond hydrochloric acid.

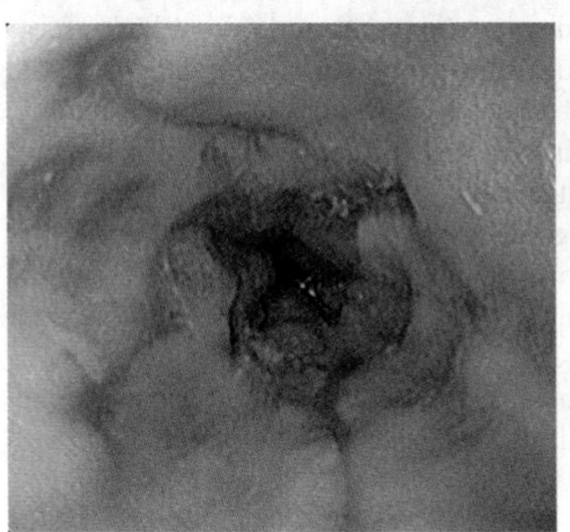

A Erosive esophagitis

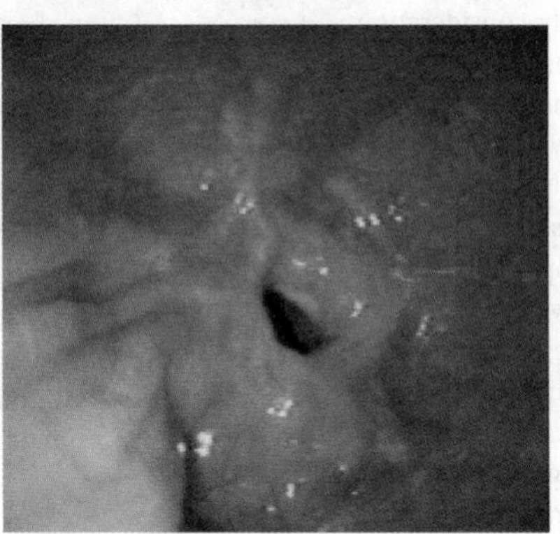

B Esophageal stricture with chronic erosive esophagitis

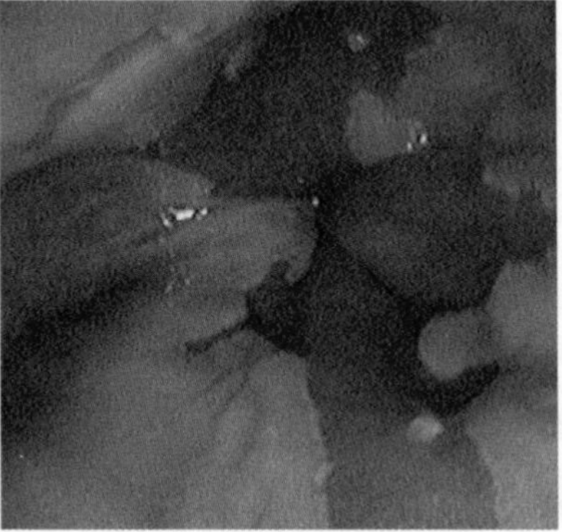

C Barrett's esophagus

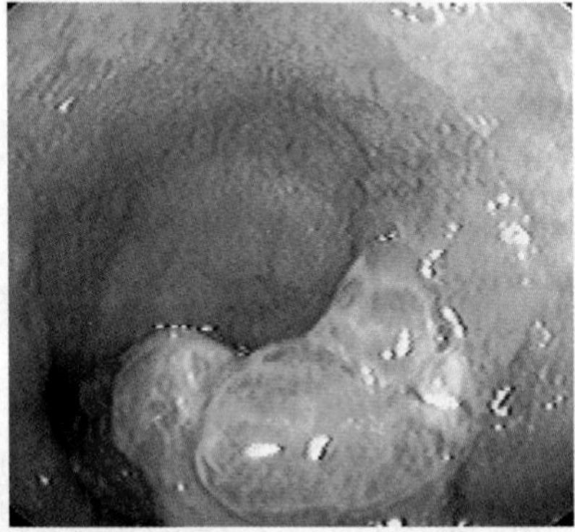

D Esophageal adenocarcinoma with Barrett's esophagus

Figure 292-9 Endoscopic appearance of (*A*) peptic esophagitis, (*B*) a peptic stricture, (*C*) Barrett's metaplasia, and (*D*) adenocarcinoma developing within an area of Barrett's esophagus.

SYMPTOMS

Heartburn and regurgitation are the typical symptoms of GERD. Somewhat less common are dysphagia and chest pain. In each case, multiple potential mechanisms for symptom genesis operate that extend beyond the basic concepts of mucosal erosion and activation of afferent sensory nerves. Specifically, hypersensitivity and functional pain are increasingly recognized as confounding factors. Nonetheless the dominant clinical strategy is of empirical treatment with acid inhibitors, reserving further evaluation for those who fail to respond. Important exceptions to this are patients with chest pain or persistent dysphagia, each of which may be indicative of more morbid conditions. With chest pain, cardiac disease must be carefully considered. In the case of persistent dysphagia, chronic reflux can lead to the development of a peptic stricture or adenocarcinoma, each of which benefits from early detection and/or specific therapy.

Extraesophageal syndromes with an established association to GERD include chronic cough, laryngitis, asthma, and dental erosions. A multitude of other conditions including pharyngitis, chronic bronchitis, pulmonary fibrosis, chronic sinusitis, cardiac arrhythmias, sleep apnea, and recurrent aspiration pneumonia have proposed associations with GERD. However, in both cases it is important to emphasize the word association as opposed to causation. In many instances the disorders likely coexist because of shared pathogenetic mechanisms rather than strict causality. Potential mechanisms for extraesophageal GERD manifestations are of either regurgitation with direct contact between the refluxate and supraesophageal structures or via a vagovagal reflex wherein reflux activation of esophageal afferent nerves triggers efferent vagal reflexes such as bronchospasm, cough, or arrhythmias.

DIFFERENTIAL DIAGNOSIS

Although generally quite characteristic, symptoms from GERD need to be distinguished from symptoms related to infectious, pill, or eosinophilic esophagitis, peptic ulcer disease, dyspepsia, biliary colic, coronary artery disease, and esophageal motility disorders. It is especially important that coronary artery disease be given early consideration because of its potentially lethal implications. The remaining elements of the differential diagnosis can be addressed by endoscopy, upper gastrointestinal series, or biliary tract ultrasonography as appropriate. The distinction among etiologies of esophagitis is usually easily made by endoscopy with mucosal biopsies, which are necessary to evaluate for eosinophilic inflammation. In terms of endoscopic appearance, infectious esophagitis is diffuse and tends to involve the proximal esophagus far more frequently than does reflux esophagitis. The ulcerations seen in peptic esophagitis are usually solitary and distal, whereas infectious ulcerations are punctate and diffuse. Eosinophilic esophagitis characteristically exhibits multiple esophageal rings, linear furrows, or white punctate exudate. Esophageal ulcerations from pill esophagitis are usually singular and deep at points of luminal narrowing, especially near the carina, with sparing of the distal esophagus.

COMPLICATIONS

The complications of GERD are related to chronic esophagitis (bleeding and stricture) and the relationship between GERD and esophageal adenocarcinoma. However, both esophagitis and peptic strictures have become increasingly rare in the era of potent antisecretory medications. Conversely, the most severe histologic consequence of GERD is Barrett's metaplasia with the associated risk of esophageal adenocarcinoma, and the incidence of these lesions has increased, not decreased in the era of potent acid suppression. Barrett's metaplasia, endoscopically recognized by tongues of reddish mucosa extending proximally from the gastroesophageal junction (Fig. 292-9) or histopathologically by the finding of specialized columnar metaplasia, is associated with at least a 20-fold increased risk for development of esophageal adenocarcinoma.

Barrett's metaplasia can progress to adenocarcinoma through the intermediate stages of low- and high-grade dysplasia (Fig. 292-10). Owing to this risk, areas of Barrett's and especially any included areas of mucosal irregularity should be extensively biopsied. The rate of cancer development is estimated at 0.5% per year, but vagaries in definition and of the extent of Barrett's metaplasia requisite to establish the diagnosis have contributed to variability and inconsistency in this risk assessment. The group at greatest risk is obese white males in their sixth decade of life. However, despite common practice, the utility of endoscopic screening and surveillance programs intended to control the adenocarcinoma risk has not been established. Also of note, no high-level evidence confirms that aggressive antisecretory therapy or antireflux surgery causes regression of Barrett's esophagus or prevents adenocarcinoma.

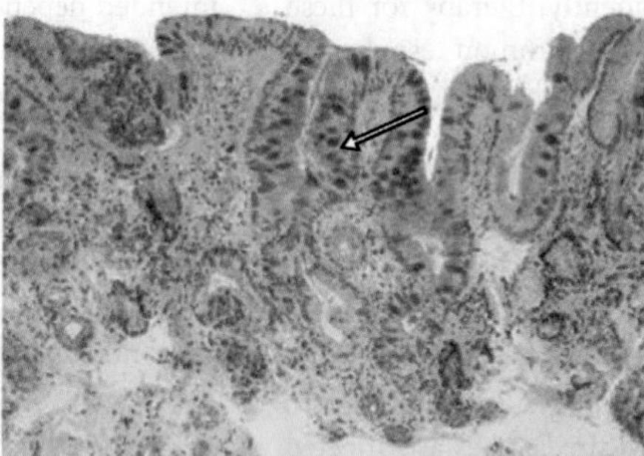

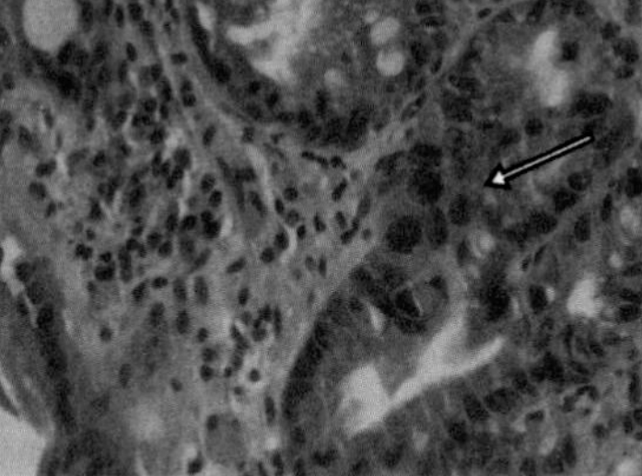

Figure 292-10 Histopathology of Barrett's metaplasia and Barrett's with high-grade dysplasia. H&E, hematoxylin and eosin.

Although the management of Barrett's esophagus remains controversial, the finding of dysplasia in Barrett's, particularly high-grade dysplasia, mandates further intervention. In addition to the high rate of progression to adenocarcinoma, there is also a high prevalence of unrecognized coexisting cancer with high-grade dysplasia. Nonetheless, treatment remains controversial. Esophagectomy, intensive endoscopic surveillance, and mucosal ablation have all been advocated. Currently, most experts advocate esophagectomy as treatment for high-grade dysplasia in an otherwise healthy patient with minimal surgical risk. However, esophagectomy has a mortality ranging from 3–10%, along with substantial morbidity. That, along with increasing evidence of the effectiveness of endoscopic therapy with purpose-built radio frequency ablation devices, has led many to favor this therapy as a preferable alternative.

TREATMENT Gastroesophageal Reflux Disease (GERD)

Lifestyle modifications are routinely advocated as GERD therapy. Broadly speaking, these fall into three categories: (1) avoidance of foods that reduce lower esophageal sphincter pressure, making them "refluxogenic" (these commonly include fatty foods, alcohol, spearmint, peppermint, tomato-based foods, possibly coffee and tea); (2) avoidance of acidic foods that are inherently irritating; and (3) adoption of behaviors to minimize reflux and/or heartburn. In general, minimal evidence supports the efficacy of these measures. However, clinical experience dictates that subsets of patients are benefitted by specific recommendations, based on their unique history and symptom profile. A patient with sleep disturbance from nighttime heartburn is likely to benefit from elevation of the head of the bed and avoidance of eating before retiring, but those recommendations are superfluous for a patient without nighttime symptoms. The most broadly applicable recommendation is for weight reduction. Even though the benefit with respect to reflux cannot be assured, the strong epidemiologic association between obesity and GERD and the secondary health gains of weight reduction are beyond dispute.

The dominant pharmacologic approach to GERD management is with inhibitors of gastric acid secretion and abundant data support the effectiveness of this approach. Pharmacologically reducing the acidity of gastric juice does not prevent reflux, but it ameliorates reflux symptoms and allows esophagitis to heal. The hierarchy of effectiveness among pharmaceuticals parallels their antisecretory potency. Proton pump inhibitors (PPIs) are more efficacious than histamine$_2$ receptor antagonists (H_2RAs), and both are superior to placebo. No major differences exist among PPIs and only modest gain is achieved by increased dosage.

Paradoxically, the perceived frequency and severity of heartburn correlate poorly with the presence or severity of esophagitis. When GERD treatments are assessed in terms of resolving heartburn, both efficacy and differences among pharmaceuticals are less clear-cut than with the objective of healing esophagitis. Although the same overall hierarchy of effectiveness exists, observed efficacy rates are lower and vary widely, likely reflective of patient heterogeneity.

Reflux symptoms tend to be chronic, irrespective of esophagitis. Thus, a common management strategy is indefinite treatment with PPIs or H_2RAs as necessary for symptom control. The side effects of PPI therapy are generally minimal. Vitamin B_{12}, calcium, and iron absorption may be compromised and susceptibility to enteric infections, particularly *Clostridium difficile* colitis increased with treatment. Consequently, as with any medication, dosage should be minimized to that necessary.

Laparoscopic Nissen fundoplication, wherein the proximal stomach is wrapped around the distal esophagus to create an antireflux barrier, is a surgical alternative to the management of chronic GERD. Just as with PPI therapy, evidence on the utility of fundoplication is strongest for treating esophagitis and controlled trials suggest similar efficacy to PPI therapy. However, the benefits of fundoplication must be weighed against potential deleterious effects, including surgical morbidity and mortality, postoperative dysphagia, failure or breakdown requiring reoperation, an inability to belch, and increased bloating, flatulence, and bowel symptoms after surgery.

EOSINOPHILIC ESOPHAGITIS

Eosinophilic esophagitis (EoE) is increasingly recognized in adults and children around the world. Population-based studies suggest the prevalence to be in excess of 1:1000 with a predilection for white males. The increasing prevalence of EoE is attributable to a combination of an increasing incidence and a growing awareness of the condition. There is also an incompletely understood, but important, overlap between EoE and GERD that delays or confuses diagnosis of the disease in many cases.

EoE is diagnosed based on the combination of typical esophageal symptoms and esophageal mucosal biopsies demonstrating esophageal squamous epithelial infiltration with eosinophils. Secondary etiologies of esophageal eosinophilia including GERD, drug hypersensitivity, connective tissue disorders, hypereosinophilic syndrome and infection are excluded. Current evidence indicates that EoE is an allergic disorder induced by antigen sensitization in susceptible individuals. Studies have demonstrated an important role for dietary allergens in both the pathogenesis and treatment of EoE. Aeroallergens may also contribute but there is much less evidence in this regard. The natural history of the disorder is uncertain as are the consequences of not treating asymptomatic or minimally symptomatic patients.

EoE should be strongly considered in children and adults with dysphagia and food impactions, regardless of the presence or absence of heartburn. Other symptoms may include atypical chest pain and heartburn, particularly heartburn that is refractory to PPI therapy. An atopic history of food allergy, asthma, eczema, or allergic rhinitis is present in the majority of patients. Cytokines such as IL-5, eotaxin, and thymus and activation-related chemokine (TARC) may be elevated in the serum. The characteristic endoscopic findings include multiple esophageal rings, linear furrows, and punctate exudates (Fig. 292-11). Histologic confirmation is made with the demonstration of increased eosinophils in the

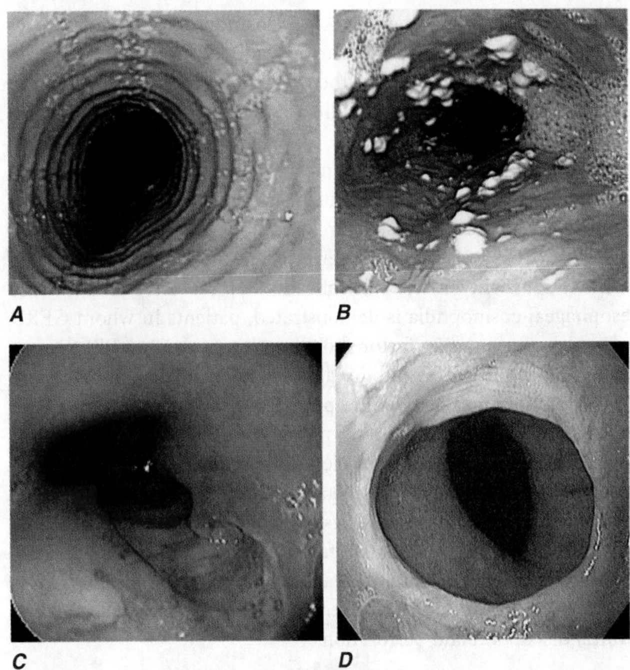

Figure 292-11 Endoscopic features of (*A*) eosinophilic esophagitis (EoE), (*B*) *Candida* esophagitis, (*C*) giant ulcer associated with HIV, (*D*) and a Schatzki ring.

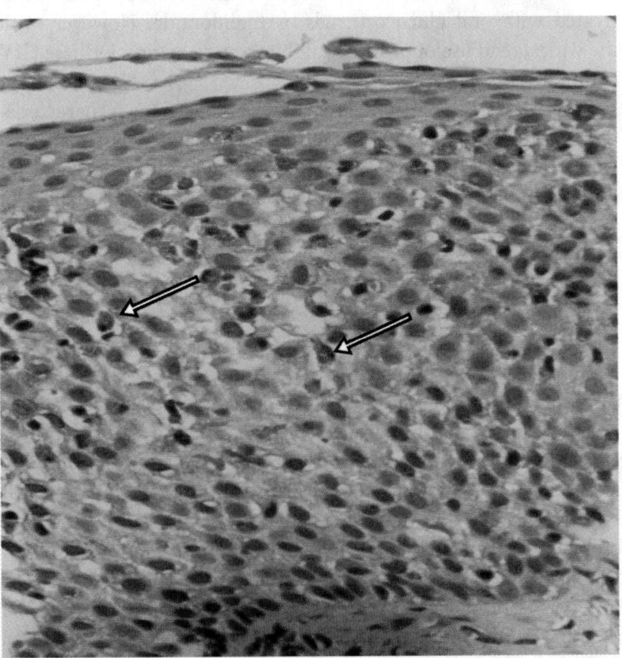

Figure 292-12 Histopathology of eosinophilic esophagitis (EoE) showing dense infiltration of the esophageal squamous epithelium with eosinophils. Eosinophilic inflammation can also be seen with gastroesophageal reflux disease (GERD); the optimal discriminatory threshold for EoE is greater than 15 eosinophils per high-power field.

esophagal mucosa (generally ≥ 15 eosinophils per high-power field) (Fig. 292-12). Fibrosis, narrow caliber esophagus, and stricture can occur with EoE, but the predictive variables for these are not known. Complications of disease include food impaction and esophageal perforation.

Treatments for EoE include dietary restrictions, PPIs, systemic or topical glucocorticoids, montelukast, immunomodulators, and endoscopic dilatation of strictures. Notably, allergy testing [radioallergosorbent test (RAST), skin prick testing] has demonstrated limited specificity in the identification of causative foods. Once esophageal eosinophilia is demonstrated, patients in whom GERD may be a confounding factor should undergo a trial of PPI therapy to determine if this results in clinical or histologic improvement. If symptoms and eosinophilia persist despite PPI therapy, other treatment options should be pursued. Topical glucocorticoids (fluticasone propionate or budesonide) are the most commonly used treatment in adults, but dietary restriction has proven effective primarily in pediatric studies. Systemic glucocorticoids are reserved for severely afflicted patients refractory to less morbid treatments. Esophageal dilation should be approached cautiously in patients with stricturing because of concerns for increased risk of esophageal mural disruption and perforation.

INFECTIOUS ESOPHAGITIS

With the increased use of immunosuppression for organ transplantation as well as chronic inflammatory diseases and chemotherapy along with the AIDS epidemic, infections with *Candida* species, *Herpesvirus,* and cytomegalovirus (CMV) have become relatively common. Although rare, infectious esophagitis also occurs among the nonimmunocompromised, with herpes simplex and *Candida albicans* being the most common pathogens. Among AIDS patients, infectious esophagitis becomes more common as the CD4 count declines; cases are rare with the CD4 count >200 and common when <100. HIV itself may also be associated with a self-limited syndrome of acute esophageal ulceration with oral ulcers and a maculopapular skin rash at the time of seroconversion. Additionally, some patients with advanced disease have deep, persistent esophageal ulcers treated with oral glucocorticoids or thalidomide. However, with the widespread use of protease inhibitors, a reduction in these HIV complications has been noted.

Regardless of the infectious agent, odynophagia is a characteristic symptom of infectious esophagitis; dysphagia, chest pain, and hemorrhage are also common. Odynophagia is uncommon with reflux esophagitis, so its presence should always raise suspicion of an alternative etiology.

CANDIDA ESOPHAGITIS

Candida is normally found in the throat, but can become pathogenic and produce esophagitis in a compromised host; *C. albicans* is most common. *Candida* esophagitis also occurs with esophageal stasis secondary to esophageal motor disorders and diverticula. Patients complain of odynophagia and dysphagia. If oral thrush is present, empirical therapy is appropriate, but coinfection is common, and persistent symptoms should lead to prompt endoscopy with biopsy, which is the most useful diagnostic evaluation. *Candida* esophagitis has a characteristic appearance of white plaques with friability. Rarely, *Candida* esophagitis is complicated by bleeding, perforation, stricture, or systemic invasion. Oral fluconazole (200 mg on the first day, followed by 100 mg daily) for 7–14 days is the preferred treatment. Patients refractory to fluconazole may respond to itraconazole. Alternatively, poorly responsive patients or those who cannot swallow medications can be treated with an intravenous echinocandin (caspofungin 50 mg daily for 7–21 days). Amphotericin B (10–15 mg IV infusion for 6 h daily to a total dose of 300–500 mg) is used in severe cases.

HERPETIC ESOPHAGITIS

Herpes simplex virus type 1 or 2 may cause esophagitis. Vesicles on the nose and lips may coexist and are suggestive of a herpetic etiology. Varicella-zoster virus can also cause esophagitis in children with chickenpox or adults with zoster. The characteristic endoscopic findings are vesicles and small, punched-out ulcerations. Because herpes simplex infections are limited to squamous epithelium, biopsies from the ulcer margins are most likely to reveal the characteristic ground glass nuclei, eosinophilic Cowdry's type A inclusion bodies, and giant cells. Culture or polymerase chain reaction (PCR) assays are helpful to identify acyclovir-resistant strains. The infection is often self-limited after a 1–2 week period. Acyclovir (400 mg orally 5 times a day for 14–21 days) or valacyclovir (1 g orally tid for 7 days) reduces this morbidity. In patients with severe odynophagia, intravenous acyclovir, 5 mg/kg every 8 h for 7–14 days, foscarnet (90 mg/kg intravenously bid for 2–4 weeks) or oral famciclovir are used.

CYTOMEGALOVIRUS

CMV esophagitis occurs only in immunocompromised patients, particularly transplant recipients. CMV is usually activated from a latent stage or may be acquired from transfusions. Endoscopically, CMV lesions appear as serpiginous ulcers in an otherwise normal mucosa, particularly in the distal esophagus. Biopsies of the ulcer bases have the highest diagnostic yield for finding the pathognomonic large nuclear or cytoplasmic inclusion bodies. Immunohistology with monoclonal antibodies to CMV and in situ hybridization tests are useful for early diagnosis. Ganciclovir, 5 mg/kg every 12 h intravenously, is the treatment of choice. Valganciclovir (900 mg bid), an oral formulation of ganciclovir, or foscarnet (90 mg/kg every 12 h intravenously) can also be used. Therapy is continued until healing, which may take 3–6 weeks.

MECHANICAL TRAUMA AND IATROGENIC INJURY

ESOPHAGEAL PERFORATION

Most cases of esophageal perforation are from instrumentation of the esophagus or trauma. Alternatively, forceful vomiting or retching can lead to spontaneous rupture at the gastroesophageal junction (Boerhaave's syndrome). More rarely, corrosive esophagitis or neoplasms lead to perforation. Instrumental perforation from endoscopy or nasogastric tube placement typically occurs in the hypopharynx or at the gastroesophageal junction. Perforation may also result at the site of stricture in the setting of endoscopic food disimpaction or esophageal dilation. Esophageal perforation causes pleuritic retrosternal pain that can be associated with pneumomediastinum and subcutaneous emphysema. Mediastinitis is a major complication of esophageal perforation, and prompt recognition is key to optimizing outcome. CT of the chest is most sensitive in detecting mediastinal air. Esophageal perforation is confirmed by a contrast swallow; usually Gastrografin followed by thin barium. Treatment includes nasogastric suction and parenteral broad-spectrum antibiotics with prompt surgical drainage and repair in noncontained leaks. Conservative therapy with NPO status and antibiotics without surgery may be appropriate in cases of minor instrumental perforation that are detected early. Endoscopic clipping or stent placement may be indicated in nonoperable cases such as perforated tumors.

MALLORY-WEISS TEAR

Vomiting, retching, or vigorous coughing can cause a nontransmural tear at the gastroesophageal junction that is a common cause of upper gastrointestinal bleeding. Most patients present with hematemesis. Antecedent vomiting is anticipated but not always evident. Bleeding usually abates spontaneously, but protracted bleeding may respond to local epinephrine or cauterization therapy, endoscopic clipping, or angiographic embolization. Surgery is rarely needed.

RADIATION ESOPHAGITIS

Radiation esophagitis can complicate treatment for thoracic cancers, especially breast and lung, with the risk proportional to radiation dosage. Radiosensitizing drugs such as doxorubicin, bleomycin, cyclophosphamide, and cisplatin also increase the risk. Dysphagia and odynophagia may last weeks to months after therapy. The esophageal mucosa becomes erythematous, edematous, and friable. Submucosal fibrosis and degenerative tissue changes and stricturing may occur years after the radiation exposure. Radiation exposure in excess of 5000 cGY has been associated with increased risk of esophageal stricture. Treatment for acute radiation esophagitis is supportive. Chronic strictures are managed with esophageal dilation.

CORROSIVE ESOPHAGITIS

Caustic esophageal injury from ingestion of alkali or, less commonly, acid can be accidental or from attempted suicide. Absence of oral injury does not exclude possible esophageal involvement. Thus, early endoscopic evaluation is recommended to assess and grade the injury to the esophageal mucosa. Severe corrosive injury may lead to esophageal perforation, bleeding, stricture, and death. Glucocorticoids have not been shown to improve the clinical outcome of acute corrosive esophagitis and are not recommended. Healing of more severe grades of caustic injury is commonly associated with severe stricture formation and often requires repeated dilatation.

PILL ESOPHAGITIS

Pill-induced esophagitis occurs when a swallowed pill fails to traverses the entire esophagus and lodges within the lumen. Generally, this is attributed to poor "pill taking habits": inadequate liquid with the pill, or lying down immediately after taking a pill. The most common location for the pill to lodge is in the mid-esophagus near the crossing of the aorta or carina. Extrinsic compression from these structures halts the movement of the pill or capsule. Since initially reported in 1970, more than 1000 cases of pill esophagitis have been reported, suggesting that this is not an unusual occurrence. A wide variety of medications are implicated with the most common being doxycycline, tetracycline, quinidine, phenytoin, potassium chloride, ferrous sulfate, nonsteroidal anti-inflammatory drugs (NSAIDs), and bisphosphonates. However, virtually any pill can result in pill esophagitis if taken carelessly.

Typical symptoms of pill esophagitis are the sudden onset of chest pain and odynophagia. Characteristically, the pain will develop over a period of hours or will awaken the individual from sleep. A classic history in the setting of ingestion of recognized pill offenders obviates the need for diagnostic testing in most patients. When endoscopy is performed, localized ulceration or inflammation is evident. Histologically, acute inflammation is typical. Chest CT imaging will sometimes reveal esophageal thickening consistent with transmural inflammation. Although the condition usually resolves within days to weeks, symptoms may persist for months and stricture can develop in severe cases. No specific therapy is known to hasten the healing process, but antisecretory medications are frequently prescribed to remove concomitant reflux as an aggravating factor. When healing results in stricture formation, dilatation is indicated.

FOREIGN BODIES AND FOOD IMPACTION

Food or foreign bodies may lodge in the esophagus causing complete obstruction, causing an inability to handle secretions (foaming at the mouth) and severe chest pain. Food impaction may occur due to stricture, carcinoma, Schatzki ring, eosinophilic esophagitis, or simply inattentive eating. If it does not spontaneously resolve, impacted food is dislodged endoscopically. Use of meat tenderizer enzymes to facilitate passage of a meat bolus is discouraged because of potential esophageal injury. Glucagon (1 mg IV) is sometimes tried before endoscopic dislodgement. After emergent treatment patients should be evaluated for potential causes of the impaction with treatment rendered as indicated.

ESOPHAGEAL MANIFESTATIONS OF SYSTEMIC DISEASE

SCLERODERMA AND COLLAGEN VASCULAR DISEASES

Scleroderma esophagus (hypotensive LES and absent esophageal peristalsis) was initially described as a manifestation of scleroderma or other collagen vascular diseases and thought to be specific for these disorders. However, this nomenclature subsequently proved unfortunate and has been discarded because an estimated half of qualifying patients do not have an identifiable systemic disease, and reflux disease is often the only identifiable association. When scleroderma esophagus occurs as a manifestation of a collagen vascular disease, the histopathologic findings are of infiltration and destruction of the esophageal muscularis propria with collagen deposition and fibrosis. The pathogenesis of absent peristalsis and LES hypotension in the absence of a collagen vascular disease is unknown. Regardless of the underlying cause, the manometric abnormalities predispose patients to severe GERD due to inadequate LES barrier function combined with poor esophageal clearance of refluxed acid. Dysphagia may also be manifest but is generally mild and alleviated by eating in an upright position and using liquids to facilitate solid emptying.

DERMATOLOGIC DISEASES

A host of dermatologic disorders (pemphigus vulgaris, bullous pemphigoid, cicatricial pemphigoid, Behçet's syndrome, epidermolysis bullosa) can affect the oropharynx and esophagus, particularly the proximal esophagus with blisters, bullae, webs, and strictures. Glucocorticoid treatment is usually effective. Erosive lichen planus, Stevens-Johnson syndrome, and graft-versus-host disease can also involve the esophagus. Esophageal dilatation may be necessary to treat strictures.

FURTHER READINGS

Furuta GT et al: Eosinophilic esophagitis in children and adults: A systematic review and consensus recommendations for diagnosis and treatment. Gastroenterology 133:1342, 2007

Jacobsen B et al: Body-mass index and symptoms of gastroesophageal reflux in women. N Engl J Med 354:2340, 2006

Kahrilas PJ: Clinical practice. Gastroesophageal reflux disease. N Engl J Med 359:1700, 2008

———: Esophageal motor disorders in terms of high resolution esophageal pressure topography: What has changed? Am J Gastroenterol 105:981, 2010

———, Pandolfino JE: Hiatus hernia. GI Motility Online, *http://www.nature.com/gimo/contents/pt1/full/gimo48.html*, 2006

——— et al: AGAI medical position statement: Management of gastroesophageal reflux disease. Gastroenterology 135:1383, 2008

Sampliner RE, Sharma P (eds): *Barrett's Esophagus and Esophageal Adenocarcinoma*, 2nd ed. Malden, MA, Blackwell, 2006

Shaheen NJ et al: Radiofrequency ablation in Barrett's esophagus with dysplasia. N Engl J Med 360:2277, 2009

Walzer N, Hirano I: Achalasia. Gastroenterol Clin North Am 37:807, 2008

CHAPTER 293
Peptic Ulcer Disease and Related Disorders

John Del Valle

PEPTIC ULCER DISEASE

Burning epigastric pain exacerbated by fasting and improved with meals is a symptom complex associated with peptic ulcer disease (PUD). An *ulcer* is defined as disruption of the mucosal integrity of the stomach and/or duodenum leading to a local defect or excavation due to active inflammation. Ulcers occur within the stomach and/or duodenum and are often chronic in nature. Acid peptic disorders are very common in the United States, with 4 million individuals (new cases and recurrences) affected per year. Lifetime prevalence of PUD in the United States is ~12% in men and 10% in women. Moreover, an estimated 15,000 deaths per year occur as a consequence of complicated PUD. The financial impact of these common disorders has been substantial, with an estimated burden on direct and indirect health care costs of ~$10 billion per year in the United States.

GASTRIC PHYSIOLOGY

Despite the constant attack on the gastroduodenal mucosa by a host of noxious agents (acid, pepsin, bile acids, pancreatic enzymes, drugs, and bacteria), integrity is maintained by an intricate system that provides mucosal defense and repair.

Gastric anatomy

The gastric epithelial lining consists of rugae that contain microscopic gastric pits, each branching into four or five gastric glands made up of highly specialized epithelial cells. The makeup of gastric glands varies with their anatomic location. Glands within the gastric cardia comprise <5% of the gastric gland area and contain mucous and endocrine cells. The 75% of gastric glands are found within the oxyntic mucosa and contain mucous neck, parietal, chief, endocrine, enterochromaffin, and enterochromaffin-like (ECL) cells (Fig. 293-1). Pyloric glands contain mucous and endocrine cells (including gastrin cells) and are found in the antrum.

The parietal cell, also known as the oxyntic cell, is usually found in the neck, or isthmus, or in the oxyntic gland. The resting, or unstimulated, parietal cell has prominent cytoplasmic tubulovesicles and intracellular canaliculi containing short microvilli along its apical surface (Fig. 293-2). H^+,K^+-adenosine triphosphatase (ATPase) is expressed in the tubulovesicle membrane; upon cell stimulation, this membrane, along with apical membranes, transforms into a dense network of apical intracellular canaliculi containing long microvilli. Acid secretion, a process requiring high energy, occurs at the apical canalicular surface. Numerous mitochondria (30–40% of total cell volume) generate the energy required for secretion.

Gastroduodenal mucosal defense

The gastric epithelium is under constant assault by a series of endogenous noxious factors, including hydrochloric acid (HCl), pepsinogen/pepsin, and bile salts. In addition, a steady flow of exogenous substances such as medications, alcohol, and bacteria encounter the gastric mucosa. A highly intricate biologic system is

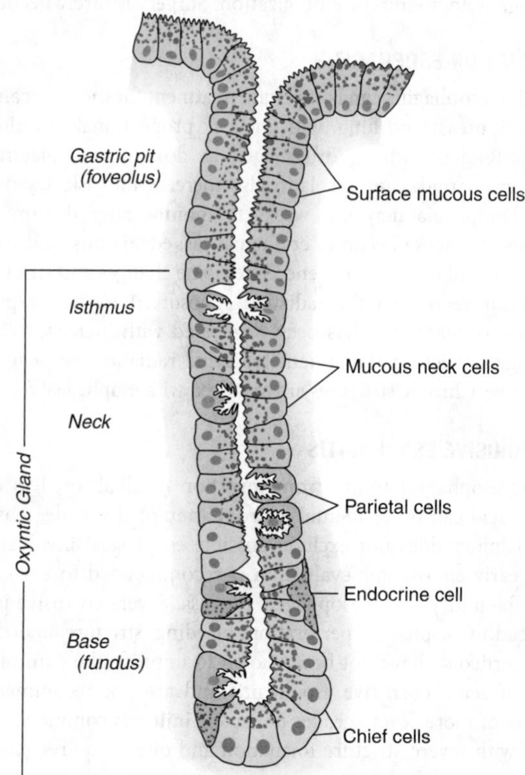

Figure 293-1 Diagrammatic representation of the oxyntic gastric gland. *(Adapted from S Ito, RJ Winchester: Cell Biol 16:541, 1963. © The Rockefeller University Press.)*

in place to provide defense from mucosal injury and to repair any injury that may occur.

The mucosal defense system can be envisioned as a three-level barrier, composed of preepithelial, epithelial, and subepithelial elements (Fig. 293-3). The first line of defense is a mucus-bicarbonate-phospholipid layer, which serves as a physicochemical barrier to multiple molecules, including hydrogen ions. Mucus is secreted in a regulated fashion by gastroduodenal surface epithelial cells. It consists primarily of water (95%) and a mixture of phospholipids and glycoproteins (mucin). The mucous gel functions as a nonstirred water layer impeding diffusion of ions and molecules such as pepsin. Bicarbonate, secreted in a regulated manner by surface

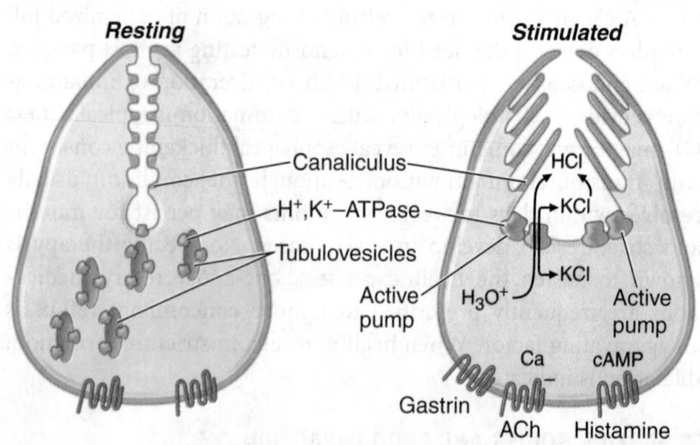

Figure 293-2 Gastric parietal cell undergoing transformation after secretagogue-mediated stimulation. cAMP, cyclic adenosine monophosphate. *(Adapted from SJ Hersey, G Sachs: Physiol Rev 75:155, 1995.)*

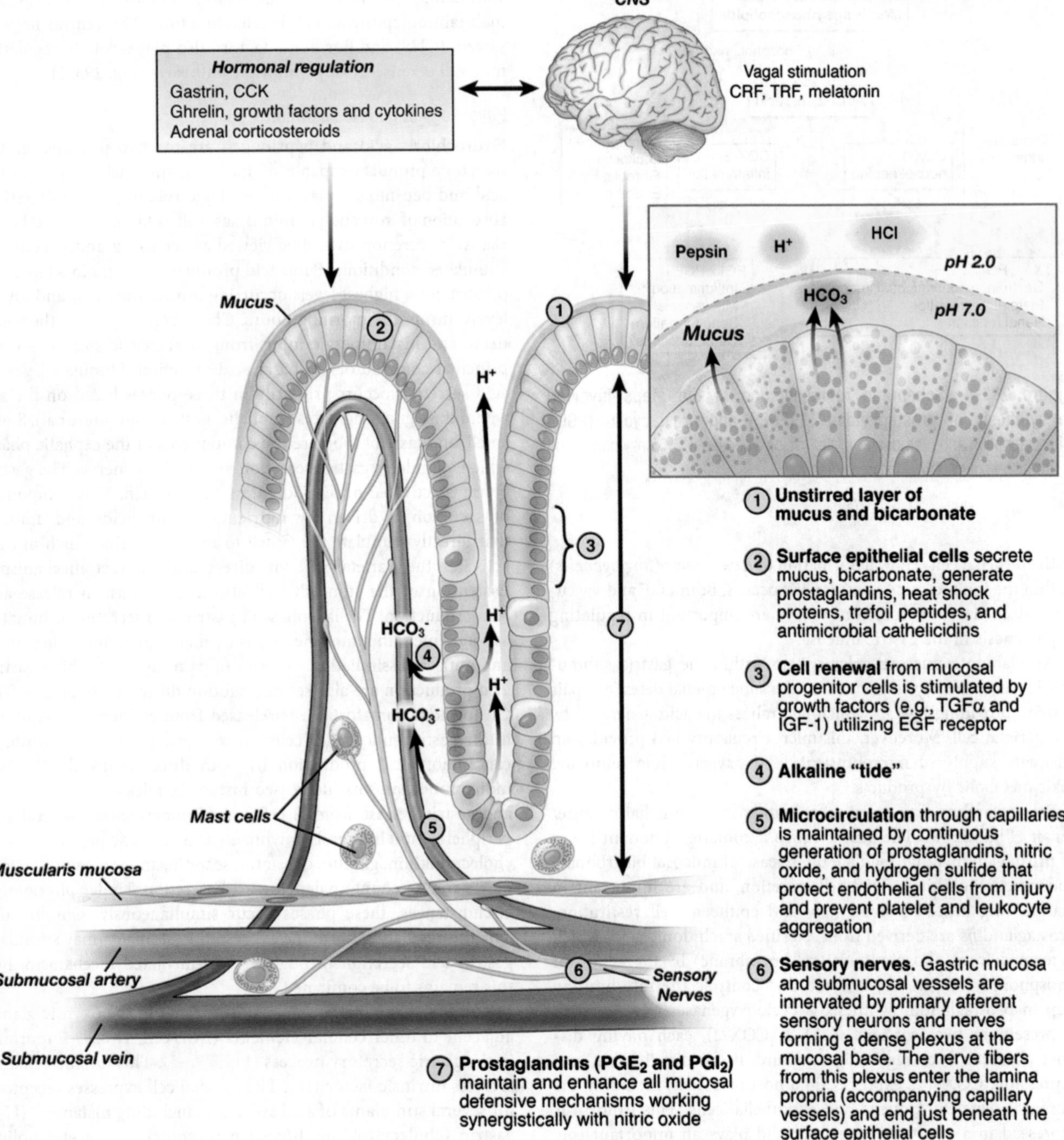

Figure 293-3 Components involved in providing gastroduodenal mucosal defense and repair. CCK, cholecystokinin; CRF, corticotropin-releasing factor; EGF, epidermal growth factor; HCl, hydrochloride; IGF, insulin-like growth factor; TGFα, transforming growth factor α; TRF, thyrotropin releasing factor. *(Modified and updated from Tarnawski A. Cellular and molecular mechanisms of mucosal defense and repair. In: Yoshikawa T, Arakawa T. Bioregulation and Its Disorders in the Gastrointestinal Tract. Tokyo, Japan: Blackwell Science, 1998:3–17.)*

epithelial cells of the gastroduodenal mucosa into the mucous gel, forms a pH gradient ranging from 1 to 2 at the gastric luminal surface and reaching 6 to 7 along the epithelial cell surface.

Surface epithelial cells provide the next line of defense through several factors, including mucus production, epithelial cell ionic transporters that maintain intracellular pH and bicarbonate production, and intracellular tight junctions. Surface epithelial cells generate heat shock proteins that prevent protein denaturation and protect cells from certain factors such as increased temperature, cytotoxic agents, or oxidative stress. Epithelial cells also generate trefoil factor family peptides and cathelicidins, which also play a role in surface cell protection and regeneration. If the preepithelial barrier were breached, gastric epithelial cells bordering a site of injury can migrate to restore a damaged region (*restitution*). This process occurs independent of cell division and requires uninterrupted blood flow and an alkaline pH in the surrounding environment. Several growth factors, including epidermal growth factor (EGF), transforming growth factor (TGF) α, and basic fibroblast growth factor (FGF), modulate the process of restitution. Larger defects that are not effectively repaired by restitution require cell proliferation. Epithelial cell regeneration is regulated by prostaglandins and growth factors such as EGF and TGF-α. In tandem

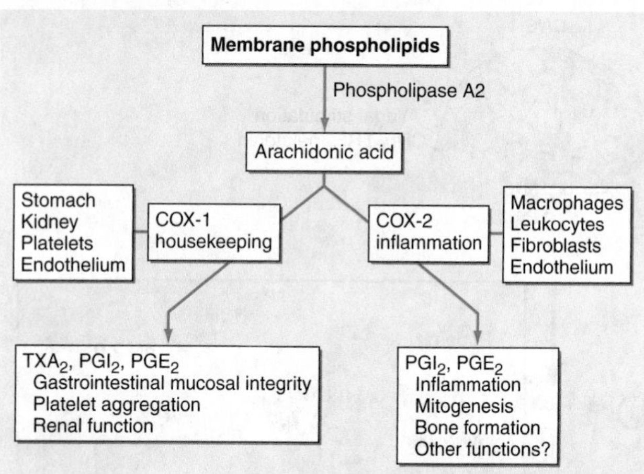

Figure 293-4 Schematic representation of the steps involved in synthesis of prostaglandin E_2 (PGE_2) and prostacyclin (PGI_2). Characteristics and distribution of the cyclooxygenase (COX) enzymes 1 and 2 are also shown. TXA_2, thromboxane A_2.

with epithelial cell renewal, formation of new vessels (*angiogenesis*) within the injured microvascular bed occurs. Both FGF and vascular endothelial growth factor (VEGF) are important in regulating angiogenesis in the gastric mucosa.

An elaborate microvascular system within the gastric submucosal layer is the key component of the subepithelial defense/repair system, providing HCO_3^-, which neutralizes the acid generated by the parietal cell. Moreover, this microcirculatory bed provides an adequate supply of micronutrients and oxygen while removing toxic metabolic by-products.

Prostaglandins play a central role in gastric epithelial defense/repair (Fig. 293-4). The gastric mucosa contains abundant levels of prostaglandins that regulate the release of mucosal bicarbonate and mucus, inhibit parietal cell secretion, and are important in maintaining mucosal blood flow and epithelial cell restitution. Prostaglandins are derived from esterified arachidonic acid, which is formed from phospholipids (cell membrane) by the action of phospholipase A_2. A key enzyme that controls the rate-limiting step in prostaglandin synthesis is cyclooxygenase (COX), which is present in two isoforms (COX-1, COX-2), each having distinct characteristics regarding structure, tissue distribution, and expression. COX-1 is expressed in a host of tissues, including the stomach, platelets, kidneys, and endothelial cells. This isoform is expressed in a constitutive manner and plays an important role in maintaining the integrity of renal function, platelet aggregation, and gastrointestinal (GI) mucosal integrity. In contrast, the expression of COX-2 is inducible by inflammatory stimuli, and it is expressed in macrophages, leukocytes, fibroblasts, and synovial cells. The beneficial effects of nonsteroidal anti-inflammatory drugs (NSAIDs) on tissue inflammation are due to inhibition of COX-2; the toxicity of these drugs (e.g., GI mucosal ulceration and renal dysfunction) is related to inhibition of the COX-1 isoform. The highly COX-2–selective NSAIDs have the potential to provide the beneficial effect of decreasing tissue inflammation while minimizing toxicity in the GI tract. Selective COX-2 inhibitors have had adverse effects on the cardiovascular system, leading to increased risk of myocardial infarction. Therefore, the FDA has removed two of these agents (valdecoxib and rofecoxib) from the market (see below).

Nitric oxide (NO) is important in the maintenance of gastric mucosal integrity. The key enzyme NO synthase is constitutively expressed in the mucosa and contributes to cytoprotection by stimulating gastric mucus, increasing mucosal blood flow and maintaining epithelial cell barrier function. The central nervous system (CNS) and hormonal factors also play a role in regulating mucosal defense through multiple pathways (Fig. 293-3).

Physiology of gastric secretion

Hydrochloric acid and pepsinogen are the two principal gastric secretory products capable of inducing mucosal injury. Gastric acid and pepsinogen play a physiologic role in protein digestion, absorption of iron and vitamin B_{12} as well as killing ingested bacteria. Acid secretion should be viewed as occurring under basal and stimulated conditions. Basal acid production occurs in a circadian pattern, with highest levels occurring during the night and lowest levels during the morning hours. Cholinergic input via the vagus nerve and histaminergic input from local gastric sources are the principal contributors to basal acid secretion. Stimulated gastric acid secretion occurs primarily in three phases based on the site where the signal originates (cephalic, gastric, and intestinal). Sight, smell, and taste of food are the components of the cephalic phase, which stimulates gastric secretion via the vagus nerve. The gastric phase is activated once food enters the stomach. This component of secretion is driven by nutrients (amino acids and amines) that directly stimulate the G cell to release gastrin, which in turn activates the parietal cell via direct and indirect mechanisms. Distention of the stomach wall also leads to gastrin release and acid production. The last phase of gastric acid secretion is initiated as food enters the intestine and is mediated by luminal distention and nutrient assimilation. A series of pathways that inhibit gastric acid production are also set into motion during these phases. The GI hormone somatostatin is released from endocrine cells found in the gastric mucosa (D cells) in response to HCl. Somatostatin can inhibit acid production by both direct (parietal cell) and indirect mechanisms (decreased histamine release from ECL cells and gastrin release from G cells). Additional neural (central and peripheral) and humoral [amylin, atrial natriuretic peptide (ANP), cholecystokinin, ghrelin, obestatin, secretin, and serotonin] factors play a role in counterbalancing acid secretion. Under physiologic circumstances, these phases occur simultaneously. Ghrelin, the appetite-regulating hormone expressed in stomach, may stimulate gastric acid secretion through a vagal-mediated mechanism, but this remains to be confirmed.

The acid-secreting parietal cell is located in the oxyntic gland, adjacent to other cellular elements (ECL cell, D cell) important in the gastric secretory process (Fig. 293-5). This unique cell also secretes intrinsic factor (IF). The parietal cell expresses receptors for several stimulants of acid secretion, including histamine (H_2), gastrin (cholecystokinin B/gastrin receptor), and acetylcholine (muscarinic, M_3). Binding of histamine to the H_2 receptor leads to activation of adenylate cyclase and an increase in cyclic adenosine monophosphate (AMP). Activation of the gastrin and muscarinic receptors results in activation of the protein kinase C/phosphoinositide signaling pathway. Each of these signaling pathways in turn regulates a series of downstream kinase cascades that control the acid-secreting pump, H^+,K^+-ATPase. The discovery that different ligands and their corresponding receptors lead to activation of different signaling pathways explains the potentiation of acid secretion that occurs when histamine and gastrin or acetylcholine are combined. More importantly, this observation explains why blocking one receptor type (H_2) decreases acid secretion stimulated by agents that activate a different pathway (gastrin, acetylcholine). Parietal cells also express receptors for ligands that inhibit acid production (prostaglandins, somatostatin, and EGF). Histamine also stimulates gastric acid secretion indirectly by activating the histamine H_3 receptor on D-cells, which inhibits somatostatin release.

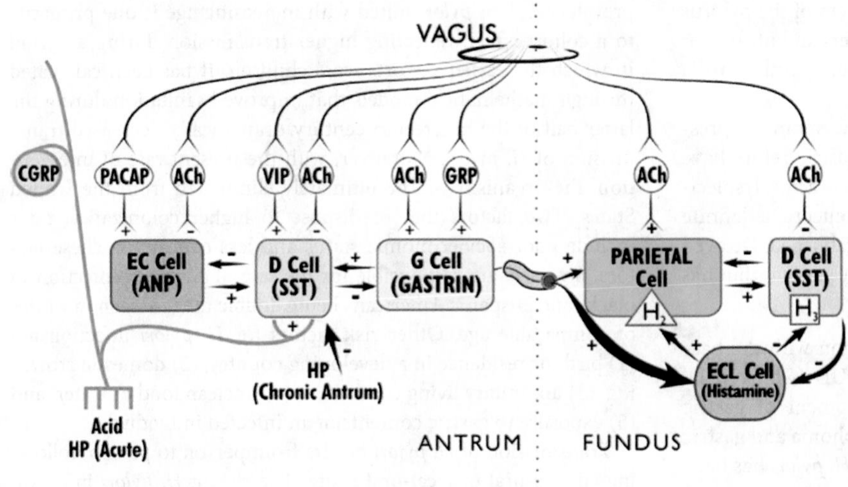

Figure 293-5 Regulation of gastric acid secretion at the cellular level. ACh, acetylcholine; ANP, atrial natriuretic peptide; CGRP, calcitonin gene-related peptide; EC, enterochromaffin; ECL, enterochromaffin-like; GRP, gastrin-releasing peptide; PACAP, pituitary adenylate-cyclase activating peptide; SST, somatostatin; VIP, vasoactive intestinal peptide.

The enzyme H^+,K^+-ATPase is responsible for generating the large concentration of H^+. It is a membrane-bound protein that consists of two subunits, α and β. The active catalytic site is found within the α subunit; the function of the β subunit is unclear. This enzyme uses the chemical energy of adenosine triphosphate (ATP) to transfer H^+ ions from parietal cell cytoplasm to the secretory canaliculi in exchange for K^+. The H^+,K^+-ATPase is located within the secretory canaliculus and in nonsecretory cytoplasmic tubulovesicles. The tubulovesicles are impermeable to K^+, which leads to an inactive pump in this location. The distribution of pumps between the nonsecretory vesicles and the secretory canaliculus varies according to parietal cell activity (Fig. 293-2). Proton pumps are recycled back to the inactive state in cytoplasmic vesicles once parietal cell activation ceases.

The chief cell, found primarily in the gastric fundus, synthesizes and secretes pepsinogen, the inactive precursor of the proteolytic enzyme pepsin. The acid environment within the stomach leads to cleavage of the inactive precursor to pepsin and provides the low pH (<2) required for pepsin activity. Pepsin activity is significantly diminished at a pH of 4 and irreversibly inactivated and denatured at a pH of ≥7. Many of the secretagogues that stimulate acid secretion also stimulate pepsinogen release. The precise role of pepsin in the pathogenesis of PUD remains to be established.

PATHOPHYSIOLOGIC BASIS OF PEPTIC ULCER DISEASE

PUD encompasses both gastric and duodenal ulcers. *Ulcers* are defined as breaks in the mucosal surface >5 mm in size, with depth to the submucosa. Duodenal ulcers (DUs) and gastric ulcers (GUs); share many common features in terms of pathogenesis, diagnosis, and treatment, but several factors distinguish them from one another.

Epidemiology

Duodenal ulcers DUs are estimated to occur in 6–15% of the Western population. The incidence of DUs declined steadily from 1960 to 1980 and has remained stable since then. The death rates, need for surgery, and physician visits have decreased by >50% over the past 30 years. The reason for the reduction in the frequency of DUs is likely related to the decreasing frequency of *Helicobacter pylori.* Before the discovery of *H. pylori,* the natural history of DUs was typified by frequent recurrences after initial therapy. Eradication of *H. pylori* has greatly reduced these recurrence rates.

Gastric ulcers GUs tend to occur later in life than duodenal lesions, with a peak incidence reported in the sixth decade. More than one-half of GUs occur in males and are less common than DUs, perhaps due to the higher likelihood of GUs being silent and presenting only after a complication develops. Autopsy studies suggest a similar incidence of DUs and GUs.

Pathology

Duodenal ulcers DUs occur most often in the first portion of the duodenum (>95%), with ~90% located within 3 cm of the pylorus. They are usually ≤1 cm in diameter but can occasionally reach 3–6 cm (giant ulcer). Ulcers are sharply demarcated, with depth at times reaching the muscularis propria. The base of the ulcer often consists of a zone of eosinophilic necrosis with surrounding fibrosis. Malignant DUs are extremely rare.

Gastric ulcers In contrast to DUs, GUs can represent a malignancy and should be biopsied upon discovery. Benign GUs are most often found distal to the junction between the antrum and the acid secretory mucosa. Benign GUs are quite rare in the gastric fundus and are histologically similar to DUs. Benign GUs associated with *H. pylori* are also associated with antral gastritis. In contrast, NSAID-related GUs are not accompanied by chronic active gastritis but may instead have evidence of a chemical gastropathy, typified by foveolar hyperplasia, edema of the lamina propria, and epithelial regeneration in the absence of *H. pylori.* Extension of smooth-muscle fibers into the upper portions of the mucosa, where they are not typically found, may also occur.

Pathophysiology

Duodenal ulcers *H. pylori* and NSAID-induced injury account for the majority of DUs. Many acid secretory abnormalities have been described in DU patients. Of these, average basal and nocturnal gastric acid secretion appears to be increased in DU patients as compared to controls; however, the level of overlap between DU patients and control subjects is substantial. The reason for this altered secretory process is unclear, but *H. pylori* infection may contribute. Accelerated gastric emptying of liquids has been noted in some DU patients, but its role in DU formation, if any, is unclear. Bicarbonate secretion is significantly decreased in the duodenal bulb of patients with an active DU as compared to control subjects. *H. pylori* infection may also play a role in this process (see below).

Gastric ulcers As in DUs, the majority of GUs can be attributed to either *H. pylori* or NSAID-induced mucosal damage. GUs that occur in the prepyloric area or those in the body associated with a DU or a duodenal scar are similar in pathogenesis to DUs. Gastric acid output (basal and stimulated) tends to be normal or decreased in GU patients. When GUs develop in the presence of minimal acid levels, impairment of mucosal defense factors may be present. Gastric ulcers have been classified based on their location: Type I occur in the gastric body and tend to be associated with low gastric acid production; type II occur in the antrum and gastric acid can vary from low to normal; type III occur within 3 cm of the pylorus and are commonly accompanied by duodenal ulcers and normal or high gastric acid production; and type IV are found in the cardia and are associated with low gastric acid production.

Abnormalities in resting and stimulated pyloric sphincter pressure with a concomitant increase in duodenal gastric reflux have been implicated in some GU patients. Although bile acids, lysolecithin, and pancreatic enzymes may injure gastric mucosa, a definite role for these in GU pathogenesis has not been established. Delayed gastric emptying of solids has been described in GU patients but has not been reported consistently

H. pylori and acid peptic disorders Gastric infection with the bacterium *H. pylori* accounts for the majority of PUD (Chap. 151). This organism also plays a role in the development of gastric mucosa-associated lymphoid tissue (MALT) lymphoma and gastric adenocarcinoma. Although the entire genome of *H. pylori* has been sequenced, it is still not clear how this organism, which resides in the stomach, causes ulceration in the duodenum, or whether its eradication will lead to a decrease in gastric cancer.

The bacterium The bacterium, initially named *Campylobacter pyloridis,* is a gram-negative microaerophilic rod found most commonly in the deeper portions of the mucous gel coating the gastric mucosa or between the mucous layer and the gastric epithelium. It may attach to gastric epithelium but under normal circumstances does not appear to invade cells. It is strategically designed to live within the aggressive environment of the stomach. It is S-shaped (~0.5–3 μm in size) and contains multiple sheathed flagella. Initially, *H. pylori* resides in the antrum but, over time, migrates toward the more proximal segments of the stomach. The organism is capable of transforming into a coccoid form, which represents a dormant state that may facilitate survival in adverse conditions. The genome of *H. pylori* (1.65 million base pairs) encodes ~1500 proteins. Among this multitude of proteins there are factors that are essential determinants of *H. pylori*–mediated pathogenesis and colonization such as the outer membrane protein (Hop proteins), urease, and the vacuolating cytotoxin (Vac A). Moreover, the majority of *H. pylori* strains contain a genomic fragment that encodes the cag pathogenicity island (cag-PAI). Several of the genes that make up cag-PAI encode components of a type IV secretion island that translocates Cag A into host cells. Once in the cell, Cag A activates a series of cellular events important in cell growth and cytokine production. *H. pylori* also has extensive genetic diversity that in turn enhances its ability to promote disease. The first step in infection by *H. pylori* is dependent on the bacteria's motility and its ability to produce urease. Urease produces ammonia from urea, an essential step in alkalinizing the surrounding pH. Additional bacterial factors include catalase, lipase, adhesins, platelet-activating factor, and pic B (induces cytokines). Multiple strains of *H. pylori* exist and are characterized by their ability to express several of these factors (Cag A, Vac A, etc.). It is possible that the different diseases related to *H. pylori* infection can be attributed to different strains of the organism with distinct pathogenic features.

Epidemiology The prevalence of *H. pylori* varies throughout the world and depends largely on the overall standard of living in the region. In developing parts of the world, 80% of the population may be infected by the age of 20, whereas the prevalence is 20–50% in industrialized countries. In contrast, in the United States this organism is rare in childhood. The overall prevalence of *H. pylori* in the United States is ~30%, with individuals born before 1950 having a higher rate of infection than those born later. About 10% of Americans <30 years of age are colonized with the bacteria. The rate of infection with *H. pylori* in industrialized countries has decreased substantially in recent decades. The steady increase in the prevalence of *H. pylori* noted with increasing age is due primarily to a cohort effect, reflecting higher transmission during a period in which the earlier cohorts were children. It has been calculated through mathematical models that improved sanitation during the latter half of the nineteenth century dramatically decreased transmission of *H. pylori.* Moreover, with the present rate of intervention, the organism will be ultimately eliminated from the United States. Two factors that predispose to higher colonization rates include poor socioeconomic status and less education. These factors, not race, are responsible for the rate of *H. pylori* infection in blacks and Hispanic Americans being double the rate seen in whites of comparable age. Other risk factors for *H. pylori* infection are (1) birth or residence in a developing country, (2) domestic crowding, (3) unsanitary living conditions, (4) unclean food or water, and (5) exposure to gastric contents of an infected individual.

Transmission of *H. pylori* occurs from person to person, following an oral-oral or fecal-oral route. The risk of *H. pylori* infection is declining in developing countries. The rate of infection in the United States has fallen by >50% when compared to 30 years ago.

Pathophysiology *H. pylori* infection is virtually always associated with a chronic active gastritis, but only 10–15% of infected individuals develop frank peptic ulceration. The basis for this difference is unknown, but is likely due to a combination of host and bacterial factors some of which are outlined below. Initial studies suggested that >90% of all DUs were associated with *H. pylori,* but *H. pylori* is present in only 30–60% of individuals with GUs and 50–70% of patients with DUs. The pathophysiology of ulcers not associated with *H. pylori* or NSAID ingestion [or the rare Zollinger-Ellison syndrome (ZES)] is becoming more relevant as the incidence of *H. pylori* is dropping, particularly in the Western world (see below).

The particular end result of *H. pylori* infection (gastritis, PUD, gastric MALT lymphoma, gastric cancer) is determined by a complex interplay between bacterial and host factors (Fig. 293-6).

1. *Bacterial factors: H. pylori* is able to facilitate gastric residence, induce mucosal injury, and avoid host defense. Different strains of *H. pylori* produce different virulence factors. A specific region of the bacterial genome, the pathogenicity island (cag-PAI), encodes the virulence factors Cag A and pic B. Vac A also contributes to pathogenicity, although it is not encoded within the pathogenicity island. These virulence factors, in conjunction

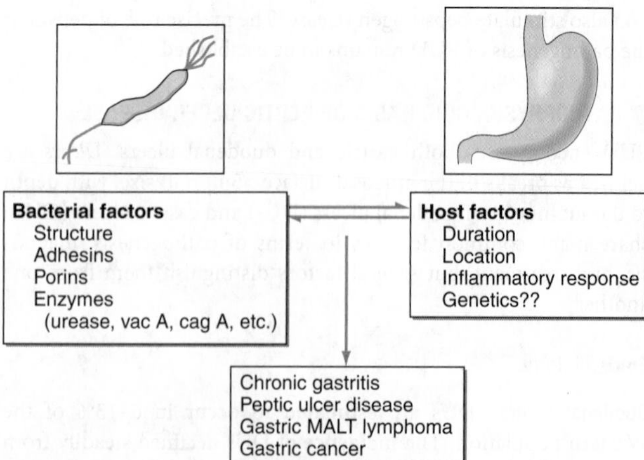

Figure 293-6 Outline of the bacterial and host factors important in determining *H. pylori*–induced gastrointestinal disease. MALT, mucosal-associated lymphoid tissue.

with additional bacterial constituents, can cause mucosal damage, in part through their ability to target the host immune cells. For example, Vac A targets human CD4 T cells, inhibiting their proliferation and in addition can disrupt normal function of B cells, CD8 T cells, macrophages and mast cells. Multiple studies have demonstrated that *H. pylori* strains that are cag-PAI positive are associated with a higher risk of peptic ulcer disease, premalignant gastric lesions and gastric cancer than are strains that lack the cag-PAI. Urease, which allows the bacteria to reside in the acidic stomach, generates NH_3, which can damage epithelial cells. The bacteria produce surface factors that are chemotactic for neutrophils and monocytes, which in turn contribute to epithelial cell injury (see below). *H. pylori* makes proteases and phospholipases that break down the glycoprotein lipid complex of the mucous gel, thus reducing the efficacy of this first line of mucosal defense. *H. pylori* expresses adhesins (OMPs like BabA), which facilitate attachment of the bacteria to gastric epithelial cells. Although lipopolysaccharide (LPS) of gram-negative bacteria often plays an important role in the infection, *H. pylori* LPS has low immunologic activity compared to that of other organisms. It may promote a smoldering chronic inflammation.

2. *Host factors:* Studies in twins suggest that there may be genetic predisposition to acquire *H. pylori.* The inflammatory response to *H. pylori* includes recruitment of neutrophils, lymphocytes (T and B), macrophages, and plasma cells. The pathogen leads to local injury by binding to class II major histocompatability complex (MHC) molecules expressed on gastric epithelial cells, leading to cell death (*apoptosis*). Moreover, bacterial strains that encode cag-PAI can introduce Cag A into the host cells, leading to further cell injury and activation of cellular pathways involved in cytokine production. Elevated concentrations of multiple cytokines are found in the gastric epithelium of *H. pylori*–infected individuals, including interleukin (IL) 1α/β, IL-2, IL-6, IL-8, tumor necrosis factor (TNF) α, and interferon (IFN-γ). *H. pylori* infection also leads to both a mucosal and a systemic humoral response, which does not lead to eradication of the bacteria but further compounds epithelial cell injury. Additional mechanisms by which *H. pylori* may cause epithelial cell injury include (1) activated neutrophil-mediated production of reactive oxygen or nitrogen species and enhanced epithelial cell turnover and (2) apoptosis related to interaction with T cells (T helper 1, or T_H1, cells) and IFN-γ.

The reason for *H. pylori*–mediated duodenal ulceration remains unclear. Studies suggest that *H. pylori* associated with duodenal ulceration may be more virulent. In addition, certain specific bacterial factors such as the duodenal ulcer-promoting gene A (*dupA*), may be associated with the development of duodenal ulcers. Another potential contributing factor is that gastric metaplasia in the duodenum of DU patients, which may be due to high acid exposure (see below), permits *H. pylori* to bind to it and produce local injury secondary to the host response. Another hypothesis is that *H. pylori* antral infection could lead to increased acid production, increased duodenal acid, and mucosal injury. Basal and stimulated [meal, gastrin-releasing peptide (GRP)] gastrin release are increased in *H. pylori*–infected individuals, and somatostatin-secreting D cells may be decreased. *H. pylori* infection might induce increased acid secretion through both direct and indirect actions of *H. pylori* and proinflammatory cytokines (IL-8, TNF, and IL-1) on G, D, and parietal cells (Fig. 293-7). Gastric ulcers, in contrast, are associated with *H. pylori* induced pangastritis and normal or low gastric acid secretion. *H. pylori* infection has also been associated with decreased duodenal mucosal bicarbonate production. Data supporting and contradicting each of these interesting theories have been demonstrated. Thus, the mechanism by which *H. pylori*

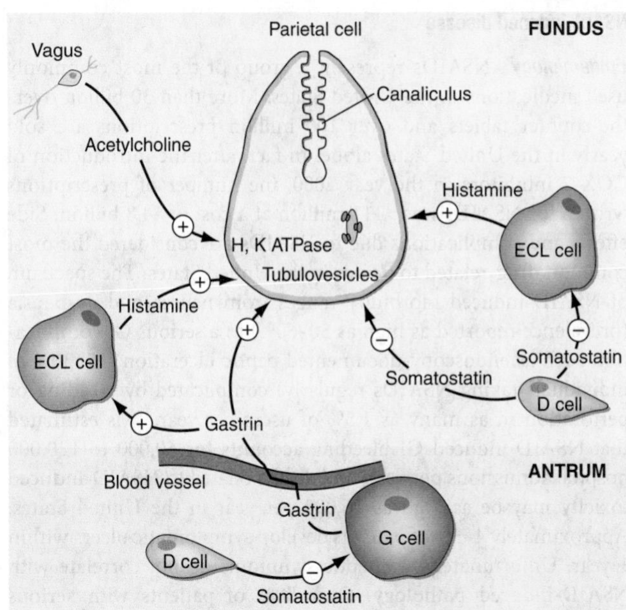

Figure 293-7 Summary of potential mechanisms by which *H. pylori* may lead to gastric secretory abnormalities. D, somatostatin cell; ECL, enterochromaffin-like cell; G, G cell. *(Adapted from J Calam et al: Gastroenterology 113:543, 1997.)*

infection of the stomach leads to duodenal ulceration remains to be established.

In summary, the final effect of *H. pylori* on the GI tract is variable and determined by microbial and host factors. The type and distribution of gastritis correlate with the ultimate gastric and duodenal pathology observed. Specifically, the presence of antral-predominant gastritis is associated with DU formation; gastritis involving primarily the corpus predisposes to the development of GUs, gastric atrophy, and ultimately gastric carcinoma (Fig. 293-8).

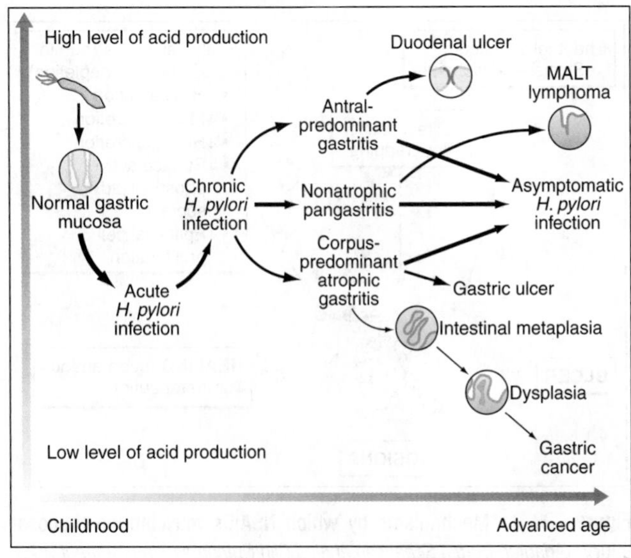

Figure 293-8 Natural history of *H. pylori*-infection. *(Used with permission from S Suerbaum, P Michetti: N Engl J Med 347:1175, 2002.)*

NSAID-induced disease

Epidemiology NSAIDs represent a group of the most commonly used medications in the United States. More than 30 billion over-the-counter tablets and over 100 million prescriptions are sold yearly in the United States alone. In fact, after the introduction of COX-2 inhibitors in the year 2000, the number of prescriptions written for NSAIDs was >111 million at a cost of $4.8 billion. Side effects and complications due to NSAIDs are considered the most common drug-related toxicities in the United States. The spectrum of NSAID-induced morbidity ranges from nausea and dyspepsia (prevalence reported as high as 50–60%) to a serious GI complication such as endoscopy-documented peptic ulceration (15–30% of individuals taking NSAIDs regularly) complicated by bleeding or perforation in as many as 1.5% of users per year. It is estimated that NSAID-induced GI bleeding accounts for 60,000 to 120,000 hospital admissions per year, and deaths related to NSAID-induced toxicity may be as high as 16,000 per year in the United States. Approximately 4–5% of patients develop symptomatic ulcers within 1 year. Unfortunately, dyspeptic symptoms do not correlate with NSAID-induced pathology. Over 80% of patients with serious NSAID-related complications did not have preceding dyspepsia. In view of the lack of warning signs, it is important to identify patients who are at increased risk for morbidity and mortality related to NSAID usage. Even 75 mg/d of aspirin may lead to serious GI ulceration; thus, no dose of NSAID is completely safe. Established risk factors include advanced age, history of ulcer, concomitant use of glucocorticoids, high-dose NSAIDs, multiple NSAIDs, concomitant use of anticoagulants, clopidogrel, and serious or multisystem disease. Possible risk factors include concomitant infection with *H. pylori*, cigarette smoking, and alcohol consumption.

Pathophysiology Prostaglandins play a critical role in maintaining gastroduodenal mucosal integrity and repair. It therefore follows that interruption of prostaglandin synthesis can impair mucosal defense and repair, thus facilitating mucosal injury via a systemic mechanism. Animal studies have demonstrated that neutrophil adherence to the gastric microcirculation plays an essential role in the initiation of NSAID-induced mucosal injury. A summary of the pathogenetic pathways by which systemically administered NSAIDs may lead to mucosal injury is shown in Fig. 293-9.

Injury to the mucosa also occurs as a result of the topical encounter with NSAIDs. Aspirin and many NSAIDs are weak acids that remain in a nonionized lipophilic form when found within the acid environment of the stomach. Under these conditions, NSAIDs migrate across lipid membranes of epithelial cells, leading to cell injury once trapped intracellularly in an ionized form. Topical NSAIDs can also alter the surface mucous layer, permitting back diffusion of H^+ and pepsin, leading to further epithelial cell damage. Moreover, enteric-coated or buffered preparations are also associated with risk of peptic ulceration.

The interplay between *H. pylori* and NSAIDs in the pathogenesis of PUD is complex. Meta-analysis supports the conclusion that each of these aggressive factors is independent and synergistic risk factors for PUD and its complications such as GI bleeding. For example, eradication of *H. pylori* reduces the likelihood of GI complications in high-risk individuals to levels observed in individuals with average risk of NSAID-induced complications.

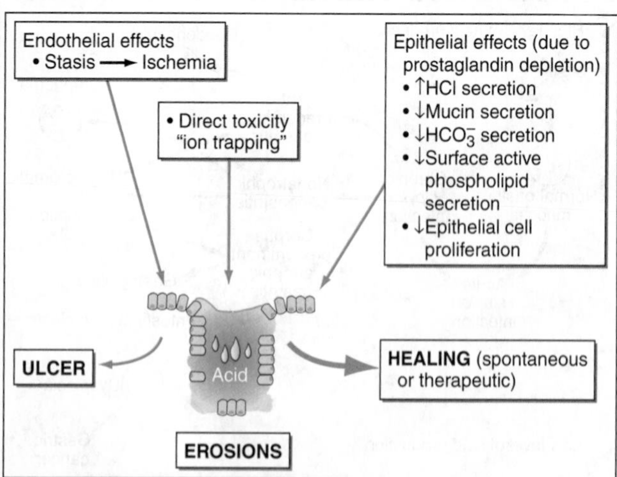

Figure 293-9 Mechanisms by which NSAIDs may induce mucosal injury. *(Adapted from J Scheiman et al: J Clin Outcomes Management 3:23, 1996. Copyright 2003 Turner White Communications, Inc., www.turner-white.com. Used with permission.)*

Pathogenetic factors unrelated to *H. Pylori* and NSAID in acid peptic disease Cigarette smoking has been implicated in the pathogenesis of PUD. Not only have smokers been found to have ulcers more frequently than do nonsmokers, but smoking appears to decrease healing rates, impair response to therapy, and increase ulcer-related complications such as perforation. The mechanism responsible for increased ulcer diathesis in smokers is unknown. Theories have included altered gastric emptying, decreased proximal duodenal bicarbonate production, increased risk for *H. pylori* infection, and cigarette-induced generation of noxious mucosal free radicals. Genetic predisposition may play a role in ulcer development. First-degree relatives of DU patients are three times as likely to develop an ulcer; however, the potential role of *H. pylori* infection in contacts is a major consideration. Increased frequency of blood group O and of the nonsecretor status have also been implicated as genetic risk factors for peptic diathesis. However, *H. pylori* preferentially binds to group O antigens. Psychological stress has been thought to contribute to PUD, but studies examining the role of psychological factors in its pathogenesis have generated conflicting results. Although PUD is associated with certain personality traits (neuroticism), these same traits are also present in individuals with nonulcer dyspepsia (NUD) and other functional and organic disorders.

Diet has also been thought to play a role in peptic diseases. Certain foods and beverages can cause dyspepsia, but no convincing studies indicate an association between ulcer formation and a specific diet. Specific chronic disorders have been shown to have a strong association with PUD: (1) systemic mastocytosis, (2) chronic pulmonary disease, (3) chronic renal failure, (4) cirrhosis, (5) nephrolithiasis, and (6) α_1-antitrypsin deficiency. Those with a possible association are (1) hyperparathyroidism, (2) coronary artery disease, (3) polycythemia vera, and (4) chronic pancreatitis.

Multiple factors play a role in the pathogenesis of PUD. The two predominant causes are *H. pylori* infection and NSAID ingestion. PUD not related to *H. pylori* or NSAIDs is increasing. Other less common causes of PUD are shown in Table 293-1. These etiologic agents should be considered as the incidence of *H. pylori* is decreasing. Independent of the inciting or injurious agent, peptic ulcers develop as a result of an imbalance between mucosal protection/repair and aggressive factors. Gastric acid plays an essential role in mucosal injury.

CLINICAL FEATURES

History

Abdominal pain is common to many GI disorders, including DU and GU, but has a poor predictive value for the presence of either DU or GU. Up to 10% of patients with NSAID-induced mucosal disease can present with a complication (bleeding, perforation, and obstruction) without antecedent symptoms. Despite this poor

TABLE 293-1 Causes of Ulcers Not Caused by *Helicobacter pylori* and NSAIDs

Pathogenesis of Non-Hp and Non-NSAID Ulcer Disease
Infection
Cytomegalovirus
Herpes simplex virus
H. heilmannii
Drug/Toxin
Bisphosphonates
Chemotherapy
Clopidogrel
Crack cocaine
Glucocorticoids (when combined with NSAIDs)
Mycophenolate mofetil
Potassium chloride
Miscellaneous
Basophilia in myeloproliferative disease
Duodenal obstruction (e.g., annular pancreas)
Infiltrating disease
Ischemia
Radiation therapy
Sarcoidosis
Crohn's disease
Idiopathic hypersecretory state

Abbreviations: Hp, *H. pylori;* NSAIDs, nonsteroidal anti-inflammatory drugs.

correlation, a careful history and physical examination are essential components of the approach to a patient suspected of having peptic ulcers.

Epigastric pain described as a burning or gnawing discomfort can be present in both DU and GU. The discomfort is also described as an ill-defined, aching sensation or as hunger pain. The typical pain pattern in DU occurs 90 minutes to 3 hours after a meal and is frequently relieved by antacids or food. Pain that awakes the patient from sleep (between midnight and 3 A.M.) is the most discriminating symptom, with two-thirds of DU patients describing this complaint. Unfortunately, this symptom is also present in one-third of patients with NUD. The pain pattern in GU patients may be different from that in DU patients, where discomfort may actually be precipitated by food. Nausea and weight loss occur more commonly in GU patients. Endoscopy detects ulcers in <30% of patients who have dyspepsia.

The mechanism for development of abdominal pain in ulcer patients is unknown. Several possible explanations include acid-induced activation of chemical receptors in the duodenum, enhanced duodenal sensitivity to bile acids and pepsin, or altered gastroduodenal motility.

Variation in the intensity or distribution of the abdominal pain, as well as the onset of associated symptoms such as nausea and/or vomiting, may be indicative of an ulcer complication. Dyspepsia that becomes constant, is no longer relieved by food or antacids, or radiates to the back may indicate a penetrating ulcer (pancreas). Sudden onset of severe, generalized abdominal pain may indicate perforation. Pain worsening with meals, nausea, and vomiting of undigested food suggest gastric outlet obstruction. Tarry stools or coffee-ground emesis indicate bleeding.

Physical examination

Epigastric tenderness is the most frequent finding in patients with GU or DU. Pain may be found to the right of the midline in 20% of patients. Unfortunately, the predictive value of this finding is rather low. Physical examination is critically important for discovering evidence of ulcer complication. Tachycardia and orthostasis suggest dehydration secondary to vomiting or active GI blood loss. A severely tender, board like abdomen suggests a perforation. Presence of a succussion splash indicates retained fluid in the stomach, suggesting gastric outlet obstruction.

PUD-related complications

Gastrointestinal bleeding GI bleeding is the most common complication observed in PUD. It occurs in ~15% of patients and more often in individuals >60 years of age. The mortality rate is as high as 5–10%. The higher incidence in the elderly is likely due to the increased use of NSAIDs in this group. Up to 20% of patients with ulcer-related hemorrhage bleed without any preceding warning signs or symptoms.

Perforation The second most common ulcer-related complication is perforation, being reported in as many as 6–7% of PUD patients. As in the case of bleeding, the incidence of perforation in the elderly appears to be increasing secondary to increased use of NSAIDs. *Penetration* is a form of perforation in which the ulcer bed tunnels into an adjacent organ. DUs tend to penetrate posteriorly into the pancreas, leading to pancreatitis, whereas GUs tend to penetrate into the left hepatic lobe. Gastrocolic fistulas associated with GUs have also been described.

Gastric outlet obstruction Gastric outlet obstruction is the least common ulcer-related complication, occurring in 1–2% of patients. A patient may have relative obstruction secondary to ulcer-related inflammation and edema in the peripyloric region. This process often resolves with ulcer healing. A fixed, mechanical obstruction secondary to scar formation in the peripyloric areas is also possible. The latter requires endoscopic (balloon dilation) or surgical intervention. Signs and symptoms relative to mechanical obstruction may develop insidiously. New onset of early satiety, nausea, vomiting, increase of postprandial abdominal pain, and weight loss should make gastric outlet obstruction a possible diagnosis.

Differential diagnosis

The list of gastrointestinal and nongastrointestinal disorders that can mimic ulceration of the stomach or duodenum is quite extensive. The most commonly encountered diagnosis among patients seen for upper abdominal discomfort is NUD. NUD, also known as *functional dyspepsia* or *essential dyspepsia,* refers to a group of heterogeneous disorders typified by upper abdominal pain without the presence of an ulcer. Dyspepsia has been reported to occur in up to 30% of the U.S. population. Up to 60% of patients seeking medical care for dyspepsia have a negative diagnostic evaluation. The etiology of NUD is not established, and the potential role of *H. pylori* in NUD remains controversial.

Several additional disease processes that may present with "ulcer-like" symptoms include proximal GI tumors, gastroesophageal reflux, vascular disease, pancreaticobiliary disease (biliary colic, chronic pancreatitis), and gastroduodenal Crohn's disease.

Diagnostic evaluation

In view of the poor predictive value of abdominal pain for the presence of a gastroduodenal ulcer and the multiple disease processes

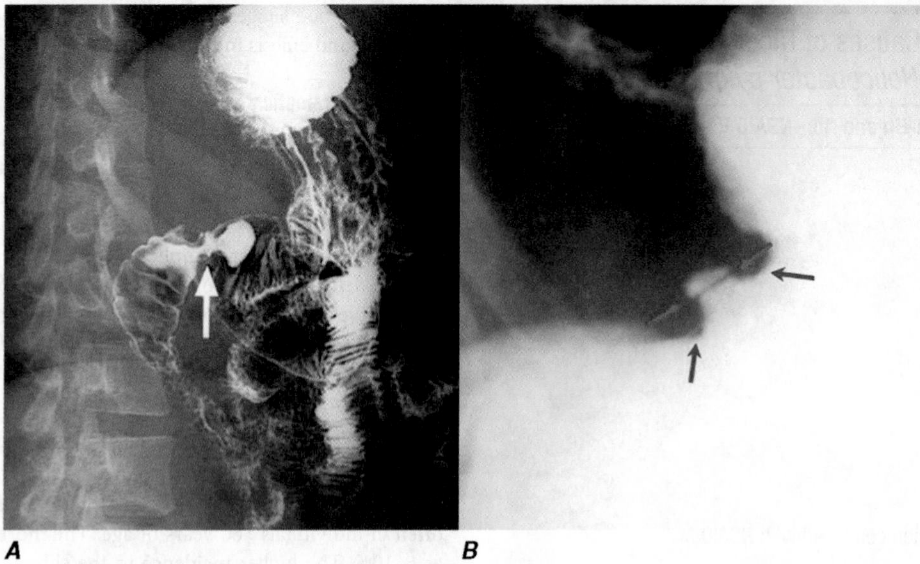

Figure 293-10 Barium study demonstrating: *A.* a benign duodenal ulcer; ***B.*** a benign gastric ulcer.

that can mimic this disease, the clinician is often confronted with having to establish the presence of an ulcer. Documentation of an ulcer requires either a radiographic (barium study) or an endoscopic procedure. However, a large percentage of patients with symptoms suggestive of an ulcer have NUD; empirical therapy is appropriate for individuals who are otherwise healthy and <45 years of age, before embarking on a diagnostic evaluation (Chap. 39).

Barium studies of the proximal GI tract are still commonly used as a first test for documenting an ulcer. The sensitivity of older single-contrast barium meals for detecting a DU is as high as 80%, with a double-contrast study providing detection rates as high as 90%. Sensitivity for detection is decreased in small ulcers (<0.5 cm), presence of previous scarring, or in postoperative patients. A DU appears as a well-demarcated crater, most often seen in the bulb (Fig. 293-10*A*). A GU may represent benign or malignant disease. Typically, a benign GU also appears as a discrete crater with radiating mucosal folds originating from the ulcer margin (Fig. 293-10*B*). Ulcers >3 cm in size or those associated with a mass are more often malignant. Unfortunately, up to 8% of GUs that appear to be benign by radiographic appearance are malignant by endoscopy or surgery. Radiographic studies that show a GU must be followed by endoscopy and biopsy.

Endoscopy provides the most sensitive and specific approach for examining the upper GI tract (Fig. 293-11). In addition to permitting direct visualization of the mucosa, endoscopy facilitates photographic documentation of a mucosal defect and tissue biopsy to rule out malignancy (GU) or *H. pylori.* Endoscopic examination is particularly helpful in identifying lesions too small to detect by radiographic examination, for evaluation of atypical radiographic abnormalities, or to determine if an ulcer is a source of blood loss.

Although the methods for diagnosing *H. pylori* are outlined in Chap. 144, a brief summary will be included here (Table 293-2). Several biopsy urease tests have been developed (PyloriTek, CLOtest, Hpfast, Pronto Dry) that have a sensitivity and specificity of >90–95%. Several noninvasive methods for detecting this organism have been developed. Three types of studies routinely used include serologic testing, the ^{13}C- or ^{14}C-urea breath test, and the fecal *H. pylori* (Hp) antigen test. A urinary Hp antigen test, as well as a refined monoclonal antibody stool antigen test, appears promising.

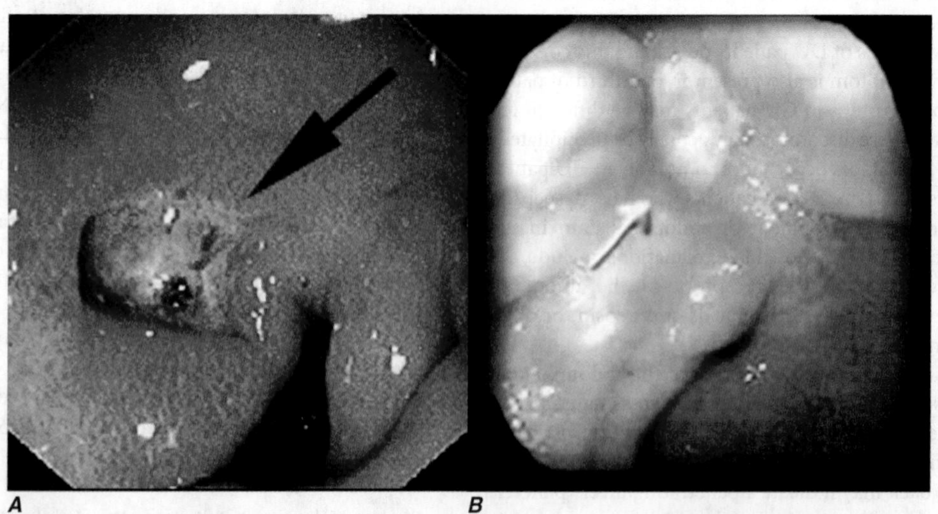

Figure 293-11 Endoscopy demonstrating: *A.* a benign duodenal ulcer; ***B.*** a benign gastric ulcer.

TABLE 293-2 Tests for Detection of *H. Pylori*

Test	Sensitivity/ Specificity, %	Comments
Invasive (Endoscopy/Biopsy Required)		
Rapid urease	80–95/95–100	Simple, false negative with recent use of PPIs, antibiotics, or bismuth compounds
Histology	80–90/>95	Requires pathology processing and staining; provides histologic information
Culture	—/—	Time-consuming, expensive, dependent on experience; allows determination of antibiotic susceptibility
Noninvasive		
Serology	>80/>90	Inexpensive, convenient; not useful for early follow-up
Urea breath test	>90/>90	Simple, rapid; useful for early follow-up; false negatives with recent therapy (see rapid urease test); exposure to low-dose radiation with ^{14}C test
Stool antigen	>90/>90	Inexpensive, convenient; not established for eradication but promising

Abbreviation: PPIs, proton pump inhibitors.

TABLE 293-3 Drugs Used in the Treatment of Peptic Ulcer Disease

Drug Type/Mechanism	Examples	Dose
Acid-suppressing drugs		
Antacids	Mylanta, Maalox, Tums, Gaviscon	100–140 meq/L 1 and 3 h after meals and hs
H_2 receptor antagonists	Cimetidine	400 mg bid
	Ranitidine	300 mg hs
	Famotidine	40 mg hs
	Nizatidine	300 mg hs
Proton pump inhibitors	Omeprazole	20 mg/d
	Lansoprazole	30 mg/d
	Rabeprazole	20 mg/d
	Pantoprazole	40 mg/d
	Esomeprazole	20 mg/d
Mucosal protective agents		
Sucralfate	Sucralfate	1 g qid
Prostaglandin analogue	Misoprostol	200 µg qid
Bismuth-containing compounds	Bismuth subsalicylate (BSS)	See anti-*H. pylori* regimens (Table 293-4)

Abbreviation: hs, at bedtime (*hora somni*).

Occasionally, specialized testing such as serum gastrin and gastric acid analysis or sham feeding may be needed in individuals with complicated or refractory PUD [see "Zollinger-Ellison Syndrome (ZES)," below]. Screening for aspirin or NSAIDs (blood or urine) may also be necessary in refractory *H. pylori*–negative PUD patients.

TREATMENT Peptic Ulcer Disease

Before the discovery of *H. pylori,* the therapy of PUD was centered on the old dictum by Schwartz of "no acid, no ulcer." Although acid secretion is still important in the pathogenesis of PUD, eradication of *H. pylori* and therapy/prevention of NSAID-induced disease is the mainstay of treatment. A summary of commonly used drugs for treatment of acid peptic disorders is shown in Table 293-3.

ACID NEUTRALIZING/INHIBITORY DRUGS

Antacids Before we understood the important role of histamine in stimulating parietal cell activity, neutralization of secreted acid with antacids constituted the main form of therapy for peptic ulcers. They are now rarely, if ever, used as the primary therapeutic agent but instead are often used by patients for symptomatic relief of dyspepsia. The most commonly used agents are mixtures of aluminum hydroxide and magnesium hydroxide. Aluminum hydroxide can produce constipation and phosphate depletion; magnesium hydroxide may cause loose stools. Many of the commonly used antacids (e.g., Maalox, Mylanta) have a combination of both aluminum and magnesium hydroxide in order to avoid these side effects. The magnesium-containing preparation should not be used in chronic renal failure patients because of possible hypermagnesemia, and aluminum may cause chronic neurotoxicity in these patients.

Calcium carbonate and sodium bicarbonate are potent antacids with varying levels of potential problems. The long-term use of calcium carbonate (converts to calcium chloride in the stomach) can lead to milk-alkali syndrome (hypercalcemia, hyperphosphatemia with possible renal calcinosis and progression to renal insufficiency). Sodium bicarbonate may induce systemic alkalosis.

H_2 Receptor Antagonists Four of these agents are presently available (cimetidine, ranitidine, famotidine, and nizatidine), and their structures share homology with histamine. Although each has different potency, all will significantly inhibit basal and stimulated acid secretion to comparable levels when used at therapeutic doses. Moreover, similar ulcer-healing rates are achieved with each drug when used at the correct dosage. Presently, this class of drug is often used for treatment of active ulcers (4–6 weeks) in combination with antibiotics directed at eradicating *H. pylori* (see below).

Cimetidine was the first H_2 receptor antagonist used for the treatment of acid peptic disorders. The initial recommended dosing profile for cimetidine was 300 mg qid. Subsequent studies have documented the efficacy of using 800 mg at bedtime for treatment of active ulcer, with healing rates approaching 80% at 4 weeks. Cimetidine may have weak antiandrogenic side effects resulting in reversible gynecomastia and impotence, primarily in patients receiving high doses for prolonged periods of time (months to years, as in ZES). In view of cimetidine's ability to inhibit cytochrome P450, careful monitoring of drugs such as warfarin, phenytoin, and theophylline is indicated with long-term usage. Other rare reversible adverse effects reported with cimetidine include confusion and elevated levels of serum aminotransferases, creatinine, and serum prolactin. Ranitidine, famotidine, and nizatidine are more potent H_2 receptor antagonists than cimetidine. Each can be used once a day at bedtime for ulcer prevention, which was commonly done before the discovery of *H. pylori* and the development of proton pump inhibitors (PPIs). Patients may develop tolerance to H_2 blockers, a rare event with PPIs (see below). Comparable nighttime dosing regimens are ranitidine 300 mg, famotidine 40 mg, and nizatidine 300 mg.

Additional rare, reversible systemic toxicities reported with H_2 receptor antagonists include pancytopenia, neutropenia, anemia, and thrombocytopenia, with a prevalence rate varying from 0.01–0.2%. Cimetidine and ranitidine (to a lesser extent) can bind to hepatic cytochrome P450; famotidine and nizatidine do not.

Proton Pump (H^+,K^+-ATPase) Inhibitors Omeprazole, esomeprazole, lansoprazole, rabeprazole, and pantoprazole are substituted benzimidazole derivatives that covalently bind and irreversibly inhibit H^+,K^+-ATPase. Esomeprazole, the newest member of this drug class, is the S-enantiomer of omeprazole, which is a racemic mixture of both S- and R-optical isomers. These are the most potent acid inhibitory agents available. Omeprazole and lansoprazole are the PPIs that have been used for the longest time. Both are acid-labile and are administered as enteric-coated granules in a sustained-release capsule that dissolves within the small intestine at a pH of 6. Lansoprazole is available in an orally disintegrating tablet that can be taken with or without water, an advantage for individuals who have significant dysphagia. Absorption kinetics are similar to the capsule. In addition, a lansoprazole-naproxen combination preparation that has been made available is targeted at decreasing NSAID-related GI injury (see below). Omeprazole is available as nonenteric-coated granules mixed with sodium bicarbonate in a powder form that can be administered orally or via gastric tube. The sodium bicarbonate has two purposes: to protect the omeprazole from acid degradation and to promote rapid gastric alkalinization and subsequent proton pump activation, which facilitates rapid action of the PPI. Pantoprazole and rabeprazole are available as enteric-coated tablets. Pantoprazole is also available as a parenteral formulation for intravenous use. These agents are lipophilic compounds; upon entering the parietal cell, they are protonated and trapped within the acid environment of the tubulovesicular and canalicular system. These agents potently inhibit all phases of gastric acid secretion. Onset of action is rapid, with a maximum acid inhibitory effect between 2 and 6 hours after administration and duration of inhibition lasting up to 72–96 hours. With repeated daily dosing, progressive acid inhibitory effects are observed, with basal and secretagogue-stimulated acid production being inhibited by >95% after 1 week of therapy. The half-life of PPIs is ~18 hours; thus, it can take between 2 and 5 days for gastric acid secretion to return to normal levels once these drugs have been discontinued. Because the pumps need to be activated for these agents to be effective, their efficacy is maximized if they are administered before a meal (except for the immediate-release formulation of omeprazole) (e.g., in the morning before breakfast). Mild to moderate hypergastrinemia has been observed in patients taking these drugs. Carcinoid tumors developed in some animals given the drugs preclinically; however, extensive experience has failed to demonstrate gastric carcinoid tumor development in humans. Serum gastrin levels return to normal levels within 1–2 weeks after drug cessation. Rebound gastric acid hypersecretion has been described in *H. pylori* negative individuals after discontinuation of PPIs. It occurs even after relatively short-term usage (2 months) and may last for up to 2 months after the PPI has been discontinued. The mechanism involves gastrin-induced hyperplasia and hypertrophy of histamine-secreting ECL cells. The clinical relevance of this observation is that individuals may have worsening symptoms of gastroesophageal reflux disease (GERD) or dyspepsia upon stopping the PPI. Gradual tapering of the PPI and switching to an H_2 receptor antagonist may prevent this from occurring. *H. pylori*-induced inflammation and concomitant decrease in acid production may explain why this does not occur in *H. pylori*-positive patients. IF production is also inhibited, but vitamin B_{12}-deficiency anemia is uncommon, probably because of the large stores of the vitamin. As with any agent that leads to significant hypochlorhydria, PPIs may interfere with absorption of drugs such as ketoconazole, ampicillin, iron, and digoxin. Hepatic cytochrome P450 can be inhibited by the earlier PPIs (omeprazole, lansoprazole). Rabeprazole, pantoprazole, and esomeprazole do not appear to interact significantly with drugs metabolized by the cytochrome P450 system. The overall clinical significance of this observation is not definitely established. Caution should be taken when using theophylline, warfarin, diazepam, atazanavir, and phenytoin concomitantly with PPIs. Long-term acid suppression, especially with PPIs, has been associated with a higher incidence of community-acquired pneumonia as well as community and hospital acquired *Clostridium difficile*-associated disease. These observations require confirmation but should alert the practitioner to take caution when recommending these agents for long-term use, especially in elderly patients at risk for developing pneumonia or *C. difficile* infection. A population-based study revealed that long-term use of PPIs was associated with the development of hip fractures in older women. The absolute risk of fracture remained low despite an observed increase associated with the dose and duration of acid suppression. The mechanism for this observation is not clear and this finding must be confirmed before making broad recommendations regarding the discontinuation of these agents in patients who benefit from them. PPIs may exert a negative effect on the anti-platelet effect of clopidogrel. Although the evidence is mixed and inconclusive, a small increase in mortality and readmission rate for coronary events is seen in patients receiving a PPI while on clopidogrel. The mechanism involves the competition of the PPI and clopidogrel with the same cytochrome p450 (CYP2C19). Whether this is a class effect of PPIs is unclear; there appears to be at least a theoretical advantage of pantoprazole over the other PPIs, but this has not been confirmed. This drug interaction is particularly relevant in light of the common use of aspirin and clopidogrel for prevention of coronary events and the efficacy of PPIs in preventing GI bleeding in these patients. The FDA has made several recommendations while awaiting further evidence to clarify the impact of PPI therapy on clopidogrel use. Health care providers should continue to prescribe clopidogrel to patients who require it and should reevaluate the need for starting or continuing treatment with a PPI. From a practical standpoint additional recommendations to consider include: Patients taking clopidogrel with aspirin, especially with other GI risk factors for bleeding, should receive GI protective therapy. Although high-dose H_2 blockers have been considered an option these do not appear to be as effective as PPIs. If PPIs are to be given, there should be a 12-h separation between administration of the PPI and clopidogrel to minimize competition of the two agents with the involved cytochrome p450. One option is to give the PPI 30 min before breakfast and the clopidogrel at bedtime. Insufficient data are available to firmly recommend one PPI over another.

Two new formulations of acid inhibitory agents are being developed. Tenatoprazole is a PPI containing an imidazopyridine ring instead of a benzimidazole ring, which promotes irreversible proton pump inhibition. This agent has a longer half-life than the other PPIs and may be beneficial for inhibiting nocturnal acid secretion, which has significant relevance in GERD. A second new class of agents is the potassium-competitive acid pump antagonists (P-CABs). These compounds inhibit gastric acid secretion via potassium competitive binding of the H^+,K^+-ATPase.

CYTOPROTECTIVE AGENTS

Sucralfate Sucralfate is a complex sucrose salt in which the hydroxyl groups have been substituted by aluminum hydroxide and sulfate. This compound is insoluble in water and becomes a viscous paste within the stomach and duodenum, binding primarily to sites of active ulceration. Sucralfate may act by several mechanisms: serving as a physicochemical barrier, promoting a trophic action by binding growth factors such as EGF, enhancing prostaglandin synthesis, stimulating mucus and bicarbonate secretion, and enhancing mucosal defense and repair. Toxicity from this drug is rare, with constipation being most common (2–3%). It should be avoided in patients with chronic renal insufficiency to prevent aluminum-induced neurotoxicity. Hypophosphatemia and gastric bezoar formation have also been reported rarely. Standard dosing of sucralfate is 1 g qid.

Bismuth-Containing Preparations Sir William Osler considered bismuth-containing compounds the drug of choice for treating PUD. The resurgence in the use of these agents is due to their effect against *H. pylori*. Colloidal bismuth subcitrate (CBS) and bismuth subsalicylate (BSS, Pepto-Bismol) are the most widely used preparations. The mechanism by which these agents induce ulcer healing is unclear. Adverse effects with short-term usage include black stools, constipation, and darkening of the tongue. Long-term usage with high doses, especially with the avidly absorbed CBS, may lead to neurotoxicity. These compounds are commonly used as one of the agents in an anti-*H. pylori* regimen (see below).

Prostaglandin Analogues In view of their central role in maintaining mucosal integrity and repair, stable prostaglandin analogues were developed for the treatment of PUD. The mechanism by which this rapidly absorbed drug provides its therapeutic effect is through enhancement of mucosal defense and repair. The most common toxicity noted with this drug is diarrhea (10–30% incidence). Other major toxicities include uterine bleeding and contractions; misoprostol is contraindicated in women who may be pregnant, and women of childbearing age must be made clearly aware of this potential drug toxicity. The standard therapeutic dose is 200 μg qid.

Miscellaneous Drugs A number of drugs including anticholinergic agents and tricyclic antidepressants were used for treating acid peptic disorders but in light of their toxicity and the development of potent antisecretory agents, these are rarely, if ever, used today.

THERAPY OF *H. PYLORI* Extensive effort has been made in determining who of the many individuals with *H. pylori* infection should be treated. The common conclusion arrived at by multiple consensus conferences around the world is that *H. pylori* should be eradicated in patients with documented PUD. This holds true independent of time of presentation (first episode or not), severity of symptoms, presence of confounding factors such as ingestion of NSAIDs, or whether the ulcer is in remission. Some have advocated treating patients with a history of documented PUD who are found to be *H. pylori*–positive by serology or breath testing. Over one-half of patients with gastric MALT lymphoma experience complete remission of the tumor in response to *H. pylori* eradication. Treating patients with NUD, to prevent gastric cancer or patients with GERD requiring long-term acid suppression, remains controversial. Guidelines from the American College of Gastroenterology suggest eradication of *H. pylori* in patients who have undergone resection of early gastric cancer. The role of *H. pylori* eradication as a means to prevent gastric cancer is still controversial although data suggest a benefit of early eradication of *H. pylori* for prevention of gastric cancer in patients with peptic ulcer disease.

Multiple drugs have been evaluated in the therapy of *H. pylori*. No single agent is effective in eradicating the organism. Combination therapy for 14 days provides the greatest efficacy. A shorter course administration (7–10 days), although attractive, has not proved as successful as the 14-days regimens. The agents used with the greatest frequency include amoxicillin, metronidazole, tetracycline, clarithromycin, and bismuth compounds.

The physician's goal in treating PUD is to provide relief of symptoms (pain or dyspepsia), promote ulcer healing, and ultimately prevent ulcer recurrence and complications. The greatest impact of understanding the role of *H. pylori* in peptic disease has been the ability to prevent recurrence. Documented eradication of *H. pylori* in patients with PUD is associated with a dramatic decrease in ulcer recurrence to <10–20% as compared to 59% in GU patients and 67% in DU patients when the organism is not eliminated. Eradication of the organism may lead to diminished recurrent ulcer bleeding. The impact of its eradication on ulcer perforation is unclear.

Suggested treatment regimens for *H. pylori* are outlined in Table 293-4. Choice of a particular regimen will be influenced by several factors, including efficacy, patient tolerance, existing

TABLE 293-4 Regimens Recommended for Eradication of *H. Pylori* Infection

Drug	Dose
Triple Therapy	
1. Bismuth subsalicylate *plus*	2 tablets qid
Metronidazole *plus*	250 mg qid
Tetracycline[a]	500 mg qid
2. Ranitidine bismuth citrate *plus*	400 mg bid
Tetracycline *plus*	500 mg bid
Clarithromycin or metronidazole	500 mg bid
3. Omeprazole (lansoprazole) *plus*	20 mg bid (30 mg bid)
Clarithromycin *plus*	250 or 500 mg bid
Metronidazole[b] *or*	500 mg bid
Amoxicillin[c]	1 g bid
Quadruple Therapy	
Omeprazole (lansoprazole)	20 mg (30 mg) daily
Bismuth subsalicylate	2 tablets qid
Metronidazole	250 mg qid
Tetracycline	500 mg qid

[a]Alternative: use prepacked Helidac (see text).
[b]Alternative: use prepacked Prevpac (see text).
[c]Use either metronidazole or amoxicillin, not both.

antibiotic resistance, and cost of the drugs. The aim for initial eradication rates should be 85–90%. Dual therapy [PPI plus amoxicillin, PPI plus clarithromycin, ranitidine bismuth citrate (Tritec) plus clarithromycin] are not recommended in view of studies demonstrating eradication rates of <80–85%. The combination of bismuth, metronidazole, and tetracycline was the first triple regimen found effective against *H. pylori.* The combination of two antibiotics plus either a PPI, H_2 blocker, or bismuth compound has comparable success rates. Addition of acid suppression assists in providing early symptom relief and may enhance bacterial eradication.

Triple therapy, although effective, has several drawbacks, including the potential for poor patient compliance and drug-induced side effects. Compliance is being addressed by simplifying the regimens so that patients can take the medications twice a day. Simpler (dual therapy) and shorter regimens (7 and 10 days) are not as effective as triple therapy for 14 days. Two anti-*H. pylori* regimens are available in prepackaged formulation: Prevpac (lansoprazole, clarithromycin, and amoxicillin) and Helidac (BSS, tetracycline, and metronidazole). The contents of the Prevpac are to be taken twice per day for 14 days, whereas Helidac constituents are taken four times per day with an antisecretory agent (PPI or H_2 blocker), also for at least 14 days.

Side effects have been reported in up to 20–30% of patients on triple therapy. Bismuth may cause black stools, constipation, or darkening of the tongue. The most feared complication with amoxicillin is pseudomembranous colitis, but this occurs in <1–2% of patients. Amoxicillin can also lead to antibiotic-associated diarrhea, nausea, vomiting, skin rash, and allergic reaction. Tetracycline has been reported to cause rashes and, very rarely, hepatotoxicity and anaphylaxis.

One important concern with treating patients who may not need therapy is the potential for development of antibiotic-resistant strains. The incidence and type of antibiotic-resistant *H. pylori* strains vary worldwide. Strains resistant to metronidazole, clarithromycin, amoxicillin, and tetracycline have been described, with the latter two being uncommon. Antibiotic-resistant strains are the most common cause for treatment failure in compliant patients. Unfortunately, in vitro resistance does not predict outcome in patients. Culture and sensitivity testing of *H. pylori* is not performed routinely. Although resistance to metronidazole has been found in as many as 30% of isolates in North America and 80% in developing countries, triple therapy is effective in eradicating the organism in >50% of patients infected with a resistant strain. Clarithromycin resistance is seen in 13% of individuals in the United States, with resistance to amoxicillin being <1% and resistance to both metronidazole and clarithromycin in the 5% range.

Failure of *H. pylori* eradication with triple therapy in a compliant patient is usually due to infection with a resistant organism. Quadruple therapy (Table 293-4), where clarithromycin is substituted for metronidazole (or vice versa), should be the next step. The combination of pantoprazole, amoxicillin, and rifabutin for 10 days has also been used successfully (86% cure rate) in patients infected with resistant strains. Additional regimens considered for second-line therapy include levofloxacin-based triple therapy (levofloxacin, amoxicillin, PPI) for 10 days and furazolidone-based triple therapy (furazolidone, amoxicillin, PPI) for 14 days. Unfortunately, there is no universally accepted treatment regimen recommended for patients who have failed two courses of antibiotics. If eradication is still not achieved in a compliant patient, then culture and sensitivity of the organism should be considered. Additional factors that may lower eradication rates include the patient's country of origin (higher in Northeast Asia than other parts of Asia or Europe) and cigarette smoking. In addition, meta-analysis suggests that even the most effective regimens (quadruple therapy including PPI, bismuth, tetracycline, and metronidazole and triple therapy including PPI, clarithromycin, and amoxicillin) may have suboptimal eradication rates (<80%), thus demonstrating the need for the development of more efficacious treatments.

In view of the observation that 15–25% of patients treated with first-line therapy may still remain infected with the organism, new approaches to treatment have been explored. One promising approach is sequential therapy. This regimen consists of 5 days of amoxicillin and a PPI, followed by an additional 5 days of PPI plus tinidazole and clarithromycin. Initial studies have demonstrated eradication rates of >90% with good patient tolerance. Confirmation of these findings and applicability of this approach in the United States are needed.

Reinfection after successful eradication of *H. pylori* is rare in the United States (<1% per year). If recurrent infection occurs within the first 6 months after completing therapy, the most likely explanation is recrudescence as opposed to reinfection.

THERAPY OF NSAID-RELATED GASTRIC OR DUODENAL INJURY

Medical intervention for NSAID-related mucosal injury includes treatment of an active ulcer and primary prevention of future injury. Recommendations for the treatment and primary prevention of NSAID-related mucosal injury are listed in Table 293-5. Ideally, the injurious agent should be stopped as the first step in the therapy of an active NSAID-induced ulcer. If that is possible, then treatment with one of the acid inhibitory agents (H_2 blockers, PPIs) is indicated. Cessation of NSAIDs is not always possible because of the patient's severe underlying disease. Only PPIs can heal GUs or DUs, independent of whether NSAIDs are discontinued.

The approach to primary prevention has included avoiding the agent, using NSAIDs that are theoretically less injurious, and/or the use of concomitant medical therapy to prevent NSAID-induced injury. Several nonselective NSAIDs that are associated with a lower likelihood of GI toxicity include diclofenac, aceclofenac, and ibuprofen, although the beneficial effect may be eliminated if higher dosages of the agents are used. Primary prevention of NSAID-induced ulceration can be accomplished by misoprostol (200 μg qid) or a PPI. High-dose H_2 blockers (famotidine, 40 mg bid) have also shown some promise in preventing endoscopically documented ulcers, although PPIs are superior. The highly selective COX-2 inhibitors, celecoxib and

TABLE 293-5 Recommendations for Treatment of NSAID-Related Mucosal Injury

Clinical Setting	Recommendation
Active ulcer	
NSAID discontinued	H_2 receptor antagonist or PPI
NSAID continued	PPI
Prophylactic therapy	Misoprostol
	PPI
	Selective COX-2 inhibitor
H. pylori infection	Eradication if active ulcer present or there is a past history of peptic ulcer disease

Abbreviations: COX-2, isoenzyme of cyclooxygenase; PPI, proton pump inhibitor.

rofecoxib, are 100 times more selective inhibitors of COX-2 than standard NSAIDs, leading to gastric or duodenal mucosal injury that is comparable to placebo; their utilization led to an increase in cardiovascular events and withdrawal from the market. Additional caution was engendered when the CLASS study demonstrated that the advantage of celecoxib in preventing GI complications was offset when low-dose aspirin was used simultaneously. Therefore, gastric protection therapy is required in individuals taking COX-2 inhibitors and aspirin prophylaxis. Finally, much of the work demonstrating the benefit of COX-2 inhibitors and PPIs on GI injury has been performed in individuals of average risk; it is unclear if the same level of benefit will be achieved in high-risk patients. For example, concomitant use of warfarin and a COX-2 inhibitor was associated with rates of GI bleeding similar to those observed in patients taking nonselective NSAIDs. A combination of factors, including withdrawal of the majority of COX-2 inhibitors from the market, the observation that low-dose aspirin appears to diminish the beneficial effect of COX-2 selective inhibitors, and the growing use of aspirin for prophylaxis of cardiovascular events, have significantly altered the approach to gastric protective therapy during the use of NSAIDs. A set of guidelines for the approach to the use of NSAIDs was published by the American College of Gastroenterology and is shown in Table 293-6. Individuals who are not at risk for cardiovascular events, do not use aspirin, and are without risk for GI complications can receive nonselective NSAIDs without gastric protection. In those without cardiovascular risk factors but with a high potential risk (prior GI bleeding or multiple GI risk factors) for NSAID-induced GI toxicity, cautious use of a selective COX-2 inhibitor and co-therapy with misoprostol or high-dose PPI is recommended. Individuals at moderate GI risk without cardiac risk factors can be treated with a COX-2 inhibitor alone or with a nonselective NSAID with misoprostol or a PPI. Individuals with cardiovascular risk factors, who require low-dose aspirin and have low potential for NSAID-induced toxicity, should be considered for a non-NSAID agent or use of a traditional NSAID in combination with gastric protection, if warranted. Finally, individuals with cardiovascular and GI risks, who require aspirin must be considered for non-NSAID therapy, but if that is not an option, then gastric protection with any type of NSAID must be considered. Any patient, regardless of risk status, who is being considered for long-term traditional NSAID therapy, should also be considered for *H. pylori* testing and treatment if positive.

APPROACH AND THERAPY: SUMMARY Controversy continues regarding the best approach to the patient who presents with dyspepsia (Chap. 39). The discovery of *H. pylori* and its role in pathogenesis of ulcers has added a new variable to the equation. Previously, if a patient <50 years of age presented with dyspepsia and without alarming signs or symptoms suggestive of an ulcer complication or malignancy, an empirical therapeutic trial with acid suppression was commonly recommended. Although this approach is practiced by some today, an approach presently gaining approval for the treatment of patients with dyspepsia is outlined in Fig. 293-12. The referral to a gastroenterologist is for the potential need of endoscopy and subsequent evaluation and treatment if the endoscopy is negative.

Once an ulcer (GU or DU) is documented, the main issue at stake is whether *H. pylori* or an NSAID is involved. With *H. pylori* present, independent of the NSAID status, triple therapy is recommended for 14 days, followed by continued acid-suppressing drugs (H_2 receptor antagonist or PPIs) for a total of 4–6 weeks. Selection of patients for documentation of *H. pylori* eradication (organisms gone at least 4 weeks after completing antibiotics) is an area of some debate. The test of choice for documenting eradication is the urea breath test (UBT). The stool antigen assay may also hold promise for this purpose, but the data have not been as clear cut as in the case of using the stool antigen test for primary diagnosis, especially if one considers patients who live in areas of low *H. pylori* prevalence. Further studies are warranted, but if the UBT is not available, a stool antigen should be considered to document eradication. The patient must be off antisecretory agents when being tested for eradication of *H. pylori* with UBT or stool antigen. Serologic testing is not useful for the purpose of documenting eradication since antibody titers fall slowly and often do not become undetectable. Two approaches toward documentation of eradication

TABLE 293-6 Guide to NSAID Therapy

	No/Low NSAID GI Risk	NSAID GI Risk
No CV risk (no aspirin)	Traditional NSAID	Coxib *or* Traditional NSAID + PPI *or* misoprostol Consider non-NSAID therapy
CV risk (consider aspirin)	Traditional NSAID + PPI *or* misoprostol if GI risk warrants gastroprotection Consider non-NSAID therapy	A gastroprotective agent must be added if a traditional NSAID is prescribed Consider non-NSAID therapy

Abbreviations: CV, cardiovascular; GI, gastrointestinal; NSAID, nonsteroidal anti-inflammatory drug; PPI, proton pump inhibitor.

Source: Adapted from AM Fendrick: Am J Manag Care 10:740, 2004. Reproduced with permission of INTELLISPHERE, LLC via Copyright Clearance Center.

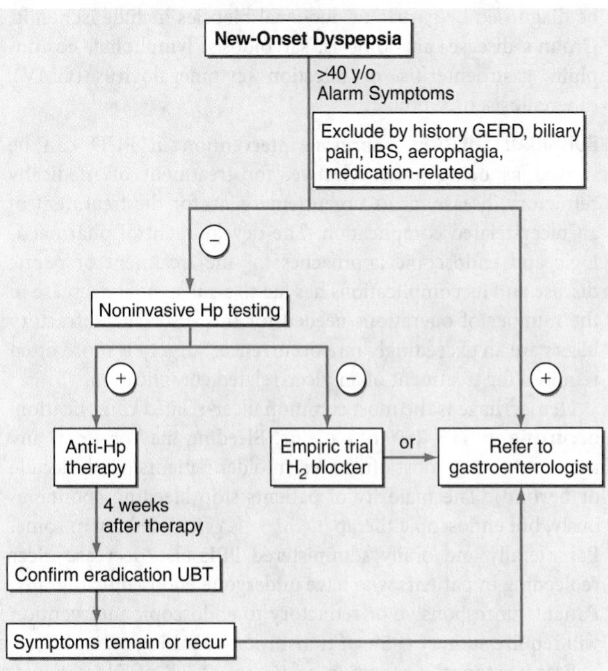

Figure 293-12 Overview of new-onset dyspepsia. Hp, *Helicobacter pylori;* UBT, urea breath test; IBS, irritable bowel syndrome. *(Adapted from BS Anand and DY Graham: Endoscopy 31:215, 1999.)*

exist: (1) Test for eradication only in individuals with a complicated course or in individuals who are frail or with multisystem disease who would do poorly with an ulcer recurrence, and (2) test all patients for successful eradication. Some recommend that patients with complicated ulcer disease, or who are frail, should be treated with long-term acid suppression, thus making documentation of *H. pylori* eradication a moot point. In view of this discrepancy in practice, it would be best to discuss with the patient the different options available.

Several issues differentiate the approach to a GU versus a DU. GUs, especially of the body and fundus, have the potential of being malignant. Multiple biopsies of a GU should be taken initially; even if these are negative for neoplasm, repeat endoscopy to document healing at 8–12 weeks should be performed, with biopsy if the ulcer is still present. About 70% of GUs eventually found to be malignant undergo significant (usually incomplete) healing.

The majority (>90%) of GUs and DUs heal with the conventional therapy outlined above. A GU that fails to heal after 12 weeks and a DU that does not heal after 8 weeks of therapy should be considered refractory. Once poor compliance and persistent *H. pylori* infection have been excluded, NSAID use, either inadvertent or surreptitious, must be excluded. In addition, cigarette smoking must be eliminated. For a GU, malignancy must be meticulously excluded. Next, consideration should be given to a gastric acid hypersecretory state such as ZES (see "Zollinger-Ellison Syndrome," below) or the idiopathic form, which can be excluded with gastric acid analysis. Although a subset of patients have gastric acid hypersecretion of unclear etiology as a contributing factor to refractory ulcers, ZES should be excluded with a fasting gastrin or secretin stimulation test (see below). More than 90% of refractory ulcers (either DUs or GUs) heal after 8 weeks of treatment with higher doses of PPI (omeprazole, 40 mg/d; lansoprazole 30–60 mg/d). This higher dose is also effective in maintaining remission. Surgical intervention may be a consideration at this point; however, other rare causes of refractory ulcers must be excluded before recommending surgery. Rare etiologies of refractory ulcers that may be diagnosed by gastric or duodenal biopsies include ischemia, Crohn's disease, amyloidosis, sarcoidosis, lymphoma, eosinophilic gastroenteritis, or infection [cytomegalovirus (CMV), tuberculosis, or syphilis].

SURGICAL THERAPY Surgical intervention in PUD can be viewed as being either elective, for treatment of medically refractory disease, or as urgent/emergent, for the treatment of an ulcer-related complication. The development of pharmacologic and endoscopic approaches for the treatment of peptic disease and its complications has led to a substantial decrease in the number of operations needed for this disorder. Refractory ulcers are an exceedingly rare occurrence. Surgery is more often required for treatment of an ulcer-related complication.

Hemorrhage is the most common ulcer-related complication, occurring in ~15–25% of patients. Bleeding may occur in any age group but is most often seen in older patients (sixth decade or beyond). The majority of patients stop bleeding spontaneously, but endoscopic therapy (Chap. 291) is necessary in some. Parenterally and orally administered PPIs also decrease ulcer rebleeding in patients who have undergone endoscopic therapy. Patients unresponsive or refractory to endoscopic intervention will require surgery (~5% of transfusion-requiring patients).

Free peritoneal perforation occurs in ~2–3% of DU patients. As in the case of bleeding, up to 10% of these patients will not have antecedent ulcer symptoms. Concomitant bleeding may occur in up to 10% of patients with perforation, with mortality being increased substantially. Peptic ulcer can also penetrate into adjacent organs, especially with a posterior DU, which can penetrate into the pancreas, colon, liver, or biliary tree.

Pyloric channel ulcers or DUs can lead to gastric outlet obstruction in ~2–3% of patients. This can result from chronic scarring or from impaired motility due to inflammation and/or edema with pylorospasm. Patients may present with early satiety, nausea, vomiting of undigested food, and weight loss. Conservative management with nasogastric suction, intravenous hydration/nutrition, and antisecretory agents is indicated for 7–10 days with the hope that a functional obstruction will reverse. If a mechanical obstruction persists, endoscopic intervention with balloon dilation may be effective. Surgery should be considered if all else fails.

SPECIFIC OPERATIONS FOR DUODENAL ULCERS Surgical treatment is designed to decrease gastric acid secretion. Operations most commonly performed include (1) vagotomy and drainage (by pyloroplasty, gastroduodenostomy, or gastrojejunostomy), (2) highly selective vagotomy (which does not require a drainage procedure), and (3) vagotomy with antrectomy. The specific procedure performed is dictated by the underlying circumstances: elective vs. emergency, the degree and extent of duodenal ulceration, and the expertise of the surgeon. Moreover, the trend has been toward minimally invasive and anatomy-preserving operations.

Vagotomy is a component of each of these procedures and is aimed at decreasing acid secretion through ablating cholinergic input to the stomach. Unfortunately, both truncal and selective vagotomy (preserves the celiac and hepatic branches) result in gastric atony despite successful reduction of both basal acid output (BAO, decreased by 85%) and maximal acid output (MAO, decreased by 50%). Drainage through pyloroplasty or gastroduodenostomy is required in an effort to compensate for the vagotomy-induced gastric motility disorder. This procedure has an intermediate complication rate and a 10% ulcer recurrence rate. To minimize gastric dysmotility, highly selective vagotomy (also known as parietal cell, super-selective, or proximal vagotomy) was developed. Only the vagal fibers innervating the portion of the stomach that contains parietal cells is transected, thus leaving fibers important for regulating gastric motility intact. Although this procedure leads to an immediate decrease in both BAO and stimulated acid output, acid secretion recovers over time. By the end of the first postoperative year, basal and stimulated acid output are ~30 and 50%, respectively, of preoperative levels. Ulcer recurrence rates are higher with highly selective vagotomy (≥10%), although the overall complication rates are the lowest of the three procedures.

The procedure that provides the lowest rates of ulcer recurrence (1%) but has the highest complication rate is vagotomy (truncal or selective) in combination with antrectomy. Antrectomy is aimed at eliminating an additional stimulant of gastric acid secretion, gastrin. Two principal types of reanastomoses are used after antrectomy: gastroduodenostomy (Billroth I) or gastrojejunostomy (Billroth II) (Fig. 293-13). Although Billroth I is often preferred over II, severe duodenal inflammation or scarring may preclude its performance. Prospective, randomized studies confirm that partial gastrectomy followed by Roux-en-Y reconstruction leads to a significantly better clinical, endoscopic, and histologic outcome than Billroth II reconstruction.

Of these procedures, highly selective vagotomy may be the one of choice in the elective setting, except in situations where ulcer recurrence rates are high (prepyloric ulcers and those refractory to medical therapy). Selection of vagotomy and antrectomy may be more appropriate in these circumstances.

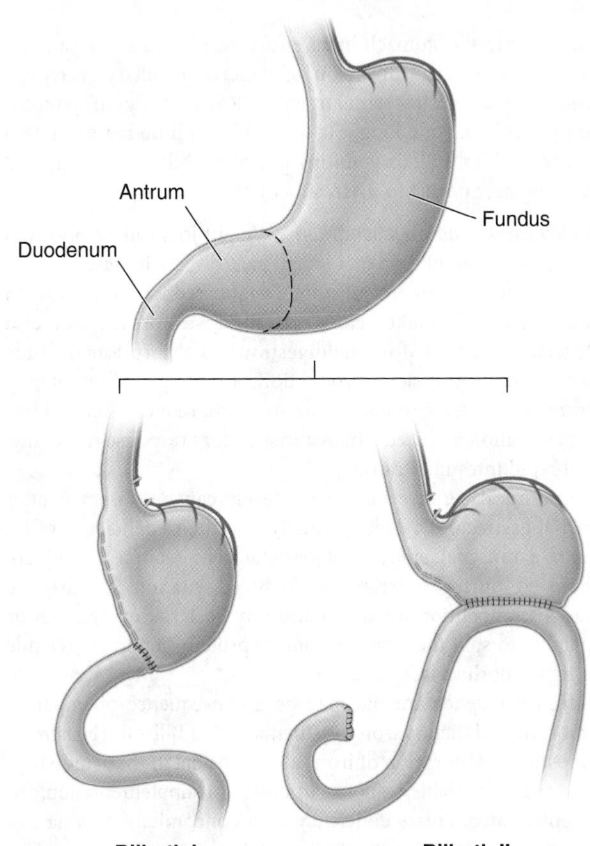

Figure 293-13 Schematic representation of Billroth I and II procedures.

These procedures have been traditionally performed by standard laparotomy. The advent of laparoscopic surgery has led several surgical teams to successfully perform highly selective vagotomy, truncal vagotomy/pyloroplasty, and truncal vagotomy/antrectomy through this approach. An increase in the number of laparoscopic procedures for treatment of PUD has occurred. Laparoscopic repair of perforated peptic ulcers is safe, feasible for the experienced surgeon and is associated with decreased postoperative pain although it does take longer than an open approach. Moreover, no difference between the two approaches is noted in postoperative complications or length of hospital stay.

Specific Operations for Gastric Ulcers The location and the presence of a concomitant DU dictate the operative procedure performed for a GU. Antrectomy (including the ulcer) with a Billroth I anastomosis is the treatment of choice for an antral ulcer. Vagotomy is performed only if a DU is present. Although ulcer excision with vagotomy and drainage procedure has been proposed, the higher incidence of ulcer recurrence makes this a less desirable approach. Ulcers located near the esophagogastric junction may require a more radical approach, a subtotal gastrectomy with a Roux-en-Y esophagogastrojejunostomy (Csende's procedure). A less aggressive approach, including antrectomy, intraoperative ulcer biopsy, and vagotomy (Kelling-Madlener procedure), may be indicated in fragile patients with a high GU. Ulcer recurrence approaches 30% with this procedure.

Surgery-Related Complications Complications seen after surgery for PUD are related primarily to the extent of the anatomic modification performed. Minimal alteration (highly selective vagotomy) is associated with higher rates of ulcer recurrence and less GI disturbance. More aggressive surgical procedures have a lower rate of ulcer recurrence but a greater incidence of GI dysfunction. Overall, morbidity and mortality related to these procedures are quite low. Morbidity associated with vagotomy and antrectomy or pyloroplasty is ≤5%, with mortality ~1%. Highly selective vagotomy has lower morbidity and mortality rates of 1 and 0.3%, respectively.

In addition to the potential early consequences of any intraabdominal procedure (bleeding, infection, thromboembolism), gastroparesis, duodenal stump leak, and efferent loop obstruction can be observed.

Recurrent ulceration The risk of ulcer recurrence is directly related to the procedure performed. Ulcers that recur after partial gastric resection tend to develop at the anastomosis (stomal or marginal ulcer). Epigastric abdominal pain is the most frequent presenting complaint (>90%). Severity and duration of pain tend to be more progressive than observed with DUs before surgery.

Ulcers may recur for several reasons, including incomplete vagotomy, inadequate drainage, retained antrum, and, less likely, persistent or recurrent *H. pylori* infection. ZES should have been excluded preoperatively. Surreptitious use of NSAIDs is an important reason for recurrent ulcers after surgery, especially if the initial procedure was done for an NSAID-induced ulcer. Once *H. pylori* and NSAIDs have been excluded as etiologic factors, the question of incomplete vagotomy or retained gastric antrum should be explored. For the latter, fasting plasma gastrin levels should be determined. If elevated, retained antrum or ZES (see below) should be considered. Incomplete vagotomy can be ruled out by gastric acid analysis coupled with sham feeding. In this test, gastric acid output is measured while the patient sees, smells, and chews a meal (without swallowing). The cephalic phase of gastric secretion, which is mediated by the vagus, is being assessed with this study. An increase in gastric acid output in response to sham feeding is evidence that the vagus nerve is intact. A rise in serum pancreatic polypeptide >50% within 30 min of sham feeding is also suggestive of an intact vagus nerve.

Medical therapy with H_2 blockers will heal postoperative ulceration in 70–90% of patients. The efficacy of PPIs has not been fully assessed in this group, but one may anticipate greater rates of ulcer healing compared to those obtained with H_2 blockers. Repeat operation (complete vagotomy, partial gastrectomy) may be required in a small subgroup of patients who have not responded to aggressive medical management.

Afferent loop syndromes Two types of afferent loop syndrome can occur in patients who have undergone partial gastric resection with Billroth II anastomosis. The more common of the two is bacterial overgrowth in the afferent limb secondary to stasis. Patients may experience postprandial abdominal pain, bloating, and diarrhea with concomitant malabsorption of fats and vitamin B_{12}. Cases refractory to antibiotics may require surgical revision of the loop. The less common afferent loop syndrome can present with severe abdominal pain and bloating that occur 20–60 minutes after meals. Pain is often followed by nausea and vomiting of bile-containing material. The pain and bloating may improve after emesis. The cause of this clinical picture is theorized to be incomplete drainage of bile and pancreatic secretions from an afferent loop that is partially obstructed. Cases refractory to dietary measures may need surgical revision.

Dumping syndrome Dumping syndrome consists of a series of vasomotor and GI signs and symptoms and occurs in patients who have undergone vagotomy and drainage (especially Billroth procedures). Two phases of dumping, early and late, can occur. Early dumping takes place 15–30 minutes after meals and consists of crampy abdominal discomfort, nausea, diarrhea, belching, tachycardia, palpitations, diaphoresis, light-headedness, and, rarely, syncope. These signs and symptoms arise from the rapid emptying of hyperosmolar gastric contents into the small intestine, resulting in a fluid shift into the gut lumen with plasma volume contraction and acute intestinal distention. Release of vasoactive GI hormones (vasoactive intestinal polypeptide, neurotensin, motilin) is also theorized to play a role in early dumping.

The late phase of dumping typically occurs 90 min to 3 h after meals. Vasomotor symptoms (light-headedness, diaphoresis, palpitations, tachycardia, and syncope) predominate during this phase. This component of dumping is thought to be secondary to hypoglycemia from excessive insulin release.

Dumping syndrome is most noticeable after meals rich in simple carbohydrates (especially sucrose) and high osmolarity. Ingestion of large amounts of fluids may also contribute. Up to 50% of postvagotomy and drainage patients will experience dumping syndrome to some degree. Signs and symptoms often improve with time, but a severe protracted picture can occur in up to 1% of patients.

Dietary modification is the cornerstone of therapy for patients with dumping syndrome. Small, multiple (six) meals devoid of simple carbohydrates coupled with elimination of liquids during meals is important. Antidiarrheals and anticholinergic agents are complementary to diet. Guar and pectin, which increase the viscosity of intraluminal contents, may be beneficial in more symptomatic individuals. Acarbose, an α-glucosidase inhibitor that delays digestion of ingested carbohydrates, has also been shown to be beneficial in the treatment of the late phases of dumping. The somatostatin analogue octreotide has been successful in diet-refractory cases. This drug is administered subcutaneously (50 μg tid), titrated according to clinical response. A long-acting depot formulation of octreotide can be administered once every 28 days and provides symptom relief comparable to the short-acting agent. In addition, patient weight gain and quality of life appear to be superior with the long-acting form.

Postvagotomy diarrhea Up to 10% of patients may seek medical attention for the treatment of postvagotomy diarrhea. This complication is most commonly observed after truncal vagotomy. Patients may complain of intermittent diarrhea that occurs typically 1–2 hours after meals. Occasionally the symptoms may be severe and relentless. This is due to a motility disorder from interruption of the vagal fibers supplying the luminal gut. Other contributing factors may include decreased absorption of nutrients (see below), increased excretion of bile acids, and release of luminal factors that promote secretion. Diphenoxylate or loperamide is often useful in symptom control. The bile salt–binding agent cholestyramine may be helpful in severe cases. Surgical reversal of a 10-cm segment of jejunum may yield a substantial improvement in bowel frequency in a subset of patients.

Bile reflux gastropathy A subset of postpartial gastrectomy patients who present with abdominal pain, early satiety, nausea, and vomiting will have mucosal erythema of the gastric remnant as the only finding. Histologic examination of the gastric mucosa reveals minimal inflammation but the presence of epithelial cell injury. This clinical picture is categorized as bile or alkaline reflux gastropathy/gastritis. Although reflux of bile is implicated as the reason for this disorder, the mechanism is unknown. Prokinetic agents, cholestyramine, and sucralfate have been somewhat effective treatments. Severe refractory symptoms may require using either nuclear scanning with ^{99m}Tc-HIDA to document reflux or an alkaline challenge test, where 0.1 *N* NaOH is infused into the stomach in an effort to reproduce the patient's symptoms. Surgical diversion of pancreaticobiliary secretions away from the gastric remnant with a Roux-en-Y gastrojejunostomy consisting of a long (50–60 cm) Roux limb has been used in severe cases. Bilious vomiting improves, but early satiety and bloating may persist in up to 50% of patients.

Maldigestion and malabsorption Weight loss can be observed in up to 60% of patients after partial gastric resection. A significant component of this weight reduction is due to decreased oral intake. However, mild steatorrhea can also develop. Reasons for maldigestion/malabsorption include decreased gastric acid production, rapid gastric emptying, decreased food dispersion in the stomach, reduced luminal bile concentration, reduced pancreatic secretory response to feeding, and rapid intestinal transit.

Decreased serum vitamin B_{12} levels can be observed after partial gastrectomy. This is usually not due to deficiency of IF, since a minimal amount of parietal cells (source of IF) are removed during antrectomy. Reduced vitamin B_{12} may be due to competition for the vitamin by bacterial overgrowth or inability to split the vitamin from its protein-bound source due to hypochlorhydria.

Iron-deficiency anemia may be a consequence of impaired absorption of dietary iron in patients with a Billroth II gastrojejunostomy. Absorption of iron salts is normal in these individuals; thus, a favorable response to oral iron supplementation can be anticipated. Folate deficiency with concomitant anemia can also develop in these patients. This deficiency may be secondary to decreased absorption or diminished oral intake.

Malabsorption of vitamin D and calcium resulting in osteoporosis and osteomalacia is common after partial gastrectomy and gastrojejunostomy (Billroth II). Osteomalacia can occur as a late complication in up to 25% of postpartial gastrectomy patients. Bone fractures occur twice as commonly in men after gastric surgery as in a control population. It may take years before x-ray findings demonstrate diminished bone density. Elevated alkaline phosphatase, reduced serum calcium, bone pain, and pathologic fractures may be seen in patients with osteomalacia. The high incidence of these abnormalities in this subgroup of patients justifies treating them with vitamin D and calcium supplementation indefinitely. Therapy is especially important in females.

Gastric adenocarcinoma The incidence of adenocarcinoma in the gastric stump is increased 15 years after resection. Some have reported a four- to fivefold increase in gastric cancer 20–25 years after resection. The pathogenesis is unclear but may involve alkaline reflux, bacterial proliferation, or hypochlorhydria. The role of endoscopic screening is not clear, and most guidelines do not support its use.

RELATED CONDITIONS

ZOLLINGER–ELLISON SYNDROME

Severe peptic ulcer diathesis secondary to gastric acid hypersecretion due to unregulated gastrin release from a non-β cell endocrine tumor (gastrinoma) defines the components of ZES. Initially, ZES was typified by aggressive and refractory ulceration in which total gastrectomy provided the only chance for enhancing survival. Today it can be cured by surgical resection in up to 30% of patients.

Epidemiology

The incidence of ZES varies from 0.1–1% of individuals presenting with PUD. Males are more commonly affected than females, and the majority of patients are diagnosed between ages 30 and 50. Gastrinomas are classified into sporadic tumors (more common) and those associated with multiple endocrine neoplasia (MEN) type I (see below). The widespread availability and use of PPIs has led to a decreased patient referral for gastrinoma evaluation, delay in diagnosis, and an increase in false-positive diagnoses of ZES.

Pathophysiology

Hypergastrinemia originating from an autonomous neoplasm is the driving force responsible for the clinical manifestations in ZES. Gastrin stimulates acid secretion through gastrin receptors on parietal cells and by inducing histamine release from ECL cells. Gastrin also has a trophic action on gastric epithelial cells. Long-standing hypergastrinemia leads to markedly increased gastric acid secretion through both parietal cell stimulation and increased parietal cell mass. The increased gastric acid output leads to peptic ulcer diathesis, erosive esophagitis, and diarrhea.

Tumor distribution

Although early studies suggested that the vast majority of gastrinomas occurred within the pancreas, a significant number of these lesions are extrapancreatic. Over 80% of these tumors are found within the hypothetical gastrinoma triangle (confluence of the cystic and common bile ducts superiorly, junction of the second and third portions of the duodenum inferiorly, and junction of the neck and body of the pancreas medially). Duodenal tumors constitute the most common nonpancreatic lesion; between 50 and 75% of gastrinomas are found here. Duodenal tumors are smaller, slower growing, and less likely to metastasize than pancreatic lesions. Less-common extrapancreatic sites include stomach, bones, ovaries, heart, liver, and lymph nodes. More than 60% of tumors are considered malignant, with up to 30–50% of patients having multiple lesions or metastatic disease at presentation. Histologically, gastrin-producing cells appear well-differentiated, expressing markers typically found in endocrine neoplasms (chromogranin, neuron-specific enolase).

Clinical manifestations

Gastric acid hypersecretion is responsible for the signs and symptoms observed in patients with ZES. Peptic ulcer is the most common clinical manifestation, occurring in >90% of gastrinoma patients. Initial presentation and ulcer location (duodenal bulb) may be indistinguishable from common PUD. Clinical situations that should create suspicion of gastrinoma are ulcers in unusual locations (second part of the duodenum and beyond), ulcers refractory to standard medical therapy, ulcer recurrence after acid-reducing surgery, ulcers presenting with frank complications (bleeding, obstruction, and perforation), or ulcers in the absence of *H. pylori* or NSAID ingestion. Symptoms of esophageal origin are present in up to two-thirds of patients with ZES, with a spectrum ranging from mild esophagitis to frank ulceration with stricture and Barrett's mucosa.

Diarrhea, the next most common clinical manifestation, is found in up to 50% of patients. Although diarrhea often occurs concomitantly with acid peptic disease, it may also occur independent of an ulcer. Etiology of the diarrhea is multifactorial, resulting from marked volume overload to the small bowel, pancreatic enzyme inactivation by acid, and damage of the intestinal epithelial surface by acid. The epithelial damage can lead to a mild degree of maldigestion and malabsorption of nutrients. The diarrhea may also have a secretory component due to the direct stimulatory effect of gastrin on enterocytes or the co-secretion of additional hormones from the tumor such as vasoactive intestinal peptide.

Gastrinomas can develop in the presence of MEN I syndrome (Chaps. 350, 351) in ~25% of patients. This autosomal dominant disorder involves primarily three organ sites: the parathyroid glands (80–90%), pancreas (40–80%), and pituitary gland (30–60%). The genetic defect in MEN I is in the long arm of chromosome 11 (11q11-q13). In view of the stimulatory effect of calcium on gastric secretion, the hyperparathyroidism and hypercalcemia seen in MEN I patients may have a direct effect on ulcer disease. Resolution of hypercalcemia by parathyroidectomy reduces gastrin and gastric acid output in gastrinoma patients. An additional distinguishing feature in ZES patients with MEN I is the higher incidence of gastric carcinoid tumor development (as compared to patients with sporadic gastrinomas). Gastrinomas tend to be smaller, multiple, and located in the duodenal wall more often than is seen in patients with sporadic ZES. Establishing the diagnosis of MEN I is critical not only from the standpoint of providing genetic counseling to the patient and his or her family but also to the surgical approach recommended.

Diagnosis

The first step in the evaluation of a patient suspected of having ZES is to obtain a fasting gastrin level. A list of clinical scenarios that should arouse suspicion regarding this diagnosis is shown in Table 293-7. Fasting gastrin levels are usually <150 pg/mL. Virtually all gastrinoma patients will have a gastrin level >150–200 pg/mL. Measurement of fasting gastrin should be repeated to confirm the clinical suspicion.

Multiple processes can lead to an elevated fasting gastrin level: gastric hypochlorhydria or achlorhydria (the most frequent), with or without pernicious anemia; retained gastric antrum; G cell hyperplasia; gastric outlet obstruction; renal insufficiency; massive small-bowel obstruction; and conditions such as rheumatoid arthritis, vitiligo, diabetes mellitus, and pheochromocytoma. Gastric acid induces feedback inhibition of gastrin release. A decrease in acid production will subsequently lead to failure of the feedback inhibitory pathway, resulting in net hypergastrinemia. Gastrin levels will thus be high in patients using antisecretory agents for the treatment of acid peptic disorders and dyspepsia. *H. pylori* infection can also cause hypergastrinemia. Although a fasting gastrin >10 times normal is highly suggestive of ZES, two-thirds of patients will have fasting gastrin levels that overlap with levels found in the more common disorders outlined above.

The next step in establishing a biochemical diagnosis of gastrinoma is to assess acid secretion. Nothing further needs to be done if decreased acid output is observed. In contrast, normal or elevated gastric acid output suggests a need for additional tests. Up to 12% of patients with common PUD may have comparable levels of acid

TABLE 293-7 When to Obtain a Fasting Serum Gastrin Level

Multiple ulcers
Ulcers in unusual locations; associated with severe esophagitis; resistant to therapy with frequent recurrences; in the absence of NSAID ingestion or *H. pylori* infection
Ulcer patients awaiting surgery
Extensive family history for peptic ulcer disease
Postoperative ulcer recurrence
Basal hyperchlorhydria
Unexplained diarrhea or steatorrhea
Hypercalcemia
Family history of pancreatic islet, pituitary, or parathyroid tumor
Prominent gastric or duodenal folds

secretion. A BAO/MAO ratio >0.6 is highly suggestive of ZES, but a ratio <0.6 does not exclude the diagnosis. Pentagastrin is no longer available in the United States, making measurement of MAO virtually impossible. An endoscopic method for measuring gastric acid output has been developed but requires further validation. If the technology for measuring gastric acid secretion is not available, a basal gastric pH ≥3 virtually excludes a gastrinoma.

Gastrin provocative tests have been developed in an effort to differentiate between the causes of hypergastrinemia and are especially helpful in patients with indeterminate acid secretory studies. The tests are the secretin stimulation test and the calcium infusion study. The most sensitive and specific gastrin provocative test for the diagnosis of gastrinoma is the secretin study. An increase in gastrin of ≥120 pg within 15 minutes of secretin injection has a sensitivity and specificity of >90% for ZES. PPI induced hypochlorhydria or achlorhydria may lead to a false-positive secretin test, thus this agent must be stopped for 1 week before testing.

The calcium infusion study is less sensitive and specific than the secretin test, which coupled with it being a more cumbersome study with greater potential for adverse effects, relegates it to rare utilization in the cases where the patient's clinical characteristics are highly suggestive of ZES, but the secretin stimulation is inconclusive.

Tumor localization

Once the biochemical diagnosis of gastrinoma has been confirmed, the tumor must be located. Multiple imaging studies have been utilized in an effort to enhance tumor localization (Table 293-8). The broad range of sensitivity is due to the variable success rates achieved by the different investigative groups. Endoscopic ultrasound (EUS) permits imaging of the pancreas with a high degree of resolution (<5 mm). This modality is particularly helpful in excluding small neoplasms within the pancreas and in assessing the presence of surrounding lymph nodes and vascular involvement, but it is not very sensitive for finding duodenal lesions. Several types of endocrine tumors express cell-surface receptors for somatostatin. This permits the localization of gastrinomas by measuring the uptake of the stable somatostatin analogue ^{111}In-pentreotide (OctreoScan) with sensitivity and specificity rates of >85%.

Up to 50% of patients have metastatic disease at diagnosis. Success in controlling gastric acid hypersecretion has shifted the emphasis of therapy toward providing a surgical cure. Detecting the primary tumor and excluding metastatic disease are critical in view of this paradigm shift. Once a biochemical diagnosis has been confirmed, the patient should first undergo an abdominal CT scan, MRI, or OctreoScan (depending on availability) to exclude metastatic disease. Once metastatic disease has been excluded, an experienced endocrine surgeon may opt for exploratory laparotomy with intraoperative ultrasound or transillumination. In other centers, careful examination of the peripancreatic area with EUS, accompanied by endoscopic exploration of the duodenum for primary tumors, will be performed before surgery. Selective arterial secretin injection may be a useful adjuvant for localizing tumors in a subset of patients.

TABLE 293-8 Sensitivity of Imaging Studies in Zollinger-Ellison Syndrome

	Sensitivity, %	
Study	Primary Gastrinoma	Metastatic Gastrinoma
Ultrasound	21–28	14
CT scan	55–70	>85
Selective angiography	35–68	33–86
Portal venous sampling	70–90	N/A
SASI	55–78	41
MRI	55–70	>85
OctreoScan	67–86	80–100
EUS	80–100	N/A

Note: CT, computed tomography; EUS, endoscopic ultrasonography; MRI, magnetic resonance imaging; OctreoScan, imaging with ^{111}In-pentreotide; SASI, selective arterial secretin injection.

TREATMENT Zollinger-Ellison Syndrome

Treatment of functional endocrine tumors is directed at ameliorating the signs and symptoms related to hormone overproduction, curative resection of the neoplasm, and attempts to control tumor growth in metastatic disease.

PPIs are the treatment of choice and have decreased the need for total gastrectomy. Initial PPI doses tend to be higher than those used for treatment of GERD or PUD. The initial dose of omeprazole, lansoprazole, rabeprazole or esomeprazole should be in the range of 60 mg in divided doses in a 24-hour period. Dosing can be adjusted to achieve a BAO <10 meq/h (at the drug trough) in surgery-naive patients and to <5 meq/h in individuals who have previously undergone an acid-reducing operation. Although the somatostatin analogue has inhibitory effects on gastrin release from receptor-bearing tumors and inhibits gastric acid secretion to some extent, PPIs have the advantage of reducing parietal cell activity to a greater degree. Despite this, octreotide may be considered as adjunctive therapy to the PPI in patients with tumors that express somatostatin receptors and have peptic symptoms that are difficult to control with high-dose PPI.

The ultimate goal of surgery would be to provide a definitive cure. Improved understanding of tumor distribution has led to immediate cure rates as high as 60% with 10-year disease-free intervals as high as 34% in sporadic gastrinoma patients undergoing surgery. A positive outcome is highly dependent on the experience of the surgical team treating these rare tumors. Surgical therapy of gastrinoma patients with MEN I remains controversial because of the difficulty in rendering these patients disease-free with surgery. In contrast to the encouraging postoperative results observed in patients with sporadic disease, only 6% of MEN I patients are disease free 5 years after an operation. Some groups suggest surgery only if a clearly identifiable, nonmetastatic lesion is documented by structural studies. Others advocate a more aggressive approach, where all patients free of hepatic metastasis are explored and all detected tumors in the duodenum are resected; this is followed by enucleation of lesions in the pancreatic head, with a distal pancreatectomy to follow. The outcome of the two approaches has not been clearly defined. Laparoscopic surgical interventions may provide attractive approaches in the future.

Therapy of metastatic endocrine tumors in general remains suboptimal; gastrinomas are no exception. In light of the observation that in many instances tumor growth is indolent and that many individuals with metastatic disease remain relatively stable for significant periods of time, many advocate not instituting systemic tumor targeted therapy until evidence of tumor progression or refractory symptoms not controlled with PPIs are noted. Medical approaches including biological therapy (IFN-α, long acting somatostatin analogues, peptide receptor radionuclides), systemic chemotherapy (streptozotocin, 5-fluorouracil, and doxorubicin), and hepatic artery embolization may lead to significant toxicity without a substantial improvement in overall survival. ^{111}In-pentetreotide has been used in the therapy of metastatic neuroendocrine tumors; further studies are needed. Several novel therapies are being explored, including radiofrequency or cryoablation of liver lesions and use of agents that block the vascular endothelial growth receptor pathway (bevacizumab, sunitinib) or the mammalian target of rapamycin (Chap. 350).

Surgical approaches including debulking surgery and liver transplantation for hepatic metastasis have also produced limited benefit.

The overall 5- and 10-year survival rates for gastrinoma patients are 62–75% and 47–53%, respectively. Individuals with the entire tumor resected or those with a negative laparotomy have 5- and 10-year survival rates >90%. Patients with incompletely resected tumors have 5- and 10-year survival rates of 43% and 25%, respectively. Patients with hepatic metastasis have <20% survival at 5 years. Favorable prognostic indicators include primary duodenal wall tumors, isolated lymph node tumor, and undetectable tumor upon surgical exploration. Poor outcome is seen in patients with shorter disease duration; higher gastrin levels (>10,000 pg/mL); large pancreatic primary tumors (>3 cm); metastatic disease to lymph nodes, liver, and bone; and Cushing's syndrome. Rapid growth of hepatic metastases is also predictive of poor outcome.

STRESS-RELATED MUCOSAL INJURY

Patients suffering from shock, sepsis, massive burns, severe trauma, or head injury can develop acute erosive gastric mucosal changes or frank ulceration with bleeding. Classified as stress-induced gastritis or ulcers, injury is most commonly observed in the acid-producing (fundus and body) portions of the stomach. The most common presentation is GI bleeding, which is usually minimal but can occasionally be life threatening. Respiratory failure requiring mechanical ventilation and underlying coagulopathy are risk factors for bleeding, which tends to occur 48–72 hours after the acute injury or insult.

Histologically, stress injury does not contain inflammation or *H. pylori*; thus, "gastritis" is a misnomer. Although elevated gastric acid secretion may be noted in patients with stress ulceration after head trauma (Cushing's ulcer) and severe burns (Curling's ulcer), mucosal ischemia and breakdown of the normal protective barriers of the stomach also play an important role in the pathogenesis. Acid must contribute to injury in view of the significant drop in bleeding noted when acid inhibitors are used as prophylaxis for stress gastritis.

Improvement in the general management of intensive care unit patients has led to a significant decrease in the incidence of GI bleeding due to stress ulceration. The estimated decrease in bleeding is from 20–30% to <5%. This improvement has led to some debate regarding the need for prophylactic therapy. The limited benefit of medical (endoscopic, angiographic) and surgical therapy in a patient with hemodynamically compromising bleeding associated with stress ulcer/gastritis supports the use of preventive measures in high-risk patients (mechanically ventilated, coagulopathy, multiorgan failure, or severe burns). Maintenance of gastric pH >3.5 with continuous infusion of H_2 blockers or liquid antacids administered every 2–3 hours are viable options. Tolerance to the H_2 blocker is likely to develop; thus, careful monitoring of the gastric pH and dose adjustment is important if H_2 blockers are used. Sucralfate slurry (1 g every 4–6 hours) has also been somewhat successful but requires a gastric tube and may lead to constipation and aluminum toxicity. Sucralfate use in endotracheal intubated patients has also been associated with aspiration pneumonia. PPIs are the treatment of choice for stress prophylaxis. Oral PPI is the best option if the patient can tolerate enteral administration. Pantoprazole is available as an intravenous formulation for individuals in whom enteral administration is not possible. If bleeding occurs despite these measures, endoscopy, intraarterial vasopressin, or embolization are options. If all else fails, then surgery should be considered. Although vagotomy and antrectomy may be used, the better approach would be a total gastrectomy, which has an exceedingly high mortality rate in this setting.

GASTRITIS

The term *gastritis* should be reserved for histologically documented inflammation of the gastric mucosa. Gastritis is not the mucosal erythema seen during endoscopy and is not interchangeable with "dyspepsia." The etiologic factors leading to gastritis are broad and heterogeneous. Gastritis has been classified based on time course (acute versus chronic), histologic features, and anatomic distribution or proposed pathogenic mechanism (Table 293-9).

The correlation between the histologic findings of gastritis, the clinical picture of abdominal pain or dyspepsia, and endoscopic findings noted on gross inspection of the gastric mucosa is poor. Therefore, there is no typical clinical manifestation of gastritis.

Acute gastritis

The most common causes of acute gastritis are infectious. Acute infection with *H. pylori* induces gastritis. However, *H. pylori* acute gastritis has not been extensively studied. It is reported as presenting with sudden onset of epigastric pain, nausea, and vomiting, and limited mucosal histologic studies demonstrate a marked infiltrate of neutrophils with edema and hyperemia. If not treated, this picture will evolve into one of chronic gastritis. Hypochlorhydria lasting for up to 1 year may follow acute *H. pylori* infection.

Bacterial infection of the stomach or phlegmonous gastritis is a rare, potentially life-threatening disorder characterized by marked and diffuse acute inflammatory infiltrates of the entire gastric wall, at times accompanied by necrosis. Elderly individuals, alcoholics, and AIDS patients may be affected. Potential iatrogenic causes include polypectomy and mucosal injection with India ink. Organisms associated with this entity include streptococci, staphylococci, *Escherichia coli, Proteus,* and *Haemophilus* species Failure of supportive measures and antibiotics may result in gastrectomy.

TABLE 293-9 Classification of Gastritis

I. Acute gastritis	II. Chronic atrophic gastritis
A. Acute *H. pylori* infection	A. Type A: Autoimmune, body-predominant
B. Other acute infectious gastritides	B. Type B: *H. pylori*–related, antral-predominant
1. Bacterial (other than *H. pylori*)	C. Indeterminant
2. *H. heilmannii*	III. Uncommon forms of gastritis
3. Phlegmonous	A. Lymphocytic
4. Mycobacterial	B. Eosinophilic
5. Syphilitic	C. Crohn's disease
6. Viral	D. Sarcoidosis
7. Parasitic	E. Isolated granulomatous gastritis
8. Fungal	

Other types of infectious gastritis may occur in immunocompromised individuals such as AIDS patients. Examples include herpetic (herpes simplex) or CMV gastritis. The histologic finding of intranuclear inclusions would be observed in the latter.

Chronic gastritis

Chronic gastritis is identified histologically by an inflammatory cell infiltrate consisting primarily of lymphocytes and plasma cells, with very scant neutrophil involvement. Distribution of the inflammation may be patchy, initially involving superficial and glandular portions of the gastric mucosa. This picture may progress to more severe glandular destruction, with atrophy and metaplasia. Chronic gastritis has been classified according to histologic characteristics. These include superficial atrophic changes and gastric atrophy.

The early phase of chronic gastritis is *superficial gastritis.* The inflammatory changes are limited to the lamina propria of the surface mucosa, with edema and cellular infiltrates separating intact gastric glands. The next stage is *atrophic gastritis.* The inflammatory infiltrate extends deeper into the mucosa, with progressive distortion and destruction of the glands. The final stage of chronic gastritis is *gastric atrophy.* Glandular structures are lost, and there is a paucity of inflammatory infiltrates. Endoscopically, the mucosa may be substantially thin, permitting clear visualization of the underlying blood vessels.

Gastric glands may undergo morphologic transformation in chronic gastritis. Intestinal metaplasia denotes the conversion of gastric glands to a small intestinal phenotype with small-bowel mucosal glands containing goblet cells. The metaplastic changes may vary in distribution from patchy to fairly extensive gastric involvement. Intestinal metaplasia is an important predisposing factor for gastric cancer (Chap. 91).

Chronic gastritis is also classified according to the predominant site of involvement. Type A refers to the body-predominant form (autoimmune) and type B is the antral-predominant form (*H. pylori*–related). This classification is artificial in view of the difficulty in distinguishing between these two entities. The term *AB gastritis* has been used to refer to a mixed antral/body picture.

Type a gastritis The less common of the two forms involves primarily the fundus and body, with antral sparing. Traditionally, this form of gastritis has been associated with pernicious anemia (Chap. 105) in the presence of circulating antibodies against parietal cells and IF; thus, it is also called *autoimmune gastritis. H. pylori* infection can lead to a similar distribution of gastritis. The characteristics of an autoimmune picture are not always present.

Antibodies to parietal cells have been detected in >90% of patients with pernicious anemia and in up to 50% of patients with type A gastritis. The parietal cell antibody is directed against H^+,K^+-ATPase. T cells are also implicated in the injury pattern of this form of gastritis. A subset of patients infected with *H. pylori* develop antibodies against H^+,K^+-ATPase, potentially leading to the atrophic gastritis pattern seen in some patients infected with this organism. The mechanism is thought to involve molecular mimicry between *H. pylori* LPS and H^+,K^+-ATPase.

Parietal cell antibodies and atrophic gastritis are observed in family members of patients with pernicious anemia. These antibodies are observed in up to 20% of individuals over age 60 and in ~20% of patients with vitiligo and Addison's disease. About one-half of patients with pernicious anemia have antibodies to thyroid antigens, and about 30% of patients with thyroid disease have circulating antiparietal cell antibodies. Anti-IF antibodies are more specific than parietal cell antibodies for type A gastritis, being present in ~40% of patients with pernicious anemia. Another parameter consistent with this form of gastritis being autoimmune in origin is the higher incidence of specific familial histocompatibility haplotypes such as HLA-B8 and HLA-DR3.

The parietal cell–containing gastric gland is preferentially targeted in this form of gastritis, and achlorhydria results. Parietal cells are the source of IF, the lack of which will lead to vitamin B_{12} deficiency and its sequelae (megaloblastic anemia, neurologic dysfunction).

Gastric acid plays an important role in feedback inhibition of gastrin release from G cells. Achlorhydria, coupled with relative sparing of the antral mucosa (site of G cells), leads to hypergastrinemia. Gastrin levels can be markedly elevated (>500 pg/mL) in patients with pernicious anemia. ECL cell hyperplasia with frank development of gastric carcinoid tumors may result from gastrin trophic effects. Hypergastrinemia and achlorhydria may also be seen in nonpernicious anemia–associated type A gastritis.

Type b gastritis Type B, or antral-predominant, gastritis is the more common form of chronic gastritis. *H. pylori* infection is the cause of this entity. Although described as "antral-predominant," this is likely a misnomer in view of studies documenting the progression of the inflammatory process toward the body and fundus of infected individuals. The conversion to a pangastritis is time-dependent–estimated to require 15–20 years. This form of gastritis increases with age, being present in up to 100% of persons over age 70. Histology improves after *H. pylori* eradication. The number of *H. pylori* organisms decreases dramatically with progression to gastric atrophy, and the degree of inflammation correlates with the level of these organisms. Early on, with antral-predominant findings, the quantity of *H. pylori* is highest and a dense chronic inflammatory infiltrate of the lamina propria is noted, accompanied by epithelial cell infiltration with polymorphonuclear leukocytes (Fig. 293-14).

Multifocal atrophic gastritis, gastric atrophy with subsequent metaplasia, has been observed in chronic *H. pylori*–induced gastritis. This may ultimately lead to development of gastric adenocarcinoma (Fig. 293-8; Chap. 91). *H. pylori* infection is now considered an independent risk factor for gastric cancer. Worldwide epidemiologic studies have documented a higher incidence of *H. pylori* infection in patients with adenocarcinoma of the stomach as compared to control subjects. Seropositivity for *H. pylori* is associated with a three- to sixfold increased risk of gastric cancer. This risk may be as high as ninefold after adjusting for the inaccuracy of serologic testing in the elderly. The mechanism by which *H. pylori* infection leads to cancer is unknown, but it appears to be related to the chronic inflammation induced by the organism. Eradication of *H. pylori* as a general preventative measure for gastric cancer is being evaluated but is not yet recommended.

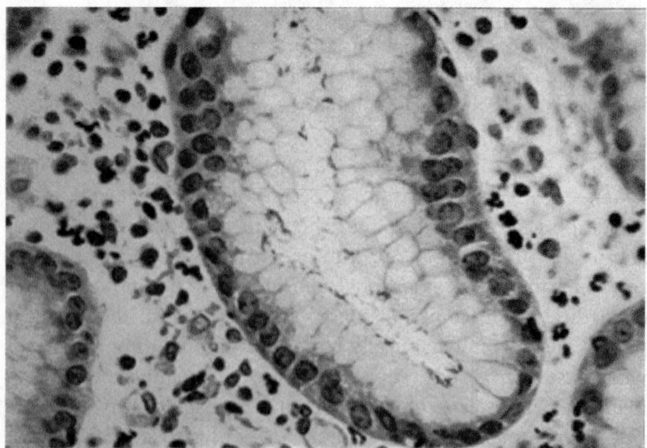

Figure 293-14 Chronic gastritis and *H. pylori* organisms. Steiner silver stain of superficial gastric mucosa, showing abundant darkly stained microorganisms layered over the apical portion of the surface epithelium. Note that there is no tissue invasion.

Infection with *H. pylori* is also associated with development of a low-grade B cell lymphoma, gastric MALT lymphoma (Chap. 110). The chronic T cell stimulation caused by the infection leads to production of cytokines that promote the B cell tumor. The tumor should be initially staged with a CT scan of the abdomen and EUS. Tumor growth remains dependent on the presence of *H. pylori*, and its eradication is often associated with complete regression of the tumor. The tumor may take more than a year to regress after treating the infection. Such patients should be followed by EUS every 2–3 months. If the tumor is stable or decreasing in size, no other therapy is necessary. If the tumor grows, it may have become a high-grade B cell lymphoma. When the tumor becomes a high-grade aggressive lymphoma histologically, it loses responsiveness to *H. pylori* eradication.

TREATMENT Chronic Gastritis

Treatment in chronic gastritis is aimed at the sequelae and not the underlying inflammation. Patients with pernicious anemia will require parenteral vitamin B_{12} supplementation on a long-term basis. Eradication of *H. pylori* is not routinely recommended unless PUD or a low-grade MALT lymphoma is present.

Miscellaneous forms of gastritis

Lymphocytic gastritis is characterized histologically by intense infiltration of the surface epithelium with lymphocytes. The infiltrative process is primarily in the body of the stomach and consists of mature T cells and plasmacytes. The etiology of this form of chronic gastritis is unknown. It has been described in patients with celiac sprue, but whether there is a common factor associating these two entities is unknown. No specific symptoms suggest lymphocytic gastritis. A subgroup of patients have thickened folds noted on endoscopy. These folds are often capped by small nodules that contain a central depression or erosion; this form of the disease is called *varioliform gastritis. H. pylori* probably plays no significant role in lymphocytic gastritis. Therapy with glucocorticoids or sodium cromoglycate has obtained unclear results.

Marked eosinophilic infiltration involving any layer of the stomach (mucosa, muscularis propria, and serosa) is characteristic of *eosinophilic gastritis.* Affected individuals will often have circulating eosinophilia with clinical manifestation of systemic allergy. Involvement may range from isolated gastric disease to diffuse eosinophilic gastroenteritis. Antral involvement predominates, with prominent edematous folds being observed on endoscopy. These prominent antral folds can lead to outlet obstruction. Patients can present with epigastric discomfort, nausea, and vomiting. Treatment with glucocorticoids has been successful.

Several systemic disorders may be associated with *granulomatous gastritis.* Gastric involvement has been observed in Crohn's disease. Involvement may range from granulomatous infiltrates noted only on gastric biopsies to frank ulceration and stricture formation. Gastric Crohn's disease usually occurs in the presence of small-intestinal disease. Several rare infectious processes can lead to granulomatous gastritis, including histoplasmosis, candidiasis, syphilis, and tuberculosis. Other unusual causes of this form of gastritis include sarcoidosis, idiopathic granulomatous gastritis, and eosinophilic granulomas involving the stomach. Establishing the specific etiologic agent in this form of gastritis can be difficult, at times requiring repeat endoscopy with biopsy and cytology. Occasionally, a surgically obtained full-thickness biopsy of the stomach may be required to exclude malignancy.

MÉNÉTRIER'S DISEASE

Ménétrier's disease is a rare entity characterized by large, tortuous gastric mucosal folds. The differential diagnosis of large gastric folds includes ZES, malignancy, infectious etiologies (CMV, histoplasmosis, syphilis), and infiltrative disorders such as sarcoidosis. The mucosal folds in Ménétrier's disease are often most prominent in the body and fundus. Histologically, massive foveolar hyperplasia (hyperplasia of surface and glandular mucous cells) is noted, which replaces most of the chief and parietal cells. This hyperplasia produces the prominent folds observed. The pits of the gastric glands elongate and may become extremely tortuous. Although the lamina propria may contain a mild chronic inflammatory infiltrate, Ménétrier's disease is not considered a form of gastritis. The etiology of this unusual clinical picture is unknown. Overexpression of growth factors such as TGF-α may be involved in the process.

Epigastric pain, at times accompanied by nausea, vomiting, anorexia, and weight loss, are signs and symptoms in patients with Ménétrier's disease. Occult GI bleeding may occur, but overt bleeding is unusual and, when present, is due to superficial mucosal erosions. Twenty to 100% of patients (depending on time of presentation) develop a protein-losing gastropathy accompanied by hypoalbuminemia and edema. Gastric acid secretion is usually reduced or absent because of the replacement of parietal cells. Large gastric folds are readily detectable by either radiographic (barium meal) or endoscopic methods. Endoscopy with deep mucosal biopsy (and cytology) is required to establish the diagnosis and exclude other entities that may present similarly. A nondiagnostic biopsy may lead to a surgically obtained full-thickness biopsy to exclude malignancy.

TREATMENT Ménétrier's Disease

Medical therapy with anticholinergic agents, prostaglandins, PPIs, prednisone, and H_2 receptor antagonists yields varying results. Anticholinergics decrease protein loss. A high-protein diet should be recommended to replace protein loss in patients with hypoalbuminemia. Ulcers should be treated with a standard approach. Severe disease with persistent and substantial protein loss may require total gastrectomy. Subtotal gastrectomy is performed by some; it may be associated with higher morbidity and mortality secondary to the difficulty in obtaining a patent and long-lasting anastomosis between normal and hyperplastic tissues.

ACKNOWLEDGMENTS

The author acknowledges the contribution of material to this chapter by Dr. Lawrence Friedman and Dr. Walter Peterson from their chapter on this subject in the 14th edition of Harrison's.

FURTHER READINGS

Ali A et al: Long-term safety concerns with proton pump inhibitors. Am J Med 122:896, 2009

Amieva M, El-Omar E: Host-bacterial interactions in *Helicobacter pylori* infection. Gastroenterology 134:306, 2008

Atherton J, Blaser M: Coadaptation of *Helicobacter pylori* and humans: Ancient history, modern implications. J Clin Invest 119:2475, 2009

Cover T, Blaser M: *Helicobacter pylori* in health and disease. Gastroenterology 136:1863, 2009

Fox JG, Wang TC: Inflammation, atrophy, and gastric cancer. J Clin Invest 117:60, 2007

JONES R et al: Gastrointestinal and cardiovascular risks of nonsteroidal anti-inflammatory drugs. Am J Med 121:464, 2008

JUHÁSZ M et al: Current standings of the proton pump inhibitor and clopidogrel co-therapy: Review on an evolving field with the eyes of the gastroenterologist. Digestion 81:10, 2010

JUURLINK D: Proton pump inhibitors and clopidogrel: Putting the interaction in perspective. Circulation 120:2310, 2009

LANAS A: Nonsteroidal anti-inflammatory drugs and cyclooxygenase inhibition in the gastrointestinal tract: A trip from peptic ulcer to colon cancer. Am J Med Sci 338:96, 2009

LANZA F et al: Guidelines for prevention of NSAID-related ulcer complications. Am J Gastroenterol 104:728, 2009

MALFERTHEINER P et al: Peptic ulcer disease. Lancet 374:1449, 2009

METZ D, JENSEN R: Gastrointestinal neuroendocrine tumors: pancreatic endocrine tumors. Gastroenterology 135:1469, 2008

SCHUBERT M, PEURA D: Control of gastric acid secretion in health and disease. Gastroenterology 134:1842, 2008

WU C et al: Early *Helicobacter pylori* eradication decreases risk of gastric cancer in patients with peptic ulcer disease. Gastroenterology 137:1641, 2009

ZAGARI R et al: Investigating dyspepsia. BMJ 337:a1400, 2008

CHAPTER 294

Disorders of Absorption

Henry J. Binder

Disorders of absorption constitute a broad spectrum of conditions with multiple etiologies and varied clinical manifestations. Almost all of these clinical problems are associated with *diminished* intestinal absorption of one or more dietary nutrients and are often referred to as the *malabsorption syndrome.* This term is not ideal as it represents a pathophysiologic state, does *not* provide an etiologic explanation for the underlying problem, and should not be considered an adequate final diagnosis. The only clinical situations in which absorption is *increased* are hemochromatosis and Wilson's disease, in which absorption of iron and copper, respectively, are increased.

Most, but not all, malabsorption syndromes are associated with *steatorrhea,* an increase in stool fat excretion of >6% of dietary fat intake. Some malabsorption disorders are not associated with steatorrhea: primary lactase deficiency, a congenital absence of the small intestinal brush border disaccharidase enzyme lactase, is associated with lactose "malabsorption," and pernicious anemia is associated with a marked decrease in intestinal absorption of cobalamin (vitamin B_{12}) due to an absence of gastric parietal cell intrinsic factor required for cobalamin absorption.

Disorders of absorption must be included in the differential diagnosis of diarrhea (Chap. 40). First, diarrhea is frequently associated with and/or is a consequence of the diminished absorption of one or more dietary nutrients. The diarrhea may be secondary either to the intestinal process that is responsible for the steatorrhea or to steatorrhea per se. Thus, celiac disease (see below) is associated with both extensive morphologic changes in the small intestinal mucosa and reduced absorption of several dietary nutrients; in contrast, the diarrhea of steatorrhea is the result of the effect of nonabsorbed dietary fatty acids on intestinal, usually colonic, ion transport. For example, oleic acid and ricinoleic acid (a bacterially hydroxylated fatty acid that is also the active ingredient in castor oil, a widely used laxative) induce active colonic Cl ion secretion, most likely secondary to increasing intracellular Ca. In addition, diarrhea per se may result in mild steatorrhea (<11 g fat excretion while on a 100-g fat diet). Second, most patients will indicate that they have diarrhea, not that they have fat malabsorption. Third, many intestinal disorders that have diarrhea as a prominent symptom (e.g., ulcerative colitis, traveler's diarrhea secondary to an enterotoxin produced by *Escherichia coli*) do not necessarily have diminished absorption of any dietary nutrient.

Diarrhea as a *symptom* (i.e., when used by patients to describe their bowel movement pattern) may be a decrease in stool consistency, an increase in stool volume, an increase in number of bowel movements, or any combination of these three changes. In contrast, diarrhea as a *sign* is a quantitative increase in stool water or weight of >200–225 mL or gram per 24 h, when a Western-type diet is consumed. Individuals consuming a diet with higher fiber content may normally have a stool weight of up to 400 g/24 h. Thus, the clinician must clarify what an individual patient means by diarrhea. Some 10% of patients referred to gastroenterologists for further evaluation of unexplained diarrhea do not have an increase in stool water when it is determined quantitatively. Such patients may have small, frequent, somewhat loose bowel movements with stool urgency that is indicative of proctitis but do not have an increase in stool weight or volume.

It is also critical to establish whether a patient's diarrhea is secondary to diminished absorption of one or more dietary nutrients, in contrast to diarrhea that is due to small- and/or large-intestinal fluid and electrolyte secretion. The former has often been termed *osmotic diarrhea,* while the latter has been referred to as *secretory diarrhea.* Unfortunately, both secretory and osmotic elements can be present simultaneously in the same disorder; thus, this separation is not always precise. Nonetheless, two studies—determination of stool electrolytes and observation of the effect of a fast on stool output—can help make this distinction.

The demonstration of the effect of prolonged (>24 h) fasting on stool output can be very effective in suggesting that a *dietary nutrient* is responsible for the individual's diarrhea. A secretory diarrhea associated with enterotoxin-induced traveler's diarrhea would not be affected by prolonged fasting, as enterotoxin-induced stimulation of intestinal fluid and electrolyte secretion is not altered by eating. In contrast, diarrhea secondary to lactose malabsorption in primary lactase deficiency would undoubtedly cease during a prolonged fast. Thus, a substantial decrease in stool output while fasting during a quantitative stool collection of at least 24 h is presumptive evidence that the diarrhea is related to malabsorption of a dietary nutrient. The persistence of stool output while fasting indicates that the diarrhea is likely secretory and that the cause of diarrhea is *not* a dietary nutrient. Either a luminal (e.g., *E. coli* enterotoxin) or circulating (e.g., vasoactive intestinal peptide) secretagogue could be responsible for the patient's diarrhea persisting unaltered during a prolonged fast. The observed effects of fasting can be compared and correlated with stool electrolyte and osmolality determinations.

Measurement of stool electrolytes and osmolality requires the comparison of stool Na^+ and K^+ concentrations determined in liquid stool to the stool osmolality to determine the presence or absence of a so-called stool osmotic gap. The following formula is used:

$$2 \times (\text{stool } [Na^+] + \text{stool } [K^+]) \leq \text{stool osmolality}$$

The cation concentrations are doubled to estimate stool anion concentrations. The presence of a significant osmotic gap suggests the presence in stool water of a substance (or substances) other than Na/K anions that is presumably responsible for the patient's diarrhea. Originally, stool osmolality was measured, but it is almost invariably greater than the required 290–300 mosmol/kg H_2O, reflecting bacterial degradation of nonabsorbed carbohydrate either immediately before defecation or in the stool jar while awaiting chemical analysis, even when the stool is refrigerated. As a result, the stool osmolality should be assumed to be 300 mosmol/kg H_2O. A low stool osmolality (<290 mosmol/kg H_2O) reflects the addition of either dilute urine or water indicating either collection of urine and stool together or so-called factitious diarrhea, a form of Münchausen's syndrome. When the calculated difference is >50, an osmotic gap is present, suggesting that the diarrhea is due to a nonabsorbed dietary nutrient, e.g., a fatty acid and/or carbohydrate. When this difference is <25, it is presumed that a dietary nutrient is not responsible for the diarrhea. Since elements of both osmotic (i.e., malabsorption of a dietary nutrient) and secretory diarrhea may be present, this separation at times is less clear-cut at the bedside than when used as a teaching example. Ideally, the presence of an osmotic gap will be associated with a marked decrease in stool output during a prolonged fast, while the absence of an osmotic gap will likely be present in an individual whose stool output had not been reduced substantially during a period of fasting.

NUTRIENT DIGESTION AND ABSORPTION

The lengths of the small intestine and colon are ~300 cm and ~80 cm, respectively. However, the effective functional surface area is approximately 600-fold greater than that of a hollow tube as a result of the presence of folds, villi (in the small intestine), and microvilli. The functional surface area of the small intestine is somewhat greater than that of a doubles tennis court. In addition to nutrient digestion and absorption, the intestinal epithelia have several other functions:

1. *Barrier and immune defense.* The intestine is exposed to a large number of potential antigens and enteric and invasive microorganisms, and it is extremely effective preventing the entry of almost all these agents. The intestinal mucosa also synthesizes and secretes secretory IgA.
2. *Fluid and electrolyte absorption and secretion.* The intestine absorbs ~7–8 L of fluid daily, comprising dietary fluid intake (1–2 L/d) and salivary, gastric, pancreatic, biliary, and intestinal fluid (6–7 L/d). Several stimuli, especially bacteria and bacterial enterotoxins, induce fluid and electrolyte secretion that may lead to diarrhea (Chap. 128).
3. *Synthesis and secretion of several proteins.* The intestinal mucosa is a major site for the production of proteins, including apolipoproteins.
4. *Production of several bioactive amines and peptides.* The intestine is one of the largest endocrine organs in the body and produces several amines (e.g., 5-hydroxytryptophan) and peptides that serve as paracrine and hormonal mediators of intestinal function.

The small and large intestines are distinct anatomically (villi are present in the small intestine but are absent in the colon) and functionally (nutrient digestion and absorption take place in the small intestine but not in the colon). No precise anatomic characteristics separate duodenum, jejunum, and ileum, although certain nutrients are absorbed exclusively in specific areas of the small intestine. However, villous cells in the small intestine (and surface epithelial cells in the colon) and crypt cells have distinct anatomic and functional characteristics. Intestinal epithelial cells are continuously renewed, with new proliferating epithelial cells at the base of the crypt migrating over 48–72 h to the tip of the villus (or surface of the colon), where they are well-developed epithelial cells with digestive and absorptive function. This high rate of cell turnover explains the relatively rapid resolution of diarrhea and other digestive tract side effects during chemotherapy as new cells not exposed to these toxic agents are produced. Equally important is the paradigm of separation of villous/surface cell and crypt cell function: Digestive hydrolytic enzymes are present primarily in the brush border of villous epithelial cells. Absorptive and secretory functions are also separated, with villous/surface cells primarily, but not exclusively, being the site for absorptive function, while secretory function is present in crypts of both the small and large intestine.

Nutrients, minerals, and vitamins are absorbed by one or more active transport mechanisms. Active transport mechanisms are energy-dependent and mediated by membrane transport proteins. These processes will result in the *net* movement of a substance against or in the absence of an electrochemical concentration gradient. Intestinal absorption of amino acids and monosaccharides, e.g., glucose, is also a specialized form of active transport—*secondary active transport.* The movement of these actively transported nutrients against a concentration gradient is Na^+-dependent and is due to a Na^+ gradient across the apical membrane. The Na^+ gradient is maintained by Na^+, K^+-adenosine triphosphatase (ATPase), the so-called Na^+ pump located on the basolateral membrane, which extrudes Na^+ and maintains low intracellular [Na] as well as the Na^+ gradient across the apical membrane. As a result, active glucose absorption and glucose-stimulated Na^+ absorption require both the apical membrane transport protein, SGLT1, and the basolateral Na^+, K^+-ATPase. In addition to glucose absorption being Na^+-dependent, glucose also stimulates Na^+ and fluid absorption, which is the physiologic basis of oral rehydration therapy for the treatment of diarrhea (Chap. 40).

The mechanisms of intestinal fluid and electrolyte absorption and secretion are discussed in Chap. 40.

Although the intestinal epithelial cells are crucial mediators of absorption and ion and water flow, the several cell types in the lamina propria (e.g., mast cells, macrophages, myofibroblasts) and the enteric nervous system interact with the epithelium to regulate mucosal cell function. The function of the intestine is the result of the integrated responses of and interactions between both intestinal epithelial cells and intestinal muscle.

ENTEROHEPATIC CIRCULATION OF BILE ACIDS

Bile acids are not present in the diet but are synthesized in the liver by a series of enzymatic steps that also include cholesterol catabolism. Indeed, interruption of the enterohepatic circulation of bile acids can reduce serum cholesterol levels by 10% before a new steady state is established. Bile acids are either primary or secondary: Primary bile acids are synthesized in the liver from cholesterol, and secondary bile acids are synthesized from primary bile acids in the intestine by colonic bacterial enzymes. The two primary bile acids in humans are cholic acid and chenodeoxycholic acid; the two most abundant secondary bile acids are deoxycholic acid and lithocholic acid. Approximately 500 mg bile acids are synthesized in the liver daily, conjugated to either taurine or glycine to form tauroconjugated or glycoconjugated bile acids, respectively, and are

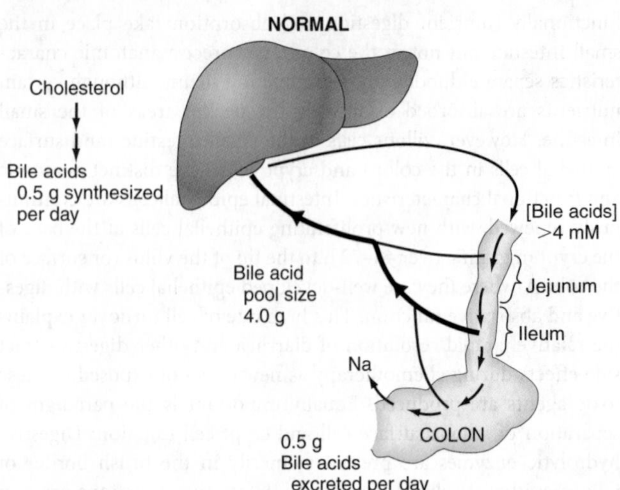

Figure 294-1 Schematic representation of the enterohepatic circulation of bile acids. Bile acid synthesis is cholesterol catabolism and occurs in the liver. Bile acids are secreted in bile and are stored in the gallbladder between meals and at night. Food in the duodenum induces the release of cholecystokinin, a potent stimulus for gallbladder contraction resulting in bile acid entry into the duodenum. Bile acids are primarily absorbed via a Na-dependent transport process that is located only in the ileum. A relatively small quantity of bile acids (~500 mg) is not absorbed in a 24-h period and is lost in stool. Fecal bile acid losses are matched by bile acid synthesis. The bile acid pool (the total amount of bile acids in the body) is ~4 g and is circulated twice during each meal or six to eight times in a 24-h period.

secreted into the duodenum in bile. The primary functions of bile acids are (1) to promote bile flow, (2) to solubilize cholesterol and phospholipid in the gallbladder by mixed micelle formation, and (3) to enhance dietary lipid digestion and absorption by forming mixed micelles in the proximal small intestine.

Bile acids are primarily absorbed by an active, Na^+-dependent process that is located exclusively in the ileum, though bile acids can also be absorbed to a lesser extent by non-carrier-mediated transport processes in the jejunum, ileum, and colon. Conjugated bile acids that enter the colon are deconjugated by colonic bacterial enzymes to unconjugated bile acids and are rapidly absorbed by nonionic diffusion. Colonic bacterial enzymes also dehydroxylate bile acids to secondary bile acids.

Bile acids absorbed from the intestine return to the liver via the portal vein where they are re-secreted (Fig. 294-1). Bile acid synthesis is largely autoregulated by 7α-hydroxylase, the initial enzyme in cholesterol degradation. A decrease in the amount of bile acids returning to the liver from the intestine is associated with an increase in bile acid synthesis/cholesterol catabolism, which helps keep the bile acid pool size relatively constant. However, the capacity to increase bile acid synthesis is limited to about two to two and a half-fold (see below). The bile acid pool size is approximately 4 g and is circulated via the enterohepatic circulation about twice during each meal, or six to eight times during a 24-h period. A relatively small quantity of bile acids is not absorbed and is excreted in stool daily; this fecal loss is matched by hepatic bile acid synthesis.

Defects in any of the steps of the enterohepatic circulation of bile acids can result in a decrease in duodenal concentration of conjugated bile acids and, as a result, steatorrhea. Thus, steatorrhea can be caused by abnormalities in bile acid synthesis and excretion, their physical state in the intestinal lumen, and reabsorption (Table 294-1).

TABLE 294-1 Defects in Enterohepatic Circulation of Bile Acids

Process	Pathophysiologic Defect	Disease Example
Synthesis	Decreased hepatic function	Cirrhosis
Biliary secretion	Altered canalicular function	Primary biliary cirrhosis
Maintenance of conjugated bile acids	Bacterial overgrowth	Jejunal diverticulosis
Reabsorption	Abnormal ileal function	Crohn's disease

Synthesis

Decreased bile acid synthesis and steatorrhea have been demonstrated in chronic liver disease, but steatorrhea is often not a major component of the illness of these patients.

Secretion

Although bile acid secretion may be reduced or absent in biliary obstruction, steatorrhea is rarely a significant medical problem in these patients. In contrast, primary biliary cirrhosis represents a defect in canalicular excretion of organic anions, including bile acids, and not infrequently is associated with steatorrhea and its consequences, e.g., chronic bone disease. Thus, the osteopenia/osteomalacia and other chronic bone abnormalities often present in patients with primary biliary cirrhosis and other cholestatic syndromes are secondary to steatorrhea that then leads to calcium and vitamin D malabsorption as well as to the effects of cholestasis (e.g., bile acids and inflammatory cytokines).

Maintenance of conjugated bile acids

In bacterial overgrowth syndromes associated with diarrhea, steatorrhea, and macrocytic anemia, a colonic type of bacterial flora is increased in the small intestine. The steatorrhea is primarily a result of the decrease in conjugated bile acids secondary to their deconjugation by colonic-type bacteria. Two complementary explanations account for the resulting impairment of micelle formation: (1) unconjugated bile acids are rapidly absorbed in the jejunum by nonionic diffusion, resulting in a reduced concentration of duodenal bile acids; and (2) the critical micellar concentration (CMC) of unconjugated bile acids is higher than that of conjugated bile acids, and therefore unconjugated bile acids are less effective than conjugated bile acids in micelle formation.

Reabsorption

Ileal dysfunction caused by either Crohn's disease or surgical resection results in a decrease in bile acid reabsorption in the ileum and an *increase* in the delivery of bile acids to the large intestine. The resulting clinical consequences—diarrhea with or without steatorrhea—are determined by the *degree* of ileal dysfunction and the *response* of the enterohepatic circulation to bile acid losses (Table 294-2). Patients with limited ileal disease or resection will often have diarrhea but not steatorrhea. The diarrhea, a result of bile acids in the colon stimulating active Cl secretion, has been called *bile acid diarrhea,* or choleretic enteropathy, and responds promptly to cholestyramine, an anion-binding resin. Such patients do not develop steatorrhea because hepatic synthesis of bile acids increases to compensate for the rate of fecal bile acid losses, resulting in maintenance of both the bile acid pool size and the intraduodenal concentrations of bile acids.

TABLE 294-2 Comparison of Bile Acid and Fatty Acid Diarrhea

	Bile Acid Diarrhea	Fatty Acid Diarrhea
Extent of ileal disease	Limited	Extensive
Ileal bile acid absorption	Reduced	Reduced
Fecal bile acid excretion	Increased	Increased
Fecal bile acid loss compensated by hepatic synthesis	Yes	No
Bile acid pool size	Normal	Reduced
Intraduodenal [bile acid]	Normal	Reduced
Steatorrhea	None or mild	>20 g
Response to cholestyramine	Yes	No
Response to low-fat diet	No	Yes

In contrast, patients with greater degrees of ileal disease and/or resection will often have diarrhea and steatorrhea that do not respond to cholestyramine. In this situation, ileal disease is also associated with increased amounts of bile acids entering the colon; however, hepatic synthesis can no longer increase sufficiently to maintain the bile acid pool size. As a consequence, the intraduodenal concentration of bile acids is also reduced to less than the CMC, resulting in impaired micelle formation and steatorrhea. This second situation is often called *fatty acid diarrhea*. Cholestyramine may not be effective (and may even increase the diarrhea by further depleting the intraduodenal bile acid concentration); however, a low-fat diet to reduce fatty acids entering the colon can be effective. Two clinical features, the length of ileum removed and the degree of steatorrhea, can predict whether an individual patient will respond to cholestyramine. Unfortunately, these predictors are imperfect, and a therapeutic trial of cholestyramine is often necessary to establish whether an individual patient will benefit from cholestyramine. Table 294-2 contrasts the characteristics of bile acid diarrhea (small ileal dysfunction) and fatty acid diarrhea (large ileal dysfunction).

LIPIDS

Steatorrhea is caused by one or more defects in the digestion and absorption of dietary fat. Average intake of dietary fat in the United States is approximately 120–150 g/d, and fat absorption is linear to dietary fat intake. The total load of fat presented to the small intestine is considerably greater, as substantial amounts of lipid are secreted in bile each day. (See above for discussion of enterohepatic circulation of bile acids.) Three types of fatty acids compose fats: long-chain fatty acids (LCFAs), medium-chain fatty acids (MCFAs), and short-chain fatty acids (SCFAs) (Table 294-3). Dietary fat is exclusively composed of long-chain triglycerides (LCTs), i.e., glycerol that is bound via ester-linkages to three LCFAs. While the majority of dietary LCFAs have carbon chain lengths of 16 or 18, fatty acids of carbon chain length >12 are metabolized in the same manner; saturated and unsaturated fatty acids are handled identically.

Assimilation of dietary lipid requires three integrated processes: (1) an intraluminal, or digestive, phase; (2) a mucosal, or absorptive, phase; and (3) a delivery, or postabsorptive, phase. An abnormality at any site of this process can cause steatorrhea (Table 294-4). Therefore, it is essential that any patient with steatorrhea be evaluated to identify the specific physiologic defect in overall lipid digestion-absorption, as therapy will be determined by the specific cause of the steatorrhea.

TABLE 294-3 Comparison of Different Types of Fatty Acids

	Long-Chain	Medium-Chain	Short-Chain
Carbon chain length	>12	8–12	<8
Present in diet	In large amounts	In small amounts	No
Origin	In diet as triglycerides	Only in small amounts in diet as triglycerides	Bacterial degradation in colon of nonabsorbed carbohydrate to fatty acids
Primary site of absorption	Small intestine	Small intestine	Colon
Requires pancreatic lipolysis	Yes	No	No
Requires micelle formation	Yes	No	No
Presence in stool	Minimal	No	Substantial

The digestive phase has two components, *lipolysis* and *micellar formation*. Although dietary lipid is in the form of LCTs, the intestinal mucosa does not absorb triglycerides; they must first be hydrolyzed (Fig. 294-2). The initial step in lipid digestion is the formation of emulsions of finely dispersed lipid, which is accomplished by mastication and gastric contractions. Lipolysis, the hydrolysis of triglycerides to free fatty acids, monoglycerides, and glycerol by lipase, is initiated in the stomach by lingual and gastric lipases that have a pH optimum of 4.5–6.0. About 20–30% of total lipolysis occurs in the stomach. Lipolysis is completed in the duodenum and jejunum by pancreatic lipase, which is inactivated by a pH <7.0. Pancreatic lipolysis is greatly enhanced by the presence of a second pancreatic enzyme, colipase, which facilitates the movement of lipase to the triglyceride.

TABLE 294-4 Defects in Lipid Digestion and Absorption in Steatorrhea

Phase: Process	Pathophysiologic Defect	Disease Example
Digestive		
Lipolysis formation	Decreased lipase secretion	Chronic pancreatitis
Micelle formation	Decreased intraduodenal bile acids	See Table 294-1
Absorptive		
Mucosal uptake and reesterification	Mucosal dysfunction	Celiac disease
Postabsorptive		
Chylomicron formation	Absent betalipoproteins	Abetalipoproteinemia
Delivery from intestine	Abnormal lymphatics	Intestinal lymphangiectasia

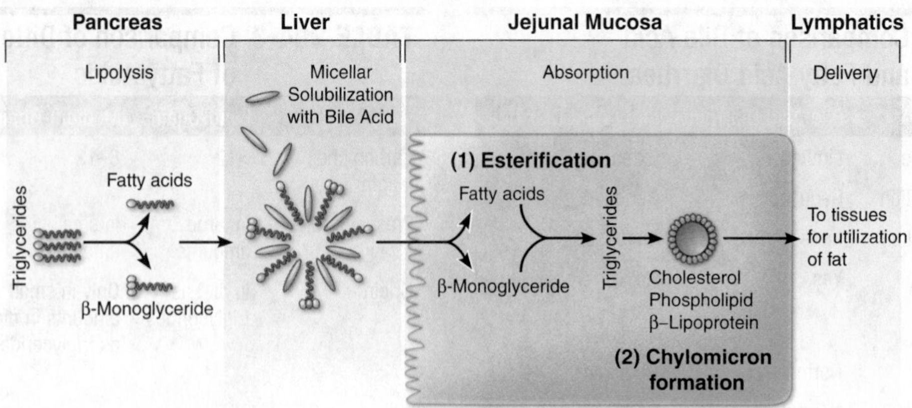

Figure 294-2 Schematic representation of lipid digestion and absorption. Dietary lipid is in the form of long-chain triglycerides (LCTs). The overall process can be divided into (1) a digestive phase that includes both lipolysis and micelle formation requiring pancreatic lipase and conjugated bile acids, respectively, in the duodenum; (2) an absorptive phase for mucosal uptake and reesterification; and (3) a postabsorptive phase that includes chylomicron formation and exit from the intestinal epithelial cell via lymphatics. *(Courtesy of John M. Dietschy, MD; with permission.)*

Impaired lipolysis can lead to steatorrhea and can occur in the presence of pancreatic insufficiency due to chronic pancreatitis in adults or cystic fibrosis in children and adolescents. Normal lipolysis can be maintained by approximately 5% of maximal pancreatic lipase secretion; thus, steatorrhea is a late manifestation of these disorders. A reduction in intraduodenal pH can also result in altered lipolysis as pancreatic lipase is inactivated at pH <7. Thus, ~15% of patients with gastrinoma (Chap. 293) with substantial increases in gastric acid secretion from ectopic production of gastrin (usually from an islet cell adenoma) have diarrhea, and some will have steatorrhea believed secondary to acid-inactivation of pancreatic lipase. Similarly, patients with chronic pancreatitis (who have reduced lipase secretion) often have a decrease in pancreatic bicarbonate secretion, which will also result in a decrease in intraduodenal pH and inactivation of endogenous pancreatic lipase or of therapeutically administered lipase.

Overlying the microvillus membrane of the small intestine is the so-called unstirred water layer, a relatively stagnant aqueous phase that must be traversed by the products of lipolysis that are primarily water-insoluble. Water-soluble mixed micelles provide a mechanism for the water-insoluble products of lipolysis to reach the luminal plasma membrane of villous epithelial cells, the site for lipid absorption. Mixed micelles are molecular aggregates composed of fatty acids, monoglycerides, phospholipids, cholesterol, and conjugated bile acids. Mixed micelles are formed when the concentration of conjugated bile acids is greater than its CMC, which differs among the several bile acids present in the small intestinal lumen. Conjugated bile acids, synthesized in the liver and excreted into the duodenum in bile, are regulated by the enterohepatic circulation (see above). Steatorrhea can result from impaired movement of fatty acids across the unstirred aqueous fluid layer in two situations: (1) an increase in the relative thickness of the unstirred water layer that occurs in bacterial overgrowth syndromes (see below) secondary to functional stasis (e.g., scleroderma); and (2) a decrease in the *duodenal* concentration of conjugated bile acids below its CMC, resulting in impaired micelle formation. Thus, steatorrhea can be caused by one or more defects in the enterohepatic circulation of bile acids.

Uptake and reesterification constitute the *absorptive phase* of lipid digestion-absorption. Although passive diffusion has been thought responsible, a carrier-mediated process may mediate fatty acid and monoglyceride uptake. Regardless of the uptake process, fatty acids and monoglycerides are reesterified by a series of enzymatic steps in the endoplasmic reticulum to form triglycerides, the form in which lipid exits from the intestinal epithelial cell. Impaired lipid absorption as a result of either mucosal inflammation (e.g., celiac disease) and/or intestinal resection can also lead to steatorrhea.

The reesterified triglycerides require the formation of *chylomicrons* to permit their exit from the small-intestinal epithelial cell and their delivery to the liver via the *lymphatics.* Chylomicrons are composed of β-lipoprotein and contain triglycerides, cholesterol, cholesterol esters, and phospholipids and enter the lymphatics, not the portal vein. Defects in the *postabsorptive phase* of lipid digestion-absorption can also result in steatorrhea, but these disorders are uncommon. Abetalipoproteinemia, or acanthocytosis, is a rare disorder of impaired synthesis of β-lipoprotein associated with abnormal erythrocytes (acanthocytes), neurologic problems, and steatorrhea. Lipolysis, micelle formation, and lipid uptake are all normal in patients with abetalipoproteinemia, but the reesterified triglyceride cannot exit from the epithelial cell because of the failure to produce chylomicrons. Small-intestinal biopsies of these rare patients in the postprandial state reveal lipid-laden small-intestinal epithelial cells that become perfectly normal in appearance following a 72–96 h fast. Similarly, abnormalities of intestinal lymphatics (e.g., intestinal lymphangiectasia) may also be associated with steatorrhea as well as protein loss (see below). Steatorrhea can result from defects at any of the several steps in lipid digestion-absorption.

The mechanism of lipid digestion-absorption outlined above is limited to *dietary* lipid that is almost exclusively in the form of LCTs (Table 294-3). Medium-chain triglycerides (MCTs), composed of fatty acids with carbon chain lengths of 8–12, are present in large amounts in coconut oil and are used as a nutritional supplement. MCTs can be digested and absorbed by a different pathway from LCTs and at one time held promise as an important treatment of steatorrhea of almost all etiologies. Unfortunately, their therapeutic effects have been less than expected because their use is often not associated with an increase in body weight for reasons that are not completely understood.

MCTs, in contrast to LCTs, do not require pancreatic lipolysis as the triglyceride can be absorbed intact by the intestinal epithelial cell. Further, micelle formation is not necessary for the absorption of MCTs or medium-chain fatty acids, if hydrolyzed by pancreatic lipase. MCTs are absorbed more efficiently than LCTs for the following reasons: (1) The rate of MCT absorption is greater than that of long-chain fatty acids; (2) medium-chain fatty acids following absorption are not reesterified; (3) following absorption, MCTs are hydrolyzed to medium-chain fatty acids; (4) MCTs do not require chylomicron formation for their exit from the intestinal epithelial cells; and (5) their route of exit is via the portal vein and not via lymphatics. Thus, the absorption of MCTs is greater than that of LCTs in pancreatic insufficiency, conditions with reduced intraduodenal bile acid concentrations, small-intestinal mucosal disease, abetalipoproteinemia, and intestinal lymphangiectasia.

SCFAs are not dietary lipids but are synthesized by colonic bacterial enzymes from nonabsorbed carbohydrate and are the anions in highest concentration in stool (between 80 and 130 m*M*). The SCFAs present in stool are primarily acetate, propionate, and butyrate, whose carbon chain lengths are 2, 3, and 4, respectively. Butyrate is the primary nutrient for colonic epithelial cells, and its deficiency may be associated with one or more colitides. SCFAs conserve calories and carbohydrate, because carbohydrates not completely absorbed in the small intestine will not be absorbed in the large intestine due to the absence of both disaccharidases and SGLT1, the transport protein that mediates monosaccharide absorption. In contrast, SCFAs are rapidly absorbed and stimulate colonic Na-Cl and fluid absorption. Most non–*Clostridium difficile* antibiotic-associated diarrhea is due to antibiotic suppression of colonic microbiota, with a resulting decrease in SCFA production. As *C. difficile* accounts for about 15–20% of all antibiotic-associated diarrhea, a relative decrease in colonic production of SCFA is likely the cause of most antibiotic-associated diarrhea.

The clinical manifestations of steatorrhea are a consequence of both the underlying disorder responsible for the development of steatorrhea and steatorrhea per se. Depending on the degree of steatorrhea and the level of dietary intake, significant fat malabsorption may lead to weight loss. Steatorrhea per se can be responsible for diarrhea; if the primary cause of the steatorrhea has not been identified, a low-fat diet can often ameliorate the diarrhea by decreasing fecal fat excretion. Steatorrhea is often associated with fat-soluble vitamin deficiency, which will require replacement with water-soluble preparations of these vitamins.

Disorders of absorption may also be associated with malabsorption of other dietary nutrients, most often carbohydrates, with or without a decrease in dietary lipid digestion and absorption. Therefore, knowledge of the mechanism of the digestion and absorption of carbohydrates, proteins, and other minerals and vitamins is useful in the evaluation of patients with altered intestinal nutrient absorption.

CARBOHYDRATES

Carbohydrates in the diet are present in the form of starch, disaccharides (sucrose and lactose), and glucose. Carbohydrates are absorbed only in the small intestine and only in the form of monosaccharides. Therefore, before their absorption, starch and disaccharides must first be digested by pancreatic amylase and intestinal brush border disaccharidases to monosaccharides. Monosaccharide absorption occurs by a Na-dependent process mediated by the brush border transport protein SGLT1.

Lactose malabsorption is the only clinically important disorder of carbohydrate absorption. Lactose, the disaccharide present in milk, requires digestion by brush border lactase to its two constituent monosaccharides, glucose and galactose. Lactase is present in almost all species in the postnatal period but then disappears throughout the animal kingdom, except in humans. Lactase activity persists in many individuals throughout life. Two different types of lactase deficiency exist—primary and secondary. In *primary lactase deficiency*, a genetically determined decrease or absence of lactase is noted, while all other aspects of both intestinal absorption and brush border enzymes are normal. In a number of non-white groups, primary lactase deficiency is common in adulthood. Table 294-5 presents the incidence of primary lactase deficiency in several ethnic groups. Northern European and North American whites are the only groups to maintain small-intestinal lactase activity throughout adult life. The persistence of lactase is the abnormality due to a defect in the regulation of its maturation. In contrast, *secondary lactase deficiency* occurs in association with small-intestinal mucosal disease with abnormalities in both structure and function of other brush border enzymes and transport processes. Secondary lactase deficiency is often seen in celiac disease.

TABLE 294-5 Primary Lactase Deficiency in Different Adult Ethnic Groups

Ethnic Group	Prevalence of Lactase Deficiency, %
Northern European	5–15
Mediterranean	60–85
African black	85–100
American black	45–80
American white	10–25
Native American	50–95
Mexican American	40–75
Asian	90–100

Source: From FJ Simons: Am J Dig Dis 23:963, 1978.

As lactose digestion is rate-limiting compared to glucose/galactose absorption, lactase deficiency is associated with significant lactose malabsorption. Some individuals with lactose malabsorption develop symptoms such as diarrhea, abdominal pain, cramps, and/or flatus. Most individuals with primary lactase deficiency do not have symptoms. Since lactose intolerance may be associated with symptoms suggestive of irritable bowel syndrome, persistence of such symptoms in an individual with lactose intolerance while on a strict lactose-free diet would suggest that the individual's symptoms were related to irritable bowel syndrome.

Development of symptoms of lactose intolerance is related to several factors:

1. *Amount of lactose in the diet.*
2. *Rate of gastric emptying.* Symptoms are more likely when gastric emptying is rapid than when gastric emptying is slower. Therefore, it is more likely that skim milk will be associated with symptoms of lactose intolerance than will whole milk, as the rate of gastric emptying following skim milk intake is more rapid. Similarly, the diarrhea observed following subtotal gastrectomy is often a result of lactose intolerance, as gastric emptying is accelerated in patients with a gastrojejunostomy.
3. *Small-intestinal transit time.* Although the small and large intestine contribute to the development of symptoms, many of the symptoms of lactase deficiency are related to the interaction of colonic bacteria and nonabsorbed lactose. More rapid small-intestinal transit makes symptoms more likely.
4. *Colonic compensation by production of SCFAs from nonabsorbed lactose.* Reduced levels of colonic microflora, which can occur following antibiotic use, will also be associated with increased symptoms following lactose ingestion, especially in a lactase-deficient individual.

Glucose-galactose or monosaccharide malabsorption may also be associated with diarrhea and is due to a congenital absence of SGLT1. Diarrhea is present when individuals with this disorder ingest carbohydrates that contain actively transported monosaccharides (e.g., glucose, galactose) but not monosaccharides that are not actively transported (e.g., fructose). Fructose is absorbed by the brush border transport protein GLUT 5, a facilitated diffusion process that is not Na-dependent and is distinct from SGLT1. In contrast, some individuals develop diarrhea as a result of consuming large quantities of sorbitol, a sugar used in diabetic candy; sorbitol is only minimally absorbed due to the absence of an intestinal absorptive transport mechanism for sorbitol.

PROTEINS

Protein is present in food almost exclusively as polypeptides and requires extensive hydrolysis to di- and tripeptides and amino acids before absorption. Proteolysis occurs in both the stomach and small intestine; it is mediated by pepsin secreted as pepsinogen by gastric chief cells and trypsinogen and other peptidases from pancreatic acinar cells. These proenzymes, pepsinogen and trypsinogen, must be activated to pepsin (by pepsin in the presence of a pH <5) and to trypsin (by the intestinal brush border enzyme enterokinase and subsequently by trypsin), respectively. Proteins are absorbed by separate transport systems for di- and tripeptides and for different types of amino acids, e.g., neutral and dibasic. Alterations in either protein or amino acid digestion and absorption are rarely observed clinically, even in the presence of extensive small-intestinal mucosal inflammation. However, three rare genetic disorders involve protein digestion-absorption: (1) *Enterokinase deficiency* is due to an absence of the brush border enzyme that converts the proenzyme trypsinogen to trypsin and is associated with diarrhea, growth retardation, and hypoproteinemia. (2) *Hartnup syndrome,* a defect in neutral amino acid transport, is characterized by a pellagra-like rash and neuropsychiatric symptoms. (3) *Cystinuria,* a defect in dibasic amino acid transport, is associated with renal calculi and chronic pancreatitis.

APPROACH TO THE PATIENT Malabsorption

The clues provided by the history, symptoms, and initial preliminary observations will serve to limit extensive, ill-focused, and expensive laboratory and imaging studies. For example, a clinician evaluating a patient with symptoms suggestive of malabsorption, who recently had extensive small-intestinal resection for mesenteric ischemia, should direct the initial assessment almost exclusively to define whether a short bowel syndrome might explain the entire clinical picture. Similarly, the development of a pattern of bowel movements suggestive of steatorrhea in a patient with long-standing alcohol abuse and chronic pancreatitis should lead toward assessing pancreatic exocrine function.

The classic picture of malabsorption is rarely seen today in most parts of the United States. As a consequence, diseases with malabsorption must be suspected in individuals with less severe symptoms and signs and with subtle evidence of the altered absorption of only a *single* nutrient rather than obvious evidence of the malabsorption of multiple nutrients.

Although diarrhea can be caused by changes in fluid and electrolyte movement in either the small or the large intestine, dietary nutrients are absorbed almost exclusively in the small intestine. Therefore, the demonstration of diminished absorption of a dietary nutrient provides unequivocal evidence of small-intestinal disease, although colonic dysfunction may also be present (e.g., Crohn's disease may involve both small and large intestine). Dietary nutrient absorption may be segmental or diffuse along the small intestine and is site-specific. Thus, for example, calcium, iron, and folic acid are exclusively absorbed by active transport processes in the proximal small intestine, especially the duodenum; in contrast, the active transport mechanisms for both cobalamin and bile acids are present only in the ileum. Therefore, in an individual who years previously had had an intestinal resection, the details of which are not presently available, a presentation with evidence of calcium, folic acid, and/or iron malabsorption but without cobalamin deficiency would make it likely that the duodenum and proximal jejunum, but not ileum, had been resected.

Some nutrients, e.g., glucose, amino acids, and lipids, are absorbed throughout the small intestine, though their rate of absorption is greater in the proximal than in the distal segments. However, following segmental resection of the small intestine, the remaining segments undergo both morphologic and functional "adaptation" to enhance absorption. Such adaptation is secondary to the presence of luminal nutrients and hormonal stimuli and may not be complete in humans for several months following the resection. Adaptation is critical for survival in individuals who have undergone massive resection of the small intestine and/or colon.

Establishing the presence of steatorrhea and identifying its specific cause are often quite difficult. The "gold standard" still remains a timed, quantitative stool fat determination. On a practical basis, stool collections are invariably difficult and often incomplete, as nobody wants to handle stool. A qualitative test—Sudan III stain—has long been available to establish the presence of an increase in stool fat. This test is rapid and inexpensive but, as a qualitative test, does not establish the degree of fat malabsorption and is best used as a preliminary screening study. Many of the blood, breath, and isotopic tests that have been developed (1) do not directly measure fat absorption; (2) have excellent sensitivity when steatorrhea is obvious and severe but have poor sensitivity when steatorrhea is mild (e.g., stool chymotrypsin, elastase, that can potentially distinguish pancreatic from nonpancreatic etiologies of steatorrhea); or (3) have not survived the transition from the research laboratory to commercial application.

Despite this situation, the use of routine laboratory studies (i.e., complete blood count, prothrombin time, serum protein determination, alkaline phosphatase) may suggest the presence of dietary nutrient depletion, especially iron, folate, cobalamin, and vitamins D and K. Additional studies include measurement of serum carotene, cholesterol, albumin, iron, folate, and cobalamin levels. The serum carotene level can also be reduced if the patient has poor dietary intake of leafy vegetables.

If steatorrhea and/or altered absorption of other nutrients are suspected, the history, clinical observations, and laboratory testing can help detect deficiency of a nutrient, especially the fat-soluble vitamins A, D, E, or K. Thus, evidence of metabolic bone disease with elevated alkaline phosphatase and/or reduced serum calcium levels would suggest vitamin D malabsorption. A deficiency of vitamin K would be suggested by an elevated prothrombin time in an individual without liver disease who was not taking anticoagulants. Macrocytic anemia would lead to evaluation of whether cobalamin or folic acid malabsorption was present. The presence of iron-deficiency anemia in the absence of occult bleeding from the gastrointestinal tract in either a male or a nonmenstruating female would require evaluation of iron malabsorption and the exclusion of celiac disease, as iron is absorbed exclusively in the proximal small intestine.

At times, however, a timed (72 h) quantitative stool collection, preferably on a defined diet, must be obtained to determine stool fat content and establish the presence of steatorrhea. The presence of steatorrhea then requires further assessment to establish the pathophysiologic process(es) responsible for the defect in dietary lipid digestion-absorption (Table 294-4). Some of the other studies include the Schilling test, D-xylose test, duodenal mucosal biopsy, small-intestinal radiologic examination, and tests of pancreatic exocrine function.

THE SCHILLING TEST This test is performed to determine the cause of cobalamin malabsorption. Unfortunately, the Schilling test has not been available commercially in the United States for the past few years. Since understanding the physiology and pathophysiology of cobalamin absorption is very valuable to enhance one's understanding of aspects of gastric, pancreatic, and ileal function, discussion of the Schilling test is provided in Chap. e37.

URINARY D-XYLOSE TEST The urinary D-xylose test for carbohydrate absorption provides an assessment of proximal small-intestinal mucosal function. D-Xylose, a pentose, is absorbed almost exclusively in the proximal small intestine. The D-xylose test is usually performed by giving 25 g D-xylose and collecting urine for 5 h. An abnormal test (<4.5 g excretion) primarily reflects the presence of duodenal/jejunal mucosal disease. The D-xylose test can also be abnormal in patients with blind loop syndrome (as a consequence primarily of abnormal intestinal mucosa) and, as a false-positive study, in patients with large collections of fluid in a third space (i.e., ascites, pleural fluid). The ease of obtaining a mucosal biopsy of the small intestine by endoscopy and the false-negative rate of the D-xylose test have led to its diminished use. When small-intestinal mucosal disease is suspected, a small-intestinal mucosal biopsy should be performed.

RADIOLOGIC EXAMINATION Radiologic examination of the small intestine using barium contrast (small-bowel series or study) can provide important information in the evaluation of the patient with presumed or suspected malabsorption. These studies are most often performed in conjunction with the examination of the esophagus, stomach, and duodenal bulb, and insufficient barium is given to the patient to permit an adequate examination of the small-intestinal mucosa, especially the ileum. As a result, many gastrointestinal radiologists alter the procedure of a barium contrast examination of the small intestine by performing either a small-bowel series in which a large amount of barium is given by mouth without concurrent examination of the esophagus and stomach or an enteroclysis study in which a large amount of barium is introduced into the duodenum via a fluoroscopically placed tube. In addition, many of the diagnostic features initially described by radiologists to denote the presence of small-intestinal disease (e.g., flocculation, segmentation) are rarely seen with current barium suspensions. Nonetheless, in skilled hands barium contrast examination of the small intestine can yield important information. For example, with extensive mucosal disease, dilation of intestine can be seen, as dilution of barium from increased intestinal fluid secretion (Fig. 294-3). A normal barium contrast study does *not* exclude the possibility of small-intestinal disease. However, a small-bowel series remains a useful examination to look for anatomic abnormalities, such as strictures and fistulas (as in Crohn's disease) or blind loop

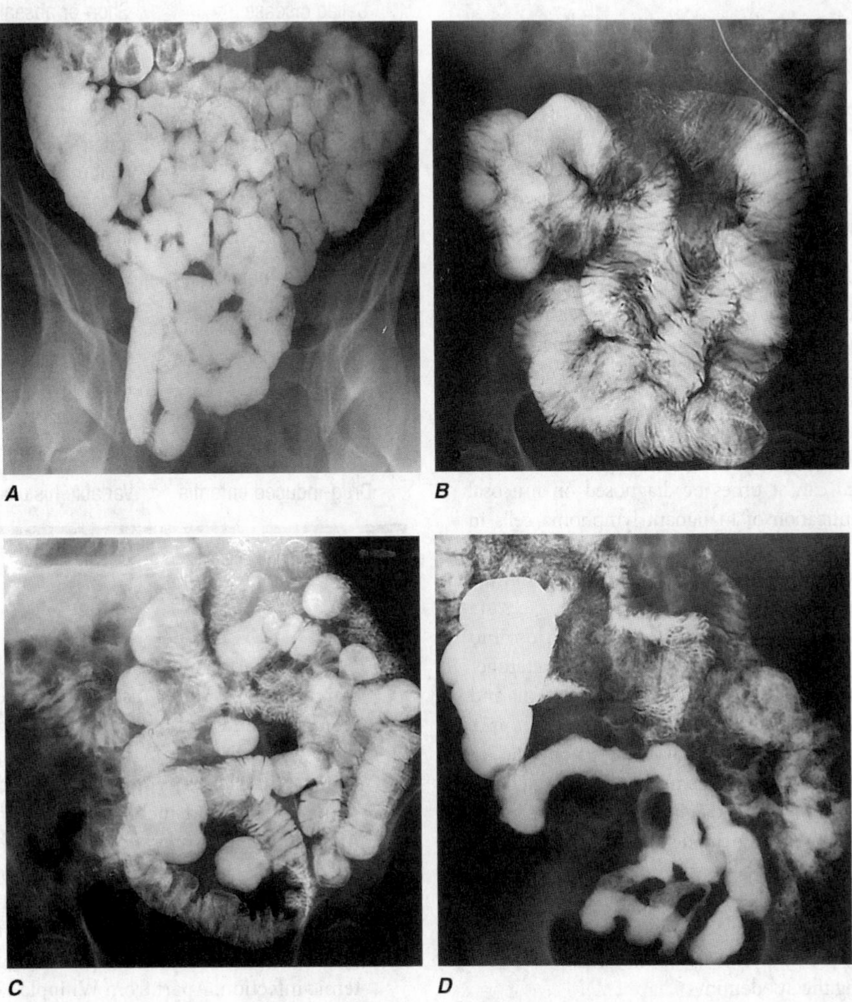

Figure 294-3 Barium contrast small-intestinal radiologic examinations. ***A.*** Normal individual. ***B.*** Celiac sprue. ***C.*** Jejunal diverticulosis. ***D.*** Crohn's disease. *(Courtesy of Morton Burrell, MD, Yale University; with permission.)*

syndrome (e.g., multiple jejunal diverticula), and to define the extent of a previous surgical resection. Other imaging studies to assess the integrity of small intestinal morphology are CT enteroclysis and magnetic resonance (MR) enteroclysis, while capsule endoscopy and double-barrel enteroscopy are other useful aids in the diagnostic assessment of small intestinal pathology.

BIOPSY OF SMALL-INTESTINAL MUCOSA A small-intestinal mucosal biopsy is essential in the evaluation of a patient with documented steatorrhea or chronic diarrhea (lasting >3 weeks) (Chap. 40). The ready availability of endoscopic equipment to examine the stomach and duodenum has led to its almost uniform use as the preferred method to obtain histologic material of proximal small-intestinal mucosa. The primary indications for a small-intestinal biopsy are (1) evaluation of a patient either with documented or suspected steatorrhea or with chronic diarrhea, and (2) diffuse or focal abnormalities of the small intestine defined on a small-intestinal series. Lesions seen on small-bowel biopsy can be classified into three different categories (Table 294-6):

1. *Diffuse, specific lesions.* Relatively few diseases associated with altered nutrient absorption have specific histopathologic abnormalities on small-intestinal mucosal biopsy, and they are uncommon. Whipple's disease is characterized by the presence of periodic acid–Schiff (PAS)–positive macrophages in the lamina propria, while the bacilli that are also present may require electron-microscopic examination for identification (Fig. 294-4). *Abetalipoproteinemia* is characterized by a normal mucosal appearance except for the presence of mucosal absorptive cells that contain lipid postprandially and disappear following a prolonged period of either fat-free intake or fasting. *Immune globulin deficiency* is associated with a variety of histopathologic findings on small-intestinal mucosal biopsy. The characteristic feature is the absence of or substantial reduction in the number of plasma cells in the lamina propria; the mucosal architecture may be either perfectly normal or flat (i.e., villous atrophy). As patients with immune globulin deficiency are often infected with *Giardia lamblia, Giardia* trophozoites may also be seen in the biopsy.
2. *Patchy, specific lesions.* Several diseases show abnormal small-intestinal mucosa with a patchy distribution. As a result, biopsies obtained randomly or in the absence of abnormalities visualized endoscopically may not reveal the diagnostic features. Intestinal *lymphoma* can at times be diagnosed on mucosal biopsy by the identification of malignant lymphoma cells in the lamina propria and submucosa (Chap. 110). The presence of dilated lymphatics in the submucosa and sometimes in the lamina propria indicates the presence of *lymphangiectasia* associated with hypoproteinemia secondary to protein loss into the intestine. *Eosinophilic gastroenteritis* comprises a heterogeneous group of disorders with a spectrum of presentations and symptoms with an eosinophilic infiltrate of the lamina propria, with or without peripheral eosinophilia. The patchy nature of the infiltrate as well as its presence in the submucosa often leads to an absence of histopathologic findings on mucosal biopsy. As the involvement of the duodenum in *Crohn's disease* is also submucosal and not necessarily continuous, mucosal biopsies are not the most direct approach to the diagnosis of duodenal Crohn's disease (Chap. 295). Amyloid deposition can be identified by Congo Red stain in some patients with *amyloidosis* involving the duodenum (Chap. 111).
3. Several microorganisms can be identified on small-intestinal biopsies, establishing a correct diagnosis. At times the small biopsy is performed to establish the diagnosis of the infection, e.g., Whipple's disease or giardiasis. In most other instances the infection is picked up incidentally during the workup of diarrhea or other abdominal symptoms. Many of these infections occur in immunocompromised patients with diarrhea and include *Cryptosporidium, Isospora belli, Microsporidia, Cyclospora, Toxoplasma,* cytomegalovirus, adenovirus, *Mycobacterium avium-intracellulare,* and *G. lamblia.* In immunocompromised patients, when *Candida, Aspergillus, Cryptococcus,* or *Histoplasma* organisms are seen on duodenal biopsy, their presence generally reflects systemic infection. Apart from Whipple's disease and infections in the immunocompromised host, the small bowel biopsy is seldom used as the primary mode to diagnose infection.

TABLE 294-6 Disease That Can Be Diagnosed by Small-Intestinal Mucosal Biopsies

Lesions	Pathologic Findings
Diffuse, Specific	
Whipple's disease	Lamina propria contains macrophages containing PAS+ material
Agammaglobulinemia	No plasma cells; either normal or absent villi ("flat mucosa")
Abetalipoproteinemia	Normal villi; epithelial cells vacuolated with fat postprandially
Patchy, Specific	
Intestinal lymphoma	Malignant cells in lamina propria and submucosa
Intestinal lymphangiectasia	Dilated lymphatics; clubbed villi
Eosinophilic gastroenteritis	Eosinophil infiltration of lamina propria and mucosa
Amyloidosis	Amyloid deposits
Crohn's disease	Noncaseating granulomas
Infection by one or more microorganisms (see text)	Specific organisms
Mastocytosis	Mast cell infiltration of lamina propria
Diffuse, Nonspecific	
Celiac disease	Short or absent villi; mononuclear infiltrate; epithelial cell damage; hypertrophy of crypts
Tropical sprue	Similar to celiac disease
Bacterial overgrowth	Patchy damage to villi; lymphocyte infiltration
Folate deficiency	Short villi; decreased mitosis in crypts; megalocytosis
Vitamin B_{12} deficiency	Similar to folate deficiency
Radiation enteritis	Similar to folate deficiency
Zollinger-Ellison syndrome	Mucosal ulceration and erosion from acid
Protein-calorie malnutrition	Villous atrophy; secondary bacterial overgrowth
Drug-induced enteritis	Variable histology

Abbreviation: PAS+, periodic acid–Schiff positive.

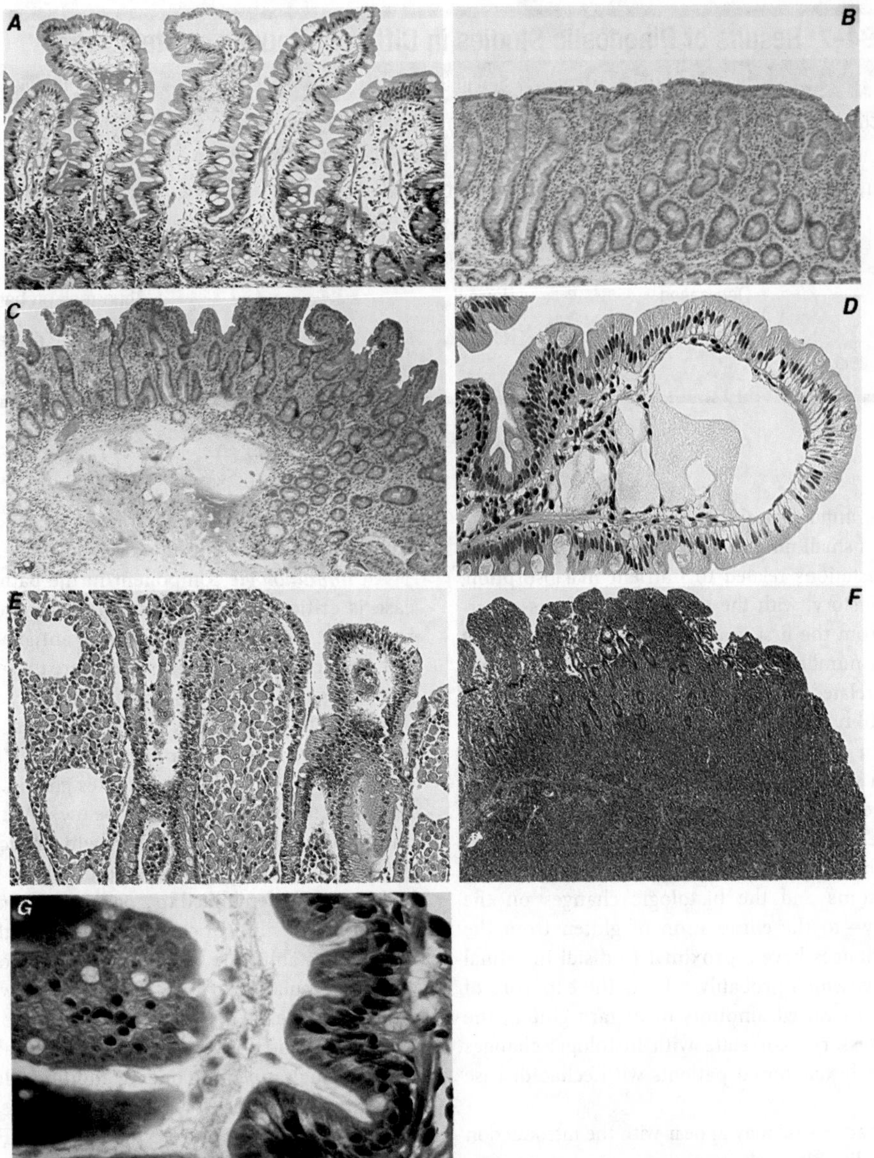

Figure 294-4 Small-intestinal mucosal biopsies. ***A.*** Normal individual. ***B.*** Untreated celiac sprue. ***C.*** Treated celiac sprue. ***D.*** Intestinal lymphangiectasia. ***E.*** Whipple's disease. ***F.*** Lymphoma. ***G.*** Giardiasis. *(Courtesy of Marie Robert, MD, Yale University; with permission.)*

Even giardiasis is more easily diagnosed with duodenal aspirates and/or stool antigen studies than by duodenal biopsy.

4. *Diffuse, nonspecific lesions. Celiac disease* presents with a characteristic mucosal appearance on duodenal/proximal jejunal mucosal biopsy that is *not* diagnostic of the disease. The diagnosis of celiac disease is established by clinical, histologic, and immunologic response to a gluten-free diet. *Tropical sprue* is associated with histologic findings similar to those of celiac disease after a tropical or subtropical exposure but does not respond to gluten restriction; most often symptoms improve with antibiotics and folate administration.

Patients with steatorrhea require assessment of *pancreatic exocrine function,* which is often abnormal in chronic pancreatitis. The secretin test that collects pancreatic secretions by duodenal intubation following intravenous administration of secretin is the only test that directly measures pancreatic exocrine function but is available only at few specialized centers. Endoscopic approaches provide excellent assessment of pancreatic duct anatomy but do *not* assess exocrine function (Chap. 312).

Table 294-7 summarizes the results of the D-xylose test, Schilling test, and small-intestinal mucosal biopsy in patients with five different causes of steatorrhea.

SPECIFIC DISEASE ENTITIES

CELIAC DISEASE

Celiac disease is a common cause of malabsorption of one or more nutrients. Though originally considered largely a disease in whites, especially those of European descent, recent observations have established that celiac disease is a common disease with protean manifestations, a worldwide distribution, and an estimated incidence in the United States that is as high as 1:113 people. Its incidence has increased over the past 50 years. Celiac disease has had several other names, including nontropical sprue, celiac sprue, adult celiac disease, and gluten-sensitive enteropathy. The etiology of celiac disease is not known, but environmental, immunologic,

TABLE 294-7 Results of Diagnostic Studies in Different Causes of Steatorrhea

	D-Xylose Test	Schilling Test	Duodenal Mucosal Biopsy
Chronic pancreatitis	Normal	50% abnormal; if abnormal, normal with pancreatic enzymes	Normal
Bacterial overgrowth syndrome	Normal or only modestly abnormal	Often abnormal; if abnormal, normal after antibiotics	Usually normal
Ileal disease	Normal	Abnormal	Normal
Celiac disease	Decreased	Normal	Abnormal: probably "flat"
Intestinal lymphangiectasia	Normal	Normal	Abnormal: "dilated lymphatics"

and genetic factors are important. Celiac disease is considered an "iceberg" disease with a small number of individuals with classical symptoms and manifestations related to nutrient malabsorption, and a varied natural history, with the onset of symptoms occurring at ages ranging from the first year of life through the eighth decade. A much larger number of individuals have manifestations that are not obviously related to intestinal malabsorption, e.g., anemia, osteopenia, infertility, neurologic symptoms ("atypical celiac disease"); while an even larger group are essentially asymptomatic though with abnormal small intestinal histopathology and serologies (see below) and are referred to as "silent' celiac disease.

The hallmark of celiac disease is the presence of an abnormal small-intestinal biopsy (Fig. 294-4) and the response of the condition—symptoms and the histologic changes on the small-intestinal biopsy—to the elimination of gluten from the diet. The histologic changes have a proximal-to-distal intestinal distribution of severity, which probably reflects the exposure of the intestinal mucosa to varied amounts of dietary gluten; the symptoms do not necessarily correlate with histologic changes especially as many newly diagnosed patients with celiac disease may be asymptomatic.

The symptoms of celiac disease may appear with the introduction of cereals in an infant's diet, although spontaneous remissions often occur during the second decade of life that may be either permanent or followed by the reappearance of symptoms over several years. Alternatively, the symptoms of celiac disease may first become evident at almost any age throughout adulthood. In many patients, frequent spontaneous remissions and exacerbations occur. The symptoms range from significant malabsorption of multiple nutrients, with diarrhea, steatorrhea, weight loss, and the consequences of nutrient depletion (i.e., anemia and metabolic bone disease), to the absence of any gastrointestinal symptoms but with evidence of the depletion of a single nutrient (e.g., iron or folate deficiency, osteomalacia, edema from protein loss). Asymptomatic relatives of patients with celiac disease have been identified as having this disease either by small-intestinal biopsy or by serologic studies [e.g., antiendomysial antibodies, tissue transglutaminase (tTG)]. The availability of these "celiac serologies" has led to a substantial increase in the diagnosis of celiac disease, and the diagnosis is now being made primarily in patients without "classic" symptoms but with atypical and subclinical presentations.

Etiology

The etiology of celiac disease is not known, but environmental, immunologic, and genetic factors all appear to contribute to the disease. One *environmental* factor is the clear association of the disease with gliadin, a component of gluten that is present in wheat, barley, and rye. In addition to the role of gluten restriction in treatment, the instillation of gluten into both normal-appearing rectum and distal ileum of patients with celiac disease results in morphologic changes within hours.

An *immunologic* component in the pathogenesis of celiac disease is critical and involves both adaptive and innate immune responses. Serum antibodies—IgA antigliadin, IgA antiendomysial, and IgA anti-tTG antibodies—are present, but it is not known whether such antibodies are primary or secondary to the tissue damage. The antiendomysial antibody has 90–95% sensitivity and 90–95% specificity; the antigen recognized by the antiendomysial antibody is tTG, which deaminates gliadin, which is presented to HLA-DQ2 or HLA-DQ8 (see below). Antibody studies are frequently used to identify patients with celiac disease; patients with these antibodies should undergo duodenal biopsy. This autoantibody has not been linked to a pathogenetic mechanism (or mechanisms) responsible for celiac disease. Nonetheless, this antibody is useful in establishing the true prevalence of celiac disease in the general population. A 4-week treatment with prednisolone of a patient with celiac disease who continues to eat gluten will induce a remission and convert the "flat" abnormal duodenal biopsy to a more normal-appearing one. In addition, gliadin peptides interact with gliadin-specific T cells that mediate tissue injury and induce the release of one or more cytokines (e.g., IFN-γ) that cause tissue injury.

Genetic factor(s) are also involved in celiac disease. The incidence of symptomatic celiac disease varies widely in different population groups (high in whites, low in blacks and Asians) and is 10% in first-degree relatives of celiac disease patients; however, serologic studies provide clear evidence that celiac disease is present worldwide. Furthermore, all patients with celiac disease express the HLA-DQ2 or HLA-DQ8 allele, though only a minority of people expressing DQ2/DQ8 have celiac disease. Absence of DQ2/DQ8 excludes the diagnosis of celiac disease.

Diagnosis

A small-intestinal biopsy is required to establish a diagnosis of celiac disease (Fig. 294-4). A biopsy should be performed in patients with symptoms and laboratory findings suggestive of nutrient malabsorption and/or deficiency and with a positive endomysial antibody test. Since the presentation of celiac disease is often subtle, without overt evidence of malabsorption or nutrient deficiency, a relatively low threshold to perform a biopsy is important. It is more prudent to perform a biopsy than to obtain another test of intestinal absorption, which can never completely exclude or establish this diagnosis.

The diagnosis of celiac disease requires the presence of characteristic histologic changes on small-intestinal biopsy together with a prompt clinical and histologic response following the institution of a gluten-free diet. If serologic studies have detected the presence of IgA antiendomysial or tTG antibodies, they too should disappear after a gluten-free diet is started. With the increase in number of patients diagnosed with celiac disease that have been largely identified by serologic studies, the spectrum of histologic changes seen on duodenal biopsy has increased and includes findings that are not as severe as the classic changes shown in Fig. 294-4. The classical changes seen on duodenal/jejunal biopsy are restricted to the mucosa and include (1) an increase in the number of intraepithelial lymphocytes; (2) absence or reduced height of villi, resulting in a flat appearance with increased crypt cell proliferation, resulting in crypt hyperplasia and loss of villous structure, with consequent villous, but not mucosal, atrophy; (3) cuboidal appearance and nuclei that are no longer oriented basally in surface epithelial cells; and (4) increased lymphocytes and plasma cells in the lamina propria (Fig. 294-4*B*). Although these features are characteristic of celiac disease, they are *not* diagnostic because a similar appearance can be seen in tropical sprue, eosinophilic enteritis, and milk-protein intolerance in children and occasionally in lymphoma, bacterial overgrowth, Crohn's disease, and gastrinoma with acid hypersecretion. However, the presence of a characteristic histologic appearance that reverts toward normal following the initiation of a gluten-free diet establishes the diagnosis of celiac disease (Fig. 294-4*C*). Readministration of gluten with or without an additional small-intestinal biopsy is not necessary.

Failure to respond to gluten restriction

The most common cause of persistent symptoms in a patient who fulfills all the criteria for the diagnosis of celiac disease is continued intake of gluten. Gluten is ubiquitous, and significant effort must be made to exclude all gluten from the diet. Use of rice in place of wheat flour is very helpful, and several support groups provide important aid to patients with celiac disease and to their families. More than 90% of patients who have the characteristic findings of celiac disease will respond to complete dietary gluten restriction. The remainder constitute a heterogeneous group (whose condition is often called *refractory celiac disease or refractory sprue*) that includes some patients who (1) respond to restriction of other dietary protein, e.g., soy; (2) respond to glucocorticoids; (3) are "temporary" (i.e., the clinical and morphologic findings disappear after several months or years); or (4) fail to respond to all measures and have a fatal outcome, with or without documented complications of celiac disease, such as development of intestinal T cell lymphoma.

Mechanism of diarrhea

The diarrhea in celiac disease has several pathogenetic mechanisms. Diarrhea may be secondary to (1) steatorrhea, which is primarily a result of the changes in jejunal mucosal function; (2) secondary lactase deficiency, a consequence of changes in jejunal brush border enzymatic function; (3) bile acid malabsorption resulting in bile acid–induced fluid secretion in the colon, in cases with more extensive disease involving the ileum; and (4) endogenous fluid secretion resulting from crypt hyperplasia. Patients with more severe involvement with celiac disease may obtain temporary improvement with *dietary lactose and fat restriction* while awaiting the full effects of total gluten restriction, which is primary therapy.

Associated diseases

Celiac disease is associated with dermatitis herpetiformis (DH), though the association has not been explained. Patients with DH have characteristic papulovesicular lesions that respond to dapsone. Almost all patients with DH have histologic changes in the small intestine consistent with celiac disease, although usually much milder and less diffuse in distribution. Most patients with DH have mild or no gastrointestinal symptoms. In contrast, relatively few patients with celiac disease have DH.

Celiac disease is also associated with diabetes mellitus type 1; IgA deficiency; Down syndrome; and Turner's syndrome. The clinical importance of the association with diabetes is that although severe watery diarrhea without evidence of malabsorption is most often diagnosed as "diabetic diarrhea" (Chap. 344), assay of antiendomysial antibodies and/or a small-intestinal biopsy must be considered to exclude celiac disease.

Complications

The most important complication of celiac disease is the development of cancer. An increased incidence of both gastrointestinal and nongastrointestinal neoplasms as well as intestinal lymphoma exists in patients with celiac disease. For unexplained reasons the occurrence of lymphoma in patients with celiac disease is higher in Ireland and the United Kingdom than in the United States. The possibility of lymphoma must be considered whenever a patient with celiac disease previously doing well on a gluten-free diet is no longer responsive to gluten restriction or a patient who presents with clinical and histologic features consistent with celiac disease does not respond to a gluten-free diet. Other complications of celiac disease include the development of intestinal ulceration independent of lymphoma and so-called refractory sprue (see above) and collagenous sprue. In *collagenous sprue,* a layer of collagen-like material is present beneath the basement membrane; patients with collagenous sprue generally do not respond to a gluten-free diet and often have a poor prognosis.

■ TROPICAL SPRUE

Tropical sprue is a poorly understood syndrome that affects both expatriates and natives in certain but not all tropical areas and is manifested by chronic diarrhea, steatorrhea, weight loss, and nutritional deficiencies, including those of both folate and cobalamin. This disease affects 5–10% of the population in some tropical areas.

Chronic diarrhea in a tropical environment is most often caused by infectious agents including *G. lamblia, Yersinia enterocolitica, C. difficile, Cryptosporidium parvum,* and *Cyclospora cayetanensis,* among other organisms. Tropical sprue should not be entertained as a possible diagnosis until the presence of cysts and trophozoites has been excluded in three stool samples.

Chronic infections of the gastrointestinal tract and diarrhea in patients with or without AIDS are discussed in Chaps. 128 and 189.

The small-intestinal mucosa in individuals living in tropical areas is not identical to that of individuals who reside in temperate climates. Biopsies reveal a mild alteration of villous architecture with a modest increase in mononuclear cells in the lamina propria, which on occasion can be as severe as that seen in celiac disease. These changes are observed both in native residents and in expatriates living in tropical regions and are usually associated with mild decreases in absorptive function, but they revert to "normal" when an individual moves or returns to a temperate area. Some have suggested that the changes seen in tropical enteropathy and in tropical sprue represent different ends of the spectrum of a single entity, but convincing evidence to support this concept is lacking.

Etiology

Because tropical sprue responds to antibiotics, the consensus is that it may be caused by one or more infectious agents. Nonetheless, the etiology and pathogenesis of tropical sprue are uncertain. First, its occurrence is not evenly distributed in all tropical areas; rather, it is found in specific locations, including southern India, the Philippines, and several Caribbean islands (e.g., Puerto Rico, Haiti), but is rarely observed in Africa, Jamaica, or Southeast Asia. Second, an occasional individual will not develop symptoms of tropical sprue until long after having left an endemic area. This is the reason why the original term for celiac disease (often referred to as celiac sprue) was *nontropical sprue* to distinguish it from tropical sprue. Third, multiple microorganisms have been identified on jejunal aspirate with relatively little consistency among studies. *Klebsiella pneumoniae, Enterobacter cloacae,* or *E. coli* have been implicated in some studies of tropical sprue, while other studies have favored a role for a toxin produced by one or more of these bacteria. Fourth, the incidence of tropical sprue appears to have decreased substantially during the past two or three decades, perhaps related to improved sanitation in many tropical countries during this time. One speculation for the reduced occurrence is the wider use of antibiotics in acute diarrhea, especially in travelers to tropical areas from temperate countries. Fifth, the role of folic acid deficiency in the pathogenesis of tropical sprue requires clarification. Folic acid is absorbed exclusively in the duodenum and proximal jejunum, and most patients with tropical sprue have evidence of folate malabsorption and depletion. Although folate deficiency can cause changes in small-intestinal mucosa that are corrected by folate replacement, several earlier studies reporting that tropical sprue could be cured by folic acid did not provide an explanation for the "insult" that was initially responsible for folate malabsorption.

The clinical pattern of tropical sprue varies in different areas of the world (e.g., India vs. Puerto Rico). Not infrequently, individuals in South India initially will report the occurrence of an acute enteritis before the development of steatorrhea and malabsorption. In contrast, in Puerto Rico a most insidious onset of symptoms and a more dramatic response to antibiotics is seen when compared to some other locations. Tropical sprue in different areas of the world may not be the same disease, and similar clinical entities may have different etiologies.

Diagnosis

The diagnosis of tropical sprue is best made by the presence of an abnormal small-intestinal mucosal biopsy in an individual with chronic diarrhea and evidence of malabsorption who is either residing or has recently lived in a tropical country. The small-intestinal biopsy in tropical sprue does not have pathognomonic features but resembles, and can often be indistinguishable from, that seen in celiac disease (Fig. 294-4). The biopsy in tropical sprue will have less villous architectural alteration and more mononuclear cell infiltrate in the lamina propria. In contrast to celiac disease, the histologic features of tropical sprue are present with a similar degree of severity throughout the small intestine, and a gluten-free diet does not result in either clinical or histologic improvement in tropical sprue.

TREATMENT Tropical Sprue

Broad-spectrum antibiotics and folic acid are most often curative, especially if the patient leaves the tropical area and does not return. Tetracycline should be used for up to 6 months and may be associated with improvement within 1–2 weeks. Folic acid alone will induce a hematologic remission as well as improvement in appetite, weight gain, and some morphologic changes in small intestinal biopsy. Because of the presence of marked folate deficiency, folic acid is most often given together with antibiotics.

SHORT BOWEL SYNDROME

This is a descriptive term for the myriad clinical problems that occur following resection of varying lengths of small intestine; or on rare occasions may be congenital, e.g., microvillous inclusion disease. The factors that determine both the type and degree of symptoms include (1) the specific segment (jejunum vs. ileum) resected, (2) the length of the resected segment, (3) the integrity of the ileocecal valve, (4) whether any large intestine has also been removed, (5) residual disease in the remaining small and/or large intestine (e.g., Crohn's disease, mesenteric artery disease), and (6) the degree of adaptation in the remaining intestine. Short bowel syndrome can occur at any age from neonates through the elderly. *Intestinal failure* is the inability to maintain nutrition without parenteral support.

Three different situations in adults demand intestinal resections: (1) mesenteric vascular disease, including atherosclerosis, thrombotic phenomena, and vasculitides; (2) primary mucosal and submucosal disease, e.g., Crohn's disease; and (3) operations without preexisting small intestinal disease, such as trauma.

Following resection of the small intestine, the residual intestine undergoes adaptation of both structure and function that may last for up to 6–12 months. Continued intake of dietary nutrients and calories is required to stimulate adaptation via direct contact with intestinal mucosa, the release of one or more intestinal hormones, and pancreatic and biliary secretions. Thus, enteral nutrition with calorie administration must be maintained, especially in the early postoperative period, even if an extensive intestinal resection requiring parenteral nutrition (PN) had been performed. The subsequent ability of such patients to absorb nutrients will not be known for several months, until adaptation is completed.

Multiple factors besides the absence of intestinal mucosa (required for lipid, fluid, and electrolyte absorption) contribute to the diarrhea and steatorrhea in these patients. Removal of the ileum and especially the ileocecal valve is often associated with more severe diarrhea than jejunal resection. Without part or all of the ileum, diarrhea can be caused by an increase in bile acids entering the colon, leading to their stimulation of colonic fluid and electrolyte secretion. Absence of the ileocecal valve is also associated with a decrease in intestinal transit time and bacterial overgrowth from the colon. The presence of the colon (or a major portion) is associated with substantially less diarrhea and lower likelihood of intestinal failure as a result of fermentation of nonabsorbed carbohydrates to SCFAs. The latter are absorbed in the colon and stimulate Na and water absorption, improving overall fluid balance. Lactose intolerance as a result of the removal of lactase-containing mucosa as well as gastric hypersecretion may also contribute to the diarrhea.

In addition to diarrhea and/or steatorrhea, a range of nonintestinal symptoms is also observed in some patients. A significant increase in renal calcium oxalate calculi is observed in patients with a small-intestinal resection with an intact colon and is due to an increase in oxalate absorption by the large intestine, with subsequent hyperoxaluria (called *enteric hyperoxaluria*). Two possible mechanisms for the increase in oxalate absorption in the colon have been suggested: (1) bile acids and fatty acids that increase colonic mucosal permeability, resulting in increased oxalate absorption; and (2) increased fatty acids that bind calcium, resulting in increased soluble oxalate that is then absorbed. Since oxalate is high in relatively few foods (e.g., spinach, rhubarb, tea), dietary restrictions alone are not adequate treatment. Cholestyramine, an anion-binding resin, and calcium have proved useful in reducing the hyperoxaluria. Similarly, an increase in cholesterol gallstones is related to a decrease in the bile acid pool size, which results in the generation of cholesterol supersaturation in gallbladder bile. Gastric hypersecretion of acid occurs in many patients following large resections of the small intestine. The etiology is unclear but may be related to either reduced hormonal inhibition of acid secretion or increased gastrin levels due to reduced small-intestinal catabolism of circulating gastrin. The resulting gastric acid secretion may be an important factor contributing to the diarrhea and steatorrhea. A reduced pH in the duodenum can inactivate pancreatic lipase and/or precipitate duodenal bile acids, thereby increasing steatorrhea, and an increase in gastric secretion can create a volume overload relative to the reduced small-intestinal absorptive capacity. Inhibition of gastric acid secretion with proton pump inhibitors can help in reducing the diarrhea and steatorrhea but only for the first six months.

TREATMENT Short Bowel Syndrome

Treatment of short bowel syndrome depends on the severity of symptoms and whether the individual is able to maintain caloric and electrolyte balance with oral intake alone. Initial treatment includes judicious use of opiates (including codeine) to reduce stool output and to establish an effective diet. An initial diet should be low-fat and high-carbohydrate, if the colon is in situ, to minimize the diarrhea from fatty acid stimulation of colonic fluid secretion. MCTs (see above), a low-lactose diet, and various soluble fiber-containing diets should also be tried. In the absence of an ileocecal valve, the possibility of bacterial overgrowth must be considered and treated. If gastric acid hypersecretion is contributing to the diarrhea and steatorrhea, a proton pump inhibitor may be helpful. Usually none of these therapeutic approaches will provide an instant solution, but they can reduce disabling diarrhea.

The patient's vitamin and mineral status must also be monitored; replacement therapy should be initiated if indicated. Fat-soluble vitamins, folate, cobalamin, calcium, iron, magnesium, and zinc are the most critical factors to monitor on a regular basis. If these approaches are not successful, home PN is an established therapy that can be maintained for many years. Small intestinal transplantation is becoming established as a possible approach for individuals with extensive intestinal resection who cannot be maintained without PN, i.e., "intestinal failure." Considerable attention has been directed to the potential effectiveness of trophic hormones, e.g., glucagon-like peptide 2 (GLP-2), to improve absorptive function.

BACTERIAL OVERGROWTH SYNDROME

Bacterial overgrowth syndrome comprises a group of disorders with diarrhea, steatorrhea, and macrocytic anemia whose common feature is the proliferation of colonic-type bacteria within the small intestine. This bacterial proliferation is due to stasis caused by impaired peristalsis (*functional stasis*), changes in intestinal anatomy (*anatomic stasis*), or direct communication between the small and large intestine. These conditions have also been referred to as *stagnant bowel syndrome* or *blind loop syndrome.*

Pathogenesis

The manifestations of bacterial overgrowth syndromes are a direct consequence of the presence of increased amounts of a colonic-type bacterial flora, such as *E. coli* or *Bacteroides,* in the small intestine. *Macrocytic anemia* is due to cobalamin, not folate, deficiency. Most bacteria require cobalamin for growth, and increasing concentrations of bacteria use up the relatively small amounts of dietary cobalamin. *Steatorrhea* is due to impaired micelle formation as a consequence of a reduced intraduodenal concentration of conjugated bile acids and the presence of unconjugated bile acids. Certain bacteria, e.g., *Bacteroides,* deconjugate conjugated bile acids to unconjugated bile acids. Unconjugated bile acids will be absorbed more rapidly than conjugated bile acids, and, as a result, the intraduodenal concentration of bile acids will be reduced. In addition, the CMC of unconjugated bile acids is higher than that of conjugated bile acids, resulting in a decrease in micelle formation. *Diarrhea* is due, at least in part, to the steatorrhea, when it is present. However, some patients manifest diarrhea *without* steatorrhea, and it is assumed that the colonic-type bacteria in these patients are producing one or more bacterial enterotoxins that are responsible for fluid secretion and diarrhea.

Etiology

The etiology of these different disorders is bacterial proliferation in the small intestinal lumen secondary to either anatomic or functional stasis or to a communication between the relatively sterile small intestine and the colon with its high levels of aerobic and anaerobic bacteria. Several examples of *anatomic* stasis have been identified: (1) one or more diverticula (both duodenal and jejunal) (Fig. 294-3*C*); (2) fistulas and strictures related to Crohn's disease (Fig. 294-3*D*); (3) a proximal duodenal afferent loop following a subtotal gastrectomy and gastrojejunostomy; (4) a bypass of the intestine, e.g., jejunoileal bypass for obesity; and (5) dilation at the site of a previous intestinal anastomosis. These anatomic derangements are often associated with the presence of a segment (or segments) of intestine out of continuity of propagated peristalsis, resulting in stasis and bacterial proliferation. Bacterial overgrowth syndromes can also occur in the *absence* of an anatomic blind loop when *functional* stasis is present. Impaired peristalsis and bacterial overgrowth in the absence of a blind loop occur in scleroderma, where motility abnormalities exist in both the esophagus and small intestine (Chap. 323). Functional stasis and bacterial overgrowth can also occur in association with diabetes mellitus and in the small intestine when a direct connection exists between the small and large intestine, including an ileocolonic resection, or occasionally following an enterocolic anastomosis that permits entry of bacteria into the small intestine as a result of bypassing the ileocecal valve.

Diagnosis

The diagnosis may be suspected from the combination of a low serum cobalamin level and an elevated serum folate level, as enteric bacteria frequently produce folate compounds that will be absorbed in the duodenum. Ideally, the diagnosis of the bacterial overgrowth syndrome is the demonstration of increased levels of aerobic and/or anaerobic colonic-type bacteria in a jejunal aspirate obtained by intubation. This specialized test is rarely available. Breath hydrogen testing with lactulose (a nondigestible disaccharide) administration has also been used to detect bacterial overgrowth. The Schilling test can also diagnose bacterial overgrowth (see supplementary material) but is also not available routinely. Often the diagnosis is suspected clinically and confirmed by response to treatment.

TREATMENT Bacterial Overgrowth Syndrome

Primary treatment should be directed, if at all possible, to the surgical correction of an anatomic blind loop. In the absence of functional stasis, it is important to define the anatomic relationships responsible for stasis and bacterial overgrowth. For example, bacterial overgrowth secondary to strictures, one or more diverticula, or a proximal afferent loop can potentially be cured by surgical correction of the anatomic state. In contrast, the functional stasis of scleroderma or certain anatomic stasis states (e.g., multiple jejunal diverticula) cannot be corrected surgically, and these conditions should be treated with broad-spectrum antibiotics. Tetracycline used to be the initial treatment of choice; due to increasing resistance, however, other antibiotics such as metronidazole, amoxicillin/clavulanic acid, and cephalosporins have been employed. The antibiotic should be given for approximately 3 weeks or until symptoms remit. Although the natural history of these conditions is chronic, antibiotics should not be given continuously. Symptoms usually remit within 2–3 weeks of initial antibiotic therapy. Therapy need not be repeated until symptoms recur. In the presence of frequent recurrences, several treatment strategies exist, but the use of antibiotics for 1 week per month, whether or not symptoms are present, is often most effective.

Unfortunately, therapy for bacterial overgrowth syndrome is largely empirical, with an absence of clinical trials on which to base rational decisions regarding the antibiotic choice, the duration of treatment, and/or the best approach for treating recurrences. Bacterial overgrowth may also occur as a component of another chronic disease, e.g., Crohn's disease, radiation enteritis, or short bowel syndrome. Treatment of the bacterial overgrowth in these settings will not cure the underlying problem but may be very important in ameliorating a subset of clinical problems that are related to bacterial overgrowth.

WHIPPLE'S DISEASE

Whipple's disease is a chronic multisystem disease associated with diarrhea, steatorrhea, weight loss, arthralgia, and central nervous system (CNS) and cardiac problems; it is caused by the bacteria *Tropheryma whipplei.* Until the identification of *T. whipplei* by polymerase chain reaction, the hallmark of Whipple's disease had been the presence of PAS-positive macrophages in the small intestine (Fig. 294-4*E*) and other organs with evidence of disease.

Etiology

Whipple's disease is caused by a small gram-positive bacillus, *T. whipplei.* The bacillus, an Actinobacteria, has low virulence but high infectivity, and relatively minimal symptoms are observed compared to the extent of the bacilli in multiple tissues.

Clinical presentation

The onset of Whipple's disease is insidious and is characterized by diarrhea, steatorrhea, abdominal pain, weight loss, migratory large-joint arthropathy, and fever as well as ophthalmologic and CNS symptoms. The development of dementia is a relatively late symptom and an extremely poor prognostic sign, especially in patients who relapse following the induction of a remission with antibiotics. For unexplained reasons, the disease occurs primarily in middle-aged white men. The steatorrhea in these patients is generally believed secondary to both small-intestinal mucosal injury and lymphatic obstruction secondary to the increased number of PAS-positive macrophages in the lamina propria of the small intestine.

Diagnosis

The diagnosis of Whipple's disease is suggested by a multisystem disease in a patient with diarrhea and steatorrhea. Obtaining tissue biopsies from the small intestine and/or other organs that may be involved (e.g., liver, lymph nodes, heart, eyes, CNS, or synovial membranes), based on the patient's symptoms, is the primary approach to establish the diagnosis of Whipple's disease. The presence of PAS-positive macrophages containing the characteristic small (0.25—1–2 mm) bacilli is suggestive of this diagnosis. However, Whipple's disease can be confused with the PAS-positive macrophages containing *M. avium* complex, which may be a cause of diarrhea in AIDS. The presence of the *T. whipplei* bacillus outside of macrophages is a more important indicator of active disease than is their presence within the macrophages. *T. whipplei* has now been successfully grown in culture.

TREATMENT Whipple's Disease

The treatment for Whipple's disease is prolonged use of antibiotics. The current drug of choice is double-strength trimethoprim/sulfamethoxazole for approximately 1 year. PAS-positive macrophages can persist following successful treatment, and the presence of bacilli outside of macrophages is indicative of persistent infection or an early sign of recurrence. Recurrence of disease activity, especially with dementia, is an extremely poor prognostic sign and requires an antibiotic that crosses the blood-brain barrier. If trimethoprim/sulfamethoxazole is not tolerated, chloramphenicol is an appropriate second choice.

PROTEIN-LOSING ENTEROPATHY

Protein-losing enteropathy is not a specific disease but rather a group of gastrointestinal and nongastrointestinal disorders with hypoproteinemia and edema in the absence of either proteinuria or defects in protein synthesis, e.g., chronic liver disease. These diseases are characterized by excess protein loss into the gastrointestinal tract. Normally, about 10% of total protein catabolism occurs via the gastrointestinal tract. Evidence of increased protein loss into the gastrointestinal tract occurs in more than 65 different diseases, which can be classified into three groups: (1) mucosal ulceration, such that the protein loss primarily represents exudation across damaged mucosa, e.g., ulcerative colitis, gastrointestinal carcinomas, and peptic ulcer; (2) nonulcerated mucosa, but with evidence of mucosal damage so that the protein loss represents loss across epithelia with altered permeability, e.g., celiac disease and Ménétrier's disease in the small intestine and stomach, respectively; and (3) lymphatic dysfunction, representing either primary lymphatic disease or secondary to partial lymphatic obstruction that may occur as a result of enlarged lymph nodes or cardiac disease.

Diagnosis

The diagnosis of protein-losing enteropathy is suggested by the presence of peripheral edema and low serum albumin and globulin levels in the absence of renal and hepatic disease. An individual with protein-losing enteropathy only rarely has selective loss of *only* albumin or *only* globulins. Therefore, marked reduction of serum albumin with normal serum globulins should not initiate an evaluation for protein-losing enteropathy but should suggest the presence of renal and/or hepatic disease. Likewise, reduced serum globulins with normal serum albumin levels are more likely a result of reduced globulin synthesis rather than enhanced globulin loss into the intestine. Documentation of an increase in protein loss into the gastrointestinal tract has been established by the administration of one of several radiolabeled proteins and its quantitation in stool during a 24- or 48-h period. Unfortunately, none of these radiolabeled proteins is available for routine clinical use. α_1-Antitrypsin, a protein that accounts for ~4% of total serum proteins and is resistant to proteolysis, can be used to document enhanced rates of serum protein loss into the intestinal tract but cannot be used to assess gastric protein loss due to its degradation in an acid milieu. α_1-Antitrypsin clearance is measured by determining stool volume and both stool and plasma α_1-antitrypsin concentrations. In addition to the loss of protein via abnormal and distended lymphatics, peripheral lymphocytes may also be lost via lymphatics, resulting in a relative lymphopenia. Thus, the presence of lymphopenia in a patient with hypoproteinemia supports the presence of increased loss of protein into the gastrointestinal tract.

Patients with increased protein loss into the gastrointestinal tract from lymphatic obstruction often have steatorrhea and diarrhea. The steatorrhea is a result of altered lymphatic flow as lipid-containing chylomicrons exit from intestinal epithelial cells via intestinal lymphatics (Table 294-4; Fig. 294-4). In the absence of mechanical or anatomic lymphatic obstruction, intrinsic intestinal lymphatic dysfunction, with or without lymphatic dysfunction in the peripheral extremities, has been named *intestinal lymphangiectasia.* Similarly, about 50% of individuals with intrinsic peripheral lymphatic disease (Milroy's disease) will also have intestinal lymphangiectasia and hypoproteinemia. Other than steatorrhea and enhanced protein loss into the gastrointestinal tract, all other aspects of intestinal absorptive function are normal in intestinal lymphangiectasia.

Other causes

Patients who appear to have idiopathic protein-losing enteropathy without any evidence of gastrointestinal disease should be examined for cardiac disease—especially right-sided valvular disease and chronic pericarditis (Chaps. 237 and 239). On occasion, hypoproteinemia can be the only presentation for these two types of heart disease. Ménétrier's disease (also called *hypertrophic gastropathy*) is an uncommon entity that involves the body and fundus of the stomach and is characterized by large gastric folds, reduced gastric acid secretion, and, at times, enhanced protein loss into the stomach.

TREATMENT Protein-Losing Enteropathy

As excess protein loss into the gastrointestinal tract is most often secondary to a specific disease, treatment should be directed primarily to the underlying disease process and not to the hypoproteinemia. For example, if significant hypoproteinemia with resulting peripheral edema is secondary to either celiac disease or ulcerative colitis, a gluten-free diet or mesalamine, respectively, would be the initial therapy. When enhanced protein loss is secondary to lymphatic obstruction, it is critical to establish the nature of this obstruction. Identification of mesenteric nodes or lymphoma may be possible by imaging studies. Similarly, it is important to exclude cardiac disease as a cause of protein-losing enteropathy either by echosonography or, on occasion, by a right-heart catheterization.

The increased protein loss that occurs in intestinal lymphangiectasia is a result of distended lymphatics associated with lipid malabsorption. Treatment of the hypoproteinemia is accomplished by a low-fat diet and the administration of MCTs (Table 294-3), which do not exit from the intestinal epithelial cells via lymphatics but are delivered to the body via the portal vein.

SUMMARY

A pathophysiologic classification of the many conditions that can produce malabsorption is given in Table 294-8. A summary of the pathophysiology of the various clinical manifestations of malabsorption is given in Table 294-9.

TABLE 294-8 Classification of Malabsorption Syndromes

Inadequate digestion	
Postgastrectomy[a]	
Deficiency or inactivation of pancreatic lipase	
Exocrine pancreatic insufficiency	
Chronic pancreatitis	
Pancreatic carcinoma	
Cystic fibrosis	
Pancreatic insufficiency—congenital or acquired	
Gastrinoma—acid inactivation of lipase[a]	
Drugs—orlistat	
Reduced intraduodenal bile acid concentration/impaired micelle formation	
Liver disease	
Parenchymal liver disease	
Cholestatic liver disease	
Bacterial overgrowth in small intestine:	
Anatomic stasis	Functional stasis
Afferent loop	Diabetes[a]
Stasis/blind	Scleroderma[a]
Loop/strictures/fistulae	Intestinal pseudoobstruction
Interrupted enterohepatic circulation of bile salts	
Ileal resection	
Crohn's disease[a]	
Drugs (bind or precipitate bile salts)—neomycin, cholestyramine, calcium carbonate	
Impaired mucosal absorption/mucosal loss or defect	
Intestinal resection or bypass[a]	
Inflammation, infiltration, or infection:	
Crohn's disease[a]	Celiac disease
Amyloidosis	Collagenous sprue
Scleroderma[a]	Whipple's disease[a]
Lymphoma[a]	Radiation enteritis[a]
Eosinophilic enteritis	Folate and vitamin B_{12} deficiency
Mastocytosis	Infections—giardiasis
Tropical sprue	Graft versus host disease
Genetic disorders	
Disaccharidase deficiency	
Agammaglobulinemia	
Abetalipoproteinemia	
Hartnup's disease	
Cystinuria	
Impaired nutrient delivery to and/or from intestine:	
Lymphatic obstruction	Circulatory disorders
Lymphoma[a]	Congestive heart failure
Lymphangiectasia	Constrictive pericarditis
	Mesenteric artery atherosclerosis
	Vasculitis
Endocrine and metabolic disorders	
Diabetes[a]	
Hypoparathyroidism	
Adrenal insufficiency	
Hyperthyroidism	
Carcinoid syndrome	

[a]Malabsorption caused by more than one mechanism.

TABLE 294-9 Pathophysiology of Clinical Manifestations of Malabsorption Disorders

Symptom or Sign	Mechanism
Weight loss/malnutrition	Anorexia, malabsorption of nutrients
Diarrhea	Impaired absorption or secretion of water and electrolytes; colonic fluid secretion secondary to unabsorbed dihydroxy bile acids and fatty acids
Flatus	Bacterial fermentation of unabsorbed carbohydrate
Glossitis, cheilosis, stomatitis	Deficiency of iron, vitamin B_{12}, folate, and vitamin A
Abdominal pain	Bowel distention or inflammation, pancreatitis
Bone pain	Calcium, vitamin D malabsorption, protein deficiency, osteoporosis
Tetany, paresthesia	Calcium and magnesium malabsorption
Weakness	Anemia, electrolyte depletion (particularly K^+)
Azotemia, hypotension	Fluid and electrolyte depletion
Amenorrhea, decreased libido	Protein depletion, decreased calories, secondary hypopituitarism
Anemia	Impaired absorption of iron, folate, vitamin B_{12}
Bleeding	Vitamin K malabsorption, hypoprothrombinemia
Night blindness/xerophthalmia	Vitamin A malabsorption
Peripheral neuropathy	Vitamin B_{12} and thiamine deficiency
Dermatitis	Deficiency of vitamin A, zinc, and essential fatty acid

FURTHER READINGS

American Gastroenterological Association: AGA technical review on the evaluation and management of chronic diarrhea. Gastroenterology 116:1464, 1999

Binder HJ: Role of colonic short-chain fatty acid transport in diarrhea. Annu Rev Physiol 72:297, 2010

Buchman AL: Etiology and initial management of short bowel syndrome. Gastroenterology 130:S5, 2006

Fenoller F et al: Whipple's disease. N Engl J Med 356:55, 2007

Green PH, Cellier C: Celiac disease. N Engl J Med 357:1731, 2007

Hammer HF: Pancreatic exocrine insufficiency: Diagnostic evaluation and replacement therapy with pancreatic enzymes. Dig Dis 28:339, 2010

Kagnoff MF: Celiac disease: Pathogenesis of a model immunogenetic disease. J Clin Invest 117:41, 2007

Schulzke JD et al: Disorders of intestinal secretion and absorption. Best Pract Res Clin Gastroenterol 23:395, 2009

Suchy FJ et al: National Institutes of Health Consensus Development Conference: Lactose intolerance and health. Ann Intern Med 152:792, 2010

CHAPTER 295
Inflammatory Bowel Disease

Sonia Friedman
Richard S. Blumberg

Inflammatory bowel disease (IBD) is an immune-mediated chronic intestinal condition. Ulcerative colitis (UC) and Crohn's disease (CD) are the two major types of IBD.

EPIDEMIOLOGY

The incidence of IBD varies within different geographic areas. CD and UC both occur at the highest incidence in Europe, the United Kingdom, and North America. In North America, incidence rates range from 2.2–14.3 cases per 100,000 person-years for UC and from 3.1–14.6 cases per 100,000 person-years for CD (Table 295-1). Prevalence ranges from 37–246 cases per 100,000 person-years for UC and from 26–199 cases per 100,000 person-years for CD. In Europe, incidence ranges from 1.5–20.3 cases per 100,000 person-years for UC and from 0.7–9.8 cases for CD; prevalence ranges from 21.4–243 cases for UC and from 8.3–214 cases per 100,000 person-years for CD. IBD has been rare in other areas except Israel, Australia, and South Africa. The incidence of IBD, especially UC, is rising in Japan, South Korea, Singapore, northern India, and Latin America, areas previously thought to have low incidence. The incidence of UC has increased sixfold in the past two decades in Hong Kong. Reports from the United States, Poland, Denmark, and South Korea indicate that the incidence of pediatric IBD is increasing rapidly as well. The highest mortality is during the first years of disease and in long-duration disease due to the risk of colon cancer. In a Danish population study, the standardized mortality ratios for CD and UC were 1.31 and 1.1, respectively.

The peak age of onset of UC and CD is between 15 and 30 years. A second peak occurs between the ages of 60 and 80. The male to female ratio for UC is 1:1 and for CD is 1.1–1.8:1. UC and CD have two- to fourfold increased frequency in Jewish populations in the United States, Europe, and South Africa. Furthermore, disease frequency differs within the Jewish populations. The prevalence of IBD in Ashkenazi Jews is about twice that of Israeli-born, Sephardic, or Asian Jews. The prevalence decreases progressively in non-Jewish white, African-American, Hispanic, and Asian populations. Urban areas have a higher prevalence of IBD than rural areas, and high socioeconomic classes have a higher prevalence than lower socioeconomic classes.

The effects of cigarette smoking are different in UC and CD. The risk of UC in smokers is 40% that of nonsmokers. Additionally, former smokers have a 1.7-fold increased risk for UC than people who have never smoked. In contrast, smoking is associated with a twofold increased risk of CD. Oral contraceptives are also linked to CD; the odds ratio of CD for oral contraceptive users is about 1.4. Appendectomy is protective against UC but is associated with an increased risk of CD. This elevated risk in CD is observed early after an appendectomy, which is diminished thereafter, making it likely that it reflects diagnostic problems in patients with incipient CD.

IBD is a familial disease in 5–10% of patients. Some of these patients may exhibit early onset disease during the first decade of life and, in CD, a concordance of anatomic site and clinical type within families. In the remainder of patients, IBD is observed in the absence of a family history (i.e., sporadic disease). If a patient has IBD, the lifetime risk that a first-degree relative will be affected is ~10%. If two parents have IBD, each child has a 36% chance of being affected. In twin studies, 58% of monozygotic twins are concordant for CD and 6% are concordant for UC, whereas 4% of dizygotic twins are concordant for CD and none are concordant for UC. In a recent twin study from Germany, the relative risk of a monozygotic twin developing Crohn's disease if his or her twin was affected was 738. The risks of developing IBD are higher in first-degree relatives of Jewish versus non-Jewish patients: 7.8% versus 5.2% for CD and 4.5% versus 1.6% for UC.

Additional evidence for genetic predisposition to IBD comes from its association with certain genetic syndromes. UC and CD are both associated with Turner's syndrome, and Hermansky-Pudlak syndrome is associated with granulomatous colitis. Glycogen storage disease type 1b can present with Crohn's-like lesions of the large and small bowel. Severe immunodeficiency disorders such as Wiskott-Aldrich syndrome and chronic granulomatous disease are associated with IBD. Immune dysregulation, polyendocrinopathy, enteropathy, X-linked (IPEX) syndrome is associated with a severe enteropathy and autoimmunity (Table 295-2). Other immunodeficiency disorders such as hypogammaglobulinemia, selective IgA deficiency, and hereditary angioedema, also exhibit an increased association with IBD.

TABLE 295-1 Epidemiology of IBD

	Ulcerative Colitis	Crohn's Disease
Incidence (North America) per person-years	2.2–14.3:100,000	3.1–14.6:100,000
Age of onset	15–30 & 60–80	15–30 & 60–80
Ethnicity	Jewish > non-Jewish white > African American > Hispanic > Asian	
Male/female ratio	1:1	1.1–1.8:1
Smoking	May prevent disease	May cause disease
Oral contraceptives	No increased risk	Odds ratio 1.4
Appendectomy	Protective	Not protective
Monozygotic twins	6% concordance	58% concordance
Dizygotic twins	0% concordance	4% concordance

ETIOLOGY AND PATHOGENESIS

A consensus hypothesis is that in genetically predisposed individuals, both exogenous factors (e.g., composition of normal intestinal microbiota) and endogenous host factors (e.g., intestinal epithelial cell barrier function, innate and adaptive immune function) interact to cause a chronic state of dysregulated mucosal immune function that is further modified by specific environmental factors (e.g., smoking, enteropathogens). Although chronic activation of the mucosal immune system may represent an appropriate response to an unidentified infectious agent, a search for such an agent has thus far been unrewarding in IBD. As such, IBD is currently considered an inappropriate immune response to the endogenous commensal microbiota within the intestines, with or without some component of autoimmunity. Importantly, the normal intestines contain a large number of immune cells in a chronic state of so-called physiologic

TABLE 295-2 Primary Genetic Disorders Associated With IBD

Name	Genetic Association	Phenotype
Turner's syndrome	Loss of part or all of X chromosome	Associated with UC and colonic CD
Hermansky-Pudlak	Autosomal recessive chromosome 10q23	Granulomatous colitis, oculocutaneous albinism, platelet dysfunction, pulmonary fibrosis
Wiskott-Aldrich syndrome (WAS)	X-linked recessive disorder, loss of WAS protein function	Colitis, immunodeficiency, severely dysfunctional platelets, and thrombocytopenia
Glycogen Storage disease	Deficiency of the glucose-6-phosphate transport protein type B1	Granulomatous colitis, presents in infancy with hypoglycemia, growth failure, hepatomegaly, and neutropenia
Immune dysregulation polyendocrinopathy, enteropathy X-linked (IPEX)	Loss of FoxP3 transcription factor and T regulatory cell function	UC-like autoimmune enteropathy, with endocrinopathy (neonatal type 1 diabetes or thyroiditis), dermatitis
Early onset IBD	Deficient IL-10 receptor function	Severe, refractory IBD in early life

Abbreviations: CD, Crohn's disease; IBD, inflammatory bowel disease; IL, interleukin; UC, ulcerative colitis; WASP, Wiskott-Aldrich syndrome protein.

inflammation, in which the gut is restrained from full immunologic responses to the commensal microbiota and dietary antigens by very powerful regulatory pathways that function within the immune system (e.g., FoxP3$^+$ T regulatory cells). During the course of infections in the normal host, full activation of the gut-associated lymphoid tissues occurs but is rapidly superseded by dampening of the immune response and tissue repair. In IBD this process may not be regulated normally.

GENETIC CONSIDERATIONS

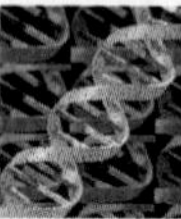

IBD is a polygenic disorder that gives rise to multiple clinical subgroups within UC and CD. A variety of genetic approaches including candidate gene studies, linkage analysis and genome-wide association studies that focus on the identification of disease-associated, single-nucleotide polymorphisms (SNP) within the human genome have identified Approximately 100 disease-associated loci on many different chromosomes (Table 295-3). About one-third of these genetic risk factors are shared between CD and UC accounting for the overlapping immunopathogenesis and consequently epidemiologic observations of both diseases in the same families and similarities in response to therapies. Because the specific causal variants for each gene or locus are largely unknown, it is not clear whether the similarities in the genetic risk factors associated with CD and UC that are observed are shared at structural or functional levels. Similarly, many of the genetic risk factors identified are also observed to be associated with risk for other immune-mediated diseases suggesting that related immunogenetic pathways are involved in the pathogenesis of multiple different disorders accounting for the common responsiveness to similar types of biologic therapies (e.g., anti-tumor necrosis factor therapies) and possibly the simultaneous occurrence of these disorders. The diseases and the genetic risk factors that are shared with IBD include rheumatoid arthritis (*TNFAIP3*), psoriasis (*IL23R, IL12B*), ankylosing spondylitis (*IL23R*), type 1 diabetes mellitus (*IL10, PTPN2*), asthma (*ORMDL3*), and systemic lupus erythematosus (*TNFAIP3, IL10*).

The genetic factors defined to date that are recognized to mediate risk for IBD have highlighted the importance of several common mechanisms of disease (Table 295-3). These include the following: Those genes that are associated with innate immunity and autophagy (e.g., *NOD2, ATG16L1, IRGM, JAK2, STAT3*) that function in innate immune cells (both parenchymal and hematopoietic) to respond to and clear bacteria, mycobacteria and viruses; those that are associated with endoplasmic reticulum (ER) and metabolic stress (e.g., *XBP1, ORMDL3, OCTN*), which serve to regulate the secretory activity of cells involved in responses to the commensal microbiota such as Paneth and goblet cells and the manner in which intestinal cells respond to the metabolic products of bacteria; those that are associated with the regulation of adaptive immunity (e.g., *IL23R, IL12B, IL10, PTPN2*), which regulate the balance between inflammatory and regulatory cytokines; and, finally, those that are involved in the development and resolution of inflammation (e.g., *MST1, CCR6, TNFAIP3, PTGER4*) and ultimately leukocyte recruitment and inflammatory mediator production. Some of these loci are associated with specific subtypes of disease such as the association between *NOD2* polymorphisms and fibrostenosing CD, especially within the ileum. However, the clinical utility of these genetic risk factors for the diagnosis or determination of prognosis and therapeutic responses remains to be defined.

DEFECTIVE IMMUNE REGULATION IN IBD

The mucosal immune system is normally unreactive to luminal contents due to oral (mucosal) tolerance. When soluble antigens are administered orally rather than subcutaneously or intramuscularly, antigen-specific nonresponsiveness is induced. Multiple mechanisms are involved in the induction of oral tolerance and include deletion or anergy of antigen-reactive T cells or induction of CD4$^+$ T cells that suppress gut inflammation (e.g., T regulatory cells expressing the FoxP3 transcription factor) that secrete anti-inflammatory cytokines such as interleukin (IL) 10 and transforming growth factor β (TGF-β). Oral tolerance may be responsible for the lack of immune responsiveness to dietary antigens and the commensal microbiota in the intestinal lumen. In IBD this suppression of inflammation is altered, leading to uncontrolled inflammation. The mechanisms of this regulated immune suppression are incompletely known.

Gene knockout ($^{-/-}$) or transgenic (Tg) mouse models of IBD have revealed that deleting specific cytokines (e.g., IL-2, IL-10, TGF-β) or their receptors, deleting molecules associated with T cell antigen recognition (e.g., T cell antigen receptors) or interfering with intestinal epithelial cell barrier function and the regulation of responses to commensal bacteria (e.g., XBP1, N-cadherin, mucus glycoprotein or NFκB) leads to spontaneous colitis or enteritis. In the majority of circumstances, intestinal inflammation in these animal models requires the presence of the commensal microbiota. Thus, a variety of specific alterations can lead to immune activation by commensal microbiota and inflammation directed at the intestines in mice. How these relate to human IBD remains to be defined but are consistent with inappropriate responses of the genetically susceptible host to the commensal bacteria.

In both UC and CD, an inflammatory pathway thus likely emerges from the genetic predisposition that is associated with inappropriate innate immune sensing and reactivity to commensal

TABLE 295-3 Genetic Loci Associated With CD and/or UC

Chr	Putative Gene	Gene Name	Protein Function	CD	UC
Innate Immunity and Autophagy					
1q23	*ITLN1*	Intelectin 1	Bacterial binding	+	
2q37	*ATG16L1*	ATG16 autophagy related 16-like 1	Autophagy	+	
5q33	*IRGM*	Immunity-related GTPase family, M	Autophagy	+	
9p24	*JAK2*	Janus kinase 2	IL-6R & IL-23R signaling	+	+
12q12	*LRRK2*	Leucine-rich repeat kinase 2	Autophagy ?	+	
16q12	*NOD2*	Nucleotide-binding oligomerization domain containing 2	Bacterial sensing	+	
17q21	*STAT3*	Signal transducer and activator of transcription 3	IL-6R, IL-23R & IL-10R signaling	+	+
ER Stress and Metabolism					
5q31	*SLC22A5*	Solute carrier family 22, member 5	β carnitine transporter	+	
7p21	*AGR2*	Anterior gradient 2	ER stress	+	+
17q21	*ORMDL3*	Orosomucoid related member 1-like 3	ER stress	+	+
22q12	*XBP1*	X-box binding protein 1	ER stress	+	+
Adaptive Immunity					
1p31	*IL23R*	Interleukin 23 receptor	Th17 cell stimulation	+	+
1q32	*IL10*	Interleukin-10	Treg associated cytokine		+
5q33	*IL12B*	Interleukin 12B	IL-12 p40 chain of IL-12/IL-23	+	+
18p11	*PTPN2*	Protein tyrosine phosphatase, nonreceptor type 2	T cell regulation	+	
Inflammation					
3p21	*MST1*	Macrophage stimulating 1	Macrophage activation	+	+
5p13	*PTGER4*	Prostaglandin E receptor 4	PGE2 receptor	+	+
6q23	*TNFAIP3*	Tumor necrosis factor, alpha-induced protein 3 (A20)	Toll-like receptor regulation	+	
6q27	*CCR6*	Chemokine (C-C motif) receptor 6	Dendritic cell migration	+	

Abbreviations: CD, Crohn's disease; ER, endoplasmic reticulum; GTPase, guanosine triphosphatase; IL, interleukin; UC, ulcerative colitis.
Source: Adapted from Kaser et al, Ann Rev Immunol 2010

bacteria together with inadequate regulatory pathways that lead to activated CD4⁺ T cells in the lamina propria that secrete excessive quantities of inflammatory cytokines relative to anti-inflammatory cytokines. Some cytokines activate other inflammatory cells (macrophages and B cells) and others act indirectly to recruit other lymphocytes, inflammatory leukocytes, and mononuclear cells from the bloodstream into the gut through interactions between homing receptors on leukocytes (e.g., $\alpha^4\beta_7$ integrin) and addressins on vascular endothelium (e.g., MadCAM1). $CD4^+$ T helper (T_H) cells that promote inflammation are of three major types, all of which may be associated with colitis in animal models and perhaps humans: T_H1 cells [secrete interferon (IFN) γ], T_H2 cells (secrete IL-4, IL-5, IL-13), and T_H17 cells (secrete IL-17, IL-21). T_H1 cells induce transmural granulomatous inflammation that resembles CD, T_H2 cells, and related natural killer T cells that secrete IL-13 induce superficial mucosal inflammation resembling UC, and T_H17 cells may be responsible for neutrophilic recruitment. Each of these T cell subsets cross-regulate each other. The T_H1 cytokine pathway is initiated by IL-12, a key cytokine in the pathogenesis of experimental models of mucosal inflammation. IL-4 and IL-23, together with IL-6 and TGF-β, induce T_H2 and T_H17 cells, respectively. Activated macrophages secrete tumor necrosis factor (TNF and IL-6). Thus, use of antibodies to block proinflammatory cytokines (e.g., anti-TNF, anti-IL-12, anti-IL-23, anti-IL-6, anti-IFN-γ) or molecules associated with leukocyte recruitment (e.g., anti-$\alpha^4\beta_7$) or use of cytokines that inhibit inflammation and promote regulatory T cells (e.g., IL-10) or promote intestinal barrier function may be beneficial to humans with intestinal inflammation.

THE INFLAMMATORY CASCADE IN IBD

Once initiated in IBD by abnormal innate immune sensing of bacteria by parenchymal cells (e.g., intestinal epithelial cells) and hematopoietic cells (e.g., dendritic cells), the immune inflammatory response is perpetuated by T-cell activation. A sequential cascade of inflammatory mediators extends the response; each step is a potential target for therapy. Inflammatory cytokines such as IL-1, IL-6, and TNF, have diverse effects on tissues. They promote fibrogenesis, collagen production, activation of tissue metalloproteinases, and the production of other inflammatory mediators; they also activate the coagulation cascade in local blood vessels (e.g., increased production of von Willebrand's factor). These cytokines are normally produced in response to infection but are usually turned off or inhibited at the appropriate time to limit tissue damage. In IBD their activity is not regulated, resulting in an imbalance between the proinflammatory and anti-inflammatory mediators. Therapies such as the 5-aminosalicylic acid (5-ASA) compounds are potent inhibitors of these inflammatory mediators through inhibition of transcription factors such as NFκB that regulate their expression.

■ EXOGENOUS FACTORS

IBD may have an as yet undefined infectious etiology. Observational studies suggest that multiple pathogens (e.g., *Salmonella, Shigella, Campylobacter, Clostridium difficile* spp.) may initiate IBD by triggering an inflammatory response that the mucosal immune system may fail to control. However, in an IBD patient, the normal microbiota is likely perceived inappropriately as if it were a pathogen. Alterations in the composition of the commensal microbiota are observed in both CD and UC. However, whether these changes are primary or secondary to inflammation is unknown. Anaerobic organisms, particularly *Bacteroides* and *Clostridia* species, and some aerobic species such as *Escherichia* may be responsible for the induction of inflammation. This notion is supported by the immune response in patients with CD to a number of bacterial antigens. In addition, agents that alter the intestinal flora such as metronidazole, ciprofloxacin, and elemental diets, may improve CD. CD also responds to fecal diversion, demonstrating the ability of luminal contents to exacerbate disease. Conversely, other organisms, so-called probiotics (e.g., *Faecalibacterium prausnitzii, Lactobacillus, Bifidobacterium, Taenia suis,* and *Saccharomyces boulardii* spp.), may inhibit inflammation in animal models and humans.

Psychosocial factors can contribute to worsening of symptoms. Major life events such as illness or death in the family, divorce or separation, interpersonal conflict, or other major loss are associated with an increase in IBD symptoms such as pain, bowel dysfunction, and bleeding. Acute daily stress can worsen bowel symptoms even after controlling for major life events. When measured with validated psychological scales, patients with active IBD have lower psychological well-being and mastery as well as higher distress than non-IBD controls.

PATHOLOGY

■ ULCERATIVE COLITIS: MACROSCOPIC FEATURES

UC is a mucosal disease that usually involves the rectum and extends proximally to involve all or part of the colon. About 40–50% of patients have disease limited to the rectum and rectosigmoid, 30–40% have disease extending beyond the sigmoid but not involving the whole colon, and 20% have a total colitis. Proximal spread occurs in continuity without areas of uninvolved mucosa. When the whole colon is involved, the inflammation extends 2–3 cm into the terminal ileum in 10–20% of patients. The endoscopic changes of *backwash ileitis* are superficial and mild and are of little clinical significance. Although variations in macroscopic activity may suggest skip areas, biopsies from normal-appearing mucosa are usually abnormal. Thus, it is important to obtain multiple biopsies from apparently uninvolved mucosa, whether proximal or distal, during endoscopy. One caveat is that effective medical therapy can change the appearance of the mucosa such that either skip areas or the entire colon can be microscopically normal.

With mild inflammation, the mucosa is erythematous and has a fine granular surface that resembles sandpaper. In more severe disease, the mucosa is hemorrhagic, edematous, and ulcerated (Fig. 295-1) In long-standing disease, inflammatory polyps (pseudopolyps) may be present as a result of epithelial regeneration. The mucosa may appear normal in remission, but in patients with many years of disease it appears atrophic and featureless, and the entire colon becomes narrowed and shortened. Patients with fulminant disease can develop a toxic colitis or megacolon where the bowel wall thins and the mucosa is severely ulcerated; this may lead to perforation.

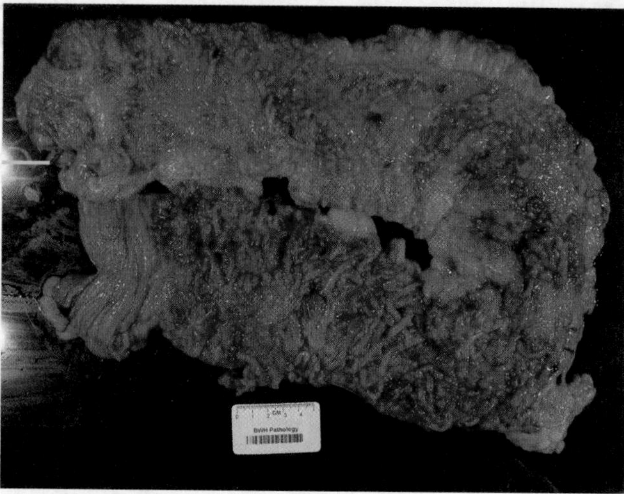

Figure 295-1 Ulcerative colitis. Diffuse (nonsegmental) mucosal disease, with broad areas of ulceration. The bowel wall is not thickened, and there is no cobblestoning. *(Courtesy of Dr. R Odze, Division of Gastrointestinal Pathology, Department of Pathology, Brigham and Women's Hospital, Boston, Massachusetts; with permission.)*

■ ULCERATIVE COLITIS: MICROSCOPIC FEATURES

Histologic findings correlate well with the endoscopic appearance and clinical course of UC. The process is limited to the mucosa and superficial submucosa, with deeper layers unaffected except in fulminant disease. In UC, two major histologic features suggest chronicity and help distinguish it from infectious or acute self-limited colitis. First, the crypt architecture of the colon is distorted; crypts may be bifid and reduced in number, often with a gap between the crypt bases and the muscularis mucosae. Second, some patients have basal plasma cells and multiple basal lymphoid aggregates. Mucosal vascular congestion, with edema and focal hemorrhage, and an inflammatory cell infiltrate of neutrophils, lymphocytes, plasma cells, and macrophages may be present. The neutrophils invade the epithelium, usually in the crypts, giving rise to cryptitis and, ultimately, to crypt abscesses (Fig. 295-2). Ileal changes in patients with backwash ileitis include villous atrophy and crypt regeneration with increased inflammation, increased neutrophil and mononuclear inflammation in the lamina propria, and patchy cryptitis and crypt abscesses.

■ CROHN'S DISEASE: MACROSCOPIC FEATURES

CD can affect any part of the gastrointestinal (GI) tract from the mouth to the anus. Some 30–40% of patients have smallbowel disease alone, 40–55% have disease involving both the small and large intestines, and 15–25% have colitis alone. In the 75% of patients with smallintestinal disease, the terminal ileum is involved in 90%. Unlike UC, which almost always involves the rectum, the rectum is often spared in CD. CD is segmental with skip areas in the midst of diseased intestine (Fig. 295-3) Perirectal fistulas, fissures, abscesses, and anal stenosis are present in one-third of patients with CD, particularly those with colonic involvement. Rarely, CD may also involve the liver and the pancreas.

Unlike UC, CD is a transmural process. Endoscopically, aphthous or small superficial ulcerations characterize mild disease; in more active disease, stellate ulcerations fuse longitudinally and

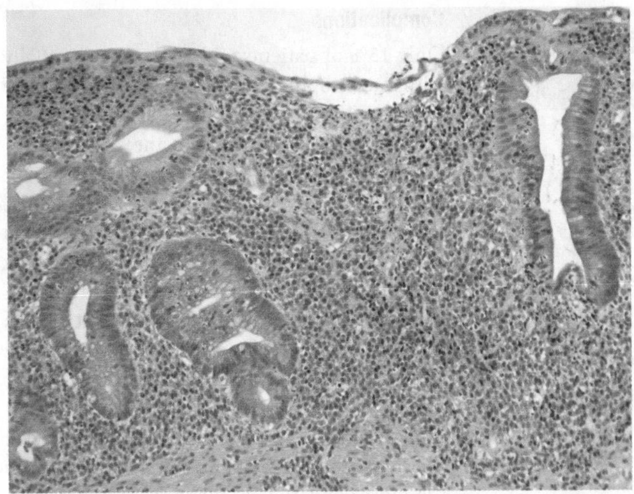

Figure 295-2 Medium power view of colonic mucosa in ulcerative colitis showing diffuse mixed inflammation, basal lymphoplasmacytosis, crypt atrophy and irregularity and superficial erosion. These features are typical of chronic active ulcerative colitis. *(Courtesy of Dr. R Odze, Division of Gastrointestinal Pathology, Department of Pathology, Brigham and Women's Hospital, Boston, Massachusetts; with permission.)*

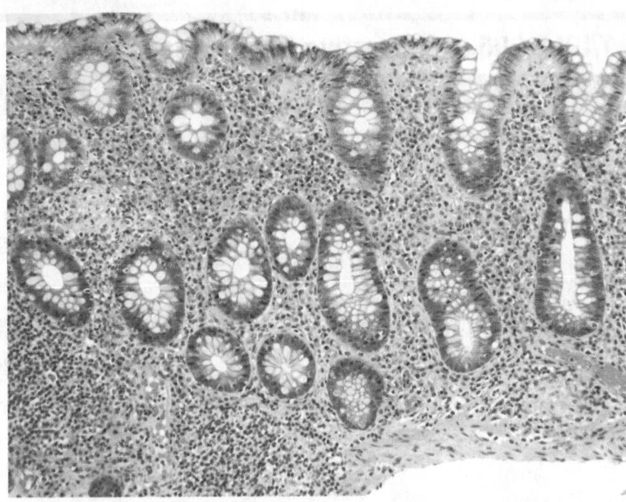

Figure 295-4 Medium power view of Crohn's colitis showing mixed acute and chronic inflammation, crypt atrophy, and multiple small epithelioid granulomas in the mucosa. *(Courtesy of Dr. R Odze, Division of Gastrointestinal Pathology, Department of Pathology, Brigham and Women's Hospital, Boston, Massachusetts; with permission.)*

transversely to demarcate islands of mucosa that frequently are histologically normal. This "cobblestone" appearance is characteristic of CD, both endoscopically and by barium radiography. As in UC, pseudopolyps can form in CD.

Active CD is characterized by focal inflammation and formation of fistula tracts, which resolve by fibrosis and stricturing of the bowel. The bowel wall thickens and becomes narrowed and fibrotic, leading to chronic, recurrent bowel obstructions. Projections of thickened mesentery encase the bowel ("creeping fat"), and serosal and mesenteric inflammation promotes adhesions and fistula formation.

■ CROHN'S DISEASE: MICROSCOPIC FEATURES

The earliest lesions are aphthoid ulcerations and focal crypt abscesses with loose aggregations of macrophages, which form noncaseating granulomas in all layers of the bowel wall (Fig. 295-4).

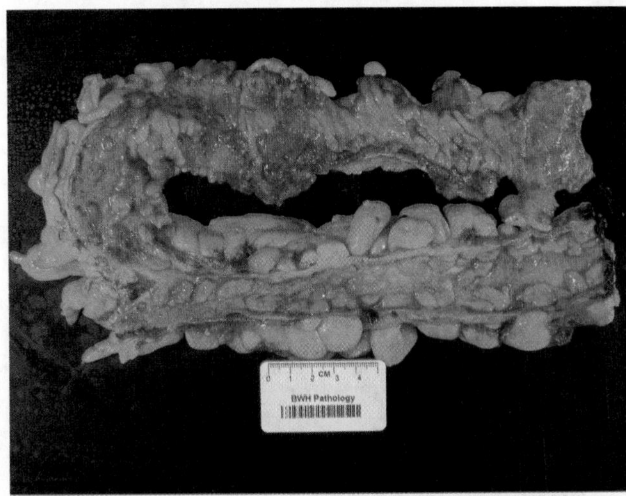

Figure 295-3 Crohn's disease of the colon showing thickening of the wall, with stenosis, linear serpiginous ulcers and cobblestoning of the mucosa. *(Courtesy of Dr. R Odze, Division of Gastrointestinal Pathology, Department of Pathology, Brigham and Women's Hospital, Boston, Massachusetts; with permission.)*

Granulomas can be seen in lymph nodes, mesentery, peritoneum, liver, and pancreas. Although granulomas are a pathognomonic feature of CD, they are rarely found on mucosal biopsies. Surgical resection reveals granulomas in about one-half of cases. Other histologic features of CD include submucosal or subserosal lymphoid aggregates, particularly away from areas of ulceration, gross and microscopic skip areas, and transmural inflammation that is accompanied by fissures that penetrate deeply into the bowel wall and sometimes form fistulous tracts or local abscesses.

CLINICAL PRESENTATION

■ ULCERATIVE COLITIS

Signs and symptoms

The major symptoms of UC are diarrhea, rectal bleeding, tenesmus, passage of mucus, and crampy abdominal pain. The severity of symptoms correlates with the extent of disease. Although UC can present acutely, symptoms usually have been present for weeks to months. Occasionally, diarrhea and bleeding are so intermittent and mild that the patient does not seek medical attention.

Patients with proctitis usually pass fresh blood or blood-stained mucus, either mixed with stool or streaked onto the surface of a normal or hard stool. They also have tenesmus, or urgency with a feeling of incomplete evacuation, but rarely have abdominal pain. With proctitis or proctosigmoiditis, proximal transit slows, which may account for the constipation commonly seen in patients with distal disease.

When the disease extends beyond the rectum, blood is usually mixed with stool or grossly bloody diarrhea may be noted. Colonic motility is altered by inflammation with rapid transit through the inflamed intestine. When the disease is severe, patients pass a liquid stool containing blood, pus, and fecal matter. Diarrhea is often nocturnal and/or postprandial. Although severe pain is not a prominent symptom, some patients with active disease may experience vague lower abdominal discomfort or mild central abdominal cramping. Severe cramping and abdominal pain can occur with severe attacks of the disease. Other symptoms in moderate to severe disease include anorexia, nausea, vomiting, fever, and weight loss.

Physical signs of proctitis include a tender anal canal and blood on rectal examination. With more extensive disease, patients have tenderness to palpation directly over the colon. Patients with a toxic

TABLE 295-4 Ulcerative Colitis: Disease Presentation

	Mild	Moderate	Severe
Bowel movements	<4 per day	4–6 per day	>6 per day
Blood in stool	Small	Moderate	Severe
Fever	None	<37.5°C mean (<99.5°F)	>37.5°C mean (>99.5°F)
Tachycardia	None	<90 mean pulse	>90 mean pulse
Anemia	Mild	>75%	≤75%
Sedimentation rate	<30 mm		>30 mm
Endoscopic appearance	Erythema, decreased vascular pattern, fine granularity	Marked erythema, coarse granularity, absent vascular markings, contact bleeding, no ulcerations	Spontaneous bleeding, ulcerations

colitis have severe pain and bleeding, and those with megacolon have hepatic tympany. Both may have signs of peritonitis if a perforation has occurred. The classification of disease activity is shown in Table 295-4.

Laboratory, endoscopic, and radiographic features

Active disease can be associated with a rise in acute-phase reactants [C-reactive protein (CRP)], platelet count, erythrocyte sedimentation rate (ESR), and a decrease in hemoglobin. Fecal lactoferrin is a highly sensitive and specific marker for detecting intestinal inflammation. Fecal calprotectin levels correlate well with histologic inflammation, predict relapses, and detect pouchitis. In severely ill patients, the serum albumin level will fall rather quickly. Leukocytosis may be present but is not a specific indicator of disease activity. Proctitis or proctosigmoiditis rarely causes a rise in CRP. Diagnosis relies upon the patient's history; clinical symptoms; negative stool examination for bacteria, *C. difficile* toxin, and ova and parasites; sigmoidoscopic appearance (see Fig. 291-4*A*); and histology of rectal or colonic biopsy specimens.

Sigmoidoscopy is used to assess disease activity and is usually performed before treatment. If the patient is not having an acute flare, colonoscopy is used to assess disease extent and activity (Fig. 295-5). Endoscopically mild disease is characterized by erythema, decreased vascular pattern, and mild friability. Moderate disease is characterized by marked erythema, absent vascular pattern, friability and erosions, and severe disease by spontaneous bleeding and ulcerations. Histologic features change more slowly than clinical features but can also be used to grade disease activity.

The earliest radiologic change of UC seen on single-contrast barium enema is a fine mucosal granularity. With increasing severity, the mucosa becomes thickened, and superficial ulcers are seen. Deep ulcerations can appear as "collar-button" ulcers, which indicate that the ulceration has penetrated the mucosa. Haustral folds may be normal in mild disease, but as activity progresses they become edematous and thickened. Loss of haustration can occur, especially in patients with long-standing disease. In addition, the colon becomes shortened and narrowed. Polyps in the colon may be postinflammatory polyps or pseudopolyps, adenomatous polyps, or carcinoma.

CT scanning is not as helpful as endoscopy and barium enema in making the diagnosis of UC, but typical findings include mild mural thickening (<1.5 cm), inhomogeneous wall density, absence of small bowel thickening, increased perirectal and presacral fat, target appearance of the rectum, and adenopathy.

Complications

Only 15% of patients with UC present initially with catastrophic illness. Massive hemorrhage occurs with severe attacks of disease in 1% of patients, and treatment for the disease usually stops the bleeding. However, if a patient requires 6–8 units of blood within 24–48 hours, colectomy is indicated. *Toxic megacolon* is defined as a transverse or right colon with a diameter of >6 cm, with loss of haustration in patients with severe attacks of UC. It occurs in about 5% of attacks and can be triggered by electrolyte abnormalities and narcotics. About 50% of acute dilations will resolve with medical therapy alone, but urgent colectomy is required for those that do not improve. Perforation is the most dangerous of the local complications, and the physical signs of peritonitis may not be obvious, especially if the patient is receiving glucocorticoids. Although perforation is rare, the mortality rate for perforation complicating a toxic megacolon is about 15%. In addition, patients can develop a toxic colitis and such severe ulcerations that the bowel may perforate without first dilating.

Strictures occur in 5–10% of patients and are always a concern in UC because of the possibility of underlying neoplasia. Although benign strictures can form from the inflammation and fibrosis of UC, strictures that are impassable with the colonoscope should be presumed malignant until proven otherwise. A stricture that prevents passage of the colonoscope is an indication for surgery. UC patients occasionally develop anal fissures, perianal abscesses, or hemorrhoids, but the occurrence of extensive perianal lesions should suggest CD.

CROHN'S DISEASE

Signs and symptoms

Although CD usually presents as acute or chronic bowel inflammation, the inflammatory process evolves toward one of two patterns of disease: a fibrostenotic obstructing pattern or a penetrating fistulous

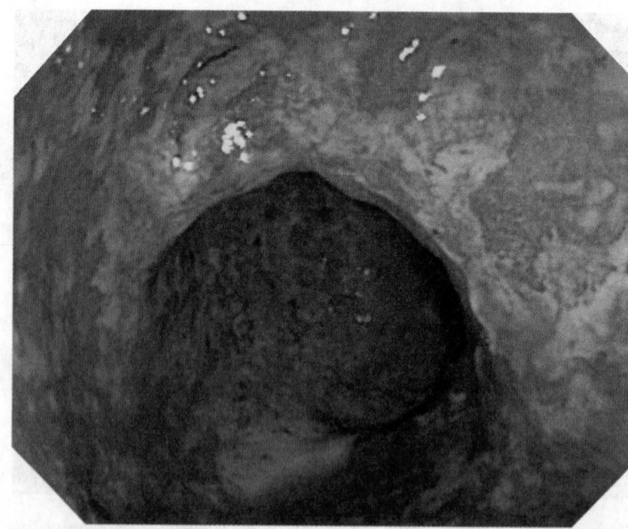

Figure 295-5 Colonoscopy with acute ulcerative colitis: Severe colon inflammation with erythema, friability, and exudates. *(Courtesy of Dr. M. Hamilton, Gastroenterology Division, Department of Medicine, Brigham and Women's Hospital, Boston, Massachusetts; with permission.)*

pattern, each with different treatments and prognoses. The site of disease influences the clinical manifestations.

Ileocolitis Because the most common site of inflammation is the terminal ileum, the usual presentation of ileocolitis is a chronic history of recurrent episodes of right lower quadrant pain and diarrhea. Sometimes the initial presentation mimics acute appendicitis with pronounced right lower quadrant pain, a palpable mass, fever, and leukocytosis. Pain is usually colicky; it precedes and is relieved by defecation. A low-grade fever is usually noted. High-spiking fever suggests intraabdominal abscess formation. Weight loss is common—typically 10–20% of body weight—and develops as a consequence of diarrhea, anorexia, and fear of eating.

An inflammatory mass may be palpated in the right lower quadrant of the abdomen. The mass is composed of inflamed bowel, adherent and indurated mesentery, and enlarged abdominal lymph nodes. Extension of the mass can cause obstruction of the right ureter or bladder inflammation, manifested by dysuria and fever. Edema, bowel wall thickening, and fibrosis of the bowel wall within the mass account for the radiographic "string sign" of a narrowed intestinal lumen.

Bowel obstruction may take several forms. In the early stages of disease, bowel wall edema and spasm produce intermittent obstructive manifestations and increasing symptoms of postprandial pain. Over several years, persistent inflammation gradually progresses to fibrostenotic narrowing and stricture. Diarrhea will decrease and be replaced by chronic bowel obstruction. Acute episodes of obstruction occur as well, precipitated by bowel inflammation and spasm or sometimes by impaction of undigested food or medication. These episodes usually resolve with intravenous fluids and gastric decompression.

Severe inflammation of the ileocecal region may lead to localized wall thinning, with microperforation and fistula formation to the adjacent bowel, the skin, or the urinary bladder, or to an abscess cavity in the mesentery. Enterovesical fistulas typically present as dysuria or recurrent bladder infections or, less commonly, as pneumaturia or fecaluria. Enterocutaneous fistulas follow tissue planes of least resistance, usually draining through abdominal surgical scars. Enterovaginal fistulas are rare and present as dyspareunia or as a feculent or foul-smelling, often painful vaginal discharge. They are unlikely to develop without a prior hysterectomy.

Jejunoileitis Extensive inflammatory disease is associated with a loss of digestive and absorptive surface, resulting in malabsorption and steatorrhea. Nutritional deficiencies can also result from poor intake and enteric losses of protein and other nutrients. Intestinal malabsorption can cause anemia, hypoalbuminemia, hypocalcemia, hypomagnesemia, coagulopathy, and hyperoxaluria with nephrolithiasis in patients with an intact colon. Many patients need to take oral and often intravenous iron. Vertebral fractures are caused by a combination of vitamin D deficiency, hypocalcemia, and prolonged glucocorticoid use. Pellagra from niacin deficiency can occur in extensive small bowel disease, and malabsorption of vitamin B_{12} can lead to megaloblastic anemia and neurologic symptoms. Other important nutrients to measure and replete if low are folate and vitamins A, E, and K. Levels of minerals such as zinc, selenium, copper, and magnesium are often low in patients with extensive small bowel inflammation or resections and these should be repleted as well. Most patients should take a daily multivitamin, calcium, and vitamin D supplements.

Diarrhea is characteristic of active disease; its causes include (1) bacterial overgrowth in obstructive stasis or fistulization, (2) bile-acid malabsorption due to a diseased or resected terminal ileum, and (3) intestinal inflammation with decreased water absorption and increased secretion of electrolytes.

Colitis and perianal disease Patients with colitis present with low-grade fevers, malaise, diarrhea, crampy abdominal pain, and sometimes hematochezia. Gross bleeding is not as common as in UC and appears in about one-half of patients with exclusively colonic disease. Only 1–2% bleed massively. Pain is caused by passage of fecal material through narrowed and inflamed segments of the large bowel. Decreased rectal compliance is another cause for diarrhea in Crohn's colitis patients. Toxic megacolon is rare but may be seen with severe inflammation and short duration disease.

Stricturing can occur in the colon in 4–16% of patients and produce symptoms of bowel obstruction. If the endoscopist is unable to traverse a stricture in Crohn's colitis, surgical resection should be considered, especially if the patient has symptoms of chronic obstruction. Colonic disease may fistulize into the stomach or duodenum, causing feculent vomiting, or to the proximal or mid-small bowel, causing malabsorption by "short circuiting" and bacterial overgrowth. Ten percent of women with Crohn's colitis will develop a rectovaginal fistula.

Perianal disease affects about one-third of patients with Crohn's colitis and is manifested by incontinence, large hemorrhoidal tags, anal strictures, anorectal fistulae, and perirectal abscesses. Not all patients with perianal fistula will have endoscopic evidence of colonic inflammation.

Gastroduodenal disease Symptoms and signs of upper GI tract disease include nausea, vomiting, and epigastric pain. Patients usually have an *Helicobacter pylori*–negative gastritis. The second portion of the duodenum is more commonly involved than the bulb. Fistulas involving the stomach or duodenum arise from the small or large bowel and do not necessarily signify the presence of upper GI tract involvement. Patients with advanced gastroduodenal CD may develop a chronic gastric outlet obstruction.

Laboratory, endoscopic, and radiographic features

Laboratory abnormalities include elevated ESR and CRP. In more severe disease, findings include hypoalbuminemia, anemia, and leukocytosis.

Endoscopic features of CD include rectal sparing, aphthous ulcerations, fistulas, and skip lesions. Colonoscopy allows examination and biopsy of mass lesions or strictures and biopsy of the terminal ileum. Upper endoscopy is useful in diagnosing gastroduodenal involvement in patients with upper tract symptoms. Ileal or colonic strictures may be dilated with balloons introduced through the colonoscope. Strictures ≤ 4 cm and those at a anastomotic sites respond better to endoscopic dilation. The perforation rate is as high as 10%. Most endoscopists dilate only fibrotic strictures and not those associated with active inflammation. Wireless capsule endoscopy (WCE) allows direct visualization of the entire small bowel mucosa (Fig. 295-6). The diagnostic yield of detecting lesions suggestive of active CD is higher with WCE than CT enterography or small bowel series. WCE cannot be used in the setting of a small bowel stricture. Capsule retention occurs in <1% of patients with suspected CD, but retention rates of 4–6% are seen in patients with established CD.

In CD, early radiographic findings in the small bowel include thickened folds and aphthous ulcerations. "Cobblestoning" from longitudinal and transverse ulcerations most frequently involves the small bowel. In more advanced disease, strictures, fistulas, inflammatory masses, and abscesses may be detected. The earliest macroscopic findings of colonic CD are aphthous ulcers. These small ulcers are often multiple and separated by normal intervening mucosa. As the disease progresses, aphthous ulcers become enlarged, deeper, and occasionally connected to one another, forming longitudinal stellate, serpiginous, and linear ulcers (see Fig. 291-4*B*).

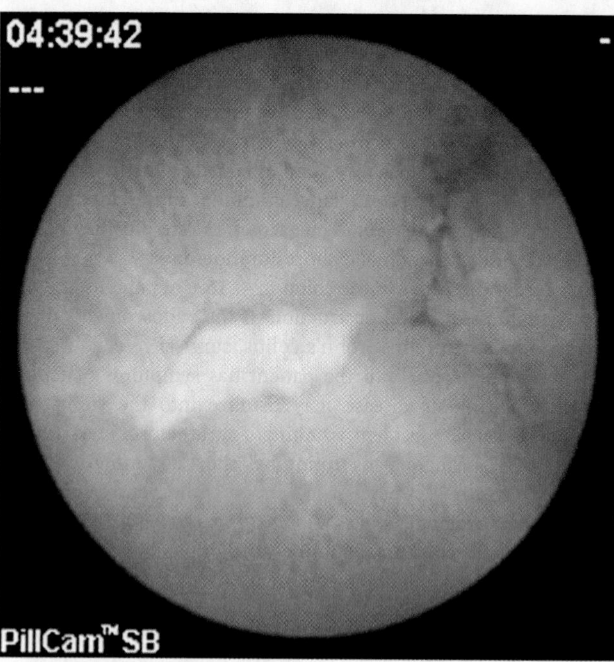

Figure 295-6 Wireless capsule endoscopy image in a patient with Crohn's disease of the ileum shows ulcerations and narrowing of the intestinal lumen. *(Courtesy of Dr. S Reddy, Gastroenterology Division, Department of Medicine, Brigham and Women's Hospital, Boston, Massachusetts; with permission.)*

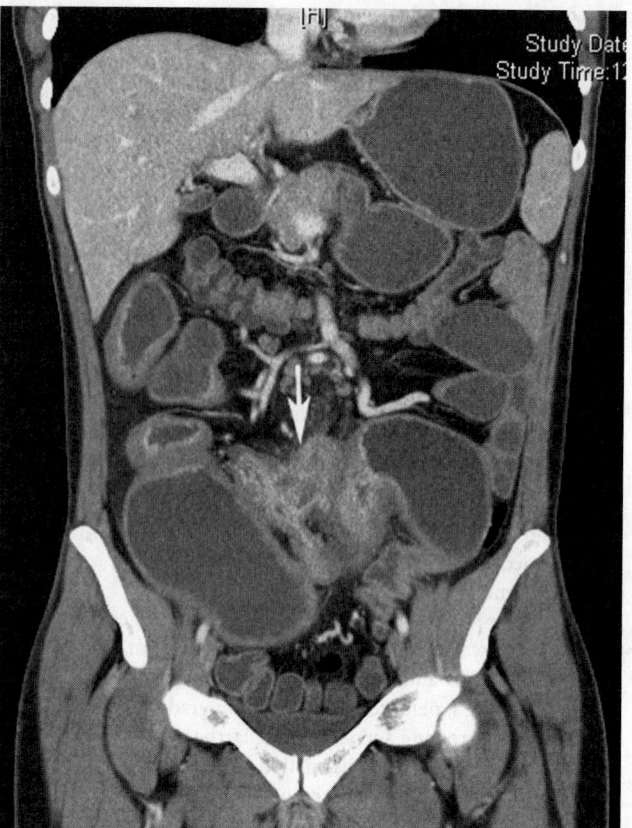

Figure 295-7 Coronal contrast-enhanced multidetector computed tomography (MDCT) image obtained after oral administration of 1350 cc of neutral oral contrast material shows dilation of small bowel loops, segmental mucosal hyperenhancement, and interloop sinus tracts (*white arrow*) and mesenteric fat stranding. *(Courtesy of Dr. K Mortele, Gastrointestinal Radiology, Department of Radiology, Brigham and Women's Hospital, Boston, Massachusetts; with permission.)*

The transmural inflammation of CD leads to decreased luminal diameter and limited distensibility. As ulcers progress deeper, they can lead to fistula formation. The radiographic "string sign" represents long areas of circumferential inflammation and fibrosis, resulting in long segments of luminal narrowing. The segmental nature of CD results in wide gaps of normal or dilated bowel between involved segments.

CT enterography combines the improved spatial and temporal resolution of multidetector-row CT with large volumes of ingested neutral enteric contrast material to permit visualization of the entire small bowel and lumen. Unlike routine CT, which is used to detect the extraenteric complications of CD such as fistula and abscess, CT enterography clearly depicts the small bowel inflammation associated with CD by displaying mural hyperenhancement, stratification, and thickening; engorged vasa recta; and perienteric inflammatory changes (Figs. 295-7 and 295-8). CT enterography is the first-line test for the evaluation of suspected CD and its complications. As an initial test in children or in adults with multiple radiation exposures, MR enterography is comparable to CT in diagnostic accuracy. Pelvic MRI is superior to CT for demonstrating pelvic lesions such as ischiorectal abscesses and perianal fistulae (Fig. 295-9).

Complications

Because CD is a transmural process, serosal adhesions develop that provide direct pathways for fistula formation and reduce the incidence of free perforation. Perforation occurs in 1–2% of patients, usually in the ileum but occasionally in the jejunum or as a complication of toxic megacolon. The peritonitis of free perforation, especially colonic, may be fatal. Intraabdominal and pelvic abscesses occur in 10–30% of patients with Crohn's disease at some time in the course of their illness. CT-guided percutaneous drainage of the abscess is standard therapy. Despite adequate drainage, most patients need resection of the offending bowel segment. Percutaneous drainage has an especially high failure rate in abdominal wall abscesses. Systemic glucocorticoid therapy increases

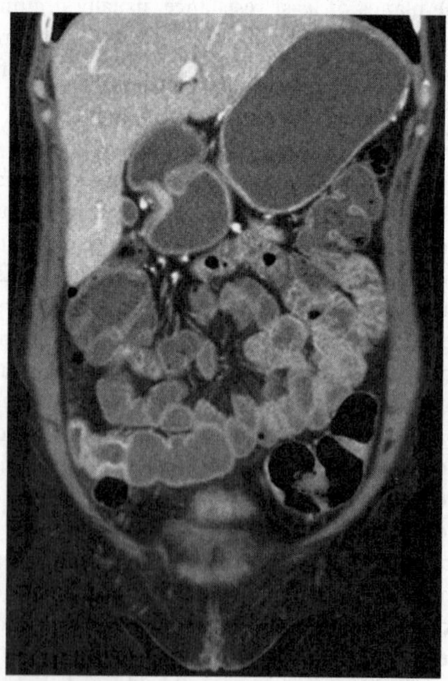

Figure 295-8 Coronal contrast-enhanced multidetector computed tomography (MDCT) image obtained after oral administration of 1350 cc of neutral oral contrast material shows mucosal hyperenhancement of the terminal ileum with narrowing and mild prestenotic dilatation. *(Courtesy of Dr. K Mortele, Gastrointestinal Radiology, Department of Radiology, Brigham and Women's Hospital, Boston, Massachusetts; with permission.)*

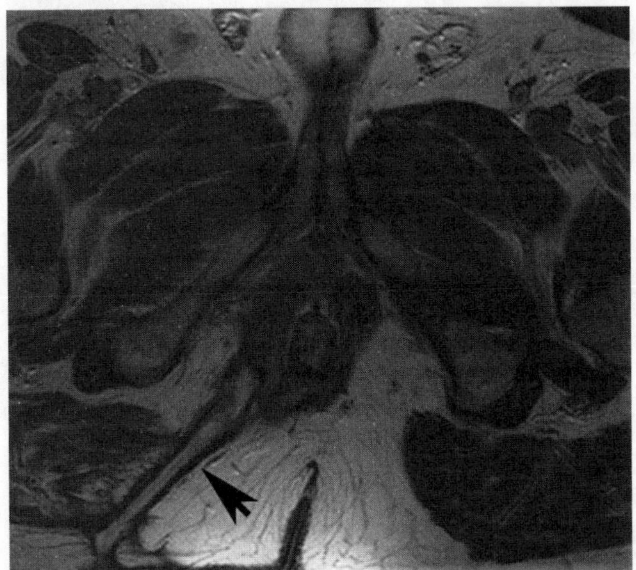

Figure 295-9 **Axial T2-weighted MR image** obtained in a 37-year-old man with Crohn's disease shows a linear fluid-filled perianal fistula (***arrow***) in the right ischioanal fossa. *(Courtesy of Dr. K Mortele, Gastrointestinal Radiology, Department of Radiology, Brigham and Women's Hospital, Boston, Massachusetts; with permission.)*

the risk of intraabdominal and pelvic abscesses in CD patients who have never had an operation. Other complications include intestinal obstruction in 40%, massive hemorrhage, malabsorption, and severe perianal disease.

Serologic markers

Patients with Crohn's disease show a wide variation in the way they present and progress over time. Some patients present with mild disease activity and do well with generally safe and mild medications, but many others exhibit more severe disease and can develop serious complications that will require surgery. Current and developing biologic therapies can help halt progression of disease and give patients with moderate to severe Crohn's disease a better quality of life. There are potential risks of biologic therapies such as infection and malignancy, and it would be optimal to determine at the time of diagnosis which patients will require more aggressive medical therapy. This same argument holds true for UC patients as well.

Subsets of patients with differing immune responses to microbial antigens have been described. These include antibodies to *Escherichia coli* (*E. coli*) outer membrane porin protein C (OmpC), which is found in 55% of CD patients, an antibody to I_2, a homologue of the bacterial transcription-factor families from a *Pseudomonas fluorescens*–associated sequence that is found in 50–54% of CD patients, as well as anti-*Saccharomyces cerevisiae* (ASCA) and autoantigens [perinuclear antineutrophil antibody (pANCA)]. A novel immune response, antiflagellin (anti-CBir1) has been identified in approximately 50% of Crohn's patients and has been suggested to represent a unique subgroup of CD patients.

Unfortunately, these serologic markers are only marginally useful in helping to make the diagnosis of UC or CD and in predicting the course of disease. For success in diagnosing IBD and in differentiating between CD and UC, the efficacy of these serologic tests depends upon the prevalence of IBD in a specific population. pANCA positivity is found in about 60–70% of UC patients and 5–10% of CD patients; 5–15% of first-degree relatives of UC patients are pANCA positive, whereas only 2–3% of the general population is pANCA positive.

Sixty to seventy percent of CD patients, 10–15% of UC patients, and up to 5% of non-IBD controls are ASCA-positive. In a patient population with a combined prevalence of UC and CD of 62%, pANCA/ASCA serology showed a sensitivity of 64% and a specificity of 94%. Positive and negative predictive values (PPVs and NPVs) for pANCA/ASCA also vary based on the prevalence of IBD in a given population. For the patient population with a prevalence of IBD of 62%, the PPV is 94%, and the NPV is 63%.

Combining these diagnostic assays may improve the ability to diagnose CD. In a referral population of CD patients, 85% had an antibody to at least one antigen (pANCA, ASCA, OmpC, and I_2); only 4% responded to all four. Some evidence suggests that antibody positivity may help predict disease phenotype. ASCA positivity is associated with an increased rate of early CD complications; OmpC–positive patients are more likely to have internal perforating disease; and I_2 positive patients are more likely to have fibrostenosing disease. Patients positive for I_2, OmpC, and ASCA are the most likely to have undergone small bowel surgery.

Anti-Cbir1 expression is associated with small-bowel disease, fibrostenosing, and internal penetrating disease. Children with CD positive for all four immune responses (ASCA+, OmpC+, I_2+, and anti-Cbir1+) may have more aggressive disease and a shorter time to progression to internal perforating and/or stricturing disease. However, larger prospective studies in both children and adults have not yet been performed and compared to CRP or other markers.

Clinical factors described at diagnosis are more helpful than serologies at predicting the natural history of Crohn's disease. The initial requirement for glucocorticoid use, an age at diagnosis below 40 years and the presence of perianal disease at diagnosis, have been shown to be independently associated with subsequent disabling CD after 5 years. Except in special circumstances [such as before consideration of an ileoanal pouch anastomosis (IPAA) in a patient with indeterminate colitis], serologic markers have only minimal clinical utility.

DIFFERENTIAL DIAGNOSIS OF UC AND CD

UC and CD have similar features to many other diseases. In the absence of a key diagnostic test, a combination of features is used (Table 295-5). Once a diagnosis of IBD is made, distinguishing between UC and CD is impossible initially in up to 15% of cases. These are termed *indeterminate colitis.* Fortunately, in most cases, the true nature of the underlying colitis becomes evident later in the course of the patient's disease. Approximately 5% (range 1–20%) of colon resection specimens are difficult to classify as either UC or CD because they exhibit overlapping histologic features.

■ INFECTIOUS DISEASE

Infections of the small intestines and colon can mimic CD or UC. They may be bacterial, fungal, viral, or protozoal in origin (Table 295-6). *Campylobacter* colitis can mimic the endoscopic appearance of severe UC and can cause a relapse of established UC. *Salmonella* can cause watery or bloody diarrhea, nausea, and vomiting. Shigellosis causes watery diarrhea, abdominal pain, and fever followed by rectal tenesmus and by the passage of blood and mucus per rectum. All three are usually self-limited, but 1% of patients infected with *Salmonella* become asymptomatic carriers. *Yersinia enterocolitica* infection occurs mainly in the terminal ileum and causes mucosal ulceration, neutrophil invasion, and thickening of the ileal wall. Other bacterial infections that may mimic IBD include *C. difficile,* which presents with watery diarrhea, tenesmus, nausea, and vomiting; and *E. coli,* three categories of which can cause colitis. These are enterohemorrhagic, enteroinvasive, and enteroadherent *E. coli,* all of which can cause bloody

TABLE 295-5 Different Clinical, Endoscopic, and Radiographic Features

	Ulcerative Colitis	Crohn's Disease
Clinical		
Gross blood in stool	Yes	Occasionally
Mucus	Yes	Occasionally
Systemic symptoms	Occasionally	Frequently
Pain	Occasionally	Frequently
Abdominal mass	Rarely	Yes
Significant perineal disease	No	Frequently
Fistulas	No	Yes
Small intestinal obstruction	No	Frequently
Colonic obstruction	Rarely	Frequently
Response to antibiotics	No	Yes
Recurrence after surgery	No	Yes
ANCA-positive	Frequently	Rarely
ASCA-positive	Rarely	Frequently
Endoscopic		
Rectal sparing	Rarely	Frequently
Continuous disease	Yes	Occasionally
"Cobblestoning"	No	Yes
Granuloma on biopsy	No	Occasionally
Radiographic		
Small bowel significantly abnormal	No	Yes
Abnormal terminal ileum	No	Yes
Segmental colitis	No	Yes
Asymmetric colitis	No	Yes
Stricture	Occasionally	Frequently

Abbreviations: ANCA, antineutrophil cytoplasm antibody; ASCA, anti-*Saccharomyces cerevisiae* antibody.

TABLE 295-6 Diseases That Mimic IBD

Infectious Etiologies		
Bacterial	**Mycobacterial**	**Viral**
Salmonella	Tuberculosis	Cytomegalovirus
Shigella	*Mycobacterium avium*	Herpes simplex
Toxigenic *Escherichia coli*	**Parasitic**	HIV
Campylobacter	Amebiasis	**Fungal**
Yersinia	*Isospora*	Histoplasmosis
Clostridium difficile	*Trichuris trichiura*	*Candida*
Gonorrhea	Hookworm	*Aspergillus*
Chlamydia trachomatis	*Strongyloides*	
Noninfectious Etiologies		
Inflammatory	**Neoplastic**	**Drugs and Chemicals**
Appendicitis	Lymphoma	NSAIDs
Diverticulitis	Metastatic carcinoma	Phosphosoda
Diversion colitis	Carcinoma of the ileum	Cathartic colon
Collagenous/lymphocytic colitis	Carcinoid	Gold
Ischemic colitis	Familial polyposis	Oral contraceptives
Radiation colitis/enteritis		Cocaine
Solitary rectal ulcer syndrome		Chemotherapy
Eosinophilic gastroenteritis		
Neutropenic colitis		
Behçet's syndrome		
Graft-versus-host disease		

Abbreviation: NSAIDs, nonsteroidal anti-inflammatory drugs.

diarrhea and abdominal tenderness. Diagnosis of bacterial colitis is made by sending stool specimens for bacterial culture and *C. difficile* toxin analysis. Gonorrhea, *Chlamydia*, and syphilis can also cause proctitis.

GI involvement with mycobacterial infection occurs primarily in the immunosuppressed patient but may occur in patients with normal immunity. Distal ileal and cecal involvement predominates, and patients present with symptoms of small bowel obstruction and a tender abdominal mass. The diagnosis is made most directly by colonoscopy with biopsy and culture. *Mycobacterium avium-intracellulare* complex infection occurs in advanced stages of HIV infection and in other immunocompromised states; it usually manifests as a systemic infection with diarrhea, abdominal pain, weight loss, fever, and malabsorption. Diagnosis is established by acid-fast smear and culture of mucosal biopsies.

Although most of the patients with viral colitis are immunosuppressed, cytomegalovirus (CMV) and herpes simplex proctitis may occur in immunocompetent individuals. CMV occurs most commonly in the esophagus, colon, and rectum but may also involve the small intestine. Symptoms include abdominal pain, bloody diarrhea, fever, and weight loss. With severe disease, necrosis and perforation can occur. Diagnosis is made by identification of characteristic intranuclear inclusions in mucosal cells on biopsy. Herpes simplex infection of the GI tract is limited to the oropharynx, anorectum, and perianal areas. Symptoms include anorectal pain, tenesmus, constipation, inguinal adenopathy, difficulty with urinary voiding, and sacral paresthesias. Diagnosis is made by rectal biopsy with identification of characteristic cellular inclusions and viral culture. HIV itself can cause diarrhea, nausea, vomiting, and anorexia. Small intestinal biopsies show partial villous atrophy; small bowel bacterial overgrowth and fat malabsorption may also be noted.

Protozoan parasites include *Isospora belli,* which can cause a self-limited infection in healthy hosts but causes a chronic profuse, watery diarrhea, and weight loss in AIDS patients. *Entamoeba histolytica* or related species infect about 10% of the world's population; symptoms include abdominal pain, tenesmus, frequent loose stools containing blood and mucus, and abdominal tenderness. Colonoscopy reveals focal punctate ulcers with normal intervening mucosa; diagnosis is made by biopsy or serum amebic antibodies. Fulminant amebic colitis is rare but has a mortality rate of >50%.

Other parasitic infections that may mimic IBD include hookworm (*Necator americanus*), whipworm (*T. trichiura*), and *Strongyloides stercoralis.* In severely immunocompromised patients, *Candida* or *Aspergillus* can be identified in the submucosa. Disseminated histoplasmosis can involve the ileocecal area.

NONINFECTIOUS DISEASE

Diverticulitis can be confused with CD clinically and radiographically. Both diseases cause fever, abdominal pain, tender abdominal mass, leukocytosis, elevated ESR, partial obstruction, and fistulas. Perianal disease or ileitis on small bowel series favors the diagnosis of CD. Significant endoscopic mucosal abnormalities are more likely in CD than in diverticulitis. Endoscopic or clinical recurrence following segmental resection favors CD. Diverticular-associated colitis is similar to CD, but mucosal abnormalities are limited to the sigmoid and descending colon.

Ischemic colitis is commonly confused with IBD. The ischemic process can be chronic and diffuse, as in UC, or segmental, as in CD. Colonic inflammation due to ischemia may resolve quickly or may persist and result in transmural scarring and stricture formation. Ischemic bowel disease should be considered in the elderly following abdominal aortic aneurysm repair or when a patient has a hypercoagulable state or a severe cardiac or peripheral vascular disorder. Patients usually present with sudden onset of left lower quadrant pain, urgency to defecate, and the passage of bright red blood per rectum. Endoscopic examination often demonstrates a normal-appearing rectum and a sharp transition to an area of inflammation in the descending colon and splenic flexure.

The effects of radiotherapy on the GI tract can be difficult to distinguish from IBD. Acute symptoms can occur within 1–2 weeks of starting radiotherapy. When the rectum and sigmoid are irradiated, patients develop bloody, mucoid diarrhea and tenesmus, as in distal UC. With small bowel involvement, diarrhea is common. Late symptoms include malabsorption and weight loss. Stricturing with obstruction and bacterial overgrowth may occur. Fistulas can penetrate the bladder, vagina, or abdominal wall. Flexible sigmoidoscopy reveals mucosal granularity, friability, numerous telangiectasias, and occasionally discrete ulcerations. Biopsy can be diagnostic.

Solitary rectal ulcer syndrome is uncommon and can be confused with IBD. It occurs in persons of all ages and may be caused by impaired evacuation and failure of relaxation of the puborectalis muscle. Single or multiple ulcerations may arise from anal sphincter overactivity, higher intrarectal pressures during defecation, and digital removal of stool. Patients complain of constipation with straining and pass blood and mucus per rectum. Other symptoms include abdominal pain, diarrhea, tenesmus, and perineal pain. Ulceration as large as 5 cm in diameter is usually seen anteriorly or anterior-laterally 3–15 cm from the anal verge. Biopsies can be diagnostic.

Several types of colitis are associated with nonsteroidal anti-inflammatory drugs (NSAIDs), including de novo colitis, reactivation of IBD, and proctitis caused by use of suppositories. Most patients with NSAID-related colitis present with diarrhea and abdominal pain, and complications include stricture, bleeding, obstruction, perforation, and fistulization. Withdrawal of these agents is crucial, and in cases of reactivated IBD, standard therapies are indicated.

THE ATYPICAL COLITIDES

Two atypical colitides—collagenous colitis and lymphocytic colitis—have completely normal endoscopic appearances. Collagenous colitis has two main histologic components: increased subepithelial collagen deposition and colitis with increased intraepithelial lymphocytes. The female to male ratio is 9:1, and most patients present in the sixth or seventh decades of life. The main symptom is chronic watery diarrhea. Treatments range from sulfasalazine or mesalamine and Lomotil to bismuth to budesonide to prednisone for refractory disease.

Lymphocytic colitis has features similar to collagenous colitis, including age at onset and clinical presentation, but it has almost equal incidence in men and women and no subepithelial collagen deposition on pathologic section. However, intraepithelial lymphocytes are increased. The frequency of celiac disease is increased in lymphocytic colitis and ranges from 9 to 27%. Celiac disease should be excluded in all patients with lymphocytic colitis, particularly if diarrhea does not respond to conventional therapy. Treatment is similar to that of collagenous colitis with the exception of a gluten-free diet for those who have celiac disease.

Diversion colitis is an inflammatory process that arises in segments of the large intestine that are excluded from the fecal stream. It usually occurs in patients with ileostomy or colostomy when a mucus fistula or a Hartmann's pouch has been created. Clinically, patients have mucus or bloody discharge from the rectum. Erythema, granularity, friability, and, in more severe cases, ulceration can be seen on endoscopy. Histopathology shows areas of active inflammation with foci of cryptitis and crypt abscesses. Crypt architecture is normal, which differentiates it from UC. It may be impossible to distinguish from CD. Short-chain fatty acid enemas may help in diversion colitis, but the definitive therapy is surgical reanastomosis.

EXTRAINTESTINAL MANIFESTATIONS

Up to one-third of IBD patients have at least one extraintestinal disease manifestation.

DERMATOLOGIC

Erythema nodosum (EN) occurs in up to 15% of CD patients and 10% of UC patients. Attacks usually correlate with bowel activity; skin lesions develop after the onset of bowel symptoms, and patients frequently have concomitant active peripheral arthritis. The lesions of EN are hot, red, tender nodules measuring 1–5 cm in diameter and are found on the anterior surface of the lower legs, ankles, calves, thighs, and arms. Therapy is directed toward the underlying bowel disease.

Pyoderma gangrenosum (PG) is seen in 1–12% of UC patients and less commonly in Crohn's colitis. Although it usually presents after the diagnosis of IBD, PG may occur years before the onset of bowel symptoms, run a course independent of the bowel disease, respond poorly to colectomy, and even develop years after proctocolectomy. It is usually associated with severe disease. Lesions are commonly found on the dorsal surface of the feet and legs but may occur on the arms, chest, stoma, and even the face. PG usually begins as a pustule and then spreads concentrically to rapidly undermine healthy skin. Lesions then ulcerate, with violaceous edges surrounded by a margin of erythema. Centrally, they contain necrotic tissue with blood and exudates. Lesions may be single or multiple and grow as large as 30 cm. They are sometimes very difficult to treat and often require intravenous (IV) antibiotics, intravenous, glucocorticoids, dapsone, azathioprine, thalidomide, IV cyclosporine, or infliximab.

Other dermatologic manifestations include pyoderma vegetans, which occurs in intertriginous areas; pyostomatitis vegetans, which involves the mucous membranes; Sweet's syndrome, a neutrophilic dermatosis; and metastatic CD, a rare disorder defined by cutaneous granuloma formation. Psoriasis affects 5–10% of patients with IBD and is unrelated to bowel activity consistent with the potential shared immunogenetic basis of these diseases. Perianal skin tags are found in 75–80% of patients with CD, especially those with colon involvement. Oral mucosal lesions, seen often in CD and rarely in UC, include aphthous stomatitis and "cobblestone" lesions of the buccal mucosa.

RHEUMATOLOGIC

Peripheral arthritis develops in 15–20% of IBD patients, is more common in CD, and worsens with exacerbations of bowel activity. It is asymmetric, polyarticular, and migratory and most often affects large joints of the upper and lower extremities. Treatment is directed at reducing bowel inflammation. In severe UC, colectomy frequently cures the arthritis.

Ankylosing spondylitis (AS) occurs in about 10% of IBD patients and is more common in CD than UC. About two-thirds of IBD patients with AS express the HLA-B27 antigen. The AS activity is not related to bowel activity and does not remit with glucocorticoids or colectomy. It most often affects the spine and pelvis, producing symptoms of diffuse low-back pain, buttock pain, and morning stiffness. The course is continuous and progressive, leading to permanent skeletal damage and deformity. Infliximab reduces spinal inflammation and improves functional status and quality of life.

Sacroiliitis is symmetric, occurs equally in UC and CD, is often asymptomatic, does not correlate with bowel activity, and does not always progress to AS. Other rheumatic manifestations include hypertrophic osteoarthropathy, pelvic/femoral osteomyelitis, and relapsing polychondritis.

OCULAR

The incidence of ocular complications in IBD patients is 1–10%. The most common are conjunctivitis, anterior uveitis/iritis, and episcleritis. Uveitis is associated with both UC and Crohn's colitis, may be found during periods of remission, and may develop in patients following bowel resection. Symptoms include ocular pain, photophobia, blurred vision, and headache. Prompt intervention, sometimes with systemic glucocorticoids, is required to prevent scarring and visual impairment. Episcleritis is a benign disorder that presents with symptoms of mild ocular burning. It occurs in 3–4% of IBD patients, more commonly in Crohn's colitis, and is treated with topical glucocorticoids.

HEPATOBILIARY

Hepatic steatosis is detectable in about one-half of the abnormal liver biopsies from patients with CD and UC; patients usually present with hepatomegaly. Fatty liver usually results from a combination of chronic debilitating illness, malnutrition, and glucocorticoid therapy. Cholelithiasis occurs in 10–35% of CD patients with ileitis or ileal resection. Gallstone formation is caused by malabsorption of bile acids, resulting in depletion of the bile salt pool and the secretion of lithogenic bile.

Primary sclerosing cholangitis (PSC) is a disorder characterized by both intrahepatic and extrahepatic bile duct inflammation and fibrosis, frequently leading to biliary cirrhosis and hepatic failure; approximately 5% of patients with UC have PSC, but 50–75% of patients with PSC have IBD. PSC occurs less often in patients with CD. Although it can be recognized after the diagnosis of IBD, PSC can be detected earlier or even years after proctocolectomy. Consistent with this, the immunogenetic basis for PSC appears to be overlapping but distinct from UC based upon genome-wide association studies (GWAS) although both IBD and PSC are commonly pANCA positive. Most patients have no symptoms at the time of diagnosis; when symptoms are present, they consist of fatigue, jaundice, abdominal pain, fever, anorexia, and malaise. The traditional gold-standard diagnostic test is endoscopic retrograde cholangiopancreatography (ERCP), but magnetic resonance cholangiopancreatography (MRCP) is also sensitive and specific. MRCP is reasonable as an initial diagnostic test in children and can visualize irregularities, multifocal strictures, and dilatations of all levels of the biliary tree. In patients with PSC, both ERCP and MRCP demonstrate multiple bile duct strictures alternating with relatively normal segments.

The bile acid ursodeoxycholic acid (ursodiol) may reduce alkaline phosphatase and serum aminotransferase levels, but histologic improvement has been marginal. High doses (25–30 mg/kg per day) may decrease the risk of colorectal dysplasia and cancer in patients with UC and PSC. Endoscopic stenting may be palliative for cholestasis secondary to bile duct obstruction. Patients with symptomatic disease develop cirrhosis and liver failure over 5–10 years and eventually require liver transplantation. PSC patients have a 10–15% lifetime risk of developing cholangiocarcinoma and then cannot be transplanted. Patients with IBD and PSC are at increased risk of colon cancer and should be surveyed yearly by colonoscopy and biopsy.

In addition, cholangiography is normal in a small percentage of patients who have a variant of PSC known as *small duct primary sclerosing cholangitis*. This variant (sometimes referred to as "pericholangitis") is probably a form of PSC involving small caliber bile ducts. It has similar biochemical and histologic features to classic PSC. It appears to have a significantly better prognosis than classic PSC, although it may evolve into classic PSC. Granulomatous hepatitis and hepatic amyloidosis are much rarer extraintestinal manifestations of IBD.

UROLOGIC

The most frequent genitourinary complications are calculi, ureteral obstruction, and ileal bladder fistulas. The highest frequency of nephrolithiasis (10–20%) occurs in patients with CD following small bowel resection. Calcium oxalate stones develop secondary to hyperoxaluria, which results from increased absorption of dietary oxalate. Normally, dietary calcium combines with luminal oxalate to form insoluble calcium oxalate, which is eliminated in the stool. In patients with ileal dysfunction, however, nonabsorbed fatty acids bind calcium and leave oxalate unbound. The unbound oxalate is then delivered to the colon, where it is readily absorbed, especially in the presence of inflammation.

METABOLIC BONE DISORDERS

Low bone mass occurs in 3–30% of IBD patients. The risk is increased by glucocorticoids, cyclosporine, methotrexate and total parenteral nutrition (TPN). Malabsorption and inflammation mediated by IL-1, IL-6, TNF and other inflammatory mediators also contribute to low bone density. An increased incidence of hip, spine, wrist, and rib fractures has been noted: 36% in CD and 45% in UC. The absolute risk of an osteoporotic fracture is about 1% per person per year. Fracture rates, particularly in the spine and hip, were highest among the elderly (age >60). One study noted an odds ratio of vertebral fracture to be 1.72 and hip fracture 1.59. The disease severity predicted the risk of a fracture. Only 13% of IBD patients who had a fracture were on any kind of antifracture treatment. Up to 20% of bone mass can be lost per year with chronic glucocorticoid use. The effect is dosage-dependent. Budesonide may also suppress the pituitary-adrenal axis and thus carries a risk of causing osteoporosis.

Osteonecrosis is characterized by death of osteocytes and adipocytes and eventual bone collapse. The pain is aggravated by motion and swelling of the joints. It affects the hips more often than knees and shoulders, and in one series 4.3% of patients developed osteonecrosis within 6 months of starting glucocorticoids. Diagnosis is made by bone scan or MRI, and treatment consists of pain control, cord decompression, osteotomy, and joint replacement.

THROMBOEMBOLIC DISORDERS

Patients with IBD have an increased risk of both venous and arterial thrombosis even if the disease is not active. Factors responsible for the hypercoagulable state have included abnormalities of the platelet-endothelial interaction, hyperhomocysteinemia, alterations in the coagulation cascade, impaired fibrinolysis, involvement of tissue factor-bearing microvesicles, disruption of the normal coagulation system by autoantibodies, as well as a genetic predisposition. A spectrum of vasculitides involving small, medium, and large vessels has also been observed.

OTHER DISORDERS

More common cardiopulmonary manifestations include endocarditis, myocarditis, pleuropericarditis, and interstitial lung disease. A secondary or reactive amyloidosis can occur in patients with long-standing IBD, especially in patients with CD. Amyloid material is deposited systemically and can cause diarrhea, constipation, and renal failure. The renal disease can be successfully treated with colchicine. Pancreatitis is a rare extraintestinal manifestation of IBD and results from duodenal fistulas; ampullary CD; gallstones; PSC; drugs such as 6-mercaptopurine, azathioprine, or, very rarely, 5-ASA agents; autoimmune pancreatitis; and primary CD of the pancreas.

TREATMENT Inflammatory Bowel Disease Treatment

5-ASA AGENTS The mainstay of therapy for mild to moderate UC is sulfasalazine and the other 5-ASA agents. These agents are effective at inducing and maintaining remission in UC. They may have a limited role in inducing remission in CD but no clear role in maintenance of CD. The most convincing evidence for the use of sulfasalazine is treatment of active Crohn's disease involving the colon. Sulfasalazine was originally developed to deliver both antibacterial (sulfapyridine) and anti-inflammatory (5-ASA) therapy into the connective tissues of joints and the colonic mucosa. The molecular structure provides a convenient delivery system to the colon by allowing the intact molecule to pass through the small intestine after only partial absorption, and to be broken down in the colon by bacterial azo reductases that cleave the azo bond linking the sulfa and 5-ASA moieties. Sulfasalazine is effective treatment for mild to moderate UC, but its high rate of side effects limits its use. Although sulfasalazine is more effective at higher doses, at 6 or 8 g/d up to 30% of patients experience allergic reactions or intolerable side effects such as headache, anorexia, nausea, and vomiting that are attributable to the sulfapyridine moiety. Hypersensitivity reactions, independent of sulfapyridine levels, include rash, fever, hepatitis, agranulocytosis, hypersensitivity pneumonitis, pancreatitis, worsening of colitis, and reversible sperm abnormalities. Sulfasalazine can also impair folate absorption, and patients should be given folic acid supplements.

Newer sulfa-free aminosalicylate preparations deliver increased amounts of the pharmacologically active ingredient of sulfasalazine (5-ASA, mesalamine) to the site of active bowel disease while limiting systemic toxicity. Peroxisome proliferator activated receptor γ (PPAR-γ) may mediate 5-ASA therapeutic action by decreasing nuclear localization of NF κB. Sulfa-free aminosalicylate formulations include alternative azo-bonded carriers, 5-ASA dimers, pH-dependent tablets, delayed-release and controlled-release preparations. Each has the same efficacy as sulfasalazine when equimolar concentrations are used. Olsalazine is composed of two 5-ASA radicals linked by an azo bond, which is split in the colon by bacterial reduction, and two 5-ASA molecules are released. Olsalazine is similar in effectiveness to sulfasalazine in treating UC, but up to 17% of patients experience nonbloody diarrhea caused by increased secretion of fluid in the small bowel. Balsalazide contains an azo bond binding mesalamine to the carrier molecule 4-aminobenzoyl-β-alanine; it is effective in the colon.

Asacol is an enteric-coated form of mesalamine with the 5-ASA being released at pH >7. The disintegration of Asacol is variable, with complete breakup of the tablet occurring in many different parts of the gut ranging from the small intestine to the splenic flexure; it has increased gastric residence when taken with a meal. Pentasa is another mesalamine formulation that uses an ethylcellulose coating to allow water absorption into small beads containing the mesalamine. Water dissolves the 5-ASA, which then diffuses out of the bead into the lumen. Disintegration of the capsule occurs in the stomach. The microspheres then disperse throughout the entire tract from the small intestine through the distal colon in both fasted and fed conditions. Additional formulations of mesalamine continue to be developed. A once-a-day formulation of mesalamine [Multi-Matrix System (MMX), marketed in the United States as Lialda] is designed to release mesalamine in the colon. The MMX technology incorporates mesalamine into a lipophilic matrix within a hydrophilic matrix encapsulated in a polymer resistant to degradation at a low pH (<7) to delay release throughout the colon. The safety profile appears to be comparable to other 5-ASA formulations. A formulation containing encapsulated mesalamine granules (Apriso) was approved for use in the United States. Apriso delivers mesalamine to the terminal ileum and colon via a proprietary extended-release mechanism (Intellicor). The outer coating (Eudragit L) dissolves at a pH >6. In addition, there is a polymer matrix core that aids in sustained release throughout the colon. Since Lialda and Apriso are given once daily, an anticipated benefit is improved compliance compared with two to four daily doses required for other mesalamine preparations. Unencapsulated versions of mesalamine (Salofalk® Granu-Stix) have been in use in Europe for induction and maintenance of remission for several years.

Appropriate doses of Asacol and other 5-ASA compounds are shown in Table 295-7. Some 50–75% of patients with mild to moderate UC improve when treated with 5-ASA doses equivalent to 2 g/d of mesalamine; the dose response continues up to at least 4.8 g/d. As a general rule, 5-ASA agents act within 2–4 weeks. 5-ASA doses equivalent to 1.5–4 g/d of mesalamine maintain remission in 50–75% of patients with UC.

Topical mesalamine enemas are effective in mild-to-moderate distal UC. Clinical response occurs in up to 80% of UC patients with colitis distal to the splenic flexure. Combination therapy with mesalamine in both oral and enema form is more effective than either treatment alone for both distal and extensive UC. Mesalamine suppositories are effective in treating proctitis.

GLUCOCORTICOIDS The majority of patients with moderate-to-severe UC benefit from oral or parenteral glucocorticoids. Prednisone is usually started at doses of 40–60 mg/d for active UC that is unresponsive to 5-ASA therapy. Parenteral glucocorticoids may be administered as hydrocortisone, 300 mg/d, or methylprednisolone, 40–60 mg/d. Topically applied glucocorticoids are also beneficial for distal colitis and may serve as an adjunct in those who have rectal involvement plus more proximal disease. Hydrocortisone enemas or foam may control active disease, although they have no proven role as maintenance therapy. These glucocorticoids are significantly absorbed from the rectum and can lead to adrenal suppression with prolonged administration. Topical 5-ASA therapy is more effective than topical steroid therapy in the treatment of distal UC.

TABLE 295-7 Oral 5-ASA Preparations

Preparation	Formulation	Delivery	Dosing Per Day
Azo-Bond			
Sulfasalazine (500 mg) (Azulfidine)	Sulfapyridine-5-ASA	Colon	3–6 g (acute) 2–4 g (maintenance)
Olsalazine (250 mg) (Dipentum)	5-ASA-5-ASA	Colon	1–3 g
Balsalazide (750 mg) (Colazal)	Aminobenzoyl-alanine-5-ASA	Colon	6.75–9 g
Delayed-Release			
Mesalamine (400, 800 mg) (Asacol)	Eudragit S (pH 7)	Distal ileum-colon	2.4–4.8 g (acute) 1.6–4.8 g (maintenance)
Mesalamine (1.2 g) (Lialda)	MMX mesalamine (SPD476)	Ileum-colon	2.4–4.8 g
Controlled-Release			
Mesalamine (250, 500, 1000 mg) (Pentasa)	Ethylcellulose microgranules	Stomach-colon	2–4 g (acute) 1.5–4 g (maintenance)
Delayed and Extended-Release			
Mesalamine (.375 g) (Apriso)	Intellicor extended-release mechanism	Ileum-colon	1.5 g (maintenance)

Glucocorticoids are also effective for treatment of moderate-to-severe CD and induce a 60–70% remission rate compared to a 30% placebo response. The systemic effects of standard glucocorticoid formulations have led to the development of more potent formulations that are less well-absorbed and have increased first-pass metabolism. Controlled ileal-release budesonide has been nearly equal to prednisone for ileocolonic CD with fewer glucocorticoid side effects. Budesonide is used for 2–3 months at a dose of 9 mg/d, then tapered. Budesonide 6 mg/d is effective in reducing relapse rates at 3–6 months but not at 12 months in CD patients with a medically induced remission.

Glucocorticoids play no role in maintenance therapy in either UC or CD. Once clinical remission has been induced, they should be tapered according to the clinical activity, normally at a rate of no more than 5 mg/week. They can usually be tapered to 20 mg/d within 4–5 weeks but often take several months to be discontinued altogether. The side effects are numerous, including fluid retention, abdominal striae, fat redistribution, hyperglycemia, subcapsular cataracts, osteonecrosis, osteoporosis, myopathy, emotional disturbances, and withdrawal symptoms. Most of these side effects, aside from osteonecrosis, are related to the dose and duration of therapy.

ANTIBIOTICS Antibiotics have no role in the treatment of active or quiescent UC. However, pouchitis, which occurs in about a third of UC patients after colectomy and IPAA, usually responds to treatment with metronidazole and/or ciprofloxacin.

Metronidazole is effective in active inflammatory, fistulous, and perianal CD and may prevent recurrence after ileal resection. The most effective dose is 15–20 mg/kg per day in three divided doses; it is usually continued for several months. Common side effects include nausea, metallic taste, and disulfiram-like reaction. Peripheral neuropathy can occur with prolonged administration (several months) and on rare occasions is permanent despite discontinuation. Ciprofloxacin (500 mg bid) is also beneficial for inflammatory, perianal, and fistulous CD but has recently been associated with Achilles tendinitis and rupture. Both ciprofloxacin and metronidazole antibiotics can be used as first-line drugs for short periods of time in active inflammatory, fistulizing and perianal CD.

AZATHIOPRINE AND 6-MERCAPTOPURINE Azathioprine and 6-mercaptopurine (6-MP) are purine analogues commonly employed in the management of glucocorticoid-dependent IBD. Azathioprine is rapidly absorbed and converted to 6-MP, which is then metabolized to the active end product, thioinosinic acid, an inhibitor of purine ribonucleotide synthesis and cell proliferation. These agents also inhibit the immune response. Efficacy can be seen as early as 3–4 weeks but can take up to 4–6 months. Adherence can be monitored by measuring the levels of 6-thioguanine and 6-methyl-mercaptopurine, end products of 6-MP metabolism. Azathioprine (2–3 mg/kg per day) or 6-MP (1–1.5 mg/kg per day) have been employed successfully as glucocorticoid-sparing agents in up to two-thirds of UC and CD patients previously unable to be weaned from glucocorticoids. The role of these immunomodulators as maintenance therapy in UC and CD and for treating active perianal disease and fistulas in CD appears promising. In addition, 6-MP or azathioprine is effective for postoperative prophylaxis of CD.

Although azathioprine and 6-MP are usually well tolerated, pancreatitis occurs in 3–4% of patients, typically presents within the first few weeks of therapy, and is completely reversible when the drug is stopped. Other side effects include nausea, fever, rash, and hepatitis. Bone marrow suppression (particularly leukopenia) is dose-related and often delayed, necessitating regular monitoring of the complete blood cell count (CBC). Additionally, 1 in 300 individuals lacks thiopurine methyltransferase, the enzyme responsible for drug metabolism; an additional 11% of the population are heterozygotes with intermediate enzyme activity. Both are at increased risk of toxicity because of increased accumulation of thioguanine metabolites. Although 6-thioguanine and 6-methylmercaptopurine levels can be followed to determine correct drug dosing and reduce toxicity, weight-based dosing is an acceptable alternative. CBCs and liver function tests should be monitored frequently regardless of dosing strategy. IBD patients treated with azathioprine/6-MP are at a fourfold increased risk of developing a lymphoma. This increased risk could be a result of the medications, the underlying disease, or both.

METHOTREXATE Methotrexate (MTX) inhibits dihydrofolate reductase, resulting in impaired DNA synthesis. Additional anti-inflammatory properties may be related to decreased IL-1 production. Intramuscular (IM) or subcutaneous (SC) MTX (25 mg/week) is effective in inducing remission and reducing glucocorticoid dosage; 15 mg/week is effective in maintaining remission in active CD. Potential toxicities include leukopenia and hepatic fibrosis, necessitating periodic evaluation of CBCs and liver enzymes. The role of liver biopsy in patients on long-term MTX is uncertain but is probably limited to those with increased liver enzymes. Hypersensitivity pneumonitis is a rare but serious complication of therapy.

CYCLOSPORINE Cyclosporine (CSA) is a lipophilic peptide with inhibitory effects on both the cellular and humoral immune systems. CSA blocks the production of IL-2 by T-helper lymphocytes. CSA binds to cyclophilin, and this complex inhibits calcineurin, a cytoplasmic phosphatase enzyme involved in the activation of T cells. CSA also indirectly inhibits B cell function by blocking helper T cells. CSA has a more rapid onset of action than 6-MP and azathioprine.

CSA is most effective when given at 2–4 mg/kg per day IV in severe UC that is refractory to IV glucocorticoids, with 82% of patients responding. CSA can be an alternative to colectomy. The long-term success of oral CSA is not as dramatic, but if patients are started on 6-MP or azathioprine at the time of hospital discharge, remission can be maintained. For the 2 mg/kg dose, levels as measured by monoclonal radioimmunoassay or by the high performance liquid chromatography assay should be maintained between 150 and 350 ng/mL.

CSA may cause significant toxicity; renal function should be monitored frequently. Hypertension, gingival hyperplasia, hypertrichosis, paresthesias, tremors, headaches, and electrolyte abnormalities are common side effects. Creatinine elevation calls for dose reduction or discontinuation. Seizures may also complicate therapy, especially if the patient is hypomagnesemic or if serum cholesterol levels are <3.1 mmol/L (<120 mg/dL). Opportunistic infections, most notably *Pneumocystis carinii* pneumonia, may occur with combination immunosuppressive treatment; prophylaxis should be given. Major adverse events occurred in 15% of patients in one large study including nephrotoxicity not responding to dose adjustment, serious infections, seizures, anaphylaxis, and death of two patients. This high incidence suggests that vigorous monitoring by experienced clinicians at tertiary care centers may be required.

TACROLIMUS Tacrolimus is a macrolide antibiotic with immunomodulatory properties similar to CSA. It is 100 times as potent as CSA and is not dependent on bile or mucosal integrity for absorption. These pharmacologic properties enable tacrolimus to have good oral absorption despite proximal small bowel Crohn's involvement. It has shown efficacy in children with refractory IBD and in adults with extensive involvement of the small bowel. It is also effective in adults with steroid-dependent or refractory UC and CD as well as refractory fistulizing CD.

BIOLOGIC THERAPIES Biologic therapy is often reserved for moderately to severely ill patients with Crohn's disease, who have failed other therapies. Patients who respond to biologic therapies enjoy an improvement in clinical symptoms, a better quality of life, less disability, fatigue and depression, and fewer surgeries and hospitalizations.

Anti-TNF Therapy The first biologic therapy approved for Crohn's disease was infliximab, a chimeric IgG1 antibody against TNF-alpha, which is now also approved for treatment of moderately to severely active ulcerative colitis. Of active CD patients refractory to glucocorticoids, 6-MP, or 5-ASA, 65% will respond to IV infliximab (5 mg/kg); one-third will enter complete remission. The ACCENT I (A Crohn's Disease Clinical Trial Evaluating Infliximab in a New Long Term Treatment Regimen) study showed that of the patients who experience an initial response, 40% of these will maintain remission for at least 1 year with repeated infusions of infliximab every 8 weeks.

Infliximab is also effective in CD patients with refractory perianal and enterocutaneous fistulas, with the ACCENT II trial showing a 68% response rate (50% reduction in fistula drainage) and a 50% complete remission rate. Reinfusion, typically every 8 weeks, is necessary to continue therapeutic benefits in many patients.

The development of antibodies to infliximab (ATI) is associated with an increased risk of infusion reactions and a decreased response to treatment. Current practice does not include giving on-demand or episodic infusions rather than periodic (every 8 weeks) infusions because patients are more likely to develop ATI. ATI are generally present when the quality of response or the response duration to infliximab infusion decreases. Decreasing the dosing intervals or increasing the dosage to 10 mg/kg may restore the efficacy of the drug.

The SONIC (Study of Biologic and Immunomodulator-Naïve Patients with Crohn's Disease) Trial compared infliximab plus azathioprine, infliximab alone and azathioprine alone in immunomodulator and biologic naïve patients with moderate-to-severe Crohn's disease. At one year, of 508 randomized patients, the infliximab plus azathioprine group exhibited a steroid-free remission rate of 46% compared with 35% (infliximab alone) and 24% (azathioprine alone). There was also increased complete mucosal healing at week 26 with the combined approach relative to either infliximab or azathioprine alone (44% vs. 30% vs. 17%). The adverse events were equal between groups.

The annual risk of lymphoma (e.g., Hodgkin's and non-Hodgkin's lymphoma) with infliximab has been estimated to be anywhere from 5:10,000 to 20:10,000. The annual risk of lymphoma in the general population is 2:10,000. Forty-eight cases of malignancy were identified by the FDA in children and adolescents with the use of TNF blockers. Etanercept and infliximab were the only TNF blockers included in the analysis. Of the 48 cases, about 50% were lymphomas. Other malignancies such as leukemia, melanoma, and solid organ tumors were reported; malignancies rarely seen in children (e.g., leiomyosarcoma, hepatic malignancies, and renal cell carcinoma) were also observed. Of note, most of these cases (88%) were receiving other immunosuppressive medications (e.g., azathioprine and methotrexate).

Hepatosplenic T cell lymphoma is a nearly universally fatal lymphoma in patients with Crohn's disease. At least 12 cases involved immunomodulators alone, and 19 cases received combination therapy. There have been three reports in patients taking adalimumab alone without an immunomodulator. Patients tend to be young and almost all male.

The FDA also reviewed 147 postmarketing reports of leukemia (including acute myeloid leukemia, chronic lymphocytic leukemia, and chronic myeloid leukemia) and 69 cases of new-onset psoriasis (including pustular, palmoplantar) occurring in patients using TNF blockers. The FDA concluded that there is a possible association with both leukemia and new-onset psoriasis with the use of TNF blockers.

Other morbidities of infliximab include acute infusion reactions and severe serum sickness. All of the anti-TNF drugs are associated with an increased risk of infections, particularly reactivation of latent tuberculosis and opportunistic fungal infections including disseminated histoplasmosis and coccidioidomycosis. Rarely, infliximab and the other anti-TNF drugs have been associated with optic neuritis, seizures, new-onset or exacerbation of clinical symptoms, and radiographic evidence of central nervous system demyelinating disorders, including multiple sclerosis. They may exacerbate symptoms in patients with New York Heart Association functional class III/IV heart failure.

Infliximab has also shown efficacy in UC. In two large randomized, placebo-controlled trials, 37–49% of patients responded to infliximab and 22% and 20% of patients were able to maintain remission after 30 and 54 weeks, respectively. Patients received infliximab at 0, 2, and 6 weeks and then every 8 weeks until the end of the study.

Some patients losing response or not tolerating infliximab can be switched to adalimumab or certolizumab pegol. The GAIN (Gauging Infliximab Efficacy in Infliximab Non-Responders) trial evaluated patients who were previously treated with infliximab and became intolerant or who initially responded and lost response. Three-hundred and twenty-five patients were randomized to adalimumab or placebo. At 4 weeks, 21% of the adalimumab group and 7% of the placebo group were in remission. In clinical practice, this remission rate in the adalimumab group increases over time with a dose increase to 40 mg weekly instead of every other week.

Adalimumab is a recombinant human monoclonal IgG1 antibody containing only human peptide sequences and is injected subcutaneously. Adalimumab binds TNF and neutralizes its function by blocking the interaction between TNF and its cell-surface receptor. Therefore, it seems to have a similar mechanism of action to infliximab but with less immunogenicity. Adalimumab has been approved for treatment of moderate to severe CD. CHARM (Crohn's Trial of the Fully Human Adalimumab for Remission Maintenance) is an adalimumab maintenance study in patients who responded to adalimumab induction therapy. About 50% of the patients in this trial were previously treated with infliximab. Remission rates ranged from 42–48% of infliximab naïve patients at 1 year compared with remission rates of 31–34% in the patients who had previously received infliximab. Certolizumab pegol is a PEGylated form of an anti-TNF antibody administered SC once monthly. SC certolizumab pegol was effective for induction of clinical response in patients with active inflammatory CD. In the PRECISE II (The PEGylated Antibody Fragment Evaluation in Crohn's Disease) trial of maintenance therapy with certolizumab in patients who responded to certolizumab induction, the results were similar to the CHARM trial. At week 26, the subgroup of patients who were infliximab naïve had a response of 69% as compared to 44% in patients who had previously received infliximab.

At least one-third of patients do not respond to infliximab, but no published controlled trial has examined infliximab nonresponders for a response to other anti-TNF agents. If a patient does not have an initial response to any anti-TNF therapy, currently it must be considered futile to try another. Before the approval of natalizumab, the only option for this group of patients was surgery.

Natalizumab Integrins are expressed on the surface of leukocytes and serve as mediators of leukocyte adhesion to vascular endothelium. Alpha4 (α4) integrin along with its beta1 (β1) or beta7 (β7) subunit interact with endothelial ligands, termed adhesion molecules or vascular addressins. Interaction between α4β7 and mucosal addressin cellular adhesion molecule (MAdCAM-1) is important in lymphocyte tracking to gut mucosa. Natalizumab is a recombinant humanized immunoglobulin G4 antibody against α4 integrin that is effective in the induction and maintenance of remission in CD patients. It was approved February 2008 for the treatment of patients with CD refractory or intolerant to anti-TNF therapy. In the ENACT-2 (Evaluation of Natalizumab in Active Crohn's Disease Therapy) study, 354 patients who had a response to natalizumab in ENACT-1 were enrolled into maintenance therapy with an infusion of natalizumab or placebo every 4 weeks through week 56. Natalizumab patients were more likely to have a response (61% vs. 28% placebo) and remission 44% versus 26% placebo. However, 3 cases of progressive multifocal leukoencephalopathy (PML) associated with the JC polyoma virus in the clinical trials and 102 cases in the postmarketing setting have been reported to date. One case occurred in a patient with Crohn's disease and 104 in patients with multiple sclerosis. The annual risk of PML associated with natalizumab is approximately 1:1000. Patients and caregivers must now adhere to the TOUCH Treatment Program, which details strict criteria including no concomitant 6-MP, azathioprine or MTX, no glucocorticoids for longer than 6 months, the signing of consent forms and a monthly check by nurses for symptoms of PML.

THERAPIES IN DEVELOPMENT Other therapies currently in development include monoclonal antibodies against IL-12 and IL-23. IL-12, derived from intestinal antigen presenting cells, initiates T_H1 mediated inflammation. IL-23 is a cytokine composed of a unique p19 subunit together with the p40 subunit of IL-12, which is also upregulated in CD mucosa and promotes T_H17 cells and inhibits T regulatory cells. Therefore, both IL-12 and IL-23 biologic activity can be inhibited by neutralizing IL-12 p40 with specific antibodies. The discovery of IL-23R as an IBD susceptibility gene strengthens the case for the use of IL-23 directed immunotherapy in IBD. Clinical trials are under way. Other promising therapies included those directed at IL-6 and the class of selective adhesion molecule inhibitors (e.g., anti-α4β7 and anti-MadCAM1 antibodies).

NUTRITIONAL THERAPIES Dietary antigens may stimulate the mucosal immune response. Patients with active CD respond to bowel rest, along with TPN. Bowel rest and TPN are as effective as glucocorticoids at inducing remission of active CD but are not effective as maintenance therapy. Enteral nutrition in the form of elemental or peptide-based preparations is also as effective as glucocorticoids or TPN, but these diets are not palatable. Enteral diets may provide the small intestine with nutrients vital to cell growth and do not have the complications of TPN. In contrast to CD, dietary intervention does not reduce inflammation in UC. Standard medical management of UC and CD is shown in Fig. 295-10.

SURGICAL THERAPY

Ulcerative Colitis Nearly one-half of patients with extensive chronic UC undergo surgery within the first 10 years of their illness. The indications for surgery are listed in Table 295-8. Morbidity is about 20% in elective, 30% for urgent, and 40% for emergency proctocolectomy. The risks are primarily hemorrhage, contamination and sepsis, and neural injury. The operation of choice is an IPAA.

Because UC is a mucosal disease, the rectal mucosa can be dissected and removed down to the dentate line of the anus or about 2 cm proximal to this landmark. The ileum is fashioned into a pouch that serves as a neorectum. This ileal pouch is then

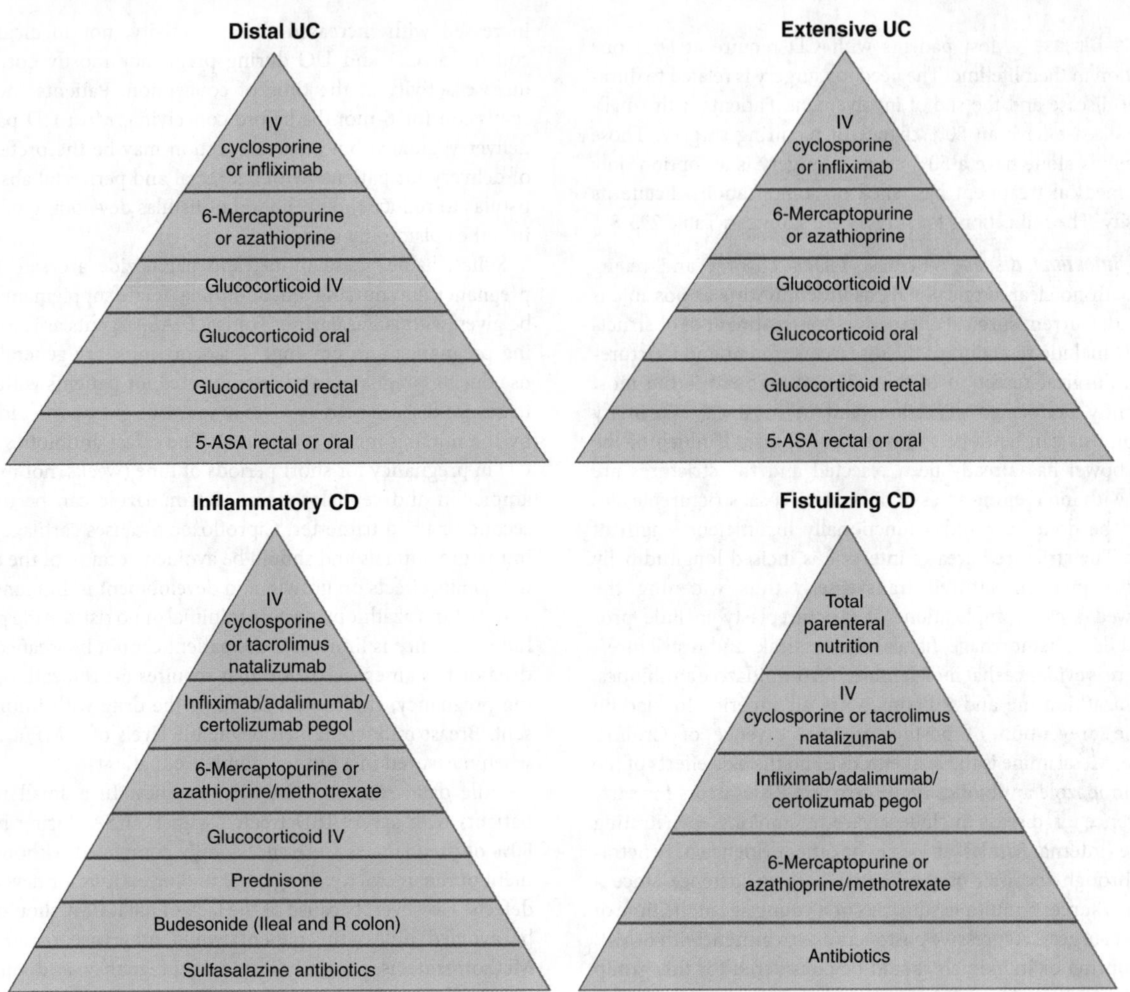

Figure 295-10 Medical management of IBD. 5-ASA, 5-aminosalicylic acid; CD, Crohn's disease; UC, ulcerative colitis.

TABLE 295-8 Indications for Surgery

Ulcerative Colitis	Crohn's Disease
Intractable disease	Small Intestine
Fulminant disease	Stricture and obstruction unresponsive to medical therapy
Toxic megacolon	Massive hemorrhage
Colonic perforation	Refractory fistula
Massive colonic hemorrhage	Abscess
Extracolonic disease	Colon and rectum
Colonic obstruction	Intractable disease
Colon cancer prophylaxis	Fulminant disease
Colon dysplasia or cancer	Perianal disease unresponsive to medical therapy
	Refractory fistula
	Colonic obstruction
	Cancer prophylaxis
	Colon dysplasia or cancer

sutured circumferentially to the anus in an end-to-end fashion. If performed carefully, this operation preserves the anal sphincter and maintains continence. The overall operative morbidity is 10%, with the major complication being bowel obstruction. Pouch failure necessitating conversion to permanent ileostomy occurs in 5–10% of patients. Some inflamed rectal mucosa is usually left behind, and thus endoscopic surveillance is necessary. Primary dysplasia of the ileal mucosa of the pouch has occurred rarely.

Patients with IPAA usually have about 6–10 bowel movements a day. On validated quality-of-life indices, they report better performance in sports and sexual activities than ileostomy patients. The most frequent complication of IPAA is pouchitis in about 30–50% of patients with UC. This syndrome consists of increased stool frequency, watery stools, cramping, urgency, nocturnal leakage of stool, arthralgias, malaise, and fever. Pouch biopsies may distinguish true pouchitis from underlying CD. Although pouchitis usually responds to antibiotics, 3–5% of patients remain refractory and may require steroids, immunomodulators, anti-TNF therapy or even pouch removal. A highly concentrated probiotic preparation with four strains of *Lactobacillus*, three strains of *Bifidobacterium*, and one strain of *Streptococcus salivarius* can prevent the recurrence of pouchitis when taken daily.

Crohn's Disease Most patients with CD require at least one operation in their lifetime. The need for surgery is related to duration of disease and the site of involvement. Patients with small-bowel disease have an 80% chance of requiring surgery. Those with colitis alone have a 50% chance. Surgery is an option only when medical treatment has failed or complications dictate its necessity. The indications for surgery are shown in Table 295-8.

Small intestinal disease Because CD is chronic and recurrent, with no clear surgical cure, as little intestine as possible is resected. Current surgical alternatives for treatment of obstructing CD include resection of the diseased segment and strictureplasty. Surgical resection of the diseased segment is the most frequently performed operation, and in most cases primary anastomosis can be done to restore continuity. If much of the small bowel has already been resected and the strictures are short, with intervening areas of normal mucosa, strictureplasties should be done to avoid a functionally insufficient length of bowel. The strictured area of intestine is incised longitudinally and the incision sutured transversely, thus widening the narrowed area. Complications of strictureplasty include prolonged ileus, hemorrhage, fistula, abscess, leak, and restricture.

There is evidence that mesalamine, nitro-imidazole antibiotics, 6-MP/azathioprine and infliximab are all superior to placebo for the prevention of postoperative recurrence of Crohn's disease. Mesalamine is the least effective and the side effects of the nitro-imidazole antibiotics limit their use. Risk factors for early recurrence of disease include cigarette smoking, penetrating disease (internal fistulas, abscesses or other evidence of penetration through the wall of the bowel), early recurrence since a previous surgery, multiple surgeries or a young age at the time of the first surgery. Aggressive postoperative treatment with 6-MP/azathioprine or infliximab should be considered for this group of patients. It is also recommended to evaluate for endoscopic recurrence of Crohn's disease via a colonoscopy, if possible, 6 months after surgery.

Colorectal disease A greater percentage of patients with Crohn's colitis require surgery for intractability, fulminant disease, and anorectal disease. Several alternatives are available, ranging from the use of a temporary loop ileostomy to resection of segments of diseased colon or even the entire colon and rectum. For patients with segmental involvement, segmental colon resection with primary anastomosis can be performed. In 20–25% of patients with extensive colitis, the rectum is spared sufficiently to consider rectal preservation. Most surgeons believe that an IPAA is contraindicated in CD due to the high incidence of pouch failure. A diverting colostomy may help heal severe perianal disease or rectovaginal fistulas, but disease almost always recurs with reanastomosis. These patients often require a total proctocolectomy and ileostomy.

INFLAMMATORY BOWEL DISEASE AND PREGNANCY

Patients with quiescent UC and CD have normal fertility rates; the fallopian tubes can be scarred by the inflammatory process of CD, especially on the right side because of the proximity of the terminal ileum. In addition, perirectal, perineal, and rectovaginal abscesses and fistulae can result in dyspareunia. Infertility in men can be caused by sulfasalazine but reverses when treatment is stopped. In women who have had pouch surgery, most studies show that the fertility rate is reduced to about one-third of normal. This is due to scarring or occlusion of the fallopian tubes secondary to pelvic inflammation.

In mild or quiescent UC and CD, fetal outcome is nearly normal. Spontaneous abortions, stillbirths, and developmental defects are increased with increased disease activity, not medications. The courses of CD and UC during pregnancy mostly correlate with disease activity at the time of conception. Patients should be in remission for 6 months before conceiving. Most CD patients can deliver vaginally, but cesarean section may be the preferred route of delivery for patients with anorectal and perirectal abscesses and fistulas to reduce the likelihood of fistulas developing or extending into the episiotomy scar.

Sulfasalazine, mesalamine, and balsalazide are safe for use in pregnancy and nursing, but additional folate supplementation must be given with sulfasalazine. Topical 5-ASA agents are also safe during pregnancy and nursing. Glucocorticoids are generally safe for use during pregnancy and are indicated for patients with moderate to severe disease activity. The amount of glucocorticoids received by the nursing infant is minimal. The safest antibiotics to use for CD in pregnancy for short periods of time (weeks, not months) are ampicillin and cephalosporin. Metronidazole can be used in the second or third trimester. Ciprofloxacin causes cartilage lesions in immature animals and should be avoided because of the absence of data on its effects on growth and development in humans.

6-MP and azathioprine pose minimal or no risk during pregnancy, but experience is limited. If the patient cannot be weaned from the drug or has an exacerbation that requires 6-MP/azathioprine during pregnancy, she should continue the drug with informed consent. Breast milk contained negligible levels of 6-MP/azathioprine when measured in a limited number of patients.

Little data exist on CSA in pregnancy. In a small number of patients with severe IBD treated with IV CSA during pregnancy, 80% of pregnancies were successfully completed without development of renal toxicity, congenital malformations, or developmental defects. However, because of the lack of data, CSA should probably be avoided unless the patient would otherwise require surgery. Methotrexate is contraindicated in pregnancy and nursing. No increased risk of stillbirths, miscarriages, or spontaneous abortions has been seen with infliximab, adalimumab or certolizumab, all class B drugs. The anti-TNF drugs are relatively safe in nursing as well because they do not pass into breast milk. Natalizumab is a class C drug, and there is limited data on pregnancy.

Surgery in UC should be performed only for emergency indications, including severe hemorrhage, perforation, and megacolon refractory to medical therapy. Total colectomy and ileostomy carry a 50–60% risk of postoperative spontaneous abortion. Fetal mortality is also high in CD requiring surgery. Patients with IPAAs have increased nighttime stool frequency during pregnancy that resolves postpartum. Transient small bowel obstruction or ileus has been noted in up to 8% of patients with ileostomies.

CANCER IN INFLAMMATORY BOWEL DISEASE

ULCERATIVE COLITIS

Patients with long-standing UC are at increased risk for developing colonic epithelial dysplasia and carcinoma (Fig. 295-11).

The risk of neoplasia in chronic UC increases with duration and extent of disease. The risk of cancer, as measured in tertiary referral centers, rises 0.5–1% per year after 8–10 years of disease in patients with pancolitis. The only prospective surveillance study reported a lower rate of cancer; 2.5% at 20 years of disease, 7.6% at 30 years of disease, and 10.8% at 40 years. The rates of colon cancer are higher than in the general population, and colonoscopic surveillance is the standard of care.

Annual or biennial colonoscopy with multiple biopsies is recommended for patients with >8–10 years of pancolitis or 12–15 years of left-sided colitis and has been widely employed to screen and survey for subsequent dysplasia and carcinoma. Risk factors for cancer in UC include long-duration disease, extensive

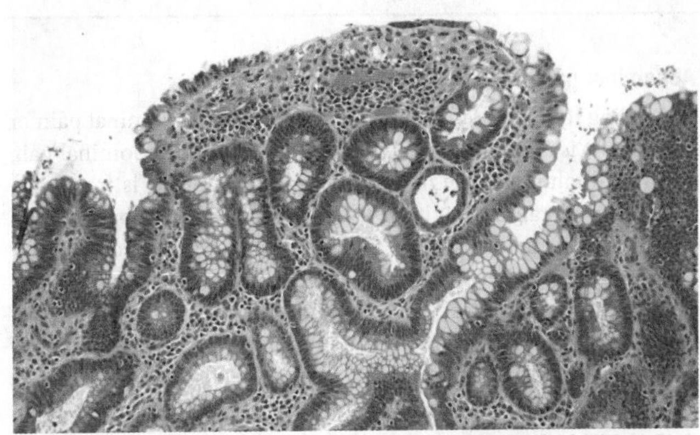

Figure 295-11 Medium power view of low-grade dysplasia in a patient with chronic ulcerative colitis. Low-grade dysplastic crypts are interspersed among regenerating crypts. *(Courtesy of Dr. R Odze, Division of Gastrointestinal Pathology, Department of Pathology, Brigham and Women's Hospital, Boston, Massachusetts; with permission.)*

disease, family history of colon cancer, PSC, a colon stricture, and the presence of postinflammatory pseudopolyps on colonoscopy.

■ CROHN'S DISEASE

Risk factors for developing cancer in Crohn's colitis are long-duration and extensive disease, bypassed colon segments, colon strictures, PSC, and family history of colon cancer. The cancer risks in CD and UC are probably equivalent for similar extent and duration of disease. In patients with extensive Crohn's colitis, the cumulative risk of detecting an initial finding of any definite dysplasia or cancer after a negative screening colonoscopy is 25% by the tenth surveillance examination. The cumulative risk of detecting an initial finding of flat high-grade dysplasia (HGD) or cancer after a negative screening colonoscopy is 7% by the ninth surveillance examination. Thus, the same endoscopic surveillance strategy used for UC is recommended for patients with chronic Crohn's colitis. A pediatric colonoscope can be used to pass narrow strictures in CD patients, but surgery should be considered in symptomatic patients with impassable strictures.

■ MANAGEMENT OF DYSPLASIA AND CANCER

Dysplasia can be flat or polypoid. If flat HGD is encountered on colonoscopic surveillance, the usual treatment for UC is colectomy and for CD is either colectomy or segmental resection. If flat low-grade dysplasia (LGD) is found (Fig. 295-11), most investigators recommend immediate colectomy. Adenomas may occur coincidently in UC and CD patients with chronic colitis and can be removed endoscopically provided that biopsies of the surrounding mucosa are free of dysplasia. New techniques such as high definition and magnification colonoscopes and dye sprays have increased the rate of dysplasia detection. In the future, endoscopists may be able to do targeted rather than segmental biopsies in patients with chronic Crohn's or ulcerative colitis.

IBD patients are also at greater risk for other malignancies. Patients with CD may have an increased risk of non-Hodgkin's lymphoma, leukemia, and myelodysplastic syndromes. Severe chronic, complicated perianal disease in CD patients may be associated with an increased risk of cancer in the lower rectum and anal canal (squamous cell cancers). Although the absolute risk of small-bowel adenocarcinoma in CD is low (2.2% at 25 years in one study), patients with long-standing, extensive, small-bowel disease should consider screening.

FURTHER READINGS

Farraye FA et al: AGA medical position statement on the diagnosis and management of colorectal neoplasia in inflammatory bowel disease. Gastroenterology 138:738, 2010

Colombel JF et al: Infliximab, azathioprine, or combination therapy for Crohn's disease. N Engl J Med 362:1383, 2010

Glocker EO et al: Inflammatory bowel disease and mutations affecting the interleukin-10 receptor. N Engl J Med 361:2033, 2009

Kane SV, Acquah LA: Placental transport of immunoglobulins: A clinical review for gastroenterologists who prescribe therapeutic monoclonal antibodies to women during conception and pregnancy. Am J Gastroenterol 104:228, 2009

Kaser A et al: Inflammatory bowel disease. Annu Rev Immunol 28:573, 2010

Kornbluth A, Sachar DB: Ulcerative colitis practice guidelines in adults: American College of Gastroenterology, Practice Parameters Committee. Am J Gastroenterol 105:501, 2010

Lichtenstein GR et al: Practice Parameters Committee of American College of Gastroenterology. Management of Crohn's disease in adults. Am J Gastroenterol 104:465, 2009

Moscandrew ME, Loftus EV Jr: Diagnostic advances in inflammatory bowel disease (imaging and laboratory). Curr Gastroenterol Rep 11:488, 2009

Rutgeerts P et al: Biological therapies for inflammatory bowel diseases. Gastroenterology 136:1182, 2009

Rutter MD et al: Thirty-year analysis of a colonoscopic surveillance program for neoplasia in ulcerative colitis. Gastroenterology 130:1030, 2006

Targan SR et al: International Efficacy of Natalizumab in Crohn's Disease Response and Remission (ENCORE) Trial Group. Natalizumab for the treatment of active Crohn's disease: Results of the ENCORE Trial. Gastroenterology 132:1672, 2007

CHAPTER 296 Irritable Bowel Syndrome

Chung Owyang

Irritable bowel syndrome (IBS) is a functional bowel disorder characterized by abdominal pain or discomfort and altered bowel habits in the absence of detectable structural abnormalities. No clear diagnostic markers exist for IBS, thus the diagnosis of the disorder is based on clinical presentation. In 2006, the Rome II criteria for the diagnosis of IBS were revised (Table 296-1). Throughout the world, about 10–20% of adults and adolescents have symptoms consistent with IBS, and most studies show a female predominance. IBS symptoms tend to come and go over time and often overlap with other functional disorders such as fibromyalgia, headache, backache, and genitourinary symptoms. Severity of symptoms varies and can significantly impair quality of life, resulting in high health care costs. Advances in basic, mechanistic, and clinical investigations have improved our understanding of this disorder and its physiologic and psychosocial determinants. Altered gastrointestinal (GI) motility, visceral hyperalgesia, disturbance of brain-gut interaction, abnormal central processing, autonomic and hormonal events, genetic and environmental factors, and psychosocial disturbances are variably involved, depending on the individual. This progress may result in improved methods of treatment.

CLINICAL FEATURES

IBS is a disorder that affects all ages, although most patients have their first symptoms before age 45. Older individuals have a lower reporting frequency. Women are diagnosed with IBS two to three times as often as men and make up 80% of the population with severe IBS. As indicated in Table 296-1, pain or abdominal discomfort is a key symptom for the diagnosis of IBS. These symptoms should be improved with defecation and/or have their onset associated with a change in frequency or form of stool. Painless diarrhea or constipation does not fulfill the diagnostic criteria to be classified as IBS. Supportive symptoms that are not part of the diagnostic criteria include defecation straining, urgency or a feeling of incomplete bowel movement, passing mucus, and bloating.

TABLE 296-1 Diagnostic Criteria for Irritable Bowel Syndrome[a]

Recurrent abdominal pain or discomfort[b] at least 3 days per month in the last 3 months associated with *two or more* of the following:

1. Improvement with defecation
2. Onset associated with a change in frequency of stool
3. Onset associated with a change in form (appearance) of stool

[a]Criteria fulfilled for the last 3 months with symptom onset at least 6 months prior to diagnosis.

[b]Discomfort means an uncomfortable sensation not described as pain. In pathophysiology research and clinical trials, a pain/discomfort frequency of at least 2 days a week during screening evaluation is required for subject eligibility.

Source: Adapted from Longstreth et al.

Abdominal pain

According to the current IBS diagnostic criteria, abdominal pain or discomfort is a prerequisite clinical feature of IBS. Abdominal pain in IBS is highly variable in intensity and location. It is frequently episodic and crampy, but it may be superimposed on a background of constant ache. Pain may be mild enough to be ignored or it may interfere with daily activities. Despite this, malnutrition due to inadequate caloric intake is exceedingly rare with IBS. Sleep deprivation is also unusual because abdominal pain is almost uniformly present only during waking hours. However, patients with severe IBS frequently wake repeatedly during the night; thus, nocturnal pain is a poor discriminating factor between organic and functional bowel disease. Pain is often exacerbated by eating or emotional stress and improved by passage of flatus or stools. In addition, female patients with IBS commonly report worsening symptoms during the premenstrual and menstrual phases.

Altered bowel habits

Alteration in bowel habits is the most consistent clinical feature in IBS. The most common pattern is constipation alternating with diarrhea, usually with one of these symptoms predominating. At first, constipation may be episodic, but eventually it becomes continuous and increasingly intractable to treatment with laxatives. Stools are usually hard with narrowed caliber, possibly reflecting excessive dehydration caused by prolonged colonic retention and spasm. Most patients also experience a sense of incomplete evacuation, thus leading to repeated attempts at defecation in a short time span. Patients whose predominant symptom is constipation may have weeks or months of constipation interrupted with brief periods of diarrhea. In other patients, diarrhea may be the predominant symptom. Diarrhea resulting from IBS usually consists of small volumes of loose stools. Most patients have stool volumes of <200 mL. Nocturnal diarrhea does not occur in IBS. Diarrhea may be aggravated by emotional stress or eating. Stool may be accompanied by passage of large amounts of mucus. Bleeding is not a feature of IBS unless hemorrhoids are present, and malabsorption or weight loss does not occur.

Bowel pattern subtypes are highly unstable. In a patient population with ~33% prevalence rates of IBS-diarrhea predominant (IBS-D), IBS-constipation predominant (IBS-C), and IBS-mixed (IBS-M) forms, 75% of patients change subtypes and 29% switch between IBS-C and IBS-D over 1 year. The heterogeneity and variable natural history of bowel habits in IBS increase the difficulty of conducting pathophysiology studies and clinical trials.

Gas and flatulence

Patients with IBS frequently complain of abdominal distention and increased belching or flatulence, all of which they attribute to increased gas. Although some patients with these symptoms actually may have a larger amount of gas, quantitative measurements reveal that most patients who complain of increased gas generate no more than a normal amount of intestinal gas. Most IBS patients have impaired transit and tolerance of intestinal gas loads. In addition, patients with IBS tend to reflux gas from the distal to the more proximal intestine, which may explain the belching.

Some patients with bloating may also experience visible distention with increase in abdominal girth. Both symptoms are more common among female patients and in those with higher overall Somatic Symptom Checklist scores. IBS patients who experienced bloating alone have been shown to have lower thresholds for pain and desire to defecate compared to those with concomitant distention irrespective of bowel habit. When patients were grouped according to sensory threshold, hyposensitive individuals had distention significantly more than those with hypersensitivity and this was observed more in the constipation subgroup. This suggests that the pathogenesis of bloating and distention may not be the same.

Upper gastrointestinal symptoms

Between 25 and 50% of patients with IBS complain of dyspepsia, heartburn, nausea, and vomiting. This suggests that other areas of the gut apart from the colon may be involved. Prolonged ambulant recordings of small-bowel motility in patients with IBS show a high incidence of abnormalities in the small bowel during the diurnal (waking) period; nocturnal motor patterns are not different from those of healthy controls. The overlap between dyspepsia and IBS is great. The prevalence of IBS is higher among patients with dyspepsia (31.7%) than among those who reported no symptoms of dyspepsia (7.9%). Conversely, among patients with IBS, 55.6% reported symptoms of dyspepsia. In addition, the functional abdominal symptoms can change over time. Those with predominant dyspepsia or IBS can flux between the two. Although the prevalence of functional gastrointestinal disorders is stable over time, the turnover in symptom status is high. Many episodes of symptom disappearance are due to subjects changing symptoms rather than total symptom resolution. Thus it is conceivable that functional dyspepsia and IBS are two manifestations of a single, more extensive digestive system disorder. Furthermore, IBS symptoms are prevalent in noncardiac chest pain patients, suggesting overlap with other functional gut disorders.

■ PATHOPHYSIOLOGY

The pathogenesis of IBS is poorly understood, although roles of abnormal gut motor and sensory activity, central neural dysfunction, psychological disturbances, mucosal inflammation, stress, and luminal factors have been proposed.

Gastrointestinal motor abnormalities

Studies of colonic myoelectrical and motor activity under unstimulated conditions have not shown consistent abnormalities in IBS. In contrast, colonic motor abnormalities are more prominent under stimulated conditions in IBS. IBS patients may exhibit increased rectosigmoid motor activity for up to 3 h after eating. Similarly, inflation of rectal balloons both in IBS-D and IBS-C patients leads to marked and prolonged distention-evoked contractile activity. Recordings from the transverse, descending, and sigmoid colon showed that the motility index and peak amplitude of high-amplitude propagating contractions (HAPCs) in diarrhea-prone IBS patients were greatly increased compared to those in healthy subjects and were associated with rapid colonic transit and accompanied by abdominal pain.

Visceral hypersensitivity

As with studies of motor activity, IBS patients frequently exhibit exaggerated sensory responses to visceral stimulation. Postprandial pain has been temporally related to entry of the food bolus into the cecum in 74% of patients. Rectal balloon inflation produces nonpainful and painful sensations at lower volumes in IBS patients than in healthy controls without altering rectal tension, suggestive of visceral afferent dysfunction in IBS. Similar studies show gastric and esophageal hypersensitivity in patients with nonulcer dyspepsia and noncardiac chest pain, raising the possibility that these conditions have a similar pathophysiologic basis. Lipids lower the thresholds for the first sensation of gas, discomfort, and pain in IBS patients. Hence, postprandial symptoms in IBS patients may be explained in part by a nutrient-dependent exaggerated sensory component of the gastrocolonic response. In contrast to enhanced gut sensitivity, IBS patients do not exhibit heightened sensitivity elsewhere in the body. Thus, the afferent pathway disturbances in IBS appear to be selective for visceral innervation with sparing of somatic pathways. The mechanisms responsible for visceral hypersensitivity are still under investigation. It has been proposed that these exaggerated responses may be due to (1) increased end-organ sensitivity with recruitment of "silent" nociceptors; (2) spinal hyperexcitability with activation of nitric oxide and possibly other neurotransmitters; (3) endogenous (cortical and brainstem) modulation of caudad nociceptive transmission; and (4) over time, the possible development of long-term hyperalgesia due to development of neuroplasticity, resulting in permanent or semipermanent changes in neural responses to chronic or recurrent visceral stimulation (Table 296-2).

TABLE 296-2 Proposed Mechanisms for Visceral Hypersensitivity

End-organ sensitivity	Long-term hyperalgesia
"Silent" nociceptors	Tonic cortical regulation
CNS modulation	Neuroplasticity
Cortex	
Brainstem	

Abbreviation: CNS, central nervous system.

Central neural dysregulation

The role of central nervous system (CNS) factors in the pathogenesis of IBS is strongly suggested by the clinical association of emotional disorders and stress with symptom exacerbation and the therapeutic response to therapies that act on cerebral cortical sites. Functional brain imaging studies such as MRI have shown that in response to distal colonic stimulation, the mid-cingulate cortex—a brain region concerned with attention processes and response selection—shows greater activation in IBS patients. Modulation of this region is associated with changes in the subjective unpleasantness of pain. In addition, IBS patients also show preferential activation of the prefrontal lobe, which contains a vigilance network within the brain that increases alertness. These may represent a form of cerebral dysfunction leading to the increased perception of visceral pain.

Abnormal psychological features

Abnormal psychiatric features are recorded in up to 80% of IBS patients, especially in referral centers; however, no single psychiatric diagnosis predominates. Most of these patients demonstrated exaggerated symptoms in response to visceral distention, and this abnormality persists even after exclusion of psychological factors.

Psychological factors influence pain thresholds in IBS patients, as stress alters sensory thresholds. An association between prior sexual or physical abuse and development of IBS has been reported. Abuse is associated with greater pain reporting, psychological distress, and poor health outcome. Brain functional MRI studies show greater activation of the posterior and middle dorsal cingulate cortex, which is implicated in affect processing in IBS patients with a past history of sexual abuse.

Thus, patients with IBS frequently demonstrate increased motor reactivity of the colon and small bowel to a variety of stimuli and altered visceral sensation associated with lowered sensation thresholds. These may result from CNS—enteric nervous system dysregulation (Fig. 296-1).

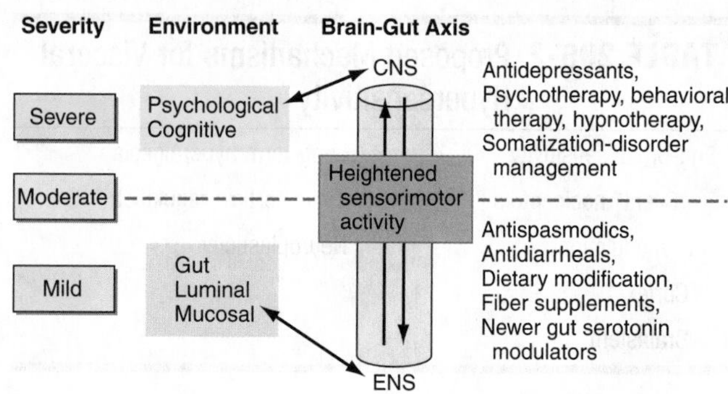

Figure 296-1 Therapeutic targets for irritable bowel syndrome. Patients with mild to moderate symptoms usually have intermittent symptoms that correlate with altered gut physiology. Treatments include gut-acting pharmacologic agents such as antispasmodics, antidiarrheals, fiber supplements, and gut serotonin modulators. Patients who have severe symptoms usually have constant pain and psychosocial difficulties. This group of patients is best managed with antidepressants and other psychosocial treatments. CNS, central nervous system; ENS, enteric nervous system.

Post-infectious IBS

IBS may be induced by GI infection. In an investigation of 544 patients with confirmed bacterial gastroenteritis, one-quarter developed IBS subsequently. Conversely, about a third of IBS patients experienced an acute "gastroenteritis-like" illness at the onset of their chronic IBS symptomatology. This group of "postinfective" IBS occurs more commonly in females and affects younger rather than older patients. Risk factors for developing post-infectious IBS include, in order of importance, prolonged duration of initial illness, toxicity of infecting bacterial strain, smoking, mucosal markers of inflammation, female gender, depression, hypochondriasis, and adverse-life events in the preceding 3 months. Age older than 60 years might protect against post-infectious IBS, whereas treatment with antibiotics has been associated with increased risk. The microbes involved in the initial infection are *Campylobacter*, *Salmonella*, and *Shigella*. Those patients with *Campylobacter* infection who are toxin-positive are more likely to develop postinfective IBS. Increased rectal mucosal enteroendocrine cells, T lymphocytes, and increased gut permeability are acute changes following *Campylobacter* enteritis that could persist for more than a year and may contribute to postinfective IBS.

Immune activation and mucosal inflammation

Some patients with IBS display persistent signs of low-grade mucosal inflammation with activated lymphocytes, mast cells, and enhanced expression of proinflammatory cytokines. These abnormalities may contribute to abnormal epithelial secretion and visceral hypersensitivity. Interestingly, clinical studies have shown increased intestinal permeability in patients with IBS-D. Psychological stress and anxiety can increase the release of proinflammatory cytokine and this in turn may alter intestinal permeability. This provides a functional link between psychological stress, immune activation, and symptom generation in patients with IBS.

Altered gut flora

A high prevalence of small intestinal bacterial overgrowth in IBS patients has been noted based on positive lactulose hydrogen breath test. This finding, however, has been challenged by a number of other studies that found no increased incidence of bacterial overgrowth based on jejunal aspirate culture. Abnormal H_2 breath test can occur because of small bowel rapid transit and may lead to erroneous interpretation. Hence, the role of testing for small intestinal bacterial overgrowth in IBS patients remains unclear.

A number of studies found significant differences between the molecular profile of the fecal microbiota of IBS patients compared with that of healthy subjects. Several bacterial genera with *Lactobacillus* sequence appear to be absent from IBS, and *Collinsella* sequences were greatly reduced in this group of patients. Currently it is unclear whether such changes are causal, consequential, or merely the result of constipation and diarrhea. In addition, the stability of the changes in the microbiota needs to be determined.

Abnormal serotonin pathways

The serotonin (5HT)-containing enterochromaffin cells in the colon are increased in a subset of IBS-D patients compared to healthy individuals or patients with ulcerative colitis. Furthermore, postprandial plasma 5HT levels were significantly higher in this group of patients compared to healthy controls. Since serotonin plays an important role in the regulation of GI motility and visceral perception, the increased release of serotonin may contribute to the postprandial symptoms of these patients and provides a rationale for the use of serotonin antagonists in the treatment of this disorder.

APPROACH TO THE PATIENT Irritable Bowel Syndrome

Because IBS is a disorder for which no pathognomonic abnormalities have been identified, its diagnosis relies on recognition of positive clinical features and elimination of other organic diseases. A careful history and physical examination are frequently helpful in establishing the diagnosis. Clinical features suggestive of IBS include the following: recurrence of lower abdominal pain with altered bowel habits over a period of time without progressive deterioration, onset of symptoms during periods of stress or emotional upset, absence of other systemic symptoms such as fever and weight loss, and small-volume stool without any evidence of blood.

On the other hand, the appearance of the disorder for the first time in old age, progressive course from time of onset, persistent diarrhea after a 48-h fast, and presence of nocturnal diarrhea or steatorrheal stools argue against the diagnosis of IBS.

Because the major symptoms of IBS—abdominal pain, abdominal bloating, and alteration in bowel habits—are common complaints of many GI organic disorders, the list of differential diagnoses is a long one. The quality, location, and timing of pain may be helpful to suggest specific disorders. Pain due to IBS that occurs in the epigastric or periumbilical area must be differentiated from biliary tract disease, peptic ulcer disorders, intestinal ischemia, and carcinoma of the stomach and pancreas. If pain occurs mainly in the lower abdomen, the possibility of diverticular disease of the colon, inflammatory bowel disease (including ulcerative colitis and Crohn's disease), and carcinoma of the colon must be considered. Postprandial pain accompanied by bloating, nausea, and vomiting suggests gastroparesis or partial intestinal obstruction. Intestinal infestation with *Giardia lamblia* or other parasites may cause similar symptoms. When diarrhea is the major complaint, the possibility of lactase deficiency, laxative abuse, malabsorption, celiac sprue, hyperthyroidism, inflammatory bowel disease, and infectious diarrhea must be ruled out. On the other hand, constipation may be a side effect of many different drugs, such as anticholinergic, antihypertensive, and antidepressant medications. Endocrinopathies such as hypothyroidism and hypoparathyroidism must also be considered in the differential diagnosis of constipation, particularly if other systemic signs or symptoms of these endocrinopathies are present. In addition, acute intermittent porphyria and lead poisoning may present in a fashion similar to IBS, with painful constipation as the major complaint. These possibilities are suspected on the basis of their clinical presentations and are confirmed by appropriate serum and urine tests.

Few tests are required for patients who have typical IBS symptoms and no alarm features. Unnecessary investigations may be costly and even harmful. The American Gastroenterological Association has delineated factors to be considered when determining the aggressiveness of the diagnostic evaluation. These include the duration of symptoms, the change in symptoms over time, the age and sex of the patient, the referral status of the patient, prior diagnostic studies, a family history of colorectal malignancy, and the degree of psychosocial dysfunction. Thus, a younger individual with mild symptoms requires a minimal diagnostic evaluation, while an older person or an individual with rapidly progressive symptoms should undergo a more thorough exclusion of organic disease. Most patients should have a complete blood count and sigmoidoscopic examination; in addition, stool specimens should be examined for ova and parasites in those who have diarrhea. In patients with persistent diarrhea not responding to simple anti-diarrhea agents, a sigmoid colon biopsy should be performed to rule out microscopic colitis. In those aged >40 years, an air-contrast barium enema or colonoscopy should also be performed. If the main symptoms are diarrhea and increased gas, the possibility of lactase deficiency should be ruled out with a hydrogen breath test or with evaluation after a 3-week lactose-free diet. Some patients with IBS-D may have undiagnosed celiac sprue. Because the symptoms of celiac sprue respond to a gluten-free diet, testing for celiac sprue in IBS may prevent years of morbidity and attendant expense. Decision-analysis studies show that serology testing for celiac sprue in patients with IBS-D has an acceptable cost when the prevalence of celiac sprue is >1% and is the dominant strategy when the prevalence is >8%. In patients with concurrent symptoms of dyspepsia, upper GI radiographs or esophagogastroduodenoscopy may be advisable. In patients with postprandial right upper quadrant pain, an ultrasonogram of the gallbladder should be obtained. Laboratory features that argue against IBS include evidence of anemia, elevated sedimentation rate, presence of leukocytes or blood in stool, and stool volume >200–300 mL/d. These findings would necessitate other diagnostic considerations.

TREATMENT Irritable Bowel Syndrome

PATIENT COUNSELING AND DIETARY ALTERATIONS Reassurance and careful explanation of the functional nature of the disorder and of how to avoid obvious food precipitants are important first steps in patient counseling and dietary change. Occasionally, a meticulous dietary history may reveal substances (such as coffee, disaccharides, legumes, and cabbage) that aggravate symptoms. Excessive fructose and artificial sweeteners, such as sorbitol or mannitol, may cause diarrhea, bloating, cramping or flatulence. As a therapeutic trial, patients should be encouraged to eliminate any foodstuffs that appear to produce symptoms. However patients should avoid nutritionally depleted diets. Patients with IBS-D anecdotally report symptom improvement after initiating a low-carbohydrate diet. A prospective study has shown marked symptomatic improvement in stool frequency, consistency, pain scores, and quality of life following 4 weeks of a very-low-carbohydrate (CHO) diet (20 g CHO/day). This diet may be tried in IBS patients who report intolerance to certain carbohydrates.

Stool-Bulking Agents High-fiber diets and bulking agents, such as bran or hydrophilic colloid, are frequently used in treating IBS. The water-holding action of fibers may contribute to increased stool bulk because of the ability of fiber to increase fecal output of bacteria. Fiber also speeds up colonic transit in most persons. In diarrhea-prone patients, whole-colonic transit is faster than average; however, dietary fiber can delay transit. Furthermore, because of their hydrophilic properties, stool-bulking agents bind water and thus prevent both excessive hydration and dehydration of stool. The latter observation may explain the clinical experience that a high-fiber diet relieves diarrhea in some IBS patients. Fiber supplementation with psyllium has been shown to reduce perception of rectal distention, indicating that fiber may have a positive effect on visceral afferent function.

The beneficial effects of dietary fiber on colonic physiology suggest that dietary fiber should be an effective treatment for IBS patients, but controlled trials of dietary fiber have produced variable results. This is not surprising since IBS is a heterogeneous disorder, with some patients being constipated and other having predominant diarrhea. Most investigations report increases in stool weight, decreases in colonic transit times, and improvement in constipation. Others have noted benefits in patients with alternating diarrhea and constipation, pain, and bloating. However, most studies observe no responses in patients with diarrhea- or pain-predominant IBS. It is possible that different fiber preparations may have dissimilar effects on selected symptoms in IBS. A cross-over comparison of different fiber preparations found that psyllium produced greater improvements in stool pattern and abdominal pain than bran. Furthermore, psyllium preparations tend to produce less bloating and distention. Despite the equivocal data regarding efficacy, most gastroenterologists consider stool-bulking agents worth trying in patients with IBS-C.

Antispasmodics Clinicians have observed that anticholinergic drugs may provide temporary relief for symptoms such as painful cramps related to intestinal spasm. Although controlled clinical trials have produced mixed results, evidence generally supports beneficial effects of anticholinergic drugs for pain. A meta-analysis of 26 double-blind clinical trials of antispasmodic agents in IBS reported better global improvement (62%) and abdominal pain reductions (64%) compared to placebo (35% and 45%, respectively), suggesting efficacy in some patients. The drugs are most effective when prescribed in anticipation of predictable pain. Physiologic studies demonstrate that anticholinergic drugs inhibit the gastrocolic reflex; hence, postprandial pain is best managed by giving antispasmodics 30 min before meals so that effective blood levels are achieved shortly before the anticipated onset of pain. Most anticholinergics contain natural belladonna alkaloids, which may cause xerostomia, urinary hesitancy and retention, blurred vision, and drowsiness. They should be used in the elderly with caution. Some physicians prefer to use synthetic anticholinergics such as dicyclomine that have less effect on mucous membrane secretions and produce fewer undesirable side effects.

Antidiarrheal Agents Peripherally acting opiate-based agents are the initial therapy of choice for IBS-D. Physiologic studies demonstrate increases in segmenting colonic contractions, delays in fecal transit, increases in anal pressures, and reductions in rectal perception with these drugs. When diarrhea is severe, especially in the painless diarrhea variant of IBS, small doses of loperamide, 2–4 mg every 4–6 h up to a maximum of 12 g/d, can be prescribed. These agents are less addictive than paregoric, codeine, or tincture of opium. In general, the intestines do not become tolerant of the antidiarrheal effect of opiates, and increasing doses are not required to maintain antidiarrheal potency. These agents are most useful if taken before anticipated stressful events that are known to cause diarrhea. However, not infrequently, a high dose of loperamide may cause cramping because of increases in segmenting colonic contractions. Another anti-diarrhea agent that may be used in IBS patients is the bile acid binder cholestyramine resin.

Antidepressant Drugs In addition to their mood-elevating effects, antidepressant medications have several physiologic effects that suggest they may be beneficial in IBS. In IBS-D patients, the tricyclic antidepressant imipramine slows jejunal migrating motor complex transit propagation and delays orocecal and whole-gut transit, indicative of a motor inhibitory effect. Some studies also suggest that tricyclic agents may alter visceral afferent neural function.

A number of studies indicate that tricyclic antidepressants may be effective in some IBS patients. In a 2-month study of desipramine, abdominal pain improved in 86% of patients compared to 59% given placebo. Another study of desipramine in 28 IBS patients showed improvement in stool frequency, diarrhea, pain, and depression. When stratified according to the predominant symptoms, improvements were observed in IBS-D patients, with no improvement being noted in IBS-C patients. The beneficial effects of the tricyclic compounds in the treatment of IBS appear to be independent of their effects on depression. The therapeutic benefits for the bowel symptoms occur faster and at a lower dosage. The efficacy of antidepressant agents in other chemical classes in the management of IBS is less well evaluated. In contrast to tricyclic agents, the selective serotonin reuptake inhibitor (SSRI) paroxetine accelerates orocecal transit, raising the possibility that this drug class may be useful in IBS-C patients. The SSRI citalopram blunts perception of rectal distention and reduces the magnitude of the gastrocolonic response in healthy volunteers. A small placebo-controlled study of citalopram in IBS patients reported reductions in pain. However, these findings could not be confirmed in another randomized controlled trial which showed that citalopram at 20 mg/day for 4 weeks was not superior to placebo in treating non-depressed IBS patients. Hence, the efficacy of SSRIs in the treatment of IBS needs further confirmation.

Antiflatulence Therapy The management of excessive gas is seldom satisfactory, except when there is obvious aerophagia or disaccharidase deficiency. Patients should be advised to eat slowly and not chew gum or drink carbonated beverages. Bloating may decrease if an associated gut syndrome such as IBS or constipation is improved. If bloating is accompanied by diarrhea and worsens after ingesting dairy products, fresh fruits, vegetables, or juices, further investigation or a dietary exclusion trial may be worthwhile. Avoiding flatogenic foods, exercising, losing excess weight, and taking activated charcoal are safe but unproven remedies. Data regarding the use of surfactants such as simethicone are conflicting. Antibiotics may help in a subgroup of IBS patients with predominant symptoms of bloating. Beano, an over-the-counter oral β-glycosidase solution, may reduce rectal passage of gas without decreasing bloating and pain. Pancreatic enzymes reduce bloating, gas, and fullness during and after high-calorie, high-fat meal ingestion.

Modulation of Gut Flora Antibiotic treatment benefits a subset of IBS patients. In a double-blind randomized placebo controlled study, neomycin dosed at 500 mg twice daily for 10 days was more effective than placebo at improving symptom scores among IBS patients. The non-absorbed oral antibiotic rifaximin is the most thoroughly studied antibiotic for the treatment of IBS. Patients receiving rifaximin at a dose of 400 mg three times daily experienced substantial improvement of global IBS symptoms over placebo. Rifaximin is the only antibiotic with demonstrated sustained benefit beyond therapy cessation in IBS patients. The drug has a favorable safety and tolerability profile compared with systemic antibiotics. However, currently there is still insufficient data to recommend routine use of this antibiotic in the treatment of IBS.

Since altered colonic flora may contribute to the pathogenesis of IBS, this has led to great interest in using probiotics to naturally alter the flora. *Bifidobacterium infantis* 35624 showed significant improvement in the composite score for abdominal pain, bloating/distention, and/or bowel movement compared with placebo in two placebo-controlled trials. Currently, there are inadequate data to comment on the efficacy of other probiotics.

Serotonin Receptor Agonist and Antagonists Serotonin receptor antagonists have been evaluated as therapies for IBS-D. Serotonin acting on 5-HT3 receptors enhances the sensitivity of afferent neurons projecting from the gut. In humans, a 5-HT3 receptor antagonist such as alosetron reduces perception of painful visceral stimulation in IBS. It also induces rectal relaxation, increases rectal compliance, and delays colonic transit. Meta-analysis of 14 randomized controlled trials of alosetron or cilansetron showed that these antagonists are more effective than placebo in achieving global improvement in IBS symptoms and relief of abdominal pain and discomfort. These agents are more likely to cause constipation in IBS patients with diarrhea alternating with constipation. 0.2% of patients using $5HT_3$ antagonist developed ischemic colitis versus none in the control group. In postrelease surveillance, 84 cases of ischemic colitis were observed, including 44 cases that required surgery and 4 deaths. As a consequence, the medication was voluntarily withdrawn by the manufacturer in 2000. Alosetron has been reintroduced under a new risk-management program where patients have to sign a patient-physician agreement. This has significantly limited its usage.

Novel 5-HT4 receptor agonists such as tegaserod exhibit prokinetic activity by stimulating peristalsis. In IBS patients with constipation, tegaserod accelerated intestinal and ascending colon transit. Clinical trials involving >4000 IBS-C patients reported reductions in discomfort and improvements in constipation and bloating, compared to placebo. Diarrhea is the major side effect. However, tegaserod has been withdrawn from the market; a meta-analysis revealed an increase in serious cardiovascular events.

Chloride Channel Activators Lubiprostone is a bicyclic fatty acid that stimulates chloride channels in the apical membrane of intestinal epithelial cells. Chloride secretion induces passive movement of sodium and water into the bowel lumen and improves bowel function. Oral lubiprostone was effective in the treatment of patients with constipation-predominant IBS in large phase II and phase III randomized double-blinded placebo-controlled multicenter trials. Responses were significantly greater in patients receiving lubiprostone 8 μg twice daily for 3 months than in those receiving placebo. In general, the drug was quite well tolerated. The major side effects are nausea and diarrhea. Lubiprostone is a new class of compounds for treatment of chronic constipation with or without IBS.

TABLE 296-3 Spectrum of Severity in IBS

	Mild	Moderate	Severe
Clinical Features			
Prevalence	70%	25%	5%
Correlations with gut physiology	+++	++	+
Symptoms constant	0	+	+++
Psychosocial difficulties	0	+	+++
Health care issues	+	++	+++
Practice type	Primary	Specialty	Referral

SUMMARY The treatment strategy of IBS depends on the severity of the disorder (Table 296-3). Most of the IBS patients have mild symptoms. They are usually cared for in primary care practices, have little or no psychosocial difficulties, and do not seek health care often. Treatment usually involves education, reassurance, and dietary/lifestyle changes. A smaller portion have moderate symptoms that are usually intermittent and correlate with altered gut physiology, e.g., worsened with eating or stress and relieved by defecation. Treatments include gut-acting pharmacologic agents such as antispasmodics, antidiarrheals, fiber supplements, and the newer gut serotonin modulators (Table 296-4). A small proportion of IBS patients have severe and refractory symptoms, are usually seen in referral centers, and frequently have constant pain and psychosocial difficulties (Fig. 296-1). This group of patients is best managed with antidepressants and other psychological treatments (Table 296-4).

TABLE 296-4 Possible Drugs for a Dominant Symptom in IBS

Symptom	Drug	Dose
Diarrhea	Loperamide	2–4 mg when necessary/maximum 12 g/d
	Cholestyramine resin	4 g with meals
	Alosetron[a]	0.5–1 mg bid (for severe IBS, women)
Constipation	Psyllium husk	3–4 g bid with meals, then adjust
	Methylcellulose	2 g bid with meals, then adjust
	Calcium polycarbophil	1 g qd to qid
	Lactulose syrup	10–20 g bid
	70% sorbitol	15 mL bid
	Polyethylene glycol 3350	17 g in 250 mL water qd
	Lubiprostone (Amitiza)	24 mg bid
	Magnesium hydroxide	30–60 mL qd
Abdominal pain	Smooth-muscle relaxant	qd to qid ac
	Tricyclic antidepressants	Start 25–50 mg hs, then adjust
	Selective serotonin reuptake inhibitors	Begin small dose, increase as needed

[a]Available only in the United States.

Source: Adapted from Longstreth et al.

FURTHER READINGS

Ford AC et al: Efficacy of antidepressants and psychological therapies in irritable bowel syndrome: Systematic review and meta-analysis. Gut 58:367, 2009

——— et al: Yield of diagnostic tests for celiac disease in individuals with symptoms suggestive of irritable bowel syndrome. Arch Intern Med 169:651, 2009

Gershon MD, Jack J: The serotonin signaling system: From basic understanding to drug development for functional GI disorders. Gastroenterology 132:397, 2007

Kassinen A et al: The fecal microbiota of irritable bowel syndrome patients differs significantly from that of healthy subjects. Gastroenterology 133:24, 2007

Longstreth GF et al: Functional bowel disorders. Gastroenterology 130:1480, 2006

Mayer EA et al: Neuroimaging of the brain-gut axis: From basic understanding to treatment of functional GI disorders. Gastroenterology 131:1925, 2006

Owyang C: Irritable bowel syndrome, in *Textbook of Gastroenterology*, 5th ed, T Yamada (ed). Oxford, UK: Wiley-Blackwell, 2009, pp 1536–73

Preidis GA, Versalovic J: Targeting the human microbiome with antibiotics, probiotics, and prebiotics: Gastrocenterology enters the metagenomics era. Gastroenterology 136:2015, 2009

Spiller R, Garsed K: Postinfectious irritable bowel syndrome. Gastroenterology 136:1979, 2009

CHAPTER 297

Diverticular Disease and Common Anorectal Disorders

Susan L. Gearhart

DIVERTICULAR DISEASE

Incidence and epidemiology

Among Western populations, diverticulosis of the colon affects nearly one-half of individuals older than age 60 years. Fortunately, only 20% of patients with diverticulosis develop symptomatic disease. However, in the United States, diverticular disease results in >200,000 hospitalizations annually, making it the fifth most costly gastrointestinal disorder. The incidence of the disease is on the rise, mainly among young patients. The mean age at presentation of the disease is 59 years. Although the prevalence among females and males is similar, males tend to present at a younger age. Diverticulosis is rare in underdeveloped countries, where diets include more fiber and roughage. However, shortly following migration to the United States, immigrants will develop diverticular disease at the same rate as U.S. natives.

Anatomy and pathophysiology

Two types of diverticula occur in the intestine: true and false (or pseudodiverticula). A true diverticulum is a saclike herniation of the entire bowel wall, whereas a pseudodiverticulum involves only a protrusion of the mucosa through the muscularis propria of the colon (Fig. 297-1). The type of diverticulum affecting the colon is the pseudodiverticulum. The protrusion occurs at the point where the nutrient artery, or *vasa recti*, penetrates through the muscularis propria, resulting in a break in the integrity of the colonic wall. Diverticula commonly affect the sigmoid colon; only 5% of persons exhibit pancolonic diverticula. This anatomic restriction may be a result of the relative high-pressure zone within the muscular sigmoid colon. Thus, higher-amplitude contractions combined with constipated, high-fat-content stool within the sigmoid lumen results in the creation of these diverticula. *Diverticulitis* is inflammation of a diverticulum. The cause is not well understood and is probably multifactorial. The predominant theory is the retention of particulate material within the diverticular sac and the formation of a fecalith. Consequently, the vasa recti is either compressed or eroded, leading to either perforation or bleeding.

Presentation, evaluation, and management of diverticular bleeding

Hemorrhage from a colonic diverticulum is the most common cause of hematochezia in patients >60 years, yet only 20% of patients with diverticulosis will have gastrointestinal bleeding. Patients at increased risk for bleeding tend to be hypertensive, have atherosclerosis, and regularly use nonsteroidal anti-inflammatory agents. Most bleeds are self-limited and stop spontaneously with bowel rest. The lifetime risk of rebleeding is 25%.

Localization of diverticular bleeding should include colonoscopy, which may be both diagnostic and therapeutic in the management of mild to moderate diverticular bleeding. If the patient is stable, massive bleeding is best managed by angiography. Mesenteric angiography can localize the bleeding site and occlude the bleeding vessel successfully with a coil in 80% of cases. The patient can then be followed closely with repetitive colonoscopy, if necessary, looking for evidence of colonic ischemia. Alternatively, a segmental resection of the colon can be undertaken to eliminate the risk of further bleeding. This may be advantageous in patients on chronic blood thinners. However, with newer techniques of highly selective coil embolization, the rate of colonic ischemia is <10% and the risk of acute rebleeding is <25%. Long-term results (40 months) indicate that more than 50% of patients with acute diverticular bleeds have had definitive treatment with highly selective angiography.

As another alternative, a selective infusion of vasopressin can be given to stop the hemorrhage, although this has been associated with significant complications, including myocardial infarction and intestinal ischemia. Furthermore, bleeding recurs in 50% of patients once the infusion is stopped. Localization studies indicate that bleeding as a result of colonic diverticulosis is more often seen

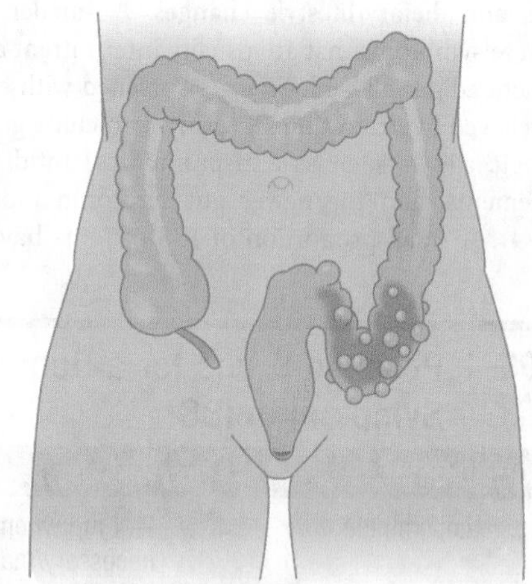

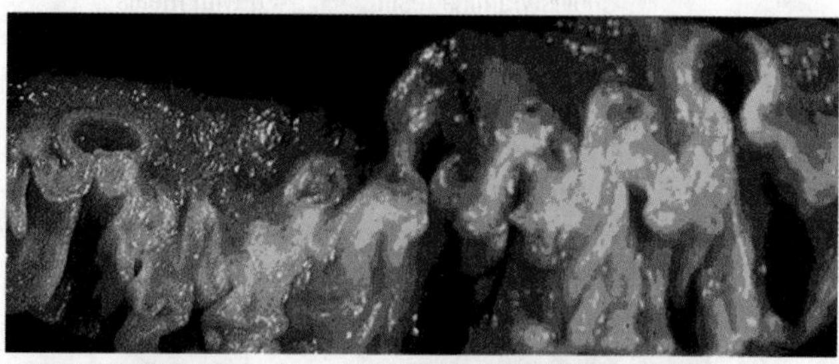

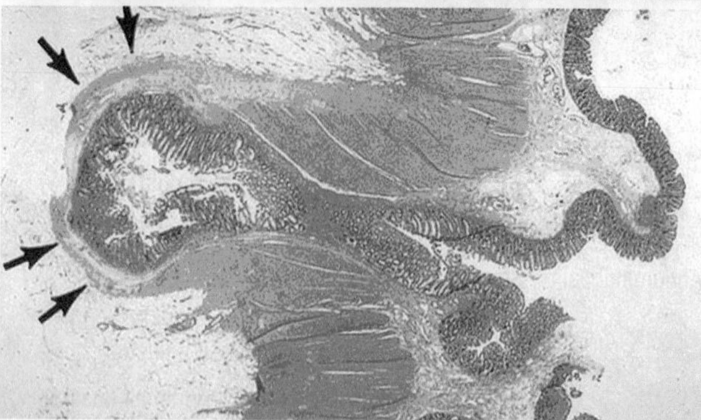

Figure 297-1 Gross and microscopic view of sigmoid diverticular disease. Arrows mark an inflamed diverticulum with the diverticular wall made up only of mucosa.

from the right colon. For this reason, patients with presumed bleeding from diverticular disease requiring emergent surgery without localization should undergo a total abdominal colectomy. If the patient is unstable or has had a 6-unit bleed within 24 h, current recommendations are that surgery should be performed. In patients without severe comorbidities, surgical resection can be performed with a primary anastomosis. A higher anastomotic leak rate has been reported in patients who received >10 units of blood.

Presentation, evaluation, and staging of diverticulitis

Acute uncomplicated diverticulitis characteristically presents with fever, anorexia, left lower quadrant abdominal pain, and obstipation (Table 297-1). In <25% of cases, patients may present with generalized peritonitis indicating the presence of a diverticular perforation. If a pericolonic abscess has formed, the patient may have abdominal distention and signs of localized peritonitis. Laboratory investigations will demonstrate a leukocytosis. Rarely, a patient may present with an air-fluid level in the left lower quadrant on plain abdominal film. This is a giant diverticulum of the sigmoid colon and is managed with resection to avoid impending perforation.

The diagnosis of diverticulitis is best made on CT with the following findings: sigmoid diverticula, thickened colonic wall >4 mm, and inflammation within the pericolic fat ± the collection of contrast material or fluid. In 16% of patients, an abdominal abscess may be present. Symptoms of irritable bowel syndrome (IBS) may mimic those of diverticulitis. Therefore, suspected diverticulitis that does not meet CT criteria or is not associated with a leukocytosis or fever is not diverticular disease. Other conditions that can mimic diverticular disease include an ovarian cyst, endometriosis, acute appendicitis, and pelvic inflammatory disease.

Barium enema or colonoscopy should not be performed in the acute setting because of the higher risk of colonic perforation associated with insufflation or insertion of barium-based contrast material under pressure. A sigmoid malignancy can masquerade as diverticular disease. Therefore, a colonoscopy should be performed ~6 weeks after an attack of diverticular disease.

Complicated diverticular disease is defined as diverticular disease associated with an abscess or perforation and less commonly with a fistula (Table 297-1). Perforated diverticular disease is staged using the Hinchey classification system (Fig. 297-2). This staging system was developed to predict outcomes following the surgical management of complicated diverticular disease. In complicated diverticular disease with fistula formation, common locations include cutaneous, vaginal, or vesicle fistulas. These conditions present with either passage of stool through the skin or vagina or the presence of air in the urinary stream (pneumaturia). Colovaginal fistulas are more common in women who have undergone a hysterectomy.

TABLE 297-1 Presentation of Diverticular Disease

Uncomplicated Diverticular Disease—75%
Abdominal pain
Fever
Leukocytosis
Anorexia/obstipation
Complicated Diverticular Disease—25%
Abscess 16%
Perforation 10%
Stricture 5%
Fistula 2%

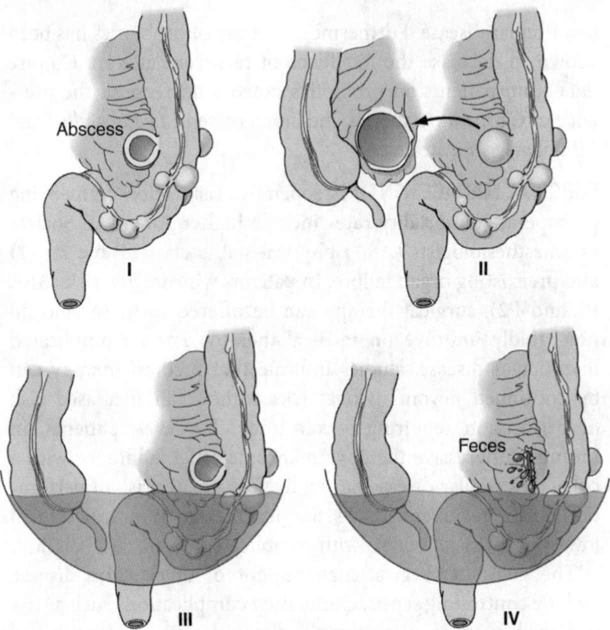

Figure 297-2 Hinchey classification of diverticulitis. Stage I: Perforated diverticulitis with a confined paracolic abscess. Stage II: Perforated diverticulitis that has closed spontaneously with distant abscess formation. Stage III: Noncommunicating perforated diverticulitis with fecal peritonitis (the diverticular neck is closed off and therefore contrast will not freely expel on radiographic images). Stage IV: Perforation and free communication with the peritoneum, resulting in fecal peritonitis.

TREATMENT Diverticular Disease

MEDICAL MANAGEMENT Asymptomatic diverticular disease discovered on imaging studies or at the time of colonoscopy is best managed by diet alterations. Patients should be instructed to eat a fiber-enriched diet that includes 30 g of fiber each day. Supplementary fiber products such as Metamucil, Fibercon, or Citrucel are useful. The incidence of complicated diverticular disease appears to be increased in patients who smoke. Therefore, patients should be encouraged to refrain from smoking. The historical recommendation to avoid eating nuts is not based on more than anecdotal data.

Symptomatic uncomplicated diverticular disease with confirmation of inflammation and infection within the colon should be treated initially with antibiotics and bowel rest. Nearly 75% of patients hospitalized for acute diverticulitis will respond to nonoperative treatment with a suitable antimicrobial regimen. The current recommended antimicrobial coverage is trimethoprim/sulfamethoxazole or ciprofloxacin and metronidazole targeting aerobic gram-negative rods and anaerobic bacteria. Unfortunately, these agents do not cover enterococci, and the addition of ampicillin to this regimen for nonresponders is recommended. Alternatively, single-agent therapy with a third-generation penicillin such as IV piperacillin or oral penicillin/clavulanic acid may be effective. The usual course of antibiotics is 7–10 days. Patients should remain on a limited diet until their pain resolves.

For long-term medical management of uncomplicated diverticular disease, rifaximin (a poorly absorbed broad-spectrum antibiotic), when compared to fiber alone, is associated with 30% less frequent recurrent symptoms from uncomplicated diverticular disease. Furthermore, the use of probiotics has been shown to decrease the incidence of recurrent attacks. Culture data from patients on probiotics noted a decrease in the presence of *Clostridium* species and an increase in *Lactobacillus* and *Bifidobacterium* strains.

SURGICAL MANAGEMENT Preoperative risk factors influencing postoperative mortality rates include higher American Society of Anesthesiologists (ASA) physical status class (Table 297-2) and preexisting organ failure. In patients who are low risk (ASA P1 and P2), surgical therapy can be offered to those who do not rapidly improve on medical therapy. For uncomplicated diverticular disease, studies indicate that medical therapy can be continued beyond two attacks without an increased risk of perforation requiring a colostomy. However, patients on immunosuppressive therapy, in chronic renal failure, or with a collagen-vascular disease have a fivefold greater risk of perforation during recurrent attacks. Surgical therapy is indicated in all low-surgical-risk patients with complicated diverticular disease.

The goals of surgical management of diverticular disease include controlling sepsis, eliminating complications such as fistula or obstruction, removing the diseased colonic segment, and restoring intestinal continuity. These goals must be obtained while minimizing morbidity rate, length of hospitalization, and cost in addition to maximizing survival and quality of life. Table 297-3 lists the operations most commonly indicated based upon Hinchey classification and the predicted morbidity and mortality rates. Surgical objectives include removal of the diseased sigmoid down to the rectosigmoid junction. Failure to do this may result in recurrent disease. The current options for uncomplicated diverticular disease include an open sigmoid resection or a laparoscopic sigmoid resection. The benefits of laparoscopic resection over open surgical techniques include early discharge (by at least 1 day), less narcotic use, less postoperative complications, and an earlier return to work.

The options for the surgical management of complicated diverticular disease (Fig. 297-3) include the following: (1) proximal diversion of the fecal stream with an ileostomy or colostomy and sutured omental patch with drainage, (2) resection with colostomy and mucous fistula or closure of distal bowel with formation of a Hartmann's pouch, (3) resection with anastomosis (coloproctostomy), or (4) resection with anastomosis and diversion (coloproctostomy with loop ileostomy or colostomy). Laparoscopic techniques have been employed for complicated diverticular disease; however, higher conversion rates to open techniques have been reported.

Patients with Hinchey stages I and II disease are managed with percutaneous drainage followed by resection with anastomosis about 6 weeks later. Percutaneous drainage is recommended for abscesses ≥5 cm with a well-defined wall that is accessible. Paracolic abscesses <5 cm in size may resolve with antibiotics alone. Contraindications to percutaneous drainage are no percutaneous access route, pneumoperitoneum, and fecal peritonitis. Urgent operative intervention is undertaken if patients develop generalized peritonitis, and most will need to be managed with a Hartmann's procedure. In selected cases, nonoperative therapy may be considered. In one nonrandomized study, nonoperative management of isolated paracolic abscesses (Hinchey stage I) was associated with only a 20% recurrence rate at 2 years. More than 80% of patients with distant abscesses (Hinchey stage II) required surgical resection for recurrent symptoms.

Hinchey stage III disease is managed with a Hartmann's procedure or with primary anastomosis and proximal diversion. If the patient has significant comorbidities, making operative intervention risky, a limited procedure including intraoperative peritoneal lavage (irrigation), omental patch to the oversewn perforation, and proximal diversion of the fecal stream with either an ileostomy or transverse colostomy can be performed. No anastomosis of any type should be attempted in Hinchey stage IV disease. A limited approach to these patients is associated with a decreased mortality rate.

TABLE 297-2 American Society of Anesthesiologists Physical Status Classification System

P1	A normal healthy patient
P2	A patient with mild systemic disease
P3	A patient with severe systemic disease
P4	A patient with severe systemic disease that is a constant threat to life
P5	A moribund patient who is not expected to survive without the operation
P6	A declared brain-dead patient whose organs are being removed for donor purposes

Recurrent symptoms

Recurrent abdominal symptoms following surgical resection for diverticular disease occurs in 10% of patients. Recurrent diverticular disease develops in patients following inadequate surgical resection. A retained segment of diseased rectosigmoid colon is associated with twice the incidence of recurrence. IBS may also cause recurrence of initial symptoms. Patients undergoing surgical resection for presumed diverticulitis and symptoms of abdominal cramping and irregular loose bowel movements consistent with IBS have functionally poorer outcomes.

TABLE 297-3 Outcome Following Surgical Therapy for Complicated Diverticular Disease

Hinchey Stage	Operative Procedure	Anastomotic Leak Rate, %	Overall Morbidity rate, %
I	Resection with primary anastomosis without diverting stoma	3.8	22
II	Resection with primary anastomosis +/− diversion	3.8	30
III	Hartmann's procedure vs. diverting colostomy and omental pedal graft	—	0 vs. 6 mortality
IV	Hartmann's procedure vs. diverting colostomy and omental pedicle graft	—	6 vs. 2 mortality

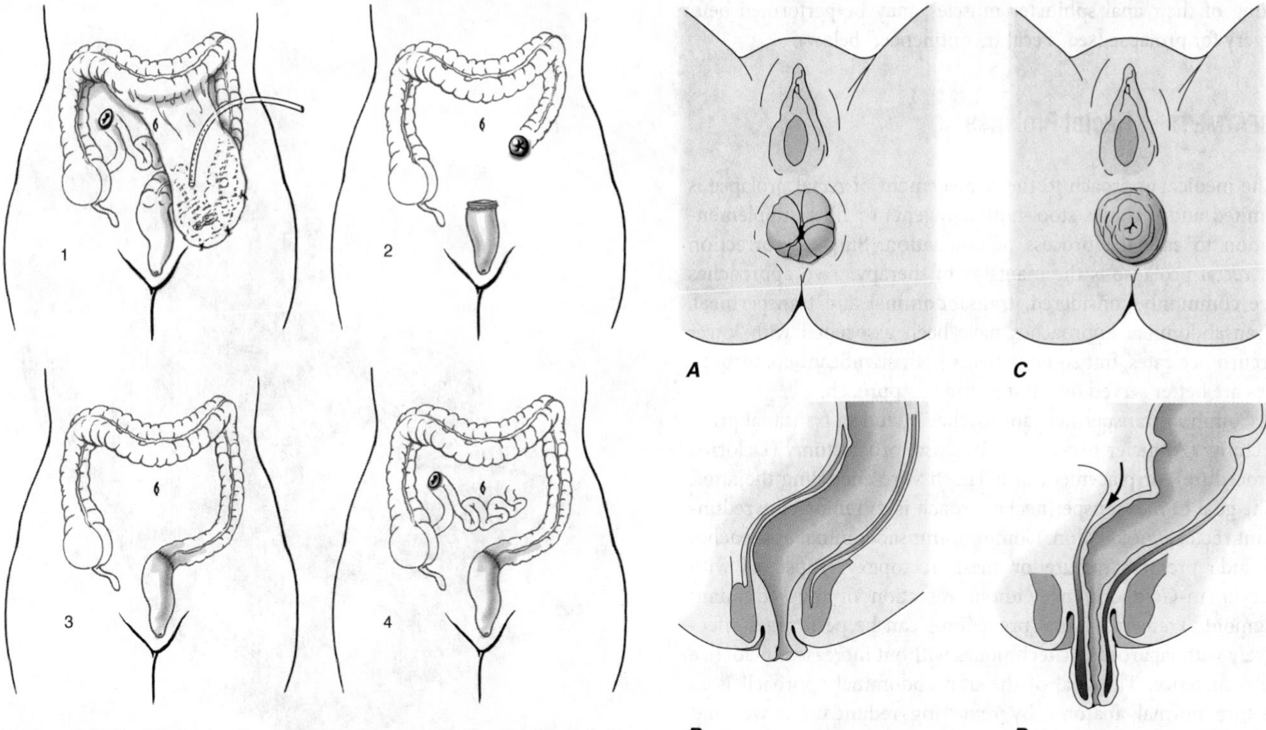

Figure 297-3 Methods of surgical management of complicated diverticular disease. ***(1)*** Drainage, omental pedicle graft, and proximal diversion. ***(2)*** Hartmann's procedure. ***(3)*** Sigmoid resection with coloproctostomy. ***(4)*** Sigmoid resection with coloproctostomy and proximal diversion.

Figure 297-4 Degree of rectal prolapse. Mucosal prolapse only (***A, B,*** sagittal view). Full-thickness prolapse associated with redundant rectosigmoid and deep pouch of Douglas (***C, D,*** sagittal view).

COMMON DISEASES OF THE ANORECTUM

RECTAL PROLAPSE (PROCIDENTIA)

Incidence and epidemiology

Rectal prolapse is six times more common in women than in men. The incidence of rectal prolapse peaks in women >60 years. Women with rectal prolapse have a higher incidence of associated pelvic floor disorders including urinary incontinence, rectocele, cystocele, and enterocele. About 20% of children with rectal prolapse will have cystic fibrosis. All children presenting with prolapse should undergo a sweat chloride test. Less common associations include Ehlers-Danlos syndrome, solitary rectal ulcer syndrome, congenital hypothyroidism, and Hirschsprung's disease.

Anatomy and pathophysiology

Rectal prolapse (procidentia) is a circumferential, full-thickness protrusion of the rectal wall through the anal orifice. It is often associated with a redundant sigmoid colon, pelvic laxity, and a deep rectovaginal septum (pouch of Douglas). Initially, rectal prolapse was felt to be the result of early internal rectal intussusception, which occurs in the upper to mid rectum. This was considered to be the first step in an inevitable progression to full-thickness external prolapse. However, only 1 of 38 patients with internal prolapse followed for >5 years developed full-thickness prolapse. Others have suggested that full-thickness prolapse is the result of damage to the nerve supply to the pelvic floor muscles or pudendal nerves from repeated stretching with straining to defecate. Damage to the pudendal nerves would weaken the pelvic floor muscles, including the external anal sphincter muscles. Bilateral pudendal nerve injury is more significantly associated with prolapse and incontinence than unilateral injury.

Presentation and evaluation

In external prolapse, the majority of patient complaints include anal mass, bleeding per rectum, and poor perianal hygiene. Prolapse of the rectum usually occurs following defecation and will spontaneously reduce or require the patient to manually reduce the prolapse. Constipation occurs in ~30–67% of patients with rectal prolapse. Differing degrees of fecal incontinence occur in 50–70% of patients. Patients with internal rectal prolapse will present with symptoms of both constipation and incontinence. Other associated findings include outlet obstruction (anismus) in 30%, colonic inertia in 10%, and solitary rectal ulcer syndrome in 12%.

Office evaluation is best performed after the patient has been given an enema, which enables the prolapse to protrude. An important distinction should be made between full-thickness rectal prolapse and isolated mucosal prolapse associated with hemorrhoidal disease (Fig. 297-4). Mucosal prolapse is known for radial grooves rather than circumferential folds around the anus and is due to increased laxity of the connective tissue between the submucosa and underlying muscle of the anal canal. The evaluation of prolapse should also include cystoproctography and colonoscopy. These examinations evaluate for associated pelvic floor disorders and rule out a malignancy or a polyp as the lead point for prolapse. If rectal prolapse is associated with chronic constipation, the patient should undergo a defecating proctogram and a sitzmark study. This will evaluate for the presence of anismus or colonic inertia. Anismus is the result of attempting to defecate against a closed pelvic floor and is also known as *nonrelaxing puborectalis*. This can be seen when straightening of the rectum fails to occur on fluoroscopy while the patient is attempting to defecate. In colonic inertia, a sitzmark study will demonstrate retention of >20% of markers on abdominal x-ray 5 days after swallowing. For patients with fecal incontinence, endoanal ultrasound and manometric evaluation, including pudendal nerve testing of their anal sphincter muscles, may be performed before surgery for prolapse (see "Fecal Incontinence," below).

TREATMENT Rectal Prolapse

The medical approach to the management of rectal prolapse is limited and includes stool-bulking agents or fiber supplementation to ease the process of evacuation. Surgical correction of rectal prolapse is the mainstay of therapy. Two approaches are commonly considered, transabdominal and transperineal. Transabdominal approaches have been associated with lower recurrence rates, but some patients with significant comorbidities are better served by a transperineal approach.

Common transperineal approaches include a transanal proctectomy (Altmeier procedure), mucosal proctectomy (Delorme procedure), or placement of a Tirsch wire encircling the anus. The goal of the transperineal approach is to remove the redundant rectosigmoid colon. Common transabdominal approaches include presacral suture or mesh rectopexy (Ripstein) with (Frykman-Goldberg) or without resection of the redundant sigmoid. Transabdominal procedures can be performed effectively with laparoscopic techniques without increased incidence of recurrence. The goal of the transabdominal approach is to restore normal anatomy by removing redundant bowel and reattaching the supportive tissue of the rectum to the presacral fascia. The final alternative is abdominal proctectomy with end-sigmoid colostomy. Colon resection, in general, is reserved for patients with constipation and outlet obstruction. If total colonic inertia is present, as defined by a history of constipation and a positive sitzmark study, a subtotal colectomy with an ileosigmoid or rectal anastomosis may be required at the time of rectopexy.

Previously, the presence of internal rectal prolapse identified on imaging studies has been considered a nonsurgical disorder and biofeedback was recommended. However, only one-third of patients will have successful resolution of symptoms from biofeedback. Two surgical procedures have been shown to be more effective than biofeedback. The STARR (stapled transanal rectal resection) procedure (Fig. 297-5) is performed through the anus in patients with internal prolapse. A circular stapling device is inserted through the anus; the internal prolapse is identified and ligated with the stapling device. The Laparoscopic Ventral Rectopexy (LVR) (Fig. 297-6) is performed by creating an opening in the peritoneum on the left side of the rectosigmoid and carrying this opening down anterior on the rectum into the pouch of Douglas. No rectal mobilization is performed, thus avoiding any autonomic nerve injury. Mesh is secured to the anterior and lateral portion of the rectum, the vaginal fornix, and the sacral promontory, allowing for closure of the rectovaginal septum and correction of the internal prolapse. In both procedures, recurrence at 1 year was low (<10%) and symptoms improved in more than three-fourths of patients.

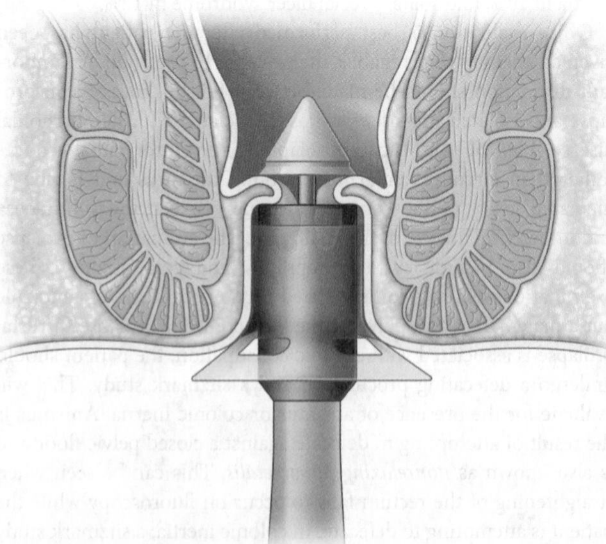

Figure 297-5 Stapled transanal rectal resection. Schematic of placement of the circular stapling device.

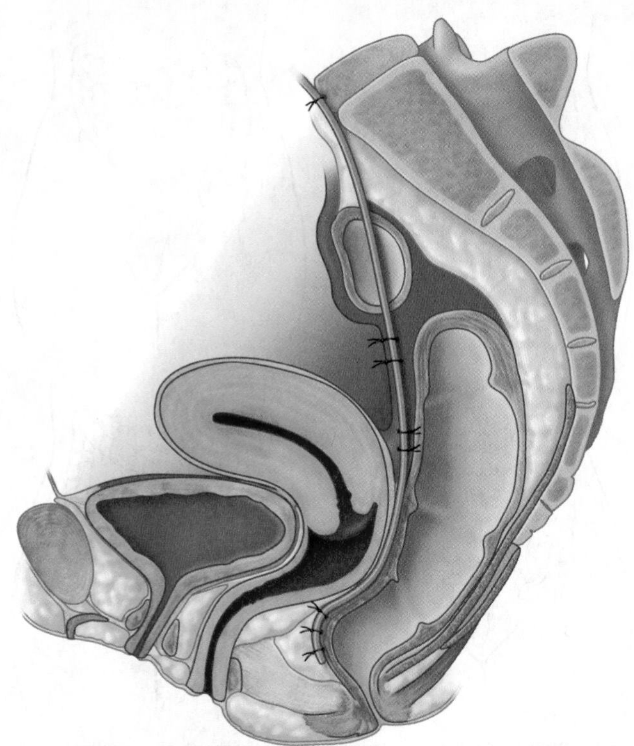

Figure 297-6 Laparoscopic Ventral Rectopexy (LVR). To reduce the internal prolapse and close any rectovaginal septal defect, the pouch of Douglas is opened and mesh is secured to the anterolateral rectum, vaginal fornix, and sacrum. (*From D'Hoore et al: Br J Surg 91:1500, 2004.*)

FECAL INCONTINENCE

Incidence and epidemiology

Fecal incontinence is the involuntary passage of fecal material >10 mL for at least 1 month. The prevalence of fecal incontinence in the United States is 0.5–11%. The majority of patients are women. A higher incidence of incontinence is seen among parous women. One-half of patients with fecal incontinence also suffer from urinary incontinence. The majority of incontinence is a result of obstetric injury to the pelvic floor, either while carrying a fetus or during the delivery. An anatomic sphincter defect may occur in up to 32% of women following childbirth regardless of visible damage to the perineum. Risk factors at the time of delivery include prolonged labor, the use of forceps, and the need for an episiotomy. Medical conditions known to contribute to the development of fecal incontinence are listed in Table 297-4.

TABLE 297-4 Medical Conditions That Contribute to Symptoms of Fecal Incontinence

Neurologic Disorders
• Dementia
• Brain tumor
• Stroke
• Multiple sclerosis
• Tabes dorsalis
• Cauda equina lesions
Skeletal Muscle Disorders
• Myasthenia gravis
• Myopathies, muscular dystrophy
Miscellaneous
• Hypothyroidism
• Irritable bowel syndrome
• Sedation
• Severe diarrhea

Anatomy and pathophysiology

The anal sphincter complex is made up of the internal and external anal sphincter. The internal sphincter is smooth muscle and a continuation of the circular fibers of the rectal wall. It is innervated by the intestinal myenteric plexus and is therefore not under voluntary control. The external anal sphincter is formed in continuation with the levator ani muscles and is under voluntary control. The pudendal nerve supplies motor innervation to the external anal sphincter. Obstetric injury may result in tearing of the muscle fibers anteriorly at the time of the delivery. This results in an obvious anterior defect on endoanal ultrasound. Injury may also be the result of stretching of the pudendal nerves. The majority of patients who suffer from fecal incontinence following obstetric injury do so several years following the birth of their last child.

Presentation and evaluation

Patients may suffer with varying degrees of fecal incontinence. Minor incontinence includes incontinence to flatus and occasional seepage of liquid stool. Major incontinence is frequent inability to control solid waste. As a result of fecal incontinence, patients suffer from poor perianal hygiene. Beyond the immediate problems associated with fecal incontinence, these patients are often withdrawn and suffer from depression. For this reason, quality-of-life measures have become an important component in the evaluation of patients with fecal incontinence.

The evaluation of fecal incontinence should include a thorough history and physical examination, anal manometry, pudendal nerve terminal motor latency (PNTML), and endoanal ultrasound. Unfortunately, all of these investigations are user-dependent. Centers that care for patients with fecal incontinence will have an anorectal physiology laboratory that uses standardized methods of evaluating anorectal physiology. Anal manometry measures resting and squeeze pressures within the anal canal using an intraluminal water-perfused catheter. Pudendal nerve studies evaluate the function of the nerves innervating the anal canal using a finger electrode placed in the anal canal. Stretch injuries to these nerves will result in a delayed response of the sphincter muscle to a stimulus, indicating a prolonged latency. Finally, ultrasound will evaluate the extent of the injury to the sphincter muscles before surgical repair. Only PNTML has been shown to consistently predict outcome following surgical intervention.

Rarely does a pelvic floor disorder exist alone. The majority of patients with fecal incontinence will have a degree of urinary incontinence. Similarly, fecal incontinence is a part of the spectrum of pelvic organ prolapse. For this reason, patients may present with symptoms of obstructed defecation as well as fecal incontinence. Careful evaluation including cinedefecography should be performed to search for other associated defects. Surgical repair of incontinence without attention to other associated defects may decrease the success of the repair.

TREATMENT Fecal Incontinence

The "gold standard" for the treatment of fecal incontinence with an isolated sphincter defect is overlapping sphincteroplasty. The external anal sphincter muscle and scar tissue as well as any identifiable internal sphincter muscle are dissected free from the surrounding adipose and connective tissue and then an overlapping repair is performed in an attempt to rebuild the muscular ring and restore its function. Other newer approaches include radio frequency therapy to the anal canal to aid in the development of collagen fibers and provide tensile strength to the sphincter muscles. Sacral nerve stimulation and the artificial bowel sphincter are both adaptations of procedures developed for the management of urinary incontinence. Sacral nerve stimulation is ideally suited for patients with intact but weak anal sphincters. A temporary nerve stimulator is placed on the third sacral nerve. If there is at least a 50% improvement in symptoms, a permanent nerve stimulator is placed under the skin. The artificial bowel sphincter is a cuff and reservoir apparatus that allows for manual inflation of a cuff placed around the anus, increasing anal tone. This allows the patient to manually close off the anal canal until defecation is necessary.

Long-term results following overlapping sphincteroplasty show about a 50% failure rate over 5 years. Poorer outcome has been seen in patients with prolonged PNTML. Long-term results for sacral stimulation have been promising; however, the indications for this procedure are presently limited in the United States. Unfortunately, the artificial bowel sphincter has been associated with a 30% infection rate.

■ HEMORRHOIDAL DISEASE

Incidence and epidemiology

Symptomatic hemorrhoids affect >1 million individuals in the Western world per year. The prevalence of hemorrhoidal disease is not selective for age or sex. However, age is known to have a deleterious effect on the anal canal. The prevalence of hemorrhoidal disease is less in underdeveloped countries. The typical low-fiber, high-fat Western diet is associated with constipation and straining and the development of symptomatic hemorrhoids.

Anatomy and pathophysiology

Hemorrhoidal cushions are a normal part of the anal canal. The vascular structures contained within this tissue aid in continence by preventing damage to the sphincter muscle. Three main hemorrhoidal complexes traverse the anal canal—the left lateral, the right anterior, and the right posterior. Engorgement and straining leads to prolapse of this tissue into the anal canal. Over time, the anatomic support system of the hemorrhoidal complex weakens, exposing this tissue to the outside of the anal canal where it is susceptible to injury. Hemorrhoids are commonly classified as internal or external. Although small external cushions do exist, the standard classification of hemorrhoidal disease is based on the progression

TABLE 297-5 The Staging and Treatment of Hemorrhoids

Stage	Description of Classification	Treatment
I	Enlargement with bleeding	Fiber supplementation Cortisone suppository Sclerotherapy
II	Protrusion with spontaneous reduction	Fiber supplementation Cortisone suppository
III	Protrusion requiring manual reduction	Fiber supplementation Cortisone suppository Banding Operative hemorrhoidectomy (stapled or traditional)
IV	Irreducible protrusion	Fiber supplementation Cortisone suppository Operative hemorrhoidectomy

of the disease from their normal internal location to the prolapsing external position (Table 297-5).

Presentation and evaluation

Patients commonly present to a physician for two reasons: bleeding and protrusion. Pain is less common than with fissures and, if present, is described as a dull ache from engorgement of the hemorrhoidal tissue. Severe pain may indicate a thrombosed hemorrhoid. Hemorrhoidal bleeding is described as bright red blood seen either in the toilet or upon wiping. Occasional patients can present with significant bleeding, which may be a cause of anemia; however, the presence of a colonic neoplasm must be ruled out. Patients who present with a protruding mass complain about inability to maintain perianal hygiene and are often concerned about the presence of a malignancy.

The diagnosis of hemorrhoidal disease is made on physical examination. Inspection of the perianal region for evidence of thrombosis or excoriation is performed, followed by a careful digital examination. Anoscopy is performed paying particular attention to the known position of hemorrhoidal disease. The patient is asked to strain. If this is difficult for the patient, the maneuver can be performed while sitting on a toilet. The physician is notified when the tissue prolapses. It is important to differentiate the circumferential appearance of a full-thickness rectal prolapse from the radial nature of prolapsing hemorrhoids (see "Rectal Prolapse," above). The stage and location of the hemorrhoidal complexes are defined.

TREATMENT Hemorrhoidal Disease

The treatment for bleeding hemorrhoids is based upon the stage of the disease (Table 297-5). In all patients with bleeding, the possibility of other causes must be considered. In young patients without a family history of colorectal cancer, the hemorrhoidal disease may be treated first and a colonoscopic examination performed if the bleeding continues. Older patients who have not had colorectal cancer screening should undergo colonoscopy or flexible sigmoidoscopy.

With rare exceptions, the acutely thrombosed hemorrhoid can be excised within the first 72 h by performing an elliptical excision. Sitz baths, fiber, and stool softeners are prescribed. Additional therapy for bleeding hemorrhoids includes banding, sclerotherapy, excisional hemorrhoidectomy, and stapled hemorrhoidectomy. Sensation begins at the dentate line; therefore, banding or sclerotherapy can be performed without discomfort in the office. Bands are placed around the engorged tissue, causing ischemia and fibrosis. This aids in fixing the tissue proximally in the anal canal. Patients may complain of a dull ache for 24 h following band application. During sclerotherapy, 1–2 mL of a sclerosant (usually sodium tetradecyl sulfate) is injected using a 25-gauge needle into the submucosa of the hemorrhoidal complex. Care must be taken not to inject the anal canal circumferentially, or stenosis may occur. The sutured and stapled hemorrhoidectomies are equally effective in the treatment of symptomatic third- and fourth-degree hemorrhoids. However, because the sutured hemorrhoidectomy involves the removal of redundant tissue down to the anal verge, unpleasant anal skin tags are removed as well. The stapled hemorrhoidectomy is associated with less discomfort; however, this procedure does not remove anal skin tags. No procedures on hemorrhoids should be done in patients who are immunocompromised or who have active proctitis. Furthermore, emergent hemorrhoidectomy for bleeding hemorrhoids is associated with a higher complication rate.

Acute complications associated with the treatment of hemorrhoids include pain, infection, recurrent bleeding, and urinary retention. Care should be taken to place bands properly and to avoid overhydration in patients undergoing operative hemorrhoidectomy. Late complications include fecal incontinence as a result of injury to the sphincter during the dissection. Anal stenosis may develop from overzealous excision, with loss of mucosal skin bridges for reepithelialization. Finally, an *ectropion* (prolapse of rectal mucosa from the anal canal) may develop. Patients with an ectropion complain of a "wet" anus as a result of inability to prevent soiling once the rectal mucosa is exposed below the dentate line.

ANORECTAL ABSCESS

Incidence and epidemiology

The development of a perianal abscess is more common in men than women by a ratio of 3:1. The peak incidence is in the third to fifth decade of life. Perianal pain associated with the presence of an abscess accounts for 15% of office visits to a colorectal surgeon. The disease is more prevalent in immunocompromised patients such as those with diabetes, hematologic disorders, or inflammatory bowel disease (IBD) and persons who are HIV. positive. These disorders should be considered in patients with recurrent perianal infections.

Anatomy and pathophysiology

An anorectal abscess is an abnormal fluid-containing cavity in the anorectal region. Anorectal abscess results from an infection involving the glands surrounding the anal canal. Normally, these glands release mucus into the anal canal, which aids in defecation. When stool accidentally enters the anal glands, the glands become infected and an abscess develops. Anorectal abscesses are perianal in 40–50% of patients, ischiorectal in 20–25%, intersphincteric in 2–5%, and supralevator in 2.5% (Fig. 297-7).

Presentation and evaluation

Perianal pain and fever are the hallmarks of an abscess. Patients may have difficulty voiding and have blood in the stool. A prostatic abscess may present with similar complaints, including dysuria. Patients with a prostatic abscess will often have a history of recurrent sexually transmitted diseases. On physical examination, a large

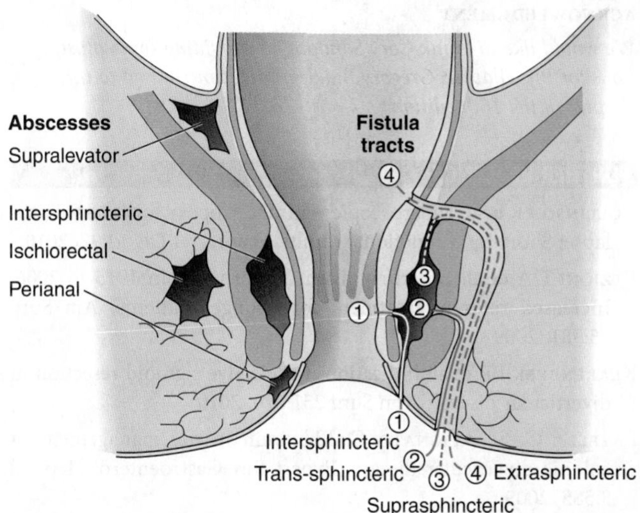

Figure 297-7 Common locations of anorectal abscess *(left)* and fistula in ano *(right).*

fluctuant area is usually readily visible. Routine laboratory evaluation shows an elevated white blood cell count. Diagnostic procedures are rarely necessary unless evaluating a recurrent abscess. A CT scan or MRI has an accuracy of 80% in determining incomplete drainage. If there is a concern about the presence of IBD, a rigid or flexible sigmoidoscopic examination may be done at the time of drainage to evaluate for inflammation within the rectosigmoid region. A more complete evaluation for Crohn's disease would include a full colonoscopy and small-bowel series.

TREATMENT Anorectal Abscess

Office drainage of an uncomplicated anorectal abscess may suffice. A small incision close to the anal verge is made and a Mallenkot drain is advanced into the abscess cavity. For patients who have a complicated abscess or who are diabetic or immunocompromised, drainage should be performed in an operating room under anesthesia. These patients are at greater risk for developing necrotizing fasciitis. The course of antibiotics is controversial but should be at least 2 weeks in patients who are immunocompromised or have prosthetic heart valves, artificial joints, diabetes, or IBD.

FISTULA IN ANO

Incidence and epidemiology

The incidence and prevalence of fistulating perianal disease parallels the incidence of anorectal abscess. Some 30–40% of abscesses will give rise to fistula in ano. While the majority of the fistulas are cryptoglandular in origin, 10% are associated with IBD, tuberculosis, malignancy, and radiation.

Anatomy and pathophysiology

A fistula in ano is defined as a communication of an abscess cavity with an identifiable internal opening within the anal canal. This identifiable opening is most commonly located at the dentate line where the anal glands enter the anal canal. Patients experiencing continuous drainage following the treatment of a perianal abscess likely have a fistula in ano. These fistulas are classified by their relationship to the anal sphincter muscles, with 70% being intersphincteric, 23% transsphincteric, 5% suprasphincteric, and 2% extrasphincteric (Fig. 297-7).

Presentation and evaluation

A patient with a fistula in ano will complain of constant drainage from the perianal region. The drainage may increase with defecation. Perianal hygiene is difficult to maintain. Examination under anesthesia is the best way to evaluate a fistula. At the time of the examination, anoscopy is performed to look for an internal opening. Diluted hydrogen peroxide will aid in identifying such an opening. In lieu of anesthesia, MRI with an endoanal coil will also identify tracts in 80% of the cases. After drainage of an abscess with insertion of a Mallenkot catheter, a fistulagram through the catheter can be obtained in search of an occult fistula tract. Goodsall's rule states that a posterior external fistula will enter the anal canal in the posterior midline, whereas an anterior fistula will enter at the nearest crypt. A fistula exiting >3 cm from the anal verge may have a complicated upward extension and may not obey Goodsall's rule.

TREATMENT Fistula In Ano

A newly diagnosed draining fistula is best managed with placement of a seton, a vessel loop or silk tie placed through the fistula tract, which maintains the tract open and quiets down the surrounding inflammation that occurs from repeated blockage of the tract. Once the inflammation is less, the exact relationship of the fistula tract to the anal sphincters can be ascertained. A simple fistulotomy can be performed for intersphincteric and low (less than one-third of the muscle) transsphincteric fistulas without compromising continence. For a higher transsphincteric fistula, an anorectal advancement flap in combination with a drainage catheter or fibrin glue may be used. Very long (>2 cm) and narrow tracts respond better to fibrin glue than shorter tracts. Simple ligation of the internal fistula tract (LIFT procedure) has also been used in the management of simple fistula with good success.

Patients should be maintained on stool-bulking agents, nonnarcotic pain medication, and sitz baths following surgery for a fistula. Early complications from these procedures include urinary retention and bleeding. Later complications are rare (<10%) and include temporary and permanent incontinence. Recurrence following fistulotomy is 0–18% and following anorectal advancement flap and the LIFT procedure is 20–30%.

ANAL FISSURE

Incidence and epidemiology

Anal fissures occur at all ages but are more common in the third through the fifth decades. A fissure is the most common cause of rectal bleeding in infancy. The prevalence is equal in males and females. It is associated with constipation, diarrhea, infectious etiologies, perianal trauma, and Crohn's disease.

Anatomy and pathophysiology

Trauma to the anal canal occurs following defecation. This injury occurs in the anterior or, more commonly, the posterior anal canal. Irritation caused by the trauma to the anal canal results in an increased resting pressure of the internal sphincter. The blood supply to the sphincter and anal mucosa enters laterally. Therefore, increased anal sphincter tone results in a relative ischemia in the region of the fissure and leads to poor healing of the anal injury. A fissure that is not in the posterior or anterior position should raise suspicion for other causes, including tuberculosis, syphilis, Crohn's disease, and malignancy.

Presentation and evaluation

A fissure can be easily diagnosed on history alone. The classic complaint is pain, which is strongly associated with defecation and is relentless. The bright red bleeding that can be associated with a fissure is less extensive than that associated with hemorrhoids. On examination, most fissures are located in either the posterior or anterior position. A lateral fissure is worrisome as it may have a less benign nature, and systemic disorders should be ruled out. A chronic fissure is indicated by the presence of a hypertrophied anal papilla at the proximal end of the fissure and a sentinel pile or skin tag at the distal end. Often the circular fibers of the hypertrophied internal sphincter are visible within the base of the fissure. If anal manometry is performed, elevation in anal resting pressure and a sawtooth deformity with paradoxical contractions of the sphincter muscles are pathognomonic.

TREATMENT Anal Fissure

The management of the acute fissure is conservative. Stool softeners for those with constipation, increased dietary fiber, topical anesthetics, glucocorticoids, and sitz baths are prescribed and will heal 60–90% of fissures. Chronic fissures are those present for >6 weeks. These can be treated with modalities aimed at decreasing the anal canal resting pressure including nifedipine or nitroglycerin ointment applied three times a day, and botulinum toxin type A, up to 20 units, injected into the internal sphincter on each side of the fissure. Surgical management includes anal dilatation and lateral internal sphincterotomy. Usually, one-third of the internal sphincter muscle is divided; it is easily identified because it is hypertrophied. Recurrence rates from medical therapy are higher, but this is offset by a risk of incontinence following sphincterotomy. Lateral internal sphincterotomy may lead to incontinence more commonly in women.

ACKNOWLEDGMENT

We would like to thank Cory Sandore for providing some illustrations for this chapter. Gregory Bulkley, MD, contributed to this chapter in the 16th edition.

FURTHER READINGS

Collinson R et al: Laparoscopic ventral rectopexy for internal prolapse: Short-term functional results. Colorectal Dis 12:97, 2010

Etzioni DA et al: Diverticulitis in California from 1995 to 2006: Increased rates of treatment for younger patients. Am Surg 75:981, 2009

Klarenbeek BR et al: Indications for elective sigmoid resection in diverticular disease. Ann Surg 251:670, 2010

Latella G, Scarpignato C: Rifaximin in the management of colonic diverticular disease. Expert Rev Gastroenterol Hepatol 3:585, 2009

Pinto R, Sands D: Surgery and sacral nerve stimulation for constipation and fecal incontinence. Gastrointest Endosc Clin North Am 19:83, 2009

Russ AJ et al: Laparoscopy improves short-term outcomes after surgery for diverticular disease. Gastroenterology 138:2213, 2010

Sajid MS et al: Open vs laparoscopic repair of full-thickness rectal prolapse: A re-meta-analysis. Colorectal Dis 12:515, 2010

Schwander O et al: Assessing the safety, effectiveness, and quality of life after the STARR procedure for obstructed defecation: Results of the German STARR registry. Langenbecks Arch Surg 395:505, 2010

Shanwani A et al: Ligation of the intersphincteric fistula tract (LIFT): A sphincter-saving technique for fistula-in-ano. Dis Colon Rectum 53:39, 2010

Touzios J, Dozois E: Diverticulosis and acute diverticulitis. Gastroenterol Clin North Am 38:513, 2009

CHAPTER 298

Mesenteric Vascular Insufficiency

Susan L. Gearhart

INTESTINAL ISCHEMIA

INCIDENCE AND EPIDEMIOLOGY

Intestinal ischemia is an uncommon vascular disease associated with a high mortality. It is categorized according to etiology: (1) arteriocclusive mesenteric ischemia (AOMI), (2) nonocclusive mesenteric ischemia (NOMI), and (3) mesenteric venous thrombosis (MVT). Acute intestinal ischemia is more common than its counterpart, chronic arterial ischemia. Risk factors for acute arterial ischemia include atrial fibrillation, recent myocardial infarction, valvular heart disease, and recent cardiac or vascular catheterization. The increased incidence of intestinal ischemia seen in Western countries parallels the incidence of atherosclerosis and the aging population. With the exception of strangulated small-bowel obstruction, ischemic colitis is the most common form of acute ischemia and the most prevalent gastrointestinal disease complicating cardiovascular surgery. The incidence of ischemic colitis following elective aortic repair is 5–9%, and the incidence triples in patients following emergent repair. Other less common forms of intestinal ischemia include chronic mesenteric angina associated with atherosclerotic disease and MVT. The latter is associated with the presence of a hypercoagulable state including protein C or S deficiency, antithrombin III deficiency, polycythemia vera, and carcinoma.

ANATOMY AND PATHOPHYSIOLOGY

Intestinal ischemia occurs when insufficient perfusion to intestinal tissue produces ischemic tissue injury. The blood supply to the intestines is depicted in Fig. 298-1. To prevent ischemic injury, extensive collateralization occurs between major mesenteric trunks and branches of the mesenteric arcades (Table 298-1). Collateral vessels within the small bowel are numerous and meet within the duodenum and the bed of the pancreas. Collateral vessels within the colon meet at the splenic flexure and descending/sigmoid colon. These areas, which are inherently at risk for decreased blood flow, are known as *Griffiths' point* and *Sudeck's point*, respectively, and are the most common locations for colonic ischemia (Fig. 298-1, shaded areas). The splanchnic circulation can receive up to 30% of the cardiac output. Protective responses to prevent intestinal

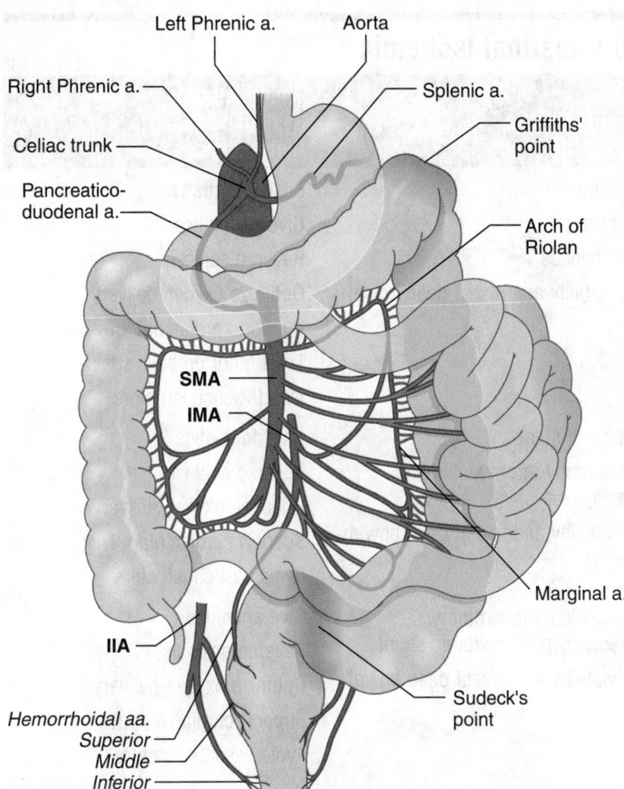

Figure 298-1 **Blood supply to the intestines** includes the celiac artery, superior mesenteric artery (SMA), inferior mesenteric artery (IMA), and branches of the internal iliac artery (IIA). Griffiths' and Sudeck's points, indicated by shaded areas, are watershed areas within the colonic blood supply and common locations for ischemia.

ischemia include abundant collateralization, autoregulation of blood flow, and the ability to increase oxygen extraction from the blood.

Occlusive ischemia is a result of disruption of blood flow by an embolus or progressive thrombosis in a major artery supplying the intestine. Emboli originate from the heart in >75% of cases and lodge preferentially just distal to the origin of the middle colic artery from the superior mesenteric artery. Progressive thrombosis of at least two of the major vessels supplying the intestine is required for the development of chronic intestinal angina. Nonocclusive ischemia is disproportionate mesenteric vasoconstriction (arteriolar vasospasm) in response to a severe physiologic stress such as dehydration or shock. If left untreated, early mucosal stress ulceration will progress to full-thickness injury.

TABLE 298-1 Collateral Arterial Intestinal Blood Flow

Involved Circulation	Mesenteric Artery	Adjoining Artery	Collateral Artery
Systemic	Celiac	Descending aorta	Phrenic
Systemic	IMA	Hypogastric	Middle hemorrhoidal
Mesenteric	Celiac	SMA	Superior/inferior pancreaticoduodenal
Mesenteric	SMA	IMA	Arch of Riolan
Mesenteric	SMA	Celiac/IMA	Intramesenteric
Mesenteric	SMA	IMA	Marginal

Abbreviations: IMA, inferior mesenteric artery; SMA, superior mesenteric artery.

PRESENTATION, EVALUATION, AND MANAGEMENT

Intestinal ischemia remains one of the most challenging diagnoses. The mortality rate is >50%. The most significant indicator of survival is the timeliness of diagnosis and treatment. An overview of diagnosis and management of each form of intestinal ischemia is given in Table 298-2.

Acute mesenteric ischemia resulting from arterial embolus or thrombosis presents with severe acute, nonremitting abdominal pain strikingly out of proportion to the physical findings. Associated symptoms may include nausea and vomiting, transient diarrhea, and bloody stools. With the exception of minimal abdominal distention and hypoactive bowel sounds, early abdominal examination is unimpressive. Later findings will demonstrate peritonitis and cardiovascular collapse. In the evaluation of acute intestinal ischemia, routine laboratory tests should be obtained, including complete blood count, serum chemistry, coagulation profile, arterial blood gas, amylase, lipase, lactic acid, blood type and cross match, and cardiac enzymes. Regardless of the need for urgent surgery, emergent admission to a monitored bed or intensive care unit is recommended for resuscitation and further evaluation. If the diagnosis of intestinal ischemia is being considered, consultation with a surgical service is necessary.

Other diagnostic modalities that may be useful in diagnosis but should not delay surgical therapy include electrocardiogram (ECG), abdominal radiographs, CT, and mesenteric angiography. More recently, mesentery duplex scanning and visible light spectroscopy during colonoscopy have been demonstrated to be beneficial. The ECG may demonstrate an arrhythmia, indicating the possible source of the emboli. A plain abdominal film may show evidence of free intraperitoneal air, indicating a perforated viscus and the need for emergent exploration. Earlier features of intestinal ischemia seen on abdominal radiographs include bowel-wall edema, known as "thumbprinting." If the ischemia progresses, air can be seen within the bowel wall (*pneumatosis intestinalis*) and within the portal venous system. Other features include calcifications of the aorta and its tributaries, indicating atherosclerotic disease. With the administration of oral and IV contrast, dynamic CT with three-dimensional reconstruction is a highly sensitive test for intestinal ischemia. In acute embolic disease, mesenteric angiography is best performed intraoperatively. A mesenteric duplex scan demonstrating a high peak velocity of flow in the superior mesenteric artery (SMA) is associated with an ~80% positive predictive value of mesenteric ischemia. More significantly, a negative duplex scan virtually precludes the diagnosis of mesenteric ischemia. Duplex imaging serves as a screening test; further investigations with angiography are needed. Endoscopic techniques using visible light spectroscopy can be used in the diagnosis of chronic ischemia.

The "gold standard" for the diagnosis and management of acute arterial occlusive disease is laparotomy. Surgical exploration should not be delayed if suspicion of acute occlusive mesenteric ischemia is high or evidence of clinical deterioration or frank peritonitis is present. The goal of operative exploration is to resect compromised bowel and restore blood supply. Intraoperative or preoperative arteriography and systemic heparinization may assist the vascular surgeon in restoring blood supply to the compromised bowel. The entire length of the small and large bowel beginning at the ligament of Treitz should be evaluated. The pattern of intestinal ischemia may indicate the level of arterial occlusion. In the case of SMA occlusion where the embolus usually lies just proximal to the origin of the middle colic artery, the proximal jejunum is often spared while the remainder of the small bowel to the transverse colon will be ischemic.

TABLE 298-2 Overview of the Management of Acute Intestinal Ischemia

Condition	Key to Early Diagnosis	Treatment of Underlying Cause	Treatment of Specific Lesion	Treatment of Systemic Consequences
Arterial embolus	Early laparotomy	Anticoagulation Cardioversion Proximal thrombectomy Aneurysmectomy	Laparotomy Embolectomy Vascular bypass Assess viability and resect dead bowel	Ensure hydration Give antibiotics Reverse acidosis Optimize oxygen delivery Support cardiac output Treat other embolic sites Avoid vasoconstrictors
Arterial thrombosis	Duplex ultrasound Angiography	Anticoagulation Hydration	Endovascular stent Endarterectomy/thrombectomy or vascular bypass Assess viability and resect dead bowel	Give antibiotics Reverse acidosis Optimize oxygen delivery Support cardiac output Avoid vasoconstrictors
Venous thrombosis	Spiral CT	Anticoagulation Massive hydration	Anticoagulation ± laparotomy/thrombectomy/portasystemic shunt Assess viability and resect dead bowel	Give antibiotics Reverse acidosis Optimize oxygen delivery Support cardiac output Avoid vasoconstrictors
Nonocclusive mesenteric ischemia	Vasospasm: Angiography Hypoperfusion: Spiral CT or colonoscopy	Ensure hydration Support cardiac output Avoid vasoconstrictors Ablate renin-angiotensin axis	Vasospasm Intraarterial vasodilators Hypoperfusion Delayed laparotomy Assess viability and resect dead bowel	Ensure hydration Give antibiotics Reverse acidosis Optimize oxygen delivery Support cardiac output Avoid vasoconstrictors

Source: Modified from GB Bulkley, in JL Cameron (ed): *Current Surgical Therapy*, 2nd ed. Toronto, BC Decker, 1986.

The surgical management of acute mesenteric ischemia of the small bowel is attempted embolectomy via intraoperative angiography or arteriotomy. Although more commonly applied to chronic disease, acute thrombosis may be managed with angioplasty, with or without endovascular stent placement. If this is unsuccessful, a bypass from the aorta to the superior mesenteric artery is performed.

Nonocclusive or vasospastic mesenteric ischemia presents with generalized abdominal pain, anorexia, bloody stools, and abdominal distention. Often these patients are obtunded, and physical findings may not assist in the diagnosis. The presence of a leukocytosis, metabolic acidosis, elevated amylase or creatinine phosphokinase levels, and/or lactic acidosis are useful in support of the diagnosis of advanced intestinal ischemia; however, these markers may not be indicative of either reversible ischemia or frank necrosis. Investigational markers for intestinal ischemia include D-dimer, glutathione S-transferase, platelet-activating factor (PAF), and mucosal pH monitoring. Regardless of the need for urgent surgery, emergent admission to a monitored bed or intensive care unit is recommended for resuscitation and further evaluation. Early manifestations of intestinal ischemia include fluid sequestration within the bowel wall leading to a loss of interstitial volume. Aggressive fluid resuscitation may be necessary. To optimize oxygen delivery, nasal O_2 and blood transfusions may be given. Broad-spectrum antibiotics should be given to provide sufficient coverage for enteric pathogens, including gram-negative and anaerobic organisms. Frequent monitoring of the patient's vital signs, urine output, blood gases, and lactate levels is paramount, as is frequent abdominal examination. All vasoconstricting agents should be avoided; fluid resuscitation is the intervention of choice to maintain hemodynamics.

If ischemic colitis is a concern, colonoscopy should be performed to assess the integrity of the colon mucosa. Visualization of the rectosigmoid region may demonstrate decreased mucosal integrity, associated more commonly with nonocclusive mesenteric ischemia, or, on occasion, occlusive disease as a result of acute loss of inferior mesenteric arterial flow following aortic surgery. Ischemia of the colonic mucosa is graded as *mild* with minimal mucosal erythema or as *moderate* with pale mucosal ulcerations and evidence of extension to the muscular layer of the bowel wall. *Severe* ischemic colitis presents with severe ulcerations resulting in black or green discoloration of the mucosa, consistent with full-thickness bowel-wall necrosis. The degree of reversibility can be predicted from the mucosal findings: Mild erythema is nearly 100% reversible, moderate ~50%, and frank necrosis is simply dead bowel. Follow-up colonoscopy can be performed to rule out progression of ischemic colitis.

Laparotomy for nonocclusive mesenteric ischemia is warranted for signs of peritonitis or worsening endoscopic findings and if the patient's condition does not improve with aggressive resuscitation. Ischemic colitis is optimally treated with resection of the ischemic bowel and formation of a proximal stoma. Primary anastomosis should not be performed in patients with acute intestinal ischemia.

Patients with MVT may present with a gradual or sudden onset. Symptoms include vague abdominal pain, nausea, and vomiting. Examination findings include abdominal distention with mild to moderate tenderness and signs of dehydration. The diagnosis of mesenteric thrombosis is frequently made on abdominal spiral CT with oral and IV contrast. Findings on CT include bowel-wall thickening and ascites. Intravenous contrast will demonstrate a delayed arterial phase and clot within the superior mesenteric vein. The goal of management is to optimize hemodynamics and correct electrolyte abnormalities with massive fluid resuscitation. Intravenous antibiotics as well as anticoagulation should be initiated. If laparotomy is performed and MVT is suspected, heparin anticoagulation is immediately initiated and compromised bowel is resected. Of all acute intestinal disorders, mesenteric venous insufficiency is associated with the best prognosis.

Chronic intestinal ischemia presents with intestinal angina or abdominal pain associated with need for increased blood flow to the intestine. Patients report abdominal cramping and pain following ingestion of a meal. Weight loss and chronic diarrhea may also be noted. Abdominal pain without weight loss is not chronic mesenteric angina. Physical examination will often reveal the presence of an abdominal bruit as well as other manifestations of atherosclerosis. Duplex ultrasound evaluation of the mesenteric vessels has gained in popularity. In the absence of obesity and an increased bowel gas pattern, the radiologist may be able to identify flow disturbances within the vessels or the lack of a vasodilation response to feeding. This tool is frequently used as a screening test for patients with symptoms suggestive of chronic mesenteric ischemia. The gold standard for confirmation of mesenteric arterial occlusion is mesenteric angiography. Evaluation with mesenteric angiography allows for identification and possible intervention for the treatment of thrombus within the vessel lumen and will also evaluate the patency of remaining mesenteric vessels. The use of mesenteric angiography may be limited in the presence of renal failure or contrast allergy. Magnetic resonance angiography is an alternative if the administration of contrast dye is contraindicated.

The management of chronic intestinal ischemia includes medical management of atherosclerotic disease by lipid-lowering medications, exercise, and cessation of smoking. A full cardiac evaluation should be performed before intervention. Newer endovascular procedures may avoid an operative intervention in selected patient populations. Angioplasty with endovascular stenting in the treatment of chronic mesenteric ischemia is associated with an 80% long-term success rate. In patients requiring surgical exploration, the approach used is determined by the mesenteric angiogram. The entire length of the small and large bowel should be evaluated, beginning at the ligament of Treitz. Restoration of blood flow at the time of laparotomy is accomplished with mesenteric bypass.

Determination of intestinal viability intraoperatively in patients with suspected intestinal ischemia can be challenging. After revascularization, the bowel wall should be observed for return of a pink color and peristalsis. Palpation of major arterial vessels can be performed as well as applying a doppler flowmeter to the antimesenteric border of the bowel wall, but neither is a definitive indicator of viability. In equivocal cases, 1 g of IV sodium fluorescein is administered and the pattern of bowel reperfusion is observed under ultraviolet illumination with a standard (3600 A) Wood's lamp. An area of nonfluorescence >5 mm in diameter suggests nonviability. If doubt persists, reexploration performed 24–48 h following surgery will allow demarcation of nonviable bowel. Primary intestinal anastomosis in patients with ischemic bowel is always worrisome, and reanastomosis should be deferred to the time of second-look laparotomy.

ACKNOWLEDGMENTS

We thank Cory Sandore for providing some illustrations for this chapter. Gregory Bulkley contributed to this chapter in the 16th edition.

FURTHER READINGS

Hsu H et al: Impact of etiological factors and APACHE II and POSSUM scores in management and clinical outcomes of acute intestinal ischemic disease after surgical treatment. World J Surg 30:2152, 2006

Matsumoto AH et al: Percutaneous transluminal angioplasty and stenting in the treatment of chronic mesenteric ischemia: Results and long-term follow-up. J Am Coll Surg 194:S22, 2002

Mitchell EL, Moneta GL: Mesenteric duplex scanning. Perspect Vasc Surg Endovasc Ther 18:175, 2006

Shih MC et al: CTA and MRA in mesenteric ischemia: Part 2, normal findings and complications after surgical and endovascular treatment. AJR Am J Roentgenol 188:462, 2007

Sise MJ: Mesenteric ischemia: the whole spectrum. Scand J Surg 99:106, 2010

Wyers MC: Acute mesenteric ischemia: Diagnostic approach and surgical treatment. Semin Vasc Surg 23:9, 2010

CHAPTER 299

Acute Intestinal Obstruction

William Silen

ETIOLOGY AND CLASSIFICATION

In 75% of patients, acute intestinal obstruction results from adhesive bands or internal hernias secondary to previous abdominal surgery or from external hernias. The incidence of acute intestinal obstruction requiring hospital admission within the first few postoperative weeks is 5–25%, and 10–50% of these patients will require surgical intervention. The incidence of postoperative intestinal obstruction may be lower following laparoscopic surgery than open procedures. However, the laparoscopic gastric bypass procedure may be associated with an unexpected high rate of intestinal obstruction, with a higher reoperative rate. Other causes of intestinal obstruction not related to previous abdominal surgery include lesions *intrinsic* to the wall of the intestine, e.g., diverticulitis, carcinoma, and regional enteritis; and luminal obstruction, e.g., gallstone obstruction, intussusception.

Two other conditions that must be differentiated from acute intestinal obstruction include *adynamic ileus* and *primary intestinal pseudo-obstruction.* Adynamic ileus is mediated via the hormonal component of the sympathoadrenal system and may occur after any peritoneal insult; its severity and duration will be dependent to some degree on the type of peritoneal injury. Hydrochloric acid, colonic contents, and pancreatic enzymes are among the most irritating to the peritoneum, whereas blood and urine are less so.

Adynamic ileus occurs to some degree after any abdominal operation. Retroperitoneal hematoma, particularly associated with vertebral fracture, may cause severe adynamic ileus, and the latter may occur with other retroperitoneal conditions, such as ureteral calculus or severe pyelonephritis. Thoracic diseases, including lower-lobe pneumonia, fractured ribs, and myocardial infarction, frequently produce adynamic ileus, as do electrolyte disturbances, particularly potassium depletion. Finally, intestinal ischemia, whether from vascular occlusion or intestinal distention itself, may perpetuate an adynamic ileus. Intestinal pseudo-obstruction is a chronic motility disorder that frequently mimics mechanical obstruction. This condition is often exacerbated by narcotic use.

PATHOPHYSIOLOGY

Distention of the intestine is caused by the accumulation of gas and fluid proximal to and within the obstructed segment. Between 70 and 80% of intestinal gas consists of swallowed air, and because this is composed mainly of nitrogen, which is poorly absorbed from the intestinal lumen, removal of air by continuous gastric suction is a useful adjunct in the treatment of intestinal distention. The accumulation of fluid proximal to the obstructing mechanism results not only from ingested fluid, swallowed saliva, gastric juice, and biliary and pancreatic secretions but also from interference with normal sodium and water transport. During the first 12–24 h of obstruction, a marked depression of flux from lumen to blood of sodium and water occurs in the distended proximal intestine. After 24 h, sodium and water move into the lumen, contributing further to the distention and fluid losses. Intraluminal pressure rises from a normal of 2–4 cmH_2O to 8–10 cmH_2O. The loss of fluids and electrolytes may be extreme, and unless replacement is prompt, hypovolemia, renal insufficiency, and shock may result. Vomiting, accumulation of fluids within the lumen, and the sequestration of fluid into the edematous intestinal wall and peritoneal cavity as a result of impairment of venous return from the intestine all contribute to massive loss of fluid and electrolytes.

A "closed loop" is the most feared complication of acute intestinal obstruction. Closed-loop obstruction results when the lumen is occluded at two points by a single mechanism such as a fascial hernia or adhesive band, thus producing a closed loop, the blood supply of which is also often occluded by the hernia or band. During peristalsis, when a "closed loop" is present, pressures reach 30–60 cmH_2O. Strangulation of the closed loop is common in association with marked distention proximal to the involved loop. A form of closed-loop obstruction is encountered when complete obstruction of the colon exists in the presence of a competent ileocecal valve (85% of individuals). Although the blood supply of the colon is not entrapped within the obstructing mechanism, distention of the cecum is extreme because of its greater diameter (Laplace's law), and impairment of the intramural blood supply is considerable, with consequent gangrene of the cecal wall. Once impairment of blood supply to the gastrointestinal tract occurs, bacterial invasion supervenes, and peritonitis develops. The systemic effects of extreme distention include elevation of the diaphragm with restricted ventilation and subsequent atelectasis. Venous return via the inferior vena cava may also be impaired.

SYMPTOMS

Mechanical intestinal obstruction is characterized by cramping midabdominal pain, which tends to be more severe the higher the obstruction. The pain occurs in paroxysms, and the patient is relatively comfortable in the intervals between the pains. Audible borborygmi are often noted by the patient simultaneously with the paroxysms of pain. The pain may become less severe as distention progresses, probably because motility is impaired in the edematous intestine. When strangulation is present, the pain is usually more localized and may be steady and severe without a colicky component, a fact that often causes delay in diagnosis of obstruction. Vomiting is almost invariable, and it is earlier and more profuse the higher the obstruction. The vomitus initially contains bile and mucus and remains as such if the obstruction is high in the intestine. With low ileal obstruction, the vomitus becomes feculent, i.e., orange-brown in color with a foul odor, which results from the overgrowth of bacteria proximal to the obstruction. Hiccups (singultus) are common. Obstipation and failure to pass gas by rectum are invariably present when the obstruction is complete, although some stool and gas may be passed spontaneously or after an enema shortly after onset of the complete obstruction. Diarrhea is occasionally observed in partial obstruction. Blood in the stool is rare but does occur in cases of intussusception.

In *adynamic ileus* as well as *colonic pseudo-obstruction*, colicky pain is absent and only discomfort from distention is evident. Vomiting may be frequent but is rarely profuse. Complete obstipation may or may not occur. Singultus (hiccups) is common.

PHYSICAL FINDINGS

Abdominal distention is the hallmark of all forms of intestinal obstruction. It is least marked in cases of obstruction high in the small intestine and most marked in colonic obstruction. In early obstruction of the small and large intestine, tenderness and rigidity are usually minimal; the temperature is rarely >37.8°C (100°F). The appearance of shock, tenderness, rigidity, and fever indicates that contamination of the peritoneum with infected intestinal content has occurred. Hernial orifices should always be carefully examined for the presence of a mass. Auscultation may reveal loud, high-pitched borborygmi coincident with colicky pain, but this finding is often absent late in strangulating or nonstrangulating obstruction. A quiet abdomen does not eliminate the possibility of obstruction, nor does it necessarily establish the diagnosis of adynamic ileus. The presence of a palpable abdominal mass usually signifies a closed-loop strangulating small-bowel obstruction; the tense fluid-filled loop is the palpable lesion.

LABORATORY AND X-RAY FINDINGS

Laboratory and radiographic studies are used to help differentiate the two important clinical aspects of this disorder: strangulation vs. nonstrangulation and partial vs. complete obstruction. Leukocytosis, with shift to the left, usually occurs when strangulation is present, but a normal white blood cell count does not exclude strangulation. Elevation of the serum amylase level is encountered occasionally in all forms of intestinal obstruction. Radiographic images demonstrating distention of fluid- and gas-filled loops of small intestine usually arranged in a "stepladder" pattern with air-fluid levels and an absence or paucity of colonic gas are pathognomonic for small-bowel obstruction. Complete obstruction is suggested when passage of gas or stool per rectum has ceased and when gas is absent in the distal intestine by x-ray. A general haze due to peritoneal fluid and sometimes a "coffee bean"–shaped mass are seen in strangulating closed loop obstruction. A thin barium upper gastrointestinal series may help to differentiate partial from complete obstruction. However, thick barium given by mouth should be avoided when the obstruction is considered to be high grade or complete since retained barium sulfate may become inspissated and either make an incomplete obstruction complete or be aspirated into the tracheobronchial tree. CT is the most commonly used modality to evaluate patients for intestinal obstruction but differentiating adynamic ileus, partial obstruction, and complete obstruction may be difficult (Fig. 299-1). The sensitivity and specificity of CT for strangulating obstruction are low (50 and 80%, respectively).

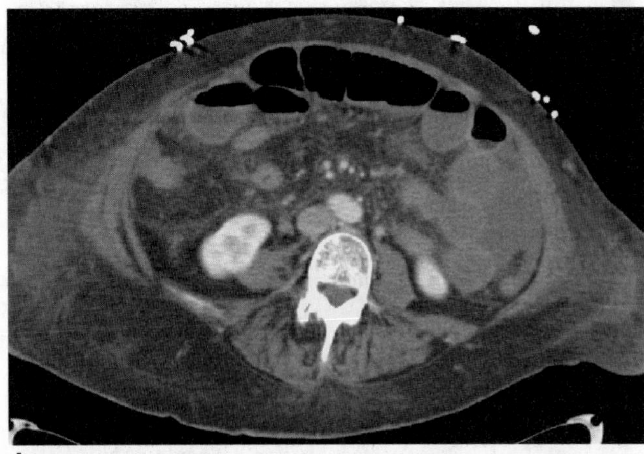

A

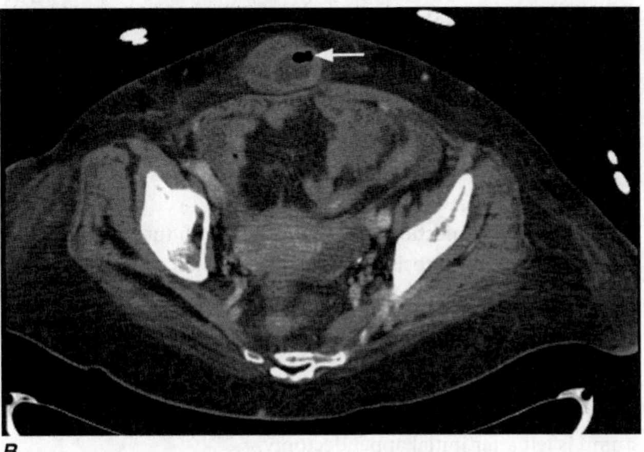

B

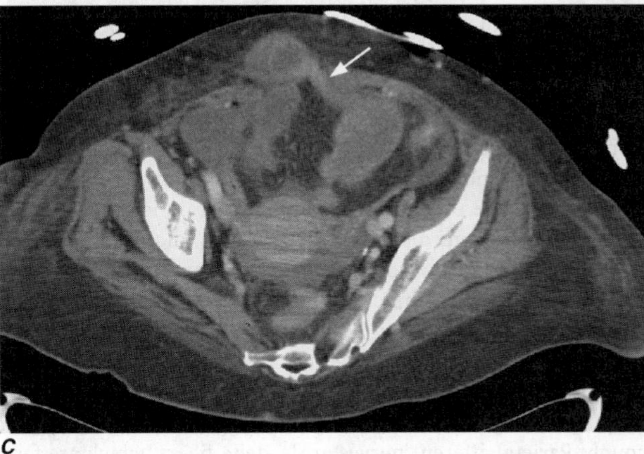

C

Figure 299-1 CT with oral and intravenous contrast demonstrating (*A*) evidence of small-bowel dilatation with air-fluid levels consistent with a small-bowel obstruction; (*B*) a partial small-bowel obstruction from an incarcerated ventral hernia (*arrow*); and (*C*) decompressed bowel seen distal to the hernia (*arrow*).

Common causes of colonic obstruction can be seen on abdominal radiographic series. These films may demonstrate a "bird's beak" sign when a sigmoid volvulus has occurred or an enlarged cecum when a cecal torsion or bascule is present. Colonic obstruction with a competent ileocecal valve is easily recognized because distention with gas is mainly confined to the colon. Gastrografin enema may help in demonstrating a complete colonic obstruction. Furthermore, *barium should never be given by mouth to a patient with a possible colonic obstruction* until that possibility has been excluded.

TREATMENT Acute Intestinal Obstruction

SMALL-INTESTINAL OBSTRUCTION The overall mortality rate for obstruction of the small intestine is about 10%. While the mortality rate for nonstrangulating obstruction is 5–8%, the mortality rate for a strangulating obstruction ranges from 20 to 75%. Since strangulating small-bowel obstruction is always complete, surgical interventions should always be undertaken in such patients after suitable preparation. Before operating, fluid and electrolyte balance should be restored and decompression instituted by means of a nasogastric tube. Replacement of potassium is especially important because intake is nil and losses in vomitus are large. A long intestinal tube is not indicated. Operative intervention may be undertaken successfully by laparoscopic techniques with a decreased incidence of wound complications. However, laparoscopic lysis of adhesions is associated with a longer operative time and higher conversion to open rate when compared to other laparoscopic procedures. Alternatively, lysis of adhesions can be achieved through an open abdominal incision. In general, >50% of adhesions that occur are found at the previous incision site. Purely nonoperative therapy is safe only in the presence of incomplete obstruction and is best used in patients without increasing abdominal pain or leukocytosis. The overall recurrence of small-bowel obstruction is 16%. Population-based studies show that although the surgical management of small-bowel obstruction is associated with longer hospital stays, the rate of readmission for obstruction is lower. However, regardless of treatment type, following the index admission, only 20% of patients required readmission within a 5-year follow-up period.

COLONIC OBSTRUCTION The mortality rate for colonic obstruction is about 20%. As in small-bowel obstruction, nonoperative treatment is contraindicated unless the obstruction is incomplete. Incomplete obstruction can be treated with colonoscopic decompression and placement of a metallic stent if a malignant lesion is present. The success rate approaches 90% depending on the location of the obstruction, with left-sided lesions being more successfully stented than right-sided lesions. In general, the colonic stent is considered to be a temporary solution or a "bridge to surgery," which allows for colonic preparation before surgical intervention. When obstruction is complete, early operation is mandatory, especially when the ileocecal valve is competent, because of the concern for cecal perforation. Cecal perforation is more likely if the cecal diameter is >10 cm on plain abdominal film.

Decisions regarding the operative management of colonic obstruction are based on the cause of the obstruction and the patient's overall well-being. For obstruction on the left side of the colon, operative management strategies include either decompression by cecostomy or transverse colostomy or resection with end-colostomy formation (Hartmann's procedure). Primary resection of obstructing left-sided lesions with on-table washout of the colon has also been accomplished safely. For a lesion of the right or transverse colon, primary resection and anastomosis can be performed safely because distention of the ileum with consequent discrepancy in size and hazard in suture are usually not present. Furthermore, the bacterial and stool content is less on the right side of the colon, decreasing the chance of infection.

ADYNAMIC ILEUS This type of ileus usually responds to nonoperative decompression and treatment of the primary disease. The prognosis is usually good. Correction of electrolyte abnormalities should be instituted (i.e., potassium, magnesium). Successful decompression of a colonic ileus has been accomplished by repetitive colonoscopy. Neostigmine is also effective in cases of colonic ileus that have not responded to other conservative treatment. Rarely, adynamic colonic distention may become so great that cecostomy is required if cecal gangrene is feared.

FURTHER READINGS

Dubois A et al: Postoperative ileus: Physiopathology, etiology and treatment. Ann Surg 178:781, 1973

Eskelinen M et al: Contributions of history-taking, physical examination, and computer assistance to diagnosis of acute small-bowel obstruction. A prospective study of 1333 patients with acute abdominal pain. Scand J Gastroenterol 29:715, 1994

Fevang BT et al: Complications and death after surgical treatment of small bowel obstruction: A 35-year institutional experience. Ann Surg 231:529, 2000

Jackson BR: The diagnosis of colonic obstruction. Dis Colon Rectum 25:603, 1982

Kucukmetin A et al: Palliative surgery versus medical management for bowel obstruction in ovarian cancer. Cochrane Database Syst Rev 7:CD007792, 2010

Silen W: *Cope's Early Diagnosis of the Acute Abdomen*, 21st ed. London, Oxford, 2005

CHAPTER 300 Acute Appendicitis and Peritonitis

William Silen

ACUTE APPENDICITIS

INCIDENCE AND EPIDEMIOLOGY

With more than 250,000 appendectomies performed annually, appendicitis is the most common abdominal surgical emergency in the United States. The peak incidence of acute appendicitis is in the second and third decades of life; it is relatively rare at the extremes of age. However, perforation is more common in infancy and in the elderly, during which periods mortality rates are highest. Males and females are equally affected, except between puberty and age 25, when males predominate in a 3:2 ratio. The incidence of appendicitis has remained stable in the United States over the last 30 years, while the incidence of appendicitis is much lower in underdeveloped countries, especially parts of Africa, and in lower socioeconomic groups. The mortality rate in the United States decreased eightfold between 1941 and 1970 but has remained at <1 per 100,000 since then.

PATHOGENESIS

Appendicitis is believed to occur as a result of appendiceal luminal obstruction. Obstruction is most commonly caused by a fecalith, which results from accumulation and inspissation of fecal matter around vegetable fibers. Enlarged lymphoid follicles associated with viral infections (e.g., measles), inspissated barium, worms (e.g., pinworms, *Ascaris*, and *Taenia*), and tumors (e.g., carcinoid or carcinoma) may also obstruct the lumen. Other common pathologic findings include appendiceal ulceration. The cause of the ulceration is unknown, although a viral etiology has been postulated. Infection with *Yersinia* organisms may cause the disease, since high complement fixation antibody titers have been found in up to 30% of cases of proven appendicitis. Luminal bacteria multiply and invade the appendiceal wall as venous engorgement and subsequent arterial compromise result from the high intraluminal pressures. Finally, gangrene and perforation occur. If the process evolves slowly, adjacent organs such as the terminal ileum, cecum, and omentum may wall off the appendiceal area so that a localized abscess will develop, whereas rapid progression of vascular impairment may cause perforation with free access to the peritoneal cavity. Subsequent rupture of primary appendiceal abscesses may produce fistulas between the appendix and bladder, small intestine, sigmoid, or cecum. Occasionally, acute appendicitis may be the first manifestation of Crohn's disease.

While chronic infection of the appendix with tuberculosis, amebiasis, and actinomycosis may occur, a useful clinical aphorism states that *chronic appendiceal inflammation is not usually the cause of prolonged abdominal pain of weeks' or months' duration.* In contrast, recurrent acute appendicitis does occur, often with complete resolution of inflammation and symptoms between attacks. Recurrent acute appendicitis may also occur if a long appendiceal stump is left after initial appendectomy.

CLINICAL MANIFESTATIONS

The sequence of abdominal discomfort and anorexia associated with acute appendicitis is pathognomonic. The pain is described as being located in the periumbilical region initially and then migrating to the right lower quadrant. This classic sequence of symptoms occurs in only 66% of patients. The differential diagnoses for periumbilical and right lower quadrant pain is listed in Table 300-1. The periumbilical abdominal pain is of the visceral type, resulting from distention of the appendiceal lumen. This pain is carried on slow-conducting C fibers and is usually poorly localized in the periumbilical or epigastric region. In general, this visceral pain is mild, often cramping and usually lasting 4–6 h, but it may not be noted by stoic individuals. As inflammation spreads to the parietal peritoneal surfaces, the pain becomes somatic, steady, and more severe and aggravated by motion or cough. Parietal afferent nerves are A delta fibers, which are fast-conducting and unilateral. These fibers localize the pain to the *right lower quadrant. Anorexia* is very common; a hungry patient almost invariably does not have acute appendicitis. *Nausea* and *vomiting* occur in 50–60% of cases, but vomiting is usually self-limited. Change in bowel habit is of little diagnostic value, since any or no alteration may be observed, although the presence of diarrhea caused by an inflamed appendix in juxtaposition to the sigmoid may cause diagnostic difficulties. Urinary frequency and dysuria occur if the appendix lies adjacent to the bladder.

Physical findings vary with time after onset of the illness and according to the location of the appendix, which may be situated deep in the pelvic cul-de-sac; in the right lower quadrant in any relation to the peritoneum, cecum, and small intestine; in the right upper quadrant (especially during pregnancy); or even in the left lower quadrant. *The diagnosis cannot be established unless tenderness can be elicited.* While tenderness is sometimes absent in the

TABLE 300-1 The Anatomic Origin of Periumbilical and Right Lower Quadrant Pain in the Differential Diagnosis of Appendicitis

Periumbilical	
Appendicitis	
Small-bowel obstruction	
Gastroenteritis	
Mesenteric ischemia	
Right Lower Quadrant	
Gastrointestinal causes	Gynecologic causes
Appendicitis	Ovarian tumor/torsion
Inflammatory bowel disease	Pelvic inflammatory disease
Right-sided diverticulitis	Renal causes
Gastroenteritis	Pyelonephritis
Inguinal hernia	Perinephritic abscess
	Nephrolithiasis

early visceral stage of the disease, it ultimately always develops and is found in any location corresponding to the position of the appendix. Typically, tenderness to palpation will often occur at McBurney's point, anatomically located on a line one-third of the way between the anterior iliac spine and the umbilicus. Abdominal tenderness may be completely absent if a retrocecal or pelvic appendix is present, in which case the sole physical finding may be tenderness in the flank or on rectal or pelvic examination. Referred rebound tenderness is often present and is most likely to be absent early in the illness. Flexion of the right hip and guarded movement by the patient are due to parietal peritoneal involvement. Hyperesthesia of the skin of the right lower quadrant and a positive psoas or obturator sign are often late findings and are rarely of diagnostic value.

The temperature is usually normal or slightly elevated [37.2°–38°C (99°–100.5°F)], but a temperature >38.3°C (101°F) should suggest perforation. Tachycardia is commensurate with the elevation of the temperature. Rigidity and tenderness become more marked as the disease progresses to perforation and localized or diffuse peritonitis. Distention is rare unless severe diffuse peritonitis has developed. A mass may develop if localized perforation has occurred but will not usually be detectable before 3 days after onset. Earlier presence of a mass suggests carcinoma of the cecum or Crohn's disease. Perforation is rare before 24 h after onset of symptoms, but the rate may be as high as 80% after 48 h.

Although moderate leukocytosis of 10,000–18,000 cells/μL is frequent (with a concomitant left shift), the absence of leukocytosis does not rule out acute appendicitis. Leukocytosis of >20,000 cells/μL suggests probable perforation. Anemia and blood in the stool suggest a primary diagnosis of carcinoma of the cecum, especially in elderly individuals. The urine may contain a few white or red blood cells without bacteria if the appendix lies close to the right ureter or bladder. Urinalysis is most useful in excluding genitourinary conditions that may mimic acute appendicitis.

Radiographs are rarely of value except when an opaque fecalith (5% of patients) is observed in the right lower quadrant (especially in children). Consequently, abdominal films are not routinely

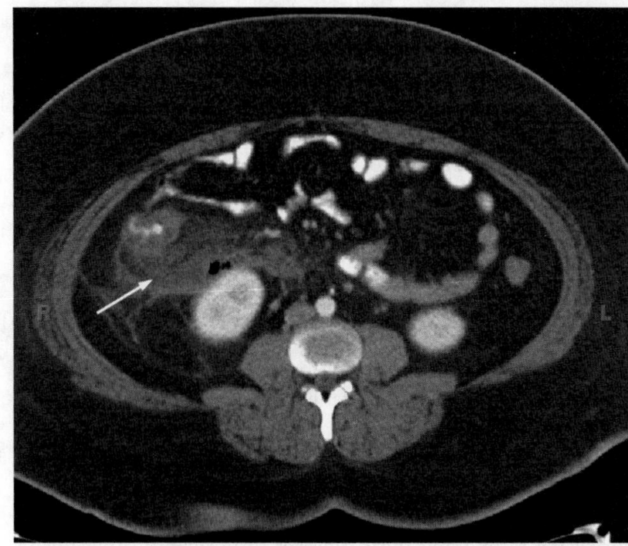

Figure 300-1 CT with oral and intravenous contrast of acute appendicitis. There is thickening of the wall of the appendix and periappendiceal stranding *(arrow)*.

obtained unless other conditions such as intestinal obstruction or ureteral calculus may be present. The diagnosis may also be established by the ultrasonic demonstration of an enlarged and thick-walled appendix. Ultrasound is most useful to exclude ovarian cysts, ectopic pregnancy, or tuboovarian abscess. Several studies have recently demonstrated the benefit of contrast-enhanced or nonenhanced CT over ultrasound and plain radiographs in the diagnosis of acute appendicitis. The findings on CT will include a thickened appendix with periappendiceal stranding and often the presence of a fecalith (Figs. 300-1 and 300-2). The reported positive predictive value of CT is 95–97% and the overall accuracy is 90–98%. Furthermore, nonvisualization of the appendix on CT is associated with the findings of a normal appendix 98% of the time. Free peritoneal air is uncommon, even in perforated appendicitis.

While the typical historic sequence and physical findings are present in 50–60% of cases, a wide variety of atypical patterns of disease are encountered, especially at the age extremes and during

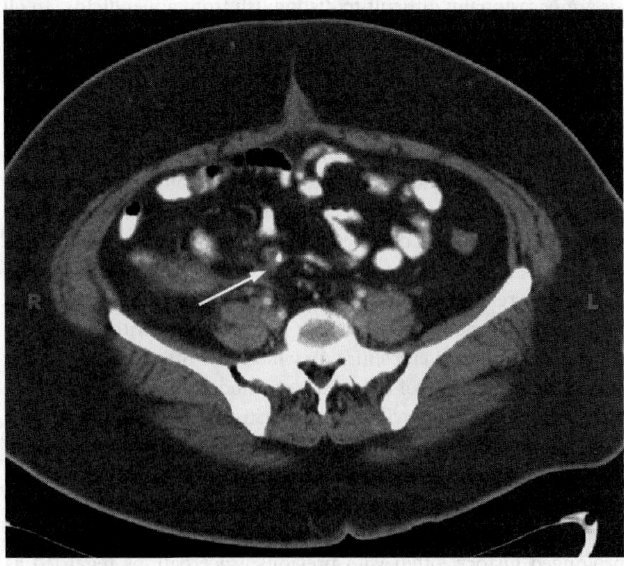

Figure 300-2 Appendiceal fecolith *(arrow)*.

pregnancy. Infants under 2 years of age have a 70–80% incidence of perforation and generalized peritonitis. This is thought to be the result of a delay in diagnosis. Any infant or child with diarrhea, vomiting, and abdominal pain is highly suspect. Fever is much more common in this age group, and abdominal distention is often the only physical finding. In the elderly, pain and tenderness are often blunted, and thus the diagnosis is also frequently delayed and leads to a 30% incidence of perforation in patients older than age 70 years. Elderly patients often present initially with a slightly painful mass (a primary appendiceal abscess) or with adhesive intestinal obstruction 5 or 6 days after a previously undetected perforated appendix.

Appendicitis occurs about once in every 500–2000 pregnancies and is the most common extrauterine condition requiring abdominal operation. The diagnosis may be missed or delayed because of the frequent occurrence of mild abdominal discomfort and nausea and vomiting during pregnancy, and because of the gradual shift of the appendix from the right lower quadrant to the right upper quadrant during the second and third trimester of pregnancy. Appendicitis tends to be most common during the second trimester. The diagnosis is best made with ultrasound, which is 80% accurate; however, if perforation has already occurred, the accuracy of ultrasound decreases to 30%. Early intervention is warranted because the incidence of fetal loss with a normal appendix is 1.5%. With perforation, the incidence of fetal loss is 20–35%.

DIFFERENTIAL DIAGNOSIS

Acute appendicitis has been labeled the *masquerader*, and the diagnosis is often more difficult to make in young females. Obtaining a good history, including sexual activity and the presence of a vaginal discharge, will help differentiate acute appendicitis from pelvic inflammatory disease (PID). The presence of a malodorous vaginal discharge and gram-negative intracellular diplococci are pathognomonic for PID. Pain on movement of the cervix is also more specific for PID but may occur in appendicitis if perforation has occurred or if the appendix lies adjacent to the uterus or adnexa. *Rupture of a graafian follicle* (mittelschmerz) occurs at midcycle and will produce pain and tenderness more diffuse and usually of a less severe degree than in appendicitis. *Rupture of a corpus luteum cyst* is identical clinically to rupture of a graafian follicle but develops about the time of menstruation. The presence of an adnexal mass, evidence of blood loss, and a positive pregnancy test help differentiate *ruptured tubal pregnancy*. *Twisted ovarian cyst* and *endometriosis* are occasionally difficult to distinguish from appendicitis. In all these female conditions, ultrasonography and laparoscopy may be of great value.

Acute mesenteric lymphadenitis and *acute gastroenteritis* are the diagnoses usually given when enlarged, slightly reddened lymph nodes at the root of the mesentery and a normal appendix are encountered at operation in a patient who usually has right lower quadrant tenderness. Retrospectively, these patients may have had a higher temperature, diarrhea, more diffuse pain and abdominal tenderness, and a lymphocytosis. Between cramps, the abdomen is completely relaxed. Children seem to be affected more frequently than adults. Some of these patients have infection with *Y. pseudotuberculosis* or *Y. enterocolitica*, in which case the diagnosis can be established by culture of the mesenteric nodes or by serologic titers (Chap. 159). In *Salmonella* gastroenteritis, the abdominal findings are similar, although the pain may be more severe and more localized, and fever and chills are common. The occurrence of similar symptoms among other members of the family may be helpful. *Regional enteritis* (Crohn's disease) is usually associated with a more prolonged history, often with previous exacerbations regarded as episodes of gastroenteritis unless the diagnosis has been established previously. Often an inflammatory mass is palpable. In addition, acute cholecystitis, perforated ulcer, acute pancreatitis, acute diverticulitis, strangulating intestinal obstruction, ureteral calculus, and pyelonephritis may present diagnostic difficulties.

TREATMENT Acute Appendicitis

If the diagnosis is in question, 4–6 h of observation with serial abdominal exams is always more beneficial than harmful. Antibiotics should not be administered when the diagnosis is in question, since they will only mask the perforation. The treatment of presumed acute appendicitis is early operation and appendectomy as soon as the patient can be prepared. Appendectomy is frequently accomplished laparoscopically and is associated with less postoperative narcotic use and earlier discharge. It is acceptable to have a 15–20% incidence of a normal appendix at the time of appendectomy to avoid perforation. The use of early laparoscopy instead of close clinical observation has not shown a clinical benefit in the management of patients with nonspecific abdominal pain.

A different approach is indicated if a palpable mass is found 3–5 days after the onset of symptoms. This finding usually represents the presence of a phlegmon or abscess, and complications from attempted surgical excision are frequent. Such patients treated with broad-spectrum antibiotics, drainage of abscesses >3 cm, parenteral fluids, and bowel rest usually show resolution of symptoms within 1 week. *Interval appendectomy* can be performed safely 6–12 weeks later. A randomized clinical trial has demonstrated that antibiotics alone can effectively treat acute, nonperforated appendicitis in 86% of male patients. However, antibiotics alone were associated with a higher recurrence rate than when followed by surgical intervention. If the mass enlarges or the patient becomes more toxic, the abscess should be drained. Free perforation is associated with generalized peritonitis and its complications, including subphrenic, pelvic, or other abscesses, and can be avoided by early diagnosis. The mortality rate for nonperforated appendicitis is 0.1%, little more than the risk of general anesthesia; for perforated appendicitis, mortality is 3% (and can reach 15% in the elderly).

ACUTE PERITONITIS

Peritonitis is an inflammation of the peritoneum; it may be localized or diffuse in location, acute or chronic in natural history, and infectious or aseptic in pathogenesis. Acute peritonitis is most often infectious and is usually related to a perforated viscus (and called *secondary peritonitis*). When no intraabdominal source is identified, infectious peritonitis is called *primary* or *spontaneous*. Acute peritonitis is associated with decreased intestinal motor activity, resulting in distention of the intestinal lumen with gas and fluid (adynamic ileus). The accumulation of fluid in the bowel together with the lack of oral intake leads to rapid intravascular volume depletion with effects on cardiac, renal, and other systems.

ETIOLOGY

Infectious agents gain access to the peritoneal cavity through a perforated viscus, a penetrating wound of the abdominal wall, or external introduction of a foreign object that is or becomes infected (e.g., a chronic peritoneal dialysis catheter). In the absence of immune compromise, host defenses are capable of eradicating small contaminations. The conditions that most commonly result in the introduction of bacteria into the peritoneum are ruptured appendix, ruptured diverticulum, perforated peptic ulcer, incarcerated hernia, gangre-

TABLE 300-2 Conditions Leading to Secondary Bacterial Peritonitis

Perforations of bowel	Perforations or leaking of other organs
Trauma, blunt or penetrating	Pancreas—pancreatitis
Inflammation	Gallbladder—cholecystitis
Appendicitis	Urinary bladder—trauma, rupture
Diverticulitis	Liver—bile leak after biopsy
Peptic ulcer disease	Fallopian tubes—salpingitis
Inflammatory bowel disease	Bleeding into the peritoneal cavity
Iatrogenic	**Disruption of integrity of peritoneal cavity**
Endoscopic perforation	Trauma
Anastomotic leaks	Continuous ambulatory peritoneal dialysis (indwelling catheter)
Catheter perforation	Intraperitoneal chemotherapy
Vascular	Perinephric abscess
Embolus	Iatrogenic—postoperative, foreign body
Ischemia	
Obstructions	
Adhesions	
Strangulated hernias	
Volvulus	
Intussusception	
Neoplasms	
Ingested foreign body, toothpick, fish bone	

nous gall bladder, volvulus, bowel infarction, cancer, inflammatory bowel disease, or intestinal obstruction. However, a wide range of mechanisms may play a role (Table 300-2). Bacterial peritonitis can also occur in the apparent absence of an intraperitoneal source of bacteria (primary or spontaneous bacterial peritonitis). This condition occurs in the setting of ascites and liver cirrhosis in 90% of the cases, usually in patients with ascites with low protein concentration (<1 g/L) (Chap. 308). Bacterial peritonitis is discussed in detail in Chap. 127.

Aseptic peritonitis may be due to peritoneal irritation by abnormal presence of physiologic fluids (e.g., gastric juice, bile, pancreatic enzymes, blood, or urine) or sterile foreign bodies (e.g., surgical sponges or instruments, starch from surgical gloves) in the peritoneal cavity or as a complication of rare systemic diseases such as lupus erythematosus, porphyria, or familial Mediterranean fever (Chap. 330). Chemical irritation of the peritoneum is greatest for acidic gastric juice and pancreatic enzymes. Secondary bacterial infection is common in chemical peritonitis.

CLINICAL FEATURES

The cardinal manifestations of peritonitis are acute abdominal pain and tenderness, usually with fever. The location of the pain depends on the underlying cause and whether the inflammation is localized or generalized. Localized peritonitis is most common in uncomplicated appendicitis and diverticulitis, and physical findings are limited to the area of inflammation. Generalized peritonitis is associated with widespread inflammation and diffuse abdominal tenderness and rebound. Rigidity of the abdominal wall is common in both localized and generalized peritonitis. Bowel sounds are usually but not always absent. Tachycardia, hypotension, and signs of dehydration are common. Leukocytosis and marked acidosis are common laboratory findings. Plain abdominal films may show dilation of large and small bowel with edema of the bowel wall. Free air under the diaphragm is associated with a perforated viscus. CT and/or ultrasonography can identify the presence of free fluid or an abscess. When ascites is present, diagnostic paracentesis with cell count (>250 neutrophils/μL is usual in peritonitis), protein and lactate dehydrogenase levels, and culture is essential. In elderly and immunosuppressed patients, signs of peritoneal irritation may be more difficult to detect.

THERAPY AND PROGNOSIS

Treatment relies on rehydration, correction of electrolyte abnormalities, antibiotics, and surgical correction of the underlying defect. Mortality rates are <10% for uncomplicated peritonitis associated with a perforated ulcer or ruptured appendix or diverticulum in an otherwise healthy person. Mortality rates of ≥40% have been reported for elderly people, those with underlying illnesses, and when peritonitis has been present for >48 h.

FURTHER READINGS

Anderson RE: The natural history and traditional management of appendicitis revisited: Spontaneous resolution and predominance of prehospital perforations imply that a correct diagnosis is more important than an early diagnosis. World J Surg 31:86, 2007

Flum DR et al: Has misdiagnosis of appendicitis decreased over time? A population-based analysis. JAMA 286:1748, 2001

Merlin MA et al: Evidence-based appendicitis: The initial work-up. Postgrad Med 122:189, 2010

Morino M et al: Acute non-specific abdominal pain: A randomized controlled study comparing early laparoscopy vs. clinical observation. Ann Surg 241:881, 2006

Solomkin JS, Mazuski J: Intra-abdominal sepsis: Newer interventional and antimicrobial therapies. Infect Dis Clin North Am 23:595, 2009

Styrud J et al: Appendectomy vs. antibiotic treatment in acute appendectomy: A prospective multicenter randomized controlled trial. World J Surg 30:1033, 2006

CHAPTER 301 Approach to the Patient With Liver Disease

Marc Ghany
Jay H. Hoofnagle

A diagnosis of liver disease usually can be made accurately by a careful history, physical examination, and application of a few laboratory tests. In some circumstances, radiologic examinations are helpful or, indeed, diagnostic. Liver biopsy is considered the criterion standard in evaluation of liver disease but is now needed less for diagnosis than for grading and staging of disease. This chapter provides an introduction to diagnosis and management of liver disease, briefly reviewing the structure and function of the liver; the major clinical manifestations of liver disease; and the use of clinical history, physical examination, laboratory tests, imaging studies, and liver biopsy.

LIVER STRUCTURE AND FUNCTION

The liver is the largest organ of the body, weighing 1–1.5 kg and representing 1.5–2.5% of the lean body mass. The size and shape of the liver vary and generally match the general body shape—long and lean or squat and square. The liver is located in the right upper quadrant of the abdomen under the right lower rib cage against the diaphragm and projects for a variable extent into the left upper quadrant. The liver is held in place by ligamentous attachments to the diaphragm, peritoneum, great vessels, and upper gastrointestinal organs. It receives a dual blood supply; ~20% of the blood flow is oxygen-rich blood from the hepatic artery, and 80% is nutrient-rich blood from the portal vein arising from the stomach, intestines, pancreas, and spleen.

The majority of cells in the liver are hepatocytes, which constitute two-thirds of the mass of the liver. The remaining cell types are Kupffer cells (members of the reticuloendothelial system), stellate (Ito or fat-storing) cells, endothelial cells and blood vessels, bile ductular cells, and supporting structures. Viewed by light microscopy, the liver appears to be organized in lobules, with portal areas at the periphery and central veins in the center of each lobule. However, from a functional point of view, the liver is organized into acini, with both hepatic arterial and portal venous blood entering the acinus from the portal areas (zone 1) and then flowing through the sinusoids to the terminal hepatic veins (zone 3); the intervening hepatocytes constituting zone 2. The advantage of viewing the acinus as the physiologic unit of the liver is that it helps to explain the morphologic patterns and zonality of many vascular and biliary diseases not explained by the lobular arrangement.

Portal areas of the liver consist of small veins, arteries, bile ducts, and lymphatics organized in a loose stroma of supporting matrix and small amounts of collagen. Blood flowing into the portal areas is distributed through the sinusoids, passing from zone 1 to zone 3 of the acinus and draining into the terminal hepatic veins ("central veins"). Secreted bile flows in the opposite direction, in a counter-current pattern from zone 3 to zone 1. The sinusoids are lined by unique endothelial cells that have prominent fenestrae of variable size, allowing the free flow of plasma but not cellular elements. The plasma is thus in direct contact with hepatocytes in the subendothelial space of Disse.

Hepatocytes have distinct polarity. The basolateral side of the hepatocyte lines the space of Disse and is richly lined with microvilli; it demonstrates endocytotic and pinocytotic activity, with passive and active uptake of nutrients, proteins, and other molecules. The apical pole of the hepatocyte forms the canalicular membranes through which bile components are secreted. The canaliculi of hepatocytes form a fine network, which fuses into the bile ductular elements near the portal areas. Kupffer cells usually lie within the sinusoidal vascular space and represent the largest group of fixed macrophages in the body. The stellate cells are located in the space of Disse but are not usually prominent unless activated, when they produce collagen and matrix. Red blood cells stay in the sinusoidal space as blood flows through the lobules, but white blood cells can migrate through or around endothelial cells into the space of Disse and from there to portal areas, where they can return to the circulation through lymphatics.

Hepatocytes perform numerous and vital roles in maintaining homeostasis and health. These functions include the synthesis of most essential serum proteins (albumin, carrier proteins, coagulation factors, many hormonal and growth factors), the production of bile and its carriers (bile acids, cholesterol, lecithin, phospholipids), the regulation of nutrients (glucose, glycogen, lipids, cholesterol, amino acids), and metabolism and conjugation of lipophilic compounds (bilirubin, anions, cations, drugs) for excretion in the bile or urine. Measurement of these activities to assess liver function is complicated by the multiplicity and variability of these functions. The most commonly used liver "function" tests are measurements of serum bilirubin, albumin, and prothrombin time. The serum bilirubin level is a measure of hepatic conjugation and excretion, and the serum albumin level and prothrombin time are measures of protein synthesis. Abnormalities of bilirubin, albumin, and prothrombin time are typical of hepatic dysfunction. Frank liver failure is incompatible with life, and the functions of the liver are too complex and diverse to be subserved by a mechanical pump; dialysis membrane; or concoction of infused hormones, proteins, and growth factors.

LIVER DISEASES

While there are many causes of liver disease (Table 301-1), they generally present clinically in a few distinct patterns, usually classified as hepatocellular, cholestatic (obstructive), or mixed. In *hepatocellular diseases* (such as viral hepatitis or alcoholic liver disease), features of liver injury, inflammation, and necrosis predominate. In *cholestatic diseases* (such as gallstone or malignant obstruction, primary biliary cirrhosis, some drug-induced liver diseases), features of inhibition of bile flow predominate. In a mixed pattern, features of both hepatocellular and cholestatic injury are present (such as in cholestatic forms of viral hepatitis and many drug-induced liver diseases). The pattern of onset and prominence of symptoms can rapidly suggest a diagnosis, particularly if major risk factors are considered such as the age and sex of the patient and a history of exposure or risk behaviors.

TABLE 301-1 Liver Diseases

Inherited hyperbilirubinemia	**Liver involvement in systemic diseases**
Gilbert's syndrome	Sarcoidosis
Crigler-Najjar syndrome, types I and II	Amyloidosis
Dubin-Johnson syndrome	Glycogen storage diseases
Rotor syndrome	Celiac disease
Viral hepatitis	Tuberculosis
Hepatitis A	*Mycobacterium avium intracellulare*
Hepatitis B	**Cholestatic syndromes**
Hepatitis C	Benign postoperative cholestasis
Hepatitis D	Jaundice of sepsis
Hepatitis E	Total parenteral nutrition (TPN)–induced jaundice
Others (mononucleosis, herpes, adenovirus hepatitis)	Cholestasis of pregnancy
Cryptogenic hepatitis	Cholangitis and cholecystitis
Immune and autoimmune liver diseases	Extrahepatic biliary obstruction (stone, stricture, cancer)
Primary biliary cirrhosis	Biliary atresia
Autoimmune hepatitis	Caroli's disease
Sclerosing cholangitis	Cryptosporidiosis
Overlap syndromes	**Drug-induced liver disease**
Graft-versus-host disease	Hepatocellular patterns (isoniazid, acetaminophen)
Allograft rejection	Cholestatic patterns (methyltestosterone)
Genetic liver diseases	Mixed patterns (sulfonamides, phenytoin)
α_1 Antitrypsin deficiency	Micro- and macrovesicular steatosis (methotrexate, fialuridine)
Hemochromatosis	**Vascular injury**
Wilson's disease	Venoocclusive disease
Benign recurrent intrahepatic cholestasis (BRIC)	Budd-Chiari syndrome
Progressive familial intrahepatic cholestasis (PFIC), types I–III	Ischemic hepatitis
Others (galactosemia, tyrosinemia, cystic fibrosis, Newman-Pick disease, Gaucher's disease)	Passive congestion
Alcoholic liver disease	Portal vein thrombosis
Acute fatty liver	Nodular regenerative hyperplasia
Acute alcoholic hepatitis	**Mass lesions**
Laënnec's cirrhosis	Hepatocellular carcinoma
Nonalcoholic fatty liver	Cholangiocarcinoma
Steatosis	Adenoma
Steatohepatitis	Focal nodular hyperplasia
Acute fatty liver of pregnancy	Metastatic tumors
	Abscess
	Cysts
	Hemangioma

Typical presenting symptoms of liver disease include jaundice, fatigue, itching, right upper quadrant pain, nausea, poor appetite, abdominal distention, and intestinal bleeding. At present, however, many patients are diagnosed with liver disease who have no symptoms and who have been found to have abnormalities in biochemical liver tests as a part of a routine physical examination or screening for blood donation or for insurance or employment. The wide availability of batteries of liver tests makes it relatively simple to demonstrate the presence of liver injury as well as to rule it out in someone suspected of liver disease.

Evaluation of patients with liver disease should be directed at (1) establishing the etiologic diagnosis, (2) estimating the disease severity (grading), and (3) establishing the disease stage (staging).

Diagnosis should focus on the category of disease such as hepatocellular, cholestatic, or mixed injury, as well as on the specific etiologic diagnosis. *Grading* refers to assessing the severity or activity of disease—active or inactive, and mild, moderate, or severe. *Staging* refers to estimating the place in the course of the natural history of the disease, whether acute or chronic; early or late; precirrhotic, cirrhotic, or end-stage.

The goal of this chapter is to introduce general, salient concepts in the evaluation of patients with liver disease that help lead to the diagnoses discussed in subsequent chapters.

CLINICAL HISTORY

The clinical history should focus on the symptoms of liver disease—their nature, patterns of onset, and progression—and on potential risk factors for liver disease. The symptoms of liver disease include constitutional symptoms such as fatigue, weakness, nausea, poor appetite, and malaise and the more liver-specific symptoms of jaundice, dark urine, light stools, itching, abdominal pain, and bloating. Symptoms can also suggest the presence of cirrhosis, end-stage liver disease, or complications of cirrhosis such as portal hypertension. Generally, the constellation of symptoms and their patterns of onset rather than a specific symptom points to an etiology.

Fatigue is the most common and most characteristic symptom of liver disease. It is variously described as lethargy, weakness, listlessness, malaise, increased need for sleep, lack of stamina, and poor energy. The fatigue of liver disease typically arises after activity or exercise and is rarely present or severe in the morning after adequate rest (afternoon versus morning fatigue). Fatigue in liver disease is often intermittent and variable in severity from hour to hour and day to day. In some patients, it may not be clear whether fatigue is due to the liver disease or to other problems such as stress, anxiety, sleep disturbance, or a concurrent illness.

Nausea occurs with more severe liver disease and may accompany fatigue or be provoked by odors of food or eating fatty foods. Vomiting can occur but is rarely persistent or prominent. Poor appetite with weight loss occurs commonly in acute liver diseases but is rare in chronic disease, except when cirrhosis is present and advanced. Diarrhea is uncommon in liver disease, except with severe jaundice, where lack of bile acids reaching the intestine can lead to steatorrhea.

Right upper quadrant discomfort or ache ("liver pain") occurs in many liver diseases and is usually marked by tenderness over the liver area. The pain arises from stretching or irritation of Glisson's capsule, which surrounds the liver and is rich in nerve endings. Severe pain is most typical of gallbladder disease, liver abscess, and severe venoocclusive disease but is an occasional accompaniment of acute hepatitis.

Itching occurs with acute liver disease, appearing early in obstructive jaundice (from biliary obstruction or drug-induced cholestasis) and somewhat later in hepatocellular disease (acute hepatitis). Itching also occurs in chronic liver diseases, typically the cholestatic forms such as primary biliary cirrhosis and sclerosing cholangitis where it is often the presenting symptom, occurring before the onset of jaundice. However, itching can occur in any liver disease, particularly once cirrhosis is present.

Jaundice is the hallmark symptom of liver disease and perhaps the most reliable marker of severity. Patients usually report darkening of the urine before they notice scleral icterus. Jaundice is rarely detectable with a bilirubin level <43 μmol/L (2.5 mg/dL). With severe cholestasis there will also be lightening of the color of the stools and steatorrhea. Jaundice without dark urine usually indicates indirect (unconjugated) hyperbilirubinemia and is typical of hemolytic anemia and the genetic disorders of bilirubin conjugation, the common and benign form being Gilbert's syndrome and the rare and severe form being Crigler-Najjar syndrome. Gilbert's syndrome affects up to 5% of the population; the jaundice is more noticeable after fasting and with stress.

Major risk factors for liver disease that should be sought in the clinical history include details of alcohol use, medications (including herbal compounds, birth control pills, and over-the-counter medications), personal habits, sexual activity, travel, exposure to jaundiced or other high-risk persons, injection drug use, recent surgery, remote or recent transfusion with blood and blood products, occupation, accidental exposure to blood or needlestick, and familial history of liver disease.

For assessing the risk of viral hepatitis, a careful history of sexual activity is of particular importance and should include the number of lifetime sexual partners and, for men, a history of having sex with men. Sexual exposure is a common mode of spread of hepatitis B but is rare for hepatitis C. A family history of hepatitis, liver disease, and liver cancer is also important. Maternal-infant transmission occurs with both hepatitis B and C. Vertical spread of hepatitis B can now be prevented by passive and active immunization of the infant at birth. Vertical spread of hepatitis C is uncommon, but there are no reliable means of prevention. Transmission is more common in HIV-co-infected mothers and is also linked to prolonged and difficult labor and delivery, early rupture of membranes, and internal fetal monitoring. A history of injection drug use, even in the remote past, is of great importance in assessing the risk for hepatitis B and C. Injection drug use is now the single most common risk factor for hepatitis C. Transfusion with blood or blood products is no longer an important risk factor for acute viral hepatitis. However, blood transfusions received before the introduction of sensitive enzyme immunoassays for antibody to hepatitis C virus (anti-HCV) in 1992 is an important risk factor for chronic hepatitis C. Blood transfusion before 1986, when screening for antibody to hepatitis B core antigen (anti-HBc) was introduced, is also a risk factor for hepatitis B. Travel to an underdeveloped area of the world, exposure to persons with jaundice, and exposure to young children in day-care centers are risk factors for hepatitis A. Hepatitis E is one of the more common causes of jaundice in Asia and Africa but is uncommon in developed nations, although mild cases have been associated with eating raw or undercooked pork or game (deer and wild boars). Tattooing and body piercing (for hepatitis B and C) and eating shellfish (for hepatitis A) are frequently mentioned but are actually quite rare types of exposure for acquiring hepatitis.

A history of alcohol intake is important in assessing the cause of liver disease and also in planning management and recommendations. In the United States, for example, at least 70% of adults drink alcohol to some degree, but significant alcohol intake is less common; in population-based surveys, only 5% have more than two drinks per day, the average drink representing 11–15 g alcohol. Alcohol consumption associated with an increased rate of alcoholic liver disease is probably more than two drinks (22–30 g) per day in women and three drinks (33–45 g) in men. Most patients with alcoholic cirrhosis have a much higher daily intake and have drunk excessively for ≥10 years before onset of liver disease. In assessing alcohol intake, the history should also focus on whether alcohol abuse or dependence is present. Alcoholism is usually defined by the behavioral patterns and consequences of alcohol intake, not on the basis of the amount of alcohol intake. *Abuse* is defined by a repetitive pattern of drinking alcohol that has adverse effects on social, family, occupational, or health status. *Dependence* is defined by alcohol-seeking behavior, despite its adverse effects. Many alcoholics demonstrate both dependence and abuse, and dependence is considered the more serious and advanced form of alcoholism. A clinically helpful approach to diagnosis of alcohol dependence and abuse is the use of the CAGE questionnaire (Table 301-2), which is recommended in all medical history-taking.

TABLE 301-2 CAGE Questions*

Acronym	Question
C	Have you ever felt you ought to *C*ut down on your drinking?
A	Have people *A*nnoyed you by criticizing your drinking?
G	Have you ever felt *G*uilty or bad about your drinking?
E	Have you ever had a drink first thing in the morning to steady your nerves or get rid of a hangover (*E*yeopener)?

*One "yes" response should raise suspicion of an alcohol use problem, and more than one is a strong indication that abuse or dependence exists.

Family history can be helpful in assessing liver disease. Familial causes of liver disease include Wilson's disease; hemochromatosis and α_1 antitrypsin (α_1AT) deficiency; and the more uncommon inherited pediatric liver diseases of familial intrahepatic cholestasis, benign recurrent intrahepatic cholestasis, and Alagille syndrome. Onset of severe liver disease in childhood or adolescence with a family history of liver disease or neuropsychiatric disturbance should lead to investigation for Wilson's disease. A family history of cirrhosis, diabetes, or endocrine failure and the appearance of liver disease in adulthood should suggest hemochromatosis and lead to investigation of iron status. Adult patients with abnormal iron studies warrant genotyping of the *HFE* gene for the C282Y and H63D mutations typical of genetic hemochromatosis. In children and adolescents with iron overload, other non-*HFE* causes of hemochromatosis should be sought. A family history of emphysema should provoke investigation of α_1AT levels and, if low, for Pi genotype.

PHYSICAL EXAMINATION

The physical examination rarely demonstrates evidence of liver dysfunction in a patient without symptoms or laboratory findings, nor are most signs of liver disease specific to one diagnosis. Thus, the physical examination complements rather than replaces the need for other diagnostic approaches. In many patients, the physical examination is normal unless the disease is acute or severe and advanced. Nevertheless, the physical examination is important in that it can be the first evidence for the presence of hepatic failure, portal hypertension, and liver decompensation. In addition, the physical examination can reveal signs that point to a specific diagnosis, either in risk factors or in associated diseases or findings.

Typical physical findings in liver disease are icterus, hepatomegaly, hepatic tenderness, splenomegaly, spider angiomata, palmar erythema, and excoriations. Signs of advanced disease include muscle wasting, ascites, edema, dilated abdominal veins, hepatic fetor, asterixis, mental confusion, stupor, and coma. In males with cirrhosis, particularly when related to alcohol, signs of hyperestrogenemia such as gynecomastia, testicular atrophy, and loss of male-pattern hair distribution may be found.

Icterus is best appreciated by inspecting the sclera under natural light. In fair-skinned individuals, a yellow color of the skin may be obvious. In dark-skinned individuals, the mucous membranes below the tongue can demonstrate jaundice. Jaundice is rarely detectable if the serum bilirubin level is <43 μmol/L (2.5 mg/dL) but may remain detectable below this level during recovery from jaundice (because of protein and tissue binding of conjugated bilirubin).

Spider angiomata and palmar erythema occur in both acute and chronic liver disease and may be especially prominent in persons with cirrhosis, but they can occur in normal individuals and are frequently present during pregnancy. Spider angiomata are superficial, tortuous arterioles and, unlike simple telangiectases, typically fill from the center outward. Spider angiomata occur only on the arms, face, and upper torso; they can be pulsatile and may be difficult to detect in dark-skinned individuals.

Hepatomegaly is not a very reliable sign of liver disease, because of the variability of the size and shape of the liver and the physical impediments to assessing liver size by percussion and palpation. Marked hepatomegaly is typical of cirrhosis, venoocclusive disease, infiltrative disorders such as amyloidosis, metastatic or primary cancers of the liver, and alcoholic hepatitis. Careful assessment of the liver edge may also demonstrate unusual firmness, irregularity of the surface, or frank nodules. Perhaps the most reliable physical finding in examining the liver is hepatic tenderness. Discomfort on touching or pressing on the liver should be carefully sought with percussive comparison of the right and left upper quadrants.

Splenomegaly occurs in many medical conditions but can be a subtle but significant physical finding in liver disease. The availability of ultrasound (US) assessment of the spleen allows for confirmation of the physical finding.

Signs of advanced liver disease include muscle-wasting and weight loss as well as hepatomegaly, bruising, ascites, and edema. Ascites is best appreciated by attempts to detect shifting dullness by careful percussion. US examination will confirm the finding of ascites in equivocal cases. Peripheral edema can occur with or without ascites. In patients with advanced liver disease, other factors frequently contribute to edema formation, including hypoalbuminemia, venous insufficiency, heart failure, and medications.

Hepatic failure is defined as the occurrence of signs or symptoms of hepatic encephalopathy in a person with severe acute or chronic liver disease. The first signs of hepatic encephalopathy can be subtle and nonspecific—change in sleep patterns, change in personality, irritability, and mental dullness. Thereafter, confusion, disorientation, stupor, and eventually coma supervene. In acute liver failure, excitability and mania may be present. Physical findings include asterixis and flapping tremors of the body and tongue. *Fetor hepaticus* refers to the slightly sweet, ammoniacal odor that can occur in patients with liver failure, particularly if there is portal-venous shunting of blood around the liver. Other causes of coma and disorientation should be excluded, mainly electrolyte imbalances, sedative use, and renal or respiratory failure. The appearance of hepatic encephalopathy during acute hepatitis is the major criterion for diagnosis of fulminant hepatitis and indicates a poor prognosis. In chronic liver disease, encephalopathy is usually triggered by a medical complication such as gastrointestinal bleeding, over-diuresis, uremia, dehydration, electrolyte imbalance, infection, constipation, or use of narcotic analgesics.

A helpful measure of hepatic encephalopathy is a careful mental status examination and use of the trail-making test, which consists of a series of 25 numbered circles that the patient is asked to connect as rapidly as possible using a pencil. The normal range for the connect-the-dot test is 15–30 seconds; it is considerably delayed in patients with early hepatic encephalopathy. Other tests include drawing abstract objects or comparison of a signature to previous examples. More sophisticated testing such as with electroencephalography and visual evoked potentials can detect mild forms of encephalopathy, but are rarely clinically useful.

Other signs of advanced liver disease include umbilical hernia from ascites, hydrothorax, prominent veins over the abdomen, and *caput medusa*, which consists of collateral veins seen radiating from the umbilicus and resulting from the recanulation of the umbilical vein. Widened pulse pressure and signs of a hyperdynamic circulation can occur in patients with cirrhosis as a result of fluid and sodium retention, increased cardiac output, and reduced peripheral resistance. Patients with long-standing cirrhosis and portal hypertension are prone to develop the hepatopulmonary syndrome, defined by the triad of liver disease, hypoxemia, and pulmonary arteriovenous shunting. The hepatopulmonary syndrome is characterized by platypnea and orthodeoxia, representing shortness of breath and oxygen desaturation that occur paradoxically upon assuming an upright position. Measurement of oxygen saturation by pulse oximetry is a reliable screening test for the presence of hepatopulmonary syndrome.

Several skin disorders and changes occur commonly in liver disease. Hyperpigmentation is typical of advanced chronic cholestatic diseases such as primary biliary cirrhosis and sclerosing cholangitis. In these same conditions, xanthelasma and tendon xanthomata occur as a result of retention and high serum levels of lipids and cholesterol. A slate-gray pigmentation to the skin also occurs with hemochromatosis if iron levels are high for a prolonged period. Mucocutaneous vasculitis with palpable purpura, especially on the lower extremities, is typical of cryoglobulinemia of chronic hepatitis C but can also occur in chronic hepatitis B.

Some physical signs point to specific liver diseases. Kayser-Fleischer rings occur in Wilson's disease and consist of a golden-brown copper pigment deposited in Descemet's membrane at the periphery of the cornea; they are best seen by slit-lamp examination. Dupuytren contracture and parotid enlargement are suggestive of chronic alcoholism and alcoholic liver disease. In metastatic liver disease or primary hepatocellular carcinoma, signs of cachexia and wasting may be prominent, as well as firm hepatomegaly and a hepatic bruit.

LABORATORY TESTING

Diagnosis in liver disease is greatly aided by the availability of reliable and sensitive tests of liver injury and function. A typical battery of blood tests used for initial assessment of liver disease includes measuring levels of serum alanine and aspartate aminotransferases (ALT and AST), alkaline phosphatase (AlkP), direct and total serum bilirubin, and albumin and assessing prothrombin time. The pattern of abnormalities generally points to hepatocellular versus cholestatic liver disease and will help to decide whether the disease is acute or chronic and whether cirrhosis and hepatic failure are present. Based on these results, further testing over time may be necessary. Other laboratory tests may be helpful, such as γ-glutamyl transpeptidase (gGT) to define whether alkaline phosphatase elevations are due to liver disease; hepatitis serology to define the type of viral hepatitis; and autoimmune markers to diagnose primary biliary cirrhosis (antimitochondrial antibody; AMA), sclerosing cholangitis (peripheral antineutrophil cytoplasmic antibody; P-ANCA), and autoimmune hepatitis (antinuclear, smooth-muscle, and liver-kidney microsomal antibody). A simple delineation of laboratory abnormalities and common liver diseases is given in Table 301-3.

The use and interpretation of liver function tests is summarized in Chap. 302.

DIAGNOSTIC IMAGING

There have been great advances made in hepatic imaging, although no method is suitably accurate in demonstrating underlying cirrhosis. There are many modalities available for imaging the liver. US, CT, and MRI are the most commonly employed and are complementary to each other. In general, US and CT have a high sensitivity for detecting biliary duct dilatation and are the first-line options for investigating the patient with suspected obstructive jaundice. All three modalities can detect a fatty liver, which appears bright on imaging studies. Modifications of CT and MRI can be used to quantify liver fat, which may ultimately be valuable in monitoring therapy in patients with fatty liver disease. Magnetic resonance cholangiopancreatography (MRCP) and endoscopic retrograde cholangiopancreatography (ERCP) are the procedures of choice for visualization of the biliary tree. MRCP offers several advantages over ERCP; there is no need for contrast media or ionizing radiation, images can be acquired faster, it is less operator dependent, and it carries no risk of pancreatitis. MRCP is superior to US and CT for detecting choledocholithiasis but less specific. It is useful in the diagnosis of bile duct obstruction and congenital biliary abnormalities, but ERCP is more valuable in evaluating ampullary lesions and primary sclerosing cholangitis. ERCP allows for biopsy, direct visualization of the ampulla and common bile duct, and intraductal ultrasonography. It also provides several therapeutic options in patients with obstructive jaundice such as sphincterotomy, stone extraction, and placement of nasobiliary catheters and biliary stents. Doppler US and MRI are used to assess hepatic vasculature and hemodynamics and to monitor surgically or radiologically placed vascular shunts such as transjugular intrahepatic portosystemic shunts. CT and MRI are indicated for the identification and evaluation of hepatic masses, staging of liver tumors, and preoperative assessment. With regard to mass lesions, sensitivity of hepatic imaging continues to increase; unfortunately, specificity remains a problem, and often two and sometimes three studies are needed before a diagnosis can be reached. Recently, methods using elastography have been developed to measure hepatic stiffness as a means of assessing hepatic fibrosis. US and MR elastrography are now

TABLE 301-3 Important Diagnostic Tests in Common Liver Diseases

Disease	Diagnostic Test
Hepatitis A	Anti-HAV IgM
Hepatitis B	
Acute	HBsAg and anti-HBc IgM
Chronic	HBsAg and HBeAg and/or HBV DNA
Hepatitis C	Anti-HCV and HCV RNA
Hepatitis D (delta)	HBsAg and anti-HDV
Hepatitis E	Anti-HEV
Autoimmune hepatitis	ANA or SMA, elevated IgG levels, and compatible histology
Primary biliary cirrhosis	Mitochondrial antibody, elevated IgM levels, and compatible histology
Primary sclerosing cholangitis	P-ANCA, cholangiography
Drug-induced liver disease	History of drug ingestion
Alcoholic liver disease	History of excessive alcohol intake and compatible histology
Nonalcoholic steatohepatitis	Ultrasound or CT evidence of fatty liver and compatible histology
α_1 Antitrypsin disease	Reduced α_1 antitrypsin levels, phenotypes PiZZ or PiSZ
Wilson's disease	Decreased serum ceruloplasmin and increased urinary copper; increased hepatic copper level
Hemochromatosis	Elevated iron saturation and serum ferritin; genetic testing for *HFE* gene mutations
Hepatocellular cancer	Elevated α-fetoprotein level >500; US or CT image of mass

Abbreviations: HAV, HBV, HCV, HDV, HEV: hepatitis A, B, C, D, or E virus; HBsAg, hepatitis B surface antigen; anti-HBc, antibody to hepatitis B core (antigen); HBeAg, hepatitis e antigen; ANA, antinuclear antibodies; SMA, smooth-muscle antibody; P-ANCA, peripheral antineutrophil cytoplasmic antibody.

undergoing evaluation for their ability to detect different degrees of hepatic fibrosis and to obviate the need for liver biopsy in assessing disease stage. If found to be reliable, hepatic elastography may be an appropriate means of monitoring fibrosis and disease progression. Finally, interventional radiologic techniques allow the biopsy of solitary lesions, performance of radiofrequency ablation and chemoembolization of cancerous lesions, insertion of drains into hepatic abscesses, measurement of portal pressure, and creation of vascular shunts in patients with portal hypertension. Which modality to use depends on factors such as availability, cost, and experience of the radiologist with each technique.

LIVER BIOPSY

Liver biopsy remains the criterion standard in the evaluation of patients with liver disease, particularly in patients with chronic liver diseases. In selected instances, liver biopsy is necessary for diagnosis but is more often useful in assessing the severity (grade) and stage of liver damage, in predicting prognosis, and in monitoring response to treatment. The size of the liver biopsy is an important determinant of its reliability; a length of 1.5–2 cm being necessary for accurate assessment of fibrosis. In the future, noninvasive means of assessing disease activity (batteries of blood tests) and fibrosis (elastography and fibrosis markers) may replace liver biopsy in assessing stage and grade of disease.

DIAGNOSIS OF LIVER DISEASE

The major causes of liver disease and key diagnostic features are outlined in Table 301-3, and an algorithm for evaluation of the patient with suspected liver disease is given in Fig. 301-1. Specifics of diagnosis are discussed in later chapters. The most common causes of acute liver disease are viral hepatitis (particularly hepatitis A, B, and C), drug-induced liver injury, cholangitis, and alcoholic liver disease. Liver biopsy is usually not needed in the diagnosis and management of acute liver disease, exceptions being situations where the diagnosis remains unclear despite thorough clinical and laboratory investigation. Liver biopsy can be helpful in the diagnosis of drug-induced liver disease and in establishing the diagnosis of acute alcoholic hepatitis.

The most common causes of chronic liver disease in general order of frequency are chronic hepatitis C, alcoholic liver disease, nonalcoholic steatohepatitis, chronic hepatitis B, autoimmune hepatitis, sclerosing cholangitis, primary biliary cirrhosis, hemochromatosis, and Wilson's disease. Strict diagnostic criteria have not been developed for most liver diseases, but liver biopsy plays an important role in the diagnosis of autoimmune hepatitis, primary biliary cirrhosis, nonalcoholic and alcoholic steatohepatitis, and Wilson's disease (with a quantitative hepatic copper level).

GRADING AND STAGING OF LIVER DISEASE

Grading refers to an assessment of the severity or activity of liver disease, whether acute or chronic; active or inactive; and mild, moderate, or severe. Liver biopsy is the most accurate means of assessing severity, particularly in chronic liver disease. Serum aminotransferase levels are used as convenient and noninvasive means to follow disease activity, but aminotransferase levels are not always reliable in reflecting disease severity. Thus, normal serum aminotransferase levels in patients with hepatitis B surface antigen (HBsAg) in serum may indicate the inactive HBsAg carrier state or may reflect mild chronic hepatitis B or hepatitis B with fluctuating disease activity. Serum testing for hepatitis B e antigen and hepatitis B virus DNA can help resolve these different patterns, but these markers can also fluctuate and change over time. Similarly, in chronic hepatitis C, serum aminotransferase levels can be normal despite moderate activity of disease. Finally, in both alcoholic and nonalcoholic steatohepatitis, aminotransferase levels are quite

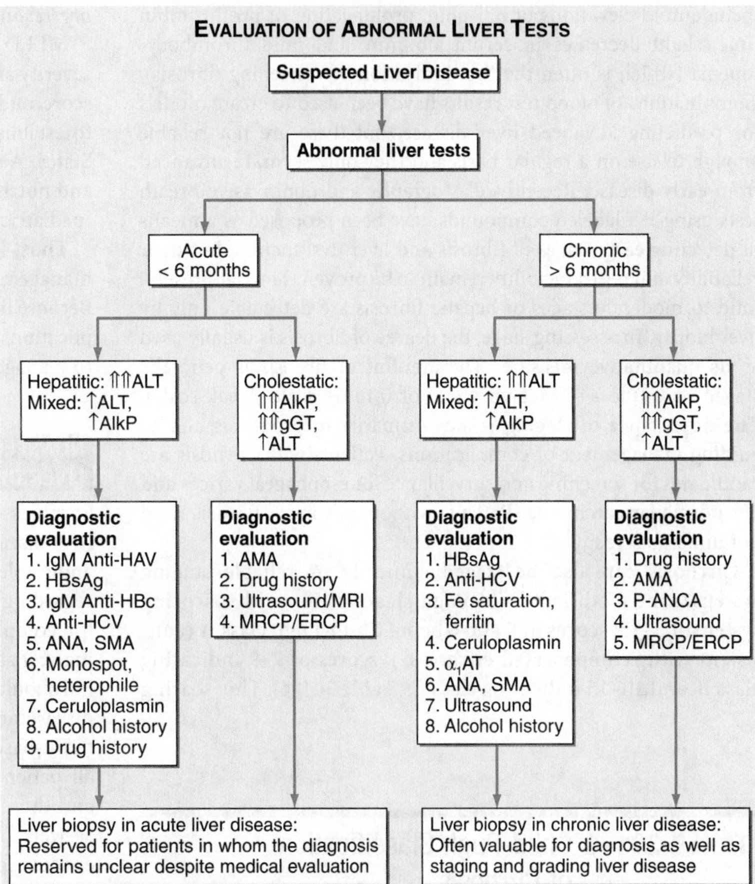

Figure 301-1 Algorithm for evaluation of abnormal liver tests. For patients with suspected liver disease, an appropriate approach to evaluation is initial testing for routine liver tests such as bilirubin, albumin, alanine aminotransferase (ALT), aspartate aminotransferase (AST), and alkaline phosphatase (AlkP). These results (sometimes complemented by testing of γ-glutamyl transpeptidase; gGT) will establish whether the pattern of abnormalities is hepatic, cholestatic, or mixed. In addition, the duration of symptoms or abnormalities will show whether the disease is acute or chronic. If the disease is acute and if history, laboratory tests, and imaging studies do not reveal a diagnosis, liver biopsy is appropriate to help establish the diagnosis. If the disease is chronic, liver biopsy can be helpful not only for diagnosis but also to grade the activity and stage the progression of disease. This approach is largely applicable to patients without immune deficiency. In patients with HIV infection or after bone marrow or solid organ transplantation, diagnostic evaluation should also include evaluation of opportunistic infections (adenovirus, cytomegalovirus, coccidioidomycosis, etc.) as well as vascular and immunologic conditions (venoocclusive disease, graft-versus-host disease). HAV, HCV: hepatitis A or C virus; HBsAg, hepatitis B surface antigen; anti-HBc, antibody to hepatitis B core (antigen); ANA, antinuclear antibodies; SMA, smooth-muscle antibody; MRCP, magnetic resonance cholangiopancreatography; ERCP, endoscopic retrograde cholangiopancreatography; α_1AT, α_1 antitrypsin; AMA; antimitochondrial antibody; P-ANCA, peripheral antineutrophil cytoplasmic antibody.

unreliable in reflecting severity. In these conditions, liver biopsy is helpful in guiding management and recommending therapy, particularly if therapy is difficult, prolonged, and expensive as is often the case in chronic viral hepatitis. There are several well-verified numerical scales for grading activity in chronic liver disease, the most common being the histology activity index and the Ishak histology scale.

Liver biopsy is also the most accurate means of assessing stage of disease as early or advanced, precirrhotic, and cirrhotic. Staging of disease pertains largely to chronic liver diseases in which progression to cirrhosis and end-stage liver disease can occur, but which may require years or decades to develop. Clinical features, biochemical tests, and hepatic imaging studies are helpful in assessing stage but generally become abnormal only in the middle to late stages of cirrhosis. Noninvasive tests that suggest advanced fibrosis include mild elevations of bilirubin, prolongation of prothrombin time, slight decreases in serum albumin, and mild thrombocytopenia (which is often the first indication of worsening fibrosis). Combinations of blood test results have been used to create models for predicting advanced liver disease, but these are not reliable enough to use on a regular basis and they only separate advanced from early disease. Recently, elastography and noninvasive breath tests using ^{13}C-labeled compounds have been proposed as a means of detecting early stages of fibrosis and liver dysfunction, but their reliability and reproducibility remain to be proven. Thus, at present, mild to moderate stages of hepatic fibrosis are detectable only by liver biopsy. In assessing stage, the degree of fibrosis is usually used as its quantitative measure. The amount of fibrosis is generally staged on a 0 to 4+ (Metavir scale) or 0 to 6+ scale (Ishak scale). The importance of staging relates primarily to prognosis and to guiding management of complications. Patients with cirrhosis are candidates for screening and surveillance for esophageal varices and hepatocellular carcinoma. Patients without advanced fibrosis need not undergo screening.

Cirrhosis can also be staged clinically. A reliable staging system is the modified Child-Pugh classification with a scoring system of 5–15: scores of 5 and 6 being Child-Pugh class A (consistent with "compensated cirrhosis"), scores of 7–9 indicating class B, and 10–15 indicating class C (Table 301-4). This scoring system was initially devised to stratify patients into risk groups prior to undergoing portal decompressive surgery. The Child-Pugh score is a reasonably reliable predictor of survival in many liver diseases and predicts the likelihood of major complications of cirrhosis such as bleeding from varices and spontaneous bacterial peritonitis. It was used to assess prognosis in cirrhosis and to provide the standard criteria for listing liver transplantation (Child-Pugh class B). Recently the Child-Pugh system has been replaced by the model for end-stage liver disease (MELD) score for assessing the need for liver transplantation. The MELD score is a prospectively derived scoring system designed to predict prognosis of patients with liver disease and portal hypertension. It is calculated using three noninvasive variables—the prothrombin time expressed as international normalized ratio (INR), serum bilirubin, and serum creatinine (*http://www.unos.org/resources/meldPeldCalculator.asp*).

MELD provides a more objective means of assessing disease severity and has less center-to-center variation than the Child-Pugh score and has a wider range of values. MELD is currently used to establish priority listing for liver transplantation in the United States. A similar system using bilirubin, INR, serum albumin, age, and nutritional status is used for children below the age of 12 years [pediatric end-stage liver disease (PELD)].

Thus, liver biopsy is helpful not only in diagnosis but also in management of chronic liver disease and assessment of prognosis. Because liver biopsy is an invasive procedure and not without complications, it should be used only when it will contribute materially to management and therapeutic decisions.

TABLE 301-4 Child-Pugh Classification of Cirrhosis

Factor	Units	1	2	3
Serum bilirubin	μmol/L	<34	34–51	>51
	mg/dL	<2.0	2.0–3.0	>3.0
Serum albumin	g/L	>35	30–35	<30
	g/dL	>3.5	3.0–3.5	<3.0
Prothrombin time	seconds prolonged	0–4	4–6	>6
	INR	<1.7	1.7–2.3	>2.3
Ascites		None	Easily controlled	Poorly controlled
Hepatic encephalopathy		None	Minimal	Advanced

Note: The Child-Pugh score is calculated by adding the scores of the five factors and can range from 5 to 15. Child-Pugh class can be A (a score of 5–6), B (7–9), or C (10 or above). Decompensation indicates cirrhosis with a Child-Pugh score of ≥7 (class B). This level has been the accepted criterion for listing liver transplantation.

NONSPECIFIC ISSUES IN MANAGEMENT OF PATIENTS WITH LIVER DISEASE

Specifics on management of different forms of acute or chronic liver disease are given in subsequent chapters, but certain issues are applicable to any patient with liver disease. These include advice regarding alcohol use, medications, vaccination, and surveillance for complications of liver disease. Alcohol should be used sparingly, if at all, by patients with liver disease. Abstinence from alcohol should be encouraged for all patients with alcohol-related liver disease and in patients with cirrhosis and those receiving interferon-based therapy for hepatitis B or C. Regarding vaccinations, all patients with liver disease should receive hepatitis A vaccine and those with risk factors should receive hepatitis B vaccination as well. Influenza and pneumococcal vaccination should also be encouraged. Patients with liver disease should be careful using any medications, other than the most necessary. Drug-induced hepatotoxicity can mimic many forms of liver disease and can cause exacerbations of chronic hepatitis and cirrhosis; drugs should be suspected in any situation in which the cause of exacerbation is unknown. Finally, consideration should be given to surveillance for complications of chronic liver disease such as variceal hemorrhage and hepatocellular carcinoma. Patients with cirrhosis warrant upper endoscopy to assess the presence of varices and should be given chronic therapy with beta blockers or offered endoscopic obliteration if large varices are found. Patients with cirrhosis also warrant screening and long-term surveillance for development of hepatocellular carcinoma. While the optimal regimen for such surveillance has not been established, an appropriate approach is US of the liver at 6- to 12-month intervals.

FURTHER READINGS

Boyer TD et al (eds): *Zakim and Boyer's Hepatology: A Textbook of Liver Disease*, 6th ed. Philadelphia, Saunders, 2011

Castera L: Transient elastography and other noninvasive tests to assess hepatic fibrosis in patients with viral hepatitis. J Viral Hepat 16:300, 2009

Freeman RB Jr: Model for end-stage liver disease (MELD) for liver allocation: A 5-year score card. Hepatology 47:1052, 2008

Hamer OW et al: Technology insight: Advances in liver imaging. Nature Gastroenterol Hepatol 4:216: 2007

Kaplowitz N, DeLeve LD (eds): *Drug-Induced Liver Disease*. New York, Informa Healthcare, 2007

Rockey DC et al: Liver biopsy. Hepatology 49: 1017, 2009

CHAPTER 302

Evaluation of Liver Function

Daniel S. Pratt

Marshall M. Kaplan

Several biochemical tests are useful in the evaluation and management of patients with hepatic dysfunction. These tests can be used to (1) detect the presence of liver disease, (2) distinguish among different types of liver disorders, (3) gauge the extent of known liver damage, and (4) follow the response to treatment.

Liver tests have shortcomings. They can be normal in patients with serious liver disease and abnormal in patients with diseases that do not affect the liver. Liver tests rarely suggest a specific diagnosis; rather, they suggest a general category of liver disease, such as hepatocellular or cholestatic, which then further directs the evaluation.

The liver carries out thousands of biochemical functions, most of which cannot be easily measured by blood tests. Laboratory tests measure only a limited number of these functions. In fact, many tests, such as the aminotransferases or alkaline phosphatase, do not measure liver function at all. Rather, they detect liver cell damage or interference with bile flow. Thus, no one test enables the clinician to accurately assess the liver's total functional capacity.

To increase both the sensitivity and the specificity of laboratory tests in the detection of liver disease, it is best to use them as a battery. Tests usually employed in clinical practice include the bilirubin, aminotransferases, alkaline phosphatase, albumin, and prothrombin time tests. When more than one of these tests provide abnormal findings or the findings are persistently abnormal on serial determinations, the probability of liver disease is high. When all test results are normal, the probability of missing occult liver disease is low.

When evaluating patients with liver disorders, it is helpful to group these tests into general categories. The classification we have found most useful is given below.

TESTS BASED ON DETOXIFICATION AND EXCRETORY FUNCTIONS

Serum bilirubin

(See also Chap. 42) Bilirubin, a breakdown product of the porphyrin ring of heme-containing proteins, is found in the blood in two fractions—conjugated and unconjugated. The unconjugated fraction, also termed the *indirect fraction*, is insoluble in water and is bound to albumin in the blood. The conjugated (direct) bilirubin fraction is water soluble and can therefore be excreted by the kidney. When measured by modifications of the original van den Bergh method, normal values of total serum bilirubin are reported between 1 and 1.5 mg/dL with 95% of a normal population falling between 0.2 and 0.9 mg/dL. If the direct-acting fraction is less than 15% of the total, the bilirubin can be considered to all be indirect. The most frequently reported upper limit of normal for conjugated bilirubin is 0.3 mg/dL.

Elevation of the unconjugated fraction of bilirubin is rarely due to liver disease. An isolated elevation of unconjugated bilirubin is seen primarily in hemolytic disorders and in a number of genetic conditions such as Crigler-Najjar and Gilbert's syndromes (Chap. 42). Isolated unconjugated hyperbilirubinemia (bilirubin elevated but <15% direct) should prompt a workup for hemolysis (Fig. 302-1). In the absence of hemolysis, an isolated, unconjugated hyperbilirubinemia in an otherwise healthy patient can be attributed to Gilbert's syndrome, and no further evaluation is required.

In contrast, conjugated hyperbilirubinemia almost always implies liver or biliary tract disease. The rate-limiting step in bilirubin metabolism is not conjugation of bilirubin, but rather the transport of conjugated bilirubin into the bile canaliculi. Thus, elevation of the conjugated fraction may be seen in any type of liver disease. In most liver diseases, both conjugated and unconjugated fractions of the bilirubin tend to be elevated. Except in the presence of a purely unconjugated hyperbilirubinemia, fractionation of the bilirubin is rarely helpful in determining the cause of jaundice.

While the degree of elevation of the serum bilirubin has not been critically assessed as a prognostic marker, it important in a number of conditions. In viral hepatitis, the higher the serum bilirubin, the greater the hepatocellular damage. Total serum bilirubin correlates with poor outcomes in alcoholic hepatitis. It is also a critical component of the Model for Endstage Liver Disease (MELD) score, a tool used to estimate survival of patients with end-stage liver disease. An elevated total serum bilirubin in patients with drug-induced liver disease indicates more severe injury.

Urine bilirubin

Unconjugated bilirubin always binds to albumin in the serum and is not filtered by the kidney. Therefore, any bilirubin found in the urine is conjugated bilirubin; the presence of bilirubinuria implies the presence of liver disease. A urine dipstick test can theoretically give the same information as fractionation of the serum bilirubin. This test is almost 100% accurate. Phenothiazines may give a false-positive reading with the Ictotest tablet. In patients recovering from jaundice, the urine bilirubin clears prior to the serum bilirubin.

Blood ammonia

Ammonia is produced in the body during normal protein metabolism and by intestinal bacteria, primarily those in the colon. The liver plays a role in the detoxification of ammonia by converting it to urea, which is excreted by the kidneys. Striated muscle also plays a role in detoxification of ammonia, which is combined

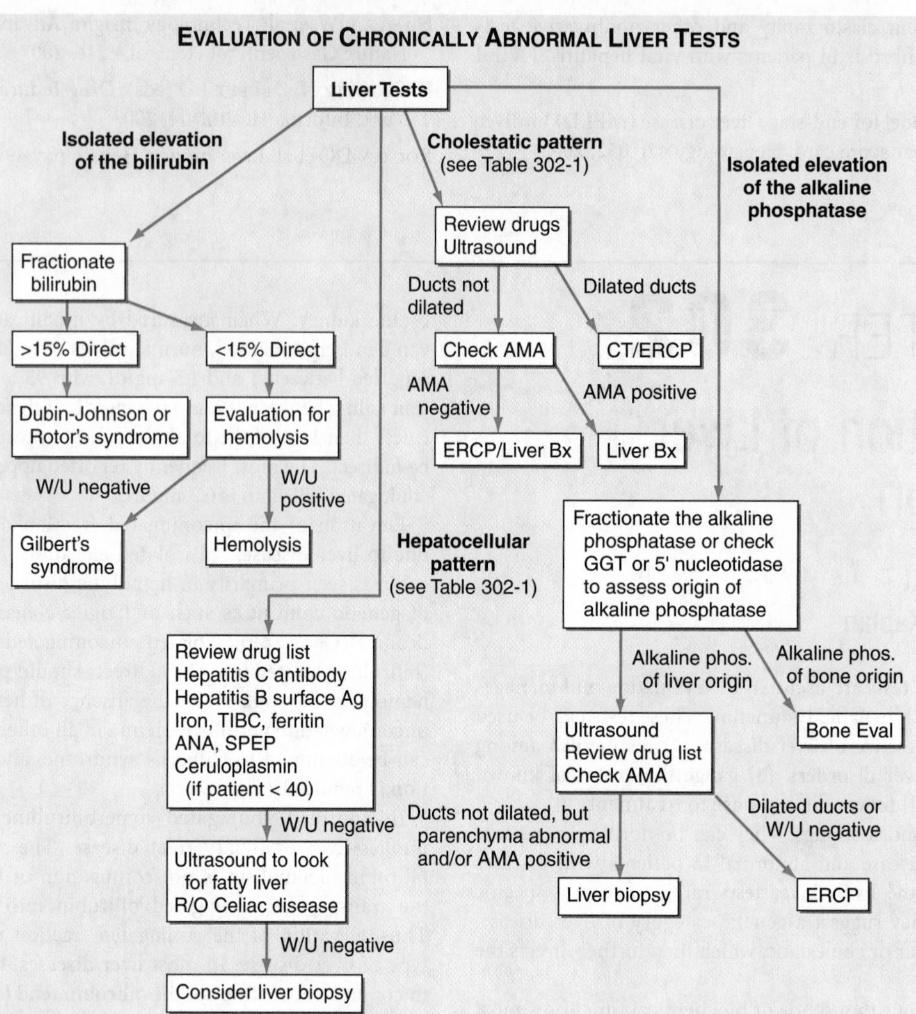

Figure 302-1 Algorithm for the evaluation of chronically abnormal liver tests. ERCP, endoscopic retrograde cholangiopancreatography; CT, computed tomography; AMA, antimitochondrial antibody; ANA, antinuclear antibody; SPEP, serum protein electrophoresis; TIBC, total iron-binding capacity; GGT, γ glutamyl transpeptidase; W/U, work up.

with glutamic acid to form glutamine. Patients with advanced liver disease typically have significant muscle wasting, which likely contributes to hyperammonemia in these patients. Some physicians use the blood ammonia for detecting encephalopathy or for monitoring hepatic synthetic function, although its use for either of these indications has problems. There is very poor correlation between either the presence or the severity of acute encephalopathy and elevation of blood ammonia; it can be occasionally useful for identifying occult liver disease in patients with mental status changes. There is also a poor correlation of the blood serum ammonia and hepatic function. The ammonia can be elevated in patients with severe portal hypertension and portal blood shunting around the liver even in the presence of normal or near-normal hepatic function. Elevated arterial ammonia levels have been shown to correlate with outcome in fulminant hepatic failure.

Serum enzymes

The liver contains thousands of enzymes, some of which are also present in the serum in very low concentrations. These enzymes have no known function in the serum and behave like other serum proteins. They are distributed in the plasma and in interstitial fluid and have characteristic half-lives, which are usually measured in days. Very little is known about the catabolism of serum enzymes, although they are probably cleared by cells in the reticuloendothelial system. The elevation of a given enzyme activity in the serum is thought to primarily reflect its increased rate of entrance into serum from damaged liver cells.

Serum enzyme tests can be grouped into three categories: (1) enzymes whose elevation in serum reflects damage to hepatocytes, (2) enzymes whose elevation in serum reflects cholestasis, and (3) enzyme tests that do not fit precisely into either pattern.

Enzymes that reflect damage to hepatocytes The aminotransferases (transaminases) are sensitive indicators of liver cell injury and are most helpful in recognizing acute hepatocellular diseases such as hepatitis. They include the aspartate aminotransferase (AST) and the alanine aminotransferase (ALT). AST is found in the liver, cardiac muscle, skeletal muscle, kidneys, brain, pancreas, lungs, leukocytes, and erythrocytes in decreasing order of concentration. ALT is found primarily in the liver and is therefore a more specific indicator of liver injury. The aminotransferases are normally present in the serum in low concentrations. These enzymes are released into the blood in greater amounts when there is damage to the liver cell membrane resulting in increased permeability. Liver cell necrosis is not required for the release of the aminotransferases, and there is a poor correlation between the degree of liver cell damage and the level of the aminotransferases. Thus, the absolute elevation of the aminotransferases is of no prognostic significance in acute hepatocellular disorders.

The normal range for aminotransferases varies widely among laboratories, but generally ranges from 10-40 U/L. The inter-laboratory variation in normal range is due to technical reasons; no reference standards exist to establish upper limits of normal for ALT and AST. Some have recommended revisions of normal limits of the aminotransferases adjustments for sex and BMI, but others have noted the potential costs and unclear benefits of implementing this change.

Any type of liver cell injury can cause modest elevations in the serum aminotransferases. Levels of up to 300 U/L are nonspecific and may be found in any type of liver disorder. Minimal ALT elevations in asymptomatic blood donors rarely indicate severe liver disease; studies have shown that fatty liver disease is the most likely explanation. Striking elevations—i.e., aminotransferases >1000 U/L—occur almost exclusively in disorders associated with extensive hepatocellular injury such as (1) viral hepatitis, (2) ischemic liver injury (prolonged hypotension or acute heart failure), or (3) toxin- or drug-induced liver injury.

The pattern of the aminotransferase elevation can be helpful diagnostically. In most acute hepatocellular disorders, the ALT is higher than or equal to the AST. While the AST:ALT ratio is typically less than 1 in patients with chronic viral hepatitis and non-alcoholic fatty liver disease, a number of groups have noted that as cirrhosis develops this ratio rises to greater than 1. An AST:ALT ratio >2:1 is suggestive, while a ratio >3:1 is highly suggestive of alcoholic liver disease. The AST in alcoholic liver disease is rarely >300 U/L, and the ALT is often normal. A low level of ALT in the serum is due to an alcohol-induced deficiency of pyridoxal phosphate.

The aminotransferases are usually not greatly elevated in obstructive jaundice. One notable exception occurs during the acute phase of biliary obstruction caused by the passage of a gallstone into the common bile duct. In this setting, the aminotransferases can briefly be in the 1000–2000 U/L range. However, aminotransferase levels decrease quickly, and the liver-function tests rapidly evolve into one typical of cholestasis.

Enzymes that reflect cholestasis The activities of three enzymes—alkaline phosphatase, 5′-nucleotidase, and γ-glutamyl transpeptidase (GGT)—are usually elevated in cholestasis. Alkaline phosphatase and 5′-nucleotidase are found in or near the bile canalicular membrane of hepatocytes, while GGT is located in the endoplasmic reticulum and in bile duct epithelial cells. Reflecting its more diffuse localization in the liver, GGT elevation in serum is less specific for cholestasis than are elevations of alkaline phosphatase or 5′-nucleotidase. Some have advocated the use of GGT to identify patients with occult alcohol use. Its lack of specificity makes its use in this setting questionable.

The normal serum alkaline phosphatase consists of many distinct isoenzymes found in the liver; bone; placenta; and, less commonly, small intestine. Patients over age 60 can have a mildly elevated alkaline phosphatase ($1\text{–}1^1/_2$ times normal), while individuals with blood types O and B can have an elevation of the serum alkaline phosphatase after eating a fatty meal due to the influx of intestinal alkaline phosphatase into the blood. It is also nonpathologically elevated in children and adolescents undergoing rapid bone growth, because of bone alkaline phosphatase, and late in normal pregnancies due to the influx of placental alkaline phosphatase.

Elevation of liver-derived alkaline phosphatase is not totally specific for cholestasis, and a less than threefold elevation can be seen in almost any type of liver disease. Alkaline phosphatase elevations greater than four times normal occur primarily in patients with cholestatic liver disorders, infiltrative liver diseases such as cancer and amyloidosis, and bone conditions characterized by rapid bone turnover (e.g., Paget's disease). In bone diseases, the elevation is due to increased amounts of the bone isoenzymes. In liver diseases, the elevation is almost always due to increased amounts of the liver isoenzyme.

If an elevated serum alkaline phosphatase is the only abnormal finding in an apparently healthy person, or if the degree of elevation is higher than expected in the clinical setting, identification of the source of elevated isoenzymes is helpful (Fig. 302-1). This problem can be approached in several ways. First, and most precise, is the fractionation of the alkaline phosphatase by electrophoresis. The second approach is based on the observation that alkaline phosphatases from individual tissues differ in susceptibility to inactivation by heat. The finding of an elevated serum alkaline phosphatase level in a patient with a heat-stable fraction strongly suggests that the placenta or a tumor is the source of the elevated enzyme in serum. Susceptibility to inactivation by heat increases, respectively, for the intestinal, liver, and bone alkaline phosphatases, bone being by far the most sensitive. The third, best substantiated, and most available approach involves the measurement of serum 5′-nucleotidase or GGT. These enzymes are rarely elevated in conditions other than liver disease.

In the absence of jaundice or elevated aminotransferases, an elevated alkaline phosphatase of liver origin often, but not always, suggests early cholestasis and, less often, hepatic infiltration by tumor or granulomata. Other conditions that cause isolated elevations of the alkaline phosphatase include Hodgkin's disease, diabetes, hyperthyroidism, congestive heart failure, amyloidosis, and inflammatory bowel disease.

The level of serum alkaline phosphatase elevation is not helpful in distinguishing between intrahepatic and extrahepatic cholestasis. There is essentially no difference among the values found in obstructive jaundice due to cancer, common duct stone, sclerosing cholangitis, or bile duct stricture. Values are similarly increased in patients with intrahepatic cholestasis due to drug-induced hepatitis; primary biliary cirrhosis; rejection of transplanted livers; and, rarely, alcohol-induced steatohepatitis. Values are also greatly elevated in hepatobiliary disorders seen in patients with AIDS (e.g., AIDS cholangiopathy due to cytomegalovirus or cryptosporidial infection and tuberculosis with hepatic involvement).

TESTS THAT MEASURE BIOSYNTHETIC FUNCTION OF THE LIVER

Serum albumin

Serum albumin is synthesized exclusively by hepatocytes. Serum albumin has a long half-life: 18–20 days, with ~4% degraded per day. Because of this slow turnover, the serum albumin is not a good indicator of acute or mild hepatic dysfunction; only minimal changes in the serum albumin are seen in acute liver conditions such as viral hepatitis, drug-related hepatoxicity, and obstructive jaundice. In hepatitis, albumin levels <3 g/dL should raise the possibility of chronic liver disease. Hypoalbuminemia is more common in chronic liver disorders such as cirrhosis and usually reflects severe liver damage and decreased albumin synthesis. One exception is the patient with ascites in whom synthesis may be normal or even increased, but levels are low because of the increased volume of distribution. However, hypoalbuminemia is not specific for liver disease and may occur in protein malnutrition of any cause, as well as protein-losing enteropathies, nephrotic syndrome, and chronic infections that are associated with prolonged increases in levels of serum interleukin 1 and/or tumor necrosis factor, cytokines that inhibit albumin synthesis. Serum albumin should not be measured for screening in patients in whom there is no suspicion of liver disease. A general medical clinic study of consecutive patients in whom no indications were present for albumin measurement showed that while 12% of patients had abnormal test results, the finding was of clinical importance in only 0.4%.

Serum globulins

Serum globulins are a group of proteins made up of γ globulins (immunoglobulins) produced by B lymphocytes and α and β globulins produced primarily in hepatocytes. γ Globulins are increased in chronic liver disease, such as chronic hepatitis and cirrhosis. In cirrhosis, the increased serum gamma globulin concentration is due to the increased synthesis of antibodies, some of which are directed against intestinal bacteria. This occurs because the cirrhotic liver fails to clear bacterial antigens that normally reach the liver through the hepatic circulation.

Increases in the concentration of specific isotypes of γ globulins are often helpful in the recognition of certain chronic liver diseases. Diffuse polyclonal increases in IgG levels are common in autoimmune hepatitis; increases >100% should alert the clinician to this possibility. Increases in the IgM levels are common in primary biliary cirrhosis, while increases in the IgA levels occur in alcoholic liver disease.

■ COAGULATION FACTORS

With the exception of factor VIII, which is produced by vascular endothelial cells, the blood clotting factors are made exclusively in hepatocytes. Their serum half-lives are much shorter than albumin, ranging from 6 h for factor VII to 5 days for fibrinogen. Because of their rapid turnover, measurement of the clotting factors is the single best acute measure of hepatic synthetic function and helpful in both the diagnosis and assessing the prognosis of acute parenchymal liver disease. Useful for this purpose is the *serum prothrombin time*, which collectively measures factors II, V, VII, and X. Biosynthesis of factors II, VII, IX, and X depends on vitamin K. The international normalized ratio (INR) is used to express the degree of anticoagulation on warfarin therapy. The INR standardizes prothrombin time measurement according to the characteristics of the thromboplastin reagent used in a particular lab which is expressed as an International Sensitivity Index (ISI); the ISI is then used in calculating the INR. Because the ISI is validated only for patients on vitamin K antagonists, there has been concern regarding the validity of using it for patients with chronic liver disease.

The prothrombin time may be elevated in hepatitis and cirrhosis as well as in disorders that lead to vitamin K deficiency such as obstructive jaundice or fat malabsorption of any kind. Marked prolongation of the prothrombin time, >5 s above control and not corrected by parenteral vitamin K administration, is a poor prognostic sign in acute viral hepatitis and other acute and chronic liver diseases. The INR, along with the total serum bilirubin and creatinine, are components of the MELD score which is used to allocate organs for liver transplantation.

■ OTHER DIAGNOSTIC TESTS

While tests may direct the physician to a category of liver disease, additional radiologic testing and procedures are often necessary to make the proper diagnosis, as shown in Fig. 302-1. The two most commonly used ancillary tests are reviewed here.

Percutaneous liver biopsy

Percutaneous biopsy of the liver is a safe procedure that can be easily performed at the bedside with local anesthesia and ultrasound guidance. Liver biopsy is of proven value in the following situations: (1) hepatocellular disease of uncertain cause, (2) prolonged hepatitis with the possibility of chronic active hepatitis, (3) unexplained

TABLE 302-1 Liver Test Patterns in Hepatobiliary Disorders

Type of Disorder	Bilirubin	Aminotransferases	Alkaline Phosphatase	Albumin	Prothrombin Time
Hemolysis/Gilbert's syndrome	Normal to 86 μmol/L (5 mg/dL) 85% due to indirect fractions No bilirubinuria	Normal	Normal	Normal	Normal
Acute hepatocellular necrosis (viral and drug hepatitis, hepatotoxins, acute heart failure)	Both fractions may be elevated Peak usually follows aminotransferases Bilirubinuria	Elevated, often >500 IU ALT >AST	Normal to <3 times normal elevation	Normal	Usually normal. If >5X above control and not corrected by parenteral vitamin K, suggests poor prognosis
Chronic hepatocellular disorders	Both fractions may be elevated Bilirubinuria	Elevated, but usually <300 IU	Normal to <3 times normal elevation	Often decreased	Often prolonged Fails to correct with parenteral vitamin K
Alcoholic hepatitis Cirrhosis	Both fractions may be elevated Bilirubinuria	AST:ALT > 2 suggests alcoholic hepatitis or cirrhosis	Normal to <3 times normal elevation	Often decreased	Often prolonged Fails to correct with parenteral vitamin K
Intra- and extra-hepatic cholestasis (Obstructive jaundice)	Both fractions may be elevated Bilirubinuria	Normal to moderate elevation Rarely >500 IU	Elevated, often >4 times normal elevation	Normal, unless chronic	Normal If prolonged, will correct with parenteral vitamin K
Infiltrative diseases (tumor, granulomata); partial bile duct obstruction	Usually normal	Normal to slight elevation	Elevated, often >4 times normal elevation Fractionate, or confirm liver origin with 5′ nucleotidase or γ glutamyl transpeptidase	Normal	Normal

hepatomegaly, (4) unexplained splenomegaly, (5) hepatic filling defects by radiologic imaging, (6) fever of unknown origin, (7) staging of malignant lymphoma. Liver biopsy is most accurate in disorders causing diffuse changes throughout the liver and is subject to sampling error in focal infiltrative disorders such as hepatic metastases. Liver biopsy should not be the initial procedure in the diagnosis of cholestasis. The biliary tree should first be assessed for signs of obstruction. Contraindications to performing a percutaneous liver biopsy include significant ascites and prolonged INR. Under these circumstances, the biopsy can be performed via the transjugular approach.

Ultrasonography

Ultrasonography is the first diagnostic test to use in patients whose liver tests suggest cholestasis, to look for the presence of a dilated intrahepatic or extrahepatic biliary tree or to identify gallstones. In addition, it shows space-occupying lesions within the liver, enables the clinician to distinguish between cystic and solid masses, and helps direct percutaneous biopsies. Ultrasound with Doppler imaging can detect the patency of the portal vein, hepatic artery, and hepatic veins and determine the direction of blood flow. This is the first test ordered in patients suspected of having Budd-Chiari syndrome.

USE OF LIVER TESTS

As previously noted, the best way to increase the sensitivity and specificity of laboratory tests in the detection of liver disease is to employ a battery of tests that includes the aminotransferases, alkaline phosphatase, bilirubin, albumin, and prothrombin time along with the judicious use of the other tests described in this chapter. Table 302-1 shows how patterns of liver tests can lead the clinician to a category of disease that will direct further evaluation. However, it is important to remember that no single set of liver tests will necessarily provide a diagnosis. It is often necessary to repeat these tests on several occasions over days to weeks for a diagnostic pattern to emerge. Figure 302-1 is an algorithm for the evaluation of chronically abnormal liver tests.

FURTHER READINGS

Bhatia V et al: Predictive value of arterial ammonia for complications and outcome in acute liver failure. Gut 55:98, 2006

Bosma PJ et al: The genetic basis of the reduced expression of bilirubin UDP-glucuronosyltransferase 1 in Gilbert's syndrome. N Engl J Med 333:1171, 1995

Kim HC et al: Normal serum aminotransferase concentration and risk of mortality from liver diseases: Prospective cohort study. BMJ 328:983, 2004

Prati D et al: Updated definitions of healthy ranges for serum alanine aminotranferase levels. Ann Intern Med 137:1, 2002

Pratt DS, Kaplan MM: Evaluation of abnormal liver-enzyme tests in the asymptomatic patient. N Engl J Med 342:1266, 2000

———: Laboratory tests, in *Schiff's Diseases of the Liver*, 10th ed, ER Schiff et al (eds). Philadelphia, Lippincott Williams & Wilkins, 2006

Torezan-Filho MA et al: Clinical significance of elevated alanine aminotransferase in blood donors: A follow-up study. Liver Int 24:575, 2004

CHAPTER 303 The Hyperbilirubinemias

Allan W. Wolkoff

BILIRUBIN METABOLISM

The details of bilirubin metabolism are presented in Chap. 42. However, the hyperbilirubinemias are best understood in terms of perturbations of specific aspects of bilirubin metabolism and transport, and these will be briefly reviewed here as depicted in Fig. 303-1.

Bilirubin is the end product of heme degradation. Some 70–90% of bilirubin is derived from degradation of the hemoglobin of senescent red blood cells. Bilirubin produced in the periphery is transported to the liver within the plasma, where, due to its insolubility in aqueous solutions, it is tightly bound to albumin. Under normal circumstances, bilirubin is removed from the circulation rapidly and efficiently by hepatocytes. Transfer of bilirubin from blood to bile involves four distinct but interrelated steps (Fig. 303-1).

1. *Hepatocellular uptake:* Uptake of bilirubin by the hepatocyte has carrier-mediated kinetics. Although a number of candidate bilirubin transporters have been proposed, the actual transporter remains elusive.
2. *Intracellular binding:* Within the hepatocyte, bilirubin is kept in solution by binding as a nonsubstrate ligand to several of the glutathione-S-transferases, formerly called ligandins.
3. *Conjugation:* Bilirubin is conjugated with one or two glucuronic acid moieties by a specific UDP-glucuronosyltransferase to form bilirubin mono- and diglucuronide, respectively. Conjugation disrupts the internal hydrogen bonding that limits aqueous solubility of bilirubin, and the resulting glucuronide conjugates are

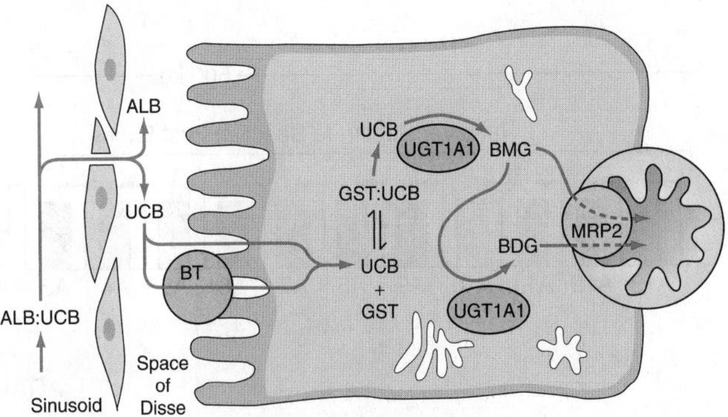

Figure 303-1 Hepatocellular bilirubin transport. Albumin-bound bilirubin in sinusoidal blood passes through endothelial cell fenestrae to reach the hepatocyte surface, entering the cell by both facilitated and simple diffusional processes. Within the cell it is bound to glutathione-S-transferases and conjugated by bilirubin-UDP-glucuronosyltransferase (UGT1A1) to mono- and diglucuronides, which are actively transported across the canalicular membrane into the bile. ALB, albumin; BDG, bilirubin diglucuronide; BMG, bilirubin monoglucuronide; BT, proposed bilirubin transporter; GST, glutathione-S-transferase; MRP2, multidrug resistance–associated protein 2; UCB, unconjugated bilirubin; UGT1A1, bilirubin-UDP-glucuronosyltransferase.

highly soluble in water. Conjugation is obligatory for excretion of bilirubin across the bile canalicular membrane into bile. The UDP-glucuronosyltransferases have been classified into gene families based on the degree of homology among the mRNAs for the various isoforms. Those that conjugate bilirubin and certain other substrates have been designated the *UGT1* family. These are expressed from a single gene complex by alternative promoter usage. This gene complex contains multiple substrate-specific first exons, designated A1, A2, etc. (Fig. 303-2), each with its own promoter and each encoding the amino-terminal half of a specific isoform. In addition, there are four common exons (exons 2–5) that encode the shared carboxyl-terminal half of all of the *UGT1* isoforms. The various first exons encode the specific aglycone substrate binding sites for each isoform, while the shared exons encode the binding site for the sugar donor, UDP-glucuronic acid, and the transmembrane domain. Exon A1 and the four common exons, collectively designated the *UGT1A1* gene (Fig. 303-2), encode the physiologically critical enzyme bilirubin-UDP-glucuronosyltransferase (UGT1A1). A functional corollary of the organization of the *UGT1* gene is that a mutation in one of the first exons will affect only a single enzyme isoform. By contrast, a mutation in exons 2–5 will alter all isoforms encoded by the *UGT1* gene complex.

4. *Biliary excretion:* Bilirubin mono- and diglucuronides are excreted across the canalicular plasma membrane into the bile canaliculus by an ATP-dependent transport process mediated by a canalicular membrane protein called *multidrug resistance–associated protein 2* (MRP2). Mutations of MRP2 result in the Dubin-Johnson syndrome (see below).

EXTRAHEPATIC ASPECTS OF BILIRUBIN DISPOSITION

Bilirubin in the gut

Following secretion into bile, conjugated bilirubin reaches the duodenum and passes down the gastrointestinal tract without reabsorption by the intestinal mucosa. An appreciable fraction is converted by bacterial metabolism in the gut to the water-soluble colorless compound urobilinogen. Urobilinogen undergoes enterohepatic cycling. Urobilinogen not taken up by the liver reaches the systemic circulation, from which some is cleared by the kidneys. Unconjugated bilirubin ordinarily does not reach the gut except in neonates or, by ill-defined alternative pathways, in the presence of severe unconjugated hyperbilirubinemia [e.g., Crigler-Najjar syndrome, type I (CN-I)]. Unconjugated bilirubin that reaches the gut is partly reabsorbed, amplifying any underlying hyperbilirubinemia. Recent reports suggest that oral administration of calcium phosphate with or without the lipase inhibitor orlistat may be an efficient means to interrupt bilirubin enterohepatic cycling to reduce serum bilirubin levels in this situation. Although orlistat administration for 4–6 weeks to 16 patients with Crigler-Najjar syndrome was associated with a 10-20% decrease in serum bilirubin in 7 patients, the cost and side effects (i.e., diarrhea) may obviate the small benefit achievable with this treatment.

Renal excretion of bilirubin conjugates

Unconjugated bilirubin is not excreted in urine, as it is too tightly bound to albumin for effective glomerular filtration and there is no tubular mechanism for its renal secretion. In contrast, the bilirubin conjugates are readily filtered at the glomerulus and can appear in urine in disorders characterized by increased bilirubin conjugates in the circulation.

DISORDERS OF BILIRUBIN METABOLISM LEADING TO UNCONJUGATED HYPERBILIRUBINEMIA

INCREASED BILIRUBIN PRODUCTION

Hemolysis

Increased destruction of erythrocytes leads to increased bilirubin turnover and unconjugated hyperbilirubinemia; the hyperbilirubinemia is usually modest in the presence of normal liver function. In particular, the bone marrow is only capable of a sustained eightfold increase in erythrocyte production in response to a hemolytic stress. Therefore, hemolysis alone cannot result in a sustained hyperbilirubinemia of more than ~68 μmol/L (4 mg/dL). Higher values imply concomitant hepatic dysfunction. When hemolysis is the only abnormality in an otherwise healthy individual, the result is a purely unconjugated hyperbilirubinemia, with the direct-reacting fraction as measured in a typical clinical laboratory being ≤15% of the total serum bilirubin. In the presence of systemic disease, which may include a degree of hepatic dysfunction, hemolysis may produce a component of conjugated hyperbilirubinemia in addition to an elevated unconjugated bilirubin concentration. Prolonged hemolysis may lead to the precipitation of bilirubin salts within the gallbladder or biliary tree, resulting in the formation of gallstones in which bilirubin, rather than cholesterol, is the major component. Such pigment stones may lead to acute or chronic cholecystitis, biliary obstruction, or any other biliary tract consequence of calculous disease.

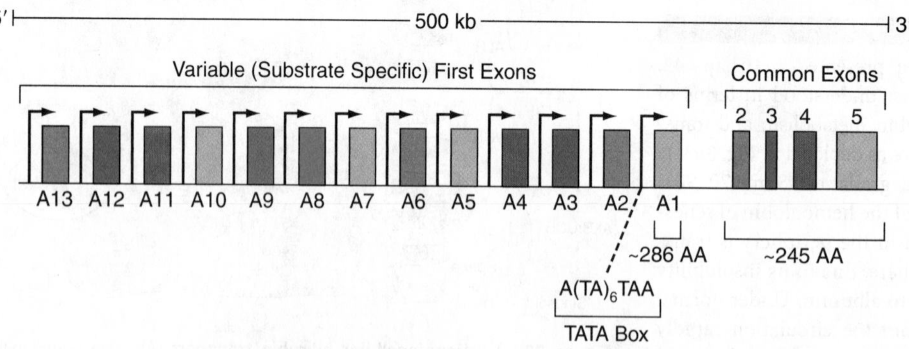

Figure 303-2 Structural organization of the human *UGT1* gene complex. This large complex on chromosome 2 contains at least 13 substrate-specific first exons (A1, A2, etc.). Since four of these are pseudogenes, nine UGT1 isoforms with differing substrate specificities are expressed. Each exon 1 has its own promoter and encodes the amino-terminal substrate-specific ~286 amino acids of the various *UGT1*-encoded isoforms, and common exons 2–5 that encode the 245 carboxyl-terminal amino acids common to all of the isoforms. mRNAs for specific isoforms are assembled by splicing a particular first exon such as the bilirubin-specific exon A1 to exons 2 to 5. The resulting message encodes a complete enzyme, in this particular case bilirubin-UDP-glucuronosyltransferase (UGT1A1). Mutations in a first exon affect only a single isoform. Those in exons 2–5 affect all enzymes encoded by the UGT1 complex.

Ineffective erythropoiesis

During erythroid maturation, small amounts of hemoglobin may be lost at the time of nuclear extrusion, and a fraction of developing erythroid cells is destroyed within the marrow. These processes normally account for a small proportion of bilirubin that is produced. In various disorders, including thalassemia major, megaloblastic anemias due to folate or vitamin B_{12} deficiency, congenital erythropoietic porphyria, lead poisoning, and various congenital and acquired dyserythropoietic anemias, the fraction of total bilirubin production derived from ineffective erythropoiesis is increased, reaching as much as 70% of the total. This may be sufficient to produce modest degrees of unconjugated hyperbilirubinemia.

Miscellaneous

Degradation of the hemoglobin of extravascular collections of erythrocytes, such as those seen in massive tissue infarctions or large hematomas, may lead transiently to unconjugated hyperbilirubinemia.

DECREASED HEPATIC BILIRUBIN CLEARANCE

Decreased hepatic uptake

Decreased hepatic bilirubin uptake is believed to contribute to the unconjugated hyperbilirubinemia of Gilbert's syndrome (GS), although the molecular basis for this finding remains unclear (see below). Several drugs, including flavaspidic acid, novobiocin, and rifampin, as well as various cholecystographic contrast agents, have been reported to inhibit bilirubin uptake. The resulting unconjugated hyperbilirubinemia resolves with cessation of the medication.

Impaired conjugation

Physiologic neonatal jaundice Bilirubin produced by the fetus is cleared by the placenta and eliminated by the maternal liver. Immediately after birth, the neonatal liver must assume responsibility for bilirubin clearance and excretion. However, many hepatic physiologic processes are incompletely developed at birth. Levels of UGT1A1 are low, and alternative excretory pathways allow passage of unconjugated bilirubin into the gut. Since the intestinal flora that convert bilirubin to urobilinogen are also undeveloped, an enterohepatic circulation of unconjugated bilirubin ensues. As a consequence, most neonates develop mild unconjugated hyperbilirubinemia between days 2 and 5 after birth. Peak levels are typically <85–170 μmol/L (5–10 mg/dL) and decline to normal adult concentrations within 2 weeks, as mechanisms required for bilirubin disposition mature. Prematurity, often associated with more profound immaturity of hepatic function and hemolysis, can result in higher levels of unconjugated hyperbilirubinemia. A rapidly rising unconjugated bilirubin concentration, or absolute levels >340 μmol/L (20 mg/dL), puts the infant at risk for bilirubin encephalopathy, or kernicterus. Under these circumstances, bilirubin crosses an immature blood-brain barrier and precipitates in the basal ganglia and other areas of the brain. The consequences range from appreciable neurologic deficits to death. Treatment options include phototherapy, which converts bilirubin into water-soluble photoisomers that are excreted directly into bile, and exchange transfusion. The canalicular mechanisms responsible for bilirubin excretion are also immature at birth, and their maturation may lag behind that of UGT1A1; this can lead to transient conjugated neonatal hyperbilirubinemia, especially in infants with hemolysis.

Acquired conjugation defects A modest reduction in bilirubin-conjugating capacity may be observed in advanced hepatitis or cirrhosis. However, in this setting, conjugation is better preserved than other aspects of bilirubin disposition, such as canalicular excretion. Various drugs, including pregnanediol, novobiocin, chloramphenicol, and gentamicin, may produce unconjugated hyperbilirubinemia by inhibiting UGT1A1 activity. Bilirubin conjugation may be inhibited by certain fatty acids that are present in breast milk but not serum of mothers whose infants have excessive neonatal hyperbilirubinemia (*breast milk jaundice*). Alternatively, there may be increased enterohepatic circulation of bilirubin in these infants. A recent study has correlated epidermal growth factor (EGF) content of breast milk with elevated bilirubin levels in these infants; however, a cause and effect relationship remains to be established. The pathogenesis of breast milk jaundice appears to differ from that of transient familial neonatal hyperbilirubinemia (Lucey-Driscoll syndrome), in which there is a UGT1A1 inhibitor in maternal serum.

HEREDITARY DEFECTS IN BILIRUBIN CONJUGATION

Three familial disorders characterized by differing degrees of unconjugated hyperbilirubinemia have long been recognized. The defining clinical features of each are described below (Table 303-1). While these disorders have been recognized for decades to reflect

TABLE 303-1 Principal Differential Characteristics of Gilbert's and Crigler-Najjar Syndromes

	Crigler-Najjar Syndrome		
Feature	**Type I**	**Type II**	**Gilbert's Syndrome**
Total serum bilirubin, μmol/L (mg/dL)	310–755 (usually >345) [18–45 (usually >20)]	100–430 (usually ≤345) [6–25 (usually ≤20)]	Typically ≤70 μmol/L (≤4 mg/dL) in absence of fasting or hemolysis
Routine liver tests	Normal	Normal	Normal
Response to phenobarbital	None	Decreases bilirubin by >25%	Decreases bilirubin to normal
Kernicterus	Usual	Rare	No
Hepatic histology	Normal	Normal	Usually normal; increased lipofuscin pigment in some
Bile characteristics			
Color	Pale or colorless	Pigmented	Normal dark color
Bilirubin fractions	>90% unconjugated	Largest fraction (mean: 57%) monoconjugates	Mainly diconjugates but monoconjugates increased (mean: 23%)
Bilirubin UDP-glucuronosyltransferase activity	Typically absent; traces in some patients	Markedly reduced: 0–10% of normal	Reduced: typically 10–33% of normal
Inheritance (all autosomal)	Recessive	Predominantly recessive	Promoter mutation: recessive Missense mutations: 7 of 8 dominant; 1 reportedly recessive

differing degrees of deficiency in the ability to conjugate bilirubin, recent advances in the molecular biology of the *UGT1* gene complex have elucidated their interrelationships and clarified previously puzzling features.

Crigler-Najjar syndrome, type I

CN-I is characterized by striking unconjugated hyperbilirubinemia of about 340–765 μmol/L (20–45 mg/dL) that appears in the neonatal period and persists for life. Other conventional hepatic biochemical tests such as serum aminotransferases and alkaline phosphatase are normal, and there is no evidence of hemolysis. Hepatic histology is also essentially normal except for the occasional presence of bile plugs within canaliculi. Bilirubin glucuronides are virtually absent from the bile, and there is no detectable constitutive expression of UGT1A1 activity in hepatic tissue. Neither UGT1A1 activity nor the serum bilirubin concentration responds to administration of phenobarbital or other enzyme inducers. In the absence of conjugation, unconjugated bilirubin accumulates in plasma, from which it is eliminated very slowly by alternative pathways that include direct passage into the bile and small intestine. These account for the small amounts of urobilinogen found in feces. No bilirubin is found in the urine. First described in 1952, the disorder is rare (estimated prevalence, 0.6–1.0 per million). Many patients are from geographically or socially isolated communities in which consanguinity is common, and pedigree analyses show an autosomal recessive pattern of inheritance. The majority of patients (type IA) exhibit defects in the glucuronide conjugation of a spectrum of substrates in addition to bilirubin, including various drugs and other xenobiotics. These individuals have mutations in one of the common exons (2–5) of the *UGT1* gene (Fig. 303-2). In a smaller subset (type IB), the defect is limited largely to bilirubin conjugation, and the causative mutation is in the bilirubin-specific exon A1. Estrogen glucuronidation is mediated by UGT1A1 and is defective in all CN-I patients. More than 30 different genetic lesions of *UGT1A1* responsible for CN-I have been identified, including deletions, insertions, alterations in intron splice donor and acceptor sites, exon skipping, and point mutations that introduce premature stop codons or alter critical amino acids. Their common feature is that they all encode proteins with absent or, at most, traces of bilirubin-UDP-glucuronosyltransferase enzymatic activity.

Prior to the availability of phototherapy, most patients with CN-I died of bilirubin encephalopathy (*kernicterus*) in infancy or early childhood. A few lived as long as early adult life without overt neurologic damage, although more subtle testing usually indicated mild but progressive brain damage. In the absence of liver transplantation, death eventually supervened from late-onset bilirubin encephalopathy, which often followed a nonspecific febrile illness. Although isolated hepatocyte transplantation has been used in a small number of cases of CN-I, early liver transplantation (Chap. 310) remains the best hope to prevent brain injury and death.

Crigler-Najjar syndrome, type II (CN-II)

This condition was recognized as a distinct entity in 1962 and is characterized by marked unconjugated hyperbilirubinemia in the absence of abnormalities of other conventional hepatic biochemical tests, hepatic histology, or hemolysis. It differs from CN-I in several specific ways (Table 303-1): (1) Although there is considerable overlap, average bilirubin concentrations are lower in CN-II; (2) accordingly, CN-II is only infrequently associated with kernicterus; (3) bile is deeply colored, and bilirubin glucuronides are present, with a striking, characteristic increase in the proportion of monoglucuronides; (4) UGT1A1 in liver is usually present at reduced levels (typically ≤10% of normal) but may be undetectable by older, less sensitive assays; (5) while typically detected in infancy, hyperbilirubinemia was not recognized in some cases until later in life and, in one instance, at age 34. As with CN-I, most CN-II cases exhibit abnormalities in the conjugation of other compounds, such as salicylamide and menthol, but in some instances the defect appears limited to bilirubin. Reduction of serum bilirubin concentrations by >25% in response to enzyme inducers such as phenobarbital distinguishes CN-II from CN-I, although this response may not be elicited in early infancy and often is not accompanied by measurable UGT1A1 induction. Bilirubin concentrations during phenobarbital administration do not return to normal but are typically in the range of 51–86 μmol/L (3–5 mg/dL). Although the incidence of kernicterus in CN-II is low, instances have occurred, not only in infants but also in adolescents and adults, often in the setting of an intercurrent illness, fasting, or another factor that temporarily raises the serum bilirubin concentration above baseline and reduces serum albumin levels. For this reason, phenobarbital therapy is widely recommended, a single bedtime dose often sufficing to maintain clinically safe plasma bilirubin concentrations.

Over 77 different mutations in the *UGT1* gene have been identified as causing CN-I or CN-II. It was found that missense mutations are more common in CN-II patients, as would be expected in this less severe phenotype. Their common feature is that they encode for a bilirubin-UDP-glucuronosyltransferase with markedly reduced, but detectable, enzymatic activity. The spectrum of residual enzyme activity explains the spectrum of phenotypic severity of the resulting hyperbilirubinemia. Molecular analysis has established that a large majority of CN-II patients are either homozygotes or compound heterozygotes for CN-II mutations and that individuals carrying one mutated and one entirely normal allele have normal bilirubin concentrations.

Gilbert's syndrome

This syndrome is characterized by mild unconjugated hyperbilirubinemia, normal values for standard hepatic biochemical tests, and normal hepatic histology other than a modest increase of lipofuscin pigment in some patients. Serum bilirubin concentrations are most often <51 μmol/L (<3 mg/dL), although both higher and lower values are frequent. The clinical spectrum of hyperbilirubinemia fades into that of CN-II at serum bilirubin concentrations of 86–136 μmol/L (5–8 mg/dL). At the other end of the scale, the distinction between mild cases of GS and a normal state is often blurred. Bilirubin concentrations may fluctuate substantially in any given individual, and at least 25% of patients will exhibit temporarily normal values during prolonged follow-up. More elevated values are associated with stress, fatigue, alcohol use, reduced caloric intake, and intercurrent illness, while increased caloric intake or administration of enzyme-inducing agents produces lower bilirubin levels. GS is most often diagnosed at or shortly after puberty or in adult life during routine examinations that include multichannel biochemical analyses. UGT1A1 activity is typically reduced to 10–35% of normal, and bile pigments exhibit a characteristic increase in bilirubin monoglucuronides. Studies of radiobilirubin kinetics indicate that hepatic bilirubin clearance is reduced to an average of one-third of normal. Administration of phenobarbital normalizes both the serum bilirubin concentration and hepatic bilirubin clearance; however, failure of UGT1A1 activity to improve in many such instances suggests the possible coexistence of an additional defect. Compartmental analysis of bilirubin kinetic data suggests that GS patients have a defect in bilirubin uptake as well as in conjugation. Defect(s) in the hepatic uptake of other organic anions that at least partially share an uptake mechanism with bilirubin, such as sulfobromophthalein and indocyanine green (ICG), are observed in a minority of patients. The metabolism and transport of bile acids that do not utilize the bilirubin uptake mechanism, are normal.

The magnitude of changes in the plasma bilirubin concentration induced by provocation tests such as 48 hours of fasting or the IV administration of nicotinic acid have been reported to be of help in separating GS patients from normal individuals. Other studies dispute this assertion. Moreover, on theoretical grounds, the results of such studies should provide no more information than simple measurements of the baseline plasma bilirubin concentration. Family studies indicate that GS and hereditary hemolytic anemias such as hereditary spherocytosis, glucose-6-phosphate dehydrogenase deficiency, and β-thalassemia trait sort independently. Reports of hemolysis in up to 50% of GS patients are believed to reflect better case finding, since patients with both GS and hemolysis have higher bilirubin concentrations, and are more likely to be jaundiced, than patients with either defect alone.

GS is common, with many series placing its prevalence at ≥8%. Males predominate over females by reported ratios ranging from 1.5:1 to >7:1. However, these ratios may have a large artifactual component since normal males have higher mean bilirubin levels than normal females, but the diagnosis of GS is often based on comparison to normal ranges established in men. The high prevalence of GS in the general population may explain the reported frequency of mild unconjugated hyperbilirubinemia in liver transplant recipients. The disposition of most xenobiotics metabolized by glucuronidation appears to be normal in GS, as is oxidative drug metabolism in the majority of reported studies. The principal exception is the metabolism of the antitumor agent irinotecan (CPT-11), whose active metabolite (SN-38) is glucuronidated specifically by bilirubin-UDP-glucuronosyltransferase. Administration of CPT-11 to patients with GS has resulted in several toxicities, including intractable diarrhea and myelosuppression. Some reports also suggest abnormal disposition of menthol, estradiol benzoate, acetaminophen, tolbutamide, and rifamycin SV. Although some of these studies have been disputed, and there have been no reports of clinical complications from use of these agents in GS, prudence should be exercised in prescribing them, or any agents metabolized primarily by glucuronidation, in this condition. It should also be noted that the HIV protease inhibitors indinavir and atazanavir (Chap. 189) can inhibit UGT1A1, resulting in hyperbilirubinemia that is most pronounced in patients with preexisting GS.

Most older pedigree studies of GS were consistent with autosomal dominant inheritance with variable expressivity. However, studies of the *UGT1* gene in GS have indicated a variety of molecular genetic bases for the phenotypic picture and several different patterns of inheritance. Studies in Europe and the United States found that nearly all patients had normal coding regions for UGT1A1 but were homozygous for the insertion of an extra TA (i.e., $A[TA]_7TAA$ rather than $A[TA]_6TAA$) in the promoter region of the first exon. This appeared to be necessary, but not sufficient, for clinically expressed GS, since 15% of normal controls were also homozygous for this variant. While normal by standard criteria, these individuals had somewhat higher bilirubin concentrations than the rest of the controls studied. Heterozygotes for this abnormality had bilirubin concentrations identical to those homozygous for the normal $A[TA]_6TAA$ allele. The prevalence of the $A[TA]_7TAA$ allele in a general Western population is 30%, in which case 9% would be homozygotes. This is slightly higher than the prevalence of GS based on purely phenotypic parameters. It was suggested that additional variables, such as mild hemolysis or a defect in bilirubin uptake, might be among the factors enhancing phenotypic expression of the defect.

Phenotypic expression of GS due solely to the $A[TA]_7TAA$ promoter abnormality is inherited as an autosomal recessive trait. A number of CN-II kindreds have been identified in whom there is also an allele containing a normal coding region but the $A[TA]_7TAA$ promoter abnormality. CN-II heterozygotes who have the $A[TA]_6TAA$ promoter are phenotypically normal, whereas those with the $A[TA]_7TAA$ promoter express the phenotypic picture of GS. GS in such kindreds may also result from homozygosity for the $A[TA]_7TAA$ promoter abnormality. Seven different missense mutations in the *UGT1* gene that reportedly cause GS with dominant inheritance have been found in Japanese individuals. Another Japanese patient with mild unconjugated hyperbilirubinemia was homozygous for a missense mutation in exon 5. GS in her family appeared to be recessive. Missense mutations causing GS have not been reported outside of certain Asian populations.

DISORDERS OF BILIRUBIN METABOLISM LEADING TO MIXED OR PREDOMINANTLY CONJUGATED HYPERBILIRUBINEMIA

In hyperbilirubinemia due to acquired liver disease (e.g., acute hepatitis, common bile duct stone), there are usually elevations in the serum concentrations of both conjugated and unconjugated bilirubin. Although biliary tract obstruction or hepatocellular cholestatic injury may present on occasion with a predominantly conjugated hyperbilirubinemia, it is generally not possible to differentiate intrahepatic from extrahepatic causes of jaundice based on the serum levels or relative proportions of unconjugated and conjugated bilirubin. The major reason for determining the amounts of conjugated and unconjugated bilirubin in the serum is for the initial differentiation of hepatic parenchymal and obstructive disorders (mixed conjugated and unconjugated hyperbilirubinemia) from the inheritable and hemolytic disorders discussed above that are associated with unconjugated hyperbilirubinemia.

FAMILIAL DEFECTS IN HEPATIC EXCRETORY FUNCTION

Dubin-Johnson syndrome (DJS)

This benign, relatively rare disorder is characterized by low-grade, predominantly conjugated hyperbilirubinemia (Table 303-2). Total bilirubin concentrations are typically between 34 and 85 μmol/L (2 and 5 mg/dL) but on occasion can be in the normal range or as high as 340–430 μmol/L (20–25 mg/dL) and can fluctuate widely in any given patient. The degree of hyperbilirubinemia may be increased by intercurrent illness, oral contraceptive use, and pregnancy. As the hyperbilirubinemia is due to a predominant rise in conjugated bilirubin, bilirubinuria is characteristically present. Aside from elevated serum bilirubin levels, other routine laboratory tests are normal. Physical examination is usually normal except for jaundice, although an occasional patient may have hepatosplenomegaly.

Patients with DJS are usually asymptomatic, although some may have vague constitutional symptoms. These latter patients have usually undergone extensive and often unnecessary diagnostic examinations for unexplained jaundice and have high levels of anxiety. In women, the condition may be subclinical until the patient becomes pregnant or receives oral contraceptives, at which time chemical hyperbilirubinemia becomes frank jaundice. Even in these situations, other routine liver function tests, including serum alkaline phosphatase and transaminase activities, are normal.

A cardinal feature of DJS is the accumulation in the lysosomes of centrilobular hepatocytes of dark, coarsely granular pigment. As a result, the liver may be grossly black in appearance. This pigment is thought to be derived from epinephrine metabolites that are not excreted normally. The pigment may disappear during bouts of viral hepatitis, only to reaccumulate slowly after recovery.

Biliary excretion of a number of anionic compounds is compromised in DJS. These include various cholecystographic agents, as well as sulfobromophthalein (Bromsulphalein, BSP), a synthetic dye formerly used in a test of liver function. In this test, the rate of disappearance of BSP from plasma was determined following bolus IV administration. BSP is conjugated with glutathione in the hepatocyte; the resulting conjugate is normally excreted rapidly into

TABLE 303-2 Principal Differential Characteristics of Inheritable Disorders of Bile Canalicular Function

	DJS	Rotor	PFIC1	BRIC1	PFIC2	BRIC2	PFIC3
Gene	*ABCCA*	?	*ATP8B1*	*ATP8B1*	*ABCB11*	*ABCB11*	*ABCB4*
Protein	MRP2	?	FIC1	FIC1	BSEP	BSEP	MDR3
Cholestasis	No	No	Yes	Episodic	Yes	Episodic	Yes
Serum γ-GT	Normal	Normal	Normal	Normal	Normal	Normal	↑↑
Serum bile acids	Normal	Normal	↑↑	↑↑ during episodes	↑↑	↑↑ during episodes	↑↑
Clinical features	Mild conjugated hyperbilirubinemia; otherwise normal liver function; dark pigment in liver; characteristic pattern of urinary coproporphyrins	Mild conjugated hyperbilirubinemia; otherwise normal liver function; liver without abnormal pigmentation	Severe cholestasis beginning in childhood	Recurrent episodes of cholestasis beginning at any age	Severe cholestasis beginning in childhood	Recurrent episodes of cholestasis beginning at any age	Severe cholestasis beginning in childhood; decreased phospholipids in bile

Abbreviations: BRIC, benign recurrent intrahepatic cholestasis; BSEP, bile salt excretory protein; DJS, Dubin-Johnson syndrome; γ-GT, γ-glutamyltransferase; MRP2, multidrug resistance–associated protein 2; PFIC, progressive familial intrahepatic cholestasis; ↑↑, increased.

the bile canaliculus. Patients with DJS exhibit characteristic rises in plasma concentrations at 90 minutes after injection, due to reflux of conjugated BSP into the circulation from the hepatocyte. Dyes such as ICG that are taken up by hepatocytes but are not further metabolized prior to biliary excretion do not show this reflux phenomenon. Continuous BSP infusion studies suggest a reduction in the t_{max} for biliary excretion. Bile acid disposition, including hepatocellular uptake and biliary excretion, is normal in DJS. These patients have normal serum and biliary bile acid concentrations and do not have pruritus.

By analogy with findings in several mutant rat strains, the selective defect in biliary excretion of bilirubin conjugates and certain other classes of organic compounds, but not of bile acids, that characterizes DJS in humans was found to reflect defective expression of MRP2, an ATP-dependent canalicular membrane transporter. Several different mutations in the *MRP2* gene produce the Dubin-Johnson phenotype, which has an autosomal recessive pattern of inheritance. Although MRP2 is undoubtedly important in the biliary excretion of conjugated bilirubin, the fact that this pigment is still excreted in the absence of MRP2 suggests that other, as yet uncharacterized, transport proteins may serve in a secondary role in this process.

Patients with DJS also have a diagnostic abnormality in urinary coproporphyrin excretion. There are two naturally occurring coproporphyrin isomers, I and III. Normally, ~75% of the coproporphyrin in urine is isomer III. In urine from DJS patients, total coproporphyrin content is normal, but >80% is isomer I. Heterozygotes for the syndrome show an intermediate pattern. The molecular basis for this phenomenon remains unclear.

Rotor syndrome

This benign, autosomal recessive disorder is clinically similar to DJS (Table 303-2), although it is seen even less frequently. A major phenotypic difference is that the liver in patients with Rotor syndrome has no increased pigmentation and appears totally normal. The only abnormality in routine laboratory tests is an elevation of total serum bilirubin, due to a predominant rise in conjugated bilirubin. This is accompanied by bilirubinuria. Several additional features differentiate Rotor syndrome from DJS. In Rotor syndrome, the gallbladder is usually visualized on oral cholecystography, in contrast to the nonvisualization that is typical of DJS. The pattern of urinary coproporphyrin excretion also differs. The pattern in Rotor syndrome resembles that of many acquired disorders of hepatobiliary function, in which coproporphyrin I, the major coproporphyrin isomer in bile, refluxes from the hepatocyte back into the circulation and is excreted in urine. Thus, total urinary coproporphyrin excretion is substantially increased in Rotor syndrome, in contrast to the normal levels seen in DJS. Although the fraction of coproporphyrin I in urine is elevated, it is usually <70% of the total, compared with ≥80% in DJS. The disorders also can be distinguished by their patterns of BSP excretion. Although clearance of BSP from plasma is delayed in Rotor syndrome, there is no reflux of conjugated BSP back into the circulation as seen in DJS. Kinetic analysis of plasma BSP infusion studies suggests the presence of a defect in intrahepatocellular storage of this compound. This has never been demonstrated directly, and the molecular basis of Rotor syndrome remains unknown.

Benign recurrent intrahepatic cholestasis (BRIC)

This rare disorder is characterized by recurrent attacks of pruritus and jaundice. The typical episode begins with mild malaise and elevations in serum aminotransferase levels, followed rapidly by rises in alkaline phosphatase and conjugated bilirubin and onset of jaundice and itching. The first one or two episodes may be misdiagnosed as acute viral hepatitis. The cholestatic episodes, which may begin in childhood or adulthood, can vary in duration from several weeks to months, followed by a complete clinical and biochemical resolution. Intervals between attacks may vary from several months to years. Between episodes, physical examination is normal, as are serum levels of bile acids, bilirubin, transaminases, and alkaline phosphatase. The disorder is familial and has an autosomal recessive pattern of inheritance. BRIC is considered a benign disorder in that it does not lead to cirrhosis or end-stage liver disease. However, the episodes of jaundice and pruritus can be prolonged and debilitating, and some patients have undergone liver transplantation to relieve the intractable and disabling symptoms. Treatment during the cholestatic episodes is symptomatic; there is no specific treatment to prevent or shorten the occurrence of episodes.

A gene termed *FIC1* was recently identified and found to be mutated in patients with BRIC. Curiously, this gene is expressed strongly in the small intestine but only weakly in the liver. The protein encoded by *FIC1* shows little similarity to those that have been shown to play a role in bile canalicular excretion of various compounds. Rather, it appears to be a member of a P-type ATPase family that transports aminophospholipids from the outer to the inner leaflet of a variety of cell membranes. Its relationship to the pathobiology of this disorder remains unclear. A second phenotypically identical form of BRIC, termed BRIC type 2, has been described resulting from mutations in the bile salt excretory protein (BSEP), the protein that is defective in progressive familial intrahepatic cholestasis type 2 (Table 303-2). How some mutations in this protein result in the episodic BRIC phenotype is unknown.

Progressive familial intrahepatic cholestasis (FIC)

This name is applied to three phenotypically related syndromes (Table 303-2). Progressive FIC type 1 (Byler disease) presents in early infancy as cholestasis that may be initially episodic. However, in contrast to BRIC, Byler's disease progresses to malnutrition, growth retardation, and end-stage liver disease during childhood. This disorder is also a consequence of an *FIC1* mutation. The functional relationship of the FIC1 protein to the pathogenesis of cholestasis in these disorders is unknown. Two other types of progressive FIC (types 2 and 3) have been described. Progressive FIC type 2 is associated with a mutation in the protein named *sister of p-glycoprotein,* which is the major bile canalicular exporter of bile acids and is also known as *bile salt excretory protein.* As noted above, some mutations of this protein are associated with BRIC type 2, rather than the progressive FIC type 2 phenotype. Progressive FIC type 3 has been associated with a mutation of MDR3, a protein that is essential for normal hepatocellular excretion of phospholipids across the bile canaliculus. Although all three types of progressive FIC have similar clinical phenotypes, only type 3 is associated with high serum levels of γ-glutamyltransferase activity. In contrast, activity of this enzyme is normal or only mildly elevated in symptomatic BRIC and progressive FIC types 1 and 2.

FURTHER READINGS

Davit-Spraul A et al: ATP8B1 and ABCB11 analysis in 62 children with normal gamma-glutamyl transferase progressive familial intrahepatic cholestasis (PFIC): Phenotypic differences between PFIC1 and PFIC2 and natural history. Hepatology 51: 1645, 2010

Fevery J: Bilirubin in clinical practice: A review. Liver Int 28:592, 2008

Kagawa T et al: Phenotypic differences in PFIC2 and BRIC2 correlate with protein stability of mutant BSEP and impaired taurocholate secretion in MDCK II cells. Am J Physiol Gastrointest Liver Physiol 294:G58, 2008

Strassburg, CP: Pharmacogenetics of Gilbert's syndrome. Pharmacogenomics 9:703, 2008.

Strauss KA et al: Management of hyperbilirubinemia and prevention of kernicterus in 20 patients with Crigler-Najjar disease. Eur J Pediatr 165:306, 2006

CHAPTER 304 Acute Viral Hepatitis

Jules L. Dienstag

Acute viral hepatitis is a systemic infection affecting the liver predominantly. Almost all cases of acute viral hepatitis are caused by one of five viral agents: hepatitis A virus (HAV), hepatitis B virus (HBV), hepatitis C virus (HCV), the HBV-associated delta agent or hepatitis D virus (HDV), and hepatitis E virus (HEV). Other transfusion-transmitted agents (e.g., "hepatitis G" virus and "TT" virus, have been identified but do not cause hepatitis). All these human hepatitis viruses are RNA viruses, except for hepatitis B, which is a DNA virus. Although these agents can be distinguished by their molecular and antigenic properties, all types of viral hepatitis produce clinically similar illnesses. These range from asymptomatic and inapparent to fulminant and fatal acute infections common to all types, on the one hand, and from subclinical persistent infections to rapidly progressive chronic liver disease with cirrhosis and even hepatocellular carcinoma, common to the bloodborne types (HBV, HCV, and HDV), on the other.

VIROLOGY AND ETIOLOGY

Hepatitis A

Hepatitis A virus is a nonenveloped 27-nm, heat-, acid-, and ether-resistant RNA virus in the *Hepatovirus* genus of the picornavirus family (Fig. 304-1). Its virion contains four capsid polypeptides, designated VP1 to VP4, which are cleaved posttranslationally from the polyprotein product of a 7500-nucleotide genome. Inactivation of viral activity can be achieved by boiling for 1 minute, by contact with formaldehyde and chlorine, or by ultraviolet irradiation. Despite nucleotide sequence variation of up to 20% among isolates of HAV,

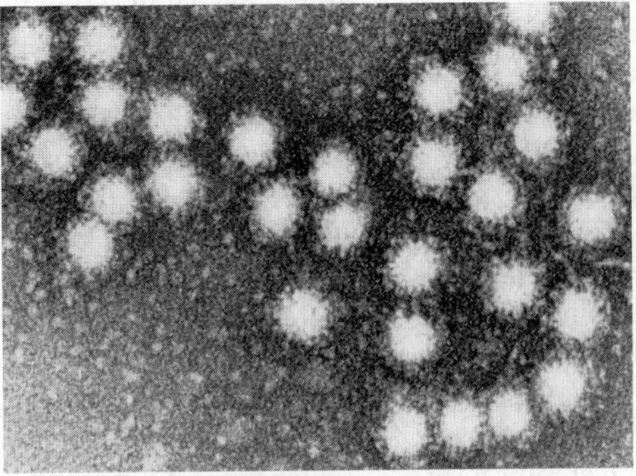
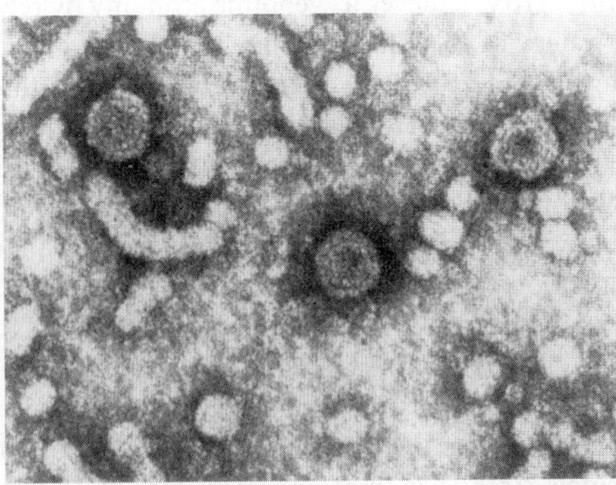

Figure 304-1 Electron micrographs of hepatitis A virus particles and serum from a patient with hepatitis B. ***Left:*** 27-nm hepatitis A virus particles purified from stool of a patient with acute hepatitis A and aggregated by antibody to hepatitis A virus. ***Right:*** Concentrated serum from a patient with hepatitis B, demonstrating the 42-nm virions, tubular forms, and spherical 22-nm particles of hepatitis B surface antigen. 132,000×. (Hepatitis D resembles 42-nm virions of hepatitis B but is smaller, 35–37 nm; hepatitis E resembles hepatitis A virus but is slightly larger, 32–34 nm; hepatitis C has been visualized as a 55-nm particle.)

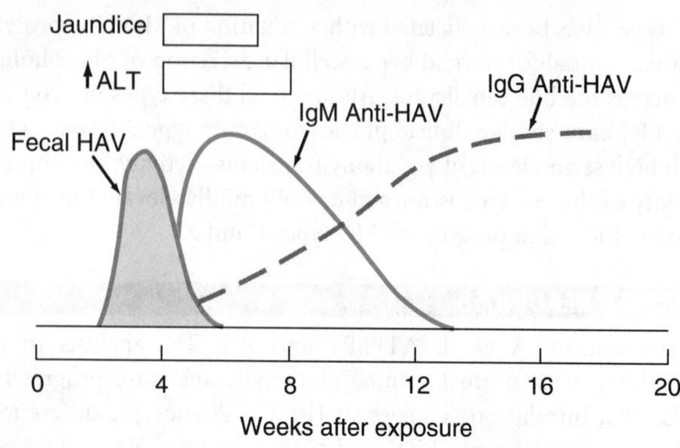

Figure 304-2 Scheme of typical clinical and laboratory features of hepatitis A.

and despite the recognition of four genotypes affecting humans, all strains of this virus are immunologically indistinguishable and belong to one serotype. Hepatitis A has an incubation period of ~4 weeks. Its replication is limited to the liver, but the virus is present in the liver, bile, stools, and blood during the late incubation period and acute preicteric phase of illness. Despite persistence of virus in the liver, viral shedding in feces, viremia, and infectivity diminish rapidly once jaundice becomes apparent. HAV can be cultivated reproducibly in vitro.

Antibodies to HAV (anti-HAV) can be detected during acute illness when serum aminotransferase activity is elevated and fecal HAV shedding is still occurring. This early antibody response is predominantly of the IgM class and persists for several months, rarely for 6–12 months. During convalescence, however, anti-HAV of the IgG class becomes the predominant antibody (Fig. 304-2). Therefore, the diagnosis of hepatitis A is made during acute illness by demonstrating anti-HAV of the IgM class. After acute illness, anti-HAV of the IgG class remains detectable indefinitely, and patients with serum anti-HAV are immune to reinfection. Neutralizing antibody activity parallels the appearance of anti-HAV, and the IgG anti-HAV present in immune globulin accounts for the protection it affords against HAV infection.

Hepatitis B

Hepatitis B virus is a DNA virus with a remarkably compact genomic structure; despite its small, circular, 3200-bp size, HBV DNA codes for four sets of viral products with a complex, multiparticle structure. HBV achieves its genomic economy by relying on an efficient strategy of encoding proteins from four overlapping genes: S, C, P, and X (Fig. 304-3), as detailed below. Once thought to be unique among viruses, HBV is now recognized as one of a family of animal viruses, hepadnaviruses (hepatotropic DNA viruses), and is classified as hepadnavirus type 1. Similar viruses infect certain species of woodchucks, ground and tree squirrels, and Pekin ducks, to mention the most carefully characterized. Like HBV, all have the same distinctive three morphologic forms, have counterparts to the envelope and nucleocapsid virus antigens of HBV, replicate in the liver but exist in extrahepatic sites, contain their own endogenous DNA polymerase, have partially double-strand and partially single-strand genomes, are associated with acute and chronic hepatitis and hepatocellular carcinoma, and rely on a replicative strategy unique among DNA viruses but typical of retroviruses. Instead of DNA replication directly from a DNA template, hepadnaviruses rely on reverse transcription (effected by the DNA polymerase) of minus-strand DNA from a "pregenomic" RNA intermediate. Then plus-strand DNA is transcribed from the minus-strand DNA

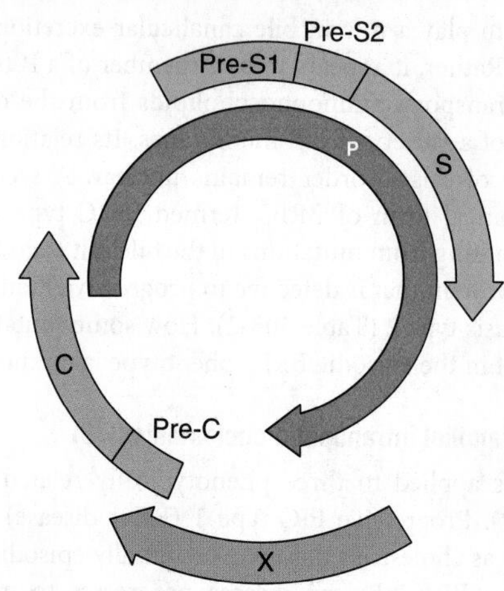

Figure 304-3 Compact genomic structure of HBV. This structure, with overlapping genes, permits HBV to code for multiple proteins. The S gene codes for the "major" envelope protein, HBsAg. Pre-S1 and pre-S2, upstream of S, combine with S to code for two larger proteins, "middle" protein, the product of pre-S2 + S, and "large" protein, the product of pre-S1 + pre-S2 + S. The largest gene, P, codes for DNA polymerase. The C gene codes for two nucleocapsid proteins, HBeAg, a soluble, secreted protein (initiation from the pre-C region of the gene) and HBcAg, the intracellular core protein (initiation after pre-C). The X gene codes for HBxAg, which can transactivate the transcription of cellular and viral genes; its clinical relevance is not known, but it may contribute to carcinogenesis by binding to p53.

template by the DNA-dependent DNA polymerase and converted in the hepatocyte nucleus to a covalently closed circular DNA, which serves as a template for messenger RNA and pregenomic RNA. Viral proteins are translated by the messenger RNA, and the proteins and genome are packaged into virions and secreted from the hepatocyte. Although HBV is difficult to cultivate in vitro in the conventional sense from clinical material, several cell lines have been transfected with HBV DNA. Such transfected cells support in vitro replication of the intact virus and its component proteins.

Viral proteins and particles Of the three particulate forms of HBV (Table 304-1), the most numerous are the 22-nm particles, which appear as spherical or long filamentous forms; these are antigenically indistinguishable from the outer surface or envelope protein of HBV and are thought to represent excess viral envelope protein. Outnumbered in serum by a factor of 100 or 1000 to 1 compared with the spheres and tubules are large, 42-nm, double-shelled spherical particles, which represent the intact hepatitis B virion (Fig. 304-1). The envelope protein expressed on the outer surface of the virion and on the smaller spherical and tubular structures is referred to as *hepatitis B surface antigen* (HBsAg). The concentration of HBsAg and virus particles in the blood may reach 500 μg/mL and 10 trillion particles per milliliter, respectively. The envelope protein, HBsAg, is the product of the S gene of HBV.

A number of different HBsAg subdeterminants have been identified. There is a common group-reactive antigen, *a*, shared by all HBsAg isolates. In addition, HBsAg may contain one of several subtype-specific antigens—namely, *d* or *y*, *w* or *r*—as well as other more recently characterized specificities. Hepatitis B isolates fall into one of at least eight subtypes and eight genotypes (A–H). Geographic distribution of genotypes and subtypes varies; genotypes A (corresponding to subtype *adw*) and D (*ayw*) predominate in the United States and Europe, while genotypes B (*adw*) and C (*adr*) predominate in Asia. Clinical course and outcome are independent of subtype, but

TABLE 304-1 Nomenclature and Features of Hepatitis Viruses

Hepatitis Type	Virus Particle, nm	Morphology	Genome*	Classification	Antigen(s)	Antibodies	Remarks
HAV	27	Icosahedral nonenveloped	7.5-kb RNA, linear, ss, +	Hepatovirus	HAV	Anti-HAV	Early fecal shedding Diagnosis: IgM anti-HAV Previous infection: IgG anti-HAV
HBV	42	Double-shelled virion (surface and core) spherical	3.2-kb DNA, circular, ss/ds	Hepadnavirus	HBsAg HBcAg HBeAg	Anti-HBs Anti-HBc Anti-HBe	Bloodborne virus; carrier state Acute diagnosis: HBsAg, IgM anti-HBc Chronic diagnosis: IgG anti-HBc, HBsAg Markers of replication: HBeAg, HBV DNA Liver, lymphocytes, other organs
	27	Nucleocapsid core			HBcAg HBeAg	Anti-HBc Anti-HBe	Nucleocapsid contains DNA and DNA polymerase; present in hepatocyte nucleus; HBcAg does not circulate; HBeAg (soluble, nonparticulate) and HBV DNA circulate—correlate with infectivity and complete virions
	22	Spherical and filamentous; represents excess virus coat material			HBsAg	Anti-HBs	HBsAg detectable in >95% of patients with acute hepatitis B; found in serum, body fluids, hepatocyte cytoplasm; anti-HBs appears following infection—protective antibody
HCV	Approx. 40–60	Enveloped	9.4-kb RNA, linear, ss, +	Hepacivirus	HCV C100-3 C33c C22-3 NS5	Anti-HCV	Bloodborne agent, formerly labeled non-A, non-B hepatitis Acute diagnosis: anti-HCV (C33c, C22-3, NS5), HCV RNA Chronic diagnosis: anti-HCV (C100-3, C33c, C22-3, NS5) and HCV RNA; cytoplasmic location in hepatocytes
HDV	35–37	Enveloped hybrid particle with HBsAg coat and HDV core	1.7-kb RNA, circular, ss, –	Resembles viroids and plant satellite viruses	HBsAg HDV antigen	Anti-HBs Anti-HDV	Defective RNA virus, requires helper function of HBV (hepadnaviruses); HDV antigen present in hepatocyte nucleus Diagnosis: anti-HDV, HDV RNA; HBV/HDV coinfection—IgM anti-HBc and anti-HDV; HDV superinfection—IgG anti-HBc and anti-HDV
HEV	32–34	Nonenveloped icosahedral	7.6-kb RNA, linear, ss, +	Hepevirus	HEV antigen	Anti-HEV	Agent of enterically transmitted hepatitis; rare in USA; occurs in Asia, Mediterranean countries, Central America Diagnosis: IgM/IgG anti-HEV (assays not routinely available); virus in stool, bile, hepatocyte cytoplasm

*ss, single-strand; ss/ds, partially single-strand, partially double-strand; –, minus-strand; +, plus-strand.

preliminary reports suggest that genotype B is associated with less rapidly progressive liver disease and a lower likelihood, or delayed appearance, of hepatocellular carcinoma than genotype C. Patients with genotype A appear to be more likely to clear circulating viremia and to achieve HBsAg seroconversion, both spontaneously and in response to antiviral therapy. In addition, "precore" mutations are favored by certain genotypes (see below).

Upstream of the S gene are the pre-S genes (Fig. 304-3), which code for pre-S gene products, including receptors on the HBV surface for polymerized human serum albumin and for hepatocyte membrane proteins. The pre-S region actually consists of both pre-S1 and pre-S2. Depending on where translation is initiated, three potential HBsAg gene products are synthesized. The protein product of the S gene is HBsAg (*major protein*), the product of the S region plus the adjacent pre-S2 region is the *middle protein*, and the product of the pre-S1 plus pre-S2 plus S regions is the *large protein*. Compared with the smaller spherical and tubular particles of HBV, complete 42-nm virions are enriched in the large protein. Both pre-S proteins and their respective antibodies can be detected during HBV infection, and the period of pre-S antigenemia appears to coincide with other markers of virus replication, as detailed below.

The intact 42-nm virion contains a 27-nm nucleocapsid core particle. Nucleocapsid proteins are coded for by the C gene. The antigen expressed on the surface of the nucleocapsid core is referred to as *hepatitis B core antigen* (HBcAg), and its corresponding antibody is anti-HBc. A third HBV antigen is *hepatitis B e antigen* (HBeAg), a soluble, nonparticulate, nucleocapsid protein that is immunologically distinct from intact HBcAg but is a product of the same C gene. The C gene has two initiation codons, a precore and a core region (Fig. 304-3). If translation is initiated at the precore region, the protein product is HBeAg, which has a signal peptide that binds it to the smooth endoplasmic reticulum and leads to its secretion into the circulation. If translation begins with the core region, HBcAg is the protein product; it has no signal peptide, it is not secreted, but it assembles into nucleocapsid particles, which bind to and incorporate RNA, and which, ultimately, contain HBV DNA. Also packaged within the nucleocapsid core is a DNA polymerase, which directs replication and repair of HBV DNA. When packaging within viral proteins is complete, synthesis of the incomplete plus strand stops; this accounts for the single-strand gap and for differences in the size of the gap. HBcAg particles remain in the hepatocyte, where they are readily detectable by immunohistochemical staining, and are exported after encapsidation by an envelope of HBsAg. Therefore, naked core particles do not circulate in the serum. The secreted nucleocapsid protein, HBeAg, provides a convenient, readily detectable, qualitative marker of HBV replication and relative infectivity.

HBsAg-positive serum containing HBeAg is more likely to be highly infectious and to be associated with the presence of hepatitis B virions (and detectable HBV DNA, see below) than HBeAg-negative or anti-HBe-positive serum. For example, HBsAg carrier mothers who are HBeAg-positive almost invariably (>90%) transmit hepatitis B infection to their offspring, whereas HBsAg carrier mothers with anti-HBe rarely (10–15%) infect their offspring.

Early during the course of acute hepatitis B, HBeAg appears transiently; its disappearance may be a harbinger of clinical improvement and resolution of infection. Persistence of HBeAg in serum beyond the first three months of acute infection may be predictive of the development of chronic infection, and the presence of HBeAg during chronic hepatitis B is associated with ongoing viral replication, infectivity, and inflammatory liver injury.

The third of the HBV genes is the largest, the P gene (Fig. 304-3), which codes for the DNA polymerase; as noted above, this enzyme has both DNA-dependent DNA polymerase and RNA-dependent reverse transcriptase activities. The fourth gene, X, codes for a small, nonparticulate protein, *hepatitis B x antigen* (HBxAg), that is capable of transactivating the transcription of both viral and cellular genes (Fig. 304-3). In the cytoplasm, HBxAg effects calcium release (possibly from mitochondria), which activates signal-transduction pathways that lead to stimulation of HBV reverse transcription and HBV DNA replication. Such transactivation may enhance the replication of HBV, leading to the clinical association observed between the expression of HBxAg and antibodies to it in patients with severe chronic hepatitis and hepatocellular carcinoma. The transactivating activity can enhance the transcription and replication of other viruses besides HBV, such as HIV. Cellular processes transactivated by X include the human interferon γ gene and class I major histocompatibility genes; potentially, these effects could contribute to enhanced susceptibility of HBV-infected hepatocytes to cytolytic T cells. The expression of X can also induce programmed cell death (apoptosis).

Serologic and virologic markers After a person is infected with HBV, the first virologic marker detectable in serum within 1–12 weeks, usually between 8–12 weeks, is HBsAg (Fig. 304-4). Circulating HBsAg precedes elevations of serum aminotransferase activity and clinical symptoms by 2–6 weeks and remains detectable during the entire icteric or symptomatic phase of acute hepatitis B and beyond. In typical cases, HBsAg becomes undetectable 1–2 months after the onset of jaundice and rarely persists beyond 6 months. After HBsAg disappears, antibody to HBsAg (anti-HBs) becomes detectable in serum and remains detectable indefinitely thereafter. Because HBcAg is intracellular and, when in the serum, sequestered within an HBsAg coat, naked core particles do not circulate in serum and, therefore, HBcAg is not detectable routinely in the serum of patients with HBV

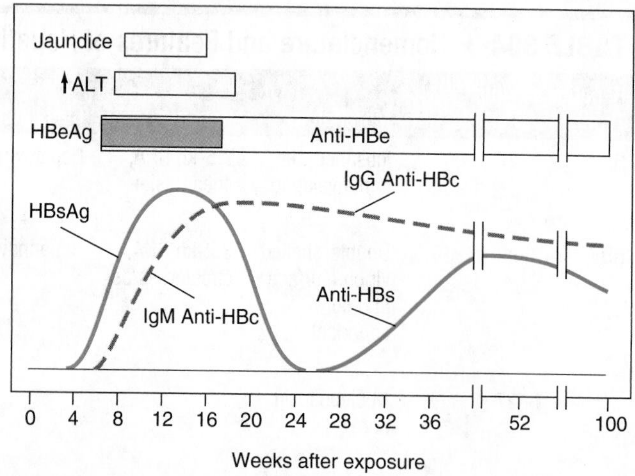

Figure 304-4 Scheme of typical clinical and laboratory features of acute hepatitis B.

infection. By contrast, anti-HBc is readily demonstrable in serum, beginning within the first 1–2 weeks after the appearance of HBsAg and preceding detectable levels of anti-HBs by weeks to months. Because variability exists in the time of appearance of anti-HBs after HBV infection, occasionally a gap of several weeks or longer may separate the disappearance of HBsAg and the appearance of anti-HBs. During this "gap" or "window" period, anti-HBc may represent the only serologic evidence of current or recent HBV infection, and blood containing anti-HBc in the absence of HBsAg and anti-HBs has been implicated in the development of transfusion-associated hepatitis B. In part because the sensitivity of immunoassays for HBsAg and anti-HBs has increased, however, this window period is rarely encountered. In some persons, years after HBV infection, anti-HBc may persist in the circulation longer than anti-HBs. Therefore, isolated anti-HBc does not necessarily indicate active virus replication; most instances of isolated anti-HBc represent hepatitis B infection in the remote past. Rarely, however, isolated anti-HBc represents low-level hepatitis B viremia, with HBsAg below the detection threshold; occasionally, isolated anti-HBc represents a cross-reacting or false-positive immunologic specificity. Recent and remote HBV infections can be distinguished by determination of the immunoglobulin class of anti-HBc. Anti-HBc of the IgM class (IgM anti-HBc) predominates during the first six months after acute infection, whereas IgG anti-HBc is the predominant class of anti-HBc beyond six months. Therefore, patients with current or recent acute hepatitis B, including those in the anti-HBc window, have IgM anti-HBc in their serum. In patients who have recovered from hepatitis B in the remote past as well as those with chronic HBV infection, anti-HBc is predominantly of the IgG class. Infrequently, in ≤1–5% of patients with acute HBV infection, levels of HBsAg are too low to be detected; in such cases, the presence of IgM anti-HBc establishes the diagnosis of acute hepatitis B. When isolated anti-HBc occurs in the rare patient with chronic hepatitis B whose HBsAg level is below the sensitivity threshold of contemporary immunoassays (a low-level carrier), the anti-HBc is of the IgG class. Generally, in persons who have recovered from hepatitis B, anti-HBs and anti-HBc persist indefinitely.

The temporal association between the appearance of anti-HBs and resolution of HBV infection as well as the observation that persons with anti-HBs in serum are protected against reinfection with HBV suggests that *anti-HBs is the protective antibody*. Therefore, strategies for prevention of HBV infection are based on providing susceptible persons with circulating anti-HBs (see below). Occasionally, in 10–20% of patients with chronic hepatitis B, low-level, low-affinity anti-HBs can be detected. This antibody is directed against a subtype determinant different from that represented by the patient's HBsAg; its presence is thought to reflect the stimulation of a related clone of antibody-forming cells, but it has no clinical relevance and does not signal imminent clearance of hepatitis B. These patients with HBsAg and such nonneutralizing anti-HBs should be categorized as having chronic HBV infection.

The other readily detectable serologic marker of HBV infection, HBeAg, appears concurrently with or shortly after HBsAg. Its appearance coincides temporally with high levels of virus replication and reflects the presence of circulating intact virions and detectable HBV DNA (with the notable exception of patients with precore mutations who cannot synthesize HBeAg—see "Molecular Variants"). Pre-S1 and pre-S2 proteins are also expressed during periods of peak replication, but assays for these gene products are not routinely available. In self-limited HBV infections, HBeAg becomes undetectable shortly after peak elevations in aminotransferase activity, before the disappearance of HBsAg, and anti-HBe then becomes detectable, coinciding with a period of relatively lower infectivity (Fig. 304-4). Because markers of HBV replication appear transiently during acute infection, testing for such markers is of little clinical utility in typical cases of acute HBV infection. In contrast, markers of HBV replication provide valuable information in patients with protracted infections.

Departing from the pattern typical of acute HBV infections, in chronic HBV infection, HBsAg remains detectable beyond six months, anti-HBc is primarily of the IgG class, and anti-HBs is either undetectable or detectable at low levels (see "Laboratory Features") (Fig. 304-5). During early chronic HBV infection, HBV DNA can be detected both in serum and in hepatocyte nuclei, where it is present in free or episomal form. This *replicative stage* of HBV infection is the time of maximal infectivity and liver injury; HBeAg is a qualitative marker and HBV DNA a quantitative marker of this replicative phase, during which all three forms of HBV circulate, including intact virions. Over time, the replicative phase of chronic HBV infection gives way to a relatively *nonreplicative phase.* This

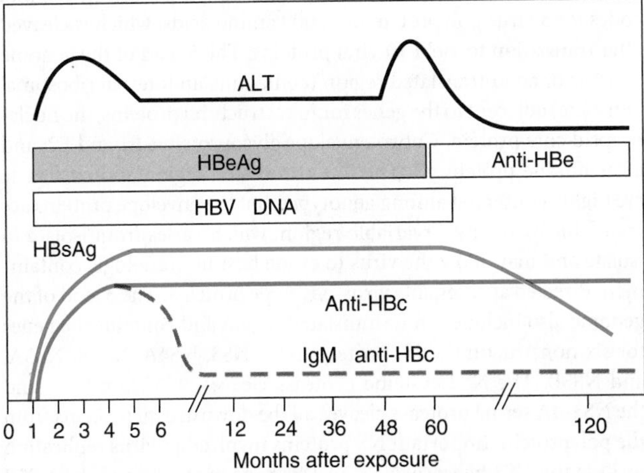

Figure 304-5 Scheme of typical laboratory features of wild-type chronic hepatitis B. HBeAg and HBV DNA can be detected in serum during the *replicative phase* of chronic infection, which is associated with infectivity and liver injury. Seroconversion from the replicative phase to the *nonreplicative phase* occurs at a rate of ~10% per year and is heralded by an acute hepatitis–like elevation of ALT activity; during the nonreplicative phase, infectivity and liver injury are limited. In HBeAg-negative chronic hepatitis B associated with mutations in the precore region of the HBV genome, replicative chronic hepatitis B occurs in the absence of HBeAg.

occurs at a rate of ~10% per year and is accompanied by seroconversion from HBeAg-positive to anti-HBe-positive. In most cases, this seroconversion coincides with a transient, acute hepatitis-like elevation in aminotransferase activity, believed to reflect cell-mediated immune clearance of virus-infected hepatocytes. In the nonreplicative phase of chronic infection, when HBV DNA is demonstrable in hepatocyte nuclei, it tends to be integrated into the host genome. In this phase, only spherical and tubular forms of HBV, *not intact virions*, circulate, and liver injury tends to subside. Most such patients would be characterized as *inactive HBV carriers*. In reality, the designations *replicative* and *nonreplicative* are only relative; even in the so-called nonreplicative phase, HBV replication can be detected at levels of ~$\leq 10^3$ virions with highly sensitive amplification probes such as the polymerase chain reaction (PCR); below this replication threshold, liver injury and infectivity of HBV are limited to negligible. Still, the distinctions are pathophysiologically and clinically meaningful. Occasionally, nonreplicative HBV infection converts back to replicative infection. Such spontaneous reactivations are accompanied by re-expression of HBeAg and HBV DNA, and sometimes of IgM anti-HBc, as well as by exacerbations of liver injury. Because high-titer IgM anti-HBc can reappear during acute exacerbations of chronic hepatitis B, relying on IgM anti-HBc versus IgG anti-HBc to distinguish between acute and chronic hepatitis B infection, respectively, may not always be reliable; in such cases, patient history is invaluable in helping to distinguish de novo acute hepatitis B infection from acute exacerbation of chronic hepatitis B infection.

Molecular variants Variation occurs throughout the HBV genome, and clinical isolates of HBV that do not express typical viral proteins have been attributed to mutations in individual or even multiple gene locations. For example, variants have been described that lack nucleocapsid proteins, envelope proteins, or both. Two categories of naturally occurring HBV variants have attracted the most attention. One of these was identified initially in Mediterranean countries among patients with an unusual serologic clinical profile. They have severe chronic HBV infection and detectable HBV DNA but with anti-HBe instead of HBeAg. These patients were found to be infected with an HBV mutant that contained an alteration in the precore region rendering the virus incapable of encoding HBeAg. Although several potential mutation sites exist in the pre-C region, the region of the C gene necessary for the expression of HBeAg (see "Virology and Etiology"), the most commonly encountered in such patients is a single base substitution, from G to A, which occurs in the second to last codon of the pre-C gene at nucleotide 1896. This substitution results in the replacement of the TGG tryptophan codon by a stop codon (TAG), which prevents the translation of HBeAg. Another mutation, in the core-promoter region, prevents transcription of the coding region for HBeAg and yields an HBeAg-negative phenotype. Patients with such mutations in the precore region and who are unable to secrete HBeAg tend to have severe liver disease that progresses more rapidly to cirrhosis or, alternatively, they are identified clinically later in the course of the natural history of chronic hepatitis B, when the disease is more advanced. Both "wild-type" HBV and precore-mutant HBV can coexist in the same patient, or mutant HBV may arise late during wild-type HBV infection. In addition, clusters of fulminant hepatitis B in Israel and Japan have been attributed to common-source infection with a precore mutant. Fulminant hepatitis B in North America and western Europe, however, occurs in patients infected with wild-type HBV, in the absence of precore mutants, and both precore mutants and other mutations throughout the HBV genome occur commonly, even in patients with typical, self-limited, milder forms of HBV infection. HBeAg-negative chronic hepatitis with mutations in the precore region is now the most frequently encountered form of hepatitis B in Mediterranean countries and in Europe. In the United States, where HBV genotype A (less prone to G1896A mutation) is prevalent, precore-mutant HBV is much less common; however, as a result of immigration from Asia and Europe, the proportion of HBeAg-negative hepatitis B–infected individuals has increased in the United States, and they now represent approximately one-third of patients with chronic hepatitis B. Characteristic of such HBeAg-negative chronic hepatitis B are lower levels of HBV DNA (usually $\leq 10^5$ copies/mL) and one of several patterns of aminotransferase activity—persistent elevations, periodic fluctuations above the normal range, and periodic fluctuations between the normal and elevated range.

The second important category of HBV mutants consists of *escape mutants*, in which a single amino acid substitution, from glycine to arginine, occurs at position 145 of the immunodominant *a* determinant common to all subtypes of HBsAg. This change in HBsAg leads to a critical conformational change that results in a loss of neutralizing activity by anti-HBs. This specific HBV/*a* mutant has been observed in two situations, active and passive immunization, in which humoral immunologic pressure may favor evolutionary change ("escape") in the virus—in a small number of hepatitis B vaccine recipients who acquired HBV infection despite the prior appearance of neutralizing anti-HBs and in liver transplant recipients who underwent the procedure for hepatitis B and who were treated with a high-potency human monoclonal anti-HBs preparation. Although such mutants have not been recognized frequently, their existence raises a concern that may complicate vaccination strategies and serologic diagnosis.

Different types of mutations emerge during antiviral therapy of chronic hepatitis B with nucleoside analogues; such "YMDD" and similar mutations in the polymerase motif of HBV are described in Chap. 306.

Extrahepatic sites Hepatitis B antigens and HBV DNA have been identified in extrahepatic sites, including lymph nodes, bone marrow, circulating lymphocytes, spleen, and pancreas. Although the virus does not appear to be associated with tissue injury in any of these extrahepatic sites, its presence in these "remote" reservoirs has been invoked (but is not necessary) to explain the recurrence of HBV infection after orthotopic liver transplantation. A more complete understanding of the clinical relevance of extrahepatic HBV remains to be defined.

Hepatitis D

The delta hepatitis agent, or HDV, the only member of the genus *Deltavirus*, is a defective RNA virus that coinfects with and requires the helper function of HBV (or other hepadnaviruses) for its replication and expression. Slightly smaller than HBV, delta is a formalin-sensitive, 35- to 37-nm virus with a hybrid structure. Its nucleocapsid expresses delta antigen, which bears no antigenic homology with any of the HBV antigens, and contains the virus genome. The delta core is "encapsidated" by an outer envelope of HBsAg, indistinguishable from that of HBV except in its relative compositions of major, middle, and large HBsAg component proteins. The genome is a small, 1700-nucleotide, circular, single-strand RNA of negative polarity that is nonhomologous with HBV DNA (except for a small area of the polymerase gene) but that has features and the rolling circle model of replication common to genomes of plant satellite viruses or viroids. HDV RNA contains many areas of internal complementarity; therefore, it can fold on itself by internal base pairing to form an unusual, very stable, rodlike structure that contains a very stable, self-cleaving and self-ligating ribozyme. HDV RNA requires host RNA polymerase II for its replication via RNA-directed RNA synthesis by transcription of genomic RNA to a complementary antigenomic (plus strand) RNA; the antigenomic RNA, in turn, serves as a template for subsequent genomic RNA synthesis. HDV RNA has only one open reading frame, and delta antigen (HDAg), a product of the antigenomic strand is the only known HDV protein; HDAg exists in two forms: a small, 195-amino-acid species, which plays a role in facilitating HDV RNA replication, and a large, 214-amino-acid species, which appears to suppress replication but is required for assembly of the antigen into virions. Delta antigens have been shown to bind directly to RNA polymerase II, resulting in stimulation of transcription. Although complete hepatitis D virions and liver injury require the cooperative helper function of HBV, intracellular replication of HDV RNA can occur without HBV. Genomic heterogeneity among HDV isolates has been described; however, pathophysiologic and clinical consequences of this genetic diversity have not been recognized. The clinical spectrum of hepatitis D is common to all seven genotypes identified, the predominant of which is genotype 1.

HDV can either infect a person simultaneously with HBV (*co-infection*) or superinfect a person already infected with HBV (*super-infection*); when HDV infection is transmitted from a donor with one HBsAg subtype to an HBsAg-positive recipient with a different subtype, the HDV agent assumes the HBsAg subtype of the recipient, rather than the donor. Because HDV relies absolutely on HBV, the duration of HDV infection is determined by the duration of (and cannot outlast) HBV infection. HDV antigen is expressed primarily in hepatocyte nuclei and is occasionally detectable in serum. During acute HDV infection, anti-HDV of the IgM class predominates, and 30–40 days may elapse after symptoms appear before anti-HDV can be detected. In self-limited infection, anti-HDV is low-titer and transient, rarely remaining detectable beyond the clearance of HBsAg and HDV antigen. In chronic HDV infection, anti-HDV circulates in high titer, and both IgM and IgG anti-HDV can be detected. HDV antigen in the liver and HDV RNA in serum and liver can be detected during HDV replication.

Hepatitis C

Hepatitis C virus, which, before its identification was labeled "non-A, non-B hepatitis," is a linear, single-strand, positive-sense, 9600-nucleotide RNA virus, the genome of which is similar in organization to that of flaviviruses and pestiviruses; HCV is the only member of the genus *Hepacivirus* in the family Flaviviridae. The HCV genome contains a single, large open reading frame (gene) that codes for a virus polyprotein of ~3000 amino acids, which is cleaved after translation to yield 10 viral proteins. The 5′ end of the genome consists of an untranslated region (containing an internal ribosomal entry site) adjacent to the genes for four structural proteins, the nucleocapsid core protein, C; two envelope glycoproteins, E1 and E2; and a membrane protein p7. The 5′ untranslated region and core gene are highly conserved among genotypes, but the envelope proteins are coded for by the hypervariable region, which varies from isolate to isolate and may allow the virus to evade host immunologic containment directed at accessible virus-envelope proteins. The 3′ end of the genome also includes an untranslated region and contains the genes for six nonstructural (NS) proteins NS2, NS3, NS4A, NS4B, NS5A, and NS5B. The NS2 cysteine protease cleaves NS3 from NS2, and the NS3-4A serine protease cleaves all the downstream proteins from the polyprotein. Important NS proteins involved in virus replication include the NS3 helicase, NS3-NS4A serine protease, and the NS5B RNA-dependent RNA polymerase (Fig. 304-6). Because HCV does not replicate via a DNA intermediate, it does not integrate into the host genome. Because HCV tends to circulate in relatively low titer, 10^3–10^7 virions/mL, visualization of virus particles, estimated to be 40–60 nm in diameter, remains difficult. Still, the replication rate of HCV is very high, 10^{12} virions per day; its half-life is 2.7 hours. The chimpanzee is a helpful but cumbersome animal model. Although a robust, reproducible, small animal model is lacking, HCV replication has been documented in an immunodeficient mouse model containing

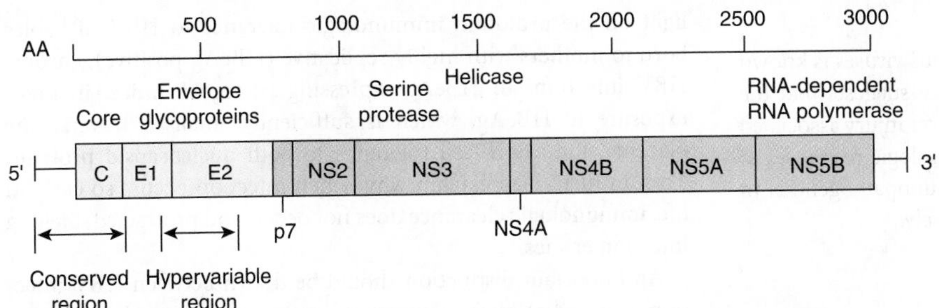

Figure 304-6 Organization of the hepatitis C virus genome and its associated, 3000 amino-acid (AA) proteins. The three structural genes at the 5′ end are the core region, C, which codes for the nucleocapsid, and the envelope regions, E1 and E2, which code for envelope glycoproteins. The 5′ untranslated region and the C region are highly conserved among isolates, while the envelope domain E2 contains the hypervariable region. Adjacent to the structural proteins is p7, a membrane protein that appears to function as an ion channel. At the 3′ end are six nonstructural (NS) regions, NS2, which codes for a cysteine protease; NS3, which codes for a serine protease and an RNA helicase; NS4 and NS4B; NS5A; and NS5B, which codes for an RNA-dependent RNA polymerase. After translation of the entire polyprotein, individual proteins are cleaved by both host and viral proteases.

explants of human liver and in transgenic mouse and rat models. Although in vitro replication has been difficult, hepatocellular carcinoma–derived cell lines have been described (replicon systems) that support replication of genetically manipulated, truncated, or full-length HCV RNA (but not intact virions). Recently, complete replication of HCV and intact 55-nm virions have been described in cell culture systems. HCV gains entry into the hepatocyte via the nonliver-specific CD81 receptor and the liver-specific tight junction protein claudin-1. Relying on the same assembly and secretion pathway as low-density lipoproteins (LPLs), HCV masquerades as a lipoprotein, which may limit its visibility to the adaptive immune system and which may explain its ability to evade immune containment and clearance.

At least six distinct major genotypes, as well as >50 subtypes within genotypes, of HCV have been identified by nucleotide sequencing. Genotypes differ one from another in sequence homology by ≥30%. Because divergence of HCV isolates within a genotype or subtype and, within the same host, may vary insufficiently to define a distinct genotype, these intragenotypic differences are referred to as *quasispecies* and differ in sequence homology by only a few percent. The genotypic and quasispecies diversity of HCV, resulting from its high mutation rate, interferes with effective humoral immunity. Neutralizing antibodies to HCV have been demonstrated, but they tend to be short lived, and HCV infection does not induce lasting immunity against reinfection with different virus isolates or even the same virus isolate. Thus, neither *heterologous* nor *homologous* immunity appears to develop commonly after acute HCV infection. Some HCV genotypes are distributed worldwide, while others are more geographically confined (see "Epidemiology and Global Features"). In addition, differences exist among genotypes in responsiveness to antiviral therapy; however, early reports of differences in pathogenicity among genotypes have not been corroborated.

Currently available, third-generation immunoassays, which incorporate proteins from the core, NS3, and NS5 regions, detect anti-HCV antibodies during acute infection. The most sensitive indicator of HCV infection is the presence of HCV RNA, which requires molecular amplification by PCR or transcription-mediated amplification (TMA) (Fig. 304-7). To allow standardization of the quantification of HCV RNA among laboratories and commercial assays, HCV RNA is reported as international units (IUs) per milliliter; quantitative assays are available that allow detection of HCV RNA with a sensitivity as low as 5 IU/mL. HCV RNA can be detected within a few days of exposure to HCV—well before the appearance of anti-HCV— and tends to persist for the duration of HCV infection; however, occasionally in patients with chronic HCV infection, HCV RNA may be detectable only intermittently. Application of sensitive molecular probes for HCV RNA has revealed the presence of replicative HCV in peripheral blood lymphocytes of infected persons; however, as is the case for HBV in lymphocytes, the clinical relevance of HCV lymphocyte infection is not known.

Hepatitis E

Previously labeled *epidemic* or *enterically transmitted non-A, non-B hepatitis,* HEV is an enterically transmitted virus that occurs primarily in India, Asia, Africa, and Central America; in those geographic areas, HEV is the most common cause of acute hepatitis. This agent, with epidemiologic features resembling those of hepatitis A, is a 32- to 34-nm, nonenveloped, HAV-like virus with a 7600-nucleotide, single-strand, positive-sense RNA genome. HEV has three open reading frames (ORF) (genes), the largest of which, *ORF1*, encodes nonstructural proteins involved in virus replication. A middle-sized gene, *ORF2*, encodes the nucleocapsid protein, the major nonstructural protein, and the smallest, *ORF3*, encodes a structural protein whose function remains undetermined. All HEV isolates appear to belong to a single serotype, despite genomic heterogeneity of up to 25% and the existence of five genotypes, only four of which have been detected in humans; genotypes 1 and 2 appear to be more virulent, while genotypes 3 and 4 are more attenuated and account for subclinical infections. Contributing to the perpetuation of this virus are animal reservoirs, most notably in swine. There is no genomic or antigenic homology, however, between HEV and HAV or other picornaviruses; and HEV, although resembling caliciviruses, is sufficiently distinct from any known agent to merit a new classification of its own as a unique genus, *Hepevirus*, within the family Hepeviridae. The virus has been detected in stool, bile, and liver and is excreted in the stool during the late incubation period; immune responses to viral antigens occur very early during the course of acute infection. Both IgM anti-HEV and IgG anti-HEV can be detected, but both fall rapidly after acute infection, reaching low levels within 9–12 months. Currently, serologic testing for HEV infection is not available routinely.

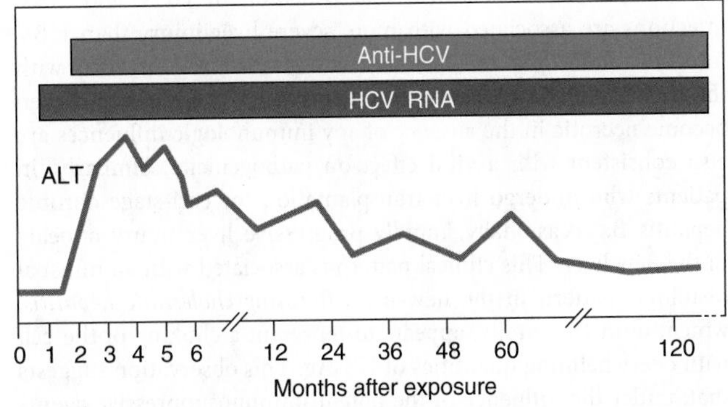

Figure 304-7 Scheme of typical laboratory features during acute hepatitis C progressing to chronicity. HCV RNA is the first detectable event, preceding alanine aminotrans ferase (ALT) elevation and the appearance of anti-HCV.

PATHOGENESIS

Under ordinary circumstances, none of the hepatitis viruses is known to be directly cytopathic to hepatocytes. Evidence suggests that the clinical manifestations and outcomes after acute liver injury associated with viral hepatitis are determined by the immunologic responses of the host. Among the viral hepatitides, the immunopathogenesis of hepatitis B and C have been studied most extensively.

Hepatitis B

For HBV, the existence of inactive hepatitis B carriers with normal liver histology and function suggests that the virus is not directly cytopathic. The fact that patients with defects in cellular immune competence are more likely to remain chronically infected rather than to clear HBV supports the role of cellular immune responses in the pathogenesis of hepatitis B–related liver injury. The model that has the most experimental support involves cytolytic T cells sensitized specifically to recognize host and hepatitis B viral antigens on the liver cell surface. Nucleocapsid proteins (HBcAg and possibly HBeAg), present on the cell membrane in minute quantities, are the viral target antigens that, with host antigens, invite cytolytic T cells to destroy HBV-infected hepatocytes. Differences in the robustness and broad polyclonality of CD8+ cytolytic T cell responsiveness and in the elaboration of antiviral cytokines by T cells have been invoked to explain differences in outcomes between those who recover after acute hepatitis, and those who progress to chronic hepatitis, or between those with mild and those with severe (fulminant) acute HBV infection.

Although a robust cytolytic T cell response occurs and eliminates virus-infected liver cells during acute hepatitis B, >90% of HBV DNA has been found in experimentally infected chimpanzees to disappear from the liver and blood before maximal T cell infiltration of the liver and before most of the biochemical and histologic evidence of liver injury. This observation suggests that components of the innate immune system and inflammatory cytokines, independent of cytopathic antiviral mechanisms, participate in the early immune response to HBV infection; this effect has been shown to represent elimination of HBV replicative intermediates from the cytoplasm and covalently closed circular viral DNA from the nucleus of infected hepatocytes. Ultimately, HBV-HLA-specific cytolytic T cell responses of the adaptive immune system are felt to be responsible for recovery from HBV infection.

Debate continues over the relative importance of viral and host factors in the pathogenesis of HBV-associated liver injury and its outcome. As noted above, precore genetic mutants of HBV have been associated with the more severe outcomes of HBV infection (severe chronic and fulminant hepatitis), suggesting that, under certain circumstances, relative pathogenicity is a property of the virus, not the host. The fact that concomitant HDV and HBV infections are associated with more severe liver injury than HBV infection alone and the fact that cells transfected in vitro with the gene for HDV (delta) antigen express HDV antigen and then become necrotic in the absence of any immunologic influences are also consistent with a viral effect on pathogenicity. Similarly, in patients who undergo liver transplantation for end-stage chronic hepatitis B, occasionally, rapidly progressive liver injury appears in the new liver. This clinical pattern is associated with an unusual histologic pattern in the new liver, *fibrosing cholestatic hepatitis*, which, ultrastructurally, appears to represent a choking of the cell with overwhelming quantities of HBsAg. This observation suggests that, under the influence of the potent immunosuppressive agents required to prevent allograft rejection, HBV may have a direct cytopathic effect on liver cells, independent of the immune system.

Although the precise mechanism of liver injury in HBV infection remains elusive, studies of nucleocapsid proteins have shed light on the profound immunologic tolerance to HBV of babies born to mothers with highly replicative (HBeAg-positive), chronic HBV infection. In HBeAg-expressing transgenic mice, in utero exposure to HBeAg, which is sufficiently small to traverse the placenta, induces T cell tolerance to both nucleocapsid proteins. This, in turn, may explain why, when infection occurs so early in life, immunologic clearance does not occur, and protracted, lifelong infection ensues.

An important distinction should be drawn between HBV infection acquired at birth, common in endemic areas, such as the Far East, and infection acquired in adulthood, common in the west. Infection in the neonatal period is associated with the acquisition of immunologic tolerance to HBV, absence of an acute hepatitis illness, but the almost invariable establishment of chronic, often lifelong infection. Neonatally acquired HBV infection can culminate decades later in cirrhosis and hepatocellular carcinoma (see "Complications and Sequelae"). In contrast, when HBV infection is acquired during adolescence or early adulthood, the host immune response to HBV infected hepatocytes tends to be robust, an acute hepatitis-like illness is the rule, and failure to recover is the exception. After adulthood acquired infection, chronicity is uncommon, and the risk of hepatocellular carcinoma is very low. Based on these observations, some authorities categorize HBV infection into an "immunotolerant" phase, an "immunoreactive" phase, and an "inactive" phase. This somewhat simplistic formulation does not apply at all to the typical adult in the west with self-limited acute hepatitis B, in whom no period of immunologic tolerance occurs. Even among those with neonatally acquired HBV infection, in whom immunologic tolerance is established definitively, intermittent bursts of hepatic necroinflammatory activity punctuate the period during the early decades of life during which liver injury appears to be quiescent (labeled by some as the "immunotolerant" phase). In addition, even when clinically apparent, liver injury and progressive fibrosis emerge during later decades (the so-called immunoreactive, or immunointolerant phase), the level of immunologic tolerance to HBV remains substantial. More accurately, in patients with neonatally acquired HBV infection, a dynamic equilibrium exists between tolerance and intolerance, the outcome of which determines the clinical expression of chronic infection. Those individuals who are infected as neonates tend to have a relatively higher level of immunologic tolerance during the early decades of life and a relatively lower level (but only rarely a loss) of tolerance in the later decades of life.

Hepatitis C

Cell-mediated immune responses and elaboration by T cells of antiviral cytokines contribute to the containment of infection and pathogenesis of liver injury associated with hepatitis C. Perhaps HCV infection of lymphoid cells plays a role in moderating immune responsiveness to the virus, as well. Intrahepatic HLA class I restricted cytolytic T cells directed at nucleocapsid, envelope, and nonstructural viral protein antigens have been demonstrated in patients with chronic hepatitis C; however, such virus-specific cytolytic T cell responses do not correlate adequately with the degree of liver injury or with recovery. Yet, a consensus has emerged supporting a role in the pathogenesis of HCV-associated liver injury of virus-activated CD4 helper T cells that stimulate, via the cytokines they elaborate, HCV-specific CD8 cytotoxic T cells. These responses appear to be more robust (higher in number, more diverse in viral antigen specificity, more functionally effective, and more long lasting) in those who recover from HCV than in those who have chronic infection. Several HLA alleles have been linked with self-limited hepatitis C, the most convincing of which is the C/C haplotype of the IL28B gene. Although attention has focused on adaptive immunity, HCV proteins have been shown to interfere with innate immunity by resulting in blocking of type 1 interferon responses and inhibition of interferon signaling and effector molecules in the interferon signaling cascade. Also shown to contribute to limiting HCV infection are natural killer cells of the innate immune system that function when HLA class 1 molecules required for successful adaptive immunity are underexpressed. Of note, the emergence of substantial viral quasispecies diversity and HCV sequence variation allow the virus to evade attempts by the host to contain HCV infection by both humoral and cellular immunity.

Finally, cross-reactivity between viral antigens (HCV NS3 and NS5A) and host autoantigens (cytochrome P450 2D6) has been invoked to explain the association between hepatitis C and a subset of patients with autoimmune hepatitis and antibodies to liver-kidney microsomal (LKM) antigen (anti-LKM) (Chap. 306).

■ EXTRAHEPATIC MANIFESTATIONS

Immune complex–mediated tissue damage appears to play a pathogenetic role in the extrahepatic manifestations of acute hepatitis B. The occasional prodromal serum sickness–like syndrome observed in acute hepatitis B appears to be related to the deposition in tissue blood vessel walls of HBsAg-anti-HBs circulating immune complexes, leading to activation of the complement system and depressed serum complement levels.

In patients with chronic hepatitis B, other types of immune-complex disease may be seen. Glomerulonephritis with the nephrotic syndrome is observed occasionally; HBsAg, immunoglobulin, and C3 deposition has been found in the glomerular basement membrane. While generalized vasculitis (polyarteritis nodosa) develops in considerably fewer than 1% of patients with chronic HBV infection, 20–30% of patients with polyarteritis nodosa have HBsAg in serum (Chap. 326). In these patients, the affected small- and medium-size arterioles contain HBsAg, immunoglobulins, and complement components. Another extrahepatic manifestation of viral hepatitis, essential mixed cryoglobulinemia (EMC), was reported initially to be associated with hepatitis B. The disorder is characterized clinically by arthritis; cutaneous vasculitis (palpable purpura); and, occasionally, with glomerulonephritis and serologically by the presence of circulating cryoprecipitable immune complexes of more than one immunoglobulin class (Chaps. 283 and 326). Many patients with this syndrome have chronic liver disease, but the association with HBV infection is limited; instead, a substantial proportion has chronic HCV infection, with circulating immune complexes containing HCV RNA. Immune-complex glomerulonephritis is another recognized extrahepatic manifestation of chronic hepatitis C.

■ PATHOLOGY

The typical morphologic lesions of all types of viral hepatitis are similar and consist of panlobular infiltration with mononuclear cells, hepatic cell necrosis, hyperplasia of Kupffer cells, and variable degrees of cholestasis. Hepatic cell regeneration is present, as evidenced by numerous mitotic figures, multinucleated cells, and "rosette" or "pseudoacinar" formation. The mononuclear infiltration consists primarily of small lymphocytes, although plasma cells and eosinophils occasionally are present. Liver cell damage consists of hepatic cell degeneration and necrosis, cell dropout, ballooning of cells, and acidophilic degeneration of hepatocytes (forming so-called Councilman or apoptotic bodies). Large hepatocytes with a ground-glass appearance of the cytoplasm may be seen in chronic but not in acute HBV infection; these cells contain HBsAg and can be identified histochemically with orcein or aldehyde fuchsin. In uncomplicated viral hepatitis, the reticulin framework is preserved.

In hepatitis C, the histologic lesion is often remarkable for a relative paucity of inflammation, a marked increase in activation of sinusoidal lining cells, lymphoid aggregates, the presence of fat (more frequent in genotype 3 and linked to increased fibrosis), and, occasionally, bile duct lesions in which biliary epithelial cells appear to be piled up without interruption of the basement membrane. Occasionally, microvesicular steatosis occurs in hepatitis D. In hepatitis E, a common histologic feature is marked cholestasis. A cholestatic variant of slowly resolving acute hepatitis A also has been described.

A more severe histologic lesion, *bridging hepatic necrosis*, also termed *subacute* or *confluent necrosis* or *interface hepatitis*, is observed occasionally in acute hepatitis. "Bridging" between lobules results from large areas of hepatic cell dropout, with collapse of the reticulin framework. Characteristically, the bridge consists of condensed reticulum, inflammatory debris, and degenerating liver cells that span adjacent portal areas, portal to central veins, or central vein to central vein. This lesion had been thought to have prognostic significance; in many of the originally described patients with this lesion, a subacute course terminated in death within several weeks to months, or severe chronic hepatitis and cirrhosis developed; however, the association between bridging necrosis and a poor prognosis in patients with acute hepatitis has not been upheld. Therefore, although demonstration of this lesion in patients with chronic hepatitis has prognostic significance (Chap. 306), its demonstration during acute hepatitis is less meaningful, and liver biopsies to identify this lesion are no longer undertaken routinely in patients with acute hepatitis. In *massive hepatic necrosis* (fulminant hepatitis, "acute yellow atrophy"), the striking feature at postmortem examination is the finding of a small, shrunken, soft liver. Histologic examination reveals massive necrosis and dropout of liver cells of most lobules with extensive collapse and condensation of the reticulin framework. When histologic documentation is required in the management of fulminant or very severe hepatitis, a biopsy can be done by the angiographically guided transjugular route, which permits the performance of this invasive procedure in the presence of severe coagulopathy.

Immunohistochemical and electron-microscopic studies have localized HBsAg to the cytoplasm and plasma membrane of infected liver cells. In contrast, HBcAg predominates in the nucleus, but, occasionally, scant amounts are also seen in the cytoplasm and on the cell membrane. HDV antigen is localized to the hepatocyte nucleus, while HAV, HCV, and HEV antigens are localized to the cytoplasm.

■ EPIDEMIOLOGY AND GLOBAL FEATURES

Before the availability of serologic tests for hepatitis viruses, all viral hepatitis cases were labeled either as "infectious" or "serum" hepatitis. Modes of transmission overlap, however, and *a clear distinction among the different types of viral hepatitis cannot be made solely on the basis of clinical or epidemiologic features* (Table 304-2). The most accurate means to distinguish the various types of viral hepatitis involves specific serologic testing.

Hepatitis A

This agent is transmitted almost exclusively by the fecal-oral route. Person-to-person spread of HAV is enhanced by poor personal hygiene and overcrowding; large outbreaks as well as sporadic cases have been traced to contaminated food, water, milk, frozen raspberries and strawberries, green onions imported from Mexico, and shellfish. Intrafamily and intrainstitutional spread are also common. Early epidemiologic observations supported a predilection for hepatitis A to occur in late fall and early winter. In temperate zones, epidemic waves have been recorded every 5–20 years as new segments of nonimmune population appeared; however, in developed countries, the incidence of hepatitis A has been declining, presumably as a function of improved sanitation, and these cyclic patterns are no longer observed. No HAV carrier state has been identified after acute hepatitis A; perpetuation of the virus in nature

TABLE 304-2 Clinical and Epidemiologic Features of Viral Hepatitis

Feature	HAV	HBV	HCV	HDV	HEV
Incubation (days)	15–45, mean 30	30–180, mean 60–90	15–160, mean 50	30–180, mean 60–90	14–60, mean 40
Onset	Acute	Insidious or acute	Insidious	Insidious or acute	Acute
Age preference	Children, young adults	Young adults (sexual and percutaneous), babies, toddlers	Any age, but more common in adults	Any age (similar to HBV)	Young adults (20–40 years)
Transmission					
Fecal-oral	+++	–	–	–	+++
Percutaneous	Unusual	+++	+++	+++	–
Perinatal	–	+++	±[a]	+	–
Sexual	±	++	±[a]	++	–
Clinical					
Severity	Mild	Occasionally severe	Moderate	Occasionally severe	Mild
Fulminant	0.1%	0.1–1%	0.1%	5–20%[b]	1–2%[e]
Progression to chronicity	None	Occasional (1–10%) (90% of neonates)	Common (85%)	Common[d]	None
Carrier	None	0.1–30%[c]	1.5–3.2%	Variable[f]	None
Cancer	None	+ (Neonatal infection)	+	±	None
Prognosis	Excellent	Worse with age, debility	Moderate	Acute, good Chronic, poor	Good
Prophylaxis	IG, inactivated vaccine	HBIG, recombinant vaccine	None	HBV vaccine (none for HBV carriers)	Vaccine
Therapy	None	Interferon Lamivudine Adefovir Pegylated interferon Entecavir Telbivudine Tenofovir	Pegylated interferon plus ribavirin telaprevir boceprevir	Interferon ±	None

[a]Primarily with HIV co-infection and high-level viremia in index case; risk ~5%.
[b]Up to 5% in acute HBV/HDV co-infection; up to 20% in HDV superinfection of chronic HBV infection.
[c]Varies considerably throughout the world and in subpopulations within countries; see text.
[d]In acute HBV/HDV co-infection, the frequency of chronicity is the same as that for HBV; in HDV superinfection, chronicity is invariable.
[e]10–20% in pregnant women.
[f]Common in Mediterranean countries, rare in North America and western Europe.
Abbreviation: HBIG, hepatitis B immunoglobulin.

depends presumably on nonepidemic, inapparent subclinical infection, ingestion of contaminated food or water in, or imported from, endemic areas, and/or contamination linked to environmental reservoirs.

In the general population, anti-HAV, a marker for previous HAV infection, increases in prevalence as a function of increasing age and of decreasing socioeconomic status. In the 1970s, serologic evidence of prior hepatitis A infection occurred in ~40% of urban populations in the United States, most of whose members never recalled having had a symptomatic case of hepatitis. In subsequent decades, however, the prevalence of anti-HAV has been declining in the United States. In developing countries, exposure, infection, and subsequent immunity are almost universal in childhood. As the frequency of subclinical childhood infections declines in developed countries, a susceptible cohort of adults emerges. Hepatitis A tends to be more symptomatic in adults; therefore, paradoxically, as the frequency of HAV infection declines, the likelihood of clinically apparent, even severe, HAV illnesses increases in the susceptible adult population. Travel to endemic areas is a common source of infection for adults from nonendemic areas. More recently recognized epidemiologic foci of HAV infection include child-care centers, neonatal intensive care units, promiscuous men who have sex with men, and injection drug users. Although hepatitis A is rarely bloodborne, several outbreaks have been recognized in recipients of clotting-factor concentrates. In the United States, the introduction of hepatitis A vaccination programs among children from high-incidence states has resulted in a >70% reduction in the annual incidence of new HAV infections and has shifted the burden of new infections from children to young adults.

Hepatitis B

Percutaneous inoculation has long been recognized as a major route of hepatitis B transmission, but the outmoded designation "serum hepatitis" is an inaccurate label for the epidemiologic spectrum of HBV infection recognized today. As detailed below, most of the hepatitis transmitted by blood transfusion is not caused by HBV; moreover, in approximately two-thirds of patients with acute type B hepatitis, no history of an identifiable percutaneous exposure can be elicited. We now recognize that many cases of hepatitis B result from less obvious modes of nonpercutaneous or covert percutaneous transmission. HBsAg has been identified in almost every body fluid from infected persons, and at least some of these body fluids—most notably semen and saliva—are infectious, albeit less so than serum, when administered percutaneously or nonpercutaneously to experimental animals. Among the nonpercutaneous modes of HBV transmission, oral ingestion has been documented as a potential but inefficient route of exposure. By contrast, the two nonpercutaneous routes considered to have the greatest impact are intimate (especially sexual) contact and perinatal transmission.

In sub-Saharan Africa, intimate contact among toddlers is considered instrumental in contributing to the maintenance of the high frequency of hepatitis B in the population. Perinatal transmission occurs primarily in infants born to HBsAg carrier mothers or mothers with acute hepatitis B during the third trimester of pregnancy or during the early postpartum period. Perinatal transmission is uncommon in North America and western Europe but occurs with great frequency and is the most important mode of HBV perpetuation in the Far East and developing countries. Although the precise mode of perinatal transmission is unknown, and although ~10% of infections may be acquired in utero, epidemiologic evidence suggests that most infections occur approximately at the time of delivery and are not related to breast-feeding. The likelihood of perinatal transmission of HBV correlates with the presence of HBeAg and high-level viral replication; 90% of HBeAg-positive mothers but only 10–15% of anti-HBe-positive mothers transmit HBV infection to their offspring. In most cases, acute infection in the neonate is clinically asymptomatic, but the child is very likely to remain chronically infected.

The >350–400 million HBsAg carriers in the world constitute the main reservoir of hepatitis B in human beings. Whereas serum HBsAg is infrequent (0.1–0.5%) in normal populations in the United States and western Europe, a prevalence of up to 5–20% has been found in the Far East and in some tropical countries; in persons with Down's syndrome, lepromatous leprosy, leukemia, Hodgkin's disease, polyarteritis nodosa; in patients with chronic renal disease on hemodialysis; and in injection drug users.

Other groups with high rates of HBV infection include spouses of acutely infected persons; sexually promiscuous persons (especially promiscuous men who have sex with men); health care workers exposed to blood; persons who require repeated transfusions especially with pooled blood-product concentrates (e.g., hemophiliacs); residents and staff of custodial institutions for the developmentally handicapped; prisoners; and, to a lesser extent, family members of chronically infected patients. In volunteer blood donors, the prevalence of anti-HBs, a reflection of previous HBV infection, ranges from 5–10%, but the prevalence is higher in lower socioeconomic strata, older age groups, and persons—including those mentioned above—exposed to blood products. Because of highly sensitive virologic screening of donor blood, the risk of acquiring HBV infection from a blood transfusion is 1 in 230,000.

Prevalence of infection, modes of transmission, and human behavior conspire to mold geographically different epidemiologic patterns of HBV infection. In the Far East and Africa, hepatitis B, a disease of the newborn and young children, is perpetuated by a cycle of maternal-neonatal spread. In North America and western Europe, hepatitis B is primarily a disease of adolescence and early adulthood, the time of life when intimate sexual contact as well as recreational and occupational percutaneous exposures tend to occur. To some degree, however, this dichotomy between high-prevalence and low-prevalence geographic regions has been minimized by immigration from high-prevalence to low-prevalence areas. The introduction of hepatitis B vaccine in the early 1980s and adoption of universal childhood vaccination policies in many countries resulted in a dramatic, ~90%, decline in the incidence of new HBV infections in those countries as well as in the dire consequences of chronic infection, including hepatocellular carcinoma. Populations and groups for whom HBV-infection screening is recommended are listed in Table 304-3.

TABLE 304-3 High-Risk Populations for Which HBV-Infection Screening Is Recommended

Persons born in countries/regions with a high (>8%) and intermediate (>2%) prevalence of HBV infection including immigrants and adopted children and including persons born in the United States who were not vaccinated as infants and whose parents immigrated from areas of high HBV endemicity.
Household and sexual contacts of persons with hepatitis B
Persons who have used injection drugs
Persons with multiple sexual contacts or a history of sexually transmitted disease
Men who have sex with men
Inmates of correctional facilities
Persons with elevated alanine or aspartate aminotransferase levels
Persons with HCV or HIV infection
Hemodialysis patients
Pregnant women
Persons who require immunosuppressive or cytotoxic therapy

Hepatitis D

Infection with HDV has a worldwide distribution, but two epidemiologic patterns exist. In Mediterranean countries (northern Africa, southern Europe, the Middle East), HDV infection is endemic among those with hepatitis B, and the disease is transmitted predominantly by nonpercutaneous means, especially close personal contact. In nonendemic areas, such as the United States and northern Europe, HDV infection is confined to persons exposed frequently to blood and blood products, primarily injection drug users and hemophiliacs. HDV infection can be introduced into a population through drug users or by migration of persons from endemic to nonendemic areas. Thus, patterns of population migration and human behavior facilitating percutaneous contact play important roles in the introduction and amplification of HDV infection. Occasionally, the migrating epidemiology of hepatitis D is expressed in explosive outbreaks of severe hepatitis, such as those that have occurred in remote South American villages as well as in urban centers in the United States. Ultimately, such outbreaks of hepatitis D—either of co-infections with acute hepatitis B or of superinfections in those already infected with HBV—may blur the distinctions between endemic and nonendemic areas. On a global scale, HDV infection declined at the end of the 1990s. Even in Italy, an HDV-endemic area, public health measures introduced to control HBV infection resulted during the 1990s in a 1.5%/year reduction in the prevalence of HDV infection. Still, the frequency of HDV infection during the first decade of the twenty-first century has not fallen below levels reached during the 1990s; the reservoir has been sustained by survivors infected during 1970–1980 and recent immigrants from still-endemic to less-endemic countries.

Hepatitis C

Routine screening of blood donors for HBsAg and the elimination of commercial blood sources in the early 1970s reduced the frequency of, but did not eliminate, transfusion-associated hepatitis. During the 1970s, the likelihood of acquiring hepatitis after transfusion of voluntarily donated, HBsAg-screened blood was ~10% per patient (up to 0.9% per unit transfused); 90–95% of these cases were classified, based on serologic exclusion of hepatitis A and B, as "non-A, non-B" hepatitis. For patients requiring transfusion of pooled products, such as clotting factor concentrates, the risk was even higher, up to 20–30%.

During the 1980s, voluntary self-exclusion of blood donors with risk factors for AIDS and then the introduction of donor screening for anti-HIV reduced further the likelihood of transfusion-associated hepatitis to <5%. During the late 1980s and early 1990s, the introduction first of "surrogate" screening tests for non-A, non-B hepatitis [alanine aminotransferase (ALT) and anti-HBc, both shown to identify blood donors with a higher likelihood of transmitting non-A, non-B hepatitis to recipients] and, subsequently, after the discovery of HCV, first-generation immunoassays for anti-HCV reduced the frequency of transfusion-associated hepatitis even further. A prospective analysis of transfusion-associated hepatitis conducted between 1986 and 1990 showed that the frequency of transfusion-associated hepatitis at one urban university hospital fell from a baseline of 3.8% per patient (0.45% per unit transfused) to 1.5% per patient (0.19% per unit) after the introduction of surrogate testing and to 0.6% per patient (0.03% per unit) after the introduction of first-generation anti-HCV assays. The introduction of second-generation anti-HCV assays reduced the frequency of transfusion-associated hepatitis C to almost imperceptible levels—1 in 100,000—and these gains were reinforced by the application of third-generation anti-HCV assays and of automated PCR testing of donated blood for HCV RNA, which has resulted in a reduction in the risk of transfusion-associated HCV infection to 1 in 2.3 million transfusions.

In addition to being transmitted by transfusion, hepatitis C can be transmitted by other percutaneous routes, such as injection drug use. In addition, this virus can be transmitted by occupational exposure to blood, and the likelihood of infection is increased in hemodialysis units. Although the frequency of transfusion-associated hepatitis C fell as a result of blood-donor screening, the overall frequency of hepatitis C remained the same until the early 1990s, when the overall frequency fell by 80%, in parallel with a reduction in the number of new cases in injection drug users. After the exclusion of anti-HCV-positive plasma units from the donor pool, rare, sporadic instances have occurred of hepatitis C among recipients of immunoglobulin (IG) preparations for intravenous (but not intramuscular) use.

Serologic evidence for HCV infection occurs in 90% of patients with a history of transfusion-associated hepatitis (almost all occurring before 1992, when second-generation HCV-screening tests were introduced); hemophiliacs and others treated with clotting factors; injection drug users; 60–70% of patients with sporadic "non-A, non-B" hepatitis who lack identifiable risk factors; 0.5% of volunteer blood donors; and, in the most recent survey conducted in the United States between 1999 and 2000, 1.6% of the general population in the United States, which translates into 4.1 million persons (3.2 million with viremia). Comparable frequencies of HCV infection occur in most countries around the world, with 170 million persons infected worldwide, but extraordinarily high prevalences of HCV infection occur in certain countries such as Egypt, where >20% of the population in some cities is infected. The high frequency in Egypt is attributable to contaminated equipment used for medical procedures and unsafe injection practices in the 1970s. In the United States, African Americans and Mexican Americans have higher frequencies of HCV infection than whites. Between 1988 and 1994, 30- to 40-year-old adult males had the highest prevalence of HCV infection; however, in a survey conducted between 1999 and 2000, the peak age decile had shifted to those age 40–49 years; an increase in hepatitis C–related mortality has paralleled this secular trend, increasing since 1995 predominantly in the 55- to 64-year age group. Thus, despite an 80% reduction in new HCV infections during the 1990s, the prevalence of HCV infection in the population was sustained by an aging cohort that had acquired their infections 2 to 3 decades earlier, during the 1960s and 1970s, as a result predominantly of self-inoculation with recreational drugs. Hepatitis C accounts for 40% of chronic liver disease, is the most frequent indication for liver transplantation, and is estimated to account for 8000–10,000 deaths per year in the United States.

The distribution of HCV genotypes varies in different parts of the world. Worldwide, genotype 1 is the most common. In the United States, genotype 1 accounts for 70% of HCV infections, while genotypes 2 and 3 account for the remaining 30%; among African Americans, the frequency of genotype 1 is even higher (i.e., 90%). Genotype 4 predominates in Egypt; genotype 5 is localized to South Africa, and genotype 6 to Hong Kong.

Most asymptomatic blood donors found to have anti-HCV and ~20–30% of persons with reported cases of acute hepatitis C do not fall into a recognized risk group; however, many such blood donors do recall risk-associated behaviors when questioned carefully.

As a bloodborne infection, HCV potentially can be transmitted sexually and perinatally; however, both of these modes of transmission are inefficient for hepatitis C. Although 10–15% of patients with acute hepatitis C report having potential sexual sources of infection, most studies have failed to identify sexual transmission of this agent. The chances of sexual and perinatal transmission have been estimated to be ~5%, well below comparable rates for HIV and HBV infections. Moreover, sexual transmission appears to be confined to such subgroups as persons with multiple sexual partners and sexually transmitted diseases; transmission of HCV infection is rare between stable, monogamous sexual partners. Breast-feeding does not increase the risk of HCV infection between an infected mother and her infant. Infection of health workers is not dramatically higher than among the general population; however, health workers are more likely to acquire HCV infection through accidental needle punctures, the efficiency of which is ~3%. Infection of household contacts is rare as well.

Other groups with an increased frequency of HCV infection include patients who require hemodialysis and organ transplantation, those who require transfusions in the setting of cancer chemotherapy, HIV-infected persons, and persons with unexplained serum aminotransferase elevations. In immunosuppressed individuals, levels of anti-HCV may be undetectable, and a diagnosis may require testing for HCV RNA. Although new acute cases of hepatitis C are rare, newly diagnosed cases are common among otherwise healthy persons who experimented briefly with injection drugs, as noted above, 2 or 3 decades earlier. Such instances usually remain unrecognized for years, until unearthed by laboratory screening for routine medical examinations, insurance applications, and attempted blood donation. Populations groups for whom HCV-infection screening is recommended are listed in Table 304-4.

Hepatitis E

This type of hepatitis, identified in India, Asia, Africa, the Middle East, and Central America, resembles hepatitis A in its primarily enteric mode of spread. The commonly recognized cases occur after contamination of water supplies such as after monsoon flooding, but sporadic, isolated cases occur. An epidemiologic feature that distinguishes HEV from other enteric agents is the rarity of secondary person-to-person spread from infected persons to their close contacts. Infections arise in populations that are immune to HAV and favor young adults. In endemic areas, the prevalence of antibodies to HEV is ≤40%. In nonendemic areas of the world, such as the United States, clinically apparent acute hepatitis E is extremely rare; however, the prevalence of antibodies to HEV can be as high as 20% in such areas. In nonendemic areas, HEV does not account for any of the sporadic "non-A, non-B" cases of hepatitis; however, cases

TABLE 304-4 High-Risk Populations for Which HCV-Infection Screening Is Recommended

Persons who have used injection drugs or those who have used illicit drugs by noninjection routes
Persons with HIV infection
Hemophiliacs treated with clotting factor concentrates prior to 1987
Hemodialysis patients
Persons with unexplained elevations of aminotransferase levels
Transfusion or transplantation recipients prior to July 1992
Children born to women with hepatitis C
Health care, public safety, and emergency medical personnel following needle injury or mucosal exposure to HCV-contaminated blood
Sexual partners of persons with hepatitis C infection

imported from endemic areas have been found in the United States. Several reports suggest a zoonotic reservoir for HEV in swine.

CLINICAL AND LABORATORY FEATURES

Symptoms and signs

Acute viral hepatitis occurs after an incubation period that varies according to the responsible agent. Generally, incubation periods for hepatitis A range from 15–45 days (mean, 4 weeks), for hepatitis B and D from 30–180 days (mean, 8–12 weeks), for hepatitis C from 15–160 days (mean, 7 weeks), and for hepatitis E from 14–60 days (mean, 5–6 weeks). The *prodromal symptoms* of acute viral hepatitis are systemic and quite variable. Constitutional symptoms of anorexia, nausea and vomiting, fatigue, malaise, arthralgias, myalgias, headache, photophobia, pharyngitis, cough, and coryza may precede the onset of jaundice by 1–2 weeks. The nausea, vomiting, and anorexia are frequently associated with alterations in olfaction and taste. A low-grade fever between 38° and 39°C (100°–102°F) is more often present in hepatitis A and E than in hepatitis B or C, except when hepatitis B is heralded by a serum sickness–like syndrome; rarely, a fever of 39.5°–40°C (103°–104°F) may accompany the constitutional symptoms. Dark urine and clay-colored stools may be noticed by the patient from 1–5 days before the onset of clinical jaundice.

With the onset of *clinical jaundice*, the constitutional prodromal symptoms usually diminish, but in some patients mild weight loss (2.5–5 kg) is common and may continue during the entire icteric phase. The liver becomes enlarged and tender and may be associated with right upper quadrant pain and discomfort. Infrequently, patients present with a cholestatic picture, suggesting extrahepatic biliary obstruction. Splenomegaly and cervical adenopathy are present in 10–20% of patients with acute hepatitis. Rarely, a few spider angiomas appear during the icteric phase and disappear during convalescence. During the *recovery phase*, constitutional symptoms disappear, but usually some liver enlargement and abnormalities in liver biochemical tests are still evident. The duration of the posticteric phase is variable, ranging 2–12 weeks, and is usually more prolonged in acute hepatitis B and C. Complete clinical and biochemical recovery is to be expected 1–2 months after all cases of hepatitis A and E and 3–4 months after the onset of jaundice in three-quarters of uncomplicated, self-limited cases of hepatitis B and C (among healthy adults, acute hepatitis B is self-limited in 95–99% while hepatitis C is self-limited in only ~15%). In the remainder, biochemical recovery may be delayed. A substantial proportion of patients with viral hepatitis never become icteric.

Infection with HDV can occur in the presence of acute or chronic HBV infection; the duration of HBV infection determines the duration of HDV infection. When acute HDV and HBV infection occur simultaneously, clinical and biochemical features may be indistinguishable from those of HBV infection alone, although occasionally they are more severe. As opposed to patients with *acute* HBV infection, patients with *chronic* HBV infection can support HDV replication indefinitely. This can happen when acute HDV infection occurs in the presence of a nonresolving acute HBV infection. More commonly, acute HDV infection becomes chronic when it is superimposed on an underlying chronic HBV infection. In such cases, the HDV superinfection appears as a clinical exacerbation or an episode resembling acute viral hepatitis in someone already chronically infected with HBV. Superinfection with HDV in a patient with chronic hepatitis B often leads to clinical deterioration (see below).

In addition to superinfections with other hepatitis agents, acute hepatitis-like clinical events in persons with chronic hepatitis B may accompany spontaneous HBeAg to anti-HBe seroconversion or spontaneous reactivation (i.e., reversion from nonreplicative to replicative infection). Such reactivations can occur as well in therapeutically immunosuppressed patients with chronic HBV infection when cytotoxic/immunosuppressive drugs are withdrawn; in these cases, restoration of immune competence is thought to allow resumption of previously checked cell-mediated immune cytolysis of HBV-infected hepatocytes. Occasionally, acute clinical exacerbations of chronic hepatitis B may represent the emergence of a precore mutant (see "Virology and Etiology"), and the subsequent course in such patients may be characterized by periodic exacerbations.

Laboratory features

The serum aminotransferases aspartate aminotransferase (AST) and ALT (previously designated SGOT and SGPT) show a variable increase during the prodromal phase of acute viral hepatitis and precede the rise in bilirubin level (Figs. 304-2 and 304-4). The acute level of these enzymes, however, does not correlate well with the degree of liver cell damage. Peak levels vary from 400–4000 IU or more; these levels are usually reached at the time the patient is clinically icteric and diminish progressively during the recovery phase of acute hepatitis. The diagnosis of anicteric hepatitis is based on clinical features and on aminotransferase elevations.

Jaundice is usually visible in the sclera or skin when the serum bilirubin value is >43 μmol/L (2.5 mg/dL). When jaundice appears, the serum bilirubin typically rises to levels ranging from 85–340 μmol/L (5–20 mg/dL). The serum bilirubin may continue to rise despite falling serum aminotransferase levels. In most instances, the total bilirubin is equally divided between the conjugated and unconjugated fractions. Bilirubin levels >340 μmol/L (20 mg/dL) extending and persisting late into the course of viral hepatitis are more likely to be associated with severe disease. In certain patients with underlying hemolytic anemia, however, such as glucose-6-phosphate dehydrogenase deficiency and sickle cell anemia, a high serum bilirubin level is common, resulting from superimposed hemolysis. In such patients, bilirubin levels >513 μmol/L (30 mg/dL) have been observed and are not necessarily associated with a poor prognosis.

Neutropenia and lymphopenia are transient and are followed by a relative lymphocytosis. Atypical lymphocytes (varying between 2 and 20%) are common during the acute phase. Measurement of the prothrombin time (PT) is important in patients with acute viral hepatitis, for a prolonged value may reflect a severe hepatic synthetic defect, signify extensive hepatocellular necrosis, and indicate a worse prognosis. Occasionally, a prolonged PT may occur with only mild increases in the serum bilirubin and aminotransferase levels. Prolonged nausea and vomiting, inadequate carbohydrate intake, and poor hepatic glycogen reserves may contribute to hypoglycemia noted occasionally in patients with severe viral hepatitis. Serum alkaline phosphatase may be normal or only mildly elevated, while a fall in serum albumin is uncommon in uncomplicated acute viral hepatitis. In some patients, mild and transient steatorrhea has been noted as well as slight microscopic hematuria and minimal proteinuria.

A diffuse but mild elevation of the γ globulin fraction is common during acute viral hepatitis. Serum IgG and IgM levels are elevated in about one-third of patients during the acute phase of viral hepatitis, but the serum IgM level is elevated more characteristically during acute hepatitis A. During the acute phase of viral hepatitis, antibodies to smooth muscle and other cell constituents may be present, and low titers of rheumatoid factor, nuclear antibody, and heterophil antibody can also be found occasionally. In hepatitis C and D, antibodies to LKM may occur; however, the species of LKM antibodies in the two types of hepatitis are different from each other as well as from the LKM antibody species characteristic of autoimmune hepatitis type 2 (Chap. 306). The autoantibodies in viral hepatitis are nonspecific and can also be associated with other viral and systemic diseases. In contrast, virus-specific antibodies, which appear during and after hepatitis virus infection, are serologic markers of diagnostic importance.

As described above, serologic tests are available with which to establish a diagnosis of hepatitis A, B, D, and C. Tests for fecal or serum HAV are not routinely available. Therefore, a diagnosis of hepatitis A is based on detection of IgM anti-HAV during acute illness (Fig. 304-2). Rheumatoid factor can give rise to false-positive results in this test.

A diagnosis of HBV infection can usually be made by detection of HBsAg in serum. Infrequently, levels of HBsAg are too low to be detected during acute HBV infection, even with contemporary, highly sensitive immunoassays. In such cases, the diagnosis can be established by the presence of IgM anti-HBc.

The titer of HBsAg bears little relation to the severity of clinical disease. Indeed, an inverse correlation exists between the serum concentration of HBsAg and the degree of liver cell damage. For example, titers are highest in immunosuppressed patients, lower in patients with chronic liver disease (but higher in mild chronic than in severe chronic hepatitis), and very low in patients with acute fulminant hepatitis. These observations suggest that, in hepatitis B, the degree of liver cell damage and the clinical course are related to variations in the patient's immune response to HBV rather than to the amount of circulating HBsAg. In immunocompetent persons, however, a correlation exists between markers of HBV *replication* and liver injury (see below).

Another serologic marker that may be of value in patients with hepatitis B is HBeAg. Its principal clinical usefulness is as an indicator of relative infectivity. Because HBeAg is invariably present during early acute hepatitis B, HBeAg testing is indicated primarily during follow-up of chronic infection.

In patients with hepatitis B surface antigenemia of unknown duration (e.g., blood donors found to be HBsAg-positive and referred to a physician for evaluation), testing for IgM anti-HBc may be useful to distinguish between acute or recent infection (IgM anti-HBc-positive) and chronic HBV infection (IgM anti-HBc-negative, IgG anti-HBc-positive). A false-positive test for IgM anti-HBc may be encountered in patients with high-titer rheumatoid factor.

Anti-HBs is rarely detectable in the presence of HBsAg in patients with *acute* hepatitis B, but 10–20% of persons with *chronic* HBV infection may harbor low-level anti-HBs. This antibody is directed not against the common group determinant, *a*, but against the heterotypic subtype determinant (e.g., HBsAg of subtype *ad* with anti-HBs of subtype *y*). In most cases, this serologic pattern cannot be attributed to infection with two different HBV subtypes, and the presence of this antibody is not a harbinger of imminent HBsAg clearance. When such antibody is detected, its presence is of no recognized clinical significance (see "Virology and Etiology").

After immunization with hepatitis B vaccine, which consists of HBsAg alone, anti-HBs is the only serologic marker to appear. The commonly encountered serologic patterns of hepatitis B and their interpretations are summarized in Table 304-5. Tests for the detection of HBV DNA in liver and serum are now available. Like HBeAg, serum HBV DNA is an indicator of HBV replication, but tests for HBV DNA are more sensitive and quantitative. First-generation hybridization assays for HBV DNA had a sensitivity of 10^5–10^6 virions/mL, a relative threshold below which infectivity and liver injury are limited and HBeAg is usually undetectable. Currently, testing for HBV DNA has shifted from insensitive hybridization assays to amplification assays (e.g., the PCR-based assay, which can detect as few as 10 or 100 virions/mL); among the commercially available PCR assays, the most useful are those with the highest sensitivity (5–10 IU/mL) and the largest dynamic range (10^0–10^9 IU/mL). With increased sensitivity, amplification assays remain reactive well below the threshold for infectivity and liver injury. These markers are useful in following the course of HBV replication in patients with chronic hepatitis B receiving antiviral chemotherapy

TABLE 304-5 Commonly Encountered Serologic Patterns of Hepatitis B Infection

HBsAg	Anti-HBs	Anti-HBc	HBeAg	Anti-HBe	Interpretation
+	–	IgM	+	–	Acute hepatitis B, high infectivity
+	–	IgG	+	–	Chronic hepatitis B, high infectivity
+	–	IgG	–	+	1. Late acute or chronic hepatitis B, low infectivity
					2. HBeAg-negative ("precore-mutant") hepatitis B (chronic or, rarely, acute)
+	+	+	+/–	+/–	1. HBsAg of one subtype and heterotypic anti-HBs (common)
					2. Process of seroconversion from HBsAg to anti-HBs (rare)
–	–	IgM	+/–	+/–	1. Acute hepatitis B
					2. Anti-HBc "window"
–	–	IgG	–	+/–	1. Low-level hepatitis B carrier
					2. Hepatitis B in remote past
–	+	IgG	–	+/–	Recovery from hepatitis B
–	+	–	–	–	1. Immunization with HBsAg (after vaccination)
					2. Hepatitis B in the remote past (?)
					3. False-positive

(e.g., with interferon or nucleoside analogues) (Chap. 306). In immunocompetent persons with chronic hepatitis B, a general correlation does appear to exist between the level of HBV replication, as reflected by the level of HBV DNA in serum, and the degree of liver injury. High-serum HBV DNA levels, increased expression of viral antigens, and necroinflammatory activity in the liver go hand in hand unless immunosuppression interferes with cytolytic T cell responses to virus-infected cells; reduction of HBV replication with antiviral drugs tends to be accompanied by an improvement in liver histology. Among patients with chronic hepatitis B, high levels of HBV DNA increase the risk of cirrhosis, hepatic decompensation, and hepatocellular carcinoma (see "Complications and Sequelae").

In patients with hepatitis C, an episodic pattern of aminotransferase elevation is common. A specific serologic diagnosis of hepatitis C can be made by demonstrating the presence in serum of anti-HCV. When contemporary immunoassays are used, anti-HCV can be detected in acute hepatitis C during the initial phase of elevated aminotransferase activity. This antibody may never become detectable in 5–10% of patients with acute hepatitis C, and levels of anti-HCV may become undetectable after recovery (albeit rare) from acute hepatitis C. In patients with chronic hepatitis C, anti-HCV is detectable in >95% of cases. Nonspecificity can confound immunoassays for anti-HCV, especially in persons with a low prior probability of infection, such as volunteer blood donors, or in persons with circulating rheumatoid factor, which can bind nonspecifically to assay reagents; testing for HCV RNA can be used in such settings to distinguish between true-positive and false-positive anti-HCV determinations. Assays for HCV RNA are the most sensitive tests for HCV infection and represent the "gold standard" in establishing a diagnosis of hepatitis C. HCV RNA can be detected even before acute elevation of aminotransferase activity and before the appearance of anti-HCV in patients with acute hepatitis C. In addition, HCV RNA remains detectable indefinitely, continuously in most but intermittently in some, in patients with chronic hepatitis C (detectable as well in some persons with normal liver tests (i.e., inactive carriers). In the small minority of patients with hepatitis C who lack anti-HCV, a diagnosis can be supported by detection of HCV RNA. If all these tests are negative and the patient has a well-characterized case of hepatitis after percutaneous exposure to blood or blood products, a diagnosis of hepatitis caused by an unidentified agent can be entertained.

Amplification techniques are required to detect HCV RNA, and two types are available. One is a branched-chain complementary DNA (bDNA) assay, in which the detection signal (a colorimetrically detectable enzyme bound to a complementary DNA probe) is amplified. The other involves target amplification (i.e., synthesis of multiple copies of the viral genome). This can be done by PCR or TMA, in which the viral RNA is reverse transcribed to complementary DNA and then amplified by repeated cycles of DNA synthesis. Both can be used as quantitative assays and a measurement of relative "viral load"; PCR and TMA, with a sensitivity of 10–10^2 IU/mL, are more sensitive than bDNA, with a sensitivity of 10^3 IU/mL; assays are available with a wide dynamic range (10–10^7 IU/mL). Determination of HCV RNA level is not a reliable marker of disease severity or prognosis but is helpful in predicting relative responsiveness to antiviral therapy. The same is true for determinations of HCV genotype (Chap. 306).

A proportion of patients with hepatitis C have isolated anti-HBc in their blood, a reflection of a common risk in certain populations of exposure to multiple bloodborne hepatitis agents. The anti-HBc in such cases is almost invariably of the IgG class and usually represents HBV infection in the remote past (HBV DNA undetectable), rarely current HBV infection with low-level virus carriage.

The presence of HDV infection can be identified by demonstrating intrahepatic HDV antigen or, more practically, an anti-HDV seroconversion (a rise in titer of anti-HDV or de novo appearance of anti-HDV). Circulating HDV antigen, also diagnostic of acute infection, is detectable only briefly, if at all. Because anti-HDV is often undetectable once HBsAg disappears, retrospective serodiagnosis of acute self-limited, simultaneous HBV and HDV infection is difficult. Early diagnosis of acute infection may be hampered by a delay of up to 30–40 days in the appearance of anti-HDV.

When a patient presents with acute hepatitis and has HBsAg and anti-HDV in serum, determination of the class of anti-HBc is helpful in establishing the relationship between infection with HBV and HDV. Although IgM anti-HBc does not distinguish *absolutely* between acute and chronic HBV infection, its presence is a reliable indicator of recent infection and its absence a reliable indicator of infection in the remote past. In simultaneous acute HBV and HDV infections, IgM anti-HBc will be detectable, while in acute HDV infection superimposed on chronic HBV infection, anti-HBc will be of the IgG class.

Tests for the presence of HDV RNA are useful for determining the presence of ongoing HDV replication and relative infectivity. Diagnostic tests for hepatitis E are commercially available in several countries outside the United States; in the United States, diagnostic assays can be performed at the Centers for Disease Control and Prevention.

Liver biopsy is rarely necessary or indicated in acute viral hepatitis, except when the diagnosis is questionable or when clinical evidence suggests a diagnosis of chronic hepatitis.

A diagnostic algorithm can be applied in the evaluation of cases of acute viral hepatitis. A patient with acute hepatitis should undergo four serologic tests, HBsAg, IgM anti-HAV, IgM anti-HBc, and anti-HCV (Table 304-6). The presence of HBsAg, with or without IgM anti-HBc, represents HBV infection. If IgM anti-HBc is present, the HBV infection is considered acute; if IgM anti-HBc is absent, the HBV infection is considered chronic. A diagnosis of acute hepatitis B can be made in the absence of HBsAg when IgM anti-HBc is detectable. A diagnosis of acute hepatitis A is based on the presence of IgM anti-HAV. If IgM anti-HAV coexists with HBsAg, a diagnosis of simultaneous HAV and HBV infections can be made; if IgM anti-HBc (with or without HBsAg) is detectable, the patient has simultaneous acute hepatitis A and B, and if IgM anti-HBc is undetectable, the patient has acute hepatitis A superimposed

TABLE 304-6 Simplified Diagnostic Approach in Patients Presenting With Acute Hepatitis

Serologic Tests of Patient's Serum				
HBsAg	IgM Anti-HAV	IgM Anti-HBc	Anti-HCV	Diagnostic Interpretation
+	–	+	–	Acute hepatitis B
+	–	–	–	Chronic hepatitis B
+	+	–	–	Acute hepatitis A superimposed on chronic hepatitis B
+	+	+	–	Acute hepatitis A and B
–	+	–	–	Acute hepatitis A
–	+	+	–	Acute hepatitis A and B (HBsAg below detection threshold)
–	–	+	–	Acute hepatitis B (HBsAg below detection threshold)
–	–	–	+	Acute hepatitis C

on chronic HBV infection. The presence of anti-HCV supports a diagnosis of acute hepatitis C. Occasionally, testing for HCV RNA or repeat anti-HCV testing later during the illness is necessary to establish the diagnosis. Absence of all serologic markers is consistent with a diagnosis of "non-A, non-B, non-C" hepatitis, if the epidemiologic setting is appropriate.

In patients with chronic hepatitis, initial testing should consist of HBsAg and anti-HCV. Anti-HCV supports and HCV RNA testing establishes the diagnosis of chronic hepatitis C. If a serologic diagnosis of chronic hepatitis B is made, testing for HBeAg and anti-HBe is indicated to evaluate relative infectivity. Testing for HBV DNA in such patients provides a more quantitative and sensitive measure of the level of virus replication and, therefore, is very helpful during antiviral therapy (Chap. 306). In patients with chronic hepatitis B and normal aminotransferase activity in the absence of HBeAg, serial testing over time is often required to distinguish between inactive carriage and HBeAg-negative chronic hepatitis B with fluctuating virologic and necroinflammatory activity. In persons with hepatitis B, testing for anti-HDV is useful in those with severe and fulminant disease, with severe chronic disease, with chronic hepatitis B and acute hepatitis-like exacerbations, with frequent percutaneous exposures, and from areas where HDV infection is endemic.

PROGNOSIS

Virtually all previously healthy patients with hepatitis A recover completely with no clinical sequelae. Similarly, in acute hepatitis B, 95–99% of previously healthy adults have a favorable course and recover completely. Certain clinical and laboratory features, however, suggest a more complicated and protracted course. Patients of advanced age and with serious underlying medical disorders may have a prolonged course and are more likely to experience severe hepatitis. Initial presenting features such as ascites, peripheral edema, and symptoms of hepatic encephalopathy suggest a poorer prognosis. In addition, a prolonged PT, low-serum albumin level, hypoglycemia, and very high-serum bilirubin values suggest severe hepatocellular disease. Patients with these clinical and laboratory features deserve prompt hospital admission. The case fatality rate in hepatitis A and B is very low (~0.1%) but is increased by advanced age and underlying debilitating disorders. Among patients ill enough to be hospitalized for acute hepatitis B, the fatality rate is 1%. Hepatitis C is less severe during the acute phase than hepatitis B and is more likely to be anicteric; fatalities are rare, but the precise case fatality rate is not known. In outbreaks of waterborne hepatitis E in India and Asia, the case fatality rate is 1–2% and up to 10–20% in pregnant women. Patients with simultaneous acute hepatitis B and hepatitis D do not necessarily experience a higher mortality rate than do patients with acute hepatitis B alone; however, in several recent outbreaks of acute simultaneous HBV and HDV infection among injection drug users, the case fatality rate has been ~5%. In the case of HDV superinfection of a person with chronic hepatitis B, the likelihood of fulminant hepatitis and death is increased substantially. Although the case fatality rate for hepatitis D has not been defined adequately, in outbreaks of severe HDV superinfection in isolated populations with a high hepatitis B carrier rate, the mortality rate has been recorded in excess of 20%.

COMPLICATIONS AND SEQUELAE

A small proportion of patients with hepatitis A experience *relapsing hepatitis* weeks to months after apparent recovery from acute hepatitis. Relapses are characterized by recurrence of symptoms, aminotransferase elevations, occasionally jaundice, and fecal excretion of HAV. Another unusual variant of acute hepatitis A is *cholestatic hepatitis*, characterized by protracted cholestatic jaundice and pruritus. Rarely, liver test abnormalities persist for many months, even up to a year. Even when these complications occur, hepatitis A remains self-limited and does not progress to chronic liver disease. During the prodromal phase of acute hepatitis B, a serum sickness-like syndrome characterized by arthralgia or arthritis, rash, angioedema, and rarely, hematuria and proteinuria may develop in 5–10% of patients. This syndrome occurs before the onset of clinical jaundice, and these patients are often diagnosed erroneously as having rheumatologic diseases. The diagnosis can be established by measuring serum aminotransferase levels, which are almost invariably elevated, and serum HBsAg. As noted above, EMC is an immune-complex disease that can complicate chronic hepatitis C and is part of a spectrum of B cell lymphoproliferative disorders, which, in rare instances, can evolve to B cell lymphoma (Chap. 110). Attention has been drawn as well to associations between hepatitis C and such cutaneous disorders as porphyria cutanea tarda and lichen planus. A mechanism for these associations is unknown. Finally, related to the reliance of HCV on lipoprotein secretion and assembly pathways and on interactions of HCV with glucose metabolism, HCV infection may be complicated by hepatic steatosis, hypercholesterolemia, insulin resistance (and other manifestations of the metabolic syndrome), and type 2 diabetes mellitus; both hepatic steatosis and insulin resistance appear to accelerate hepatic fibrosis and blunt responsiveness to antiviral therapy (Chap. 306).

The most feared complication of viral hepatitis is *fulminant hepatitis* (massive hepatic necrosis); fortunately, this is a rare event. Fulminant hepatitis is primarily seen in hepatitis B and D, as well as hepatitis E, but rare fulminant cases of hepatitis A occur primarily in older adults and in persons with underlying chronic liver disease, including, according to some reports, chronic hepatitis B and C. Hepatitis B accounts for >50% of fulminant cases of viral hepatitis, a sizable proportion of which are associated with HDV infection and another proportion with underlying chronic hepatitis C. Fulminant hepatitis is hardly ever seen in hepatitis C, but hepatitis E, as noted above, can be complicated by fatal fulminant hepatitis in 1–2% of all cases and in up to 20% of cases in pregnant women. Patients usually present with signs and symptoms of encephalopathy that may evolve to deep coma. The liver is usually small and the PT excessively prolonged. The combination of rapidly shrinking liver size, rapidly rising bilirubin level, and marked prolongation of the PT, even as aminotransferase levels fall, together with clinical signs of confusion, disorientation, somnolence, ascites, and edema, indicates that the patient has hepatic failure with encephalopathy. Cerebral edema is common; brainstem compression, gastrointestinal bleeding, sepsis, respiratory failure, cardiovascular collapse, and renal failure are terminal events. The mortality rate is exceedingly high (>80% in patients with deep coma), but patients who survive may have a complete biochemical and histologic recovery. If a donor liver can be located in time, liver transplantation may be lifesaving in patients with fulminant hepatitis (Chap. 310).

Documenting the disappearance of HBsAg after apparent clinical recovery from acute hepatitis B is particularly important. Before laboratory methods were available to distinguish between acute hepatitis and acute hepatitis-like exacerbations (*spontaneous reactivations*) of chronic hepatitis B, observations suggested that ~10% of previously healthy patients remained HBsAg-positive for >6 months after the onset of clinically apparent acute hepatitis B. One-half of these persons cleared the antigen from their circulations during the next several years, but the other 5% remained chronically HBsAg-positive. More recent observations suggest that the true rate of chronic infection after clinically apparent acute hepatitis B is as low as 1% in normal, immunocompetent, young adults. Earlier, higher estimates may have been confounded by inadvertent inclusion of acute exacerbations in chronically infected patients; these patients, chronically HBsAg-positive before exacerbation, were unlikely to seroconvert to HBsAg-negative thereafter. Whether the rate of chronicity is 10% or 1%, such patients have anti-HBc in serum; anti-HBs is either undetected or detected at low titer against the opposite subtype specificity of the antigen (see "Laboratory Features"). These patients may (1) be inactive carriers; (2) have low-grade, mild chronic hepatitis; or (3) have moderate to severe chronic hepatitis with or without cirrhosis. The likelihood of remaining chronically infected after acute HBV infection is especially high among neonates, persons with Down's syndrome, chronically hemodialyzed patients, and immunosuppressed patients, including persons with HIV infection.

Chronic hepatitis is an important late complication of acute hepatitis B occurring in a small proportion of patients with acute disease but more common in those who present with chronic infection without having experienced an acute illness, as occurs typically after neonatal infection or after infection in an immunosuppressed host (Chap. 306). Certain clinical and laboratory features suggest progression of acute hepatitis to chronic hepatitis: (1) lack of complete resolution of clinical symptoms of anorexia, weight loss, fatigue, and the persistence of hepatomegaly; (2) the presence of bridging/interface or multilobular hepatic necrosis on liver biopsy during protracted, severe acute viral hepatitis; (3) failure of the serum aminotransferase, bilirubin, and globulin levels to return to normal within 6–12 months after the acute illness; and (4) the persistence of HBeAg for >3 months or HBsAg for >6 months after acute hepatitis.

Although acute hepatitis D infection does not increase the likelihood of chronicity of simultaneous acute hepatitis B, hepatitis D has the potential for contributing to the severity of chronic hepatitis B. Hepatitis D superinfection can transform inactive or mild chronic hepatitis B into severe, progressive chronic hepatitis and cirrhosis; it also can accelerate the course of chronic hepatitis B. Some HDV superinfections in patients with chronic hepatitis B lead to fulminant hepatitis. As defined in longitudinal studies over 3 decades, the annual rates of cirrhosis and hepatocellular carcinoma in patients with chronic hepatitis D are 4% and 2.8%, respectively. Although HDV and HBV infections are associated with severe liver disease, mild hepatitis and even inactive carriage have been identified in some patients, and the disease may become indolent beyond the early years of infection.

After acute HCV infection, the likelihood of remaining chronically *infected* approaches 85–90%. Although many patients with chronic hepatitis C have no symptoms, cirrhosis may develop in as many as 20% within 10–20 years of acute illness; in some series of cases reported by referral centers, cirrhosis has been reported in as many as 50% of patients with chronic hepatitis C. Although chronic hepatitis C accounts for at least 40% of cases of chronic liver disease and of patients undergoing liver transplantation for end-stage liver disease in the United States and Europe, in the majority of patients with chronic hepatitis C, morbidity and mortality are limited during the initial 20 years after the onset of infection. Progression of chronic hepatitis C may be influenced by age of acquisition, duration of infection, immunosuppression, coexisting excessive alcohol use, concomitant hepatic steatosis, other hepatitis virus infection, or HIV co-infection. In fact, instances of severe and rapidly progressive chronic hepatitis B and C are being recognized with increasing frequency in patients with HIV infection (Chap. 189). In contrast, neither HAV nor HEV causes chronic liver disease.

Rare complications of viral hepatitis include pancreatitis, myocarditis, atypical pneumonia, aplastic anemia, transverse myelitis, and peripheral neuropathy. Persons with chronic hepatitis B, particularly those infected in infancy or early childhood and especially those with HBeAg and/or high-level HBV DNA, have an enhanced risk of hepatocellular carcinoma. The risk of hepatocellular carcinoma is increased as well in patients with chronic hepatitis C, almost exclusively in patients with cirrhosis, and almost always after at least several decades, usually after 3 decades of disease (Chap. 92). In children, hepatitis B may present rarely with anicteric hepatitis, a nonpruritic papular rash of the face, buttocks, and limbs, and lymphadenopathy (papular acrodermatitis of childhood or Gianotti-Crosti syndrome).

Rarely, autoimmune hepatitis (Chap. 306) can be triggered by a bout of otherwise self-limited acute hepatitis, as reported after acute hepatitis A, B, and C.

DIFFERENTIAL DIAGNOSIS

Viral diseases such as infectious mononucleosis; those due to cytomegalovirus, herpes simplex, and coxsackieviruses; and toxoplasmosis may share certain clinical features with viral hepatitis and cause elevations in serum aminotransferase and, less commonly, in serum bilirubin levels. Tests such as the differential heterophile and serologic tests for these agents may be helpful in the differential diagnosis if HBsAg, anti-HBc, IgM anti-HAV, and anti-HCV determinations are negative. Aminotransferase elevations can accompany almost any systemic viral infection; other rare causes of liver injury confused with viral hepatitis are infections with *Leptospira*, *Candida*, *Brucella*, *Mycobacteria*, and *Pneumocystis*. A complete drug history is particularly important, for many drugs and certain anesthetic agents can produce a picture of either acute hepatitis or cholestasis (Chap. 305). Equally important is a past history of unexplained "repeated episodes" of acute hepatitis. This history should alert the physician to the possibility that the underlying disorder is chronic hepatitis. Alcoholic hepatitis must also be considered, but usually the serum aminotransferase levels are not as markedly elevated and other stigmata of alcoholism may be present. The finding on liver biopsy of fatty infiltration, a neutrophilic inflammatory reaction, and "alcoholic hyaline" would be consistent with alcohol-induced rather than viral liver injury. Because acute hepatitis may present with right upper quadrant abdominal pain, nausea and vomiting, fever, and icterus, it is often confused with acute cholecystitis, common duct stone, or ascending cholangitis. Patients with acute viral hepatitis may tolerate surgery poorly; therefore, it is important to exclude this diagnosis, and in confusing cases, a percutaneous liver biopsy may be necessary before laparotomy. Viral hepatitis in the elderly is often misdiagnosed as obstructive jaundice resulting from a common duct stone or carcinoma of the pancreas. Because acute hepatitis in the elderly may be quite severe and the operative mortality high, a thorough evaluation including biochemical tests, radiographic studies of the biliary tree, and even liver biopsy may be necessary to exclude primary parenchymal liver disease. Another clinical constellation that may mimic acute hepatitis is right ventricular failure with passive hepatic congestion or hypoperfusion syndromes, such as those associated with shock, severe hypotension, and severe left ventricular failure. Also included in this general category is any disorder that interferes with venous return to the heart, such as right atrial myxoma, constrictive pericarditis, hepatic vein occlusion (Budd-Chiari syndrome), or veno-occlusive disease. Clinical features are usually sufficient to distinguish among these vascular disorders and viral hepatitis. Acute fatty liver of pregnancy, cholestasis of pregnancy, eclampsia, and the HELLP (*h*emolysis, *e*levated *l*iver tests, and *l*ow *p*latelets) syndrome can be confused with viral hepatitis during pregnancy. Very rarely, malignancies metastatic to the liver can mimic acute or even fulminant viral hepatitis. Occasionally, genetic or metabolic liver disorders (e.g., Wilson's disease, α_1-antitrypsin deficiency) as well as nonalcoholic fatty liver disease are confused with viral hepatitis.

TREATMENT Acute Viral Hepatitis

In hepatitis B, among previously healthy adults who present with clinically apparent acute hepatitis, recovery occurs in ~99%; therefore, antiviral therapy is not likely to improve the rate of recovery and is not required. In rare instances of severe acute hepatitis B, treatment with a nucleoside analogue at oral doses used to treat chronic hepatitis B (Chap. 306) has been attempted successfully. Although clinical trials have not been done to establish the efficacy of this approach; although severe acute hepatitis B is not an approved indication for therapy; and although the duration of therapy has not been determined; nonetheless, most authorities would recommend institution of antiviral therapy with a nucleoside analogue for severe, but not mild–moderate, acute hepatitis B. In typical cases of acute hepatitis C, recovery is rare, progression to chronic hepatitis is the rule, and meta-analyses of small clinical trials suggest that antiviral therapy with interferon alfa monotherapy (3 million units SC three times a week) is beneficial, reducing the rate of chronicity considerably by inducing sustained responses in 30–70% of patients. In a German multicenter study of 44 patients with acute symptomatic hepatitis C, initiation of intensive interferon alfa therapy (5 million units SC daily for 4 weeks, then three times a week for another 20 weeks) within an average of 3 months after infection resulted in a sustained virologic response rate of 98%. Although treatment of acute hepatitis C is recommended, the optimum regimen, duration of therapy, and time to initiate therapy remain to be determined. Many authorities now opt for a 24-week course (beginning within 2–3 months after onset) of the best regimen identified for the treatment of chronic hepatitis C, long-acting pegylated interferon plus the nucleoside analogue ribavirin, although the value of adding ribavirin has not been demonstrated (see Chap. 306 for doses). Because of the marked reduction over the past 2 decades in the frequency of acute hepatitis C, opportunities to identify and treat patients with acute hepatitis C are rare, except in injection drug users. Hospital epidemiologists, however, will encounter health workers who sustain hepatitis C-contaminated needle sticks; when monitoring for ALT elevations and HCV, RNA after these accidents identifies acute hepatitis C (risk only ~3%), therapy should be initiated.

Notwithstanding these specific therapeutic considerations, in most cases of typical acute viral hepatitis, specific treatment generally is not necessary. Although hospitalization may be required for clinically severe illness, most patients do not require hospital care. Forced and prolonged bed rest is not essential for full recovery, but many patients will feel better with restricted physical activity. A high-calorie diet is desirable, and because many patients may experience nausea late in the day, the major caloric intake is best tolerated in the morning. Intravenous feeding is necessary in the acute stage if the patient has persistent vomiting and cannot maintain oral intake. Drugs capable of producing adverse reactions such as cholestasis and drugs metabolized by the liver should be avoided. If severe pruritus is present, the use of the bile salt-sequestering resin cholestyramine is helpful. Glucocorticoid therapy has no value in acute viral hepatitis, even in severe cases associated with *bridging necrosis*, and may be deleterious, even increasing the risk of chronicity (e.g., of acute hepatitis B).

Physical isolation of patients with hepatitis to a single room and bathroom is rarely necessary except in the case of fecal incontinence for hepatitis A and E or uncontrolled, voluminous bleeding for hepatitis B (with or without concomitant hepatitis D) and hepatitis C. Because most patients hospitalized with hepatitis A excrete little, if any, HAV, the likelihood of HAV transmission from these patients during their hospitalization is low. Therefore, burdensome *enteric precautions are no longer recommended.* Although gloves should be worn when the bedpans or fecal material of patients with hepatitis A are handled, these precautions do not represent a departure from sensible procedure and contemporary universal precautions for all hospitalized patients. For patients with hepatitis B and hepatitis C, emphasis should be placed on blood precautions (i.e., avoiding direct, ungloved hand contact with blood and other body fluids). Enteric precautions are unnecessary. The importance of simple hygienic precautions such as hand washing cannot be overemphasized. Universal precautions that have been adopted for all patients apply to patients with viral hepatitis.

Hospitalized patients may be discharged following substantial symptomatic improvement, a significant downward trend in the serum aminotransferase and bilirubin values, and a return to normal of the PT. Mild aminotransferase elevations should not be considered contraindications to the gradual resumption of normal activity.

In *fulminant hepatitis*, the goal of therapy is to support the patient by maintenance of fluid balance, support of circulation and respiration, control of bleeding, correction of hypoglycemia, and treatment of other complications of the comatose state in anticipation of liver regeneration and repair. Protein intake should be restricted, and oral lactulose or neomycin administered. Glucocorticoid therapy has been shown in controlled trials to be ineffective. Likewise, exchange transfusion, plasmapheresis, human cross-circulation, porcine liver cross-perfusion, hemoperfusion, and extracorporeal liver-assist devices have not been proven to enhance survival. Meticulous intensive care that includes prophylactic antibiotic coverage is the one factor that does appear to improve survival. Orthotopic liver transplantation is resorted to with increasing frequency, with excellent results, in patients with fulminant hepatitis (Chap. 310).

PROPHYLAXIS

Because application of therapy for acute viral hepatitis is limited and because antiviral therapy for chronic viral hepatitis is cumbersome and costly but effective in only a proportion of patients (Chap. 306), emphasis is placed on prevention through immunization. The prophylactic approach differs for each of the types of viral hepatitis. In the past, immunoprophylaxis relied exclusively on passive immunization with antibody-containing globulin preparations purified by cold ethanol fractionation from the plasma of hundreds of normal donors. Currently, for hepatitis A and B, active immunization with vaccines is the preferable approach to prevention.

Hepatitis A

Both passive immunization with IG and active immunization with killed vaccines are available. All preparations of IG contain anti-HAV concentrations sufficient to be protective. When administered before exposure or during the early incubation period, IG is effective in preventing clinically apparent hepatitis A. For postexposure prophylaxis of intimate contacts (household, sexual, institutional) of persons with hepatitis A, the administration of 0.02 mL/kg is recommended as early after exposure as possible; it may be effective even when administered as late as 2 weeks after exposure. Prophylaxis is not necessary for those who have already received hepatitis A vaccine, casual contacts (office, factory, school, or hospital), for most elderly persons, who are very likely to be immune, or for those known to have anti-HAV in their serum. In day-care centers, recognition of hepatitis A in children or staff should provide a stimulus for immunoprophylaxis in the center and in the children's family members. By the time most common-source outbreaks of hepatitis A are recognized, it is usually too late in the incubation period for IG to be effective; however, prophylaxis may limit the frequency of secondary cases. For travelers to tropical countries, developing countries, and other areas outside standard tourist routes, IG prophylaxis had been recommended before a vaccine became available. When such travel lasted <3 months, 0.02 mL/kg was given; for longer travel or residence in these areas, a dose of 0.06 mL/kg every 4–6 months was recommended. Administration of plasma-derived globulin is safe; all contemporary lots of IG are subjected to viral inactivation steps and must be free of HCV RNA as determined by PCR testing. Administration of IM lots of IG has not been associated with transmission of HBV, HCV, or HIV.

Formalin-inactivated vaccines made from strains of HAV attenuated in tissue culture have been shown to be safe, immunogenic, and effective in preventing hepatitis A. Hepatitis A vaccines are approved for use in persons who are at least one year old and appear to provide adequate protection beginning 4 weeks after a primary inoculation. If it can be given within 4 weeks of an expected exposure, such as by travel to an endemic area, hepatitis A vaccine is the preferred approach to *pre-exposure* immunoprophylaxis. If travel is more imminent, IG (0.02 mL/kg) should be administered at a different injection site, along with the first dose of vaccine. Because vaccination provides long-lasting protection (protective levels of anti-HAV should last 20 years after vaccination), persons whose risk will be sustained (e.g., frequent travelers or those remaining in endemic areas for prolonged periods) should be vaccinated, and vaccine should supplant the need for repeated IG injections. Shortly after its introduction, hepatitis A vaccine was recommended for children living in communities with a high incidence of HAV infection; in 1999, this recommendation was extended to include all children living in states, counties, and communities with high rates of HAV infection. As of 2006, the Advisory Committee on Immunization Practices of the U.S. Public Health Service recommended *routine hepatitis A vaccination of all children*. Other groups considered to be at increased risk for HAV infection and who are candidates for hepatitis A vaccination include military personnel, populations with cyclic outbreaks of hepatitis A (e.g., Alaskan natives), employees of day-care centers, primate handlers, laboratory workers exposed to hepatitis A or fecal specimens, and patients with chronic liver disease. Because of an increased risk of fulminant hepatitis A—observed in some experiences but not confirmed in others—among patients with chronic hepatitis C, patients with chronic hepatitis C are candidates for hepatitis A vaccination, as are persons with chronic hepatitis B. Other populations whose recognized risk of hepatitis A is increased should be vaccinated, including men who have sex with men, injection drug users, persons with clotting disorders who require frequent administration of clotting-factor concentrates, persons traveling from the United States to countries with high or intermediate hepatitis A endemicity, postexposure prophylaxis for contacts of persons with hepatitis A, and household members and other close contacts of adopted children arriving from countries with high and moderate hepatitis A endemicity. Recommendations for dose and frequency differ for the two approved vaccine preparations (Table 304-7); all injections are IM. Hepatitis A vaccine has been reported to be effective in preventing secondary household cases of acute hepatitis A, but its role in other instances of postexposure prophylaxis remains to be demonstrated. In the United States, reported mortality resulting from hepatitis A declined in parallel with hepatitis A vaccine-associated reductions in the annual incidence of new infections.

TABLE 304-7 Hepatitis A Vaccination Schedules

Age, years	No. of Doses	Dose	Schedule, months
HAVRIX (GlaxoSmithKline)[a]			
1–18	2	720 ELU[b] (0.5 mL)	0, 6–12
≥19	2	1440 ELU (1 mL)	0, 6–12
VAQTA (Merck)			
1–18	2	25 units (0.5 mL)	0, 6–18
≥19	2	50 units (1 mL)	0, 6–18

[a]A combination of this hepatitis A vaccine and hepatitis B vaccine, TWINRIX, is licensed for simultaneous protection against both of these viruses among adults (age ≥18 years). Each 1-mL dose contains 720 ELU of hepatitis A vaccine and 20 μg of hepatitis B vaccine. These doses are recommended at months 0, 1, and 6.
[b]Enzyme-linked immunoassay units.
Abbreviation: ELU, enzyme-linked immunoassay unit.

Hepatitis B

Until 1982, prevention of hepatitis B was based on *passive* immunoprophylaxis either with standard IG, containing modest levels of anti-HBs, or hepatitis B immunoglobulin (HBIG), containing high-titer anti-HBs. The efficacy of standard IG has never been established and remains questionable; even the efficacy of HBIG, demonstrated in several clinical trials, has been challenged, and its contribution appears to be in reducing the frequency of clinical *illness*, not in preventing *infection*. The first vaccine for *active* immunization, introduced in 1982, was prepared from purified, noninfectious 22-nm spherical forms of HBsAg derived from the plasma of healthy HBsAg carriers. In 1987, the plasma-derived vaccine was supplanted by a genetically engineered vaccine derived from recombinant yeast. The latter vaccine consists of HBsAg particles that are nonglycosylated but are otherwise indistinguishable from natural HBsAg; two recombinant vaccines are licensed for use in the United States. Current recommendations can be divided into those for pre-exposure and postexposure prophylaxis.

For *pre-exposure* prophylaxis against hepatitis B in settings of frequent exposure (health workers exposed to blood; hemodialysis patients and staff; residents and staff of custodial institutions for the developmentally handicapped; injection drug users; inmates of long-term correctional facilities; persons with multiple sexual partners; persons such as hemophiliacs who require long-term, high-volume therapy with blood derivatives; household and sexual contacts of HBsAg carriers; persons living in or traveling extensively in endemic areas; unvaccinated children under the age of 18; and unvaccinated children who are Alaskan natives, Pacific Islanders, or residents in households of first-generation immigrants from endemic countries), three IM (deltoid, not gluteal) injections of hepatitis B vaccine are recommended at 0, 1, and 6 months (other, optional schedules are summarized in Table 304-8). Pregnancy is *not* a contraindication to vaccination. In areas of low HBV endemicity such as the United States, despite the availability of safe and effective hepatitis B vaccines, a strategy of vaccinating persons in high-risk groups has not been effective. The incidence of new hepatitis B cases continued to increase in the United States after the introduction of vaccines; <10% of all targeted persons in high-risk groups have actually been vaccinated, and ~30% of persons with sporadic acute hepatitis B do not fall into any high-risk-group category. Therefore, to have an impact on the frequency of HBV infection in an area of low endemicity such as the United States, universal hepatitis B vaccination in childhood has been recommended. For unvaccinated children born after the implementation of

TABLE 304-8 Preexposure Hepatitis B Vaccination Schedules

Target Group	No. of Doses	Dose	Schedule, months
RECOMBIVAX-HB (Merck)[a]			
Infants, children (<1–10 years)	3	5 μg (0.5 mL)	0, 1–2, 4–6
Adolescents (11–19 years)	3 or 4	5 μg (0.5 mL)	0–2, 1–4, 4–6 *or* 0, 12, 24 *or* 0, 1, 2, 12
	or		
	2	10 μg (1 mL)	0, 4–6 (age 11–15)
Adults (≥20 years)	3	10 μg (1 mL)	0–2, 1–4, 4–6
Hemodialysis patients[b]			
<20 years	3	5 μg (0.5 mL)	0, 1, 6
≥20 years	3	40 μg (4 mL)	0, 1, 6
ENGERIX-B (GlaxoSmithKline)[c]			
Infants, children (<1–10 years)	3 or 4	10 μg (0.5 mL)	0, 1–2, 4–6 *or* 0, 1, 2,12
Adolescents (10–19 years)	3 or 4	10 μg (0.5 mL)	0, 1–2, 4–6 *or* 0, 12, 24 *or* 0, 1, 2, 12
Adults (≥20 years)	3 or 4	20 μg (1 mL)	0–2, 1–4, 4–60, 1, 2, 12
Hemodialysis patients[b]			
<20 years	4	10 μg (0.5 mL)	0, 1, 2, 6
≥20 years	4	40 μg (2 mL)	0, 1, 2, 6

[a]This manufacturer produces a licensed combination of hepatitis B vaccine and vaccines against *Haemophilus influenzae* type b and *Neisseria meningitides*, Comvax, for use in infants and young children. Please consult product insert for dose and schedule.
[b]This group also includes other immunocompromised persons.
[c]This manufacturer produces two licensed combination hepatitis B vaccines: (1) Twinrix, recombinant hepatitis B vaccine plus inactivated hepatitis A vaccine, is licensed for simultaneous protection against both of these viruses among adults (age ≥ 18 years). Each 1-mL dose contains 720 ELU of hepatitis A vaccine and 20 μg of hepatitis B vaccine. These doses are recommended at months 0, 1, and 6. (2) Pediatrix, recombinant hepatitis B vaccine plus diphtheria and tetanus toxoid, pertussis, and inactivated poliovirus, is licensed for use in infants and young children. Please consult product insert for doses and schedules.

universal infant vaccination, vaccination during early adolescence, at age 11–12 years, was recommended, and this recommendation has been extended to include all unvaccinated children age 0–19 years. In HBV-hyperendemic areas (e.g., Asia), universal vaccination of children has resulted in a marked 10- to 15-year decline in hepatitis B and its complications, including hepatocellular carcinoma.

The two available recombinant hepatitis B vaccines are comparable, one containing 10 μg of HBsAg (Recombivax-HB) and the other containing 20 μg of HBsAg (Engerix-B), and recommended doses for each injection vary for the two preparations (Table 304-8). Combinations of hepatitis B vaccine with other childhood vaccines are available as well (Table 304-8).

For unvaccinated persons sustaining an exposure to HBV, *postexposure* prophylaxis with a combination of HBIG (for rapid achievement of high-titer circulating anti-HBs) and hepatitis B vaccine (for achievement of long-lasting immunity as well as its apparent efficacy in attenuating clinical illness after exposure) is recommended. For *perinatal* exposure of infants born to HBsAg-positive mothers, a single dose of HBIG, 0.5 mL, should be administered IM in the thigh *immediately after birth*, followed by a complete course of three injections of recombinant hepatitis B vaccine (see doses above) to be started within the first 12 hours of life. For those experiencing a direct percutaneous inoculation or transmucosal exposure to HBsAg-positive blood or body fluids (e.g., accidental *needle stick*, other mucosal penetration, or ingestion), a single IM dose of HBIG, 0.06 mL/kg, administered as soon after exposure as possible, is followed by a complete course of hepatitis B vaccine to begin within the first week. For those exposed by *sexual* contact to a patient with acute hepatitis B, a single IM dose of HBIG, 0.06 mL/kg, should be given within 14 days of exposure, to be followed by a complete course of hepatitis B vaccine. When both HBIG and hepatitis B vaccine are recommended, they may be given at the same time but at separate sites.

The precise duration of protection afforded by hepatitis B vaccine is unknown; however, ~80–90% of immunocompetent vaccinees retain protective levels of anti-HBs for at least 5 years, and 60–80% for 10 years. Thereafter and even after anti-HBs becomes undetectable, protection persists against clinical hepatitis B, hepatitis B surface antigenemia, and chronic HBV infection. Currently, *booster* immunizations are not recommended routinely, except in immunosuppressed persons who have lost detectable anti-HBs or immunocompetent persons who sustain percutaneous HBsAg-positive inoculations after losing detectable antibody. Specifically, for hemodialysis patients, annual anti-HBs testing is recommended after vaccination; booster doses are recommended when anti-HBs levels fall to <10 mIU/mL. As noted above, for persons at risk of both hepatitis A and B, a combined vaccine is available containing 720 enzyme-linked immunoassay units (ELUs) of inactivated HAV and 20 μg of recombinant HBsAg (at 0, 1, and 6 months).

Hepatitis D

Infection with hepatitis D can be prevented by vaccinating susceptible persons with hepatitis B vaccine. No product is available for immunoprophylaxis to prevent HDV superinfection in HBsAg carriers; for them, avoidance of percutaneous exposures and limitation of intimate contact with persons who have HDV infection are recommended.

Hepatitis C

IG is ineffective in preventing hepatitis C and is no longer recommended for postexposure prophylaxis in cases of perinatal, needle stick, or sexual exposure. Although prototype vaccines that induce antibodies to HCV envelope proteins have been developed, currently, hepatitis C vaccination is not feasible practically. Genotype and quasispecies viral heterogeneity, as well as rapid evasion of neutralizing antibodies by this rapidly mutating virus, conspire to render HCV a difficult target for immunoprophylaxis with a vaccine. Prevention of transfusion-associated hepatitis C has been accomplished by the following successively introduced measures: exclusion of commercial blood donors and reliance on a volunteer blood supply; screening donor blood with surrogate markers such as ALT (no longer recommended) and anti-HBc, markers that identify segments of the blood donor population with an increased risk of bloodborne infections; exclusion of blood donors in high-risk groups for AIDS and the introduction of anti-HIV screening tests; and progressively sensitive serologic and virologic screening tests for HCV infection.

In the absence of active or passive immunization, prevention of hepatitis C includes behavior changes and precautions to limit exposures to infected persons. Recommendations designed to identify patients with clinically inapparent hepatitis as candidates for medical management have as a secondary benefit the identification of persons whose contacts could be at risk of becoming infected. A so-called look-back program has been recommended to identify persons who were transfused before 1992 with blood from a donor found subsequently to have hepatitis C. In addition, anti-HCV testing is recommended for anyone who received a blood transfusion or a transplanted organ before the introduction of second-generation screening tests in 1992, those who ever used injection drugs (or took other illicit drugs by noninjection routes), chronically hemodialyzed patients, persons with clotting disorders who received clotting factors made before 1987 from pooled blood products, persons with elevated aminotransferase levels, health workers exposed to HCV-positive blood or contaminated needles, persons with HIV infection, health care and public safety personnel following a needle-stick or other nonpercutaneous exposure to HCV-infected material, sexual partners of persons with hepatitis C, and children born to HCV-positive mothers (Table 304-4).

For stable, monogamous sexual partners, sexual transmission of hepatitis C is unlikely, and sexual barrier precautions are not recommended. For persons with multiple sexual partners or with sexually transmitted diseases, the risk of sexual transmission of hepatitis C is increased, and barrier precautions (latex condoms) are recommended. A person with hepatitis C should avoid sharing such items as razors, toothbrushes, and nail clippers with sexual partners and family members. No special precautions are recommended for babies born to mothers with hepatitis C, and breast-feeding does not have to be restricted.

Hepatitis E

Whether IG prevents hepatitis E remains undetermined. A safe and effective recombinant vaccine has been developed and is available in endemic areas but not in the United States.

FURTHER READINGS

Blum HE, Marcellin P: EASL Consensus Conference on Hepatitis B. J Hepatol 39(Suppl 1):1, 2003

Centers For Disease Control and Prevention: Updated U.S. Public Health Service guidelines for the management of occupational exposures to HBV, HCV, and HIV and recommendations for postexposure prophylaxis. MMWR 50(RR-11):1, 2001

———: A comprehensive immunization strategy to eliminate transmission of hepatitis B virus infection in the United States: Recommendations of the Advisory Committee on Immunization Practices (ACIP) part 1: Immunization of infants, children, and adolescents. MMWR 54 (RR-16):1, 2005

———: A comprehensive immunization strategy to eliminate transmission of hepatitis B virus infection in the United States: Recommendations of the Advisory Committee on Immunization Practices (ACIP) part II: Immunization of adults. MMWR 55(RR-16):1, 2006

———: Prevention of hepatitis A through active or passive immunization: Recommendations of the Advisory Committee on Immunization Practices (ACIP). MMWR 55 (RR-7):1, 2006

———: Recommendations for identification and public health management of persons with chronic hepatitis B virus infection. MMWR 57(RR-8):1, 2008

———: Updated recommendations from the Advisory Committee on Immunization Practices (ACIP) for use of hepatitis A vaccine in close contacts of newly arriving international adoptees. MMWR 58:1006, 2009

Chen CJ et al: Risk of hepatocellular carcinoma across a biological gradient of serum hepatitis B virus DNA level. JAMA 295:65, 2006

Dienstag JL: Hepatitis B virus infection. N Engl J Med 359:1486, 2008

Dienstag JL, McHutchison JG: American Gastroenterological Association technical review on the management of hepatitis C. Gastroenterology 130:231, 2006

Ferrari C et al: Immunopathogenesis of hepatitis B. J Hepatol 39(Suppl 1):S36, 2003

Ganem D, Prince AM: Hepatitis B virus infection—natural history and clinical consequences. N Engl J Med 350:1118, 2004

Ghany MG et al: Diagnosis, management, and treatment of hepatitis C: An update. Hepatology 49:1335, 2009

Gish RG, Locarnini SA: Chronic hepatitis B: Current testing strategies. Clin Gastroenterol Hepatol 4:666, 2006

Hadziyannis SJ, Vassilopoulos D: Hepatitis B e antigen-negative chronic hepatitis B. Hepatology 34:617, 2001

Jaeckel E et al: Treatment of acute hepatitis C with interferon alfa-2b. N Engl J Med 345:1452, 2001

Lauer GM, Walker BD: Medical progress: Hepatitis C virus infection. N Engl J Med 345:41, 2001

Lok ASF, McMahon BJ: Chronic hepatitis B: Hepatology 45:507, 2007

———: Chronic hepatitis B: Update 2009. Hepatology 50: 661, 2009

National Institutes of Health Consensus Development Conference: Management of hepatitis B. Hepatology 49 (Suppl 5):S1, 2009

Pawlotsky J-M: Molecular diagnosis of viral hepatitis. Gastroenterology 122:1554, 2002

Rehermann B: Immune response in hepatitis B virus infection. Semin Liver Dis 23:21, 2003

Rizzetto M: Hepatitis D: Thirty years after. J Hepatol 50:1043, 2009

Romeo R et al: A 28-year study of the course of hepatitis Delta infection: A risk factor for cirrhosis and hepatocellular carcinoma. Gastroenterology 136:1629, 2009

Schreiber GB et al: The risk of transfusion-transmitted viral infection. N Engl J Med 334:1685, 1996

Thimme R et al: Viral and immunological determinants of hepatitis C virus clearance, persistence, and disease. Proc Natl Acad Sci USA 99:15661, 2002

Thomas D, Seeff LB: Natural history of hepatitis C. Clin Liver Dis 9:383, 2005

——— et al: Genetic variation in IL28B and spontaneous clearance of hepatitis C virus Nature 461:798, 2009

Von Hahn T et al: Hepatitis C virus continuously escapes from neutralizing antibody and T-cell responses during chronic infection in vivo. Gastroenterology 132:667, 2007

Yang H-I et al: Hepatitis B e antigen and the risk of hepatocellular carcinoma. N Engl J Med 347:168, 2002

CHAPTER 305 Toxic and Drug-Induced Hepatitis

Jules L. Dienstag

Liver injury may follow the inhalation, ingestion, or parenteral administration of a number of pharmacologic and chemical agents. These include industrial toxins (e.g., carbon tetrachloride, trichloroethylene, and yellow phosphorus); the heat-stable toxic bicyclic octapeptides of certain species of *Amanita* and *Galerina* (hepatotoxic mushroom poisoning); and, more commonly, pharmacologic agents used in medical therapy. Among patients with acute liver failure, drug-induced liver injury is the cause in a majority of all cases, and liver toxicity accounts for the abandonment of many new drugs during their development. It is essential that any patient presenting with jaundice or altered biochemical liver tests be questioned carefully about exposure to chemicals used in work or at home, drugs taken by prescription or bought over the counter, and herbal or alternative medicines. Hepatotoxic drugs can injure the hepatocyte directly (e.g., via a free-radical or metabolic intermediate that causes peroxidation of membrane lipids and that results in liver cell injury). Alternatively, the drug or its metabolite can distort cell membranes or other cellular molecules, bind covalently to intracellular proteins, activate apoptotic pathways, interfere with bile salt export proteins, or block biochemical pathways or cellular integrity (Figure 305-1). Interference with bile canalicular pumps can allow endogenous bile acids, which can injure the liver, to accumulate. Such injuries, in turn, may lead to necrosis of hepatocytes; injure bile ducts, producing cholestasis; or block pathways of lipid movement, inhibit protein synthesis, or impair mitochondrial oxidation of fatty acids, resulting in lactic acidosis and intracellular triglyceride accumulation (expressed histologically as microvesicular steatosis). In some cases, drug metabolites sensitize hepatocytes to toxic cytokines, and differences between susceptible and nonsusceptible drug recipients may be attributable to polymorphisms in elaboration of competing, protective cytokines, as has been suggested for acetaminophen hepatotoxicity (see below). Immunologically mediated liver injury has been postulated to represent another mechanism of drug hepatotoxicity (see below). In addition, a role has been shown for activation of nuclear transporters, such as the constitutive androstane receptor (CAR), in the induction of drug hepatotoxicity.

Most drugs, which are water-insoluble, undergo a series of hepatic metabolic transformation steps, culminating in a water-soluble form appropriate for renal or biliary excretion. This process begins with oxidation or methylation initially mediated by the microsomal mixed-function oxygenases cytochrome P450 (phase I reaction) followed by glucuronidation or sulfation (phase II reaction) or inactivation by glutathione. Most drug hepatotoxicity is mediated by a phase I toxic metabolite, but glutathione depletion, precluding inactivation of harmful compounds by glutathione S-transferase, can contribute as well.

In general, two major types of chemical hepatotoxicity have been recognized: (1) direct toxic and (2) idiosyncratic. As shown in Table 305-1, direct toxic hepatitis occurs with predictable regularity in individuals exposed to the offending agent and is dose-dependent. The latent period between exposure and liver injury is usually short (often several hours), although clinical manifestations may be delayed for 24–48 hours. Agents producing toxic hepatitis are generally systemic poisons or are converted in the liver to toxic metabolites. The direct hepatotoxins result in morphologic abnormalities that are reasonably characteristic and reproducible for each toxin. For example, carbon tetrachloride and trichloroethylene characteristically produce a centrilobular zonal necrosis, whereas yellow phosphorus poisoning typically results in periportal injury. The hepatotoxic octapeptides of *Amanita phalloides* usually produce massive hepatic necrosis; the lethal dose of the toxin is ~10 mg, the amount found in a single deathcap mushroom. Tetracycline, when administered in IV doses >1.5 g daily, leads to microvesicular fat deposits in the liver. Liver injury, which is often only one facet of the toxicity produced by the direct hepatotoxins, may go unrecognized until jaundice appears.

In idiosyncratic drug reactions, the occurrence of hepatitis is usually infrequent (1 in 10^3–10^5 patients) and unpredictable; the response is not as clearly dose-dependent as is injury associated with direct hepatotoxins, and liver injury may occur at any time during or shortly after exposure to the drug. Adding to the difficulty of predicting or identifying idiosyncratic drug hepatotoxicity is the occurrence of mild, transient, nonprogressive serum aminotransferase elevations that resolve with continued drug use. Such "adaptation," the mechanism of which is unknown, occurs in such drugs as isoniazid, valproate, phenytoin, and HMG-CoA reductase inhibitors (statins). Extrahepatic manifestations of hypersensitivity, such as rash, arthralgias, fever, leukocytosis, and eosinophilia, occur in about one-quarter of patients with idiosyncratic hepatotoxic drug reactions; this observation and the unpredictability of idiosyncratic drug hepatotoxicity contributed to the hypothesis that this category of drug reactions is immunologically mediated. More recent evidence, however, suggests that, in most cases, even idiosyncratic reactions represent direct hepatotoxicity but are caused by drug metabolites rather than by the intact compound. Even the prototypes of idiosyncratic hepatotoxicity reactions, halothane hepatitis and isoniazid hepatotoxicity, associated frequently with hypersensitivity manifestations, are now recognized to be mediated by toxic metabolites that damage liver cells directly. Currently, most idiosyncratic reactions are thought to result from differences in metabolic reactivity to specific agents; host susceptibility is mediated by the kinetics of toxic metabolite generation, which differs among individuals, probably mediated by genetic polymorphisms in drug-metabolizing pathways (e.g., differences in cytochrome C450 enzyme isotypes or in acetylation). Associations between certain HLA haplotypes have been drawn with hepatotoxicity of such drugs as amoxicillin/clavulanate, statins, halothane, nitrofurantoin, chlorpromazine, and flucloxacillin. Occasionally, however, the clinical features of an allergic reaction (prominent tissue eosinophilia, autoantibodies, etc.) are difficult to ignore. In vitro models have been described in which lymphocyte cytotoxicity can be demonstrated against rabbit hepatocytes altered by incubation with the potential offending drug. Furthermore, several instances of drug hepatotoxicity are associated with the appearance of autoantibodies, including a class of antibodies to liver-kidney microsomes, anti-LKM2, directed against a cytochrome P450 enzyme. Similarly, in selected cases, a drug or its metabolite has been shown to bind to a host cellular component forming a hapten; the immune response to this "neoantigen" is postulated to play a role in the pathogenesis of liver injury. Therefore, some authorities subdivide idiosyncratic drug hepatotoxicity into hypersensitivity (allergic) and "metabolic" categories. Several unusual exceptions notwithstanding, true drug allergy is difficult to support in most cases of idiosyncratic drug-induced liver injury.

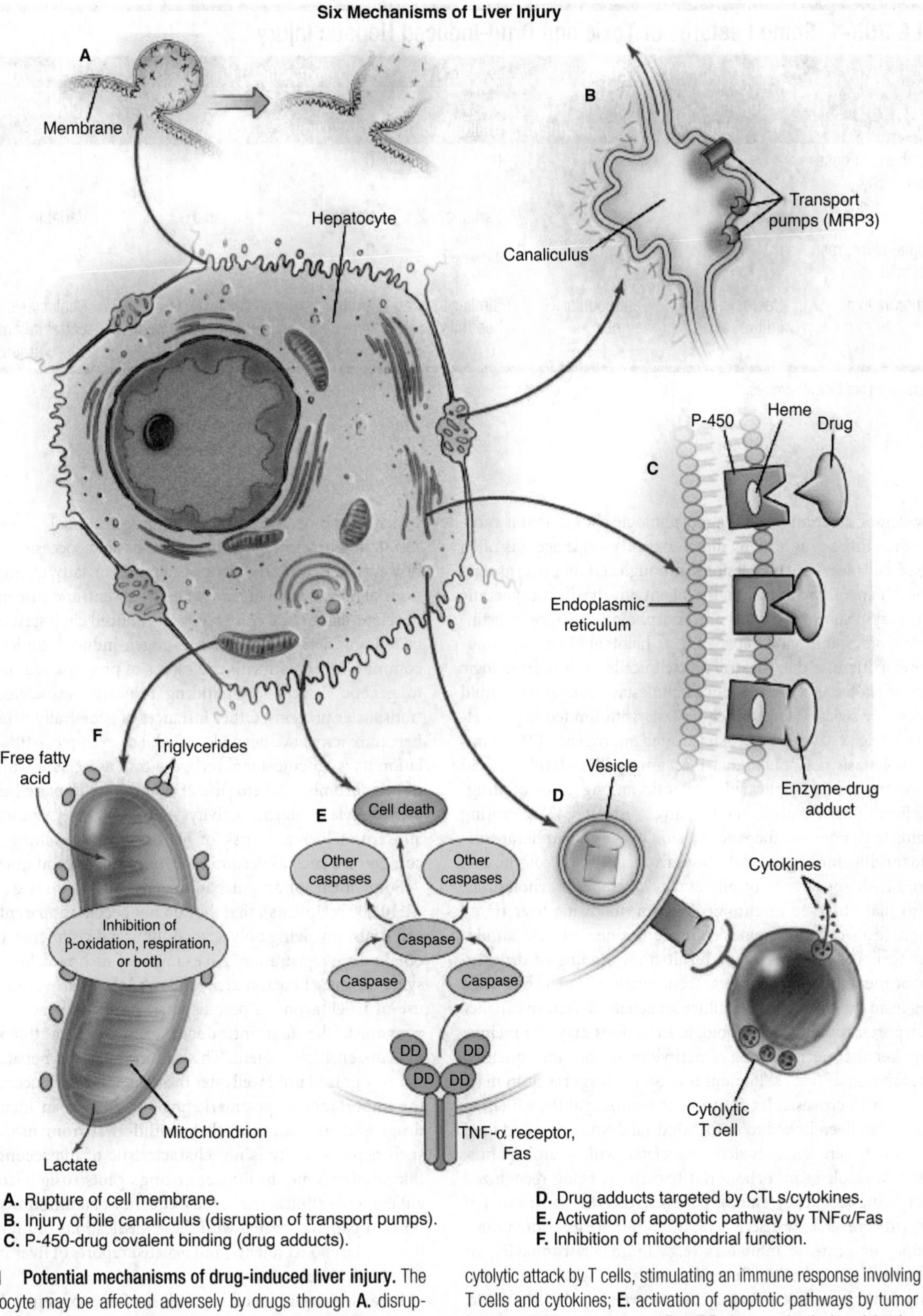

Figure 305-1 Potential mechanisms of drug-induced liver injury. The normal hepatocyte may be affected adversely by drugs through **A.** disruption of intracellular calcium homeostasis that leads to the disassembly of actin fibrils at the surface of the hepatocyte, resulting in blebbing of the cell membrane, rupture, and cell lysis; **B.** disruption of actin filaments next to the canaliculus (the specialized portion of the cell responsible for bile excretion), leading to loss of villous processes and interruption of transport pumps such as multidrug resistance–associated protein 3 (MRP3), which, in turn, prevents the excretion of bilirubin and other organic compounds; **C.** covalent binding of the heme-containing cytochrome P-450 enzyme to the drug, thus creating nonfunctioning adducts; **D.** migration of these enzyme-drug adducts to the cell surface in vesicles to serve as target immunogens for cytolytic attack by T cells, stimulating an immune response involving cytolytic T cells and cytokines; **E.** activation of apoptotic pathways by tumor necrosis factor α (TNF-α) receptor or Fas (DD denotes death domain), triggering the cascade of intercellular caspases, resulting in programmed cell death; or **F.** inhibition of mitochondrial function by a dual effect on both β-oxidation and the respiratory-chain enzymes, leading to failure of free fatty acid metabolism, a lack of aerobic respiration, and accumulation of lactate and reactive oxygen species (which may disrupt mitochondrial DNA). Toxic metabolites excreted in bile may damage bile-duct epithelium (not shown). CTLs, cytolytic T lymphocytes. *(Reproduced from Lee WM: Drug-induced hepatotoxicity. N Engl J Med 349:474, 2003, with permission.)*

TABLE 305-1 Some Features of Toxic and Drug-Induced Hepatic Injury

	Direct Toxic Effect*		Idiosyncratic*			Other*
Features	(Carbon Tetrachloride)	(Acetaminophen)	(Halothane)	(Isoniazid)	(Chlorpromazine)	(Oral Contraceptive Agents)
Predictable and dose-related toxicity	+	+	0	0	0	+
Latent period	Short	Short	Variable	Variable	Variable	Variable
Arthralgia, fever, rash, eosinophilia	0	0	+	0	+	0
Liver morphology	Necrosis, fatty infiltration	Centrilobular necrosis	Similar to viral hepatitis	Similar to viral hepatitis	Cholestasis *with* portal inflammation	Cholestasis *without* portal inflammation, vascular lesions

*The drugs listed are typical samples.

Idiosyncratic reactions lead to a morphologic pattern that is more variable than those produced by direct toxins; a single agent is often capable of causing a variety of lesions, although certain patterns tend to predominate. Depending on the agent involved, idiosyncratic hepatitis may result in a clinical and morphologic picture indistinguishable from that of viral hepatitis (e.g., halothane) or may simulate extrahepatic bile duct obstruction clinically with morphologic evidence of cholestasis. Drug-induced cholestasis ranges from mild to increasingly severe: (1) bland cholestasis with limited hepatocellular injury (e.g., estrogens, 17,α-substituted androgens); (2) inflammatory cholestasis [e.g., phenothiazines, amoxicillin-clavulanic acid (the most frequently implicated antibiotic among cases of drug-induced liver injury), oxacillin, erythromycin estolate]; (3) sclerosing cholangitis (e.g., after intrahepatic infusion of the chemotherapeutic agent floxuridine for hepatic metastases from a primary colonic carcinoma); (4) disappearance of bile ducts, "ductopenic" cholestasis, similar to that observed in chronic rejection following liver transplantation (e.g., carbamazepine, chlorpromazine, tricyclic antidepressant agents). Cholestasis may result from binding of drugs to canalicular membrane transporters, accumulation of toxic bile acids resulting from canalicular pump failure, or genetic defects in canalicular transporter proteins. Morphologic alterations may also include bridging hepatic necrosis (e.g., methyldopa), or, infrequently, hepatic granulomas (e.g., sulfonamides). Some drugs result in macrovesicular or microvesicular steatosis or steatohepatitis, which, in some cases, has been linked to mitochondrial dysfunction and lipid peroxidation. Severe hepatotoxicity associated with steatohepatitis, most likely a result of mitochondrial toxicity, is being recognized with increasing frequency among patients receiving antiretroviral therapy with reverse transcriptase inhibitors (e.g., zidovudine, didanosine) or protease inhibitors (e.g., indinavir, ritonavir) for HIV infection (Chap. 189). Generally, such mitochondrial hepatotoxicity of these antiretroviral agents is reversible, but dramatic, nonreversible hepatotoxicity associated with mitochondrial injury (inhibition of DNA polymerase γ) was the cause of acute liver failure encountered during early clinical trials of now-abandoned fialuridine, a fluorinated pyrimidine analogue with potent antiviral activity against hepatitis B virus. Another potential target for idiosyncratic drug hepatotoxicity is sinusoidal lining cells; when these are injured, such as by high-dose chemotherapeutic agents (e.g., cyclophosphamide, melphalan, busulfan) administered prior to bone marrow transplantation, venoocclusive disease can result.

Not all adverse hepatic drug reactions can be classified as either toxic or idiosyncratic in type. For example, oral contraceptives, which combine estrogenic and progestational compounds, may result in impairment of hepatic tests and, occasionally, jaundice; however, they do not produce necrosis or fatty change, manifestations of hypersensitivity are generally absent, and susceptibility to the development of oral contraceptive–induced cholestasis appears to be genetically determined. Such estrogen-induced cholestasis is more common in women with cholestasis of pregnancy, a disorder linked to genetic defects in multidrug resistance–associated canalicular transporter proteins. Other instances of genetically determined drug hepatotoxicity have been identified. For example, ~10% of the population have an autosomal recessive trait associated with the absence of cytochrome P450 enzyme 2D6 and have impaired debrisoquine-4-hydroxylase enzyme activity. As a result, they cannot metabolize, and are at increased risk of hepatotoxicity resulting from certain compounds such as desipramine, propranolol, and quinidine.

Some forms of drug hepatotoxicity are so rare (e.g., occurring in <1:10,000 recipients), that they do not become apparent during clinical trials, involving only several thousand recipients, conducted to obtain drug registration. An example of such rare, but serious, idiosyncratic drug hepatotoxicity followed the approval and generalized use of troglitazone, a peroxisomal, proliferator activator–receptor γ agonist, the first introduced example of a thiazolidinedione insulin-sensitizing agent. This instance of drug hepatotoxicity was not recognized until well after the drug was introduced, underlining the importance of postmarketing surveillance in identifying toxic drugs and in leading to their withdrawal from use. Fortunately, such hepatotoxicity is not characteristic of the second-generation thiazolidinedione insulin-sensitizing agents rosiglitazone and pioglitazone; in clinical trials, the frequency of aminotransferase elevations in patients treated with these medications did not differ from that in placebo recipients, and isolated reports of liver injury among recipients are extremely rare.

Because drug-induced hepatitis is often a presumptive diagnosis and many other disorders produce a similar clinicopathologic picture, evidence of a causal relationship between the use of a drug and subsequent liver injury may be difficult to establish. The relationship is most convincing for the direct hepatotoxins, which lead to a high frequency of hepatic impairment after a short latent period. Idiosyncratic reactions may be reproduced, in some instances, when rechallenge, after an asymptomatic period, results in a recurrence of signs, symptoms, and morphologic and biochemical abnormalities. Rechallenge, however, is often ethically unfeasible, because severe reactions may occur. Causality-assessment methodologies [scoring systematically based on a checklist of such variables as index of suspicion, time of onset, clinical-biochemical features, type of injury (direct, idiosyncratic), extrahepatic features, course, histologic features, drug serum levels, genetic markers and polymorphisms, and exclusion of other potential causes] have been adopted to add objectivity to diagnoses of drug-induced liver injury; however, even these approaches have their limitations and yield residual uncertainty.

Generally, drug hepatotoxicity is not more frequent in persons with underlying chronic liver disease. Reported exceptions include hepatotoxicity of aspirin, methotrexate, isoniazid (only in certain experiences), and antiretroviral therapy for HIV infection.

TREATMENT Toxic and Drug-Induced Hepatic Disease

Treatment is largely supportive, except in acetaminophen hepatotoxicity (see below). In patients with fulminant hepatitis resulting from drug hepatotoxicity, liver transplantation may be lifesaving (Chap. 310). Withdrawal of the suspected agent is indicated at the first sign of an adverse reaction. In the case of the direct toxins, liver involvement should not divert attention from renal or other organ involvement, which may also threaten survival. Glucocorticoids for drug hepatotoxicity with allergic features, silibinin for hepatotoxic mushroom poisoning, and ursodeoxycholic acid for cholestatic drug hepatotoxicity have never been shown to be effective and are not recommended.

In Table 305-2, several classes of chemical agents are listed together with examples of the pattern of liver injury produced by them. Certain drugs appear to be responsible for the development of chronic as well as acute hepatic injury. For example, oxyphenisatin, methyldopa, and isoniazid have been associated with moderate to severe chronic hepatitis, and halothane and methotrexate have been implicated in the development of cirrhosis. A syndrome resembling primary biliary cirrhosis has been described following treatment with chlorpromazine, methyl testosterone, tolbutamide, and other drugs. Portal hypertension in the absence of cirrhosis may result from alterations in hepatic architecture produced by vitamin A or arsenic intoxication, industrial exposure to vinyl chloride, or administration of thorium dioxide. The latter three agents have also been associated with angiosarcoma of the liver. Oral contraceptives have been implicated in the development of hepatic adenoma and, rarely, hepatocellular carcinoma and hepatic vein occlusion (Budd-Chiari syndrome). Another unusual lesion, peliosis hepatis (blood cysts of the liver), has been observed in some patients treated with anabolic steroids. The existence of these hepatic disorders expands the spectrum of liver injury induced by chemical agents and emphasizes the need for a thorough drug history in all patients with liver dysfunction.

The following are patterns of adverse hepatic reactions for some prototypic agents.

ACETAMINOPHEN HEPATOTOXICITY (DIRECT TOXIN)

Acetaminophen can cause severe centrilobular hepatic necrosis when ingested in large amounts in suicide attempts or accidentally by children. In the United States and England, acetaminophen hepatotoxicity is the most common culprit among patients presenting with acute liver failure and the leading indication for liver transplantation among patients with drug-induced liver failure. A single dose of 10–15 g, occasionally less, may produce clinical evidence of liver injury. Fatal fulminant disease is usually (although not invariably) associated with ingestion of ≥25 g. Blood levels of acetaminophen correlate with the severity of hepatic injury (levels >300 μg/mL 4 h after ingestion are predictive of the development of severe damage; levels <150 μg/mL suggest that hepatic injury is highly unlikely). Nausea, vomiting, diarrhea, abdominal pain, and shock are early manifestations occurring 4–12 hours after ingestion. Then 24–48 hours later, when these features are abating, hepatic injury becomes apparent. Maximal abnormalities and hepatic failure may not be evident until 4–6 days after ingestion, and aminotransferase levels approaching 10,000 units are not uncommon (i.e., levels far exceeding those in patients with viral hepatitis). Renal failure and myocardial injury may be present.

Acetaminophen is metabolized predominantly by a phase II reaction to innocuous sulfate and glucuronide metabolites; however, a small proportion of acetaminophen is metabolized by a phase I reaction to a hepatotoxic metabolite formed from the parent compound by the cytochrome P450 CYP2E1. This metabolite, *N*-acetyl-p-benzoquinone-imine (NAPQI), is detoxified by binding to "hepatoprotective" glutathione to become harmless, water-soluble mercapturic acid, which undergoes renal excretion. When excessive amounts of NAPQI are formed, or when glutathione levels are low, glutathione levels are depleted and overwhelmed, permitting covalent binding to nucleophilic hepatocyte macromolecules forming acetaminophen-protein "adducts." These adducts, which can be measured in serum by high-performance liquid chromatography, hold promise as diagnostic markers of acetaminophen hepatotoxicity. The binding of acetaminophen to hepatocyte macromolecules is believed to lead to hepatocyte necrosis; the precise sequence and mechanism are unknown. Hepatic injury may be potentiated by prior administration of alcohol, phenobarbital, isoniazid, or other drugs; by conditions that stimulate the mixed-function oxidase system; or by conditions such as starvation that reduce hepatic glutathione levels. The xenobiotic (environmental, exogenous substance) receptor CAR has been shown in a mouse model of acetaminophen hepatotoxicity to induce acetaminophen-metabolizing enzymes and, thereby, regulate and increase hepatotoxicity. Cimetidine, which inhibits P450 enzymes, has the potential to reduce generation of the toxic metabolite. Alcohol induces cytochrome P450 CYP2E1; consequently, increased levels of the toxic metabolite NAPQI are produced in chronic alcoholics after acetaminophen ingestion. In addition, alcohol suppresses hepatic glutathione production. Therefore, in chronic alcoholics, the toxic dose of acetaminophen may be as low as 2 g, and alcoholic patients should be warned specifically about the dangers of even standard doses of this commonly used drug. Such "therapeutic misadventures" also occur occasionally in patients with severe, febrile illnesses or pain syndromes; in such a setting, several days of anorexia and near-fasting coupled with regular administration of extra-strength acetaminophen formulations result in a combination of glutathione depletion and relatively high NAPQI levels in the absence of a history of recognized acetaminophen overdose. In a 2006 study, aminotransferase elevations were identified in 31–44% of normal subjects treated for 14 days with the maximal recommended dose of acetaminophen, 4 g daily (administered alone or as part of an acetaminophen/opioid combination); because these changes were transient and never associated with bilirubin elevation, the clinical relevance of these findings remains to be determined. Although underlying HCV infection was found to be associated with an increased risk of acute liver injury in patients hospitalized for acetaminophen overdose, generally, in patients with nonalcoholic liver disease, acetaminophen taken in recommended doses, may be the safest analgesic/antipyretic. In this vein, acetaminophen use in cirrhotic patients has not been associated with hepatic decompensation. On the other hand, because of the link between acetaminophen use and liver injury, and because of the limited safety margin between safe and toxic doses, the Food and Drug Administration (FDA) has recommended that the daily dose of acetaminophen be reduced from 4 g

TABLE 305-2 Principal Alterations of Hepatic Morphology Produced by Some Commonly Used Drugs and Chemicals[a]

Principal Morphologic Change	Class of Agent	Example
Cholestasis	Anabolic steroid	Methyl testosterone
	Antibiotic	Erythromycin estolate, nitrofurantoin, rifampin, amoxicillin-clavulanic acid, oxacillin
	Anticonvulsant	Carbamazine
	Antidepressant	Duloxetine, mirtazapine, tricyclic antidepressants
	Anti-inflammatory	Sulindac
	Antiplatelet	Clopidogrel
	Antihypertensive	Irbesartan, fosinopril
	Antithyroid	Methimazole
	Calcium channel blocker	Nifedipine, verapamil
	Immunosuppressive	Cyclosporine
	Lipid-lowering	Ezetimibe
	Oncotherapeutic	Anabolic steroids, busulfan, tamoxifen, irinotecan, cytarabine
	Oral contraceptive	Norethynodrel with mestranol
	Oral hypoglycemic	Chlorpropamide
	Tranquilizer	Chlorpromazine[b]
Fatty liver	Antiarrhythmic	Amiodarone
	Antibiotic	Tetracycline (high-dose, IV)
	Anticonvulsant	Valproic acid
	Antiviral	Dideoxynucleosides (e.g., zidovudine), protease inhibitors (e.g., indinavir, ritonavir)
	Oncotherapeutic	Asparaginase, methotrexate
Hepatitis	Anesthetic	Halothane[c]
	Antiandrogen	Flutamide
	Antibiotic	Isoniazid,[c] rifampicin, nitrofurantoin, telithromycin, minocycline,[d] pyrazinamide, trovafloxacin[e]
	Anticonvulsant	Phenytoin, carbamazine, valproic acid, phenobarbital
	Antidepressant	Iproniazid, amitriptyline, imipramine, trazodone, venlafaxine, fluoxetine, paroxetine, duloxetine, sertraline, nefazodone,[e] bupropion
	Antifungal	Ketoconazole, fluconazole, itraconazole
	Antihypertensive	Methyldopa,[c] captopril, enalapril, lisinopril, losartan
	Anti-inflammatory	Ibuprofen, indomethacin, diclofenac, sulindac, bromfenac
	Antipsychotic	Risperidone
	Antiviral	Zidovudine, didanosine, stavudine, nevirapine, ritonavir, indinavir, tipranavir, zalcitabine
	Calcium channel blocker	Nifedipine, verapamil, diltiazem
	Cholinesterase inhibitor	Tacrine
	Diuretic	Chlorothiazide
	Laxative	Oxyphenisatin[c,e]
	Norepinephrine-reuptake inhibitor	Atomoxetine
	Oral hypoglycemic	Troglitazone,[e] acarbose
Mixed hepatitis/ cholestatic	Antibiotic	Amoxicillin-clavulanic acid, trimethoprim-sulfamethoxazole
	Antibacterial	Clindamycin
	Antifungal	Terbinafine
	Antihistamine	Cyproheptadine
	Immunosuppressive	Azathioprine
	Lipid-lowering	Nicotinic acid, lovastatin, ezetimide
Toxic (necrosis)	Analgesic	Acetaminophen
	Hydrocarbon	Carbon tetrachloride
	Metal	Yellow phosphorus
	Mushroom	*Amanita phalloides*
	Solvent	Dimethylformamide
Granulomas	Antiarrhythmic	Quinidine, diltiazem
	Antibiotic	Sulfonamides
	Anticonvulsant	Carbamazine
	Anti-inflammatory	Phenylbutazone
	Xanthine oxidase inhibitor	Allopurinol

[a]Several agents cause more than one type of liver lesion and appear under more than one category.

[b]Rarely associated with primary biliary cirrhosis-like lesion.

[c]Occasionally associated with chronic hepatitis or bridging hepatic necrosis or cirrhosis.

[d]Associated with an autoimmune hepatitis-like syndrome.

[e]Withdrawn from use because of severe hepatotoxicity.

to 3.25 g (even lower for persons with chronic alcohol use), that all acetaminophen-containing products be labeled prominently as containing acetaminophen, and that the potential for liver injury be prominent in the packaging of acetaminophen and acetaminophen-containing products.

TREATMENT Acetaminophen Overdosage

Treatment includes gastric lavage, supportive measures, and oral administration of activated charcoal or cholestyramine to prevent absorption of residual drug. Neither charcoal nor cholestyramine appears to be effective if given >30 min after acetaminophen ingestion; if they are used, the stomach lavage should be done before other agents are administered orally. The chances of possible, probable, and high-risk hepatotoxicity can be derived from a nomogram plot (Fig. 305-2), readily available in emergency departments as a function of measuring acetaminophen plasma levels 8 h after ingestion. In patients with high acetaminophen blood levels (>200 μg/mL measured at 4 h or >100 μg/mL at 8 h after ingestion), the administration of sulfhydryl compounds (e.g., cysteamine, cysteine, or *N*-acetylcysteine) reduces the severity of hepatic necrosis. These agents appear to act by providing a reservoir of sulfhydryl groups to bind the toxic metabolites or by stimulating synthesis and repletion of hepatic glutathione. Therapy should be begun within 8 h of ingestion but may be effective even if given as late as 24–36 h after overdose. Later administration of sulfhydryl compounds is of uncertain value. Routine use of *N*-acetylcysteine has substantially reduced the occurrence of fatal acetaminophen hepatotoxicity. When given orally, *N*-acetylcysteine is diluted to yield a 5% solution. A loading dose of 140 mg/kg is given, followed by 70 mg/kg every 4 h for 15–20 doses. Whenever a patient with potential acetaminophen hepatotoxicity is encountered, a local poison control center should be contacted. Treatment can be stopped when plasma acetaminophen levels indicate that the risk of liver damage is low. If signs of hepatic failure (e.g., progressive jaundice, coagulopathy, confusion) occur despite *N*-acetylcysteine therapy for acetaminophen hepatotoxicity, liver transplantation may be the only option. Early arterial blood lactate levels among such patients with acute liver failure may distinguish patients highly likely to require liver transplantation (lactate levels >3.5 mmol/L) from those likely to survive without liver replacement.

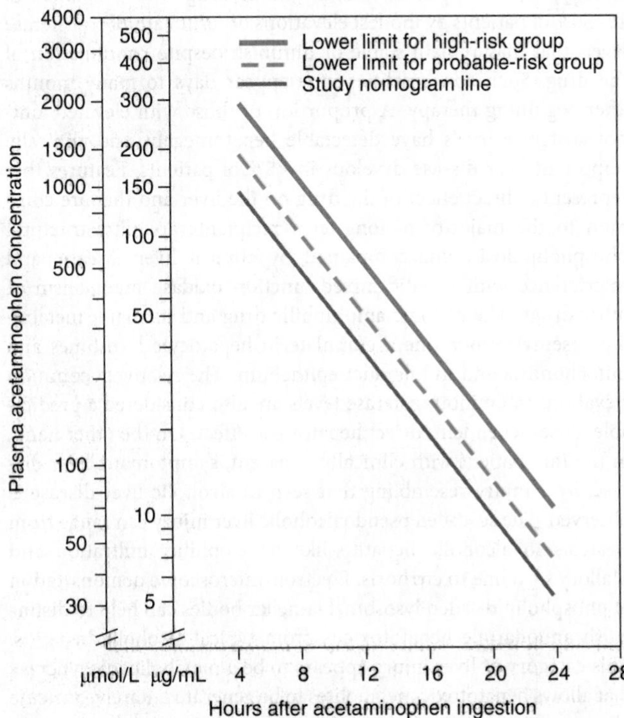

Figure 305-2 Nomogram to define risk of acetaminophen hepatotoxicity according to initial plasma acetaminophen concentration. *(After BH Rumack, H Matthew: Pediatrics 55:871, 1975.)*

Survivors of acute acetaminophen overdose usually have no hepatic sequelae. In a few patients, prolonged or repeated administration of acetaminophen in therapeutic doses appears to have led to the development of chronic hepatitis and cirrhosis.

HALOTHANE HEPATOTOXICITY (IDIOSYNCRATIC REACTION)

Although, currently, halothane anesthesia is administered in only rare situations, halothane hepatotoxicity was one of the prototypical, and most intensively studied, examples of idiosyncratic drug hepatotoxicity. Administration of halothane, a nonexplosive fluorinated hydrocarbon anesthetic agent that is structurally similar to chloroform, results in severe hepatic necrosis in a small number of individuals, many of whom have previously been exposed to this agent. The failure to produce similar hepatic lesions reliably in animals, the rarity of hepatic impairment in human beings, and the delayed appearance of hepatic injury suggest that halothane is not a direct hepatotoxin but rather a sensitizing agent; however, manifestations of hypersensitivity are seen in <25% of cases. A genetic predisposition leading to an idiosyncratic metabolic reactivity has been postulated and appears to be the most likely mechanism of halothane hepatotoxicity. Adults (rather than children), obese people, and women appear to be particularly susceptible. Fever, moderate leukocytosis, and eosinophilia may occur in the first week following halothane administration. Jaundice is usually noted 7–10 days after exposure but may occur earlier in previously exposed patients. Nausea and vomiting may precede the onset of jaundice. Hepatomegaly is often mild, but liver tenderness is common, and serum aminotransferase levels are elevated. The pathologic changes at autopsy are indistinguishable from massive hepatic necrosis resulting from viral hepatitis. The case-fatality rate of halothane hepatitis is not known but may vary from 20–40% in cases with severe liver involvement. Patients in whom unexplained spiking fever, especially delayed fever, or jaundice develops after halothane anesthesia should not receive this agent again. Because cross-reactions between halothane and methoxyflurane have been reported, the latter agent should not be used after halothane reactions. Later-generation halogenated hydrocarbon anesthetics that have supplanted halothane except in rare instances (e.g., certain types of thoracic surgery), are believed to be associated with a lower risk of hepatotoxicity.

METHYLDOPA HEPATOTOXICITY (TOXIC AND IDIOSYNCRATIC REACTION)

Minor alterations in liver tests are reported in ~5% of patients treated with this antihypertensive agent. These trivial abnormalities typically resolve despite continued drug administration. In <1% of patients, acute liver injury resembling viral or chronic hepatitis or, rarely, a cholestatic reaction is seen 1–20 weeks after methyldopa is started. In 50% of cases the interval is <4 weeks. A prodrome of fever, anorexia, and malaise may be noted for a few days before the onset of jaundice. Rash, lymphadenopathy, arthralgia, and eosinophilia are rare. Serologic markers of autoimmunity are detected infrequently, and <5% of patients have a Coombs-positive hemolytic anemia.

In ~15% of patients with methyldopa hepatotoxicity, the clinical, biochemical, and histologic features are those of moderate to severe chronic hepatitis, with or without bridging necrosis and macronodular cirrhosis. With discontinuation of the drug, the disorder usually resolves. Although methyldopa is currently used infrequently, its hepatotoxicity is very well characterized. Among the currently popular antihypertensive agents, angiotensin-converting enzyme (ACE) inhibitors, such as captopril and enalapril, have been blamed, albeit rarely, for hepatotoxicity (primarily cholestasis and cholestatic hepatitis, but also hepatocellular injury). Angiotensin-II receptor antagonists, such as losartan, are unlikely hepatotoxins, although rare reports of liver injury in their recipients have appeared.

ISONIAZID HEPATOTOXICITY (TOXIC AND IDIOSYNCRATIC REACTION)

In ~10% of adults treated with the antituberculosis agent isoniazid, elevated serum aminotransferase levels develop during the first few weeks of therapy; this appears to represent an adaptive response to a toxic metabolite of the drug. Whether or not isoniazid is continued, these values (usually <200 units) return to normal in a few weeks. In ~1% of treated patients, an illness develops that is indistinguishable from viral hepatitis; approximately one-half of these cases occur within the first 2 months of treatment; in the remainder, clinical disease may be delayed for many months. Liver biopsy reveals morphologic changes similar to those of viral hepatitis or bridging hepatic necrosis. The disease may be severe, with a case-fatality rate of 10%. Important liver injury appears to be age-related, increasing substantially after age 35; the highest frequency is in patients over age 50, the lowest under the age of 20. Even for patients >50 years of age monitored carefully during therapy, hepatotoxicity occurs in only ~2%, well below the risk estimate derived from earlier experiences. Isoniazid hepatotoxicity is enhanced by alcohol, rifampin, and pyrazinamide. Fever, rash, eosinophilia, and other manifestations of drug allergy are distinctly unusual. A reactive metabolite of acetylhydrazine, a metabolite of isoniazid, may be responsible for liver injury, and patients who are rapid acetylators would be more prone to such injury. Counterintuitively, in some reports, the opposite is true; slow acetylators are more likely to experience hepatotoxicity and more severe hepatotoxicity than rapid acetylators. Contrary to past reports, more recent studies suggest that hepatotoxicity due to isoniazid as well as to combination antituberculous therapy that includes isoniazid is more likely in patients with underlying chronic hepatitis B. A picture resembling chronic hepatitis has been observed in a few patients. Careful liver-test monitoring is advisable in patients being treated with isoniazid.

SODIUM VALPROATE HEPATOTOXICITY (TOXIC AND IDIOSYNCRATIC REACTION)

Sodium valproate, an anticonvulsant useful in the treatment of petit mal and other seizure disorders, has been associated with the development of severe hepatic toxicity and, rarely, fatalities, predominantly in children but also in adults. Among children listed as candidates for liver transplantation, valproate is the most common antiepileptic drug implicated. Asymptomatic elevations of serum aminotransferase levels have been recognized in as many as 45% of treated patients. These "adaptive" changes, however, appear to have no clinical importance, because major hepatotoxicity is not seen in the majority of patients despite continuation of drug therapy. In the rare patients in whom jaundice, encephalopathy, and evidence of hepatic failure are found, examination of liver tissue reveals microvesicular fat and bridging hepatic necrosis, predominantly in the centrilobular zone. Bile duct injury may also be apparent. Most likely, sodium valproate is not directly hepatotoxic, but its metabolite, 4-pentenoic acid, may be responsible for hepatic injury. Valproate hepatotoxicity is more common in persons with mitochondrial enzyme deficiencies and may be ameliorated by IV administration of carnitine, which valproate therapy can deplete.

PHENYTOIN HEPATOTOXICITY (IDIOSYNCRATIC REACTION)

Phenytoin, formerly diphenylhydantoin, a mainstay in the treatment of seizure disorders, has been associated in rare instances with the development of severe hepatitis-like liver injury leading to fulminant hepatic failure. In many patients, the hepatitis is associated with striking fever, lymphadenopathy, rash (Stevens-Johnson syndrome or exfoliative dermatitis), leukocytosis, and eosinophilia, suggesting an immunologically mediated hypersensitivity mechanism. Despite these observations, evidence suggests that metabolic idiosyncrasy may be responsible for hepatic injury. In the liver, phenytoin is converted by cytochrome P450 to metabolites, including the highly reactive electrophilic arene oxides. These metabolites are normally metabolized further by epoxide hydrolases. A defect (genetic or acquired) in epoxide hydrolase activity could permit covalent binding of arene oxides to hepatic macromolecules, thereby leading to hepatic injury. Hepatic injury is usually manifest within the first 2 months after beginning phenytoin therapy. With the exception of an abundance of eosinophils in the liver, the clinical, biochemical, and histologic picture resembles that of viral hepatitis. In rare instances, bile duct injury may be the salient feature of phenytoin hepatotoxicity, with striking features of intrahepatic cholestasis. Asymptomatic elevations of aminotransferase and alkaline phosphatase levels have been observed in a sizable proportion of patients receiving long-term phenytoin therapy. These liver changes are believed by some authorities to represent the potent hepatic enzyme-inducing properties of phenytoin and are accompanied histologically by swelling of hepatocytes in the absence of necroinflammatory activity or evidence of chronic liver disease.

AMIODARONE HEPATOTOXICITY (TOXIC AND IDIOSYNCRATIC REACTION)

Therapy with this potent antiarrhythmic drug is accompanied in 15–50% of patients by modest elevations of serum aminotransferase levels that may remain stable or diminish despite continuation of the drug. Such abnormalities may appear days to many months after beginning therapy. A proportion of those with elevated aminotransferase levels have detectable hepatomegaly, and clinically important liver disease develops in <5% of patients. Features that represent a direct effect of the drug on the liver and that are common to the majority of long-term recipients are ultrastructural phospholipidosis, unaccompanied by clinical liver disease, and interference with hepatic mixed-function oxidase metabolism of other drugs. The cationic amphiphilic drug and its major metabolite desethylamiodarone accumulate in hepatocyte lysosomes and mitochondria and in bile duct epithelium. The relatively common elevations in aminotransferase levels are also considered a predictable, dose-dependent, direct hepatotoxic effect. On the other hand, in the rare patient with clinically apparent, symptomatic liver disease, liver injury resembling that seen in alcoholic liver disease is observed. The so-called pseudoalcoholic liver injury can range from steatosis to alcoholic hepatitis-like neutrophilic infiltration and Mallory's hyaline to cirrhosis. Electron-microscopic demonstration of phospholipid-laden lysosomal lamellar bodies can help to distinguish amiodarone hepatotoxicity from typical alcoholic hepatitis. This category of liver injury appears to be a metabolic idiosyncrasy that allows hepatotoxic metabolites to be generated. Rarely, an acute idiosyncratic hepatocellular injury resembling viral hepatitis or cholestatic hepatitis occurs. Hepatic granulomas have occasionally been observed. Because amiodarone has a long half-life, liver injury may persist for months after the drug is stopped.

■ ERYTHROMYCIN HEPATOTOXICITY (CHOLESTATIC IDIOSYNCRATIC REACTION)

The most important adverse effect associated with erythromycin, more common in children than adults, is the infrequent occurrence of a cholestatic reaction. Although most of these reactions have been associated with erythromycin estolate, other erythromycins may also be responsible. The reaction usually begins during the first 2 or 3 weeks of therapy and includes nausea, vomiting, fever, right upper quadrant abdominal pain, jaundice, leukocytosis, and moderately elevated aminotransferase and alkaline phosphatase levels. The clinical picture can resemble acute cholecystitis or bacterial cholangitis. Liver biopsy reveals variable cholestasis; portal inflammation comprising lymphocytes, polymorphonuclear leukocytes, and eosinophils; and scattered foci of hepatocyte necrosis. Symptoms and laboratory findings usually subside within a few days of drug withdrawal, and evidence of chronic liver disease has not been found on follow-up. The precise mechanism remains ill-defined.

■ ORAL CONTRACEPTIVE HEPATOTOXICITY (CHOLESTATIC REACTION)

The administration of oral contraceptive combinations of estrogenic and progestational steroids leads to intrahepatic cholestasis with pruritus and jaundice in a small number of patients weeks to months after taking these agents. Especially susceptible seem to be patients with recurrent idiopathic jaundice of pregnancy, severe pruritus of pregnancy, or a family history of these disorders. With the exception of liver biochemical tests, laboratory studies are normal, and extrahepatic manifestations of hypersensitivity are absent. Liver biopsy reveals cholestasis with bile plugs in dilated canaliculi and striking bilirubin staining of liver cells. In contrast to chlorpromazine-induced cholestasis, portal inflammation is absent. The lesion is reversible on withdrawal of the agent. The two steroid components appear to act synergistically on hepatic function, although the estrogen may be primarily responsible. Oral contraceptives are contraindicated in patients with a history of recurrent jaundice of pregnancy. Primarily benign, but rarely malignant, neoplasms of the liver, hepatic vein occlusion, and peripheral sinusoidal dilatation have also been associated with oral contraceptive therapy. Focal nodular hyperplasia of the liver is not more frequent among users of oral contraceptives.

■ 17,α-ALKYL-SUBSTITUTED ANABOLIC STEROIDS (CHOLESTATIC REACTION)

In the majority of patients receiving these agents, used therapeutically mainly in the treatment of bone marrow failure but used surreptitiously and without medical indication (or unknowingly when included in nutritional supplements) by athletes to improve their performance, mild hepatic dysfunction develops. Impaired excretory function is the predominant defect, but the precise mechanism is uncertain. Jaundice, which appears to be dose-related, develops in only a minority of patients and may be the sole clinical manifestation of hepatotoxicity, although anorexia, nausea, and malaise may occur. Pruritus is not a prominent feature. Serum aminotransferase levels are usually <100 units, and serum alkaline phosphatase levels are normal; mildly elevated; or, in <5% of patients, three or more times the upper limit of normal. Examination of liver tissue reveals cholestasis without inflammation or necrosis. Hepatic sinusoidal dilatation and peliosis hepatis have been found in a few patients. The cholestatic disorder is usually reversible on cessation of treatment, although fatalities have been linked to peliosis. An association with hepatic adenoma and hepatocellular carcinoma has been reported.

■ TRIMETHOPRIM-SULFAMETHOXAZOLE HEPATOTOXICITY (IDIOSYNCRATIC REACTION)

This antibiotic combination is used routinely for urinary tract infections in immunocompetent persons and for prophylaxis against and therapy of *Pneumocystis carinii* pneumonia in immunosuppressed persons (transplant recipients, patients with AIDS). With its increasing use, its occasional hepatotoxicity is being recognized with growing frequency. Its likelihood is unpredictable, but when it occurs, trimethoprim-sulfamethoxazole hepatotoxicity follows a relatively uniform latency period of several weeks and is often accompanied by eosinophilia, rash, and other features of a hypersensitivity reaction. Biochemically and histologically, acute hepatocellular necrosis predominates, but cholestatic features are quite frequent. Occasionally, cholestasis without necrosis occurs, and, very rarely, a severe cholangiolytic pattern of liver injury is observed. In most cases, liver injury is self-limited, but rare fatalities have been recorded. The hepatotoxicity is attributable to the sulfamethoxazole component of the drug and is similar in features to that seen with other sulfonamides; tissue eosinophilia and granulomas may be seen. The risk of trimethoprim-sulfamethoxazole hepatotoxicity is increased in persons with HIV infection.

■ HMG-COA REDUCTASE INHIBITORS (STATINS) (IDIOSYNCRATIC MIXED HEPATOCELLULAR AND CHOLESTATIC REACTION)

Between 1 and 2% of patients taking lovastatin, simvastatin, pravastatin, fluvastatin, or one of the newer statin drugs for the treatment of hypercholesterolemia experience asymptomatic, reversible elevations (>threefold) of aminotransferase activity. Acute hepatitis-like histologic changes, centrilobular necrosis, and centrilobular cholestasis have been described in several cases. In a larger proportion, minor aminotransferase elevations appear during the first several weeks of therapy. Careful laboratory monitoring can distinguish between patients with minor, transitory changes; who may continue therapy; and those with more profound and sustained abnormalities, who should discontinue therapy. Because clinically meaningful aminotransferase elevations are so rare after statin use and do not differ in meta-analyses from the frequency of such laboratory abnormalities in placebo recipients, a panel of liver experts recommended to the National Lipid Association's Safety Task Force that liver-test monitoring was not necessary in patients treated with statins and that statin therapy need not be discontinued in patients found to have asymptomatic isolated aminotransferase elevations during therapy. Statin hepatotoxicity is not increased in patients with chronic hepatitis C, hepatic steatosis, or other underlying liver diseases, and statins can be used safely in these patients.

■ TOTAL PARENTERAL NUTRITION (STEATOSIS, CHOLESTASIS)

Total parenteral nutrition (TPN) is often complicated by cholestatic hepatitis attributable to either steatosis, cholestasis, or gallstones (or gallbladder sludge). Steatosis or steatohepatitis may result from the excess carbohydrate calories in these nutritional supplements and is the predominant form of TPN-associated liver disorder in adults. The frequency of this complication has been reduced substantially by the introduction of balanced TPN formulas that rely on lipid as an alternative caloric source. Cholestasis and cholelithiasis, caused by the absence of stimulation of bile flow and secretion resulting from the lack of oral intake, is the predominant form of TPN-associated liver disease in infants, especially in premature neonates. Often, cholestasis in such neonates is multifactorial, contributed to by other factors such as sepsis, hypoxemia, and hypotension; occasionally, TPN-induced cholestasis in neonates culminates in chronic liver disease and liver failure. When TPN-associated liver-test abnormalities occur in adults, balancing the TPN formula with more lipid is the intervention of first recourse. In infants with TPN-associated cholestasis, the addition of oral feeding may ameliorate the problem. Therapeutic interventions suggested, but not shown, to be of proven benefit, include cholecystokinin, ursodeoxycholic acid, *S*-adenosyl methionine, and taurine.

"ALTERNATIVE AND COMPLEMENTARY MEDICINES" (IDIOSYNCRATIC HEPATITIS, STEATOSIS)

The misguided popularity of herbal medications that are of scientifically unproven efficacy and that lack prospective safety oversight by regulatory agencies has resulted in occasional instances of hepatotoxicity. Included among the herbal remedies associated with toxic hepatitis are Jin Bu Huan, xiao-chai-hu-tang, germander, chaparral, senna, mistletoe, skullcap, gentian, comfrey (containing pyrrolizidine alkaloids), Ma huang, bee pollen, valerian root, pennyroyal oil, kava, celandine, Impila (*Callilepsis laureaola*), LipoKinetix, Hyroxycut, herbal nutritional supplements, and herbal teas. Well characterized are the acute hepatitis-like histologic lesions following Jin Bu Huan use: focal hepatocellular necrosis, mixed mononuclear portal tract infiltration, coagulative necrosis, apoptotic hepatocyte degeneration, tissue eosinophilia, and microvesicular steatosis. Megadoses of vitamin A can injure the liver, as can pyrrolizidine alkaloids, which often contaminate Chinese herbal preparations and can cause a venoocclusive injury leading to sinusoidal hepatic vein obstruction. Because some alternative medicines induce toxicity via active metabolites, alcohol and drugs that stimulate cytochrome P450 enzymes may enhance the toxicity of some of these products. Conversely, some alternative medicines also stimulate cytochrome P450 and may result in or amplify the toxicity of recognized drug hepatotoxins. Given the widespread use of such poorly defined herbal preparations, hepatotoxicity is likely to be encountered with increasing frequency; therefore, a drug history in patients with acute and chronic liver disease should include use of "alternative medicines" and other nonprescription preparations sold in so-called health food stores.

HIGHLY ACTIVE ANTIRETROVIRAL THERAPY (HAART) FOR HIV INFECTION (MITOCHONDRIAL TOXIC, IDIOSYNCRATIC, STEATOSIS; HEPATOCELLULAR, CHOLESTATIC, AND MIXED)

The recognition of drug hepatotoxicity in persons with HIV infection is complicated in this population by the many alternative causes of liver injury (chronic viral hepatitis, fatty infiltration, infiltrative disorders, mycobacterial infection, etc.), but drug hepatotoxicity associated with HAART is an emerging and common type of liver injury in HIV-infected persons (Chap. 189). Although no one antiviral agent is recognized as a potent hepatotoxin, combination regimens including reverse transcriptase and protease inhibitors cause hepatotoxicity in ~10% of treated patients. Implicated most frequently are combinations including nucleoside analogue reverse transcriptase inhibitors zidovudine, didanosine, and, to a lesser extent, stavudine; protease inhibitors ritonavir and indinavir (and amprenavir when used together with ritonavir) as well as tipranavir; and nonnucleoside reverse transcriptase inhibitors nevirapine and, to a lesser extent, efavirenz. These drugs cause predominantly hepatocellular injury but cholestatic injury as well, and prolonged (>6 months) use of reverse transcriptase inhibitors has been associated with mitochondrial injury, steatosis, and lactic acidosis. Indirect hyperbilirubinemia, resulting from direct inhibition of bilirubin-conjugating activity by UDP-glucuronosyltransferase, usually without elevation of aminotransferase or alkaline phosphatase activities, occurs in ~10% of patients treated with the protease inhibitor indinavir. Distinguishing the impact of HAART hepatotoxicity in patients with HIV and hepatitis virus co-infection is made challenging by the following: (1) both chronic hepatitis B and hepatitis C can affect the natural history of HIV infection and the response to HAART, and (2) HAART can have an impact on chronic viral hepatitis. For example, immunologic reconstitution with HAART can result in immunologically mediated liver-cell injury in patients with chronic hepatitis B co-infection if treatment with an antiviral agent for hepatitis B, e.g., the nucleoside analogue lamivudine, is withdrawn or if nucleoside analogue resistance emerges. Infection with HIV, especially with low CD4+ T cell counts, has been reported to increase the rate of hepatic fibrosis associated with chronic hepatitis C, and HAART therapy can increase levels of serum aminotransferases and hepatitis C virus RNA in patients with hepatitis C co-infection. Didanosine or stavudine should not be used with ribavirin in patients with HIV/hepatitis C virus co-infection, because of an increased risk of severe mitochondrial toxicity and lactic acidosis.

ACKNOWLEDGEMENT

Kurt J. Isselbacher, MD, contributed to this chapter in previous editions of Harrison's.

FURTHER READINGS

Chalasani et al: Causes, clinical features, and outcomes from a prospective study of drug-induced liver injury in the United States. Gastroenterology 135:1924, 2008

Chang CY, Schiano TD: Review article: drug hepatotoxicity. Aliment Pharmacol Ther 25:1135, 2007

Daly AK et al: *HLA-B*5701* genotype is a major determinant of drug-induced liver injury due to flucloxacillin. Nature Genetics 41:816, 2009

Kaplowitz N, Deleve LD (eds): *Drug-Induced Liver Disease*. 2nd ed, New York, Informa Healthcare, 2007

Lee WM: Drug-induced hepatotoxicity. N Engl J Med 349:474, 2003

Lucena MI et al: Mitochondrial superoxide dismutase and glutathione peroxidase in idiosyncratic drug-induced liver injury. Hepatology 52:303, 2010

Mindikoglu AL et al: Outcome of liver transplantation for drug-induced acute liver failure in the United States: Analysis of the United Network for Organ Sharing database. Liver Transpl 15:719, 2009

Navarro VJ, Senior JR: Drug-related hepatotoxicity. N Engl J Med 354:731, 2006

Nunez M: Hepatotoxicity of antiretrovirals: Incidence, mechanisms and management. J Hepatol 44:S132, 2006

Schmidt LE et al: Acute versus chronic alcohol consumption in acetaminophen-induced hepatotoxicity. Hepatology 35:876, 2002

Zhang J et al: Modulation of acetaminophen-induced hepatotoxicity by the xenobiotic receptor CAR. Science 298:422, 2002

CHAPTER 306

Chronic Hepatitis

Jules L. Dienstag

Chronic hepatitis represents a series of liver disorders of varying causes and severity in which hepatic inflammation and necrosis continue for at least 6 months. Milder forms are nonprogressive or only slowly progressive, while more severe forms may be associated with scarring and architectural reorganization, which, when advanced, lead ultimately to cirrhosis. Several categories of chronic hepatitis have been recognized. These include chronic viral hepatitis, drug-induced chronic hepatitis (Chap. 305), and autoimmune chronic hepatitis. In many cases, clinical and laboratory features are insufficient to allow assignment into one of these three categories; these "idiopathic" cases are also believed to represent autoimmune chronic hepatitis. Finally, clinical and laboratory features of chronic hepatitis are observed occasionally in patients with such hereditary/metabolic disorders as Wilson's disease (copper overload) (Chaps. 308 and 360) and nonalcoholic fatty liver disease (Chap. 309) and even occasionally in patients with alcoholic liver injury (Chap. 307). Although all types of chronic hepatitis share certain clinical, laboratory, and histopathologic features, chronic viral and chronic autoimmune hepatitis are sufficiently distinct to merit separate discussions. For discussion of acute hepatitis, see Chap. 304.

CLASSIFICATION OF CHRONIC HEPATITIS

Common to all forms of chronic hepatitis are histopathologic distinctions based on localization and extent of liver injury. These vary from the milder forms, previously labeled *chronic persistent hepatitis* and *chronic lobular hepatitis*, to the more severe form, formerly called *chronic active hepatitis*. When first defined, these designations were believed to have prognostic implications, which have been challenged by more recent observations. Categorization of chronic hepatitis based primarily on histopathologic features has been replaced by a more informative classification based on a combination of clinical, serologic, and histologic variables. Classification of chronic hepatitis is based on (1) its *cause*; (2) its histologic activity, or *grade*; and (3) its degree of progression, or *stage*. Thus, neither clinical features alone nor histologic features—requiring liver biopsy—alone are sufficient to characterize and distinguish among the several categories of chronic hepatitis.

CLASSIFICATION BY CAUSE

Clinical and serologic features allow the establishment of a diagnosis of *chronic viral hepatitis*, caused by hepatitis B, hepatitis B plus D, or hepatitis C; *autoimmune hepatitis*, including several subcategories, I and II (perhaps III), based on serologic distinctions; *drug-associated chronic hepatitis*; and a category of unknown cause, or *cryptogenic chronic hepatitis* (Table 306-1). These are addressed in more detail below.

CLASSIFICATION BY GRADE

Grade, a histologic assessment of necroinflammatory activity, is based on examination of the liver biopsy. An assessment of important histologic features includes the degree of *periportal necrosis* and the disruption of the limiting plate of periportal hepatocytes by inflammatory cells (so-called *piecemeal necrosis* or *interface hepatitis*); the degree of confluent necrosis that links or forms bridges between vascular structures—between portal tract and portal tract or even more important bridges between portal tract and central vein—referred to as *bridging necrosis*; the degree of hepatocyte degeneration and focal necrosis within the lobule; and the degree of *portal inflammation*. Several scoring systems that take these histologic features into account have been devised, and the most popular are the histologic activity index (HAI), used commonly in the United States, and the METAVIR score, used in Europe (Table 306-2). Based on the presence and degree of these features of histologic activity, chronic hepatitis can be graded as mild, moderate, or severe.

CLASSIFICATION BY STAGE

The stage of chronic hepatitis, which reflects the level of progression of the disease, is based on the degree of hepatic fibrosis. When fibrosis is so extensive that fibrous septa surround parenchymal nodules and alter the normal architecture of the liver lobule, the histologic lesion is defined as *cirrhosis*. Staging is based on the degree of fibrosis as categorized on a numerical scale from 0–6 (HAI) or 0–4 (METAVIR) (Table 306-2).

TABLE 306-1 Clinical and Laboratory Features of Chronic Hepatitis

Type of hepatitis	Diagnostic test(s)	Autoantibodies	Therapy
Chronic hepatitis B	HBsAg, IgG anti-HBc, HBeAg, HBV DNA	Uncommon	IFN-α, PEG IFN-α lamivudine adefovir entecavir telbivudine tenofovir
Chronic hepatitis C	Anti-HCV, HCV RNA	Anti-LKM1[a]	PEG IFN-α plus ribavirin Telaprevir[d] Boceprevir[d]
Chronic hepatitis D	Anti-HDV, HDV RNA, HBsAg, IgG anti-HBc	Anti-LKM3	IFN-α, PEG IFN-α[c]
Autoimmune hepatitis	ANA[b] (homogeneous), anti-LKM1 (±) Hyperglobulinemia	ANA, anti-LKM1 anti-SLA[e]	Prednisone, azathioprine
Drug-associated	—	Uncommon	Withdraw drug
Cryptogenic	All negative	None	Prednisone (?), azathioprine (?)

[a]Antibodies to liver-kidney microsomes type 1 (autoimmune hepatitis type II and some cases of hepatitis C)

[b]Antinuclear antibody (autoimmune hepatitis type I)

[c]Clinical trials suggest benefit of IFN-α therapy; PEG IFN-α is as effective, if not more so.

[d]Expected approval date 2011.

[e]Antibodies to soluble liver antigen (autoimmune hepatitis type III)

Abbreviations: HBc, hepatitis B core; HBeAg, hepatitis B e antigen; HBsAg, hepatitis B surface antigen; HBV, hepatitis B virus; HCV, hepatitis C virus; HDV, hepatitis D virus; IFN-α, interferon-α; IgG, immunoglobulin G; LKM, liver-kidney microsome; PEG-IFN-α, pegylated interferon-α; SLA, soluble liver antigen.

TABLE 306-2 Histologic Grading and Staging of Chronic Hepatitis

	Histologic Activity Index (HAI)[a]		METAVIR[b]	
Histologic Feature	**Severity**	**Score**	**Severity**	**Score**
Necroinflammatory Activity (grade)				
Periportal necrosis, including piecemeal necrosis and/or bridging necrosis (BN)	None	0	None	0
	Mild	1	Mild	1
	Mild/Moderate	2	Moderate	2
	Moderate	3	Severe	3
	Severe	4		
			Bridging necrosis	Yes
				No
Intralobular Confluent necrosis	—none	0	None or mild	0
	—focal	1	Moderate	1
	—Zone 3 some	2	Severe	2
	—Zone 3 most	3		
	—Zone 3 + BN few	4		
	—Zone 3 + BN multiple	5		
	—Panacinar/multiacinar	6		
Focal	—none	0		
	—≤1 focus/10x field	1		
	—2–4 foci/10x field	2		
	—5–10 foci/10x field	3		
	—>10 foci/10x field	4		
Portal Inflammation	None	0		
	Mild	1		
	Moderate	2		
	Moderate/marked	3		
	Marked	4		
	Total	0–18		A0–A3[c]
Fibrosis (stage)				
None		0		F0
Portal fibrosis—some		1		F1
Portal fibrosis—most		2		F1
Bridging fibrosis—few		3		F2
Bridging fibrosis—many		4		F3
Incomplete cirrhosis		5		F4
Cirrhosis		6		F4
	Total	6		4

[a]J Hepatol 22:696, 1995
[b]Hepatology 24:289, 1996
[c]Necroinflammatory grade: A0 = none; A1 = mild; A2 = moderate; A3 = severe

CHRONIC VIRAL HEPATITIS

Both the enterically transmitted forms of viral hepatitis, hepatitis A and E, are self-limited and do not cause chronic hepatitis (rare reports notwithstanding in which acute hepatitis A serves as a trigger for the onset of autoimmune hepatitis in genetically susceptible patients). In contrast, the entire clinicopathologic spectrum of chronic hepatitis occurs in patients with chronic viral hepatitis B and C as well as in patients with chronic hepatitis D superimposed on chronic hepatitis B.

CHRONIC HEPATITIS B

The likelihood of chronicity after acute hepatitis B varies as a function of age. Infection at birth is associated with clinically silent acute infection but a 90% chance of chronic infection, while infection in young adulthood in immunocompetent persons is typically associated with clinically apparent acute hepatitis but a risk of chronicity of only approximately 1%. Most cases of chronic hepatitis B among adults, however, occur in patients who never had a recognized episode of clinically apparent acute viral hepatitis. The degree of liver injury (grade) in patients with chronic hepatitis B is variable, ranging from none in inactive carriers to mild to moderate to severe. Among adults with chronic hepatitis B, histologic features are of prognostic importance. In one long-term study of patients with chronic hepatitis B, investigators found a 5-year survival rate of 97% for patients with mild chronic hepatitis, 86% for patients with moderate to severe chronic hepatitis, and only 55% for patients with chronic hepatitis and postnecrotic cirrhosis. The 15-year survival in these cohorts was 77, 66, and 40%, respectively. On the other hand, more recent observations do not allow us to be so sanguine about the prognosis in patients with mild chronic hepatitis; among such patients followed for 1–13 years, progression to more severe chronic hepatitis and cirrhosis has been observed in more than a quarter of cases.

More important to consider than histology alone in patients with chronic hepatitis B is the degree of hepatitis B virus (HBV) replication. As reviewed in Chap. 304, chronic HBV infection can occur in the presence or absence of serum hepatitis B e antigen (HBeAg), and generally, for both HBeAg-reactive and HBeAg-negative chronic hepatitis B, the level of HBV DNA correlates with the level of liver injury and risk of progression. In *HBeAg-reactive chronic hepatitis B*, two phases have been recognized based on the relative level of HBV replication. The relatively *replicative phase* is characterized by the presence in the serum of HBeAg and HBV DNA levels well in excess of 10^5–10^6 virions/mL, by the presence in the liver of detectable intrahepatocyte nucleocapsid antigens [primarily hepatitis B core antigen (HBcAg)], by high infectivity, and by accompanying liver injury. In contrast, the relatively *nonreplicative phase* is characterized by the absence of the conventional serum marker of HBV replication (HBeAg), the appearance of anti-HBe, levels of HBV DNA below a threshold of ~10^3 virions/mL, the absence of intrahepatocytic HBcAg, limited infectivity, and minimal liver injury. Those patients in the replicative phase tend to have more severe chronic hepatitis, while those in the nonreplicative phase tend to have minimal or mild chronic hepatitis or to be inactive hepatitis B carriers; however, distinctions in HBV replication and in histologic category do not always coincide. The likelihood in a patient with HBeAg-reactive chronic hepatitis B of converting spontaneously from relatively replicative to nonreplicative infection is approximately 10–15% per year. In patients with HBeAg-reactive chronic HBV infection, especially when acquired at birth or in early childhood, as recognized commonly in Asian countries, a dichotomy is common between very high levels of HBV replication and negligible levels of liver injury. Yet despite the relatively immediate, apparently benign nature of liver disease for many decades in this population, patients with childhood-acquired HBV infection are the ones at ultimately increased risk later in life of cirrhosis and hepatocellular carcinoma (HCC) (Chap. 92). A discussion of the pathogenesis of liver injury in patients with chronic hepatitis B appears in Chap. 304.

HBeAg-negative chronic hepatitis B [i.e., chronic HBV infection with active virus replication, readily detectable HBV DNA but without HBeAg (anti-HBe-reactive)], is more common than HBeAg-reactive chronic hepatitis B in Mediterranean and European countries and in Asia (and, correspondingly, in HBV genotypes other than A). Compared to patients with HBeAg-reactive chronic hepatitis B, patients with HBeAg-negative chronic hepatitis B have levels of HBV DNA that are several orders of magnitude lower (no more than 10^5–10^6 virions/mL) than those observed in the HBeAg-reactive subset. Most such cases represent precore or core-promoter mutations acquired late in the natural history of the disease (mostly early-life onset; age range 40–55 years, older than that for HBeAg-reactive chronic hepatitis B); these mutations prevent translation of HBeAg from the precore component of the HBV genome (precore mutants) or are characterized by down-regulated transcription of precore mRNA (core-promoter mutants; Chap. 304). Although their levels of HBV DNA tend to be lower than among patients with HBeAg-reactive chronic hepatitis B, patients with HBeAg-negative chronic hepatitis B can have progressive liver injury (complicated by cirrhosis and HCC) and experience episodic reactivation of liver disease reflected in fluctuating levels of aminotransferase activity ("flares"). The biochemical and histologic activity of HBeAg-negative disease tends to correlate closely with levels of HBV replication, unlike the case mentioned above of Asian patients with HBeAg-reactive chronic hepatitis B during the early decades of their HBV infection. An important point worth reiterating is the observation that the level of HBV replication is the most important risk factor for the ultimate development of cirrhosis and HCC in both HBeAg-reactive and HBeAg-negative patients. Although levels of HBV DNA are lower and more readily suppressed by therapy to undetectable levels in HBeAg-negative (compared to HBeAg-reactive) chronic hepatitis B, achieving sustained responses that permit discontinuation of antiviral therapy is less likely in HBeAg-negative patients (see below). Inactive carriers are patients with circulating hepatitis B surface antigen (HBsAg), normal serum aminotransferase levels, undetectable HBeAg, and levels of HBV DNA that are either undetectable or present at levels $\leq 10^3$ virions/mL. This serologic profile can occur not only in inactive carriers but also in patients with HBeAg-negative chronic hepatitis B during periods of relative inactivity; distinguishing between the two requires sequential biochemical and virologic monitoring over many months.

The spectrum of *clinical features* of chronic hepatitis B is broad, ranging from asymptomatic infection to debilitating disease or even end-stage, fatal hepatic failure. As noted above, the onset of the disease tends to be insidious in most patients, with the exception of the very few in whom chronic disease follows failure of resolution of clinically apparent acute hepatitis B. The clinical and laboratory features associated with progression from acute to chronic hepatitis B are discussed in Chap. 304.

Fatigue is a common symptom, and persistent or intermittent *jaundice* is a common feature in severe or advanced cases. Intermittent deepening of jaundice and recurrence of malaise and anorexia, as well as worsening fatigue, are reminiscent of acute hepatitis; such exacerbations may occur spontaneously, often coinciding with evidence of virologic reactivation; may lead to progressive liver injury; and, when superimposed on well-established cirrhosis, may cause hepatic decompensation. Complications of cirrhosis occur in end-stage chronic hepatitis and include ascites, edema, bleeding gastroesophageal varices, hepatic encephalopathy, coagulopathy, or hypersplenism. Occasionally, these complications bring the patient to initial clinical attention. Extrahepatic complications of chronic hepatitis B, similar to those seen during the prodromal phase of acute hepatitis B, are associated with deposition of circulating hepatitis B antigen–antibody immune complexes. These include arthralgias and arthritis, which are common, and the more rare purpuric cutaneous lesions (leukocytoclastic vasculitis), immune-complex glomerulonephritis, and generalized vasculitis (polyarteritis nodosa) (Chaps. 304 and 326).

Laboratory features of chronic hepatitis B do not distinguish adequately between histologically mild and severe hepatitis. Aminotransferase elevations tend to be modest for chronic hepatitis B but may fluctuate in the range of 100–1000 units. As is true for acute viral hepatitis B, alanine aminotransferase (ALT) tends to be more elevated than aspartate aminotransferase (AST); however, once cirrhosis is established, AST tends to exceed ALT. Levels of alkaline phosphatase activity tend to be normal or only marginally elevated. In severe cases, moderate elevations in serum bilirubin [51.3–171 μmol/L (3–10 mg/dL)] occur. Hypoalbuminemia and prolongation of the prothrombin time occur in severe or end-stage cases. Hyperglobulinemia and detectable circulating autoantibodies are distinctly absent in chronic hepatitis B (in contrast to autoimmune hepatitis). Viral markers of chronic HBV infection are discussed in Chap. 304.

TREATMENT Chronic Hepatitis B

Although progression to cirrhosis is more likely in severe than in mild or moderate chronic hepatitis B, all forms of chronic hepatitis B can be progressive, and progression occurs primarily in patients with active HBV replication. Moreover, in populations of patients with chronic hepatitis B who are at risk for HCC (Chap. 92), the risk is highest for those with continued, high-level HBV replication and lower for persons in whom initially high-level HBV DNA falls spontaneously over time. Therefore, management of chronic hepatitis B is directed at suppressing the level of virus replication. Although clinical trials tend to focus on clinical endpoints achieved over 1–2 years (e.g., suppression of HBV DNA to undetectable levels, loss of HBeAg/HBsAg, improvement in histology, normalization of ALT), these short-term gains translate into reductions in the risk of clinical progression, hepatic decompensation, and death. To date, seven drugs have been approved for treatment of chronic hepatitis B: injectable interferon (IFN) α; pegylated interferon [long-acting IFN bound to polyethylene glycol (PEG), known as *PEG IFN*]; and the oral agents lamivudine, adefovir dipivoxil, entecavir, telbivudine, and tenofovir.

Antiviral therapy for hepatitis B has evolved rapidly since the mid-1990s, as has the sensitivity of tests for HBV DNA. When IFN and lamivudine were evaluated in clinical trials, HBV DNA was measured by insensitive hybridization assays with detection thresholds of 10^5–10^6 virions/mL; when adefovir, entecavir, telbivudine, tenofovir, and PEG IFN were studied in clinical trials, HBV DNA was measured by sensitive amplification assays [polymerase chain reaction [(PCR)] with detection thresholds of 10^1–10^3 virions/mL. Recognition of these distinctions is helpful when comparing results of clinical trials that established the efficacy of these therapies (reviewed below in chronological order of publication of these efficacy trials).

INTERFERON IFN-α was the first approved therapy for chronic hepatitis B. Although it is no longer used to treat hepatitis B, standard IFN is important historically, having provided important lessons about antiviral therapy in general. For immunocompetent adults with HBeAg-reactive chronic hepatitis B [who tend to have high-level HBV DNA (>10^5–10^6 virions/mL) and histologic evidence of chronic hepatitis on liver biopsy], a 16-week course of IFN given subcutaneously at a daily dose of 5 million units, or three times a week at a dose of 10 million units, results in a loss of HBeAg and hybridization-detectable HBV DNA (i.e., a reduction to levels below 10^5–10^6 virions/mL) in ~30% of patients, with a concomitant improvement in liver histology. Seroconversion from HBeAg to anti-HBe occurs in approximately 20%, and, in early trials, approximately 8% lost HBsAg. Successful IFN therapy and seroconversion are often accompanied by an acute hepatitis-like elevation in aminotransferase activity, which has been postulated to result from enhanced cytolytic T cell clearance of HBV-infected hepatocytes. Relapse after successful therapy is rare (1 or 2%). The likelihood of responding to IFN is higher in patients with lower levels of HBV DNA and substantial elevations of ALT. Although children can respond as well as adults, IFN therapy has not been effective in very young children infected at birth. Similarly, IFN therapy has not been effective in immunosuppressed persons, Asian patients with minimal-to-mild ALT elevations, or patients with decompensated chronic hepatitis B (in whom such therapy can actually be detrimental, sometimes precipitating decompensation, often associated with severe adverse effects). Among patients with HBeAg loss during therapy, long-term follow-up has demonstrated that 80% experience eventual loss of HBsAg [i.e., all serologic markers of infection, and normalization of ALT over a 9-year posttreatment period]. In addition, improved long-term and complication-free survival as well as a reduction in the frequency of HCC have been documented among interferon responders, supporting the conclusion that successful interferon therapy improves the natural history of chronic hepatitis B.

Initial trials of brief-duration IFN therapy in patients with *HBeAg-negative chronic hepatitis B* were disappointing, suppressing HBV replication transiently during therapy but almost never resulting in sustained antiviral responses. In subsequent IFN trials among patients with HBeAg-negative chronic hepatitis B, however, more protracted courses, lasting up to 1½ years, have been reported to result in sustained remissions documented to last for several years, with suppressed HBV DNA and aminotransferase activity, in ~20%.

Complications of IFN therapy include systemic "flu-like" symptoms; marrow suppression; emotional lability (irritability, depression, anxiety); autoimmune reactions (especially autoimmune thyroiditis); and miscellaneous side effects such as alopecia, rashes, diarrhea, and numbness and tingling of the extremities. With the possible exception of autoimmune thyroiditis, all these side effects are reversible upon dose lowering or cessation of therapy.

Although no longer competitive with the newer generation of antivirals, IFN did represent the first successful antiviral approach and set a standard against which to measure subsequent drugs in the achievement of durable virologic, serologic, biochemical, and histologic responses; consolidation of virologic and biochemical benefit in the ensuing years after therapy; and improvement in the natural history of chronic hepatitis B. Standard IFN has been supplanted by long-acting PEG IFN (see below), and IFN nonresponders are now treated with one of the newer oral nucleoside analogues.

LAMIVUDINE The first of the nucleoside analogues to be approved, the dideoxynucleoside lamivudine, inhibits reverse transcriptase activity of both HIV and HBV and is a potent and effective agent for patients with chronic hepatitis B. Although generally superseded by newer, more potent agents, lamivudine is still used in regions of the world where newer agents are not yet approved are or not affordable. In clinical trials among patients with HBeAg-reactive chronic hepatitis B, lamivudine therapy at daily doses of 100 mg for 48–52 weeks suppressed HBV DNA by a median of approximately 5.5 $\log_{10}$ copies/mL and to undetectable levels, as measured by PCR amplification assays, in approximately 40% of patients. Therapy was associated with HBeAg loss in 32–33%; HBeAg seroconversion (i.e., conversion from HBeAg-reactive to anti-HBe-reactive) in 16–21%; normalization of ALT in 40–75%; improvement in histology in 50–60%; retardation in fibrosis in 20–30%; and prevention of progression to cirrhosis. HBeAg responses can occur even in subgroups who are resistant to IFN (e.g., those with high-level HBV DNA) or who failed in the past to respond to it. As is true for IFN therapy of chronic hepatitis B, patients with near-normal ALT activity tend not to experience HBeAg responses (despite suppression of HBV DNA), and those with ALT levels exceeding five times the upper limit of normal can expect 1-year HBeAg seroconversion rates of 50–60%. Generally, HBeAg seroconversions are confined to patients who achieve suppression of HBV DNA to <10^4 genomes/mL. Among patients who undergo HBeAg responses during a year-long course of therapy and in whom the response is sustained for 4–6 months after cessation of therapy, the response is durable thereafter in the vast majority, >80%; therefore, the achievement of an HBeAg response represents a viable stopping point in therapy. Reduced durability has been reported in some Asian experiences; however, in most western and Asian patient study populations, long-term durability of HBeAg responses is the rule, which, at least in western patients, is accompanied by a posttreatment HBsAg seroconversion rate comparable to that seen after IFN-induced HBeAg responses. To support the durability of HBeAg responses, patients receive a period of consolidation therapy (at least 6 months in western patients, at least 1 year in Asian patients) after HBeAg seroconversion; close posttreatment monitoring is necessary to identify HBV reactivation promptly and to resume therapy. If HBeAg is unaffected by lamivudine therapy, the current approach is to continue therapy until an HBeAg response occurs, but long-term therapy may be required to suppress HBV replication and, in turn, limit liver injury; HBeAg seroconversions can increase to a level of 50% after 5 years of therapy. Histologic improvement continues to accrue with therapy beyond the first year; after a cumulative course of 3 years of lamivudine therapy, necroinflammatory activity is reduced in the majority of patients, and even cirrhosis has been shown to regress to precirrhotic stages.

Losses of HBsAg have been few during the first year of lamivudine therapy, and this observation had been cited as an advantage of IFN-based over lamivudine therapy; however, in head-to-head comparisons between standard IFN and lamivudine monotherapy, HBsAg losses were rare in both groups. Trials in which lamivudine and IFN were administered in combination failed to show a benefit of combination therapy over lamivudine monotherapy for either treatment-naïve patients or prior IFN nonresponders.

In patients with *HBeAg-negative chronic hepatitis B* (i.e., in those with precore and core-promoter HBV mutations), 1 year of lamivudine therapy results in HBV DNA suppression and normalization of ALT in three-quarters of patients and in histologic improvement in approximately two-thirds. Therapy has been shown to suppress HBV DNA by approximately 4.5 $\log_{10}$ copies/mL (baseline HBV DNA levels are lower than in patients with HBeAg-reactive hepatitis B) and to undetectable levels in approximately 70%, as measured by sensitive PCR amplification assays. Lacking HBeAg at the outset, patients with HBeAg-negative chronic hepatitis B cannot achieve an HBeAg response—a stopping point in HBeAg-reactive patients; almost invariably, when therapy is discontinued, reactivation is the rule. Therefore, these patients require long-term therapy; with successive years, the proportion with suppressed HBV DNA and normal ALT increases.

Clinical and laboratory side effects of lamivudine are negligible, indistinguishable from those observed in placebo recipients. Still, lamivudine doses should be reduced in patients with reduced creatinine clearance. During lamivudine therapy, transient ALT elevations, resembling those seen during IFN therapy and during spontaneous HBeAg-to-anti-HBe seroconversions, occur in one-fourth of patients. These ALT elevations may result from restored cytolytic T cell activation permitted by suppression of HBV replication. Similar ALT elevations, however, occur at an identical frequency in placebo recipients, but ALT elevations associated with HBeAg seroconversion are confined to lamivudine-treated patients. When therapy is stopped after a year of therapy, two- to threefold ALT elevations occur in 20–30% of lamivudine-treated patients, representing renewed liver-cell injury as HBV replication returns. Although these posttreatment flares are almost always transient and mild, rare severe exacerbations, especially in cirrhotic patients, have been observed, mandating close and careful clinical and virologic monitoring after discontinuation of treatment. Many authorities caution against discontinuing therapy in patients with cirrhosis, in whom posttreatment flares could precipitate decompensation.

Long-term monotherapy with lamivudine is associated with methionine-to-valine (M204V) or methionine-to-isoleucine (M204I) mutations, primarily at amino acid 204 in the tyrosine-methionine-aspartate-aspartate (YMDD) motif of HBV DNA polymerase, analogous to mutations that occur in HIV-infected patients treated with this drug. During a year of therapy, YMDD mutations occur in 15–30% of patients; the frequency increases with each year of therapy, reaching 70% at year 5. Ultimately, patients with YMDD mutants experience degradation of clinical, biochemical, and histologic responses; therefore, if treatment is begun with lamivudine monotherapy, the emergence of lamivudine resistance, reflected clinically by a breakthrough from suppressed levels of HBV DNA and ALT, is managed by adding another antiviral to which YMDD variants are sensitive (e.g., adefovir, tenofovir; see below).

Currently, although lamivudine is very safe and still used widely in other parts of the world, in the United States and Europe, lamivudine has been eclipsed by more potent antivirals that have superior resistance profiles (see below). Still, as the first successful oral antiviral agent for use in hepatitis B, lamivudine has provided proof of the concept that polymerase inhibitors can achieve virologic, serologic, biochemical, and histologic benefits. In addition, lamivudine has been shown to be effective in the treatment of patients with decompensated hepatitis B (for whom IFN is contraindicated), in some of whom decompensation can be reversed. Moreover, among patients with cirrhosis or advanced fibrosis, lamivudine has been shown to be effective in reducing the risk of progression to hepatic decompensation and, marginally, the risk of HCC.

Because lamivudine monotherapy can result universally in the rapid emergence of YMDD variants in persons with HIV infection, patients with chronic hepatitis B should be tested for anti-HIV prior to therapy; if HIV infection is identified, lamivudine monotherapy at the HBV daily dose of 100 mg is contraindicated. These patients should be treated for both HIV and HBV with an HIV drug regimen that includes or is supplemented by at least two drugs active against HBV; highly active antiretroviral therapy (HAART) often contains two drugs with antiviral activity against HBV (e.g., tenofovir and emtricitabine), but if lamivudine is part of the regimen, the daily dose should be 300 mg (Chap. 189). The safety of lamivudine during pregnancy has not been established; however, the drug is not teratogenic in rodents and has been used safely in pregnant women with HIV infection and with HBV infection. Limited data even suggest that administration of lamivudine during the last months of pregnancy to mothers with high-level hepatitis B viremia ($\geq 10^8$ IU/ml) can reduce the likelihood of perinatal transmission of hepatitis B.

ADEFOVIR DIPIVOXIL At an oral daily dose of 10 mg, the acyclic nucleotide analogue adefovir dipivoxil, the prodrug of adefovir, reduces HBV DNA by approximately 3.5–4 $\log_{10}$ copies/mL and is equally effective in treatment-naïve patients and IFN nonresponders. In HBeAg-reactive chronic hepatitis B, a 48-week course of adefovir dipivoxil was shown to achieve histologic improvement (and reduce the progression of fibrosis) and normalization of ALT in just over one-half of patients, HBeAg seroconversion in 12%, HBeAg loss in 23%, and suppression to an undetectable level of HBV DNA in 13–21%, as measured by PCR. Similar to IFN and lamivudine, adefovir dipivoxil is more likely to achieve an HBeAg response in patients with high baseline ALT (e.g., among adefovir-treated patients with ALT level >5 times the upper limit of normal), HBeAg seroconversions occurred in 25%. The durability of adefovir-induced HBeAg responses is high (91% in one study); therefore, HBeAg response can be relied upon as a stopping point for adefovir therapy, after a period of consolidation therapy, as outlined above. Although data on the impact of additional therapy beyond 1 year are limited, biochemical, serologic, and virologic outcomes improve progressively as therapy is continued.

In patients with *HBeAg-negative chronic hepatitis B*, a 48-week course of 10 mg/d of adefovir dipivoxil resulted in histologic improvement in two-thirds, normalization of ALT in three-fourths, and suppression of HBV DNA to PCR-undetectable levels in one-half to two-thirds. As was true for lamivudine, because HBeAg responses—a potential stopping point—cannot be achieved in this group, reactivation is the rule when adefovir therapy is discontinued, and indefinite, long-term therapy is required. Treatment beyond the first year consolidates the gain of the first year; after 5 years of therapy, improvement in hepatic inflammation and regression of fibrosis was observed in three-fourths of patients, ALT was normal in 70%, and HBV DNA was undetectable in almost 70%.

Adefovir contains a flexible acyclic linker instead of the L-nucleoside ring of lamivudine, avoiding steric hindrance by mutated amino acids. In addition, the molecular structure of phosphorylated adefovir is very similar to that of its natural substrate; therefore mutations to adefovir would also affect binding of the natural substrate, dATP. Hypothetically, these are among the reasons that resistance to adefovir dipivoxil is much less likely than resistance to lamivudine; no resistance was encountered in 1 year of clinical-trial therapy. In subsequent years, however, adefovir resistance begins to emerge [asparagine to threonine at amino acid 236 (N236T) and alanine to valine or threonine at amino acid 181 (A181V/T), primarily], occurring in 2.5% after 2 years, but in 29% after 5 years of therapy (reported in HBeAg-negative patients). Among patients co-infected with HBV and HIV and who have normal CD4+ T cell counts, adefovir dipivoxil is effective in suppressing HBV dramatically (by 5 $\log_{10}$ in one study). Moreover, adefovir dipivoxil is effective in lamivudine-resistant, YMDD-mutant HBV and can be used when such lamivudine-induced variants emerge. When lamivudine resistance occurs, adding adefovir (i.e., maintaining lamivudine to preempt the emergence of adefovir resistance), is superior to switching to adefovir. Almost invariably, patients with adefovir-mutant HBV respond to lamivudine (or newer agents, such as entecavir, see below). When, in the past, adefovir had been evaluated as therapy for HIV infection, doses of 60–120 mg were required to suppress HIV, and, at these doses, the drug was nephrotoxic. Even at 30 mg/d, creatinine elevations of 44 μmol/L (0.5 mg/dL) occur in 10% of patients; however, at the HBV-effective dose of 10 mg, such elevations of creatinine are rarely encountered. If any nephrotoxicity does occur, it rarely appears before 6–8 months of therapy. Although renal tubular injury is a rare potential side effect, and although creatinine monitoring is recommended during treatment, the therapeutic index of adefovir dipivoxil is high, and the nephrotoxicity observed in clinical trials at higher doses was reversible. For patients with underlying renal disease, frequency of administration of adefovir dipivoxil should be reduced to every 48 h for creatinine clearances of 20–49 mL/min; to every 72 h for creatinine clearances of 10–19 mL/min; and once a week, following dialysis, for patients undergoing hemodialysis. Adefovir dipivoxil is very well tolerated, and ALT elevations during and after withdrawal of therapy are similar to those observed and described above in clinical trials of lamivudine. An advantage of adefovir is its relatively favorable resistance profile; however, it is not as potent as the other approved oral agents, it does not suppress HBV DNA as rapidly or as uniformly as the others, it is the least likely of all agents to result in HBeAg seroconversion, and 20–50% of patients fail to suppress HBV DNA by 2 $\log_{10}$ ("primary nonresponders"). For these reasons, adefovir has been supplanted in both treatment-naïve and lamivudine-resistant patients by the more potent, less resistance-prone nucleotide analogue tenofovir (see below).

PEGYLATED INTERFERON After long-acting PEG IFN was shown to be effective in the treatment of hepatitis C (see below), this more convenient drug was evaluated in the treatment of chronic hepatitis B. Once-a-week PEG IFN is more effective than the more frequently administered, standard IFN, and several large-scale trials of PEG IFN versus oral nucleoside analogues have been conducted among patients with HBeAg-reactive and HBeAg-negative chronic hepatitis B.

In HBeAg-reactive chronic hepatitis B, two large-scale studies were done, one with PEG IFN-α 2b (100 μg weekly for 32 weeks, then 50 μg weekly for another 20 weeks for a total of 52 weeks, with a comparison arm of combination PEG IFN with oral lamivudine) in 307 subjects; the other involved PEG IFN-α 2a (180 μg weekly for 48 weeks) in 814 primarily Asian patients, three-fourths of whom had ALT ≥2 × the upper limit of normal, with comparison arms of lamivudine monotherapy and combination PEG IFN plus lamivudine. At the end of therapy (48–52 weeks) in the PEG IFN monotherapy arms, HBeAg loss occurred in approximately 30%, HBeAg seroconversion in 22–27%, undetectable HBV DNA (<400 copies/mL by PCR) in 10–25%, normal ALT in 34–39%, and a mean reduction in HBV DNA of 2 $\log_{10}$ copies/mL (PEG IFN-α 2b) to 4.5 $\log_{10}$ copies/mL (PEG IFN-α 2a). Six months after completing PEG IFN monotherapy in these trials, HBeAg losses were present in approximately 35%, HBeAg seroconversion in approximately 30%, undetectable HBV DNA in 7–14%, normal ALT in 32–41%, and a mean reduction in HBV DNA of 2–2.4 $\log_{10}$ copies/mL. Although the combination of PEG IFN and lamivudine was superior at the end of therapy in one or more serologic, virologic, or biochemical outcomes, neither the combination arm (in both studies) nor the lamivudine monotherapy arm (in the PEG IFN-α 2a trial) demonstrated any benefit compared to the PEG IFN monotherapy arms 6 months after therapy. Moreover, HBsAg seroconversion occurred in 3–7% of PEG IFN recipients (with or without lamivudine); some of these seroconversions were identified by the end of therapy, but many were identified during the posttreatment follow-up period. The likelihood of HBeAg loss in PEG IFN–treated HBeAg-reactive patients is associated with HBV genotype A > B > C > D (shown for PEG IFN α-2b but not for α-2a).

Based on these results, some authorities concluded that PEG IFN monotherapy should be the first-line therapy of choice in HBeAg-reactive chronic hepatitis B; however, this conclusion has been challenged. Although a finite, 1-year course of PEG IFN results in a higher rate of sustained response (6 months after treatment) than is achieved with oral nucleoside/nucleotide analogue therapy, the comparison is confounded by the fact that oral agents are not discontinued at the end of 1 year. Instead, taken orally and free of side effects, therapy with oral agents is extended indefinitely or until after the occurrence of an HBeAg response. The rate of HBeAg responses after 2 years of oral-agent nucleoside analogue therapy is at least as high as, if not higher than, that achieved with PEG IFN after 1 year; favoring oral agents is the absence of injections and difficult-to-tolerate side effects as well as lower direct and indirect medical costs and inconvenience. The association of HBsAg responses with PEG IFN therapy occurs in such a small proportion of patients that subjecting everyone to PEG IFN for the marginal gain of HBsAg responses during or immediately after therapy in such a very small minority is questionable. Moreover, HBsAg responses occur in a comparable proportion of patients treated with early-generation nucleoside/nucleotide analogues in the years after therapy, and, with the newer, more potent nucleoside analogues, the frequency of HBsAg loss during the first year of therapy equals that of PEG IFN and is exceeded during year 2 (see below). Of course, resistance is not an issue during PEG IFN therapy, but the risk of resistance is much lower with new agents (≤1% up to 3–5 years in previously treatment-naïve, entecavir-treated and tenofovir-treated patients; see below). Finally, the level of HBV DNA inhibition that can be achieved with the newer agents, and even with lamivudine, exceeds that which can be achieved with PEG IFN, in some cases by several orders of magnitude.

In HBeAg-negative chronic hepatitis B, a trial of PEG IFN-α 2a (180 μg weekly for 48 weeks versus comparison arms of lamivudine monotherapy and of combination therapy) in 564 patients showed that PEG IFN monotherapy resulted at the end of therapy in suppression of HBV DNA by a mean of 4.1 $\log_{10}$ copies/mL, undetectable HBV DNA (<400 copies/mL by PCR) in 63%, normal ALT in 38%, and loss of HBsAg in 4%. Although lamivudine monotherapy and combination lamivudine–PEG IFN therapy were both superior to PEG IFN at the end of therapy, no advantage of lamivudine monotherapy or combination therapy was apparent over PEG IFN monotherapy 6 months after therapy—suppression of HBV DNA by a mean of 2.3 $\log_{10}$ copies/mL, undetectable HBV DNA in 19%, and normal ALT in 59%. In subjects involved in this trial followed for up to 5 years, among the two-thirds followed who had been treated initially with PEG IFN, 17% maintained HBV DNA suppression to <400 copies/ml, but ALT remained normal in only 22%; HBsAg loss increased gradually to 12%. Among the half followed who had been treated initially with lamivudine monotherapy, HBV DNA remained <400 copies/ml in 7% and ALT normal in 16%; by year 5, 3.5% had lost HBsAg. As was the case for standard IFN therapy in HBeAg-negative patients, longer after PEG IFN treatment, although a small subset maintained their responses, the proportion who benefited was very small, raising questions about the relative value of a finite period of PEG IFN, versus a longer course with a potent, low-resistance oral nucleoside analogue in these patients.

ENTECAVIR Entecavir, an oral cyclopentyl guanosine analogue polymerase inhibitor, appears to be the most potent of the HBV antivirals and is just as well tolerated as lamivudine. In a 709-subject clinical trial among HBeAg-reactive patients, oral entecavir, 0.5 mg daily, was compared to lamivudine, 100 mg daily. At 48 weeks, entecavir was superior to lamivudine in suppression of HBV DNA, mean 6.9 versus 5.5 $\log_{10}$ copies/mL and in percent with undetectable HBV DNA (<300 copies/mL by PCR), 67% versus 36%; histologic improvement (≥2-point improvement in necroinflammatory HAI score), 72% versus 62%; and normal ALT (68% versus 60%). The two treatments were indistinguishable in percent with HBeAg loss (22% versus 20%) and seroconversion (21% versus 18%). Among patients treated with entecavir for 96 weeks, HBV DNA was undetectable cumulatively in 80% (versus 39% for lamivudine), and HBeAg seroconversions had occurred in 31% (versus 26% for lamivudine); the HBeAg seroconversion rate after 3 years of entecavir in this cohort was 39%. Similarly, in a 638-subject clinical trial among HBeAg-negative patients, at week 48, oral entecavir, 0.5 mg daily, was superior to lamivudine, 100 mg daily, in suppression of HBV DNA, mean 5.0 versus 4.5 $\log_{10}$ copies/mL and in percent with undetectable HBV DNA, 90% versus 72%; histologic improvement, 70% versus 61% and normal ALT, 78% versus 71%. No resistance mutations were encountered in previously treatment-naïve, entecavir-treated patients during 96 weeks of therapy, and in a cohort of subjects treated for up to 5 years, resistance emerged in 1.2%. Its high barrier to resistance coupled with its high potency renders entecavir a first-line drug for patients with chronic hepatitis B.

Entecavir is also effective against lamivudine-resistant HBV infection. In a trial of 286 lamivudine-resistant patients, entecavir, at a higher daily dose of 1 mg, was superior to lamivudine, as measured at week 48, in achieving suppression of HBV DNA (mean 5.1 versus 0.48 $\log_{10}$ copies/mL); undetectable HBV DNA, in 72% versus 19%; normal ALT, in 61% versus 15%; HBeAg loss, in 10% versus 3%; and HBeAg seroconversion, in 8% versus 3%. In this population of lamivudine-experienced patients, however, entecavir resistance emerged in 7% at 48 weeks. Although entecavir resistance requires both a YMDD mutation and a second mutation at one of several other sites (e.g., T184A, S202G/I, or M250V), resistance to entecavir in lamivudine-resistant chronic hepatitis B has been recorded to increase progressively to 43% at 4 years; therefore, entecavir is not as attractive a choice as adefovir or tenofovir for patients with lamivudine-resistant hepatitis B.

At the end of 2 years of entecavir therapy in clinical trials among HBeAg-reactive patients, HBsAg seroconversion was observed in 5% (≤2% during the first year). In addition, on-treatment and posttreatment ALT flares are relatively uncommon and relatively mild in entecavir-treated patients. In clinical trials, entecavir has had an excellent safety profile; doses should be reduced for patients with reduced creatinine clearance. Entecavir does have low-level antiviral activity against HIV and cannot be used as monotherapy to treat HBV infection in HIV-HBV co-infected persons.

TELBIVUDINE Telbivudine, a cytosine analogue, appears to be similar in efficacy to entecavir; however, it is slightly less potent in suppressing HBV DNA (a slightly more profound median 6.4 $\log_{10}$ reduction in HBeAg-reactive disease, a similar 5.2 $\log_{10}$ reduction in HBeAg-negative disease). In its registration trial, telbivudine at an oral daily dose of 600 mg suppressed HBV DNA to <300 copies/ml in 60% of HBeAg-positive and 88% of HBeAg-negative patients, reduced ALT to normal in 77% of HBeAg-positive and 74% of HBeAg-negative patients, and improved histology in 65% of HBeAg-positive and 67% HBeAg-negative patients. Although resistance to telbivudine (M204I, not M204V mutations) was less frequent than resistance to lamivudine at the end of 1 year, resistance mutations after 2 years of treatment occurred in up to 22%. Generally well tolerated, telbivudine has been associated with a low frequency of asymptomatic creatine kinase elevations and with a very low frequency of peripheral neuropathy; frequency of administration should be reduced for patients with impaired creatinine clearance. Its excellent potency notwithstanding, the inferior resistance profile of telbivudine has limited its appeal; telbivudine is neither recommended as first-line therapy nor widely used.

TENOFOVIR Tenofovir disoproxil fumarate, an acyclic nucleotide analogue and potent antiretroviral agent used to treat HIV infection, is similar to adefovir but more potent in suppressing HBV DNA and inducing HBeAg responses; it is highly active against both wild-type and lamivudine-resistant HBV and active in patients whose response to adefovir is slow and/or limited. At an oral once-daily dose of 300 mg for 48 weeks, tenofovir suppressed HBV DNA by 6.2 $\log_{10}$ [to undetectable levels (<400 copies/ml) in 76%] in HBeAg-positive and 4.6 $\log_{10}$ (to undetectable levels in 93%) in HBeAg-negative patients; reduced ALT to normal in 68% of HBeAg-positive and 76% of HBeAg-negative patients; and improved histology in 74% of HBeAg-positive and 72% of HBeAg-negative patients. In HBeAg-positive patients, HBeAg seroconversions occurred in 21% by the end of year 1 and in 27% by the end of year 2 of tenofovir treatment; HBsAg loss occurred in 3% by the end of year 1 and 6% by the end of year 2. The safety (negligible renal toxicity and mild reduction in bone density) and resistance profile (none recorded through 3 years) of tenofovir are very favorable as well; therefore, tenofovir has supplanted adefovir both as first-line therapy for chronic hepatitis B and as add-on therapy for lamivudine-resistant chronic hepatitis B. Frequency of tenofovir administration should be reduced for patients with impaired creatinine clearance.

A comparison of the six antiviral therapies in current use appears in Table 306-3; their relative potencies in suppressing HBV DNA are shown in Fig. 306-1.

COMBINATION THERAPY Although the combination of lamivudine and PEG IFN suppresses HBV DNA more profoundly

TABLE 306-3 Comparison of Pegylated Interferon (PEG IFN), Lamivudine, Adefovir, Entecavir, Telbivudine, and Tenofovir Therapy for Chronic Hepatitis B[a]

Feature	PEG IFN[b]	Lamivudine	Adefovir	Entecavir	Telbivudine	Tenofovir
Route of administration	Subcutaneous Injection	Oral	Oral	Oral	Oral	Oral
Duration of therapy[c]	48–52 weeks	≥52 weeks	≥48 weeks	≥48 weeks	≥52 weeks	≥48 weeks
Tolerability	Poorly tolerated	Well tolerated	Well tolerated; creatinine monitoring recommended	Well tolerated	Well tolerated	Well tolerated creatinine monitoring recommended
HBeAg seroconversion						
1 yr Rx	18–20%	16–21%	12%	21%	22%	21%
>1 yr Rx	NA	up to 50% @ 5 yrs	43% @ 3 yrs[d]	31% @ 2 yrs 39% @ 3 yrs	30% @ 2 yrs	27% @ 2 yrs
Log_{10} HBV DNA reduction (mean copies/ml)						
HBeAg-reactive	4.5	5.5	median 3.5–5	6.9	6.4	6.2
HBeAg-negative	4.1	4.4–4.7	median 3.5–3.9	5.0	5.2	4.6
HBV DNA PCR negative (<300–400 copies/ml; <1,000 copies/ml for adefovir) end of yr 1						
HBeAg-reactive	10–25%	36–44%	13–21%	67% (91% @ 4 yrs)	60%	76%
HBeAg-negative	63%	60–73%	48–77%	90%	88%	93%
ALT normalization at end of yr 1						
HBeAg-reactive	39%	41–75%	48–61%	68%	77%	68%
HBeAg-negative	34–38%	62–79%	48–77%	78%	74%	76%
HBsAg loss yr 1	3–4%	≤1%	0%	2%	<1%	3%
yr 2	12% 5 yr after 1 yr of Rx	no data	5% at yr 5	5%	no data	6%
Histologic improvement (≥2 point reduction in HAI) at yr 1						
HBeAg-reactive	38% 6 months after	49–62%	53–68%	72%	65%	74%
HBeAg-negative	48% 6 months after	61–66%	64%	70%	67%	72%
Viral resistance	None	15-30% @ 1 yr 70% @ 5 yrs	None @ 1 yr 29% at 5 yrs	≤1% @ 1 yr[e] 1.2% @ 5 yr[e]	up to 5% @ yr 1 up to 22% @ yr 2	0% @ yr 1 0% through yr 3
Cost (US$) for 1 yr	~$18,000	~$2,500	~$6,500	~$8,700[f]	~$6,000	~$6,000

[a]Generally, these comparisons are based on data on each drug tested individually versus placebo in registration clinical trials; because, with rare exception, these comparisons are not based on head-to-head testing of these drugs, relative advantages and disadvantages should be interpreted cautiously.

[b]Although standard interferon α administered daily or three times a week is approved as therapy for chronic hepatitis B, it has been supplanted by PEG IFN, which is administered once a week and is more effective. Standard interferon has no advantages over PEG IFN.

[c]Duration of therapy in clinical efficacy trials; use in clinical practice may vary.

[d]Because of a computer-generated randomization error that resulted in misallocation of drug versus placebo during the second year of clinical-trial treatment, the frequency of HBeAg seroconversion beyond the first year is an estimate (Kaplan-Meier analysis) based on the small subset in whom adefovir was administered correctly.

[e]7% during a year of therapy (43% at year 4) in lamivudine-resistant patients.

[f]~17,400 for lamivudine-refractory patients.

Abbreviations: ALT, alanine aminotransferase; HAI, histologic activity index; HBeAg, hepatitis B e antigen; HBsAg, hepatitis B surface antigen; HBV, hepatitis B virus; NA, not applicable; PEG IFN, pegylated interferon; PCR, polymerase chain reaction; Rx, therapy; yr, year.

during therapy than does monotherapy with either drug alone (and is much less likely to be associated with lamivudine resistance), this combination used for a year is no better than a year of PEG IFN in achieving sustained responses. To date, combinations of oral nucleoside/nucleotide agents have not achieved an enhancement in virologic, serologic, or biochemical efficacy over that achieved by the more potent of the combined drugs given individually. On the other hand, combining agents that are not cross-resistant (e.g., lamivudine and adefovir or tenofovir) has the potential to reduce the risk or perhaps even to

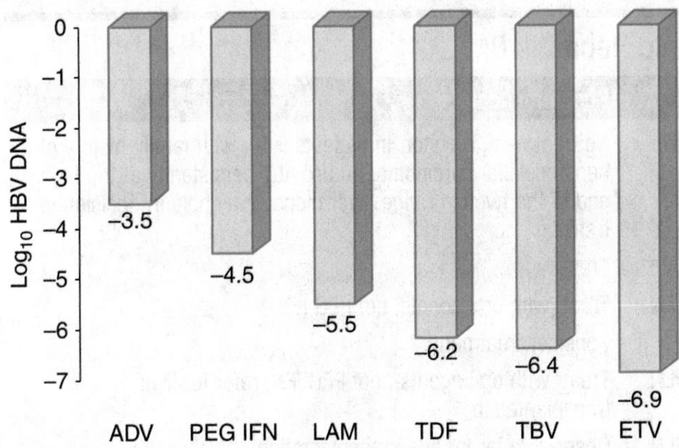

Figure 306-1 Relative potency of antiviral drugs for hepatitis B, as reflected by median $\log_{10}$ HBV DNA reduction in HBeAg-positive chronic hepatitis B. These data are from individual reports of large, randomized controlled registration trials that were the basis for approval of the drugs. In most instances, these data do not represent direct comparisons among the drugs, because study populations were different, baseline patient variables were not always uniform, and the sensitivity and dynamic range of the HBV DNA assays used in the trials varied. ADV, adefovir dipivoxil; PEG IFN, pegylated interferon α-2a; LAM, lamivudine; TDF, tenofovir disoproxil fumarate; TBV, telbivudine; ETV, entecavir.

preempt entirely the emergence of drug resistance. In the future, the treatment paradigm may shift from the current approach of sequential monotherapy to preemptive combination therapy; however, designing and executing clinical trials that demonstrate superior efficacy and resistance profile of combination therapy over monotherapy with entecavir or tenofovir will be very challenging.

NOVEL ANTIVIRALS AND STRATEGIES In addition to the seven approved antiviral drugs for hepatitis B, emtricitabine, a fluorinated cytosine analogue very similar to lamivudine in structure, efficacy, and resistance profile, offers no advantage over lamivudine. A combination of emtricitabine and tenofovir is approved for the treatment of HIV infection and is an appealing combination therapy for hepatitis B; however, neither emtricitabine nor the combination are approved yet for hepatitis B. Several initially promising antiviral agents have been abandoned because of toxicity (e.g., clevudine, which was linked to myopathy during its clinical development). Because direct-acting antivirals have been so successful in the management of chronic hepatitis B, more unconventional approaches—e.g., immunologic or genetic manipulation—are not likely to be competitive. Finally, initial emphasis in the development of antiviral therapy for hepatitis B was placed on monotherapy; whether combination regimens will yield additive or synergistic efficacy remains to be determined).

TREATMENT RECOMMENDATIONS Several learned societies and groups of expert physicians have issued treatment recommendations for patients with chronic hepatitis B; the most authoritative and updated (and free of financial support by pharmaceutical companies) are those of the American Association for the Study of Liver Diseases (AASLD) and of the European Association for the Study of the Liver (EASL). Although the recommendations differ slightly, a consensus has emerged on most of the important points (Table 306-4). No treatment is recommended or available for inactive "nonreplicative" hepatitis B carriers (undetectable HBeAg with normal ALT and HBV DNA $\leq 10^3$ IU/ml documented serially over time). In patients with detectable HBeAg and HBV DNA levels $>2 \times 10^4$ IU/ml, treatment is recommended by the AASLD for those with ALT levels above 2 × the upper limit of normal. (The EASL recommends treatment in HBeAg-positive patients for HBV DNA levels $>2 \times 10^3$ IU/ml and ALT above the upper limit of normal.) For HBeAg-positive patients with ALT ≤2 × the upper limit of normal, in whom sustained responses are not likely and who would require multiyear therapy, antiviral therapy is not recommended currently. This pattern is common during the early decades of life among Asian patients infected at birth; even in this group, therapy would be considered for those >40 years of age, ALT persistently at the high end of the twofold range, and/or with a family history of hepatocellular carcinoma, especially if the liver biopsy shows moderate to severe necroinflammatory activity or fibrosis. In this group, when, eventually, ALT becomes elevated later in life, antiviral therapy should be instituted. For patients with HBeAg-negative chronic hepatitis B, ALT >2 × the upper limit of normal (above the upper limit of normal according to EASL) and HBV DNA $>2 \times 10^3$ IU/ml, antiviral therapy is recommended. If HBV DNA is $>2 \times 10^3$ IU/ml and ALT is 1 to >2 × the upper limit of normal, liver biopsy should be considered to help in arriving at a decision to treat if substantial liver injury is present (treatment in this subset would be recommended according to EASL guidelines, because ALT is elevated).

For patients with compensated cirrhosis, because antiviral therapy has been shown to retard clinical progression, treatment is recommended regardless of HBeAg status and ALT as long as HBV DNA is detectable at $>2 \times 10^3$ IU/ml (detectable at any level according to the EASL); monitoring without therapy is recommended for those with HBV DNA $<2 \times 10^3$ IU/ml, unless ALT is elevated. For patients with decompensated cirrhosis, treatment is recommended regardless of serologic and biochemical status, as long as HBV DNA is detectable. Patients with decompensated cirrhosis should be evaluated as candidates for liver transplantation.

Among the seven available drugs for hepatitis B, PEG IFN has supplanted standard IFN, entecavir has supplanted lamivudine, and tenofovir has supplanted adefovir. PEG IFN, entecavir, or tenofovir are recommended as first-line therapy (Table 306-3). PEG IFN requires finite-duration therapy, achieves the highest rate of HBeAg responses after a year of therapy, and does not support viral mutations, but it requires subcutaneous injections and is associated with inconvenience and intolerability. Oral nucleoside analogues require long-term therapy in most patients, and when used alone, lamivudine and telbivudine foster the emergence of viral mutations, adefovir somewhat less so, and entecavir (except in lamivudine-experienced patients) and tenofovir rarely at all. Oral agents do not require injections, are very well tolerated, lead to improved histology in 50–90% of patients, suppress HBV DNA more profoundly than PEG IFN, and are effective even in patients who fail to respond to IFN-based therapy. Although oral agents are less likely to result in HBeAg responses during the first year of therapy, as compared to PEG IFN, treatment with oral agents tends to be extended beyond the first year and, by the end of the second year, yields HBeAg responses (and even HBsAg responses) comparable in frequency to those achieved after 1 year of PEG IFN (and without the associated side effects) (Table 306-5). Although adefovir and tenofovir are safe, creatinine monitoring is recommended. Substantial experience with lamivudine during pregnancy (see above) has identified no teratogenicity. Although interferons

TABLE 306-4 Recommendations for Treatment of Chronic Hepatitis B[a]

HBeAg status	Clinical	HBV DNA (IU/ml)	ALT	Recommendation
HBeAg-reactive	[b]	$>2 \times 10^4$	$\leq 2 \times$ ULN[c]	No treatment; monitor. In patients >40, with family history of hepatocellular carcinoma, and/or ALT persistently at the high end of the twofold range, liver biopsy may help in decision to treat
	Chronic hepatitis	$>2 \times 10^4$ [d]	$>2 \times$ ULN [d]	Treat[e]
	Cirrhosis compensated	$>2 \times 10^3$	< or > ULN	Treat[e] with oral agents, not PEG IFN
		$<2 \times 10^3$	>ULN	Consider treatment[f]
	Cirrhosis decompensated	Detectable	< or > ULN	Treat[e] with oral agents[g], not PEG IFN; refer for liver transplantation
		Undetectable	< or > ULN	Observe; refer for liver transplantation
HBeAg-negative	[b]	$\leq 2 \times 10^3$	≤ULN	Inactive carrier; treatment not necessary
	Chronic hepatitis	$>10^3$	$1\text{->}2 \times$ ULN[d]	Consider liver biopsy; treat[h] if biopsy shows moderate to severe inflammation or fibrosis
	Chronic hepatitis	$>10^4$	$>2 \times$ ULN[d]	Treat[h,i]
	Cirrhosis compensated	$>2 \times 10^3$	< or > ULN	Treat[e] with oral agents, not PEG IFN
		$<2 \times 10^3$	>ULN	Consider treatment[f]
	Cirrhosis decompensated	Detectable	< or > ULN	Treat[h] with oral agents[g], not PEG IFN; refer for liver transplantation
		Undetectable	< or > ULN	Observe; refer for liver transplantation

[a]Based on practice guidelines of the American Association for the Study of Liver Diseases (AASLD). Except as indicated in footnotes, these guidelines are similar to those issued by the European Association for the Study of the Liver (EASL).

[b]Liver disease tends to be mild or inactive clinically; most such patients do not undergo liver biopsy.

[c]This pattern is common during early decades of life in Asian patients infected at birth.

[d]According to the EASL guidelines, treat if HBV DNA is $>2 \times 10^3$ IU/ml and ALT >ULN.

[e]One of the potent oral drugs with a high barrier to resistance (entecavir or tenofovir) or PEG IFN can be used as first-line therapy (see text). These oral agents, but not PEG IFN, should be used for interferon-refractory/intolerant and immunocompromised patients. PEG IFN is administered weekly by subcutaneous injection for a year; the oral agents are administered daily for at least a year and continued indefinitely or until at least 6 months after HBeAg seroconversion.

[f]According to EASL guidelines, patients with compensated cirrhosis and detectable HBV DNA at any level, even with normal ALT, are candidates for therapy. Most authorities would treat indefinitely, even in HBeAg-positive disease after HBeAg seroconversion.

[g]Because the emergence of resistance can lead to loss of antiviral benefit and further deterioration in decompensated cirrhosis, a low-resistance regimen is recommended—entecavir or tenofovir monotherapy or combination therapy with the more resistance-prone lamivudine (or telbivudine) plus adefovir. Therapy should be instituted urgently.

[h]Because HBeAg seroconversion is not an option, the goal of therapy is to suppress HBV DNA and maintain a normal ALT. PEG IFN is administered by subcutaneous injection weekly for a year; caution is warranted in relying on a 6-month posttreatment interval to define a sustained response, because the majority of such responses are lost thereafter. Oral agents, entecavir or tenofovir, are administered daily, usually indefinitely or, until as very rarely occurs, virologic and biochemical responses are accompanied by HBsAg seroconversion.

[i]For older patients and those with advanced fibrosis, consider lowering the HBV DNA threshold to $>2 \times 10^3$ IU/ml.

Abbreviations: ALT, alanine aminotransferase; AASLD, American Association for the Study of Liver Diseases; EASL, European Association for the Study of the Liver; HBeAg, hepatitis B e antigen; HBsAg, hepatitis B surface antigen; HBV, hepatitis B virus; PEG IFN, pegylated interferon; ULN, upper limits of normal.

do not appear to cause congenital anomalies, interferons have antiproliferative properties and should not be used during pregnancy. Adefovir during pregnancy has not been associated with birth defects; however, there may be an increased risk of spontaneous abortion. Data on the safety of entecavir during pregnancy have not been published. Sufficient data in animals and limited data in humans suggest that telbivudine and tenofovir can be used safely during pregnancy. In general, except perhaps for lamivudine, and until additional data become available, the other antivirals for hepatitis B should be avoided or used with extreme caution during pregnancy.

As noted above, some physicians prefer to begin with PEG IFN, while other physicians and patients prefer oral agents as first-line therapy. For patients with decompensated cirrhosis, the emergence of resistance can result in further deterioration and loss of antiviral effectiveness. Therefore, in this patient subset, the threshold for relying on therapy with a very favorable resistance profile (e.g., entecavir or tenofovir) or on combination therapy (e.g., lamivudine or telbivudine with adefovir) is low. PEG IFN should not be used in patients with compensated or decompensated cirrhosis.

For patients with end-stage chronic hepatitis B who undergo liver transplantation, reinfection of the new liver is almost universal in the absence of antiviral therapy. The majority of patients become high-level viremic carriers with minimal liver injury. Before the availability of antiviral therapy, an unpredictable proportion experienced severe hepatitis B–related liver injury, sometimes a fulminant-like hepatitis, sometimes a rapid recapitulation of the original severe chronic hepatitis B (Chap. 304). Currently, however, prevention of recurrent hepatitis B after liver transplantation has been achieved definitively by *combining* hepatitis B immune globulin with one of the oral nucleoside or nucleotide analogues (Chap. 310).

TABLE 306-5 Pegylated Interferon Versus Oral Nucleoside Analogues for the Treatment of Chronic Hepatitis B

	PEG IFN	Nucleoside Analogues
Administration	Weekly injection	Daily, orally
Tolerability	Poorly tolerated, intensive monitoring	Well tolerated, limited monitoring
Duration of therapy	Finite 48 weeks	≥1 year, indefinite in most patients
Maximum mean HBV DNA suppression	4.5 $\log_{10}$	6.9 $\log_{10}$
Effective in high-level HBV DNA (≥10^9 IU/ml)	No	Yes
HBeAg seroconversion		
During 1 year of therapy	~30%	~20%
During >1 year of therapy	Not applicable	30% (year 2)–50% (year 5)
HBeAg-negative posttreatment HBV DNA suppression	17% @ 5 years	7% @ 4 years (lamivudine)
HBsAg loss		
During 1 year of therapy	3–4%	0–3%
During >1 year of therapy	Not applicable	3–6% @ 2 years of therapy
After 1 year of therapy–HBeAg-negative	12% @ 5 years	3.5% @ 5 years
Antiviral resistance	None	Lamivudine: ~30% year 1, ~70% year 5 Adefovir: 0% year 1, ~30% year 5 Telbivudine: up to 4% year 1, 22% year 2 Entecavir: ≤1.2% through year 5 Tenofovir: 0% through year 3
Use in cirrhosis, transplantation, immunosuppressed	No	Yes
Cost, 1 year of therapy	++++	+ to ++

Abbreviations: HBV, hepatitis B virus; HBeAg, hepatitis B e antigen; HBsAg, hepatitis B surface antigen; IU/ml, international units per milliliter; PEG IFN, pegylated interferon.

For patients treated with the more resistance-prone (lamivudine, telbivudine) or less potent (adefovir) oral agents, assessment of response at 24 weeks (48 weeks for adefovir) can identify those at high risk for inadequate response and breakthrough resistance (i.e., the presence of residual detectable viremia). When such inadequate responses are identified, a second, non-cross-resistant agent can be added or the initial agent can be replaced by a more potent agent. This "roadmap" approach has been rendered irrelevant by the use of the current generation of highly potent, low-resistant agents entecavir and tenofovir. Still, at 24 weeks, if HBV DNA exceeds 2×10^3 IU/ml, switching to a different agent or adding a second agent is advisable.

Patients with HBV-HIV co-infection can have progressive HBV-associated liver disease and, occasionally, a severe exacerbation of hepatitis B resulting from immunologic reconstitution following highly active antiretroviral therapy. Lamivudine should never be used as monotherapy in patients with HBV-HIV infection because HIV resistance emerges rapidly to both viruses. Adefovir has been used successfully to treat chronic hepatitis B in HBV-HIV co-infected patients but is no longer considered a first-line agent for HBV. Entecavir has low-level activity against HIV and can result in selection of HIV resistance; therefore, it should be avoided in HBV-HIV co-infection. Tenofovir and the combination of tenofovir and emtricitabine in one pill are approved therapies for HIV and represent excellent choices for treating HBV infection in HBV-HIV co-infected patients. Generally, even for HBV-HIV co-infected patients who do not yet meet treatment criteria for HIV infection, treating for both HBV and HIV is recommended.

Patients with chronic hepatitis B who undergo cytotoxic chemotherapy for treatment of malignancies as well as patients treated with immunosuppressive, anticytokine, or antitumor necrosis factor therapies experience enhanced HBV replication and viral expression on hepatocyte membranes during chemotherapy coupled with suppression of cellular immunity. When chemotherapy is withdrawn, such patients are at risk for reactivation of hepatitis B, often severe and occasionally fatal. Such rebound reactivation represents restoration of cytolytic T cell function against a target organ enriched in HBV expression. Preemptive treatment with lamivudine prior to the initiation of chemotherapy has been shown to reduce the risk of such reactivation. In all likelihood, the newer, more potent oral antiviral agents will work as well and with a lower risk of antiviral drug resistance. The optimal duration of antiviral therapy after completion of chemotherapy is not known, but a suggested approach is 6 months for inactive hepatitis B carriers and longer-duration therapy in patients with baseline HBV DNA levels >2×10^3 IU/ml, until standard clinical endpoints are met (Table 306-4).

CHRONIC HEPATITIS D (DELTA HEPATITIS)

Chronic hepatitis D (HDV) may follow acute co-infection with HBV but at a rate no higher than the rate of chronicity of acute hepatitis B. That is, although HDV co-infection can increase the severity of acute hepatitis B, HDV does not increase the likelihood of progression to chronic hepatitis B. When, however, HDV superinfection occurs in a person who is already chronically infected with HBV, long-term HDV infection is the rule and a worsening of the liver disease the expected consequence. Except for severity, chronic hepatitis B plus D has similar clinical and laboratory features to those seen in chronic hepatitis B alone. Relatively severe and progressive chronic hepatitis, with or without cirrhosis, is the rule, and mild chronic hepatitis is the exception. Occasionally, mild hepatitis or even, rarely, inactive carriage occurs in patients with chronic hepatitis B plus D, and the disease may become indolent after several years of infection. A distinguishing serologic feature of chronic hepatitis D is the presence in the circulation of antibodies to liver-kidney microsomes (anti-LKM); however, the anti-LKM seen in hepatitis D, anti-LKM3, are directed against uridine diphosphate glucuronosyltransferase and are distinct from anti-LKM1 seen in patients with autoimmune hepatitis and in a subset of patients with chronic hepatitis C (see below). The clinical and laboratory features of chronic HDV infection are summarized in Chap. 304.

TREATMENT Chronic Hepatitis D

Management is not well defined. Glucocorticoids are ineffective and are not used. Preliminary experimental trials of IFN-α suggested that conventional doses and durations of therapy lower levels of HDV RNA and aminotransferase activity only transiently during treatment but have no impact on the natural history of the disease. In contrast, high-dose IFN-α (9 million units three times a week) for 12 months may be associated with a sustained loss of HDV replication and clinical improvement in up to 50% of patients. Moreover, the beneficial impact of treatment has been observed to persist for 15 years and to be associated with a reduction in grade of hepatic necrosis and inflammation, reversion of advanced fibrosis (improved stage), and clearance of HDV RNA in some patients. A suggested approach to therapy has been high-dose, long-term IFN for at least a year and, in responders, extension of therapy until HDV RNA and HBsAg clearance. PEG IFN has also been shown to be effective in the treatment of chronic hepatitis D and is likely to become a more convenient replacement for standard IFN. None of the nucleoside analogue antiviral agents for hepatitis B is effective in hepatitis D. In patients with end-stage liver disease secondary to chronic hepatitis D, liver transplantation has been effective. If hepatitis D recurs in the new liver without the expression of hepatitis B (an unusual serologic profile in immunocompetent persons but common in transplant patients), liver injury is limited. In fact, the outcome of transplantation for chronic hepatitis D is superior to that for chronic hepatitis B; in such patients, combination hepatitis B immune globulin and nucleoside analogue therapy for hepatitis B is indicated (Chap. 310).

CHRONIC HEPATITIS C

Regardless of the epidemiologic mode of acquisition of hepatitis C virus (HCV) infection, chronic hepatitis follows acute hepatitis C in 50–70% of cases; chronic infection is common even in those with a return to normal in aminotransferase levels after acute hepatitis C, adding up to an 85% likelihood of chronic HCV infection after acute hepatitis C. Few clues had emerged to explain host differences associated with chronic infection until recently, when variation in a single nucleotide polymorphism (SNP) on chromosome 19, IL28B (which codes for interferon-λ3), was identified that distinguished between responders and nonresponders to antiviral therapy (see below). The same variants correlated with spontaneous resolution after acute infection: 53% in genotype C/C, 30% in genotype C/T, but only 23% in genotype T/T.

In patients with chronic hepatitis C followed for 20 years, progression to cirrhosis occurs in about 20–25%. Such is the case even for patients with relatively clinically mild chronic hepatitis, including those without symptoms, with only modest elevations of aminotransferase activity and with mild chronic hepatitis on liver biopsy. Even in cohorts of well-compensated patients with chronic hepatitis C referred for clinical research trials (no complications of chronic liver disease and with normal hepatic synthetic function), the prevalence of cirrhosis may be as high as 50%. Most cases of hepatitis C are identified initially in asymptomatic patients who have no history of acute hepatitis C (e.g., those discovered while attempting to donate blood, while undergoing lab testing as part of an application for life insurance, or as a result of routine laboratory tests). The source of HCV infection in many of these cases is not defined, although a long-forgotten percutaneous exposure in the remote past can be elicited in a substantial proportion and probably accounts for most infections; most of these infections were acquired in the 1960s and 1970s, coming to clinical attention decades later.

Approximately one-third of patients with chronic hepatitis C have normal or near-normal aminotransferase activity; although one-third to one-half of these patients have chronic hepatitis on liver biopsy, the grade of liver injury and stage of fibrosis tend to be mild in the vast majority. In some cases, more severe liver injury has been reported—even, rarely, cirrhosis, most likely the result of previous histologic activity. Among patients with persistent normal aminotransferase activity sustained over ≥5–10 years, histologic progression has been shown to be rare; however, approximately one-fourth of patients with normal aminotransferase activity experience subsequent aminotransferase elevations, and histologic injury can be progressive once abnormal biochemical activity resumes. Therefore, continued clinical monitoring is indicated, even for patients with normal aminotransferase activity.

Despite this substantial rate of progression of chronic hepatitis C, and despite the fact that liver failure can result from end-stage chronic hepatitis C, the long-term prognosis for chronic hepatitis C in a majority of patients is relatively benign. Mortality over 10–20 years among patients with transfusion-associated chronic hepatitis C has been shown not to differ from mortality in a matched population of transfused patients in whom hepatitis C did not develop. Although death in the hepatitis group is more likely to result from liver failure, and although hepatic decompensation may occur in ~15% of such patients over the course of a decade, the majority (almost 60%) of patients remain asymptomatic and well compensated, with no clinical sequelae of chronic liver disease. Overall, chronic hepatitis C tends to be very slowly and insidiously progressive, if at all, in the vast majority of patients, while in approximately one-fourth of cases, chronic hepatitis C will progress eventually to end-stage cirrhosis. In fact, because HCV infection is so prevalent, and because a proportion of patients progress inexorably to end-stage liver disease, hepatitis C is the most frequent indication for liver transplantation (Chap. 310). Referral bias may account for the more severe outcomes described in cohorts of patients reported from tertiary care centers (20-year progression of ≥20%) versus the more benign outcomes in cohorts of patients monitored from initial blood-product-associated acute hepatitis or identified in community settings (20-year progression of only 4–7%). Still unexplained, however, are the wide ranges in reported progression to cirrhosis, from 2% over 17 years in a population of women with hepatitis C infection acquired from contaminated anti-D immune globulin to 30% over ≤11 years in recipients of contaminated intravenous immune globulin.

Progression of liver disease in patients with chronic hepatitis C has been reported to be more likely in patients with older age, longer duration of infection, advanced histologic stage and grade, genotype 1, more complex quasispecies diversity, increased hepatic iron, concomitant other liver disorders (alcoholic liver disease, chronic hepatitis B, hemochromatosis, α_1-antitrypsin deficiency, and steatohepatitis), HIV infection, and obesity. Among these variables, however, duration of infection appears to be one of the most important, and some of the others probably reflect disease duration to some extent (e.g., quasispecies diversity, hepatic iron accumulation). No other epidemiologic or clinical features of chronic hepatitis C (e.g., severity of acute hepatitis, level of aminotransferase activity, level of HCV RNA, presence or absence of jaundice during acute hepatitis) are predictive of eventual outcome. Despite the relatively benign nature of chronic hepatitis C over time in many patients, cirrhosis following chronic hepatitis C has been associated with the late development, after several decades, of HCC (Chap. 88); the annual rate of HCC in cirrhotic patients with hepatitis C is 1–4%, occurring primarily in patients who have had HCV infection for 30 years or more.

Perhaps the best prognostic indicator in chronic hepatitis C is liver histology; the rate of hepatic fibrosis may be slow, moderate, or rapid. Patients with mild necrosis and inflammation as well as those with limited fibrosis have an excellent prognosis and limited progression to cirrhosis. In contrast, among patients with moderate to severe necroinflammatory activity or fibrosis, including septal or bridging fibrosis, progression to cirrhosis is highly likely over the course of 10–20 years. Among patients with compensated cirrhosis associated with hepatitis C, the 10-year survival rate is close to 80%; mortality occurs at a rate of 2–6% per year; decompensation at a rate of 4–5% per year; and, as noted above, HCC at a rate of 1–4% per year. A discussion of the pathogenesis of liver injury in patients with chronic hepatitis C appears in Chap. 304.

Clinical features of chronic hepatitis C are similar to those described above for chronic hepatitis B. Generally, fatigue is the most common symptom; jaundice is rare. Immune complex–mediated extrahepatic complications of chronic hepatitis C are less common than in chronic hepatitis B (despite the fact that assays for immune complexes are often positive in patients with chronic hepatitis C), with the exception of essential mixed cryoglobulinemia (Chap. 304), which is linked to cutaneous vasculitis and membranoproliferative glomerulonephritis as well as lymphoproliferative disorders such as B-cell lymphoma and unexplained monoclonal gammopathy. In addition, chronic hepatitis C has been associated with extrahepatic complications unrelated to immune-complex injury. These include Sjögren's syndrome, lichen planus, porphyria cutanea tarda, type-II diabetes mellitus and the metabolic syndrome (including insulin resistance and steatohepatitis).

Laboratory features of chronic hepatitis C are similar to those in patients with chronic hepatitis B, but aminotransferase levels tend to fluctuate more (the characteristic episodic pattern of aminotransferase activity) and to be lower, especially in patients with long-standing disease. An interesting and occasionally confusing finding in patients with chronic hepatitis C is the presence of autoantibodies. Rarely, patients with autoimmune hepatitis (see below) and hyperglobulinemia have false-positive immunoassays for anti-HCV. On the other hand, some patients with serologically confirmable chronic hepatitis C have circulating anti-LKM. These antibodies are anti-LKM1, as seen in patients with autoimmune hepatitis type 2 (see below), and are directed against a 33-amino-acid sequence of cytochrome P450 IID6. The occurrence of anti-LKM1 in some patients with chronic hepatitis C may result from the partial sequence homology between the epitope recognized by anti-LKM1 and two segments of the HCV polyprotein. In addition, the presence of this autoantibody in some patients with chronic hepatitis C suggests that autoimmunity may be playing a role in the pathogenesis of chronic hepatitis C.

Histopathologic features of chronic hepatitis C, especially those that distinguish hepatitis C from hepatitis B, are described in Chap. 304.

TREATMENT Chronic Hepatitis C

Therapy for chronic hepatitis C has evolved substantially in the two decades since IFN-α was introduced for this indication. When first approved, IFN-α was administered via subcutaneous injection three times a week for 6 months but achieved a sustained virologic response, SVR (Fig. 306-2) (a reduction of HCV RNA to undetectable levels by PCR when measured ≥6 months after completion of therapy) below 10%. Doubling the duration of therapy—but not increasing the dose or changing IFN preparations—increased the SVR rate to ~20%, and addition to the regimen of daily ribavirin, an oral guanosine nucleoside, increased the SVR rate to 40%. When used alone, ribavirin is ineffective and does not reduce HCV RNA levels, but ribavirin enhances the efficacy of IFN by reducing the likelihood of virologic relapse after the achievement of an end-treatment response (ETR) (Fig. 306-2) (response measured during, and maintained to the end of, treatment). Proposed mechanisms to explain the role of ribavirin include subtle direct reduction of HCV replication, inhibition of host inosine monophosphate dehydrogenase activity (and associated depletion of guanosine pools), immune modulation, induction of virologic mutational catastrophe, and enhancement of interferon-stimulated gene expression. Interferon therapy results in activation of the JAK-STAT signal transduction pathway, which culminates in the intracellular elaboration of genes and their protein products that have antiviral properties. Hepatitis C proteins inhibit JAK-STAT signaling at several steps along the pathway, and exogenous interferon restores expression of interferon-stimulated genes and their antiviral effects.

The current standard of care is the combination of long-acting pegylated IFN (PEG IFN) and ribavirin, which has increased responsiveness (frequency of SVR) to as high as 55% overall, >40% in genotypes 1 and 4 and to >80% in genotypes 2 and 3. Still, many important lessons about antiviral therapy for chronic hepatitis C were learned from the experience with IFN monotherapy and combination IFN-ribavirin therapy. Even in the absence of biochemical and virologic responses, histologic improvement occurs in approximately three-fourths of all treated patients. In chronic hepatitis C, unlike the case in hepatitis B, responses to therapy are not accompanied by transient, acute hepatitis-like aminotransferase elevations. Instead, ALT levels fall precipitously during therapy. Up to 90% of virologic

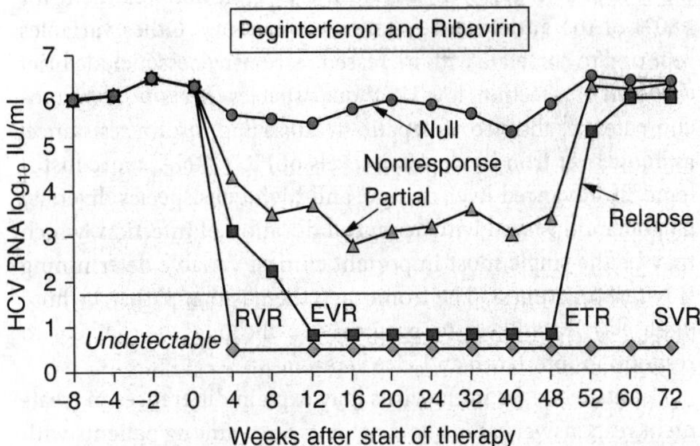

Figure 306-2 Virologic responses during a 48-week course of antiviral therapy in patients with hepatitis C, genotype 1 or 4 (for genotypes 2 or 3, the course would be 24 weeks). Nonresponders can be classified as null responders (HCV RNA reduction of <2 log_{10} IU/ml) or partial responders (HCV RNA reduction ≥2 log_{10} IU/ml but not suppressed to undetectable) by week 24 of therapy. In responders, HCV RNA can become undetectable, as shown with sensitive amplification assays, within 4 weeks (RVR, rapid virologic response); can be reduced by ≥2 log_{10} IU/ml within 12 weeks (early virologic response, EVR; if HCV RNA is undetectable at 12 weeks, the designation is "complete" EVR); or at the end of therapy, 48 weeks (ETR, end-treatment response). In responders, if HCV RNA remains undetectable for 24 weeks after ETR, week 72, the patient has a sustained virologic response (SVR), but if HCV RNA becomes detectable again, the patient is considered to have relapsed. *(Reproduced with permission, courtesy of Marc G. Ghany, National Institute of Diabetes and Digestive and Kidney Diseases, National Institutes of Health and the American Association for the Study of Liver Diseases Hepatology 49:1335, 2009.)*

responses are achieved within the first 12 weeks of therapy; responses thereafter are rare. Most relapses occur within the first 12 weeks after treatment. Sustained virologic responses are very durable; normal ALT, improved histology, and absence of HCV RNA in serum and liver have been documented a decade after successful therapy, and "relapses" 2 years after sustained responses are almost unheard of. Thus, an SVR to antiviral therapy of chronic hepatitis C is tantamount to a cure.

Patient variables that tend to correlate with sustained virologic responsiveness to IFN-based therapy include favorable genotype (genotypes 2 and 3 as opposed to genotypes 1 and 4), low baseline HCV RNA level (<2 million copies/mL, which is equivalent to ~800,000 IU/ml, the current convention of quantitation), histologically mild hepatitis and minimal fibrosis, age <40, absence of obesity as well as insulin resistance and type-II diabetes mellitus, and female gender. Patients with cirrhosis can respond, but they are less likely to do so. Studies of combination IFN-ribavirin therapy have shown that in patients with genotype 1, therapy should last a full 48 weeks, while in those with genotypes 2 and 3, a 24-week course of therapy suffices (although more recent observations allow refined tailoring of treatment duration based on rapidity of response, see below). The response rate in African Americans is disappointingly low for reasons that are not fully understood. Potentially contributing to, but not explaining entirely, low responsiveness in African Americans are a higher proportion with genotype 1, slower early viral kinetics during therapy, impaired HCV-specific immunity, and recently recognized host genetic differences in IL28B alleles, described below. The response rate in Latino patients is also low, despite the fact that the frequency of the favorable IL28B C allele is as common in Hispanic patients as in whites. Moreover, the likelihood of a sustained response is best if adherence to the treatment regimen is high (i.e., if patients receive ≥80% of the IFN and ribavirin doses and if they continue treatment for ≥80% of the anticipated duration of therapy). Other variables reported to correlate with increased responsiveness include brief duration of infection, low HCV quasispecies diversity, immunocompetence, absence of hepatic steatosis and insulin resistance, and low liver iron levels. High levels of HCV RNA, more histologically advanced liver disease, and high quasispecies diversity all go hand in hand with advanced duration of infection, which may be the single most important clinical variable determining IFN responsiveness. The ironic fact, then, is that patients whose disease is least likely to progress are the ones *most* likely to respond to interferon and vice versa.

Genetic changes in the virus may explain differences in treatment responsiveness in some patients (e.g., among patients with genotype 1b, responsiveness to IFN is enhanced in those with amino-acid-substitution mutations in the nonstructural protein 5A gene). As described above in the discussion of spontaneous recovery from acute hepatitis C, interferon gene variants discovered recently in gene-wide association studies have been shown to have a substantial impact on responsiveness of patients with genotype 1 to antiviral therapy. In studies of patients treated with PEG IFN and ribavirin, variants of the IL28B SNP that code for IFN-λ3 (a type-III IFN, the receptors for which are more discretely distributed than IFN α receptors and more concentrated in hepatocytes) correlate significantly with responsiveness. Patients homozygous for the C allele at this locus have the highest frequency of achieving an SVR (~80%), those homozygous for the T allele at this locus are least likely to achieve an SVR (~25%), and those heterozygous at this locus (C/T) have an intermediate level of responsiveness (SVRs in ~35%). The fact that C/C is common in whites of European ancestry and even more so in Japanese persons but rare in African Americans helps explain the differences in observed responsiveness among these population groups.

Side effects of IFN therapy are described above in the section on treatment of chronic hepatitis B. The most pronounced side effect of ribavirin therapy is hemolysis; a reduction in hemoglobin of up to 2–3 g or in hematocrit of 5–10% can be anticipated. A small, unpredictable proportion of patients experience profound, brisk hemolysis, resulting in symptomatic anemia; therefore, close monitoring of blood counts is crucial, and ribavirin should be avoided in patients with anemia or hemoglobinopathies and in patients with coronary artery disease or cerebrovascular disease, in whom anemia can precipitate an ischemic event. When symptomatic anemia occurs, ribavirin dose reductions or addition of erythropoietin to boost red blood cell levels may be required; erythropoietin has been shown to improve patients' quality of life but not the likelihood of achieving an SVR. If ribavirin is stopped during therapy, SVR rates fall, but responsiveness can be maintained as long as the ribavirin is not stopped and the total ribavirin dose exceed 60% of the planned dose. In addition, ribavirin, which is renally excreted, should not be used in patients with renal insufficiency; the drug is teratogenic, precluding its use during pregnancy and mandating the scrupulous use of efficient contraception during therapy (interferons, too, because of their antiproliferative properties, are contraindicated during pregnancy).

Ribavirin can also cause nasal and chest congestion, pruritus, and precipitation of gout. Combination IFN-ribavirin therapy is more difficult to tolerate than IFN monotherapy. In one large clinical trial of combination therapy versus monotherapy, among those in the 1-year treatment group, 21% of the combination group (but only 14% of the monotherapy group) had to discontinue treatment, while 26% of the combination group (but only 9% of the monotherapy group) required dose reductions.

Studies of viral kinetics have shown that despite a virion half-life in serum of only 2–3 h, the level of HCV is maintained by a high replication rate of 10^{12} hepatitis C virions per day. IFN-α blocks virion production or release with an efficacy that increases with increasing drug doses; moreover, the calculated death rate for infected cells during IFN therapy is inversely related to viral load; patients with the most rapid death rate of infected hepatocytes are more likely to achieve undetectable HCV RNA at 3 months; in practice, failure to achieve an early virologic response (EVR), a ≥2-$\log_{10}$ reduction in HCV RNA by week 12, predicts failure to experience a subsequent SVR. Similarly, patients in whom HCV RNA becomes undetectable within 4 weeks [i.e., who achieve a rapid virologic response (RVR)], have a very high likelihood of achieving a sustained virologic response (Fig. 306-2). Therefore, to achieve rapid viral clearance from serum and the liver, *high-dose induction therapy* has been advocated. In practice, however, high-dose induction with IFN-based therapy has not yielded higher sustained response rates.

TREATMENT OF CHOICE For the treatment of chronic hepatitis C, standard IFNs have now been supplanted by PEG IFNs. These have elimination times up to sevenfold longer than standard IFNs (i.e., a substantially longer half-life), and achieve prolonged concentrations, permitting administration once (rather than three times) a week. Instead of the frequent drug peaks (linked to side effects) and troughs (when drug is absent) associated with frequent administration of short-acting IFNs, administration of PEG IFNs results in drug concentrations that are more stable and sustained over time. Once-a-week PEG IFN monotherapy is twice as effective as monotherapy with its standard

IFN counterpart, approaches the efficacy of combination standard IFN plus ribavirin, and is as well tolerated as standard IFNs, without more difficult-to-manage thrombocytopenia and leukopenia than standard IFNs. The current standard of care, however, is a combination of PEG IFN plus ribavirin.

Two PEG IFNs are available: PEG IFN α-2b and α-2a. PEG IFN α-2b consists of a 12-kD, linear PEG molecule bound to IFN α-2b, while PEG IFN α-2a consists of a larger, 40kD, branched PEG molecule bound to IFN α-2a; because of its larger size and smaller volume of extravascular distribution, PEG IFN α-2a can be given at a uniform dose independent of weight, while the dose of the smaller PEG IFN α-2b, which has a much wider volume distribution, must be weight-based (Table 306-6). In the registration trial for PEG IFN α-2b plus ribavirin, the best regimen was 48 weeks of 1.5 μg/kg of PEG IFN once a week plus 800 mg of ribavirin daily. A post hoc analysis suggested that weight-based dosing of ribavirin would have been more effective than the fixed 800-mg dose used in the study. In the first registration trial for PEG IFN α-2a plus ribavirin, the best regimen was 48 weeks of 180 μg of PEG IFN plus 1000 mg (for patients <75 kg) to 1200 mg (for patients ≥75 kg) of ribavirin. Sustained virologic responses of 54 and 56% were reported in these two studies, respectively. A subsequent study of PEG IFN α-2a plus ribavirin showed that, for patients with genotypes 2 and 3, a duration of 24 weeks and a ribavirin dose of 800 mg was sufficient. Among the three studies, for patients in the optimal treatment arm, SVR rates for patients with genotype 1 were 42–51% and for patients with genotypes 2 and 3 rates were 76–82%. Between genotypes 2 and 3, genotype 3 is somewhat more refractory, and some authorities would extend therapy for a full 48 weeks in patients with genotype 3, especially if they have advanced hepatic fibrosis or cirrhosis and/or high-level HCV RNA.

In the initial registration trials for combination PEG IFN plus ribavirin, both combination PEG IFN regimens were compared to standard IFN α-2b plus ribavirin. Side effects of the combination PEG IFN α-2b regimen were comparable to those for the combination standard IFN regimen; however, when the combination PEG IFN α-2a regimen was compared to the combination standard IFN α-2b regimen, flu-like symptoms and depression were less common in the combination PEG IFN group. Although ascertainment of side effects differed between studies of the two drugs, when each was tested against standard IFN α-2b plus ribavirin, combination PEG IFN α-2a plus ribavirin appeared to be better tolerated. In a recent head-to-head trial of the two PEG IFNs (the "IDEAL" trial), the two PEG IFNs were found to be comparable in efficacy (achievement of SVR) (Fig. 306-3) and tolerability, although headache, nausea, fever, myalgia, depression, and drug discontinuation for any reason were less frequent in patients treated with PEG IFN α-2a than standard-dose PEG IFN α-2b. In contrast, neutropenia and rash were more frequent in patients treated with PEG IFN α-2a than standard-dose PEG IFN α-2b. In two subsequent head-to-head trials and a systematic review of randomized trials, PEG IFN α–2a was more effective than α–2b (SVR in genotype 1-4: 48–55% versus 32–40%, respectively). In trials of PEG IFN α-2b among patients with HCV genotype 1, a broader range of weight-based daily ribavirin doses has been validated: 800 mg for weight <65 kg, 1000 mg for weight 65–85 kg, 1200 mg for weight >85–105 kg, and 1400 mg for weight >105 kg. Recommended doses for the two PEG IFNs plus ribavirin and other comparisons between the two therapies are shown in Table 306-6.

Unless ribavirin is contraindicated (see above), combination PEG IFN plus ribavirin is the recommended course of therapy—24 weeks for genotypes 2 and 3 and 48 weeks for genotype 1. Measurement of quantitative HCV RNA levels at 12 weeks is helpful in guiding therapy; if a 2-$\log_{10}$ drop in HCV RNA has not been achieved by this time, chances for an SVR are negligible. If the 12-week HCV RNA has fallen by two $\log_{10}$ (EVR), the chances for an SVR at the end of therapy are approximately two-thirds; if the 12-week HCV RNA is undetectable ("complete" EVR),

TABLE 306-6 Pegylated Interferon α-2a and α-2b for Chronic Hepatitis C

	PEG IFN α-2b	PEG IFN α-2a
PEG size	12 kD linear	40 kD branched
Elimination half-life	54 hours	65 hours
Clearance	725 mL/hour	60 mL/hour
Dose	1.5 μg/kg (weight-based)	180 μg
Storage	Room temperature	Refrigerated
Ribavirin dose		
Genotype 1	800–1400 mg[a]	1000–1200 mg[b]
Genotype 2/3	800 mg	800 mg
Duration of therapy		
Genotype 1	48 weeks	48 weeks
Genotype 2/3	48 weeks[c]	24 weeks
Efficacy of combination Rx[d]	54%	56%
Genotype 1	40–42%	41–51%
Genotype 2/3	82%	76–78%

[a] In the registration trial for PEG IFN α-2b plus ribavirin, the optimal regimen was 1.5 μg of PEG IFN plus 800 mg of ribavirin; however, a posthoc analysis of this study suggested that higher ribavirin doses are better. In subsequent trials of PEG IFN α-2b with ribavirin in patients with genotype 1, the following daily ribavirin doses have been validated: 800 mg for patients weighing <65 kg, 1000 mg for patients weighing >65-85 kg, 1200 for patients weighing >85–105 kg, and 1400 mg for patients weighing >105 kg.

[b] 1000 mg for patients weighing <75 kg; 1200 mg for patients weighing ≥75 kg.

[c] In the registration trial for PEG IFN α-2b plus ribavirin, all patients were treated for 48 weeks; however, data from other trials of standard interferons and the other PEG IFN demonstrated that 24 weeks suffices for patients with genotypes 2 and 3. For patients with genotype 3 who have advanced fibrosis/cirrhosis and/or high-level HCV RNA, a full 48 weeks is preferable.

[d] Attempts to compare the two PEG IFN preparations based on the results of registration clinical trials are confounded by differences between trials of the two agents in methodological details (different ribavirin doses, different methods for recording depression, and other side effects) and study-population composition (different proportion with bridging fibrosis/cirrhosis, proportion from the United States versus international, mean weight, proportion with genotype 1, and proportion with high-level HCV RNA). In the head-to-head comparison of the two PEG IFN preparations in the "IDEAL" trial reported in 2009, the two drugs were comparable in tolerability and efficacy. PEG IFN α-2b was administered at [a] weekly weight-based dose of 1.0 μg/kg or 1.5 μg/kg, and PEG IFN α-2a was administered at a weekly fixed dose of 180 μg. For PEG IFN α-2b, daily ribavirin weight-based doses ranged between 800–1400 mg based on weight criteria (see footnote a, above), while for PEG IFN α-2a, daily ribavirin weight-based doses ranged between 1000–1200 mg (footnote b, above). For the two PEG IFN α-2b study arms, ribavirin dose reductions for ribavirin-associated adverse effects were done in 200–400-mg decrements; for PEG IFN α-2a, the ribavirin dose was reduced to 600 mg for intolerability. Sustained virologic responses occurred in 38.0% of the low-dose PEG IFN α-2b group, 39.8% of the standard, full-dose PEG IFN α-2b group, and 40.9% of the PEG IFN α-2a group.

Abbreviations: PEG, polyethylene glycol; PEG IFN, pegylated interferon; HCV RNA, hepatitis C virus RNA.

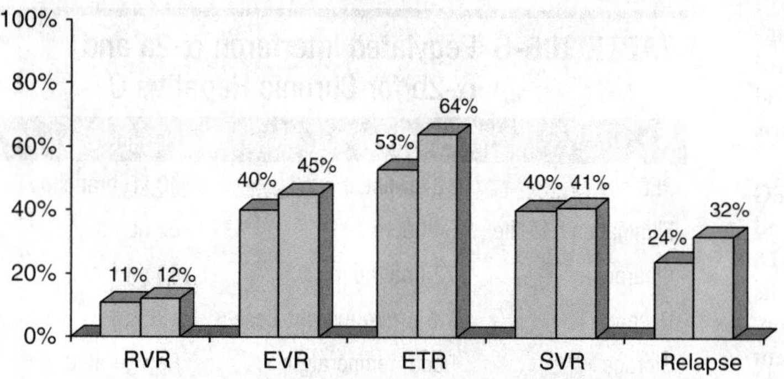

Figure 306-3 Head-to-head comparison of standard-dose PEG IFN α-2b 1.5 μg/kg weekly and PEG IFN α-2a 180 μg weekly administered with daily ribavirin in the "IDEAL" trial. Percent achieving treatment milestones for PEG IFN α-2b (green boxes) and PEG IFN α-2a (orange boxes). RVR, rapid virologic response, HCV RNA undetectable at week 4; EVR, early virologic response, HCV RNA undetectable at week 12; ETR, end-treatment response, HCV RNA undetectable at end of treatment week 48; SVR, sustained virologic response, HCV RNA remaining undetectable 24 weeks after completing 48 weeks of therapy. Relapse, reappearance of detectable HCV RNA by week 72 in patients with an end-treatment response at week 48. PEG IFN α-2a suppressed HCV RNA in a higher proportion of patients at weeks 12 and 48 but, because of a higher relapse rate at week 72, resulted in the same SVR rate as PEG IFN α-2b.

the chances for a sustained virologic response exceed 80% (Fig. 306-2). Because absence of an EVR is such a strong predictor of the absence of an ultimate sustained virologic response, failure to achieve a 12-week 2-$\log_{10}$ drop in HCV RNA (EVR) may be used as a signal to discontinue therapy.

Studies have suggested that the frequency of an SVR to PEG IFN/ribavirin therapy can be increased in patients with baseline variables weighing against a response (e.g., HCV RNA $>8 \times 10^5$ IU/ml, weight >85 kg) by raising the dose of PEG IFN (e.g., to as high as 270 μg of PEG IFN α-2a) and/or the dose of ribavirin to as high as 1600 mg daily (if tolerated or supplemented by erythropoietin) or by tailoring treatment based on viral response to prolong the duration of viral clearance before discontinuing therapy, i.e., extending therapy from 48 to 72 weeks for patients with genotype 1 and a slow virologic response, i.e., those whose HCV RNA has not fallen rapidly to undetectable levels within 4 weeks (absence of "rapid virologic response"). Tailoring therapy based on the kinetics of HCV RNA reduction has also been applied to abbreviating the duration of therapy in patients with genotype 1 (and 4). The results of several clinical trials suggest that, in patients with genotype 1 (and 4) who have a 4-week RVR (which occurs in ≤20%), especially in the subset with a baseline low level of HCV RNA, 24 weeks of therapy with PEG IFN and weight-based ribavirin suffices, yielding SVR rates of ~90% and comparable to those achieved in this cohort with 48 weeks of therapy. Although initial reports suggested that, for patients with genotype 2 and (somewhat less so) genotype 3, in rapid virologic responders with undetectable HCV RNA at week 4, the total duration of therapy required to achieve an SVR could be as short as 12–16 weeks, a very sizable, definitive subsequent trial showed that relapse is increased if treatment duration is curtailed and that a full 24 weeks is superior for these genotypes (except for the minority with very low baseline levels of HCV RNA).

Persons with chronic HCV infection have been shown to suffer increased liver-related mortality. On the other hand, successful antiviral therapy of chronic hepatitis C resulting in an SVR has been shown to improve survival, to lower the risk of liver failure and liver-related death, to slow the progression of chronic hepatitis C, and to reverse fibrosis and even cirrhosis. Although successful treatment reduces mortality in cirrhotic patients (and those with advanced fibrosis) and reduces the likelihood of hepatocellular carcinoma, the risk of decompensation, death, and liver cancer persists, albeit at a much reduced level, necessitating continued clinical monitoring and cancer surveillance after SVR in cirrhotics. On the other hand, in the absence of an SVR, IFN-based therapy does not reduce the risk of hepatocellular carcinoma. Similarly, for nonresponders to PEG IFN/ribavirin therapy, three trials of long-term maintenance therapy with PEG IFN have shown no benefit in reducing the risk of histologic progression or clinical decompensation, including the development of hepatocellular carcinoma. For PEG IFN/ribavirin nonresponders who have had a full, adequate course of therapy, the benefit of retreatment—with higher doses or a longer course of the original PEG IFN regimen or the alternative PEG IFN regimen or with a different type of IFN preparation (e.g., consensus IFN)—is marginal at best.

INDICATIONS FOR ANTIVIRAL THERAPY Patients with chronic hepatitis C who have detectable HCV RNA in serum, whether or not aminotransferase levels are increased, and chronic hepatitis of at least moderate grade and stage (portal or bridging fibrosis) are candidates for antiviral therapy with PEG IFN plus ribavirin. Most authorities recommend 800 mg of ribavirin for patients with genotypes 2 and 3 for both types of PEG IFN and weight-based 1000–1200 mg (when used with PEG IFN α-2a) or 800–1400 mg (when used with PEG IFN α-2b) ribavirin for patients with genotype 1 (and 4), unless ribavirin is contraindicated (Table 306-7). Although patients with persistently normal ALT activity tend to progress histologically very slowly or not at all, they respond to antiviral therapy just as well as do patients with elevated ALT levels; therefore, while observation without therapy is an option, such patients are potential candidates for antiviral therapy. As noted above, therapy with IFN has been shown to improve survival and complication-free survival and to slow progression of fibrosis.

Prior to therapy, HCV genotype should be determined, and the genotype dictates the duration of therapy: 48 weeks for patients with genotype 1, 24 weeks for those with genotypes 2 and 3. For patients with genotype 1 (and 4), especially those with low baseline HCV RNA, 24 weeks of PEG IFN/ribavirin therapy may suffice if HCV RNA becomes undetectable within 4 weeks (RVR); for patients with genotypes 2 and 3, a full, 24-week course is most effective, although the duration may be reduced to 12–16 weeks for patients with genotype 2, a low baseline level of viremia, and an RVR, especially to be considered for patients who tolerate therapy poorly. As noted above, the absence of a 2-$\log_{10}$ drop in HCV RNA at week 12 (EVR) weighs heavily against the likelihood of an SVR; therefore, measuring HCV RNA at 12 weeks is recommended routinely (Fig. 306-2), especially for patients with genotype 1, and therapy can be discontinued if an EVR is not achieved. Among patients with an EVR (≥2-$\log_{10}$ HCV RNA reduction) but with HCV RNA still detectable at week 24, an SVR is unlikely, and therapy can be discontinued. Although response rates are lower in patients with certain pretreatment variables, selection for treatment should not be based on symptoms, genotype, HCV RNA level, mode of acquisition of hepatitis C, or advanced hepatic fibrosis. Patients with cirrhosis can respond and should not be excluded as candidates for therapy.

TABLE 306-7 Indications and Recommendations for Antiviral Therapy of Chronic Hepatitis C

Standard Indications for Therapy
Detectable HCV RNA (with or without elevated ALT)
Portal/bridging fibrosis or moderate to severe hepatitis on liver biopsy (the necessity of a pretreatment biopsy is being debated).
These indications apply to adults as well as to children aged 2–17, in whom treatment may be considered at reduced weight-based doses (see product inserts).
Retreatment Recommended
Relapsers after a previous course of standard interferon monotherapy or combination standard interferon/ribavirin therapy.
A course of PEG IFN plus ribavirin (retreatment not recommended with PEG IFN/ribavirin if relapse occurred after a full course of PEG IFN/ribavirin).
Nonresponders to a previous course of standard IFN monotherapy or combination standard IFN/ribavirin therapy.
A course of PEG IFN plus ribavirin—more likely to achieve a sustained virologic response in white patients without previous ribavirin therapy, with low baseline HCV RNA levels, with a ≥2-$\log_{10}$ reduction in HCV RNA during previous therapy, with genotypes 2 and 3, and without reduction in ribavirin dose. (Retreatment not recommended with PEG IFN/ribavirin if nonresponse occurred to a full course of PEG IFN/ribavirin.)
Antiviral Therapy not Recommended Routinely but Management Decisions Made on an Individual Basis
Age >60
Mild hepatitis on liver biopsy.
Persons with severe renal insufficiency (glomerular filtration rate <60 ml/min) who do not require hemodialysis (reduced-dose PEG IFN and ribavirin). Antiviral therapy in patients requiring hemodialysis is more complicated, less successful, and associated with more adverse effects; if treatment is pursued, either standard doses of standard interferon 3 times a week or reduced doses of weekly PEG IFN in combination with reduced doses of daily ribavirin should be used.
Long-Term Maintenance Therapy Recommended
Cutaneous vasculitis and glomerulonephritis associated with chronic hepatitis C.
Long-Term Maintenance Therapy in Nonresponders not Recommended
Antiviral Therapy not Recommended
Decompensated cirrhosis (except, perhaps, in transplantation centers with experience in graded escalation, low-dose treatment to achieve undetectable HCV RNA prior to transplantation; results are mixed).
Pregnancy (teratogenicity of ribavirin).
Contraindications to use of interferon or ribavirin.
Standard Therapeutic Regimens
First-line treatment: PEG IFN subcutaneously once a week plus daily ribavirin orally
HCV genotypes 1 and 4—48 weeks of therapy
PEG IFN α-2a 180 μg weekly plus ribavirin 1000 mg/day (weight <75 kg) to 1200 mg/day (weight <75 kg) or
PEG IFN α-2b 1.5 μg/kg weekly plus daily oral ribavirin 800 mg for weight <65 kg, 1000 mg for weight 65–85 kg, 1200 mg for weight >85–105 kg, and 1400 mg for weight >105 kg
HCV genotypes 2 and 3—24 weeks of therapy
PEG IFN α-2a 180 μg weekly plus ribavirin 800 mg/day or
PEG IFN α-2b 1.5 μg/kg weekly plus ribavirin 800 mg/day (For patients with genotype 3 who have advanced fibrosis and/or high-level HCV RNA, a full 48 weeks of therapy may be preferable.)
Alternative regimen: PEG IFN (α-2a 180 μg or α-2b 1.0 μg/kg) subcutaneously once a week (primarily for patients in whom ribavirin is contraindicated or not tolerated) for 24 (genotypes 2 and 3) or 48 (genotypes 1 and 4) weeks.
Early discontinuation: Failure to achieve an EVR, i.e., ≥2 $\log_{10}$ HCV RNA reduction by week 12 or, if EVR is achieved, failure to achieve suppression of HCV RNA to undetectable by week 24.
"Tailored" Therapeutic Regimens Based on Rapid Treatment Milestones
HCV genotypes 1 and 4.
For RVR, i.e., undetectable HCV RNA at week 4, especially in patients with low baseline HCV RNA, consider truncating the course of therapy to 24 weeks.
For patients with slow, delayed response, i.e., who clear detectable HCV RNA between weeks 12 and 24, consider prolonging the course of therapy to 72 weeks.
"Tailored" Therapeutic Regimens Based on Baseline Variables Associated with Reduced Responsiveness
HCV genotypes 1 and 4
For patients with HCV RNA >8 × 10^5 IU/ml and weighing >85 kg, consider increasing the weekly PEG IFN dose (e.g., for PEG IFN α-2a up to 270 μg) and the daily ribavirin dose (e.g., up to 1600 mg).
For HCV-HIV co-infected patients: 48 weeks, regardless of genotype, of weekly PEG IFN α-2a (180 μg) or PEG IFN α-2b (1.5 μg/kg) plus a daily ribavirin dose of at least 600–800 mg, up to full weight-based dosing, at doses comparable to those for HCV-monoinfected patients, if tolerated.

(*continued*)

TABLE 306-7 Indications and Recommendations for Antiviral Therapy of Chronic Hepatitis C (*Continued*)

Features Associated with Reduced Responsiveness
Single nucleotide polymorphism (SNP) T allele (as opposed to C allele) at IL28B locus
Genotype 1
High-level HCV RNA (>2 × 10^6 copies/ml or >8 × 10^5 IU/ml)
Advanced fibrosis (bridging fibrosis, cirrhosis)
Long-duration disease
Age >40
High HCV quasispecies diversity
Immunosuppression
African-American ethnicity
Latino ethnicity
Obesity
Hepatic steatosis
Insulin resistance, type-II diabetes mellitus
Reduced adherence (lower drug doses and reduced duration of therapy)

Abbreviations: ALT, alanine aminotransferase; HCV, hepatitis C virus; IFN, interferon; PEG IFN, pegylated interferon; IU, international units (1 IU/ml is equivalent to ~2.5 copies/ml).

Patients who have relapsed (Fig. 306-2) after a course of IFN monotherapy are candidates for retreatment with PEG IFN plus ribavirin (i.e., a more effective treatment regimen is required). For nonresponders to a prior course of IFN monotherapy, retreatment with IFN monotherapy or combination IFN plus ribavirin therapy is unlikely to achieve a sustained virologic response; however, a trial of combination PEG IFN plus ribavirin may be worthwhile. End-treatment virologic responses as high as 40% can occur in this setting, but an SVR is the outcome in <15–20% of patients. Sustained virologic responses to retreatment of nonresponders are more frequent in those who had never received ribavirin in the past, those with genotypes 2 and 3, those with low pretreatment HCV RNA levels, and noncirrhotics, but less frequent in African Americans, those who failed to achieve a substantial reduction in HCV RNA during their previous course of therapy (null responders, Fig. 306-2), and those who required ribavirin-dose reductions. Potential approaches to improving responsiveness to PEG IFN/ribavirin in prior nonresponders include longer duration of treatment; higher doses of either PEG IFN, ribavirin, or both; and switching to a different IFN preparation; however, as noted above, none of these approaches achieves more than a marginal benefit.

Early treatment is indicated for persons with acute hepatitis C (Chap. 304). In patients with biochemically and histologically mild chronic hepatitis C, the rate of progression is slow, and monitoring without therapy is an option; however, such patients respond just as well to combination PEG IFN plus ribavirin therapy as those with elevated ALT and more histologically severe hepatitis. Therefore, therapy for these patients should be considered and the decision made based on such factors as patient motivation, genotype, stage of fibrosis, age, and comorbid conditions. A pretreatment liver biopsy to assess histologic grade and stage provides substantial information about progression of hepatitis C in the past, has prognostic value for future progression, and can identify such histologic factors as steatosis and stage of fibrosis, which can influence responsiveness to therapy. As therapy has improved for patients with a broad range of histologic severity, and as noninvasive laboratory markers and imaging correlates of fibrosis have gained popularity, some authorities, especially in Europe, have placed less value on, and do not recommend, pretreatment liver biopsies. On the other hand, serum markers of fibrosis are not considered sufficiently accurate, and histologic findings provide important prognostic information to physician and patient. Therefore, although the contemporary role of a pretreatment liver biopsy commands less of a consensus, a pretreatment liver biopsy still provides useful information and should be considered.

Patients with compensated cirrhosis can respond to therapy, although their likelihood of a sustained response is lower than in noncirrhotics; moreover, survival has been shown to improve after successful antiviral therapy in cirrhotics. Similarly, although several retrospective studies have suggested that antiviral therapy in cirrhotics with chronic hepatitis C, independent of treatment outcome per se, reduces the frequency of HCC, less advanced disease in the treated cirrhotics, not treatment itself (i.e., lead-time bias), may have accounted for the reduced frequency of HCC observed in the treated cohorts in these reports; prospective studies to address this question have failed to demonstrate benefit, unless a sustained virologic response is achieved. Patients with decompensated cirrhosis are not candidates for IFN-based antiviral therapy but should be referred for liver transplantation. Some liver-transplantation centers have evaluated progressively escalated, low-dose antiviral therapy in an attempt to eradicate hepatitis C viremia prior to transplantation; however, such therapy has been shown to reduce but not to prevent the risk of HCV reinfection after transplantation. After liver transplantation for end-stage liver disease caused by hepatitis C, recurrent hepatitis C is the rule, and the pace of disease progression is more accelerated than in immunocompetent patients (Chap. 310). Current therapy with PEG IFN and ribavirin after liver transplantation is unsatisfactory in most patients, but attempts to minimize immunosuppression are beneficial. The cutaneous and renal vasculitis of HCV-associated essential mixed cryoglobulinemia (Chap. 304) may respond to antiviral therapy, but sustained responses are rare after discontinuation of therapy; therefore, prolonged, perhaps indefinite, therapy is recommended in this group. Anecdotal reports suggest that antiviral therapy may be effective in porphyria cutanea tarda or lichen planus associated with hepatitis C.

In patients with HCV/HIV co-infection, hepatitis C is more progressive and severe than in HCV-monoinfected patients. Although patients with HCV/HIV co-infection respond to antiviral therapy for hepatitis C, they do not respond as well as patients with HCV infection alone. Four large national and international trials of antiviral therapy among patients with HCV/HIV co-infection have shown that PEG IFN (both α-2a and α-2b) plus ribavirin (daily doses ranging from flat-dosed 600–800 mg to weight-based 1000/1200 mg) is superior to standard IFN regimens; however, SVR rates were lower than in HCV-monoinfected patients, ranging from 14 to 38% for patients with genotypes 1 and 4 and from 44 to 73% for patients with genotypes 2 and 3. In the three largest trials, all patients, including those with genotypes 2 and 3, were treated for a full 48 weeks. In addition, tolerability of therapy was lower than in HCV-monoinfected patients; therapy was discontinued because of side effects in 12–39% of patients in these clinical trials. Based on these trials, weekly PEG IFN plus daily ribavirin at a daily dose of at least 600–800 mg, up to full weight-based doses, at doses recommended for HCV-monoinfected patients, if tolerated, is recommended for a full 48 weeks, regardless of genotype. An alternative recommendation for ribavirin doses was issued by a European Consensus Conference and consisted of standard, weight-based 1000–1200 mg for genotypes 1 and 4, but 800 mg for genotypes 2 and 3. A head-to-head trial of combination PEG IFN/ribavirin therapy in HCV/HIV co-infection demonstrated statistically indistinguishable efficacy of the two types of PEG IFN, despite a small advantage for PEG IFN α-2a: for PEG IFN α-2b and α-2a, SVRs occurred in 28% versus 32%, respectively, of patients with genotypes 1 and 4 and in 62% versus 71%, respectively, of patients with genotypes 2 and 3. In HCV/HIV-infected patients, ribavirin can potentiate the toxicity of didanosine (e.g., lactic acidosis) and the lipoatrophy of stavudine, and zidovudine can exacerbate ribavirin-associated hemolytic anemia; therefore, these drug combinations should be avoided.

Patients with a history of injection-drug use and alcoholism can be treated successfully for chronic hepatitis C, preferably in conjunction with drug- and alcohol-treatment programs. Because ribavirin is excreted renally, patients with end-stage renal disease, including those undergoing dialysis (which does not clear ribavirin), are not ideal candidates for ribavirin therapy. Rare reports suggest that reduced-dose ribavirin can be used, but the frequency of anemia is very high and data on efficacy are limited. If patients with renal failure (glomerular filtration rate <60 ml/min) are treated, the PEG IFN α-2a dose should be reduced from 180 to 135 μg weekly and the PEG IFN α-2b dose reduced from 1.5 to 1 μg/kg weekly; similarly, the daily ribavirin dose in this population should be reduced to 200–800 mg (but not used or used cautiously at very low doses) if hemodialysis is required. Neither the optimal regimen nor the efficacy of therapy is well established in this population.

NOVEL ANTIVIRALS To date, attempts to develop better-tolerated ribavirin successors or improved types of IFN α or longer acting IFNs than PEG IFN have not been successful. The demonstration that responsiveness to antiviral therapy is influenced by genetic variation in IL28B, which codes for IFN-λ (as noted above), raises the possibility that IFN-λ might be an effective or even more effective IFN for treating hepatitis C; early trials are in progress. Among the most exciting new approaches to antiviral therapy are orally administered direct antivirals that target HCV polymerase or protease. Two protease inhibitors that are in late stages of development, are expected to be approved in 2011. The NS3-4A serine protease inhibitors telaprevir and boceprevir suppress HCV RNA profoundly and, when used together with PEG IFN and ribavirin in patients with genotype-1 HCV infection, can increase RVR rates to as high as 80% (telaprevir) and SVR rates from those achieved with current standard-of-care therapy by 20–30% to ~65–75%, in most patients with only half the duration of current therapy. These triple-drug combinations appear to yield even higher rates of SVR in >50% of prior relapsers (>70–90%) but also to achieve SVR in prior nonresponders, even in null responders to PEG IFN/ribavirin therapy (~30%). Although these new drugs add elements of additional toxicity (severe rash in ~5% of telaprevir-treated patients and anemia in half of boceprevir-treated patients), they represent an opportunity for curing a substantially larger proportion of patients with shorter treatment courses. Because resistance to these oral agents used alone has been both anticipated and observed, polymerase and protease inhibitors are being evaluated in combinations with PEG IFN and ribavirin to preempt the emergence of resistance. Potentially, in the future, combinations of direct antiviral agents will be used in drug cocktails that may replace IFN-based regimens entirely.

AUTOIMMUNE HEPATITIS

DEFINITION

Autoimmune hepatitis is a chronic disorder characterized by continuing hepatocellular necrosis and inflammation, usually with fibrosis, which can progress to cirrhosis and liver failure. When fulfilling criteria of severity, this type of chronic hepatitis, when untreated, may have a 6-month mortality of as high as 40%. Based on contemporary estimates of the natural history of treated autoimmune hepatitis, the 10-year survival is 80–90%. The prominence of extrahepatic features of autoimmunity as well as seroimmunologic abnormalities in this disorder supports an autoimmune process in its pathogenesis; this concept is reflected in the labels *lupoid, plasma cell*, or *autoimmune hepatitis.* Autoantibodies and other typical features of autoimmunity, however, do not occur in all cases; among the broader categories of "idiopathic" or cryptogenic chronic hepatitis, many, perhaps the majority, are probably autoimmune in origin. Cases in which hepatotropic viruses, metabolic/genetic derangements, and hepatotoxic drugs have been excluded represent a spectrum of heterogeneous liver disorders of unknown cause, a proportion of which are most likely autoimmune hepatitis.

IMMUNOPATHOGENESIS

The weight of evidence suggests that the progressive liver injury in patients with autoimmune hepatitis is the result of a cell-mediated immunologic attack directed against liver cells. In all likelihood, predisposition to autoimmunity is inherited, while the liver specificity of this injury is triggered by environmental (e.g., chemical or viral) factors. For example, patients have been described in whom apparently self-limited cases of acute hepatitis A, B, or C led to autoimmune hepatitis, presumably because of genetic susceptibility or predisposition. Evidence to support an autoimmune pathogenesis in this type of hepatitis includes the following: (1) In the liver, the histopathologic lesions are composed predominantly of cytotoxic T cells and plasma cells; (2) circulating autoantibodies (nuclear, smooth muscle, thyroid, etc.; see below), rheumatoid factor, and hyperglobulinemia are common; (3) other autoimmune disorders—such as thyroiditis, rheumatoid arthritis, autoimmune hemolytic anemia, ulcerative colitis, membranoproliferative glomerulonephritis, juvenile diabetes mellitus, celiac disease, and

Sjögren's syndrome—occur with increased frequency in patients and in their relatives who have autoimmune hepatitis; (4) histocompatibility haplotypes associated with autoimmune diseases, such as HLA-B1, -B8, -DR3, and -DR4 as well as extended haplotype DRB1 alleles, are common in patients with autoimmune hepatitis; and (5) this type of chronic hepatitis is responsive to glucocorticoid/immunosuppressive therapy, effective in a variety of autoimmune disorders.

Cellular immune mechanisms appear to be important in the pathogenesis of autoimmune hepatitis. In vitro studies have suggested that in patients with this disorder, lymphocytes are capable of becoming sensitized to hepatocyte membrane proteins and of destroying liver cells. Abnormalities of immunoregulatory control over cytotoxic lymphocytes (impaired regulatory CD4+CD25+ T cell influences) may play a role as well. Studies of genetic predisposition to autoimmune hepatitis demonstrate that certain haplotypes are associated with the disorder, as enumerated above. The precise triggering factors, genetic influences, and cytotoxic and immunoregulatory mechanisms involved in this type of liver injury remain incompletely defined.

Intriguing clues into the pathogenesis of autoimmune hepatitis come from the observation that circulating autoantibodies are prevalent in patients with this disorder. Among the autoantibodies described in these patients are antibodies to nuclei [so-called antinuclear antibodies (ANAs), primarily in a homogeneous pattern] and smooth muscle (so-called anti-smooth-muscle antibodies, directed at actin), anti-LKM (see below), antibodies to "soluble liver antigen/liver pancreas antigen" (directed against a uracil-guanine-adenine transfer RNA suppressor protein), as well as antibodies to the liver-specific asialoglycoprotein receptor (or "hepatic lectin") and other hepatocyte membrane proteins. Although some of these provide helpful diagnostic markers, their involvement in the pathogenesis of autoimmune hepatitis has not been established.

Humoral immune mechanisms have been shown to play a role in the extrahepatic manifestations of autoimmune and idiopathic hepatitis. Arthralgias, arthritis, cutaneous vasculitis, and glomerulonephritis occurring in patients with autoimmune hepatitis appear to be mediated by the deposition of circulating immune complexes in affected tissue vessels, followed by complement activation, inflammation, and tissue injury. While specific viral antigen-antibody complexes can be identified in acute and chronic viral hepatitis, the nature of the immune complexes in autoimmune hepatitis has not been defined.

Many of the *clinical features* of autoimmune hepatitis are similar to those described for chronic viral hepatitis. The onset of disease may be insidious or abrupt; the disease may present initially like, and be confused with, acute viral hepatitis; a history of recurrent bouts of what had been labeled *acute hepatitis* is not uncommon. A subset of patients with autoimmune hepatitis has distinct features. Such patients are predominantly young to middle-aged women with marked hyperglobulinemia and high-titer circulating ANAs. This is the group with positive lupus erythematosus (LE) preparations (initially labeled "lupoid" hepatitis) in whom other autoimmune features are common. Fatigue, malaise, anorexia, amenorrhea, acne, arthralgias, and jaundice are common. Occasionally arthritis, maculopapular eruptions (including cutaneous vasculitis), erythema nodosum, colitis, pleurisy, pericarditis, anemia, azotemia, and sicca syndrome (keratoconjunctivitis, xerostomia) occur. In some patients, complications of cirrhosis, such as ascites and edema (associated with hypoalbuminemia), encephalopathy, hypersplenism, coagulopathy, or variceal bleeding may bring the patient to initial medical attention.

The course of autoimmune hepatitis may be variable. In those with mild disease or limited histologic lesions (e.g., piecemeal necrosis without bridging), progression to cirrhosis is limited. In those with severe symptomatic autoimmune hepatitis (aminotransferase levels >10 times normal, marked hyperglobulinemia, "aggressive" histologic lesions—bridging necrosis or multilobular collapse, cirrhosis), the 6-month mortality without therapy may be as high as 40%. Such severe disease accounts for only 20% of cases; the natural history of milder disease is variable, often accentuated by spontaneous remissions and exacerbations. Especially poor prognostic signs include the presence histologically of multilobular collapse at the time of initial presentation and failure of the bilirubin to improve after 2 weeks of therapy. Death may result from hepatic failure, hepatic coma, other complications of cirrhosis (e.g., variceal hemorrhage), and intercurrent infection. In patients with established cirrhosis, HCC may be a late complication (Chap. 92) but occurs less frequently than in cirrhosis associated with viral hepatitis.

Laboratory features of autoimmune hepatitis are similar to those seen in chronic viral hepatitis. Liver biochemical tests are invariably abnormal but may not correlate with the clinical severity or histopathologic features in individual cases. Many patients with autoimmune hepatitis have normal serum bilirubin, alkaline phosphatase, and globulin levels with only minimal aminotransferase elevations. Serum AST and ALT levels are increased and fluctuate in the range of 100–1000 units. In severe cases, the serum bilirubin level is moderately elevated [51–171 μmol/L (3–10 mg/dL)]. Hypoalbuminemia occurs in patients with very active or advanced disease. Serum alkaline phosphatase levels may be moderately elevated or near normal. In a small proportion of patients, marked elevations of alkaline phosphatase activity occur; in such patients, clinical and laboratory features overlap with those of primary biliary cirrhosis (Chap. 308). The prothrombin time is often prolonged, particularly late in the disease or during active phases.

Hypergammaglobulinemia (>2.5 g/dL) is common in autoimmune hepatitis. Rheumatoid factor is common as well. As noted above, circulating autoantibodies are also prevalent. The most characteristic are ANAs in a homogeneous staining pattern. Smooth-muscle antibodies are less specific, seen just as frequently in chronic viral hepatitis. Because of the high levels of globulins achieved in the circulation of some patients with autoimmune hepatitis, occasionally the globulins may bind nonspecifically in solid-phase binding immunoassays for viral antibodies. This has been recognized most commonly in tests for antibodies to hepatitis C virus, as noted above. In fact, studies of autoantibodies in autoimmune hepatitis have led to the recognition of new categories of autoimmune hepatitis. *Type I autoimmune hepatitis* is the classic syndrome occurring in young women, associated with marked hyperglobulinemia, lupoid features, circulating ANAs, and HLA-DR3 or HLA-DR4 (especially B8-DRB1*03). Also associated with type I autoimmune hepatitis are autoantibodies against actin as well as atypical perinuclear antineutrophilic cytoplasmic antibodies (pANCA).

Type II autoimmune hepatitis, often seen in children, more common in Mediterranean populations, and linked to HLA-DRB1 and HLA-DQB1 haplotypes, is associated not with ANA but with anti-LKM. Actually, anti-LKM represent a heterogeneous group of antibodies. In type II autoimmune hepatitis, the antibody is anti-LKM1, directed against cytochrome P450 2D6. This is the same anti-LKM seen in some patients with chronic hepatitis C. Anti-LKM2 is seen in drug-induced hepatitis, and anti-LKM3 is seen in patients with chronic hepatitis D. Another autoantibody observed in type II autoimmune hepatitis is directed against liver cytosol formiminotransferase cyclodeaminase (anti-liver cytosol 1). More controversial is whether or not a third category of autoimmune hepatitis exists, *type III autoimmune hepatitis*. These patients lack ANA and anti-LKM1 but have circulating antibodies to soluble liver antigen/liver pancreas antigen. Most of these patients are women and have clinical features similar to, perhaps more severe than, those of patients with type I autoimmune hepatitis.

Type III autoimmune hepatitis does not appear to represent a distinct category but, instead, is part of the spectrum of type I autoimmune hepatitis; this subcategory has not been adopted by a consensus of international experts.

Liver biopsy abnormalities are similar to those described for chronic viral hepatitis. Expanding portal tracts and extending beyond the plate of periportal hepatocytes into the parenchyma (designated *interface hepatitis* or *piecemeal necrosis*) is a mononuclear cell infiltrate that, in autoimmune hepatitis, may include the presence of plasma cells. Necroinflammatory activity characterizes the lobular parenchyma, and evidence of hepatocellular regeneration is reflected by "rosette" formation, the occurrence of thickened liver cell plates, and regenerative "pseudolobules." Septal fibrosis, bridging fibrosis, and cirrhosis are frequent. Bile duct injury and granulomas are uncommon; however, a subgroup of patients with autoimmune hepatitis has histologic, biochemical, and serologic features overlapping those of primary biliary cirrhosis (Chap. 308).

DIAGNOSTIC CRITERIA

An international group has suggested a set of criteria for establishing a diagnosis of autoimmune hepatitis. Exclusion of liver disease caused by genetic disorders, viral hepatitis, drug hepatotoxicity, and alcohol are linked with such inclusive diagnostic criteria as hyperglobulinemia, autoantibodies, and characteristic histologic features. This international group has also suggested a comprehensive diagnostic scoring system that, rarely required for typical cases, may be helpful when typical features are not present. Factors that weigh in favor of the diagnosis include female gender; predominant aminotransferase elevation; presence and level of globulin elevation; presence of nuclear, smooth muscle, LKM1, and other autoantibodies; concurrent other autoimmune diseases; characteristic histologic features (interface hepatitis, plasma cells, rosettes); HLA DR3 or DR4 markers; and response to treatment (see below). Weighing against the diagnosis are predominant alkaline phosphatase elevation, mitochondrial antibodies, markers of viral hepatitis, history of hepatotoxic drugs or excessive alcohol, histologic evidence of bile duct injury, or such atypical histologic features as fatty infiltration, iron overload, and viral inclusions.

DIFFERENTIAL DIAGNOSIS

Early during the course of chronic hepatitis, autoimmune hepatitis may resemble typical *acute viral hepatitis* (Chap. 304). Without histologic assessment, severe chronic hepatitis cannot be readily distinguished based on clinical or biochemical criteria from mild chronic hepatitis. In adolescence, *Wilson's disease* (Chaps. 308 and 360) may present with features of chronic hepatitis long before neurologic manifestations become apparent and before the formation of Kayser-Fleischer rings. In this age group, serum ceruloplasmin and serum and urinary copper determinations plus measurement of liver copper levels will establish the correct diagnosis. *Postnecrotic* or *cryptogenic cirrhosis* and *primary biliary cirrhosis* (Chap. 308) share clinical features with autoimmune hepatitis, and both alcoholic hepatitis (Chap. 307) and nonalcoholic steatohepatitis (Chap. 309) may present with many features common to autoimmune hepatitis; historic, biochemical, serologic, and histologic assessments are usually sufficient to allow these entities to be distinguished from autoimmune hepatitis. Of course, the distinction between autoimmune and chronic viral hepatitis is not always straightforward, especially when viral antibodies occur in patients with autoimmune disease or when autoantibodies occur in patients with viral disease. Furthermore, the presence of extrahepatic features such as arthritis, cutaneous vasculitis, or pleuritis—not to mention the presence of circulating autoantibodies—may cause confusion with *rheumatologic disorders* such as rheumatoid arthritis and systemic lupus erythematosus. The existence of clinical and biochemical features of progressive necroinflammatory liver disease distinguishes chronic hepatitis from these other disorders, which are not associated with severe liver disease.

Finally, occasionally, features of autoimmune hepatitis overlap with features of autoimmune biliary disorders such as primary biliary cirrhosis, primary sclerosing cholangitis (Chaps. 308 and 311), or, even more rarely, mitochondrial antibody-negative autoimmune cholangitis. Such overlap syndromes are difficult to categorize, and often response to therapy may be the distinguishing factor that establishes the diagnosis.

TREATMENT Autoimmune Hepatitis

The mainstay of management in autoimmune hepatitis is glucocorticoid therapy. Several controlled clinical trials have documented that such therapy leads to symptomatic, clinical, biochemical, and histologic improvement as well as increased survival. A therapeutic response can be expected in up to 80% of patients. Unfortunately, therapy has not been shown to prevent ultimate progression to cirrhosis; however, instances of reversal of fibrosis and cirrhosis have been reported in patients responding to treatment. Although some advocate the use of prednisolone (the hepatic metabolite of prednisone), prednisone is just as effective and is favored by most authorities. Therapy may be initiated at 20 mg/d, but a popular regimen in the United States relies on an initiation dose of 60 mg/d. This high dose is tapered successively over the course of a month down to a maintenance level of 20 mg/d. An alternative, but equally effective, approach is to begin with half the prednisone dose (30 mg/d) along with azathioprine (50 mg/d). With azathioprine maintained at 50 mg/d, the prednisone dose is tapered over the course of a month down to a maintenance level of 10 mg/d. The advantage of the combination approach is a reduction, over the span of an 18-month course of therapy, in serious, life-threatening complications of steroid therapy from 66% down to under 20%. In combination regimens, 6-mercaptopurine may be substituted for its prodrug azathioprine, but this is rarely required. Azathioprine alone, however, is not effective in achieving remission, nor is alternate-day glucocorticoid therapy. Limited experience with budesonide in noncirrhotic patients suggests that this steroid side effect–sparing drug may be effective. Although therapy has been shown to be effective for severe autoimmune hepatitis (AST ≥10 times the upper limit of normal or ≥5 times the upper limit of normal in conjunction with serum globulin greater than or equal to twice normal; bridging necrosis or multilobular necrosis on liver biopsy; presence of symptoms), therapy is not indicated for mild forms of chronic hepatitis, and the efficacy of therapy in mild or asymptomatic autoimmune hepatitis has not been established.

Improvement of fatigue, anorexia, malaise, and jaundice tends to occur within days to several weeks; biochemical improvement occurs over the course of several weeks to months, with a fall in serum bilirubin and globulin levels and an increase in serum albumin. Serum aminotransferase levels usually drop promptly, but improvements in AST and ALT alone do not appear to be reliable markers of recovery in individual patients; histologic improvement, characterized by a decrease in mononuclear infiltration and in hepatocellular necrosis, may be delayed for 6–24 months. Still, if interpreted cautiously, aminotransferase levels are valuable indicators of relative disease activity, and many authorities do *not* advocate for serial liver biopsies to assess therapeutic success or to guide decisions to alter or stop therapy. Rapidity of response is more common in older patients

(≥69 years) and those with HLA DBR1*04; although rapid responders may progress less slowly to cirrhosis and liver transplantation, they are no less likely than slower responders to relapse after therapy. Therapy should continue for at least 12–18 months. After tapering and cessation of therapy, the likelihood of relapse is at least 50%, even if posttreatment histology has improved to show mild chronic hepatitis, and the majority of patients require therapy at maintenance doses indefinitely. Continuing azathioprine alone (2 mg/kg body weight daily) after cessation of prednisone therapy may reduce the frequency of relapse.

In medically refractory cases, an attempt should be made to intensify treatment with high-dose glucocorticoid monotherapy (60 mg daily) or combination glucocorticoid (30 mg daily) plus high-dose azathioprine (150 mg daily) therapy. After a month, doses of prednisone can be reduced by 10 mg a month, and doses of azathioprine can be reduced by 50 mg a month toward ultimate, conventional maintenance doses. Patients refractory to this regimen may be treated with cyclosporine, tacrolimus, or mycophenolate mofetil; however, to date, only limited anecdotal reports support these approaches. If medical therapy fails, or when chronic hepatitis progresses to cirrhosis and is associated with life-threatening complications of liver decompensation, liver transplantation is the only recourse (Chap. 310); failure of the bilirubin to improve after 2 weeks of therapy should prompt early consideration of the patient for liver transplantation. Recurrence of autoimmune hepatitis in the new liver occurs rarely in most experiences but in as many as 35–40% of cases in others.

ACKNOWLEDGMENT

Kurt J. Isselbacher, MD, contributed to this chapter in previous editions of Harrison's.

FURTHER READINGS

Benhamou Y, Salmon D (guest ed): Proceedings of the 1st European consensus conference on the treatment of chronic hepatitis B and C in HIV co-infected patients. J Hepatol 44(Suppl 1): S1, 2006

Chang T-T et al: A comparison of entecavir and lamivudine for HBeAg-positive chronic hepatitis B. N Engl J Med 354:1001, 2006

Czaja AJ, Freese DK: AASLD practice guidelines: Diagnosis and treatment of autoimmune hepatitis. Hepatology 36:479, 2002

——, Manns MP: Advances in the diagnosis, pathogenesis, and management of autoimmune hepatitis. Gastroenterology 139:58, 2010

Di Bisceglie AM et al: Prolonged therapy of advanced chronic hepatitis C with low dose peginterferon. N Engl J Med 359:2429, 2008

Dienstag JL, McHutchison JG: American Gastroenterological Association medical position statement on the management of hepatitis C. Gastroenterology 130:225, 2006

——: American Gastroenterological Association technical review on the management of hepatitis C. Gastroenterology 130:231, 2006

——: Hepatitis B virus infection. N Engl J Med 359:1486, 2008

European Association for the Study of the Liver: EASL Consensus Conference on Hepatitis B. J Hepatol 39(Suppl 1):S1, 2003

——: EASL practice guidelines: Management of chronic hepatitis B. J Hepatol 50:227, 2009

Fung SK, Lok ASF: Treatment of chronic hepatitis B: Who to treat, what to use, and for how long? Clin Gastroenterol Hepatol 2:839, 2004

Gale MJ, Foy EM: Evasion of intracellular host defence by hepatitis C virus. Nature 436:939, 2005

Ge D et al: Genetic Variation in IL28B predicts hepatitis C treatment-induced viral clearance. Nature 461:399, 2009

Ghany MG et al: AASLD practice guidelines: Diagnosis, management, and treatment of hepatitis C: An update. Hepatology 49:1335, 2009

Hézode C et al: Telaprevir and peginterferon with or without ribavirin for chronic HCV infection. N Engl J Med 360:1839, 2009

Krawitt EL: Autoimmune hepatitis. N Engl J Med 354:54, 2006

Lai C-L et al: Entecavir versus lamivudine for patients with HBeAg-negative chronic hepatitis B. N Engl J Med 354:1011, 2006

Liaw Y-F et al: Asian-Pacific consensus statement on the management of chronic hepatitis B: A 2008 update. Hepatol International 2:263, 2008

Locarnini SA (guest ed): The control of hepatitis B: The role for chemoprevention. Semin Liver Dis 26:1, 2006

Lok ASF, McMahon BJ: AASLD practice guidelines: Chronic hepatitis B: An update. Hepatology 45:507, 2007

——: AASLD practice guideline update: Chronic hepatitis B: Update 2009. Hepatology 50:661, 2009 (full version accessible at *http://publish.aasld.org/practiceguidelines/Documents/Bookmarked%20Practice%20Guidelines/Chronic_Hep_B_Update_2009%208_24_2009.pdf*, accessed December 14, 2011)

McHutchison JG et al: Peginterferon alfa-2b or alfa-2a with ribavirin for treatment of hepatitis C infection. N Engl J Med 361:580, 2009

——: Telaprevir with peginterferon and ribavirin for chronic HCV genotype 1 infection. N Engl J Med 360:1827, 2009

National Institutes of Health Consensus Development Conference: Management of hepatitis C. Hepatology 36:1S, 2002

——: Management of hepatitis B. Hepatology 49 L:S1, 2009

O'Brien TR: Interferon-alfa, interferon-λ and hepatitis C. Nature Genet 41:1048, 2009

Pawlotsky J-M et al: The hepatitis C virus life cycle as a target for new antiviral therapies. Gastroenterology 132:1979, 2007

Pearlman BL: Chronic hepatitis C therapy: Changing the rules of duration. Clin Gastroenterol Hepatol 4:963, 2006

Thomas DL et al: Genetic variation in IL28B and spontaneous clearance of hepatitis C virus. Nature 461:798, 2009

Toy M et al: Potential impact of long-term nucleoside therapy on the mortality and morbidity of active chronic hepatitis B. Hepatology 50:743, 2009

Wong WW-S et al: Surrogate end points and long-term outcome in patients with chronic hepatitis B. Clin Gastroenterol Hepatol 7:1113, 2009

CHAPTER 307
Alcoholic Liver Disease

Mark E. Mailliard
Michael F. Sorrell

Chronic and excessive alcohol ingestion is one of the major causes of liver disease. Per capita, alcohol consumption and cirrhosis have risen in the last decade in United Kingdom and Russia but has decreased in many developed countries including the United States. The pathology of alcoholic liver disease consists of three major lesions, with the injury rarely existing in a pure form: (1) fatty liver, (2) alcoholic hepatitis, and (3) cirrhosis. Fatty liver is present in >90% of binge and chronic drinkers. A much smaller percentage of heavy drinkers will progress to alcoholic hepatitis, thought to be a precursor to cirrhosis. The prognosis of severe alcoholic liver disease is dismal; the mortality of patients with alcoholic hepatitis concurrent with cirrhosis is nearly 60% at 4 years. Although alcohol is considered a direct hepatotoxin, only between 10 and 20% of alcoholics will develop alcoholic hepatitis. The explanation for this apparent paradox is unclear but involves the complex interaction of facilitating factors, such as intake frequency, diet, and gender.

ETIOLOGY AND PATHOGENESIS

Quantity and duration of alcohol intake are the most important risk factors involved in the development of alcoholic liver disease (Table 307-1). The roles of beverage type(s), i.e. wine, beer, or spirits, and pattern of drinking (daily versus binge drinking) are less clear. Progress of the hepatic injury beyond the fatty liver stage seems to require additional risk factors that remain incompletely defined. Although there are genetic predispositions for alcoholism (Chapter 392), and candidate genes for liver steatosis and fibrosis, gender is a strong determinant for alcoholic liver disease. Women are more susceptible to alcoholic liver injury when compared to men. They develop advanced liver disease with substantially less alcohol intake. In general, the time it takes to develop liver disease is directly related to the amount of alcohol consumed. It is useful in estimating alcohol consumption to understand that one beer, four ounces of wine, or one ounce of 80% spirits all contain ~12 g of alcohol. The threshold for developing alcoholic liver disease in men is an intake of >60–80 g/d of alcohol for 10 years, while women are at increased risk for developing similar degrees of liver injury by consuming 20–40 g/d. Ingestion of 160 g/d is associated with a 25-fold increased risk of developing alcoholic cirrhosis. Gender-dependent differences result from poorly understood effects of estrogen and the metabolism of alcohol. Diet, particularly an increase in liver injury from high fat or the protective effect of coffee, has been postulated to play a part in the development of the pathogenic process.

TABLE 307-1 Risk Factors for Alcoholic Liver Disease

Risk Factor	Comment
Quantity	In men, 40–80 g/d of ethanol produces fatty liver; 160 g/d for 10–20 years causes hepatitis or cirrhosis. Only 15% of alcoholics develop alcoholic liver disease.
Gender	Women exhibit increased susceptibility to alcoholic liver disease at amounts >20 g/d; two drinks per day is probably safe.
Hepatitis C	HCV infection concurrent with alcoholic liver disease is associated with younger age for severity, more advanced histology, decreased survival.
Genetics	Gene polymorphisms may include alcohol dehydrogenase, cytochrome P4502E1, and those associated with alcoholism (twin studies).
Malnutrition	Alcohol injury does not require malnutrition, but obesity and fatty liver from the effect of carbohydrate on the transcriptional control of lipid synthesis and transport may be factors. Patients should receive vigorous attention to nutritional support.

Chronic infection with hepatitis C (HCV) (Chap. 306) is an important comorbidity in the progression of alcoholic liver disease to cirrhosis in chronic and excessive drinkers. Even moderate alcohol intake of 20–50 g/d increases the risk of cirrhosis and hepatocellular cancer in HCV-infected individuals. Patients with both alcoholic liver injury and HCV infection develop decompensated liver disease at a younger age and have poorer overall survival. Increased liver iron stores and, rarely, porphyria cutanea tarda can occur as a consequence of the overlapping injurious processes secondary to alcohol abuse and HCV infection. In addition, alcohol intake of >50 g/d by HCV-infected patients decreases the efficacy of interferon-based antiviral therapy.

Our understanding of the pathogenesis of alcoholic liver injury is incomplete. Alcohol is a direct hepatotoxin, but ingestion of alcohol initiates a variety of metabolic responses that influence the final hepatotoxic response. The initial concept of malnutrition as the major pathogenic mechanism has been replaced by the understanding that the hepatic metabolism of alcohol initiates a pathogenic process including the production of toxic protein-aldehyde adducts, the generation of reducing equivalents that promotes lipogenesis, and the inhibition of fatty-acid oxidation. Endotoxins, oxidative stress, immunologic activity, and pro-inflammatory cytokine release contribute to the resulting liver injury (Fig. 307-1). The complex interaction of intestinal and hepatic cells is crucial to alcohol-mediated liver injury. Tumor necrosis factor α (TNF-α) and intestine-derived endotoxemia facilitate hepatocyte apoptosis and necrosis. Stellate cell activation and collagen production are key events in hepatic fibrogenesis. The resulting fibrosis determines the architectural derangement of the liver following chronic alcohol ingestion.

PATHOLOGY

The liver has a limited repertoire in response to injury. Fatty liver is the initial and most common histologic response to hepatotoxic stimuli, including excessive alcohol ingestion. The accumulation of fat within the perivenular hepatocytes coincides with the location of alcohol dehydrogenase, the major enzyme responsible for alcohol metabolism. Continuing alcohol ingestion results in fat accumulation throughout the entire hepatic lobule. Despite extensive fatty change and distortion of the hepatocytes with macrovesicular fat, the cessation of drinking results in normalization of hepatic architecture and fat content within the liver. Alcoholic fatty liver has traditionally been regarded as entirely benign, but similar to the spectrum of nonalcoholic fatty-liver disease (Chap. 309), the

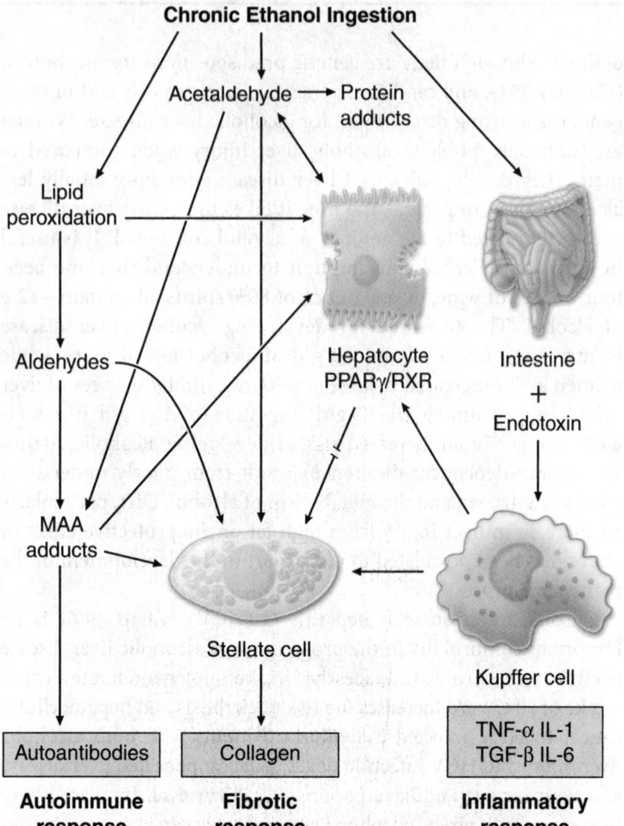

Figure 307-1 Biomedical and cellular pathogenesis of liver injury secondary to chronic ethanol ingestion. MAA, malondialdehyde-acetaldehyde; TNF, tumor necrosis factor; TGF, transforming growth factor; IL, interleukin; PPAR, peroxisome proliferator-activated receptor; RXR, retinoid X receptor.

appearance of steatohepatitis and certain pathologic features such as giant mitochondria, perivenular fibrosis, and macrovesicular fat may be associated with progressive liver injury.

The transition between fatty liver and the development of alcoholic hepatitis is blurred. The hallmark of alcoholic hepatitis is hepatocyte injury characterized by ballooning degeneration, spotty necrosis, polymorphonuclear infiltrate, and fibrosis in the perivenular and perisinusoidal space of Disse. Mallory bodies are often present in florid cases but are neither specific nor necessary to establishing the diagnosis. Alcoholic hepatitis is thought to be a precursor to the development of cirrhosis. However, like fatty liver, it is potentially reversible with cessation of drinking. Cirrhosis is present in up to 50% of patients with biopsy-proven alcoholic hepatitis and its regression is uncertain, even with abstention.

CLINICAL FEATURES

The clinical manifestations of alcoholic fatty liver are subtle and characteristically detected as a consequence of the patient's visit for a seemingly unrelated matter. Previously unsuspected hepatomegaly is often the only clinical finding. Occasionally, patients with fatty liver will present with right upper quadrant discomfort, nausea, and, rarely, jaundice. Differentiation of alcoholic fatty liver from nonalcoholic fatty liver is difficult unless an accurate drinking history is ascertained. In every instance where liver disease is present, a thoughtful and sensitive drinking history should be obtained. Standard, validated questions accurately detect alcohol-related problems (Chap. 392). Alcoholic hepatitis is associated with a wide gamut of clinical features. Fever, spider nevi, jaundice, and abdominal pain simulating an acute abdomen represent the extreme end of the spectrum, while many patients will be entirely asymptomatic. Portal hypertension, ascites, or variceal bleeding can occur in the absence of cirrhosis. Recognition of the clinical features of alcoholic hepatitis is central to the initiation of an effective and appropriate diagnostic and therapeutic strategy. It is important to recognize that patients with alcoholic cirrhosis often exhibit clinical features identical to other causes of cirrhosis.

LABORATORY FEATURES

Patients with alcoholic liver disease are often identified through routine screening tests. The typical laboratory abnormalities seen in fatty liver are nonspecific and include modest elevations of the aspartate aminotransferase (AST), alanine aminotransferase (ALT), and γ-glutamyl transpeptidase (GGTP), accompanied by hypertriglyceridemia, hypercholesterolemia, and, occasionally, hyperbilirubinemia. In alcoholic hepatitis and in contrast to other causes of fatty liver, the AST and ALT are usually elevated two- to sevenfold. They are rarely >400 IU, and the AST/ALT ratio >1 (Table 307-2). Hyperbilirubinemia is common and is accompanied by modest increases in the alkaline phosphatase level. Derangement in hepatocyte synthetic function indicates more serious disease. Hypoalbuminemia and coagulopathy are common in advanced liver injury. Ultrasonography is useful in detecting fatty infiltration of the liver and determining liver size. The demonstration by ultrasound of portal vein flow reversal, ascites, and intraabdominal collaterals indicates serious liver injury with less potential for complete reversal of liver disease.

PROGNOSIS

Critically ill patients with alcoholic hepatitis have short-term (30-day) mortality rates >50%. Severe alcoholic hepatitis is heralded by coagulopathy (prothrombin time increased >5 s), anemia, serum albumin concentrations <25 g/L (2.5 mg/dL), serum bilirubin levels >137 μmol/L (8 mg/dL), renal failure, and ascites. A discriminant function calculated as 4.6 X [the prolongation of the prothrombin time above control (seconds)] + serum bilirubin (mg/dL) can identify patients with a poor prognosis (discriminant function >32). A Model for End-Stage Liver Disease score (MELD, Chap. 310) ≥21 also is associated with significant mortality in alcoholic hepatitis. The presence of ascites, variceal hemorrhage, deep encephalopathy, or hepatorenal syndrome predicts a dismal prognosis. The pathologic

TABLE 307-2 Laboratory Diagnosis of Alcoholic Fatty Liver and Alcoholic Hepatitis

Test	Comment
AST	Increased two- to sevenfold, <400 U/L, greater than ALT
ALT	Increased two- to sevenfold, <400 U/L
AST/ALT	Usually >1
GGTP	Not specific to alcohol, easily inducible, elevated in all forms of fatty liver
Bilirubin	May be markedly increased in alcoholic hepatitis despite modest elevation in alkaline phosphatase
PMN	If >5500/μL, predicts severe alcoholic hepatitis when discriminant function >32

Note: AST, aspartate aminotransferase; ALT, alanine aminotransferase; GGTP, gamma-glutamyl transpeptidase; PMN, polymorphonuclear cells.

stage of the injury can be helpful in predicting prognosis. Liver biopsy should be performed whenever possible to confirm the diagnosis, to establish potential reversibility of the liver disease, and to guide the therapeutic decisions.

TREATMENT Alcoholic Liver Disease

Complete abstinence from alcohol is the cornerstone in the treatment of alcoholic liver disease. Improved survival and the potential for reversal of histologic injury regardless of the initial clinical presentation are associated with total avoidance of alcohol ingestion. Referral of patients to experienced alcohol counselors and/or alcohol treatment programs should be routine in the management of patients with alcoholic liver disease. Attention should be directed to the nutritional and psychosocial states during the evaluation and treatment periods. Because of data suggesting that the pathogenic mechanisms in alcoholic hepatitis involve cytokine release and the perpetuation of injury by immunologic processes, glucocorticoids have been extensively evaluated in the treatment of alcoholic hepatitis. Patients with severe alcoholic hepatitis, defined as a discriminant function >32 or MELD >20, should be given prednisone, 40 mg/d, or prednisolone, 32 mg/d, for 4 weeks, followed by a steroid taper (Fig. 307-2). Exclusion criteria include active gastrointestinal bleeding, renal failure, or pancreatitis. Women with encephalopathy from severe alcoholic hepatitis may be particularly good candidates for glucocorticoids. A Lille score >0.45, at *http://www.lillemodel.com*, uses pretreatment variables plus the change in total bilirubin at day seven of glucocorticoids to identify patients unresponsive to therapy.

The role of TNF-α expression and receptor activity in alcoholic liver injury has led to an examination of TNF inhibition as an alternative to glucocorticoids for severe alcoholic hepatitis.

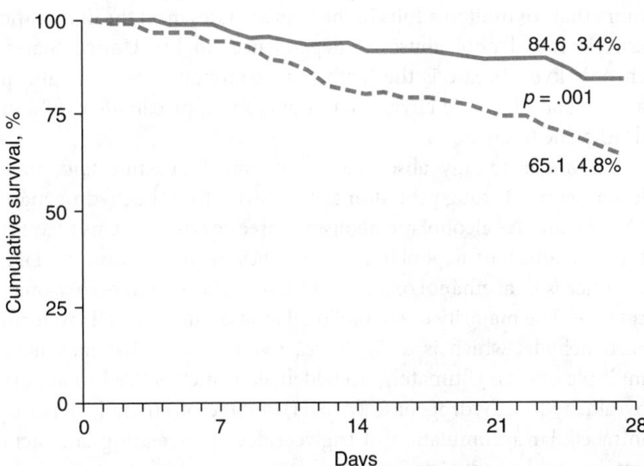

Figure 307-2 Effect of glucocorticoid therapy of severe alcoholic hepatitis on short-term survival: the result of a meta-analysis of individual data from three studies. Prednisolone, solid line; placebo, dotted line. *(Adapted from Mathurin et al., with permission from Elsevier Science.)*

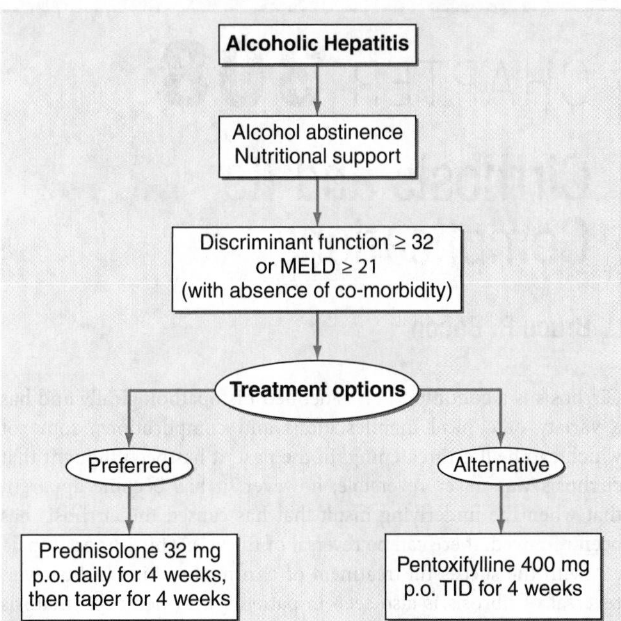

Figure 307-3 Treatment algorithm for alcoholic hepatitis. As identified by a calculated discriminant function >32 (see text), patients with severe alcoholic hepatitis, without the presence of gastrointestinal bleeding or infection, would be candidates for either glucocorticoids or pentoxifylline administration.

The nonspecific TNF inhibitor, pentoxifylline, demonstrated improved survival in the therapy of severe alcoholic hepatitis (Fig. 307-3). Monoclonal antibodies that neutralize serum TNF-α should not be used in alcoholic hepatitis because of recent studies reporting increased deaths secondary to infection and renal failure. Because of inordinate surgical mortality and the high rates of recidivism following transplantation, patients with alcoholic hepatitis are not candidates for immediate liver transplantation. The transplant candidacy of these patients should be reevaluated after a defined period of sobriety.

FURTHER READINGS

Akriviadis E et al: Pentoxifylline improves short-term survival in severe acute alcoholic hepatitis: A double blind placebo controlled trial. Gastroenterology 119:1637, 2000

Luvet A et al: The Lille model: A new tool for therapeutic strategy in patients with severe alcoholic hepatitis treated with steroids. Hepatology 45: 1348, 2007

Mathurin P et al: Corticosteroids improve short-term survival in patients with severe alcoholic hepatitis (AH): Individual data analysis of the last three randomized placebo controlled double blind trials of corticosteroids in severe AH. J Hepatol 36:480, 2002

Zakhari S, Li Ting-Kai: Determinants of alcohol use and abuse: Impact of quantity and frequency patterns on liver disease. Hepatology 46: 2032, 2007

CHAPTER 308 Cirrhosis and Its Complications

Bruce R. Bacon

Cirrhosis is a condition that is defined histopathologically and has a variety of clinical manifestations and complications, some of which can be life-threatening. In the past, it has been thought that cirrhosis was never reversible; however, it has become apparent that when the underlying insult that has caused the cirrhosis has been removed, there can be reversal of fibrosis. This is most apparent with the successful treatment of chronic hepatitis C; however, reversal of fibrosis is also seen in patients with hemochromatosis who have been successfully treated and in patients with alcoholic liver disease who have discontinued alcohol use.

Regardless of the cause of cirrhosis, the pathologic features consist of the development of fibrosis to the point that there is architectural distortion with the formation of regenerative nodules. This results in a decrease in hepatocellular mass, and thus function, and an alteration of blood flow. The induction of fibrosis occurs with activation of hepatic stellate cells, resulting in the formation of increased amounts of collagen and other components of the extracellular matrix.

Clinical features of cirrhosis are the result of pathologic changes and mirror the severity of the liver disease. Most hepatic pathologists provide an assessment of grading and staging when evaluating liver biopsy samples. These grading and staging schemes vary between disease states and have been developed for most conditions, including chronic viral hepatitis, nonalcoholic fatty liver disease, and primary biliary cirrhosis. Advanced fibrosis usually includes bridging fibrosis with nodularity designated as stage 3 and cirrhosis designated as stage 4. Patients who have cirrhosis have varying degrees of compensated liver function, and clinicians need to differentiate between those who have stable, compensated cirrhosis and those who have decompensated cirrhosis. Patients who have developed complications of their liver disease and have become decompensated should be considered for liver transplantation. Many of the complications of cirrhosis will require specific therapy. *Portal hypertension* is a significant complicating feature of decompensated cirrhosis and is responsible for the development of ascites and bleeding from esophagogastric varices, two complications that signify decompensated cirrhosis. Loss of hepatocellular function results in jaundice, coagulation disorders, and hypoalbuminemia and contributes to the causes of portosystemic encephalopathy. The complications of cirrhosis are basically the same regardless of the etiology. Nonetheless, it is useful to classify patients by the cause of their liver disease (Table 308-1); patients can be divided into broad groups with alcoholic cirrhosis, cirrhosis due to chronic viral hepatitis, biliary cirrhosis, and other, less-common causes such as cardiac cirrhosis, cryptogenic cirrhosis, and other miscellaneous causes.

TABLE 308-1 Causes of Cirrhosis

Alcoholism	Cardiac cirrhosis
Chronic viral hepatitis	Inherited metabolic liver disease
Hepatitis B	Hemochromatosis
Hepatitis C	Wilson's disease
Autoimmune hepatitis	α_1 Antitrypsin deficiency
Nonalcoholic steatohepatitis	Cystic fibrosis
Biliary cirrhosis	Cryptogenic cirrhosis
Primary biliary cirrhosis	
Primary sclerosing cholangitis	
Autoimmune cholangiopathy	

ALCOHOLIC CIRRHOSIS

Excessive chronic alcohol use can cause several different types of chronic liver disease, including alcoholic fatty liver, alcoholic hepatitis, and alcoholic cirrhosis. Furthermore, use of excessive alcohol can contribute to liver damage in patients with other liver diseases, such as hepatitis C, hemochromatosis, and those patients who have fatty liver disease related to obesity. Chronic alcohol use can produce fibrosis in the absence of accompanying inflammation and/or necrosis. Fibrosis can be centrilobular, pericellular, or periportal. When fibrosis reaches a certain degree, there is disruption of the normal liver architecture and replacement of liver cells by regenerative nodules. In alcoholic cirrhosis, the nodules are usually <3 mm in diameter; this form of cirrhosis is referred to as *micronodular*. With cessation of alcohol use, larger nodules may form, resulting in a mixed micronodular and macronodular cirrhosis.

Pathogenesis

Alcohol is the most commonly used drug in the United States, and more than two-thirds of adults drink alcohol each year. Thirty percent have had a binge within the past month, and over 7% of adults regularly consume more than two drinks per day. Unfortunately, more than 14 million adults in the United States meet the diagnostic criteria for alcohol abuse or dependence. In the United States, chronic liver disease is the tenth most common cause of death in adults, and alcoholic cirrhosis accounts for approximately 40% of deaths due to cirrhosis.

Ethanol is mainly absorbed by the small intestine and, to a lesser degree, through the stomach. Gastric alcohol dehydrogenase (ADH) initiates alcohol metabolism. Three enzyme systems account for metabolism of alcohol in the liver. These include cytosolic ADH, the microsomal ethanol oxidizing system (MEOS), and peroxisomal catalase. The majority of ethanol oxidation occurs via ADH to form acetaldehyde, which is a highly reactive molecule that may have multiple effects. Ultimately, acetaldehyde is metabolized to acetate by aldehyde dehydrogenase (ALDH). Intake of ethanol increases intracellular accumulation of triglycerides by increasing fatty acid uptake and by reducing fatty acid oxidation and lipoprotein secretion. Protein synthesis, glycosylation, and secretion are impaired. Oxidative damage to hepatocyte membranes occurs due to the formation of reactive oxygen species; acetaldehyde is a highly reactive molecule that combines with proteins to form protein-acetaldehyde adducts. These adducts may interfere with specific enzyme activities, including microtubular formation and hepatic protein trafficking. With acetaldehyde-mediated hepatocyte damage, certain reactive oxygen species can result in Kupffer cell activation. As a result, profibrogenic cytokines are produced that initiate and perpetuate stellate cell activation, with the resultant production of excess collagen and extracellular matrix. Connective tissue appears in both periportal and pericentral zones and eventually connects portal triads with central veins forming regenerative nodules. Hepatocyte loss occurs, and with increased collagen production and deposition, together with continuing hepatocyte destruction, the liver contracts and shrinks in size. This process generally takes from years to decades to occur and requires repeated insults.

Clinical features

The diagnosis of alcoholic liver disease requires an accurate history regarding both amount and duration of alcohol consumption. Patients with alcoholic liver disease can present with nonspecific symptoms such as vague right upper quadrant pain, fever, nausea and vomiting, diarrhea, anorexia, and malaise. Alternatively, they may present with more specific complications of chronic liver disease, including ascites, edema, or upper gastrointestinal (GI) hemorrhage. Many cases present incidentally at the time of autopsy or elective surgery. Other clinical manifestations include the development of jaundice or encephalopathy. The abrupt onset of any of these complications may be the first event prompting the patient to seek medical attention. Other patients may be identified in the course of an evaluation of routine laboratory studies that are found to be abnormal. On physical examination, the liver and spleen may be enlarged, with the liver edge being firm and nodular. Other frequent findings include scleral icterus, palmar erythema (Fig. 308-1), spider angiomas (Fig. 308-2), parotid gland enlargement, digital clubbing, muscle wasting, or the development of edema and ascites. Men may have decreased body hair and gynecomastia as well as testicular atrophy, which may be a consequence of hormonal abnormalities or a direct toxic effect of alcohol on the testes. In women with advanced alcoholic cirrhosis, menstrual irregularities usually occur, and some women may be amenorrheic. These changes are often reversible following cessation of alcohol.

Laboratory tests may be completely normal in patients with early compensated alcoholic cirrhosis. Alternatively, in advanced liver disease, many abnormalities usually are present. Patients may be anemic either from chronic GI blood loss, nutritional deficiencies, or hypersplenism related to portal hypertension, or as a direct suppressive effect of alcohol on the bone marrow. A unique form of hemolytic anemia (with spur cells and acanthocytes) called *Zieve's syndrome* can occur in patients with severe alcoholic hepatitis. Platelet counts are often reduced early in the disease, reflective of portal hypertension with hypersplenism. Serum total bilirubin can be normal or elevated with advanced disease. Direct bilirubin is frequently mildly elevated in patients with a normal total bilirubin, but the abnormality typically progresses as the disease worsens. Prothrombin times are often prolonged and usually do not respond to administration of parenteral vitamin K. Serum sodium levels are usually normal unless patients have ascites and then can be depressed, largely due to ingestion of excess free water. Serum alanine and aspartate aminotransferases (ALT, AST) are typically elevated, particularly in patients who continue to drink, with AST levels being higher than ALT levels, usually by a 2:1 ratio.

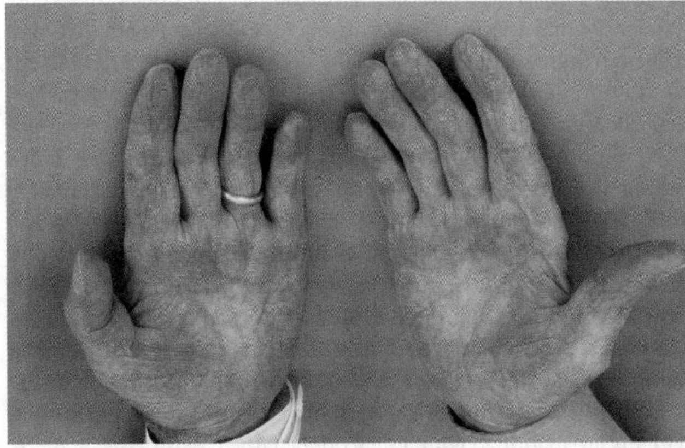

Figure 308-1 Palmar erythema. This figure shows palmar erythema in a patient with alcoholic cirrhosis. The erythema is peripheral over the palm with central pallor.

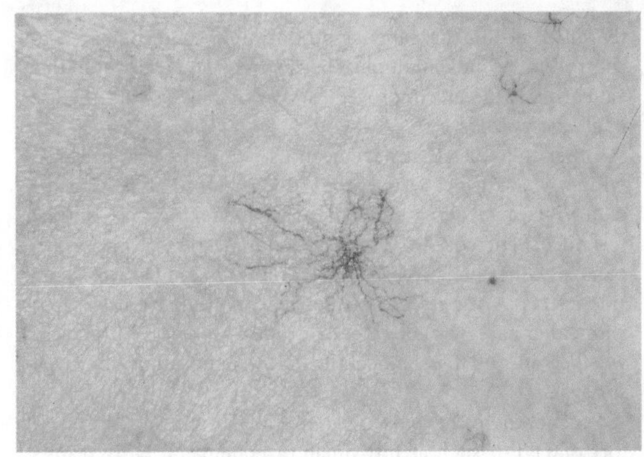

Figure 308-2 Spider angioma. This figure shows a spider angioma in a patient with hepatitis C cirrhosis. With release of central compression, the arteriole fills from the center and spreads out peripherally.

Diagnosis

Patients who have any of the above-mentioned clinical features, physical examination findings, or laboratory studies should be considered to have alcoholic liver disease. The diagnosis, however, requires accurate knowledge that the patient is continuing to use and abuse alcohol. Furthermore, other forms of chronic liver disease (e.g., chronic viral hepatitis or metabolic or autoimmune liver diseases) must be considered or ruled out or, if present, an estimate of relative causality along with the alcohol use should be determined. Liver biopsy can be helpful to confirm a diagnosis, but generally when patients present with alcoholic hepatitis and are still drinking, liver biopsy is withheld until abstinence has been maintained for at least 6 months to determine residual, nonreversible disease.

In patients who have had complications of cirrhosis and who continue to drink, there is a <50% 5-year survival. In contrast, in those patients who are able to remain abstinent, the prognosis is significantly improved. In patients with advanced liver disease, the prognosis remains poor; however, in those individuals who are able to remain abstinent, liver transplantation is a viable option.

TREATMENT Alcoholic Cirrhosis

Abstinence is the cornerstone of therapy for patients with alcoholic liver disease. In addition, patients require good nutrition and long-term medical supervision to manage underlying complications that may develop. Complications such as the development of ascites and edema, variceal hemorrhage, or portosystemic encephalopathy all require specific management and treatment. Glucocorticoids are occasionally used in patients with severe alcoholic hepatitis in the absence of infection. Survival has been shown to improve in certain studies. Treatment is restricted to patients with a discriminant function (DF) value of >32. The DF is calculated as the serum total bilirubin plus the difference in the patient's prothrombin time compared to control (in seconds) multiplied by 4.6. In patients for whom this value is >32, there is improved survival at 28 days with the use of glucocorticoids.

Other therapies that have been used include oral pentoxifylline, which decreases the production of tumor necrosis factor α (TNF-α) and other proinflammatory cytokines. In contrast to glucocorticoids, with which complications can occur, pentoxifylline is relatively easy to administer and has few if any side effects. A variety of nutritional therapies have been tried with either parenteral or enteral feedings; however, it is unclear whether any of these modalities have significantly improved survival.

Recent studies have used parenterally administered inhibitors of TNF-α such as infliximab or etanercept. Early results have shown no adverse events; however, there was no clear-cut improvement in survival. Anabolic steroids, propylthiouracil, antioxidants, colchicine, and penicillamine have all been used but do not show clear-cut benefits and are not recommended.

As mentioned above, the cornerstone to treatment is cessation of alcohol use. Recent experience with medications that reduce craving for alcohol such as acamprosate calcium has been favorable. Patients may take other necessary medications even in the presence of cirrhosis. Acetaminophen use is often discouraged in patients with liver disease; however, if no more than 2 g of acetaminophen per day are consumed, there generally are no problems.

CIRRHOSIS DUE TO CHRONIC VIRAL HEPATITIS B OR C

Of patients exposed to the hepatitis C virus (HCV), approximately 80% develop chronic hepatitis C, and of those, about 20–30% will develop cirrhosis over 20–30 years. Many of these patients have had concomitant alcohol use, and the true incidence of cirrhosis due to hepatitis C alone is unknown. Nonetheless, this represents a significant number of patients. It is expected that an even higher percentage will go on to develop cirrhosis over longer periods of time. In the United States, approximately 5 million people have been exposed to the hepatitis C virus, with about 3.5 to 4 million who are chronically viremic. Worldwide, about 170 million individuals have hepatitis C, with some areas of the world (e.g., Egypt) having up to 15% of the population infected. HCV is a noncytopathic virus, and liver damage is probably immune-mediated. Progression of liver disease due to chronic hepatitis C is characterized by portal-based fibrosis with bridging fibrosis and nodularity developing, ultimately culminating in the development of cirrhosis. In cirrhosis due to chronic hepatitis C, the liver is small and shrunken with characteristic features of a mixed micro- and macronodular cirrhosis seen on liver biopsy. In addition to the increased fibrosis that is seen in cirrhosis due to hepatitis C, an inflammatory infiltrate is found in portal areas with interface hepatitis and occasionally some lobular hepatocellular injury and inflammation. In patients with HCV genotype 3, steatosis is often present.

Similar findings are seen in patients with cirrhosis due to chronic hepatitis B. Of adult patients exposed to hepatitis B, about 5% develop chronic hepatitis B, and about 20% of those patients will go on to develop cirrhosis. Special stains for hepatitis B core (HBc) and hepatitis B surface (HBs) antigen will be positive, and ground-glass hepatocytes signifying hepatitis B surface antigen (HBsAg) may be present. In the United States, there are about 2 million carriers of hepatitis B, whereas in other parts of the world where hepatitis B virus (HBV) is endemic (i.e., Asia, Southeast Asia, sub-Saharan Africa), up to 15% of the population may be infected having acquired the infection vertically at the time of birth. Thus, over 300–400 million individuals are thought to have hepatitis B worldwide. Approximately 25% of these individuals may ultimately develop cirrhosis.

Clinical features and diagnosis

Patients with cirrhosis due to either chronic hepatitis C or B can present with the usual symptoms and signs of chronic liver disease. Fatigue, malaise, vague right upper quadrant pain, and laboratory abnormalities are frequent presenting features. Diagnosis requires a thorough laboratory evaluation, including quantitative HCV RNA testing and analysis for HCV genotype, or hepatitis B serologies to include HBsAg, anti-HBs, HBeAg (hepatitis B e antigen), anti-HBe, and quantitative HBV DNA levels.

TREATMENT Cirrhosis Due to Chronic Viral Hepatitis B or C

Management of complications of cirrhosis revolves around specific therapy for treatment of whatever complications occur, whether they be esophageal variceal hemorrhage, development of ascites and edema, or encephalopathy. In patients with chronic hepatitis B, numerous studies have shown beneficial effects of antiviral therapy, which is effective at viral suppression, as evidenced by reducing aminotransferase levels and HBV DNA levels, and improving histology by reducing inflammation and fibrosis. Several clinical trials and case series have demonstrated that patients with decompensated liver disease can become compensated with the use of antiviral therapy directed against hepatitis B. Currently available therapy includes lamivudine, adefovir, telbivudine, entecavir, and tenofovir. Interferon α can also be used for treating hepatitis B, but it should not be used in cirrhotics.

Treatment of patients with cirrhosis due to hepatitis C is a little more difficult because the side effects of pegylated interferon and ribavirin therapy are oftentimes difficult to manage. Dose-limiting cytopenias (platelets, white blood cells, red blood cells) or severe side effects can result in discontinuation of treatment. Nonetheless, if patients can tolerate treatment, and if it is successful, the benefit is great and disease progression is reduced.

CIRRHOSIS FROM AUTOIMMUNE HEPATITIS AND NONALCOHOLIC FATTY LIVER DISEASE

Other causes of posthepatitic cirrhosis include autoimmune hepatitis and cirrhosis due to nonalcoholic steatohepatitis. Many patients with autoimmune hepatitis (AIH) present with cirrhosis that is already established. Typically, these patients will not benefit from immunosuppressive therapy with glucocorticoids or azathioprine because the AIH is "burned out." In this situation, liver biopsy does not show a significant inflammatory infiltrate. Diagnosis in this setting requires positive autoimmune markers such as antinuclear antibody (ANA) or anti-smooth-muscle antibody (ASMA). When patients with AIH present with cirrhosis and active inflammation accompanied by elevated liver enzymes, there can be considerable benefit from the use of immunosuppressive therapy.

Patients with nonalcoholic steatohepatitis are increasingly being found to have progressed to cirrhosis. With the epidemic of obesity that continues in Western countries, more and more patients are identified with nonalcoholic fatty liver disease. Of these, a significant subset have nonalcoholic steatohepatitis and can progress to increased fibrosis and cirrhosis. Over the past several years, it has been increasingly recognized that many patients who were thought to have cryptogenic cirrhosis in fact have nonalcoholic steatohepatitis. As their cirrhosis progresses, they become catabolic and then lose the telltale signs of steatosis seen on biopsy. Management of complications of cirrhosis due to either AIH or nonalcoholic steatohepatitis is similar to that for other forms of cirrhosis.

BILIARY CIRRHOSIS

Biliary cirrhosis has pathologic features that are different from either alcoholic cirrhosis or posthepatitic cirrhosis, yet the manifestations of end-stage liver disease are the same. Cholestatic liver disease may result from necroinflammatory lesions, congenital or metabolic processes, or external bile duct compression. Thus, two broad categories reflect the anatomic sites of abnormal bile retention: *intrahepatic* and *extrahepatic*. The distinction is important for obvious therapeutic reasons. Extrahepatic obstruction may benefit from surgical or endoscopic biliary tract decompression, whereas intrahepatic cholestatic processes will not improve with such interventions and require a different approach.

The major causes of chronic cholestatic syndromes are primary biliary cirrhosis (PBC), autoimmune cholangitis (AIC), primary sclerosing cholangitis (PSC), and idiopathic adulthood ductopenia. These syndromes are usually clinically distinguished from each other by antibody testing, cholangiographic findings, and clinical presentation. However, they all share the histopathologic features of chronic cholestasis, such as cholate stasis; copper deposition; xanthomatous transformation of hepatocytes; and irregular, so-called biliary fibrosis. In addition, there may be chronic portal inflammation, interface activity, and chronic lobular inflammation. Ductopenia is a result of this progressive disease as patients develop cirrhosis.

PRIMARY BILIARY CIRRHOSIS

PBC is seen in about 100–200 individuals per million, with a strong female preponderance and a median age of around 50 years at the time of diagnosis. The cause of PBC is unknown; it is characterized by portal inflammation and necrosis of cholangiocytes in small- and medium-sized bile ducts. Cholestatic features prevail, and biliary cirrhosis is characterized by an elevated bilirubin level and progressive liver failure. Liver transplantation is the treatment of choice for patients with decompensated cirrhosis due to PBC. A variety of therapies have been proposed, but ursodeoxycholic acid (UDCA) is the only approved treatment that has some degree of efficacy by slowing the rate of progression of the disease.

Antimitochondrial antibodies (AMA) are present in about 90% of patients with PBC. These autoantibodies recognize intermitochondrial membrane proteins that are enzymes of the pyruvate dehydrogenase complex (PDC), the branched-chain 2-oxoacid dehydrogenase complex, and the 2-oxogluterate dehydrogenase complex. Most relate to pyruvate dehydrogenase. These autoantibodies are not pathogenic but rather are useful markers for making a diagnosis of PBC.

Pathology

Histopathologic analyses of liver biopsies of patients with PBC have resulted in identifying four distinct stages of the disease as it progresses. The earliest lesion is termed *chronic nonsuppurative destructive cholangitis* and is a necrotizing inflammatory process of the portal tracts. Medium and small bile ducts are infiltrated with lymphocytes and undergo duct destruction. Mild fibrosis and sometimes bile stasis can occur. With progression, the inflammatory infiltrate becomes less prominent, but the number of bile ducts is reduced and there is proliferation of smaller bile ductules. Increased fibrosis ensues with the expansion of periportal fibrosis to bridging fibrosis. Finally, cirrhosis, which may be micronodular or macronodular, develops.

Clinical features

Currently, most patients with PBC are diagnosed well before the end-stage manifestations of the disease are present, and, as such, most patients are actually asymptomatic. When symptoms are present, they most prominently include a significant degree of fatigue out of proportion to what would be expected for either the severity of the liver disease or the age of the patient. Pruritus is seen in approximately 50% of patients at the time of diagnosis, and it can be debilitating. It might be intermittent and usually is most bothersome in the evening. In some patients, pruritus can develop toward the end of pregnancy, and there are examples of patients having been diagnosed with cholestasis of pregnancy rather than PBC. Pruritus that presents prior to the development of jaundice indicates severe disease and a poor prognosis.

Physical examination can show jaundice and other complications of chronic liver disease, including hepatomegaly, splenomegaly, ascites, and edema. Other features that are unique to PBC include hyperpigmentation, xanthelasma, and xanthomata, which are related to the altered cholesterol metabolism seen in this disease. Hyperpigmentation is evident on the trunk and the arms and is seen in areas of exfoliation and lichenification associated with progressive scratching related to the pruritus. Bone pain resulting from osteopenia or osteoporosis is occasionally seen at the time of diagnosis.

Laboratory findings

Laboratory findings in PBC show cholestatic liver enzyme abnormalities with an elevation in γ-glutamyl transpeptidase and alkaline phosphatase (ALP) along with mild elevations in aminotransferases (ALT and AST). Immunoglobulins, particularly IgM, are typically increased. Hyperbilirubinemia usually is seen once cirrhosis has developed. Thrombocytopenia, leukopenia, and anemia may be seen in patients with portal hypertension and hypersplenism. Liver biopsy shows characteristic features as described above and should be evident to any experienced hepatopathologist. Up to 10% of patients with characteristic PBC will have features of AIH as well and are defined as having "overlap" syndrome. These patients are treated as PBC patients and may progress to cirrhosis with the same frequency as typical PBC patients.

Diagnosis

PBC should be considered in patients with chronic cholestatic liver enzyme abnormalities. It is most often seen in middle-aged women. AMA testing may be negative, and it should be remembered that as many as 10% of patients with PBC may be AMA-negative. Liver biopsy is most important in this setting of AMA-negative PBC. In patients who are AMA-negative with cholestatic liver enzymes, PSC should be ruled out by way of cholangiography.

TREATMENT Primary Biliary Cirrhosis

Treatment of the typical manifestations of cirrhosis are no different for PBC than for other forms of cirrhosis. UDCA has been shown to improve both biochemical and histologic features of the disease. Improvement is greatest when therapy is initiated early; the likelihood of significant improvement with UDCA is low in patients with PBC who present with manifestations of cirrhosis. UDCA is given in doses of 13–15 mg/kg per day; the medication is usually well-tolerated, although some patients have worsening pruritus with initiation of therapy. A small proportion of patients may have diarrhea or headache as a side effect of the drug. UDCA has been shown to slow the rate of progression of PBC, but it does not reverse or cure the disease. Patients with PBC require long-term follow-up by a physician experienced with the disease. Certain patients may need to be considered for liver transplantation should their liver disease decompensate.

The main symptoms of PBC are fatigue and pruritus, and symptom management is important. Several therapies have been tried for treatment of fatigue, but none of them have been successful; frequent naps should be encouraged. Pruritus is treated with antihistamines, narcotic receptor antagonists (naltrexone), and rifampin. Cholestyramine, a bile salt-sequestering agent, has been helpful in some patients but is somewhat tedious and difficult to take. Plasmapheresis has been used rarely in patients with severe intractable pruritus. There is an increased incidence of osteopenia and osteoporosis in patients with cholestatic liver disease, and bone density testing should be performed. Treatment with a bisphosphonate should be instituted when bone disease is identified.

PRIMARY SCLEROSING CHOLANGITIS

As in PBC, the cause of PSC remains unknown. PSC is a chronic cholestatic syndrome that is characterized by diffuse inflammation and fibrosis involving the entire biliary tree, resulting in chronic cholestasis. This pathologic process ultimately results in obliteration of both the intra- and extrahepatic biliary tree, leading to biliary cirrhosis, portal hypertension, and liver failure. The cause of PSC remains unknown despite extensive investigation into various mechanisms related to bacterial and viral infections, toxins, genetic predisposition, and immunologic mechanisms, all of which have been postulated to contribute to the pathogenesis and progression of this syndrome.

Pathologic changes that can occur in PSC show bile duct proliferation as well as ductopenia and fibrous cholangitis (pericholangitis). Often, liver biopsy changes in PSC are not pathognomonic, and establishing the diagnosis of PSC must involve imaging of the biliary tree. Periductal fibrosis is occasionally seen on biopsy specimens and can be quite helpful in making the diagnosis. As the disease progresses, biliary cirrhosis is the final, end-stage manifestation of PSC.

Clinical features

The usual clinical features of PSC are those found in cholestatic liver disease, with fatigue, pruritus, steatorrhea, deficiencies of fat-soluble vitamins, and the associated consequences. As in PBC, the fatigue is profound and nonspecific. Pruritus can often be debilitating and is related to the cholestasis. The severity of pruritus does not correlate with the severity of the disease. Metabolic bone disease, as seen in PBC, can occur with PSC and should be treated (see above).

Laboratory findings

Patients with PSC typically are identified in the course of an evaluation of abnormal liver enzymes. Most patients have at least a twofold increase in ALP and may have elevated aminotransferases as well. Albumin levels may be decreased, and prothrombin times are prolonged in a substantial proportion of patients at the time of diagnosis. Some degree of correction of a prolonged prothrombin time may occur with parenteral vitamin K. A small subset of patients have aminotransferase elevations greater than five times the upper limit of normal and may have features of AIH on biopsy. These individuals are thought to have an overlap syndrome between PSC and AIH. Autoantibodies are frequently positive in patients with the overlap syndrome but are typically negative in patients who only have PSC. One autoantibody, the perinuclear antineutrophil cytoplasmic antibody (p-ANCA), is positive in about 65% of patients with PSC. Over 50% of patients with PSC also have ulcerative colitis (UC); accordingly, once a diagnosis of PSC is established, colonoscopy should be performed to look for evidence of UC.

Diagnosis

The definitive diagnosis of PSC requires cholangiographic imaging. Over the last several years, MRI with magnetic resonance cholangiopancreatography (MRCP) has been used as the imaging technique of choice for initial evaluation. Once patients are screened in this manner, some investigators feel that endoscopic retrograde cholangiopancreatography (ERCP) should also be performed to be certain whether or not a dominant stricture is present. Typical cholangiographic findings in PSC are multifocal stricturing and beading involving both the intrahepatic and extrahepatic biliary tree. However, though involvement may be of the intrahepatic bile ducts alone or of the extrahepatic bile ducts alone, more commonly, both are involved. These strictures are typically short and with intervening segments of normal or slightly dilated bile ducts that are distributed diffusely, producing the classic beaded appearance. The gallbladder and cystic duct can be involved in up to 15% of cases. Patients with high-grade, diffuse stricturing of the intrahepatic bile ducts have an overall poor prognosis. Gradually, biliary cirrhosis develops, and patients will progress to decompensated liver disease with all the manifestations of ascites, esophageal variceal hemorrhage, and encephalopathy.

TREATMENT Primary Sclerosing Cholangitis

There is no specific proven treatment for PSC, although studies are currently ongoing using high-dose (20 mg/kg per day) UDCA to determine its benefit. Endoscopic dilatation of dominant strictures can be helpful, but the ultimate treatment is liver transplantation. A dreaded complication of PSC is the development of cholangiocarcinoma, which is a relative contraindication to liver transplantation. Symptoms of pruritus are common, and the approach is as mentioned previously for this problem in patients with PBC (see above).

CARDIAC CIRRHOSIS

Definition

Patients with long-standing right-sided congestive heart failure may develop chronic liver injury and cardiac cirrhosis. This is an increasingly uncommon, if not rare, cause of chronic liver disease given the advances made in the care of patients with heart failure.

Etiology and pathology

In the case of long-term right-sided heart failure, there is an elevated venous pressure transmitted via the inferior vena cava and hepatic veins to the sinusoids of the liver, which become dilated and engorged with blood. The liver becomes enlarged and swollen, and with long-term passive congestion and relative ischemia due to poor circulation, centrilobular hepatocytes can become necrotic, leading to pericentral fibrosis. This fibrotic pattern can extend to the periphery of the lobule outward until a unique pattern of fibrosis causing cirrhosis can occur.

Clinical features

Patients typically have signs of congestive heart failure and will manifest an enlarged firm liver on physical examination. ALP levels are characteristically elevated, and aminotransferases may be normal or slightly increased with AST usually higher than ALT. It is unlikely that patients will develop variceal hemorrhage or encephalopathy.

Diagnosis

The diagnosis is usually made in someone with clear-cut cardiac disease who has an elevated ALP and an enlarged liver. Liver biopsy shows a pattern of fibrosis that can be recognized by an experienced hepatopathologist. Differentiation from Budd-Chiari syndrome (BCS) can be made by seeing extravasation of red blood cells in BCS, but not in cardiac hepatopathy. Venoocclusive disease can also affect hepatic outflow and has characteristic features on liver biopsy. Venoocclusive disease can be seen under the circumstances of conditioning for bone marrow transplant with radiation and chemotherapy; it can also be seen with the ingestion of certain herbal teas as well as pyrrolizidine alkaloids. This is typically seen in Caribbean countries and rarely in the United States. Treatment is based on management of the underlying cardiac disease.

OTHER TYPES OF CIRRHOSIS

There are several other less-common causes of chronic liver disease that can progress to cirrhosis. These include inherited metabolic liver diseases such as hemochromatosis, Wilson's disease, α_1 antitrypsin (α_1AT) deficiency, and cystic fibrosis. For all of these disorders, the manifestations of cirrhosis are similar, with some minor variations, to those seen in other patients with other causes of cirrhosis.

Hemochromatosis is an inherited disorder of iron metabolism that results in a progressive increase in hepatic iron deposition, which, over time, can lead to a portal-based fibrosis progressing to cirrhosis, liver failure, and hepatocellular cancer. While the frequency of hemochromatosis is relatively common, with genetic susceptibility occurring in 1 in 250 individuals, the frequency of end-stage manifestations due to the disease is relatively low, and fewer than 5% of those patients who are genotypically susceptible will go on to develop severe liver disease from hemochromatosis. Diagnosis is made with serum iron studies showing an elevated transferrin saturation and an elevated ferritin level, along with abnormalities identified by *HFE* mutation analysis. Treatment is straightforward, with regular therapeutic phlebotomy.

Wilson's disease is an inherited disorder of copper homeostasis with failure to excrete excess amounts of copper, leading to an accumulation in the liver. This disorder is relatively uncommon, affecting 1 in 30,000 individuals. Wilson's disease typically affects adolescents and young adults. Prompt diagnosis before end-stage manifestations become irreversible can lead to significant clinical improvement. Diagnosis requires determination of ceruloplasmin levels, which are low; 24-hour urine copper levels, which are elevated; typical physical examination findings, including Kayser-Fleischer corneal rings, and characteristic liver biopsy findings. Treatment consists of copper-chelating medications.

α_1AT deficiency results from an inherited disorder that causes abnormal folding of the α_1AT protein, resulting in failure of secretion of that protein from the liver. It is unknown how the retained protein leads to liver disease. Patients with α_1AT deficiency at greatest risk for developing chronic liver disease have the ZZ phenotype, but only about 10–20% of such individuals will develop chronic liver disease. Diagnosis is made by determining α_1AT levels and phenotype. Characteristic periodic acid–Schiff (PAS)-positive, diastase-resistant globules are seen on liver biopsy. The only effective treatment is liver transplantation, which is curative.

Cystic fibrosis is an uncommon inherited disorder affecting Caucasians of Northern European descent. A biliary-type cirrhosis can occur, and some patients derive benefit from the chronic use of UDCA.

MAJOR COMPLICATIONS OF CIRRHOSIS

The clinical course of patients with advanced cirrhosis is often complicated by a number of important sequelae that can occur regardless of the underlying cause of the liver disease. These include portal hypertension and its consequences of gastroesophageal variceal hemorrhage, splenomegaly, ascites, hepatic encephalopathy, spontaneous bacterial peritonitis (SBP), hepatorenal syndrome, and hepatocellular carcinoma (Table 308-2).

PORTAL HYPERTENSION

Portal hypertension is defined as the elevation of the hepatic venous pressure gradient (HVPG) to >5 mmHg. Portal hypertension is caused by a combination of two simultaneously occurring hemodynamic processes: (1) increased intrahepatic resistance to the passage of blood flow through the liver due to cirrhosis and regenerative nodules, and (2) increased splanchnic blood flow secondary to vasodilation within the splanchnic vascular bed. Portal hypertension is directly responsible for the two major complications of cirrhosis: variceal hemorrhage and ascites. *Variceal hemorrhage* is an immediate life-threatening problem with a 20–30% mortality rate associated with each episode of bleeding. The portal venous system normally drains blood from the stomach, intestines, spleen, pancreas, and gallbladder, and the portal vein is formed by the confluence of the superior mesenteric and splenic veins. Deoxygenated blood from the small bowel drains into the superior mesenteric vein along with blood from the head of the pancreas, the ascending colon, and part of the transverse colon. Conversely, the splenic vein drains the spleen and the pancreas and is joined by the inferior mesenteric vein, which brings blood from the transverse and descending colon as well as from the superior two-thirds of the rectum. Thus, the portal vein normally receives blood from almost the entire GI tract.

The causes of portal hypertension are usually subcategorized as prehepatic, intrahepatic, and posthepatic (Table 308-3). Prehepatic causes of portal hypertension are those affecting the portal venous system before it enters the liver; they include portal vein thrombosis and splenic vein thrombosis. Posthepatic causes encompass those affecting the hepatic veins and venous drainage to the heart; they

TABLE 308-2 Complications of Cirrhosis

Portal hypertension	Coagulopathy
Gastroesophageal varices	Factor deficiency
Portal hypertensive gastropathy	Fibrinolysis
Splenomegaly, hypersplenism	Thrombocytopenia
Ascites	Bone disease
Spontaneous bacterial peritonitis	Osteopenia
Hepatorenal syndrome	Osteoporosis
Type 1	Osteomalacia
Type 2	Hematologic abnormalities
Hepatic encephalopathy	Anemia
Hepatopulmonary syndrome	Hemolysis
Portopulmonary hypertension	Thrombocytopenia
Malnutrition	Neutropenia

TABLE 308-3 Classification of Portal Hypertension

Prehepatic
Portal vein thrombosis
Splenic vein thrombosis
Massive splenomegaly (Banti's syndrome)
Hepatic
Presinusoidal
Schistosomiasis
Congenital hepatic fibrosis
Sinusoidal
Cirrhosis—many causes
Alcoholic hepatitis
Postsinusoidal
Hepatic sinusoidal obstruction (venoocclusive syndrome)
Posthepatic
Budd-Chiari syndrome
Inferior vena caval webs
Cardiac causes
Restrictive cardiomyopathy
Constrictive pericarditis
Severe congestive heart failure

include BCS, venoocclusive disease, and chronic right-sided cardiac congestion. Intrahepatic causes account for over 95% of cases of portal hypertension and are represented by the major forms of cirrhosis. Intrahepatic causes of portal hypertension can be further subdivided into presinusoidal, sinusoidal, and postsinusoidal causes. Postsinusoidal causes include venoocclusive disease, while presinusoidal causes include congenital hepatic fibrosis and schistosomiasis. Sinusoidal causes are related to cirrhosis from various causes.

Cirrhosis is the most common cause of portal hypertension in the United States, and clinically significant portal hypertension is present in >60% of patients with cirrhosis. Portal vein obstruction may be idiopathic or can occur in association with cirrhosis or with infection, pancreatitis, or abdominal trauma.

Coagulation disorders that can lead to the development of portal vein thrombosis include polycythemia vera; essential thrombocytosis; deficiencies in protein C, protein S, antithrombin 3, and factor V Leiden; and abnormalities in the gene-regulating prothrombin production. Some patients may have a subclinical myeloproliferative disorder.

Clinical features

The three primary complications of portal hypertension are gastroesophageal varices with hemorrhage, ascites, and hypersplenism. Thus, patients may present with upper GI bleeding, which, on endoscopy, is found to be due to esophageal or gastric varices, with the development of ascites along with peripheral edema, or with an enlarged spleen with associated reduction in platelets and white blood cells on routine laboratory testing.

Esophageal varices Over the last decade, it has become common practice to screen known cirrhotics with endoscopy to look for esophageal varices. Such screening studies have shown that approximately one-third of patients with histologically confirmed cirrhosis have varices. Approximately 5–15% of cirrhotics per year develop varices, and it is estimated that the majority of patients with cirrhosis will develop varices over their lifetimes. Furthermore, it is anticipated that roughly one-third of patients with varices will develop bleeding. Several factors predict the risk of bleeding, including the severity of cirrhosis (Child's class, MELD score); the height of wedged-hepatic vein pressure; the size of the varix; the location of the varix; and certain endoscopic stigmata, including red wale signs, hematocystic spots, diffuse erythema, bluish color, cherry red spots, or white-nipple spots. Patients with tense ascites are also at increased risk for bleeding from varices.

Diagnosis

In patients with cirrhosis who are being followed chronically, the development of portal hypertension is usually revealed by the presence of thrombocytopenia; the appearance of an enlarged spleen; or the development of ascites, encephalopathy, and/or esophageal varices with or without bleeding. In previously undiagnosed patients, any of these features should prompt further evaluation to determine the presence of portal hypertension and liver disease. Varices should be identified by endoscopy. Abdominal imaging, either by CT or MRI, can be helpful in demonstrating a nodular liver and in finding changes of portal hypertension with intraabdominal collateral circulation. If necessary, interventional radiologic procedures can be performed to determine wedged and free hepatic vein pressures that will allow for the calculation of a wedged-to-free gradient, which is equivalent to the portal pressure. The average normal wedged-to-free gradient is 5 mmHg, and patients with a gradient >12 mmHg are at risk for variceal hemorrhage.

TREATMENT Variceal Hemorrhage

Treatment for variceal hemorrhage as a complication of portal hypertension is divided into two main categories: (1) primary prophylaxis and (2) prevention of re-bleeding once there has been an initial variceal hemorrhage. Primary prophylaxis requires routine screening by endoscopy of all patients with cirrhosis. Once varices that are at increased risk for bleeding are identified, primary prophylaxis can be achieved either through nonselective beta blockade or by variceal band ligation. Numerous placebo-controlled clinical trials of either propranolol or nadolol have been reported in the literature. The most rigorous studies were those that only included patients with significantly enlarged varices or with hepatic vein pressure gradients >12 mmHg. Patients treated with beta blockers have a lower risk of variceal hemorrhage than those treated with placebo over 1 and 2 years of follow-up. There is also a decrease in mortality related to variceal hemorrhage. Unfortunately, overall survival was improved in only one study. Further studies have demonstrated that the degree of reduction of portal pressure is a significant feature to determine success of therapy. Therefore, it has been suggested that repeat measurements of hepatic vein pressure gradients may be used to guide pharmacologic therapy; however, this may be cost-prohibitive. Several studies have evaluated variceal band ligation and variceal sclerotherapy as methods for providing primary prophylaxis.

Endoscopic variceal ligation (EVL) has achieved a level of success and comfort with most gastroenterologists who see patients with these complications of portal hypertension. Thus, in patients with cirrhosis who are screened for portal hypertension and are found to have large varices, it is recommended that they receive either beta blockade or primary prophylaxis with EVL.

The approach to patients once they have had a variceal bleed is first to treat the acute bleed, which can be life-threatening, and then to prevent further bleeding. Prevention of further bleeding is usually accomplished with repeated variceal band ligation until varices are obliterated. Treatment of acute bleeding requires both fluid and blood-product replacement as well as prevention of subsequent bleeding with EVL.

The medical management of acute variceal hemorrhage includes the use of vasoconstricting agents, usually somatostatin or Octreotide. Vasopressin was used in the past but is no longer commonly used. Balloon tamponade (Sengstaken-Blakemore tube or Minnesota tube) can be used in patients who cannot get endoscopic therapy immediately or who need stabilization prior to endoscopic therapy. Control of bleeding can be achieved in the vast majority of cases; however, bleeding recurs in the majority of patients if definitive endoscopic therapy has not been instituted. Octreotide, a direct splanchnic vasoconstrictor, is given at dosages of 50–100 μg/h by continuous infusion. Endoscopic intervention is employed as first-line treatment to control bleeding acutely. Some endoscopists will use variceal injection therapy (sclerotherapy) as initial therapy, particularly when bleeding is vigorous. Variceal band ligation is used to control acute bleeding in over 90% of cases and should be repeated until obliteration of all varices is accomplished. When esophageal varices extend into the proximal stomach, band ligation is less successful. In these situations, when bleeding continues from gastric varices, consideration for transjugular intrahepatic portosystemic shunt (TIPS) should be made. This technique creates a portosystemic shunt by a percutaneous approach using an expandable metal stent, which is advanced under angiographic guidance to the hepatic veins and then through the substance of the liver to create a direct portocaval shunt. This offers an alternative to surgery for acute decompression of portal hypertension. Encephalopathy can occur in as many as 20% of patients after TIPS and is particularly problematic in elderly patients and in those patients with preexisting encephalopathy. TIPS should be reserved for those individuals who fail endoscopic or medical management or who are poor surgical risks. TIPS can sometimes be used as a bridge to transplantation. Surgical esophageal transsection is a procedure that is rarely used and generally is associated with a poor outcome.

PREVENTION OF RECURRENT BLEEDING (Fig. 308-3) Once patients have had an acute bleed and have been managed successfully, attention should be paid to preventing recurrent bleeding. This usually requires repeated variceal band ligation until varices are obliterated. Beta blockade may be of adjunctive benefit in patients who are having recurrent variceal band ligation; however, once varices have been obliterated, the need for beta blockade is lessened. Despite successful variceal obliteration, many patients will still have portal hypertensive gastropathy from which bleeding can occur. Nonselective beta blockade may be helpful to prevent further bleeding from portal hypertensive gastropathy once varices have been obliterated.

Portosystemic shunt surgery is less commonly performed with the advent of TIPS; nonetheless, this procedure should be considered for patients with good hepatic synthetic function who could benefit by having portal decompressive surgery.

SPLENOMEGALY AND HYPERSPLENISM

Congestive splenomegaly is common in patients with portal hypertension. Clinical features include the presence of an enlarged spleen on physical examination and the development of thrombocytopenia and leukopenia in patients who have cirrhosis. Some patients will

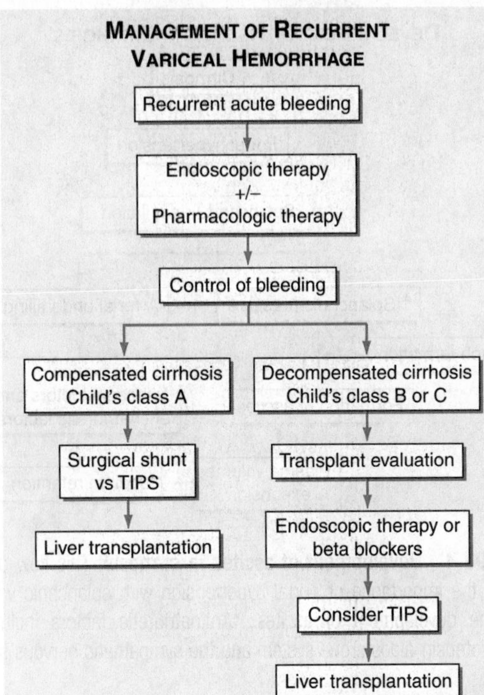

Figure 308-3 Management of recurrent variceal hemorrhage. This algorithm describes an approach to management of patients who have recurrent bleeding from esophageal varices. Initial therapy is generally with endoscopic therapy often supplemented by pharmacologic therapy. With control of bleeding, a decision needs to be made as to whether patients should go on to a surgical shunt or TIPS (if they are Child's class A) and be considered for transplant, or if they should have TIPS and be considered for transplant (if they are Child's class B or C). TIPS, transjugular intrahepatic portosystemic shunt.

have fairly significant left-sided and left upper quadrant abdominal pain related to an enlarged and engorged spleen. Splenomegaly itself usually requires no specific treatment, although splenectomy can be successfully performed under very special circumstances.

Hypersplenism with the development of thrombocytopenia is a common feature of patients with cirrhosis and is usually the first indication of portal hypertension.

ASCITES

Definition

Ascites is the accumulation of fluid within the peritoneal cavity. Overwhelmingly, the most common cause of ascites is portal hypertension related to cirrhosis; however, clinicians should remember that malignant or infectious causes of ascites can be present as well, and careful differentiation of these other causes are obviously important for patient care.

Pathogenesis

The presence of portal hypertension contributes to the development of ascites in patients who have cirrhosis (Fig. 308-4). There is an increase in intrahepatic resistance, causing increased portal pressure, but there is also vasodilation of the splanchnic arterial system, which, in turn, results in an increase in portal venous inflow. Both of these abnormalities result in increased production of splanchnic lymph. Vasodilating factors such as nitric oxide are responsible for the vasodilatory effect. These hemodynamic changes result in sodium retention by causing activation of the

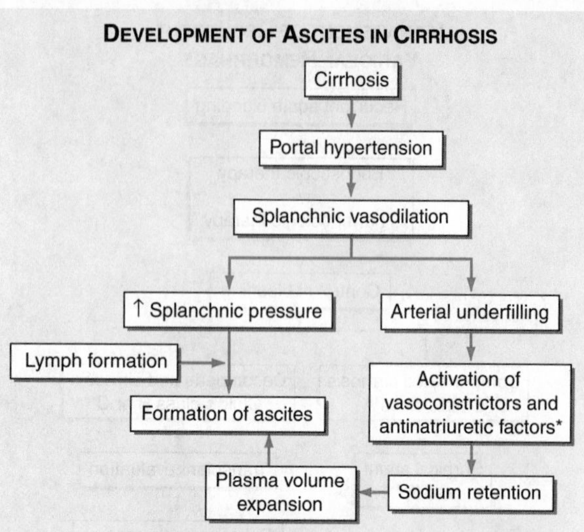

Figure 308-4 Development of ascites in cirrhosis. This flow diagram illustrates the importance of portal hypertension with splanchnic vasodilation in the development of ascites. *Antinatriuretic factors include the renin-angiotensin-aldosterone system and the sympathetic nervous system.

renin-angiotensin-aldosterone system with the development of hyperaldosteronism. The renal effects of increased aldosterone leading to sodium retention also contribute to the development of ascites. Sodium retention causes fluid accumulation and expansion of the extracellular fluid volume, which results in the formation of peripheral edema and ascites. Sodium retention is the consequence of a homeostatic response caused by underfilling of the arterial circulation secondary to arterial vasodilation in the splanchnic vascular bed. Because the retained fluid is constantly leaking out of the intravascular compartment into the peritoneal cavity, the sensation of vascular filling is not achieved, and the process continues. Hypoalbuminemia and reduced plasma oncotic pressure also contribute to the loss of fluid from the vascular compartment into the peritoneal cavity. Hypoalbuminemia is due to decreased synthetic function in a cirrhotic liver.

Clinical features

Patients typically note an increase in abdominal girth that is often accompanied by the development of peripheral edema. The development of ascites is often insidious, and it is surprising that some patients wait so long and become so distended before seeking medical attention. Patients usually have at least 1–2 L of fluid in the abdomen before they are aware that there is an increase. If ascitic fluid is massive, respiratory function can be compromised, and patients will complain of shortness of breath. Hepatic hydrothorax may also occur in this setting, contributing to respiratory symptoms. Patients with massive ascites are often malnourished and have muscle wasting and excessive fatigue and weakness.

Diagnosis

Diagnosis of ascites is by physical examination and is often aided by abdominal imaging. Patients will have bulging flanks, may have a fluid wave, or may have the presence of shifting dullness. This is determined by taking patients from a supine position to lying on either their left or right side and noting the movement of the dullness to percussion. Subtle amounts of ascites can be detected by ultrasound or CT scanning. Hepatic hydrothorax is more common on the right side and implicates a rent in the diaphragm with free flow of ascitic fluid into the thoracic cavity.

When patients present with ascites for the first time, it is recommended that a diagnostic paracentesis be performed to characterize the fluid. This should include the determination of total protein and albumin content, blood cell counts with differential, and cultures. In the appropriate setting, amylase may be measured and cytology performed. In patients with cirrhosis, the protein concentration of the ascitic fluid is quite low, with the majority of patients having an ascitic fluid protein concentration <1 g/dL. The development of the serum ascites-to-albumin gradient (SAAG) has replaced the description of exudative or transudative fluid. When the gradient between the serum albumin level and the ascitic fluid albumin level is >1.1 g/dL, the cause of the ascites is most likely due to portal hypertension; this is usually in the setting of cirrhosis. When the gradient is <1.1 g/dL, infectious or malignant causes of ascites should be considered. When levels of ascitic fluid proteins are very low, patients are at increased risk for developing SBP. A high level of red blood cells in the ascitic fluid signifies a traumatic tap or perhaps a hepatocellular cancer or a ruptured omental varix. When the absolute level of polymorphonuclear leukocytes is >250/μL, the question of ascitic fluid infection should be strongly considered. Ascitic fluid cultures should be obtained using bedside inoculation of culture media.

TREATMENT Ascites

Patients with small amounts of ascites can usually be managed with dietary sodium restriction alone. Most average diets in the United States contain 6 to 8 g of sodium per day, and if patients eat at restaurants or fast-food outlets, the amount of sodium in their diet can exceed this amount. Thus, it is often extremely difficult to get patients to change their dietary habits to ingest <2 g of sodium per day, which is the recommended amount. Patients are frequently surprised to realize how much sodium is in the standard U.S. diet; thus, it is important to make educational pamphlets available to the patient. Often, a simple recommendation is to eat fresh or frozen foods, avoiding canned or processed foods, which are usually preserved with sodium. When a moderate amount of ascites is present, diuretic therapy is usually necessary. Traditionally, spironolactone at 100–200 mg/d as a single dose is started, and furosemide may be added at 40–80 mg/d, particularly in patients who have peripheral edema. In patients who have never received diuretics before, the failure of the above-mentioned dosages suggests that they are not being compliant with a low-sodium diet. If compliance is confirmed and ascitic fluid is not being mobilized, spironolactone can be increased to 400–600 mg/d and furosemide increased to 120–160 mg/d. If ascites is still present with these dosages of diuretics in patients who are compliant with a low-sodium diet, then they are defined as having *refractory ascites*, and alternative treatment modalities including repeated large-volume paracentesis, or a TIPS procedure should be considered (Fig. 308-5). Recent studies have shown that TIPS, while managing the ascites, does not improve survival in these patients. Unfortunately, TIPS is often associated with an increased frequency of hepatic encephalopathy and must be considered carefully on a case-by-case basis. The prognosis for patients with cirrhosis with ascites is poor, and some studies have shown that <50% of patients survive 2 years after the onset of ascites. Thus, there should be consideration for liver transplantation in patients with the onset of ascites.

■ SPONTANEOUS BACTERIAL PERITONITIS

SBP is a common and severe complication of ascites characterized by spontaneous infection of the ascitic fluid without an intraabdominal

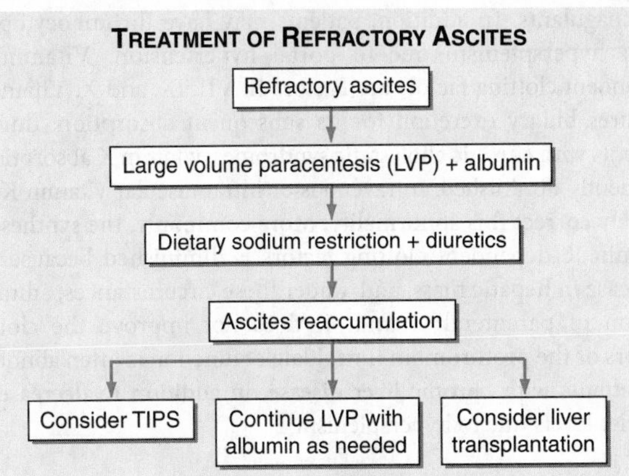

Figure 308-5 Treatment of refractory ascites. In patients who develop azotemia in the course of receiving diuretics in the management of their ascites, some will require repeated large-volume paracentesis (LVP), some may be considered for transjugular intrahepatic portosystemic shunt (TIPS), and some would be good candidates for liver transplantation. These decisions are all individualized.

source. In patients with cirrhosis and ascites severe enough for hospitalization, SBP can occur in up to 30% of individuals and can have a 25% in-hospital mortality rate. Bacterial translocation is the presumed mechanism for development of SBP, with gut flora traversing the intestine into mesenteric lymph nodes, leading to bacteremia and seeding of the ascitic fluid. The most common organisms are *Escherichia coli* and other gut bacteria; however, gram-positive bacteria, including *Streptococcus viridans, Staphylococcus aureus,* and *Enterococcus* sp., can also be found. If more than two organisms are identified, secondary bacterial peritonitis due to a perforated viscus should be considered. The diagnosis of SBP is made when the fluid sample has an absolute neutrophil count >250/μL. Bedside cultures should be obtained when ascitic fluid is tapped. Patients with ascites may present with fever, altered mental status, elevated white blood cell count, and abdominal pain or discomfort, or they may present without any of these features. Therefore, it is necessary to have a high degree of clinical suspicion, and peritoneal taps are important for making the diagnosis. Treatment is with a second-generation cephalosporin, with cefotaxime being the most commonly used antibiotic. In patients with variceal hemorrhage, the frequency of SBP is significantly increased, and prophylaxis against SBP is recommended when a patient presents with upper GI bleeding. Furthermore, in patients who have had an episode(s) of SBP and recovered, once-weekly administration of antibiotics is used as prophylaxis for recurrent SBP.

HEPATORENAL SYNDROME

The hepatorenal syndrome (HRS) is a form of functional renal failure without renal pathology that occurs in about 10% of patients with advanced cirrhosis or acute liver failure. There are marked disturbances in the arterial renal circulation in patients with HRS; these include an increase in vascular resistance accompanied by a reduction in systemic vascular resistance. The reason for renal vasoconstriction is most likely multifactorial and is poorly understood. The diagnosis is made usually in the presence of a large amount of ascites in patients who have a stepwise progressive increase in creatinine. Type 1 HRS is characterized by a progressive impairment in renal function and a significant reduction in creatinine clearance within 1–2 weeks of presentation. Type 2 HRS is characterized by a reduction in glomerular filtration rate with an elevation of serum creatinine level, but it is fairly stable and is associated with a better outcome than that of Type 1 HRS.

HRS is often seen in patients with refractory ascites and requires exclusion of other causes of acute renal failure. Treatment has, unfortunately, been difficult, and in the past, dopamine or prostaglandin analogues were used as renal vasodilating medications. Carefully performed studies have failed to show clear-cut benefit from these therapeutic approaches. Currently, patients are treated with midodrine, an α-agonist, along with octreotide and intravenous albumin. The best therapy for HRS is liver transplantation; recovery of renal function is typical in this setting. In patients with either type 1 or type 2 HRS, the prognosis is poor unless transplant can be achieved within a short period of time.

HEPATIC ENCEPHALOPATHY

Portosystemic encephalopathy is a serious complication of chronic liver disease and is broadly defined as an alteration in mental status and cognitive function occurring in the presence of liver failure. In acute liver injury with fulminant hepatic failure, the development of encephalopathy is a requirement for a diagnosis of fulminant failure. Encephalopathy is much more commonly seen in patients with chronic liver disease. Gut-derived neurotoxins that are not removed by the liver because of vascular shunting and decreased hepatic mass get to the brain and cause the symptoms that we know of as hepatic encephalopathy. Ammonia levels are typically elevated in patients with hepatic encephalopathy, but the correlation between severity of liver disease and height of ammonia levels is often poor, and most hepatologists do not rely on ammonia levels to make a diagnosis. Other compounds and metabolites that may contribute to the development of encephalopathy include certain false neurotransmitters and mercaptans.

Clinical features

In acute liver failure, changes in mental status can occur within weeks to months. Brain edema can be seen in these patients, with severe encephalopathy associated with swelling of the gray matter. Cerebral herniation is a feared complication of brain edema in acute liver failure, and treatment is meant to decrease edema with mannitol and judicious use of intravenous fluids.

In patients with cirrhosis, encephalopathy is often found as a result of certain precipitating events such as hypokalemia, infection, an increased dietary protein load, or electrolyte disturbances. Patients may be confused or exhibit a change in personality. They may actually be quite violent and difficult to manage; alternatively, patients may be very sleepy and difficult to rouse. Because precipitating events are so commonly found, they should be sought carefully. If patients have ascites, this should be tapped to rule out infection. Evidence of GI bleeding should be sought, and patients should be appropriately hydrated. Electrolytes should be measured and abnormalities corrected. In patients presenting with encephalopathy, asterixis is often present. Asterixis can be elicited by having patients extend their arms and bend their wrists back. In this maneuver, patients who are encephalopathic have a "liver flap"—i.e., a sudden forward movement of the wrist. This requires patients to be able to cooperate with the examiner and obviously cannot be elicited in patients who are severely encephalopathic or in hepatic coma.

The diagnosis of hepatic encephalopathy is clinical and requires an experienced clinician to recognize and put together all of the various features. Often when patients have encephalopathy for the first time, they are unaware of what is transpiring, but once they have been through the experience for the first time, they can identify when this is developing in subsequent situations and can often self-medicate to impair the development or worsening of encephalopathy.

TREATMENT Hepatic Encephalopathy

Treatment is multifactorial and includes management of the above-mentioned precipitating factors. Sometimes hydration and correction of electrolyte imbalance is all that is necessary. In the past, restriction of dietary protein was considered for patients with encephalopathy; however, the negative impact of that maneuver on overall nutrition is thought to outweigh the benefit when treating encephalopathy, and it is thus discouraged. There may be some benefit to replacing animal-based protein with vegetable-based protein in some patients with encephalopathy that is difficult to manage. The mainstay of treatment for encephalopathy, in addition to correcting precipitating factors, is to use lactulose, a nonabsorbable disaccharide, which results in colonic acidification. Catharsis ensues, contributing to the elimination of nitrogenous products in the gut that are responsible for the development of encephalopathy. The goal of lactulose therapy is to promote 2–3 soft stools per day. Patients are asked to titrate their amount of ingested lactulose to achieve the desired effect. Poorly absorbed antibiotics are often used as adjunctive therapies for patients who have had a difficult time with lactulose. The alternating administration of neomycin and metronidazole has commonly been employed to reduce the individual side effects of each: neomycin for renal insufficiency and ototoxicity and metronidazole for peripheral neuropathy. More recently, rifaximin at 550 mg twice daily has been very effective in treating encephalopathy without the known side effects of neomycin or metronidazole. Zinc supplementation is sometimes helpful in patients with encephalopathy and is relatively harmless. The development of encephalopathy in patients with chronic liver disease is a poor prognostic sign, but this complication can be managed in the vast majority of patients.

MALNUTRITION IN CIRRHOSIS

Because the liver is principally involved in the regulation of protein and energy metabolism in the body, it is not surprising that patients with advanced liver disease are commonly malnourished. Once patients become cirrhotic, they are more catabolic, and muscle protein is metabolized. There are multiple factors that contribute to the malnutrition of cirrhosis, including poor dietary intake, alterations in gut nutrient absorption, and alterations in protein metabolism. Dietary supplementation for patients with cirrhosis is helpful in preventing patients from becoming catabolic.

ABNORMALITIES IN COAGULATION

Coagulopathy is almost universal in patients with cirrhosis. There is decreased synthesis of clotting factors and impaired clearance of anticoagulants. In addition, patients may have thrombocytopenia from hypersplenism due to portal hypertension. Vitamin K–dependent clotting factors are Factors II, VII, IX, and X. Vitamin K requires biliary excretion for its subsequent absorption; thus, in patients with chronic cholestatic syndromes, vitamin K absorption is frequently diminished. Intravenous or intramuscular vitamin K can quickly correct this abnormality. More commonly, the synthesis of vitamin K–dependent clotting factors is diminished because of a decrease in hepatic mass, and, under these circumstances, administration of parenteral vitamin K does not improve the clotting factors or the prothrombin time. Platelet function is often abnormal in patients with chronic liver disease, in addition to decreases in platelet levels due to hypersplenism.

BONE DISEASE IN CIRRHOSIS

Osteoporosis is common in patients with chronic cholestatic liver disease because of malabsorption of vitamin D and decreased calcium ingestion. The rate of bone resorption exceeds that of new bone formation in patients with cirrhosis resulting in bone loss. Dual x-ray absorptiometry (DEXA) is a useful method for determining osteoporosis or osteopenia in patients with chronic liver disease. When a DEXA scan shows decreased bone mass, treatment should be administered with bisphosphonates that are effective at inhibiting resorption of bone and efficacious in the treatment of osteoporosis.

HEMATOLOGIC ABNORMALITIES IN CIRRHOSIS

Numerous hematologic manifestations of cirrhosis are present, including anemia from a variety of causes including hypersplenism, hemolysis, iron deficiency, and perhaps folate deficiency from malnutrition. Macrocytosis is a common abnormality in red blood cell morphology seen in patients with chronic liver disease, and neutropenia may be seen as a result of hypersplenism.

FURTHER READINGS

Arroyo V et al: Pathogenesis and treatment of hepatorenal syndrome. Semin Liver Dis 28:81, 2008

Bass NM et al: Rifaximin treatment in hepatic encephalopathy. N Engl J Med 362:1071, 2010

Friedman SL: Mechanisms of hepatic fibrogenesis. Gastroenterology 134:1655, 2008

Krowka MJ et al: Hepatopulmonary syndrome and portopulmonary hypertension: A report of the multicenter liver transplant database. Liver Transpl 10:174, 2004

O'Brien AO, Williams R: Nutrition and endstage liver disease: Principles and practice. Gastroenterology 134:1729, 2008

CHAPTER 309

Genetic, Metabolic, and Infiltrative Diseases Affecting the Liver

Bruce R. Bacon

There are a number of disorders of the liver that fit within the categories of genetic, metabolic, and infiltrative disorders. Inherited disorders include hemochromatosis, Wilson's disease, α_1 antitrypsin (α_1AT) deficiency, and cystic fibrosis (CF). Hemochromatosis is the most common inherited disorder affecting Caucasian populations, with the genetic susceptibility for the disease being identified in 1 in 250 individuals. Over the past 15 years, it has become increasingly apparent that nonalcoholic fatty liver disease (NAFLD) is the most common cause of elevated liver enzymes found in the U.S. population. With the obesity epidemic in the United States, it is estimated that 20% of the population may have abnormal liver enzymes on the basis of NAFLD and 3% may have nonalcoholic steatohepatitis (NASH). Infiltrative disorders of the liver are relatively rare.

GENETIC LIVER DISEASES

Hereditary hemochromatosis

Hereditary hemochromatosis (HH) is a common inherited disorder of iron metabolism (Chap. 357). Our knowledge of the disease and its phenotypic expression has changed since 1996, when the gene for HH, called *HFE*, was identified, allowing for genetic testing for the two major mutations (C282Y and H63D) that are responsible for *HFE*-related HH. Subsequently, several additional genes/proteins involved in the regulation of iron homeostasis have been identified, contributing to a better understanding of cellular iron uptake and release and the characterization of additional causes of inherited iron overload (Table 309-1).

Most patients with HH are asymptomatic; however, when patients present with symptoms, they are frequently nonspecific and include weakness, fatigue, lethargy, and weight loss. Specific, organ-related symptoms include abdominal pain, arthralgias, and symptoms and signs of chronic liver disease. Increasingly, most patients are now identified before they have symptoms, either through family studies or from the performance of screening iron studies. Several prospective population studies have shown that C282Y homozygosity is found in about 1 in 250 individuals of Northern European descent, with the heterozygote frequency seen in approximately 1 in 10 individuals. It is important to consider HH in patients who present with the symptoms and signs known to occur in established HH. When confronted with abnormal serum iron studies, clinicians should not wait for typical symptoms or findings of HH to appear before considering the diagnosis. However, once the diagnosis of HH is considered, either by an evaluation of abnormal screening iron studies, in the context of family studies, in a patient with an abnormal genetic test, or in the evaluation of a patient with any of the typical symptoms or clinical findings, definitive diagnosis is relatively straightforward. Transferrin saturation [serum iron divided by total iron-binding capacity (TIBC) or transferrin, times 100%] and ferritin levels should be obtained. Both of these will be elevated in a symptomatic patient. It must be remembered that ferritin is an acute-phase reactant and can be elevated in a number of other inflammatory disorders, such as rheumatoid arthritis, or in various neoplastic diseases, such as lymphoma or other cancers. Also, serum ferritin is elevated in a majority of patients with NASH, in the absence of iron overload.

TABLE 309-1 Classification of Iron Overload Syndromes

Hereditary Hemochromatosis (HH)
HFE-related (type 1)
C282Y/C282Y
C282Y/H63D
Other *HFE* mutations
Non-*HFE*-related
Juvenile HH
HJV—hemojuvelin (type 2a)
HAMP—hepcidin (type 2b)
TfR2-related HH (type 3)
Ferroportin-related HH (type 4)
African iron overload
Secondary Iron Overload
Iron-loading anemias
Parenteral iron overload
Chronic liver disease
Miscellaneous
Neonatal iron overload
Aceruloplasminemia
Congenital atransferrinemia

Abbreviations: HJV, hemojuvelin; HAMP, hepcidin; TfR2, transferrin receptor 2.

At present, if patients have an elevated transferrin saturation or ferritin level, genetic testing should be performed; if they are a C282Y homozygote or a compound heterozygote (C282Y/H63D), the diagnosis is confirmed. If the ferritin is >1000 μg/L, the patient should be considered for liver biopsy because there is an increased frequency of advanced fibrosis in these individuals. If liver biopsy is performed, iron deposition is found in a periportal distribution with a periportal to pericentral gradient; iron is found predominantly in parenchymal cells, and Kupffer cells are spared.

TREATMENT Hereditary Hemochromatosis

Treatment of HH is relatively straightforward with weekly phlebotomy aimed to reduce iron stores, recognizing that each unit of blood contains 200 to 250 mg of iron. If patients are diagnosed and treated before the development of hepatic fibrosis, all complications of the disease can be avoided. Maintenance phlebotomy is required in most patients and usually can be achieved with 1 unit of blood removed every 2–3 months. Family studies should be performed with transferrin saturation, ferritin, and genetic testing offered to all first-degree relatives.

Wilson's disease

Wilson's disease is an inherited disorder of copper homeostasis first described in 1912 (Chap. 360). The Wilson's disease gene was discovered in 1993, with the identification of *ATP7B*. This P-type ATPase is involved in copper transport and is necessary for the export of copper from the hepatocyte. Thus, in patients with mutations in *ATP7B*, copper is retained in the liver, leading to increased copper storage and ultimately liver disease as a result.

The clinical presentation of Wilson's disease is variable and includes chronic hepatitis, hepatic steatosis, and cirrhosis in adolescents and young adults. Neurologic manifestations indicate that liver disease is present and include speech disorders and various movement disorders. Diagnosis includes the demonstration of a reduced ceruloplasmin level, increased urinary excretion of copper, the presence of Kayser-Fleischer rings in the corneas of the eyes, and an elevated hepatic copper level, in the appropriate clinical setting. The genetic diagnosis of Wilson's disease is difficult because >200 mutations in *ATP7B* have been described with different degrees of frequency and penetration in certain populations.

TREATMENT Wilson's Disease

Treatment consists of copper-chelating medications such as D-penicillamine and trientine. A role for zinc acetate has also been established. Medical treatment is lifelong, and severe relapses leading to liver failure and death can occur with cessation of therapy. Liver transplantation is curative with respect to the underlying metabolic defect and restores the normal phenotype with respect to copper homeostasis.

α_1 Antitrypsin deficiency

Alpha-1-antitrypsin (AAT) deficiency was first described in the late 1960s in patients with severe pulmonary disease. AAT is a 52 kD glycoprotein produced in hepatocytes, phagocytes, and epithelial cells in the lungs, which inhibits serine proteases, primarily neutrophil elastase. In AAT deficiency, increased amounts of neutrophil elastase can result in progressive lung injury from degradation of elastin leading to premature emphysema. In the 1970s, AAT deficiency was discovered as a cause of neonatal liver disease, so-called "neonatal hepatitis." It is now known to be a cause of liver disease in infancy, early childhood, adolescence, and in adults.

In AAT deficiency, variants in the proteinase inhibitor (Pi) gene located on chromosome 14, alters AAT structure interfering with hepatocellular export. Aggregated, deformed polymers of AAT accumulate in the hepatocyte endoplasmic reticulum. There are over 75 different AAT variants. Conventional nomenclature identifies normal variants as PiMM; these individuals have normal blood levels of AAT. The most common abnormal variants are called S and Z. Individuals homozygous for the Z mutation (PiZZ) have low levels of AAT (about 15% of normal) and these patients are susceptible to liver and/or lung disease, yet only a proportion (about 25%) of PiZZ patients develop disease manifestations. Null variants have undetectable levels of AAT and are susceptible to premature lung disease.

AAT deficiency has been identified in all populations; however, the disorder is most common in patients of Northern European and Iberian descent. The disorder affects about 1 in 1500 to 2000 individuals in North America. The natural history of AAT deficiency is quite variable because many individuals with the PiZZ variant never develop disease, whereas others can develop childhood cirrhosis leading to liver transplantation.

In adults, the diagnosis often comes in the course of evaluation of patients with abnormal liver test abnormalities or in a work-up for cirrhosis. A hint to diagnosis may be coexistent lung disease at a relatively young age or a family history of liver and/or lung disease. Patients may have symptoms of pulmonary disease with cough and dyspnea. Liver disease may be asymptomatic other than fatigue, or patients may present with complications of decompensated liver disease.

Diagnosis of AAT deficiency is confirmed by blood tests showing reduced levels of serum AAT, accompanied by Pi determinations. Most patients with liver disease have either PiZZ or PiSZ; occasionally, patients with PiMZ have reduced levels of AAT, but they usually do not have a low enough level to cause disease. Liver biopsy is often performed to determine stage of hepatic fibrosis and shows characteristic PAS-positive, diastase-resistant globules in the periphery of the hepatic lobule.

TREATMENT α_1 Antitrypsin Deficiency

Treatment of AAT deficiency is usually nonspecific and supportive. For patients with liver involvement, other sources of liver injury, such as alcohol, should be avoided. Evidence for other liver diseases (e.g., viral hepatitis B and C, hemochromatosis, NAFLD, etc.) should be sought and treated if possible. Smoking can worsen lung disease progression in AAT and should be discontinued. Patients with lung disease may be eligible to receive infusions of AT, which has been shown to halt further damage to the lungs. If liver disease becomes decompensated, transplantation should be pursued and is curative. Following transplant, patients express the Pi phenotype of the donor. Finally, risk of hepatocellular carcinoma is significantly increased in patients with cirrhosis due to AAT deficiency.

Cystic fibrosis

CF should also be considered as an inherited form of chronic liver disease, although the principal manifestations of CF include chronic lung disease and pancreatic insufficiency (Chap. 259). A small percentage of patients with CF who survive to adulthood have a form of biliary cirrhosis characterized by cholestatic liver enzyme abnormalities and the development of chronic liver disease. Ursodeoxycholic acid is occasionally helpful in improving liver test abnormalities and in reducing symptoms. The disease is slowly progressive.

■ METABOLIC LIVER DISEASES

Nonalcoholic fatty liver disease

NAFLD was first described in the 1950s when fatty liver was characterized in a group of obese patients. In 1980, Ludwig and colleagues at the Mayo Clinic described 20 obese, diabetic, nonalcoholic patients who had similar findings on liver biopsy to patients with alcoholic liver disease, and the term nonalcoholic steatohepatitis was introduced. The prevalence of NAFLD in the United States and Europe ranges from 14–20%. This increased prevalence relates directly to the obesity epidemic seen in these populations. In the United States, NASH is thought to occur in ~3% of the general population, with fibrosis due to NASH being seen in >40% of obese patients. The spectrum of NAFLD includes simple hepatic steatosis, which, over time, can progress to NASH, with the subsequent development of fibrosis and cirrhosis. Causes of macrovesicular steatosis are listed in Table 309-2. It is now known that many patients with hitherto identified "cryptogenic" cirrhosis in fact have liver disease on the basis of NASH, with the resolution of the steatosis once patients become catabolic due to cirrhosis.

TABLE 309-2 Causes of Macrovesicular Steatosis

Insulin resistance, hyperinsulinemia
Centripetal obesity
Type 2 diabetes
Medications
Glucocorticoids
Estrogens
Tamoxifen
Amiodarone
Nutritional
Starvation
Protein deficiency (Kwashiorkor)
Choline deficiency
Liver disease
Wilson disease
Chronic hepatitis C—genotype 3
Indian childhood cirrhosis
Jejunoileal bypass

Most patients who come to medical attention with NAFLD are identified as a result of incidentally discovered elevated liver enzymes (ALT, AST). When patients are symptomatic, symptoms include fatigue or a vague right upper quadrant discomfort. ALT is generally higher than AST, and aminotransferases are only mildly (1.5–2 times the upper limit of normal) elevated. Recent studies have shown that many patients can have advanced fibrosis with NASH and even cirrhosis due to NASH with normal liver enzymes, indicating that the prevalence of the disease is likely to be even greater than was previously suspected. NASH is frequently seen in conjunction with other components of the metabolic syndrome (hypertension, diabetes mellitus, elevated lipids, and obesity), with NAFLD being considered the hepatic manifestation of this syndrome (Chap. 242). Insulin resistance is the underlying link between these various disorders and numerous studies have shown that virtually all patients with NASH have insulin resistance. Abnormal ferritin values are seen in ~50% of patients with NASH, and an elevated ferritin level may be a marker of insulin resistance in NASH.

The diagnosis of NAFLD requires a careful history to determine the amount of alcohol used. Most investigators in the field of fatty liver disease require that <20 g/d of alcohol be consumed to exclude alcoholic liver disease. Laboratory testing for other liver diseases such as hepatitis B and C, iron studies, ceruloplasmin, α-1 antitrypsin levels, and autoimmune serologies should also be determined. Imaging studies can show characteristic features of a fatty liver, but the ultimate diagnosis of either hepatic steatosis or NASH requires liver biopsy. Liver biopsy shows characteristic macrovesicular steatosis with occasional microvesicular fat being identified. A mixed inflammatory infiltrate is found in a lobular distribution. The histologic features of NASH are very similar to those seen in alcoholic liver disease; Mallory's hyaline can be seen in both disorders, although the number of hepatocytes containing Mallory's hyaline and the size of the deposits are frequently greater in alcoholic liver disease than in NASH. The fibrosis that occurs in NASH has a characteristic perivenular and perisinusoidal distribution. Most cross-sectional studies show that up to 30–40% of NASH patients can develop advanced fibrosis, with cirrhosis being identified in 10–15% of individuals in series. Increasingly, patients are being identified with cryptogenic cirrhosis who have most likely had NASH for decades. These patients can develop liver failure and require liver transplantation, and some patients can progress to the development of hepatocellular cancer. Often, when cirrhotic, these patients will not have steatosis on biopsy, but following transplant, NAFLD will frequently recur.

TREATMENT Nonalcoholic Fatty Liver Disease

The mainstay of treatment of fatty liver disease is weight loss and exercise, which is often difficult to achieve in this population. As an aid to weight loss, orlistat, which is a reversible inhibitor of gastric and pancreatic lipase, has been shown to result in a small decrease in body weight and is usually fairly well tolerated. This medication is now available over-the-counter. Bariatric surgery has been used and shows striking success, but is obviously a fairly drastic maneuver for induction of weight loss. Recent studies have focused on the presence of insulin resistance at the center of the pathophysiologic mechanisms of NAFLD. The thiazolidinedione medications are PPAR gamma inhibitors, which improve insulin sensitivity within the adipocyte and skeletal muscle by upregulating specific protein kinases involved in decreasing fatty acid synthesis. Two drugs—pioglitizone and rosiglitizone—are currently available and are being evaluated as potential therapeutic options in the treatment of NASH. Antioxidants have also been used, and a recent large multicenter study has shown benefit from vitamin E supplementation. Treatment of hyperlipidemia with statin-type agents has shown improvement in liver enzymes, but they have not been assessed for effects on histology. Ursodeoxycholic acid has been used and improves liver enzymes in patients with many liver diseases, but it has not been definitively helpful for fatty liver disease. At present, efforts should be directed to encouraging patients with NAFLD to lose weight and exercise.

Lipid storage diseases

There are a number of rare lipid storage diseases that involve the liver, including the inherited disorders of Gaucher's and Niemann-Pick disease (Chap. 362). Other rare disorders include abetalipoproteinemia, Tangier disease, Fabray's disease, and types I and V hyperlipoproteinemia. Hepatomegaly is present due to increased fat deposition and increased glycogen found in the liver.

Porphyrias

The porphyrias are a group of metabolic disorders in which there are defects in the biosynthesis of heme necessary for incorporation into numerous hemoproteins such as hemoglobin, myoglobin, catalase, and the cytochromes (Chap. 358). Porphyrias can present as either acute or chronic diseases, with the acute disorder causing recurring bouts of abdominal pain, and the chronic disorders characterized by painful skin lesions. Porphyria cutanea tarda (PCT) is the most commonly encountered porphyria. Patients present with characteristic vesicular lesions on sun-exposed areas of the skin, principally the dorsum of the hands, the tips of the ears, or the cheeks. About 40% of patients with PCT have mutations in the gene for hemochromatosis (*HFE*), and ~50% have hepatitis C; thus, iron studies and *HFE* mutation analysis as well as hepatitis C testing should be considered in all patients who present with PCT. PCT is also associated with excess alcohol use and some medications, most notably estrogens.

TREATMENT Porphyrias

The mainstay of treatment of PCT is iron reduction by therapeutic phlebotomy, which is successful in reversing the skin lesions in the majority of patients. If hepatitis C is present, this should be treated as well. Acute intermittent porphyria presents with abdominal pain, with the diagnosis made by avoidance of certain precipitating factors such as starvation or certain diets. Intravenous heme as hematin has been used for treatment.

INFILTRATIVE DISORDERS

Amyloidosis

Amyloidosis is a metabolic storage disease that results from deposition of insoluble proteins that are aberrantly folded and assembled and then deposited in a variety of tissues (Chap. 111). Amyloidosis is divided into two types, primary and secondary, based on the broad concepts of association with myeloma (primary) or chronic inflammatory illnesses (secondary). The disease is generally considered rare, although, in certain disease states or in certain populations, it can be more common. For example, when associated with familial Mediterranean fever, it is seen in high frequency in Sephardic Jews and Armenians living in Armenia and less frequently in Ashkenazi Jews, Turks, and Arabs. Amyloidosis frequently affects patients suffering from tuberculosis and leprosy and can be seen in upwards of 10–15% of patients with ankylosing spondylitis, rheumatoid arthritis, or Crohn's disease. In one surgical pathology series, amyloid was found in <1% of cases. The liver is commonly involved in cases of systemic amyloidosis, but it is frequently inapparent clinically and only documented at autopsy. Pathologic findings in the liver include positive staining with the Congo red histochemical stain where there is an apple-green birefringence noted under polarizing light.

Granulomas

Granulomas are frequently found in the liver when patients are being evaluated for cholestatic liver enzyme abnormalities. Granulomas can be seen in primary biliary cirrhosis, but there are other characteristic clinical (e.g., pruritus, fatigue) and laboratory findings (cholestatic liver tests, antimitochondrial antibody) that allow for a definitive diagnosis of that disorder. Granulomatous infiltration can also be seen as the principal hepatic manifestation of sarcoidosis, and this is the most common presentation of hepatic granulomas (Chap. 329). The vast majority of these patients do not require any specific treatment other than what would normally be used for treatment of their sarcoidosis. A small subset, however, can develop a particularly bothersome desmoplastic reaction with a significant increase in fibrosis, which can progress to cirrhosis and liver failure. These patients may require treatment with immunosuppressive therapy and may require liver transplantation. In patients who have granulomas in the liver not associated with sarcoidosis, treatment is rarely needed.

Diagnosis requires liver biopsy, and it is important to establish a diagnosis so that a cause for the elevated liver enzymes is carefully identified. Some medications can cause granulomatous infiltration of the liver, the most notable of which is allopurinol.

Lymphoma

Involvement of the liver with lymphoma can sometimes be with bulky mass lesions but can also be as a difficult-to-diagnose infiltrative disorder that does not show any characteristic findings on abdominal imaging studies (Chap. 110). Patients may present with severe liver disease, jaundice, hypoalbuminemia, mild to moderately elevated aminotransferases, and an elevated alkaline phosphatase.

A liver biopsy is required for diagnosis and should be considered when routine blood testing does not lead to a diagnosis of the liver dysfunction.

FURTHER READINGS

PIETRANGELO A: Hereditary hemochromatosis: Pathogenesis, diagnosis, and treatment. Gastroenterology 139:393, 2010

ROBERTS EA et al: Diagnosis and treatment of Wilson disease: An update. Hepatology 47:2089, 2008

SANYAL AJ et al: Pioglitazone, vitamin E, or placebo for nonalcoholic steatohepatitis. N Engl J Med 362:1675, 2010

SILVERMAN EK, SANDHAUS RA: Clinical practice. Alpha 1-antitrypsin deficiency. N Engl J Med 360:2749, 2009

CHAPTER 310

Liver Transplantation

Jules L. Dienstag
Raymond T. Chung

Liver transplantation—the replacement of the native, diseased liver by a normal organ (allograft)—has matured from an experimental procedure reserved for desperately ill patients to an accepted, lifesaving operation applied more optimally in the natural history of end-stage liver disease. The preferred and technically most advanced approach is *orthotopic transplantation*, in which the native organ is removed and the donor organ is inserted in the same anatomic location. Pioneered in the 1960s by Thomas Starzl at the University of Colorado and, later, at the University of Pittsburgh and by Roy Calne in Cambridge, England, liver transplantation is now performed routinely worldwide. Success measured as 1-year survival has improved from ~30% in the 1970s to ~90% today. These improved prospects for prolonged survival, dating back to the early 1980s, resulted from refinements in operative technique, improvements in organ procurement and preservation, advances in immunosuppressive therapy, and, perhaps most influentially, more enlightened patient selection and timing. Despite the perioperative morbidity and mortality, the technical and management challenges of the procedure, and its costs, liver transplantation has become the approach of choice for selected patients whose chronic or acute liver disease is progressive, life-threatening, and unresponsive to medical therapy. Based on the current level of success, the number of liver transplants has continued to grow each year; in 2009, 6320 patients received liver allografts in the United States. Still, the demand for new livers continues to outpace availability; as of mid-2010, 16,785 patients in the United States were on a waiting list for a donor liver.

In response to this drastic shortage of donor organs, many transplantation centers supplement cadaver-organ liver transplantation with living-donor transplantation.

INDICATIONS

Potential candidates for liver transplantation are children and adults who, in the absence of contraindications (see below), suffer from severe, irreversible liver disease for which alternative medical or surgical treatments have been exhausted or are unavailable. *Timing of the operation is of critical importance.* Indeed, improved timing and better patient selection are felt to have contributed more to the increased success of liver transplantation in the 1980s and beyond than all the impressive technical and immunologic advances combined. Although the disease should be advanced, and although opportunities for spontaneous or medically induced stabilization or recovery should be allowed, the procedure should be done sufficiently early to give the surgical procedure a fair chance for success. Ideally, transplantation should be considered in patients with end-stage liver disease who are experiencing or have experienced a life-threatening complication of hepatic decompensation or whose quality of life has deteriorated to unacceptable levels. Although patients with well-compensated cirrhosis can survive for many years, many patients with quasi-stable chronic liver disease have much more advanced disease than may be apparent. As discussed below, the better the status of the patient prior to transplantation, the higher will be the anticipated success rate of transplantation. The decision about *when* to transplant is complex and requires the combined judgment of an experienced team of hepatologists, transplant surgeons, anesthesiologists, and specialists in support services, not to mention the well-informed consent of the patient and the patient's family.

TABLE 310-1 Indications for Liver Transplantation

Children	Adults
Biliary atresia	Primary biliary cirrhosis
Neonatal hepatitis	Secondary biliary cirrhosis
Congenital hepatic fibrosis	Primary sclerosing cholangitis
Alagille's syndrome[a]	Autoimmune hepatitis
Byler's disease[b]	Caroli's disease[c]
α_1-Antitrypsin deficiency	Cryptogenic cirrhosis
Inherited disorders of metabolism	Chronic hepatitis with cirrhosis
Wilson's disease	Hepatic vein thrombosis
Tyrosinemia	Fulminant hepatitis
Glycogen storage diseases	Alcoholic cirrhosis
Lysosomal storage diseases	Chronic viral hepatitis
Protoporphyria	Primary hepatocellular malignancies
Crigler-Najjar disease type I	Hepatic adenomas
Familial hypercholesterolemia	Nonalcoholic steatohepatitis
Primary hyperoxaluria type I	Familial amyloid polyneuropathy
Hemophilia	

[a]Arteriohepatic dysplasia, with paucity of bile ducts, and congenital malformations, including pulmonary stenosis.
[b]Intrahepatic cholestasis, progressive liver failure, mental and growth retardation.
[c]Multiple cystic dilatations of the intrahepatic biliary tree.

TRANSPLANTATION IN CHILDREN

Indications for transplantation in children are listed in Table 310-1. The most common is *biliary atresia. Inherited or genetic disorders of metabolism* associated with liver failure constitute another major indication for transplantation in children and adolescents. In Crigler-Najjar disease type I and in certain hereditary disorders of the urea cycle and of amino acid or lactate-pyruvate metabolism, transplantation may be the only way to prevent impending deterioration of central nervous system function, despite the fact that the native liver is structurally normal. Combined heart and liver transplantation has yielded dramatic improvement in cardiac function and in cholesterol levels in children with homozygous familial hypercholesterolemia; combined liver and kidney transplantation has been successful in patients with primary hyperoxaluria type I. In hemophiliacs with transfusion-associated hepatitis and liver failure, liver transplantation has been associated with recovery of normal Factor VIII synthesis.

TRANSPLANTATION IN ADULTS

Liver transplantation is indicated for end-stage *cirrhosis* of all causes (Table 310-1). In *sclerosing cholangitis* and *Caroli's disease* (multiple cystic dilatations of the intrahepatic biliary tree), recurrent infections and sepsis associated with inflammatory and fibrotic obstruction of the biliary tree may be an indication for transplantation. Because prior biliary surgery complicates and is a relative contraindication for liver transplantation, surgical diversion of the biliary tree has been all but abandoned for patients with sclerosing cholangitis. In patients who undergo transplantation for *hepatic vein thrombosis (Budd-Chiari syndrome)*, postoperative anticoagulation is essential; underlying myeloproliferative disorders may have to be treated but are not a contraindication to liver transplantation. If a donor organ can be located quickly, before life-threatening complications—including cerebral edema—set in, patients with acute liver failure are candidates for liver transplantation. Routine candidates for liver transplantation are patients with *alcoholic cirrhosis, chronic viral hepatitis,* and *primary hepatocellular malignancies.* Although all three of these categories are considered to be high risk, liver transplantation can be offered to carefully selected patients. Currently, chronic hepatitis C and alcoholic liver disease are the most common indications for liver transplantation, accounting for over 40% of all adult candidates who undergo the procedure. Patients with alcoholic cirrhosis can be considered as candidates for transplantation if they meet strict criteria for abstinence and reform; however, these criteria still do not prevent recidivism in up to a quarter of cases. Patients with chronic hepatitis C have early allograft and patient survival comparable to those of other subsets of patients after transplantation; however, reinfection in the donor organ is universal, recurrent hepatitis C is insidiously progressive, the impact of antiviral therapy is limited, allograft cirrhosis develops in 20–30% at 5 years, and cirrhosis and late organ failure are being recognized with increasing frequency beyond 5 years. In patients with chronic hepatitis B, in the absence of measures to prevent recurrent hepatitis B, survival after transplantation is reduced by approximately 10–20%; however, prophylactic use of hepatitis B immune globulin (HBIg) during and after transplantation increases the success of transplantation to a level comparable to that seen in patients with nonviral causes of liver decompensation. Specific oral antiviral drugs (e.g., lamivudine, adefovir, entecavir, and tenofovir disoproxil fumarate (Chap. 306), can be used both for prophylaxis against and for treatment of recurrent hepatitis B, facilitating further the management of patients undergoing liver transplantation for end-stage hepatitis B; most transplantation centers rely on a combination of HBIg and antiviral drugs to manage patients with hepatitis B. Issues of disease recurrence are discussed in more detail below. Patients with nonmetastatic primary hepatobiliary tumors—primary hepatocellular carcinoma (HCC), cholangiocarcinoma, hepatoblastoma, angiosarcoma, epithelioid hemangioendothelioma, and multiple or massive hepatic adenomata—have undergone liver transplantation; however, for some hepatobiliary malignancies, overall survival is significantly lower than that for other categories of liver disease. Most transplantation centers have reported 5-year recurrence-free survival rates in patients with unresectable HCC for single tumors <5 cm in diameter or for three or fewer lesions all <3 cm comparable to those seen in patients undergoing transplantation for nonmalignant indications. Consequently, liver transplantation is currently restricted to patients whose hepatic malignancies meet these criteria. Expanded criteria for patients with HCC are being evaluated. Because the likelihood of recurrent cholangiocarcinoma is very high, only highly selected patients with limited disease are being evaluated for transplantation after intensive chemotherapy and radiation.

CONTRAINDICATIONS

Absolute contraindications for transplantation include life-threatening systemic diseases, uncontrolled extrahepatic bacterial or fungal infections, preexisting advanced cardiovascular or pulmonary disease, multiple uncorrectable life-threatening congenital anomalies, metastatic malignancy, and active drug or alcohol abuse (Table 310-2). Because carefully selected patients in their sixties and even seventies have undergone transplantation successfully, advanced age per se is no longer considered an absolute contraindication; however, in older patients a more thorough preoperative evaluation should be undertaken to exclude ischemic cardiac disease and other comorbid conditions. Advanced age (>70 years), however, should be considered a *relative contraindication*—that is, a factor to be taken into account with other relative contraindications. Other relative contraindications include portal vein thrombosis, HIV infection, preexisting renal disease not associated with liver disease (which may prompt consideration of combined liver and kidney transplantation), intrahepatic or biliary sepsis, severe hypoxemia (Po_2 <50 mmHg) resulting from right-to-left intrapulmonary shunts, portopulmonary hypertension with high mean pulmonary artery pressures (>35 mmHg), previous extensive hepatobiliary surgery, any uncontrolled serious psychiatric disorder, and lack of sufficient social supports. Any one of these relative contraindications is insufficient in and of itself to preclude transplantation. For example, the problem of portal vein thrombosis can be overcome by constructing a graft from the donor liver portal vein to the recipient's superior mesenteric vein. Now that highly active antiretroviral therapy has dramatically improved the survival of persons with HIV infection (Chap. 189), and because end-stage liver disease caused by chronic hepatitis C and B has emerged as a serious source of morbidity and mortality in the HIV-infected population, liver transplantation has now been performed successfully in selected HIV-positive persons who have excellent control of HIV infection. Selected patients with CD4+ T cell counts >100/μL and with pharmacologic suppression of HIV viremia have undergone transplantation for end-stage liver disease. HIV-infected persons who have received liver allografts for end-stage liver disease resulting from chronic hepatitis B have experienced survival rates compared to those of HIV-negative persons undergoing transplantation for the same indication. In contrast, recurrent hepatitis C virus (HCV) in the allograft has limited long-term success in persons with HCV-related end-stage liver disease.

TABLE 310-2 Contraindications to Liver Transplantation

Absolute	Relative
Uncontrolled extrahepatobiliary infection	Age >70
Active, untreated sepsis	Prior extensive hepatobiliary surgery
Uncorrectable, life-limiting congenital anomalies	Portal vein thrombosis
Active substance or alcohol abuse	Renal failure not attributable to liver disease
Advanced cardiopulmonary disease	Previous extrahepatic malignancy (not including nonmelanoma skin cancer)
Extrahepatobiliary malignancy (not including nonmelanoma skin cancer)	Severe obesity
Metastatic malignancy to the liver	Severe malnutrition/wasting
Cholangiocarcinoma	Medical noncompliance
AIDS	HIV seropositivity with failure to control HIV viremia or CD4 <100/μL
Life-threatening systemic diseases	Intrahepatic sepsis Severe hypoxemia secondary to right-to-left intrapulmonary shunts (Po_2<50 mmHg) Severe pulmonary hypertension (mean pulmonary artery pressure >35 mmHg) Uncontrolled psychiatric disorder

TECHNICAL CONSIDERATIONS

CADAVER DONOR SELECTION

Cadaver donor livers for transplantation are procured primarily from victims of head trauma. Organs from brain-dead donors up to age 60 are acceptable if the following criteria are met: hemodynamic stability, adequate oxygenation, absence of bacterial or fungal infection, absence of abdominal trauma, absence of hepatic dysfunction, and serologic exclusion of hepatitis B (HBV) and C viruses and HIV. Occasionally, organs from donors with hepatitis B and C are used (e.g., for recipients with prior hepatitis B and C, respectively). Organs from donors with antibodies to hepatitis B core antigen (anti-HBc) can also be used when the need is especially urgent, and recipients of these organs are treated prophylactically with HBIg and other antiviral drugs. Cardiovascular and respiratory functions are maintained artificially until the liver can be removed. Transplantation of organs procured from deceased donors who have succumbed to cardiac death can be performed successfully under selected circumstances, when ischemic time is minimized and liver histology preserved. Compatibility in ABO blood group and organ size between donor and recipient are important considerations in donor selection; however, ABO-incompatible, split liver, or reduced-donor-organ transplants can be performed in emergencies or marked donor scarcity. Tissue typing for human leukocyte antigen (HLA) matching is not required, and preformed cytotoxic HLA antibodies do not preclude liver transplantation. Following perfusion with cold electrolyte solution, the donor liver is removed and packed in ice. The use of University of Wisconsin (UW) solution, rich in lactobionate and raffinose, has permitted the extension of cold ischemic time up to 20 hours; however, 12 hours may be a more reasonable limit. Improved techniques for harvesting multiple organs from the same donor have increased the availability of donor livers, but the availability of donor livers is far outstripped by the demand. Currently in the United States, all donor livers are distributed through a nationwide organ-sharing network [United Network for Organ Sharing (UNOS)] designed to allocate available organs based on regional considerations and recipient acuity. Recipients who have the highest disease severity generally have the highest priority, but allocation strategies that balance highest urgency against best outcomes continue to evolve to distribute cadaver organs most effectively. Allocation based on the Child-Turcotte-Pugh (CTP) score, which uses five clinical variables (encephalopathy stage, ascites, bilirubin, albumin, and prothrombin time) and waiting time, has been replaced by allocation based on urgency alone, calculated by the Model for End-Stage Liver Disease (MELD) score. The MELD score is based on a mathematical model that includes bilirubin, creatinine, and prothrombin time expressed as international normalized ratio (INR) (Table 310-3). Neither waiting time (except as a tie breaker between two potential recipients with the same MELD scores) nor posttransplantation outcome is taken into account, but the MELD score has been shown to reduce waiting list mortality, to reduce waiting time prior to transplantation, to be the best predictor of pretransplantation mortality, to satisfy the prevailing view that medical need should be the decisive determinant, and to eliminate both the subjectivity inherent in the CTP scoring system (presence and degree of ascites and hepatic encephalopathy) and the differences in waiting times among different regions of the country. Recent data indicate that liver recipients with MELD scores <15 experienced higher posttransplantation mortality rates than similarly classified patients who remained on the wait list. This observation has led to the modification of UNOS policy to allocate donor organs to candidates with MELD scores exceeding 15 within the local or regional procurement organization before offering the organ to local patients whose scores are <15. In addition, serum sodium, another important predictor of survival in liver transplantation candidates, is taken into consideration in allocating donor livers.

TABLE 310-3 United Network for Organ Sharing (UNOS) Liver Transplantation Waiting List Criteria

Status 1	Fulminant hepatic failure (including primary graft nonfunction and hepatic artery thrombosis within 7 days after transplantation as well as acute decompensated Wilson's disease)[a]

The Model for End-Stage Liver Disease (MELD) score, on a continuous scale,[b] determines allocation of the remainder of donor organs. This model is based on the following calculation:

$3.78 \times \log_e$ bilirubin (mg/100 mL) $+ 11.2 \times \log_e$ international normalized ratio (INR) $+ 9.57 \times \log_e$ creatinine (mg/100 mL) $+ 6.43$ ($\times 0$ for alcoholic and cholestatic liver disease, $\times 1$ for all other types of liver disease).[c,d,e]

Online calculators to determine MELD scores are available, such as the following: *http://optn.transplant.hrsa.gov/resources/professionalresources.asp?index=9.*

[a]For children <18 years of age, Status 1 includes acute or chronic liver failure plus hospitalization in an intensive care unit or inborn errors of metabolism. Status 1 is retained for those persons with fulminant hepatic failure and supersedes the MELD score.

[b]The MELD scale is continuous, with 34 levels ranging between 6 and 40. Donor organs usually do not become available unless the MELD score exceeds 20.

[c]Patients with stage T2 hepatocellular carcinoma receive 22 disease-specific points. An α-fetoprotein level = 500 ng/mL is considered as Stage I hepatocellular carcinoma even without evidence for a tumor on imaging.

[d]Creatinine is included because renal function is a validated predictor of survival in patients with liver disease. For adults undergoing dialysis twice a week, the creatinine in the equation is set to 4 mg/100 mL.

[e]For children <18 years of age, the Pediatric End-Stage Liver Disease (PELD) scale is used. This scale is based on albumin, bilirubin, INR, growth failure, and age. Status 1 is retained.

The highest priority (status 1) continues to be reserved for patients with fulminant hepatic failure or primary graft nonfunction. Because candidates for liver transplantation who have HCC may not be sufficiently decompensated to compete for donor organs based on urgency criteria alone, and because protracted waiting for cadaver donor organs often results in tumor growth beyond acceptable limits for transplantation, such patients are assigned disease-specific MELD points (Table 310-3).

LIVING DONOR TRANSPLANTATION

Occasionally, especially for liver transplantation in children, one cadaver organ can be split between two recipients (one adult and one child). A more viable alternative, transplantation of the right lobe of the liver from a healthy adult donor into an adult recipient, has gained increased popularity. Living donor transplantation of the left lobe (left lateral segment), introduced in the early 1990s to alleviate the extreme shortage of donor organs for small children, accounts currently for approximately one-third of all liver transplantation procedures in children. Driven by the shortage of cadaver organs, living donor transplantation involving the more sizable right lobe is being considered with increasing frequency in adults; however, living donor liver transplantation cannot be expected to solve the donor organ shortage; 219 such procedures were done in 2009, representing only about 4% of all liver transplant operations done in the United States.

Living donor transplantation can reduce waiting time and cold-ischemia time; is done under elective, rather than emergency, circumstances; and may be lifesaving in recipients who cannot afford to wait for a cadaver donor. The downside, of course, is the risk to the healthy donor (a mean of 10 weeks of medical disability; biliary complications in ~5%; postoperative complications such as wound infection, small-bowel obstruction, and incisional hernias in 9–19%; and even, in 0.2–0.4%, death) as well as the increased frequency of biliary (15–32%) and vascular (10%) complications in the recipient. Potential donors must participate voluntarily without coercion, and transplantation teams should go to great lengths to exclude subtle coercive or inappropriate psychological factors as well as outline carefully to both donor and recipient the potential benefits and risks of the procedure. Donors for the procedure should be 18–60 years old; have a compatible blood type with the recipient; have no chronic medical problems or history of major abdominal surgery; be related genetically or emotionally to the recipient; and pass an exhaustive series of clinical, biochemical, and serologic evaluations to unearth disqualifying medical disorders. The recipient should meet the same UNOS criteria for liver transplantation as recipients of a cadaver donor allograft. Comprehensive outcome data on adult-to-adult living donor liver transplantation are being collected (*www.nih-a2all.org*).

SURGICAL TECHNIQUE

Removal of the recipient's native liver is technically difficult, particularly in the presence of portal hypertension with its associated collateral circulation and extensive varices and especially in the presence of scarring from previous abdominal operations. The combination of portal hypertension and coagulopathy (elevated prothrombin time and thrombocytopenia) may translate into large blood product transfusion requirements. After the portal vein and infrahepatic and suprahepatic inferior vena cavae are dissected, the hepatic artery and common bile duct are dissected. Then the native liver is removed and the donor organ inserted. During the anhepatic phase, coagulopathy, hypoglycemia, hypocalcemia, and hypothermia are encountered and must be managed by the anesthesiology team. Caval, portal vein, hepatic artery, and bile duct anastomoses are performed in succession, the last by end-to-end suturing of the donor and recipient common bile ducts or by choledochojejunostomy to a Roux-en-Y loop if the recipient common bile duct cannot be used for reconstruction (e.g., in sclerosing cholangitis). A typical transplant operation lasts 8 hours, with a range of 6–18 hours. Because of excessive bleeding, large volumes of blood, blood products, and volume expanders may be required during surgery; however, blood requirements have fallen sharply with improvements in surgical technique and experience.

As noted above, emerging alternatives to orthotopic liver transplantation include split-liver grafts, in which one donor organ is divided and inserted into two recipients; and living donor procedures, in which part of the left (for children), the left (for children or small adults), or the right (for adults) lobe of the liver is harvested from a living donor for transplantation into the recipient. In the adult procedure, once the right lobe is removed from the donor, the donor right hepatic vein is anastomosed to the recipient right hepatic vein remnant, followed by donor-to-recipient anastomoses of the portal vein and then the hepatic artery. Finally, the biliary anastomosis is performed, duct-to-duct if practical or via Roux-en-Y anastomosis. Heterotopic liver transplantation, in which the donor liver is inserted without removal of the native liver, has met with very limited success and acceptance, except in a very small number of centers. In attempts to support desperately ill patients until a suitable donor organ can be identified, several transplantation centers are studying extracorporeal perfusion with bioartificial liver cartridges constructed from hepatocytes bound to hollow fiber systems and used as temporary hepatic-assist devices, but their efficacy remains to be established. Areas of research with the potential to overcome the shortage of donor organs include hepatocyte transplantation and xenotransplantation with genetically modified organs of nonhuman origin (e.g., swine).

POSTOPERATIVE COURSE AND MANAGEMENT

IMMUNOSUPPRESSIVE THERAPY

The introduction in 1980 of cyclosporine as an immunosuppressive agent contributed substantially to the improvement in survival after liver transplantation. Cyclosporine, a calcineurin inhibitor (CNI), blocks early activation of T cells and is specific for T cell functions that result from the interaction of the T cell with its receptor and that involve the calcium-dependent signal transduction pathway. As a result, the activity of cyclosporine leads to inhibition of lymphokine gene activation, blocking interleukins 2, 3, and 4, tumor necrosis factor α, and other lymphokines. Cyclosporine also inhibits B cell functions. This process occurs without affecting rapidly dividing cells in the bone marrow, which may account for the reduced frequency of posttransplantation systemic infections. The most common and important side effect of cyclosporine therapy is nephrotoxicity. Cyclosporine causes dose-dependent renal tubular injury and direct renal artery vasospasm. Following renal function is therefore important in monitoring cyclosporine therapy, perhaps even a more reliable indicator than blood levels of the drug. Nephrotoxicity is reversible and can be managed by dose reduction. Other adverse effects of cyclosporine therapy include hypertension, hyperkalemia, tremor, hirsutism, glucose intolerance, and gingival hyperplasia.

Tacrolimus, a macrolide lactone antibiotic isolated from a Japanese soil fungus, *Streptomyces tsukubaensis*, has the same mechanism of action as cyclosporine but is 10–100 times more potent. Initially applied as "rescue" therapy for patients in whom rejection occurred despite the use of cyclosporine, tacrolimus was shown to be associated with a reduced frequency of acute, refractory, and chronic rejection. Although patient and graft survival are the same with these two drugs, the advantage of tacrolimus in minimizing episodes of rejection, reducing the need for additional glucocorticoid doses, and reducing the likelihood of bacterial and cytomegalovirus (CMV) infection has simplified the management of patients undergoing liver transplantation. In addition, the oral absorption of tacrolimus is more predictable than that of cyclosporine, especially during the early postoperative period when T-tube drainage interferes with the enterohepatic circulation of cyclosporine. As a result, in most transplantation centers tacrolimus has now supplanted cyclosporine for primary immunosuppression, and many centers rely on oral rather than IV administration from the outset. For transplantation centers that prefer cyclosporine, a better-absorbed microemulsion preparation is now available.

Although more potent than cyclosporine, tacrolimus is also more toxic and more likely to be discontinued for adverse events. The toxicity of tacrolimus is similar to that of cyclosporine; nephrotoxicity and neurotoxicity are the most commonly encountered adverse effects, and neurotoxicity (tremor, seizures, hallucinations, psychoses, coma) is more likely and more severe in tacrolimus-treated patients. Both drugs can cause diabetes mellitus, but tacrolimus does not cause hirsutism or gingival hyperplasia. Because of overlapping toxicity between cyclosporine and tacrolimus, especially nephrotoxicity, and because tacrolimus reduces cyclosporine clearance, these two drugs should not be used together. Because 99% of tacrolimus is metabolized by the liver, hepatic dysfunction reduces its clearance; in primary graft nonfunction (when, for technical reasons or because of ischemic damage prior to its insertion, the allograft is defective and does not function normally from the outset), tacrolimus doses have to be reduced substantially, especially in children. Both cyclosporine and tacrolimus are metabolized by the cytochrome P450 IIIA system, and, therefore, drugs that induce cytochrome P450 (e.g., phenytoin, phenobarbital, carbamazepine, rifampin) reduce available levels of cyclosporine and tacrolimus; drugs that inhibit cytochrome P450 (e.g., erythromycin, fluconazole, ketoconazole, clotrimazole, itraconazole, verapamil, diltiazem, nicardipine, cimetidine, danazol, metoclopramide, bromocriptine, and the HIV protease inhibitor ritonavir) increase cyclosporine and tacrolimus blood levels. Indeed, itraconazole is used occasionally to help boost tacrolimus levels. Like azathioprine, cyclosporine and tacrolimus appear to be associated with a risk of lymphoproliferative malignancies (see below), which may occur earlier after cyclosporine or tacrolimus than after azathioprine therapy. Because of these side effects, combinations of cyclosporine or tacrolimus with prednisone and an antimetabolite (azathioprine or mycophenolic acid, see below)—all at reduced doses—are preferable regimens for immunosuppressive therapy.

Mycophenolic acid, a nonnucleoside purine metabolism inhibitor derived as a fermentation product from several *Penicillium* species, is another immunosuppressive drug being used increasingly for patients undergoing liver transplantation. Mycophenolate has been shown to be better than azathioprine, when used with other standard immunosuppressive drugs, in preventing rejection after renal transplantation and has been adopted widely as well for use in liver transplantation. The most common adverse effects of mycophenolate are bone marrow suppression and gastrointestinal complaints.

In patients with pretransplantation renal dysfunction or renal deterioration that occurs intraoperatively or immediately postoperatively, tacrolimus or cyclosporine therapy may not be practical; under these circumstances, induction or maintenance of immunosuppression with antithymocyte globulin (ATG, thymoglobulin) or monoclonal antibodies to T cells, OKT3, may be appropriate. Therapy with these agents has been especially effective in reversing acute rejection in the posttransplant period and is the standard treatment for acute rejection that fails to respond to methylprednisolone boluses. Available data support the use of thymoglobulin induction to delay CNI use and its attendant nephrotoxicity. IV infusions of thymoglobulin may be complicated by fever and chills, which can be ameliorated by premedication with antipyretics and a low dose of glucocorticoids. Infusions of OKT3 may be complicated by fever, chills, and diarrhea, or by pulmonary edema, which can be fatal. Because OKT3 is such a potent immunosuppressive agent, its use is also more likely to be complicated by opportunistic infection or lymphoproliferative disorders; therefore, because of the availability of alternative immunosuppressive drugs, OKT3 is used less often nowadays.

Rapamycin, an inhibitor of later events in T cell activation, is approved for use in kidney transplantation but is not approved for use in liver transplant recipients because of the reported association with an increased frequency of hepatic artery thrombosis in the first month posttransplantation. In patients with CNI-related nephrotoxicity, conversion to rapamycin has been demonstrated to be effective in preventing rejection with accompanying improvements in renal function. Because of its profound antiproliferative effects, rapamycin has also been suggested to be a useful immunosuppressive agent in patients with a prior or current history of malignancy, such as HCC. Side effects include hyperlipidemia, peripheral edema, oral ulcers, and interstitial pneumonitis.

The most important principle of immunosuppression is that the ideal approach strikes a balance between immunosuppression and immunologic competence. In general, given sufficient immunosuppression, acute liver allograft rejection is nearly always reversible. On one hand, incompletely treated acute rejection predisposes to the development of chronic rejection, which can threaten graft survival. On the other hand, if the cumulative dose of immunosuppressive therapy is too large, the patient may succumb to opportunistic infection. In hepatitis C, pulse glucocorticoids or OKT3 use accelerate recurrent allograft hepatitis. Further complicating matters, acute rejection can be difficult to distinguish histologically from recurrent hepatitis C. Therefore, immunosuppressive drugs must be used judiciously, with strict attention to the infectious consequences of such therapy and careful confirmation of the diagnosis of acute rejection. In this vein, efforts have been made to minimize the use of glucocorticoids, a mainstay of immunosuppressive regimens, and steroid-free immunosuppression can be achieved in some instances. Patients who undergo liver transplantation for autoimmune diseases such as primary biliary cirrhosis, autoimmune hepatitis, and primary sclerosing cholangitis are less likely to achieve freedom from glucocorticoids.

POSTOPERATIVE COMPLICATIONS

Complications of liver transplantation can be divided into nonhepatic and hepatic categories (Tables 310-4 and 310-5). In addition, both immediate postoperative and late complications are encountered. As a rule, patients who undergo liver transplantation have been chronically ill for protracted periods and may be malnourished and wasted. The impact of such chronic illness and the multisystem failure that accompanies liver failure continue to require attention in the postoperative period. Because of the massive fluid losses and fluid shifts that occur during the operation, patients may remain fluid-overloaded during the immediate postoperative period, straining cardiovascular reserve; this effect can be amplified in the face of transient renal dysfunction and pulmonary capillary vascular permeability. Continuous monitoring of cardiovascular and pulmonary function, measures to maintain the integrity of the intravascular compartment and to treat extravascular volume overload, and scrupulous attention to potential sources and sites of

TABLE 310-4 Nonhepatic Complications of Liver Transplantation

Fluid overload	
Cardiovascular instability	Arrhythmias
	Congestive heart failure
	Cardiomyopathy
Pulmonary compromise	Pneumonia
	Pulmonary capillary vascular permeability
	Fluid overload
Renal dysfunction	Prerenal azotemia
	Hypoperfusion injury (acute tubular necrosis)
	Drug nephrotoxicity
	↓ Renal blood flow secondary to ↑ intraabdominal pressure
Hematologic	Anemia 2° to gastrointestinal and/or intraabdominal bleeding
	Hemolytic anemia, aplastic anemia
	Thrombocytopenia
Infection	Bacterial: early, common postoperative infections
	Fungal/parasitic: late, opportunistic infections
	Viral: late, opportunistic infections, recurrent hepatitis
Neuropsychiatric	Seizures
	Metabolic encephalopathy
	Depression
	Difficult psychosocial adjustment
Diseases of donor	Infectious
	Malignant
Malignancy	B cell lymphoma (posttransplantation lymphoproliferative disorders)
	De novo neoplasms (particularly squamous cell skin carcinoma)

infection are of paramount importance. Cardiovascular instability may also result from the electrolyte imbalance that may accompany reperfusion of the donor liver as well as from restoration of systemic vascular resistance following implantation. Pulmonary function may be compromised further by paralysis of the right hemidiaphragm associated with phrenic nerve injury. The hyperdynamic state with increased cardiac output that is characteristic of patients with liver failure reverses rapidly after successful liver transplantation.

Other immediate management issues include renal dysfunction. Prerenal azotemia, acute kidney injury associated with hypoperfusion (acute tubular necrosis), and renal toxicity caused by antibiotics, tacrolimus, or cyclosporine are encountered frequently in the postoperative period, sometimes necessitating dialysis. Hemolytic uremic syndrome can be associated with cyclosporine, tacrolimus, or OKT3. Occasionally, postoperative intraperitoneal bleeding may be sufficient to increase intraabdominal pressure, which, in turn, may reduce renal blood flow; this effect is rapidly reversible when abdominal distention is relieved by exploratory laparotomy to identify and ligate the bleeding site and to remove intraperitoneal clot.

PART 14 Disorders of the Gastrointestinal System

TABLE 310-5 Hepatic Complications of Liver Transplantation

Hepatic Dysfunction Common after Major Surgery	
Prehepatic	Pigment load
	Hemolysis
	Blood collections (hematomas, abdominal collections)
Intrahepatic	
Early	Hepatotoxic drugs and anesthesia
	Hypoperfusion (hypotension, shock, sepsis)
	Benign postoperative cholestasis
Late	Transfusion-associated hepatitis
	Exacerbation of primary hepatic disease
Posthepatic	Biliary obstruction
	↓ Renal clearance of conjugated bilirubin (renal dysfunction)
Hepatic Dysfunction Unique to Liver Transplantation	
Primary graft nonfunction	
Vascular compromise	Portal vein obstruction
	Hepatic artery thrombosis
	Anastomotic leak with intraabdominal bleeding
Bile duct disorder	Stenosis, obstruction, leak
Rejection	
Recurrent primary hepatic disease	

Anemia may also result from acute upper gastrointestinal bleeding or from transient hemolytic anemia, which may be autoimmune, especially when blood group O livers are transplanted into blood group A or B recipients. This autoimmune hemolytic anemia is mediated by donor intrahepatic lymphocytes that recognize red blood cell A or B antigens on recipient erythrocytes. Transient in nature, this process resolves once the donor liver is repopulated by recipient bone marrow–derived lymphocytes; the hemolysis can be treated by transfusing blood group O red blood cells and/or by administering higher doses of glucocorticoids. Transient thrombocytopenia is also commonly encountered. Aplastic anemia, a late occurrence, is rare but has been reported in almost 30% of patients who underwent liver transplantation for acute, severe hepatitis of unknown cause.

Bacterial, fungal, or viral infections are common and may be life-threatening postoperatively. Early after transplant surgery, common postoperative infections predominate—pneumonia, wound infections, infected intraabdominal collections, urinary tract infections, and IV line infections—rather than opportunistic infections; these infections may involve the biliary tree and liver as well. Beyond the first postoperative month, the toll of immunosuppression becomes evident, and opportunistic infections—CMV, herpes viruses, fungal infections (*Aspergillus*, *Candida*, cryptococcal disease), mycobacterial infections, parasitic infections (*Pneumocystis*, *Toxoplasma*), bacterial infections (*Nocardia*, *Legionella*, and *Listeria*)—predominate. Rarely, early infections represent those transmitted with the donor liver, either infections present in the donor or infections acquired during procurement processing. De novo viral hepatitis infections acquired from the donor organ or, almost unheard of nowadays, from transfused blood products occur after typical incubation periods for these agents (well beyond the first month). Obviously, infections in an immunosuppressed host demand early recognition and prompt management; prophylactic antibiotic therapy is administered routinely in the immediate postoperative period. Use of sulfamethoxazole with trimethoprim reduces the incidence of postoperative *Pneumocystis carinii* pneumonia. Antiviral prophylaxis for CMV with ganciclovir should be administered in patients at high risk (e.g., when a CMV-seropositive donor organ is implanted into a CMV-seronegative recipient).

Neuropsychiatric complications include seizures (commonly associated with cyclosporine and tacrolimus toxicity), metabolic encephalopathy, depression, and difficult psychosocial adjustment. Rarely, diseases are transmitted by the allograft from the donor to the recipient. In addition to viral and bacterial infections, malignancies of donor origin have occurred. Posttransplantation lymphoproliferative disorders, especially B cell lymphoma, are a recognized complication associated with immunosuppressive drugs such as azathioprine, tacrolimus, and cyclosporine (see above). Epstein-Barr virus has been shown to play a contributory role in some of these tumors, which may regress when immunosuppressive therapy is reduced. De novo neoplasms appear at increased frequency after liver transplantation, particularly squamous cell carcinomas of the skin. Routine screening should be performed.

Long-term complications after liver transplantation attributable primarily to immunosuppressive medications include diabetes mellitus (associated with glucocorticoids) as well as hypertension, hyperlipidemia, and chronic renal insufficiency (associated with cyclosporine and tacrolimus). Monitoring and treating these disorders is a routine component of posttransplantation care; in some cases, they respond to changes in immunosuppressive regimen, while in others, specific treatment of the disorder is introduced.

HEPATIC COMPLICATIONS

Hepatic dysfunction after liver transplantation is similar to the hepatic complications encountered after major abdominal and cardiothoracic surgery; however, in addition, hepatic complications include primary graft failure, vascular compromise, failure or stricture of the biliary anastomoses, and rejection. As in nontransplant surgery, postoperative jaundice may result from prehepatic, intrahepatic, and posthepatic sources. *Prehepatic* sources represent the massive hemoglobin pigment load from transfusions, hemolysis, hematomas, ecchymoses, and other collections of blood. *Early intrahepatic* liver injury includes effects of hepatotoxic drugs and anesthesia; hypoperfusion injury associated with hypotension, sepsis, and shock; and benign postoperative cholestasis. *Late intrahepatic* sources of liver injury include posttransfusion hepatitis and exacerbation of primary disease. *Posthepatic* sources of hepatic dysfunction include biliary obstruction and reduced renal clearance of conjugated bilirubin. Hepatic complications unique to liver transplantation include primary graft failure associated with ischemic injury to the organ during harvesting; vascular compromise associated with thrombosis or stenosis of the portal vein or hepatic artery anastomoses; vascular anastomotic leak; stenosis, obstruction, or leakage of the anastomosed common bile duct; recurrence of primary hepatic disorder (see below); and rejection.

TRANSPLANT REJECTION

Despite the use of immunosuppressive drugs, rejection of the transplanted liver still occurs in a proportion of patients, beginning 1–2 weeks after surgery. Clinical signs suggesting rejection are fever, right upper quadrant pain, and reduced bile pigment and volume. Leukocytosis may occur, but the most reliable indicators are increases in serum bilirubin and aminotransferase levels. Because these tests lack specificity, distinguishing among rejection, biliary obstruction, primary graft nonfunction, vascular compromise, viral hepatitis, CMV infection, drug hepatotoxicity, and recurrent primary disease may be difficult. Radiographic visualization of the biliary tree and/or percutaneous liver biopsy often help to establish the correct diagnosis. Morphologic features of acute rejection include a mixed portal cellular infiltrate, bile duct injury, and/or endothelial inflammation ("endothelialitis"); some of these findings are reminiscent of graft-versus-host disease, primary biliary cirrhosis, or recurrent allograft hepatitis C. As soon as transplant rejection is suspected, treatment consists of IV methylprednisolone in repeated boluses; if this fails to abort rejection, many centers use thymoglobulin or OKT3. Caution should be exercised when managing acute rejection with pulse glucocorticoids or OKT3 in patients with HCV infection, because of the high risk of triggering recurrent allograft hepatitis C.

Chronic rejection is a relatively rare outcome that can follow repeated bouts of acute rejection or that occurs unrelated to preceding rejection episodes. Morphologically, chronic rejection is characterized by progressive cholestasis, focal parenchymal necrosis, mononuclear infiltration, vascular lesions (intimal fibrosis, subintimal foam cells, fibrinoid necrosis), and fibrosis. This process may be reflected as ductopenia—the vanishing bile duct syndrome. Reversibility of chronic rejection is limited; in patients with therapy-resistant chronic rejection, retransplantation has yielded encouraging results.

OUTCOME

SURVIVAL

The survival rate for patients undergoing liver transplantation has improved steadily since 1983. One-year survival rates have increased from ~70% in the early 1980s to 85–90% from 2003 to 2009. Currently the 5-year survival rate exceeds 60%. An important observation is the relationship between clinical status before transplantation and outcome. For patients who undergo liver transplantation when their level of compensation is high (e.g., still working or only partially disabled), a 1-year survival rate of >85% is common. For those whose level of decompensation mandates continuous in-hospital care prior to transplantation, the 1-year survival rate is about 70%, while for those who are so decompensated that they require life support in an intensive care unit, the 1-year survival rate is ~50%. Since UNOS's adoption in 2002 of the MELD system for organ allocation, posttransplantation survival has been found to be affected adversely for candidates with MELD scores >25, considered high disease severity. Thus, irrespective of allocation scheme, high disease severity pretransplantation corresponds to diminished post-transplantation survival. Another important distinction in survival has been drawn between high- and low-risk patient categories. For patients who do not fit any "high-risk" designations, 1-year and 5-year survival rates of 85 and 80%, respectively, have been recorded. In contrast, among patients in high-risk categories—cancer, fulminant hepatitis, age >65, concurrent renal failure, respirator dependence, portal vein thrombosis, and history of a portacaval shunt or multiple right upper quadrant operations—survival statistics fall into the range of 60% at 1 year and 35% at 5 years. Survival after retransplantation for primary graft nonfunction is ~50%. Causes of failure of liver transplantation vary with time. Failures within the first 3 months result primarily from technical complications, postoperative infections, and hemorrhage. Transplant failures after the first 3 months are more likely to result from infection, rejection, or recurrent disease (such as malignancy or viral hepatitis).

RECURRENCE OF PRIMARY DISEASE

Features of autoimmune hepatitis, primary sclerosing cholangitis, and primary biliary cirrhosis overlap with those of rejection or posttransplantation bile duct injury. Whether autoimmune hepatitis and sclerosing choangitis recur after liver transplantation is controversial; data supporting recurrent autoimmune hepatitis (in up to one-third of patients in some series) are more convincing than those supporting recurrent sclerosing cholangitis. Similarly, reports of recurrent primary biliary cirrhosis after liver transplantation have appeared; however, the histologic features of primary biliary cirrhosis and chronic rejection are virtually indistinguishable and occur as frequently in patients with primary biliary cirrhosis as in patients undergoing transplantation for other reasons. The presence of a florid inflammatory bile duct lesion is highly suggestive of the recurrence of primary biliary cirrhosis, but even this lesion can be observed in acute rejection. Hereditary disorders such as Wilson's disease and α_1 antitrypsin deficiency have not recurred after liver transplantation; however, recurrence of disordered iron metabolism has been observed in some patients with hemochromatosis. Hepatic vein thrombosis (Budd-Chiari syndrome) may recur; this can be minimized by treating underlying myeloproliferative disorders and by anticoagulation. Because cholangiocarcinoma recurs almost invariably, few centers now offer transplantation to such patients; however, a few highly selected patients with operatively confirmed stage I or II cholangiocarcinoma who undergo liver transplantation combined with neoadjuvant chemoradiation may experience excellent outcomes. In patients with intrahepatic hepatocellular carcinoma who meet criteria for transplantation, 1- and 5-year survivals are similar to those observed in patients undergoing liver transplantation for nonmalignant disease. Finally, metabolic disorders such as nonalcoholic steatohepatitis recur frequently, especially if the underlying metabolic predisposition is not altered. The metabolic syndrome occurs commonly after liver transplantation as a result of recurrent nonalcoholic fatty liver, immunosuppressive medications, and/or, in patients with hepatitis C related to the impact of HCV infection on insulin resistance, diabetes, and fatty liver.

Hepatitis A can recur after transplantation for fulminant hepatitis A, but such acute reinfection has no serious clinical sequelae. In fulminant hepatitis B, recurrence is not the rule; however, in the absence of any prophylactic measures, hepatitis B usually recurs after transplantation for end-stage chronic hepatitis B. Before the introduction of prophylactic antiviral therapy, immunosuppressive therapy sufficient to prevent allograft rejection led inevitably to marked increases in hepatitis B viremia, regardless of pretransplantation levels. Overall graft and patient survival were poor, and some patients experienced a rapid recapitulation of severe injury—severe chronic hepatitis or even fulminant hepatitis—after transplantation. Also recognized in the era before availability of antiviral regimens was *fibrosing cholestatic hepatitis,* rapidly progressive liver injury associated with marked hyperbilirubinemia, substantial prolongation of the prothrombin time (both out of proportion to relatively modest elevations of aminotransferase activity), and rapidly progressive liver failure. This lesion has been suggested to represent a "choking off" of the hepatocyte by an overwhelming density of HBV proteins. Complications such as sepsis and pancreatitis were also observed more frequently in patients undergoing liver transplantation for hepatitis B prior to the introduction of antiviral therapy. The introduction of long-term prophylaxis with HBIg revolutionized liver transplantation for chronic hepatitis B. Preoperative hepatitis B vaccination, preoperative or postoperative interferon (IFN) therapy, or short-term (≤2 months) HBIg prophylaxis has not been shown to be effective, but a retrospective analysis of data from several hundred European patients followed for 3 years after transplantation has shown that long-term (≥6 months) prophylaxis with HBIg is associated with a lowering of the risk of HBV reinfection from ~75% to 35% and a reduction in mortality from ~50% to 20%.

As a result of long-term HBIg use following liver transplantation for chronic hepatitis B, similar improvements in outcome have been observed in the United States, with 1-year survival rates between 75% and 90%. Currently, with HBIg prophylaxis, the outcome of liver transplantation for chronic hepatitis B is indistinguishable from that for chronic liver disease unassociated with chronic hepatitis B; essentially, medical concerns regarding liver transplantation for chronic hepatitis B have been eliminated. Passive immunoprophylaxis with HBIg is begun during the anhepatic stage of surgery, repeated daily for the first 6 postoperative days, then continued with infusions that are given either at regular intervals of 4–6 weeks or, alternatively, when anti-hepatitis B surface (HBs) levels fall below a threshold of 100 mIU/mL. The current approach in most centers is to continue HBIg indefinitely, which can add approximately $20,000 per year to the cost of care; some centers are evaluating regimens that shift to less frequent administration or to IM administration in the late posttransplantation period or, in low-risk patients, maintenance with antiviral therapy (see below) alone. Still, "breakthrough" HBV infection occasionally occurs.

Further improving the outcome of liver transplantation for chronic hepatitis B is the current availability of such antiviral drugs as lamivudine, adefovir, entecavir, and tenofovir disoproxil fumarate (Chap. 306). When these drugs are administered to patients with decompensated liver disease, a proportion improve sufficiently to postpone imminent liver transplantation. In addition, lamivudine can be used to prevent recurrence of HBV infection when administered *prior* to transplantation; to treat hepatitis B that recurs *after* transplantation, including in patients who break through HBIg prophylaxis; and to reverse the course of otherwise fatal fibrosing cholestatic hepatitis. Clinical trials have shown that lamivudine antiviral therapy reduces the level of HBV replication substantially, sometimes even resulting in clearance of hepatitis B surface antigen (HBsAg); reduces alanine aminotransferase (ALT) levels; and improves histologic features of necrosis and inflammation. Long-term use of lamivudine is safe and effective, but after several months a proportion of patients become resistant to lamivudine, resulting from YMDD (tyrosine-methionine-aspartate-aspartate) mutations in the HBV polymerase motif (Chap. 306). In approximately one-half of such resistant patients, hepatic deterioration may ensue. Fortunately, adefovir or tenofovir disoproxil fumarate are available as well and can be used to treat lamivudine-associated YMDD variants, effectively "rescuing" patients experiencing hepatic decompensation after lamivudine breakthrough. Currently, most liver transplantation centers combine HBIg plus lamivudine, adefovir, entecavir, or tenofovir disoproxil fumarate. Clinical trials are underway to define the optimal application of these antiviral agents in the management of patients undergoing liver transplantation for chronic hepatitis B; conceivably, in the future, combinations of oral antiviral drugs may supplant HBIg.

Prophylactic approaches applied to patients undergoing liver transplantation for chronic hepatitis B are being used as well for patients without hepatitis B who receive organs from donors with anti-hepatitis B core (HBc). Patients who undergo liver transplantation for chronic hepatitis B plus D are less likely to experience recurrent liver injury than patients undergoing liver transplantation for hepatitis B alone; still, such co-infected patients would also be offered standard posttransplantation prophylactic therapy for hepatitis B.

Accounting for up to 40% of all liver transplantation procedures, the most common indication for liver transplantation is end-stage liver disease resulting from chronic hepatitis C. Recurrence of HCV infection after liver transplantation can be documented in almost every patient. The clinical consequences of recurrent hepatitis C are limited during the first 5 years after transplantation. Nonetheless, despite the relative clinical benignity of recurrent hepatitis C in the early years after liver transplantation, and despite the negligible impact on patient survival during these early years, histologic studies have documented the presence of moderate to severe chronic hepatitis in more than one-half of all patients and bridging fibrosis or cirrhosis in ~10%. Moreover, progression to cirrhosis within 5 years is even more common, occurring in up to two-thirds of patients if moderate hepatitis is detected in a 1-year biopsy. Not surprisingly, then, for patients undergoing transplantation for hepatitis C, allograft and patient survival are diminished substantially between 5 and 10 years after transplantation. In a proportion of patients, even during the early posttransplantation period, recurrent hepatitis C may be sufficiently severe biochemically and histologically to merit antiviral therapy. Treatment with pegylated interferon (IFN) can *suppress* HCV-associated liver injury but rarely leads to *sustained* benefit. Sustained virologic responses are the exception, and reduced tolerability is often dose-limiting. Preemptive combination antiviral therapy with pegylated IFN and the nucleoside analogue ribavirin immediately after transplantation does not appear to provide any advantage over therapy introduced after clinical hepatitis has occurred. Similarly, although IFN-based antiviral therapy is not recommended for patients with decompensated liver disease, some centers have experimented with pretransplantation antiviral therapy in an attempt to eradicate HCV replication prior to transplantation; preliminary results are promising, but IFN treatment of patients with end-stage liver disease can lead to worsening of hepatic decompensation, and HCV infection has recurred after transplantation in some of these recipients. Trials of hepatitis C immune globulin preparations to prevent recurrent hepatitis C after liver transplantation have not been successful.

A small number succumb to early HCV-associated liver injury, and a syndrome reminiscent of fibrosing cholestatic hepatitis (see above) has been observed rarely. Because patients with more episodes of rejection receive more immunosuppressive therapy, and because immunosuppressive therapy enhances HCV replication, patients with severe or multiple episodes of rejection are more likely to experience early recurrence of hepatitis C after transplantation. Both high viral levels and older donor age have been linked to recurrent HCV-induced liver disease and to earlier disease recurrence after transplantation.

Patients who undergo liver transplantation for end-stage alcoholic cirrhosis are at risk of resorting to drinking again after transplantation, a potential source of recurrent alcoholic liver injury. Currently, alcoholic liver disease is one of the more common indications for liver transplantation, accounting for 20–25% of all liver transplantation procedures, and most transplantation centers screen candidates carefully for predictors of continued abstinence. Recidivism is more likely in patients whose sobriety prior to transplantation was <6 months. For abstinent patients with alcoholic cirrhosis, liver transplantation can be undertaken successfully, with outcomes comparable to those for other categories of patients with chronic liver disease, when coordinated by a team approach that includes substance abuse counseling.

■ POSTTRANSPLANTATION QUALITY OF LIFE

Full rehabilitation is achieved in the majority of patients who survive the early postoperative months and escape chronic rejection or unmanageable infection. Psychosocial maladjustment interferes with medical compliance in a small number of patients, but most manage to adhere to immunosuppressive regimens, which must be continued indefinitely. In one study, 85% of patients who survived their transplant operations returned to gainful activities. In fact, some women have conceived and carried pregnancies to term after transplantation without demonstrable injury to their infants.

FURTHER READINGS

Angus PW et al: A randomized study of adefovir dipivoxil in place of HBIG in combination with lamivudine as post-liver transplantation hepatitis B prophylaxis. Hepatology 48:1460, 2008

Berenguer M: Systematic review of the treatment of established recurrent hepatitis C with pegylated interferon in combination with ribavirin. J Hepatol 49:274, 2008

Berg CL et al: Improvement in survival associated with adult-to-adult living donor liver transplantation. Gastroenterology 133:1806, 2007

Cholongitas E et al: A systematic review of the performance of the model for end-stage liver disease (MELD) in the setting of liver transplantation. Liver Transpl 12:1049, 2006

Dharancy S et al: Mycophenolate mofetil monotherapy for severe side effects of calcineurin inhibitors following liver transplantation. Am J Transplant 40:2985, 2008

Fishman JA: Infection in solid-organ transplant recipients. N Engl J Med 357:2601, 2007

Gallegos-Orozco JF, Vargas HE: Liver transplantation: From Child to MELD. Med Clin North Am 93:931, 2009

Gane EJ et al: Lamivudine plus low-dose hepatitis B immunoglobulin to prevent recurrent hepatitis B following liver transplantation. Gastroenterology 132:931, 2007

Kim WR et al: Hyponatremia and mortality among patients on the liver-transplant waiting list. N Engl J Med 359:1018, 2008

Murray KF, Carithers RL Jr: AASLD practice guidelines: Evaluation of the patient for liver transplantation. Hepatology 41:1407, 2005

O'Leary JG et al: Indications for liver transplantation. Gastroenterology 134:1764, 2008

Pillai AA, Levitsky J: Overview of immunosuppression in liver transplantation. World J Gastroenterol 15:4225, 2009

Roland ME, Stock PG: Liver transplantation in HIV-infected recipients. Semin Liver Dis 26:273, 2006

Starzl TE, Fung JJ: Themes of liver transplantation. Hepatology 51:1869, 2010

Terrault NA, Berenguer M: Treating hepatitis C infection in liver transplant recipients. Liver Transpl 12:1192, 2006

Watt KDS, Charlton MR: Metabolic syndrome and liver transplantation: A review and guide to management. J Hepatol 53:199, 2010

Webb K et al: Transplantation for alcoholic liver disease: Report of a consensus meeting. Liver Transpl 12:301, 2006

CHAPTER 311

Diseases of the Gallbladder and Bile Ducts

Norton J. Greenberger
Gustav Paumgartner

PHYSIOLOGY OF BILE PRODUCTION AND FLOW

BILE SECRETION AND COMPOSITION

Bile formed in the hepatic lobules is secreted into a complex network of canaliculi, small bile ductules, and larger bile ducts that run with lymphatics and branches of the portal vein and hepatic artery in portal tracts situated between hepatic lobules. These interlobular bile ducts coalesce to form larger septal bile ducts that join to form the right and left hepatic ducts, which in turn, unite to form the common hepatic duct. The common hepatic duct is joined by the cystic duct of the gallbladder to form the common bile duct (CBD), which enters the duodenum (often after joining the main pancreatic duct) through the ampulla of Vater.

Hepatic bile is an isotonic fluid with an electrolyte composition resembling blood plasma. The electrolyte composition of gallbladder bile differs from that of hepatic bile because most of the inorganic anions, chloride and bicarbonate, have been removed by reabsorption across the gallbladder epithelium. As a result of water reabsorption, total solute concentration of bile increases from 3–4 g/dL in hepatic bile to 10–15 g/dL in gallbladder bile.

Major solute components of bile by moles percent include bile acids (80%), lecithin and traces of other phospholipids (16%), and unesterified cholesterol (4.0%). In the lithogenic state, the cholesterol value can be as high as 8–10%. Other constituents include conjugated bilirubin; proteins (all immunoglobulins, albumin, metabolites of hormones, and other proteins metabolized in the liver); electrolytes; mucus; and, often, drugs and their metabolites.

The total daily basal secretion of hepatic bile is ~500–600 mL. Many substances taken up or synthesized by the hepatocyte are secreted into the bile canaliculi. The canalicular membrane forms microvilli and is associated with microfilaments of actin, microtubules, and other contractile elements. Prior to their secretion into the bile, many substances are taken up into the hepatocyte, while others, such as phospholipids, a portion of primary bile acids, and some cholesterol are synthesized de novo in the hepatocyte. Three mechanisms are important in regulating bile flow: (1) active transport of bile acids from hepatocytes into the bile canaliculi, (2) active transport of other organic anions, and (3) cholangiocellular secretion. The last is a secretin-mediated and cyclic AMP–dependent mechanism that results in the secretion of a sodium- and bicarbonate-rich fluid into the bile ducts.

Active vectorial secretion of biliary constituents from the portal blood into the bile canaliculi is driven by a set of polarized transport systems at the basolateral (sinusoidal) and the canalicular apical plasma membrane domains of the hepatocyte. Two sinusoidal bile salt uptake systems have been cloned in humans, the Na^+/taurocholate cotransporter (NTCP, SLC10A1) and the organic anion–transporting proteins (OATPs), which also transport a large variety of non-bile salt organic anions. Several ATP-dependent canalicular transport systems, "export pumps," (ATP-binding cassette transport proteins, also known as ABC transporters) have been identified, the most important of which are: the bile salt export pump (BSEP, ABCB11); the anionic conjugate export pump (MRP2, ABCC2), which mediates the canalicular excretion of various amphiphilic conjugates formed by phase II conjugation (e.g., bilirubin mono- and diglucuronides and drugs); the multidrug export pump (MDR1, ABCB1) for hydrophobic cationic compounds; and the phospholipid export pump

(MDR3, ABCB4). Two hemitransporters ABCG5/G8, functioning as a couple, constitute the canalicular cholesterol and phytosterol transporter. F1C1 (ATP8B1) is an aminophospholipid transferase ("flippase") essential for maintaining the lipid asymmetry of the canalicular membrane. The canalicular membrane also contains ATP-independent transport systems such as the Cl/HCO_3 anion exchanger isoform 2 (AE2, SLC4A2) for canalicular bicarbonate secretion. For most of these transporters, genetic defects have been identified that are associated with various forms of cholestasis or defects of biliary excretion. F1C1 is defective in progressive familial intrahepatic cholestasis type 1 (PFIC1) and benign recurrent intrahepatic cholestasis type 1 (BRIC1) and results in ablation of all other ATP-dependent transporter functions. BSEP is defective in PFIC2 and BRIC2. Mutations of MRP2 (ABCC2) cause the Dubin-Johnson syndrome, an inherited form of conjugated hyperbilirubinemia (Chap. 303). A defective MDR3 (ABCB4) results in PFIC3. ABCG5/G8, the canalicular half transporters for cholesterol and other neutral sterols, are defective in sitosterolemia. The cystic fibrosis transmembrane regulator (CFTR, ABCC7) located on bile duct epithelial cells but not on canalicular membranes is defective in cystic fibrosis, which is associated with impaired cholangiocellular pH regulation during ductular bile formation and chronic cholestatic liver disease, occasionally resulting in biliary cirrhosis.

■ THE BILE ACIDS

The primary bile acids, cholic acid and chenodeoxycholic acid (CDCA), are synthesized from cholesterol in the liver, conjugated with glycine or taurine, and secreted into the bile. Secondary bile acids, including deoxycholate and lithocholate, are formed in the colon as bacterial metabolites of the primary bile acids. However, lithocholic acid is much less efficiently absorbed from the colon than deoxycholic acid. Another secondary bile acid, found in low concentration, is ursodeoxycholic acid (UDCA), a stereoisomer of CDCA. In healthy subjects, the ratio of glycine to taurine conjugates in bile is ~3:1.

Bile acids are detergent-like molecules that in aqueous solutions and above a critical concentration of about 2 m*M* form molecular aggregates called *micelles*. Cholesterol alone is sparingly soluble in aqueous environments, and its solubility in bile depends on both the total lipid concentration and the relative molar percentages of bile acids and lecithin. Normal ratios of these constituents favor the formation of solubilizing *mixed micelles*, while abnormal ratios promote the precipitation of cholesterol crystals in bile via an intermediate liquid crystal phase.

In addition to facilitating the biliary excretion of cholesterol, bile acids facilitate the normal intestinal absorption of dietary fats, mainly cholesterol and fat-soluble vitamins, via a micellar transport mechanism (Chap. 294). Bile acids also serve as a major physiologic driving force for hepatic bile flow and aid in water and electrolyte transport in the small bowel and colon.

■ ENTEROHEPATIC CIRCULATION

Bile acids are efficiently conserved under normal conditions. Unconjugated, and to a lesser degree also conjugated, bile acids are absorbed by *passive diffusion* along the entire gut. Quantitatively much more important for bile salt recirculation, however, is the *active transport* mechanism for conjugated bile acids in the distal ileum (Chap. 294). The reabsorbed bile acids enter the portal bloodstream and are taken up rapidly by hepatocytes, reconjugated, and resecreted into bile (enterohepatic circulation).

The normal bile acid pool size is approximately 2–4 g. During digestion of a meal, the bile acid pool undergoes at least one or more enterohepatic cycles, depending on the size and composition of the meal. Normally, the bile acid pool circulates ~5–10 times daily. Intestinal absorption of the pool is about 95% efficient; therefore, fecal loss of bile acids is in the range of 0.2–0.4 g/d. In the steady state, this fecal loss is compensated by an equal daily synthesis of bile acids by the liver, and, thus, the size of the bile acid pool is maintained. Bile acids returning to the liver suppress de novo hepatic synthesis of primary bile acids from cholesterol by inhibiting the rate-limiting enzyme cholesterol 7-hydroxylase. While the loss of bile salts in stool is usually matched by increased hepatic synthesis, the maximum rate of synthesis is ~5 g/d, which may be insufficient to replete the bile acid pool size when there is pronounced impairment of intestinal bile salt reabsorption.

The expression of ABC transporters in the enterohepatic circulation and of the rate-limiting enzymes of bile acid and cholesterol synthesis are regulated in a coordinated fashion by nuclear receptors, which are ligand-activated transcription factors. The hepatic bile salt export pump (BSEP, ABCB11) is upregulated by the farnesoid X receptor (FXR), a bile acid sensor that also represses bile acid synthesis. The expression of the cholesterol transporter, ABCG5/G8, is upregulated by the liver X receptor (LXR), which is an oxysterol sensor.

■ GALLBLADDER AND SPHINCTERIC FUNCTIONS

In the fasting state, the sphincter of Oddi offers a high-pressure zone of resistance to bile flow from the CBD into the duodenum. This tonic contraction serves to (1) prevent reflux of duodenal contents into the pancreatic and bile ducts and (2) promote filling of the gallbladder. The major factor controlling the evacuation of the gallbladder is the peptide hormone cholecystokinin (CCK), which is released from the duodenal mucosa in response to the ingestion of fats and amino acids. CCK produces (1) powerful contraction of the gallbladder, (2) decreased resistance of the sphincter of Oddi, and (3) enhanced flow of biliary contents into the duodenum.

Hepatic bile is "concentrated" within the gallbladder by energy-dependent transmucosal absorption of water and electrolytes. Almost the entire bile acid pool may be sequestered in the gallbladder following an overnight fast for delivery into the duodenum with the first meal of the day. The normal capacity of the gallbladder is ~30 mL of bile.

DISEASES OF THE GALLBLADDER

■ CONGENITAL ANOMALIES

Anomalies of the biliary tract are not uncommon and include abnormalities in number, size, and shape (e.g., agenesis of the gallbladder, duplications, rudimentary or oversized "giant" gallbladders, and diverticula). *Phrygian cap* is a clinically innocuous entity in which a partial or complete septum (or fold) separates the fundus from the body. Anomalies of position or suspension are not uncommon and include left-sided gallbladder, intrahepatic gallbladder, retrodisplacement of the gallbladder, and "floating" gallbladder. The latter condition predisposes to acute torsion, volvulus, or herniation of the gallbladder.

■ GALLSTONES

Epidemiology and pathogenesis

Gallstones are quite prevalent in most western countries. In the United States, the third National Health and Nutrition Examination Survey (NHANES III) has revealed an overall prevalence of gallstones of 7.9% in men and 16.6% in women. The prevalence was high in Mexican Americans (8.9% in men, 26.7% in women), intermediate for non-Hispanic whites (8.6% in men, 16.6% in women), and low for African Americans (5.3% in men, 13.9% in women).

Gallstones are formed because of abnormal bile composition. They are divided into two major types: cholesterol stones account for more than 80% of the total, with pigment stones comprising less than 20%. Cholesterol gallstones usually contain >50% cholesterol monohydrate plus an admixture of calcium salts, bile pigments, and proteins. Pigment stones are composed primarily of calcium bilirubinate; they contain <20% cholesterol and are classified into "black" and "brown" types, the latter forming secondary to chronic biliary infection.

Cholesterol stones and biliary sludge Cholesterol is essentially water insoluble and requires aqueous dispersion into either micelles or vesicles, both of which require the presence of a second lipid to solubilize the cholesterol. Cholesterol and phospholipids are secreted into bile as unilamellar bilayered vesicles, which are converted into mixed micelles consisting of bile acids, phospholipids, and cholesterol by the action of bile acids. If there is an excess of cholesterol in relation to phospholipids and bile acids, unstable, cholesterol-rich vesicles remain, which aggregate into large multilamellar vesicles from which cholesterol crystals precipitate (Fig. 311-1).

There are several important mechanisms in the formation of lithogenic (stone-forming) bile. The most important is increased biliary secretion of cholesterol. This may occur in association with obesity, the metabolic syndrome, high-caloric and cholesterol-rich diets, or drugs (e.g., clofibrate) and may result from increased activity

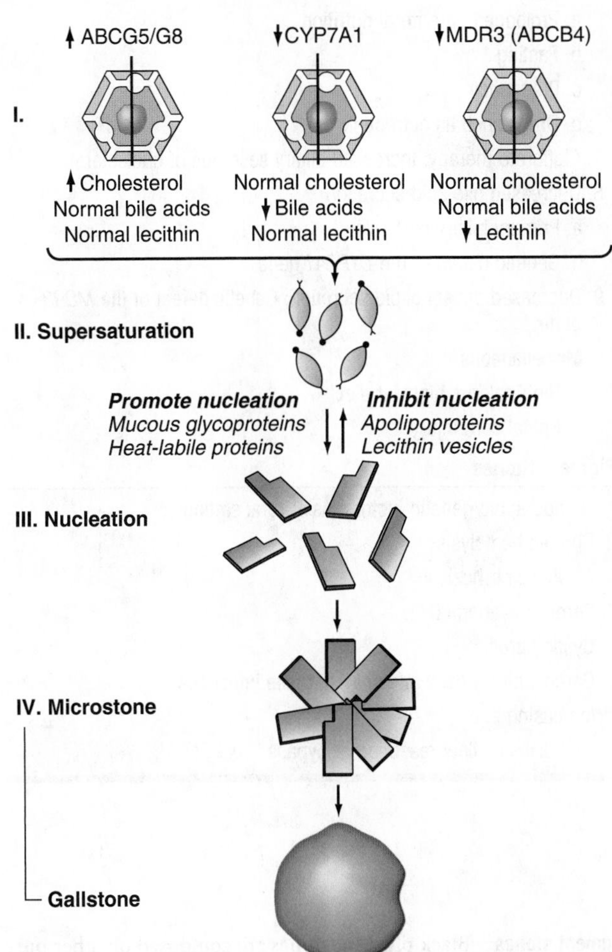

Figure 311-1 Scheme showing pathogenesis of cholesterol gallstone formation. Conditions or factors that increase the ratio of cholesterol to bile acids and phospholipids (lecithin) favor gallstone formation. ABCB4, ATP-binding cassette transporter; ABCG5/8, ATP-binding cassette (ABC) transporter G5/G8; CYP7A1, cytochrome P-450 7A1; MDR3, multidrug resistance protein 3, also called phospholipid export pump.

of hydroxymethylglutaryl-coenzyme A (HMG-CoA) reductase, the rate-limiting enzyme of hepatic cholesterol synthesis, and increased hepatic uptake of cholesterol from blood. In patients with gallstones, dietary cholesterol *increases* biliary cholesterol secretion. This does not occur in non-gallstone patients on high-cholesterol diets. In addition to environmental factors such as high-caloric and cholesterol-rich diets, genetic factors play an important role in gallstone disease. A large study of symptomatic gallstones in Swedish twins provided strong evidence for a role of genetic factors in gallstone pathogenesis. Genetic factors accounted for 25%, shared environmental factors for 13%, and individual environmental factors for 62% of the phenotypic variation among monozygotic twins. A single nucleotide polymorphism of the gene encoding the hepatic cholesterol transporter ABCG5/G8 has been found in 21% of patients with gallstones, but only in 9% of the general population. It is thought to cause a gain of function of the cholesterol transporter and to contribute to cholesterol hypersecretion. A high prevalence of gallstones is found among first-degree relatives of gallstone carriers and in certain ethnic populations such as American Indians as well as Chilean Indians and Chilean Hispanics. A common genetic trait has been identified for some of these populations by mitochondrial DNA analysis. In some patients, impaired hepatic conversion of cholesterol to bile acids may also occur, resulting in an increase of the lithogenic cholesterol/bile acid ratio. Although most cholesterol stones have a polygenic basis, there are rare monogenic (mendelian) causes. Recently, a mutation in the *CYP7A1* gene has been described that results in a deficiency of the enzyme cholesterol 7-hydroxylase, which catalyzes the initial step in cholesterol catabolism and bile acid synthesis. The homozygous state is associated with hypercholesterolemia and gallstones. Because the phenotype is expressed in the heterozygote state, mutations in the *CYP7A1* gene may contribute to the susceptibility to cholesterol gallstone disease in the population. Mutations in the *MDR3* (ABCB4) gene, which encodes the phospholipid export pump in the canalicular membrane of the hepatocyte, may cause defective phospholipid secretion into bile, resulting in cholesterol supersaturation of bile and formation of cholesterol gallstones in the gallbladder and in the bile ducts. Thus, an excess of biliary cholesterol in relation to bile acids and phospholipids is primarily due to hypersecretion of cholesterol, but hyposecretion of bile acids or phospholipids may contribute. An additional disturbance of bile acid metabolism that is likely to contribute to supersaturation of bile with cholesterol is enhanced conversion of cholic acid to deoxycholic acid, with replacement of the cholic acid pool by an expanded deoxycholic acid pool. It may result from enhanced dehydroxylation of cholic acid and increased absorption of newly formed deoxycholic acid. An increased deoxycholate secretion is associated with hypersecretion of cholesterol into bile.

While supersaturation of bile with cholesterol is an important prerequisite for gallstone formation, it is generally not sufficient by itself to produce cholesterol precipitation in vivo. Most individuals with supersaturated bile do not develop stones because the time required for cholesterol crystals to nucleate and grow is longer than the time bile spends in the gallbladder.

An important mechanism is *nucleation* of cholesterol monohydrate crystals, which is greatly accelerated in human lithogenic bile. Accelerated nucleation of cholesterol monohydrate in bile may be due to either an *excess of pronucleating factors* or a *deficiency of antinucleating factors*. Mucin and certain non-mucin glycoproteins, principally immunoglobulins, appear to be pronucleating factors, while apolipoproteins A-I and A-II and other glycoproteins appear to be antinucleating factors. Cholesterol monohydrate crystal nucleation and crystal growth probably occur within the mucin gel layer. Vesicle fusion leads to liquid crystals, which, in turn, nucleate into solid cholesterol monohydrate crystals. Continued growth of the crystals occurs by direct nucleation of cholesterol molecules from supersaturated unilamellar or multilamellar biliary vesicles.

A third important mechanism in cholesterol gallstone formation is *gallbladder hypomotility*. If the gallbladder emptied all supersaturated or crystal-containing bile completely, stones would not be able to grow. A high percentage of patients with gallstones exhibit abnormalities of gallbladder emptying. Ultrasonographic studies show that gallstone patients display an increased gallbladder volume during fasting and also after a test meal (residual volume) and that fractional emptying after gallbladder stimulation is decreased.

Biliary sludge is a thick, mucous material that, upon microscopic examination, reveals lecithin-cholesterol liquid crystals, cholesterol monohydrate crystals, calcium bilirubinate, and mucin gels. Biliary sludge typically forms a crescent-like layer in the most dependent portion of the gallbladder and is recognized by characteristic echoes on ultrasonography (see below). The presence of biliary sludge implies two abnormalities: (1) the normal balance between gallbladder mucin secretion and elimination has become deranged and (2) nucleation of biliary solutes has occurred. That biliary sludge may be a precursor form of gallstone disease is evident from several observations. In one study, 96 patients with gallbladder sludge were followed prospectively by serial ultrasound studies. In 18%, biliary sludge disappeared and did not recur for at least 2 years. In 60%, biliary sludge disappeared and reappeared; in 14%, gallstones (8% asymptomatic, 6% symptomatic) developed; and in 6%, severe biliary pain with or without acute pancreatitis occurred. In 12 patients, cholecystectomies were performed, 6 for gallstone-associated biliary pain and 3 in symptomatic patients with sludge but without gallstones who had prior attacks of pancreatitis; the latter did not recur after cholecystectomy. It should be emphasized that biliary sludge can develop with disorders that cause gallbladder hypomotility; i.e., surgery, burns, total parenteral nutrition, pregnancy, and oral contraceptives—all of which are associated with gallstone formation. However, the presence of biliary sludge implies supersaturation of bile with either cholesterol or calcium bilirubinate.

Two other conditions are associated with cholesterol-stone or biliary-sludge formation: pregnancy and rapid weight reduction through a very low-calorie diet. There appear to be two key changes during pregnancy that contribute to a "cholelithogenic state": (1) a marked increase in cholesterol saturation of bile during the third trimester and (2) sluggish gallbladder contraction in response to a standard meal, resulting in impaired gallbladder emptying. That these changes are related to pregnancy per se is supported by several studies that show reversal of these abnormalities quite rapidly after delivery. During pregnancy, gallbladder sludge develops in 20–30% of women and gallstones in 5–12%. Although biliary sludge is a common finding during pregnancy, it is usually asymptomatic and often resolves spontaneously after delivery. Gallstones, which are less common than sludge and frequently associated with biliary colic, may also disappear after delivery because of spontaneous dissolution related to bile becoming unsaturated with cholesterol postpartum.

Approximately 10–20% of persons with rapid weight reduction achieved through very low calorie dieting develop gallstones. In a study involving 600 patients who completed a 16-week, 520-kcal/d diet, UDCA in a dosage of 600 mg/d proved highly effective in preventing gallstone formation; gallstones developed in only 3% of UDCA recipients, compared to 28% of placebo-treated patients.

To summarize, cholesterol gallstone disease occurs because of several defects, which include (1) bile supersaturation with cholesterol, (2) nucleation of cholesterol monohydrate with subsequent crystal retention and stone growth, and (3) abnormal gallbladder motor function with delayed emptying and stasis. Other important factors known to predispose to cholesterol-stone formation are summarized in Table 311-1.

TABLE 311-1 Predisposing Factors for Cholesterol and Pigment Gallstone Formation

Cholesterol Stones

1. Demographic/genetic factors: Prevalence highest in North American Indians, Chilean Indians, and Chilean Hispanics, greater in Northern Europe and North America than in Asia, lowest in Japan; familial disposition; hereditary aspects
2. Obesity, metabolic syndrome: Normal bile acid pool and secretion but increased biliary secretion of cholesterol
3. Weight loss: Mobilization of tissue cholesterol leads to increased biliary cholesterol secretion while enterohepatic circulation of bile acids is decreased
4. Female sex hormones
    a. Estrogens stimulate hepatic lipoprotein receptors, increase uptake of dietary cholesterol, and increase biliary cholesterol secretion
    b. Natural estrogens, other estrogens, and oral contraceptives lead to decreased bile salt secretion and decreased conversion of cholesterol to cholesteryl esters
5. Increasing age: Increased biliary secretion of cholesterol, decreased size of bile acid pool, decreased secretion of bile salts
6. Gallbladder hypomotility leading to stasis and formation of sludge
    a. Prolonged parenteral nutrition
    b. Fasting
    c. Pregnancy
    d. Drugs such as octreotide
7. Clofibrate therapy: Increased biliary secretion of cholesterol
8. Decreased bile acid secretion
    a. Primary biliary cirrhosis
    b. Genetic defect of the *CYP7A1* gene
9. Decreased phospholipid secretion: Genetic defect of the *MDR3* gene
10. Miscellaneous
    a. High-calorie, high-fat diet
    b. Spinal cord injury

Pigment Stones

1. Demographic/genetic factors: Asia, rural setting
2. Chronic hemolysis
3. Alcoholic cirrhosis
4. Pernicious anemia
5. Cystic fibrosis
6. Chronic biliary tract infection, parasite infections
7. Increasing age
8. Ileal disease, ileal resection or bypass

Pigment stones Black pigment stones are composed of either pure calcium bilirubinate or polymer-like complexes with calcium and mucin glycoproteins. They are more common in patients who have chronic hemolytic states (with increased conjugated bilirubin in bile), liver cirrhosis, Gilbert's syndrome, or cystic fibrosis. Gallbladder stones in patients with ileal diseases, ileal resection, or ileal bypass generally are also black pigment stones. Enterohepatic recycling of bilirubin in ileal disease states contributes to their pathogenesis. Brown pigment stones are composed of calcium salts of unconjugated bilirubin with varying amounts of cholesterol and protein. They are caused by the presence of increased amounts of unconjugated, insoluble bilirubin in bile that precipitates to form stones. Deconjugation of an excess of soluble bilirubin mono- and diglucuronides may be mediated by endogenous β-glucuronidase but may also occur by spontaneous hydrolysis. Sometimes, the enzyme is also produced when bile is chronically infected by bacteria, and such stones are brown. Pigment stone formation is especially prominent in Asians and is often associated with infections in the gallbladder and biliary tree (Table 311-1).

Diagnosis

Procedures of potential use in the diagnosis of cholelithiasis and other diseases of the gallbladder are detailed in Table 311-2. Ultrasonography of the gallbladder is very accurate in the identification of cholelithiasis and has replaced oral cholecystography (Fig. 311-2*A*). Stones as small as 1.5 mm in diameter may be confidently identified provided that firm criteria are used [e.g., acoustic "shadowing" of opacities that are within the gallbladder lumen and that change with the patient's position (by gravity)]. In major medical centers, the false-negative and false-positive rates for ultrasound in gallstone patients are ~2–4%. Biliary sludge is material of low echogenic activity that typically forms a layer in the most dependent position of the gallbladder. This layer shifts with postural changes but fails to produce acoustic shadowing; these two characteristics distinguish sludges from gallstones. Ultrasound can also be used to assess the emptying function of the gallbladder.

The plain abdominal film may detect gallstones containing sufficient calcium to be radiopaque (10–15% of cholesterol and ~50% of pigment stones). Plain radiography may also be of use in the diagnosis of emphysematous cholecystitis, porcelain gallbladder, limey bile, and gallstone ileus.

Oral cholecystography (OCG) has historically been a useful procedure for the diagnosis of gallstones but has been replaced by ultrasound and is regarded as obsolete. It may be used to assess the patency of the cystic duct and gallbladder emptying function. Further, OCG can also delineate the size and number of gallstones and determine whether they are calcified.

Radiopharmaceuticals such as ^{99m}Tc-labeled *N*-substituted iminodiacetic acids (HIDA, DIDA, DISIDA, etc.) are rapidly extracted from the blood and are excreted into the biliary tree in high concentration even in the presence of mild to moderate serum bilirubin elevations. Failure to image the gallbladder in the presence of biliary ductal visualization may indicate cystic duct obstruction, acute or chronic cholecystitis, or surgical absence of the organ. Such scans have some application in the diagnosis of acute cholecystitis.

Symptoms of gallstone disease

Gallstones usually produce symptoms by causing inflammation or obstruction following their migration into the cystic duct or CBD. The most specific and characteristic symptom of gallstone disease is biliary colic that is a constant and often long-lasting pain (see below). Obstruction of the cystic duct or CBD by a stone produces increased intraluminal pressure and distention of the viscus that cannot be relieved by repetitive biliary contractions. The resultant visceral pain is characteristically a severe, steady ache or fullness in the epigastrium or right upper quadrant (RUQ) of the abdomen with frequent radiation to the interscapular area, right scapula, or shoulder.

Biliary colic begins quite suddenly and may persist with severe intensity for 15 min to 5 h, subsiding gradually or rapidly. It is steady rather than intermittent as would be suggested by the word

TABLE 311-2 Diagnostic Evaluation of the Gallbladder

Diagnostic Advantages	Diagnostic Limitations	Comment
Gallbladder Ultrasound		
Rapid	Bowel gas	Procedure of choice for detection of stones
Accurate identification of gallstones (>95%)	Massive obesity	
Simultaneous scanning of GB, liver, bile ducts, pancreas	Ascites	
"Real-time" scanning allows assessment of GB volume, contractility		
Not limited by jaundice, pregnancy		
May detect very small stones		
Plain Abdominal x-ray		
Low cost	Relatively low yield	Pathognomonic findings in: calcified gallstones
Readily available	? Contraindicated in pregnancy	Limey bile, porcelain GB
		Emphysematous cholecystitis
		Gallstone ileus
Radioisotope Scans (HIDA, DIDA, etc.)		
Accurate identification of cystic duct obstruction	? Contraindicated in pregnancy	Indicated for confirmation of suspected acute cholecystitis; less sensitive and less specific in chronic cholecystitis; useful in diagnosis of acalculous cholecystopathy, especially if given with CCK to assess gallbladder emptying
Simultaneous assessment of bile ducts	Serum bilirubin >103–205 μmol/L (6–12 mg/dL)	
	Cholecystogram of low resolution	

Abbreviations: CCK, cholecystokinin; GB, gallbladder; GBUS, gallbladder ultrasound.

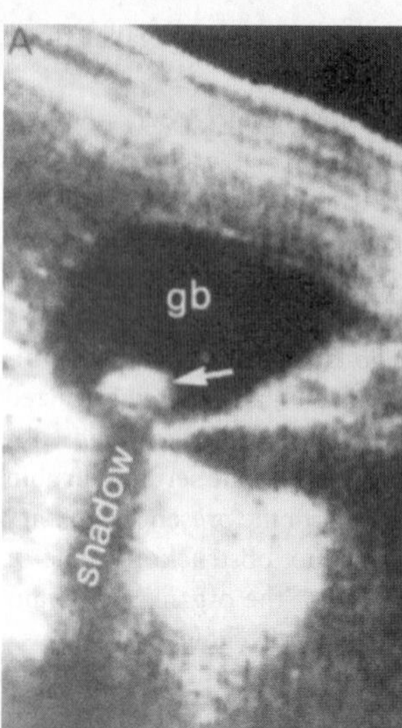

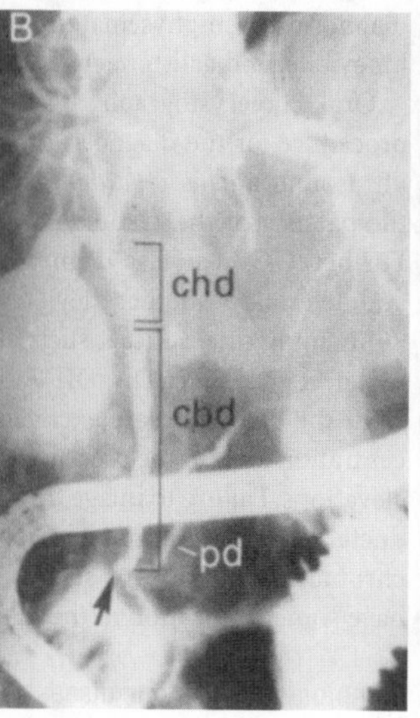

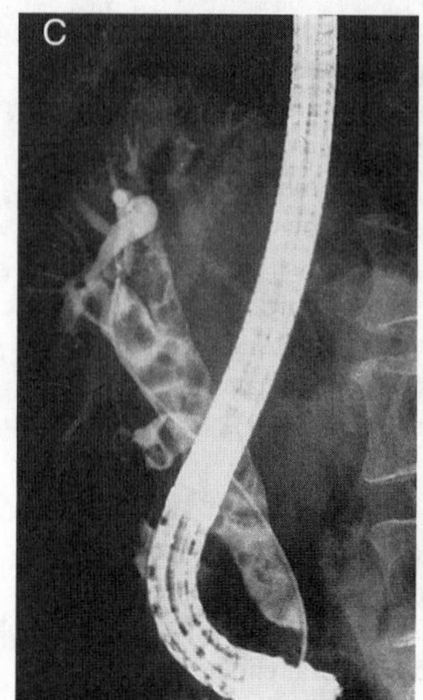

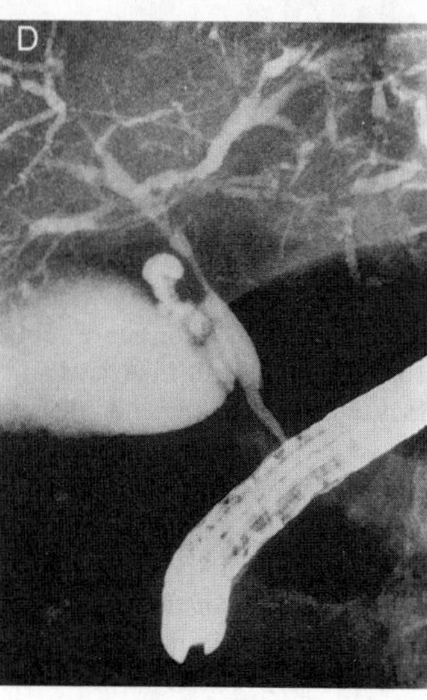

Figure 311-2 Examples of ultrasound and radiologic studies of the biliary tract. ***A.*** An ultrasound study showing a distended gallbladder containing a single large stone (*arrow*), which casts an acoustic shadow. ***B.*** Endoscopic retrograde cholangiopancreatogram (ERCP) showing normal biliary tract anatomy. In addition to the endoscope and large vertical gallbladder filled with contrast dye, the common hepatic duct (CHD), common bile duct (CBD), and pancreatic duct (PD) are shown. The arrow points to the ampulla of Vater. ***C.*** Endoscopic retrograde cholangiogram (ERC) showing choledocholithiasis. The biliary tract is dilatated and contains multiple radiolucent calculi. ***D.*** ERCP showing sclerosing cholangitis. The common bile duct shows areas that are strictured and narrowed.

colic, which must be regarded as a misnomer, although it is in widespread use. An episode of biliary pain persisting beyond 5 h should raise the suspicion of acute cholecystitis (see below). Nausea and vomiting frequently accompany episodes of biliary pain. An elevated level of serum bilirubin and/or alkaline phosphatase suggests a common duct stone. Fever or chills (rigors) with biliary pain usually imply a complication, i.e., cholecystitis, pancreatitis, or cholangitis. Complaints of vague epigastric fullness, dyspepsia, eructation, or flatulence, especially following a fatty meal, should not be confused with biliary pain. Such symptoms are frequently elicited from patients with or without gallstone disease but are not specific for biliary calculi. Biliary colic may be precipitated by eating a fatty meal, by consumption of a large meal following a period of prolonged fasting, or by eating a normal meal; it is frequently nocturnal, occurring within a few hours of retiring.

Natural history

Gallstone disease discovered in an asymptomatic patient or in a patient whose symptoms are not referable to cholelithiasis is a common clinical problem. The natural history of "silent," or asymptomatic, gallstones has occasioned much debate. A study of predominantly male silent gallstone patients suggests that the cumulative risk for the development of symptoms or complications is relatively low—10% at 5 years, 15% at 10 years, and 18% at 15 years. Patients remaining asymptomatic for 15 years were found to be unlikely to develop symptoms during further follow-up, and most patients who did develop complications from their gallstones experienced *prior* warning symptoms. Similar conclusions apply to diabetic patients with silent gallstones. Decision analysis has suggested that (1) the cumulative risk of death due to gallstone disease while on expectant management is small, and (2) prophylactic cholecystectomy is not warranted.

Complications requiring cholecystectomy are much more common in gallstone patients who have developed symptoms of biliary pain. Patients found to have gallstones at a young age are more likely to develop symptoms from cholelithiasis than are patients >60 years at the time of initial diagnosis. Patients with diabetes mellitus and gallstones may be somewhat more susceptible to septic complications, but the magnitude of risk of septic biliary complications in diabetic patients is incompletely defined.

TREATMENT Gallstones

SURGICAL THERAPY In asymptomatic gallstone patients, the risk of developing symptoms or complications requiring surgery is quite small (in the range of 1–2% per year). Thus, a recommendation for cholecystectomy in a patient with gallstones should probably be based on assessment of three factors: (1) the presence of symptoms that are frequent enough or severe enough to interfere with the patient's general routine; (2) the presence of a prior complication of gallstone disease, i.e., history of acute cholecystitis, pancreatitis, gallstone fistula, etc.; or (3) the presence of an underlying condition predisposing the patient to increased risk of gallstone complications (e.g., calcified or porcelain gallbladder and/or a previous attack of acute cholecystitis regardless of current symptomatic status). Patients with very large gallstones (>3 cm in diameter) and patients having gallstones in a congenitally anomalous gallbladder might also be considered for prophylactic cholecystectomy. Although young age is a worrisome factor in asymptomatic gallstone patients, few authorities would now recommend routine cholecystectomy in all young patients with silent stones. Laparoscopic cholecystectomy is a minimal-access approach for the removal of the gallbladder together with its stones. Its advantages include a markedly shortened hospital stay, minimal disability, as well as decreased cost, and it is the procedure of choice for most patients referred for elective cholecystectomy.

From several studies involving >4000 patients undergoing laparoscopic cholecystectomy, the following key points emerge: (1) complications develop in ~4% of patients, (2) conversion to laparotomy occurs in 5%, (3) the death rate is remarkably low (i.e., <0.1%), and (4) bile duct injuries are unusual (i.e.,

0.2–0.5%) but more frequent than with open cholecystectomy. These data indicate why laparoscopic cholecystectomy has become the "gold standard" for treating symptomatic cholelithiasis.

MEDICAL THERAPY—GALLSTONE DISSOLUTION Ursodeoxycholic acid (UDCA) decreases cholesterol saturation of bile and also appears to produce a lamellar liquid crystalline phase in bile that allows a dispersion of cholesterol from stones by physical-chemical means. UDCA may also retard cholesterol crystal nucleation. In carefully selected patients with a functioning gallbladder and with radiolucent stones <10 mm in diameter, complete dissolution can be achieved in ~50% of patients within 6 months to 2 years. For good results within a reasonable time period, this therapy should be limited to radiolucent stones smaller than 5 mm in diameter. The dose of UDCA should be 10–15 mg/kg per day. Stones larger than 15 mm in size rarely dissolve. Pigment stones are not responsive to UDCA therapy. The highest success rate (i.e., >70%) occurs in patients with small (<5 mm) floating radiolucent gallstones. Probably ≤10% of patients with *symptomatic* cholelithiasis are candidates for such treatment. However, in addition to the vexing problem of recurrent stones (30–50% over 3–5 years of follow-up), there is also the factor of taking an expensive drug for up to 2 years. The advantages and success of laparoscopic cholecystectomy have largely reduced the role of gallstone dissolution to patients who wish to avoid or are not candidates for elective cholecystectomy. However, patients with cholesterol gallstone disease who develop recurrent choledocholithiasis after cholecystectomy should be on long-term treatment with ursodeoxycholic acid.

ACUTE AND CHRONIC CHOLECYSTITIS

Acute cholecystitis

Acute inflammation of the gallbladder wall usually follows obstruction of the cystic duct by a stone. Inflammatory response can be evoked by three factors: (1) *mechanical inflammation* produced by increased intraluminal pressure and distention with resulting ischemia of the gallbladder mucosa and wall, (2) *chemical inflammation* caused by the release of lysolecithin (due to the action of phospholipase on lecithin in bile) and other local tissue factors, and (3) *bacterial inflammation*, which may play a role in 50–85% of patients with acute cholecystitis. The organisms most frequently isolated by culture of gallbladder bile in these patients include *Escherichia coli*, *Klebsiella* spp., *Streptococcus* spp., and *Clostridium* spp.

Acute cholecystitis often begins as an attack of biliary pain that progressively worsens. Approximately 60–70% of patients report having experienced prior attacks that resolved spontaneously. As the episode progresses, however, the pain of acute cholecystitis becomes more generalized in the right upper abdomen. As with biliary colic, the pain of cholecystitis may radiate to the interscapular area, right scapula, or shoulder. Peritoneal signs of inflammation such as increased pain with jarring or on deep respiration may be apparent. The patient is anorectic and often nauseated. Vomiting is relatively common and may produce symptoms and signs of vascular and extracellular volume depletion. Jaundice is unusual early in the course of acute cholecystitis but may occur when edematous inflammatory changes involve the bile ducts and surrounding lymph nodes.

A low-grade fever is characteristically present, but shaking chills or rigors are not uncommon. The RUQ of the abdomen is almost invariably tender to palpation. An enlarged, tense gallbladder is palpable in 25–50% of patients. Deep inspiration or cough during subcostal palpation of the RUQ usually produces increased pain and inspiratory arrest (Murphy's sign). Localized rebound tenderness in the RUQ is common, as are abdominal distention and hypoactive bowel sounds from paralytic ileus, but generalized peritoneal signs and abdominal rigidity are usually lacking, in the absence of perforation.

The diagnosis of acute cholecystitis is usually made on the basis of a characteristic history and physical examination. The triad of sudden onset of RUQ tenderness, fever, and leukocytosis is highly suggestive. Typically, leukocytosis in the range of 10,000–15,000 cells per microliter with a left shift on differential count is found. The serum bilirubin is mildly elevated [<85.5 μmol/L (5 mg/dL)] in fewer than half of patients, while about one-fourth have modest elevations in serum aminotransferases (usually less than a fivefold elevation). Ultrasound will demonstrate calculi in 90–95% of cases and is useful for detection of signs of gallbladder inflammation including thickening of the wall, pericholecystic fluid, and dilation of the bile duct. The radionuclide (e.g., HIDA) biliary scan may be confirmatory if bile duct imaging is seen without visualization of the gallbladder.

Approximately 75% of patients treated medically have remission of acute symptoms within 2–7 days following hospitalization. In 25%, however, a complication of acute cholecystitis will occur despite conservative treatment (see below). In this setting, prompt surgical intervention is required. Of the 75% of patients with acute cholecystitis who undergo remission of symptoms, ~25% will experience a recurrence of cholecystitis within 1 year, and 60% will have at least one recurrent bout within 6 years. In view of the natural history of the disease, acute cholecystitis is best treated by early surgery whenever possible.

Mirizzi's syndrome is a rare complication in which a gallstone becomes impacted in the cystic duct or neck of the gallbladder causing compression of the CBD, resulting in CBD obstruction and jaundice. Ultrasound shows gallstone(s) lying outside the hepatic duct. Endoscopic retrograde cholangiopancreatography (ERCP) (Fig. 311-2*B*) or percutaneous transhepatic cholangiography (PTC) or magnetic resonance cholangiopancreatography (MRCP) will usually demonstrate the characteristic extrinsic compression of the CBD. Surgery consists of removing the cystic duct, diseased gallbladder, and the impacted stone. The preoperative diagnosis of Mirizzi's syndrome is important to avoid CBD injury.

Acalculous cholecystitis In 5–10% of patients with acute cholecystitis, calculi obstructing the cystic duct are not found at surgery. In >50% of such cases, an underlying explanation for acalculous inflammation is not found. An increased risk for the development of acalculous cholecystitis is especially associated with serious trauma or burns, with the postpartum period following prolonged labor, and with orthopedic and other nonbiliary major surgical operations in the postoperative period. It may possibly complicate periods of prolonged parenteral hyperalimentation. For some of these cases, biliary sludge in the cystic duct may be responsible. Other precipitating factors include vasculitis, obstructing adenocarcinoma of the gallbladder, diabetes mellitus, torsion of the gallbladder, "unusual" bacterial infections of the gallbladder (e.g., *Leptospira*, *Streptococcus*, *Salmonella*, or *Vibrio cholerae*), and parasitic infestation of the gallbladder. Acalculous cholecystitis may also be seen with a variety of other systemic disease processes (sarcoidosis, cardiovascular disease, tuberculosis, syphilis, actinomycosis, etc.).

Although the clinical manifestations of acalculous cholecystitis are indistinguishable from those of calculous cholecystitis, the setting of acute gallbladder inflammation complicating severe underlying illness is characteristic of acalculous disease. Ultrasound, CT, or radionuclide examinations demonstrating a large, tense, static gallbladder without stones and with evidence of poor emptying over a prolonged period may be diagnostically useful in some cases. The complication rate for acalculous cholecystitis exceeds that for calculous cholecystitis. Successful management of acute acalculous cholecystitis appears to depend primarily on early diagnosis and surgical intervention, with meticulous attention to postoperative care.

Acalculous cholecystopathy Disordered motility of the gallbladder can produce recurrent biliary pain in patients without gallstones. Infusion of an octapeptide of CCK can be used to measure the gallbladder ejection fraction during cholescintigraphy. The surgical findings have included abnormalities such as chronic cholecystitis, gallbladder muscle hypertrophy, and/or a markedly narrowed cystic duct. Some of these patients may well have had antecedent gallbladder disease. The following criteria can be used to identify patients with acalculous cholecystopathy: (1) recurrent episodes of typical RUQ pain characteristic of biliary tract pain, (2) abnormal CCK cholescintigraphy demonstrating a gallbladder ejection fraction of <40%, and (3) infusion of CCK reproduces the patient's pain. An additional clue would be the identification of a large gallbladder on ultrasound examination. Finally, it should be noted that sphincter of Oddi dysfunction can also give rise to recurrent RUQ pain and CCK-scintigraphic abnormalities.

Emphysematous cholecystitis So-called emphysematous cholecystitis is thought to begin with acute cholecystitis (calculous or acalculous) followed by ischemia or gangrene of the gallbladder wall and infection by gas-producing organisms. Bacteria most frequently cultured in this setting include anaerobes, such as *C. welchii* or *C. perfringens*, and aerobes, such as *E. coli*. This condition occurs most frequently in elderly men and in patients with diabetes mellitus. The clinical manifestations are essentially indistinguishable from those of nongaseous cholecystitis. The diagnosis is usually made on plain abdominal film by finding gas within the gallbladder lumen, dissecting within the gallbladder wall to form a gaseous ring, or in the pericholecystic tissues. The morbidity and mortality rates with emphysematous cholecystitis are considerable. Prompt surgical intervention coupled with appropriate antibiotics is mandatory.

Chronic cholecystitis

Chronic inflammation of the gallbladder wall is almost always associated with the presence of gallstones and is thought to result from repeated bouts of subacute or acute cholecystitis or from persistent mechanical irritation of the gallbladder wall by gallstones. The presence of bacteria in the bile occurs in >25% of patients with chronic cholecystitis. The presence of infected bile in a patient with *chronic* cholecystitis undergoing elective cholecystectomy probably adds little to the operative risk. Chronic cholecystitis may be asymptomatic for years, may progress to symptomatic gallbladder disease or to acute cholecystitis, or may present with complications (see below).

Complications of cholecystitis

Empyema and hydrops Empyema of the gallbladder usually results from progression of acute cholecystitis with persistent cystic duct obstruction to superinfection of the stagnant bile with a pus-forming bacterial organism. The clinical picture resembles that of cholangitis with high fever; severe RUQ pain; marked leukocytosis; and often, prostration. Empyema of the gallbladder carries a high risk of gram-negative sepsis and/or perforation. Emergency surgical intervention with proper antibiotic coverage is required as soon as the diagnosis is suspected.

Hydrops or mucocele of the gallbladder may also result from prolonged obstruction of the cystic duct, usually by a large solitary calculus. In this instance, the obstructed gallbladder lumen is progressively distended, over a period of time, by mucus (mucocele) or by a clear transudate (hydrops) produced by mucosal epithelial cells. A visible, easily palpable, nontender mass sometimes extending from the RUQ into the right iliac fossa may be found on physical examination. The patient with hydrops of the gallbladder frequently remains asymptomatic, although chronic RUQ pain may also occur. Cholecystectomy is indicated, because empyema, perforation, or gangrene may complicate the condition.

Gangrene and perforation Gangrene of the gallbladder results from ischemia of the wall and patchy or complete tissue necrosis. Underlying conditions often include marked distention of the gallbladder, vasculitis, diabetes mellitus, empyema, or torsion resulting in arterial occlusion. Gangrene usually predisposes to perforation of the gallbladder, but perforation may also occur in chronic cholecystitis without premonitory warning symptoms. *Localized perforations* are usually contained by the omentum or by adhesions produced by recurrent inflammation of the gallbladder. Bacterial superinfection of the walled-off gallbladder contents results in abscess formation. Most patients are best treated with cholecystectomy, but some seriously ill patients may be managed with cholecystostomy and drainage of the abscess. *Free perforation* is less common but is associated with a mortality rate of ~30%. Such patients may experience a sudden transient relief of RUQ pain as the distended gallbladder decompresses; this is followed by signs of generalized peritonitis.

Fistula formation and gallstone ileus *Fistulization* into an adjacent organ adherent to the gallbladder wall may result from inflammation and adhesion formation. Fistulas into the duodenum are most common, followed in frequency by those involving the hepatic flexure of the colon, stomach or jejunum, abdominal wall, and renal pelvis. Clinically "silent" biliary-enteric fistulas occurring as a complication of acute cholecystitis have been found in up to 5% of patients undergoing cholecystectomy. Asymptomatic cholecystoenteric fistulas may sometimes be diagnosed by finding gas in the biliary tree on plain abdominal films. Barium contrast studies or endoscopy of the upper gastrointestinal tract or colon may demonstrate the fistula. Treatment in the symptomatic patient usually consists of cholecystectomy, CBD exploration, and closure of the fistulous tract.

Gallstone ileus refers to mechanical intestinal obstruction resulting from the passage of a large gallstone into the bowel lumen. The stone customarily enters the duodenum through a cholecystoenteric fistula at that level. The site of obstruction by the impacted gallstone is usually at the ileocecal valve, provided that the more proximal small bowel is of normal caliber. The majority of patients do not give a history of either prior biliary tract symptoms or complaints suggestive of acute cholecystitis or fistulization. Large stones, >2.5 cm in diameter, are thought to predispose to fistula formation by gradual erosion through the gallbladder fundus. Diagnostic confirmation may occasionally be found on the plain abdominal film (e.g., small-intestinal obstruction with gas in the biliary tree and a calcified, ectopic gallstone) or following an upper gastrointestinal series (cholecystoduodenal fistula with small-bowel obstruction at the ileocecal valve). Laparotomy with stone extraction (or propulsion into the colon) remains the procedure of choice to relieve obstruction. Evacuation of large stones within the gallbladder should also be performed. In general, the gallbladder and its attachment to the intestines should be left alone.

Limey (milk of calcium) bile and porcelain gallbladder Calcium salts in the lumen of the gallbladder in sufficient concentration may produce calcium precipitation and diffuse, hazy opacification of bile or a layering effect on plain abdominal roentgenography. This so-called limey bile, or milk of calcium bile, is usually clinically innocuous, but cholecystectomy is recommended, especially when it occurs in a hydropic gallbladder. In the entity called *porcelain gallbladder*, calcium salt deposition within the wall of a chronically inflamed gallbladder may be detected on the plain abdominal film.

Cholecystectomy is advised in all patients with porcelain gallbladder because in a high percentage of cases this finding appears to be associated with the development of carcinoma of the gallbladder.

TREATMENT Acute Cholecystitis

MEDICAL THERAPY Although surgical intervention remains the mainstay of therapy for acute cholecystitis and its complications, a period of in-hospital stabilization may be required before cholecystectomy. Oral intake is eliminated, nasogastric suction may be indicated, and extracellular volume depletion and electrolyte abnormalities are repaired. Meperidine or nonsteroidal anti-inflammatory drugs (NSAIDs) are usually employed for analgesia because they may produce less spasm of the sphincter of Oddi than drugs such as morphine. Intravenous antibiotic therapy is usually indicated in patients with severe acute cholecystitis, even though bacterial superinfection of bile may not have occurred in the early stages of the inflammatory process. Antibiotic therapy is guided by the most common organisms likely to be present, which are *E. coli*, *Klebsiella* spp., and *Streptococcus* spp. Effective antibiotics include ureidopenicillins such as piperacillin or mezlocillin, ampicillin sulbactam, ciprofloxacin, moxifloxacin, and third-generation cephalosporins. Anaerobic coverage by a drug such as metronidazole should be added if gangrenous or emphysematous cholecystitis is suspected. Imipenem/meropenem represent potent parenteral antibiotics that cover the whole spectrum of bacteria causing ascending cholangitis. They should, however, be reserved for the most severe, life-threatening infections when other regimens have failed (Chap. 149). Postoperative complications of wound infection, abscess formation, or sepsis are reduced in antibiotic-treated patients.

SURGICAL THERAPY The optimal timing of surgical intervention in patients with acute cholecystitis depends on stabilization of the patient. The clear trend is toward earlier surgery, and this is due in part to requirements for shorter hospital stays. Urgent (emergency) cholecystectomy or cholecystostomy is probably appropriate in most patients in whom a complication of acute cholecystitis such as empyema, emphysematous cholecystitis, or perforation is suspected or confirmed. Patients with uncomplicated acute cholecystitis should undergo early elective laparoscopic cholecystectomy, ideally within 72 hours after diagnosis. The complication rate is not increased in patients undergoing early as opposed to delayed (>6 weeks after diagnosis) cholecystectomy. Delayed surgical intervention is probably best reserved for (1) patients in whom the overall medical condition imposes an unacceptable risk for early surgery and (2) patients in whom the diagnosis of acute cholecystitis is in doubt. Early cholecystectomy (within 72 hours) is the treatment of choice for most patients with acute cholecystitis. Mortality figures for emergency cholecystectomy in most centers approach 3%, while the mortality risk for early elective cholecystectomy is ~0.5% in patients under age 60. Of course, the operative risks increase with age-related diseases of other organ systems and with the presence of long- or short-term complications of gallbladder disease. Seriously ill or debilitated patients with cholecystitis may be managed with cholecystostomy and tube drainage of the gallbladder. Elective cholecystectomy may then be done at a later date.

Postcholecystectomy complications

Early complications following cholecystectomy include atelectasis and other pulmonary disorders, abscess formation (often subphrenic), external or internal hemorrhage, biliary-enteric fistula, and bile leaks. Jaundice may indicate absorption of bile from an intraabdominal collection following a biliary leak or mechanical obstruction of the CBD by retained calculi, intraductal blood clots, or extrinsic compression.

Overall, cholecystectomy is a very successful operation that provides total or near-total relief of preoperative symptoms in 75–90% of patients. The most common cause of persistent postcholecystectomy symptoms is an overlooked symptomatic nonbiliary disorder (e.g., reflux esophagitis, peptic ulceration, pancreatitis, or—most often—irritable bowel syndrome). In a small percentage of patients, however, a disorder of the extrahepatic bile ducts may result in persistent symptomatology. These so-called postcholecystectomy syndromes may be due to (1) biliary strictures, (2) retained biliary calculi, (3) cystic duct stump syndrome, (4) stenosis or dyskinesia of the sphincter of Oddi, or (5) bile salt–induced diarrhea or gastritis.

Cystic duct stump syndrome In the absence of cholangiographically demonstrable retained stones, symptoms resembling biliary pain or cholecystitis in the postcholecystectomy patient have frequently been attributed to disease in a long (>1 cm) cystic duct remnant (cystic duct stump syndrome). Careful analysis, however, reveals that postcholecystectomy complaints are attributable to other causes in almost all patients in whom the symptom complex was originally thought to result from the existence of a long cystic duct stump. Accordingly, considerable care should be taken to investigate the possible role of other factors in the production of postcholecystectomy symptoms before attributing them to cystic duct stump syndrome.

Papillary dysfunction, papillary stenosis, spasm of the sphincter of Oddi, and biliary dyskinesia Symptoms of biliary colic accompanied by signs of recurrent, intermittent biliary obstruction may be produced by papillary stenosis, papillary dysfunction, spasm of the sphincter of Oddi, and biliary dyskinesia. Papillary stenosis is thought to result from acute or chronic inflammation of the papilla of Vater or from glandular hyperplasia of the papillary segment. Five criteria have been used to define papillary stenosis: (1) upper abdominal pain, usually RUQ or epigastric; (2) abnormal liver tests; (3) dilatation of the common bile duct upon ERCP examination; (4) delayed (>45 min) drainage of contrast material from the duct; and (5) increased basal pressure of the sphincter of Oddi, a finding that may be of only minor significance. An alternative to ERCP is magnetic resonance cholangiography (MRC) if ERCP and/or biliary manometry are either unavailable or not feasible. In patients with papillary stenosis, quantitative hepatobiliary scintigraphy has revealed delayed transit from the common bile duct to the bowel, ductal dilatation, and abnormal time-activity dynamics. This technique can also be used before and after sphincterotomy to document improvement in biliary emptying. Treatment consists of endoscopic or surgical sphincteroplasty to ensure wide patency of the distal portions of both the bile and pancreatic ducts. The greater the number of the preceding criteria present, the greater the likelihood that a patient does have a degree of papillary stenosis sufficient to justify correction. The factors usually considered as indications for sphincterotomy include (1) prolonged duration of symptoms, (2) lack of response to symptomatic treatment, (3) presence of severe disability, and (4) the patient's choice of sphincterotomy over surgery (given a clear understanding on his or her part of the risks involved in both procedures).

Criteria for diagnosing dyskinesia of the sphincter of Oddi are even more controversial than those for papillary stenosis. Proposed mechanisms include spasm of the sphincter, denervation sensitivity resulting in hypertonicity, and abnormalities of the sequencing or frequency rates of sphincteric-contraction waves. When thorough evaluation has failed to demonstrate another cause for the pain, and when cholangiographic and manometric criteria suggest a diagnosis of biliary dyskinesia, medical treatment with nitrites or anticholinergics to attempt pharmacologic relaxation of the sphincter has been proposed. Endoscopic biliary sphincterotomy (EBS) or surgical sphincteroplasty may be indicated in patients who fail to respond to a 2- to 3-month trial of medical therapy, especially if basal sphincter of Oddi pressures are elevated. EBS has become the procedure of choice for removing bile duct stones and for other biliary and pancreatic problems.

Bile salt–induced diarrhea and gastritis Postcholecystectomy patients may develop symptoms of dyspepsia, which have been attributed to duodenogastric reflux of bile. However, firm data linking these symptoms to bile gastritis after surgical removal of the gallbladder are lacking. Cholecystectomy induces persistent changes in gut transit, and these changes effect a noticeable modification of bowel habits. Cholecystectomy shortens gut transit time by accelerating passage of the fecal bolus through the colon with marked acceleration in the right colon, thus causing an increase in colonic bile acid output and a shift in bile acid composition toward the more diarrheagenic secondary bile acids. Diarrhea that is severe enough, i.e., three or more watery movements per day, can be classified as postcholecystectomy diarrhea, and this occurs in 5–10% of patients undergoing elective cholecystectomy. Treatment with bile acid–sequestering agents such as cholestyramine or colestipol is often effective in ameliorating troublesome diarrhea.

THE HYPERPLASTIC CHOLECYSTOSES

The term *hyperplastic cholecystoses* is used to denote a group of disorders of the gallbladder characterized by excessive proliferation of normal tissue components.

Adenomyomatosis is characterized by a benign proliferation of gallbladder surface epithelium with glandlike formations, extramural sinuses, transverse strictures, and/or fundal nodule ("adenoma" or "adenomyoma") formation.

Cholesterolosis is characterized by abnormal deposition of lipid, especially cholesteryl esters within macrophages in the lamina propria of the gallbladder wall. In its diffuse form ("strawberry gallbladder"), the gallbladder mucosa is brick red and speckled with bright yellow flecks of lipid. The localized form shows solitary or multiple "cholesterol polyps" studding the gallbladder wall. Cholesterol stones of the gallbladder are found in nearly half the cases. Cholecystectomy is indicated in both adenomyomatosis and cholesterolosis when symptomatic or when cholelithiasis is present.

The prevalence of gallbladder polyps in the adult population is ~5%, with a marked male predominance. Few significant changes have been found over a 5-year period in asymptomatic patients with gallbladder polyps <10 mm in diameter. Cholecystectomy is recommended in symptomatic patients, as well as in asymptomatic patients >50 years of age, or in those whose polyps are >10 mm in diameter or associated with gallstones or polyp growth on serial ultrasonography.

DISEASES OF THE BILE DUCTS

CONGENITAL ANOMALIES

Biliary atresia and hypoplasia

Atretic and hypoplastic lesions of the extrahepatic and large intrahepatic bile ducts are the most common biliary anomalies of clinical relevance encountered in infancy. The clinical picture is one of severe obstructive jaundice during the first month of life, with pale stools. When biliary atresia is suspected on the basis of clinical, laboratory, and imaging findings the diagnosis is confirmed by surgical exploration and operative cholangiography. Approximately 10% of cases of biliary atresia are treatable with roux-en-Y choledochojejunostomy, with the Kasai procedure (hepatic portoenterostomy) being attempted in the remainder in an effort to restore some bile flow. Most patients, even those having successful biliary-enteric anastomoses, eventually develop chronic cholangitis, extensive hepatic fibrosis, and portal hypertension.

Choledochal cysts

Cystic dilatation may involve the free portion of the CBD, i.e., choledochal cyst, or may present as diverticulum formation in the intraduodenal segment. In the latter situation, chronic reflux of pancreatic juice into the biliary tree can produce inflammation and stenosis of the extrahepatic bile ducts leading to cholangitis or biliary obstruction. Because the process may be gradual, ~50% of patients present with onset of symptoms after age 10. The diagnosis may be made by ultrasound, abdominal CT, MRC, or cholangiography. Only one-third of patients show the classic triad of abdominal pain, jaundice, and an abdominal mass. Ultrasonographic detection of a cyst separate from the gallbladder should suggest the diagnosis of choledochal cyst, which can be confirmed by demonstrating the entrance of extrahepatic bile ducts into the cyst. Surgical treatment involves excision of the "cyst" and biliary-enteric anastomosis. Patients with choledochal cysts are at increased risk for the subsequent development of cholangiocarcinoma.

Congenital biliary ectasia

Dilatation of intrahepatic bile ducts may involve either the major intrahepatic radicles (Caroli's disease), the inter- and intralobular ducts (congenital hepatic fibrosis), or both. In Caroli's disease, clinical manifestations include recurrent cholangitis, abscess formation in and around the affected ducts, and, often, gallstone formation within portions of ectatic intrahepatic biliary radicles. Ultrasound, MRC, and CT are of great diagnostic value in demonstrating cystic dilatation of the intrahepatic bile ducts. Treatment with ongoing antibiotic therapy is usually undertaken in an effort to limit the frequency and severity of recurrent bouts of cholangitis. Progression to secondary biliary cirrhosis with portal hypertension, extrahepatic biliary obstruction, cholangiocarcinoma, or recurrent episodes of sepsis with hepatic abscess formation is common.

CHOLEDOCHOLITHIASIS

Pathophysiology and clinical manifestations

Passage of gallstones into the CBD occurs in ~10–15% of patients with cholelithiasis. The incidence of common duct stones increases with increasing age of the patient, so that up to 25% of elderly patients may have calculi in the common duct at the time of cholecystectomy. Undetected duct stones are left behind in ~1–5% of cholecystectomy patients. The overwhelming majority of bile duct stones are cholesterol stones formed in the gallbladder, which then migrate into the extrahepatic biliary tree through the cystic duct. Primary calculi arising de novo in the ducts are usually pigment stones developing in patients with (1) hepatobiliary parasitism or chronic, recurrent cholangitis; (2) congenital anomalies of the bile ducts (especially Caroli's disease); (3) dilated, sclerosed, or strictured ducts; or (4) an *MDR3* (ABCB4) gene defect leading to impaired biliary phospholipids secretion (low phospholipid–associated cholelithiasis). Common duct stones may remain asymptomatic for years, may pass spontaneously into the duodenum, or (most often) may present with biliary colic or a complication.

Complications

Cholangitis Cholangitis may be acute or chronic, and symptoms result from inflammation, which usually is caused by at least partial obstruction to the flow of bile. Bacteria are present on bile culture in ~75% of patients with acute cholangitis early in the symptomatic course. The characteristic presentation of acute cholangitis involves biliary pain, jaundice, and spiking fevers with chills (Charcot's triad). Blood cultures are frequently positive, and leukocytosis is typical. *Nonsuppurative acute cholangitis* is most common and may respond relatively rapidly to supportive measures and to treatment with antibiotics. In *suppurative acute cholangitis*, however, the presence of pus under pressure in a completely obstructed ductal system leads to symptoms of severe toxicity—mental confusion, bacteremia, and septic shock. Response to antibiotics alone in this setting is relatively poor, multiple hepatic abscesses are often present, and the mortality rate approaches 100% unless prompt endoscopic or surgical relief of the obstruction and drainage of infected bile are carried out. Endoscopic management of bacterial cholangitis is as effective as surgical intervention. ERCP with endoscopic sphincterotomy is safe and the preferred initial procedure for both establishing a definitive diagnosis and providing effective therapy.

Obstructive jaundice Gradual obstruction of the CBD over a period of weeks or months usually leads to initial manifestations of jaundice or pruritus without associated symptoms of biliary colic or cholangitis. Painless jaundice may occur in patients with choledocholithiasis, but is much more characteristic of biliary obstruction secondary to malignancy of the head of the pancreas, bile ducts, or ampulla of Vater.

In patients whose obstruction is secondary to choledocholithiasis, associated chronic calculous cholecystitis is very common, and the gallbladder in this setting may be relatively indistensible. The absence of a palpable gallbladder in most patients with biliary obstruction from duct stones is the basis for Courvoisier's law, i.e., that the presence of a palpably enlarged gallbladder suggests that the biliary obstruction is secondary to an underlying malignancy rather than to calculous disease. Biliary obstruction causes progressive dilatation of the intrahepatic bile ducts as intrabiliary pressures rise. Hepatic bile flow is suppressed, and reabsorption and regurgitation of conjugated bilirubin into the bloodstream lead to jaundice accompanied by dark urine (bilirubinuria) and light-colored (acholic) stools.

CBD stones should be suspected in any patient with cholecystitis whose serum bilirubin level is >85.5 μmol/L (5 mg/dL). The maximum bilirubin level is seldom >256.5 μmol/L (15.0 mg/dL) in patients with choledocholithiasis unless concomitant hepatic disease or another factor leading to marked hyperbilirubinemia exists. Serum bilirubin levels ≥342.0 μmol/L (20 mg/dL) should suggest the possibility of neoplastic obstruction. The serum alkaline phosphatase level is almost always elevated in biliary obstruction. A rise in alkaline phosphatase often precedes clinical jaundice and may be the only abnormality in routine liver function tests. There may be a two- to tenfold elevation of serum aminotransferases, especially in association with acute obstruction. Following relief of the obstructing process, serum aminotransferase elevations usually return rapidly to normal, while the serum bilirubin level may take 1–2 weeks to return to normal. The alkaline phosphatase level usually falls slowly, lagging behind the decrease in serum bilirubin.

Pancreatitis The most common associated entity discovered in patients with nonalcoholic acute pancreatitis is biliary tract disease. Biochemical evidence of pancreatic inflammation complicates acute cholecystitis in 15% of cases and choledocholithiasis in >30%, and the common factor appears to be the passage of gallstones through the common duct. Coexisting pancreatitis should be suspected in patients with symptoms of cholecystitis who develop (1) back pain or pain to the left of the abdominal midline, (2) prolonged vomiting with paralytic ileus, or (3) a pleural effusion, especially on the left side. Surgical treatment of gallstone disease is usually associated with resolution of the pancreatitis.

Secondary biliary cirrhosis Secondary biliary cirrhosis may complicate prolonged or intermittent duct obstruction with or without recurrent cholangitis. Although this complication may be seen in patients with choledocholithiasis, it is more common in cases of prolonged obstruction from stricture or neoplasm. Once established, secondary biliary cirrhosis may be progressive even after correction of the obstructing process, and increasingly severe hepatic cirrhosis may lead to portal hypertension or to hepatic failure and death. Prolonged biliary obstruction may also be associated with clinically relevant deficiencies of the fat-soluble vitamins A, D, E, and K.

Diagnosis and treatment

The diagnosis of choledocholithiasis is usually made by cholangiography (Table 311-3), either preoperatively by endoscopic retrograde cholangiogram (ERC) (Fig. 311-2C) or MRCP or intraoperatively at the time of cholecystectomy. As many as 15% of patients undergoing cholecystectomy will prove to have CBD stones. When CBD stones are suspected prior to laparoscopic cholecystectomy, preoperative ERCP with endoscopic papillotomy and stone extraction is the preferred approach. It not only provides stone clearance but also defines the anatomy of the biliary tree in relationship to the cystic duct. CBD stones should be suspected in gallstone patients who have any of the following risk factors: (1) a history of jaundice or pancreatitis, (2) abnormal tests of liver function, and (3) ultrasonographic or MRCP evidence of a dilated CBD or stones in the duct. Alternatively, if intraoperative cholangiography reveals retained stones, postoperative ERCP can be carried out. The need for preoperative ERCP is expected to decrease further as laparoscopic techniques for bile duct exploration improve.

The widespread use of laparoscopic cholecystectomy and ERCP has decreased the incidence of complicated biliary tract disease and the need for choledocholithotomy and T-tube drainage of the bile ducts. EBS followed by spontaneous passage or stone extraction is the treatment of choice in the management of patients with common duct stones, especially in elderly or poor-risk patients.

TRAUMA, STRICTURES, AND HEMOBILIA

Most benign strictures of the extrahepatic bile ducts result from surgical trauma and occur in about 1 in 500 cholecystectomies. Strictures may present with bile leak or abscess formation in the immediate postoperative period or with biliary obstruction or cholangitis as long as 2 years or more following the inciting trauma. The diagnosis is established by percutaneous or endoscopic cholangiography. Endoscopic brushing of biliary strictures may be helpful in establishing the nature of the lesion and is more accurate than bile cytology alone. When positive exfoliative cytology is obtained, the diagnosis of a neoplastic stricture is established. This procedure is especially important in patients with primary sclerosing cholangitis (PSC) who are predisposed to the development of cholangiocarcinomas. Successful operative correction of non-PSC bile duct strictures by a skillful surgeon with duct-to-bowel anastomosis is usually possible, although mortality rates from surgical complications, recurrent cholangitis, or secondary biliary cirrhosis are high.

Hemobilia may follow traumatic or operative injury to the liver or bile ducts, intraductal rupture of a hepatic abscess or aneurysm of the hepatic artery, biliary or hepatic tumor hemorrhage, or mechanical complications of choledocholithiasis or hepatobiliary parasitism. Diagnostic procedures such as liver biopsy, PTC, and transhepatic biliary drainage catheter placement may also be complicated by hemobilia. Patients often present with a classic triad of biliary pain, obstructive jaundice, and melena or occult blood in the stools. The diagnosis is sometimes made by cholangiographic evidence of blood clot in the biliary tree, but selective angiographic verification may be required. Although minor episodes of hemobilia may resolve without operative intervention, surgical ligation of the bleeding vessel is frequently required.

TABLE 311-3 Diagnostic Evaluation of the Bile Ducts

Diagnostic Advantages	Diagnostic Limitations	Contraindications	Complications	Comment
Hepatobiliary Ultrasound				
Rapid Simultaneous scanning of GB, liver, bile ducts, pancreas Accurate identification of dilated bile ducts Not limited by jaundice, pregnancy Guidance for fine-needle biopsy	Bowel gas Massive obesity Ascites Barium Partial bile duct obstruction Poor visualization of distal CBD	None	None	Initial procedure of choice in investigating possible biliary tract obstruction
Computed Tomography				
Simultaneous scanning of GB, liver, bile ducts, pancreas Accurate identification of dilated bile ducts, masses Not limited by jaundice, gas, obesity, ascites High-resolution image Guidance for fine-needle biopsy	Extreme cachexia Movement artifact Ileus Partial bile duct obstruction	Pregnancy	Reaction to iodinated contrast, if used	Indicated for evaluation of hepatic or pancreatic masses Procedure of choice in investigating possible biliary obstruction if diagnostic limitations prevent HBUS
Magnetic Resonance Cholangiopancreatography				
Useful modality for visualizing pancreatic and biliary ducts Has excellent sensitivity for bile duct dilatation, biliary stricture, and intraductal abnormalities Can identify pancreatic duct dilatation or stricture, pancreatic duct stenosis, and pancreas divisum	Cannot offer therapeutic intervention High cost	Claustrophobia Certain metals (iron)	None	
Endoscopic Retrograde Cholangiopancreatography				
Simultaneous pancreatography Best visualization of distal biliary tract Bile or pancreatic cytology Endoscopic sphincterotomy and stone removal Biliary manometry	Gastroduodenal obstruction ? Roux-en-Y biliary-enteric anastomosis	Pregnancy ? Acute pancreatitis ? Severe cardiopulmonary disease	Pancreatitis Cholangitis, sepsis Infected pancreatic pseudocyst Perforation (rare) Hypoxemia, aspiration	Cholangiogram of choice in: Absence of dilated ducts ? Pancreatic, ampullary or gastroduodenal disease Prior biliary surgery Endoscopic sphincterotomy a treatment possibility
Percutaneous Transhepatic Cholangiogram				
Extremely successful when bile ducts dilated Best visualization of proximal biliary tract Bile cytology/culture Percutaneous transhepatic drainage	Nondilated or sclerosed ducts	Pregnancy Uncorrectable coagulopathy Massive ascites ? Hepatic abscess	Bleeding Hemobilia Bile peritonitis Bacteremia, sepsis	Indicated when ERCP is contraindicated or failed
Endoscopic Ultrasound				
Most sensitive method to detect ampullary stones				

Abbreviations: CBD, common bile duct; ERCP, endoscopic retrograde cholangiopancreatography; GB, gallbladder; HBUS, hepatobiliary ultrasound.

■ EXTRINSIC COMPRESSION OF THE BILE DUCTS

Partial or complete biliary obstruction may be produced by extrinsic compression of the ducts. The most common cause of this form of obstructive jaundice is carcinoma of the head of the pancreas. Biliary obstruction may also occur as a complication of either acute or chronic pancreatitis or involvement of lymph nodes in the porta hepatis by lymphoma or metastatic carcinoma. The latter should be distinguished from cholestasis resulting from massive replacement of the liver by tumor.

■ HEPATOBILIARY PARASITISM

Infestation of the biliary tract by adult helminths or their ova may produce a chronic, recurrent pyogenic cholangitis with or without multiple hepatic abscesses, ductal stones, or biliary obstruction. This condition is relatively rare but does occur in inhabitants of southern China and elsewhere in Southeast Asia. The organisms most commonly involved are trematodes or flukes, including *Clonorchis sinensis*, *Opisthorchis viverrini* or *O. felineus*, and *Fasciola hepatica*. The biliary tract also may be involved by intraductal migration of adult *Ascaris lumbricoides* from the duodenum or by intrabiliary rupture of hydatid cysts of the liver produced by *Echinococcus* spp. The diagnosis is made by cholangiography and the presence of characteristic ova on stool examination. When obstruction is present, the treatment of choice is laparotomy under antibiotic coverage, with common duct exploration and a biliary drainage procedure.

■ SCLEROSING CHOLANGITIS

Primary or idiopathic sclerosing cholangitis is characterized by a progressive, inflammatory, sclerosing, and obliterative process affecting the extrahepatic and/or the intrahepatic bile ducts. The disorder occurs up to 75% in association with inflammatory bowel disease, especially ulcerative colitis. It may also be associated with autoimmune pancreatitis; multifocal fibrosclerosis syndromes such as retroperitoneal, mediastinal, and/or periureteral fibrosis; Riedel's struma; or pseudotumor of the orbit.

Immunoglobulin G4–associated cholangitis is a recently described biliary disease of unknown etiology that presents with biochemical and cholangiographic features indistinguishable from PSC, is often associated with autoimmune pancreatitis and other fibrosing conditions, and is characterized by elevated serum IgG4 and infiltration of IgG4-positive plasma cells in bile ducts and liver tissue. In contrast to PSC, it is not associated with inflammatory bowel disease and should be suspected if associated with increased serum IgG4 and unexplained pancreatic disease. Glucocorticoids are regarded as the initial treatment of choice. Relapse is common after steroid withdrawal especially with proximal strictures. Long-term treatment with glucocorticoids and/or azathioprine may be needed after relapse or for inadequate response (Chap. 313).

Patients with primary sclerosing cholangitis often present with signs and symptoms of chronic or intermittent biliary obstruction: RUQ abdominal pain, pruritus, jaundice, or acute cholangitis. Late in the course, complete biliary obstruction, secondary biliary cirrhosis, hepatic failure, or portal hypertension with bleeding varices may occur. The diagnosis is usually established by finding multifocal, diffusely distributed strictures with intervening segments of normal or dilated ducts, producing a beaded appearance on cholangiography (Fig. 311-2*D*). The cholangiographic techniques of choice in suspected cases are MRCP and ERCP. When a diagnosis of sclerosing cholangitis has been established, a search for associated diseases, especially for chronic inflammatory bowel disease, should be carried out.

A recent study describes the natural history and outcome for 305 patients of Swedish descent with primary sclerosing cholangitis; 134 (44%) of the patients were asymptomatic at the time of diagnosis and, not surprisingly, had a significantly higher survival rate. The independent predictors of a bad prognosis were age, serum bilirubin concentration, and liver histologic changes. Cholangiocarcinoma was found in 24 patients (8%). Inflammatory bowel disease was closely associated with primary sclerosing cholangitis and had a prevalence of 81% in this study population.

Small duct PSC is defined by the presence of chronic cholestasis and hepatic histology consistent with PSC but with normal findings on cholangiography. Small duct PSC is found in ~5% of patients with PSC and may represent an earlier stage of PSC associated with a significantly better long-term prognosis. However, such patients may progress to classic PSC and/or end-stage liver disease with consequent necessity of liver transplantation.

In patients with AIDS, cholangiopancreatography may demonstrate a broad range of biliary tract changes as well as pancreatic duct obstruction and occasionally pancreatitis (Chap. 189). Further, biliary tract lesions in AIDS include infection and cholangiopancreatographic changes similar to those of PSC. Changes noted include: (1) diffuse involvement of intrahepatic bile ducts alone, (2) involvement of both intra- and extrahepatic bile ducts, (3) ampullary stenosis, (4) stricture of the intrapancreatic portion of the common bile duct, and (5) pancreatic duct involvement. Associated infectious organisms include *Cryptosporidium*, *Mycobacterium avium-intracellulare*, cytomegalovirus, *Microsporidia*, and *Isospora*. In addition, acalculous cholecystitis occurs in up to 10% of patients. ERCP sphincterotomy, while not without risk, provides significant pain reduction in patients with AIDS-associated papillary stenosis. Secondary sclerosing cholangitis may occur as a long-term complication of choledocholithiasis, cholangiocarcinoma, operative or traumatic biliary injury, or contiguous inflammatory processes.

TREATMENT Sclerosing Cholangitis

Therapy with cholestyramine may help control symptoms of pruritus, and antibiotics are useful when cholangitis complicates the clinical picture. Vitamin D and calcium supplementation may help prevent the loss of bone mass frequently seen in patients with chronic cholestasis. Glucocorticoids, methotrexate, and cyclosporine have not been shown to be efficacious in PSC. UDCA in high dosage (20 mg/kg) improves serum liver tests, but an effect on survival has not been documented. In cases where high-grade biliary obstruction (dominant strictures) has occurred, balloon dilatation or stenting may be appropriate. Only rarely is surgical intervention indicated. Efforts at biliary-enteric anastomosis or stent placement may, however, be complicated by recurrent cholangitis and further progression of the stenosing process. The prognosis is unfavorable, with a median survival of 9 to 12 years following the diagnosis, regardless of therapy. Four variables (age, serum bilirubin level, histologic stage, and splenomegaly) predict survival in patients with PSC and serve as the basis for a risk score. PSC is one of the most common indications for liver transplantation.

FURTHER READINGS

Apstein MD, Carey MC: Pathogenesis of cholesterol gallstones: A parsimonious hypothesis. Eur J Clin Invest 26:343, 1996

Ghazale A et al: Immunoglobuline G4-associated cholangitis: Clinical profile and response to therapy. Gastroenterol 134:706, 2008

Johansson M et al: Randomized clinical trial of open versus laparoscopic cholecystectomy for acute cholecystitis. Br J Surg 92:44, 2005

Lammert F, Miquel J-F: Gallstone disease: From genes to evidence-based therapy. J Hepatol 48:S124, 2008

Papi C et al: Timing of cholecystectomy for acute calculous cholecystitis: a meta-analysis. Am J Gastroenterol 99:147, 2004

Portincasa P et al: Cholesterol gallstone disease. Lancet 368:230, 2006

Ransohoff DF, Gracie WA: Treatment of gallstones. Ann Intern Med 119:606, 1993

Tischendorf JJW et al: Characterization, outcome, and prognosis in 273 patients with primary sclerosing cholangitis: a single center study. Am J Gastroenterol 102:107, 2007

CHAPTER 312

Approach to the Patient With Pancreatic Disease

Norton J. Greenberger
Darwin L. Conwell
Peter A. Banks

GENERAL CONSIDERATIONS

As emphasized in Chap. 313, the etiologies as well as the clinical manifestations of pancreatitis are quite varied. Although it is well-appreciated that pancreatitis is frequently secondary to biliary tract disease and alcohol abuse, it can also be caused by drugs, trauma, and viral infections and is associated with metabolic and connective tissue disorders. In ~30% of patients with acute pancreatitis and 25–40% of patients with chronic pancreatitis, the etiology initially can be obscure.

Although good data exist concerning the incidence of acute pancreatitis (about 5–35/100,000 new cases per year worldwide, with a mortality rate of about 3%), the number of patients who suffer with acute pancreatitis is largely increasing and is now estimated to be 70 hospitalizations/100,000 persons annually, resulting in >200,000 new cases of acute pancreatitis per year in the United States. Only one prospective study on the incidence of chronic pancreatitis is available; it showed an incidence of 8.2 new cases per 100,000 per year and a prevalence of 26.4 cases per 100,000. These numbers probably underestimate considerably the true incidence and prevalence, because non alcohol–induced pancreatitis has been largely ignored. At autopsy, the prevalence of chronic pancreatitis ranges from 0.04 to 5%. The relative inaccessibility of the pancreas to direct examination and the nonspecificity of the abdominal pain associated with pancreatitis make the diagnosis of pancreatitis difficult and usually dependent on elevation of blood amylase and/or lipase levels. Many patients with chronic pancreatitis do not have elevated blood amylase or lipase levels. Some patients with chronic pancreatitis develop signs and symptoms of pancreatic exocrine insufficiency, and, thus, objective evidence for pancreatic disease can be demonstrated. However, there is a very large reservoir of pancreatic exocrine function. More than 90% of the pancreas must be damaged before maldigestion of fat and protein is manifested. Noninvasive, indirect tests of pancreatic exocrine function (fecal elastase) are much more likely to give abnormal results in patients with obvious pancreatic disease (i.e., pancreatic calcification, steatorrhea, or diabetes mellitus, than in patients with occult disease). Thus, the number of patients who have subclinical exocrine dysfunction (<90% loss of function) is unknown.

TESTS USEFUL IN THE DIAGNOSIS OF PANCREATIC DISEASE

Several tests have proved of value in the evaluation of pancreatic disease. Examples of specific tests and their usefulness in the diagnosis of acute and chronic pancreatitis are summarized in Table 312-1 and Fig. 312-1. At some institutions, pancreatic-function tests are available and performed if the diagnosis of pancreatic disease remains a possibility after noninvasive tests [ultrasound, CT, magnetic resonance cholangiopancreatography (MRCP)] or invasive tests [endoscopic retrograde cholangiopancreatography (ERCP), endoscopic

TABLE 312-1 Tests Useful in the Diagnosis of Acute and Chronic Pancreatitis and Pancreatic Tumors

Test	Principle	Comment
Pancreatic Enzymes in Body Fluids		
Amylase		
1. Serum	Pancreatic inflammation leads to increased enzyme levels	Simple; 20–40% false negatives and positives; reliable if test results are three times the upper limit of normal
2. Urine	Renal clearance of amylase is increased in acute pancreatitis	Infrequently used
3. Ascitic fluid	Disruption of gland or main pancreatic duct leads to increased amylase concentration	Can help establish diagnosis of acute pancreatitis; false positives occur with intestinal obstruction and perforated ulcer
4. Pleural fluid	Exudative pleural effusion with pancreatitis	False positives occur with carcinoma of the lung and esophageal perforation
Serum lipase	Pancreatic inflammation leads to increased enzyme levels	New methods have greatly simplified determination; positive in 70–85% of cases

(continued)

TABLE 312-1 Tests Useful in the Diagnosis of Acute and Chronic Pancreatitis and Pancreatic Tumors (*Continued*)

Test	Principle	Comment
Studies Pertaining to Pancreatic Structure		
Radiologic and radionuclide tests		
1. Plain film of the abdomen	Can be abnormal in acute and chronic pancreatitis	Simple; normal in >50% of cases of both acute and chronic pancreatitis
2. Upper GI x rays		Now obsolete
3. Ultrasonography (US)	Can provide information on edema, inflammation, calcification, pseudocysts, and mass lesions	Simple, noninvasive; sequential studies quite feasible; useful in diagnosis of pseudocyst limited by interference by bowel gas
4. CT scan	Permits detailed visualization of pancreas and surrounding structures, pancreatic fluid collection, pseudocyst, degree of necrosis	Useful in the diagnosis of pancreatic calcification, dilated pancreatic ducts, and pancreatic tumors; may not be able to distinguish between inflammatory and neoplastic mass lesions
5. Endoscopic retrograde cholangiopancreatography (ERCP)	Cannulation of pancreatic and common bile duct permits visualization of pancreatic-biliary ductal system	Can provide diagnostic data in 60–85% of cases; differentiation of chronic pancreatitis from pancreatic carcinoma may be difficult; now considered primarily a therapeutic procedure
6. Endoscopic ultrasonography (EUS)	High-frequency transducer employed with EUS can produce very high-resolution images and depict changes in the pancreatic duct and parenchyma with great detail	Can be used to assess chronic pancreatitis and pancreatic carcinoma
7. Magnetic resonance cholangiopancreatography	Three-dimensional rendering has been used to produce very good images of the pancreatic duct by a noninvasive technique	Has largely replaced ERCP as a diagnostic test
Pancreatic biopsy with US or CT guidance	Percutaneous aspiration biopsy with skinny needle and localization of lesion by US	High diagnostic yield; laparotomy avoided; can be done with EUS requires special technical skills
Tests of Exocrine Pancreatic Function		
Direct stimulation of the pancreas with analysis of duodenal contents		
1. Secretin-pancreozymin (CCK) test	Secretin leads to increased output of pancreatic juice and HCO_3^-; CCK leads to increased output of pancreatic enzymes; pancreatic secretory response is related to the functional mass of pancreatic tissue	Sensitive enough to detect occult disease; involves duodenal intubation and fluoroscopy; poorly defined normal enzyme response; overlap in chronic pancreatitis; large secretory reserve capacity of the pancreas, currently done at only a few medical centers
2. Endoscopic secretin—CCK test	Replaces need for tube placement duodenum	Sensitive enough to detect occult disease; avoids intubation and fluoroscopy; requires sedation
Measurement of intraluminal digestion products		
1. Microscopic examination of stool for undigested meat fibers and fat	Lack of proteolytic and lipolytic enzymes causes decreased digestion of meat fibers and triglycerides	Simple, reliable; not sensitive enough to detect milder cases of pancreatic insufficiency
2. Quantitative stool fat determination	Lack of lipolytic enzymes brings about impaired fat digestion	Reliable, reference standard for defining severity of malabsorption; does not distinguish between maldigestion and malabsorption
3. Fecal nitrogen	Lack of proteolytic enzymes leads to impaired protein digestion, resulting in an increase in stool nitrogen	Does not distinguish between maldigestion and malabsorption; low sensitivity
Measurement of pancreatic enzymes in feces		
1. Elastase	Pancreatic secretion of proteolytic enzymes; not degraded in intestine	Good sensitivity if stools not liquid

Abbreviation: CCK, cholecystokinin.

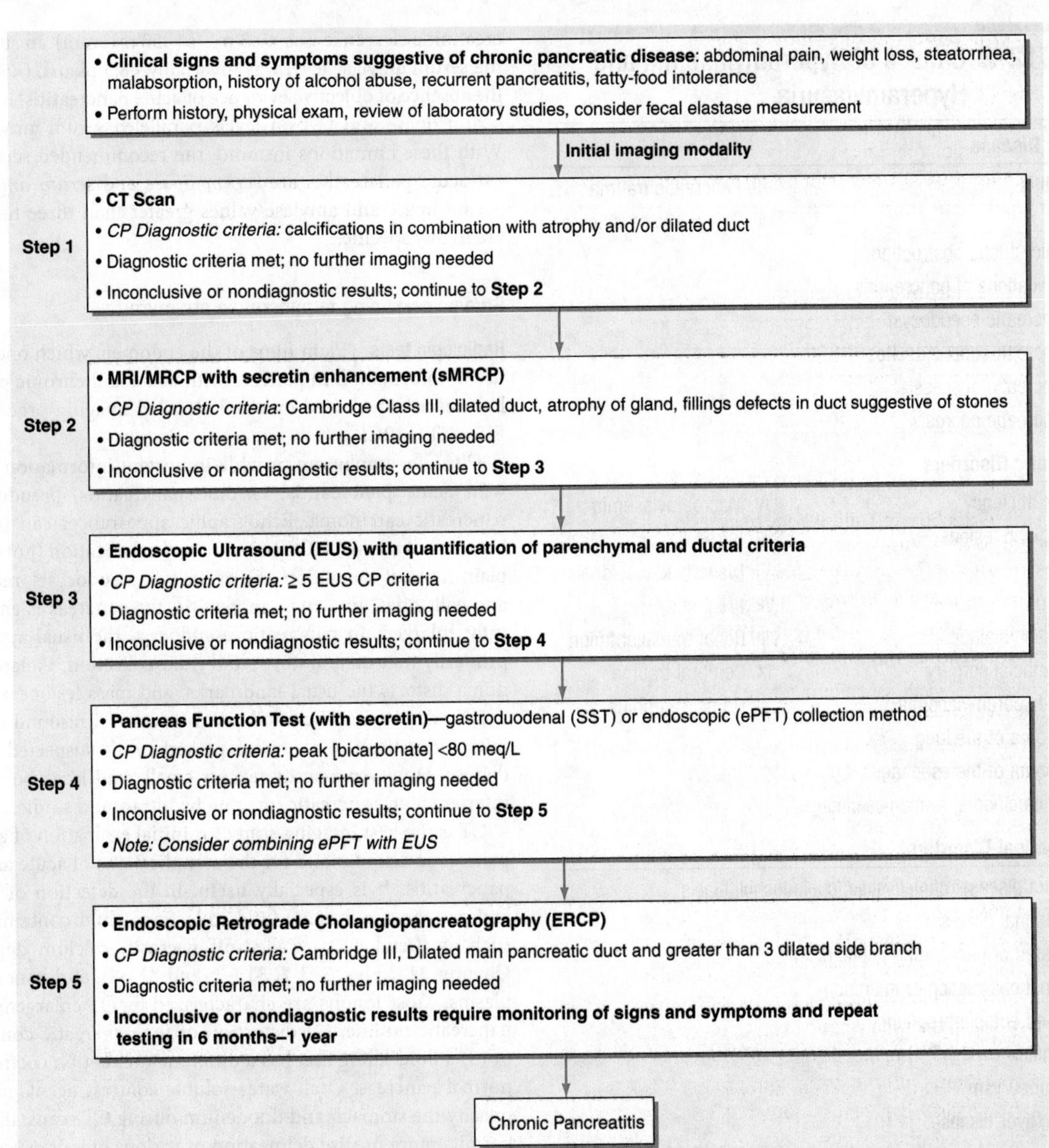
• Clinical signs and symptoms suggestive of chronic pancreatic disease: abdominal pain, weight loss, steatorrhea, malabsorption, history of alcohol abuse, recurrent pancreatitis, fatty-food intolerance
• Perform history, physical exam, review of laboratory studies, consider fecal elastase measurement
Initial imaging modality
Step 1
• CT Scan
• CP Diagnostic criteria: calcifications in combination with atrophy and/or dilated duct
• Diagnostic criteria met; no further imaging needed
• Inconclusive or nondiagnostic results; continue to Step 2
Step 2
• MRI/MRCP with secretin enhancement (sMRCP)
• CP Diagnostic criteria: Cambridge Class III, dilated duct, atrophy of gland, fillings defects in duct suggestive of stones
• Diagnostic criteria met; no further imaging needed
• Inconclusive or nondiagnostic results; continue to Step 3
Step 3
• Endoscopic Ultrasound (EUS) with quantification of parenchymal and ductal criteria
• CP Diagnostic criteria: ≥ 5 EUS CP criteria
• Diagnostic criteria met; no further imaging needed
• Inconclusive or nondiagnostic results; continue to Step 4
Step 4
• Pancreas Function Test (with secretin)—gastroduodenal (SST) or endoscopic (ePFT) collection method
• CP Diagnostic criteria: peak [bicarbonate] <80 meq/L
• Diagnostic criteria met; no further imaging needed
• Inconclusive or nondiagnostic results; continue to Step 5
• Note: Consider combining ePFT with EUS
Step 5
• Endoscopic Retrograde Cholangiopancreatography (ERCP)
• CP Diagnostic criteria: Cambridge III, Dilated main pancreatic duct and greater than 3 dilated side branch
• Diagnostic criteria met; no further imaging needed
• Inconclusive or nondiagnostic results require monitoring of signs and symptoms and repeat testing in 6 months–1 year
Chronic Pancreatitis

Figure 312-1 A step-wise diagnostic approach to the patient with suspected chronic pancreatitis (CP). Endoscopic ultrasonography (EUS) and magnetic resonance cholangiopancreatography (sMRCP/MRCP) are appropriate diagnostic alternatives to endoscopic retrograde cholangiopancreatography (ERCP).

ultrasonography (EUS)] have given normal or inconclusive results. In this regard, tests employing *direct* stimulation of the pancreas are the most sensitive.

Pancreatic enzymes in body fluids

The serum amylase and lipase levels are widely used as screening tests for acute pancreatitis in the patient with acute abdominal pain or back pain. Values greater than three times the upper limit of normal virtually clinch the diagnosis if gut perforation or infarction is excluded. In acute pancreatitis, the serum amylase and lipase are usually elevated within 24 hours of onset and remains so for 3–7 days. Levels usually return to normal within 7 days unless there is pancreatic ductal disruption, ductal obstruction, or pseudocyst formation. Approximately 85% of patients with acute pancreatitis have a threefold or greater elevated serum amylase and lipase levels. The values may be normal if (1) there is a delay (of 2–5 days) before blood samples are obtained, (2) the underlying disorder is chronic pancreatitis rather than acute pancreatitis, or (3) hypertriglyceridemia is present. Patients with hypertriglyceridemia and proven pancreatitis have been found to have spuriously low levels of amylase and perhaps lipase activity. In the absence of objective evidence of pancreatitis by abdominal ultrasound, CT scan, MRCP, or EUS, mild to moderate elevations of amylase, and/or lipase are not helpful in making a diagnosis of chronic pancreatitis.

The serum amylase can be elevated in other conditions (Table 312-2), in part because the enzyme is found in many organs. In addition to the pancreas and salivary glands, small quantities of amylase are found in the tissues of the fallopian tubes, lung, thyroid, and tonsils and can be produced by various tumors (carcinomas of the lung, esophagus, breast, and ovary). Urinary amylase measurements, including the amylase/creatinine clearance ratio, are no more sensitive or specific than blood amylase levels and are rarely employed. Isoamylase determinations do not accurately distinguish elevated blood amylase levels due to bona fide pancreatitis from

TABLE 312-2 Causes of Hyperamylasemia and Hyperamylasuria

Pancreatic Disease	
I. Pancreatitis	II. Pancreatic trauma
A. Acute	III. Pancreatic carcinoma
B. Chronic: ductal obstruction	
C. Complications of pancreatitis	
1. Pancreatic pseudocyst	
2. Pancreatogenous ascites	
3. Pancreatic abscess	
4. Pancreatic necrosis	
Nonpancreatic Disorders	
I. Renal insufficiency	IV. Macroamylasemia
II. Salivary gland lesions	V. Burns
A. Mumps	VI. Diabetic ketoacidosis
B. Calculus	VII. Pregnancy
C. Irradiation sialadenitis	VIII. Renal transplantation
D. Maxillofacial surgery	IX. Cerebral trauma
III. "Tumor" hyperamylasemia	X. Drugs: morphine
A. Carcinoma of the lung	
B. Carcinoma of the esophagus	
C. Breast carcinoma, ovarian carcinoma	
Other Abdominal Disorders	
I. Biliary tract disease: cholecystitis, choledocholithiasis	
II. Intraabdominal disease	
A. Perforated or penetrating peptic ulcer	
B. Intestinal obstruction or infarction	
C. Ruptured ectopic pregnancy	
D. Peritonitis	
E. Aortic aneurysm	
F. Chronic liver disease	
G. Postoperative hyperamylasemia	

elevated blood amylase levels due to a nonpancreatic source of amylase, especially when the blood amylase level is only moderately elevated.

Elevation of ascitic fluid amylase occurs in acute pancreatitis as well as in (1) pancreatogenous ascites due to disruption of the main pancreatic duct or a leaking pseudocyst and (2) other abdominal disorders that simulate pancreatitis (e.g., intestinal obstruction, intestinal infarction, or perforated peptic ulcer). Elevation of pleural fluid amylase can occur in acute pancreatitis, chronic pancreatitis, carcinoma of the lung, and esophageal perforation.

Lipase may now be the single best enzyme to measure for the diagnosis of acute pancreatitis. Improvements in substrates and technology offer clinicians improved options, especially when a turbidimetric assay is used. The newer lipase assays have colipase as a cofactor and are fully automated.

No single blood test is reliable for the diagnosis of acute pancreatitis in patients with renal failure. Determining whether a patient with renal failure and abdominal pain has pancreatitis remains a difficult clinical problem. One study found that serum amylase levels were elevated in patients with renal dysfunction only when creatinine clearance was <0.8 mL/s (<50 mL/min). In such patients, the serum amylase level was invariably <8.3 μkat/L (<500 IU/L) in the absence of objective evidence of acute pancreatitis. In that study, serum lipase and trypsin levels paralleled serum amylase values. With these limitations in mind, the recommended screening tests for acute pancreatitis are *serum lipase* and *serum amylase levels.* Serum lipase and amylase values greater than three times normal are highly specific.

Studies pertaining to pancreatic structure

Radiologic tests Plain films of the abdomen, which once provided useful information in patients with acute and chronic pancreatitis, have been superceded by other detailed imaging procedures (US, EUS, CT, MRCP).

Ultrasonography can provide important information in patients with acute pancreatitis, chronic pancreatitis, pseudocysts, and pancreatic carcinoma. Echographic appearances can indicate the presence of edema, inflammation, and calcification (not obvious on plain films of the abdomen), as well as pseudocysts, mass lesions, and gallstones. In acute pancreatitis, the pancreas is characteristically enlarged. In pancreatic pseudocyst, the usual appearance is primarily that of smooth, round fluid collection. Pancreatic carcinoma distorts the usual landmarks, and mass lesions >3.0 cm are usually detected as localized, solid lesions. Ultrasound is often the initial investigation for most patients with suspected pancreatic disease. However, obesity, excess small- and large-bowel gas can interfere with pancreatic imaging by ultrasound studies.

CT is the best imaging study for initial evaluation of a suspected pancreatic disorder and for the complications of acute and chronic pancreatitis. It is especially useful in the detection of pancreatic and peripancreatic acute fluid collections, fluid-containing lesions such as pseudocysts, walled-off necrosis, calcium deposits (see Chapter 313, Figs. 313-1, 313-2, and 313-4), and pancreatic neoplasms. Most lesions are characterized by (1) enlargement of the pancreatic outline, (2) distortion of the pancreatic contour, and/or (3) a fluid filling that has a different attenuation coefficient than normal pancreas. Oral, water-soluble contrast agents are used to opacify the stomach and duodenum during CT scans; this strategy permits more precise delineation of various organs as well as mass lesions. Dynamic CT (using rapid IV administration of contrast) is useful in estimating the extent of pancreatic necrosis and in predicting morbidity and mortality. Spiral (helical) CT provides clear images much more rapidly and essentially negates artifact caused by patient movement.

EUS produces high-resolution images of the pancreatic parenchyma and pancreatic duct with a transducer fixed to an endoscope that can be directed onto the surface of the pancreas through the stomach or duodenum. EUS and MRCP have largely replaced ERCP for diagnostic purposes in many centers. EUS allows one to obtain information about the pancreatic duct as well as the parenchyma and has few procedure-related complications associated with it, in contrast to the 5–20% of post-ERCP pancreatitis observed. EUS is also helpful in detecting common bile duct stones. Pancreatic masses can be biopsied via EUS and one can deliver nerve-blocking agents through EUS fine-needle injection. Criteria for abnormalities on EUS in severe chronic pancreatic disease have been developed. Currently, chronic pancreatitis is considered diagnosed by EUS if five or more criteria listed in Table 312-3 are present. Recent studies comparing EUS and ERCP to the secretin test in patients with unexplained abdominal pain suspected of having chronic pancreatitis show equivalent diagnostic accuracy in detecting early changes of chronic pancreatitis. The exact role of EUS versus CT, ERCP, or function testing in the early diagnosis of chronic pancreatitis has yet to be clearly defined.

TABLE 312-3 Endoscopic Ultrasonographic Criteria for Chronic Pancreatitis

Ductal	Parenchymal
Stones	Echogenic strands
Echogenic ductal walls	Echogenic foci
Irregular ductal walls	Calcifications
Stricture	Lobular contour
Visible side branches	Cyst
Ductular dilatation	

MRCP/ MRI is now being used to view the bile ducts, pancreatic duct, and the pancreas parenchyma. Non breath–holding and three-dimensional turbo spin-echo techniques are being used to produce superb MRCP images. The main pancreatic duct and common bile duct can be seen well, but there is still a question as to whether changes can be detected consistently in the secondary ducts. The secondary ducts are not visualized in a normal pancreas. MRCP may be particularly useful to evaluate the pancreatic duct in high-risk patients such as the elderly because this is a noninvasive procedure. Secretin enhanced MRCP is currently under investigation but is emerging as a method to better evaluate ductal changes.

Both EUS and MRCP have largely replaced diagnostic ERCP in most patients. As these techniques become more refined, they may well be the diagnostic tests of choice to evaluate the pancreatic duct. ERCP is still needed for treatment of bile duct and pancreatic duct lesions. ERCP is primarily of therapeutic value after CT, EUS, or MRCP have detected abnormalities requiring invasive endoscopic treatment. ERCP can also be helpful at clarification of equivocal findings discovered with other imaging techniques (see Chap. 313, Figs. 313-1*C*, 313-3*D*, and 313-4*B*). Pancreatic carcinoma is characterized by stenosis or obstruction of either the pancreatic duct or the common bile duct; both ductal systems are often abnormal. In chronic pancreatitis, ERCP abnormalities include (1) luminal narrowing; (2) irregularities in the ductal system with stenosis, dilation, sacculation, and ectasia; and (3) blockage of the pancreatic duct by calcium deposits. The presence of ductal stenosis and irregularity can make it difficult to distinguish chronic pancreatitis from carcinoma. It is important to be aware that ERCP changes interpreted as indicating chronic pancreatitis actually may be due to the effects of aging on the pancreatic duct or to the fact that the procedure was performed within several weeks of an attack of acute pancreatitis. Although aging may cause impressive ductal alterations, it does not affect the results of pancreatic function tests (i.e., the secretin test). Elevated serum amylase levels after ERCP have been reported in 25–75% of patients, and clinical pancreatitis in 5–20% of patients. There are no satisfactory means to pharmacologically prevent ERCP-induced pancreatitis, despite many agents such as octreotide and nitroglycerin having been suggested and evaluated. The best way to prevent ERCP-induced pancreatitis is to not perform this procedure for diagnostic purposes in high-risk patients, especially in women with acute relapsing pancreatitis in whom there is no evidence of biliary obstruction and patients with unexplained abdominal pain but no other abnormalities. If no lesion is found in the biliary and/or pancreatic ducts in a patient with repeated attacks of acute pancreatitis, manometric studies of the sphincter of Oddi may be indicated. Such studies, however, do increase the risk of post-ERCP/manometry acute pancreatitis. Such pancreatitis appears to be more common in patients with a nondilated pancreatic duct.

Pancreatic biopsy with radiologic guidance Percutaneous aspiration biopsy or a trucut biopsy of a pancreatic mass often distinguishes a pancreatic inflammatory mass from a pancreatic neoplasm.

TESTS OF EXOCRINE PANCREATIC FUNCTION

Pancreatic function tests (Table 312-1) can be divided into the following:

1. *Direct stimulation of the pancreas* by IV infusion of secretin or secretin plus cholecystokinin (CCK) followed by collection and measurement of duodenal contents
2. Study of *intraluminal digestion products*, such as undigested meat fibers, stool fat, and fecal nitrogen
3. *Measurement of fecal pancreatic enzymes* such as elastase

The secretin test, used to detect diffuse pancreatic disease, is based on the physiologic principle that the pancreatic secretory response is directly related to the functional mass of pancreatic tissue. In the standard assay, secretin is given IV in a dose of 0.2 μg/kg of synthetic human secretin as a bolus. Normal values for the standard secretin test are (1) volume output >2 mL/kg per hour, (2) bicarbonate (HCO_3^-) concentration >80 mmol/L, and (3) HCO_3^- output >10 mmol/L in 1 hour. The most reproducible measurement, giving the highest level of discrimination between normal subjects and patients with chronic pancreatic exocrine insufficiency, appears to be the maximal bicarbonate concentration.

There may be a dissociation between the results of the secretin test and other tests of absorptive function. For example, patients with chronic pancreatitis often have abnormally low outputs of HCO_3^- after secretin but have normal fecal fat excretion. Thus the secretin test measures the secretory capacity of ductular epithelium, while fecal fat excretion indirectly reflects intraluminal lipolytic activity. Steatorrhea does not occur until intraluminal levels of lipase are markedly reduced, underscoring the fact that only small amounts of enzymes are necessary for intraluminal digestive activities. It must be noted that, an abnormal secretin test result suggests only that chronic pancreatic damage is present.

Measurement of *intraluminal digestion products* (i.e., undigested muscle fibers, stool fat, and fecal nitrogen) is discussed in Chap. 294. The amount of human elastase in stool reflects the pancreatic output of this proteolytic enzyme. Decreased elastase activity in stool is an excellent test to detect severe pancreatic exocrine insufficiency in patients with chronic pancreatitis and cystic fibrosis provided that the stool specimen is solid.

Tests useful in the diagnosis of exocrine pancreatic insufficiency and the differential diagnosis of malabsorption are also discussed in Chaps. 294 and 313.

PART 14 Disorders of the Gastrointestinal System

CHAPTER 313
Acute and Chronic Pancreatitis

Norton J. Greenberger
Darwin L. Conwell
Bechien U. Wu
Peter A. Banks

BIOCHEMISTRY AND PHYSIOLOGY OF PANCREATIC EXOCRINE SECRETION

GENERAL CONSIDERATIONS

The pancreas secretes 1500–3000 mL of isosmotic alkaline (pH >8) fluid per day containing about 20 enzymes. The pancreatic secretions provide the enzymes needed to effect the major digestive activity of the gastrointestinal tract and provide an optimal pH for the function of these enzymes.

REGULATION OF PANCREATIC SECRETION

The exocrine pancreas is influenced by intimately interacting hormonal and neural systems. *Gastric acid* is the stimulus for the release of secretin from the duodenum, which stimulates the secretion of water and electrolytes from pancreatic ductal cells. Release of cholecystokinin (CCK) from the duodenum and proximal jejunum is largely triggered by long-chain fatty acids, certain essential amino acids (tryptophan, phenylalanine, valine, methionine), and gastric acid itself. CCK evokes an enzyme-rich secretion from acinar cells in the pancreas. The *parasympathetic nervous system* (via the vagus nerve) exerts significant control over pancreatic secretion. Secretion evoked by secretin and CCK depends on permissive roles of vagal afferent and efferent pathways. This is particularly true for enzyme secretion, whereas water and bicarbonate secretions are heavily dependent on the hormonal effects of secretin and to a lesser extent CCK. Also, vagal stimulation effects the release of vasoactive intestinal peptide (VIP), a secretin agonist.

Pancreatic exocrine secretion is influenced by inhibitory neuropeptides such as somatostatin, pancreatic polypeptide, peptide YY, neuropeptide Y, enkephalin, pancreastatin, calcitonin gene–related peptides, glucagon, and galanin. Although pancreatic polypeptide and peptide YY may act primarily on nerves outside the pancreas, somatostatin acts at multiple sites. Nitric oxide (NO) is also an important neurotransmitter. The mechanism of action of these various factors has not been fully defined.

WATER AND ELECTROLYTE SECRETION

Bicarbonate is the ion of primary physiologic importance within pancreatic secretion. The ductal cells secrete bicarbonate predominantly derived from plasma (93%) more than from intracellular metabolism (7%). Bicarbonate enters through the sodium bicarbonate cotransporter with depolarization caused by chloride efflux through the cystic fibrosis transmembrane conductance regulator (CFTR). Secretin and VIP, both of which increase intracellular cyclic AMP, act on the ductal cells opening the CFTR in promoting secretion. CCK, acting as a neuromodulator, markedly potentiates the stimulatory effects of secretin. Acetylcholine also plays an important role in ductal cell secretion. Bicarbonate helps neutralize gastric acid and creates the appropriate pH for the activity of pancreatic enzymes and bile salts.

ENZYME SECRETION

The acinar cell is highly compartmentalized and is concerned with the secretion of pancreatic enzymes. Proteins synthesized by the rough endoplasmic reticulum are processed in the Golgi and then targeted to the appropriate site, whether that be zymogen granules, lysosomes, or other cell compartments. The pancreas secretes amylolytic, lipolytic, and proteolytic enzymes. *Amylolytic enzymes* such as amylase, hydrolyze starch to oligosaccharides and to the disaccharide maltose. The *lipolytic enzymes* include lipase, phospholipase A_2, and cholesterol esterase. Bile salts inhibit lipase in isolation, but colipase, another constituent of pancreatic secretion, binds to lipase and prevents this inhibition. Bile salts activate phospholipase A and cholesterol esterase. *Proteolytic enzymes* include endopeptidases (trypsin, chymotrypsin), which act on internal peptide bonds of proteins and polypeptides; exopeptidases (carboxypeptidases, aminopeptidases), which act on the free carboxyl- and amino-terminal ends of peptides, respectively; and elastase. The proteolytic enzymes are secreted as inactive precursors and packaged as zymogens. Ribonucleases (deoxyribonucleases, ribonuclease) are also secreted. *Enterokinase*, an enzyme found in the duodenal mucosa, cleaves the lysine-isoleucine bond of trypsinogen to form trypsin. Trypsin then activates the other proteolytic zymogens and phospholipase A_2 in a cascade phenomenon. All pancreatic enzymes have pH optima in the alkaline range. The nervous system initiates pancreatic enzyme secretion. The neurologic stimulation is cholinergic, involving extrinsic innervation by the vagus nerve and subsequent innervation by intrapancreatic cholinergic nerves. The stimulatory neurotransmitters are acetylcholine and gastrin-releasing peptides. These neurotransmitters activate calcium-dependent second messenger systems, resulting in the release of zymogen granules. VIP is present in intrapancreatic nerves and potentiates the effect of acetylcholine. In contrast to other species, there are no CCK receptors on acinar cells in humans. CCK in physiologic concentrations stimulates pancreatic secretion by stimulating afferent vagal and intrapancreatic nerves.

AUTOPROTECTION OF THE PANCREAS

Autodigestion of the pancreas is prevented by the packaging of pancreatic proteases in precursor form and by the synthesis of protease inhibitor [i.e., pancreatic secretory trypsin inhibitor (PSTI) or SPINK1], which can bind and inactivate about 20% of trypsin activity. Mesotrypsin, chymotrypsin c, and enzyme y can also lyse and inactivate trypsin. These protease inhibitors are found in the acinar cell, the pancreatic secretions, and the α_1- and α_2-globulin fractions of plasma. In addition, low calcium concentration within the cytosol of acinar cells in the normal pancreas promotes the destruction of spontaneously activated trypsin. Loss of any of these protective mechanisms leads to zymogen activation, autodigestion, and acute pancreatitis.

EXOCRINE-ENDOCRINE RELATIONSHIPS

Insulin appears to be needed locally for secretin and CCK to promote exocrine secretion; thus, it acts in a permissive role for these two hormones.

ENTEROPANCREATIC AXIS AND FEEDBACK INHIBITION

Pancreatic enzyme secretion is controlled, at least in part, by a negative feedback mechanism induced by the presence of active serine proteases in the duodenum. To illustrate, perfusion of the duodenal lumen with phenylalanine causes a prompt result in increased plasma CCK levels as well as increased secretion of chymotrypsin and other pancreatic enzymes. However, simultaneous perfusion with trypsin blunts both responses. Conversely, perfusion of the duodenal lumen with protease inhibitors actually leads to enzyme hypersecretion. The available evidence supports the concept that the duodenum contains a peptide called *CCK-releasing factor* (CCK-RF) that is involved in stimulating CCK release. It appears that serine proteases inhibit pancreatic secretion by inactivating a CCK-releasing peptide in the lumen of the small intestine. Thus, the integrative result of both bicarbonate and enzyme secretion depends on a feedback process for both bicarbonate and pancreatic enzymes. Acidification of the duodenum releases secretin, which stimulates vagal and other neural pathways to activate pancreatic duct cells, which secrete bicarbonate. This bicarbonate then neutralizes the duodenal acid, and the feedback loop is completed. Dietary proteins bind proteases, thereby leading to an increase in free CCK-RF. CCK is then released into the blood in physiologic concentrations, acting primarily through the neural pathways (vagal-vagal). This leads to acetylcholine-mediated pancreatic enzyme secretion. Proteases continue to be secreted from the pancreas until the protein within the duodenum is digested. At this point, pancreatic protease secretion is reduced to basic levels, thus completing this step in the feedback process.

ACUTE PANCREATITIS

GENERAL CONSIDERATIONS

Pancreatic inflammatory disease may be classified as (1) acute pancreatitis or (2) chronic pancreatitis. The pathologic spectrum of acute pancreatitis varies from *interstitial pancreatitis*, which is usually a mild and self-limited disorder, to *necrotizing pancreatitis*, in which the extent of pancreatic necrosis may correlate with the severity of the attack and its systemic manifestations.

The incidence of pancreatitis varies in different countries and depends on cause [e.g., alcohol, gallstones, metabolic factors, and drugs (Table 313-1)]. The estimated incidence in the United States is increasing and is now estimated to be 70 hospitalizations/100,000 persons annually, thus resulting in >200,000 new cases of acute pancreatitis per year.

ETIOLOGY AND PATHOGENESIS

There are many causes of acute pancreatitis (Table 313-1), but the mechanisms by which these conditions trigger pancreatic inflammation have not been fully elucidated. Gallstones continue to be the leading cause of acute pancreatitis in most series (30–60%). The risk of acute pancreatitis in patients with at least one gallstone <5 mm in diameter is fourfold greater than that in patients with larger stones. Alcohol is the second most common cause, responsible for 15–30% of cases in the United States. The incidence of pancreatitis in alcoholics is surprisingly low (5/100,000), indicating that in addition to the amount of alcohol ingested unknown factors affect a person's susceptibility to pancreatic injury. The mechanism of injury is incompletely understood. Acute pancreatitis occurs in 5–20% of patients following endoscopic retrograde cholangiopancreatography (ERCP). Despite extensive research into the medical and endoscopic prevention of post-ERCP pancreatitis, there has been little decline in incidence. Use of prophylactic pancreatic duct stent after retrograde pancreatogram or pancreatic sphincterotomy has shown promise in reducing pancreatitis but requires further prospective evaluation. Risk factors for post-ERCP pancreatitis include minor papilla sphincterotomy, sphincter of Oddi dysfunction, prior history of post-ERCP pancreatitis, age <60 years, >2 contrast injections into the pancreatic duct, and endoscopic trainee involvement.

TABLE 313-1 Causes of Acute Pancreatitis

Common Causes
Gallstones (including microlithiasis)
Alcohol (acute and chronic alcoholism)
Hypertriglyceridemia
Endoscopic retrograde cholangiopancreatography (ERCP), especially after biliary manometry
Trauma (especially blunt abdominal trauma)
Postoperative (abdominal and nonabdominal operations)
Drugs (azathioprine, 6-mercaptopurine, sulfonamides, estrogens, tetracycline, valproic acid, anti-HIV medications)
Sphincter of Oddi dysfunction
Uncommon Causes
Vascular causes and vasculitis (ischemic-hypoperfusion states after cardiac surgery)
Connective tissue disorders and thrombotic thrombocytopenic purpura (TTP)
Cancer of the pancreas
Hypercalcemia
Periampullary diverticulum
Pancreas divisum
Hereditary pancreatitis
Cystic fibrosis
Renal failure
Rare Causes
Infections (mumps, coxsackievirus, cytomegalovirus, echovirus, parasites)
Autoimmune (e.g., Sjögren's syndrome)
Causes to Consider in Patients with Recurrent Bouts of Acute Pancreatitis without an Obvious Etiology
Occult disease of the biliary tree or pancreatic ducts, especially microlithiasis, sludge
Drugs
Hypertriglyceridemia
Pancreas divisum
Pancreatic cancer
Sphincter of Oddi dysfunction
Cystic fibrosis
Idiopathic

Hypertriglyceridemia is the cause of acute pancreatitis in 1.3–3.8% of cases; serum triglyceride levels are usually >11.3 mmol/L (>1000 mg/dL). Most patients with hypertriglyceridemia, when subsequently examined, show evidence of an underlying derangement in lipid metabolism, probably unrelated to pancreatitis. Such patients are prone to recurrent episodes of pancreatitis. Any factor (e.g., drugs or alcohol) that causes an abrupt increase in serum triglycerides to levels >11 mmol/L (1000 mg/dL) can precipitate a bout of acute pancreatitis. Finally, patients with a deficiency of apolipoprotein CII have an increased incidence of pancreatitis; apolipoprotein CII activates lipoprotein lipase, which is important in clearing chylomicrons from the bloodstream. Patients with diabetes mellitus who have developed ketoacidosis and patients who are on certain medications such as oral contraceptives may also develop high triglyceride levels. Approximately 2–5% of cases of acute pancreatitis are drug related. Drugs cause pancreatitis either by a hypersensitivity reaction or by the generation of a toxic metabolite, although in some cases it is not clear which of these mechanisms is operative (Table 313-1).

Autodigestion is a currently accepted pathogenic theory; according to it, pancreatitis results when proteolytic enzymes (e.g., trypsinogen, chymotrypsinogen, proelastase, and lipolytic enzymes such as phospholipase A_2) are activated in the pancreas rather than in the intestinal lumen. A number of factors (e.g., endotoxins, exotoxins, viral infections, ischemia, anoxia, lysosomal calcium, and direct trauma) are believed to facilitate activation of trypsin. Activated proteolytic enzymes, especially trypsin, not only digest pancreatic and peripancreatic tissues but also can activate other enzymes, such as elastase and phospholipase A_2. Spontaneous activation of trypsin also can occur.

ACTIVATION OF PANCREATIC ENZYMES IN THE PATHOGENESIS OF ACUTE PANCREATITIS

Several recent studies have suggested that pancreatitis is a disease that evolves in three phases. The initial phase is characterized by intrapancreatic digestive enzyme activation and acinar cell injury. Trypsin activation appears to be mediated by lysosomal hydrolases such as cathepsin B that become colocalized with digestive enzymes in intracellular organelles; it is currently believed that acinar cell injury is the consequence of trypsin activation. The second phase of pancreatitis involves the activation, chemoattraction, and sequestration of leukocytes and macrophages in the pancreas, resulting in an enhanced intrapancreatic inflammatory reaction. Neutrophil depletion induced by prior administration of an antineutrophil serum has been shown to reduce the severity of experimentally induced pancreatitis. There is also evidence to support the concept that neutrophil sequestration can activate trypsinogen. Thus, intrapancreatic acinar cell activation of trypsinogen could be a two-step process (i.e., an early neutrophil-independent and a later neutrophil-dependent phase). The third phase of pancreatitis is due to the effects of activated proteolytic enzymes and cytokines, released by the inflamed pancreas, on distant organs. Activated proteolytic enzymes, especially trypsin, not only digest pancreatic and peripancreatic tissues but also activate other enzymes such as elastase and phospholipase A_2. The active enzymes and cytokines then digest cellular membranes and cause proteolysis, edema, interstitial hemorrhage, vascular damage, coagulation necrosis, fat necrosis, and parenchymal cell necrosis. Cellular injury and death result in the liberation of bradykinin peptides, vasoactive substances, and histamine that can produce vasodilation, increased vascular permeability, and edema with profound effects on many organs, most notably the lung. The systemic inflammatory response syndrome (SIRS) and acute respiratory distress syndrome (ARDS) as well as multiorgan failure may occur as a result of this cascade of local as well as distant effects.

There appear to be a number of genetic factors that can increase the susceptibility and/or modify the severity of pancreatic injury in acute pancreatitis. Four susceptibility genes have been identified: (1) cationic trypsinogen mutations (PRSS1m, R122Hm, and N291), (2) pancreatic secretory trypsin inhibitor (SPINK1), (3) CFTR, and (4) monocyte chemotactic protein (MCP-1). Experimental and clinical data indicate that MCP-1 may be an important inflammatory mediator in the early pathologic process of acute pancreatitis, a determinant of the severity of the inflammatory response, and a promoter of organ failure.

APPROACH TO THE PATIENT Abdominal Pain

Abdominal pain is the major symptom of acute pancreatitis. Pain may vary from a mild and tolerable discomfort and more commonly to severe, constant, and incapacitating distress. Characteristically, the pain, which is steady and boring in character, is located in the epigastrium and periumbilical region and often radiates to the back as well as to the chest, flanks, and lower abdomen. The pain is frequently more intense when the patient is supine, and patients may obtain some relief by sitting with the trunk flexed and knees drawn up. Nausea, vomiting, and abdominal distention due to gastric and intestinal hypomotility and chemical peritonitis are also frequent complaints.

Physical examination frequently reveals a distressed and anxious patient. Low-grade fever, tachycardia, and hypotension are fairly common. Shock is not unusual and may result from (1) hypovolemia secondary to exudation of blood and plasma proteins into the retroperitoneal space and a "retroperitoneal burn" due to activated proteolytic enzymes; (2) increased formation and release of kinin peptides, which cause vasodilation and increased vascular permeability; and (3) systemic effects of proteolytic and lipolytic enzymes released into the circulation. Jaundice occurs infrequently; when present, it usually is due to edema of the head of the pancreas with compression of the intrapancreatic portion of the common bile duct. Erythematous skin nodules due to subcutaneous fat necrosis may occur. In 10–20% of patients, there are pulmonary findings, including basilar rales, atelectasis, and pleural effusion, the latter most frequently left sided. Abdominal tenderness and muscle rigidity are present to a variable degree, but, compared with the intense pain, these signs may be unimpressive. Bowel sounds are usually diminished or absent. An enlarged pancreas with walled off necrosis or a pseudocyst may be palpable in the upper abdomen later in the disease course (i.e., four to six weeks). A faint blue discoloration around the umbilicus (Cullen's sign) may occur as the result of hemoperitoneum, and a blue-red-purple or green-brown discoloration of the flanks (Turner's sign) reflects tissue catabolism of hemoglobin. The latter two findings, which are uncommon, indicate the presence of a severe necrotizing pancreatitis.

LABORATORY DATA

The diagnosis of acute pancreatitis is usually established by the detection of an increased level of serum amylase and lipase. Values threefold or more above normal virtually clinch the diagnosis if gut perforation, ischemia, and infarction are excluded. However, there appears to be no definite correlation between the severity of pancreatitis and the degree of serum lipase and amylase elevations. After three to seven days, even with continuing evidence of pancreatitis, total serum amylase values tend to return toward normal. However, pancreatic isoamylase and lipase levels may remain elevated for 7 to 14 days. It will be recalled that amylase elevations in serum and urine occur in many conditions other than pancreatitis (see Chap. 312, Table 312-2). Importantly, patients with *acidemia* (arterial pH ≤7.32) may have spurious elevations in serum amylase. In one study, 12 of 33 patients with acidemia had elevated serum amylase, but only 1 had an elevated lipase value; in 9, salivary-type amylase was the predominant serum isoamylase. This finding explains why patients with diabetic ketoacidosis may have marked elevations in serum amylase without any other evidence of acute pancreatitis. Serum lipase activity increases in parallel with amylase activity. A threefold elevated serum lipase value is usually diagnostic of acute pancreatitis; these tests are especially helpful in patients with nonpancreatic causes of hyperamylasemia (see Chap. 312, Table 312-2).

Leukocytosis (15,000–20,000 leukocytes per μL) occurs frequently. Patients with more severe disease may show hemoconcentration with hematocrit values >44% and/or azotemia with a blood urea nitrogen (BUN) level >22 mg/dL because of loss of plasma into the retroperitoneal space and peritoneal cavity.

TABLE 313-2 Severe Acute Pancreatitis

Risk Factors for Severity
• Age >60 years
• Obesity, BMI >30
• Comorbid disease
Markers of Severity within 24 Hours
• SIRS [temperature >38° or <36°C (>100.4° or 96.8°F), Pulse >90, Tachypnea >24, ↑ WBC >12,000]
• Hemoconcentration (Hct >44%)
• BISAP
• (B) Blood urea nitrogen (BUN) >22 mg%
• (I) Impaired mental status
• (S) SIRS: 2/4 present
• (A) Age >60 years
• (P) Pleural effusion
• Organ Failure
• Cardiovascular: systolic BP <90 mmHg, heartrate >130
• Pulmonary: Pa_{O_2} <60 mmHg
• Renal serum creatinine >2.0 mg%
Markers of Severity during Hospitalization
• Persistent organ failure
• Pancreatic necrosis
• Hospital-acquired infection

Abbreviation: BISAP, bedside index of severity in acute pancreatitis.

TABLE 313-3 CT Findings and Grading of Acute Pancreatitis [CT Severity Index (CTSI)]

Grade	Findings	Score
A	Normal pancreas: normal size, sharply defined, smooth contour, homogeneous enhancement, retroperitoneal peripancreatic fat without enhancement	0
B	Focal or diffuse enlargement of the pancreas, contour may show irregularity, enhancement may be inhomogeneous but there is no peri-pancreatic inflammation	1
C	Peripancreatic inflammation with intrinsic pancreatic abnormalities	2
D	Intrapancreatic or extrapancreatic fluid collections	3
E	Two or more large collections or gas in the pancreas or retroperitoneum	4
Necrosis score based on contrast-enhanced CT		
Necrosis, %		Score
0		0
<33		2
33–50		4
≥50		6

Note: CT severity index equals unenhanced CT score plus necrosis score: maximum = 10; ≥6 = severe disease.

Source: Modified from EJ Balthazar et al: Radiology 1990;174:331.

Hemoconcentration may be the harbinger of more severe disease (i.e., pancreatic necrosis), while azotemia is a significant risk factor for mortality. *Hyperglycemia* is common and is due to multiple factors, including decreased insulin release, increased glucagon release, and an increased output of adrenal glucocorticoids and catecholamines. *Hypocalcemia* occurs in ~25% of patients, and its pathogenesis is incompletely understood. Although earlier studies suggested that the response of the parathyroid gland to a decrease in serum calcium is impaired, subsequent observations have failed to confirm this phenomenon. Intraperitoneal saponification of calcium by fatty acids in areas of fat necrosis occurs occasionally, with large amounts (up to 6.0 g) dissolved or suspended in ascitic fluid. Such "soap formation" may also be significant in patients with pancreatitis, mild hypocalcemia, and little or no obvious ascites. *Hyperbilirubinemia* [serum bilirubin >68 μmol/L (>4.0 mg/dL)] occurs in ~10% of patients. However, jaundice is transient, and serum bilirubin levels return to normal in four to seven days. Serum alkaline phosphatase and aspartate aminotransferase levels are also transiently elevated and they parallel serum bilirubin values and may point to gallbladder-related disease. Markedly elevated serum lactic dehydrogenase levels [>8.5 μmol/L (>500 U/dL)] suggest a poor prognosis. *Hypertriglyceridemia* occurs in 5–10% of patients, and serum amylase levels in these individuals are often spuriously normal (Chap. 312). Approximately 5–10% of patients have *hypoxemia* (arterial P_{O_2} ≤ 60 mmHg), which may herald the onset of ARDS. Finally, the electrocardiogram is occasionally abnormal in acute pancreatitis with ST-segment and T-wave abnormalities simulating myocardial ischemia.

A CT scan can confirm the clinical impression of acute pancreatitis even with less than a threefold increase in serum amylase and lipase levels. Importantly, CT can be helpful in indicating the severity of acute pancreatitis and the risk of morbidity and mortality and in evaluating the complications of acute pancreatitis (Table 313-3). However, a CT scan obtained within the first several days of symptom onset may underestimate the extent of tissue injury. What may appear to be intestinal pancreatitis on initial CT scan may evolve to pancreatic necrosis on repeat CT scan three to five days later (Fig. 313-1). Sonography is useful in acute pancreatitis to evaluate the gallbladder if gallstone disease is suspected. Radiologic studies useful in the diagnosis of acute pancreatitis are discussed in Chap. 312, and listed in Table 312-1, and depicted in Figs. 313-1 to 313-3.

DIAGNOSIS

Any severe acute pain in the abdomen or back should suggest the possibility acute pancreatitis. The diagnosis is usually entertained when a patient with a possible predisposition to pancreatitis presents with severe and constant abdominal pain, frequently associated with nausea, emesis, fever, tachycardia, and abnormal findings on abdominal examination. Laboratory studies may reveal leukocytosis, hypocalcemia, and hyperglycemia. The diagnosis of acute pancreatitis requires two of the following: typical abdominal pain, threefold or greater elevation in serum amylase and/or lipase level, and/or confirmatory findings on cross-sectional abdominal imaging. Although not required for diagnosis, markers of severity include hemoconcentration (hematocrit >44%), azotemia (BUN >22 mg/dL), and signs of organ failure (Table 313-2).

The *differential diagnosis* should include the following disorders: (1) perforated viscus, especially peptic ulcer; (2) acute cholecystitis and biliary colic; (3) acute intestinal obstruction; (4) mesenteric vascular occlusion; (5) renal colic; (6) myocardial infarction; (7) dissecting aortic aneurysm; (8) connective tissue disorders with vasculitis; (9) pneumonia; and (10) diabetic ketoacidosis.

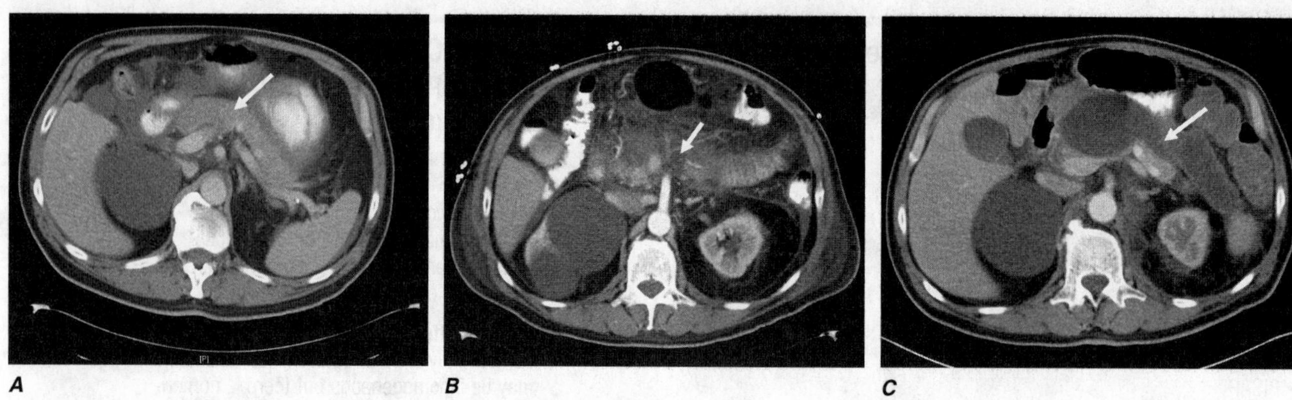

Figure 313-1 Acute pancreatitis: CT evolution. *A.* Contrast-enhanced CT scan of the abdomen performed on admission for a patient with clinical and biochemical parameters suggestive of acute pancreatitis. Note the abnormal enhancement of the pancreatic parenchyma (arrow) suggestive of interstitial pancreatitis. *B.* Contrast-enhanced CT scan of the abdomen performed on the same patient six days later for persistent fever and systemic inflammatory response syndrome. The pancreas now demonstrates significant areas of nonenhancement consistent with development of necrosis, particularly in the body and neck region (arrow). Note that an early CT scan obtained within the first 48 hours of hospitalization may underestimate or miss necrosis. *C.* Contrast-enhanced CT scan of the abdomen performed on the same patient two months after the initial episode of acute pancreatitis. CT now demonstrates evidence of a fluid collection consistent with walled-off pancreatic necrosis (arrow). *(Courtesy of Dr. KJ Mortele, Brigham and Women's Hospital; with permission.)*

A penetrating duodenal ulcer can usually be identified by imaging studies or endoscopy. A perforated duodenal ulcer is readily diagnosed by the presence of free intraperitoneal air on abdominal imaging. It may be difficult to differentiate acute cholecystitis from acute pancreatitis, since an elevated serum amylase may be found in both disorders. Pain of biliary tract origin is more right sided or epigastric than periumbilical and can be more severe; ileus is usually absent. Sonography is helpful in establishing the diagnosis of cholelithiasis and cholecystitis. Intestinal obstruction due to mechanical factors can be differentiated from pancreatitis by the

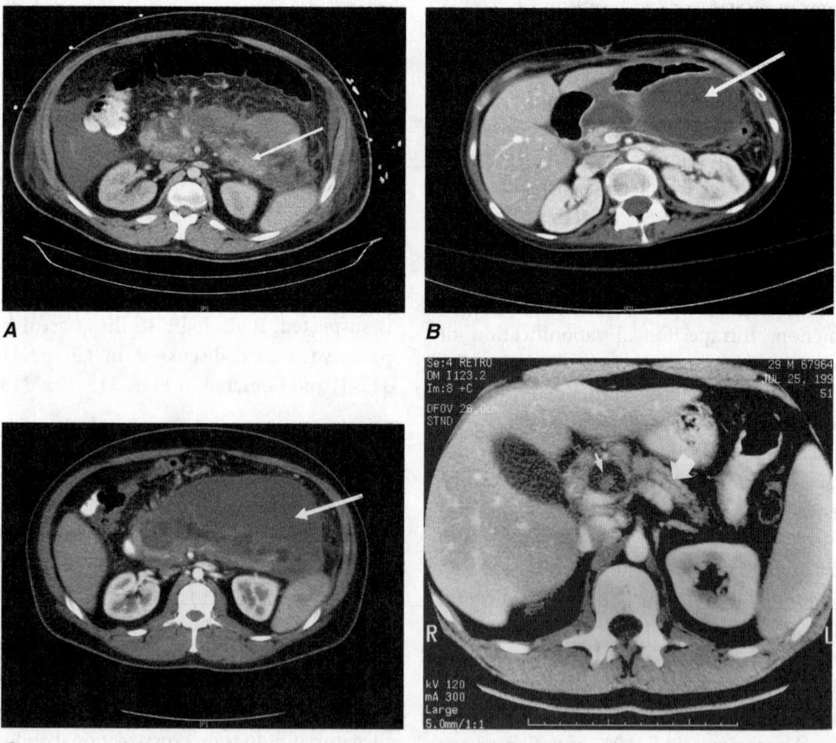

Figure 313-2 *A.* Acute necrotizing pancreatitis: CT scan. Contrast-enhanced CT scan showing acute pancreatitis with necrosis. Arrow shows partially enhancing body/tail of pancreas surrounded by fluid with decreased enhancement in the neck/body of the pancreas. *B.* Acute fluid collection: CT scan. Contrast-enhanced CT scan showing fluid collection in the retroperitoneum (arrow) compressing the air-filled stomach arising from the pancreas in a patient with asparaginase-induced acute necrotizing pancreatitis. *C.* Walled-off pancreatic necrosis: CT scan. CT scan showing marked walled-off necrosis of the pancreas and peripancreatic area (arrow) in a patient with necrotizing pancreatitis. Addendum: In past years, both of these CT findings (Figs. 313-2B and 313-2C) would have been misinterpreted as pseudocysts. *D.* Spiral CT showing a pseudocyst (small arrow) with a pseudoaneurysm (light area in pseudocyst). Note the demonstration of the main pancreatic duct (big arrow), even though this duct is minimally dilated by ERCP. *(A, B, C, courtesy of Dr. KJ Mortele, Brigham and Women's Hospital; D, courtesy of Dr. PR Ros, Brigham and Women's Hospital; with permission.)*

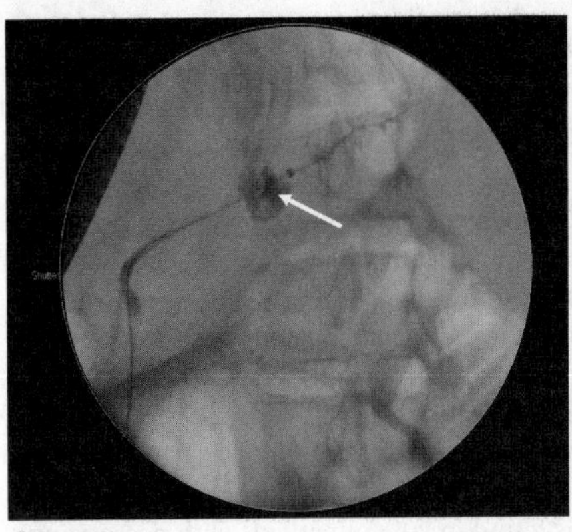

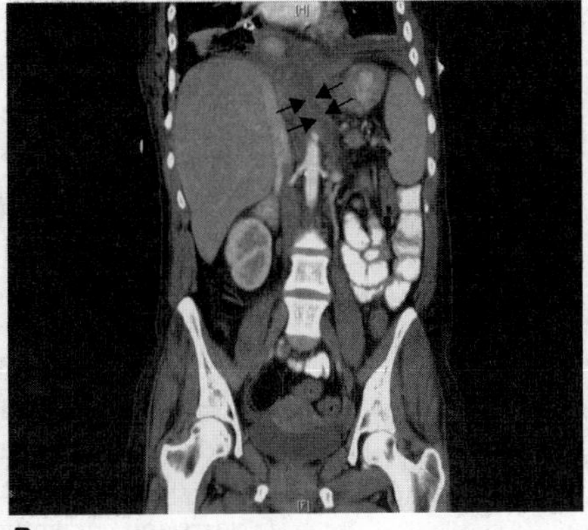

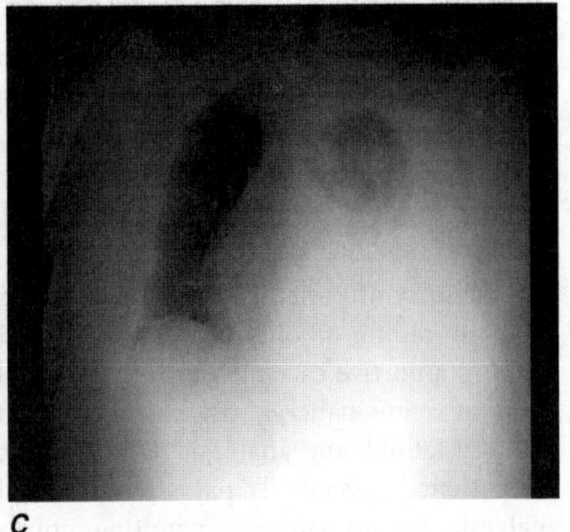

Figure 313-3 *A.* **Pancreaticopleural fistula: pancreatic duct leak on ERCP.** Pancreatic duct leak demonstrated (arrow) at the time of retrograde pancreatogram in a patient with acute exacerbation of alcohol-induced acute or chronic pancreatitis. *B.* Pancreaticopleural fistula: CT Scan. Contrast-enhanced CT scan (coronal view) with arrows showing fistula tract from pancreatic duct disruption in the pancreatic pleural fistula. *C.* Pancreaticopleural fistula: Chest x-ray. Large pleural effusion in the left hemithorax from a disrupted pancreatic duct. Analysis of pleural fluid revealed elevated amylase concentration. *(Courtesy of Dr. KJ Mortele, Brigham and Women's Hospital; with permission.)*

history of crescendo-decrescendo pain, findings on abdominal examination, and CT of the abdomen showing changes characteristic of mechanical obstruction. Acute mesenteric vascular occlusion is usually suspected in elderly debilitated patients with brisk leukocytosis, abdominal distention, and bloody diarrhea, confirmed by CT or MR angiography. Systemic lupus erythematosus and polyarteritis nodosa may be confused with pancreatitis, especially since pancreatitis may develop as a complication of these diseases. Diabetic ketoacidosis is often accompanied by abdominal pain and elevated total serum amylase levels, thus closely mimicking acute pancreatitis. However, the serum lipase level is not elevated in diabetic ketoacidosis.

■ COURSE OF THE DISEASE AND COMPLICATIONS

The initial assessment of severity in acute pancreatitis is critical for the appropriate triage and management of patients. The basis for the classification, severity, and complications of acute pancreatitis was initially established at the International Symposium held in Atlanta in 1992. While the definitions have come under greater scrutiny in recent years, it still serves as the common language for clinical care and research in acute pancreatitis. The criteria for severity in acute pancreatitis was defined as organ failure of at least one organ system (defined as a systolic blood pressure <90 mmHg, Pao_2 ≤60 mmHg, creatinine >2.0 mg/dL after rehydration, and gastrointestinal bleeding >500 mL/24 hours) and the presence of a local complication such as necrosis, pseudocyst, and abscess.

Early predictors of severity at 48 hours included ≥3 Ranson's signs and APACHE II score ≥8. Traditional severity indices such as APACHE II and Ranson's criteria have not been clinically useful since they are cumbersome, require collection of a large amount of clinical and laboratory data over time, and do not have acceptable positive and negative predictive value for severe acute pancreatitis. A recent simplified scoring system for the early prediction of mortality was developed from a large cohort of patients with acute pancreatitis. This scoring system, referred to as the Bedside Index of Severity in Acute Pancreatitis (BISAP), incorporates five clinical and laboratory parameters obtained within the first 24 hours of hospitalization: (Table 313-2) (*B*UN >25, *I*mpaired mental status, *S*IRS, *A*ge >60 years, *P*leural effusion on radiography). Presence of three or more of these factors was associated with substantially increased risk for in-hospital mortality among patients with acute pancreatitis.

Apart from the severity indices, there are additional factors that can be used to assess severity in acute pancreatitis. They are best separated into risk factors for severity and markers of severity within 24 hours of admission and during hospitalization. Risk factors for severe acute pancreatitis on admission include older age (>60 years), obesity (BMI ≥30), and comorbid disease. There is also evidence to support initial episode and alcohol use as additional risk factors for severity. At admission and during the first 24 hours, markers of severity in acute pancreatitis include scoring systems such as BISAP score and APACHE II, SIRS, azotemia, hemoconcentration, and organ failure. During hospitalization, markers of severity include persistent organ failure lasting more than 48 hours and pancreatic necrosis.

The course of acute pancreatitis is defined by two phases. In the first phase, which lasts one to two weeks, severity is defined by clinical parameters rather than morphologic findings. The most important clinical parameter is persistent organ failure (i.e., lasting longer than 48 hours), which is the usual cause of death. Severity in the second phase is defined by both clinical parameters and morphologic criteria. The important clinical parameter of severity, as in the first phase, is persistent organ failure. The morphologic criteria of greatest interest is the development of necrotizing pancreatitis, especially when it prolongs hospitalization and/or it requires active intervention such as operative, endoscopic, or percutaneous therapy or requires supportive measures such as renal dialysis, ventilator support, or need for nasoenteric feeding.

The importance of the recognition of interstitial versus necrotizing acute pancreatitis has lead to the development of a CT severity index (Table 313-3) as another measure of severity that is best evaluated three to five days into hospitalization because it may not be possible to distinguish interstitial from necrotizing pancreatitis on contrast-enhanced CT scan on the day of admission. CT identification of local complications, particularly necrosis, is critical because patients with infected and sterile necrosis are at greatest risk of mortality (Figs. 313-1, 313-2). The median prevalence of organ failure is 54% in necrotizing pancreatitis. The prevalence of organ failure is perhaps slightly higher in infected versus sterile necrosis. With single organ system failure, the mortality is 3–10% but increases to 47% with multisystem organ failure. These data serve to highlight that a patient found to have pancreatic necrosis with multisystem organ failure is the most likely to die.

However, it should be noted that necrotizing pancreatitis is uncommon (10% of all patients with acute pancreatitis), and the far greater proportion of patients presenting in clinical practice have interstitial pancreatitis, which also is associated with organ failure in 10% and death in 3% of cases. This roughly translates to similar absolute mortality figures in the interstitial and necrotizing pancreatitis populations since interstitial disease is far more prevalent.

Mild acute pancreatitis

The majority of patients with mild acute pancreatitis and either no organ failure or only transient organ failure will respond to simple supportive care measures that form the hallmark of treatment in acute pancreatitis: bowel rest, intravenous hydration with crystalloid, and analgesia. Oral intake can be resumed once the patient is essentially pain free in the absence of parenteral analgesia, has no nausea or vomiting, normal bowel sounds, and is hungry. Typically, a clear or full liquid diet has been recommended for the initial meal, but a low-fat solid diet is a reasonable choice following recovery from mild acute pancreatitis. Patients with gallstone pancreatitis are at increased risk of recurrence. Therefore, following recovery from mild pancreatitis, consideration should be given to performing a laparoscopic cholecystectomy during the same admission. An alternative for patients who are not surgical candidates would be to perform an endoscopic biliary sphincterotomy.

Severe acute pancreatitis (See Figs. 313-1, 313-2)

Patients with predictive markers of severity on admission such as obesity or hemoconcentration are also managed with supportive measures outlined as above. It is recommended that vigorous fluid resuscitation take place. Measurement of hematocrit and BUN every 12 hours is recommended to ensure adequacy of fluid resuscitation. A decrease in hematocrit and BUN during the first 12 to 24 hours is strong evidence that sufficient fluids are being administered. If the hematocrit remains elevated or increases further (particularly among those whose hematocrit on admission are >44), fluid resuscitation is inadequate.

Patients with persistent organ failure that does not respond to increased fluids (to counteract hypotension and increased serum creatinine) and/or nasal oxygen to overcome hypoxemia as well as those patients with labored respirations that may herald respiratory failure should be transferred to an intensive care unit for aggressive hydration and close monitoring for the possible need of intubation with mechanical ventilation, hemodialysis, and support of blood pressure.

TREATMENT Acute Pancreatitis

In most patients (85–90%) with acute pancreatitis, the disease is self-limited and subsides spontaneously, usually within three to seven days after treatment is instituted. Conventional measures include (1) analgesics for pain, (2) IV fluids and colloids to maintain normal intravascular volume, and (3) no oral alimentation.

Once it is clear that a patient will not be able to tolerate oral feeding (a determination that can usually be made within 48–72 hours), enteral nutrition should be considered [rather than total parenteral nutrition (TPN)] since it maintains gut barrier integrity, thereby preventing bacterial translocation, is less expensive, and has fewer complications than TPN. The route through which enteral feeding is administered is under debate. Nasogastric access is easier to establish and may be as safe as nasojejunal enteral nutrition. However, enteral nutrition that bypasses the stomach and duodenum stimulates pancreatic secretions less and this rationale theoretically supports the use of the nasojejunal route. It has not been demonstrated whether either route is superior in altering morbidity and mortality. When patients with necrotizing pancreatitis begin oral intake of food, consideration should also be given to the addition of pancreatic enzyme supplementation and proton pump inhibitor therapy to assist with fat digestion and reduce gastric acid.

ROLE OF ANTIBIOTICS There is currently no role for prophylactic antibiotics in either interstitial or necrotizing pancreatitis. Although several early studies suggested a role for prophylactic antibiotics in patients with necrotizing pancreatitis, two recent double-blind, randomized controlled trials failed to demonstrate a reduction in pancreatic infection with use of antibiotic prophylaxis. However, it should also be noted that the overall rate of infected necrosis has been in decline over the past 10–15 years and currently is found in 20% of patients with necrotizing pancreatitis. It is reasonable to start antibiotics in a patient who appears septic while awaiting the results of cultures. If cultures are negative, the antibiotics should be discontinued to minimize the risk of developing fungal superinfection.

Percutaneous aspiration of necrosis with Gram stain and culture should generally not be performed until at least 7–10 days after establishing a diagnosis of necrotizing pancreatitis and only if there are ongoing signs of possible pancreatic infection such as sustained leukocytosis, fever, or organ failure. Once a diagnosis of infected necrosis is established, appropriate antibiotics should be instituted and surgical debridement should be undertaken. There exist minimally invasive alternative therapies such as endoscopic, percutaneous catheter, and retroperitoneal techniques for necrosectomy. However, there are currently no randomized studies supporting the use of one over another modality. For patients with sterile necrosis, medical management is usually maintained indefinitely unless patients develop serious complications such as compartment syndrome, intestinal perforation, pseudoaneurysms not responding to embolization, or inability to resume oral intake after four to six weeks of treatment (Fig. 313-2).

There are several clearly defined roles for ERCP in acute pancreatitis. Urgent ERCP (within 24 hours) is indicated in patients who have severe acute biliary pancreatitis with organ failure and/or cholangitis. Elective ERCP with sphincterotomy can be considered in patients with persistent or incipient biliary obstruction, those deemed to be poor candidates for cholecystectomy, and for those in whom there is strong suspicion for bile duct stones after cholecystectomy. ERCP with stent placement is also indicated for pancreatic ductal disruptions that occur as part of the inflammatory process and result in peripancreatic fluid collections (Fig. 313-3*A*).

Several drugs have been evaluated by prospective controlled trials and found ineffective in the treatment of acute pancreatitis. The list, by no means complete, includes glucagon, H_2 blockers, protease inhibitors such as aprotinin, glucocorticoids, calcitonin, nonsteroidal anti-inflammatory drugs (NSAIDs), and lexipafant, a platelet-activating factor inhibitor. A recent meta-analysis of somatostatin, octreotide, and the antiprotease gabexate mesylate in the therapy of acute pancreatitis suggested (1) a reduced mortality rate but no change in complications with octreotide and (2) no effect on the mortality rate but reduced pancreatic damage with gabexate.

A dynamic contrast-enhanced CT (CECT) scan performed three to five days after hospitalization provides valuable information on the severity and prognosis of acute pancreatitis (Fig. 313-1). In particular, a CECT scan allows estimation of the presence and extent of pancreatic necrosis. Recent studies suggest that the likelihood of prolonged pancreatitis or a serious complication is negligible when the CT severity index is 1 or 2 and low with scores of 3–6. However, patients with scores of 7–10 had a 92%

morbidity rate and a 17% mortality rate (Table 313-3). A few retrospective studies have raised concern that the use of IV contrast early in the course of acute pancreatitis might intensify pancreatic necrosis. However, since prospective human studies are not available, it is recommended that a CECT scan be obtained only after vigorous initial fluid resuscitation.

Elevation of serum amylase/lipase or persistent inflammatory changes seen on CT scans should not discourage feeding a hungry asymptomatic patient. In this regard, persistence of inflammatory changes on CT scans or persistent elevations in serum amylase/lipase may not resolve for weeks to months. The patient with unremitting severe necrotizing pancreatitis requires vigorous fluid resuscitation and close attention to complications such as cardiovascular collapse, respiratory insufficiency, and pancreatic infection. A useful indicator of severe/complicated forms of acute pancreatitis is the persistence of the systemic SIRS beyond 48 hours. SIRS was defined in 1992 in a joint conference of the American College of Chest Physicians and Society of Critical Care Medicine as a standardized clinical syndrome to indicate the presence of systemic inflammation irrespective of etiology. Several studies have linked persistent SIRS with an increased risk of organ failure and death in acute pancreatitis. Complications from acute pancreatitis should be managed by a combination of radiologic and surgical means (see below). Although sterile necrosis is most often managed conservatively, surgical pancreatic debridement (necrosectomy) should be considered for definitive management of infected necrosis. Such decisions are influenced by response to antibiotic treatment. Multiple operations may be required. A recent study compared the step-up approach, i.e., percutaneous or endoscopic transgastric drainage with open necrosectomy for necrotizing pancreatitis. One third of the patients successfully treated with the step-up approach did not require major abdominal surgery. Enteral-feeding with a nasojejunal tube has been demonstrated to have fewer infectious complications than with total parenteral nutrition (TPN) and is the preferred method of nutritional support. In addition to nutritional support, enteral feeding helps to maintain integrity of the intestinal tract during severe acute pancreatitis.

Patients with severe gallstone-induced pancreatitis, complicated by cholangitis, may improve dramatically if papillotomy is carried out within the first 36–72 hours of the attack. Studies indicate that only those patients with gallstone pancreatitis who are in the very severe group should be considered for urgent ERCP. Finally, the treatment for patients with hypertriglyceridemia-associated pancreatitis includes (1) weight loss to ideal weight, (2) a lipid-restricted diet, (3) exercise, (4) avoidance of alcohol and of drugs that can elevate serum triglycerides (i.e., estrogens, vitamin A, thiazides, and propranolol), and (5) control of diabetes.

Recurrent pancreatitis

Approximately 25% of patients who have had an attack of acute pancreatitis have a recurrence. The two most common etiologic factors are alcohol and cholelithiasis. In patients with recurrent pancreatitis without an obvious cause the differential diagnosis should encompass occult biliary tract disease including microlithiasis, hypertriglyceridemia, drugs, pancreatic cancer, sphincter of Oddi dysfunction, pancreas divisum, cystic fibrosis, and pancreatic cancer (Table 313-1). In one series of 31 patients diagnosed initially as having idiopathic or recurrent acute pancreatitis, 23 were found to have occult gallstone disease. Thus, approximately two-thirds of patients with recurrent acute pancreatitis without an obvious cause actually have occult gallstone disease due to microlithiasis. Genetic defects as in hereditary pancreatitis can result in recurrent pancreatitis. Other diseases of the biliary tree and pancreatic ducts that can cause acute pancreatitis include choledochocele; ampullary tumors; pancreas divisum; and pancreatic duct stones, stricture, and tumor. Approximately 2–4% of patients with pancreatic carcinoma present with acute pancreatitis.

■ INFECTED PANCREATIC NECROSIS AND PSEUDOCYST

Pancreatic necrosis does not usually become secondarily infected until at least 7–10 days after the onset of acute pancreatitis. Approximately one-half of cases of infected necrosis can be diagnosed between the 7th and 21st day, the remainder after 21 days. The diagnosis of pancreatic infection can be accomplished by CT-guided needle aspiration with Gram stain and culture. The organisms are most frequently gram-negative bacteria of intestinal origin. Clinical clues that should alert the clinician to the possibility of infected necrosis are persistent fever, leukocytosis, and organ failure in a patient with necrotizing pancreatitis. Some reports suggest that patients who have more than 50% pancreatic necrosis are more likely to have infected pancreatic necrosis than those who have lesser amounts of necrosis. Choices of treatment in infected pancreatic necrosis include surgical debridement; endoscopic debridement, if the pancreatic necrosis has been circumscribed into the entity termed *walled-off necrosis* that affects the posterior wall of the stomach; and, on occasion, radiologic catheter drainage with irrigation in an effort to eliminate at least some infected semisolid material as well as the infected liquid material. Radiologic approach is usually suggested to treat a patient who is too ill to undergo surgical debridement.

Walled-off necrosis

In necrotizing pancreatitis, there is invariably an intense inflammatory response involving the fat around the pancreas. This inflammatory process frequently results in peripancreatic necrosis. Eventually, after three to six weeks, there is coalescence of the pancreatic necrosis and peripancreatic fat necrosis into a structure that is encapsulated by fibrous tissue. The name that was originally used to describe this entity was "organized necrosis." New terminology now refers to it as "walled-off necrosis."

The walled-off necrosis contains semisolid necrotic tissue together with a considerable amount of dark fluid representing liquefaction of devitalized pancreatic and peripancreatic tissue as well as some blood.

Walled-off necrosis and a pancreatic pseudocyst may look very similar on first inspection of a contrast-enhanced CT scan. Both show a low attenuation nonenhancing round structure enclosed by a capsule containing fibrous tissue that enhances due to small blood vessels within the capsule. On closer inspection, a distinction can be made. In walled-off necrosis, serial images clearly show that a portion of the pancreas as well as variable amounts of peripancreatic tissue are necrotic. In interstitial pancreatitis, the pancreas enhances normally in response to intravenous contrast, thereby confirming that the process is interstitial pancreatitis. The encapsulated structure is readily seen to be adjacent to the pancreas.

Pseudocysts

Pseudocysts of the pancreas are extrapancreatic collections of pancreatic fluid containing pancreatic enzymes and a small amount of debris. In contrast to true cysts, pseudocysts do not have an epithelial lining. The walls consist of necrotic tissue, granulation tissue, and fibrous tissue.

A pseudocyst should be distinguished from a postnecrotic fluid collection that contains heterogeneous material including residual necrotic debris. Disruption of the pancreatic ductal system is common. However, the subsequent course of this disruption varies widely, ranging from spontaneous healing to continuous leakage of pancreatic juice, which results in tense ascites. Pseudocysts are preceded by pancreatitis in 90% of cases and by trauma in 10%. Approximately 85% are located in the body or tail of the pancreas and 15% in the head. Some patients have two or more pseudocysts. Abdominal pain, with or without radiation to the back, is the usual presenting complaint. A palpable, tender mass may be found in the middle or left upper abdomen.

On imaging studies, 75% of pseudocysts can be seen to displace some portion of the gastrointestinal tract. Sonography, however, is reliable in detecting pseudocysts. Sonography also permits differentiation between an edematous, inflamed pancreas, which can give rise to a palpable mass, and an actual pseudocyst. Furthermore, serial ultrasound studies will indicate whether a pseudocyst has resolved. CT or MRI complements ultrasonography in the diagnosis of pancreatic pseudocyst, especially when the pseudocyst is infected as suggested by the rare finding of gas within the fluid collection.

In earlier studies with sonography, lesions thought to be pseudocysts were seen to resolve in 25–40% of patients. However, it is now recognized that it is important to distinguish between walled-off necrosis and pseudocysts that typically develop later in the course of acute pancreatitis. Pseudocysts that are >5 cm in diameter may persist for >6 weeks. Recent natural history studies have suggested that noninterventional, expectant management is the best course in selected patients with minimal symptoms and no evidence of active alcohol use in whom the pseudocyst appears mature by radiography and does not resemble a cystic neoplasm. A significant number of these pseudocysts resolve spontaneously in >6 weeks after their formation. Also, these studies demonstrate that large pseudocyst size is not an absolute indication for interventional therapy and that many peripancreatic fluid collections detected on CT in cases of acute pancreatitis resolve spontaneously. A pseudocyst that does not resolve spontaneously can occasionally lead to serious complications, such as (1) pain caused by expansion of the lesion and pressure on other viscera, (2) rupture, (3) hemorrhage, and (4) abscess. Rupture of a pancreatic pseudocyst is a particularly serious complication. In this case, shock almost always supervenes, and mortality rates range from 14% if the rupture is not associated with hemorrhage to >60% if hemorrhage has occurred. Rupture and hemorrhage are the prime causes of death from pancreatic pseudocyst. A triad of findings—an increase in the size of the mass, a localized bruit over the mass, and a sudden decrease in hemoglobin level and hematocrit without obvious external blood loss—should alert one to the possibility of hemorrhage from a pseudocyst. Thus, in patients who are stable and free of complications and in whom serial ultrasound studies show that the pseudocyst is shrinking, conservative therapy is indicated. Conversely, if the pseudocyst is expanding and is complicated by severe pain, hemorrhage, or abscess, the patient should be operated on. Chronic pseudocysts can be treated safely and drainage can be accomplished by endoscopic, radiologic, or surgical means.

Pseudoaneurysms develop in up to 10% of patients with acute pancreatitis at sites reflecting the distribution of pseudocysts and fluid collections (Fig. 313-2*D*). The splenic artery is most frequently involved, followed by the inferior and superior pancreatic duodenal arteries. This diagnosis should be suspected in patients with pancreatitis who develop upper gastrointestinal bleeding without an obvious cause or in whom thin-cut CT scanning reveals a contrast-enhanced lesion within or adjacent to a suspected pseudocyst. CT angiography can identify the lesion, which can then be treated with angiographic embolization.

The local and systemic complications of acute pancreatitis are summarized in Table 313-4. Systemic complications include pulmonary, cardiovascular, hematologic, renal, metabolic, and central nervous system (CNS) abnormalities. *Purtscher's retinopathy*, a relatively unusual complication, is manifested by a sudden and severe loss of vision in a patient with acute pancreatitis. It is characterized by a peculiar funduscopic appearance with cotton-wool spots and hemorrhages confined to an area limited by the optic disc and macula; it is believed to be due to occlusion of the posterior retinal artery with aggregated granulocytes.

TABLE 313-4 Complications of Acute Pancreatitis

Local	
Necrosis	Pancreatic ascites
Sterile	Disruption of main pancreatic duct
Infected	Leaking pseudocyst
Walled-off necrosis	Involvement of contiguous organs by necrotizing pancreatitis
Pancreatic fluid collections	Massive intraperitoneal hemorrhage
Pancreatic abscess	Thrombosis of blood vessels (splenic vein, portal vein)
Pancreatic pseudocyst	Bowel infarction
Pain	Obstructive jaundice
Rupture	
Hemorrhage	
Infection	
Obstruction of gastrointestinal tract (stomach, duodenum, colon)	
Systemic	
Pulmonary	Renal
Pleural effusion	Oliguria
Atelectasis	Azotemia
Mediastinal abscess	Renal artery and/or renal vein thrombosis
Pneumonitis	Acute tubular necrosis
Acute respiratory distress syndrome	Metabolic
Cardiovascular	Hyperglycemia
Hypotension	Hypertriglyceridemia
Hypovolemia	Hypocalcemia
Sudden death	Encephalopathy
Nonspecific ST-T changes in electrocardiogram simulating myocardial infarction	Sudden blindness (Purtscher's retinopathy)
Pericardial effusion	Central nervous system
Hematologic	Psychosis
Disseminated intravascular coagulation	Fat emboli
Gastrointestinal hemorrhage	Fat necrosis
Peptic ulcer disease	Subcutaneous tissues (erythematous nodules)
Erosive gastritis	Bone
Hemorrhagic pancreatic necrosis with erosion into major blood vessels	Miscellaneous (mediastinum, pleura, nervous system)
Portal vein thrombosis, variceal hemorrhage	

Pancreatitis in patients with AIDS

The incidence of acute pancreatitis is increased in patients with AIDS for two reasons: (1) the high incidence of infections involving the pancreas such as infections with cytomegalovirus, *Cryptosporidium*, and the *Mycobacterium avium* complex; and (2) the frequent use by patients with AIDS of medications such as didanosine, pentamidine, trimethoprim-sulfamethoxazole, and protease inhibitors (Chap. 189).

PANCREATIC ASCITES AND PANCREATIC PLEURAL EFFUSIONS

Pancreatic ascites or pancreatic pleural effusion are initially identified based on CT or MRI imaging and are usually due to disruption of the main pancreatic duct, often by an internal fistula between the duct and the peritoneal cavity or a leaking pseudocyst (Fig. 313-3*A*). This diagnosis is suggested in a patient with a history of acute pancreatitis in whom the ascites or pleural fluid has both increased levels of albumin [>30 g/L (>3 g/dL)] and a markedly elevated level of amylase. An ERCP or magnetic resonance cholangio pancreatography (MRCP) confirms the clinical suspicion and radiologic findings and often demonstrates passage of contrast material from a disrupted major pancreatic duct or a pseudocyst into the peritoneal cavity. The differential diagnosis of pancreatic ascites should include intraperitoneal carcinomatosis, tuberculous peritonitis, constrictive pericarditis, and Budd-Chiari syndrome.

TREATMENT Pancreatic Ascites and Pancreatic Pleural Effusions

If the pancreatic duct disruption is posterior, an internal fistula may develop between the pancreatic duct and the pleural space, producing a pleural effusion (pancreaticopleural fistula) that is usually left-sided and often massive (Fig. 313-3). If the pancreatic duct disruption is anterior, amylase- and lipase-rich peritoneal fluid accumulate (pancreatic ascites). A leaking, disrupted pancreatic duct is best treated by ERCP and "bridging" stent placement and infrequently requires thoracentesis or chest tube drainage.

Treatment may also require enteral or parenteral alimentation to improve nutrition. If ascites or pleural fluid persists after two to three weeks of medical management, and the disruption is unable to be stented, the patient should be considered for surgical intervention after retrograde pancreatography to define the anatomy of the disrupted duct.

CHRONIC PANCREATITIS AND PANCREATIC EXOCRINE INSUFFICIENCY

PATHOPHYSIOLOGY

Chronic pancreatitis is a disease process characterized by irreversible damage to the pancreas as distinct from the reversible changes noted in acute pancreatitis. The condition is best defined by the presence of histologic abnormalities, including chronic inflammation, fibrosis, and progressive destruction of both exocrine and eventually endocrine tissue. A number of etiologies may result in chronic pancreatitis, and may result in the cardinal complications of chronic pancreatitis such as abdominal pain, steatorrhea, weight loss, and diabetes mellitus (Table 313-5).

The events that initiate the inflammatory process in the pancreas are incompletely understood. Current experimental and clinical observations have shown that alcohol has a direct toxic effect on the pancreas. While patients with alcohol-induced pancreatitis generally consume large amounts of alcohol, some consume as little as ≤50 g/d. Prolonged consumption of socially acceptable amounts of alcohol is compatible with the development of chronic pancreatitis. Findings of extensive pancreatic fibrosis in patients who died during their first attack of clinical acute alcohol-induced pancreatitis support the concept that such patients already had chronic pancreatitis.

There is a strong association of smoking and chronic pancreatitis. Cigarette smoke leads to an increased susceptibility to pancreatic self-digestion and predisposes to dysregulation of duct cell CFTR function.

TABLE 313-5 Chronic Pancreatitis and Pancreatic Exocrine Insufficiency: TIGAR-O Classification System

Toxic-metabolic	**Autoimmune**
Alcoholic	Isolated autoimmune chronic pancreatitis
Tobacco smoking	Autoimmune chronic pancreatitis associated with Sjögren's syndrome
Hypercalcemia	Inflammatory bowel disease
Hyperlipidemia	Primary biliary cirrhosis
Chronic renal failure	
Medications—phenacetin abuse	**Recurrent and Severe Acute Pancreatitis**
Toxins—organotin compounds (e.g., DBTC)	Postnecrotic (severe acute pancreatitis)
Idiopathic	Recurrent acute pancreatitis
Early onset	Vascular diseases/ischemia
Late onset	Postirradiation
Tropical	
Genetic	**Obstructive**
Hereditary pancreatitis	Pancreas divisum
Cationic trypsinogen	Sphincter of Oddi disorders (controversial)
$PRSS_1$	Duct obstruction (e.g., tumor)
$PRSS_2$	Preampullary duodenal wall cysts
CFTR mutations	Posttraumatic pancreatic duct scars
SPINK1 mutations	

Abbreviations: DBTC, dibutylin dichloride; TIGAR-O, toxic-metabolic, idiopathic, genetic, autoimmune, recurrent and severe acute pancreatitis, obstructive.

It has become increasingly apparent that smoking is an independent, dose-dependent risk factor for chronic pancreatitis and recurrent acute pancreatitis. Smoking is clearly associated with progression of disease in late-onset idiopathic chronic pancreatitis and with increased disease severity in alcohol-induced chronic pancreatitis.

Recent characterization of pancreatic stellate cells (PSC) has added insight to the underlying cellular responses behind development of chronic pancreatitis. Specifically, PSCs are believed to play a role in maintaining normal pancreatic architecture that can shift toward fibrogenesis in the case of chronic pancreatitis. The sentinel acute pancreatitis event (SAPE) hypothesis uniformly describes the events in the pathogenesis of chronic pancreatitis. It is believed that alcohol or additional stimuli lead to matrix metalloproteinase–mediated destruction of normal collagen in pancreatic parenchyma, which later allows for pancreatic remodeling. Proinflammatory cytokines, tumor necrosis factor α (TNF-α), interleukin 1 (IL-1), and interleukin 6 (IL-6) as well as oxidant complexes are able to induce PSC activity with subsequent new collagen synthesis. In addition to being stimulated by cytokines, oxidants, or growth factors, PSCs also possess transforming growth factor β (TGF-β)–mediated self-activating autocrine pathways that may explain disease progression in chronic pancreatitis even after removal of noxious stimuli.

ETIOLOGIC CONSIDERATIONS

Among adults in the United States, alcoholism is the most common cause of clinically apparent chronic pancreatitis, while cystic fibrosis is the most frequent cause in children. In up to 25% of adults in the United States with chronic pancreatitis, the cause is not known. That is, they are labeled as *idiopathic chronic pancreatitis.* Recent investigations have indicated that up to 15% of patients with idiopathic pancreatitis may have pancreatitis due to genetic defects (Table 313-5).

Whitcomb and associates studied several large families with hereditary chronic pancreatitis and were able to identify a genetic defect that affects the gene encoding for trypsinogen. Several additional defects of this gene have also been described. The defect prevents the destruction of trypsinogen and allows it to be resistant to the effect of trypsin inhibitor, become spontaneously activated, and to remain activated. It is hypothesized that this continual activation of digestive enzymes within the gland leads to acute injury and, finally, chronic pancreatitis. This group of investigators has also reported that another form of hereditary chronic pancreatitis tends to present later in life, has a female predominance, and frequently leads to chronic pancreatitis.

Several other groups of investigators have documented mutations of *CFTR*. This gene functions as a cyclic AMP–regulated chloride channel. In patients with cystic fibrosis, the high concentration of macromolecules can block the pancreatic ducts. It must be appreciated, however, that there is a great deal of heterogeneity in relationship to the *CFTR* gene defect. More than 1000 putative mutations of the *CFTR* gene have been identified. Attempts to elucidate the relationship between the genotype and pancreatic manifestations have been hampered by the number of mutations. The ability to detect *CFTR* mutations has led to the recognition that the clinical spectrum of the disease is broader than previously thought. Two recent studies have clarified the association between mutations of the *CFTR* gene and another monosymptomatic form of cystic fibrosis (i.e., chronic pancreatitis). It is estimated that in patients with idiopathic pancreatitis, the frequency of a single *CFTR* mutation is 11 times the expected frequency and the frequency of two mutant alleles is 80 times the expected frequency. In these studies, the patients were adults when the diagnosis of pancreatitis was made; none had any clinical evidence of pulmonary disease, and sweat test results were not diagnostic of cystic fibrosis. The prevalence of such mutations is unclear, and further studies are certainly needed. In addition, the therapeutic and prognostic implication of these findings with respect to managing pancreatitis remains to be determined. Long-term follow-up of affected patients is needed. *CFTR* mutations are common in the general population. It is unclear whether the *CFTR* mutation alone can lead to pancreatitis as an autosomal recessive disease. A recent study evaluated 39 patients with idiopathic chronic pancreatitis to assess the risk associated with these mutations. Patients with two *CFTR* mutations (compound heterozygotes) demonstrated *CFTR* function at a level between that seen in typical cystic fibrosis and cystic fibrosis carriers and had a fortyfold increased risk of pancreatitis. The presence of an *N34S SPINK1* mutation increased the risk twentyfold. A combination of two *CFTR* mutations and an *N34S SPINK1* mutation increased the risk of pancreatitis 900-fold. Table 313-5 lists recognized causes of chronic pancreatitis and pancreatic exocrine insufficiency.

■ AUTOIMMUNE PANCREATITIS (TABLE 313-6)

Autoimmune pancreatitis (AIP) is an uncommon disorder of presumed autoimmune causation with characteristic laboratory, histologic, and morphologic findings. AIP has been described as a primary pancreatic disorder; however, it is also associated with other disorders of presumed autoimmune etiology, including primary sclerosing cholangitis, primary biliary sclerosis, rheumatoid arthritis, Sjögren's syndrome, ulcerative colitis, mediastinal adenopathy, autoimmune thyroiditis, tubulointerstitial nephritis, and retroperitoneal fibrosis. Mild symptoms, usually abdominal pain, are present but attacks of acute pancreatitis are unusual. Furthermore, AIP is not a common cause of idiopathic recurrent pancreatitis. In the United States, 50–75% of patients with AIP present with obstructive jaundice.

TABLE 313-6 Clinical Features of Autoimmune Pancreatitis (AIP)

- Mild symptoms usually abdominal pain, but without frequent attacks of pancreatitis, which are unusual
- Presentation with obstructive jaundice
- Diffuse swelling and enlargement of the pancreas, especially the head, the latter mimicking carcinoma of the pancreas
- Diffuse irregular narrowing of the pancreatic duct in ERCP
- Increased levels of serum gamma globulins especially IgG4
- Presence of other autoantibodies (ANA), rheumatoid factor (RF)
- Can occur with other autoimmune diseases: Sjögren's syndrome, primary sclerosing cholangitis, ulcerative colitis, rheumatoid arthritis
- Extra pancreatic bile duct changes such as stricture of the common bile duct and intrahepatic ducts
- Absence of pancreatic calcifications or cysts
- Pancreatic biopsies reveal extensive fibrosis and lymphoplasmacytic infiltration
- Glucocorticoids are effective in alleviating symptoms, decreasing size of the pancreas, and reversing histopathologic changes
- Two-thirds of patients present with either obstructive jaundice or a "mass" in the head of the pancreas mimicking carcinoma

Weight loss and new onset of diabetes may also occur. An obstructive pattern on liver tests is common (i.e., disproportionately elevated serum alkaline phosphatase and minimally elevated serum aminotransferases). Elevated serum levels of immunoglobulin G4 (IgG4) provide a marker for the disease, particularly in Western populations. Serum IgG4 normally accounts for only 5–6% of the total IgG4 in healthy patients but is elevated at least twofold higher than 135 mg/dL in those with AIP. CT scans reveal abnormalities in the majority of patients and include diffuse enlargement, focal enlargement, and a distinct enlargement at the head of the pancreas. ERCP or MRCP reveals strictures in the bile duct in more than one-third of patients with AIP; these may be common bile duct strictures, intrahepatic bile duct strictures, or proximal bile duct strictures, with accompanying narrowing of the pancreatic bile duct. This has been termed autoimmune cholangitis. Characteristic histologic findings include extensive lymphoplasmacytic infiltrates with dense fibrosis around pancreatic ducts, as well as a lymphoplasmacytic infiltration, resulting in an obliterative phlebitis.

The Mayo Clinic criteria indicate that AIP can be diagnosed with at least one of three abnormalities: (1) diagnostic histology; (2) characteristic findings on CT and pancreatography combined with elevated IgG4 levels; and (3) response to glucocorticoid therapy, with improvement in pancreatic and extrapancreatic manifestations.

Glucocorticoids have shown efficacy in alleviating symptoms, decreasing the size of the pancreas, and reversing histopathologic features in patients with AIP. Patients may respond dramatically to glucocorticoid therapy within a two- to four-week period. Prednisone is usually administered at an initial dose of 40 mg/d for four weeks followed by a taper of the daily dosage by 5 mg/week based on monitoring of clinical parameters. Relief of symptoms, serial changes in abdominal imaging of the pancreas and bile ducts, decreased serum γ-globulin and IgG4 levels, and improvements in liver tests are parameters to follow. A poor response to glucocorticoids over a two- to four-week period should raise suspicion of pancreatic cancer or other forms of chronic pancreatitis. In most reports, 50–70% of patients responded to glucocorticoids, but about 25% required a second course of treatment while a smaller number required maintenance treatment with prednisone at a dosage of 5–10 mg/d. Patients with bile duct strictures are less likely to have a sustained response to glucocorticoids and may require immunosuppressive therapy with azathioprine or 6-mercaptopurine.

Clinical features of chronic pancreatitis

Patients with chronic pancreatitis seek medical attention predominantly because of two symptoms: abdominal pain or maldigestion and weight loss. The abdominal pain may be quite variable in location, severity, and frequency. The pain can be constant or intermittent with frequent pain-free intervals. Eating may exacerbate the pain, leading to a fear of eating with consequent weight loss. The spectrum of abdominal pain ranges from mild to quite severe, with narcotic dependence as a frequent consequence. Maldigestion is manifested as chronic diarrhea, steatorrhea, weight loss, and fatigue. Patients with chronic abdominal pain may or may not progress to maldigestion, and ~20% of patients will present with symptoms of maldigestion without a history of abdominal pain. Patients with chronic pancreatitis have significant morbidity and mortality and utilize appreciable amounts of societal resources. Despite the steatorrhea, clinically apparent deficiencies of fat-soluble vitamins are surprisingly uncommon. Physical findings in these patients are usually unimpressive so that there is a disparity between the severity of abdominal pain and the physical signs that usually consist of some mild tenderness.

In contrast to acute pancreatitis, the serum amylase and lipase levels are usually not strikingly elevated in chronic pancreatitis. Elevation of serum bilirubin and alkaline phosphatase may indicate cholestasis secondary to common bile duct stricture caused by chronic inflammation. Many patients have impaired glucose tolerance with elevated fasting blood glucose levels. The diagnostic test with the best sensitivity and specificity is the hormone stimulation test utilizing secretin. It becomes abnormal when ≥60% of the pancreatic exocrine function has been lost. This usually correlates well with the onset of chronic abdominal pain. In earlier studies, approximately 40% of patients with chronic pancreatitis had cobalamin (vitamin B_{12}) malabsorption. This can be corrected by the administration of oral pancreatic enzymes. The fecal elastase-1 and small bowel biopsy are useful in the evaluation of patients with suspected pancreatic steatorrhea. The fecal elastase level will be abnormal and small bowel histology will be normal in such patients. A decrease of fecal elastase level to <100 μg per gram of stool strongly suggests severe pancreatic exocrine insufficiency.

Utilizing radiographic techniques (Fig. 313-4), it can be shown that diffuse calcifications noted on plain film of the abdomen usually indicate significant damage to the pancreas. While alcohol is by far the most common cause of pancreatic calcification such calcification may also be noted in hereditary pancreatitis, posttraumatic pancreatitis, hypercalcemic pancreatitis, islet cell tumors, idiopathic chronic pancreatitis, and tropical pancreatitis. Abdominal ultrasonography, CT scanning, and MRCP greatly aid in the diagnosis of pancreatic disease (Fig. 313-4). In addition to excluding a pseudocyst and pancreatic cancer, CT may show calcification, dilated ducts, or an atrophic pancreas. MRCP provides a direct view of the pancreatic duct and is now the diagnostic procedure of choice. The role of endoscopic ultrasonography (EUS) in diagnosing early chronic pancreatitis is still being defined. A total of nine endosonographic features have been described in chronic pancreatitis. The presence of five or more features is considered diagnostic of chronic pancreatitis. EUS complements pancreatic function tests, and a combination of a hormone-stimulation function test and EUS is a modality to evaluate the pancreatic duct morphology, parenchymal

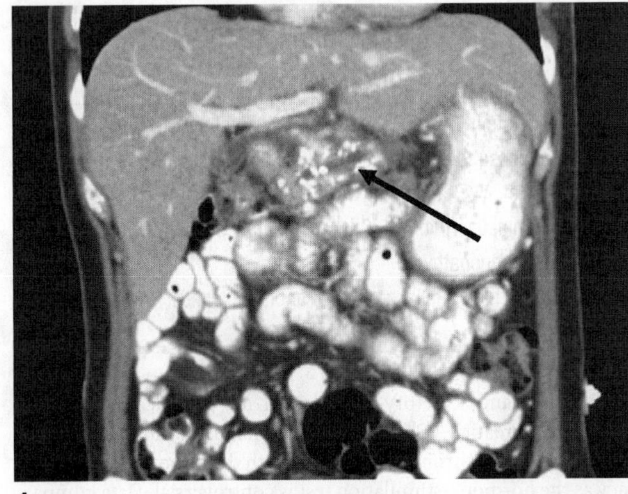

A

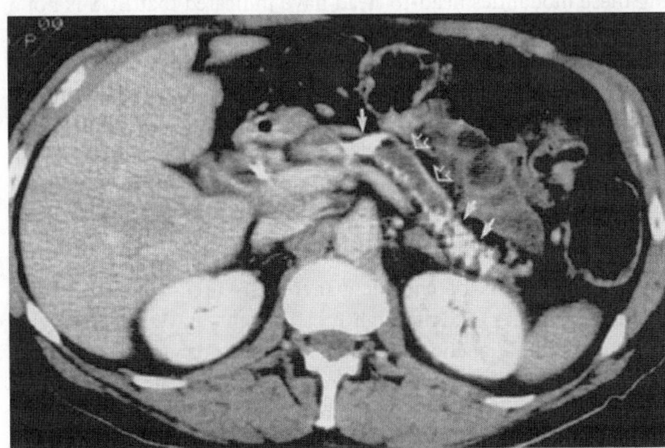

B

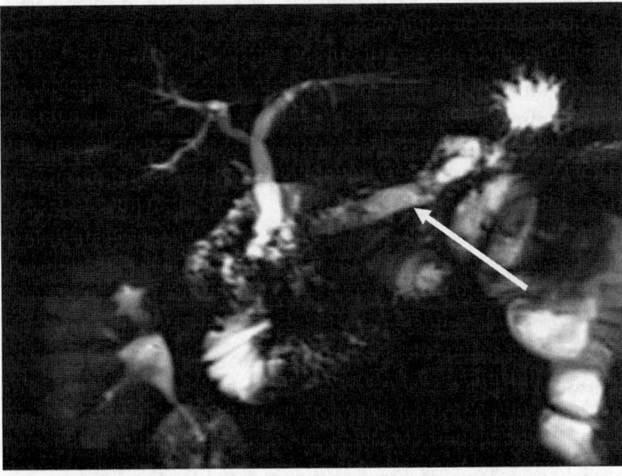

C

Figure 313-4 *A.* Chronic pancreatitis and pancreatic calculi: CT scan. In this contrast-enhanced CT scan of the abdomen, there is evidence of an atrophic pancreas with multiple calcifications and stones in the parenchyma and dilated pancreatic duct (arrow). *B.* In this contrast-enhanced CT scan of the abdomen, there is evidence of an atrophic pancreas with multiple calcifications (*arrows*). Note the markedly dilated pancreatic duct seen in this section through the body and tail (*open arrows*). *C.* Chronic pancreatitis on MRCP: dilated duct with filling defects. Gadolinium-enhanced MRI/MRCP reveals a dilated pancreatic duct (arrow) in chronic pancreatitis with multiple filling defects suggestive of pancreatic duct calculi. *(A, C, courtesy of Dr. KJ Mortele, Brigham and Women's Hospital; with permission.)*

TABLE 313-7 Complications of Chronic Pancreatitis

Narcotic addiction	Gastrointestinal bleeding
Impaired glucose tolerance	Jaundice
Gastroparesis	Cholangitis and/or biliary cirrhosis
Cobalamin malabsorption	Subcutaneous fat necrosis
Nondiabetic retinopathy	Bone pain
Effusions with high amylase content	Pancreatic cancer

architecture, and secretory function for the presence or extent of chronic pancreatitis (Chap. 312). Whether EUS alone can detect early, noncalcific chronic pancreatitis with the same degree of accuracy as the hormone-stimulation test is controversial. Data comparing these modalities head-to-head have indicated that EUS is not a sensitive enough test for detecting early chronic pancreatitis (Chap. 312) and may show positive features in patients who have dyspepsia or even in normal controls. However, recent data suggest that EUS can be combined with endoscopic pancreatic function testing (EUS-ePFT) during a single endoscopy to screen for chronic pancreatitis in patients with chronic abdominal pain.

Complications of chronic pancreatitis

The complications of chronic pancreatitis are protean and are listed in Table 313-7. Although most patients have impaired glucose tolerance, diabetic ketoacidosis and coma are uncommon. Likewise, end-organ damage (retinopathy, neuropathy, nephropathy) is also uncommon. A nondiabetic retinopathy may be due to either vitamin A and/or zinc deficiency. Gastrointestinal bleeding may occur from peptic ulceration, gastritis, a pseudocyst eroding into the duodenum, or ruptured varices secondary to splenic vein thrombosis due to chronic inflammation of the tail of the pancreas. Jaundice, cholestasis, and biliary cirrhosis may occur from the chronic inflammatory reaction around the intrapancreatic portion of the common bile duct. Twenty years after the diagnosis of calcific chronic pancreatitis, the cumulative risk of pancreatic carcinoma is 4%. Patients with hereditary pancreatitis are at a tenfold higher risk for pancreatic cancer.

TREATMENT Chronic Pancreatitis

The treatment of steatorrhea with pancreatic enzymes is straightforward even though complete correction of steatorrhea is unusual. Enzyme therapy usually brings diarrhea under control and restores absorption of fat to an acceptable level and effects weight gain. Thus, pancreatic enzymes have been the cornerstone of pancreatic therapy. In treating steatorrhea, it is important to use a potent pancreatic formulation that will deliver sufficient lipase into the duodenum to correct maldigestion and decrease steatorrhea (Table 313-8). In an attempt to standardize the enzyme activity, potency and bioavailability, the Food and Drug Administration (FDA) required that all pancreas enzyme drugs in the United States obtain a New Drug Application (NDA) by April 2008. Table 313-8 lists frequently utilized formulations but availability will be based on compliance with the FDA mandate. Recent data suggests that dosages up to 80,000–100,000 units of lipase per meal may be necessary to normalize nutritional parameters in malnourished chronic pancreatitis patients.

The management of pain in patients with chronic pancreatitis is problematic.

Recent meta-analyses have shown no consistent benefit of enzyme therapy at reducing pain in chronic pancreatitis. In some patients with idiopathic chronic pancreatitis, conventional nonenteric coated enzyme preparations containing high concentrations of serine proteases may relieve mild abdominal pain or discomfort. The pain relief experienced by these patients actually may be due to improvements in the dyspepsia from maldigestion. Table 313-8 lists the frequently utilized pancreatic enzyme preparations in the United States.

Oxidative stress has also been implicated in the pathophysiology of the pain of chronic pancreatitis. A recent randomized prospective study from India showed antioxidant therapy to be beneficial at reducing pain in mild chronic pancreatitis. Gastroparesis is also quite common in patients with chronic pancreatitis. It is important to recognize this because treatment with enzymes may fail simply because gastroparesis is preventing the appropriate delivery of enzymes into the upper intestine where the enzymes can then act via a feedback inhibition process. In patients with painful chronic pancreatitis, it is important to evaluate gastric emptying and, if gastric emptying is impaired, to effect proper emptying with prokinetic agents. In this setting, enzyme therapy is more apt to be successful.

Endoscopic treatment of chronic pancreatitis pain may involve sphincterotomy, stenting, stone extraction, and drainage of a pancreatic pseudocyst. Therapy directed to the pancreatic duct would seem to be most appropriate in the setting of a dominant stricture, if a ductal stone has led to obstruction. The use of endoscopic stenting for patients with chronic pain, but without a dominant stricture, has not been subjected to any controlled trials. It is now appreciated that significant complications can occur from stenting (i.e., bleeding, cholangitis, stent migration, and stent clogging). All of these may lead to pancreatitis. Importantly, damage to the pancreatic duct and the pancreatic parenchyma can occur following stenting. In patients with large-duct disease usually from alcohol-induced chronic pancreatitis, ductal decompression has been the therapy of choice. Among such patients, 80% seem to obtain immediate relief; however, at the end of three years, one-half the patients have recurrence of pain. Two randomized prospective trials comparing endoscopic to surgical therapy for chronic pancreatitis demonstrated that surgical therapy was superior to endoscopy at decreasing pain and improving quality of life in selected patients with dilated ducts and abdominal pain. This would suggest that chronic pancreatitis patients with dilated ducts and pain should be considered for surgical intervention. The role of preoperative stenting prior to surgery as a predictor of response has yet to be proven.

A Whipple procedure as well as total pancreatectomy and autologous islet cell transplantation have been used in selected patients with chronic pancreatitis and abdominal pain refractory to conventional therapy. The patients who have benefited the most from total pancreatectomy have chronic pancreatitis without prior pancreatic surgery or evidence of islet cell insufficiency. The role of this procedure remains to be fully defined but may be an option in lieu of ductal decompression surgery or pancreatic resection in patients with intractable, painful small-duct disease, particularly as the standard surgical procedures tend to decrease islet cell yield. Celiac plexus block has not been demonstrated to provide long-lasting pain relief.

HEREDITARY PANCREATITIS

Hereditary pancreatitis is a rare disease that is similar to chronic pancreatitis except for an early age of onset and evidence of hereditary factors (involving an autosomal dominant gene with incomplete penetrance). A genomewide search using genetic

TABLE 313-8 Frequently Utilized Pancreatic Enzyme Preparations

Enzyme Preparations	Manufacturer, Location	Lipase*	Protease*	Amylase*
Enteric Coated (EC)				
Ultrase	Axcan Pharma, Birmingham, AL			
[EC microspheres in capsules]				
Ultrase		4,500	25,000	20,000
Ultrase 12		12,000	39,000	39,000
Ultrase 18		18,000	58,500	58,500
Ultrase 20		20,000	65,000	65,000
Creon	Solvay Pharmaceuticals, Marietta, GA			
[delayed-release capsules containing EC spheres]				
Creon 6		6,000	19,000	30,000
Creon 12		12,000	38,000	60,000
Creon 24		24,000	76,000	120,000
Pancrease	Ortho-McNeil Pharmaceuticals, Riritan, NJ			
[EC microtablets in capsule]				
Pancrease MT 4		4,000	12,000	12,000
Pancrease MT 10		10,000	30,000	30,000
Pancrease MT 16		16,000	48,000	48,000
Pancrease MT 20		20,000	44,000	56,000
Pancreacarb	Digestive Care, Inc., Bethlehem, PA			
[EC microspheres (buffered) in delayed-release capsule]				
Pancreacarb MS-8		8,000	45,000	40,000
Nonenteric Coated				
Viokase	Axcan Scandipharm, Birmingham, AL			
(pancrelipase, USP) Tablets, Powder				
Viokase 8		8,000	30,000	30,000
Viokase 16		16,000	60,000	60,000
Viokase Powder: Lactose, sodium chloride, each 0.7 g (1/4 teaspoonful)		16,800	70,000	70,000
Kuzyme/Ku-trase	UCB Inc., Rochester, NY			
Ku-zyme		1,200	15,000	15,000
Kutrase		1,200	30,000	30,000

*United States Pharmacopeia (USP) units per tablet or capsule

Note: FDA has mandated all enzyme manufacturers to submit new drug applications (NDAs) for all pancreatic extract drug products after reviewing data that showed substantial variations among currently marketed products. Numerous manufacturers have investigations underway to seek FDA approval for the treatment of exocrine pancreatic insufficiency (EPI) due to cystic fibrosis (CF) or other conditions under the new guidelines for this class of drugs (www.fda.gov).

linkage analysis identified the hereditary pancreatitis gene on chromosome 7. Mutations in ion codons 29 (exon 2) and 122 (exon 3) of the cationic trypsinogen gene cause autosomal dominant forms of hereditary pancreatitis. The codon 122 mutations lead to a substitution of the corresponding arginine with another amino acid, usually histidine. This substitution, when it occurs, eliminates a fail-safe trypsin self-destruction site necessary to eliminate trypsin that is prematurely activated within the acinar cell. These patients have recurring attacks of severe abdominal pain that may last from a few days to a few weeks. The serum amylase and lipase levels may be elevated during acute attacks but are usually normal. Patients frequently develop pancreatic calcification, diabetes mellitus, and steatorrhea; in addition, they have an increased incidence of pancreatic carcinoma, with the cumulative incidence being as high as 40% by age 70 years. A recent natural history study of hereditary pancreatitis in more than 200 patients from France reported that abdominal pain started in childhood at age 10 years, steatorrhea developed at age 29 years, diabetes at age 38 years, and pancreatic carcinoma at age 55 years. Such patients often require surgical ductal decompression for pain relief. Abdominal complaints in relatives of patients with hereditary pancreatitis should raise the question of pancreatic disease.

Pancreatic secretory trypsin inhibitor (PSTI) gene mutations

PSTI, or SPINK1, is a 56-amino-acid peptide that specifically inhibits trypsin by physically blocking its active site. SPINK1 acts as the first line of defense against prematurely activated trypsinogen in the acinar cell. Recently, it has been shown that the frequency of SPINK1 mutations in patients with idiopathic chronic pancreatitis is markedly increased, suggesting that these mutations may be associated with pancreatitis.

PANCREATIC ENDOCRINE TUMORS

Pancreatic endocrine tumors are discussed in Chap. 350.

OTHER CONDITIONS

ANNULAR PANCREAS

When the ventral pancreatic anlage fails to migrate correctly to make contact with the dorsal anlage, the result may be a ring of pancreatic tissue encircling the duodenum. Such an annular pancreas may cause intestinal obstruction in the neonate or the adult. Symptoms of postprandial fullness, epigastric pain, nausea, and vomiting may be present for years before the diagnosis is entertained. The radiographic findings are symmetric dilation of the proximal duodenum with bulging of the recesses on either side of the annular band, effacement but not destruction of the duodenal mucosa, accentuation of the findings in the right anterior oblique position, and lack of change on repeated examinations. The differential diagnosis should include duodenal webs, tumors of the pancreas or duodenum, postbulbar peptic ulcer, regional enteritis, and adhesions. Patients with annular pancreas have an increased incidence of pancreatitis and peptic ulcer. Because of these and other potential complications, the treatment is surgical even if the condition has been present for years. Retrocolic duodenojejunostomy is the procedure of choice, although some surgeons advocate Billroth II gastrectomy, gastroenterostomy, and vagotomy.

PANCREAS DIVISUM

Pancreas divisum occurs when the embryologic ventral and dorsal pancreatic anlagen fail to fuse, so that pancreatic drainage is accomplished mainly through the accessory papilla. Pancreas divisum is the most common congenital anatomic variant of the human pancreas. Current evidence indicates that this anomaly does not predispose to the development of pancreatitis in the great majority of patients who harbor it. However, the combination of pancreas divisum and a small accessory orifice could result in dorsal duct obstruction. The challenge is to identify this subset of patients with dorsal duct pathology. Cannulation of the dorsal duct by ERCP is not as easily done as is cannulation of the ventral duct. Patients with pancreatitis and pancreas divisum demonstrated by MRCP or ERCP should be treated with conservative measures. In many of these patients, pancreatitis is idiopathic and unrelated to the pancreas divisum. Endoscopic or surgical intervention is indicated only if pancreatitis recurs and no other cause can be found. If marked dilation of the dorsal duct can be demonstrated, surgical ductal decompression should be performed. It should be stressed that the ERCP appearance of pancreas divisum (i.e., a small-caliber ventral duct with an arborizing pattern) may be mistaken as representing an obstructed main pancreatic duct secondary to a mass lesion.

MACROAMYLASEMIA

In macroamylasemia, amylase circulates in the blood in a polymer form too large to be easily excreted by the kidney. Patients with this condition demonstrate an elevated serum amylase value, a low urinary amylase value, and a C_{am}/C_{cr} ratio of <1%. The presence of macroamylase can be documented by chromatography of the serum. The prevalence of macroamylasemia is 1.5% of the nonalcoholic general adult hospital population. Usually macroamylasemia is an incidental finding and is not related to disease of the pancreas or other organs.

Macrolipasemia has now been documented in a few patients with cirrhosis or non-Hodgkin's lymphoma. In these patients, the pancreas appeared normal on ultrasound and CT examination. Lipase was shown to be complexed with immunoglobulin A. Thus, the possibility of *both* macroamylasemia and macrolipasemia should be considered in patients with elevated blood levels of these enzymes.

ACKNOWLEDGMENTS

This chapter represents a revised version of the chapter by Dr. Norton J. Greenberger and Dr. Phillip P. Toskes that was in the previous editions of Harrison's.

FURTHER READINGS

Banks PA, Freeman M: Practice guidelines in acute pancreatitis. Am J Gastroenterol 101:2379, 2006

Conwell DL et al: An endoscopic pancreatic function test with synthetic porcine secretin for the evaluation of chronic abdominal pain and suspected chronic pancreatitis. Gastrointest Endosc 57:37, 2003

Forsmark CE: The early diagnosis of chronic pancreatitis. Clin Gastroenterol Hepatol 6:1291, 2008

Pandol SJ et al: Acute pancreatitis: Bench to the bedside. Gastroenterology 132:1127, 2007

Rebours V et al: The natural history of hereditary pancreatitis: A national series. Gut 58:97, 2009

Thomson A: Enteral versus parenteral nutritional support in acute pancreatitis: A clinical review. J Gastroenterol Hepatol 21:22, 2006

van Santvoort HC et al: A step-up approach or open necrosectomy for necrotizing pancreatitis. N Engl J Med 362:1491, 2010

Waljee AK et al: Systematic review: Pancreatic enzyme treatment of malabsorption associated with chronic pancreatitis. Aliment Pharmacol Ther 29:235, 2008

Whitcomb DC et al: Hereditary pancreatitis is caused by a mutation in the cationic trypsinogen gene. Nat Genet 14:141, 1996

Witt H et al: Chronic pancreatitis: Challenges and advances in pathogenesis, genetics, diagnosis, and therapy. Gastroenterology 132:1557, 2007

Wu BU, Conwell DL: Acute pancreatitis part I: Approach to early management. Clin Gastroenterol Hepatol 8:410, 2010

——— et al: The early prediction of mortality in acute pancreatitis: A large population-based study. Gut 57:1698, 2008

——— et al: Early changes in blood urea nitrogen mortality in acute pancreatitis. Gastroenterology 137:129, 2009

PART 15

Disorders of the Joints and Adjacent Tissues

SECTION 1 The Immune System in Health and Disease

SECTION 2 Disorders of Immune-Mediated Injury

SECTION 3 Disorders of the Joints and Adjacent Tissues

CHAPTER 314

Introduction to the Immune System

Barton F. Haynes
Kelly A. Soderberg
Anthony S. Fauci

DEFINITIONS

- *Adaptive immune system*—recently evolved system of immune responses mediated by T and B lymphocytes. Immune responses by these cells are based on specific antigen recognition by clonotypic receptors that are products of genes that rearrange during development and throughout the life of the organism. Additional cells of the adaptive immune system include various types of antigen-presenting cells.
- *Antibody*—B cell–produced molecules encoded by genes that rearrange during B cell development consisting of immunoglobulin heavy and light chains that together form the central component of the B cell receptor for antigen. Antibody can exist as B cell–surface antigen-recognition molecules or as secreted molecules in plasma and other body fluids (Table 314-13).
- *Antigens*—foreign or self-molecules that are recognized by the adaptive and innate immune systems resulting in immune cell triggering, T cell activation, and/or B cell antibody production.
- *Antimicrobial peptides*—small peptides <100 amino acids in length that are produced by cells of the innate immune system and have anti-infectious agent activity (Table 314-2).
- *Apoptosis*—the process of *programmed cell death* whereby signaling through various "death receptors" on the surface of cells [e.g., tumor necrosis factor (TNF) receptors, CD95] leads to a signaling cascade that involves activation of the caspase family of molecules and leads to DNA cleavage and cell death. Apoptosis, which does not lead to induction of inordinate inflammation, is to be contrasted with *cell necrosis*, which does lead to induction of inflammatory responses.
- *Autoimmune diseases*—diseases such as systemic lupus erythematosus and rheumatoid arthritis in which cells of the adaptive immune system such as autoreactive T and B cells become overreactive and produce self-reactive T cell and antibody responses.
- *Autoinflammatory diseases*—hereditary disorders such as hereditary periodic fevers (HPFs) characterized by recurrent episodes of severe inflammation and fever due to mutations in controls of the innate inflammatory response, i.e., the inflammasome (see below and Table 314-6). Patients with HPFs also have rashes and serosal and joint inflammation and some can have neurologic symptoms. Autoinflammatory diseases are different from autoimmune diseases in that evidence for activation of adaptive immune cells such as autoreactive B cells is not present.
- *B cell receptor for antigen*—complex of surface molecules that rearrange during postnatal B cell development, made up of surface immunoglobulin (Ig) and associated Ig αβ chain molecules that recognize nominal antigen via Ig heavy- and light-chain variable regions, and signal the B cell to terminally differentiate to make antigen-specific antibody (Fig. 314-8).
- *B lymphocytes*—bone marrow–derived or bursal-equivalent lymphocytes that express surface immunoglobulin (the B cell receptor for antigen) and secrete specific antibody after interaction with antigen (Figs. 314-2 and 314-6).
- *CD classification of human lymphocyte differentiation antigens*—the development of monoclonal antibody technology led to the discovery of a large number of new leukocyte surface molecules. In 1982, the First International Workshop on Leukocyte Differentiation Antigens was held to establish a nomenclature for cell-surface molecules of human leukocytes. From this and subsequent leukocyte differentiation workshops has come the *cluster of differentiation* (CD) classification of leukocyte antigens (Table 314-1).
- *Chemokines*—soluble molecules that direct and determine immune cell movement and circulation pathways.
- *Complement*—cascading series of plasma enzymes and effector proteins whose function is to lyse pathogens and/or target them to be phagocytized by neutrophils and monocyte/macrophage lineage cells of the reticuloendothelial system (Fig. 314-5).
- *Co-stimulatory molecules*—molecules of antigen-presenting cells (such as B7-1 and B7-2 or CD40) that lead to T cell activation when bound by ligands on activated T cells (such as CD28 or CD40 ligand) (Fig. 314-7).
- *Cytokines*—soluble proteins that interact with specific cellular receptors that are involved in the regulation of the growth and activation of immune cells and mediate normal and pathologic inflammatory and immune responses (Tables 314-7, 314-9, and 314-10).
- *Dendritic cells*—myeloid and/or lymphoid lineage antigen-presenting cells of the adaptive immune system. Immature dendritic cells, or dendritic cell precursors, are key components of the innate immune system by responding to infections with production of high levels of cytokines. Dendritic cells are key initiators both of innate immune responses via cytokine production and of adaptive immune responses via presentation of antigen to T lymphocytes (Figs. 314-2 and 314-3, Table 314-5).
- *Inflammasome*—large cytoplasmic complexes of intracellular proteins that link the sensing of microbial products and cellular stress to the proteolytic activation of interleukin (IL)-1β and IL-18 inflammatory cytokines. Activation of molecules in the inflammasome is a key step in the response of the innate immune system for intracellular recognition of microbial and other danger signals in both health and pathologic states (Table 314-6).
- *Innate immune system*—ancient immune recognition system of host cells bearing germ line–encoded pattern recognition receptors (PRRs) that recognize pathogens and trigger a variety of mechanisms of pathogen elimination. Cells of the innate immune system include natural killer cell lymphocytes, monocytes/macrophages, dendritic cells, neutrophils, basophils, eosinophils, tissue mast cells, and epithelial cells (Tables 314-2 to 314-5 and 314-12).

- *Large granular lymphocytes*—lymphocytes of the innate immune system with azurophilic cytotoxic granules that have natural killer cell activity capable of killing foreign and host cells with few or no self–major histocompatibility complex (MHC) class I molecules (Fig. 314-4).
- *Natural killer cells*—large granular lymphocytes that kill target cells expressing few or no human leukocyte antigen (HLA) class I molecules, such as malignantly transformed cells and virally infected cells. Natural killer cells express receptors that inhibit killer cell function when self–major histocompatibility complex class I is present (Fig. 314-4).
- *Natural killer (NK) T cells* —innate-like lymphocytes that use an invariant T cell receptor (TCR)-α chain combined with a limited set of TCR-β chains and coexpress receptors commonly found on NK cells. NK T cells recognize lipid antigens of bacterial, viral, fungal, and protozoal infectious agents.
- *Pathogen-associated molecular patterns* (PAMPs)—Invariant molecular structures expressed by large groups of microorganisms that are recognized by host cellular pattern recognition receptors in the mediation of innate immunity (Fig. 314-1).
- *Pattern recognition receptors* (PRRs)—germ line–encoded receptors expressed by cells of the innate immune system that recognize pathogen-associated molecular patterns (Table 314-3).
- *Polyreactive natural antibodies*—preexisting low-affinity antibodies produced by innate B cells that cross-react with multiple antigens and are available at the time of infection to bind to and coat the invading pathogen and harness innate responses to slow the infection until an adaptive high-affinity protective antibody response can be made.
- *T cell receptor (TCR) for antigen*—complex of surface molecules that rearrange during postnatal T cell development made up of clonotypic TCR-α and -β chains that are associated with the CD3 complex composed of invariant γ, δ, ε, ζ, and η chains. TCR-α and -β chains recognize peptide fragments of protein antigen physically bound in antigen-presenting cell major histocompatibility complex class I or II molecules, leading to signaling via the CD3 complex to mediate effector functions (Fig. 314-7).
- *T cells*—thymus-derived lymphocytes that mediate adaptive cellular immune responses including T helper, T regulatory, and cytotoxic T lymphocyte effector cell functions (Figs. 314-2, 314-3, and 314-7).
- *Tolerance*—B and T cell nonresponsiveness to antigens that results from encounter with foreign or self-antigens by B and T lymphocytes in the absence of expression of antigen-presenting cell co-stimulatory molecules. Tolerance to antigens may be induced and maintained by multiple mechanisms either centrally (in the thymus for T cells or bone marrow for B cells) or peripherally at sites throughout the peripheral immune system.

INTRODUCTION

The human immune system has evolved over millions of years from both invertebrate and vertebrate organisms to develop sophisticated defense mechanisms to protect the host from microbes and their virulence factors. The normal immune system has three key properties: a highly diverse repertoire of antigen receptors that enables recognition of a nearly infinite range of pathogens; immune memory, to mount rapid recall immune responses; and immunologic tolerance, to avoid immune damage to normal self-tissues. From invertebrates, humans have inherited the *innate immune system*, an ancient defense system that uses germ line–encoded proteins to recognize pathogens. Cells of the innate immune system, such as macrophages, dendritic cells, and natural killer (NK) lymphocytes, recognize pathogen-associated molecular patterns (PAMPs) that are highly conserved among many microbes and use a diverse set of pattern recognition receptor molecules (PRRs). Important components of the recognition of microbes by the innate immune system include (1) recognition by germ line–encoded host molecules, (2) recognition of key microbe virulence factors but not recognition of self-molecules, and (3) nonrecognition of benign foreign molecules or microbes. Upon contact with pathogens, macrophages and NK cells may kill pathogens directly or, in concert with dendritic cells, may activate a series of events that both slow the infection and recruit the more recently evolved arm of the human immune system, the *adaptive immune system.*

Adaptive immunity is found only in vertebrates and is based on the generation of antigen receptors on T and B lymphocytes by gene rearrangements, such that individual T or B cells express unique antigen receptors on their surface capable of specifically recognizing diverse antigens of the myriad infectious agents in the environment. Coupled with finely tuned specific recognition mechanisms that maintain tolerance (nonreactivity) to self-antigens, T and B lymphocytes bring both *specificity* and *immune memory* to vertebrate host defenses.

This chapter describes the cellular components, key molecules (Table 314-1), and mechanisms that make up the innate and adaptive immune systems and describes how adaptive immunity is recruited to the defense of the host by innate immune responses. An appreciation of the cellular and molecular bases of innate and adaptive immune responses is critical to understanding the pathogenesis of inflammatory, autoimmune, infectious, and immunodeficiency diseases.

THE INNATE IMMUNE SYSTEM

All multicellular organisms, including humans, have developed the use of a limited number of surface and intracellular germ line–encoded molecules that recognize large groups of pathogens. Because of the myriad human pathogens, host molecules of the human innate immune system sense "danger signals" and either recognize PAMPs, the common molecular structures shared by many pathogens, or recognize host cell molecules produced in response to infection such as heat shock proteins and fragments of the extracellular matrix. PAMPs must be conserved structures vital to pathogen virulence and survival, such as bacterial endotoxin, so that pathogens cannot mutate molecules of PAMPs to evade human innate immune responses. PRRs are host proteins of the innate immune system that recognize PAMPs as host danger signal molecules (Tables 314-2 and 314-3). Thus, recognition of pathogen molecules by hematopoietic and nonhematopoietic cell types leads to activation/production of the complement cascade, cytokines, and antimicrobial peptides as effector molecules. In addition, pathogen PAMPs as host danger signal molecules activate dendritic cells to mature and to express molecules on the dendritic cell surface that optimize antigen presentation to respond to foreign antigens.

PATTERN RECOGNITION

Major PRR families of proteins include C-type lectins, leucine-rich proteins, macrophage scavenger receptor proteins, plasma pentraxins, lipid transferases, and integrins (Table 314-3). A major group of PRR collagenous glycoproteins with C-type lectin domains are termed *collectins* and include the serum protein mannose-binding lectin (MBL). MBL and other collectins, as well as two other protein families—the pentraxins (such as C-reactive protein and serum amyloid P) and macrophage scavenger receptors—all have the property of opsonizing (coating) bacteria for phagocytosis by macrophages and can also activate the complement cascade to lyse bacteria. Integrins are cell-surface adhesion molecules that signal after cells bind bacterial lipopolysaccharide (LPS) and activate phagocytic cells to ingest pathogens.

TABLE 314-1 Human Leukocyte Surface Antigens—The CD Classification of Leukocyte Differentiation Antigens

Surface Antigen (Other Names)	Family	Molecular Mass, kDa	Distribution	Ligand(s)	Function
CD1a (T6, HTA-1)	Ig	49	CD, cortical thymocytes, Langerhans type of dendritic cells	TCRγδ T cells	CD1 molecules present lipid antigens of intracellular bacteria such as *Mycobacterium leprae* and *M. tuberculosis* to TCRγδ T cells.
CD1b	Ig	45	CD, cortical thymocytes, Langerhans type of dendritic cells	TCRγδ T cells	
CD1c	Ig	43	DC, cortical thymocytes, subset of B cells, Langerhans type of dendritic cells	TCRγδ T cells	
CD1d	Ig	?	Cortical thymocytes, intestinal epithelium, Langerhans type of dendritic cells	TCRγδ T cells	
CD2 (T12, LFA-2)	Ig	50	T, NK	CD58, CD48, CD59, CD15	Alternative T cell activation, T cell anergy, T cell cytokine production, T- or NK-mediated cytolysis, T cell apoptosis, cell adhesion
CD3 (T3, Leu-4)	Ig	γ:25–28, δ:21–28, ε:20–25, η:21–22, ζ:16	T	Associates with the TCR	T cell activation and function; ζ is the signal transduction component of the CD3 complex
CD4 (T4, Leu-3)	Ig	55	T, myeloid	MHC-II, HIV, gp120, IL-16, SABP	T cell selection, T cell activation, signal transduction with p56*lck*, primary receptor for HIV
CD7 (3A1, Leu-9)	Ig	40	T, NK	K-12 (CD7L)	T and NK cell signal transduction and regulation of IFN-γ, TNF-α production
CD8 (T8, Leu-2)	Ig	34	T	MHC-I	T cell selection, T cell activation, signal transduction with p56*lck*
CD14 (LPS-receptor)	LRG	53–55	M, G (weak), not by myeloid progenitors	Endotoxin (lipopolysaccharide), lipoteichoic acid, PI	TLR4 mediates with LPS and other PAMP activation of innate immunity
CD19 B4	Ig	95	B (except plasma cells), FDC	Not known	Associates with CD21 and CD81 to form a complex involved in signal transduction in B cell development, activation, and differentiation
CD20 (B1)	Unassigned	33–37	B (except plasma cells)	Not known	Cell signaling, may be important for B cell activation and proliferation
CD21 (B2, CR2, EBV-R, C3dR)	RCA	145	Mature B, FDC, subset of thymocytes	C3d, C3dg, iC3b, CD23, EBV	Associates with CD19 and CD81 to form a complex involved in signal transduction in B cell development, activation, and differentiation; Epstein-Barr virus receptor
CD22 (BL-CAM)	Ig	130–140	Mature B	CDw75	Cell adhesion, signaling through association with p72*sky*, p53/56*lyn*, PI3 kinase, SHP1, fLCγ
CD23 (FcεRII, B6, Leu-20, BLAST-2)	C-type lectin	45	B, M, FDC	IgE, CD21, CD11b, CD11c	Regulates IgE synthesis, cytokine release by monocytes
CD28	Ig	44	T, plasma cells	CD80, CD86	Co-stimulatory for T cell activation; involved in the decision between T cell activation and anergy

(*continued*)

TABLE 314-1 Human Leukocyte Surface Antigens—The CD Classification of Leukocyte Differentiation Antigens (*Continued*)

Surface Antigen (Other Names)	Family	Molecular Mass, kDa	Distribution	Ligand(s)	Function
CD40	TNFR	48–50	B, DC, EC, thymic epithelium, MP, cancers	CD154	B cell activation, proliferation, and differentiation; formation of GCs; isotype switching; rescue from apoptosis
CD45 (LCA, T200, B220)	PTP	180, 200, 210, 220	All leukocytes	Galectin-1, CD2, CD3, CD4	T and B activation, thymocyte development, signal transduction, apoptosis
CD45RA	PTP	210, 220	Subset T, medullary thymocytes, "naive" T	Galectin-1, CD2, CD3, CD4	Isoforms of CD45 containing exon 4 (A), restricted to a subset of T cells
CD45RB	PTP	200, 210, 220	All leukocytes	Galectin-1, CD2, CD3, CD4	Isoforms of CD45 containing exon 5 (B)
CD45RC	PTP	210, 220	Subset T, medullary thymocytes, "naive" T	Galectin-1, CD2, CD3, CD4	Isoforms of CD45 containing exon 6 (C), restricted to a subset of T cells
CD45RO	PTP	180	Subset T, cortical thymocytes, "memory" T	Galectin-1, CD2, CD3, CD4	Isoforms of CD45 containing no differentially spliced exons, restricted to a subset of T cells
CD80 (B7-1, BB1)	Ig	60	Activated B and T, MP, DC	CD28, CD152	Co-regulator of T cell activation; signaling through CD28 stimulates and through CD152 inhibits T cell activation
CD86 (B7-2, B70)	Ig	80	Subset B, DC, EC, activated T, thymic epithelium	CD28, CD152	Co-regulator of T cell activation; signaling through CD28 stimulates and through CD152 inhibits T cell activation
CD95 (APO-1, Fas)	TNFR	135	Activated T and B	Fas ligand	Mediates apoptosis
CD152 (CTLA-4)	Ig	30–33	Activated T	CD80, CD86	Inhibits T cell proliferation
CD154 (CD40L)	TNF	33	Activated CD4+ T, subset CD8+ T, NK, M, basophil	CD40	Co-stimulatory for T cell activation, B cell proliferation and differentiation

Abbreviations: CTLA, cytotoxic T lymphocyte–associated protein; DC, dendritic cells; EBV, Epstein-Barr virus; EC, endothelial cells; ECM, extracellular matrix; Fcγ RIIIA, low-affinity IgG receptor isoform A; FDC, follicular dendritic cells; G, granulocytes; GC, germinal center; GPI, glycosyl phosphatidylinositol; HTA, human thymocyte antigen; IgG, immunoglobulin G; LCA, leukocyte common antigen; LPS, lipopolysaccharide; MHC-I, major histocompatibility complex class I; MP, macrophages; Mr, relative molecular mass; NK, natural killer cells; P, platelets; PBT, peripheral blood T cells; PI, phosphatidylinositol; PI3K, phosphatidylinositol 3-kinase; PLC, phospholipase C; PTP, protein tyrosine phosphatase; TCR, T cell receptor; TNF, tumor necrosis factor; TNFR, tumor necrosis factor receptor. For an expanded list of cluster of differentiation (CD) human antigens, see Harrison's Online at *http://www.accessmedicine.com;* and for a full list of CD human antigens from the most recent Human Workshop on Leukocyte Differentiation Antigens (VII), see *http://mpr.nci.nih.gov/prow/.*

Source: Compiled from T Kishimoto et al (eds): *Leukocyte Typing VI*, New York, Garland Publishing 1997; R Brines et al: Immunology Today 18S:1, 1997; and S Shaw (ed): *Protein Reviews on the Web, http://mpr.nci.nih.gov/prow/.*

There are multiple connections between the innate and adaptive immune systems; these include (1) a plasma protein, LPS-binding protein, which binds and transfers LPS to the macrophage LPS receptor, CD14; (2) a human family of proteins called *Toll-like receptor proteins* (TLRs), some of which are associated with CD14, bind LPS, and signal epithelial cells, dendritic cells, and macrophages to produce cytokines and upregulate cell-surface molecules that signal the initiation of adaptive immune responses (Fig. 314-1, Tables 314-3 and 314-4), and (3) families of intracellular microbial sensors called NOD-like receptors (NLRs) and RIG-like helicases (RLHs). Proteins in the Toll family can be expressed on macrophages, dendritic cells, and B cells as well as on a variety of nonhematopoietic cell types, including respiratory epithelial cells. Ten TLRs have been identified in humans and 13 TLRs in mice (Tables 314-4 and 314-5). Upon ligation, TLRs activate a series of intracellular events that lead to the killing of bacteria- and viral-infected cells as well as to the recruitment and ultimate activation of antigen-specific T and B lymphocytes (Fig. 314-1). Importantly, signaling by massive amounts of LPS through TLR4 leads to the release of large amounts of cytokines that mediate LPS-induced shock. Mutations in TLR4 proteins in mice protect from LPS shock, and TLR mutations in humans protect from LPS-induced inflammatory diseases such as LPS-induced asthma (Fig. 314-1).

Two other families of intracellular PRRs are the NLRs (NOD-like receptors) and the RLHs (RIG-like helicases). These families, unlike the TLRs, are composed primarily of soluble intracellular proteins that scan the cytoplasm for intracellular pathogens (Tables 314-2 and 314-3).

TABLE 314-2 Major Components of the Innate Immune System

Pattern recognition receptors (PRR)	C-type lectins, leucine-rich proteins, scavenger receptors, pentraxins, lipid transferases, integrins, inflammasome proteins
Antimicrobial peptides	α-Defensins, β-defensins, cathelin, protegrin, granulysin, histatin, secretory leukoprotease inhibitor, and probiotics
Cells	Macrophages, dendritic cells, NK cells, NK-T cells, neutrophils, eosinophils, mast cells, basophils, and epithelial cells
Complement components	Classic and alternative complement pathway, and proteins that bind complement components
Cytokines	Autocrine, paracrine, endocrine cytokines that mediate host defense and inflammation, as well as recruit, direct, and regulate adaptive immune responses

Abbreviation: NK cells, natural killer cells.

The intracellular microbial sensors, NLRs, after triggering, form large cytoplasmic complexes termed *inflammasomes*, which are aggregates of molecules including NOD-like receptor pyrin (NLRP) proteins that are members of the NLR family (Table 314-3). Inflammasomes activate inflammatory caspases and IL-1β in the presence of nonbacterial danger signals (cell stress) and bacterial PAMPs. Mutations in inflammasome proteins can lead to chronic inflammation in a group of periodic febrile diseases called *autoinflammatory syndromes* (Table 314-6).

■ EFFECTOR CELLS OF INNATE IMMUNITY

Cells of the innate immune system and their roles in the first line of host defense are listed in Table 314-5. Equally important as their roles in the mediation of innate immune responses are the roles that each cell type plays in recruiting T and B lymphocytes of the adaptive immune system to engage in specific antipathogen responses.

Monocytes-macrophages

Monocytes arise from precursor cells within bone marrow (Fig. 314-2) and circulate with a half-life ranging from 1 to 3 days. Monocytes leave the peripheral circulation by marginating in capillaries and migrating into a vast extravascular pool. Tissue macrophages arise from monocytes that have migrated out of the circulation and by in situ proliferation of macrophage precursors in tissue. Common locations where tissue macrophages (and certain of their specialized forms) are found are lymph node, spleen, bone marrow, perivascular connective tissue, serous cavities such as the peritoneum, pleura, skin connective tissue, lung (alveolar macrophages), liver (Kupffer cells), bone (osteoclasts), central nervous system (microglia cells), and synovium (type A lining cells).

In general, monocytes-macrophages are on the first line of defense associated with innate immunity and ingest and destroy microorganisms through the release of toxic products such as hydrogen peroxide (H_2O_2) and nitric oxide (NO). Inflammatory mediators

TABLE 314-3 Major Pattern Recognition Receptors (PRR) of the Innate Immune System

PRR Protein Family	Sites of Expression	Examples	Ligands (PAMPs)	Functions of PRR
Toll-like receptors	Multiple cell types	TLR2-10	Bacterial and viral carbohydrates	Activate innate immune cells to respond to multiple pathogens and initiate adaptive immune responses
C-type Lectins	Plasma proteins	Collectins		Opsonization of bacteria and virus, activation of complement
Humoral			Terminal mannose	
Cellular	Macrophages, dendritic cell	Macrophage mannose receptor	Carbohydrate on HLA molecules	Phagocytosis of pathogens
	Natural killer (NK) cells	NKG2-A		Inhibits killing of host cells expressing HLA + self-peptides
Leucine-rich proteins	Macrophages, dendritic cells, epithelial cells	CD14	Lipopolysaccharide (LPS)	Binds LPS and Toll proteins
Scavenger receptors	Macrophage	Macrophage scavenger receptors	Bacterial cell walls	Phagocytosis of bacteria
Pentraxins	Plasma protein	C-reactive proteins	Phosphatidyl choline	Opsonization of bacteria, activation of complement
	Plasma protein	Serum amyloid P	Bacterial cell walls	Opsonization of bacteria, activation of complement
Lipid transferases	Plasma protein	LPS binding protein	LPS	Binds LPS, transfers LPS to CD14
Integrins	Macrophages, dendritic cells, NK cells	CD11b,c; CD18	LPS	Signals cells, activates phagocytosis
NOD-like Receptors	Innate cells	NALP-3	Viral DNA Bacterial muramyl dipeptide	Cytosolic proteins involved in innate sensing

Abbreviation: PAMPs, pathogen-associated molecular patterns.

Source: Adapted from R Medzhitov, CA Janeway: Curr Opin Immunol 9:4, 1997. Copyright 1997, with permission from Elsevier.

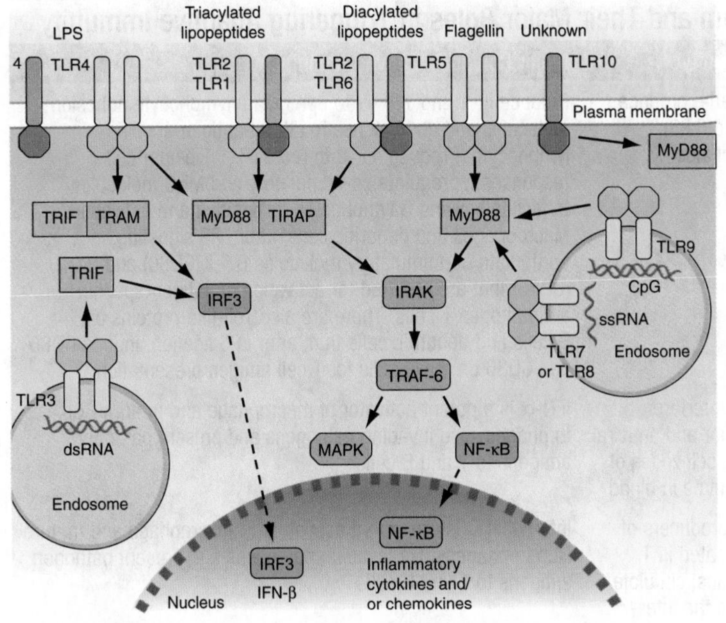

Figure 314-1 Overview of major TLR signaling pathways. All TLRs signal through MyD88, with the exception of TLR3. TLR4 and the TLR2 subfamily (TLR1, TLR2, TLR6) also engage TIRAP. TLR3 signals through TRIF. TRIF is also used in conjunction with TRAM in the TLR4–MyD88-independent pathway. Dashed arrrows indicate translocation into the nucleus. LPS, lipopolysaccharide; dsRNA, double-strand RNA; ssRNA, single-strand RNA; MAPK, mitogen-activated protein kinases; NF-κB, nuclear factor-κB; IFN, interferon; IRF3, interferon regulatory factor 3; TLR, Toll-like receptor. *(Adapted from D van Duin et al., with permission.)*

TABLE 314-4 The Role of Pattern Recognition Receptors (PRRs) in Modulation of Adaptive Immune Responses

PRR Family	PRRs	Ligand	DC or Macrophage Cytokine Response	Adaptive Immune Response
TLRs	TLR2 (heterodimer with TLR1 or 6)	Lipopeptides Pam-3-cys (TLR 2/1) MALP (TLR 2/6)	Low IL-12p70 High IL-10 IL-6	T_H1 T_H2 T regulatory
	TLR3	dsRNA	IL-12p70 IFN-α IL-6	T_H1
	TLR4	*E. coli* LPS	High IL-12p70 Intermediate IL-10 IL-6	T_H1
	TLR5	Flagellin	High IL-12p70 Low IL-12p70	T_H1 T_H2
	TLR7/8	ssRNA Imidazoquinolines	High IL-12p70 IFN-α IL-6	T_H1
	TLR9	CpG DNA	High IL-12p70 Low IL-10 IL-6 IFN-α	T_H1
	TLR10	?	?	?
C-type lectins	DC-SIGN	Env of HIV; core protein of HCV; components of *Mycobacterium tuberculosis; Helicobacter pylori*, Lewis Ag	*H. pylori*, Lewis Ag Suppresses IL-12p70 Suppresses TLR signaling in DCs	T_H2 T regulatory
NOD	NOD2	Muramyl dipeptide of peptidoglycan	Induces IL-10 in DCs	Weak T cell response (tolerogenic?)
Mannose receptor	Mannose receptor	Mannosylated lipoarabinomannans from bacillus Calmette-Guerin and *M. tuberculosis*	Suppresses IL-12 and TLR signaling in DCs	Weak T cell response? (tolerogenic?)

Abbreviations: dsRNA, double-strand RNA; ssRNA, single-strand RNA; LPS, lipopolysaccharide; T_H2, helper T cell; T_H1, helper T cell; CpG, sequences in DNA recognized by TLR-9; MALP, macrophage-activating lipopeptide; DC-SIGN, DC-specific C-type lectin; NOD, NOTCH protein domain; TLR, Toll-like receptor; HCV, hepatitis C.

Source: B Pulendran: J Immunol 174:2457, 2005. Copyright 2005 The American Association of Immunologists, Inc., with permission.

TABLE 314-5 Cells of the Innate Immune System and Their Major Roles in Triggering Adaptive Immunity

Cell Type	Major Role in Innate Immunity	Major Role in Adaptive Immunity
Macrophages	Phagocytose and kill bacteria; produce antimicrobial peptides; bind (LPS); produce inflammatory cytokines	Produce IL-1 and TNF-α to upregulate lymphocyte adhesion molecules and chemokines to attract antigen-specific lymphocyte. Produce IL-12 to recruit T_H1 T helper cell responses; upregulate co-stimulatory and MHC molecules to facilitate T and B lymphocyte recognition and activation. Macrophages and dendritic cells, after LPS signaling, upregulate co-stimulatory molecules B7-1 (CD80) and B7-2 (CD86) that are required for activation of antigen-specific antipathogen T cells. There are also Toll-like proteins on B cells and dendritic cells that, after LPS ligation, induce CD80 and CD86 on these cells for T cell antigen presentation.
Plasmacytoid f dendritic cells (DCs) of lymphoid lineage	Produce large amounts of interferon-α (IFN-α), which has antitumor and antiviral activity, and are found in T cell zones of lymphoid organs; they circulate in blood	IFN-α is a potent activator of macrophage and mature DCs to phagocytose invading pathogens and present pathogen antigens to T and B cells
Myeloid dendritic cells are of two types; interstitial and Langerhans-derived	Interstitial DCs are strong producers of IL-12 and IL-10 and are located in T cell zones of lymphoid organs, circulate in blood, and are present in the interstices of the lung, heart, and kidney; Langerhans DCs are strong producers of IL-12; are located in T cell zones of lymph nodes, skin epithelia, and the thymic medulla; and circulate in blood	Interstitial DCs are potent activators of macrophage and mature DCs to phagocytose invading pathogens and present pathogen antigens to T and B cells
Natural killer (NK) cells	Kill foreign and host cells that have low levels of MHC+ self-peptides. Express NK receptors that inhibit NK function in the presence of high expression of self-MHC.	Produce TNF-α and IFN-γ, which recruit T_H1 helper T cell responses
NK-T cells	Lymphocytes with both T cell and NK surface markers that recognize lipid antigens of intracellular bacteria such as *Mycobacterium tuberculosis* by CD1 molecules and kill host cells infected with intracellular bacteria.	Produce IL-4 to recruit T_H2 helper T cell responses, IgG1 and IgE production
Neutrophils	Phagocytose and kill bacteria, produce antimicrobial peptides	Produce nitric oxide synthase and nitric oxide, which inhibit apoptosis in lymphocytes and can prolong adaptive immune responses
Eosinophils	Kill invading parasites	Produce IL-5, which recruits Ig-specific antibody responses
Mast cells and basophils	Release TNF-α, IL-6, and IFN-γ in response to a variety of bacterial PAMPs	Produce IL-4, which recruits T_H2 helper T cell responses and recruit IgG1- and IgE-specific antibody responses
Epithelial cells	Produce antimicrobial peptides; tissue-specific epithelia produce mediator of local innate immunity; e.g., lung epithelial cells produce surfactant proteins (proteins within the collectin family) that bind and promote clearance of lung-invading microbes	Produces TGF-β, which triggers IgA-specific antibody responses

Abbreviations: LPS, lipopolysaccharide; PAMP, pathogen-associated molecular patterns; TNF-α, tumor necrosis factor-alpha; IL-4, IL-5, IL-6, IL-10, and IL-12, interleukin 4, 5, 6, 10, and 12, respectively.

Source: Adapted from R Medzhitov, CA Janeway: Curr Opinion Immunol 9:4, 1997. Copyright 1997, with permission from Elsevier.

produced by macrophages attract additional effector cells such as neutrophils to the site of infection. Macrophage mediators include prostaglandins; leukotrienes; platelet activating factor; cytokines such as interleukin (IL)-1, tumor necrosis factor (TNF)-α, IL-6, and IL-12; and chemokines (Tables 314-7 to 314-10).

Although monocytes-macrophages were originally thought to be the major antigen-presenting cells (APCs) of the immune system, it is now clear that cell types called dendritic cells are the most potent and effective APCs in the body (see below). Monocytes-macrophages mediate innate immune effector functions such as destruction of antibody-coated bacteria, tumor cells, or even normal hematopoietic cells in certain types of autoimmune cytopenias. Monocytes-macrophages ingest bacteria or are infected by viruses, and in doing so, they frequently undergo programmed

TABLE 314-6 Diseases Associated With Inflammasome Activity

Disease	Clinical Features	Gene Mutated	Etiologic Agent	Inflammasome Involvement	*Anakinra Response
Familial cold autoinflammatory syndrome (FCAS)	Fever, arthralgia, cold-induced urticaria	NALP3		Overactive	Yes
Muckle-Wells syndrome (MWS)	Fever, arthralgia, urticaria, sensorineural deafness, amyloidosis	NAPL3		Overactive	Yes
Chronic infantile neurologic cutaneous and articular syndrome (CINCA, NOMID)	Fever, severe arthralgia, urticaria, neurologic problems, severe amyloidosis	NALP3		Overactive	Yes
Familial Mediterranean fever (FMF)	Fever, peritonitis, pleuritis, amyloidosis	Pyrin		Overactive	Partial
Pyogenic arthritis, pyoderma gangrenosum, and acne syndrome (PAPA)	Pyogenic sterile arthritis	PSTPIP1		Overactive	Yes
Hyperimmunoglobulin D syndrome (HIDS)	Arthralgia, abdominal pain, lymphadenopathy	Mevalonate kinase		To be demonstrated	Yes
Tumor necrosis factor receptor-1–associated syndrome (TRAPS)	Fever, abdominal pain, skin lesions	TNF-R1		To be demonstrated	Yes
Systemic onset juvenile idiopathic arthritis (SOJIA)	Chronic joint inflammation		Unknown	To be demonstrated	Yes
Adult-onset Still's disease (AOSD)	Arthralgia, fever		Unknown	To be demonstrated	Yes
Behçet's disease	Arthralgia, uveitis, ulcers		Unknown	To be demonstrated	Yes
Schnitzler's syndrome	Urticaria, fever, arthralgia		Unknown	To be demonstrated	Yes
Gout	Metabolic arthritis, pain		Uric acid (MSU)	Activated	Yes
Pseudogout	Arthritis		CPPD	Activated	Yes
Contact dermatitis	Urticaria		Irritants	Activated	Unknown
Fever syndrome	Fever	NALP12		Unknown	Unknown
Hydatidiform mole	Hydatid mole	NALP7		Unknown	Unknown
Vitiligo	Skin depigmentation, autoimmunity	NALP1		Unknown	Unknown

*Anakinra is a recombinant IL-1 receptor antagonist that functions to block the biologic activity of naturally occuring interleukin-1 (IL-1).

Source: From F Martinon et al: Ann Rev Immunol 27:229, 2009. Copyright 2009. Reproduced with permission from Annual Reviews Inc.

cell death or *apoptosis*. Macrophages that are infected by intracellular infectious agents are recognized by dendritic cells as infected and apoptotic cells and are phagocytosed by dendritic cells. In this manner, dendritic cells "cross-present" infectious agent antigens of macrophages to T cells. Activated macrophages can also mediate antigen-nonspecific lytic activity and eliminate cell types such as tumor cells in the absence of antibody. This activity is largely mediated by cytokines (i.e., TNF-α and IL-1). Monocytes-macrophages express lineage-specific molecules (e.g., the cell-surface LPS receptor, CD14) as well as surface receptors for a number of molecules, including the Fc region of IgG, activated complement components, and various cytokines (Table 314-7).

Dendritic cells

Human dendritic cells (DCs) are heterogenous and contain several subsets, including myeloid DCs and plasmacytoid DCs. Myeloid DCs can differentiate into either macrophages-monocytes or tissue-specific DCs. In contrast to myeloid DCs, plasmacytoid DCs are inefficient antigen-presenting cells but are potent producers of type I interferon (IFN) (e.g., IFN-α) in response to viral infections. The maturation of DCs is regulated through cell-to-cell contact and soluble factors, and DCs attract immune effectors through secretion of chemokines. When DCs come in contact with bacterial products, viral proteins, or host proteins released as danger signals from distressed host cells (Figs. 314-2 and 314-3), infectious agent molecules bind to various TLRs and activate DCs to release cytokines and chemokines that drive cells of the innate immune system to become activated to respond to the invading organism, and recruit T and B cells of the adaptive immune system to respond. Plasmacytoid DCs produce antiviral IFN-α that activates NK cell killing of pathogen-infected cells; IFN-α also activates T cells to mature into antipathogen cytotoxic (killer) T cells. Following contact with pathogens, both plasmacytoid and myeloid DCs produce chemokines that attract helper and cytotoxic T cells, B cells, polymorphonuclear cells, and naïve and memory T cells as well as regulatory T cells to ultimately

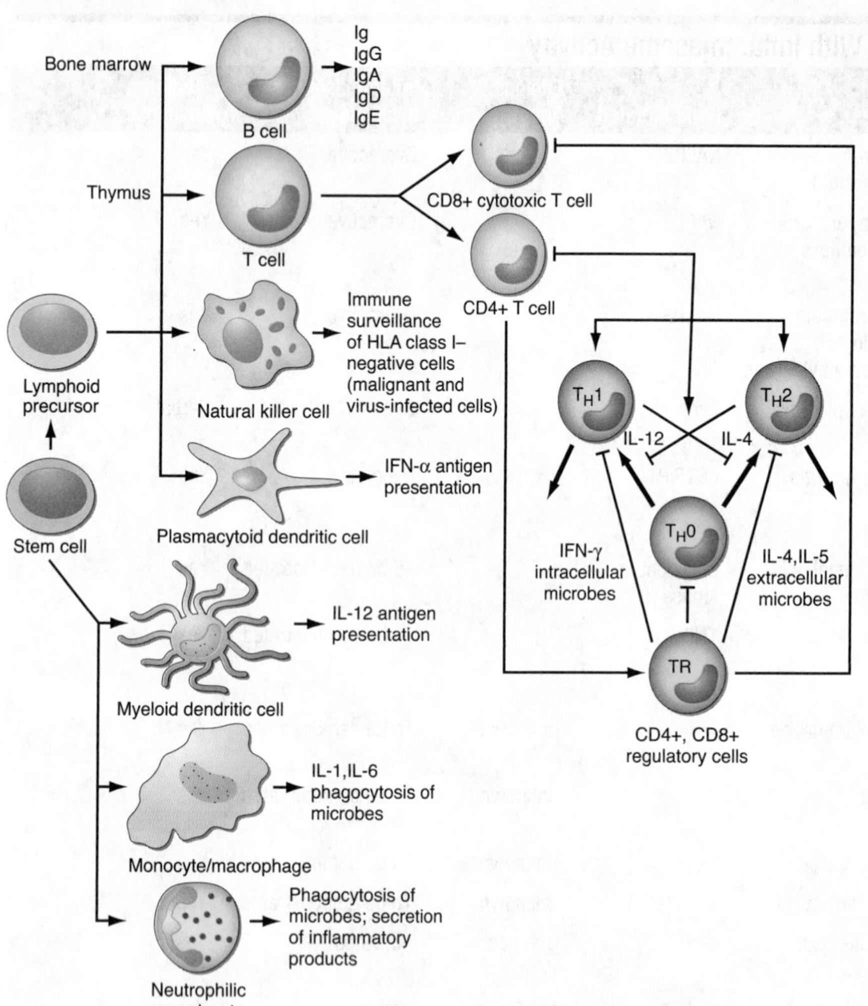

Figure 314-2 Schematic model of intercellular interactions of adaptive immune system cells. In this figure, the arrows denote that cells develop from precursor cells or produce cytokines or antibodies; lines ending with bars indicate suppressive intercellular interactions. Stem cells differentiate into either T cells, antigen-presenting dendritic cells, natural killer cells, macrophages, granulocytes, or B cells. Foreign antigen is processed by dendritic cells, and peptide fragments of foreign antigen are presented to CD4+ and/or CD8+ T cells. CD8+ T cell activation leads to induction of cytotoxic T lymphocyte (CTL) or killer T cell generation, as well as induction of cytokine-producing CD8+ cytotoxic T cells. For antibody production against the same antigen, active antigen is bound to sIg within the B cell receptor complex and drives B cell maturation into plasma cells that secrete Ig. T_H1 or T_H2 CD4+ T cells producing interleukin (IL) 4, IL-5, or interferon (IFN)γ regulate the Ig class switching and determine the type of antibody produced. T_H17 cells secrete IL-17, IL-22, IL-26, which contribute to host defense against extracellular bacteria and fungi, particularly at mucosal surfaces. CD4+, CD25+ T regulatory cells produce IL-10 and downregulate T and B cell responses once the microbe has been eliminated. GM-CSF, granulocyte-macrophage colony stimulating factor; TNF, tumor necrosis factor.

dampen the immune response once the pathogen is controlled. TLR engagement on DCs upregulates MHC class II, B7-1 (CD80), and B7-2 (CD86), which enhance DC-specific antigen presentation and induce cytokine production (Table 314-7). Thus, DCs are important bridges between early (innate) and later (adaptive) immunity. DCs also modulate and determine the types of immune responses induced by pathogens via the TLRs expressed on DCs (TLR7-9 on plasmacytoid DCs, TLR4 on monocytoid DCs) and via the TLR adapter proteins that are induced to associate with TLRs (Fig. 314-1, Table 314-4). In addition, other PRRs, such as C-type lectins, NLRs, and mannose receptors, upon ligation by pathogen products, activate cells of the adaptive immune system and, like TLR stimulation, by a variety of factors, determine the type and quality of the adaptive immune response that is triggered (Table 314-4).

Large granular lymphocytes/natural killer cells

Large granular lymphocytes (LGLs) or NK cells account for ~5–15% of peripheral blood lymphocytes. NK cells are nonadherent, nonphagocytic cells with large azurophilic cytoplasmic granules. NK cells express surface receptors for the Fc portion of IgG (CD16) and for NCAM-I (CD56), and many NK cells express T lineage markers, particularly CD8, and proliferate in response to IL-2. NK cells arise in both bone marrow and thymic microenvironments.

Functionally, NK cells share features with both monocytes-macrophages and neutrophils in that they mediate both antibody-dependent cellular cytotoxicity (ADCC) and NK cell activity. ADCC is the binding of an opsonized (antibody-coated) target cell to an Fc receptor–bearing effector cell via the Fc region of antibody, resulting in lysis of the target by the effector cell. NK cell cytotoxicity is the nonimmune (i.e., effector cell never having had previous contact with the target), MHC-unrestricted, non-antibody-mediated killing of target cells, which are usually malignant cell types, transplanted foreign cells, or virus-infected cells. Thus, NK cell cytotoxicity may play an important role in immune surveillance and destruction of malignant and virally infected host cells. NK cell hyporesponsiveness is also observed in patients with *Chédiak-Higashi syndrome*, an autosomal recessive disease associated with fusion of cytoplasmic granules and defective degranulation of neutrophil lysosomes.

NK cells have a variety of surface receptors that have inhibitory or activating functions and belong to two structural families. These families include the immunoglobulin superfamily and the lectin-like type II transmembrane proteins. NK immunoglobulin superfamily receptors include the killer cell immunoglobulin-like activating or inhibitory receptors (KIRs), many of which have been shown to have HLA class I ligands. The KIRs are made up proteins with either two (KIR2D) or three (KIR3D) extracellular immunoglobulin domains (D). Moreover, their nomenclature designates their function as either inhibitory KIRs with a long (L) cytoplasmic tail and immunoreceptor tyrosine-based inhibitory motif (ITIM) (KIRDL) or activating KIRs with a short (S) cytoplasmic tail (KIRDS). NK cell inactivation by KIRs is a central mechanism to prevent damage to normal host cells. Genetic studies have demonstrated the association of KIRs with viral infection outcome and autoimmune disease (Table 314-11).

In addition to the KIRs, a second set of immunoglobulin superfamily receptors include the natural cytotoxicity receptors (NCRs), which include NKp46, NKp30, and NKp44. These receptors help to

TABLE 314-7 Cytokines and Cytokine Receptors

Cytokine	Receptor	Cell Source	Cell Target	Biologic Activity
IL-1α,β	Type I IL-1r, Type II IL-1r	Monocytes/macrophages, B cells, fibroblasts, most epithelial cells including thymic epithelium, endothelial cells	All cells	Upregulates adhesion molecule expression, neutrophil and macrophage emigration, mimics shock, fever, upregulates hepatic acute-phase protein production, facilitates hematopoiesis
IL-2	IL-2r α,β, common γ	T cells	T cells, B cells, NK cells, monocytes-macrophages	Promotes T cell activation and proliferation, B cell growth, NK cell proliferation and activation, enhanced monocyte/macrophage cytolytic activity
IL-3	IL-3r, common β	T cells, NK cells, mast cells	Monocytes-macrophages, mast cells, eosinophils, bone marrow progenitors	Stimulates hematopoietic progenitors
IL-4	IL-4r α, common γ	T cells, mast cells, basophils	T cells, B cells, NK cells, monocytes-macrophages, neutrophils, eosinophils, endothelial cells, fibroblasts	Stimulates T_H2 helper T cell differentiation and proliferation. Stimulates B cell Ig class switch to IgG1 and IgE anti-inflammatory action on T cells, monocytes
IL-5	IL-5r α, common γ	T cells, mast cells, eosinophils	Eosinophils, basophils, murine B cells	Regulates eosinophil migration and activation
IL-6	IL-6r, gp130	Monocytes-macrophages, B cells, fibroblasts, most epithelium including thymic epithelium, endothelial cells	T cells, B cells, epithelial cells, hepatocytes, monocytes-macrophages	Induces acute-phase protein production, T and B cell differentiation and growth, myeloma cell growth, and osteoclast growth and activation
IL-7	IL-7r α, common γ	Bone marrow, thymic epithelial cells	T cells, B cells, bone marrow cells	Differentiates B, T, and NK cell precursors, activates T and NK cells
IL-8	CXCR1, CXCR2	Monocytes-macrophages, T cells, neutrophils, fibroblasts, endothelial cells, epithelial cells	Neutrophils, T cells, monocytes-macrophages, endothelial cells, basophils	Induces neutrophil, monocyte, and T cell migration, induces neutrophil adherence to endothelial cells and histamine release from basophils, and stimulates angiogenesis. Suppresses proliferation of hepatic precursors
IL-9	IL-9r α, common γ	T cells	Bone marrow progenitors, B cells, T cells, mast cells	Induces mast cell proliferation and function, synergizes with IL-4 in IgG and IgE production and T cell growth, activation, and differentiation
IL-10	IL-10r	Monocytes-macrophages, T cells, B cells, keratinocytes, mast cells	Monocytes-macrophages, T cells, B cells, NK cells, mast cells	Inhibits macrophage proinflammatory cytokine production, downregulates cytokine class II antigen and B7-1 and B7-2 expression, inhibits differentiation of T_H1 helper T cells, inhibits NK cell function, stimulates mast cell proliferation and function, B cell activation, and differentiation
IL-11	IL-11, gp130	Bone marrow stromal cells	Megakaryocytes, B cells, hepatocytes	Induces megakaryocyte colony formation and maturation, enhances antibody responses, stimulates acute-phase protein production
IL-12 (35-kD and 40-kD subunits)	IL-12r	Activated macrophages, dendritic cells, neutrophils	T cells, NK cells	Induces T_H1 T helper cell formation and lymphokine-activated killer cell formation. Increases CD8+ CTL cytolytic activity; ↓IL-17, ↑IFN-γ.
IL-13	IL-13/IL-4	T cells (T_H2)	Monocytes-macrophages, B cells, endothelial cells, keratinocytes	Upregulates VCAM-1 and C-C chemokine expression on endothelial cells and B cell activation and differentiation, and inhibits macrophage proinflammatory cytokine production
IL-14	Unknown	T cells	Normal and malignant B cells	Induces B cell proliferation

(*continued*)

TABLE 314-7 Cytokines and Cytokine Receptors (*Continued*)

Cytokine	Receptor	Cell Source	Cell Target	Biologic Activity
IL-15	IL-15r α, common γ, IL2r β	Monocytes-macrophages, epithelial cells, fibroblasts	T cells, NK cells	Promotes T cell activation and proliferation, angiogenesis, and NK cells
IL-16	CD4	Mast cells, eosinophils, CD8+ T cells, respiratory epithelium	CD4+ T cells, monocytes-macrophages, eosinophils	Promotes chemoattraction of CD4+ T cells, monocytes, and eosinophils. Inhibits HIV replication. Inhibits T cell activation through CD3/T cell receptor
IL-17	IL17r	CD4+ T cells	Fibroblasts, endothelium, epithelium	Enhances cytokine secretion
IL-18	IL-18r (IL-1R-related protein)	Keratinocytes, macrophages	T cells, B cells, NK cells	Upregulates IFN-γ production, enhances NK cell cytotoxicity
IL-21	IL-δγ chain/IL-21R	CD4 T cells	NK cells	Downregulates NK cell–activating molecules, NKG2D/DAP10
IL-23	IL-12Rb1/IL23R	Macrophages, other cell types	T cells	Opposite effects of IL-12 (↑IL-17, ↑IFN-γ)
IFN-α	Type I interferon receptor	All cells	All cells	Promotes antiviral activity. Stimulates T cell, macrophage, and NK cell activity. Direct antitumor effects. Upregulates MHC class I antigen expression. Used therapeutically in viral and autoimmune conditions
IFN-β	Type I interferon receptor	All cells	All cells	Antiviral activity. Stimulates T cell, macrophage, and NK cell activity. Direct antitumor effects. Upregulates MHC class I antigen expression. Used therapeutically in viral and autoimmune conditions
IFN-γ	Type II interferon receptor	T cells, NK cells	All cells	Regulates macrophage and NK cell activations. Stimulates immunoglobulin secretion by B cells. Induction of class II histocompatibility antigens. T_H1 T cell differentiation.
TNF-α	TNFrI, TNFrII	Monocytes-macrophages, mast cells, basophils, eosinophils, NK cells, B cells, T cells, keratinocytes, fibroblasts, thymic epithelial cells	All cells except erythrocytes	Fever, anorexia, shock, capillary leak syndrome, enhanced leukocyte cytotoxicity, enhanced NK cell function, acute phase protein synthesis, proinflammatory cytokine induction.
TNF-β	TNFrI, TNFrII	T cells, B cells	All cells except erythrocytes	Cell cytotoxicity, lymph node and spleen development.
LT-β	LTβR	T cells	All cells except erythrocytes	Cell cytotoxicity, normal lymph node development
G-CSF	G-CSFr; gp130	Monocytes-macrophages, fibroblasts, endothelial cells, thymic epithelial cells, stromal cells	Myeloid cells, endothelial cells	Regulates myelopoiesis. Enhances survival and function of neutrophils. Clinical use in reversing neutropenia after cytotoxic chemotherapy.
GM-CSF	GM-CSFr, common β	T cells, monocytes-macrophages, fibroblasts, endothelial cells, thymic epithelial cells	Monocytes-macrophages, neutrophils, eosinophils, fibroblasts, endothelial cells	Regulates myelopoiesis. Enhances macrophage bactericidal and tumoricidal activity. Mediator of dendritic cell maturation and function. Upregulates NK cell function. Clinical use in reversing neutropenia after cytotoxic chemotherapy.
M-CSF	M-CSFr (*c-fms* protooncogene)	Fibroblasts, endothelial cells, monocytes-macrophages, T cells, B cells, epithelial cells including thymic epithelium	Monocytes-macrophages	Regulates monocyte-macrophage production and function.
LIF	LIFr; gp130	Activated T cells, bone marrow stromal cells, thymic epithelium	Megakaryocytes, monocytes, hepatocytes, possibly lymphocyte subpopulations	Induces hepatic acute-phase protein production. Stimulates macrophage differentiation. Promotes growth of myeloma cells and hematopoietic progenitors. Stimulates thrombopoiesis.

(*continued*)

TABLE 314-7 Cytokines and Cytokine Receptors (*Continued*)

Cytokine	Receptor	Cell Source	Cell Target	Biologic Activity
OSM	OSMr; LIFr; gp130	Activated monocytes-macrophages and T cells, bone marrow stromal cells, some breast carcinoma cell lines, myeloma cells	Neurons, hepatocytes, monocytes-macrophages, adipocytes, alveolar epithelial cells, embryonic stem cells, melanocytes, endothelial cells, fibroblasts, myeloma cells	Induces hepatic acute-phase protein production. Stimulates macrophage differentiation. Promotes growth of myeloma cells and hematopoietic progenitors. Stimulates thrombopoiesis. Stimulates growth of Kaposi's sarcoma cells.
SCF	SCFr (*c-kit* protooncogene)	Bone marrow stromal cells and fibroblasts	Embryonic stem cells, myeloid and lymphoid precursors, mast cells.	Stimulates hematopoietic progenitor cell growth, mast cell growth, promotes embryonic stem cell migration.
TGF-β (3 isoforms)	Type I, II, III TGF-β receptor	Most cell types	Most cell types	Downregulates T cell, macrophage, and granulocyte responses. Stimulates synthesis of matrix proteins. Stimulates angiogenesis.
Lymphotactin/SCM-1	Unknown	NK cells, mast cells, double negative thymocytes, activated CD8+ T cells	T cells, NK cells	Chemoattractant for lymphocytes. Only known chemokine of C class.
MCP-1	CCR2	Fibroblasts, smooth-muscle cells, activated PBMCs	Monocytes-macrophages, NK cells, memory T cells, basophils	Chemoattractant for monocytes, activated memory T cells, and NK cells. Induces granule release from CD8+ T cells and NK cells. Potent histamine-releasing factor for basophils. Suppresses proliferation of hematopoietic precursors. Regulates monocyte protease production.
MCP-2	CCR1, CCR2	Fibroblasts, activated PBMCs	Monocytes-macrophages, T cells, eosinophils, basophils, NK cells	Chemoattractant for monocytes, memory and naïve T cells, eosinophils, ?NK cells. Activates basophils and eosinophils. Regulates monocyte protease production.
MCP-3	CCR1, CCR2	Fibroblasts, activated PBMCs	Monocytes-macrophages, T cells, eosinophils, basophils, NK cells, dendritic cells	Chemoattractant for monocytes, memory and naïve T cells, dendritic cells, eosinophils, ?NK cells. Activates basophils and eosinophils. Regulates monocyte protease production.
MCP-4	CCR2, CCR3	Lung, colon, small intestinal epithelial cells, activated endothelial cells	Monocytes-macrophages, T cells, eosinophils, basophils	Chemoattractant for monocytes, T cells, eosinophils, and basophils
Eotaxin	CCR3	Pulmonary epithelial cells, heart	Eosinophils, basophils	Potent chemoattractant for eosinophils and basophils. Induces allergic airways disease. Acts in concert with IL-5 to activate eosinophils. Antibodies to eotaxin inhibit airway inflammation.
TARC	CCR4	Thymus, dendritic cells, activated T cells	T cells, NK cells	Chemoattractant for T and NK cells.
MDC	CCR4	Monocytes-macrophages, dendritic cells, thymus	Activated T cells	Chemoattractant for activated T cells. Inhibits infection with T cell tropic HIV.
MIP-1α	CCR1, CCR5	Monocytes-macrophages, T cells	Monocytes-macrophages, T cells, dendritic cells, NK cells, eosinophils, basophils	Chemoattractant for monocytes, T cells, dendritic cells, NK cells, and weak chemoattractant for eosinophils and basophils. Activates NK cell function. Suppresses proliferation of hematopoietic precursors. Necessary for myocarditis associated with Coxsackie virus infection. Inhibits infection with monocytotropic HIV.
MIP-1β	CCR5	Monocytes-macrophages, T cells	Monocytes-macrophages, T cells, NK cells, dendritic cells	Chemoattractant for monocytes, T cells, and NK cells. Activates NK cell function. Inhibits infection with monocytotropic HIV.

(*continued*)

TABLE 314-7 Cytokines and Cytokine Receptors (*Continued*)

Cytokine	Receptor	Cell Source	Cell Target	Biologic Activity
RANTES	CCR1, CCR2, CCR5	Monocytes-macrophages, T cells, fibroblasts, eosinophils	Monocytes-macrophages, T cells, NK cells, dendritic cells, eosinophils, basophils	Chemoattractant for monocytes-macrophages, CD4+, CD45Ro+T cells, CD8+ T cells, NK cells, eosinophils, and basophils. Induces histamine release from basophils. Inhibits infections with monocytotropic HIV.
LARC/MIP-3α/ Exodus-1	CCR6	Dendritic cells, fetal liver cells, activated T cells	T cells, B cells	Chemoattractant for lymphocytes.
ELC/MIP-3β	CCR7	Thymus, lymph node, appendix	Activated T cells and B cells	Chemoattractant for B and T cells. Receptor upregulated on EBV-infected B cells and HSV-infected T cells.
I-309/TCA-3	CCR8	Activated T cells	Monocytes-macrophages, T cells	Chemoattractant for monocytes. Prevents glucocorticoid-induced apoptosis in some T cell lines.
SLC/TCA-4/ Exodus-2	Unknown	Thymic epithelial cells, lymph node, appendix and spleen	T cells	Chemoattractant for T lymphocytes. Inhibits hematopoiesis.
DC-CK1/PARC	Unknown	Dendritic cells in secondary lymphoid tissues	Naïve T cells	May have a role in induction of immune responses.
TECK	Unknown	Dendritic cells, thymus, liver, small intestine	T cells, monocytes-macrophages, dendritic cells	Thymic dendritic cell–derived cytokine, possibly involved in T cell development
GRO-α/MGSA	CXCR2	Activated granulocytes, monocyte-macrophages, and epithelial cells.	Neutrophils, epithelial cells, ?endothelial cells	Neutrophil chemoattractant and activator. Mitogenic for some melanoma cell lines. Suppresses proliferation of hematopoietic precursors. Angiogenic activity.
GRO-β/MIP-2α	CXCR2	Activated granulocytes and monocyte-macrophages	Neutrophils and ?endothelial cells.	Neutrophil chemoattractant and activator. Angiogenic activity.
NAP-2	CXCR2	Platelets	Neutrophils, basophils	Derived from platelet basic protein. Neutrophil chemoattractant and activator.
IP-10	CXCR3	Monocytes-macrophages, T cells, fibroblasts, endothelial cells, epithelial cells	Activated T cells, tumor-infiltrating lymphocytes, ?endothelial cells, ?NK cells	IFN-γ-inducible protein that is a chemoattractant for T cells. Suppresses proliferation of hematopoietic precursors.
MIG	CXCR3	Monocytes-macrophages, T cells, fibroblasts	Activated T cells, tumor-infiltrating lymphocytes	IFN-γ-inducible protein that is a chemoattractant for T cells. Suppresses proliferation of hematopoietic precursors.
SDF-1	CXCR4	Fibroblasts	T cells, dendritic cells, ?basophils, ?endothelial cells	Low-potency, high-efficacy T cell chemoattractant. Required for B-lymphocyte development. Prevents infection of CD4+, CXCR4+ cells by T cell tropic HIV.
Fractalkine	CX3CR1	Activated endothelial cells	NK cells, T cells, monocytes-macrophages	Cell-surface chemokine/mucin hybrid molecule that functions as a chemoattractant, leukocyte activator, and cell adhesion molecule.
PF-4	Unknown	Platelets, megakaryocytes	Fibroblasts, endothelial cells	Chemoattractant for fibroblasts. Suppresses proliferation of hematopoietic precursors. Inhibits endothelial cell proliferation and angiogenesis.

Abbreviations: IL, interleukin; NK, natural killer; T_H1 and T_H2, helper T cell subsets; Ig, immunoglobulin; CXCR, CXC-type chemokine receptor; B7-1, CD80, B7-2, CD86; PBMC, peripheral blood mononuclear cells; VCAM, vascular cell adhesion molecule; IFN, interferon; MHC, major histocompatibility complex; TNF, tumor necrosis factor; G-CSF, granulocyte colony-stimulating factor; GM-CSF, granulocyte-macrophage CSF; M-CSF, macrophage CSF; LIF, leukemia inhibitory factor; OSM, oncostatin M; SCF, stem cell factor; TGF, transforming growth factor; MCP, monocyte chemotactic protein; CCR, CC-type chemokine receptor; TARC, thymus- and activation-regulated chemokine; MDC, macrophage-derived chemokine; MIP, macrophage inflammatory protein; RANTES, regulated on activation, normally T cell–expressed and –secreted; LARC, liver- and activation-regulated chemokine; EBV, Epstein-Barr virus; ELC, EB11 ligand chemokine (MIP-1b); HSV, herpes simplex virus; TCA, T-cell activation protein; DC-CK, dendritic cell chemokine; PARC, pulmonary- and activation-regulated chemokine; SLC, secondary lymphoid tissue chemokine; TECK, thymus expressed chemokine; GRP, growth-related peptide; MGSA, melanoma growth-stimulating activity; NAP, neutrophil-activating protein; IP-10, IFN-γ-inducible protein-10; MIG, monokine induced by IFN-γ; SDF, stromal cell-derived factor; PF, platelet factor.

Source: Data from JS Sundy et al: Appendix B, in *Inflammation, Basic Principles and Clinical Correlates,* 3rd ed, J Gallin and R Snyderman (eds). Philadelphia, Lippincott Williams and Wilkins, 1999.

TABLE 314-8 CC, CXC_1, CX_3, C_1 and XC Families of Chemokines and Chemokine Receptors

Chemokine Receptor	Chemokine Ligands	Cell Types	Disease Connection
CCR1	CCL3 (MIP-1α), CCL5 (RANTES), CCL7 (MCP-3), CCL14 (HCC1)	T cells, monocytes, eosinophils, basophils	Rheumatoid arthritis, multiple sclerosis
CCR2	CCL2 (MCP-1), CCL8 (MCP-2), CCL7 (MCP-3), CCL13 (MCP-4), CCL16 (HCC4)	Monocytes, dendritic cells (immature), memory T cells	Atherosclerosis, rheumatoid arthritis, multiple sclerosis, resistance to intracellular pathogens, type 2 diabetes mellitus
CCR3	CCL11 (eotaxin), CCL13 (eotaxin-2), CCL7 (MCP-3), CCL5 (RANTES), CCL8 (MCP-2), CCL13 (MCP-4)	Eosinophils, basophils, mast cells, T_H2, platelets	Allergic asthma and rhinitis
CCR4	CCL17 (TARC), CCL22 (MDC)	T cells (T_H2) dendritic cells (mature), basophils, macrophages, platelets	Parasitic infection, graft rejection, T cell homing to skin
CCR5	CCL3 (MIP-1α), CCL4 (MIP-1α), CCL5 (RANTES), CCL11 (eotaxin), CCL14 (HCC1), CCL16 (HCC4)	T cells, monocytes	HIV-1 co-receptor (T cell–tropic strains), transplant rejection
CCR6	CCL20 (MIP-3α, LARC)	T cells (T regulatory and memory), B cells, dendritic cells	Mucosal humoral immunity, allergic asthma, intestinal T cell homing
CCR7	CCL19 (ELC), CCL21 (SLC)	T cells, dendritic cells (mature)	Transport of T cells and dendritic cells to lymph nodes, antigen presentation, and cellular immunity
CCR8	CCL1 (1309)	T cells (T_H2), monocytes, dendritic cells	Dendritic cell migration to lymph node, type 2 cellular immunity, granuloma formation
CCR9	CCL25 (TECK)	T cells, IgA+ plasma cells	Homing of T cells and IgA+ plasma cells to the intestine, inflammatory bowel disease
CCR10	CCL27 (CTACK), CCL28 (MEC)	T cells	T cell homing to intestine and skin
CXCR1	CXCL8 (interleukin-8), CXCL6 (GCP2)	Neutrophils, monocytes	Inflammatory lung disease, COPD
CXCR2	CXCL8, CXCL1 (GROα), CXCL2 (GROα), CXCL3 (GROα), CXCL5 (ENA-78), CXCL6	Neutrophils, monocytes, microvascular endothelial cells	Inflammatory lung disease, COPD, angiogenic for tumor growth
CXCR3-A	CXCL9 (MIG), CXCL10 (IP-10), CXCL11 (I-TAC)	Type 1 helper cells, mast cells, mesangial cells	Inflammatory skin disease, multiple sclerosis, transplant rejection
CXCR3-B	CXCL4 (PF4), CXCL9 (MIG), CXCL10 (IP-10), CXCL11 (I-TAC)	Microvascular endothelial cells, neoplastic cells	Angiostatic for tumor growth
CXCR4	CXCL12 (SDF-1)	Widely expressed	HIV-1 co-receptor (T cell–tropic), tumor metastases, hematopoiesis
CXCR5	CXCL13 (BCA-1)	B cells, follicular helper T cells	Formation of B cell follicles
CXCR6	CXCL16 (SR-PSOX)	CD8+ T cells, natural killer cells, and memory CD4+ T cells	Inflammatory liver disease, atherosclerosis (CXCL16)
CX_3CR1	CX3CL1 (fractalkine)	Macrophages, endothelial cells, smooth-muscle cells	Atherosclerosis
XCR1	XCL1 (lymphotactin), XCL2	T cells, natural killer cells	Rheumatoid arthritis, IgA nephropathy, tumor response

Abbreviations: MIP, macrophage inflammatory protein; MCP, monocyte chemoattractant protein; HCC, hemofiltrate chemokine; T_H2, type 2 helper T cells; TARC, thymus- and activation-regulated chemokine; MDC, macrophage-derived chemokine; LARC, liver- and activation-regulated chemokine; ELC, Epstein-Barr I1-ligand chemokine; SLC, secondary lymphoid-tissue chemokine; TECK, thymus-expressed chemokine; CTACK, cutaneous T cell–attracting chemokine; MEC, mammary-enriched chemokine; GCP, granulocyte chemotactic protein; COPD, chronic obstructive pulmonary disease; GRO, growth-regulated oncogene; ENA, epithelial-cell–derived neutrophil-activating peptide; MIG, monokine induced by interferon-γ; IP-10, interferon inducible 10; I-TAC, interferon-inducible T-cell alpha chemoattractant; PF, platelet factor; SDF, stromal-cell–derived factor; BCA-1, B-cell chemoattractant 1; SR-PSOX, scavenger receptor for phosphatidylserine-containing oxidized lipids.

Source: From IF Charo, RM Ranshohoff: N Engl J Med 354:610, 2006, with permission.

CHAPTER 314 Introduction to the Immune System

TABLE 314-9 Major Structural Families of Cytokines

Four α-helix-bundle family interleukins	Interleukin-2 (IL-2) Subfamily:
	Interleukins: IL-2, IL-3, IL-4, IL-5, IL-6, IL-7, IL-9, IL-11, IL-12, IL-13, IL-15, IL-21, IL-23
	Not called interleukins: Colony-stimulating factor-1 (CSF1), granulocyte–macrophage colony-stimulating factor (CSF2), Flt-3 ligand, erythropoietin (EPO), thrombopoietin (THPO), leukocyte inhibitory factor (LIF)
	Not interleukins: Growth hormone (GH1), prolactin (PRL), leptin (LEP), cardiotrophin (CTF1), ciliary neurotrophic factor (CNTF), cytokine receptor-like factor 1 (CLC or CLF) Interferon (IFN) subfamily: IFN-β, IFN-α
	IL-10 subfamily: IL-10, IL-19, IL-20, IL-22, IL-24, and IL-26
IL-1 family	IL-1α (IL1A), IL-1β (IL1B), IL-18 (IL18), and paralogues, IL-17A, IL-17B, IL-17C, IL-17D, IL-17E, IL-17F
Chemokines	IL-8, MCP-1, MCP-2, MCP-3, MCP-4, eotaxin, TARC, LARC/MIP-3α, MDC, MIP-1α, MIP-1β, RANTES, MIP-3β, I-309, SLC, PARC, TECK, GROα, GROβ, NAP-2, IP-19, MIG, SDF-1, PF4

Abbreviations: GRO, growth-related peptide; IL, interleukin; IP, INF-γ-inducible protein; LARC, liver- and activation-regulated chemokine; MCP, monocyte chemotactic protein; MDC, macrophage-derived chemokine; MIG, monokine induced by IFN-γ; MIP, macrophage inflammatory protein; NAP, neutrophil-activating protein; PARC, pulmonary- and activation-regulated chemokine; PF4, platelet factor; RANTES, regulated on activation, normally T cell–expressed and –secreted; SDF, stromal cell–derived factor; SLC, secondary lymphoid tissue.

Source: Adapted from JW Schrader: Trends Immunol 23:573, 2002. Copyright 2002, with permission from Elsevier.

mediate NK cell activation against target cells. The ligands to which NCRs bind on target cells remain largely undefined.

NK cell signaling is, therefore, a highly coordinated series of inhibiting and activating signals that prevent NK cells from responding to uninfected, nonmalignant self-cells; however, they are activated to attack malignant and virally infected cells (Fig. 314-4). Recent evidence suggests that NK cells, although not possessing rearranging immune recognition genes, may be able to mediate recall for NK cell responses to viruses and for immune responses such as contact hypersensitivity.

Some NK cells express CD3 and invariant T cell receptor (TCR) alpha chains and are termed *NK T cells*. TCRs of NK T cells recognize lipid molecules of intracellular bacteria when presented in the context of CD1d molecules on APCs. Upon activation, NK T cells secrete effector cytokines such as IL-4 and IFNγ. This mode of recognition of intracellular bacteria such as *Listeria monocytogenes* and *Mycobacterium tuberculosis* by NK T cells leads to induction of activation of DCs and is thought to be an important innate defense mechanism against these organisms.

Neutrophils, eosinophils, and basophils

Granulocytes are present in nearly all forms of inflammation and are amplifiers and effectors of innate immune responses (Figs. 314-2 and 314-3). Unchecked accumulation and activation of granulocytes can lead to host tissue damage, as seen in neutrophil- and eosinophil-mediated *systemic necrotizing vasculitis*. Granulocytes are derived from stem cells in bone marrow. Each type of granulocyte (neutrophil, eosinophil, or basophil) is derived from a different subclass of progenitor cell that is stimulated to proliferate by colony-stimulating factors (Table 314-7). During terminal maturation of granulocytes, class-specific nuclear morphology and cytoplasmic granules appear that allow for histologic identification of granulocyte type.

TABLE 314-10 Cytokine Families Grouped by Structural Similarity

Hematopoietins	IL-2, IL-3, IL-4, IL-5, IL-6, IL-7, IL-9, IL-11, IL-12, IL-15, IL-16, IL-17, IL-21, IL-23, EPO, LIF, GM-CSF, G-CSF, OSM, CNTF, GH, and TPO
	TNF-α, LT-α, LT-β, CD40L, CD30L, CD27L, 4-1BBL, OX40, OPG, and FasL
IL-1	IL-1α, IL-1β, IL-1ra, IL-18, bFGF, aFGF, and ECGF
PDGF	PDGF A, PDGF B, and M-CSF
TGF-β	TGF-β and BMPs (1,2,4 etc.)
C-X-C chemokines	IL-8, Gro-α/β/γ, NAP-2, ENA78, GCP-2, PF4, CTAP-3, MIG, and IP-10
C-C chemokines	MCP-1, MCP-2, MCP-3, MIP-1α, MIP-1β, RANTES

Abbreviations: aFGF, acidic fibroblast growth factor; 4-1BBL, 401 BB ligand; bFGF, basic fibroblast growth factor; BMP, bone marrow morphogenetic proteins; C-C, cysteine-cysteine; CD, cluster of differentiation; CNTF, ciliary neurotrophic factor; CTAP, connective tissue–activating peptide; C-X-C, cysteine-x-cysteine; ECGF, endothelial cell growth factor; EPO, erythropoietin; FasL, Fas ligand; GCP-2, granulocyte chemotactic protein 2; G-CSF, granulocyte colony-stimulating factor; GH, growth hormone; GM-CSF, granulocyte-macrophage colony-stimulating factor; Gro, growth-related gene products; IFN, interferon; IL, interleukin; IP, interferon-γ inducible protein; LIF, leukemia inhibitory factor; LT, lymphotoxin; MCP, monocyte chemoattractant; M-CSF, macrophage colony-stimulating factor; MIG, monokine induced by interferon-γ; MIP, macrophage inflammatory protein; NAP-2, neutrophil activating protein 2; OPG, osteoprotegerin; OSM, oncostatin M; PDGF, platelet-derived growth factor; PF, platelet factor; R, receptor; RANTES, regulated on activation, normal T cell–expressed and –secreted; TGF, transforming growth factor; TNF, tumor necrosis factor; TPO, thyroperoxidase.

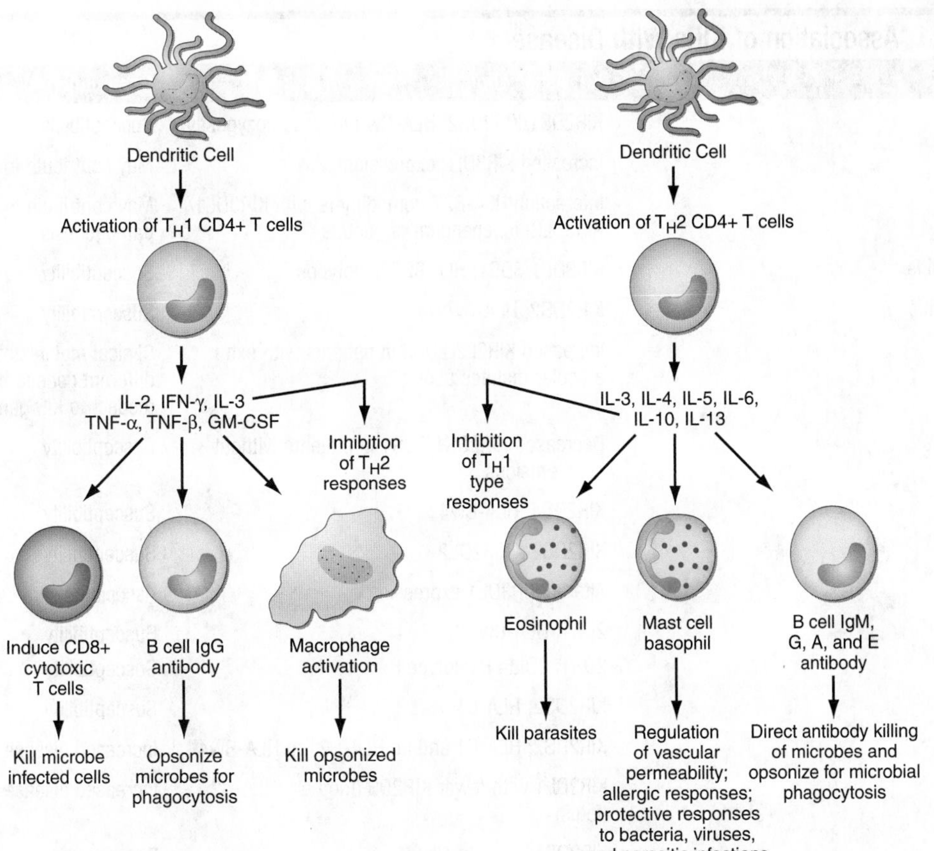

Figure 314-3 CD4+ helper T1 (T_H1) cells and T_H2 T cells secrete distinct but overlapping sets of cytokines. T_H1 CD4+ cells are frequently activated in immune and inflammatory reactions against intracellular bacteria or viruses, while T_H2 CD4+ cells are frequently activated for certain types of antibody production against parasites and extracellular encapsulated bacteria; they are also activated in allergic diseases. GM-CSF, granulocyte-macrophage colony-stimulating factor; IFN, interferon; IL, interleukin; TNF, tumor necrosis factor. *(Adapted from Romagnani; with permission.)*

Neutrophils express Fc receptors for IgG (CD16) and receptors for activated complement components (C3b or CD35). Upon interaction of neutrophils with opsonized bacteria or immune complexes, azurophilic granules (containing myeloperoxidase, lysozyme, elastase, and other enzymes) and specific granules (containing lactoferrin, lysozyme, collagenase, and other enzymes) are released, and microbicidal superoxide radicals (O_2^-) are generated at the neutrophil surface. The generation of superoxide leads to inflammation by direct injury to tissue and by alteration of macromolecules such as collagen and DNA.

Eosinophils express Fc receptors for IgG (CD32) and are potent cytotoxic effector cells for various parasitic organisms. In *Nippostrongylus brasiliensis* helminth infection, eosinophils are important cytotoxic effector cells for removal of these parasites. Key to regulation of eosinophil cytotoxicity to *N. brasiliensis* worms are antigen-specific T helper cells that produce IL-4, thus providing an example of regulation of innate immune responses by adaptive immunity antigen-specific T cells. Intracytoplasmic contents of eosinophils, such as major basic protein, eosinophil cationic protein, and eosinophil-derived neurotoxin, are capable of directly damaging tissues and may be responsible in part for the organ system dysfunction in the *hypereosinophilic syndromes* (Chap. 60). Since the eosinophil granule contains anti-inflammatory types of enzymes (histaminase, arylsulfatase, phospholipase D), eosinophils may homeostatically downregulate or terminate ongoing inflammatory responses.

Basophils and tissue mast cells are potent reservoirs of cytokines such as IL-4 and can respond to bacteria and viruses with antipathogen cytokine production through multiple TLRs expressed on their surface. Mast cells and basophils can also mediate immunity through the binding of antipathogen antibodies. This is a particularly important host defense mechanism against parasitic diseases. Basophils express high-affinity surface receptors for IgE (FcRI) and, upon cross-linking of basophil-bound IgE by antigen, can release histamine, eosinophil chemotactic factor of anaphylaxis, and neutral protease—all mediators of allergic immediate (anaphylaxis) hypersensitivity responses (Table 314-12). In addition, basophils express surface receptors for activated complement components (C3a, C5a), through which mediator release can be directly effected. Thus, basophils, like most cells of the immune system, can be activated in the service of host defense against pathogens, or they can be activated for mediation release and cause pathogenic responses in allergic and inflammatory diseases. For further discussion of tissue mast cells, see Chap. 317.

The complement system

The complement system, an important soluble component of the innate immune system, is a series of plasma enzymes, regulatory proteins, and proteins that are activated in a cascading fashion, resulting in cell lysis. There are four pathways of the complement system: the classic activation pathway activated by antigen/antibody immune complexes, the MBL (a serum collectin; Table 314-3) activation pathway activated by microbes with terminal mannose groups, the alternative activation pathway activated by microbes or tumor cells, and the terminal pathway that is common to the first three pathways and leads to the membrane attack complex that lyses

TABLE 314-11 Association of KIRs With Disease

Disease	KIR Association	Observation
Psoriatic arthritis	KIR2DS1/KIR2DS2; HLA-Cw group homozygosity	Susceptibility
Spondylarthritides	Increased KIR3DL2 expression	May contribute to disease pathology
	Interaction HLA-B27 homodimers with KIR3DL1/ KIR3DL2; independent of peptide	May contribute to disease pathogenesis
Ankylosing spondylitis	KIR3DL1/3DS1; HLA B27 genotypes	Susceptibility
Rheumatoid vasculitis	KIR2DS2; HLA-Cw*03	Susceptibility
	Increased KIR2L2/2DS2 in patients with extra articular manifestations	Clinical manifestations may have different genetic backgrounds with respect to KIR genotype
Rheumatoid arthritis	Decreased KIR2DS1/3DS1 in patients without bone erosions	Susceptibility
	KIR2DS4; HLA-Cw4	Susceptibility
Scleroderma	KIR2DS2+/KIR2DL2-	Susceptibility
Behçet's disease	Altered KIR3DL1 expression	Associated with severe eye disease
Psoriasis vulgaris	2DS1; HLA-Cw*06	Susceptibility
	2DS1; 2DL5; Haplotype B	Susceptibility
IDDM	KIR2DS2; HLA-C1	Susceptibility
Type 1 diabetes	KIR2DS2; HLA-C1 and no HLA-C2, no HLA-Bw4	Increased disease progression
Preeclampsia	KIR2DL1 with fewer KIR2DS (mother); HLA-C2 (fetus)	Increased disease progression
AIDS	KIR3DS1; HLA-Bw4Ile80	Decreased disease progression
	KIR3DS1 homozygous; No HLA-Bw4Ile^{80}	Increased disease progression
HCV infection	KIR2DL3 homozygous; HLA-C1 homozygous	Decreased disease progression
Cervical neoplasia (HPV induced)	KIR3DS1; HLA-C1 homozygous and no HLA-Bw4	Increased disease progression
Malignant melanoma	KIR2DL2 and/or KIR2DL3; HLA-C1	Increased disease progression

Abbreviations: HCV, hepatitis C virus; HLA, human leukocyte antigen; HPV, human papillomavirus; IDDM, insulin-dependent diabetes mellitus; KIR, killer cell immunoglobulin-like receptor.
Source: Adapted from Diaz-Pena et al.

cells (Fig. 314-5). The series of enzymes of the complement system are serine proteases.

Activation of the classic complement pathway via immune complex binding to C1q links the innate and adaptive immune systems via specific antibody in the immune complex. The alternative complement activation pathway is antibody-independent and is activated by binding of C3 directly to pathogens and "altered self" such as tumor cells. In the renal glomerular inflammatory disease *IgA nephropathy*, IgA activates the alternative complement pathway and causes glomerular damage and decreased renal function. Activation of the classic complement pathway via C1, C4, and C2 and activation of the alternative pathway via factor D, C3, and factor B both lead to cleavage and activation of C3. C3 activation fragments, when bound to target surfaces such as bacteria and other foreign antigens, are critical for opsonization (coating by antibody and complement) in preparation for phagocytosis. The MBL pathway substitutes MBL-associated serine proteases (MASPs) 1 and 2 for C1q, C1r, and C1s to activate C4. The MBL activation pathway is activated by mannose on the surface of bacteria and viruses.

The three pathways of complement activation all converge on the final common terminal pathway. C3 cleavage by each pathway results in activation of C5, C6, C7, C8, and C9, resulting in the membrane attack complex that physically inserts into the membranes of target cells or bacteria and lyses them.

Thus, complement activation is a critical component of innate immunity for responding to microbial infection. The functional consequences of complement activation by the three initiating pathways and the terminal pathway are shown in Fig. 314-5. In general the cleavage products of complement components facilitate microbe or damaged cell clearance (C1q, C4, C3), promote activation and enhancement of inflammation (anaphylatoxins, C3a, C5a), and promote microbe or opsonized cell lysis (membrane attack complex).

■ CYTOKINES

Cytokines are soluble proteins produced by a wide variety of hematopoietic and nonhematopoietic cell types (Tables 314-7 to 314-10). They are critical for both normal innate and adaptive immune responses, and their expression may be perturbed in most immune, inflammatory, and infectious disease states.

Cytokines are involved in the regulation of the growth, development, and activation of immune system cells and in the mediation of the inflammatory response. In general, cytokines are characterized by considerable redundancy; different cytokines have similar functions. In addition, many cytokines are pleiotropic in that they are capable of acting on many different cell types. This pleiotropism results from the expression on multiple cell types of receptors for

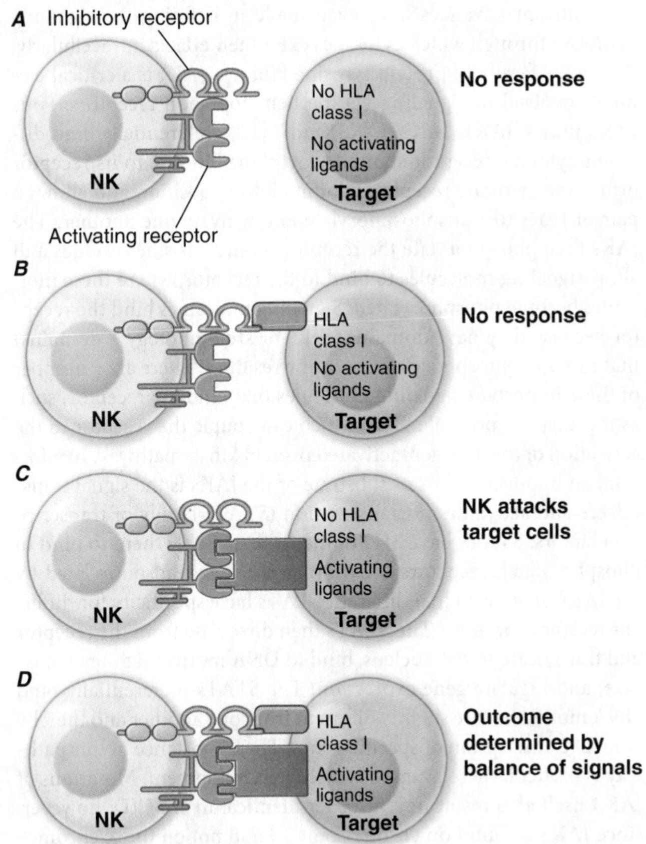

Figure 314-4 Encounters between NK cells: potential targets and possible outcomes. The amount of activating and inhibitory receptors on the NK cells and the amount of ligands on the target cell, as well as the qualitative differences in the signals transduced, determine the extent of the NK response. *A.* When target cells have no HLA class I nor activating ligands, NK cells cannot kill target cells. *B.* When target cells bear self-HLA, NK cells cannot kill targets. *C.* When target cells are pathogen infected and have downregulated HLA and express activating ligands, NK cells kill target cells. *D.* When NK cells encounter targets with both self-HLA and activating receptors, then the level of target killing is determined by the balance of inhibitory and activating signals to the NK cell. HLA, human leukocyte antigen; NK, natural killer. *(Adapted from Lanier; reproduced with permission from Annual Reviews Inc. Copyright 2011 by Annual Reviews Inc.)*

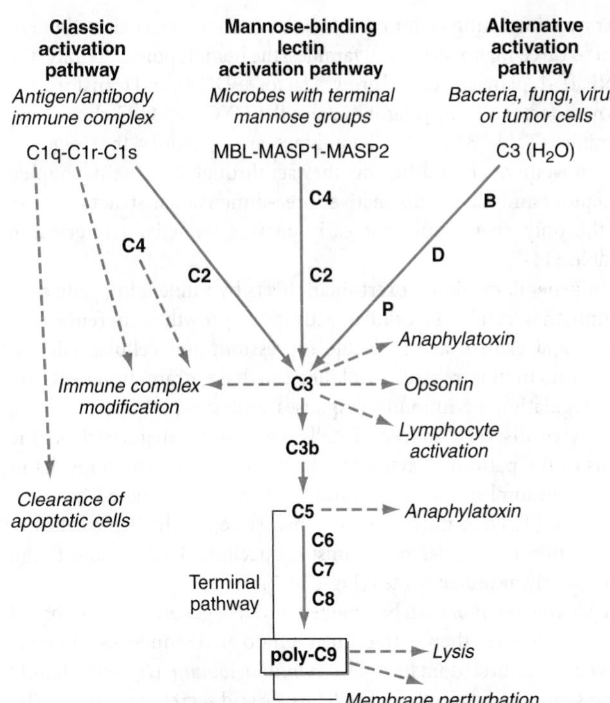

Figure 314-5 The four pathways and the effector mechanisms of the complement system. Dashed arrows indicate the functions of pathway components. *(After Morley and Walport; with permission. Copyright Academic Press, London, 2000.)*

the same cytokine (see below), leading to the formation of "cytokine networks." The action of cytokines may be (1) autocrine when the target cell is the same cell that secretes the cytokine, (2) paracrine when the target cell is nearby, and (3) endocrine when the cytokine is secreted into the circulation and acts distal to the source.

Cytokines have been named based on presumed targets or based on presumed functions. Those cytokines that are thought to primarily target leukocytes have been named interleukins (IL-1, -2, -3, etc.). Many cytokines that were originally described as having a certain function have retained those names (granulocyte

TABLE 314-12 Examples of Mediators Released From Human Cells and Basophils

Mediator	Actions
Histamine	Smooth-muscle contraction, increased vascular permeability
Slow reacting substance of anaphylaxis (SRSA) (leukotriene C4, D4, E4)	Smooth-muscle contraction
Eosinophil chemotactic factor of anaphylaxis (ECF-A)	Chemotactic attraction of eosinophils
Platelet-activating factor	Activates platelets to secrete serotonin and other mediators: smooth-muscle contraction; induces vascular permeability
Neutrophil chemotactic factor (NCF)	Chemotactic attraction of neutrophils
Leukotactic activity (leukotriene B4)	Chemotactic attraction of neutrophils
Heparin	Anticoagulant
Basophil kallikrein of anaphylaxis (BK-A)	Cleaves kininogen to form bradykinin

colony-stimulating factor or G-CSF, etc.). Cytokines belong in general to three major structural families: the hematopoietin family; the TNF, IL-1, platelet-derived growth factor (PDGF), and transforming growth factor (TGF) β families; and the CXC and C-C chemokine families (Table 314-10). Chemokines are cytokines that regulate cell movement and trafficking; they act through G protein–coupled receptors and have a distinctive three-dimensional structure. IL-8 is the only chemokine that early on was named an interleukin (Table 314-7).

In general, cytokines exert their effects by influencing gene activation that results in cellular activation, growth, differentiation, functional cell-surface molecule expression, and cellular effector function. In this regard, cytokines can have dramatic effects on the regulation of immune responses and the pathogenesis of a variety of diseases. Indeed, T cells have been categorized on the basis of the pattern of cytokines that they secrete, which results in either humoral immune response (T_H2) or cell-mediated immune response (T_H1). A third type of T helper cell is the T_H17 cell that contributes to host defense against extracellular bacteria and fungi, particularly at mucosal sites (Fig. 314-2).

Cytokine receptors can be grouped into five general families based on similarities in their extracellular amino acid sequences and conserved structural domains. The *immunoglobulin (Ig) superfamily* represents a large number of cell-surface and secreted proteins. The IL-1 receptors (type 1, type 2) are examples of cytokine receptors with extracellular Ig domains.

The hallmark of the *hematopoietic growth factor (type 1) receptor* family is that the extracellular regions of each receptor contain two conserved motifs. One motif, located at the N terminus, is rich in cysteine residues. The other motif is located at the C terminus proximal to the transmembrane region and comprises five amino acid residues, tryptophan-serine-X-tryptophan-serine (WSXWS). This family can be grouped on the basis of the number of receptor subunits they have and on the utilization of shared subunits. A number of cytokine receptors, i.e., IL-6, IL-11, IL-12, and leukemia inhibitory factor, are paired with gp130. There is also a common 150-kDa subunit shared by IL-3, IL-5, and granulocyte-macrophage colony-stimulating factor (GM-CSF) receptors. The gamma chain (γ_c) of the IL-2 receptor is common to the IL-2, IL-4, IL-7, IL-9, and IL-15 receptors. Thus, the specific cytokine receptor is responsible for ligand-specific binding, while the subunits such as gp130, the 150-kDa subunit, and γ_c are important in signal transduction. The γ_c gene is on the X chromosome, and mutations in the γ_c protein result in the *X-linked form of severe combined immune deficiency syndrome (X-SCID)* (Chap. 316).

The members of the *interferon (type II) receptor* family include the receptors for IFN-γ and -β, which share a similar 210-amino-acid binding domain with conserved cysteine pairs at both the amino and carboxy termini. The members of the *TNF (type III) receptor family* share a common binding domain composed of repeated cysteine-rich regions. Members of this family include the p55 and p75 receptors for TNF (TNF-R1 and TNF-R2, respectively); CD40 antigen, which is an important B cell–surface marker involved in immunoglobulin isotype switching; fas/Apo-1, whose triggering induces apoptosis; CD27 and CD30, which are found on activated T cells and B cells; and nerve growth factor receptor.

The common motif for the *seven transmembrane helix family* was originally found in receptors linked to GTP-binding proteins. This family includes receptors for chemokines (Table 314-8), β-adrenergic receptors, and retinal rhodopsin. It is important to note that two members of the chemokine receptor family, CXC chemokine receptor type 4 (CXCR4) and β chemokine receptor type 5 (CCR5), have been found to serve as the two major co-receptors for binding and entry of HIV into CD4-expressing host cells (Chap. 189).

Significant advances have been made in defining the signaling pathways through which cytokines exert their effects intracellularly. The Janus family of protein tyrosine kinases (JAK) is a critical element involved in signaling via the hematopoietin receptors. Four JAK kinases, JAK1, JAK2, JAK3, and Tyk2, preferentially bind different cytokine receptor subunits. Cytokine binding to its receptor brings the cytokine receptor subunits into apposition and allows a pair of JAKs to transphosphorylate and activate one another. The JAKs then phosphorylate the receptor on the tyrosine residues and allow signaling molecules to bind to the receptor, where these molecules become phosphorylated. Signaling molecules bind the receptor because they have domains (SH2, or src homology 2 domains) that can bind phosphorylated tyrosine residues. There are a number of these important signaling molecules that bind the receptor, such as the adapter molecule SHC, which can couple the receptor to the activation of the mitogen-activated protein kinase pathway. In addition, an important class of substrate of the JAKs is the signal transducers and activators of transcription (STAT) family of transcription factors. STATs have SH2 domains that enable them to bind to phosphorylated receptors, where they are then phosphorylated by the JAKs. It appears that different STATs have specificity for different receptor subunits. The STATs then dissociate from the receptor and translocate to the nucleus, bind to DNA motifs that they recognize, and regulate gene expression. The STATs preferentially bind DNA motifs that are slightly different from one another and thereby control transcription of specific genes. The importance of this pathway is particularly relevant to lymphoid development. Mutations of JAK3 itself also result in a disorder identical to X-SCID; however, since JAK3 is found on chromosome 19 and not on the X chromosome, JAK3 deficiency occurs in boys and girls (Chap. 316).

THE ADAPTIVE IMMUNE SYSTEM

Adaptive immunity is characterized by antigen-specific responses to a foreign antigen or pathogen. A key feature of adaptive immunity is that following the initial contact with antigen (*immunologic priming*), subsequent antigen exposure leads to more rapid and vigorous immune responses (*immunologic memory*). The adaptive immune system consists of dual limbs of cellular and humoral immunity. The principal effectors of cellular immunity are T lymphocytes, while the principal effectors of humoral immunity are B lymphocytes. Both B and T lymphocytes derive from a common stem cell (Fig. 314-6).

The proportion and distribution of immunocompetent cells in various tissues reflect cell traffic, homing patterns, and functional capabilities. Bone marrow is the major site of maturation of B cells, monocytes-macrophages, dendritic cells, and granulocytes and contains pluripotent stem cells that, under the influence of various colony-stimulating factors, are capable of giving rise to all hematopoietic cell types. T cell precursors also arise from hematopoietic stem cells and home to the thymus for maturation. Mature T lymphocytes, B lymphocytes, monocytes, and dendritic cells enter the circulation and home to peripheral lymphoid organs (lymph nodes, spleen) and mucosal surface-associated lymphoid tissue (gut, genitourinary, and respiratory tracts) as well as the skin and mucous membranes and await activation by foreign antigen.

T cells

The pool of effector T cells is established in the thymus early in life and is maintained throughout life both by new T cell production in the thymus and by antigen-driven expansion of virgin peripheral T cells into "memory" T cells that reside in peripheral lymphoid organs. The thymus exports ~2% of the total number of thymocytes per day throughout life, with the total number of daily thymic emigrants decreasing by ~3% per year during the first four decades of life.

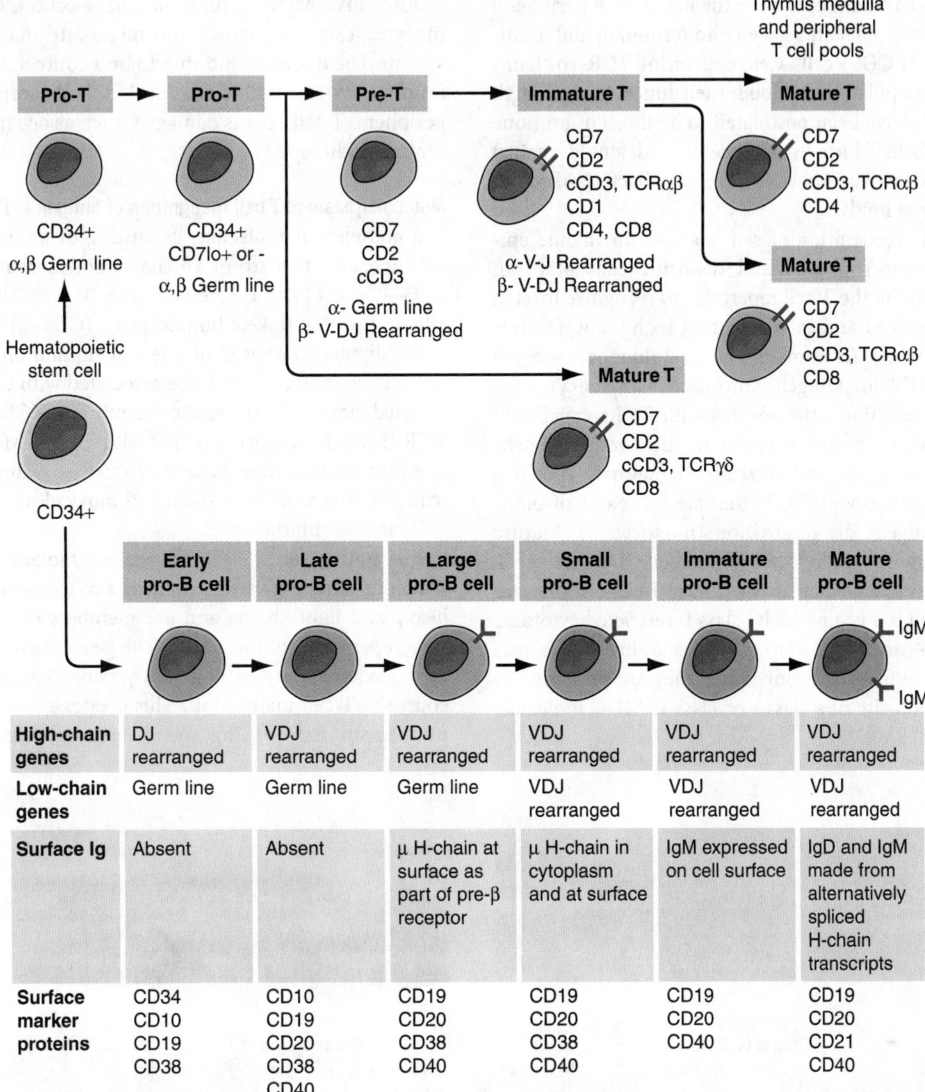

	Early pro-B cell	Late pro-B cell	Large pro-B cell	Small pro-B cell	Immature pro-B cell	Mature pro-B cell
High-chain genes	DJ rearranged	VDJ rearranged	VDJ rearranged	VDJ rearranged	VDJ rearranged	VDJ rearranged
Low-chain genes	Germ line	Germ line	Germ line	VDJ rearranged	VDJ rearranged	VDJ rearranged
Surface Ig	Absent	Absent	μ H-chain at surface as part of pre-β receptor	μ H-chain in cytoplasm and at surface	IgM expressed on cell surface	IgD and IgM made from alternatively spliced H-chain transcripts
Surface marker proteins	CD34 CD10 CD19 CD38	CD10 CD19 CD20 CD38 CD40	CD19 CD20 CD38 CD40	CD19 CD20 CD38 CD40	CD19 CD20 CD40	CD19 CD20 CD21 CD40

Figure 314-6 Development stages of T and B cells. Elements of the developing T and B cell receptor for antigen are shown schematically. The classification into the various stages of B cell development is primarily defined by rearrangement of the immunoglobulin (Ig), heavy (H), and light (L) chain genes and by the absence or presence of specific surface markers. *[Adapted from CA Janeway et al (eds): Immunobiology. The Immune Systemic Health and Disease, 4th ed. New York, Garland, 1999; with permission.]* The classification of stages of T cell development is primarily defined by cell-surface marker protein expression (sCD3, surface CD3 expression, cCD3, cytoplasmic CD3 expression; TCR, T cell receptor).

Mature T lymphocytes constitute 70–80% of normal peripheral blood lymphocytes (only 2% of the total-body lymphocytes are contained in peripheral blood), 90% of thoracic duct lymphocytes, 30–40% of lymph node cells, and 20–30% of spleen lymphoid cells. In lymph nodes, T cells occupy deep paracortical areas around B cell germinal centers, and in the spleen, they are located in periarteriolar areas of white pulp (Chap. 59). T cells are the primary effectors of cell-mediated immunity, with subsets of T cells maturing into CD8+ cytotoxic T cells capable of lysis of virus-infected or foreign cells (short-lived effector T cells). Two populations of long-lived memory T cells are triggered by infections: effector memory and central memory T cells. Effector memory T cells reside in nonlymphoid organs and respond rapidly to repeated pathogenic infections with cytokine production and cytotoxic functions to kill virus-infected cells. Central memory T cells home to lymphoid organs where they replenish long- and short-lived and effector memory T cells as needed.

In general, CD4+ T cells are also the primary regulatory cells of T and B lymphocyte and monocyte function by the production of cytokines and by direct cell contact (Fig. 314-2). In addition, T cells regulate erythroid cell maturation in bone marrow and, through cell contact (CD40 ligand), have an important role in activation of B cells and induction of Ig isotype switching.

Human T cells express cell-surface proteins that mark stages of intrathymic T cell maturation or identify specific functional subpopulations of mature T cells. Many of these molecules mediate or participate in important T cell functions (Table 314-1, Fig. 314-6).

The earliest identifiable T cell precursors in bone marrow are CD34+ pro-T cells (i.e., cells in which TCR genes are neither rearranged nor expressed). In the thymus, CD34+ T cell precursors begin cytoplasmic (c) synthesis of components of the CD3 complex of TCR-associated molecules (Fig. 314-6). Within T cell precursors, TCR for antigen gene rearrangement yields two T cell lineages, expressing either TCR-αβ chains or TCR-γδ chains. T cells expressing the TCR-αβ chains constitute the majority of peripheral T cells in blood, lymph node, and spleen and terminally differentiate into either CD4+ or CD8+ cells. Cells expressing TCR-γδ chains circulate as a minor population in blood; their functions, although not fully understood, have been postulated to be those of immune surveillance at epithelial surfaces and cellular defenses against mycobacterial organisms and other intracellular bacteria through recognition of bacterial lipids.

In the thymus, the recognition of self-peptides on thymic epithelial cells, thymic macrophages, and dendritic cells plays an important role in shaping the T cell repertoire to recognize foreign antigen (*positive selection*) and in eliminating highly autoreactive T cells (*negative selection*). As immature cortical thymocytes begin to express surface TCR for antigen, autoreactive thymocytes are destroyed (negative selection), thymocytes with TCRs capable of interacting with foreign antigen peptides in the context of self-MHC antigens are activated and develop to maturity (positive selection), and thymocytes with TCRs that are incapable of binding to self-MHC antigens die of attrition (*no selection*). Mature thymocytes that are positively selected are either CD4+ helper T cells or MHC class II–restricted cytotoxic (killer) T cells, or they are CD8+ T cells destined to become MHC class I–restricted cytotoxic T cells. *MHC class I–* or *class II–restricted* means that T cells recognize antigen peptide fragments only when they are presented in the antigen-recognition site of a class I or class II MHC molecule, respectively (Chap. 315).

After thymocyte maturation and selection, CD4 and CD8 thymocytes leave the thymus and migrate to the peripheral immune system. The thymus continues to be a contributor to the peripheral immune system, well into adult life, both normally and when the peripheral T cell pool is damaged, such as occurs in AIDS and cancer chemotherapy.

Molecular basis of T cell recognition of antigen The TCR for antigen is a complex of molecules consisting of an antigen-binding heterodimer of either αβ or γδ chains noncovalently linked with five CD3 subunits (γ, δ, ε, ζ, and η) (Fig. 314-7). The CD3 ζ chains are either disulfide-linked homodimers (CD3-ζ_2) or disulfide-linked heterodimers composed of one ζ chain and one η chain. TCR-αβ or TCR-γδ molecules must be associated with CD3 molecules to be inserted into the T cell–surface membrane, TCRα being paired with TCR-β and TCR-γ being paired with TCR-δ. Molecules of the CD3 complex mediate transduction of T cell activation signals via TCRs, while TCR-α and -β or -γ and -δ molecules combine to form the TCR antigen-binding site.

The α, β, γ, and δ TCR for antigen molecules have amino acid sequence homology and structural similarities to immunoglobulin heavy and light chains and are members of the *immunoglobulin gene superfamily* of molecules. The genes encoding TCR molecules are encoded as clusters of gene segments that rearrange during the course of T cell maturation. This creates an efficient and compact mechanism for housing the diversity requirements of antigen

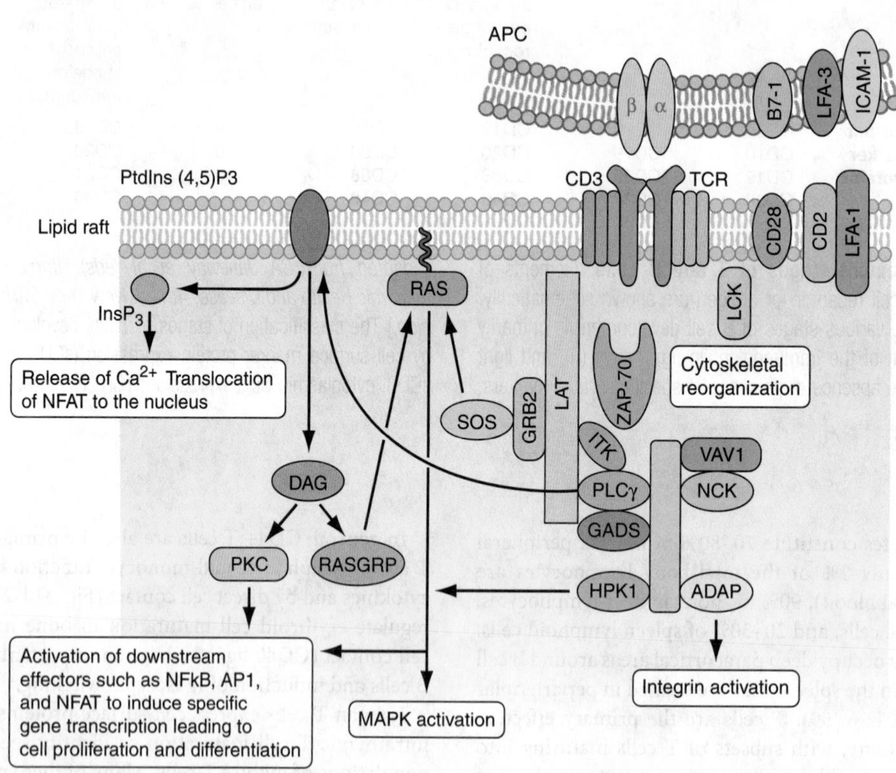

Figure 314-7 Signaling through the T cell receptor. Activation signals are mediated via immunoreceptor tyrosine-based activation (ITAM) sequences in LAT and CD3 chains (blue bars) that bind to enzymes and transduce activation signals to the nucleus via the indicated intracellular activation pathways. Ligation of the T-cell receptor (TCR) by MHC complexed with antigen results in sequential activation of LCK and γ-chain-associated protein kinase of 70 kDa (ZAP-70). ZAP-70 phosphorylates several downstream targets, including LAT (linker for activation of T cells) and SLP76 [SCR homology 2 (SH2) domain-containing leukocyte protein of 76 kDa]. SLP76 is recruited to membrane-bound LAT through its constitutive interaction with GADS (GRB2-related adaptor protein). Together, SLP76 and LAT nucleate a multimolecular signaling complex, which induces a host of downstream responses, including calcium flux, mitogen-activated protein kinase (MAPK) activation, integrin activation, and cytoskeletal reorganization. APC denotes antigen-presenting cell. *(Adapted from Koretzky et al; with permission from Macmillan Publishers Ltd. Copyright 2006.)*

receptor molecules. The TCR-α chain is on chromosome 14 and consists of a series of V (variable), J (joining), and C (constant) regions. The TCR-β chain is on chromosome 7 and consists of multiple V, D (diversity), J, and C TCR-β loci. The TCR-γ chain is on chromosome 7, and the TCR-δ chain is in the middle of the TCR-α locus on chromosome 14. Thus, molecules of the TCR for antigen have constant (framework) and variable regions, and the gene segments encoding the α, β, γ, and δ chains of these molecules are recombined and selected in the thymus, culminating in synthesis of the completed molecule. In both T and B cell precursors (see below), DNA rearrangements of antigen receptor genes involve the same enzymes, recombinase activating gene (RAG)1 and RAG2, both DNA-dependent protein kinases.

TCR diversity is created by the different V, D, and J segments that are possible for each receptor chain by the many permutations of V, D, and J segment combinations, by "N-region diversification" due to the addition of nucleotides at the junction of rearranged gene segments, and by the pairing of individual chains to form a TCR dimer. As T cells mature in the thymus, the repertoire of antigen-reactive T cells is modified by selection processes that eliminate many autoreactive T cells, enhance the proliferation of cells that function appropriately with self-MHC molecules and antigen, and allow T cells with nonproductive TCR rearrangements to die.

TCR-αβ cells do not recognize native protein or carbohydrate antigens. Instead, T cells recognize only short (~9–13 amino acids) peptide fragments derived from protein antigens taken up or produced in APCs. Foreign antigens may be taken up by endocytosis into acidified intracellular vesicles or by phagocytosis and degraded into small peptides that associate with MHC class II molecules (exogenous antigen-presentation pathway). Other foreign antigens arise endogenously in the cytosol (such as from replicating viruses) and are broken down into small peptides that associate with MHC class I molecules (endogenous antigen-presenting pathway). Thus, APCs proteolytically degrade foreign proteins and display peptide fragments embedded in the MHC class I or II antigen-recognition site on the MHC molecule surface, where foreign peptide fragments are available to bind to TCR-αβ or TCR-γδ chains of reactive T cells. CD4 molecules act as adhesives and, by direct binding to MHC class II (DR, DQ, or DP) molecules, stabilize the interaction of TCR with peptide antigen (Fig. 314-7). Similarly, CD8 molecules also act as adhesives to stabilize the TCR-antigen interaction by direct CD8 molecule binding to MHC class I (A, B, or C) molecules.

Antigens that arise in the cytosol and are processed via the endogenous antigen-presentation pathway are cleaved into small peptides by a complex of proteases called the *proteasome*. From the proteasome, antigen peptide fragments are transported from the cytosol into the lumen of the endoplasmic reticulum by a heterodimeric complex termed *transporters associated with antigen processing*, or TAP proteins. There, MHC class I molecules in the endoplasmic reticulum membrane physically associate with processed cytosolic peptides. Following peptide association with class I molecules, peptide–class I complexes are exported to the Golgi apparatus, and then to the cell surface, for recognition by CD8+ T cells.

Antigens taken up from the extracellular space via endocytosis into intracellular acidified vesicles are degraded by vesicle proteases into peptide fragments. Intracellular vesicles containing MHC class II molecules fuse with peptide-containing vesicles, thus allowing peptide fragments to physically bind to MHC class II molecules. Peptide–MHC class II complexes are then transported to the cell surface for recognition by CD4+ T cells (Chap. 315).

Whereas it is generally agreed that the TCR-αβ receptor recognizes peptide antigens in the context of MHC class I or class II molecules, lipids in the cell wall of intracellular bacteria such as *M. tuberculosis* can also be presented to a wide variety of T cells, including subsets of TCR-γδ T cells, and a subset of CD8+ TCR-αβ T cells. Importantly, bacterial lipid antigens are not presented in the context of MHC class I or II molecules, but rather are presented in the context of MHC-related CD1 molecules. Some γδ T cells that recognize lipid antigens via CD1 molecules have very restricted TCR usage, do not need antigen priming to respond to bacterial lipids, and may actually be a form of innate rather than acquired immunity to intracellular bacteria.

Just as foreign antigens are degraded and their peptide fragments presented in the context of MHC class I or class II molecules on APCs, endogenous self-proteins also are degraded and self-peptide fragments are presented to T cells in the context of MHC class I or class II molecules on APCs. In peripheral lymphoid organs, there are T cells that are capable of recognizing self-protein fragments but normally are *anergic* or *tolerant*, i.e., nonresponsive to self-antigenic stimulation, due to lack of self-antigen upregulating APC *co-stimulatory molecules* such as B7-1 (CD80) and B7-2 (CD86) (see below).

Once engagement of mature T cell TCR by foreign peptide occurs in the context of self–MHC class I or class II molecules, binding of non-antigen-specific adhesion ligand pairs such as CD54-CD11/CD18 and CD58-CD2 stabilizes MHC peptide–TCR binding, and the expression of these adhesion molecules is upregulated (Fig. 314-7). Once antigen ligation of the TCR occurs, the T cell membrane is partitioned into *lipid membrane microdomains*, or *lipid rafts*, that coalesce the key signaling molecules TCR/CD3 complex, CD28, CD2, LAT (linker for activation of T cells), intracellular activated (dephosphorylated) src family protein tyrosine kinases (PTKs), and the key CD3ζ-associated protein-70 (ZAP-70) PTK (Fig. 314-7). Importantly, during T cell activation, the CD45 molecule, with protein tyrosine phosphatase activity is partitioned away from the TCR complex to allow activating phosphorylation events to occur. The coalescence of signaling molecules of activated T lymphocytes in *microdomains* has suggested that T cell–APC interactions can be considered *immunologic synapses*, analogous in function to neuronal synapses.

After TCR-MHC binding is stabilized, activation signals are transmitted through the cell to the nucleus and lead to the expression of gene products important in mediating the wide diversity of T cell functions such as the secretion of IL-2. The TCR does not have intrinsic signaling activity but is linked to a variety of signaling pathways via immunoreceptor tyrosine-based activation motifs (ITAMs) expressed on the various CD3 chains that bind to proteins that mediate signal transduction. Each of the pathways results in the activation of particular transcription factors that control the expression of cytokine and cytokine receptor genes. Thus, antigen-MHC binding to the TCR induces the activation of the src family of PTKs, fyn and lck (lck is associated with CD4 or CD8 co-stimulatory molecules); phosphorylation of CD3ζ chain; activation of the related tyrosine kinases ZAP-70 and syk; and downstream activation of the calcium-dependent calcineurin pathway, the ras pathway, and the protein kinase C pathway. Each of these pathways leads to activation of specific families of transcription factors (including NF-AT, fos and jun, and rel/NF-κB) that form heteromultimers capable of inducing expression of IL-2, IL-2 receptor, IL-4, TNF-α, and other T cell mediators.

In addition to the signals delivered to the T cell from the TCR complex and CD4 and CD8, molecules on the T cell such as CD28 and inducible co-stimulator (ICOS) and molecules on dendritic cells such as B7-1 (CD80) and B7-2 (CD86) also deliver important co-stimulatory signals that upregulate T cell cytokine production and are essential for T cell activation. If signaling through CD28 or ICOS does not occur, or if CD28 is blocked, the T cell becomes anergic rather than activated (see "Immune Tolerance and Autoimmunity" below).

T cell superantigens Conventional antigens bind to MHC class I or II molecules in the groove of the αβ heterodimer and bind to

T cells via the V regions of the TCR-α and -β chains. In contrast, superantigens bind directly to the lateral portion of the TCR-β chain and MHC class II β chain and stimulate T cells based solely on the Vβ gene segment utilized independent of the D, J, and Vα sequences present. *Superantigens* are protein molecules capable of activating up to 20% of the peripheral T cell pool, whereas conventional antigens activate <1 in 10,000 T cells. T cell superantigens include staphylococcal enterotoxins and other bacterial products. Superantigen stimulation of human peripheral T cells occurs in the clinical setting of *staphylococcal toxic shock syndrome*, leading to massive overproduction of T cell cytokines that leads to hypotension and shock (Chap. 135).

B cells Mature B cells constitute 10–15% of human peripheral blood lymphocytes, 20–30% of lymph node cells, 50% of splenic lymphocytes, and ~10% of bone marrow lymphocytes. B cells express on their surface intramembrane immunoglobulin (Ig) molecules that function as B cell receptors (BCRs) for antigen in a complex of Ig-associated α and β signaling molecules with properties similar to those described in T cells (Fig. 314-8). Unlike T cells, which recognize only processed peptide fragments of conventional antigens embedded in the notches of MHC class I and class II antigens of APCs, B cells are capable of recognizing and proliferating to whole unprocessed native antigens via antigen binding to B cell–surface Ig (sIg) receptors. B cells also express surface receptors for the Fc region of IgG molecules (CD32) as well as receptors for activated complement components (C3d or CD21, C3b or CD35). The primary function of B cells is to produce antibodies. B cells also serve as APCs and are highly efficient at antigen processing. Their antigen-presenting function is enhanced by a variety of cytokines. Mature B cells are derived from bone marrow precursor cells that arise continuously throughout life (Fig. 314-6).

B lymphocyte development can be separated into antigen-independent and antigen-dependent phases. Antigen-independent B cell development occurs in primary lymphoid organs and includes all stages of B cell maturation up to the sIg+ mature B cell. Antigen-dependent B cell maturation is driven by the interaction of antigen with the mature B cell sIg, leading to memory B cell induction, Ig class switching, and plasma cell formation. Antigen-dependent stages of B cell maturation occur in secondary lymphoid organs, including lymph node, spleen, and gut Peyer's patches. In contrast to the T cell repertoire that is generated intrathymically before contact with foreign antigen, the repertoire of B cells expressing diverse antigen-reactive sites is modified by further alteration of Ig genes after stimulation by antigen—a process called *somatic hypermutation*—which occurs in lymph node germinal centers.

During B cell development, diversity of the antigen-binding variable region of Ig is generated by an ordered set of Ig gene rearrangements that are similar to the rearrangements undergone by TCR α, β, γ, and δ genes. For the heavy chain, there is first a rearrangement

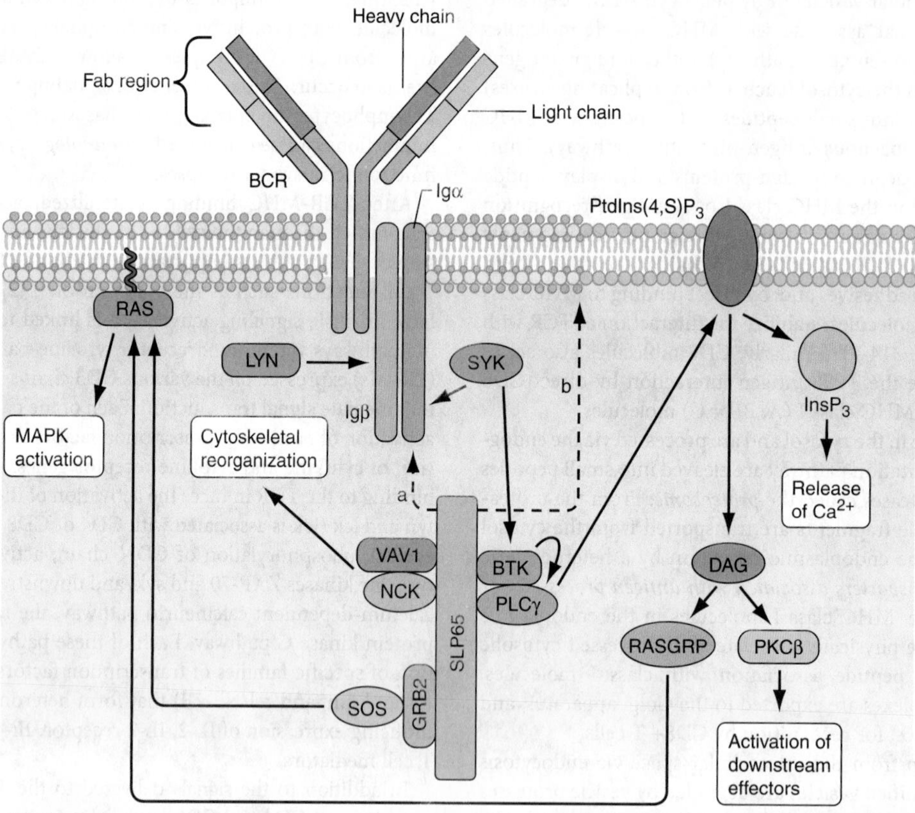

Figure 314-8 B cell receptor (BCR) activation results in the sequential activation of protein tyrosine kinases, which results in the formation of a signaling complex and activation of downstream pathways as shown. Whereas SLP76 is recruited to the membrane through GADS and LAT, the mechanism of SLP65 recruitment is unclear. Studies have indicated two mechanisms: (a) direct binding by the SH2 domain of SLP65 to immunoglobulin (Ig) of the BCR complex or (b) membrane recruitment through a leucine zipper in the amino terminus of SLP65 and an unknown binding partner. ADAP, adhesion- and degranulation-promoting adaptor protein; AP1, activator protein 1; BTK, Bruton's tyrosine kinase; DAG, diacylglycerol; GRB2, growth factor receptor–bound protein 2; HPK1, hematopoietic progenitor kinase 1; $InsP_3$, inositol-1,4,5-trisphosphate; ITK, interleukin-2-inducible T cell kinase; NCK, noncatalytic region of tyrosine kinase; NF-B, nuclear factor B; PKC, protein kinase C; PLC, phospholipase C; $PtdIns(4,5)P_2$, phosphatidylinositol-4,5-bisphosphate; RASGRP, RAS guanyl-releasing protein; SOS, son of sevenless homologue; SYK, spleen tyrosine kinase. *(Adapted from Koretzky et al; with permission from Macmillan Publishers Ltd. Copyright 2006.)*

of D segments to J segments, followed by a second rearrangement between a V gene segment and the newly formed D-J sequence; the C segment is aligned to the V-D-J complex to yield a functional Ig heavy chain gene (V-D-J-C). During later stages, a functional κ or γ light chain gene is generated by rearrangement of a V segment to a J segment, ultimately yielding an intact Ig molecule composed of heavy and light chains.

The process of Ig gene rearrangement is regulated and results in a single antibody specificity produced by each B cell, with each Ig molecule comprising one type of heavy chain and one type of light chain. Although each B cell contains two copies of Ig light and heavy chain genes, only one gene of each type is productively rearranged and expressed in each B cell, a process termed *allelic exclusion*.

There are ~300 $V_κ$ genes and 5 $J_κ$ genes, resulting in the pairing of $V_κ$ and $J_κ$ genes to create >1500 different light chain combinations. The number of distinct κ light chains that can be generated is increased by somatic mutations within the $V_κ$ and $J_κ$ genes, thus creating large numbers of possible specificities from a limited amount of germ-line genetic information. As noted above, in heavy chain Ig gene rearrangement, the VH domain is created by the joining of three types of germ-line genes called V_H, D_H, and J_H, thus allowing for even greater diversity in the variable region of heavy chains than of light chains.

The most immature B cell precursors (early pro-B cells) lack cytoplasmic Ig (cIg) and sIg (Fig. 314-6). The large pre-B cell is marked by the acquisition of the surface pre-BCR composed of μ heavy (H) chains and a pre-B light chain, termed ψLC. ψLC is a surrogate light chain receptor encoded by the nonrearranged V pre-B and the γ5 light chain locus (the pre-BCR). Pro- and pre-B cells are driven to proliferate and mature by signals from bone marrow stroma—in particular, IL-7. Light chain rearrangement occurs in the small pre-B cell stage such that the full BCR is expressed at the immature B cell stage. Immature B cells have rearranged Ig light chain genes and express sIgM. As immature B cells develop into mature B cells, sIgD is expressed as well as sIgM. At this point, B lineage development in bone marrow is complete, and B cells exit into the peripheral circulation and migrate to secondary lymphoid organs to encounter specific antigens.

Random rearrangements of Ig genes occasionally generate self-reactive antibodies, and mechanisms must be in place to correct these mistakes. One such mechanism is BCR editing, whereby autoreactive BCRs are mutated to not react with self-antigens. If receptor editing is unsuccessful in eliminating autoreactive B cells, then autoreactive B cells undergo negative selection in the bone marrow through induction of apoptosis after BCR engagement of self-antigen.

After leaving the bone marrow, B cells populate peripheral B cell sites, such as lymph node and spleen, and await contact with foreign antigens that react with each B cell's clonotypic receptor. Antigen-driven B cell activation occurs through the BCR, and a process known as *somatic hypermutation* takes place whereby point mutations in rearranged H- and L-genes give rise to mutant sIg molecules, some of which bind antigen better than the original sIg molecules. Somatic hypermutation, therefore, is a process whereby memory B cells in peripheral lymph organs have the best binding, or the highest-affinity antibodies. This overall process of generating the best antibodies is called *affinity maturation of antibody*.

Lymphocytes that synthesize IgG, IgA, and IgE are derived from sIgM+, sIgD+ mature B cells. Ig class switching occurs in lymph node and other peripheral lymphoid tissue germinal centers. CD40 on B cells and CD40 ligand on T cells constitute a critical co-stimulatory receptor-ligand pair of immune-stimulatory molecules. Pairs of CD40+ B cells and CD40 ligand+ T cells bind and drive B cell Ig class switching via T cell–produced cytokines such as IL-4 and TGF-β. IL-1, -2, -4, -5, and -6 synergize to drive mature B cells to proliferate and differentiate into Ig-secreting cells.

Humoral mediators of adaptive immunity: Immunoglobulins

Immunoglobulins are the products of differentiated B cells and mediate the humoral arm of the immune response. The primary functions of antibodies are to bind specifically to antigen and bring about the inactivation or removal of the offending toxin, microbe, parasite, or other foreign substance from the body. The structural basis of Ig molecule function and Ig gene organization has provided insight into the role of antibodies in normal protective immunity, pathologic immune-mediated damage by immune complexes, and autoantibody formation against host determinants.

All immunoglobulins have the basic structure of two heavy and two light chains (Fig. 314-8). Immunoglobulin isotype (i.e., G, M, A, D, E) is determined by the type of Ig heavy chain present. IgG and IgA isotypes can be divided further into subclasses (G1, G2, G3, G4, and A1, A2) based on specific antigenic determinants on Ig heavy chains. The characteristics of human immunoglobulins are outlined in Table 314-13. The four chains are covalently linked by disulfide bonds. Each chain is made up of a V region and C regions (also called *domains*), themselves made up of units of ~110 amino acids. Light chains have one variable (V_L) and one constant (C_L) unit; heavy chains have one variable unit (V_H) and three or four constant (C_H) units, depending on isotype. As the name suggests, the constant, or C, regions of Ig molecules are made up of homologous sequences and share the same primary structure as all other Ig chains of the same isotype and subclass. Constant regions are involved in biologic functions of Ig molecules. The C_H2 domain of IgG and the C_H4 units of IgM are involved with the binding of the C1q portion of C1 during complement activation. The C_H region at the carboxy-terminal end of the IgG molecule, the Fc region, binds to surface Fc receptors (CD16, CD32, CD64) of macrophages, dendritic cells, NK cells, B cells, neutrophils, and eosinophils.

Variable regions (V_L and V_H) constitute the antibody-binding (Fab) region of the molecule. Within the V_L and V_H regions are hypervariable regions (extreme sequence variability) that constitute the antigen-binding site unique to each Ig molecule. The idiotype is defined as the specific region of the Fab portion of the Ig molecule to which antigen binds. Antibodies against the idiotype portion of an antibody molecule are called *anti-idiotype antibodies*. The formation of such antibodies in vivo during a normal B cell antibody response may generate a negative (or "off") signal to B cells to terminate antibody production.

IgG constitutes ~75–85% of total serum immunoglobulin. The four IgG subclasses are numbered in order of their level in serum, IgG1 being found in greatest amounts and IgG4 the least. IgG subclasses have clinical relevance in their varying ability to bind macrophage and neutrophil Fc receptors and to activate complement (Table 314-13). Moreover, selective deficiencies of certain IgG subclasses give rise to clinical syndromes in which the patient is inordinately susceptible to bacterial infections. IgG antibodies are frequently the predominant antibody made after rechallenge of the host with antigen (secondary antibody response).

IgM antibodies normally circulate as a 950-kDa pentamer with 160-kDa bivalent monomers joined by a molecule called the *J chain*, a 15-kDa nonimmunoglobulin molecule that also effects polymerization of IgA molecules. IgM is the first immunoglobulin to appear in the immune response (primary antibody response) and is the initial type of antibody made by neonates. Membrane IgM in the monomeric form also functions as a major antigen receptor on the surface of mature B cells (Table 314-13). IgM is an important component of immune complexes in autoimmune diseases. For example, IgM antibodies against IgG molecules (rheumatoid factors) are present in high titers in *rheumatoid arthritis*, other collagen diseases, and some infectious diseases (*subacute bacterial endocarditis*).

IgA constitutes only 7–15% of total serum immunoglobulin but is the predominant class of immunoglobulin in secretions. IgA in secretions

TABLE 314-13 Physical, Chemical, and Biologic Properties of Human Immunoglobulins

Property	IgG	IgA	IgM	IgD	IgE
Usual molecular form	Monomer	Monomer, dimer	Pentamer, hexamer	Monomer	Monomer
Other chains	None	J chain, SC	J chain	None	None
Subclasses	G1, G2, G3, G4	A1, A2	None	None	None
Heavy chain allotypes	Gm (=30)	No A1, A2m (2)	None	None	None
Molecular mass, kDa	150	160, 400	950, 1150	175	190
Serum level in average adult, mg/mL	9.5–12.5	1.5–2.6	0.7–1.7	0.04	0.0003
Percentage of total serum Ig	75–85	7–15	5–10	0.3	0.019
Serum half-life, days	23	6	5	3	2.5
Synthesis rate, mg/kg per day	33	65	7	0.4	0.016
Antibody valence	2	2,4	10, 12	2	2
Classical complement activation	+(G1, 2?, 3)	–	++	–	–
Alternate complement activation	+(G4)	+	–	+	–
Binding cells via Fc	Macrophages, neutrophils, large granular lymphocytes	Lymphocytes	Lymphocytes	None	Mast cells, basophils, B cells
Biologic properties	Placental transfer, secondary Ab for most antipathogen responses	Secretory immunoglobulin	Primary Ab responses	Marker for mature B cells	Allergy, antiparasite responses

Source: After L Carayannopoulos, JD Capra, in WE Paul (ed): *Fundamental Immunology*, 3rd ed. New York, Raven, 1993; with permission.

(tears, saliva, nasal secretions, gastrointestinal tract fluid, and human milk) is in the form of secretory IgA (sIgA), a polymer consisting of two IgA monomers, a joining molecule, again called the J chain, and a glycoprotein called the *secretory protein*. Of the two IgA subclasses, IgA1 is primarily found in serum, whereas IgA2 is more prevalent in secretions. IgA fixes complement via the alternative complement pathway and has potent antiviral activity in humans by prevention of virus binding to respiratory and gastrointestinal epithelial cells.

IgD is found in minute quantities in serum and, together with IgM, is a major receptor for antigen on the B cell surface. IgE, which is present in serum in very low concentrations, is the major class of immunoglobulin involved in arming mast cells and basophils by binding to these cells via the Fc region. Antigen cross-linking of IgE molecules on basophil and mast cell surfaces results in release of mediators of the immediate hypersensitivity (allergic) response (Table 314-13).

■ CELLULAR INTERACTIONS IN REGULATION OF NORMAL IMMUNE RESPONSES

The net result of activation of the humoral (B cell) and cellular (T cell) arms of the adaptive immune system by foreign antigen is the elimination of antigen directly by specific effector T cells or in concert with specific antibody. Figure 314-2 is a simplified schematic diagram of the T and B cell responses indicating some of these cellular interactions.

The expression of adaptive immune cell function is the result of a complex series of immunoregulatory events that occur in phases. Both T and B lymphocytes mediate immune functions, and each of these cell types, when given appropriate signals, passes through stages, from activation and induction through proliferation, differentiation, and ultimately effector functions. The effector function expressed may be at the end point of a response, such as secretion of antibody by a differentiated plasma cell, or it might serve a regulatory function that modulates other functions, such as is seen with CD4+ and CD8+ T lymphocytes that modulate both differentiation of B cells and activation of CD8+ cytotoxic T cells.

CD4 helper T cells can be subdivided on the basis of cytokines produced (Fig. 314-2). Activated T_H1-type helper T cells secrete IL-2, IFN-γ, IL-3, TNF-α, GM-CSF, and TNF-β, while activated T_H2-type helper T cells secrete IL-3, -4, -5, -6, -10, and -13. T_H1 CD4+ T cells, through elaboration of IFN-γ, have a central role in mediating intracellular killing by a variety of pathogens. T_H1 CD4+ T cells also provide T cell help for generation of cytotoxic T cells and some types of opsonizing antibody, and they generally respond to antigens that lead to delayed hypersensitivity types of immune responses for many intracellular viruses and bacteria (such as HIV or *M. tuberculosis*). In contrast, T_H2 cells have a primary role in regulatory humoral immunity and isotype switching. T_H2 cells, through production of IL-4 and IL-10, have a regulatory role in limiting proinflammatory responses mediated by T_H1 cells (Fig. 314-2). In addition, T_H2 CD4+ T cells provide help to B cells for specific Ig production and respond to antigens that require high antibody levels for foreign antigen elimination (extracellular encapsulated bacteria such as *Streptococcus pneumoniae* and certain parasite infections). More recently, a new subset of the T_H family has been described termed T_H17 characterized by these cells to secrete cytokines such as IL-17, -22, and -26. T_H17 cells have been shown to play a role in autoimmune inflammatory disorders in addition to defense against extracellular bacteria and fungi, particularly at mucosal surfaces (Fig. 314-3). In summary, the type of T cell response generated in an immune response is determined by the microbe PAMPs presented to the DCs, the TLRs on the DCs that become activated, the types of DCs that are activated, and the cytokines that are produced (Table 314-4). Commonly, myeloid DCs produce IL-12 and activate T_H1 T cell responses that result in IFN-γ and cytotoxic T cell induction, and plasmacytoid DCs produce IFN-α and lead to T_H2 responses that result in IL-4 production and enhanced antibody responses.

As shown in Figs. 314-2 and 314-3, upon activation by DCs, T cell subsets that produce IL-2, IL-3, IFN-γ, and/or IL-4, -5, -6, -10, and -13 are generated and exert positive and negative influences on effector T and B cells. For B cells, trophic effects are mediated by a variety of cytokines, particularly T cell–derived IL-3, -4, -5, and -6, that act at sequential stages of B cell maturation, resulting in B cell proliferation, differentiation, and ultimately antibody secretion. For cytotoxic T cells, trophic factors include inducer T cell secretion of IL-2, IFN-γ, and IL-12.

An important type of immunomodulatory T cell that controls immune responses is *CD4+* and *CD8+ T regulatory cells.* These cells constitutively express the α chain of the IL-2 receptor (CD25), produce large amounts of IL-10, and can suppress both T and B cell responses. T regulatory cells are induced by immature dendritic cells and play key roles in maintaining tolerance to self-antigens in the periphery. Loss of T regulatory cells is the cause of organ-specific autoimmune disease in mice such as autoimmune thyroiditis, adrenalitis, and oophoritis (see "Immune Tolerance and Autoimmunity" below). T regulatory cells also play key roles in controlling the magnitude and duration of immune responses to microbes. Normally, after the initial immune response to a microbe has eliminated the invader, T regulatory cells are activated to suppress the antimicrobe response and prevent host injury. Some microbes have adapted to induce T regulatory cell activation at the site of infection to promote parasite infection and survival. In *Leishmania* infection, the parasite locally induces T regulatory cell accumulation at skin infection sites that dampens anti-*Leishmania* T cell responses and prevents elimination of the parasite. It is thought that many chronic infections such as by *M. tuberculosis* are associated with abnormal T regulatory cell activation that prevents elimination of the microbe.

Although B cells recognize native antigen via B cell–surface Ig receptors, B cells require T cell help to produce high-affinity antibody of multiple isotypes that are the most effective in eliminating foreign antigen. This T cell dependence likely functions in the regulation of B cell responses and in protection against excessive autoantibody production. T cell–B cell interactions that lead to high-affinity antibody production require (1) processing of native antigen by B cells and expression of peptide fragments on the B cell surface for presentation to T_H cells, (2) the ligation of B cells by both the TCR complex and the CD40 ligand, (3) induction of the process termed *antibody isotype switching* in antigen-specific B cell clones, and (4) induction of the process of affinity maturation of antibody in the germinal centers of B cell follicles of lymph node and spleen.

Naïve B cells express cell-surface IgD and IgM, and initial contact of naïve B cells with antigen is via binding of native antigen to B cell–surface IgM. T cell cytokines, released following T_H2 cell contact with B cells or by a "bystander" effect, induce changes in Ig gene conformation that promote recombination of Ig genes. These events then result in the "switching" of expression of heavy chain exons in a triggered B cell, leading to the secretion of IgG, IgA, or, in some cases, IgE antibody with the same V region antigen specificity as the original IgM antibody, for response to a wide variety of extracellular bacteria, protozoa, and helminths. CD40 ligand expression by activated T cells is critical for induction of B cell antibody isotype switching and for B cell responsiveness to cytokines. Patients with mutations in T cell CD40 ligand have B cells that are unable to undergo isotype switching, resulting in lack of memory B cell generation and the immunodeficiency syndrome of *X-linked hyper-IgM syndrome* (Chap. 316).

IMMUNE TOLERANCE AND AUTOIMMUNITY

Immune tolerance is defined as the absence of activation of pathogenic autoreactivity. *Autoimmune diseases* are syndromes caused by the activation of T or B cells or both, with no evidence of other causes such as infections or malignancies (Chap. 318). Once thought to be mutually exclusive, immune tolerance and autoimmunity are now both recognized to be present normally in health; when abnormal, they represent extremes from the normal state. For example, it is now known that low levels of autoreactivity of T and B cells with self-antigens in the periphery are critical to their survival. Similarly, low levels of autoreactivity and thymocyte recognition of self-antigens in the thymus are the mechanisms whereby (1) normal T cells are positively selected to survive and leave the thymus to respond to foreign microbes in the periphery and (2) T cells highly reactive to self-antigens are negatively selected and die to prevent overly self-reactive T cells from getting into the periphery (central tolerance). However, not all self-antigens are expressed in the thymus to delete highly self-reactive T cells, and there are mechanisms for peripheral tolerance induction of T cells as well. Unlike the presentation of microbial antigens by mature dendritic cells, the presentation of self-antigens by immature dendritic cells neither activates nor matures the dendritic cells to express high levels of co-stimulatory molecules such as B7-1 (CD80) or B7-2 (CD86). When peripheral T cells are stimulated by dendritic cells expressing self-antigens in the context of HLA molecules, sufficient stimulation of T cells occurs to keep them alive, but otherwise they remain anergic, or nonresponsive, until they contact a dendritic cell with high levels of co-stimulatory molecules expressing microbial antigens. In the latter setting, normal T cells then become activated to respond to the microbe. If B cells have high-self-reactivity BCRs, they normally undergo either deletion in the bone marrow or receptor editing to express a less autoreactive receptor. Although many autoimmune diseases are characterized by abnormal or pathogenic autoantibody production (Table 314-14), most autoimmune diseases are caused by a combination of excess T and B cell reactivity.

Multiple factors contribute to the genesis of clinical autoimmune disease syndromes, including genetic susceptibility (Table 314-14), environmental immune stimulants such as drugs [e.g., procainamide and phenytoin (Dilantin) with drug-induced systemic lupus erythematosus], infectious agent triggers (such as Epstein-Barr virus and autoantibody production against red blood cells and platelets), and loss of T regulatory cells (leading to thyroiditis, adrenalitis, and oophoritis).

Immunity at mucosal surfaces

Mucosa covering the respiratory, digestive, and urogenital tracts; the eye conjunctiva; the inner ear; and the ducts of all exocrine glands contain cells of the innate and adaptive mucosal immune system that protect these surfaces against pathogens. In the healthy adult, mucosa-associated lymphoid tissue (MALT) contains 80% of all immune cells within the body and constitutes the largest mammalian lymphoid organ system.

MALT has three main functions: (1) to protect the mucous membranes from invasive pathogens; (2) to prevent uptake of foreign antigens from food, commensal organisms, and airborne pathogens and particulate matter; and (3) to prevent pathologic immune responses from foreign antigens if they do cross the mucosal barriers of the body (Fig. 314-9).

MALT is a compartmentalized system of immune cells that functions independently from systemic immune organs. Whereas the systemic immune organs are essentially sterile under normal conditions and respond vigorously to pathogens, MALT immune cells are continuously bathed in foreign proteins and commensal bacteria, and they must select those pathogenic antigens that must be eliminated. MALT contains anatomically defined foci of immune cells in the intestine, tonsil, appendix, and peribronchial areas that are inductive sites for mucosal immune responses. From these sites, immune T and B cells migrate to effector sites in mucosal parenchyma and exocrine glands where mucosal immune cells eliminate pathogen-infected cells. In addition to mucosal immune responses, all mucosal sites have strong mechanical and chemical barriers and cleansing functions to repel pathogens.

TABLE 314-14 Recombinant or Purified Autoantigens Recognized by Autoantibodies Associated With Human Autoimmune Disorders

Autoantigen	Autoimmune Diseases	Autoantigen	Autoimmune Diseases
Cell- or Organ-Specific Autoimmunity			
Acetylcholine receptor	Myasthenia gravis	Insulin receptor	Type B insulin resistance, acanthosis, systemic lupus erythematosus (SLE)
Actin	Chronic active hepatitis, primary biliary cirrhosis	Intrinsic factor type 1	Pernicious anemia
Adenine nucleotide translator (ANT)	Dilated cardiomyopathy, myocarditis	Leukocyte function-associated antigen (LFA-1)	Treatment-resistant Lyme arthritis
β-Adrenoreceptor	Dilated cardiomyopathy		
Aromatic L-amino acid decarboxylase	Autoimmune polyendocrine syndrome type 1 (APS-1)	Myelin-associated glycoprotein (MAG)	Polyneuropathy
Asialoglycoprotein receptor	Autoimmune hepatitis	Myelin-basic protein	Multiple sclerosis, demyelinating diseases
Bactericidal/permeability-increasing protein (Bpi)	Cystic fibrosis vasculitides	Myelin oligodendrocyte glycoprotein (MOG)	Multiple sclerosis
Calcium-sensing receptor	Acquired hypoparathyroidism	Myosin	Rheumatic fever
Cholesterol side-chain cleavage enzyme (CYPIIa)	Autoimmune polyglandular syndrome-1	p-80-Collin	Atopic dermatitis
Collagen type IV-α3-chain	Goodpasture syndrome	Pyruvate dehydrogenase complex-E2 (PDC-E2)	Primary biliary cirrhosis
Cytochrome P450 2D6 (CYP2D6)	Autoimmune hepatitis		
Desmin	Crohn's disease, coronary artery disease	Sodium iodide symporter (NIS)	Graves' disease, autoimmune hypothyroidism
Desmoglein 1	Pemphigus foliaceus		
Desmoglein 3	Pemphigus vulgaris	SOX-10	Vitiligo
F-actin	Autoimmune hepatitis	Thyroid and eye muscle shared protein	Thyroid-associated ophthalmopathy
GM gangliosides	Guillain-Barré syndrome		
Glutamate decarboxylase (GAD65)	Type 1 diabetes, stiff-person syndrome	Thyroglobulin	Autoimmune thyroiditis
Glutamate receptor (GLUR)	Rasmussen encephalitis	Thyroid peroxidase	Autoimmune Hashimoto thyroiditis
H/K ATPase	Autoimmune gastritis	Thyrotropin receptor	Graves' disease
17-α-Hydroxylase (CYP17)	Autoimmune polyglandular syndrome-1	Tissue transglutaminase	Celiac disease
21-Hydroxylase (CYP21)	Addison disease	Transcription coactivator p75	Atopic dermatitis
IA-2 (ICA512)	Type 1 diabetes	Tryptophan hydroxylase	Autoimmune polyglandular syndrome-1
Insulin	Type 1 diabetes, insulin hypoglycemic syndrome (Hirata disease)	Tyrosinase Tyrosine hydroxylase	Vitiligo, metastatic melanoma Autoimmune polyglandular syndrome-1
Systemic Autoimmunity			
ACTH	ACTH deficiency	Histone H2A-H2B-DNA	SLE
Aminoacyl-tRAN histidyl synthetase	Myositis, dermatomyositis	IgE receptor	Chronic idiopathic urticaria
Aminoacyl-tRNA synthetase (several)	Polymyositis, dermatomyositis	Keratin	RA
Cardiolipin	SLE, anti-phospholipid syndrome	Ku-DNA-protein kinase	SLE
Carbonic anhydrase II	SLE, Sjögren's syndrome, systemic sclerosis	Ku-nucleoprotein La phosphoprotein (La 55-B)	Connective tissue syndrome Sjögren's syndrome
Collagen (multiple types)	Rheumatoid arthritis (RA), SLE, progressive systemic sclerosis	Myeloperoxidase	Necrotizing and crescentic glomerulonephritis (NCGN), systemic vasculitis

(continued)

PART 15 Disorders of the Joints and Adjacent Tissues

TABLE 314-14 Recombinant or Purified Autoantigens Recognized by Autoantibodies Associated With Human Autoimmune Disorders (*Continued*)

Autoantigen	Autoimmune Diseases	Autoantigen	Autoimmune Diseases
Systemic Autoimmunity			
Centromere-associated proteins	Systemic sclerosis	Proteinase 3 (PR3)	Granulomatosis with polyangiitis (Wegener's), Churg-Strauss syndrome
DNA-dependent nucleoside-stimulated ATPase	Dermatomyositis	RNA polymerase I–III (RNP)	Systemic sclerosis, SLE
Fibrillarin	Scleroderma	Signal recognition protein (SRP54)	Polymyositis
Fibronectin	SLE, RA, morphea	Topoisomerase-1 (Scl-70)	Scleroderma, Raynaud syndrome
Glucose-6-phosphate isomerase	RA	Tublin	Chronic liver disease, visceral leishmaniasis
β2-Glycoprotein I (B2-GPI)	Primary antiphospholipid syndrome		
Golgin (95, 97, 160, 180) Heat shock protein	Sjögren's syndrome, SLE, RA Various immune-related disorders	Vimentin	Systemic autoimmune disease
Hemidesmosomal protein 180	Bullous pemphigoid, herpes gestationis, cicatricial pemphigoid		
Plasma Protein and Cytokine Autoimmunity			
C1 inhibitor	Autoimmune C1 deficiency	Glycoprotein IIb/IIIg and Ib/IX	Autoimmune thrombocytopenia purpura
C1q	SLE, membrane proliferative glomerulonephritis (MPGN)	IgA	Immunodeficiency associated with SLE, pernicious anemia, thyroiditis, Sjögren's syndrome and chronic active hepatitis
Cytokines (IL-1α, IL-1β, IL-6, IL-10, LIF)	RA, systemic sclerosis, normal subjects		
Factor II, factor V, factor VII, factor VIII, factor IX, factor X, factor XI, thrombin vWF	Prolonged coagulation time	Oxidized LDL (OxLDL)	Atherosclerosis
Cancer and Paraneoplastic Autoimmunity			
Amphiphysin	Neuropathy, small cell lung cancer	p62 (IGF-II mRNA-binding protein)	Hepatocellular carcinoma (China)
Cyclin B1	Hepatocellular carcinoma	Recoverin	Cancer-associated retinopathy
DNA topoisomerase II	Liver cancer	Ri protein	Paraneoplastic opsoclonus myoclonus ataxia
Desmoplakin	Paraneoplastic pemphigus		
Gephyrin	Paraneoplastic stiff-person syndrome	βIV spectrin	Lower motor neuron syndrome
Hu proteins	Paraneoplastic encephalomyelitis	Synaptotagmin	Lambert-Eaton myasthenic syndrome
Neuronal nicotinic acetylcholine receptor	Subacute autonomic neuropathy, cancer	Voltage-gated calcium channels	Lambert-Eaton myasthenic syndrome
p53	Cancer, SLE	Yo protein	Paraneoplastic cerebellar degeneration

Source: From A Lernmark et al: J Clin Invest 108:1091, 2001; with permission.

Key components of MALT include specialized epithelial cells called "membrane" or "M" cells that take up antigens and deliver them to dendritic cells or other APCs. Effector cells in MALT include B cells producing antipathogen neutralizing antibodies of secretory IgA as well as IgG isotype, T cells producing similar cytokines as in systemic immune system response, and T helper and cytotoxic T cells that respond to pathogen-infected cells.

Secretory IgA is produced in amounts of >50 mg/kg of body weight per 24 h and functions to inhibit bacterial adhesion, inhibit macromolecule absorption in the gut, neutralize viruses, and enhance antigen elimination in tissue through binding to IgA and receptor-mediated transport of immune complexes through epithelial cells.

Recent studies have demonstrated the importance of commensal gut and other mucosal bacteria to the health of the human immune

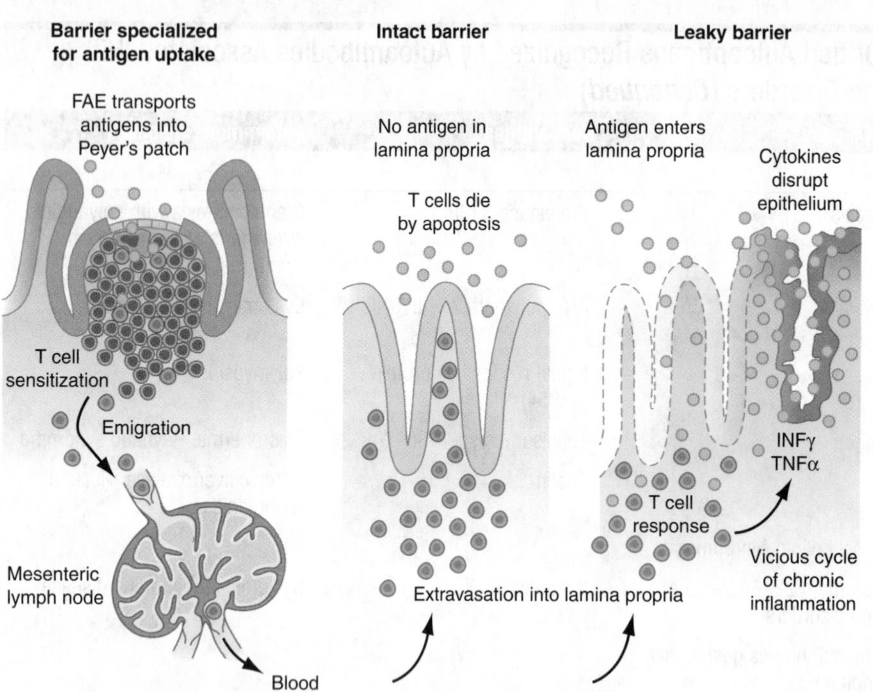

Figure 314-9 Increased epithelial permeability may be important in the development of chronic gut T cell–mediated inflammation. CD4 T cells activated by gut antigens in Peyer's patches migrate to the LP. In healthy individuals, these cells die by apoptosis. Increased epithelial permeability may allow sufficient antigen to enter the LP to trigger T cell activation, breaking tolerance mediated by immunosuppressive cytokines and perhaps T regulatory cells. Proinflammatory cytokines then further increase epithelial permeability, setting up a vicious cycle of chronic inflammation. *(From MacDonald and Monteleone; with permission.)*

system. Normal commensal flora induces anti-inflammatory events in the gut and protects epithelial cells from pathogens through TLRs and other PRR signaling. When the gut is depleted of normal commensal flora, the immune system becomes abnormal, with loss of T_H1 T cell function. Restoration of the normal gut flora can reestablish the balance in T helper cell ratios characteristic of the normal immune system. When the gut barrier is intact, either antigens do not transverse the gut epithelium or, when pathogens are present, a self-limited, protective MALT immune response eliminates the pathogen (Fig. 314-9). However, when the gut barrier breaks down, immune responses to commensal flora antigens can cause inflammatory bowel diseases such as *Crohn's disease* and, perhaps, *ulcerative colitis* (Fig. 314-9) (Chap. 295). Uncontrolled MALT immune responses to food antigens, such as gluten, can cause *celiac disease* (Chap. 295).

THE CELLULAR AND MOLECULAR CONTROL OF PROGRAMMED CELL DEATH

The process of apoptosis (programmed cell death) plays a crucial role in regulating normal immune responses to antigen. In general, a wide variety of stimuli trigger one of several apoptotic pathways to eliminate microbe-infected cells, eliminate cells with damaged DNA, or eliminate activated immune cells that are no longer needed (Fig. 314-10). The largest known family of "death receptors" is the tumor necrosis factor receptor (TNF-R) family [TNF-R1, TNF-R2, Fas (CD95), death receptor 3 (DR3), death receptor 4 [DR4, TNF-related apoptosis-including ligand receptor 1 (TRAIL-R1)], and death receptor 5 (DR5, TRAIL-R2)]; their ligands are all in the TNF-α family. Binding of ligands to these death receptors leads to a signaling cascade that involves activation of the *caspase* family of molecules that leads to DNA cleavage and cell death. Two other pathways of programmed cell death involve nuclear *p53* in the elimination of cells with abnormal DNA and *mitochondrial cytochrome c* to induce cell death in damaged cells (Fig. 314-10). A number of human diseases have now been described that result from, or are associated with, mutated apoptosis genes (Table 314-15). These include mutations in the Fas and Fas ligand genes in autoimmune and lymphoproliferation syndromes, and multiple associations of mutations in genes in the apoptotic pathway with malignant syndromes.

MECHANISMS OF IMMUNE-MEDIATED DAMAGE TO MICROBES OR HOST TISSUES

Several responses by the host innate and adaptive immune systems to foreign microbes culminate in rapid and efficient elimination of microbes. In these scenarios, the classic weapons of the adaptive immune system (T cells, B cells) interface with cells (macrophages, dendritic cells, NK cells, neutrophils, eosinophils, basophils) and soluble products (microbial peptides, pentraxins, complement and coagulation systems) of the innate immune system (Chaps. 60 and 317).

There are five general phases of host defenses: (1) migration of leukocytes to sites of antigen localization; (2) antigen-nonspecific recognition of pathogens by macrophages and other cells and systems of the innate immune system; (3) specific recognition of foreign antigens mediated by T and B lymphocytes; (4) amplification of the inflammatory response with recruitment of specific and nonspecific effector cells by complement components, cytokines, kinins, arachidonic acid metabolites, and mast cell–basophil products; and (5) macrophage, neutrophil, and lymphocyte participation in destruction of antigen with ultimate removal of antigen particles by phagocytosis (by macrophages or neutrophils) or by direct cytotoxic mechanisms (involving macrophages, neutrophils, DCs, and lymphocytes). Under normal circumstances, orderly progression of host defenses through these phases results in a well-controlled immune and inflammatory response that protects the host from the offending antigen. However, dysfunction of any of the host defense systems can damage host tissue and produce clinical disease. Furthermore, for certain pathogens or antigens, the normal immune response itself might contribute substantially to the tissue damage. For example, the immune and inflammatory response in the brain to certain pathogens such as *M. tuberculosis* may be responsible for much of the morbidity rate of this disease in that organ system (Chap. 165). In addition, the morbidity rate associated with certain pneumonias such as that caused by *Pneumocystis jiroveci* may be associated more with inflammatory infiltrates than with the tissue-destructive effects of the microorganism itself (Chap. 207).

The molecular basis of lymphocyte–endothelial cell interactions

The control of lymphocyte circulatory patterns between the bloodstream and peripheral lymphoid organs operates at the level of lymphocyte–endothelial cell interactions to control the specificity of lymphocyte subset entry into organs. Similarly, lymphocyte–endothelial cell interactions regulate the entry of lymphocytes into inflamed tissue. Adhesion molecule expression on lymphocytes and endothelial cells regulates the retention and subsequent egress of lymphocytes within tissue sites of antigenic stimulation, delaying

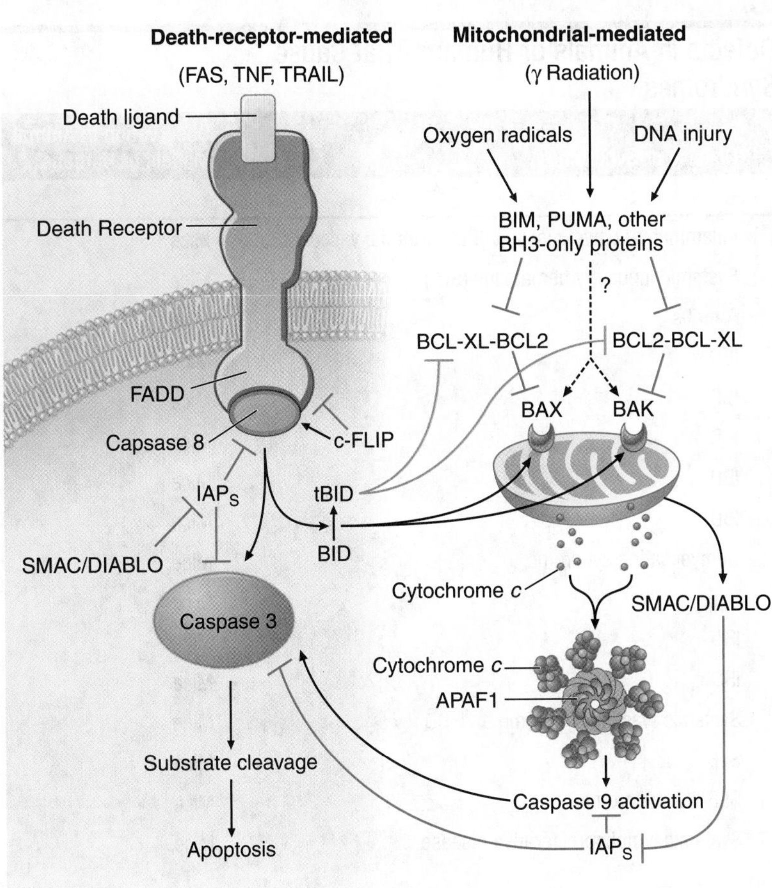

Figure 314-10 Pathways of Cellular Apoptosis. There are two major pathways of apoptosis: the death-receptor pathway, which is mediated by activation of death receptors, and the BCL2-regulated mitochondrial pathway, which is mediated by noxious stimuli that ultimately lead to mitochondrial injury. Ligation of death receptors recruits the adaptor protein FAS-associated death domain (FADD). FADD in turn recruits caspase 8, which ultimately activates caspase 3, the key "executioner" caspase. Cellular FLICE-inhibitory protein (c-FLIP) can either inhibit or potentiate binding of FADD and caspase 8, depending on its concentration. In the intrinsic pathway, proapoptotic BH3 proteins are activated by noxious stimuli, which interact with and inhibit antiapoptotic BCL2 or BCL-XL. Thus, BAX and BAK are free to induce mitochondrial permeabilization with release of cytochrome *c*, which ultimately results in the activation of caspase 9 through the apoptosome. Caspase 9 then activates caspase 3. SMAC/DIABLO is also released after mitochondrial permeabilization and acts to block the action of inhibitors of apoptosis protein (IAPs), which inhibit caspase activation. There is potential cross-talk between the two pathways, which is mediated by the truncated form of BID (tBID) that is produced by caspase 8–mediated BID cleavage; tBID acts to inhibit the BCL2-BCL-XL pathway and to activate BAX and BAK. There is debate (indicated by the question mark) as to whether proapoptotic BH3 molecules (e.g., BIM and PUMA) act directly on BAX and BAK to induce mitochondrial permeability or whether they act only on BCL2-BCL-XL. APAF1, apoptotic protease-activating factor 1; BH3, BCL homologue; TNF, tumor necrosis factor; TRAIL, TNF-related apoptosis-inducing ligand. *(From Hotchkiss et al; with permission.)*

cell exit from tissue and preventing reentry into the circulating lymphocyte pool (Fig. 314-11). All types of lymphocyte migration begin with lymphocyte attachment to specialized regions of vessels, termed *high endothelial venules* (HEVs). An important concept is that adhesion molecules do not generally bind their ligand until a conformational change (ligand activation) occurs in the adhesion molecule that allows ligand binding. Induction of a conformation-dependent determinant on an adhesion molecule can be accomplished by cytokines or via ligation of other adhesion molecules on the cell.

The first stage of lymphocyte–endothelial cell interactions, *attachment and rolling*, occurs when lymphocytes leave the stream of flowing blood cells in a postcapillary venule and roll along venule endothelial cells (Fig. 314-11). Lymphocyte rolling is mediated by the L-selectin molecule (LECAM-1, LAM-1, CD62L) and slows cell transit time through venules, allowing time for activation of adherent cells.

The second stage of lymphocyte–endothelial cell interactions, *firm adhesion with activation-dependent stable arrest*, requires stimulation of lymphocytes by chemoattractants or by endothelial cell–derived cytokines. Cytokines thought to participate in adherent cell activation include members of the IL-8 family, platelet-activation factor, leukotriene B_4, and C5a. In addition, HEVs express chemokines, SLC (CCL21) and ELC (CCL19), which participate in this process. Following activation by chemoattractants, lymphocytes shed L-selectin from the cell surface and upregulate cell CD11b/18 (MAC-1) or CD11a/18 (LFA-1) molecules, resulting in firm attachment of lymphocytes to HEVs.

Lymphocyte homing to peripheral lymph nodes involves adhesion of L-selectin to glycoprotein HEV ligands collectively referred to as *peripheral node addressin (PNAd)*, whereas homing of lymphocytes to intestine Peyer's patches primarily involves adhesion of the α4,β7 integrin to mucosal addressin cell adhesion molecule-1 (MAdCAM-1) on the Peyer's patch HEVs. However, for migration to mucosal Peyer's patch lymphoid aggregates, naïve lymphocytes primarily use L-selectin, whereas memory lymphocytes use α4,β7 integrin. α4,β1 Integrin (CD49d/CD29, VLA-4)–VCAM-1 interactions are important in the initial interaction of memory lymphocytes with HEVs of multiple organs in sites of inflammation (Table 314-16).

The third stage of leukocyte emigration in HEVs is *sticking and arrest*. Sticking of the lymphocyte to endothelial cells and arrest at the site of sticking are mediated predominantly by ligation of α1,β2 integrin LFA-1 to the integrin ligand ICAM-1 on HEVs. While the first three stages of lymphocyte attachment to HEVs take only a few seconds, the fourth stage of lymphocyte emigration, *transendothelial migration*, takes ~10 min. Although the molecular mechanisms that control lymphocyte transendothelial migration are not fully characterized, the HEV CD44 molecule and molecules of the HEV glycocalyx (extracellular matrix) are thought to play important regulatory roles in this process (Fig. 314-11). Finally, expression of matrix metalloproteases capable of digesting the subendothelial basement membrane, rich in nonfibrillar collagen, appears to be required for the penetration of lymphoid cells into the extravascular sites.

Abnormal induction of HEV formation and use of the molecules discussed above have been implicated in the induction and maintenance of inflammation in a number of chronic inflammatory diseases. In animal models of Type 1 diabetes mellitus, MAdCAM-1 and GlyCAM-1 have been shown to be highly expressed on HEVs in inflamed pancreatic islets, and treatment of these animals with inhibitors of L-selectin and α4 integrin function blocked the development of Type 1 diabetes mellitus (Chap. 344). A similar role

TABLE 314-15 Immune System Molecule Defects in Animals or Humans That Cause Autoimmune or Malignant Syndromes

Protein	Defect	Disease or Syndrome	Observation in Animal Models or Humans
Cytokines and Signaling Proteins			
Tumor necrosis factor (TNF) α	Overexpression	Inflammatory bowel disease (IBD), arthritis, vasculitis	Mice
TNF-α	Underexpression	Systemic lupus erythematosus (SLE)	Mice
Interleukin-1-receptor antagonist	Underexpression	Arthritis	Mice
IL-2	Overexpression	IBD	Mice
IL-7	Overexpression	IBD	Mice
IL-10	Overexpression	IBD	Mice
IL-2 receptor	Overexpression	IBD	Mice
IL-10 receptor	Overexpression	IBD	Mice
IL-3	Overexpression	Demyelinating syndrome	Mice
Interferon-δ	Overexpression in skin	SLE	Mice
STAT-3	Underexpression	IBD	Mice
STAT-4	Overexpression	IBD	Mice
Transforming growth factor (TGF) β	Underexpression	Systemic wasting syndrome and IBD	Mice
TGF-β receptor in T cells	Underexpression	SLE	Mice
Programmed death (PD-1)	Underexpression	SLE-like syndrome	Mice
Cytotoxic T lymphocyte, antigen-4 (CTLA-4)	Underexpression	Systemic lymphoproliferative disease	Mice
IL-10	Underexpression	IBD (mouse) Type 1 diabetes, thyroid disease, primary (human)	Mice and humans
Major Histocompatibility Locus Molecules*			
HLA B27	Allele expression or overexpression	Inflammatory bowel disease	Rats and humans
Complement deficiency of C1, 2, 3 or 4	Underexpression		Humans
LIGHT (TNF superfamily 14)	Overexpression	Systemic lymphoproliferative (mouse) and autoimmunity	Mice
HLA class II DQB10301, DQB10302	Allele expression	Juvenile-onset diabetes	Humans
HLA class II DQB10401, DQB10402	Allele expression	Rheumatoid arthritis	Humans
HLA class I B27	Allele expression	Ankylosing spondylitis, IBD	Rats and humans
Apoptosis Proteins			
TNF receptor 1 (TNF-R1)	Underexpression	Familial periodic fever syndrome	Humans
Fas (CD95; Apo-1)	Underexpression	Autoimmune lymphoproliferative syndrome type 1 (ALPS 1); malignant lymphoma; bladder cancer	Humans
Fas ligand	Underexpression	SLE (only one case identified)	Humans
Perforin	Underexpression	Familial hemophagocytic lymphohistiocytosis (FHL)	Humans
Caspase 10	Underexpression	Autoimmune lymphoproliferative syndrome type II (ALPS II)	Humans
bcl-10	Underexpression	Non-Hodgkin's lymphoma	Humans
P53	Underexpression	Various malignant neoplasms	Humans
Bax	Underexpression	Colon cancer; hematopoietic malignancies	Humans
bcl-2	Underexpression	Non-Hodgkin's lymphoma	Humans
c-IAP2	Underexpression	Low-grade MALT lymphoma	Humans
NAIP1	Underexpression	Spinal muscular atrophy	Humans

*Many autoimmune diseases are associated with a myriad of major compatibility complex gene allele (HLA) types. They are presented here as examples.

Abbreviation: MALT, mucosa-associated lymphoid tissue.

Source: Adapted from Mullauer and from Davidson and Diamond; with permission.

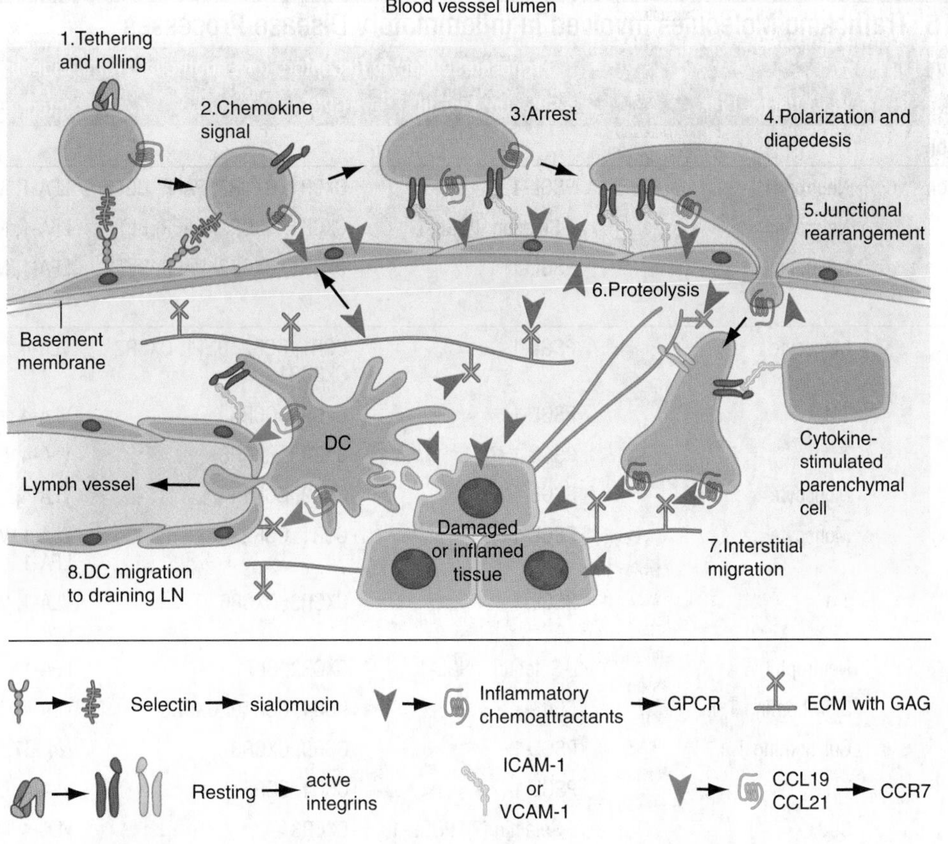

Figure 314-11 Key migration steps of immune cells at sites of inflammation. Inflammation due to tissue damage or infection induces the release of cytokines (not shown) and inflammatory chemoattractants (red arrowheads) from distressed stromal cells and "professional" sentinels, such as mast cells and macrophages (not shown). The inflammatory signals induce upregulation of endothelial selectins and immunoglobulin "superfamily" members, particularly ICAM-1 and/or VCAM-1. Chemoattractants, particularly chemokines, are produced by or translocated across venular endothelial cells (red arrow) and are displayed in the lumen to rolling leukocytes. Those leukocytes that express the appropriate set of trafficking molecules undergo a multistep adhesion cascade (steps 1–3) and then polarize and move by diapedesis across the venular wall (steps 4 and 5). Diapedesis involves transient disassembly of endothelial junctions and penetration through the underlying basement membrane (step 6). Once in the extravascular (interstitial) space, the migrating cell uses different integrins to gain "footholds" on collagen fibers and other ECM molecules, such as laminin and fibronectin, and on inflammation-induced ICAM-1 on the surface of parenchymal cells (step 7). The migrating cell receives guidance cues from distinct sets of chemoattractants, particularly chemokines, which may be immobilized on glycosaminoglycans (GAG) that "decorate" many ECM molecules and stromal cells. Inflammatory signals also induce tissue DCs to undergo maturation. Once DCs process material from damaged tissues and invading pathogens, they upregulate CCR7, which allows them to enter draining lymph vessels that express the CCR7 ligand CCL21 (and CCL19). In lymph nodes (LN), these antigen-loaded mature DCs activate naïve T cells and expand pools of effector lymphocytes, which enter the blood and migrate back to the site of inflammation. T cells in tissue also use this CCR7-dependent route to migrate from peripheral sites to draining lymph nodes through afferent lymphatics. *(Adapted from AD Luster et al: Nat Immunol 6:1182, 2005; with permission from Macmillan Publishers Ltd. Copyright 2005.)*

for abnormal induction of the adhesion molecules of lymphocyte emigration has been suggested in *rheumatoid arthritis* (Chap. 321), *Hashimoto's thyroiditis* (Chap. 341), *Graves' disease* (Chap. 341), *multiple sclerosis* (Chap. 380), *Crohn's disease* (Chap. 295), and *ulcerative colitis* (Chap. 295).

Immune-complex formation

Clearance of antigen by immune-complex formation between antigen, complement, and antibody is a highly effective mechanism of host defense. However, depending on the level of immune complexes formed and their physicochemical properties, immune complexes may or may not result in host and foreign cell damage. After antigen exposure, certain types of soluble antigen-antibody complexes freely circulate and, if not cleared by the reticuloendothelial system, can be deposited in blood vessel walls and in other tissues such as renal glomeruli and cause *vasculitis* or *glomerulonephritis* syndromes (Chaps. 283 and 326). Deficiencies of early complement components are associated with inefficient clearance of immune complexes and immune complex mediated tissue damage in autoimmune syndromes, while deficiencies of the later complement components are associated with susceptibility to recurrent *neisseria* infections (Table 314-17).

Immediate-type hypersensitivity

Helper T cells that drive antiallergen IgE responses are usually T_H2-type inducer T cells that secrete IL-4, IL-5, IL-6, and IL-10. Mast cells and basophils have high-affinity receptors for the Fc portion of IgE (FcRI), and cell-bound antiallergen IgE effectively "arms"

TABLE 314-16 Trafficking Molecules Involved in Inflammatory Disease Processes

Disease	Key Effector Cell	Proposed Leukocyte Receptors for Endothelial Traffic Signals		
		L-Selectin, Ligand	GPCR	Integrin[a]
Acute Inflammation				
Myocardial infarction	Neutrophil	PSGL-1	CXCR1, CXCR2, PAFR, BLT1	LFA-1, Mac-1
Stroke	Neutrophil	L-Selectin, PSGL-1	CXCR1, CXCR2, PAFR, BLT1	LFA-1, Mac-1
Ischemia-reperfusion	Neutrophil	PSGL-1	CXCR1, CXCR2, PAFR, BLT1	LFA-1, Mac-1
T_H1 Inflammation				
Atherosclerosis	Monocyte	PSGL-1	CCR1, CCR2, BLT1, CXCR2, CX3CR1	VLA-4
	T_H1	PSGL-1	CXCR3, CCR5	VLA-4
Multiple sclerosis	T_H1	PSGL-1 (?)	CXCR3, CXCR6	VLA-4, LFA-1
	Monocyte	PSGL-1 (?)	CCR2, CCR1	VLA-4, LFA-1
Rheumatoid arthritis	Monocyte	PSGL-1	CCR1, CCR2	VLA-1, VLA-2, VLA-4, LFA-1
	T_H1	PSGL-1	CXCR3, CXCR6	VLA-1, VLA-2, VLA-4, LFA-1
	Neutrophil	L-Selectin, PSGL-1	CXCR2, BLT1	LFA-1[b]
Psoriasis	Skin-homing T_H1	CLA	CCR4, CCR10, CXCR3	VLA-4[c], LFA-1
Crohn disease	Gut-homing T_H1	PSGL-1	CCR9, CXCR3	$\alpha4$, $\beta7$, LFA-1
Type I diabetes	T_H1	PSGL-1 (?)	CCR4, CCR5	VLA-4, LFA-1
	CD8	L-Selectin (?), PSGL-1 (?)	CXCR3	VLA-4, LFA-1
Allograft rejection	CD8	PSGL-1	CXCR3, CX3CR1, BLT1	VLA-4, LFA-1
	B cell	L-Selectin, PSGL-1	CXCR5, CXCR4	VLA-4, LFA-1
Hepatitis	CD8	PSGL-1	CXCR3, CCR5, CXCR6	VLA-4
Lupus	T_H1	None	CXCR6	VLA-4[d]
	Plasmacytoid DC	L-Selectin, CLA	CCR7, CXCR3, ChemR23	LFA-1, Mac-1
	B cell	CLA (?)	CXCR5, CXCR4	LFA-1
T_H2 Inflammation				
Asthma	T_H2	PSGL-1	CCR4, CCR8, BLT1	LFA-1
	Eosinophil	PSGL-1	CCR3, PAFR, BLT1	VLA-4, LFA-1
	Mast cells	PSGL-1	CCR2, CCR3, BLT1	VLA-4, LFA-1
Atopic dermatitis	Skin-homing T_H2	CLA	CCR4, CCR10	VLA-4, LFA-1

[a]Various β_1 integrins have been linked in different ways in basal lamina and interstitial migration of distinct cell types and inflammatory settings.
[b]In some settings, Mac-1 has been linked to transmigration.
[c]CD44 can act in concert with VLA-4 in particular models of leukocyte arrest.
[d]T_H2 cells require VAP-1 to traffic to inflamed liver.

Source: From AD Luster et al: Nat Immunol 6:1182, 2005; with permission from Macmillan Publishers Ltd. Copyright 2005.

basophils and mast cells. Mediator release is triggered by antigen (allergen) interaction with Fc receptor–bound IgE, the mediators released are responsible for the pathophysiologic changes of *allergic diseases* (Table 314-12). Mediators released from mast cells and basophils can be divided into three broad functional types: (1) those that increase vascular permeability and contract smooth muscle (histamine, platelet-activating factor, SRS-A, BK-A), (2) those that are chemotactic for or activate other inflammatory cells (ECF-A, NCF, leukotriene B_4), and (3) those that modulate the release of other mediators (BK-A, platelet-activating factor) (Chap. 317).

Cytotoxic reactions of antibody

In this type of immunologic injury, complement-fixing (C1-binding) antibodies against normal or foreign cells or tissues (IgM, IgG1, IgG2, IgG3) bind complement via the classic pathway and initiate a sequence of events similar to that initiated by immune-complex deposition, resulting in cell lysis or

TABLE 314-17 Complement Deficiencies and Associated Diseases

Component	Associated Diseases
Classic Pathway	
Clq, Clr, Cls, C4	Immune-complex syndromes,* pyogenic infections
C2	Immune-complex syndromes,* few with pyogenic infections
C1 Inhibitor	Rare immune-complex disease, few with pyogenic infections
C3 and Alternative Pathway C3	
C3	Immune-complex syndromes,* pyogenic infections
D	Pyogenic infections
Properdin	*Neisseria* infections
I	Pyogenic infections
H	Hemolytic uremic syndrome
Membrane Attack Complex	
C5, C6, C7, C8	Recurrent *Neisseria* infections, immune-complex disease
C9	Rare *Neisseria* infections

*Immune-complex syndromes include systemic lupus erythematosus (SLE) and SLE-like syndromes, glomerulonephritis, and vasculitis syndromes.

Source: After JA Schifferli, DK Peters: Lancet 88:957, 1983. Copyright 1983, with permission from Elsevier.

tissue injury. Examples of antibody-mediated cytotoxic reactions include red cell lysis in *transfusion reactions*, *Goodpasture's syndrome* with anti–glomerular basement membrane antibody formation, and *pemphigus vulgaris* with antiepidermal antibodies inducing blistering skin disease.

Classic delayed-type hypersensitivity reactions

Inflammatory reactions initiated by mononuclear leukocytes and not by antibody alone have been termed *delayed-type hypersensitivity reactions*. The term *delayed* has been used to contrast a secondary cellular response that appears 48–72 h after antigen exposure with an *immediate* hypersensitivity response generally seen within 12 h of antigen challenge and initiated by basophil mediator release or preformed antibody. For example, in an individual previously infected with *M. tuberculosis* organisms, intradermal placement of tuberculin purified-protein derivative as a skin test challenge results in an indurated area of skin at 48–72 h, indicating previous exposure to tuberculosis.

The cellular events that result in classic delayed-type hypersensitivity responses are centered around T cells (predominantly, though not exclusively, IFN-γ, IL-2, and TNF-α-secreting T_H1-type helper T cells) and macrophages. Recently NK cells have been suggested to play a major role in the form of delayed hypersensitivity that occurs following skin contact with immunogens. First, local immune and inflammatory responses at the site of foreign antigen upregulate endothelial cell adhesion molecule expression, promoting the accumulation of lymphocytes at the tissue site. In the general schemes outlined in Figs. 314-2 and 314-3, antigen is processed by dendritic cells and presented to small numbers of CD4+ T cells expressing a TCR specific for the antigen. IL-12 produced by APCs induces T cells to produce IFN-γ (T_H1 response). Macrophages frequently undergo epithelioid cell transformation and fuse to form multinucleated giant cells in response to IFN-γ. This type of mononuclear cell infiltrate is termed *granulomatous inflammation*. Examples of diseases in which delayed-type hypersensitivity plays a major role are fungal infections (*histoplasmosis*; Chap. 199), mycobacterial infections (*tuberculosis, leprosy*; Chaps. 165 and 166), chlamydial infections (*lymphogranuloma venereum*; Chap. 176), helminth infections (*schistosomiasis*; Chap. 219), reactions to toxins (*berylliosis*; Chap. 256), and hypersensitivity reactions to organic dusts (*hypersensitivity pneumonitis*; Chap. 255). In addition, delayed-type hypersensitivity responses play important roles in tissue damage in autoimmune diseases such as *rheumatoid arthritis, temporal arteritis*, and granulomatosis with polyangiitis (Wegener's) (Chaps. 321 and 326).

CLINICAL EVALUATION OF IMMUNE FUNCTION

Clinical assessment of immunity requires investigation of the four major components of the immune system that participate in host defense and in the pathogenesis of autoimmune diseases: (1) humoral immunity (B cells); (2) cell-mediated immunity (T cells, monocytes); (3) phagocytic cells of the reticuloendothelial system (macrophages), as well as polymorphonuclear leukocytes; and (4) complement. Clinical problems that require an evaluation of immunity include chronic infections, recurrent infections, unusual infecting agents, and certain autoimmune syndromes. The type of clinical syndrome under evaluation can provide information regarding possible immune defects (Chap. 316). Defects in cellular immunity generally result in viral, mycobacterial, and fungal infections. An extreme example of deficiency in cellular immunity is AIDS (Chap. 189). Antibody deficiencies result in recurrent bacterial infections, frequently with organisms such as *S. pneumoniae* and *Haemophilus influenzae* (Chap. 316). Disorders of phagocyte function are frequently manifested by recurrent skin infections, often due to *Staphylococcus aureus* (Chap. 60). Finally, deficiencies of early and late complement components are associated with autoimmune phenomena and recurrent *Neisseria* infections (Table 314-17). For further discussion of useful initial screening tests of immune function, see Chap. 316.

IMMUNOTHERAPY

Many therapies for autoimmune and inflammatory diseases involve the use of nonspecific immune-modulating or immunosuppressive agents such as glucocorticoids or cytotoxic drugs. The goal of development of new treatments for immune-mediated diseases is to design ways to specifically interrupt pathologic immune responses, leaving nonpathologic immune responses intact. Novel ways to interrupt pathologic immune responses that are under investigation include the use of anti-inflammatory cytokines or specific cytokine inhibitors as anti-inflammatory agents, the use of monoclonal antibodies against T or B lymphocytes as therapeutic agents, the induction of anergy by administration of soluble CTLA-4 protein, the use of intravenous Ig for certain infections and immune complex–mediated diseases, the use of specific cytokines to reconstitute components of the immune system, and bone marrow transplantation to replace the pathogenic immune system with a more normal immune system (Chaps. 60, 316, and 189). In particular, the use of a monoclonal antibody to B cells (rituximab, anti-CD20 MAb) is approved in the United States for the treatment of non-Hodgkin's lymphoma (Chap. 110) and, in combination with methotrexate, for treatment of adult patients with severe rheumatoid arthritis resistant to TNF-α inhibitors (Chap. 321).

Cytokines and cytokine inhibitors

Recently, a humanized mouse anti-TNF-α monoclonal antibody (MAb) has been shown to be effective in both rheumatoid arthritis and ulcerative colitis. Use of anti-TNF-α antibody therapy has resulted in clinical improvement in patients with these diseases and has opened the way for targeting TNF-α to treat other severe forms of autoimmune and/or inflammatory disease. Blockage of TNF-α has been effective in *rheumatoid arthritis*, *psoriasis*, *Crohn's disease*, and *ankylosing spondylitis*. Anti-TNF-α MAb (infliximab) has been approved by the FDA for treatment of patients with rheumatoid arthritis.

Other cytokine inhibitors are recombinant soluble TNF-α receptor (R) fused to human Ig and Anakinra (soluble *IL-1 receptor antagonist*, or IL-1 ra). The treatment of autoinflammatory syndromes (Table 314-6) with recombinant IL-1 receptor antagonist can prevent symptoms in these syndromes, since the overproduction of IL-1β is a hallmark of these diseases.

Soluble TNF-αR (etanercept) and IL-1 ra act to inhibit the activity of pathogenic cytokines in rheumatoid arthritis, i.e., TNF-α and IL-1, respectively. Similarly, anti-IL-6, IFN-β, and IL-11 act to inhibit pathogenic proinflammatory cytokines. Anti-IL-6 inhibits IL-6 activity, while IFN-β and IL-11 decrease IL-1 and TNF-α production.

Of particular note has been the successful use of IFN-γ in the treatment of the phagocytic cell defect in *chronic granulomatous disease* (Chap. 60).

Monoclonal antibodies to T and B cells

The OKT3 MAb against human T cells has been used for several years as a T cell–specific immunosuppressive agent that can substitute for horse anti-thymocyte globulin (ATG) in the treatment of solid organ transplant rejection. OKT3 produces fewer allergic reactions than ATG but does induce human anti-mouse Ig antibody—thus limiting its use. Anti-CD4 MAb therapy has been used in trials to treat patients with rheumatoid arthritis. While inducing profound immunosuppression, anti-CD4 MAb treatment also induces susceptibility to severe infections. Treatment of patients with a MAb against the T cell molecule CD40 ligand (CD154) is under investigation to induce tolerance to organ transplants, with promising results reported in animal studies. Monoclonal antibodies to the CD25 (IL-2α) receptor (Basiliximab) are being used for treatment of graft-versus-host disease in bone marrow transplantation, and anti-CD20 MAb (rituximab) is used to treat hematologic neoplasms, autoimmune diseases, and kidney transplant rejection. The anti-IgE monoclonal antibody (omalizumab) is used for blocking antigen-specific IgE that causes *hay fever* and *allergic rhinitis* (Chap. 317); however, side effects of anti-IgE include increased risk of anaphylaxis. Studies have shown that T_H17 cells, in addition to T_H1, are mediators of inflammation in Crohn's disease, and anti–IL-12/IL-23p40 antibody therapy has been studied as a treatment.

It is important to realize the potential risks for these immunosuppressive monoclonal antibodies. Natalizumab is a humanized IgG antibody against an α4 integrin that inhibits leukocyte migration into tissues, and has been approved for treatment of multiple sclerosis in the United States. Both it and anti-CD20 (rituximab) have been associated with the onset of progressive multifocal leukoencephalopathy (PML)—a serious and usually fatal CNS infection caused by JC polyoma virus. Efalizumab, a humanized IgG monoclonal antibody previously approved for treatment of plaque psoriasis, has now been taken off the market due to reactivation of JC virus leading to fatal PML. Thus, use of any currently approved immunosuppressant immunotherapies should be undertaken with caution and with careful monitoring of patients according to FDA guidelines.

Tolerance induction

Specific immunotherapy has moved into a new era with the introduction of soluble CTLA-4 protein into clinical trials. Use of this molecule to block T cell activation via TCR/CD28 ligation during organ or bone marrow transplantation has showed promising results in animals and in early human clinical trials. Specifically, treatment of bone marrow with CTLA-4 protein reduces rejection of the graft in HLA-mismatched bone marrow transplantation. In addition, promising results with soluble CTLA-4 have been reported in the downmodulation of autoimmune T cell responses in the treatment of psoriasis; and it is being studied for treatment of systemic lupus erythematosus (Chap. 319).

Intravenous immunoglobulin (IVIg)

IVIg has been used successfully to block reticuloendothelial cell function and immune complex clearance in various immune cytopenias such as immune thrombocytopenia (Chap. 115). In addition, IVIg is useful for prevention of tissue damage in certain inflammatory syndromes such as Kawasaki disease (Chap. 326) and as Ig replacement therapy for certain types of immunoglobulin deficiencies (Chap. 316). In addition, controlled clinical trials support the use of IVIg in selected patients with graft-versus-host disease, multiple sclerosis, myasthenia gravis, Guillain-Barré syndrome, and chronic demyelinating polyneuropathy.

Stem cell transplantation

Hematopoietic stem cell transplantation (SCT) is now being comprehensively studied to treat several autoimmune diseases, including systemic lupus erythematosus, multiple sclerosis, and scleroderma. The goal of immune reconstitution in autoimmune disease syndromes is to replace a dysfunctional immune system with a normally reactive immune cell repertoire. Preliminary results in patients with scleroderma and lupus have showed encouraging results. Controlled clinical trials in these three diseases are now being launched in the United States and Europe to compare the toxicity and efficacy of conventional immunosuppression therapy with that of myeloablative autologous SCT.

Thus, a number of recent insights into immune system function have spawned a new field of interventional immunotherapy and have enhanced the prospect for development of specific and nontoxic therapies for immune and inflammatory diseases.

FURTHER READINGS

Andreakos ETH et al: Role of cytokines, in *Rheumatoid Arthritis*, EW St. Clair et al (eds). Philadelphia, Lippincott Williams & Wilkins, 2004, pp 134–149

Berger JR et al: Monoclonal antibodies and progressive multifocal leukoencephalopathy. MAbs 1:583, 2009

Blander JM et al: Toll-dependent selection of microbial antigens for presentation by dendritic cells. Nature 440:808, 2006

Carson KR et al: Monoclonal antibody-associated progressive multifocal leucoencephalopathy in patients treated with rituximab, natalizumab, and efalizumab: A review from the Research on Adverse Drug Events and Reports (RADAR) Project. Lancet Oncol 10:816, 2009

Davidson A, Diamond B: Autoimmune diseases. N Engl J Med 345:340, 2001

Diaz-Pena R et al: KIR genes and their role in spondyloarthropathies. Adv Exp Med Biol 649:286, 2009

Falschlehner C et al: Following TRAIL's path in the immune system. Immunology 127:145, 2009

Franchi L et al: The inflammasome: A caspase-1-activation platform that regulates immune responses. Nat Immunol 10:241, 2009

Hotchkiss RS et al: Cell death. N Engl J Med 361:1570, 2009

Iwasaki A, Medzhitov R: Regulation of adaptive immunity by the innate immune system. Science 327:291, 2010

Kelley WN et al (eds): *Textbook of Rheumatology*, 4th ed. Philadelphia, Saunders, 1993, chaps. 6, 7, 10, 13, 15, 16

Koretzky GA et al: SLP76 and SLP65: Complex regulation of signaling in lymphocytes and beyond. Nat Rev Immunol 6:67, 2006

Korman BD et al: Progressive multifocal leukoencephalopathy, efalizumab, and immunosuppression: A cautionary tale for dermatologists. Arch Dermatol 145:937, 2009

Kronenberg M et al: Innate-like recognition of microbes by invariant natural killer T cells. Curr Opin Immunol 21:391, 2009

Lanier L: NK cell recognition. Annu Rev Immunol 23:225, 2005

Lernmark A: Autoimmune diseases: Are markers ready for prediction? J Clin Invest 108:1091, 2001

Louten J et al: Development and function of Th17 cells in health and disease. J Allergy Clin Immunol 123:1004, 2009

MacDonald TT et al: Immunity, inflammation, and allergy in the gut. Science 307:1920, 2005

Martinon F et al: The inflammasomes: Guardians of the body. Annu Rev Immunol 27:229, 2009

Middendorp S et al: NKT cells in mucosal immunity. Mucosal Immunol 2(5):393, 2009

Morley BJ, Walport MJ: *The Complement Facts Books*. London, Academic Press, 2000, chap. 2

Mullauer L et al: Mutations in apoptosis genes: A pathogenetic factor for human disease. Mutat Res 488:211, 2001

Paust S et al: Adaptive immune responses mediated by natural killer cells. Immunol Rev 235:286, 2010

Rajagopalan S et al: Understanding how combinations of HLA and KIR genes influence disease. J Exp Med 201:1025, 2005

Ramaswamy M et al: Harnessing programmed cell death as a therapeutic strategy in rheumatic diseases. Nat Rev Rheumatol 2011 [epub ahead of print]

Rinaudo C et al: Vaccinology in the Genome Era. J Clin Invest 119:2515, 2009

Rivera J et al: Molecular regulation of mast cell activation. J Allergy Clin Immunol 6:1214, 2006

Romagnani S: CD4 effector cells, in *Inflammation: Basic Principles and Clinical Correlates*, 3rd ed, J Gallin, R Snyderman (eds). Philadelphia, Lippincott Williams & Wilkins, 1999, pp 177

Schroder K et al: The NLRP3 inflammasome: a sensor for metabolic danger? Science 327:296, 2010

Steinman RM, Banchereau J: Taking dendritic cells into medicine. Nature 449:419, 2007

Ting JPY et al: How the noninflammasome NLRs function in the innate immune system. Science 327:286, 2010

Ueno H et al: Targeting human dendritic cell subsets for improved vaccines. Semin Immunol 23:21, 2011

van Duin D et al: Triggering TLR signaling in vaccination. Trends Immunol 27:49, 2006

Weaver C et al: Interplay between the Th17 and Treg cell lineages: a co-evolutionary perspective. Nat Rev Immunol 9:883, 2009

Whelan B et al: mAbs in nonlupus autoimmune rheumatic disease. Curr Opin Hemat 16:280, 2009

Williams AP et al: Hanging in the balance. Mol Interv 5:226, 2005

CHAPTER 315

The Major Histocompatibility Complex

Gerald T. Nepom

THE HLA COMPLEX AND ITS PRODUCTS

The human major histocompatibility complex (MHC), commonly called the human leukocyte antigen (HLA) complex, is a 4-megabase (Mb) region on chromosome 6 (6p21.3) that is densely packed with expressed genes. The best known of these genes are the HLA class I and class II genes, whose products are critical for immunologic specificity and transplantation histocompatibility, and they play a major role in susceptibility to a number of autoimmune diseases. Many other genes in the HLA region are also essential to the innate and antigen-specific functioning of the immune system. The HLA region shows extensive conservation with the MHC of other mammals in terms of genomic organization, gene sequence, and protein structure and function.

The *HLA class I genes* are located in a 2-Mb stretch of DNA at the telomeric end of the HLA region (Fig. 315-1). The classic (MHC class Ia) HLA-A, -B, and -C loci, the products of which are integral participants in the immune response to intracellular infections, tumors, and allografts, are expressed in all nucleated cells and are highly polymorphic in the population. *Polymorphism* refers to a high degree of allelic variation within a genetic locus that leads to extensive variation between different individuals expressing different alleles. More than 650 alleles at HLA-A, 1000 at HLA-B, and 360 at HLA-C have been identified in different human populations, making this the most highly polymorphic segment known within the human genome. Each of the alleles at these loci encodes a *heavy chain* (also called an *α chain*) that associates noncovalently with the nonpolymorphic light chain *β_2-microglobulin*, encoded on chromosome 15.

The nomenclature of HLA genes and their products reflects the grafting of newer DNA sequence information on an older system based on serology. Among class I genes, alleles of the HLA-A, -B, and -C loci were originally identified in the 1950s, 1960s, and 1970s by alloantisera, derived primarily from multiparous women, who in the course of normal pregnancy produce antibodies against paternal antigens expressed on fetal cells. The serologic allotypes were designated by consecutive numbers (e.g., HLA-A1, HLA-B8).

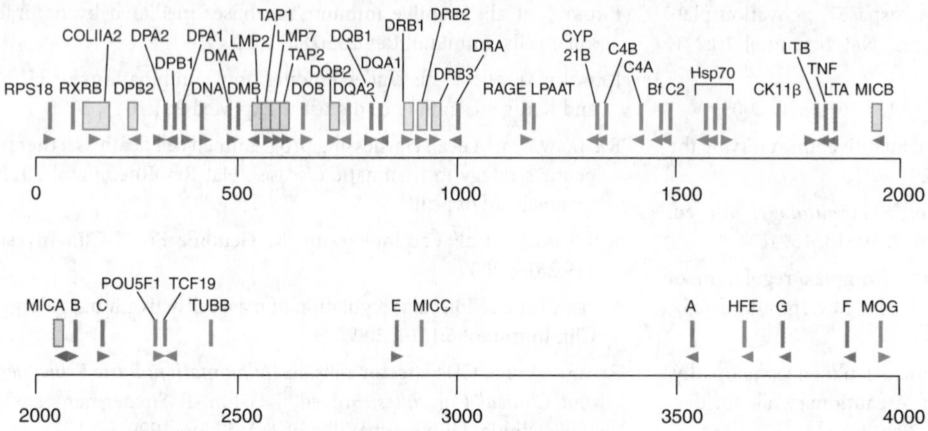

Figure 315-1 Physical map of the HLA region, showing the class I and class II loci, other immunologically important loci, and a sampling of other genes mapped to this region. Gene orientation is indicated by arrowheads. Scale is in kilobase (kb). The approximate genetic distance from DP to A is 3.2 cM. This includes 0.8 cM between A and B (including 0.2 cM between C and B), 0.4–0.8 cM between B and DR-DQ, and 1.6–2.0 cM between DR-DQ and DP.

Currently, under World Health Organization (WHO) nomenclature, class I alleles are given a single designation that indicates locus, serologic specificity, and sequence-based subtype. For example, HLA-A*0201 indicates subtype 1 of the serologically defined allele HLA-A2. Subtypes that differ from each other at the nucleotide but not the amino acid sequence level are designated by an extra numeral (e.g., HLA-B*07021 and HLA-B*07022 are two variants of the HLA-B702 subtype of HLA-B*07). The nomenclature of class II genes, discussed below, is made more complicated by the fact that both chains of a class II molecule are encoded by closely linked HLA-encoded loci, both of which may be polymorphic, and by the presence of differing numbers of isotypic DRB loci in different individuals. It has become clear that accurate HLA genotyping requires DNA sequence analysis, and the identification of alleles at the DNA sequence level has contributed greatly to the understanding of the role of HLA molecules as peptide-binding ligands, to the analysis of associations of HLA alleles with certain diseases, to the study of the population genetics of HLA, and to a clearer understanding of the contribution of HLA differences to allograft rejection and graft-versus-host disease. Current databases of HLA class I and class II sequences can be accessed by the Internet (e.g., from the IMGT/HLA Database, *http://www.ebi.ac.uk/imgt/hla*), and frequent updates of HLA gene lists are published in several journals.

The biologic significance of this MHC genetic diversity, resulting in extreme variation in the human population, is evident from the perspective of the structure of MHC molecules. As shown in Fig. 315-2, the MHC class I and class II genes encode MHC molecules that bind small peptides, and together this complex (pMHC; peptide-MHC) forms the ligand for recognition by T lymphocytes, through the antigen-specific T cell receptor (TCR). There is a direct link between the genetic variation and this structural interaction: The allelic changes in genetic sequence result in diversification of the peptide-binding capabilities of each MHC molecule and in differences for specific TCR binding. Thus, different pMHC complexes bind different antigens and are targets for recognition by different T cells.

The class I MHC and class II MHC structures, shown in Fig. 315-2*B*, *C*, are structurally closely related; however, there are a few key differences. While both bind peptides and present them to T cells, the binding pockets have different shapes, which influence the types of immune responses that result (discussed below). In addition, there are structural contact sites for T cell molecules known as CD8

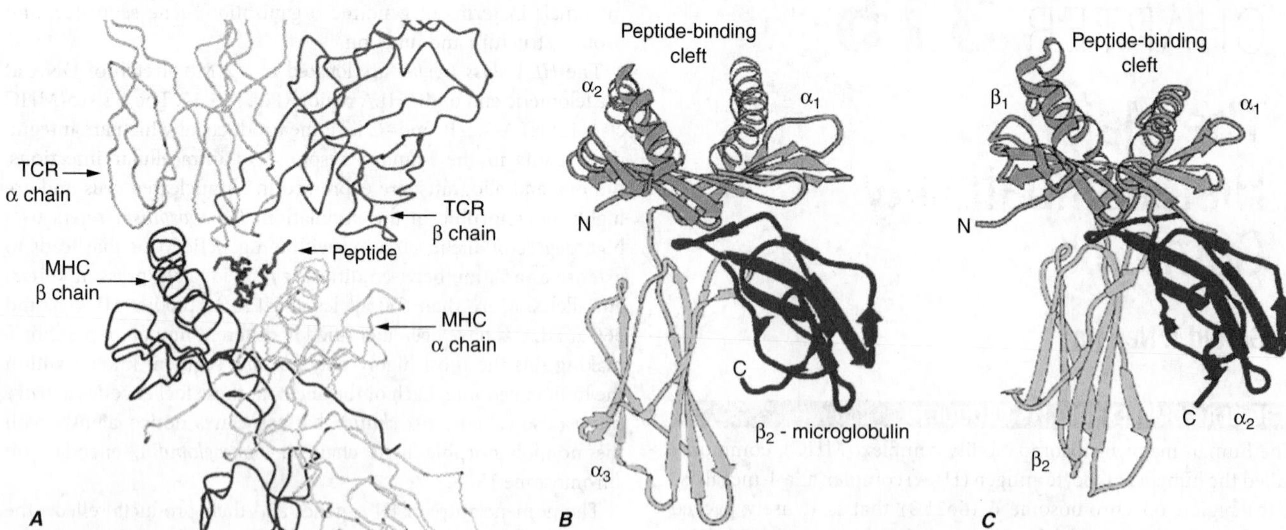

Figure 315-2 ***A.* The trimolecular complex of TCR (top), MHC molecule (bottom)** and a bound peptide form the structural determinants of specific antigen recognition. Other panels (***B.*** and ***C.***) show the domain structure of MHC class I (*B*) and class II (*C*) molecules. The α_1 and α_2 domains of class I and the α_1 and β_1 domains of class II form a β-sheet platform that forms the floor of the peptide-binding groove, and α helices that form the sides of the groove. The α_3 (*B*) and β_2 domains (*C*) project from the cell surface and form the contact sites for CD8 and CD4, respectively. *(Adapted from EL Reinhertz et al: Science 286:1913, 1999; and C Janeway et al: Immunobiology Bookshelf, 2nd ed, Garland Publishing, New York, 1997; with permission.)*

and CD4, expressed on the class I or class II membrane-proximal domains, respectively. This ensures that when peptide antigens are presented by class I molecules, the responding T cells are predominantly of the CD8 class, and similarly, that T cells responding to class II pMHC complexes are predominantly CD4.

The nonclassic, or class Ib, MHC molecules, HLA-E, -F, and -G, are much less polymorphic than MHC Ia and appear to have distinct functions. The HLA-E molecule has a peptide repertoire displaying signal peptides cleaved from classic MHC class I molecules and is the major self-recognition target for the natural killer (NK) cell–inhibitory receptors NKG2A or NKG2C paired with CD94 (see below and Chap. 314). This appears to be a function of immune surveillance, as loss of MHC class I signal peptides serves as a surrogate marker for injured or infected cells, leading to release of the inhibitory signal and subsequent activation of NK cells. HLA-E can also bind and present peptides to CD8 T cells, albeit with a limited scope, as only three HLA-E alleles are known. HLA-G is expressed selectively in extravillous trophoblasts, the fetal cell population directly in contact with maternal tissues. It binds a wide array of peptides, is expressed in six different alternatively spliced forms, and provides inhibitory signals to both NK cells and T cells, presumably in the service of maintaining maternofetal tolerance; 14 HLA-G alleles have been identified. The protein product of HLA-F is found mainly intracellularly, and the function of this locus, which encodes four alleles, remains largely unknown.

Additional class I–like genes have been identified, some HLA-linked and some encoded on other chromosomes, that show only distant homology to the class Ia and Ib molecules but share the three-dimensional class I structure. Those on chromosome 6p21 include MIC-A and MIC-B, which are encoded centromeric to HLA-B, and HLA-HFE, located 3 to 4 cM (centi-Morgan) telomeric of HLA-F. MIC-A and MIC-B do not bind peptide but are expressed on gut and other epithelium in a stress-inducible manner and serve as activation signals for certain γδ T cells, NK cells, CD8 T cells, and activated macrophages, acting through the activating NKG2D receptors. Sixty-seven MIC-A and 30 MIC-B alleles are known, and additional diversification comes from variable alanine repeat sequences in the transmembrane domain. Due to this structural diversity, MIC-A can be recognized as a foreign tissue target during organ transplantation, contributing to graft failure. HLA-HFE encodes the gene defective in hereditary hemochromatosis (Chap. 357). Among the non-HLA, class I–like genes, CD1 refers to a family of molecules that present glycolipids or other nonpeptide ligands to certain T cells, including T cells with NK activity; FcRn binds IgG within lysosomes and protects it from catabolism (Chap. 314); and Zn-α_2-glycoprotein 1 binds a nonpeptide ligand and promotes catabolism of triglycerides in adipose tissue. Like the HLA-A, -B, -C, -E, -F, and -G heavy chains, each of which forms a heterodimer with β_2-microglobulin (Fig. 315-2), the class I–like molecules, HLA-HFE, FcRn, and CD1 also bind to β_2-microglobulin, but MIC-A, MIC-B, and Zn-α_2-glycoprotein 1 do not.

The *HLA class II region* is also illustrated in Fig. 315-1. Multiple class II genes are arrayed within the centromeric 1 Mb of the HLA region, forming distinct haplotypes. A *haplotype* refers to an array of alleles at polymorphic loci along a chromosomal segment. Multiple class II genes are present on a single haplotype, clustered into three major subregions: HLA-DR, -DQ, and -DP. Each of these subregions contains at least one functional alpha (A) locus and one functional beta (B) locus. Together these encode proteins that form the α and β polypeptide chains of a mature class II HLA molecule. Thus, the DRA and DRB genes encode an HLA-DR molecule; products of the *DQAl* and *DQBl* genes form an HLA-DQ molecule; and the *DPAl* and *DPBl* genes encode an HLA-DP molecule. There are several DRB genes (*DRB1*, *DRB2*, *DRB3*, etc.), so that two expressed DR molecules are encoded on most haplotypes by combining the α-chain product of the DRA gene with separate β chains. More than 530 alleles have been identified at the HLA-DRB1 locus, with most of the variation occurring within limited segments encoding residues that interact with antigens. Detailed analysis of sequences and population distribution of these alleles strongly suggest that this diversity is actively selected by environmental pressures associated with pathogen diversity.

In the DQ region, both DQA1 and DQB1 are polymorphic, with 34 DQA1 alleles and 72 DQB1 alleles. The current nomenclature is largely analogous to that discussed above for class I, using the convention "locus * allele." Thus, for example, subtypes of the serologically defined specificity DR4, encoded by the DRB1 locus, are termed DRB1*0401, *0402, etc. In addition to allelic polymorphism, products of different DQA1 alleles can, with some limitations, pair with products of different DQB1 alleles through both *cis* and *trans* pairing to create combinatorial complexity and expand the number of expressed class II molecules. Because of the enormous allelic diversity in the general population, most individuals are heterozygous at all of the class I and class II loci. Thus, most individuals express six classic class I molecules (two each of HLA-A, -B, and -C) and around eight class II molecules—two DP, two DR (more in the case of haplotypes with additional functional DRB genes), and up to four DQ (two *cis* and two *trans*).

OTHER GENES IN THE MHC

In addition to the class I and class II genes themselves, there are numerous genes interspersed among the HLA loci that have interesting and important immunologic functions. Our current concept of the function of MHC genes now encompasses many of these additional genes, some of which are also highly polymorphic. Indeed, direct comparison of the complete DNA sequences for eight of the entire 4-Mb MHC regions from different haplotypes show >44,000 nucleotide variations, encoding an extremely high potential for biologic diversity, and at least 97 genes located in this region are known to have coding region sequence variation. Specific examples include the TAP and LMP genes, as discussed in more detail below, which encode molecules that participate in intermediate steps in the HLA class I biosynthetic pathway. Another set of HLA genes, DMA and DMB, perform an analogous function for the class II pathway. These genes encode an intracellular molecule that facilitates the proper complexing of HLA class II molecules with antigen (see below). The *HLA class III region* is a name given to a cluster of genes between the class I and class II complexes, which includes genes for the two closely related cytokines tumor necrosis factor (TNF)-α and lymphotoxin (TNF-β); the complement components C2, C4, and Bf; heat shock protein (HSP)70; and the enzyme 21-hydroxylase.

The class I genes HLA-A, -B, and -C are expressed in all nucleated cells, although generally to a higher degree on leukocytes than on nonleukocytes. In contrast, the class II genes show a more restricted distribution: HLA-DR and HLA-DP genes are constitutively expressed on most cells of the myeloid cell lineage, whereas all three class II gene families (HLA-DR, -DQ, and -DP) are inducible by certain stimuli provided by inflammatory cytokines such as interferon γ. Within the lymphoid lineage, expression of these class II genes is constitutive on B cells and inducible on human T cells. Most endothelial and epithelial cells in the body, including the vascular endothelium and the intestinal epithelium, are also inducible for class II gene expression. Thus, while these somatic tissues normally express only class I and not class II genes, during times of local inflammation they are recruited by cytokine stimuli to express class II genes as well, thereby becoming active participants in ongoing immune responses. Class II expression is controlled largely at the transcriptional level through a conserved set of promoter elements that interact with a protein known as *CIITA*. Cytokine-mediated induction of CIITA is a principal method by which tissue-specific expression of HLA gene expression is controlled. Other HLA genes involved in the immune response such as TAP and LMP, are also susceptible to upregulation by signals such as interferon γ. Sequence data for the entire HLA region can be accessed on the Internet (e.g., *http://www.sanger.ac.uk/HGP/Chr6/MHC*).

LINKAGE DISEQUILIBRIUM

In addition to extensive polymorphism at the class I and class II loci, another characteristic feature of the HLA complex is *linkage disequilibrium*. This is formally defined as a deviation from Hardy-Weinberg equilibrium for alleles at linked loci. This is reflected in the very low recombination rates between certain loci within the HLA complex. For example, recombination between DR and DQ loci is almost never observed in family studies, and characteristic haplotypes with particular arrays of DR and DQ alleles are found in every population. Similarly, the complement components C2, C4, and Bf are almost invariably inherited together, and the alleles at these loci are found in characteristic haplotypes. In contrast, there is a recombinational hotspot between DQ and DP, which are separated by 1–2 cM of genetic distance, despite their close physical proximity. Certain extended haplotypes encompassing the interval from DQ into the class I region are commonly found, the most notable being the haplotype DR3-B8-A1, which is found, in whole or in part, in 10–30% of northern European whites. It has been hypothesized that selective pressures may maintain linkage disequilibrium in HLA, but this remains to be determined. As discussed below under HLA and immunologic disease, one consequence of the phenomenon of linkage disequilibrium has been the resulting difficulty in assigning HLA-disease associations to a single allele at a single locus.

MHC STRUCTURE AND FUNCTION

Class I and class II molecules display a distinctive structural architecture, which contains specialized functional domains responsible for the unique genetic and immunologic properties of the HLA complex. The principal known function of both class I and class II HLA molecules is to bind antigenic peptides in order to present antigen to an appropriate T cell. The ability of a particular peptide to satisfactorily bind to an individual HLA molecule is a direct function of the molecular fit between the amino acid residues on the peptide with respect to the amino acid residues of the HLA molecule. The bound peptide forms a tertiary structure called the *MHC-peptide complex*, which communicates with T lymphocytes through binding to the TCR molecule. The first site of TCR-MHC-peptide interaction in the life of a T cell occurs in the thymus, where self-peptides are presented to developing thymocytes by MHC molecules expressed on thymic epithelium and hematopoietically derived antigen-presenting cells, which are primarily responsible for positive and negative selection, respectively (Chap. 314). Thus, the population of MHC–T cell complexes expressed in the thymus shapes the TCR repertoire. Mature T cells encounter MHC molecules in the periphery both in the maintenance of tolerance (Chap. 318) and in the initiation of immune responses. The MHC-peptide-TCR interaction is the central event in the initiation of most antigen-specific immune responses, since it is the structural determinant of the specificity. For potentially immunogenetic peptides, the ability of a given peptide to be generated and bound by an HLA molecule is a primary feature of whether or not an immune response to that peptide can be generated, and the repertoire of peptides that a particular individual's HLA molecules can bind exerts a major influence over the specificity of that individual's immune response.

When a TCR molecule binds to an HLA-peptide complex, it forms intermolecular contacts with both the antigenic peptide and with the HLA molecule itself. The outcome of this recognition event depends on the density and duration of the binding interaction, accounting for a dual specificity requirement for activation of the T cell. That is, the TCR must be specific both for the antigenic peptide and for the HLA molecule. The polymorphic nature of the presenting molecules, and the influence that this exerts on the peptide repertoire of each molecule, results in the phenomenon of *MHC restriction* of the T cell specificity for a given peptide. The binding of CD8 or CD4 molecules to the class I or class II molecule, respectively, also contributes to the interaction between T cell and the HLA-peptide complex, by providing for the selective activation of the appropriate T cell.

CLASS I STRUCTURE

(Fig. 315-2*B*) As noted above, MHC class I molecules provide a cell-surface display of peptides derived from intracellular proteins, and they also provide the signal for self-recognition by NK cells. Surface-expressed class I molecules consist of an MHC-encoded 44-kD glycoprotein heavy chain, a non-MHC-encoded 12-kD light chain β_2-microglobulin, and an antigenic peptide, typically 8–11 amino acids in length and derived from intracellularly produced protein. The heavy chain displays a prominent peptide-binding groove. In HLA-A and -B molecules, the groove is ~3 nm in length by 1.2 nm in maximum width (30 Å × 12 Å), whereas it is apparently somewhat wider in HLA-C. Antigenic peptides are noncovalently bound in an extended conformation within the peptide-binding groove, with both N- and C-terminal ends anchored in pockets within the groove (A and F pockets, respectively) and, in many cases, with a prominent kink, or arch, approximately one-third of the way from the N-terminus that elevates the peptide main chain off the floor of the groove.

A remarkable property of peptide binding by MHC molecules is the ability to form highly stable complexes with a wide array of peptide sequences. This is accomplished by a combination of peptide sequence–independent and peptide sequence–dependent bonding. The former consists of hydrogen bond and van der Waals interactions between conserved residues in the peptide-binding groove and charged or polar atoms along the peptide backbone. The latter is dependent upon the six side pockets that are formed by the irregular surface produced by protrusion of amino acid side chains from within the binding groove. The side chains lining the pockets interact with some of the peptide side chains. The sequence polymorphism among different class I alleles and isotypes predominantly affects the residues that line these pockets, and the interactions of these residues with peptide residues constitute the sequence-dependent bonding that confers a particular sequence "motif" on the range of peptides that can bind any given MHC molecule.

CLASS I BIOSYNTHESIS

(Fig. 315-3*A*) The biosynthesis of the classic MHC class I molecules reflects their role in presenting endogenous peptides. The heavy chain is cotranslationally inserted into the membrane of the endoplasmic reticulum (ER), where it becomes glycosylated and associates sequentially with the chaperone proteins calnexin and ERp57. It then forms a complex with β_2-microglobulin, and this complex associates with the chaperone calreticulin and the MHC-encoded molecule tapasin, which physically links the class I complex to TAP, the MHC-encoded transporter associated with antigen processing. Meanwhile, peptides generated within the cytosol from intracellular proteins by the multisubunit, multicatalytic proteasome complex are actively transported into the ER by TAP, where they are trimmed by a peptidase known as *ERAAP* (ER aminopeptidase associated with antigen processing). At this point, peptides with appropriate

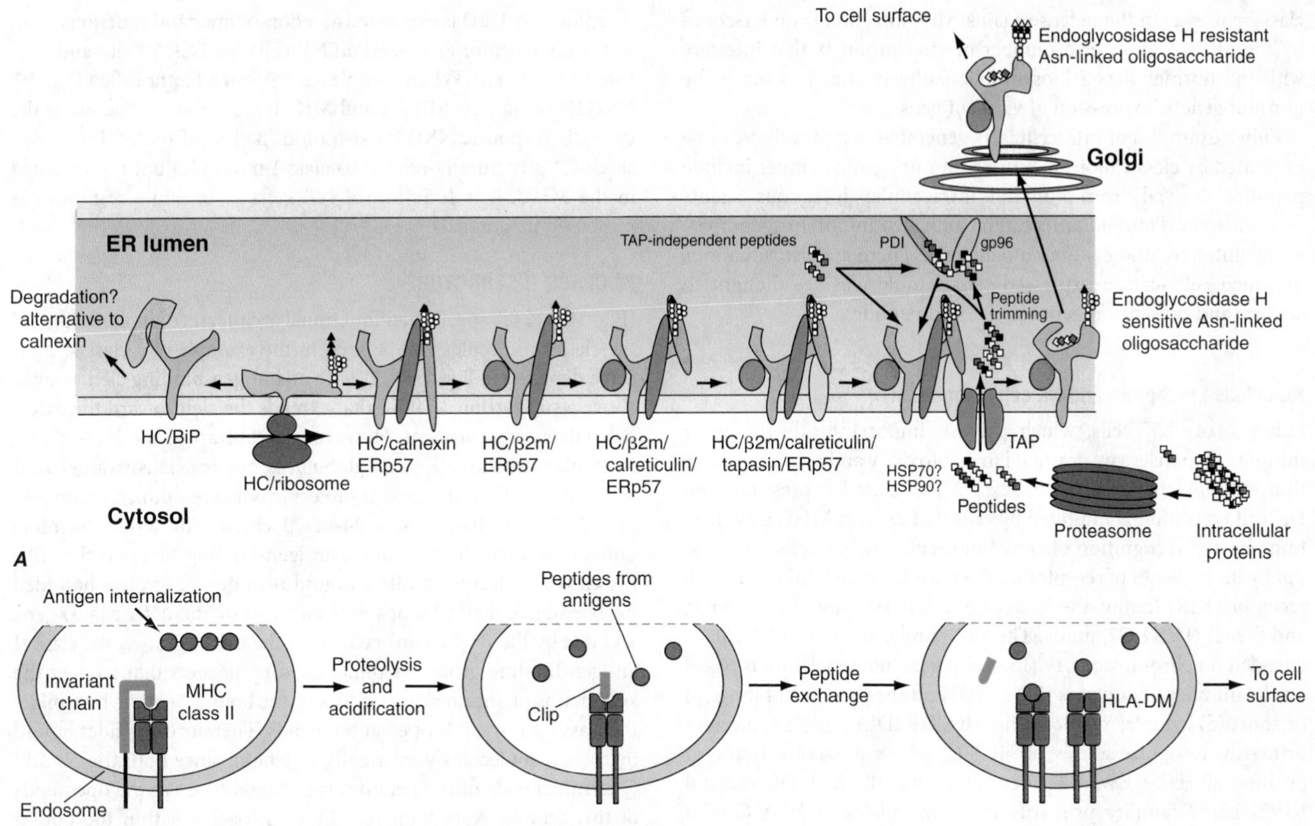

Figure 315-3 Biosynthesis of class I *(A)* and class II *(B)* molecules. ***A.*** Nascent heavy chain (HC) becomes associated with β_2-microglobulin (β2m) and peptide through interactions with a series of chaperones. Peptides generated by the proteasome are transported into the endoplasmic reticulum (ER) by TAP. Peptides undergo N-terminal trimming in the ER and become associated with chaperones, including gp96 and PDI. Once peptide binds to HC-β2m, the HC-β2m-peptide trimeric complex exits the ER and is transported by the secretory pathway to the cell surface. In the Golgi, the N-linked oligosaccharide undergoes maturation, with addition of sialic acid residues. Molecules are not necessarily drawn to scale. ***B.*** Pathway of HLA class II molecule assembly and antigen processing. After transport through the Golgi and post-Golgi compartment, the class II–invariant chain complex moves to an acidic endosome, where the invariant chain is proteolytically cleaved into fragments and displaced by antigenic peptides, facilitated by interactions with the DMA-DMB chaperone protein. This class II molecule–peptide complex is then transported to the cell surface.

sequence complementarity bind specific class I molecules to form complete, folded heavy chain–β_2-microglobulin–peptide trimer complexes. These are transported rapidly from the ER, through the *cis*- and *trans*-Golgi where the N-linked oligosaccharide is further processed, and thence to the cell surface.

Most of the peptides transported by TAP are produced in the cytosol by proteolytic cleavage of intracellular proteins by the multisubunit, multicatalytic proteasome, and inhibitors of the proteasome dramatically reduce expression of class I–presented antigenic peptides. A thiol-dependent oxidoreductase Erp57, which mediates disulfide bond rearrangements, also appears to play an important role in folding the class I–peptide complex into a stable multicomponent molecule. The MHC-encoded proteasome subunits LMP2 and LMP7 may influence the spectrum of peptides produced but are not essential for proteasome function.

■ CLASS I FUNCTION

Peptide antigen presentation

On any given cell, a class I molecule occurs in 100,000–200,000 copies and binds several hundred to several thousand distinct peptide species. The vast majority of these peptides are self-peptides to which the host immune system is tolerant by one or more of the mechanisms that maintain tolerance [e.g., clonal deletion in the thymus or clonal anergy or clonal ignorance in the periphery (Chaps. 314 and 318)]. However, class I molecules bearing foreign peptides expressed in a permissive immunologic context activate CD8 T cells, which, if naïve, will then differentiate into cytolytic T lymphocytes (CTLs). These T cells and their progeny, through their αβ TCRs, are then capable of Fas/CD95- and/or perforin-mediated cytotoxicity and/or cytokine secretion (Chap. 314) upon further encounter with the class I–peptide combination that originally activated it, and also with other combinations of class I molecule plus peptide that present a similar immunochemical stimulus to the TCR. As alluded to above, this phenomenon by which T cells recognize foreign antigens in the context of specific MHC alleles is termed *MHC restriction*, and the specific MHC molecule is termed the *restriction element*. The most common source of foreign peptides presented by class I molecules is viral infection, in the course of which peptides from viral proteins enter the class I pathway. The generation of a strong CTL response that destroys virally infected cells represents an important antigen-specific defense against many viral infections (Chap. 314). In the case of some viral infections—hepatitis B, for example—CTL-induced target cell apoptosis is thought to be a more important mechanism of tissue damage than any direct cytopathic effect of the virus itself. The importance of the class I pathway in the defense against viral infection is underscored by the identification of a number of viral products that interfere with the normal class I biosynthetic pathway and thus block the immunogenetic expression of viral antigens.

Other examples of intracellularly generated peptides that can be presented by class I molecules in an immunogenic manner include peptides derived from nonviral intracellular infectious agents (e.g., *Listeria, Plasmodium*), tumor antigens, minor histocompatibility antigens, and certain autoantigens. There are also situations in which cell surface–expressed class I molecules are thought to acquire and present exogenously derived peptides.

HLA class I receptors and NK cell recognition

(Chap. 314) NK cells, which play an important role in innate immune responses, are activated to cytotoxicity and cytokine secretion by contact with cells that lack MHC class I expression, and NK cell activation is inhibited by cells that express MHC class I. In humans, the recognition of class I molecules by NK cells is carried out by three classes of receptor families, the killer cell–inhibitory cell receptor (KIR) family, the leukocyte Ig-like receptor (LIR) family, and the CD94/NKG2 family. The KIR family, also called CD158, is encoded on chromosome 19q13.4. KIR gene nomenclature is based on the number of domains (2D or 3D) and the presence of long (L) or short (S) cytoplasmic domains. The KIR2DL1 and S1 molecules primarily recognize alleles of HLA-C, which possess a lysine at position 80 (HLA-Cw2, -4, -5 and -6), while the KIR2DL2/S2 and KIR2DL3/S3 families primarily recognize alleles of HLA-C with asparagine at this position (HLA-Cw1,-3, -7 and -8). The KIR3D L1 and S1 molecules predominantly recognize HLA-B alleles that fall into the HLA-Bw4 class determined by residues 77–83 in the α_1 domain of the heavy chain, while the KIR3DL2 molecule is an inhibitory receptor for HLA-A*03. One of the KIR products, KIR2DL4, is known to be an activating receptor for HLA-G. The most common KIR haplotype in whites contains one activating KIR and six inhibitory KIR genes, although there is a great deal of diversity in the population, with >100 different combinations. It appears that most individuals have at least one inhibitory KIR for a self-HLA class I molecule, providing a structural basis for NK cell target specificity, which helps prevent NK cells from attacking normal cells. The importance of KIR-HLA interactions to many immune responses is illustrated by studies associating KIR3DL1 or S1 with multiple sclerosis (Chapter 380), an autoimmune disease, but also with partial protection against HIV (Chap. 189); in both cases consistent with a role for HLA-KIR mediated NK activation.

The LIR gene family (CD85, also called ILT) is encoded centromeric of the KIR locus on 19q13.4, and it encodes a variety of inhibitory immunoglobulin-like receptors expressed on many lymphocyte and other hematopoietic lineages. Interaction of LIR-1 (ILT2) with NK or T cells inhibits activation and cytotoxicity, mediated by many different HLA class I molecules, including HLA-G. HLA-F also appears to interact with LIR molecules, although the functional context for this is not understood.

The third family of NK receptors for HLA is encoded in the NK complex on chromosome 12p12.3-13.1 and consists of CD94 and five NKG2 genes, A/B, C, E/H, D, and F. These molecules are C-type (calcium-binding) lectins, and most function as disulfide-bonded heterodimers between CD94 and one of the NKG2 glycoproteins. The principal ligand of CD94/NKG2A receptors is the HLA-E molecule, complexed to a peptide derived from the signal sequence of classic HLA class I molecules and HLA-G. Thus, analogous to the way in which KIR receptors recognize HLA-C, the NKG2 receptor monitors self–class I expression, albeit indirectly through peptide recognition in the context of HLA-E. NKG2C, -E, and -H appear to have similar specificities but act as activating receptors. NKG2D is expressed as a homodimer and functions as an activating receptor expressed on NK cells, γδ TCR T cells, and activated CD8 T cells. When complexed with an adaptor called DAP10, NKG2D recognizes MIC-A and MIC-B molecules and activates the cytolytic response. NKG2D also binds a class of molecules known as *ULBP*, structurally related to class I molecules but not encoded in the MHC. The function of NK cells in immune responses is discussed in Chap. 314.

CLASS II STRUCTURE

(Fig. 315-2*C*) A specialized functional architecture similar to that of the class I molecules can be seen in the example of a class II molecule depicted in Fig. 315-2*C*, with an antigen-binding cleft arrayed above a supporting scaffold that extends the cleft toward the external cellular environment. However, in contrast to the HLA class I molecular structure, β_2-microglobulin is not associated with class II molecules. Rather, the class II molecule is a heterodimer, composed of a 29-kD α chain and a 34-kD β chain. The amino-terminal domains of each chain form the antigen-binding elements that, like the class I molecule, cradle a bound peptide in a groove bounded by extended α-helical loops, one encoded by the A (α chain) gene and one by the B (β chain) gene. Like the class I groove, the class II antigen-binding groove is punctuated by pockets that contact the side chains of amino acid residues of the bound peptide, but unlike the class I groove, it is open at both ends. Therefore, peptides bound by class II molecules vary greatly in length, since both the N- and C-terminal ends of the peptides can extend through the open ends of this groove. Approximately 11 amino acids within the bound peptide form intimate contacts with the class II molecule itself, with backbone hydrogen bonds and specific side chain interactions combining to provide, respectively, stability and specificity to the binding (Fig. 315-4).

The genetic polymorphisms that distinguish different class II genes correspond to changes in the amino acid composition of the class II molecule, and these variable sites are clustered predominantly around the pocket structures within the antigen-binding groove. As with class I, this is a critically important feature of the class II molecule, which explains how genetically different individuals have functionally different HLA molecules.

BIOSYNTHESIS AND FUNCTION OF CLASS II MOLECULES

(Fig. 315-3*B*) The intracellular assembly of class II molecules occurs within a specialized compartmentalized pathway that differs dramatically from the class I pathway described above. As illustrated in Fig. 315-3*B*, the class II molecule assembles in the ER in association with a chaperone molecule, known as the *invariant chain*. The invariant chain performs at least two roles. First, it binds to the class II molecule and blocks the peptide-binding groove, thus preventing antigenic peptides from binding. This role of the invariant chain appears to account for one of the important differences between class I and class II MHC pathways, since it can explain why class I molecules present endogenous peptides from proteins newly synthesized in the ER but class II molecules generally do not. Second, the invariant chain contains molecular localization signals that direct the class II molecule to traffic into post-Golgi compartments known as *endosomes*, which develop into specialized acidic compartments where proteases cleave the invariant chain, and antigenic peptides can now occupy the class II groove. The specificity and tissue distribution of these proteases appear to be an important way in which the immune system regulates access to the peptide-binding groove and T cells become exposed to specific self-antigens. Differences in protease expression in the thymus and in the periphery may

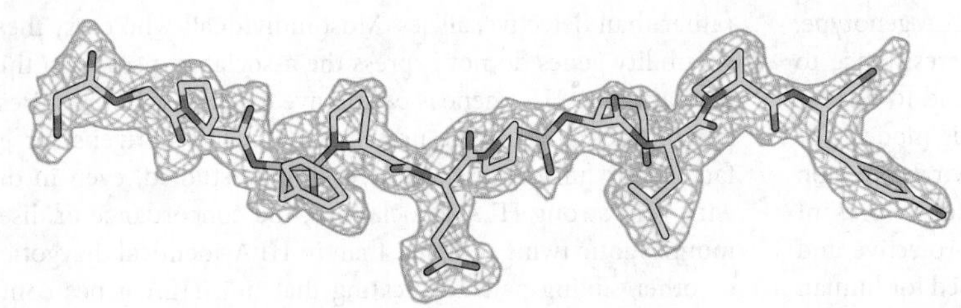

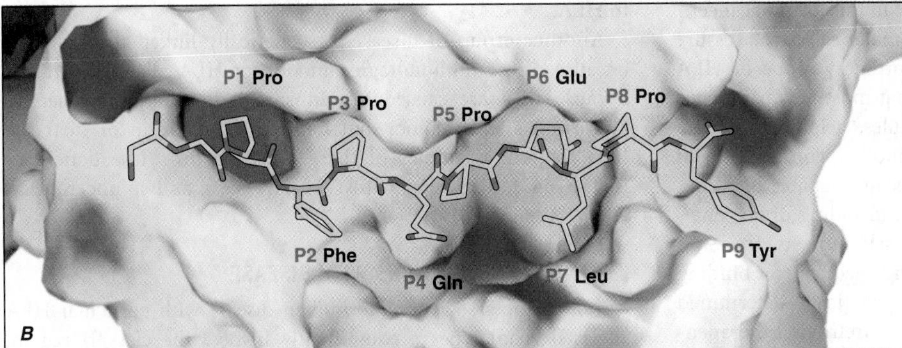

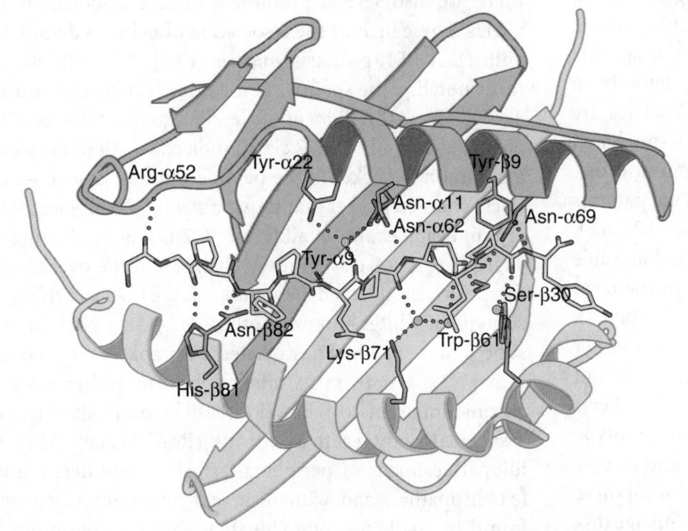

Figure 315-4 Specific intermolecular interactions determine peptide binding to MHC class II molecules. A short peptide sequence derived from alpha-gliadin ***(A.)*** is accommodated within the MHC class II binding groove by specific interactions between peptide side chains (the P1–P9 residues illustrated in ***(B.)*** and corresponding pockets in the MHC class II structure. The latter are determined by the genetic polymorphisms of the MHC gene, in this case encoding an HLA-DQ2 molecule ***(C.)***. This shows the extensive hydrogen bond and salt bridge network, which tightly constrains the pMHC complex and presents the complex of antigen and restriction element for CD4 T cell recognition. *(From Kim C et al: Structural basis for HLA-DQ2-mediated presentation of gluten epitopes in celiac disease. Proc Natl Acad Sci USA 101:4175, 2004.)*

in part determine which specific peptide sequences comprise the peripheral repertoire for T cell recognition. It is at this stage in the intracellular pathway, after cleavage of the invariant chain, that the MHC-encoded DM molecule catalytically facilitates the exchange of peptides within the class II groove to help optimize the specificity and stability of the MHC-peptide complex.

Once this MHC-peptide complex is deposited in the outer cell membrane it becomes the target for T cell recognition via a specific TCR expressed on lymphocytes. Because the endosome environment contains internalized proteins retrieved from the extracellular environment, the class II–peptide complex often contains bound antigens that were originally derived from extracellular proteins. In this way, the class II peptide–loading pathway provides a mechanism for immune surveillance of the extracellular space. This appears to be an important feature that permits the class II molecule to bind foreign peptides, distinct from the endogenous pathway of class I–mediated presentation.

ROLE OF HLA IN TRANSPLANTATION

The development of modern clinical transplantation in the decades since the 1950s provided a major impetus for elucidation of the HLA system, as allograft survival is highest when donor and recipient are HLA-identical. Although many molecular events participate in transplantation rejection, allogeneic differences at class I and class II loci play a major role. Class I molecules can promote T cell responses in several different ways. In the cases of allografts in which the host and donor are mismatched at one or more class I loci, host T cells can be activated by classic *direct alloreactivity*, in which the antigen receptors on the host T cells react with the foreign class I molecule expressed on the allograft. In this situation, the response of any given TCR may be dominated by the allogeneic MHC molecule, the peptide bound to it, or some combination of the two. Another type of host antigraft T cell response involves the uptake and processing of donor MHC antigens by host antigen-presenting cells and the subsequent presentation of the resulting peptides by host MHC molecules. This mechanism is termed *indirect alloreactivity*.

In the case of class I molecules on allografts that are shared by the host and the donor, a host T cell response may still be triggered because of peptides that are presented by the class I molecules of the graft but not of the host. The most common basis for the existence of these endogenous antigen peptides, called *minor histocompatibility antigens*, is a genetic difference between donor and host at a non-MHC locus encoding the structural gene for the protein from which the peptide is derived. These loci are termed *minor histocompatibility loci*, and nonidentical individuals typically differ at many such loci. CD4 T cells react to analogous class II variation, both direct and indirect, and class II differences alone are sufficient to drive allograft rejection.

ASSOCIATION OF HLA ALLELES WITH SUSCEPTIBILITY TO DISEASE

It has long been postulated that infectious agents provide the driving force for the allelic diversification seen in the HLA system. An important corollary of this hypothesis is that resistance to specific pathogens may differ between individuals, based on HLA genotype. Observations of specific HLA genes associated with resistance to malaria or dengue fever, persistence of hepatitis B, and to disease progression in HIV infection are consistent with this model. For example, failure to clear persistent hepatitis B or C viral infection may reflect the inability of particular HLA molecules to present viral antigens effectively to T cells. Similarly, both protective and susceptible HLA allelic associations have been described for human papilloma virus–associated cervical neoplasia, implicating the MHC as an influence in mediating viral clearance in this form of cancer.

Pathogen diversity is probably also the major selective pressure favoring HLA heterozygosity. The extraordinary scope of HLA allelic diversity increases the likelihood that most new pathogens will be recognized by some HLA molecules, helping to ensure immune fitness to the host. However, another consequence of diversification is that some alleles may become capable of recognition of "innocent bystander" molecules, including drugs, environmental molecules, and tissue-derived self-antigens. In a few instances, single HLA alleles display a strong selectivity for binding of a particular agent that accounts for a genetically determined response: hypersensitivity to abacavir, an antiretroviral therapeutic, is directly linked to binding of abacavir in the antigen-binding pockets of HLA-B*5701, and chronic beryllium toxicity is linked to binding of beryllium by HLA-DP molecules with a specific glutamic acid polymorphic residue on the class II beta chain. Even in the case of more complex diseases, particular HLA alleles are strongly associated with certain inappropriate immune-mediated disease states, particularly for some common autoimmune disorders (Chap. 318). By comparing allele frequencies in patients with any particular disease and in control populations, >100 such associations have been identified, some of which are listed in Table 315-1. The strength of genetic association is reflected in the term *relative risk*, which is a statistical odds ratio representing the risk of disease for an individual carrying a particular genetic marker compared with the risk for individuals in that population without that marker. The nomenclature shown in Table 315-1 reflects both the HLA serotype (e.g., DR3, DR4) and the HLA genotype (e.g., DRB1*0301, DRB1*0401). It very likely the class I and class II alleles themselves are the true susceptibility alleles for most of these associations. However, because of the extremely strong linkage disequilibrium between the DR and DQ loci, in some cases it has been difficult to determine the specific locus or combination of class II loci involved. In some cases, the susceptibility gene may be one of the HLA-linked genes located near the class I or class II region, but not the HLA gene itself, and in other cases the susceptibility gene may be a non-HLA gene such as TNF-α, which is nearby. Indeed, since linkage disequilibrium of some haplotypes extends across large segments of the MHC region, it is quite possible that combinations of genes may account for the particular associations of HLA haplotypes with disease. For example, on some haplotypes associated with rheumatoid arthritis, both HLA-DRB1 alleles and a particular polymorphism associated with the TNF locus may be contributory to disease risk. Other candidates for similar epistatic effects include the IKBL gene and the MICA locus, potentially in combination with classic HLA class II risk alleles.

As might be predicted from the known function of the class I and class II gene products, almost all of the diseases associated with specific HLA alleles have an immunologic component to their pathogenesis. The recent development of soluble HLA-peptide recombinant molecules as biological probes of T cell function, often in multivalent complexes referred to as "MHC tetramers," represents an opportunity to use HLA genetic associations to develop biomarkers for detection of early disease progression. However, it should be stressed that even the strong HLA associations with disease (those associations with relative risk of ≥10) implicate normal, rather than defective, alleles. Most individuals who carry these susceptibility genes do not express the associated disease; in this way, the particular HLA gene is permissive for disease but requires other environmental (e.g., the presence of specific antigens) or genetic factors for full penetrance. In each case studied, even in diseases with very strong HLA associations, the concordance of disease in monozygotic twins is higher than in HLA-identical dizygotic twins or other sibling pairs, indicating that non-HLA genes contribute to susceptibility and can significantly modify the risk attributable to HLA.

Another group of diseases is genetically linked to HLA, not because of the immunologic function of HLA alleles but rather because they are caused by autosomal dominant or recessive abnormal alleles at loci that happen to reside in or near the HLA region. Examples of these are 21-hydroxylase deficiency (Chap. 342), hemochromatosis (Chap. 357), and spinocerebellar ataxia (Chap. 374).

CLASS I ASSOCIATIONS WITH DISEASE

Although the associations of human disease with particular HLA alleles or haplotypes predominantly involve the class II region, there are also several prominent disease associations with class I alleles. These include the association of Behçet's disease (Chap. 327) with HLA-B51, psoriasis vulgaris (Chap. 52) with HLA-Cw6, and, most notably, the spondyloarthritides (Chap. 325) with HLA-B27. Twenty-five HLA-B locus alleles, designated HLA-B*2701–B*2725, encode the family of B27 class I molecules. All of the subtypes share a common B pocket in the peptide-binding groove—a deep, negatively charged pocket that shows a strong preference for binding the arginine side chain. In addition, B27 is among the most negatively charged of HLA class I heavy chains, and the overall preference is for positively charged peptides. HLA-B*2705 is the predominant subtype in whites and most other non-Asian populations, and this subtype is very highly associated with ankylosing spondylitis (AS) (Chap. 325), both in its idiopathic form and in association with chronic inflammatory bowel disease or psoriasis vulgaris. It is also associated with reactive arthritis (ReA) (Chap. 325), with other idiopathic forms of peripheral arthritis (undifferentiated spondyloarthropathy), and with recurrent acute anterior uveitis. B27 is found in 50–90% of individuals with these conditions, compared with a prevalence of ~7% in North American whites.

It can be concluded that the B27 molecule itself is involved in disease pathogenesis, based on strong evidence from clinical epidemiology and on the occurrence of a spondyloarthropathy-like disease in HLA-B27 transgenic rats. The association of B27 with these diseases may derive from the specificity of a particular peptide or family of peptides bound to B27 or through another mechanism that is independent of the peptide specificity of B27. In particular, HLA-B27 has been shown to form heavy chain homodimers, utilizing the cysteine residue at position 67 of the B57 α chain, in the absence of β_2-microglobulin. These homodimers are expressed on the surface of lymphocytes and monocytes from patients with AS, and receptors including KIR3DL1, KIR3DL2, and ILT4 are capable of binding to them, promoting the activation and survival of cells expressing these receptors. Alternatively, this dimerization "misfolding" of B27 may initiate an intracellular stress signalling response, called the unfolded protein response (UPR), capable of modulating immune cell function. Whether these interactions contribute to disease susceptibility or pathogenesis is currently unknown.

CLASS II DISEASE ASSOCIATIONS

As can be seen in Table 315-1, the majority of associations of HLA and disease are with class II alleles. Several diseases have complex HLA genetic associations.

TABLE 315-1 Significant HLA Class I and Class II Associations With Disease

	Marker	Gene	Strength of Association
Spondyloarthropathies			
Ankylosing spondylitis	B27	B*2702, –04, –05	++++
Reactive arthritis (Reiter's)	B27		++++
Acute anterior uveitis	B27		+++
Reactive arthritis *(Yersinia, Salmonella, Shigella, Chlamydia)*	B27		+++
Psoriatic spondylitis	B27		+++
Collagen-Vascular Diseases			
Juvenile arthritis, pauciarticular	DR8		++
	DR5		++
Rheumatoid arthritis	DR4	DRB1*0401, –04, –05	+++
Sjögren's syndrome	DR3		++
Systemic lupus erythematosus			
White	DR3		+
Japanese	DR2		++
Autoimmune Gut and Skin			
Gluten-sensitive enteropathy (celiac disease)	DQ2	DQA1*0501 DQB1*0201	+++
Chronic active hepatitis	DR3		++
Dermatitis herpetiformis	DR3		+++
Psoriasis vulgaris	Cw6		++
Pemphigus vulgaris	DR4	DRB1*0402	+++
	DQ1	DQB1*0503	
Bullous pemphigoid variant	DQ7	DQB1*0301	+
Autoimmune Endocrine			
Type 1 diabetes mellitus	DQ8	DQB1*0302	+++
	DR4	DRB1*0401, –04	
	DR3		++
	DR2	DQB1*0602	—[a]
Hyperthyroidism (Graves')	B8		+
	DR3		+
Hyperthyroidism (Japanese)	B35		+
Adrenal insufficiency	DR3		++
Autoimmune Neurologic			
Myasthenia gravis	B8		+
	DR3		+
Multiple sclerosis	DR2	DRB1*1501 DRB5*0101	++
Other			
Behçet's disease	B51		++
Congenital adrenal hyperplasia	B47	21-OH (Cyp21B)	+++
Narcolepsy	DR2	DQB1*0602	++++
Goodpasture's syndrome (anti-GBM)	DR2		++
Abacavir hypersensitivity	B57	B*5701	++++

[a]Strong negative association; i.e., genetic association with protection from diabetes.

Celiac disease

In the case of celiac disease (Chap. 294), it is probable that the HLA-DQ genes are the primary basis for the disease association. HLA-DQ genes present on both the celiac-associated DR3 and DR7 haplotypes include the *DQB1*0201* gene, and further detailed studies have documented a specific class II αβ dimer encoded by the *DQA1*0501* and *DQB1*0201* genes, which appears to account for most of the HLA genetic contribution to celiac disease susceptibility. This specific HLA association with celiac disease may have a straightforward explanation: peptides derived from the wheat gluten component gliaden are bound to the molecule encoded by *DQA1*0501* and *DQB1*0201* and presented to T cells. Gliaden-derived peptides that are implicated in this immune activation bind the DQ class II dimer best when the peptide contains a glutamine to glutamic acid substitution. It has been proposed that tissue transglutaminase, an enzyme present at increased levels in the intestinal cells of celiac patients, converts glutamine to glutamic acid in gliadin, creating peptides that are capable of being bound by the DQ2 molecule and presented to T cells.

Pemphigus vulgaris

In the case of pemphigus vulgaris (Chap. 54), there are two HLA genes associated with disease, *DRB1*0402* and *DQB1*0503*. Peptides derived from desmoglien3, an epidermal autoantigen, bind to the DRB1*0402- and DQB1*0503-encoded HLA molecules, and this combination of specific peptide binding and disease-associated class II molecule is sufficient to stimulate desmoglien-specific T cells. A bullous pemphigoid clinical variant, not involving desmoglien recognition, has been found to be associated with HLA-DQB1*0301.

Juvenile arthritis

Pauciarticular juvenile arthritis (Chap. 321) is an autoimmune disease associated with genes at the DRB1 locus and also with genes at the DPB1 locus. Patients with both DPB1*0201 and a DRB1 susceptibility allele (usually DRB1*08 or -*05) have a higher relative risk than expected from the additive effect of those genes alone. In juvenile patients with rheumatoid factor–positive polyarticular disease, heterozygotes carrying both DRB1*0401 and -*0404 have a relative risk > 100, reflecting an apparent synergy in individuals inheriting both of these susceptibility genes.

Type 1 diabetes mellitus

Type 1 (autoimmune) diabetes mellitus (Chap. 344) is associated with MHC genes on more than one haplotype. The presence of both the DR3 and DR4 haplotypes in one individual confers a twentyfold increased risk for type 1 diabetes; the strongest single association is with DQB1*0302, and all haplotypes that carry a *DQB1*0302* gene are associated with type 1 diabetes, whereas related haplotypes that carry a different DQB1 gene are not. However, the relative risk associated with inheritance of this gene can be modified, depending on other HLA genes present either on the same or a second haplotype. For example, the presence of a DR2-positive haplotype containing a *DQB1*0602* gene is associated with decreased risk. This gene, *DQB1*0602*, is considered "protective" for type 1 diabetes. Even some DRB1 genes that can occur on the same haplotype as DQB1*0302 may modulate risk, so that individuals with the DR4 haplotype that contains DRB1*0403 are less susceptible to type 1 diabetes than individuals with other DR4-DQB1*0302 haplotypes.

Although the presence of a DR3 haplotype in combination with the DR4-DQB1*0302 haplotype is a very high-risk combination for diabetes susceptibility, the specific gene on the DR3 haplotype that is responsible for this synergy is not yet identified. There are some characteristic structural features of the diabetes-associated DQ molecule encoded by DQB1*0302, particularly the capability for binding peptides that have negatively charged amino acids near their C-termini. This may indicate a role for specific antigenic peptides or T cell interactions in the immune response to islet-associated proteins.

HLA and rheumatoid arthritis

The HLA genes associated with rheumatoid arthritis (RA) (Chap. 321) encode a distinctive sequence of amino acids from codons 67–74 of the DRβ molecule: RA-associated class II molecules carry the sequence LeuLeuGluGlnArgArgAlaAla or LeuLeuGluGlnLysArgAlaAla in this region, while non-RA-associated genes carry one or more differences in this region. These residues form a portion of the molecule that lies in the middle of the α-helical portion of the DRB1-encoded class II molecule, termed the *shared epitope*.

The highest risk for susceptibility to RA comes in individuals who carry both a *DRB1*0401* and *DRB1*0404* gene. These DR4-positive RA-associated alleles are most frequent among patients with more severe, erosive disease. Several mechanisms have been proposed that link the shared epitope to immune reactivity in RA. This portion of the class II molecule may allow preferential binding of an arthritogenic peptide, it may favor the expansion of a type of self-reactive T lymphocyte, or it may itself form part of the pMHC ligand recognized by TCR that initiates synovial tissue recognition.

■ MOLECULAR MECHANISMS FOR HLA-DISEASE ASSOCIATIONS

As noted above, HLA molecules play a key role in the selection and establishment of the antigen-specific T cell repertoire and a major role in the subsequent activation of those T cells during the initiation of an immune response. Precise genetic polymorphisms characteristic of individual alleles dictate the specificity of these interactions and thereby instruct and guide antigen-specific immune events. These same genetically determined pathways are therefore implicated in disease pathogenesis when specific HLA genes are responsible for autoimmune disease susceptibility.

The fate of developing T cells within the thymus is determined by the affinity of interaction between T cell receptor and HLA molecules bearing self-peptides, and thus the particular HLA types of each individual control the precise specificity of the T cell repertoire (Chap. 314). The primary basis for HLA-associated disease susceptibility may well lie within this thymic maturation pathway. The positive selection of potentially autoreactive T cells, based on the presence of specific HLA susceptibility genes, may establish the threshold for disease risk in a particular individual.

At the time of onset of a subsequent immune response, the primary role of the HLA molecule is to bind peptide and present it to antigen-specific T cells. The HLA complex can therefore be viewed as encoding genetic determinants of precise immunologic activation events. Antigenic peptides that bind particular HLA molecules are capable of stimulating T cell immune responses; peptides that do not bind are not presented to T cells and are not immunogenic. This genetic control of the immune response is mediated by the polymorphic sites within the HLA antigen–binding groove that interact with the bound peptides. In autoimmune and immune-mediated diseases, it is likely that specific tissue antigens that are targets for pathogenic lymphocytes are complexed with the HLA molecules encoded by specific susceptibility alleles. In autoimmune diseases with an infectious etiology, it is likely that immune responses to peptides derived from the initiating pathogen are bound and presented by particular HLA molecules to activate T lymphocytes that play a triggering or contributory role in disease pathogenesis. The concept that early events in disease initiation are triggered by specific HLA-peptide complexes offers some prospects for therapeutic intervention, since it may be possible to design compounds that interfere with the formation or function of specific HLA-peptide–T cell receptor interactions.

When considering mechanisms of HLA associations with immune response and disease, it is well to remember that just as HLA genetics are complex, so are the mechanisms likely to be heterogeneous. Immune-mediated disease is a multistep process in which one of the HLA-associated functions is to establish a repertoire of potentially reactive T cells, while another HLA-associated function is to provide the essential peptide-binding specificity for T cell recognition. For diseases with multiple HLA genetic associations, it is possible that both of these interactions occur and synergize to advance an accelerated pathway of disease.

FURTHER READINGS

Caillat-Zucman S: Molecular mechanisms of HLA association with autoimmune diseases. Tissue Antigens 73:1, 2008

Carrington M et al: KIR-HLA intercourse in HIV disease. Trends Immunol 16:620, 2008

Horton R et al: Variation analysis and gene annotation of eight MHC haplotypes: The MHC Haplotype Project. Immunogenetics 60:1, 2008

Jones EY et al: MHC class II proteins and disease: A structural perspective. Nat Rev Immunol 6:271, 2006

Nepom GT: Major histocompatibility complex-directed susceptibility to rheumatoid arthritis. Adv Immunol 68:315, 1998

———: Tetramer analysis of human autoreactive CD4-positive T cells. Adv Immunol 88:51, 2005

Shiina T et al: The HLA genomic loci map: Expression, interaction, diversity and disease. J Hum Genet 54:15, 2009

CHAPTER 316

Primary Immune Deficiency Diseases

Alain Fischer

Immunity is intrinsic to life and an important tool in the fight for survival against pathogenic microorganisms. The human immune system can be divided into two major components: the innate immune system and the adaptive immune system (Chap. 314). The innate immune system provides the rapid triggering of inflammatory responses based on the recognition (at the cell surface or within cells) of either molecules expressed by microorganisms or molecules that serve as "danger signals" released by cells under attack. These receptor/ligand interactions trigger signaling events that ultimately lead to inflammation. Virtually all cell lineages (not just immune cells) are involved in innate immune responses; however, myeloid cells (i.e., neutrophils and macrophages) play a major role because of their phagocytic capacity. The adaptive immune system operates by clonal recognition of antigens followed by a dramatic expansion of antigen-reactive cells and execution of an immune effector program. Most of the effector cells die off rapidly, whereas memory cells persist. Although both T and B lymphocytes recognize distinct chemical moieties and execute distinct adaptive immune responses, the latter is largely dependent on the former in generating long-lived humoral immunity. Adaptive responses utilize components of the innate immune system; for example, the antigen-presentation capabilities of dendritic cells help to determine the type of effector response. Not surprisingly, immune responses are controlled by a series of regulatory mechanisms.

Hundreds of gene products have been characterized as effectors or mediators of the immune system (Chap. 314). Whenever the expression or function of one of these products is genetically impaired (provided the function is nonredundant), a primary immunodeficiency (PID) occurs.

Primary immunodeficiencies are genetic diseases with primarily Mendelian inheritance. More than 200 conditions have now been described and deleterious mutations in approximately 150 genes have been identified. The overall prevalence of PIDs has been estimated in various countries at 5 per 100,000 individuals; however, given the difficulty in diagnosing these rare and complex diseases, this figure is probably an underestimate. Primary immunodeficiencies can involve all possible aspects of immune responses, from innate through adaptive, cell differentiation, and effector function and regulation. For the sake of clarity, PIDs should be classified according to (1) the arm of the immune system that is defective and (2) the mechanism of the defect (when known). Table 316-1 classifies the most prevalent PIDs according to this manner of classification; however, one should bear in mind that the classification of PIDs sometimes involves arbitrary decisions because of overlap and, in some cases, lack of data.

The consequences of PIDs vary widely as a function of the molecules that are defective. This concept translates into multiple levels of vulnerability to infection by pathogenic and opportunistic microorganisms, ranging from extremely broad [as in severe combined immunodeficiency (SCID)] to narrowly restricted to a single microorganism [as in Mendelian susceptibility to mycobacterial disease (MSMD)]. The locations of the sites of infection and the causal microorganisms involved will thus help physicians arrive at proper diagnoses. Primary immunodeficiencies can also lead to immunopathologic responses such as allergy (as in Wiskott-Aldrich syndrome), lymphoproliferation, and autoimmunity. A combination of recurrent infections, inflammation, and autoimmunity can be observed in a number of PIDs, thus creating obvious therapeutic challenges. Finally, some PIDs increase the risk of cancer, notably but not exclusively lymphocytic cancers, e.g., lymphoma.

DIAGNOSIS OF PRIMARY IMMUNODEFICIENCIES

The most frequent symptom prompting the diagnosis of a PID is the presence of recurrent or unusually severe infections. As mentioned above, recurrent allergic or autoimmune manifestations may also alert the physician to a possible diagnosis of PID. In such cases, a detailed account of the subject's personal and family medical history should be obtained. It is of the utmost importance to gather as much medical information as possible on relatives and up to several generations of ancestors. In addition to the obvious focus on primary symptoms, the clinical examination should evaluate the size of lymphoid organs and, when appropriate, look for the characteristic signs of a number of complex syndromes that may be associated with a PID.

The performance of laboratory tests should be guided to some extent by the clinical findings. Infections of the respiratory tract (bronchi, sinuses) mostly suggest a defective antibody response. In general, invasive bacterial infections can result from complement deficiencies, signaling defects of innate immune responses, asplenia, or defective antibody responses. Viral infections, recurrent *Candida* infections, and opportunistic infections are generally suggestive of impaired T cell immunity. Skin infections and deep-seated abscesses primarily reflect innate immune defects (such as chronic granulomatous disease); however, they may also appear in the autosomal dominant hyper-IgE syndrome. Table 316-2 summarizes the laboratory tests that are most frequently used to diagnose a PID. More specific tests (notably genetic tests) are then used to make a definitive diagnosis.

The primary immunodeficiencies discussed below have been grouped together according to the affected cells and the mechanisms involved (Table 316-1, Fig. 316-1).

PRIMARY IMMUNODEFICIENCIES OF THE INNATE IMMUNE SYSTEM

Primary immunodeficiencies of the innate immune system are relatively rare and account for approximately 10% of all PIDs.

SEVERE CONGENITAL NEUTROPENIA

Severe congenital neutropenia (SCN) consists of a group of inherited diseases that are characterized by severely impaired neutrophil counts [<500 polymorphonuclear leukocytes (PMN)/μL of blood]. The condition is usually manifested from birth. Severe congenital neutropenia may also be cyclic (with a 3-week periodicity), and other neutropenia syndromes can also be intermittent. Although the most frequent inheritance pattern for SCN is autosomal dominant, autosomal recessive and X-linked recessive conditions also exist. Bacterial infections at the interface between the body and the external milieu (e.g., the orifices, wounds, and the respiratory tract) are common manifestations. Bacterial infections can rapidly progress through soft tissue and are followed by dissemination in the bloodstream. Severe visceral fungal infections can also ensue. The absence of pus is a hallmark of this condition.

Diagnosis of SCN requires examination of the bone marrow. Most SCNs are associated with a block in granulopoiesis at the promyelocytic stage (Fig. 316-1). Severe congenital neutropenia

TABLE 316-1 Classification of Primary Immune Deficiency Diseases

Deficiencies of the Innate Immune System	
• Phagocytic cells:	
- Impaired production: severe congenital neutropenia (SCN)	
- Asplenia	
- Impaired adhesion: leukocyte adhesion deficiency (LAD)	
- Impaired killing: chronic granulomatous disease (CGD)	
• Innate immunity receptors and signal transduction:	
- Defects in Toll-like receptor signaling	
- Mendelian susceptibility to mycobacterial disease	
• Complement deficiencies:	
- Classical, alternative, and lectin pathways	
- Lytic phase	
Deficiencies of the Adaptive Immune System	
• T lymphocytes:	
- Impaired development	Severe combined immune deficiencies (SCIDs) DiGeorge syndrome
- Impaired survival, migration, function	Severe combined immunodeficiencies Hyper-IgE syndrome (autosomal dominant) CD40 ligand deficiency Wiskott-Aldrich syndrome Ataxia-telangiectasia and other DNA repair deficiencies
• B lymphocytes:	
- Impaired development	XL and AR agammaglobulinemia
- Impaired function	Hyper-IgM syndrome Common variable immunodeficiency (CVID) IgA deficiency
Regulatory Defects	
• Innate immunity	Autoinflammatory syndromes (outside the scope of this chapter) Severe colitis
• Adaptive immunity	Hemophagocytic lymphohistiocytosis (HLH) Autoimmune lymphoproliferation syndrome (ALPS) Autoimmunity and inflammatory diseases (IPEX, APECED)

Abbreviations: APECED, autoimmune polyendocrinopathy candidiasis ectodermal dysplasia; AR, autosomal recessive; IPEX, immunodysregulation polyendocrinopathy enteropathy X-linked syndrome; XL, X-linked.

has multiple etiologies, and to date mutations in 11 different genes have been identified. Most of these mutations result in isolated SCN, whereas others are syndromic (Chap. 60). The most frequent forms of SCN are caused by the premature cell death of granulocyte precursors, as observed in deficiencies of GFI1, HAX1, and elastase 2 (ELA2), with the latter accounting for 50% of SCN sufferers. Certain ELA2 mutations cause cyclic neutropenia syndrome. A gain-of-function mutation in the *WASP* gene (see the section on "Wiskott-Aldrich syndrome" below) causes X-linked SCN, which is also associated with monocytopenia.

As mentioned above, SCN exposes the patient to life-threatening, disseminated bacterial and fungal infections. Treatment requires careful hygiene measures, notably in infants. Later in life, special oral and dental care is essential, along with the prevention of bacterial infection by prophylactic administration of trimethoprim/sulfamethoxazole. Subcutaneous injection of the cytokine granulocyte colony-stimulating factor (G-CSF) usually improves neutrophil development and thus prevents infection in most SCN diseases. However, there are two caveats: (1) a few cases of SCN with ELA2 mutation are refractory to G-CSF and may require curative treatment via allogeneic hematopoietic stem cell transplantation (HSCT) and (2) a subset of G-CSF-treated patients carrying ELA2 mutations are at a greater risk of developing acute myelogenous leukemia associated (in most cases) with somatic gain-of-function mutations of the G-CSF receptor gene.

■ ASPLENIA

Primary failure of the development of a spleen is an extremely rare disease that can be either syndromic (in Ivemark syndrome) or isolated with an autosomal dominant expression; in the latter case, the gene remains to be identified. Due to the absence of natural filtration of microbes in the blood, asplenia predisposes affected individuals to fulminant infections by encapsulated bacteria. Although most infections occur in the first years of life, cases may also arise in adulthood. The diagnosis is confirmed by abdominal ultrasonography and the detection of Howell-Jolly bodies in red blood cells. Effective prophylactic measures (twice-daily oral penicillin and appropriate vaccination programs) usually prevent fatal outcomes. The genetic causes of asplenia remain unknown.

■ LEUKOCYTE ADHESION DEFICIENCY (LAD)

Leukocyte adhesion deficiency consists of three autosomal recessive conditions (LAD I, II, and III) (Chap. 60). The most frequent condition (LAD I) is caused by mutations in the β2 integrin gene; following leukocyte activation, β2 integrins mediate adhesion to inflamed endothelium expressing cognate ligands. LAD III results from a defect in a regulatory protein (kindlin, also known as Fermt 3) involved in activating the ligand affinity of β2 integrins. The extremely rare LAD II condition is the end result of a defect in selectin-mediated leukocyte rolling that occurs prior to β2 integrin binding. There is a primary defect in fucose transporter such that oligosaccharide selectin ligands are missing in this syndromic condition.

Given that neutrophils are not able to reach infected tissues, LAD renders the individual susceptible to bacterial and fungal infections in a way that is similar to that of patients with SCN. LAD also causes impaired wound healing and delayed loss of the umbilical cord. A diagnosis can be suspected in cases of pus-free skin/tissue infections and massive hyperleukocytosis (>30,000/μL) in the blood (mostly granulocytes). Patients with LAD III also develop bleeding because the β2 integrin in platelets is not functional. Use of

TABLE 316-2 Test Most Frequently Used to Diagnose a Primary Immune Deficiency (PID)

Test	Information	PID Disease
• Blood cell counts and cell morphology	Neutrophil counts	↓Severe congenital neutropenia, ↑↑ LAD
	Lymphocyte counts*	T cell ID
	Eosinophilia	WAS, Hyper-IgE syndrome
	Howell-Jolly bodies	Asplenia
• Chest x-ray	Thymic shadow	SCID, DiGeorge syndrome
	Costochondral junctions	Adenosine deaminase deficiency
• Bone x-ray	Metaphyseal ends	Cartilage hair hypoplasia
• Immunoglobulin serum levels	IgG, IgA, IgM	B cell ID
	IgE	Hyper-IgE syndrome, WAS, T cell ID
• Lymphocyte phenotype	T, B lymphocyte counts	T cell ID, agammaglobulinemia
• Dihydrorhodamine fluorescence (DHR) assay Nitroblue tetrazolium (NBT) assay	Reactive oxygen species production by PMN	Chronic granulomatous disease
• CH50, AP50	Classic and alternative complement pathways	Complement deficiencies
• Ultrasonography of the abdomen	Spleen size	Asplenia

*Normal counts vary with age. For example, the lymphocyte count is between 3000 and 9000/μL of blood below the age of 3 months and between 1500 and 2500/μL in adults.

Abbreviations: ID, immunodeficiency; LAD, leukocyte adhesion deficiency; PMNs, polymorphonuclear leukocytes; SCID, severe combined immunodeficiency; WAS, Wiskott-Aldrich syndrome.

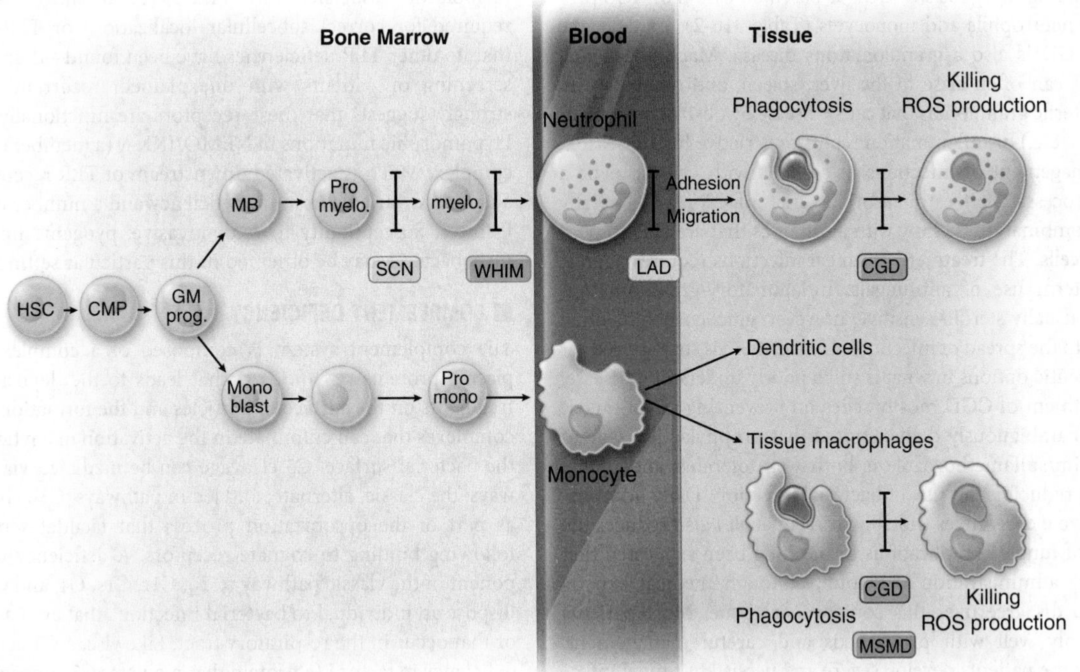

Figure 316-1 Differentiation of phagocytic cells and related primary immunodeficiencies (PIDs). Hematopoietic stem cells (HSCs) differentiate into common myeloid progenitors (CMPs) and then granulocyte-monocyte progenitors (GM-prog.), which, in turn, differentiate into neutrophils (MB: myeloblasts; Promyelo: promyelocytes; myelo: myelocytes) or monocytes (monoblasts and promonocytes). Upon activation, neutrophils adhere to the vascular endothelium, transmigrate, and phagocytose the targets. Reactive oxygen species (ROS) are delivered to the microorganism-containing phagosomes. Macrophages in tissues kill using the same mechanism. Following activation by interferon γ (not shown here), macrophages can be armed to kill intracellular pathogens such as mycobacteria. For sake of simplicity, not all cell differentiation stages are shown. The abbreviations for PIDs are contained in boxes placed at corresponding stages of the pathway. SCN, severe congenital neutropenia; WHIM, warts, hypogammaglobulinemia, immunodeficiency myelokathexis; LAD, leukocyte adhesion deficiencies; CGD, chronic granulomatous diseases; MSMD, Mendelian susceptibility to mycobacterial disease.

immunofluorescence and functional assays to detect β2 integrin can help form a diagnosis. Severe forms of LAD may require hematopoietic stem cell transplantation (HSCT), although gene therapy is also now being considered. Neutrophil-specific granule deficiency (a very rare condition caused by a mutation in the gene for transcription factor C/EBPα) results in a condition that is clinically similar to LAD.

■ CHRONIC GRANULOMATOUS DISEASES

Chronic granulomatous diseases (CGDs) are characterized by impaired phagocytic killing of microorganisms by neutrophils and macrophages (Chap. 60). The incidence is approximately 1 per 200,000 live births. About 70% of cases are associated with X-linked recessive inheritance versus autosomal inheritance in the remaining 30%. CGD causes deep-tissue bacterial and fungal abscesses in macrophage-rich organs such as the lymph nodes, liver, and lungs. Recurrent skin infections (such as folliculitis) are common and can prompt an early diagnosis of CGD. The infectious agents are typically catalase-positive bacteria (such as *Staphylococcus aureus* and *Serratia marcescens*) but also include *Burkholderia cepacia*, pathogenic mycobacteria (in certain regions of the world), and fungi (mainly filamentous molds, such as *Aspergillus*).

CGD is caused by defective production of reactive oxygen species (ROS) in the phagolysosome membrane following phagocytosis of microorganisms. It results from the lack of a component of NADPH oxidase (gp91phox or p22phox) or of the associated adapter/activating proteins (p47phox, p67phox, or p40phox) that mediate the transport of electrons into the phagolysosome for creating ROS by interaction with O_2. Under normal circumstances, these ROS either directly kill engulfed microorganisms or enable the rise in pH needed to activate the phagosomal proteases that contribute to microbial killing. Diagnosis of CGD is based on assays of ROS production in neutrophils and monocytes (Table 316-2). As its name suggests, CGD is also a granulomatous disease. Macrophage-rich granulomas can often arise in the liver, spleen, and other organs. These are sterile granulomas that cause disease by obstruction (bladder, pylorus, etc.) or inflammation (colitis, restrictive lung disease).

The management of infections in patients with CGD can be a complex process. The treatment of bacterial infections is generally based on combination therapy with antibiotics that are able to penetrate into cells. The treatment of fungal infections requires aggressive, long-term use of antifungals. Inflammatory/granulomatous lesions are usually steroid-sensitive; however, glucocorticoids often contribute to the spread of infections. Hence, there is strong need for new therapeutic options in what is still a poorly understood disease.

The treatment of CGD mostly relies on preventing infections. It has been unambiguously demonstrated that prophylactic usage of trimethoprim/sulfamethoxazole is both well tolerated and highly effective in reducing the risk of bacterial infection. Daily administration of azole derivatives (notably intraconazole) also reduces the frequency of fungal complications. It has long been suggested that interferon-γ administration is helpful, although medical experts continue to disagree over this controversial issue. Most patients do reasonably well with prophylaxis and careful management. However, some patients develop severe and persistent fungal infections and/or chronic inflammatory complications that ultimately require HSCT. The latter is an established curative approach for CGD; however, the risk-versus-benefit ratio must be carefully assessed on a case-by-case basis. Gene therapy approaches are also being evaluated.

■ MENDELIAN SUSCEPTIBILITY TO MYCOBACTERIAL DISEASE (MSMD)

This group of diseases is characterized by a defect in the IL-12 interferon (IFN)-γ axis (including IL-12p40, IL-12 receptor (R) β_1, interferon-γ R_1 and R_2, and STAT1 deficiencies), which ultimately leads to impaired IFN-γ-dependent macrophage activation. Both recessive and dominant inheritance modes have been observed. The hallmark of this PID is a specific and narrow vulnerability to tuberculous and nontuberculous mycobacteria. The most severe phenotype (as observed in complete IFN-γ receptor deficiency) is characterized by disseminated infection that can be fatal even when aggressive and appropriate antimycobacterial therapy is applied. In addition to mycobacterial infections, MSMD patients (and particularly those with an IL-12/IL-12 R deficiency) are prone to developing *Salmonella* infections. Although MSMDs are very rare, they should be considered in any patient with persistent mycobacterial infection. Treatment with interferon γ may efficiently bypass an IL-12/IL-12 R deficiency.

■ TOLL-LIKE RECEPTOR (TLR) PATHWAY DEFICIENCIES

In a certain group of patients with early-onset, invasive *Streptococcus pneumoniae* infections or (less frequently) *Staphylococcus aureus* or other pyogenic infections, conventional screening for PIDs does not identify the cause of the defect in host defense. It has been established that these patients carry recessive mutations in genes that encode essential adaptor molecules (IRAK4 and MYD88) involved in the signaling pathways of the majority of known Toll-like receptors (TLRs) (Chap. 314). Remarkably, susceptibility to infection appears to decrease after the first few years of life—perhaps an indication that adaptive immunity (once triggered by an initial microbial challenge) is then able to prevent recurrent infections.

Certain TLRs (TLR-3, -7, -8, and -9) are involved in the recognition of RNA and DNA and usually become engaged during viral infections. Very specific susceptibility to herpes simplex encephalitis has been described in patients with a deficiency in Unc93b (a molecule associated with TLR-3, -7, -8, and -9 and probably required for correct subcellular localization) or TLR-3. The fact that no other TLR deficiencies have been found—despite extensive screening of patients with unexplained, recurrent infections—strongly suggests that these receptors are functionally redundant. Hypomorphic mutations in NEMO/IKK-γ (a member of the NF-κB complex, which is activated downstream of TLR receptors) lead to a complex, variable immunodeficiency and a number of associated features. Susceptibility to both invasive, pyogenic infections and mycobacteria may be observed in this particular setting.

■ COMPLEMENT DEFICIENCY

The complement system is composed of a complex cascade of plasma proteins (Chap. 314) that leads to the deposition of C3b fragments on the surface of particles and the formation of immune complexes that can culminate in the activation of a lytic complex at the bacterial surface. C3 cleavage can be mediated via three pathways: the classic, alternate, and lectin pathways. C3b coats particles as part of the opsonization process that facilitates phagocytosis following binding to cognate receptors. A deficiency in any component of the classic pathway (C1q, C1r, C1s, C4, and C2) can predispose an individual to bacterial infections that are tissue-invasive or that occur in the respiratory tract. Likewise, a C3 deficiency or a deficiency in factor I (a protein that regulates C3 consumption, thus leading to a C3 deficiency due to its absence) also results in the same type of vulnerability to infection. It has recently been reported that a very rare deficiency in Ficolin-3 predisposes affected individuals to bacterial infections. Deficiencies in the alternative pathway (factors D and properdin) are associated with the occurrence of invasive *Neisseria* infections.

Lastly, deficiencies of any complement component involved in the lytic phase (C5, C6, C7, C8, and, to a lesser extent, C9) predispose affected individuals to systemic infection by *Neisseria*. This is explained by the critical role of complement in the lysis of the thick cell wall possessed by this class of bacteria.

Diagnosis of a complement deficiency relies primarily on testing the status of the classic and alternate pathway via functional assays, i.e., the CH50 and AP50 tests, respectively. When either pathway is profoundly impaired, determination of the status of the relevant components in that pathway enables a precise diagnosis. Appropriate vaccinations and daily administration of oral penicillin are efficient means of preventing recurrent infections. It is noteworthy that several complement deficiencies (in the classic pathway and the lytic phase) may also predispose affected individuals to autoimmune diseases (notably systemic lupus erythematosus; Chap. 319).

PRIMARY IMMUNODEFICIENCIES OF THE ADAPTIVE IMMUNE SYSTEM

■ T LYMPHOCYTE DEFICIENCIES (TABLE 316-1, FIGS. 316-2 AND 316-3)

Given the central role of T lymphocytes in adaptive immune responses (Chap. 314), PIDs involving T cells generally have severe pathologic consequences; this explains the poor overall prognosis and the need for early diagnosis and the early intervention with appropriate therapy. Several differentiation pathways of T cell effectors have been described, one or all of which may be affected by a given PID (Fig. 316-2). Follicular helper CD4+ T cells in germinal centers are required for T-dependent antibody production, including the generation of Ig class-switched, high-affinity antibodies. CD4+ T_{H1} cells provide cytokine-dependent (mostly interferon-γ-dependent) help to macrophages for intracellular killing of various microorganisms, including mycobacteria and *Salmonella*. CD4+ T_{H2} cells produce IL-4, IL-5, and IL-13 and thus recruit and activate eosinophils and other cells required to fight helminth infections. CD4+ T_{H17} cells produce IL-17 and IL-22 cytokines that recruit neutrophils to the skin and lungs to fight bacterial and fungal infections. Cytotoxic CD8+ T cells can kill infected cells, notably in the context of viral infections. In addition, certain T cell deficiencies predispose affected individuals to *Pneumocystis jiroveci* lung infections early in life and to chronic gut/biliary duct/liver infections by *Cryptosporidia* and related genera later on in life. Lastly, naturally occuring or induced regulatory T cells are essential for controlling inflammation (notably reactivity to commensal bacteria in the gut) and autoimmunity. The role of other T cell subsets with limited T cell receptor (TCR) diversity [such as γδTCR T cells or natural killer T (NKT) cells] in PIDs is less well known; however, these subsets can be defective in certain PIDs and this finding can sometimes contribute to the diagnosis (e.g., NKT cell deficiency in X-linked proliferative syndrome). T cell deficiencies account for approximately 20% of all cases of PID.

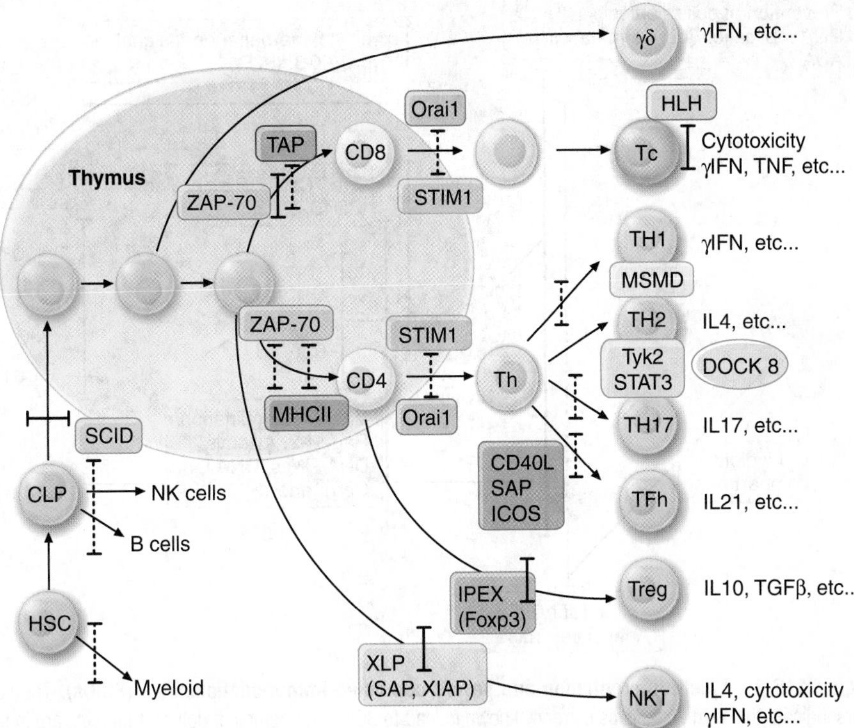

Figure 316-2 T cell differentiation, effector pathways, and related primary immunodeficiencies (PIDs). Hematopoietic stem cells (HSCs) differentiate into common lymphoid progenitors (CLPs), which, in turn, give rise to the T cell precursors that migrate to the thymus. The development of CD4+ and CD8+ T cells is shown. Known T cell effector pathways are indicated, i.e., γδ cells, cytotoxic T cells (Tc), TH1, TH2, TH17, TFh (follicular helper) CD4 effector T cells, regulatory T cells (Treg), and natural killer T cells (NKTs); abbreviations for PIDs are contained in boxes. Vertical bars indicate a complete deficiency; broken bars a partial deficiency. SCID, severe combined immunodeficiency; ZAP 70, zeta-associated protein deficiency, MHCII, major histocompatibility complex class II deficiency; TAP, TAP1 and 2 deficiencies; Orai1, Stim1 deficiencies; HLH, hematopoietic lymphohistiocytosis; MSMD, Mendelian susceptibility to mycobacterial disease; Tyk2, DOCK8, autosomal recessive form of hyper-IgE syndrome; STAT3, autosomal dominant form of hyper-IgE syndrome; CD40L, ICOS, SAP deficiencies; IPEX, immunodysregulation polyendocrinopathy enteropathy X-linked syndrome; XLP, X-linked proliferative syndromes.

Severe combined immunodeficiencies

Severe combined immunodeficiencies (SCIDs) constitute a group of rare PIDs characterized by a profound block in T cell development and thus the complete absence of these cells. The developmental block is always the consequence of an intrinsic deficiency. The incidence of SCID is estimated to be 1 in 50,000 to 100,000 live births. Given the severity of the T cell deficiency, clinical consequences occur early in life (usually within 3 to 6 months of birth). The most frequent clinical manifestations are recurrent oral candidiasis, failure to thrive, and protracted diarrhea and/or acute interstitial pneumonitis caused by *Pneumocystis jiroveci* (although the latter can also be observed in the first year of life in children with B cell deficiencies). Severe viral infections or invasive bacterial infections can also occur. Patients may also experience complications related to infections caused by live vaccines (notably bacille Calmette-Guérin; BCG) that may lead not only to local and regional infection but also to disseminated infection manifested by fever, splenomegaly, and skin and lytic bone lesions. A scaly skin eruption can be observed in a context of maternal T cell engraftment (see below). A diagnosis of SCID can be suspected on the basis of the patient's clinical history and, possibly, a family history of deaths in very young children (suggestive of either X-linked or recessive inheritance). Lymphocytopenia is strongly suggestive of SCID in more than 90% of cases (Table 316-2). The absence of a thymic shadow on a chest x-ray can also be suggestive of SCID. An accurate diagnosis relies on precise determination of the number of circulating T, B, and NK lymphocytes and their subsets. T cell lymphopenia may be masked in some patients by the presence of maternal T

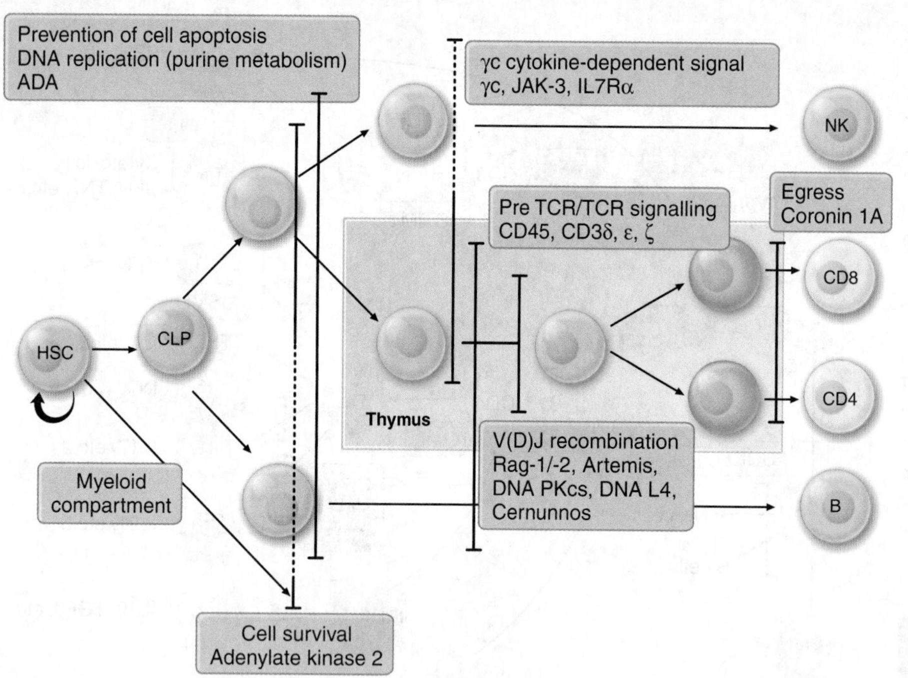

Figure 316-3 T cell differentiation and severe combined immunodeficiencies (SCIDs). The vertical bars indicate the six mechanisms currently known to lead to SCID. The names of deficient proteins are indicated in the boxes adjacent to the vertical bars. A broken line means that deficiency is partial or involves only some of the indicated immunodeficiencies. HSCs, hematopoietic stem cells; CLPs, common lymphoid progenitors; ADA, adenosine deaminase deficiency; NKs, natural killer cells; TCR, T cell receptor; DNAL4, DNA ligase 4.

cells (derived from maternal-fetal blood transfers) that cannot be eliminated. Although counts are usually low (<500/μL of blood), higher maternal T cell counts may, under some circumstances, initially mask the presence of SCID. Thus, screening for maternal cells by using adequate genetic markers should be performed whenever necessary. Inheritance pattern analysis and lymphocyte phenotyping can discriminate between various forms of SCID and provide guidance in the choice of accurate molecular diagnostic tests (see below). To date, six distinct causative mechanisms for SCID (Fig. 316-3) have been identified:

Severe combined immunodeficiency caused by a cytokine-signaling deficiency The most frequent SCID phenotype (accounting for 40–50% of all cases) is the absence of both T and NK cells. This outcome results from a deficiency in either the common γ chain (γc) receptor (γc) that is shared by several cytokine receptors (the IL-2, -4, -7, -9, -15, and -21 receptors) or Jak-associated kinase (JAK) 3 that binds to the cytoplasmic portion of the γc chain receptor and induces signal transduction following cytokine binding. The former form of SCID (γc deficiency) has an X-linked inheritance mode, while the second is autosomal recessive. A lack of the IL-7Rα chain (which, together with γc, forms the IL-7 receptor) induces a selective T cell deficiency.

Purine metabolism deficiency Ten to 20% of SCID patients exhibit a deficiency in adenosine deaminase (ADA), an enzyme of purine metabolism that deaminates adenosine (ado) and deoxyadenosine (dAdo). An ADA deficiency results in the accumulation of ado and dAdo metabolites that induce premature cell death of lymphocyte progenitors. The condition results in the absence of B and NK lymphocytes as well as T cells. The clinical expression of complete ADA deficiency typically occurs very early in life. Since ADA is a ubiquitous enzyme, its deficiency can also cause bone dysplasia with abnormal costochondral junctions and metaphyses (found in 50% of cases) and neurologic defects. The very rare purine nucleoside phosphorylase (PNP) deficiency causes a profound although incomplete T cell deficiency that is often associated with severe neurologic impairments.

Defective rearrangements of T and B cell receptors A series of SCID conditions are characterized by a selective deficiency in T and B lymphocytes with autosomal recessive inheritance. These conditions account for 20–30% of SCID cases and result from mutations in genes encoding proteins that mediate the recombination of V(D)J gene elements in T and B cell antigen receptor genes (required for the generation of diversity in antigen recognition). The main deficiencies involve RAG-1, RAG-2, DNA-dependent protein kinase, and Artemis. A less severe (albeit variable) immunologic phenotype can result from other deficiencies in the same pathway, i.e., DNA ligase 4 and Cernunnos deficiencies. Given that these latter factors are involved in DNA repair, these deficiencies also cause developmental defects.

Defective (pre-)T cell receptor signaling in the thymus A selective T cell defect can be caused by a series of rare deficiencies in molecules involved in signaling via the pre-TCR or the TCR. These include deficiencies in CD3 subunits associated with the (pre)TCR (i.e., CD3δ, ε, and ζ) and CD45.

Reticular dysgenesis Reticular dysgenesis is an extremely rare form of SCID that causes T and NK deficiencies with severe neutropenia and sensorineural deafness. It results from an adenylate kinase 2 deficiency.

Defective egress of lymphocytes Defective egress of lymphocytes from the thymus has been found in a patient with very low T cell counts but a normal thymic shadow. This condition was found to result from a deficiency in coronin-1A.

Patients with SCID require appropriate care with aggressive anti-infective therapies, immunoglobulin replacement, and (when necessary) parenteral nutrition support. In most cases, curative treatment relies on HSCT. Today, HSCT provides a very high curative potential for SCID patients who are otherwise in reasonably good condition. In this regard, the feasibility of neonatal screening is now being evaluated. Gene therapy has been found to be successful for cases of X-linked SCID (γc deficiency) and SCID caused by an ADA deficiency, although toxicity has become an issue in the treatment of the former disease. Lastly, a third option for the treatment of ADA deficiency consists of enzyme substitution with a pegylated enzyme.

Thymic defects

A profound T cell defect can also result from faulty development of the thymus, as is most often observed in rare cases of DiGeorge syndrome—a relatively common condition leading to a constellation of developmental defects. In approximately 1% of such cases, the thymus is completely absent, leading to virtually no mature T cells. However, expansion of oligoclonal T cells can occur and is associated with skin lesions. Diagnosis (using immunofluorescence in situ hybridization) is based on the identification of a hemizygous deletion in the long arm of chromosome 22. To recover the capability for T cell differentiation, these cases require a thymic graft. CHARGE (*c*oloboma of the eye, *h*eart anomaly, choanal *a*tresia, *r*etardation, *g*enital and *e*ar anomalies) syndrome (CHD7 deficiency) is a less frequent cause of impaired thymus development. Lastly, the very rare "nude" defect is characterized by the absence of both hair and the thymus.

Omenn syndrome

Omenn syndrome consists of a subset of T cell deficiencies that present with a unique phenotype, including early-onset erythrodermia, alopecia, hepatosplenomegaly, and failure to thrive. These patients usually display T cell lymphocytosis, eosinophilia, and low B cell counts. It has been found that the T cells of these patients exhibit a low TCR heterogeneity. This peculiar syndrome is the consequence of hypomorphic mutations in genes usually associated with SCID, i.e., RAG-1, RAG-2, or (less frequently) Artemis or IL-7Rα. The impaired homeostasis of differentiating T cells thus causes this immune system–associated disease. These patients are very fragile, requiring simultaneous anti-infective therapy, nutritional support, and immunosuppression. HSCT provides a curative approach.

Functional T cell defects (Fig. 316-2)

A subset of T cell PIDs with autosomal inheritance is characterized by partially preserved T cell differentiation but defective activation resulting in abnormal effector function. There are many causes of these defects, but all lead to susceptibility to viral and opportunistic infections, chronic diarrhea, and failure to thrive, with onset during childhood. Careful phenotyping and in vitro functional assays are required to identify these diseases, the best characterized of which are the following.

Zeta-associated protein 70 (ZAP70) deficiency Zeta-associated protein 70 is recruited to the TCR following antigen recognition. A ZAP70 deficiency leads typically to an almost complete absence of CD8+ T cells; CD4+ T cells are present but cannot be activated in vitro by TCR stimulation.

Calcium signaling defects A small number of patients have been reported who exhibit a profound defect in in vitro T and B cell activation as a result of defective antigen receptor-mediated Ca^{2+} influx. This defect is caused by a mutation in the calcium channel gene (ORAI-) or its activator (STIM-1). It is noteworthy that these patients are also prone to autoimmune manifestations (blood cytopenias) and exhibit a nonprogressive muscle disease.

Human leukocyteantigen (HLA) class II deficiency Defective expression of HLA class II molecules is the hallmark of a group of four recessive genetic defects all of which affect molecules (RFX5, RFXAP, RFXANK, and CIITA) involved in the transactivation of the genes coding for HLA class II. As a result, low but variable CD4+ T cell counts are observed in addition to defective antigen-specific T and B cell responses. These patients are particularly susceptible to herpesvirus, adenovirus, and enterovirus infections and chronic gut/liver *Cryptosporidium* infections.

HLA class I deficiency Defective expression of molecules involved in antigen presentation by HLA class I molecules (i.e., TAP-1, TAP-2, and Tapasin) leads to reduced CD8+ T cell counts, loss of HLA class I antigen expression, and a particular phenotype consisting of chronic obstructive pulmonary disease and severe vasculitis.

Other defects A variety of other T cell PIDs have been described, some of which are associated with a precise molecular defect [e.g., IL-2-inducible T cell kinase (ITK) deficiency]. These conditions are also characterized by profound vulnerability to infections, such as severe Epstein-Barr virus (EBV)–induced B cell proliferation and autoimmune disorders in ITK deficiency. Milder phenotypes are associated with CD8 and CD3γ deficiencies.

HSCT is indicated for most of these diseases, although the prognosis is worse than in SCID because many patients are chronically infected at the time of diagnosis. Fairly aggressive immunosuppression and myeloablation may be necessary to achieve engraftment of allogeneic stem cells.

T cell primary immunodeficiencies with DNA repair defects

This is a group of PIDs characterized by a combination of T and B cell defects of variable intensity, together with a number of nonimmunologic features resulting from DNA fragility. The autosomal recessive disorder *ataxia-telangiectasia* (AT) is the most frequently encountered condition in this group. It has an incidence of 1:40,000 live births and causes B cell defects (low IgA, IgG2 deficiency, and low antibody production), which often require immunoglobulin replacement. Ataxia telangiectasia is associated with a progressive T cell immunodeficiency. As the name suggests, the hallmark features of AT are telangiectasia and cerebellar ataxia. The latter manifestations may not be detectable before the age of 3–4 years, so that AT should be considered in young children with IgA deficiency and recurrent and problematic infections. Diagnosis is based on a cytogenetic analysis showing excessive chromosomal rearrangements (mostly affecting chromosomes 7 and 14) in lymphocytes. Ataxia telangiectasia is caused by a mutation in the gene encoding the ATM protein—a kinase that plays an important role in the detection and repair of DNA lesions (or cell death if the lesions are too numerous) by triggering several different pathways. Overall, AT is a progressive disease that carries a very high risk of lymphoma, leukemia, and (during adulthood) carcinomas. A variant of AT ("AT-like disease") is caused by mutation in the *MRE11* gene.

Nijmegen breakage syndrome (NBS) is a less common condition that also results from chromosome instability (with the same cytogenetic abnormalities as in AT). NBS is characterized by a severe T and B cell combined immune deficiency with autosomal recessive inheritance. Individuals with NBS exhibit microcephaly and a bird-like face, but have neither ataxia nor telangiectasia. The risk of malignancies is very high. Nijmegen breakage syndrome results from a deficiency in Nibrin (NBSI, a protein associated with MRE11 and Rad50 that is involved in checking DNA lesions) caused by hypomorphic mutations.

Severe forms of *dyskeratosis congenita* (also known as Hoyeraal-Hreidarsson syndrome) combine a progressive immunodeficiency that can also include an absence of B and NK lymphocytes, progressive bone marrow failure, microcephaly, in utero growth retardation, and gastrointestinal disease. The disease can be X-linked or, more rarely, autosomal recessive. It is caused by the mutation of genes encoding telomere maintenance proteins, including dyskerin (DKC1).

Finally, the *immunodeficiency with centromeric and facial anomalies* (ICF) is a complex syndrome of autosomal recessive inheritance that variably combines a mild T cell immune deficiency with a more severe B cell immune deficiency, coarse face, digestive disease, and mild mental retardation. A diagnostic feature is the detection by cytogenetic analysis of multiradial aspects in multiple chromosomes (most frequently 1, 9, and 16) corresponding to an abnormal DNA structure secondary to defective DNA methylation. It is the consequence of a deficiency in the DNA methyltransferase DNMT3B.

T cell primary immunodeficiencies with hyper-IgE

Several T cell PIDs are associated with elevated serum IgE levels (as in Omenn syndrome). A condition sometimes referred to as *autosomal recessive hyper-IgE syndrome* is notably characterized by recurrent bacterial infections in the skin and respiratory tract and severe skin and mucosal infections by pox viruses and human papillomaviruses, together with severe allergic manifestations. T and B lymphocyte counts are low. Mutations in the *DOCK8* gene have been found in a subset of these patients.

A very rare, related condition with autosomal recessive inheritance that causes a similar susceptibility to infection with various microbes (see above), including mycobacteria, reportedly results from a deficiency in Tyk-2, a JAK family kinase involved in the signaling of many different cytokine receptors.

Autosomal dominant hyper-IgE syndrome (HIES)

This unique condition, the *autosomal dominant hyper-IgE syndrome*, is usually diagnosed by the combination of recurrent skin and lung infections that can be complicated by pneumatoceles. Infections are caused by pyogenic bacteria and fungi. Several other manifestations characterize HIES, including facial dysmorphy, defective loss of primary teeth, hyperextensibility, scoliosis, and osteoporosis. Elevated serum IgE levels are typical of this syndrome. Recently, defective TH17 effector responses have been shown to account at least in part for the specific patterns of susceptibility to particular microbes. This condition is caused by a heterozygous (dominant) mutation in the gene encoding the transcription factor STAT3 that is required in a number of signaling pathways following binding of cytokine to cytokine receptors (such as that of IL-6 and the IL-6 receptor).

Cartilage hair hypoplasia

The autosomal recessive *cartilage hair hypoplasia* (CHH) disease is characterized by short-limb dwarfism, metaphyseal dysostosis, and sparse hair, together with a combined T and B cell PID of extremely variable intensity (ranging from quasi-SCID to no clinically significant immune defects). The condition can predispose to erythroblastopenia, autoimmunity, and tumors. It is caused by mutations in the *RMRP* gene for a noncoding ribosome-associated RNA.

CD40 ligand and CD40 deficiencies

Hyper-IgM syndrome (HIGM) is a well-known PID that is usually classified as a B cell immune deficiency (see Fig. 316-4 and below). It results from defective immunoglobulin class switch recombination (CSR) in germinal centers and leads to profound deficiency in production of IgG, IgA, and IgE (although IgM production is maintained). Approximately half of HIGM sufferers are also prone to opportunistic infections, e.g., interstitial pneumonitis caused by *Pneumocystis jiroveci* (in young children), protracted diarrhea and cholangitis caused by *Cryptosporidium*, and infection of the brain with *Toxoplasma gondii*.

In the majority of cases, this condition has an X-linked inheritance and is caused by a deficiency in CD40 ligand (L). CD40L induces signaling events in B cells that are necessary for both CSR and adequate activation of other CD40-expressing cells that are involved in innate immune responses against the above-mentioned microorganisms. More rarely, the condition is caused by a deficiency in CD40 itself. The poorer prognosis of CD40L and CD40 deficiencies (relative to most other HIGM conditions) implies that (1) thorough investigations have to be performed in all cases of HIGM and (2) potentially curative HSCT should be discussed on a case-by-case basis for this group of patients.

Wiskott-Aldrich syndrome

Wiskott-Aldrich syndrome (WAS) is a complex, recessive, X-linked disease with an incidence of approximately 1 in 200,000 live births. It is caused by mutations in the *WASP* gene that affect not only T lymphocytes but also the other lymphocyte subsets, dendritic cells, and platelets. WAS is typically characterized by the following clinical manifestations: recurrent bacterial infections, eczema, and

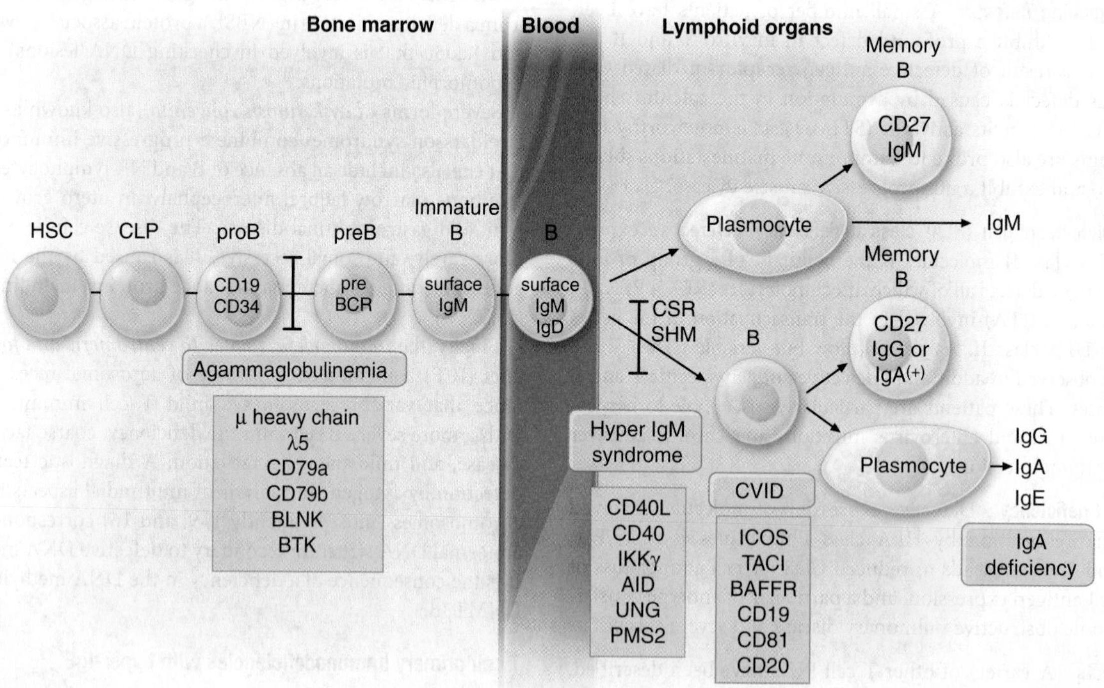

Figure 316-4 B cell differentiation and related primary immunodeficiencies (PIDs). Hematopoietic stem cells (HSCs) differentiate into common lymphoid progenitors (CLPs), which give rise to pre-B cells. The B cell differentiation pathway goes through the pre–B cell stage (expression of the μ heavy chain and surrogate light chain), the immature B cell stage (expression of surface IgM), and the mature B cell stage (expression of surface IgM and IgD). The main phenotypic characteristics of these cells are indicated. In lymphoid organs, B cells can differentiate into plasma cells and produce IgM or undergo (in germinal centers) Ig class switch recombination (CSR) and somatic mutation of the variable region of V genes (SHM) that enable selection of high-affinity antibodies. These B cells produce antibodies of various isotypes and generate memory B cells. PIDs are indicated in the purple boxes. CVID: common variable immunodeficiency.

bleeding caused by thrombocytopenia. However, these manifestations are highly variable—mostly as a consequence of the many different *WASP* mutations that have been observed. Null mutations predispose affected individuals to invasive and bronchopulmonary infections, viral infections, severe eczema, and autoimmune manifestations. The latter include autoantibody-mediated blood cytopenia, glomerulonephritis, skin and visceral vasculitis (including brain vasculitis), erythema nodosum, and arthritis. Another possible consequence of WAS is lymphoma, which may be virally induced (e.g., by EBV or Kaposi's sarcoma–associated herpesvirus). Thrombocytopenia can be severe and compounded by the peripheral destruction of platelets associated with autoimmune disorders. Hypomorphic mutations usually lead to milder outcomes that are generally limited to thrombocytopenia. It is noteworthy that even patients with "isolated" X-linked thrombocytopenia can develop severe autoimmune disease or lymphoma later in life. The immunologic workup is not very informative; there can be a relative CD8+ T cell deficiency, frequently accompanied by low serum IgM levels and decreased antigen-specific antibody responses. A typical feature is reduced-sized platelets on a blood smear. Diagnosis is based on intracellular immunofluorescence analysis of WAS protein (WASp) expression in blood cells. WASp regulates the actin cytoskeleton and thus plays an important role in many lymphocyte functions, including cell adhesion and migration and the formation of synapses between antigen-presenting and target cells. Predisposition to autoimmune disorders may (at least in part) be related to defective regulatory T cells. The treatment of WAS should match the severity of disease expression. Prophylactic antibiotics, immunoglobulin G (IgG) supplementation, and careful topical treatment of eczema are indicated. Although splenectomy improves platelet count in a majority of cases, this intervention is associated with a significant risk of infection (both pre- and post-HSCT). Allogeneic HSCT is curative, with fairly good results overall. Gene therapy trials are also under way.

A few other complex PIDs are worth mentioning. *Sp110 deficiency* causes a T cell PID with liver venoocclusive disease and hypogammaglobulinemia. *Chronic mucocutaneous candidiasis* (CMC) is probably a heterogeneous disease, considering the different inheritance patterns that have been observed. In some cases, chronic candidiasis is associated with late-onset bronchopulmonary infections, bronchiectasis, and brain aneurysms. Moderate forms of CMC are related to autoimmunity and AIRE deficiency (see below). In this setting, predisposition to candida infection is associated with the detection of autoantibodies to TH17 cytokines. Recently, innate immunodeficiencies (CARD9 and possibly Dectin-1) have been found in a few families with CMC.

■ B LYMPHOCYTE DEFICIENCIES (TABLE 316-1, FIG. 316-4)

Deficiencies that predominantly affect B lymphocytes are the most frequent PIDs and account for 60–70% of all cases. B lymphocytes make antibodies. Pentameric IgMs are found in the vascular compartment and are also secreted at mucosal surfaces. IgG antibodies diffuse freely into extravascular spaces, whereas IgA antibodies are produced and secreted predominantly from mucosa-associated lymphoid tissues. Although Ig isotypes have distinct effector functions, including Fc receptor–mediated and (indirectly) C_3 receptor–dependent phagocytosis of microorganisms, they share the ability to recognize and neutralize a given pathogen. Defective antibody production therefore allows the establishment of invasive, pyogenic bacterial infections as well as recurrent sinus and pulmonary infections (mostly caused by *Streptococcus pneumoniae, Haemophilus influenzae, Moraxella catarrhalis*, and, less frequently, by gram-negative bacteria). If left untreated, recurrent bronchial infections lead to bronchiectasis and, ultimately, cor pulmonale and death. Parasitic infections such as caused by *Giardia lambliasis* as well as bacterial infections caused by *Helicobacter and Campylobacter* of the gut are also observed. A complete lack of antibody production (namely agammaglobulinemia) can also predispose affected individuals to severe, chronic, disseminated enteroviral infections causing meningoencephalitis, hepatitis, and a dermatomyositis-like disease.

Even with the most profound of B cell deficiencies, infections rarely occur before the age of 6 months; this is because of transient protection provided by the transplacental passage of immunoglobulins during the last trimester of pregnancy. Conversely, a genetically nonimmunodeficient child born to a mother with hypogammaglobulinemia is, in the absence of maternal Ig substitution, usually prone to severe bacterial infections in utero and for several months after birth.

Diagnosis of B cell PIDs relies on the determination of serum Ig levels (Table 316-2). Determination of antibody production following immunization with tetanus toxoid vaccine or nonconjugated pneumococcal polysaccharide antigens can also help diagnose more subtle deficiencies. Another useful test is B cell phenotype determination in switched μ–S– CD27+ and nonswitched memory B cells (μ+S+ CD27+). In agammaglobulinemic patients, examination of bone marrow B cell precursors (Fig. 316-4) can help obtain a precise diagnosis and guide the choice of genetic tests.

Agammaglobulinemia

Agammaglobulinemia is characterized by a profound defect in B cell development (<1% of the normal B cell blood count). In most patients, very low residual Ig isotypes can be detected in the serum. In 85% of cases, agammaglobulinemia is caused by a mutation in the *BTK* gene that is located on the X-chromosome. The *BTK* gene product is a kinase that participates in (pre) B cell receptor signaling. When the kinase is defective, there is a block (albeit a leaky one) at the pre-B to B cell stage (Fig. 316-4). Detection of *BTK* by intracellular immunofluorescence of monocytes, and lack thereof in patients with X-linked agammaglobulinemia, is a useful diagnostic test. Not all of the mutations in *BTK* result in agammaglobulinemia, since some patients have a milder form of hypogammaglobulinemia and low but detectable B cell counts. These cases should not be confused with common variable immunodeficiency (CVID, see below). About 10% of agammaglobulinemia cases are caused by alterations in genes encoding elements of the pre-B cell receptor, i.e., the μ heavy chain, the λ5 surrogate light chain, Igα or Igβ, and the scaffold protein BLNK. In 5% of cases, the defect is unknown. It is noteworthy that agammaglobulinemia can be observed in patients with ICF syndrome, despite the presence of normal peripheral B cell counts. Lastly, agammaglobulinemia can be a manifestation of a myelodysplastic syndrome (associated or not with neutropenia). Treatment of agammaglobulinemic patients is based on immunoglobulin replacement (see below). Profound hypogammaglobulinemia is also observed in adults, in association with thymoma.

Hyper-IgM (HIGM) syndromes

Hyper-IgM syndrome is a rare B cell PID characterized by defective Ig CSR. It results in very low serum levels of IgG and IgA and elevated or normal serum IgM levels. The clinical severity is similar to that seen in agammaglobulinemia, although chronic lung disease and sinusitis are less frequent and enteroviral infections are uncommon. As discussed above, a diagnosis of HIGM involves screening for an X-linked CD40L deficiency and an autosomal recessive CD40 deficiency, which affect both B and T cells. In 50% of cases affecting only B cells, these isolated HIGM syndromes result from mutations in the gene encoding activation-induced deaminase, the protein that induces CSR in B cell germinal centers. These patients usually have enlarged lymphoid organs. In the other 50% of cases, the etiology is unknown (except for rare UNG and PMS2 deficiencies). Furthermore, IgM-mediated autoimmunity and lymphomas can occur in HIGM syndrome. It is noteworthy that HIGM can result from fetal rubella syndrome or can be a predominant immunologic feature of other PIDs, such as the immunodeficiency associated with ectodermic anhydrotic hypoplasia X-linked NEMO deficiency and the combined T and B cell PIDs caused by DNA repair defects such as ataxia-telangectasia and Cernunnos deficiency.

Common variable immunodeficiency (CVID)

CVID is an ill-defined condition characterized by low serum levels of one or more Ig isotypes. Its prevalence is estimated to be 1 in 20,000. The condition is recognized predominantly in adults, although clinical manifestations can occur earlier in life. Hypogammaglobulinemia is associated with at least partially defective antibody production in response to vaccine antigens. B lymphocyte counts are often normal but can be low. Besides infections, CVID patients may develop lymphoproliferation (splenomegaly), granulomatous lesions, colitis, antibody-mediated autoimmune disease, and lymphomas. A family history is found in 10% of cases. A clear-cut dominant inheritance pattern is found in some families, whereas recessive inheritance is observed more rarely. In most cases, no molecular cause can be identified. A small number of patients in Germany were found to carry mutations in the *ICOS* gene encoding a T cell-membrane protein that contributes to B cell activation and survival. In 10% of patients with CVID, monoallelic or biallelic mutations of the gene encoding TACI (a member of the TNF receptor family that is expressed on B cells) have been found. In fact, heterozygous TACI mutations correspond to a genetic susceptibility factor, since similar heterozygous mutations are found in 1% of controls. The BAFF receptor was found to be defective in a kindred with CVID, although not all individuals carrying the mutation have CVID.

A diagnosis of CVID should be made after excluding the presence of hypomorphic mutations associated with agammaglobulinemia or more subtle T cell defects; this is particularly the case in children. It is possible that many cases of CVID result from a constellation of factors, rather than a single genetic defect. Recently, rare cases of hypogammaglobulinemia were found to be associated with CD19 and CD81 deficiencies. These patients have B cells that can be identified by typing for other B cell markers.

Selective Ig isotype deficiencies

IgA deficiency and CVID represent polar ends of a clinical spectrum due to the same underlying gene defect(s) in a large subset of these patients. IgA deficiency is the most common PID; it can be found in 1 in every 600 individuals. It is asymptomatic in most cases; however, individuals may present with increased numbers of acute and chronic respiratory infections that may lead to bronchiectasis. In addition, over their lifetime, these patients experience an increased susceptibility to drug allergies, atopic disorders, and autoimmune diseases. Symptomatic IgA deficiency is probably related to CVID, since it can be found in relatives of patients with CVID. Furthermore, IgA deficiency may progress to CVID. It is thus important to assess serum Ig levels in IgA-deficient patients (especially when infections occur frequently) in order to detect changes that should prompt the initiation of immunoglobulin replacement. Selective IgG2 (+G4) deficiency (which in some cases may be associated with IgA deficiency) can also result in recurrent sinopulmonary infections and should thus be specifically sought in this clinical setting. These conditions are ill-defined and a pathophysiologic explanation has not been found.

Selective antibody deficiency to polysaccharide antigens

Some patients with normal serum Ig levels are prone to *S. pneumoniae* and *H. influenzae* infections of the respiratory tract. Defective production of antibodies against polysaccharide antigens (such as those in the *S. pneumoniae* cell wall) can be observed and is probably causative. This condition may correspond to a defect in marginal zone B cells, a B cell subpopulation involved in T-independent antibody responses.

Immunoglobulin replacement

IgG antibodies have a half-life of 21–28 days. Thus, injection of plasma-derived polyclonal IgG containing a myriad of high-affinity antibodies can provide protection against disease-causing microorganisms in patients with defective IgG antibody production. This form of therapy should not be based on laboratory data alone (i.e., IgG and/or antibody deficiency) but should be guided by the occurrence or not of infections; otherwise, patients might be subjected to unjustified IgG infusions. Immunoglobulin replacement can be performed by IV or subcutaneous routes. In the former case, injections have to be repeated every 3–4 weeks, with a residual target level of 800 mg/mL in patients who had very low IgG levels prior to therapy. Subcutaneous injections are typically performed once a week, although the frequency can be adjusted on a case-by-case basis. A trough level of 800 mg/mL is desirable. Whatever the mode of administration, the main goal is to reduce the frequency of the respiratory tract infections and prevent chronic lung and sinus disease. The two routes appear to be equally safe and efficacious and so the choice should be left to the preference of the patient.

In patients with chronic lung disease, chest physical therapy with good pulmonary toilet and the cyclic use of antibiotics are also needed. Immunoglobulin replacement is well tolerated by most patients, although the selection of the best-tolerated Ig preparation may be necessary in certain cases. Since IgG preparations contain a small proportion of IgAs, caution should be taken in patients with residual antibody production capacity and a complete IgA deficiency, as these subjects may develop anti-IgA antibodies that can trigger anaphylactic shock. These patients should be treated with IgA-free IgG preparations. Immunoglobulin replacement is a lifelong therapy; its rationale and procedures have to be fully understood and mastered by the patient and his or her family, in order to guarantee the strict observance required for efficacy.

PRIMARY IMMUNODEFICIENCIES AFFECTING REGULATORY PATHWAYS (TABLE 316-1)

An increasing number of PIDs have been found to cause homeostatic dysregulation of the immune system, either alone or in association with increased vulnerability to infections. Defects of this type affecting the innate immune system and autoinflammatory syndromes will not be covered in this chapter. However, three specific entities (hemophagocytic lymphohistiocytosis, lymphoproliferation, and autoimmunity) will be described below.

■ HEMOPHAGOCYTIC LYMPHOHISTIOCYTOSIS

Hemophagocytic lymphohistiocytosis (HLH) is characterized by an unremitting activation of CD8+ T lymphocytes and macrophages that leads to organ damage (notably in the liver, bone marrow, and central nervous system). This syndrome results from a broad set of inherited diseases, all of which impair T and NK lymphocyte cytotoxicity. The manifestations of HLH are often induced by a viral infection. EBV is the most frequent trigger. In severe forms of HLH, disease onset may start during the first year of life or even (in rare cases) at birth.

Diagnosis relies on the identification of the characteristic symptoms of HLH (fever, hepatosplenomegay, edema, neurologic diseases, blood cytopenia, increased liver enzymes, hypofibrinogenemia, high triglyceride levels, elevated markers of T cell activation, and hemophagocytic features in the bone marrow or cerebrospinal fluid). Functional assays of postactivation cytotoxic granule exocytosis (CD107 fluorescence at the cell membrane) can suggest genetically determined HLH. The conditions can be classified into three subsets:

1. Familial HLH with autosomal recessive inheritance, including perforin deficiency (30% of cases) that can be recognized by assessing intracellular perforin expression; Munc13-4 deficiency (30% of cases); syntaxin 11 deficiency (10% of cases); Munc18-2 deficiency (20% of cases); and a few residual cases that lack a known molecular defect.
2. HLH with partial albinism. Three conditions combine HLH and abnormal pigmentation, where hair examination can help in the diagnosis: Chediak-Higashi syndrome, Griscelli syndrome, and Hermansky Pudlak syndrome type II. Chediak-Higashi syndrome is also characterized by the presence of giant lysosomes within leukocytes (Chap. 60), in addition to a primary neurologic disorder with slow progression of symptoms over time.
3. X-linked proliferative syndrome (XLP) is characterized in most patients by the induction of HLH following EBV infection, while other patients develop progressive hypogammaglobulinemia similar to what is observed in CVID and/or certain lymphomas. XLP is caused by a mutation in the *SH2DIA* gene that encodes the adaptor protein SAP (associated with a SLAM family receptor). Several immunologic abnormalities have been described, including low 2B4-mediated NK cell cytotoxicity, impaired differentiation of NKT cells, defective antigen-induced T cell death, and defective T cell helper activity for B cells. A related disorder (XLP2) has recently been described. It is also X-linked and induces HLH (frequently after EBV infection), although the clinical manifestation may be less pronounced. The condition is associated with a deficiency of the antiapoptotic molecule XIAP. The pathophysiology of XLP2 and its relationship to XLP1 remain unclear.

HLH is a life-threatening complication. The treatment of this condition requires aggressive immunosuppression with either the cytotoxic agent VP-16 or anti-T cell antibodies. Once remission has been achieved, HSCT should be performed, since it provides the only curative form of therapy.

AUTOIMMUNE LYMPHOPROLIFERATIVE SYNDROME

Autoimmune lymphoproliferative syndrome (ALPS) is characterized by nonmalignant T and B lymphoproliferation causing splenomegaly and enlarged lymph nodes; 70% of patients also display autoimmune manifestations such as autoimmune cytopenias, Guillain-Barré syndrome, uveitis, and hepatitis (Chaps. 59 and 314). A hallmark of ALPS is the presence of CD4 -CD8- TCRαβ+ T cells (2–50%) in the blood of affected individuals. Hypergammaglobulinemia involving IgG and IgA is also frequently observed. The syndrome is caused by a defect in Fas-mediated apoptosis of lymphocytes, which can thus accumulate and mediate autoimmunity. Furthermore, ALPS can lead to malignancies.

Most patients carry a heterozygous mutation in the gene encoding Fas that is characterized by dominant inheritance and variable penetrance, depending on the nature of the mutation. A rare and severe form of the disease with early onset can be observed in patients carrying a biallelic mutation of Fas, which profoundly impairs the protein's expression and/or function. Fas-ligand, caspase 10, caspase 8, and neuroblastoma RAS viral oncogene homologue (NRAS) mutations have also been reported in a few cases of ALPS. Many cases of ALPS have not been precisely delineated at the molecular level. Treatment of ALPS is essentially based on the use of proapoptotic drugs, which need to be carefully administered in order to avoid toxicity.

COLITIS, AUTOIMMUNITY, AND PRIMARY IMMUNODEFICIENCIES

Several PIDs (most of which are T cell-related) can cause severe gut inflammation. The prototypic example is *immunodysregulation polyendocrinopathy enteropathy X-linked syndrome* (IPEX), characterized by a widespread inflammatory enteropathy, food intolerance, skin rashes, autoimmune cytopenias, and diabetes. The syndrome is caused by loss-of-function mutations in the gene encoding the transcription factor FOXP3, which is required for the acquisition of effector function by regulatory T cells. In most cases of IPEX, CD4+CD25+ regulatory T cells are absent from the blood. This condition has a poor prognosis and requires aggressive immunosuppression. The only possible curative approach is allogeneic HSCT. IPEX-like syndromes that lack a FOXP3 mutation have also been described. In some cases, a CD25 deficiency has been found. Defective CD25 expression also impairs regulatory cell expansion/function. This functional T cell deficiency means that CD25-deficient patients are also at increased risk of opportunistic infections. It is noteworthy that abnormalities in regulatory T cells have been described in other PID settings, such as in Omenn syndrome, STAT5b deficiency, STIM1 (Ca flux) deficiency, and WAS; these abnormalities may account (at least in part) for the occurrence of inflammation and autoimmunity. The autoimmune features observed in a small fraction of patients with DiGeorge syndrome may have the same cause. Recently, severe inflammatory gut disease has been described in patients with a deficiency in the IL-10 receptor.

A distinct autoimmune entity is observed in *autoimmune polyendocrinopathy candidiasis ectodermal dysplasia* (APECED) syndrome, which is characterized by autosomal recessive inheritance. It consists of multiple autoimmune manifestations that can affect solid organs in general and endocrine glands in particular. Mild, chronic *Candida* infection is often associated with this syndrome. The condition is due to mutations in the autoimmune regulator (AIRE) gene and results in impaired thymic expression of self-antigens by medullary epithelial cells and impaired negative selection of self-reactive T cells that leads to autoimmune manifestations.

CONCLUSION

The variety and complexity of the clinical manifestations of the many different PIDs strongly indicate that it is important to raise awareness of these diseases. Indeed, early diagnosis is essential for establishing an appropriate therapeutic regimen. Hence, patients with suspected PIDs must always be referred to experienced clinical centers that are able to perform appropriate molecular and genetic tests. A precise molecular diagnosis is not only necessary for initiating the most suitable treatment but it is also important for genetic counseling and prenatal diagnosis.

One pitfall that may hamper diagnosis is the high variability that is associated with many PIDs. Variable disease expression can result from the differing consequences of various mutations associated with a given condition, as exemplified by WAS and, to a lesser extent, X-linked agammaglobulinemia (XLA). There can also be effects of modifier genes (as also suspected in XLA) and environmental factors such as EBV infection that can be the main trigger of disease in X-linked lymphoproliferative (XLP) conditions. Furthermore, it has recently been established that somatic mutations in an affected gene can attenuate the phenotype of a number of T cell PIDs. This has been described for ADA deficiency, X-linked SCID, RAG deficiencies, NF-κB essential modulator (NEMO) deficiency, and, most frequently, in WAS. In contrast, somatic mutations can create disease states analogous to PID, as reported for ALPS. Lastly, cytokine-neutralizing autoantibodies can mimic a PID, as shown for interferon γ.

Many aspects of the pathophysiology of PIDs are still unknown, and the disease-causing gene mutations have not been identified in all cases (as illustrated by CVID and IgA deficiency). However, our medical understanding of PIDs has now reached the stage where scientifically based approaches to the diagnosis and treatment of these diseases can be implemented.

FURTHER READINGS

Boztug K, Klein C: Novel genetic etiologies of severe congenital neutropenia. Curr Opin Immunol 21:472, 2009

Browne SK, Holland SM: Anticytokine autoantibodies in infectious diseases: Pathogenesis and mechanisms. Lancet Infect Dis 10:875, 2010

Fischer A: Human primary immunodeficiency diseases. Immunity 27:835, 2007

Nelson KS, Lewis DB: Adult-onset presentations of genetic immunodeficiencies: Genes can throw slow curves. Curr Opin Infect Dis 23:359, 2010

Notarangelo LD, et al: Primary immunodeficiencies: 2009 update. J Allergy Clin Immunol 124:1161, 2009

Ochs HD et al: *Primary Immunodeficiency Diseases. A Molecular and Genetic Approach*. New York, Oxford University Press, 1999

Seger RA: Modern management of chronic granulomatous disease. Br J Haematol 140:255, 2008

Stiehm ER et al: *Immunologic Disorders in Infants and Children*. Philadelphia, Elsevier Saunders, 2004

Wood P et al: Recognition, clinical diagnosis and management of patients with primary antibody deficiencies: A systematic review. Clin Exp Immunol 149:410, 2007

CHAPTER 317

Allergies, Anaphylaxis, and Systemic Mastocytosis

K. Frank Austen

The term *atopic allergy* implies a familial tendency to manifest such conditions as asthma, rhinitis, urticaria, and eczematous dermatitis (atopic dermatitis) alone or in combination, and in association with the presence of IgE. However, individuals without an atopic background may also develop hypersensitivity reactions, particularly urticaria and anaphylaxis, associated with the presence of IgE. Inasmuch as the mast cell is the key effector cell of the biologic response in allergic rhinitis, urticaria, anaphylaxis, and systemic mastocytosis, its developmental biology, activation pathway, product profile, and target tissues will be considered in the introduction to these clinical disorders.

The binding of IgE to human mast cells and basophils, a process termed *sensitization*, prepares these cells for subsequent antigen-specific activation. The sensitization of the high-affinity Fc receptor for IgE, designated FcεRI, also stabilizes the cellular expression of the receptor. FcεRI is composed of one α, one β, and two disulfide-linked γ chains, which together cross the plasma membrane seven times. The α chain is responsible for IgE binding, and the β and γ chains provide for signal transduction that follows the aggregation of the sensitized tetrameric receptors by polymeric antigen. Signal transduction is initiated through the action of an Src family–related tyrosine kinase, termed *Lyn*, that is constitutively associated with the β chain. Lyn transphosphorylates the canonical immunoreceptor tyrosine-based activation motifs (ITAMs) of the β and γ chains of the receptor, resulting in recruitment of more active Lyn to the β chain and of Syk tyrosine kinase. The phosphorylated tyrosines in the ITAMs function as binding sites for the tandem *src* homology two (SH2) domains within Syk. Syk activates not only phospholipase Cγ, which associates with the Linker of Activated T Cells at the plasma membrane, but also phosphatidylinositol 3-kinase to provide phosphatidylinositol-3,4,5-trisphosphate, which allows membrane targeting of the Tec family kinase Btk and its activation by Lyn. In addition, the Src family tyrosine kinase Fyn becomes activated after aggregation of IgE receptors and phosphorylates the adapter protein Gab2 that enhances activation of phosphatidylinositol 3-kinase. Indeed, this additional input is essential for mast cell activation, but it can be partially inhibited by Lyn, indicating that the extent of mast cell activation is in part regulated by the interplay between these Src family kinases. Activated phospholipase Cγ cleaves phospholipid membrane substrates to provide inositol-1,4,5-trisphosphate (IP_3) and 1,2-diacylglycerols (1,2-DAGs) so as to mobilize intracellular calcium and activate protein kinase C, respectively. The subsequent opening of calcium-regulated activated channels provides the sustained elevations of intracellular calcium required to recruit the mitogen-activated protein kinases, ERK, JNK, and p38 (serine/threonine kinases), which provide cascades to augment arachidonic acid release and to mediate nuclear translocation of transcription factors for various cytokines. The calcium ion–dependent activation of phospholipases cleaves membrane phospholipids to generate lysophospholipids, which, like 1,2-DAG, may facilitate the fusion of the secretory granule perigranular membrane with the cell membrane, a step that releases the membrane-free granules containing the preformed mediators of mast cell effects.

The secretory granule of the human mast cell has a crystalline structure, unlike mast cells of lower species. IgE-dependent cell activation results in solubilization and swelling of the granule contents within the first minute of receptor perturbation; this reaction is followed by the ordering of intermediate filaments about the swollen granule, movement of the granule toward the cell surface, and fusion of the perigranular membrane with that of other granules and with the plasmalemma to form extracellular channels for mediator release while maintaining cell viability.

In addition to exocytosis, aggregation of FcεRI initiates two other pathways for generation of bioactive products, namely, lipid mediators and cytokines. The biochemical steps involved in expression of such cytokines as tumor necrosis factor α (TNF-α), interleukin (IL) 1, IL-6, IL-4, IL-5, IL-13, granulocyte-macrophage colony-stimulating factor (GM-CSF), and others, including an array of chemokines, have not been specifically defined for mast cells. Inhibition studies of cytokine production (IL-1β, TNF-α, and IL-6) in mouse mast cells with cyclosporine or FK506 reveal binding to the ligand-specific immunophilin and attenuation of the calcium ion- and calmodulin-dependent serine/threonine phosphatase, calcineurin.

Lipid mediator generation (Fig. 317-1) involves translocation of calcium ion–dependent cytosolic phospholipase A_2 to the outer nuclear membrane, with subsequent release of arachidonic acid for metabolic processing by the distinct prostanoid and leukotriene pathways. The constitutive prostaglandin endoperoxide synthase-1 (PGHS-1/cyclooxygenase-1) and the de novo inducible PGHS-2 (cyclooxygenase-2) convert released arachidonic acid to the sequential intermediates, prostaglandins G_2 and H_2. The glutathione-dependent hematopoietic prostaglandin D_2 (PGD_2) synthase then converts PGH_2 to PGD_2, the predominant mast cell prostanoid. The PGD_2 receptors, DP_1 and DP_2, are distributed to smooth muscle as well as to T_H2 lymphocytes, eosinophils, and basophils implicated in allergic inflammation.

For the leukotriene biosynthetic pathway, the released arachidonic acid is metabolized by 5-lipoxygenase (5-LO) in the presence of an integral nuclear membrane protein, the 5-LO activating protein (FLAP). The calcium ion–dependent translocation of 5-LO to the nuclear membrane converts the arachidonic acid to the sequential intermediates, 5-hydroperoxyeicosatetraenoic acid (5-HPETE) and leukotriene (LT) A_4. LTA_4 is conjugated with reduced glutathione by LTC_4 synthase, an integral nuclear membrane protein homologous to FLAP. Intracellular LTC_4 is released by a carrier-specific export step for extracellular metabolism to the additional cysteinyl leukotrienes, LTD_4 and LTE_4, by the sequential removal of glutamic acid and glycine. Alternatively, cytosolic LTA_4 hydrolase converts some LTA_4 to the dihydroxy leukotriene LTB_4, which also undergoes specific export. Two receptors for LTB_4, BLT_1 and BLT_2, mediate chemotaxis

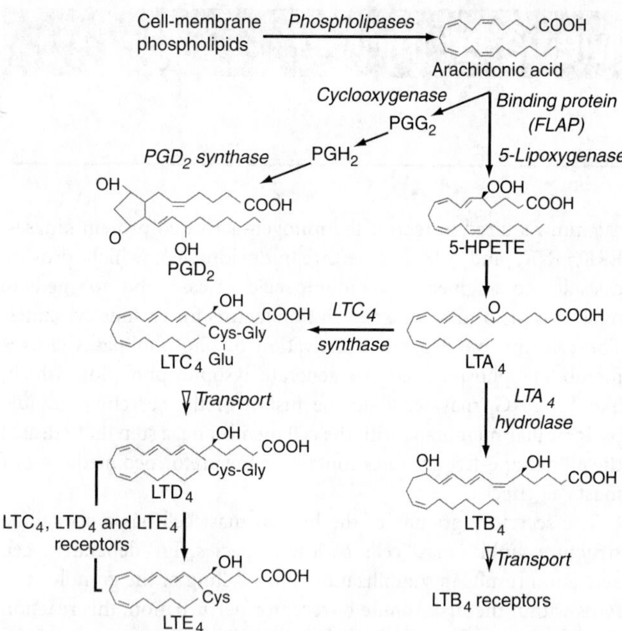

Figure 317-1 Pathways for biosynthesis and release of membrane-derived lipid mediators from mast cells. In the 5-lipoxygenase pathway leukotriene A_4 (LTA_4) is the intermediate from which the terminal-pathway enzymes generate the distinct final products, leukotriene C_4 (LTC_4) and leukotriene B_4 (LTB_4), which leave the cell by separate saturable transport systems. Gamma glutamyl transpeptidase and a dipeptidase then cleave glutamic acid and glycine from LTC_4 to form LTD_4 and LTE_4, respectively. The major mast cell product of the cyclooxygenase system is PGD_2.

of human neutrophils. Two receptors for the cysteinyl leukotrienes, $CysLT_1$ and $CysLT_2$, are present on smooth muscle of the airways and the microvasculature and on hematopoietic cells such as macrophages, eosinophils, and mast cells. Whereas the $CysLT_1$ receptor has a preference for LTD_4 and is blocked by the receptor antagonists in clinical use, the $CysLT_2$ receptor is equally responsive to LTD_4 and LTC_4, is unaffected by these antagonists, and is a negative regulator of the function of the $CysLT_1$ receptor. The lysophospholipid formed during the release of arachidonic acid from 1-*O*-alkyl-2-acyl-*sn*-glyceryl-3-phosphorylcholine can be acetylated in the second position to form platelet-activating factor (PAF).

Unlike most other cells of bone marrow origin, mast cells leave the marrow and circulate as committed progenitors lacking their definitive secretory granules and characteristic FcεRI. These committed progenitors express the receptor, c-*kit*, for stem cell factor (SCF), and unlike other lineages, they retain and increase its expression with maturation. The SCF interaction with c-*kit* is an absolute requirement for the development of constitutive tissue mast cells residing in skin and connective tissue sites and for the T_H2 cell–dependent comitogenesis providing mast cells to mucosal surfaces. Indeed, in clinical T cell deficiencies, mast cells are absent from the intestinal mucosa but are present in the submucosa. Based on the immunodetection of secretory granule neutral proteases, mast cells in the lung parenchyma and intestinal mucosa selectively express tryptase, and those in the intestinal and airway submucosa, skin, lymph nodes, and breast parenchyma express tryptase, chymase, and carboxypeptidase A (CPA). The secretory granules of mast cells selectively positive for tryptase exhibit closed scrolls with a periodicity suggestive of a crystalline structure by electron microscopy; whereas the secretory granules of mast cells with multiple proteases are scroll-poor, with an amorphous or lattice-like appearance.

Mast cells are distributed at cutaneous and mucosal surfaces and in submucosal tissues about venules and could influence the entry of foreign substances by their rapid response capability (Fig. 317-2). Upon stimulus-specific activation and secretory granule exocytosis, histamine and acid hydrolases are solubilized, whereas the neutral proteases, which are cationic, remain largely bound to the anionic proteoglycans, heparin and chrondroitin sulfate E, with which they function as a complex. Histamine and the various lipid mediators (PGD_2, $LTC_4/D_4/E_4$, PAF) alter venular permeability, thereby allowing influx of plasma proteins such as complement and immunoglobulins, whereas LTB_4 mediates leukocyte–endothelial cell adhesion and subsequent directed migration (chemotaxis). The accumulation of leukocytes and plasma opsonins would facilitate defense of the microenvironment. The inflammatory response can also be detrimental, as in bronchial asthma, where the smooth-muscle constrictor activity of the cysteinyl leukotrienes is evident and much more potent than that of histamine.

The cellular component of the mast cell–mediated inflammatory response would be augmented and sustained by cytokines and chemokines of mast cell origin. IgE-dependent activation of human skin mast cells in situ elicits TNF-α production and release, which in turn induces endothelial cell responses favoring leukocyte adhesion. Similarly, activation of purified human lung mast cells or cord blood–derived cultured mast cells in vitro results in substantial production of proinflammatory (TNF-α) and immunomodulatory cytokines (IL-4, IL-5, IL-13) and chemokines. Bronchial biopsy specimens from patients with bronchial asthma reveal that mast cells are immunohistochemically positive for IL-4 and IL-5, but that the predominant localization of IL-4, IL-5, and GM-CSF is to T cells, defined as T_H2 by this profile. IL-4 modulates the T cell phenotype to the T_H2 subtype, determines the isotype switch to IgE (as does IL-13), and upregulates FcεRI-mediated expression of cytokines by mast cells.

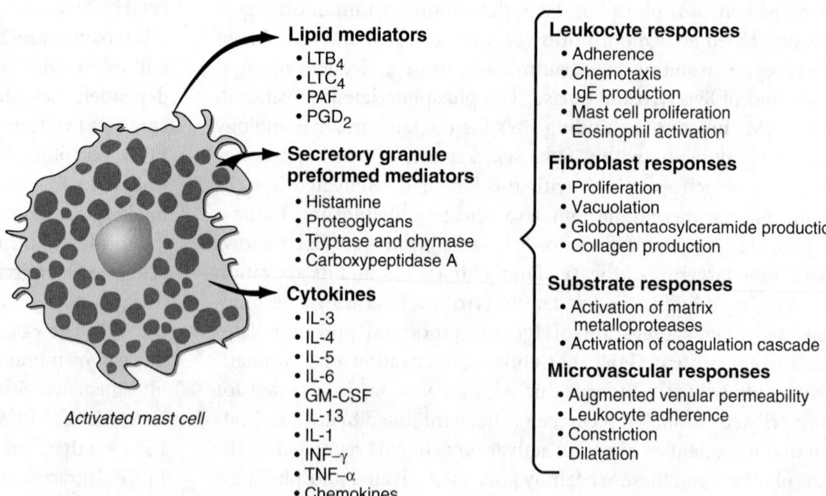

Figure 317-2 Bioactive mediators of three categories generated by IgE-dependent activation of murine mast cells can elicit common but sequential target cell effects leading to acute and sustained inflammatory responses. LT, leukotriene; PAF, platelet-activating factor; PGD_2, prostaglandin D_2; IL, interleukin; GM-CSF, granulocyte-macrophage colony-stimulating factor; INF, interferon; TNF, tumor necrosis factor.

An immediate and late cellular phase of allergic inflammation can be induced in the skin, nose, or lung of some allergic humans with local allergen challenge. In the immediate phase of a local challenge, there is pruritus and watery discharge from the nose, bronchospasm and mucus secretion in the lungs, and a wheal-and-flare response with pruritus in the skin. The reduced nasal patency, reduced pulmonary function, or evident erythema with swelling at the skin site in a late-phase response at 6–8 hours is associated with biopsy findings of infiltrating and activated T_H2 cells, eosinophils, basophils, and even some neutrophils. This allergic inflammation proceeding from early mast cell activation to late cellular infiltration has been used as an experimental surrogate of perennial rhinitis or bronchial asthma. However, in bronchial asthma, there is an intrinsic hyperreactivity of the airways independent of the associated inflammation.

Consideration of the mechanism of immediate-type hypersensitivity diseases in the human has focused largely on the IgE-dependent recognition of otherwise nontoxic substances. A region of chromosome 5 (5q23-31) contains genes implicated in the control of IgE levels including IL-4 and IL-13, as well as IL-3 and IL-9, which are involved in mucosal mast cell hyperplasia, and IL-5 and GM-CSF, which are central to eosinophil development and their enhanced tissue viability. Genes with linkage to the specific IgE response to particular allergens include those encoding the major histocompatibility complex (MHC) and certain chains of the T cell receptor (TCR-αδ). The complexity of atopy and the associated diseases includes susceptibility, severity, and therapeutic responses, each of which is among the separate variables modulated by both innate and adaptive immune stimuli.

The induction of allergic disease requires sensitization of a predisposed individual to a specific allergen. The greatest propensity for the development of atopic allergy occurs in childhood and early adolescence. The allergen is processed by antigen-presenting cells of the monocytic lineage located throughout the body at surfaces that contact the outside environment, such as the nose, lungs, eyes, skin, and intestine. These antigen-presenting cells present the epitope-bearing peptides via their MHC to T helper cells and their subsets. The T cell response depends both on cognate recognition and on the cytokine microenvironment provided by the antigen-presenting dendritic cells, with IL-4 directing a T_H2 subset, interferon (IFN) γ a T_H1 profile, and IL-6 with transforming growth factor β (TGFβ) a T_H17 subset. Allergens not only present antigenic epitopes via dendritic cells but also contain pattern recognition ligands that facilitate the immune response by direct initiation of cytokine generation from innate cell types such as basophils, mast cells, eosinophils, and others. The T_H2 response is associated with activation of specific B cells that can also present allergens or that transform into plasma cells for antibody production. Synthesis and release into the plasma of allergen-specific IgE results in sensitization of FcεR1-bearing cells such as mast cells and basophils, which become activated on exposure to the specific allergen. In certain diseases, including those associated with atopy, the monocyte and eosinophil populations can express a trimeric FcεR1, which lacks the β chain, and yet respond to its aggregation.

ANAPHYLAXIS

DEFINITION

The life-threatening anaphylactic response of a sensitized human appears within minutes after systemic exposure to specific antigen and is manifested by respiratory distress due to laryngeal edema and/or intense bronchospasm, often followed by vascular collapse, or by shock without antecedent respiratory difficulty. Cutaneous manifestations exemplified by pruritus and urticaria with or without angioedema are characteristic of such systemic anaphylactic reactions. Gastrointestinal manifestations include nausea, vomiting, crampy abdominal pain, and diarrhea.

PREDISPOSING FACTORS AND ETIOLOGY

There is no convincing evidence that age, sex, race, or geographic location predisposes a human to anaphylaxis except through exposure to some immunogen. According to most studies, atopy does not predispose individuals to anaphylaxis from penicillin therapy or venom of a stinging insect but is a risk factor for allergens in food or latex.

The materials capable of eliciting the systemic anaphylactic reaction in humans include the following: heterologous proteins in the form of hormones (insulin, vasopressin, parathormone); enzymes (trypsin, chymotrypsin, penicillinase, streptokinase); pollen extracts (ragweed, grass, trees); nonpollen allergen extracts (dust mites, dander of cats, dogs, horses, and laboratory animals); food (peanuts, milk, eggs, seafood, nuts, grains, beans, gelatin in capsules); monoclonal antibodies; occupation-related products (latex rubber products); Hymenoptera venom (yellow jacket, yellow and baldfaced hornets, paper wasp, honey bee, imported fire ants); polysaccharides such as dextran and thiomersal as a vaccine preservative; drugs such as protamine; antibiotics (penicillins, cephalosporins, amphotericin B, nitrofurantoin, quinolones); chemotherapy agents (carboplatin, paclitaxel, doxorubicin); local anesthetics (procaine, lidocaine); muscle relaxants (suxamethonium, gallamine, pancuronium); vitamins (thiamine, folic acid); diagnostic agents (sodium dehydrocholate, sulfobromophthalein); and occupation-related chemicals (ethylene oxide). Drugs are considered to function as haptens that form immunogenic conjugates with host proteins. The conjugating hapten may be the parent compound, a nonenzymatically derived storage product, or a metabolite formed in the host.

PATHOPHYSIOLOGY AND MANIFESTATIONS

Individuals differ in the time of appearance of symptoms and signs, but the hallmark of the anaphylactic reaction is the onset of some manifestation within seconds to minutes after introduction of the antigen, generally by injection or less commonly by ingestion. There may be upper or lower airway obstruction or both. Laryngeal edema may be experienced as a "lump" in the throat, hoarseness, or stridor, while bronchial obstruction is associated with a feeling of tightness in the chest and/or audible wheezing. Patients with bronchial asthma are predisposed to severe involvement of the lower airways. Flushing with diffuse erythema and a feeling of warmth may occur. A characteristic feature is the eruption of well-circumscribed, discrete cutaneous wheals with erythematous, raised, serpiginous borders and blanched centers. These urticarial eruptions are intensely pruritic and may be localized or disseminated. They may coalesce to form giant hives, and they seldom persist beyond 48 h. A localized, nonpitting, deeper edematous cutaneous process, angioedema, may also be present. It may be asymptomatic or cause a burning or stinging sensation.

In fatal cases with clinical bronchial obstruction, the lungs show marked hyperinflation on gross and microscopic examination. The microscopic findings in the bronchi, however, are limited to luminal secretions, peribronchial congestion, submucosal edema, and eosinophilic infiltration, and the acute emphysema is attributed to intractable bronchospasm that subsides with death. The angioedema resulting in death by mechanical obstruction occurs in the epiglottis and larynx, but the process also is evident in the hypopharynx and to some extent in the trachea. On microscopic examination, there is wide separation of the collagen fibers and the glandular elements; vascular congestion and eosinophilic infiltration also are present. Patients dying of vascular collapse without antecedent hypoxia from respiratory insufficiency have visceral congestion with a presumptive loss of intravascular blood volume. The associated electrocardiographic abnormalities, with or without infarction, in some patients may reflect a primary cardiac event mediated by mast cells or may be secondary to a critical reduction in blood volume.

The angioedematous and urticarial manifestations of the anaphylactic syndrome have been attributed to the release of endogenous histamine. A role for the cysteinyl leukotrienes in causing marked bronchiolar constriction seems likely. Vascular collapse without respiratory distress in response to experimental challenge with the sting of a hymenopteran was associated with marked and prolonged elevations in blood histamine and intravascular coagulation and kinin generation. The finding that patients with systemic mastocytosis and episodic vascular collapse excrete large amounts of PGD_2 metabolites in addition to histamine suggests that PGD_2 is also of importance in the hypotensive anaphylactic reactions. The PAF level can be elevated in the serum of patients with anaphylaxis, and its concentration is correlated inversely with the constitutive level of the acetylhydrolase involved in its inactivation. The actions of the array of mast cell–derived mediators are likely additive or synergistic at the target tissues.

DIAGNOSIS

The diagnosis of an anaphylactic reaction depends on a history revealing the onset of symptoms and signs within minutes after the responsible material is encountered. It is appropriate to rule out a complement-mediated immune complex reaction, an idiosyncratic response to a nonsteroidal anti-inflammatory drug (NSAID), or the direct effect of certain drugs or diagnostic agents on mast cells. Intravenous administration of a chemical mast cell–degranulating agent, including opiate derivatives and radiographic contrast media, may elicit generalized urticaria, angioedema, and a sensation of retrosternal oppression with or without clinically detectable bronchoconstriction or hypotension. Aspirin and other NSAIDs such as indomethacin, aminopyrine, and mefenamic acid may precipitate a life-threatening episode of obstruction of upper or lower airways, especially in patients with asthma, that is clinically indistinguishable from anaphylaxis but is not associated with the presence of specific IgE or elevation of blood tryptase. This syndrome, which is commonly associated with nasal polyposis, is due to inhibition of PGHS-1 with corresponding unregulated, amplified generation of the cysteinyl leukotrienes via the 5-LO/LTC_4 synthase pathway. In the transfusion anaphylactic reaction that occurs in patients with IgA deficiency, the responsible specificity resides in IgG or IgE anti-IgA; the mechanism of the reaction mediated by IgG anti-IgA is presumed to be complement activation with secondary mast cell participation.

The presence of specific IgE in the blood of patients with systemic anaphylaxis was demonstrated historically by passive transfer of the serum intradermally into a normal recipient, followed 24 h later by antigen challenge into the same site, with subsequent development of a wheal and flare (the *Prausnitz-Küstner reaction*). In current clinical practice, immunoassays using purified antigens can demonstrate the presence of specific IgE in the serum of patients with anaphylactic reactions, and intracutaneous skin testing may be performed after the patient has recovered to elicit a local wheal and flare in response to the putative antigen. Elevations of tryptase levels in serum implicate mast cell activation in a systemic reaction and are particularly informative for anaphylaxis with episodes of hypotension during general anesthesia or when there has been a fatal outcome. However, because of the short half-life of tryptase, elevated levels are best detected within 4 hours of a systemic reaction.

TREATMENT Anaphylaxis

Early recognition of an anaphylactic reaction is mandatory, since death occurs within minutes to hours after the first symptoms. Mild symptoms such as pruritus and urticaria can be controlled by administration of 0.3 to 0.5 mL of 1:1000 (1 mg/mL) epinephrine SC or IM, with repeated doses as required at 5- to 20-min intervals for a severe reaction. If the antigenic material was injected into an extremity, the rate of absorption may be reduced by prompt application of a tourniquet proximal to the reaction site, administration of 0.2 mL of 1:1000 epinephrine into the site, and removal without compression of an insect stinger, if present. An IV infusion should be initiated to provide a route for administration of 2.5 mL epinephrine, diluted 1:10,000, at 5- to 10-min intervals, volume expanders such as normal saline, and vasopressor agents such as dopamine if intractable hypotension occurs. Replacement of intravascular volume due to postcapillary venular leakage may require several liters of saline. Epinephrine provides both α- and β-adrenergic effects, resulting in vasoconstriction, bronchial smooth-muscle relaxation, and attenuation of enhanced venular permeability. When epinephrine fails to control the anaphylactic reaction, hypoxia due to airway obstruction or related to a cardiac arrhythmia, or both, must be considered. Oxygen alone via a nasal catheter or with nebulized albuterol may be helpful, but either endotracheal intubation or a tracheostomy is mandatory for oxygen delivery if progressive hypoxia develops. Ancillary agents such as the antihistamine diphenhydramine, 50–100 mg IM or IV, and aminophylline, 0.25–0.5 g IV, are appropriate for urticaria-angioedema and bronchospasm, respectively. Intravenous glucocorticoids, 0.5–1 mg/kg of medrol, are not effective for the acute event but may alleviate later recurrence of bronchospasm, hypotension, or urticaria.

PREVENTION

Prevention of anaphylaxis must take into account the sensitivity of the recipient, the dose and character of the diagnostic or therapeutic agent, and the effect of the route of administration on the rate of absorption. Beta blockers are relatively contraindicated in persons at risk for anaphylactic reactions, especially those sensitive to Hymenoptera venom or those undergoing immunotherapy for respiratory system allergy. If there is a definite history of a past anaphylactic reaction to a medication, even though mild, it is advisable to select a structurally unrelated agent. A knowledge of cross-reactivity among agents is critical since, for example, cephalosporins have a cross-reactive ring structure with the penicillins. When skin testing, a prick or scratch skin test should precede an intradermal test, since the latter has a higher risk of causing anaphylaxis. These tests should be performed before the administration of certain materials that are likely to elicit anaphylactic reactions, such as allergenic extracts. Skin testing for antibiotics or chemotherapeutic agents should be performed only on patients with a positive clinical history consistent with an IgE-mediated reaction and in imminent need of the antibiotic in question; skin testing is of no value for non-IgE-mediated eruptions. With regard to penicillin, two-thirds of patients with a positive reaction history and positive skin tests to benzylpenicilloyl-polylysine (BPL) and/or the minor determinant mixture (MDM) of benzylpenicillin products experience allergic reactions with treatment, and these reactions are almost uniformly of the anaphylactic type in those patients with minor determinant reactivity. Even patients without a history of previous clinical reactions have a 2–6% incidence of positive skin tests to the two test materials, and about 3 per 1000 with a negative history experience anaphylaxis with therapy, with a mortality of about 1 per 100,000.

If an agent carrying a risk of an anaphylactic response is required because a non-cross-reactive alternative is not available, desensitization can be performed with most antibiotics and other classes of therapeutic agents by the IV, SC, or oral route. Typically, graded quantities of the drug are given by the selected route starting below the threshold dose for an adverse reaction and then doubling each dose until a therapeutic dosage is achieved. Due to the risk of systemic anaphylaxis during the course of desensitization, such a procedure should be performed under the supervision of a specialist and in a setting in which resuscitation equipment is at hand and an IV line is in place. Once a desensitized state is achieved, it is critical to continue administration of the therapeutic agent at regular intervals throughout the treatment period to prevent the reestablishment of a significant pool of sensitized cells.

A different form of protection involves the development of blocking antibody of the IgG class, which protects against Hymenoptera venom–induced anaphylaxis by interacting with antigen so that less reaches the sensitized tissue mast cells. The maximal risk for systemic anaphylactic reactions in persons with Hymenoptera sensitivity occurs in association with a currently positive skin test. Although there is only low-grade cross-reactivity between honey bee and yellow jacket venoms, there is a high degree of cross-reactivity between yellow jacket venom and the rest of the vespid venoms (yellow or baldfaced hornets and wasps). Prevention involves modification of outdoor activities to exclude bare feet, wearing perfumed toiletries, eating in areas attractive to insects, clipping hedges or grass, and hauling away trash or fallen fruit. As with each anaphylactic sensitivity, the individual should wear an informational bracelet and have immediate access to an unexpired autoinjectable epinephrine kit. The limitations of lifestyle and the psychological duress can be addressed by venom immunotherapy. Although it has been recommended that venom therapy be continued indefinitely or until the skin and specific serum IgE tests are unremarkable, there is evidence that 5 years of treatment induces a state of resistance to sting reactions that is independent of serum levels of specific IgG or IgE. For children with a systemic reaction limited to skin, the likelihood of progression to more serious respiratory or vascular manifestations is low, and thus immunotherapy is not recommended.

URTICARIA AND ANGIOEDEMA

DEFINITION

Urticaria and angioedema may appear separately or together as cutaneous manifestations of localized nonpitting edema; a similar process may occur at mucosal surfaces of the upper respiratory or gastrointestinal tract. *Urticaria* involves only the superficial portion of the dermis, presenting as well-circumscribed wheals with erythematous raised serpiginous borders and blanched centers that may coalesce to become giant wheals. *Angioedema* is a well-demarcated localized edema involving the deeper layers of the skin, including the subcutaneous tissue. Recurrent episodes of urticaria and/or angioedema of less than 6 weeks' duration are considered acute, whereas attacks persisting beyond this period are designated chronic.

PREDISPOSING FACTORS AND ETIOLOGY

Urticaria and angioedema probably occur more frequently than usually described because of the evanescent, self-limited nature of such eruptions, which seldom require medical attention when limited to the skin. Although persons in any age group may experience acute or chronic urticaria and/or angioedema, these lesions increase in frequency after adolescence, with the highest incidence occurring in persons in the third decade of life; indeed, one survey of college students indicated that 15–20% had experienced a pruritic wheal reaction.

TABLE 317-1 Classification of Urticaria and/or Angioedema

1. IgE-dependent
- a. Specific antigen sensitivity (pollens, foods, drugs, fungi, molds, Hymenoptera venom, helminths)
- b. Physical: dermographism, cold, solar
- c. Autoimmune

2. Bradykinin-mediated
- a. Hereditary angioedema: C1 inhibitor deficiency: null (type 1) and dysfunctional (type 2)
- b. Acquired angioedema: C1 inhibitor deficiency: anti-idiotype and anti-C1 inhibitor
- c. Angiotensin-converting enzyme inhibitors

3. Complement-mediated
- a. Necrotizing vasculitis
- b. Serum sickness
- c. Reactions to blood products

4. Nonimmunologic
- a. Direct mast cell–releasing agents (opiates, antibiotics, curare, D-tubocurarine, radiocontrast media)
- b. Agents that alter arachidonic acid metabolism (aspirin and nonsteroidal anti-inflammatory agents, azo dyes, and benzoates)

5. Idiopathic

The classification of urticaria-angioedema presented in Table 317-1 focuses on the different mechanisms for eliciting clinical disease and can be useful for differential diagnosis; nonetheless, most cases of chronic urticaria are idiopathic. Urticaria and/or angioedema occurring during the appropriate season in patients with seasonal respiratory allergy or as a result of exposure to animals or molds is attributed to inhalation or physical contact with pollens, animal dander, and mold spores, respectively. However, urticaria and angioedema secondary to inhalation are relatively uncommon compared to urticaria and angioedema elicited by ingestion of fresh fruits, shellfish, fish, milk products, chocolate, legumes including peanuts, and various drugs that may elicit not only the anaphylactic syndrome with prominent gastrointestinal complaints but also chronic urticaria.

Additional etiologies include physical stimuli such as cold, heat, solar rays, exercise, and mechanical irritation. The physical urticarias can be distinguished by the precipitating event and other aspects of the clinical presentation. *Dermographism*, which occurs in 1–4% of the population, is defined by the appearance of a linear wheal at the site of a brisk stroke with a firm object or by any configuration appropriate to the eliciting event (Fig. 317-3). Dermographism has a prevalence that peaks in the second to third decades. It is not influenced by an atopic diathesis and has a duration generally of <5 years. *Pressure urticaria*, which often accompanies chronic idiopathic urticaria, presents in response to a sustained stimulus such as a shoulder strap or belt, running (feet), or manual labor (hands). *Cholinergic urticaria* is distinctive in that the pruritic wheals are of small size (1–2 mm) and are surrounded by a large area of erythema; attacks are precipitated by fever, a hot bath or shower, or exercise and are presumptively attributed to a rise in core body temperature. *Exercise-related anaphylaxis* can be precipitated by exertion alone or can be dependent on prior food ingestion. The clinical

Dermographism

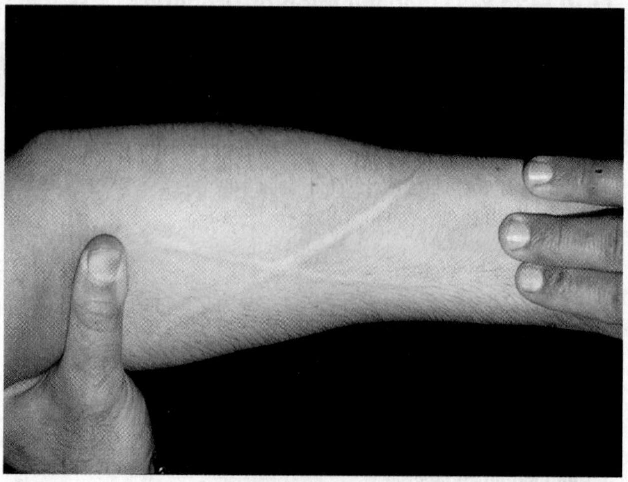

Figure 317-3 Dermographic urticarial lesion induced by stroking the forearm lightly with the edge of a tongue blade. The photograph, taken after 2 minutes, demonstrates a prominent wheal and flare reaction in the shape of an *X*. *(Photograph provided by Allen P. Kaplan, MD, Medical University of South Carolina.)*

presentation can be limited to flushing, erythema, and pruritic urticaria but may progress to angioedema of the face, oropharynx, larynx, or intestine or to vascular collapse; it is distinguished from cholinergic urticaria by presenting with wheals of conventional size and by not occurring with fever or a hot bath. *Cold urticaria* is local at body areas exposed to low ambient temperature or cold objects (ice cube) but can progress to vascular collapse with immersion in cold water (swimming). *Solar urticaria* is subdivided into six groups by the response to specific portions of the light spectrum. *Vibratory angioedema* may occur after years of occupational exposure or can be idiopathic; it may be accompanied by cholinergic urticaria. Other rare forms of physical allergy, always defined by stimulus-specific elicitation, include *local heat urticaria*, *aquagenic urticaria* from contact with water of any temperature (sometimes associated with polycythemia vera), and *contact urticaria* from direct interaction with some chemical substance.

Angioedema without urticaria due to the generation of bradykinin occurs with C1 inhibitor (C1INH) deficiency that may be inborn as an autosomal dominant characteristic or may be acquired through the appearance of an autoantibody. The angiotensin-converting enzyme (ACE) inhibitors can provoke a similar clinical presentation in 0.1–0.5% of hypertensive patients due to attenuated degradation of bradykinin. The urticaria and angioedema associated with classic serum sickness or with hypocomplementemic cutaneous necrotizing angiitis are believed to be immune-complex diseases. The drug reactions to mast cell granule–releasing agents and to NSAIDs may be systemic, resembling anaphylaxis, or limited to cutaneous sites.

PATHOPHYSIOLOGY AND MANIFESTATIONS

Urticarial eruptions are distinctly pruritic, may involve any area of the body from the scalp to the soles of the feet, and appear in crops of 12- to 36-hour duration, with old lesions fading as new ones appear. Most of the physical urticarias (cold, cholinergic, dermatographism) are an exception, with individual lesions lasting less than 2 hours. The most common sites for urticaria are the extremities and face, with angioedema often being periorbital and in the lips. Although self-limited in duration, angioedema of the upper respiratory tract may be life-threatening due to laryngeal obstruction, while gastrointestinal involvement may present with abdominal colic, with or without nausea and vomiting, and may result in unnecessary surgical intervention. No residual discoloration occurs with either urticaria or angioedema unless there is an underlying process leading to superimposed extravasation of erythrocytes.

The pathology is characterized by edema of the superficial dermis in urticaria and of the subcutaneous tissue and deep dermis in angioedema. Collagen bundles in affected areas are widely separated, and the venules are sometimes dilated. Any perivenular infiltrate consists of lymphocytes, monocytes, eosinophils, and neutrophils that are present in varying combination and numbers.

Perhaps the best-studied example of IgE- and mast cell–mediated urticaria and angioedema is *cold urticaria*. Cryoglobulins or cold agglutinins may be recognized in up to 5% of these patients. Immersion of an extremity in an ice bath precipitates angioedema of the distal portion with urticaria at the air interface within minutes of the challenge. Histologic studies reveal marked mast cell degranulation with associated edema of the dermis and subcutaneous tissues. The histamine level in the plasma of venous effluent of the cold-challenged and angioedematous extremity is markedly increased, but no such increase appears in the plasma of effluent of the contralateral normal extremity. Elevated levels of histamine have been found in the plasma of venous effluent and in the fluid of suction blisters at experimentally induced lesional sites in patients with dermographism, pressure urticaria, vibratory angioedema, light urticaria, and heat urticaria. By ultrastructural analysis, the pattern of mast cell degranulation in cold urticaria resembles an IgE-mediated response with solubilization of granule contents, fusion of the perigranular and cell membranes, and discharge of granule contents, whereas in a dermographic lesion there is additional superimposed zonal (piecemeal) degranulation. Elevations of plasma histamine levels with biopsy-proven mast cell degranulation have also been demonstrated with generalized attacks of *cholinergic urticaria* and *exercise-related anaphylaxis* precipitated experimentally in subjects exercising on a treadmill while wearing a wet suit; however, only subjects with cholinergic urticaria have a concomitant decrease in pulmonary function.

Up to 40% of patients with chronic urticaria have an autoimmune cause for their disease including autoantibodies to IgE (5–10%) or, more commonly, to the α chain of FcεRI (35–45%). In these patients, autologous serum injected into their own skin can induce a wheal and flare reaction involving mast cell activation. The presence of these antibodies can also be recognized by their capacity to release histamine or induce activation markers such as CD63 or CD203 on basophils. An association with antibodies to microsomal peroxidase and/or thyroglobulin has been observed often with clinically significant Hashimoto's thyroiditis. In vitro studies reveal that these autoantibodies can mediate basophil degranulation with enhancement by serum as a source of the anaphylatoxic fragment, C5a.

Hereditary angioedema is an autosomal dominant disease due to a deficiency of C1INH (type 1) in about 85% of patients and to a dysfunctional protein (type 2) in the remainder. In the acquired form of C1INH deficiency, there is excessive consumption due either to immune complexes formed between anti-idiotypic antibody and monoclonal IgG presented by B cell lymphomas or to an autoantibody directed to C1INH. C1INH blocks the catalytic function of activated factor XII (Hageman factor) and of kallikrein, as well as the C1r/C1s components of C1. During clinical attacks of angioedema, C1INH-deficient patients have elevated plasma levels of bradykinin, particularly in the venous effluent of an involved extremity, and reduced levels of prekallikrein and high-molecular-weight kininogen, from which bradykinin is cleaved. The parallel decline in the complement substrates C4 and C2 reflects the action of activated C1 during such attacks. Mice with targeted disruption of the gene for C1INH exhibit a chronic increase in vascular permeability. The pathobiology is aggravated by administration of an ACE inhibitor (captopril) and is attenuated by breeding the C1INH null strain to a bradykinin 2 receptor (Bk2R) null strain. As ACE is also described as kininase II, the use of blockers results in impaired bradykinin degradation and explains the angioedema that occurs idiosyncratically in hypertensive patients with a normal C1INH.

DIAGNOSIS

The rapid onset and self-limited nature of urticarial and angioedematous eruptions are distinguishing features. Additional characteristics are the occurrence of the urticarial crops in various stages of evolution and the asymmetric distribution of the angioedema. Urticaria and/or angioedema involving IgE-dependent mechanisms are often appreciated by historic considerations implicating specific allergens or physical stimuli, by seasonal incidence, and by exposure to certain environments. Direct reproduction of the lesion with physical stimuli is particularly valuable because it so often establishes the cause of the lesion. The diagnosis of an environmental allergen based on the clinical history can be confirmed by skin testing or assay for allergen-specific IgE in serum. IgE-mediated urticaria and/or angioedema may or may not be associated with an elevation of total IgE or with peripheral eosinophilia. Fever, leukocytosis, and an elevated sedimentation rate are absent.

The classification of urticarial and angioedematous states presented in Table 317-1 in terms of possible mechanisms necessarily includes some differential diagnostic points. Hypocomplementemia is not observed in IgE-mediated mast cell disease and may reflect either an acquired abnormality generally attributed to the formation of immune complexes or a genetic deficiency of C1INH. Chronic recurrent urticaria, generally in females, associated with arthralgias, an elevated sedimentation rate, and normo- or hypocomplementemia suggests an underlying cutaneous necrotizing angiitis. Vasculitic urticaria typically persists longer than 72 hours, whereas conventional urticaria often has a duration of 12–36 hours. Confirmation depends on a biopsy that reveals cellular infiltration, nuclear debris, and fibrinoid necrosis of the venules. The same pathobiologic process accounts for the urticaria in association with such diseases as systemic lupus erythematosus or viral hepatitis with or without associated arteritis. Serum sickness per se or a similar clinical entity due to drugs includes not only urticaria but also pyrexia, lymphadenopathy, myalgia, and arthralgia or arthritis. Urticarial reactions to blood products or intravenous administration of immunoglobulin are defined by the event and generally are not progressive unless the recipient is IgA-deficient in the former case or the reagent is aggregated in the latter.

The diagnosis of hereditary angioedema is suggested not only by family history but also by the lack of pruritus and of urticarial lesions, the prominence of recurrent gastrointestinal attacks of colic, and episodes of laryngeal edema. Laboratory diagnosis depends on demonstrating a deficiency of C1INH antigen (type 1) or a nonfunctional protein (type 2) by a catalytic inhibition assay. While levels of C1 are normal, its substrates, C4 and C2, are chronically depleted and fall further during attacks due to the activation of additional C1. Patients with the acquired forms of C1INH deficiency have the same clinical manifestations but differ in the lack of a familial element. Furthermore, their sera exhibit a reduction of C1 function and C1q protein as well as C1INH, C4, and C2. Inborn C1INH deficiency and ACE inhibitor–elicited angioedema are associated with elevated levels of bradykinin.

Urticaria and angioedema can be differentiated from contact sensitivity, a vesicular eruption that progresses to chronic thickening of the skin with continued allergenic exposure. They can also be differentiated from atopic dermatitis, a condition that may present as erythema, edema, papules, vesiculation, and oozing proceeding to a subacute and chronic stage in which vesiculation is less marked or absent and scaling, fissuring, and lichenification predominate in a distribution that characteristically involves the flexor surfaces. In cutaneous mastocytosis, the reddish brown macules and papules, characteristic of urticaria pigmentosa, urticate with pruritus upon trauma; and in systemic mastocytosis, without or with urticaria pigmentosa, there is episodic systemic flushing with or without urtication but no angioedema.

TREATMENT Urticaria and Angioedema

Identification of the etiologic factor(s) and subsequent elimination provide the most satisfactory therapeutic program; this approach is feasible to varying degrees with IgE-mediated reactions to allergens or physical stimuli. For most forms of urticaria, H_1 antihistamines such as chlorpheniramine or diphenhydramine effectively attenuate both urtication and pruritus, but because of their side effects, nonsedating agents such as loratadine, desloratadine, and fexofenadine, or low-sedating agents such as cetirizine or levocetirizine generally are used first. Cyproheptadine in dosages beginning at 8 mg and ranging up to 32 mg daily and especially hydroxyzine in dosages beginning at 40 mg and ranging up to 200 mg daily have proven effective when H_1 antihistamines fail. The addition of an H_2 antagonist such as cimetidine, ranitidine, or famotidine in conventional dosages may add benefit when H_1 antihistamines are inadequate. Doxepin, a dibenzoxepin tricyclic compound with both H_1 and H_2 receptor antagonist activity, is yet another alternative. A $CysLT_1$ receptor antagonist such as montelukast, 10 mg/d, or zafirlukast, 20 mg twice a day, can be important add-on therapy. Topical glucocorticoids are of no value, and systemic glucocorticoids are generally avoided in idiopathic, allergen-induced, or physical urticarias due to their long-term toxicity. Systemic glucocorticoids are useful in the management of patients with pressure urticaria, vasculitic urticaria (especially with eosinophil prominence), idiopathic angioedema with or without urticaria, or chronic urticaria that responds poorly to conventional treatment. With persistent vasculitic urticaria, hydroxychloroquine, dapsone, or colchicine may be added to the regimen after hydroxyzine and before or along with systemic glucocorticoids. Cyclosporine can be efficacious for patients with chronic idiopathic or chronic autoimmune urticaria that is severe and poorly responsive to other modalities and/or where a glucocorticoid requirement is excessive. For chronic urticaria induced by autoantibody activation of mast cells and basophils, monoclonal anti-IgE antibodies such as omalizumab may be considered.

The therapy of inborn C1INH deficiency has been simplified by the finding that attenuated androgens correct the biochemical defect and afford prophylactic protection; their efficacy is attributed to production by the normal gene of an amount of functional C1INH sufficient to control the spontaneous activation of C1. The antifibrinolytic agent ε-aminocaproic acid may be used for preoperative prophylaxis but is contraindicated in patients with thrombotic tendencies or ischemia due to arterial atherosclerosis. Infusion of isolated C1INH protein may be used for prophylaxis or treatment of an acute attack; a bradykinin 2 receptor antagonist and ecallantide, a kallikrein inhibitor, which are administered SC, are each being assessed for amelioration of attacks. For acquired C1INH deficiency, treatment of the underlying hematologic malignancy is recommended.

SYSTEMIC MASTOCYTOSIS

DEFINITION

Systemic mastocytosis is defined by a clonal expansion of mast cells that in most instances is indolent and nonneoplastic. The mast cell expansion is generally recognized only in bone marrow and in the normal peripheral distribution sites of the cells, such as skin, gastrointestinal mucosa, liver, and spleen. Mastocytosis occurs at any age and has a slight preponderance in males. The prevalence of systemic mastocytosis is not known, a familial occurrence is rare, and atopy is not increased.

CLASSIFICATION AND PATHOPHYSIOLOGY

A consensus classification for mastocytosis recognizes cutaneous mastocytosis with variants and four systemic forms (Table 317-2). The form designated as *indolent systemic mastocytosis* (ISM) accounts for the majority of patients; it implies that there is no evidence of an associated hematologic disorder, liver disease, or lymphadenopathy and is not known to alter life expectancy. In *systemic mastocytosis associated with clonal hematologic non-mast cell lineage disease* (SM-AHNMD), the prognosis is determined by the nature of the associated disorder, which can range from dysmyelopoiesis to leukemia. In *aggressive systemic mastocytosis* (ASM), mast cell infiltration/proliferation in multiple organs such as liver, spleen, gut, CNS, and/or bone results in a poor prognosis; a subset of patients with this form has prominent eosinophilia with hepatosplenomegaly and lymphadenopathy. *Mast cell leukemia* is the rarest form of the disease and is invariably fatal at present; the peripheral blood contains circulating, metachromatically staining, atypical mast cells.

A point mutation of A to T at codon 816 of c-*kit* that causes an aspartic acid to valine substitution is found in multiple cell lineages in patients with mastocytosis, resulting in a somatic gain-in-function mutation. This substitution, as well as other rare mutations of c-*kit*, is characteristic of adults with SM-AHNMD but is also present in patients with ISM or cutaneous mastocytosis, as might be anticipated because mast cells are of bone marrow lineage. The prognosis for patients with cutaneous mastocytosis and for almost all with ISM is a normal life expectancy, while that for patients with SM-AHNMD is determined by a non-mast cell component. In infants and children with cutaneous manifestations, namely, urticaria pigmentosa or bullous lesions, visceral involvement is usually lacking, and resolution is common because gain-in-function mutations are infrequent.

TABLE 317-2 Classification of Mastocytosis

Cutaneous mastocytosis (CM)
Urticaria pigmentosa (UP)/maculopapular cutaneous mastocytosis (MPCM)
Variants: plaque form, nodular form; telangiectasia macularis eruptiva perstans (TMEP); diffuse cutaneous mastocytosis (DCM)
Solitary mastocytoma of skin
Indolent systemic mastocytosis (ISM)
Systemic mastocytosis with an associated clonal hematologic non-mast cell lineage disease (SM-AHNMD)
Aggressive systemic mastocytosis (ASM)
Variant: lymphadenopathic mastocytosis with eosinophilia
Mast cell leukemia (MCL)
Mast cell sarcoma (MCS)

Source: Modified from SH Swerdlow et al (eds): *World Health Organization Classification of Tumors: Pathology and Genetics in Tumors of Hematopoietic and Lymphoid Tissues.* Lyon, IARC Press, 2008.

CLINICAL MANIFESTATIONS

The clinical manifestations of systemic mastocytosis, distinct from a leukemic complication, are due to tissue occupancy by the mast cell mass, the tissue response to that mass, and the release of bioactive substances acting at both local and distal sites. The pharmacologically induced manifestations are pruritus, flushing, palpitations and vascular collapse, gastric distress, lower abdominal crampy pain, and recurrent headache. The increase in local cell burden is evidenced by the lesions of urticaria pigmentosa at skin sites and is a direct cause of bone pain and/or malabsorption. Mast cell–mediated fibrotic changes occur in liver, spleen, and bone marrow but not in gastrointestinal tissue or skin. Immunofluorescent analysis of bone marrow and skin lesions in ISM and of spleen, lymph node, and skin in ASM has revealed only one mast cell phenotype, namely, scroll-poor cells expressing tryptase, chymase, and CPA.

The cutaneous lesions of urticaria pigmentosa are reddish-brown macules or papules that respond to trauma with urtication and erythema (Darier's sign). The apparent incidence of these lesions is ≤90% in patients with ISM and <50% in those with SM-AHNMD or ASM. Approximately 1% of patients with ISM have skin lesions that appear as tan-brown macules with striking patchy erythema and associated telangiectasia (telangiectasia macularis eruptiva perstans). In the upper gastrointestinal tract, gastritis and peptic ulcer are significant problems. In the lower intestinal tract, the occurrence of diarrhea and abdominal pain is attributed to increased motility due to mast cell mediators; this problem can be aggravated by malabsorption, which can also cause secondary nutritional insufficiency and osteomalacia. The periportal fibrosis associated with mast cell infiltration and a prominence of eosinophils may lead to portal hypertension and ascites. In some patients, flushing and recurrent vascular collapse are markedly aggravated by an idiosyncratic response to a minimal dosage of NSAIDs. The neuropsychiatric disturbances are clinically most evident as impaired recent memory, decreased attention span, and "migraine-like" headaches. Patients may experience exacerbation of a specific clinical sign or symptom with alcohol ingestion, use of mast cell–interactive narcotics, or ingestion of NSAIDs.

DIAGNOSIS

Although the diagnosis of mastocytosis is generally suspected on the basis of the clinical history and physical findings, and can be supported by laboratory procedures, it can be established only by a tissue diagnosis. By convention, the diagnosis of systemic mastocytosis depends heavily on bone marrow biopsy to meet the criteria of one major plus one minor or three minor findings (Table 317-3). The bone marrow provides the major criterion by revealing aggregates

TABLE 317-3 Diagnostic Criteria for Systemic Mastocytosis*

Major: Multifocal dense infiltrates of mast cells in bone marrow or other extracutaneous tissues with confirmation by immunodetection of tryptase or metachromasia
Minor: Abnormal mast cell morphology with a spindle shape and/or multilobed or eccentric nucleus
Aberrant mast cell surface phenotype with expression of CD25 (IL-2 receptor) and CD2 in addition to C117 (c-*kit*)
Detection of codon 816 mutation in peripheral blood cells, bone marrow cells, or lesional tissue
Total serum tryptase (mostly alpha) greater than 20 ng/mL

*Diagnosis requires either the major and one minor or three minor criteria.

of mast cells, often in paratrabecular and perivascular locations with lymphocytes and eosinophils, as well as the minor criteria of an abnormal mast cell morphology, an aberrant mast cell membrane immunophenotype, or a codon 816 mutation in any cell type. A serum total tryptase level and/or a 24-hour urine collection for measurement of histamine, histamine metabolites, or metabolites of PGD_2 are noninvasive approaches to consider before bone marrow biopsy. The α form of tryptase is elevated in more than one-half of patients with systemic mastocytosis and provides a minor criterion; the β form is increased in patients undergoing an anaphylactic reaction. Additional studies directed by the presentation include a bone scan or skeletal survey; contrast studies of the upper gastrointestinal tract with small-bowel follow-through, CT scan, or endoscopy; and a neuropsychiatric evaluation, including an electroencephalogram.

The differential diagnosis requires the exclusion of other flushing disorders. The 24-hour urine assessment of 5-hydroxy-indoleacetic acid and metanephrines should exclude a carcinoid tumor or a pheochromocytoma. Most patients with recurrent anaphylaxis, including the idiopathic group, present with angioedema and/or wheezing, which are not manifestations of systemic mastocytosis.

TREATMENT Systemic Mastocytosis

The management of systemic mastocytosis uses a stepwise and symptom/sign–directed approach that includes an H_1 antihistamine for flushing and pruritus, an H_2 antihistamine or proton pump inhibitor for gastric acid hypersecretion, oral cromolyn sodium for diarrhea and abdominal pain, and aspirin for severe flushing with or without associated vascular collapse, despite use of H_1 and H_2 antihistamines, to block biosynthesis of PGD_2. Systemic glucocorticoids appear to alleviate the malabsorption. Headaches are generally managed with tricyclic antidepressants and other neurotransmitter-modifying agents. Ketotifen has been used to alleviate flushing in patients with gastric intolerance to NSAIDs and in patients with bone pain or intractable headaches. The efficacy of IFN-α in ASM is controversial, perhaps because of dosage limitations due to side effects. Treatment with hydroxyurea to reduce the mast cell lineage progenitors has a benefit in ASM. Chemotherapy is appropriate for the frank leukemias. Although c-*kit* is a receptor tyrosine kinase, the gain-in-function mutation of codon 816 is not susceptible to inhibition by imatinib mesylate.

ALLERGIC RHINITIS

DEFINITION

Allergic rhinitis is characterized by sneezing; rhinorrhea; obstruction of the nasal passages; conjunctival, nasal, and pharyngeal itching; and lacrimation, all occurring in a temporal relationship to allergen exposure. Although commonly seasonal due to elicitation by airborne pollens, it can be perennial in an environment of chronic exposure. In North America, the incidence of allergic rhinitis is about 7%. The overall prevalence in North America is nearly 20%, with the peak prevalence of nearly 40% occurring in childhood and adolescence.

PREDISPOSING FACTORS AND ETIOLOGY

Allergic rhinitis generally occurs in atopic individuals, i.e., in persons with a family history of a similar or related symptom complex and a personal history of collateral allergy expressed as eczematous dermatitis, urticaria, and/or asthma (Chap. 254). Up to 40% of patients with rhinitis manifest asthma, whereas ~70% of individuals with asthma experience rhinitis. Symptoms generally appear before the fourth decade of life and tend to diminish gradually with aging, although complete spontaneous remissions are uncommon. A relatively small number of weeds that depend on wind rather than insects for cross-pollination, as well as grasses and some trees, produce sufficient quantities of pollen suitable for wide distribution by air currents to elicit seasonal allergic rhinitis. The dates of pollination of these species generally vary little from year to year in a particular locale but may be quite different in another climate. In the temperate areas of North America, trees typically pollinate from March through May, grasses in June and early July, and ragweed from mid-August to early October. Molds, which are widespread in nature because they occur in soil or decaying organic matter, may propagate spores in a pattern that depends on climatic conditions. Perennial allergic rhinitis occurs in response to allergens that are present throughout the year, including desquamating epithelium in animal dander, cockroach-derived proteins, mold spores, or dust, which has mites such as *Dermatophagoides farinae* and *D. pteronyssinus*. Dust mites are scavengers of flecks of human skin and coat the digestate with mite-specific protein for excretion. In up to one-half of patients with perennial rhinitis, no clear-cut allergen can be demonstrated as causative. The ability of allergens to cause rhinitis rather than lower respiratory tract symptoms may be attributed to their large size, 10–100 μm, and retention within the nose.

PATHOPHYSIOLOGY AND MANIFESTATIONS

Episodic rhinorrhea, sneezing, obstruction of the nasal passages with lacrimation, and pruritus of the conjunctiva, nasal mucosa, and oropharynx are the hallmarks of allergic rhinitis. The nasal mucosa is pale and boggy, the conjunctiva congested and edematous, and the pharynx generally unremarkable. Swelling of the turbinates and mucous membranes with obstruction of the sinus ostia and eustachian tubes precipitates secondary infections of the sinuses and middle ear, respectively. Nasal polyps, representing mucosal protrusions containing edema fluid with variable numbers of eosinophils, can increase obstructive symptoms and can concurrently arise within the nasopharynx or sinuses. Nasal polyps may occur independent of allergic rhinitis in patients with the aspirin-intolerant triad of rhinosinusitis and asthma and in patients with chronic staphylococcal colonization, which produces superantigens leading to an intense T_H2 inflammatory response.

The nose presents a large mucosal surface area through the folds of the turbinates and serves to adjust the temperature and moisture content of inhaled air and to filter out particulate materials >10 μm in size by impingement in a mucous blanket; ciliary action moves the entrapped particles toward the pharynx. Entrapment of pollen and digestion of the outer coat by mucosal enzymes such as lysozymes release protein allergens generally of 10,000–40,000 molecular weight. The initial interaction occurs between the allergen and intraepithelial mast cells and then proceeds to involve deeper perivenular mast cells, both of which are sensitized with specific IgE. During the symptomatic season when the mucosae are already swollen and hyperemic, there is enhanced adverse reactivity to the seasonal pollen. Biopsy specimens of nasal mucosa during seasonal rhinitis show submucosal edema with infiltration by eosinophils, along with some basophils and neutrophils.

The mucosal surface fluid contains IgA that is present because of its secretory piece and also IgE, which apparently arrives by diffusion from plasma cells in proximity to mucosal surfaces. IgE fixes to mucosal and submucosal mast cells, and the intensity of the clinical response to inhaled allergens is quantitatively related to the naturally occurring pollen dose. In sensitive individuals, the introduction of allergen into the nose is associated with sneezing, "stuffiness," and discharge, and the fluid contains histamine, PGD_2, and leukotrienes. Thus the mast cells of the nasal mucosa and submucosa generate and release mediators through IgE-dependent reactions that are capable of producing tissue edema and eosinophilic infiltration.

DIAGNOSIS

The diagnosis of seasonal allergic rhinitis depends largely on an accurate history of occurrence coincident with the pollination of the offending weeds, grasses, or trees. The continuous character of perennial allergic rhinitis due to contamination of the home or place of work makes historic analysis difficult, but there may be a variability in symptoms that can be related to exposure to animal dander, dust mite and/or cockroach allergens, fungal spores, or work-related allergens such as latex. Patients with perennial rhinitis commonly develop the problem in adult life, and manifest nasal congestion and a postnasal discharge, often associated with thickening of the sinus membranes demonstrated by radiography. Perennial nonallergic rhinitis with eosinophilia syndrome (NARES) occurs in the middle decades of life and is characterized by nasal obstruction, anosmia, chronic sinusitis, and frequent aspirin intolerance. The term *vasomotor rhinitis* or *perennial nonallergic rhinitis* designates a condition of enhanced reactivity of the nasopharynx in which a symptom complex resembling perennial allergic rhinitis occurs with nonspecific stimuli, including chemical odors, temperature and humidity variations, and position changes but occurs without tissue eosinophilia or an allergic etiology. Other entities to be excluded are structural abnormalities of the nasopharynx; exposure to irritants; gustatory rhinitis associated with cholinergic activation that occurs while eating or ingesting alcohol; hypothyroidism; upper respiratory tract infection; pregnancy with prominent nasal mucosal edema; prolonged topical use of α-adrenergic agents in the form of nose drops (rhinitis medicamentosa); and the use of certain therapeutic agents such as rauwolfia, β-adrenergic antagonists, estrogens, progesterone, ACE inhibitors, aspirin and other NSAIDS, and drugs for erectile dysfunction (phosphodiesterase-5 inhibitors).

The nasal secretions of allergic patients are rich in eosinophils, and a modest peripheral eosinophilia is a common feature. Local or systemic neutrophilia implies infection. Total serum IgE is frequently elevated, but the demonstration of immunologic specificity for IgE is critical to an etiologic diagnosis. A skin test by the intracutaneous route (puncture or prick) with the allergens of interest provides a rapid and reliable approach to identifying allergen-specific IgE that has sensitized cutaneous mast cells. A positive intracutaneous skin test with 1:10–1:20 weight/volume of extract has a high predictive value for the presence of allergy. An intradermal test with a 1:500–1:1000 dilution of 0.05 mL may follow if indicated by history when the intracutaneous test is negative, but while more sensitive, it is less reliable due to the reactivity of some asymptomatic individuals at the test dose. Skin testing by the intracutaneous route for food allergens can be supportive of the clinical history. A double-blind, placebo-controlled challenge may document a food allergy, but such a procedure does bear the risk of an anaphylactic reaction. An elimination diet is safer but is tedious and less definitive. Food allergy is uncommon as a cause of allergic rhinitis.

Newer methodology for detecting total IgE, including the development of enzyme-linked immunosorbent assays (ELISA) employing anti-IgE bound to either a solid-phase or a liquid-phase particle, provides rapid and cost-effective determinations. Measurements of specific anti-IgE in serum are obtained by its binding to an allergen and quantitation by subsequent uptake of labeled anti-IgE. As compared to the skin test, the assay of specific IgE in serum is less sensitive but has high specificity.

PREVENTION

Avoidance of exposure to the offending allergen is the most effective means of controlling allergic diseases; removal of pets from the home to avoid animal danders, utilization of air-filtration devices to minimize the concentrations of airborne pollens, elimination of cockroach-derived proteins by chemical destruction of the pest and careful food storage, travel to areas where the allergen is not being generated, and even a change of domicile to eliminate a mold spore problem may be necessary. Control of dust mites by allergen avoidance includes use of plastic-lined covers for mattresses, pillows, and comforters; using a filter-equipped vacuum cleaner; washing bedding and clothes at temperatures >54.5°C (above 130°F); and elimination of carpets and drapes.

TREATMENT Allergic Rhinitis

Although allergen avoidance is the most cost-effective means of managing allergic rhinitis, treatment with pharmacologic agents represents the standard approach to seasonal or perennial allergic rhinitis. Oral antihistamines of the H_1 class are effective for nasopharyngeal itching, sneezing, and watery rhinorrhea and for such ocular manifestations as itching, tearing, and erythema, but they are not efficacious for the nasal congestion. The older antihistamines are sedating, and they induce psychomotor impairment, including reduced eye-hand coordination and impaired automobile driving skills. Their anticholinergic (muscarinic) effects include visual disturbance, urinary retention, and constipation. Because the newer H_1 antihistamines such as fexofenadine, loratadine, desloradine, cetirizine, levocetirizine, olopatadine, bilastine, and azelastine are less lipophilic and more H_1 selective, their ability to cross the blood-brain barrier is reduced, and thus their sedating and anticholinergic side effects are minimized. These newer antihistamines do not differ appreciably in efficacy for relief of rhinitis and/or sneezing. Azelastine nasal spray may benefit individuals with nonallergic vasomotor rhinitis, but it has an adverse effect of dysgeusia (taste perversion) in some patients. Because antihistamines have little effect on congestion, α-adrenergic agents such as phenylephrine or oximetazoline are generally used topically to alleviate nasal congestion and obstruction. However, the duration of their efficacy is limited because of rebound rhinitis (i.e., 7- to 14-day use can lead to rhinitis medicamentosa) and such systemic responses as hypertension. Oral α-adrenergic agonist decongestants containing pseudoephedrine are standard for the management of nasal congestion, generally in combination with an antihistamine. While oral antihistamines typically reduce nasal and ocular symptoms by about one third, pseudoephedrine must be added to achieve a similar reduction in nasal congestion. These pseudoephedrine combination products can cause insomnia and are precluded from use in patients with narrow angle glaucoma, urinary retention, severe hypertension, marked coronary artery disease, or a first trimester pregnancy. The $CysLT_1$ blocker montelukast is approved for treatment of both seasonal and perennial rhinitis, and it reduces both nasal and ocular symptoms by about 20%. Cromolyn sodium, a nasal spray, is essentially without side effects and is used prophylactically on a continuous basis during the season. The clinical efficacy of cromolyn sodium used prophylactically is less than that of second-generation oral antihistamines and less than that of intranasal glucocorticoids. Intranasal high-potency glucocorticoids are the most potent drugs available for the relief of established rhinitis, seasonal or perennial, and are effective in relieving nasal congestion. They provide

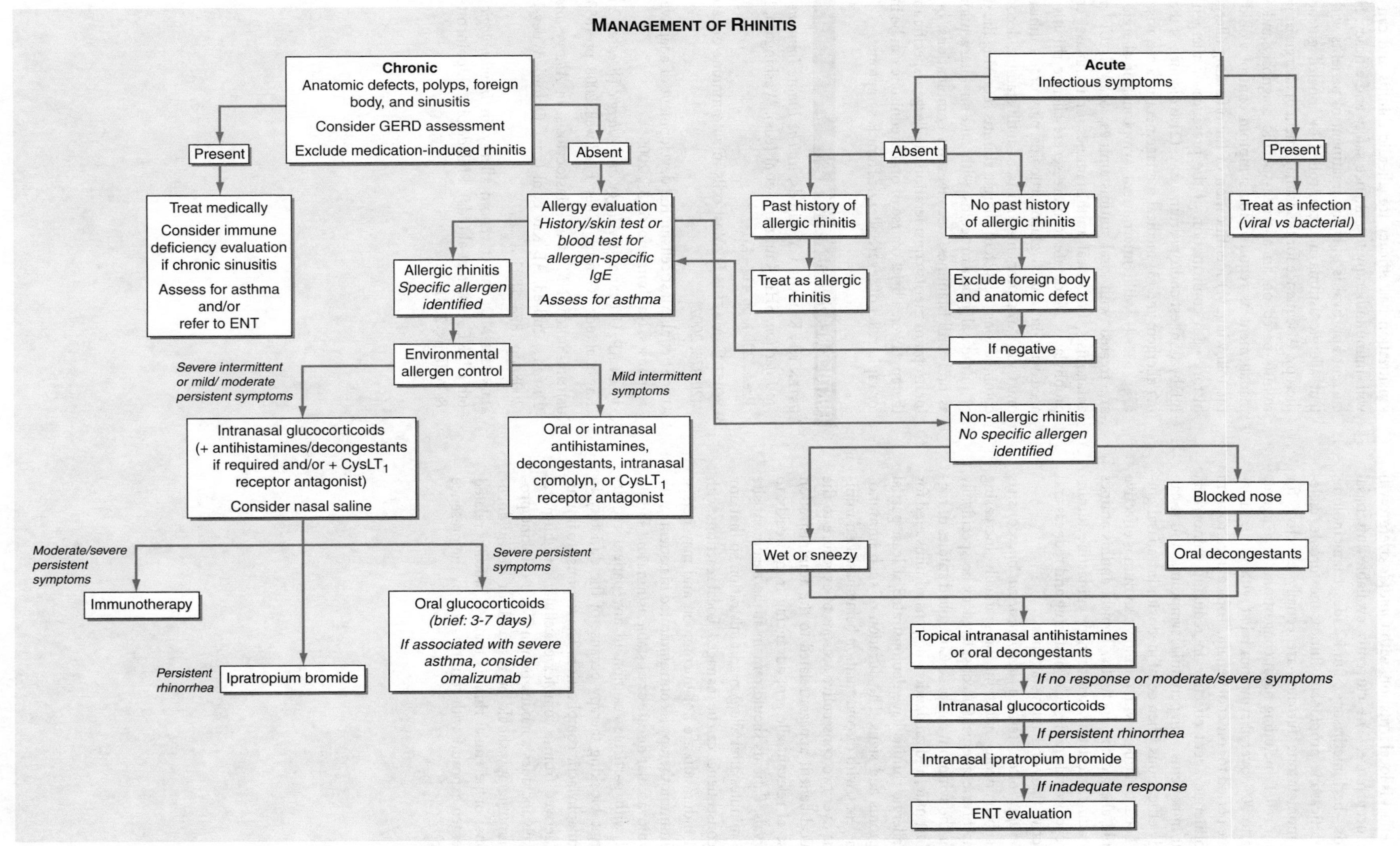

Figure 317-4 Algorithm for the diagnosis and management of rhinitis. ENT, ear, nose, and throat; GERD, gastroesophageal reflux disease.

efficacy with substantially reduced side effects as compared with this same class of agent administered orally. Their most frequent side effect is local irritation, with *Candida* overgrowth being a rare occurrence. The currently available intranasal glucocorticoids—beclomethasone, flunisolide, triamcinolone, budesonide, fluticasone propionate, fluticasone furoate, ciclesonide, and mometasone furoate—are equally effective for nasal symptom relief, including nasal congestion; these agents all achieve up to 70% overall symptom relief with some variation in the time period for onset of benefit. Topical ipratropium is an anticholinergic agent effective in reducing rhinorrhea, including that in patients with perennial symptoms, and it can be additionally efficacious when combined with intranasal glucocorticoids. Local treatment with cromolyn sodium is effective in treating mild allergic conjunctivitis. Topical antihistamines such as olopatadine, azelastine, ketotifen, or epinastine administered to the eye provide rapid relief of itching and redness and are more effective than oral antihistamines.

Immunotherapy, often termed *hyposensitization*, consists of repeated subcutaneous injections of gradually increasing concentrations of the allergen(s) considered to be specifically responsible for the symptom complex. Controlled studies of ragweed, grass, dust mite, and cat dander allergens administered for treatment of allergic rhinitis have demonstrated at least partial relief of symptoms and signs. The duration of such immunotherapy is 3–5 years, with discontinuation being based on minimal symptoms over two consecutive seasons of exposure to the allergen. Clinical benefit appears related to the administration of a high dose of relevant allergen, advancing from weekly to monthly intervals. Patients should remain at the treatment site for at least 20 minutes after allergen administration so that any anaphylactic consequence can be managed. Local reactions with erythema and induration are not uncommon and may persist for 1–3 days. Immunotherapy is contraindicated in patients with significant cardiovascular disease or unstable asthma and should be conducted with particular caution in any patient requiring β-adrenergic blocking therapy because of the difficulty in managing an anaphylactic complication. The response to immunotherapy is derived from a complex of cellular and humoral effects that likely includes a modulation in T cell cytokine production. Immunotherapy should be reserved for clearly documented seasonal or perennial rhinitis that is clinically related to defined allergen exposure with confirmation by the presence of allergen-specific IgE. Systemic treatment with a monoclonal antibody to IgE (omalizumab) that blocks mast cell and basophil sensitization has efficacy for allergic rhinitis and can be used with immunotherapy to enhance safety and efficacy. However, current approval is only for treatment of patients with persistent allergic asthma not controlled by inhaled glucocorticoid therapy. A sequence for the management of allergic or perennial rhinitis based on an allergen-specific diagnosis and stepwise management as required for symptom control would include the following: (1) identification of the offending allergen(s) by history with confirmation of the presence of allergen-specific IgE by skin test and/or serum assay; (2) avoidance of the offending allergen; and (3) medical management in a stepwise fashion (Fig. 317-4). Mild intermittent symptoms of allergic rhinitis are treated with oral antihistamines, oral $CysLT_1$ receptor antagonists, intranasal antihistamines, or intranasal cromolyn prophylaxis. Moderate to more severe allergic rhinitis is managed with intranasal glucocorticoids plus oral antihistamines, oral $CysLT_1$ receptor antagonists, or antihistamine-decongestant combinations. Persistent allergic rhinitis requiring the daily use of intranasal glucocorticoids with add-on interventions such as oral antihistamines, decongestant combinations, or topical ipratropium merits consideration of allergen-specific immunotherapy. Even a brief course of oral prednisone can be indicated for rapid relief of severe allergic rhinitis symptoms.

FURTHER READINGS

Austen KF, Kanaoka Y: Lipids, in *The Innate Immune Response to Infection*, SHE Kaufmann et al (eds). Washington, DC, ASM Press, 2004, pp 417–431

Benoist C, Mathis D: Mast cells in autoimmune disease. Nature 420:875, 2002

Galli SJ et al: Mast cells in the development of adaptive immune responses. Nat Immunol 6:135, 2005

Kaplan AP: Urticaria, in *Allergy and Allergic Diseases*, 2nd ed, AB Kay et al (eds). Oxford, Wiley-Blackwell, 2008, pp 1853–1875

Kushnir-Sukov NM et al: Mastocytosis, in *Allergy and Allergic Diseases*, 2nd ed, AB Kay et al (eds). Oxford, Wiley-Blackwell, 2008, pp 1878–1893

Valentine MD: Insect venom allergy, in *Immunologic Diseases*, 6th ed, KF Austen et al (eds). Philadelphia, Lippincott Williams & Wilkins, 2001

CHAPTER 318

Autoimmunity and Autoimmune Diseases

Betty Diamond
Peter E. Lipsky

One of the central features of the immune system is the capacity to mount an inflammatory response to nonself while avoiding harm to self tissues. While recognition of self plays an important role in shaping the repertoires of immune receptors on both T and B cells, and in the clearance of apoptotic debris from tissues throughout the body, the development of potentially harmful immune responses to self-antigens is, in general, precluded. The essential feature of an autoimmune disease is that tissue injury is caused by the immunologic reaction of the organism against its own tissues. Autoimmunity, on the other hand, refers merely to the presence of antibodies or T lymphocytes that react with self-antigens and does not necessarily imply that the self-reactivity has pathogenic consequences. Autoimmunity is present in all individuals; however, autoimmune disease represents the end result of the breakdown of one or more of the basic mechanisms regulating immune tolerance.

Autoimmunity is seen in normal individuals and in higher frequency in normal older people. Polyreactive autoantibodies that recognize many host antigens are present throughout life. Expression of these antibodies may be increased following some inciting events. These are usually of the IgM heavy chain isotype and are encoded by nonmutated germline immunoglobulin variable region genes. When autoimmunity is induced by an inciting event, such as infection or tissue damage from trauma or ischemia, the autoreactivity is in general self-limited. Such autoimmunity may, however, be persistent, and then may or may not result in ensuing pathology. Even in the presence of organ pathology, it may be difficult to determine whether the damage is mediated by autoreactivity. Following an inciting event, the development of self-reactivity may be the consequence of an ongoing pathologic process, and be nonpathogenic, or may contribute to tissue inflammation and damage.

MECHANISMS OF AUTOIMMUNITY

Since Ehrlich first postulated the existence of mechanisms to prevent the generation of self-reactivity in 1900, ideas concerning the nature of this inhibition have developed in parallel with a progressive increase in understanding of the immune system. Burnet's clonal selection theory included the idea that interaction of lymphoid cells with their specific antigens during fetal or early postnatal life would lead to elimination of such "forbidden clones." This idea became untenable, however, when it was shown that autoimmune diseases could be induced in experimental animals by simple immunization procedures, that autoantigen-binding cells could be demonstrated easily in the circulation of normal individuals, and that self-limited autoimmune phenomena frequently developed following tissue damage from infection or trauma. These observations indicated that clones of cells capable of responding to autoantigens were present in the repertoire of antigen-reactive cells in normal adults and suggested that mechanisms in addition to clonal deletion were responsible for preventing their activation.

TABLE 318-1 Mechanisms Preventing Autoimmunity

1. Sequestration of self-antigen
2. Generation and maintenance of tolerance
   a. Central deletion of autoreactive lymphocytes
   b. Peripheral anergy of autoreactive lymphocytes
   c. Receptor replacement in autoreactive lymphocytes
3. Regulatory mechanisms

Currently, three general processes are thought to be involved in the maintenance of selective unresponsiveness to autoantigens (Table 318-1): (1) sequestration of self-antigens, rendering them inaccessible to the immune system; (2) specific unresponsiveness (tolerance or anergy) of relevant T or B cells; and (3) limitation of potential reactivity by regulatory mechanisms.

Derangements of these normal processes may predispose to the development of autoimmunity (Table 318-2). In general, these abnormal responses require an exogenous trigger such as bacterial or viral infection or cigarette smoking and require the presence of endogenous abnormalities in the cells of the immune system. Microbial superantigens, such as staphylococcal protein A and staphylococcal enterotoxins, are substances that can stimulate a broad range of T and B cells based upon specific interactions with selected families of immune receptors, irrespective of their antigen specificity. If autoantigen-reactive T and/or B cells express these receptors, autoimmunity might develop. Alternatively, molecular

TABLE 318-2 Mechanisms of Autoimmunity

I. Exogenous
   A. Molecular mimicry
   B. Superantigenic stimulation
   C. Microbial adjuvanticity
II. Endogenous
   A. Altered antigen presentation
      1. Loss of immunologic privilege
      2. Presentation of novel or cryptic epitopes (epitope spreading)
      3. Alteration of self-antigen
      4. Enhanced function of antigen-presenting cells
         a. Co-stimulatory molecule expression
         b. Cytokine production
   B. Increased T cell help
      1. Cytokine production
      2. Co-stimulatory molecules
   C. Increased B cell function
   D. Apoptotic defects
   E. Cytokine imbalance
   F. Altered immunoregulation

mimicry or cross-reactivity between a microbial product and a self-antigen might lead to activation of autoreactive lymphocytes. One of the best examples of autoreactivity and autoimmune disease resulting from molecular mimicry is rheumatic fever, in which antibodies to the M protein of streptococci cross-react with myosin, laminin, and other matrix proteins as well as neuronal antigens. Deposition of these autoantibodies in the heart initiates an inflammatory response, whereas penetration of these antibodies into the brain can result in Sydenham's chorea. Molecular mimicry between microbial proteins and host tissues has been reported in type 1 diabetes mellitus, rheumatoid arthritis, and multiple sclerosis. It is presumed that infectious agents may be able to overcome self-tolerance because they possess molecules, such as bacterial endotoxin, RNA, or DNA, that have adjuvant-like effects on the immune system that increase the immunogenicity of the microbial antigens. The adjuvants activate dendritic cells through pattern recognition receptors and stimulate the activation of previously quiescent lymphocytes that recognize both microbial and self antigen.

Endogenous derangements of the immune system may also contribute to the loss of immunologic tolerance to self-antigens and the development of autoimmunity (Table 318-2). Some autoantigens reside in immunologically privileged sites, such as the brain or the anterior chamber of the eye. These sites are characterized by the inability of engrafted tissue to elicit immune responses. Immunologic privilege results from a number of events, including the limited entry of proteins from those sites into lymphatics, the local production of immunosuppressive cytokines such as transforming growth factor β, and the local expression of molecules such as Fas ligand that can induce apoptosis of activated T cells. Lymphoid cells remain in a state of immunologic ignorance (neither activated nor anergized) to proteins expressed uniquely in immunologically privileged sites. If the privileged site is damaged by trauma or inflammation, or if T cells are activated elsewhere, proteins expressed at this site can become the targets of immunologic assault. Such an event may occur in multiple sclerosis and sympathetic ophthalmia, in which antigens uniquely expressed in the brain and eye, respectively, become the target of activated T cells.

Alterations in antigen presentation may also contribute to autoimmunity. Peptide determinants (*epitopes*) of a self antigen that are not routinely presented to lymphocytes may be recognized as a result of altered proteolytic processing of the molecule and the ensuing presentation of novel peptides (cryptic epitopes). When B cells rather than dendritic cells present self antigen, they may also present cryptic epitopes that can activate autoreactive T cells. These cryptic epitopes will not have previously been available to effect the silencing of autoreactive lymphocytes. Furthermore, once there is immunologic recognition of one protein component of a multimolecular complex, reactivity may be induced to other components of the complex following internalization and presentation of all molecules within the complex (epitope spreading). Finally, inflammation, drug exposure, or normal senescence may cause a primary chemical alteration in proteins, resulting in the generation of immune responses that cross-react with normal self-proteins. For example, the induction and/or release of protein arginine deaminase enzymes results in the conversion of arginine residues to citrullines in a variety of proteins, thereby altering their capacity to induce immune responses. Production of anticitrullinated protein antibodies has been observed in rheumatoid arthritis, chronic lung disease, as well as normal smokers and may contribute to organ pathology. Alterations in the availability and presentation of autoantigens may be important components of immunoreactivity in certain models of organ-specific autoimmune diseases. In addition, these factors may be relevant in understanding the pathogenesis of various drug-induced autoimmune conditions. However, the diversity of autoreactivity manifest in non-organ-specific systemic autoimmune diseases suggests that these conditions might result from a more general activation of the immune system rather than from an alteration in individual self-antigens.

Many autoimmune diseases are characterized by the presence of antibodies that react with apoptotic material. Defects in the clearance of apoptotic material have been shown to elicit autoimmunity and autoimmune disease in a number of animal models. Moreover, defects in the clearance of apoptotic material have been found in subjects with systemic lupus erythematosus (SLE). Apoptotic debris not quickly cleared by the immune system can function as endogenous ligands for a number of pattern recognition receptors on dendritic cells. Under such circumstances, there is activation of dendritic cells, and an immune response to apoptotic debris can develop. In addition, the presence of extracellular apoptotic material within germinal centers of secondary lymphoid organs may facilitate the direct activation of autoimmune B cell clones or function to select autoimmune B cell clones during immune responses.

A number of experimental models have suggested that intense stimulation of T lymphocytes can produce nonspecific signals that bypass the need for antigen-specific helper T cells and lead to polyclonal B cell activation with the formation of multiple autoantibodies. For example, antinuclear, antierythrocyte, and antilymphocyte antibodies are produced during the chronic graft-versus-host reaction. In addition, true autoimmune diseases, including autoimmune hemolytic anemia and immune complex–mediated glomerulonephritis, can also be induced in this manner. While it is clear that such diffuse activation of helper T cell activity can cause autoimmunity, nonspecific stimulation of B lymphocytes can also lead to the production of autoantibodies. Thus, the administration of polyclonal B cell activators, such as bacterial endotoxin, to normal mice leads to the production of a number of autoantibodies, including those directed to DNA and IgG (rheumatoid factor). Moreover, excess BAFF can also cause T cell–independent B cell activation and heavy chain class switching and the development of autoimmunity. SLE, for example, can be induced in mice through exuberant dendritic cell activation, a redundancy of TLR7 on the y chromosome (BXSByaa mice) or through exposure to CpG, a ligand for TLR 9. The ensuing induction of inflammatory mediators can cause a switch from production of nonpathogenic IgM autoantibodies to pathogenic IgG autoantibodies in the absence of antigen-specific T cell help.

Aberrant selection of the B or T cell repertoire at the time of antigen receptor expression can also predispose to autoimmunity. For example, B cell immunodeficiency caused by an absence of the B cell receptor–associated kinase, Bruton's tyrosine kinase, leads to X-linked agammaglobulinemia. This syndrome is characterized by reduced B cell activation, but also by diminished negative selection of autoreactive B cells probably caused by high levels of BAFF, resulting in increased autoreactivity within a diminished B cell repertoire. Likewise, negative selection of autoreactive T cells in the thymus requires expression of the autoimmune regulator (AIRE) gene that enables the expression of tissue-specific proteins in thymic medullary epithelial cells. Peptides from these proteins are expressed in the context of major histocompatibility complex (MHC) molecules and mediate the elimination of autoreactive T cells. The absence of AIRE gene expression leads to a failure of negative selection of autoreactive cells, autoantibody production, and severe inflammatory destruction of multiple organs. Individuals deficient in AIRE gene expression develop autoimmune polyendocrinopathy-candidiasis-ectodermal dystrophy (APECED).

Primary alterations in the activity of T and/or B cells, cytokine imbalances, or defective immunoregulatory circuits may also contribute to the emergence of autoimmunity. Diminished production of tumor necrosis factor (TNF) and interleukin (IL) 10 has been reported to be associated with the development of autoimmunity. Overproduction of type 1 interferon has also been associated with autoimmunity. Overexpression of co-stimulatory molecules on T cells similarly can lead to autoantibody production.

Autoimmunity may also result from an abnormality of immunoregulatory mechanisms. Observations made in both human autoimmune disease and animal models suggest that defects in the generation and expression of regulatory T cell activity may allow for the production of autoimmunity. It has recently been appreciated that the IPEX (immunodysregulation, polyendocrinopathy, enteropathy X-linked) syndrome results from the failure to express the FOXP3 gene, which encodes a molecule critical in the differentiation of regulatory T cells. Administration of normal regulatory T cells or factors derived from them can prevent the development of autoimmune disease in rodent models of autoimmunity. Abnormalities in the function of regulatory T cells have been noted in a number of human autoimmune diseases, although it remains uncertain whether these are causative or are secondary abnormalities owing to inflammation. Finally, recent data indicate that B cells may also exert regulatory function, largely through the production of the cytokine IL-10. Deficiency of IL-10-producing regulatory B cells can prolong the course of an animal model of multiple sclerosis.

It should be apparent that no single mechanism can explain all the varied manifestations of autoimmunity. Furthermore, genetic evaluation has shown that a number of abnormalities often need to converge to induce an autoimmune disease. Additional factors that appear to be important determinants in the induction of autoimmunity include age, sex (many autoimmune diseases are far more common in women), genetic background, exposure to infectious agents, and environmental contacts. How all of these disparate factors affect the capacity to develop self-reactivity is currently being investigated intensively.

GENETIC CONSIDERATIONS

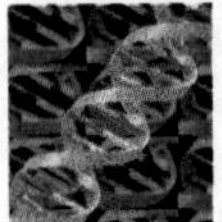

Evidence in humans that there are susceptibility genes for autoimmunity comes from family studies and especially from studies of twins. Studies in type 1 diabetes mellitus, rheumatoid arthritis, multiple sclerosis, and SLE have shown that approximately 15–30% of pairs of monozygotic twins show disease concordance, compared with <5% of dizygotic twins. The occurrence of different autoimmune diseases within the same family has suggested that certain susceptibility genes may predispose to a variety of autoimmune diseases. Genetic mapping has begun to identify chromosomal regions that predispose to specific autoimmune diseases. It is notable that some genes are associated with multiple autoimmune diseases, whereas others are more specifically associated with only one autoimmune condition. The gene encoding PTPN22 is associated with multiple autoimmune diseases. Its product is a phosphatase expressed by a variety of hematopoietic cells that downregulates antigen receptor–mediated stimulation of T and B cells. A gain-of-function polymorphism of this gene is associated with type 1 diabetes mellitus, rheumatoid arthritis, and SLE in some populations. The explanation of the association of this polymorphism with autoimmune disease is uncertain, but it is likely that it diminishes antigen receptor signaling during lymphocyte development permitting escape of autoreactive clones or decreased activation-induced apoptosis of autoantigen-reactive lymphocytes in the periphery. In recent years, genomewide association studies have demonstrated a variety of other genes that are involved in human autoimmune diseases. Most genes individually confer a relatively low risk for autoimmune diseases and are found in normal individuals. No gene has been identified that is essential for autoimmune diseases. In addition to this evidence from humans, certain inbred mouse strains reproducibly develop specific spontaneous or experimentally induced autoimmune diseases, whereas others do not. These findings have led to an extensive search for genes that determine susceptibility to autoimmune disease.

The strongest consistent association for susceptibility to autoimmune disease has been found with particular alleles of the MHC. It has been suggested that the association of MHC genotype with autoimmune disease relates to differences in the ability of different allelic variations of MHC molecules to present autoantigenic peptides to autoreactive T cells. An alternative hypothesis involves the role of MHC alleles in shaping the T cell receptor repertoire during T cell ontogeny in the thymus. Additionally, specific MHC gene products may themselves be the source of peptides that can be recognized by T cells. Cross-reactivity between such MHC peptides and peptides derived from proteins produced by common microbes may trigger autoimmunity by molecular mimicry. However, MHC genotype alone does not determine the development of autoimmunity. Identical twins are far more likely to develop the same autoimmune disease than MHC-identical nontwin siblings, suggesting that genetic factors other than the MHC also affect disease susceptibility. Recent studies of the genetics of type 1 diabetes mellitus, SLE, rheumatoid arthritis, and multiple sclerosis in humans and mice have shown that there are several independently segregating disease susceptibility loci in addition to the MHC. Genes that encode molecules of the innate immune response are also involved in autoimmunity. In humans, inherited homozygous deficiency of the early proteins of the classic pathway of complement (C1q, C4, or C2) as well as genes involved in the type 1 interferon pathway are very strongly associated with the development of SLE.

IMMUNOPATHOGENIC MECHANISMS IN AUTOIMMUNE DISEASES

The mechanisms of tissue injury in autoimmune diseases can be divided into antibody-mediated and cell-mediated processes. Representative examples are listed in Table 318-3.

The pathogenicity of autoantibodies can be mediated through several mechanisms, including opsonization of soluble factors or cells, activation of an inflammatory cascade via the complement system, and interference with the physiologic function of soluble molecules or cells.

In autoimmune thrombocytopenic purpura, opsonization of platelets targets them for elimination by phagocytes. Likewise, in autoimmune hemolytic anemia, binding of immunoglobulin to red cell membranes leads to phagocytosis and lysis of the opsonized cell. Goodpasture's syndrome, a disease characterized by lung hemorrhage and severe glomerulonephritis, represents an example of antibody binding leading to local activation of complement and neutrophil accumulation and activation. The autoantibody in this disease binds to the α_3 chain of type IV collagen in the basement membrane. In SLE, activation of the complement cascade at sites of immunoglobulin deposition in renal glomeruli is considered to be a major mechanism of renal damage. Moreover, the DNA- and RNA-containing immune complexes in SLE activate TLR 9 and 7, respectively, in dendritic cells and promote a proinflammatory, immunogenic milieu conducive to amplifying the autoimmune response.

Autoantibodies can also interfere with normal physiologic functions of cells or soluble factors. Autoantibodies against hormone receptors can lead to stimulation of cells or to inhibition of cell function through interference with receptor signaling. For example,

TABLE 318-3 Mechanisms of Tissue Damage in Autoimmune Disease

Effector	Mechanism	Target	Disease
Autoantibody	Blocking or inactivation	α Chain of the nicotinic acetylcholine receptor	Myasthenia gravis
		Phospholipid–β_2-glycoprotein 1 complex	Antiphospholipid syndrome
		Insulin receptor	Insulin-resistant diabetes mellitus
		Intrinsic factor	Pernicious anemia
	Stimulation	TSH receptor (LATS)	Graves' disease
		Proteinase-3 (ANCA)	Granulomatosis with polyangiitis (Wegener's)
		Epidermal cadherin$_1$ Desmoglein 3	Pemphigus vulgaris
	Complement activation	α_3 Chain of collagen IV	Goodpasture's syndrome
	Immune-complex formation	Double-stranded DNA	Systemic lupus erythematosus
		Ig	Rheumatoid arthritis
	Opsonization	Platelet GpIIb:IIIa	Autoimmune thrombocytopenic purpura
		Rh antigens, I antigen	Autoimmune hemolytic anemia
	Antibody-dependent cellular cytotoxicity	Thyroid peroxidase, thyroglobulin	Hashimoto's thyroiditis
T cells	Cytokine production	?	Rheumatoid arthritis, multiple sclerosis, type 1 diabetes mellitus
	Cellular cytotoxicity	?	Type 1 diabetes mellitus

Abbreviations: ANCA, antineutrophil cytoplasmic antibody; LATS, long-acting thyroid stimulator; TSH, thyroid-stimulating hormone.

long-acting thyroid stimulators, which are autoantibodies that bind to the receptor for thyroid-stimulating hormone (TSH), are present in Graves' disease and function as agonists, causing the thyroid to respond as if there were an excess of TSH. Alternatively, antibodies to the insulin receptor can cause insulin-resistant diabetes mellitus through receptor blockade. In myasthenia gravis, autoantibodies to the acetylcholine receptor can be detected in 85–90% of patients and are responsible for muscle weakness. The exact location of the antigenic epitope, the valence and affinity of the antibody, and perhaps other characteristics determine whether activation or blockade results from antibody binding.

Antiphospholipid antibodies are associated with thromboembolic events in primary and secondary antiphospholipid syndrome and have also been associated with fetal wastage. The major antibody is directed to the phospholipid–β_2-glycoprotein I complex and appears to exert a procoagulant effect. In pemphigus vulgaris, autoantibodies bind to a component of the epidermal cell desmosome, desmoglein 3, and play a role in the induction of the disease. They exert their pathologic effect by disrupting cell-cell junctions through stimulation of the production of epithelial proteases, leading to blister formation. Cytoplasmic antineutrophil cytoplasmic antibody (c-ANCA), found in granulomatosis with polyangiitis (Wegener's), is an antibody to an intracellular antigen, the 29-kDa serine protease (proteinase-3). In vitro experiments have shown that IgG anti-c-ANCA causes cellular activation and degranulation of primed neutrophils.

It is important to note that autoantibodies of a given specificity may cause disease only in genetically susceptible hosts, as has been shown in experimental models of myasthenia gravis, SLE, rheumatic fever and rheumatoid arthritis. It is also important to be aware that once organ damage is initiated, new inflammatory cascades are initiated that can sustain and amplify the autoimmune process. Finally, some autoantibodies seem to be markers for disease but have as yet no known pathogenic potential.

■ AUTOIMMUNE DISEASES

Manifestations of autoimmunity are found in a large number of pathologic conditions. However, their presence does not necessarily imply that the pathologic process is an autoimmune disease. A number of attempts to establish formal criteria for the diagnosis of autoimmune diseases have been made, but none is universally accepted. One set of criteria is shown in Table 318-4; however, this should be viewed merely as a guide in consideration of the problem.

To classify a disease as autoimmune, it is necessary to demonstrate that the immune response to a self-antigen causes the observed pathology. Initially, the demonstration that antibodies against the affected tissue could be detected in the serum of patients suffering from various diseases was taken as evidence that these diseases had an autoimmune basis. However, such autoantibodies are also found when tissue damage is caused by trauma or infection, and the autoantibody is secondary to tissue damage. Thus, it is necessary to show that autoimmunity is pathogenic before classifying a disease as autoimmune.

If the autoantibodies are pathogenic, it may be possible to transfer disease to experimental animals by the administration of autoantibodies, with the subsequent development of pathology in the recipient similar to that seen in the patient from whom the antibodies were obtained. This has been shown, for example, in Graves' disease. Some autoimmune diseases can be transferred from mother to fetus and are observed in the newborn babies of diseased mothers. The symptoms of the disease in the newborn

TABLE 318-4 Human Autoimmune Disease: Presumptive Evidence for an Immunologic Pathogenesis

Major Criteria

1. Presence of autoantibodies or evidence of cellular reactivity to self
2. Documentation of relevant autoantibody or lymphocytic infiltrate in the pathologic lesion
3. Demonstration that relevant autoantibody or T cells can cause tissue pathology
   a. Transplacental transmission
   b. Adaptive transfer into animals
   c. In vitro impact on cellular function

Supportive Evidence

1. Reasonable animal model
2. Beneficial effect from immunosuppressive agents
3. Association with other evidence of autoimmunity
4. No evidence of infection or other obvious cause

TABLE 318-5 Some Autoimmune Diseases

Organ Specific	
Graves' disease	Vitiligo
Hashimoto's thyroiditis	Autoimmune hemolytic anemia
Autoimmune polyglandular syndrome	Autoimmune thrombocytopenic purpura
Type 1 diabetes mellitus	Pernicious anemia
Insulin-resistant diabetes mellitus	Myasthenia gravis
Immune-mediated infertility	Multiple sclerosis
Autoimmune Addison's disease	Guillain-Barré syndrome
Pemphigus vulgaris	Stiff-man syndrome
Pemphigus foliaceus	Acute rheumatic fever
Dermatitis herpetiformis	Sympathetic ophthalmia
Autoimmune alopecia	Goodpasture's syndrome
Organ Nonspecific (Systemic)	
Systemic lupus erythematosus	Granulomatosis with polyangiitis (Wegener's)
Rheumatoid arthritis	Antiphospholipid syndrome
Systemic necrotizing vasculitis	Sjögren's syndrome

usually disappear as the levels of the maternal antibody decrease. An exception, however, is congenital heart block, in which damage to the developing conducting system of the heart follows in utero transfer of anti-Ro antibody from the mother to the fetus. This can result in a permanent developmental defect in the heart.

In most situations, the critical factors that determine when the development of autoimmunity results in autoimmune disease have not been delineated. The relationship of autoimmunity to the development of autoimmune disease may relate to the fine specificity of the antibodies or T cells or their specific effector capabilities. In many circumstances, a mechanistic understanding of the pathogenic potential of autoantibodies has not been established. In some autoimmune diseases, biased production of cytokines by helper T (T_H) cells may play a role in pathogenesis. In this regard, T cells can differentiate into specialized effector cells that predominantly produce interferon γ (T_H1), IL-4 (T_H2), IL-17 (T_H17) or provide help to B cells (T follicular helper, T_{FH}) (Chap. 314). T_H1 cells facilitate macrophage activation and classic cell-mediated immunity, whereas T_H2 cells are thought to have regulatory functions and are involved in the resolution of normal immune responses and also the development of responses to a variety of parasites; T_H17 cells produce a number of inflammatory cytokines, including IL-17 and IL-22, and T_{FH} cells help B cells by constitutively producing IL-21. In a number of autoimmune diseases, such as rheumatoid arthritis, multiple sclerosis, type 1 diabetes mellitus, and Crohn's disease, there appears to be biased differentiation of T_H1 cells, with resultant organ damage. More recently, studies suggest accentuated differentiation of T_H17 cells associated with animal models of inflammatory arthritis and also rheumatoid arthritis, whereas increased differentiation of T_{FH} cells has been associated with animal models of SLE.

■ ORGAN-SPECIFIC VERSUS SYSTEMIC AUTOIMMUNE DISEASES

Autoimmune diseases form a spectrum, from those specifically affecting a single organ to systemic disorders with involvement of many organs (Table 318-5). Hashimoto's autoimmune thyroiditis is an example of an organ-specific autoimmune disease (Chap. 341). In this disorder, there is a specific lesion in the thyroid associated with infiltration of mononuclear cells and damage to follicular cells. Antibody to thyroid constituents can be demonstrated in nearly all cases. Other organ- or tissue-specific autoimmune disorders include pemphigus vulgaris, autoimmune hemolytic anemia, idiopathic thrombocytopenic purpura, Goodpasture's syndrome, myasthenia gravis, and sympathetic ophthalmia. One important feature of some organ-specific autoimmune diseases is the tendency for overlap, such that an individual with one specific syndrome is more likely to develop a second syndrome. For example, there is a high incidence of pernicious anemia in individuals with autoimmune thyroiditis. More striking is the tendency for individuals with an organ-specific autoimmune disease to develop multiple other manifestations of autoimmunity without the development of associated organ pathology. Thus, as many as 50% of individuals with pernicious anemia have non-cross-reacting antibodies to thyroid constituents, whereas patients with myasthenia gravis may develop antinuclear antibodies, antithyroid antibodies, rheumatoid factor, antilymphocyte antibodies, and polyclonal hypergammaglobulinemia. Part of the explanation for this may relate to the genetic elements shared by individuals with these different diseases.

Systemic autoimmune diseases differ from organ-specific diseases in that pathologic lesions are found in multiple diverse organs and tissues. The hallmark of these conditions is the demonstration of associated relevant autoimmune manifestations that are likely to be etiologic in the organ pathology. SLE represents the prototype of these disorders because of its abundance of autoimmune manifestations.

SLE is a disease of protean manifestations that characteristically involves the kidneys, joints, skin, serosal surfaces, blood vessels, and central nervous system (Chap. 319). The disease is associated with a vast array of autoantibodies whose production appears to be a part of a generalized hyperreactivity of the humoral immune system. Other features of SLE include generalized B cell hyperresponsiveness and polyclonal hypergammaglobulinemia. Current evidence suggests that both hypo- and hyperresponsiveness to antigen can lead to survival and activation of autoreactive B cells in SLE.

TREATMENT Autoimmune Diseases

Treatment of autoimmune diseases can focus on either suppressing the induction of autoimmunity, restoring normal regulatory mechanisms, or inhibiting the effector mechanisms. To eliminate autoreactive cells, immunosuppressive or ablative therapies are most commonly used. In recent years, cytokine blockade has been demonstrated to be effective in preventing immune activation in some diseases. New therapies have also been developed to target lymphoid cells more specifically, either by blocking a co-stimulatory signal needed for T or B cell activation, by blocking the migratory capacity of lymphocytes, or by eliminating the effector T cells or B cells. The efficacy of these therapies is not yet demonstrated. Newer trials are testing the possibility of using autoantigen itself to induce tolerance. One major advance in inhibiting effector mechanisms has been the introduction of cytokine blockade, targeting TNF or IL-1, that appears to limit organ damage in some diseases. Biologicals that interface with T cell activation (CTLA-4Ig) or delete B cells (anti-CD20 antibody) have also recently been approved for the treatment of rheumatoid arthritis. Therapies that prevent target organ damage or support target organ function remain an important therapeutic approach to autoimmune disease.

FURTHER READINGS

Annunziato F et al: Type 17 T helper cells—Origins, features and possible roles in rheumatic disease. Nat Rev 5:325, 2009

Baechler EC et al: Gene expression profiling in human autoimmunity. Immunol Rev 210:120, 2006

Drexler SK, Foxwell BM: The role of Toll-like receptors in chronic inflammation. Int J Biochem Cell Biol 42:506, 2010

Fujinami RS et al: Molecular mimicry, bystander activation, or viral persistence: Infections and autoimmune disease. Clin Microbiol Rev 19:80, 2006

Gauld SB et al: Silencing of autoreactive B cells by anergy: A fresh perspective. Curr Opin Immunol 18:292, 2006

Mackay IR: Clustering and commonalities among autoimmune diseases. J Autoimmun 33:170, 2009

Maier LM, Hafler DA: Autoimmunity risk alleles in costimulation pathways. Immunol Rev 229:322, 2009

Pisetsky DS: The role of innate immunity in the induction of autoimmunity. Autoimmun Rev 8:69, 2008

Podojil JR, Miller SD: Molecular mechanisms of T-cell receptor and costimulatory molecule ligation/blockade in autoimmune disease therapy. Immunol Rev 229:337, 2009

Rosen A, Casciola-Rosen L: Autoantigens in systemic autoimmunity: Critical partner in pathogenesis. J Intern Med 265:625, 2009

CHAPTER 319

Systemic Lupus Erythematosus

Bevra Hannahs Hahn

DEFINITION AND PREVALENCE

Systemic lupus erythematosus (SLE) is an autoimmune disease in which organs and cells undergo damage initially mediated by tissue-binding autoantibodies and immune complexes. In most patients, autoantibodies are present for a few years before the first clinical symptom appears; clinical manifestations are heterogeneous. Ninety percent of patients at diagnosis are women of childbearing years; people of all genders, ages, and ethnic groups are susceptible. Prevalence of SLE in the United States is 10 to 400 per 100,000 depending on race and gender; highest prevalence is in black women and lowest is in white men.

PATHOGENESIS AND ETIOLOGY

The proposed pathogenic mechanisms of SLE are illustrated in Fig. 319-1. Interactions between susceptibility genes and environmental factors result in abnormal immune responses, which vary among different patients. Those responses may include (1) activation of innate immunity (dendritic cells, monocyte/macrophages) by CpG DNA, DNA in immune complexes, viral RNA, and RNA in RNA/protein self-antigens; (2) lowered activation thresholds and abnormal activation pathways in adaptive immunity cells (T and B lymphocytes); (3) ineffective regulatory CD4+ and CD8+ T cells; and (4) reduced clearance of immune complexes and of apoptotic cells. Self-antigens (nucleosomal DNA/protein; RNA/protein in Sm, Ro, and La; phospholipids) are available for recognition by the immune system in surface blebs of apoptotic cells; thus antigens, autoantibodies, and immune complexes persist for prolonged periods of time, allowing inflammation and disease to develop. Immune cell activation is accompanied by increased secretion of proinflammatory type 1 and 2 interferons (IFNs), tumor necrosis factor α (TNF-α), interleukin (IL)-17 and B cell–maturation/survival cytokines B lymphocyte stimulator (BLyS/BAFF), and IL-10. Upregulation of genes induced by interferons is a genetic "signature" in peripheral blood cells of SLE in approximately 50% of patients. Decreased production of other cytokines also contributes to SLE: Lupus T and natural killer (NK) cells fail to produce enough IL-2 and transforming growth factor β (TGF-β) to induce and sustain regulatory CD4+ and CD8+ T cells. The result of these abnormalities is sustained production of autoantibodies (referred to in Fig. 319-1 and described in Table 319-1) and immune complexes; pathogenic subsets bind target tissues, with activation of complement, leading to release of cytokines, chemokines, vasoactive peptides, oxidants, and destructive enzymes. This is accompanied by influx into target tissues of T cells, monocyte/macrophages, and dendritic cells, as well as activation of resident macrophages and dendritic cells. In the setting of chronic inflammation, accumulation of growth factors and products of chronic oxidation contribute to irreversible tissue damage, including fibrosis/sclerosis, in glomeruli, arteries, brain, lungs, and other tissues.

SLE is a multigenic disease. Rare single-gene defects confer high hazard ratios (HR) for SLE (5–25), including homozygous deficiencies of early components of complement (C1q,r,s; C2; C4) and a mutation in TREX1 on the X chromosome. In most genetically susceptible individuals, normal alleles of multiple genes each contribute a small amount to abnormal immune/inflammation/tissue

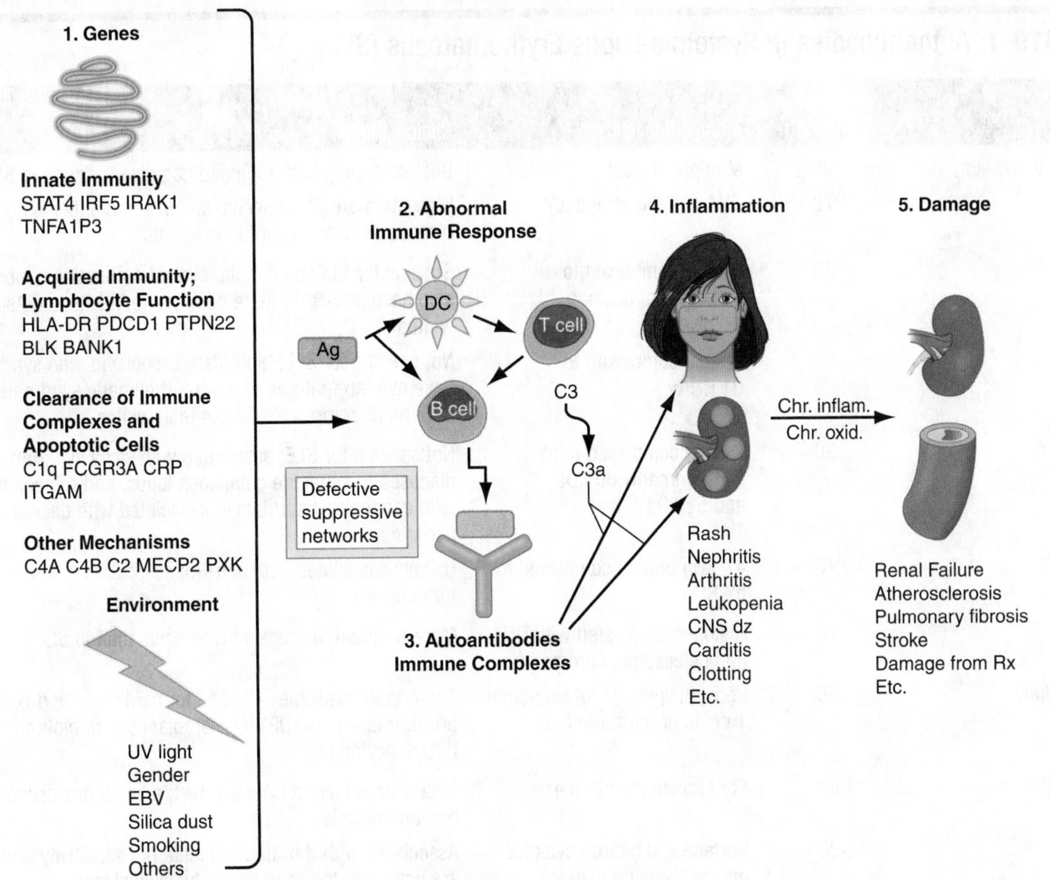

Figure 319-1 Pathogenesis of SLE. Genes confirmed in more than one genome-wide association analysis in Northern European whites as increasing susceptibility to SLE or lupus nephritis are listed (reviewed in Moser KL et al, Recent insights into the genetic basis of SLE. Genes Immun 2009:10:373). Gene-environment interactions result in abnormal immune responses that generate pathogenic autoantibodies and immune complexes that deposit in tissue, activate complement, cause inflammation, and over time lead to irreversible organ damage. Ag, antigen; C1q, complement system; C3, complement component; CNS, central nervous system; DC, dendritic cell; EBV, Epstein-Barr virus; HLA, human leukocyte antigen; FcR, immunoglobulin Fc-binding receptor; IL, interleukin; MCP, monocyte chemotactic protein; PTPN, phosphotyrosine phosphatase; UV, ultraviolet.

damage responses; if enough predisposing variations are present, disease results. Thirty to forty predisposing genes (examples listed in Fig 319-1) have been identified in recent genome-wide association studies in thousands of Northern European white patients and controls. They confer HR for SLE of 1.5–3. Such relatively weak gene polymorphisms that increase risk for SLE can be classified by their potential role in pathogenesis. Predisposing, antigen-presenting human leukocyte antigen (HLA)-molecules are most commonly found, in multiple ethnic groups (HLA DRB1 *0301 and *1501, as well as multiple genes across the 120-gene region). Other genetic factors in whites include innate immunity pathway gene polymorphisms, especially associated with interferon alpha (STAT4, IRF5, IRAK1. TNFAIP3, PTPN22), genes in lymphocyte signaling pathways (PTPN22, PDCD-1, Ox40L, BANK-1, LYN, BLK), genes that affect clearance of apoptotic cells or immune complexes (C1q, FCRG IIA and IIIA, CRP, ITGAM), and genes that influence neutrophil adherence (ITGAM), and endothelial cell function (TREX-1). Some polymorphisms influence clinical manifestations; such as single nucleotide polymorphisms (SNPs) of STAT 4 that associate with severe disease, anti-DNA, nephritis, and anti-phospholipid syndrome (Chap. 320), and an allele of FCGRIIA encoding a receptor that binds immune complexes poorly and predisposes to nephritis. Some gene effects are in promoter regions (e.g., IL-10) and others are conferred by copy numbers (e.g., C4A). In addition to genome-encoded susceptibility and protective genes, the influence of certain micro (mi) RNAs on gene transcription, as well as posttranscriptional epigenetic modification of DNA, which is hypomethylated in SLE, also contribute to disease susceptibility.

Some gene polymorphisms contribute to several autoimmune diseases, such as STAT4 and CTLA4. All these gene polymorphisms/transcription/epigenetic combinations influence immune responses to the external and internal environment; when such responses are too high and/or too prolonged and/or inadequately regulated, autoimmune disease results.

Female sex is permissive for SLE with evidence for hormone effects, genes on the X chromosome, and epigenetic differences between genders playing a role. Females of many mammalian species make higher antibody responses than males. Women exposed to estrogen-containing oral contraceptives or hormone replacement have an increased risk of developing SLE (1.2–2-fold). Estradiol binds to receptors on T and B lymphocytes, increasing activation and survival of those cells, thus favoring prolonged immune responses. Genes on the X chromosome that influence SLE, such as TREX-1, may play a role in gender predisposition—possibly because some genes on the second X in females are not silent. People with XXY karyotype (Klinefelter's syndrome) have a significantly increased risk for SLE.

Several environmental stimuli may influence SLE (Fig. 319-1). Exposure to ultraviolet light causes flares of SLE in approximately 70% of patients, possibly by increasing apoptosis in skin cells or by

TABLE 319-1 Autoantibodies in Systemic Lupus Erythematosus (SLE)

Antibody	Prevalence, %	Antigen Recognized	Clinical Utility
Antinuclear antibodies	98	Multiple nuclear	Best screening test; repeated negative tests make SLE unlikely
Anti-dsDNA	70	DNA (double-stranded)	High titers are SLE-specific and in some patients correlate with disease activity, nephritis, vasculitis
Anti-Sm	25	Protein complexed to 6 species of nuclear U1 RNA	Specific for SLE; no definite clinical correlations; most patients also have anti-RNP; more common in blacks and Asians than whites
Anti-RNP	40	Protein complexed to U1 RNAγ	Not specific for SLE; high titers associated with syndromes that have overlap features of several rheumatic syndromes including SLE; more common in blacks than whites
Anti-Ro (SS-A)	30	Protein complexed to hY RNA, primarily 60 kDa and 52 kDa	Not specific for SLE; associated with sicca syndrome, predisposes to subacute cutaneous lupus, and to neonatal lupus with congenital heart block; associated with decreased risk for nephritis
Anti-La (SS-B)	10	47-kDa protein complexed to hY RNA	Usually associated with anti-Ro; associated with decreased risk for nephritis
Antihistone	70	Histones associated with DNA (in nucleosome, chromatin)	More frequent in drug-induced lupus than in SLE
Antiphospholipid	50	Phospholipids, β_2 glycoprotein 1 cofactor, prothrombin	Three tests available—ELISAs for cardiolipin and β_2G1, sensitive prothrombin time (DRVVT); predisposes to clotting, fetal loss, thrombocytopenia
Antierythrocyte	60	Erythrocyte membrane	Measured as direct Coombs' test; a small proportion develops overt hemolysis
Antiplatelet	30	Surface and altered cytoplasmic antigens on platelets	Associated with thrombocytopenia but sensitivity and specificity are not good; this is not a useful clinical test
Antineuronal (includes anti-glutamate receptor)	60	Neuronal and lymphocyte surface antigens	In some series a positive test in CSF correlates with active CNS lupus.
Antiribosomal P	20	Protein in ribosomes	In some series a positive test in serum correlates with depression or psychosis due to CNS lupus

Abbreviations: CNS, central nervous system; CSF, cerebrospinal fluid; DRVVT, dilute Russell viper venom time; ELISA, enzyme-linked immunosorbent assay.

altering DNA and intracellular proteins to make them antigenic. It is likely that some infections induce a normal immune response that matures to contain some T and B cells that recognize self-antigens; such cells are not appropriately regulated, and autoantibody production occurs. Most SLE patients have autoantibodies for 3 years or more before the first symptoms of disease, suggesting that regulation controls the degree of autoimmunity for years before quantities and qualities of autoantibodies and pathogenic B and T cells cause clinical disease. Epstein-Barr virus (EBV) may be one infectious agent that can trigger SLE in susceptible individuals. Children and adults with SLE are more likely to be infected by EBV than age-, sex-, and ethnicity-matched controls. EBV contains amino acid sequences that mimic sequences on human spliceosomes (RNA/protein antigens) often recognized by autoantibodies in people with SLE. Current tobacco smoking increases risk for SLE [odds ratio (OR) 1.5]. Prolonged occupational exposure to silica (e.g., inhalation of soap powder dust) increases risk (OR 4.3) in black women. Thus, interplay between genetic susceptibility, environment, gender, and abnormal immune responses results in autoimmunity (Chap. 318).

PATHOLOGY

In SLE, biopsies of affected skin show deposition of Ig at the dermal-epidermal junction (DEJ), injury to basal keratinocytes, and inflammation dominated by T lymphocytes in the DEJ and around blood vessels and dermal appendages. Clinically unaffected skin may also show Ig deposition at the DEJ.

In renal biopsies, the pattern and severity of injury are important in diagnosis and in selecting the best therapy. Many clinical studies of lupus nephritis have used the World Health Organization (WHO) classification of lupus nephritis. However, the International Society of Nephrology (ISN) and the Renal Pathology Society (RPS) have published a newer, similar classification (Table 319-2) that is replacing WHO standards. An advantage of the ISN/RPS classification is the addition of "a" for active and "c" for chronic changes, giving the physician information regarding the potential reversibility of disease. All the classification systems focus on glomerular disease, although the presence of tubular interstitial and vascular disease is important to clinical outcomes. In general, class III and IV disease, as well as class V accompanied by III or IV disease, should be treated with aggressive immunosuppression if possible, because there is a high risk for end-stage renal disease (ESRD) if patients are untreated or undertreated. Treatment for lupus nephritis is not recommended in patients with class I or II disease or with extensive irreversible changes. In children, a diagnosis of SLE can be established on the basis of renal histology without meeting additional diagnostic criteria (Table 319-3).

Histologic abnormalities in blood vessels may also determine therapy. Patterns of vasculitis are not specific for SLE but may

TABLE 319-2 Classification of Lupus Nephritis (International Society of Nephrology and Renal Pathology Society)

Class I: Minimal Mesangial Lupus Nephritis
Normal glomeruli by light microscopy, but mesangial immune deposits by immunofluorescence.
Class II: Mesangial Proliferative Lupus Nephritis
Purely mesangial hypercellularity of any degree or mesangial matrix expansion by light microscopy, with mesangial immune deposits. A few isolated subepithelial or subendothelial deposits may be visible by immunofluorescence or electron microscopy, but not by light microscopy.
Class III: Focal Lupus Nephritis
Active or inactive focal, segmental or global endo- or extracapillary glomerulonephritis involving <50% of all glomeruli, typically with focal subendothelial immune deposits, with or without mesangial alterations.
Class III (A): Active lesions—focal proliferative lupus nephritis
Class III (A/C): Active and chronic lesions—focal proliferative and sclerosing lupus nephritis
Class III (C): Chronic inactive lesions with glomerular scars—focal sclerosing lupus nephritis
Class IV: Diffuse Lupus Nephritis
Active or inactive diffuse, segmental or global endo- or extracapillary glomerulonephritis involving ≥50% of all glomeruli, typically with diffuse subendothelial immune deposits, with or without mesangial alterations. This class is divided into diffuse segmental (IV-S) lupus nephritis when √50% of the involved glomeruli have segmental lesions, and diffuse global (IV-G) lupus nephritis when ≥50% of the involved glomeruli have global lesions. Segmental is defined as a glomerular lesion that involves less than one-half of the glomerular tuft. This class includes cases with diffuse wire loop deposits but with little or no glomerular proliferation.
Class IV-S (A): Active lesions—diffuse segmental proliferative lupus nephritis
Class IV-G (A): Active lesions—diffuse global proliferative lupus nephritis
Class IV-S (A/C): Active and chronic lesions—diffuse segmental proliferative and sclerosing lupus nephritis
Class IV-G (A/C): Active and chronic lesions—diffuse global proliferative and sclerosing lupus nephritis
Class IV-S (C): Chronic inactive lesions with scars—diffuse segmental sclerosing lupus nephritis
Class IV-G (C): Chronic inactive lesions with scars—diffuse global sclerosing lupus nephritis
Class V: Membranous Lupus Nephritis
Global or segmental subepithelial immune deposits or their morphologic sequelae by light microscopy and by immunofluorescence or electron microscopy, with or without mesangial alterations. Class V lupus nephritis may occur in combination with class III or IV, in which case both will be diagnosed. Class V lupus nephritis may show advanced sclerosis.
Class VI: Advanced Sclerotic Lupus Nephritis
≥90% of glomeruli globally sclerosed without residual activity.

Note: Indicate and grade (mild, moderate, severe) tubular atrophy, interstitial inflammation and fibrosis, severity of arteriosclerosis or other vascular lesions.
Source: JJ Weening et al: Kidney Int 65:521, 2004. Reprinted by permission from Macmillan Publishers Ltd., Copyright 2004.

indicate active disease: leukocytoclastic vasculitis is most common (Chap. 326).

Lymph node biopsies are usually performed to rule out infection or malignancies. In SLE, they show nonspecific diffuse chronic inflammation.

DIAGNOSIS

The diagnosis of SLE is based on characteristic clinical features and autoantibodies. Current criteria for classification are listed in Table 319-3, and an algorithm for diagnosis and initial therapy is shown in Fig. 319-2. The criteria are intended for confirming the diagnosis of SLE in patients included in studies; the author uses them in individual patients for estimating the probability that a disease is SLE. Any combination of ≥4 of 11 criteria, well documented at any time during an individual's history, makes it likely that the patient has SLE. (Specificity and sensitivity are ~95% and ~75%, respectively.) In many patients, criteria accrue over time. Antinuclear antibodies (ANA) are positive in >98% of patients during the course of disease; repeated negative tests suggest that the diagnosis is not SLE, unless other autoantibodies are present (Fig. 319-2). High-titer IgG antibodies to double-stranded DNA and antibodies to the Sm antigen are both specific for SLE and, therefore, favor the diagnosis in the presence of compatible clinical manifestations. The presence in an individual of multiple autoantibodies without clinical symptoms should not be considered diagnostic for SLE, although such persons are at increased risk.

INTERPRETATION OF CLINICAL MANIFESTATIONS

When a diagnosis of SLE is made, it is important to establish the severity and potential reversibility of the illness and to estimate the possible consequences of various therapeutic interventions. In the following sections, descriptions of some disease manifestations begin with relatively mild problems and progress to those more life-threatening.

OVERVIEW AND SYSTEMIC MANIFESTATIONS

At its onset, SLE may involve one or several organ systems; over time, additional manifestations may occur (Tables 319-3 and 319-4). Most of the autoantibodies characteristic of each person are

TABLE 319-3 Diagnostic Criteria for Systemic Lupus Erythematosus

Malar rash	Fixed erythema, flat or raised, over the malar eminences
Discoid rash	Erythematous circular raised patches with adherent keratotic scaling and follicular plugging; atrophic scarring may occur
Photosensitivity	Exposure to ultraviolet light causes rash
Oral ulcers	Includes oral and nasopharyngeal ulcers, observed by physician
Arthritis	Nonerosive arthritis of two or more peripheral joints, with tenderness, swelling, or effusion
Serositis	Pleuritis or pericarditis documented by ECG or rub or evidence of effusion
Renal disorder	Proteinuria >0.5 g/d or $\sqrt{3}$+, or cellular casts
Neurologic disorder	Seizures or psychosis without other causes
Hematologic disorder	Hemolytic anemia or leukopenia (<4000/μL) or lymphopenia (<1500/μL) or thrombocytopenia (<100,000/μL) in the absence of offending drugs
Immunologic disorder	Anti-dsDNA, anti-Sm, and/or anti-phospholipid
Antinuclear antibodies	An abnormal titer of ANA by immunofluorescence or an equivalent assay at any point in time in the absence of drugs known to induce ANAs

If ≥4 of these criteria, well documented, are present at any time in a patient's history, the diagnosis is likely to be SLE. Specificity is ~95%; sensitivity is ~75%.
Abbreviations: ANA, antinuclear antibodies; dsDNA, double-strand DNA; ECG, electrocardiography.
Source: Criteria published by EM Tan et al: Arthritis Rheum 25:1271, 1982; update by MC Hochberg, Arthritis Rheum 40:1725, 1997.

present at the time clinical manifestations appear (Tables 319-1 and 319-3). Severity of SLE varies from mild and intermittent to severe and fulminant. Most patients experience exacerbations interspersed with periods of relative quiescence; permanent complete remissions (absence of symptoms with no treatment) are rare. Systemic symptoms, particularly fatigue and myalgias/arthralgias, are present most of the time. Severe systemic illness requiring glucocorticoid therapy can occur with fever, prostration, weight loss, and anemia with or without other organ-targeted manifestations.

■ MUSCULOSKELETAL MANIFESTATIONS

Most people with SLE have intermittent polyarthritis, varying from mild to disabling, characterized by soft tissue swelling and tenderness in joints, most commonly in hands, wrists, and knees. Joint deformities (hands and feet) develop in only 10% of patients. Erosions on joint x-rays are rare; their presence suggests a non-lupus inflammatory arthropathy such as rheumatoid arthritis (Chap. 321); some experts think that erosions can occur in SLE. If pain persists in a single joint, such as knee, shoulder, or hip, a diagnosis of ischemic necrosis of bone should be considered, particularly if there are no other manifestations of active SLE. The prevalence of ischemic necrosis of bone is increased in SLE, especially in patients treated with systemic glucocorticoids. Myositis with clinical muscle weakness, elevated creatine kinase levels, positive MRI scan, and muscle necrosis and inflammation on biopsy can occur, although most patients have myalgias without frank myositis. Glucocorticoid therapies (commonly) and antimalarial therapies (rarely) can also cause muscle weakness; these adverse effects must be distinguished from active disease.

■ CUTANEOUS MANIFESTATIONS

Lupus dermatitis can be classified as discoid lupus erythematosus (DLE), systemic rash, subacute cutaneous lupus erythematosus (SCLE), or "other." Discoid lesions are roughly circular with slightly raised, scaly hyperpigmented erythematous rims and depigmented, atrophic centers in which all dermal appendages are permanently destroyed. Lesions can be disfiguring, particularly on the face and scalp. Treatment consists primarily of topical or locally injected glucocorticoids and systemic antimalarials. Only 5% of people with DLE have SLE (although one-half have positive ANA); however, among individuals with SLE, as many as 20% have DLE. The most common SLE rash is a photosensitive, slightly raised erythema, occasionally scaly, on the face (particularly the cheeks and nose—the "butterfly" rash), ears, chin, V region of the neck and chest, upper back, and extensor surfaces of the arms. Worsening of this rash often accompanies flare of systemic disease. SCLE consists of scaly red patches similar to psoriasis, or circular flat red-rimmed lesions. Patients with these manifestations are exquisitely photosensitive; most have antibodies to Ro (SS-A). Other SLE rashes include recurring urticaria, lichen planus–like dermatitis, bullae, and panniculitis ("lupus profundus"). Rashes can be minor or severe; they may be the major disease manifestation. Small, painful ulcerations on the oral or nasal mucosa are common in SLE; the lesions resemble aphthous ulcers.

■ RENAL MANIFESTATIONS

Nephritis is usually the most serious manifestation of SLE, particularly since nephritis and infection are the leading causes of mortality in the first decade of disease. Since nephritis is asymptomatic in most lupus patients, urinalysis should be ordered in any person suspected of having SLE. The classification of lupus nephritis is primarily histologic (see "Pathology," above, and Table 319-2). Renal biopsy is useful in planning current and near-future therapies. Patients with dangerous proliferative forms of glomerular damage (ISN III and IV) usually have microscopic hematuria and proteinuria (>500 mg per 24 h); approximately one-half develop nephrotic syndrome, and most develop hypertension. If diffuse proliferative glomerulonephritis (DPGN) is untreated, virtually all patients develop ESRD within 2 years of diagnosis. Therefore, aggressive immunosuppression is indicated (usually systemic glucocorticoids plus a cytotoxic drug), unless 90% of glomeruli have irreversible damage (Fig. 319-2, Table 319-5). Blacks are more likely to develop ESRD than are whites, even with the most current therapies. Overall in the United States, ~20% of individuals with lupus DPGN die or develop ESRD within 10 years of diagnosis. Such individuals require aggressive control of SLE and of the complications of renal disease and of therapy. A small proportion of SLE patients with proteinuria (usually nephrotic) have membranous glomerular changes without proliferation on renal biopsy. Their outcome is better than for those with DPGN. Lupus nephritis tends to be an ongoing disease, with flares requiring retreatment or intensification of treatment over many years. For most people with lupus nephritis, accelerated atherosclerosis becomes important after several years of disease; attention must be given to control of systemic inflammation, blood pressure, hyperlipidemia, and hyperglycemia.

■ NERVOUS SYSTEM MANIFESTATIONS

There are many central nervous system (CNS) and peripheral nervous system manifestations of SLE; in some patients these are the major cause of morbidity and mortality. It is useful to approach

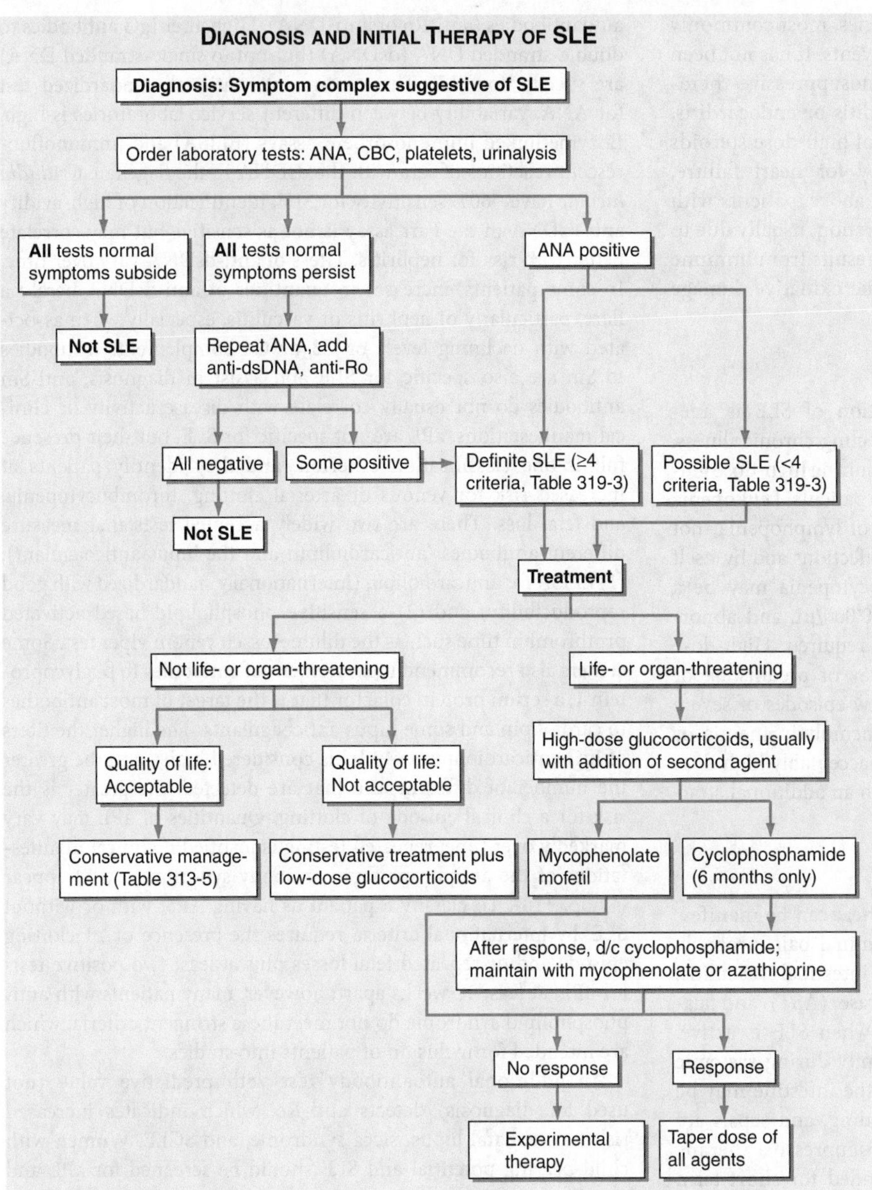

Figure 319-2 Algorithm for diagnosis and initial therapy of SLE. ANA, antinuclear antibodies; CBC, complete blood count.

this diagnostically by asking first whether the symptoms result from SLE or another condition (such as infection in immunosuppressed individuals). If symptoms are related to SLE, it should be determined whether they are caused by a diffuse process (requiring immunosuppression) or vascular occlusive disease (requiring anticoagulation). The most common manifestation of diffuse CNS lupus is cognitive dysfunction, including difficulties with memory and reasoning. Headaches are also common. When excruciating, they often indicate SLE flare; when milder, they are difficult to distinguish from migraine or tension headaches. Seizures of any type may be caused by lupus; treatment often requires both antiseizure and immunosuppressive therapies. Psychosis can be the dominant manifestation of SLE; it must be distinguished from glucocorticoid-induced psychosis. The latter usually occurs in the first weeks of glucocorticoid therapy, at daily doses of ≥40 mg of prednisone or equivalent; psychosis resolves over several days after glucocorticoids are decreased or stopped. Myelopathy is not rare and is often disabling; rapid immunosuppressive therapy starting with glucocorticoids is standard of care.

VASCULAR OCCLUSIONS

The prevalence of transient ischemic attacks, strokes, and myocardial infarctions is increased in patients with SLE. These vascular events are increased in, but not exclusive to, SLE patients with antibodies to phospholipids (aPL). Antiphospholipid antibodies are associated with hypercoagulability and acute thrombotic events, whereas chronic disease is associated with accelerated atherosclerosis (Chap. 320). Ischemia in the brain can be caused by focal occlusion (either noninflammatory or associated with vasculitis) or by embolization from carotid artery plaque or from fibrinous vegetations of Libman-Sacks endocarditis. Appropriate tests for aPL (see below) and for sources of emboli should be ordered in such patients to estimate the need for, intensity of, and duration of anti-inflammatory and/or anticoagulant therapies. In SLE, myocardial infarctions are primarily manifestations of accelerated atherosclerosis. The increased risk for vascular events is seven- to tenfold overall, and higher in women <45 years old with SLE. Characteristics associated with increased risk for atherosclerosis include older age, hypertension, dyslipidemia, dysfunctional proinflammatory high-density lipoproteins, repeated high scores for disease activity, high cumulative or daily doses of glucocorticoids, and high levels of homocysteine. When it is most likely that an event results from clotting, long-term anticoagulation is the therapy of choice. Two processes can occur at once—vasculitis plus bland vascular occlusions—in which case it is appropriate to treat with anticoagulation plus immunosuppression. Statin therapies reduce levels of low-density lipoproteins (LDL) in SLE patients; reduction of cardiac events by statins has been shown in SLE patients with renal transplants but not in other SLE cohorts to date.

PULMONARY MANIFESTATIONS

The most common pulmonary manifestation of SLE is pleuritis with or without pleural effusion. This manifestation, when mild, may respond to treatment with nonsteroidal anti-inflammatory drugs (NSAIDs); when more severe, patients require a brief course of glucocorticoid therapy. Pulmonary infiltrates also occur as a manifestation of active SLE and are difficult to distinguish from infection on imaging studies. Life-threatening pulmonary manifestations include interstitial inflammation leading to fibrosis, shrinking lung syndrome, and intra-alveolar hemorrhage; all of these probably require early aggressive immunosuppressive therapy as well as supportive care.

CARDIAC MANIFESTATIONS

Pericarditis is the most frequent cardiac manifestation; it usually responds to anti-inflammatory therapy and infrequently leads to tamponade. More serious cardiac manifestations are myocarditis and fibrinous endocarditis of Libman-Sacks. The endocardial involvement can lead to valvular insufficiencies, most commonly of the mitral or aortic valves, or to embolic events. It has not been proven that glucocorticoid or other immunosuppressive therapies lead to improvement of lupus myocarditis or endocarditis, but it is usual practice to administer a trial of high-dose steroids along with appropriate supportive therapy for heart failure, arrhythmia, or embolic events. As discussed above, patients with SLE are at increased risk for myocardial infarction, usually due to accelerated atherosclerosis, which probably results from immune attack, chronic inflammation, and/or chronic oxidative damage to arteries.

■ HEMATOLOGIC MANIFESTATIONS

The most frequent hematologic manifestation of SLE is anemia, usually normochromic normocytic, reflecting chronic illness. Hemolysis can be rapid in onset and severe, requiring high-dose glucocorticoid therapy, which is effective in most patients. Leukopenia is also common and almost always consists of lymphopenia, not granulocytopenia; this rarely predisposes to infections and by itself usually does not require therapy. Thrombocytopenia may be a recurring problem. If platelet counts are >40,000/μL and abnormal bleeding is absent, therapy may not be required. High-dose glucocorticoid therapy (e.g., 1 mg/kg per day of prednisone or equivalent) is usually effective for the first few episodes of severe thrombocytopenia. Recurring or prolonged hemolytic anemia or thrombocytopenia, or disease requiring an unacceptably high dose of daily glucocorticoids, should be treated with an additional strategy (see "Treatment," below).

■ GASTROINTESTINAL MANIFESTATIONS

Nausea, sometimes with vomiting and diarrhea, can be manifestations of an SLE flare, as can diffuse abdominal pain probably caused by autoimmune peritonitis and/or intestinal vasculitis. Increases in serum aspartate aminotransferase (AST) and alanine aminotransferase (ALT) are common when SLE is active. These manifestations usually improve promptly during systemic glucocorticoid therapy. Vasculitis involving the intestine may be life-threatening; perforations, ischemia, bleeding, and sepsis are frequent complications. Aggressive immunosuppressive therapy with high-dose glucocorticoids is recommended for short-term control; evidence of recurrence is an indication for additional therapies.

■ OCULAR MANIFESTATIONS

Sicca syndrome (Sjögren's syndrome; Chap. 324) and nonspecific conjunctivitis are common in SLE and rarely threaten vision. In contrast, retinal vasculitis and optic neuritis are serious manifestations: blindness can develop over days to weeks. Aggressive immunosuppression is recommended, although there are no controlled trials to prove effectiveness. Complications of glucocorticoid therapy include cataracts (common) and glaucoma.

LABORATORY TESTS

Laboratory tests serve (1) to establish or rule out the diagnosis; (2) to follow the course of disease, particularly to suggest that a flare is occurring or organ damage is developing; and (3) to identify adverse effects of therapies.

■ TESTS FOR AUTOANTIBODIES (TABLES 319-1 AND 319-3)

Diagnostically, the most important autoantibodies to detect are ANA as the test is positive in >95% of patients, usually at the onset of symptoms. A few patients develop ANA within 1 year of symptom onset; repeated testing may thus be useful. ANA-negative lupus exists but is rare in adults and is usually associated with other autoantibodies (anti-Ro or anti-DNA). High-titer IgG antibodies to double-stranded DNA (dsDNA) (but not to single-stranded DNA) are specific for SLE. There is no international standardized test for ANA; variability between different service laboratories is high. Enzyme-linked immunosorbent assays (ELISA) and immunofluorescent reactions of sera with the dsDNA in the flagellate *Crithidia luciliae* have ~60% sensitivity for SLE; identification of high-avidity anti-dsDNA in the Farr assay is not as sensitive but may correlate better with risk for nephritis. Titers of anti-dsDNA vary over time. In some patients, increases in quantities of anti-dsDNA herald a flare, particularly of nephritis or vasculitis, especially when associated with declining levels of C3 or C4 complement. Antibodies to Sm are also specific for SLE and assist in diagnosis; anti-Sm antibodies do not usually correlate with disease activity or clinical manifestations. aPL are not specific for SLE, but their presence fulfills one classification criterion, and they identify patients at increased risk for venous or arterial clotting, thrombocytopenia, and fetal loss. There are two widely accepted tests that measure different antibodies (anticardiolipin and the lupus anticoagulant): (1) ELISA for anticardiolipin (internationally standardized with good reproducibility) and (2) a sensitive phospholipid-based activated prothrombin time such as the dilute Russell venom viper test. Some centers also recommend measurement of antibodies to β_2 glycoprotein 1, a serum protein cofactor that is the target of most antibodies to cardiolipin and some lupus anticoagulants. The higher the titers of IgG anticardiolipin (>40 IU is considered high), and the greater the number of different aPL that are detected, the greater is the risk for a clinical episode of clotting. Quantities of aPL may vary markedly over time; repeated testing is justified if clinical manifestations of the antiphospholipid antibody syndrome (APS) appear (Chap. 320). To classify a patient as having APS, with or without SLE, by international criteria requires the presence of ≥1 clotting episode and/or repeated fetal losses plus at least two positive tests for aPL, at least 12 weeks apart; however, many patients with antiphospholipid syndrome do not meet these stringent criteria, which are intended for inclusion of patients into studies.

An additional autoantibody test with predictive value (not used for diagnosis) detects anti-Ro, which indicates increased risk for neonatal lupus, sicca syndrome, and SCLE. Women with child-bearing potential and SLE should be screened for aPL and anti-Ro.

■ STANDARD TESTS FOR DIAGNOSIS

Screening tests for complete blood count, platelet count, and urinalysis may detect abnormalities that contribute to the diagnosis and influence management decisions.

■ TESTS FOR FOLLOWING DISEASE COURSE

It is useful to follow tests that indicate the status of organ involvement known to be present during SLE flares. These might include urinalysis for hematuria and proteinuria, hemoglobin levels, platelet counts, and serum levels of creatinine or albumin. There is great interest in identification of additional markers of disease activity. Candidates include levels of anti-DNA antibodies, several components of complement (C3 is most widely available), activated complement products (including those that bind to the C4d receptor on erythrocytes), IFN-inducible gene expression in peripheral blood cells, soluble IL-2 levels, and urinary levels of TNF-like weak inducer of apoptosis (TWEAK), neutrophil gelatinase-associated lipocalin (NGAL), or monocyte chemotactic protein 1 (MCP-1). None is uniformly agreed upon as a reliable indicator of flare or of response to therapeutic interventions. The physician should determine for each patient whether certain laboratory test changes predict flare. If so, altering therapy in response to these changes may be advisable

TABLE 319-4 Clinical Manifestations of SLE and Prevalence Over the Entire Course of Disease*

Manifestation	Prevalence, %
Systemic: Fatigue, malaise, fever, anorexia, weight loss	95
Musculoskeletal	95
Arthralgias/myalgias	95
Nonerosive polyarthritis	60
Hand deformities	10
Myopathy/myositis	25/5
Ischemic necrosis of bone	15
Cutaneous	80
Photosensitivity	70
Malar rash	50
Oral ulcers	40
Alopecia	40
Discoid rash	20
Vasculitis rash	20
Other (e.g., urticaria, subacute cutaneous lupus)	15
Hematologic	85
Anemia (chronic disease)	70
Leukopenia (<4000/μL)	65
Lymphopenia (<1500/μL)	50
Thrombocytopenia (<100,000/μL)	15
Lymphadenopathy	15
Splenomegaly	15
Hemolytic anemia	10
Neurologic	60
Cognitive disorder	50
Mood disorder	40
Headache	25
Seizures	20
Mono-, polyneuropathy	15
Stroke, TIA	10
Acute confusional state or movement disorder	2–5
Aseptic meningitis, myelopathy	<1
Cardiopulmonary	60
Pleurisy, pericarditis, effusions	30–50
Myocarditis, endocarditis	10
Lupus pneumonitis	10
Coronary artery disease	10
Interstitial fibrosis	5
Pulmonary hypertension, ARDS, hemorrhage	<5
Shrinking lung syndrome	<5
Renal	30–50
Proteinuria >500 mg/24 h, cellular casts	30–50
Nephrotic syndrome	25
End-stage renal disease	5–10
Gastrointestinal	40
Nonspecific (nausea, mild pain, diarrhea)	30
Abnormal liver enzymes	40
Vasculitis	5
Thrombosis	15
Venous	10
Arterial	5
Ocular	15
Sicca syndrome	15
Conjunctivitis, episcleritis	10
Vasculitis	5

*Numbers indicate percent of patients who have the manifestation at some time during the course of illness.
Abbreviations: ARDS, acute respiratory distress syndrome; TIA, transient ischemic attack.

(30 mg of prednisone daily for 2 weeks has been shown to prevent flares in patients with rising anti-DNA plus falling complement). In addition, given the increased prevalence of atherosclerosis in SLE, it is advisable to follow the recommendations of the National Cholesterol Education Program for testing and treatment, including scoring of SLE as an independent risk factor, similar to diabetes mellitus.

TREATMENT Systemic Lupus Erythematosus

There is no cure for SLE, and complete sustained remissions are rare. Therefore, the physician should plan to induce improvement of acute flares and then maintain improvements with strategies that suppress symptoms to an acceptable level and prevent organ damage. Usually patients will endure some adverse effects of medications. Therapeutic choices depend on (1) whether disease manifestations are life-threatening or likely to cause organ damage, justifying aggressive therapies; (2) whether manifestations are potentially reversible; and (3) the best approaches to preventing complications of disease and its treatments. Therapies, doses, and adverse effects are listed in Table 319-5.

CONSERVATIVE THERAPIES FOR MANAGEMENT OF NON-LIFE-THREATENING DISEASE Among patients with fatigue, pain, and autoantibodies of SLE, but without major organ involvement, management can be directed to suppression of symptoms. Analgesics and antimalarials are mainstays. NSAIDs are useful analgesics/anti-inflammatories, particularly for arthritis/arthralgias. However, two major issues currently indicate caution in using NSAIDs. First, SLE patients compared with the general population are at increased risk for NSAID-induced aseptic meningitis, elevated serum transaminases, hypertension, and renal dysfunction. Second, all NSAIDs, particularly those that inhibit cyclooxygenase-2 specifically, may increase risk for myocardial infarction. Acetaminophen to control pain may be a good strategy,

TABLE 319-5 Medications for the Management of SLE

Medication	Dose Range	Drug Interactions	Serious or Common Adverse Effects
NSAIDs, salicylates (Ecotrin[a] and St. Joseph's aspirin[a] approved by FDA for use in SLE)	Doses toward upper limit of recommended range usually required	A2R/ACE inhibitors, glucocorticoids, fluconazole, methotrexate, thiazides	NSAIDs: Higher incidence of aseptic meningitis, transaminitis, decreased renal function, vasculitis of skin; entire class, especially COX-2-specific inhibitors, may increase risk for myocardial infarction Salicylates: ototoxicity, tinnitus Both: GI events and symptoms, allergic reactions, dermatitis, dizziness, acute renal failure, edema, hypertension
Topical glucocorticoids	Mid-potency for face; mid to high potency other areas	None known	Atrophy of skin, contact dermatitis, folliculitis, hypopigmentation, infection
Topical sunscreens	SPF 15 at least; 30+ preferred	None known	Contact dermatitis
Hydroxychloroquine[a] (quinacrine can be added or substituted)	200–400 mg qd (100 mg qd)	None known	Retinal damage, agranulocytosis, aplastic anemia, ataxia, cardiomyopathy, dizziness, myopathy, ototoxicity, peripheral neuropathy, pigmentation of skin, seizures, thrombocytopenia. Use in pregnancy may be acceptable. Pregnancy category D Quinacrine usually causes diffuse yellow skin coloration
DHEA (dehydroepiandrosterone)	200 mg qd	Unclear	Acne, menstrual irregularities, high serum levels of testosterone
Methotrexate (for dermatitis, arthritis)	10–25 mg once a week, PO or SC, with folic acid; decrease dose if CrCl <60 mL/min	Acitretin, leflunomide, NSAIDs and salicylates, penicillins, probenecid, sulfonamides, trimethoprim	Anemia, bone marrow suppression, leukopenia, thrombocytopenia, hepatotoxicity, nephrotoxicity, infections, neurotoxicity, pulmonary fibrosis, pneumonitis, severe dermatitis, seizures. Teratogenic. Pregnancy category X
Glucocorticoids, oral[a] (several specific brands are approved by FDA for use in SLE)	Prednisone, prednisolone: 0.5–1 mg/kg per day for severe SLE 0.07–0.3 mg/kg per day or qod for milder disease	A2R/ACE antagonists, antiarrhythmics class III, β_2, cyclosporine, NSAIDs and salicylates, phenothiazines, phenytoins, quinolones, rifampin, risperidone, thiazides, sulfonylureas, warfarin	Infection, VZV infection, hypertension, hyperglycemia, hypokalemia, acne, allergic reactions, anxiety, aseptic necrosis of bone, cushingoid changes, CHF, fragile skin, insomnia, menstrual irregularities, mood swings, osteoporosis, psychosis
Methylprednisolone sodium succinate, IV[a] (FDA approved for lupus nephritis)	For severe disease, 1 g IV qd × 3 days	As for oral glucocorticoids	As for oral glucocorticoids (if used repeatedly); anaphylaxis
Cyclophosphamide[b,c] IV	7–25 mg/kg q month × 6; consider mesna administration with dose	Allopurinol, bone marrow suppressants, colony-stimulating factors, doxorubicin, rituximab, succinylcholine, zidovudine	Infection, VZV infection, bone marrow suppression, leukopenia, anemia, thrombocytopenia, hemorrhagic cystitis (less with IV), carcinoma of the bladder, alopecia, nausea, diarrhea, malaise, malignancy, ovarian and testicular failure. Teratogenic. Pregnancy category D
Mycophenolate mofetil[b] or mycophenolic acid	MMF: 2–3 g/d PO; max 1 g bid if CrCl <25 mL/min. MPA: 360–1080 mg bid. Caution if CrCl <25 mL/min	Acyclovir, antacids, azathioprine, bile acid–binding resins, ganciclovir, iron, salts, probenecid, oral contraceptives	Infection, leukopenia, anemia, thrombocytopenia, lymphoma, lymphoproliferative disorders, malignancy, alopecia, cough, diarrhea, fever, GI symptoms, headache, hypertension, hypercholesterolemia, hypokalemia, insomnia, peripheral edema, transaminitis, tremor, rash. Teratogenic. Pregnancy category D
Azathioprine[b]	2–3 mg/kg per day PO; decrease frequency of dose if CrCl <50 mL/min	ACE inhibitors, allopurinol, bone marrow suppressants, interferons, mycophenolate mofetil, rituximab, warfarin, zidovudine	Infection, VZV infection, bone marrow suppression, leukopenia, anemia, thrombocytopenia, pancreatitis, hepatotoxicity, malignancy, alopecia, fever, flulike illness, GI symptoms. Use in pregnancy may be acceptable. Pregnancy category D
Belimumab	10 mg/kg i.v.	wk 0,2,4 then monthly	Infusion reactions Allergy Infections probable
Rituximab (for patients resistant to above therapies)	375 mg/M2 q wk × 4 or 1 g q 2 wks × 2	IVIg	Infection (including PML), infusion reactions, headache, arrythmias, allergic responses. Pregnancy category C
Belimumab	10 mg/kg i.v.	IV Ig	Infec

[a]Indicates medication is approved for use in SLE by the U.S. Food and Drug Administration.
[b]Indicates the medication has been used with glucocorticoids in the trials showing efficacy.
[c]See text for low dose regimen.

Abbreviations: A2R, angiotensin 2 receptor; ACE, angiotensin-converting enzyme; CHF, congestive heart failure; CrCl, creatinine clearance; FDA, U.S. Food and Drug Administration; GI, gastrointestinal; NSAIDs, nonsteroidal anti-inflammatory drugs; SPF, sun protection factor; VZV, varicella-zoster virus.

but NSAIDs are more effective in some patients. The relative hazards of NSAIDs compared with low-dose glucocorticoid therapy have not been established. Antimalarials (hydroxychloroquine, chloroquine, and quinacrine) often reduce dermatitis, arthritis, and fatigue. A randomized, placebo-controlled, prospective trial has shown that withdrawal of hydroxychloroquine results in increased numbers of disease flares. Hydroxychloroquine reduces accrual of tissue damage over time. Because of potential retinal toxicity, patients receiving antimalarials should undergo ophthalmologic examinations annually. A placebo-controlled prospective trial suggests that administration of dehydroepiandrosterone may reduce disease activity. If quality of life is inadequate in spite of these conservative measures, treatment with low doses of systemic glucocorticoids may be necessary. Dermatitis should be managed with topical sunscreens, antimalarials, and topical glucocorticoids and/or tacrolimus. Since recent data show that mycophenolate mofetil, and belimumab (added to background therapies of glucocorticoids-plus-antimalarial-plus immunosuppressive) reduce disease activity in nonrenal manifestations of SLE, it is reasonable to consider these interventions in patients with persistent disease activity despite standard therapies. Azathioprine or methotrexate may also be considered for such patients (Table 319-5).

LIFE-THREATENING SLE: PROLIFERATIVE FORMS OF LUPUS NEPHRITIS The mainstay of treatment for any inflammatory life-threatening or organ-threatening manifestations of SLE is systemic glucocorticoids (0.5–1 mg/kg per day PO or 1000 mg of methylprednisolone sodium succinate IV daily for 3 days followed by 0.5–1 mg/kg of daily prednisone or equivalent). Evidence that glucocorticoid therapy is lifesaving comes from retrospective studies from the predialysis era; survival is significantly better in people with DPGN treated with high-dose daily glucocorticoids (40–60 mg of prednisone daily for 4–6 months) versus lower doses. Currently, high doses are recommended for much shorter periods; recent trials of interventions for severe SLE employ 4–6 weeks of 0.5 to 1 mg/kg/day of prednisone or equivalent. Thereafter, doses are tapered as rapidly as the clinical situation permits, usually to a maintenance dose varying from 5–10 mg of prednisone or equivalent per day or from 10–20 mg every other day. Most patients with an episode of severe lupus require many years of maintenance therapy with low-dose glucocorticoids, which can be increased to prevent or treat disease flares. Frequent attempts to gradually reduce the glucocorticoid requirement are recommended since virtually everyone develops important adverse effects (Table 319-5). Prospective controlled trials in active lupus nephritis show that induction of improvement by administration of high doses of glucocorticoids (1000 mg of methylprednisolone daily for 3 days) by IV routes compared with daily oral routes shortens the time to maximal improvement by a few weeks but ultimately improvements are similar. It has become standard practice to initiate therapy for active, potentially life-threatening SLE with high-dose IV glucocorticoid pulses, based on studies in lupus nephritis. This approach must be tempered by safety considerations, such as the presence of conditions adversely affected by glucocorticoids (infection, hyperglycemia, hypertension, osteoporosis, etc.).

Cytotoxic/immunosuppressive agents added to glucocorticoids are recommended to treat serious SLE. Almost all prospective controlled trials in SLE involving cytotoxic agents have been conducted in combination with glucocorticoids in patients with lupus nephritis. Therefore, the following recommendations apply to treatment of nephritis. Either cyclophosphamide (an alkylating agent) or mycophenolate mofetil (a relatively lymphocyte-specific inhibitor of inosine monophosphatase and therefore of purine synthesis) is an acceptable choice for induction of improvement in severely ill patients; azathioprine (a purine analogue and cycle-specific antimetabolite) is probably less effective but may be used if the other immunosuppressives are not tolerated or not available. In patients whose renal biopsies show ISN grade III or IV disease, early treatment with combinations of glucocorticoids and cyclophosphamide reduces progression to ESRD and improves survival; this difference can be seen after approximately 5 years of therapy. Shorter-term studies with glucocorticoids plus mycophenolate mofetil (prospective randomized trials of 6 months) show that this regimen is similar to cyclophosphamide in inducing improvement. Comparisons are complicated by effects of race, since higher proportions of blacks (and other non-Asian, non-white races) respond to mycophenolate than to cyclophosphamide, whereas similar proportions of whites and Asians respond to each drug. Regarding toxicity, diarrhea is more common with mycophenolate while herpetic infections, amenorrhea, and leukopenia are more common with cyclophosphamide; rates of severe infections and death are similar in some studies, although mycophenolate is less toxic than cyclophosphamide in others. Therapeutic responses to cyclophosphamide and mycophenolate begin 3–16 weeks after treatment is initiated, whereas glucocorticoid responses may begin within 24 h. For maintenance therapy, mycophenolate may be better than azathioprine in preventing flares and progression of lupus nephritis; either drug is acceptable and both are safer than cyclophosphamide. If cyclophosphamide is used for induction therapy, the recommended "National Institutes of Health (NIH)" dose (based on clinical trials at that institution) is 500–750 mg/m^2 intravenously, monthly for 6 months, followed by maintenance with daily oral mycophenolate or azathioprine. The incidence of ovarian failure, a common effect of cyclophosphamide therapy, can be reduced by treatment with a gonadotropin-releasing hormone agonist (e.g., Lupron 3.75 mg IM) prior to each monthly cyclophosphamide dose. Since cyclophosphamide has many adverse effects and is generally disliked by patients, alternative approaches using lower doses have been tested. European studies have shown that IV cyclophosphamide at doses of 500 mg every 2 weeks for six doses ("low dose") is as effective as the recommended higher dose given for a longer duration in the NIH regimen ("high dose"). All patients were maintained on azathioprine after the course of cyclophosphamide was completed. Ten-year follow-up has shown no differences in the high-dose and low-dose groups (death or ESRD in 9–20% in each group). The majority of the European patients were white; it is not clear that the data apply to U.S. populations. Patients with high serum creatinine levels [e.g., ≥265 μmol/L (≥3 mg/dL)] many months in duration and high chronicity scores on renal biopsy are not likely to respond to immunosuppression. In general, it may be better to induce improvement in a black or Hispanic patient with proliferative glomerulonephritis with mycophenolate (2–3 g daily) rather than with cyclophosphamide, with the option to switch if no evidence of response is detectable after 3–6 months of treatment. For whites and Asians, induction with either mycophenolate or cyclophosphamide is acceptable. Cyclophosphamide may be discontinued when it is clear that a patient is improving; the number of SLE flares is reduced by maintenance therapy with mycophenolate (1.5–2 g daily) or azathioprine (2 mg/kg/d). Both cyclophosphamide and mycophenolate are potentially teratogenic; patients should be off either medication for at least 3 months before attempting to conceive. If azathioprine is used either for induction or maintenance therapy, patients may be prescreened for homozygous deficiency of the TMPT enzyme (which is required to metabolize the 6-mercaptopurine product of azathioprine) since they are at higher risk for bone marrow suppression.

Good improvement occurs in ~80% of lupus nephritis patients receiving either cyclophosphamide or mycophenolate at 1–2 years of follow-up. However, at least 50% of these individuals have flares of nephritis over the next 5 years, and retreatment is required; such individuals are more likely to progress to ESRD. Long-term outcome of lupus nephritis to most interventions is better in whites than in blacks. Chlorambucil is an alkylating agent that can be substituted for cyclophosphamide; the risk of irreversible bone marrow suppression may be greater with this agent. Methotrexate (a folinic acid antagonist) may have a role in the treatment of arthritis and dermatitis, but probably not in nephritis or other life-threatening disease. Small controlled trials (in Asia) of leflunomide, a relatively lymphocyte-specific pyrimidine antagonist licensed for use in rheumatoid arthritis, have suggested it can suppress disease activity in some SLE patients. Cyclosporine and tacrolimus, which inhibit production of IL-2 and T lymphocyte functions, are used by some clinicians particularly for membranous lupus nephritis. Since they have potential nephrotoxicity, but little bone marrow toxicity, the author uses them for periods of only a few months in patients with steroid-resistant cytopenias of SLE, or in steroid-resistant patients who have developed bone marrow suppression from standard cytotoxic agents.

Use of biologicals directed against B cells for active SLE is under intense study. Use of anti-CD20 (Rituximab), particularly in those patients with SLE who are resistant to the more standard combination therapies discussed above, is controversial. Several open trials have shown efficacy in a majority of such patients—both for nephritis and for extrarenal lupus. However, recent prospective placebo-controlled randomized trials did not show a difference between anti-CD20 and placebo when added to standard combination therapies. In contrast, recent trials of anti-BLyS (belimumab, directed against the ligand of the BLyS/BAFF receptor on B cells that promotes B cell survival and differentiation to plasmablasts) showed a small, but statistically significant, better suppression of disease activity in comparison to placebo, when added to standard combhnation therapies. The US FDA has approved belimumab for treatment of SLE: it has not been studied in active nephritis or central nervous system lupus.

It is important to note that there are few if any randomized, controlled, prospective studies of any agents in life-threatening SLE that do not include nephritis. Therefore, use of glucocorticoids plus byclophosphamide or mycophenolate in other life-threatening conditions is based on studies in nephritis.

SPECIAL CONDITIONS IN SLE THAT MAY REQUIRE ADDITIONAL OR DIFFERENT THERAPIES **Crescentic Lupus Nephritis** The presence of cellular or fibrotic crescents in glomeruli with proliferative glomerulonephritis (INS-IVG)] indicates a worse prognosis than in patients without this feature. There are few large prospective controlled trials showing efficacy of cyclophosphamide, mycophenolate, or cyclosporine in such cases. Most authorities currently recommend that cyclophosphamide in the NIH-recommended high dose or high doses of mycophenolate are the induction therapies of choice, in addition to glucocorticoids.

Membranous Lupus Nephritis Most SLE patients with membranous (INS-V) nephritis also have proliferative changes and should be treated for proliferative disease; however, some have pure membranous changes. Treatment for this group is less well defined; recent prospective controlled trials suggest that alternate-day glucocorticoids plus cyclophosphamide or mycophenolate or cyclosporine are all effective in the majority of patients in reducing proteinuria; whether they preserve renal function over the lonf term is more controversial.

Pregnancy and Lupus Fertility rates for men and women with SLE are probably normal. However, rate of fetal loss is increased (approximately two- to threefold) in women with SLE. Fetal demise is higher in mothers with high disease activity, antiphospholipid antibodies, and/or active nephritis. Suppression of disease activity can be achieved by administration of systemic glucocorticoids. A placental enzyme, 11-β-dehydrogenase 2, deactivates glucocorticoids; it is more effective in deactivating prednisone and prednisolone than the fluorinated glucocorticoids dexamethasone and betamethasone. Glucocorticoids are listed by the FDA as pregnancy category A (no evidence of teratogenicity in human studies); cyclosporine, tacrolimus, and rituximab are listed as category C (may be teratogenic in animals but no good evidence in humans); azathioprine, hydroxychloroquine, mycophenolate mofetil, and cyclophosphamide are category D (there is evidence of teratogenicity in humans. but benefits might outweigh risks in certain situations); and methotrexate is category X (risks outweigh benefits). Therefore, active SLE in pregnant women should be controlled with prednisone/prednisolone at the lowest effective doses for the shortest time required. Adverse effects of prenatal glucocorticoid exposure (primarily betamethasone) on offspring may include low birth weight, developmental abnormalities in the CNS, and predilection toward adult metabolic syndrome. It is likely that each of these glucocorticoids and immunosuppressive medications get into breast milk, at least in low levels; patients should consider not breast-feeding if they need therapy for SLE. In SLE patients with aPL (on at least two occasions) and prior fetal losses, treatment with heparin (usually low-molecular-weight) plus low-dose aspirin has been shown in prospective controlled trials to increase significantly the proportion of live births; however, a recent prospective trial showed no differences in fetal outcomes in women taking aspirin compared to those on aspirin plus low-molecular-weight heparin. An additional potential problem for the fetus is the presence of antibodies to Ro, sometimes associated with neonatal lupus consisting of rash and congenital heart block. The latter can be life-threatening; therefore, the presence of anti-Ro requires vigilant monitoring of fetal heart rates with prompt intervention (delivery if possible) if distress occurs. To date, treatments of mother to reverse established heart block in the fetus, newborn, or infant (other than insertion of a pacemaker) have not been successful. Women with SLE usually tolerate pregnancy without disease flares. However, a small proportion develops severe flares requiring aggressive glucocorticoid therapy or early delivery. Poor maternal outcomes are highest in women with active nephritis or irreversible organ damage in kidneys, brain, or heart.

Lupus and Antiphospholipid Antibody Syndrome (Chap. 20) Patients with SLE who have venous or arterial clotting, and/or repeated fetal losses, and at least two positive tests for aPL have APS and should be managed with long-term anticoagulation. A target international normalized ratio (INR) of 2–2.5 is recommended for patients with one episode of venous clotting; an INR of 3–3.5 is recommended for patients with recurring clots or arterial clotting, particularly in the central nervous system. Recommendations are based on both retrospective and prospective studies of posttreatment clotting events and adverse effects from anticoagulation.

Microvascular Thrombotic Crisis (Thrombotic Thrombocytopenic Purpura, Hemolytic-Uremic Syndrome) This syndrome of hemolysis, thrombocytopenia, and microvascular thrombosis in kidneys, brain, and other tissues carries a high mortality rate and occurs most commonly in young individuals with lupus nephritis. The most useful laboratory tests are identification of schistocytes on peripheral blood smears, elevated serum levels of lactate dehydrogenase, and antibodies to ADAMS13. Plasma exchange or extensive plasmapheresis is usually life-saving; most authorities recommend concomitant glucocorticoid therapy; there is no evidence that cytotoxic drugs are effective.

Lupus Dermatitis Patients with any form of lupus dermatitis should minimize exposure to ultraviolet light, employing appropriate clothing and sunscreens with a sun protection factor of at least 15. Topical glucocorticoids and antimalarials (such as hydroxychloroquine) are effective in reducing lesion severity in most patients and are relatively safe. Systemic treatment with retinoic acid is a useful strategy in patients with inadequate improvement on topical glucocorticoids and antimalarials; adverse effects are potentially severe (particularly fetal abnormalities), and there are stringent reporting requirements for its use in the United States. Extensive, pruritic, bullous, or ulcerating dermatitides usually improve promptly after institution of systemic glucocorticoids; tapering may be accompanied by flare of lesions, thus necessitating use of a second medication such as hydroxychloroquine, retinoids, or cytotoxic medications such as methotrexate or azathioprine. In therapy-resistant lupus dermatitis there are reports of success with topical tacrolimus (caution must be exerted because of the possible increased risk for malignancies) or with systemic dapsone or thalidomide (the extreme danger of fetal deformities from thalidomide requires permission from and supervision by the supplier).

PREVENTIVE THERAPIES Prevention of complications of SLE and its therapy include providing appropriate vaccinations (the administration of influenza and pneumococcal vaccines has been studied in patients with SLE; flare rates are similar to those receiving placebo) and suppressing recurrent urinary tract infections. In addition, strategies to prevent osteoporosis should be initiated in most patients likely to require long-term glucocorticoid therapy and/or with other predisposing factors. Control of hypertension and appropriate prevention strategies for atherosclerosis, including monitoring and treatment of dyslipidemias, management of hyperglycemia, and obesity, are recommended.

EXPERIMENTAL THERAPIES Studies of highly targeted experimental therapies for SLE are in progress. They include targeting (1) activated B lymphocytes with anti-BLyS, or TACI-Ig; (2) inhibition of IFNα; (3) inhibition of B/T cell second signal co-activation with CTLA-Ig; and (4) inhibition of innate immune activation via TLR7 or TLR7 and 9, and induction of regulatory T cells with peptides from immunoglobulins or autoantigens. A few studies have employed vigorous untargeted immunosuppression with high-dose cyclophosphamide plus anti–T cell strategies, with rescue by transplantation of autologous hematopoietic stem cells for the treatment of severe and refractory SLE. One U.S. report showed an estimated mortality rate over 5 years of 15% and sustained remission in 50%. It is hoped that the next edition of this text will recommend more effective and less toxic approaches to treatment of SLE based on some of these strategies.

PATIENT OUTCOMES, PROGNOSIS, AND SURVIVAL

Survival in patients with SLE in the United States, Canada, Europe, and China is approximately 95% at 5 years, 90% at 10 years, and 78% at 20 years. In the United States, African Americans and Hispanic Americans with a mestizo heritage have a worse prognosis than whites, whereas Africans in Africa and Hispanic Americans with a Puerto Rican origin do not. The relative importance of gene mixtures and environmental differences accounting for ethnic differences is not known. Poor prognosis (~50% mortality in 10 years) in most series is associated with (at the time of diagnosis) high serum creatinine levels [>124 μmol/L (>1.4 mg/dL)], hypertension, nephrotic syndrome (24-h urine protein excretion >2.6 g), anemia [hemoglobin <124 g/L (<12.4 g/dL)], hypoalbuminemia, hypocomplementemia, aPL, male sex, and ethnicity (African American, Hispanic with mestizo heritage). Data regarding outcomes in SLE patients with renal transplants show mixed results: some series have a twofold increase in graft rejection compared to patients with other causes of ESRD, whereas others show no differences. Overall patient survival is comparable (85% at 2 years). Lupus nephritis occurs in approximately 10% of transplanted kidneys. Disability in patients with SLE is common due primarily to chronic fatigue, arthritis, and pain, as well as renal disease. As many as 25% of patients may experience remissions, sometimes for a few years, but these are rarely permanent. The leading causes of death in the first decade of disease are systemic disease activity, renal failure, and infections; subsequently, thromboembolic events become increasingly frequent causes of mortality.

DRUG-INDUCED LUPUS

This is a syndrome of positive ANA associated with symptoms such as fever, malaise, arthritis or intense arthralgias/myalgias, serositis, and/or rash. The syndrome appears during therapy with certain medications and biologic agents, occurs predominantly in whites, has less female predilection than SLE, rarely involves kidneys or brain, is rarely associated with anti-dsDNA, is commonly associated with antibodies to histones, and usually resolves over several weeks after discontinuation of the offending medication. The list of substances that can induce lupus-like disease is long. Among the most frequent are the antiarrhythmics procainamide, disopyramide, and propafenone; the antihypertensive hydralazine; several angiotensin-converting enzyme inhibitors and beta blockers; the antithyroid propylthiouracil; the antipsychotics chlorpromazine and lithium; the anticonvulsants carbamazepine and phenytoin; the antibiotics isoniazid, minocycline, and macrodantin; the antirheumatic sulfasalazine; the diuretic hydrochlorothiazide; the antihyperlipidemics lovastatin and simvastatin; and interferons and TNF inhibitors. ANA usually appears before symptoms; however, many of the medications mentioned above induce ANA in patients who never develop symptoms of drug-induced lupus. It is appropriate to test for ANA at the first hint of relevant symptoms and to use test results to help decide whether to withdraw the suspect agent.

FURTHER READINGS

Falk RJ et al: Therapy of diffuse and proliferative lupus nephritis. UpToDate, October 2010

Helmick CG et al: Estimates of the prevalence of arthritis and other rheumatic conditions in the United States. Part 1. Arthritis Rheum 58:15, 2008

Kasitanon N et al: Predictors of survival in systemic lupus erythematosus. Medicine (Baltimore) 85:147, 2006

Rahman A, Isenberg D: Systemic lupus erythematosus. New Engl J Med 358:929, 2008

Schur PH, Wallace DJ: Overview of the therapy and prognosis of systemic lupus erythematosus in adults. UpToDate, October 2010

Wallace DJ, Hahn BH (eds): *Dubois' Lupus Erythematosus*, 8th ed. Philadelphia, Lippincott, 2008

CHAPTER 320

Antiphospholipid Antibody Syndrome

Haralampos M. Moutsopoulos
Panayiotis G. Vlachoyiannopoulos

DEFINITION

Antiphospholipid antibody syndrome (APS) is an autoantibody-mediated acquired thrombophilia characterized by recurrent arterial or venous thrombosis and/or pregnancy morbidity in the presence of autoantibodies against phospholipid (PL)-binding plasma proteins, mainly a plasma apolipoprotein known as β2 glycoprotein I (β2GPI) and prothrombin (Table 320-1). Another group of antibodies termed *lupus anticoagulant* (LA) prolong clotting times in vitro; this prolongation is not corrected by adding normal plasma to the detection system. APS may occur alone (primary), or in association with any other autoimmune disease (secondary). Catastrophic APS (CAPS) is defined as a rapidly progressive thromboembolic disease involving simultaneously three or more organs, organ systems, or tissues leading to corresponding functional defects.

EPIDEMIOLOGY

Anti-PL (aPL)-binding plasma protein antibodies occur in 1–5% of general population. Their prevalence increases with age; however, it is questionable whether they induce thrombotic events in elderly individuals. One-third of patients with systemic lupus erythematosus (SLE) (Chap. 319) possess these antibodies while their prevalence in other autoimmune connective tissue disorders such as systemic sclerosis (scleroderma), Sjögren's syndrome, dermatomyositis, rheumatoid arthritis, and early undifferentiated connective tissue disease, ranges from 6% to 15%. One-third of aPL positive individuals experience thrombotic events or pregnancy morbidity.

TABLE 320-1 Classification and Nomenclature of Antiphospholipid Antibodies

- Antibodies against cardiolipin (aCL), a negatively charged phospholipid, detected by enzyme-linked immunosorbent assay (ELISA)
- Antibodies against β2GPI, (anti-β2GPI) detected by ELISA in the absence of PL.
- LA detected by clotting assays. LA constitutes a heterogeneous group of antibodies directed also against PL binding proteins, mainly β2GPI and prothrombin. LA antibodies induce elongation in vitro of the following clotting times:

Activated partial thromboplastin time (aPTT), kaolin clotting time (KCT), dilute Russel viper venom test (dRVVT)

- Antibodies against phospholipids/cholesterol complexes detected as biologic false-positive serologic test for syphilis (BFP-STS) and Venereal Disease Research Laboratory Test (VDRL)

PATHOGENESIS

The trigger for the induction of antibodies to PL-binding proteins is not known. Preceding infections, however, have been proposed as the initiating event. These antibodies are pathogenic since anti-β2GPI/β2GPI complexes inactivate natural anticoagulants such as protein C, activate cells involved in the coagulation cascade to a prothrombotic phenotype, activate complement, and inhibit syncytium-trophoblast differentiation. Activated protein C (APC) binds the pro-coagulant factors Va and VIIIa and inactivates them. Anti-β2GPI/β2GPI complexes inhibit the APC activity in vivo by competing with the components of the APC/Va/VIIIa complexes for binding to a number of PL-binding sites, or by disrupting these complexes. Domain V of β2GPI can interact with apolipoprotein E receptor 2′ (apoER2′) and/or with the GPIbα subunit of the GPIb/IX/V receptor of platelets. Furthermore platelet factor 4 (PF4) tetramers dimerize β2GPI and the resulting complexes are recognized by anti-β2GPI antibodies, eventually activating the p38 mitogen-activated protein (p38 MAP) kinase phosphorylation, and leading to thromboxane B_2 (TXB_2) production in vitro. In fact, increased levels of 11-dehydro-TXB_2, have been found in the urine of patients with APS. Anti-β2GPI antibodies activate nuclear factor kappa B (NF-κB) in monocytes and endothelial cells by interacting with surface receptors not yet identified, leading to the secretion of pro-inflammatory cytokines, such as interleukins -1,-6, and -8; the expression of adhesion molecules such as intercellular adhesion molecule (ICAM-1), vascular cell adhesion molecule 1 (VCAM-1), and E-selectin; inhibition of cell-surface plasminogen activation; and the expressions of tissue factor, changing the phenotype of these cells to a prothrombotic form. As shown in mouse models, anti-β2GPI antibodies induce fetal injury through complement activation, since C4-deficient mice were protected from fetal injury.

CLINICAL MANIFESTATIONS AND LABORATORY FINDINGS

Clinical manifestations represent mainly a direct or indirect expression of venous or arterial thrombosis and/or pregnancy morbidity (Table 320-2). Clinical features associated with venous thrombosis are superficial and deep vein thrombosis, cerebral venous thrombosis, signs and symptoms of intracranial hypertension, retinal vein thrombosis, pulmonary emboli, pulmonary arterial hypertension, and Budd-Chiari syndrome. Livedo reticularis consists of a mottled reticular vascular pattern that appears as a lace-like, purplish discoloration of the skin. It is probably caused by swelling of the venules owing to obstruction of capillaries by thrombi. This clinical manifestation correlates with vascular lesions such as those in the central nervous system as well as aseptic bone necrosis. Arterial thrombosis is manifested as migraines, cognitive dysfunction, transient ischemic attacks, stroke, myocardial infarction, arterial thrombosis of upper and lower extremities, ischemic leg ulcers, digital gangrene, avascular necrosis of bone, retinal artery occlusion leading to painless monocular loss of vision (amaurosis fugax), renal artery stenosis, and glomerular lesions, as well as infarcts of spleen, pancreas, and adrenals. Libman-Sacks endocarditis consists of very small vegetations, histologically characterized by organized platelet-fibrin microthrombi surrounded by growing fibroblasts and macrophages. Glomerular lesions are manifested with hypertension, mildly elevated serum creatinine levels, proteinuria, and mild hematuria. Histologically, these lesions are characterized in an acute phase by thrombotic microangiopathy involving glomerular capillaries, and in a chronic phase with fibrous intima hyperplasia, fibrous and/or fibrocellular occlusions of arterioles and focal cortical atrophy (Table 320-2). Premature atherosclerosis has been

TABLE 320-2 Clinical Features of Antiphospholipid Antibody Syndrome

Manifestation	%
Venous Thrombosis and Related Consequences	
Deep vein thrombosis	39
Livedo reticularis	24
Pulmonary embolism	14
Superficial thrombophlebitis	12
Thrombosis in various other sites	11
Arterial Thrombosis and Related Consequences	
Stroke	20
Cardiac valve thickening/dysfunction and/or Libman-Sacks vegetations	14
Transient ischemic attack	11
Myocardial ischemia (infarction or angina) and coronary bypass thrombosis	10
Leg ulcers and/or digital gangrene	9
Arterial thrombosis in the extremities	7
Retinal artery thrombosis/amaurosis fugax	7
Ischemia of visceral organs or avascular necrosis of bone	6
Multi-infarct dementia	3
Neurologic Manifestations of Uncertain Etiology	
Migraine	20
Epilepsy	7
Chorea	1
Cerebellar ataxia	1
Transverse myelopathy	0.5
Renal Manifestations Due to Various Reasons (Renal Artery/Renal Vein/Glomerular Thrombosis, Fibrous Intima Hyperplasia)	3
Osteoarticular Manifestations	
Arthralgia	39
Arthritis	27
Obstetric Manifestations (Referred to the Number of Pregnancies)	
Preeclampsia	10
Eclampsia	4
Fetal Manifestations (Referred to the Number of Pregnancies)	
Early fetal loss (<10 weeks)	35
Late fetal loss (≥10 weeks)	17
Premature birth among the live births	11
Hematologic Manifestations	
Thrombocytopenia	30
Autoimmune hemolytic anemia	10

Source: Adapted from R Cervera et al.

recognized as a rare feature of APS. Coombs-positive hemolytic anemia and thrombocytopenia are laboratory findings associated with APS. Discontinuation of therapy, major surgery, infection, and trauma may trigger CAPS.

DIAGNOSIS AND DIFFERENTIAL DIAGNOSIS

The diagnosis of APS should be seriously considered in cases of thrombosis, cerebral vascular accidents in individuals younger than 55 years of age, or pregnancy morbidity in the presence of livedo reticularis or thrombocytopenia. In these cases aPL antibodies should be measured. The presence of at least one clinical and one laboratory criterion ensures the diagnosis even in the presence of other causes of thrombophilia. Clinical criteria include: (1) vascular thrombosis defined as one or more clinical episodes of arterial, venous, or small vessel thrombosis in any tissue or organ; and (2) pregnancy morbidity, defined as (a) one or more unexplained deaths of a morphologically normal fetus at or beyond the tenth week of gestation, or (b) one or more premature births of a morphologically normal neonate before the thirty-fourth week of gestation because of eclampsia, severe preeclampsia, or placental insufficiency; or (c) three or more unexplained consecutive spontaneous abortions before the 10th week of gestation. Laboratory criteria include (1) LA, (2) anticardiolipin (aCL) and/or (3) anti-β2GPI antibodies, at intermediate or high titers on two occasions, 12 weeks apart.

Differential diagnosis is based on the exclusion of other inherited or acquired causes of thrombophilia (Chap. 116), Coombs positive hemolytic anemia (Chap. 106), and thrombocytopenia (Chap. 115). Livedo reticularis with or without a painful ulceration on the lower extremities also may be a manifestation of disorders affecting (1) the vascular wall such as polyarteritis nodosa, SLE, cryoglobulinemia, and lymphomas; or (2) the vascular lumen, such as myeloproliferative disorders, atherosclerosis, hypercholesterolemia, or other causes of thrombophilia.

TREATMENT Antiphospholipid Antibody Syndrome

After the first thrombotic event, APS patients should be placed on warfarin for life aiming to achieve an international normalized ratio (INR) ranging from 2.5 to 3.5, alone or in combination with 80 mg of aspirin daily. Pregnancy morbidity is prevented by a combination of heparin with aspirin 80 mg daily. Intravenous immunoglobulin (IVIg) 400 mg/kg qd for 5 days may also prevent abortions, while glucocorticoids are ineffective. Evidence-based treatment of patients with aPL in the absence of any clinical event is not available; however, aspirin 80 mg daily protects patients with SLE positive for aPL antibodies from developing thrombotic events.

Some patients with APS and patients with CAPS have recurrent thrombotic events despite appropriate anticoagulation. In these cases IVIg 400 mg/kg qd for 5 days or anti-CD20 monoclonal antibody 375 mg/m^2 per week for 4 weeks may be of benefit. Patients with CAPS, who are treated in the intensive care unit, are unable to receive warfarin; in this situation therapeutic doses of low-molecular-weight heparin should be administered. In cases of heparin- induced thrombocytopenia and thrombosis syndrome, inhibitors of phospholipid-bound activated factor X (FXa), such as fondaparinux 7.5 mg SC daily or rivaroxaban 10 mg PO daily are effective. The above drugs are administered by fixed doses and do not require close monitoring; their safety during the first trimester of pregnancy has not been clearly established.

FURTHER READINGS

Cervera R et al: Antiphospholipid syndrome: Clinical and immunologic manifestations and patterns of disease expression in a cohort of 1,000 patients. Arthritis Rheum 46:1019, 2002

Crowther MA et al: A comparison of two intensities of warfarin for the prevention of recurrent thrombosis in patients with the antiphospholipid antibody syndrome. N Engl J Med 349:1133, 2003

George D, Erkan D: Antiphospholipid syndrome. Prog Cardiovasc Dis 52:115, 2009

Miyakis S et al: International consensus statement on an update of the classification criteria for definite antiphospholipid syndrome (APS). J Thromb Haemost 295:4, 2006

Ruiz-Irastorza G et al: Antiphospholipid syndrome. Lancet 376:1498, 2010

Sikara MP et al: β2 glycoprotein I (β2GPI) binds platelet factor 4 (PF4): Implications for the pathogenesis of Antiphospholipid syndrome. Blood 115:713, 2010

Tektonidou M et al: Risk factors for thrombosis and primary thrombosis prevention in patients with systemic lupus erythematosus with or without antiphospholipid antibodies. Arthritis Rheum 61:29, 2009

Vlachoyiannopoulos PG et al: Antiphospholipid antibodies: Laboratory and pathogenetic aspects. Crit Rev Clin Lab Sci 271:44, 2007

CHAPTER 321 Rheumatoid Arthritis

Ankoor Shah

E. William St. Clair

INTRODUCTION

Rheumatoid arthritis (RA) is a chronic inflammatory disease of unknown etiology marked by a symmetric, peripheral polyarthritis. It is the most common form of chronic inflammatory arthritis and often results in joint damage and physical disability. Because it is a systemic disease, RA may result in a variety of extraarticular manifestations, including fatigue, subcutaneous nodules, lung involvement, pericarditis, peripheral neuropathy, vasculitis, and hematologic abnormalities.

Insights gained by a wealth of basic and clinical research over the past two decades have revolutionized the contemporary paradigms for the diagnosis and management of RA. Serum antibodies to cyclic citrullinated peptides (anti-CCPs) are now recognized to be a valuable biomarker of diagnostic and prognostic significance. Advances in ultrasound and magnetic resonance imaging have improved our ability to detect joint inflammation and destruction in RA. The science of RA has taken a major leap forward with the identification of new disease-related genes and further deciphering of the molecular pathways of disease pathogenesis. The relative importance of these different mechanisms has been highlighted by the observed benefits of the new class of highly targeted biologic therapies. Despite these gains, incomplete understanding of the initiating pathogenic pathways of RA remains a sizable barrier to its cure and prevention.

The last two decades have witnessed a remarkable improvement in the outcomes of RA. The historic descriptions of crippling arthritis are currently encountered much less frequently. Much of this progress can be traced to the expanded therapeutic armamentarium and the adoption of early treatment intervention. The shift in treatment strategy dictates a new mind-set for primary care practitioners—namely, one that demands early referral of patients with inflammatory arthritis to a rheumatologist for prompt diagnosis and initiation of therapy. Only then will patients achieve their best outcomes.

CLINICAL FEATURES

The incidence of RA increases between 25 and 55 years of age, after which it plateaus until the age of 75 and then decreases. The presenting symptoms of RA typically result from inflammation of the joints, tendons, and bursae. Patients often complain of early morning joint stiffness lasting more than 1 hour and easing with physical activity. The earliest involved joints are typically the small joints of the hands and feet. The initial pattern of joint involvement may be monoarticular, oligoarticular (≤4 joints), or polyarticular (>5 joints), usually in a symmetric distribution. Some patients with an inflammatory arthritis will present with too few affected joints and other characteristic features to be classified as having RA—so-called undifferentiated inflammatory arthritis. Those with an undifferentiated arthritis, who are most likely to be diagnosed later with RA, have a higher number of tender and swollen joints, test positive for serum rheumatoid factor (RF) or anti-CCP antibodies, and have higher scores for physical disability.

Once the disease process of RA is established, the wrists, metacarpophalangeal (MCP), and proximal interphalangeal (PIP) joints stand out as the most frequently involved joints (Fig. 321-1). Distal interphalangeal (DIP) joint involvement may occur in RA, but it usually is a manifestation of coexistent osteoarthritis. Flexor tendon tenosynovitis is a frequent hallmark of RA and leads to decreased range of motion, reduced grip strength, and "trigger" fingers. Progressive destruction of the joints and soft tissues may lead to chronic, irreversible deformities. Ulnar deviation results from subluxation of the MCP joints, with subluxation of the proximal phalanx to the volar side of the hand. Hyperextension of the PIP joint with flexion of the DIP joint ("swan-neck deformity"), flexion of the PIP joint with hyperextension of the DIP joint ("boutonnière deformity"), and subluxation of the first MCP joint with hyperextension of the first interphalangeal (IP) joint ("Z-line deformity") also may result from damage to the tendons, joint capsule, and other soft tissues in these small joints. Inflammation about the ulnar styloid and tenosynovitis of the extensor carpi ulnaris may cause subluxation of the distal ulna, resulting in a "piano-key movement" of the ulnar styloid. While metatarsophalangeal joint (MTP) involvement is a feature of early disease in the feet, the ankle and midtarsal regions are usually affected later in the course of disease and often predispose to pes planovalgus ("flat feet"). Large joints, including the knees and shoulders, are often affected in established disease, although these joints may remain asymptomatic for many years after onset.

Atlantoaxial involvement of the cervical spine is clinically noteworthy because of its potential to cause compressive myelopathy and neurologic dysfunction. Neurologic manifestations are rarely

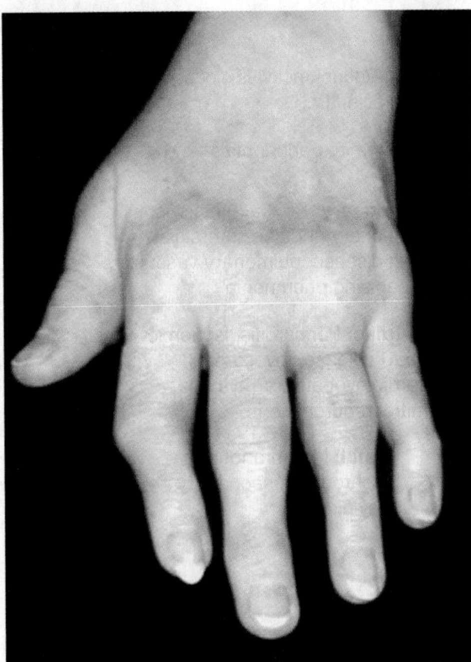

Figure 321-1 Metacarpophalangeal and proximal interphalangeal joint swelling in rheumatoid arthritis. *(Courtesy of the American College of Rheumatology Image Bank.)*

a presenting sign or symptom of atlantoaxial disease, but they may evolve over time with progressive instability of C1 on C2. The prevalence of atlantoaxial subluxation has been declining in recent years, and occurs now in less than 10% of patients. Unlike the spondyloarthritides (Chap. 325), RA does not affect the thoracic and lumbar spine except in very unusual circumstances. Radiographic abnormalities of the temporomandibular joint occur commonly in patients with RA, but they are rarely associated with significant symptoms or functional impairment.

Extraarticular manifestations may develop during the clinical course of RA, even prior to the onset of arthritis (Fig. 321-2). Patients most likely to develop extraarticular disease have a history of smoking, early onset of significant physical disability, and test positive for serum RF. Subcutaneous nodules, secondary Sjögren's syndrome, pulmonary nodules, and anemia are among the most frequently observed extraarticular manifestations. Recent studies have shown a decrease in the incidence and severity of at least some extraarticular manifestations, particularly Felty's syndrome and vasculitis.

The most common systemic and extraarticular features of RA are described in more detail in the sections below.

CONSTITUTIONAL

These signs and symptoms include weight loss, fever, fatigue, malaise, depression, and in the most severe cases, cachexia; they generally reflect a high degree of inflammation and may even precede the onset of joint symptoms. In general, the presence of a fever of >38.3°C (101°F) at any time during the clinical course should raise suspicion of systemic vasculitis (see below) or infection.

NODULES

Subcutaneous nodules occur in 30–40% of patients and more commonly in those with the highest levels of disease activity, the disease-related shared epitope (see below), a positive test for serum RF, and radiographic evidence of joint erosions. When palpated, the nodules are generally firm; nontender; and adherent to periosteum, tendons, or bursae; developing in areas of the skeleton subject to repeated trauma or irritation such as the forearm, sacral prominences, and the Achilles tendon. They may also occur in the lungs, pleura, pericardium, and peritoneum. Nodules are typically benign, although they can be associated with infection, ulceration, and gangrene.

SJÖGREN'S SYNDROME

Secondary Sjögren's syndrome (Chap. 324) is defined by the presence of either keratoconjunctivitis sicca (dry eyes) or xerostomia (dry mouth) in association with another connective tissue disease, such as RA. Approximately 10% of patients with RA have secondary Sjögren's syndrome.

PULMONARY

Pleural disease, the most common pulmonary manifestation of RA, may produce pleuritic chest pain and dyspnea, as well as a pleural friction rub and effusion. Pleural effusions tend to be exudative with increased numbers of monocytes and neutrophils. Interstitial lung disease (ILD) may also occur in patients with RA and is heralded by symptoms of dry cough and progressive shortness of breath. Diagnosis is readily made by high-resolution chest CT scan. Pulmonary function testing shows a restrictive pattern (e.g., reduced total lung capacity) with a reduced diffusing capacity for carbon monoxide (D_{LCO}). The presence of ILD confers a poor prognosis. The prognosis is not quite as poor as that of idiopathic pulmonary fibrosis (e.g., usual interstitial pneumonitis) because ILD secondary to RA responds more favorably than idiopathic ILD to immunosuppressive therapy (Chap. 261). Pulmonary nodules may be solitary or multiple. Caplan's syndrome is a rare subset of pulmonary nodulosis characterized by the development of nodules and pneumoconiosis following silica exposure. Other less common pulmonary findings include respiratory bronchiolitis and bronchiectasis.

CARDIAC

The most frequent site of cardiac involvement in RA is the pericardium. However, clinical manifestations of pericarditis occur in less than 10% of patients with RA despite the fact that pericardial involvement may be detected in nearly one-half of the these patients by echocardiogram or autopsy studies. Cardiomyopathy, another clinically important manifestation of RA, may result from necrotizing or granulomatous myocarditis, coronary artery disease, or diastolic dysfunction. This involvement too may be subclinical and only identified by echocardiography or cardiac MRI. Rarely, the heart muscle may contain rheumatoid nodules or be infiltrated with amyloid. Mitral regurgitation is the most common valvular abnormality in RA, occurring at a higher frequency than the general population.

VASCULITIS

Rheumatoid vasculitis (Chap. 326) is seen most commonly in patients with long-standing disease, a positive test for serum RF, and hypocomplementemia; the overall incidence is quite rare, occurring in no more than 1% of cases. The cutaneous signs vary and include petechiae, purpura, digital infarcts, gangrene, livedo reticularis, and in severe cases large, painful lower extremity ulcerations. Vasculitic ulcers, which may be difficult to distinguish from those caused by venous insufficiency, may be treated successfully with immunosuppressive agents (requiring cytotoxic treatment in severe cases) as well as skin grafting. Sensorimotor polyneuropathies, such as mononeuritis multiplex, may occur in association with systemic rheumatoid vasculitis.

HEMATOLOGIC

A normochromic, normocytic anemia often develops in patients with RA and is the most common hematologic abnormality. The

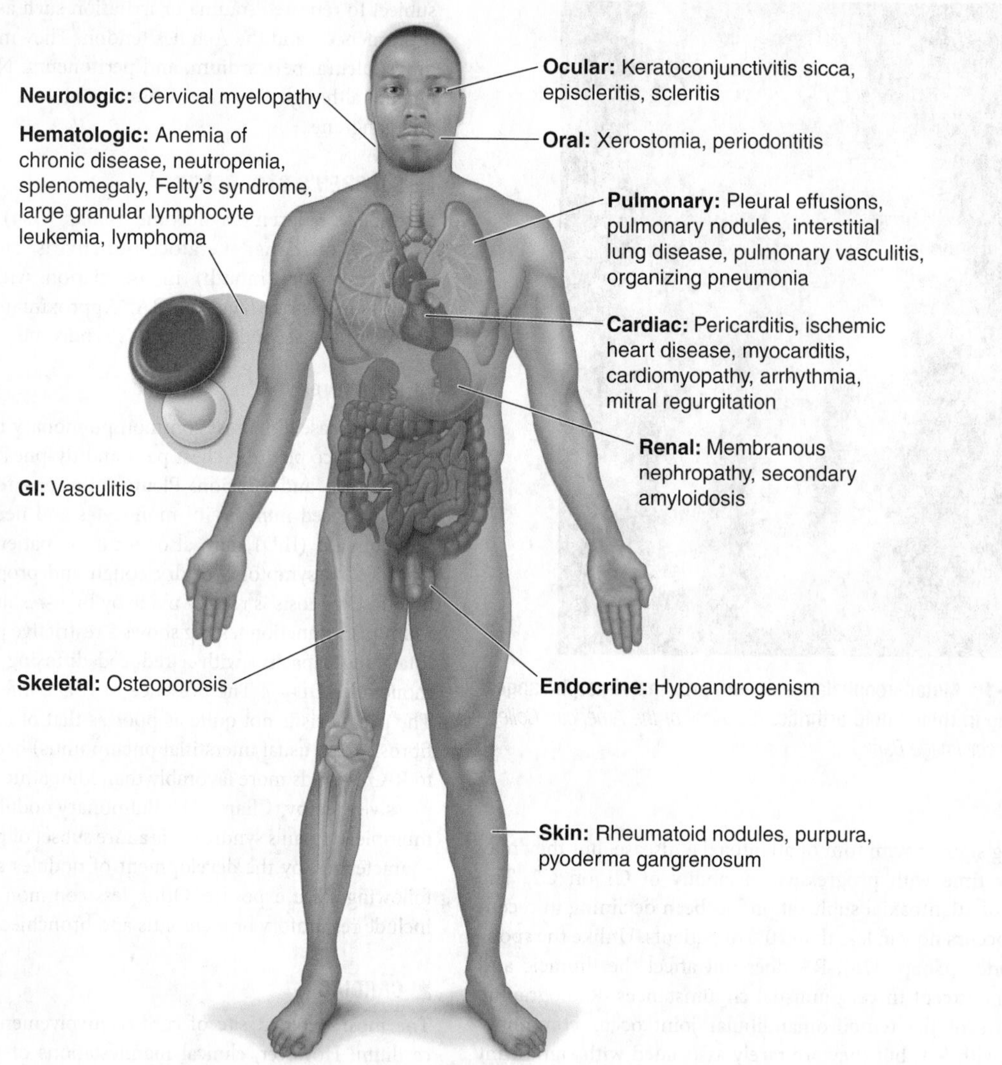

Figure 321-2 Extraarticular manifestations of rheumatoid arthritis.

degree of anemia parallels the degree of inflammation, correlating with the levels of serum C-reactive protein (CRP) and erythrocyte sedimentation rate (ESR). Platelet counts may also be elevated in RA as an acute-phase reactant. Immune-mediated thrombocytopenia is rare in this disease.

Felty's syndrome is defined by the clinical triad of neutropenia, splenomegaly, and nodular RA and is seen in less than 1% of patients, although its incidence appears to be declining in the face of more aggressive treatment of the joint disease. It typically occurs in white patients in the late stages of severe RA. T cell large granular lymphocyte leukemia (T-LGL) may have a similar clinical presentation and often occurs in association with RA. T-LGL is characterized by a chronic, indolent clonal growth of LGL cells, leading to neutropenia and splenomegaly. As opposed to Felty's syndrome, T-LGL may develop early in the course of RA. Leukopenia apart from these disorders is uncommon and most often due to drug therapy.

LYMPHOMA

Large cohort studies have shown a two- to fourfold increased risk of lymphoma in RA patients compared with the general population. The most common histopathologic type of lymphoma is a diffuse large B-cell lymphoma. The risk of developing lymphoma increases if the patient has high levels of disease activity or Felty's syndrome.

ASSOCIATED CONDITIONS

In addition to extraarticular manifestations, several conditions associated with RA contribute to disease morbidity and mortality rates. They are worthy of mention because they affect chronic disease management.

Cardiovascular disease

The most common cause of death in patients with RA is cardiovascular disease. The incidence of coronary artery disease and carotid atherosclerosis is higher in RA patients than in the general population even when controlling for traditional cardiac risk factors, such as hypertension, obesity, hypercholesterolemia, diabetes, and cigarette smoking. Furthermore, congestive heart failure (including both systolic and diastolic dysfunction) occurs at an approximately twofold higher rate in RA than in the general population. The presence of elevated serum inflammatory markers appears to confer an increased risk of cardiovascular disease in this population.

Osteoporosis

Osteoporosis is more common in patients with RA than an age- and sex-matched population, with prevalence rates of 20–30%. The inflammatory milieu of the joint probably spills over into the rest of the body and promotes generalized bone loss by activating osteoclasts. Chronic use of glucocorticoids and disability-related immobility also contributes to osteoporosis. Hip fractures are more likely to occur in patients with RA and are significant predictors of increased disability and mortality rate in this disease.

Hypoandrogenism

Men and postmenopausal women with RA have lower mean serum testosterone, luteinizing hormone (LH) and dehydroepiandrosterone (DHEA) levels than control populations. It has thus been hypothesized that hypoandrogenism may play a role in the pathogenesis of RA or arise as a consequence of the chronic inflammatory response. In fact, some studies suggest that higher testosterone levels offer some protection from RA in younger males. The idea that the low serum testosterone levels associated with RA arise from the chronic inflammatory state comes from observations that clinical improvement following successful treatment correlates with an increase in serum testosterone levels. From a clinical perspective, it is important to realize that patients receiving chronic glucocorticoid therapy may develop hypoandrogenism owing to inhibition of LH and follicle-stimulating hormone (FSH) secretion from the pituitary gland. Since low testosterone levels may lead to osteoporosis, men with serum testosterone levels below the physiologic range should be considered for androgen replacement therapy.

EPIDEMIOLOGY

RA affects approximately 0.5–1% of the adult population worldwide. There is evidence that the overall incidence of RA has been decreasing in recent decades, whereas the prevalence has remained the same because individuals with RA are living longer. The incidence and prevalence of RA varies based on geographic location, both globally and among certain ethnic groups within a country (Fig. 321-3). For example, the Native American Yakima, Pima, and Chippewa tribes of North America have reported prevalence rates in some studies of nearly 7%. In contrast, many population studies from Africa and Asia show lower prevalence rates for RA in the range of 0.2–0.4%.

Like many other autoimmune diseases, RA occurs more commonly in females than in males, with a 2–3:1 ratio. Interestingly, studies of RA from some of the Latin American and African countries show an even greater predominance of disease in females compared to males, with ratios of 6–8:1. Given this preponderance of females, various theories have been proposed to explain the possible role of estrogen in disease pathogenesis. Most of the theories center on the role of estrogens in enhancing the immune response. For example, some experimental studies have shown that estrogen can stimulate production of tumor necrosis factor α (TNF-α), a major cytokine in the pathogenesis of RA.

GENETIC CONSIDERATIONS

It has been recognized for over 30 years that genetic factors contribute to the occurrence of RA as well as to its severity. The likelihood that a first-degree relative of a patient will share the diagnosis of RA is 2–10 times greater than in the general population. There remains, however, some uncertainty in the extent to which genetics plays a role in the causative mechanisms of RA. While twin studies imply that genetic factors may explain up to 60% of the occurrence of RA, the more commonly stated estimate falls in the range of 10–25%. The estimate of genetic influence may vary across studies due to gene–environment interactions.

The alleles known to confer the greatest risk of RA are located within the major histocompatibility complex (MHC). It has been estimated that one-third of the genetic risk for RA resides within this locus. Most, but probably not all, of this risk is associated with allelic variation in the HLA-DRB1 gene, which encodes the MHC II β-chain molecule. The disease-associated HLA-DRB1 alleles share an amino acid sequence at positions 70–74 in the third hypervariable regions of the HLA-DR β-chain, termed the *shared epitope (SE)*. Carriership of the SE alleles is associated with production of anti-CCP antibodies and worse disease outcomes. Some of these HLA-DRB1 alleles bestow a high risk of disease (*0401), whereas others confer a more moderate risk (*0101, *0404, *1001, and *0901). In Greece, for example, where RA tends to be milder than in western European countries, RA susceptibility has been associated with

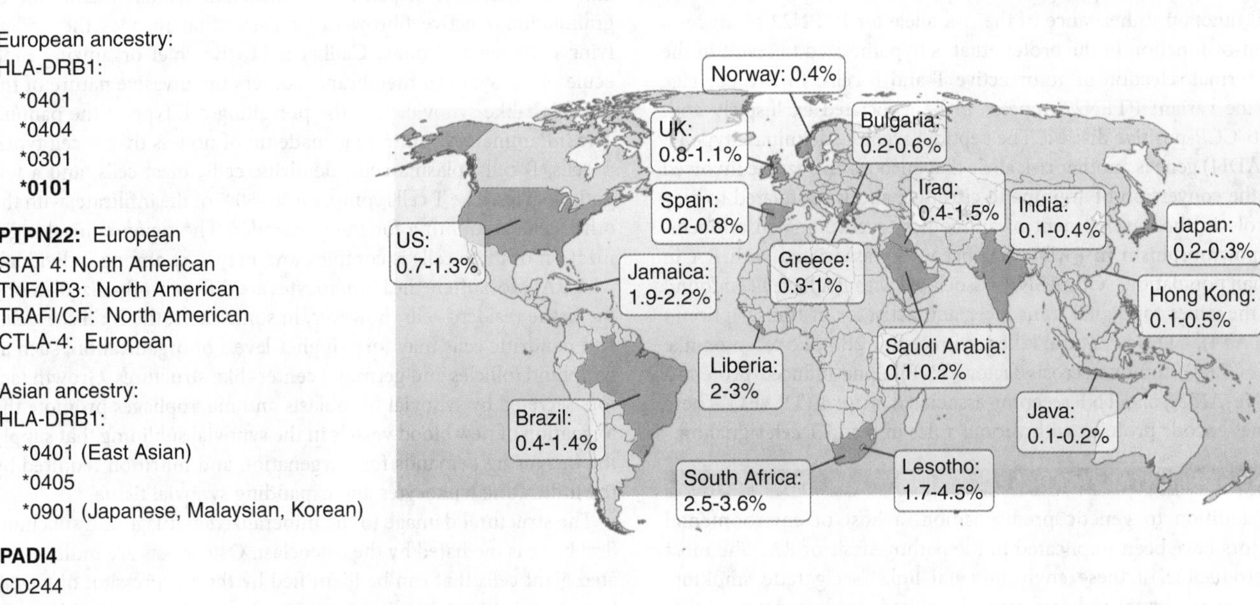

Figure 321-3 Global prevalence rates of rheumatoid arthritis (RA) with genetic associations. Listed are the major genetic alleles associated with RA. While human leukocyte antigen (HLA)-DRB1 mutations are found globally, some alleles have been associated with RA in only certain ethnic groups.

the *0101 SE allele. By comparison, the *0401 or *0404 alleles are found in approximately 50–70% of Northern Europeans and are the predominant risk alleles in this group. The most common disease susceptibility SE alleles in Asians, namely the Japanese, Koreans, and Chinese, are *0405 and *0901. Lastly, disease susceptibility of Native American populations such as the Pima and Tlingit Indians, where the prevalence of RA can be as high as 7%, is associated with the SE allele *1042. The risk of RA conferred by these SE alleles is less in African and Hispanic Americans than in individuals of European ancestry.

Genome-wide association studies (GWAS) have made possible the identification of several non-MHC-related genes that contribute to RA susceptibility. GWAS are based on the detection of single-nucleotide polymorphisms (SNPs), which allow for examination of the genetic architecture of complex diseases such as RA. There are approximately 10 million common SNPs within a human genome consisting of 3 billion base pairs. As a rule, GWAS identify only common variants, namely, those with a frequency of more than 5% in the general population.

Overall, several themes have emerged from GWAS in RA. First, several of the non-MHC loci identified as risk alleles for RA have only a modest effect on risk; they also contribute to the risk for developing other autoimmune diseases, such as Type 1 diabetes mellitus, systemic lupus erythematosus, and multiple sclerosis. Second, most of the associations are described in patients with anti-CCP antibody-positive disease. Third, risk alleles vary among ethnic groups. Fourth, the risk loci mostly reside in genes encoding proteins involved in the regulation of the immune response, such as the signaling pathway for the nuclear factor kappa-light-chain-enhancer of activated B cells (NF-κB). However, the risk alleles identified by GWAS only account at present for approximately 5% of the genetic risk, suggesting that rare variants or other classes of DNA variants, such as variants in copy number, may be yet found that significantly contribute to the overall risk model.

Among the best examples of the non-MHC genes contributing to the risk of RA is the gene encoding protein tyrosine phosphatase non-receptor 22 (PTPN22). This gene varies in frequency among patients from different parts of Europe (e.g., 3–10%), but is absent in patients of East Asian ancestry. PTPN22 encodes lymphoid tyrosine phosphatase, a protein that regulates T and B cell function. Inheritance of the risk allele for PTPN22 produces a gain-of-function in the protein that is hypothesized to result in the abnormal selection of autoreactive T and B cells. In RA, carriage of the variant PTPN22 appears to be associated exclusively with anti-CCP-positive disease. The peptidyl arginine deiminase type IV (PADI4) gene is another risk allele that encodes an enzyme involved in the conversion of arginine to citrulline and is postulated to play a role in the development of antibodies to citrullinated antigens. A polymorphism in PADI4 has been only associated with RA in Asian populations. Other SNPs associated with RA have been found in the genes for signal transducer and activator of transcription 4 (STAT4), CD244 (natural killer cell receptor 2B4), Fc receptor-like 3 (FCLR3), tumor necrosis factor (TNF) alpha-induced protein 3 (TNF-AIP3), and TNF receptor-associated factor 1 (TRAF1). These genes encode proteins with various roles in B and T cell signaling.

ENVIRONMENTAL FACTORS

In addition to genetic predisposition, a host of environmental factors have been implicated in the pathogenesis of RA. The most reproducible of these environmental links is cigarette smoking. Numerous cohort and case control studies have demonstrated that smoking confers a relative risk for developing RA of 1.5–3.5. A twin who smokes will have a significantly higher risk for RA than his or her monozygotic co-twin, theoretically with the same genetic risk, who does not smoke. Interestingly, the risk from smoking is almost exclusively related to RF- and anti-CCP antibody-positive disease.

Researchers began to aggressively seek an infectious etiology for RA after the discovery in 1931 that sera from patients with this disease could agglutinate strains of streptococci. Certain viruses such as Epstein-Barr virus (EBV) have garnered the most interest over the past 30 years given their ubiquity, ability to persist for many years in the host, and frequent association with arthritic complaints. For example, titers of IgG antibodies against EBV antigens in the peripheral blood and saliva are significantly higher in patients with RA than the general population. EBV DNA has also been found in synovial fluid and synovial cells of RA patients. Blood and synovial fluid analyses have also suggested a possible link with mycoplasma and parvovirus B19 infection. Since the evidence for these links is largely circumstantial, it has not been possible to directly implicate infection as a causative factor in RA.

PATHOLOGY

RA affects the synovial tissue and underlying cartilage and bone. The synovial membrane, which covers most articular surfaces, tendon sheaths, and bursae, normally is a thin layer of connective tissue. In joints, it faces the bone and cartilage, bridging the opposing bony surfaces and inserting at periosteal regions close to the articular cartilage. It consists primarily of two cell types—type A synoviocytes (macrophage-derived) and type B synoviocytes (fibroblast-derived). The synovial fibroblasts are the most abundant and produce the structural components of joints, including collagen, fibronectin, and laminin, as well as other extracellular constituents of the synovial matrix. The sublining layer consists of blood vessels and a sparse population of mononuclear cells within a loose network of connective tissue. Synovial fluid, an ultrafiltrate of blood, diffuses through the subsynovial lining tissue across the synovial membrane and into the joint cavity. Its main constituents are hyaluronan and lubricin. Hyaluronan is a glycosaminoglycan that contributes to the viscous nature of synovial fluid, which along with lubricin, lubricates the surface of the articular cartilage.

The pathologic hallmarks of RA are synovial inflammation and proliferation, focal bone erosions, and thinning of articular cartilage. Chronic inflammation leads to synovial lining hyperplasia and the formation of pannus, a thickened cellular membrane of granulation–reactive fibrovascular tissue that invades the underlying cartilage and bone. Cadherin-11, the chief organizing molecule of the synovial membrane, confers the invasive nature of the fibroblast-like synoviocytes, the prevailing cell type of the pannus. The inflammatory infiltrate is made up of no less than 6 cell types: T cells, B cells, plasma cells, dendritic cells, mast cells, and a few granulocytes. The T cells comprise 30–50% of the infiltrate, with the other cells accounting for the remainder. The topographical organization of these cells is complex and may vary among individuals with RA. Most often, the lymphocytes are diffusely organized among the tissue resident cells; however, in some cases, the B cells, T cells, and dendritic cells may form higher levels of organization, such as lymphoid follicles and germinal center–like structures. Growth factors secreted by synovial fibroblasts and macrophages promote the formation of new blood vessels in the synovial sublining that supply the increasing demands for oxygenation and nutrition required by the infiltrating leukocytes and expanding synovial tissue.

The structural damage to the mineralized cartilage and subchondral bone is mediated by the osteoclast. Osteoclasts are multinucleated giant cells that can be identified by their expression of CD68, tartrate-resistant acid phosphatase, cathepsin K, and the calcitonin receptor. They appear at the pannus-bone interface where they eventually form resorption lacunae. These lesions typically localize where the synovial membrane inserts into the periosteal surface at the edges of bones close to the rim of articular cartilage and at the attachment sites of ligaments and tendon sheaths. This process most likely explains why bone erosions usually develop at the radial sites of the MCP joints juxtaposed to the insertion sites of the tendons, collateral ligaments, and synovial membrane. Another form of bone loss is periarticular osteopenia that occurs in joints with active inflammation. It is associated with substantial thinning of the bony trabeculae along the metaphyses of bones, and likely results from inflammation of the bone marrow cavity. These lesions can be visualized on MRI scans, where they appear as signal alterations in the bone marrow adjacent to inflamed joints. Their signal characteristics show they are water-rich with a low fat content, and consistent with highly vascularized inflammatory tissue. These bone marrow lesions are often the forerunner of bone erosions.

The cortical bone layer that separates the bone marrow from the invading pannus is relatively thin and susceptible to penetration by the inflamed synovium. The bone marrow lesions seen on MRI scans are associated with an endosteal bone response characterized by the accumulation of osteoblasts and deposition of osteoid. Thus, in recent years, the concept of joint pathology in RA has been extended to include the bone marrow cavity. Finally, a third form of bone loss is generalized osteoporosis, which results in the thinning of trabecular bone throughout the body.

Articular cartilage is an avascular tissue comprised of a specialized matrix of collagens, proteoglycans, and other proteins. It is organized in four distinct regions (superficial, middle, deep, and calcified cartilage zones)—chondrocytes constitute the unique cellular component in these layers. Originally, cartilage was considered to be an inert tissue, but it is now known to be a highly responsive tissue that reacts to inflammatory mediators and mechanical factors, which in turn, alter the balance between cartilage anabolism and catabolism. In RA, the initial areas of cartilage degradation are juxtaposed to the synovial pannus. The cartilage matrix is characterized by a generalized loss of proteoglycan, most evident in the superficial zones adjacent to the synovial fluid. Degradation of cartilage may also take place in the perichondrocytic zone and in regions adjacent to the subchondral bone.

PATHOGENESIS

The pathogenic mechanisms of synovial inflammation are likely to result from a complex interplay of genetic, environmental, and immunologic factors that produces dysregulation of the immune system and a breakdown in self-tolerance (Fig. 321-4). Precisely what triggers these initiating events and what genetic and environmental factors disrupt the immune system remain a mystery. However, a detailed molecular picture is emerging of the mechanisms underlying the chronic inflammatory response and the destruction of the articular cartilage and bone.

In RA, the earliest detectable preclinical stage is a breakdown in self-tolerance. This idea is supported by the finding that autoantibodies, such as RF and anti-CCP antibodies, may be found in sera from patients long before clinical disease. However, the antigenic targets of anti-CCP antibodies and RF are not restricted to the joint, and their role in disease pathogenesis remains speculative. Anti-CCP antibodies are directed against deiminated peptides, which result from posttranslational modification by the enzyme PADI4. They recognize citrulline-containing regions of several different matrix proteins, including filaggrin, keratin, fibrinogen, and vimentin. Other autoantibodies have been found in a minority of patients with RA, but they also occur in the setting of other types of arthritis. They bind to a diverse array of autoantigens, including type II collagen, human cartilage gp-39, aggrecan, calpastatin, BiP (immunoglobulin binding protein), and glucose-6-phosphate isomerase.

In theory, environmental stimulants may synergize with other factors to bring about inflammation in RA. People who smoke display higher citrullination of proteins in bronchoalveolar fluid than those who do not smoke. Thus, it has been speculated that long-term exposure to tobacco smoke might induce citrullination of cellular proteins in the lungs and enhance the expression of a neoepitope capable of inducing self-reactivity. Exposure to silicone dust and mineral oil, which has adjuvant effects, has also been linked to an increased risk for anti-CCP antibody-positive RA.

How might microbes or their products be involved in the initiating events of RA? The immune system is alerted to the presence of microbial infections through Toll-like receptors (TLRs). There are 10 TLRs in humans that recognize a variety of microbial products, including bacterial cell-surface lipopolysaccharides and heat-shock proteins (TLR4), lipoproteins (TLR2), double-strand RNA viruses (TLR3), and unmethylated CpG DNA from bacteria (TLR9). TLR2, -3, and -4 are abundantly expressed by synovial fibroblasts in early RA, and when bound by their ligands upregulate production of proinflammatory cytokines. Although such events could amplify inflammatory pathways in RA, a specific role for TLRs in disease pathogenesis has not been elucidated.

The pathogenesis of RA is built upon the concept that self-reactive T cells drive the chronic inflammatory response. In theory, self-reactive T cells might arise in RA from abnormal central (thymic) selection due to defects in DNA repair leading to an imbalance of T cell death and life, or defects in the cell signaling apparatus lowering the threshold for T cell activation. Similarly, abnormal selection of the T cell repertoire in the periphery might lead to a breakdown in T cell tolerance. The support for these theories comes mainly from studies of arthritis in mouse models. It has not been shown that patients with RA have abnormal thymic selection of T cells or defective apoptotic pathways regulating cell death. At least some antigen stimulation inside the joint seems likely, owing to the fact that T cells in the synovium express a cell-surface phenotype indicating prior antigen exposure and show evidence of clonal expansion. Of interest, peripheral blood T cells from patients with RA have been shown to display a fingerprint of premature aging that mostly affects inexperienced naïve T cells. In these studies, the most glaring findings have been the loss of telomeric sequences and a decrease in the thymic output of new T cells. While intriguing, it is not clear how generalized T cell abnormalities might provoke a systemic disease dominated by synovitis.

There is substantial evidence supporting a role for CD4+ T cells in the pathogenesis of RA. First, the co-receptor CD4 on the surface of T cells binds to invariant sites on MHC class II molecules, stabilizing the MHC-peptide–T cell receptor complex during T cell activation. Since the SE on MHC class II molecules is a risk factor for RA, it may be speculated that CD4+ T cell activation plays a role in the pathogenesis of this disease. Second, CD4+ memory T cells are enriched in the synovial tissue from patients with RA, and can be implicated through "guilt by association." Third, CD4+ T cells have been shown to be important in the initiation of arthritis in animal models. Fourth, T cell–directed therapies, such as cyclosporine and abatacept (CTLA4-Ig), have shown clinical efficacy in this disease. Taken together, these lines of evidence suggest that CD4+ T cells play an important role in orchestrating the chronic inflammatory response in RA. However, other cell types, such as CD8+ T cells, natural killer (NK) cells, and B cells are present in synovial tissue and may also influence pathogenic responses.

In the rheumatoid joint, by mechanisms of cell-cell contact and release of soluble mediators, activated T cells stimulate macrophages and fibroblast-like synoviocytes to generate proinflammatory mediators and proteases that drive the synovial inflammatory response and destroy the cartilage and bone. CD4+ T cells also provide help to B cells, which in turn, produce antibodies that may promote further inflammation in the joint. The previous T cell–centric model for the pathogenesis of RA was based on a T_H1-driven paradigm, which came from studies indicating that CD4+

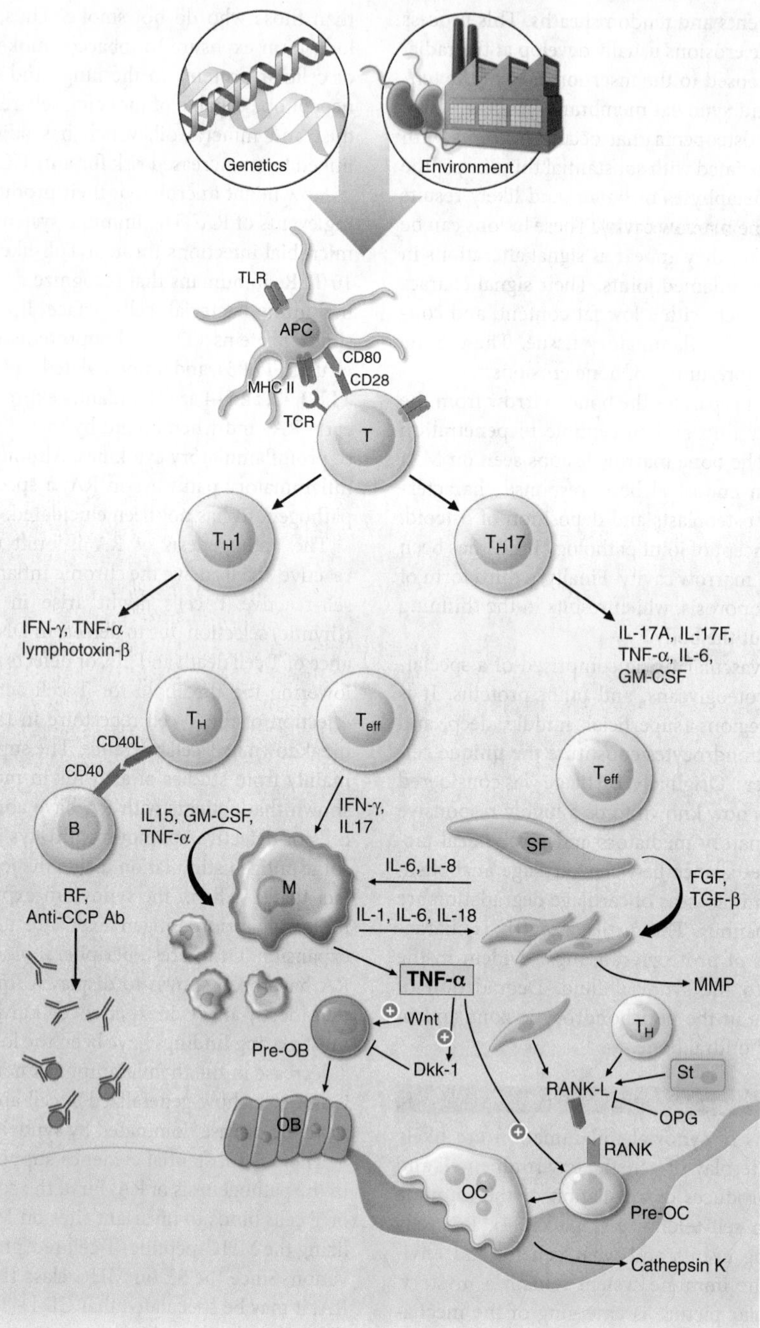

Figure 321-4 Pathophysiologic mechanisms of inflammation and joint destruction. Genetic predisposition along with environmental factors may trigger the development of rheumatoid arthritis (RA), with subsequent synovial T cell activation. CD4+ T cells become activated by antigen-presenting cells (APCs) through interactions between the T cell receptor and class II major histocompatibility complex (MHC)-peptide antigen (signal 1) with co-stimulation through the CD28-CD80/86 pathway, as well as other pathways (signal 2). In theory, ligands binding Toll-like receptors (TLRs) may further stimulate activation of APCs inside the joint. Synovial CD4+ T cells differentiate into T_H1 and T_H17 cells, each with their distinctive cytokine profile. CD4+ T_H cells in turn activate B cells, some of which are destined to differentiate into autoantibody-producing plasma cells. Immune complexes, possibly comprised of rheumatoid factors (RFs) and anti–cyclic citrullinated peptides (CCP) antibodies, may form inside the joint, activating the complement pathway and amplifying inflammation. T effector cells stimulate synovial macrophages (M) and fibroblasts (SF) to secrete proinflammatory mediators, among which is tumor necrosis factor α (TNF-α). TNF-α upregulates adhesion molecules on endothelial cells, promoting leukocyte influx into the joint. It also stimulates the production of other inflammatory mediators, such as interleukin 1 (IL-1), IL-6, and granulocyte-macrophage colony-stimulating factor (GM-CSF). TNF-α has a critically important function in regulating the balance between bone destruction and formation. It upregulates the expression of dickkopf-1 (DKK-1), which can then internalize Wnt receptors on osteoblast precursors. Wnt is a soluble mediator that promotes osteoblastogenesis and bone formation. In RA, bone formation is inhibited through the Wnt pathway, presumably due to the action of elevated levels of DKK-1. In addition to inhibiting bone formation, TNF-α stimulates osteoclastogenesis. However, it is not sufficient by itself to induce the differentiation of osteoclast precursors (Pre-OC) into activated osteoclasts capable of eroding bone. Osteoclast differentiation requires the presence of macrophage colony-stimulating factor (M-CSF) and receptor activator of nuclear factor κB (RANK) ligand, which binds to RANK on the surface of Pre-OC. Inside the joint, RANKL is mainly derived from stromal cells, synovial fibroblasts, and T cells. Osteoprotegerin (OPG) acts as a decoy receptor for RANKL, thereby inhibiting osteoclastogenesis and bone loss. FGF, fibroblast growth factor; IFN, interferon; TGF, transforming growth factor.

T helper (T_H) cells differentiated into T_H1 and T_H2 subsets, each with their distinctive cytokine profiles. T_H1 cells were found to mainly produce interferon γ (IFN-γ), lymphotoxin β, and TNF-α, while T_H2 cells predominately secreted interleukin (IL)-4, IL-5, IL-6, IL-10, and IL-13. The recent discovery of another subset of T_H cells, namely the T_H17 lineage, has revolutionized our concepts concerning the pathogenesis of RA. In humans, naïve T cells are induced to differentiate into T_H17 cells by exposure to transforming growth factor β (TGF-β), IL-1, IL-6, and IL-23. Upon activation, T_H17 cells secrete a variety of proinflammatory mediators such as IL-17, IL-21, IL-22, TNF-α, IL-26, IL-6, and granulocyte-macrophage colony-stimulating factor (GM-CSF). Substantial evidence now exists from both animal models and humans that IL-17 plays an important role not only in promoting joint inflammation but also in destroying cartilage and subchondral bone.

Activated B cells are also important players in the chronic inflammatory response. B cells give rise to plasma cells, which in turn, produce antibodies, including RF and anti-CCP antibodies. RFs may form large immune complexes inside the joint that contribute to the pathogenic process by fixing complement and promoting the release of proinflammatory chemokines and chemoattractants. In mouse models of arthritis, RF-containing immune complexes as well as anti-CCP-containing immune complexes synergize with other mechanisms to exacerbate the synovial inflammatory response.

RA is often considered to be a macrophage-driven disease because this cell type is the predominant source of proinflammatory cytokines inside the joint. Key proinflammatory cytokines released by synovial macrophages include TNF-α, IL-1, IL-6, IL-12, IL-15, IL-18, and IL-23. Synovial fibroblasts, the other major cell type in this microenvironment, produce the cytokines IL-1 and IL-6 as well as TNF-α. TNF-α is a pivotal cytokine in the pathobiology of synovial inflammation. It upregulates adhesion molecules on endothelial cells, promoting the influx of leukocytes into the synovial microenvironment. It also activates synovial fibroblasts, stimulates angiogenesis, promotes pain receptor sensitizing pathways, and drives osteoclastogenesis. Fibroblasts secrete matrix metalloproteinases (MMPs) as well as other proteases that are chiefly responsible for the breakdown of articular cartilage.

Osteoclast activation at the site of the pannus is closely tied to the presence of focal bone erosion. Receptor activator of nuclear factor κB ligand (RANKL) is expressed by stromal cells, synovial fibroblasts, and T cells. Upon binding to its receptor RANK on osteoclast progenitors, RANKL stimulates osteoclast differentiation and bone resorption. RANKL activity is regulated by osteoprotegerin (OPG), a decoy receptor of RANKL that blocks osteoclast formation. Monocytic cells in the synovium serve as the precursors of osteoclasts and, when exposed to macrophage colony-stimulating factor (M-CSF) and RANKL, fuse to form polykaryons termed *preosteoclasts*. These precursor cells undergo further differentiation into osteoclasts with the characteristic ruffled membrane. Cytokines such as TNF-α, IL-1, IL-6, and IL-17 increase the expression of RANKL in the joint and thus promote osteoclastogenesis. Osteoclasts also secrete cathepsin K, which is a cysteine protease that degrades the bone matrix by cleaving collagen.

Increased bone loss is only part of the story in RA, as decreased bone formation plays a crucial role in bone remodeling at sites of inflammation. Recent evidence shows that inflammation suppresses bone formation. The proinflammatory cytokine TNF-α plays a key role in actively suppressing bone formation by enhancing the expression of dickkopf-1 (DKK-1). DKK-1 is an important inhibitor of the Wnt pathway, which acts to promote osteoblast differentiation and bone formation. The Wnt system is a family of soluble glycoproteins that bind to cell-surface receptors known as frizzled (fz) and low-density lipoprotein (LDL) receptor–related proteins (LRPs) and promote cell growth. In animal models, increased levels of DKK-1 are associated with decreased bone formation, while inhibition of DKK-1 protects against structural damage in the joint. Wnt proteins also induce the formation of OPG and thereby shut down bone resorption, emphasizing their key role in tightly regulating the balance between bone resorption and formation.

DIAGNOSIS

The clinical diagnosis of RA is largely based on signs and symptoms of a chronic inflammatory arthritis, with laboratory and radiographic results providing important supplemental information. In 2010, a collaborative effort between the American College of Rheumatology (ACR) and the European League Against Rheumatism (EULAR) revised the 1987 ACR classification criteria for RA in an effort to improve early diagnosis with the goal of identifying patients who would benefit from early introduction of disease-modifying therapy (Table 321-1). Application of the newly revised criteria yields a score of 0–10, with a score of ≥6 fulfilling the requirements for definite RA. The new classification criteria differ in several ways from the older criteria set. The new criteria include a positive test for serum anti-cyclic citrullinated peptide antibodies as an item, which carries greater specificity for the diagnosis of RA than a positive test for rheumatoid factor. The newer classification criteria also do not take into account if the patient has rheumatoid nodules or radiographic joint damage because these findings occur rarely in early RA. It is important to emphasize that the new 2010 ACR-EULAR criteria are "classification criteria" as opposed to "diagnostic criteria" and serve to distinguish patients at the onset of

TABLE 321-1 Classification Criteria for Rheumatoid Arthritis

		Score
Joint involvement	1 large joint (shoulder, elbow, hip, knee, ankle)	0
	2–10 large joints	1
	1–3 small joints (MCP, PIP, Thumb IP, MTP, wrists)	2
	4–10 small joints	3
	>10 joints (at least 1 small joint)	5
Serology	Negative RF and negative ACPA	0
	Low-positive RF or low-positive anti-CCP antibodies (≤3 times ULN)	2
	High-positive RF or high-positive anti-CCP antibodies (>3 times ULN)	3
Acute-phase reactants	Normal CRP and normal ESR	0
	Abnormal CRP or abnormal ESR	1
Duration of symptoms	<6 weeks	0
	≥6 weeks	1

Note: These criteria are aimed at classification of newly presenting patients who have at least 1 joint with definite clinical synovitis that is not better explained by another disease.

Abbreviations: CCP, cyclic citrullinated peptides; CRP, C-reactive protein; ESR, erythrocyte sedimentation rate; IP, interphalangeal joint; MCP, metacarpophalangeal joint; MTP, metatarsophalangeal joint; PIP, proximal interphalangeal joint; RF, rheumatoid factor; ULN, upper limit of normal.

Source: Neogi et al: Arthritis Rheum 62:2569, 2010.

disease with a high likelihood of evolving into a chronic disease with persistent synovitis and joint damage. The presence of radiographic joint erosions or subcutaneous nodules may inform the diagnosis in the later stages of the disease.

■ LABORATORY FEATURES

IgM, IgG, and IgA isotypes of RF occur in sera from patients with RA, although the IgM isotype is the one most frequently measured by commercial laboratories. Serum IgM RF has been found in 75–80% of patients with RA; therefore, a negative result does not exclude the presence of this disease. It is also found in other connective tissue diseases, such as primary Sjögren's syndrome, systemic lupus erythematosus, and type II mixed essential cryoglobulinemia, as well as chronic infections such as subacute bacterial endocarditis and hepatitis B and C. Serum RF may also be detected in 1–5% of the healthy population.

The presence of serum anti-CCP antibodies has about the same sensitivity as serum RF for the diagnosis of RA. However, its diagnostic specificity approaches 95%, so a positive test for anti-CCP antibodies in the setting of an early inflammatory arthritis is useful for distinguishing RA from other forms of arthritis. There is some incremental value in testing for the presence of both RF and anti-CCP, as some patients with RA are positive for RF but negative for anti-CCP and visa versa. The presence of RF or anti-CCP antibodies also has prognostic significance, with anti-CCP antibodies showing the most value for predicting worse outcomes.

■ SYNOVIAL FLUID ANALYSIS

Typically, synovial fluid from patients with RA reflects an inflammatory state. Synovial fluid white blood cell (WBC) counts can vary widely, but generally range between 5000 and 50,000 WBC/μ^3 compared to <2000 WBC/μ for a non-inflammatory condition such as osteoarthritis. In contrast to the synovial tissue, the overwhelming cell type in the synovial fluid is the neutrophil. Synovial fluid also contains RF and anti-CCP antibodies and immune complexes, as well as by-products of complement activation. Clinically, the analysis of synovial fluid is most useful for confirming an inflammatory arthritis (as opposed to osteoarthritis), while at the same time excluding infection or a crystal-induced arthritis such as gout or pseudogout (Chap. 333).

■ JOINT IMAGING

Joint imaging is a valuable tool not only for diagnosing RA, but also for tracking progression of any joint damage. Plain x-ray is the most common imaging modality, but it is limited to visualization of the bony structures and inferences about the state of the articular cartilage based on the amount of narrowing of the joint space. MRI and ultrasound techniques offer the added value of detecting changes in the soft tissues such as synovitis, tenosynovitis, and effusions as well as greater sensitivity for identifying bony abnormalities. Plain radiographs are usually relied upon in clinical practice for the purpose of diagnosis and monitoring of affected joints. However, in selected cases, MRI and ultrasound can provide additional diagnostic information that may guide clinical decision-making.

Plain radiography

Classically in RA, the initial radiographic finding is juxtaarticular osteopenia. Practically speaking, however, this finding is difficult to appreciate on plain films, and in particular, on the newer digitalized x-rays. Other findings on plain radiographs include soft tissue swelling, symmetric joint space loss, and subchondral erosions, most frequently in the wrists and hands (MCPs and PIPs) and the feet (MTPs). In the feet, the lateral aspect of the fifth MTP is often targeted first, but other MTP joints may be involved at the same time. X-ray imaging of advanced RA may reveal signs of severe destruction, including joint subluxation and collapse (Fig. 321-5).

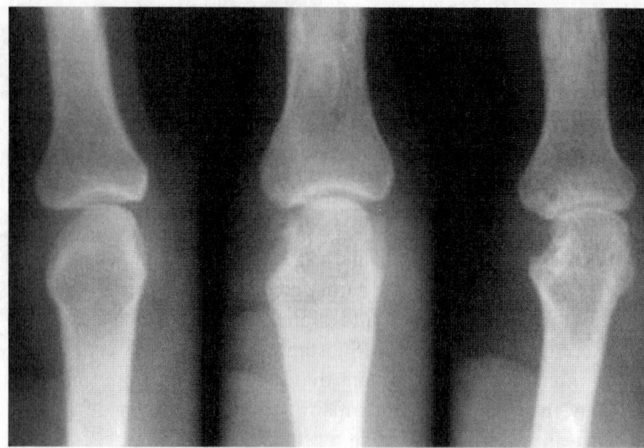

Figure 321-5 X-ray demonstrating progression of erosions on the proximal interphalangeal joint. *(Courtesy of the American College of Rheumatology.)*

MRI

MRI offers the greatest sensitivity for detecting synovitis and joint effusions, as well as early bone and bone marrow changes. These soft tissue abnormalities often occur before osseous changes are noted on x-ray. Presence of bone marrow edema has been recognized to be an early sign of inflammatory joint disease, and can predict the subsequent development of erosions on plain radiographs as well as MRI scans. Cost and availability of MRI are the main factors limiting its routine clinical use.

Ultrasound

Ultrasound, including power color Doppler, has the ability to detect more erosions than plain radiography, especially in easily accessible joints. Less clear, however, is the ability of ultrasound to reliably detect synovitis, including increased joint vascularity indicative of inflammation. The usefulness of ultrasound is dependent on the experience of the sonographer; however, it does offer the advantages of portability, lack of radiation, and low expense relative to MRI, factors that make it attractive as a clinical tool.

CLINICAL COURSE

The natural history of RA is complex and affected by a number of factors including age of onset, gender, genotype, phenotype (i.e., extraarticular manifestations or variants of RA), and comorbid conditions, which make for a truly heterogeneous disease. There is no simple way to predict the clinical course. It is important to realize that as many as 10% of patients with inflammatory arthritis fulfilling ACR classification criteria for RA will undergo a spontaneous remission within 6 months (particularly seronegative patients). However, the vast majority of patients will exhibit a pattern of persistent and progressive disease activity that waxes and wanes in intensity over time. A minority of patients will show intermittent and recurrent explosive attacks of inflammatory arthritis interspersed with periods of disease quiescence. Finally, an aggressive form of RA may occur in an unfortunate few with inexorable progression of severe erosive joint disease, although this highly destructive course is less common in the modern treatment era of biologics.

Disability, as measured by the Health Assessment Questionnaire (HAQ), shows gradual worsening of disability over time in the face of poorly controlled disease activity and disease progression. Disability may result from both a disease activity–related component that is potentially reversible with therapy and a joint damage–related component owing to the cumulative and largely irreversible effects of cartilage and bone breakdown. Early in the course of disease, the extent of joint inflammation is the primary determinant of disability, while in the later stages of disease, the amount of joint damage is the dominant contributing factor. Previous studies have shown that more than one-half of patients with RA are unable to work 10 years after the onset of their disease; however, increased employability and less work absenteeism has been reported recently with the use of newer therapies and earlier treatment intervention.

The overall mortality rate in RA is two times greater than the general population, with ischemic heart disease being the most common cause of death followed by infection. Median life expectancy is shortened by an average of 7 years for men and 3 years for women compared to control populations. Patients at higher risk for shortened survival are those with systemic extraarticular involvement, low functional capacity, low socioeconomic status, low education, and chronic prednisone use.

TREATMENT Rheumatoid Arthritis

The amount of clinical disease activity in patients with RA reflects the overall burden of inflammation and is the variable most influencing treatment decisions. Joint inflammation is the main driver of joint damage and is the most important cause of functional disability in the early stages of disease. Several composite indices have been developed to assess clinical disease activity. The ACR 20, 50, and 70 improvement criteria [which corresponds to a 20%, 50%, and 70% improvement in joint counts, physician/patient assessment of disease severity, pain scale, serum levels of acute-phase reactants (ESR or CRP), and a functional assessment of disability using a self-administered patient questionnaire] are a composite index with a dichotomous response variable. The ACR improvement criteria are commonly used in clinical trials as an endpoint for comparing the proportion of responders between treatment groups. In contrast, the Disease Activity Score (DAS), Simplified Disease Activity Index (SDAI), and the Clinical Disease Activity Index (CDAI) are continuous measures of disease activity. These scales are increasingly used in clinical practice for tracking disease status, and in particular, for documenting treatment response.

Several developments during the past two decades have changed the therapeutic landscape in RA. They include: (1) the emergence of methotrexate as the disease-modifying antirheumatic drug (DMARD) of first choice for the treatment of early RA; (2) the development of novel highly efficacious biologicals that can be used alone or in combination with methotrexate; and (3) the proven superiority of combination DMARD regimens over methotrexate alone. The medications used for the treatment of RA may be divided into broad categories: nonsteroidal anti-inflammatory drugs (NSAIDs); glucocorticoids, such as prednisone and methylprednisolone; conventional disease-modifying anti-rheumatic drugs (DMARDs); and biologic DMARDs (Table 321-2). While disease for some patients with RA is managed adequately with a single DMARD, such as methotrexate, the situation entails in most cases the use of a combination DMARD regimen that may vary in its components over the treatment course depending on fluctuations in disease activity and emergence of drug-related toxicities and comorbidities.

NSAIDS NSAIDs were formally viewed as the core of all other RA therapy, but they are now considered to be adjunctive therapy for management of symptoms uncontrolled by other measures. NSAIDs exhibit both analgesic and anti-inflammatory properties. The anti-inflammatory effects of NSAIDs derive from their ability to nonselectively inhibit cyclooxygenase (COX)-1 and COX-2. Although the results of clinical trials suggest NSAIDs are roughly equivalent in their efficacy, experience suggests that some individuals may preferentially respond to a particular NSAID. Chronic use should be minimized due to the possibility of side effects, including gastritis and peptic ulcer disease as well as impairment of renal function.

GLUCOCORTICOIDS Glucocorticoids may serve in several ways to control disease activity in RA. First, they may be administered in low-to-moderate doses to achieve rapid disease control before the onset of fully effective DMARD therapy, which often takes several weeks or even months. Second, a 1–2 week burst of glucocorticoids may be prescribed for the management of acute disease flares, with dose and duration guided by the severity of the exacerbation. Chronic administration of low doses (5–10 mg/d) of prednisone (or its equivalent) may also be warranted to control disease activity in patients with an inadequate response to DMARD therapy. Low-dose prednisone therapy has been shown in prospective studies to retard radiographic progression of joint disease; however, the benefits of this approach must be carefully weighed against the risks. Best practices minimize chronic use of low-dose prednisone therapy owing to the risk of osteoporosis and other long-term complications; however, the use of chronic prednisone therapy is unavoidable in many cases. Finally, if a patient exhibits one or a few actively inflamed joints, the clinician may consider intraarticular injection of an intermediate-acting glucocorticoid such as triamcinolone acetonide. This approach may allow for rapid control of inflammation in the setting of a limited number of affected joints. Caution must be exercised to appropriately exclude joint infection, as it often mimics an RA flare.

Osteoporosis ranks as an important long-term complication of chronic prednisone use. The ACR recommends primary prevention of glucocorticoid-induced osteoporosis with a bisphosphonate in any patient receiving 5 mg/d or more of prednisone for greater than 3 months. While prednisone use is known to increase the risk of peptic ulcer disease, especially with concomitant NSAID use, no evidence-based guidelines have been published regarding the use of gastrointestinal ulcer prophylaxis in this situation.

DMARDs DMARDs are so named because of their ability to slow or prevent structural progression of RA. The conventional DMARDs include hydroxychloroquine, sulfasalazine, methotrexate, and leflunomide; they exhibit a delayed onset of action of approximately 6–12 weeks. Methotrexate is the DMARD of choice for the treatment of RA and is the anchor drug for most combination therapies. It was approved for the treatment of RA in 1986 and remains the benchmark for the efficacy and safety of new disease-modifying therapies. At the dosages used for the treatment of RA, methotrexate has been shown to stimulate adenosine release from cells, producing an anti-inflammatory effect. The clinical efficacy of leflunomide, an inhibitor of pyrimidine synthesis, appears similar to that of methotrexate; it has been shown in well-designed trials to be effective for the treatment of RA as monotherapy or in combination with methotrexate and other DMARDs.

Although similar to the other DMARDs in its slow onset of action, hydroxychloroquine has not been shown to delay radiographic progression of disease and thus is not considered to be a true DMARD. In clinical practice, hydroxychloroquine is generally used for treatment of early, mild disease or as adjunctive therapy in combination with other DMARDs. Sulfasalazine is utilized in a similar manner and has been shown in randomized, controlled trials to reduce radiographic progression of disease. Minocycline,

TABLE 321-2 DMARDs Used for the Treatment of Rheumatoid Arthritis

Drug	Dosage	Serious Toxicities	Other Common Side Effects	Initial Evaluation	Monitoring
Hydroxychloroquine	200–400 mg/d orally (≤6.5 mg/kg)	Irreversible retinal damage Cardiotoxicity Blood dyscrasia	Nausea Diarrhea Headache Rash	Eye examination if > 40 years old or prior ocular disease	Funduscopic and visual field testing every 12 months
Sulfasalazine	Initial: 500 mg orally twice daily Maintenance: 1000–1500 mg twice daily	Granulocytopenia Hemolytic anemia (with G6PD deficiency)	Nausea Diarrhea Headache	CBC, LFTs G6PD level	CBC every 2–4 weeks for first 3 months, then every 3 months
Methotrexate	10–25 mg/week orally or SQ Folic acid 1 mg/d to reduce toxicities	Hepatotoxicity Myelosuppression Infection Interstitial pneumonitis Pregnancy category X	Nausea Diarrhea Stomatitis/mouth ulcers Alopecia Fatigue	CBC, LFTs Viral hepatitis panel* Chest x-ray	CBC, creatinine, LFTs every 2–3 months
Leflunomide	10–20 mg/d	Hepatotoxicity Myelosuppression Infection Pregnancy category X	Alopecia Diarrhea	CBC, LFTs Viral hepatitis panel*	CBC, creatinine, LFTs every 2–3 months
TNF-α Inhibitors	Infliximab: 3 mg/kg IV at weeks 0, 2, 6, then every 8 weeks. May increase dose up to 10 mg/kg every 4 weeks	↑ Risk bacterial, fungal infections Reactivation of latent TB ↑ Lymphoma risk (controversial) Drug-induced lupus Neurologic deficits	Infusion reaction ↑ LFTs	PPD skin test	LFTs periodically
	Etanercept: 50 mg SQ weekly, or 25 mg SQ biweekly	As above	Injection site reaction	PPD skin test	Monitor for injection site reactions
	Adalimumab: 40 mg SQ every other week	As above	Injection site reaction	PPD skin test	Monitor for injection site reactions
	Golimumab: 50 mg SQ monthly	As above	Injection site reaction	PPD skin test	Monitor for injection site reactions
	Certolizumab: 400 mg SQ weeks 0, 2, 4 then 200 mg every other week	As above	Injection site reaction	PPD skin test	Monitor for injection site reactions
Abatacept	Weight based: <60 kg: 500 mg 60–100 kg: 750 mg >100 kg: 1000 mg IV dose at week 0, 2 and 4, and then every 4 weeks	↑ Risk bacterial, viral infections	Headache Nausea	PPD skin test	Monitor for infusion reactions
Anakinra	100 mg SQ daily	↑ Risk bacterial, viral infections Reactivation of latent TB Neutropenia	Injection site reaction Headache	PPD skin test CBC with differential	CBC every month for 3 months, then every 4 months for 1 year Monitor for injection site reactions

(continued)

TABLE 321-2 DMARDs Used for the Treatment of Rheumatoid Arthritis (*Continued*)

Drug	Dosage	Serious Toxicities	Other Common Side Effects	Initial Evaluation	Monitoring
Rituximab	1000 mg IV × 2, day 0 and 14 May repeat course every 24 weeks or more Premedicate with methylprednisolone 100 mg to decrease infusion reaction	↑ Risk bacterial, viral infections Infusion reaction Cytopenia Hepatitis B reactivation	Rash Fever	CBC Viral hepatitis panel*	CBC at regular intervals
Tocilizumab	4–8 mg/kg 8 mg/kg IV monthly	Risk of infection Infusion reaction LFT elevation Dyslipidemia Cytopenias		PPD skin test	CBC and LFTs at regular intervals

*Viral hepatitis panel: hepatitis B surface antigen, hepatitis C viral antibody.

Abbreviations: CBC, complete blood count; DMARDs, disease-modifying anti-rheumatic drugs; G6PD, glucose-6-phosphate dehydrogenase; IV, intravenous; LFTs, liver function tests; PPD, purified peptide derivative; SQ, subcutaneous; TB, tuberculosis.

gold salts, penicillamine, azathioprine, and cyclosporine have all been used for the treatment of RA with varying degrees of success; however, they are used sparingly now due to their inconsistent clinical efficacy or unfavorable toxicity profile.

BIOLOGICALS Biologic DMARDs have revolutionized the treatment of RA over the past decade (Table 321-2). They are protein therapeutics designed mostly to target cytokines and cell-surface molecules. The TNF inhibitors were the first biologicals approved for the treatment of RA. Anakinra, an IL-1 receptor antagonist, was approved shortly thereafter; however, its benefits have proved to be relatively modest compared with the other biologicals. Abatacept, rituximab, and tocilizumab are the newest members of this class.

Anti-TNF Agents The development of TNF inhibitors was originally spurred by the experimental finding that TNF is a critical upstream mediator of joint inflammation. Currently, five agents that inhibit TNF-α are approved for the treatment of RA. There are three different anti-TNF monoclonal antibodies. Infliximab is a chimeric (part mouse and human) monoclonal antibody, while adalimumab and golimumab are humanized monoclonal antibodies. Certolizumab pegol is a pegylated Fc-free fragment of a humanized monoclonal antibody with binding specificity for TNF-α. Lastly, etanercept is a soluble fusion protein comprising the TNF receptor 2 in covalent linkage with the Fc portion of IgG1. All of the TNF inhibitors have been shown in randomized controlled clinical trials to reduce the signs and symptoms of RA, slow radiographic progression of joint damage, and improve physical function and quality of life. Anti-TNF drugs are typically used in combination with background methotrexate therapy. This combination regimen, which affords maximal benefit in many cases, is often the next step for treatment of patients with an inadequate response to methotrexate therapy. Etanercept, adalimumab, certolizumab pegol, and golimumab have also been approved for use as monotherapy.

Anti-TNF agents should be avoided in patients with active infection or a history of hypersensitivity to these agents. A major concern is the increased risk for infection, especially opportunistic fungal infection and reactivation of latent tuberculosis. For this reason, all patients are screened for latent tuberculosis according to national guidelines prior to starting anti-TNF therapy (Chap. 165). In the United States, patients are skin tested using an intradermal injection of purified peptide derivative (PPD); individuals with skin reactions of more than 5 mm are presumed to have had previous exposure to TB and are evaluated for active disease and treated accordingly.

Anakinra Anakinra, the recombinant form of the naturally occurring IL-1 receptor antagonist, has seen limited use for the treatment of RA owing to its modest clinical efficacy. However, anakinra has enjoyed a resurgence of late for the treatment of some rare syndromes dependent on IL-1 production, including neonatal-onset inflammatory disease, Muckle-Wells syndrome, and familial cold urticaria, systemic juvenile-onset inflammatory arthritis, and adult-onset Still's disease. Anakinra should not be combined with an anti-TNF drug due to the high rate of serious infections as observed with this regimen in a clinical trial.

Abatacept Abatacept is a soluble fusion protein consisting of the extracellular domain of human cytotoxic T lymphocyte–associated antigen 4 (CTLA-4) linked to the modified portion of human IgG. It inhibits the co-stimulation of T cells by blocking CD28-CD80/86 interactions and may also inhibit the function of antigen-presenting cells by reverse signaling through CD80 and CD86. Abatacept has been shown in clinical trials to reduce disease activity, slow radiographic progression of damage, and improve functional disability. Most patients receive abatacept in combination with methotrexate or another DMARD such as leflunomide. Its onset of action is usually slower than that of the anti-TNF agents. Abatacept therapy has been associated with an increased risk of infection but is usually well tolerated otherwise.

Rituximab Rituximab is a chimeric monoclonal antibody directed against CD20, a cell-surface molecule expressed by most mature B-lymphocytes. It works by depleting B cells, which in turn, leads to a reduction in the inflammatory response by unknown mechanisms. Rituximab has been approved for the treatment of refractory RA in combination with methotrexate and has been shown to be more effective for patients with seropositive than seronegative disease. Rituximab therapy has been associated with mild-to-moderate infusion reactions as well as an increased risk of infection. Notably, there have been isolated reports of a potentially lethal brain disorder, progressive multifocal leukoencephalopathy (PML), in association with rituximab therapy, although the absolute risk of this complication appears to be very low in patients with RA. Most of these cases have occurred on a background of previous or current exposure to other potent immunosuppressive drugs.

Tocilizumab Tocilizumab is a humanized monoclonal antibody directed against the membrane and soluble forms of the IL-6 receptor. IL-6 is a proinflammatory cytokine implicated in the pathogenesis of RA, with detrimental effects on both joint inflammation and damage. IL-6 binding to its receptor activates intracellular signaling pathways that affect the acute-phase response, cytokine production, and osteoclast activation. Clinical trials have attested to the clinical efficacy of tocilizumab therapy for RA, both as monotherapy and in combination with methotrexate and other DMARDs. Tocilizumab has been associated with an increased risk of infection, neutropenia, and thrombocytopenia; however, the hematologic abnormalities appear to be reversible upon stopping the drug. In addition, this agent has been shown to increase LDL cholesterol; however, it is not known as yet if this effect on lipid levels increases the risk for development of atherosclerotic disease.

APPROACH TO THE PATIENT Rheumatoid Arthritis

The original treatment pyramid for RA is now considered to be obsolete and has evolved into a new strategy that focuses on several goals: (1) early, aggressive therapy to prevent joint damage and disability; (2) frequent modification of therapy with utilization of combination therapy where appropriate; (3) individualization of therapy in an attempt to maximize response and minimize side effects; and (4) achieving, whenever possible, remission of clinical disease activity. A considerable amount of evidence supports this intensive treatment approach.

As mentioned earlier, methotrexate is the DMARD of first choice for initial treatment of moderate-to-severe RA. Failure to achieve adequate improvement with methotrexate therapy calls for consideration of an effective combination regimen. Effective combinations include: methotrexate, sulfasalazine, and hydroxychloroquine (triple therapy); methotrexate and leflunomide; and methotrexate plus a biological. The combination of methotrexate and an anti-TNF agent, for example, has been shown in randomized, controlled trials to be superior to methotrexate alone not only for reducing signs and symptoms of disease, but also for retarding the progression of structural joint damage. The caveat of these studies, however, is that the protection against structural damage afforded by combining an anti-TNF drug with methotrexate appears to be restricted to a subset of patients with a high risk for disease progression. This subset corresponds to approximately 25% of patients enrolled in clinical trials. The remaining patients do not show significant progression in joint damage over 12 months while receiving methotrexate alone. Predicting which patients will ultimately show radiologic joint damage is imprecise at best, although some factors such as an elevated serum level of acute-phase reactants, high burden of joint inflammation, and the presence of erosive disease are associated with increased likelihood of developing structural injury.

Some patients may not respond to an anti-TNF drug or be intolerant of its side effects. Initial responders to an anti-TNF agent that later worsen may benefit from switching to another anti-TNF agent. Other biologicals, such as abatacept and rituximab, may also be considered for the treatment of patients whose disease is refractory to anti-TNF therapy. The addition of abatacept or rituximab to background methotrexate therapy has been shown in well-designed clinical trials to be effective for reducing the signs and symptoms of joint inflammation and slowing radiographic progression of disease. Early in the treatment course, abatacept may also be considered in lieu of an anti-TNF drug depending on the clinical circumstances (e.g., relative contraindication for the use of an anti-TNF agent).

A clinical state defined as low disease activity or remission is the optimal goal of therapy, although most patients never achieve remission despite every effort to achieve it. Composite indices, such as the Disease Activity Score -28 or DAS28, are useful for classifying states of low disease activity and remission; however, they are imperfect tools due to the limitations of the clinical joint examination in which low-grade synovitis may escape detection. Complete remission has been stringently defined as the total absence of all articular and extraarticular inflammation and immunologic activity related to RA. However, evidence for this state can be difficult to demonstrate in clinical practice. In an effort to standardize and simplify the definition of remission for clinical trials, the ACR and EULAR developed two provisional operational definitions of remission in RA (Table 321-3). A patient may be considered in remission if he or she 1) meets all of the clinical and laboratory criteria listed in Table 321-3 or 2) has a composite Simplified Disease Activity Index (SDAI) score of <3.3. The SDAI is calculated by taking the sum of a tender joint and swollen joint count (using 28 joints), patient global assessment (0–10 scale), physician global assessment (0–10 scale), and C-reactive protein (in mg/dL). This definition of remission does not take into account the possibility of subclinical synovitis or that damage alone may produce a tender or swollen joint. Ignoring the semantics of these definitions, the aforementioned remission criteria are nonetheless useful for setting a level of disease control that will likely result in minimal or no progression of structural damage and disability.

PHYSICAL THERAPY AND ASSISTIVE DEVICES All patients should receive a prescription for exercise and physical activity. Dynamic strength training, community-based comprehensive

TABLE 321-3 ACR/EULAR Provisional Definition of Remission in Rheumatoid Arthritis

At any time point, patient must satisfy all of the following:

- Tender joint count ≤1
- Swollen joint count ≤1
- C-reactive protein ≤1 mg/dL
- Patient global assessment ≤1 (on a 0–10 scale)

OR

At any time point, patient must have a Simplified Disease Activity Index score of ≤3.3

Source: Adapted from Felson et al.

physical therapy, and physical-activity coaching (emphasizing 30 minutes of moderately intensive activity most days a week) have all been shown to improve muscle strength and perceived health status. Foot orthotics for painful valgus deformity decreases foot pain and resulting disability and functional limitations. Judicious use of wrist splints can also decrease pain; however, their benefits may be offset by decreased dexterity and a variable effect on grip strength.

SURGERY Surgical procedures may improve pain and disability in RA—most notably the hands, wrists, and feet, typically after the failure of medical therapy with varying degrees of reported long-term success. For large joints, such as the knee, hip, shoulder, or elbow, total joint arthroplasty is an option for advanced joint disease. A few surgical options exist for dealing with the smaller hand joints. Silicone implants are the most common prosthetic for MCP arthroplasty, and are generally implanted in patients with severe decreased arc of motion, marked flexion contractures, MCP joint pain with radiographic abnormalities and severe ulnar drift. Synovectomy and limited fusion are offered for the early rheumatoid wrist, but they are used much less frequently now compared to the past because of the availability of improved DMARD therapies. Arthrodesis and total wrist arthroplasty are reserved for patients with severe disease that have substantial pain and functional impairment. These two procedures appear to have equal efficacy in terms of pain control and patient satisfaction. Numerous surgical options exist for correction of hallux valgus in the forefoot, including arthrodesis and arthroplasty, as well as primarily arthrodesis for refractory hindfoot pain.

OTHER MANAGEMENT CONSIDERATIONS **Pregnancy** Up to 75% of female RA patients will note overall improvement in symptoms during pregnancy, but often will flare post-delivery. Flares during pregnancy are generally treated with low doses of prednisone; hydroxychloroquine and sulfasalazine are probably the safest DMARDs to use during pregnancy. Methotrexate and leflunomide therapy are contraindicated during pregnancy due to their teratogenicity in animals and humans. The experience with biologic agents has been insufficient to make specific recommendations for their use during pregnancy. Most rheumatologists avoid their use in this setting; however, exceptions are considered depending on the circumstances.

Elderly Patients RA presents in up to one-third of patients after the age of 60; however, it has been recognized that older individuals receive less aggressive treatment due to concerns about increased risks of drug toxicity. Studies suggest that conventional DMARDs as well as biologic agents are equally effective and safe in younger and older patients. Due to comorbidities, many elderly patients have an increased risk of infection. Aging also leads to a gradual decline in renal function that may raise the risk for side effects from NSAIDs and some DMARDS, such as methotrexate. Renal function must be taken into consideration before prescribing methotrexate, which is mostly cleared by the kidneys. To reduce the risks of side effects, methotrexate doses may need to be adjusted downward for the drop in renal function that usually comes with the seventh and eighth decades of life. Methotrexate is usually not prescribed for patients with a serum creatinine greater than 2 mg/dl.

GLOBAL CHALLENGES

Developing countries are finding an increase in the incidence of noncommunicable, chronic diseases such as diabetes, cardiovascular disease, and RA in the face of ongoing poverty, rampant infectious disease, and poor access to modern health care facilities. In these areas, patients tend to have a greater delay in diagnosis and limited access to specialists, and thus greater disease activity and disability at presentation. In addition, infection risk remains a significant issue for the treatment of RA in developing countries because of the immunosuppression associated with the use of glucocorticoids and most DMARDs. For example, in some developing countries, patients undergoing treatment for RA have a substantial increase in the incidence of tuberculosis, which demands the implementation of far more comprehensive screening practices and liberal use of isoniazid prophylaxis than in developed countries. The increased prevalence of hepatitis B and C, as well as human immunodeficiency virus (HIV), in these developing countries also poses challenges. Reactivation of viral hepatitis has been observed in association with some of the DMARDs, such as rituximab. Also, reduced access to antiretroviral therapy may limit the control of HIV infection and therefore the choice of DMARD therapies.

Despite these challenges, one should attempt to implement early treatment of RA in the developing countries with the resources at hand. Sulfasalazine and methotrexate are all reasonably accessible throughout the world where they can be utilized as both monotherapy and in combination with other drugs. The use of biologic agents is increasing in the developed countries as well as in other areas around the world, although their use is limited by high cost; national protocols restrict their use, and concerns remain about the risk for opportunistic infections.

SUMMARY

Improved understanding of the pathogenesis of RA and its treatment has dramatically revolutionized the management of this disease. The outcomes of patients with RA are vastly superior to those of the prebiologic modifier era; more patients than in years past are able to avoid significant disability and continue working, albeit with some job modifications in many cases. The need for early and aggressive treatment of RA as well as frequent follow-up visits for monitoring of drug therapy has implications for our health care system. Primary care physicians and rheumatologists must be prepared to work together as a team to reach the ambitious goals of best practice. In many settings, rheumatologists have reengineered their practice in a way that places high priority on consultations for any new patient with early inflammatory arthritis.

The therapeutic regimens for RA are becoming increasingly complex with the rapidly expanding therapeutic armamentarium. Patients receiving these therapies must be carefully monitored by both the primary care physician and the rheumatologist to minimize the risk of side effects and identify quickly any complications of chronic immunosuppression. Also, prevention and treatment of RA-associated conditions such as ischemic heart disease and osteoporosis will likely benefit from a team approach owing to the value of multidisciplinary care.

Research will continue to search for new therapies with superior efficacy and safety profiles and investigate treatment strategies that can bring the disease under control more rapidly and nearer to remission. However, prevention and cure of RA will likely require new breakthroughs in our understanding of disease pathogenesis. These insights may come from genetic studies illuminating critical pathways in the mechanisms of joint inflammation. Equally ambitious is the lofty goal of biomarker discovery that will open the door to personalized medicine for the care of patients with RA.

FURTHER READINGS

Felson DT et al: American College of Rheumatology/European League Against Rheumatism provisional definition of remission in rheumatoid arthritis for clinical trials. Arthritis Rheum 63:573, 2011

Goldring MB, Marcu KB: Cartilage homeostasis in health and rheumatic diseases. Arthritis Res Ther 11:224, 2009

GOLDRING SR, GOLDRING MB: Eating bone or adding it: The Wnt pathway decides. Nat Med 13:133, 2007

GORONZY JJ, WEYAND CM: Developments in the scientific understanding of rheumatoid arthritis. Arthritis Res Ther 11:249, 2009

GRAVALLESE EM et al: Identification of cell types responsible for bone resorption in rheumatoid arthritis and juvenile rheumatoid arthritis. Am J Pathol 152:943, 1998

HOLERS VM: Antibodies to citrullinated proteins: pathogenic and diagnostic significance. Curr Rheumatol Rep 9:396, 2007

MCINNES IB, SCHETT G: Cytokines in the pathogenesis of rheumatoid arthritis. Nat Rev Immunol 7: 429, 2007

MICHOU L et al: Associations between genetic factors, tobacco smoking and autoantibodies in familial and sporadic rheumatoid arthritis. Ann Rheum Dis 67:466, 2008

MODY GM, CARDIEL MH: Challenges in the management of rheumatoid arthritis in developing countries. Best Pract Res Clin Rheumatol 22:621, 2008

MYASOEDOVA E et al: Epidemiology of rheumatiod arthritis: Rheumatoid arthritis and mortality. Curr Rheumatol Rep 12:379, 2010

NEOGI T et al: 2010 Rheumatoid arthritis classification criteria: An American College of Rheumatology/European League Against Rheumatism collaborative initiative. Arthritis Rheum 62:2569, 2010

PLENGE RM: Rheumatoid arthritis genetics: 2009 update. Curr Rheumatol Rep 11:351, 2009

SCOTT DL, KINGSLEY GH: Tumor necrosis factor inhibitors for rheumatoid arthritis. N Engl J Med 355:704, 2006

———, STEER S. The course of established rheumatoid arthritis. Best Pract Res Clin Rheumatol 21:943, 2007

SMOLEN JS, et al: New therapies for treatment of rheumatoid arthritis. Lancet 370:1861, 2007

TURESSON C et al: Extra-articular disease manifestations in rheumatoid arthritis: incidence trends and risk factors over 46 years. Ann Rheum Dis 62:722, 2003

CHAPTER 322

Acute Rheumatic Fever

Jonathan R. Carapetis

Acute rheumatic fever (ARF) is a multisystem disease resulting from an autoimmune reaction to infection with group A streptococcus. Although many parts of the body may be affected, almost all of the manifestations resolve completely. The exception is cardiac valvular damage [rheumatic heart disease (RHD)], which may persist after the other features have disappeared.

GLOBAL CONSIDERATIONS

ARF and RHD are diseases of poverty. They were common in all countries until the early twentieth century, when their incidence began to decline in industrialized nations. This decline was largely attributable to improved living conditions—particularly less crowded housing and better hygiene—which resulted in reduced transmission of group A streptococci. The introduction of antibiotics and improved systems of medical care had a supplemental effect. Recurrent outbreaks of ARF began in the 1980s in the Rocky Mountain states of the United States, where elevated rates persist.

The virtual disappearance of ARF and reduction in the incidence of RHD in industrialized countries during the twentieth century unfortunately was not replicated in developing countries, where these diseases continue unabated. RHD is the most common cause of heart disease in children in developing countries and is a major cause of mortality and morbidity in adults as well. It has been estimated that between 15 and 19 million people worldwide are affected by RHD, with approximately one-quarter of a million deaths occurring each year. Some 95% of ARF cases and RHD deaths now occur in developing countries.

Although ARF and RHD are relatively common in all developing countries, they occur at particularly elevated rates in certain regions. These "hot spots" are sub-Saharan Africa, Pacific nations, Australasia, and the Indian subcontinent (Fig. 322-1). Unfortunately, most developing countries do not currently have coordinated, register-based RHD control programs, which are proven to be cost-effective in reducing the burden of RHD. Enhancing awareness of RHD and mobilizing resources for its control in developing countries is an issue requiring international attention.

EPIDEMIOLOGY

ARF is mainly a disease of children aged 5–14 years. Initial episodes become less common in older adolescents and young adults and are rare in persons aged >30 years. By contrast, recurrent episodes of ARF remain relatively common in adolescents and young adults. This pattern contrasts with the prevalence of RHD, which peaks between 25 and 40 years. There is no clear gender association for ARF, but RHD more commonly affects females, sometimes up to twice as frequently as males.

PATHOGENESIS

ORGANISM FACTORS

Based on currently available evidence, ARF is exclusively caused by infection of the upper respiratory tract with group A streptococci (see Chap. 136). Although classically, certain M-serotypes (particularly types 1, 3, 5, 6, 14, 18, 19, 24, 27, and 29) were associated with ARF, in high-incidence regions, it is now thought that any strain of group A streptococcus has the potential to cause ARF. Potential role of skin infection and of groups C and G streptococci are currently being investigated.

HOST FACTORS

Approximately 3–6% of any population may be susceptible to ARF, and this proportion does not vary dramatically between populations. Findings of familial clustering of cases and concordance in monozygotic twins—particularly for chorea—confirm that susceptibility to ARF is an inherited characteristic. Particular human leukocyte antigen (HLA) class II alleles appear to be strongly associated with susceptibility. Associations have also been described with high levels of circulating mannose-binding lectin and polymorphisms of transforming growth factor β_1 gene and immunoglobulin genes. High-level expression of a particular alloantigen present on B cells, D8-17, has been found in patients with a history of ARF in many

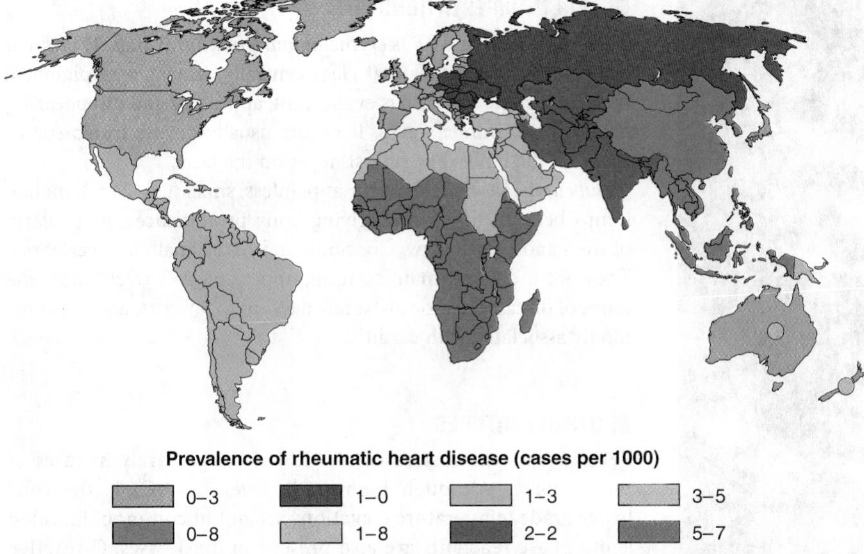

Figure 322-1 Prevalence of rheumatic heart disease in children aged 5–14 years. Circles within Australia and New Zealand represent indigenous populations, and also Pacific Islanders in New Zealand. *(From JR Carapetis et al: Lancet Infect Dis. Copyright 2005, with permission from Elsevier.)*

populations, with intermediate-level expression in first-degree family members, suggesting that this may be a marker of inherited susceptibility.

THE IMMUNE RESPONSE

When a susceptible host encounters a group A streptococcus, an autoimmune reaction results, which leads to damage to human tissues as a result of cross-reactivity between epitopes on the organism and the host (Fig. 322-2). Cross-reactive epitopes are present in the streptococcal M protein and the *N*-acetylglucosamine of group A streptococcal carbohydrate and are immunologically similar to molecules in human myosin, tropomyosin, keratin, actin, laminin, vimentin, and *N*-acetylglucosamine. It is currently thought that the initial damage is due to cross-reactive antibodies attaching at the cardiac valve endothelium, allowing the entry of primed CD4+ T cells, leading to subsequent T cell-mediated inflammation.

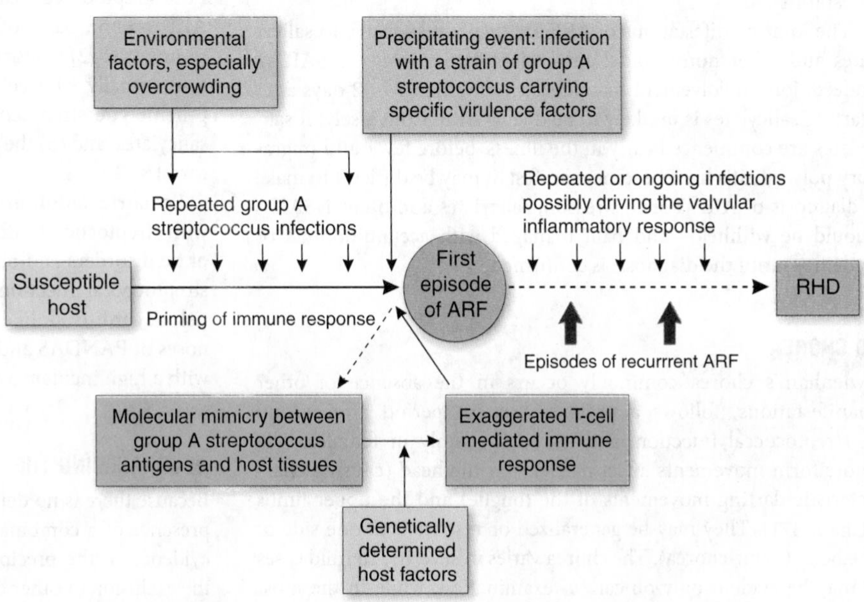

Figure 322-2 Pathogenetic pathway for acute rheumatic fever and rheumatic heart disease. *(From JR Carapetis et al: Lancet 366:155, 2005. Copyright 2005, with permission from Elsevier.)*

CLINICAL FEATURES

There is a latent period of ~3 weeks (1–5 weeks) between the precipitating group A streptococcal infection and the appearance of the clinical features of ARF. The exceptions are chorea and indolent carditis, which may follow prolonged latent periods lasting up to 6 months. Although many patients report a prior sore throat, the preceding group A streptococcal infection is commonly subclinical; in these cases it can only be confirmed using streptococcal antibody testing. The most common clinical presentation of ARF is polyarthritis and fever. Polyarthritis is present in 60–75% of cases and carditis in 50–60%. The prevalence of chorea in ARF varies substantially between populations, ranging from <2% to 30%. Erythema marginatum and subcutaneous nodules are now rare, being found in <5% of cases.

HEART INVOLVEMENT

Up to 60% of patients with ARF progress to RHD. The endocardium, pericardium, or myocardium may be affected. Valvular damage is the hallmark of rheumatic carditis. The mitral valve is almost always affected, sometimes together with the aortic valve; isolated aortic valve involvement is rare. Early valvular damage leads to regurgitation. Over ensuing years, usually as a result of recurrent episodes, leaflet thickening, scarring, calcification, and valvular stenosis may develop (Fig. 322-3). See Videos 322-1 and 322-2 on the DVD. Therefore the characteristic manifestation of carditis in previously unaffected individuals is mitral regurgitation, sometimes accompanied by aortic regurgitation. Myocardial inflammation may affect electrical conduction pathways, leading to P-R interval prolongation (first-degree AV block or rarely higher-level block) and softening of the first heart sound.

JOINT INVOLVEMENT

To qualify as a major manifestation, joint involvement in ARF must be arthritic, i.e., objective evidence of inflammation, with hot, swollen, red and/or tender joints, and involvement of more than one joint (i.e., polyarthritis). The typical arthritis is migratory, moving from one joint to another over a period of hours. ARF almost always affects the large joints—most commonly the knees, ankles, hips, and

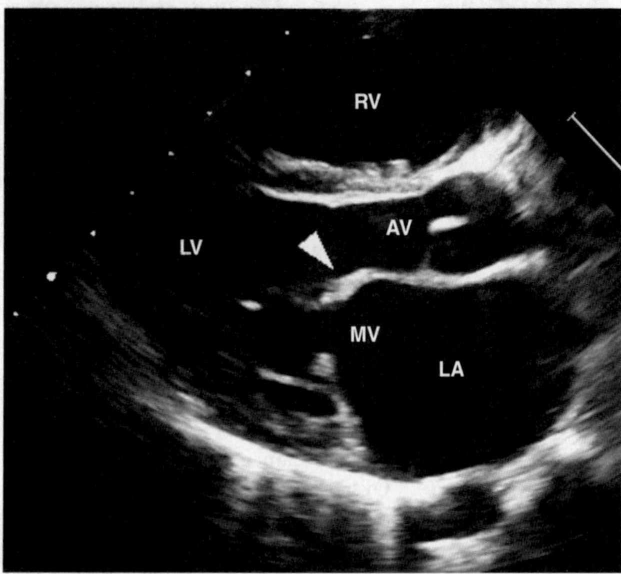

Figure 322-3 Transthoracic echocardiographic image from a 5-year-old boy with chronic rheumatic heart disease. This diastolic image demonstrates leaflet thickening, restriction of the anterior mitral valve leaflet tip, and doming of the body of the leaflet toward the interventricular septum. This appearance (marked by the arrowhead) is commonly described as a "hockey stick" or an "elbow" deformity. AV, aortic valve; LA, left atrium; LV, left ventricle; MV, mitral valve; RV, right ventricle. (*Courtesy of Dr. Bo Remenyi, Department of Paediatric and Congential Cardiac Services, Starship Children's Hospital, Auckland, New Zealand.*)

elbows—and is asymmetric. The pain is severe and usually disabling until anti-inflammatory medication is commenced.

Less severe joint involvement is also relatively common but qualifies only as a minor manifestation. Arthralgia without objective joint inflammation usually affects large joints in the same migratory pattern as polyarthritis. In some populations, aseptic monoarthritis may be a presenting feature of ARF. This may occur because of early commencement of anti-inflammatory medication before the typical migratory pattern is established.

The joint manifestations of ARF are highly responsive to salicylates and other nonsteroidal anti-inflammatory drugs (NSAIDs). Indeed, joint involvement that persists more than 1 or 2 days after starting salicylates is unlikely to be due to ARF. Conversely, if salicylates are commenced early in the illness, before fever and migratory polyarthritis have become manifest, it may be difficult to make a diagnosis of ARF. For this reason, salicylates and other NSAIDs should be withheld—and pain managed with acetaminophen or codeine—until the diagnosis is confirmed.

■ CHOREA

Sydenham's chorea commonly occurs in the absence of other manifestations, follows a prolonged latent period after group A streptococcal infection, and is found mainly in females. The choreiform movements affect particularly the head (causing characteristic darting movements of the tongue) and the upper limbs (Chap. 371). They may be generalized or restricted to one side of the body (hemi-chorea). The chorea varies in severity. In mild cases it may be evident only on careful examination, while in the most severe cases the affected individuals are unable to perform activities of daily living and are at risk of injuring themselves. Chorea eventually resolves completely, usually within 6 weeks.

■ SKIN MANIFESTATIONS

The classic rash of ARF is *erythema marginatum* (Chap. 17), which begins as pink macules that clear centrally, leaving a serpiginous, spreading edge. The rash is evanescent, appearing and disappearing before the examiner's eyes. It occurs usually on the trunk, sometimes on the limbs, but almost never on the face.

Subcutaneous nodules occur as painless, small (0.5–2 cm), mobile lumps beneath the skin overlying bony prominences, particularly of the hands, feet, elbows, occiput, and occasionally the vertebrae. They are a delayed manifestation, appearing 2–3 weeks after the onset of disease, last for just a few days up to 3 weeks, and are commonly associated with carditis.

■ OTHER FEATURES

Fever occurs in most cases of ARF, although rarely in cases of pure chorea. Although high-grade fever (≥39°C) is the rule, lower grade temperature elevations are not uncommon. Elevated acute-phase reactants are also present in most cases. C-reactive protein (CRP) and erythrocyte sedimentation rate (ESR) are often dramatically elevated. Occasionally the peripheral leukocyte count is mildly elevated.

■ EVIDENCE OF A PRECEDING GROUP A STREPTOCOCCAL INFECTION

With the exception of chorea and low-grade carditis, both of which may become manifest many months later, evidence of a preceding group A streptococcal infection is essential in making the diagnosis of ARF. As most cases do not have a positive throat swab culture or rapid antigen test, serologic evidence is usually needed. The most common serologic tests are the anti-streptolysin O (ASO) and anti-DNase B (ADB) titers. Where possible, age-specific reference ranges should be determined in a local population of healthy people without a recent group A streptococcal infection.

■ OTHER POST-STREPTOCOCCAL SYNDROMES THAT MAY BE CONFUSED WITH RHEUMATIC FEVER

Post-streptococcal reactive arthritis (PSRA) is differentiated from ARF on the basis of: (1) small-joint involvement that is often symmetric; (2) a short latent period following streptococcal infection (usually <1 week); (3) occasional causation by nongroup A β-hemolytic streptococcal infection; (4) slower responsiveness to salicylates; and (5) the absence of other features of ARF, particularly carditis.

Pediatric autoimmune neuropsychiatric disorders associated with streptococcal infection (PANDAS) is a term that links a range of tic disorders and obsessive-compulsive symptoms with group A streptococcal infections. People with PANDAS are said not to be at risk of carditis, unlike patients with Sydenham's chorea. The diagnoses of PANDAS and PSRA should rarely be made in populations with a high incidence of ARF.

■ CONFIRMING THE DIAGNOSIS

Because there is no definitive test, the diagnosis of ARF relies on the presence of a combination of typical clinical features together with evidence of the precipitating group A streptococcal infection, and the exclusion of other diagnoses. This uncertainty led Dr. T. Duckett Jones in 1944 to develop a set of criteria (subsequently known as the *Jones criteria*) to aid in the diagnosis. An expert panel convened by the World Health Organization (WHO) clarified the use of the Jones criteria in ARF recurrences (Table 322-1). Because each revision of the Jones criteria since 1944 has reduced sensitivity and increased specificity, in response to the decline in incidence of ARF in high-income countries, there is now concern that they may be too insensitive for countries where ARF incidence remains high. As a result, some countries (e.g., Australia and New Zealand) have developed their own, more sensitive, diagnostic criteria for ARF in their populations (links available at the *RHDnet* website *www.worldheart.org/rhd*).

TREATMENT Acute Rheumatic Fever

Patients with possible ARF should be followed closely to ensure that the diagnosis is confirmed, treatment of heart failure and other symptoms is undertaken, and preventive measures including commencement of secondary prophylaxis, inclusion on an ARF registry, and health education are commenced. Echocardiography should be performed on all possible cases to aid in making the diagnosis and to determine the severity at baseline of any carditis. Other tests that should be performed are listed in Table 322-2.

There is no treatment for ARF that has been proven to alter the likelihood of developing, or the severity of, RHD. With the exception of treatment of heart failure, which may be life-saving in cases of severe carditis, the treatment of ARF is symptomatic.

ANTIBIOTICS All patients with ARF should receive antibiotics sufficient to treat the precipitating group A streptococcal infection (Chap. 136). Penicillin is the drug of choice and can be given orally [as phenoxymethyl penicillin, 500 mg (250 mg for children ≤27 kg) PO twice daily, or amoxicillin 50 mg/kg (max 1 g) daily, for 10 days] or as a single dose of 1.2 million units (600,000 units for children ≤27 kg) IM benzathine penicillin G.

SALICYLATES AND NSAIDS These may be used for the treatment of arthritis, arthralgia, and fever, once the diagnosis is confirmed. They are of no proven value in the treatment of carditis or chorea. Aspirin is the drug of choice. An initial dose of 80–100 mg/kg per day in children (4–8 g/d in adults) in 4–5 divided doses is often needed for the first few days up to 2 weeks. A lower dose should be used if symptoms of salicylate toxicity emerge, such as nausea, vomiting, or tinnitus. When the acute symptoms are substantially resolved, the dose can be reduced to 60–70 mg/kg per day for a further 2–4 weeks. Fever, joint manifestations, and elevated acute-phase reactants sometimes recur up to 3 weeks after the medication is discontinued. This does not indicate a recurrence and can be managed by recommencing salicylates for a brief period. Although less well studied, naproxen at a dose of 10–20 mg/kg per day has been reported to lead to good symptomatic response.

CONGESTIVE HEART FAILURE Glucocorticoids The use of glucocorticoids in ARF remains controversial. Two meta-analyses have failed to demonstrate a benefit of glucocorticoids compared to placebo or salicylates in improving the short- or longer term outcome of carditis. However, the studies included in these meta-analyses all took place >40 years ago and did not use medications in common usage today. Many clinicians treat cases of severe carditis (causing heart failure) with glucocorticoids in the belief that they may reduce the acute inflammation and result in more rapid resolution of failure. However, the potential benefits of this treatment should be balanced against

TABLE 322-1 2002–2003 World Health Organization Criteria for the Diagnosis of Rheumatic Fever and Rheumatic Heart Disease (Based on the 1992 Revised Jones Criteria)

Diagnostic Categories	Criteria
Primary episode of rheumatic fever[a]	Two major or one major and two minor manifestations plus evidence of preceding group A streptococcal infection
Recurrent attack of rheumatic fever in a patient without established rheumatic heart disease	Two major or one major and two minor manifestations plus evidence of preceding group A streptococcal infection
Recurrent attack of rheumatic fever in a patient with established rheumatic heart disease[b]	Two minor manifestations plus evidence of preceding group A streptococcal infection[c]
Rheumatic chorea Insidious onset rheumatic carditis[b]	Other major manifestations or evidence of group A streptococcal infection not required
Chronic valve lesions of rheumatic heart disease (patients presenting for the first time with pure mitral stenosis or mixed mitral valve disease and/or aortic valve disease)[d]	Do not require any other criteria to be diagnosed as having rheumatic heart disease
Major manifestations	Carditis Polyarthritis Chorea Erythema marginatum Subcutaneous nodules
Minor manifestations	Clinical: fever, polyarthralgia Laboratory: elevated erythrocyte sedimentation rate or leukocyte count[e] Electrocardiogram: prolonged P-R interval
Supporting evidence of a preceding streptococcal infection within the last 45 days	Elevated or rising anti-streptolysin O or other streptococcal antibody, *or* A positive throat culture, *or* Rapid antigen test for group A streptococcus, *or* Recent scarlet fever[e]

[a]Patients may present with polyarthritis (or with only polyarthralgia or monoarthritis) and with several (three or more) other minor manifestations, together with evidence of recent group A streptococcal infection. Some of these cases may later turn out to be rheumatic fever. It is prudent to consider them as cases of "probable rheumatic fever" (once other diagnoses are excluded) and advise regular secondary prophylaxis. Such patients require close follow-up and regular examination of the heart. This cautious approach is particularly suitable for patients in vulnerable age groups in high incidence settings.

[b]Infective endocarditis should be excluded.

[c]Some patients with recurrent attacks may not fulfill these criteria.

[d]Congenital heart disease should be excluded.

[e]1992 Revised Jones criteria do not include elevated leukocyte count as a laboratory minor manifestation (but do include elevated C-reactive protein), and do not include recent scarlet fever as supporting evidence of a recent streptococcal infection.

Source: Reprinted with permission from WHO Expert Consultation on Rheumatic Fever and Rheumatic Heart Disease (2001: Geneva, Switzerland): *Rheumatic Fever and Rheumatic Heart Disease: Report of a WHO Expert Consultation* (WHO Tech Rep Ser, 923). Geneva, World Health Organization, 2004.

TABLE 322-2 Recommended Tests in Cases of Possible Acute Rheumatic Fever

Recommended for all cases
White blood cell count
Erythrocyte sedimentation rate
C-reactive protein
Blood cultures if febrile
Electrocardiogram (repeat in 2 weeks and 2 months if prolonged P-R interval or other rhythm abnormality)
Chest x-ray if clinical or echocardiographic evidence of carditis
Echocardiogram (consider repeating after 1 month if negative)
Throat swab (preferably before giving antibiotics)—culture for group A streptococcus
Anti-streptococcal serology: both anti-streptolysin O and anti-DNase B titres, if available (repeat 10–14 days later if 1st test not confirmatory)
Tests for alternative diagnoses, depending on clinical features
Repeated blood cultures if possible endocarditis
Joint aspirate (microscopy and culture) for possible septic arthritis
Copper, ceruloplasmin, anti-nuclear antibody, drug screen for choreiform movements
Serology and auto-immune markers for arboviral, auto-immune or reactive arthritis

Source: Reprinted with permission from National Heart Foundation of Australia.

the possible adverse effects, including gastrointestinal bleeding and fluid retention. If used, prednisone or prednisolone are recommended at doses of 1–2 mg/kg per day (maximum, 80 mg). Glucocorticoids are often only required for a few days or up to a maximum of 3 weeks.

MANAGEMENT OF HEART FAILURE See Chap. 234.

BED REST Traditional recommendations for long-term bed rest, once the cornerstone of management, are no longer widely practiced. Instead, bed rest should be prescribed as needed while arthritis and arthralgia are present, and for patients with heart failure. Once symptoms are well controlled, gradual mobilization can commence as tolerated.

CHOREA Medications to control the abnormal movements do not alter the duration or outcome of chorea. Milder cases can usually be managed by providing a calm environment. In patients with severe chorea, carbamazepine or sodium valproate are preferred to haloperidol. A response may not be seen for 1–2 weeks, and a successful response may only be to reduce rather than resolve the abnormal movements. Medication should be continued for 1–2 weeks after symptoms subside.

INTRAVENOUS IMMUNOGLOBULIN (IVIG) Small studies have suggested that IVIg may lead to more rapid resolution of chorea but has shown no benefit on the short- or long-term outcome of carditis in ARF without chorea. In the absence of better data, IVIg is *not* recommended except in cases of severe chorea refractory to other treatments.

PROGNOSIS

Untreated, ARF lasts on average 12 weeks. With treatment, patients are usually discharged from hospital within 1–2 weeks. Inflammatory markers should be monitored every 1–2 weeks until they have normalized (usually within 4–6 weeks), and an echocardiogram should be performed after 1 month to determine if there has been progression of carditis. Cases with more severe carditis need close clinical and echocardiographic monitoring in the longer term.

Once the acute episode has resolved, the priority in management is to ensure long-term clinical follow-up and adherence to a regimen of secondary prophylaxis. Patients should be entered onto the local ARF registry (if present) and contact made with primary care practitioners to ensure a plan for follow-up and administration of secondary prophylaxis before the patient is discharged. Patients and their families should also be educated about their disease, emphasizing the importance of adherence to secondary prophylaxis. If carditis is present, they should also be informed of the need for antibiotic prophylaxis against endocarditis for dental and surgical procedures.

PREVENTION

PRIMARY PREVENTION

Ideally, primary prevention would entail elimination of the major risk factors for streptococcal infection, particularly overcrowded housing. This is difficult to achieve in most places where ARF is common.

Therefore, the mainstay of primary prevention for ARF remains primary prophylaxis (i.e., the timely and complete treatment of group A streptococcal sore throat with antibiotics). If commenced within 9 days of sore throat onset, a course of penicillin (as outlined above for treatment of ARF) will prevent almost all cases of ARF that would otherwise have developed. This important strategy relies on individuals presenting for medical care when they have a sore throat, the availability of trained health and microbiology staff along with the materials and infrastructure to take throat swabs, and a reliable supply of penicillin. Unfortunately, many of these elements are not available in developing countries.

SECONDARY PREVENTION

The mainstay of controlling ARF and RHD is secondary prevention. Because patients with ARF are at dramatically higher risk than the general population of developing a further episode of ARF after a group A streptococcal infection, they should receive long-term penicillin prophylaxis to prevent recurrences. The best antibiotic for secondary prophylaxis is benzathine penicillin G (1.2 million units, or 600,000 units if ≤27 kg) delivered every 4 weeks. It can be given every 3 weeks, or even every 2 weeks, to persons considered to be at particularly high risk, although in settings where good compliance with 4-weekly dosing can be achieved, more frequent dosing is rarely needed. Oral penicillin V (250 mg) can be given twice-daily instead but is somewhat less effective than benzathine penicillin G. Penicillin allergic patients can receive erythromycin (250 mg) twice daily.

The duration of secondary prophylaxis is determined by many factors, in particular the duration since the last episode of ARF (recurrences become less likely with increasing time), age (recurrences are less likely with increasing age), and the severity of RHD (if severe, it may be prudent to avoid even a very small risk of recurrence because of the potentially serious consequences) (Table 322-3). Secondary prophylaxis is best delivered as part of a coordinated RHD control program, based around a registry of patients. Registries improve the ability to follow patients and identify those who default from prophylaxis and institute strategies to improve adherence.

TABLE 322-3 American Heart Association Recommendations for Duration of Secondary Prophylaxis*

Category of Patient	Duration of Prophylaxis
Rheumatic fever without carditis	For 5 years after the last attack or 21 years of age (whichever is longer)
Rheumatic fever with carditis but no residual valvular disease	For 10 years after the last attack, or 21 years of age (whichever is longer)
Rheumatic fever with persistent valvular disease, evident clinically or on echocardiography	For 10 years after the last attack, or 40 years of age (whichever is longer). Sometimes lifelong prophylaxis.

*These are only recommendations and must be modified by individual circumstances as warranted. Note that other organizations have slightly different recommendations (see *www.worldheart.org/rhd* for links).

Source: Adapted from AHA Scientific Statement Prevention of Rheumatic Fever and Diagnosis and Treatment of Acute Streptococcal Pharyngitis. Circulation 119:1541, 2009.

FURTHER READINGS

Carapetis JR et al: Acute rheumatic fever. Lancet 366:155, 2005

———et al: The global burden of group A streptococcal diseases. Lancet Infect Dis 5:685, 2005

Gerber MA et al: Prevention of rheumatic fever and diagnosis and treatment of acute Streptococcal pharyngitis: A scientific statement from the American Heart Association Rheumatic Fever, Endocarditis, and Kawasaki Disease Committee of the Council on Cardiovascular Disease in the Young, the Interdisciplinary Council on Functional Genomics and Translational Biology, and the Interdisciplinary Council on Quality of Care and Outcomes Research: Endorsed by the American Academy of Pediatrics. Circulation 119:1541, 2009

Lennon D et al: School-based prevention of acute rheumatic fever: A group randomized trial in New Zealand. Pediatr Infect Dis J 28:787, 2009

National Heart Foundation of Australia: *Diagnosis and Management of Acute Rheumatic Fever and Rheumatic Heart Disease in Australia: Complete Evidence-Based Review and Guideline.* Melbourne, National Heart Foundation of Australia, 2006

Paar JA et al: Prevalence of rheumatic heart disease in children and young adults in Nicaragua. Am J Cardiol 105:1809, 2010

Special Writing Group of the Committee on Rheumatic Fever, Endocarditis and Kawasaki Disease of the American Heart Association: Guidelines for the diagnosis of acute rheumatic fever: Jones criteria, 1992 update. JAMA 268:2069, 1992

Steer A et al: Group A streptococcal vaccines: facts versus fantasy. Curr Opin Infect Dis 22:544, 2009

Steer AC, Carapetis JR: Acute rheumatic fever and rheumatic heart disease in indigenous populations. Pediatr Clin North Am 56:1401, 2009

CHAPTER 323

Systemic Sclerosis (Scleroderma) and Related Disorders

John Varga

DEFINITION

Systemic sclerosis (SSc) is a connective tissue disorder of unknown etiology, heterogeneous clinical manifestations, and chronic and often progressive course. The diffuse cutaneous form of SSc (dcSSc) is characterized by thickening of the skin (scleroderma) and distinctive involvement of multiple internal organs, most notably the lungs, gastrointestinal tract, heart, and kidneys. The early stage of the disease is associated with prominent inflammatory features. Over time, patients develop functional and structural alterations in multiple vascular beds and progressive visceral organ dysfunction due to fibrosis. Although the presence of thickened skin (scleroderma) distinguishes SSc from other connective tissue diseases, scleroderma-like skin induration can occur in localized forms of scleroderma and other disorders (Table 323-1). Patients can be classified into two principal subsets defined largely by the pattern of skin involvement, as well as clinical and laboratory manifestations (Table 323-2). Diffuse cutaneous SSc is associated with progressive skin induration, starting in the fingers and ascending from distal to proximal extremities, the face, and the trunk. These patients are at risk for early pulmonary fibrosis and acute renal involvement. Patients with limited cutaneous SSc (lcSSc) generally have long-standing Raynaud's phenomenon before other manifestations of SSc appear. Skin involvement in lcSSc is slowly progressive and remains limited to the fingers (sclerodactyly), distal extremities, and face, but the trunk is not affected. A subset of patients with lcSSc have prominent calcinosis cutis, Raynaud's phenomenon, esophageal dysmotility, sclerodactyly, and telangiectasia, a constellation termed *CREST syndrome.* However, these features may also be seen in patients with dcSSc. Visceral organ involvement in lcSSc tends to show insidious progression. Although the long-term prognosis of lcSSc is better than that of dcSSc, pulmonary arterial hypertension (PAH), interstitial lung disease, hypothyroidism, and primary biliary cirrhosis may develop in the late stage of lcSSc. In some patients, Raynaud's phenomenon and other typical features of SSc occur in the absence of detectable skin thickening. This syndrome has been termed *SSc sine scleroderma.*

EPIDEMIOLOGY

SSc is an acquired sporadic disease with a worldwide distribution and affecting all races. In the United States, the incidence is estimated at 9–19 cases per million per year. The only community-based survey of SSc yielded a prevalence of 286 cases per million population. There are an estimated 100,000 cases in the United States, although this number may be significantly higher if patients who do not meet strict classification criteria are also included. Studies from England, Australia, and Japan showed rates of SSc that were

TABLE 323-1 Conditions Associated With Scleroderma-Like Induration

Systemic sclerosis (SSc)
Limited cutaneous SSc
Diffuse cutaneous SSc
Localized scleroderma
Guttate morphea, diffuse morphea
Linear scleroderma, coup de sabre, hemifacial atrophy
Pansclerotic morphea
Overlap syndromes
Mixed connective tissue disease
SSc/polymyositis
Stiff Skin Syndrome
Undifferentiated connective tissue disease
Scleredema and diabetic scleredema
Scleromyxedema (papular mucinosis)
Nephrogenic systemic fibrosis (nephrogenic fibrosing dermatopathy)
Chronic graft-versus-host disease
Diffuse fasciitis with eosinophilia (Shulman disease, eosinophilic fasciitis)
Eosinophilia-myalgia syndrome
Chemically induced scleroderma-like conditions
Vinyl chloride–induced disease
Pentazocine-induced skin fibrosis
Paraneoplastic syndrome

TABLE 323-2 Subsets of Systemic Sclerosis (SSc): Limited Cutaneous SSc Versus Diffuse Cutaneous SSc

Features	Limited Cutaneous SSc	Diffuse Cutaneous SSc
Skin involvement	Indolent onset. Limited to fingers, distal to elbows, face; slow progression	Rapid onset. Diffuse: fingers, extremities, face, trunk; rapid progression
Raynaud's phenomenon	Precedes skin involvement; associated with critical ischemia	Onset coincident with skin involvement, may be mild
Musculoskeletal	Early arthralgia, fatigue	Severe arthralgia, carpal tunnel syndrome, tendon friction rubs
Pulmonary fibrosis	Occasional, moderate	Frequent, early and severe
Pulmonary arterial hypertension	Frequent, late, may be isolated	May occur, often in association with pulmonary fibrosis
Scleroderma renal crisis	Very rare	Occurs in 15%; early
Calcinosis cutis	Frequent, prominent	May occur, mild
Characteristic autoantibodies	Anticentromere	Antitopoisomerase I (Scl-70), anti-RNA polymerase III

lower than in the United States. Age, gender, and ethnicity are important factors determining disease susceptibility. Like other connective tissue diseases, SSc shows a female predominance that is most pronounced in the childbearing years and declines after menopause. While SSc can present at any age, the most common age of onset for both limited and diffuse cutaneous forms is in the range of 30–50 years. The incidence is higher in blacks than whites, and disease onset occurs at an earlier age. Furthermore, blacks are more likely to have the diffuse cutaneous form of SSc associated with interstitial lung involvement and a worse prognosis.

GENETIC CONSIDERATIONS

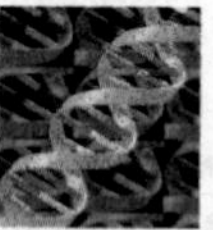

SSc shows a non-Mendelian pattern of inheritance. Monozygotic twins have a relatively low concordance rate for SSc (4.7%), although concordance for antinuclear antibodies is significantly greater. A genetic contribution to disease susceptibility is indicated by the fact that 1.6% of SSc patients have a first-degree relative with SSc, a prevalence rate substantially higher than in the general population. The risk of other autoimmune diseases, including systemic lupus erythematosus (SLE) (Chap. 319) and rheumatoid arthritis (Chap. 321), is also increased. Among Choctaw Indians from Oklahoma, SSc prevalence as high as 4690 per million has been reported. Genetic investigations in SSc have focused on candidate gene polymorphisms. Small studies have shown associations with the genes encoding angiotensin-converting enzyme (ACE); endothelin-1 and nitric oxide synthase; B cell markers (CD19); chemokines (monocyte chemoattractant protein-1) and chemokine receptors; interferon signaling mediators STAT4 and IRF5; migration inhibitory factor; cytokines [interleukin 1α (IL-1α, IL-4, and tumor necrosis factor α (TNF-α)]; growth factors and their receptors [connective tissue growth factor (CTGF) and transforming growth factor β (TGF-β)]; and extracellular matrix proteins [fibronectin, fibrillin, and secreted protein acidic-rich in cysteine (SPARC)]. To date, these genetic studies indicate that as in other complex diseases, multiple genetic loci are involved in SSc, and their individual contributions to disease susceptibility are modest. Genome-wise association studies to identify additional genetic susceptibility loci in SSc are currently underway.

ENVIRONMENTAL AND OCCUPATIONAL RISK FACTORS

Patients with SSc have increased serum antibodies to human cytomegalovirus (hCMV), and antitopoisomerase-I (Scl-70) autoantibodies recognize antigenic epitopes present on the hCMV-derived proteins, suggesting molecular mimicry as a possible mechanistic link between hCMV infection and SSc. Evidence of human parvovirus B19 infection in SSc patients has also been presented; however, the etiologic role of viruses remains unproven. Reports of geographic clustering of SSc cases suggesting shared environmental exposures have not been substantiated by careful investigation. An epidemic of a novel syndrome with features suggestive of SSc occurred in Spain in the 1980s. The outbreak, termed *toxic oil syndrome* and affecting over 20,000 individuals, was linked to contaminated rapeseed oils used for cooking. A similar epidemic outbreak, termed *eosinophilia-myalgia syndrome* (EMS), occurred a decade later in the United States. Affected individuals presented with marked eosinophilia and severe myalgia, followed by the development of scleroderma-like chronic skin lesions. The EMS epidemic was linked to the consumption of imported batches of L-tryptophan used as dietary supplements. While both of these apparently novel toxic-epidemic syndromes were characterized by scleroderma-like chronic skin changes and variable visceral organ involvement they were associated with clinical, pathologic, and laboratory features that clearly distinguished them from SSc. The incidence of SSc is increased among miners exposed to silica. Other occupational exposures tentatively linked with SSc include polyvinyl chloride, epoxy resins, and aromatic hydrocarbons including toluene and trichloroethylene. Drugs implicated in SSc-like illnesses include bleomycin, pentazocine and cocaine, and appetite suppressants linked with pulmonary hypertension. As yet unknown inhaled factors may play a role in the development of SSc-associated interstitial lung disease. Case reports and series describing SSc in women with silicone breast implants had raised concern regarding a possible causal role of silicone in SSc. However, large-scale epidemiologic investigations found no evidence of increased risk of SSc.

PATHOGENESIS

A comprehensive view of the pathogenesis of SSc must incorporate the three cardinal features of the disease: (1) vasculopathy, (2) cellular and humoral auto immunity, and (3) progressive visceral and vascular fibrosis in multiple organs (Fig. 323-1). Autoimmunity and altered vascular reactivity may be the earliest manifestations of SSc. Complex interplay between these processes is thought to initiate and then amplify the fibrotic process.

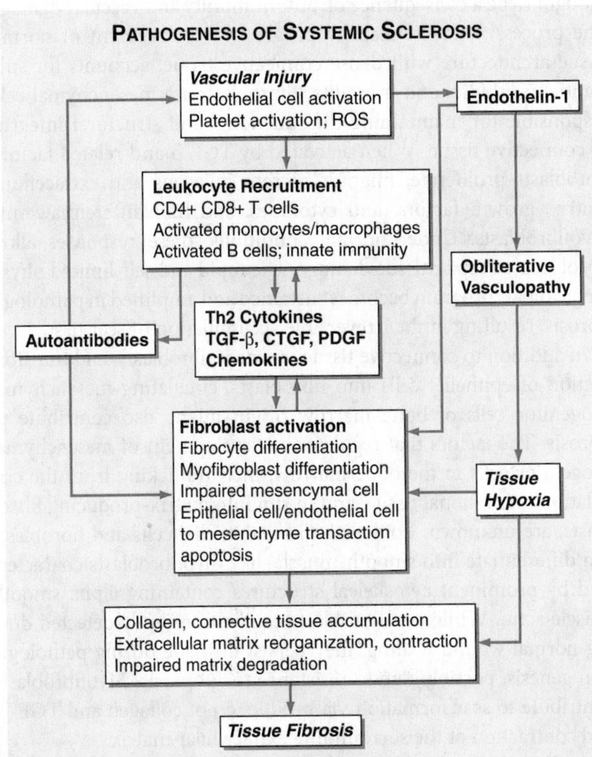

Figure 323-1 Initial vascular injury in a genetically susceptible individual leads to functional and structural vascular alterations, inflammation, and autoimmunity. The inflammatory and immune responses initiate and sustain fibroblast activation and differentiation, resulting in pathologic fibrogenesis and irreversible tissue damage. Vascular damage results in tissue ischemia that further contributes to progressive fibrosis and atrophy. CTGF, connective tissue growth factor; PDGF, platelet-derived growth factor; TGF-β, transforming growth factor-β.

ANIMAL MODELS OF DISEASE

There is no single animal model of SSc that reproduces the three cardinal processes that underlie the pathogenesis, but some models recapitulate selected disease characteristics. The tight-skin mouse (Tsk1) is a naturally occurring fibrosis model characterized by spontaneous skin thickening. The mutation responsible for the phenotype, a duplication in the fibrillin-1 gene, gives rise to an abnormally large fibrillin-1 protein that contributes to defective extracellular matrix assembly and aberrant activation of TGF-β. Mutations in the fibrillin-1 gene are associated with Marfan's disease and the stiff skin syndrome but have not been described in patients with SSc. Fibrosis in the skin and lungs can be induced in mice by bleomycin injections or by transplantation of human leukocyte antigen (HLA)-mismatched bone marrow or spleen cells. Increasingly, manipulation of mice via mutagenesis or targeted genetic modification such as knock-out or transgenesis are utilized to create new disease models and for dissecting the roles of individual molecules in the underlying processes. For example, genetic targeting of Smad3, an intracellular TGF-β signal transducer, or of the nuclear receptor peroxisome proliferator-activated receptor (PPAR) gamma, yielded mice that were resistant or hypersensitive to bleomycin-induced scleroderma. These mouse models become increasingly useful for preclinical testing of novel treatments.

MICROANGIOPATHY

Vascular involvement in SSc is extensive, involves multiple vascular beds, and has important clinical consequences. Raynaud's phenomenon, an early manifestation, is characterized by an altered blood-flow response to cold challenge. This initially reversible functional vascular abnormality is associated with alterations in the autonomic and peripheral nervous systems, with impaired production of neuropeptides such as calcitonin gene-related peptide from sensory afferent nerves and heightened sensitivity of α_2-adrenergic receptors on vascular smooth-muscle cells. While isolated Raynaud's phenomenon is common, relatively benign, and nonprogressive, SSc-associated Raynaud's phenomenon is frequently complicated by irreversible structural and functional changes. Viruses, superoxide radicals, vascular cytotoxic factors, and immune responses such as complement and circulating autoantibodies to endothelial cells may each contribute to endothelial cell injury in early SSc. Endothelial injury results in dysregulated production of endothelium-derived vasodilatory (nitric oxide and prostacyclin) and vasoconstricting (endothelin-1) substances, as well as increased expression of intercellular adhesion molecule 1 (ICAM-1) and other surface adhesion molecules. Microvessels show enhanced permeability and transendothelial leukocyte diapedesis, activation of coagulation and fibrinolytic cascades, and platelet aggregation. Smooth muscle cell–like myointimal cells proliferate, the basement membrane is thickened and reduplicated, and fibrosis of the adventitial layers develops. The vasculopathic process affects capillaries, as well as arterioles, and even large vessels in many organs, resulting in reduced blood flow, tissue ischemia, and generation of profibrotic factors. Progressive luminal occlusion due to intimal and medial hypertrophy, combined with persistent endothelial cell damage and adventitial fibrosis, establish a vicious cycle culminating in the striking absence of blood vessels seen on angiograms of the hands and kidneys in late-stage disease. Damaged endothelium promotes platelet aggregation with release of serotonin and platelet alpha granules including thromboxane, a potent vasoconstrictor, and of platelet-derived growth factor (PDGF). Vascular compromise is aggravated by defective fibrinolysis. Oxidative stress due to ischemia-reperfusion is associated with generation of reactive oxygen species (ROS) that further damage the endothelium through peroxidation of membrane lipids. Paradoxically, the process of revascularization that normally reestablishes blood flow to ischemic tissue is defective in SSc despite elevated levels of vascular endothelial growth factor (VEGF) and other angiogenic factors. The number of bone marrow–derived CD34+ CD133+ endothelial progenitor cells is markedly reduced in the circulation, and their differentiation in vitro into mature endothelial cells is impaired. Thus, widespread capillary malformation and loss, obliterative vasculopathy of small and medium-sized arteries, and failure to repair damaged vessels are hallmarks of SSc.

INFLAMMATION AND CELLULAR IMMUNITY

In the early stages of SSc, activated T cells and monocytes/macrophages accumulate in lesional skin, lungs, and other affected organs. Infiltrating T cells express CD45 and HLA-DR activation markers and display restricted T cell receptor signatures indicative of oligoclonal expansion in response to (unknown) antigen. Circulating CD4+ T cells have elevated levels of chemokine receptors and α_1 integrin adhesion molecules, accounting for their enhanced ability to bind to endothelium and to fibroblasts. Endothelial cells express ICAM-1 and other adhesion molecules that facilitate leukocyte diapedesis. Activated macrophages and T cells show a T_H2-polarized immune response and secrete IL-4 and IL-13. T_H2 cytokines induce the production of TGF-β and promote collagen synthesis and other profibrotic responses, whereas the T_H1 cytokine interferon γ (IFN-γ) inhibits collagen synthesis and blocks cytokine-mediated fibroblast activation. Because TGF-β stimulates its own synthesis, as well as that of CTGF (also termed CCN2) and other cytokines, TGF-β establishes an autocrine/paracrine stimulatory loop that sustains activation of fibroblasts and other effector cells (Chaps. 314 and 318). Regulatory T cells (Tregs) are essential for maintaining normal immune tolerance. While the frequency of Tregs in the peripheral blood is elevated in SSc, their immunosuppressive function is defective.

Humoral autoimmunity

Antinuclear antibodies occur in virtually all patients with SSc. In addition, a number of mutually exclusive autoantibodies that are highly specific for SSc have been described. These antibodies show strong association with specific disease phenotypes and genetically determined HLA haplotypes (Table 323-3). Autoantibody levels correlate with disease severity, and titers fluctuate with disease activity. While some SSc-specific autoantibodies are antinuclear and directed against intracellular proteins such as topoisomerase-I, and the RNA polymerases, others are directed against cell-surface antigens or secreted proteins. Functional autoantibodies have well-established clinical utility as diagnostic and prognostic markers in SSc, although their pathogenetic role in the disease manifestations remains uncertain. Autoantibodies to fibroblasts, endothelial cells, PDGF cell-surface receptors, fibrillin-1, and matrix metalloproteinase enzymes have been described in SSc. The direct pathogenetic role of these self antibodies in SSc remains to be firmly established.

A variety of mechanisms have been proposed for the occurrence of autoantibodies in SSc. Proteolytic cleavage, increased expression, or altered subcellular localization of certain cellular proteins in SSc could lead to their recognition as neoepitopes by the immune system. For example, cytotoxic T cells release the protease granzyme B that cleaves peptides, and generates neoepitopes that can break immune tolerance. Recent studies implicate B cells in both the autoimmune and fibrotic responses in SSc. In addition to their well-recognized role in antibody production, B cells can also present antigen, produce IL-6 and TGF-β, and modulate T cell and dendritic cell function. In SSc, B cells show elevated CD19 expression, and reduced numbers of memory B cells and early plasma cells. Gene expression profiling of lesional skin has identified mRNA expression signatures characteristic of B cell activation.

TABLE 323-3 Autoantibodies and Associated Features in Systemic Sclerosis (SSc)

Target Antigen	SSc Subset	Characteristic Clinical Association
Topoisomerase-I	dcSSc	Tendon friction rubs, ILD, cardiac involvement, scleroderma renal crisis
Centromere proteins	lcSSc	Digital ischemia, calcinosis, isolated PAH; renal crisis rare
RNA polymerase III	dcSSc	Extensive skin, tendon friction rubs, renal crisis
U3-RNP	dcSSc	PAH, ILD, scleroderma renal crisis, myositis
Th/TO	lcSSc	ILD, PAH
PM/Scl	lcSSc	Calcinosis, myositis
U1-RNP	MCTD	PAH

Abbreviations: dcSSc, diffuse cutaneous SSc; ILD, interstitial lung disease; lcSSc, limited cutaneous SSc; MCTD, mixed connective tissue disease; PAH, pulmonary arterial hypertension.

FIBROSIS

Fibrosis affecting multiple organs distinguishes SSc from other connective tissue diseases. Fibrosis characteristically follows, and is thought to be a consequence of, autoimmunity and vascular damage. The process, characterized by progressive replacement of normal tissue architecture with dense connective tissue, accounts for substantial morbidity and mortality. Fibroblasts are mesenchymal cells responsible for maintaining the functional and structural integrity of connective tissue. When activated by TGF-β and related factors, fibroblasts proliferate, migrate, secrete collagens and extracellular matrix, growth factors, and cytokines, and transdifferentiate into myofibroblasts. Under normal conditions, these responses allow fibroblasts to repair tissue damage. The rapid and self-limited physiologic repair program becomes sustained and amplified in pathologic fibrosis, resulting in the irreversible accumulation of scar tissue.

In addition to connective tissue–resident fibroblasts, and transformation of epithelial cells into fibroblasts, circulating mesenchymal progenitor cells of bone marrow origin might also contribute to fibrosis. The factors that regulate the development of mesenchymal progenitor cells in the bone marrow, their trafficking from the circulation into lesional tissue, and in situ into matrix-producing fibroblasts, are unknown. Epithelial and endothelial cells and fibroblasts can differentiate into smooth-muscle–like myofibroblasts characterized by prominent cytoskeleal structures containing alpha smooth muscle actin. While myofibroblasts can be transiently detected during normal wound healing, they persist in tissue during pathologic fibrogenesis, possibly due to resistance to apoptosis. Myofibroblasts contribute to scar formation via production of collagen and TGF-β, and contraction of the surrounding extracellular matrix.

Explanted fibroblasts display an abnormally activated phenotype in culture. Compared to normal fibroblasts, SSc fibroblasts have variably increased rates of collagen gene transcription and display smooth-muscle actin stress fibers. Furthermore, they show enhanced secretion of extracellular matrix molecules, cytokines, and growth factors; expression of chemokine receptors and cell surface adhesion molecules; resistance to apoptosis; spontaneously generate ROS; and autocrine TGF-β signaling. The abnormal "scleroderma phenotype" of these cells persists during their serial passage in vitro.

Factors contributing to the autonomously activated phenotype include autocrine TGF-β stimulatory loops, hypoxia, deregulated microRNA expressions and other epigenetic modifications, and altered cell-matrix interaction. Global transcriptome analyses show differential expression of many extracellular matrix genes, including collagens, fibronectin, and fibrillins in SSc fibroblasts. A majority of the abnormally expressed genes could be linked to TGF-β responses, but other fibrogenic signaling pathways involving CTGF, endothelin-1m hypoxia, PDGF and Wnts are also operative in SSc.

PATHOLOGY

The distinguishing pathologic hallmark of SSc is the combination of widespread capillary loss and obliterative vasculopathy of small arteries and arterioles, together with fibrosis in the skin and internal organs. In early disease, perivascular cellular infiltrates composed of CD4+ and CD8+ T lymphocytes, monocytes/macrophages, plasma cells, mast cells, and occasionally B cells may be detected in multiple organs prior to the appearance of fibrosis. The vascular lesion is characterized by intimal proliferation in the small and medium-sized arteries, resulting in luminal narrowing. Obliterative vasculopathy as a late finding is prominent in the heart, lungs, kidneys, and intestinal tract. Fibrosis is found in the skin, lungs, gastrointestinal tract, heart, tendon sheath, perifascicular tissue surrounding skeletal muscle, and some endocrine organs. In these tissues, accumulation of connective tissue composed of endothelin-1m collagens, fibronectin, proteoglycans, and other structural macromolecules progressively disrupts normal architecture, resulting in functional impairment of affected organs.

SKIN

In the skin, fibrosis causes dermal expansion and obliteration of the hair follicles, sweat glands, and other appendages (Fig. 323-2A). Collagen fiber accumulation is most prominent in the reticular dermis, and the fibrotic process invades the subjacent adipose layer with entrapment of fat cells. The epidermis is atrophic, and the rete pegs are effaced.

LUNGS

Patchy infiltration of the alveolar walls with T lymphocytes, macrophages, and eosinophils occurs in early disease. With progression, interstitial fibrosis and vascular damage dominate the pathologic picture, often coexisting within the same lesions in patients with dcSSc. Pulmonary fibrosis is characterized by expansion of the alveolar interstitium, with accumulation of collagen and other connective tissue proteins. The most common histologic pattern in SSc is fibrotic nonspecific interstitial pneumonia (Fig. 323-2B). Progressive thickening of the alveolar septae results in obliteration of the airspaces and honeycombing, as well as loss of pulmonary blood vessels. This process impairs gas exchange and contributes to worsening of pulmonary hypertension. Intimal thickening of the pulmonary arteries, best seen with elastin stain, underlies pulmonary hypertension (Fig. 323-2C) and, at autopsy, is often associated with multiple pulmonary emboli and evidence of myocardial fibrosis.

GASTROINTESTINAL TRACT

Pathologic changes can be found at any level from the mouth to the rectum. The lower esophagus is frequently involved, with prominent atrophy of the muscular layers; striated muscle in the upper third of the esophagus is generally spared. Characteristic vascular lesions are often present. Replacement of the normal intestinal tract architecture results in diminished peristaltic activity, with gastroesophageal reflux, dysmotility, and small-bowel obstruction. Chronic reflux is associated with esophageal inflammation, ulcerations, and stricture formation and may lead to Barrett's metaplasia.

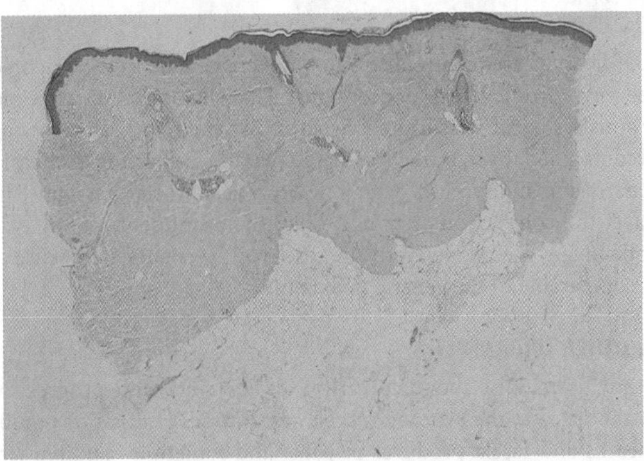

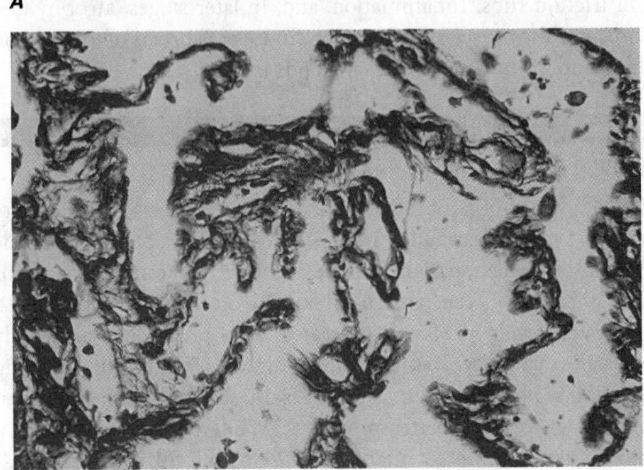

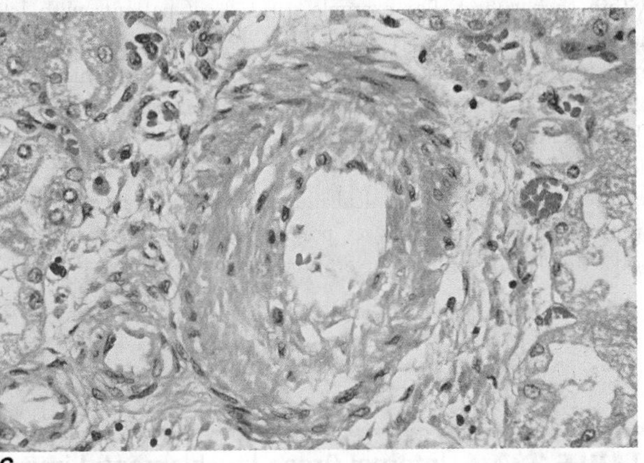

Figure 323-2 Pathologic findings in systemic sclerosis (SSc). ***A.*** Dermal sclerosis. The skin is thickened due to marked expansion of the dermis. Thick bundles of densely packed collagen replace skin appendages. ***B.*** Early interstitial lung disease. Diffuse fibrosis of the alveolar septae and a chronic inflammatory cell infiltrate. Trichrome stain. ***C.*** Pulmonary arterial obliterative vasculopathy. Striking intimal hyperplasia and narrowing of the lumen of a small pulmonary artery, with minimal interstitial fibrosis, in a patient with limited cutaneous SSc.

KIDNEYS

In the kidneys, lesions in the interlobular and arcuate arteries predominate, whereas glomerulonephritis is rare. Chronic renal ischemia is associated with shrunken glomeruli. Patients with scleroderma renal crisis show dramatic changes in small renal arteries with reduplication of elastic lamina, marked intimal proliferation, and narrowing of the lumen, often accompanied by thrombosis and microangiopathic hemolysis.

■ HEART

The heart is frequently affected, with prominent involvement of the myocardium and pericardium. The characteristic arteriolar lesions are concentric intimal hypertrophy and luminal narrowing, accompanied by contraction band necrosis reflecting ischemia-reperfusion injury, and patchy myocardial fibrosis that may also affect the conduction system. Despite the prominent role of ischemia in SSc, the frequency of atherosclerotic coronary artery disease is comparable to the general population.

■ OTHER ORGANS

Synovitis may be found in early SSc; however, with progression of the disease, the synovium becomes fibrotic. Fibrosis of tendon sheaths and fascia produces palpable and sometimes audible tendon friction rubs. Inflammation, and, in later stages, atrophy and fibrosis of the muscles are common findings. Fibrosis of the thyroid gland and of the minor salivary glands may be seen.

CLINICAL FEATURES

■ OVERVIEW

Virtually every organ is affected in SSc (Table 323-4). While there is a great deal of variability in the clinical manifestations from one patient to the next, patients can be classified into one of two major subsets based on the pattern of skin involvement (Table 323-2). Moreover, while dcSSc is associated with prominent and early internal organ involvement, lcSSc presents with long-standing Raynaud's phenomenon, indolent skin, limited internal organ involvement, and a better prognosis. While patient stratification into diffuse and limited cutaneous subsets is useful, disease expression is far more complex, and several distinct phenotypes exist within each subset. For example, 10–15% of patients with lcSSc develop severe pulmonary arterial hypertension without significant interstitial lung disease (ILD). Other patients have systemic features of SSc without appreciable skin involvement (SSc sine scleroderma). Unique clinical phenotypes of SSc associate with specific autoantibodies (Table 323-3). Patients with "overlap" have typical SSc features coexisting with clinical and laboratory evidence of another autoimmune disease such as polymyositis, Sjögren's syndrome, polyarthritis, autoimmune liver disease, or SLE.

TABLE 323-4 Internal Organ Involvement: Limited Cutaneous and Diffuse Cutaneous Forms of Systemic Sclerosis

Features	Limited Cutaneous SSc (%)	Diffuse Cutaneous SSc (%)
Skin involvement	90*	100
Raynaud's phenomenon	99	98
Esophageal involvement	90	80
Pulmonary fibrosis	35	65
Pulmonary arterial hypertension	15	15
Myopathy	11	23
Cardiac involvement	9	12
Scleroderma renal crisis	2	15

*10% of lcSSc patients have SSc sine scleroderma.

The term *scleroderma* refers to localized scleroderma and is used to describe a group of localized skin disorders that primarily affect children (Table 323-1). In contrast to SSc, localized scleroderma is rarely associated with Raynaud's phenomenon or internal organ involvement. Morphea presents as solitary or multiple circular patches of thickened skin and, less commonly, widespread induration (generalized or pansclerotic morphea); the fingers are spared. Linear scleroderma—streaks of thickened skin, typically in one or both lower extremities—may affect the subcutaneous tissues with fibrosis and atrophy of supporting structures, muscle, and bone. In children, the growth of affected long bones can be retarded. When linear scleroderma lesions cross joints, significant contractures can develop.

■ INITIAL CLINICAL PRESENTATION

The initial presentation is quite different in the diffuse and the limited cutaneous forms of the disease. In patients with dcSSc, the interval between Raynaud's phenomenon and appearance of other manifestations is generally brief (weeks to months). Soft tissue swelling and intense pruritus are signs of the early inflammatory "edematous" phase of dcSSc. The fingers, hands, distal limbs, and face are usually affected first. Diffuse hyperpigmentation and carpal tunnel syndrome can occur. Arthralgias, muscle weakness and decreased joint mobility are common. During the ensuing weeks to months, the inflammatory edematous phase evolves into the "fibrotic" phase, with skin induration that is associated with loss of body hair, reduced production of skin oils, and a decline in sweating capacity. The subcutaneous tissue becomes affected, with fat atrophy and fibrosis of underlying fascia, muscle, and other soft tissue structures. Progressive flexion contractures of the fingers ensue. The wrists, elbows, shoulders, hip girdles, knees, and ankles become stiff due to fibrosis of the supporting joint structures. While advancing skin involvement is the most visible manifestation of early dcSSc, important internal organ involvement develops during this stage. The initial 4 years from disease onset is the period of rapidly evolving systemic involvement and greatest risk for pulmonary and renal damage. If organ failure does not occur during this period, the systemic process may stabilize.

Compared to dcSSc, the course of lcSSc is generally more indolent. The period between the onset of Raynaud's phenomenon and manifestations such as gastroesophageal reflux, telangiectasia, or calcinosis can be several years. Raynaud's phenomenon tends to be more severe than in dcSSc, and can be associated with critical ischemia, ulcerations, and autoamputation of the fingers. On the other hand, significant renal involvement and pulmonary fibrosis are uncommon in lcSSc patients. Cardiac involvement and isolated pulmonary arterial hypertension develop in 10–15%. Overlap of SSc with the sicca complex, polyarthritis, cutaneous vasculitis, and biliary cirrhosis is seen primarily in the lcSSc subset.

ORGAN INVOLVEMENT

■ RAYNAUD'S PHENOMENON

Raynaud's phenomenon is an episodic vasoconstriction in the fingers and toes that occurs in virtually every patient with SSc. Vasoconstriction may also affect the tip of the nose and earlobes. Attacks are triggered by exposure to cold, a decrease in temperature, emotional stress, and vibration. Typical attacks start with pallor, followed by cyanosis of variable duration. Eventually erythema develops spontaneously or with rewarming of the digit. The progression of the three color phases reflects the underlying pathogenic mechanisms of vasoconstriction, ischemia, and reperfusion.

As much as 3–5% of the general population has Raynaud's phenomenon, and it is more frequent in women. In the absence of

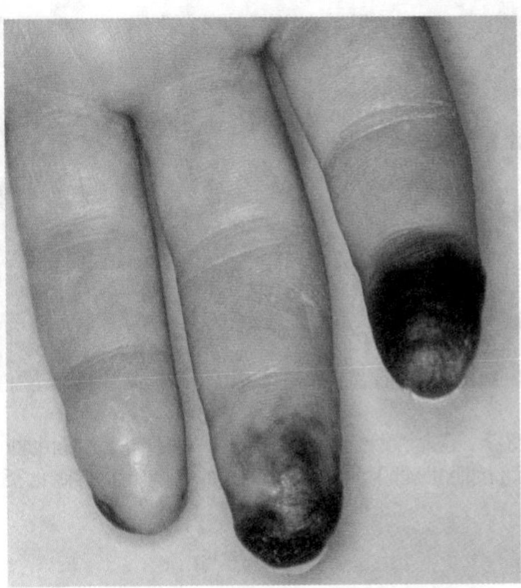

Figure 323-3 Digital necrosis. Sharply demarcated necrosis of the fingertip in a patient with limited cutaneous systemic sclerosis (SSc) associated with severe Raynaud's phenomenon.

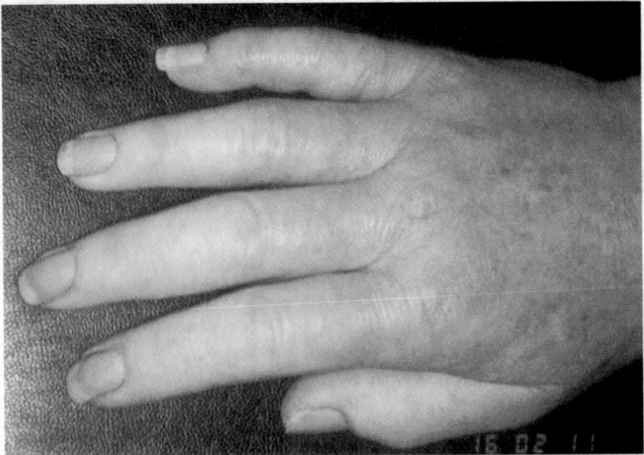

Figure 323-4 Sclerodactyly. Note skin induration on the fingers, and fixed flexion contractures at the proximal interphalangeal joints in a patient with limited cutaneous systemic sclerosis (SSc).

associated signs or symptoms of an underlying condition, Raynaud's phenomenon is classified as primary, and represents an exaggerated physiologic response to cold. Secondary Raynaud's phenomenon can occur as a complication of SSc and other connective tissue diseases, hematologic and endocrine conditions, and occupational disorders, and with the use of drugs such as the beta blocker atenolol and anticancer drugs such as cisplatin and bleomycin. Distinguishing primary versus secondary Raynaud's phenomenon can present a diagnostic challenge. The diagnosis of primary Raynaud's phenomenon is supported by the following: absence of an underlying cause on history and physical examination; a family history of Raynaud's phenomenon; absence of digital tissue necrosis, ulceration, or gangrene; and a negative test for antinuclear antibodies. Secondary Raynaud's phenomenon tends to develop at an older age (>30 years), is clinically more severe (episodes more frequent, prolonged, and painful), and is frequently associated with ischemic lesions and infarction in the digits (Fig. 323-3). The cutaneous capillaries at the nail bed can be viewed under a drop of grade B immersion oil using a low-power stereoscopic microscope. Nailfold capillaroscopy can be helpful in the evaluation of Raynaud's phenomenon; patients with primary Raynaud's phenomenon have normal capillaries that appear as regularly spaced parallel vascular loops, whereas in SSc and other connective tissue diseases, nailfold capillaries are distorted with widened and irregular loops, dilated lumen, and areas of vascular "dropout." In SSc, abnormal vascular reactivity may involve multiple vascular beds, and cold-induced Raynaud's-like episodic vasospasm has been documented in the pulmonary, renal, gastrointestinal, and coronary circulations.

■ SKIN FEATURES

While early-stage SSc is associated with edematous skin changes, skin thickening is the hallmark that distinguishes SSc from other connective tissue diseases. The distribution of skin thickening is invariably symmetric and bilateral. It typically starts in the fingers, and then characteristically advances from distal to proximal extremities in an ascending fashion. The involved skin is firm, coarse, and thickened, and the extremities and trunk may be darkly pigmented. In some patients, diffuse tanning in the absence of sun exposure is a very early manifestation of skin involvement. In dark-skinned patients, vitiligo-like hypopigmentation may occur. Because pigment loss spares the perifollicular areas, the skin may have a "salt-and-pepper" appearance, most prominently on the scalp, upper back, and chest. Dermal sclerosis due to collagen accumulation causes obliteration of hair follicles, sweat glands, and eccrine and sebaceous glands, resulting in hair loss, decreased sweating, and dry skin. Transverse creases on the dorsum of the fingers disappear (Fig. 323-4). Fixed flexion contractures of the fingers cause reduced hand mobility and lead to muscle atrophy. Skin thickening in combination with fibrosis of the subjacent tendons accounts for contractures of the wrists, elbows, and knees. Thick ridges at the neck due to firm adherence of skin to the underlying platysma muscle interfere with neck extension. The face assumes a characteristic "mauskopf" appearance with taut and shiny skin, loss of wrinkles, and occasionally an expressionless facies due to reduced mobility of the eyelids, cheeks, and mouth. Thinning of the lips with accentuation of the central incisor teeth and fine wrinkles (radial furrowing) around the mouth complete the picture. Reduced oral aperture (microstomia) interferes with eating and oral hygiene. The nose assumes a pinched, beak-like appearance.

In established SSc, the skin is firmly bound to the subcutaneous fat (tethering) and undergoes thinning and atrophy. Telangiectasia are dilated skin capillaries 2–20 mm in diameter frequently seen in lcSSc. These lesions, reminiscent of hereditary hemorrhagic telangiectasia, are prominent on the face, hands, lips, and oral mucosa (Fig. 323-5). Breakdown of atrophic skin leads to chronic ulcerations at the extensor surfaces of the proximal interphalangeal joints, the volar pads of the fingertips, and bony prominences such as the elbows and malleoli. Ulcers are painful and may become secondarily infected, resulting in osteomyelitis. Healing of ischemic fingertip ulcerations leaves characteristic fixed digital "pits." Loss of soft tissue at the fingertips due to ischemia is frequent and may be associated with striking resorption of the terminal phalanges (acro-osteolysis) (Fig. 323-6).

Calcium deposits occur in the skin and soft tissues. Calcinosis cutis is most common in patients with lcSSc who are positive for anticentromere antibodies. The deposits, varying in size from tiny punctate lesions to large conglomerate masses, are composed of calcium hydroxyapatite crystals and can be readily visualized on plain x-rays. Frequent locations include the finger pads, palms, extensor surfaces of the forearms, and the olecranon and prepatellar bursae (Fig. 323-7). Paraspinal calcifications may cause neurologic complications. Calcific deposits appears as persistent firm, nontender

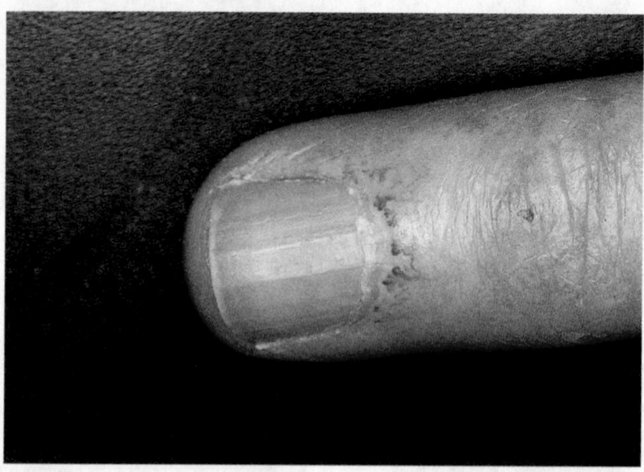

A

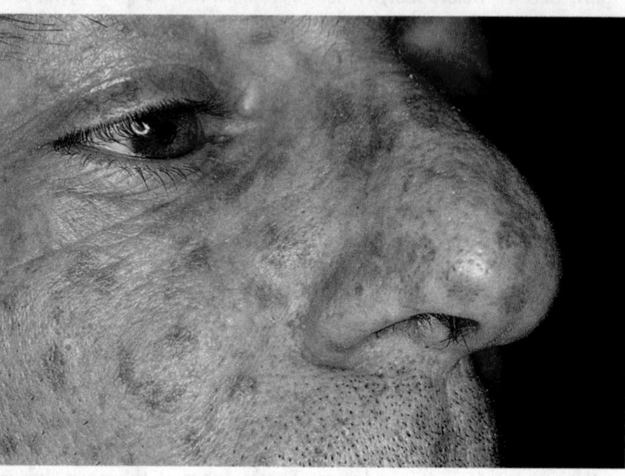

B

Figure 323-5 **Cutaneous vascular changes.** *A.* Capillary changes at the nailfold in a patient with limited cutaneous systemic sclerosis (lcSSc). *B.* Telangiectasia on the face.

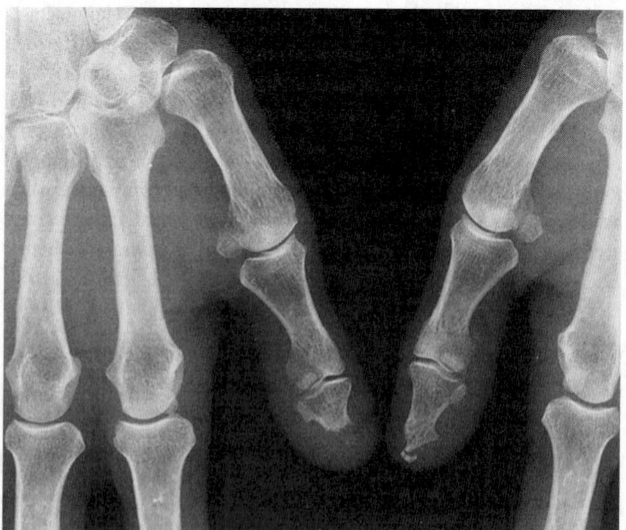

Figure 323-6 Acro-osteolysis. Note dissolution of terminal phalanges in a patient with long-standing limited cutaneous systemic sclerosis (lcSSc) and Raynaud's phenomenon.

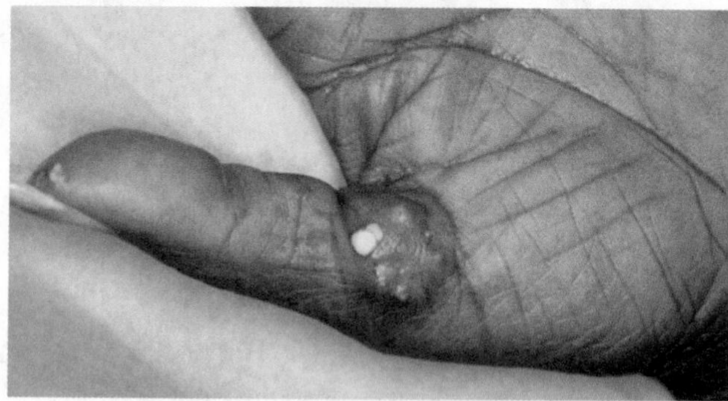

Figure 323-7 Calcinosis cutis. Note large calcific deposit breaking through the skin in a patient with limited cutaneous systemic sclerosis (lcSSc).

subcutaneous lumps. They may occasionally ulcerate through the overlying skin, producing drainage of chalky white material, pain, and local inflammation.

■ PULMONARY FEATURES

Pulmonary involvement can be documented in most patients with SSc and is now the leading cause of death. There are two main types of significant pulmonary involvement: ILD and PAH. Many patients with SSc develop some degree of both complications. Less frequent pulmonary manifestations of SSc include aspiration pneumonitis complicating gastroesophageal reflux, pulmonary hemorrhage due to endobronchial telangiectasia, obliterative bronchiolitis, pleural reactions, restrictive ventilatory defect due to chest wall fibrosis, spontaneous pneumothorax, and drug-induced lung toxicity. The incidence of lung cancer, particularly bronchioloalveolar carcinoma, may be increased.

Pulmonary involvement can remain asymptomatic until it is advanced. The most frequent presenting respiratory symptoms—exertional dyspnea, fatigue, and reduced exercise tolerance—are often subtle and slowly progressive. A chronic dry cough may be present. Physical examination may reveal "Velcro" crackles at the lung bases. Pulmonary function testing (PFT) is a sensitive method for detecting early pulmonary involvement. The most common abnormalities are reductions in forced vital capacity (FVC) or single breath diffusing capacity of the lung for carbon monoxide (DLco). A reduction in DLco that is significantly out of proportion to the reduction in FVC suggests pulmonary vascular disease, but may also be due to anemia. With exercise, patients show a decrease in PO_2.

Interstitial lung disease (ILD)

Some evidence of ILD can be found in up to 90% of patients with SSc at autopsy and 85% by thin-section high-resolution computed tomography (HRCT). ILD and pulmonary fibrosis cause restrictive pulmonary function defect with impaired gas exchange, characterized on PFT by decreased FVC and DLco but unaffected flow rates. Clinically significant ILD develops in 16–43% of patients with SSc; the frequency varies depending on the detection method used. Risk factors include male gender, African American race, diffuse skin involvement, severe gastroesophageal reflux, and the presence of topoisomerase-I autoantibodies, as well as a low FVC or DLco at initial presentation. In patients who develop significant ILD, the most rapid progression in lung disease occurs early in the course of the disease (within the first 3 years), when the FVC can decline by 30% per year.

Chest radiography is useful for ruling out infection and other causes of pulmonary involvement, but compared to HRCT it is

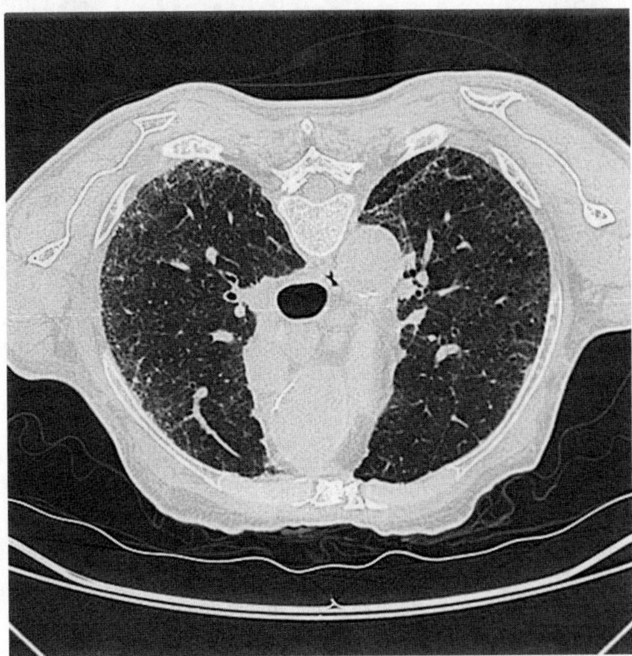

Figure 323-8 High-resolution CT scan of the lungs: interstitial lung disease. Note bilateral reticulonodular opacifications in a peripheral distribution in the lower lobes of the lungs in a patient with diffuse cutaneous systemic sclerosis (dcSSc).

relatively insensitive for detection of early ILD. HRCT may show subpleural reticular linear opacities, predominantly in the lower lobes, even in asymptomatic patients (Fig. 323-8). Additional findings include mediastinal lymphadenopathy, nodules, traction bronchiectasis and in some cases, honeycomb cystic changes. Ground-glass opacification, alone or in combination with a reticular pattern, is seen in 50% of patients. Ground-glass opacification on HRCT is indicative of fine fibrosis, and does not identify alveolitis or predict rapid progression. The extent of lung disease on HRCT is a predictor of mortality in SSc. Bronchoalveolar lavage (BAL) can demonstrate inflammation in the lower respiratory tract and may be useful for ruling out infection., While an elevated proportion of neutrophils (>2%) and/or eosinophils (>3%) in the BAL fluid is correlated with more extensive lung disease on HRCT, and is associated with more rapid decline in FVC and reduced survival, BAL is not useful for identifying reversible alveolitis. Lung biopsy is indicated only in patients with atypical findings on chest radiographs and should be thoracoscopically guided. The histologic pattern on lung biopsy may be helpful in predicting the risk of progression of ILD. The most common pattern in SSc, nonspecific interstitial pneumnia, carries a better prognosis than usual interstitial pneumnia. Recent studies suggest that measurement of serum factors such as KL-6, a glycoprotein found in type II pneumocytes and alveolar macrophages, may have utility as biomarkers for the detection and serial monitoring of ILD in patients with SSc.

Pulmonary arterial hypertension (PAH)

PAH, defined as a mean pulmonary arterial pressure >25mmHg with a pulmonary capillary wedge pressure <15 mmHg, is a major complication of SSc. Approximately 15% of SSc patients have PAH that can occur in association with ILD or as an isolated pulmonary abnormality. The natural history of SSc-associated PAH is variable, but in many patients it follows a downhill course with development of right heart failure and significant mortality. Risk factors for PAH include limited cutaneous disease with anticentromere antibodies, late age at disease onset, severe Raynaud's phenomenon, and the presence of antibodies to U1-RNP, U3-RNP (fibrillarin), and B23.

Patients with early PAH are generally asymptomatic. The initial symptom is typically exertional dyspnea and reduced exercise capacity. With progression, angina, exertional near-syncope, and symptoms and signs of right-sided heart failure appear. Physical examination shows tachypnea, a prominent pulmonic S_2 heart sound, palpable right ventricular heave, elevated jugular venous pressure, and dependent edema. Doppler echocardiography provides a noninvasive method for estimating the pulmonary arterial pressure is widely used to screen and for pulmonary hypertension. Echocardiographic estimates of pulmonary arterial systolic pressures exceeding 40 mmHg at rest suggest PAH. Pulmonary function testing may show a reduced DLco in isolation or combined with a restrictive pattern. Because echocardiography can result in over- or underestimation of pulmonary arterial pressures in SSc, right heart catheterization is always required to confirm the presence of PAH and accurately assess its severity, including the degree of right heart dysfunction. Serum levels of brain natriuretic peptide (BNP) and N-terminal pro-BNP correlate with the presence and severity of PAH in SSc, as well as survival. Therefore, BNP measurements can be useful in screening SSc patients and in monitoring the response to treatment. The prognosis of PAH is determined by the degree of pulmonary arterial pressure elevation.

■ GASTROINTESTINAL INVOLVEMENT

The gastrointestinal tract is affected in up to 90% of SSc patients with both limited and diffuse cutaneous forms of the disease. The pathologic features of atrophy of smooth muscle, intact mucosa, and obliterative small-vessel vasculopathy are similar throughout the length of the gastrointestinal tract.

Upper gastrointestinal tract involvement

Oropharyngeal manifestations due to a combination of xerostomia, reduced oral aperture, periodontal disease and resorption of the mandibular condyles are frequent. The frenulum of the tongue may be shortened. Symptoms of gastroesophageal reflux disease (GERD) develop early. Most patients have heartburn, regurgitation, and dysphagia. A combination of reduced lower esophageal sphincter pressure resulting in gastroesophageal reflux, impaired esophageal clearance of refluxed gastric contents due to diminished motility in the distal two-thirds of the esophagus, and delayed gastric emptying accounts for GERD. Chest CT scan characteristically shows a dilated esophagus with intraluminal air. Severe erosive esophagitis may be found on endoscopy in patients with minimal symptoms. Endoscopy may be necessary to rule out opportunistic infections with candida, herpes virus, and cytomegalovirus. Esophageal strictures and Barrett's esophagus may complicate chronic GERD. Because Barrett's esophagus is associated with an increased risk of adenocarcinoma, SSc patients with this lesion need to undergo periodic endoscopy and biopsy. Extraesophageal manifestations of GERD such as hoarseness and chronic cough may occur. Aspiration pneumonitis also may occur, aggravating underlying ILD.

Gastroparesis with early satiety, abdominal distention, and aggravated reflux symptoms is common. The presence and severity of gastroparesis can be assessed by radionuclide gastric emptying studies. Gastric antral vascular ectasia (GAVE) in the antrum may occur. These subepithelial lesions, reflecting the diffuse small-vessel vasculopathy of SSc, are described as "watermelon stomach" due to their endoscopic appearance. Patients with GAVE can have recurrent episodes of gastrointestinal bleeding, resulting in chronic unexplained anemia. Manometric testing shows abnormalities in the upper small intestines of most patients with SSc.

Lower gastrointestinal tract involvement

Impaired intestinal motility may result in malabsorption and chronic diarrhea secondary to bacterial overgrowth. Fat and protein malabsorption and B_{12} and vitamin D deficiency ensue, sometimes culminating in severe malnutrition. Disturbed intestinal motor function can also cause intestinal pseudoobstruction, with symptoms of nausea and abdominal distension that are indistinguishable from those of delayed gastric emptying. Patients present with recurrent episodes of acute abdominal pain, nausea, and vomiting. Radiographic studies show acute intestinal obstruction, and the major diagnostic challenge is to differentiate pseudoobstruction, which responds to supportive care and intravenous nutritional supplementation, from mechanical obstruction. Colonic involvement may cause severe constipation, fecal incontinence, gastrointestinal bleeding from telangiectasia, and rectal prolapse. In late-stage SSc, wide-mouth sacculations or diverticula occur in the colon, occasionally causing perforation and bleeding. An occasional radiologic finding is pneumatosis cystoides intestinalis due to air trapping in the bowel wall that may rarely rupture and cause benign pneumoperitoneum. Although the liver is rarely affected, primary biliary cirrhosis may coexist with SSc.

■ RENAL INVOLVEMENT: SCLERODERMA RENAL CRISIS

Scleroderma renal crisis, the most dreaded complication of SSc, occurs in 10–15% of patients, and almost always within 4 years of the onset of the disease. Prior to the advent of ACE inhibitors, short-term survival in scleroderma renal crisis was <10%. The pathogenesis involves obliterative vasculopathy and luminal narrowing of the renal arcuate and interlobular arteries. Progressive reduction in renal blood flow, aggravated by vasospasm, leads to juxtaglomerular hyperplasia, increased renin secretion, and activation of angiotensin, with further renal vasoconstriction resulting in a vicious cycle that culminates in malignant hypertension. Risk factors for scleroderma renal crisis include African American race, male gender, diffuse cutaneous SSc with extensive and progressive skin involvement, and autoantibodies to RNA polymerases I and III. Palpable tendon friction rubs, pericardial effusion, new unexplained anemia, and thrombocytopenia may be harbingers of impending scleroderma renal crisis. High-risk patients with early SSc should be counseled to check their blood pressure daily. Patients with lcSSc infrequently develop scleroderma renal crisis. Because there is an association between glucocorticoid use and the onset of scleroderma renal crisis, prednisone should be used in high-risk SSc patients only when absolutely required, and at low doses (<10 mg/d).

Patients characteristically present with accelerated hypertension and progressive renal insufficiency. However, in approximately 10% of patients, blood pressure remains normal. Normotensive renal crisis is generally associated with a poor outcome. Headache, blurred vision, and chest pain may accompany elevation of blood pressure. Urinalysis typically shows mild proteinuria, granular casts, and microscopic hematuria; thrombocytopenia and microangiopathic hemolysis with fragmented red blood cells can be seen. Progressive oliguric renal failure over several days generally follows. In some cases, scleroderma renal crisis is misdiagnosed as thrombotic thrombocytopenic purpura. The value of kidney biopsy in this setting is uncertain. Oliguria or a creatinine >3 mg/dL at presentation predicts poor outcome, with permanent hemodialysis and high mortality. Prompt aggressive intervention with short-acting ACE inhibitors to achieve adequate blood pressure control before the onset of renal failure results in improved prognosis. In contrast, there is no evidence to support the practice of "prophylactic" use of ACE inhibitors in normotensive SSc patients. Rarely, crescentic glomerulonephritis occurs in the setting of SSc.

■ CARDIAC INVOLVEMENT

Although cardiac involvement is often clinically silent, it is frequently detected when sensitive diagnostic tools are used. Cardiac disease occurs more frequently in patients with dcSSc than in those with lcSSc, and generally develops within 3 years of the onset of skin thickening. Clinically evident cardiac involvement in SSc is a poor prognostic factor. The endocardium, myocardium, and pericardium may be affected separately or together. Manifestations include pericardial effusions, atrial and ventricular tachycardias, conduction abnormalities, valvular regurgitation, hypertrophy, and heart failure. Systemic and pulmonary hypertension and lung and renal involvement may also impact on the heart. Despite the presence of widespread obliterative vasculopathy, the frequency of clinical or pathologic epicardial coronary artery disease in SSc is not increased. While conventional echocardiography has low sensitivity for detecting SSc preclinical heart involvement, newer modalities such as tissue Doppler echocardiography (TDE) and cardiac magnetic resonance imaging (MRI) reveal a high prevalence of abnormal myocardial function. Thallium perfusion studies document abnormal cardiac perfusion in a majority of patients. The serum level of N-terminal pro-brain natriuretic peptide (NT-pro-BNP), a ventricular hormone, is a sensitive and specific diagnostic marker for increased pulmonary artery pressure in SSc, but may also have utility as a marker of primary cardiac involvement. Myocarditis can occur in association with inflammatory polymyositis, and can be diagnosed using cardiac MRI. Pericardial effusions occur in over 15% of patients and, rarely, may cause tamponade.

■ MUSCULOSKELETAL COMPLICATIONS

Carpal tunnel syndrome occurs frequently and may be a presenting manifestation of SSc. Generalized arthralgia and stiffness are prominent in early disease. Joint mobility is progressively impaired, especially in patients with dcSSc. Most commonly affected are the hands. Contractures develop at the proximal interphalangeal joints and wrists. In patients with dcSSc, large joint contractures can be accompanied by tendon friction rubs characterized by leathery crepitation that can be heard or palpated upon passive movement. Tendon rubs are due to extensive fibrosis and adhesion of the tendon sheaths and fascial planes at the affected joint. Movement at the elbows, shoulders, and knees is frequently reduced. True joint inflammation is uncommon; however, occasional patients develop erosive polyarthritis in the hands. Muscle weakness is common, and may indicate deconditioning, disuse atrophy, and malnutrition. Less commonly, inflammatory myositis indistinguishable from idiopathic polymyositis may occur. A chronic noninflammatory myopathy characterized by atrophy and fibrosis in the absence of elevated muscle enzyme levels can be seen in late-stage SSc. Bone resorption occurs most commonly in the terminal phalanges, where it causes loss of the distal tufts (acro-osteolysis) (Fig. 323-5). Resorption of the mandibular condyles can lead to bite difficulties. Osteolysis can also affect the ribs and distal clavicles.

■ OTHER DISEASE MANIFESTATIONS

Many SSc patients develop dry eyes and dry mouth (sicca complex). Biopsy of the minor salivary glands shows fibrosis rather than focal lymphocytic infiltration characteristic of primary Sjögren's syndrome (Chap. 324). Hypothyroidism is common and generally due to fibrosis of the thyroid gland. Whereas the central nervous system is generally spared in SSc, sensory trigeminal neuropathy due to fibrosis or vasculopathy can occur, presenting with gradual onset of pain and numbness. Pregnancy in women with SSc is associated with an increased rate of adverse fetal outcomes. Furthermore, cardiopulmonary involvement may worsen during pregnancy, and new onset of scleroderma renal crisis has been described. Erectile dysfunction is frequent in men with SSc and may be the initial disease manifestation. Inability to attain or maintain penile erection is due to vascular insufficiency and fibrosis. The risk of certain malignancies is increased in SSc. Some studies have indicated that cancers of the lung, tongue, and breast occur more frequently in patients with SSc. Barrett's metaplasia is associated with increased risk for adenocarcinoma of the esophagus.

LABORATORY FEATURES

A mild normocytic or microcytic anemia due to chronic inflammation is frequent in patients with SSc. Iron deficiency anemia may indicate gastrointestinal bleeding caused by GAVE or chronic esophagitis. Macrocytic anemia, indicating a maturation disorder, may be caused by folate and vitamin B_{12} deficiency due to small bowel bacterial overgrowth and malabsorption, or by drugs such as methotrexate or alkylating agents. Microangiopathic hemolytic anemia, caused by mechanical trauma and fragmentation of red blood cells during their passage through microvessels coated with fibrin or platelet thrombi, is a hallmark of scleroderma renal crisis. Thrombocytopenia and leukopenia generally indicate drug toxicity. In contrast to other connective tissue diseases, the erythrocyte sedimentation rate (ESR) is generally normal; an elevation may signal coexisting myositis or malignancy.

Antinuclear autoantibodies are present in almost all patients with SSc and can be detected at disease onset. Autoantibodies against topoisomerase-I (Scl-70) and centromere are specific for SSc and are mutually exclusive. Topoisomerase-I antibodies are detected in 31% of patients with dcSSc, but in only 13% of patients with lcSSc; conversely, anticentromere antibodies are detected in 38% of patients with lcSSc, but in only 2% of patients with dcSSc. Anticentromere antibodies are commonly associated with lcSSc and PAH, and only rarely with cardiac or renal involvement or significant ILD. Topoisomerase-I-positive patients have reduced survival compared to those without this antibody; whereas anticentromere antibody-positive patients have improved survival compared to those without this antibody. Nucleolar immunofluorescence pattern on serologic testing reflects antibodies to U3-RNP (fibrillarin), Th/To, or PM/Scl, whereas a speckled immunofluorescence pattern indicates antibodies to RNA polymerase III. Although antibodies to β2GPI occur in antiphospholipid antibody syndrome and are not specific for SSc, their presence in SSc is associated with an increased risk of ischemic lesions in the fingers. No direct pathogenic role has been firmly established for any of the SSc-associated autoantibodies; however, antibody titers can correlate with disease severity and fluctuate with disease activity.

DIAGNOSIS

The diagnosis of SSc is made primarily on clinical grounds and is generally straightforward in patients with established disease. The presence of skin induration, with a characteristic symmetric distribution pattern associated with typical visceral organ manifestations, establishes the diagnosis with a high degree of certainty. While the conditions listed in Table 323-1 can be associated with skin induration, the distribution pattern of skin lesions, together with the absence of Raynaud's phenomenon or typical visceral organ manifestations or SSc-specific autoantibodies, differentiates these conditions from SSc. Occasionally, full-thickness biopsy of the skin is required for establishing the diagnosis of scleredema, scleromyxedema, or nephrogenic systemic fibrosis. In lcSSc a history of antecedent Raynaud's phenomenon and gastroesophageal reflux symptoms, coupled with the presence of sclerodactyly and capillary changes on nailfold capillaroscopy, often in combinations with telangiectasia and calcinosis cutis, helps to establish the diagnosis. The finding of digital tip pitting scars and radiologic evidence of pulmonary fibrosis in the lower lobes are particularly helpful diagnostically. Primary Raynaud's phenomenon is a common benign condition that must be differentiated from early or limited SSc. Nailfold microscopy is particularly helpful in this situation, because in primary Raynaud's phenomenon the nailfold capillaries are normal, whereas in SSc capillary abnormalities, as well as serum autoantibodies can be detected even before other disease manifestations.

Establishing the diagnosis of SSc in early disease may be a challenge. In dcSSc, initial symptoms are often nonspecific and relate to inflammation. Patients complain of fatigue, swelling, aching, and stiffness, and Raynaud's phenomenon may initially be absent. Physical examination may reveal diffuse upper extremity edema and puffy fingers. Patients at this stage are sometimes diagnosed as early rheumatoid arthritis, systemic lupus erythematosus, myositis, or, most commonly, undifferentiated connective tissue disease. Within weeks to months, Raynaud's phenomenon and characteristic clinical features appear accompanied by advancing induration of the skin. The presence of antinuclear and SSc-specific autoantibodies provides a high degree of diagnostic specificity. Raynaud's phenomenon with fingertip ulcerations or other evidence of digital ischemia, coupled with telangiectasia, distal esophageal dysmotility, unexplained ILD or PAH, or accelerated hypertension with renal failure in the absence of skin induration, suggests the diagnosis of SSc sine scleroderma. These patients may have anticentromere antibodies.

TREATMENT Systemic Sclerosis

OVERVIEW To date, no therapy has been shown to significantly alter the natural history of SSc. In contrast, multiple interventions are highly effective in alleviating the symptoms and in slowing the progression of the cumulative organ damage. A significant reduction in disease-related mortality has been noted during the past 25 years. Because of the marked heterogeneity in clinical presentations, patients need careful investigation at baseline, and evaluation and treatment approaches must be individually tailored according to each patient's unique needs. Optimal management incorporates the following principles: prompt and accurate diagnosis; classification and risk stratification based on clinical and laboratory evaluation; early recognition of organ-based complications and assessment of their extent, severity, and likelihood of deterioration; regular monitoring for progression, disease activity, and response to therapy; and continuing patient education. In order to minimize irreversible organ damage, the management of life-threatening complications must be proactive, with regular screening and initiation of appropriate intervention at the earliest possible opportunity. In light of the complex, multisystemic nature of the disease, an integrated team-based approach is optimal. Most patients are treated with combinations of drugs that act upon different aspects of the disease. Patients should become familiar with the spectrum of potential complications, have an understanding of the therapeutic options and natural history of the disease, and be empowered to partner with their physicians. This typically requires a long-term relationship between patient and physician, with ongoing counseling and encouragement.

DISEASE-MODIFYING THERAPY: IMMUNOSUPPRESSIVE AGENTS Immunosuppressive agents effective in other connective tissue diseases have generally shown modest or no benefit in the treatment of SSc. Glucocorticoids may be useful for alleviating stiffness and aching in early-stage dcSSc, but do not influence the progression of skin or internal organ involvement. Furthermore, their use in high doses is associated with an increased risk of scleroderma renal crisis. Therefore, glucocorticoids should be avoided if possible; when absolutely necessary, they should be given at the lowest dose possible and for brief periods only. The use of cyclophosphamide has been extensively studied in light of its efficacy in the treatment of vasculitis (Chap. 326), systemic lupus erythematosus (Chap. 319), and other autoimmune diseases (Chap. 318).

Cyclophosphamide has been evaluated in the treatment of SSc in retrospective and prospective controlled clinical trials. Both oral and intermittent intravenous cyclophosphamide were shown to reduce the progression of ILD in SSc patients with early symptomatic disease, with stabilization, and, rarely, modest improvement of pulmonary function and HRCT after 1 year of treatment. Improvement in respiratory symptoms and the extent of skin induration was also noted. The beneficial effect of cyclophosphamide on lung function wanes upon discontinuation of therapy. The benefits of cyclophosphamide need to be balanced against its potential toxicity, including bone marrow suppression, opportunistic infections, hemorrhagic cystitis and bladder cancer, premature ovarian failure, and late secondary malignancies.

In small clinical trials in SSc, methotrexate treatment was associated with a modest improvement in skin scores. Mycophenolate mofetil treatment was associated with improved skin induration in uncontrolled studies and was generally well tolerated. The use of immunomodulatory agents such as cyclosporine, azathioprine, rituximab, extracorporeal photophoresis, imatinib, thalidomide, or rapamycin for the treatment of SSc is currently not well supported by the literature. Immune ablation using high-dose chemotherapy with or without irradiation, followed by autologous stem cell reconstitution, is undergoing evaluation in randomized clinical trials in SSc. In light of its potential morbidity and mortality, as well as cost, autologous stem cell transplantation in SSc is still considered experimental.

Anti-Fibrotic Therapy Because widespread tissue fibrosis causes progressive organ damage in dcSSc, drugs that interfere with the fibrotic process represent a rational approach to therapy. D-Penicillamine has been extensively used as an antifibrotic agent. Retrospective studies in SSc indicated that D-penicillamine stabilized and improved skin induration, prevented new internal organ involvement, and improved survival. However, a randomized controlled clinical trial in early active SSc found no difference in the extent of skin involvement between patients treated with standard-dose (750 mg/d) or very low-dose (125 mg every other day) D-penicillamine. Minocycline, recombinant relaxin, interferon (INF)-γ, and inhibitors of tumor necrosis factor have failed to show meaningful clinical benefit in SSc.

Vascular Therapy The goal of vascular therapy is to control Raynaud's phenomenon, prevent the development and enhance the healing of ischemic complications, and slow the progression of obliterative vasculopathy. Patients with Raynaud's phenomenon should dress warmly, minimize cold exposure or stress, and avoid drugs that could precipitate or exacerbate vasospastic episodes. Some patients may respond to biofeedback therapy. Calcium channel blockers such as nifedipine or diltiazem are commonly used but show only moderate benefit, and their use is often limited by side effects (palpitations, dependent edema, light-headedness). While ACE inhibitors do not reduce the frequency or severity of episodes, angiotensin II receptor blockers such as losartan are effective and generally well tolerated. Some patients with Raynaud's phenomenon may require α_1-adrenergic receptor blockers (e.g., prazosin), 5-phosphodiesterase inhibitors (e.g., sildenafil), serotonin reuptake inhibitors (e.g., fluoxetine), topical nitroglycerine, and intravenous prostaglandins. Low-dose aspirin and dipyridamole prevent platelet aggregation and may have a role as adjunctive agents. In patients with ischemic finger ulcerations, the endothelin-1 receptor antagonist bosentan reduces the development of new ulcers. Digital sympathectomy and local injections of botulinum type A (botox) into the digits are options in some patients with severe Raynaud's phenomenon associated with ischemia. Empirical long-term therapy with statins and antioxidants may delay the progression of vascular damage and obliteration. The use of calcium channel blockers has been associated with improved cardiac perfusion and cardiac function in SSc patients with cardiac involvement.

TREATMENT OF GASTROINTESTINAL COMPLICATIONS Because gastroesophageal reflux is very common, all patients with SSc should be treated for this complication. Significant reflux may occur in the absence of symptoms. Patients should be instructed to elevate the head of the bed and eat frequent small meals. Proton pump inhibitors reduce acid reflux and may need to be given in relatively high doses. Recurrent gastrointestinal bleeding from vascular ectasia in the gastric antrum (watermelon stomach) is amenable to treatment with laser photocoagulation. Bacterial overgrowth due to small-bowel dysmotility causes abdominal bloating and diarrhea and may lead to malabsorption and severe malnutrition. Treatment with short courses of rotating broad-spectrum antibiotics such as metronidazole, erythromycin, and tetracycline can eradicate bacterial overgrowth. Parenteral hyperalimentation is indicated if malnutrition develops. Chronic hypomotility of the small bowel may respond to octreotide.

TREATMENT OF PULMONARY ARTERIAL HYPERTENSION (PAH) Because PAH is asymptomatic until it is advanced, patients with SSc should be screened for the presence of PAH on a regular basis. When PAH is symptomatic, treatment should be started with an oral endothelin-1 receptor antagonist or a phosphodiesterase inhibitor such as sildenafil. Patients may also require diuretics, oral anticoagulation, and digoxin when appropriate. If hypoxemia is documented, supplemental oxygen should be given by nasal cannula in order to avoid hypoxia-induced secondary pulmonary vasoconstriction. Inhibitors of phosphodiesterase type 5 (e.g., sildenafil) have been shown to have short-term efficacy in PAH and may be used in combination with bosentan. Prostacyclin analogues such as epoprostenol or treprostinil can be administered intravenously or by continuous subcutaneous infusion, or frequent inhalations via nebulizer. Lung transplantation remains an option for patients with SSc-associated PAH who fail medical therapy.

TREATMENT OF RENAL CRISIS Scleroderma renal crisis is a medical emergency because the outcome is largely determined by the extent of renal damage present at the time that aggressive therapy is initiated. Prompt recognition of impending or early scleroderma renal crisis is therefore essential, and efforts should be made to avoid its occurrence. High risk patients with early SSc and extensive and progressive skin involvement should be instructed to monitor their blood pressure daily and report significant alterations immediately. Potentially nephrotoxic drugs should be avoided, and glucocorticoids used only when absolutely necessary, and at low doses. When scleroderma renal crisis occurs, treatment should be started promptly with short-acting ACE inhibitors, with the goal of achieving rapid normalization of the blood pressure. Kidney biopsy is rarely useful in this setting. Up to two-thirds of patients require dialysis. However, substantial renal recovery can occur following renal crisis, and up to one-half of the patients may be able to discontinue dialysis. Kidney transplantation is appropriate for patients who are unable to discontinue dialysis after 2 years. Survival of SSc patients with with renal transplantation is comparable to that in other connective tissue diseases, and recurrence of renal crisis is rare.

SKIN CARE Because skin involvement in SSc is never life-threatening, and it stabilizes, and may even regress spontaneously over time, the overall management of the disease should not be dictated by its cutaneous manifestations. The inflammatory symptoms of early skin involvement can be effectively controlled with systemic antihistamines and cautious and short-term use of low-dose glucocorticoids (<5 mg/d of prednisone). Retrospective studies have shown that D-penicillamine reduced the extent and progression of skin induration; however, these benefits could not be substantiated in a controlled prospective trial. Cyclophosphamide and methotrexate have also been shown to have modest effects on skin induration. Because induration is associated with dryness, patients should use hydrophilic ointments and bath oils. Regular skin massage is helpful. Telangiectasia may present a cosmetic problem, especially when they occur on the face. Treatment with pulsed dye laser may have short-term benefit. Fingertip ulcerations should be protected by occlusive dressing to promote healing and prevent infection. Infected skin ulcers are treated with topical antibiotics. Surgical debridement may be indicated. No therapy has been shown to be effective in preventing the formation of calcific soft tissue deposits or in promoting their dissolution.

COURSE

The natural history of SSc is highly variable and difficult to predict, especially in early stages when the specific disease subset—diffuse or limited cutaneous form—is not clear. Patient with dcSSc have a more rapidly progressive disease and worse prognosis than those with lcSSc.

In dcSSc, early inflammatory symptoms such as fatigue, edema, arthralgia, and pruritus tend to subside 2–4 years after the onset of disease, and the extent of skin thickening reaches a plateau after which it generally shows slow regression. It is during the early edematous stage, generally lasting <3 years, that visceral organ involvement develops and progresses. While existing visceral organ involvement, such as pulmonary fibrosis, may continue to progress, new organ involvement is rare after the skin involvement reaches its peak. Scleroderma renal crisis almost invariably occurs within the first 4 years of disease. In dcSSc patients with late-stage disease (>6 years), the skin is usually soft and atrophic. Skin regression characteristically occurs in an order that is the reverse of initial involvement, with softening on the trunks followed by proximal and then distal extremities. Sclerodactyly and finger contractures generally persist. Cutaneous telangiectasia and calcinosis are common, making it difficult to differentiate late-stage dcSSc from lcSSc. Relapse or recurrence of skin thickening after the peak of skin involvement has been reached is rare. Patients with lcSSc follow a clinical course that is markedly different than that of dcSSc. In this subset of SSc, Raynaud's phenomenon typically precedes other disease manifestations by years or even decades. Visceral organ complications such as PAH and ILD generally develop late and tend to be slowly progressive.

PROGNOSIS

SSc confers a substantial increase in the risk of premature death, with age- and gender-adjusted mortality rates that are fivefold to eightfold higher compared to the general population. In one population-based study of SSc patients with all forms of the disease, the median survival was 11 years. In patients with dcSSc, 5- and 10-year survivals are 70% and 55%, respectively, whereas in patients with lcSSc, 5- and 10-year survivals are 90% and 75%, respectively. The prognosis of SSc correlates with the extent of skin involvement, which itself is a surrogate for visceral organ involvement. Major causes of death are PAH, pulmonary fibrosis, gastrointestinal involvement, and cardiac disease. Scleroderma renal crisis is associated with a 30% 3-year mortality. Lung cancer and excess cardiovascular deaths also contribute to increased mortality. Markers of worse prognosis include male gender, African American race, older age of disease onset, extensive skin thickening with truncal involvement, evidence of significant or progressive visceral organ involvement, and the presence of anti-topoisomerase-I and anti-RNA polymerase III antibodies. Additional predictors of increased mortality at initial evaluation include an elevated ESR, anemia, and proteinuria. In one study, SSc patients with extensive skin involvement, lung vital capacity <55% predicted, significant gastrointestinal involvement (pseudoobstruction or malabsorption), evidence of cardiac involvement (arrhythmias or congestive heart failure), or scleroderma renal crisis had a cumulative 9-year survival <40%. The severity of PAH is itself strongly associated with mortality, and SSc patients who had a mean pulmonary arterial pressure ≥45 mmHg had a 33% 3-year survival. The advent of ACE inhibitor therapy for scleroderma renal crisis had a dramatic impact on survival, increasing from a <10% 1-year survival in the pre-ACE inhibitor era to a >70% 3-year survival at the present time.

MIXED CONNECTIVE TISSUE DISEASE

Patients who have lcSSc coexisting with features of SLE, polymyositis, and rheumatoid arthritis may have mixed connective tissue disease (MCTD). This overlap syndrome is generally associated with the presence of high titers of autoantibodies to U1-RNP. The characteristic initial presentation is Raynaud's phenomenon associated with puffy fingers and myalgia. Gradually, lcSSc features of sclerodactyly, calcinosis, and cutaneous telangiectasia develop. Skin rashes suggestive of systemic lupus erythematosus (malar rash, photosensitivity) or of dermatomyositis (heliotrope rash on the eyelids, erythematous rash on the knuckles) occur. Arthralgia is common, and some patients develop erosive polyarthritis. Pulmonary fibrosis and isolated or secondary PAH may develop. Other manifestations include esophageal dysmotility, pericarditis, Sjögren's syndrome, and renal disease, especially membranous glomerulonephritis. Laboratory evaluation indicates features of inflammation with elevated ESR and hypergammaglobulinemia. While anti-U1RNP antibodies are detected in the serum in high titers, SSc-specific autoantibodies are not found. In contrast to SSc, patients with MCTD often show a good response to treatment with glucocorticoids, and the long-term prognosis is better than that of SSc. Whether MCTD is a truly distinct entity or is, rather, a subset of SLE or SSc remains controversial.

EOSINOPHILIC FASCIITIS

Eosinophilic fasciitis is a rare idiopathic disorder associated with induration of the skin that generally develops rapidly. Adults are primarily affected. The skin has a coarse cobblestone "peau d'orange" appearance. In contrast to SSc, internal organ involvement is rare, and Raynaud's phenomenon and SSc-associated autoantibodies are absent. Furthermore, skin involvement spares the fingers. Full-thickness excisional biopsy of the lesional skin reveals fibrosis of the subcutaneous fascia, and is generally required for diagnosis. Inflammation and eosinophil infiltration in the fascia are variably present. In the acute phase of the illness, peripheral blood eosinophilia may be prominent. MRI appears to be a sensitive tool for the diagnosis of eosinophilic fasciitis. In some patients, eosinophilic fasciitis occurs in association with, or preceding, myelodysplastic syndromes or multiple myeloma. Treatment with glucocorticoids leads to prompt resolution of the eosinophilia. In contrast, skin changes generally show slow and variable improvement. The prognosis of patients with eosinophilic fasciitis is good.

FURTHER READINGS

Feghali-Bostwick C et al: Analysis of systemic sclerosis in twins reveals low concordance for disease and high concordance for the presence of antinuclear antibodies. Arthritis Rheum 48:1956, 2003

Kuwana M et al: Defective vasculogenesis in systemic sclerosis. Lancet 364:603, 2004

Mayes MD et al: Prevalence, incidence, survival, and disease characteristics of systemic sclerosis in a large US population. Arthritis Rheum 48:2246, 2003

Milano A et al: Molecular subsets in the gene expression signatures of scleroderma skin. PLoS ONE 3:e2696, 2008; erratum: PLoS ONE 3:doi: 10.1371/annotation/05bed72c-c6f6-4685-a732-02-c78e5f66c2, 2008

Scussel-Lonzetti L et al: Predicting mortality in systemic sclerosis: Analysis of a cohort of 309 French Canadian patients with emphasis on features at diagnosis as predictive factors for survival. Medicine (Baltimore) 81:154, 2002

Tashkin DP et al: Cyclophosphamide versus placebo in scleroderma lung disease. N Engl J Med 354:2655, 2006

———: Effects of 1-year treatment with cyclophosphamide on outcomes at 2 years in scleroderma lung disease. Am J Respir Crit Care Med 176:1026, 2007

Varga J, Abraham D: Systemic sclerosis: A prototypic multisystem fibrotic disorder. J Clin Invest 117:557, 2007

Whitfield ML et al: Systemic and cell type-specific gene expression patterns in SSc skin. Proc Natl Acad Sci U S A 100:12319, 2003

CHAPTER 324
Sjögren's Syndrome

Haralampos M. Moutsopoulos
Athanasios G. Tzioufas

DEFINITION, INCIDENCE, AND PREVALENCE

Sjögren's syndrome is a chronic, slowly progressive autoimmune disease characterized by lymphocytic infiltration of the exocrine glands resulting in xerostomia and dry eyes. Approximately one-third of patients present with systemic manifestations; a small but significant number of patients may develop malignant lymphoma. The disease presents alone (primary Sjögren's syndrome) or in association with other autoimmune rheumatic diseases (secondary Sjögren's syndrome) (Table 324-1).

Middle-aged women (female-to-male ratio, 9:1) are primarily affected, although it may occur in all ages, including childhood. The prevalence of primary Sjögren's syndrome is approximately 0.5–1%, while 30% of patients with autoimmune rheumatic diseases suffer from secondary Sjögren's syndrome.

PATHOGENESIS

Sjögren's syndrome is characterized by both lymphocytic infiltration of the exocrine glands and B lymphocyte hyperreactivity. An oligomonoclonal B cell process, which is characterized by cryoprecipitable monoclonal immunoglobulins (IgMκ) with rheumatoid factor activity, is evident in up to 25% of patients.

Sera of patients with Sjögren's syndrome often contain autoantibodies directed against non-organ-specific antigens such as immunoglobulins (rheumatoid factors) and extractable nuclear and cytoplasmic antigens (Ro/SS-A, La/SS-B). Ro/SS-A autoantigen consists of two polypeptides (52 and 60 kDa) in conjunction with cytoplasmic RNAs, whereas the 48-kDa La/SS-B protein is bound to RNA III polymerase transcripts. Autoantibodies to Ro/SS-A and La/SS-B antigens are usually detected at the time of diagnosis and are associated with earlier disease onset, longer disease duration, salivary gland enlargement, more severe lymphocytic infiltration of minor salivary glands, and certain extraglandular manifestations. Antibodies to α-fodrin (120 kDa), a salivary gland–specific protein, as well as muscarinic receptor 3 (M3R) also have been found in sera of patients with Sjögren's syndrome. The major infiltrating cells in the affected exocrine glands are activated T and B lymphocytes. T cells predominate in mild lesions, whereas B-cells in more severe lesions. T regulatory cells also have been detected. Macrophages and dendritic cells also are found. The number of interleukin (IL)-18 positive macrophages has been shown to correlate with parotid gland enlargement and low levels of the C4 component of complement, both adverse predictors for lymphoma development. Glandular epithelial cells undergo apoptotic death by signals provided from T cells. Infiltrating lymphocytes not only provide apoptotic messages to epithelial cells but also tend to be resistant to apoptosis. Ductal and acinar epithelial cells appear to play a significant role in the initiation and perpetuation of the autoimmune injury. They express class II major histocompatibility complex (MHC), costimulatory molecules, and intracellular autoantigens expressed on cell membranes, thus being able to provide signals essential for lymphocytic activation. Finally, they inappropriately produce proinflammatory cytokines and lymphoattractant chemokines necessary for sustaining the autoimmune lesion and progressing to more sophisticated ectopic germinal center formation, that occurs in one-fifth of patients. They also express functional receptors of innate immunity, particularly TLR 3, 7, and 9, that may account for the perpetuation of the autoimmune response. Similar to T cells, CD40+ B cells also have a tendency to be resistant to apoptosis. B-cell activating factor (BAFF) has been found to be elevated in patients with Sjögren's syndrome, especially those with hypergammaglobulinemia, and probably accounts for this

TABLE 324-1 Association of Sjögren's Syndrome With Other Autoimmune Diseases

Rheumatoid arthritis
Systemic lupus erythematosus
Scleroderma
Mixed connective tissue disease
Primary biliary cirrhosis
Vasculitis
Chronic active hepatitis

antiapoptotic effect. Glandular epithelial cells seem to have an active role in the production of BAFF, since it may be expressed and secreted after stimulation with type I interferon, as well as with viral or synthetic dsRNA. The triggering factor for epithelial activation appears to be a persistent enteroviral infection (possibly by coxsackievirus strains).

A defect in cholinergic activity mediated through the M3 receptor and redistribution of the water-channel protein aquaporin-5, both leading to neuroepithelial dysfunction and diminished glandular secretions, have been proposed.

Molecular analysis of human leukocyte antigen (HLA) class II genes has revealed that patients with Sjögren's syndrome, regardless of their ethnic origin, are highly associated with the HLA DQA1*0501 allele. Recent genome-wide association studies, disclosed increased prevalence of single nucleotide polymorphisms in genes of IRF-5 and STAT-4, participating in the activation of the type I interferon pathway.

CLINICAL MANIFESTATIONS

The majority of Sjögren's syndrome patients have symptoms related to diminished lacrimal and salivary gland function. In most patients, the primary syndrome runs a slow and benign course. The initial manifestations can be mucosal or nonspecific dryness, and 8–10 years may elapse from the initial symptoms to full-blown development of the disease.

The principal oral symptom of Sjögren's syndrome is dryness (xerostomia). Patients complain of difficulty in swallowing dry food, inability to speak continuously, a burning sensation, increase in dental caries, and problems in wearing complete dentures. Physical examination shows a dry, erythematous, sticky oral mucosa. There is atrophy of the filiform papillae on the dorsum of the tongue, and saliva from the major glands is either not expressible or cloudy. Enlargement of the parotid or other major salivary glands occurs in two-thirds of patients with primary Sjögren's syndrome but is uncommon in those with the secondary syndrome. Diagnostic tests include sialometry, sialography, and scintigraphy. Newer imaging techniques including ultrasound, MRI or MR sialography of the major salivary glands are also being used. The labial minor salivary gland biopsy permits histopathologic confirmation of the focal lymphocytic infiltrates.

Ocular involvement is the other major manifestation of Sjögren's syndrome. Patients usually complain of a sandy or gritty feeling under the eyelids. Other symptoms include burning, accumulation of thick strands at the inner canthi, decreased tearing, redness, itching, eye fatigue, and increased photosensitivity. These symptoms are attributed to the destruction of corneal and bulbar conjunctival epithelium, defined as *keratoconjunctivitis sicca.* Diagnostic evaluation of keratoconjunctivitis sicca includes measurement of tear flow by Schirmer's I test and tear composition as assessed by the tear breakup time or tear lysozyme content. Slit-lamp examination of the cornea and conjunctiva after rose Bengal staining reveals punctuate corneal ulcerations and attached filaments of corneal epithelium.

Involvement of other exocrine glands occurs less frequently and includes a decrease in mucous gland secretions of the upper and lower respiratory tree, resulting in dry nose, throat, and trachea (xerotrachea), and diminished secretion of the exocrine glands of the gastrointestinal tract, leading to esophageal mucosal atrophy, atrophic gastritis, and subclinical pancreatitis. Dyspareunia due to dryness of the external genitalia and dry skin also may occur.

Extraglandular (systemic) manifestations are seen in one-third of patients with Sjögren's syndrome (Table 324-2), while they are very rare in patients with Sjögren's syndrome associated with rheumatoid arthritis. These patients complain more often of easy fatigability, low-grade fever, Raynaud's phenomenon, myalgias, and arthralgias. Most patients with primary Sjögren's syndrome experience at least one episode of nonerosive arthritis during the course of their disease. Manifestations of pulmonary involvement are frequently evident histologically but rarely clinically important. Dry cough is the major manifestation that is attributed to small airway disease. Renal involvement includes interstitial nephritis, clinically manifested by hyposthenuria and renal tubular dysfunction with or without acidosis. Untreated acidosis may lead to nephrocalcinosis. Glomerulonephritis is a rare finding that occurs in patients with mixed cryoglobulinemia, or systemic lupus erythematosus overlapping with Sjögren's syndrome. Vasculitis affects small and medium-sized vessels. The most common clinical features are purpura, recurrent urticaria, skin ulcerations, glomerulonephritis, and mononeuritis multiplex. Sensorineural hearing loss was found in one-half of patients with Sjögren's syndrome and correlated with the presence of anticardiolipin antibodies.

TABLE 324-2 Prevalence of Extraglandular Manifestations in Primary Sjögren's Syndrome

Clinical Manifestation	Percent
Arthralgias/arthritis	60
Raynaud's phenomenon	37
Lymphadenopathy	14
Lung involvement	14
Vasculitis	11
Kidney involvement	9
Liver involvement	6
Lymphoma	6
Splenomegaly	3
Peripheral neuropathy	2
Myositis	1

It has been suggested that primary Sjögren's syndrome with vasculitis may also present with multifocal, recurrent, and progressive nervous system disease, such as hemiparesis, transverse myelopathy, hemisensory deficits, seizures, and movement disorders. Aseptic meningitis and multiple sclerosis also have been reported in these patients.

Lymphoma is a well-known manifestation of Sjögren's syndrome that usually presents later in the illness. Persistent parotid gland enlargement, purpura, leukopenia, cryoglobulinemia, and low C4 complement levels are manifestations suggesting the development of lymphoma. Interestingly, the same risk factors account for glomerulonephritis and lymphoma and are those that confer increased mortality. Most lymphomas are extranodal, low-grade marginal zone B cell lymphomas and are usually detected incidentally upon evaluating the labial biopsy. The affected lymph nodes are usually peripheral. Survival is decreased in patients with B symptoms, lymph node mass >7 cm in diameter, and high or intermediate histologic grade.

Routine laboratory tests reveal mild normochromic, normocytic anemia. An elevated erythrocyte sedimentation rate is found in approximately 70% of patients.

TABLE 324-3 Differential Diagnosis of Sicca Symptoms

Xerostomia	Dry Eye	Bilateral Parotid Gland Enlargement
Viral infections	Inflammation	Viral infections
Drugs	Stevens-Johnson syndrome	Mumps
Psychotherapeutic	Pemphigoid	Influenza
Parasympatholytic	Chronic conjunctivitis	Epstein-Barr
Antihypertensive	Chronic blepharitis	Coxsackievirus A
Psychogenic	Sjögren's syndrome	Cytomegalovirus
Irradiation	Toxicity	HIV
Diabetes mellitus	Burns	Sarcoidosis
Trauma	Drugs	Amyloidosis
Sjögren's syndrome	Neurologic conditions	Sjögren's syndrome
	Impaired lacrimal gland function	Metabolic
	Impaired eyelid function	Diabetes mellitus
	Miscellaneous	Hyperlipoproteinemias
	Trauma	Chronic pancreatitis
	Hypovitaminosis A	Hepatic cirrhosis
	Blink abnormality	Endocrine
	Anesthetic cornea	Acromegaly
	Lid scarring	Gonadal hypofunction
	Epithelial irregularity	

DIAGNOSIS AND DIFFERENTIAL DIAGNOSIS

The diagnosis of primary Sjögren's syndrome is obtained if the patient presents with eye and/or mouth dryness, the eye tests disclose keratoconjunctivitis sicca, the mouth evaluation reveals the classic manifestations of the syndrome, and the patient's serum reacts with Ro/SS-A and/or La/SS-B autoantigens. Labial biopsy is needed when the diagnosis is uncertain or to rule out other conditions that may cause dry mouth or eyes or parotid gland enlargement (Tables 324-3, 324-4). Validated diagnostic criteria have been established by a European study and have now been further improved by a European-American study group (Table 324-5). Hepatitis C virus infection should be ruled out since, apart from serologic tests, the remainder of the clinicopathologic picture is almost identical to that of Sjögren's syndrome.

TREATMENT Sjögren's Syndrome

Treatment of Sjögren's syndrome is aimed at symptomatic relief and limiting the damaging local effects of chronic xerostomia and keratoconjunctivitis sicca by substituting or simulating the missing secretions (Fig. 324-1).

To replace deficient tears, there are several readily available ophthalmic preparations (Tearisol; Liquifilm; 0.5% methylcellulose; Hypo Tears). If corneal ulcerations are present, eye patching and boric acid ointments are recommended. Certain drugs that may decrease lacrimal and salivary secretion such as diuretics, antihypertensive drugs, anticholinergics, and antidepressants should be avoided.

TABLE 324-4 Differential Diagnosis of Sjögren's Syndrome

HIV Infection and Sicca Syndrome	Sjögren's Syndrome	Sarcoidosis
Predominant in young males	Predominant in middle-aged women	Invariable
Lack of autoantibodies to Ro/SS-A and/or La/SS-B	Presence of autoantibodies	Lack of autoantibodies to Ro/SS-A and/or La/SS-B
Lymphoid infiltrates of salivary glands by CD8+ lymphocytes	Lymphoid infiltrates of salivary glands by CD4+ lymphocytes	Granulomas in salivary glands
Association with HLA-DR5	Association with HLA-DR3 and -DRw52	Unknown
Positive serologic tests for HIV	Negative serologic tests for HIV	Negative serologic tests for HIV

TABLE 324-5 Revised International Classification Criteria for Sjögren's Syndrome[a,b,c]

I. Ocular symptoms: a positive response to at least one of three validated questions.
   1. Have you had daily, persistent, troublesome dry eyes for more than 3 months?
   2. Do you have a recurrent sensation of sand or gravel in the eyes?
   3. Do you use tear substitutes more than three times a day?

II. Oral symptoms: a positive response to at least one of three validated questions.
   1. Have you had a daily feeling of dry mouth for more than 3 months?
   2. Have you had recurrent or persistently swollen salivary glands as an adult?
   3. Do you frequently drink liquids to aid in swallowing dry foods?

III. Ocular signs: objective evidence of ocular involvement defined as a positive result to at least one of the following two tests:
   1. Shirmer's I test, performed without anesthesia (≤5 mm in 5 min)
   2. Rose Bengal score or other ocular dye score (≥4 according to van Bijsterveld's scoring system)

IV. Histopathology: In minor salivary glands focal lymphocytic sialoadenitis, with a focus score ≥1.

V. Salivary gland involvement: objective evidence of salivary gland involvement defined by a positive result to at least one of the following diagnostic tests:
   1. Unstimulated whole salivary flow (≤1.5 mL in 15 min)
   2. Parotid sialography
   3. Salivary scintigraphy

VI. Antibodies in the serum to Ro/SS-A or La/SS-B antigens, or both.

[a]Exclusion criteria: Past head and neck radiation treatment, hepatitis C infection, AIDS, preexisting lymphoma, sarcoidosis, graft-versus-host disease, use of anticholinergic drugs.

[b]Primary Sjögren's syndrome: any four of the six items, as long as item IV (histopathology) or VI (serology) is positive, or any three of the four objective criteria items (items III, IV, V, VI).

[c]In patients with a potentially associated disease (e.g., another well-defined connective tissue disease), the presence of item I or item II plus any two from among items III, IV, and V may be considered as indicative of secondary Sjögren's syndrome.

Source: From C Vitali et al: Ann Rheum Dis 61: 554, 2002. Copyright 2002 with permission from BMJ Publishing Group Ltd.

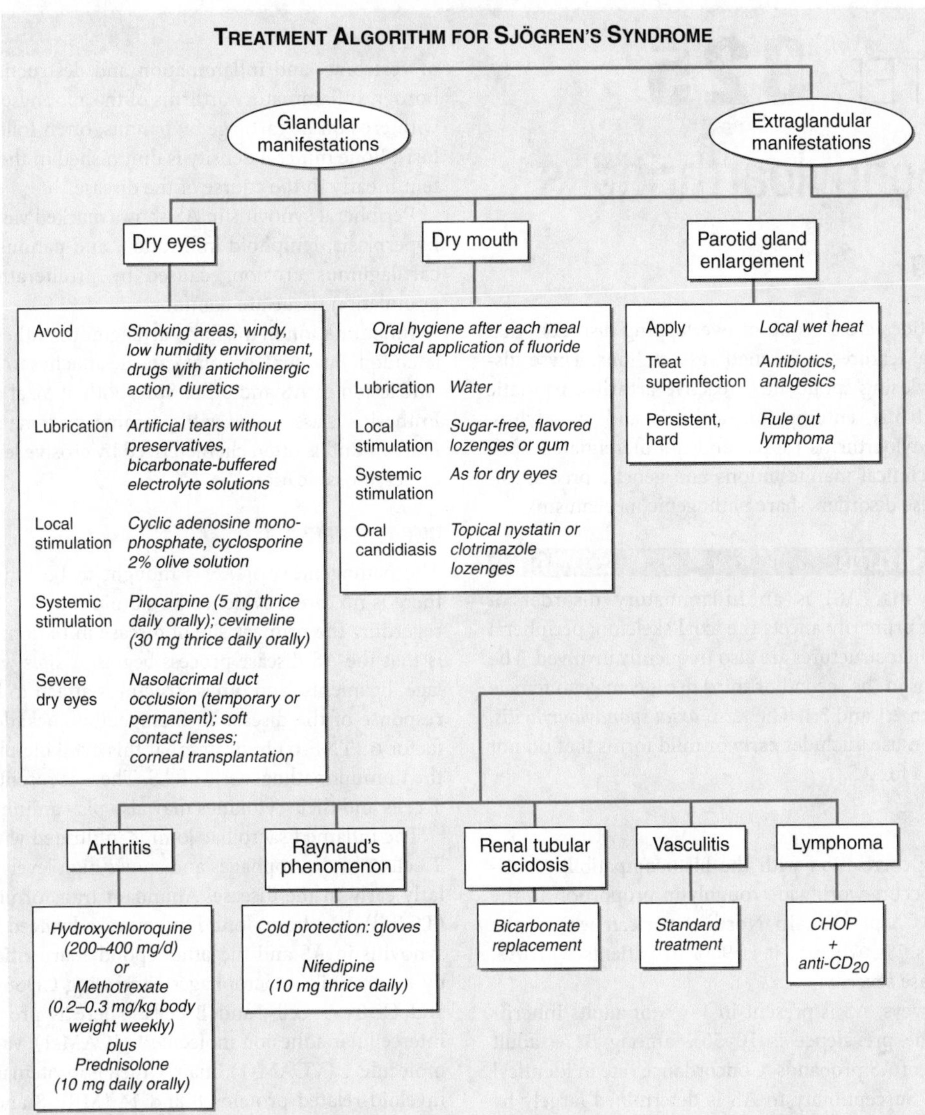

Figure 324-1 **Treatment algorithm** for Sjögren's syndrome.

For xerostomia the best replacement is water. Propionic acid gels may be used to treat vaginal dryness. To stimulate secretions, pilocarpine (5 mg thrice daily) or cevimeline (30 mg thrice daily) administered orally appears to improve sicca manifestations, and both are well tolerated. Hydroxychloroquine (200 mg) is helpful for arthralgias.

Patients with renal tubular acidosis should receive sodium bicarbonate orally (0.5–2 mmol/kg in four divided doses). Glucocorticoids (1 mg/kg per day) and/or immunosuppressive agents (e.g., cyclophosphamide) are indicated only for the treatment of systemic vasculitis. Anti–tumor necrosis factor agents are ineffective. Anti-CD20 monoclonal antibody therapy appears to be effective in patients with systemic disease and particularly with vasculitis, arthritis and fatigability. Combination of anti CD-20 with a classic CHOP regimen leads to increased survival in patients with high-grade lymphomas.

FURTHER READINGS

Christodoulou MI et al: Foxp3 T-regulatory cells in Sjögren's syndrome: Correlation with the grade of the autoimmune lesion and certain adverse prognostic factors. Am J Pathol 173:1389, 2008

Kassan S, Moutsopoulos HM: Clinical manifestations and early diagnosis of Sjögren syndrome. Arch Intern Med 164:1275, 2004

Manoussakis MN et al: Rates of infiltration by macrophages and dendritic cells and expression of interleukin-18 and interleukin-12 in the chronic inflammatory lesions of Sjögren's syndrome: Correlation with certain features of immune hyperactivity and factors associated with high risk of lymphoma development. Arthritis Rheum 56:3977, 2007

Mavragani CP et al: The management of Sjögren's syndrome. Nat Clin Pract Rheum 2:252, 2006

Ramos-casals M, et al: Treatment of primary Sjögren syndrome: a systematic review. Jama 304:452, 2010

Voulgarelis M, Tzioufas AG: Pathogenetic mechanisms in the initiation and perpetuation of Sjögren's syndrome. Nat Rev Rheumatol 6:529, 2010

CHAPTER 325

The Spondyloarthritides

Joel D. Taurog

The spondyloarthritides are a group of overlapping disorders that share certain clinical features and genetic associations. These disorders include ankylosing spondylitis, reactive arthritis, psoriatic arthritis and spondylitis, enteropathic arthritis and spondylitis, juvenile-onset spondyloarthritis (SpA), and undifferentiated SpA. The similarities in clinical manifestations and genetic predisposition suggest that these disorders share pathogenic mechanisms.

ANKYLOSING SPONDYLITIS

Ankylosing spondylitis (AS) is an inflammatory disorder of unknown cause that primarily affects the axial skeleton; peripheral joints and extraarticular structures are also frequently involved. The disease usually begins in the second or third decade; male to female prevalence is between 2:1 and 3:1. The term *axial spondyloarthritis*, coming into common use, includes early or mild forms that do not meet classical criteria for AS.

EPIDEMIOLOGY

AS shows a striking correlation with the histocompatibility antigen HLA-B27 and occurs worldwide roughly in proportion to the prevalence of B27 (Chap. 315). In North American whites, the prevalence of B27 is 7%, whereas it is 90% in patients with AS, independent of disease severity.

In population surveys, AS is present in 1–6% of adults inheriting B27, whereas the prevalence is 10–30% among B27+ adult first-degree relatives of AS probands. Concordance rate in identical twins is about 65%. Susceptibility to AS is determined largely by genetic factors, with B27 comprising up to one-half of the genetic component. Other HLA-linked genes may also contribute to susceptibility to AS. Genome-wide single-nucleotide polymorphism (SNP) analysis has identified additional susceptibility alleles in the genes encoding ERAP1 (chromosome 5q15) and IL-23R (chromosome 1p31.3). The genes encoding TNFSF15, TNFSF1A, STAT3, ANTXR2, and IL1R2, and at least six other chromosomal regions have also been implicated.

PATHOLOGY

The sites of axial inflammation in AS are inaccessible to routine biopsy and are rarely approached surgically. Knowledge of the axial histopathology is therefore based mostly on advanced cases. Sacroiliitis is often the earliest manifestations of AS. Synovitis, pannus, myxoid marrow, subchondral granulation tissue and marrow edema, enthesitis, and chondroid differentiation are found. Macrophages, T cells, and osteoclasts are prevalent. Eventually the eroded joint margins are gradually replaced by fibrocartilage regeneration and then by ossification. The joint may become totally obliterated.

In the spine, there is inflammatory granulation tissue at the junction of annulus fibrosis and vertebral bone. The outer annular fibers are eroded and eventually replaced by bone, forming the beginning of a syndesmophyte, which then grows by continued endochondral ossification, ultimately bridging the adjacent vertebral bodies. Ascending progression of this process leads to the "bamboo spine." Other lesions in the spine include diffuse osteoporosis, erosion of vertebral bodies at the disk margin, "squaring" or "barreling" of vertebrae, and inflammation and destruction of the disk-bone border. Inflammatory arthritis of the apophyseal joints is common, with erosion of cartilage by pannus, often followed by bony ankylosis. Bone mineral density is diminished in the spine and proximal femur early in the course of the disease.

Peripheral synovitis in AS shows marked vascularity, lining layer hyperplasia, lymphoid infiltration, and pannus formation. Central cartilaginous erosions caused by proliferation of subchondral granulation tissue are common.

Inflammation in the fibrocartilaginous enthesis, the region where a tendon, ligament, or joint capsule attaches to bone, is a characteristic lesion in AS and other SpA, both at axial and peripheral sites. Enthesitis is associated with prominent edema of the adjacent bone marrow and is often characterized by erosive lesions that eventually undergo ossification.

PATHOGENESIS

The pathogenesis of AS is thought to be immune-mediated, but there is no direct evidence for autoimmunity. There is uncertainty regarding the primary site of disease initiation. A unifying concept is that the AS disease process begins at sites where articular cartilage, ligaments, and other structures attach to bone. The dramatic response of the disease to therapeutic blockade of tumor necrosis factor α (TNF-α) indicates that this cytokine plays a central role in the immunopathogenesis of AS. There is recent evidence that T_H17 T cells and their cytokines may also play an important role.

The inflamed sacroiliac joint is infiltrated with CD4+ and CD8+ T cells and macrophages and shows high levels of TNF-α, particularly early in the disease. Abundant transforming growth factor β (TGF-β) has been found in more advanced lesions. Peripheral synovitis in AS and the other spondyloarthritides is characterized by neutrophils, macrophages expressing CD68 and CD163, CD4+ and CD8+ T cells, and B cells. There is prominent staining for intercellular adhesion molecule 1 (ICAM-1), vascular cell adhesion molecule 1 (VCAM-1), matrix metalloproteinase 3 (MMP-3), and myeloid-related proteins 8 and 14 (MRP-8 and MRP-14). Unlike rheumatoid arthritis (RA) synovium, citrullinated proteins and cartilage gp39 peptide–major histocompatibility complexes (MHCs) are absent. No specific event or exogenous agent that triggers the onset of disease has been identified, although overlapping features with reactive arthritis and inflammatory bowel disease (IBD) suggest that enteric bacteria may play a role. Triggering of innate immunity by microdamage at entheseal sites has recently been emphasized. Strong evidence that B27 plays a direct role is provided by genetic epidemiology studies and by the finding that rats transgenic for B27 spontaneously develop dramatic arthritis and spondylitis. However, the role of B27 remains unresolved. Since B27 rats lacking CD8+ T cells still develop arthritis and spondylitis, classical peptide antigen presentation to CD8+ T cells is probably not the primary disease mechanism. However, the association of AS with ERAP1, which strongly influences the MHC class I peptide repertoire, is only found in B27+ patients and suggests that peptide binding to B27 is nonetheless important. The B27 heavy chain has an unusual tendency to misfold, a process that may be proinflammatory. Genetic and functional studies in humans have suggested a role for natural killer (NK) cells in AS, possibly through interaction with B27. Defective dendritic cell function is a consistent feature of SpA-prone B27 rats not yet well investigated in patients.

CLINICAL MANIFESTATIONS

The symptoms of the disease are usually first noticed in late adolescence or early adulthood; the median age in Western countries is 23. In 5% of patients, symptoms begin after age 40. The initial symptom is usually dull pain, insidious in onset, felt deep in the lower lumbar or gluteal region, accompanied by low-back morning stiffness of up to a few hours' duration that improves with activity and returns following inactivity. Within a few months, the pain has usually become persistent and bilateral. Nocturnal exacerbation of pain often forces the patient to rise and move around.

In some patients, bony tenderness (presumably reflecting enthesitis or osteitis) may accompany back pain or stiffness, while in others it may be the predominant complaint. Common sites include the costosternal junctions, spinous processes, iliac crests, greater trochanters, ischial tuberosities, tibial tubercles, and heels. Arthritis in the hips and shoulders ("root" joints) occurs in 25–35% of patients. Severe isolated hip arthritis or bony chest pain may be the presenting complaint. Arthritis of peripheral joints other than the hips and shoulders, usually asymmetric, occurs in up to 30% of patients. Neck pain and stiffness from involvement of the cervical spine are usually relatively late manifestations but are occasionally dominant symptoms. Rare patients, particularly in the older age group, present with predominantly constitutional symptoms.

AS often has a juvenile onset in developing countries. Peripheral arthritis and enthesitis usually predominate, with axial symptoms supervening in late adolescence.

Initially, physical findings mirror the inflammatory process. The most specific findings involve loss of spinal mobility, with limitation of anterior and lateral flexion and extension of the lumbar spine and of chest expansion. Limitation of motion is usually out of proportion to the degree of bony ankylosis, reflecting muscle spasm secondary to pain and inflammation. Pain in the sacroiliac joints may be elicited either with direct pressure or with stress on the joints. In addition, there is commonly tenderness upon palpation at the sites of symptomatic bony tenderness and paraspinous muscle spasm.

The modified Schober test is a useful measure of lumbar spine flexion. The patient stands erect, with heels together, and marks are made on the spine at the lumbosacral junction (identified by a horizontal line between the posterosuperior iliac spines) and 10 cm above. The patient then bends forward maximally with knees fully extended, and the distance between the two marks is measured. This distance increases by ≥5 cm in the case of normal mobility and by <4 cm in the case of decreased mobility. Chest expansion is measured as the difference between maximal inspiration and maximal forced expiration in the fourth intercostal space in males or just below the breasts in females, with the patient's hands resting on or just behind the head. Normal chest expansion is ≥5 cm.

Limitation or pain with motion of the hips or shoulders is usually present if these joints are involved. It should be emphasized that early in the course of mild cases, symptoms may be subtle and nonspecific, and the physical examination may be completely normal.

The course of the disease is extremely variable, ranging from the individual with mild stiffness and normal radiographs to the patient with a totally fused spine and severe bilateral hip arthritis, accompanied by severe peripheral arthritis and extraarticular manifestations. Pain tends to be persistent early in the disease and then becomes intermittent, with alternating exacerbations and quiescent periods. In a typical severe untreated case with progression of the spondylitis to syndesmophyte formation, the patient's posture undergoes characteristic changes, with obliterated lumbar lordosis, buttock atrophy, and accentuated thoracic kyphosis. There may be a forward stoop of the neck or flexion contractures at the hips, compensated by flexion at the knees. Disease progression can be estimated clinically from loss of height, limitation of chest expansion and spinal flexion, and occiput-to-wall distance. Occasional individuals are encountered with advanced deformities who report having never had significant symptoms.

There is little consensus regarding the factors that predict disease progression and functional outcome. In some but not all studies, onset of AS in adolescence and early hip involvement correlate with a worse prognosis. AS in women tends to progress less frequently to total spinal ankylosis, although there is some evidence for an increased prevalence of isolated cervical ankylosis and peripheral arthritis in women. In industrialized countries, peripheral arthritis (distal to hips and shoulders) occurs in less than one-half of patients with AS, usually as a late manifestation, whereas in developing countries, the prevalence is much higher, with onset typically early in the disease course. Pregnancy has no consistent effect on AS, with symptoms improving, remaining the same, or deteriorating in about one-third of pregnant patients, respectively. Smoking correlates with adverse outcome.

The most serious complication of the spinal disease is spinal fracture, which can occur with even minor trauma to the rigid, osteoporotic spine. The lower cervical spine is most commonly involved. These fractures are often displaced and cause spinal cord injury. A recent survey suggested a >10% lifetime risk of fracture. Occasionally, fracture through a diskovertebral junction and adjacent neural arch, termed *pseudoarthrosis*, most common in the thoracolumbar spine, can be an unrecognized source of persistent localized pain and/or neurologic dysfunction. Wedging of thoracic vertebrae is common and correlates with accentuated kyphosis.

The most common extraarticular manifestation is acute anterior uveitis, which occurs in 40% of patients and can antedate the spondylitis. Attacks are typically unilateral, causing pain, photophobia, and increased lacrimation. These tend to recur, often in the opposite eye. Cataracts and secondary glaucoma are not uncommon sequelae. Up to 60% of patients have inflammation in the colon or ileum. This is usually asymptomatic, but frank IBD occurs in 5–10% of patients with AS (see "Enteropathic Arthritis," below). About 10% of patients meeting criteria for AS have psoriasis (see "Psoriatic Arthritis," below). Aortic insufficiency, sometimes leading to congestive heart failure, occurs in a few percent of patients, occasionally early in the course of the spinal disease but usually after prolonged disease. Third-degree heart block may occur alone or together with aortic insufficiency. Subclinical pulmonary lesions and cardiac dysfunction may be relatively common. Cauda equina syndrome and upper pulmonary lobe fibrosis are rare late complications. Retroperitoneal fibrosis is a rare associated condition. Prostatitis has been reported to have an increased prevalence. Amyloidosis is rare (Chap. 112).

Several validated measures of disease activity and functional outcome are in widespread use in the study and management of AS, particularly the Bath Ankylosing Spondylitis Disease Activity Index (BASDAI), a measure of disease activity; the Bath Ankylosing Spondylitis Functional Index (BASFI), a measure of limitation in activities of daily living; and several measures of radiographic changes. Despite persistence of the disease, most patients remain gainfully employed. Some but not all studies of survival in AS have suggested that AS shortens life span, compared with the general population. Mortality attributable to AS is largely the result of spinal trauma, aortic insufficiency, respiratory failure, amyloid nephropathy, or complications of therapy such as upper gastrointestinal hemorrhage. The impact of anti-TNF therapy on outcome and mortality is not yet known, but there is evidence for significantly improved work productivity.

■ LABORATORY FINDINGS

No laboratory test is diagnostic of AS. In most ethnic groups, HLA-B27 is present in 80–90% of patients. Erythrocyte sedimentation rate (ESR) and C-reactive protein (CRP) are often, but not always, elevated. Mild anemia may be present. Patients with severe disease may show an elevated alkaline phosphatase level. Elevated serum IgA levels are common. Rheumatoid factor, anti-cyclic citrullinated peptide (CCP), and antinuclear antibodies (ANAs) are largely absent unless caused by a coexistent disease, although ANAs may appear with anti-TNF therapy. Synovial fluid from peripheral joints in AS is nonspecifically inflammatory. In cases with restriction of chest wall motion, decreased vital capacity and increased functional residual capacity are common, but airflow is normal and ventilatory function is usually well maintained.

RADIOGRAPHIC FINDINGS

Radiographically demonstrable sacroiliitis is eventually present in AS. The earliest changes by standard radiography are blurring of the cortical margins of the subchondral bone, followed by erosions and sclerosis. Progression of the erosions leads to "pseudowidening" of the joint space; as fibrous and then bony ankylosis supervene, the joints may become obliterated. The changes and progression of the lesions are usually symmetric.

In the lumbar spine, progression of the disease leads to straightening, caused by loss of lordosis, and reactive sclerosis, caused by osteitis of the anterior corners of the vertebral bodies with subsequent erosion, leading to "squaring" or even "barreling" of one or more vertebral bodies. Progressive ossification leads to eventual formation of marginal syndesmophytes, visible on plain films as bony bridges connecting successive vertebral bodies anteriorly and laterally.

In many cases, years may elapse before unequivocal sacroiliac abnormalities are evident on plain radiographs, and consequently magnetic resonance imaging (MRI) is being increasingly used in diagnosing AS. Active sacroiliitis is best visualized by dynamic MRI with fat saturation, either T2-weighed turbo spin-echo sequence or short tau inversion recovery (STIR) with high resolution, or T1-weighted images with contrast enhancement. These techniques are much more sensitive than conventional radiography for identifying early intraarticular inflammation, cartilage changes, and underlying bone marrow edema in sacroiliitis (Fig. 325-1). They are also highly sensitive for evaluation of acute and chronic spinal changes (Fig. 325-2).

Reduced bone mineral density can be detected by dual-energy x-ray absorptiometry of the femoral neck and the lumbar spine. By using a lateral projection of the L3 vertebral body, falsely elevated readings related to spinal ossification can be avoided.

DIAGNOSIS

It is important to establish the diagnosis of early AS before the development of irreversible deformity. This goal presents a challenge for several reasons: (1) Back pain is very common, but AS is much less common; (2) an early presumptive diagnosis often relies on clinical grounds requiring considerable expertise; and (3) young individuals with early AS are often reluctant to seek medical care. The widely used modified New York criteria (1984) are based on the presence of definite radiographic sacroiliitis and are too insensitive in early or mild cases. In 2009, new criteria for axial SpA were proposed by the Assessment of Spondyloarthritis International Society (ASAS) (Table 325-1). They are applicable to individuals with ≥3 months of back pain with age of onset <45 years old. Active inflammation of the sacroiliac (SI) joints as determined by dynamic MRI is considered equivalent to the older criterion of definite radiographic sacroiliitis (see below).

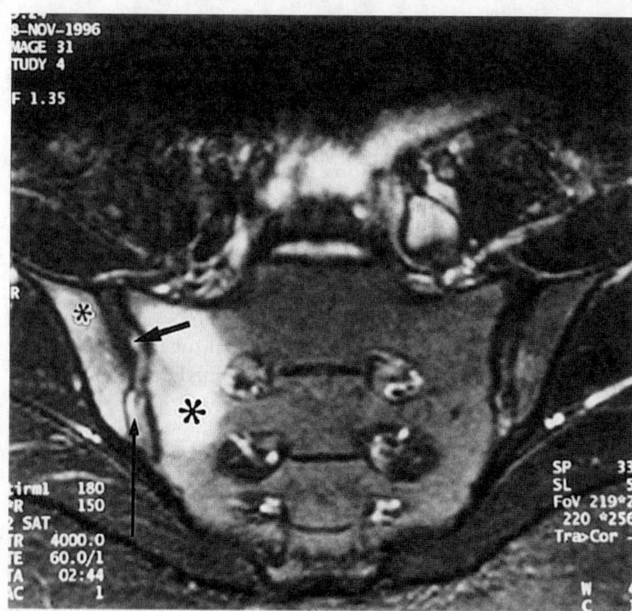

Figure 325-1 Early sacroiliitis in a patient with AS, indicated by prominent edema in the juxtaarticular bone marrow (asterisks), synovium and joint capsule (thin arrow), and interosseous ligaments (thick arrow) on a STIR (short tau inversion recovery) magnetic resonance image. *(From M. Bollow et al. Zeitschrift für Rheumatologie 58:61, 1999. Reproduced with permission.)*

AS must be differentiated from numerous other causes of low-back pain, some far more common than AS. To qualify as the criterion for inflammatory back pain of axial SpA (Table 325-1), the chronic (≥3 months) back pain should have four or more of these characteristic features: (1) age of onset below 40 years old, (2) insidious onset, (3) improvement with exercise and (4) no improvement with rest, and (5) pain at night with improvement upon getting up. Other common features of inflammatory back pain include morning stiffness >30 min, awakening from back pain during

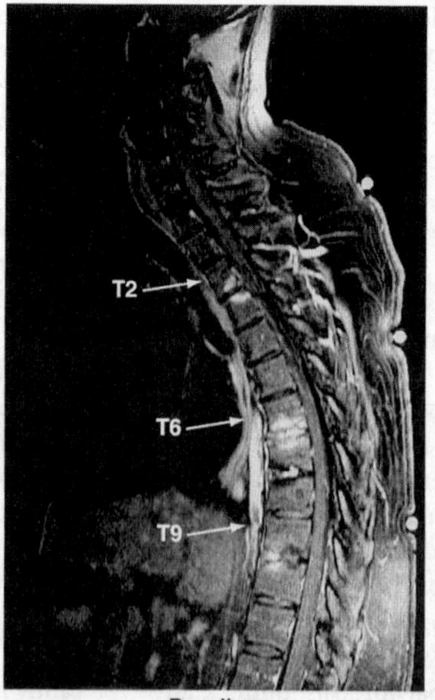

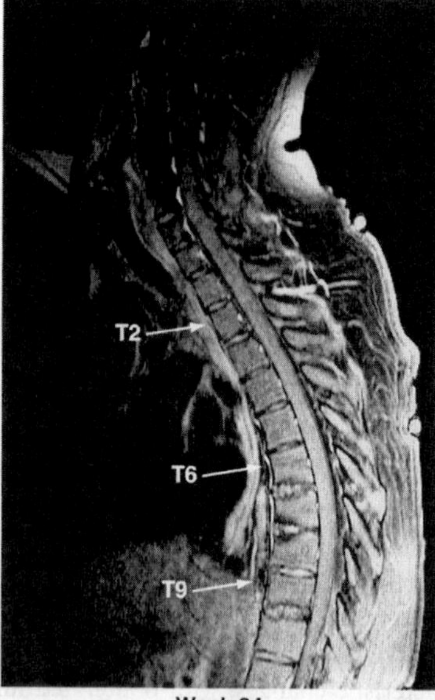

Figure 325-2 Spinal inflammation (spondylodiskitis) in a patient with AS and its dramatic response to treatment with infliximab. Gadolinium-enhanced T1-weighted magnetic resonance images, with fat saturation, at baseline and after 24 weeks of infliximab therapy. *(From J Braun et al.)*

TABLE 325-1 ASAS Criteria for Classification of Axial Spondyloarthritis (To Be Applied for Patients With Back Pain ≥3 Months and Age of Onset <45 years)[a]

Sacroiliitis on imaging plus ≥1 SpA feature	or	HLA-B27 plus ≥2 other SpA features
Sacroiliitis on imaging		**SpA features**
• Active (acute) inflammation on MRI highly suggestive of SpA-associated sacroiliitis[b] and/or • Definite radiographic sacroiliitis according to modified New York criteria[c]		• Inflammatory back pain[d] • Arthritis[e] • Enthesitis (heel)[f] • Anterior uveitis[g] • Dactylitis[e] • Psoriasis[e] • Crohn's disease or ulcerative colitis[e] • Good response to NSAIDs[h] • Family history of SpA[i] • HLA-B27 • Elevated CRP[j]

[a]Sensitivity 83%, specificity 84%. The imaging arm (sacroiliitis) alone has a sensitivity of 66% and a specificity of 97%.
[b]Bone marrow edema and/or osteitis on short tau inversion recovery (STIR) or gadolinium-enhanced T1 image.
[c]Bilateral grade ≥2 or unilateral grade 3 or 4.
[d]See text for criteria.
[e]Past or present, diagnosed by a physician.
[f]Past or present pain or tenderness on examination at calcaneus insertion of Achilles tendon or plantar fascia.
[g]Past or present, confirmed by an ophthalmologist.
[h]Substantial relief of back pain at 24–48 h after a full dose of NSAID.
[i]First- or second-degree relatives with ankylosing spondylitis (AS), psoriasis, uveitis, reactive arthritis (ReA), or inflammatory bowel disease (IBD).
[j]After exclusion of other causes of elevated CRP.
Abbreviations: ASAS, Assessment of Spondyloarthritis International Society; CRP, C-reactive protein; NSAIDs, nonsteroidal anti-inflammatory drugs; SpA, spondyloarthritis.
Source: From M Rudwaleit et al: Ann Rheum Dis 68:777, 2009. Copyright 2009, with permission from BMJ Publishing Group Ltd.

only the second half of the night, and alternating buttock pain. In clinical decision-making, all of these features are additive. The most common causes of back pain other than AS are primarily mechanical or degenerative rather than primarily inflammatory and tend not to show clustering of these features.

Less-common metabolic, infectious, and malignant causes of back pain must also be differentiated from AS, including infectious spondylitis, spondylodiskitis, and sacroiliitis, and primary or metastatic tumor. Ochronosis can produce a phenotype that is clinically and radiographically similar to AS. Calcification and ossification of paraspinous ligaments occur in *diffuse idiopathic skeletal hyperostosis* (DISH), which occurs in the middle-aged and elderly and is usually not symptomatic. Ligamentous calcification gives the appearance of "flowing wax" on the anterior bodies of the vertebrae. Intervertebral disk spaces are preserved, and sacroiliac and apophyseal joints appear normal, helping to differentiate DISH from spondylosis and from AS, respectively.

TREATMENT Ankylosing Spondylitis

All management of AS should include an exercise program designed to maintain posture and range of motion. Nonsteroidal anti-inflammatory drugs (NSAIDs) are the first line of pharmacologic therapy for AS. These agents reduce pain and tenderness and increase mobility in many patients with AS. There is evidence that daily NSAID therapy slows radiographic progression. However, many patients with AS have continued symptoms and develop deformity despite NSAID therapy. Beginning in 2000, dramatic responses to anti-TNF-α therapy were reported in patients with AS and other spondyloarthritides. Patients with AS treated with either infliximab (chimeric human/mouse anti-TNF-α monoclonal antibody), etanercept (soluble p75 TNF-α receptor–IgG fusion protein), or adalimumab or golimumab (human anti-TNF-α monoclonal antibodies) have shown rapid, profound, and sustained reductions in all clinical and laboratory measures of disease activity. Patients with long-standing disease and even some with complete spinal ankylosis have shown significant improvement in both objective and subjective indicators of disease activity and function, including morning stiffness, pain, spinal mobility, peripheral joint swelling, CRP, and ESR. MRI studies indicate substantial resolution of bone marrow edema, enthesitis, and joint effusions in the sacroiliac joints, spine, and peripheral joints (Fig. 325-2). Similar results have been obtained in large randomized controlled trials of all four agents and many open-label studies. About one-half of the patients achieve a ≥50% reduction in the BASDAI. The response tends to be stable over time, and partial or full remissions are common. Increased bone mineral density is found as early as 24 weeks after onset of therapy. There is evidence that anti-TNF therapy does not prevent syndesmophyte formation, although the practical clinical significance of this is not yet clear. A mechanism for this has been proposed based on the observation that TNF-α inhibits new bone formation by upregulating DKK-1, a negative regulator of the wingless (Wnt) signaling pathway that promotes osteoblast activity. Serum DKK-1 levels are inappropriately low in AS patients and are also suppressed by anti-TNF therapy.

The dosages of anti-TNF agents used in AS patients have usually been similar to those in RA. Infliximab is given intravenously, 3–5 mg/kg body weight, and then repeated 2 weeks later, again 6 weeks later, and then at 8-week intervals. Etanercept is given by subcutaneous injection, 50 mg once weekly. Adalimumab is given by subcutaneous injection, 40 mg biweekly. Golimumab is given by subcutaneous injection, 50 or 100 mg every 4 weeks.

Although these potent immunosuppressive agents have so far been relatively safe, seven types of side effects are not rare: (1) serious infections, including disseminated tuberculosis; (2) hematologic disorders, such as pancytopenia; (3) demyelinating disorders; (4) exacerbation of congestive heart failure; (5) systemic lupus erythematosus–related autoantibodies and clinical features; (6) hypersensitivity infusion or injection site reactions; and (7) severe liver disease. No increased incidence of malignancy has been observed in AS patients treated for over 5 years.

Because of the expense, potentially serious side effects, and unknown long-term effects of these agents, their use should be restricted to patients with a definite diagnosis and active disease (BASDAI ≥4 out of 10 and expert opinion) that is inadequately responsive to therapy with at least two different NSAIDs. Before initiation of anti-TNF therapy, all patients should be tested for tuberculin (TB) reactivity, and reactors (≥5 mm) should be treated with anti-TB agents. Contraindications include active infection or high risk of infection; malignancy or premalignancy;

and history of systemic lupus erythematosus, multiple sclerosis, or related autoimmunity. Pregnancy and breast-feeding are relative contraindications. Continuation beyond 12 weeks of therapy requires either a 50% reduction in BASDAI or absolute reduction of ≥2 out of 10, and favorable expert opinion. Sulfasalazine, in doses of 2–3 g/d, has been shown to be of modest benefit, primarily for peripheral arthritis. A therapeutic trial of this agent should precede any use of anti-TNF agents in patients with predominantly peripheral arthritis. Methotrexate, although widely used, has not been shown to be of benefit in AS, nor has any therapeutic role for gold or oral glucocorticoids been documented. Potential benefit in AS has been reported for thalidomide, 200 mg/d, perhaps acting through inhibition of TNF-α.

The most common indication for surgery in patients with AS is severe hip joint arthritis, the pain and stiffness of which are usually dramatically relieved by total hip arthroplasty. Rare patients may benefit from surgical correction of extreme flexion deformities of the spine or of atlantoaxial subluxation.

Attacks of uveitis are usually managed effectively with local glucocorticoid administration in conjunction with mydriatic agents, although systemic glucocorticoids, immunosuppressive drugs, or anti-TNF therapy may be required. TNF inhibitors reduce the frequency of attacks of uveitis in patients with AS, although cases of new or recurrent uveitis after use of a TNF inhibitor have been observed, especially with etanercept.

Coexistent cardiac disease may require pacemaker implantation and/or aortic valve replacement. Management of axial osteoporosis is at present similar to that used for primary osteoporosis, since data specific for AS are not available.

REACTIVE ARTHRITIS

Reactive arthritis (ReA) refers to acute nonpurulent arthritis complicating an infection elsewhere in the body. In recent years, the term has been used primarily to refer to SpA following enteric or urogenital infections.

Other forms of reactive and infection-related arthritis not associated with B27 and showing a spectrum of clinical features different from SpA, such as Lyme disease and rheumatic fever, are discussed in Chaps. 173 and 322.

HISTORIC BACKGROUND

The association of acute arthritis with episodes of diarrhea or urethritis has been recognized for centuries. A large number of cases during World Wars I and II focused attention on the triad of arthritis, urethritis, and conjunctivitis, often with additional mucocutaneous lesions, which became widely known by eponyms that are now of historic interest only.

The identification of bacterial species capable of triggering the clinical syndrome and the finding that many patients possess the B27 antigen led to the unifying concept of ReA as a clinical syndrome triggered by specific etiologic agents in a genetically susceptible host. A similar spectrum of clinical manifestations can be triggered by enteric infection with any of several *Shigella*, *Salmonella*, *Yersinia*, and *Campylobacter* species; by genital infection with *Chlamydia trachomatis*; and by other agents as well. The triad of arthritis, urethritis, and conjunctivitis represents a small part of the spectrum of the clinical manifestations of ReA. For the purposes of this chapter, the use of the term *ReA* will be restricted to those cases of SpA in which there is at least presumptive evidence for a related antecedent infection. Patients with clinical features of ReA who lack evidence of an antecedent infection will be considered to have *undifferentiated spondyloarthritis*, discussed below.

EPIDEMIOLOGY

Following the first reports of association of ReA with HLA-B27, in most hospital-based series in which *Shigella*, *Yersinia*, or *Chlamydia* were the triggering infectious agents, 60–85% of patients were found to be B27-positive, with a lower prevalence in ReA triggered by *Salmonella* and *Campylobacter*. In more recent community-based or common-source epidemic studies, the prevalence of B27 in ReA has often been below 50%, and in some instances not elevated at all. The most common age range is 18–40 years, but ReA can occur in children over 5 years of age and in older adults.

The gender ratio in ReA following enteric infection is nearly 1:1, whereas venereally acquired ReA occurs mainly in men. The overall prevalence and incidence of ReA are difficult to assess because of the variable prevalence of triggering infections and genetic susceptibility factors in different populations. In Scandinavia, an annual incidence of 10–28:100,000 has been reported. The spondyloarthritides were formerly almost unknown in sub-Saharan Africa. However, ReA and other peripheral SpA have now become the most common rheumatic diseases in Africans in the wake of the AIDS epidemic, without association to B27, which is very rare in these populations. SpA in Africans with HIV infection usually occurs in individuals with stage I disease (as classified by the World Health Organization). It is often the first manifestation of infection and often remits with disease progression. In contrast, Western white patients with HIV and SpA are usually B27-positive, and the arthritis flares as AIDS advances.

PATHOLOGY

Synovial histology is similar to that of other SpA. Enthesitis shows increased vascularity and macrophage infiltration of fibrocartilage. Microscopic histopathologic evidence of inflammation has occasionally been noted in the colon and ileum of patients with postvenereal ReA, but much less commonly than in postenteric ReA. The skin lesions of keratoderma blenorrhagica, associated mainly with venereally acquired ReA, are histologically indistinguishable from psoriatic lesions.

ETIOLOGY AND PATHOGENESIS

Of the four *Shigella* species *S. sonnei*, *S. boydii*, *S. flexneri*, and *S. dysenteriae*, *S. flexneri* has most often been implicated in cases of ReA, both sporadic and epidemic. *S. sonnei* and *S. dysenteriae* trigger some cases of ReA.

Other bacteria identified definitively as triggers of ReA include several *Salmonella* spp., *Yersinia enterocolitica*, *Y. pseudotuberculosis*, *Campylobacter jejuni*, and *Chlamydia trachomatis*. There is also evidence implicating *Clostridium difficile*, *Campylobacter coli*, certain toxigenic *E. coli*, and possibly *Ureaplasma urealyticum* and *Mycoplasma genitalium*. Respiratory infection with *Chlamydia pneumoniae* has also been implicated. There are also numerous isolated reports of acute arthritis preceded by other bacterial, viral, or parasitic infections, and even following intravesicular bacillus Calmette-Guérin (BCG) treatment for bladder cancer.

It has not been determined whether ReA occurs by the same pathogenic mechanism following infection with each of these microorganisms, nor has the mechanism been elucidated in the case of any one of the known bacterial triggers. Most, if not all, of the organisms well established to be triggers produce lipopolysaccharide (LPS) and share a capacity to attack mucosal surfaces, to invade host cells, and to survive intracellularly. Antigens from *Chlamydia*, *Yersinia*, *Salmonella*, and *Shigella* have been shown to be present in the synovium and/or synovial fluid leukocytes of patients with ReA for long periods following the acute attack. In ReA triggered by *Y. enterocolitica*, bacterial LPS and heat-shock protein antigens have been found in peripheral blood cells years after the triggering infection. *Yersinia* DNA and *C. trachomatis* DNA and RNA have been detected in synovial tissue from ReA patients, suggesting the presence of viable organisms despite uniform failure to culture the organism from these specimens. The specificity of these findings is unclear, however, since chromosomal bacterial DNA has also been found in synovium in other rheumatic diseases, and 16S rRNA from a very wide variety of bacteria has been found in ReA synovium. In several older studies, synovial T cells that specifically responded to antigens of the inciting organism were reported and characterized as predominantly CD4+ with a T_H2 or T regulatory phenotype. More recent work has documented high levels of IL-17 in ReA synovial fluid, but the source has not been identified. HLA-B27 seems to be associated with more severe and chronic forms of ReA, but its pathogenic role remains to be determined. HLA-B27 significantly prolongs the intracellular survival of *Y. enterocolitica* and *S. enteritidis* in human and mouse cell lines. Prolonged intracellular bacterial survival, promoted by B27, other factors, or both, may permit trafficking of infected leukocytes from the site of primary infection to joints, where an innate and/or adaptive immune response to persistent bacterial antigens may then promote arthritis.

■ CLINICAL FEATURES

The clinical manifestations of ReA constitute a spectrum that ranges from an isolated, transient monarthritis or enthesitis to severe multisystem disease. A careful history will usually elicit evidence of an antecedent infection 1–4 weeks before onset of symptoms of the reactive disease. However, in a sizable minority, no clinical or laboratory evidence of an antecedent infection can be found. In cases of presumed venereally acquired reactive disease, there is often a history of a recent new sexual partner, even without laboratory evidence of infection.

Constitutional symptoms are common, including fatigue, malaise, fever, and weight loss. The musculoskeletal symptoms are usually acute in onset. Arthritis is usually asymmetric and additive, with involvement of new joints occurring over a few days to 1–2 weeks. The joints of the lower extremities, especially the knee, ankle, and subtalar, metatarsophalangeal, and toe interphalangeal joints, are most commonly involved, but the wrist and fingers can be involved as well. The arthritis is usually quite painful, and tense joint effusions are not uncommon, especially in the knee. Patients often cannot walk without support. Dactylitis, or "sausage digit," a diffuse swelling of a solitary finger or toe, is a distinctive feature of ReA and other peripheral spondyloarthritides but can be seen in polyarticular gout and sarcoidosis. Tendinitis and fasciitis are particularly characteristic lesions, producing pain at multiple insertion sites (entheses), especially the Achilles insertion, the plantar fascia, and sites along the axial skeleton. Spinal and low-back pain are quite common and may be caused by insertional inflammation, muscle spasm, acute sacroiliitis, or, presumably, arthritis in intervertebral joints.

Urogenital lesions may occur throughout the course of the disease. In males, urethritis may be marked or relatively asymptomatic and may be either an accompaniment of the triggering infection or a result of the reactive phase of the disease. Prostatitis is also common. Similarly, in females, cervicitis or salpingitis may be caused either by the infectious trigger or by the sterile reactive process.

Ocular disease is common, ranging from transient, asymptomatic conjunctivitis to an aggressive anterior uveitis that occasionally proves refractory to treatment and may result in blindness.

Mucocutaneous lesions are frequent. Oral ulcers tend to be superficial, transient, and often asymptomatic. The characteristic skin lesions, *keratoderma blenorrhagica*, consist of vesicles that become hyperkeratotic, ultimately forming a crust before disappearing. They are most common on the palms and soles but may occur elsewhere as well. In patients with HIV infection, these lesions are often extremely severe and extensive, sometimes dominating the clinical picture (Chap. 189). Lesions may occur on the glans penis, termed *circinate balanitis*; these consist of vesicles that quickly rupture to form painless superficial erosions, which in circumcised individuals can form crusts similar to those of keratoderma blenorrhagica. Nail changes are common and consist of onycholysis, distal yellowish discoloration, and/or heaped-up hyperkeratosis.

Less-frequent or rare manifestations of ReA include cardiac conduction defects, aortic insufficiency, central or peripheral nervous system lesions, and pleuropulmonary infiltrates.

Arthritis typically persists 3–5 months, but courses up to 1 year can occur. Chronic joint symptoms persist in about 15% of patients and in up to 60% in hospital-based series. Recurrences of the acute syndrome are also common. Work disability or forced change in occupation are common in those with persistent joint symptoms. Chronic heel pain is often particularly distressing. Low-back pain, sacroiliitis, and frank AS are also common sequelae. In most studies, HLA-B27–positive patients have shown a worse outcome than B27-negative patients. Patients with *Yersinia*- or *Salmonella*-induced arthritis have less chronic disease than those whose initial episode follows epidemic shigellosis.

■ LABORATORY AND RADIOGRAPHIC FINDINGS

The ESR and acute-phase reactants are usually elevated during the acute phase of the disease. Mild anemia may be present. Synovial fluid is nonspecifically inflammatory. In most ethnic groups, about one-half of the patients are B27-positive. The triggering infection usually does not persist at the site of primary mucosal infection through the time of onset of the reactive disease, but it may be possible to culture the organism, e.g., in the case of *Yersinia*- or *Chlamydia*-induced disease. Serologic evidence of a recent infection may be present, such as a marked elevation of antibodies to *Yersinia*, *Salmonella*, or *Chlamydia*. Polymerase chain reaction (PCR) for chlamydial DNA in first-voided urine specimens is said to have high sensitivity.

In early or mild disease, radiographic changes may be absent or confined to juxtaarticular osteoporosis. With long-standing persistent disease, marginal erosions and loss of joint space can be seen in affected joints. Periostitis with reactive new bone formation is characteristic, as in all the SpA. Spurs at the insertion of the plantar fascia are common.

Sacroiliitis and spondylitis may be seen as late sequelae. Sacroiliitis is more commonly asymmetric than in AS, and spondylitis, rather than ascending symmetrically, can begin anywhere along the lumbar spine. The syndesmophytes may be asymmetric, coarse and nonmarginal, arising from the middle of a vertebral body, a pattern less commonly seen in primary AS. Progression to spinal fusion is uncommon.

■ DIAGNOSIS

ReA is a clinical diagnosis with no definitively diagnostic laboratory test or radiographic finding. The diagnosis should be entertained in any patient with an acute inflammatory, asymmetric, additive arthritis or tendinitis. The evaluation should include questioning regarding possible triggering events such as an episode of diarrhea or dysuria. On physical examination, attention must be paid to the distribution of the joint and tendon involvement and to possible sites of extraarticular involvement, such as the eyes, mucous membranes, skin, nails, and genitalia. Synovial fluid analysis may be helpful in excluding septic or crystal-induced arthritis. Culture, serology, or molecular methods may help to identify a triggering infection.

Although typing for B27 has low negative predictive value in ReA, it may have prognostic significance in terms of severity, chronicity, and the propensity for spondylitis and uveitis. Furthermore, if positive, it can be helpful diagnostically in atypical cases. HIV testing is often indicated and may be necessary in order to select appropriate therapy.

It is important to differentiate ReA from disseminated gonococcal disease (Chap. 144), both of which can be venereally acquired and associated with urethritis. Unlike ReA, gonococcal arthritis and tenosynovitis tend to involve both upper and lower extremities equally, to lack back symptoms, and to be associated with characteristic vesicular skin lesions. A positive gonococcal culture from the urethra or cervix does not exclude a diagnosis of ReA; however, culturing gonococci from blood, skin lesion, or synovium establishes the diagnosis of disseminated gonococcal disease. PCR assay for *N. gonorrhoeae* and *C. trachomatis* may be helpful. Occasionally, only a therapeutic trial of antibiotics can distinguish the two.

ReA shares many features in common with psoriatic arthropathy. However, psoriatic arthritis is usually gradual in onset; the arthritis tends to affect primarily the upper extremities; there is less associated periarthritis; and there are usually no associated mouth ulcers, urethritis, or bowel symptoms.

TREATMENT Reactive Arthritis

Most patients with ReA benefit to some degree from high-dose NSAIDs, although acute symptoms are rarely completely ameliorated, and some patients fail to respond at all. Indomethacin, 75–150 mg/d in divided doses, is the initial treatment of choice, but other NSAIDs may be tried.

Prompt, appropriate antibiotic treatment of acute chlamydial urethritis or enteric infection may prevent the emergence of ReA. However, several controlled trials have failed to demonstrate any benefit for antibiotic therapy that is initiated after onset of arthritis. One long-term follow-up study suggested that although antibiotic therapy had no effect on the acute episode of ReA, it helped prevent subsequent chronic SpA. Another such study failed to demonstrate any long-term benefit. A promising recent double-blind placebo-controlled study showed that a majority of patients with chronic ReA due to *Chlamydia* benefited significantly from a 6-month course of rifampin 300 mg daily plus azithromycin 500 mg daily for 5 days then twice weekly, or 6 months of rifampin 300 mg daily plus doxycycline 100 mg twice daily.

Multicenter trials have suggested that sulfasalazine, up to 3 g/d in divided doses, may be beneficial to patients with persistent ReA.[1] Patients with persistent disease may respond to azathioprine, 1–2 mg/kg per day, or to methotrexate, up to 20 mg per week. Although no controlled trials of anti-TNF-α in ReA have been reported, anecdotal evidence supports the use of these agents in severe chronic cases, although lack of response has also been observed.[1]

Tendinitis and other enthesitic lesions may benefit from intralesional glucocorticoids. Uveitis may require aggressive treatment to prevent serious sequelae (see above). Skin lesions ordinarily require only symptomatic treatment. In patients with HIV infection and ReA, many of whom have severe skin lesions, the skin lesions in particular respond to antiretroviral therapy. Cardiac complications are managed conventionally; management of neurologic complications is symptomatic.

Comprehensive management includes counseling of patients in the avoidance of sexually transmitted disease and exposure to enteropathogens, as well as appropriate use of physical therapy, vocational counseling, and continued surveillance for long-term complications such as ankylosing spondylitis.

[1]Azathioprine, methotrexate, sulfasalazine, pamidronate, and thalido-mide have not been approved for this purpose by the U.S. Food and Drug Administration at the time of publication.

PSORIATIC ARTHRITIS

Psoriatic arthritis (PsA) refers to an inflammatory arthritis that characteristically occurs in individuals with psoriasis.

HISTORIC BACKGROUND

The association between arthritis and psoriasis was noted in the nineteenth century. In the 1960s, on the basis of epidemiologic and clinical studies, it became clear that unlike RA the arthritis associated with psoriasis was usually seronegative, often involved the distal interphalangeal (DIP) joints of the fingers and the spine and sacroiliac joints, had distinctive radiographic features, and showed considerable familial aggregation. In the 1970s, PsA was included in the broader category of the spondyloarthritides because of features similar to those of AS and ReA.

EPIDEMIOLOGY

Estimates of the prevalence of PsA among individuals with psoriasis range from 5 to 30%. In white populations, psoriasis is estimated to have a prevalence of 1–3%. Psoriasis and PsA are less common in other races in the absence of HIV infection, and the prevalence of PsA in individuals with psoriasis may be less common. First-degree relatives of PsA patients have an elevated risk for psoriasis, for PsA itself, and for other forms of SpA. Of patients with psoriasis, up to 30% have an affected first-degree relative. In monozygotic twins, the reported concordance for psoriasis varies from 35 to 72%, and for PsA from 10 to 30%. A variety of HLA associations have been found. The HLA-Cw6 gene is directly associated with psoriasis, particularly familial juvenile-onset (type I) psoriasis. HLA-B27 is associated with psoriatic spondylitis (see below). HLA-DR7, -DQ3, and -B57 are associated with PsA because of linkage disequilibrium with Cw6. Other associations with PsA include HLA-B13, -B37, -B38, -B39, and DR4. A recent genome-wide scan found association of both psoriasis and PsA with a polymorphism at the HCP5 locus closely linked to HLA-B, and also to IL-23R, IL-12B (chromosome 5q31), and several other chromosomal regions.

PATHOLOGY

The inflamed synovium in PsA resembles that of RA, although with somewhat less hyperplasia and cellularity than in RA, and somewhat greater vascularity. Some studies have indicated a higher tendency to synovial fibrosis in PsA. Unlike RA, PsA shows prominent enthesitis, with histology similar to that of the other spondyloarthritides.

PATHOGENESIS

PsA is almost certainly immune-mediated and probably shares pathogenic mechanisms with psoriasis. PsA synovium shows infiltration with T cells, B cells, macrophages, and NK receptor–expressing cells, with upregulation of leukocyte homing receptors. Clonally expanded CD8+ T cells are frequent in PsA. Plasmacytoid dendritic cells are thought to play a key role in psoriasis, and there is some evidence for their participation in psoriatic arthritis. There is abundant synovial overexpression of proinflammatory cytokines. Interleukin 2, interferon-γ, TNF-α, and IL-1β, -6, -8, -10, -12, -13, and -15 are found in PsA synovium or synovial fluid. T_H17 derived cytokines are likely to be important in PsA, given their prominence in psoriasis and in other spondyloarthritides, the genetic association with genes in the IL-12/IL-23 axis, and the therapeutic response to an antibody to the shared IL-12/23 p40 subunit (see below). Consistent with the extensive bone lesions in PsA, patients with PsA have been found to have a marked increase in osteoclastic precursors in peripheral blood and upregulation of receptor activator of nuclear factor κβ ligand (RANKL) in the synovial lining layer.

CLINICAL FEATURES

In 60–70% of cases, psoriasis precedes joint disease. In 15–20% of cases, the two manifestations appear within 1 year of each other. In about 15–20% of cases, the arthritis precedes the onset of psoriasis and can present a diagnostic challenge. The frequency in men and women is almost equal, although the frequency of disease patterns differs somewhat in the two sexes. The disease can begin in childhood or late in life but typically begins in the fourth or fifth decade, at an average age of 37 years.

The spectrum of arthropathy associated with psoriasis is quite broad. Many classification schemes have been proposed. In the original scheme of Wright and Moll, five patterns are described: (1) arthritis of the DIP joints; (2) asymmetric oligoarthritis; (3) symmetric polyarthritis similar to RA; (4) axial involvement (spine and sacroiliac joints); and (5) arthritis mutilans, a highly destructive form of disease. These patterns are not fixed, and the pattern that persists chronically often differs from that of the initial presentation. A simpler scheme in recent use contains three patterns: oligoarthritis, polyarthritis, and axial arthritis.

Nail changes in the fingers or toes occur in 90% of patients with PsA, compared with 40% of psoriatic patients without arthritis, and pustular psoriasis is said to be associated with more severe arthritis. Several articular features distinguish PsA from other joint disorders. Dactylitis occurs in >30%; enthesitis and tenosynovitis are also common and are probably present in most patients, although often not appreciated on physical examination. Shortening of digits because of underlying osteolysis is particularly characteristic of PsA (Fig. 325-3), and there is a much greater tendency than in RA for both fibrous and bony ankylosis of small joints. Rapid ankylosis of one or more proximal interphalangeal (PIP) joints early in the course of disease is not uncommon. Back and neck pain and stiffness are also common in PsA.

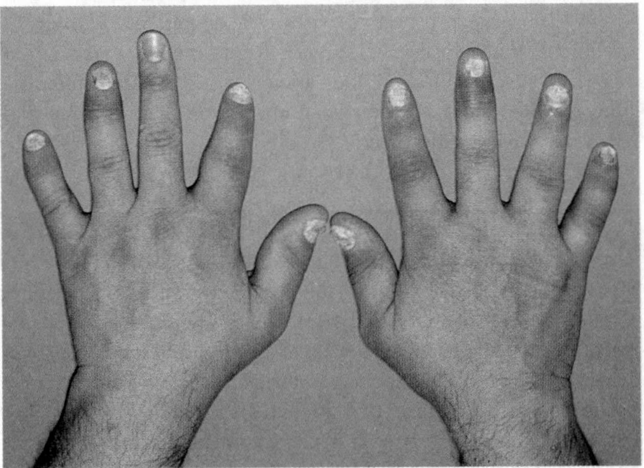

Figure 325-3 Characteristic lesions of psoriatic arthritis. Inflammation is prominent in the DIP joints (left 5th, 4th, 2nd; right 2nd, 3rd, and 5th) and PIP joints (left 2nd, right 2nd, 4th, and 5th). There is dactylitis in the left 2nd finger and thumb, with pronounced telescoping of the left 2nd finger. Nail dystrophy (hyperkeratosis and onycholysis) affects each of the fingers except the left 3rd finger, the only finger without arthritis. *(Courtesy of Donald Raddatz, MD; with permission.)*

Arthropathy confined to the DIP joints predominates in about 15% of cases. Accompanying nail changes in the affected digits are almost always present. These joints are also often affected in the other patterns of PsA. Approximately 30% of patients have asymmetric oligoarthritis. This pattern commonly involves a knee or another large joint with a few small joints in the fingers or toes, often with dactylitis. Symmetric polyarthritis occurs in about 40% of PsA patients at presentation. It may be indistinguishable from RA in terms of the joints involved, but other features characteristic of PsA are usually also present. In general, peripheral joints in PsA tend to be somewhat less tender than in RA, although signs of inflammation are usually present. Almost any peripheral joint can be involved. Axial arthropathy without peripheral involvement is found in about 5% of PsA patients. It may be indistinguishable from idiopathic AS, although more neck involvement and less thoracolumbar spinal involvement is characteristic, and nail changes are not found in idiopathic AS. A small percentage of PsA patients have arthritis mutilans, in which there can be widespread shortening of digits ("telescoping"), sometimes coexisting with ankylosis and contractures in other digits.

Six patterns of nail involvement are identified: pitting, horizontal ridging, onycholysis, yellowish discoloration of the nail margins, dystrophic hyperkeratosis, and combinations of these findings. Other extraarticular manifestations of the spondyloarthritides are common. Eye involvement, either conjunctivitis or uveitis, is reported in 7–33% of PsA patients. Unlike the uveitis associated with AS, the uveitis in PsA is more often bilateral, chronic, and/or posterior. Aortic valve insufficiency has been found in <4% of patients, usually after long-standing disease.

Widely varying estimates of clinical outcome have been reported in PsA. At its worst, severe PsA with arthritis mutilans is at least as crippling and ultimately fatal as severe RA. Unlike RA, however, many patients with PsA experience temporary remissions. Overall, erosive disease develops in the majority of patients, progressive disease with deformity and disability is common, and in some large published series, mortality was found to be significantly increased compared with the general population.

The psoriasis and associated arthropathy seen with HIV infection both tend to be severe and can occur in populations with very little psoriasis in noninfected individuals. Severe enthesopathy, dactylitis, and rapidly progressive joint destruction are seen, but axial involvement is very rare. This condition is prevented by or responds well to antiretroviral therapy.

LABORATORY AND RADIOGRAPHIC FINDINGS

There are no laboratory tests diagnostic of PsA. ESR and CRP are often elevated. A small percentage of patients may have low titers of rheumatoid factor or antinuclear antibodies. About 10% of patients have anti-CCP antibodies. Uric acid may be elevated in the presence of extensive psoriasis. HLA-B27 is found in 50–70% of patients with axial disease, but ≤20% in patients with only peripheral joint involvement.

The peripheral and axial arthropathies in PsA show a number of radiographic features that distinguish them from RA and AS, respectively. Characteristics of peripheral PsA include DIP involvement, including the classic "pencil-in-cup" deformity; marginal erosions with adjacent bony proliferation ("whiskering"); small-joint ankylosis; osteolysis of phalangeal and metacarpal bone, with telescoping of digits; and periostitis and proliferative new bone at sites of enthesitis. Characteristics of axial PsA include asymmetric sacroiliitis; compared with idiopathic AS, less zygapophyseal joint arthritis, fewer and less symmetric and delicate syndesmophytes;

fluffy hyperperiostosis on anterior vertebral bodies; severe cervical spine involvement, with a tendency to atlantoaxial subluxation but relative sparing of the thoracolumbar spine; and paravertebral ossification. Ultrasound and MRI both readily demonstrate enthesitis and tendon sheath effusions that can be difficult to assess on physical examination. A recent MRI study of 68 PsA patients found sacroiliitis in 35%, unrelated to B27 but correlated with restricted spinal movement.

DIAGNOSIS

Classification criteria for PsA were published in 2006 [Classification of Psoriatic Arthritis (CASPAR) criteria] that have been widely accepted (Table 325-2). The sensitivity and specificity of these criteria exceed 90%, and they are useful for early diagnosis. The criteria are based on the history, presence of psoriasis, characteristic peripheral or spinal joint symptoms, signs, and imaging. Diagnosis can be challenging when the arthritis precedes psoriasis, the psoriasis is undiagnosed or obscure, or the joint involvement closely resembles another form of arthritis. A high index of suspicion is needed in any patient with an undiagnosed inflammatory arthropathy. The history should include inquiry about psoriasis in the patient and family members. Patients should be asked to disrobe for the physical examination, and psoriasiform lesions should be sought in the scalp, ears, umbilicus, and gluteal folds in addition to more accessible sites; the finger and toe nails should also be carefully examined. Axial symptoms or signs, dactylitis, enthesitis, ankylosis, the pattern of joint involvement, and characteristic radiographic changes can be helpful clues. The differential diagnosis includes all other forms of arthritis, which can occur coincidentally in individuals with psoriasis. The differential diagnosis of isolated DIP involvement is short. Osteoarthritis (Heberden's nodes) is usually not inflammatory; gout involving more than one DIP joint often involves other sites and may be accompanied by tophi; the very rare entity multicentric reticulohistiocytosis involves other joints and has characteristic small pearly periungual skin nodules; and the uncommon entity inflammatory osteoarthritis, like the others, lacks the nail changes of PsA. Radiography can be helpful in all of these cases and in distinguishing between psoriatic spondylitis and idiopathic AS. A history of trauma to an affected joint preceding the onset of arthritis is said to occur more frequently in PsA than in other types of arthritis, perhaps reflecting the Koebner phenomenon in which psoriatic skin lesions can arise at sites of the skin trauma.

TABLE 325-2 The CASPAR (*Cl*assification Criteria for *P*soriatic *Ar*thritis) Criteria[a]

To meet the CASPAR criteria, a patient must have inflammatory articular disease (joint, spine, or entheseal) with ≥3 points from any of the following five categories:

1. Evidence of current psoriasis,[b, c] a personal history of psoriasis, or a family history of psoriasis[d]
2. Typical psoriatic nail dystrophy[e] observed on current physical examination
3. A negative test result for rheumatoid factor
4. Either current dactylitis[f] or a history of dactylitis recorded by a rheumatologist
5. Radiographic evidence of juxtaarticular new bone formation[g] in the hand or foot

[a]Specificity of 99% and sensitivity of 91%.
[b]Current psoriasis is assigned 2 points; all other features are assigned 1 point.
[c]Psoriatic skin or scalp disease present at the time of examination, as judged by a rheumatologist or dermatologist.
[d]History of psoriasis in a first- or second-degree relative.
[e]Onycholysis, pitting, or hyperkeratosis.
[f]Swelling of an entire digit.
[g]Ill-defined ossification near joint margins, excluding osteophyte formation.
Source: From W Taylor et al.

TREATMENT Psoriatic Arthritis

Ideally, coordinated therapy is directed at both the skin and joints in PsA. As described above for AS, use of the anti-TNF-α agents has revolutionized the treatment of PsA. Prompt and dramatic resolution of both arthritis and skin lesions has been observed in large, randomized controlled trials of etanercept, infliximab, adalimumab, and golimumab. Many of the responding patients had long-standing disease that was resistant to all previous therapy, as well as extensive skin disease. The clinical response is more dramatic than in RA, and delay of disease progression has been demonstrated radiographically. Paradoxically, rare cases have been reported of exacerbation or de novo appearance of psoriasis precipitated by anti-TNF therapy for a variety of conditions. In some cases, the therapy can nevertheless be continued.

The anti-T cell biologic agent alefacept, in combination with methotrexate, has shown benefit in both psoriatic arthritis and psoriasis. Ustekinumab, a monoclonal antibody to the shared IL-23/IL-12p40 subunit, has shown promise in treating both psoriasis and PsA in early clinical trials.

Other treatment for PsA has been based on drugs that have efficacy in RA and/or in psoriasis. Although methotrexate in doses of 15–25 mg/week and sulfasalazine (usually given in doses of 2–3 g/d) have each been found to have clinical efficacy in controlled trials, neither effectively halts progression of erosive joint disease. Other agents with efficacy in psoriasis reported to benefit PsA are cyclosporine, retinoic acid derivatives, and psoralens plus ultraviolet A light (PUVA). There is controversy regarding the efficacy in PsA of gold and antimalarials, which have been widely used in RA. The pyrimidine synthetase inhibitor leflunomide has been shown in a randomized controlled trial to be beneficial in both psoriasis and psoriatic arthritis.

All of these treatments require careful monitoring. Immunosuppressive therapy may be used cautiously in HIV-associated PsA if the HIV infection is well controlled.

In one large prospective series, 7% of patients with PsA required musculoskeletal surgery beginning at a mean of 13 years' disease duration. Indications for surgery are similar to those in RA, although there is an impression that outcomes in PsA may be less satisfactory.

UNDIFFERENTIATED AND JUVENILE-ONSET SPONDYLOARTHRITIS

Many patients, usually young adults, present with some features of one or more of the spondyloarthritides discussed above. Until recently, these patients were said to have undifferentiated spondyloarthritis, or simply spondyloarthritis, as defined by the 1991 European Spondyloarthropathy Study Group criteria (Table 325-3). For example, a patient may present with inflammatory synovitis of one knee, Achilles tendinitis, and dactylitis of one digit. Some of these patients may have ReA in which the triggering infection remains clinically silent. In some other cases, the patient subsequently develops IBD or psoriasis or the process eventually meets criteria for AS. This diagnosis of undifferentiated SpA was also commonly applied to patients with inflammatory back pain, who did meet modified New York criteria for AS. Most of these would now be classified under the new category of axial spondyloarthritis (Table 325-1).

TABLE 325-3 European Spondyloarthropathy Study Group (ESSG) Criteria for Spondyloarthritis[a]

Inflammatory Back Pain[b]	*or*	Synovitis • Asymmetric *or* • Predominantly in lower extremities
	and	

One or more of the following:

- Family history of SpA[b]
- Psoriasis[b]
- Crohn's disease or ulcerative colitis[c]
- Nongonococcal urethritis, cervicitis, or acute diarrhea within 1 month before arthritis
- Alternating buttock pain[d]
- Enthesitis[b]
- Radiographic sacroiliitis[b]

[a]Sensitivity >85%, specificity >85%.
[b]See definition in Table 325-1.
[c]Past or present, diagnosed by a physician and confirmed by endoscopy or radiography.
[d]Past or present pain alternating between the right and left gluteal regions.
SpA, spondyloarthritis.
Source: From M Dougados et al; J Sieper J et al. Copyright 2009, with permission from BMJ Publishing Group Ltd.

Approximately one-half of the patients with undifferentiated SpA are HLA-B27-positive, and thus the absence of B27 is not useful in establishing or excluding the diagnosis. In familial cases, which are much more frequently B27-positive, there is often eventual progression to classical AS.

In juvenile-onset SpA, which begins between ages 7 and 16, most commonly in boys (60–80%), an asymmetric, predominantly lower-extremity oligoarthritis and enthesitis without extraarticular features is the typical mode of presentation. The prevalence of B27 in this condition, which has been termed the *seronegative enthesopathy and arthropathy (SEA) syndrome*, is approximately 80%. Many, but not all, of these patients go on to develop AS in late adolescence or adulthood.

Management of undifferentiated SpA is similar to that of the other spondyloarthritides. Response to anti-TNF-α therapy has been documented, and this therapy is indicated in severe, persistent cases not responsive to other treatment. One 2004 publication reported significant benefit in patients with long-standing undifferentiated spondyloarthropathy treated for 9 months with doxycycline and rifampin. These data await confirmation.

Current pediatric textbooks and journals should be consulted for information on management of juvenile-onset SpA.

ENTEROPATHIC ARTHRITIS

HISTORIC BACKGROUND

A relationship between arthritis and IBD was observed in the 1930s. The relationship was further defined by the epidemiologic studies in the 1950s and 1960s and included in the concept of the spondyloarthritides in the 1970s.

EPIDEMIOLOGY

Both of the common forms of IBD, ulcerative colitis (UC) and Crohn's disease (CD) (Chap. 295), are associated with SpA. UC and CD both have an estimated prevalence of 0.05–0.1%, and the incidence of each is thought to have increased in recent decades. AS and peripheral arthritis are both associated with UC and with CD. Wide variations have been reported in the estimated frequencies of these associations. In recent series, AS was diagnosed in 1–10%, and peripheral arthritis in 10–50% of patients with IBD. Inflammatory back pain and enthesopathy are common, and many patients have sacroiliitis on imaging studies.

The prevalence of UC or CD in patients with AS is thought to be 5–10%. However, investigation of unselected SpA patients by ileocolonoscopy has revealed that from one-third to two-thirds of patients with AS have subclinical intestinal inflammation that is evident either macroscopically or histologically. These lesions have also been found in patients with undifferentiated SpA or ReA (both enterically and urogenitally acquired).

Both UC and CD have a tendency to familial aggregation, more so for CD. HLA associations have been weak and inconsistent. HLA-B27 is found in up to 70% of patients with IBD and AS, but in ≤15% of patients with IBD and peripheral arthritis or IBD alone. Three alleles of the *NOD2/CARD15* gene on chromosome 16 have been found in approximately one-half of patients with CD. These alleles are not associated with the spondyloarthritides per se. However, they are found significantly more often in (1) CD patients with sacroiliitis than in those without sacroiliitis, and (2) SpA patients with chronic inflammatory gut lesions than in those with normal gut histology. These associations are independent of HLA-B27.

Genome studies have shown that CD and UC have some susceptibility genes in common and some specific to each condition. Among these, IL-23R (highly associated with CD and to a lesser degree with UC) is shared with AS and psoriasis. TNFSF15, associated with CD, has also been found linked to SpA.

PATHOLOGY

Available data for IBD-associated peripheral arthritis suggest a synovial histology similar to other spondyloarthritides. Association with arthropathy does not affect the gut histology of UC or CD (Chap. 295). The subclinical inflammatory lesions in the colon and distal ileum associated with SpA have been classified as either acute or chronic. The former resemble acute bacterial enteritis, with largely intact architecture and neutrophilic infiltration in the lamina propria. The latter resemble the lesions of CD, with distortion of villi and crypts, aphthoid ulceration, and mononuclear cell infiltration in the lamina propria.

PATHOGENESIS

Both IBD and SpA are immune-mediated, but the specific pathogenic mechanisms are poorly understood, and the connection between the two is obscure. The shared genetics could reflect either shared pathogenetic mechanisms, close genetic linkage of separate susceptibility alleles, or both. IBD is a common phenotype in a number of rodent lines with transgenic overexpression or targeted deletion of genes involved in immune processes. Arthritis is an accompanying prominent feature in two of these IBD models, B27 transgenic rats and mice with constitutive overexpression of TNF-α, and immune dysregulation is prominent in both. Several lines of evidence indicate trafficking of leukocytes between the gut and the joint. Mucosal leukocytes from IBD patients have been shown to bind avidly to synovial vasculature through several different adhesion molecules. Macrophages expressing CD163 are prominent in the inflammatory lesions of both gut and synovium in the spondyloarthritides.

CLINICAL FEATURES

AS associated with IBD is clinically indistinguishable from idiopathic AS. It runs a course independent of the bowel disease, and in many patients it precedes the onset of IBD, sometimes by many years. Peripheral arthritis not infrequently begins before onset of overt bowel disease. The spectrum of peripheral arthritis includes acute self-limited attacks of oligoarthritis that often coincide with relapses of IBD, and more chronic and symmetric polyarticular arthritis that runs a course independent of IBD activity. The patterns of joint involvement are similar in UC and CD. In general, erosions and deformities are infrequent in IBD-associated peripheral arthritis, and joint surgery is infrequently required. Isolated destructive hip arthritis is a rare complication of CD, apparently distinct from osteonecrosis and septic arthritis. Dactylitis and enthesopathy are occasionally found. In addition to the ~20% of IBD patients with SpA, a comparable percentage have arthralgias or fibromyalgia symptoms.

Other extraintestinal manifestations of IBD are seen in addition to arthropathy, including uveitis, pyoderma gangrenosum, erythema nodosum, and finger clubbing, all somewhat more commonly in CD than UC. The uveitis shares the features described above for PsA-associated uveitis.

LABORATORY AND RADIOGRAPHIC FINDINGS

Laboratory findings reflect the inflammatory and metabolic manifestations of IBD. Joint fluid is usually at least mildly inflammatory. Of patients with AS and IBD, 30–70% carry the HLA-B27 gene, compared with >90% of patients with AS alone and 50–70% of those with AS and psoriasis. Hence, definite or probable AS in a B27-negative individual in the absence of psoriasis should prompt a search for occult IBD. Radiographic changes in the axial skeleton are the same as in uncomplicated AS. Erosions are uncommon in peripheral arthritis but may occur, particularly in the metatarsophalangeal joints. Isolated destructive hip disease has been described.

DIAGNOSIS

Diarrhea and arthritis are both common conditions that can coexist for a variety of reasons. When etiopathogenically related, reactive arthritis and IBD-associated arthritis are the most common causes. Rare causes include celiac disease, blind loop syndromes, and Whipple's disease. In most cases, diagnosis depends upon investigation of the bowel disease.

TREATMENT Enteropathic Arthritis

Treatment of CD has been improved by therapy with anti-TNF agents. Infliximab and adalimumab are effective for induction and maintenance of clinical remission in CD, and infliximab has been shown to be effective in fistulizing CD. IBD-associated arthritis also responds to these agents. Other treatment for IBD, including sulfasalazine and related drugs, systemic glucocorticoids, and immunosuppressive drugs, are also usually of benefit for associated peripheral arthritis. NSAIDs are generally helpful and well tolerated, but they can precipitate flares of IBD. Rare cases of IBD, usually UC, have apparently been precipitated by anti-TNF therapy, usually etanercept, given for any of several rheumatic diseases.

SAPHO SYNDROME

The syndrome of synovitis, acne, pustulosis, hyperostosis, and osteitis (SAPHO) is characterized by a variety of skin and musculoskeletal manifestations. Dermatologic manifestations include palmoplantar pustulosis, acne conglobata, acne fulminans, and hidradenitis suppurativa. The main musculoskeletal findings are sternoclavicular and spinal hyperostosis, chronic recurrent foci of sterile osteomyelitis, and axial or peripheral arthritis. Cases with one or a few manifestations are probably the rule. The ESR is usually elevated, sometimes dramatically. In some cases, bacteria, most often *Propionibacterium acnes*, have been cultured from bone biopsy specimens and occasionally other sites. Inflammatory bowel disease was coexistent in 8% of patients in one large series. B27 is not associated. Either bone scan or CT scan is helpful diagnostically. A recent MRI report described a characteristic vertebral body corner cortical erosions in 12 out of 12 patients. High-dose NSAIDs may provide relief from bone pain. A number of uncontrolled series and case reports describe successful therapy with pamidronate or other bisphosphonates. Response to anti-TNF-α therapy has also been observed, although in a few cases this has been associated with a flare of skin manifestations. Successful prolonged antibiotic therapy has also been reported.

WHIPPLE'S DISEASE

Whipple's disease (Chap. 294) is a rare chronic bacterial infection, mostly of middle-aged white men, caused by *Tropheryma whipplei*. At least 75% of affected individuals develop an oligo- or polyarthritis. The joint manifestations usually precede other symptoms of the disease by 5 years or more; they are thus particularly important because appropriate antibiotic therapy is curative, whereas the untreated disease is fatal. Large and small peripheral joints and sacroiliac joints may be involved. The arthritis is abrupt in onset, migratory, usually lasts hours to a few days, and then resolves completely. Chronic polyarthritis can occur but is not typical. Eventually prolonged diarrhea, malabsorption, and weight loss occur. Other manifestations of systemic disease include fever, edema, serositis, endocarditis, pneumonia, hypotension, lymphadenopathy, hyperpigmentation, subcutaneous nodules, clubbing, and uveitis. Central nervous system involvement eventually develops in 80% of untreated patients, with cognitive changes, headache, diplopia, and papilledema, and may be detectable on MRI. Oculomasticatory and oculofacial-skeletal myorhythmia with supranuclear vertical gaze palsy are said to be pathognomonic. Laboratory abnormalities include anemia and changes from malabsorption. Synovial fluid is usually inflammatory. Radiography rarely shows joint erosions but may show sacroiliitis. Abdominal CT may reveal lymphadenopathy. Foamy macrophages containing periodic acid–Schiff (PAS)-staining bacterial remnants can be seen in biopsies of small intestine, synovium, lymph node, and other tissues.

The complete genome sequence of *T. whipplei* was published in 2003. Diagnosis is facilitated by PCR amplification of sequences of the 16S ribosomal gene or other genes of *T. whipplei* in biopsied tissue. In the future, this may be supplanted or complemented by serologic tests. The organism is ubiquitous in the environment and is found in some healthy individuals, so the mere presence of DNA does not establish a diagnosis. The syndrome responds to therapy with penicillin (or ceftriaxone) and streptomycin for 2 weeks followed by trimethoprim-sulfamethoxazole for 1–2 years, but other antibiotic regimens may be preferable, and infectious disease consultation is strongly advised. Monitoring for central nervous system relapse is critical. Recently, nonclassical infections with *T. whipplei* have been described, including endocarditis.

FURTHER READINGS

Australo-Anglo-American Spondyloarthritis Consortium (TASC) et al: Genome-wide association study of ankylosing spondylitis identifies non-MHC susceptibility loci. Nat Genet 42:123, 2010

Benjamin M et al: Microdamage and altered vascularity at the enthesis-bone interface provides an anatomic explanation for bone involvement in the HLA-B27-associated spondylarthritides and allied disorders. Arthritis Rheum 56:224, 2007

Braun J et al: Persistent clinical efficacy and safety of anti-tumour necrosis factor alpha therapy with infliximab in patients with ankylosing spondylitis over 5 years: Evidence for different types of response. Ann Rheum Dis 67:340, 2008

BROWN MA: Genetics and the pathogenesis of ankylosing spondylitis. Curr Opin Rheumatol 21:318, 2009

BURTON PR et al: Association scan of 14,500 nonsynonymous SNPs in four diseases identifies autoimmunity variants. Nat Genet 39:1329, 2007

CARTER J et al: Combination antibiotics as a treatment for chronic *Chlamydia*-induced reactive arthritis. Arthritis Rheum 62:1298, 2010

CHANDRAN V et al: Sensitivity of the classification of psoriatic arthritis criteria in early psoriatic arthritis. Arthritis Rheum 57:1560, 2007

DAVIS JC, Jr et al: Efficacy and safety of up to 192 weeks of etanercept therapy in patients with ankylosing spondylitis. Ann Rheum Dis 67:346, 2008

DIARRA D et al: Dickkopf-1 is a master regulator of joint remodeling. Nat Med 13:156, 2007

DOUGADOS M et al: The European Spondyloarthropathy Study Group preliminary criteria for the classification of spondyloarthropathy. Arthritis Rheum 34:1218, 1991

FITZGERALD O, WINCHESTER R: Psoriatic arthritis: From pathogenesis to therapy. Arthritis Res Ther 11:214, 2009

INMAN RD et al: Efficacy and safety of golimumab in patients with ankylosing spondylitis: Results of a randomized, double-blind, placebo-controlled, phase III trial. Arthritis Rheum 58:3402, 2008

LÓPEZ-LARREA C, DIAZ-PEÑA R (eds): Molecular mechanisms of spondyloarthropathies, in *Advances in Experimental Medicine and Biology*, vol. 649. Austin, TX, Springer Science+Business Media and Landes Bioscience, 2009

MAGREY M, KHAN MA: New insights into synovitis, acne, pustulosis, hyperostosis, and osteitis (SAPHO) syndrome. Curr Rheumatol Rep 11:329, 2009

MAKSYMOWYCH WP et al: Inflammatory lesions of the spine on magnetic resonance imaging predict the development of new syndesmophytes in ankylosing spondylitis: evidence of a relationship between inflammation and new bone formation. Arthritis Rheum 60:93, 2009

RUDWALEIT M et al: The early disease stage in axial spondylarthritis: Results from the German Spondyloarthritis Inception Cohort. Arthritis Rheum 60:717, 2009

———: The development of Assessment of Spondyloarthritis International Society classification criteria for axial spondyloarthritis (pt. I): Classification of paper patients by expert opinion including uncertainty appraisal. Ann Rheum Dis 68:770, 2009

———: The development of Assessment of Spondyloarthritis International Society classification criteria for axial spondyloarthritis (pt. II): Validation and final selection. Ann Rheum Dis 68:777, 2009

SCHNEIDER T et al: Whipple's disease: New aspects of pathogenesis and treatment. Lancet Infect Dis 8:179, 2008

SIEPER J et al: The Assessment of Spondyloarthritis International Society (ASAS) handbook: A guide to assess spondyloarthritis. Ann Rheum Dis 68:ii1, 2009

SINGH R et al: Th1/Th17 cytokine profiles in patients with reactive arthritis/undifferentiated spondyloarthropathy. J Rheumatol 34:2285, 2007

TAYLOR W et al: Classification criteria for psoriatic arthritis. Development of new criteria from a large international study. Arthritis Rheum, 54:2665, 2006

ZINOVIEVA E et al: Comprehensive linkage and association analyses identify haplotype, near to the TNFSF15 gene, significantly associated with spondyloarthritis. PLoS Genet 5:e1000528, 2009

CHAPTER 326 The Vasculitis Syndromes

Carol A. Langford
Anthony S. Fauci

DEFINITION

Vasculitis is a clinicopathologic process characterized by inflammation of and damage to blood vessels. The vessel lumen is usually compromised, and this is associated with ischemia of the tissues supplied by the involved vessel. A broad and heterogeneous group of syndromes may result from this process, since any type, size, and location of blood vessel may be involved. Vasculitis and its consequences may be the primary or sole manifestation of a disease; alternatively, vasculitis may be a secondary component of another primary disease. Vasculitis may be confined to a single organ, such as the skin, or it may simultaneously involve several organ systems.

CLASSIFICATION

A major feature of the vasculitic syndromes as a group is the fact that there is a great deal of heterogeneity at the same time as there is considerable overlap among them. This heterogeneity and overlap in addition to a lack of understanding of the pathogenesis of these syndromes have been major impediments to the development of a coherent classification system for these diseases. Table 326-1 lists the major vasculitis syndromes. The distinguishing and overlapping features of these syndromes are discussed below.

PATHOPHYSIOLOGY AND PATHOGENESIS

Generally, most of the vasculitic syndromes are assumed to be mediated at least in part by immunopathogenic mechanisms that occur in response to certain antigenic stimuli (Table 326-2). However, evidence supporting this hypothesis is for the most part indirect and may reflect epiphenomena as opposed to true causality. Furthermore, it is unknown why some individuals might develop vasculitis in response to certain antigenic stimuli, whereas others do not. It is likely that a number of factors are involved in the ultimate expression of a vasculitic syndrome. These include the genetic predisposition, environmental exposures, and the regulatory mechanisms associated with immune response to certain antigens.

TABLE 326-1 Vasculitis Syndromes

Primary Vasculitis Syndromes	Secondary Vasculitis Syndromes
Granulomatosis with polyangiitis (Wegener's)	Drug-induced vasculitis
Churg-Strauss syndrome	Serum sickness
Polyarteritis nodosa	Vasculitis associated with other primary diseases
Microscopic polyangiitis	
Giant cell arteritis	Infection
Takayasu's arteritis	Malignancy
Henoch-Schönlein purpura	Rheumatic disease
Idiopathic cutaneous vasculitis	
Cryoglobulinemic vasculitis	
Behçet's syndrome	
Isolated vasculitis of the central nervous system	
Cogan's syndrome	
Kawasaki disease	

PATHOGENIC IMMUNE-COMPLEX FORMATION

Vasculitis is generally considered within the broader category of *immune-complex diseases* that include serum sickness and certain of the connective tissue diseases, of which systemic lupus erythematosus (Chap. 319) is the prototype. Although deposition of immune complexes in vessel walls is the most widely accepted pathogenic mechanism of vasculitis, the causal role of immune complexes has not been clearly established in most of the vasculitic syndromes. Circulating immune complexes need not result in deposition of the complexes in blood vessels with ensuing vasculitis, and many patients with active vasculitis do not have demonstrable circulating or deposited immune complexes. The actual antigen contained in the immune complex has only rarely been identified in vasculitic syndromes. In this regard, hepatitis B antigen has been identified in both the circulating and deposited immune complexes in a subset of patients who have features of a systemic vasculitis, most notably in polyarteritis nodosa (PAN; see "Polyarteritis Nodosa"). Cryoglobulinemic vasculitis is strongly associated with hepatitis C virus infection; hepatitis C virions and hepatitis C virus antigen-antibody complexes have been identified in the cryoprecipitates of these patients (see "Cryoglobulinemic Vasculitis").

The mechanisms of tissue damage in immune complex-mediated vasculitis resemble those described for serum sickness. In this model, antigen-antibody complexes are formed in antigen excess and are deposited in vessel walls whose permeability has been increased by vasoactive amines such as histamine, bradykinin, and leukotrienes released from platelets or from mast cells as a result of IgE-triggered mechanisms. The deposition of complexes results in activation of complement components, particularly C5a, which is strongly chemotactic for neutrophils. These cells then infiltrate the vessel wall, phagocytose the immune complexes, and release their intracytoplasmic enzymes, which damage the vessel wall. As the process becomes subacute or chronic, mononuclear cells infiltrate the vessel wall. The common denominator of the resulting syndrome is compromise of the vessel lumen with ischemic changes in the tissues supplied by the involved vessel. Several variables may explain why only certain types of immune complexes cause vasculitis and why only certain vessels are affected in individual patients. These include the ability of the reticuloendothelial system to clear circulating complexes from the blood, the size and physicochemical properties of immune complexes, the relative degree of turbulence of blood flow, the intravascular hydrostatic pressure in different vessels, and the preexisting integrity of the vessel endothelium.

TABLE 326-2 Potential Mechanisms of Vessel Damage in Vasculitis Syndromes

Pathogenic immune complex formation and/or deposition
Henoch-Schönlein purpura
Vasculitis associated with collagen vascular diseases
Serum sickness and cutaneous vasculitis syndromes
Hepatitis C–associated cryoglobulinemic vasculitis
Polyarteritis nodosa–like vasculitis associated with hepatitis B
Production of antineutrophilic cytoplasmic antibodies
Granulomatosis with polyangiitis (Wegener's)
Churg-Strauss syndrome
Microscopic polyangiitis
Pathogenic T lymphocyte responses and granuloma formation
Giant cell arteritis
Takayasu's arteritis
Granulomatosis with polyangiitis (Wegener's)
Churg-Strauss syndrome

Source: Adapted from Sneller and Fauci.

ANTINEUTROPHIL CYTOPLASMIC ANTIBODIES (ANCA)

ANCA are antibodies directed against certain proteins in the cytoplasmic granules of neutrophils and monocytes. These autoantibodies are present in a high percentage of patients with active granulomatosis with polyangiitis (Wegener's) and microscopic polyangiitis, and in a lower percentage of patients with Churg-Strauss syndrome. Because these diseases share the presence of ANCA and small-vessel vasculitis, some investigators have come to refer to them collectively as "ANCA-associated vasculitis." However, as these diseases possess unique clinical phenotypes in which ANCA may be absent, it remains our opinion that granulomatosis with polyangiitis (Wegener's), microscopic polyangiitis, and Churg-Strauss syndrome should continue to be viewed as separate entities.

There are two major categories of ANCA based on different targets for the antibodies. The terminology of *cytoplasmic ANCA* (cANCA) refers to the diffuse, granular cytoplasmic staining pattern observed by immunofluorescence microscopy when serum antibodies bind to indicator neutrophils. Proteinase-3, a 29-kDa neutral serine proteinase present in neutrophil azurophilic granules, is the major cANCA antigen. More than 90% of patients with typical active granulomatosis with polyangiitis (Wegener's) have detectable antibodies to proteinase-3 (see below). The terminology of *perinuclear ANCA* (pANCA) refers to the more localized perinuclear or nuclear staining pattern of the indicator neutrophils. The major target for pANCA is the enzyme myeloperoxidase; other targets that can produce a pANCA pattern of staining include elastase, cathepsin G, lactoferrin, lysozyme, and bactericidal/permeability-increasing protein. However, only antibodies to myeloperoxidase have been convincingly associated with vasculitis. Antimyeloperoxidase antibodies have been reported to occur in variable percentages of patients with microscopic polyangiitis, Churg-Strauss syndrome, crescentic glomerulonephritis, and granulomatosis with polyangiitis (Wegener's) (see below). A pANCA pattern of staining that is not due to antimyeloperoxidase antibodies has been associated with nonvasculitic entities such as rheumatic and nonrheumatic autoimmune diseases, inflammatory bowel disease, certain drugs, and infections such as endocarditis and bacterial airway infections in patients with cystic fibrosis.

It is unclear why patients with these vasculitis syndromes develop antibodies to myeloperoxidase or proteinase-3, whereas such antibodies are rare in other inflammatory diseases and autoimmune diseases. It is also unclear what role these antibodies play in disease pathogenesis. There are a number of in vitro observations that suggest possible mechanisms whereby these antibodies can contribute to the pathogenesis of the vasculitis syndromes. Proteinase-3 and myeloperoxidase reside in the azurophilic granules and lysosomes of resting neutrophils and monocytes, where they are apparently inaccessible to serum antibodies. However, when neutrophils or monocytes are primed by tumor necrosis factor α (TNF-α) or interleukin 1 (IL-1), proteinase-3 and myeloperoxidase translocate to the cell membrane, where they can interact with extracellular ANCA. The neutrophils then degranulate and produce reactive oxygen species that can cause tissue damage. Furthermore, ANCA-activated neutrophils can adhere to and kill endothelial cells in vitro. Activation of neutrophils and monocytes by ANCA also induces the release of proinflammatory cytokines such as IL-1 and IL-8. Recent adoptive transfer experiments in genetically engineered mice provide further evidence for a direct pathogenic role of ANCA in vivo. In contradiction, however, a number of clinical and laboratory observations argue against a primary pathogenic role for ANCA. Patients may have active granulomatosis with polyangiitis (Wegener's) in the absence of ANCA; the absolute height of the antibody titers does not correlate well with disease activity; and patients with granulomatosis with polyangiitis (Wegener's) in remission may continue to have high antiproteinase-3 (cANCA) titers for years (see below). Thus, the role of these autoantibodies in the pathogenesis of systemic vasculitis remains unclear.

PATHOGENIC T LYMPHOCYTE RESPONSES AND GRANULOMA FORMATION

In addition to the classic immune complex–mediated mechanisms of vasculitis as well as ANCA, other immunopathogenic mechanisms may be involved in damage to vessels. The most prominent of these are delayed hypersensitivity and cell-mediated immune injury as reflected in the histopathologic feature of granulomatous vasculitis. However, immune complexes themselves may induce granulomatous responses. Vascular endothelial cells can express HLA class II molecules following activation by cytokines such as interferon (IFN) γ. This allows these cells to participate in immunologic reactions such as interaction with CD4+ T lymphocytes in a manner similar to antigen-presenting macrophages. Endothelial cells can secrete IL-1, which may activate T lymphocytes and initiate or propagate in situ immunologic processes within the blood vessel. In addition, IL-1 and TNF-α are potent inducers of endothelial-leukocyte adhesion molecule 1 (ELAM-1) and vascular cell adhesion molecule 1 (VCAM-1), which may enhance the adhesion of leukocytes to endothelial cells in the blood vessel wall. Other mechanisms such as direct cellular cytotoxicity, antibody directed against vessel components, or antibody-dependent cellular cytotoxicity have been suggested in certain types of vessel damage. However, there is no convincing evidence to support their causal contribution to the pathogenesis of any of the recognized vasculitic syndromes.

APPROACH TO THE PATIENT: General Principles of Diagnosis

The diagnosis of vasculitis is often considered in any patient with an unexplained systemic illness. However, there are certain clinical abnormalities that when present alone or in combination should suggest a diagnosis of vasculitis. These include palpable purpura, pulmonary infiltrates and microscopic hematuria, chronic inflammatory sinusitis, mononeuritis multiplex, unexplained ischemic events, and glomerulonephritis with evidence of multisystem disease. A number of nonvasculitic diseases may also produce some or all of these abnormalities. Thus, the first step in the workup of a patient with suspected vasculitis is to exclude other diseases that produce clinical manifestations that can mimic vasculitis (Table 326-3). It is particularly important to exclude infectious diseases with features that overlap those of vasculitis, especially if the patient's clinical condition is deteriorating rapidly and empirical immunosuppressive treatment is being contemplated.

Once diseases that mimic vasculitis have been excluded, the workup should follow a series of progressive steps that establish the diagnosis of vasculitis and determine, where possible, the category of the vasculitis syndrome (Fig. 326-1). This approach is of considerable importance since several of the vasculitis syndromes require aggressive therapy with glucocorticoids and cytotoxic agents, while other syndromes usually resolve spontaneously and require symptomatic treatment only. The definitive diagnosis of vasculitis is made upon biopsy of involved tissue. The yield of "blind" biopsies of organs with no subjective or objective evidence of involvement is very low and should be avoided. When syndromes such as PAN, Takayasu's arteritis, or isolated central nervous system (CNS) vasculitis are suspected, arteriogram of organs with suspected involvement should be performed. However, arteriograms should not be performed routinely when patients present with localized cutaneous vasculitis with no clinical indication of visceral involvement.

GENERAL PRINCIPLES OF TREATMENT Once a diagnosis of vasculitis has been established, a decision regarding therapeutic strategy

TABLE 326-3 Conditions That Can Mimic Vasculitis

Infectious diseases
Bacterial endocarditis
Disseminated gonococcal infection
Pulmonary histoplasmosis
Coccidioidomycosis
Syphilis
Lyme disease
Rocky Mountain spotted fever
Whipple's disease
Coagulopathies/thrombotic microangiopathies
Antiphospholipid antibody syndrome
Thrombotic thrombocytopenic purpura
Neoplasms
Atrial myxoma
Lymphoma
Carcinomatosis
Drug toxicity
Cocaine
Amphetamines
Ergot alkaloids
Methysergide
Arsenic
Sarcoidosis
Atheroembolic disease
Antiglomerular basement membrane disease (Goodpasture's syndrome)
Amyloidosis
Migraine

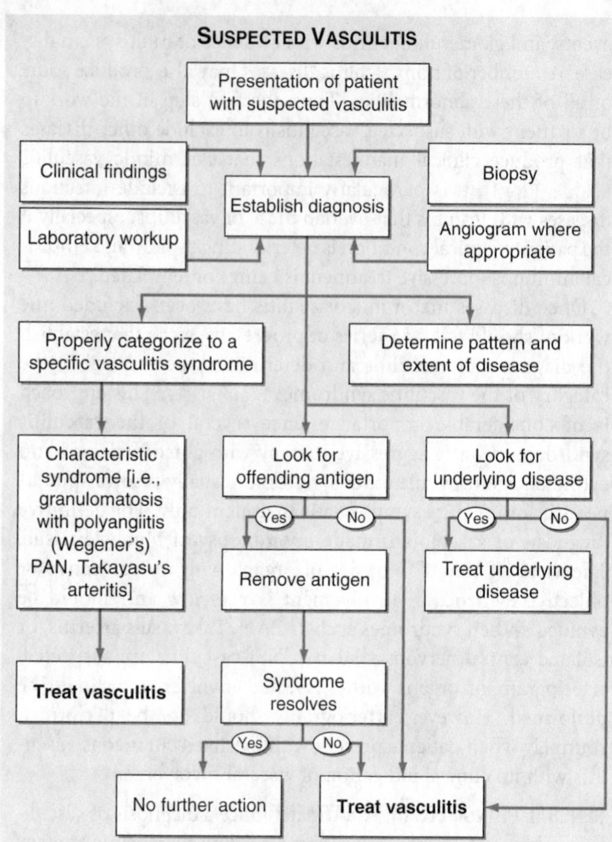

Figure 326-1 Algorithm for the approach to a patient with suspected diagnosis of vasculitis. PAN, polyarteritis nodosa.

must be made (Fig. 326-1). If an offending antigen that precipitates the vasculitis is recognized, the antigen should be removed where possible. If the vasculitis is associated with an underlying disease such as an infection, neoplasm, or connective tissue disease, the underlying disease should be treated. If the syndrome represents a primary vasculitic disease, treatment should be initiated according to the category of the vasculitis syndrome. Specific therapeutic regimens are discussed below for the individual vasculitis syndromes; however, certain general principles regarding therapy should be considered. Decisions regarding treatment should be based upon the use of regimens for which there has been published literature supporting efficacy for that particular vasculitic disease. Since the potential toxic side effects of certain therapeutic regimens may be substantial, the risk-versus-benefit ratio of any therapeutic approach should be weighed carefully. On the one hand, glucocorticoids and/or cytotoxic therapy should be instituted immediately in diseases where irreversible organ system dysfunction and high morbidity and mortality rates have been clearly established. Granulomatosis with polyangiitis (Wegener's) is the prototype of a severe systemic vasculitis requiring such a therapeutic approach (see below). On the other hand, when feasible, aggressive therapy should be avoided for vasculitic manifestations that rarely result in irreversible organ system dysfunction and that usually do not respond to such therapy. For example, idiopathic cutaneous vasculitis usually resolves with symptomatic treatment, and prolonged courses of glucocorticoids uncommonly result in clinical benefit. Cytotoxic agents have not proved to be beneficial in idiopathic cutaneous vasculitis, and their toxic side effects generally outweigh any potential beneficial effects. Glucocorticoids should be initiated in those systemic vasculitides that cannot be specifically categorized or for which there is no established standard therapy; cytotoxic therapy should be added in these diseases only if an adequate response does not result or if remission can only be achieved and maintained with an unacceptably toxic regimen of glucocorticoids. When remission is achieved, one should continually attempt to taper glucocorticoids and discontinue when possible. When using cytotoxic regimens, one should base the choice of agent upon the available therapeutic data supporting efficacy in that disease, the site and severity of organ involvement, and the toxicity profile of the drug.

Physicians should be thoroughly aware of the toxic side effects of therapeutic agents employed that can include both acute and long-term complications (Table 326-4). Morbidity and mortality can occur as a result of treatment and strategies to monitor for and prevent toxicity represent an essential part of patient care. Glucocorticoids are an important part of treatment for most vasculitides but are associated with substantial toxicities. Monitoring and prevention of glucocorticoid-induced bone loss is important in all patients. With the use of daily cyclophosphamide, strategies are particularly important and are directed toward minimization of bladder toxicity and prevention of leukopenia. Instructing the patient to take cyclophosphamide all at once in the morning with a large amount of fluid throughout the day in order to maintain a dilute urine can reduce the risk of bladder injury. Bladder cancer

TABLE 326-4 Major Toxic Side Effects of Drugs Commonly Used in the Treatment of Systemic Vasculitis

Glucocorticoids	
Osteoporosis	Growth suppression in children
Cataracts	Hypertension
Glaucoma	Avascular necrosis of bone
Diabetes mellitus	Myopathy
Electrolyte abnormalities	Alterations in mood
Metabolic abnormalities	Psychosis
Suppression of inflammatory and immune responses leading to opportunistic infections	Pseudotumor cerebri Peptic ulcer diathesis Pancreatitis
Cushingoid features	
Cyclophosphamide	
Bone marrow suppression	Hypogammaglobulinemia
Cystitis	Pulmonary fibrosis
Bladder carcinoma	Myelodysplasia
Gonadal suppression	Oncogenesis
Gastrointestinal intolerance	Teratogenicity
	Opportunistic infections
Methotrexate	
Gastrointestinal intolerance	Pneumonitis
Stomatitis	Teratogenicity
Bone marrow suppression	Opportunistic infections
Hepatotoxicity (may lead to fibrosis or cirrhosis)	
Azathioprine	
Gastrointestinal intolerance	Opportunistic infections
Bone marrow suppression	Hypersensitivity
Hepatotoxicity	

can occur several years after discontinuation of cyclophosphamide therapy; therefore, monitoring for bladder cancer should continue indefinitely in patients who have received cyclophosphamide. Bone marrow suppression is an important toxicity of cyclophosphamide and can be observed during glucocorticoid tapering or over time, even after periods of stable measurements. Monitoring of the complete blood count every 1–2 weeks for as long as the patient receives cyclophosphamide can effectively prevent cytopenias. Maintaining the white blood count (WBC) at >3000/μL and the neutrophil count >1500/μL is essential to reduce the risk of life-threatening infections.

Methotrexate and azathioprine are also associated with bone marrow suppression, and complete blood counts should be obtained every 1–2 weeks for the first 1–2 months after their initiation and once a month thereafter. To lessen toxicity, methotrexate is often given together with folic acid, 1 mg daily, or folinic acid, 5–10 mg once a week 24 h following methotrexate. Prior to initiation of azathioprine, thiopurine methyltransferase (TPMT), an enzyme involved in the metabolism of azathioprine, should be assayed because inadequate levels may result in severe cytopenia.

Infection represents a significant toxicity for all vasculitis patients treated with immunosuppressive therapy. Infections with *Pneumocystis jiroveci* and certain fungi can be seen even in the face of WBCs that are within normal limits, particularly in patients receiving glucocorticoids. All vasculitis patients who are receiving daily glucocorticoids in combination with a cytotoxic drug should receive trimethoprim-sulfamethoxazole (TMP-SMX) or another prophylactic therapy to prevent *P. jiroveci* infection.

Finally, it should be emphasized that each patient is unique and requires individual decision-making. The above outline should serve as a framework to guide therapeutic approaches; however, flexibility should be practiced in order to provide maximal therapeutic efficacy with minimal toxic side effects in each patient.

GRANULOMATOSIS WITH POLYANGIITIS (WEGENER'S)

DEFINITION

Granulomatosis with polyangiitis (Wegener's) is a distinct clinicopathologic entity characterized by granulomatous vasculitis of the upper and lower respiratory tracts together with glomerulonephritis. In addition, variable degrees of disseminated vasculitis involving both small arteries and veins may occur.

INCIDENCE AND PREVALENCE

Granulomatosis with polyangiitis (Wegener's) is an uncommon disease with an estimated prevalence of 3 per 100,000. It is extremely rare in blacks compared with whites; the male-to-female ratio is 1:1. The disease can be seen at any age; ~15% of patients are <19 years of age, but only rarely does the disease occur before adolescence; the mean age of onset is ~40 years.

PATHOLOGY AND PATHOGENESIS

The histopathologic hallmarks of granulomatosis with polyangiitis (Wegener's) are necrotizing vasculitis of small arteries and veins together with granuloma formation, which may be either intravascular or extravascular (Fig. 326-2). Lung involvement typically appears as multiple, bilateral, nodular cavitary infiltrates (Fig. 326-3), which on biopsy almost invariably reveal the typical necrotizing granulomatous vasculitis. Upper airway lesions, particularly those in the sinuses and nasopharynx, typically reveal inflammation, necrosis, and granuloma formation, with or without vasculitis.

In its earliest form, renal involvement is characterized by a focal and segmental glomerulitis that may evolve into a rapidly progressive crescentic glomerulonephritis. Granuloma formation is only rarely seen on renal biopsy. In contrast to other forms of glomerulonephritis, evidence of immune complex deposition is not found in the renal lesion of granulomatosis with polyangiitis (Wegener's). In addition to the classic triad of disease of the upper and lower respiratory tracts and kidney, virtually any organ can be involved with vasculitis, granuloma, or both.

The immunopathogenesis of this disease is unclear, although the involvement of upper airways and lungs with granulomatous vasculitis suggests an aberrant cell-mediated immune response to an exogenous or even endogenous antigen that enters through or resides in the upper airway. Chronic nasal carriage of *Staphylococcus aureus* has been reported to be associated with a higher relapse rate of granulomatosis with polyangiitis (Wegener's); however, there is no evidence for a role of this organism in the pathogenesis of the disease.

Peripheral blood mononuclear cells obtained from patients with granulomatosis with polyangiitis (Wegener's) manifest increased secretion of IFN-γ but not of IL-4, IL-5, or IL-10 compared to normal controls. In addition, TNF-α production from peripheral blood mononuclear cells and CD4+ T cells is elevated. Furthermore, monocytes from patients with granulomatosis with polyangiitis (Wegener's) produce increased amounts of IL-12. These findings indicate an unbalanced T_H1-type T cell cytokine pattern in this disease that may have pathogenic and perhaps ultimately therapeutic implications.

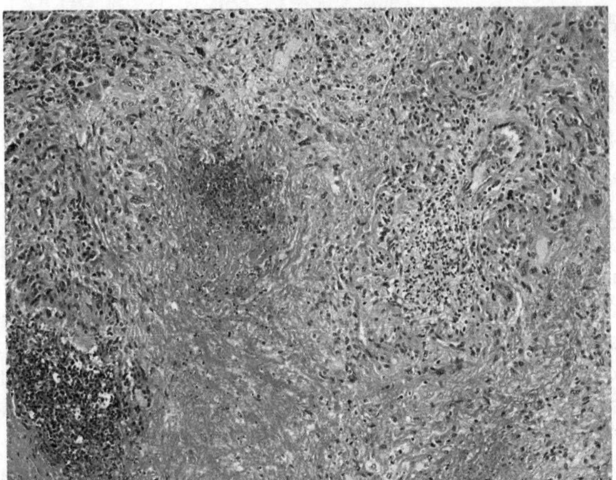

Figure 326-2 Lung histology in granulomatosis with polyangiitis (Wegener's). This area of geographic necrosis has a serpiginous border of histiocytes and giant cells surrounding a central necrotic zone. Vasculitis is also present with neutrophils and lymphocytes infiltrating the wall of a small arteriole (*upper right*). *(Courtesy of William D. Travis, MD; with permission.)*

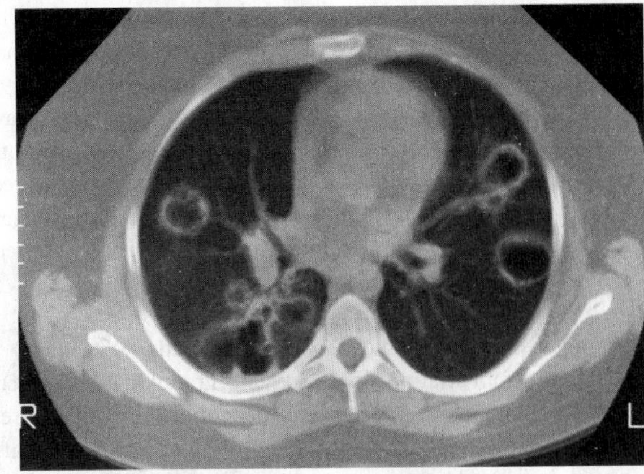

Figure 326-3 Computed tomography scan of a patient with granulomatosis with polyangiitis (Wegener's). The patient developed multiple, bilateral, and cavitary infiltrates.

A high percentage of patients with granulomatosis with polyangiitis (Wegener's) develop ANCA, and these autoantibodies may play a role in the pathogenesis of this disease (see above).

CLINICAL AND LABORATORY MANIFESTATIONS

Involvement of the upper airways occurs in 95% of patients with granulomatosis with polyangiitis (Wegener's). Patients often present with severe upper respiratory tract findings such as paranasal sinus pain and drainage and purulent or bloody nasal discharge, with or without nasal mucosal ulceration (Table 326-5). Nasal septal perforation may follow, leading to saddle nose deformity. Serous otitis media may occur as a result of eustachian tube blockage. Subglottic tracheal stenosis resulting from active disease or scarring occurs in ~16% of patients and may result in severe airway obstruction.

Pulmonary involvement may be manifested as asymptomatic infiltrates or may be clinically expressed as cough, hemoptysis, dyspnea, and chest discomfort. It is present in 85–90% of patients. Endobronchial disease, either in its active form or as a result of fibrous scarring, may lead to obstruction with atelectasis.

Eye involvement (52% of patients) may range from a mild conjunctivitis to dacryocystitis, episcleritis, scleritis, granulomatous sclerouveitis, ciliary vessel vasculitis, and retroorbital mass lesions leading to proptosis.

Skin lesions (46% of patients) appear as papules, vesicles, palpable purpura, ulcers, or subcutaneous nodules; biopsy reveals vasculitis, granuloma, or both. Cardiac involvement (8% of patients) manifests as pericarditis, coronary vasculitis, or, rarely, cardiomyopathy. Nervous system manifestations (23% of patients) include cranial neuritis, mononeuritis multiplex, or, rarely, cerebral vasculitis and/or granuloma.

Renal disease (77% of patients) generally dominates the clinical picture and, if left untreated, accounts directly or indirectly for most of the mortality rate in this disease. Although it may smolder in some cases as a mild glomerulitis with proteinuria, hematuria, and red blood cell casts, it is clear that once clinically detectable renal functional impairment occurs, rapidly progressive renal failure usually ensues unless appropriate treatment is instituted.

While the disease is active, most patients have nonspecific symptoms and signs such as malaise, weakness, arthralgias, anorexia, and weight loss. Fever may indicate activity of the underlying disease but more often reflects secondary infection, usually of the upper airway.

Characteristic laboratory findings include a markedly elevated erythrocyte sedimentation rate (ESR), mild anemia and leukocytosis, mild hypergammaglobulinemia (particularly of the IgA class), and mildly elevated rheumatoid factor. Thrombocytosis may be seen as an acute-phase reactant. Approximately 90% of patients with active granulomatosis with polyangiitis (Wegener's) have a positive antiproteinase-3 ANCA. However, in the absence of active disease, the sensitivity drops to ~60–70%. A small percentage of patients with granulomatosis with polyangiitis (Wegener's) may have antimyeloperoxidase rather than antiproteinase-3 antibodies, and up to 20% may lack ANCA.

Patients with granulomatosis with polyangiitis (Wegener's) have been found to have an increased incidence of venous thrombotic events. Although routine anticoagulation for all patients is not recommended, a heightened awareness for any clinical features suggestive of deep venous thrombosis or pulmonary emboli is warranted.

DIAGNOSIS

The diagnosis of granulomatosis with polyangiitis (Wegener's) is made by the demonstration of necrotizing granulomatous vasculitis on tissue biopsy in a patient with compatible clinical features. Pulmonary tissue offers the highest diagnostic yield, almost invariably revealing granulomatous vasculitis. Biopsy of upper airway tissue usually reveals granulomatous inflammation with necrosis but may not show vasculitis. Renal biopsy can confirm the presence of pauci-immune glomerulonephritis.

TABLE 326-5 Granulomatosis With Polyangiitis (Wegener's): Frequency of Clinical Manifestations in 158 Patients Studied at the National Institutes of Health

Manifestation	Percent at Disease Onset	Percent Throughout Course of Disease
Kidney		
Glomerulonephritis	18	77
Ear/nose/throat	73	92
Sinusitis	51	85
Nasal disease	36	68
Otitis media	25	44
Hearing loss	14	42
Subglottic stenosis	1	16
Ear pain	9	14
Oral lesions	3	10
Lung	45	85
Pulmonary infiltrates	25	66
Pulmonary nodules	24	58
Hemoptysis	12	30
Pleuritis	10	28
Eyes		
Conjunctivitis	5	18
Dacryocystitis	1	18
Scleritis	6	16
Proptosis	2	15
Eye pain	3	11
Visual loss	0	8
Retinal lesions	0	4
Corneal lesions	0	1
Iritis	0	2
Other[a]		
Arthralgias/arthritis	32	67
Fever	23	50
Cough	19	46
Skin abnormalities	13	46
Weight loss (>10% body weight)	15	35
Peripheral neuropathy	1	15
Central nervous system disease	1	8
Pericarditis	2	6
Hyperthyroidism	1	3

[a]Fewer than 1% had parotid, pulmonary artery, breast, or lower genitourinary (urethra, cervix, vagina, testicular) involvement.

Source: Hoffman et al.

The specificity of a positive antiproteinase-3 ANCA for granulomatosis with polyangiitis (Wegener's) is very high, especially if active glomerulonephritis is present. However, the presence of ANCA should be adjunctive and, with rare exceptions, should not substitute for a tissue diagnosis. False-positive ANCA titers have been reported in certain infectious and neoplastic diseases.

In its typical presentation, the clinicopathologic complex of granulomatosis with polyangiitis (Wegener's) usually provides ready differentiation from other disorders. However, if all the typical features are not present at once, it needs to be differentiated from the other vasculitides, antiglomerular basement membrane disease (Goodpasture's syndrome) (Chap. 283), relapsing polychondritis (Chap. 328), tumors of the upper airway or lung, and infectious diseases such as histoplasmosis (Chap. 199), mucocutaneous leishmaniasis (Chap. 212), and rhinoscleroma (Chap. 31) as well as noninfectious granulomatous diseases.

Of particular note is the differentiation from *midline granuloma* and *upper airway neoplasms*, which are part of the spectrum of *midline destructive diseases*. These diseases lead to extreme tissue destruction and mutilation localized to the midline upper airway structures including the sinuses; erosion through the skin of the face commonly occurs, a feature that is extremely rare in granulomatosis with polyangiitis (Wegener's). Although blood vessels may be involved in the intense inflammatory reaction and necrosis, primary vasculitis is not seen. Midline granuloma is part of the spectrum of *angiocentric immunoproliferative lesions* that are considered to represent a spectrum of postthymic T cell proliferative lesions and should be treated as such (Chap. 110). The term *idiopathic* has been applied to midline granuloma when extensive diagnostic workup including multiple biopsies has failed to reveal anything other than inflammation and necrosis. Under these circumstances, it is possible that the tumor cells were masked by the intensive inflammatory response. Such cases have responded to local irradiation with 50 Gy (5000 rad). Upper airway lesions should never be irradiated in granulomatosis with polyangiitis (Wegener's). Cocaine-induced tissue injury can be another important mimic of granulomatosis with polyangiitis (Wegener's) in patients who present with isolated midline destructive disease. ANCA that target human neutrophil elastase can be found in patients with cocaine-induced midline destructive lesions and can confound the differentiation from granulomatosis with polyangiitis (Wegener's).

Granulomatosis with polyangiitis (Wegener's) must also be differentiated from *lymphomatoid granulomatosis*, which is an Epstein-Barr virus–positive B cell proliferation that is associated with an exuberant T cell reaction. Lymphomatoid granulomatosis is characterized by lung, skin, CNS, and kidney involvement in which atypical lymphocytoid and plasmacytoid cells infiltrate nonlymphoid tissue in an angioinvasive manner. In this regard, it clearly differs from granulomatosis with polyangiitis (Wegener's) in that it is not an inflammatory vasculitis in the classic sense but an infiltration of vessels with atypical mononuclear cells; granuloma may be present in involved tissues. Up to 50% of patients may develop a true malignant lymphoma.

TREATMENT Granulomatosis With Polyangiitis (Wegener's)

Prior to the introduction of effective therapy, granulomatosis with polyangiitis (Wegener's) was universally fatal within a few months of diagnosis. Glucocorticoids alone led to some symptomatic improvement, with little effect on the ultimate course of the disease. The development of treatment with cyclophophamide dramatically changed patient outcome such that marked improvement was seen in >90% of patients, complete remission in 75% of patients, and 5-year patient survival was seen in over 80%.

Despite the ability to successfully induce remission, 50–70% of remissions are later associated with one or more relapses. The determination of relapse should be based on objective evidence of disease activity, taking care to rule out other features that may have a similar appearance such as infection, medication toxicity, or chronic disease sequelae. The ANCA titer can be misleading and should not be used to assess disease activity. Many patients who achieve remission continue to have elevated titers for years. Results from a large prospective study found that increases in ANCA were not associated with relapse and that only 43% relapsed within 1 year of an increase in ANCA levels. Thus, a rise in ANCA by itself is not a harbinger of immediate disease relapse and should not lead to reinstitution or increase in immunosuppressive therapy.

Reinduction of remission after relapse is almost always achieved; however, a high percentage of patients ultimately have some degree of damage from irreversible features of their disease, such as varying degrees of renal insufficiency, hearing loss, tracheal stenosis, saddle nose deformity, and chronically impaired sinus function. Patients who developed irreversible renal failure but who achieved subsequent remission have undergone successful renal transplantation.

Because long-term cyclophosphamide is associated with substantial toxicity, approaches have been developed that seek to minimize the duration of exposure to cyclophosphamide while still taking advantage of its efficacy for severe disease. Treatment of granulomatosis with polyangiitis (Wegener's) is currently viewed as having two phases: *induction*, where active disease is put into remission, followed by *maintenance*. The decision regarding which agents to use for induction and maintenance is based upon disease severity together with individual patient factors that include contraindication, relapse history, and comorbidities.

CYCLOPHOSPHAMIDE INDUCTION FOR SEVERE DISEASE For patients with severe disease, daily cyclophosphamide combined with glucocorticoids has been repeatedly proved to effectively induce remission and prolong survival. At the initiation of therapy, glucocorticoids are usually given as prednisone, 1 mg/kg per day for the first month, followed by gradual tapering on an alternate-day or daily schedule with discontinuation after ~6–9 months. Cyclophosphamide is given in doses of 2 mg/kg per day orally, but as it is renally eliminated, dosage reduction should be considered in patients with renal insufficiency. Some reports have indicated therapeutic success with less frequent and severe toxic side effects using IV cyclophosphamide. In a recent randomized trial, IV cyclophosphamide 15 mg/kg, three infusions given every 2 weeks, then every 3 weeks thereafter, was compared to cyclophosphamide 2 mg/kg daily given for 3 months followed by 1.5 mg/kg daily. Although IV cyclophosphamide was found to have a comparable rate of remission with a lower cumulative cyclophosphamide dose and occurrence of leukopenia, the use of a consolidation phase and an insufficient frequency of blood count monitoring may have negatively influenced the results in those who received daily cyclophosphamide. Of note in this study was that relapse occurred in 19% of those who received IV cyclophosphamide as compared to 9% who received daily oral administration. We continue to strongly favor daily cyclophosphamide with utilization of blood count monitoring every 1–2 weeks (as discussed above) and limiting the duration of induction exposure to 3–6 months.

In patients with imminently life-threatening disease, such as rapidly progressive glomerulonephritis or pulmonary hemorrhage requiring mechanical ventilation, a regimen of daily cyclophosphamide and glucocorticoids is the treatment of choice to induce remission. Adjunctive plasmapheresis was found to further improve renal recovery in a study of patients with rapidly progressive glomerulonephritis who had a creatinine of greater than 5.8 mg/dL.

REMISSION MAINTENANCE AFTER CYCLOPHOSPHAMIDE After 3–6 months of induction treatment, cyclophosphamide should be stopped and switched to another agent for remission maintenance. The agents with which there has been the greatest published experience are methotrexate and azathioprine. Methotrexate is administered orally or subcutaneously starting at a dosage of 0.3 mg/kg as a single weekly dose, not to exceed 15 mg/week. If the treatment is well tolerated after 1–2 weeks, the dosage should be increased by 2.5 mg weekly up to a dosage of 20–25 mg/week and maintained at that level. Azathioprine, 2 mg/kg per day, has also proved effective in maintaining remission following induction with daily cyclophosphamide. In a randomized trial comparing methotrexate to azathioprine for remission maintenance, comparable rates of toxicity and relapse were seen. Therefore, the choice of agent is often based on toxicity profile, as methotrexate cannot be given to patients with renal insufficiency or chronic liver disease, as well as on other individual patient factors. In patients who are unable to receive methotrexate or azathioprine or who have relapsed through such treatment, mycophenolate mofetil, 1000 mg twice a day, may also sustain remission following cyclophosphamide induction.

The optimal duration of maintenance therapy is uncertain. In the absence of toxicity, maintenance therapy is usually given for a minimum of 2 years past remission, after which time consideration can be given for tapering over a 6–12 month period until discontinuation. Some patients with significant organ damage or a history of relapse may benefit from longer-term continuation of a maintenance agent.

METHOTREXATE INDUCTION FOR NONSEVERE DISEASE For selected patients whose disease is not immediately life threatening or in those patients who have experienced significant cyclophosphamide toxicity, methotrexate together with glucocorticoids given at the dosages described above may be considered as an alternative for induction therapy, which is then continued for maintenance.

RITUXIMAB INDUCTION FOR SEVERE DISEASE Rituximab is a chimeric monoclonal antibody directed against CD20 present on normal and malignant B lymphocytes that is FDA approved for the treatment of non-Hodgkin's lymphoma, chronic lymphocytic lymphoma, and rheumatoid arthritis. In two recent randomized trials that enrolled ANCA positive patients with severe active granulomatosis with polyangiitis (Wegener's) or microscopic polyangiitis, rituximab 375 mg/m^2 once a week for 4 weeks in combination with glucocorticoids was found to be as effective as cyclophosphamide with glucocorticoids for inducing disease remission. In the trial which also enrolled patients with relapsing disease, rituximab was found to be statistically superior to cyclophosphamide.

While the data supports that rituximab is effective for remission induction severe active granulomatosis with polyangiitis (Wegener's) or microscopic polyangiitis, there remain a number of ongoing questions regarding rituximab that must be considered in weighing its use in the individual patient. These include that there are no long-term data regarding relapse risk or long-term safety with rituximab, it is unclear how often rituximab needs to be given, and as all patients in the randomized trials were ANCA positive, its efficacy in ANCA negative patients is unknown. It is also uncertain whether the use of other maintenance agents after rituximab would provide any additional benefit in prolonging remission or increase toxicity as these were not used in either randomized trial.

While rituximab does not have the bladder toxicity or infertility concerns, as can occur with cyclophosphamide, in both of the randomized trials, the rate of adverse events was similar in the rituximab and cyclophosphamide arms. Serious side effects of rituximab include infusion reactions, severe mucocutaneous reactions, and rare reports of progressive multifocal leukoencephalopathy. As rituximab can bring about reactivation of hepatitis B, all patients should undergo hepatitis screening prior to treatment with rituximab.

OTHER BIOLOGIC THERAPIES Etanercept, a dimeric fusion protein containing the 75-kDa TNF receptor bound to human IgG1, was not found to sustain remission when used adjunctively to standard therapy and should not be used in the treatment of granulomatosis with polyangiitis (Wegener's).

TRIMETHOPRIM-SULFAMETHOXAZOLE Although certain reports have indicated that TMP-SMX may be of benefit in the treatment of granulomatosis with polyangiitis (Wegener's) isolated to the sinonasal tissues, it should never be used alone to treat active granulomatosis with polyangiitis (Wegener's) outside of the upper airway such as in patients with renal or pulmonary disease. In a study examining the effect of TMP-SMX on relapse, decreased relapses were shown only with regard to upper airway disease, and no differences in major organ relapses were observed.

ORGAN-SPECIFIC TREATMENT Not all manifestations of granulomatosis with polyangiitis (Wegener's) require or respond to cytotoxic therapy. In managing non-major organ disease, such as that isolated to the sinus, joints, or skin, the risks of treatment should be carefully weighed against the benefits. Treatment with cyclophosphamide is rarely if ever justified for the treatment of isolated sinus disease in granulomatosis with polyangiitis (Wegener's). Although patients with non-major organ disease may be effectively treated without cytotoxic therapy, these individuals must be monitored closely for the development of disease activity affecting the lungs, kidneys, or other major organs. Subglottic tracheal stenosis and endobronchial stenosis are examples of disease manifestations that do not typically respond to systemic immunosuppressive treatment.

MICROSCOPIC POLYANGIITIS

DEFINITION

The term *microscopic polyarteritis* was introduced into the literature by Davson in 1948 in recognition of the presence of glomerulonephritis in patients with PAN. In 1992, the Chapel Hill Consensus Conference on the Nomenclature of Systemic Vasculitis adopted the term *microscopic polyangiitis* to connote a necrotizing vasculitis with few or no immune complexes affecting small vessels (capillaries, venules, or arterioles). Glomerulonephritis is very common in microscopic polyangiitis, and pulmonary capillaritis often occurs. The absence of granulomatous inflammation in microscopic polyangiitis is said to differentiate it from granulomatosis with polyangiitis (Wegener's).

INCIDENCE AND PREVALENCE

The incidence of microscopic polyangiitis has not yet been reliably established due to its previous inclusion as part of PAN. The mean age of onset is ~57 years of age, and males are slightly more frequently affected than females.

PATHOLOGY AND PATHOGENESIS

The vasculitis seen in microscopic polyangiitis has a predilection to involve capillaries and venules in addition to small and medium-sized arteries. Immunohistochemical staining reveals a paucity of immunoglobulin deposition in the vascular lesion of microscopic polyangiitis, suggesting that immune-complex formation does not play a role in the pathogenesis of this syndrome. The renal lesion seen in microscopic polyangiitis is identical to that of granulomatosis with polyangiitis (Wegener's). Like granulomatosis with polyangiitis (Wegener's), microscopic polyangiitis is highly associated with the presence of ANCA, which may play a role in pathogenesis of this syndrome (see above).

CLINICAL AND LABORATORY MANIFESTATIONS

Because of its predilection to involve the small vessels, microscopic polyangiitis and granulomatosis with polyangiitis (Wegener's) share similar clinical features. Disease onset may be gradual, with initial symptoms of fever, weight loss, and musculoskeletal pain; however, it is often acute. Glomerulonephritis occurs in at least 79% of patients and can be rapidly progressive, leading to renal failure. Hemoptysis may be the first symptom of alveolar hemorrhage, which occurs in 12% of patients. Other manifestations include mononeuritis multiplex and gastrointestinal tract and cutaneous vasculitis. Upper airway disease and pulmonary nodules are not typically found in microscopic polyangiitis and, if present, suggest granulomatosis with polyangiitis (Wegener's).

Features of inflammation may be seen, including an elevated ESR, anemia, leukocytosis, and thrombocytosis. ANCA are present in 75% of patients with microscopic polyangiitis, with antimyeloperoxidase antibodies being the predominant ANCA associated with this disease.

DIAGNOSIS

The diagnosis is based on histologic evidence of vasculitis or pauci-immune glomerulonephritis in a patient with compatible clinical features of multisystem disease. Although microscopic polyangiitis is strongly ANCA-associated, no studies have as yet established the sensitivity and specificity of ANCA in this disease.

TREATMENT Microscopic Polyangiitis

The 5-year survival rate for patients with treated microscopic polyangiitis is 74%, with disease-related mortality occurring from alveolar hemorrhage or gastrointestinal, cardiac, or renal disease. Studies on treatment have come from trials that have included patients with granulomatosis with polyangiitis (Wegener's) or microscopic polyangiitis. Currently, the treatment approach for microscopic polyangiitis is the same as is used for granulomatosis with polyangiitis (Wegener's) [see "Granulomatosis With Polyangiitis (Wegener's)" for a detailed description of this therapeutic regimen), and patients with immediately life-threatening disease should be treated with the combination of prednisone and daily cyclophosphamide. Recent studies with rituximab also included ANCA positive patients with microscopic polyangiitis. Disease relapse has been observed in at least 34% of patients. Treatment for such relapses would be similar to that used at the time of initial presentation and based upon site and severity of disease.

CHURG-STRAUSS SYNDROME

DEFINITION

Churg-Strauss syndrome, also referred to as *allergic angiitis and granulomatosis*, was described in 1951 by Churg and Strauss and is characterized by asthma, peripheral and tissue eosinophilia, extravascular granuloma formation, and vasculitis of multiple organ systems.

INCIDENCE AND PREVALENCE

Churg-Strauss syndrome is an uncommon disease with an estimated annual incidence of 1–3 per million. The disease can occur at any age with the possible exception of infants. The mean age of onset is 48 years, with a female-to-male ratio of 1.2:1.

PATHOLOGY AND PATHOGENESIS

The necrotizing vasculitis of Churg-Strauss syndrome involves small and medium-sized muscular arteries, capillaries, veins, and venules. A characteristic histopathologic feature of Churg-Strauss syndrome is granulomatous reactions that may be present in the tissues or even within the walls of the vessels themselves. These are usually associated with infiltration of the tissues with eosinophils. This process can occur in any organ in the body; lung involvement is predominant, with skin, cardiovascular system, kidney, peripheral nervous system, and gastrointestinal tract also commonly involved. Although the precise pathogenesis of this disease is uncertain, its strong association with asthma and its clinicopathologic manifestations, including eosinophilia, granuloma, and vasculitis, point to aberrant immunologic phenomena.

CLINICAL AND LABORATORY MANIFESTATIONS

Patients with Churg-Strauss syndrome often exhibit nonspecific manifestations such as fever, malaise, anorexia, and weight loss, which are characteristic of a multisystem disease. The pulmonary findings in Churg-Strauss syndrome clearly dominate the clinical picture with severe asthmatic attacks and the presence of pulmonary infiltrates. Mononeuritis multiplex is the second most common manifestation and occurs in up to 72% of patients. Allergic rhinitis and sinusitis develop in up to 61% of patients and are often observed early in the course of disease. Clinically recognizable heart disease occurs in ~14% of patients and is an important cause of mortality. Skin lesions occur in ~51% of patients and include purpura in addition to cutaneous and subcutaneous nodules. The renal disease in Churg-Strauss syndrome is less common and generally less severe than that of granulomatosis with polyangiitis (Wegener's) and microscopic polyangiitis.

The characteristic laboratory finding in virtually all patients with Churg-Strauss syndrome is a striking eosinophilia, which reaches levels >1000 cells/μL in >80% of patients. Evidence of inflammation as evidenced by elevated ESR, fibrinogen, or α_2-globulins can be found in 81% of patients. The other laboratory findings reflect the organ systems involved. Approximately 48% of patients with Churg-Strauss syndrome have circulating ANCA that is usually antimyeloperoxidase.

DIAGNOSIS

Although the diagnosis of Churg-Strauss syndrome is optimally made by biopsy in a patient with the characteristic clinical manifestations (see above), histologic confirmation can be challenging as the pathognomonic features often do not occur simultaneously. In order to be diagnosed with Churg-Strauss syndrome, a patient should have evidence of asthma, peripheral blood eosinophilia, and clinical features consistent with vasculitis.

TREATMENT Churg-Strauss Syndrome

The prognosis of untreated Churg-Strauss syndrome is poor, with a reported 5-year survival of 25%. With treatment, prognosis is favorable, with one study finding a 78-month actuarial survival rate of 72%. Myocardial involvement is the most frequent cause of death and is responsible for 39% of patient mortality. Glucocorticoids alone appear to be effective in many patients. Dosage tapering is often limited by asthma, and many patients require low-dose prednisone for persistent asthma many years after clinical recovery from vasculitis. In glucocorticoid failure or in patients who present with fulminant multisystem disease, the treatment of choice is a combined regimen of daily cyclophosphamide and prednisone (see "Granulomatosis With Polyangiitis (Wegener's)" for a detailed description of this therapeutic regimen).

POLYARTERITIS NODOSA

■ DEFINITION

PAN, also referred to as *classic PAN*, was described in 1866 by Kussmaul and Maier. It is a multisystem, necrotizing vasculitis of small and medium-sized muscular arteries in which involvement of the renal and visceral arteries is characteristic. PAN does not involve pulmonary arteries, although bronchial vessels may be involved; granulomas, significant eosinophilia, and an allergic diathesis are not observed.

■ INCIDENCE AND PREVALENCE

It is difficult to establish an accurate incidence of PAN because previous reports have included PAN and microscopic polyangiitis as well as other related vasculitides. PAN, as currently defined, is felt to be a very uncommon disease.

■ PATHOLOGY AND PATHOGENESIS

The vascular lesion in PAN is a necrotizing inflammation of small and medium-sized muscular arteries. The lesions are segmental and tend to involve bifurcations and branchings of arteries. They may spread circumferentially to involve adjacent veins. However, involvement of venules is not seen in PAN and, if present, suggests microscopic polyangiitis (see below). In the acute stages of disease, polymorphonuclear neutrophils infiltrate all layers of the vessel wall and perivascular areas, which results in intimal proliferation and degeneration of the vessel wall. Mononuclear cells infiltrate the area as the lesions progress to the subacute and chronic stages. Fibrinoid necrosis of the vessels ensues with compromise of the lumen, thrombosis, infarction of the tissues supplied by the involved vessel, and, in some cases, hemorrhage. As the lesions heal, there is collagen deposition, which may lead to further occlusion of the vessel lumen. Aneurysmal dilations up to 1 cm in size along the involved arteries are characteristic of PAN. Granulomas and substantial eosinophilia with eosinophilic tissue infiltrations are not characteristically found and suggest Churg-Strauss syndrome (see above).

Multiple organ systems are involved, and the clinicopathologic findings reflect the degree and location of vessel involvement and the resulting ischemic changes. As mentioned above, pulmonary arteries are not involved in PAN, and bronchial artery involvement is uncommon. The pathology in the kidney in classic PAN is that of arteritis without glomerulonephritis. In patients with significant hypertension, typical pathologic features of glomerulosclerosis may be seen. In addition, pathologic sequelae of hypertension may be found elsewhere in the body.

The presence of a PAN-like vasculitis in patients with hepatitis B together with the isolation of circulating immune complexes composed of hepatitis B antigen and immunoglobulin, and the demonstration by immunofluorescence of hepatitis B antigen, IgM, and complement in the blood vessel walls, strongly suggest the role of immunologic phenomena in the pathogenesis of this disease. Hairy cell leukemia can be associated with PAN; the pathogenic mechanisms of this association are unclear.

■ CLINICAL AND LABORATORY MANIFESTATIONS

Nonspecific signs and symptoms are the hallmarks of PAN. Fever, weight loss, and malaise are present in over one-half of cases. Patients usually present with vague symptoms such as weakness, malaise, headache, abdominal pain, and myalgias that can rapidly progress to a fulminant illness. Specific complaints related to the vascular involvement within a particular organ system may also dominate the presenting clinical picture as well as the entire course of the illness (Table 326-6). In PAN, renal involvement most commonly manifests as hypertension, renal insufficiency, or hemorrhage due to microaneurysms.

TABLE 326-6 Clinical Manifestations Related to Organ System Involvement in Classic Polyarteritis Nodosa

Organ System	Percent Incidence	Clinical Manifestations
Renal	60	Renal failure, hypertension
Musculoskeletal	64	Arthritis, arthralgia, myalgia
Peripheral nervous system	51	Peripheral neuropathy, mononeuritis multiplex
Gastrointestinal tract	44	Abdominal pain, nausea and vomiting, bleeding, bowel infarction and perforation, cholecystitis, hepatic infarction, pancreatic infarction
Skin	43	Rash, purpura, nodules, cutaneous infarcts, livedo reticularis, Raynaud's phenomenon
Cardiac	36	Congestive heart failure, myocardial infarction, pericarditis
Genitourinary	25	Testicular, ovarian, or epididymal pain
Central nervous system	23	Cerebral vascular accident, altered mental status, seizure

Source: From TR Cupps, AS Fauci: *The Vasculitides*. Philadelphia, Saunders, 1981.

There are no diagnostic serologic tests for PAN. In >75% of patients, the leukocyte count is elevated with a predominance of neutrophils. Eosinophilia is seen only rarely and, when present at high levels, suggests the diagnosis of Churg-Strauss syndrome. The anemia of chronic disease may be seen, and an elevated ESR is almost always present. Other common laboratory findings reflect the particular organ involved. Hypergammaglobulinemia may be present, and all patients should be screened for hepatitis B. Antibodies against myeloperoxidase or proteinase-3 (ANCA) are rarely found in patients with PAN.

■ DIAGNOSIS

The diagnosis of PAN is based on the demonstration of characteristic findings of vasculitis on biopsy material of involved organs. In the absence of easily accessible tissue for biopsy, the arteriographic demonstration of involved vessels, particularly in the form of aneurysms of small and medium-sized arteries in the renal, hepatic, and visceral vasculature, is sufficient to make the diagnosis. Aneurysms of vessels are not pathognomonic of PAN; furthermore, aneurysms need not always be present, and arteriographic findings may be limited to stenotic segments and obliteration of vessels. Biopsy of symptomatic organs such as nodular skin lesions, painful testes, and nerve/muscle provides the highest diagnostic yields.

TREATMENT Polyarteritis Nodosa

The prognosis of untreated PAN is extremely poor, with a reported 5-year survival rate between 10 and 20%. Death usually results from gastrointestinal complications, particularly bowel infarcts and perforation, and cardiovascular causes. Intractable hypertension often compounds dysfunction in other organ systems, such as the kidneys, heart, and CNS, leading to additional late morbidity and mortality in PAN. With the introduction of treatment, survival rate has increased substantially. Favorable therapeutic results have been reported in PAN with the combination of prednisone and cyclophosphamide (see "Granulomatosis With Polyangiitis (Wegener's)" for a detailed description of this therapeutic regimen). In less severe cases of PAN, glucocorticoids alone have resulted in disease remission. In patients with hepatitis B who have a PAN-like vasculitis, antiviral therapy represents an important part of therapy and has been used in combination with glucocorticoids and plasma exchange. Careful attention to the treatment of hypertension can lessen the acute and late morbidity and mortality rates associated with renal, cardiac, and CNS complications of PAN. Following successful treatment, relapse of PAN has been estimated to occur in 10–20% of patients.

GIANT CELL ARTERITIS AND POLYMYALGIA RHEUMATICA

DEFINITION

Giant cell arteritis, also referred to as *cranial arteritis* or *temporal arteritis*, is an inflammation of medium- and large-sized arteries. It characteristically involves one or more branches of the carotid artery, particularly the temporal artery. However, it is a systemic disease that can involve arteries in multiple locations, particularly the aorta and its main branches.

Giant cell arteritis is closely associated with *polymyalgia rheumatica*, which is characterized by stiffness, aching, and pain in the muscles of the neck, shoulders, lower back, hips, and thighs. Most commonly, polymyalgia rheumatica occurs in isolation, but it may be seen in 40–50% of patients with giant cell arteritis. In addition, ~10–20% of patients who initially present with features of isolated polymyalgia rheumatica later go on to develop giant cell arteritis. This strong clinical association together with data from pathophysiologic studies has increasingly supported that giant cell arteritis and polymyalgia rheumatica represent differing clinical spectrums of a single disease process.

INCIDENCE AND PREVALENCE

Giant cell arteritis occurs almost exclusively in individuals >50 years. It is more common in women than in men and is rare in blacks. The incidence of giant cell arteritis varies widely in different studies and in different geographic regions. A high incidence has been found in Scandinavia and in regions of the United States with large Scandinavian populations, compared to a lower incidence in southern Europe. The annual incidence rates in individuals ≥50 years range from 6.9 to 32.8 per 100,000 population. Familial aggregation has been reported, as has an association with HLA-DR4. In addition, genetic linkage studies have demonstrated an association of giant cell arteritis with alleles at the HLA-DRB1 locus, particularly HLA-DRB1*04 variants. In Olmsted County, Minnesota, the annual incidence of polymyalgia rheumatica in individuals ≥50 years is 58.7 per 100,000 population.

PATHOLOGY AND PATHOGENESIS

Although the temporal artery is most frequently involved in giant cell arteritis, patients often have a systemic vasculitis of multiple medium- and large-sized arteries, which may go undetected. Histopathologically, the disease is a panarteritis with inflammatory mononuclear cell infiltrates within the vessel wall with frequent giant cell formation. There is proliferation of the intima and fragmentation of the internal elastic lamina. Pathophysiologic findings in organs result from the ischemia related to the involved vessels.

Experimental data support that giant cell arteritis is an antigen-driven disease in which activated T lymphocytes, macrophages, and dendritic cells play a critical role in the disease pathogenesis. Sequence analysis of the T cell receptor of tissue-infiltrating T cells in lesions of giant cell arteritis indicates restricted clonal expansion, suggesting the presence of an antigen residing in the arterial wall. Giant cell arteritis is believed to be initiated in the adventitia where CD4+ T cells enter through the vasa vasorum, become activated, and orchestrate macrophage differentiation. T cells recruited to vasculitic lesions in patients with giant cell arteritis produce predominantly IL-2 and IFN-γ, and the latter has been suggested to be involved in the progression to overt arteritis.

CLINICAL AND LABORATORY MANIFESTATIONS

Giant cell arteritis is most commonly characterized clinically by the complex of fever, anemia, high ESR, and headaches in a patient over the age of 50 years. Other phenotypic manifestations include features of systemic inflammation including malaise, fatigue, anorexia, weight loss, sweats, arthralgias, polymyalgia rheumatica, or large-vessel disease.

In patients with involvement of the cranial arteries, headache is the predominant symptom and may be associated with a tender, thickened, or nodular artery, which may pulsate early in the disease but may become occluded later. Scalp pain and claudication of the jaw and tongue may occur. A well-recognized and dreaded complication of giant cell arteritis, particularly in untreated patients, is ischemic optic neuropathy, which may lead to serious visual symptoms, even sudden blindness in some patients. However, most patients have complaints relating to the head or eyes before visual loss. Attention to such symptoms with institution of appropriate therapy (see below) will usually avoid this complication. Other cranial ischemic complications include strokes, scalp or tongue infarction.

Up to one-third of patients can have large-vessel disease that can be the primary presentation of giant cell arteritis or can emerge at a later point in patients who have had previous cranial arteritis features or polymyalgia rheumatica. Manifestations of large-vessel disease can include subclavian artery stenosis that can present as arm claudication or aortic aneurysms involving the thoracic and to a lesser degree the abdominal aorta, which carry risks of rupture or dissection.

Characteristic laboratory findings in addition to the elevated ESR include a normochromic or slightly hypochromic anemia. Liver function abnormalities are common, particularly increased alkaline phosphatase levels. Increased levels of IgG and complement have been reported. Levels of enzymes indicative of muscle damage such as serum creatine kinase are not elevated.

DIAGNOSIS

The diagnosis of giant cell arteritis and its associated clinicopathologic syndrome can often be suggested clinically by the demonstration of the complex of fever, anemia, and high ESR with or without symptoms of polymyalgia rheumatica in a patient >50 years. The diagnosis is confirmed by biopsy of the temporal artery. Since involvement of the vessel may be segmental, positive yield is increased by obtaining a biopsy segment of 3–5 cm together with serial sectioning of biopsy specimens. Ultrasonography of the temporal artery has been reported to be helpful in diagnosis. A temporal artery biopsy should be obtained as quickly as possible in the setting of ocular signs and symptoms, and under these circumstances therapy should not be delayed pending a biopsy. In this regard, it has been reported that temporal artery biopsies may show vasculitis even after ~14 days of glucocorticoid therapy. A dramatic clinical response to a trial of glucocorticoid therapy can further support the diagnosis.

Large vessel disease may be suggested by symptoms and findings on physical examination such as diminished pulses or bruits. It is confirmed by vascular imaging, most commonly through magnetic resonance or computed tomography.

Isolated polymyalgia rheumatica is a clinical diagnosis made by the presence of typical symptoms of stiffness, aching, and pain in the muscles of the hip and shoulder girdle, an increased ESR, the absence of clinical features suggestive of giant cell arteritis, and a prompt therapeutic response to low-dose prednisone.

TREATMENT Giant Cell Arteritis and Polymyalgia Rheumatica

Acute disease-related mortality directly from giant cell arteritis is very uncommon with fatalities occurring from cerebrovascular events or myocardial infarction. However, patients are at risk of late mortality from aortic aneurysm rupture or dissection as patients with giant cell arteritis are 18 times more likely to develop thoracic aortic aneurysms than the general population.

The goals of treatment in giant cell arteritis are to reduce symptoms and, most importantly, to prevent visual loss. The treatment approach for cranial and large-vessel disease in giant cell arteritis is currently the same. Giant cell arteritis and its associated symptoms are exquisitely sensitive to glucocorticoid therapy. Treatment should begin with prednisone, 40–60 mg/d for ~1 month, followed by a gradual tapering. When ocular signs and symptoms occur, consideration should be given for the use of methylprednisolone 1000 mg daily for 3 days to protect remaining vision. Although the optimal duration of glucocorticoid therapy has not been established, most series have found that patients require treatment for ≥2 years. Symptom recurrence during prednisone tapering develops in 60–85% of patients with giant cell arteritis, requiring a dosage increase. The ESR can serve as a useful indicator of inflammatory disease activity in monitoring and tapering therapy and can be used to judge the pace of the tapering schedule. However, minor increases in the ESR can occur as glucocorticoids are being tapered and do not necessarily reflect an exacerbation of arteritis, particularly if the patient remains symptom-free. Under these circumstances, the tapering should continue with caution. Glucocorticoid toxicity occurs in 35–65% of patients and represents an important cause of patient morbidity. Aspirin 81 mg daily has been found to reduce the occurrence of cranial ischemic complications in giant cell arteritis and should be given in addition to glucocorticoids in patients who do not have contraindications. The use of weekly methotrexate as a glucocorticoid-sparing agent has been examined in two randomized placebo-controlled trials that reached conflicting conclusions. Infliximab, a monoclonal antibody to TNF, was studied in a randomized trial and was not found to provide benefit.

Patients with isolated polymyalgia rheumatica respond promptly to prednisone, which can be started at a lower dose of 10–20 mg/d. Similar to giant cell arteritis, the ESR can serve as a useful indicator in monitoring and prednisone reduction. Recurrent polymyalgia symptoms develop in the majority of patients during prednisone tapering. One study of weekly methotrexate found that the use of this drug reduced the prednisone dose on average by only 1 mg and did not decrease prednisone-related side effects. A randomized trial in polymyalgia rheumatica did not find infliximab to lessen relapse or glucocorticoid requirements.

TAKAYASU'S ARTERITIS

DEFINITION

Takayasu's arteritis is an inflammatory and stenotic disease of medium- and large-sized arteries characterized by a strong predilection for the aortic arch and its branches. For this reason, it is often referred to as the *aortic arch syndrome.*

INCIDENCE AND PREVALENCE

Takayasu's arteritis is an uncommon disease with an estimated annual incidence rate of 1.2–2.6 cases per million. It is most prevalent in adolescent girls and young women. Although it is more common in Asia, it is neither racially nor geographically restricted.

PATHOLOGY AND PATHOGENESIS

The disease involves medium- and large-sized arteries, with a strong predilection for the aortic arch and its branches; the pulmonary artery may also be involved. The most commonly affected arteries seen by arteriography are listed in Table 326-7. The involvement of the major branches of the aorta is much more marked at their origin than distally. The disease is a panarteritis with inflammatory mononuclear cell infiltrates and occasionally giant cells. There are marked intimal proliferation and fibrosis, scarring and vascularization of the media, and disruption and degeneration of the elastic lamina. Narrowing of the lumen occurs with or without thrombosis. The vasa vasorum are frequently involved. Pathologic changes in various organs reflect the compromise of blood flow through the involved vessels.

Immunopathogenic mechanisms, the precise nature of which is uncertain, are suspected in this disease. As with several of the vasculitis syndromes, circulating immune complexes have been demonstrated, but their pathogenic significance is unclear.

TABLE 326-7 Frequency of Arteriographic Abnormalities and Potential Clinical Manifestations of Arterial Involvement in Takayasu's Arteritis

Artery	Percent of Arteriographic Abnormalities	Potential Clinical Manifestations
Subclavian	93	Arm claudication, Raynaud's phenomenon
Common carotid	58	Visual changes, syncope, transient ischemic attacks, stroke
Abdominal aorta[a]	47	Abdominal pain, nausea, vomiting
Renal	38	Hypertension, renal failure
Aortic arch or root	35	Aortic insufficiency, congestive heart failure
Vertebral	35	Visual changes, dizziness
Coeliac axis[a]	18	Abdominal pain, nausea, vomiting
Superior mesenteric[a]	18	Abdominal pain, nausea, vomiting
Iliac	17	Leg claudication
Pulmonary	10–40	Atypical chest pain, dyspnea
Coronary	<10	Chest pain, myocardial infarction

[a]Arteriographic lesions at these locations are usually asymptomatic but may potentially cause these symptoms.
Source: Kerr et al.

■ CLINICAL AND LABORATORY MANIFESTATIONS

Takayasu's arteritis is a systemic disease with generalized as well as vascular symptoms. The generalized symptoms include malaise, fever, night sweats, arthralgias, anorexia, and weight loss, which may occur months before vessel involvement is apparent. These symptoms may merge into those related to vascular compromise and organ ischemia. Pulses are commonly absent in the involved vessels, particularly the subclavian artery. The frequency of arteriographic abnormalities and the potentially associated clinical manifestations are listed in Table 326-7. Hypertension occurs in 32–93% of patients and contributes to renal, cardiac, and cerebral injury.

Characteristic laboratory findings include an elevated ESR, mild anemia, and elevated immunoglobulin levels.

■ DIAGNOSIS

The diagnosis of Takayasu's arteritis should be suspected strongly in a young woman who develops a decrease or absence of peripheral pulses, discrepancies in blood pressure, and arterial bruits. The diagnosis is confirmed by the characteristic pattern on arteriography, which includes irregular vessel walls, stenosis, poststenotic dilation, aneurysm formation, occlusion, and evidence of increased collateral circulation. Complete aortic arteriography by catheter-directed dye arteriography or magnetic resonance arteriography should be obtained in order to fully delineate the distribution and degree of arterial disease. Histopathologic demonstration of inflamed vessels adds confirmatory data; however, tissue is rarely readily available for examination.

TREATMENT Takayasu's Arteritis

The long-term outcome of patients with Takayasu's arteritis has varied widely between studies. Although two North American reports found overall survival to be ≥94%, the 5-year mortality rate from other studies has ranged from 0 to 35%. Disease-related mortality most often occurs from congestive heart failure, cerebrovascular events, myocardial infarction, aneurysm rupture, or renal failure. Even in the absence of life-threatening disease, Takayasu's arteritis can be associated with significant morbidity. The course of the disease is variable, and although spontaneous remissions may occur, Takayasu's arteritis is most often chronic and relapsing. Although glucocorticoid therapy in doses of 40–60 mg prednisone per day alleviates symptoms, there are no convincing studies that indicate that they increase survival. The combination of glucocorticoid therapy for acute signs and symptoms and an aggressive surgical and/or arterioplastic approach to stenosed vessels has markedly improved outcome and decreased morbidity by lessening the risk of stroke, correcting hypertension due to renal artery stenosis, and improving blood flow to ischemic viscera and limbs. Unless it is urgently required, surgical correction of stenosed arteries should be undertaken only when the vascular inflammatory process is well controlled with medical therapy. In individuals who are refractory to or unable to taper glucocorticoids, methotrexate in doses up to 25 mg per week has yielded encouraging results. Preliminary results with anti-TNF therapies have been encouraging, but will require further study through randomized trials to determine efficacy.

HENOCH-SCHÖNLEIN PURPURA

■ DEFINITION

Henoch-Schönlein purpura, also referred to as *anaphylactoid purpura*, is a small-vessel vasculitis characterized by palpable purpura (most commonly distributed over the buttocks and lower extremities), arthralgias, gastrointestinal signs and symptoms, and glomerulonephritis.

■ INCIDENCE AND PREVALENCE

Henoch-Schönlein purpura is usually seen in children; most patients range in age from 4 to 7 years; however, the disease may also be seen in infants and adults. It is not a rare disease; in one series it accounted for between 5 and 24 admissions per year at a pediatric hospital. The male-to-female ratio is 1.5:1. A seasonal variation with a peak incidence in spring has been noted.

■ PATHOLOGY AND PATHOGENESIS

The presumptive pathogenic mechanism for Henoch-Schönlein purpura is immune-complex deposition. A number of inciting antigens have been suggested including upper respiratory tract infections, various drugs, foods, insect bites, and immunizations. IgA is the antibody class most often seen in the immune complexes and has been demonstrated in the renal biopsies of these patients.

■ CLINICAL AND LABORATORY MANIFESTATIONS

In pediatric patients, palpable purpura is seen in virtually all patients; most patients develop polyarthralgias in the absence of frank arthritis. Gastrointestinal involvement, which is seen in almost 70% of pediatric patients, is characterized by colicky abdominal pain usually associated with nausea, vomiting, diarrhea, or constipation and is frequently accompanied by the passage of blood and mucus per rectum; bowel intussusception may occur. Renal involvement occurs in 10–50% of patients and is usually characterized by mild glomerulonephritis leading to proteinuria and microscopic hematuria, with red blood cell casts in the majority of patients (Chap. 283); it usually resolves spontaneously without therapy. Rarely, a progressive glomerulonephritis will develop. In adults, presenting symptoms are most frequently related to the skin and joints, while initial complaints related to the gut are less common. Although certain studies have found that renal disease is more frequent and more severe in adults, this has not been a consistent finding. However, the course of renal disease in adults may be more insidious and thus requires close follow-up. Myocardial involvement can occur in adults but is rare in children.

Laboratory studies generally show a mild leukocytosis, a normal platelet count, and occasionally eosinophilia. Serum complement components are normal, and IgA levels are elevated in about one-half of patients.

■ DIAGNOSIS

The diagnosis of Henoch-Schönlein purpura is based on clinical signs and symptoms. Skin biopsy specimen can be useful in confirming leukocytoclastic vasculitis with IgA and C3 deposition by immunofluorescence. Renal biopsy is rarely needed for diagnosis but may provide prognostic information in some patients.

TREATMENT Henoch-Schönlein Purpura

The prognosis of Henoch-Schönlein purpura is excellent. Mortality is exceedingly rare, and 1–5% of children progress to end-stage renal disease. Most patients recover completely, and some do not require therapy. Treatment is similar for adults and children. When glucocorticoid therapy is required, prednisone, in doses of 1 mg/kg per day and tapered according to clinical response, has been shown to be useful in decreasing tissue edema, arthralgias, and abdominal discomfort; however, it has not proved beneficial in the treatment of skin or renal disease and does not appear to shorten the duration of active disease or lessen the chance of recurrence. Patients with rapidly progressive glomerulonephritis have been anecdotally reported to benefit from intensive plasma exchange combined with cytotoxic drugs. Disease recurrences have been reported in 10–40% of patients.

IDIOPATHIC CUTANEOUS VASCULITIS

DEFINITION

The term *cutaneous vasculitis* is defined broadly as inflammation of the blood vessels of the dermis. Due to its heterogeneity, cutaneous vasculitis has been described by a variety of terms including *hypersensitivity vasculitis* and *cutaneous leukocytoclastic angiitis*. However, cutaneous vasculitis is not one specific disease but a manifestation that can be seen in a variety of settings. In >70% of cases, cutaneous vasculitis occurs either as part of a primary systemic vasculitis or as a secondary vasculitis related to an inciting agent or an underlying disease (see "Secondary Vasculitis," below). In the remaining 30% of cases, cutaneous vasculitis occurs idiopathically.

INCIDENCE AND PREVALENCE

Cutaneous vasculitis represents the most commonly encountered vasculitis in clinical practice. The exact incidence of idiopathic cutaneous vasculitis has not been determined due to the predilection for cutaneous vasculitis to be associated with an underlying process and the variability of its clinical course.

PATHOLOGY AND PATHOGENESIS

The typical histopathologic feature of cutaneous vasculitis is the presence of vasculitis of small vessels. Postcapillary venules are the most commonly involved vessels; capillaries and arterioles may be involved less frequently. This vasculitis is characterized by a *leukocytoclasis*, a term that refers to the nuclear debris remaining from the neutrophils that have infiltrated in and around the vessels during the acute stages. In the subacute or chronic stages, mononuclear cells predominate; in certain subgroups, eosinophilic infiltration is seen. Erythrocytes often extravasate from the involved vessels, leading to palpable purpura.

CLINICAL AND LABORATORY MANIFESTATIONS

The hallmark of idiopathic cutaneous vasculitis is the predominance of skin involvement. Skin lesions may appear typically as palpable purpura; however, other cutaneous manifestations of the vasculitis may occur, including macules, papules, vesicles, bullae, subcutaneous nodules, ulcers, and recurrent or chronic urticaria. The skin lesions may be pruritic or even quite painful, with a burning or stinging sensation. Lesions most commonly occur in the lower extremities in ambulatory patients or in the sacral area in bedridden patients due to the effects of hydrostatic forces on the postcapillary venules. Edema may accompany certain lesions, and hyperpigmentation often occurs in areas of recurrent or chronic lesions.

There are no specific laboratory tests diagnostic of idiopathic cutaneous vasculitis. A mild leukocytosis with or without eosinophilia is characteristic, as is an elevated ESR. Laboratory studies should be aimed toward ruling out features to suggest an underlying disease or a systemic vasculitis.

DIAGNOSIS

The diagnosis of cutaneous vasculitis is made by the demonstration of vasculitis on biopsy. An important diagnostic principle in patients with cutaneous vasculitis is to search for an etiology of the vasculitis—be it an exogenous agent, such as a drug or an infection, or an endogenous condition, such as an underlying disease (Fig. 326-1). In addition, a careful physical and laboratory examination should be performed to rule out the possibility of systemic vasculitis. This should start with the least invasive diagnostic approach and proceed to the more invasive only if clinically indicated.

TREATMENT Idiopathic Cutaneous Vasculitis

When an antigenic stimulus is recognized as the precipitating factor in the cutaneous vasculitis, it should be removed; if this is a microbe, appropriate antimicrobial therapy should be instituted. If the vasculitis is associated with another underlying disease, treatment of the latter often results in resolution of the former. In situations where disease is apparently self-limited, no therapy, except possibly symptomatic therapy, is indicated. When cutaneous vasculitis persists and when there is no evidence of an inciting agent, an associated disease, or an underlying systemic vasculitis, the decision to treat should be based on weighing the balance between the degree of symptoms and the risk of treatment. Some cases of idiopathic cutaneous vasculitis resolve spontaneously, while others remit and relapse. In those patients with persistent vasculitis, a variety of therapeutic regimens have been tried with variable results. In general, the treatment of idiopathic cutaneous vasculitis has not been satisfactory. Fortunately, since the disease is generally limited to the skin, this lack of consistent response to therapy usually does not lead to a life-threatening situation. Agents with which there have been anecdotal reports of success include dapsone, colchicine, hydroxychloroquine, and nonsteroidal anti-inflammatory agents. Glucocorticoids are often used in the treatment of idiopathic cutaneous vasculitis. Therapy is usually instituted as prednisone, 1 mg/kg per day, with rapid tapering where possible, either directly to discontinuation or by conversion to an alternate-day regimen followed by ultimate discontinuation. In cases that prove refractory to glucocorticoids, a trial of a cytotoxic agent may be indicated. Patients with chronic vasculitis isolated to cutaneous venules rarely respond dramatically to any therapeutic regimen, and cytotoxic agents should be used only as a last resort in these patients. Methotrexate and azathioprine have been used in such situations in anecdotal reports. Although cyclophosphamide is the most effective therapy for the systemic vasculitides, it should almost never be used for idiopathic cutaneous vasculitis because of the potential toxicity.

CRYOGLOBULINEMIC VASCULITIS

DEFINITION

Cryoglobulins are cold-precipitable monoclonal or polyclonal immunoglobulins. Cryoglobulinemia may be associated with a systemic vasculitis characterized by palpable purpura, arthralgias, weakness, neuropathy, and glomerulonephritis. Although this can be observed in association with a variety of underlying disorders including multiple myeloma, lymphoproliferative disorders, connective tissue diseases, infection, and liver disease, in many instances it appeared to be idiopathic. Because of the apparent absence of an underlying disease and the presence of cryoprecipitate containing oligoclonal/polyclonal immunoglobulins, this entity was referred to as *essential mixed cryoglobulinemia*. Since the discovery of hepatitis C, it has been established that the vast majority of patients who were considered to have essential mixed cryoglobulinemia have cryoglobulinemic vasculitis related to hepatitis C infection.

INCIDENCE AND PREVALENCE

The incidence of cryoglobulinemic vasculitis has not been established. It has been estimated, however, that 5% of patients with chronic hepatitis C will develop cryoglobulinemic vasculitis.

PATHOLOGY AND PATHOGENESIS

Skin biopsies in cryoglobulinemic vasculitis reveal an inflammatory infiltrate surrounding and involving blood vessel walls, with fibrinoid necrosis, endothelial cell hyperplasia, and hemorrhage. Deposition of immunoglobulin and complement is common. Abnormalities of uninvolved skin including basement membrane alterations and deposits in vessel walls may be found. Membranoproliferative glomerulonephritis is responsible for 80% of all renal lesions in cryoglobulinemic vasculitis.

The association between hepatitis C and cryoglobulinemic vasculitis has been supported by the high frequency of documented hepatitis C infection, the presence of hepatitis C RNA and anti–hepatitis C antibodies in serum cryoprecipitates, evidence of hepatitis C antigens in vasculitic skin lesions, and the effectiveness of antiviral therapy (see below). Current evidence suggests that in the majority of cases, cryoglobulinemic vasculitis occurs when an aberrant immune response to hepatitis C infection leads to the formation of immune complexes consisting of hepatitis C antigens, polyclonal hepatitis C–specific IgG, and monoclonal IgM rheumatoid factor. The deposition of these immune complexes in blood vessel walls triggers an inflammatory cascade that results in cryoglobulinemic vasculitis.

CLINICAL AND LABORATORY MANIFESTATIONS

The most common clinical manifestations of cryoglobulinemic vasculitis are cutaneous vasculitis, arthritis, peripheral neuropathy, and glomerulonephritis. Renal disease develops in 10–30% of patients. Life-threatening rapidly progressive glomerulonephritis or vasculitis of the CNS, gastrointestinal tract, or heart occurs infrequently.

The presence of circulating cryoprecipitates is the fundamental finding in cryoglobulinemic vasculitis. Rheumatoid factor is almost always found and may be a useful clue to the disease when cryoglobulins are not detected. Hypocomplementemia occurs in 90% of patients. An elevated ESR and anemia occur frequently. Evidence for hepatitis C infection must be sought in all patients by testing for hepatitis C antibodies and hepatitis C RNA.

TREATMENT Cryoglobulinemic Vasculitis

Acute mortality directly from cryoglobulinemic vasculitis is uncommon, but the presence of glomerulonephritis is a poor prognostic sign for overall outcome. In such patients, 15% progress to end-stage renal disease, with 40% later experiencing fatal cardiovascular disease, infection, or liver failure. As indicated above, the majority of cases are associated with hepatitis C infection. In such patients, treatment with IFN-α and ribavirin (Chap. 304) can prove beneficial. Clinical improvement with antiviral therapy is dependent on the virologic response. Patients who clear hepatitis C from the blood have objective improvement in their vasculitis along with significant reductions in levels of circulating cryoglobulins, IgM, and rheumatoid factor. However, substantial portions of patients with hepatitis C do not have a sustained virologic response to such therapy, and the vasculitis typically relapses with the return of viremia. While transient improvement can be observed with glucocorticoids, a complete response is seen in only 7% of patients. Plasmapheresis and cytotoxic agents have been used in anecdotal reports. These observations have not been confirmed, and such therapies carry significant risks.

BEHÇET'S SYNDROME

Behçet's syndrome is a clinicopathologic entity characterized by recurrent episodes of oral and genital ulcers, iritis, and cutaneous lesions. The underlying pathologic process is a leukocytoclastic venulitis, although vessels of any size and in any organ can be involved. This disorder is described in detail in Chap. 327.

ISOLATED VASCULITIS OF THE CENTRAL NERVOUS SYSTEM

Isolated vasculitis of the CNS, which is also called *primary angiitis of the CNS* (PACNS), is an uncommon clinicopathologic entity characterized by vasculitis restricted to the vessels of the CNS without other apparent systemic vasculitis. The inflammatory process is usually composed of mononuclear cell infiltrates with or without granuloma formation.

Patients may present with headaches, altered mental function, and focal neurologic defects. Systemic symptoms are generally absent. Devastating neurologic abnormalities may occur depending on the extent of vessel involvement. The diagnosis can be suggested by abnormal MRI of the brain, an abnormal lumbar puncture, and/or demonstration of characteristic vessel abnormalities on arteriography (Fig. 326-4), but it is confirmed by biopsy of the brain parenchyma and leptomeninges. In the absence of a brain biopsy, care should be taken not to misinterpret as true primary vasculitis arteriographic abnormalities that might actually be related to another cause. An important entity in the differential diagnosis is reversible cerebral vasoconstrictive syndrome, which typically presents with "thunderclap" headache and is associated with arteriographic abnormalities that mimic PACNS that are reversible. Other diagnostic considerations include infection, atherosclerosis, emboli, connective tissue disease, sarcoidosis, malignancy, and drug-associated causes. The prognosis of granulomatous PACNS is poor; however, some reports indicate that glucocorticoid therapy, alone or together with cyclophosphamide administered as described above, has induced clinical remissions.

COGAN'S SYNDROME

Cogan's syndrome is characterized by interstitial keratitis together with vestibuloauditory symptoms. It may be associated with a systemic vasculitis, particularly aortitis with involvement of the aortic

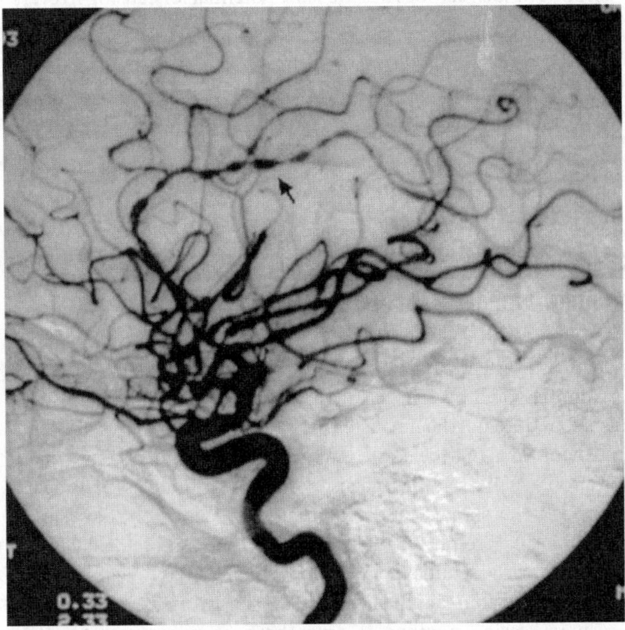

Figure 326-4 Cerebral arteriogram from a 32-year-old male with central nervous system vasculitis. Dramatic beading (*arrow*) typical of vasculitis is seen.

valve. Glucocorticoids are the mainstay of treatment. Initiation of treatment as early as possible after the onset of hearing loss improves the likelihood of a favorable outcome.

KAWASAKI DISEASE

Kawasaki disease, also referred to as *mucocutaneous lymph node syndrome,* is an acute, febrile, multisystem disease of children. Some 80% of cases occur prior to the age of 5, with the peak incidence occurring at ≤2 years. It is characterized by nonsuppurative cervical adenitis and changes in the skin and mucous membranes such as edema; congested conjunctivae; erythema of the oral cavity, lips, and palms; and desquamation of the skin of the fingertips. Although the disease is generally benign and self-limited, it is associated with coronary artery aneurysms in ~25% of cases, with an overall case-fatality rate of 0.5–2.8%. These complications usually occur between the third and fourth weeks of illness during the convalescent stage. Vasculitis of the coronary arteries is seen in almost all the fatal cases that have been autopsied. There is typical intimal proliferation and infiltration of the vessel wall with mononuclear cells. Beadlike aneurysms and thromboses may be seen along the artery. Other manifestations include pericarditis, myocarditis, myocardial ischemia and infarction, and cardiomegaly.

Apart from the up to 2.8% of patients who develop fatal complications, the prognosis of this disease for uneventful recovery is excellent. High-dose IV γ globulin (2 g/kg as a single infusion over 10 h) together with aspirin (100 mg/kg per day for 14 days followed by 3–5 mg/kg per day for several weeks) have been shown to be effective in reducing the prevalence of coronary artery abnormalities when administered early in the course of the disease. Surgery may be necessary for Kawasaki disease patients that have giant coronary artery aneurysms or other coronary complications. Surgical treatment most commonly includes thromboendarterectomy, thrombus clearing, aneurysmal reconstruction, and coronary artery bypass grafting.

POLYANGIITIS OVERLAP SYNDROMES

Some patients with systemic vasculitis manifest clinicopathologic characteristics that do not fit precisely into any specific disease but have overlapping features of different vasculitides. Active systemic vasculitis in such settings has the same potential for causing irreversible organ system damage as when it occurs in one of the defined syndromes listed in Table 326-1. The diagnostic and therapeutic considerations as well as the prognosis for these patients depend on the sites and severity of active vasculitis. Patients with vasculitis that could potentially cause irreversible damage to a major organ system should be treated as described under "Granulomatosis With Polyangiitis (Wegener's)."

SECONDARY VASCULITIS

■ DRUG-INDUCED VASCULITIS

Vasculitis associated with drug reactions usually presents as palpable purpura that may be generalized or limited to the lower extremities or other dependent areas; however, urticarial lesions, ulcers, and hemorrhagic blisters may also occur (Chap. 55). Signs and symptoms may be limited to the skin, although systemic manifestations such as fever, malaise, and polyarthralgias may occur. Although the skin is the predominant organ involved, systemic vasculitis may result from drug reactions. Drugs that have been implicated in vasculitis include allopurinol, thiazides, gold, sulfonamides, phenytoin, and penicillin (Chap. 55).

An increasing number of drugs have been reported to cause vasculitis associated with antimyeloperoxidase ANCA. Of these, the best evidence of causality exists for hydralazine and propylthiouracil. The clinical manifestations in ANCA-positive drug-induced vasculitis can range from cutaneous lesions to glomerulonephritis and pulmonary hemorrhage. Outside of drug discontinuation, treatment should be based on the severity of the vasculitis. Patients with immediately life-threatening small-vessel vasculitis should initially be treated with glucocorticoids and cyclophosphamide as described for granulomatosis with polyangiitis (Wegener's). Following clinical improvement, consideration may be given for tapering such agents along a more rapid schedule.

■ SERUM SICKNESS AND SERUM SICKNESS–LIKE REACTIONS

These reactions are characterized by the occurrence of fever, urticaria, polyarthralgias, and lymphadenopathy 7–10 days after primary exposure and 2–4 days after secondary exposure to a heterologous protein (classic serum sickness) or a nonprotein drug such as penicillin or sulfa (serum sickness–like reaction). Most of the manifestations are not due to a vasculitis; however, occasional patients will have typical cutaneous venulitis that may progress rarely to a systemic vasculitis.

■ VASCULITIS ASSOCIATED WITH OTHER UNDERLYING DISEASES

Certain *infections* may directly trigger an inflammatory vasculitic process. For example, rickettsias can invade and proliferate in the endothelial cells of small blood vessels causing a vasculitis (Chap. 174). In addition, the inflammatory response around blood vessels associated with certain systemic fungal diseases such as histoplasmosis (Chap. 199) may mimic a primary vasculitic process. A leukocytoclastic vasculitis predominantly involving the skin with occasional involvement of other organ systems may be a minor component of many other infections. These include *subacute bacterial endocarditis, Epstein-Barr virus infection, HIV infection,* as well as a number of other infections.

Vasculitis can be associated with certain *malignancies,* particularly lymphoid or reticuloendothelial neoplasms. Leukocytoclastic venulitis confined to the skin is the most common finding; however, widespread systemic vasculitis may occur. Of particular note is the association of *hairy cell leukemia* (Chap. 110) with PAN.

A number of *connective tissue diseases* have vasculitis as a secondary manifestation of the underlying primary process. Foremost among these are *systemic lupus erythematosus* (Chap. 319), *rheumatoid arthritis* (Chap. 321), *inflammatory myositis* (Chap. 388), *relapsing polychondritis* (Chap. 328), and *Sjögren's syndrome* (Chap. 324). The most common form of vasculitis in these conditions is the small-vessel venulitis isolated to the skin. However, certain patients may develop a fulminant systemic necrotizing vasculitis.

Secondary vasculitis has also been observed in association with *ulcerative colitis, congenital deficiencies of various complement components, retroperitoneal fibrosis, primary biliary cirrhosis,* α_1*-antitrypsin deficiency,* and *intestinal bypass surgery.*

FURTHER READINGS

de Groot K et al: Randomized trial of cyclophosphamide versus methotrexate for induction of remission in early systemic antineutrophil cytoplasmic antibody-associated vasculitis. Arthritis Rheum 52:2461, 2005

Finkielman JD et al: Antiproteinase 3 antineutrophil cytoplasmic antibodies and disease activity in Wegener granulomatosis. Ann Intern Med 147:611, 2007

Guillevin L et al: Microscopic polyangiitis. Clinical and laboratory findings in eighty-five patients. Arthritis Rheum 42:421, 1999

Hoffman GS, Specks U: Antineutrophil cytoplasmic antibodies. Arthritis Rheum 41:1521, 1998

——— et al: Wegener's granulomatosis: An analysis of 158 patients. Ann Intern Med 116:488, 1992

Jayne D et al: A randomized trial of maintenance therapy for vasculitis associated with antineutrophil cytoplasmic autoantibodies. N Engl J Med 349:36, 2003

Jennette JC et al: Nomenclature of systemic vasculitis. Proposal of an international consensus conference. Arthritis Rheum 37:187, 1994

Kerr G et al: Takayasu arteritis. Ann Intern Med 120:919, 1994

Langford CA et al: Use of a cyclophosphamide-induction methotrexate-maintenance regimen for the treatment of Wegener's granulomatosis: Extended follow-up and rate of relapse. Am J Med 114:463, 2003

Ludviksson BR et al: Active Wegener's granulomatosis is associated with HLA-DR+ CD4+ T cells exhibiting an unbalanced Th-1 type T cell cytokine pattern: Reversal with IL-10. J Immunol 160:3602, 1998

Sneller MC, Fauci AS: Pathogenesis of vasculitis syndromes. Med Clin North Am 81:221, 1997

Stone JH et al: Rituximab versus cyclophosphamide for ANCA-associated vasculitis. N Engl J Med 363:221, 2010

CHAPTER 327

Behçet's Syndrome

Haralampos M. Moutsopoulos

DEFINITION, INCIDENCE, AND PREVALENCE

Behçet's syndrome is a multisystem disorder presenting with recurrent oral and genital ulcerations as well as ocular involvement. The diagnosis is clinical and based on internationally agreed diagnostic criteria (Table 327-1).

The syndrome affects young males and females from the Mediterranean region, the Middle East, and the Far East, suggesting a link with the ancient Silk Route. Males and females are affected equally, but males often have more severe disease. Blacks are very infrequently affected.

PATHOGENESIS

The etiology and pathogenesis of this syndrome remain obscure. The main pathologic lesion is systemic perivasculitis with early neutrophil infiltration and endothelial swelling. In some patients, diffuse inflammatory disease, involving all layers of large vessels and resulting to formation of pseudoaneurysms, suggests vasculitis of vasa vasorum. Apart from neutrophils, increased numbers of infiltrating CD4+ T cells are observed. Circulating autoantibodies against α-enolase of endothelial cells, selenium binding protein and anti-*Saccharomyces cerevisiae antibodies* (ASCA—characteristic of Crohn's A recent genome-wide association study, confirmed the known association of Behçet's disease with HLA-B*51 and identified a second, independent association within the MHC Class I region. In addition, an association with IL10 and the IL23R-IL12RB2 locus were also observed. Interestingly, the disease-associated IL10 variant was correlated with diminished mRNA expression and low protein production.

TABLE 327-1 Diagnostic Criteria of Behçet's Disease

Recurrent oral ulceration plus two of the following:
Recurrent genital ulceration
Eye lesions
Skin lesions
Pathergy test

CLINICAL FEATURES

The recurrent aphthous ulcerations are a sine qua non for the diagnosis. The ulcers are usually painful, are shallow or deep with a central yellowish necrotic base, appear singly or in crops, and are located anywhere in the oral cavity. Small ulcers, less than 10 mm in diameter are seen in 85% of patients, while large or herpetiform lesions are less frequent. The ulcers persist for 1–2 weeks and subside without leaving scars. The genital ulcers are less common but more specific, are painful, do not affect the glans penis or urethra, and produce scrotal scars.

Skin involvement is observed in 80% of patients and includes folliculitis, erythema nodosum, an acne-like exanthem, and, infrequently, vasculitis, Sweet's syndrome, and pyoderma gangrenosum. Nonspecific skin inflammatory reactivity to any scratches or intradermal saline injection (pathergy test) is a common and specific manifestation.

Eye involvement with scarring and bilateral panuveitis is the most dreaded complication, since it occasionally progresses rapidly to blindness. The eye disease, occurring in 50% of patients, is usually present at the onset but may also develop within the first few years. In addition to iritis, posterior uveitis, retinal vessel occlusions, and optic neuritis can be seen in some patients with the syndrome.

Non-deforming arthritis or arthralgias are seen in a 50% of patients and affects the knees and ankles.

Superficial or deep peripheral vein thrombosis is seen in 30% of patients. Pulmonary emboli are a rare complication. The superior vena cava is obstructed occasionally, producing a dramatic clinical picture. Arterial involvement occurs in less than 5% of patients and presents with aortitis or peripheral arterial aneurysm and arterial thrombosis. Pulmonary artery vasculitis presenting with dyspnea, cough, chest pain, hemoptysis, and infiltrates on chest roentgenograms has been reported in 5% of patients and should be differentiated from thromboembolic disease since it warrants anti-inflammatory and not thrombolytic therapy.

Neurologic involvement (5–10%) appears mainly in the parenchymal form (80%); it is associated with brainstem involvement and has a serious prognosis (*CNS-Behçet's syndrome*). IL-6 is persistently raised in cerebrospinal fluid of these patients. Dural sinus thrombi (20%) are associated with headache and increased intracranial pressure. MRI and/or proton magnetic resonance spectroscopy (MRS) are very sensitive and should be employed if CNS-Behçet's syndrome is suspected.

Gastrointestinal involvement is seen more frequently in patients from Japan and consists of mucosal ulcerations of the gut, resembling Crohn's disease.

Epididymitis is seen in 5% of patients, while amyloidosis of AA type and glomerulonephritis are uncommon.

Laboratory findings are mainly nonspecific indices of inflammation, such as leukocytosis and elevated erythrocyte sedimentation rate, as well as C-reactive protein levels.

TREATMENT Behçet's Syndrome

The severity of the syndrome usually abates with time. Apart from the patients with CNS-Behçet's syndrome and major vessel disease, the life expectancy seems to be normal and the only serious complication is blindness.

Mucous membrane involvement may respond to topical glucocorticoids in the form of mouthwash or paste. In more serious cases, thalidomide (100 mg/d) is effective. Thrombophlebitis is treated with aspirin, 325 mg/d. Colchicine can be beneficial for the mucocutaneous manifestations and arthritis. Uveitis and CNS-Behçet's syndrome require systemic glucocorticoid therapy (prednisone, 1 mg/kg per day) and azathioprine (2–3 mg/kg per day). Cyclosporin (5mg/kg) has been used for sight-threatening uveitis, alone or in combination with azathioprine. Pulse doses of cyclophosphamide are useful early in the course of the disease, for pulmonary or peripheral arterial aneurysms. Recent recommendations for anti–tumor necrosis factor therapy suggest that they may serve as an add-on immunosuppressive therapy in patients with panuveitis refractory or intolerant to other immunosuppressives.

FURTHER READINGS

Al-Araji A, Kidd DP: Neuro- Behçet's disease: Epidemiology, clinical characteristics, and management. Lancet Neurol 8:192, 2009

Hatemi G et al: Eular recommendations for the management of Behçet's disease. Ann Rheum Dis 67:1656, 2008

Kural-Seyahi E et al: The long-term mortality and morbidity of Behçet syndrome: A 2-decade outcome survey of 387 patients followed at a dedicated center. Medicine (Baltimore) 82:60, 2003

Lee KH et al: Human alpha-enolase from endothelial cells as a target antigen of anti-endothelial cell antibody in Behçet's disease. Arthritis Rheum 48:2025, 2003

Remmers EF et al Genome-wide association study identifies variants in the MHC class I, IL10, and IL23R-IL12RB2 regions associated with Behçet's disease. Nat Genet 42:698, 2010

Yurdakul S, Yazizi H: Behçet's syndrome. Best Pract Res Clin Rheumatol 22:793, 2008

CHAPTER 328 Relapsing Polychondritis

Carol A. Langford

Relapsing polychondritis is an uncommon disorder of unknown cause characterized by inflammation of cartilage predominantly affecting the ears, nose, and laryngotracheobronchial tree. Other manifestations include scleritis, neurosensory hearing loss, polyarthritis, cardiac abnormalities, skin lesions, and glomerulonephritis. Relapsing polychondritis has been estimated to have an incidence of 3.5 per million population per year. The peak age of onset is between the ages of 40–50 years, but relapsing polychondritis may affect children and the elderly. It is found in all races, and both sexes are equally affected. No familial tendency is apparent. A significantly higher frequency of HLA-DR4 has been found in patients with relapsing polychondritis than in healthy individuals. A predominant subtype allele(s) of HLA-DR4 was not found. Approximately 30% of patients with relapsing polychondritis will have another rheumatologic disorder, the most frequent being systemic vasculitis, followed by rheumatoid arthritis, systemic lupus erythematosus (SLE), Sjögren's syndrome, or the spondyloarthritides. Nonrheumatic disorders associated with relapsing polychondritis include inflammatory bowel disease, primary biliary cirrhosis, and myelodysplastic syndrome (Table 328-1). In most cases, these disorders antedate the appearance of relapsing polychondritis, usually by months or years.

TABLE 328-1 Disorders Associated With Relapsing Polychondritis[a]

Systemic vasculitis
Rheumatoid arthritis
Systemic lupus erythematosus
Sjögren's syndrome
Spondyloarthritides
Behçet's disease
Inflammatory bowel disease
Primary biliary cirrhosis
Myelodysplastic syndrome

[a]Systemic vasculitis is the most common association followed by rheumatoid arthritis, systemic lupus erythematosus, and Sjögren's syndrome.

Source: Modified from Michet.

PATHOLOGY AND PATHOPHYSIOLOGY

The earliest abnormality of hyaline and elastic cartilage noted histologically is a focal or diffuse loss of basophilic staining indicating depletion of proteoglycan from the cartilage matrix. Inflammatory infiltrates are found adjacent to involved cartilage and consist predominantly of mononuclear cells and occasional plasma cells. In acute disease, polymorphonuclear white cells may also be present. Destruction of cartilage begins at the outer edges and advances centrally. There is lacunar breakdown and loss of chondrocytes. Degenerating cartilage is replaced by granulation tissue and later by fibrosis and focal areas of calcification. Small loci of cartilage regeneration may be present. Immunofluorescence studies have shown immunoglobulins and complement at sites of involvement. Extracellular granular material observed in the degenerating cartilage matrix by electron microscopy has been interpreted to be enzymes, immunoglobulins, or proteoglycans.

Immunologic mechanisms play a role in the pathogenesis of relapsing polychondritis. The accumulating data strongly suggest that both humoral and cell-mediated immunity play an important role in the pathogenesis of relapsing polychondritis. Immunoglobulin and complement deposits are found at sites of inflammation. In addition, antibodies to type II collagen and to matrilin-1 and immune complexes are detected in the sera of some patients. The possibility that an immune response to type II collagen may be important in the pathogenesis is supported experimentally by the occurrence of auricular chondritis in rats immunized with type II collagen. Antibodies to type II collagen are found in the sera of these animals, and immune deposits are detected at sites of ear inflammation. Humoral immune responses to type IX and type XI collagen, matrilin-1, and cartilage oligomeric matrix protein have been demonstrated in some patients. In a study, rats immunized with matrilin-1 were found to develop severe inspiratory stridor and swelling of the nasal septum. The rats had severe inflammation with erosions of the involved cartilage, which was characterized by increased numbers of CD4+ and CD8+ T cells in the lesions. The cartilage of the joints and ear pinna was not involved. All had IgG antibodies to matrilin-1. Matrilin-1 is a noncollagenous protein present in the extracellular matrix in cartilage. It is present in high concentrations in the trachea and is also present in the nasal septum but not in articular cartilage. A subsequent study demonstrated serum anti-matrilin-1 antibodies in approximately 13% of patients with relapsing polychondritis; approximately 70% of these patients had respiratory symptoms. Cell-mediated immunity may also be operative in causing tissue injury, since lymphocyte transformation can be demonstrated when lymphocytes of patients are exposed to cartilage extracts. T cells specific for type II collagen have been found in some patients, and CD4+ T cells have been observed at sites of cartilage inflammation.

CLINICAL MANIFESTATIONS

The onset of relapsing polychondritis is frequently abrupt with the appearance of one or two sites of cartilaginous inflammation. The pattern of cartilaginous involvement and the frequency of episodes vary widely among patients. Non-cartilaginous presentations may also occur. Systemic inflammatory features such as fever, fatigue, and weight loss occur and may precede the clinical signs of relapsing polychondritis by several weeks. Relapsing polychondritis may go unrecognized for several months or even years in patients who only initially manifest intermittent joint pain and/or swelling, or who have unexplained eye inflammation, hearing loss, valvular heart disease, or pulmonary symptoms.

Auricular chondritis is the most frequent presenting manifestation of relapsing polychondritis occurring in 40% of patients and eventually affecting about 85% of patients (Table 328-2). One or both ears are involved, either sequentially or simultaneously. Patients experience the sudden onset of pain, tenderness, and swelling of the cartilaginous portion of the ear (Fig. 328-1). This typically involves the pinna of the ears, sparing the earlobes because they do not contain cartilage. The overlying skin has a beefy red or violaceous color. Prolonged or recurrent episodes lead to cartilage destruction and result in a flabby or droopy ear. Swelling may close off the eustachian tube or the external auditory meatus, either of which can impair hearing. Inflammation of the internal auditory artery or its cochlear branch produces hearing loss, vertigo, ataxia, nausea, and vomiting. Vertigo is almost always accompanied by hearing loss.

Approximately 61% of patients will develop nasal involvement, with 21% having this at the time of presentation. Patients may experience nasal stuffiness, rhinorrhea, and epistaxis. The bridge of the nose and surrounding tissue becomes red, swollen, and tender and may collapse, producing a saddlenose deformity (Fig. 328-2). In some patients, nasal deformity develops insidiously without overt inflammation. Saddlenose is observed more frequently in younger patients, especially in women.

TABLE 328-2 Clinical Manifestations of Relapsing Polychondritis

Clinical Feature	Presenting	Cumulative
	Frequency, %	
Auricular chondritis	43	89
Arthritis	32	72
Nasal chondritis	21	61
Ocular inflammation	18	59
Laryngotracheal symptoms	23	55
Reduced hearing	7	40
Saddle nose deformity	11	25
Cutaneous	4	25
Laryngotracheal stricture	15	23
Vasculitis	2	14
Elevated creatinine	7	13
Aortic or mitral regurgitation	0	12

Source: Modified from Kent et al.

Joint involvement is the presenting manifestation in relapsing polychondritis in approximately one-third of patients and may be present for several months before other features appear. Eventually, more than one-half of the patients will have arthralgias or arthritis. The arthritis is usually asymmetric and oligo- or polyarticular, and it involves both large and small peripheral joints. An episode of arthritis lasts from a few days to several weeks and resolves spontaneously without joint erosion or deformity. Attacks of arthritis may not be temporally related to other manifestations of relapsing polychondritis. Joint fluid has been reported to be noninflammatory.

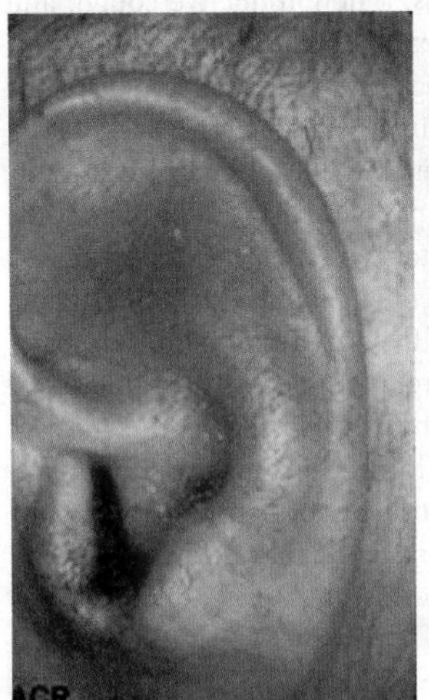

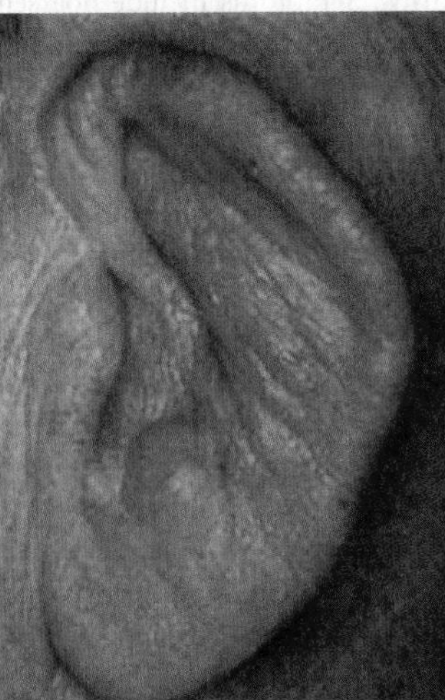

Figure 328-1 ***Left.*** The pinna is erythematous, swollen, and tender. Not shown is the ear lobule that is spared as there is no underlying cartilage. ***Right.*** The pinna is thickened and deformed. The destruction of the underlying cartilage results in a floppy ear. *(Reprinted from the Clinical Slide Collection on the Rheumatic Diseases, ©1991, 1995, 1997, 1998, 1999. Used by permission of the American College of Rheumatology.)*

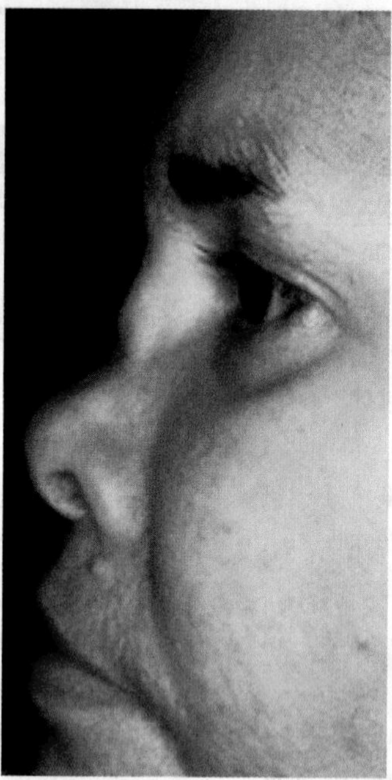

Figure 328-2 Saddlenose results from destruction and collapse of the nasal cartilage. *(Reprinted from the Clinical Slide Collection on the Rheumatic Diseases, ©1991, 1995, 1997, 1998, 1999. Used by permission of the American College of Rheumatology.)*

In addition to peripheral joints, inflammation may involve the costochondral, sternomanubrial, and sternoclavicular cartilages. Destruction of these cartilages may result in a pectus excavatum deformity or even a flail anterior chest wall.

Eye manifestations occur in more than one-half of patients and include conjunctivitis, episcleritis, scleritis, iritis, uveitis, and keratitis. Ocular inflammation can be severe and visually threatening. Other manifestations include eyelid and periorbital edema, proptosis, optic neuritis, extraocular muscle palsies, retinal vasculitis, and renal vein occlusion.

Laryngotracheobronchial involvement occurs in ~50% of patients and is among the most serious manifestations of relapsing polychondritis. Symptoms include hoarseness, a nonproductive cough, and tenderness over the larynx and proximal trachea. Mucosal edema, strictures, and/or collapse of laryngeal or tracheal cartilage may cause stridor and life-threatening airway obstruction necessitating tracheostomy. Involvement can extend into the lower airways resulting in tracheobronchomalacia. Collapse of cartilage in bronchi leads to pneumonia and, when extensive, to respiratory insufficiency.

Cardiac valvular regurgitation occurs in about 5–10% of patients and is due to progressive dilation of the valvular ring or to destruction of the valve cusps. Aortic regurgitation occurs in about 7% of patients with the mitral and other heart valves being affected less often. Other cardiac manifestations include pericarditis, myocarditis, coronary vasculitis, and conduction abnormalities. Aneurysms of the proximal, thoracic, or abdominal aorta may occur even in the absence of active chondritis and occasionally rupture.

Renal disease occurs in about 10% of patients. The most common renal lesions include mesangial expansion or segmental necrotizing glomerulonephritis, which have been reported to have small amounts of electron-dense deposits in the mesangium where there is also faint deposition of C3 and/or IgG or IgM. Tubulointerstitial disease and IgA nephropathy have also been reported.

Approximately 25% of patients have skin lesions, which can include purpura, erythema nodosum, erythema multiforme, angioedema/urticaria, livedo reticularis, and panniculitis.

Features of vasculitis are seen in up to 25% of patients and can affect any size vessel. Large vessel vasculitis may present with aortic aneurysms and medium vessel disease may affect the coronary, hepatic, mesenteric, or renal arteries or vessel supplying nerves. Skin vessel disease and involvement of the postcapillary venules can also occur. A variety of primary vasculitides have also been reported to occur in association with relapsing polychondritis (Chap. 326). One specific overlap is the "MAGIC" syndrome (*m*outh *a*nd *g*enital ulcers with *i*nflamed *c*artilage) in which patients present with features of both relapsing polychondritis and Behçet's disease (Chap. 327).

LABORATORY FINDINGS AND DIAGNOSTIC IMAGING

There are no laboratory features that are diagnostic for relapsing polychondritis. Mild leukocytosis and normocytic, normochromic anemia are often present. Eosinophilia is observed in 10% of patients. The erythrocyte sedimentation rate and C-reactive protein are usually elevated. Rheumatoid factor and antinuclear antibody tests are occasionally positive in low titers and complement levels are normal. Antibodies to type II collagen are present in fewer than one-half of the patients and are not specific. Circulating immune complexes may be detected, especially in patients with early active disease. Elevated levels of γ globulin may be present. Antineutrophil cytoplasmic antibodies (ANCA), either cytoplasmic (cANCA) or perinuclear (pANCA), are found in some patients with active disease. However, on target antigen specific testing, there are only occasional reports of positive myeloperoxidase-ANCA and proteinase 3-ANCA are very rarely found in relapsing polychondritis.

The upper and lower airways can be evaluated by imaging techniques such as computed tomography and magnetic resonance imaging. Bronchoscopy provides direct visualization of the airways but can be a high-risk procedure in patients with airway compromise. Pulmonary function testing with flow-volume loops can show inspiratory and/or expiratory obstruction. Imaging can also be useful to detect extracartilaginous disease. The chest film may show widening of the ascending or descending aorta due to an aneurysm, and cardiomegaly when aortic insufficiency is present. MRI can assess aortic aneurysmal dilatation. Electrocardiography and echocardiography can be useful in further evaluating for cardiac features of disease.

DIAGNOSIS

Diagnosis is based on recognition of the typical clinical features. Biopsies of the involved cartilage from the ear, nose, or respiratory tract will confirm the diagnosis but are only necessary when clinical features are not typical. Diagnostic criteria were suggested in 1976 by McAdam et al and modified by Damiani and Levine in 1979. These criteria continue to be generally used in clinical practice. McAdam et al proposed the following: (1) recurrent chondritis of both auricles; (2) nonerosive inflammatory arthritis; (3) chondritis of nasal cartilage; (4) inflammation of ocular structures, including conjunctivitis, keratitis, scleritis/episcleritis, and/or uveitis; (5) chondritis of the laryngeal and/or tracheal cartilages; and (6) cochlear and/or vestibular damage manifested by neurosensory hearing loss, tinnitus, and/or vertigo. The diagnosis is certain when three or more of these features are present along with a positive biopsy from the ear, nasal, or respiratory cartilage. Damiani and Levine later suggested that the diagnosis could be made when one or more of the above features and a positive biopsy were present, when two or more separate sites of cartilage inflammation were present that responded to glucocorticoids or dapsone, or when three or more of the above features were present.

The differential diagnosis of relapsing polychondritis is centered around its sites of clinical involvement. Patients with granulomatosis with polyangiitis (Wegener's) may have a saddlenose and tracheal involvement but can be distinguished by the primary inflammation occurring in the mucosa at these sites, the absence of auricular involvement, and the presence of pulmonary parenchymal disease. Patients with Cogan's syndrome have interstitial keratitis and vestibular and auditory abnormalities, but this syndrome does not involve the respiratory tract or ears. Reactive arthritis may initially resemble relapsing polychondritis because of oligoarticular arthritis and eye involvement, but it is distinguished in time by the appearance of urethritis and typical mucocutaneous lesions and the absence of nose or ear cartilage involvement. Rheumatoid arthritis may initially suggest relapsing polychondritis because of arthritis and eye inflammation. The arthritis in rheumatoid arthritis, however, is erosive and symmetric. In addition, rheumatoid factor titers are usually high compared with those in relapsing polychondritis and anti-cyclic citrullinated peptide is usually not seen. Bacterial infection of the pinna may be mistaken for relapsing polychondritis but differs by usually involving only one ear, including the earlobe. Auricular cartilage may also be damaged by trauma or frostbite.

TREATMENT Relapsing Polychondritis

In patients with active chondritis, prednisone, 40–60 mg/d, is often effective in suppressing disease activity; it is tapered gradually once disease is controlled. In some patients, prednisone can be stopped, while in others low doses in the range of 5–10 mg/d are required for continued suppression of disease. Dapsone 50–100 mg/d has been effective for cartilage inflammation and joint features in some patients. Other immunosuppressive drugs such as cyclophosphamide, methotrexate, azathioprine, or cyclosporine should be reserved for patients who have severe organ-threatening disease, fail to respond to prednisone, or who require high doses for control of disease activity. Patients with significant ocular inflammation often require intraocular glucocorticoids as well as high doses of prednisone. There are a small number of reports on the use of tumor necrosis factor antagonists, which are too few in number to assess efficacy. A small retrospective series of nine patients did not find anti-CD20 (rituximab) to provide benefit although this experience remains too small to draw firm conclusions. Heart valve replacement or repair of an aortic aneurysm may be necessary. When obstruction is severe, tracheostomy is required. Stents may be necessary in patients with tracheobronchial collapse.

PATIENT OUTCOME, PROGNOSIS, AND SURVIVAL

The course of relapsing polychondritis is highly variable, with inflammatory episodes lasting from a few days to several weeks and then subsiding spontaneously. Attacks may recur at intervals varying from weeks to months. In other patients, the disease has a chronic, smoldering course. In a few patients, the disease may be limited to one or two episodes of cartilage inflammation. In one study, the 5-year estimated survival rate was 74% and the 10-year survival rate 55%. In contrast to earlier series, only about one-half of the deaths could be attributed to relapsing polychondritis or complications of treatment. Pulmonary complications accounted for only 10% of all fatalities. In general, patients with more widespread disease have a worse prognosis.

ACKNOWLEDGMENT

This chapter represents a revised version of the text authored by Dr. Bruce C. Gilliland that appeared in previous editions of Harrison's Principles of Internal Medicine. Dr. Gilliland passed away on February 17, 2007, and had been a contributor to Harrison's since the 11th edition.

FURTHER READINGS

Ernst A et al: Relapsing polychondritis and airway involvement. Chest 135:1024, 2009

Kent PD et al: Relapsing polychondritis. Curr Opin Rheumatol 16:56, 2004

Letko E et al: Relapsing polychondritis: A clinical review. Semin Arthritis Rheum 31:384, 2002

Michet CJ et al: Relapsing polychondritis. Survival and predictive role of early disease manifestations. Ann Intern Med 104:74, 1986

Staats BA et al: Relapsing polychondritis. Semin Respir Crit Care Med 23:145, 2002

Trentham DE, Le CH: Relapsing polychondritis. Ann Intern Med 129:114, 1998

CHAPTER 329 Sarcoidosis

Robert P. Baughman
Elyse E. Lower

DEFINITION

Sarcoidosis is an inflammatory disease characterized by the presence of noncaseating granulomas. The disease is often multisystem and requires the presence of involvement in two or more organs for a specific diagnosis. The finding of granulomas is not specific for sarcoidosis, and other conditions known to cause granulomas must be ruled out. These conditions include mycobacterial and fungal infections, malignancy, and environmental agents such as beryllium. While sarcoidosis can affect virtually every organ of the body, the lung is most commonly affected. Other organs commonly affected are the liver, skin, and eye. The clinical outcome of sarcoidosis varies, with remission occurring in over one-half of the patients within a few years of diagnosis; however, the remaining patients may develop a chronic disease that lasts for decades.

ETIOLOGY

Despite multiple investigations, the cause of sarcoidosis remains unknown. Currently, the most likely etiology is an infectious or noninfectious environmental agent that triggers an inflammatory response in a genetically susceptible host. Among the possible infectious agents, careful studies have shown a much higher incidence of *Propionibacter acnes* in the lymph nodes of sarcoidosis patients compared to controls. An animal model has shown that *P. acnes* can induce a granulomatous response in mice similar to sarcoidosis. Others have demonstrated the presence of a mycobacterial protein [*Mycobacterium tuberculosis* catalase-peroxidase (mKatG)] in the granulomas of some sarcoidosis patients. This protein is very resistant to degradation and may represent the persistent antigen in sarcoidosis. Immune response to this and other mycobacterial proteins has been documented by another laboratory. These studies suggest that a mycobacterium similar to *M. tuberculosis* could be responsible for sarcoidosis. The mechanism exposure/infection with such agents has been the focus of other studies. Environmental exposures to insecticides and mold have been associated with an increased risk for disease. In addition, health care workers appear to have an increased risk. Also, sarcoidosis in a donor organ has occurred after transplantation into a sarcoidosis patient. Some authors have suggested that sarcoidosis is not due to a single agent but represents a particular host response to multiple agents. Some studies have been able to correlate the environmental exposures to genetic markers. These studies have supported the hypothesis that a genetically susceptible host is a key factor in the disease.

INCIDENCE AND PREVALENCE

Sarcoidosis is seen worldwide, with the highest prevalence reported in the Nordic population. In the United States, the disease has been reported more commonly in African Americans than whites, with the ratio of African Americans to whites ranging from 3:1 to 17:0. Women appear to be slightly more susceptible than men. The lower estimate is from a large health maintenance organization in Detroit. The earlier American studies finding the higher incidence in African Americans may have been influenced by the fact that African Americans seem to develop more extensive and chronic pulmonary disease. Since most sarcoidosis clinics are run by pulmonologists, a selection bias may have occurred. Worldwide, the prevalence of the disease varies from 20–60 per 100,000 for many groups such as Japanese, Italians, and American whites. Higher rate occurs in Ireland and Nordic countries. In one closely observed community in Sweden, the lifetime risk for developing sarcoidosis was 3%.

Sarcoidosis often occurs in young, otherwise healthy adults. It is uncommon to diagnose the disease in someone under age 18. However, it has become clear that a second peak in incidence develops around age 60. In a study of >700 newly diagnosed sarcoidosis patients in the United States, one-half of the patients were ≥40 years at the time of diagnosis.

Although most cases of sarcoidosis are sporadic, a familial form of the disease exists. At least 5% of patients with sarcoidosis will have a family member with sarcoidosis. Sarcoidosis patients who are Irish or African American seem to have a two to three times higher rate of familial disease.

PATHOPHYSIOLOGY AND IMMUNOPATHOGENESIS

The granuloma is the pathologic hallmark of sarcoidosis. A distinct feature of sarcoidosis is the local accumulation of inflammatory cells. Extensive studies in the lung using bronchoalveolar lavage (BAL) have demonstrated that the initial inflammatory response is an influx of T helper cells. In addition, there is an accumulation of activated monocytes. Figure 329-1 is a proposed model for sarcoidosis. Using the HLA-CD4 complex, antigen-presenting cells present an unknown antigen to the helper T cell. Studies have clarified that specific HLA haplotypes such as HLA-DRB1*1101 are associated with an increased risk for developing sarcoidosis. In addition, different HLA haplotypes are associated with different clinical outcomes.

The macrophage/helper T cell cluster leads to activation with the increased release of several cytokines. These include interleukin (IL)-2 released from the T cell and interferon γ and tumor necrosis factor (TNF) released by the macrophage. The T cell is a necessary part of the initial inflammatory response. In advanced, untreated HIV infection, patients who lack helper T cells rarely develop sarcoidosis. In contrast, several reports confirm that sarcoidosis becomes unmasked as HIV-infected individuals receive antiretroviral therapy, with subsequent restoration of their immune system. In contrast, treatment of established pulmonary sarcoidosis with cyclosporine, a drug that downregulates helper T cell responses, seems to have little impact on sarcoidosis.

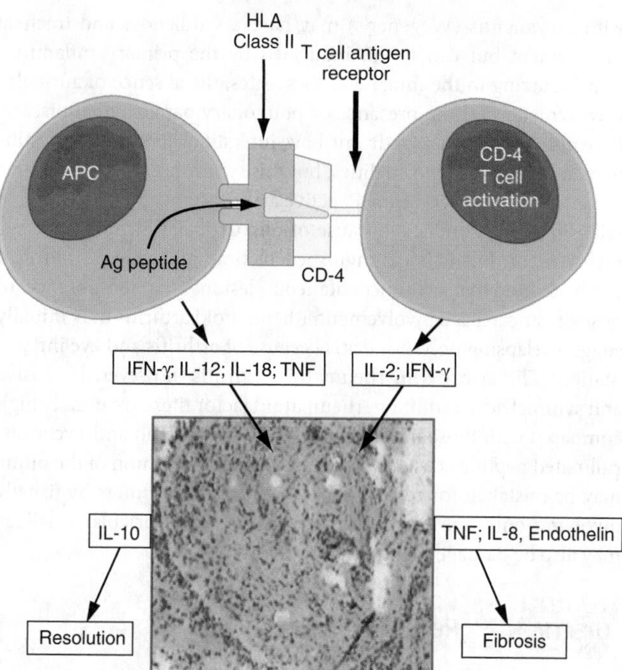

Figure 329-1 Schematic representation of initial events of sarcoidosis. The antigen-presenting cell and helper T cell complex leads to the release of multiple cytokines. This forms a granuloma. Over time, the granuloma may resolve or lead to chronic disease, including fibrosis. APC, antigen-presenting cell; HLA, human leukocyte antigen; IFN, interferon; IL, interleukin; TNF, tumor necrosis factor.

The granulomatous response of sarcoidosis can resolve with or without therapy. However, in at least 20% of patients with sarcoidosis, a chronic form of the disease develops. This persistent form of the disease is associated with the secretion of high levels of IL-8. Also, studies have reported that in patients with this chronic form of disease excessive amounts of TNF are released in the areas of inflammation.

It is sometimes difficult to determine early on the ultimate clinical outcome of sarcoidosis. One form of the disease, *Löfgren's syndrome*, consists of erythema nodosum, hilar adenopathy on chest roentgenogram, and uveitis. Löfgren's syndrome is associated with a good prognosis, with >90% of patients experiencing disease resolution within 2 years. A recently proposed expansion of the term Lofgren's syndrome includes periarticular arthritis without erythema nodosum. Recent studies have demonstrated that the HLA-DRB1*03 was found in two-thirds of Scandinavian patients with Löfgren's syndrome. More than 95% of those patients who were HLA-DRB1*03 positive had resolution of their disease within 2 years, while nearly one-half of the remaining patients had disease for more than 2 years. It remains to be determined whether these observations can be applied to a non-Scandinavian population.

CLINICAL MANIFESTATIONS

The presentation of sarcoidosis ranges from patients who are asymptomatic to those with organ failure. It is unclear how often sarcoidosis is asymptomatic. In countries where routine chest roentgenogram screening is performed, 20–30% of pulmonary cases are detected in asymptomatic individuals. The inability to screen for other asymptomatic forms of the disease would suggest that as many as one-third of sarcoidosis patients are asymptomatic.

Respiratory complaints including cough and dyspnea are the most common presenting symptoms. In many cases, the patient presents with a 2–4 week history of these symptoms. Unfortunately, due to the nonspecific nature of pulmonary symptoms, the patient may see physicians for up to a year before a diagnosis is confirmed. For these patients, the diagnosis of sarcoidosis is usually only suggested when a chest roentgenogram is performed.

Symptoms related to cutaneous and ocular disease are the next two most common complaints. Skin lesions are often nonspecific. However, since these lesions are readily observed, the patient and treating physician are often led to a diagnosis. In contrast to patients with pulmonary disease, patients with cutaneous lesions are more likely to be diagnosed within 6 months of symptoms.

Nonspecific constitutional symptoms include fatigue, fever, night sweats, and weight loss. Fatigue is perhaps the most common constitutional symptom that affects these patients. Given its insidious nature, patients are usually not aware of the association with their sarcoidosis until their disease resolves.

The overall incidence of sarcoidosis at the time of diagnosis and eventual common organ involvement are summarized in Table 329-1. Over time, skin, eye, and neurologic involvement seem more apparent. In the United States, the frequency of specific organ involvement appears to be affected by age, race, and gender. For example, eye disease is more common among African Americans. Under the age of 40, it occurs more frequently in women. However, in those diagnosed over the age of 40, eye disease is more common in men.

LUNG

Lung involvement occurs in >90% of sarcoidosis patients. The most commonly used method for detecting lung disease is still the chest roentgenogram. Figure 329-2 illustrates the chest roentgenogram from a sarcoidosis patient with bilateral hilar adenopathy. Although the CT scan has changed the diagnostic approach to interstitial lung disease, the CT scan is not usually considered a monitoring tool for patients with sarcoidosis. Figure 329-3 demonstrates some of the characteristic CT features, including peribronchial thickening and reticular nodular changes, which are predominantly subpleural.

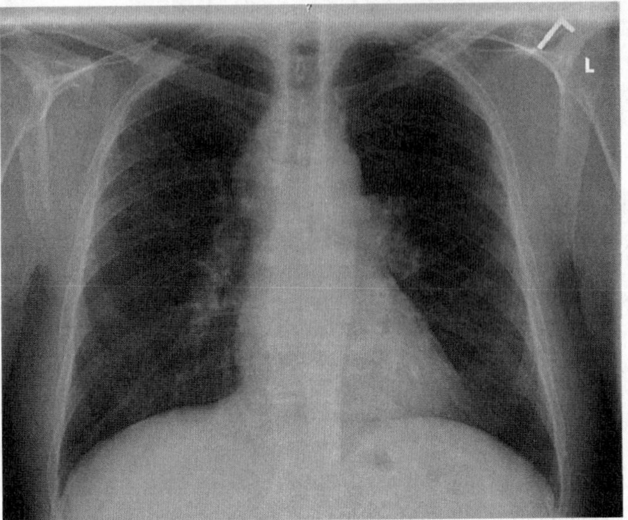

Figure 329-2 Posterior-anterior chest roentgenogram demonstrating bilateral hilar adenopathy, stage 1 disease.

The peribronchial thickening seen on CT scan seems to explain the high yield of granulomas from bronchial biopsies performed for diagnosis.

While the CT scan is more sensitive, the standard scoring system described by Scadding in 1961 for chest roentgenograms remains the preferred method of characterizing the chest involvement. Stage 1 is hilar adenopathy alone (Fig. 329-2), often with right paratracheal involvement. Stage 2 is a combination of adenopathy plus infiltrates, whereas stage 3 reveals infiltrates alone. Stage 4 consists of fibrosis. Usually the infiltrates in sarcoidosis are predominantly an upper lobe process. Only in a few noninfectious diseases is an upper lobe predominance noted. In addition to sarcoidosis, the differential diagnosis of upper lobe disease includes hypersensitivity pneumonitis, silicosis, and Langerhans cell histiocytosis. For infectious diseases, tuberculosis and *Pneumocystis* pneumonia can often present as upper lobe diseases.

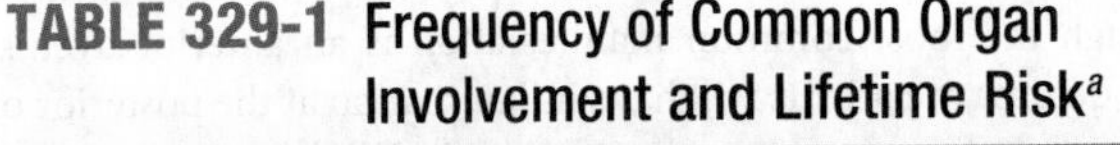

TABLE 329-1 Frequency of Common Organ Involvement and Lifetime Risk[a]

	Presentation, %[b]	Follow-up, %[c]
Lung	95	94
Skin	24	43
Eye	12	29
Extrathoracic lymph node	15	16
Liver	12	14
Spleen	7	8
Neurologic	5	16
Cardiac	2	3

[a]Patients could have more than one organ involved.

[b]From ACCESS study of 736 patients evaluated. within 6 months of diagnosis.

[c]From follow-up of 1024 sarcoidosis patients seen at the University of Cincinnati Interstitial Lung Disease and Sarcoidosis Clinic from 2002–2006.

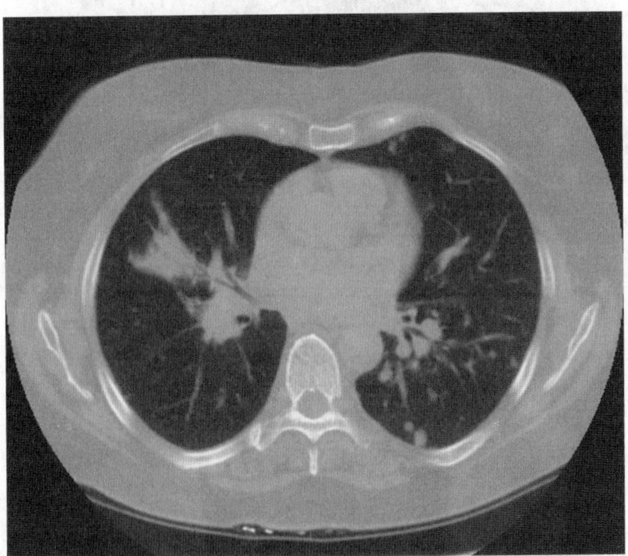

Figure 329-3 High-resolution CT scan of chest demonstrating patchy reticular nodularity, including areas of confluence.

Lung volumes, mechanics, and diffusion all are useful in evaluating interstitial lung diseases such as sarcoidosis. The diffusion of carbon monoxide (DLCO) is the most sensitive test for an interstitial lung disease. Reduced lung volumes are a reflection of the restrictive lung disease seen in sarcoidosis. However, a third of the patients presenting with sarcoidosis still have lung volumes within the normal range, despite abnormal chest roentgenograms and dyspnea.

Approximately one-half of sarcoidosis patients present with obstructive disease, reflected by a reduced ratio of forced vital capacity expired in one second (FEV_1/FVC). Cough is a very common symptom. Airway involvement causing varying degrees of obstruction underlies the cough in most sarcoidosis patients. Airway hyperreactivity as determined by methacholine challenge will be positive in some of these patients. A few patients with cough will respond to traditional bronchodilators as the only form of treatment. In some cases, high-dose inhaled glucocorticoids alone are useful.

Pulmonary arterial hypertension is reported in at least 5% of sarcoidosis patients. Either direct vascular involvement or the consequence of fibrotic changes in the lung can lead to pulmonary arterial hypertension. In sarcoidosis patients with end-stage fibrosis awaiting lung transplant, 70% will have pulmonary arterial hypertension. This is a much higher incidence than that reported for other fibrotic lung diseases. In less advanced, but still symptomatic, patients pulmonary arterial hypertension has been noted in up to 50% of the cases. Because sarcoidosis-associated pulmonary arterial hypertension may respond to therapy, evaluation for this should be considered in persistently symptomatic patients.

SKIN

Skin involvement is eventually identified in over a third of patients with sarcoidosis. The classic cutaneous lesions include erythema nodosum, maculopapular lesions, hyper- and hypopigmentation, keloid formation, and subcutaneous nodules. A specific complex of involvement of the bridge of the nose, the area beneath the eyes, and the cheeks is referred to as *lupus pernio* (Fig. 329-4) and is diagnostic for a chronic form of sarcoidosis.

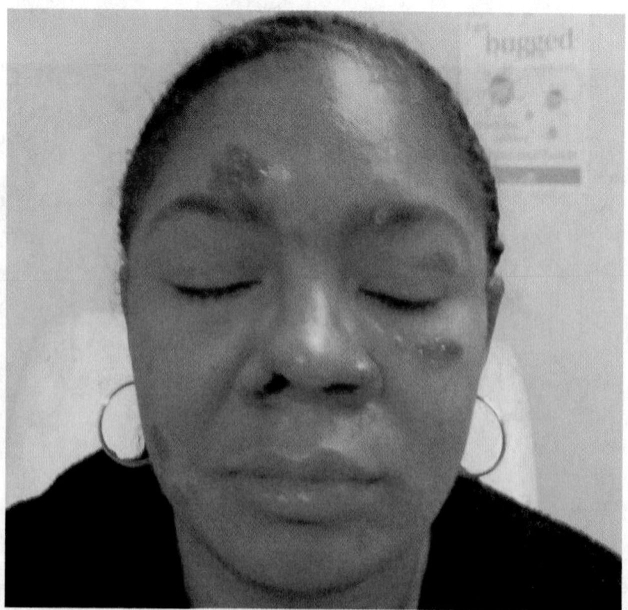

Figure 329-4 Chronic inflammatory lesions around nose, eyes, and cheeks, referred to as lupus pernio.

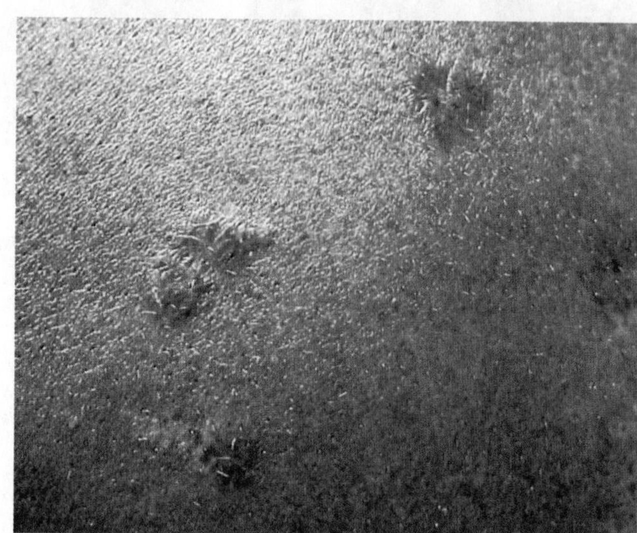

Figure 329-5 Maculopapular lesions on the trunk of a sarcoidosis patient.

In contrast, erythema nodosum is a transient rash that can be seen in association with hilar adenopathy and uveitis (Löfgren's syndrome). Erythema nodosum is more common in women and in certain self-described demographic groups including whites and Puerto Ricans. In the United States, the other manifestations of skin sarcoidosis, especially lupus pernio, are more common in African Americans than whites.

The maculopapular lesions from sarcoidosis are the most common chronic form of the disease (Fig. 329-5). These are often overlooked by the patient and physician, since they are chronic and not painful. Initially, these lesions are usually purplish papules and are often indurated. They can become confluent and infiltrate large areas of the skin. With treatment, the color and induration may fade. Because these lesions are caused by noncaseating granulomas, the diagnosis of sarcoidosis can be readily made by a skin biopsy.

EYE

The frequency of ocular manifestations for sarcoidosis varies depending on race. In Japan, >70% of sarcoidosis patients develop ocular disease, while in the United States only 30% have eye disease, with problems more common in African Americans than whites. Although the most common manifestation is an anterior uveitis, over a quarter of patients will have inflammation at the posterior of the eye, including retinitis and pars planitis. While symptoms such as photophobia, blurred vision, and increased tearing can occur, some asymptomatic patients still have active inflammation. Initially asymptomatic patients with ocular sarcoidosis can eventually develop blindness. Therefore, it is recommended that all patients with sarcoidosis receive a dedicated ophthalmologic examination. Sicca is seen in over one-half of the chronic sarcoidosis patients. Dry eyes appear to be a reflection of prior lacrimal gland disease. Although the patient may no longer have active inflammation, the dry eyes may require natural tears or other lubricants.

LIVER

Using biopsies to detect granulomatous disease, liver involvement can be identified in over one-half of sarcoidosis patients. However, using liver function studies, only 20–30% of patients will have evidence of liver involvement. The most common abnormality of liver function is an elevation of the alkaline phosphatase level, consistent with an obstructive pattern. In addition, elevated transaminase levels can occur. An elevated bilirubin level is a marker for more advanced liver disease. Overall, only 5% of sarcoidosis patients have sufficient symptoms from their liver disease to require specific therapy. Although symptoms can be due to hepatomegaly, more frequently symptoms result from extensive intrahepatic cholestasis leading to portal hypertension. In this case, ascites and esophageal varices can occur. It is rare that a sarcoidosis patient will require a liver transplant, because even the patient with cirrhosis due to sarcoidosis can respond to systemic therapy. On a cautionary note, patients with both sarcoidosis and hepatitis C should avoid therapy with interferon α because of its association with the development or worsening of granulomatous disease.

BONE MARROW AND SPLEEN

One or more bone marrow manifestations can be identified in many sarcoidosis patients. The most common hematologic problem is lymphopenia, which is a reflection of sequestration of the lymphocytes into the areas of inflammation. Anemia occurs in 20% of patients and leukopenia is less common. Bone marrow examination will reveal granulomas in about a third of patients. Splenomegaly can be detected in 5–10% of patients, but splenic biopsy reveals granulomas in 60% of patients. The CT scan can be relatively specific for sarcoidosis involvement of the spleen (Fig. 329-6). Both bone marrow and spleen involvement are more common in African Americans than whites. These manifestations alone are rarely an indication for therapy. On occasion, splenectomy may be indicated for massive symptomatic splenomegaly or profound pancytopenia.

CALCIUM METABOLISM

Hypercalcemia and/or hypercalciuria occurs in about 10% of sarcoidosis patients. It is more common in whites than African Americans and in men. The mechanism of abnormal calcium metabolism is increased production of 1,25-dihydroxyvitamin D by the granuloma itself. The 1,25-dihydroxyvitamin D causes increased intestinal absorption of calcium, leading to hypercalcemia with a suppressed parathyroid hormone (PTH) level (Chap. 353). Increased exogenous vitamin D from diet or sunlight exposure may exacerbate this problem. Serum calcium should be determined

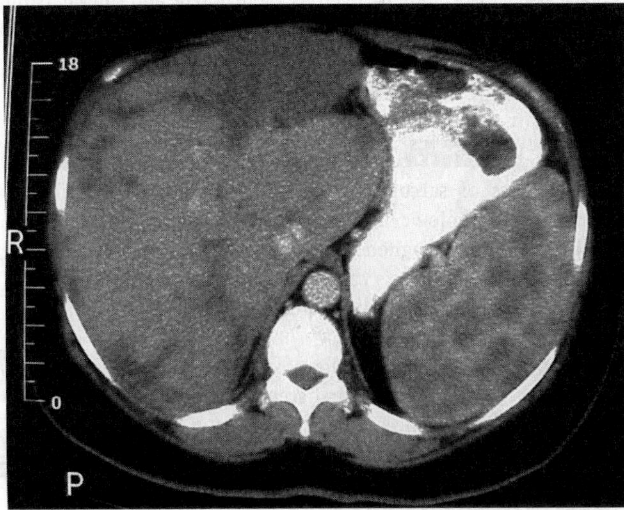

Figure 329-6 CT scan of the abdomen after oral and intravenous contrast. The stomach is compressed by the enlarged spleen. Within the spleen, areas of hypo- and hyperdensity are identified.

as part of the initial evaluation of all sarcoidosis patients, and a repeat determination may be useful during the summer months with increased sun exposure. In patients with a history of renal calculi, a 24-h urine calcium measurement should be obtained. If a sarcoidosis patient with a history of renal calculi is to be placed on calcium supplements, a follow-up 24-h urine calcium level should be measured.

RENAL DISEASE

Direct kidney involvement occurs in <5% of sarcoidosis patients. It is associated with granulomas in the kidney itself and can lead to nephritis. However, hypercalcemia is the most likely cause of sarcoidosis-associated renal disease. In 1–2% of sarcoidosis patients, acute renal failure has been encountered as a result of hypercalcemia. Treatment of the hypercalcemia with glucocorticoids and other therapies often improves, but does not totally resolve, the renal dysfunction.

NERVOUS SYSTEM

Neurologic disease is reported in 5–10% of sarcoidosis patients and appears to be of equal frequency across all ethnic groups. Any part of the central or peripheral nervous system can be affected. The presence of granulomatous inflammation is often visible on MRI studies. The MRI with gadolinium enhancement may demonstrate space-occupying lesions, but the MRI can be negative due to small lesions or the effect of systemic therapy in reducing the inflammation. The cerebral spinal fluid (CSF) findings include lymphocytic meningitis with a mild increase in protein. The CSF glucose is usually normal but can be low. Certain areas of the nervous system are more commonly affected in neurosarcoidosis. These include cranial nerve involvement, basilar meningitis, myelopathy, and anterior hypothalamic disease with associated diabetes insipidus (Chap. 340). Seizures and cognitive changes also occur. Of the cranial nerves, seventh nerve paralysis can be transient and mistaken for Bell's palsy (idiopathic seventh nerve paralysis). Since this form of neurosarcoidosis often resolves within weeks and may not recur, it may have occurred prior to a definitive diagnosis of sarcoidosis. Optic neuritis is another cranial nerve manifestation of sarcoidosis. This manifestation is more chronic and usually requires long-term systemic therapy. It can be associated with both anterior and posterior uveitis. Differentiating between neurosarcoidosis and multiple sclerosis can be difficult at times. Optic neuritis can occur in both diseases. In some patients with sarcoidosis, multiple enhancing white matter abnormalities may be detected by MRI, suggesting multiple sclerosis. In such cases, the presence of meningeal enhancement or hypothalamic involvement suggests neurosarcoidosis, as does evidence of extraneurologic disease such as pulmonary or skin involvement, which also suggests sarcoidosis. Since the response of neurosarcoidosis to glucocorticoids and cytotoxic therapy is different from that of multiple sclerosis, differentiating between these disease entities is important.

CARDIAC

The presence of cardiac involvement is influenced by race. Over a quarter of Japanese sarcoidosis patients develop cardiac disease, whereas only 5% of sarcoidosis patients in the United States and Europe develop cardiac disease. However, there is no apparent difference between whites and African Americans. Cardiac disease usually presents as either congestive heart failure or cardiac arrhythmias. Both manifestations result from infiltration of the heart muscle by granulomas. Diffuse granulomatous involvement of the heart muscle can lead to ejection fractions below 10%. Even in this situation, improvement in the ejection fraction can occur with systemic therapy. Arrhythmias can also occur with diffuse infiltration or with more patchy cardiac involvement. If the atrioventricular (AV) node is infiltrated, heart block can occur. This can be detected by routine electrocardiography. Ventricular arrhythmias and sudden death due to ventricular tachycardia are common causes of death. Arrhythmias are best detected using 24-h ambulatory monitoring. Because ventricular arrhythmias are usually multifocal due to patchy multiple granulomas in the heart, ablation therapy is not useful. Patients with significant ventricular arrhythmias should be considered for an implanted defibrillator, which appears to have reduced the rate of death in cardiac sarcoidosis. While systemic therapy can be useful in treating the arrhythmias, patients may still have malignant arrhythmias up to 6 months after starting successful treatment, and the risk for recurrent arrhythmias occurs whenever medications are tapered.

MUSCULOSKELETAL SYSTEM

Direct granulomatous bone and muscle involvement as documented by x-ray, MRI (Fig. 329-7), gallium scan, or biopsy can be seen in about 10% of sarcoidosis patients. However, a larger percentage of sarcoidosis patients complain of myalgias and arthralgias. These complaints are similar to those reported by patients with other inflammatory diseases, including chronic infections such as mononucleosis. Fatigue associated with sarcoidosis may be overwhelming for many patients. Recent studies have demonstrated a link between fatigue and small peripheral nerve fiber disease in sarcoidosis.

OTHER ORGAN INVOLVEMENT

Although sarcoidosis can affect any organ of the body, rarely does it involve the breast, testes, ovary, or stomach. Because of the rarity of involvement, a mass in one of these areas requires a biopsy to rule out other diseases including cancer. For example, in a study of breast problems in female sarcoidosis patients, a breast lesion was more likely to be granulomas from sarcoidosis than from breast cancer. However, findings on the physical examination or mammogram cannot reliably differentiate between these lesions. More importantly, as women with sarcoidosis age, breast cancer becomes more common. Therefore, it is recommended that routine screening including mammography be performed along with other imaging studies (ultrasound, MRI) or biopsy as clinically indicated.

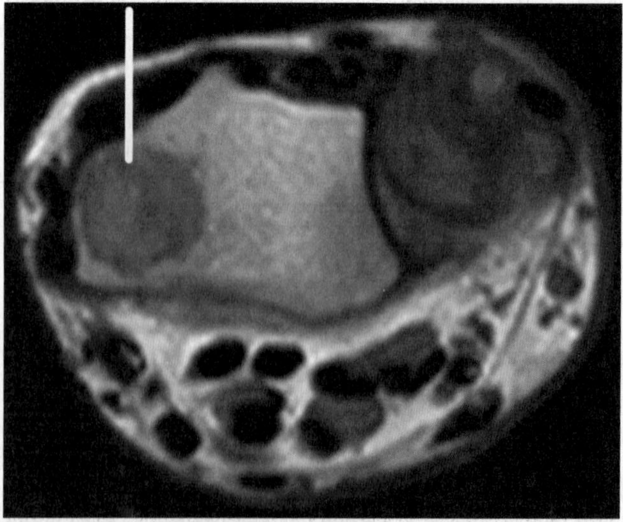

Figure 329-7 MRI of wrist demonstrating large cyst in a sarcoidosis patient (*line*).

COMPLICATIONS

Sarcoidosis is usually a self-limited, non-life-threatening disease. However, organ-threatening disease can occur. These complications can include blindness, paraplegia, or renal failure. Death from sarcoidosis occurs in about 5% of patients seen in sarcoidosis referral clinics. The usual causes of death related to sarcoidosis are from lung, cardiac, neurologic, or liver involvement. In respiratory failure, an elevation of the right atrial pressure is a poor prognostic finding. Lung complications can also include infections such as mycetoma, which can subsequently lead to massive bleeding. In addition, the use of immunosuppressive agents can increase the incidence of serious infections.

LABORATORY FINDINGS

The chest roentgenogram remains the most commonly used tool to assess lung involvement in sarcoidosis. As noted above, the chest roentgenogram classifies involvement into four stages, with stages 1 and 2 having hilar and paratracheal adenopathy. The CT scan has been used increasingly in evaluating interstitial lung disease. In sarcoidosis, the presence of adenopathy and a nodular infiltrate is not specific for sarcoidosis. Adenopathy up to 2 cm can be seen in other inflammatory lung diseases such as idiopathic pulmonary fibrosis. However, adenopathy >2 cm in the short axis supports the diagnosis of sarcoidosis over other interstitial lung diseases.

The positive emission tomography (PET) scan has increasingly replaced gallium 67 scanning to identify areas of sarcoidosis in the chest and other parts of the body. Both tests can be used to identify potential areas for biopsy. Cardiac PET scanning has also proved useful in assessing cardiac sarcoidosis. A positive PET scan may be due to the granulomas from sarcoidosis and not to disseminated malignancy.

Serum levels of angiotensin-converting enzyme (ACE) can be helpful in the diagnosis of sarcoidosis. However, the test has somewhat low sensitivity and specificity. Elevated levels of ACE are reported in 60% of patients with acute disease and only 20% of patients with chronic disease. Although there are several causes for mild elevation of ACE, including diabetes, elevations of >50% of the upper limit of normal are seen in only a few conditions including sarcoidosis, leprosy, Gaucher's disease, hyperthyroidism, and disseminated granulomatous infections such as miliary tuberculosis. There is an insertion/deletion (I/D) polymorphism of the *ACE* gene on what is felt to be in the noncritical part of the gene. There is a phenotypic difference for ACE levels, with II polymorphism having the lowest and DD polymorphism the highest levels of ACE for both sarcoidosis patients and healthy controls. There is no clear-cut association between ACE phenotype and clinical manifestation of disease. Because the ACE level is determined by a biologic assay, the concurrent use of an ACE inhibitor such as lisinopril will lead to a very low ACE level.

DIAGNOSIS

The diagnosis of sarcoidosis requires both compatible clinical features and pathologic findings. Since the cause of sarcoidosis remains elusive, the diagnosis cannot be made with 100% certainty. Nevertheless, the diagnosis can be made with reasonable certainty based on history and physical features along with laboratory and pathologic findings.

Patients are usually evaluated for possible sarcoidosis based on two scenarios (Fig. 329-8). In the first scenario, a patient may undergo a biopsy revealing a noncaseating granuloma in either a pulmonary or an extrapulmonary organ. If the clinical presentation is consistent with sarcoidosis and there is no alternative cause for the granulomas identified, then the patient is felt to have sarcoidosis.

In the second scenario, signs or symptoms suggesting sarcoidosis such as the presence of bilateral adenopathy may be present in an otherwise asymptomatic patient or a patient with uveitis or a rash

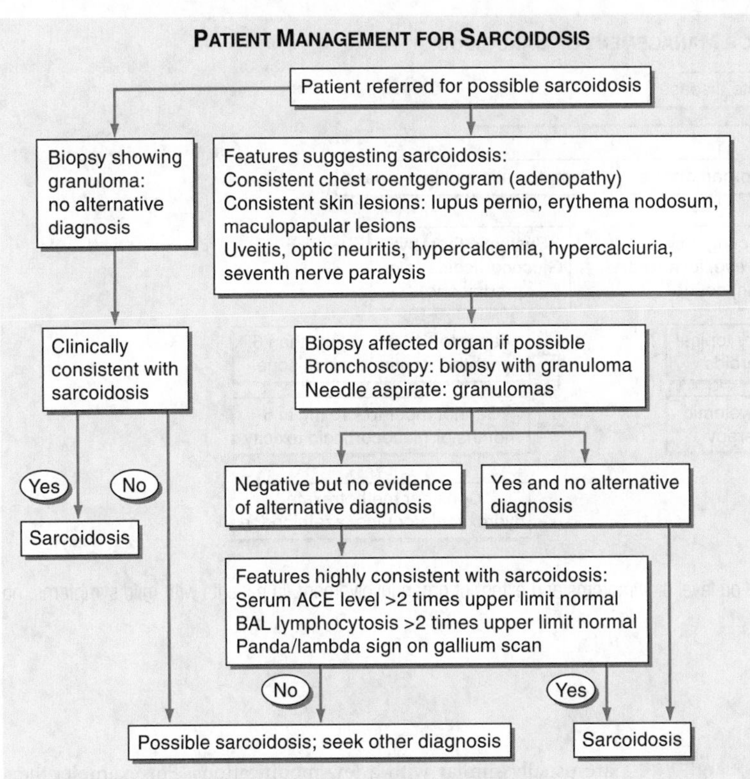

Figure 329-8 Proposed approach to management of patient with possible sarcoidosis. Presence of one or more of these features supports the diagnosis of sarcoidosis: uveitis, optic neuritis, hypercalcemia, hypercalciuria, seventh cranial nerve paralysis, diabetes insipidus.

consistent with sarcoidosis. At this point, a diagnostic procedure should be performed. For the patient with a compatible skin lesion, a skin biopsy should be considered. Other biopsies to consider could include liver, extrathoracic lymph node, or muscle. In some cases, a biopsy of the affected organ may not be easy to perform (such as a brain or spinal cord lesion). In other cases, such as an endomyocardial biopsy, the likelihood of a positive biopsy is low. Because of the high rate of pulmonary involvement in these cases, the lung may be easier to approach by bronchoscopy. During the bronchoscopy, a transbronchial biopsy, bronchial biopsy, or transbronchial needle aspirate of an enlarged mediastinal lymph node can be performed. The endobronchial ultrasonography-guided transbronchial needle aspirate may be particularly useful in the patient with stage 1 disease (i.e., adenopathy without infiltrates).

If the biopsy reveals granulomas, an alternative diagnosis such as infection or malignancy must be excluded. Bronchoscopic washings can be sent for cultures for fungi and tuberculosis. For the pathologist, the more tissue that is provided, the more comfortable is the diagnosis of sarcoidosis. A needle aspirate may be adequate in an otherwise classic case of sarcoidosis, but may be insufficient in a patient in whom lymphoma or fungal infection is a likely alternative diagnosis. Since granulomas can be seen on the edge of a lymphoma, the presence of a few granulomas from a needle aspirate may not be sufficient to clarify the diagnosis. Mediastinoscopy remains the procedure of choice to confirm the presence or absence of lymphoma in the mediastinum. Alternatively, for most patients, evidence of extrathoracic disease (e.g., eye involvement) may further support the diagnosis of sarcoidosis.

For patients with negative pathology, positive supportive tests may increase the likelihood of the diagnosis of sarcoidosis. These tests include an elevated ACE level, which can also be elevated in other granulomatous diseases but not in malignancy. A positive gallium scan can support the diagnosis if increased activity is noted in the parotids and lacrimal glands (*panda sign*) or in the right paratracheal and left hilar area (*lambda sign*). A BAL is often performed during the bronchoscopy. An increase in the percentage of lymphocytes supports the diagnosis of sarcoidosis. The use of the lymphocyte markers CD4 and CD8 can be used to determine the CD4/CD8 ratio of these increased lymphocytes in the BAL fluid. A ratio of >3.5 is strongly supportive of sarcoidosis but is less sensitive than an increase in lymphocytes alone. Although in general, an increase in BAL lymphocytes is supportive of the diagnosis, other conditions must be considered.

These supportive tests when combined with commonly associated clinical features of the disease, which are not diagnostic of sarcoidosis, can enhance the diagnostic probability. These nondiagnostic features include uveitis, renal stones, hypercalcemia, seventh cranial nerve paralysis, or erythema nodosum.

The *Kviem-Siltzbach procedure* is a specific diagnostic test for sarcoidosis. An intradermal injection of specially prepared tissue derived from the spleen of a known sarcoidosis patient is biopsied 4–6 weeks after injection. If noncaseating granulomas are seen, this is highly specific for the diagnosis of sarcoidosis. Unfortunately, there is no commercially available Kviem-Siltzbach reagent, and some locally prepared batches have lower specificity. Thus, this test is of historic interest and is rarely used in current clinical practice.

Because the diagnosis of sarcoidosis can never be certain, over time other features may arise that lead to an alternative diagnosis. Conversely, evidence for new organ involvement may eventually confirm the diagnosis of sarcoidosis.

PROGNOSIS

The risk of death or loss of organ function remains low in sarcoidosis. Poor outcomes usually occur in patients who present with advanced disease in whom treatment seems to have little impact. In these cases, irreversible fibrotic changes have frequently occurred.

For the majority of patients, initial presentation occurs during the granulomatous phase of the disease as depicted in Fig. 329-1. It is clear that many patients resolve their disease within 2–5 years. These patients are felt to have acute, self-limiting sarcoidosis. However, there is a form of the disease that does not resolve within the first 2–5 years. These chronic patients can be identified at presentation by certain risk factors at presentation such as fibrosis on chest roentgenogram, presence of lupus pernio, bone cysts, cardiac or neurologic disease (except isolated seventh nerve paralysis), and presence of renal calculi due to hypercalciuria. Recent studies also indicate that patients who require glucocorticoids for any manifestation of their disease in the first 6 months of presentation have a >50% chance of having chronic disease. In contrast, <10% of patients who require no systemic therapy in the first 6 months will require chronic therapy.

TREATMENT Sarcoidosis

The indications for therapy should be based on symptoms. The patient with elevated liver function tests or an abnormal chest roentgenogram probably does not benefit from treatment. However, these patients should be monitored for evidence of progressive, symptomatic disease.

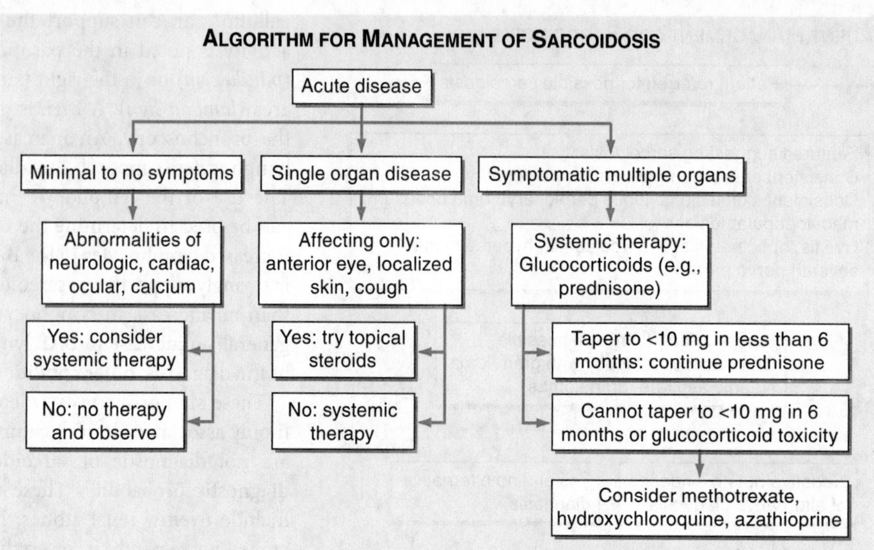

Figure 329-9 The management of acute sarcoidosis is based on level of symptoms and extent of organ involvement. In patients with mild symptoms, no therapy may be needed unless specified manifestations are noted.

One approach to therapy is summarized in Figs. 329-9 and 329-10. We have divided the approach into treating acute versus chronic disease. For acute disease, no therapy remains a viable option for patients with no or mild symptoms. For symptoms confined to only one organ, topical therapy is preferable. For multiorgan disease or disease too extensive for topical therapy, an approach to systemic therapy is outlined. Glucocorticoids remain the drugs of choice for this disease. However, the decision to continue to treat with glucocorticoids or to add steroid-sparing agents depends on the tolerability, duration, and dosage of glucocorticoids. Table 329-2 summarizes the dosage and monitoring of several commonly used drugs. According to the available trials, evidence-based recommendations are made. Most of these recommendations are for pulmonary disease because most of the trials were performed only in pulmonary disease. Treatment recommendations for extrapulmonary disease are usually similar with a few modifications. For example, the dosage of glucocorticoids is usually higher for neurosarcoidosis and lower for cutaneous disease. There was some suggestion that higher doses would be beneficial for cardiac sarcoidosis, but one study found that initial doses >40 mg/d prednisone were associated with a worse outcome because of toxicity.

While most patients receive glucocorticoids as their initial systemic therapy, toxicity associated with prolonged therapy often leads to steroid-sparing alternatives. The antimalarial drugs such as hydroxychloroquine are more effective for skin than pulmonary disease. Minocycline may also be useful for cutaneous sarcoidosis. For pulmonary and other extra-pulmonary disease, cytotoxic agents are often employed. These include methotrexate, azathioprine, chlorambucil, and cyclophosphamide. The most widely studied cytotoxic agent has been methotrexate. This agent works in approximately two-thirds

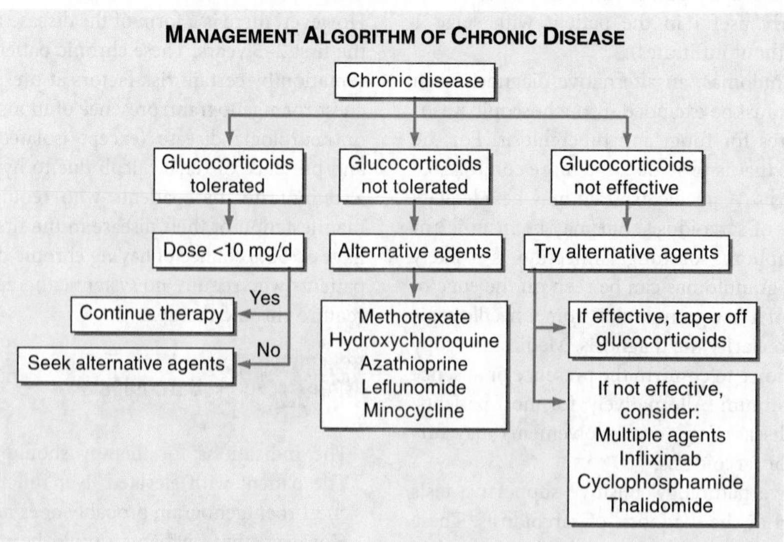

Figure 329-10 Approach to chronic disease is based on whether glucocorticoid therapy is tolerated or not.

TABLE 329-2 Commonly Used Drugs to Treat Sarcoidosis

Drug	Initial Dose	Maintenance Dose	Monitoring	Toxicity	Support Therapy[a]	Support Monitoring[a]
Prednisone	20–40 mg qd	Taper to 5–10 mg	Glucose, blood pressure, bone density	Diabetes, osteoporosis	A: Acute pulmonary D: Extrapulmonary	
Hydroxychloroquine	200–400 mg qd	400 mg qd	Eye exam q6–12 mo	Ocular	B: Some forms of disease	D: Routine eye exam
Methotrexate	10 mg qw	2.5–15 mg qw	CBC, renal, hepatic q2mo	Hematologic, nausea, hepatic, pulmonary	B: Steroid sparing C: Some forms chronic disease	D: Routine hematologic, renal, and hepatic monitoring
Azathioprine	50–150 mg qd	50–200 mg qd	CBC, renal q2mo	Hematologic, nausea	C: Some forms chronic disease	D: Routine hematologic monitoring
Infliximab	3–5 mg/kg q2wk for 2 doses	3–10 mg/kg q4–8 wk	Initial PPD	Infections, allergic reaction, carcinogen	A: Chronic pulmonary disease	B: Caution in patients with latent tuberculosis or advanced congestive heart failure

[a]Grade A: supported by at least two double-blind randomized control trials; grade B: supported by prospective cohort studies; grade C: supported primarily by two or more retrospective studies; grade D: only one retrospective study or based on experience in other diseases.

Abbreviations: CBC, complete blood count; PPD, purified protein derivative test for tuberculosis.

Source: Adapted from Baughman and Selroos.

of sarcoidosis patients, regardless of the disease manifestation. As noted in Table 329-2, specific guidelines for monitoring therapy have been recommended. Cytokine modulators such as thalidomide and pentoxifylline have also been used in a limited number of cases.

The anti-TNF agents have recently been studied in sarcoidosis, with prospective randomized trials of both etanercept and infliximab completed. Etanercept has a limited role as a steroid-sparing agent. Conversely, infliximab significantly improved lung function when given to patients with chronic disease already on glucocorticoids and cytotoxic agents. The difference in response for these two agents is similar to that observed in Crohn's disease, where infliximab is effective and etanercept is not. In addition, there is a higher risk for reactivation of tuberculosis with infliximab compared to etanercept. The differential response rate could be explained by differences in mechanism of action since etanercept is a TNF receptor antagonist and infliximab is a monoclonal antibody against TNF. In contrast to etanercept, infliximab also binds to TNF on the surface of some cells that are releasing TNF and this can lead to cell lysis. This effect has been documented in Crohn's disease. There is currently limited information about the dose and effectiveness of adalimumab, another anti-TNF antibody, versus infliximab in sarcoidosis. The role of the newer therapeutic agents for sarcoidosis is still evolving. However, these targeted therapies confirm that TNF may be an important target, especially in the treatment of chronic disease. However, these agents are not a panacea, since sarcoidosis-like disease has occurred in patients treated with anti-TNF agents for nonsarcoidosis indications.

FURTHER READINGS

Baughman RP, Selroos O: Evidence-based approach to treatment of sarcoidosis, in PG Gibson et al (eds): *Evidence-Based Respiratory Medicine*. Oxford, BMJ Books Blackwell, 2005, pp 491–508

de Kleijn WP et al: Fatigue in sarcoidosis: a systematic review. Curr Opin Pulm Med 15:499, 2009

Drake WP et al: Cellular recognition of Mycobacterium tuberculosis ESAT-6 and KatG peptides in systemic sarcoidosis. Infect Immun 75:527, 2007

Grunewald J, Eklund A: Löfgren's syndrome: Human leukocyte antigen strongly influences the disease course. Am J Respir Crit Care Med 179:307, 2009

Hunninghake GW et al: ATS/ERS/WASOG statement on sarcoidosis. American Thoracic Society/European Respiratory Society/World Association of Sarcoidosis and other Granulomatous Disorders. Sarcoidosis Vasc Diffuse Lung Dis 16:149, 1999

Iannuzzi MC et al: Sarcoidosis. N Engl J Med 357:2153, 2007

Judson MA et al: Efficacy of infliximab in extrapulmonary sarcoidosis: Results from a randomised trial. Eur Respir J 31:1189, 2008

Newman LS et al: A case control etiologic study of sarcoidosis: Environmental and occupational risk factors. Am J Respir Crit Care Med 170:1324, 2004

Rossman MD et al: HLA-DRB1*1101: A significant risk factor for sarcoidosis in blacks and whites. Am J Hum Genet 73:720, 2003

Ziegenhagen MW et al: Exaggerated TNF-alpha release of alveolar macrophages in corticosteroid resistant sarcoidosis. Sarcoidosis Vasc Diffuse Lung Dis 19:185, 2002

CHAPTER 330

Familial Mediterranean Fever and Other Hereditary Recurrent Fevers

Daniel L. Kastner

Familial Mediterranean fever (FMF) is the prototype of a group of inherited diseases (Table 330-1) that are characterized by recurrent episodes of fever with serosal, synovial, or cutaneous inflammation and, in some individuals, the eventual development of systemic AA amyloidosis (Chap. 112). Because of the relative infrequency of high-titer autoantibodies or antigen-specific T cells, the term *autoinflammatory* has been proposed to describe these disorders, rather than autoimmune. The innate immune system, with its myeloid effector cells and germline receptors for pathogen-associated molecular patterns and endogenous danger signals, plays a predominant role in the pathogenesis of the autoinflammatory diseases.

BACKGROUND AND PATHOPHYSIOLOGY

FMF was first recognized among Armenians, Arabs, Turks, and non-Ashkenazi (primarily North African and Iraqi) Jews. With the advent of genetic testing, FMF has been documented with increasing frequency among Ashkenazi Jews, Italians, and other Mediterranean populations, and occasional cases have been confirmed even in the absence of known Mediterranean ancestry. FMF is recessively inherited, but, particularly in countries where families are small, a positive family history can only be elicited in ~50% of cases. DNA testing demonstrates carrier frequencies as high as 1:3 among affected populations, suggesting a heterozygote advantage.

The FMF gene encodes a 781-amino acid, ~95 kDa protein denoted *pyrin* (or *marenostrin*) that is expressed in granulocytes, eosinophils, monocytes, dendritic cells, and synovial and peritoneal fibroblasts. The N-terminal 92 amino acids of pyrin define a motif, the PYRIN domain, that is similar in structure to death domains, death effector domains, and caspase recruitment domains. PYRIN domains mediate homotypic protein-protein interactions and have been found in several other proteins, including cryopyrin, which is mutated in three other recurrent fever syndromes. Through a number of mechanisms, including the interaction of the PYRIN domain with an intermediary adaptor protein, pyrin regulates caspase-1 [interleukin (IL) 1β-converting enzyme], and thereby IL-1β secretion. Mice bearing FMF-associated pyrin mutations exhibit inflammation and excessive IL-1 production.

ACUTE ATTACKS

Febrile episodes in FMF may begin even in early infancy; 90% of patients have had their first attack by age 20. Typical FMF episodes generally last 24–72 hours, with arthritic attacks tending to last somewhat longer. In some patients the episodes occur with great regularity, but more often the frequency of attacks varies over time, ranging from as often as once every few days to remissions lasting several years. Attacks are often unpredictable, although some patients relate them to physical exertion, emotional stress, or menses; pregnancy may be associated with remission.

If measured, fever is nearly always present throughout FMF attacks. Severe hyperpyrexia and even febrile seizures may be seen in infants, and fever is sometimes the only manifestation of FMF in young children.

Over 90% of FMF patients experience abdominal attacks at some time. Episodes range in severity from dull, aching pain and distention with mild tenderness on direct palpation to severe generalized pain with absent bowel sounds, rigidity, rebound tenderness, and air-fluid levels on upright radiographs. CT scanning may demonstrate a small amount of fluid in the abdominal cavity. If such patients undergo exploratory laparotomy, a sterile, neutrophil-rich peritoneal exudate is present, sometimes with adhesions from previous episodes. Ascites is rare.

Pleural attacks are usually manifested by unilateral, sharp, stabbing chest pain. Radiographs may show atelectasis and sometimes an effusion. If performed, thoracentesis demonstrates an exudative fluid rich in neutrophils. After repeated attacks, pleural thickening may develop.

FMF arthritis is most frequent among individuals homozygous for the M694V mutation, which is especially common in the non-Ashkenazi Jewish population. Acute arthritis in FMF is usually monoarticular, affecting the knee, ankle, or hip, although other patterns can be seen, particularly in children. Large sterile effusions rich in neutrophils are frequent, without commensurate erythema or warmth. Even after repeated arthritic attacks, radiographic changes are rare. Before the advent of colchicine prophylaxis, chronic arthritis of the knee or hip were seen in ~5% of FMF patients with arthritis. Chronic sacroiliitis can occur in FMF irrespective of the HLA-B27 antigen, even in the face of colchicine therapy. In the United States, FMF patients are much more likely to have arthralgia than arthritis.

The most characteristic cutaneous manifestation of FMF is erysipelas-like erythema, a raised erythematous rash that most commonly occurs on the dorsum of the foot, ankle, or lower leg alone or in combination with abdominal pain, pleurisy, or arthritis. Biopsy demonstrates perivascular infiltrates of granulocytes and monocytes. This rash is seen most often in M694V homozygotes and is relatively rare in the United States.

Exercise-induced (nonfebrile) myalgia is common in FMF, and a small percentage of patients develop a protracted febrile myalgia that can last several weeks. Symptomatic pericardial disease is rare, although some patients have small pericardial effusions as an incidental echocardiographic finding. Unilateral acute scrotal inflammation may occur in prepubertal boys. Aseptic meningitis has been reported in FMF, but the causal connection is controversial. Vasculitis, including Henoch-Schönlein purpura and polyarteritis nodosum (Chap. 326) may be seen at increased frequency in FMF.

Laboratory features of FMF attacks are consistent with acute inflammation and include an elevated erythrocyte sedimentation rate, leukocytosis, thrombocytosis (in children), and elevations in C-reactive protein, fibrinogen, haptoglobin, and serum immunoglobulins. Transient albuminuria and hematuria may also be seen.

AMYLOIDOSIS

Before the advent of colchicine prophylaxis, systemic amyloidosis was a common complication of FMF. It is caused by deposition

TABLE 330-1 The Hereditary Recurrent Fever Syndromes

	FMF	TRAPS	HIDS	MWS	FCAS	NOMID
Ethnicity	Jewish, Arab, Turkish, Armenian, Italian	Any ethnic group	Predominantly Dutch, northern European	Any ethnic group	Any ethnic group	Any ethnic group
Inheritance	Recessive[a]	Dominant	Recessive	Dominant	Dominant	Usually de novo mutations
Gene/chromosome	*MEFV*/16p13.3	*TNFRSF1A*/12p13	*MVK*/12q24	*NLRP3*/1q44	*NLRP3*/1q44	*NLRP3*/1q44
Protein	Pyrin	p55 TNF receptor	Mevalonate kinase	Cryopyrin	Cryopyrin	Cryopyrin
Attack length	1–3 days	Often > 7 days	3–7 days	1–2 days	Minutes–3 days	Continuous, with flares
Serosa	Pleurisy, peritonitis; asymptomatic pericardial effusions	Pleurisy, peritonitis, pericarditis	Abd pain, but seldom peritonitis; pleurisy, pericarditis uncommon	Abd pain common; pleurisy, pericarditis rare	Rare	Rare
Skin	Erysipeloid erythema	Centrifugally migrating erythema	Diffuse maculopapular rash; oral ulcers	Diffuse urticaria-like rash	Cold-induced urticaria-like rash	Diffuse urticaria-like rash
Joints	Acute monoarthritis; chronic hip arthritis (rare)	Acute monoarthritis, arthralgia	Arthralgia, oligoarthritis	Arthralgia, large joint oligoarthritis	Polyarthralgia	Epiphyseal, patellar overgrowth, clubbing
Muscle	Exercise-induced myalgia common; protracted febrile myalgia rare	Migratory myalgia	Uncommon	Myalgia common	Sometimes myalgia	Sometimes myalgia
Eyes, ears	Uncommon	Periorbital edema, conjunctivitis, rarely uveitis	Uncommon	Conjunctivitis, episcleritis, optic disc edema; sensorineural hearing loss	Conjunctivitis	Conjunctivitis, uveitis, optic disc edema, blindness, sensorineural hearing loss
CNS	Aseptic meningitis rare	Headache	Headache	Headache	Headache	Aseptic meningitis, seizures
Amyloidosis	Most common in M694V homozygotes	~15% of cases	Uncommon	~25% of cases	Uncommon	Late complication
Treatment	Oral colchicine prophylaxis	Glucocorticoids, etanercept, anakinra (IL-1 receptor antagonist)	NSAIDs for fever; IL-1β and TNF inhibitors investigational	Anakinra, rilonacept, canakinumab	Anakinra, rilonacept, canakinumab	Anakinra

[a]A substantial percentage of patients with clinical FMF have only a single demonstrable *MEFV* mutation on DNA sequencing.

Abbreviations: FCAS, familial cold autoinflammatory syndrome; FMF, familial Mediterranean fever; HIDS, hyperimmunoglobulinemia D with periodic fever syndrome; IL, interleukin; MWS, Muckle-Wells syndrome; NOMID, neonatal-onset multisystem inflammatory disease; NSAIDs, nonsteroidal anti-inflammatories; TNF, tumor necrosis factor; TRAPS, TNF receptor-associated periodic syndrome.

of a fragment of serum amyloid A, an acute-phase reactant, in the kidneys, adrenals, intestine, spleen, lung, and testes (Chap. 112). Amyloidosis should be suspected in patients who have proteinuria between attacks; renal or rectal biopsy are used most often to establish the diagnosis. Risk factors include the M694V homozygous genotype, positive family history (independent of FMF mutational status), the SAA 1 genotype, male gender, noncompliance with colchicine therapy, and having grown up in the Middle East.

DIAGNOSIS

For typical cases, physicians experienced with FMF can often make the diagnosis on clinical grounds alone. Clinical criteria sets for FMF have been shown to have high sensitivity and specificity in parts of the world where the pretest probability of FMF is high. Genetic testing can provide a useful adjunct in ambiguous cases or for physicians not experienced in FMF. Most of the more severe disease-associated FMF mutations are in exon 10 of the gene, with a smaller group of milder variants in exon 2. An updated list of mutations for FMF and other hereditary recurrent fevers can be found online at *http://fmf.igh.cnrs.fr/infevers/*.

Genetic testing has permitted a broadening of the clinical spectrum and geographic distribution of FMF and may be of prognostic value. Most studies indicate that M694V homozygotes have an earlier age of onset and a higher frequency of arthritis, rash, and amyloidosis. In contrast, the E148Q variant is usually associated with milder disease. E148Q is sometimes found in *cis* with exon 10 mutations, which complicates the interpretation of genetic test results. Only ~70% of patients with clinically typical FMF have two identifiable mutations in *trans*, suggesting either that current screening methods do not detect all of the relevant mutations or that one mutation may be sufficient to cause disease under some circumstances. In these cases clinical judgment is very important, and sometimes a therapeutic trial of colchicine may help to confirm the diagnosis. Genetic testing of unaffected individuals is usually inadvisable, because of the possibility of nonpenetrance and the potential impact of a positive test on future insurability.

If a patient is seen during his or her first attack, the differential diagnosis may be broad, although delimited by the specific organ involvement. After several attacks the differential diagnosis may include the other hereditary recurrent fever syndromes (Table 330-1); the syndrome of periodic fever with aphthous ulcers, pharyngitis, and cervical adenopathy (PFAPA); systemic-onset juvenile rheumatoid arthritis or adult Still's disease; porphyria; hereditary angioedema; inflammatory bowel disease; and, in women, gynecologic disorders.

TREATMENT Familial Mediterranean Fever

The treatment of choice for FMF is daily oral colchicine, which decreases the frequency and intensity of attacks and prevents the development of amyloidosis in compliant patients. Intermittent dosing at the onset of attacks is not as effective as daily prophylaxis and is of unproven value in preventing amyloidosis. The usual adult dose of colchicine is 1.2–1.8 mg/d, which causes substantial reduction in symptoms in two-thirds of patients and some improvement in >90%. Children may require lower doses, although not proportionately to body weight.

Common side effects of colchicine include bloating, abdominal cramps, lactose intolerance, and diarrhea. They can be minimized by starting at a low dose and gradually advancing as tolerated, splitting the dose, use of simethecone for flatulence, and avoidance of dairy products. If taken by either parent at the time of conception, colchicine may cause a small increase in the risk of trisomy 21 (Down syndrome). In elderly patients with renal insufficiency, colchicine can cause a myoneuropathy characterized by proximal muscle weakness and elevation of the creatine kinase. Cyclosporine inhibits hepatic excretion of colchicine by its effects on the MDR-1 transport system, sometimes leading to colchicine toxicity in patients who have undergone renal transplantation for amyloidosis. Intravenous colchicine should generally not be administered to patients already taking oral colchicine, because severe, sometimes fatal, toxicity can occur in this setting.

There are no established alternatives for the small number of patients who do not respond to colchicine or cannot tolerate therapeutic dosages, although the IL-1 receptor antagonist and inhibitors of tumor necrosis factor (TNF) are investigational. Bone marrow transplantation has been suggested for refractory FMF, but the risk-benefit ratio is currently regarded as unacceptable.

OTHER HEREDITARY RECURRENT FEVERS

Within 5 years of the discovery of the FMF gene, three additional genes causing five other hereditary recurrent fever syndromes were identified, catalyzing a paradigm shift in diagnosis and treatment of these disorders.

TNF RECEPTOR–ASSOCIATED PERIODIC SYNDROME (TRAPS)

TRAPS is caused by dominantly inherited mutations in the extracellular domains of the 55-kDa TNF receptor (TNFRSF1A, p55). Although originally described in a large Irish family (and hence the name *familial Hibernian fever*), TRAPS has a broad ethnic distribution. TRAPS episodes often begin in childhood. The duration of attacks ranges from 1–2 days to as long as several weeks, and in severe cases symptoms may be nearly continuous. In addition to peritoneal, pleural, and synovial attacks similar to FMF, TRAPS patients frequently have ocular inflammation (most often conjunctivitis and/or periorbital edema), and a distinctive migratory myalgia with overlying painful erythema may be present. TRAPS patients generally respond better to glucocorticoids than to prophylactic colchicine. About 15% develop amyloidosis. The diagnosis of TRAPS is based on the demonstration of *TNFRSF1A* mutations in the presence of characteristic symptoms. Leukocytes from patients with certain TRAPS mutations exhibit a defect in TNF receptor-shedding, possibly impairing normal homeostasis. However, a more complex picture is emerging, with a number of functional abnormalities, some of which are ligand-independent, contributing to the autoinflammatory phenotype. Etanercept, a TNF inhibitor, ameliorates TRAPS attacks, although its effect on amyloidosis is unproven. Perhaps because of the ligand-independent signaling abnormalities in TRAPS, IL-1 inhibition has been beneficial in some patients.

HYPERIMMUNOGLOBULINEMIA D WITH PERIODIC FEVER SYNDROME (HIDS)

HIDS is a recessively inherited recurrent fever syndrome found primarily in individuals of northern European ancestry. It is caused by mutations in mevalonate kinase (*MVK*), encoding an enzyme involved in the synthesis of cholesterol and nonsterol isoprenoids. Attacks usually begin in infancy, and last 3–5 days. Clinically distinctive features include painful cervical adenopathy, a diffuse maculopapular rash sometimes affecting the palms and soles, and aphthous ulcers; pleurisy is rare, as is amyloidosis. Although originally defined by the persistent elevation of serum IgD, disease activity is not related to IgD levels, and some patients with FMF or TRAPS may have modestly increased serum IgD. Moreover, occasional patients with *MVK* mutations and recurrent fever have normal IgD levels. All patients with mutations have markedly elevated urinary mevalonate levels during their febrile attacks, although the inflammatory manifestations are likely to be due to a deficiency of isoprenoids rather than an excess of mevalonate. There is currently no established treatment for HIDS, although intermittent or continuous IL-1 inhibition are investigational.

THE CRYOPYRINOPATHIES, OR CRYOPYRIN-ASSOCIATED PERIODIC SYNDROMES (CAPS)

Three hereditary febrile syndromes, familial cold autoinflammatory syndrome (FCAS), Muckle-Wells syndrome (MWS), and neonatal-onset multisystem inflammatory disease (NOMID), are all caused by mutations in *NLRP3* (formerly known as *CIAS1)*, the gene encoding cryopyrin (or NLRP3), and represent a clinical spectrum of disease. FCAS patients develop chills, fever, headache, arthralgia, conjunctivitis, and an urticaria-like rash in response to generalized cold exposure. In MWS, an urticarial rash is noted, but it is not usually induced by cold; MWS patients also develop fevers, abdominal pain, limb pain, arthritis, conjunctivitis, and, over time, sensorineural hearing loss. NOMID is the most severe of the three disorders, with chronic aseptic meningitis, a characteristic arthropathy, and rash. Like the FMF protein, pyrin, cryopyrin has an N-terminal PYRIN domain. Cryopyrin regulates IL-1β production through the formation of a macromolecular complex termed the *inflammasome*. Peripheral blood leukocytes from patients with FCAS, MWS, and NOMID release increased amounts of IL-1β upon in vitro stimulation, relative to healthy controls. Macrophages from cryopyrin-deficient mice exhibit decreased IL-1β production in response to certain gram-positive bacteria, bacterial RNA, and monosodium urate crystals. Patients with all three cryopyrinopathies show a dramatic response to injections of IL-1 inhibitors. Increased IL-1 signaling is also a feature of the recently-described deficiency in the interleukin-1 receptor antagonist (DIRA), a recessively inherited disorder similarly responsive to anakinra treatment. In contrast to the cryopyrinopathies, DIRA presents with pustular skin lesions and multifocal sterile osteomyelitis, and fever is often not a prominent feature.

FURTHER READINGS

Aksentijevich I et al: An autoinflammatory disease with deficiency of the interleukin-1-receptor antagonist. N Engl J Med 360:2426, 2009

Dinarello CA: Interleukin-1β and the autoinflammatory diseases. N Engl J Med 360:2467, 2009

Goldbach-Mansky R et al: Neonatal-onset multisystem inflammatory disease responsive to interleukin-1β inhibition. N Engl J Med 355:581, 2006

Hoffman HM et al: Prevention of cold-associated acute inflammation in familial cold autoinflammatory syndrome by interleukin-1 receptor antagonist. Lancet 364:1779, 2004

Hull KM et al: The TNF receptor–associated periodic syndrome (TRAPS). Emerging concepts of an autoinflammatory disorder. Medicine (Baltimore) 81:349, 2002

Kastner DL et al: Autoinflammatory disease reloaded: a clinical perspective. Cell 140:784, 2010

Kuijk LM et al: HMG-CoA reductase inhibition induces IL-1β release through Rac1/PI3K/PKB-dependent caspase-1 activation. Blood 112:3563, 2008

Lachmann HJ et al: In vivo regulation of interleukin 1β in patients with cryopyrin-associated periodic syndromes. J Exp Med 206:1029, 2009

Masters SL et al: *Horror autoinflammaticus:* The molecular pathophysiology of autoinflammatory disease. Annu Rev Immunol 27:621, 2009

Schroder K, Tschopp J: The inflammasomes. Cell 140: 140:821, 2010

SECTION 3 Disorders of the Joints and Adjacent Tissues

CHAPTER 331 Approach to Articular and Musculoskeletal Disorders

John J. Cush
Peter E. Lipsky

Musculoskeletal complaints account for >315 million outpatient visits per year and nearly 20% of all outpatient visits in the United States. The Centers for Disease Control and Prevention estimate that 22% (46 million) of the U.S. population has physician-diagnosed arthritis and 19 million have significant functional limitation. While many patients will have self-limited conditions requiring minimal evaluation and only symptomatic therapy and reassurance, specific musculoskeletal presentations or their persistence may herald a more serious condition that requires further evaluation or laboratory testing to establish a diagnosis. The goal of the musculoskeletal evaluation is to formulate a differential diagnosis that leads to an accurate diagnosis and timely therapy, while avoiding excessive diagnostic testing and unnecessary treatment (Table 331-1). There are several urgent conditions that must be diagnosed promptly to avoid significant morbid or mortal sequelae. These "red flag" diagnoses include septic arthritis, acute crystal-induced arthritis (e.g., gout), and fracture. Each may be suspected by its acute onset and monarticular or focal musculoskeletal pain (see below).

Individuals with musculoskeletal complaints should be evaluated with a thorough history, a comprehensive physical and musculoskeletal examination, and, if appropriate, laboratory testing. The initial encounter should determine whether the musculoskeletal complaint signals a red flag condition (septic arthritis, gout, or fracture) or not. The evaluation should proceed to ascertain if the complaint is (1) *articular* or *nonarticular* in origin, (2) *inflammatory* or *noninflammatory* in nature, (3) *acute* or *chronic* in duration, and (4) *localized (monarticular)* or *widespread (polyarticular)* in distribution.

TABLE 331-1 Evaluation of Patients With Musculoskeletal Complaints

Goals
Accurate diagnosis
Timely provision of therapy
Avoidance of unnecessary diagnostic testing
Approach
Anatomic localization of complaint (articular vs. nonarticular)
Determination of the nature of the pathologic process (inflammatory vs. noninflammatory)
Determination of the extent of involvement (monarticular, polyarticular, focal, widespread)
Determination of chronology (acute vs. chronic)
Consider the most common disorders first
Formulation of a differential diagnosis

With such an approach and an understanding of the pathophysiologic processes, the musculoskeletal complaint or presentation can be characterized (e.g., acute inflammatory monarthritis or a chronic noninflammatory, nonarticular widespread pain) to narrow the diagnostic possibilities. A diagnosis can be made in the vast majority of individuals. However, some patients will not fit immediately into an established diagnostic category. Many musculoskeletal disorders resemble each other at the outset, and some may take weeks or months to evolve into a readily recognizable diagnostic entity. This consideration should temper the desire to establish a definitive diagnosis at the first encounter.

ARTICULAR VERSUS NONARTICULAR

The musculoskeletal evaluation must discriminate the anatomic origin(s) of the patient's complaint. For example, ankle pain can result from a variety of pathologic conditions involving disparate anatomic structures, including gonococcal arthritis, calcaneal fracture, Achilles tendinitis, plantar fasciitis, cellulitis, and peripheral or entrapment neuropathy. Distinguishing between articular and nonarticular conditions requires a careful and detailed examination. Articular structures include the synovium, synovial fluid, articular cartilage, intraarticular ligaments, joint capsule, and juxtaarticular bone. Nonarticular (or periarticular) structures, such as supportive extraarticular ligaments, tendons, bursae, muscle, fascia, bone, nerve, and overlying skin, may be involved in the pathologic process. Although musculoskeletal complaints are often ascribed to the joints, nonarticular disorders more frequently underlie such complaints. Distinguishing between these potential sources of pain may be challenging to the unskilled examiner. Articular disorders may be characterized by deep or diffuse pain, pain or limited range of motion on active and passive movement, and swelling (caused by synovial proliferation, effusion, or bony enlargement), crepitation, instability, "locking," or deformity. By contrast, nonarticular disorders tend to be painful on active, but not passive (or assisted), range of motion. Periarticular conditions often demonstrate point or focal tenderness in regions adjacent to articular structures, and have physical findings remote from the joint capsule. Moreover, nonarticular disorders seldom demonstrate swelling, crepitus, instability, or deformity of the joint itself.

INFLAMMATORY VERSUS NONINFLAMMATORY DISORDERS

In the course of a musculoskeletal evaluation, the examiner should determine the nature of the underlying pathologic process and whether inflammatory or noninflammatory findings exist. Inflammatory disorders may be infectious (infection with *Neisseria gonorrhoea* or *Mycobacterium tuberculosis*), crystal-induced (gout, pseudogout), immune-related [rheumatoid arthritis (RA), systemic lupus erythematosus (SLE)], reactive (rheumatic fever, reactive arthritis), or idiopathic. Inflammatory disorders may be identified by any of the four cardinal signs of inflammation (erythema, warmth, pain, or swelling), systemic symptoms (fatigue, fever, rash, weight loss), or laboratory evidence of inflammation [elevated erythrocyte sedimentation rate (ESR) or C-reactive protein (CRP), thrombocytosis, anemia of chronic disease, or hypoalbuminemia]. Articular stiffness commonly accompanies chronic musculoskeletal disorders and can extend beyond the joint. However, the severity and duration of stiffness may be diagnostically important. Morning stiffness related to inflammatory disorders (such as RA or polymyalgia rheumatica) is precipitated by prolonged rest, is described as severe, lasts for hours, and may improve with activity or anti-inflammatory medications. By contrast, intermittent stiffness (also known as gel phenomenon), associated with noninflammatory conditions [such as osteoarthritis (OA)], is precipitated by brief periods of rest, usually lasts less than 60 minutes, and is exacerbated by activity. Fatigue may accompany inflammation (as seen in RA and polymyalgia rheumatica) but may also be a consequence of fibromyalgia (a noninflammatory disorder), anemia, cardiac failure, endocrinopathy, poor nutrition, chronic pain, poor sleep, or depression. Noninflammatory disorders may be related to trauma (rotator cuff tear), repetitive use (bursitis, tendinitis), degeneration or ineffective repair (OA), neoplasm (pigmented villonodular synovitis), or pain amplification (fibromyalgia). Noninflammatory disorders are often characterized by pain without synovial swelling or warmth, absence of inflammatory or systemic features, daytime gel phenomena rather than morning stiffness, and normal (for age) or negative laboratory investigations.

Identification of the nature of the underlying process and the site of the complaint will enable the examiner to characterize the musculoskeletal presentation (e.g., acute inflammatory monarthritis, chronic noninflammatory, nonarticular widespread pain), narrow the diagnostic considerations, and assess the need for immediate diagnostic or therapeutic intervention or for continued observation. Figure 331-1 presents an algorithmic approach to the evaluation of patients with musculoskeletal complaints. This approach is remarkably effective and relies on clinical and historic features, rather than laboratory testing, to diagnose many common rheumatic disorders.

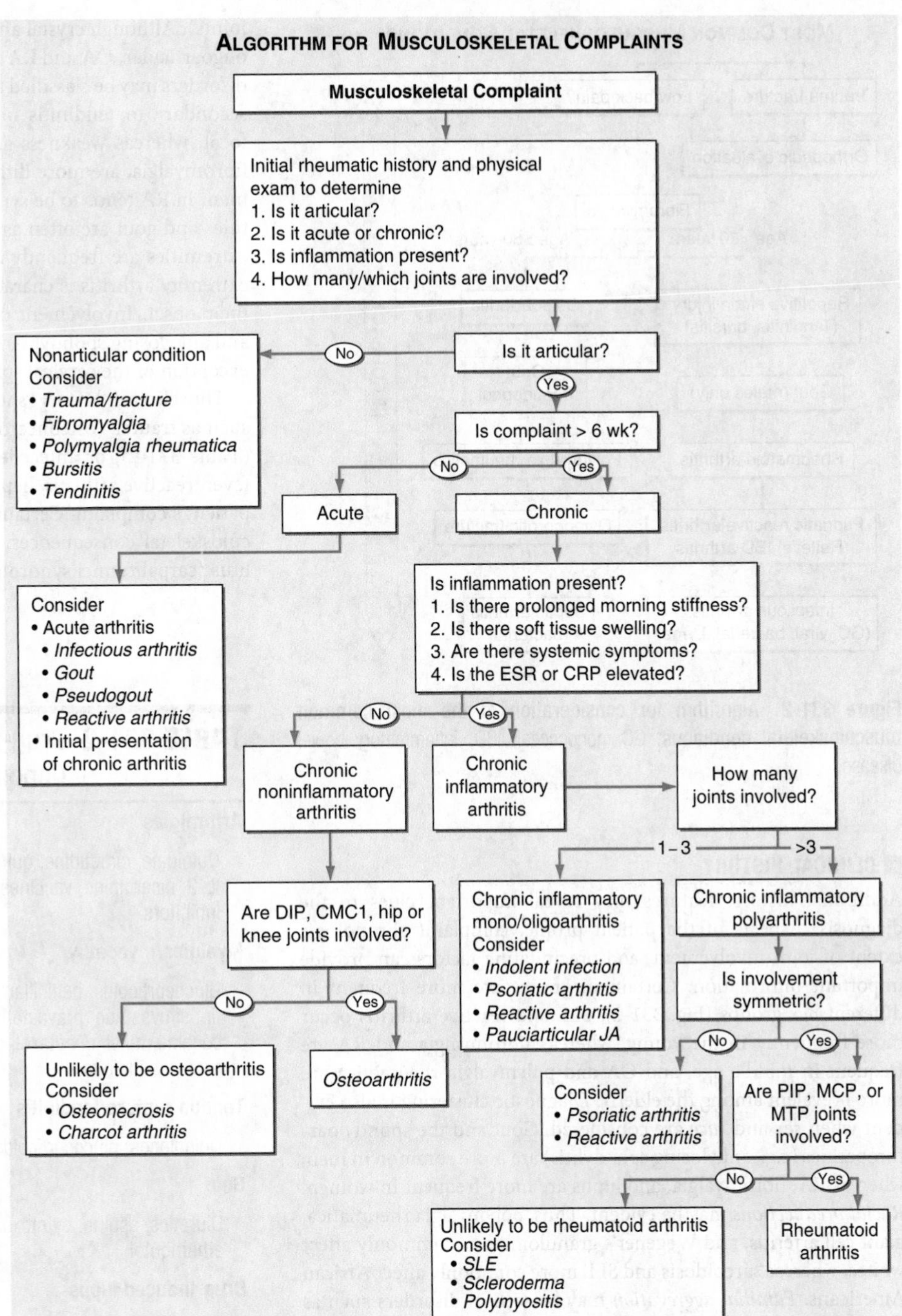

Figure 331-1 Algorithm for the diagnosis of musculoskeletal complaints. An approach to formulating a differential diagnosis (shown in italics). CMC, carpometacarpal; CRP, C-reactive protein; DIP, distal interphalangeal; ESR, erythrocyte sedimentation rate; JA, juvenile arthritis; MCP, metacarpophalangeal; MTP, metatarsophalangeal; PIP, proximal interphalangeal; PMR, polymyalgia rheumatica; SLE, systemic lupus erythematosus.

The algorithmic approach may be unnecessary in patients with the most commonly encountered ailments; as these can also be considered based on frequency and characteristic presentations. The most prevalent causes of musculoskeletal complaints are shown in Fig. 331-2. As trauma, fracture, overuse syndromes, and fibromyalgia are among the most common causes of presentation, these should be considered during the initial encounter. If these possibilities are excluded, other frequently occurring disorders should be considered according to the patient's age. Hence, those younger than 60 years are commonly affected by repetitive use/strain disorders, gout (men only), RA, spondyloarthritis, and uncommonly, infectious arthritis. Patients over age 60 years are frequently affected by OA, crystal (gout and pseudogout) arthritis, polymyalgia rheumatica, osteoporotic fracture, and uncommonly, septic arthritis. These conditions are between 10 and 100 times more prevalent than other serious autoimmune conditions, such as systemic lupus erythematosus, scleroderma, polymyositis, and vasculitis.

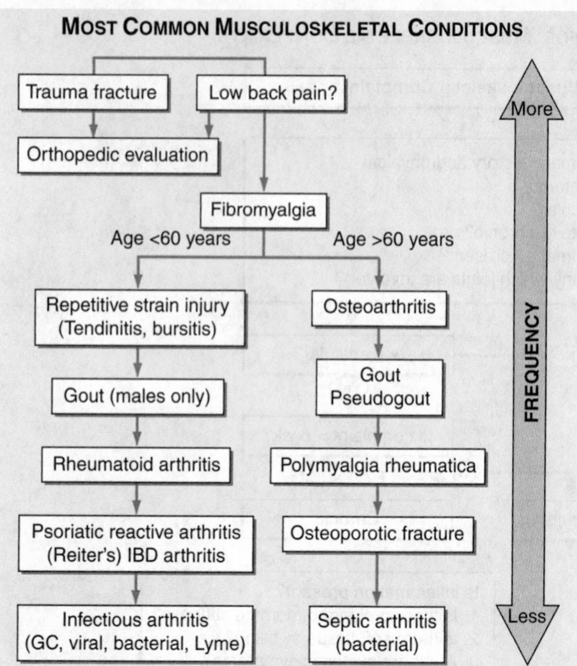

Figure 331-2 Algorithm for consideration of the most common musculoskeletal conditions. GC, gonococcal; IBD, inflammatory bowel disease.

CLINICAL HISTORY

Additional historic features may reveal important clues to the diagnosis. Aspects of the patient profile, complaint chronology, extent of joint involvement, and precipitating factors can provide important information. Certain diagnoses are more frequent in different *age* groups (Fig. 331-2). SLE and reactive arthritis occur more frequently in the young, whereas fibromyalgia and RA are frequent in middle age, and OA and polymyalgia rheumatica are more prevalent among the elderly. Diagnostic clustering is also evident when *sex* and *race* are considered. Gout and the spondyloarthropathies (e.g., ankylosing spondylitis) are more common in men, whereas RA, fibromyalgia, and lupus are more frequent in women. *Racial predilections* may be evident. Thus, polymyalgia rheumatica, giant cell arteritis, and Wegener's granulomatosis commonly affect whites, whereas sarcoidosis and SLE more commonly affect African Americans. *Familial aggregation* may be seen in disorders such as ankylosing spondylitis, gout, and Heberden's nodes of OA.

The chronology of the complaint is an important diagnostic feature and can be divided into the *onset, evolution,* and *duration.* The onset of disorders such as septic arthritis or gout tends to be abrupt, whereas OA, RA, and fibromyalgia may have more indolent presentations. The patients' complaints may evolve differently and be classified as chronic (OA), intermittent (crystal or Lyme arthritis), migratory (rheumatic fever, gonococcal or viral arthritis), or additive (RA, psoriatic arthritis). Musculoskeletal disorders are typically classified as acute or chronic based upon a symptom duration that is either less than or greater than 6 weeks, respectively. Acute arthropathies tend to be infectious, crystal-induced, or reactive. Chronic conditions include noninflammatory or immunologic arthritides (e.g., OA, RA) and nonarticular disorders (e.g., fibromyalgia).

The *extent* or *distribution* of articular involvement is often informative. Articular disorders are classified based on the number of joints involved, as either *monarticular* (one joint), *oligoarticular* or *pauciarticular* (two or three joints), or *polyarticular* (four or more joints). Although crystal and infectious arthritis are often mono- or oligoarticular, OA and RA are polyarticular disorders. Nonarticular disorders may be classified as either focal or widespread. Complaints secondary to tendinitis or carpal tunnel syndrome are typically focal, whereas weakness and myalgia, caused by polymyositis or fibromyalgia, are more diffuse in their presentation. Joint involvement in RA tends to be symmetric, whereas the spondyloarthropathies and gout are often asymmetric and oligoarticular. The upper extremities are frequently involved in RA and OA, whereas lower extremity arthritis is characteristic of reactive arthritis and gout at their onset. Involvement of the axial skeleton is common in OA and ankylosing spondylitis but is infrequent in RA, with the notable exception of the cervical spine.

The clinical history should also identify *precipitating events,* such as trauma (osteonecrosis, meniscal tear), drug administration (Table 331-2), or antecedent or intercurrent illnesses (rheumatic fever, reactive arthritis, hepatitis), that may have contributed to the patient's complaint. Certain comorbidities may predispose to musculoskeletal consequences. This is especially so for diabetes mellitus (carpal tunnel syndrome), renal insufficiency (gout), psoriasis

TABLE 331-2 Drug-Induced Musculoskeletal Conditions

Arthralgias
Quinidine, cimetidine, quinolones, chronic acyclovir, interferon, IL-2, nicardipine, vaccines, rifabutin, aromatase and HIV protease inhibitors
Myalgias/myopathy
Glucocorticoids, penicillamine, hydroxychloroquine, AZT, lovastatin, simvastatin, pravastatin, clofibrate, interferon, IL-2, alcohol, cocaine, taxol, docetaxel, colchicine, quinolones, cyclosporine, protease inhibitors
Tendon rupture/tendinitis
Quinolones, glucocorticoids, isotretinoin
Gout
Diuretics, aspirin, cytotoxics, cyclosporine, alcohol, moonshine, ethambutol
Drug-induced lupus
Hydralazine, procainamide, quinidine, phenytoin, carbamazepine, methyldopa, isoniazid, chlorpromazine, lithium, penicillamine, tetracyclines, TNF inhibitors, ACE inhibitors, ticlopidine
Osteonecrosis
Glucocorticoids, alcohol, radiation, bisphosphonates
Osteopenia
Glucocorticoids, chronic heparin, phenytoin, methotrexate
Scleroderma
Vinyl chloride, bleomycin, pentazocine, organic solvents, carbidopa, tryptophan, rapeseed oil
Vasculitis
Allopurinol, amphetamines, cocaine, thiazides, penicillamine, propylthiouracil, montelukast, TNF inhibitors, hepatitis B vaccine, trimethoprim/sulfamethoxazole

Abbreviations: ACE, angiotensin-converting enzyme; IL-2, interleukin 2; TNF, tumor necrosis factor.

(psoriatic arthritis), myeloma (low back pain), cancer (myositis), and osteoporosis (fracture) or when using certain drugs such as glucocorticoids (osteonecrosis, septic arthritis) and diuretics or chemotherapy (gout) (Table 331-2).

Lastly, a thorough *rheumatic review of systems* may disclose useful diagnostic information. A variety of musculoskeletal disorders may be associated with systemic features such as fever (SLE, infection), rash (SLE, psoriatic arthritis), nail abnormalities (psoriatic or reactive arthritis), myalgias (fibromyalgia, statin- or drug-induced myopathy), or weakness (polymyositis, neuropathy). In addition, some conditions are associated with involvement of other organ systems including the eyes (Behçet's disease, sarcoidosis, spondyloarthritis), gastrointestinal tract (scleroderma, inflammatory bowel disease), genitourinary tract (reactive arthritis, gonococcemia), or the nervous system (Lyme disease, vasculitis).

RHEUMATOLOGIC EVALUATION OF THE ELDERLY

The incidence of rheumatic diseases rises with age, such that 58% of those >65 years will have joint complaints. Musculoskeletal disorders in elderly patients are often not diagnosed because the signs and symptoms may be insidious, overlooked, or overshadowed by comorbidities. These difficulties are compounded by the diminished reliability of laboratory testing in the elderly, who often manifest nonpathologic abnormal results. For example, the ESR may be misleadingly elevated, and low-titer positive tests for rheumatoid factor and antinuclear antibodies (ANAs) may be seen in up to 15% of elderly patients. Although nearly all rheumatic disorders afflict the elderly, certain diseases and drug-induced disorders (Table 331-2) are more common in this age group. The elderly should be approached in the same manner as other patients with musculoskeletal complaints, but with an emphasis on identifying the potential rheumatic consequences of medical comorbidities and therapies. OA, osteoporosis, gout, pseudogout, polymyalgia rheumatica, vasculitis, and drug-induced disorders are all more common in the elderly than in other individuals. The physical examination should identify the nature of the musculoskeletal complaint as well as coexisting diseases that may influence diagnosis and choice of treatment.

RHEUMATOLOGIC EVALUATION OF THE HOSPITALIZED PATIENT

Inpatient and outpatient evaluations and diagnostic considerations may differ, owing to greater symptom severity, more acute presentations, and greater interplay of comorbidities with the hospitalized patient. Patients with rheumatic disorders tend to be admitted for one of several reasons: (1) acute onset of inflammatory arthritis; (2) undiagnosed systemic or febrile illness; (3) musculoskeletal trauma; or (4) exacerbation or deterioration of an existing autoimmune disorder (e.g., SLE); or (5) new medical comorbidities (e.g., thrombotic event, lymphoma, infection) arising in patients with articular or connective tissue disorders. Notably, in the United States, rheumatic patients are seldom if ever admitted because of widespread pain, serologic abnormalities, or for the initiation of new therapies, although this is routinely done in other parts of the world.

Acute monarticular inflammatory arthritis may be a "red flag condition" (e.g., septic arthritis, gout, pseudogout) that will require arthrocentesis. However, new-onset polyarticular inflammatory arthritis will have a wider differential diagnosis (e.g., RA, hepatitis-related arthritis, serum sickness, drug-induced lupus, polyarticular septic arthritis) and may require targeted laboratory investigations rather than synovial fluid analysis. Patients with febrile, multisystem disorders will require exclusion of infectious or neoplastic etiologies and an evaluation driven by dominant symptoms with the greatest specificity. Conditions worthy of consideration may include vasculitis (giant cell arteritis in the elderly or polyarteritis nodosa in younger patients), adult-onset Still's disease, SLE, antiphospholipid antibody syndrome, and sarcoidosis. As misdiagnosis of connective tissue disorders is common, patients who present with a reported preexisting rheumatic condition (e.g., SLE, RA, ankylosing spondylitis) should have their diagnosis confirmed by careful history, physical and musculoskeletal examination, and detailed review of their medical records. It is important to note that when rheumatic disease patients are admitted to the hospital, it is usually for medical problems unrelated to their autoimmune disease, but rather because of either a comorbid condition or complication of drug therapy. Patients with chronic inflammatory disorders (e.g., RA, SLE, psoriasis, etc.) have an augmented risk of infection, cardiovascular events, and neoplasia.

Certain conditions, such as acute gout, can be precipitated in hospitalized patients by surgery, dehydration, or other events and should be considered when hospitalized patients are evaluated for the acute onset of a musculoskeletal condition. It is also common for positive results obtained from overly aggressive and unfocused laboratory testing to generate the need for a full rheumatologic evaluation.

PHYSICAL EXAMINATION

The goal of the physical examination is to ascertain the structures involved, the nature of the underlying pathology, the functional consequences of the process, and the presence of systemic or extraarticular manifestations. A knowledge of topographic anatomy is necessary to identify the primary site(s) of involvement and differentiate articular from nonarticular disorders. The musculoskeletal examination depends largely on careful inspection, palpation, and a variety of specific physical maneuvers to elicit diagnostic signs (Table 331-3). Although most articulations of the appendicular skeleton can be examined in this manner, adequate inspection and palpation are not possible for many axial (e.g., zygapophyseal) and inaccessible (e.g., sacroiliac or hip) joints. For such joints, there is a greater reliance upon specific maneuvers and imaging for assessment.

Examination of involved and uninvolved joints will determine whether *pain*, *warmth*, *erythema*, or *swelling* is present. The locale and level of pain elicited by palpation or movement should be quantified. One example would be to count the number of tender joints on palpation of 28 easily examined joints [proximal interphalangeals (PIPs), metacarpophalangeals (MCPs), wrists, elbows, shoulders, and knees] (with a range of 0–28). Similarly, the number of swollen joints (0–28) can be counted and recorded. Careful examination should distinguish between true articular swelling (caused by synovial effusion or synovial proliferation) and nonarticular (or periarticular) involvement, which usually extends beyond the normal joint margins. Synovial effusion can be distinguished from synovial hypertrophy or bony hypertrophy by palpation or specific maneuvers. For example, small to moderate knee effusions may be identified by the "bulge sign" or "ballottement of the patellae." Bursal effusions (e.g., effusions of the olecranon or prepatellar bursa) are often focal, periarticular, overlie bony prominences, and are fluctuant with sharply defined borders. Joint *stability* can be assessed by palpation and by the application of manual stress. *Subluxation* or *dislocation*, which may be secondary to traumatic, mechanical, or inflammatory causes, can be assessed by inspection and palpation. Joint *swelling* or *volume* can be assessed by palpation. Distention of the articular capsule usually causes pain and evident swelling. The patient will attempt to minimize the pain by maintaining the joint in the position of least intraarticular pressure and greatest volume, usually partial flexion. For this reason, inflammatory effusions may give rise to flexion contractures. Clinically, this

TABLE 331-3 Glossary of Musculoskeletal Terms

Crepitus

A palpable (less commonly audible) vibratory or crackling sensation elicited with joint motion; fine joint crepitus is common and often insignificant in large joints; coarse joint crepitus indicates advanced cartilaginous and degenerative changes (as in osteoarthritis)

Subluxation

Alteration of joint alignment such that articulating surfaces incompletely approximate each other

Dislocation

Abnormal displacement of articulating surfaces such that the surfaces are not in contact

Range of motion

For diarthrodial joints, the arc of measurable movement through which the joint moves in a single plane

Contracture

Loss of full movement resulting from a fixed resistance caused either by tonic spasm of muscle (reversible) or by fibrosis of periarticular structures (permanent)

Deformity

Abnormal shape or size of a structure; may result from bony hypertrophy, malalignment of articulating structures, or damage to periarticular supportive structures

Enthesitis

Inflammation of the entheses (tendinous or ligamentous insertions on bone)

Epicondylitis

Infection or inflammation involving an epicondyle

may be detected as fluctuant or "squishy" swelling, with grapelike compressibility. Inflammation may result in fixed flexion deformities, or diminished range of motion—especially on extension, when joint volumes are decreased. Active and passive *range of motion* should be assessed in all planes, with contralateral comparison. Serial evaluations of the joints should record the number of tender and swollen joints and loss of a normal range of motion, using a goniometer to quantify the arc of movement. Each joint should be passively manipulated through its full range of motion (including, as appropriate, flexion, extension, rotation, abduction, adduction, lateral bending, inversion, eversion, supination, pronation, medial/lateral deviation, plantar- or dorsiflexion). Limitation of motion is frequently caused by effusion, pain, deformity, or contracture. If passive motion exceeds active motion, a periarticular process (e.g., tendinitis, tendon rupture, or myopathy) should be considered. *Contractures* may reflect antecedent synovial inflammation or trauma. Minor joint *crepitus* is common during joint palpation and maneuvers, but may indicate significant cartilage degeneration as it becomes coarser (e.g., OA). Joint *deformity* usually indicates a long-standing or aggressive pathologic process. Deformities may result from ligamentous destruction, soft tissue contracture, bony enlargement, ankylosis, erosive disease, or subluxation. Examination of the musculature will document strength, atrophy, pain, or spasm. Appendicular muscle weakness should be characterized as proximal or distal. Muscle strength should be assessed by observing the patient's performance (e.g., walking, rising from a chair, grasping, writing). Strength may also be graded on a 5-point scale: 0 for no movement; 1 for trace movement or twitch; 2 for movement with gravity eliminated; 3 for movement against gravity only; 4 for movement against gravity and resistance; and 5 for normal strength. The examiner should assess for often-overlooked nonarticular or periarticular involvement, especially when articular complaints are not supported by objective findings referable to the joint capsule. The identification of soft tissue/nonarticular pain will prevent unwarranted and often expensive additional evaluations. Specific maneuvers may reveal common nonarticular abnormalities, such as a carpal tunnel syndrome (which can be identified by Tinel's or Phalen's sign). Other examples of soft tissue abnormalities include olecranon bursitis, epicondylitis (e.g., tennis elbow), enthesitis (e.g., Achilles tendinitis), and tender trigger points associated with fibromyalgia.

APPROACH TO REGIONAL RHEUMATIC COMPLAINTS

Although all patients should be evaluated in a logical and thorough manner, many cases with focal musculoskeletal complaints are caused by commonly encountered disorders that exhibit a predictable pattern of onset, evolution, and localization; they can often be diagnosed immediately on the basis of limited historic information and selected maneuvers or tests. Although nearly every joint could be approached in this manner, the evaluation of four common involved anatomic regions—the hand, shoulder, hip, and knee—are reviewed here.

HAND PAIN

Focal or unilateral hand pain may result from trauma, overuse, infection, or a reactive or crystal-induced arthritis. By contrast, bilateral hand complaints commonly suggest a degenerative (e.g., OA), systemic, or inflammatory/immune (e.g., RA) etiology. The distribution or pattern of joint involvement is highly suggestive of certain disorders (Fig. 331-3). Thus, OA (or degenerative

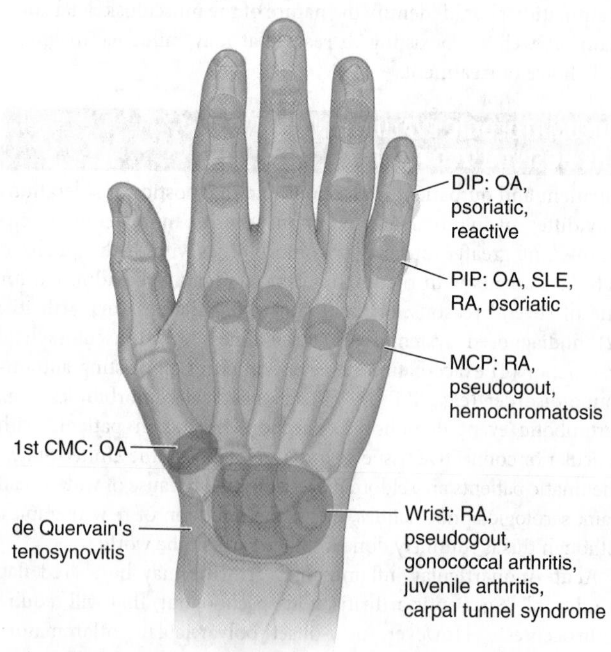

Figure 331-3 Sites of hand or wrist involvement and their potential disease associations. CMC, carpometacarpal; DIP, distal interphalangeal; MCP, metacarpophalangeal; OA, osteoarthritis; PIP, proximal interphalangeal; RA, rheumatoid arthritis; SLE, systemic lupus erythematosus. *(From Cush et al, with permission.)*

arthritis) may manifest as distal interphalangeal (DIP) and PIP joint pain with bony hypertrophy sufficient to produce Heberden's and Bouchard's nodes, respectively. Pain, with or without bony swelling, involving the base of the thumb (first carpometacarpal joint) is also highly suggestive of OA. By contrast, RA tends to involve the PIP, MCP, intercarpal, and carpometacarpal joints (wrist) with pain, prolonged stiffness, and palpable synovial tissue hypertrophy. Psoriatic arthritis may mimic the pattern of joint involvement seen in OA (DIP and PIP joints), but can be distinguished by the presence of inflammatory signs (erythema, warmth, synovial swelling), with or without carpal involvement, nail pitting, or onycholysis. Hemochromatosis should be considered when degenerative changes (bony hypertrophy) are seen at the second and third MCP joints with associated chondrocalcinosis or episodic, inflammatory wrist arthritis.

Soft tissue swelling over the dorsum of the hand and wrist may suggest an inflammatory extensor tendon tenosynovitis possibly caused by gonococcal infection, gout, or inflammatory arthritis (e.g., RA). Tenosynovitis is suggested by localized warmth, swelling, or pitting edema and may be confirmed when the soft tissue swelling tracks with tendon movement, such as flexion and extension of fingers or when pain is induced while stretching the extensor tendon sheaths (flexing the digits distal to the MCP joints and maintaining the wrist in a fixed, neutral position).

Focal wrist pain localized to the radial aspect may be caused by de Quervain's tenosynovitis resulting from inflammation of the tendon sheath(s) involving the abductor pollicis longus or extensor pollicis brevis (Fig. 331-3). This commonly results from overuse or follows pregnancy and may be diagnosed with Finkelstein's test. A positive result is present when radial wrist pain is induced after the thumb is flexed and placed inside a clenched fist and the patient actively deviates the hand downward with ulnar deviation at the wrist. Carpal tunnel syndrome is another common disorder of the upper extremity and results from compression of the median nerve within the carpal tunnel. Manifestations include pain in the wrist that may radiate with paresthesia to the thumb, second and third fingers, and radial half of the fourth finger and, at times, atrophy of thenar musculature. Carpal tunnel syndrome is commonly associated with pregnancy, edema, trauma, OA, inflammatory arthritis, and infiltrative disorders (e.g., amyloidosis). The diagnosis may be suggested by a positive Tinel's or Phalen's sign. With each test, paresthesia in a median nerve distribution is induced or increased by either "thumping" the volar aspect of the wrist (Tinel's sign) or pressing the extensor surfaces of both flexed wrists against each other (Phalen's sign). The variable sensitivity of these tests may require nerve conduction velocity testing to confirm a suspected diagnosis.

■ SHOULDER PAIN

During the evaluation of shoulder disorders, the examiner should carefully note any history of trauma, fibromyalgia, infection, inflammatory disease, occupational hazards, or previous cervical disease. In addition, the patient should be questioned as to the activities or movement(s) that elicit shoulder pain. While arthritis is suggested by pain on movement in all planes, pain with specific active motion suggests a periarticular (nonarticular) process. Shoulder pain may originate in the glenohumeral or acromioclavicular joints, subacromial (subdeltoid) bursa, periarticular soft tissues (e.g., fibromyalgia, rotator cuff tear/tendinitis), or cervical spine (Fig. 331-4). Shoulder pain is referred frequently from the cervical spine but may also be referred from intrathoracic lesions (e.g., a Pancoast tumor) or from gall bladder, hepatic, or diaphragmatic disease. Fibromyalgia should be suspected when glenohumeral pain is accompanied by diffuse periarticular (i.e., subacromial, bicipital) pain and tender points (i.e., trapezius or supraspinatus). The shoulder should be put through its full range of motion both actively and passively (with examiner assistance): forward flexion, extension, abduction, adduction, and internal and external rotation. Manual inspection of the periarticular structures will often provide important diagnostic information. Glenohumeral involvement is best detected by placing the thumb over the glenohumeral joint and applying pressure anteriorly while internally and externally rotating the humeral head. The examiner should apply direct manual pressure over the subacromial bursa that lies lateral to and immediately beneath the acromion (Fig. 331-4). Subacromial bursitis is a frequent cause of shoulder pain. Anterior to the subacromial bursa, the bicipital tendon traverses the bicipital groove. This tendon is best identified by palpating it in its groove as the patient rotates the humerus internally and externally. Direct pressure over the tendon may reveal pain indicative of bicipital tendinitis. Palpation of the acromioclavicular joint may disclose local pain, bony hypertrophy, or, uncommonly, synovial swelling. Whereas OA and RA commonly affect the acromioclavicular joint, OA seldom involves the glenohumeral joint, unless there is a traumatic or occupational cause. The glenohumeral joint is best palpated anteriorly by placing the thumb over the humeral head (just medial and inferior to the coracoid process) and having the patient rotate the humerus internally and externally. Pain localized to this region is indicative of glenohumeral pathology. Synovial effusion or tissue is seldom palpable but, if present, may suggest infection, RA, or an acute tear of the rotator cuff.

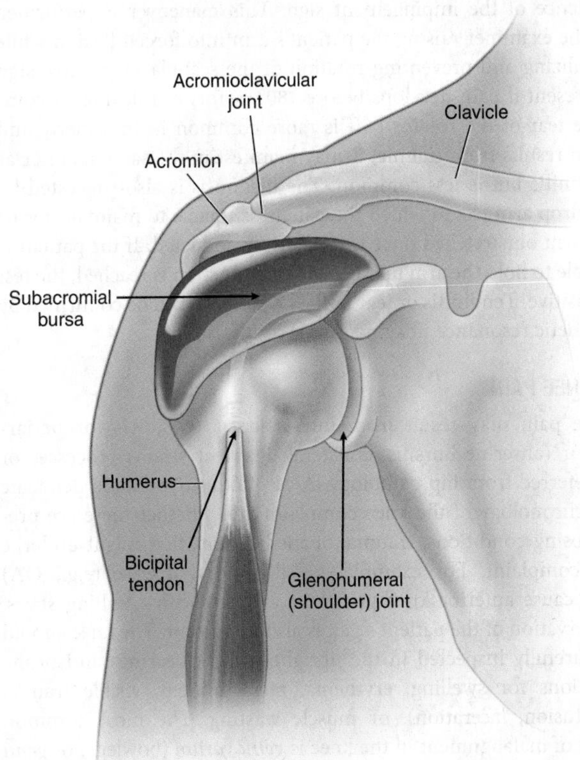

Figure 331-4 Origins of shoulder pain. The schematic diagram of the shoulder indicates with arrows the most common causes and locations of shoulder pain.

Rotator cuff tendinitis or tear is a very common cause of shoulder pain. The rotator cuff is formed by the tendons of the supraspinatus, infraspinatus, teres minor, and subscapularis muscles. Rotator cuff tendinitis is suggested by pain on active abduction (but not passive abduction), pain over the lateral deltoid muscle, night pain, and evidence of the impingement sign. This maneuver is performed by the examiner raising the patient's arm into forced flexion while stabilizing and preventing rotation of the scapula. A positive sign is present if pain develops before 180° of forward flexion. A complete tear of the rotator cuff is more common in the elderly and often results from trauma; it may manifest in the same manner as tendinitis but is less common. The diagnosis is also suggested by the drop arm test in which the patient is unable to maintain his or her arm outstretched once it is passively abducted. If the patient is unable to hold the arm up once 90° of abduction is reached, the test is positive. Tendinitis or tear of the rotator cuff can be confirmed by magnetic resonance imaging (MRI) or ultrasound.

KNEE PAIN

Knee pain may result from intraarticular (OA, RA) or periarticular (anserine bursitis, collateral ligament strain) processes or be referred from hip pathology. A careful history should delineate the chronology of the knee complaint and whether there are predisposing conditions, trauma, or medications that might underlie the complaint. For example, patellofemoral disease (e.g., OA) may cause anterior knee pain that worsens with climbing stairs. Observation of the patient's gait is also important. The knee should be carefully inspected in the upright (weight-bearing) and prone positions for swelling, erythema, malalignment, visible trauma (contusion, laceration), or muscle wasting. The most common form of malalignment in the knee is *genu varum* (bowlegs) or *genu valgum* (knock-knees). Bony swelling of the knee joint commonly results from hypertrophic osseous changes seen with disorders such as OA and neuropathic arthropathy. Swelling caused by hypertrophy of the synovium or synovial effusion may manifest as a fluctuant, ballotable, or soft tissue enlargement in the suprapatellar pouch (suprapatellar reflection of the synovial cavity) or regions lateral and medial to the patella. Synovial effusions may also be detected by balloting the patella downward toward the femoral groove or by eliciting a "bulge sign." With the knee extended the examiner should manually compress, or "milk," synovial fluid down from the suprapatellar pouch and lateral to the patellae. The application of manual pressure lateral to the patella may cause an observable shift in synovial fluid (bulge) to the medial aspect. The examiner should note that this maneuver is only effective in detecting small to moderate effusions (<100 mL). Inflammatory disorders such as RA, gout, pseudogout, and reactive arthritis may involve the knee joint and produce significant pain, stiffness, swelling, or warmth. A popliteal or *Baker's cyst* is best palpated with the knee partially flexed and is best viewed posteriorly with the patient standing and knees fully extended to visualize isolated or unilateral popliteal swelling or fullness.

Anserine bursitis is an often missed periarticular cause of knee pain in adults. The pes anserine bursa underlies the insertion of the conjoined tendons (sartorius, gracilis, semitendinosis) on the anteromedial proximal tibia and may be painful following trauma, overuse, or inflammation. It is often tender in patients with fibromyalgia, obesity, and knee osteoarthritis. Other forms of bursitis may also present as knee pain. The prepatellar bursa is superficial and is located over the inferior portion of the patella. The infrapatellar bursa is deeper and lies beneath the patellar ligament before its insertion on the tibial tubercle.

Internal derangement of the knee may result from trauma or degenerative processes. Damage to the meniscal cartilage (medial or lateral) frequently presents as chronic or intermittent knee pain. Such an injury should be suspected when there is a history of trauma, athletic activity, or chronic knee arthritis, and when the patient relates symptoms of "locking," clicking, or "giving way" of the joint. With the knee flexed 90° and the patient's foot on the table, pain elicited during palpation over the joint line or when the knee is stressed laterally or medially may suggest a meniscal tear. A positive McMurray test may also indicate a meniscal tear. To perform this test, the knee is first flexed at 90°, and the leg is then extended while the lower extremity is simultaneously torqued medially or laterally. A painful click during inward rotation may indicate a lateral meniscus tear, and pain during outward rotation may indicate a tear in the medial meniscus. Lastly, damage to the cruciate ligaments should be suspected with acute onset of pain, possibly with swelling, a history of trauma, or a synovial fluid aspirate that is grossly bloody. Examination of the cruciate ligaments is best accomplished by eliciting a drawer sign. With the patient recumbent, the knee should be partially flexed and the foot stabilized on the examining surface. The examiner should manually attempt to displace the tibia anteriorly or posteriorly with respect to the femur. If anterior movement is detected, then anterior cruciate ligament damage is likely. Conversely, significant posterior movement may indicate posterior cruciate damage. Contralateral comparison will assist the examiner in detecting significant anterior or posterior movement.

HIP PAIN

The hip is best evaluated by observing the patient's gait and assessing range of motion. The vast majority of patients reporting "hip pain" localize their pain unilaterally to the posterior gluteal musculature (Fig. 331-5). Such pain tends to radiate down the posterolateral aspect of the thigh and may or may not be associated with complaints of low back pain. This presentation frequently results from degenerative arthritis of the lumbosacral spine or disks and commonly follows a dermatomal distribution with involvement of nerve roots between L4 and S1. Sciatica is caused by impingement of

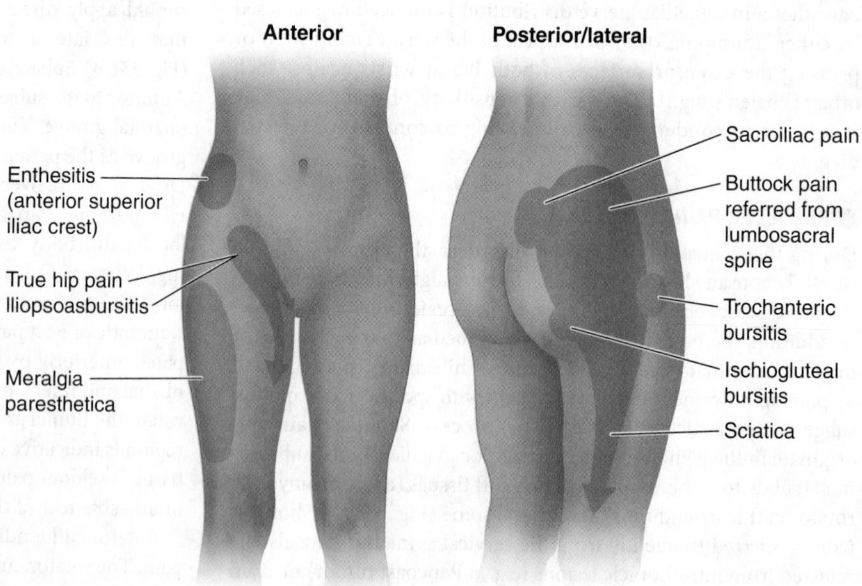

Figure 331-5 Origins of hip pain and dysesthesias. *(From Cush et al, with permission.)*

the L4, L5, or S1 nerve (i.e., from a herniated disk) and manifests as unilateral neuropathic pain extending from the gluteal region down the posterolateral leg to the foot. Some individuals instead localize their "hip pain" laterally to the area overlying the trochanteric bursa. Because of the depth of this bursa, swelling and warmth are usually absent. Diagnosis of trochanteric bursitis can be confirmed by inducing point tenderness over the trochanteric bursa. Gluteal and trochanteric pain may also indicate underlying fibromyalgia. Range of movement may be limited by pain. Pain in the hip joint is less common and tends to be located anteriorly, over the inguinal ligament; it may radiate medially to the groin. Uncommonly, iliopsoas bursitis may mimic true hip joint pain. Diagnosis of iliopsoas bursitis may be suggested by a history of trauma or inflammatory arthritis. Pain associated with iliopsoas bursitis is localized to the groin or anterior thigh and tends to worsen with hyperextension of the hip; many patients prefer to flex and externally rotate the hip to reduce the pain from a distended bursa.

LABORATORY INVESTIGATIONS

The vast majority of musculoskeletal disorders can be easily diagnosed by a complete history and physical examination. An additional objective of the initial encounter is to determine whether additional investigations or immediate therapy is required. A number of features indicate the need for additional evaluation. Monarticular conditions require additional evaluation, as do traumatic or inflammatory conditions and conditions accompanied by neurologic changes or systemic manifestations of serious disease. Finally, individuals with chronic symptoms (>6 weeks), especially when there has been a lack of response to symptomatic measures, are candidates for additional evaluation. The extent and nature of the additional investigation should be dictated by the clinical features and suspected pathologic process. Laboratory tests should be used to confirm a specific clinical diagnosis and not be used to screen or evaluate patients with vague rheumatic complaints. Indiscriminate use of broad batteries of diagnostic tests and radiographic procedures is rarely a useful or cost-effective means to establish a diagnosis.

Besides a complete blood count, including a white blood cell (WBC) and differential count, the routine evaluation should include a determination of an acute-phase reactant such as the ESR or CRP, which can be useful in discriminating inflammatory from noninflammatory disorders. Both are inexpensive, easily obtained, and may be elevated with infection, inflammation, autoimmune disorders, neoplasia, pregnancy, renal insufficiency, advanced age, and hyperlipidemia. Extreme elevation of the acute-phase reactants (CRP, ESR) is seldom seen without evidence of serious illness (e.g., sepsis, pleuropericarditis, polymyalgia rheumatica, giant cell arteritis, adult Still's disease).

Serum uric acid determinations are useful in the diagnosis of gout and in monitoring the response to urate-lowering therapy. Uric acid, the end product of purine metabolism, is primarily excreted in the urine. Serum values range from 238 to 516 μmol/L (4.0–8.6 mg/dL) in men; the lower values [178–351 μmol/L (3.0–5.9 mg/dL)] seen in women are caused by the uricosuric effects of estrogen. Urinary uric acid levels are normally <750 mg per 24 h. Although hyperuricemia [especially levels >535 μmol/L (9 mg/dL)] is associated with an increased incidence of gout and nephrolithiasis, levels may not correlate with the severity of articular disease. Uric acid levels (and the risk of gout) may be increased by inborn errors of metabolism (Lesch-Nyhan syndrome), disease states (renal insufficiency, myeloproliferative disease, psoriasis), or drugs (alcohol, cytotoxic therapy, thiazides). Although nearly all patients with gout will demonstrate hyperuricemia at some time during their illness, up to 5% of patients with an acute gouty attack will have normal serum uric acid levels, presumably from acute inflammation augmented excretion of uric acid. Monitoring serum uric acid may be useful in assessing the response to hypouricemic therapy or chemotherapy as the goal of therapy is to lower serum urate below 6 mg/dL.

Serologic tests for rheumatoid factor (RF), cyclic citrullinated peptide (CCP) antibodies, antinuclear antibodies (ANA), complement levels, Lyme and antineutrophil cytoplasmic antibodies (ANCA), or antistreptolysin O (ASO) titer should be carried out only when there is clinical evidence to suggest an associated diagnosis, as these have poor predictive value when used for screening, especially when the pretest probability is low. Although 4–5% of a healthy population will have positive tests for RF and ANAs, only 1% and <0.4% of the population will have RA or SLE, respectively. IgM RF (autoantibodies against the Fc portion of IgG) is found in 80% of patients with RA and may also be seen in low titers in patients with chronic infections (tuberculosis, leprosy, hepatitis); other autoimmune diseases (SLE, Sjögren's syndrome); and chronic pulmonary, hepatic, or renal diseases. When considering RA, both serum RF and anti-CCP antibodies should be obtained as these are complementary. Both are comparably sensitive but CCP antibodies are more specific than RF. In RA, the presence of anti-CCP and rheumatoid factor antibodies may indicate a greater risk for more severe, erosive polyarthritis. ANAs are found in nearly all patients with SLE and may also be seen in patients with other autoimmune diseases (polymyositis, scleroderma, antiphospholipid syndrome, Sjogren's syndrome), drug-induced lupus (resulting from hydralazine, procainamide, quinidine, tetracyclines, tumor necrosis factor inhibitors), chronic liver or renal disorders, and advanced age. Positive ANAs are found in 5% of adults and in up to 14% of elderly or chronically ill individuals. The ANA test is very sensitive but poorly specific for lupus, as <5% of all positive results will be caused by lupus alone. The interpretation of a positive ANA test may depend on the magnitude of the titer and the pattern observed by immunofluorescence microscopy (Table 331-4). Diffuse and

TABLE 331-4 Antinuclear Antibody (ANA) Patterns and Clinical Associations

ANA Pattern	Antigen Identified	Clinical Correlate
Diffuse	Deoxyribonucleoprotein	Nonspecific
	Histones	Drug-induced lupus, lupus
Peripheral (rim)	ds-DNA	50% of SLE (specific)
Speckled	U1-RNP	>90% of MCTD
	Sm	30% of SLE (specific)
	Ro (SS-A)	Sjögrens 60%, SCLE, neonatal lupus, ANA(–) lupus
	La (SS-B)	50% of Sjögrens, 15% lupus
	Scl-70	40% of diffuse scleroderma
	PM-1	Polymyositis (PM), dermatomyositis
	Jo-1	PM w/pneumonitis + arthritis
Nucleolar	RNA polymerase I, others	40% of PSS
Centromere	Kinetochore	75% CREST (limited scleroderma)

Abbreviations: ANA, antinuclear antibody; CREST, *c*alcinosis, *R*aynaud phenomenon, *e*sophageal involvement; *s*clerodactyly; and *t*elangiectasia; MCTD, mixed connective tissue disease; PSS, progressive systemic sclerosis; SCLE, subacute cutaneous lupus erythematosus; SLE, systemic lupus erythematosus.

speckled patterns are least specific, whereas a peripheral, or rim, pattern [related to autoantibodies against double-strand (native) DNA] is highly specific and suggestive of lupus. Centromeric patterns are seen in patients with limited scleroderma [*c*alcinosis, *R*aynaud's phenomenon, *e*sophageal involvement, *s*clerodactyly, *t*elangiectasia (CREST) syndrome] or primary biliary sclerosis, and nucleolar patterns may be seen in patients with diffuse systemic sclerosis or inflammatory myositis.

Aspiration and analysis of synovial fluid are always indicated in acute monarthritis or when an infectious or crystal-induced arthropathy is suspected. Synovial fluid may distinguish between noninflammatory and inflammatory processes by analysis of the appearance, viscosity, and cell count. Tests for synovial fluid glucose, protein, lactate dehydrogenase, lactic acid, or autoantibodies are not recommended as they have no diagnostic value. Normal synovial fluid is clear or a pale straw color and is viscous, primarily because of the high levels of hyaluronate. Noninflammatory synovial fluid is clear, viscous, and amber-colored, with a white blood cell count of <2000/μL and a predominance of mononuclear cells. The viscosity of synovial fluid is assessed by expressing fluid from the syringe one drop at a time. Normally, there is a stringing effect, with a long tail behind each synovial drop. Effusions caused by OA or trauma will have normal viscosity. Inflammatory fluid is turbid and yellow, with an increased white cell count (2000–50,000/μL) and a polymorphonuclear leukocyte predominance. Inflammatory fluid has reduced viscosity, diminished hyaluronate, and little or no tail following each drop of synovial fluid. Such effusions are found in RA, gout, and other inflammatory arthritides. Septic fluid is opaque and purulent, with a WBC count usually >50,000/μL, a predominance of polymorphonuclear leukocytes (>75%), and low viscosity. Such effusions are typical of septic arthritis but may occur with RA or gout. In addition, hemorrhagic synovial fluid may be seen with trauma, hemarthrosis, or neuropathic arthritis. An algorithm for synovial fluid aspiration and analysis is shown in Fig. 331-6. Synovial fluid should be analyzed immediately for appearance, viscosity, and cell count. Monosodium urate crystals (observed in gout) are seen by polarized microscopy and are long, needle-shaped, negatively birefringent, and usually intracellular. In chondrocalcinosis and pseudogout, calcium pyrophosphate dihydrate crystals are usually short, rhomboid-shaped, and positively birefringent. Whenever infection is suspected, synovial fluid should be Gram-stained and cultured appropriately. If gonococcal arthritis is suspected, immediate plating of the fluid on appropriate culture medium is indicated. Synovial fluid from patients with chronic monarthritis should also be cultured for *M. tuberculosis* and fungi. Last, it should be noted that crystal-induced and septic arthritis occasionally occur together in the same joint.

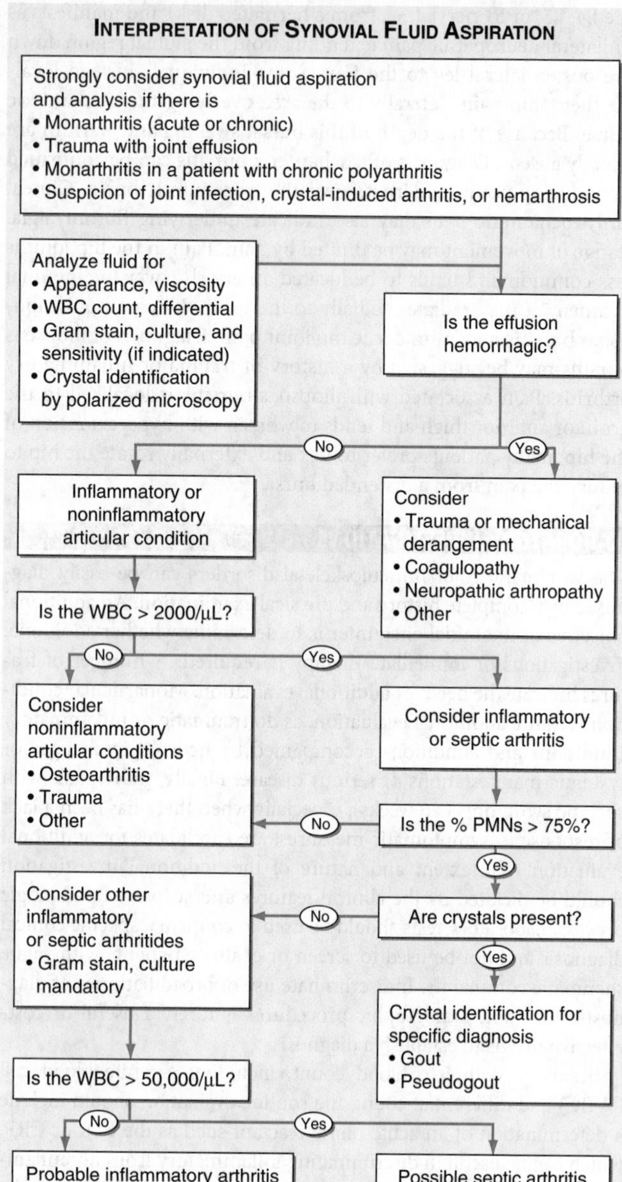

Figure 331-6 Algorithmic approach to the use and interpretation of synovial fluid aspiration and analysis. PMNs, polymorphonuclear (leukocytes); WBC, white blood cell (count).

DIAGNOSTIC IMAGING IN JOINT DISEASES

Conventional radiography has been a valuable tool in the diagnosis and staging of articular disorders. Plain x-rays are most appropriate when there is a history of trauma, suspected chronic infection, progressive disability, or monarticular involvement; when therapeutic alterations are considered; or when a baseline assessment is desired for what appears to be a chronic process. However, in acute inflammatory arthritis, early radiography is rarely helpful in establishing a diagnosis and may only reveal soft tissue swelling or juxtaarticular demineralization. As the disease progresses, calcification (of soft tissues, cartilage, or bone), joint space narrowing, erosions, bony ankylosis, new bone formation (sclerosis, osteophytes, or periostitis), or subchondral cysts may develop and suggest specific clinical entities. Consultation with a radiologist will help define the optimal imaging modality, technique, or positioning and prevent the need for further studies.

Additional imaging techniques may possess greater diagnostic sensitivity and facilitate early diagnosis in a limited number of articular disorders and in selected circumstances and are indicated when conventional radiography is inadequate or nondiagnostic (Table 331-5). *Ultrasonography* is useful in the detection of soft tissue abnormalities, such as tenosynovitis, that cannot be fully appreciated by clinical examination. Owing to low cost, portability, and wider use, ultrasound use has grown and is the preferred method for the evaluation of synovial (Baker's) cysts, rotator cuff tears, tendinitis and tendon injury, and suspected early synovitis. Its utility is enhanced by operator experience. *Radionuclide scintigraphy* provides useful information regarding the metabolic status of bone and, along with radiography, is well suited for total-body assessment of the extent and distribution of skeletal involvement.

TABLE 331-5 Diagnostic Imaging Techniques for Musculoskeletal Disorders

Method	Imaging Time, h	Cost[a]	Current Indications
Ultrasound[b]	<1	++	Synovial cysts
			Rotator cuff tears
			Tendon injury
Radionuclide scintigraphy			
^{99m}Tc	1–4	++	Metastatic bone survey
			Evaluation of Paget's disease
			Acute and chronic osteomyelitis
^{111}In-WBC	24	+++	Acute infection
			Prosthetic infection
			Acute osteomyelitis
^{67}Ga	24–48	++++	Acute and chronic infection
			Acute osteomyelitis
Computed tomography	<1	+++	Herniated intervertebral disk
			Sacroiliitis
			Spinal stenosis
			Spinal trauma
			Osteoid osteoma
			Stress fracture
Magnetic resonance imaging	1/2–2	++++	Avascular necrosis
			Osteomyelitis
			Intraarticular derangement and soft tissue injury
			Derangements of axial skeleton and spinal cord
			Herniated intervertebral disk
			Pigmented villonodular synovitis
			Inflammatory and metabolic muscle pathology

[a]Relative cost for imaging study.
[b]Results depend on operator.

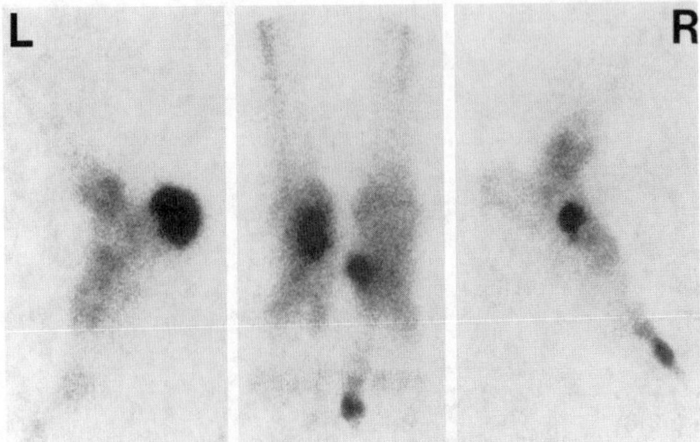

Figure 331-7 [^{99m}Tc]Diphosphonate scintigraphy of the feet of a 33-year-old African-American male with reactive arthritis, manifested by sacroiliitis, urethritis, uveitis, asymmetric oligoarthritis, and enthesitis. This bone scan demonstrates increased uptake indicative of enthesitis involving the insertions of the left Achilles tendon, plantar aponeurosis, and right tibialis posterior tendon as well as arthritis of the right first interphalangeal joint.

Radionuclide imaging is a very sensitive, but poorly specific, means of detecting inflammatory or metabolic alterations in bone or periarticular soft tissue structures. The limited tissue contrast resolution of scintigraphy may obscure the distinction between a bony or periarticular process and may necessitate the additional use of MRI. Scintigraphy, using ^{99m}Tc, ^{67}Ga, or ^{111}In-labeled WBCs has been applied to a variety of articular disorders with variable success (Table 331-5). Although [^{99m}Tc] pertechnate or diphosphate scintigraphy (Fig. 331-7) may be useful in identifying osseous infection, neoplasia, inflammation, increased blood flow, bone remodeling, heterotopic bone formation, or avascular necrosis, MRI is preferred in most instances. The poor specificity of ^{99m}Tc scanning has largely limited its use to surveys for bone metastases and Paget's disease of bone. Gallium scanning utilizes ^{67}Ga, which binds serum and cellular transferrin and lactoferrin, and is preferentially taken up by neutrophils, macrophages, bacteria, and tumor tissue (e.g., lymphoma). As such, it is primarily used in the identification of occult infection or malignancy. Scanning with ^{111}In-labeled WBCs has been used to detect osteomyelitis and infectious or inflammatory arthritis. Nevertheless, the use of ^{111}In-labeled WBC or ^{67}Ga scanning has largely been replaced by MRI, except when there is a suspicion of prosthetic joint infections.

CT provides detailed visualization of the axial skeleton. Articulations previously considered difficult to visualize by radiography (e.g., zygapophyseal, sacroiliac, sternoclavicular, hip joints) can be effectively evaluated using CT. CT has been demonstrated to be useful in the diagnosis of low back pain syndromes (e.g., spinal stenosis vs. herniated disk), sacroiliitis, osteoid osteoma, and stress fractures. Helical or spiral CT (with or without contrast angiography) is a novel technique that is rapid, cost-effective, and sensitive in diagnosing pulmonary embolism or obscure fractures, often in the setting of initially equivocal findings. High-resolution CT can be advocated in the evaluation of suspected or established infiltrative lung disease (e.g., scleroderma or rheumatoid lung). The recent use of hybrid [positron emission tomography (PET)/CT or single-photon emission CT (SPECT)] scans in metastatic evaluations have incorporated CT to provide better anatomic localization of scintigraphic abnormalities.

MRI has significantly advanced the ability to image musculoskeletal structures. MRI has the advantages of providing multiplanar images with fine anatomic detail and contrast resolution (Fig. 331-8) that allows for the superior ability to visualize bone marrow and soft tissue periarticular structures. Although more costly with a longer procedural time than CT, the MRI has become the preferred technique when evaluating complex musculoskeletal disorders.

MRI can image fascia, vessels, nerve, muscle, cartilage, ligaments, tendons, pannus, synovial effusions, and bone marrow. Visualization of particular structures can be enhanced by altering the pulse sequence to produce either T1- or T2-weighted spin echo, gradient echo, or inversion recovery [including short tau inversion recovery (STIR)] images. Because of its sensitivity to changes in marrow fat, MRI is a sensitive but nonspecific means of detecting osteonecrosis, osteomyelitis, and marrow inflammation indicating overlying synovitis or osteitis (Fig. 331-8). Because of its enhanced soft tissue resolution, MRI is more sensitive than arthrography or CT in the diagnosis of soft tissue injuries (e.g., meniscal and rotator cuff tears); intraarticular derangements; marrow abnormalities (osteonecrosis, myeloma); and spinal cord or nerve root damage or synovitis.

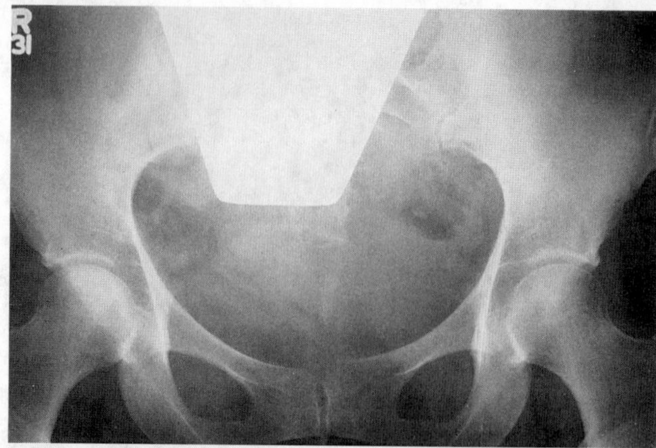

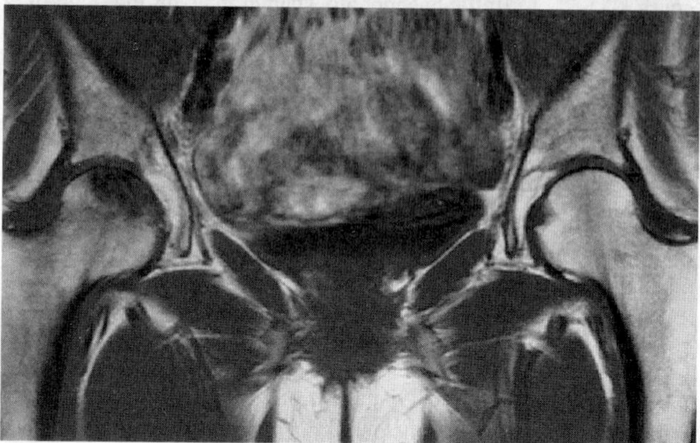

Figure 331-8 Superior sensitivity of MRI in the diagnosis of osteonecrosis of the femoral head. A 45-year-old woman receiving high-dose glucocorticoids developed right hip pain. Conventional x-rays (*top*) demonstrated only mild sclerosis of the right femoral head. T1-weighted MRI (*bottom*) demonstrated low-density signal in the right femoral head, diagnostic of osteonecrosis.

FURTHER READINGS

American College of Rheumatology Ad Hoc Committee on Clinical Guidelines: Guidelines for the initial evaluation of the adult patient with acute musculoskeletal symptoms. Arthritis Rheum 39:1, 1996

Avouac J et al: Diagnostic and predictive value of anti-cyclic citrullinated protein antibodies in rheumatoid arthritis: A systematic literature review. Ann Rheum Dis 65:845, 2006

Cush JJ et al: Evaluation of musculoskeletal complaints, in *Rheumatology: Diagnosis and Therapeutics,* 2nd ed, JJ Cush et al (eds). Philadelphia, Lippincott Williams & Wilkins, 2005, pp 3–20

Hootman JM, Helmick CG: Projections of US prevalence of arthritis and associated activity limitations. Arthritis Rheum 54:226, 2006

Kavanaugh A: The utility of immunologic laboratory tests in patients with rheumatic diseases. Arthritis Rheum 44:2221, 2001

Ory PA: Radiography in the assessment of musculoskeletal conditions. Best Pract Res Clin Rheumatol 17:495, 2003

Rudwaleit M et al: How to diagnose axial spondyloarthritis early. Ann Rheum Dis 63:535, 2004

Shmerling RH et al: Synovial fluid tests: What should be ordered? JAMA 264:1009, 1990

CHAPTER 332 Osteoarthritis

David T. Felson

Osteoarthritis (OA) is the most common type of arthritis. Its high prevalence, especially in the elderly, and the high rate of disability related to disease make it a leading cause of disability in the elderly. Because of the aging of Western populations and because obesity, a major risk factor, is increasing in prevalence, the occurrence of osteoarthritis is on the rise. In the United States, osteoarthritis prevalence will increase by 66–100% by 2020.

OA affects certain joints, yet spares others (Fig. 332-1). Commonly affected joints include the cervical and lumbosacral spine, hip, knee, and first metatarsal phalangeal joint (MTP). In the hands, the distal and proximal interphalangeal joints and the base of the thumb are often affected. Usually spared are the wrist, elbow, and ankle. Our joints were designed, in an evolutionary sense, for brachiating apes, animals that still walked on four limbs. We thus develop OA in joints that were ill designed for human tasks such as pincer grip (OA in the thumb base) and walking upright (OA in knees and hips) Some joints, like the ankles, may be spared because their articular cartilage may be uniquely resistant to loading stresses.

OA can be diagnosed based on structural abnormalities or on the symptoms these abnormalities evoke. According to cadaveric studies, by elderly years, structural changes of OA are nearly universal. These include cartilage loss (seen as joint space loss on x-rays) and osteophytes. Many persons with x-ray evidence of OA have no joint symptoms and, while the prevalence of structural abnormalities is of interest in understanding disease pathogenesis, what matters more from a clinical perspective is the prevalence of symptomatic OA. Symptoms, usually joint pain, determine disability, visits to clinicians, and disease costs.

Symptomatic OA of the knee (pain on most days of a recent month in a knee plus x-ray evidence of OA in that knee) occurs in ~12% of persons age ≥60 in the United States and 6% of all adults age ≥30. Symptomatic hip OA is roughly one-third as common as disease in the knee. While radiographically evident hand OA and the appearance of bony enlargement in affected hand joints (Fig. 332-2) are extremely common in older persons, most cases are often not symptomatic. Even so, symptomatic hand OA occurs in ~10% of elderly individuals and often produces measurable limitation in function.

The prevalence of OA rises strikingly with age. Regardless of how it is defined, OA is uncommon in adults under age 40 and highly

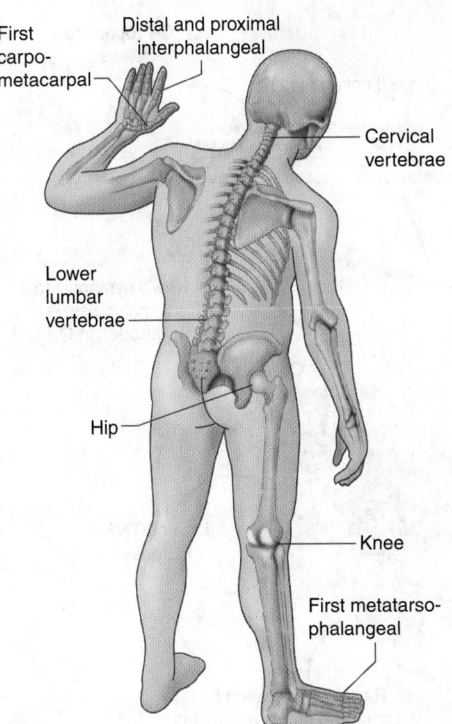

Figure 332-1 Joints affected by osteoarthritis.

prevalent in those over age 60. It is also a disease that, at least in middle-aged and elderly persons, is much more common in women than in men, and sex differences in prevalence increase with age.

X-ray evidence of OA is common in the lower back and neck, but back pain and neck pain have not been tied to findings of OA on x-ray. Thus, back pain and neck pain are treated separately (Chap. 15).

DEFINITION

OA is joint failure, a disease in which all structures of the joint have undergone pathologic change, often in concert. The pathologic sine qua non of disease is hyaline articular cartilage loss, present in a focal and, initially, nonuniform manner. This is accompanied by increasing thickness and sclerosis of the subchondral bony plate, by outgrowth of osteophytes at the joint margin, by stretching of the articular capsule, by mild synovitis in many affected joints, and by weakness of muscles bridging the joint. In knees, meniscal degeneration is part of the disease. There are numerous pathways that lead to joint failure, but the initial step is often joint injury in the setting of a failure of protective mechanisms.

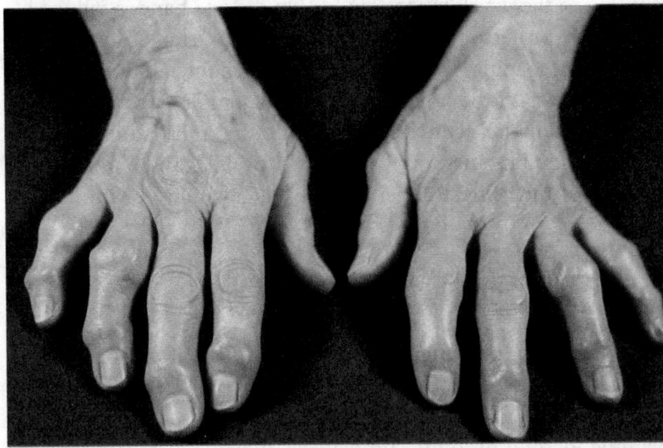

Figure 332-2 Severe osteoarthritis of the hands affecting the distal interphalangeal joints (Heberden's nodes) and the proximal interphalangeal joints (Bouchard's nodes). There is no clear bony enlargement of the other common site in the hands, the thumb base.

JOINT PROTECTIVE MECHANISMS AND THEIR FAILURE

Joint protectors include: joint capsule and ligaments, muscle, sensory afferents, and underlying bone. Joint capsule and ligaments serve as joint protectors by providing a limit to excursion, thereby fixing the range of joint motion.

Synovial fluid reduces friction between articulating cartilage surfaces, thereby serving as a major protector against friction-induced cartilage wear. This lubrication function depends on the molecule *lubricin*, a mucinous glycoprotein secreted by synovial fibroblasts whose concentration diminishes after joint injury and in the face of synovial inflammation.

The ligaments, along with overlying skin and tendons, contain mechanoreceptor sensory afferent nerves. These mechanoreceptors fire at different frequencies throughout a joint's range of motion, providing feedback by way of the spinal cord to muscles and tendons. As a consequence, these muscles and tendons can assume the right tension at appropriate points in joint excursion to act as optimal joint protectors, anticipating joint loading.

Muscles and tendons that bridge the joint are key joint protectors. Their contractions at the appropriate time in joint movement provide the appropriate power and acceleration for the limb to accomplish its tasks. Focal stress across the joint is minimized by muscle contraction that decelerates the joint before impact and assures that when joint impact arrives, it is distributed broadly across the joint surface.

Failure of these joint protectors increases the risk of joint injury and OA. For example, in animals, OA develops rapidly when a sensory nerve to the joint is sectioned and joint injury induced. Similarly, in humans, Charcot arthropathy, a severe and rapidly progressive OA, develops when minor joint injury occurs in the presence of posterior column peripheral neuropathy. Another example of joint protector failure is rupture of ligaments, a well-known cause of the early development of OA.

CARTILAGE AND ITS ROLE IN JOINT FAILURE

In addition to being a primary target tissue for disease, cartilage also functions as a joint protector. A thin rim of tissue at the ends of two opposing bones, cartilage is lubricated by synovial fluid to provide an almost frictionless surface across which these two bones move. The compressible stiffness of cartilage compared to bone provides the joint with impact-absorbing capacity.

Since the earliest changes of OA may occur in cartilage and abnormalities there can accelerate disease development, understanding the structure and physiology of cartilage is critical to an appreciation of disease pathogenesis. The two major macromolecules in cartilage are type 2 collagen, which provides cartilage its tensile strength, and aggrecan, a proteoglycan macromolecule linked with hyaluronic acid, which consists of highly negatively charged glycosaminoglycans. In normal cartilage, type 2 collagen is woven tightly, constraining the aggrecan molecules in the interstices between collagen strands, forcing these highly negatively charged molecules into close proximity with one another. The aggrecan molecule, through electrostatic repulsion of its negative charges, gives cartilage its compressive stiffness. Chondrocytes, the cells within this avascular tissue, synthesize all elements of the matrix. In addition, they produce enzymes that break down the matrix and cytokines and growth factors, which in turn provide autocrine/paracrine feedback that modulates synthesis of matrix molecules (Fig. 332-3). Cartilage matrix synthesis and catabolism are in a dynamic equilibrium influenced by the cytokine and growth factor

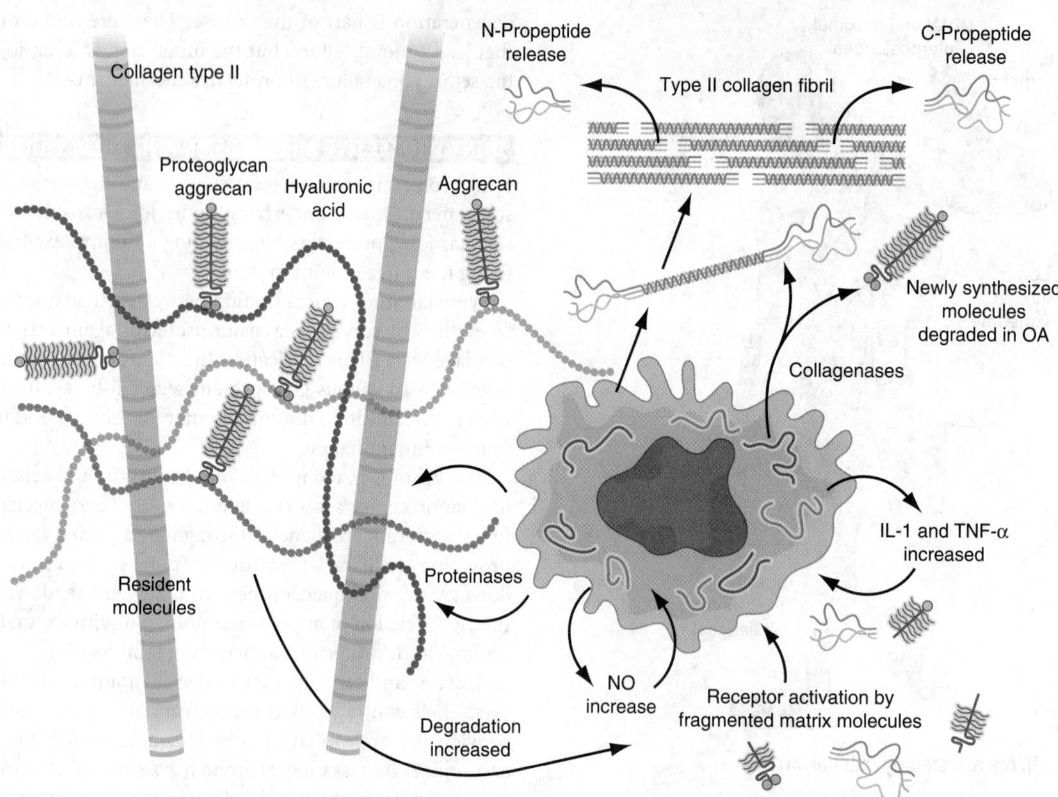

Figure 332-3 The chondrocyte and its products, type II collagen, aggrecan, and enzymes, which degrade these structures along with molecules stimulating chondrocytes. IL, interleukin; NO, nitric oxide; OA, osteoarthritis; TNF, tumor necrosis factor. *(From AR Poole et al: Ann Rheum Dis 61(S):ii78, 2002.)*

environment. Mechanical and osmotic stress on chondrocytes induces these cells to alter gene expression and increase production of inflammatory cytokines and matrix-degrading enzymes. While chondrocytes synthesize numerous enzymes, especially matrix metalloproteinases (MMP), only a few of these enzymes are critical in regulating cartilage breakdown. Type 2 cartilage is degraded primarily by MMP-13 (collagenase 3), with other collagenases playing a minor role. Aggrecan degradation is a consequence, in part, of activation of two aggrecanases (ADAMTS-4 and ADAMTS-5) and perhaps of MMPs. Both collagenase and aggrecanases act primarily in the territorial matrix surrounding chondrocytes; however, as the osteoarthritic process develops, their activities and effects spread throughout the matrix, especially in the superficial layers of cartilage.

The synovium and chondrocytes synthesize numerous growth factors and cytokines. Chief among them is interleukin (IL) 1, which exerts transcriptional effects on chondrocytes, stimulating production of proteinases and suppressing cartilage matrix synthesis. In animal models of OA, IL-1 blockade prevents cartilage loss. Tumor necrosis factor (TNF) α may play a similar role to that of IL-1. These cytokines also induce chondrocytes to synthesize prostaglandin E_2, nitric oxide, and bone morphogenic protein 2 (BMP-2), which together have complex effects on matrix synthesis and degradation. Nitric oxide inhibits aggrecan synthesis and enhances proteinase activity, whereas BMP-2 stimulates anabolic activity. At early stages in the matrix response to injury and in the healthy response to loading, the net effect of cytokine stimulation may be matrix synthesis but, ultimately, excess IL-1 triggers matrix degradation. Enzymes in the matrix are held in check by activation inhibitors, including tissue inhibitor of metalloproteinase (TIMP). Growth factors are also part of this complex network, with insulin-like growth factor type 1 and transforming growth factor β playing prominent roles in stimulating anabolism by chondrocytes.

Whereas healthy cartilage is metabolically sluggish, with slow matrix turnover and synthesis and degradation in balance, cartilage in early OA or after an injury is highly metabolically active. In the latter situation, stimulated chondrocytes synthesize enzymes and new matrix molecules, with those enzymes becoming activated in the matrix, causing release of degraded aggrecan and type 2 collagen into cartilage and into the synovial fluid. OA cartilage is characterized by gradual depletion of aggrecan, an unfurling of the tightly woven collagen matrix, and loss of type 2 collagen. With these changes comes increasing vulnerability of cartilage, which loses its compressive stiffness.

RISK FACTORS

Joint vulnerability and joint loading are the two major factors contributing to the development of OA. On the one hand, a vulnerable joint whose protectors are dysfunctional can develop OA with minimal levels of loading, perhaps even levels encountered during everyday activities. On the other hand, in a young joint with competent protectors, a major acute injury or long-term overloading is necessary to precipitate disease. Risk factors for OA can be understood in terms of their effect either on joint vulnerability or on loading (Fig. 332-4).

SYSTEMIC RISK FACTORS

Age is the most potent risk factor for OA. Radiographic evidence of OA is rare in individuals under age 40; however, in some joints, such as the hands, OA occurs in >50% of persons over age 70. Aging increases joint vulnerability through several mechanisms. Whereas dynamic loading of joints stimulates cartilage matrix synthesis by chondrocytes in young cartilage, aged cartilage is less responsive to these stimuli. Indeed, because of the poor responsiveness of older cartilage to such stimulation, cartilage transplant operations are far more challenging in older than in younger persons. Partly

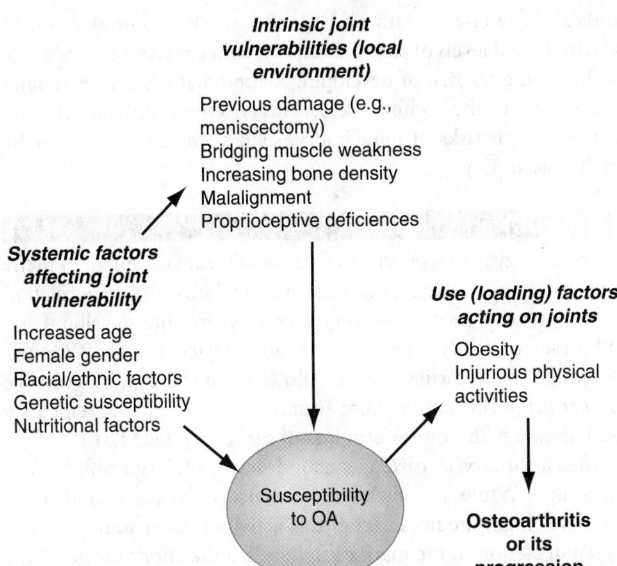

Figure 332-4 Risk factors for osteoarthritis either contribute to the susceptibility of the joint (systemic factors or factors in the local joint environment) or increase risk by the load they put on the joint. Usually a combination of loading and susceptibility factors is required to cause disease or its progression.

because of this failure to synthesize matrix with loading, cartilage thins with age, and thinner cartilage experiences higher shear stress at basal layers and is at greater risk of cartilage damage. Also, joint protectors fail more often with age. Muscles that bridge the joint become weaker with age and also respond less quickly to oncoming impulses. Sensory nerve input slows with age, retarding the feedback loop of mechanoreceptors to muscles and tendons related to their tension and position. Ligaments stretch with age, making them less able to absorb impulses. These factors work in concert to increase the vulnerability of older joints to OA.

Older women are at high risk of OA in all joints, a risk that emerges as women reach their sixth decade. While hormone loss with menopause may contribute to this risk, there is little understanding of the unique vulnerability of older women vs. men to OA.

HERITABILITY AND GENETICS

OA is a highly heritable disease, but its heritability varies by joint. Fifty percent of the hand and hip OA in the community is attributable to inheritance, i.e., to disease present in other members of the family. However, the heritable proportion of knee OA is at most 30%, with some studies suggesting no heritability at all. Whereas many people with OA have disease in multiple joints, this "generalized OA" phenotype is rarely inherited and is more often a consequence of aging.

Emerging evidence has identified genetic mutations that confer a high risk of OA, one of which is a polymorphism within the growth differentiation factor 5 gene. This polymorphism diminishes the quantity of GDF5, which normally has anabolic effects on the synthesis of cartilage matrix.

GLOBAL CONSIDERATIONS

Hip OA is rare in China and in immigrants from China to the United States. However, OA in the knees is at least as common, if not more so, in Chinese than in whites from the United States, and knee OA represents a major cause of disability in China, especially in rural areas. Anatomic differences between Chinese and white hips may account for much of the difference in hip OA prevalence, with white hips having a higher prevalence of anatomic predispositions to the development of OA. Persons from Africa, but not African Americans, may also have a very low rate of hip OA.

RISK FACTORS IN THE JOINT ENVIRONMENT

Some risk factors increase vulnerability of the joint through local effects on the joint environment. With changes in joint anatomy, for example, load across the joint is no longer distributed evenly across the joint surface, but rather shows an increase in focal stress. In the hip, three uncommon developmental abnormalities occurring in utero or childhood, congenital dysplasia, Legg-Perthes disease, and slipped capital femoral epiphysis, leave a child with distortions of hip joint anatomy that often lead to OA later in life. Girls are predominantly affected by acetabular dysplasia, a mild form of congenital dislocation, whereas the other abnormalities more often affect boys. Depending on the severity of the anatomic abnormalities, hip OA occurs either in young adulthood (severe abnormalities) or middle age (mild abnormalities).

Major injuries to a joint also can produce anatomic abnormalities that leave the joint susceptible to OA. For example, a fracture through the joint surface often causes OA in joints in which the disease is otherwise rare such as the ankle and the wrist. Avascular necrosis can lead to collapse of dead bone at the articular surface, producing anatomic irregularities and subsequent OA.

Tears of ligamentous and fibrocartilaginous structures that protect the joints, such as the anterior cruciate ligament and the meniscus in the knee and the labrum in the hip, increase joint susceptibility and can lead to premature OA. Meniscal tears increase with age and when chronic are often asymptomatic but lead to adjacent cartilage damage and accelerated osteoarthritis. Even injuries that do not produce diagnosed joint injuries may increase risk of OA, perhaps because the structural injury was not detected at the time. For example, in the Framingham Study subjects, men with a history of major knee injury, but no surgery, had a 3.5-fold increased risk for subsequent knee OA.

Another source of anatomic abnormality is malalignment across the joint (Fig. 332-5). This factor has been best studied in the knee, which is the fulcrum of the longest lever arm in the body. Varus (bowlegged) knees with OA are at exceedingly high risk of cartilage loss in the medial or inner compartment of the knee, whereas valgus (knock-kneed) malalignment predisposes to rapid cartilage loss in the lateral compartment. Malalignment causes this effect by decreasing contact area during loading, increasing stress on a focal area of cartilage, which then breaks down. There is evidence that

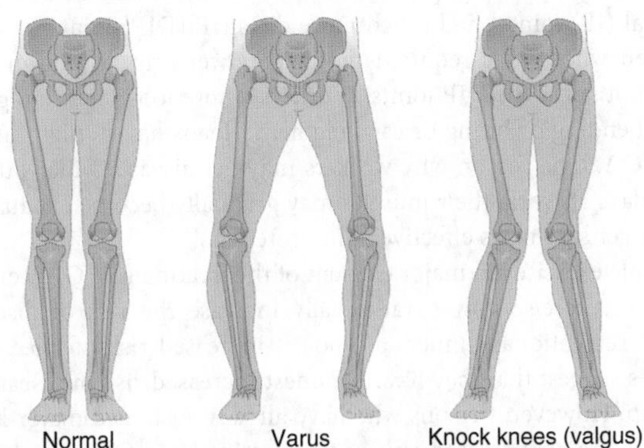

Figure 332-5 The two types of limb malalignment in the frontal plane: varus, in which the stress is placed across the medial compartment of the knee joint, and valgus, which places excess stress across the lateral compartment of the knee.

malalignment in the knee not only causes cartilage loss but leads to underlying bone damage, producing bone marrow lesions seen on MRI. Malalignment in the knee often produces such a substantial increase in focal stress within the knee (as evidenced by its destructive effects on subchondral bone) that severely malaligned knees may be destined to progress regardless of the status of other risk factors.

Weakness in the quadriceps muscles bridging the knee increases the risk of the development of painful OA in the knee.

Patients with knee OA have impaired proprioception across their knees, and this may predispose them to further disease progression. The role of bone in serving as a shock absorber for impact load is not well understood, but persons with increased bone density are at high risk of OA, suggesting that the resistance of bone to impact during joint use may play a role in disease development.

LOADING FACTORS

Obesity

Three to six times body weight is transmitted across the knee during single-leg stance. Any increase in weight may be multiplied by this factor to reveal the excess force across the knee in overweight persons during walking. Obesity is a well-recognized and potent risk factor for the development of knee OA and, less so, for hip OA. Obesity precedes the development of disease and is not just a consequence of the inactivity present in those with disease. It is a stronger risk factor for disease in women than in men, and in women, the relationship of weight to the risk of disease is linear, so that with each increase in weight, there is a commensurate increase in risk. Weight loss in women lowers the risk of developing symptomatic disease. Not only is obesity a risk factor for OA in weight-bearing joints, but obese persons have more severe symptoms from the disease.

Obesity's effect on the development and progression of disease is mediated mostly through the increased loading in weight-bearing joints that occurs in overweight persons. However, a modest association of obesity with an increased risk of hand OA suggests that there may be a systemic metabolic factor circulating in obese persons that affects disease risk also.

Repeated use of joint

There are two categories of repetitive joint use, occupational use and leisure time physical activities. Workers performing repetitive tasks as part of their occupations for many years are at high risk of developing OA in the joints they use repeatedly. For example, farmers are at high risk for hip OA, and miners have high rates of OA in knees and spine, Even within a textile mill, women whose jobs required fine pincer grip [increasing the stress across the interphalangeal (IP) joints] had much more distal IP (DIP) joint OA than women whose jobs required repeated power grip, a motion that does not stress the DIP joints. Workers whose jobs require regular knee bending or lifting or carrying heavy loads have a high rate of knee OA. One reason why workers may get disease is that during long days at work, their muscles may gradually become exhausted, no longer serving as effective joint protectors.

While exercise is a major element of the treatment of OA, certain types of exercise may paradoxically increase the risk of disease. While recreational runners are not at increased risk of knee OA, studies suggest that they have a modest increased risk of disease in the hip. However, persons who have already sustained major knee injuries are at increased risk of progressive knee OA as a consequence of running. Compared to nonrunners, elite runners (professional runners and those on Olympic teams) have high risks of both knee and hip OA. Given the widespread recommendation to adopt a healthier, more exercise-filled lifestyle; longitudinal epidemiologic studies of exercise contain cautionary notes. For example, women with increased levels of physical activity, either as teenagers or at age 50, had a higher risk of developing symptomatic hip disease later in life than women who were sedentary. Other athletic activities that pose high risks of joint injury, such as football, may thereby predispose to OA.

PATHOLOGY

The pathology of OA provides evidence of the involvement of many joint structures in disease. Cartilage initially shows surface fibrillation and irregularity. As disease progresses, focal erosions develop there, and these eventually extend down to the subjacent bone. With further progression, cartilage erosion down to bone expands to involve a larger proportion of the joint surface, even though OA remains a focal disease with nonuniform loss of cartilage (Fig. 332-6).

After an injury to cartilage, chondrocytes undergo mitosis and clustering. While the metabolic activity of these chondrocyte clusters is high, the net effect of this activity is to promote proteoglycan depletion in the matrix surrounding the chondrocytes. This is because the catabolic is greater than the synthetic activity. As disease develops, collagen matrix becomes damaged, the negative charges of proteoglycans get exposed, and cartilage swells from ionic attraction to water molecules. Because in damaged cartilage proteoglycans are no longer forced into close proximity, cartilage does not bounce back after loading as it did when healthy, and cartilage becomes vulnerable to further injury. Chondrocytes at the basal level of cartilage undergo apoptosis.

With loss of cartilage come alterations in subchondral bone. Stimulated by growth factors and cytokines, osteoclasts and osteoblasts in the subchondral bony plate, just underneath cartilage, become activated. Bone formation produces a thickening and stiffness of the subchondral plate that occurs even before cartilage ulcerates. Trauma to bone during joint loading may be the primary factor driving this bone response, with healing from injury (including microcracks) producing stiffness. Small areas of osteonecrosis usually exist in joints with advanced disease. Bone death may also be caused by bone trauma with shearing of microvasculature, leading to a cutoff of vascular supply to some bone areas.

At the margin of the joint, near areas of cartilage loss, osteophytes form. These start as outgrowths of new cartilage and, with neurovascular invasion from the bone, this cartilage ossifies. Osteophytes

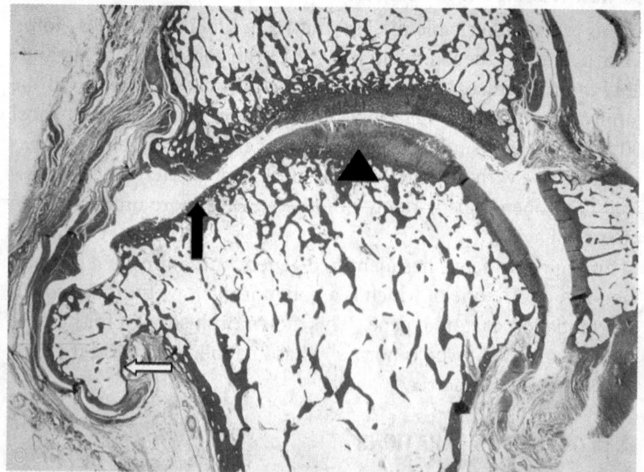

Figure 332-6 Pathologic changes of osteoarthritis in a toe joint. Note the nonuniform loss of cartilage (*arrowhead* vs. *solid arrow*), the increased thickness of the subchondral bone envelope (*solid arrow*), and the osteophyte (*open arrow*). *(From the American College of Rheumatology slide collection.)*

are an important radiographic hallmark of OA. In malaligned joints, osteophytes grow larger on the side of the joint subject to most loading stress (e.g., in varus knees, osteophytes grow larger on the medial side).

The synovium produces lubricating fluids that minimize shear stress during motion. In healthy joints, the synovium consists of a single discontinuous layer filled with fat and containing two types of cells, macrophages and fibroblasts, but in OA, it can sometimes become edematous and inflamed. There is a migration of macrophages from the periphery into the tissue, and cells lining the synovium proliferate. Enzymes secreted by the synovium digest cartilage matrix that has been sheared from the surface of the cartilage.

Additional pathologic changes occur in the capsule, which stretches, becomes edematous, and can become fibrotic.

The pathology of OA is not identical across joints. In hand joints with severe OA, for example, there are often cartilage erosions in the center of the joint probably produced by bony pressure from the opposite side of the joint. In hand OA, pathology has also been noted in ligament site insertions, which may help propagate disease.

Basic calcium phosphate and calcium pyrophosphate dihydrate crystals are present microscopically in most joints with end-stage OA. Their role in osteoarthritic cartilage is unclear, but their release from cartilage into the joint space and joint fluid likely triggers synovial inflammation, which can, in turn, produce release of enzymes and trigger nociceptive stimulation.

SOURCES OF PAIN

Because cartilage is aneural, cartilage loss in a joint is not accompanied by pain. Thus, pain in OA likely arises from structures outside the cartilage. Innervated structures in the joint include the synovium, ligaments, joint capsule, muscles, and subchondral bone. Most of these are not visualized by the x-ray, and the severity of x-ray changes in OA correlates poorly with pain severity.

Based on MRI studies in osteoarthritic knees comparing those with and without pain and on studies mapping tenderness in unanesthetized joints, likely sources of pain include synovial inflammation, joint effusions, and bone marrow edema. Modest synovitis develops in many but not all osteoarthritic joints. Some diseased joints have no synovitis, whereas others have synovial inflammation that approaches the severity of joints with rheumatoid arthritis (Chap. 321). The presence of synovitis on MRI is correlated with the presence and severity of knee pain. Capsular stretching from fluid in the joint stimulates nociceptive fibers there, inducing pain. Increased focal loading as part of the disease not only damages cartilage but probably also injures the underlying bone. As a consequence, bone marrow edema appears on the MRI; histologically, this edema signals the presence of microcracks and scar, which are the consequences of trauma. These lesions may stimulate bone nociceptive fibers. Also, hemostatic pressure within bone rises in OA, and the increased pressure itself may stimulate nociceptive fibers, causing pain. Lastly, osteophytes themselves may be a source of pain. When osteophytes grow, neurovascular innervation penetrates through the base of the bone into the cartilage and into the developing osteophyte.

Pain may arise from outside the joint also, including bursae near the joints. Common sources of pain near the knee are anserine bursitis and iliotibial band syndrome.

CLINICAL FEATURES

Joint pain from OA is activity-related. Pain comes on either during or just after joint use and then gradually resolves. Examples include knee or hip pain with going up or down stairs, pain in weight-bearing joints when walking, and, for hand OA, pain when cooking. Early in disease, pain is episodic, triggered often by a day or two of overactive use of a diseased joint, such as a person with knee OA taking a long run and noticing a few days of pain thereafter. As disease progresses, the pain becomes continuous and even begins to be bothersome at night. Stiffness of the affected joint may be prominent, but morning stiffness is usually brief (<30 min).

In knees, buckling may occur, in part, due to weakness of muscles crossing the joint. Mechanical symptoms, such as buckling, catching, or locking, could also signify internal derangement, such as meniscal tears, and need to be evaluated. In the knee, pain with activities requiring knee flexion, such as stair climbing and arising from a chair, often emanates from the patellofemoral compartment of the knee, which does not actively articulate until the knee is bent ~35°.

OA is the most common cause of chronic knee pain in persons over age 45, but the differential diagnosis is long. Inflammatory arthritis is likely if there is prominent morning stiffness and many other joints are affected. Bursitis occurs commonly around knees and hips. A physical examination should focus on whether tenderness is over the joint line (at the junction of the two bones around which the joint is articulating) or is outside of it. Anserine bursitis, medial and distal to the knee, is an extremely common cause of chronic knee pain that may respond to a glucocorticoid injection. Prominent nocturnal pain in the absence of end-stage OA merits a distinct workup. For hip pain, OA can be detected by loss of internal rotation on passive movement, and pain isolated to an area lateral to the hip joint usually reflects the presence of trochanteric bursitis.

No blood tests are routinely indicated for workup of patients with OA unless symptoms and signs suggest inflammatory arthritis. Examination of the synovial fluid is often more helpful diagnostically than an x-ray. If the synovial fluid white count is >1000 per μL, inflammatory arthritis or gout or pseudogout are likely, the latter two being also identified by the presence of crystals.

X-rays are indicated to evaluate chronic hand pain and hip pain thought to be due to OA, as the diagnosis is often unclear without confirming radiographs. For knee pain, x-rays should be obtained if symptoms or signs are not typical of OA or if knee pain persists after inauguration of effective treatment. In OA, radiographic findings (Fig. 332-7) correlate poorly with the presence and severity of pain. Further, radiographs may be normal in early disease as they are insensitive to cartilage loss and other early findings.

While MRI may reveal the extent of pathology in an osteoarthritic joint, it is not indicated as part of the diagnostic workup.

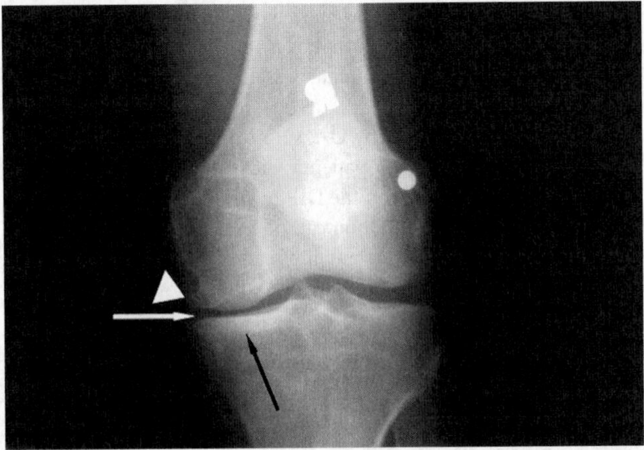

Figure 332-7 X-ray of knee with medial osteoarthritis. Note the narrowed joint space on medial side of the joint only (*white arrow*), the sclerosis of the bone in the medial compartment providing evidence of cortical thickening (*black arrow*), and the osteophytes in the medial femur (*white wedge*).

Findings such as meniscal tears in cartilage and bone lesions occur in most patients with OA in the knee, but almost never warrant a change in therapy.

TREATMENT Osteoarthritis

The goals of the treatment of OA are to alleviate pain and minimize loss of physical function. To the extent that pain and loss of function are consequences of inflammation, of weakness across the joint, and of laxity and instability, the treatment of OA involves addressing each of these impairments. Comprehensive therapy consists of a multimodality approach including nonpharmacologic and pharmacologic elements.

Patients with mild and intermittent symptoms may need only reassurance or nonpharmacologic treatments. Patients with ongoing, disabling pain are likely to need both nonpharmaco- and pharmacotherapy.

Treatments for knee OA have been more completely evaluated than those for hip and hand OA or for disease in other joints. Thus, while the principles of treatment are identical for OA in all joints, we shall focus below on the treatment of knee OA, noting specific recommendations for disease in other joints, especially when they differ from those for disease in the knee.

NONPHARMACOTHERAPY Since OA is a mechanically driven disease, the mainstay of treatment involves altering loading across the painful joint and improving the function of joint protectors, so they can better distribute load across the joint. Ways of lessening focal load across the joint include

(1) avoiding activities that overload the joint, as evidenced by their causing pain;
(2) improving the strength and conditioning of muscles that bridge the joint, so as to optimize their function; and
(3) unloading the joint, either by redistributing load within the joint with a brace or a splint or by unloading the joint during weight bearing with a cane or a crutch.

The simplest effective treatment for many patients is to avoid activities that precipitate pain. For example, for the middle-aged patient whose long-distance running brings on symptoms of knee OA, a less demanding form of weight-bearing activity may alleviate all symptoms. For an older person whose daily constitutionals up and down hills bring on knee pain, routing the constitutional away from hills might eliminate symptoms.

Each pound of weight increases the loading across the knee three- to sixfold. Weight loss may have a commensurate multiplier effect, unloading both knees and hips. Thus, weight loss, especially if substantial, may lessen symptoms of knee and hip OA.

In hand joints affected by OA, splinting, by limiting motion, often minimizes pain for patients with involvement either in the base of the thumb or in the DIP or proximal IP joints. With an appropriate splint, function can often be preserved. Weight-bearing joints such as knees and hips can be unloaded by using a cane in the hand opposite to the affected joint for partial weight bearing. A physical therapist can help teach the patient how to use the cane optimally, including ensuring that its height is optimal for unloading. Crutches or walkers can serve a similar beneficial function.

Exercise Osteoarthritic pain in knees or hips during weight bearing results in lack of activity and poor mobility and, because OA is so common, the inactivity that results represents a public health concern, increasing the risk of cardiovascular disease and of obesity. Aerobic capacity is poor in most elders with symptomatic knee OA, worse than others of the same age.

The development of weakness in muscles that bridge osteoarthritic joints is multifactorial in etiology. First, there is a decline in strength with age. Second, with limited mobility comes disuse muscle atrophy. Third, patients with painful knee or hip OA alter their gait so as to lessen loading across the affected joint, and this further diminishes muscle use. Fourth, "arthrogenous inhibition" may occur, whereby contraction of muscles bridging the joint is inhibited by a nerve afferent feedback loop emanating in a swollen and stretched joint capsule; this prevents maximal attainment of voluntary maximal strength. Since adequate muscle strength and conditioning are critical to joint protection, weakness in a muscle that bridges a diseased joint makes the joint more susceptible to further damage and pain. The degree of weakness correlates strongly with the severity of joint pain and the degree of physical limitation. One of the cardinal elements of the treatment of OA is to improve the functioning of muscles surrounding the joint.

For knee and hip OA, trials have shown that exercise lessens pain and improves physical function. Most effective exercise regimens consist of aerobic and/or resistance training, the latter of which focuses on strengthening muscles across the joint. Exercises are likely to be effective, especially if they train muscles for the activities a person performs daily. Some exercises may actually increase pain in the joint; these should be avoided, and the regimen needs to be individualized to optimize effectiveness and minimize discomfort. Range-of-motion exercises, which do not strengthen muscles, and isometric exercises that strengthen muscles, but not through range of motion, are unlikely to be effective by themselves. Isokinetic and isotonic strengthening (strengthening that occurs when a person flexes or extends the knees against resistance) have been shown consistently to be efficacious. Low-impact exercises, including water aerobics and water resistance training, are often better tolerated by patients than exercises involving impact loading, such as running or treadmill exercises. A patient should be referred to an exercise class or to a therapist who can create an individualized regimen, and then an individualized home-based regimen can be crafted.

There is no strong evidence that patients with hand OA benefit from therapeutic exercise, although for any patient with OA, individualized exercise programs should be tried. Adherence to exercise over the long term is the major challenge to an exercise prescription. In trials involving patients with knee OA, who are interested in exercise treatment, a third to over a half of patients stopped exercising by 6 months. Less than 50% continued regular exercise at 1 year. The strongest predictor of continued exercise in a patient is a previous personal history of successful exercise. Physicians should reinforce the exercise prescription at each clinic visit, help the patient recognize barriers to ongoing exercise, and identify convenient times for exercise to be done routinely. The combination of exercise with calorie restriction is especially effective in lessening pain.

One clinical trial has suggested that, among those with very early OA, participating in a strengthening and multimodality exercise program led to improvement in cartilage biochemistry, as evidenced by MRI imaging. There is little other evidence, however, that strengthening or other exercise has an effect on joint structure.

Correction of Malalignment Malalignment in the frontal plane (varus-valgus) markedly increases the stress across the joint, which can lead to progression of disease and to pain and disability (Fig. 332-5). Correcting malalignment, either surgically or with bracing, may relieve pain in persons whose knees are maligned. Malalignment develops over years as a consequence of gradual anatomic alterations of the joint and bone, and correcting it is often very challenging. One way is with a fitted brace, which takes an often varus osteoarthritic knee and straightens it by putting valgus stress across the knee. Unfortunately, many patients are unwilling to wear a realigning knee brace, plus in patients with obese legs, braces may slip with usage and lose their realigning effect. They are indicated for willing patients who can learn to put them on correctly and on whom they do not slip.

Other ways of correcting malalignment across the knee include the use of orthotics in footwear. Unfortunately, while they may have modest effects on knee alignment, trials have heretofore not demonstrated efficacy of a lateral wedge orthotic vs. placebo wedges.

Pain from the patellofemoral compartment of the knee can be caused by tilting of the patella or patellar malalignment with the patella riding laterally (or less often, medially) in the femoral trochlear groove. Using a brace to realign the patella, or tape to pull the patella back into the trochlear sulcus or reduce its tilt, has been shown, when compared to placebo taping in clinical trials, to lessen patellofemoral pain. However, patients may find it difficult to apply tape, and skin irritation from the tape is common. Commercial patellar braces may be a solution, but they have not been tested.

While their effect on malalignment is questionable, neoprene sleeves pulled to cover the knee lessen pain and are easy to use and popular among patients. The explanation for their therapeutic effect on pain is unclear.

In patients with knee OA, acupuncture produces modest pain relief compared to placebo needles and may be an adjunctive treatment.

PHARMACOTHERAPY While nonpharmacologic approaches to therapy constitute its mainstay, pharmacotherapy serves an important adjunctive role in OA treatment. Available drugs are administered using oral, topical, and intraarticular routes.

Acetaminophen, Nonsteroidal Anti-inflammatory Drugs (NSAIDs), and COX-2 Inhibitors Acetaminophen (paracetamol) is the initial analgesic of choice for patients with OA in knee, hip, or hands. For some patients, it is adequate to control symptoms, in which case more toxic drugs such as NSAIDs can be avoided. Doses up to 1 g 4 times daily can be used (Table 332-1).

NSAIDs are the most popular drugs to treat osteoarthritic pain. They can be administered either topically or orally. In clinical trials, oral NSAIDs produce ~30% greater improvement in pain than high-dose acetaminophen. Occasional patients treated with NSAIDs experience dramatic pain relief, whereas others experience little improvement. Initially, NSAIDs should be administered topically or taken orally on an "as needed" basis because side effects are less frequent with low intermittent doses, which may be highly efficacious. If occasional medication use is insufficiently effective, then daily treatment may be indicated, with an anti-inflammatory dose selected (Table 332-1). Patients should be reminded to take low-dose aspirin and ibuprofen at different times to eliminate a drug interaction.

NSAIDs taken orally have substantial and frequent side effects, the most common of which is upper gastrointestinal toxicity, including dyspepsia, nausea, bloating, gastrointestinal bleeding, and ulcer disease. Some 30–40% of patients experience upper gastrointestinal (GI) side effects so severe as to require discontinuation of medication. To minimize the risk of nonsteroidal-related GI side effects, patients should not take two NSAIDs, and

TABLE 332-1 Pharmacologic Treatment for Osteoarthritis

Treatment	Dosage	Comments
Acetaminophen	Up to 1 g qid	Prolongs half-life of warfarin
Oral NSAIDs and COX-2 inhibitors[a]		Take with food. Increased risk of myocardial infarction and stroke for some NSAIDs and especially COX-2 inhibitors. High rates of gastrointestinal side effects, including ulcers and bleeding, occur. Patients at high risk for gastrointestinal side effects should also take either a proton pump inhibitor or misoprostol.[b] There is an increased gastrointestinal side effects or bleeding when taken with acetylsalicylic acid. Can also cause edema and renal insufficiency.
Naproxen	375–500 mg bid	
Salsalate	1500 mg bid	
Ibuprofen	600–800 mg 3–4 times a day	
Topical NSAIDs		Rub onto joint. Few systemic side effects. Skin irritation common.
Diclofenac Na 1% gel	4gm qid (for knees)	
Opiates	Various	Common side effects include dizziness, sedation, nausea or vomiting, dry mouth, constipation, urinary retention, and pruritis. Respiratory and central nervous system depression can occur.
Capsaicin	0.025–0.075% cream 3–4 times a day	Can irritate mucous membranes.
Intraarticular injections		
Steroids		
Hyaluronans	Varies from 3–5 weekly injections depending on preparation	Mild to moderate pain at injection site. Controversy exists re: efficacy.

[a]COX-2, cyclooxygenase 2; NSAIDs, nonsteroidal anti-inflammatory drugs.

[b]Patients at high risk include those with previous gastrointestinal events, persons ≥60 years, and persons taking glucocorticoids. Trials have shown the efficacy of proton pump inhibitors and misoprostol in the prevention of ulcers and bleeding. Misoprostol is associated with a high rate of diarrhea and cramping; therefore, proton pump inhibitors are more widely used to reduce NSAID-related gastrointestinal symptoms.

Source: Adapted from Felson 2006.

should take medications after food; if risk is high, patients should take a gastroprotective agent, such as a proton pump inhibitor. Certain oral agents are safer to the stomach than others including nonacetylated salicylates and nabumetone. Major NSAID-related GI side effects can occur in patients who do not complain of upper GI symptoms. In one study of patients hospitalized for GI bleeding, 81% had no premonitory symptoms.

Because of the increased rates of cardiovascular events associated with cyclooxygenase 2 (COX-2) inhibitors and with some conventional NSAIDs such as diclofenac, many of these drugs are not appropriate long-term treatment choices for older persons with osteoarthritis, especially those at high risk of heart disease or stroke. The American Heart Association has identified rofecoxib and all other COX-2 inhibitors as putting patients at high risk, although low doses of celecoxib, such as 200 mg/d, may not be associated with an elevation of risk. The only conventional NSAID that appears safe from a cardiovascular perspective is naproxen, but it does have gastrointestinal toxicity.

There are other common side effects of NSAIDs, including the tendency to develop edema, because of prostaglandin inhibition of afferent blood supply to glomeruli in the kidneys and, for similar reasons, a predilection toward reversible renal insufficiency. Blood pressure may increase modestly in some NSAID-treated patients.

With the approval by the U.S. Food and Drug Administration of topical diclofenac and the availability of these agents in Europe, clinicians have a choice of administration modality for anti-inflammatory drugs. NSAIDs can be placed into a gel or topical solution with another chemical modality that enhances penetration of the skin barrier. When absorbed through the skin, plasma concentrations are an order of magnitude lower than with the same amount of drug administered orally or parenterally. However, when these drugs are administered topically in proximity to a superficial joint, (knees, hands, but not hips), the drug can be found in joint tissues such as the synovium and cartilage. Trial results have varied but generally have found that topical NSAIDs are slightly less efficacious than oral agents, but have far fewer gastrointestinal and systemic side effects. Unfortunately, topical NSAIDs often cause local skin irritation where the medication is applied, inducing redness, burning or itching in up to 40 percent of patients (see Table 332-1).

Intraarticular Injections: Glucocorticoids and Hyaluronic Acid Since synovial inflammation is likely to be a major cause of pain in patients with OA, local anti-inflammatory treatments administered intraarticularly may be effective in ameliorating pain, at least temporarily. Glucocorticoid injections provide such efficacy, but work better than placebo injections for only 1 or 2 weeks. This may be because the disease remains mechanically driven and, when a person begins to use the joint, the loading factors that induce pain return. Glucocorticoid injections are useful to get patients over acute flares of pain and may be especially indicated if the patient has coexistent OA and crystal deposition disease, especially from calcium pyrophosphate dihydrate crystals (Chap. 333). There is no evidence that repeated glucocorticoid injections into the joint are dangerous.

Hyaluronic acid injections can be given for treatment of symptoms in knee and hip OA, but there is controversy as to whether they have efficacy vs. placebo (Table 332-1).

Optimal therapy for OA is often achieved by trial and error, with each patient having idiosyncratic responses to specific treatments. When medical therapies have failed and the patient has an unacceptable reduction in their quality of life and ongoing pain and disability, then at least for knee and hip OA, total joint arthroplasty is indicated.

SURGERY For knee OA, several operations are available. Among the most popular surgeries, at least in the United States, is arthroscopic debridement and lavage. Randomized trials evaluating this operation have showed that its efficacy is no greater than that of sham surgery or no treatment for relief of pain or disability. Even mechanical symptoms such as buckling, which are extremely common in patients with knee OA, do not respond to arthroscopic debridement. Arthroscopic meniscectomy is indicated for acute meniscal tears in which symptoms such as locking and acute pain are clearly related temporally to a knee injury that produced the tear.

For patients with knee OA isolated to the medial compartment, operations to realign the knee to lessen medial loading can relieve pain. These include a high tibial osteotomy, in which the tibia is broken just below the tibial plateau and realigned so as to load the lateral, nondiseased compartment, or a unicompartmental replacement with realignment. Each surgery may provide the patient with years of pain relief before they require a total knee replacement.

Ultimately, when the patient with knee or hip OA has failed medical treatment modalities and remains in pain, with limitations of physical function that compromise the quality of life, the patient should be referred for total knee or hip arthroplasty. These are highly efficacious operations that relieve pain and improve function in the vast majority of patients. Currently failure rates are ~1% per year, although these rates are higher in obese patients. The chance of surgical success is greater in centers where at least 25 such operations are performed yearly or with surgeons who perform multiple operations annually. The timing of knee or hip replacement is critical. If the patient suffers for many years until their functional status has declined substantially, with considerable muscle weakness, postoperative functional status may not improve to a level achieved by others who underwent operation earlier in their disease course.

Cartilage Regeneration Chondrocyte transplantation has not been found to be efficacious in OA, perhaps because OA includes pathology of joint mechanics, which is not corrected by chondrocyte transplants. Similarly, abrasion arthroplasty (chondroplasty) has not been well studied for efficacy in OA, but it produces fibrocartilage in place of damaged hyaline cartilage. Both of these surgical attempts to regenerate and reconstitute articular cartilage may be more likely to be efficacious early in disease when joint malalignment and many of the other noncartilage abnormalities that characterize OA have not yet developed.

FURTHER READINGS

Abramson SB, Attur M: Developments in the scientific understanding of osteoarthritis. Arthritis Res Ther 11:227, 2009

Bennell K, Hinman R: Exercise as a treatment for osteoarthritis. Curr Opin Rheumatol 17:634, 2005

Felson DT: Osteoarthritis of the knee. N Engl J Med 354:841, 2006

———: Developments in the clinical understanding of osteoarthritis. Arthritis Res Ther 11:203, 2009

Krohn K: Footwear alterations and bracing as treatments for knee osteoarthritis. Curr Opin Rheumatol 17:653, 2005

CHAPTER 333
Gout and Other Crystal-Associated Arthropathies

H. Ralph Schumacher
Lan X. Chen

The use of polarizing light microscopy during synovial fluid analysis in 1961 by McCarty and Hollander and the subsequent application of other crystallographic techniques, such as electron microscopy, energy-dispersive elemental analysis, and x-ray diffraction, have allowed investigators to identify the roles of different microcrystals, including monosodium urate (MSU), calcium pyrophosphate dihydrate (CPPD), calcium apatite (apatite), and calcium oxalate (CaOx), in inducing acute or chronic arthritis or periarthritis. The clinical events that result from deposition of MSU, CPPD, apatite, and CaOx have many similarities but also have important differences. Before the use of crystallographic techniques in rheumatology, much of what was considered to be gouty arthritis in fact was not. Because of often similar clinical presentations, the need to perform synovial fluid analysis to distinguish the type of crystal involved must be emphasized. Polarized light microscopy alone can identify most typical crystals; apatite, however, is an exception. Aspiration and analysis of effusions are also important to assess the possibility of infection. Apart from the identification of specific microcrystalline materials or organisms, synovial fluid characteristics in crystal-associated diseases are nonspecific, and synovial fluid can be inflammatory or noninflammatory. A list of possible musculoskeletal manifestations of crystal-associated arthritis is shown in Table 333-1.

GOUT

Gout is a metabolic disease that most often affects middle-aged to elderly men and postmenopausal women. It results from an increased body pool of urate with hyperuricemia. It typically is characterized by episodic acute and chronic arthritis caused by deposition of MSU crystals in joints and connective tissue tophi and the risk for deposition in kidney interstitium or uric acid nephrolithiasis (Chap. 359).

TABLE 333-1 Musculoskeletal Manifestations of Crystal-Induced Arthritis

Acute mono- or polyarthritis	Destructive arthropathies
Bursitis	Pseudo-rheumatoid arthritis
Tendinitis	Pseudo-ankylosing spondylitis
Enthesitis	Spinal stenosis
Tophaceous deposits	Crowned dens syndrome
Peculiar type of osteoarthritis	Carpal tunnel syndrome
Synovial osteochondromatosis	Tendon rupture

ACUTE AND CHRONIC ARTHRITIS

Acute arthritis is the most common early clinical manifestation of gout. Usually, only one joint is affected initially, but polyarticular acute gout can occur in subsequent episodes. The metatarsophalangeal joint of the first toe often is involved, but tarsal joints, ankles, and knees also are affected commonly. Especially in elderly patients or in advanced disease, finger joints may be involved. Inflamed Heberden's or Bouchard's nodes may be a first manifestation of gouty arthritis. The first episode of acute gouty arthritis frequently begins at night with dramatic joint pain and swelling. Joints rapidly become warm, red, and tender, with a clinical appearance that often mimics that of cellulitis. Early attacks tend to subside spontaneously within 3–10 days, and most patients have intervals of varying length with no residual symptoms until the next episode. Several events may precipitate acute gouty arthritis: dietary excess, trauma, surgery, excessive ethanol ingestion, hypouricemic therapy, and serious medical illnesses such as myocardial infarction and stroke.

After many acute mono- or oligoarticular attacks, a proportion of gouty patients may present with a chronic nonsymmetric synovitis, causing potential confusion with rheumatoid arthritis (Chap. 321). Less commonly, chronic gouty arthritis will be the only manifestation, and, more rarely, the disease will manifest only as periarticular tophaceous deposits in the absence of synovitis. Women represent only 5–20% of all patients with gout. Premenopausal gout is rare; it is seen mostly in individuals with a strong family history of gout. Kindreds of precocious gout in young females caused by decreased renal urate clearance and renal insufficiency have been described. Most women with gouty arthritis are postmenopausal and elderly, have osteoarthritis and arterial hypertension that cause mild renal insufficiency, and usually are receiving diuretics.

Laboratory diagnosis

Even if the clinical appearance strongly suggests gout, the presumptive diagnosis ideally should be confirmed by needle aspiration of acutely or chronically involved joints or tophaceous deposits. Acute septic arthritis, several of the other crystalline-associated arthropathies, palindromic rheumatism, and psoriatic arthritis may present with similar clinical features. During acute gouty attacks, needle-shaped MSU crystals typically are seen both intracellularly and extracellularly (Fig. 333-1). With compensated polarized light

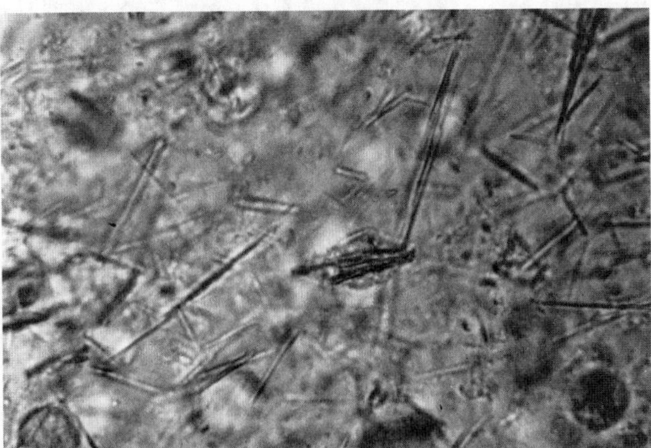

Figure 333-1 Extracellular and intracellular monosodium urate crystals, as seen in a fresh preparation of synovial fluid, illustrate needle- and rod-shaped crystals. These crystals are strongly negative birefringent crystals under compensated polarized light microscopy; 400×.

these crystals are brightly birefringent with negative elongation. Synovial fluid leukocyte counts are elevated from 2000 to 60,000/μL. Effusions appear cloudy due to the increased numbers of leukocytes. Large amounts of crystals occasionally produce a thick pasty or chalky joint fluid. Bacterial infection can coexist with urate crystals in synovial fluid; if there is any suspicion of septic arthritis, joint fluid must be cultured.

MSU crystals also can often be demonstrated in the first metatarsophalangeal joint and in knees not acutely involved with gout. Arthrocentesis of these joints is a useful technique to establish the diagnosis of gout between attacks.

Serum uric acid levels can be normal or low at the time of an acute attack, as inflammatory cytokines can be uricosuric and effective initiation of hypouricemic therapy can precipitate attacks. This limits the value of serum uric acid determinations for the diagnosis of gout. Nevertheless, serum urate levels are almost always elevated at some time and are important to use to follow the course of hypouricemic therapy. A 24-h urine collection for uric acid can, in some cases, be useful in assessing the risk of stones, elucidating overproduction or underexcretion of uric acid, and deciding whether it may be appropriate to use a uricosuric therapy (Chap. 359). Excretion of >800 mg of uric acid per 24 h on a regular diet suggests that causes of overproduction of purine should be considered. Urinalysis, serum creatinine, hemoglobin, white blood cell (WBC) count, liver function tests, and serum lipids should be obtained because of possible pathologic sequelae of gout and other associated diseases requiring treatment and as baselines because of possible adverse effects of gout treatment.

Radiographic features

Early in the disease radiographic studies may only confirm clinically evident swelling. Cystic changes, well-defined erosions with sclerotic margins (often with overhanging bony edges), and soft tissue masses are characteristic features of advanced chronic tophaceous gout. Ultrasound, CT and MRI are being studied and are likely to become more sensitive for early changes.

TREATMENT Gout

ACUTE GOUTY ARTHRITIS The mainstay of treatment during an acute attack is the administration of anti-inflammatory drugs such as nonsteroidal anti-inflammatory drugs (NSAIDs), colchicine, or glucocorticoids. NSAIDs are used most often in individuals without complicating comorbid conditions. Both colchicine and NSAIDs may be poorly tolerated and dangerous in the elderly and in the presence of renal insufficiency and gastrointestinal disorders. This was repeated later. Ice pack applications and rest of the involved joints can be helpful. Colchicine given orally is a traditional and effective treatment if used early in an attack. One useful regimen is one 0.6-mg tablet given every 8 h with subsequent tapering. This is generally better tolerated than the formerly advised hourly regimen. The drug must be stopped promptly at the first sign of loose stools, and symptomatic treatment must be given for the diarrhea. Intravenous colchicine has been taken off the market. NSAIDs given in full anti-inflammatory doses are effective in ~90% of patients, and the resolution of signs and symptoms usually occurs in 5–8 days. The most effective drugs are any of those with a short half-life and include indomethacin, 25–50 mg tid; naproxen, 500 mg bid; ibuprofen, 800 mg tid; and diclofenac, 50 mg tid. Glucocorticoids given IM or orally, for example, prednisone, 30–50 mg/d as the initial dose and gradually tapered with the resolution of the attack, can be effective in polyarticular gout. For a single joint or a few involved joints intraarticular triamcinolone acetonide, 20–40 mg, or methylprednisolone, 25–50 mg, have been effective and well tolerated. Based on recent evidence on the essential role of the inflammasome and interleukin 1 β (IL-1β) in acute gout, anakinra has been used and other inhibitors of IL-1β are under investigation.

HYPOURICEMIC THERAPY Ultimate control of gout requires correction of the basic underlying defect: the hyperuricemia. Attempts to normalize serum uric acid to <300–360 μmol/L (5.0–6.0 mg/dL) to prevent recurrent gouty attacks and eliminate tophaceous deposits entail a commitment to long-term hypouricemic regimens and medications that generally are required for life. Hypouricemic therapy should be considered when, as in most patients, the hyperuricemia cannot be corrected by simple means (control of body weight, low-purine diet, increase in liquid intake, limitation of ethanol use, decreased use of fructose-containing foods and beverages, and avoidance of diuretics). The decision to initiate hypouricemic therapy usually is made taking into consideration the number of acute attacks (urate lowering may be cost-effective after two attacks), serum uric acid levels [progression is more rapid in patients with serum uric acid >535 μmol/L (>9.0 mg/dL)], the patient's willingness to commit to lifelong therapy, or the presence of uric acid stones. Urate-lowering therapy should be initiated in any patient who already has tophi or chronic gouty arthritis. Uricosuric agents such as probenecid can be used in patients with good renal function who underexcrete uric acid, with <600 mg in a 24-h urine sample. Urine volume must be maintained by ingestion of 1500 mL of water every day. Probenecid can be started at a dose of 250 mg twice daily and increased gradually as needed up to 3 g per day to maintain a serum uric acid level <360 μmol/L (6 mg/dL). Probenecid is generally not effective in patients with serum creatinine levels >177 μmol/L (2 mg/dL). These patients may require allopurinol or benzbromarone (not available in the United States). Benzbromarone is another uricosuric drug that is more effective in patients with renal failure. Some agents used to treat common comorbidities, including losartan, fenofibrate, and amlodipine, have some mild uricosuric effects.

The xanthine oxidase inhibitor allopurinol is by far the most commonly used hypouricemic agent and is the best drug to lower serum urate in overproducers, urate stone formers, and patients with renal disease. It can be given in a single morning dose, 100–300 mg initially and increasing up to 800 mg if needed. In patients with chronic renal disease, the initial allopurinol dose should be lower and adjusted depending on the serum creatinine concentration; for example, with a creatinine clearance of 10 mL/min, one generally would use 100 mg every other day. Doses can be increased gradually to reach the target urate level of 6 mg/dL; however, more studies are needed to provide exact guidance. Toxicity of allopurinol has been recognized increasingly in patients who use thiazide diuretics and patients allergic to penicillin and ampicillin. The most serious side effects include life-threatening toxic epidermal necrolysis, systemic vasculitis, bone marrow suppression, granulomatous hepatitis, and renal failure. Patients with mild cutaneous reactions to allopurinol can reconsider the use of a uricosuric agent, undergo an attempt at desensitization to allopurinol, or take febuxostat, a new, chemically unrelated specific xanthine oxidase inhibitor. Febuxostat is approved at 40 or 80 mg once a day and does not require dose adjustment in mild to moderate renal disease. Patients can also pay increased attention to diet and should be aware of new alternative agents (see below). Urate-lowering drugs are generally not initiated during acute attacks but after the patient is stable and low-dose colchicine has been initiated to decrease the risk of the flares that often occur with urate lowering. Colchicine anti-inflammatory prophylaxis in doses of 0.6 mg one to two times daily should be given along with the hypouricemic therapy until the patient is normouricemic and without gouty attacks for 6 months or as long as tophi are present. Colchicine should not be used in dialysis patients and is given in lower doses in patients with renal disease or with P gylcoprotein or CYP3A4 inhibitors such as clarithromycin that can increase toxicity or colchicine. Pegloticase is a new urate-lowering biologic agent that can be effective in patients allergic to or failing xanthine oxidase inhibitors. New uricosurics are undergoing investigation.

CPPD DEPOSITION DISEASE

PATHOGENESIS

The deposition of CPPD crystals in articular tissues is most common in the elderly, occurring in 10–15% of persons age 65–75 years and 30–50% of those >85 years. In most cases, this process is asymptomatic and the cause of CPPD deposition is uncertain. Because >80% of patients are >60 years and 70% have preexisting joint damage from other conditions, it is likely that biochemical changes in aging or diseased cartilage favors crystal nucleation. In patients with CPPD arthritis there is increased production of inorganic pyrophosphate and decreased levels of pyrophosphatases in cartilage extracts. Mutations in the *ANKH* gene, as described in both familial and sporadic cases, can increase elaboration and extracellular transport of pyrophosphate. The increase in pyrophosphate production appears to be related to enhanced activity of ATP pyrophosphohydrolase and 5′-nucleotidase, which catalyze the reaction of ATP to adenosine and pyrophosphate. This pyrophosphate could combine with calcium to form CPPD crystals in matrix vesicles or on collagen fibers. There are decreased levels of cartilage glycosaminoglycans that normally inhibit and regulate crystal nucleation. High activities of transglutaminase enzymes also may contribute to the deposition of CPPD crystals.

Release of CPPD crystals into the joint space is followed by the phagocytosis of those crystals by monocyte-macrophages and neutrophils, which respond by releasing chemotactic and inflammatory substances and, as with MSU crystals, activate the inflammasome.

A minority of patients with CPPD arthropathy have metabolic abnormalities or hereditary CPPD disease (Table 333-2). These associations suggest that a variety of different metabolic products may enhance CPPD deposition either by directly altering cartilage or by inhibiting inorganic pyrophosphatases. Included among these conditions are hyperparathyroidism, hemochromatosis, hypophosphatasia, hypomagnesemia, and possibly myxedema. The presence of CPPD arthritis in individuals <50 years old should lead to consideration of these metabolic disorders (Table 333-2) and inherited forms of disease, including those identified in a variety of ethnic groups. Genomic DNA studies performed on different kindreds have shown a possible location of genetic defects on chromosome 8q or on chromosome 5p in a region that expresses the gene of the membrane pyrophosphate channel (*ANKH* gene). As noted above, mutations described in the *ANKH* gene in kindreds with CPPD arthritis can increase extracellular pyrophosphate and induce CPPD crystal formation. Investigation of younger patients with CPPD deposition should include inquiry for evidence of familial aggregation and evaluation of serum calcium, phosphorus, alkaline phosphatase, magnesium, serum iron, and transferrin.

TABLE 333-2 Conditions Associated With Calcium Pyrophosphate Dihydrate Disease

Aging
Disease-associated
Primary hyperparathyroidism
Hemochromatosis
Hypophosphatasia
Hypomagnesemia
Chronic gout
Postmeniscectomy
Gitelman's syndrome
Epiphyseal dysplasias

CLINICAL MANIFESTATIONS

CPPD arthropathy may be asymptomatic, acute, subacute, or chronic or may cause acute synovitis superimposed on chronically involved joints. Acute CPPD arthritis originally was termed *pseudogout* by McCarty and co-workers because of its striking similarity to gout. Other clinical manifestations of CPPD deposition include (1) induction or enhancement of peculiar forms of osteoarthritis, (2) induction of severe destructive disease that may radiographically mimic neuropathic arthritis, (3) production of symmetric synovitis that is clinically similar to rheumatoid arthritis and sometimes seen in familial forms with early onset, (4) intervertebral disk and ligament calcification with restriction of spine mobility that mimics ankylosing spondylitis (also seen in hereditary forms), (5) spinal stenosis (most commonly seen in the elderly), and (6) rarely periarticular tophus-like nodules.

The knee is the joint most frequently affected in CPPD arthropathy. Other sites include the wrist, shoulder, ankle, elbow, and hands. The temporomandibular joint and ligamentum flavum of the spinal canal may be involved. Clinical and radiographic evidence indicates that CPPD deposition is polyarticular in at least two-thirds of patients. When the clinical picture resembles that of slowly progressive osteoarthritis, diagnosis may be difficult. Joint distribution may provide important clues suggesting CPPD disease. For example, primary osteoarthritis less often involves a metacarpophalangeal, wrist, elbow, shoulder, or ankle joints. If radiographs reveal punctate and/or linear radiodense deposits in fibrocartilaginous joint menisci or articular hyaline cartilage (*chondrocalcinosis*), the diagnostic likelihood of CPPD disease is further increased. *Definitive diagnosis* requires demonstration of typical rhomboid or rodlike crystals in synovial fluid or articular tissue (Fig. 333-2). In the absence of joint effusion or indications to obtain a synovial biopsy, chondrocalcinosis is presumptive of CPPD deposition. One exception is chondrocalcinosis due to CaOx in some patients with chronic renal failure.

Acute attacks of CPPD arthritis may be precipitated by trauma. Rapid diminution of serum calcium concentration, as may occur in severe medical illness or after surgery (especially parathyroidectomy), can also lead to pseudogout attacks.

In as many as 50% of cases, episodes of CPPD-induced inflammation are associated with low-grade fever and, on occasion, temperatures as high as 40°C (104°F). Whether or not radiographic proof of chondrocalcinosis is evident in the involved joint(s), synovial fluid analysis with microbial cultures is essential to rule out the possibility of infection. In fact, infection in a joint with any microcrystalline deposition process can lead to crystal shedding and subsequent

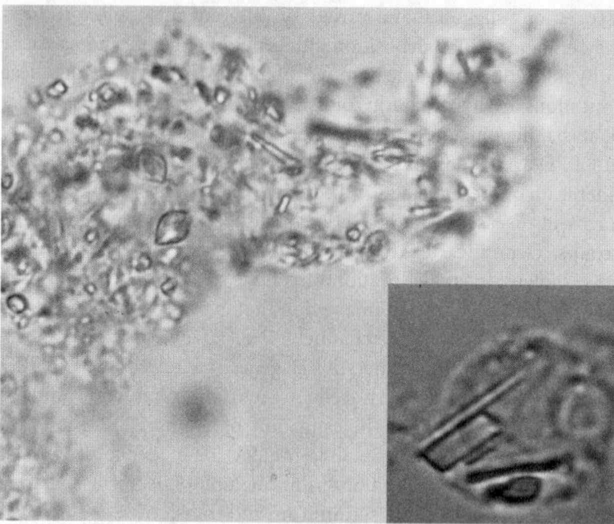

Figure 333-2 Intracellular and extracellular calcium pyrophosphate dihydrate crystals, as seen in a fresh preparation of synovial fluid, illustrate rectangular, rod-shaped, and rhomboid crystals that are weakly positive birefringent crystals (compensated polarized light microscopy; 400×).

synovitis from both crystals and microorganisms. Synovial fluid in acute CPPD disease has inflammatory characteristics. The leukocyte count can range from several thousand cells to 100,000 cells/μL, with the mean being about 24,000 cells/μL and the predominant cell being the neutrophil. Polarized light microscopy usually reveals rhomboid, square, or rodlike crystals with weak positive birefringence inside tissue fragments and fibrin clots and in neutrophils (Fig. 333-2). CPPD crystals may coexist with MSU and apatite in some cases.

TREATMENT CPPD Deposition Disease

Untreated acute attacks may last a few days to as long as a month. Treatment by joint aspiration and NSAIDs or by intraarticular glucocorticoid injection may result in return to prior status in ≤10 days. For patients with frequent recurrent attacks of pseudogout, daily prophylactic treatment with low doses of colchicine may be helpful in decreasing the frequency of the attacks. Severe polyarticular attacks usually require short courses of glucocorticoids or, as recently reported, an IL-1β antagonist, anakinra. Unfortunately, there is no effective way to remove CPPD deposits from cartilage and synovium. Uncontrolled studies suggest that the administration of antimalarial agents or even methotrexate may be helpful in controlling persistent synovitis. Patients with progressive destructive large-joint arthropathy may require joint replacement.

CALCIUM APATITE DEPOSITION DISEASE

PATHOGENESIS

Apatite is the primary mineral of normal bone and teeth. Abnormal accumulation of basic calcium phosphates, largely carbonate substituted apatite, can occur in areas of tissue damage (dystrophic calcification), hypercalcemic or hyperparathyroid states (metastatic calcification), and certain conditions of unknown cause (Table 333-3). In chronic renal failure, hyperphosphatemia can contribute to extensive apatite deposition both in and around joints. Familial aggregation is rarely seen; no association with

TABLE 333-3 Conditions Associated With Apatite Deposition Disease

Aging
Osteoarthritis
Hemorrhagic shoulder effusions in the elderly (Milwaukee shoulder)
Destructive arthropathy
Tendinitis, bursitis
Tumoral calcinosis (sporadic cases)
Disease-associated
Hyperparathyroidism
Milk-alkali syndrome
Renal failure/long-term dialysis
Connective tissue diseases (e.g., systemic sclerosis, idiopathic myositis, SLE)
Heterotopic calcification after neurologic catastrophes (e.g., stroke, spinal cord injury)
Heredity
Bursitis, arthritis
Tumoral calcinosis
Fibrodysplasia ossificans progressiva

Abbreviation: SLE, systemic lupus erythematosus.

ANKH mutations has been described thus far. Apatite crystals are deposited primarily on matrix vessels. Incompletely understood alterations in matrix proteoglycans, phosphatases, hormones, and cytokines probably can influence crystal formation.

Apatite aggregates are commonly present in synovial fluid in an extremely destructive chronic arthropathy of the elderly that occurs most often in the shoulders (Milwaukee shoulder) and in a similar process in hips, knees, and erosive osteoarthritis of fingers. Joint destruction is associated with damage to cartilage and supporting structures, leading to instability and deformity. Progression tends to be indolent, and synovial fluid leukocyte counts are usually <2000/μL. Symptoms range from minimal to severe pain and disability that may lead to joint replacement surgery. Whether severely affected patients merely represent an extreme synovial tissue response to the apatite crystals that are so common in osteoarthritis is uncertain. Synovial lining cell or fibroblast cultures exposed to apatite (or CPPD) crystals can undergo mitosis and markedly increase the release of prostaglandin E_2 and cytokines and also collagenases and neutral proteases, underscoring the destructive potential of abnormally stimulated synovial lining cells.

CLINICAL MANIFESTATIONS

Periarticular or articular deposits may occur and may be associated with acute reversible inflammation and/or chronic damage to the joint capsule, tendons, bursa, or articular surfaces. The most common sites of apatite deposition include bursae and tendons in and/or around the knees, shoulders, hips, and fingers. Clinical manifestations include asymptomatic radiographic abnormalities, acute synovitis, bursitis, tendinitis, and chronic destructive arthropathy. Although the true incidence of apatite arthritis is not known, 30–50% of patients with osteoarthritis have apatite microcrystals in their synovial fluid. Such crystals frequently can be identified in clinically stable osteoarthritic joints, but they are more likely to come to attention in persons experiencing acute or subacute worsening of joint pain and swelling. The synovial fluid leukocyte count in apatite arthritis is usually low (<2000/μL) despite dramatic symptoms, with predominance of mononuclear cells.

DIAGNOSIS

Intra- and/or periarticular calcifications with or without erosive, destructive, or hypertrophic changes may be seen on radiographs (Fig. 333-3). They should be distinguished from the linear calcifications typical of CPPD deposition disease.

Definitive diagnosis of apatite arthropathy, also called basic calcium phosphate disease, depends on identification of crystals from synovial fluid or tissue (Fig. 333-3). Individual crystals are very small and can be seen only by electron microscopy. Clumps of crystals may appear as 1- to 20-μm shiny intra- or extracellular nonbirefringent globules or aggregates that stain purplish with Wright's stain and bright red with alizarin red S. Tetracycline binding is under investigation as a labeling alternative. Absolute identification depends on electron microscopy with energy-dispersive elemental analysis, x-ray diffraction, infrared spectroscopy, or Raman microspectroscopy, but they usually are not required in clinical diagnosis.

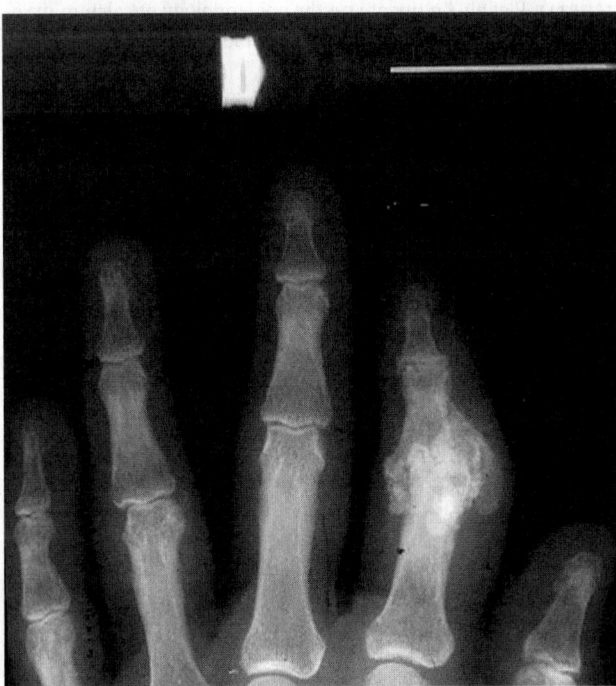

A

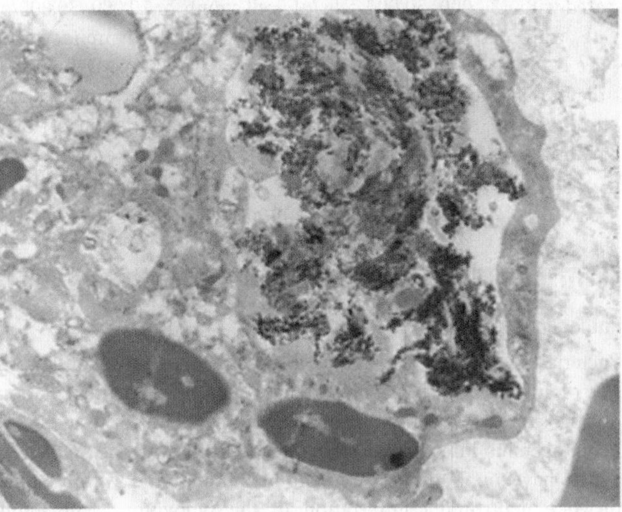

B

Figure 333-3 ***A.* Radiograph showing calcification** due to apatite crystals surrounding an eroded joint. ***B.*** An electron micrograph demonstrates dark needle-shaped apatite crystals within a vacuole of a synovial fluid mononuclear cell (30,000×).

TREATMENT Calcium Apatite Deposition Disease

Treatment of apatite arthritis or periarthritis is nonspecific. Acute attacks of bursitis or synovitis may be self-limiting, resolving in days to several weeks. Aspiration of effusions and the use of either NSAIDs or oral colchicine for 2 weeks or intra- or periarticular injection of a depot glucocorticoid appear to shorten the duration and intensity of symptoms. Local injection of disodium ethylenediaminetetraacetic acid (EDTA) was effective in one study of calcific tendinitis at the shoulder. Periarticular apatite deposits may be resorbed with resolution of attacks. Agents to lower serum phosphate levels may lead to resorption of deposits in renal failure patients receiving hemodialysis. In patients with underlying severe destructive articular changes, response to medical therapy is usually less rewarding.

CaOx DEPOSITION DISEASE

PATHOGENESIS

Primary oxalosis is a rare hereditary metabolic disorder (Chap. 364). Enhanced production of oxalic acid may result from at least two different enzyme defects, leading to hyperoxalemia and deposition of calcium oxalate crystals in tissues. Nephrocalcinosis, renal failure, and death usually occur before age 20. Acute and/or chronic CaOx arthritis and periarthritis may complicate primary oxalosis during later years of illness.

Secondary oxalosis is more common than the primary disorder. It is one of the many metabolic abnormalities that complicate end-stage renal disease. In chronic renal disease, calcium oxalate deposits have long been recognized in visceral organs, blood vessels, bones, and cartilage and are now known to be one of the causes of arthritis in chronic renal failure. Thus far, reported patients have been dependent on long-term hemodialysis or peritoneal dialysis (Chap. 281), and many had received ascorbic acid supplements. Ascorbic acid is metabolized to oxalate, which is inadequately cleared in uremia and by dialysis. Such supplements usually are avoided in dialysis programs because of the risk of enhancing hyperoxalosis and its sequelae.

CLINICAL MANIFESTATIONS AND DIAGNOSIS

CaOx aggregates can be found in bone, articular cartilage, synovium, and periarticular tissues. From these sites, crystals may be shed, causing acute synovitis. Persistent aggregates of CaOx can, like apatite and CPPD, stimulate synovial cell proliferation and enzyme release, resulting in progressive articular destruction. Deposits have been documented in fingers, wrists, elbows, knees, ankles, and feet.

Clinical features of acute CaOx arthritis may not be distinguishable from those due to sodium urate, CPPD, or apatite. Radiographs may reveal chondrocalcinosis or soft tissue calcifications. CaOx-induced synovial effusions are usually noninflammatory, with <2000 leukocytes/μL, or mildly inflammatory. Neutrophils or mononuclear cells can predominate. CaOx crystals have a variable shape and variable birefringence to polarized light. The most easily recognized forms are bipyramidal, have strong birefringence (Fig. 333-4), and stain with alizarin red S.

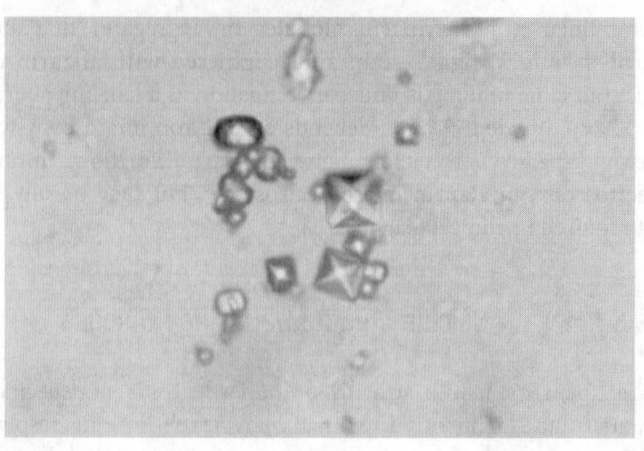

Figure 333-4 Bipyramidal and small polymorphic calcium oxalate crystals from synovial fluid are a classic finding in CaOx arthropathy (ordinary light microscopy; 400×).

TREATMENT Calcium Oxalate Deposition Disease

Treatment of CaOx arthropathy with NSAIDs, colchicine, intraarticular glucocorticoids, and/or an increased frequency of dialysis has produced only slight improvement. In primary oxalosis, liver transplantation has induced a significant reduction in crystal deposits (Chap. 364).

ACKNOWLEDGMENT

This chapter has been revised for the previous edition and this edition from an original version written by Antonio Reginato, MD, in earlier editions of Harrison's Principles of Internal Medicine.

FURTHER READINGS

Maldonado I et al: Oxalate crystal deposition disease. Curr Rheumatol Rep 4:257, 2002

Molloy ES, McCarthy GM: Basic calcium phosphate crystals: Pathways to joint destruction. Curr Opinion Rheumatol 18:187, 2006

Reiders MK et al: A randomised controlled trial on the efficacy and tolerability with dose escalation of allopurinol 300–600 mg/day versus benzbromarone 100–200 mg/day in patients with gout. Ann Rheum Dis 68:892, 2009

Richette P et al: An update on the epidemiology of calcium pyrophosphate dihydrate crystal deposition disease. Rheumatology (Oxford) 48:711, 2009

Thouverey C et al: Inorganic pyrophosphate as a regulator of hydroxyapatite or calcium pyrophosphate dihydrate mineral deposition by matrix vesicles. Osteoarthritis Cartilage 17:64, 2009

Wortmann RL et al (eds): *Crystal-Induced Arthropathies: Gout, Pseudogout and Apatite-Associated Syndromes*. New York, Taylor & Francis, 2006

CHAPTER 334

Infectious Arthritis

Lawrence C. Madoff

Although *Staphylococcus aureus*, *Neisseria gonorrhoeae*, and other bacteria are the most common causes of infectious arthritis, various mycobacteria, spirochetes, fungi, and viruses also infect joints (Table 334-1). Since acute bacterial infection can destroy articular cartilage rapidly, all inflamed joints must be evaluated without delay to exclude noninfectious processes and determine appropriate antimicrobial therapy and drainage procedures. For more detailed information on infectious arthritis caused by specific organisms, the reader is referred to the chapters on those organisms.

Acute bacterial infection typically involves a single joint or a few joints. Subacute or chronic monarthritis or oligoarthritis suggests mycobacterial or fungal infection; episodic inflammation is seen in syphilis, Lyme disease, and the reactive arthritis that follows enteric infections and chlamydial urethritis. Acute polyarticular inflammation occurs as an immunologic reaction during the course of endocarditis, rheumatic fever, disseminated neisserial infection, and acute hepatitis B. Bacteria and viruses occasionally infect multiple joints, the former most commonly in persons with rheumatoid arthritis.

APPROACH TO THE PATIENT Infectious Arthritis

Aspiration of synovial fluid—an essential element in the evaluation of potentially infected joints—can be performed without difficulty in most cases by the insertion of a large-bore needle into the site of maximal fluctuance or tenderness or by the route of easiest access. Ultrasonography or fluoroscopy may be used to guide aspiration of difficult-to-localize effusions of the hip and, occasionally, the shoulder and other joints. Normal synovial fluid contains <180 cells (predominantly mononuclear cells) per microliter. Synovial cell counts averaging 100,000/μL (range, 25,000–250,000/μL), with >90% neutrophils, are characteristic of acute bacterial infections. Crystal-induced, rheumatoid, and other noninfectious inflammatory arthritides usually are associated with <30,000–50,000 cells/μL; cell counts of 10,000–30,000/μL, with 50–70% neutrophils and the remainder lymphocytes, are common in mycobacterial and fungal infections. Definitive diagnosis of an infectious process relies on identification of the pathogen in stained smears of synovial fluid, isolation of the pathogen from cultures of synovial fluid and blood, or detection of microbial nucleic acids and proteins by nucleic acid amplification (NAA)–based assays and immunologic techniques.

ACUTE BACTERIAL ARTHRITIS

Pathogenesis

Bacteria enter the joint from the bloodstream; from a contiguous site of infection in bone or soft tissue; or by direct inoculation during surgery, injection, animal or human bite, or trauma. In hematogenous infection, bacteria escape from synovial capillaries, which have no limiting basement membrane, and within hours provoke neutrophilic infiltration of the synovium. Neutrophils and bacteria enter the joint space; later, bacteria adhere to articular cartilage. Degradation of cartilage begins within 48 h as a result of increased intraarticular pressure, release of proteases and cytokines from chondrocytes and synovial macrophages, and invasion of the cartilage by bacteria and inflammatory cells. Histologic studies

TABLE 334-1 Differential Diagnosis of Arthritis Syndromes

Acute Monarticular Arthritis	Chronic Monarticular Arthritis	Polyarticular Arthritis
Staphylococcus aureus	*Mycobacterium tuberculosis*	*Neisseria meningitidis*
Streptococcus pneumoniae	Nontuberculous mycobacteria	*N. gonorrhoeae*
β-Hemolytic streptococci	*Borrelia burgdorferi*	Nongonococcal bacterial arthritis
Gram-negative bacilli	*Treponema pallidum*	Bacterial endocarditis
Neisseria gonorrhoeae	*Candida* species	*Candida* species
Candida species	*Sporothrix schenckii*	Poncet's disease (tuberculous rheumatism)
Crystal-induced arthritis	*Coccidioides immitis*	Hepatitis B virus
Fracture	*Blastomyces dermatitidis*	Parvovirus B19
Hemarthrosis	*Aspergillus* species	HIV
Foreign body	*Cryptococcus neoformans*	Human T-lymphotropic virus type I
Osteoarthritis	*Nocardia* species	Rubella virus
Ischemic necrosis	*Brucella* species	Arthropod-borne viruses
Monarticular rheumatoid arthritis	Legg-Calvé-Perthes disease	Sickle cell disease flare
	Osteoarthritis	Reactive arthritis
		Serum sickness
		Acute rheumatic fever
		Inflammatory bowel disease
		Systemic lupus erythematosus
		Rheumatoid arthritis/Still's disease
		Other vasculitides
		Sarcoidosis

reveal bacteria lining the synovium and cartilage as well as abscesses extending into the synovium, cartilage, and—in severe cases—subchondral bone. Synovial proliferation results in the formation of a pannus over the cartilage, and thrombosis of inflamed synovial vessels develops. Bacterial factors that appear important in the pathogenesis of infective arthritis include various surface-associated adhesins in *S. aureus* that permit adherence to cartilage and endotoxins that promote chondrocyte-mediated breakdown of cartilage.

Microbiology

The hematogenous route of infection is the most common route in all age groups, and nearly every bacterial pathogen is capable of causing septic arthritis. In infants, group B streptococci, gram-negative enteric bacilli, and *S. aureus* are the most common pathogens. Since the advent of the *Haemophilus influenzae* vaccine, the predominant causes among children <5 years of age have been *S. aureus*, *Streptococcus pyogenes* (group A *Streptococcus*), and (in some centers) *Kingella kingae*. Among young adults and adolescents, *N. gonorrhoeae* is the most commonly implicated organism. *S. aureus* accounts for most nongonococcal isolates in adults of all ages; gram-negative bacilli, pneumococci, and β-hemolytic streptococci—particularly groups A and B but also groups C, G, and F—are involved in up to one-third of cases in older adults, especially those with underlying comorbid illnesses.

Infections after surgical procedures or penetrating injuries are due most often to *S. aureus* and occasionally to other gram-positive bacteria or gram-negative bacilli. Infections with coagulase-negative staphylococci are unusual except after the implantation of prosthetic joints or arthroscopy. Anaerobic organisms, often in association with aerobic or facultative bacteria, are found after human bites and when decubitus ulcers or intraabdominal abscesses spread into adjacent joints. Polymicrobial infections complicate traumatic injuries with extensive contamination. Bites and scratches from cats and other animals may introduce *Pasteurella multocida* into joints, and bites from humans may introduce *Eikenella corrodens* or other components of the oral flora.

Nongonococcal bacterial arthritis

Epidemiology Although hematogenous infections with virulent organisms such as *S. aureus*, *H. influenzae*, and pyogenic streptococci occur in healthy persons, there is an underlying host predisposition in many cases of septic arthritis. Patients with rheumatoid arthritis have the highest incidence of infective arthritis (most often secondary to *S. aureus*) because of chronically inflamed joints; glucocorticoid therapy; and frequent breakdown of rheumatoid nodules, vasculitic ulcers, and skin overlying deformed joints. Diabetes mellitus, glucocorticoid therapy, hemodialysis, and malignancy all carry an increased risk of infection with *S. aureus* and gram-negative bacilli. Tumor necrosis factor inhibitors (etanercept and infliximab), which increasingly are used for the treatment of rheumatoid arthritis, predispose to mycobacterial infections and possibly to other pyogenic bacterial infections and could be associated with septic arthritis in this population. Pneumococcal infections complicate alcoholism, deficiencies of humoral immunity, and hemoglobinopathies. Pneumococci, *Salmonella* species, and *H. influenzae* cause septic arthritis in persons infected with HIV. Persons with primary immunoglobulin deficiency are at risk for mycoplasmal arthritis, which results in permanent joint damage if tetracycline and replacement therapy with IV immunoglobulin are not administered promptly. IV drug users acquire staphylococcal and streptococcal infections from

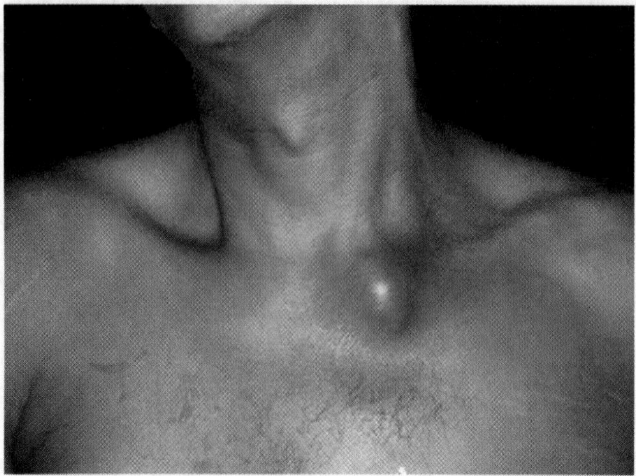

Figure 334-1 Acute septic arthritis of the sternoclavicular joint. A man in his forties with a history of cirrhosis presented with a new onset of fever and lower neck pain. He had no history of IV drug use or previous catheter placement. Jaundice and a painful swollen area over his left sternoclavicular joint were evident on physical examination. Cultures of blood drawn at admission grew group B *Streptococcus.* The patient recovered after treatment with IV penicillin. *(Courtesy of Francisco M. Marty, MD, Brigham and Women's Hospital, Boston; with permission.)*

their own flora and acquire pseudomonal and other gram-negative infections from drugs and injection paraphernalia.

Clinical manifestations Some 90% of patients present with involvement of a single joint—most commonly the knee; less frequently the hip; and still less often the shoulder, wrist, or elbow. Small joints of the hands and feet are more likely to be affected after direct inoculation or a bite. Among IV drug users, infections of the spine, sacroiliac joints, and sternoclavicular joints (Fig. 334-1) are more common than infections of the appendicular skeleton. Polyarticular infection is most common among patients with rheumatoid arthritis and may resemble a flare of the underlying disease.

The usual presentation consists of moderate to severe pain that is uniform around the joint, effusion, muscle spasm, and decreased range of motion. Fever in the range of 38.3°–38.9°C (101°–102°F) and sometimes higher is common but may not be present, especially in persons with rheumatoid arthritis, renal or hepatic insufficiency, or conditions requiring immunosuppressive therapy. The inflamed, swollen joint is usually evident on examination except in the case of a deeply situated joint such as the hip, shoulder, or sacroiliac joint. Cellulitis, bursitis, and acute osteomyelitis, which may produce a similar clinical picture, should be distinguished from septic arthritis by their greater range of motion and less than circumferential swelling. A focus of extraarticular infection such as a boil or pneumonia should be sought. Peripheral-blood leukocytosis with a left shift and elevation of the erythrocyte sedimentation rate or C-reactive protein level are common.

Plain radiographs show evidence of soft tissue swelling, joint-space widening, and displacement of tissue planes by the distended capsule. Narrowing of the joint space and bony erosions indicate advanced infection and a poor prognosis. Ultrasound is useful for detecting effusions in the hip, and CT or MRI can demonstrate infections of the sacroiliac joint, the sternoclavicular joint, and the spine very well.

Laboratory findings Specimens of peripheral blood and synovial fluid should be obtained before antibiotics are administered. Blood cultures are positive in up to 50–70% of *S. aureus* infections but are less frequently positive in infections due to other organisms. The synovial fluid is turbid, serosanguineous, or frankly purulent. Gram-stained smears confirm the presence of large numbers of neutrophils. Levels of total protein and lactate dehydrogenase in synovial fluid are elevated, and the glucose level is depressed; however, these findings are not specific for infection, and measurement of these levels is not necessary for diagnosis. The synovial fluid should be examined for crystals, because gout and pseudogout can resemble septic arthritis clinically, and infection and crystal-induced disease occasionally occur together. Organisms are seen on synovial fluid smears in nearly three-quarters of infections with *S. aureus* and streptococci and in 30–50% of infections due to gram-negative and other bacteria. Cultures of synovial fluid are positive in >90% of cases. Inoculation of synovial fluid into bottles containing liquid media for blood cultures increases the yield of a culture, especially if the pathogen is a fastidious organism or the patient is taking an antibiotic. Although not yet widely available, NAA-based assays for bacterial DNA will be useful for the diagnosis of partially treated or culture-negative bacterial arthritis.

TREATMENT Nongonococcal Bacterial Arthritis

Prompt administration of systemic antibiotics and drainage of the involved joint can prevent destruction of cartilage, postinfectious degenerative arthritis, joint instability, or deformity. Once samples of blood and synovial fluid have been obtained for culture, empirical antibiotics should be given that are directed against the bacteria visualized on smears or the pathogens that are likely in light of the patient's age and risk factors. Initial therapy should consist of IV administration of bactericidal agents; direct instillation of antibiotics into the joint is not necessary to achieve adequate levels in synovial fluid and tissue. An IV third-generation cephalosporin such as cefotaxime (1 g every 8 h) or ceftriaxone (1–2 g every 24 h) provides adequate empirical coverage for most community-acquired infections in adults when smears show no organisms. IV vancomycin (1 g every 12 h) is used if there are gram-positive cocci on the smear. If methicillin-resistant *S. aureus* is an unlikely pathogen (e.g., when it is not widespread in the community), either oxacillin or nafcillin (2 g every 4 h) should be given. In addition, an aminoglycoside or third-generation cephalosporin should be given to IV drug users or other patients in whom *Pseudomonas aeruginosa* may be the responsible agent.

Definitive therapy is based on the identity and antibiotic susceptibility of the bacteria isolated in culture. Infections due to staphylococci are treated with oxacillin, nafcillin, or vancomycin for 4 weeks. Pneumococcal and streptococcal infections due to penicillin-susceptible organisms respond to 2 weeks of therapy with penicillin G (2 million units IV every 4 h); infections caused by *H. influenzae* and by strains of *Streptococcus pneumoniae* that are resistant to penicillin are treated with cefotaxime or ceftriaxone for 2 weeks. Most enteric gram-negative infections can be cured in 3–4 weeks by a second- or third-generation cephalosporin given IV or by a fluoroquinolone such as levofloxacin (500 mg IV or PO every 24 h). *P. aeruginosa* infection should be treated for at least 2 weeks with a combination regimen of an aminoglycoside plus either an extended-spectrum penicillin such as mezlocillin (3 g IV every 4 h) or an antipseudomonal cephalosporin such as ceftazidime (1 g IV every 8 h). If tolerated, this regimen is continued for an additional 2 weeks; alternatively, a fluoroquinolone such as ciprofloxacin (750 mg PO twice daily) is given by itself or with the penicillin or cephalosporin in place of the aminoglycoside.

Timely drainage of pus and necrotic debris from the infected joint is required for a favorable outcome. Needle aspiration of readily accessible joints such as the knee may be adequate if loculations or particulate matter in the joint does not prevent its thorough decompression. Arthroscopic drainage and lavage may be employed initially or within several days if repeated needle aspiration fails to relieve symptoms, decrease the volume of the effusion and the synovial white cell count, and clear bacteria from smears and cultures. In some cases, arthrotomy is necessary to remove loculations and debride infected synovium, cartilage, or bone. Septic arthritis of the hip is best managed with arthrotomy, particularly in young children, in whom infection threatens the viability of the femoral head. Septic joints do not require immobilization except for pain control before symptoms are alleviated by treatment. Weight bearing should be avoided until signs of inflammation have subsided, but frequent passive motion of the joint is indicated to maintain full mobility. Although addition of glucocorticoids to antibiotic treatment improves the outcome of *S. aureus* arthritis in experimental animals, no clinical trials have evaluated this approach in humans.

Gonococcal arthritis

Epidemiology Although its incidence has declined in recent years, gonococcal arthritis (Chap. 144) has accounted for up to 70% of episodes of infectious arthritis in persons <40 years of age in the United States. Arthritis due to *N. gonorrhoeae* is a consequence of bacteremia arising from gonococcal infection or, more frequently, from asymptomatic gonococcal mucosal colonization of the urethra, cervix, or pharynx. Women are at greatest risk during menses and during pregnancy and overall are two to three times more likely than men to develop disseminated gonococcal infection (DGI) and arthritis. Persons with complement deficiencies, especially of the terminal components, are prone to recurrent episodes of gonococcemia. Strains of gonococci that are most likely to cause DGI include those which produce transparent colonies in culture, have the type IA outer-membrane protein, or are of the AUH-auxotroph type.

Clinical manifestations and laboratory findings The most common manifestation of DGI is a syndrome of fever, chills, rash, and articular symptoms. Small numbers of papules that progress to hemorrhagic pustules develop on the trunk and the extensor surfaces of the distal extremities. Migratory arthritis and tenosynovitis of the knees, hands, wrists, feet, and ankles are prominent. The cutaneous lesions and articular findings are believed to be the consequence of an immune reaction to circulating gonococci and immune-complex deposition in tissues. Thus, cultures of synovial fluid are consistently negative, and blood cultures are positive in <45% of patients. Synovial fluid may be difficult to obtain from inflamed joints and usually contains only 10,000–20,000 leukocytes/μL.

True gonococcal septic arthritis is less common than the DGI syndrome and always follows DGI, which is unrecognized in one-third of patients. A single joint such as the hip, knee, ankle, or wrist is usually involved. Synovial fluid, which contains >50,000 leukocytes/μL, can be obtained with ease; the gonococcus is only occasionally evident in gram-stained smears, and cultures of synovial fluid are positive in <40% of cases. Blood cultures are almost always negative.

Because it is difficult to isolate gonococci from synovial fluid and blood, specimens for culture should be obtained from potentially infected mucosal sites. Cultures and gram-stained smears of skin lesions are occasionally positive. All specimens for culture should be plated onto Thayer-Martin agar directly or in special transport media at the bedside and transferred promptly to the microbiology laboratory in an atmosphere of 5% CO_2, as generated in a candle jar. NAA-based assays are extremely sensitive in detecting gonococcal DNA in synovial fluid. A dramatic alleviation of symptoms within 12–24 h after the initiation of appropriate antibiotic therapy supports a clinical diagnosis of the DGI syndrome if cultures are negative.

TREATMENT Gonococcal Arthritis

Initial treatment consists of ceftriaxone (1 g IV or IM every 24 h) to cover possible penicillin-resistant organisms. Once local and systemic signs are clearly resolving and if the sensitivity of the isolate permits, the 7-day course of therapy can be completed with an oral agent such as ciprofloxacin (500 mg twice daily). If penicillin-susceptible organisms are isolated, amoxicillin (500 mg three times daily) may be used. Suppurative arthritis usually responds to needle aspiration of involved joints and 7–14 days of antibiotic treatment. Arthroscopic lavage or arthrotomy is rarely required. Patients with DGI should be treated for *Chlamydia trachomatis* infection unless this infection is ruled out by appropriate testing.

It is noteworthy that arthritis symptoms similar to those seen in DGI occur in meningococcemia. A dermatitis-arthritis syndrome, purulent monarthritis, and reactive polyarthritis have been described. All respond to treatment with IV penicillin.

SPIROCHETAL ARTHRITIS

Lyme disease

Lyme disease (Chap. 173) due to infection with the spirochete *Borrelia burgdorferi* causes arthritis in up to 70% of persons who are not treated. Intermittent arthralgias and myalgias—but not arthritis—occur within days or weeks of inoculation of the spirochete by the *Ixodes* tick. Later, there are three patterns of joint disease: (1) Fifty percent of untreated persons experience intermittent episodes of monarthritis or oligoarthritis involving the knee and/or other large joints. The symptoms wax and wane without treatment over months, and each year 10–20% of patients report loss of joint symptoms. (2) Twenty percent of untreated persons develop a pattern of waxing and waning arthralgias. (3) Ten percent of untreated patients develop chronic inflammatory synovitis that results in erosive lesions and destruction of the joint. Serologic tests for IgG antibodies to *B. burgdorferi* are positive in >90% of persons with Lyme arthritis, and an NAA-based assay detects *Borrelia* DNA in 85%.

TREATMENT Lyme Arthritis

Lyme arthritis generally responds well to therapy. A regimen of oral doxycycline (100 mg twice daily for 30 days), oral amoxicillin (500 mg four times daily for 30 days), or parenteral ceftriaxone (2 g/d for 2–4 weeks) is recommended. Patients who do not respond to a total of 2 months of oral therapy or 1 month of parenteral therapy are unlikely to benefit from additional antibiotic therapy and are treated with anti-inflammatory agents or synovectomy. Failure of therapy is associated with host features such as the human leukocyte antigen DR4 (HLA-DR4) genotype, persistent reactivity to OspA (outer-surface protein A), and the presence of hLFA-1 (human leukocyte function–associated antigen 1), which cross-reacts with OspA.

Syphilitic arthritis

Articular manifestations occur in different stages of syphilis (Chap. 169). In early congenital syphilis, periarticular swelling and immobilization of the involved limbs (Parrot's pseudoparalysis) complicate osteochondritis of long bones. Clutton's joint, a late manifestation of congenital syphilis that typically develops between ages 8 and 15 years, is caused by chronic painless synovitis with effusions of large joints, particularly the knees and elbows. Secondary syphilis may be associated with arthralgias, with symmetric arthritis of the knees and ankles and occasionally of the shoulders and wrists, and with sacroiliitis. The arthritis follows a subacute to chronic course with a mixed mononuclear and neutrophilic synovial-fluid pleocytosis (typical cell counts, 5000–15,000/μL). Immunologic mechanisms may contribute to the arthritis, and symptoms usually improve rapidly with penicillin therapy. In tertiary syphilis, Charcot's joint results from sensory loss due to tabes dorsalis. Penicillin is not helpful in this setting.

MYCOBACTERIAL ARTHRITIS

Tuberculous arthritis (Chap. 165) accounts for ~1% of all cases of tuberculosis and 10% of extrapulmonary cases. The most common presentation is chronic granulomatous monarthritis. An unusual syndrome, Poncet's disease, is a reactive symmetric form of polyarthritis that affects persons with visceral or disseminated tuberculosis. No mycobacteria are found in the joints, and symptoms resolve with antituberculous therapy.

Unlike tuberculous osteomyelitis (Chap. 126), which typically involves the thoracic and lumbar spine (50% of cases), tuberculous arthritis primarily involves the large weight-bearing joints, in particular the hips, knees, and ankles, and only occasionally involves smaller non-weight-bearing joints. Progressive monarticular swelling and pain develop over months or years, and systemic symptoms are seen in only half of all cases. Tuberculous arthritis occurs as part of a disseminated primary infection or through late reactivation, often in persons with HIV infection or other immunocompromised hosts. Coexistent active pulmonary tuberculosis is unusual.

Aspiration of the involved joint yields fluid with an average cell count of 20,000/μL, with ~50% neutrophils. Acid-fast staining of the fluid yields positive results in fewer than one-third of cases, and cultures are positive in 80%. Culture of synovial tissue taken at biopsy is positive in ~90% of cases and shows granulomatous inflammation in most. NAA methods can shorten the time to diagnosis to 1 or 2 days. Radiographs reveal peripheral erosions at the points of synovial attachment, periarticular osteopenia, and eventually joint-space narrowing. Therapy for tuberculous arthritis is the same as that for tuberculous pulmonary disease, requiring the administration of multiple agents for 6–9 months. Therapy is more prolonged in immunosuppressed individuals such as those infected with HIV.

Various atypical mycobacteria (Chap. 167) found in water and soil may cause chronic indolent arthritis. Such disease results from trauma and direct inoculation associated with farming, gardening, or aquatic activities. Smaller joints, such as the digits, wrists, and knees, are usually involved. Involvement of tendon sheaths and bursae is typical. The mycobacterial species involved include *Mycobacterium marinum*, *M. avium-intracellulare*, *M. terrae*, *M. kansasii*, *M. fortuitum*, and *M. chelonae*. In persons who have HIV infection or are receiving immunosuppressive therapy, hematogenous spread to the joints has been reported for *M. kansasii*, *M. avium-intracellulare*, and *M. haemophilum*. Diagnosis usually requires biopsy and culture, and therapy is based on antimicrobial susceptibility patterns.

FUNGAL ARTHRITIS

Fungi are an unusual cause of chronic monarticular arthritis. Granulomatous articular infection with the endemic dimorphic fungi *Coccidioides immitis*, *Blastomyces dermatitidis*, and (less commonly) *Histoplasma capsulatum* (Fig. 334-2) results from hematogenous seeding or direct extension from bony lesions in persons with disseminated disease. Joint involvement is an unusual complication of sporotrichosis (infection with *Sporothrix schenckii*) among gardeners and other persons who work with soil or sphagnum moss. Articular sporotrichosis is six times more common among men than among women, and alcoholics and other debilitated hosts are at risk for polyarticular infection.

Candida infection involving a single joint—usually the knee, hip, or shoulder—results from surgical procedures, intraarticular injections, or (among critically ill patients with debilitating illnesses such as diabetes mellitus or hepatic or renal insufficiency and patients receiving immunosuppressive therapy) hematogenous

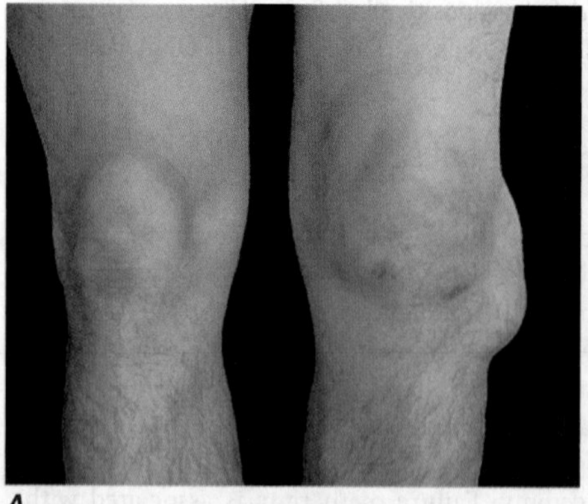
A

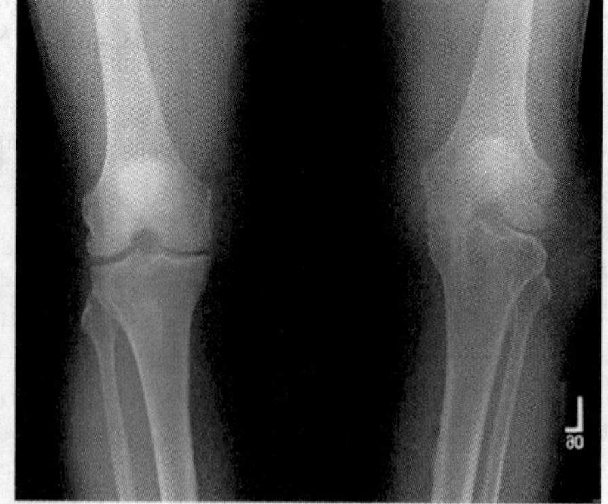
B

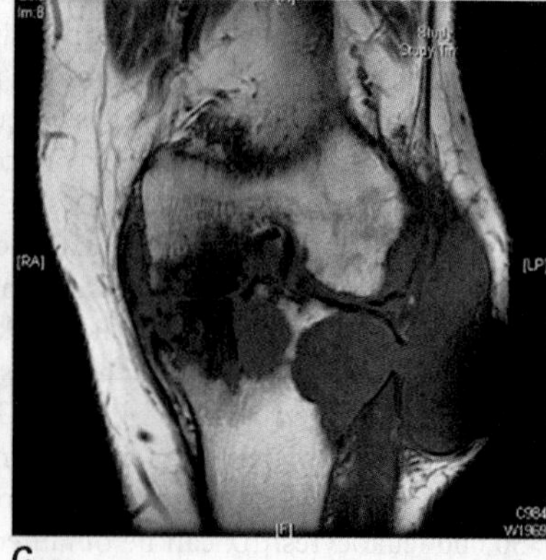

C

Figure 334-2 Chronic arthritis caused by *Histoplasma capsulatum* in the left knee. ***A.*** A man in his sixties from El Salvador presented with a history of progressive knee pain and difficulty walking for several years. He had undergone arthroscopy for a meniscal tear 7 years before presentation (without relief) and had received several intraarticular glucocorticoid injections. The patient developed significant deformity of the knee over time, including a large effusion in the lateral aspect. ***B.*** An x-ray of the knee showed multiple abnormalities, including severe medial femorotibial joint-space narrowing, several large subchondral cysts within the tibia and the patellofemoral compartment, a large suprapatellar joint effusion, and a large soft tissue mass projecting laterally over the knee. ***C.*** MRI further defined these abnormalities and demonstrated the cystic nature of the lateral knee abnormality. Synovial biopsies demonstrated chronic inflammation with giant cells, and cultures grew *H. capsulatum* after 3 weeks of incubation. All clinical cystic lesions and the effusion resolved after 1 year of treatment with itraconazole. The patient underwent a left total knee replacement for definitive treatment. *(Courtesy of Francisco M. Marty, MD, Brigham and Women's Hospital, Boston; with permission.)*

spread. *Candida* infections in IV drug users typically involve the spine, sacroiliac joints, or other fibrocartilaginous joints. Unusual cases of arthritis due to *Aspergillus* species, *Cryptococcus neoformans*, *Pseudallescheria boydii*, and the dematiaceous fungi also have resulted from direct inoculation or disseminated hematogenous infection in immunocompromised persons.

The synovial fluid in fungal arthritis usually contains 10,000–40,000 cells/μL, with ~70% neutrophils. Stained specimens and cultures of synovial tissue often confirm the diagnosis of fungal arthritis when studies of synovial fluid give negative results. Treatment consists of drainage and lavage of the joint and systemic administration of an antifungal agent directed at a specific pathogen. The doses and duration of therapy are the same as for disseminated disease (see Part 8, Section 16). Intraarticular instillation of amphotericin B has been used in addition to IV therapy.

VIRAL ARTHRITIS

Viruses produce arthritis by infecting synovial tissue during systemic infection or by provoking an immunologic reaction that involves joints. As many as 50% of women report persistent arthralgias, and 10% report frank arthritis within 3 days of the rash that follows natural infection with rubella virus and within 2–6 weeks after receipt of live-virus vaccine. Episodes of symmetric inflammation of fingers, wrists, and knees uncommonly recur for >1 year, but a syndrome of chronic fatigue, low-grade fever, headaches, and myalgias can persist for months or years. IV immunoglobulin has been helpful in selected cases. Self-limited monarticular or migratory polyarthritis may develop within 2 weeks of the parotitis of mumps; this sequela is more common among men than among women. Approximately 10% of children and 60% of women develop arthritis after infection with parvovirus B19. In adults, arthropathy sometimes occurs without fever or rash. Pain and stiffness, with less prominent swelling (primarily of the hands but also of the knees, wrists, and ankles), usually resolve within weeks, although a small proportion of patients develop chronic arthropathy.

About 2 weeks before the onset of jaundice, up to 10% of persons with acute hepatitis B develop an immune complex–mediated, serum sickness–like reaction with maculopapular rash, urticaria, fever, and arthralgias. Less common developments include symmetric arthritis involving the hands, wrists, elbows, or ankles and morning stiffness that resembles a flare of rheumatoid arthritis. Symptoms resolve at the time jaundice develops. Many persons with chronic hepatitis C infection report persistent arthralgia or arthritis, both in the presence and in the absence of cryoglobulinemia.

Painful arthritis involving larger joints often accompanies the fever and rash of several arthropod-borne viral infections, including those caused by chikungunya, O'nyong-nyong, Ross River, Mayaro, and Barmah Forest viruses (Chap. 196). Symmetric arthritis involving the hands and wrists may occur during the convalescent phase of infection with lymphocytic choriomeningitis virus. Patients infected with an enterovirus frequently report arthralgias, and echovirus has been isolated from patients with acute polyarthritis.

Several arthritis syndromes are associated with HIV infection. Reactive arthritis (Reiter's syndrome) with painful lower-extremity oligoarthritis often follows an episode of urethritis in HIV-infected persons. HIV-associated reactive arthritis appears to be extremely common among persons with the HLA-B27 haplotype, but sacroiliac joint disease is unusual and is seen mostly in the absence of HLA-B27. Up to one-third of HIV-infected persons with psoriasis develop psoriatic arthritis. Painless monarthropathy and persistent symmetric polyarthropathy occasionally complicate HIV infection. Chronic persistent oligoarthritis of the shoulders, wrists, hands, and knees occurs in women infected with human T cell lymphotropic virus type I. Synovial thickening, destruction of articular cartilage, and leukemic-appearing atypical lymphocytes in synovial fluid are characteristic, but progression to T cell leukemia is unusual.

PARASITIC ARTHRITIS

Arthritis due to parasitic infection is rare. The guinea worm *Dracunculus medinensis* may cause destructive joint lesions in the lower extremities as migrating gravid female worms invade joints or cause ulcers in adjacent soft tissues that become secondarily infected. Hydatid cysts infect bones in 1–2% of cases of infection with *Echinococcus granulosus*. The expanding destructive cystic lesions may spread to and destroy adjacent joints, particularly the hip and pelvis. In rare cases, chronic synovitis has been associated with the presence of schistosomal eggs in synovial biopsies. Monarticular arthritis in children with lymphatic filariasis appears to respond to therapy with diethylcarbamazine even in the absence of microfilariae in synovial fluid. Reactive arthritis has been attributed to hookworm, *Strongyloides*, *Cryptosporidium*, and *Giardia* infection in case reports, but confirmation is required.

POSTINFECTIOUS OR REACTIVE ARTHRITIS

Reactive polyarthritis develops several weeks after ~1% of cases of nongonococcal urethritis and 2% of enteric infections, particularly those due to *Yersinia enterocolitica*, *Shigella flexneri*, *Campylobacter jejuni*, and *Salmonella* species. Only a minority of these patients have the other findings of classic reactive arthritis, including urethritis, conjunctivitis, uveitis, oral ulcers, and rash. Studies have identified microbial DNA or antigen in synovial fluid or blood, but the pathogenesis of this condition is poorly understood.

Reactive arthritis is most common among young men (except after *Yersinia* infection) and has been linked to the HLA-B27 locus as a potential genetic predisposing factor. Patients report painful, asymmetric oligoarthritis that affects mainly the knees, ankles, and feet. Low-back pain is common, and radiographic evidence of sacroiliitis is found in patients with long-standing disease. Most patients recover within 6 months, but prolonged recurrent disease is more common in cases that follow chlamydial urethritis. Antiinflammatory agents help relieve symptoms, but the role of prolonged antibiotic therapy in eliminating microbial antigen from the synovium is controversial.

Migratory polyarthritis and fever constitute the usual presentation of acute rheumatic fever in adults (Chap. 322). This presentation is distinct from that of poststreptococcal reactive arthritis, which also follows infections with group A *Streptococcus* but is not migratory, lasts beyond the typical 3-week maximum of acute rheumatic fever, and responds poorly to aspirin.

INFECTIONS IN PROSTHETIC JOINTS

Infection complicates 1–4% of total joint replacements. The majority of infections are acquired intraoperatively or immediately postoperatively as a result of wound breakdown or infection; less commonly, these joint infections develop later after joint replacement and are the result of hematogenous spread or direct inoculation. The presentation may be acute, with fever, pain, and local signs of inflammation, especially in infections due to *S. aureus*, pyogenic streptococci, and enteric bacilli. Alternatively, infection may persist for months or years without causing constitutional symptoms when less virulent organisms, such as coagulase-negative staphylococci or diphtheroids, are involved. Such indolent infections usually are acquired during joint implantation and are discovered during evaluation of chronic unexplained pain or after a radiograph shows loosening of the prosthesis; the erythrocyte sedimentation rate and C-reactive protein level are usually elevated in such cases.

The diagnosis is best made by needle aspiration of the joint; accidental introduction of organisms during aspiration must be avoided meticulously. Synovial fluid pleocytosis with a predominance of polymorphonuclear leukocytes is highly suggestive of infection, since other inflammatory processes uncommonly affect prosthetic joints. Culture and Gram's stain usually yield the responsible pathogen. Sonication of explanted prosthetic material can improve the yield of culture, presumably by breaking up bacterial biofilms on the surfaces of prostheses. Use of special media for unusual pathogens such as fungi, atypical mycobacteria, and *Mycoplasma* may be necessary if routine and anaerobic cultures are negative.

TREATMENT Prosthetic Joint Infections

Treatment includes surgery and high doses of parenteral antibiotics, which are given for 4–6 weeks because bone is usually involved. In most cases, the prosthesis must be replaced to cure the infection. Implantation of a new prosthesis is best delayed for several weeks or months because relapses of infection occur most commonly within this time frame. In some cases, reimplantation is not possible, and the patient must manage without a joint, with a fused joint, or even with amputation. Cure of infection without removal of the prosthesis is occasionally possible in cases that are due to streptococci or pneumococci and that lack radiologic evidence of loosening of the prosthesis. In these cases, antibiotic therapy must be initiated within several days of the onset of infection, and the joint should be drained vigorously by open arthrotomy or arthroscopically. In selected patients who prefer to avoid the high morbidity rate associated with joint removal and reimplantation, suppression of the infection with antibiotics may be a reasonable goal. A high cure rate with retention of the prosthesis has been reported when the combination of oral rifampin and ciprofloxacin is given for 3–6 months to persons with staphylococcal prosthetic joint infection of short duration. This approach, which is based on the ability of rifampin to kill organisms adherent to foreign material and in the stationary growth phase, requires confirmation in prospective trials.

Prevention

To avoid the disastrous consequences of infection, candidates for joint replacement should be selected with care. Rates of infection are particularly high among patients with rheumatoid arthritis, persons who have undergone previous surgery on the joint, and persons with medical conditions requiring immunosuppressive therapy. Perioperative antibiotic prophylaxis, usually with cefazolin, and measures to decrease intraoperative contamination, such as laminar flow, have lowered the rates of perioperative infection to <1% in many centers. After implantation, measures should be taken to prevent or rapidly treat extraarticular infections that might give rise to hematogenous spread to the prosthesis. The effectiveness of prophylactic antibiotics for the prevention of hematogenous infection after dental procedures has not been demonstrated; in fact, viridans streptococci and other components of the oral flora are extremely unusual causes of prosthetic joint infection. Accordingly, the American Dental Association and the American Academy of Orthopaedic Surgeons do not recommend antibiotic prophylaxis for most dental patients with total joint replacements. They do, however, recommend prophylaxis for patients who may be at high risk of hematogenous infection, including those with inflammatory arthropathies, immunosuppression, type 1 diabetes mellitus, joint replacement within the preceding 2 years, previous prosthetic joint infection, malnourishment, or hemophilia. The recommended regimen is amoxicillin (2 g PO) 1 h before dental procedures associated with a high incidence of bacteremia. Clindamycin (600 mg PO) is suggested for patients allergic to penicillin.

ACKNOWLEDGMENTS

The contributions of James H. Maguire and the late Scott J. Thaler to this chapter in earlier editions are gratefully acknowledged.

FURTHER READINGS

Bardin T: Gonococcal arthritis. Best Pract Res Clin Rheumatol 17:201, 2003

Franssila R, Hedman K: Infection and musculoskeletal conditions: Viral causes of arthritis. Best Pract Res Clin Rheumatol 20:1139, 2006

Harrington JT: Mycobacterial and fungal arthritis. Curr Opin Rheumatol 10:335, 1998

Mathews CJ et al: Bacterial septic arthritis in adults. Lancet 375:846, 2010

Medina Rodriguez F: Rheumatic manifestations of human immunodeficiency virus infection. Rheum Dis Clin North Am 29:145, 2003

Meehan AM et al: Outcome of penicillin-susceptible streptococcal prosthetic joint infection treated with debridement and retention of the prosthesis. Clin Infect Dis 36:845, 2003

Moyad TF et al: Evaluation and management of the infected total hip and knee. Orthopedics 31:589, 2008

Shirtliff ME, Mader JT: Acute septic arthritis. Clin Microbiol Rev 15:527, 2002

Stengel D et al: Systematic review and meta-analysis of antibiotic therapy for bone and joint infections. Lancet Infect Dis 1:175, 2001

Tarkowski A: Infection and musculoskeletal conditions: Infectious arthritis. Best Pract Res Clin Rheumatol 20:1029, 2006

Trampuz A et al: Sonication of removed hip and knee prostheses for diagnosis of infection. N Engl J Med 357:654, 2007

Zimmerli W et al: Prosthetic-joint infections. N Engl J Med 351:145, 2004

CHAPTER 335

Fibromyalgia

Leslie J. Crofford

DEFINITION

Fibromyalgia (FM) is characterized by chronic widespread musculoskeletal pain and tenderness. Although it is defined primarily as a pain syndrome, FM patients also commonly complain of associated neuropsychological symptoms of fatigue, unrefreshing sleep, cognitive dysfunction, anxiety, and depression. Patients with FM have an increased prevalence of other syndromes associated with pain and fatigue, including chronic fatigue syndrome (Chap. 389), temporomandibular disorder, chronic headaches, irritable bowel syndrome, interstitial cystitis/painful bladder syndrome, and other pelvic pain syndromes. Available evidence implicates the central nervous system as key to maintaining pain and other core symptoms of FM and related conditions. The presence of FM is associated with substantial negative consequences for physical and social functioning.

EPIDEMIOLOGY

FM is far more common in women than in men, with a ratio of about 9:1. In population-based studies worldwide, there is general agreement that the prevalence rate is approximately 2–3%, with rates of closer to 5–10% in primary care practices. The prevalence data are similar across socioeconomic classes. Cultural factors may play a role in determining whether patients with FM symptoms seek medical attention; however, even in cultures in which secondary gain is not expected to play a significant role, the prevalence of FM remains in this range.

CLINICAL MANIFESTATIONS

Pain and tenderness

The most common presenting complaint of a patient with FM is "pain all over." Patients with FM have pain that is typically above and below the waist on both sides of the body and involves the axial skeleton (neck, back, or chest). The pain attributable to FM is poorly localized, difficult to ignore, severe in its intensity, and associated with a reduced functional capacity. Pain should have been present most of the day on most days for at least 3 months.

The clinical pain of FM is associated with increased evoked pain sensitivity. In clinical practice, this is determined by a tender point examination in which the examiner uses the thumbnail to exert pressure of approximately 4 kg/m², or the pressure leading to blanching of the tip of the thumbnail, on well-defined musculotendinous sites (Fig. 335-1). American College of Rheumatology classification criteria previously required that 11 of 18 sites be perceived as painful for a diagnosis of FM. In practice, tenderness is a continuous variable, and strict application of a categorical threshold for diagnosis specifics is no longer necessary. Increased pain sensitivity can be demonstrated not only for the mechanical pressure-induced pain used in the clinic but also for nonmuscular mechanical pressure, heat, cold, and other sensory stimuli; this reinforces the idea that the pathogenic mechanisms of FM are not related to specific musculoskeletal pathology but to altered pain processing. New criteria eliminate tender points and focus on clinical symptoms of widespread pain and neuropsychological symptoms.

Patients with FM often have peripheral pain generators that are thought to serve as triggers for the more widespread pain attributed to central nervous system factors. Potential pain generators such

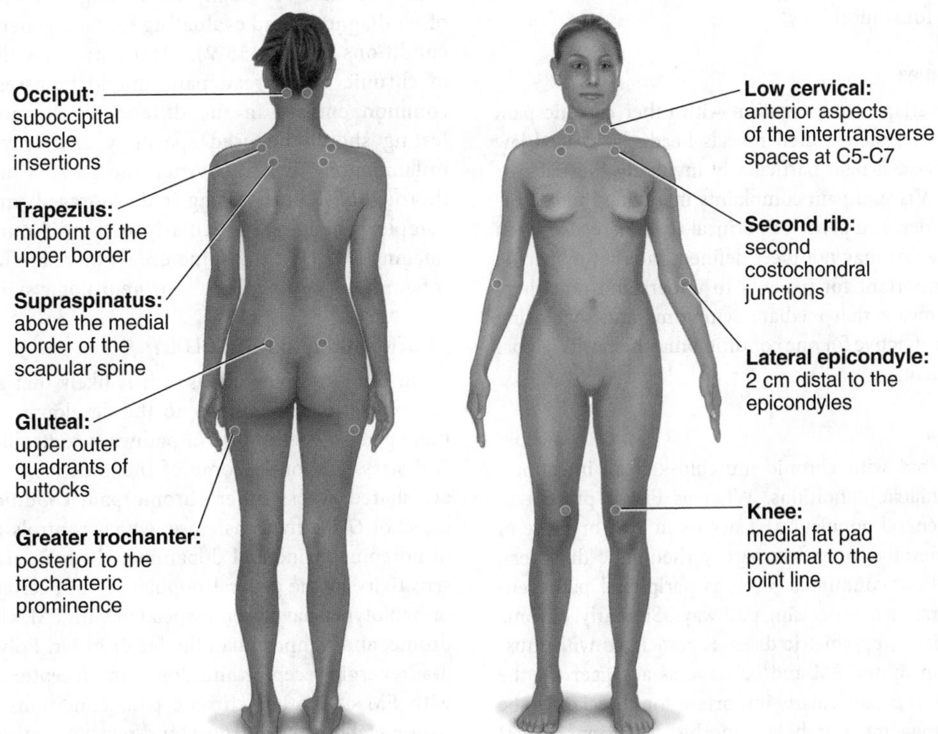

Figure 335-1 Tender point assessment in patients with fibromyalgia.

as arthritis, bursitis, tendinitis, neuropathies, and other inflammatory or degenerative conditions should be identified by history and physical examination. More subtle pain generators may include joint hypermobility and scoliosis. Patients also may have chronic myalgias triggered by infectious, metabolic, or psychiatric conditions that can serve as triggers for the development of FM. These conditions are often in the differential diagnosis of patients with FM, and a major challenge is to distinguish the ongoing activity of a triggering condition from FM as a consequence of a comorbid condition that should itself be treated.

Neuropsychological symptoms

In addition to widespread pain, FM patients typically complain of fatigue, stiffness, sleep disturbance, cognitive dysfunction, anxiety, and depression. These symptoms are present to varying degrees in most FM patients but are not present in every patient or at all times. Such symptoms may, however, have an equal or even greater impact on function and quality of life. Fatigue is highly prevalent in patients under primary care who ultimately are diagnosed with FM. Pain, stiffness, and fatigue often are worsened by exercise or unaccustomed activity (postexertional malaise). The sleep complaints include difficulty falling asleep, difficulty staying asleep, and early-morning awakening. Regardless of the specific complaint, patients awake feeling unrefreshed. Patients with FM may meet criteria for restless legs syndrome and sleep-disordered breathing; frank sleep apnea can also be present. Cognitive complaints are characterized as slowness in processing, difficulties with attention or concentration, problems with word retrieval, and short-term memory loss. Studies have demonstrated altered cognitive function in these domains in patients with FM, though speed of processing is age-appropriate. Symptoms of anxiety and depression are common, and the lifetime prevalence of mood disorders in patients with FM approaches 80%. Although depression is neither necessary nor sufficient for the diagnosis of FM, it is important to screen for major depressive disorders by querying for depressed mood and anhedonia. Analysis of genetic factors that are likely to predispose to FM reveals shared neurobiologic pathways with mood disorders, providing the basis for comorbidity.

Overlapping syndromes

Because FM can overlap in presentation with other chronic pain conditions, review of systems often reveals headaches, facial/jaw pain, regional myofascial pain particularly involving the neck or back, and arthritis. Visceral pain complaints involving the gastrointestinal tract, bladder, and pelvic or perineal region are also often present. Patients may or may not meet defined criteria for specific syndromes. It is important for patients to understand that there may be shared pathways that mediate symptoms and that using treatment strategies effective for one condition may help with global symptom management.

Comorbid conditions

FM is often comorbid with chronic musculoskeletal, infectious, metabolic, or psychiatric conditions. Whereas FM is present in only 2–5% of the general population, it occurs in 20% or more of patients with degenerative or inflammatory rheumatic disorders, probably because these conditions serve as peripheral pain generators to alter central pain-processing pathways. Similarly, chronic infectious, metabolic, or psychiatric diseases associated with musculoskeletal pain can mimic FM and/or serve as a trigger for the development of FM. It is particularly important for clinicians to be sensitive to pain management of these comorbid conditions so that when FM emerges, as characterized by pain outside the boundaries of what could reasonably be explained by the triggering condition, development of neuropsychological symptoms, or tenderness on physical examination, treatment of central pain processes will be undertaken rather than continuing to focus on treating peripheral or inflammatory causes of pain.

Psychosocial considerations

Symptoms of FM often have their onset and are exacerbated during periods of high levels of real or perceived stress. This may reflect an interaction between central stress physiology, vigilance or anxiety, and central pain-processing pathways. Understanding current psychosocial stressors will aid in patient management as many factors that exacerbate symptoms cannot be addressed by using pharmacologic approaches. Furthermore, there is a high prevalence of exposure to previous interpersonal and other forms of violence in patients with FM and related conditions. If posttraumatic stress disorder is an issue, the clinician should be aware of it and consider treatment options.

Functional impairment

It is crucial to evaluate the impact of FM symptoms on function and role fulfillment. In defining the success of a management strategy, improved function is a key measure. Functional assessment should include physical, mental, and social domains. Understanding where role functioning falls short will assist in establishing treatment goals.

DIFFERENTIAL DIAGNOSIS

Because musculoskeletal pain is such a common complaint, the differential diagnosis of FM is broad. Table 335-1 lists some of the more common conditions that should be considered. Patients with inflammatory causes for widespread pain should be identifiable on the basis of specific history, physical findings, and laboratory or radiographic tests.

LABORATORY OR RADIOGRAPHIC TESTING

Routine laboratory and radiographic tests are normal in patients with FM, and so diagnostic testing is focused on excluding other diagnoses and evaluating for pain generators or comorbid conditions (Table 335-2). Most patients with a new complaint of chronic widespread pain should be assessed for the most common entities in the differential diagnosis. Radiographic testing should be used sparingly and only for diagnosis of inflammatory arthritis. After the patient has been evaluated thoroughly, repeat testing is discouraged unless the symptom complex changes. Particularly to be discouraged is advanced imaging (MRI) of the spine unless there are features suggesting inflammatory spine disease or neurologic symptoms.

GENETICS AND PHYSIOLOGY

As in most complex diseases, it is likely that a number of genes contribute to vulnerability to the development of FM. To date, these genes appear to be in pathways controlling pain sensitivity and stress response. Some of the genetic underpinnings of FM are shared across other chronic pain conditions. For example, catechol-*O*-methyltransferase, which controls the synaptic levels of norepinephrine and dopamine, has been associated with pain sensitivity in the general population and certain polymorphisms or haplotypes have been associated with FM, chronic fatigue syndrome, and temporomandibular disorder. Polymorphisms of the β-adrenergic receptor and dopamine receptor are also associated with FM and other chronic pain conditions. Genes associated with metabolism, transport, and receptors of serotonin and other monoamines have also been implicated in FM and overlapping conditions. Taken together, the pathways in which polymorphisms

TABLE 335-1 Common Conditions in the Differential Diagnosis of Fibromyalgia

Inflammatory
Polymyalgia rheumatica
Inflammatory arthritis: rheumatoid arthritis, spondyloarthritides
Connective tissues diseases: systemic lupus erythematosus, Sjögren's syndrome
Infectious
Hepatitis C
Human immunodeficiency virus (HIV)
Lyme disease
Parvovirus B19
Epstein-Barr virus
Noninflammatory
Degenerative joint/spine/disk disease
Myofascial pain syndromes
Bursitis, tendinitis, repetitive strain injuries
Endocrine
Hypo- or hyperthyroidism
Hyperparathyroidism
Neurologic diseases
Multiple sclerosis
Neuropathic pain syndromes
Psychiatric disease
Major depressive disorder
Drugs
Statins
Aromatase inhibitors

TABLE 335-2 Laboratory and Radiographic Testing in Patients With Fibromyalgia Symptoms

Routine
Erythrocyte sedimentation rate (ESR) and C-reactive protein (CRP)
Complete blood count (CBC)
Complete metabolic panel
Thyroid-stimulating hormone (TSH)
Guided by history and physical examination
Antinuclear antibody (ANA)
Anti-SSA (anti-Sjögren's syndrome A) and anti-SSB
Rheumatoid factor and anticyclic citrullinated peptide (anti-CCP)
Creatine phosphokinase (CPK)
Viral and bacterial serologies
Spine and joint radiographs

have been identified in FM patients further implicate central factors as mediating the physiology that leads to FM clinical manifestations.

Psychophysical testing of patients with FM has demonstrated altered sensory afferent pain processing and impaired descending noxious inhibitory control leading to hyperalgesia and allodynia. Functional MRI and other research imaging procedures clearly demonstrate activation of the brain regions involved in the experience of pain in response to stimuli that are innocuous in study participants without FM. Pain perception in FM patients is influenced by the emotional and cognitive dimensions, such as catastrophizing and perceptions of control, providing a solid basis for recommendations for cognitive and behavioral treatment strategies.

APPROACH TO THE PATIENT Fibromyalgia

FM occurs commonly and has an extraordinary impact on functioning and health-related quality of life; however, symptoms and impact can be managed effectively by physicians and other health professionals. Developing a partnership with patients with a goal of understanding and implementing a treatment strategy and choosing appropriate nonpharmacologic and pharmacologic treatments are essential for improving the outcome of FM.

TREATMENT Fibromyalgia

NONPHARMACOLOGIC TREATMENT Patients with chronic pain, fatigue, and other neuropsychological symptoms require a framework for understanding the symptoms that have such an important impact on their function and quality of life. Providing explanation of the genetics, triggers, and physiology of FM can be an important adjunct in relieving the associated anxiety as well as reducing the overall cost of health care resources. In addition, patients must be educated regarding the expectations for treatment. The physician should focus on improved function and quality of life rather than elimination of pain. Illness behaviors should be discouraged, and behaviors that focus on improved function strongly encouraged.

Treatment strategies should include physical conditioning, with encouragement to begin at low levels of aerobic exercise with slow but consistent advancement. Patients who have been physically inactive or who report postexertional malaise may do best in supervised or water-based programs to start. Treatments that incorporate improved physical function with relaxation, such as yoga and Tai Chi, may also be helpful. Strength training may be recommended after a patient has reached his or her aerobic goals. Exercise programs are helpful for reductions in tenderness and for enhanced self-efficacy. Cognitive-behavioral strategies to improve sleep hygiene and reduce illness behaviors can also be helpful in management.

PHARMACOLOGIC APPROACHES It is essential for the clinician to treat any comorbid triggering condition and clearly delineate for the patient the treatment goals for each medication. For example, glucocorticoids or nonsteroidal anti-inflammatory drugs may be useful for management of inflammatory triggers but are not effective for FM-related symptoms. At present, the treatment approaches that have proved most successful in FM patients target afferent or descending pain pathways. Table 335-3 outlines the drugs with demonstrated effectiveness. It should be

TABLE 335-3 Pharmacologic Agents Effective for Treatment of Fibromyalgia

Antidepressants: balanced serotonin:norepinephrine reuptake inhibition
Amitryptiline
Duloxetine[a]
Milnacipran[a]
Anticonvulsants: ligands of the alpha-2-delta subunit of voltage-gated calcium channels
Gabapentin
Pregabalin[a]

[a]Approved for fibromyalgia by the U.S. Food and Drug Administration.

emphasized strongly that opioid analgesics are to be avoided in patients with FM. These agents have no demonstrated efficacy in FM and are associated with opioid-induced hyperalgesia that can worsen both symptoms and function. Utilization of single agents to treat multiple symptom domains is strongly encouraged. For example, if a patient's symptom complex is dominated by pain and sleep disturbance, using an agent that exerts both analgesic and sleep-promoting effects is desirable. These agents include sedating antidepressants such as amitriptyline or alpha-2-delta ligands such as gabapentin and pregabalin. For patients with pain associated with fatigue, anxiety, or depression, drugs that have both analgesic and antidepressant/anxiolytic effects, such as duloxetine or milnacipran, may be the best first choice.

FURTHER READINGS

Annemans L et al: Health economic consequences related to the diagnosis of fibromyalgia syndrome. Arthritis Rheum 58:895, 2008

Arnold LM: New therapies in fibromyalgia. Arthritis Res Ther 8:212, 2006

Boomershine CS, Crofford LJ: A symptom-based approach to pharmacologic management of fibromyalgia. Nat Rev Rheumatol 5:191, 2009

Busch AJ et al: Exercise for fibromyalgia: A systematic review. J Rheumatol 35:1130, 2008

Wolfe F et al: The American College of Rheumatology preliminary diagnostic criteria for fibromyalgia and measurement of symptom severity. Arthritis Care Res 62:600, 2010

Williams DA, Clauw DJ: Understanding fibromyalgia: Lessons from the broader pain research community. J Pain 10:777, 2009

CHAPTER 336 Arthritis Associated With Systemic Disease, and Other Arthritides

Carol A. Langford

Brian F. Mandell

ARTHRITIS ASSOCIATED WITH SYSTEMIC DISEASE

ARTHROPATHY OF ACROMEGALY

Acromegaly is the result of excessive production of growth hormone by an adenoma in the anterior pituitary gland (Chap. 339). The excessive secretion of growth hormone along with insulin-like growth factor I stimulates proliferation of cartilage, periarticular connective tissue, and bone, resulting in several musculoskeletal problems, including osteoarthritis, back pain, muscle weakness, and carpal tunnel syndrome.

Osteoarthritis is a common feature, most often affecting the knees, shoulders, hips, and hands. Single or multiple joints may be affected. Hypertrophy of cartilage initially produces radiographic widening of the joint space. The newly synthesized cartilage is abnormally susceptible to fissuring, ulceration, and destruction. Ligamental laxity of joints further contributes to the development of osteoarthritis. Cartilage degrades, the joint space narrows, and subchondral sclerosis and osteophytes develop. Joint examination reveals crepitus and laxity. Joint fluid is noninflammatory. Calcium pyrophosphate dihydrate crystals are found in the cartilage in some cases of acromegaly arthropathy and, when shed into the joint, these can elicit attacks of pseudogout. Chondrocalcinosis may be observed on radiographs. Back pain is extremely common, perhaps as a result of spine hypermobility. Spine radiographs show normal or widened intervertebral disk spaces, hypertrophic anterior osteophytes, and ligamental calcification. These changes are similar to those observed in patients with diffuse idiopathic skeletal hyperostosis. Dorsal kyphosis in conjunction with elongation of the ribs contributes to the development of the barrel chest seen in acromegalic patients. The hands and feet become enlarged, owing to soft tissue proliferation. The fingers are thickened and have spadelike distal tufts. One-third of patients have a thickened heel pad. Approximately 25% of patients have Raynaud's phenomenon. Carpal tunnel syndrome occurs in about half of patients. The median nerve is compressed by excess connective tissue in the carpal tunnel. Patients with acromegaly could develop proximal muscle weakness, which is thought to be caused by the effect of growth hormone on muscle. Serum muscle enzyme levels and electromyography are normal. Muscle biopsy specimens show muscle fibers of varying size but with no inflammation.

ARTHROPATHY OF HEMOCHROMATOSIS

Hemochromatosis is a disorder of iron storage. Excessive amounts of iron are absorbed from the intestine, leading to iron deposition in parenchymal cells, which results in impairment of organ function (Chap. 357). Symptoms of hemochromatosis usually begin between the ages of 40 and 60 but can occur earlier. Arthropathy, which occurs in 20–40% of patients, usually begins after the age of 50 and may be the first clinical feature of hemochromatosis. The arthropathy is an osteoarthritis-like disorder affecting the small joints of the hands, followed later by larger joints such as knees, ankles, shoulders, and hips. The second and third metacarpophalangeal joints of both hands are often the first and prominent joints affected; this may provide an important clue to the possibility of hemochromatosis because these joints are not predominantly affected by "routine" osteoarthritis. Patients experience some morning stiffness and pain with use of involved joints. The affected joints are enlarged and mildly tender. Radiographs show narrowing of the joint space, subchondral sclerosis, subchondral cysts, and juxtaarticular proliferation of bone with frequent hooklike osteophytes. The synovial fluid is noninflammatory. The synovium shows mild to moderate proliferation of iron containing lining cells, fibrosis, and some mononuclear cell infiltration. In approximately half of patients, there is evidence of calcium pyrophosphate deposition disease (CPPD), and some patients experience episodes of acute pseudogout.

Iron may damage the articular cartilage in several ways. Iron catalyzes superoxide-dependent lipid peroxidation, which may play a role in joint damage. In animal models, ferric iron has been shown to interfere with collagen formation and increase the release of lysosomal enzymes from cells in the synovial membrane. Iron inhibits synovial tissue pyrophosphatase in vitro and, therefore, may inhibit pyrophosphatase in vivo, resulting in chondrocalcinosis.

TREATMENT Arthropathy of Hemochromatosis

The treatment of hemochromatosis is repeated phlebotomy. Unfortunately, this treatment has little effect on established arthritis, which, along with chondrocalcinosis, may progress. Symptomatic treatment of the arthritis consists of administration of acetaminophen and nonsteroidal anti-inflammatory drugs (NSAIDs), as tolerated. Acute pseudogout attacks are treated with high doses of an NSAID or a short course of glucocorticoids. Hip or knee total joint replacement has been successful in advanced disease.

HEMOPHILIC ARTHROPATHY

Hemophilia is a sex-linked recessive genetic disorder characterized by the absence or deficiency of factor VIII (hemophilia A, or classic hemophilia) or factor IX (hemophilia B, or Christmas disease) (Chap. 116). Hemophilia A constitutes 85% of cases. Spontaneous hemarthrosis is a common problem with both types of hemophilia and can lead to a deforming arthritis. The frequency and severity of hemarthrosis are related to the degree of clotting factor deficiency. Hemarthrosis is not common in other disorders of coagulation such as von Willebrand disease, factor V deficiency, warfarin therapy, or thrombocytopenia.

Hemarthrosis occurs after one year of age, when the child begins to walk and run. In order of frequency, the joints most commonly affected are the knees, ankles, elbows, shoulders, and hips. Small joints of the hands and feet are occasionally involved.

In the initial stage of arthropathy, hemarthrosis produces a warm, tensely swollen, and painful joint. The patient holds the affected joint in flexion and guards against any movement. Blood in the joint remains liquid because of the absence of intrinsic clotting factors and the absence of tissue thromboplastin in the synovium. The synovial blood is resorbed over a period of a week or longer, depending on the size of the hemarthrosis. Joint function usually returns to normal or baseline in about two weeks. Low-grade temperature elevation may accompany hemarthrosis, but a fever >101 warrants concern for infection.

Recurrent hemarthrosis may result in chronic arthritis. The involved joints remain swollen, and flexion deformities develop. Joint motion may be restricted and function severely limited. Restricted joint motion, or laxity with subluxation, are features of end-stage disease.

Bleeding into muscle and soft tissue also causes musculoskeletal dysfunction. When bleeding into the iliopsoas muscle occurs, the hip is held in flexion because of the pain, resulting in a hip flexion contracture. Rotation of the hip is preserved, which distinguishes this problem from hemarthrosis or other causes of hip synovitis. Expansion of the hematoma may place pressure on the femoral nerve, resulting in a femoral neuropathy. Hemorrhage into a closed compartment space, such as the calf or volar compartment in the forearm, can result in muscle necrosis, neuropathy, and flexion deformities of the ankles, wrists, and fingers. When bleeding involves periosteum or bone, a painful pseudotumor forms. These occur distal to the elbows or knees in children and improve with treatment of the hemophilia. Surgical removal is indicated if the pseudotumor continues to enlarge. In adults, pseudotumors occur in the femur and pelvis and are usually refractory to treatment. When bleeding occurs in muscle, cysts may develop within the muscle. Needle aspiration of a cyst is contraindicated because it can induce further bleeding; however, if they become secondarily infected, drainage may be necessary (after factor repletion).

Septic arthritis rarely occurs in hemophilia and is difficult to distinguish from acute hemarthrosis on physical examination. If there is serious suspicion of an infected joint, the joint should be aspirated immediately, the fluid cultured, and the patient started on antibiotics that provide broad coverage, including *staphylococcus*, until the results of the culture return. Clotting-factor deficiency should be corrected before arthrocentesis to minimize the risk of traumatic bleeding.

Radiographs of joints reflect the stage of disease. In early stages, there is only capsule distention; later, juxtaarticular osteopenia, marginal erosions, and subchondral cysts develop. Late in the disease, the joint space is narrowed and there is bony overgrowth similar to osteoarthritis.

TREATMENT Hemarthrosis

The treatment of musculoskeletal bleeding is initiated with the immediate infusion of factor VIII or IX at the first sign of joint or muscle hemorrhage. Patients who have developed factor inhibitors are at greater risk for joint damage and may benefit from receiving recombinant activated factor VII or activated prothrombin complex concentrate. The joint should be rested in a position of forced extension, as tolerated, to avoid contracture. Analgesia should be provided; ideally, the nonselective NSAIDs, which can diminish platelet function, should be avoided if possible. Selective cyclooxygenase-2 inhibitors do not interfere with platelet function and may be preferable based upon a demonstrated increased risk of upper GI bleeding and theoretical risk of increased articular bleeding with nonselective NSAIDs. Synovectomy, open or arthroscopic, may be attempted in patients with chronic symptomatic synovial proliferation and recurrent hemarthrosis, although hypertrophied synovium is very vascular and subject to bleeding. Both types of synovectomy reduce the number of hemarthroses. Open surgical synovectomy, however, is associated with some loss of range of motion. Both require aggressive prophylaxis against bleeding. Radiosynovectomy with either yttrium 90 silicate or phosphorus 31 colloid has been effective and may be attempted when surgical synovectomy is not practical. Total joint replacement is indicated for severe joint destruction and incapacitating pain.

ARTHROPATHIES ASSOCIATED WITH HEMOGLOBINOPATHIES

Sickle cell disease

Sickle cell disease (Chap. 104) is associated with several musculoskeletal abnormalities (Table 336-1). Children under the age of five may develop diffuse swelling, tenderness, and warmth of the hands and feet lasting from one to three weeks. The condition,

TABLE 336-1 Musculoskeletal Abnormalities in Sickle Cell Disease

Sickle Cell Dactylitis	Avascular Necrosis
Joint effusions in sickle cell crises	Bone changes secondary to marrow hyperplasia
Osteomyelitis	Septic arthritis
Infarction of bone	Gouty arthritis
Infarction of bone marrow	

referred to as *sickle cell dactylitis* or *hand-foot syndrome*, has also been observed in sickle cell thalassemia. Dactylitis is believed to result from infarction of the bone marrow and cortical bone leading to periostitis and soft tissue swelling. Radiographs show periosteal elevation, subperiosteal new bone formation, and areas of radiolucency and increased density involving the metacarpals, metatarsals, and proximal phalanges. These bone changes disappear after several months. The syndrome leaves little or no residual damage. Because hematopoiesis ceases in the small bones of hands and feet with age, the syndrome is rarely seen after age five.

Sickle cell crisis is associated with periarticular pain and occasionally with joint effusions. The joint and periarticular area are warm and tender. Knees and elbows are most often affected, but other joints can be involved. Joint effusions are usually noninflammatory. Acute synovial infarction can cause a sterile effusion with high synovial fluid neutrophil counts. Synovial biopsies have shown mild lining cell proliferation and microvascular thrombosis with infarctions. Scintigraphic studies have shown decreased marrow uptake adjacent to the involved joint. The treatment is that for sickle cell crisis (Chap. 104).

Patients with sickle cell disease seem predisposed to osteomyelitis, which commonly involves the long tubular bones (Chap. 126) and *Salmonella* is a particularly frequent cause (Chap. 153). Radiographs of the involved site show periosteal elevation initially, followed by disruption of the cortex. Treatment of the infection results in healing of the bone lesion. Sickle cell disease is also more frequently associated with bone infarction resulting from vasoocclusion secondary to the sickling of red cells. Bone infarction also occurs in hemoglobin sickle cell disease and sickle cell thalassemia (Chap. 104). The bone pain in sickle cell crisis is due to bone and bone marrow infarction. In children, infarction of the epiphyseal growth plate interferes with normal growth of the affected extremity. Radiographically, infarction of the bone cortex results in periosteal elevation and irregular thickening of the bone cortex. Infarction in the bone marrow leads to lysis, fibrosis, and new bone formation. Clinical distinction between osteomyelitis and bone infarctions can be difficult; imaging can be helpful.

Avascular necrosis of the head of the femur occurs in ~5% of patients. It also occurs in the humeral head and less commonly in the distal femur, tibial condyles, distal radius, vertebral bodies, and other juxtaarticular sites. Irregularity of the femoral head and other articular surfaces often results in degenerative joint disease. Radiograph of the affected joint may show patchy radiolucency and density followed by flattening of the bone. MRI is a sensitive technique for detecting early avascular necrosis as well as bone infarction elsewhere. Total hip replacement and placement of prostheses in other joints may improve function and relieve the joint pain in these patients.

Septic arthritis is occasionally encountered in sickle cell disease (Chap. 334). Multiple joints may be infected. Joint infection may result from bacteremia due to splenic dysfunction or from contiguous osteomyelitis. The more common microorganisms include *Staphylococcus aureus*, *Streptococcus*, and *Salmonella*. *Salmonella* does not cause septic arthritis as frequently as osteomyelitis. Acute gouty arthritis is uncommon in sickle cell disease, even though 40% of patients are hyperuricemic. However, it may occur in patients generally not expected to get gout (younger, including female patients). Hyperuricemia is due to overproduction of uric acid secondary to increased red cell turnover as well as suboptimal renal excretion. Attacks may be polyarticular, and arthrocentesis should be performed as the diagnostic test to distinguish infection from gout or synovial infarction.

The bone marrow hyperplasia in sickle cell disease results in widening of the medullary cavities, thinning of the cortices, and coarse trabeculations and central cupping of the vertebral bodies. These changes are also seen to a lesser degree in hemoglobin sickle cell disease and sickle cell thalassemia. In normal individuals, red marrow is located mostly in the axial skeletal, but in sickle cell disease, red marrow is found in the bones of the extremities and even in the tarsal and carpal bones. Vertebral compression may lead to dorsal kyphosis, and softening of the bone in the acetabulum may result in protrusio acetabuli.

Thalassemia

β Thalassemia is a congenital disorder of hemoglobin synthesis characterized by impaired production of β chains (Chap. 104). Bone and joint abnormalities occur in β thalassemia, being most common in the major and intermedia groups. In one study, ~50% of patients with β thalassemia had evidence of symmetric ankle arthropathy, characterized by a dull aching pain aggravated by weight bearing. The onset was most often in the second or third decade of life. The degree of ankle pain in these patients varied. Some patients experienced self-limited ankle pain, which occurred only after strenuous physical activity and lasted several days to weeks. Other patients had chronic ankle pain, which became worse with walking. Symptoms eventually abated in a few patients. Compression of the ankle, calcaneus, or forefoot was painful in some patients. Synovial fluid from two patients was noninflammatory. Radiographs of ankle showed osteopenia, widened medullary spaces, thin cortices, and coarse trabeculations. These findings are largely the result of bone marrow expansion. The joint space was preserved. Specimens of bone from three patients revealed osteomalacia, osteopenia, and microfractures. Increased osteoblasts as well as increased foci of bone resorption were present on the bone surface. Iron staining was found in the bone trabeculae, in osteoid, and in the cement line. Synovium showed hyperplasia of lining cells, which contained deposits of hemosiderin. This arthropathy was considered to be related to the underlying bone pathology. The role of iron overload or abnormal bone metabolism in the pathogenesis of this arthropathy is not known. The arthropathy was treated with analgesics and splints. Patients were also transfused to decrease hematopoiesis and bone marrow expansion.

Patients with β-thalassemia major and intermedia also have involvement of other joints, including the knees, hips, and shoulders. Acquired hemochromatosis with arthropathy has been described in a patient with thalassemia. Gouty arthritis and septic arthritis can occur. Avascular necrosis is not a feature of thalassemia because there is no sickling of red cells leading to thrombosis and infarction.

β-Thalassemia minor (trait) is also associated with joint manifestations. Chronic seronegative oligoarthritis affecting predominantly ankles, wrists, and elbows has been described. These patients had mild persistent synovitis without large effusions. Joint erosions were not seen. Recurrent episodes of an acute asymmetric arthritis have also been reported; episodes last less than a week and may affect knees, ankles, shoulders, elbows, wrists, and metacarpal phalangeal joints. The mechanism for this arthropathy is unknown. Treatment with nonsteroidal drugs was not particularly effective.

MUSCULOSKELETAL DISORDERS ASSOCIATED WITH HYPERLIPIDEMIA (See also Chap. 356)

Musculoskeletal or cutaneous manifestations may be the first clinical indication of a specific hereditary disorder of lipoprotein metabolism. Patients with familial hypercholesterolemia (previously referred to as *type II hyperlipoproteinemia)* may have recurrent migratory polyarthritis involving knees and other large peripheral joints and, to a lesser degree, peripheral small joints. Pain ranges from moderate to incapacitating. The involved joints can be warm, erythematous, swollen, and tender. Arthritis usually has a sudden onset, lasts from a few days to two weeks, and does not cause joint damage. Episodes may suggest acute gout attacks. Several attacks occur per year. Synovial fluid from involved joints is not inflammatory and contains few white cells and no crystals. Joint involvement may actually represent inflammatory periarthritis or peritendinitis and not true arthritis. The recurrent, transient nature of the arthritis may suggest rheumatic fever, especially because patients with hyperlipoproteinemia may have an elevated erythrocyte sedimentation rate and elevated antistreptolysin O titers, because the latter are quite common. Attacks of tendinitis, including the large Achilles and patellar tendons, may come on gradually and last only a few days or be acute as described above. Patients may be asymptomatic between attacks. Achilles tendinitis and other joint manifestations often precede the appearance of xanthomas and may be the first clinical indication of hyperlipoproteinemia. Attacks of tendinitis may occur following treatment with a lipid-lowering drug. Patients, over time, may develop tendinous xanthomas in the Achilles, patellar, and extensor tendons of the hands and feet. Xanthomas have also been reported in the peroneal tendon, the plantar aponeurosis, and the periosteum overlying the distal tibia. These xanthomas are located within tendon fibers. Tuberous xanthomas are soft subcutaneous masses located over the extensor surfaces of the elbows, knees, and hands, as well as on the buttocks. They appear in childhood in homozygous patients and, after the age of 30, in heterozygous patients. Patients with elevated plasma levels of very low density lipoprotein (VLDL) and triglyceride (previously referred to as *type IV hyperlipoproteinemia)* may also have a mild inflammatory arthritis affecting large and small peripheral joints, usually in an asymmetric pattern, with only a few joints involved at a time. The onset of arthritis is usually in middle age. Arthritis may be persistent or recurrent, with episodes lasting a few days to weeks. Joint pain is severe in some patients. Patients may experience morning stiffness. Joint tenderness and periarticular hyperesthesia may also be present, as may synovial thickening. Joint fluid is usually noninflammatory and without crystals but may have increased white blood cell counts with predominantly mononuclear cells. Radiographs may show juxtaarticular osteopenia and cystic lesions. Large bone cysts have been noted in a few patients. Xanthoma and bone cysts are also observed in other lipoprotein disorders. The pathogenesis of arthritis in patients with familial hypercholesterolemia or with elevated levels of VLDL and triglyceride is not well understood. NSAIDs or analgesics usually provide adequate relief of symptoms when used on an as-needed basis.

Clinical improvement may occur in patients as they are treated with lipid-lowering agents; however, patients treated with an HMG-CoA reductase inhibitor may experience myalgias, and a few patients may develop a myopathy, myositis, or even rhabdomyolysis. Patients who develop myositis while on statin therapy may be susceptible to this side effect due to an underlying muscle disorder and should be reevaluated after discontinuation of the drug. Myositis has also been reported with the use of niacin (Chap. 388) but is less common than myalgias.

Musculoskeletal syndromes have not clearly been associated with the more common mixed hyperlipidemias seen in general practice.

OTHER ARTHRITIDES

NEUROPATHIC JOINT DISEASE

Neuropathic joint disease (Charcot's joint) is a progressive destructive arthritis associated with loss of pain sensation, proprioception, or both. Normal muscular reflexes that modulate joint movement are decreased. Without these protective mechanisms, joints are subjected to repeated trauma, resulting in progressive cartilage and bone damage. Neuropathic arthropathy was first described by Jean-Martin Charcot in 1868 in patients with tabes dorsalis. The term *Charcot joint* is commonly used interchangeably with *neuropathic joint*. Today, diabetes mellitus is the most frequent cause of neuropathic joint disease (Fig. 336-1). A variety of other disorders are associated with neuropathic arthritis including leprosy, yaws, syringomyelia, meningomyelocele, congenital indifference to pain, peroneal muscular atrophy (Charcot-Marie-Tooth disease), and amyloidosis. An arthritis resembling neuropathic joint disease has been reported in patients who have received frequent intraarticular glucocorticoid injections into a weight-bearing joint, but this is a rare complication. The distribution of joint involvement depends on the underlying neurologic disorder (Table 336-2). In tabes dorsalis, knees, hips, and ankles are most commonly affected; in syringomyelia, the glenohumeral joint, elbow, and wrist; and in diabetes mellitus, the tarsal and tarsometatarsal joints are most commonly affected.

Pathology and pathophysiology

The pathologic changes in the neuropathic joint are similar to those found in the severe osteoarthritic joint. There is fragmentation and eventual loss of articular cartilage with eburnation of the underlying bone. Osteophytes are found at the joint margins. With more advanced disease, erosions are present on the joint surface. Fractures, devitalized bone, intraarticular loose bodies, and microscopic fragments of cartilage and bone may be present.

At least two underlying mechanisms are believed to be involved in the pathogenesis of neuropathic arthritis. An abnormal autonomic nervous system is thought to be responsible for the dysregulated blood flow to the joint with subsequent resorption of

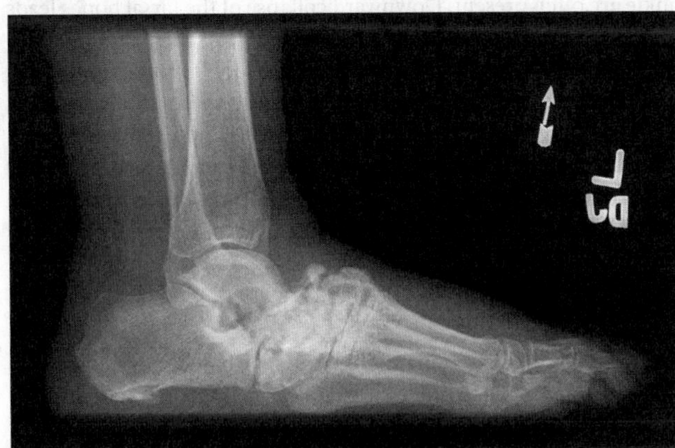

Figure 336-1 Charcot arthropathy associated with diabetes mellitus. Lateral foot radiograph demonstrating complete loss of the arch due to bony fragmentation and dislocation in the midfoot. *(Courtesy of Andrew Neckers, MD and Jean Schils, MD; with permission.)*

TABLE 336-2 Disorders Associated With Neuropathic Joint Disease

Diabetes mellitus	Amyloidosis
Tabes dorsalis	Leprosy
Meningomyelocele	Congenital indifference to pain
Syringomyelia	Peroneal muscular atrophy

bone. Loss of bone, particularly in the diabetic foot, may be the initial finding. With the loss of deep pain, proprioception, and protective neuromuscular reflexes, the joint is subjected to repeated microtrauma, resulting in ligamental tears and bone fractures. The mechanism of injury that occurs following frequent intraarticular glucocorticoid injections is thought to be due to the analgesic effect of glucocorticoids leading to overuse of an already damaged joint, which results in accelerated cartilage damage, although steroid-induced cartilage damage be more common in some animal species than in humans. It is not understood why only a few patients with neuropathy develop clinically evident neuropathic arthritis.

Clinical manifestations

Neuropathic joint disease usually begins in a single joint and then becomes apparent in other joints, depending on the underlying neurologic disorder. The involved joint progressively becomes enlarged due to bony overgrowth and synovial effusion. Loose bodies may be palpated in the joint cavity. Joint instability, subluxation, and crepitus occur as the disease progresses. Neuropathic joints may develop rapidly, and a totally disorganized joint with multiple bony fragments may evolve in a patient within weeks or months. The amount of pain experienced by the patient is less than would be anticipated based on the degree of joint damage. Patients may experience sudden joint pain from intraarticular fractures of osteophytes or condyles.

Neuropathic arthritis is encountered most often in patients with diabetes mellitus, with the incidence estimated in the range of 0.5%. The usual age of onset is ≥50 years, following several years of diabetes, but exceptions occur. The tarsal and tarsometatarsal joints are most often affected, followed by the metatarsophalangeal and talotibial joints. The knees and spine are occasionally involved. Patients often attribute the onset of foot pain to antecedent trauma such as twisting their foot. Neuropathic changes may develop rapidly following a foot fracture or dislocation. Swelling of the foot and ankle are often present. Downward collapse of the tarsal bones leads to convexity of the sole, referred to as a "rocker foot." Large osteophytes may protrude from the top of the foot. Calluses frequently form over the metatarsal heads and may lead to infected ulcers and osteomyelitis. The value of protective inserts and orthotics, as well as regular foot examination, cannot be overstated. Radiographs may show resorption and tapering of the distal metatarsal bones. The term *Lisfranc fracture-dislocation* is sometimes used to describe the destructive changes at the tarsometatarsal joints.

Diagnosis

The diagnosis of neuropathic arthritis is based on the clinical features and characteristic radiographic findings in a patient with an underlying sensory neuropathy. The differential diagnosis of neuropathic arthritis depends upon the severity of the process and includes osteomyelitis, osteonecrosis, advanced osteoarthritis, stress fractures, and CPPD. Radiographs in neuropathic arthritis initially show changes of osteoarthritis with joint space narrowing, subchondral bone sclerosis, osteophytes, and joint effusions followed later by marked destructive and hypertrophic changes. The radiographic findings of neuropathic arthritis may be difficult to differentiate from those of osteomyelitis, especially in the diabetic foot. The joint margins in a neuropathic joint tend to be distinct, while in osteomyelitis, they are blurred. Imaging studies may be helpful, but cultures of tissue from the joint are often required to exclude osteomyelitis. MRI and bone scans using indium 111–labeled white blood cells or indium 111–labeled immunoglobulin G, which will show an increased uptake in osteomyelitis but not in a neuropathic joint may be useful. A technetium bone scan will not distinguish osteomyelitis from neuropathic arthritis, as increased uptake is observed in both. The joint fluid in neuropathic arthritis is noninflammatory; may be xanthochromic or even bloody; and may contain fragments of synovium, cartilage, and bone. The finding of calcium pyrophosphate dihydrate crystals supports the diagnosis of crystal-associated arthropathy. In the absence of such crystals, an increased number of leukocytes may indicate osteomyelitis.

TREATMENT Neuropathic Joint Disease

The primary focus of treatment is to stabilize the joint. Treatment of the underlying disorder, even if successful, does not usually affect established joint disease. Braces and splints are helpful. Their use requires close surveillance, because patients may be unable to appreciate pressure from a poorly adjusted brace. In the diabetic patient, early recognition and treatment of a Charcot's foot by prohibiting weight bearing of the foot for at least eight weeks may possibly prevent severe disease from developing. Fusion of an unstable joint may improve function and reduce pain, but nonunion is frequent, especially when immobilization of the joint is inadequate.

HYPERTROPHIC OSTEOARTHROPATHY AND CLUBBING

Hypertrophic osteoarthropathy (HOA) is characterized by clubbing of digits and, in more advanced stages, by periosteal new bone formation and synovial effusions. HOA may be primary or familial and begin in childhood. Secondary HOA is associated with intrathoracic malignancies, suppurative and some hypoxemic lung diseases, congenital heart disease, and a variety of other disorders. Clubbing is almost always a feature of HOA but can occur as an isolated manifestation (Fig. 336-2). The presence of clubbing in isolation may be congenital or represent either an early stage or one

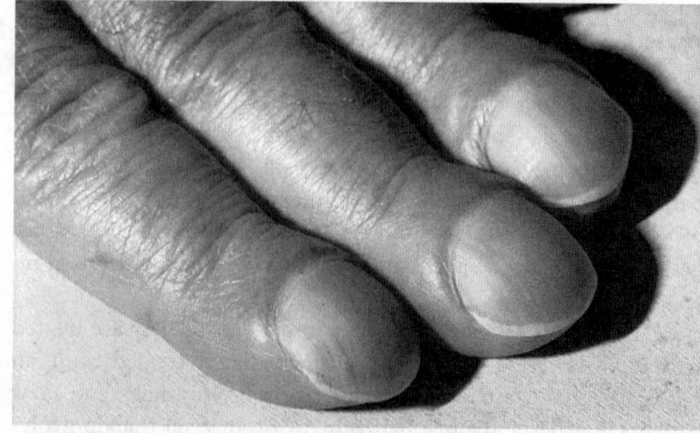

Figure 336-2 Clubbing of fingers. *(Reprinted from the Clinical Slide Collection on the Rheumatic Diseases, Copyright 1991, 1995. Used by permission of the American College of Rheumatology.)*

element in the spectrum of HOA. The presence of isolated acquired clubbing has the same clinical significance as clubbing associated with periostitis.

Pathology and pathophysiology of acquired HOA

In HOA, the bone changes in the distal extremities begin as periostitis followed by new bone formation. At this stage, a radiolucent area may be observed between the new periosteal bone and subjacent cortex. As the process progresses, multiple layers of new bone are deposited, which become contiguous with the cortex and result in cortical thickening. The outer portion of bone is laminated in appearance, with an irregular surface. Initially, the process of periosteal new bone formation involves the proximal and distal diaphyses of the tibia, fibula, radius, and ulna and, less frequently, the femur, humerus, metacarpals, metatarsals, and phalanges. Occasionally, scapulae, clavicles, ribs, and pelvic bones are also affected. The adjacent interosseous membranes may become ossified. The distribution of the bone manifestations is usually bilateral and symmetric. The soft tissue overlying the distal third of the arms and legs may be thickened. Proliferation of connective tissue occurs in the nail bed and volar pad of digits, giving the distal phalanges a clubbed appearance. Small blood vessels in the clubbed digits are dilated and have thickened walls. In addition, the number of arteriovenous anastomoses is increased.

Several theories have been suggested for the pathogenesis of HOA, but many have been disproved or have not explained the development in all clinical disorders associated with HOA. Previously proposed neurogenic and humoral theories are no longer considered likely explanations for HOA. Recent studies have suggested a role for platelets in the development of HOA. It has been observed that megakaryocytes and large platelet particles, present in venous circulation, were fragmented in their passage through normal lung. In patients with cyanotic congenital heart disease and in other disorders associated with right-to-left shunts, these large platelet particles bypass the lung and reach the distal extremities, where they can interact with endothelial cells. Platelet-endothelial activation in the distal portion of extremities may result in the release of platelet-derived growth factor (PDGF) and other factors leading to the proliferation of connective tissue and periosteum. Stimulation of fibroblasts by PDGF and transforming growth factor β results in cell growth and collagen synthesis. Elevated plasma levels of von Willebrand factor antigen have been found in patients with both primary and secondary forms of HOA, indicating endothelial activation or damage. Abnormalities of collagen synthesis have been demonstrated in the involved skin of patients with primary HOA. Other factors are undoubtedly involved in the pathogenesis of HOA, and further studies are needed to better understand this disorder.

Clinical manifestations

Primary or familial HOA, also referred to as *pachydermoperiostitis* or *Touraine-Solente-Golé syndrome*, usually begins insidiously at puberty. In a smaller number of patients, the onset is in the first year of life. The disorder is inherited as an autosomal dominant trait with variable expression and is nine times more common in boys than in girls. Approximately one-third of patients have a family history of primary HOA.

Primary HOA is characterized by clubbing, periostitis, and unusual skin features. A small number of patients with this syndrome do not express clubbing. The skin changes and periostitis are prominent features of this syndrome. The skin becomes thickened and coarse. Deep nasolabial folds develop, and the forehead may become furrowed. Patients may have heavy-appearing eyelids and ptosis. The skin is often greasy, and there may be excessive sweating of the hands and feet. Patients may also experience acne vulgaris, seborrhea, and folliculitis. In a few patients, the skin over the scalp becomes very thick and corrugated, a feature that has been descriptively termed *cutis verticis gyrata*. The distal extremities, particularly the legs, become thickened owing to proliferation of new bone and soft tissue; when the process is extensive, the distal lower extremities resemble those of an elephant. The periostitis is usually not painful, because it may be in secondary HOA. Clubbing of the fingers may be extensive, producing large, bulbous deformities and clumsiness. Clubbing also affects the toes. Patients may experience articular and periarticular pain, especially in the ankles and knees, and joint motion may be mildly restricted owing to periarticular bone overgrowth. Noninflammatory effusions occur in the wrists, knees, and ankles. Synovial hypertrophy is not found. Associated abnormalities observed in patients with primary HOA include hypertrophic gastropathy, bone marrow failure, female escutcheon, gynecomastia, and cranial suture defects. In patients with primary HOA, the symptoms disappear when adulthood is reached.

HOA secondary to an underlying disease occurs more frequently than primary HOA. It accompanies a variety of disorders and may precede clinical features of the associated disorder by months. Clubbing is more frequent than the full syndrome of HOA in patients with associated illnesses. Because clubbing evolves over months and is usually asymptomatic, it is often recognized first by the physician and not the patient. Patients may experience a burning sensation in their fingertips. Clubbing is characterized by widening of the fingertips, enlargement of the distal volar pad, convexity of the nail contour, and the loss of the normal 15° angle between the proximal nail and cuticle. The thickness of the digit at the base of the nail is greater than the thickness at the distal interphalangeal joint. An objective measurement of finger clubbing can be made by determining the diameter at the base of the nail and at the distal interphalangeal joint of all 10 digits. Clubbing is present when the sum of the individual digit ratios is >10. At the bedside, clubbing can be appreciated by having the patient place the dorsal surface of the distal phalanges of the fourth fingers together with the nails of the fourth fingers opposing each other. Normally, an open area is visible between the bases of the opposing fingernails; when clubbing is present, this open space is no longer visible. The base of the nail feels spongy when compressed, and the nail can be easily rocked on its bed. When clubbing is advanced, the finger may have a drumstick appearance, and the distal interphalangeal joint can be hyperextended. Periosteal involvement in the distal extremities may produce a burning or deep-seated aching pain. The pain can be quite incapacitating and is aggravated by dependency and relieved by elevation of the affected limbs. Pressure applied over the distal forearms and legs or gentle percussion of the distal long bones like the tibia may be quite painful.

Patients may experience joint pain, most often in the ankles, wrists, and knees. Joint effusions may be present; usually, they are small and noninflammatory. The small joints of the hands are rarely affected. Severe joint or long bone pain may be the presenting symptom of an underlying lung malignancy and may precede the appearance of clubbing. In addition, the progression of HOA tends to be more rapid when associated with malignancies, most notably bronchogenic carcinoma. Noninflammatory but variably painful knee effusions may occur prior to the appearance of clubbing and symptoms of distal periostitis. Unlike primary HOA, excessive sweating and oiliness of the skin and thickening of the facial skin are uncommon in secondary HOA.

HOA occurs in 5–10% of patients with intrathoracic malignancies, the most common being bronchogenic carcinoma and pleural tumors (Table 336-3). Lung metastases infrequently cause HOA. HOA is also seen in patients with intrathoracic infections, including lung abscesses, empyema, bronchiectasis, and chronic obstructive lung disease, but uncommonly in pulmonary tuberculosis. HOA

TABLE 336-3 Disorders Associated With Hypertrophic Osteoarthropathy

Pulmonary	Cardiovascular
Bronchogenic carcinoma and other neoplasms	Cyanotic congenital heart disease
Lung abscesses, empyema, bronchiectasis	Subacute bacterial endocarditis
Chronic interstitial pneumonitis	Infected arterial grafts[a]
Cystic fibrosis	Aortic aneurysm[b]
Chronic obstructive lung disease	Aneurysm of major extremity artery[a]
Sarcoidosis	Patent ductus arteriosus[b]
Gastrointestinal	Arteriovenous fistula of major extremity vessel[a]
Inflammatory bowel disease	Thyroid (thyroid acropachy)
Sprue	Hyperthyroidism (Graves' disease)
Neoplasms: esophagus, liver, bowel	

[a]Unilateral involvement.
[b]Bilateral lower extremity involvement.

may also accompany chronic interstitial pneumonitis, sarcoidosis, and cystic fibrosis. In the latter, clubbing is more common than the full syndrome of HOA. Other causes of clubbing include congenital heart disease with right-to-left shunts, bacterial endocarditis, Crohn's disease, ulcerative colitis, sprue, and neoplasms of the esophagus, liver, and small and large bowel. In patients with congenital heart disease with right-to-left shunts, clubbing alone occurs more often than the full syndrome of HOA.

Unilateral clubbing has been found in association with aneurysms of major extremity arteries, with infected arterial grafts, and with arteriovenous fistulas of brachial vessels. Clubbing of the toes but not fingers has been associated with an infected abdominal aortic aneurysm and patent ductus arteriosus. Clubbing of a single digit may follow trauma and has been reported in tophaceous gout and sarcoidosis. While clubbing occurs more commonly than the full syndrome in most diseases, periostitis in the absence of clubbing has been observed in the affected limb of patients with infected arterial grafts.

Hyperthyroidism (Graves' disease), treated or untreated, is occasionally associated with clubbing and periostitis of the bones of the hands and feet. This condition is referred to as *thyroid acropachy*. Periostitis may be asymptomatic and occurs in the midshaft and diaphyseal portion of the metacarpal and phalangeal bones. Significant hand joint pain may occur; this may respond to successful therapy of the thyroid dysfunction. The long bones of the extremities are seldom affected. Elevated levels of long-acting thyroid stimulator are found in the serum of these patients.

Laboratory findings

The laboratory abnormalities reflect the underlying disorder. The synovial fluid of involved joints has <500 white cells per microliter, and the cells are predominantly mononuclear. Radiographs show a faint radiolucent line beneath the new periosteal bone along the shaft of long bones at their distal end. These changes are observed most frequently at the ankles, wrists, and knees. The ends of the distal phalanges may show osseous resorption. Radionuclide studies show pericortical linear uptake along the cortical margins of long bones that may be present before any radiographic changes.

TREATMENT Hypertrophic Osteoarthropathy

The treatment of HOA is to identify the associated disorder and treat it appropriately. The symptoms and signs of HOA may disappear completely with removal or effective chemotherapy of a tumor or with antibiotic therapy and drainage of a chronic pulmonary infection. Vagotomy or percutaneous block of the vagus nerve leads to symptomatic relief in some patients. NSAIDs or analgesics may help control symptoms of HOA.

REFLEX SYMPATHETIC DYSTROPHY SYNDROME

The reflex sympathetic dystrophy syndrome is now referred to as *complex regional pain syndrome, type 1*, by the new Classification of the International Association for the Study of Pain. It is characterized by pain and swelling, usually of a distal extremity, accompanied by vasomotor instability, trophic skin changes, and the rapid development of bony demineralization. Reflex sympathetic dystrophy syndrome, including its treatment, is covered in greater detail in Chap. 376.

TIETZE SYNDROME AND COSTOCHONDRITIS

Tietze syndrome is manifested by painful swelling of one or more costochondral articulations. The age of onset is usually before 40, and both sexes are affected equally. In most patients, only one joint is involved, usually the second or third costochondral joint. The onset of anterior chest pain may be sudden or gradual. The pain may radiate to the arms or shoulders and is aggravated by sneezing, coughing, deep inspirations, or twisting motions of the chest. The term *costochondritis* is often used interchangeably with *Tietze syndrome*, but some workers restrict the former term to pain of the costochondral articulations without swelling. Costochondritis is observed in patients over age 40; tends to affect the third, fourth, and fifth costochondral joints; and occurs more often in women. Both syndromes may mimic cardiac or upper abdominal causes of pain. Rheumatoid arthritis, ankylosing spondylitis, and reactive arthritis (Reiter's syndrome) may involve costochondral joints but are distinguished easily by their other clinical features. Other skeletal causes of anterior chest wall pain are xiphoidalgia and the slipping rib syndrome, which usually involves the tenth rib. Malignancies such as breast cancer, prostate cancer, plasma cell cytoma, and sarcoma can invade the ribs, thoracic spine, or chest wall and produce symptoms suggesting Tietze syndrome. Patients with osteomalacia may have significant rib pain, with or without documented micro fractures. These conditions should be distinguishable by radiographs, bone scanning, vitamin D measurement, or biopsy. Analgesics, anti-inflammatory drugs, and local glucocorticoid injections usually relieve symptoms of costochondritis/Tietze syndrome. Care should be taken to avoid overdiagnosing these syndromes in patients with acute chest pain syndromes; many patients will be tender to overly vigorous palpation of the costochondral joints.

MYOFASCIAL PAIN SYNDROME

Myofascial pain syndrome is characterized by multiple areas of localized musculoskeletal pain and tenderness in association with tender points. The pain is deep and aching and may be accompanied by a burning sensation. Myofascial pain may be regional and follow trauma, overuse, or prolonged static contraction of a muscle or muscle group, which may occur when reading or writing at a desk or working at a computer. In addition, this syndrome may be associated with underlying osteoarthritis of the neck or low back. Pain may be referred from tender points to defined areas distant from the area of original tenderness. Palpation of the tender point reproduces or accentuates the pain. The tender points are usually located in the center of a muscle belly, but they can occur at other sites such as costosternal junctions, the xiphoid process, ligamentous and tendinous insertions, fascia, and fatty areas. Tender point sites in muscle have been described as feeling indurated and taut, and palpation may cause the muscle to twitch. These findings, however, have been shown not to be unique for myofascial pain syndrome, because in a controlled study, they were also present in some "normal" subjects. Myofascial pain most often involves the posterior neck, low back, shoulders, and chest. Chronic pain in the muscles of the posterior neck may involve referral of pain from a tender point in the erector neck muscle or upper trapezius to the head, leading to persistent headaches, which may last for days. Tender points in the paraspinal muscles of the low back may refer pain to the buttock. Pain may be referred down the leg from a tender point in the gluteus medius and can mimic sciatica. A tender point in the infraspinatus muscle may produce local and referred pain over the lateral deltoid and down the outside of the arm into the hand. Injection of a local anesthetic such as 1% lidocaine into the tender point site often results in at least transient pain relief. Another useful technique is first to spray from the tender point toward the area of referred pain with an agent such as ethyl chloride and then to stretch the muscle. This maneuver may need to be repeated several times. Massage and application of ultrasound to the affected area also may be beneficial. Patients should be instructed in methods to prevent muscle stresses related to work and recreation. Posture and resting positions are important in preventing muscle tension. The prognosis in most patients is good. In some patients, regionally localized myofascial pain syndrome may seem to evolve into more generalized fibromyalgia (Chap. 335). Abnormal or nonrestorative sleep is a common accompaniment in these patients and may need to be specifically addressed.

NEOPLASIAS AND ARTHRITIS

Primary tumors and tumor-like disorders of synovium are uncommon but should be considered in the differential diagnosis of monarticular joint disease. In addition, metastases to bone and primary bone tumors adjacent to a joint may produce joint symptoms. For further discussion, see Chap. 98.

Pigmented villonodular synovitis (PVNS) is characterized by the slowly progressive, exuberant, benign proliferation of synovial tissue, usually involving a single joint. The most common age of onset is in the third decade, and women are affected slightly more often than men. The cause of this disorder is unknown.

The synovium has a brownish color and numerous large, finger-like villi that fuse to form pedunculated nodules. There is marked hyperplasia of synovial cells in the stroma of the villi. Hemosiderin granules and lipids are found in the cytoplasm of macrophages and in the interstitial tissue. Multinucleated giant cells may be present. The proliferative synovium grows into the subsynovial tissue and invades adjacent cartilage and bone.

The clinical picture of pigmented villonodular synovitis is characterized by the insidious onset of persistent swelling and pain in affected joints, most commonly the knee. Other joints affected include the hips, ankles, calcaneocuboid joints, elbows, and small joints of the fingers or toes. The disease may also involve the common flexor sheath of the hands or fingers. Less commonly, tendon sheaths in the wrist, ankle, or foot may be involved. Symptoms of pain, a catching sensation, or stiffness may initially be mild and intermittent and may be present for years before the patient seeks medical attention. Radiographs may show joint space narrowing, erosions, and subchondral cysts. The joint fluid contains blood and is dark red or almost black in color. Lipid-containing macrophages may be present in the fluid. The joint fluid may be clear if hemorrhage has not occurred. Some patients have polyarticular involvement.

The treatment of pigmented villonodular synovitis is complete synovectomy. With incomplete synovectomy, the villonodular synovitis recurs, and the rate of tissue growth may be faster than it was originally. Irradiation of the involved joint has been successful in some patients.

Synovial chondromatosis is a disorder characterized by multiple focal metaplastic growths of normal-appearing cartilage in the synovium or tendon sheath. Segments of cartilage break loose and continue to grow as loose bodies. When calcification and ossification of loose bodies occur, the disorder is referred to as *synovial osteochondromatosis*. The disorder is usually monarticular and affects young to middle-aged individuals. The knee is most often involved, followed by hip, elbow, and shoulder. Symptoms are pain, swelling, and decreased motion of the joint. Radiographs may show several rounded calcifications within the joint cavity. Treatment is synovectomy; however, as in PVNS, the tumor may recur.

Synovial sarcoma is a malignant neoplasm often found near a large joint of both upper and lower extremities, being more common in the lower extremity. It seldom arises within the joint itself. Synovial sarcomas constitute 10% of soft tissue sarcomas. The tumor is believed to arise from primitive mesenchymal tissue that differentiates into epithelial cells and/or spindle cells. Small foci of calcification may be present in the tumor mass. It occurs most often in young adults and is more common in men. The tumor presents as a slowly growing deep-seated mass near a joint, without much pain. The area of the knee is the most common site, followed by the foot, ankle, elbow, and shoulder. Other primary sites include the buttocks, abdominal wall, retroperitoneum, and mediastinum. The tumor spreads along tissue planes. The most common site of visceral metastasis is lung. The diagnosis is made by biopsy. Treatment is wide resection of the tumor, including adjacent muscle and regional lymph nodes, followed by chemotherapy and radiation therapy. Amputation of the involved distal extremity may be required. Chemotherapy may be beneficial in some patients with metastatic disease. Isolated pulmonary metastasis can be surgically removed. The five-year survival rate with treatment is variable depending on the staging of the tumor, ranging from approximately 25% to 60% or higher. Synovial sarcomas tend to recur locally and metastasize to regional lymph nodes, lungs, and skeleton.

In addition to the rare direct metastases of solid cell tumors to the highly vascular synovium, neoplasia arising from nonarticular organ sites can affect joints in other ways. Acute leukemias in children can mimic juvenile inflammatory arthritis with severe joint pain and fever. In adults, chronic and acute myeloid leukemia can rarely infiltrate the synovium. The rarely occurring hairy cell leukemia has a peculiar tendency to cause episodic inflammatory oligoarthritis and tenosynovitis; these episodes are dramatic and mimic acute gout attacks. They respond to potent anti-inflammatory therapy with glucocorticoids; with remission of the leukemia, they may abate. Carcinomas can be associated with several paraneoplastic articular syndromes, including hypertrophic pulmonary osteoarthropathy (discussed above). Acute palmar fasciitis with polyarthritis is a well-described, but rare association with certain cancers, mainly adenocarcinomas. Clinically, this is fairly abrupt in onset with pain in the MCP and PIP joints of the hands with rapidly evolving contractures of the fingers due to thickening of the palmar (flexor) tendons. A similar syndrome can be seen in diabetics. Paraneoplastic arthritis has been described and may occur in several patterns: asymmetric predominantly lower extremity joints and symmetric, polyarthritis with hand joint involvement. Tumors were often found after the onset of the arthritis, although many patients had a preceding period of malaise or weight loss. The onset is often acute, and patients tend to be older males. These features should raise the specter of an underlying malignancy (or viral infection such as hepatitis C) as the cause of the arthritis.

In one series, the symptoms resolved with successful therapy of the malignancy but did not recur with relapse of the malignancy. Dermatomyositis is also well described as a paraneoplastic syndrome and may have joint pain and arthritis as components of the syndrome. Malignancy associated arthritis may be responsive to NSAID therapy and to treatment of the primary neoplasm.

ACKNOWLEDGMENT

This chapter represents a revised version of the chapter authored by Dr. Bruce C. Gilliland that was in the previous editions of Harrison's. *Dr. Gilliland passed away on February 17, 2007, and had been a contributor to Harrison's Principles of Internal Medicine since the 11th edition.*

FURTHER READINGS

Altman RD, Tenenbaum J: Hypertrophic osteoarthropathy, in *Kelley's Textbook of Rheumatology*, 7th ed, ED Harris et al (eds). Philadelphia, Saunders, 2005, pp 1748–1753

Cronin ME: Rheumatic aspects of endocrinopathies, in *Arthritis and Allied Conditions*, 15th ed, WJ Koopman (ed). Philadelphia, Lippincott Williams & Wilkins, 2005, pp 2559–2576

Heck LW JR: Arthritis associated with hematologic disorders, storage diseases, disorders of lipid metabolism, and dysproteinemias, in *Arthritis and Allied Conditions*, 15th ed, WJ Koopman (ed). Philadelphia, Lippincott Williams & Wilkins, 2005, pp 1969–1990

CHAPTER 337

Periarticular Disorders of the Extremities

Carol A. Langford

Bruce C. Gilliland†

A number of periarticular disorders have become increasingly common over the past two to three decades, due in part to greater participation in recreational sports by individuals of a wide range of ages. Periarticular disorders most commonly affect the knee or shoulder. With the exception of bursitis, hip pain is most often articular or is being referred from disease affecting another structure (Chap 331). This chapter discusses some of the more common periarticular disorders.

BURSITIS

Bursitis is inflammation of a bursa, which is a thin-walled sac lined with synovial tissue. The function of the bursa is to facilitate movement of tendons and muscles over bony prominences. Excessive frictional forces from overuse, trauma, systemic disease (e.g., rheumatoid arthritis, gout), or infection may cause bursitis. *Subacromial bursitis* (subdeltoid bursitis) is the most common form of bursitis. The subacromial bursa, which is contiguous with the subdeltoid bursa, is located between the undersurface of the acromion and the humeral head and is covered by the deltoid muscle. Bursitis is caused by repetitive overhead motion and often accompanies rotator cuff tendinitis. Another frequently encountered form is *trochanteric bursitis*, which involves the bursa around the insertion of the gluteus medius onto the greater trochanter of the femur. Patients experience pain over the lateral aspect of the hip and upper thigh and have tenderness over the posterior aspect of the greater trochanter. External rotation and resisted abduction of the hip elicit pain. *Olecranon bursitis* occurs over the posterior elbow, and when the area is acutely inflamed, infection or gout should be excluded by aspirating the bursa and performing a Gram stain and culture on the fluid as well as examining the fluid for urate crystals. *Achilles bursitis* involves the bursa located above the insertion of the tendon to the calcaneus and results from overuse and wearing tight shoes. *Retrocalcaneal bursitis* involves the bursa that is located between the calcaneus and posterior surface of the Achilles tendon. The pain is experienced at the back of the heel, and swelling appears on the medial and/or lateral side of the tendon. It occurs in association with spondyloarthropathies, rheumatoid arthritis, gout, or trauma. *Ischial bursitis* (weaver's bottom) affects the bursa separating the gluteus medius from the ischial tuberosity and develops from prolonged sitting and pivoting on hard surfaces. *Iliopsoas bursitis* affects the bursa that lies between the iliopsoas muscle and hip joint and is lateral to the femoral vessels. Pain is experienced over this area and is made worse by hip extension and flexion. *Anserine bursitis* is an inflammation of the sartorius bursa located over the medial side of the tibia just below the knee and under the conjoint tendon and is manifested by pain on climbing stairs. Tenderness is present over the insertion of the conjoint tendon of the sartorius, gracilis, and semitendinosus. *Prepatellar bursitis* (housemaid's knee) occurs in the bursa situated between the patella and overlying skin and is caused by kneeling on hard surfaces. Gout or infection may also occur at this site. Treatment of bursitis consists of prevention of the aggravating situation, rest of the involved part, administration of a nonsteroidal anti-inflammatory drug (NSAID) where appropriate for an individual patient, or local glucocorticoid injection.

ROTATOR CUFF TENDINITIS AND IMPINGEMENT SYNDROME

Tendinitis of the rotator cuff is the major cause of a painful shoulder and is currently thought to be caused by inflammation of the tendon(s). The rotator cuff consists of the tendons of the supraspinatus, infraspinatus, subscapularis, and teres minor muscles, and inserts on the humeral tuberosities. Of the tendons forming the rotator cuff, the supraspinatus tendon is the most often affected, probably because of its repeated impingement (*impingement syndrome*) between the humeral head and the undersurface of the anterior third of the acromion and coracoacromial ligament above as well as the reduction in its blood supply that occurs with abduction of the arm (Fig. 337-1). The tendon of the infraspinatus and that of the long head of the biceps are less commonly involved. The process begins with edema and hemorrhage of the rotator cuff, which evolves to fibrotic thickening and eventually to rotator cuff degeneration with tendon tears and bone spurs. Subacromial bursitis also accompanies this syndrome. Symptoms usually appear after injury or overuse, especially with activities involving elevation of the arm with some degree of forward flexion. Impingement syndrome occurs in persons participating in baseball, tennis, swimming, or occupations that require repeated elevation of the arm. Those over age 40 are particularly susceptible. Patients complain of

†Deceased. A contributor to HPIM since the 11th edition, Dr. Gilliland passed away on February 17, 2007.

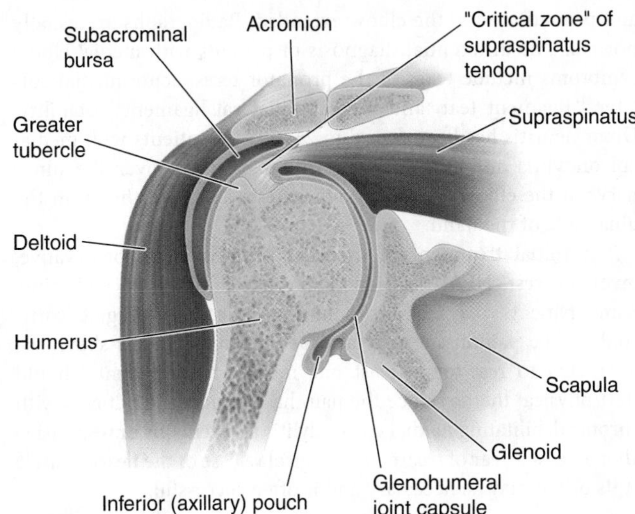

Figure 337-1 Coronal section of the shoulder illustrating the relationships of the glenohumeral joint, the joint capsule, the subacromial bursa, and the rotator cuff (supraspinatus tendon). *[From F Kozin, in Arthritis and Allied Conditions, 13th ed, WJ Koopman (ed). Baltimore, Williams & Wilkins, 1997, with permission.]*

a dull aching in the shoulder, which may interfere with sleep. Severe pain is experienced when the arm is actively abducted into an overhead position. The arc between 60° and 120° is especially painful. Tenderness is present over the lateral aspect of the humeral head just below the acromion. NSAIDs, local glucocorticoid injection, and physical therapy may relieve symptoms. Surgical decompression of the subacromial space may be necessary in patients refractory to conservative treatment.

Patients may tear the supraspinatus tendon acutely by falling on an outstretched arm or lifting a heavy object. Symptoms are pain along with weakness of abduction and external rotation of the shoulder. Atrophy of the supraspinatus muscles develops. The diagnosis is established by arthrogram, ultrasound, or MRI. Surgical repair may be necessary in patients who fail to respond to conservative measures. In patients with moderate-to-severe tears and functional loss, surgery is indicated.

CALCIFIC TENDINITIS

This condition is characterized by deposition of calcium salts, primarily hydroxyapatite, within a tendon. The exact mechanism of calcification is not known but may be initiated by ischemia or degeneration of the tendon. The supraspinatus tendon is most often affected because it is frequently impinged on and has a reduced blood supply when the arm is abducted. The condition usually develops after age 40. Calcification within the tendon may evoke acute inflammation, producing sudden and severe pain in the shoulder. However, it may be asymptomatic or not related to the patient's symptoms.

BICIPITAL TENDINITIS AND RUPTURE

Bicipital tendinitis, or tenosynovitis, is produced by friction on the tendon of the long head of the biceps as it passes through the bicipital groove. When the inflammation is acute, patients experience anterior shoulder pain that radiates down the biceps into the forearm. Abduction and external rotation of the arm are painful and limited. The bicipital groove is very tender to palpation. Pain may be elicited along the course of the tendon by resisting supination of the forearm with the elbow at 90° (Yergason's supination sign). Acute rupture of the tendon may occur with vigorous exercise of the arm and is often painful. In a young patient, it should be repaired surgically. Rupture of the tendon in an older person may be associated with little or no pain and is recognized by the presence of persistent swelling of the biceps ("Popeye" muscle) produced by the retraction of the long head of the biceps. Surgery is usually not necessary in this setting.

DE QUERVAIN'S TENOSYNOVITIS

In this condition, inflammation involves the abductor pollicis longus and the extensor pollicis brevis as these tendons pass through a fibrous sheath at the radial styloid process. The usual cause is repetitive twisting of the wrist. It may occur in pregnancy, and it also occurs in mothers who hold their babies with the thumb outstretched. Patients experience pain on grasping with their thumb, such as with pinching. Swelling and tenderness are often present over the radial styloid process. The Finkelstein sign is positive, which is elicited by having the patient place the thumb in the palm and close the fingers over it. The wrist is then ulnarly deviated, resulting in pain over the involved tendon sheath in the area of the radial styloid. Treatment consists initially of splinting the wrist and an NSAID. When severe or refractory to conservative treatment, glucocorticoid injections can be very effective.

PATELLAR TENDINITIS (JUMPER'S KNEE)

Tendinitis involves the patellar tendon at its attachment to the lower pole of the patella. Patients may experience pain when jumping during basketball or volleyball, going up stairs, or doing deep knee squats. Tenderness is noted on examination over the lower pole of the patella. Treatment consists of rest, icing, and NSAIDs, followed by strengthening and increasing flexibility.

ILIOTIBIAL BAND SYNDROME

The iliotibial band is a thick connective tissue that runs from the ilium to the fibula. Patients with iliotibial band syndrome most commonly present with aching or burning pain at the site where the band courses over the lateral femoral condyle of the knee; pain may also radiate up the thigh, toward the hip. Predisposing factors for iliotibial band syndrome include a varus alignment of the knee, excessive running distance, poorly fitted shoes, or continuous running on uneven terrain. Treatment consists of rest, NSAIDs, physical therapy, and addressing risk factors such as shoes and running surface. Glucocorticoid injection into the area of tenderness can provide relief, but running must be avoided for at least two weeks after the injection. Surgical release of the iliotibial band has been helpful in rare patients for whom conservative treatment has failed.

ADHESIVE CAPSULITIS

Often referred to as "frozen shoulder," adhesive capsulitis is characterized by pain and restricted movement of the shoulder, usually in the absence of intrinsic shoulder disease. Adhesive capsulitis may follow bursitis or tendinitis of the shoulder or be associated with systemic disorders such as chronic pulmonary disease, myocardial infarction, and diabetes mellitus. Prolonged immobility of the arm contributes to the development of adhesive capsulitis. Pathologically, the capsule of the shoulder is thickened, and a mild chronic inflammatory infiltrate and fibrosis may be present.

Adhesive capsulitis occurs more commonly in women after age 50. Pain and stiffness usually develop gradually but progress rapidly in some patients. Night pain is often present in the affected shoulder and pain may interfere with sleep. The shoulder is tender to palpation, and both active and passive movement are restricted.

Radiographs of the shoulder show osteopenia. The diagnosis is typically made by physical examination but can be confirmed if necessary by arthrography, in that only a limited amount of contrast material, usually <15 mL, can be injected under pressure into the shoulder joint.

In most patients, the condition improves spontaneously 1–3 years after onset. While pain usually improves, many patients are left with some limitation of shoulder motion. Early mobilization of the arm following an injury to the shoulder may prevent the development of this disease. Physical therapy provides the foundation of treatment for adhesive capsulitis. Local injections of glucocorticoids and NSAIDs may also provide relief of symptoms. Slow but forceful injection of contrast material into the joint may lyse adhesions and stretch the capsule, resulting in improvement of shoulder motion. Manipulation under anesthesia may be helpful in some patients.

LATERAL EPICONDYLITIS (TENNIS ELBOW)

Lateral epicondylitis, or tennis elbow, is a painful condition involving the soft tissue over the lateral aspect of the elbow. The pain originates at or near the site of attachment of the common extensors to the lateral epicondyle and may radiate into the forearm and dorsum of the wrist. The pain usually appears after work or recreational activities involving repeated motions of wrist extension and supination against resistance. Most patients with this disorder injure themselves in activities other than tennis, such as pulling weeds, carrying suitcases or briefcases, or using a screwdriver. The injury in tennis usually occurs when hitting a backhand with the elbow flexed. Shaking hands and opening doors can reproduce the pain. Striking the lateral elbow against a solid object may also induce pain.

The treatment is usually rest along with administration of an NSAID. Ultrasound, icing, and friction massage may also help relieve pain. When pain is severe, the elbow is placed in a sling or splinted at 90° of flexion. When the pain is acute and well localized, injection of a glucocorticoid using a small-gauge needle may be effective. Following injection, the patient should be advised to rest the arm for at least one month and avoid activities that would aggravate the elbow. Once symptoms have subsided, the patient should begin rehabilitation to strengthen and increase flexibility of the extensor muscles before resuming physical activity involving the arm. A forearm band placed 2.5–5.0 cm (1–2 in.) below the elbow may help to reduce tension on the extensor muscles at their attachment to the lateral epicondyle. The patient should be advised to restrict activities requiring forcible extension and supination of the wrist. Improvement may take several months. The patient may continue to experience mild pain but, with care, can usually avoid the return of debilitating pain. Occasionally, surgical release of the extensor aponeurosis may be necessary.

MEDIAL EPICONDYLITIS

Medial epicondylitis is an overuse syndrome resulting in pain over the medial side of the elbow with radiation into the forearm. The cause of this syndrome is considered to be repetitive resisted motions of wrist flexion and pronation, which lead to microtears and granulation tissue at the origin of the pronator teres and forearm flexors, particularly the flexor carpi radialis. This overuse syndrome is usually seen in patients >35 years and is much less common than lateral epicondylitis. It occurs most often in work-related repetitive activities but also occurs with recreational activities such as swinging a golf club (golfer's elbow) or throwing a baseball. On physical examination, there is tenderness just distal to the medial epicondyle over the origin of the forearm flexors. Pain can be reproduced by resisting wrist flexion and pronation with the elbow extended. Radiographs are usually normal. The differential diagnosis of patients with medial elbow symptoms include tears of the pronator teres, acute medial collateral ligament tear, and medial collateral ligament instability. Ulnar neuritis has been found in 25–50% of patients with medial epicondylitis and is associated with tenderness over the ulnar nerve at the elbow as well as hypesthesia and paresthesia on the ulnar side of the hand.

The initial treatment of medial epicondylitis is conservative, involving rest, NSAIDs, friction massage, ultrasound, and icing. Some patients may require splinting. Injections of glucocorticoids at the painful site may also be effective. Patients should be instructed to rest for at least one month. Also, patients should start physical therapy once the pain has subsided. In patients with chronic debilitating medial epicondylitis that remains unresponsive after at least a year of treatment, surgical release of the flexor muscle at its origin may be necessary and is often successful.

PLANTAR FASCIITIS

Plantar fasciitis is a common cause of foot pain in adults, with the peak incidence occurring in people between the ages of 40 and 60 years. It is also seen more frequently in a younger population consisting of runners, aerobic exercise dancers, and ballet dancers. The pain originates at or near the site of the plantar fascia attachment to the medial tuberosity of the calcaneus. Several factors that increase the risk of developing plantar fasciitis include obesity, pes planus (flat foot or absence of the foot arch when standing), pes cavus (high-arched foot), limited dorsiflexion of the ankle, prolonged standing, walking on hard surfaces, and faulty shoes. In runners, excessive running and a change to a harder running surface may precipitate plantar fasciitis.

The diagnosis of plantar fasciitis can usually be made on the basis of history and physical examination alone. Patients experience severe pain with the first steps on arising in the morning or following inactivity during the day. The pain usually lessens with weight-bearing activity during the day, only to worsen with continued activity. Pain is made worse on walking barefoot or up stairs. On examination, maximal tenderness is elicited on palpation over the inferior heel corresponding to the site of attachment of the plantar fascia.

Imaging studies may be indicated when the diagnosis is not clear. Plain radiographs may show heel spurs, which are of little diagnostic significance. Ultrasonography in plantar fasciitis can demonstrate thickening of the fascia and diffuse hypoechogenicity, indicating edema at the attachment of the plantar fascia to the calcaneus. MRI is a sensitive method for detecting plantar fasciitis, but it is usually not required for establishing the diagnosis.

The differential diagnosis of inferior heel pain includes calcaneal stress fractures, the spondyloarthritides, rheumatoid arthritis, gout, neoplastic or infiltrative bone processes, and nerve compression/entrapment syndromes.

Resolution of symptoms occurs within 12 months in more than 80% of patients with plantar fasciitis. The patient is advised to reduce or discontinue activities that can exacerbate plantar fasciitis. Initial treatment consists of ice, heat, massage, and stretching. Stretching of the plantar fascia and calf muscles are commonly employed and can be beneficial. Orthotics provide medial arch support and can be effective. Foot strapping or taping are commonly performed, and some patients may benefit by wearing a night splint designed to keep the ankle in a neutral position. A short course of NSAIDs can be given to patients when the benefits outweigh the risks. Local glucocorticoid injections have also been shown to be efficacious but may carry an increased risk for plantar fascia rupture. Plantar fasciotomy is reserved for those patients who have failed to improve after at least 6–12 months of conservative treatment.

FURTHER READINGS

Buchbinder R: Plantar fasciitis. N Engl J Med 350:2159, 2004

Husni EM, Donohue JP: Painful shoulder and reflex sympathetic dystrophy syndrome, in *Arthritis and Allied Conditions*, 15th ed, WJ Koopman (ed). Philadelphia, Lippincott Williams & Wilkins, 2005, pp 2133–2152

Martin SD, Thornhill TS: Shoulder pain, in *Kelley's Textbook of Rheumatology*, 7th ed, ED Harris et al (eds). Philadelphia, Saunders, 2005, pp 557–587

Matsen FA 3rd. Clinical practice. Rotator-cuff failure. N Engl J Med 358:2138, 2008

Neer CS II: Impingement lesions. Clin Orthop 173:70, 1983

Sheridan MA, Hannafin JA. Upper extremity: emphasis on frozen shoulder. Orthop Clin North Am 37:531, 2006

PART 16

Endocrinology and Metabolism

SECTION 1 Endocrinology

SECTION 2 Disorders of Bone and Mineral Metabolism

SECTION 3 Disorders of Intermediary Metabolism

CHAPTER 338

Principles of Endocrinology

J. Larry Jameson

The management of endocrine disorders requires a broad understanding of intermediary metabolism, reproductive physiology, bone metabolism, and growth. Accordingly, the practice of endocrinology is intimately linked to a conceptual framework for understanding hormone secretion, hormone action, and principles of feedback control. The endocrine system is evaluated primarily by measuring hormone concentrations, arming the clinician with valuable diagnostic information. Most disorders of the endocrine system are amenable to effective treatment once the correct diagnosis is determined. Endocrine deficiency disorders are treated with physiologic hormone replacement; hormone excess conditions, which usually are due to benign glandular adenomas, are managed by removing tumors surgically or reducing hormone levels medically.

SCOPE OF ENDOCRINOLOGY

The specialty of endocrinology encompasses the study of glands and the hormones they produce. The term *endocrine* was coined by Starling to contrast the actions of hormones secreted internally (*endocrine*) with those secreted externally (*exocrine*) or into a lumen, such as the gastrointestinal tract. The term *hormone*, derived from a Greek phrase meaning "to set in motion," aptly describes the dynamic actions of hormones as they elicit cellular responses and regulate physiologic processes through feedback mechanisms.

Unlike many other specialties in medicine, it is not possible to define endocrinology strictly along anatomic lines. The classic endocrine glands—pituitary, thyroid, parathyroid, pancreatic islets, adrenals, and gonads—communicate broadly with other organs through the nervous system, hormones, cytokines, and growth factors. In addition to its traditional synaptic functions, the brain produces a vast array of peptide hormones, and this has led to the discipline of neuroendocrinology. Through the production of hypothalamic releasing factors, the central nervous system (CNS) exerts a major regulatory influence over pituitary hormone secretion (Chap. 339). The peripheral nervous system stimulates the adrenal medulla. The immune and endocrine systems are also intimately intertwined. The adrenal hormone cortisol is a powerful immunosuppressant. Cytokines and interleukins (ILs) have profound effects on the functions of the pituitary, adrenal, thyroid, and gonads. Common endocrine diseases such as autoimmune thyroid disease and Type 1 diabetes mellitus are caused by dysregulation of immune surveillance and tolerance. Less common diseases such as polyglandular failure, Addison's disease, and lymphocytic hypophysitis also have an immunologic basis.

The interdigitation of endocrinology with physiologic processes in other specialties sometimes blurs the role of hormones. For example, hormones play an important role in maintenance of blood pressure, intravascular volume, and peripheral resistance in the cardiovascular system. Vasoactive substances such as catecholamines, angiotensin II, endothelin, and nitric oxide are involved in dynamic changes of vascular tone in addition to their multiple roles in other tissues. The heart is the principal source of atrial natriuretic peptide, which acts in classic endocrine fashion to induce natriuresis at a distant target organ (the kidney). Erythropoietin, a traditional circulating hormone, is made in the kidney and stimulates erythropoiesis in bone marrow (Chap. 57). The kidney is also integrally involved in the renin-angiotensin axis (Chap. 342) and is a primary target of several hormones, including parathyroid hormone (PTH), mineralocorticoids, and vasopressin. The gastrointestinal tract produces a surprising number of peptide hormones, such as cholecystokinin, ghrelin, gastrin, secretin, and vasoactive intestinal peptide, among many others. Adipose tissue produces leptin, which acts centrally to control appetite. Carcinoid and islet tumors can secrete excessive amounts of these hormones, leading to specific clinical syndromes (Chap. 350). Many of these gastrointestinal hormones are also produced in the CNS, where their functions are poorly understood. As hormones such as inhibin, ghrelin, and leptin are discovered, they become integrated into the science and practice of medicine on the basis of their functional roles rather than their tissues of origin.

Characterization of hormone receptors frequently reveals unexpected relationships to factors in nonendocrine disciplines. The growth hormone (GH) and leptin receptors, for example, are members of the cytokine receptor family. The G protein–coupled receptors (GPCRs), which mediate the actions of many peptide hormones, are used in numerous physiologic processes, including vision, smell, and neurotransmission.

NATURE OF HORMONES

Hormones can be divided into five major classes: (1) *amino acid derivatives* such as dopamine, catecholamine, and thyroid hormone; (2) *small neuropeptides* such as gonadotropin-releasing hormone (GnRH), thyrotropin-releasing hormone (TRH), somatostatin, and vasopressin; (3) *large proteins* such as insulin, luteinizing hormone (LH), and PTH produced by classic endocrine glands; (4) *steroid hormones* such as cortisol and estrogen that are synthesized from cholesterol-based precursors; and (5) *vitamin derivatives* such as retinoids (vitamin A) and vitamin D. A variety of *peptide growth factors*, most of which act locally, share actions with hormones. As a rule, amino acid derivatives and peptide hormones interact with cell-surface membrane receptors. Steroids, thyroid hormones, vitamin D, and retinoids are lipid-soluble and interact with intracellular nuclear receptors.

HORMONE AND RECEPTOR FAMILIES

Many hormones and receptors can be grouped into families, reflecting their structural similarities (Table 338-1). The evolution of these families generates diverse but highly selective pathways of hormone action. Recognition of these relationships allows extrapolation of information gleaned from one hormone or receptor to other family members.

The glycoprotein hormone family, consisting of thyroid-stimulating hormone (TSH), follicle-stimulating hormone (FSH), LH, and human chorionic gonadotropin (hCG), illustrates many features of related hormones. The glycoprotein hormones are heterodimers that have the α subunit in common; the β subunits are distinct

TABLE 338-1 Membrane Receptor Families and Signaling Pathways

Receptors	Effectors	Signaling Pathways
G Protein–Coupled Seven-Transmembrane (GPCR)		
β-Adrenergic LH, FSH, TSH	$G_s\alpha$, adenylate cyclase	Stimulation of cyclic AMP production, protein kinase A
Glucagon PTH, PTHrP ACTH, MSH GHRH, CRH	Ca^{2+} channels	Calmodulin, Ca^{2+}-dependent kinases
α-Adrenergic Somatostatin	$G_i\alpha$	Inhibition of cyclic AMP production Activation of K^+, Ca^{2+} channels
TRH, GnRH	G_q, G_{11}	Phospholipase C, diacylglycerol, IP_3, protein kinase C, voltage-dependent Ca^{2+} channels
Receptor Tyrosine Kinase		
Insulin, IGF-I	Tyrosine kinases, IRS	MAP kinases, PI 3-kinase; AKT, also known as protein kinase B, PKB
EGF, NGF	Tyrosine kinases, ras	Raf, MAP kinases, RSK
Cytokine Receptor–Linked Kinase		
GH, PRL	JAK, tyrosine kinases	STAT, MAP kinase, PI 3-kinase, IRS-1
Serine Kinase		
Activin, TGF-β, MIS	Serine kinase	Smads

Abbreviations: IP_3, inositol triphosphate; IRS, insulin receptor substrates; MAP, mitogen-activated protein; MSH, melanocyte-stimulating hormone; NGF, nerve growth factor; PI, phosphatidylinositol; RSK, ribosomal S6 kinase; TGF-β, transforming growth factor β. For all other abbreviations, see text.

and confer specific biologic actions. The overall three-dimensional architecture of the β subunits is similar, reflecting the locations of conserved disulfide bonds that restrain protein conformation. The cloning of the β-subunit genes from multiple species suggests that this family arose from a common ancestral gene, probably by gene duplication and subsequent divergence to evolve new biologic functions.

As the hormone families enlarge and diverge, their receptors must co-evolve if new biologic functions are to be derived. Related GPCRs, for example, have evolved for each of the glycoprotein hormones. These receptors are structurally similar, and each is coupled to the $G_s\alpha$ signaling pathway. However, there is minimal overlap of hormone binding. For example, TSH binds with high specificity to the TSH receptor but interacts minimally with the LH or the FSH receptor. Nonetheless, there can be subtle physiologic consequences of hormone cross-reactivity with other receptors. Very high levels of hCG during pregnancy stimulate the TSH receptor and increase thyroid hormone levels, resulting in a compensatory decrease in TSH.

Insulin and insulin-like growth factor I (IGF-I) and IGF-II have structural similarities that are most apparent when precursor forms of the proteins are compared. In contrast to the high degree of specificity seen with the glycoprotein hormones, there is moderate cross-talk among the members of the insulin/IGF family. High concentrations of an IGF-II precursor produced by certain tumors (e.g., sarcomas) can cause hypoglycemia, partly because of binding to insulin and IGF-I receptors (Chap. 100). High concentrations of insulin also bind to the IGF-I receptor, perhaps accounting for some of the clinical manifestations seen in severe insulin resistance.

Another important example of receptor cross-talk is seen with PTH and parathyroid hormone–related peptide (PTHrP) (Chap. 353). PTH is produced by the parathyroid glands, whereas PTHrP is expressed at high levels during development and by a variety of tumors (Chap. 100). These hormones have amino acid sequence similarity, particularly in their amino-terminal regions. Both hormones bind to a single PTH receptor that is expressed in bone and kidney. Hypercalcemia and hypophosphatemia therefore may result from excessive production of either hormone, making it difficult to distinguish hyperparathyroidism from hypercalcemia of malignancy solely on the basis of serum chemistries. However, sensitive and specific assays for PTH and PTHrP now allow these disorders to be distinguished more readily.

Based on their specificities for DNA binding sites, the nuclear receptor family can be subdivided into type 1 receptors (GR, MR, AR, ER, PR) that bind steroids and type 2 receptors (TR, VDR, RAR, PPAR) that bind thyroid hormone, vitamin D, retinoic acid, or lipid derivatives. Certain functional domains in nuclear receptors, such as the zinc finger DNA-binding domains, are highly conserved. However, selective amino acid differences within this domain confer DNA sequence specificity. The hormone-binding domains are more variable, providing great diversity in the array of small molecules that bind to different nuclear receptors. With few exceptions, hormone binding is highly specific for a single type of nuclear receptor. One exception involves the glucocorticoid and mineralocorticoid receptors. Because the mineralocorticoid receptor also binds glucocorticoids with high affinity, an enzyme (11β-hydroxysteroid dehydrogenase) in renal tubular cells inactivates glucocorticoids, allowing selective responses to mineralocorticoids such as aldosterone. However, when very high glucocorticoid concentrations occur, as in Cushing's syndrome, the glucocorticoid degradation pathway becomes saturated, allowing excessive cortisol levels to exert mineralocorticoid effects (sodium retention, potassium wasting). This phenomenon is particularly pronounced in ectopic adrenocorticotropic hormone (ACTH) syndromes (Chap. 342). Another example of relaxed nuclear receptor specificity involves the estrogen receptor, which can bind an array of compounds, some of which have little apparent structural similarity to the high-affinity ligand estradiol. This feature of the estrogen receptor makes it susceptible to activation by "environmental estrogens" such as resveratrol, octylphenol, and many other aromatic hydrocarbons. However, this lack of specificity provides an opportunity to synthesize a remarkable series of clinically useful antagonists (e.g., tamoxifen) and selective estrogen response modulators (SERMs) such as raloxifene. These compounds generate distinct conformations that alter receptor interactions with components of the transcription machinery (see below), thereby conferring their unique actions.

HORMONE SYNTHESIS AND PROCESSING

The synthesis of peptide hormones and their receptors occurs through a classic pathway of gene expression: transcription → mRNA → protein → posttranslational protein processing → intracellular sorting, followed by membrane integration or secretion (Chap. 61).

Many hormones are embedded within larger precursor polypeptides that are proteolytically processed to yield the biologically active hormone. Examples include proopiomelanocortin (POMC) → ACTH; proglucagon → glucagon; proinsulin → insulin; and pro-PTH → PTH, among others. In many cases, such as POMC and proglucagon, these precursors generate multiple biologically active peptides. It is provocative that hormone precursors are typically inactive, presumably adding an additional level of regulatory control. Prohormone conversion occurs not only for peptide hormones but also for certain steroids (testosterone → dihydrotestosterone) and thyroid hormone ($T_4 \rightarrow T_3$).

Hormone precursor processing is intimately linked to intracellular sorting pathways that transport proteins to appropriate vesicles and enzymes, resulting in specific cleavage steps, followed by protein folding and translocation to secretory vesicles. Hormones destined for secretion are translocated across the endoplasmic reticulum under the guidance of an amino-terminal signal sequence that subsequently is cleaved. Cell-surface receptors are inserted into the membrane via short segments of hydrophobic amino acids that remain embedded within the lipid bilayer. During translocation through the Golgi and endoplasmic reticulum, hormones and receptors are also subject to a variety of posttranslational modifications, such as glycosylation and phosphorylation, which can alter protein conformation, modify circulating half-life, and alter biologic activity.

Synthesis of most steroid hormones is based on modifications of the precursor, cholesterol. Multiple regulated enzymatic steps are required for the synthesis of testosterone (Chap. 346), estradiol (Chap. 347), cortisol (Chap. 342), and vitamin D (Chap. 352). This large number of synthetic steps predisposes to multiple genetic and acquired disorders of steroidogenesis.

Although endocrine genes contain regulatory DNA elements similar to those found in many other genes, their exquisite control by other hormones also necessitates the presence of specific hormone response elements. For example, the TSH genes are repressed directly by thyroid hormones acting through the thyroid hormone receptor (TR), a member of the nuclear receptor family. Steroidogenic enzyme gene expression requires specific transcription factors, such as steroidogenic factor-1 (SF-1), acting in conjunction with signals transmitted by trophic hormones (e.g., ACTH or LH). For some hormones, substantial regulation occurs at the level of translational efficiency. Insulin biosynthesis, although it requires ongoing gene transcription, is regulated primarily at the translational level in response to elevated levels of glucose or amino acids.

HORMONE SECRETION, TRANSPORT, AND DEGRADATION

The circulating level of a hormone is determined by its rate of secretion and its circulating half-life. After protein processing, peptide hormones (GnRH, insulin, GH) are stored in secretory granules. As these granules mature, they are poised beneath the plasma membrane for imminent release into the circulation. In most instances, the stimulus for hormone secretion is a releasing factor or neural signal that induces rapid changes in intracellular calcium concentrations, leading to secretory granule fusion with the plasma membrane and release of its contents into the extracellular environment and bloodstream. Steroid hormones, in contrast, diffuse into the circulation as they are synthesized. Thus, their secretory rates are closely aligned with rates of synthesis. For example, ACTH and LH induce steroidogenesis by stimulating the activity of *st*eroidogenic *a*cute *r*egulatory (StAR) protein (transports cholesterol into the mitochondrion) along with other rate-limiting steps (e.g., cholesterol side-chain cleavage enzyme, CYP11A1) in the steroidogenic pathway.

Hormone transport and degradation dictate the rapidity with which a hormonal signal decays. Some hormonal signals are evanescent (e.g., somatostatin), whereas others are longer-lived (e.g., TSH). Because somatostatin exerts effects in virtually every tissue, a short half-life allows its concentrations and actions to be controlled locally. Structural modifications that impair somatostatin degradation have been useful for generating long-acting therapeutic analogues such as octreotide (Chap. 339). In contrast, the actions of TSH are highly specific for the thyroid gland. Its prolonged half-life accounts for relatively constant serum levels even though TSH is secreted in discrete pulses.

An understanding of circulating hormone half-life is important for achieving physiologic hormone replacement, as the frequency of dosing and the time required to reach steady state are intimately linked to rates of hormone decay. T4, for example, has a circulating half-life of 7 days. Consequently, >1 month is required to reach a new steady state, and single daily doses are sufficient to achieve constant hormone levels. T_3, in contrast, has a half-life of 1 day. Its administration is associated with more dynamic serum levels, and it must be administered two to three times per day. Similarly, synthetic glucocorticoids vary widely in their half-lives; those with longer half-lives (e.g., dexamethasone) are associated with greater suppression of the hypothalamic-pituitary-adrenal (HPA) axis. Most protein hormones [e.g., ACTH, GH, prolactin (PRL), PTH, LH] have relatively short half-lives (<20 min), leading to sharp peaks of secretion and decay. The only accurate way to profile the pulse frequency and amplitude of these hormones is to measure levels in frequently sampled blood (every 10 min or less) over long durations (8–24 h). Because this is not practical in a clinical setting, an alternative strategy is to pool three to four samples drawn at about 30-min intervals or interpret the results in the context of a relatively wide normal range. Rapid hormone decay is useful in certain clinical settings. For example, the short half-life of PTH allows the use of intraoperative PTH determinations to confirm successful removal of an adenoma. This is particularly valuable diagnostically when there is a possibility of multicentric disease or parathyroid hyperplasia, as occurs with multiple endocrine neoplasia (MEN) or renal insufficiency.

Many hormones circulate in association with serum-binding proteins. Examples include (1) T_4 and T_3 binding to thyroxine-binding globulin (TBG), albumin, and thyroxine-binding prealbumin (TBPA); (2) cortisol binding to cortisol-binding globulin (CBG); (3) androgen and estrogen binding to sex hormone–binding globulin (SHBG) [also called testosterone-binding globulin (TeBG)]; (4) IGF-I and -II binding to multiple IGF-binding proteins (IGFBPs); (5) GH interactions with GH-binding protein (GHBP), a circulating fragment of the GH receptor extracellular domain; and (6) activin binding to follistatin. These interactions provide a hormonal reservoir, prevent otherwise rapid degradation of unbound hormones, restrict hormone access to certain sites (e.g., IGFBPs), and modulate the unbound, or "free," hormone concentrations. Although a variety of binding protein abnormalities have been identified, most have few clinical consequences aside from creating diagnostic problems. For example, TBG deficiency can reduce total thyroid hormone levels greatly, but the free concentrations of T_4 and T_3 remain normal. Liver disease and certain medications can also influence binding protein levels (e.g., estrogen increases TBG) or cause displacement of hormones from binding proteins (e.g., salsalate displaces T_4 from TBG). In general, only unbound hormone is available to interact with receptors and thus elicit a biologic response. Short-term perturbations in binding proteins change the free hormone concentration, which in turn induces compensatory adaptations through feedback loops. SHBG changes in women are an exception to this self-correcting mechanism. When SHBG decreases because of insulin resistance or androgen excess, the unbound testosterone concentration is increased, potentially leading to hirsutism (Chap. 49). The increased unbound testosterone level does not result in an adequate compensatory feedback correction because estrogen, not testosterone, is the primary regulator of the reproductive axis.

An additional exception to the unbound hormone hypothesis involves megalin, a member of the low-density lipoprotein (LDL) receptor family that serves as an endocytotic receptor for carrier-bound vitamins A and D and SHBG-bound androgens and estrogens. After internalization, the carrier proteins are degraded in lysosomes and release their bound ligands within the cells. Membrane transporters have also been identified for thyroid hormones.

Hormone degradation can be an important mechanism for regulating concentrations locally. As noted above, 11β-hydroxysteroid dehydrogenase inactivates glucocorticoids in renal tubular cells, preventing actions through the mineralocorticoid receptor. Thyroid hormone deiodinases convert T_4 to T_3 and can inactivate T_3. During development, degradation of retinoic acid by Cyp26b1 prevents primordial germ cells in the male from entering meiosis, as occurs in the female ovary.

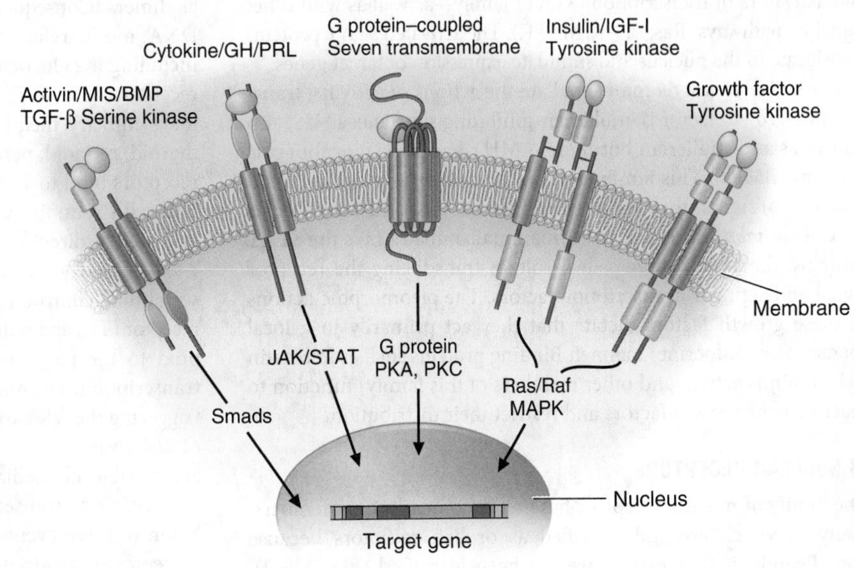

Figure 338-1 Membrane receptor signaling. MAPK, mitogen-activated protein kinase; PKA, -C, protein kinase A, C; TGF, transforming growth factor. For other abbreviations, see text.

HORMONE ACTION THROUGH RECEPTORS

Receptors for hormones are divided into two major classes: membrane and nuclear. *Membrane receptors* primarily bind peptide hormones and catecholamines. *Nuclear receptors* bind small molecules that can diffuse across the cell membrane, such as steroids and vitamin D. Certain general principles apply to hormone-receptor interactions regardless of the class of receptor. Hormones bind to receptors with specificity and an affinity that generally coincides with the dynamic range of circulating hormone concentrations. Low concentrations of free hormone (usually 10^{-12} to 10^{-9} *M*) rapidly associate and dissociate from receptors in a bimolecular reaction such that the occupancy of the receptor at any given moment is a function of hormone concentration and the receptor's affinity for the hormone. Receptor numbers vary greatly in different target tissues, providing one of the major determinants of specific cellular responses to circulating hormones. For example, ACTH receptors are located almost exclusively in the adrenal cortex, and FSH receptors are found predominantely in the gonads. In contrast, insulin and TRs are widely distributed, reflecting the need for metabolic responses in all tissues.

MEMBRANE RECEPTORS

Membrane receptors for hormones can be divided into several major groups: (1) seven transmembrane GPCRs, (2) tyrosine kinase receptors, (3) cytokine receptors, and (4) serine kinase receptors (Fig. 338-1). The *seven transmembrane GPCR family* binds a remarkable array of hormones, including large proteins (e.g., LH, PTH), small peptides (e.g., TRH, somatostatin), catecholamines (epinephrine, dopamine), and even minerals (e.g., calcium). The extracellular domains of GPCRs vary widely in size and are the major binding site for large hormones. The transmembrane-spanning regions are composed of hydrophobic α-helical domains that traverse the lipid bilayer. Like some channels, these domains are thought to circularize and form a hydrophobic pocket into which certain small ligands fit. Hormone binding induces conformational changes in these domains, transducing structural changes to the intracellular domain, which is a docking site for G proteins.

The large family of *G proteins*, so named because they bind guanine nucleotides [guanosine triphosphate (GTP), guanosine diphosphate (GDP)], provides great diversity for coupling receptors to different signaling pathways. G proteins form a heterotrimeric complex that is composed of various α and βγ subunits. The α subunit contains the guanine nucleotide–binding site and hydrolyzes GTP → GDP. The βγ subunits are tightly associated and modulate the activity of the α subunit as well as mediating their own effector signaling pathways. G protein activity is regulated by a cycle that involves GTP hydrolysis and dynamic interactions between the α and αβ subunits. Hormone binding to the receptor induces GDP dissociation, allowing Gα to bind GTP and dissociate from the αβ complex. Under these conditions, the Gα subunit is activated and mediates signal transduction through various enzymes, such as adenylate cyclase and phospholipase C. GTP hydrolysis to GDP allows reassociation with the αβ subunits and restores the inactive state. As described below, a variety of endocrinopathies result from G protein mutations or from mutations in receptors that modify their interactions with G proteins. G proteins interact with other cellular proteins, including kinases, channels, G protein–coupled receptor kinases (GRKs), and arrestins, that mediate signaling as well as receptor desensitization and recycling.

The *tyrosine kinase receptors* transduce signals for insulin and a variety of growth factors, such as IGF-I, epidermal growth factor (EGF), nerve growth factor, platelet-derived growth factor, and fibroblast growth factor. The cysteine-rich extracellular ligand-binding domains contain growth factor binding sites. After ligand binding, this class of receptors undergoes autophosphorylation, inducing interactions with intracellular adaptor proteins such as Shc and insulin receptor substrates. In the case of the insulin receptor, multiple kinases are activated, including the Raf-Ras-MAPK and the Akt/protein kinase B pathways. The tyrosine kinase receptors play a prominent role in cell growth and differentiation as well as in intermediary metabolism.

The GH and PRL receptors belong to the *cytokine receptor* family. Analogous to the tyrosine kinase receptors, ligand binding induces receptor interaction with intracellular kinases—the Janus kinases (JAKs), which phosphorylate members of the signal transduction and activators of transcription (STAT) family—as well as with other signaling pathways (Ras, PI3-K, MAPK). The activated STAT proteins translocate to the nucleus and stimulate expression of target genes.

The *serine kinase receptors* mediate the actions of activins, transforming growth factor β, müllerian-inhibiting substance (MIS, also known as anti-müllerian hormone, AMH), and bone morphogenic proteins (BMPs). This family of receptors (consisting of type I and II subunits) signals through proteins termed *smads* (fusion of terms for *Caenorhabditis elegans* sma + mammalian mad). Like the STAT proteins, the smads serve a dual role of transducing the receptor signal and acting as transcription factors. The pleomorphic actions of these growth factors dictate that they act primarily in a local (paracrine or autocrine) manner. Binding proteins such as follistatin (which binds activin and other members of this family) function to inactivate the growth factors and restrict their distribution.

NUCLEAR RECEPTORS

The family of nuclear receptors has grown to nearly 100 members, many of which are still classified as orphan receptors because their ligands, if they exist, have not been identified (Fig. 338-2). Otherwise, most nuclear receptors are classified on the basis of the nature of their ligands. Though all nuclear receptors ultimately act to increase or decrease gene transcription, some (e.g., glucocorticoid receptor) reside primarily in the cytoplasm, whereas others (e.g., thyroid hormone receptor) are always located in the nucleus. After ligand binding, the cytoplasmically localized receptors translocate to the nucleus. There is growing evidence that certain nuclear receptors (e.g., glucocorticoid, estrogen) can also act at the membrane or in the cytoplasm to activate or repress signal transduction pathways, providing a mechanism for cross-talk between membrane and nuclear receptors.

The structures of nuclear receptors have been studied extensively, including by x-ray crystallography. The DNA binding domain, consisting of two zinc fingers, contacts specific DNA recognition sequences in target genes. Most nuclear receptors bind to DNA as dimers. Consequently, each monomer recognizes an individual DNA motif, referred to as a "half-site." The steroid receptors, including the glucocorticoid, estrogen, progesterone, and androgen receptors, bind to DNA as homodimers. Consistent with this twofold symmetry, their DNA recognition half-sites are palindromic. The thyroid, retinoid, peroxisome proliferator activated, and vitamin D receptors bind to DNA preferentially as heterodimers in combination with retinoid X receptors (RXRs). Their DNA half-sites are arranged as direct repeats.

The carboxy-terminal hormone-binding domain mediates transcriptional control. For type II receptors such as thyroid hormone receptor (TR) and retinoic acid receptor (RAR), co-repressor proteins bind to the receptor in the absence of ligand and silence gene transcription. Hormone binding induces conformational changes, triggering the release of co-repressors and inducing the recruitment of coactivators that stimulate transcription. Thus, these receptors are capable of mediating dramatic changes in the level of gene activity. Certain disease states are associated with defective regulation of these events. For example, mutations in the TR prevent co-repressor dissociation, resulting in a dominant form of hormone resistance (Chap. 341). In promyelocytic leukemia, fusion of RARα to other nuclear proteins causes aberrant gene silencing and prevents normal cellular differentiation. Treatment with retinoic acid reverses this repression and allows cellular differentiation and apoptosis to occur. Most type 1 steroid receptors interact weakly with co-repressors, but ligand binding still induces interactions with an array of coactivators. X-ray crystallography shows that various SERMs induce distinct estrogen receptor conformations. The tissue-specific responses caused by these agents in breast, bone, and uterus appear to reflect distinct interactions with coactivators. The receptor-coactivator complex stimulates gene transcription by several pathways, including (1) recruitment of enzymes (histone acetyl transferases) that modify chromatin structure, (2) interactions with additional transcription factors on the target gene, and (3) direct interactions with components of the general transcription apparatus to enhance the rate of RNA polymerase II–mediated transcription. Studies of nuclear receptor-mediated transcription show that these are dynamic events that involve relatively rapid (e.g., 30–60 min) cycling of transcription complexes on any specific target gene.

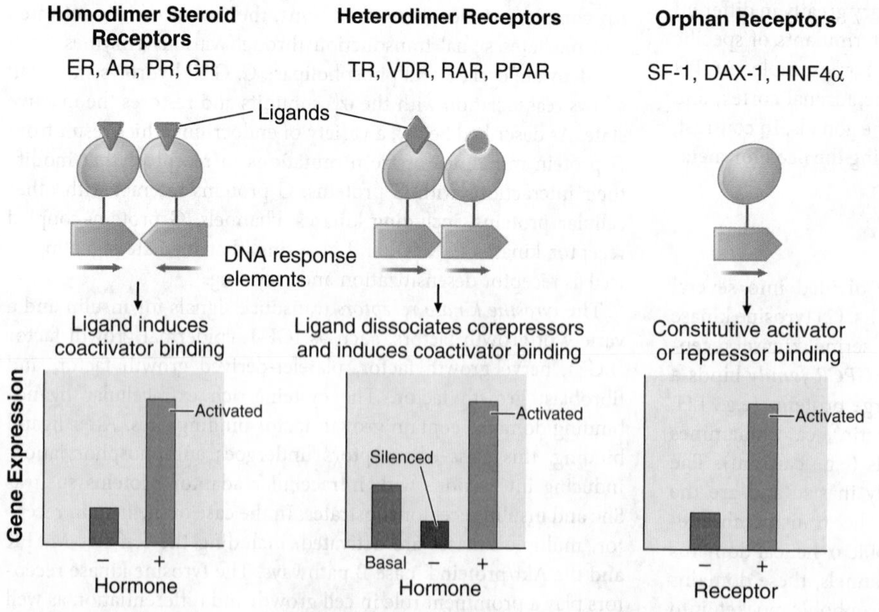

Figure 338-2 Nuclear receptor signaling. ER, estrogen receptor; AR, androgen receptor; PR, progesterone receptor; GR, glucocorticoid receptor; TR, thyroid hormone receptor; VDR, vitamin D receptor; RAR, retinoic acid receptor; PPAR, peroxisome proliferator activated receptor; SF-1, steroidogenic factor-1; DAX, *d*osage-sensitive sex-reversal, *a*drenal hypoplasia congenita, *X*-chromosome; HNF4α, hepatic nuclear factor 4α.

FUNCTIONS OF HORMONES

The functions of individual hormones are described in detail in subsequent chapters. Nevertheless, it is useful to illustrate how most biologic responses require integration of several different hormone pathways. The physiologic functions of hormones can be divided into three general areas: (1) growth and differentiation, (2) maintenance of homeostasis, and (3) reproduction.

GROWTH

Multiple hormones and nutritional factors mediate the complex phenomenon of growth (Chap. 339). Short stature may be caused by GH deficiency, hypothyroidism, Cushing's syndrome, precocious puberty, malnutrition, chronic illness, or genetic abnormalities that affect the epiphyseal growth plates (e.g., *FGFR3* and *SHOX* mutations). Many factors (GH, IGF-I, thyroid hormones) stimulate growth, whereas others (sex steroids) lead to epiphyseal closure. Understanding these hormonal interactions is important in the diagnosis and management of growth disorders. For example, delaying exposure to high levels of sex steroids may enhance the efficacy of GH treatment.

MAINTENANCE OF HOMEOSTASIS

Though virtually all hormones affect homeostasis, the most important among them are the following:

1. Thyroid hormone—controls about 25% of basal metabolism in most tissues
2. Cortisol—exerts a permissive action for many hormones in addition to its own direct effects
3. PTH—regulates calcium and phosphorus levels
4. Vasopressin—regulates serum osmolality by controlling renal free-water clearance
5. Mineralocorticoids—control vascular volume and serum electrolyte (Na^+, K^+) concentrations
6. Insulin—maintains euglycemia in the fed and fasted states

The defense against hypoglycemia is an impressive example of integrated hormone action (Chap. 345). In response to the fasted state and falling blood glucose, insulin secretion is suppressed, resulting in decreased glucose uptake and enhanced glycogenolysis, lipolysis, proteolysis, and gluconeogenesis to mobilize fuel sources. If hypoglycemia develops (usually from insulin administration or sulfonylureas), an orchestrated counterregulatory response occurs—glucagon and epinephrine rapidly stimulate glycogenolysis and gluconeogenesis, whereas GH and cortisol act over several hours to raise glucose levels and antagonize insulin action.

Although free-water clearance is controlled primarily by vasopressin, cortisol and thyroid hormone are also important for facilitating renal tubular responses to vasopressin (Chap. 340). PTH and vitamin D function in an interdependent manner to control calcium metabolism (Chap. 352). PTH stimulates renal synthesis of 1,25-dihydroxyvitamin D, which increases calcium absorption in the gastrointestinal tract and enhances PTH action in bone. Increased calcium, along with vitamin D, feeds back to suppress PTH, thus maintaining calcium balance.

Depending on the severity of a specific stress and whether it is acute or chronic, multiple endocrine and cytokine pathways are activated to mount an appropriate physiologic response. In severe acute stress such as trauma or shock, the sympathetic nervous system is activated and catecholamines are released, leading to increased cardiac output and a primed musculoskeletal system. Catecholamines also increase mean blood pressure and stimulate glucose production. Multiple stress-induced pathways converge on the hypothalamus, stimulating several hormones, including vasopressin and corticotropin-releasing hormone (CRH). These hormones, in addition to cytokines (tumor necrosis factor α, IL-2, IL-6), increase ACTH and GH production. ACTH stimulates the adrenal gland, increasing cortisol, which in turn helps sustain blood pressure and dampen the inflammatory response. Increased vasopressin acts to conserve free water.

REPRODUCTION

The stages of reproduction include (1) sex determination during fetal development (Chap. 349); (2) sexual maturation during puberty (Chaps. 346 and 347); (3) conception, pregnancy, lactation, and child rearing (Chap. 347); and (4) cessation of reproductive capability at menopause (Chap. 348). Each of these stages involves an orchestrated interplay of multiple hormones, a phenomenon well illustrated by the dynamic hormonal changes that occur during each 28-day menstrual cycle. In the early follicular phase, pulsatile secretion of LH and FSH stimulates the progressive maturation of the ovarian follicle. This results in gradually increasing estrogen and progesterone levels, leading to enhanced pituitary sensitivity to GnRH, which, when combined with accelerated GnRH secretion, triggers the LH surge and rupture of the mature follicle. Inhibin, a protein produced by the granulosa cells, enhances follicular growth and feeds back to the pituitary to selectively suppress FSH without affecting LH. Growth factors such as EGF and IGF-I modulate follicular responsiveness to gonadotropins. Vascular endothelial growth factor and prostaglandins play a role in follicle vascularization and rupture.

During pregnancy, the increased production of prolactin, in combination with placentally derived steroids (e.g., estrogen and progesterone), prepares the breast for lactation. Estrogens induce the production of progesterone receptors, allowing for increased responsiveness to progesterone. In addition to these and other hormones involved in lactation, the nervous system and oxytocin mediate the suckling response and milk release.

HORMONAL FEEDBACK REGULATORY SYSTEMS

Feedback control, both negative and positive, is a fundamental feature of endocrine systems. Each of the major hypothalamic-pituitary-hormone axes is governed by negative feedback, a process that maintains hormone levels within a relatively narrow range (Chap. 339). Examples of hypothalamic-pituitary negative feedback include (1) thyroid hormones on the TRH-TSH axis, (2) cortisol on the CRH-ACTH axis, (3) gonadal steroids on the GnRH-LH/FSH axis, and (4) IGF-I on the growth hormone–releasing hormone (GHRH)-GH axis (Fig. 338-3). These regulatory loops include both positive (e.g., TRH, TSH) and negative (e.g., T_4, T_3) components, allowing for exquisite control of hormone levels. As an example, a small reduction of thyroid hormone triggers a rapid increase of TRH and TSH secretion, resulting in thyroid gland stimulation and

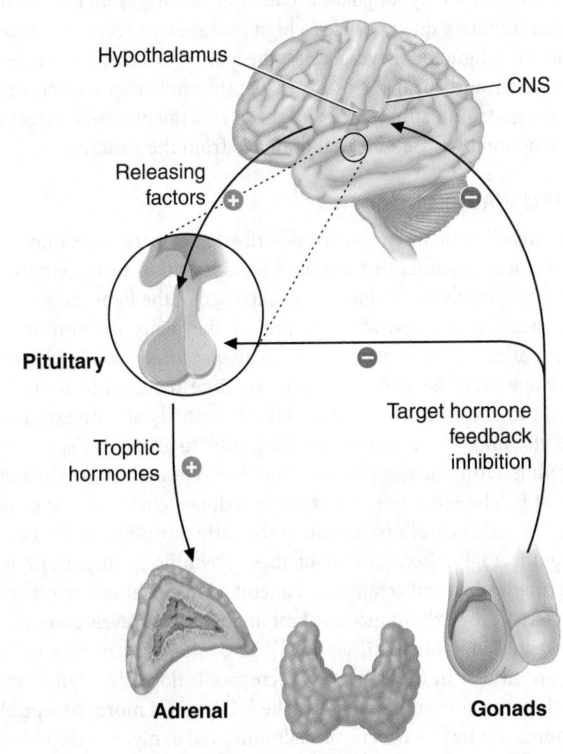

Figure 338-3 Feedback regulation of endocrine axes. CNS, central nervous system.

increased thyroid hormone production. When thyroid hormone reaches a normal level, it feeds back to suppress TRH and TSH, and a new steady state is attained. Feedback regulation also occurs for endocrine systems that do not involve the pituitary gland, such as calcium feedback on PTH, glucose inhibition of insulin secretion, and leptin feedback on the hypothalamus. An understanding of feedback regulation provides important insights into endocrine testing paradigms (see below).

Positive feedback control also occurs but is not well understood. The primary example is estrogen-mediated stimulation of the midcycle LH surge. Though chronic low levels of estrogen are inhibitory, gradually rising estrogen levels stimulate LH secretion. This effect, which is illustrative of an endocrine rhythm (see below), involves activation of the hypothalamic GnRH pulse generator. In addition, estrogen-primed gonadotropes are extraordinarily sensitive to GnRH, leading to amplification of LH release.

PARACRINE AND AUTOCRINE CONTROL

The previously mentioned examples of feedback control involve classic endocrine pathways in which hormones are released by one gland and act on a distant target gland. However, local regulatory systems, often involving growth factors, are increasingly recognized. *Paracrine regulation* refers to factors released by one cell that act on an adjacent cell in the same tissue. For example, somatostatin secretion by pancreatic islet δ cells inhibits insulin secretion from nearby β cells. *Autocrine regulation* describes the action of a factor on the same cell from which it is produced. IGF-I acts on many cells that produce it, including chondrocytes, breast epithelium, and gonadal cells. Unlike endocrine actions, paracrine and autocrine control are difficult to document because local growth factor concentrations cannot be measured readily.

Anatomic relationships of glandular systems also greatly influence hormonal exposure: the physical organization of islet cells enhances their intercellular communication; the portal vasculature of the hypothalamic-pituitary system exposes the pituitary to high concentrations of hypothalamic releasing factors; testicular seminiferous tubules gain exposure to high testosterone levels produced by the interdigitated Leydig cells; the pancreas receives nutrient information and local exposure to peptide hormones (incretins) from the gastrointestinal tract; and the liver is the proximal target of insulin action because of portal drainage from the pancreas.

HORMONAL RHYTHMS

The feedback regulatory systems described above are superimposed on hormonal rhythms that are used for adaptation to the environment. Seasonal changes, the daily occurrence of the light-dark cycle, sleep, meals, and stress are examples of the many environmental events that affect hormonal rhythms. The *menstrual cycle* is repeated on average every 28 days, reflecting the time required to follicular maturation and ovulation (Chap. 347). Essentially all pituitary hormone rhythms are entrained to sleep and to the *circadian cycle*, generating reproducible patterns that are repeated approximately every 24 h. The HPA axis, for example, exhibits characteristic peaks of ACTH and cortisol production in the early morning, with a nadir during the night. Recognition of these rhythms is important for endocrine testing and treatment. Patients with Cushing's syndrome characteristically exhibit increased midnight cortisol levels compared with normal individuals (Chap. 342). In contrast, morning cortisol levels are similar in these groups, as cortisol is normally high at this time of day in normal individuals. The HPA axis is more susceptible to suppression by glucocorticoids administered at night as they blunt the early-morning rise of ACTH. Understanding these rhythms allows glucocorticoid replacement that mimics diurnal production by administering larger doses in the morning than in the afternoon. Disrupted sleep rhythms can alter hormonal regulation. For example, sleep deprivation causes mild insulin resistance, food craving, and hypertension, which are reversible, at least in the short term.

Other endocrine rhythms occur on a more rapid time scale. Many peptide hormones are secreted in discrete bursts every few hours. LH and FSH secretion are exquisitely sensitive to GnRH pulse frequency. Intermittent pulses of GnRH are required to maintain pituitary sensitivity, whereas continuous exposure to GnRH causes pituitary gonadotrope desensitization. This feature of the hypothalamic-pituitary-gonadotrope axis forms the basis for using long-acting GnRH agonists to treat central precocious puberty or to decrease testosterone levels in the management of prostate cancer. It is important to be aware of the pulsatile nature of hormone secretion and the rhythmic patterns of hormone production in relating serum hormone measurements to normal values. For some hormones, integrated markers have been developed to circumvent hormonal fluctuations. Examples include 24-h urine collections for cortisol, IGF-I as a biologic marker of GH action, and HbA1c as an index of long-term (weeks to months) blood glucose control.

Often, one must interpret endocrine data only in the context of other hormones. For example, PTH levels typically are assessed in combination with serum calcium concentrations. A high serum calcium level in association with elevated PTH is suggestive of hyperparathyroidism, whereas a suppressed PTH in this situation is more likely to be caused by hypercalcemia of malignancy or other causes of hypercalcemia. Similarly, TSH should be elevated when T_4 and T_3 concentrations are low, reflecting reduced feedback inhibition. When this is not the case, it is important to consider secondary hypothyroidism, which is caused by a defect at the level of the pituitary.

PATHOLOGIC MECHANISMS OF ENDOCRINE DISEASE

Endocrine diseases can be divided into three major types of conditions: (1) hormone excess, (2) hormone deficiency, and (3) hormone resistance (Table 338-2).

CAUSES OF HORMONE EXCESS

Syndromes of hormone excess can be caused by neoplastic growth of endocrine cells, autoimmune disorders, and excess hormone administration. Benign endocrine tumors, including parathyroid, pituitary, and adrenal adenomas, often retain the capacity to produce hormones, perhaps reflecting the fact that they are relatively well differentiated. Many endocrine tumors exhibit subtle defects in their "set points" for feedback regulation. For example, in Cushing's disease, impaired feedback inhibition of ACTH secretion is associated with autonomous function. However, the tumor cells are not completely resistant to feedback, as evidenced by ACTH suppression by higher doses of dexamethasone (e.g., high-dose dexamethasone test) (Chap. 342). Similar set point defects are also typical of parathyroid adenomas and autonomously functioning thyroid nodules.

The molecular basis of some endocrine tumors, such as the MEN syndromes (MEN 1, 2A, 2B), have provided important insights into tumorigenesis (Chap. 351). MEN 1 is characterized primarily by the triad of parathyroid, pancreatic islet, and pituitary tumors. MEN 2 predisposes to medullary thyroid carcinoma, pheochromocytoma, and hyperparathyroidism. The *MEN1* gene, located on chromosome 11q13, encodes a putative tumor-suppressor gene, menin. Analogous to the paradigm first described for retinoblastoma, the affected individual inherits a mutant copy of the *MEN1* gene, and tumorigenesis ensues after a somatic "second hit" leads to loss of function of the normal *MEN1* gene (through deletion or point mutations).

In contrast to inactivation of a tumor-suppressor gene, as occurs in MEN 1 and most other inherited cancer syndromes, MEN 2 is caused by activating mutations in a single allele. In this case, activating mutations of the *RET* protooncogene, which encodes a receptor tyrosine kinase, leads to thyroid C cell hyperplasia in

TABLE 338-2 Causes of Endocrine Dysfunction

Type of Endocrine Disorder	Examples
Hyperfunction	
Neoplastic	
Benign	Pituitary adenomas, hyperparathyroidism, autonomous thyroid or adrenal nodules, pheochromocytoma
Malignant	Adrenal cancer, medullary thyroid cancer, carcinoid
Ectopic	Ectopic ACTH, SIADH secretion
Multiple endocrine neoplasia	MEN 1, MEN 2
Autoimmune	Graves' disease
Iatrogenic	Cushing's syndrome, hypoglycemia
Infectious/inflammatory	Subacute thyroiditis
Activating receptor mutations	LH, TSH, Ca^{2+} and PTH receptors, $G_s\alpha$
Hypofunction	
Autoimmune	Hashimoto's thyroiditis, Type 1 diabetes mellitus, Addison's disease, polyglandular failure
Iatrogenic	Radiation-induced hypopituitarism, hypothyroidism, surgical
Infectious/inflammatory	Adrenal insufficiency, hypothalamic sarcoidosis
Hormone mutations	GH, LHβ, FSHβ, vasopressin
Enzyme defects	21-Hydroxylase deficiency
Developmental defects	Kallmann syndrome, Turner syndrome, transcription factors
Nutritional/vitamin deficiency	Vitamin D deficiency, iodine deficiency
Hemorrhage/infarction	Sheehan's syndrome, adrenal insufficiency
Hormone resistance	
Receptor mutations	
Membrane	GH, vasopressin, LH, FSH, ACTH, GnRH, GHRH, PTH, leptin, Ca^{2+}
Nuclear	AR, TR, VDR, ER, GR, PPARγ
Signaling pathway mutations	Albright's hereditary osteodystrophy
Postreceptor	Type 2 diabetes mellitus, leptin resistance

Abbreviations: AR, androgen receptor; ER, estrogen receptor; GR, glucocorticoid receptor; PPAR, peroxisome proliferator activated receptor; SIADH, syndrome of inappropriate antidiuretic hormone; TR, thyroid hormone receptor; VDR, vitamin D receptor. For all other abbreviations, see text.

childhood before the development of medullary thyroid carcinoma. Elucidation of this pathogenic mechanism has allowed early genetic screening for *RET* mutations in individuals at risk for MEN 2, permitting identification of those who may benefit from prophylactic thyroidectomy and biochemical screening for pheochromocytoma and hyperparathyroidism.

Mutations that activate hormone receptor signaling have been identified in several GPCRs. For example, activating mutations of the LH receptor cause a dominantly transmitted form of male-limited precocious puberty, reflecting premature stimulation of testosterone synthesis in Leydig cells (Chap. 346). Activating mutations in these GPCRs are located predominantly in the transmembrane domains and induce receptor coupling to $G_s\alpha$ even in the absence of hormone. Consequently, adenylate cyclase is activated, and cyclic adenosine monophosphate (AMP) levels increase in a manner that mimics hormone action. A similar phenomenon results from activating mutations in $G_s\alpha$. When these mutations occur early in development, they cause McCune-Albright syndrome. When they occur only in somatotropes, the activating $G_s\alpha$ mutations cause GH-secreting tumors and acromegaly (Chap. 339).

In autoimmune Graves' disease, antibody interactions with the TSH receptor mimic TSH action, leading to hormone overproduction (Chap. 341). Analogous to the effects of activating mutations of the TSH receptor, these stimulating autoantibodies induce conformational changes that release the receptor from a constrained state, thereby triggering receptor coupling to G proteins.

■ CAUSES OF HORMONE DEFICIENCY

Most examples of hormone deficiency states can be attributed to glandular destruction caused by autoimmunity, surgery, infection, inflammation, infarction, hemorrhage, or tumor infiltration (Table 338-2). Autoimmune damage to the thyroid gland (Hashimoto's thyroiditis) and pancreatic islet β cells (Type 1 diabetes mellitus) is a prevalent cause of endocrine disease. Mutations in a number of hormones, hormone receptors, transcription factors, enzymes, and channels can also lead to hormone deficiencies.

■ HORMONE RESISTANCE

Most severe hormone resistance syndromes are due to inherited defects in membrane receptors, nuclear receptors, or the pathways that transduce receptor signals. These disorders are characterized by defective hormone action despite the presence of increased hormone levels. In complete androgen resistance, for example, mutations in the androgen receptor result in a female phenotypic appearance in genetic (XY) males, even though LH and testosterone levels are increased (Chap. 349). In addition to these relatively rare genetic disorders, more common acquired forms of functional hormone resistance include insulin resistance in Type 2 diabetes mellitus, leptin resistance in obesity, and GH resistance in catabolic states. The pathogenesis of functional resistance involves receptor downregulation and postreceptor desensitization of signaling pathways; functional forms of resistance are generally reversible.

APPROACH TO THE PATIENT — Endocrine Disease

Because most glands are relatively inaccessible, the examination usually focuses on the manifestations of hormone excess or deficiency as well as direct examination of palpable glands, such as the thyroid and gonads. For these reasons, it is important to evaluate patients in the context of their presenting symptoms, review of systems, family and social history, and exposure to medications that may affect the endocrine system. Astute clinical skills are required to detect subtle symptoms and signs suggestive of underlying endocrine disease. For example, a patient with Cushing's syndrome may manifest specific findings, such as central fat redistribution, striae, and proximal muscle weakness, in addition to features seen commonly in the general population, such as obesity, plethora, hypertension, and glucose intolerance. Similarly, the insidious onset of hypothyroidism—with mental slowing, fatigue, dry skin, and other features—can be difficult to distinguish from similar, nonspecific findings in the general population. Clinical judgment that is based on knowledge of disease prevalence and pathophysiology is required to decide when to embark on more extensive evaluation of these disorders. Laboratory testing plays an essential role in endocrinology by allowing quantitative assessment of hormone levels and dynamics. Radiologic imaging tests such as CT scan, MRI, thyroid scan, and ultrasound are also used for the diagnosis of endocrine disorders. However, these tests generally are employed only after a hormonal abnormality has been established by biochemical testing.

HORMONE MEASUREMENTS AND ENDOCRINE TESTING Immunoassays are the most important diagnostic tool in endocrinology, as they allow sensitive, specific, and quantitative determination of steady-state and dynamic changes in hormone concentrations. Immunoassays use antibodies to detect specific hormones. For many peptide hormones, these measurements are now configured to use two different antibodies to increase binding affinity and specificity. There are many variations of these assays; a common format involves using one antibody to capture the antigen (hormone) onto an immobilized surface and a second antibody, coupled to a chemiluminescent [immunochemiluminescent assay (ICMA)] or radioactive immunoradiometric assay (IRMA)] signal, to detect the antigen. These assays are sensitive enough to detect plasma hormone concentrations in the picomolar to nanomolar range, and they can readily distinguish structurally related proteins, such as PTH from PTHrP. A variety of other techniques are used to measure specific hormones, including mass spectroscopy, various forms of chromatography, and enzymatic methods; bioassays are now rarely used.

Most hormone measurements are based on plasma or serum samples. However, urinary hormone determinations remain useful for the evaluation of some conditions. Urinary collections over 24 h provide an integrated assessment of the production of a hormone or metabolite, many of which vary during the day. It is important to assure complete collections of 24-h urine samples; simultaneous measurement of creatinine provides an internal control for the adequacy of collection and can be used to normalize some hormone measurements. A 24-h urine free cortisol measurement largely reflects the amount of unbound cortisol, thus providing a reasonable index of biologically available hormone. Other commonly used urine determinations include 17-hydroxycorticosteroids, 17-ketosteroids, vanillylmandelic acid, metanephrine, catecholamines, 5-hydroxyindoleacetic acid, and calcium.

The value of quantitative hormone measurements lies in their correct interpretation in a clinical context. The normal range for most hormones is relatively broad, often varying by a factor of two- to tenfold. The normal ranges for many hormones are sex- and age-specific. Thus, using the correct normative database is an essential part of interpreting hormone tests. The pulsatile nature of hormones and factors that can affect their secretion, such as sleep, meals, and medications, must also be considered. Cortisol values increase fivefold between midnight and dawn; reproductive hormone levels vary dramatically during the female menstrual cycle.

For many endocrine systems, much information can be gained from basal hormone testing, particularly when different components of an endocrine axis are assessed simultaneously. For example, low testosterone and elevated LH levels suggest a primary gonadal problem, whereas a hypothalamic-pituitary disorder is likely if both LH and testosterone are low. Because TSH is a sensitive indicator of thyroid function, it is generally recommended as a first-line test for thyroid disorders. An elevated TSH level is almost always the result of primary hypothyroidism, whereas a low TSH is most often caused by thyrotoxicosis. These predictions can be confirmed by determining the free thyroxine level. Elevated calcium and PTH levels suggest hyperparathyroidism, whereas PTH is suppressed in hypercalcemia caused by malignancy or granulomatous diseases. A suppressed ACTH in the setting of hypercortisolemia, or increased urine free cortisol, is seen with hyperfunctioning adrenal adenomas.

It is not uncommon, however, for baseline hormone levels associated with pathologic endocrine conditions to overlap with the normal range. In this circumstance, dynamic testing is useful to separate the two groups further. There are a multitude of dynamic endocrine tests, but all are based on principles of feedback regulation, and most responses can be remembered on the basis of the pathways that govern endocrine axes. *Suppression tests* are used in the setting of suspected endocrine hyperfunction. An example is the dexamethasone suppression test used to evaluate Cushing's syndrome (Chaps. 339 and 342). *Stimulation tests* generally are used to assess endocrine hypofunction. The ACTH stimulation test, for example, is used to assess the adrenal gland response in patients with suspected adrenal insufficiency. Other stimulation tests use hypothalamic-releasing factors such as CRH and GHRH to evaluate pituitary hormone reserve (Chap. 339). Insulin-induced hypoglycemia also evokes pituitary ACTH and GH responses. Stimulation tests based on reduction or inhibition of endogenous hormones are now used infrequently. Examples include metyrapone inhibition of cortisol synthesis and clomiphene inhibition of estrogen feedback.

SCREENING AND ASSESSMENT OF COMMON ENDOCRINE DISORDERS Many endocrine disorders are prevalent in the adult population (Table 338-3) and can be diagnosed and managed by general internists, family practitioners, or other primary health care providers. The high prevalence and clinical impact of certain endocrine diseases justifies vigilance for features of these disorders during routine physical examinations; laboratory screening is indicated in selected high-risk populations.

TABLE 338-3 Examples of Prevalent Endocrine and Metabolic Disorders in the Adult

Disorder	Approx. Prevalence in Adults[a]	Screening/Testing Recommendations[b]	Chapter
Obesity	31% BMI ≥30 65% BMI ≥25	Calculate BMI Measure waist circumference Exclude secondary causes Consider comorbid complications	78
Type 2 diabetes mellitus	>7%	Beginning at age 45, screen every 3 years, or earlier in high-risk groups: Fasting plasma glucose (FPG) >126 mg/dL Random plasma glucose >200 mg/dL An elevated HbA1c Consider comorbid complications	344

(*continued*)

PART 16 Endocrinology and Metabolism

TABLE 338-3 Examples of Prevalent Endocrine and Metabolic Disorders in the Adult (*Continued*)

Disorder	Approx. Prevalence in Adults[a]	Screening/Testing Recommendations[b]	Chapter
Hyperlipidemia	20–25%	Cholesterol screening at least every 5 years; more often in high-risk groups Lipoprotein analysis (LDL, HDL) for increased cholesterol, CAD, diabetes Consider secondary causes	356
Hypothyroidism	5–10%, women 0.5–2%, men	TSH; confirm with free T_4 Screen women after age 35 and every 5 years thereafter	341
Graves' disease	1–3%, women 0.1%, men	TSH, free T_4	341
Thyroid nodules and neoplasia	2–5% palpable >25% by ultrasound	Physical examination of thyroid Fine-needle aspiration biopsy	341
Osteoporosis	5–10%, women 2–5%, men	Bone mineral density measurements in women >65 years or in postmenopausal women or men at risk Exclude secondary causes	354
Hyperparathyroidism	0.1–0.5%, women > men	Serum calcium PTH, if calcium is elevated Assess comorbid conditions	353
Infertility	10%, couples	Investigate both members of couple Semen analysis in male Assess ovulatory cycles in female Specific tests as indicated	346, 347
Polycystic ovarian syndrome	5–10%, women	Free testosterone, DHEAS Consider comorbid conditions	347
Hirsutism	5–10%	Free testosterone, DHEAS Exclude secondary causes Additional tests as indicated	49
Menopause	Median age, 51	FSH	348
Hyperprolactinemia	15% in women with amenorrhea or galactorrhea	PRL level MRI, if not medication-related	339
Erectile dysfunction	20–30%	Careful history, PRL, testosterone Consider secondary causes (e.g., diabetes)	48
Gynecomastia	15%	Often, no tests are indicated Consider Klinefelter syndrome Consider medications, hypogonadism, liver disease	346
Klinefelter syndrome	0.2%, men	Karyotype Testosterone	349
Vitamin D deficiency	40–50%	Measure serum 25-OH vitamin D Consider secondary causes	352
Turner syndrome	0.03%, women	Karyotype Consider comorbid conditions	349

[a]The prevalence of most disorders varies among ethnic groups and with aging. Data based primarily on U.S. population.

[b]See individual chapters for additional information on evaluation and treatment. Early testing is indicated in patients with signs and symptoms of disease and in those at increased risk.

Abbreviations: BMI, body mass index; CAD, coronary artery disease; DHEAS, dehydroepiandrosterone; HDL, high-density lipoprotein; LDL, low-density lipoprotein. For other abbreviations, see text.

FURTHER READINGS

Golden SH et al: Clinical review: Prevalence and incidence of endocrine and metabolic disorders in the United States: A comprehensive review. J Clin Endocrinol Metab 94:1853, 2009

Jameson JL, DeGroot LJ (eds): *Endocrinology*, 6th ed. Philadelphia, Elsevier, 2010

Kleinau G, Krause G: Thyrotropin and homologous glycoprotein hormone receptors: Structural and functional aspects of extracellular signaling mechanisms. Endocr Rev 30:133, 2009

Marx SJ, Simonds WF: Hereditary hormone excess: Genes, molecular pathways, and syndromes. Endocr Rev 26:615, 2005

Veldhuis JD et al: Motivations and methods for analyzing pulsatile hormone secretion. Endocr Rev 29:823, 2008

CHAPTER 339

Disorders of the Anterior Pituitary and Hypothalamus

Shlomo Melmed
J. Larry Jameson

The anterior pituitary often is referred to as the "master gland" because, together with the hypothalamus, it orchestrates the complex regulatory functions of many other endocrine glands. The anterior pituitary gland produces six major hormones: (1) prolactin (PRL), (2) growth hormone (GH), (3) adrenocorticotropic hormone (ACTH), (4) luteinizing hormone (LH), (5) follicle-stimulating hormone (FSH), and (6) thyroid-stimulating hormone (TSH) (Table 339-1). Pituitary hormones are secreted in a pulsatile manner, reflecting stimulation by an array of specific hypothalamic releasing factors. Each of these pituitary hormones elicits specific responses in peripheral target tissues. The hormonal products of those peripheral glands, in turn, exert feedback control at the level of the hypothalamus and pituitary to modulate pituitary function (Fig. 339-1). Pituitary tumors cause characteristic hormone-excess syndromes. Hormone deficiency may be inherited or acquired. Fortunately, there are efficacious treatments for the various pituitary hormone-excess and -deficiency syndromes. Nonetheless, these diagnoses are often elusive; this emphasizes the importance of recognizing subtle clinical manifestations and performing the correct laboratory diagnostic tests. For discussion of disorders of the posterior pituitary, or neurohypophysis, see Chap. 340.

ANATOMY AND DEVELOPMENT

ANATOMY

The pituitary gland weighs ~600 mg and is located within the sella turcica ventral to the diaphragma sella; it consists of anatomically and functionally distinct anterior and posterior lobes. The bony sella is contiguous to vascular and neurologic structures, including the cavernous sinuses, cranial nerves, and optic chiasm. Thus, expanding intrasellar pathologic processes may have significant central mass effects in addition to their endocrinologic impact.

Hypothalamic neural cells synthesize specific releasing and inhibiting hormones that are secreted directly into the portal vessels of the pituitary stalk. Blood supply of the pituitary gland comes from the superior and inferior hypophyseal arteries (Fig. 339-2). The hypothalamic-pituitary portal plexus provides the major blood source for the anterior pituitary, allowing reliable transmission of hypothalamic peptide pulses without significant systemic dilution; consequently, pituitary cells are exposed to releasing or inhibiting factors and in turn release their hormones as discrete pulses (Fig. 339-3).

The posterior pituitary is supplied by the inferior hypophyseal arteries. In contrast to the anterior pituitary, the posterior lobe is directly innervated by hypothalamic neurons (supraopticohypophyseal and tuberohypophyseal nerve tracts) via the pituitary stalk (Chap. 340). Thus, posterior pituitary production of vasopressin

TABLE 339-1 Anterior Pituitary Hormone Expression and Regulation

Cell	Corticotrope	Somatotrope	Lactotrope	Thyrotrope	Gonadotrope
Tissue-specific transcription factor	T-Pit	Prop-1, Pit-1	Prop-1, Pit-1	Prop-1, Pit-1, TEF	SF-1, DAX-1
Fetal appearance	6 weeks	8 weeks	12 weeks	12 weeks	12 weeks
Hormone	POMC	GH	PRL	TSH	FSH LH
Protein	Polypeptide	Polypeptide	Polypeptide	Glycoprotein α, β subunits	Glycoprotein α, β subunits
Amino acids	266 (ACTH 1–39)	191	199	211	210 204
Stimulators	CRH, AVP, gp-130 cytokines	GHRH, ghrelin	Estrogen, TRH, VIP	TRH	GnRH, activins, estrogen
Inhibitors	Glucocorticoids	Somatostatin, IGF-I	Dopamine	T_3, T_4, dopamine, somatostatin, glucocorticoids	Sex steroids, inhibin
Target gland	Adrenal	Liver, other tissues	Breast, other tissues	Thyroid	Ovary, testis
Trophic effect	Steroid production	IGF-I production, growth induction, insulin antagonism	Milk production	T_4 synthesis and secretion	Sex steroid production, follicle growth, germ cell maturation
Normal range	ACTH, 4–22 pg/L	<0.5 μg/L*	M < 15; F <20 μg/L	0.1–5 mU/L	M, 5–20 IU/L, F (basal), 5–20 IU/L

*Hormone secretion integrated over 24 h.

Abbreviations: M, male; F, female. For other abbreviations, see text.

Source: Adapted from I Shimon, S Melmed, in S Melmed, P Conn (eds): *Endocrinology: Basic and Clinical Principles*. Totowa, NJ, Humana, 2005.

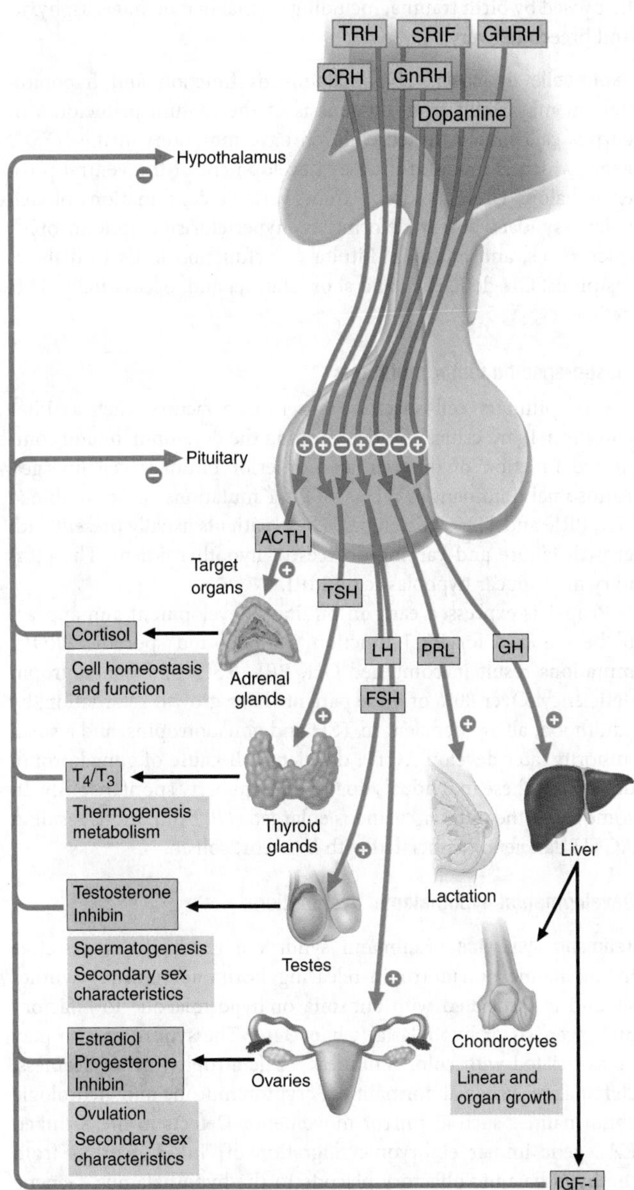

Figure 339-1 Diagram of pituitary axes. Hypothalamic hormones regulate anterior pituitary trophic hormones that in turn determine target gland secretion. Peripheral hormones feed back to regulate hypothalamic and pituitary hormones. For abbreviations, see text.

[antidiuretic hormone (ADH)] and oxytocin is particularly sensitive to neuronal damage by lesions that affect the pituitary stalk or hypothalamus.

PITUITARY DEVELOPMENT

The embryonic differentiation and maturation of anterior pituitary cells have been elucidated in considerable detail. Pituitary development from Rathke's pouch involves a complex interplay of lineage-specific transcription factors expressed in pluripotent precursor cells and gradients of locally produced growth factors (Table 339-1). The transcription factor Prop-1 induces pituitary development of Pit-1-specific lineages as well as gonadotropes. The transcription factor Pit-1 determines cell-specific expression of GH, PRL, and TSH in somatotropes, lactotropes, and thyrotropes. Expression of high levels of estrogen receptors in cells that contain Pit-1 favors PRL expression, whereas thyrotrope embryonic factor (TEF) induces TSH expression. Pit-1 binds to GH, PRL, and TSH gene regulatory elements as well as to recognition sites on its

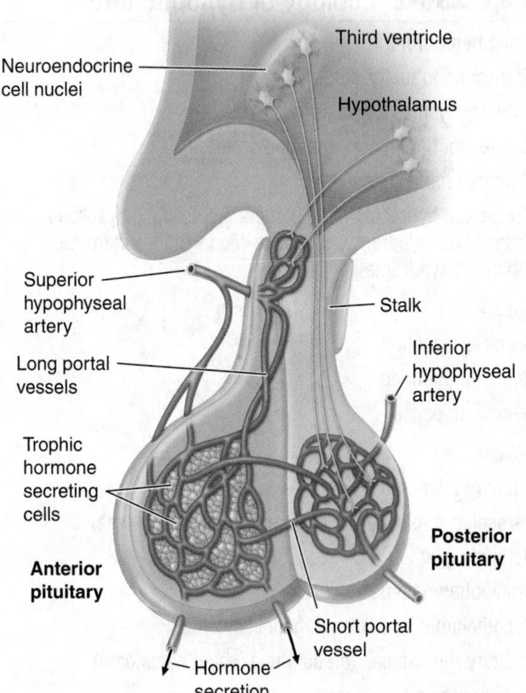

Figure 339-2 Diagram of hypothalamic-pituitary vasculature. The hypothalamic nuclei produce hormones that traverse the portal system and impinge on anterior pituitary cells to regulate pituitary hormone secretion. Posterior pituitary hormones are derived from direct neural extensions.

own promoter, providing a mechanism for maintaining specific pituitary phenotypic stability. Gonadotrope cell development is further defined by the cell-specific expression of the nuclear receptors steroidogenic factor (SF-1) and *d*osage-sensitive sex reversal, *a*drenal hypoplasia critical region, on chromosome *X*, gene *1* (DAX-1). Development of corticotrope cells, which express the proopiomelanocortin (POMC) gene, requires the T-Pit transcription factor. Abnormalities of pituitary development caused by mutations of Pit-1, Prop-1, SF-1, DAX-1, and T-Pit result in a series of rare, selective or combined pituitary hormone deficits.

HYPOTHALAMIC AND ANTERIOR PITUITARY INSUFFICIENCY

Hypopituitarism results from impaired production of one or more of the anterior pituitary trophic hormones. Reduced pituitary function can result from inherited disorders; more commonly, hypopituitarism is acquired and reflects the compressive mass effects of tumors or the consequences of inflammation or vascular damage.

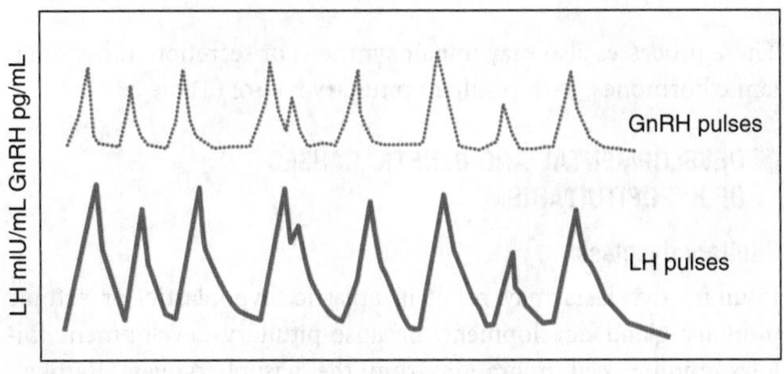

Figure 339-3 Hypothalamic gonadotropin-releasing hormone (GnRH) pulses induce secretory pulses of luteinizing hormone (LH).

TABLE 339-2 Etiology of Hypopituitarism*

Development/structural
Transcription factor defect
Pituitary dysplasia/aplasia
Congenital CNS mass, encephalocele
Primary empty sella
Congenital hypothalamic disorders (septo-optic dysplasia, Prader-Willi syndrome, Laurence-Moon-Biedl syndrome, Kallmann syndrome)
Traumatic
Surgical resection
Radiation damage
Head injuries
Neoplastic
Pituitary adenoma
Parasellar mass (germinoma, ependymoma, glioma)
Rathke's cyst
Craniopharyngioma
Hypothalamic hamartoma, gangliocytoma
Pituitary metastases (breast, lung, colon carcinoma)
Lymphoma and leukemia
Meningioma
Infiltrative/inflammatory
Lymphocytic hypophysitis
Hemochromatosis
Sarcoidosis
Histiocytosis X
Granulomatous hypophysitis
Vascular
Pituitary apoplexy
Pregnancy-related (infarction with diabetes; postpartum necrosis)
Sickle cell disease
Arteritis
Infections
Fungal (histoplasmosis)
Parasitic (toxoplasmosis)
Tuberculosis
Pneumocystis carinii

*Trophic hormone failure associated with pituitary compression or destruction usually occurs sequentially: GH > FSH > LH > TSH > ACTH. During childhood, growth retardation is often the presenting feature, and in adults, hypogonadism is the earliest symptom.

These processes also may impair synthesis or secretion of hypothalamic hormones, with resultant pituitary failure (Table 339-2).

DEVELOPMENTAL AND GENETIC CAUSES OF HYPOPITUITARISM

Pituitary dysplasia

Pituitary dysplasia may result in aplastic, hypoplastic, or ectopic pituitary gland development. Because pituitary development follows midline cell migration from the nasopharyngeal Rathke's pouch, midline craniofacial disorders may be associated with pituitary dysplasia. Acquired pituitary failure in the newborn also can be caused by birth trauma, including cranial hemorrhage, asphyxia, and breech delivery.

Septo-optic dysplasia Hypothalamic dysfunction and hypopituitarism may result from dysgenesis of the septum pellucidum or corpus callosum. Affected children have mutations in the *HESX1* gene, which is involved in early development of the ventral prosencephalon. These children exhibit variable combinations of cleft palate, syndactyly, ear deformities, hypertelorism, optic atrophy, micropenis, and anosmia. Pituitary dysfunction leads to diabetes insipidus, GH deficiency and short stature, and, occasionally, TSH deficiency.

Tissue-specific factor mutations

Several pituitary cell–specific transcription factors, such as Pit-1 and Prop-1, are critical for determining the development and committed function of differentiated anterior pituitary cell lineages. Autosomal dominant or recessive Pit-1 mutations cause combined GH, PRL, and TSH deficiencies. These patients usually present with growth failure and varying degrees of hypothyroidism. The pituitary may appear hypoplastic on MRI.

Prop-1 is expressed early in pituitary development and appears to be required for Pit-1 function. Familial and sporadic *PROP1* mutations result in combined GH, PRL, TSH, and gonadotropin deficiency. Over 80% of these patients have growth retardation; by adulthood, all are deficient in TSH and gonadotropins, and a small minority later develop ACTH deficiency. Because of gonadotropin deficiency, these individuals do not enter puberty spontaneously. In some cases, the pituitary gland is enlarged. *TPIT* mutations result in ACTH deficiency associated with hypocortisolism.

Developmental hypothalamic dysfunction

Kallmann syndrome Kallmann syndrome results from defective hypothalamic gonadotropin-releasing hormone (GnRH) synthesis and is associated with anosmia or hyposmia due to olfactory bulb agenesis or hypoplasia (Chap. 346). The syndrome also may be associated with color blindness, optic atrophy, nerve deafness, cleft palate, renal abnormalities, cryptorchidism, and neurologic abnormalities such as mirror movements. Defects in the X-linked *KAL* gene impair embryonic migration of GnRH neurons from the hypothalamic olfactory placode to the hypothalamus. Genetic abnormalities, in addition to *KAL* mutations, also can cause isolated GnRH deficiency. Autosomal recessive (i.e., *GPR54, KISS1*) and dominant (i.e., *FGFR1*) modes of transmission have been described, and there is a growing list of genes associated with GnRH deficiency (*GNRH1, PROK2, PROKR2, CH7, PCSK1, FGF8, TAC3, TACR3*). GnRH deficiency prevents progression through puberty. Males present with delayed puberty and pronounced hypogonadal features, including micropenis, probably the result of low testosterone levels during infancy. Females present with primary amenorrhea and failure of secondary sexual development.

Kallmann syndrome and other causes of congenital GnRH deficiency are characterized by low LH and FSH levels and low concentrations of sex steroids (testosterone or estradiol). In sporadic cases of isolated gonadotropin deficiency, the diagnosis is often one of exclusion after other causes of hypothalamic-pituitary dysfunction have been eliminated. Repetitive GnRH administration restores normal pituitary gonadotropin responses, pointing to a hypothalamic defect.

Long-term treatment of men with human chorionic gonadotropin (hCG) or testosterone restores pubertal development and secondary sex characteristics; women can be treated with cyclic estrogen and progestin. Fertility also may be restored by the administration of gonadotropins or by using a portable infusion pump to deliver subcutaneous, pulsatile GnRH.

Bardet-Biedl syndrome This is a rare genetically heterogeneous disorder characterized by mental retardation, renal abnormalities, obesity, and hexadactyly, brachydactyly, or syndactyly. Central diabetes insipidus may or may not be associated. GnRH deficiency occurs in 75% of males and half of affected females. Retinal degeneration begins in early childhood, and most patients are blind by age 30. Numerous subtypes of Bardet-Biedl syndrome (BBS) have been identified, with genetic linkage to at least nine different loci. Several of the loci encode genes involved in basal body cilia function, and this may account for the diverse clinical manifestations.

Leptin and leptin receptor mutations Deficiencies of leptin or its receptor cause a broad spectrum of hypothalamic abnormalities, including hyperphagia, obesity, and central hypogonadism (Chap. 77). Decreased GnRH production in these patients results in attenuated pituitary FSH and LH synthesis and release.

Prader-Willi syndrome This is a contiguous gene syndrome that results from deletion of the paternal copies of the imprinted *SNRPN* gene, the *NECDIN* gene, and possibly other genes on chromosome 15q. Prader-Willi syndrome is associated with hypogonadotropic hypogonadism, hyperphagia-obesity, chronic muscle hypotonia, mental retardation, and adult-onset diabetes mellitus (Chap. 62). Multiple somatic defects also involve the skull, eyes, ears, hands, and feet. Diminished hypothalamic oxytocin- and vasopressin-producing nuclei have been reported. Deficient GnRH synthesis is suggested by the observation that chronic GnRH treatment restores pituitary LH and FSH release.

ACQUIRED HYPOPITUITARISM

Hypopituitarism may be caused by accidental or neurosurgical trauma; vascular events such as apoplexy; pituitary or hypothalamic neoplasms, craniopharyngioma, lymphoma, or metastatic tumors; inflammatory disease such as lymphocytic hypophysitis; infiltrative disorders such as sarcoidosis, hemochromatosis (Chap. 357), and tuberculosis; or irradiation.

Increasing evidence suggests that patients with brain injury, including sports trauma, subarachnoid hemorrhage, and irradiation, have transient hypopituitarism and require intermittent long-term endocrine follow-up, as permanent hypothalamic or pituitary dysfunction will develop in 25–40% of these patients.

Hypothalamic infiltration disorders

These disorders—including sarcoidosis, histiocytosis X, amyloidosis, and hemochromatosis—frequently involve both hypothalamic and pituitary neuronal and neurochemical tracts. Consequently, diabetes insipidus occurs in half of patients with these disorders. Growth retardation is seen if attenuated GH secretion occurs before pubertal epiphyseal closure. Hypogonadotropic hypogonadism and hyperprolactinemia are also common.

Inflammatory lesions

Pituitary damage and subsequent dysfunction can be seen with chronic infections such as tuberculosis, with opportunistic fungal infections associated with AIDS, and in tertiary syphilis. Other inflammatory processes, such as granulomas and sarcoidosis, may mimic the features of a pituitary adenoma. These lesions may cause extensive hypothalamic and pituitary damage, leading to trophic hormone deficiencies.

Cranial irradiation

Cranial irradiation may result in long-term hypothalamic and pituitary dysfunction, especially in children and adolescents, as they are more susceptible to damage after whole-brain or head and neck therapeutic irradiation. The development of hormonal abnormalities correlates strongly with irradiation dosage and the time interval after completion of radiotherapy. Up to two-thirds of patients ultimately develop hormone insufficiency after a median dose of 50 Gy (5000 rad) directed at the skull base. The development of hypopituitarism occurs over 5–15 years and usually reflects hypothalamic damage rather than primary destruction of pituitary cells. Although the pattern of hormone loss is variable, GH deficiency is most common, followed by gonadotropin and ACTH deficiency. When deficiency of one or more hormones is documented, the possibility of diminished reserve of other hormones is likely. Accordingly, anterior pituitary function should be continually evaluated over the long term in previously irradiated patients, and replacement therapy instituted when appropriate (see below).

Lymphocytic hypophysitis

This occurs most often in postpartum women; it usually presents with hyperprolactinemia and MRI evidence of a prominent pituitary mass that often resembles an adenoma, with mildly elevated PRL levels. Pituitary failure caused by diffuse lymphocytic infiltration may be transient or permanent but requires immediate evaluation and treatment. Rarely, isolated pituitary hormone deficiencies have been described, suggesting a selective autoimmune process targeted to specific cell types. Most patients manifest symptoms of progressive mass effects with headache and visual disturbance. The erythrocyte sedimentation rate often is elevated. As the MRI image may be indistinguishable from that of a pituitary adenoma, hypophysitis should be considered in a postpartum woman with a newly diagnosed pituitary mass before an unnecessary surgical intervention is undertaken. The inflammatory process often resolves after several months of glucocorticoid treatment, and pituitary function may be restored, depending on the extent of damage.

Pituitary apoplexy

Acute intrapituitary hemorrhagic vascular events can cause substantial damage to the pituitary and surrounding sellar structures. Pituitary apoplexy may occur spontaneously in a preexisting adenoma; postpartum (Sheehan's syndrome); or in association with diabetes, hypertension, sickle cell anemia, or acute shock. The hyperplastic enlargement of the pituitary, which occurs normally during pregnancy, increases the risk for hemorrhage and infarction. Apoplexy is an endocrine emergency that may result in severe hypoglycemia, hypotension and shock, central nervous system (CNS) hemorrhage, and death. Acute symptoms may include severe headache with signs of meningeal irritation, bilateral visual changes, ophthalmoplegia, and, in severe cases, cardiovascular collapse and loss of consciousness. Pituitary CT or MRI may reveal signs of intratumoral or sellar hemorrhage, with deviation of the pituitary stalk and compression of pituitary tissue.

Patients with no evident visual loss or impaired consciousness can be observed and managed conservatively with high-dose glucocorticoids. Those with significant or progressive visual loss or loss of consciousness require urgent surgical decompression. Visual recovery after sellar surgery is inversely correlated with the length of time after the acute event. Therefore, severe ophthalmoplegia or visual deficits are indications for early surgery. Hypopituitarism is very common after apoplexy.

Empty sella

A partial or apparently totally empty sella is often an incidental MRI finding. These patients usually have normal pituitary function, implying that the surrounding rim of pituitary tissue is fully functional. Hypopituitarism, however, may develop insidiously. Pituitary masses also may undergo clinically silent infarction and involution with development of a partial or totally empty sella by cerebrospinal fluid (CSF) filling the dural herniation. Rarely, small but functional pituitary adenomas may arise within the rim of pituitary tissue, and they are not always visible on MRI.

PRESENTATION AND DIAGNOSIS

The clinical manifestations of hypopituitarism depend on which hormones are lost and the extent of the hormone deficiency. GH deficiency causes growth disorders in children and leads to abnormal body composition in adults (see below). Gonadotropin deficiency causes menstrual disorders and infertility in women and decreased sexual function, infertility, and loss of secondary sexual characteristics in men. TSH and ACTH deficiency usually develop later in the course of pituitary failure. TSH deficiency causes growth retardation in children and features of hypothyroidism in children and adults. The secondary form of adrenal insufficiency caused by ACTH deficiency leads to hypocortisolism with relative preservation of mineralocorticoid production. PRL deficiency causes failure of lactation. When lesions involve the posterior pituitary, polyuria and polydipsia reflect loss of vasopressin secretion. Epidemiologic studies have documented an increased mortality rate in patients with long-standing pituitary damage, primarily from increased cardiovascular and cerebrovascular disease. Previous head or neck irradiation is also a determinant of increased mortality rates in patients with hypopituitarism.

LABORATORY INVESTIGATION

Biochemical diagnosis of pituitary insufficiency is made by demonstrating low levels of trophic hormones in the setting of low levels of target hormones. For example, low free thyroxine in the setting of a low or inappropriately normal TSH level suggests secondary hypothyroidism. Similarly, a low testosterone level without elevation of gonadotropins suggests hypogonadotropic hypogonadism. Provocative tests may be required to assess pituitary reserve (Table 339-3). GH responses to insulin-induced hypoglycemia, arginine, L-dopa, growth hormone–releasing hormone (GHRH), or growth hormone–releasing peptides (GHRPs) can be used to assess GH reserve. Corticotropin-releasing hormone (CRH) administration induces ACTH release, and administration of synthetic ACTH (cosyntropin) evokes adrenal cortisol release as an indirect indicator of pituitary ACTH reserve (Chap. 342). ACTH reserve is most reliably assessed by measuring ACTH and cortisol levels during insulin-induced hypoglycemia. However, this test should be performed cautiously in patients with suspected adrenal insufficiency because of enhanced susceptibility to hypoglycemia and hypotension. Administering insulin to induce hypoglycemia is contraindicated in patients with active coronary artery disease or seizure disorders.

TREATMENT Hypopituitarism

Hormone replacement therapy, including glucocorticoids, thyroid hormone, sex steroids, growth hormone, and vasopressin, is usually safe and free of complications. Treatment regimens that mimic physiologic hormone production allow for maintenance of satisfactory clinical homeostasis. Effective dosage schedules are outlined in Table 339-4. Patients in need of glucocorticoid replacement require careful dose adjustments during stressful events such as acute illness, dental procedures, trauma, and acute hospitalization.

HYPOTHALAMIC, PITUITARY, AND OTHER SELLAR MASSES

PITUITARY TUMORS

Pituitary adenomas are the most common cause of pituitary hormone hypersecretion and hyposecretion syndromes in adults. They account for ~15% of all intracranial neoplasms and have been identified with a population prevalence of ~80/100,000. At autopsy, up to one-quarter of all pituitary glands harbor an unsuspected microadenoma (<10 mm diameter). Similarly, pituitary imaging detects small clinically inapparent pituitary lesions in at least 10% of individuals.

Pathogenesis

Pituitary adenomas are benign neoplasms that arise from one of the five anterior pituitary cell types. The clinical and biochemical phenotypes of pituitary adenomas depend on the cell type from which they are derived. Thus, tumors arising from lactotrope (PRL), somatotrope (GH), corticotrope (ACTH), thyrotrope (TSH), or gonadotrope (LH, FSH) cells hypersecrete their respective hormones (Table 339-5). Plurihormonal tumors that express combinations of GH, PRL, TSH, ACTH, and the glycoprotein hormone α or β subunit may be diagnosed by careful immunocytochemistry or may manifest as clinical syndromes that combine features of these hormonal hypersecretory syndromes. Morphologically, these tumors may arise from a single polysecreting cell type or include cells with mixed function within the same tumor.

Hormonally active tumors are characterized by autonomous hormone secretion with diminished feedback responsiveness to physiologic inhibitory pathways. Hormone production does not always correlate with tumor size. Small hormone-secreting adenomas may cause significant clinical perturbations, whereas larger adenomas that produce less hormone may be clinically silent and remain undiagnosed (if no central compressive effects occur). About one-third of all adenomas are clinically nonfunctioning and produce no distinct clinical hypersecretory syndrome. Most of them arise from gonadotrope cells and may secrete small amounts of α- and β-glycoprotein hormone subunits or, very rarely, intact circulating gonadotropins. True pituitary carcinomas with documented extracranial metastases are exceedingly rare.

Almost all pituitary adenomas are monoclonal in origin, implying the acquisition of one or more somatic mutations that confer a selective growth advantage. Consistent with their clonal origin, complete surgical resection of small pituitary adenomas usually cures hormone hypersecretion. Nevertheless, hypothalamic hormones such as GHRH and CRH also enhance mitotic activity of their respective pituitary target cells in addition to their role in pituitary hormone regulation. Thus, patients who harbor rare abdominal or chest tumors that elaborate ectopic GHRH or CRH may present with somatotrope or corticotrope hyperplasia with GH or ACTH hypersecretion.

Several etiologic genetic events have been implicated in the development of pituitary tumors. The pathogenesis of sporadic forms of acromegaly has been particularly informative as a model of tumorigenesis. GHRH, after binding to its G protein–coupled somatotrope receptor, utilizes cyclic AMP (adenosine monophosphate) as a second messenger to stimulate GH secretion and somatotrope proliferation. A subset (~35%) of GH-secreting pituitary tumors contain sporadic mutations in Gsα (Arg 201 $\rightarrow$ Cys or His; Gln 227 $\rightarrow$ Arg). These mutations attenuate intrinsic GTPase activity, resulting in constitutive elevation of cyclic AMP, Pit-1 induction, and activation of cyclic AMP response element binding protein (CREB), thereby promoting somatotrope cell proliferation and GH secretion.

Characteristic loss of heterozygosity (LOH) in various chromosomes has been documented in large or invasive macroadenomas,

TABLE 339-3 Tests of Pituitary Sufficiency

Hormone	Test	Blood Samples	Interpretation
Growth hormone	Insulin tolerance test: Regular insulin (0.05–0.15 U/kg IV)	–30, 0, 30, 60, 120 min for glucose and GH	Glucose < 40 mg/dL; GH should be >3 μg/L
	GHRH test: 1 μg/kg IV	0, 15, 30, 45, 60, 120 min for GH	Normal response is GH >3 μg/L
	L-Arginine test: 30 g IV over 30 min	0, 30, 60, 120 min for GH	Normal response is GH >3 μg/L
	L-Dopa test: 500 mg PO	0, 30, 60, 120 min for GH	Normal response is GH >3 μg/L
Prolactin	TRH test: 200–500 μg IV	0, 20, and 60 min for TSH and PRL	Normal prolactin is >2 μg/L and increase >200% of baseline
ACTH	Insulin tolerance test: regular insulin (0.05–0.15 U/kg IV)	–30, 0, 30, 60, 90 min for glucose and cortisol	Glucose <40 mg/dL Cortisol should increase by >7 μg/dL or to >20 μg/dL
	CRH test: 1 μg/kg ovine CRH IV at 8 A.M.	0, 15, 30, 60, 90, 120 min for ACTH and cortisol	Basal ACTH increases 2- to 4-fold and peaks at 20–100 pg/mL Cortisol levels >20–25 μg/dL
	Metyrapone test: Metyrapone (30 mg/kg) at midnight	Plasma 11-deoxycortisol and cortisol at 8 A.M.; ACTH can also be measured	Plasma cortisol should be <4 μg/dL to assure an adequate response Normal response is 11-deoxycortisol >7.5 μg/dL or ACTH >75 pg/mL
	Standard ACTH stimulation test: ACTH 1-24 (cosyntropin), 0.25 mg IM or IV	0, 30, 60 min for cortisol and aldosterone	Normal response is cortisol >21 μg/dL and aldosterone response of >4 ng/dL above baseline
	Low-dose ACTH test: ACTH 1-24 (cosyntropin), 1 μg IV	0, 30, 60 min for cortisol	Cortisol should be >21 μg/dL
	3-day ACTH stimulation test consists of 0.25 mg ACTH 1-24 given IV over 8 h each day		Cortisol >21 μg/dL
TSH	Basal thyroid function tests: T_4, T_3, TSH	Basal measurements	Low free thyroid hormone levels in the setting of TSH levels that are not appropriately increased indicate pituitary insufficiency
	TRH test: 200–500 μg IV	0, 20, 60 min for TSH and PRL[a]	TSH should increase by >5 mU/L unless thyroid hormone levels are increased
LH, FSH	LH, FSH, testosterone, estrogen	Basal measurements	Basal LH and FSH should be increased in postmenopausal women Low testosterone levels in the setting of low LH and FSH indicate pituitary insufficiency
	GnRH test: GnRH (100 μg) IV	0, 30, 60 min for LH and FSH	In most adults, LH should increase by 10 IU/L and FSH by 2 IU/L Normal responses are variable
Multiple hormones	Combined anterior pituitary test: GHRH (1 μg/kg), CRH (1 μg/kg), GnRH (100 μg), TRH (200 μg) are given IV	–30, 0, 15, 30, 60, 90, 120 min for GH, ACTH, cortisol, LH, FSH, and TSH	Combined or individual releasing hormone responses must be elevated in the context of basal target gland hormone values and may not be uniformly diagnostic (see text)

[a]Evoked PRL response indicates lactotrope integrity.
Note: For abbreviations, see text.

suggesting the presence of putative tumor suppressor genes at these loci. LOH of chromosome regions on 11q13, 13, and 9 is present in up to 20% of sporadic pituitary tumors, including GH-, PRL-, and ACTH-producing adenomas and some nonfunctioning tumors.

Compelling evidence also favors growth factor promotion of pituitary tumor proliferation. Basic fibroblast growth factor (bFGF) is abundant in the pituitary and has been shown to stimulate pituitary cell mitogenesis. Other factors involved in initiation and promotion of pituitary tumors include loss of negative-feedback inhibition (as seen with primary hypothyroidism or hypogonadism) and estrogen-mediated or paracrine angiogenesis. Growth characteristics and neoplastic behavior also may be influenced by several activated oncogenes, including *RAS* and pituitary tumor transforming gene (*PTTG*), or inactivation of growth suppressor genes, including *MEG3*.

Genetic syndromes associated with pituitary tumors

Several familial syndromes are associated with pituitary tumors, and the genetic mechanisms for some of them have been unraveled (Table 339-6).

TABLE 339-4 Hormone Replacement Therapy for Adult Hypopituitarism*

Trophic Hormone Deficit	Hormone Replacement
ACTH	Hydrocortisone (10–20 mg A.M.; 5–10 mg P.M.) Cortisone acetate (25 mg A.M.; 12.5 mg P.M.) Prednisone (5 mg A.M.)
TSH	L-Thyroxine (0.075–0.15 mg daily)
FSH/LH	Males Testosterone enanthate (200 mg IM every 2 weeks) Testosterone skin patch (5 mg/d) Females Conjugated estrogen (0.65–1.25 mg qd for 25 days) Progesterone (5–10 mg qd) on days 16–25 Estradiol skin patch (0.5 mg, every other day) For fertility: Menopausal gonadotropins, human chorionic gonadotropins
GH	Adults: Somatotropin (0.1–1.25 mg SC qd) Children: Somatotropin [0.02–0.05 (mg/kg per day)]
Vasopressin	Intranasal desmopressin (5–20 μg twice daily) Oral 300–600 μg qd

*All doses shown should be individualized for specific patients and should be reassessed during stress, surgery, or pregnancy. Male and female fertility requirements should be managed as discussed in Chap. 44.
Note: For abbreviations, see text.

TABLE 339-5 Classification of Pituitary Adenomas*

Adenoma Cell Origin	Hormone Product	Clinical Syndrome
Lactotrope	PRL	Hypogonadism, galactorrhea
Gonadotrope	FSH, LH, subunits	Silent or hypogonadism
Somatotrope	GH	Acromegaly/gigantism
Corticotrope	ACTH	Cushing's disease
Mixed growth hormone and prolactin cell	GH, PRL	Acromegaly, hypogonadism, galactorrhea
Other plurihormonal cell	Any	Mixed
Acidophil stem cell	PRL, GH	Hypogonadism, galactorrhea, acromegaly
Mammosomatotrope	PRL, GH	Hypogonadism, galactorrhea, acromegaly
Thyrotrope	TSH	Thyrotoxicosis
Null cell	None	Pituitary failure
Oncocytoma	None	Pituitary failure

*Hormone-secreting tumors are listed in decreasing order of frequency. All tumors may cause local pressure effects, including visual disturbances, cranial nerve palsy, and headache.
Note: For abbreviations, see text.
Source: Adapted from S Melmed, in JL Jameson (ed): *Principles of Molecular Medicine*, Totowa, NJ, Humana Press, 1998.

Multiple endocrine neoplasia (MEN) 1 is an autosomal dominant syndrome characterized primarily by a genetic predisposition to parathyroid, pancreatic islet, and pituitary adenomas (Chap. 351). MEN1 is caused by inactivating germ-line mutations in *MENIN*, a constitutively expressed tumor-suppressor gene located on chromosome 11q13. Loss of heterozygosity, or a somatic mutation of the remaining normal *MENIN* allele, leads to tumorigenesis. About half of affected patients develop prolactinomas; acromegaly and Cushing's syndrome are less commonly encountered.

Carney syndrome is characterized by spotty skin pigmentation, myxomas, and endocrine tumors, including testicular, adrenal, and pituitary adenomas. Acromegaly occurs in about 20% of these patients. A subset of patients have mutations in the R1α regulatory subunit of protein kinase A (*PRKAR1A*).

McCune-Albright syndrome consists of polyostotic fibrous dysplasia, pigmented skin patches, and a variety of endocrine disorders, including acromegaly, adrenal adenomas, and autonomous ovarian function (Chap. 347). Hormonal hypersecretion results from constitutive cyclic AMP production caused by inactivation of the GTPase activity of Gsα. The Gsα mutations occur postzygotically, leading to a mosaic pattern of mutant expression.

Familial acromegaly is a rare disorder in which family members may manifest either acromegaly or gigantism. The disorder is associated with LOH at a chromosome 11q13 locus distinct from that of *MENIN*. A subset of families with a predisposition for familial pituitary tumors, especially acromegaly, have been found to harbor inactivating mutations in the *AIP* gene, which encodes the aryl hydrocarbon receptor interacting protein.

TABLE 339-6 Familial Pituitary Tumor Syndromes

	Gene Mutated	Clinical Features
Multiple endocrine neoplasia 1 (MEN 1)	*MEN1* (11q13)	Hyperparathyroidism Pancreatic neuroendocrine tumors Foregut carcinoids Adrenal adenomas Skin lesions Pituitary adenomas (40%)
Multiple endocrine neoplasia 4 (MEN 4)	*CDKNIB* *(12p13)*	Hyperparathyroidsm Pituitary adenomas Other tumors
Carney complex	*PRKAR1A* *(17q23-24)*	Pituitary hyperplasia and adenomas (10%) Atrial myxomas Schwannomas Adrenal hyperplasia Lentigines
Familial pituitary adenomas	*AIP* *(11q13.3)*	Acromegaly/gigantism (15%)

OTHER SELLAR MASSES

Craniopharyngiomas are benign, suprasellar cystic masses that present with headaches, visual field deficits, and variable degrees of hypopituitarism. They are derived from Rathke's pouch and arise near the pituitary stalk, commonly extending into the suprasellar cistern. Craniopharyngiomas are often large, cystic, and locally invasive. Many are partially calcified, exhibiting a characteristic appearance on skull x-ray and CT images. More than half of all patients present before age 20, usually with signs of increased intracranial pressure, including headache, vomiting, papilledema, and hydrocephalus. Associated symptoms include visual field abnormalities, personality changes and cognitive deterioration, cranial nerve damage, sleep difficulties, and weight gain. Hypopituitarism can be documented in about 90%, and diabetes insipidus occurs in about 10% of patients. About half of affected children present with growth retardation. MRI is generally superior to CT for evaluating cystic structure and tissue components of craniopharyngiomas. CT is useful to define calcifications and evaluate invasion into surrounding bony structures and sinuses.

Treatment usually involves transcranial or transsphenoidal surgical resection followed by postoperative radiation of residual tumor. Surgery alone is curative in less than half of patients because of recurrences due to adherence to vital structures or because of small tumor deposits in the hypothalamus or brain parenchyma. The goal of surgery is to remove as much tumor as possible without risking complications associated with efforts to remove firmly adherent or inaccessible tissue. In the absence of radiotherapy, about 75% of craniopharyngiomas recur, and 10-year survival is less than 50%. In patients with incomplete resection, radiotherapy improves 10-year survival to 70–90% but is associated with increased risk of secondary malignancies. Most patients require lifelong pituitary hormone replacement.

Developmental failure of Rathke's pouch obliteration may lead to *Rathke's cysts*, which are small (<5 mm) cysts entrapped by squamous epithelium and are found in about 20% of individuals at autopsy. Although Rathke's cleft cysts do not usually grow and are often diagnosed incidentally, about a third present in adulthood with compressive symptoms, diabetes insipidus, and hyperprolactinemia due to stalk compression. Rarely, hydrocephalus develops. The diagnosis is suggested preoperatively by visualizing the cyst wall on MRI, which distinguishes these lesions from craniopharyngiomas. Cyst contents range from CSF-like fluid to mucoid material. *Arachnoid cysts* are rare and generate an MRI image that is isointense with cerebrospinal fluid.

Sella chordomas usually present with bony clival erosion, local invasiveness, and, on occasion, calcification. Normal pituitary tissue may be visible on MRI, distinguishing chordomas from aggressive pituitary adenomas. Mucinous material may be obtained by fine-needle aspiration.

Meningiomas arising in the sellar region may be difficult to distinguish from nonfunctioning pituitary adenomas. Meningiomas typically enhance on MRI and may show evidence of calcification or bony erosion. Meningiomas may cause compressive symptoms.

Histiocytosis X includes a variety of syndromes associated with foci of eosinophilic granulomas. Diabetes insipidus, exophthalmos, and punched-out lytic bone lesions (*Hand-Schüller-Christian disease*) are associated with granulomatous lesions visible on MRI, as well as a characteristic axillary skin rash. Rarely, the pituitary stalk may be involved.

Pituitary metastases occur in ~3% of cancer patients. Bloodborne metastatic deposits are found almost exclusively in the posterior pituitary. Accordingly, diabetes insipidus can be a presenting feature of lung, gastrointestinal, breast, and other pituitary metastases. About half of pituitary metastases originate from breast cancer; about 25% of patients with metastatic breast cancer have such deposits. Rarely, pituitary stalk involvement results in anterior pituitary insufficiency. The MRI diagnosis of a metastatic lesion may be difficult to distinguish from an aggressive pituitary adenoma; the diagnosis may require histologic examination of excised tumor tissue. Primary or metastatic lymphoma, leukemias, and plasmacytomas also occur within the sella.

Hypothalamic hamartomas and *gangliocytomas* may arise from astrocytes, oligodendrocytes, and neurons with varying degrees of differentiation. These tumors may overexpress hypothalamic neuropeptides, including GnRH, GHRH, and CRH. With GnRH-producing tumors, children present with precocious puberty, psychomotor delay, and laughing-associated seizures. Medical treatment of GnRH-producing hamartomas with long-acting GnRH analogues effectively suppresses gonadotropin secretion and controls premature pubertal development. Rarely, hamartomas also are associated with craniofacial abnormalities; imperforate anus; cardiac, renal, and lung disorders; and pituitary failure as features of *Pallister-Hall syndrome*, which is caused by mutations in the carboxy terminus of the *GLI3* gene. Hypothalamic hamartomas are often contiguous with the pituitary, and preoperative MRI diagnosis may not be possible. Histologic evidence of hypothalamic neurons in tissue resected at transsphenoidal surgery may be the first indication of a primary hypothalamic lesion.

Hypothalamic gliomas and *optic gliomas* occur mainly in childhood and usually present with visual loss. Adults have more aggressive tumors; about a third are associated with neurofibromatosis.

Brain germ-cell tumors may arise within the sellar region. They include *dysgerminomas*, which frequently are associated with diabetes insipidus and visual loss. They rarely metastasize. *Germinomas, embryonal carcinomas, teratomas*, and *choriocarcinomas* may arise in the parasellar region and produce hCG. These germ-cell tumors present with precocious puberty, diabetes insipidus, visual field defects, and thirst disorders. Many patients are GH-deficient with short stature.

METABOLIC EFFECTS OF HYPOTHALAMIC LESIONS

Lesions involving the anterior and preoptic hypothalamic regions cause paradoxical vasoconstriction, tachycardia, and hyperthermia. Acute hyperthermia usually is due to a hemorrhagic insult, but poikilothermia may also occur. Central disorders of thermoregulation result from posterior hypothalamic damage. The *periodic hypothermia syndrome* is characterized by episodic attacks of rectal temperatures <30°C (86°F), sweating, vasodilation, vomiting, and bradycardia (Chap. 19). Damage to the ventromedial hypothalamic nuclei by craniopharyngiomas, hypothalamic trauma, or inflammatory disorders may be associated with *hyperphagia* and *obesity*. This region appears to contain an energy-satiety center where melanocortin receptors are influenced by leptin, insulin, POMC products, and gastrointestinal peptides (Chap. 77). Polydipsia and hypodipsia are associated with damage to central osmoreceptors located in preoptic nuclei (Chap. 340). Slow-growing hypothalamic lesions can cause increased somnolence and disturbed sleep cycles as well as obesity, hypothermia, and emotional outbursts. Lesions of the central hypothalamus may stimulate sympathetic neurons, leading to elevated serum catecholamine and cortisol levels. These patients are predisposed to cardiac arrhythmias, hypertension, and gastric erosions.

EVALUATION

Local mass effects

Clinical manifestations of sellar lesions vary, depending on the anatomic location of the mass and the direction of its extension (Table 339-7). The dorsal sellar diaphragm presents the least resistance to soft tissue expansion from the sella; consequently, pituitary

TABLE 339-7 Features of Sellar Mass Lesions*

Impacted Structure	Clinical Impact
Pituitary	Hypogonadism
	Hypothyroidism
	Growth failure and adult hyposomatotropism
	Hypoadrenalism
Optic chiasm	Loss of red perception
	Bitemporal hemianopia
	Superior or bitemporal field defect
	Scotoma
	Blindness
Hypothalamus	Temperature dysregulation
	Appetite and thirst disorders
	Obesity
	Diabetes insipidus
	Sleep disorders
	Behavioral dysfunction
	Autonomic dysfunction
Cavernous sinus	Opthalmoplegia with or without ptosis or diplopia
	Facial numbness
Frontal lobe	Personality disorder
	Anosmia
Brain	Headache
	Hydrocephalus
	Psychosis
	Dementia
	Laughing seizures

*As the intrasellar mass expands, it first compresses intrasellar pituitary tissue, then usually invades dorsally through the dura to lift the optic chiasm or laterally to the cavernous sinuses. Bony erosion is rare, as is direct brain compression. Microadenomas may present with headache.

adenomas frequently extend in a suprasellar direction. Bony invasion may occur as well.

Headaches are common features of small intrasellar tumors, even with no demonstrable suprasellar extension. Because of the confined nature of the pituitary, small changes in intrasellar pressure stretch the dural plate; however, headache severity correlates poorly with adenoma size or extension.

Suprasellar extension can lead to visual loss by several mechanisms, the most common being compression of the optic chiasm, but rarely, direct invasion of the optic nerves or obstruction of CSF flow leading to secondary visual disturbances also occurs. Pituitary stalk compression by a hormonally active or inactive intrasellar mass may compress the portal vessels, disrupting pituitary access to hypothalamic hormones and dopamine; this results in early hyperprolactinemia and later concurrent loss of other pituitary hormones. This "stalk section" phenomenon may also be caused by trauma, whiplash injury with posterior clinoid stalk compression, or skull base fractures. Lateral mass invasion may impinge on the cavernous sinus and compress its neural contents, leading to cranial nerve III, IV, and VI palsies as well as effects on the ophthalmic and maxillary branches of the fifth cranial nerve (Chap. 376). Patients may present with diplopia, ptosis, ophthalmoplegia, and decreased facial sensation, depending on the extent of neural damage. Extension into the sphenoid sinus indicates that the pituitary mass has eroded through the sellar floor. Aggressive tumors rarely invade the palate roof and cause nasopharyngeal obstruction, infection, and CSF leakage. Temporal and frontal lobe involvement may rarely lead to uncinate seizures, personality disorders, and anosmia. Direct hypothalamic encroachment by an invasive pituitary mass may cause important metabolic sequelae, including precocious puberty or hypogonadism, diabetes insipidus, sleep disturbances, dysthermia, and appetite disorders.

MRI

Sagittal and coronal T1-weighted MRI imaging before and after administration of gadolinium allows precise visualization of the pituitary gland with clear delineation of the hypothalamus, pituitary stalk, pituitary tissue and surrounding suprasellar cisterns, cavernous sinuses, sphenoid sinus, and optic chiasm. Pituitary gland height ranges from 6 mm in children to 8 mm in adults; during pregnancy and puberty, the height may reach 10–12 mm. The upper aspect of the adult pituitary is flat or slightly concave, but in adolescent and pregnant individuals, this surface may be convex, reflecting physiologic pituitary enlargement. The stalk should be midline and vertical. CT scan is reserved to define the extent of bony erosion or the presence of calcification.

Anterior pituitary gland soft tissue consistency is slightly heterogeneous on MRI, and signal intensity resembles that of brain matter on T1-weighted imaging (Fig. 339-4). Adenoma density is usually lower than that of surrounding normal tissue on T1-weighted imaging, and the signal intensity increases with T2-weighted images. The high phospholipid content of the posterior pituitary results in a "pituitary bright spot."

Sellar masses are encountered commonly as incidental findings on MRI, and most of them are pituitary adenomas (incidentalomas). In the absence of hormone hypersecretion, these small intrasellar lesions can be monitored safely with MRI, which is performed annually and then less often if there is no evidence of further growth. Resection should be considered for incidentally discovered macroadenomas, as about one-third become invasive or cause local

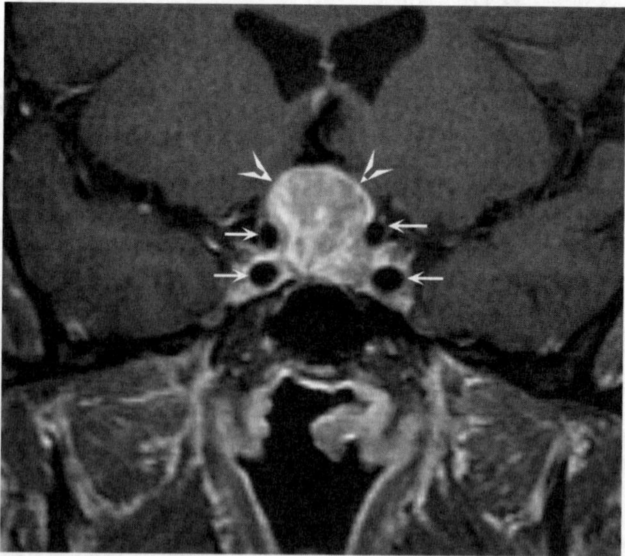

Figure 339-4 Pituitary adenoma. Coronal T1-weighted postcontrast MR image shows a homogeneously enhancing mass (*arrowheads*) in the sella turcica and suprasellar region compatible with a pituitary adenoma; the small arrows outline the carotid arteries.

pressure effects. If hormone hypersecretion is evident, specific therapies are indicated. When larger masses (>1 cm) are encountered, they should also be distinguished from nonadenomatous lesions. Meningiomas often are associated with bony hyperostosis; craniopharyngiomas may be calcified and are usually hypodense, whereas gliomas are hyperdense on T2-weighted images.

Ophthalmologic evaluation

Because optic tracts may be contiguous to an expanding pituitary mass, reproducible visual field assessment using perimetry techniques should be performed on all patients with sellar mass lesions that abut the optic chiasm (Chap. 28). Bitemporal hemianopia or superior bitemporal defects are classically observed, reflecting the location of these tracts within the inferior and posterior part of the chiasm. Homonymous cuts reflect postchiasmal lesions, and monocular field cuts prechiasmal lesions. Loss of red perception is an early sign of optic tract pressure. Early diagnosis reduces the risk of blindness, scotomas, or other visual disturbances.

Laboratory investigation

The presenting clinical features of functional pituitary adenomas (e.g., acromegaly, prolactinomas, or Cushing's syndrome) should guide the laboratory studies (Table 339-8). However, for a sellar mass with no obvious clinical features of hormone excess, laboratory studies are geared toward determining the nature of the tumor and assessing the possible presence of hypopituitarism. When a pituitary adenoma is suspected based on MRI, initial hormonal evaluation usually includes (1) basal PRL; (2) insulin-like growth factor (IGF) I; (3) 24-h urinary free cortisol (UFC) and/or overnight oral dexamethasone (1 mg) suppression test; (4) α subunit, FSH, and LH; and (5) thyroid function tests. Additional hormonal evaluation may be indicated based on the results of these tests. Pending more detailed assessment of hypopituitarism, a menstrual history, measurement of testosterone and 8 A.M. cortisol levels, and thyroid function tests usually identify patients with pituitary hormone deficiencies that require hormone replacement before further testing or surgery.

TABLE 339-8 Screening Tests for Functional Pituitary Adenomas

	Test	Comments
Acromegaly	Serum IGF-I	Interpret IGF-I relative to age- and sex-matched controls
	Oral glucose tolerance test with GH obtained at 0, 30, and 60 min	Normal subjects should suppress growth hormone to <1 μg/L
Prolactinoma	Serum PRL	Exclude medications
		MRI of the sella should be ordered if prolactin is elevated
Cushing's disease	24-h urinary free cortisol	Ensure urine collection is total and accurate
	Dexamethasone (1 mg) at 11 P.M. and fasting plasma cortisol measured at 8 A.M.	Normal subjects suppress to <5 μg/dL
	ACTH assay	Distinguishes adrenal adenoma (ACTH suppressed) from ectopic ACTH or Cushing's disease (ACTH normal or elevated)

Note: For abbreviations, see text.

Histologic evaluation

Immunohistochemical staining of pituitary tumor specimens obtained at transsphenoidal surgery confirms clinical and laboratory studies and provides a histologic diagnosis when hormone studies are equivocal and in cases of clinically nonfunctioning tumors. Occasionally, ultrastructural assessment by electron microscopy is required for diagnosis.

TREATMENT Hypothalamic, Pituitary, and Other Sellar Masses

OVERVIEW Successful management of sellar masses requires accurate diagnosis as well as selection of optimal therapeutic modalities. Most pituitary tumors are benign and slow-growing. Clinical features result from local mass effects and hormonal hypo- or hypersecretion syndromes caused directly by the adenoma or occurring as a consequence of treatment. Thus, lifelong management and follow-up are necessary for these patients.

MRI with gadolinium enhancement for pituitary visualization, new advances in transsphenoidal surgery and in stereotactic radiotherapy (including gamma-knife radiotherapy), and novel therapeutic agents have improved pituitary tumor management. The goals of pituitary tumor treatment include normalization of excess pituitary secretion, amelioration of symptoms and signs of hormonal hypersecretion syndromes, and shrinkage or ablation of large tumor masses with relief of adjacent structure compression. Residual anterior pituitary function should be preserved during treatment and sometimes can be restored by removing the tumor mass. Ideally, adenoma recurrence should be prevented.

TRANSSPHENOIDAL SURGERY Transsphenoidal rather than transfrontal resection is the desired surgical approach for pituitary tumors, except for the rare invasive suprasellar mass surrounding the frontal or middle fossa or the optic nerves or invading posteriorly behind the clivus. Intraoperative microscopy facilitates visual distinction between adenomatous and normal pituitary tissue as well as microdissection of small tumors that may not be visible by MRI (Fig. 339-5). Transsphenoidal surgery also avoids the cranial invasion and manipulation of brain tissue required by subfrontal surgical approaches. Endoscopic techniques with three-dimensional intraoperative localization have also improved visualization and access to tumor tissue.

In addition to correction of hormonal hypersecretion, pituitary surgery is indicated for mass lesions that impinge on surrounding structures. Surgical decompression and resection are required for an expanding pituitary mass accompanied by persistent headache, progressive visual field defects, cranial nerve palsies, hydrocephalus, and, occasionally, intrapituitary hemorrhage and apoplexy. Transsphenoidal surgery sometimes is used for pituitary tissue biopsy to establish a histologic diagnosis.

Whenever possible, the pituitary mass lesion should be selectively excised; normal pituitary tissue should be manipulated or resected only when critical for effective mass dissection. Nonselective hemihypophysectomy or total hypophysectomy

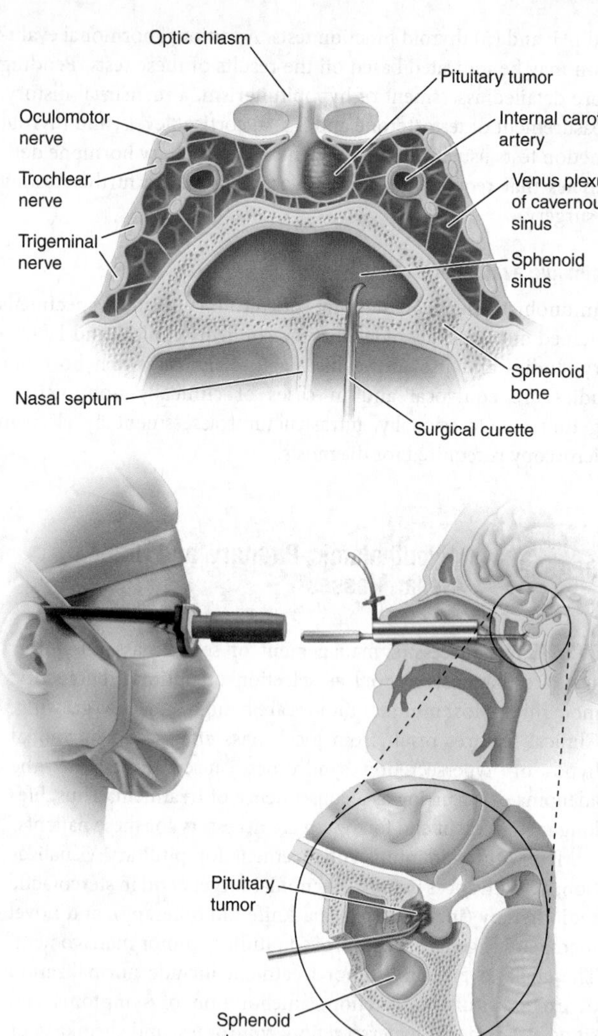

Figure 339-5 Transsphenoidal resection of pituitary mass via the endonasal approach. *(Adapted from R Fahlbusch: Endocrinol Metab Clin 21:669, 1992.)*

may be indicated if no hypersecreting mass lesion is clearly discernible, multifocal lesions are present, or the remaining nontumorous pituitary tissue is obviously necrotic. This strategy, however, increases the likelihood of hypopituitarism and the need for lifelong hormone replacement.

Preoperative mass effects, including visual field defects and compromised pituitary function, may be reversed by surgery, particularly when the deficits are not long-standing. For large and invasive tumors, it is necessary to determine the optimal balance between maximal tumor resection and preservation of anterior pituitary function, especially for preserving growth and reproductive function in younger patients. Similarly, tumor invasion outside the sella is rarely amenable to surgical cure; the surgeon must judge the risk-versus-benefit ratio of extensive tumor resection.

Side Effects Tumor size, the degree of invasiveness, and experience of the surgeon largely determine the incidence of surgical complications. Operative mortality rate is about 1%. Transient diabetes insipidus and hypopituitarism occur in up to 20% of patients. Permanent diabetes insipidus, cranial nerve damage, nasal septal perforation, or visual disturbances may be encountered in up to 10% of patients. CSF leaks occur in 4% of patients. Less common complications include carotid artery injury, loss of vision, hypothalamic damage, and meningitis. Permanent side effects are rare after surgery for microadenomas.

RADIATION Radiation is used either as a primary therapy for pituitary or parasellar masses or, more commonly, as an adjunct to surgery or medical therapy. Focused megavoltage irradiation is achieved by precise MRI localization, using a high-voltage linear accelerator and accurate isocentric rotational arcing. A major determinant of accurate irradiation is reproduction of the patient's head position during multiple visits and maintenance of absolute head immobility. A total of <50 Gy (5000 rad) is given as 180-cGy (180-rad) fractions divided over about 6 weeks. Stereotactic radiosurgery delivers a large single high-energy dose from a cobalt 60 source (gamma knife), linear accelerator, or cyclotron. Long-term effects of gamma-knife surgery are unclear but appear to be similar to those encountered with conventional radiation.

The role of radiation therapy in pituitary tumor management depends on multiple factors, including the nature of the tumor, the age of the patient, and the availability of surgical and radiation expertise. Because of its relatively slow onset of action, radiation therapy is usually reserved for postsurgical management. As an adjuvant to surgery, radiation is used to treat residual tumor and in an attempt to prevent regrowth. Irradiation offers the only means for potentially ablating significant postoperative residual nonfunctioning tumor tissue. In contrast, PRL- and GH-secreting tumor tissues are amenable to medical therapy.

Side Effects In the short term, radiation may cause transient nausea and weakness. Alopecia and loss of taste and smell may be more long-lasting. Failure of pituitary hormone synthesis is common in patients who have undergone head and neck or pituitary-directed irradiation. More than 50% of patients develop loss of GH, ACTH, TSH, and/or gonadotropin secretion within 10 years, usually due to hypothalamic damage. Lifelong follow-up with testing of anterior pituitary hormone reserve is therefore required after radiation treatment. Optic nerve damage with impaired vision due to optic neuritis is reported in about 2% of patients who undergo pituitary irradiation. Cranial nerve damage is uncommon now that radiation doses are ≤2 Gy (200 rad) at any one treatment session and the maximum dose is <50 Gy (5000 rad). The use of stereotactic radiotherapy may reduce damage to adjacent structures. Radiotherapy for pituitary tumors has been associated with adverse mortality rates, mainly from cerebrovascular disease. The cumulative risk of developing a secondary tumor after conventional radiation is 1.3% after 10 years and 1.9% after 20 years.

MEDICAL Medical therapy for pituitary tumors is highly specific and depends on tumor type. For prolactinomas, dopamine agonists are the treatment of choice. For acromegaly, somatostatin analogues and GH receptor antagonists are indicated. For TSH-secreting tumors, somatostatin analogues and occasionally dopamine agonists are indicated. ACTH-secreting tumors and nonfunctioning tumors are generally not responsive to medications and require surgery and/or irradiation.

PROLACTIN

SYNTHESIS

PRL consists of 198 amino acids and has a molecular mass of 21,500 kDa; it is weakly homologous to GH and human placental lactogen (hPL), reflecting the duplication and divergence of a common GH-PRL-hPL precursor gene. PRL is synthesized in lactotropes, which constitute about 20% of anterior pituitary cells. Lactotropes and somatotropes are derived from a common precursor cell that may give rise to a tumor that secretes both PRL and GH. Marked lactotrope cell hyperplasia develops during pregnancy and the first few months of lactation. These transient functional changes in the lactotrope population are induced by estrogen.

SECRETION

Normal adult serum PRL levels are about 10–25 μg/L in women and 10–20 μg/L in men. PRL secretion is pulsatile, with the highest secretory peaks occurring during rapid eye movement sleep. Peak serum PRL levels (up to 30 μg/L) occur between 4:00 and 6:00 A.M. The circulating half-life of PRL is about 50 min.

PRL is unique among the pituitary hormones in that the predominant central control mechanism is inhibitory, reflecting dopamine-mediated suppression of PRL release. This regulatory pathway accounts for the spontaneous PRL hypersecretion that occurs with pituitary stalk section, often a consequence of compressive mass lesions at the skull base. Pituitary dopamine type 2 (D_2) receptors mediate inhibition of PRL synthesis and secretion. Targeted disruption (gene knockout) of the murine D_2 receptor in mice results in hyperprolactinemia and lactotrope proliferation. As discussed below, dopamine agonists play a central role in the management of hyperprolactinemic disorders.

Thyrotropin-releasing hormone (TRH) (pyro Glu-His-Pro-NH_2) is a hypothalamic tripeptide that elicits prolactin release within 15–30 min after intravenous injection. The physiologic relevance of TRH for PRL regulation is unclear, and it appears primarily to regulate TSH (Chap. 341). *Vasoactive intestinal peptide* (VIP) also induces PRL release, whereas glucocorticoids and thyroid hormone weakly suppress PRL secretion.

Serum PRL levels rise transiently after exercise, meals, sexual intercourse, minor surgical procedures, general anesthesia, chest wall injury, acute myocardial infarction, and other forms of acute stress. PRL levels increase markedly (about tenfold) during pregnancy and decline rapidly within 2 weeks of parturition. If breast-feeding is initiated, basal PRL levels remain elevated; suckling stimulates reflex increases in PRL levels that last for about 30–45 min. Breast suckling activates neural afferent pathways in the hypothalamus that induce PRL release. With time, suckling-induced responses diminish and interfeeding PRL levels return to normal.

ACTION

The PRL receptor is a member of the type I cytokine receptor family that also includes GH and interleukin (IL) 6 receptors. Ligand binding induces receptor dimerization and intracellular signaling by Janus kinase (JAK), which stimulates translocation of the signal transduction and activators of transcription (STAT) family to activate target genes. In the breast, the lobuloalveolar epithelium proliferates in response to PRL, placental lactogens, estrogen, progesterone, and local paracrine growth factors, including IGF-I.

PRL acts to induce and maintain lactation, decrease reproductive function, and suppress sexual drive. These functions are geared toward ensuring that maternal lactation is sustained and not interrupted by pregnancy. PRL inhibits reproductive function by suppressing hypothalamic GnRH and pituitary gonadotropin secretion and by impairing gonadal steroidogenesis in both women and men. In the ovary, PRL blocks folliculogenesis and inhibits granulosa cell aromatase activity, leading to hypoestrogenism and anovulation. PRL also has a luteolytic effect, generating a shortened, or inadequate, luteal phase of the menstrual cycle. In men, attenuated LH secretion leads to low testosterone levels and decreased spermatogenesis. These hormonal changes decrease libido and reduce fertility in patients with hyperprolactinemia.

HYPERPROLACTINEMIA

Etiology

Hyperprolactinemia is the most common pituitary hormone hypersecretion syndrome in both men and women. PRL-secreting pituitary adenomas (prolactinomas) are the most common cause of PRL levels >200 μg/L (see below). Less pronounced PRL elevation can also be seen with microprolactinomas but is more commonly caused by drugs, pituitary stalk compression, hypothyroidism, or renal failure (Table 339-9).

Pregnancy and lactation are the important physiologic causes of hyperprolactinemia. Sleep-associated hyperprolactinemia reverts to normal within an hour of awakening. Nipple stimulation and

TABLE 339-9 Etiology of Hyperprolactinemia

I. Physiologic hypersecretion	**V. Drug-induced hypersecretion**
Pregnancy	Dopamine receptor blockers
Lactation	Atypical antipsychotics: risperidone
Chest wall stimulation	Phenothiazines: chlorpromazine, perphenazine
Sleep	Butyrophenones: haloperidol
Stress	Thioxanthenes
II. Hypothalamic–pituitary stalk damage	Metoclopramide
Tumors	Dopamine synthesis inhibitors
Craniopharyngioma	α-Methyldopa
Suprasellar pituitary mass	Catecholamine depletors
Meningioma	Reserpine
Dysgerminoma	Opiates
Metastases	H_2 antagonists
Empty sella	Cimetidine, ranitidine
Lymphocytic hypophysitis	Imipramines
Adenoma with stalk compression	Amitriptyline, amoxapine
Granulomas	Serotonin reuptake inhibitors
Rathke's cyst	Fluoxetine
Irradiation	Calcium channel blockers
Trauma	Verapamil
Pituitary stalk section	Estrogens
Suprasellar surgery	TRH
III. Pituitary hypersecretion	
Prolactinoma	
Acromegaly	
IV. Systemic disorders	
Chronic renal failure	
Hypothyroidism	
Cirrhosis	
Pseudocyesis	
Epileptic seizures	

Note: Hyperprolactinemia >200 μg/L almost invariably is indicative of a prolactin-secreting pituitary adenoma. Physiologic causes, hypothyroidism, and drug-induced hyperprolactinemia should be excluded before extensive evaluation.

sexual orgasm also may increase PRL. Chest wall stimulation or trauma (including chest surgery and herpes zoster) invoke the reflex suckling arc with resultant hyperprolactinemia. Chronic renal failure elevates PRL by decreasing peripheral clearance. Primary hypothyroidism is associated with mild hyperprolactinemia, probably because of compensatory TRH secretion.

Lesions of the hypothalamic-pituitary region that disrupt hypothalamic dopamine synthesis, portal vessel delivery, or lactotrope responses are associated with hyperprolactinemia. Thus, hypothalamic tumors, cysts, infiltrative disorders, and radiation-induced damage cause elevated PRL levels, usually in the range of 30–100 μg/L. Plurihormonal adenomas (including GH and ACTH tumors) may hypersecrete PRL directly. Pituitary masses, including clinically nonfunctioning pituitary tumors, may compress the pituitary stalk to cause hyperprolactinemia.

Drug-induced inhibition or disruption of dopaminergic receptor function is a common cause of hyperprolactinemia (Table 339-9). Thus, antipsychotics and antidepressants are a relatively common cause of mild hyperprolactinemia. Most patients receiving risperidone have elevated prolactin levels, sometimes exceeding 200 ug/L. Methyldopa inhibits dopamine synthesis and verapamil blocks dopamine release, also leading to hyperprolactinemia. Hormonal agents that induce PRL include estrogens and TRH.

Presentation and diagnosis

Amenorrhea, galactorrhea, and infertility are the hallmarks of hyperprolactinemia in women. If hyperprolactinemia develops before menarche, primary amenorrhea results. More commonly, hyperprolactinemia develops later in life and leads to oligomenorrhea and ultimately to amenorrhea. If hyperprolactinemia is sustained, vertebral bone mineral density can be reduced compared with age-matched controls, particularly when it is associated with pronounced hypoestrogenemia. Galactorrhea is present in up to 80% of hyperprolactinemic women. Although usually bilateral and spontaneous, it may be unilateral or expressed only manually. Patients also may complain of decreased libido, weight gain, and mild hirsutism.

In men with hyperprolactinemia, diminished libido, infertility, and visual loss (from optic nerve compression) are the usual presenting symptoms. Gonadotropin suppression leads to reduced testosterone, impotence, and oligospermia. True galactorrhea is uncommon in men with hyperprolactinemia. If the disorder is long-standing, secondary effects of hypogonadism are evident, including osteopenia, reduced muscle mass, and decreased beard growth.

The diagnosis of idiopathic hyperprolactinemia is made by exclusion of known causes of hyperprolactinemia in the setting of a normal pituitary MRI. Some of these patients may harbor small microadenomas below visible MRI sensitivity (~2 mm).

■ GALACTORRHEA

Galactorrhea, the inappropriate discharge of milk-containing fluid from the breast, is considered abnormal if it persists longer than 6 months after childbirth or discontinuation of breast-feeding. Postpartum galactorrhea associated with amenorrhea is a self-limiting disorder usually associated with moderately elevated PRL levels. Galactorrhea may occur spontaneously, or it may be elicited by nipple pressure. In both men and women, galactorrhea may vary in color and consistency (transparent, milky, or bloody) and arise either unilaterally or bilaterally. Mammography or ultrasound is indicated for bloody discharges (particularly from a single nipple), which may be caused by breast cancer. Galactorrhea is commonly associated with hyperprolactinemia caused by any of the conditions listed in Table 339-9. Acromegaly is associated with galactorrhea in about one-third of patients. Treatment of galactorrhea usually involves managing the underlying disorder (e.g., replacing T_4 for hypothyroidism, discontinuing a medication, treating prolactinoma).

Laboratory investigation

Basal, fasting morning PRL levels (normally <20 μg/L) should be measured to assess hypersecretion. Both false-positive and false-negative results may be encountered. In patients with markedly elevated PRL levels (>1000 μg/L), reported results may be falsely lowered because of assay artifacts; sample dilution is required to measure these high values accurately. Falsely elevated values may be caused by aggregated forms of circulating PRL, which are usually biologically inactive (macroprolactinemia). Hypothyroidism should be excluded by measuring TSH and T_4 levels.

TREATMENT Hyperprolactinemia

Treatment of hyperprolactinemia depends on the cause of elevated PRL levels. Regardless of the etiology, however, treatment should be aimed at normalizing PRL levels to alleviate suppressive effects on gonadal function, halt galactorrhea, and preserve bone mineral density. Dopamine agonists are effective for most causes of hyperprolactinemia (see the treatment section for prolactinoma, below) regardless of the underlying cause.

If the patient is taking a medication known to cause hyperprolactinemia, the drug should be withdrawn, if possible. For psychiatric patients who require neuroleptic agents, supervised dose titration or the addition of a dopamine agonist can help restore normoprolactinemia and alleviate reproductive symptoms. However, dopamine agonists sometimes worsen the underlying psychiatric condition, especially at high doses. Hyperprolactinemia usually resolves after adequate thyroid hormone replacement in hypothyroid patients or after renal transplantation in patients undergoing dialysis. Resection of hypothalamic or sellar mass lesions can reverse hyperprolactinemia caused by stalk compression and reduced dopamine tone. Granulomatous infiltrates occasionally respond to glucocorticoid administration. In patients with irreversible hypothalamic damage, no treatment may be warranted. In up to 30% of patients with hyperprolactinemia—usually without a visible pituitary microadenoma—the condition may resolve spontaneously.

■ PROLACTINOMA

Etiology and prevalence

Tumors arising from lactotrope cells account for about half of all functioning pituitary tumors, with a population prevalence of ~10/100,000 in men and ~30/100,000 in women. Mixed tumors that secrete combinations of GH and PRL, ACTH and PRL, and rarely TSH and PRL are also seen. These plurihormonal tumors are usually recognized by immunohistochemistry, sometimes without apparent clinical manifestations from the production of additional hormones. Microadenomas are classified as <1 cm in diameter and usually do not invade the parasellar region. Macroadenomas are >1 cm in diameter and may be locally invasive and impinge on adjacent structures. The female:male ratio for microprolactinomas is 20:1, whereas the sex ratio is near 1:1 for macroadenomas. Tumor size generally correlates directly with PRL concentrations; values >250 μg/L usually are associated with macroadenomas. Men tend to present with larger tumors than women, possibly because the features of male hypogonadism are less readily evident. PRL levels remain stable in most patients, reflecting the slow growth of these tumors. About 5% of microadenomas progress in the long term to macroadenomas.

Presentation and diagnosis

Women usually present with amenorrhea, infertility, and galactorrhea. If the tumor extends outside the sella, visual field defects or other mass effects may be seen. Men often present with impotence, loss of libido, infertility, or signs of central CNS compression, including headaches and visual defects. Assuming that physiologic and medication-induced causes of hyperprolactinemia are excluded (Table 339-9), the diagnosis of prolactinoma is likely with a PRL level >200 μg/L. PRL levels <100 μg/L may be caused by microadenomas, other sellar lesions that decrease dopamine inhibition, or nonneoplastic causes of hyperprolactinemia. For this reason, an MRI should be performed in all patients with hyperprolactinemia. It is important to remember that hyperprolactinemia caused secondarily by the mass effects of nonlactotrope lesions is also corrected by treatment with dopamine agonists despite failure to shrink the underlying mass. Consequently, PRL suppression by dopamine agonists does not necessarily indicate that the underlying lesion is a prolactinoma.

TREATMENT Prolactinoma

As microadenomas rarely progress to become macroadenomas, no treatment may be needed if fertility is not desired. Estrogen replacement is indicated to prevent bone loss and other consequences of hypoestrogenemia and does not appear to increase the risk of tumor enlargement; these patients should be monitored by regular serial PRL and MRI measurements.

For symptomatic microadenomas, therapeutic goals include control of hyperprolactinemia, reduction of tumor size, restoration of menses and fertility, and resolution of galactorrhea. Dopamine agonist doses should be titrated to achieve maximal PRL suppression and restoration of reproductive function (Fig. 339-6). A normalized PRL level does not ensure reduced tumor size. However, tumor shrinkage usually is not seen in those who do not respond with lowered PRL levels. For macroadenomas, formal visual field testing should be performed before initiating dopamine agonists. MRI and visual fields should be assessed at 6- to 12-month intervals until the mass shrinks and annually thereafter until maximum size reduction has occurred.

MEDICAL Oral dopamine agonists (cabergoline and bromocriptine) are the mainstay of therapy for patients with micro- or macroprolactinomas. Dopamine agonists suppress PRL secretion and synthesis as well as lactotrope cell proliferation. In patients with microadenomas who have achieved normoprolactinemia and significant reduction of tumor mass, the dopamine agonist may be withdrawn after 2 years. These patients should be monitored carefully for evidence of prolactinoma recurrence. About 20% of patients (especially males) are resistant to dopaminergic treatment; these adenomas may exhibit decreased D_2 dopamine receptor numbers or a postreceptor defect. D_2 receptor gene mutations in the pituitary have not been reported.

Cabergoline An ergoline derivative, cabergoline is a long-acting dopamine agonist with high D_2 receptor affinity. The drug effectively suppresses PRL for >14 days after a single oral dose and induces prolactinoma shrinkage in most patients. Cabergoline (0.5 to 1.0 mg twice weekly) achieves normoprolactinemia and resumption of normal gonadal function in ~80% of patients with microadenomas; galactorrhea improves or resolves in 90% of patients. Cabergoline normalizes PRL and shrinks ~70% of macroprolactinomas. Mass effect symptoms, including headaches and visual disorders, usually improve dramatically within days after cabergoline initiation; improvement of sexual function requires several weeks of treatment but may occur before complete normalization of prolactin levels. After initial control of PRL levels has been achieved, cabergoline should be reduced to the lowest effective maintenance dose.

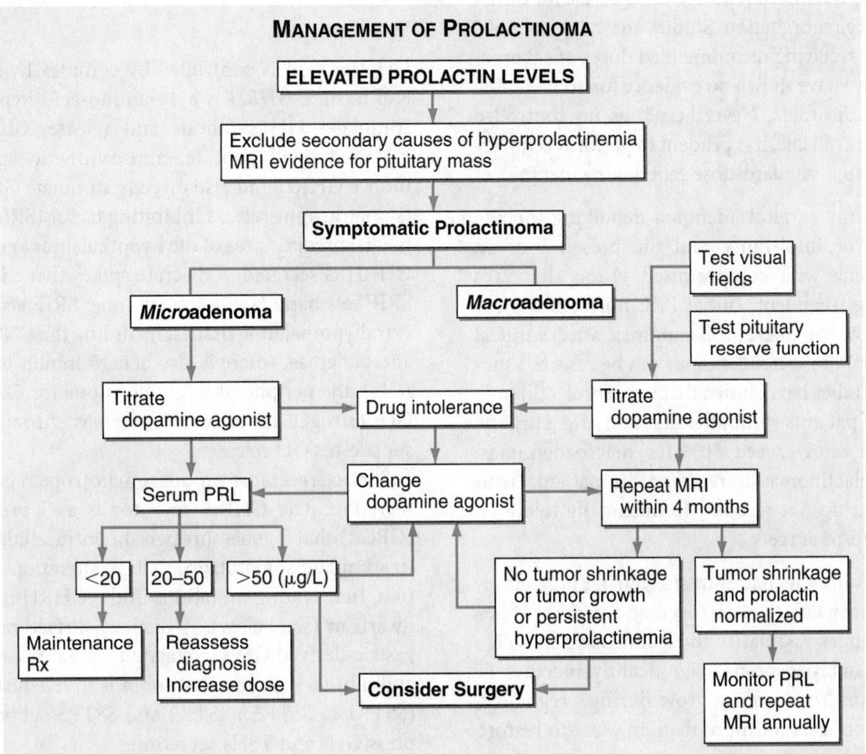

Figure 339-6 Management of prolactinoma. MRI, magnetic resonance imaging; PRL, prolactin.

In ~5% of treated patients harboring a microadenoma, hyperprolactinemia may resolve and not recur when dopamine agonists are discontinued after long-term treatment. Cabergoline also may be effective in patients resistant to bromocriptine. Adverse effects and drug intolerance are encountered less commonly than with bromocriptine.

Bromocriptine The ergot alkaloid bromocriptine mesylate is a dopamine receptor agonist that suppresses prolactin secretion. Because it is short-acting, the drug is preferred when pregnancy is desired. In microadenomas bromocriptine rapidly lowers serum prolactin levels to normal in up to 70% of patients, decreases tumor size, and restores gonadal function. In patients with macroadenomas, prolactin levels are also normalized in 70% of patients and tumor mass shrinkage (≥50%) is achieved in most patients.

Therapy is initiated by administering a low bromocriptine dose (0.625–1.25 mg) at bedtime with a snack, followed by gradually increasing the dose. Most patients are controlled with a daily dose of ≤7.5 mg (2.5 mg tid).

Side Effects Side effects of dopamine agonists include constipation, nasal stuffiness, dry mouth, nightmares, insomnia, and vertigo; decreasing the dose usually alleviates these problems. Nausea, vomiting, and postural hypotension with faintness may occur in ~25% of patients after the initial dose. These symptoms may persist in some patients. In general, fewer side effects are reported with cabergoline. For the approximately 15% of patients who are intolerant of oral bromocriptine, cabergoline may be better tolerated. Intravaginal administration of bromocriptine is often efficacious in patients with intractable gastrointestinal side effects. Auditory hallucinations, delusions, and mood swings have been reported in up to 5% of patients and may be due to the dopamine agonist properties or to the lysergic acid derivative of the compounds. Rare reports of leukopenia, thrombocytopenia, pleural fibrosis, cardiac arrhythmias, and hepatitis have been described. Patients with Parkinson's disease who receive at least 3 mg of cabergoline daily have been reported to be at risk for development of cardiac valve regurgitation. Studies analyzing over 500 prolactinoma patients receiving recommended doses of cabergoline (up to 2 mg weekly) have shown no evidence for an increased incidence of valvular disorders. Nevertheless, as no controlled prospective studies are available, it is prudent to perform echocardiograms before initiating standard-dose cabergoline therapy.

Surgery Indications for surgical adenoma debulking include dopamine resistance or intolerance and the presence of an invasive macroadenoma with compromised vision that fails to improve after drug treatment. Initial PRL normalization is achieved in about 70% of microprolactinomas after surgical resection, but only 30% of macroadenomas can be resected successfully. Follow-up studies have shown that hyperprolactinemia recurs in up to 20% of patients within the first year after surgery; long-term recurrence rates exceed 50% for macroadenomas. Radiotherapy for prolactinomas is reserved for patients with aggressive tumors that do not respond to maximally tolerated dopamine agonists and/or surgery.

PREGNANCY The pituitary increases in size during pregnancy, reflecting the stimulatory effects of estrogen and perhaps other growth factors on pituitary vascularity and lactotrope cell hyperplasia. About 5% of microadenomas significantly increase in size, but 15–30% of macroadenomas grow during pregnancy. Bromocriptine has been used for more than 30 years to restore fertility in women with hyperprolactinemia, without evidence of teratogenic effects. Nonetheless, most authorities recommend strategies to minimize fetal exposure to the drug. For women taking bromocriptine who desire pregnancy, mechanical contraception should be used through three regular menstrual cycles to allow for conception timing. When pregnancy is confirmed, bromocriptine should be discontinued and PRL levels followed serially, especially if headaches or visual symptoms occur. For women harboring macroadenomas, regular visual field testing is recommended, and the drug should be reinstituted if tumor growth is apparent. Although pituitary MRI may be safe during pregnancy, this procedure should be reserved for symptomatic patients with severe headache and/or visual field defects. Surgical decompression may be indicated if vision is threatened. Although comprehensive data support the efficacy and relative safety of bromocriptine-facilitated fertility, patients should be advised of potential unknown deleterious effects and the risk of tumor growth during pregnancy. As cabergoline is long-acting with a high D_2-receptor affinity, it is not recommended for use in women when fertility is desired.

GROWTH HORMONE

SYNTHESIS

GH is the most abundant anterior pituitary hormone, and GH-secreting somatotrope cells constitute up to 50% of the total anterior pituitary cell population. Mammosomatotrope cells, which coexpress PRL with GH, can be identified by using double immunostaining techniques. Somatotrope development and GH transcription are determined by expression of the cell-specific Pit-1 nuclear transcription factor. Five distinct genes encode GH and related proteins. The pituitary GH gene (*hGH-N*) produces two alternatively spliced products that give rise to 22-kDa GH (191 amino acids) and a less abundant 20-kDa GH molecule with similar biologic activity. Placental syncytiotrophoblast cells express a GH variant (*hGH-V*) gene; the related hormone human chorionic somatotropin (HCS) is expressed by distinct members of the gene cluster.

SECRETION

GH secretion is controlled by complex hypothalamic and peripheral factors. *GHRH* is a 44-amino-acid hypothalamic peptide that stimulates GH synthesis and release. Ghrelin, an octanoylated gastric-derived peptide, and synthetic agonists of the *GHS-R* induce GHRH and also directly stimulate GH release. *Somatostatin* [somatotropin-release inhibiting factor (SRIF)] is synthesized in the medial preoptic area of the hypothalamus and inhibits GH secretion. GHRH is secreted in discrete spikes that elicit GH pulses, whereas SRIF sets basal GH secretory tone. SRIF also is expressed in many extrahypothalamic tissues, including the CNS, gastrointestinal tract, and pancreas, where it also acts to inhibit islet hormone secretion. *IGF-I*, the peripheral target hormone for GH, feeds back to inhibit GH; estrogen induces GH, whereas chronic glucocorticoid excess suppresses GH release.

Surface receptors on the somatotrope regulate GH synthesis and secretion. The GHRH receptor is a G protein–coupled receptor (GPCR) that signals through the intracellular cyclic AMP pathway to stimulate somatotrope cell proliferation as well as GH production. Inactivating mutations of the GHRH receptor cause profound dwarfism (see below). A distinct surface receptor for ghrelin, the gastric-derived GH secretagogue, is expressed in the hypothalamus and pituitary. Somatostatin binds to five distinct receptor subtypes (SSTR1 to SSTR5); SSTR2 and SSTR5 subtypes preferentially suppress GH (and TSH) secretion.

GH secretion is pulsatile, with highest peak levels occurring at night, generally correlating with sleep onset. GH secretory rates decline markedly with age so that hormone levels in middle age are about 15% of pubertal levels. These changes are paralleled by an age-related decline in lean muscle mass. GH secretion is also reduced in obese individuals, though IGF-I levels may not be suppressed, suggesting a change in the setpoint for feedback control. Elevated GH levels occur within an hour of deep sleep onset as well as after exercise, physical stress, and trauma and during sepsis. Integrated 24-h GH secretion is higher in women and is also enhanced by estrogen replacement. Using standard assays, random GH measurements are undetectable in ~50% of daytime samples obtained from healthy subjects and are also undetectable in most obese and elderly subjects. Thus, single random GH measurements do not distinguish patients with adult GH deficiency from normal persons.

GH secretion is profoundly influenced by nutritional factors. Using newer ultrasensitive GH assays with a sensitivity of 0.002 μg/L, a glucose load suppresses GH to <0.7 μg/L in women and to <0.07 μg/L in men. Increased GH pulse frequency and peak amplitudes occur with chronic malnutrition or prolonged fasting. GH is stimulated by intravenous L-arginine, dopamine, and apomorphine (a dopamine receptor agonist), as well as by α-adrenergic pathways. β-Adrenergic blockage induces basal GH and enhances GHRH- and insulin-evoked GH release.

ACTION

The pattern of GH secretion may affect tissue responses. The higher GH pulsatility observed in men compared with the relatively continuous GH secretion in women may be an important biologic determinant of linear growth patterns and liver enzyme induction.

The 70-kDa peripheral GH receptor protein has structural homology with the cytokine/hematopoietic superfamily. A fragment of the receptor extracellular domain generates a soluble GH binding protein (GHBP) that interacts with GH in the circulation. The liver and cartilage contain the greatest number of GH receptors. GH binding to preformed receptor dimers is followed by internal rotation and subsequent signaling through the JAK/STAT pathway. Activated STAT proteins translocate to the nucleus, where they modulate expression of GH-regulated target genes. GH analogues that bind to the receptor but are incapable of mediating receptor signaling are potent antagonists of GH action. A GH receptor antagonist (pegvisomant) is approved for treatment of acromegaly.

GH induces protein synthesis and nitrogen retention and impairs glucose tolerance by antagonizing insulin action. GH also stimulates lipolysis, leading to increased circulating fatty acid levels, reduced omental fat mass, and enhanced lean body mass. GH promotes sodium, potassium, and water retention and elevates serum levels of inorganic phosphate. Linear bone growth occurs as a result of complex hormonal and growth factor actions, including those of IGF-I. GH stimulates epiphyseal prechondrocyte differentiation. These precursor cells produce IGF-I locally, and their proliferation is also responsive to the growth factor.

INSULIN-LIKE GROWTH FACTORS

Although GH exerts direct effects in target tissues, many of its physiologic effects are mediated indirectly through IGF-I, a potent growth and differentiation factor. The liver is the major source of circulating IGF-I. In peripheral tissues, IGF-I exerts local paracrine actions that appear to be both dependent on and independent of GH. Thus, GH administration induces circulating IGF-I as well as stimulating local IGF-I production in multiple tissues.

Both IGF-I and IGF-II are bound to high-affinity circulating IGF-binding proteins (IGFBPs) that regulate IGF bioactivity. Levels of IGFBP3 are GH-dependent, and it serves as the major carrier protein for circulating IGF-I. GH deficiency and malnutrition usually are associated with low IGFBP3 levels. IGFBP1 and IGFBP2 regulate local tissue IGF action but do not bind appreciable amounts of circulating IGF-I.

Serum IGF-I concentrations are profoundly affected by physiologic factors. Levels increase during puberty, peak at 16 years, and subsequently decline by >80% during the aging process. IGF-I concentrations are higher in women than in men. Because GH is the major determinant of hepatic IGF-I synthesis, abnormalities of GH synthesis or action (e.g., pituitary failure, GHRH receptor defect, GH receptor defect) reduce IGF-I levels. Hypocaloric states are associated with GH resistance; IGF-I levels are therefore low with cachexia, malnutrition, and sepsis. In acromegaly, IGF-I levels are invariably high and reflect a log-linear relationship with GH concentrations.

IGF-I physiology

IGF-I has been approved for use in patients with GH-resistance syndromes. Injected IGF-I (100 μg/kg) induces hypoglycemia, and lower doses improve insulin sensitivity in patients with severe insulin resistance and diabetes. In cachectic subjects, IGF-I infusion (12 μg/kg per hour) enhances nitrogen retention and lowers cholesterol levels. Longer-term subcutaneous IGF-I injections enhance protein synthesis and are anabolic. Although bone formation markers are induced, bone turnover also may be stimulated by IGF-I.

IGF-I side effects are dose-dependent, and overdose may result in hypoglycemia, hypotension, fluid retention, temporomandibular jaw pain, and increased intracranial pressure, all of which are reversible. Avascular femoral head necrosis has been reported. Chronic excess IGF-I administration presumably would result in features of acromegaly.

DISORDERS OF GROWTH AND DEVELOPMENT

Skeletal maturation and somatic growth

The growth plate is dependent on a variety of hormonal stimuli, including GH, IGF-I, sex steroids, thyroid hormones, paracrine growth factors, and cytokines. The growth-promoting process also requires caloric energy, amino acids, vitamins, and trace metals and consumes about 10% of normal energy production. Malnutrition impairs chondrocyte activity and reduces circulating IGF-I and IGFBP3 levels.

Linear bone growth rates are very high in infancy and are pituitary-dependent. Mean growth velocity is ~6 cm/year in later childhood and usually is maintained within a given range on a standardized percentile chart. Peak growth rates occur during midpuberty when bone age is 12 (girls) or 13 (boys). Secondary sexual development is associated with elevated sex steroids that cause progressive epiphyseal growth plate closure. *Bone age* is delayed in patients with all forms of true GH deficiency or GH receptor defects that result in attenuated GH action.

Short stature may occur as a result of constitutive intrinsic growth defects or because of acquired extrinsic factors that impair growth. In general, delayed bone age in a child with short stature is suggestive of a hormonal or systemic disorder, whereas normal bone age in a short child is more likely to be caused by a genetic cartilage dysplasia or growth plate disorder (Chap. 363).

GH deficiency in children

GH deficiency Isolated GH deficiency is characterized by short stature, micropenis, increased fat, high-pitched voice, and a propensity to hypoglycemia due to relatively unopposed insulin action. Familial modes of inheritance are seen in one-third of these individuals and may be autosomal dominant, recessive, or X-linked. About 10% of children with GH deficiency have mutations in the *GH-N* gene, including gene deletions and a wide range of point mutations. Mutations in transcription factors Pit-1 and Prop-1, which control somatotrope development result in GH deficiency in combination with other pituitary hormone deficiencies, which may become manifest only in adulthood. The diagnosis of *idiopathic GH deficiency* (IGHD) should be made only after known molecular defects have been rigorously excluded.

GHRH receptor mutations Recessive mutations of the GHRH receptor gene in subjects with severe proportionate dwarfism are associated with low basal GH levels that cannot be stimulated by exogenous GHRH, GHRP, or insulin-induced hypoglycemia, as well as anterior pituitary hypoplasia The syndrome exemplifies the importance of the GHRH receptor for somatotrope cell proliferation and hormonal responsiveness.

Growth hormone insensitivity This is caused by defects of GH receptor structure or signaling. Homozygous or heterozygous mutations of the GH receptor are associated with partial or complete GH insensitivity and growth failure (*Laron syndrome*). The diagnosis is based on normal or high GH levels, with decreased circulating GHBP, and low IGF-I levels. Very rarely, defective IGF-I, IGF-I receptor, or IGF-I signaling defects are also encountered. *STAT5B* mutations result in immunodeficiency with abrogated GH signaling, leading to short stature with normal or elevated GH levels and low IGF-I levels.

Nutritional short stature Caloric deprivation and malnutrition, uncontrolled diabetes, and chronic renal failure represent secondary causes of abrogated GH receptor function. These conditions also stimulate production of proinflammatory cytokines, which act to exacerbate the block of GH-mediated signal transduction. Children with these conditions typically exhibit features of acquired short stature with normal or elevated GH, and low IGF-I levels. Circulating GH receptor antibodies may rarely cause peripheral GH insensitivity.

Psychosocial short stature Emotional and social deprivation lead to growth retardation accompanied by delayed speech, discordant hyperphagia, and an attenuated response to administered GH. A nurturing environment restores growth rates.

Presentation and diagnosis

Short stature is commonly encountered in clinical practice, and the decision to evaluate these children requires clinical judgment in association with auxologic data and family history. Short stature should be evaluated comprehensively if a patient's height is >3 standard deviations (SD) below the mean for age or if the growth rate has decelerated. Skeletal maturation is best evaluated by measuring a radiologic bone age, which is based mainly on the degree of wrist bone growth plate fusion. Final height can be predicted using standardized scales (Bayley-Pinneau or Tanner-Whitehouse) or estimated by adding 6.5 cm (boys) or subtracting 6.5 cm (girls) from the midparental height.

Laboratory investigation

Because GH secretion is pulsatile, GH deficiency is best assessed by examining the response to provocative stimuli, including exercise, insulin-induced hypoglycemia, and other pharmacologic tests that normally increase GH to >7 μg/L in children. Random GH measurements do not distinguish normal children from those with true GH deficiency. Adequate adrenal and thyroid hormone replacement should be assured before testing. Age- and sex-matched IGF-I levels are not sufficiently sensitive or specific to make the diagnosis but can be useful to confirm GH deficiency. Pituitary MRI may reveal pituitary mass lesions or structural defects. Molecular analyses for known mutations should be undertaken when the cause of short stature remains cryptic, or when additional clinical features suggest a gentic cause.

TREATMENT Disorders of Growth and Development

Replacement therapy with recombinant GH (0.02–0.05 mg/kg per day subcutaneously) restores growth velocity in GH-deficient children to ~10 cm/year. If pituitary insufficiency is documented, other associated hormone deficits should be corrected—especially adrenal steroids. GH treatment is also moderately effective for accelerating growth rates in children with Turner syndrome and chronic renal failure.

In patients with GH insensitivity and growth retardation due to mutations of the GH receptor, treatment with IGF-I bypasses the dysfunctional GH receptor.

■ ADULT GH DEFICIENCY (AGHD)

This disorder usually is caused by hypothalamic or pituitary somatotrope damage. Acquired pituitary hormone deficiency follows a typical pattern in which loss of adequate GH reserve foreshadows subsequent hormone deficits. The sequential order of hormone loss is usually GH → FSH/LH → TSH → ACTH.

Presentation and diagnosis

The clinical features of AGHD include changes in body composition, lipid metabolism, and quality of life and cardiovascular dysfunction (Table 339-10). Body composition changes are common and include reduced lean body mass, increased fat mass with selective deposition of intraabdominal visceral fat, and increased waist-to-hip ratio. Hyperlipidemia, left ventricular dysfunction, hypertension, and increased plasma fibrinogen levels also may be present.

TABLE 339-10 Features of Adult Growth Hormone Deficiency

Clinical	Imaging
Impaired quality of life	Pituitary: mass or structural damage
Decreased energy and drive	Bone: reduced bone mineral density
Poor concentration	Abdomen: excess omental adiposity
Low self-esteem	**Laboratory**
Social isolation	Evoked GH <3 ng/mL
Body composition changes	IGF-I and IGFBP3 low or normal
Increased body fat mass	Increased LDL cholesterol
Central fat deposition	Concomitant gonadotropin, TSH, and/or ACTH reserve deficits may be present
Increased waist-hip ratio	
Decreased lean body mass	
Reduced exercise capacity	
Reduced maximum O_2 uptake	
Impaired cardiac function	
Reduced muscle mass	
Cardiovascular risk factors	
Impaired cardiac structure and function	
Abnormal lipid profile	
Decreased fibrinolytic activity	
Atherosclerosis	
Omental obesity	

Abbreviation: LDL, low-density lipoprotein. For other abbreviations, see text.

Bone mineral content is reduced, with resultant increased fracture rates. Patients may experience social isolation, depression, and difficulty maintaining gainful employment. Adult hypopituitarism is associated with a threefold increase in cardiovascular mortality rates in comparison to age- and sex-matched controls, and this may be due to GH deficiency, as patients in these studies were replaced with other deficient pituitary hormones.

Laboratory investigation

AGHD is rare, and in light of the nonspecific nature of associated clinical symptoms, patients appropriate for testing should be selected carefully on the basis of well-defined criteria. With few exceptions, testing should be restricted to patients with the following predisposing factors: (1) pituitary surgery, (2) pituitary or hypothalamic tumor or granulomas, (3) history of cranial irradiation, (4) radiologic evidence of a pituitary lesion, (5) childhood requirement for GH replacement therapy, and rarely (6) unexplained low age- and sex-matched IGF-I levels. The transition of a GH-deficient adolescent to adulthood requires retesting to document subsequent adult GH deficiency. Up to 20% of patients previously treated for childhood-onset GH deficiency are found to be GH-sufficient on repeat testing as adults.

A significant proportion (~25%) of truly GH-deficient adults have low-normal IGF-I levels. Thus, as in the evaluation of GH deficiency in children, valid age- and sex-matched IGF-I measurements provide a useful index of therapeutic responses but are not sufficiently sensitive for diagnostic purposes. The most validated test to distinguish pituitary-sufficient patients from those with AGHD is insulin-induced (0.05–0.1 U/kg) hypoglycemia. After glucose reduction to ~40 mg/dL, most individuals experience neuroglycopenic symptoms (Chap. 345), and peak GH release occurs at 60 min and remains elevated for up to 2 h. About 90% of healthy adults exhibit GH responses >5 μg/L; AGHD is defined by a peak GH response to hypoglycemia of <3 μg/L. Although insulin-induced hypoglycemia is safe when performed under appropriate supervision, it is contraindicated in patients with diabetes, ischemic heart disease, cerebrovascular disease, or epilepsy and in elderly patients. Alternative stimulatory tests include intravenous arginine (30 g), GHRH (1 μg/kg), GHRP-6 (90 μg) and in glucagon (1 mg). Combinations of these tests may evoke GH secretion in subjects who are not responsive to a single test.

TREATMENT Adult GH Deficiency

Once the diagnosis of AGHD is unequivocally established, replacement of GH may be indicated. Contraindications to therapy include the presence of an active neoplasm, intracranial hypertension, and uncontrolled diabetes and retinopathy. The starting dose of 0.1–0.2 mg/d should be titrated (up to a maximum of 1.25 mg/d) to maintain IGF-I levels in the mid-normal range for age- and sex-matched controls (Fig. 339-7). Women require higher doses than men, and elderly patients require less GH. Long-term GH maintenance sustains normal IGF-I levels and is associated with persistent body composition changes (e.g., enhanced lean body mass and lower body fat). High-density lipoprotein cholesterol increases, but total cholesterol and insulin levels do not change significantly. Lumbar spine bone mineral density increases, but this response is gradual (>1 year). Many patients note significant improvement in quality of life when evaluated by standardized questionnaires. The effect of GH replacement on mortality rates in GH-deficient patients is currently the subject of long-term prospective investigation.

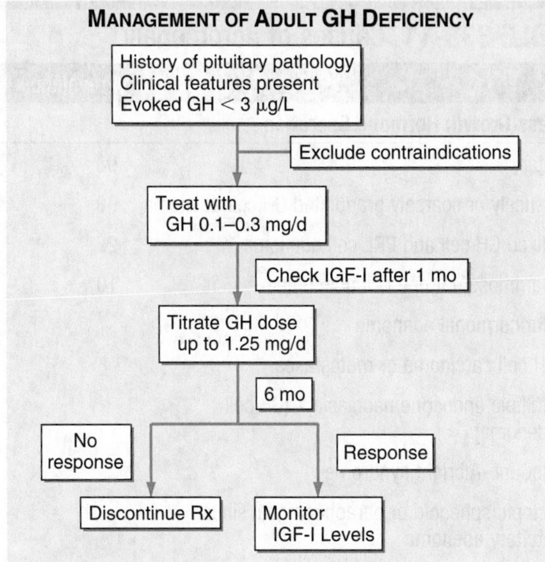

Figure 339-7 Management of adult growth hormone (GH) deficiency. IGF, insulin-like growth factor.

About 30% of patients exhibit reversible dose-related fluid retention, joint pain, and carpal tunnel syndrome, and up to 40% exhibit myalgias and paresthesia. Patients receiving insulin require careful monitoring for dosing adjustments, as GH is a potent counterregulatory hormone for insulin action. Patients with Type 2 diabetes mellitus initially develop further insulin resistance. However, glycemic control improves with the sustained loss of abdominal fat associated with long-term GH replacement. Headache, increased intracranial pressure, hypertension, and tinnitus occur rarely. Pituitary tumor regrowth and progression of skin lesions or other tumors are being assessed in long-term surveillance programs. To date, development of these potential side effects does not appear significant.

ACROMEGALY

Etiology

GH hypersecretion is usually the result of a somatotrope adenoma but may rarely be caused by extrapituitary lesions (Table 339-11). In addition to more common GH-secreting somatotrope adenomas, mixed mammosomatotrope tumors and acidophilic stem-cell adenomas secrete both GH and PRL. In patients with acidophilic stem-cell adenomas, features of hyperprolactinemia (hypogonadism and galactorrhea) predominate over the less clinically evident signs of acromegaly. Occasionally, mixed plurihormonal tumors are encountered that also secrete ACTH, the glycoprotein hormone α subunit, or TSH in addition to GH. Patients with partially empty sellas may present with GH hypersecretion due to a small GH-secreting adenoma within the compressed rim of pituitary tissue; some of these may reflect the spontaneous necrosis of tumors that were previously larger. GH-secreting tumors rarely arise from ectopic pituitary tissue remnants in the nasopharynx or midline sinuses.

There are case reports of ectopic GH secretion by tumors of pancreatic, ovarian, lung, or hematopoietic origin. Rarely, excess GHRH production may cause acromegaly because of chronic stimulation of somatotropes. These patients present with classic features of acromegaly, elevated GH levels, pituitary enlargement on MRI, and pathologic characteristics of pituitary hyperplasia. The most common cause of GHRH-mediated acromegaly is a chest or abdominal

TABLE 339-11 Causes of Acromegaly

	Prevalence, %
Excess Growth Hormone Secretion	
Pituitary	98
Densely or sparsely granulated GH cell adenoma	60
Mixed GH cell and PRL cell adenoma	25
Mammosomatrope cell adenoma	10
Plurihormonal adenoma	
GH cell carcinoma or metastases	
Multiple endocrine neoplasia 1 (GH cell adenoma)	
McCune-Albright syndrome	
Ectopic sphenoid or parapharyngeal sinus pituitary adenoma	
Extrapituitary tumor	
Pancreatic islet cell tumor	<1
Lymphoma	
Excess Growth Hormone–Releasing Hormone Secretion	
Central	<1
Hypothalamic hamartoma, choristoma, ganglioneuroma	<1
Peripheral	<1
Bronchial carcinoid, pancreatic islet cell tumor, small cell lung cancer, adrenal adenoma, medullary thyroid carcinoma, pheochromocytoma	

Source: Adapted from S Melmed: N Engl J Med 322:966, 1990.
Abbreviations: GH, growth hormone; PRL, prolactin.

carcinoid tumor. Although these tumors usually express positive GHRH immunoreactivity, clinical features of acromegaly are evident in only a minority of patients with carcinoid disease. Excessive GHRH also may be elaborated by hypothalamic tumors, usually choristomas or neuromas.

Presentation and diagnosis

Protean manifestations of GH and IGF-I hypersecretion are indolent and often are not clinically diagnosed for 10 years or more. Acral bony overgrowth results in frontal bossing, increased hand and foot size, mandibular enlargement with prognathism, and widened space between the lower incisor teeth. In children and adolescents, initiation of GH hypersecretion before epiphyseal long bone closure is associated with development of pituitary gigantism (Fig. 339-8). Soft tissue swelling results in increased heel pad thickness, increased shoe or glove size, ring tightening, characteristic coarse facial features, and a large fleshy nose. Other commonly encountered clinical features include hyperhidrosis, a deep and hollow-sounding voice, oily skin, arthropathy, kyphosis, carpal tunnel syndrome, proximal muscle weakness and fatigue, acanthosis nigricans, and skin tags. Generalized visceromegaly occurs, including cardiomegaly, macroglossia, and thyroid gland enlargement.

The most significant clinical impact of GH excess occurs with respect to the cardiovascular system. Coronary heart disease, cardiomyopathy with arrhythmias, left ventricular hypertrophy, decreased diastolic function, and hypertension ultimately occur in most patients if untreated. Upper airway obstruction with sleep apnea occurs in more than 60% of patients and is associated with both soft tissue laryngeal airway obstruction and central sleep dysfunction. Diabetes mellitus develops in 25% of patients with acromegaly, and most patients are intolerant of a glucose load (as GH counteracts the action of insulin). Acromegaly is associated with an increased risk of colon polyps and mortality from colonic malignancy; polyps are diagnosed in up to one-third of patients. Overall mortality is increased about threefold and is due primarily

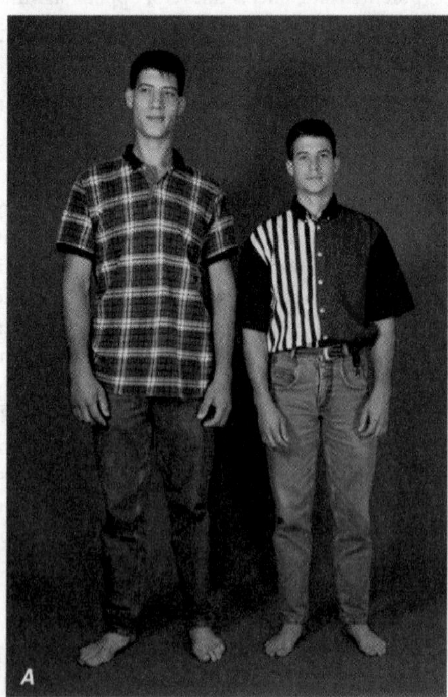

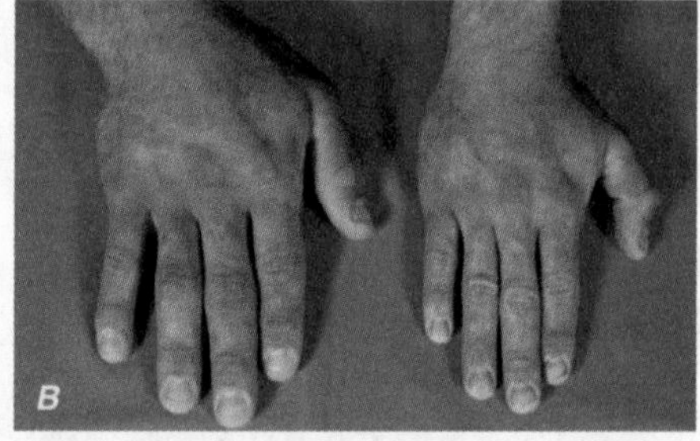

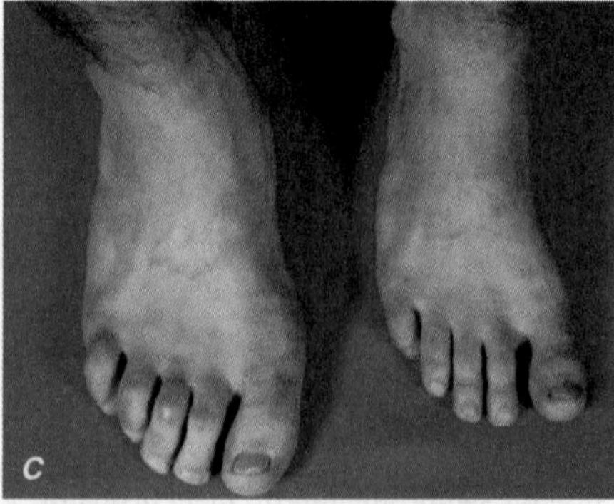

Figure 339-8 Features of acromegaly/gigantism. A 22-year-old man with gigantism due to excess growth hormone is shown to the left of his identical twin. The increased height and prognathism *(A)* and enlarged hand *(B)* and foot *(C)* of the affected twin are apparent. Their clinical features began to diverge at the age of approximately 13 years. *(Reproduced from R Gagel, IE McCutcheon: N Engl J Med 324:524, 1999; with permission.)*

to cardiovascular and cerebrovascular disorders and respiratory disease. Unless GH levels are controlled, survival is reduced by an average of 10 years compared with an age-matched control population.

Laboratory investigation

Age- and sex-matched serum IGF-I levels are elevated in acromegaly. Consequently, an IGF-I level provides a useful laboratory screening measure when clinical features raise the possibility of acromegaly. Due to the pulsatility of GH secretion, measurement of a single random GH level is not useful for the diagnosis or exclusion of acromegaly and does not correlate with disease severity. The diagnosis of acromegaly is confirmed by demonstrating the failure of GH suppression to <0.4 μg/L within 1–2 h of an oral glucose load (75 g). When newer ultrasensitive GH assays are used, normal nadir GH levels are even lower (<0.05 μg/L). About 20% of patients exhibit a paradoxical GH rise after glucose. PRL should be measured, as it is elevated in ~25% of patients with acromegaly. Thyroid function, gonadotropins, and sex steroids may be attenuated because of tumor mass effects. Because most patients will undergo surgery with glucocorticoid coverage, tests of ACTH reserve in asymptomatic patients are more efficiently deferred until after surgery.

TREATMENT Acromegaly

The goal of treatment is to control GH and IGF-I hypersecretion, ablate or arrest tumor growth, ameliorate comorbidities, restore mortality rates to normal, and preserve pituitary function.

Surgical resection of GH-secreting adenomas is the initial treatment for most patients (Fig. 339-9). Somatostatin analogues are used as adjuvant treatment for preoperative shrinkage of large invasive macroadenomas, immediate relief of debilitating symptoms, and reduction of GH hypersecretion; in frail patients experiencing morbidity; and in patients who decline surgery or, when surgery fails, to achieve biochemical control. Irradiation or repeat surgery may be required for patients who cannot tolerate or do not respond to adjunctive medical therapy. The high rate of late hypopituitarism and the slow rate (5–15 years) of biochemical response are the main disadvantages of radiotherapy. Irradiation is also relatively ineffective in normalizing IGF-I levels. Stereotactic ablation of GH-secreting adenomas by gamma-knife radiotherapy is promising, but initial reports suggest that long-term results and side effects are similar to those observed with conventional radiation. Somatostatin analogues may be required while awaiting the full benefits of radiotherapy. Systemic sequelae of acromegaly, including cardiovascular disease, diabetes, and arthritis, should be managed aggressively. Mandibular surgical repair may be indicated.

SURGERY Transsphenoidal surgical resection by an experienced surgeon is the preferred primary treatment for both microadenomas (cure rate ~70%) and macroadenomas (<50% cured). Soft tissue swelling improves immediately after tumor resection. GH levels return to normal within an hour, and IGF-I levels are normalized within 3–4 days. In ~10% of patients, acromegaly may recur several years after apparently successful surgery; hypopituitarism develops in up to 15% of patients after surgery.

SOMATOSTATIN ANALOGUES Somatostatin analogues exert their therapeutic effects through SSTR2 and SSTR5 receptors, both of which invariably are expressed by GH-secreting tumors. Octreotide acetate is an eight-amino-acid synthetic somatostatin analogue. In contrast to native somatostatin, the analogue is relatively resistant to plasma degradation. It has a 2-h serum half-life and possesses fortyfold greater potency than native somatostatin to suppress GH. Octreotide is administered by subcutaneous injection, beginning with 50 μg tid; the dose can be increased gradually up to 1500 μg/d. Fewer than 10% of patients do not

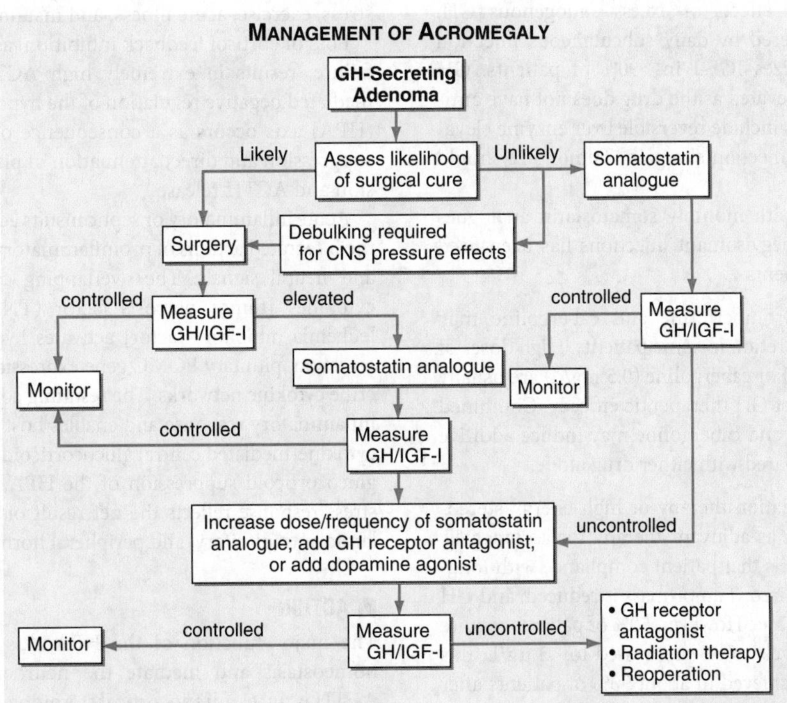

Figure 339-9 Management of acromegaly. GH, growth hormone; CNS, central nervous system; IGF, insulin-like growth factor. *(Adapted from S Melmed et al: J Clin Endocrinol Metab 94:1509–1517, 2009; © The Endocrine Society.)*

respond to the analogue. Octreotide suppresses integrated GH levels and normalizes IGF-I levels in ~75% of treated patients.

The long-acting somatostatin depot formulations, octreotide and lanreotide, are the preferred medical treatment for patients with acromegaly. *Sandostatin-LAR* is a sustained-release, long-acting formulation of octreotide incorporated into microspheres that sustain drug levels for several weeks after intramuscular injection. GH suppression occurs for as long as 6 weeks after a 30-mg intramuscular injection; long-term monthly treatment sustains GH and IGF-I suppression and also reduces pituitary tumor size in ~50% of patients. *Lanreotide* autogel, a slow-release depot somatostatin preparation, is a cyclic somatostatin octapeptide analogue that suppresses GH and IGF-I hypersecretion after a 60-mg subcutaneous injection. Long-term monthly administration controls GH hypersecretion in two-thirds of treated patients and improves patient compliance because of the long interval required between drug injections. Rapid relief of headache and soft tissue swelling occurs in ~75% of patients within days to weeks of somatostatin analogue initiation. Most patients report symptomatic improvement, including amelioration of headache, perspiration, obstructive apnea, and cardiac failure.

Side Effects Somatostatin analogues are well tolerated in most patients. Adverse effects are short-lived and mostly relate to drug-induced suppression of gastrointestinal motility and secretion. Nausea, abdominal discomfort, fat malabsorption, diarrhea, and flatulence occur in one-third of patients, and these symptoms usually remit within 2 weeks. Octreotide suppresses postprandial gallbladder contractility and delays gallbladder emptying; up to 30% of patients develop long-term echogenic sludge or asymptomatic cholesterol gallstones. Other side effects include mild glucose intolerance due to transient insulin suppression, asymptomatic bradycardia, hypothyroxinemia, and local injection site discomfort.

GH RECEPTOR ANTAGONIST Pegvisomant antagonizes endogenous GH action by blocking peripheral GH binding to its receptor. Consequently, serum IGF-I levels are suppressed, reducing the deleterious effects of excess endogenous GH. Pegvisomant is administered by daily subcutaneous injection (10–20 mg) and normalizes IGF-I in >90% of patients. GH levels, however, remain elevated as the drug does not have antitumor actions. Side effects include reversible liver enzyme elevation, lipodystrophy, and injection site pain. Tumor size should be monitored by MRI.

Combined treatment with monthly somatostatin analogues and weekly or biweekly pegvisomant injections has been used effectively in resistant patients.

DOPAMINE AGONISTS Bromocriptine and cabergoline may modestly suppress GH secretion in some patients. High doses of bromocriptine (≥20 mg/d) or cabergoline (0.5 mg/d) are usually required to achieve modest GH therapeutic efficacy. Combined treatment with octreotide and cabergoline may induce additive biochemical control compared with either drug alone.

RADIATION External radiation therapy or high-energy stereotactic techniques are used as adjuvant therapy for acromegaly. An advantage of radiation is that patient compliance with long-term treatment is not required. Tumor mass is reduced, and GH levels are attenuated over time. However, 50% of patients require at least 8 years for GH levels to be suppressed to <5 μg/L; this level of GH reduction is achieved in about 90% of patients after 18 years but represents suboptimal GH suppression. Patients may require interim medical therapy for several years before attaining maximal radiation benefits. Most patients also experience hypothalamic-pituitary damage, leading to gonadotropin, ACTH, and/or TSH deficiency within 10 years of therapy.

In summary, surgery is the preferred primary treatment for GH-secreting microadenomas (Fig. 339-9). The high frequency of GH hypersecretion after macroadenoma resection usually necessitates adjuvant or primary medical therapy for these larger tumors. Patients unable to receive or respond to unimodal medical treatment may benefit from combined treatments or can be offered radiation.

ADRENOCORTICOTROPIC HORMONE

(See also Chap. 342)

■ SYNTHESIS

ACTH-secreting corticotrope cells constitute about 20% of the pituitary cell population. ACTH (39 amino acids) is derived from the POMC precursor protein (266 amino acids) that also generates several other peptides, including β-lipotropin, β-endorphin, met-enkephalin, α-melanocyte-stimulating hormone (α-MSH), and corticotropin-like intermediate lobe protein (CLIP). The POMC gene is potently suppressed by glucocorticoids and induced by CRH, arginine vasopressin (AVP), and proinflammatory cytokines, including IL-6, as well as leukemia inhibitory factor.

CRH, a 41-amino-acid hypothalamic peptide synthesized in the paraventricular nucleus as well as in higher brain centers, is the predominant stimulator of ACTH synthesis and release. The CRH receptor is a GPCR that is expressed on the corticotrope and signals to induce POMC transcription.

■ SECRETION

ACTH secretion is pulsatile and exhibits a characteristic circadian rhythm, peaking at 6 A.M. and reaching a nadir about midnight. Adrenal glucocorticoid secretion, which is driven by ACTH, follows a parallel diurnal pattern. ACTH circadian rhythmicity is determined by variations in secretory pulse amplitude rather than changes in pulse frequency. Superimposed on this endogenous rhythm, ACTH levels are increased by physical and psychological stress, exercise, acute illness, and insulin-induced hypoglycemia.

Loss of cortisol feedback inhibition, as occurs in primary adrenal failure, results in extremely high ACTH levels. Glucocorticoid-mediated negative regulation of the hypothalamic-pituitary-adrenal (HPA) axis occurs as a consequence of both hypothalamic CRH suppression and direct attenuation of pituitary POMC gene expression and ACTH release.

Acute inflammatory or septic insults activate the HPA axis through the integrated actions of proinflammatory cytokines, bacterial toxins, and neural signals. The overlapping cascade of ACTH-inducing cytokines [tumor necrosis factor (TNF); IL-1, -2, and -6; and leukemia inhibitory factor] activates hypothalamic CRH and AVP secretion, pituitary POMC gene expression, and local pituitary paracrine cytokine networks. The resulting cortisol elevation restrains the inflammatory response and enables host protection. Concomitantly, cytokine-mediated central glucocorticoid receptor resistance impairs glucocorticoid suppression of the HPA. Thus, the neuroendocrine stress response reflects the net result of highly integrated hypothalamic, intrapituitary, and peripheral hormone and cytokine signals.

■ ACTION

The major function of the HPA axis is to maintain metabolic homeostasis and mediate the neuroendocrine stress response. ACTH induces adrenocortical steroidogenesis by sustaining adrenal cell proliferation and function. The receptor for ACTH, designated *melanocortin-2 receptor*, is a GPCR that induces steroidogenesis by stimulating a cascade of steroidogenic enzymes (Chap. 342).

ACTH DEFICIENCY

Presentation and diagnosis

Secondary adrenal insufficiency occurs as a result of pituitary ACTH deficiency. It is characterized by fatigue, weakness, anorexia, nausea, vomiting, and, occasionally, hypoglycemia. In contrast to primary adrenal failure, hypocortisolism associated with pituitary failure usually is not accompanied by hyperpigmentation or mineralocorticoid deficiency.

ACTH deficiency is commonly due to glucocorticoid withdrawal after treatment-associated suppression of the HPA axis. Isolated ACTH deficiency may occur after surgical resection of an ACTH-secreting pituitary adenoma that has suppressed the HPA axis; this phenomenon is suggestive of a surgical cure. The mass effects of other pituitary adenomas or sellar lesions may lead to ACTH deficiency, but usually in combination with other pituitary hormone deficiencies. Partial ACTH deficiency may be unmasked in the presence of an acute medical or surgical illness, when clinically significant hypocortisolism reflects diminished ACTH reserve. Rarely, *TPIT* or *POMC* mutations result in primary ACTH deficiency.

Laboratory diagnosis

Inappropriately low ACTH levels in the setting of low cortisol levels are characteristic of diminished ACTH reserve. Low basal serum cortisol levels are associated with blunted cortisol responses to ACTH stimulation and impaired cortisol response to insulin-induced hypoglycemia, or testing with metyrapone or CRH. For a description of provocative ACTH tests, see Chap. 342.

TREATMENT ACTH Deficiency

Glucocorticoid replacement therapy improves most features of ACTH deficiency. The total daily dose of hydrocortisone replacement preferably should not exceed 25 mg daily, divided into two or three doses. Prednisone (5 mg each morning) is longer-acting and has fewer mineralocorticoid effects than hydrocortisone. Some authorities advocate lower maintenance doses in an effort to avoid cushingoid side effects. Doses should be increased severalfold during periods of acute illness or stress.

CUSHING'S SYNDROME (ACTH-PRODUCING ADENOMA)

(See also Chap. 342)

Etiology and prevalence

Pituitary corticotrope adenomas account for 70% of patients with endogenous causes of Cushing's syndrome. However, it should be emphasized that iatrogenic hypercortisolism is the most common cause of cushingoid features. Ectopic tumor ACTH production, cortisol-producing adrenal adenomas, adrenal carcinoma, and adrenal hyperplasia account for the other causes; rarely, ectopic tumor CRH production is encountered.

ACTH-producing adenomas account for about 10–15% of all pituitary tumors. Because the clinical features of Cushing's syndrome often lead to early diagnosis, most ACTH-producing pituitary tumors are relatively small microadenomas. However, macroadenomas also are seen while some ACTH-expressing adenomas are clinically silent. Cushing's disease is 5–10 times more common in women than in men. These pituitary adenomas exhibit unrestrained ACTH secretion, with resultant hypercortisolemia. However, they retain partial suppressibility in the presence of high doses of administered glucocorticoids, providing the basis for dynamic testing to distinguish pituitary from nonpituitary causes of Cushing's syndrome.

Presentation and diagnosis

The diagnosis of Cushing's syndrome presents two great challenges: (1) to distinguish patients with pathologic cortisol excess from those with physiologic or other disturbances of cortisol production and (2) to determine the etiology of cortisol excess.

Typical features of chronic cortisol excess include thin skin, central obesity, hypertension, plethoric moon facies, purple striae and easy bruisability, glucose intolerance or diabetes mellitus, gonadal dysfunction, osteoporosis, proximal muscle weakness, signs of hyperandrogenism (acne, hirsutism), and psychological disturbances (depression, mania, and psychoses) (Table 339-12). Hematopoietic features of hypercortisolism include leukocytosis, lymphopenia, and eosinopenia. Immune suppression includes delayed hypersensitivity. These protean yet commonly encountered manifestations of hypercortisolism make it challenging to decide which patients mandate formal laboratory evaluation. Certain features make pathologic causes of hypercortisolism more likely; they include characteristic central redistribution of fat, thin skin with striae and bruising, and proximal muscle weakness. In children and in young females, early osteoporosis may be particularly prominent. The primary cause of death is cardiovascular disease, but infections and risk of suicide are also increased.

Rapid development of features of hypercortisolism associated with skin hyperpigmentation and severe myopathy suggests an

TABLE 339-12 Clinical Features of Cushing's Syndrome (All Ages)

Symptoms/Signs	Frequency, %
Obesity or weight gain (>115% ideal body weight)	80
Thin skin	80
Moon facies	75
Hypertension	75
Purple skin striae	65
Hirsutism	65
Menstrual disorders (usually amenorrhea)	60
Plethora	60
Abnormal glucose tolerance	55
Impotence	55
Proximal muscle weakness	50
Truncal obesity	50
Acne	45
Bruising	45
Mental changes	45
Osteoporosis	40
Edema of lower extremities	30
Hyperpigmentation	20
Hypokalemic alkalosis	15
Diabetes mellitus	15

Source: Adapted from MA Magiokou et al, in ME Wierman (ed): *Diseases of the Pituitary.* Totowa, NJ, Humana, 1997.

ectopic source of ACTH. Hypertension, hypokalemic alkalosis, glucose intolerance, and edema are also more pronounced in these patients. Serum potassium levels <3.3 mmol/L are evident in ~70% of patients with ectopic ACTH secretion but are seen in <10% of patients with pituitary-dependent Cushing's syndrome.

Laboratory investigation

The diagnosis of Cushing's syndrome is based on laboratory documentation of endogenous hypercortisolism. Measurement of 24-h urine free cortisol (UFC) is a precise and cost-effective screening test. Alternatively, the failure to suppress plasma cortisol after an overnight 1-mg dexamethasone suppression test can be used to identify patients with hypercortisolism. As nadir levels of cortisol occur at night, elevated midnight samples of cortisol are suggestive of Cushing's syndrome. Basal plasma ACTH levels often distinguish patients with ACTH-independent (adrenal or exogenous glucocorticoid) from those with ACTH-dependent (pituitary, ectopic ACTH) Cushing's syndrome. Mean basal ACTH levels are about eightfold higher in patients with ectopic ACTH secretion than in those with pituitary ACTH-secreting adenomas. However, extensive overlap of ACTH levels in these two disorders precludes using ACTH measurements to make the distinction. Instead, dynamic testing based on differential sensitivity to glucocorticoid feedback or ACTH stimulation in response to CRH or cortisol reduction is used to distinguish ectopic from pituitary sources of excess ACTH (Table 339-13). Very rarely, circulating CRH levels are elevated, reflecting ectopic tumor-derived secretion of CRH and often ACTH. For further discussion of dynamic testing for Cushing's syndrome, see Chap. 342.

Most ACTH-secreting pituitary tumors are <5 mm in diameter, and about half are undetectable by sensitive MRI. The high prevalence of incidental pituitary microadenomas diminishes the ability to distinguish ACTH-secreting pituitary tumors accurately from nonsecreting incidentalomas.

Inferior petrosal venous sampling

Because pituitary MRI with gadolinium enhancement is insufficiently sensitive to detect small (<2 mm) pituitary ACTH-secreting adenomas, bilateral inferior petrosal sinus ACTH sampling before and after CRH administration may be required to distinguish these lesions from ectopic ACTH-secreting tumors that may have similar clinical and biochemical characteristics. Simultaneous assessment of ACTH in each inferior petrosal vein and in the peripheral circulation provides a strategy for confirming and localizing pituitary ACTH production. Sampling is performed at baseline and 2, 5, and 10 min after intravenous bovine CRH (1 μg/kg) injection. An increased ratio (>2) of inferior petrosal:peripheral vein ACTH confirms pituitary Cushing's syndrome. After CRH injection, peak petrosal:peripheral ACTH ratios ≥3 confirm the presence of a pituitary ACTH-secreting tumor. The sensitivity of this test is >95%, with very rare false-positive results. False-negative results may be encountered in patients with aberrant venous drainage. Petrosal sinus catheterizations are technically difficult, and about 0.05% of patients develop neurovascular complications. The procedure should not be performed in patients with hypertension or in the presence of a well-visualized pituitary adenoma on MRI.

TABLE 339-13 Differential Diagnosis of ACTH-Dependent Cushing's Syndrome*

	ACTH-Secreting Pituitary Tumor	Ectopic ACTH Secretion
Etiology	Pituitary corticotrope adenoma	Bronchial, abdominal carcinoid
	Plurihormonal adenoma	Small cell lung cancer
		Thymoma
Sex	F > M	M > F
Clinical features	Slow onset	Rapid onset
		Pigmentation
		Severe myopathy
Serum potassium <3.3 μg/L	<10%	75%
24-h urinary free cortisol (UFC)	High	High
Basal ACTH level	Inappropriately high	Very high
Dexamethasone suppression		
1 mg overnight		
Low dose (0.5 mg q6h)	Cortisol >5 μg/dL	Cortisol >5 μg/dL
High dose (2 mg q6h)	Cortisol <5 μg/dL	Cortisol >5 μg/dL
UFC > 80% suppressed	Microadenomas: 90%	10%
	Macroadenomas: 50%	
Inferior petrosal sinus sampling (IPSS)		
Basal		
IPSS: peripheral	>2	<2
CRH-induced		
IPSS: peripheral	>3	<3

*ACTH-independent causes of Cushing's syndrome are diagnosed by suppressed ACTH levels and an adrenal mass in the setting of hypercortisolism. Iatrogenic Cushing's syndrome is excluded by history.

Abbreviations: ACTH, adrenocorticotropic hormone; CRH, corticotropin-releasing hormone; F, female; M, male.

TREATMENT Cushing's Syndrome

Selective transsphenoidal resection is the treatment of choice for Cushing's disease (Fig. 339-10). The remission rate for this procedure is ~80% for microadenomas but <50% for macroadenomas. After successful tumor resection, most patients experience a postoperative period of symptomatic ACTH deficiency that may last up to 12 months. This usually requires low-dose cortisol replacement, as patients experience both steroid withdrawal symptoms and have a suppressed HPA axis. Biochemical recurrence occurs in approximately 5% of patients in whom surgery was initially successful.

When initial surgery is unsuccessful, repeat surgery is sometimes indicated, particularly when a pituitary source for ACTH is well documented. In older patients, in whom issues of growth and fertility are less important, hemi- or total hypophysectomy may be necessary if a discrete pituitary adenoma is not recognized. Pituitary irradiation may be used after unsuccessful surgery, but

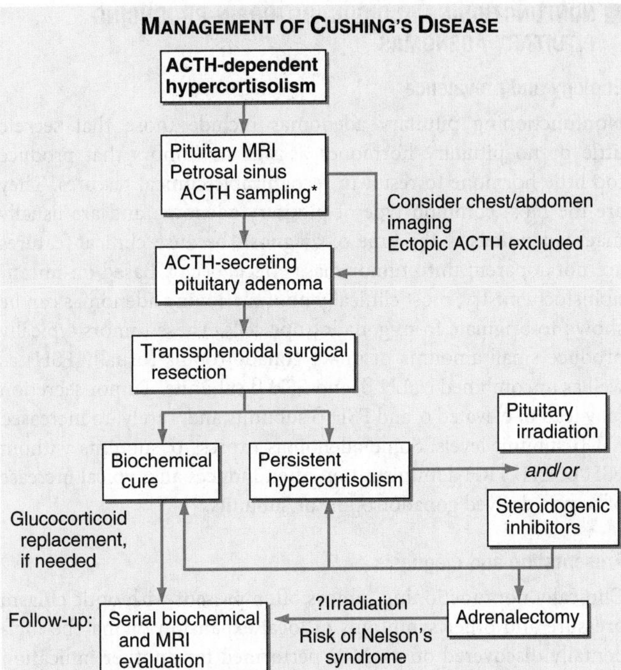

Figure 339-10 Management of Cushing's syndrome. ACTH, adrenocorticotropin hormone; MRI, magnetic resonance imaging. *, Not usually required.

it cures only about 15% of patients. Because the effects of radiation are slow and only partially effective in adults, steroidogenic inhibitors are used in combination with pituitary irradiation to block adrenal effects of persistently high ACTH levels.

Ketoconazole, an imidazole derivative antimycotic agent, inhibits several P450 enzymes and effectively lowers cortisol in most patients with Cushing's disease when administered twice daily (600–1200 mg/d). Elevated hepatic transaminases, gynecomastia, impotence, gastrointestinal upset, and edema are common side effects. *Metyrapone* (2–4 g/d) inhibits 11β-hydroxylase activity and normalizes plasma cortisol in up to 75% of patients. Side effects include nausea and vomiting, rash, and exacerbation of acne or hirsutism. *Mitotane* (*o,p*′-DDD; 3–6 g/d orally in four divided doses) suppresses cortisol hypersecretion by inhibiting 11β-hydroxylase and cholesterol side-chain cleavage enzymes and by destroying adrenocortical cells. Side effects of mitotane include gastrointestinal symptoms, dizziness, gynecomastia, hyperlipidemia, skin rash, and hepatic enzyme elevation. It also may lead to hypoaldosteronism. Other agents include *aminoglutethimide* (250 mg tid), *trilostane* (200–1000 mg/d), *cyproheptadine* (24 mg/d), and IV *etomidate* (0.3 mg/kg per hour). Glucocorticoid insufficiency is a potential side effect of agents used to block steroidogenesis.

The use of steroidogenic inhibitors has decreased the need for bilateral adrenalectomy. Removal of both adrenal glands corrects hypercortisolism but may be associated with significant morbidity rates and necessitates permanent glucocorticoid and mineralocorticoid replacement. Adrenalectomy in the setting of residual corticotrope adenoma tissue predisposes to the development of *Nelson's syndrome*, a disorder characterized by rapid pituitary tumor enlargement and increased pigmentation secondary to high ACTH levels. Radiation therapy may be indicated to prevent the development of Nelson's syndrome after adrenalectomy.

GONADOTROPINS: FSH AND LH

SYNTHESIS AND SECRETION

Gonadotrope cells constitute about 10% of anterior pituitary cells and produce two gonadotropins—LH and FSH. Like TSH and hCG, LH and FSH are glycoprotein hormones that consist of α and β subunits. The α subunit is common to these glycoprotein hormones; specificity is conferred by the β subunits, which are expressed by separate genes.

Gonadotropin synthesis and release are dynamically regulated. This is particularly true in women, in whom rapidly fluctuating gonadal steroid levels vary throughout the menstrual cycle. Hypothalamic GnRH, a 10-amino-acid peptide, regulates the synthesis and secretion of both LH and FSH. GnRH is secreted in discrete pulses every 60–120 min, and the pulses in turn elicit LH and FSH pulses (Fig. 339-3). The pulsatile mode of GnRH input is essential to its action; pulses prime gonadotrope responsiveness, whereas continuous GnRH exposure induces desensitization. Based on this phenomenon, long-acting GnRH agonists are used to suppress gonadotropin levels in children with precocious puberty and in men with prostate cancer (Chap. 95) and are used in some ovulation-induction protocols to reduce levels of endogenous gonadotropins (Chap. 347). Estrogens act at both the hypothalamus and the pituitary to modulate gonadotropin secretion. Chronic estrogen exposure is inhibitory, whereas rising estrogen levels, as occur during the preovulatory surge, exert positive feedback to increase gonadotropin pulse frequency and amplitude. Progesterone slows GnRH pulse frequency but enhances gonadotropin responses to GnRH. Testosterone feedback in men also occurs at the hypothalamic and pituitary levels and is mediated in part by its conversion to estrogens.

Although GnRH is the main regulator of LH and FSH secretion, FSH synthesis is also under separate control by the gonadal peptides inhibin and activin, which are members of the transforming growth factor β (TGF-β) family. Inhibin selectively suppresses FSH, whereas activin stimulates FSH synthesis (Chap. 347).

ACTION

The gonadotropin hormones interact with their respective GPCRs expressed in the ovary and testis, evoking germ-cell development and maturation and steroid hormone biosynthesis. In women, FSH regulates ovarian follicle development and stimulates ovarian estrogen production. LH mediates ovulation and maintenance of the corpus luteum. In men, LH induces Leydig cell testosterone synthesis and secretion and FSH stimulates seminiferous tubule development and regulates spermatogenesis.

GONADOTROPIN DEFICIENCY

Hypogonadism is the most common presenting feature of adult hypopituitarism even when other pituitary hormones are also deficient. It is often a harbinger of hypothalamic or pituitary lesions that impair GnRH production or delivery through the pituitary stalk. As noted above, hypogonadotropic hypogonadism is a common presenting feature of hyperprolactinemia.

A variety of inherited and acquired disorders are associated with *isolated hypogonadotropic hypogonadism* (IHH) (Chap. 346). Hypothalamic defects associated with GnRH deficiency include two X-linked disorders, Kallmann syndrome (see above) and mutations in the *DAX1* gene, as well as dominant mutations in *FGFR1*. Mutations in GPR54, kisspeptin, the GnRH receptor, and the LH β or FSH β subunit genes are additional causes of selective gonadotropin deficiency. Acquired forms of GnRH deficiency leading to hypogonadotropism are seen in association with anorexia nervosa (Chap. 79), stress, starvation, and extreme exercise but also may be idiopathic. Hypogonadotropic hypogonadism in these disorders is reversed by removal of the stressful stimulus or by caloric replenishment.

Presentation and diagnosis

In premenopausal women, hypogonadotropic hypogonadism presents as diminished ovarian function leading to oligomenorrhea or amenorrhea, infertility, decreased vaginal secretions, decreased libido, and breast atrophy. In hypogonadal adult men, secondary testicular failure is associated with decreased libido and potency, infertility, decreased muscle mass with weakness, reduced beard and body hair growth, soft testes, and characteristic fine facial wrinkles. Osteoporosis occurs in both untreated hypogonadal women and men.

Laboratory investigation

Central hypogonadism is associated with low or inappropriately normal serum gonadotropin levels in the setting of low sex hormone concentrations (testosterone in men, estradiol in women). Because gonadotropin secretion is pulsatile, valid assessments may require repeated measurements or the use of pooled serum samples. Men have reduced sperm counts.

Intravenous GnRH (100 μg) stimulates gonadotropes to secrete LH (which peaks within 30 min) and FSH (which plateaus during the ensuing 60 min). Normal responses vary according to menstrual cycle stage, age, and sex of the patient. Generally, LH levels increase about threefold, whereas FSH responses are less pronounced. In the setting of gonadotropin deficiency, a normal gonadotropin response to GnRH indicates intact pituitary gonadotrope function and suggests a hypothalamic abnormality. An absent response, however, cannot reliably distinguish pituitary from hypothalamic causes of hypogonadism. For this reason, GnRH testing usually adds little to the information gained from baseline evaluation of the hypothalamic-pituitary-gonadotrope axis except in cases of isolated GnRH deficiency (e.g., Kallmann syndrome).

MRI examination of the sellar region and assessment of other pituitary functions usually are indicated in patients with documented central hypogonadism.

TREATMENT Gonadotropin Deficiency

In males, testosterone replacement is necessary to achieve and maintain normal growth and development of the external genitalia, secondary sex characteristics, male sexual behavior, and androgenic anabolic effects, including maintenance of muscle function and bone mass. Testosterone may be administered by intramuscular injections every 1–4 weeks or by using skin patches that are replaced daily (Chap. 346). Testosterone gels are also available. Gonadotropin injections [hCG or human menopausal gonadotropin (hMG)] over 12–18 months are used to restore fertility. Pulsatile GnRH therapy (25–150 ng/kg every 2 h), administered by a subcutaneous infusion pump, is also effective for treatment of hypothalamic hypogonadism when fertility is desired.

In premenopausal women, cyclical replacement of estrogen and progesterone maintains secondary sexual characteristics and integrity of genitourinary tract mucosa and prevents premature osteoporosis (Chap. 347). Gonadotropin therapy is used for ovulation induction. Follicular growth and maturation are initiated using hMG or recombinant FSH; hCG or human luteinizing hormone (hLH) is subsequently injected to induce ovulation. As in men, pulsatile GnRH therapy can be used to treat hypothalamic causes of gonadotropin deficiency.

NONFUNCTIONING AND GONADOTROPIN-PRODUCING PITUITARY ADENOMAS

Etiology and prevalence

Nonfunctioning pituitary adenomas include those that secrete little or no pituitary hormones as well as tumors that produce too little hormone to result in recognizable clinical features. They are the most common type of pituitary adenoma and are usually macroadenomas at the time of diagnosis because clinical features are not apparent until tumor mass effects occur. Based on immunohistochemistry, most clinically nonfunctioning adenomas can be shown to originate from gonadotrope cells. These tumors typically produce small amounts of intact gonadotropins (usually FSH) as well as uncombined α, LH β, and FSH β subunits. Tumor secretion may lead to elevated α and FSH β subunits and, rarely, to increased LH β subunit levels. Some adenomas express α subunits without FSH or LH. TRH administration often induces an atypical increase of tumor-derived gonadotropins or subunits.

Presentation and diagnosis

Clinically nonfunctioning tumors often present with optic chiasm pressure and other symptoms of local expansion or may be incidentally discovered on an MRI performed for another indication (incidentaloma). Rarely, menstrual disturbances or ovarian hyperstimulation occur in women with large tumors that produce FSH and LH. More commonly, adenoma compression of the pituitary stalk or surrounding pituitary tissue leads to attenuated LH and features of hypogonadism. PRL levels are usually slightly increased, also because of stalk compression. It is important to distinguish this circumstance from true prolactinomas, as nonfunctioning tumors do not shrink in response to treatment with dopamine agonists.

Laboratory investigation

The goal of laboratory testing in clinically nonfunctioning tumors is to classify the type of the tumor, identify hormonal markers of tumor activity, and detect possible hypopituitarism. Free α subunit levels may be elevated in 10–15% of patients with nonfunctioning tumors. In female patients, peri- or postmenopausal basal FSH concentrations are difficult to distinguish from tumor-derived FSH elevation. Premenopausal women have cycling FSH levels, also preventing clear-cut diagnostic distinction from tumor-derived FSH. In men, gonadotropin-secreting tumors may be diagnosed because of slightly increased gonadotropins (FSH > LH) in the setting of a pituitary mass. Testosterone levels are usually low despite the normal or increased LH level, perhaps reflecting reduced LH bioactivity or the loss of normal LH pulsatility. Because this pattern of hormone test results is also seen in primary gonadal failure and, to some extent, with aging (Chap. 346), the finding of increased gonadotropins alone is insufficient for the diagnosis of a gonadotropin-secreting tumor. In the majority of patients with gonadotrope adenomas, TRH administration stimulates LH β subunit secretion; this response is not seen in normal individuals. GnRH testing, however, is not helpful for making the diagnosis. For nonfunctioning and gonadotropin-secreting tumors, the diagnosis usually rests on immunohistochemical analyses of surgically resected tumor tissue, as the mass effects of these tumors usually necessitate resection.

Although acromegaly or Cushing's syndrome usually presents with unique clinical features, clinically inapparent (silent) somatotrope or corticotrope adenomas may only be diagnosed by immunostaining of resected tumor tissue. If PRL levels are <100 μg/L in a patient harboring a pituitary mass, a nonfunctioning adenoma causing pituitary stalk compression should be considered.

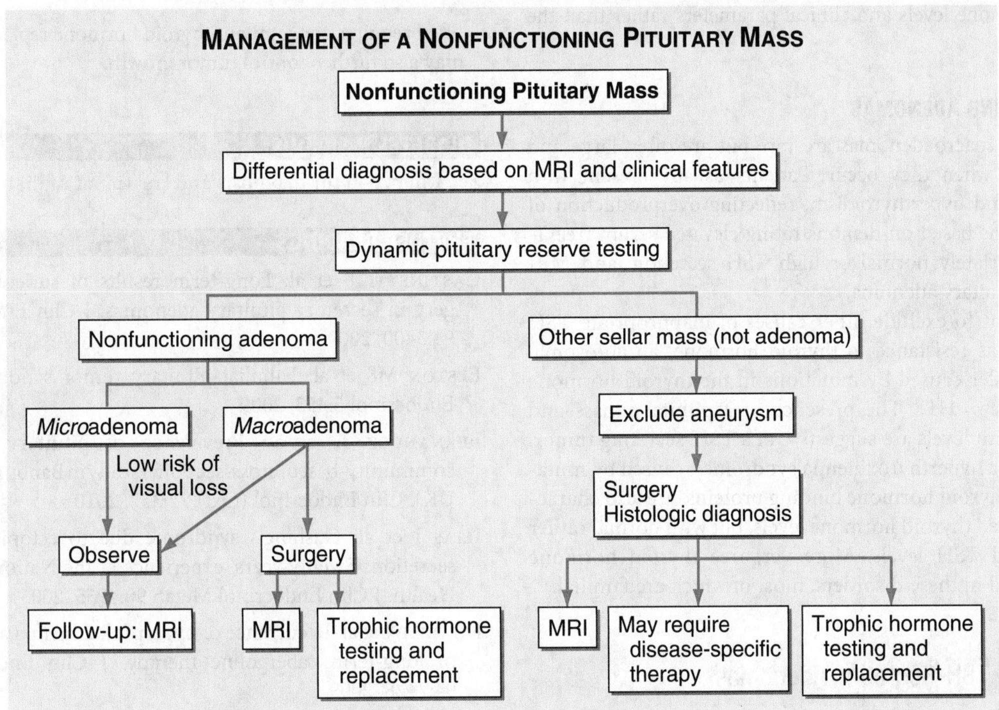

Figure 339-11 Management of a nonfunctioning pituitary mass.

TREATMENT Nonfunctioning and Gonadotropin-Producing Pituitary Adenomas

Asymptomatic small nonfunctioning microadenomas adenomas with no threat to vision may be followed with regular MRI and visual field testing without immediate intervention. However, for macroadenomas, transsphenoidal surgery is indicated to reduce tumor size and relieve mass effects (Fig. 339-11). Although it is not usually possible to remove all adenoma tissue surgically, vision improves in 70% of patients with preoperative visual field defects. Preexisting hypopituitarism that results from tumor mass effects may improve or resolve completely. Beginning about 6 months postoperatively, MRI scans should be performed yearly to detect tumor regrowth. Within 5–6 years after successful surgical resection, ~15% of nonfunctioning tumors recur. When substantial tumor remains after transsphenoidal surgery, adjuvant radiotherapy may be indicated to prevent tumor regrowth. Radiotherapy may be deferred if no postoperative residual mass is evident.

Nonfunctioning pituitary tumors respond poorly to dopamine agonist treatment and somatostatin analogues are largely ineffective for shrinking these tumors. The selective GnRH antagonist Nal-Glu GnRH suppresses FSH hypersecretion but has no effect on adenoma size.

THYROID-STIMULATING HORMONE

SYNTHESIS AND SECRETION

TSH-secreting thyrotrope cells constitute 5% of the anterior pituitary cell population. TSH is structurally related to LH and FSH. It shares a common α subunit with these hormones but contains a specific TSH β subunit. TRH is a hypothalamic tripeptide (pyroglutamyl histidylprolinamide) that acts through a GPCR to stimulate TSH synthesis and secretion; it also stimulates the lactotrope cell to secrete PRL. TSH secretion is stimulated by TRH, whereas thyroid hormones, dopamine, somatostatin, and glucocorticoids suppress TSH by overriding TRH induction.

Thyrotrope growth and TSH secretion are both induced when negative feedback inhibition by thyroid hormones is removed. Thus, thyroid damage (including surgical thyroidectomy), radiation-induced hypothyroidism, chronic thyroiditis, and prolonged goitrogen exposure are associated with increased TSH. Long-standing untreated hypothyroidism can lead to thyrotrope hyperplasia and pituitary enlargement, which may be evident on MRI.

ACTION

TSH is secreted in pulses, though the excursions are modest in comparison to other pituitary hormones because of the low amplitude of the pulses and the relatively long half-life of TSH. Consequently, single determinations of TSH suffice to assess its circulating levels. TSH binds to a GPCR on thyroid follicular cells to stimulate thyroid hormone synthesis and release (Chap. 341).

TSH DEFICIENCY

Features of central hypothyroidism due to TSH deficiency mimic those seen with primary hypothyroidism but are generally less severe. Pituitary hypothyroidism is characterized by low basal TSH levels in the setting of low free thyroid hormone. In contrast, patients with hypothyroidism of hypothalamic origin (presumably due to a lack of endogenous TRH) may exhibit normal or even slightly elevated TSH levels. The TSH produced in this circumstance appears to have reduced biologic activity because of altered glycosylation.

TRH (200 μg) injected intravenously causes a two- to threefold increase in TSH (and PRL) levels within 30 min. Although TRH testing can be used to assess TSH reserve, abnormalities of the thyroid axis usually can be detected based on basal free T_4 and TSH levels, and TRH testing is rarely indicated.

Thyroid-replacement therapy should be initiated after adequate adrenal function has been established. Dose adjustment is based on thyroid hormone levels and clinical parameters rather than the TSH level.

TSH-SECRETING ADENOMAS

TSH-producing macroadenomas are rare but are often large and locally invasive when they occur. Patients usually present with thyroid goiter and hyperthyroidism, reflecting overproduction of TSH. Diagnosis is based on demonstrating elevated serum free T_4 levels, inappropriately normal or high TSH secretion, and MRI evidence of a pituitary adenoma.

It is important to exclude other causes of inappropriate TSH secretion, such as resistance to thyroid hormone, an autosomal dominant disorder caused by mutations in the thyroid hormone β receptor (Chap. 341). The presence of a pituitary mass and elevated α subunit levels are suggestive of a TSH-secreting tumor. Dysalbuminemic hyperthyroxinemia syndromes, caused by mutations in serum thyroid hormone binding proteins, are also characterized by elevated thyroid hormone levels, but with normal rather than suppressed TSH levels. Moreover, free thyroid hormone levels are normal in these disorders, most of which are familial.

TREATMENT TSH-Secreting Adenomas

The initial therapeutic approach is to remove or debulk the tumor mass surgically, usually using a transsphenoidal approach. Total resection is not often achieved as most of these adenomas are large and locally invasive. Normal circulating thyroid hormone levels are achieved in about two-thirds of patients after surgery. Thyroid ablation or antithyroid drugs (methimazole and propylthiouracil) can be used to reduce thyroid hormone levels. Somatostatin analogue treatment effectively normalizes TSH and α subunit hypersecretion, shrinks the tumor mass in 50% of patients, and improves visual fields in 75% of patients; euthyroidism is restored in most patients. Because somatostatin analogues markedly suppress TSH, biochemical hypothyroidism often requires concomitant thyroid hormone replacement, which may also further control tumor growth.

DIABETES INSIPIDUS

See Chap. 340 for diagnosis and treatment of diabetes insipidus.

FURTHER READINGS

Castinetti F et al: Long-term results of stereotactic radiosurgery in secretory pituitary adenomas. J Clin Endocrinol Metab 94:3400, 2009

Elston MS et al: Familial pituitary tumor syndromes. Nat Rev Endocrinol 5:453, 2009

Fernandez A et al: Prevalence of pituitary adenomas: A community-based, cross-sectional study in Banbury (Oxfordshire, UK). Clin Endocrinol (Oxf) 72:377, 2010

Ilias I et al: Cushing's syndrome due to ectopic corticotropin secretion: Twenty years' experience at the National Institutes of Health. J Clin Endocrinol Metab 90:4955, 2005

Kharlip J et al: Recurrence of hyperprolactinemia after withdrawal of long-term cabergoline therapy. J Clin Endocrinol Metab 94:2428, 2009

Liu H et al: Systematic review: The safety and efficacy of growth hormone in the healthy elderly. Ann Intern Med 146:104, 2007

Melmed S: Acromegaly. N Engl J Med 355:2558, 2006

——— et al: Diagnosis and treatment of hyperprolactinemia: An Endorcine Society Clinical Practice Guideline. J Clin Endocrinol Metab 96:273, 2011

Molitch ME: Evaluation and treatment of adult growth hormone deficiency: An Endocrine Society Clinical Practice Guideline. J Clin Endocrinol Metab 91:1621, 2006

Nieman LK et al: The diagnosis of Cushing's syndrome: An Endocrine Society Clinical Practice Guideline. J Clin Endocrinol Metab 93:1526, 2008

CHAPTER 340 Disorders of the Neurohypophysis

Gary L. Robertson

The neurohypophysis, or posterior pituitary, is formed by axons that originate in large cell bodies in the supraoptic and paraventricular nuclei of the hypothalamus. It produces two hormones: (1) arginine vasopressin (AVP), also known as antidiuretic hormone, and (2) oxytocin. AVP acts on the renal tubules to reduce water loss by concentrating the urine. Oxytocin stimulates postpartum milk letdown in response to suckling. AVP deficiency causes diabetes insipidus (DI), which is characterized by the production of large amounts of dilute urine. Excessive or inappropriate AVP production predisposes to hyponatremia if water intake is not reduced in parallel with urine output.

VASOPRESSIN

SYNTHESIS AND SECRETION

AVP is a nonapeptide composed of a six-member disulfide ring and a tripeptide tail (Fig. 340-1). It is synthesized via a polypeptide precursor that includes AVP, neurophysin, and copeptin, all encoded by a single gene on chromosome 20. After preliminary processing and folding, the precursor is packaged in neurosecretory vesicles, where it is transported down the axon, further processed to AVP, and stored in neurosecretory vesicles until the hormone and other components are released by exocytosis into peripheral blood.

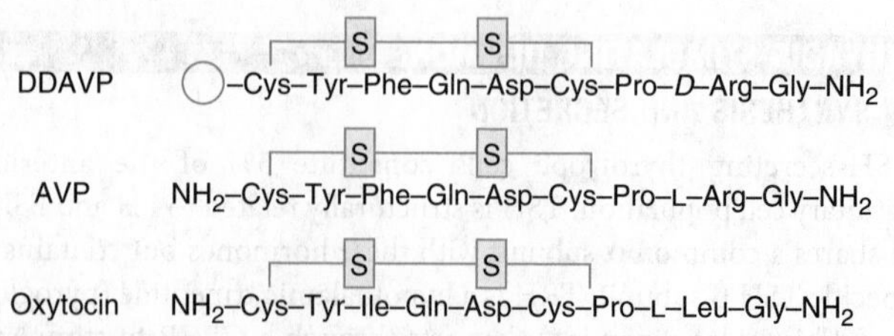

Figure 340-1 Primary structures of arginine vasopressin (AVP), oxytocin, and desmopressin.

AVP secretion is regulated primarily by the "effective" osmotic pressure of body fluids. This control is mediated by specialized hypothalamic cells known as *osmoreceptors*, which are extremely sensitive to small changes in the plasma concentration of sodium and certain other solutes but normally are insensitive to other solutes such as urea and glucose. The osmoreceptors appear to include inhibitory as well as stimulatory components that function in concert to form a threshold, or set point, control system. Below this threshold, plasma AVP is suppressed to levels that permit the development of a maximum water diuresis. Above it, plasma AVP rises steeply in direct proportion to plasma osmolarity, quickly reaching levels sufficient to effect a maximum antidiuresis. The absolute levels of plasma osmolarity/sodium at which minimally and maximally effective levels of plasma AVP occur, vary appreciably from person to person, apparently owing to genetic influences on the set and sensitivity of the system. However, the average threshold, or set point, for AVP release corresponds to a plasma osmolarity or sodium of about 280 mosmol/L or 135 meq/L, respectively; levels only 2–4% higher normally result in maximum antidiuresis.

Though it is relatively stable in a healthy adult, the set point of the osmoregulatory system can be lowered by pregnancy, the menstrual cycle, estrogen, and relatively large, acute reductions in blood pressure or volume. Those reductions are mediated largely by neuronal afferents that originate in transmural pressure receptors of the heart and large arteries and project via the vagus and glossopharyngeal nerves to the brainstem, from which postsynaptic projections ascend to the hypothalamus. These pathways maintain a tonic inhibitory tone that decreases when blood volume or pressure falls by >10–20%. This baroregulatory system is probably of minor importance in the physiology of AVP secretion because the hemodynamic changes required to effect it usually do not occur during normal activities. However, the baroregulatory system undoubtedly plays an important role in AVP secretion in patients with large, acute disturbances of hemodynamic function.

AVP secretion also can be stimulated by nausea, acute hypoglycemia, glucocorticoid deficiency, smoking, and, possibly, hyperangiotensinemia. The emetic stimuli are extremely potent since they typically elicit immediate, 50- to 100-fold increases in plasma AVP even when the nausea is transient and is not associated with vomiting or other symptoms. They appear to act via the emetic center in the medulla and can be blocked completely by treatment with antiemetics such as fluphenazine. There is no evidence that pain or other noxious stresses have any effect on AVP unless they elicit a vasovagal reaction with its associated nausea and hypotension.

■ ACTION

The most important, if not the only, physiologic action of AVP is to reduce water excretion by promoting concentration of urine. This antidiuretic effect is achieved by increasing the hydroosmotic permeability of cells that line the distal tubule and medullary collecting ducts of the kidney (Fig. 340-2). In the absence of AVP, these cells are impermeable to water and reabsorb little, if any, of the relatively large volume of dilute filtrate that enters from the proximal nephron. This results in the excretion of very large volumes (as much as 0.2 mL/kg per min) of maximally dilute urine (specific gravity and osmolarity ~1.000 and 50 mosmol/L, respectively), a condition known as *water diuresis*. In the presence of AVP, these cells become selectively permeable to water, allowing the water to diffuse back down the osmotic gradient created by the hypertonic renal medulla. As a result, the dilute fluid passing through the tubules is concentrated and the rate of urine flow decreases. The magnitude of this effect varies in direct proportion to the plasma AVP concentration and, at maximum levels, approximates a urine flow rate as low as 0.35 mL/min and a urine osmolarity as high as 1200 mosmol/L. This action is mediated via binding to G protein–coupled V_2 receptors on the serosal surface of the cell, activation of adenyl cyclase, and insertion into the luminal surface of water channels composed of a protein known as *aquaporin 2* (AQP2). The V_2 receptors and aquaporin 2 are encoded by genes on chromosomes Xq28 and 12q13, respectively.

At high concentrations, AVP also causes contraction of smooth muscle in blood vessels and in the gastrointestinal tract, induces glycogenolysis in the liver, and potentiates adrenocorticotropic hormone (ACTH) release by corticotropin-releasing factor. These effects are mediated by V_{1a} or V_{1b} receptors that are coupled to phospholipase C. Their role, if any, in human physiology/pathophysiology is uncertain.

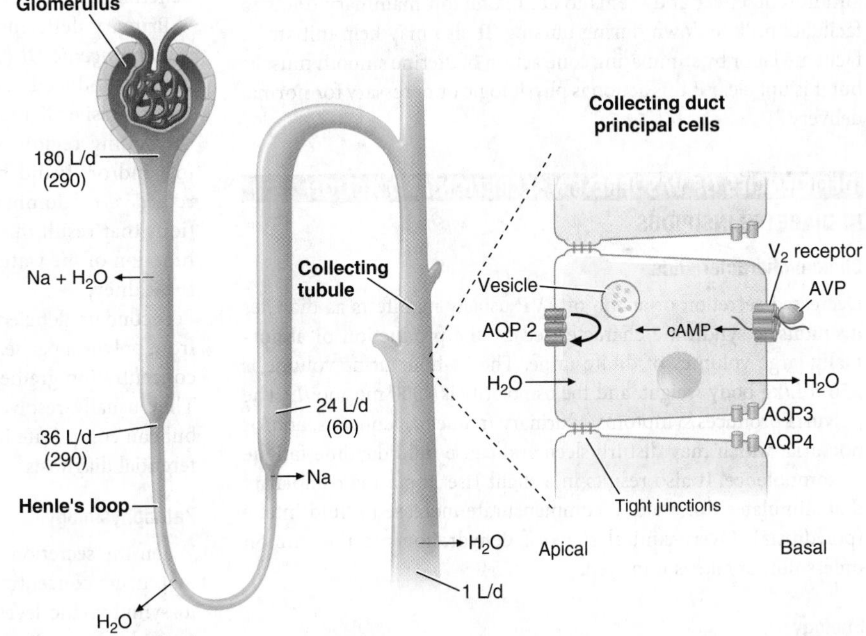

Figure 340-2 Antidiuretic effect of arginine vasopressin (AVP) in the regulation of urine volume. In a typical 70-kg adult, the kidney filters ~180 L/d of plasma. Of this, ~144 L (80%) is reabsorbed isosmotically in the proximal tubule and another 8 L (4–5%) is reabsorbed without solute in the descending limb of Henle's loop. The remainder is diluted to an osmolarity of ~60 mmol/kg by selective reabsorption of sodium and chloride in the ascending limb. In the absence of AVP, the urine issuing from the loop passes largely unmodified through the distal tubules and collecting ducts, resulting in a maximum water diuresis. In the presence of AVP, solute-free water is reabsorbed osmotically through the principal cells of the collecting ducts, resulting in the excretion of a much smaller volume of concentrated urine. This antidiuretic effect is mediated via a G protein–coupled V_2 receptor that increases intracellular cyclic AMP, thereby inducing translocation of aquaporin 2 (AQP 2) water channels into the apical membrane. The resultant increase in permeability permits an influx of water that diffuses out of the cell through AQP 3 and AQP 4 water channels on the basal-lateral surface. The net rate of flux across the cell is determined by the number of AQP 2 water channels in the apical membrane and the strength of the osmotic gradient between tubular fluid and the renal medulla. Tight junctions on the lateral surface of the cells serve to prevent unregulated water flow.

■ METABOLISM

AVP distributes rapidly into a space roughly equal to the extracellular fluid volume. It is cleared irreversibly with a $t_{1/2}$ of 10–30 minutes. Most AVP clearance is due to degradation in the liver and kidneys. During pregnancy, the metabolic clearance of AVP is increased three- to fourfold due to placental production of an N-terminal peptidase.

THIRST

Because AVP cannot reduce water loss below a certain minimum level obligated by urinary solute load and evaporation from skin and lungs, a mechanism for ensuring adequate intake is essential for preventing dehydration. This vital function is performed by the thirst mechanism. Like AVP, thirst is regulated primarily by an osmostat that is situated in the anteromedial hypothalamus and is able to detect very small changes in the plasma concentration of sodium and certain other effective solutes. The thirst osmostat appears to be "set" about 5% higher than the AVP osmostat. This arrangement ensures that thirst, polydipsia, and dilution of body fluids do not occur until plasma osmolarity/sodium start to exceed the defensive capacity of the antidiuretic mechanism.

OXYTOCIN

Oxytocin is also a nonapeptide, and it differs from AVP only at positions 3 and 8 (Fig. 340-1). However, it has relatively little antidiuretic effect and seems to act mainly on mammary ducts to facilitate milk letdown during nursing. It also may help initiate or facilitate labor by stimulating contraction of uterine smooth muscle, but it is not clear if this action is physiologic or necessary for normal delivery.

DEFICIENCIES OF VASOPRESSIN SECRETION AND ACTION

■ DIABETES INSIPIDUS

Clinical characteristics

Decreased secretion or action of AVP usually manifests as diabetes insipidus, a syndrome characterized by the production of abnormally large volumes of dilute urine. The 24-hour urine volume is >50 mL/kg body weight, and the osmolarity is <300 mosmol/L. The polyuria produces symptoms of urinary frequency, enuresis, and/or nocturia, which may disturb sleep and cause mild daytime fatigue or somnolence. It also results in a slight rise in plasma osmolarity that stimulates thirst and a commensurate increase in fluid intake (polydipsia). Overt clinical signs of dehydration are uncommon unless fluid intake is impaired.

Etiology

Deficient secretion of AVP can be primary or secondary. The primary form usually results from agenesis or irreversible destruction of the neurohypophysis and is referred to variously as *neurohypophyseal DI*, *pituitary DI*, or *central DI*. It can be caused by a variety of congenital, acquired, or genetic disorders, but in about one-half of all adult patients it is idiopathic (Table 340-1). The surgically induced forms of pituitary DI usually appear within 24 hours and then go through a 2- to 3-week interim period of inappropriate antidiuresis, after which they may or may not recur. The genetic form usually is transmitted in an autosomal dominant mode and is caused by diverse mutations in the coding region of the AVP–neurophysin II (or *AVP-NPII*) gene. All the mutations alter one or more amino acids known to be critical for correct folding of the prohormone, thus interfering with its processing and trafficking through the endoplasmic reticulum. The AVP deficiency and DI develop gradually several months to years after birth, progressing from partial to severe and permanent DI. They appear to result from accumulation of misfolded mutant precursor followed by selective degeneration of AVP-producing magnocellular neurons. An autosomal recessive form due to an inactivating mutation in the AVP portion of the gene, an X-linked recessive form due to an unidentified gene on Xq28, and an autosomal recessive form due to mutations of the *WFS 1* gene responsible for Wolfram's syndrome [diabetes insipidus, diabetes mellitus, optic atrophy, and neural deafness (DIDMOAD)] have also been described. A primary deficiency of plasma AVP also can result from increased metabolism by an N-terminal aminopeptidase produced by the placenta. It is referred to as *gestational DI* since the signs and symptoms manifest during pregnancy and usually remit several weeks after delivery.

Secondary deficiencies of AVP result from inhibition of secretion by excessive intake of fluids. They are referred to as *primary polydipsia* and can be divided into three subcategories. One of them, *dipsogenic DI*, is characterized by inappropriate thirst caused by a reduction in the set of the osmoregulatory mechanism. It sometimes occurs in association with multifocal diseases of the brain such as neurosarcoid, tuberculous meningitis, and multiple sclerosis but is often idiopathic. The second subtype, *psychogenic polydipsia*, is not associated with thirst, and the polydipsia seems to be a feature of psychosis or obsessive compulsive disorder. The third subtype, *iatrogenic polydipsia*, results from recommendations to increase fluid intake for its presumed health benefits.

Primary deficiencies in the antidiuretic action of AVP result in *nephrogenic DI* (Table 340-1). They can be genetic, acquired, or drug induced. The genetic form usually is transmitted in a semirecessive X-linked manner and is caused by mutations in the coding region of the V_2 receptor gene that impair trafficking and/or ligand binding of the mutant receptor. Autosomal recessive or dominant forms are caused by AQP2 gene mutations that result in complete or partial defects in trafficking and function of the water channels in distal and collecting tubules of the kidney.

Secondary deficiencies in the antidiuretic response to AVP result from polyuria per se. They are caused by washout of the medullary concentration gradient and/or suppression of aquaporin function. They usually resolve 24–48 hours after the polyuria is corrected but can complicate interpretation of some acute tests used for differential diagnosis.

Pathophysiology

When the secretion or action of AVP falls below 80–85% of normal, urine concentration ceases and the rate of urine output rises to symptomatic levels. If the defect is due to pituitary, gestational, or nephrogenic DI, the polyuria results in a small (1–2%) decrease in body water and a commensurate increase in plasma osmolarity and sodium concentration that stimulate thirst and a compensatory increase in water intake. As a result, *hypernatremia and other overt physical or laboratory signs of dehydration do not develop unless the patient also has a defect in thirst or fails to drink for some other reason.*

The severity of the antidiuretic defect varies markedly from patient to patient. In some, the deficiencies in AVP secretion or action are so severe that even an intense stimulus such as nausea or severe dehydration does not raise plasma AVP enough to concentrate the urine. In others, the deficiency is incomplete, and a modest stimulus such as a few hours of fluid deprivation, smoking, or a vasovagal reaction increases plasma AVP sufficiently to raise urine osmolarity as high as 800 mosmol/L. The maximum achieved is usually less than normal, but that is the case largely because

TABLE 340-1 Causes of Diabetes Insipidus

Pituitary diabetes insipidus	Nephrogenic diabetes insipidus
Acquired	Acquired
Head trauma (closed and penetrating) including pituitary surgery	Drugs
Neoplasms	Lithium
Primary	Demeclocycline
Craniopharyngioma	Methoxyflurane
Pituitary adenoma (suprasellar)	Amphotericin B
Dysgerminoma	Aminoglycosides
Meningioma	Cisplatin
Metastatic (lung, breast)	Rifampin
Hematologic (lymphoma, leukemia)	Foscarnet
Granulomas	Metabolic
Sarcoidosis	Hypercalcemia, hypercalciuria
Histiocytosis	Hypokalemia
Xanthoma disseminatum	Obstruction (ureter or urethra)
Infectious	Vascular
Chronic meningitis	Sickle cell disease and trait
Viral encephalitis	Ischemia (acute tubular necrosis)
Toxoplasmosis	Granulomas
Inflammatory	Sarcoidosis
Lymphocytic infundibuloneurohypophysitis	Neoplasms
Granulomatosis with polyangiitis (Wegener's)	Sarcoma
Lupus erythematosus	Infiltration
Scleroderma	Amyloidosis
Chemical toxins	Pregnancy
Tetrodotoxin	Idiopathic
Snake venom	Genetic
Vascular	X-linked recessive (*AVP receptor-2 gene*)
Sheehan's syndrome	Autosomal recessive (AQP2 gene)
Aneurysm (internal carotid)	Autosomal dominant (AQP2 gene)
Aortocoronary bypass	**Primary polydipsia**
Hypoxic encephalopathy	Acquired
Pregnancy (vasopressinase)	Psychogenic
Idiopathic	Schizophrenia
Congenital malformations	Obsessive compulsive disorder
Septo-optic dysplasia	Dipsogenic (abnormal thirst)
Midline craniofacial defects	Granulomas
Holoprosencephaly	Sarcoidosis
Hypogenesis, ectopia of pituitary	Infectious
Genetic	Tuberculous meningitis
Autosomal dominant (*AVP-neurophysin gene*)	Head trauma (closed and penetrating)
Autosomal recessive (*AVP-neurophysin gene*)	Demyelination
Autosomal recessive-Wolfram-(4p – *WFS 1 gene*)	Multiple sclerosis
X-linked recessive (Xq28)	Drugs
Deletion chromosome 7q	Lithium
	Carbamazepine
	Idiopathic
	Iatrogenic

maximal concentrating capacity is temporarily impaired by chronic polyuria.

In primary polydipsia, the pathogenesis of the polydipsia and polyuria is the reverse of that in pituitary, nephrogenic, and gestational DI. Thus, the excessive intake of fluids slightly increases body water, thereby reducing plasma osmolarity, AVP secretion, and urinary concentration. The latter results in a compensatory increase in urinary free-water excretion that varies in direct proportion to intake. Therefore, hyponatremia or clinically appreciable overhydration is uncommon unless the polydipsia is very severe or the compensatory water diuresis is impaired by a drug or disease that stimulates or mimics endogenous AVP.

In the dipsogenic form of primary polydipsia, fluid intake is excessive because the osmotic threshold for thirst appears to be reset to the left, often well below that for AVP release. When deprived of fluids or subjected to another acute osmotic or nonosmotic stimulus, these individuals invariably increase plasma AVP normally, but the resultant increase in urine concentration is usually subnormal because the individuals' renal capacities to concentrate the urine also are blunted temporarily by chronic polyuria. Thus, the maximum level of urine osmolarity achieved is usually indistinguishable from that in patients with partial pituitary, partial gestational, or partial nephrogenic DI. Patients with psychogenic or iatrogenic polydipsia respond similarly to fluid restriction but do not complain of thirst and usually offer other explanations for their high fluid intake.

Differential diagnosis

When symptoms of urinary frequency, enuresis, nocturia, and/or persistent thirst are present, the possibility of DI should be evaluated after excluding glucosuria by collecting a 24-hour urine on ad libitum fluid intake. If the volume exceeds 50 mL/kg per day (3500 mL in a 70-kg male) and the osmolarity is <300 mosmol/L, DI is confirmed and the patient should be evaluated further to determine the type.

In differentiating among the various types of DI, the history alone may be sufficient if it reveals a likely antecedent such as pituitary surgery. Usually, however, that type of indicator is absent, ambiguous, or misleading and other approaches are needed. Except in the rare patient with hypertonic dehydration under basal conditions, differentiation should begin with a *fluid deprivation test.* It can be performed on an outpatient basis if the necessary staff and facilities are available. To minimize patient discomfort, avoid excessive dehydration, and maximize the information obtained, the test should be started in the morning and continued with hourly monitoring of body weight, plasma osmolarity and/or sodium concentration, urine volume, and urine osmolarity until either of two endpoints is reached. If fluid deprivation does not result in urine concentration (osmolarity >300 mosmol/L, specific gravity >1.010) before body weight decreases by 5% or plasma osmolarity/sodium rise above the upper limit of normal, the patient has severe pituitary or severe nephrogenic DI. These disorders usually can be distinguished by administering desmopressin (0.03 μg/kg SC or IV) and repeating the measurement of urine osmolarity 1–2 hours later. An increase of >50% indicates severe pituitary DI, whereas a smaller or absent response is strongly suggestive of nephrogenic DI.

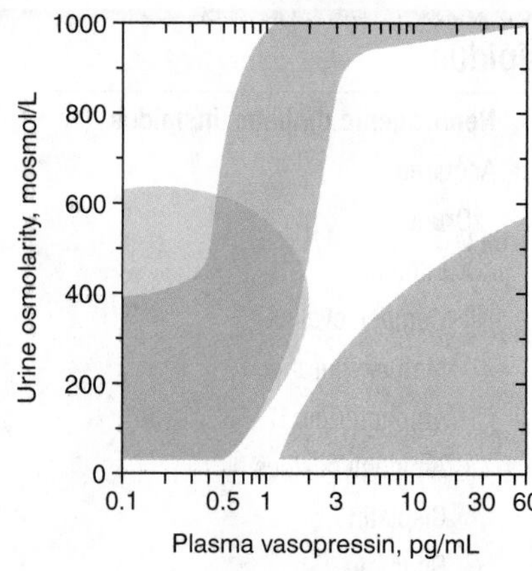

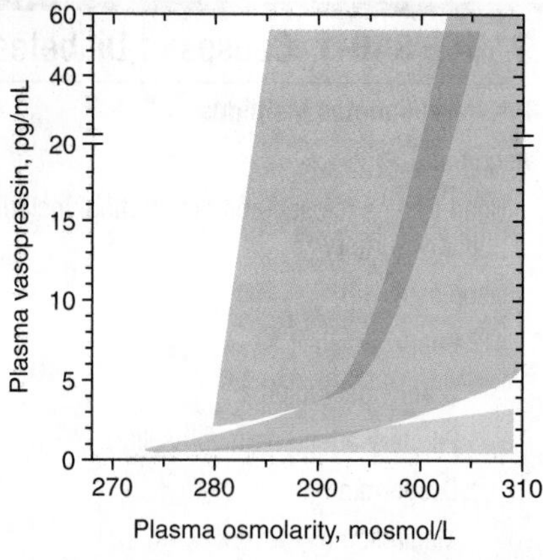

Figure 340-3 Relationship of plasma AVP to urine osmolarity (*left*) and plasma osmolarity (*right*) before and during fluid deprivation–hypertonic saline infusion test in patients who are normal or have primary polydipsia (blue zones), pituitary diabetes insipidus (green zones), or nephrogenic diabetes insipidus (pink zones).

Conversely, if fluid deprivation results in concentration of the urine, severe defects in AVP secretion and action are excluded and the question becomes whether the patient has partial pituitary DI, partial nephrogenic DI, or primary polydipsia. The maximum levels of urine osmolarity achieved before and after desmopressin injection are of no help in this regard because the values in the three groups vary widely and overlap owing to impairment of renal concentrating capacity caused by polyuria per se. Therefore, another approach is needed to differentiate among them. The easiest and least expensive method is to measure plasma AVP before and during the fluid deprivation test and analyze the results in relation to the concurrent plasma and urine osmolarity (Fig. 340-3). This approach invariably differentiates partial nephrogenic DI from partial pituitary DI and primary polydipsia. It also differentiates partial pituitary DI from primary polydipsia if plasma osmolarity and/or sodium are clearly above the normal range when the hormone is measured. However, the requisite level of hypertonic dehydration may be difficult to produce by fluid deprivation alone when urine concentration occurs. Therefore, it is usually necessary to continue the fluid deprivation and infuse hypertonic (3%) saline at a rate of 0.1 mL/kg per min until plasma osmolarity/sodium measured every 20 to 30 minutes reach or slightly exceed the upper limit of normal. At that point the plasma osmolarity/sodium, which is usually reached in 30 to 90 minutes, the measurement of plasma AVP should be repeated and the result related to plasma osmolarity/sodium is as before.

An alternative method of differential diagnosis is MRI of the pituitary and hypothalamus. In most healthy adults and children, the posterior pituitary emits a hyperintense signal in T1-weighted midsagittal images. This "bright spot" is almost always present in patients with primary polydipsia but is invariably absent or abnormally small in patients with pituitary DI. It is usually also small or absent in nephrogenic DI presumably because of high secretion and turnover of AVP. Thus, a normal bright spot virtually excludes pituitary DI, argues against nephrogenic DI, and strongly suggests primary polydipsia. Lack of the bright spot is less helpful, however, because it is absent not only in pituitary and nephrogenic DI but also in some healthy adults and patients with empty sella who do not have DI or AVP deficiency.

The other way to distinguish among the three basic types of DI is a closely monitored trial of desmopressin therapy.

TREATMENT Diabetes Insipidus

The signs and symptoms of uncomplicated pituitary DI can be eliminated completely by treatment with desmopressin (DDAVP), a synthetic analogue of AVP (Fig. 340-1). DDAVP acts selectively at V_2 receptors to increase urine concentration and decrease urine flow in a dose-dependent manner (Fig. 340-4). It is also more resistant to degradation than is AVP and has a three- to fourfold longer duration of action. Desmopressin can be given by IV or SC injection, nasal inhalation, or oral tablet. The doses required to control pituitary DI completely vary widely, depending on the patient and the route of administration. However, they usually range from 1–2 μg qd or bid by injection, 10–20 μg bid or tid by nasal spray, or 100–400 μg bid or tid orally. The onset of action is rapid, ranging from as little as 15 minutes after injection to 60 minutes after oral administration. When given in doses sufficient to normalize urinary osmolarity and flow completely, desmopressin produces a slight (1–3%) increase in total body water and a commensurate decrease in plasma osmolarity and sodium concentration that rapidly eliminates thirst and polydipsia. Consequently, water balance is maintained and hyponatremia does not develop unless the osmoregulation of thirst is also impaired or fluid intake is excessive for another reason such as a misconception about the need to prevent dehydration. Fortunately, thirst abnormalities are rare in pituitary DI, and other motivations to drink excessively usually can be eliminated by patient education. Therefore, desmopressin usually can be given safely in doses sufficient to normalize urine output completely, thereby avoiding the inconvenience and discomfort of intermittent escape otherwise needed to prevent water intoxication.

Primary polydipsia cannot be treated safely with desmopressin or any other antidiuretic drug because eliminating the polyuria does not eliminate the urge to drink. Therefore, it produces hyponatremia and/or other signs of water intoxication, usually within 24 to 48 hours if urine output is normalized completely. Patient education may eliminate iatrogenic polydipsia, but it is largely ineffective in psychogenic or dipsogenic DI. In these patients, the only help currently available is to try to prevent water intoxication by warning about the use of drugs that can impair urinary free-water excretion directly or indirectly.

The polyuria and polydipsia of nephrogenic DI are not affected by treatment with standard doses of desmopressin. If

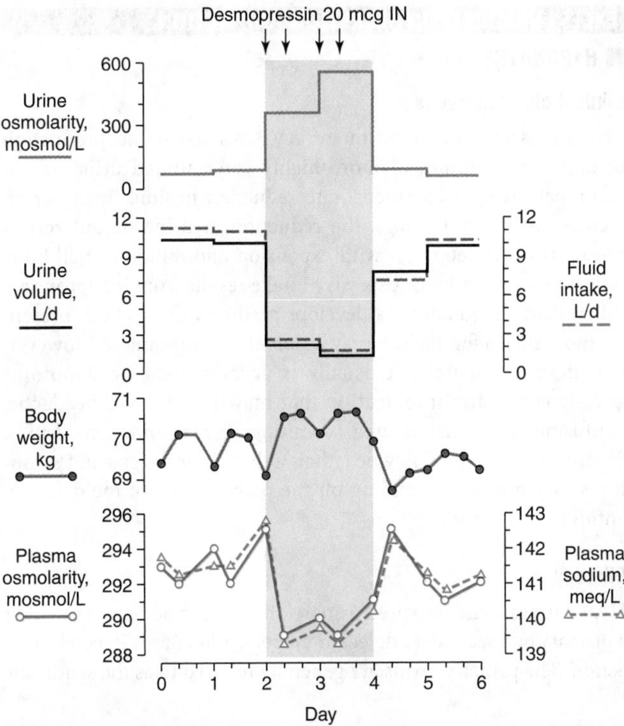

Figure 340-4 Effect of desmopressin therapy on water balance in a patient with uncomplicated pituitary diabetes insipidus. Note that treatment rapidly reduces thirst and fluid intake as well as urine output to normal, with only a slight increase in body water (weight) and a decrease in plasma osmolarity/sodium. *[From P Felig, L Frohman (eds): Endocrinology and Metabolism, 4th ed. New York, McGraw-Hill, 2001, with permission.]*

resistance is partial, it may be overcome by tenfold higher doses, but this treatment is too expensive and inconvenient to be useful chronically. However, treatment with conventional doses of a thiazide diuretic and/or amiloride in conjunction with a low-sodium diet and a prostaglandin synthesis inhibitor (e.g., indomethacin) usually reduces the polyuria and polydipsia by 30–70% and may eliminate them completely in some patients. Side effects such as hypokalemia and gastric irritation can be minimized by the use of amiloride or potassium supplements and by taking medications with meals.

ADIPSIC HYPERNATREMIA

Clinical characteristics

A defect in the thirst mechanism results in adipsic hypernatremia, a syndrome characterized by chronic or recurrent hypertonic dehydration. The hypernatremia varies widely in severity and usually is associated with signs of hypovolemia such as tachycardia, postural hypotension, azotemia, hyperuricemia, and hypokalemia. Muscle weakness, pain, rhabdomyolysis, hyperglycemia, hyperlipidemia, and acute renal failure may also occur. DI usually does not exist at presentation but may develop during rehydration.

Etiology

Deficient thirst is usually due to hypogenesis or destruction of the osmoreceptors in the anterior hypothalamus. Because of their proximity, the osmoreceptors that regulate AVP secretion also are usually impaired. These defects can result from various congenital malformations of midline brain structures or may be acquired due to diseases such as occlusions of the anterior communicating artery, primary or metastatic tumors in the hypothalamus, head trauma, surgery, granulomatous diseases such as sarcoidosis and histiocytosis, AIDS, and cytomegalovirus encephalitis.

Pathophysiology

A deficiency of thirst results in a failure to drink enough water to replenish obligatory renal and extrarenal losses, causing hypertonic dehydration. In most patients, the response of AVP to osmotic stimulation is also deficient (Fig. 340-5). If the deficiency is partial, it may not be clinically apparent at first because the hypertonicity and hypovolemia are severe enough to stimulate the release of AVP in the small amounts necessary to concentrate the urine. However, when the hypertonicity and hypovolemia are reduced, plasma AVP falls and polyuria develop, often before the dehydration is corrected fully. Patients

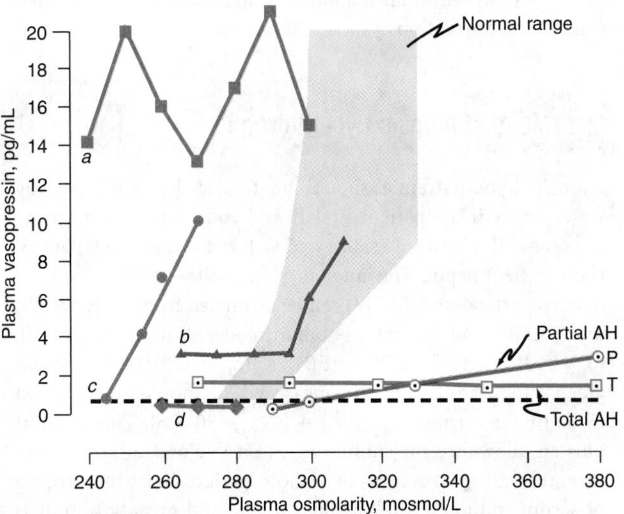

Figure 340-5 Heterogeneity of osmoregulatory dysfunction in adipsic hypernatremia (AH) and the syndrome of inappropriate antidiuresis (SIAD). Each line depicts schematically the relationship of plasma arginine vasopressin (AVP) to plasma osmolarity during water loading and/or infusion of 3% saline in a patient with either AH (open symbols) or SIAD (closed symbols). The shaded area indicates the normal range of the relationship. The horizontal broken line indicates the plasma AVP level below which the hormone is undetectable and urinary concentration usually does not occur. Lines P and T represent patients with a selective deficiency in the osmoregulation of thirst and AVP that is either partial (○) or total (□). In the latter, plasma AVP does not change in response to increases or decreases in plasma osmolarity but remains within a range sufficient to concentrate the urine even if overhydration produces hypotonic hyponatremia. In contrast, if the osmoregulatory deficiency is partial (○), rehydration of the patient suppresses plasma AVP to levels that result in urinary dilution and polyuria before plasma osmolarity and sodium are reduced to normal. Lines *a–d* represent different defects in the osmoregulation of plasma AVP observed in patients with SIAD. In *a* (■), plasma AVP is markedly elevated and fluctuates widely without relation to changes in plasma osmolarity, indicating complete loss of osmoregulation. In *b* (▲), plasma AVP remains fixed at a slightly elevated level until plasma osmolarity reaches the normal range, at which point it begins to rise appropriately, indicating a selective defect in the inhibitory component of the osmoregulatory mechanism. In *c* (●), plasma AVP rises in close correlation with plasma osmolarity before the latter reaches the normal range, indicating downward resetting of the osmostat. In *d* (◆), plasma AVP appears to be osmoregulated normally, suggesting that the inappropriate antidiuresis is caused by some other abnormality.

with a complete lack of osmoregulation do not develop DI at any level of hydration because they cannot osmotically suppress or stimulate AVP secretion. Therefore, a hyponatremic syndrome indistinguishable from inappropriate antidiuresis may develop if rehydration is excessive. In most patients, the neurohypophysis and the AVP response to hemodynamic or emetic stimuli are normal. In a few, however, the neurohypophysis is also destroyed, resulting in a combination of chronic pituitary DI and hypodipsia that is particularly difficult to manage.

Differential diagnosis

Adipsic hypernatremia usually can be distinguished clinically from other causes of inadequate fluid intake (e.g., coma, paralysis, restraints, absence of fresh water) that can also result in hypertonic dehydration. Previous episodes and/or denial of thirst and failure to drink spontaneously when the patient is conscious, unrestrained, and hypernatremic are virtually diagnostic of adipsia. The hypernatremia caused by excessive oral or intravenous intake of sodium can also be distinguished by the history and/or physical examination and laboratory signs of volume expansion rather than contraction.

TREATMENT Adipsic Hypernatremia

Adipsic hypernatremia should be treated by administering water orally if the patient is alert and cooperative or by using hypotonic fluids (0.45% saline or 5% dextrose and water) via IV if the patient is not. The amount of free water in liters required to correct the deficit (ΔFW) can be estimated from body weight in kg (BW) and the serum sodium concentration in mmol/L (S_{Na}) by the formula $\Delta FW = 0.5BW \times [(S_{Na} - 140)/140]$. If serum glucose ($S_{Glu}$) is elevated, the measured S_{Na} should be corrected (S_{Na}^*) by the formula $S_{Na}^* = S_{Na} + [(S_{Glu} - 90)/36]$. This amount plus an allowance for continuing insensible and urinary losses should be given over a 24- to 48-hour period. Close monitoring of serum sodium as well as fluid intake and urinary output is essential because, depending on the extent of osmoreceptor deficiency (Fig. 340-5), some patients will develop AVP-deficient DI, requiring desmopressin therapy to complete rehydration; others will develop hyponatremia and a syndrome of inappropriate antidiuresis (SIAD)-like picture if overhydrated. If hyperglycemia and/or hypokalemia are present, insulin and/or potassium supplements should be given with the expectation that both can be discontinued soon after rehydration is complete. Plasma urea/creatinine should be monitored closely for signs of acute renal failure.

Once the patient has been rehydrated, an MRI of the brain and tests of anterior pituitary function should be performed to look for the cause and collateral defects in other hypothalamic functions. A long-term management plan to prevent or minimize recurrence of the fluid and electrolyte imbalance also should be developed. This should include a practical method that can be used to regulate fluid intake in accordance with day-to-day variations in water balance. The most effective way to do this is to prescribe desmopressin to control DI if it is present and teach the patient how to adjust daily fluid intake in accordance with day-to-day changes in body weight or serum sodium as determined by home monitoring analyzers. Prescribing a constant fluid intake is ineffective and potentially dangerous because it does not take into account the large, uncontrolled variations in insensible loss that inevitably result from changes in ambient temperature and physical activity.

EXCESS VASOPRESSIN SECRETION AND ACTION

HYPONATREMIA (See also Chap. 45)

Clinical characteristics

Excessive secretion or action of AVP results in the production of decreased volumes of more highly concentrated urine. If not accompanied by a commensurate reduction in fluid intake or an increase in insensible loss, the reduction in urine output results in excess water retention with expansion and dilution of all body fluids. In some patients, excessive intake results from inappropriate thirst. If the hyponatremia develops gradually or has been present for more than a few days, it may be largely asymptomatic. However, if it develops acutely, it usually is accompanied by symptoms and signs of water intoxication that may include mild headache, confusion, anorexia, nausea, vomiting, coma, and convulsions. Severe hyponatremia may be lethal. Other clinical signs and symptoms vary greatly, depending on the pathogenesis of the defect in antidiuretic function.

Etiology

Hyponatremia and impaired urinary dilution can be caused by either a primary or a secondary defect in the regulation of AVP secretion or action. The primary forms are generally referred to as the syndrome

TABLE 340-2 Causes of Syndrome of Inappropriate Antidiuresis (SIAD)

Neoplasms	Neurologic
Carcinomas	Guillain-Barré syndrome
Lung	Multiple sclerosis
Duodenum	Delirium tremens
Pancreas	Amyotrophic lateral sclerosis
Ovary	Hydrocephalus
Bladder, ureter	Psychosis
Other neoplasms	Peripheral neuropathy
Thymoma	Congenital malformations
Mesothelioma	Agenesis corpus callosum
Bronchial adenoma	Cleft lip/palate
Carcinoid	Other midline defects
Gangliocytoma	Metabolic
Ewing's sarcoma	Acute intermittent porphyria
Head trauma (closed and penetrating)	Pulmonary
Infections	Asthma
Pneumonia, bacterial or viral	Pneumothorax
Abscess, lung or brain	Positive-pressure respiration
Cavitation (aspergillosis)	Drugs
Tuberculosis, lung or brain	Vasopressin or desmopressin
Meningitis, bacterial or viral	Chlorpropamide
Encephalitis	Oxytocin, high dose
AIDS	Vincristine
Vascular	Carbamazepine
Cerebrovascular occlusions, hemorrhage	Nicotine
	Phenothiazines
Cavernous sinus thrombosis	Cyclophosphamide
Genetic	Tricyclic antidepressants
X-linked recessive	Monoamine oxidase inhibitors
(V_2 receptor gene)	Serotonin reuptake inhibitors

of inappropriate antidiuresis. They have many different causes, including ectopic production of AVP by lung cancer or other neoplasms; eutopic release by various diseases or drugs; and exogenous administration of AVP, desmopressin, or large doses of oxytocin (Table 340-2). The ectopic forms result from abnormal expression of the *AVP-NPII* gene by primary or metastatic malignancies. The eutopic forms occur most often in patients with acute infections or strokes but have also been associated with many other neurologic diseases and injuries. In this case, the SIAD is usually self-limited and remits spontaneously within 2–3 weeks, but about 10% of cases are chronic. The mechanisms by which these diseases disrupt osmoregulation are not known. The defect in osmoregulation can take any of four distinct forms (Fig. 340-5). In one of the most common (reset osmostat), AVP secretion remains fully responsive to changes in plasma osmolarity/sodium but the threshold, or set point, of the osmoregulatory system is abnormally low. These patients differ from those with the other types of osmoregulatory defect in that they are able to maximally suppress plasma AVP and dilute their urine if their fluid intake is high enough to reduce their plasma osmolarity/sodium to the new set point. Another, smaller subgroup (~10% of the total) has inappropriate antidiuresis without a demonstrable defect in the osmoregulation of plasma AVP (Fig. 340-5). In some of them, all young boys, the inappropriate antidiuresis has been traced to a constitutively activating mutation of the V_2 receptor gene. This unusual variant may be referred to as familial nephrogenic SIAD to distinguish it from other possible causes of the syndrome.

The secondary forms of osmotically inappropriate antidiuresis also have multiple causes. They usually are subdivided into three types, depending on the nature of the abnormal stimulus and the state of extracellular fluid volume. Type I occurs in sodium-retaining, edema-forming states such as congestive heart failure, cirrhosis, and nephrosis. It is associated with markedly excessive retention of water and sodium that is thought to be stimulated by a large reduction in "effective" blood volume caused by low cardiac output and/or redistribution of plasma from the intravascular space to the interstitial space. Type II occurs in sodium-depleted states such as severe gastroenteritis, diuretic abuse, and mineralocorticoid deficiency. It is due to stimulation of AVP by a large reduction in blood volume and/or pressure. In both types, the increased AVP secretion appears to be due to downward resetting of the osmostat. Type III is due to nonosmotic, nonhemodynamic AVP stimuli such as nausea or isolated glucocorticoid deficiency that produce a form of euvolemic hyponatremia similar to SIAD (Table 340-3). They are differentiated because the cause of excess AVP secretion in type III can be corrected quickly and completely by treatments (antiemetics or glucocorticoids) that are not useful in SIAD.

Pathophysiology

When osmotic suppression of antidiuresis is impaired for any reason, retention of water and dilution of body fluids occur only if intake exceeds the rate of obligatory and insensible and urinary losses. The excess water intake sometimes is due to an associated defect in the osmoregulation of thirst (dipsogenic) but also can be psychogenic or iatrogenic, including IV administration of hypotonic fluids.

In SIAD, the excessive retention of water expands extracellular and intracellular volume, increases glomerular filtration and atrial natriuretic hormone, suppresses plasma renin activity, and increases urinary sodium excretion. This natriuresis reduces total body sodium, and this serves to counteract the extracellular hypervolemia but aggravates the hyponatremia. The osmotically driven increase in intracellular volume results in swelling of brain cells

TABLE 340-3 Differential Diagnosis of Hyponatremia Based on Clinical Assessment of Extracellular Fluid Volume (ECFV)

Clinical Findings	Type I, Hypervolemic	Type II, Hypovolemic	Type III, Euvolemic	SIAD Euvolemic
History				
CHF, cirrhosis, or nephrosis	Yes	No	No	No
Salt and water loss	No	Yes	No	No
ACTH–cortisol deficiency and/or nausea and vomiting	No	No	Yes	No
Physical examination				
Generalized edema, ascites	Yes	No	No	No
Postural hypotension	Maybe	Maybe	Maybe[a]	No
Laboratory				
BUN, creatinine	High-normal	High-normal	Low-normal	Low-normal
Uric acid	High-normal	High-normal	Low-normal	Low-normal
Serum potassium	Low-normal	Low-normal[b]	Normal[c]	Normal
Serum albumin	Low-normal	High-normal	Normal	Normal
Serum cortisol	Normal-high	Normal-high[d]	Low[e]	Normal
Plasma renin activity	High	High	Low[f]	Low
Urinary sodium (meq unit of time)[g]	Low	Low[h]	High[i]	High[i]

[a]Postural hypotension may occur in secondary (ACTH-dependent) adrenal insufficiency even though extracellular fluid volume and aldosterone are usually normal.

[b]Serum potassium may be high if hypovolemia is due to aldosterone deficiency.

[c]Serum potassium may be low if vomiting causes alkalosis.

[d]Serum cortisol is low if hypovolemia is due to primary adrenal insufficiency (Addison's disease).

[e]Serum cortisol will be normal or high if the cause is nausea and vomiting rather than secondary (ACTH-dependent) adrenal insufficiency.

[f]Plasma renin activity may be high if the cause is secondary (ACTH) adrenal insufficiency.

[g]Urinary sodium should be expressed as the *rate of excretion* rather than the concentration. In a hyponatremic adult, an excretion rate >25 meq/d (or 25 μeq/mg of creatinine) could be considered high.

[h]The rate of urinary sodium excretion may be high if the hypovolemia is due to diuretic abuse, primary adrenal insufficiency, or other causes of renal sodium wasting.

[i]The rate of urinary sodium excretion may be low if intake is curtailed by symptoms or treatment.

Abbreviations: ACTH, adrenocorticotropic hormone; BUN, blood urea nitrogen; CHF, congestive heart failure; SIAD, syndrome of inappropriate antidiuresis.

and increases intracranial pressure; this is probably responsible for the symptoms of acute water intoxication. Within a few days, this swelling may be counteracted by inactivation or elimination of intracellular solutes, resulting in the remission of symptoms even though the hyponatremia persists. The pathophysiology of type III (euvolemic) hyponatremia is probably similar to that of SIAD.

In type I (hypervolemic) or type II (hypovolemic) hyponatremia, the antidiuretic effect of hemodynamically induced AVP release is enhanced by decreased distal delivery of glomerular filtrate that results from increased reabsorption of sodium in proximal nephrons. If the marked reduction in urine output is not associated with a commensurate reduction in water intake or an increase in insensible loss, body fluids are expanded and diluted, resulting in hyponatremia. Unlike SIAD, however, glomerular filtration is reduced and plasma renin activity and aldosterone are elevated due to either effective hypovolemia (type I) or absolute hypovolemia (type II). Thus, urinary sodium excretion is low (unless sodium reabsorption is impaired by a diuretic), and the hyponatremia is usually accompanied by hypokalemia, azotemia, and hyperuricemia. The sodium retention is an appropriate compensatory response to severe volume and sodium depletion in type II but is inappropriate and deleterious in type I since body sodium and extracellular volume are already markedly increased, as evidenced by the presence of generalized edema.

Differential diagnosis

SIAD is a diagnosis of exclusion that usually can be made from the history, physical examination, and basic laboratory data. The possibility that hyponatremia is due to an osmotically driven shift of water from the intracellular space to the extracellular space can be excluded if plasma glucose is not high enough to account for the hyponatremia [serum sodium decreases ~1 meq/L for each rise in glucose of 2 mmol/L (36 mg/dL)] and/or plasma osmolarity is reduced in proportion to sodium (each decrease in serum sodium of 1 meq/L should reduce plasma osmolarity by ~2 mosmol/L). The type of hypotonic hyponatremia can then be determined by standard clinical indicators of the extracellular fluid volume (Table 340-3). If these findings are ambiguous or contradictory, measuring the rate of urinary sodium excretion or plasma renin activity may be helpful *provided* that the hyponatremia is not in the recovery phase or due to a primary defect in renal conservation of sodium, diuretic abuse, or hyporeninemic hypoaldosteronism. The latter may be suspected if serum potassium is elevated instead of low as it usually is in types I and II hyponatremia. Measurements of plasma AVP are currently of no value in differentiating among the three types of hyponatremia since the abnormalities are similar. In patients who fulfill the clinical criteria for type III (euvolemic) hyponatremia, morning plasma cortisol should also be measured to exclude secondary adrenal insufficiency. If it is normal and there is no history of nausea/vomiting, the diagnosis of SIAD is confirmed and a careful search for occult lung cancer or other common causes of the syndrome (Table 340-2) should be undertaken. If an activating mutation of the V_2 receptor gene is suspected, plasma AVP should be measured while the hyponatremia and antidiuresis are present. If it is undetectable, DNA should be collected for analysis of the V_2 receptor gene.

TREATMENT Hyponatremia

The management of hyponatremia differs depending not only on the type but also on the severity and duration of symptoms. In a patient with SIAD and few symptoms, the objective is to reduce body water gradually by restricting total fluid intake to less than the sum of urinary and insensible losses. Because the water derived from food (300–700 mL/d) usually approximates basal insensible losses in adults, total discretionary intake (all liquids) should be at least 500 mL less than urinary output. If achievable, this usually reduces body water and increases serum sodium by about 1–2% per day. If the symptoms or signs of water intoxication are more severe, the hyponatremia can be corrected more rapidly by supplementing the fluid restriction with IV infusion of hypertonic (3%) saline. This treatment also has the advantage of correcting the sodium deficiency that is partly responsible for the hyponatremia in SIAD and produces a solute diuresis that serves to remove some of the excess water. However, if plasma sodium is raised too rapidly or too much and the hyponatremia has been present for >24–48 hours, it also has the potential to produce central pontine myelinolysis, an acute, potentially fatal neurologic syndrome characterized by quadriparesis, ataxia, and abnormal extraocular movements. The risk of this complication can be minimized by observing several precautions: 3% saline should be infused at a rate ≤0.05 mL/kg body weight per min; the effect should be monitored continuously by STAT measurements of serum sodium at least once every 2 hours; and the infusion should be stopped as soon as serum sodium increases by 12 mmol/L or to 130 mmol/L, whichever comes first. Urinary output should be monitored continuously since SIAD can remit spontaneously at any time, resulting in an acute water diuresis that greatly accelerates the rate of rise in serum sodium produced by fluid restriction and 3% saline infusion.

In chronic SIAD, the hyponatremia can be corrected by treatment with demeclocycline, 150–300 mg PO tid or gid, or fludrocortisone, 0.05–0.2 mg PO bid. The effect of the demeclocycline manifests in 7–14 days and is due to production of a reversible form of nephrogenic DI. Potential side effects include phototoxicity and azotemia. The effect of fludrocortisone also requires 1–2 weeks and is partly due to increased retention of sodium and possibly inhibition of thirst. It also increases urinary potassium excretion, which may require replacement through dietary adjustments or supplements and may induce hypertension, occasionally necessitating discontinuation of the treatment.

Nonpeptide AVP antagonists that block the antidiuretic effect of AVP have been used experimentally to treat SIAD. They produce a dose-dependent increase in urinary free-water excretion, that, if combined with a modest restriction of fluid intake, reduces body water and corrects the hyponatremia. The antagonists appear to have no adverse side effects, but, like hypertonic saline, they probably carry the risk of inducing osmotic demyelinization if the hyponatremia is corrected too rapidly. One of them, a combined V_2/V_{1a} antagonist (Conivaptan), has been approved for short-term in-hospital IV treatment of SIAD and the hyponatremia of congestive heart failure. It is a substrate and inhibitor of cytochrome P450 and should not be used in conjunction with other drugs metabolized by these pathways. Other V_2 receptor antagonists are currently in phase III trials.

In type I hyponatremia, fluid restriction is also appropriate and somewhat effective if it can be maintained. However, infusion of hypertonic saline is contraindicated because it further increases total body sodium and edema and may precipitate cardiovascular decompensation. Preliminary studies with antagonists of V_2 receptors indicate that they are almost as effective in type I hyponatremia as they are in SIAD.

In type II hyponatremia, the defect in AVP secretion and water balance usually can be corrected easily and quickly by stopping the loss of sodium and water and/or replacing the deficits by mouth or IV infusion of normal or hypertonic saline. As with the treatment of other forms of hyponatremia, care must be taken to ensure that plasma sodium does not increase too rapidly. Fluid restriction and administration of AVP antagonists are contraindicated in type II as they would only aggravate the underlying volume depletion and could result in hemodynamic collapse.

In euvolemic hyponatremia due to protracted nausea and vomiting or isolated glucocorticoid deficiency (type III), all abnormalities can be corrected quickly and completely by giving an antiemetic or stress doses of hydrocortisone. As with other treatments, care must be taken to ensure that serum sodium does not rise too quickly or too far.

GLOBAL PERSPECTIVES The incidence, clinical characteristics, etiology, pathophysiology, differential diagnosis, and treatments of fluid and electrolyte disorders in tropical and nonindustrialized countries differ in some respects from those in the United States and other industrialized parts of the world. Hyponatremia, for example, appears to be more common and is more likely to be due to infectious diseases such as cholera, shigellosis, and other diarrheal disorders. In these circumstances, hyponatremia is probably due to gastrointestinal losses of salt and water (hypovolemia type II), but other abnormalities, including undefined infectious toxins, also may contribute. The causes of DI are similar worldwide except that malaria and venoms from snake or insect bites are much more common.

FURTHER READINGS

Bichet D: Vasopressin receptor mutations in nephrogenic diabetes insipidus. Semin Nephrol 28:245, 2008

Biswas M, Davies JS: Hyponatremia in clinical practice. Postgrad Med J 83:373, 2007

Christensen JH, Rittig S: Familial neurohypophyseal diabetes insipidus—an update. Semin Nephrol 26:209, 2006

Feldman BJ et al: Nephrogenic syndrome of inappropriate antidiuresis. N Engl J Med 352:1884, 2005

Kristof RA et al: Incidence, clinical manifestations and course of water and electrolytes metabolism disturbances following transsphenoidal pituitary adenoma surgery: A prospective observational study. J Neurosurg 111:555, 2009

Liamis G et al: A review of drug induced hyponatremia. Am J Kidney Dis 52:144, 2008

Loonen AJM et al: Aquaporin 2 mutations in nephrogenic diabetes insipidus. Semin Nephrol 28:252, 2008

Robertson GL: Antidiuretic hormone: Normal and disordered function. Endocrinol Metab Clin North Am 30:671, 2001

Sitprija V: Altered fluid, electrolyte and mineral status in tropical disease with an emphasis on malaria and leptospirosis. Nature Clin Pract Nephrol 42:91, 208

CHAPTER 341

Disorders of the Thyroid Gland

J. Larry Jameson

Anthony P. Weetman

The thyroid gland produces two related hormones, thyroxine (T_4) and triiodothyronine (T_3) (Fig. 341-1). Acting through thyroid hormone receptors α and β, these hormones play a critical role in cell differentiation during development and help maintain thermogenic and metabolic homeostasis in the adult. Autoimmune disorders of the thyroid gland can stimulate overproduction of thyroid hormones (*thyrotoxicosis*) or cause glandular destruction and hormone deficiency (*hypothyroidism*). In addition, benign nodules and various forms of thyroid cancer are relatively common and amenable to detection by physical examination.

ANATOMY AND DEVELOPMENT

The thyroid (Greek *thyreos*, shield, plus *eidos*, form) consists of two lobes connected by an isthmus. It is located anterior to the trachea between the cricoid cartilage and the suprasternal notch. The normal thyroid is 12–20 g in size, highly vascular, and soft in consistency. Four parathyroid glands, which produce parathyroid hormone (Chap. 353), are located posterior to each pole of the thyroid. The recurrent laryngeal nerves traverse the lateral borders of the thyroid gland and must be identified during thyroid surgery to avoid injury and vocal cord paralysis.

The thyroid gland develops from the floor of the primitive pharynx during the third week of gestation. The developing gland migrates along the thyroglossal duct to reach its final location in the neck. This feature accounts for the rare ectopic location of thyroid tissue at the base of the tongue (lingual thyroid) as well as the occurrence of thyroglossal duct cysts along this developmental tract. Thyroid hormone synthesis normally begins at about 11 weeks' gestation.

Neural crest derivatives from the ultimobranchial body give rise to thyroid medullary C cells that produce calcitonin, a calcium-lowering hormone. The C cells are interspersed throughout the thyroid gland, although their density is greatest in the juncture of

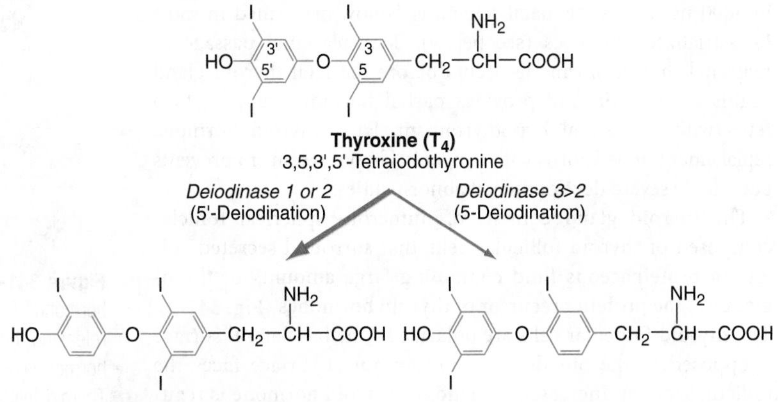

Figure 341-1 Structures of thyroid hormones. Thyroxine (T_4) contains four iodine atoms. Deiodination leads to production of the potent hormone triiodothyronine (T_3), or the inactive hormone reverse T_3.

TABLE 341-1 Genetic Causes of Congenital Hypothyroidism

Defective Gene Protein	Inheritance	Consequences
PROP-1	Autosomal recessive	Combined pituitary hormone deficiencies with preservation of adrenocorticotropic hormone
PIT-1	Autosomal recessive Autosomal dominant	Combined deficiencies of growth hormone, prolactin, thyroid-stimulating hormone (TSH)
TSHβ	Autosomal recessive	TSH deficiency
TTF-1 (TITF-1)	Autosomal dominant	Variable thyroid hypoplasia, choreoathetosis, pulmonary problems
TTF-2 (FOXE-1)	Autosomal recessive	Thyroid agenesis, choanal atresia, spiky hair
PAX-8	Autosomal dominant	Thyroid dysgenesis
TSH-receptor	Autosomal recessive	Resistance to TSH
$G_{s\alpha}$ (Albright hereditary osteodystrophy)	Autosomal dominant	Resistance to TSH
Na^+/I^- symporter	Autosomal recessive	Inability to transport iodide
THOX2	Autosomal dominant	Organification defect
Thyroid peroxidase	Autosomal recessive	Defective organification of iodide
Thyroglobulin	Autosomal recessive	Defective synthesis of thyroid hormone
Pendrin	Autosomal recessive	Pendred syndrome: sensorineural deafness and partial organification defect in thyroid
Dehalogenase 1	Autosomal recessive	Loss of iodide reutilization

the upper one-third and lower two-thirds of the gland. Calcitonin plays a minimal role in calcium homeostasis in humans but the C-cells are important because of their involvement in medullary thyroid cancer.

Thyroid gland development is orchestrated by the coordinated expression of several developmental transcription factors. Thyroid transcription factor (TTF)-1, TTF-2, and paired homeobox-8 (PAX-8) are expressed selectively, but not exclusively, in the thyroid gland. In combination, they dictate thyroid cell development and the induction of thyroid-specific genes such as thyroglobulin (Tg), thyroid peroxidase (TPO), the sodium iodide symporter (Na^+/I, NIS), and the thyroid-stimulating hormone receptor (TSH-R). Mutations in these developmental transcription factors or their downstream target genes are rare causes of thyroid agenesis or dyshormonogenesis, though the causes of most forms of congenital hypothyroidism remain unknown (Table 341-1). Because congenital hypothyroidism occurs in approximately 1 in 4000 newborns, neonatal screening is now performed in most industrialized countries (see below). Transplacental passage of maternal thyroid hormone occurs before the fetal thyroid gland begins to function and provides partial hormone support to a fetus with congenital hypothyroidism. Early thyroid hormone replacement in newborns with congenital hypothyroidism prevents potentially severe developmental abnormalities.

The thyroid gland consists of numerous spherical follicles composed of thyroid follicular cells that surround secreted colloid, a proteinaceous fluid containing large amounts of thyroglobulin, the protein precursor of thyroid hormones (Fig. 341-2). The thyroid follicular cells are polarized—the basolateral surface is apposed to the bloodstream and an apical surface faces the follicular lumen. Increased demand for thyroid hormone is regulated by thyroid-stimulating hormone (TSH), which binds to its receptor on the basolateral surface of the follicular cells, leading to Tg reabsorption from the follicular lumen, proteolysis within the cytoplasm, yielding thyroid hormones for secretion into the bloodstream.

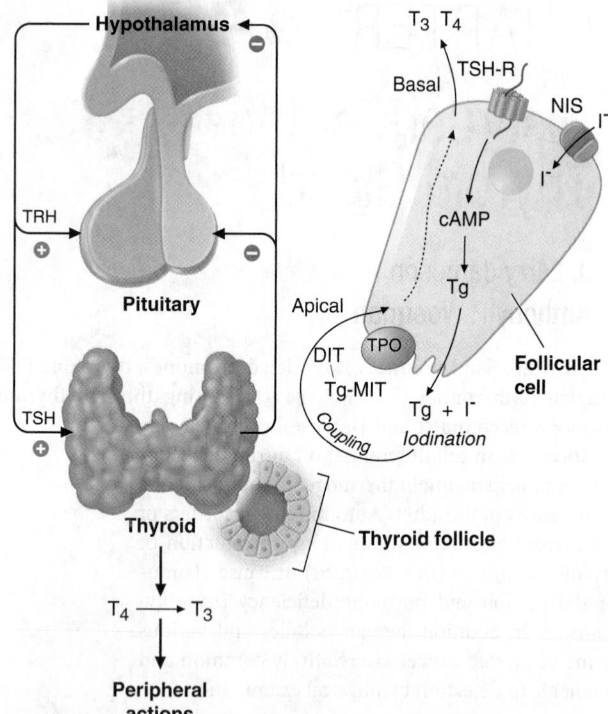

Figure 341-2 Regulation of thyroid hormone synthesis. ***Left.*** Thyroid hormones T_4 and T_3 feed back to inhibit hypothalamic production of thyrotropin-releasing hormone (TRH) and pituitary production of thyroid-stimulating hormone (TSH). TSH stimulates thyroid gland production of T_4 and T_3. ***Right.*** Thyroid follicles are formed by thyroid epithelial cells surrounding proteinaceous colloid, which contains thyroglobulin. Follicular cells, which are polarized, synthesize thyroglobulin and carry out thyroid hormone biosynthesis (see text for details). TSH-R, thyroid-stimulating hormone receptor; Tg, thyroglobulin; NIS, sodium iodide symporter; TPO, thyroid peroxidase; DIT, diiodotyrosine; MIT, monoiodotyrosine.

REGULATION OF THE THYROID AXIS

TSH, secreted by the thyrotrope cells of the anterior pituitary, plays a pivotal role in control of the thyroid axis and serves as the most useful physiologic marker of thyroid hormone action. TSH is a 31-kDa hormone composed of α and β subunits; the α subunit is common to the other glycoprotein hormones [luteinizing hormone, follicle-stimulating hormone, human chorionic gonadotropin (hCG)], whereas the TSH β subunit is unique to TSH. The extent and nature of carbohydrate modification are modulated by thyrotropin-releasing hormone (TRH) stimulation and influence the biologic activity of the hormone.

The thyroid axis is a classic example of an endocrine feedback loop. Hypothalamic TRH stimulates pituitary production of TSH, which, in turn, stimulates thyroid hormone synthesis and secretion. Thyroid hormones, acting predominantly through thyroid hormone receptor β2 (TRβ2), feed back to inhibit TRH and TSH production (Fig. 341-2). The "set-point" in this axis is established by TSH. TRH is the major positive regulator of TSH synthesis and secretion. Peak TSH secretion occurs ~15 min after administration of exogenous TRH. Dopamine, glucocorticoids, and somatostatin suppress TSH but are not of major physiologic importance except when these agents are administered in pharmacologic doses. Reduced levels of thyroid hormone increase basal TSH production and enhance TRH-mediated stimulation of TSH. High thyroid hormone levels rapidly and directly suppress TSH gene expression secretion and inhibit TRH stimulation of TSH, indicating that thyroid hormones are the dominant regulator of TSH production. Like other pituitary hormones, TSH is released in a pulsatile manner and exhibits a diurnal rhythm; its highest levels occur at night. However, these TSH excursions are modest in comparison to those of other pituitary hormones, in part, because TSH has a relatively long plasma half-life (50 minutes). Consequently, single measurements of TSH are adequate for assessing its circulating level. TSH is measured using immunoradiometric assays that are highly sensitive and specific. These assays readily distinguish between normal and suppressed TSH values; thus, TSH can be used for the diagnosis of hyperthyroidism (low TSH) as well as hypothyroidism (high TSH).

THYROID HORMONE SYNTHESIS, METABOLISM, AND ACTION

THYROID HORMONE SYNTHESIS

Thyroid hormones are derived from Tg, a large iodinated glycoprotein. After secretion into the thyroid follicle, Tg is iodinated on tyrosine residues that are subsequently coupled via an ether linkage. Reuptake of Tg into the thyroid follicular cell allows proteolysis and the release of newly synthesized T_4 and T_3.

Iodine metabolism and transport

Iodide uptake is a critical first step in thyroid hormone synthesis. Ingested iodine is bound to serum proteins, particularly albumin. Unbound iodine is excreted in the urine. The thyroid gland extracts iodine from the circulation in a highly efficient manner. For example, 10–25% of radioactive tracer (e.g., ^{123}I) is taken up by the normal thyroid gland over 24 hours; this value can rise to 70–90% in Graves' disease. Iodide uptake is mediated by NIS, which is expressed at the basolateral membrane of thyroid follicular cells. NIS is most highly expressed in the thyroid gland, but low levels are present in the salivary glands, lactating breast, and placenta. The iodide transport mechanism is highly regulated, allowing adaptation to variations in dietary supply. Low iodine levels increase the amount of NIS and stimulate uptake, whereas high iodine levels suppress NIS expression and uptake. The selective expression of NIS in the thyroid allows isotopic scanning, treatment of hyperthyroidism, and ablation of thyroid cancer with radioisotopes of iodine, without significant effects on other organs. Mutation of the *NIS* gene is a rare cause of congenital hypothyroidism, underscoring its importance in thyroid hormone synthesis. Another iodine transporter, pendrin, is located on the apical surface of thyroid cells and mediates iodine efflux into the lumen. Mutation of the *pendrin* gene causes *Pendred syndrome*, a disorder characterized by defective organification of iodine, goiter, and sensorineural deafness.

Iodine deficiency is prevalent in many mountainous regions and in central Africa, central South America, and northern Asia (Fig. 341-3). Europe remains mildly iodine deficient and health surveys indicate that iodine intake has been falling in the United States and Australia. The World Health Organization (WHO) estimates that about 2 billion people are iodine-deficient, based on urinary excretion data. In areas of relative iodine deficiency, there is an increased prevalence of goiter and, when deficiency is severe, hypothyroidism and cretinism. *Cretinism* is characterized by mental and growth retardation and occurs when children who live in iodine-deficient regions are not treated with iodine or thyroid hormone to restore normal thyroid hormone levels during early life. These children are often born to mothers with iodine deficiency, and it is likely that maternal thyroid hormone deficiency worsens the condition. Concomitant selenium deficiency may also contribute to the neurologic manifestations of cretinism. Iodine supplementation of salt, bread, and other food substances has markedly reduced the prevalence of cretinism. Unfortunately, however, iodine deficiency remains the most common cause of preventable mental deficiency, often because of societal resistance to food additives or the cost of supplementation. In addition to overt cretinism, mild iodine deficiency can lead to subtle reduction of IQ. Oversupply of iodine, through supplements or foods enriched in iodine (e.g., shellfish, kelp), is associated

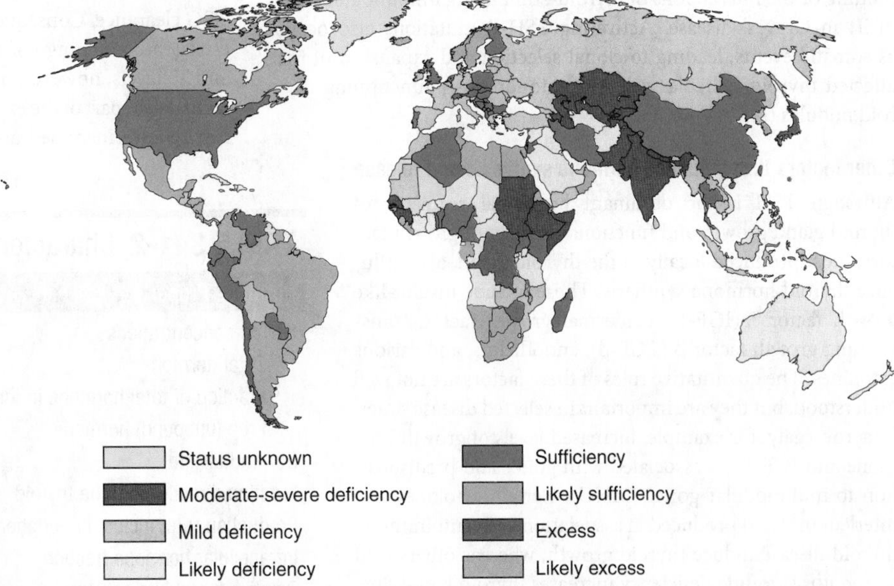

Figure 341-3 Worldwide iodine nutrition. Data are from the WHO and the International Council for the Control of Iodine Deficiency Disorders (*http://indorgs.virginia.edu/iccidd/mi/cidds.html*).

with an increased incidence of autoimmune thyroid disease. The recommended average daily intake of iodine is 150–250 μg/d for adults, 90–120 μg/d for children, and 250 μg/d for pregnant and lactating women. Urinary iodine is >10 μg/dL in iodine-sufficient populations.

Organification, coupling, storage, release

After iodide enters the thyroid, it is trapped and transported to the apical membrane of thyroid follicular cells, where it is oxidized in an organification reaction that involves TPO and hydrogen peroxide. The reactive iodine atom is added to selected tyrosyl residues within Tg, a large (660 kDa) dimeric protein that consists of 2769 amino acids. The iodotyrosines in Tg are then coupled via an ether linkage in a reaction that is also catalyzed by TPO. Either T_4 or T_3 can be produced by this reaction, depending on the number of iodine atoms present in the iodotyrosines. After coupling, Tg is taken back into the thyroid cell, where it is processed in lysosomes to release T_4 and T_3. Uncoupled mono- and diiodotyrosines (MIT, DIT) are deiodinated by the enzyme dehalogenase, thereby recycling any iodide that is not converted into thyroid hormones.

Disorders of thyroid hormone synthesis are rare causes of congenital hypothyroidism. The vast majority of these disorders are due to recessive mutations in TPO or Tg, but defects have also been identified in the TSH-R, NIS, pendrin, hydrogen peroxide generation, and dehalogenase. Because of the biosynthetic defect, the gland is incapable of synthesizing adequate amounts of hormone, leading to increased TSH and a large goiter.

TSH action

TSH regulates thyroid gland function through the TSH-R, a seven-transmembrane G protein–coupled receptor (GPCR). The TSH-R is coupled to the α subunit of stimulatory G protein ($G_s\alpha$), which activates adenylyl cyclase, leading to increased production of cyclic AMP. TSH also stimulates phosphatidylinositol turnover by activating phospholipase C. The functional role of the TSH-R is exemplified by the consequences of naturally occurring mutations. Recessive loss-of-function mutations cause thyroid hypoplasia and congenital hypothyroidism. Dominant gain-of-function mutations cause sporadic or familial hyperthyroidism that is characterized by goiter, thyroid cell hyperplasia, and autonomous function. Most of these activating mutations occur in the transmembrane domain of the receptor. They mimic the conformational changes induced by TSH binding or the interactions of thyroid-stimulating immunoglobulins (TSI) in Graves' disease. Activating TSH-R mutations also occur as somatic events, leading to clonal selection and expansion of the affected thyroid follicular cell and autonomously functioning thyroid nodules (see below).

Other factors that influence hormone synthesis and release

Although TSH is the dominant hormonal regulator of thyroid gland growth and function, a variety of growth factors, most produced locally in the thyroid gland, also influence thyroid hormone synthesis. These include insulin-like growth factor I (IGF-1), epidermal growth factor, transforming growth factor β (TGF-β), endothelins, and various cytokines. The quantitative roles of these factors are not well understood, but they are important in selected disease states. In acromegaly, for example, increased levels of growth hormone and IGF-1 are associated with goiter and predisposition to multinodular goiter (MNG). Certain cytokines and interleukins (ILs) produced in association with autoimmune thyroid disease induce thyroid growth, whereas others lead to apoptosis. Iodine deficiency increases thyroid blood flow and upregulates the NIS, stimulating more efficient iodine uptake. Excess iodide transiently inhibits thyroid iodide organification, a phenomenon known as the *Wolff-Chaikoff effect*. In individuals with a normal thyroid, the gland escapes from this inhibitory effect and iodide organification resumes; the suppressive action of high iodide may persist, however, in patients with underlying autoimmune thyroid disease.

THYROID HORMONE TRANSPORT AND METABOLISM

Serum binding proteins

T_4 is secreted from the thyroid gland in about twentyfold excess over T_3 (Table 341-2). Both hormones are bound to plasma proteins, including thyroxine-binding globulin (TBG), transthyretin (TTR, formerly known as thyroxine-binding prealbumin, or TBPA), and albumin. The plasma-binding proteins increase the pool of circulating hormone, delay hormone clearance, and may modulate hormone delivery to selected tissue sites. The concentration of TBG is relatively low (1–2 mg/dL), but because of its high affinity for thyroid hormones ($T_4 > T_3$), it carries about 80% of the bound hormones. Albumin has relatively low affinity for thyroid hormones but has a high plasma concentration (~3.5 g/dL), and it binds up to 10% of T_4 and 30% of T_3. TTR carries about 10% of T_4 but little T_3.

When the effects of the various binding proteins are combined, approximately 99.98% of T_4 and 99.7% of T_3 are protein-bound. Because T_3 is less tightly bound than T_4, the fraction of unbound T_3 is greater than unbound T_4, but there is less unbound T_3 in the circulation because it is produced in smaller amounts and cleared more rapidly than T_4. The unbound or "free" concentrations of the hormones are ~2×10^{-11} *M* for T_4 and ~6×10^{-12} *M* for T_3, which roughly correspond to the thyroid hormone receptor binding constants for these hormones (see below). The unbound hormone is thought to be biologically available to tissues. Nonetheless, the homeostatic mechanisms that regulate the thyroid axis are directed toward maintenance of normal concentrations of unbound hormones.

Abnormalities of thyroid hormone binding proteins

A number of inherited and acquired abnormalities affect thyroid hormone binding proteins. X-linked TBG deficiency is associated with very low levels of total T_4 and T_3. However, because unbound hormone levels are normal, patients are euthyroid and TSH levels are normal. It is important to recognize this disorder to avoid efforts to normalize total T_4 levels, as this leads to thyrotoxicosis and is futile because of rapid hormone clearance in the absence of TBG. TBG levels are elevated by estrogen, which increases sialylation and delays TBG clearance. Consequently, in women who are pregnant or taking estrogen-containing contraceptives, elevated TBG increases total T_4 and T_3 levels; however, unbound T_4 and T_3 levels are normal. These features are part of the explanation for why women with hypothyroidism require increased amounts of l-thyroxine replacement as TBG

TABLE 341-2 Characteristics of Circulating T_4 and T_3

Hormone Property	T_4	T_3
Serum concentrations		
Total hormone	8 μg/dL	0.14 μg/dL
Fraction of total hormone in the free form	0.02%	0.3%
Free (unbound) hormone	$21 \times 10^{-12}M$	$6 \times 10^{-12}M$
Serum half-life	7 d	0.75 d
Fraction directly from the thyroid	100%	20%
Production rate, including peripheral conversion	90 μg/d	32 μg/d
Intracellular hormone fraction	~20%	~70%
Relative metabolic potency	0.3	1
Receptor binding	$10^{-10}M$	$10^{-11}M$

TABLE 341-3 Conditions Associated With Euthyroid Hyperthyroxinemia

Disorder	Cause	Transmission	Characteristics
Familial dysalbuminemic hyperthyroxinemia (FDH)	Albumin mutations, usually R218H	AD	Increased T_4 Normal unbound T_4 Rarely increased T_3
TBG			
Familial excess	Increased TBG production	XL	Increased total T_4, T_3 Normal unbound T_4, T_3
Acquired excess	Medications (estrogen), pregnancy, cirrhosis, hepatitis	Acquired	Increased total T_4, T_3 Normal unbound T_4, T_3
Transthyretin[a]			
Excess	Islet tumors	Acquired	Usually normal T_4, T_3
Mutations	Increased affinity for T_4 or T_3	AD	Increased total T_4, T_3 Normal unbound T_4, T_3
Medications: propranolol, ipodate, iopanoic acid, amiodarone	Decreased $T_4 \rightarrow T_3$ conversion	Acquired	Increased T4 Decreased T3 Normal or increased TSH
Sick-euthyroid syndrome	Acute illness, especially psychiatric disorders	Acquired	Transiently increased unbound T_4 Decreased TSH T_4 and T_3 may also be decreased (see text)
Resistance to thyroid hormone (RTH)	Thyroid hormone receptor β mutations	AD	Increased unbound T_4, T_3 Normal or increased TSH Some patients clinically thyrotoxic

[a]Also known as thyroxine-binding prealbumin, TBPA.
Abbreviations: AD, autosomal dominant; TBG, thyroxine-binding globulin; TSH, thyroid-stimulating hormone; XL, X-linked.

levels are increased by pregnancy or estrogen treatment. Mutations in TBG, TTR, and albumin may increase the binding affinity for T_4 and/or T_3 and cause disorders known as *euthyroid hyperthyroxinemia* or *familial dysalbuminemic hyperthyroxinemia* (FDH) (Table 341-3). These disorders result in increased total T_4 and/or T_3, but unbound hormone levels are normal. The familial nature of the disorders, and the fact that TSH levels are normal rather than suppressed, should suggest this diagnosis. Unbound hormone levels (ideally measured by dialysis) are normal in FDH. The diagnosis can be confirmed by using tests that measure the affinities of radiolabeled hormone binding to specific transport proteins or by performing DNA sequence analyses of the abnormal transport protein genes.

Certain medications, such as salicylates and salsalate, can displace thyroid hormones from circulating binding proteins. Although these drugs transiently perturb the thyroid axis by increasing free thyroid hormone levels, TSH is suppressed until a new steady state is reached, thereby restoring euthyroidism. Circulating factors associated with acute illness may also displace thyroid hormone from binding proteins (see "Sick Euthyroid Syndrome," below).

Deiodinases

T_4 may be thought of as a precursor for the more potent T_3. T_4 is converted to T_3 by the deiodinase enzymes (Fig. 341-1). Type I deiodinase, which is located primarily in thyroid, liver, and kidneys, has a relatively low affinity for T_4. Type II deiodinase has a higher affinity for T_4 and is found primarily in the pituitary gland, brain, brown fat, and thyroid gland. Expression of type II deiodinase allows it to regulate T_3 concentrations locally, a property that may be important in the context of levothyroxine (T_4) replacement. Type II deiodinase is also regulated by thyroid hormone; hypothyroidism induces the enzyme, resulting in enhanced $T_4 \rightarrow T_3$ conversion in tissues such as brain and pituitary. $T_4 \rightarrow T_3$ conversion is impaired by fasting, systemic illness or acute trauma, oral contrast agents, and a variety of medications (e.g., propylthiouracil, propranolol, amiodarone, glucocorticoids). Type III deiodinase inactivates T_4 and T_3 and is the most important source of reverse T_3 (rT_3). Massive hemangiomas that express type III deiodinase are a rare cause of hypothyroidism in infants.

■ THYROID HORMONE ACTION

Thyroid hormone transport

Circulating thyroid hormones enter cells by passive diffusion and via specific transporters such as the monocarboxylate 8 (MCT8) transporter. Mutations in the *MCT8* gene have been identified in patients with X-linked psychomotor retardation and thyroid function abnormalities (low T_4, high T_3, and high TSH). After entering cells, thyroid hormones act primarily through nuclear receptors, although they also have nongenomic actions through stimulating plasma membrane and mitochondrial enzymatic responses.

Nuclear thyroid hormone receptors

Thyroid hormones bind with high affinity to nuclear *thyroid hormone receptors* (TRs) α and β. Both TRα and TRβ are expressed in most tissues, but their relative expression levels vary among organs; TRα is particularly abundant in brain, kidneys, gonads, muscle, and heart, whereas TRβ expression is relatively high in the pituitary and liver. Both receptors are variably spliced to form unique isoforms. The TRβ2 isoform, which has a unique amino terminus, is selectively expressed in the hypothalamus and pituitary, where it plays a role in feedback control of the thyroid axis (see above). The TRα2 isoform

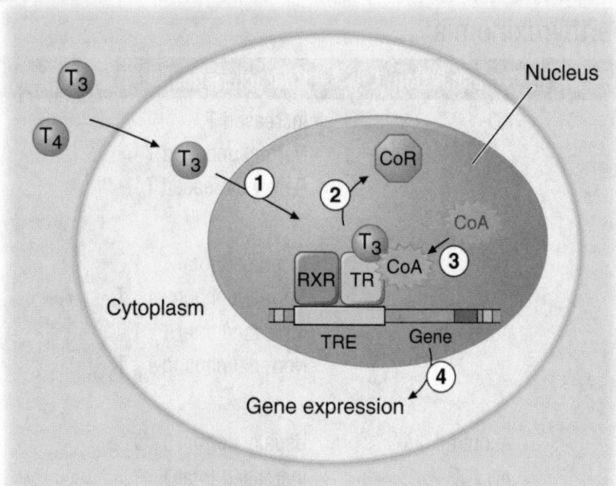

Figure 341-4 Mechanism of thyroid hormone receptor action. The thyroid hormone receptor (TR) and retinoid X receptor (RXR) form heterodimers that bind specifically to thyroid hormone response elements (TRE) in the promoter regions of target genes. In the absence of hormone, TR binds co-repressor (CoR) proteins that silence gene expression. The numbers refer to a series of ordered reactions that occur in response to thyroid hormone: (1) T_4 or T_3 enters the nucleus; (2) T_3 binding dissociates CoR from TR; (3) Coactivators (CoA) are recruited to the T_3-bound receptor; (4) gene expression is altered.

contains a unique carboxy terminus that precludes thyroid hormone binding; it may function to block the action of other TR isoforms.

The TRs contain a central DNA-binding domain and a C-terminal ligand-binding domain. They bind to specific DNA sequences, termed *thyroid response elements* (TREs), in the promoter regions of target genes (Fig. 341-4). The receptors bind as homodimers or, more commonly, as heterodimers with retinoic acid X receptors (RXRs) (Chap. 338). The activated receptor can either stimulate gene transcription (e.g., myosin heavy chain α) or inhibit transcription (e.g., TSH β-subunit gene), depending on the nature of the regulatory elements in the target gene.

Thyroid hormones (T_3 and T_4) bind with similar affinities to TRα and TRβ. However, structural differences in the ligand binding domains provide the potential for developing receptor-selective agonists or antagonists. T_3 is bound with 10–15 times greater affinity than T_4, which explains its increased hormonal potency. Though T_4 is produced in excess of T_3, receptors are occupied mainly by T_3, reflecting $T_4 \rightarrow T_3$ conversion by peripheral tissues, greater T_3 bioavailability in the plasma, and receptors' greater affinity for T_3. After binding to TRs, thyroid hormone induces conformational changes in the receptors that modify its interactions with accessory transcription factors. Importantly, in the absence of thyroid hormone binding, the aporeceptors bind to co-repressor proteins that inhibit gene transcription. Hormone binding dissociates the co-repressors and allows the recruitment of coactivators that enhance transcription. The discovery of TR interactions with corepressors explains the fact that TR silences gene expression in the absence of hormone binding. Consequently, hormone deficiency has a profound effect on gene expression because it causes gene repression as well as loss of hormone-induced stimulation. This concept has been corroborated by the finding that targeted deletion of the TR genes in mice has a less-pronounced phenotypic effect than hormone deficiency.

Thyroid hormone resistance

Resistance to thyroid hormone (RTH) is an autosomal dominant disorder characterized by elevated thyroid hormone levels and inappropriately normal or elevated TSH. Individuals with RTH do not, in general, exhibit signs and symptoms that are typical of hypothyroidism because hormone resistance is partial and is compensated by increased levels of thyroid hormone. The clinical features of RTH can include goiter, attention deficit disorder, mild reduction in IQ, delayed skeletal maturation, tachycardia, and impaired metabolic responses to thyroid hormone.

RTH is caused by mutations in the TRβ receptor gene. These mutations, located in restricted regions of the ligand-binding domain, cause loss of receptor function. However, because the mutant receptors retain the capacity to dimerize with RXRs, bind to DNA, and recruit co-repressor proteins, they function as antagonists of the remaining normal TRβ and TRα receptors. This property, referred to as "dominant negative" activity, explains the autosomal dominant mode of transmission. The diagnosis is suspected when unbound thyroid hormone levels are increased without suppression of TSH. Similar hormonal abnormalities are found in other affected family members, although the TRβ mutation arises de novo in about 20% of patients. DNA sequence analysis of the TRβ gene provides a definitive diagnosis. RTH must be distinguished from other causes of euthyroid hyperthyroxinemia (e.g., FDH) and inappropriate secretion of TSH by TSH-secreting pituitary adenomas (Chap. 339). In most patients, no treatment is indicated; the importance of making the diagnosis is to avoid inappropriate treatment of mistaken hyperthyroidism and to provide genetic counseling.

PHYSICAL EXAMINATION

In addition to the examination of the thyroid itself, the physical examination should include a search for signs of abnormal thyroid function and the extrathyroidal features of ophthalmopathy and dermopathy (see below). Examination of the neck begins by inspecting the seated patient from the front and side and noting any surgical scars, obvious masses, or distended veins. The thyroid can be palpated with both hands from behind or while facing the patient, using the thumbs to palpate each lobe. It is best to use a combination of these methods, especially when nodules are small. The patient's neck should be slightly flexed to relax the neck muscles. After locating the cricoid cartilage, the isthmus can be identified and followed laterally to locate either lobe (normally, the right lobe is slightly larger than the left). By asking the patient to swallow sips of water, thyroid consistency can be better appreciated as the gland moves beneath the examiner's fingers.

Features to be noted include thyroid size, consistency, nodularity, and any tenderness or fixation. An estimate of thyroid size (normally 12–20 g) should be made, and a drawing is often the best way to record findings. However, ultrasound is the method of choice when it is important to determine thyroid size accurately. The size, location, and consistency of any nodules should also be defined. A bruit over the gland indicates increased vascularity, as occurs in hyperthyroidism. If the lower borders of the thyroid lobes are not clearly felt, a goiter may be retrosternal. Large retrosternal goiters can cause venous distention over the neck and difficulty breathing, especially when the arms are raised (Pemberton's sign). With any central mass above the thyroid, the tongue should be extended, as thyroglossal cysts then move upward. The thyroid examination is not complete without assessment for lymphadenopathy in the supraclavicular and cervical regions of the neck.

LABORATORY EVALUATION

Measurement of thyroid hormones

The enhanced sensitivity and specificity of *TSH assays* have greatly improved laboratory assessment of thyroid function. Because TSH levels change dynamically in response to alterations of T_4 and T_3, a logical approach to thyroid testing is to first determine whether

TSH is suppressed, normal, or elevated. With rare exceptions (see below), a normal TSH level excludes a primary abnormality of thyroid function. This strategy depends on the use of immunochemiluminometric assays (ICMAs) for TSH that are sensitive enough to discriminate between the lower limit of the reference range and the suppressed values that occur with thyrotoxicosis. Extremely sensitive (fourth-generation) assays can detect TSH levels ≤0.004 mU/L, but, for practical purposes, assays sensitive to ≤0.1 mU/L are sufficient. The widespread availability of the TSH ICMA has rendered the TRH stimulation test obsolete, because the failure of TSH to rise after an intravenous bolus of 200–400 μg TRH has the same implications as a suppressed basal TSH measured by ICMA.

The finding of an abnormal TSH level must be followed by measurements of circulating thyroid hormone levels to confirm the diagnosis of hyperthyroidism (suppressed TSH) or hypothyroidism (elevated TSH). Radioimmunoassays are widely available for serum *total* T_4 and *total* T_3. T_4 and T_3 are highly protein-bound, and numerous factors (illness, medications, genetic factors) can influence protein binding. It is useful, therefore, to measure the free, or unbound, hormone levels, which correspond to the biologically available hormone pool. Two direct methods are used to measure *unbound thyroid hormones*: (1) unbound thyroid hormone competition with radiolabeled T_4 (or an analogue) for binding to a solid-phase antibody, and (2) physical separation of the unbound hormone fraction by ultracentrifugation or equilibrium dialysis. Though early unbound hormone immunoassays suffered from artifacts, newer assays correlate well with the results of the more technically demanding and expensive physical separation methods. An indirect method to estimate unbound thyroid hormone levels is to calculate the free T_3 or free T_4 index from the total T_4 or T_3 concentration and the *thyroid hormone binding ratio* (THBR). The latter is derived from the *T_3-resin uptake test*, which determines the distribution of radiolabeled T_3 between an absorbent resin and the unoccupied thyroid hormone binding proteins in the sample. The binding of the labeled T_3 to the resin is increased when there is reduced unoccupied protein binding sites (e.g., TBG deficiency) or increased total thyroid hormone in the sample; it is decreased under the opposite circumstances. The product of THBR and total T_3 or T_4 provides the *free T_3 or T_4 index*. In effect, the index corrects for anomalous total hormone values caused by abnormalities in hormone-protein binding.

Total thyroid hormone levels are *elevated* when TBG is increased due to estrogens (pregnancy, oral contraceptives, hormone therapy, tamoxifen), and *decreased* when TBG binding is reduced (androgens, nephrotic syndrome). Genetic disorders and acute illness can also cause abnormalities in thyroid hormone binding proteins, and various drugs [phenytoin, carbamazepine, salicylates, and nonsteroidal anti-inflammatory drugs (NSAIDs)] can interfere with thyroid hormone binding. Because unbound thyroid hormone levels are normal and the patient is euthyroid in all of these circumstances, assays that measure unbound hormone are preferable to those for total thyroid hormones.

For most purposes, the unbound T_4 level is sufficient to confirm thyrotoxicosis, but 2–5% of patients have only an elevated T_3 level (T_3 toxicosis). Thus, unbound T_3 levels should be measured in patients with a suppressed TSH but normal unbound T_4 levels.

There are several clinical conditions in which the use of TSH as a screening test may be misleading, particularly without simultaneous unbound T_4 determinations. Any severe nonthyroidal illness can cause abnormal TSH levels (see below). Although hypothyroidism is the most common cause of an elevated TSH level, rare causes include a TSH-secreting pituitary tumor (Chap. 339), thyroid hormone resistance, and assay artifact. Conversely, a suppressed TSH level, particularly <0.1 mU/L, usually indicates thyrotoxicosis but may also be seen during the first trimester of pregnancy (due to hCG secretion), after treatment of hyperthyroidism (because TSH can remain suppressed for several months), and in response to certain medications (e.g., high doses of glucocorticoids or dopamine). Importantly, secondary hypothyroidism, caused by hypothalamic-pituitary disease, is associated with a variable (low to high-normal) TSH level, which is inappropriate for the low T_4 level. Thus, *TSH should not be used as an isolated laboratory test to assess thyroid function in patients with suspected or known pituitary disease.*

Tests for the end-organ effects of thyroid hormone excess or depletion, such as estimation of basal metabolic rate, tendon reflex relaxation rates, or serum cholesterol, are not useful as clinical determinants of thyroid function.

Tests to determine the etiology of thyroid dysfunction

Autoimmune thyroid disease is detected most easily by measuring circulating antibodies against TPO and Tg. As antibodies to Tg alone are uncommon, it is reasonable to measure only TPO antibodies. About 5–15% of euthyroid women and up to 2% of euthyroid men have thyroid antibodies; such individuals are at increased risk of developing thyroid dysfunction. Almost all patients with autoimmune hypothyroidism, and up to 80% of those with Graves' disease, have TPO antibodies, usually at high levels.

TSI are antibodies that stimulate the TSH-R in Graves' disease. They can be measured in bioassays or indirectly in assays for TSH-binding inhibiting immunoglobulins (TBII) that detect antibody binding to the receptor. The main use of these assays is to predict neonatal thyrotoxicosis caused by high maternal levels of TSI in the last trimester of pregnancy.

Serum Tg levels are increased in all types of thyrotoxicosis except *thyrotoxicosis factitia* caused by self-administration of thyroid hormone. Tg levels are particularly increased in thyroiditis, reflecting thyroid tissue destruction and release of Tg. The main role for Tg measurement, however, is in the follow-up of thyroid cancer patients. After total thyroidectomy and radioablation, Tg levels should be undetectable; in the absence of anti-Tg antibodies, measurable levels indicate incomplete ablation or recurrent cancer.

Radioiodine uptake and thyroid scanning

The thyroid gland selectively transports radioisotopes of iodine (^{123}I, ^{125}I, ^{131}I) and ^{99m}Tc pertechnetate, allowing thyroid imaging and quantitation of radioactive tracer fractional uptake.

Nuclear imaging of Graves' disease is characterized by an enlarged gland and increased tracer uptake that is distributed homogeneously. Toxic adenomas appear as focal areas of increased uptake, with suppressed tracer uptake in the remainder of the gland. In toxic MNG, the gland is enlarged—often with distorted architecture—and there are multiple areas of relatively increased or decreased tracer uptake. Subacute thyroiditis is associated with very low uptake because of follicular cell damage and TSH suppression. Thyrotoxicosis factitia is also associated with low uptake.

Although the use of fine-needle aspiration (FNA) biopsy has diminished the use of thyroid scans in the evaluation of solitary thyroid nodules, the functional features of thyroid nodules have some prognostic significance. So-called cold nodules, which have diminished tracer uptake, are usually benign. However, these nodules are more likely to be malignant (~5–10%) than so-called hot nodules, which are almost never malignant.

Thyroid scanning is also used in the follow-up of thyroid cancer. After thyroidectomy and ablation using ^{131}I, there is diminished radioiodine uptake in the thyroid bed, allowing the detection of metastatic thyroid cancer deposits that retain the ability to transport iodine. Whole-body scans using 111–185 MBq (3–5 mCi) ^{131}I are typically performed after thyroid hormone withdrawal to raise the TSH level or after the administration of recombinant human TSH.

Thyroid ultrasound

Ultrasonography is used increasingly to assist in the diagnosis of nodular thyroid disease, a reflection of the limitations of the physical examination and improvements in ultrasound technology. Using 10-MHz instruments, spatial resolution and image quality are excellent, allowing the detection of nodules and cysts >3 mm. In addition to detecting thyroid nodules, ultrasound is useful for monitoring nodule size and for the aspiration of nodules or cystic lesions. Ultrasound-guided FNA biopsy of thyroid lesions lowers the rate of inadequate sampling. Ultrasonography is also used in the evaluation of recurrent thyroid cancer, including possible spread to cervical lymph nodes.

HYPOTHYROIDISM

Iodine deficiency remains the most common cause of hypothyroidism worldwide. In areas of iodine sufficiency, autoimmune disease (Hashimoto's thyroiditis) and iatrogenic causes (treatment of hyperthyroidism) are most common (Table 341-4).

CONGENITAL HYPOTHYROIDISM

Prevalence

Hypothyroidism occurs in about 1 in 4000 newborns. It may be transient, especially if the mother has TSH-R blocking antibodies or has received antithyroid drugs, but permanent hypothyroidism occurs in the majority. Neonatal hypothyroidism is due to thyroid gland dysgenesis in 80–85%, to inborn errors of thyroid hormone synthesis in 10–15%, and is TSH-R antibody-mediated in 5% of affected newborns. The developmental abnormalities are twice as common in girls. Mutations that cause congenital hypothyroidism are being increasingly identified, but the vast majority remain idiopathic (Table 341-1).

Clinical manifestations

The majority of infants appear normal at birth, and <10% are diagnosed based on clinical features, which include prolonged jaundice, feeding problems, hypotonia, enlarged tongue, delayed bone maturation, and umbilical hernia. Importantly, permanent neurologic damage results if treatment is delayed. Typical features of adult hypothyroidism may also be present (Table 341-5). Other congenital malformations, especially cardiac, are four times more common in congenital hypothyroidism.

Diagnosis and treatment

Because of the severe neurologic consequences of untreated congenital hypothyroidism, neonatal screening programs have been established. These are generally based on measurement of TSH or T_4 levels in heel-prick blood specimens. When the diagnosis is confirmed, T_4 is instituted at a dose of 10–15 μg/kg per day, and the dose is adjusted by close monitoring of TSH levels. T_4 requirements are relatively great during the first year of life, and a high circulating T_4 level is usually needed to normalize TSH. Early treatment with T_4 results in normal IQ levels, but subtle neurodevelopmental abnormalities may occur in those with the most severe hypothyroidism at diagnosis or when treatment is delayed or suboptimal.

AUTOIMMUNE HYPOTHYROIDISM

Classification

Autoimmune hypothyroidism may be associated with a goiter (Hashimoto's, or *goitrous thyroiditis*) or, at the later stages of the disease, minimal residual thyroid tissue (*atrophic thyroiditis*). Because the autoimmune process gradually reduces thyroid function, there is a phase of compensation when normal thyroid hormone levels are maintained by a rise in TSH. Though some patients may have minor symptoms, this state is called *subclinical hypothyroidism*. Later, unbound T_4 levels fall and TSH levels rise further; symptoms become more readily apparent at this stage (usually TSH >10 mIU/L), which is referred to as *clinical hypothyroidism* or *overt hypothyroidism*.

Prevalence

The mean annual incidence rate of autoimmune hypothyroidism is up to 4 per 1000 women and 1 per 1000 men. It is more common

TABLE 341-4 Causes of Hypothyroidism

Primary
Autoimmune hypothyroidism: Hashimoto's thyroiditis, atrophic thyroiditis
Iatrogenic: ^{131}I treatment, subtotal or total thyroidectomy, external irradiation of neck for lymphoma or cancer
Drugs: iodine excess (including iodine-containing contrast media and amiodarone), lithium, antithyroid drugs, *p*-aminosalicylic acid, interferon-α and other cytokines, aminoglutethimide, sunitinib
Congenital hypothyroidism: absent or ectopic thyroid gland, dyshormonogenesis, TSH-R mutation
Iodine deficiency
Infiltrative disorders: amyloidosis, sarcoidosis, hemochromatosis, scleroderma, cystinosis, Riedel's thyroiditis
Overexpression of type 3 deoiodinase in infantile hemangioma
Transient
Silent thyroiditis, including postpartum thyroiditis
Subacute thyroiditis
Withdrawal of thyroxine treatment in individuals with an intact thyroid
After ^{131}I treatment or subtotal thyroidectomy for Graves' disease
Secondary
Hypopituitarism: tumors, pituitary surgery or irradiation, infiltrative disorders, Sheehan's syndrome, trauma, genetic forms of combined pituitary hormone deficiencies
Isolated TSH deficiency or inactivity
Bexarotene treatment
Hypothalamic disease: tumors, trauma, infiltrative disorders, idiopathic

Abbreviations: TSH, thyroid-stimulating hormone; TSH-R, TSH receptor.

TABLE 341-5 Signs and Symptoms of Hypothyroidism (Descending Order of Frequency)

Symptoms	Signs
Tiredness, weakness	Dry coarse skin; cool peripheral extremities
Dry skin	Puffy face, hands, and feet (myxedema)
Feeling cold	Diffuse alopecia
Hair loss	Bradycardia
Difficulty concentrating and poor memory	Peripheral edema
Constipation	Delayed tendon reflex relaxation
Weight gain with poor appetite	Carpal tunnel syndrome
Dyspnea	Serous cavity effusions
Hoarse voice	
Menorrhagia (later oligomenorrhea or amenorrhea)	
Paresthesia	
Impaired hearing	

in certain populations, such as the Japanese, probably because of genetic factors and chronic exposure to a high-iodine diet. The mean age at diagnosis is 60 years, and the prevalence of overt hypothyroidism increases with age. Subclinical hypothyroidism is found in 6–8% of women (10% over the age of 60) and 3% of men. The annual risk of developing clinical hypothyroidism is about 4% when subclinical hypothyroidism is associated with positive TPO antibodies.

Pathogenesis

In Hashimoto's thyroiditis, there is a marked lymphocytic infiltration of the thyroid with germinal center formation, atrophy of the thyroid follicles accompanied by oxyphil metaplasia, absence of colloid, and mild to moderate fibrosis. In atrophic thyroiditis, the fibrosis is much more extensive, lymphocyte infiltration is less pronounced, and thyroid follicles are almost completely absent. Atrophic thyroiditis likely represents the end stage of Hashimoto's thyroiditis rather than a distinct disorder.

As with most autoimmune disorders, susceptibility to autoimmune hypothyroidism is determined by a combination of genetic and environmental factors, and the risk of either autoimmune hypothyroidism or Graves' disease is increased among siblings. HLA-DR polymorphisms are the best documented genetic risk factors for autoimmune hypothyroidism, especially HLA-DR3, -DR4, and -DR5 in Caucasians. A weak association also exists between polymorphisms in *CTLA-4*, a T cell–regulatory gene, and autoimmune hypothyroidism. Both of these genetic associations are shared by other autoimmune diseases, which may explain the relationship between autoimmune hypothyroidism and other autoimmune diseases, especially type 1 diabetes mellitus, Addison's disease, pernicious anemia, and vitiligo (Chap. 351). HLA-DR and *CTLA-4* polymorphisms account for approximately half of the genetic susceptibility to autoimmune hypothyroidism. Other contributory loci remain to be identified. A gene on chromosome 21 may be responsible for the association between autoimmune hypothyroidism and Down syndrome. The female preponderance of thyroid autoimmunity is most likely due to sex steroid effects on the immune response, but an X chromosome–related genetic factor is also possible and may account for the high frequency of autoimmune hypothyroidism in Turner's syndrome. Environmental susceptibility factors are poorly defined at present. A high iodine intake may increase the risk of autoimmune hypothyroidism by immunologic effects or direct thyroid toxicity. There is no convincing evidence for a role of infection except for the congenital rubella syndrome, in which there is a high frequency of autoimmune hypothyroidism. Viral thyroiditis does not induce subsequent autoimmune thyroid disease.

The thyroid lymphocytic infiltrate in autoimmune hypothyroidism is composed of activated CD4+ and CD8+ T cells as well as B cells. Thyroid cell destruction is primarily mediated by the CD8+ cytotoxic T cells, which destroy their targets by either perforin-induced cell necrosis or granzyme B–induced apoptosis. In addition, local T cell production of cytokines, such as tumor necrosis factor (TNF), IL-1, and interferon γ (IFN-γ), may render thyroid cells more susceptible to apoptosis mediated by death receptors, such as Fas, which are activated by their respective ligands on T cells. These cytokines also impair thyroid cell function directly and induce the expression of other proinflammatory molecules by the thyroid cells themselves, such as cytokines, HLA class I and class II molecules, adhesion molecules, CD40, and nitric oxide. Administration of high concentrations of cytokines for therapeutic purposes (especially IFN-α) is associated with increased autoimmune thyroid disease, possibly through mechanisms similar to those in sporadic disease.

Antibodies to TPO and Tg are clinically useful markers of thyroid autoimmunity, but any pathogenic effect is restricted to a secondary role in amplifying an ongoing autoimmune response. TPO antibodies fix complement, and complement membrane-attack complexes are present in the thyroid in autoimmune hypothyroidism. However, transplacental passage of Tg or TPO antibodies has no effect on the fetal thyroid, which suggests that T cell–mediated injury is required to initiate autoimmune damage to the thyroid.

Up to 20% of patients with autoimmune hypothyroidism have antibodies against the TSH-R, which, in contrast to TSI, do not stimulate the receptor but prevent the binding of TSH. These TSH-R-blocking antibodies, therefore, cause hypothyroidism and, especially in Asian patients, thyroid atrophy. Their transplacental passage may induce transient neonatal hypothyroidism. Rarely, patients have a mixture of TSI and TSH-R-blocking antibodies, and thyroid function can oscillate between hyperthyroidism and hypothyroidism as one or the other antibody becomes dominant. Predicting the course of disease in such individuals is difficult, and they require close monitoring of thyroid function. Bioassays can be used to document that TSH-R-blocking antibodies reduce the cyclic AMP–inducing effect of TSH on cultured TSH-R-expressing cells, but these assays are difficult to perform. TBII assays that measure the binding of antibodies to the receptor by competition with radiolabeled TSH do not distinguish between TSI- and TSH-R-blocking antibodies, but a positive result in a patient with spontaneous hypothyroidism is strong evidence for the presence of blocking antibodies. The use of these assays does not generally alter clinical management, although it may be useful to confirm the cause of transient neonatal hypothyroidism.

Clinical manifestations

The main clinical features of hypothyroidism are summarized in Table 341-5. The onset is usually insidious, and the patient may become aware of symptoms only when euthyroidism is restored. Patients with Hashimoto's thyroiditis may present because of goiter rather than symptoms of hypothyroidism. The goiter may not be large, but it is usually irregular and firm in consistency. It is often possible to palpate a pyramidal lobe, normally a vestigial remnant of the thyroglossal duct. Rarely is uncomplicated Hashimoto's thyroiditis associated with pain.

Patients with atrophic thyroiditis or the late stage of Hashimoto's thyroiditis present with symptoms and signs of hypothyroidism. The skin is dry, and there is decreased sweating, thinning of the epidermis, and hyperkeratosis of the stratum corneum. Increased dermal glycosaminoglycan content traps water, giving rise to skin thickening without pitting (*myxedema*). Typical features include a

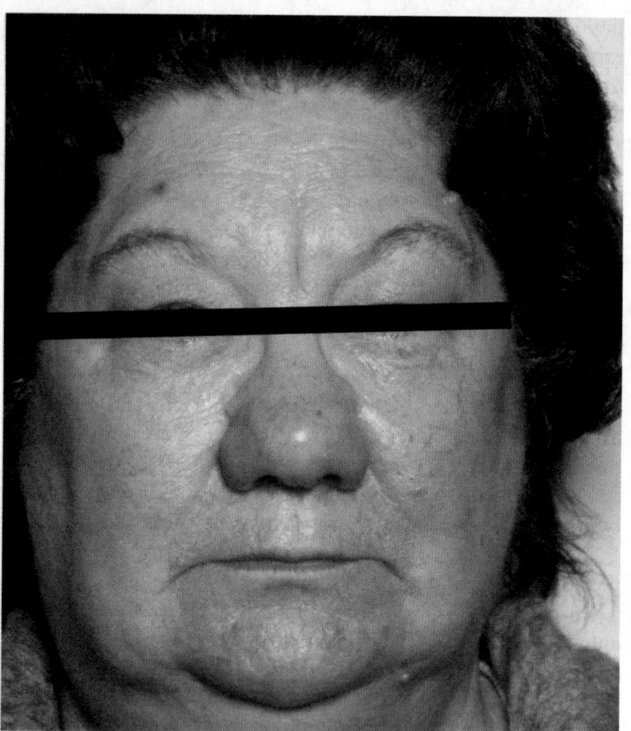

Figure 341-5 Facial appearance in hypothyroidism. Note puffy eyes and thickened skin.

puffy face with edematous eyelids and nonpitting pretibial edema (Fig. 341-5). There is pallor, often with a yellow tinge to the skin due to carotene accumulation. Nail growth is retarded, and hair is dry, brittle, difficult to manage, and falls out easily. In addition to diffuse alopecia, there is thinning of the outer third of the eyebrows, although this is not a specific sign of hypothyroidism.

Other common features include constipation and weight gain (despite a poor appetite). In contrast to popular perception, the weight gain is usually modest and due mainly to fluid retention in the myxedematous tissues. Libido is decreased in both sexes, and there may be oligomenorrhea or amenorrhea in long-standing disease, but menorrhagia is also common. Fertility is reduced, and the incidence of miscarriage is increased. Prolactin levels are often modestly increased (Chap. 339) and may contribute to alterations in libido and fertility and cause galactorrhea.

Myocardial contractility and pulse rate are reduced, leading to a reduced stroke volume and bradycardia. Increased peripheral resistance may be accompanied by hypertension, particularly diastolic. Blood flow is diverted from the skin, producing cool extremities. Pericardial effusions occur in up to 30% of patients but rarely compromise cardiac function. Though alterations in myosin heavy chain isoform expression have been documented, cardiomyopathy is unusual. Fluid may also accumulate in other serous cavities and in the middle ear, giving rise to conductive deafness. Pulmonary function is generally normal, but dyspnea may be caused by pleural effusion, impaired respiratory muscle function, diminished ventilatory drive, or sleep apnea.

Carpal tunnel and other entrapment syndromes are common, as is impairment of muscle function with stiffness, cramps, and pain. On examination, there may be slow relaxation of tendon reflexes and pseudomyotonia. Memory and concentration are impaired. Experimentally, PET scans examining glucose metabolism in hypothyroid subjects show lower regional activity in the amygdala, hippocampus, and perigenual anterior cingulated cortex, among other regions, and this activity corrects after thyroxine replacement. Rare neurologic problems include reversible cerebellar ataxia, dementia, psychosis, and myxedema coma. *Hashimoto's encephalopathy* has been defined as a steroid-responsive syndrome associated with TPO antibodies, myoclonus, and slow-wave activity on electroencephalography, but the relationship with thyroid autoimmunity or hypothyroidism is not established. The hoarse voice and occasionally clumsy speech of hypothyroidism reflect fluid accumulation in the vocal cords and tongue.

The features described above are the consequence of thyroid hormone deficiency. However, autoimmune hypothyroidism may be associated with signs or symptoms of other autoimmune diseases, particularly vitiligo, pernicious anemia, Addison's disease, alopecia areata, and type 1 diabetes mellitus. Less-common associations include celiac disease, dermatitis herpetiformis, chronic active hepatitis, rheumatoid arthritis, systemic lupus erythematosus (SLE), myasthenia gravis, and Sjögren's syndrome. Thyroid-associated ophthalmopathy, which usually occurs in Graves' disease (see below), occurs in about 5% of patients with autoimmune hypothyroidism.

Autoimmune hypothyroidism is uncommon in children and usually presents with slow growth and delayed facial maturation. The appearance of permanent teeth is also delayed. Myopathy, with muscle swelling, is more common in children than in adults. In most cases, puberty is delayed, but precocious puberty sometimes occurs. There may be intellectual impairment if the onset is before 3 years and the hormone deficiency is severe.

Laboratory evaluation

A summary of the investigations used to determine the existence and cause of hypothyroidism is provided in Fig. 341-6. A normal

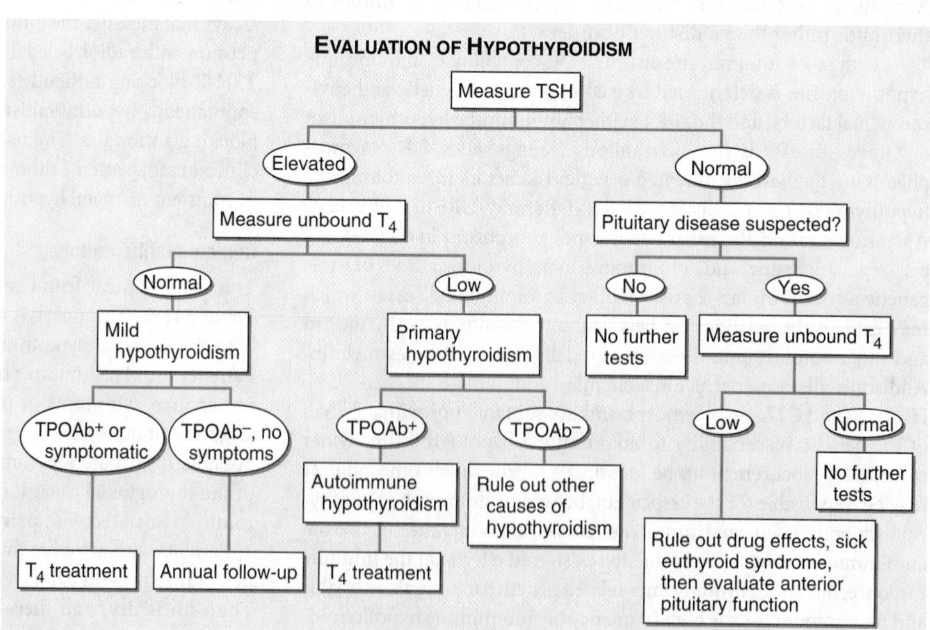

Figure 341-6 Evaluation of hypothyroidism. TPOAb+, thyroid peroxidase antibodies present; TPOAb−, thyroid peroxidase antibodies not present; TSH, thyroid-stimulating hormone.

TSH level excludes primary (but not secondary) hypothyroidism. If the TSH is elevated, an unbound T_4 level is needed to confirm the presence of clinical hypothyroidism, but T_4 is inferior to TSH when used as a screening test, because it will not detect subclinical hypothyroidism. Circulating unbound T_3 levels are normal in about 25% of patients, reflecting adaptive deiodinase responses to hypothyroidism. T_3 measurements are, therefore, not indicated.

Once clinical or subclinical hypothyroidism is confirmed, the etiology is usually easily established by demonstrating the presence of TPO antibodies, which are present in >90% of patients with autoimmune hypothyroidism. TBII can be found in 10–20% of patients, but these determinations are not needed routinely. If there is any doubt about the cause of a goiter associated with hypothyroidism, FNA biopsy can be used to confirm the presence of autoimmune thyroiditis. Other abnormal laboratory findings in hypothyroidism may include increased creatine phosphokinase, elevated cholesterol and triglycerides, and anemia (usually normocytic or macrocytic). Except when accompanied by iron deficiency, the anemia and other abnormalities gradually resolve with thyroxine replacement.

Differential diagnosis

An asymmetric goiter in Hashimoto's thyroiditis may be confused with a multinodular goiter or thyroid carcinoma, in which thyroid antibodies may also be present. Ultrasound can be used to show the presence of a solitary lesion or a multinodular goiter rather than the heterogeneous thyroid enlargement typical of Hashimoto's thyroiditis. FNA biopsy is useful in the investigation of focal nodules. Other causes of hypothyroidism are discussed below and in Table 341-4, but rarely cause diagnostic confusion.

■ OTHER CAUSES OF HYPOTHYROIDISM

Iatrogenic hypothyroidism is a common cause of hypothyroidism and can often be detected by screening before symptoms develop. In the first 3–4 months after radioiodine treatment, transient hypothyroidism may occur due to reversible radiation damage. Low-dose thyroxine treatment can be withdrawn if recovery occurs. Because TSH levels are suppressed by hyperthyroidism, unbound T_4 levels are a better measure of thyroid function than TSH in the months following radioiodine treatment. Mild hypothyroidism after subtotal thyroidectomy may also resolve after several months, as the gland remnant is stimulated by increased TSH levels.

Iodine deficiency is responsible for endemic goiter and cretinism but is an uncommon cause of adult hypothyroidism unless the iodine intake is very low or there are complicating factors, such as the consumption of thiocyanates in cassava or selenium deficiency. Though hypothyroidism due to iodine deficiency can be treated with thyroxine, public health measures to improve iodine intake should be advocated to eliminate this problem. Iodized salt or bread or a single bolus of oral or intramuscular iodized oil have all been used successfully.

Paradoxically, chronic iodine excess can also induce goiter and hypothyroidism. The intracellular events that account for this effect are unclear, but individuals with autoimmune thyroiditis are especially susceptible. Iodine excess is responsible for the hypothyroidism that occurs in up to 13% of patients treated with amiodarone (see below). Other drugs, particularly lithium, may also cause hypothyroidism. Transient hypothyroidism caused by thyroiditis is discussed below.

Secondary hypothyroidism is usually diagnosed in the context of other anterior pituitary hormone deficiencies; isolated TSH deficiency is very rare (Chap. 339). TSH levels may be low, normal, or even slightly increased in secondary hypothyroidism; the latter is due to secretion of immunoactive but bioinactive forms of TSH. The diagnosis is confirmed by detecting a low unbound T_4 level. The goal of treatment is to maintain T_4 levels in the upper half of the reference range, because TSH levels cannot be used to monitor therapy.

TREATMENT Hypothyroidism

CLINICAL HYPOTHYROIDISM If there is no residual thyroid function, the daily replacement dose of levothyroxine is usually 1.6 μg/kg body weight (typically 100–150 μg). In many patients, however, lower doses suffice until residual thyroid tissue is destroyed. In patients who develop hypothyroidism after the treatment of Graves' disease, there is often underlying autonomous function, necessitating lower replacement doses (typically 75–125 μg/d).

Adult patients under 60 without evidence of heart disease may be started on 50–100 μg levothyroxine (T_4) daily. The dose is adjusted on the basis of TSH levels, with the goal of treatment being a normal TSH, ideally in the lower half of the reference range. TSH responses are gradual and should be measured about two months after instituting treatment or after any subsequent change in levothyroxine dosage. The clinical effects of levothyroxine replacement are slow to appear. Patients may not experience full relief from symptoms until 3–6 months after normal TSH levels are restored. Adjustment of levothyroxine dosage is made in 12.5- or 25-μg increments if the TSH is high; decrements of the same magnitude should be made if the TSH is suppressed. Patients with a suppressed TSH of any cause, including T_4 overtreatment, have an increased risk of atrial fibrillation and reduced bone density.

Although dessicated animal thyroid preparations (thyroid extract USP) are available, they are not recommended because the ratio of T_3 to T_4 is nonphysiologic. The use of levothyroxine combined with liothyronine (triiodothyronine, T_3) has been investigated, but benefit has not been confirmed in prospective studies. There is no place for liothyronine alone as long-term replacement, because the short half-life necessitates three or four daily doses and is associated with fluctuating T_3 levels.

Once full replacement is achieved and TSH levels are stable, follow-up measurement of TSH is recommended at annual intervals and may be extended to every 2–3 years if a normal TSH is maintained over several years. It is important to ensure ongoing adherence, however, as patients do not feel any symptomatic difference after missing a few doses of levothyroxine, and this sometimes leads to self-discontinuation.

In patients of normal body weight who are taking ≥200 μg of levothyroxine per day, an elevated TSH level is often a sign of poor adherence to treatment. This is also the likely explanation for fluctuating TSH levels, despite a constant levothyroxine dosage. Such patients often have normal or high unbound T_4 levels, despite an elevated TSH, because they remember to take medication for a few days before testing; this is sufficient to normalize T_4, but not TSH levels. It is important to consider variable adherence, because this pattern of thyroid function tests is otherwise suggestive of disorders associated with inappropriate TSH secretion (Table 341-3). Because T_4 has a long half-life (7 days), patients who miss a dose can be advised to take two doses of the skipped tablets at once. Other causes of increased levothyroxine requirements must be excluded, particularly malabsorption (e.g., celiac disease, small-bowel surgery), estrogen therapy, and drugs that interfere with T_4 absorption or clearance such as cholestyramine, ferrous sulfate, calcium supplements, lovastatin, aluminum hydroxide, rifampicin, amiodarone, carbamazepine, and phenytoin.

SUBCLINICAL HYPOTHYROIDISM By definition, subclinical hypothyroidism refers to biochemical evidence of thyroid hormone deficiency in patients who have few or no apparent clinical features of hypothyroidism. There are no universally accepted recommendations for the management of subclinical hypothyroidism, but the most recently published guidelines do not recommend routine treatment when TSH levels are below 10 mU/L. It is important to confirm that any elevation of TSH is sustained over a 3-month period before treatment is given. As long as excessive treatment is avoided, there is no risk in correcting a slightly increased TSH. Moreover, there is a risk that patients will progress to overt hypothyroidism, particularly when the TSH level is elevated and TPO antibodies are present. Treatment is administered by starting with a low dose of levothyroxine (25–50 μg/d) with the goal of normalizing TSH. If thyroxine is not given, thyroid function should be evaluated annually.

SPECIAL TREATMENT CONSIDERATIONS Rarely, levothyroxine replacement is associated with pseudotumor cerebri in children. Presentation appears to be idiosyncratic and occurs months after treatment has begun. Women with a history or high risk of hypothyroidism should ensure that they are euthyroid prior to conception and during early pregnancy as maternal hypothyroidism may adversely affect fetal neural development and cause preterm delivery. The presence of thyroid autoantibodies alone, in a euthyroid patient, is also associated with preterm delivery, and outcome may be improved by levothyroxine treatment. Thyroid function should be evaluated immediately after pregnancy is confirmed and at the beginning of the second and third trimesters. The dose of levothyroxine may need to be increased by ≥50% during pregnancy and returned to previous levels after delivery. Elderly patients may require 20% less thyroxine than younger patients. In the elderly, especially patients with known coronary artery disease, the starting dose of levothyroxine is 12.5–25 μg/d with similar increments every 2–3 months until TSH is normalized. In some patients, it may be impossible to achieve full replacement despite optimal antianginal treatment. *Emergency surgery* is generally safe in patients with untreated hypothyroidism, although routine surgery in a hypothyroid patient should be deferred until euthyroidism is achieved.

Myxedema coma still has a high mortality rate, despite intensive treatment. Clinical manifestations include reduced level of consciousness, sometimes associated with seizures, as well as the other features of hypothyroidism (Table 341-5). Hypothermia can reach 23°C (74°F). There may be a history of treated hypothyroidism with poor compliance, or the patient may be previously undiagnosed. Myxedema coma almost always occurs in the elderly and is usually precipitated by factors that impair respiration, such as drugs (especially sedatives, anesthetics, antidepressants), pneumonia, congestive heart failure, myocardial infarction, gastrointestinal bleeding, or cerebrovascular accidents. Sepsis should also be suspected. Exposure to cold may also be a risk factor. Hypoventilation, leading to hypoxia and hypercapnia, plays a major role in pathogenesis; hypoglycemia and dilutional hyponatremia also contribute to the development of myxedema coma.

Levothyroxine can initially be administered as a single IV bolus of 500 μg, which serves as a loading dose. Although further levothyroxine is not strictly necessary for several days, it is usually continued at a dose of 50–100 μg/d. If suitable IV preparation is not available, the same initial dose of levothyroxine can be given by nasogastric tube (though absorption may be impaired in myxedema). An alternative is to give liothyronine (T_3) intravenously or via nasogastric tube, in doses ranging from 10 to 25 μg every 8–12 h. This treatment has been advocated because $T_4 \rightarrow T_3$ conversion is impaired in myxedema coma. However, excess liothyronine has the potential to provoke arrhythmias. Another option is to combine levothyroxine (200 μg) and liothyronine (25 μg) as a single, initial IV bolus followed by daily treatment with levothyroxine (50–100 μg/d) and liothyronine (10 μg every 8 h).

Supportive therapy should be provided to correct any associated metabolic disturbances. External warming is indicated only if the temperature is <30°C, as it can result in cardiovascular collapse (Chap. 19). Space blankets should be used to prevent further heat loss. Parenteral hydrocortisone (50 mg every 6 h) should be administered, because there is impaired adrenal reserve in profound hypothyroidism. Any precipitating factors should be treated, including the early use of broad-spectrum antibiotics, pending the exclusion of infection. Ventilatory support with regular blood gas analysis is usually needed during the first 48 hours. Hypertonic saline or IV glucose may be needed if there is severe hyponatremia or hypoglycemia; hypotonic IV fluids should be avoided because they may exacerbate water retention secondary to reduced renal perfusion and inappropriate vasopressin secretion. The metabolism of most medications is impaired, and sedatives should be avoided if possible or used in reduced doses. Medication blood levels should be monitored, when available, to guide dosage.

THYROTOXICOSIS

Thyrotoxicosis is defined as the state of thyroid hormone excess and is not synonymous with *hyperthyroidism*, which is the result of excessive thyroid function. However, the major etiologies of thyrotoxicosis are hyperthyroidism caused by Graves' disease, toxic MNG, and toxic adenomas. Other causes are listed in Table 341-6.

■ GRAVES' DISEASE

Epidemiology

Graves' disease accounts for 60–80% of thyrotoxicosis. The prevalence varies among populations, reflecting genetic factors and iodine

TABLE 341-6 Causes of Thyrotoxicosis

Primary hyperthyroidism
Graves' disease
Toxic multinodular goiter
Toxic adenoma
Functioning thyroid carcinoma metastases
Activating mutation of the TSH receptor
Activating mutation of $G_s\alpha$ (McCune-Albright syndrome)
Struma ovarii
Drugs: iodine excess (Jod-Basedow phenomenon)
Thyrotoxicosis without hyperthyroidism
Subacute thyroiditis
Silent thyroiditis
Other causes of thyroid destruction: amiodarone, radiation, infarction of adenoma
Ingestion of excess thyroid hormone (thyrotoxicosis factitia) or thyroid tissue
Secondary hyperthyroidism
TSH-secreting pituitary adenoma
Thyroid hormone resistance syndrome: occasional patients may have features of thyrotoxicosis
Chorionic gonadotropin-secreting tumors[a]
Gestational thyrotoxicosis[a]

[a]Circulating TSH levels are low in these forms of secondary hyperthyroidism.

Abbreviations: TSH, thyroid-stimulating hormone.

intake (high iodine intake is associated with an increased prevalence of Graves' disease). Graves' disease occurs in up to 2% of women but is one-tenth as frequent in men. The disorder rarely begins before adolescence and typically occurs between 20 and 50 years of age; it also occurs in the elderly.

Pathogenesis

As in autoimmune hypothyroidism, a combination of environmental and genetic factors, including polymorphisms in HLA-DR, *CTLA-4*, *CD25*, *PTPN22* (a T cell regulatory gene) and *TSH-R*, contribute to Graves' disease susceptibility. The concordance for Graves' disease in monozygotic twins is 20–30%, compared to <5% in dizygotic twins. Indirect evidence suggests that stress is an important environmental factor, presumably operating through neuroendocrine effects on the immune system. Smoking is a minor risk factor for Graves' disease and a major risk factor for the development of ophthalmopathy. Sudden increases in iodine intake may precipitate Graves' disease, and there is a threefold increase in the occurrence of Graves' disease in the postpartum period. Graves' disease may occur during the immune reconstitution phase after highly active antiretroviral therapy (HAART) or alemtuzumab treatment.

The hyperthyroidism of Graves' disease is caused by TSI that are synthesized in the thyroid gland as well as in bone marrow and lymph nodes. Such antibodies can be detected by bioassays or by using the more widely available TBII assays. The presence of TBII in a patient with thyrotoxicosis implies the existence of TSI, and these assays are useful in monitoring pregnant Graves' patients in whom high levels of TSI can cross the placenta and cause neonatal thyrotoxicosis. Other thyroid autoimmune responses, similar to those in autoimmune hypothyroidism (see above), occur concurrently in patients with Graves' disease. In particular, TPO antibodies occur in up to 80% of cases and serve as a readily measurable marker of autoimmunity. Because the coexisting thyroiditis can also affect thyroid function, there is no direct correlation between the level of TSI and thyroid hormone levels in Graves' disease. In the long term, spontaneous autoimmune hypothyroidism may develop in up to 15% of patients with Graves' disease.

Cytokines appear to play a major role in thyroid-associated ophthalmopathy. There is infiltration of the extraocular muscles by activated T cells; the release of cytokines such as IFN-γ, TNF, and IL-1 results in fibroblast activation and increased synthesis of glycosaminoglycans that trap water, thereby leading to characteristic muscle swelling. Late in the disease, there is irreversible fibrosis of the muscles. Orbital fibroblasts may be particularly sensitive to cytokines, perhaps explaining the anatomic localization of the immune response. Though the pathogenesis of thyroid-associated ophthalmopathy remains unclear, there is mounting evidence that the TSH-R may be a shared autoantigen that is expressed in the orbit; this would explain the close association with autoimmune thyroid disease. Increased fat is an additional cause of retrobulbar tissue expansion. The increase in intraorbital pressure can lead to proptosis, diplopia, and optic neuropathy

Clinical manifestations

Signs and symptoms include features that are common to any cause of thyrotoxicosis (Table 341-7) as well as those specific for Graves' disease. The clinical presentation depends on the severity of thyrotoxicosis, the duration of disease, individual susceptibility to excess thyroid hormone, and the patient's age. In the elderly, features of thyrotoxicosis may be subtle or masked, and patients may present mainly with fatigue and weight loss, a condition known as *apathetic thyrotoxicosis*.

Thyrotoxicosis may cause unexplained weight loss, despite an enhanced appetite, due to the increased metabolic rate. Weight gain occurs in 5% of patients, however, because of increased food intake. Other prominent features include hyperactivity, nervousness, and irritability, ultimately leading to a sense of easy fatigability in some patients. Insomnia and impaired concentration are common; apathetic thyrotoxicosis may be mistaken for depression in the elderly. Fine tremor is a frequent finding, best elicited by having patients stretch out their fingers while feeling the fingertips with the palm. Common neurologic manifestations include hyperreflexia, muscle wasting, and proximal myopathy without fasciculation. Chorea is rare. Thyrotoxicosis is sometimes associated with a form of hypokalemic periodic paralysis; this disorder is particularly common in Asian males with thyrotoxicosis, but it occurs in other ethnic groups as well.

TABLE 341-7 Signs and Symptoms of Thyrotoxicosis (Descending Order of Frequency)

Symptoms	Signs[a]
Hyperactivity, irritability, dysphoria	Tachycardia; atrial fibrillation in the elderly
Heat intolerance and sweating	Tremor
Palpitations	Goiter
Fatigue and weakness	Warm, moist skin
Weight loss with increased appetite	Muscle weakness, proximal myopathy
Diarrhea	Lid retraction or lag
Polyuria	Gynecomastia
Oligomenorrhea, loss of libido	

[a]Excludes the signs of ophthalmopathy and dermopathy specific for Graves' disease.

The most common cardiovascular manifestation is sinus tachycardia, often associated with palpitations, occasionally caused by supraventricular tachycardia. The high cardiac output produces a bounding pulse, widened pulse pressure, and an aortic systolic murmur and can lead to worsening of angina or heart failure in the elderly or those with preexisting heart disease. Atrial fibrillation is more common in patients >50 years of age. Treatment of the thyrotoxic state alone converts atrial fibrillation to normal sinus rhythm in about half of patients, suggesting the existence of an underlying cardiac problem in the remainder.

The skin is usually warm and moist, and the patient may complain of sweating and heat intolerance, particularly during warm weather. Palmar erythema, onycholysis, and, less commonly, pruritus, urticaria, and diffuse hyperpigmentation may be evident. Hair texture may become fine, and a diffuse alopecia occurs in up to 40% of patients, persisting for months after restoration of euthyroidism. Gastrointestinal transit time is decreased, leading to increased stool frequency, often with diarrhea and occasionally mild steatorrhea. Women frequently experience oligomenorrhea or amenorrhea; in men, there may be impaired sexual function and, rarely, gynecomastia. The direct effect of thyroid hormones on bone resorption leads to osteopenia in long-standing thyrotoxicosis; mild hypercalcemia occurs in up to 20% of patients, but hypercalciuria is more common. There is a small increase in fracture rate in patients with a previous history of thyrotoxicosis.

In Graves' disease, the thyroid is usually diffusely enlarged to two to three times its normal size. The consistency is firm, but less so than in MNG. There may be a thrill or bruit due to the increased vascularity of the gland and the hyperdynamic circulation.

Lid retraction, causing a staring appearance, can occur in any form of thyrotoxicosis and is the result of sympathetic overactivity. However, Graves' disease is associated with specific eye signs that comprise *Graves' ophthalmopathy* (Fig. 341-7A). This condition is also called *thyroid-associated ophthalmopathy*, as it occurs in the absence of Graves' disease in 10% of patients. Most of these

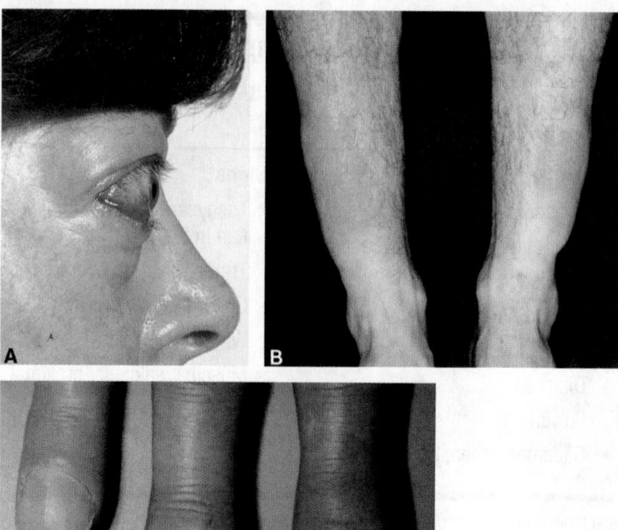

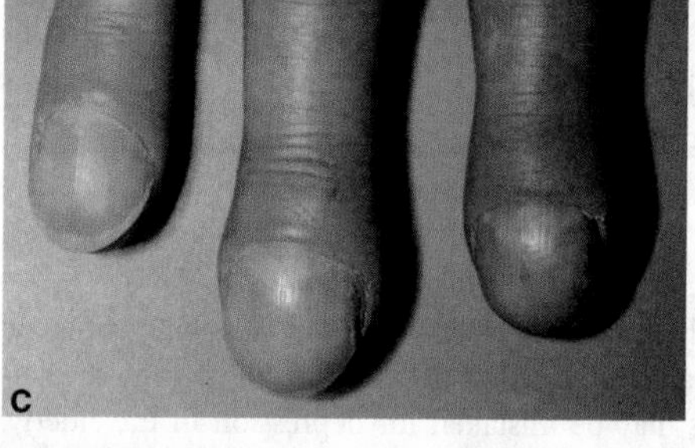

Figure 341-7 Features of Graves' disease. ***A.*** Ophthalmopathy in Graves' disease; lid retraction, periorbital edema, conjunctival injection, and proptosis are marked. ***B.*** Thyroid dermopathy over the lateral aspects of the shins. ***C.*** Thyroid acropachy.

individuals have autoimmune hypothyroidism or thyroid antibodies. The onset of Graves' ophthalmopathy occurs within the year before or after the diagnosis of thyrotoxicosis in 75% of patients but can sometimes precede or follow thyrotoxicosis by several years, accounting for some cases of euthyroid ophthalmopathy.

Some patients with Graves' disease have little clinical evidence of ophthalmopathy. However, the enlarged extraocular muscles typical of the disease, and other subtle features, can be detected in almost all patients when investigated by ultrasound or CT imaging of the orbits. Unilateral signs are found in up to 10% of patients. The earliest manifestations of ophthalmopathy are usually a sensation of grittiness, eye discomfort, and excess tearing. About one-third of patients have proptosis, best detected by visualization of the sclera between the lower border of the iris and the lower eyelid, with the eyes in the primary position. Proptosis can be measured using an exophthalmometer. In severe cases, proptosis may cause corneal exposure and damage, especially if the lids fail to close during sleep. Periorbital edema, scleral injection, and chemosis are also frequent. In 5–10% of patients, the muscle swelling is so severe that diplopia results, typically, but not exclusively, when the patient looks up and laterally. The most serious manifestation is compression of the optic nerve at the apex of the orbit, leading to papilledema; peripheral field defects; and, if left untreated, permanent loss of vision.

Many scoring systems have been used to gauge the extent and activity of the orbital changes in Graves' disease. The "NO SPECS" scheme is an acronym derived from the following eye changes:

0 = **N**o signs or symptoms
1 = **O**nly signs (lid retraction or lag), no symptoms
2 = **S**oft-tissue involvement (periorbital edema)
3 = **P**roptosis (>22 mm)
4 = **E**xtraocular-muscle involvement (diplopia)
5 = **C**orneal involvement
6 = **S**ight loss

Although useful as a mnemonic, the NO SPECS scheme is inadequate to describe the eye disease fully, and patients do not necessarily progress from one class to another. When Graves' eye disease is active and severe, referral to an ophthalmologist is indicated and objective measurements are needed, such as lid-fissure width; corneal staining with fluorescein; and evaluation of extraocular muscle function (e.g., Hess chart), intraocular pressure and visual fields, acuity, and color vision.

Thyroid dermopathy occurs in <5% of patients with Graves' disease (Fig. 341-7*B*), almost always in the presence of moderate or severe ophthalmopathy. Although most frequent over the anterior and lateral aspects of the lower leg (hence the term *pretibial myxedema*), skin changes can occur at other sites, particularly after trauma. The typical lesion is a noninflamed, indurated plaque with a deep pink or purple color and an "orange skin" appearance. Nodular involvement can occur, and the condition can rarely extend over the whole lower leg and foot, mimicking elephantiasis. *Thyroid acropachy* refers to a form of clubbing found in <1% of patients with Graves' disease (Fig. 341-7*C*). It is so strongly associated with thyroid dermopathy that an alternative cause of clubbing should be sought in a Graves' patient without coincident skin and orbital involvement.

Laboratory evaluation

Investigations used to determine the existence and cause of thyrotoxicosis are summarized in Fig. 341-8. In Graves' disease, the TSH level is suppressed and total and unbound thyroid hormone levels are increased. In 2–5% of patients (and more in areas of borderline iodine intake), only T_3 is increased (T_3 toxicosis). The converse state of T_4 toxicosis, with elevated total and unbound T_4 and normal T_3 levels, is occasionally seen when hyperthyroidism is induced by excess iodine, providing surplus substrate for thyroid hormone synthesis. Measurement of TPO antibodies or TBII may be useful if the diagnosis is unclear clinically but is not needed routinely. Associated abnormalities that may cause diagnostic confusion in thyrotoxicosis include elevation of bilirubin, liver enzymes, and ferritin. Microcytic anemia and thrombocytopenia may occur.

Differential diagnosis

Diagnosis of Graves' disease is straightforward in a patient with biochemically confirmed thyrotoxicosis, diffuse goiter on palpation, ophthalmopathy, and often a personal or family history of autoimmune disorders. For patients with thyrotoxicosis who lack these features, the most reliable diagnostic method is to measure TBII or TSI. An alternative is to undertake a radionuclide (^{99m}Tc, ^{123}I, or ^{131}I) scan of the thyroid, which will distinguish the diffuse, high uptake of Graves' disease from nodular thyroid disease, destructive thyroiditis, ectopic thyroid tissue, and factitious thyrotoxicosis. In secondary hyperthyroidism due to a TSH-secreting pituitary tumor, there is also a diffuse goiter. The presence of a nonsuppressed TSH level and the finding of a pituitary tumor on CT or MRI scan readily identify such patients.

Clinical features of thyrotoxicosis can mimic certain aspects of other disorders, including panic attacks, mania, pheochromocytoma, and weight loss associated with malignancy. The diagnosis of thyrotoxicosis can be easily excluded if the TSH and unbound T_4 and T_3 levels are normal. A normal TSH also excludes Graves' disease as a cause of diffuse goiter.

Clinical course

Clinical features generally worsen without treatment; mortality was 10–30% before the introduction of satisfactory therapy. Some patients with mild Graves' disease experience spontaneous relapses and remissions. Rarely, there may be fluctuation between hypo- and hyperthyroidism due to changes in the functional activity of TSH-R antibodies. About 15% of patients who enter remission after treatment develop hypothyroidism 10–15 years later as a result of the destructive autoimmune process.

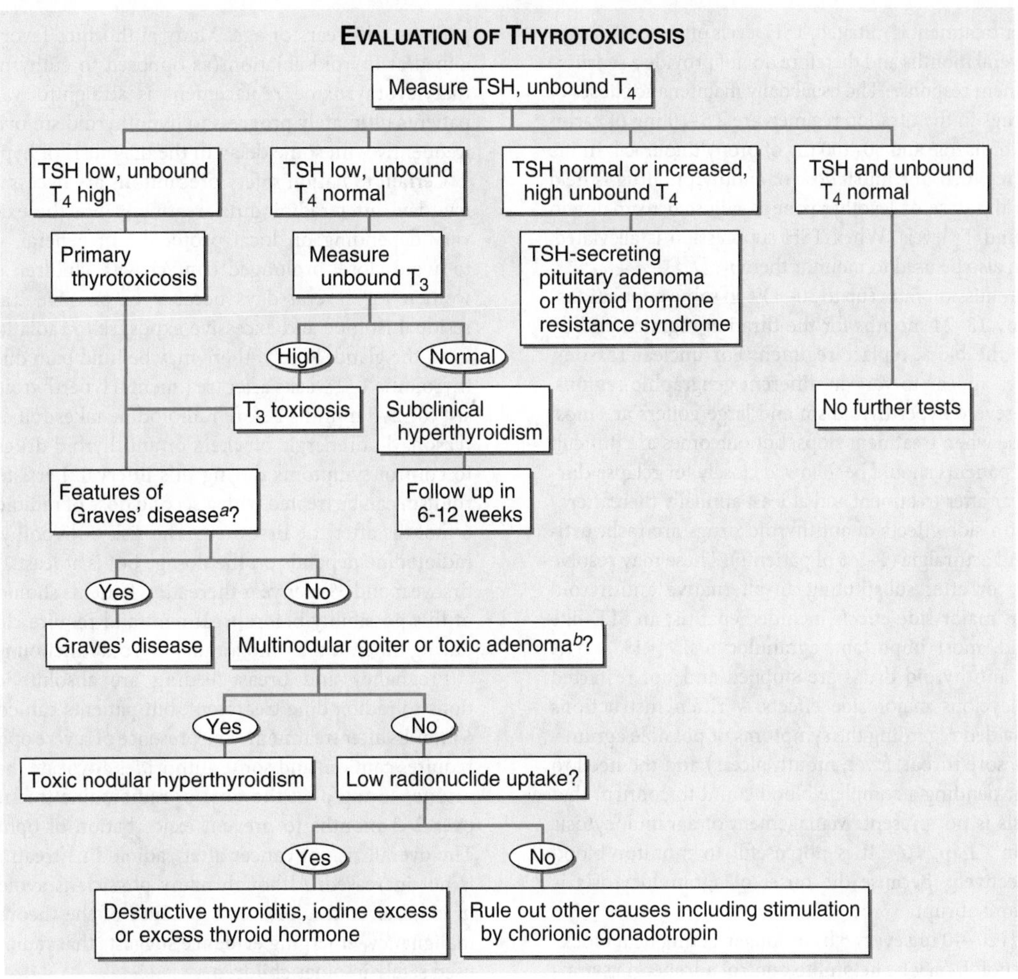

Figure 341-8 Evaluation of thyrotoxicosis. [a]Diffuse goiter, positive TPO antibodies, ophthalmopathy, dermopathy; [b]can be confirmed by radionuclide scan. TSH, thyroid-stimulating hormone.

The clinical course of ophthalmopathy does not follow that of the thyroid disease. Ophthalmopathy typically worsens over the initial 3–6 months, followed by a plateau phase over the next 12–18 months, with spontaneous improvement, particularly in the soft tissue changes. However, the course is more fulminant in up to 5% of patients, requiring intervention in the acute phase if there is optic nerve compression or corneal ulceration. Diplopia may appear late in the disease due to fibrosis of the extraocular muscles. Some studies suggest that radioiodine treatment for hyperthyroidism worsens the eye disease in a small proportion of patients (especially smokers). Antithyroid drugs or surgery have no adverse effects on the clinical course of ophthalmopathy. Thyroid dermopathy, when it occurs, usually appears 1–2 years after the development of Graves' hyperthyroidism; it may improve spontaneously.

TREATMENT Graves' Disease

The *hyperthyroidism* of Graves' disease is treated by reducing thyroid hormone synthesis, using antithyroid drugs, or reducing the amount of thyroid tissue with radioiodine (^{131}I) treatment or by thyroidectomy. Antithyroid drugs are the predominant therapy in many centers in Europe and Japan, whereas radioiodine is more often the first line of treatment in North America. These differences reflect the fact that no single approach is optimal and that patients may require multiple treatments to achieve remission.

The main *antithyroid drugs* are the thionamides, such as propylthiouracil, carbimazole, and the active metabolite of the latter, methimazole. All inhibit the function of TPO, reducing oxidation and organification of iodide. These drugs also reduce thyroid antibody levels by mechanisms that remain unclear, and they appear to enhance rates of remission. Propylthiouracil inhibits deiodination of $T_4 \rightarrow T_3$. However, this effect is of minor benefit, except in the most severe thyrotoxicosis, and is offset by the much shorter half-life of this drug (90 min) compared to methimazole (6 h).

There are many variations of antithyroid drug regimens. The initial dose of carbimazole or methimazole is usually 10–20 mg every 8 or 12 h, but once-daily dosing is possible after euthyroidism is restored. Propylthiouracil is given at a dose of 100–200 mg every 6–8 h, and divided doses are usually given throughout the course. Lower doses of each drug may suffice in areas of low iodine intake. The starting dose of antithyroid drugs can be gradually reduced (titration regimen) as thyrotoxicosis improves. Alternatively, high doses may be given combined with levothyroxine supplementation (block-replace regimen) to avoid drug-induced hypothyroidism. Initial reports suggesting superior remission rates with the block-replace regimen have not been reproduced in several other trials. The titration regimen is often preferred to minimize the dose of antithyroid drug and provide an index of treatment response.

Thyroid function tests and clinical manifestations are reviewed 3–4 weeks after starting treatment, and the dose is titrated based on unbound T_4 levels. Most patients do not achieve euthyroidism until

6–8 weeks after treatment is initiated. TSH levels often remain suppressed for several months and therefore do not provide a sensitive index of treatment response. The usual daily maintenance doses of antithyroid drugs in the titration regimen are 2.5–10 mg of carbimazole or methimazole and 50–100 mg of propylthiouracil. In the block-replace regimen, the initial dose of antithyroid drug is held constant, and the dose of levothyroxine is adjusted to maintain normal unbound T_4 levels. When TSH suppression is alleviated, TSH levels can also be used to monitor therapy.

Maximum remission rates (up to 30–50% in some populations) are achieved by 18–24 months for the titration regimen and by 6 months for the block-replace regimen. For unclear reasons, remission rates appear to vary in different geographic regions. Patients with severe hyperthyroidism and large goiters are most likely to relapse when treatment stops, but outcomes are difficult to predict. All patients should be followed closely for relapse during the first year after treatment and at least annually thereafter.

The common side effects of antithyroid drugs are rash, urticaria, fever, and arthralgia (1–5% of patients). These may resolve spontaneously or after substituting an alternative antithyroid drug. Rare but major side effects include hepatitis; an SLE-like syndrome; and, most important, agranulocytosis (<1%). It is essential that antithyroid drugs are stopped and not restarted if a patient develops major side effects. Written instructions should be provided regarding the symptoms of possible agranulocytosis (e.g., sore throat, fever, mouth ulcers) and the need to stop treatment pending a complete blood count to confirm that agranulocytosis is not present. Management of agranulocytosis is described in Chap. 107. It is not useful to monitor blood counts prospectively, because the onset of agranulocytosis is idiosyncratic and abrupt.

Propranolol (20–40 mg every 6 h) or longer-acting beta blockers such as atenolol, may be helpful to control adrenergic symptoms, especially in the early stages before antithyroid drugs take effect. Beta blockers are also useful in patients with thyrotoxic periodic paralysis, pending correction of thyrotoxicosis. The need for anticoagulation with coumadin should be considered in all patients with atrial fibrillation. If digoxin is used, increased doses are often needed in the thyrotoxic state.

Radioiodine causes progressive destruction of thyroid cells and can be used as initial treatment or for relapses after a trial of antithyroid drugs. There is a small risk of thyrotoxic crisis (see below) after radioiodine, which can be minimized by pretreatment with antithyroid drugs for at least a month before treatment. Antecedent treatment with antithyroid drugs should be considered for all elderly patients or for those with cardiac problems to deplete thyroid hormone stores before administration of radioiodine. Carbimazole or methimazole must be stopped at least 2 days before radioiodine administration to achieve optimum iodine uptake. Propylthiouracil has a prolonged radioprotective effect and should be stopped several weeks before radioiodine is given, or a larger dose of radioiodine will be necessary.

Efforts to calculate an optimal dose of radioiodine that achieves euthyroidism without a high incidence of relapse or progression to hypothyroidism have not been successful. Some patients inevitably relapse after a single dose because the biologic effects of radiation vary between individuals, and hypothyroidism cannot be uniformly avoided even using accurate dosimetry. A practical strategy is to give a fixed dose based on clinical features, such as the severity of thyrotoxicosis, the size of the goiter (increases the dose needed), and the level of radioiodine uptake (decreases the dose needed). ^{131}I dosage generally ranges between 185 MBq (5 mCi) to 555 MBq (15 mCi). Incomplete treatment or early relapse is more common in males and in patients <40 years of age. Many authorities favor an approach aimed at thyroid ablation (as opposed to euthyroidism), given that levothyroxine replacement is straightforward and most patients ultimately progress to hypothyroidism over 5–10 years, frequently with some delay in the diagnosis of hypothyroidism.

Certain radiation safety precautions are necessary in the first few days after radioiodine treatment, but the exact guidelines vary depending on local protocols. In general, patients need to avoid close, prolonged contact with children and pregnant women for several days because of possible transmission of residual isotope and excessive exposure to radiation emanating from the gland. Rarely, there may be mild pain due to radiation thyroiditis 1–2 weeks after treatment. Hyperthyroidism can persist for 2–3 months before radioiodine takes full effect. For this reason, β-adrenergic blockers or antithyroid drugs can be used to control symptoms during this interval. Persistent hyperthyroidism can be treated with a second dose of radioiodine, usually 6 months after the first dose. The risk of hypothyroidism after radioiodine depends on the dosage but is at least 10–20% in the first year and 5% per year thereafter. Patients should be informed of this possibility before treatment and require close follow-up during the first year and annual thyroid function testing.

Pregnancy and breast-feeding are absolute contraindications to radioiodine treatment, but patients can conceive safely 6 months after treatment. The presence of severe ophthalmopathy requires caution, and some authorities advocate the use of prednisone, 40 mg/d, at the time of radioiodine treatment, tapered over 2–3 months to prevent exacerbation of ophthalmopathy. The overall risk of cancer after radioiodine treatment in adults is not increased. Although many physicians avoid radioiodine in children and adolescents because of the theoretical risks of malignancy, emerging evidence suggests that radioiodine can be used safely in older children.

Subtotal or near-total thyroidectomy is an option for patients who relapse after antithyroid drugs and they prefer this treatment to radioiodine. Some experts recommend surgery in young individuals, particularly when the goiter is very large. Careful control of thyrotoxicosis with antithyroid drugs, followed by potassium iodide (3 drops SSKI orally tid), is needed prior to surgery to avoid thyrotoxic crisis and to reduce the vascularity of the gland. The major complications of surgery—bleeding, laryngeal edema, hypoparathyroidism, and damage to the recurrent laryngeal nerves—are unusual when the procedure is performed by highly experienced surgeons. Recurrence rates in the best series are <2%, but the rate of hypothyroidism is only slightly less than that following radioiodine treatment.

The titration regimen of antithyroid drugs should be used to manage Graves' disease in *pregnancy*, as blocking doses of these drugs produce fetal hypothyroidism. Propylthiouracil is usually used because of relatively low transplacental transfer and its ability to block $T_4 \rightarrow T_3$ conversion. Also, carbimazole and methimazole have been associated with rare cases of fetal *aplasia cutis* and other defects, such as choanal atresia. The lowest effective dose of propylthiouracil should be given, and it is often possible to stop treatment in the last trimester because TSI tend to decline in pregnancy. Nonetheless, the transplacental transfer of these antibodies rarely causes *fetal* or *neonatal thyrotoxicosis*. Poor intrauterine growth, a fetal heart rate of >160 beats/min, and high levels of maternal TSI in the last trimester may herald this complication. Antithyroid drugs given to the mother can be used to treat the fetus and may be needed for 1–3 months after delivery, until the maternal antibodies disappear from the baby's circulation. The postpartum period is a time of major risk for relapse of Graves' disease. Breast-feeding is safe with low doses of antithyroid drugs. Graves' disease in *children* is usually managed with antithyroid drugs, often given as a prolonged course of the titration regimen. Surgery or radioiodine may be indicated for severe disease.

Thyrotoxic crisis, or *thyroid storm*, is rare and presents as a life-threatening exacerbation of hyperthyroidism, accompanied by fever, delirium, seizures, coma, vomiting, diarrhea, and jaundice. The mortality rate due to cardiac failure, arrhythmia, or hyperthermia is as high as 30%, even with treatment. Thyrotoxic crisis is usually precipitated by acute illness (e.g., stroke, infection, trauma, diabetic ketoacidosis), surgery (especially on the thyroid), or radioiodine treatment of a patient with partially treated or untreated hyperthyroidism. Management requires intensive monitoring and supportive care, identification and treatment of the precipitating cause, and measures that reduce thyroid hormone synthesis. Large doses of propylthiouracil (600 mg loading dose and 200–300 mg every 6 h) should be given orally or by nasogastric tube or per rectum; the drug's inhibitory action on $T_4 \rightarrow T_3$ conversion makes it the antithyroid drug of choice. One hour after the first dose of propylthiouracil, stable iodide is given to block thyroid hormone synthesis via the Wolff-Chaikoff effect (the delay allows the antithyroid drug to prevent the excess iodine from being incorporated into new hormone). A saturated solution of potassium iodide (5 drops SSKI every 6 h), or ipodate or iopanoic acid (500 mg per 12 h), may be given orally. (Sodium iodide, 0.25 g IV every 6 h, is an alternative but is not generally available.) Propranolol should also be given to reduce tachycardia and other adrenergic manifestations (40–60 mg PO every 4 h; or 2 mg IV every 4 h). Although other β-adrenergic blockers can be used, high doses of propranolol decrease $T_4 \rightarrow T_3$ conversion, and the doses can be easily adjusted. Caution is needed to avoid acute negative inotropic effects, but controlling the heart rate is important, as some patients develop a form of high-output heart failure. Additional therapeutic measures include glucocorticoids (e.g., dexamethasone, 2 mg every 6 h), antibiotics if infection is present, cooling, oxygen, and intravenous fluids.

Ophthalmopathy requires no active treatment when it is mild or moderate, because there is usually spontaneous improvement. General measures include meticulous control of thyroid hormone levels, cessation of smoking, and an explanation of the natural history of ophthalmopathy. Discomfort can be relieved with artificial tears (e.g., 1% methylcellulose), eye ointment, and the use of dark glasses with side frames. Periorbital edema may respond to a more upright sleeping position or a diuretic. Corneal exposure during sleep can be avoided by using patches or taping the eyelids shut. Minor degrees of diplopia improve with prisms fitted to spectacles. Severe ophthalmopathy, with optic nerve involvement or chemosis resulting in corneal damage, is an emergency requiring joint management with an ophthalmologist. Short-term benefit can be gained in about two-thirds of patients by the use of high-dose glucocorticoids (e.g., prednisone, 40–80 mg daily), sometimes combined with cyclosporine. Glucocorticoid doses are tapered by 5 mg every 2 weeks, but the taper often results in reemergence of congestive symptoms. Pulse therapy with IV methylprednisolone (e.g., 500–1000 mg of methylprednisolone in 250 mL of saline infused over 2 h daily for 1 week) followed by an oral regimen is also used. When glucocorticoids are ineffective, orbital decompression can be achieved by removing bone from any wall of the orbit, thereby allowing displacement of fat and swollen extraocular muscles. The transantral route is used most often, because it requires no external incision. Proptosis recedes an average of 5 mm, but there may be residual or even worsened diplopia. Once the eye disease has stabilized, surgery may be indicated for relief of diplopia and correction of the appearance. External beam radiotherapy of the orbits has been used for many years, but the efficacy of this therapy remains unclear, and it is best reserved for those who have failed or are not candidates for glucocorticoid therapy.

Thyroid dermopathy does not usually require treatment, but it can cause cosmetic problems or interfere with the fit of shoes. Surgical removal is not indicated. If necessary, treatment consists of topical, high-potency glucocorticoid ointment under an occlusive dressing. Octreotide may be beneficial in some cases.

OTHER CAUSES OF THYROTOXICOSIS

Destructive thyroiditis (subacute or silent thyroiditis) typically presents with a short thyrotoxic phase due to the release of preformed thyroid hormones and catabolism of Tg (see "Subacute Thyroiditis," below). True hyperthyroidism is absent, as demonstrated by a low radionuclide uptake. Circulating Tg levels are usually increased. Other causes of thyrotoxicosis with low or absent thyroid radionuclide uptake include *thyrotoxicosis factitia*, iodine excess, and, rarely, ectopic thyroid tissue, particularly teratomas of the ovary (*struma ovarii*); and functional metastatic follicular carcinoma. Whole-body radionuclide studies can demonstrate ectopic thyroid tissue, and thyrotoxicosis factitia can be distinguished from destructive thyroiditis by the clinical features and low levels of Tg. Amiodarone treatment is associated with thyrotoxicosis in up to 10% of patients, particularly in areas of low iodine intake (see below).

TSH-secreting pituitary adenoma is a rare cause of thyrotoxicosis. It can be identified by the presence of an inappropriately normal or increased TSH level in a patient with hyperthyroidism, diffuse goiter, and elevated T_4 and T_3 levels (Chap. 339). Elevated levels of the α-subunit of TSH, released by the TSH-secreting adenoma, support this diagnosis, which can be confirmed by demonstrating the pituitary tumor on MRI or CT scan. A combination of transsphenoidal surgery, sella irradiation, and octreotide may be required to normalize TSH, because many of these tumors are large and locally invasive at the time of diagnosis. Radioiodine or antithyroid drugs can be used to control thyrotoxicosis.

Thyrotoxicosis caused by *toxic MNG* and *hyperfunctioning solitary nodules* is discussed below.

THYROIDITIS

A clinically useful classification of thyroiditis is based on the onset and duration of disease (Table 341-8).

ACUTE THYROIDITIS

Acute thyroiditis is rare and due to suppurative infection of the thyroid. In children and young adults, the most common cause is the presence of a piriform sinus, a remnant of the fourth branchial pouch that connects the oropharynx with the thyroid. Such sinuses are predominantly left-sided. A long-standing goiter and degeneration in a thyroid malignancy are risk factors in the elderly. The patient presents with thyroid pain, often referred to the throat or ears, and a small, tender goiter that may be asymmetric. Fever, dysphagia, and erythema over the thyroid are common, as are systemic symptoms of a febrile illness and lymphadenopathy.

The differential diagnosis of *thyroid pain* includes subacute or, rarely, chronic thyroiditis; hemorrhage into a cyst; malignancy including lymphoma; and, rarely, amiodarone-induced thyroiditis or amyloidosis. However, the abrupt presentation and clinical features of acute thyroiditis rarely cause confusion. The erythrocyte sedimentation rate (ESR) and white cell count are usually increased, but thyroid function is normal. FNA biopsy shows infiltration by polymorphonuclear leukocytes; culture of the sample can identify the

TABLE 341-8 Causes of Thyroiditis

Acute

Bacterial infection: especially *Staphylococcus*, *Streptococcus*, and *Enterobacter*

Fungal infection: *Aspergillus*, *Candida*, *Coccidioides*, *Histoplasma*, and *Pneumocystis*

Radiation thyroiditis after ^{131}I treatment

Amiodarone (may also be subacute or chronic)

Subacute

Viral (or granulomatous) thyroiditis

Silent thyroiditis (including postpartum thyroiditis)

Mycobacterial infection

Chronic

Autoimmunity: focal thyroiditis, Hashimoto's thyroiditis, atrophic thyroiditis

Riedel's thyroiditis

Parasitic thyroiditis: echinococcosis, strongyloidiasis, cysticercosis

Traumatic: after palpation

organism. Caution is needed in immunocompromised patients as fungal, mycobacterial, or *Pneumocystis* thyroiditis can occur in this setting. Antibiotic treatment is guided initially by Gram stain and, subsequently, by cultures of the FNA biopsy. Surgery may be needed to drain an abscess, which can be localized by CT scan or ultrasound. Tracheal obstruction, septicemia, retropharyngeal abscess, mediastinitis, and jugular venous thrombosis may complicate acute thyroiditis but are uncommon with prompt use of antibiotics.

SUBACUTE THYROIDITIS

This is also termed *de Quervain's thyroiditis*, *granulomatous thyroiditis*, or *viral thyroiditis*. Many viruses have been implicated, including mumps, coxsackie, influenza, adenoviruses, and echoviruses, but attempts to identify the virus in an individual patient are often unsuccessful and do not influence management. The diagnosis of subacute thyroiditis is often overlooked because the symptoms can mimic pharyngitis. The peak incidence occurs at 30–50 years, and women are affected three times more frequently than men.

Pathophysiology

The thyroid shows a characteristic patchy inflammatory infiltrate with disruption of the thyroid follicles and multinucleated giant cells within some follicles. The follicular changes progress to granulomas accompanied by fibrosis. Finally, the thyroid returns to normal, usually several months after onset. During the initial phase of follicular destruction, there is release of Tg and thyroid hormones, leading to increased circulating T_4 and T_3 and suppression of TSH (Fig. 341-9). During this destructive phase, radioactive iodine uptake is low or undetectable. After several weeks, the thyroid is depleted of stored thyroid hormone and a phase of hypothyroidism typically occurs, with low unbound T_4 (and sometimes T_3) and moderately increased TSH levels. Radioactive iodine uptake returns to normal or is even increased as a result of the rise in TSH. Finally, thyroid hormone and TSH levels return to normal as the disease subsides.

Clinical manifestations

The patient usually presents with a painful and enlarged thyroid, sometimes accompanied by fever. There may be features of thyrotoxicosis or hypothyroidism, depending on the phase of the illness. Malaise and symptoms of an upper respiratory tract infection may precede the thyroid-related features by several weeks. In other patients, the onset is acute, severe, and without obvious antecedent. The patient typically complains of a sore throat, and examination reveals a small goiter that is exquisitely tender. Pain is often referred to the jaw or ear. Complete resolution is the usual outcome, but permanent hypothyroidism can occur, particularly in those with coincidental thyroid autoimmunity. A prolonged course over many months, with one or more relapses, occurs in a small percentage of patients.

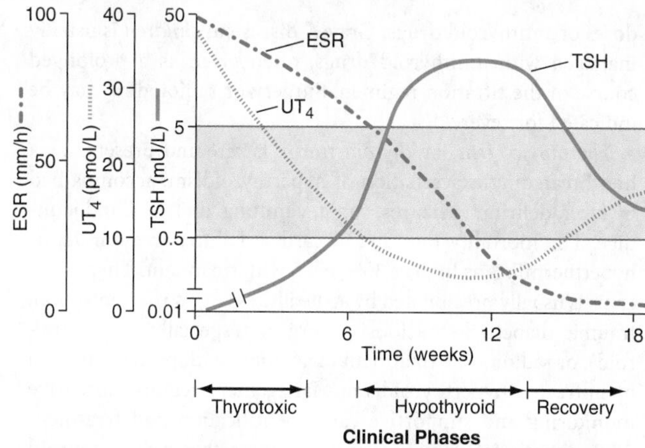

Figure 341-9 Clinical course of subacute thyroiditis. The release of thyroid hormones is initially associated with a thyrotoxic phase and suppressed thyroid-stimulating hormone (TSH). A hypothyroid phase then ensues, with low T_4 and TSH levels that are initially low but gradually increase. During the recovery phase, increased TSH levels combined with resolution of thyroid follicular injury leads to normalization of thyroid function, often several months after the beginning of the illness. ESR, erythrocyte sedimentation rate; FT_4, free or unbound T_4.

Laboratory evaluation

As depicted in Fig. 341-9, thyroid function tests characteristically evolve through three distinct phases over about 6 months: (1) thyrotoxic phase, (2) hypothyroid phase, and (3) recovery phase. In the thyrotoxic phase, T_4 and T_3 levels are increased, reflecting their discharge from the damaged thyroid cells, and TSH is suppressed. The T_4/T_3 ratio is greater than in Graves' disease or thyroid autonomy, in which T_3 is often disproportionately increased. The diagnosis is confirmed by a high ESR and low radioiodine uptake. The white blood cell count may be increased, and thyroid antibodies are negative. If the diagnosis is in doubt, FNA biopsy may be useful, particularly to distinguish unilateral involvement from bleeding into a cyst or neoplasm.

TREATMENT Subacute Thyroiditis

Relatively large doses of aspirin (e.g., 600 mg every 4–6 h) or NSAIDs are sufficient to control symptoms in many cases. If this treatment is inadequate, or if the patient has marked local or systemic symptoms, glucocorticoids should be given. The usual starting dose is 40–60 mg prednisone, depending on severity. The dose is gradually tapered over 6–8 weeks, in response to improvement in symptoms and the ESR. If a relapse occurs during glucocorticoid withdrawal, treatment should be started again and withdrawn more gradually. In these patients, it is useful to wait until the radioactive iodine uptake normalizes before stopping treatment. Thyroid function should be monitored every 2–4 weeks using TSH and unbound T_4 levels. Symptoms of thyrotoxicosis improve spontaneously but may be ameliorated by β-adrenergic blockers; antithyroid drugs play no role in treatment of the thyrotoxic phase.

Levothyroxine replacement may be needed if the hypothyroid phase is prolonged, but doses should be low enough (50 to 100 μg daily) to allow TSH-mediated recovery.

SILENT THYROIDITIS

Painless thyroiditis, or *"silent" thyroiditis*, occurs in patients with underlying autoimmune thyroid disease. It has a clinical course similar to that of subacute thyroiditis, except that there is little or no thyroid tenderness. The condition occurs in up to 5% of women 3–6 months after pregnancy and is then termed *postpartum thyroiditis*. Typically, patients have a brief phase of thyrotoxicosis lasting 2–4 weeks, followed by hypothyroidism for 4–12 weeks, and then resolution; often, however, only one phase is apparent. The condition is associated with the presence of TPO antibodies antepartum, and it is three times more common in women with type 1 diabetes mellitus. As in subacute thyroiditis, the radioactive iodine uptake is initially suppressed. In addition to the painless goiter, silent thyroiditis can be distinguished from subacute thyroiditis by a normal ESR and the presence of TPO antibodies. Glucocorticoid treatment is not indicated for silent thyroiditis. Severe thyrotoxic symptoms can be managed with a brief course of propranolol, 20–40 mg three or four times daily. Thyroxine replacement may be needed for the hypothyroid phase but should be withdrawn after 6–9 months, as recovery is the rule. Annual follow-up thereafter is recommended, because a proportion of these individuals develop permanent hypothyroidism. The condition may recur in subsequent pregnancies.

DRUG-INDUCED THYROIDITIS

Patients receiving cytokines such as IFN-α or IL-2 may develop painless thyroiditis. IFN-α, which is used to treat chronic hepatitis B or C and hematologic and skin malignancies, causes thyroid dysfunction in up to 5% of treated patients. It has been associated with painless thyroiditis, hypothyroidism, and Graves' disease, and is most common in women with TPO antibodies prior to treatment. For discussion of amiodarone, see "Amiodarone Effects on Thyroid Function," below.

CHRONIC THYROIDITIS

Focal thyroiditis is present in 20–40% of euthyroid autopsy cases and is associated with serologic evidence of autoimmunity, particularly the presence of TPO antibodies. These antibodies are 4–10 times more common in otherwise healthy women than men. The most common clinically apparent cause of chronic thyroiditis is *Hashimoto's thyroiditis*, an autoimmune disorder that often presents as a firm or hard goiter of variable size (see above). *Riedel's thyroiditis* is a rare disorder that typically occurs in middle-aged women. It presents with an insidious, painless goiter with local symptoms due to compression of the esophagus, trachea, neck veins, or recurrent laryngeal nerves. Dense fibrosis disrupts normal gland architecture and can extend outside the thyroid capsule. Despite these extensive histologic changes, thyroid dysfunction is uncommon. The goiter is hard, nontender, often asymmetric, and fixed, leading to suspicion of a malignancy. Diagnosis requires open biopsy as FNA biopsy is usually inadequate. Treatment is directed to surgical relief of compressive symptoms. Tamoxifen may also be beneficial. There is an association between Riedel's thyroiditis and idiopathic fibrosis at other sites (retroperitoneum, mediastinum, biliary tree, lung, and orbit).

SICK EUTHYROID SYNDROME

Any acute, severe illness can cause abnormalities of circulating TSH or thyroid hormone levels in the absence of underlying thyroid disease, making these measurements potentially misleading. The major cause of these hormonal changes is the release of cytokines such as IL-6. Unless a thyroid disorder is strongly suspected, the routine testing of thyroid function should be avoided in acutely ill patients.

The most common hormone pattern in sick euthyroid syndrome (SES) is a decrease in total and unbound T_3 levels (low T_3 syndrome) with normal levels of T_4 and TSH. The magnitude of the fall in T_3 correlates with the severity of the illness. T_4 conversion to T_3 via peripheral deiodination is impaired, leading to increased reverse T_3 (rT_3). Despite this effect, decreased clearance rather than increased production is the major basis for increased rT_3. Also, T_4 is alternately metabolized to the hormonally inactive T_3 sulfate. It is generally assumed that this low T_3 state is adaptive, because it can be induced in normal individuals by fasting. Teleologically, the fall in T_3 may limit catabolism in starved or ill patients.

Very sick patients may exhibit a dramatic fall in total T_4 and T_3 levels (low T_4 syndrome). This state has a poor prognosis. A key factor in the fall in T_4 levels is altered binding to TBG. T_4 assays usually demonstrate a normal unbound T_4 level in such patients, depending on the assay method used. Fluctuation in TSH levels also creates challenges in the interpretation of thyroid function in sick patients. TSH levels may range from <0.1 to >20 mIU/L; these alterations reverse after recovery, confirming the absence of underlying thyroid disease. A rise in cortisol or administration of glucocorticoids may provide a partial explanation for decreased TSH levels. The exact mechanisms underlying the subnormal TSH seen in 10% of sick patients and the increased TSH seen in 5% remain unclear but may be mediated by cytokines including IL-12 and IL-18.

Any severe illness can induce changes in thyroid hormone levels, but certain disorders exhibit a distinctive pattern of abnormalities. Acute liver disease is associated with an initial rise in total (but not unbound) T_3 and T_4 levels, due to TBG release; these levels become subnormal with progression to liver failure. A transient increase in total and unbound T_4 levels, usually with a normal T_3 level, is seen in 5–30% of acutely ill psychiatric patients. TSH values may be transiently low, normal, or high in these patients. In the early stage of HIV infection, T_3 and T_4 levels rise, even if there is weight loss. T_3 levels fall with progression to AIDS, but TSH usually remains normal. Renal disease is often accompanied by low T_3 concentrations, but with normal rather than increased rT_3 levels, due to an unknown factor that increases uptake of rT_3 into the liver.

The diagnosis of SES is challenging. Historic information may be limited, and patients often have multiple metabolic derangements. Useful features to consider include previous history of thyroid disease and thyroid function tests, evaluation of the severity and time course of the patient's acute illness, documentation of medications that may affect thyroid function or thyroid hormone levels, and measurements of rT_3 together with unbound thyroid hormones and TSH. The diagnosis of SES is frequently presumptive, given the clinical context and pattern of laboratory values; only resolution of the test results with clinical recovery can clearly establish this disorder. Treatment of SES with thyroid hormone (T_4 and/or T_3) is controversial, but most authorities recommend monitoring the patient's thyroid function tests during recovery, without administering thyroid hormone, unless there is historic or clinical evidence suggestive of hypothyroidism. Sufficiently large randomized controlled trials using thyroid hormone are unlikely to resolve this therapeutic controversy in the near future, because clinical presentations and outcomes are highly variable.

AMIODARONE EFFECTS ON THYROID FUNCTION

Amiodarone is a commonly used type III antiarrhythmic agent (Chap. 233). It is structurally related to thyroid hormone and contains 39% iodine by weight. Thus, typical doses of amiodarone (200 mg/d) are associated with very high iodine intake, leading to greater than fortyfold increases in plasma and urinary iodine levels. Moreover, because amiodarone is stored in adipose tissue, high iodine levels persist for >6 months after discontinuation of the drug. Amiodarone inhibits deiodinase activity, and its metabolites function as weak antagonists of thyroid hormone action. Amiodarone has the following effects on thyroid function: (1) acute, transient suppression of thyroid function; (2) hypothyroidism in patients susceptible to the inhibitory effects of a high iodine load; and (3) thyrotoxicosis that may be caused by either a Jod-Basedow effect from the iodine load, in the setting of MNG or incipient Graves' disease, or a thyroiditis-like condition.

The initiation of amiodarone treatment is associated with a transient decrease of T_4 levels, reflecting the inhibitory effect of iodine on T_4 release. Soon thereafter, most individuals escape from iodide-dependent suppression of the thyroid (Wolff-Chaikoff effect), and the inhibitory effects on deiodinase activity and thyroid hormone receptor action become predominant. These events lead to the following pattern of thyroid function tests: increased T_4, decreased T_3, increased rT_3, and a transient TSH increase (up to 20 mIU/L). TSH levels normalize or are slightly suppressed within 1–3 months.

The incidence of hypothyroidism from amiodarone varies geographically, apparently correlating with iodine intake. Hypothyroidism occurs in up to 13% of amiodarone-treated patients in iodine-replete countries, such as the United States, but is less common (<6% incidence) in areas of lower iodine intake, such as Italy or Spain. The pathogenesis appears to involve an inability of the thyroid gland to escape from the Wolff-Chaikoff effect in autoimmune thyroiditis. Consequently, amiodarone-associated hypothyroidism is more common in women and individuals with positive TPO antibodies. It is usually unnecessary to discontinue amiodarone for this side effect, because levothyroxine can be used to normalize thyroid function. TSH levels should be monitored, because T_4 levels are often increased for the reasons described above.

The management of amiodarone-induced thyrotoxicosis (AIT) is complicated by the fact that there are different causes of thyrotoxicosis and because the increased thyroid hormone levels exacerbate underlying arrhythmias and coronary artery disease. Amiodarone treatment causes thyrotoxicosis in 10% of patients living in areas of low iodine intake and in 2% of patients in regions of high iodine intake. There are two major forms of AIT, although some patients have features of both. Type 1 AIT is associated with an underlying thyroid abnormality (preclinical Graves' disease or nodular goiter). Thyroid hormone synthesis becomes excessive as a result of increased iodine exposure (Jod-Basedow phenomenon). Type 2 AIT occurs in individuals with no intrinsic thyroid abnormalities and is the result of drug-induced lysosomal activation leading to destructive thyroiditis with histiocyte accumulation in the thyroid; the incidence rises as cumulative amiodarone dosage increases. Mild forms of type 2 AIT can resolve spontaneously or can occasionally lead to hypothyroidism. Color-flow doppler thyroid scanning shows increased vascularity in type 1 AIT but decreased vascularity in type 2 AIT. Thyroid scintiscans are difficult to interpret in this setting because the high endogenous iodine levels diminish tracer uptake. However, the presence of normal or rarely increased uptake favors type 1 AIT.

In AIT, the drug should be stopped, if possible, although this is often impractical because of the underlying cardiac disorder. Discontinuation of amiodarone will not have an acute effect because of its storage and prolonged half-life. High doses of antithyroid drugs can be used in type 1 AIT but are often ineffective. In type 2 AIT, oral contrast agents, such as sodium ipodate (500 mg/d) or sodium tyropanoate (500 mg, 1–2 doses/d), rapidly reduce T_4 and T_3 levels, decrease $T_4 \rightarrow T_3$ conversion, and may block tissue uptake of thyroid hormones. Potassium perchlorate, 200 mg every 6 h, has been used to reduce thyroidal iodide content. Perchlorate treatment has been associated with agranulocytosis, though the risk appears relatively low with short-term use. Glucocorticoids, as administered for subacute thyroiditis, have modest benefit in type 2 AIT. Lithium blocks thyroid hormone release and can also provide some benefit. Near-total thyroidectomy rapidly decreases thyroid hormone levels and may be the most effective long-term solution if the patient can undergo the procedure safely.

THYROID FUNCTION IN PREGNANCY

Five factors alter thyroid function in pregnancy: (1) the transient increase in hCG during the first trimester, which stimulates the TSH-R; (2) the estrogen-induced rise in TBG during the first trimester, which is sustained during pregnancy; (3) alterations in the immune system, leading to the onset, exacerbation, or amelioration of an underlying autoimmune thyroid disease (see above); (4) increased thyroid hormone metabolism by the placenta; and (5) increased urinary iodide excretion, which can cause impaired thyroid hormone production in areas of marginal iodine sufficiency. Women with a precarious iodine intake (<50 μg/d) are most at risk of developing a goiter during pregnancy, and iodine supplementation should be considered to prevent maternal and fetal hypothyroidism and the development of neonatal goiter.

The rise in circulating hCG levels during the first trimester is accompanied by a reciprocal fall in TSH that persists into the middle of pregnancy. This appears to reflect weak binding of hCG, which is present at very high levels, to the TSH-R. Rare individuals have been described with variant TSH-R sequences that enhance hCG binding and TSH-R activation. Human chorionic gonadotropin-induced changes in thyroid function can result in transient gestational hyperthyroidism and/or *hyperemesis gravidarum*, a condition characterized by severe nausea and vomiting and risk of volume depletion. Antithyroid drugs are rarely needed, and parenteral fluid replacement usually suffices until the condition resolves.

Maternal hypothyroidism occurs in 2–3% of women of child-bearing age and is associated with increased risk of developmental delay in the offspring. Consequently, TSH screening for hypothyroidism is indicated in early pregnancy and should be considered in women who are planning pregnancy, particularly if they have a goiter or strong family history of autoimmune thyroid disease. Thyroid hormone requirements are increased by 25–50 μg/d during pregnancy.

GOITER AND NODULAR THYROID DISEASE

Goiter refers to an enlarged thyroid gland. Biosynthetic defects, iodine deficiency, autoimmune disease, and nodular diseases can each lead to goiter, though by different mechanisms. Biosynthetic defects and iodine deficiency are associated with reduced efficiency of thyroid hormone synthesis, leading to increased TSH, which stimulates thyroid growth as a compensatory mechanism to overcome the block in hormone synthesis. Graves' disease and Hashimoto's thyroiditis are also associated with goiter. In Graves' disease, the goiter results mainly from the TSH-R–mediated effects of TSI. The goitrous form of Hashimoto's thyroiditis occurs because of acquired defects in hormone synthesis, leading to elevated levels of TSH and its consequent growth effects. Lymphocytic infiltration and immune system–induced growth factors also contribute to thyroid enlargement in Hashimoto's thyroiditis. Nodular disease is characterized by the disordered growth of thyroid cells, often combined with the gradual development of fibrosis. Because the management of goiter depends on the etiology, the detection of thyroid enlargement on physical examination should prompt further evaluation to identify its cause.

Nodular thyroid disease is common, occurring in about 3–7% of adults when assessed by physical examination. Using more sensitive techniques, such as ultrasound, it is present in >25% of adults.

Thyroid nodules may be solitary or multiple, and they may be functional or nonfunctional.

■ DIFFUSE NONTOXIC (SIMPLE) GOITER

Etiology and pathogenesis

When diffuse enlargement of the thyroid occurs in the absence of nodules and hyperthyroidism, it is referred to as a *diffuse nontoxic goiter*. This is sometimes called *simple goiter*, because of the absence of nodules, or *colloid goiter*, because of the presence of uniform follicles that are filled with colloid. Worldwide, diffuse goiter is most commonly caused by iodine deficiency and is termed *endemic goiter* when it affects >5% of the population. In nonendemic regions, *sporadic goiter* occurs, and the cause is usually unknown. Thyroid enlargement in teenagers is sometimes referred to as *juvenile goiter*. In general, goiter is more common in women than men, probably because of the greater prevalence of underlying autoimmune disease and the increased iodine demands associated with pregnancy.

In *iodine-deficient areas*, thyroid enlargement reflects a compensatory effort to trap iodide and produce sufficient hormone under conditions in which hormone synthesis is relatively inefficient. Somewhat surprisingly, TSH levels are usually normal or only slightly increased, suggesting increased sensitivity to TSH or activation of other pathways that lead to thyroid growth. Iodide appears to have direct actions on thyroid vasculature and may indirectly affect growth through vasoactive substances such as endothelins and nitric oxide. Endemic goiter is also caused by exposure to environmental *goitrogens* such as cassava root, which contains a thiocyanate; vegetables of the Cruciferae family (known as cruciferous vegetables) (e.g., brussels sprout, cabbage, and cauliflower); and milk from regions where goitrogens are present in grass. Though relatively rare, inherited defects in thyroid hormone synthesis lead to a diffuse nontoxic goiter. Abnormalities at each step in hormone synthesis, including iodide transport (NIS), Tg synthesis, organification and coupling (TPO), and the regeneration of iodide (dehalogenase), have been described.

■ CLINICAL MANIFESTATIONS AND DIAGNOSIS

If thyroid function is preserved, most goiters are asymptomatic. Spontaneous hemorrhage into a cyst or nodule may cause the sudden onset of localized pain and swelling. Examination of a diffuse goiter reveals a symmetrically enlarged, nontender, generally soft gland without palpable nodules. Goiter is defined, somewhat arbitrarily, as a lateral lobe with a volume greater than the thumb of the individual being examined. If the thyroid is markedly enlarged, it can cause tracheal or esophageal compression. These features are unusual, however, in the absence of nodular disease and fibrosis. *Substernal goiter* may obstruct the thoracic inlet. *Pemberton's sign* refers to symptoms of faintness with evidence of facial congestion and external jugular venous obstruction when the arms are raised above the head, a maneuver that draws the thyroid into the thoracic inlet. Respiratory flow measurements and CT or MRI should be used to evaluate substernal goiter in patients with obstructive signs or symptoms.

Thyroid function tests should be performed in all patients with goiter to exclude thyrotoxicosis or hypothyroidism. It is not unusual, particularly in iodine deficiency, to find a low total T_4, with normal T_3 and TSH, reflecting enhanced $T_4 \rightarrow T_3$ conversion. A low TSH with a normal free T_3 and free T_4, particularly in older patients, suggests the possibility of thyroid autonomy or undiagnosed Graves' disease, and is termed *subclinical thyrotoxicosis*. The benefit of treatment (typically with radioiodine) in subclinical thyrotoxicosis, versus follow-up and implementing treatment if free T_3 or free T_4 levels become abnormal, is unclear, but treatment is increasingly recommended in the elderly to reduce the risk of atrial fibrillation and bone loss. TPO antibodies may be useful to identify patients at increased risk of autoimmune thyroid disease. Low urinary iodine levels (<10 μg/dL) support a diagnosis of iodine deficiency. Thyroid scanning is not generally necessary but will reveal increased uptake in iodine deficiency and most cases of dyshormonogenesis. Ultrasound is not generally indicated in the evaluation of diffuse goiter unless a nodule is palpable on physical examination.

TREATMENT Diffuse Nontoxic (Simple) Goiter

Iodine or thyroid hormone replacement induces variable regression of goiter in iodine deficiency, depending on how long it has been present and the degree of fibrosis that has developed. Because of the possibility of underlying thyroid autonomy, caution should be exercised when instituting suppressive thyroxine therapy in patients with goiter, particularly if the baseline TSH is in the low to normal range. In younger patients, the dose of levothyroxine can be started at 100 mcg/d and adjusted to suppress the TSH into the low to normal, but detectable, range. Treatment of elderly patients should be initiated at 50 mcg/d. The efficacy of suppressive treatment is greater in younger patients and for those with soft goiters. Significant regression is usually seen within 3–6 months of treatment; after this time, it is unlikely to occur. In older patients and in those with some degree of nodular disease or fibrosis, fewer than one-third demonstrate significant shrinkage of the goiter. Surgery is rarely indicated for diffuse goiter. Exceptions include documented evidence of tracheal compression or obstruction of the thoracic outlet, which are more likely to be associated with substernal multinodular goiters (see below). Subtotal or near-total thyroidectomy for these or cosmetic reasons should be performed by an experienced surgeon to minimize complication rates. Surgery should be followed by replacement with levothyroxine, with the aim of keeping the TSH level at the lower end of the reference range to prevent regrowth of the goiter. Radioiodine reduces goiter size by about 50% in the majority of patients over 6–12 months. It is rarely associated with transient acute swelling of the thyroid, which is usually inconsequential unless there is severe tracheal narrowing. If they are not treated with levothyroxine, patients should be followed after radioiodine treatment for the possible development of hypothyroidism.

■ NONTOXIC MULTINODULAR GOITER

Etiology and pathogenesis

Depending on the population studied, MNG occurs in up to 12% of adults. MNG is more common in women than men and increases in prevalence with age. It is more common in iodine-deficient regions but also occurs in regions of iodine sufficiency, reflecting multiple genetic, autoimmune, and environmental influences on the pathogenesis.

There is typically wide variation in nodule size. Histology reveals a spectrum of morphologies ranging from hypercellular regions to cystic areas filled with colloid. Fibrosis is often extensive, and areas of hemorrhage or lymphocytic infiltration may be seen. Using molecular techniques, most nodules within a MNG are polyclonal in origin, suggesting a hyperplastic response to locally produced growth factors and cytokines. TSH, which is usually not elevated, may play a permissive or contributory role. Monoclonal lesions also occur within a MNG, reflecting mutations in genes that confer a selective growth advantage to the progenitor cell.

Clinical manifestations

Most patients with nontoxic MNG are asymptomatic and euthyroid. MNG typically develops over many years and is detected on routine physical examination or when an individual notices an enlargement in the neck. If the goiter is large enough, it can ultimately lead to compressive symptoms including difficulty swallowing, respiratory distress (tracheal compression), or plethora (venous congestion); but these symptoms are uncommon. Symptomatic MNGs are usually extraordinarily large and/or develop fibrotic areas that cause compression. Sudden pain in a MNG is usually caused by hemorrhage into a nodule but should raise the possibility of invasive malignancy. Hoarseness, reflecting laryngeal nerve involvement, also suggests malignancy.

Diagnosis

On examination, thyroid architecture is distorted, and multiple nodules of varying size can be appreciated. Because many nodules are deeply embedded in thyroid tissue or reside in posterior or substernal locations, it is not possible to palpate all nodules. A TSH level should be measured to exclude subclinical hyper- or hypothyroidism, but thyroid function is usually normal. Tracheal deviation is common, but compression must usually exceed 70% of the tracheal diameter before there is significant airway compromise. Pulmonary function testing can be used to assess the functional effects of compression and to detect tracheomalacia, which characteristically causes inspiratory stridor. CT or MRI can be used to evaluate the anatomy of the goiter and the extent of substernal extension, which is often much greater than is apparent on physical examination. A barium swallow may reveal the extent of esophageal compression. The risk of malignancy in MNG is similar to that in solitary nodules. Ultrasonography can be used to identify which nodules should be biopsied, including large, dominant nodules or those with sonographic characteristics suggestive of malignancy (e.g., microcalcifications, hypoechogenicity, increased vascularity).

TREATMENT Nontoxic Multinodular Goiter

Most nontoxic MNGs can be managed conservatively. T_4 suppression is rarely effective for reducing goiter size and introduces the risk of subclinical or overt thyrotoxicosis, particularly if there is underlying autonomy or if it develops during treatment. If levothyroxine is used, it should be started at low doses (50 μg) and advanced gradually while monitoring the TSH level to avoid excessive suppression. Contrast agents and other iodine-containing substances should be avoided because of the risk of inducing the *Jod-Basedow effect*, characterized by enhanced thyroid hormone production by autonomous nodules. Radioiodine is used with increasing frequency because it can decrease goiter size and may selectively ablate regions of autonomy. Dosage of ^{131}I depends on the size of the goiter and radioiodine uptake but is usually about 3.7 MBq (0.1 mCi) per gram of tissue, corrected for uptake [typical dose 370–1070 MBq (10 to 29 mCi)]. Repeat treatment may be needed and effectiveness may be increased by concurrent administration of recombinant TSH. It is possible to achieve a 40–50% reduction in goiter size in most patients. Earlier concerns about radiation-induced thyroid swelling and tracheal compression have diminished; studies have shown this complication to be rare. When acute compression occurs, glucocorticoid treatment or surgery may be needed. Radiation-induced hypothyroidism is less common than after treatment for Graves' disease. However, posttreatment autoimmune thyrotoxicosis may occur in up to 5% of patients treated for nontoxic MNG. Surgery remains highly effective but is not without risk, particularly in older patients with underlying cardiopulmonary disease.

TOXIC MULTINODULAR GOITER

The pathogenesis of toxic MNG appears to be similar to that of nontoxic MNG; the major difference is the presence of functional autonomy in toxic MNG. The molecular basis for autonomy in toxic MNG remains unknown. As in nontoxic goiters, many nodules are polyclonal, while others are monoclonal and vary in their clonal origins. Genetic abnormalities known to confer functional autonomy, such as activating TSH-R or $G_s\alpha$ mutations (see below), are not usually found in the autonomous regions of toxic MNG goiter.

In addition to features of goiter, the clinical presentation of toxic MNG includes subclinical hyperthyroidism or mild thyrotoxicosis. The patient is usually elderly and may present with atrial fibrillation or palpitations, tachycardia, nervousness, tremor, or weight loss. Recent exposure to iodine, from contrast dyes or other sources, may precipitate or exacerbate thyrotoxicosis. The TSH level is low. The T_4 level may be normal or minimally increased; T_3 is often elevated to a greater degree than T_4. Thyroid scan shows heterogeneous uptake with multiple regions of increased and decreased uptake; 24-hour uptake of radioiodine may not be increased.

TREATMENT Toxic Multinodular Goiter

The management of toxic MNG is challenging. Antithyroid drugs, often in combination with beta blockers, can normalize thyroid function and address clinical features of thyrotoxicosis. This treatment, however, often stimulates the growth of the goiter, and in contrast to Graves' disease, spontaneous remission does not occur. Radioiodine can be used to treat areas of autonomy as well as to decrease the mass of the goiter. Usually, however, some degree of autonomy remains, presumably because multiple autonomous regions emerge as soon as others are treated. Nonetheless, a trial of radioiodine should be considered before subjecting patients, many of whom are elderly, to surgery. Surgery provides definitive treatment of underlying thyrotoxicosis as well as goiter. Patients should be rendered euthyroid using an antithyroid drug before operation.

HYPERFUNCTIONING SOLITARY NODULE

A solitary, autonomously functioning thyroid nodule is referred to as *toxic adenoma*. The pathogenesis of this disorder has been unraveled by demonstrating the functional effects of mutations that stimulate the TSH-R signaling pathway. Most patients with solitary hyperfunctioning nodules have acquired somatic, activating mutations in the TSH-R (Fig. 341-10). These mutations, located primarily in the receptor transmembrane domain, induce constitutive receptor coupling to $G_{S\alpha}$, increasing cyclic AMP levels and leading to enhanced thyroid follicular cell proliferation and function. Less commonly, somatic mutations are identified in $G_{S\alpha}$. These mutations, which are similar to those seen in McCune-Albright syndrome (Chap. 347) or in a subset of somatotrope adenomas (Chap. 339), impair GTP hydrolysis, also causing constitutive activation of the cyclic AMP signaling pathway. In most series, activating mutations in either the TSH-R or the $G_{S\alpha}$ subunit genes are identified in >90% of patients with solitary hyperfunctioning nodules.

Thyrotoxicosis is usually mild. The disorder is suggested by the presence of the thyroid nodule, which is generally large enough to be palpable, and by the absence of clinical features suggestive of Graves' disease or other causes of thyrotoxicosis. A thyroid scan

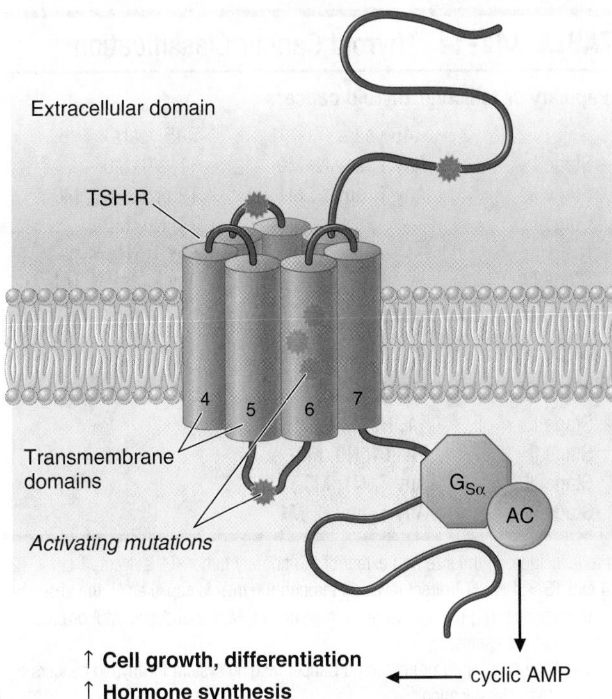

Figure 341-10 Activating mutations of the TSH-R. Mutations (*) that activate the thyroid-stimulating hormone receptor (TSH-R) reside mainly in transmembrane 5 and intracellular loop 3, though mutations have occurred in a variety of different locations. The effect of these mutations is to induce conformational changes that mimic TSH binding, thereby leading to coupling to stimulatory G protein ($G_{S\alpha}$) and activation of adenylate cyclase (AC), an enzyme that generates cyclic AMP.

provides a definitive diagnostic test, demonstrating focal uptake in the hyperfunctioning nodule and diminished uptake in the remainder of the gland, as activity of the normal thyroid is suppressed.

TREATMENT Hyperfunctioning Solitary Nodule

Radioiodine ablation is usually the treatment of choice. Because normal thyroid function is suppressed, ^{131}I is concentrated in the hyperfunctioning nodule with minimal uptake and damage to normal thyroid tissue. Relatively large radioiodine doses [e.g., 370–1110 MBq (10–29.9 mCi)^{131}I] have been shown to correct thyrotoxicosis in about 75% of patients within 3 months. Hypothyroidism occurs in <10% of those patients over the next 5 years. Surgical resection is also effective and is usually limited to enucleation of the adenoma or lobectomy, thereby preserving thyroid function and minimizing risk of hypoparathyroidism or damage to the recurrent laryngeal nerves. Medical therapy using antithyroid drugs and beta blockers can normalize thyroid function but is not an optimal long-term treatment. Using ultrasound guidance, repeated ethanol injections, or percutaneous radiofrequency thermal ablation have been used successfully in some centers to ablate hyperfunctioning nodules, and these techniques have also been used to reduce the size of nonfunctioning thyroid nodules.

BENIGN NEOPLASMS

The various types of benign thyroid nodules are listed in Table 341-9. These lesions are common (5–10% adults), particularly when assessed by sensitive techniques such as ultrasound. The risk of malignancy is

TABLE 341-9 Classification of Thyroid Neoplasms

Benign	
Follicular epithelial cell adenomas	
Macrofollicular (colloid)	
Normofollicular (simple)	
Microfollicular (fetal)	
Trabecular (embryonal)	
Hürthle cell variant (oncocytic)	
Malignant	**Approximate Prevalence, %**
Follicular epithelial cell	
Well-differentiated carcinomas	
Papillary carcinomas	80–90
Pure papillary	
Follicular variant	
Diffuse sclerosing variant	
Tall cell, columnar cell variants	
Follicular carcinomas	5–10
Minimally invasive	
Widely invasive	
Hürthle cell carcinoma (oncocytic)	
Insular carcinoma	
Undifferentiated (anaplastic) carcinomas	
C cell (calcitonin-producing)	
Medullary thyroid cancer	<10
Sporadic	
Familial	
MEN 2	
Other malignancies	
Lymphomas	1–2
Sarcomas	
Metastases	
Others	

Note: MEN, multiple endocrine neoplasia.

very low for *macrofollicular adenomas* and *normofollicular adenomas. Microfollicular, trabecular, and Hürthle cell variants* raise greater concern, and the histology is more difficult to interpret. About one-third of palpable nodules are *thyroid cysts.* These may be recognized by their ultrasound appearance or based on aspiration of large amounts of pink or straw-colored fluid (colloid). Many are mixed cystic/solid lesions, in which case it is desirable to aspirate cellular components under ultrasound or harvest cells after cytospin of cyst fluid. Cysts frequently recur, even after repeated aspiration, and may require surgical excision if they are large or if the cytology is suspicious. Sclerosis has been used with variable success but is often painful and may be complicated by infiltration of the sclerosing agent.

The treatment approach for benign nodules is similar to that for MNG. TSH suppression with levothyroxine decreases the size of about 30% of nodules and may prevent further growth. If a nodule has not decreased in size after 6–12 months of suppressive therapy, treatment should be discontinued because little benefit is likely to accrue from long-term treatment; the risk of iatrogenic subclinical thyrotoxicosis should also be considered.

THYROID CANCER

Thyroid carcinoma is the most common malignancy of the endocrine system. Malignant tumors derived from the follicular epithelium are classified according to histologic features. Differentiated tumors, such as papillary thyroid cancer (PTC) or follicular thyroid

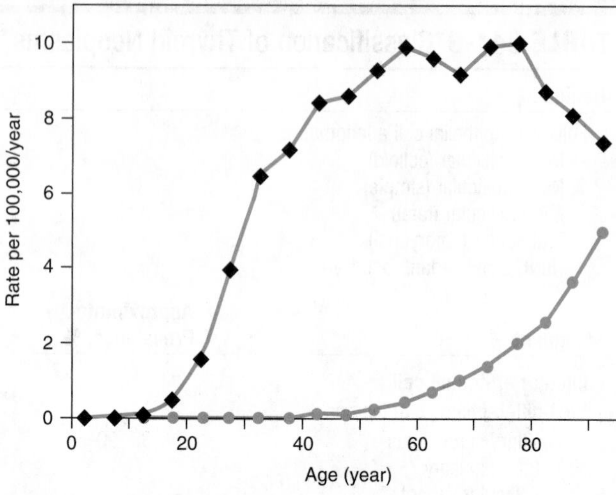

Figure 341-11 Age-associated incidence (—◆—) and mortality (—●—) rates for invasive thyroid cancer. *[Adapted from LAG Ries et al (eds): SEER Cancer Statistics Review, 1973–1996, Bethesda, National Cancer Institute, 1999.]*

cancer (FTC), are often curable, and the prognosis is good for patients identified with early-stage disease. In contrast, anaplastic thyroid cancer (ATC) is aggressive, responds poorly to treatment, and is associated with a bleak prognosis.

The incidence of thyroid cancer (~9/100,000 per year) increases with age, plateauing after about age 50 (Fig. 341-11). Age is also an important prognostic factor—thyroid cancer at a young age (<20) or in older persons (>45) is associated with a worse prognosis. Thyroid cancer is twice as common in women as men, but male gender is associated with a worse prognosis. Additional important risk factors include a history of childhood head or neck irradiation, large nodule size (≥4 cm), evidence for local tumor fixation or invasion into lymph nodes, and the presence of metastases (Table 341-10). Several unique features of thyroid cancer facilitate its management: (1) thyroid nodules are readily palpable, allowing early detection and biopsy by FNA; (2) iodine radioisotopes can be used to diagnose (^{123}I) and treat (^{131}I) differentiated thyroid cancer, reflecting the unique uptake of this anion by the thyroid gland; and (3) serum markers allow the detection of residual or recurrent disease, including the use of Tg levels for PTC and FTC and calcitonin for medullary thyroid cancer (MTC).

CLASSIFICATION

Thyroid neoplasms can arise in each of the cell types that populate the gland, including thyroid follicular cells, calcitonin-producing C cells, lymphocytes, and stromal and vascular elements, as well as metastases from other sites (Table 341-9). The American Joint Committee on Cancer (AJCC) has designated a staging system using the TNM classification (Table 341-11). Several other classification and staging systems are also widely used, some of which place greater emphasis on histologic features or risk factors such as age or gender.

TABLE 341-10 Risk Factors for Thyroid Carcinoma in Patients With Thyroid Nodule

History of head and neck irradiation	Family history of thyroid cancer or MEN 2
Age <20 or >45 years	Vocal cord paralysis, hoarse voice
Bilateral disease	Nodule fixed to adjacent structures
Increased nodule size (>4 cm)	Extrathyroidal extension
New or enlarging neck mass	Suspected lymph node involvement
Male gender	Iodine deficiency (follicular cancer)

Abbreviation: MEN, multiple endocrine neoplasia.

TABLE 341-11 Thyroid Cancer Classification[a]

Papillary or follicular thyroid cancers		
	<45 years	>45 years
Stage I	Any T, any N, M0	T1, N0, M0
Stage II	Any T, any N, M1	T2 or T3, N0, M0
Stage III	—	T4, N0, M0 Any T, N1, M0
Stage IV	—	Any T, any N, M1
Anaplastic thyroid cancer		
Stage IV	All cases are stage IV	
Medullary thyroid cancer		
Stage I	T1, N0, M0	
Stage II	T2–T4, N0, M0	
Stage III	Any T, N1, M0	
Stage IV	Any T, any N, M1	

[a]Criteria include: T, the size and extent of the primary tumor (T1 ≤ 1 cm; 1 cm < T2 ≤ 4 cm; T3 > 4 cm; T4 direct invasion through the thyroid capsule); N, the absence (N0) or presence (N1) of regional node involvement; M, the absence (M0) or presence (M1) of metastases.

Source: American Joint Committee on Cancer staging system for thyroid cancers using the TNM classification.

PATHOGENESIS AND GENETIC BASIS

Radiation

Early studies of the pathogenesis of thyroid cancer focused on the role of external radiation, which predisposes to chromosomal breaks, leading to genetic rearrangements and loss of tumor-suppressor genes. External radiation of the mediastinum, face, head, and neck region was administered in the past to treat an array of conditions, including acne and enlargement of the thymus, tonsils, and adenoids. Radiation exposure increases the risk of benign and malignant thyroid nodules, is associated with multicentric cancers, and shifts the incidence of thyroid cancer to an earlier age group. Radiation from nuclear fallout also increases the risk of thyroid cancer. Children seem more predisposed to the effects of radiation than adults. Of note, radiation derived from ^{131}I therapy appears to contribute minimal increased risk of thyroid cancer.

TSH and growth factors

Many differentiated thyroid cancers express TSH receptors and, therefore, remain responsive to TSH. This observation provides the rationale for T_4 suppression of TSH in patients with thyroid cancer. Residual expression of TSH receptors also allows TSH-stimulated uptake of ^{131}I therapy (see below).

Oncogenes and tumor-suppressor genes

Thyroid cancers are monoclonal in origin, consistent with the idea that they originate as a consequence of mutations that confer a growth advantage to a single cell. In addition to increased rates of proliferation, some thyroid cancers exhibit impaired apoptosis and features that enhance invasion, angiogenesis, and metastasis. Thyroid neoplasms have been analyzed for a variety of genetic alterations, but without clear evidence of an ordered acquisition of somatic mutations as they progress from the benign to the malignant state. On the other hand, certain mutations are relatively specific for thyroid neoplasia, some of which correlate with histologic classification (Table 341-12).

As described above, activating mutations of the TSH-R and the $G_{S\alpha}$ subunit are associated with autonomously functioning nodules. Though these mutations induce thyroid cell growth, this type of nodule is almost always benign.

Activation of the RET-RAS-BRAF signaling pathway is seen in most PTCs, though the types of mutations are heterogeneous. A variety of rearrangements involving the *RET* gene on chromosome 10 brings this receptor tyrosine kinase under the control of other promoters, leading to receptor overexpression. *RET* rearrangements occur in 20–40% of PTCs in different series and were observed with increased frequency in tumors developing after the Chernobyl radiation accident. Rearrangements in PTC have also been observed for another tyrosine kinase gene, *TRK1*, which is located on chromosome 1. To date, the identification of PTC with *RET* or *TRK1* rearrangements has not proven useful for predicting

TABLE 341-12 Genetic Alterations in Thyroid Neoplasia

Gene/Protein	Type of Gene	Chromosomal Location	Genetic Abnormality	Tumor
TSH receptor	GPCR receptor	14q31	Point mutations	Toxic adenoma, differentiated carcinomas
$G_{S\alpha}$	G protein	20q13.2	Point mutations	Toxic adenoma, differentiated carcinomas
RET/PTC	Receptor tyrosine kinase	10q11.2	Rearrangements PTC1: (inv(10)q11.2q21) PTC2: (t(10;17)(q11.2;q23)) PTC3: ELE1/TK	PTC
RET	Receptor tyrosine kinase	10q11.2	Point mutations	MEN 2, medullary thyroid cancer
BRAF	MEK kinase	7q24	Point mutations, rearrangements	PTC, ATC
TRK	Receptor tyrosine kinase	1q23-24	Rearrangements	Multinodular goiter, papillary thyroid cancer
RAS	Signal transducing p21	Hras 11p15.5Kras 12p12.1; Nras 1p13.2	Point mutations	Differentiated thyroid carcinoma, adenomas
p53	Tumor suppressor, cell cycle control, apoptosis	17p13	Point mutations Deletion, insertion	Anaplastic cancer
APC	Tumor suppressor, adenomatous polyposis coli gene	5q21-q22	Point mutations	Anaplastic cancer, also associated with familial polyposis coli
p16 (MTS1, CDKN2A)	Tumor suppressor, cell cycle control	9p21	Deletions	Differentiated carcinomas
p21/WAF	Tumor suppressor, cell cycle control	6p21.2	Overexpression	Anaplastic cancer
MET	Receptor tyrosine kinase	7q31	Overexpression	Follicular thyroid cancer
c-MYC	Receptor tyrosine kinase	8q24.12.-13	Overexpression	Differentiated carcinoma
PTEN	Phosphatase	10q23	Point mutations	PTC in Cowden's syndrome (multiple hamartomas, breast tumors, gastrointestinal polyps, thyroid tumors)
CTNNB1	β-Catenin	3p22	Point mutations	Anaplastic cancer
Loss of heterozygosity (LOH)	?Tumor suppressors	3p; 11q13, other loci	Deletions	Differentiated thyroid carcinomas, anaplastic cancer
PAX8-PPARγ 1	Transcription factor Nuclear receptor fusion	t(2;3)(q13;p25)	Translocation	Follicular adenoma or carcinoma

Abbreviations: TSH, thyroid-stimulating hormone; $G_{S\alpha}$, G-protein stimulating α-subunit; RET, rearranged during transfection proto-oncogene; PTC, papillary thyroid cancer; TRK, tyrosine kinase receptor; RAS, rat sarcoma proto-oncogene; p53, p53 tumor suppressor gene; MET, met proto-oncogene (hepatocyte growth factor receptor); c-MYC, cellular homologue of myelocytomatosis virus proto-oncogene; PTEN, phosphatase and tensin homologue; APC, adenomatous polyposis coli; MTS, multiple tumor suppressor; CDKN2A, cyclin-dependent kinase inhibitor 2A; P21, p21 tumor suppressor; WAF, wild-type p53 activated fragment; GPCR, G protein–coupled receptor; ELE1/TK, RET-activating gene ele1/tyrosine kinase; MEN 2, multiple endocrine neoplasia-2; PAX8, paired domain transcription factor; PPARγ1, peroxisome-proliferator activated receptor γ1; BRAF, v-raf homologue, B1; MEK, mitogen extracellular signal-regulated kinase.

Source: Adapted with permission from P Kopp, JL Jameson, in JL Jameson (ed): *Principles of Molecular Medicine.* Totowa, NJ, Humana Press, 1998.

prognosis or treatment responses. *BRAF* mutations appear to be the most common genetic alteration in PTC. These mutations activate the kinase, which stimulates the mitogen-activated protein MAP kinase (MAPK) cascade. *RAS* mutations, which also stimulate the MAPK cascade, are found in about 20–30% of thyroid neoplasms, including both PTC and FTC. Of note, simultaneous *RET*, *BRAF*, and *RAS* mutations do not occur in the same tumor, suggesting that activation of the MAPK cascade is critical for tumor development, independent of the step that initiates the cascade.

RAS mutations also occur in FTCs. In addition, a rearrangement of the thyroid developmental transcription factor PAX8 with the nuclear receptor PPARγ is identified in a significant fraction of FTCs. Loss of heterozygosity of 3p or 11q, consistent with deletions of tumor-suppressor genes, is also common in FTCs.

Most of the mutations seen in differentiated thyroid cancers have also been detected in ATCs. *BRAF* mutations are seen in up to 50% of ATCs. Mutations in CTNNB1, which encodes β-catenin, occur in about two-thirds of ATCs, but not in PTC or FTC. Mutations of the tumor suppressor p53 also play an important role in the development of ATC. Because p53 plays a role in cell cycle surveillance, DNA repair, and apoptosis, its loss may contribute to the rapid acquisition of genetic instability as well as poor treatment responses (Chap. 84) (Table 341-12).

The role of molecular diagnostics in the clinical management of thyroid cancer is under investigation. In principle, analyses of specific mutations might aid in classification, prognosis, or choice of treatment. However, there is no clear evidence to date that this information alters clinical decision making.

MTC, when associated with multiple endocrine neoplasia (MEN) type 2, harbors an inherited mutation of the *RET* gene. Unlike the rearrangements of *RET* seen in PTC, the mutations in MEN2 are point mutations that induce constitutive activity of the tyrosine kinase (Chap. 351). MTC is preceded by hyperplasia of the C cells, raising the likelihood that as-yet-unidentified "second hits" lead to cellular transformation. A subset of sporadic MTC contain somatic mutations that activate *RET*.

WELL-DIFFERENTIATED THYROID CANCER

Papillary

PTC is the most common type of thyroid cancer, accounting for 70–90% of well-differentiated thyroid malignancies. Microscopic PTC is present in up to 25% of thyroid glands at autopsy, but most of these lesions are very small (several millimeters) and are not clinically significant. Characteristic cytologic features of PTC help make the diagnosis by FNA or after surgical resection; these include psammoma bodies, cleaved nuclei with an "orphan-Annie" appearance caused by large nucleoli, and the formation of papillary structures.

PTC tends to be multifocal and to invade locally within the thyroid gland as well as through the thyroid capsule and into adjacent structures in the neck. It has a propensity to spread via the lymphatic system but can metastasize hematogenously as well, particularly to bone and lung. Because of the relatively slow growth of the tumor, a significant burden of pulmonary metastases may accumulate, sometimes with remarkably few symptoms. The prognostic implication of lymph node spread is debated. Lymph node involvement by thyroid cancer can be well tolerated but appears to increase the risk of recurrence and mortality, particularly in older patients. The staging of PTC by the TNM system is outlined in Table 341-11. Most papillary cancers are identified in the early stages (>80% stages I or II) and have an excellent prognosis, with survival curves similar to expected survival (Fig. 341-12*A*). Mortality is markedly increased in stage IV disease (distant metastases), but this group comprises only about 1% of patients. The treatment of PTC is described below.

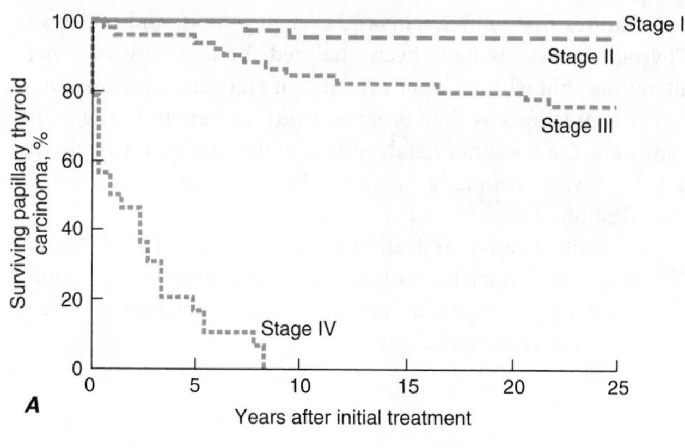

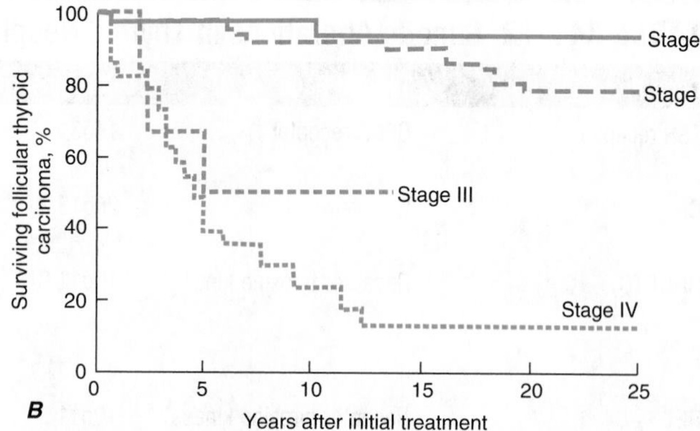

Figure 341-12 Survival rates in patients with differentiated thyroid cancer. ***A.*** Papillary cancer, cohort of 1851 patients. I, 1107 (60%); II, 408 (22%); III, 312 (17%); IV, 24 (1%); $n = 1185$. ***B.*** Follicular cancer, cohort of 153 patients. I, 42 (27%); II, 82 (54%); III, 6 (4%); IV, 23 (15%); $n = 153$. *[Adapted from PR Larsen et al: William's Textbook of Endocrinology, 9th ed, JD Wilson et al (eds). Philadelphia, Saunders, 1998, pp 389–575, with permission.]*

Follicular

The incidence of FTC varies widely in different parts of the world; it is more common in iodine-deficient regions. FTC is difficult to diagnose by FNA because the distinction between benign and malignant follicular neoplasms rests largely on evidence of invasion into vessels, nerves, or adjacent structures. FTC tends to spread by hematogenous routes leading to bone, lung, and central nervous system metastases. Mortality rates associated with FTC are less favorable than for PTC, in part because a larger proportion of patients present with stage IV disease (Fig. 341-12*B*). Poor prognostic features include distant metastases, age >50 years, primary tumor size >4 cm, Hürthle cell histology, and the presence of marked vascular invasion.

TREATMENT Well-Differentiated Thyroid Cancer

SURGERY All well-differentiated thyroid cancers should be surgically excised. In addition to removing the primary lesion, surgery allows accurate histologic diagnosis and staging, and multicentric disease is commonly found in the contralateral thyroid lobe. Lymph node spread can also be assessed at the time of surgery, and involved nodes can be removed. Recommendations about the extent of surgery vary for stage I disease, as survival rates are similar for lobectomy and near-total thyroidectomy. Lobectomy is associated with a lower incidence of hypoparathyroidism and injury to the recurrent laryngeal nerves. However, it is not possible to monitor Tg levels or to perform whole-body ^{131}I scans in the presence of the residual lobe. Moreover, if final staging or subsequent follow-up indicates the need for radioiodine scanning or treatment, repeat surgery is necessary to remove the remaining thyroid tissue. Therefore, near-total thyroidectomy is preferable in almost all patients; complication rates are acceptably low if the surgeon is highly experienced in the procedure. Postsurgical radioablation of the remnant thyroid tissue is increasingly being used because it may destroy remaining or multifocal thyroid carcinoma, and it facilitates the use of Tg determinations and radioiodine scanning for long-term follow-up by eliminating residual normal or neoplastic tissue.

TSH SUPPRESSION THERAPY As most tumors are still TSH-responsive, levothyroxine suppression of TSH is a mainstay of thyroid cancer treatment. Though TSH suppression clearly provides therapeutic benefit, there are no prospective studies that identify the optimal level of TSH suppression. A reasonable goal is to suppress TSH as much as possible without subjecting the patient to unnecessary side effects from excess thyroid hormone, such as atrial fibrillation, osteopenia, anxiety, and other manifestations of thyrotoxicosis. For patients at low risk of recurrence, TSH should be suppressed into the low but detectable range (0.1–0.5 mIU/L). For patients at high risk of recurrence or with known metastatic disease, complete TSH suppression is indicated if there are no strong contraindications to mild thyrotoxicosis. In this instance, unbound T_4 must also be monitored to avoid excessive treatment.

RADIOIODINE TREATMENT Well-differentiated thyroid cancer still incorporates radioiodine, though less efficiently than normal thyroid follicular cells. Radioiodine uptake is determined primarily by expression of the NIS and is stimulated by TSH, requiring expression of the TSH-R. The retention time for radioactivity is influenced by the extent to which the tumor retains differentiated functions such as iodide trapping and organification. After near-total thyroidectomy, substantial thyroid tissue often remains, particularly in the thyroid bed and surrounding the parathyroid glands. Consequently, ^{131}I ablation is necessary to eliminate remaining normal thyroid tissue and to treat residual tumor cells.

Indications The use of therapeutic doses of radioiodine remains an area of controversy in thyroid cancer management. However, postoperative thyroid ablation and radioiodine treatment of known residual PTC or FTC clearly reduces recurrence rates but has a smaller impact on mortality, particularly in patients at relatively low risk. This low-risk group includes most patients with stage 1 PTC with primary tumors <1.5 cm in size. For patients with larger papillary tumors, spread to the adjacent lymph nodes, FTC, or evidence of metastases, thyroid ablation and radioiodine treatment are generally indicated.

^{131}I Thyroid Ablation and Treatment As noted above, the decision to use ^{131}I for thyroid ablation should be coordinated with the surgical approach, as radioablation is much more effective when there is minimal remaining normal thyroid tissue. A typical strategy is to treat the patient for several weeks postoperatively with liothyronine (25 μg bid or tid), followed by thyroid hormone withdrawal. Ideally, the TSH level should increase to >50 mU/L over 3–4 weeks. The level to which TSH rises is dictated largely by the amount of normal thyroid tissue remaining postoperatively. Recombinant human TSH (rhTSH) has also been used to enhance ^{131}I uptake for postsurgical ablation. It appears to be at least as effective as thyroid hormone withdrawal and should be particularly useful as residual thyroid tissue prevents an adequate endogenous TSH rise.

A pretreatment scanning dose of ^{131}I [usually 111–185 MBq (3–5 mCi)] can reveal the amount of residual tissue and provides guidance about the dose needed to accomplish ablation. However, because of concerns about radioactive "stunning" that impairs subsequent treatment, there is a trend to avoid pretreatment scanning and to proceed directly to ablation, unless there is suspicion that the amount of residual tissue will alter therapy. A maximum outpatient ^{131}I dose is 1110 MBq (29.9 mCi) in the United States, though ablation is often more complete using greater doses [1850–3700 MBq (50–100 mCi)]. Patients should be placed on a low-iodine diet (<50 μg/d urinary iodine) to increase radioiodine uptake. In patients with known residual cancer, the larger doses ensure thyroid ablation and may destroy remaining tumor cells. A whole-body scan following the high-dose radioiodine treatment is useful to identify possible metastatic disease.

Follow-Up Whole-Body Thyroid Scanning and Thyroglobulin Determinations An initial whole-body scan should be performed about 6 months after thyroid ablation. The strategy for follow-up management of thyroid cancer has been altered by the availability of rhTSH to stimulate ^{131}I uptake and by the improved sensitivity of Tg assays to detect residual or recurrent disease. A scheme for using either rhTSH or thyroid hormone withdrawal for thyroid scanning is summarized in Fig. 341-13. After thyroid ablation, rhTSH can be used in follow-up to stimulate Tg and ^{131}I uptake without subjecting patients to thyroid hormone withdrawal and its associated symptoms of hypothyroidism as well as the risk of tumor growth after prolonged TSH stimulation. Alternatively, in patients who are likely to require ^{131}I treatment, the traditional approach of thyroid hormone withdrawal can be used to increase TSH. This involves switching patients from

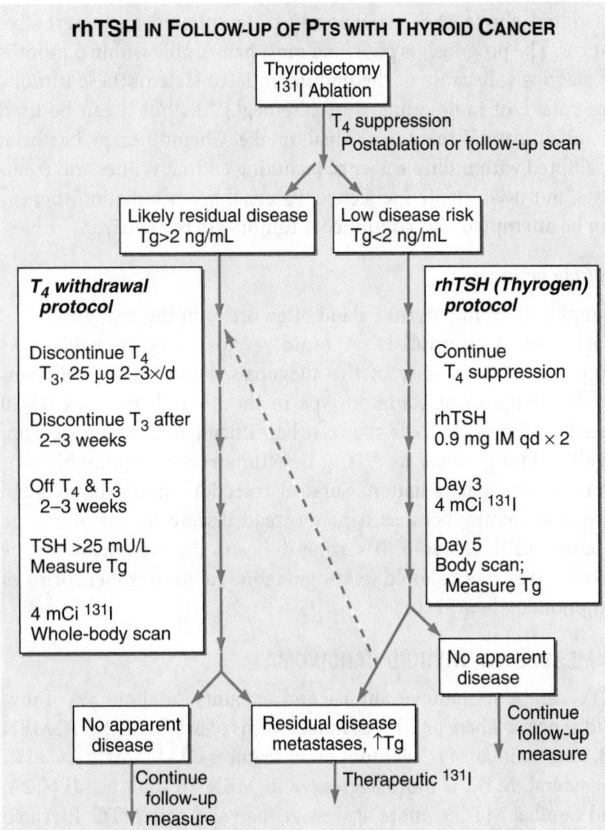

Figure 341-13 **Use of recombinant human thyroid-stimulating hormone (TSH) in the follow-up of patients with thyroid cancer.** Tg, thyroglobulin; rhTSH, recombinant human TSH.

levothyroxine (T_4) to the more rapidly cleared hormone liothyronine (T_3), thereby allowing TSH to increase more quickly. Because TSH stimulates Tg levels, Tg measurements should be obtained after administration of rhTSH or when TSH levels have risen after thyroid hormone withdrawal.

In low-risk patients who have no clinical evidence of residual disease after ablation and a basal Tg <1 ng/ml, increasing evidence supports the use of rhTSH-stimulated Tg levels one year after ablation, without the need for radioiodine scanning. If stimulated Tg levels are low (<2 ng/ml) and, ideally, undetectable, these patients can be managed with suppressive therapy and measurements of unstimulated Tg every 6–12 months. The absence of Tg antibodies should be confirmed in these patients. On the other hand, patients with residual disease on whole-body scanning or those with elevated Tg levels require additional ^{131}I therapy. In addition, most authorities advocate radioiodine treatment for scan-negative, Tg-positive (Tg >5–10 ng/mL) patients, as many derive therapeutic benefit from a large dose of ^{131}I.

In addition to radioiodine, external beam radiotherapy is also used to treat specific metastatic lesions, particularly when they cause bone pain or threaten neurologic injury (e.g., vertebral metastases).

New Potential Therapies Kinase inhibitors are being explored as a means to target pathways known to be active in thyroid cancer, including the Ras, BRAF, EGFR, VEGFR, and angiogenesis pathways. Partial responses have been seen in small trials using motesaniv, sorafenib, and other agents, but the efficacy of these agents awaits larger studies.

■ ANAPLASTIC AND OTHER FORMS OF THYROID CANCER

Anaplastic thyroid cancer

As noted above, ATC is a poorly differentiated and aggressive cancer. The prognosis is poor, and most patients die within 6 months of diagnosis. Because of the undifferentiated state of these tumors, the uptake of radioiodine is usually negligible, but it can be used therapeutically if there is residual uptake. Chemotherapy has been attempted with multiple agents, including anthracyclines and paclitaxel, but it is usually ineffective. External beam radiation therapy can be attempted and continued if tumors are responsive.

Thyroid lymphoma

Lymphoma in the thyroid gland often arises in the background of Hashimoto's thyroiditis. A rapidly expanding thyroid mass suggests the possibility of this diagnosis. Diffuse large-cell lymphoma is the most common type in the thyroid. Biopsies reveal sheets of lymphoid cells that can be difficult to distinguish from small-cell lung cancer or ATC. These tumors are often highly sensitive to external radiation. Surgical resection should be avoided as initial therapy because it may spread disease that is otherwise localized to the thyroid. If staging indicates disease outside of the thyroid, treatment should follow guidelines used for other forms of lymphoma (Chap. 110).

■ MEDULLARY THYROID CARCINOMA

MTC can be sporadic or familial and accounts for about 5% of thyroid cancers. There are three familial forms of MTC: MEN 2A, MEN 2B, and familial MTC without other features of MEN (Chap. 351). In general, MTC is more aggressive in MEN 2B than in MEN 2A, and familial MTC is more aggressive than sporadic MTC. Elevated serum calcitonin provides a marker of residual or recurrent disease. It is reasonable to test all patients with MTC for *RET* mutations, as genetic counseling and testing of family members can be offered to those individuals who test positive for mutations.

The management of MTC is primarily surgical. Unlike tumors derived from thyroid follicular cells, these tumors do not take up radioiodine. External radiation treatment and chemotherapy may provide palliation in patients with advanced disease (Chap. 351).

APPROACH TO THE PATIENT: A Thyroid Nodule

Palpable thyroid nodules are found in about 5% of adults, but the prevalence varies considerably worldwide. Given this high prevalence rate, practitioners commonly identify thyroid nodules. The main goal of this evaluation is to identify, in a cost-effective manner, the small subgroup of individuals with malignant lesions.

Nodules are more common in iodine-deficient areas, in women, and with aging. Most palpable nodules are >1 cm in diameter, but the ability to feel a nodule is influenced by its location within the gland (superficial versus deeply embedded), the anatomy of the patient's neck, and the experience of the examiner. More sensitive methods of detection, such as CT, thyroid ultrasound, and pathologic studies, reveal thyroid nodules in >20% of glands. The presence of these thyroid incidentalomas has led to much debate about how to detect nodules and which nodules to investigate further. Most authorities still rely on physical examination to detect thyroid nodules, reserving ultrasound for monitoring nodule size or as an aid in thyroid biopsy.

An approach to the evaluation of a solitary nodule is outlined in Fig. 341-14. Most patients with thyroid nodules have normal thyroid function tests. Nonetheless, thyroid function should be assessed by measuring a TSH level, which may be suppressed by one or more autonomously functioning nodules. If the TSH is suppressed, a radionuclide scan is indicated to determine if the identified nodule is "hot," as lesions with increased uptake are almost never malignant and FNA is unnecessary. Otherwise, FNA biopsy, ideally performed with ultrasound guidance, should be the first step in the evaluation of a thyroid nodule. FNA has good sensitivity and specificity when performed by physicians familiar with the procedure and when the results are interpreted by experienced cytopathologists. The technique is particularly useful for detecting PTC. The distinction of benign and malignant follicular lesions is often not possible using cytology alone.

In several large studies, FNA biopsies yielded the following findings: 70% benign, 10% malignant or suspicious for malignancy, and 20% nondiagnostic or yielding insufficient material for diagnosis. Characteristic features of malignancy mandate surgery. A diagnosis of follicular neoplasm also warrants surgery, as benign and malignant lesions cannot be distinguished based on cytopathology or frozen section. The management of patients with benign lesions is more variable. Many authorities advocate TSH suppression, whereas others monitor nodule size without suppression. With either approach, thyroid nodule size should be monitored, ideally using ultrasound. Repeat FNA is indicated if a nodule enlarges, and a second biopsy should be performed within 2–5 years to confirm the benign status of the nodule.

Nondiagnostic biopsies occur for many reasons, including a fibrotic reaction with relatively few cells available for aspiration, a cystic lesion in which cellular components reside along the cyst margin, or a nodule that may be too small for accurate aspiration. For these reasons, ultrasound-guided FNA is indicated when the FNA is repeated. Ultrasound characteristics are also useful for deciding which nodules to biopsy when multiple nodules are present. Sonographic characteristics suggestive of malignancy include microcalcifications, increased vascularity, and hypoechogenicity within the nodule.

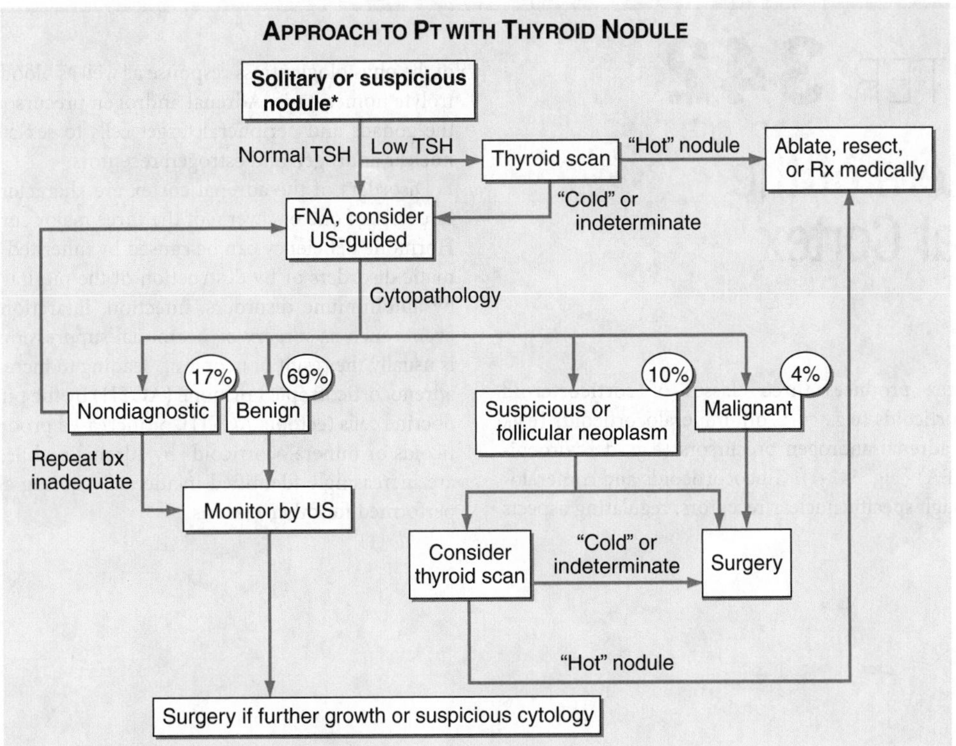

Figure 341-14 Approach to the patient with a thyroid nodule. See text and references for details. *About one-third of nodules are cystic or mixed solid-cystic. US, ultrasound; TSH, thyroid-stimulating hormone; FNA, fine-needle aspiration.

The evaluation of a thyroid nodule is stressful for most patients. They are concerned about the possibility of thyroid cancer, whether verbalized or not. It is constructive, therefore, to review the diagnostic approach and to reassure patients when no malignancy is found. When a suspicious lesion or thyroid cancer is identified, the generally favorable prognosis and available treatment options can be reassuring.

FURTHER READINGS

Abalovich M et al: Management of thyroid dysfunction during pregnancy and postpartum: An Endocrine Society Clinical Practice Guideline. J Clin Endocrinol Metab 92 (Suppl): S1, 2007

Bahn RS: Graves' ophthalmopathy. N Engl J Med 362:726, 2010

Bauer M et al: Brain glucose metabolism in hypothyroidism: a positron emission tomography study before and after thyroid hormone replacement therapy. J Clin Endocrinol Metab 94:2922, 2009

Biondi B, Cooper DS: The clinical significance of subclinical thyroid disease. Endocr Rev 29:76, 2008

———: Benefits of thyrotropin suppression versus the risks of adverse effects in differentiated thyroid cancer. Thyroid 20:135, 2010

Brent GA: Clinical practice. Graves' disease. N Engl J Med 358:2594, 2008

DeGroot LJ et al: Thyroid gland, in *Endocrinology*, 6th ed, JL Jameson, LJ DeGroot (eds). Philadelphia, Elsevier Saunders, 2009

Fagin JA, Mitsiades N: Molecular pathology of thyroid cancer: diagnostic and clinical implications. Best Pract Res Clin Endocrinol Metab. 22: 955, 2008

Hegedüs L: Treatment of Graves' hyperthyroidism: Evidence-based and emerging modalities. Endocrinol Metab Clin North Am. 38:355, 2009

Sherman SI et al: Motesanib diphosphate in progressive differentiated thyroid cancer. N Engl J Med 359:31, 2008

Stagnaro-Green A: Maternal thyroid disease and preterm delivery. J Clin Endocrinol Metab 94: 21, 2009

Zeitlin AA et al: Genetic developments in autoimmune thyroid disease: an evolutionary process. Clin Endocrinol 68:671, 2008

Zimmermann MB: Iodine deficiency. Endocr Rev 30:376, 2009

CHAPTER 342

Disorders of the Adrenal Cortex

Wiebke Arlt

The adrenal cortex produces three classes of corticosteroid hormones: glucocorticoids (e.g., cortisol), mineralocorticoids (e.g., aldosterone), and adrenal androgen precursors (e.g., dehydroepiandrosterone, DHEA) (Fig. 342-1). Glucocorticoids and mineralocorticoids act through specific nuclear receptors, regulating aspects of the physiologic stress response as well as blood pressure and electrolyte homeostasis. Adrenal androgen precursors are converted in the gonads and peripheral target cells to sex steroids that act via nuclear androgen and estrogen receptors.

Disorders of the adrenal cortex are characterized by deficiency or excess of one or several of the three major corticosteroid classes. Hormone deficiency can be caused by inherited glandular or enzymatic disorders or by destruction of the pituitary or adrenal gland by autoimmune disorders, infection, infarction, or by iatrogenic events such as surgery or hormonal suppression. Hormone excess is usually the result of neoplasia, leading to increased production of adrenocorticotropic hormone (ACTH) by the pituitary or neuroendocrine cells (ectopic ACTH), or increased production of glucocorticoids or mineralocorticoids by adrenal nodules. Adrenal nodules are increasingly identified incidentally during abdominal imaging performed for other reasons.

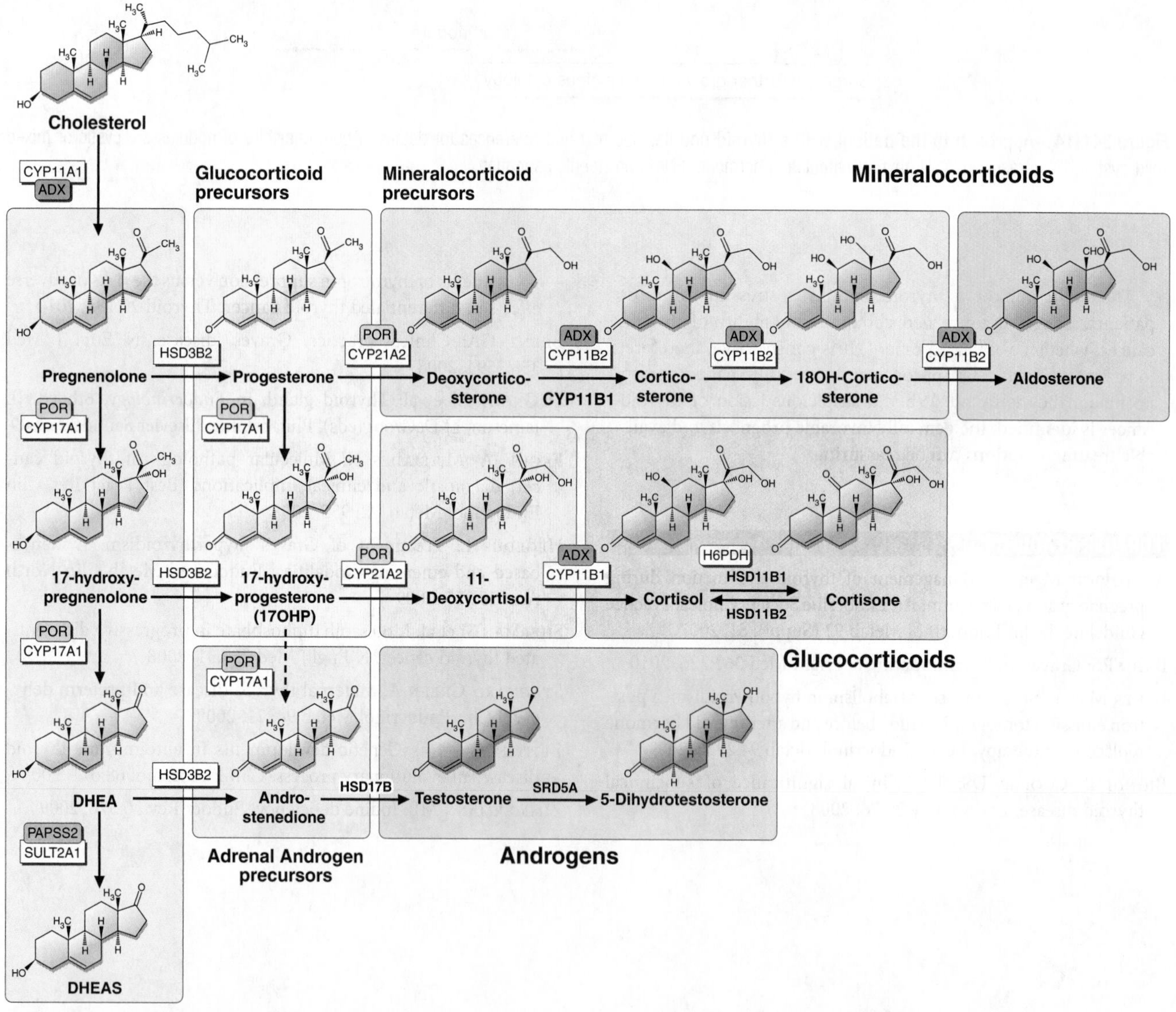

Figure 342-1 Adrenal steroidogenesis. CYP11A1, side chain cleavage enzyme; CYP17A1, 17α-hydroxylase/17,20 lyase; POR, P450 oxidoreductase; ADX, adrenodoxin; HSD3B2, 3β-hydroxysteroid dehydrogenase type 2; CYP21A2, 21-hydroxylase; CYP11B1, 11β-hydroxylase; CYP11B2, aldosterone synthase; HSD11B1, 11β-hydroxysteroid dehydrogenase type 1; HSD11B2, 11β-hydroxysteroid dehydrogenase type 2; H6PDH, hexose-6-phosphate dehydrogenase; HSD17B, 17β-hydroxysteroid dehydrogenase; SRD5A, 5α-reductase; SULT2A1, DHEA sulfotransferase; DHEA, dehydroepiandrosterone; DHEAS, dehydroepiandrosterone sulfate; PAPSS2, PAPS synthase type 2.

ADRENAL ANATOMY AND DEVELOPMENT

The normal adrenal glands weigh 6–11 g each. They are located above the kidneys and have their own blood supply. Arterial blood flows initially to the subcapsular region and then meanders from the outer cortical zona glomerulosa through the intermediate zona fasciculata to the inner zona reticularis and eventually to the adrenal medulla. The right suprarenal vein drains directly into the vena cava while the left suprarenal vein drains into the left renal vein.

During early embryonic development, the adrenals originate from the urogenital ridge and then separate from gonads and kidneys about the 6th week of gestation. Concordant with the time of sexual differentiation (seventh to ninth week of gestation, see Chap. 349), the adrenal cortex starts to produce cortisol and the adrenal sex steroid precursor DHEA. The orphan nuclear receptors SF1 (steroidogenic factor 1) and DAX1 (dosage-sensitive sex reversal gene 1), among others, play a crucial role during this period of development, as they regulate a multitude of adrenal genes involved in steroidogenesis.

REGULATORY CONTROL OF STEROIDOGENESIS

Production of glucocorticoids and adrenal androgens is under the control of the hypothalamic-pituitary-adrenal (HPA) axis, whereas mineralocorticoids are regulated by the renin-angiotensin-aldosterone (RAA) system.

Glucocorticoid synthesis is under inhibitory feedback control by the hypothalamus and the pituitary (Fig. 342-2). Hypothalamic release of corticotropin-releasing hormone (CRH) occurs in response to endogenous or exogenous stress. CRH stimulates the cleavage of the 241–amino acid polypeptide pro opiomelanocortin (POMC) by pituitary-specific prohormone convertase, yielding adrenocorticotropic hormone (ACTH). ACTH is released by the corticotrope cells of the anterior pituitary and acts as the pivotal regulator of cortisol synthesis, with additional short-term effects on mineralocorticoid and adrenal androgen synthesis. The release of CRH, and subsequently ACTH, occurs in a pulsatile fashion that follows a circadian rhythm under the control of the hypothalamus, specifically its suprachiasmatic nucleus (SCN), with additional regulation by a complex network of cell-specific clock genes. Reflecting the pattern of ACTH secretion, adrenal cortisol secretion exhibits a distinct circadian rhythm, with peak levels in the morning and low levels in the evening (Fig. 342-3).

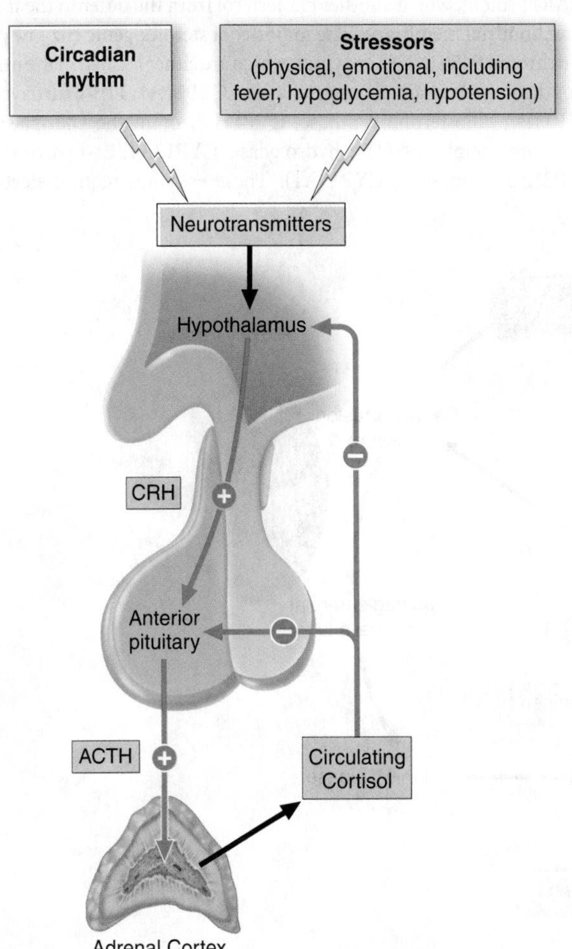

Figure 342-2 Regulation of the hypothalamic-pituitary-adrenal (HPA) axis. CRH, corticotropin-releasing hormone; ACTH, adrenocorticotropic hormone.

Diagnostic tests assessing the HPA axis make use of the fact that it is regulated by negative feedback. Glucocorticoid excess is diagnosed by employing a dexamethasone suppression test. Dexamethasone, a potent glucocorticoid, suppresses CRH/ACTH and, therefore, endogenous cortisol. Various versions of the dexamethasone suppression test are described in detail in Chap. 339. If cortisol production is autonomous (e.g., adrenal nodule), ACTH is already suppressed and dexamethasone has little additional effect. If cortisol production is driven by an ACTH-producing pituitary adenoma, dexamethasone suppression is ineffective at low doses but usually induces suppression at high doses. If cortisol production is driven by an ectopic source of ACTH, the tumors are usually resistant to dexamethasone suppression. Thus, the dexamethasone suppression test is useful to establish the diagnosis of Cushing's syndrome and to assist with the differential diagnosis of cortisol excess.

Conversely, to assess glucocorticoid deficiency, ACTH stimulation of cortisol production is used. The ACTH peptide contains 39 amino acids but the first 24 are sufficient to elicit a physiologic response. The standard ACTH stimulation test involves administration of cosyntropin (ACTH 1-24), 0.25 mg IM or IV, and collection of blood samples at 0, 30, and 60 minutes for cortisol. A normal response is defined as a cortisol level >20 μg/dL or an increment of >10 μg/dL over baseline. A low-dose (1 μg cosyntropin IV) version of this test has been advocated to avoid overstimulation of the adrenal gland. Alternatively, an insulin tolerance test (ITT) can be used to assess adrenal insufficiency. It involves injection of insulin to induce hypoglycemia, which represents a strong stress signal that triggers hypothalamic CRH release and activation of the entire HPA axis. The ITT involves administration of regular insulin 0.1 U/kg IV (dose should be lower if hypopituitarism is likely) and collection of blood samples at 0, 30, 60, and 120 minutes for glucose, cortisol, and growth hormone (GH), if also assessing the GH axis. Oral or IV glucose is administered after the patient has achieved symptomatic hypoglycemia (usually glucose <40 mg/dL). A normal response is defined as a cortisol >20 μg/dL and GH >5.1 μg/L. The ITT requires careful clinical monitoring and sequential measurements of glucose. It is contraindicated in patients with coronary disease, cerebrovascular disease, or seizure disorders, which has made the short cosyntropin test the commonly accepted first-line test.

Mineralocorticoid production is controlled by the RAA regulatory cycle, which is initiated by the release of renin from the juxtaglomerular cells in the kidney, resulting in cleavage of angiotensinogen to angiotensin I in the liver (Fig. 342-4). Angiotensin-converting enzyme (ACE) cleaves angiotensin I to angiotensin II, which binds and activates the angiotensin II receptor type 1 (AT1 receptor), resulting in increased aldosterone production and vasoconstriction. Aldosterone enhances sodium retention and potassium excretion, and increases the arterial perfusion pressure, which in turn regulates renin release. Because mineralocorticoid

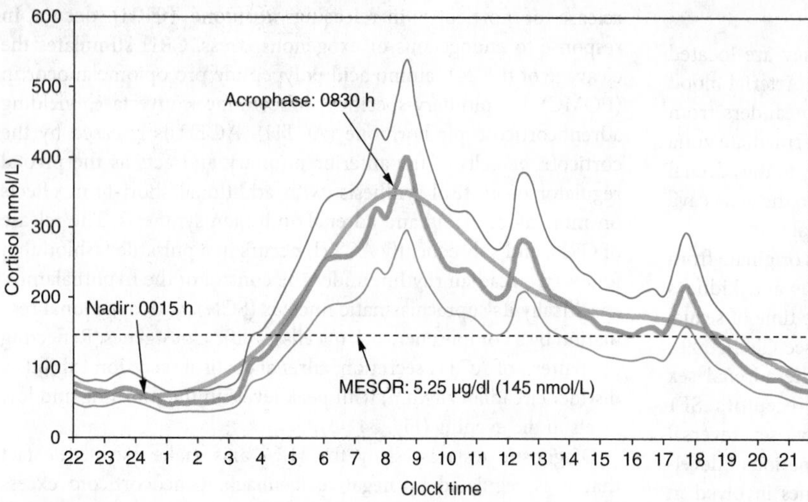

Figure 342-3 Physiologic cortisol circadian rhythm. Circulating cortisol concentrations drop under the rhythm-adjusted mean (MESOR) in the early evening hours, with nadir levels around midnight and a rise in the early morning hours; peak levels are observed ~8:30 A.M. (acrophase). *(Modified after Debono M et al: Modified-release hydrocortisone to provide circadian cortisol profiles. J Clin Endocrinol Metab 94:1548, 2009.)*

synthesis is primarily under the control of the RAA system, hypothalamic-pituitary damage does not significantly impact the capacity of the adrenal to synthesize aldosterone.

Similar to the HPA axis, the assessment of the RAA system can be used for diagnostic purposes. If mineralocorticoid excess is present, there is a counter-regulatory downregulation of plasma renin (see below for testing). Conversely, in mineralocorticoid deficiency, plasma renin is markedly increased. Physiologically, oral or IV sodium loading results in suppression of aldosterone, a response that is attenuated or absent in patients with autonomous mineralocorticoid excess.

STEROID HORMONE SYNTHESIS, METABOLISM, AND ACTION

ACTH stimulation is required for the initiation of steroidogenesis. The ACTH receptor MC2R (melanocortin 2 receptor) interacts with the MC2R-accessory protein MRAP, and the complex is transported to the adrenocortical cell membrane, where it binds to ACTH (Fig. 342-5). ACTH stimulation generates cyclic AMP (cAMP), which upregulates the protein kinase A (PKA) signaling pathway. PKA activation impacts steroidogenesis in three distinct ways: (1) increases the import of cholesterol esters; (2) increases the activity of hormone-sensitive lipase, which cleaves cholesterol esters to cholesterol for import into the mitochondrion; and (3) increases the availability and phosphorylation of CREB (cAMP response element binding), a transcription factor that enhances transcription of CYP11A1 and other enzymes required for glucocorticoid synthesis.

Adrenal steroidogenesis occurs in a zone-specific fashion, with mineralocorticoid synthesis occurring in the outer zona glomerulosa, glucocorticoid synthesis in the zona fasciculata, and adrenal androgen synthesis in the inner zona reticularis (Fig. 342-1). All steroidogenic pathways require cholesterol import into the mitochondrion, a process initiated by the action of the steroidogenic acute regulatory (StAR) protein, which shuttles cholesterol from the outer to the inner mitochondrial membrane. The majority of steroidogenic enzymes are cytochrome P450 (CYP) enzymes, which are either located in the mitochondrion (side chain cleavage enzyme, CYP11A1; 11β-hydroxylase, CYP11B1; aldosterone synthase, CYP11B2) or in the endoplasmic reticulum membrane (17α-hydroxylase, CYP17A1; 21-hydroxylase, CYP21A2; aromatase, CYP19A1). These enzymes require electron

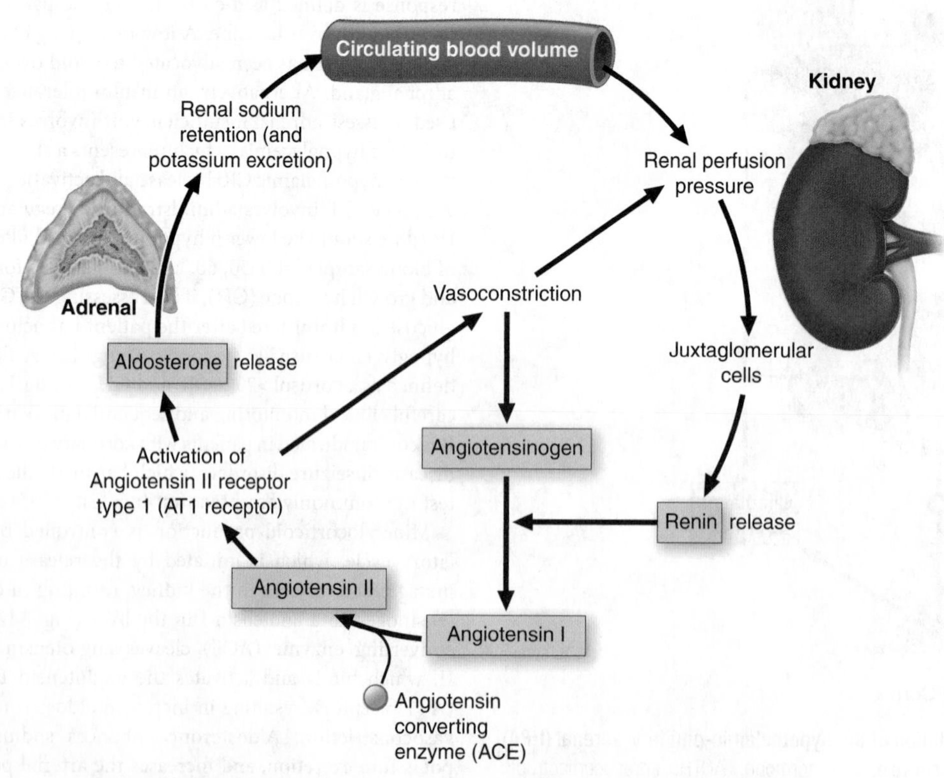

Figure 342-4 Regulation of the renin-angiotensin-aldosterone (RAA) system.

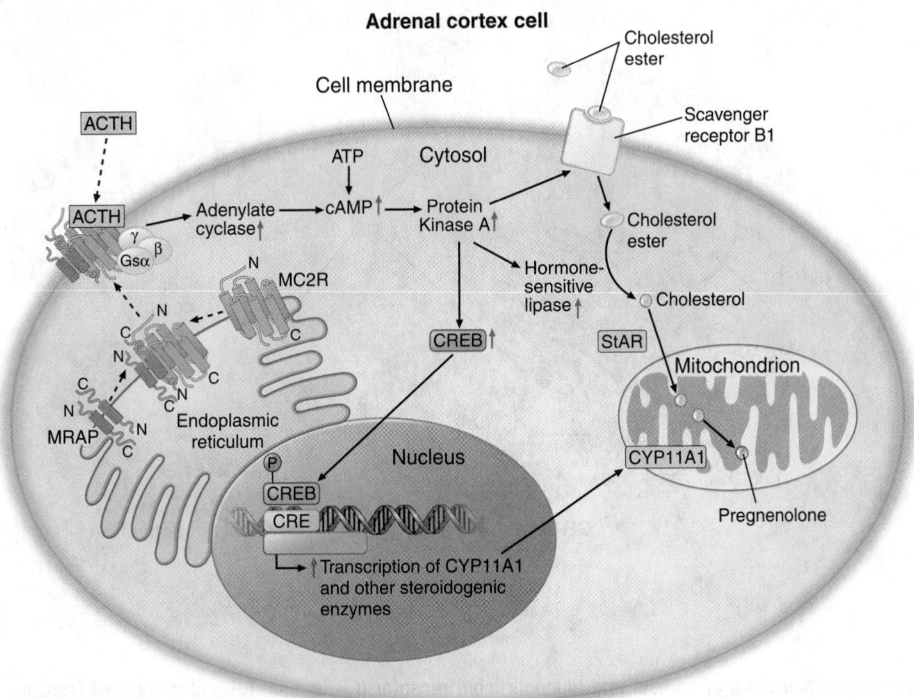

Figure 342-5 ACTH effects on adrenal steroidogenesis. ACTH, adrenocorticotropic hormone; ATP, adenosine triphosphate; CRE, cAMP response element; CREB, cAMP response element binding; MRAP, MC2R-accessory protein; StAR, steroidogenic acute regulatory [protein].

donation via specific redox cofactor enzymes, P450 oxidoreductase (POR), and adrenodoxin/adrenodoxin reductase (ADX/ADR) for the microsomal and mitochondrial CYP enzymes, respectively. In addition, the short-chain dehydrogenase 3β-hydroxysteroid dehydrogenase type 2 (3β-HSD2), also termed Δ4,Δ5 isomerase, plays a major role in adrenal steroidogenesis.

The cholesterol side chain cleavage enzyme CYP11A1 generates pregnenolone. Glucocorticoid synthesis requires conversion of pregnenolone to progesterone by 3β-HSD2, followed by conversion to 17-hydroxyprogesterone by CYP17A1, further hydroxylation at carbon 21 by 21-hydroxylase, and eventually, 11β-hydroxylation by CYP11B1 to generate active cortisol (Fig. 342-1). Mineralocorticoid synthesis also requires progesterone, which is first converted to deoxycorticosterone by CYP21A2 and then converted via corticosterone and 18-hydroxycorticosterone to aldosterone in three steps catalyzed by CYP11B2. For adrenal androgen synthesis, pregnenolone undergoes conversion by CYP17A1, which uniquely catalyzes two enzymatic reactions. Via its 17α-hydroxylase activity, CYP17A1 converts pregnenolone to 17-hydroxypregnenolone, followed by generation of the universal sex steroid precursor DHEA via CYP17A1 17,20 lyase activity. The majority of DHEA is secreted by the adrenal in the form of its sulfate ester, DHEAS, generated by DHEA sulfotransferase (SULT2A1).

Following its release from the adrenal, cortisol circulates in the bloodstream mainly bound to cortisol-binding globulin (CBG) and to a lesser extent to albumin, with only a minor fraction circulating as free, unbound hormone. Free cortisol is thought to enter cells directly, not requiring active transport. In addition, in a multitude of peripheral target tissues of glucocorticoid action, including adipose, liver, muscle, and brain, cortisol is generated from inactive cortisone within the cell by the enzyme 11β-hydroxysteroid dehydrogenase type 1 (11β-HSD1) (Fig. 342-6). Thereby, 11β-HSD1 functions as a tissue-specific prereceptor regulator of glucocorticoid action. For the conversion of inactive cortisone to active cortisol, 11β-HSD1 requires nicotinamide adenine dinucleotide phosphate [NADPH (reduced form)], which is provided by the enzyme hexose-6-phosphate dehydrogenase (H6PDH). Like the catalytic domain of 11β-HSD1, H6PDH is located in the lumen of the endoplasmic reticulum, and converts glucose-6-phosphate (G6P) to 6-phosphogluconate (6PGL), thereby regenerating NADP+ to NADPH, which drives the activation of cortisol from cortisone by 11β-HSD1.

In the cytosol of target cells, cortisol binds and activates the glucocorticoid receptor (GR), which results in dissociation of heat shock proteins (HSP) from the receptor and subsequent dimerization (Fig. 342-6). Cortisol-bound GR dimers translocate to the nucleus and activate glucocorticoid response elements (GRE) in the DNA sequence, thereby enhancing transcription of glucocorticoid-regulated genes (GR transactivation). However, cortisol-bound GR can also form heterodimers with transcription factors such as AP-1 or NF-κB, resulting in transrepression of proinflammatory genes, a mechanism of major importance for the anti-inflammatory action of glucocorticoids. It is important to note that corticosterone also exerts glucocorticoid activity, albeit much weaker than cortisol itself. However, in rodents corticosterone is the major glucocorticoid and in patients with 17-hydroxylase deficiency, lack of cortisol can be compensated for by higher concentrations of corticosterone that accumulates as a consequence of the enzymatic block.

Cortisol is inactivated to cortisone by the microsomal enzyme 11β-hydroxysteroid dehydrogenase type 2 (11β-HSD2) (Fig. 342-7), mainly in the kidney, but also in the colon, salivary glands, and other target tissues. Cortisol and aldosterone bind the mineralocorticoid receptor (MR) with equal affinity; however, cortisol circulates in the bloodstream at about a thousandfold higher concentration. Thus, only rapid inactivation of cortisol to cortisone by 11β-HSD2 prevents MR activation by excess cortisol, thereby acting as a tissue-specific modulator of the MR pathway. In addition to cortisol and aldosterone, deoxycorticosterone (DOC) (Fig. 342-1) also exerts mineralocorticoid activity. DOC accumulation due to 11β-hydroxylase deficiency or due to tumor-related excess production can result in mineralocorticoid excess.

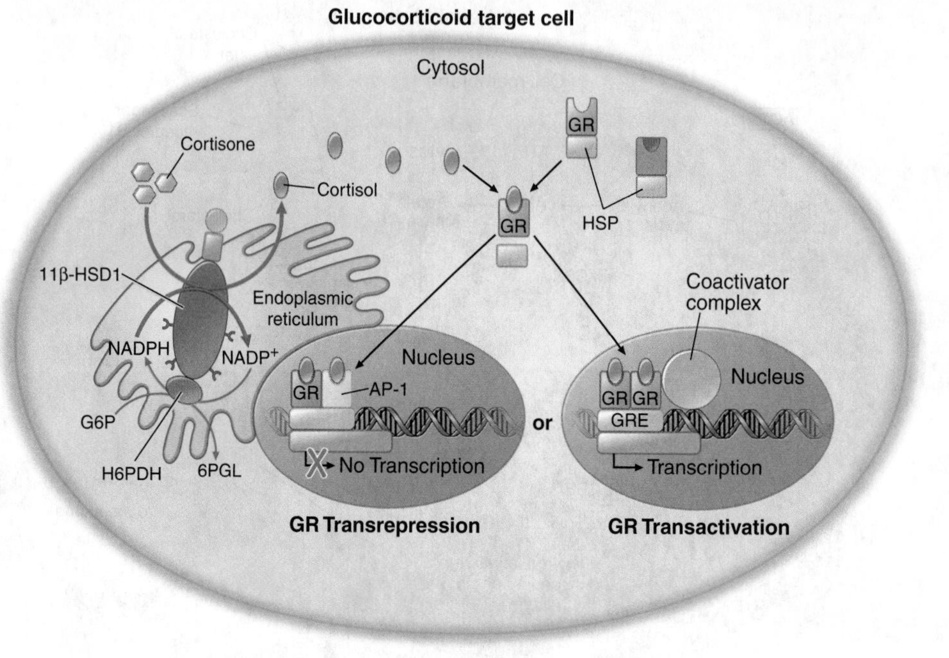

Figure 342-6 Prereceptor activation of cortisol and glucocorticoid receptor (GR) action. GRE, glucocorticoid response elements; HSP, heat shock proteins; NADPH, nicotinamide adenine dinucleotide phosphate (reduced form).

Analogous to cortisol action via the GR, aldosterone (or cortisol) binding to the MR dissociates the HSP–receptor complex, allowing homodimerization of the MR, and translocation of the hormone-bound MR dimer to the nucleus (Fig. 342-7). The activated MR enhances transcription of the epithelial sodium channel (ENaC) and serum glucocorticoid-inducible kinase 1 (SGK-1). In the cytosol, interaction of ENaC with Nedd4 prevents cell surface expression of ENaC. However, SGK-1 phosphorylates serine residues within the Nedd4 protein, reduces the interaction between Nedd4 and ENaC and consequently enhances the trafficking of ENaC to the cell surface, where it mediates sodium retention.

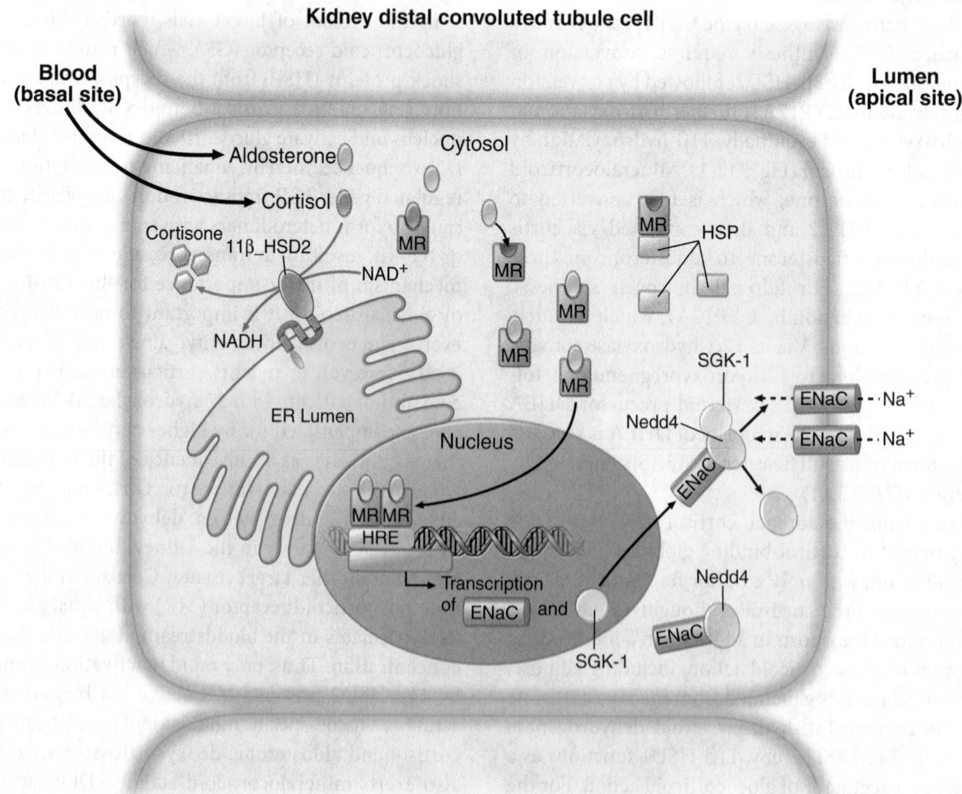

Figure 342-7 Prereceptor inactivation of cortisol and mineralocorticoid receptor action.

■ CUSHING'S SYNDROME

(See also Chap. 339) Cushing's syndrome reflects a constellation of clinical features that result from chronic exposure to excess glucocorticoids of any etiology. The disorder can be ACTH-dependent (e.g., pituitary corticotrope adenoma, ectopic secretion of ACTH by nonpituitary tumor) or ACTH-independent (e.g., adrenocortical adenoma, adrenocortical carcinoma, nodular adrenal hyperplasia), as well as iatrogenic (e.g., administration of exogenous glucocorticoids to treat various inflammatory conditions). The term *Cushing's disease* refers specifically to Cushing's syndrome caused by a pituitary corticotrope adenoma.

Epidemiology

Cushing's syndrome is generally considered a rare disease. It occurs with an incidence of 1–2 per 100,000 population per year. However, it is debated whether mild cortisol excess may be more prevalent among patients with several features of Cushing's such as centripetal obesity, type 2 diabetes, and osteoporotic vertebral fractures, recognizing that these are relatively nonspecific and common in the population.

In the overwhelming majority of patients, Cushing's syndrome is caused by an ACTH-producing corticotrope adenoma of the pituitary (Table 342-1), as initially described by Harvey Cushing in 1912. Cushing's disease more frequently affects women, with the exception of prepubertal cases, where it is more common in boys. By contrast, ectopic ACTH syndrome is more frequently identified in men. Only 10% of patients with Cushing's syndrome have a primary, adrenal cause of their disease (e.g., autonomous cortisol excess independent of ACTH), and most of these patients are women. Overall, the medical use of glucocorticoids for immunosuppression, or for the treatment of inflammatory disorders, is the most common cause of Cushing's syndrome.

Etiology

In at least 90% of patients with Cushing's disease, ACTH excess is caused by a corticotrope pituitary microadenoma, often only a few millimeters in diameter. Pituitary macroadenomas (i.e. tumors >1 cm in size), are found in only 5–10% of patients. Pituitary corticotrope adenomas usually occur sporadically, but very rarely can be found in the context of multiple endocrine neoplasia type 1 (MEN1) (Chap. 351).

Ectopic ACTH production is predominantly caused by occult carcinoid tumors, most frequently in the lung, but also in thymus or pancreas. Because of their small size, these tumors are often difficult to locate. Advanced small cell lung cancer can cause ectopic ACTH production. In rare cases, ectopic ACTH production has been found to originate from medullary thyroid carcinoma or pheochromocytoma, the latter co-secreting catecholamines and ACTH.

The majority of patients with ACTH-independent cortisol excess harbor a cortisol-producing adrenal adenoma. Adrenocortical carcinomas may also cause ACTH-independent disease and are often large, with excess production of several corticosteroid classes. A rare but notable cause of adrenal cortisol excess is ACTH-independent macronodular hyperplasia (AIMAH), generally characterized by ectopic expression of receptors not usually found in the adrenal, including receptors for luteinizing hormone, vasopressin, serotonin, interleukin-1, or gastric inhibitory peptide (GIP), the cause of food-dependent Cushing's. Activation of these receptors results in upregulation of PKA signaling, as physiologically occurs with ACTH, with a subsequent increase in cortisol production. Mutations in a regulatory subunit of PKA (PRKAR1A) are found in patients with primary pigmented nodular adrenal disease (PPNAD) as part of *Carney's complex*, an autosomal dominant multiple neoplasia condition associated with cardiac myxomas, hyperlentiginosis, Sertoli's cell tumors, and PPNAD. PPNAD can present as micronodular or macronodular hyperplasia, or both. Another rare cause of ACTH-independent Cushing's is *McCune-Albright syndrome*, also associated with polyostotic fibrous dysplasia, unilateral café-au-lait spots, and precocious puberty. McCune-Albright syndrome is caused by activating mutations in GNAS-1 (guanine nucleotide binding protein alpha stimulating activity polypeptide 1), and such mutations have also been found in bilateral macronodular hyperplasia without other McCune-Albright features (Table 342-1; see also Chap. 355).

TABLE 342-1 Causes of Cushing's Syndrome

Causes of Cushing's Syndrome	Female:Male Ratio	%
ACTH-Dependent Cushing's		**90**
Cushing's disease (= ACTH-producing pituitary adenoma)	4:1	75
Ectopic ACTH syndrome (due to ACTH secretion by bronchial or pancreatic carcinoid tumors, small cell lung cancer, medullary thyroid carcinoma, pheochromocytoma and others)	1:1	15
ACTH-Independent Cushing's	4:1	**10**
Adrenocortical adenoma		5-10
Adrenocortical carcinoma		1%
Rare causes: PPNAD, primary pigmented nodular adrenal disease; AIMAH, ACTH-independent massive adrenal hyperplasia; McCune-Albright syndrome		<1%

Abbreviations: ACTH, adrenocorticotropic hormone; AIMAH, ACTH-independent macronodular hyperplasia; PPNAD, primary pigmented nodular adrenal disease.

Clinical manifestations

Glucocorticoids affect almost all cells of the body and thus signs of cortisol excess impact multiple physiologic systems (Table 342-2), with upregulation of gluconeogenesis, lipolysis, and protein catabolism causing the most prominent features. In addition, excess glucocorticoid secretion overcomes the ability of 11β-HSD2 to rapidly inactivate cortisol to cortisone in the kidney, thereby exerting mineralocorticoid actions, manifest as diastolic hypertension, hypokalemia, and edema. Excess glucocorticoids also interfere with central regulatory systems, leading to suppression of gonadotropins with subsequent hypogonadism and amenorrhea, and suppression of the hypothalamic-pituitary-thyroid axis, resulting in decreased TSH (thyroid-stimulating hormone) secretion.

The majority of clinical signs and symptoms observed in Cushing's syndrome are relatively nonspecific and include features such as obesity, diabetes, diastolic hypertension, hirsutism, and depression that are commonly found in patients who do not have Cushing's. Therefore, careful clinical assessment is an important aspect of evaluating suspected cases. A diagnosis of Cushing's should be considered when several clinical features are found in the same patient, in particular when more specific features are found. These include fragility of the skin, with easy bruising and broad (>1 cm), purplish striae (Fig. 342-8), and signs of proximal myopathy, which becomes most obvious when trying to stand up from a chair without the use of hands or when climbing stairs. Clinical manifestations of

TABLE 342-2 Signs and Symptoms of Cushing's Syndrome

Body Compartment/System	Signs and Symptoms
Body fat	Weight gain, central obesity, rounded face, fat pad on back of neck ("buffalo hump")
Skin	Facial plethora, thin and brittle skin, easy bruising, broad and purple stretch marks, acne, hirsutism
Bone	Osteopenia, osteoporosis (vertebral fractures), decreased linear growth in children
Muscle	Weakness, proximal myopathy (prominent atrophy of gluteal and upper leg muscles)
Cardiovascular system	Hypertension, hypokalemia, edema, atherosclerosis
Metabolism	Glucose intolerance/diabetes, dyslipidemia
Reproductive system	Decreased libido, in women amenorrhea (due to cortisol-mediated inhibition of gonadotropin release)
Central nervous system	Irritability, emotional lability, depression, sometimes cognitive defects, in severe cases, paranoid psychosis
Blood and immune system	Increased susceptibility to infections, increased white blood cell count, eosinopenia, hypercoagulation with increased risk of deep vein thrombosis and pulmonary embolism

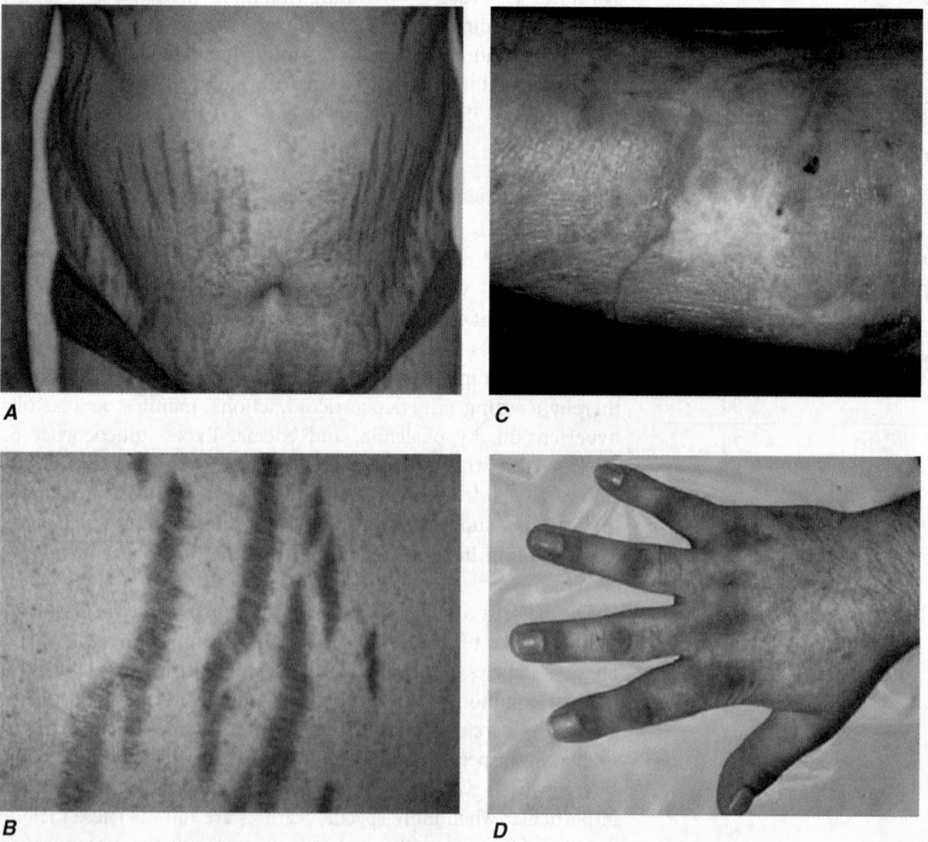

Figure 342-8 Clinical features of Cushing's syndrome. ***A.*** Note central obesity and broad, purple stretch marks (***B.*** close-up). ***C.*** Note thin and brittle skin in an elderly patient with Cushing's. ***D.*** Hyperpigmentation of the knuckles in a patient with ectopic ACTH excess.

Cushing's do not differ substantially among the different causes of Cushing's. In ectopic ACTH syndrome, hyperpigmentation of the knuckles, scars, or skin areas exposed to increased friction can be observed (Fig. 342-8), and is caused by stimulatory effects of excess ACTH and other POMC cleavage products on melanocyte pigment production. Furthermore, patients with ectopic ACTH syndrome, and some with adrenocortical carcinoma as the cause of Cushing's, may have a more brisk onset and rapid progression of clinical signs and symptoms.

Patients with Cushing's syndrome can be acutely endangered by deep vein thrombosis, with subsequent pulmonary embolism due to a hypercoagulable state associated with Cushing's. The majority of patients also experience psychiatric symptoms, mostly in the form of anxiety or depression, but acute paranoid or depressive psychosis may also occur. Even after cure, long-term health may be affected by an increased risk of cardiovascular disease and osteoporosis with vertebral fractures, depending on the duration and degree of exposure to significant cortisol excess.

Diagnosis

The most important first step in the management of patients with suspected Cushing's syndrome is to establish the correct diagnosis. Most mistakes in clinical management, leading to unnecessary imaging or surgery, are made because the diagnostic protocol is not followed (Fig. 342-9). This protocol requires establishing the diagnosis of Cushing's beyond doubt prior to employing any tests used for the differential diagnosis of the condition. In principle, after excluding exogenous glucocorticoid use as the cause of clinical signs and symptoms, suspected cases should be tested if there are multiple and progressive features of Cushing's, particularly features with a potentially higher discriminatory value. Exclusion of Cushing's is also indicated in patients with incidentally discovered adrenal masses.

A diagnosis of Cushing's can be considered as established if the results of several tests are consistently suggestive of Cushing's. These tests may include increased 24-hour urinary free cortisol excretion in three separate collections, failure to appropriately suppress morning cortisol after overnight exposure to dexamethasone, and evidence of loss of diurnal cortisol secretion with high levels at midnight, the time of the physiologically lowest secretion (Fig. 342-9). Factors potentially affecting the outcome of these diagnostic tests have to be excluded such as incomplete 24-hour urine collection or rapid inactivation of dexamethasone due to concurrent intake of CYP3A4-inducing drugs (e.g., antiepileptics, rifampicin). Concurrent intake of oral contraceptives that raise CBG and thus total cortisol can cause failure to suppress after dexamethasone. If in doubt, testing should be repeated after 4–6 weeks off estrogens. Patients with pseudo-Cushing states, i.e., alcohol-related, and those with cyclic Cushing's may require further testing to safely

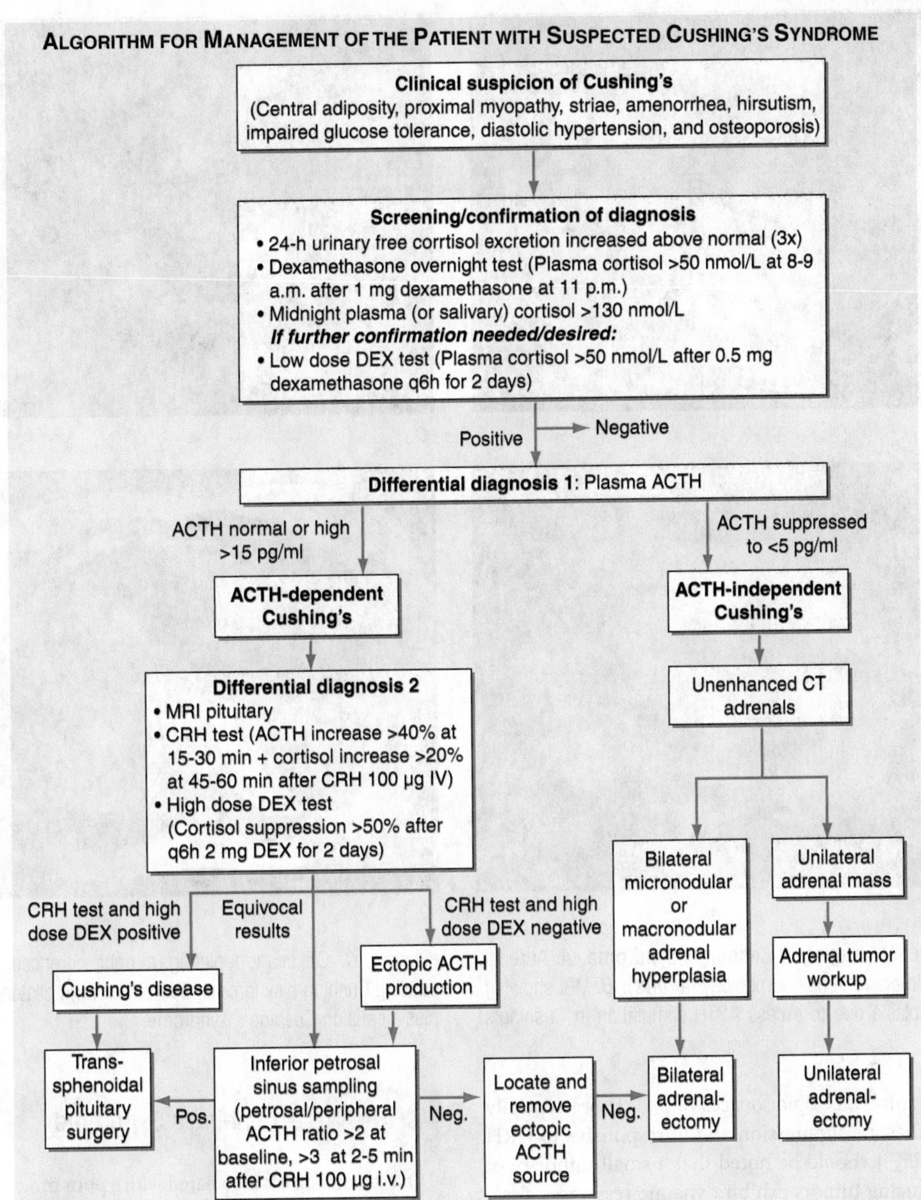

Figure 342-9 **Management of the patient with suspected Cushing's syndrome.** CHR, corticotropin-releasing hormone; DEX, dexamethasone.

confirm or exclude the diagnosis of Cushing's. In addition, the biochemical assays employed can affect the test results, with specificity representing a common problem with antibody-based assays for the measurement of urinary free cortisol. These assays have been greatly improved by the introduction of highly specific tandem mass spectrometry.

Differential diagnosis

The evaluation of patients with confirmed Cushing's should be carried out by an endocrinologist and begins with the differential diagnosis of ACTH-dependent and ACTH-independent cortisol excess (Fig. 342-9). Generally, plasma ACTH levels are suppressed in cases of autonomous adrenal cortisol excess, as a consequence of enhanced negative feedback to the hypothalamus and pituitary. By contrast, patients with ACTH-dependent Cushing's have normal or increased plasma ACTH, with very high levels being found in some patients with ectopic ACTH syndrome. Importantly, imaging should only be used after it is established whether the cortisol excess is ACTH-dependent or ACTH-independent, as nodules in the pituitary or the adrenal are a common finding in the general population. In patients with confirmed ACTH-independent excess, adrenal imaging is indicated (Fig. 342-10), preferably using an unenhanced CT scan. This allows assessment of adrenal morphology and determination of tumor density in Hounsfield Units (HU), which helps to distinguish between benign and malignant adrenal lesions.

For ACTH-dependent cortisol excess (Chap. 339), an MRI of the pituitary is the investigation of choice, but it may not show an abnormality in up to 40% of cases because small tumors are below the sensitivity of detection. Characteristically, pituitary corticotrope adenomas fail to enhance following gadolinium administration on T1-weighted MRI images. In all cases of confirmed ACTH-dependent Cushing's, further tests are required for the differential diagnosis of pituitary Cushing's disease and ectopic ACTH syndrome. These tests exploit the fact that most pituitary corticotrope adenomas still display regulatory features, including residual ACTH suppression by high-dose glucocorticoids and CRH

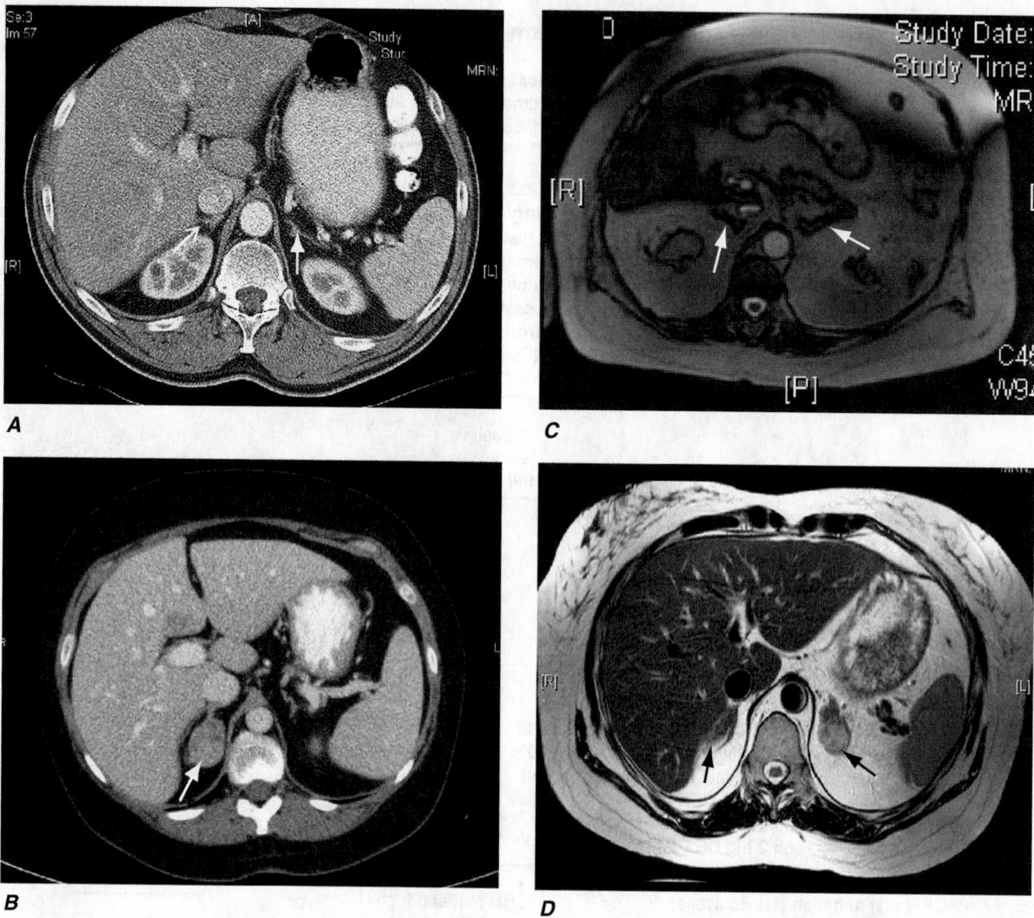

Figure 342-10 Adrenal imaging in Cushing's syndrome. ***A.*** Adrenal CT showing normal bilateral adrenal morphology (*arrows*). ***B.*** MRI showing bilateral adrenal hyperplasia due to excess ACTH stimulation in Cushing's disease. ***C.*** CT scan depicting a right adrenocortical adenoma (*arrow*) causing Cushing's syndrome. ***D.*** MRI showing bilateral macronodular hyperplasia causing Cushing's syndrome.

responsiveness. In contrast, ectopic sources of ACTH are typically resistant to dexamethasone suppression and unresponsive to CRH (Fig. 342-9). However, it should be noted that a small minority of ectopic ACTH-producing tumors exhibit dynamic responses similar to pituitary corticotrope tumors. If the two tests show discordant results, or if there is any other reason for doubt, the differential diagnosis can be further clarified by performing bilateral inferior petrosal sinus sampling (IPSS) with concurrent blood sampling for ACTH in the right and left inferior petrosal sinus and a peripheral vein. An increased central/peripheral plasma ACTH ratio >2 at baseline and >3 after CRH injection is indicative of Cushing's disease (Fig. 342-9), with very high sensitivity and specificity. Of note, the results of the IPSS cannot be reliably used for lateralization (i.e. prediction of the location of the tumor within the pituitary), because there is broad interindividual variability in the venous drainage of the pituitary region. Importantly, no cortisol-lowering agents should be used prior to IPSS.

If the differential diagnostic testing indicates ectopic ACTH syndrome, then further imaging should include high-resolution, fine-cut CT scanning of the chest and abdomen for scrutiny of the lung, thymus, and pancreas. If no lesions are identified, an MRI of the chest can be considered as carcinoid tumors usually show high signal intensity on T2-weighted images. Furthermore, octreotide scintigraphy can be helpful in some cases as ectopic ACTH-producing tumors often express somatostatin receptors. Depending on the suspected cause, patients with ectopic ACTH syndrome should also undergo blood sampling for fasting gut hormones, chromogranin A, calcitonin, and biochemical exclusion of pheochromocytoma.

TREATMENT Cushing's Syndrome

Overt Cushing's is associated with a poor prognosis if left untreated. In ACTH-independent disease, treatment consists of surgical removal of the adrenal tumor. For smaller tumors, a minimally invasive approach can be employed, whereas for larger tumors and those suspected of malignancy, an open approach is preferred.

In Cushing's disease, the treatment of choice is selective removal of the pituitary corticotrope tumor, usually via a transsphenoidal approach. This results in an initial cure rate of 70–80% when performed by a highly experienced surgeon. However, even after initial remission following surgery, long-term follow-up is important as late relapse occurs in a significant number of patients. If pituitary disease recurs, there are several options, including second surgery, radiotherapy, stereotactic radiosurgery, and bilateral adrenalectomy. These options need to be applied in a highly individualized fashion.

In some with very severe, overt Cushing's (e.g., difficult to control hypokalemic hypertension or acute psychosis), it may be necessary to introduce medical therapy to rapidly control the cortisol excess during the period leading up to surgery. Similarly, patients with metastasized, glucocorticoid-producing carcinomas may require long-term antiglucocorticoid drug treatment. In case of ectopic ACTH syndrome, in which the tumor cannot be located, one must carefully weigh whether drug treatment or bilateral adrenalectomy is the most appropriate choice, with the latter facilitating immediate cure but requiring life-long corticosteroid replacement. In this instance, it is paramount to ensure regular imaging follow-up for identification of the ectopic ACTH source.

Oral agents with established efficacy in Cushing's syndrome are metyrapone and ketoconazole. Metyrapone inhibits cortisol synthesis at the level of 11β-hydroxylase (Fig. 342-1), whereas the antimycotic drug ketoconazole inhibits the early steps of steroidogenesis. Typical starting doses are 500 mg/tid for metyrapone (maximum dose, 6 g) and 200 mg/tid for ketoconazole (maximum dose, 1200 mg). Mitotane, a derivative of the insecticide o,p'DDD, is an adrenolytic agent that is also effective for reducing cortisol. Because of its side effect profile, it is most commonly used in the context of adrenocortical carcinoma, but low-dose treatment (500–1000 mg per day) has also been used in benign Cushing's. In severe cases of cortisol excess, etomidate can be used to lower cortisol. It is administered by continuous IV infusion in low, nonanesthetic doses.

After the successful removal of an ACTH- or cortisol-producing tumor, the HPA axis will remain suppressed. Thus, hydrocortisone replacement needs to be initiated at the time of surgery and slowly tapered following recovery, to allow physiologic adaptation to normal cortisol levels. Depending on degree and duration of cortisol excess, the HPA axis may require many months or even years to resume normal function.

MINERALOCORTICOID EXCESS

Epidemiology

Following the first description of a patient with an aldosterone-producing adrenal adenoma (*Conn's syndrome*), mineralocorticoid excess was thought to represent a rare cause of hypertension. However, in studies systematically screening all patients with hypertension, a much higher prevalence is now recognized, ranging from 5 to 12%. The prevalence is higher when patients are preselected for hypokalemic hypertension.

Etiology

The most common cause of mineralocorticoid excess is primary hyperaldosteronism, reflecting excess production of aldosterone by the adrenal zona glomerulosa. Bilateral micronodular hyperplasia is somewhat more common than unilateral adrenal adenomas (Table 342-3). Bilateral adrenal hyperplasia is usually micronodular but can also contain larger nodules that might be mistaken for a unilateral adenoma. In rare instances, primary hyperaldosteronism is caused by an adrenocortical carcinoma. Carcinomas should be considered in younger patients and in those with larger tumors, as benign aldosterone-producing adenomas usually measure <1 cm in diameter.

A rare cause of aldosterone excess is glucocorticoid-remediable aldosteronism (GRA), which is caused by a chimeric gene resulting from cross-over of promoter sequences between the CYP11B1 and CYP11B2 genes that are involved in glucocorticoid and mineralocorticoid synthesis, respectively (Fig. 342-1). This rearrangement brings CYP11B2 under the control of ACTH receptor signaling; consequently, aldosterone production is regulated by ACTH rather than by renin. The family history can be helpful as there may be evidence for dominant transmission of hypertension. Recognition of the disorder is important because it can be associated with early-onset hypertension and strokes. In addition, glucocorticoid suppression can reduce aldosterone production.

Other rare causes of mineralocorticoid excess are listed in Table 342-3. An important cause is excess binding and activation of the mineralocorticoid receptor by a steroid other than aldosterone. Cortisol acts as a potent mineralocorticoid if it escapes efficient inactivation to cortisone by 11β-HSD2 in the kidney (Fig. 342-7). This can be caused by inactivating mutations in the *HSD11B2* gene resulting in the syndrome of apparent mineralocorticoid excess

TABLE 342-3 Causes of Mineralocorticoid Excess

Causes of Mineralocorticoid Excess	Mechanism	%
Primary Hyperaldosteronism		
Adrenal (Conn's) adenoma	Autonomous aldosterone excess	40
Bilateral (micronodular) adrenal hyperplasia	Autonomous aldosterone excess	60
Glucocorticoid-remediable hyperaldosteronism (dexamethasone-suppressible hyperaldosteronism)	Crossover between the *CYP11B1* and *CYP11B2* genes results in ACTH-driven aldosterone production	<1
Other Causes (Rare)		<1
Syndrome of apparent mineralocorticoid excess (AME)	Mutations in *HSD11B2* result in lack of renal activation of cortisol to cortisone, leading to excess activation of the MR by cortisol	
Cushing's syndrome	Cortisol excess overcomes the capacity of HSD11B2 to inactivate cortisol to cortisone, consequently flooding the MR	
Glucocorticoid resistance	Upregulation of cortisol production due to GR mutations results in flooding of the MR by cortisol	
Adrenocortical carcinoma	Autonomous aldosterone and/or DOC excess	
Congenital adrenal hyperplasia	Accumulation of DOC due to mutations in *CYP11B1* or *CYP17A1*	
Progesterone-induced hypertension	Progesterone acts as an abnormal ligand due to mutations in the *MR* gene	
Liddle's syndrome	Mutant ENaC β or γ subunits resulting in reduced degradation of ENaC keeping the membrane channel in open conformation for longer, enhancing mineralocorticoid action	

Abbreviations: DOC, deoxycorticosterone; ENaC, epithelial sodium channel; GR, glucocorticoid receptor; MR, mineralocorticoid receptor.

(AME) that characteristically manifests with severe hypokalemic hypertension in childhood. However, milder mutations may cause normokalemic hypertension manifesting in adulthood (Type II AME). Inhibition of 11β-HSD2 by excess licorice ingestion also results in hypokalemic hypertension, as does overwhelming of 11β-HSD2 conversion capacity by cortisol excess in Cushing's syndrome. Desoxycorticosterone (DOC) also binds and activates the mineralocorticoid receptor and can cause hypertension if its circulating concentrations are increased. This can arise through autonomous DOC secretion by an adrenocortical carcinoma, but also when DOC accumulates as a consequence of an adrenal enzymatic block, as seen in congenital adrenal hyperplasia due to CYP11B1 (11β-hydroxylase) or CYP17A1 (17α-hdyroxylase) deficiency (Fig. 342-1). Progesterone can cause hypokalemic hypertension in rare individuals who harbor a mineralocorticoid receptor mutation that enhances binding and activation by progesterone; physiologically, progesterone normally exerts antimineralocorticoid activity. Finally, excess mineralocorticoid activity can be caused by mutations in the β or γ subunits of the ENaC, disrupting its interaction with Nedd4 (Fig. 342-7), and thereby decreasing receptor internalization and degradation. The constitutively active ENAC drives hypokalemic hypertension, resulting in an autosomal dominant disorder termed *Liddle's syndrome*.

Clinical manifestations

Excess activation of the mineralocorticoid receptor leads to potassium depletion and increased sodium retention, with the latter causing an expansion of extracellular and plasma volume. Increased ENaC activity also results in hydrogen depletion that can cause metabolic alkalosis. Aldosterone also has direct effects on the vascular system, where it increases cardiac remodeling and decreases compliance. Aldosterone excess may cause direct damage to the myocardium and the kidney glomeruli, in addition to secondary damage due to systemic hypertension.

The clinical hallmark of mineralocorticoid excess is hypokalemic hypertension; serum sodium tends to be normal due to the concurrent fluid retention, which in some cases can lead to peripheral edema. Hypokalemia can be exacerbated by thiazide drug treatment, which leads to increased delivery of sodium to the distal renal tubule, thereby driving potassium excretion. Severe hypokalemia can be associated with muscle weakness, overt proximal myopathy, or even hypokalemic paralysis. Severe alkalosis contributes to muscle cramps and, in severe cases, can cause tetany.

Diagnosis

Diagnostic screening for mineralocorticoid excess is not currently recommended for all patients with hypertension, but should be restricted to those who exhibit hypertension associated with drug resistance, hypokalemia, an adrenal mass, or hypertension before the age of 40 years (Fig. 342-11). The accepted screening test is concurrent measurement of plasma renin and aldosterone with subsequent calculation of the aldosterone-renin ratio (ARR) (Fig. 342-11); serum potassium needs to be normalized prior to testing. Stopping antihypertensive medication can be cumbersome, particularly in patients with severe hypertension. Thus, for practical purposes, in the first instance the patient can remain on the usual antihypertensive medications, with the exception that mineralocorticoid receptor antagonists need to be ceased at least 4 weeks prior to ARR measurement. The remaining antihypertensive drugs usually do not affect the outcome of ARR testing, except that β-blocker treatment can cause false-positive results and ACE/AT1R inhibitors can cause false-negative results in milder cases (Table 342-4).

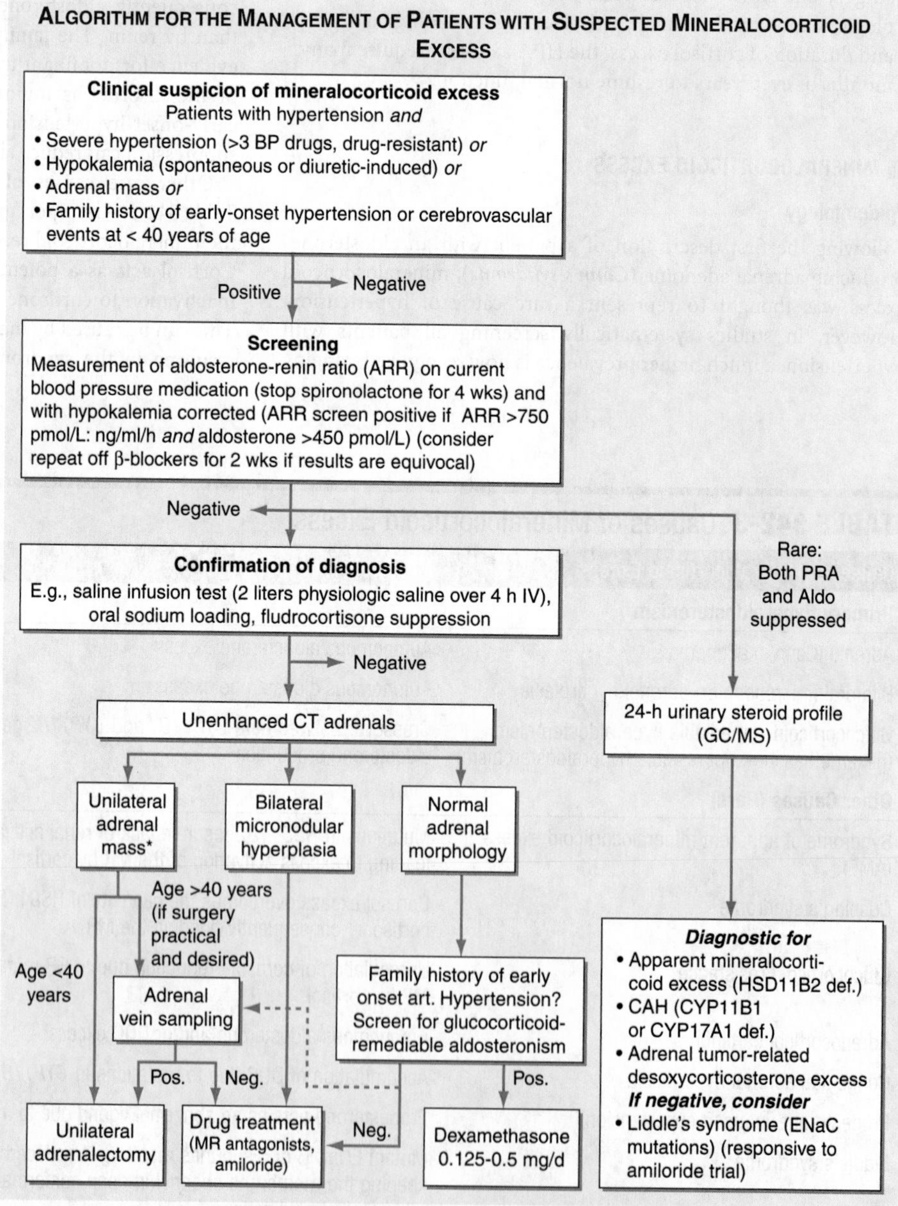

Figure 342-11 Management of patients with suspected mineralocorticoid excess. Perform adrenal tumor workup (see Fig. 342-12). GC/MS, gaschromatography/mass spectrometry.

TABLE 342-4 Effects of Antihypertensive Drugs on the Aldosterone-Renin-Ratio (ARR)

Drug	Effect on Renin	Effect on Aldosterone	Net Effect on ARR
β-Blockers	↓	↑	↑
α_1-Blockers	→	→	→
α_2-Sympathomimetics	→	→	→
ACE inhibitors	↑	↓	↓
AT1R blockers	↑	↓	↓
Calcium antagonists	→	→	→
Diuretics	(↑)	(↑)	→/(↓)

ARR screening is positive if the ratio is greater than 750 pmol/L: ng/mL per hour, with a concurrently high normal or increased aldosterone (Fig. 342-11). If one relies on the ARR only, the likelihood of a false-positive ARR becomes greater when renin levels are very low. The characteristics of the biochemical assays are also important. Some labs measure plasma renin activity whereas others measure plasma renin concentrations. Antibody-based assays for the measurement of serum aldosterone lack the reliability of tandem mass spectrometry assays but these are not yet ubiquitously available.

Diagnostic confirmation of mineralocorticoid excess in a patient with positive ARR screening result should be undertaken by an endocrinologist as the tests lack optimized validation. The most straightforward is the saline infusion test, which involves the IV administration of 2 L of physiologic saline over a 4-hour period. Failure of aldosterone to suppress below 140 pmol/L (5 ng/dL) is indicative of autonomous mineralocorticoid excess. Alternative tests are the oral sodium loading test (300 mmol NaCl/d for 3 days) or the fludrocortisone suppression test (0.1 mg q6h with 30 mmol NaCl q8h for 4 days); the latter can be difficult because of the risk of profound hypokalemia and increased hypertension. In patients with overt hypokalemic hypertension, strongly positive ARR, and concurrently increased aldosterone levels, confirmatory testing is usually not necessary.

Differential diagnosis and treatment

After the diagnosis of hyperaldosteronism is established, the next step is to use adrenal imaging to further assess the cause. Fine-cut CT scanning of the adrenal region is the method of choice as it provides excellent visualization of adrenal morphology. CT will readily identify larger tumors suspicious of malignancy but may miss lesions smaller than 5 mm. The differentiation between bilateral micronodular hyperplasia and a unilateral adenoma is only required if a surgical approach is feasible and desired. Consequently, selective adrenal vein sampling (AVS) should only be carried out in surgical candidates with either no obvious lesion on CT or evidence of a unilateral lesion in patients older than 40 years, as the latter patients have a high likelihood of harboring a coincidental, endocrine inactive adrenal adenoma (Fig. 342-11). AVS is used to compare aldosterone levels in the inferior vena cava and between the right and left adrenal veins. AVS requires concurrent measurement of cortisol to document correct placement of the catheter in the adrenal veins and should demonstrate a cortisol gradient >3 between the vena cava and each adrenal vein. Lateralization is confirmed by an aldosterone/cortisol ratio that is at least twofold higher on one side than the other. AVS is a complex procedure that requires a highly skilled interventional radiologist. Even then, the right adrenal vein can be difficult to cannulate correctly, which invalidates the procedure. There is also no agreement as to whether the two adrenal veins should be cannulated simultaneously or successively and whether ACTH stimulation enhances the diagnostic value of AVS.

Patients younger than 40 years with confirmed mineralocorticoid excess and a unilateral lesion can go straight to surgery, which is also indicated in patients with confirmed lateralization documented by a valid AVS procedure. Laparoscopic adrenalectomy is the preferred approach. Patients who are not surgical candidates, or with evidence of bilateral hyperplasia based on CT or AVS, should be treated medically (Fig. 342-11). Medical treatment, which can also be considered prior to surgery to avoid postsurgical hypoaldosteronism, consists primarily of the mineralocorticoid receptor antagonist spironolactone. It can be started at 12.5–50 mg bid and titrated up to a maximum of 400 mg/d to control blood pressure and normalize potassium. Side effects include menstrual irregularity, decreased libido, and gynecomastia. The more selective MR antagonist eplerenone can also be used. Doses start at 25 mg bid and it can be titrated up to 200 mg/d. Another useful drug is the sodium channel blocker amiloride (5–10 mg/bid).

In patients with normal adrenal morphology and family history of early-onset, severe hypertension, a diagnosis of GRA should be considered and can be evaluated using genetic testing. Treatment of GRA consists of administering dexamethasone, using the lowest dose possible to control blood pressure. Some patients also require additional MR antagonist treatment.

The diagnosis of nonaldosterone-related mineralocorticoid excess is based on documentation of suppressed renin and suppressed aldosterone in the presence of hypokalemic hypertension. This testing is best carried out by employing urinary steroid metabolite profiling by gas chromatography/mass spectrometry (GC/MS). An increased free cortisol over free cortisone ratio is suggestive of AME and can be treated with dexamethasone. Steroid profiling by GC/MS also detects the steroids associated with CYP11B1 and CYP17A1 deficiency or the irregular steroid secretion pattern in a DOC-producing adrenocortical carcinoma (Fig. 342-11). If the GC/MS profile is normal, then Liddle's syndrome should be considered. It is very sensitive to amiloride treatment but will not respond to MR antagonist treatment, as the defect is due to a constitutively active ENaC.

APPROACH TO THE PATIENT: Incidentally Discovered Adrenal Mass

Epidemiology Incidentally discovered adrenal masses, commonly termed adrenal "incidentalomas," are common, with a prevalence of at least 2% in the general population as documented in CT and autopsy series. The prevalence increases with age, with 1% of 40-year-olds and 7% of 70-year-olds harboring an adrenal mass.

Etiology Most solitary adrenal tumors are monoclonal neoplasms. Several genetic syndromes, including MEN-1 (*MEN1*), MEN-2 (*RET*), Carney's complex (*PRKAR1A*), and McCune-Albright (*GNAS1*), can have adrenal tumors as one of their features. Somatic mutations in MEN1, GNAS1, and PRKAR1A have been identified in a small proportion of sporadic adrenocortical adenomas. Aberrant expression of membrane receptors (gastric inhibitory peptide, β-adrenergic, luteinizing hormone, vasopressin V1 and interleukin-I receptors) have been identified in some sporadic cases of macronodular adrenocortical hyperplasia.

The majority of adrenal nodules are endocrine inactive adrenocortical adenomas. However, larger series suggest that

TABLE 342-5 Classification of Unilateral Adrenal Masses

Benign	Approximate Prevalence (%)
Adrenocortical adenoma	
Endocrine inactive	60–85
Cortisol-producing	5–10
Aldosterone-producing	2–5
Pheochromocytoma	5–10
Adrenal myelolipoma	<1
Adrenal ganglioneuroma	<0.1
Adrenal hemangioma	<0.1
Adrenal cyst	<1
Adrenal hematoma/hemorrhagic infarction	<1
Indeterminate	
Adrenocortical oncocytoma	<1
Malignant	
Adrenocortical carcinoma	2–5
Malignant pheochromocytoma	<1
Adrenal neuroblastoma	<0.1
Lymphomas (incl. primary adrenal lymphoma)	<1
Metastases (most frequent: breast, lung)	15

Note: Bilateral adrenal enlargement/masses may be caused by congenital adrenal hyperplasia, bilateral macronodular hyperplasia, bilateral hemorrhage (due to antiphospholipid syndrome or sepsis-associated Waterhouse-Friderichsen syndrome), granuloma, amyloidosis, infiltrative disease including tuberculosis.

up to 25% of adrenal nodules are hormonally active, due to a cortisol-or aldosterone-producing adrenocortical adenoma or a pheochromocytoma associated with catecholamine excess (Table 342-5). Adrenocortical carcinoma is rare but it is the cause of an adrenal mass in 5% of patients. However, the most common cause of a malignant adrenal mass is metastasis originating from another solid tissue tumor (Table 342-5).

Differential diagnosis and treatment Patients with an adrenal mass >1 cm require a diagnostic evaluation. Two key questions need to be addressed: (1) Does the tumor autonomously secrete hormones that could have a detrimental effect on health?, and (2) Is the adrenal mass benign or malignant?

Hormone secretion by an adrenal mass occurs along a continuum, with a gradual increase in clinical manifestations in parallel with hormone levels. Exclusion of catecholamine excess from a pheochromocytoma arising from the adrenal medulla is a mandatory part of the diagnostic workup (Fig. 342-12). Furthermore, autonomous cortisol and aldosterone secretion resulting in Cushing's syndrome or primary hyperaldosteronism, respectively, require exclusion. Adrenal incidentalomas are associated with lower levels of autonomous cortisol secretion, and patients may lack overt clinical features of Cushing's syndrome. Nonetheless, they may exhibit one or more components of the metabolic syndrome (e.g., obesity, type 2 diabetes, or hypertension). There is ongoing debate about the optimal treatment for these patients with mild or subclinical Cushing's syndrome. Overproduction of adrenal androgen precursors, DHEA and its sulfate, is rare and is most frequently seen in the context of adrenocortical carcinoma, as are increased levels of steroid precursors such as 17-hydroxyprogesterone.

For the differentiation of benign from malignant adrenal masses, imaging is relatively sensitive though specificity is suboptimal. CT is the procedure of choice for imaging the adrenal glands (Fig. 342-12). The risk of adrenocortical carcinoma, pheochromocytoma, and benign adrenal myelolipoma increases with the diameter of the adrenal mass. However, size alone is of poor predictive value, with only 80% sensitivity and 60% specificity for the differentiation of benign from malignant masses when using a 4-cm cut-off. Metastases are found with similar frequency in adrenal masses of all sizes. Tumor density on unenhanced CT is of additional diagnostic value, with most adrenocortical adenomas being lipid rich and thus presenting with low attenuation values [i.e., densities of <10 Hounsfield Units (HU)]. By contrast, adrenocortical carcinomas, but also pheochromocytomas, usually have high attenuation values (i.e. densities >20 HU on precontrast scans). Generally, benign lesions are rounded and homogenous whereas most malignant lesions appear lobulated and inhomogeneous. Pheochromocytoma and adrenomyelolipoma may also exhibit lobulated and inhomogeneous features. Additional information can be obtained from CT by assessment of contrast wash-out after 15 minutes, which is >50% in benign lesions but <40% in malignant lesions, which usually have a more extensive vascularization. MRI also allows for the visualization of the adrenal glands with somewhat lower resolution than CT. However, as it does not involve exposure to ionizing radiation, it is preferred in children, young adults, and during pregnancy. MRI has a valuable role in the characterization of indeterminate adrenal lesions using chemical shift analysis, with malignant tumors rarely showing loss of signal on opposed-phase MRI.

Fine-needle aspiration (FNA) or CT-guided biopsy of an adrenal mass is almost never indicated. FNA of a pheochromocytoma can cause a life-threatening hypertensive crisis. FNA of an adrenocortical carcinoma violates the tumor capsule. FNA should only be considered in a patient with a history of nonadrenal malignancy and a newly detected adrenal mass. FNA should be carried out only after careful exclusion of pheochromocytoma and if the outcome will influence therapeutic management. It is important to recognize that in 25% of patients with a previous history of nonadrenal malignancy, a newly detected mass on CT is not a metastasis.

Adrenal masses associated with confirmed hormone excess or suspected malignancy are usually treated surgically (Fig. 342-12) or, if adrenalectomy is not feasible or desired, with medication. Preoperative exclusion of glucocorticoid excess is particularly important for the prediction of postoperative suppression of the contralateral adrenal gland, which requires glucocorticoid replacement before surgery. If the initial decision is for observation, imaging and biochemical testing should be repeated about a year after the first assessment. However, this may be performed earlier in patients with borderline imaging or hormonal findings. There is no agreement with regard to the required long-term follow-up beyond 1 year and in patients with normal biochemistry and no evidence of increased tumor size at follow-up.

ADRENOCORTICAL CARCINOMA

Adrenocortical carcinoma (ACC) is a rare malignancy with an annual incidence of 1–2 per million population. ACC is generally considered a highly malignant tumor; however, it presents with broad interindividual variability with regard to biologic characteristics

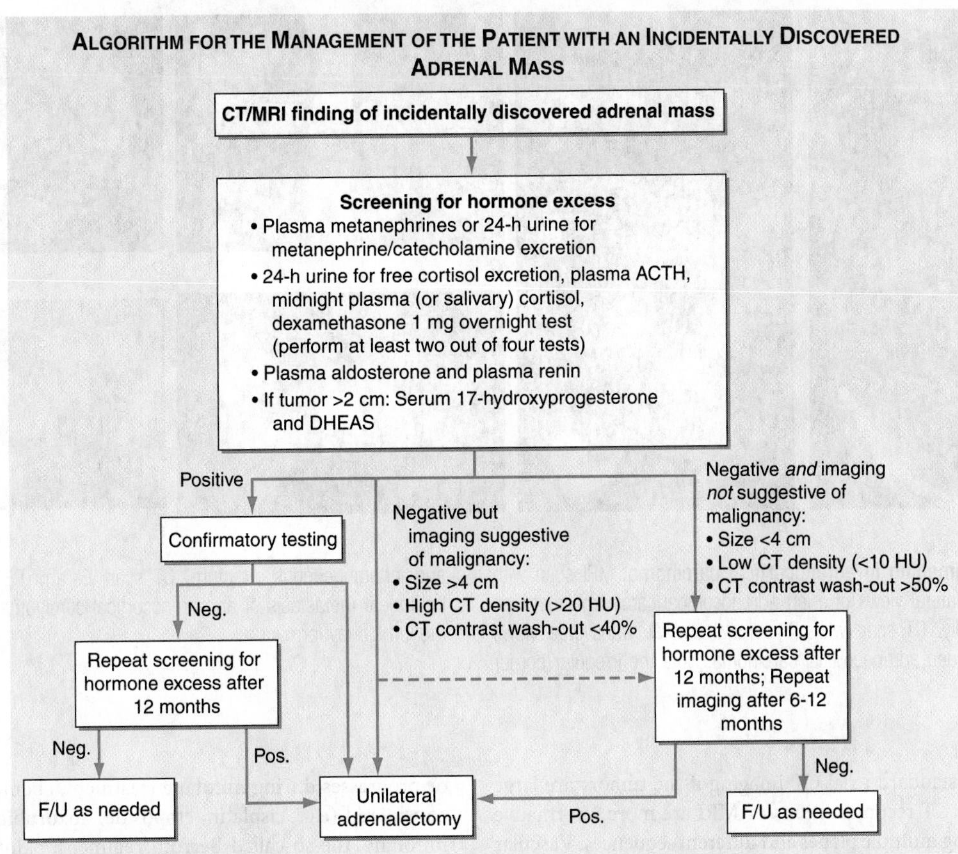

Figure 342-12 **Management of the patient with an incidentally discovered adrenal mass.** F/U, follow-up.

and clinical behavior. Somatic mutations in the tumor suppressor gene *TP53* are found in 25% of apparently sporadic ACC. Germline *TP53* mutations are the cause of the Li-Fraumeni syndrome associated with multiple solid organ cancers including ACC and are found in 25% of pediatric ACC cases; the *TP53* mutation R337H is found in almost all pediatric ACC in Brazil. Other genetic changes identified in ACC include alterations in the Wnt/β-catenin pathway and in the insulin-like growth factor 2 (IGF2) cluster; IGF2 overexpression is found in 90% of ACC.

Patients with large adrenal tumors suspicious of malignancy should be managed by a multidisciplinary specialist team, including an endocrinologist, an oncologist, a surgeon, a radiologist, and a histopathologist. FNA is not indicated in suspected ACC: first, cytology and also histopathology of a core biopsy cannot differentiate between benign and malignant primary adrenal masses; second, FNA violates the tumor capsule and may even cause needle canal metastasis. Even when the entire tumor specimen is available, the histopathologic differentiation between benign and malignant lesions is a diagnostic challenge. The most common histopathologic classification is the Weiss score, taking into account high nuclear grade; mitotic rate (>5/HPF); atypical mitosis; <25% clear cells; diffuse architecture; and presence of necrosis, venous invasion, and invasion of sinusoidal structures and tumor capsule. The presence of three or more elements suggests ACC.

Although 60–70% of ACCs are biochemically found to overproduce hormones, this is not clinically apparent in many patients due to the relatively inefficient steroid production by the adrenocortical cancer cells. Excess production of glucocorticoids and adrenal androgen precursors are most common. Mixed excess production of several corticosteroid classes by an adrenal tumor is generally indicative of malignancy.

Tumor staging at diagnosis (Table 342-6) has important prognostic implications and requires scanning of the chest and abdomen for local organ invasion, lymphadenopathy, and metastases. Intravenous contrast medium is necessary for maximum sensitivity for hepatic metastases. An adrenal origin may be difficult

TABLE 342-6 Classification System for Staging of Adrenocortical Carcinoma

Stage	ENSAT Stage	TNM Definitions
I	T1,N0, M0	T1, tumor ≤5 cm N0, no positive lymph node M0, no distant metastases
II	T2,N0,M0	T2, tumor >5 cm N0, no positive lymph node M0, no distant metastases
III	T1–T2,N1,M0 T3–T4,N0–N1,M0	N1, positive lymph node(s) M0, no distant metastases T3, tumor infiltration into surrounding tissue T4, tumor invasion into adjacent organs ***or*** venous tumor thrombus in vena cava or renal vein
IV	T1–T4,N0–N1,M1	M1, presence of distant metastases

Abbreviation: ENSAT, European Network for the Study of Adrenal Tumors.

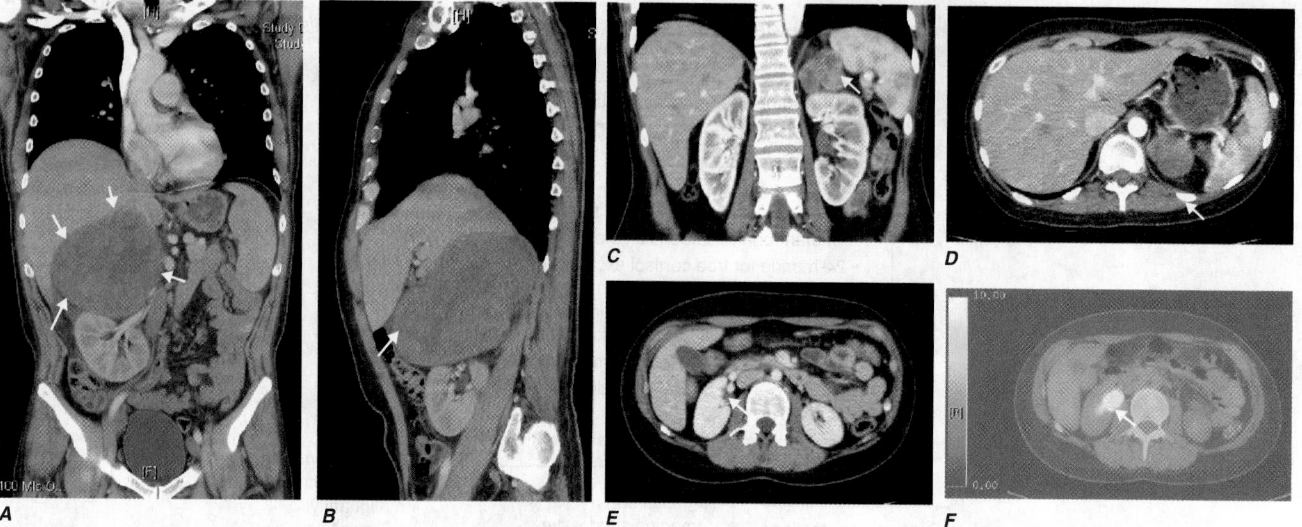

Figure 342-13 Imaging in adrenocortical carcinoma. MRI scan with ***A.*** frontal and ***B.*** lateral views of a left adrenocortical carcinoma that was detected incidentally. CT scan with ***C.*** coronal and ***D.*** transverse views depicting a right-sided adrenocortical carcinoma. Note the irregular border and inhomogeneous structure. CT scan ***E.*** and PET-CT ***F.*** visualizing a peritoneal metastasis of an adrenocortical carcinoma in close proximity to the left kidney (arrow).

to determine on standard axial CT imaging if the tumors are large and invasive, but CT reconstructions or MRI are more informative (Fig. 342-13) using multiple planes and different sequences. Vascular and adjacent organ invasion is diagnostic of malignancy. 18-Fluoro-2-deoxy-D-glucose positron emission tomography (18-FDG PET) is highly sensitive for the detection of malignancy and can be used to detect small metastases or local recurrence that may not be obvious on CT (Fig. 342-13). However, FDG PET is not specific and therefore cannot be used for differentiating benign from malignant adrenal lesions. Metastasis in ACC most frequently occurs to liver and lung.

ACC carries a poor prognosis and cure can be achieved only by complete surgical removal. Capsule violation during primary surgery, metastasis at diagnosis, and primary treatment in a non-specialist center are major determinants of poor survival. If the primary tumor invades adjacent organs, en bloc removal of kidney and spleen should be considered to reduce the risk of recurrence. Surgery can also be considered in a patient with metastases if there is severe tumor-related hormone excess. This indication needs to be carefully weighed against surgical risk, including thromboembolic complications, and the resulting delay in the introduction of other therapeutic options. Patients with confirmed ACC and successful removal of the primary tumor should receive adjuvant treatment with mitotane (o,p'DDD), particularly in patients with a high risk of recurrence as determined by tumor size >8 cm, histopathologic signs of vascular invasion, capsule invasion or violation, and a Ki67 proliferation index ≥10%. Mitotane is usually started at 500 mg qid, with doses increased by 1000 mg/d every 1–2 weeks as tolerated. The maximum tolerated dose is usually 8–10 g/m^2 per day. Adjuvant mitotane should be continued for at least 2 years, if the patient can tolerate side effects. Regular monitoring of plasma mitotane levels is mandatory (therapeutic range 14–20 mg/L; neurotoxic complications more frequent >20 mg/L), as is concurrent replacement with hydrocortisone. The latter should be given at higher doses than usually employed in adrenal insufficiency (e.g., 20 mg tid), as mitotane increases glucocorticoid inactivation due to the induction of hepatic CYP3A4 activity. It also increases circulating cortisol-binding globulin, thereby decreasing the available free cortisol fraction. Single metastases can be addressed surgically or with radiofrequency ablation as appropriate. If the tumor recurs or progresses during mitotane treatment, chemotherapy should be considered (e.g., cisplatin, etoposide, doxorubicin plus continuing mitotane, the so-called Berrutti regimen); painful bone metastasis responds to irradiation. Overall survival in ACC is still poor, with 5-year survival rates of 30–40%.

■ ADRENAL INSUFFICIENCY

Epidemiology

The prevalence of well-documented, permanent adrenal insufficiency is 5 in 10,000 in the general population. Hypothalamic-pituitary origin of disease is most frequent, with a prevalence of 3 in 10,000, whereas primary adrenal insufficiency has a prevalence of 2 in 10,000. Approximately one-half of the latter cases are acquired, mostly caused by autoimmune destruction of the adrenal glands; the other one-half are genetic, most commonly caused by distinct enzymatic blocks in adrenal steroidogenesis affecting glucocorticoid synthesis (i.e. congenital adrenal hyperplasia.)

Adrenal insufficiency arising from suppression of the HPA axis as a consequence of exogenous glucocorticoid treatment is much more common, occurring in 0.5–2% of the population in developed countries.

Etiology

Primary adrenal insufficiency is most commonly caused by autoimmune adrenalitis. Isolated autoimmune adrenalitis accounts for 30–40%, whereas 60–70% develop adrenal insufficiency as part of autoimmune polyglandular syndromes (APS) (Chap. 351) (Table 342-7). APS1, also termed APECED (autoimmune polyendocrinopathy-candidiasis-ectodermal dystrophy), is the underlying cause in 10% of patients affected by APS. APS1 is transmitted in an autosomal recessive manner and is caused by mutations in the autoimmune regulator gene *AIRE*. Associated autoimmune conditions overlap with those seen in APS2, but may also include total alopecia, primary hypoparathyroidism, and, in rare cases, lymphoma. APS1 patients invariably develop chronic mucocutaneous candidiasis, usually manifest in childhood, and preceding adrenal insufficiency by years or decades. The much more prevalent

TABLE 342-7 Causes of Primary Adrenal Insufficiency

Diagnosis	Gene	Associated Features
Autoimmune polyglandular syndrome 1 (APS1)	*AIRE*	Hypoparathyroidism, chronic mucocutaneous candidiasis, other autoimmune disorders, rarely lymphomas
Autoimmune polyglandular syndrome 2 (APS2)	Associations with HLA-DR3, CTLA-4	Hypothyroidism, hyperthyroidism, premature ovarian failure, vitiligo, type 1 diabetes mellitus, pernicious anemia
Isolated autoimmune adrenalitis	Associations with HLA-DR3, CTLA-4	
Congenital adrenal hyperplasia (CAH)	*CYP21A2, CYP11B1, CYP17A1, HSD3B2, POR*	See Table 342-10 (see also Chap. 349)
Congenital lipoid adrenal hyperplasia (CLAH)	*StAR, CYP11A1*	46,XY DSD, gonadal failure (see also Chap. 349)
Adrenal hypoplasia congenita (AHC)	*NR0B1* (DAX-1), *NR5A1* (SF-1)	46,XY DSD, gonadal failure (see also Chap. 349)
Adrenoleukodystrophy (ALD), adrenomyeloneuropathy (AMN)	*X-ALD*	Demyelination of central nervous system (ALD) or spinal cord and peripheral nerves (AMN)
Familial glucocorticoid deficiency		ACTH insensitivity syndromes due to mutations in the ACTH receptor MC2R and its accessory protein MRAP tall stature
- FGD1	*MC2R*	Alacrima, achalasia, neurologic impairment
- FGD2	*MRAP*	
- FGD3	?	
Triple A syndrome	*AAAS*	
Smith-Lemli-Opitz-Syndrome	*SLOS*	Cholesterol synthesis disorder associated with mental retardation, craniofacial malformations, growth failure
Kearns-Sayre syndrome	Mitochondrial DNA deletions	Progressive external ophthalmoplegia, pigmentary retinal degeneration, cardiac conduction defects, gonadal failure, hypoparathyroidism, type 1 diabetes
IMAGe syndrome	?	Intrauterine growth retardation, metaphyseal dysplasia, genital anomalies
Adrenal infections		Tuberculosis, HIV, CMV, cryptococcosis, histoplasmosis, coccidioidomycosis
Adrenal infiltration		Metastases, lymphomas, sarcoidosis, amyloidosis, hemochromatosis
Adrenal hemorrhage		Meningococcal sepsis (Waterhouse-Friderichsen syndrome), primary antiphospholipid syndrome
Drug-induced		Mitotane, aminoglutethimide, arbiraterone, trilostane, etomidate, ketoconazole, suramin, RU486
Bilateral adrenalectomy		E.g., in the management of Cushing's or after bilateral nephrectomy

Abbreviations: CMV, cytomegalovirus; DSD, disordered sex development.

APS2 is of polygenic inheritance, with confirmed associations with the *HLA-DR3* gene region in the major histocompatibility complex and distinct gene regions involved in immune regulation (*CTLA-4, PTPN22, CLEC16A*). Coincident autoimmune disease most frequently includes thyroid autoimmune disease, vitiligo, and premature ovarian failure. Less commonly, additional features may include type 1 diabetes and pernicious anemia caused by vitamin B_{12} deficiency.

X-linked adrenoleukodystrophy has an incidence of 1:20,000 males and is caused by mutations in the *X-ALD* gene encoding the peroxisomal membrane transporter protein ABCD1; its disruption results in accumulation of very long chain (>24 carbon atoms) fatty acids. Approximately 50% of cases manifest in early childhood with rapidly progressive white matter disease (cerebral ALD); 35% present during adolescence or in early adulthood with neurologic features indicative of myelin and peripheral nervous system involvement (adrenomyeloneuropathy, AMN). In the remaining 15%, adrenal insufficiency is the sole manifestation of disease. Of note, distinct mutations manifest with variable penetrance within affected families.

Rarer causes of adrenal insufficiency involve destruction of the adrenal glands as a consequence of infection, hemorrhage, or infiltration (Table 342-7); tuberculous adrenalitis is still a frequent cause of disease in developing countries. Adrenal metastases rarely cause adrenal insufficiency, and this occurs only with bilateral, bulky metastases.

Inborn causes of primary adrenal insufficiency other than congenital adrenal hyperplasia are rare, causing less than 1% of cases. However, their elucidation provides important insights into adrenal gland development and physiology. Mutations causing primary adrenal insufficiency (Table 342-7) include factors regulating adrenal development and steroidogenesis (DAX-1, SF-1), cholesterol synthesis, import and cleavage (DHCR7, StAR, CYP11A1), and elements of the adrenal ACTH response pathway (MC2R, MRAP) (Fig. 342-5).

Secondary adrenal insufficiency is the consequence of dysfunction of the hypothalamic-pituitary component of the HPA axis (Table 342-8). Excluding iatrogenic suppression, the overwhelming majority of cases are caused by pituitary or hypothalamic tumors, or their treatment by surgery or irradiation (Chap. 339). Rarer causes include pituitary apoplexy, either as a consequence of an infarcted pituitary adenoma or transient reduction in the blood supply of the pituitary during surgery or after rapid blood loss associated with parturition, also termed Sheehan's syndrome. Isolated ACTH deficiency is rarely caused by autoimmune disease or pituitary infiltration (Table 342-8). Mutations in the ACTH precursor POMC or in factors regulating pituitary development are genetic causes of ACTH deficiency (Table 342-8).

Clinical manifestations

In principle, the clinical features of primary adrenal insufficiency are characterized by the loss of both glucocorticoid and mineralocorticoid secretion (Table 342-9). In secondary adrenal insufficiency, only glucocorticoid deficiency is present, as the adrenal itself is intact and thus still amenable to regulation by the RAA system. Adrenal androgen secretion is disrupted in both primary and secondary adrenal insufficiency (Table 342-9). Hypothalamic-pituitary disease can lead to additional clinical manifestations due to involvement of other endocrine axes (thyroid, gonads, growth hormone, prolactin) or visual impairment with bitemporal hemianopia caused by chiasmal compression. It is important to recognize that iatrogenic adrenal insufficiency caused by exogenous glucocorticoid suppression of the HPA axis may result in all symptoms associated with glucocorticoid deficiency (Table 342-9), if exogenous glucocorticoids are stopped abruptly. However, patients will appear clinically Cushingoid as a result of the preceding overexposure to glucocorticoids.

Chronic adrenal insufficiency manifests with relatively nonspecific signs and symptoms such as fatigue and loss of energy, often resulting in delayed or missed diagnoses (e.g., as depression or anorexia). A distinguishing feature of primary adrenal insufficiency is hyperpigmentation, which is caused by excess ACTH stimulation of melanocytes. Hyperpigmentation is most pronounced in skin areas exposed to increased friction or shear stress and is increased by sunlight (Fig. 342-14). Conversely, in secondary adrenal insufficiency, the skin has an alabaster-like paleness due to lack of ACTH secretion.

Hyponatremia is a characteristic biochemical feature in primary adrenal insufficiency and is found in 80% of patients at presentation. Hyperkalemia is present in 40% of patients at initial diagnosis. Hyponatremia is primarily caused by mineralocorticoid deficiency but can also occur in secondary adrenal insufficiency due to diminished inhibition of ADH by cortisol, resulting in mild syndrome of inappropriate secretion of antidiuretic hormone (SIADH). Glucocorticoid deficiency also results in slightly increased TSH concentrations that normalize within days to weeks after initiation of glucocorticoid replacement.

TABLE 342-8 Causes of Secondary Adrenal Insufficiency

Diagnosis	Gene	Associated Features
Pituitary tumors (endocrine active and inactive adenomas, very rare: carcinoma)		Depending on tumor size and location: visual field impairment (bilateral hemianopia), hyperprolactinemia, secondary hypothyroidism, hypogonadism, growth hormone deficiency
Other mass lesions affecting the hypothalamic-pituitary region		Craniopharyngioma, meningioma, ependymoma, metastases
Pituitary irradiation		Radiotherapy administered for pituitary tumors, brain tumors, or craniospinal irradiation in leukemia
Autoimmune hypophysitis		Often associated with pregnancy; may present with panhypopituitarism or isolated ACTH deficiency; can be associated with autoimmune thyroid disease, more rarely with vitiligo, premature ovarian failure, type 1 diabetes, pernicious anemia
Pituitary apoplexy/hemorrhage		Hemorrhagic infarction of large pituitary adenomas or pituitary infarction consequent to traumatic major blood loss (e.g., surgery or pregnancy: Sheehan's syndrome)
Pituitary infiltration		Tuberculosis, actinomycosis, sarcoidosis, histiocytosis X, granulomatosis with polyangiitis (Wegener's), metastases
Drug-induced		Chronic glucocorticoid excess (endogenous or exogenous)
Congenital isolated ACTH deficiency	*TBX19* (Tpit)	
Combined pituitary hormone deficiency (CPHD)	*PROP-1*	Progressive development of CPHD in the order GH, PRL, TSH, LH/FSH, ACTH
	HESX1	CPHD and septo-optic dysplasia
	LHX3	CPHD and limited neck rotation, sensorineural deafness
	LHX4	CPHD and cerebellar abnormalities
	SOX3	CPHD and variable mental retardation
Proopiomelanocortin (POMC) deficiency	*POMC*	Early-onset obesity, red hair pigmentation

Abbreviations: ACTH, adrenocorticotropic hormone; GH, growth hormone; LH/FSH, luteinizing hormone/follicle-stimulating hormone; PRL, prolactin; TSH, thyroid-stimulating hormone.

TABLE 342-9 Signs and Symptoms of Adrenal Insufficiency

Signs and Symptoms Caused by Glucocorticoid Deficiency
Fatigue, lack of energy
Weight loss, anorexia
Myalgia, joint pain
Fever
Anemia, lymphocytosis, eosinophilia
Slightly increased TSH (due to loss of feedback inhibition of TSH release)
Hypoglycemia (more frequent in children)
Low blood pressure, postural hypotension
Hyponatremia (due to loss of feedback inhibition of AVP release)
Signs and Symptoms Caused by Mineralocorticoid Deficiency (Primary AI Only)
Abdominal pain, nausea, vomiting
Dizziness, postural hypotension
Salt craving
Low blood pressure, postural hypotension
Increased serum creatinine (due to volume depletion)
Hyponatremia
Hyperkalemia
Signs and Symptoms Caused by Adrenal Androgen Deficiency
Lack of energy
Dry and itchy skin (in women)
Loss of libido (in women)
Loss of axillary and pubic hair (in women)
Other Signs and Symptoms
Hyperpigmentation (primary AI only) [due to excess of pro-opiomelanocortin (POMC)–derived peptides]
Alabaster-colored pale skin (secondary AI only) (due to deficiency of POMC-derived peptides)

Acute adrenal insufficiency usually occurs after a prolonged period of nonspecific complaints and is more frequently observed in patients with primary adrenal insufficiency, due to the loss of both glucocorticoid and mineralocorticoid secretion. Postural hypotension may progress to hypovolemic shock. Adrenal insufficiency may mimic features of acute abdomen with abdominal tenderness, nausea, vomiting, and fever. In some cases, the primary presentation may resemble neurologic disease, with decreased responsiveness, progressing to stupor and coma. An adrenal crisis can be triggered by an intercurrent illness, surgical or other stress, or increased glucocorticoid inactivation (e.g., hyperthyroidism).

Diagnosis

The diagnosis of adrenal insufficiency is established by the short cosyntropin test, a safe and reliable tool with excellent predictive diagnostic value (Fig. 342-15). The cut-off for failure is usually defined at cortisol levels of <500–550 nmol/L (18–20 μg/dL) sampled 30–60 minutes after ACTH stimulation; the exact cut-off is dependent on the locally available assay. During the early phase of HPA disruption (e.g., within 4 weeks of pituitary insufficiency), patients may still respond to exogenous ACTH stimulation. In this circumstance, the insulin tolerance test is an alternative choice but is more invasive and should be carried out only under a specialist's supervision (see above). Induction of hypoglycemia is contraindicated in individuals with diabetes mellitus, cardiovascular disease, or history of seizures. Random serum cortisol measurements are of limited diagnostic value, as baseline cortisol levels may be coincidentally low due to the physiologic diurnal rhythm of cortisol secretion (Fig. 342-3). Similarly, many patients with secondary adrenal insufficiency have relatively normal baseline cortisol levels but fail to mount an appropriate cortisol response to ACTH, which can only be revealed by stimulation testing. Importantly, tests to establish the diagnosis of adrenal insufficiency should never delay treatment. Thus, in a patient with suspected adrenal crisis, it is reasonable to draw baseline cortisol levels, provide replacement therapy, and defer formal stimulation testing until a later time.

Once adrenal insufficiency is confirmed, measurement of plasma ACTH is the next step, with increased or inappropriately low levels defining primary and secondary origin of disease, respectively (Fig. 342-15). In primary adrenal insufficiency, increased plasma renin will confirm the presence of mineralocorticoid deficiency. At initial presentation, patients with primary adrenal insufficiency should undergo screening for steroid autoantibodies as a marker of autoimmune adrenalitis. If these tests are negative, adrenal imaging by CT is indicated to investigate possible hemorrhage, infiltration, or masses. In male patients with negative autoantibodies in the plasma, very long chain fatty acids should be measured to exclude X-ALD. Patients with inappropriately low ACTH, in the presence of confirmed cortisol deficiency, should undergo hypothalamic-pituitary imaging by MRI. Features suggestive of preceding pituitary apoplexy such as sudden-onset severe headache, or history of previous head trauma, should be carefully explored, particularly in patients with no obvious MRI lesion.

TREATMENT Acute Adrenal Insufficiency

Acute adrenal insufficiency requires immediate initiation of rehydration, usually carried out by saline infusion at initial rates of 1 L/h with continuous cardiac monitoring. Glucocorticoid replacement should be initiated by bolus injection of 100 mg hydrocortisone, followed by the administration of 100–200 mg hydrocortisone over 24 h, either by continuous infusion or provided by several IV or IM injections. Mineralocorticoid replacement can be initiated once the daily hydrocortisone dose has been reduced to <50 mg because at higher doses hydrocortisone provides sufficient stimulation of mineralocorticoid receptors.

Glucocorticoid replacement for the treatment of chronic adrenal insufficiency should be administered at a dose that replaces the physiologic daily cortisol production, which is usually achieved by the oral administration of 15–25 mg hydrocortisone in two to three divided doses. Pregnancy may require an increase in hydrocortisone dose by 50% during the last trimester. In all patients, at least one-half of the daily dose should be administered in the morning. Currently available glucocorticoid preparations fail to mimic the physiologic cortisol secretion rhythm (Fig. 342-3). Long-acting glucocorticoids such as prednisolone or dexamethasone are not preferred as they result in increased glucocorticoid exposure due to extended glucocorticoid receptor activation at times of physiologically low cortisol secretion. There are no well-established dose equivalencies, but as a guide, equipotency can be assumed for 1 mg hydrocortisone, 1.6 mg

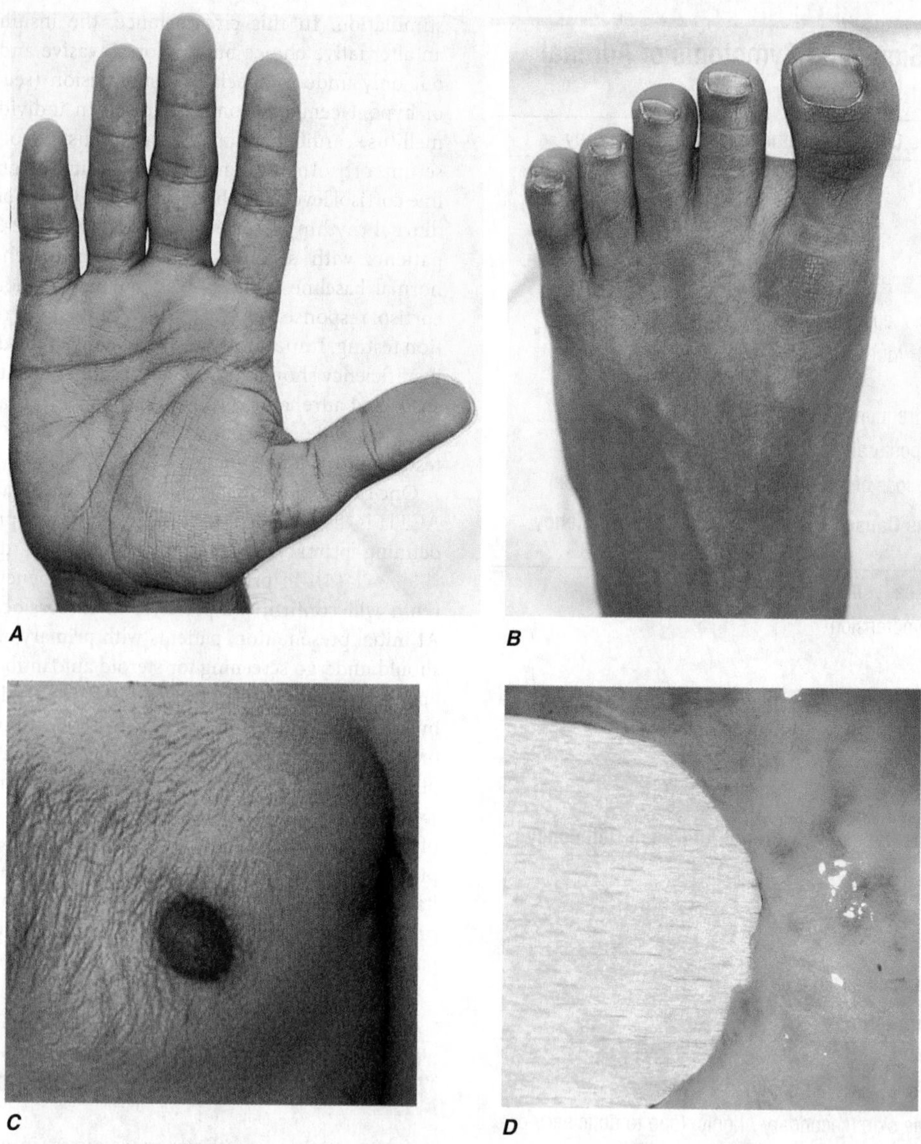

Figure 342-14 Clinical features of Addison's disease. Note the hyperpigmentation in areas of increased friction including (*A*) palmar creases, (*B*) dorsal foot, (*C*) nipples and axillary region, and (*D*) patchy hyperpigmentation of the oral mucosa.

cortisone acetate, 0.2 mg prednisolone, 0.25 mg prednisone, and 0.025 mg dexamethasone.

Monitoring of glucocorticoid replacement is mainly based on the history and examination for signs and symptoms suggestive of glucocorticoid over- or under-replacement, including assessment of body weight and blood pressure. Plasma ACTH, 24-hour urinary free cortisol, or serum cortisol day curves reflect whether hydrocortisone has been taken or not, but do not convey reliable information about replacement quality. In patients with isolated primary adrenal insufficiency, monitoring should include screening for autoimmune thyroid disease, and female patients should be made aware of the possibility of premature ovarian failure. Supraphysiologic glucocorticoid treatment with doses equivalent to 30 mg hydrocortisone or more will affect bone metabolism, and these patients should undergo regular bone mineral density evaluation. All patients with adrenal insufficiency need to be instructed about the requirement for stress-related glucocorticoid dose adjustments. These generally consist of doubling the routine oral glucocorticoid dose in the case of intercurrent illness with fever and bedrest and the need for IV hydrocortisone injection at a daily dose of 100 mg in cases of prolonged vomiting, surgery, or trauma. Patients living or traveling in regions with delayed access to acute health care should carry a hydrocortisone self-injection emergency kit, in addition to their usual steroid emergency cards and bracelets.

Mineralocorticoid replacement in primary adrenal insufficiency should be initiated at a dose of 100–150 μg fludrocortisone. The adequacy of treatment can be evaluated by measuring blood pressure, sitting and standing, to detect a postural drop indicative of hypovolemia. In addition, serum sodium, potassium, and plasma renin should be measured regularly. Renin levels should be kept in the upper normal reference range. Changes in glucocorticoid dose may also impact on mineralocorticoid replacement as cortisol also binds the mineralocorticoid receptor; 40 mg hydrocortisone is equivalent to 100 μg fludrocortisone. In patients living or traveling in areas with hot or tropical weather conditions, the fludrocortisone dose should be increased by 50–100 μg during the summer. Mineralocorticoid dose may also need to be adjusted during pregnancy, due to the antimineralocorticoid activity of

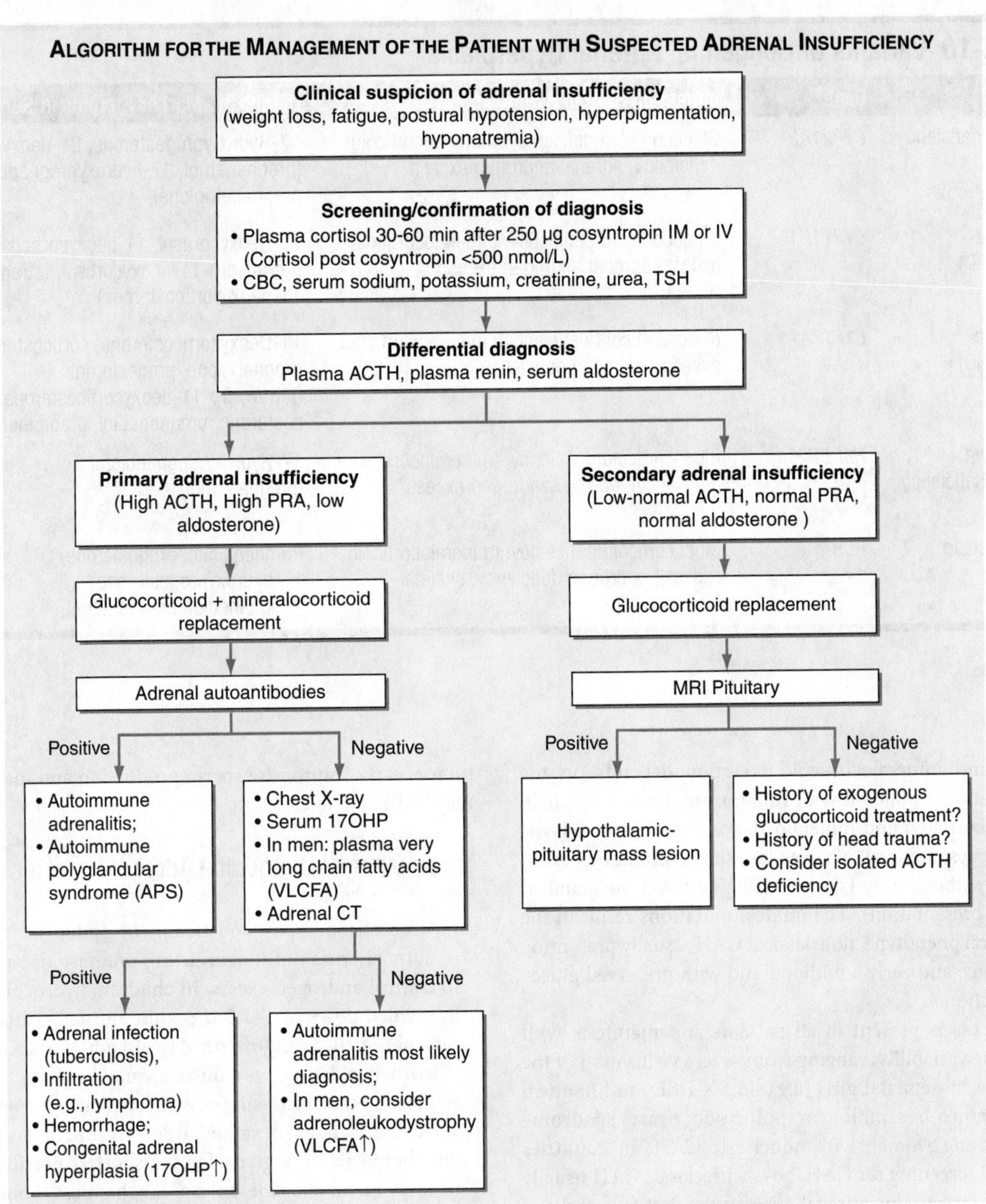

Figure 342-15 **Management of the patient with suspected adrenal insufficiency.** PRA, plasma renin activity.

progesterone, but this is less often required than hydrocortisone dose adjustment. Plasma renin cannot serve as a monitoring tool during pregnancy, as renin rises physiologically during gestation.

Adrenal androgen replacement is an option in patients with lack of energy, despite optimized glucocorticoid and mineralocorticoid replacement. It may also be indicated in women with features of androgen deficiency, including loss of libido. Adrenal androgen replacement can be achieved by once-daily administration of 25–50 mg DHEA. Treatment is monitored by measurement of DHEAS, androstenedione, testosterone, and SHBG 24 hours after the last DHEA dose.

CONGENITAL ADRENAL HYPERPLASIA

(See also Chap. 349) Congenital adrenal hyperplasia (CAH) is caused by mutations in genes encoding steroidogenic enzymes involved in glucocorticoid synthesis (CYP21A2, CYP17A1, HSD3B2, CYP11B1) or in the cofactor enzyme P450 oxidoreductase that serves as an electron donor to CYP21A2 and CYP17A1 (Fig. 342-1). Invariably, patients affected by CAH exhibit glucocorticoid deficiency. Depending on the exact step of enzymatic block, they may also have excess production mineralocorticoids or deficient production of sex steroids (Table 342-10). The diagnosis of CAH is readily established by measurement of the steroids accumulating before the distinct enzymatic block, either in serum or in urine, preferably by the use of mass spectrometry–based assays (Table 342-10).

Mutations in CYP21A2 are the most prevalent cause of CAH, responsible for 90–95% of cases. 21-Hydroxylase deficiency disrupts glucocorticoid and mineralocorticoid synthesis (Fig. 342-1), resulting in diminished negative feedback via the HPA axis. This leads to increased pituitary ACTH release, which drives increased synthesis of adrenal androgen precursors and subsequent androgen excess. The degree of impairment of

TABLE 342-10 Variants of Congenital Adrenal Hyperplasia

Variant	Gene	Impact on Steroid Synthesis	Diagnostic Marker Steroids in Serum (and Urine)
21-Hydroxylase deficiency (21OHD)	*CYP21A2*	Glucocorticoid deficiency, mineralocorticoid deficiency, adrenal androgen excess	17-Hydroxyprogesterone, 21-deoxycortisol (pregnanetriol, 17-hydroxypregnanolone, pregnanetriolone)
11β-Hydroxylase deficiency (11OHD)	*CYP11B1*	Glucocorticoid deficiency, mineralocorticoid excess, adrenal androgen excess	11-Deoxycortisol, 11-deoxycorticosterone (tetrahydro-11-deoxycortisol, tetrahydro-11-deoxycorticosterone)
17α-Hydroxylase deficiency (17OHD)	*CYP17A1*	(Glucocorticoid deficiency), mineralocorticoid excess, androgen deficiency	11-Deoxycorticosterone, corticosterone, pregnenolone, progesterone (tetrahydro-11-deoxycorticosterone, tetrahydrocorticosterone, pregnenediol, pregnanediol)
3β-Hydroxysteroid dehydrogenase deficiency (3bHSDD)	*HSD3B2*	Glucocorticoid deficiency, (mineralocorticoid deficiency), adrenal androgen excess	17-Hydroxypregnanolone (pregnanetriol)
P450 oxidoreductase deficiency (ORD)	*POR*	Glucocorticoid deficiency, (mineralocorticoid excess), androgen deficiency, skeletal malformations	Pregnenolone, progesterone, 17-hydroxyprogesterone (pregnanediol, pregnanetriol)

glucocorticoid and mineralocorticoid secretion depends on the severity of mutations. Major loss-of-function mutations result in combined glucocorticoid and mineralocorticoid deficiency (classic CAH, neonatal presentation), whereas less severe mutations affect glucocorticoid synthesis only (simple virilizing CAH, neonatal or early childhood presentation). The mildest mutations result in the least severe clinical phenotype, nonclassical CAH, usually presenting during adolescence and early adulthood and with preserved glucocorticoid production.

Androgen excess is present in all patients and manifests with broad phenotypic variability, ranging from severe virilization of the external genitalia in neonatal girls (e.g., 46,XX DSD) to hirsutism and oligomenorrhea resembling a polycystic ovary syndrome phenotype in young women with nonclassic CAH. In countries without neonatal screening for CAH, boys with classic CAH usually present with life-threatening adrenal crisis in the first few weeks of life (salt-wasting crisis); a simple-virilizing genotype manifests with precocious pseudo-puberty and advanced bone age in early childhood, whereas men with nonclassic CAH are usually detected only through family screening.

Glucocorticoid treatment is more complex than for other causes of primary adrenal insufficiency. It not only needs to replace missing glucocorticoids but also aims to suppress the increased ACTH drive and subsequent androgen excess. Current treatment is hampered by the lack of glucocorticoid preparations that mimic the diurnal cortisol secretion profile, resulting in a prolonged period of ACTH stimulation and subsequent androgen production during the early morning hours. In childhood, optimization of growth and pubertal development are important goals of glucocorticoid treatment, in addition to prevention of adrenal crisis and treatment of 46,XX DSD. In adults, the focus shifts to preserving fertility and preventing side effects of glucocorticoid overtreatment, namely, the metabolic syndrome and osteoporosis. Fertility can be compromised in women due to oligo/amenorrhea with chronic anovulation as a consequence of androgen excess. Men may develop so-called testicular adrenal rest tumors (Fig. 342-16). These consist of hyperplastic cells with adrenocortical characteristics located in the rete testis and should not be confused with testicular tumors. Testicular adrenal rest tumors can compromise sperm production and induce fibrosis that may be irreversible.

TREATMENT Congenital Adrenal Hyperplasia

Hydrocortisone is a good treatment option for the prevention of adrenal crisis but longer-acting prednisolone may be needed to control androgen excess. In children, hydrocortisone is given in divided doses at 1–1.5 times the normal cortisol production rate (about 10–13 mg/m^2 per day). In adults, intermediate-acting glucocorticoids (e.g., prednisone) may be given, using the lowest dose necessary to suppress excess androgen production. For achieving fertility, dexamethasone treatment may be required, but should be only given for the shortest possible time period to limit metabolic side effects. Biochemical monitoring should include androstenedione and testosterone, aiming for the normal sex-specific reference range. 17-Hydroxyprogesterone (17OHP) is a useful marker of overtreatment, indicated by 17OHP levels within the normal range of healthy controls. Glucocorticoid overtreatment may suppress the hypothalamic-pituitary-gonadal axis. Thus, treatment needs to be carefully titrated against clinical features of disease control. Stress dose glucocorticoids should be given at double or triple the daily dose for surgery, acute illness, or severe trauma. Poorly controlled CAH can result in adrenocortical hyperplasia, which gave the disease its name, and may present as macronodular hyperplasia subsequent to long-standing ACTH excess (Fig. 342-15). The nodular areas can develop autonomous adrenal androgen production, and may be unresponsive to glucocorticoid treatment.

Mineralocorticoid requirements change during life and are higher in children, explained by relative mineralocorticoid resistance that diminishes with ongoing maturation of the kidney. Children with CAH usually receive mineralocorticoid and salt replacement. However, young adults with CAH should undergo reassessment of their mineralocorticoid reserve. Plasma renin should be regularly monitored and kept within the upper half of the normal reference range.

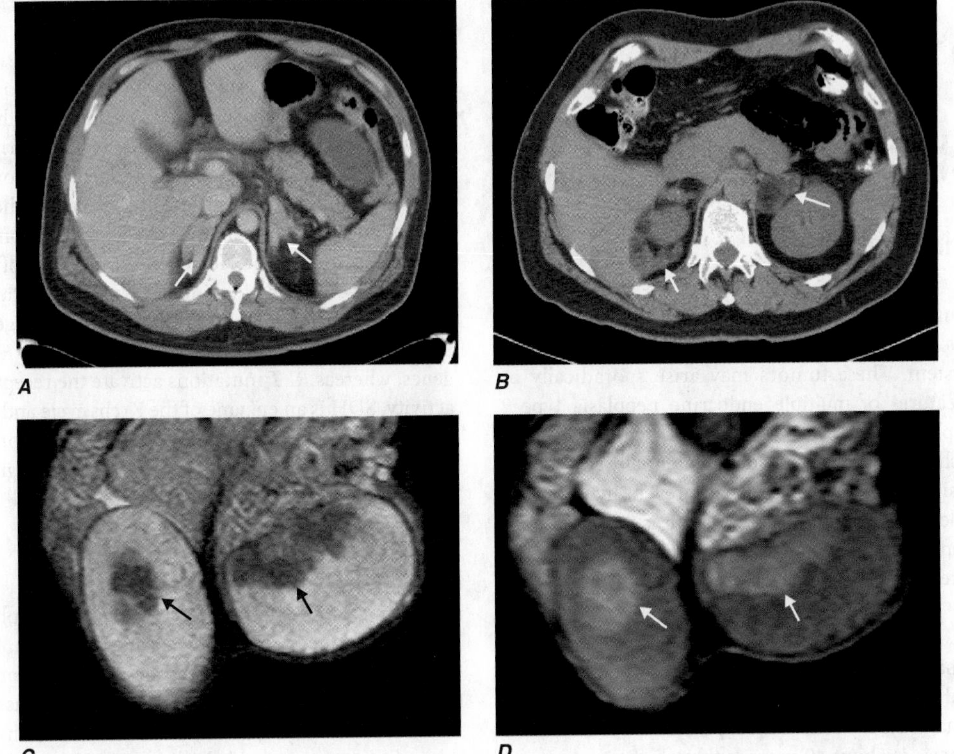

Figure 342-16 Imaging in congenital adrenal hyperplasia (CAH). Adrenal CT scans showing homogenous bilateral hyperplasia in a young patient with classic CAH ***A*** and macronodular bilateral hyperplasia ***B*** in a middle-aged classic CAH patient with longstanding poor disease control. MRI scan with T1-weighted ***C*** and T2-weighted ***D*** images showing bilateral testicular adrenal rest tumors (arrows) in a young patient with salt-wasting congenital adrenal hyperplasia. *(Courtesy of N. Reisch.)*

FURTHER READINGS

Arlt W et al: Health status of adults with congenital adrenal hyperplasia: A cohort study of 203 patients. J Clin Endocrinol Metab 95:5110, 2010

Biller BM et al: Treatment of adrenocorticotropin-dependent Cushing's syndrome: A consensus statement. J Clin Endocrinol Metab 93:2454, 2008

Debono M et al: Novel strategies for hydrocortisone replacement. Best Pract Res Clin Endocrinol Metab 23:221, 2009

Fassnacht M, Allolio B: Clinical management of adrenocortical carcinoma. Best Pract Res Clin Endocrinol Metab 23:273, 2009

Funder JW et al: Case detection, diagnosis, and treatment of patients with primary aldosteronism: An Endocrine Society Clinical Practice Guideline. J Clin Endocrinol Metab 93:3266, 2008

Krone N, Arlt W: Genetics of congenital adrenal hyperplasia. Best Pract Res Clin Endocrinol Metab 23:181, 2009

Nieman LK et al: The diagnosis of Cushing's syndrome: An Endocrine Society Clinical Practice Guideline. J Clin Endocrinol Metab 93:1526, 2008

Speiser PW et al: Congenital adrenal hyperplasia due to steroid 21-hydroxylase deficiency: An Endocrine Society clinical practice guideline. J Clin Endocrinol Metab 95:4133, 2010

Young WF Jr: Clinical practice. The incidentally discovered adrenal mass. N Engl J Med 356:601, 2007

CHAPTER 343
Pheochromocytoma

Hartmut P. H. Neumann

Pheochromocytomas and paragangliomas are catecholamine-producing tumors derived from the sympathetic or parasympathetic nervous system. These tumors may arise sporadically or be inherited as features of multiple endocrine neoplasia type 2 or several other pheochromocytoma-associated syndromes. The diagnosis of pheochromocytomas provides a potentially correctable cause of hypertension, and their removal can prevent hypertensive crises that can be lethal. The clinical presentation is variable, ranging from an adrenal incidentaloma to a patient in hypertensive crisis with associated cerebrovascular or cardiac complications.

■ EPIDEMIOLOGY

Pheochromocytoma is estimated to occur in 2–8 of 1 million persons per year, and about 0.1% of hypertensive patients harbor a pheochromocytoma. Autopsy series reveal prevalence of 0.2%. The mean age at diagnosis is about 40 years, although the tumors can occur from early childhood until late in life. The "rule of tens" for pheochromocytomas states that about 10% are bilateral, 10% are extraadrenal, and 10% are malignant. However, these percentages are higher in the inherited syndromes.

■ ETIOLOGY AND PATHOGENESIS

Pheochromocytomas and paragangliomas are well-vascularized tumors that arise from cells derived from the sympathetic (e.g., adrenal medulla) or parasympathetic (e.g., carotid body, glomus vagale) paraganglia (Fig. 343-1). The name *pheochromocytoma* reflects the black-colored staining caused by chromaffin oxidation of catecholamines. Although a variety of terms have been used to describe these tumors, most clinicians use the term *pheochromocytoma* to describe symptomatic catecholamine-producing tumors, including those in extraadrenal retroperitoneal, pelvic, and thoracic sites. The term *paraganglioma* is used to describe catecholamine-producing tumors in the head and neck. These tumors may secrete little or no catecholamines.

The etiology of sporadic pheochromocytomas and paragangliomas is unknown. However, about 25% of patients have an inherited condition, including germ-line mutations in the *RET, VHL, NF1, SDHB, SDHC, SDHD,* or *SDHAF2* genes. Biallelic gene inactivation has been demonstrated for the *VHL, NF1,* and *SDH* genes, whereas *RET* mutations activate the receptor tyrosine kinase activity. SDH is an enzyme of the Krebs cycle and the mitochondrial respiratory chain. The VHL protein is a component of a ubiquitin E3 ligase. *VHL* mutations reduce protein degradation, resulting in upregulation of components involved in cell cycle progression, glucose metabolism, and oxygen sensing.

■ CLINICAL FEATURES

The clinical presentation is so variable that pheochromocytoma has been termed "the great masquerader" (Table 343-1). Among the presenting symptoms, episodes of palpitations, headaches, and profuse sweating are typical and constitute a classic triad. The presence of all three symptoms in association with hypertension makes pheochromocytoma a likely diagnosis. However, a pheochromocytoma can be asymptomatic for years, and some tumors grow to a considerable size before patients note symptoms.

The dominant sign is hypertension. Classically, patients have episodic hypertension, but sustained hypertension is also common. Catecholamine crises can lead to heart failure, pulmonary edema, arrhythmias, and intracranial hemorrhage. During episodes of hormone release, which can occur at very divergent intervals, patients are anxious and pale, and they experience tachycardia and palpitations. These paroxysms generally last less than an hour and may be precipitated by surgery, positional changes, exercise, pregnancy, urination (particularly bladder pheochromocytomas),

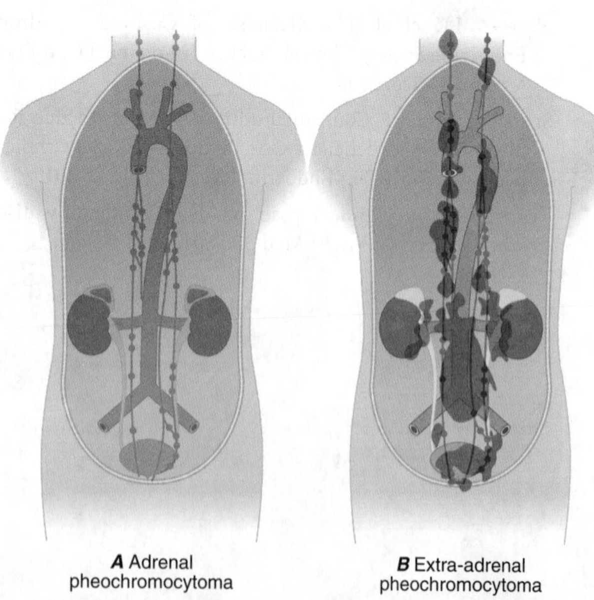

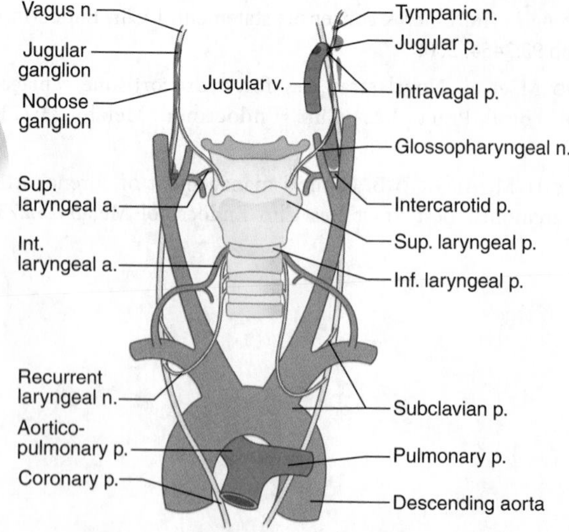

Figure 343-1 The paraganglial system and topographic sites (in red) of pheochromocytomas and paragangliomas. *[Parts* ***A,B,*** *from WM Manger, RW Gifford: Clinical and experimental pheochromocytoma. Cambridge, Blackwell Science, 1996; Part* ***C,*** *from GG Glenner, PM Grimley: Tumors of the Extra-adrenal Paraganglion System (Including Chemoreceptors), Atlas of Tumor Pathology, 2nd Series, Fascicle 9. Washington, DC, AFIP, 1974.]*

TABLE 343-1 Clinical Features Associated With Pheochromocytoma

Headaches	Weight loss
Sweating attacks	Paradoxical response to antihypertensive drugs
Palpitations and tachycardia	Polyuria and polydipsia
Hypertension, sustained or paroxysmal	Constipation
Anxiety and panic attacks	Orthostatic hypotension
Pallor	Dilated cardiomyopathy
Nausea	Erythrocytosis
Abdominal pain	Elevated blood sugar
Weakness	Hypercalcemia

and various medications (e.g., tricyclic antidepressants, opiates, metoclopramide).

■ DIAGNOSIS

The diagnosis is based on documentation of catecholamine excess by biochemical testing and localization of the tumor by imaging. Both are of equal importance, although measurement of catecholamines is traditionally the first step.

Biochemical testing

Pheochromocytomas and paragangliomas synthesize and store catecholamines, which include norepinephrine (noradrenaline), epinephrine (adrenaline), and dopamine. Elevated plasma and urinary levels of catecholamines and the methylated metabolites, metanephrines, are the cornerstone for the diagnosis. The hormonal activity of tumors fluctuates, resulting in considerable variation in serial catecholamine measurements. Thus, there is some value in obtaining tests during or soon after a symptomatic crisis. However, most tumors continuously leak O-methylated metabolites, which are detected by measurements of metanephrines.

Catecholamines and metanephrines can be measured by using different methods (e.g., high-performance liquid chromatography, enzyme-linked immunosorbent assay, and liquid chromatography/mass spectrometry). In a clinical context suspicious for pheochromocytoma, when values are increased three times the upper limit of normal, a pheochromocytoma is highly likely regardless of the assay used. However, as summarized in Table 343-2, the sensitivity and specificity of available biochemical tests vary greatly, and these differences are important in assessing patients with borderline elevations of different compounds. Urinary tests for vanillylmandelic acid (VMA), metanephrines (total or fractionated), and catecholamines are widely available and are used commonly for initial testing. Among these tests, the fractionated metanephrines and catecholamines are the most sensitive. Plasma tests are more convenient and include measurements of catecholamines and metanephrines. Measurements of plasma metanephrine are the most sensitive and are less susceptible to false-positive elevations from stress, including venipuncture. Although the incidence of false-positive test results has been reduced by the introduction of newer assays, physiologic stress responses and medications that increase catecholamines still can confound testing. Because the tumors are relatively rare, borderline elevations are likely to be false positives. In this circumstance, it is important to exclude diet or drug exposure (withdrawal of levodopa, sympathomimetics, diuretics, tricyclic antidepressants, alpha and beta blockers) that might cause false positives and then repeat testing or perform a clonidine suppression test (measurement of plasma metanephrines 3 h after oral administration of 300 μg of clonidine). Other pharmacologic tests, such as the phentolamine test and the glucagon provocation test, are of relatively low sensitivity and are not recommended.

TABLE 343-2 Biochemical and Imaging Methods Used for Pheochromocytoma and Paraganglioma Diagnosis

Diagnostic Method	Sensitivity	Specificity
24-h urinary tests		
Vanillylmandelic acid	++	++++
Catecholamines	+++	+++
Fractionated metanephrines	++++	++
Total metanephrines	+++	++++
Plasma tests		
Catecholamines	+++	++
Free metanephrines	++++	+++
CT	++++	+++
MRI	++++	+++
MIBG scintigraphy	+++	++++
Somatostatin receptor scintigraphy*	++	++
Dopa (dopamine) PET	+++	++++

*Particularly high in head and neck paragangliomas.

Abbreviations: MIBG, metaiodobenzylguanidine; PET, positron emission tomography.

Diagnostic imaging

A variety of methods have been used to localize pheochromocytomas and paragangliomas (Table 343-2). CT and MRI are similar in sensitivity. CT should be performed with contrast. T2-weighted MRI with gadolinium contrast is optimal for detecting pheochromocytomas and is somewhat better than CT for imaging extra-adrenal pheochromocytomas and paragangliomas. About 5% of adrenal incidentalomas, which usually are detected by CT or MRI, prove to be pheochromocytomas after endocrinologic evaluation.

Tumors also can be localized by using radioactive tracers, including 131I- or 123I-metaiodobenzylguanidine (MIBG), 111In-somatostatin analogues, or 18F-dopa (or dopamine) positron emission tomography (PET). Because these agents exhibit selective uptake in paragangliomas, nuclear imaging is particularly useful in the hereditary syndromes.

Differential diagnosis

When one is entertaining the possibility of a pheochromocytoma, other disorders to consider include essential hypertension, anxiety attacks, use of cocaine or amphetamines, mastocytosis or carcinoid syndrome (usually lacking hypertension), intracranial lesions, clonidine withdrawal, autonomic epilepsy, and factitious crises (usually from sympathomimetic amines). When an asymptomatic adrenal mass is identified, likely diagnoses other than pheochromocytoma include a nonfunctioning adrenal adenoma, aldosteronoma, and cortisol-producing adenoma (Cushing's syndrome).

TREATMENT Pheochromocytoma

Complete tumor removal is the ultimate therapeutic goal. Preoperative patient preparation is essential for safe surgery. α-Adrenergic blockers (phenoxybenzamine) should be initiated at relatively low doses (e.g., 5–10 mg orally three times per day) and increased as tolerated every few days. Because patients are volume-constricted, liberal salt intake and hydration are necessary to avoid orthostasis. Adequate alpha blockade generally requires 7 days, with a typical final dose of 20–30 mg phenoxybenzamine three times per day. Oral prazosin or intravenous phentolamine can be used to manage paroxysms while awaiting adequate alpha blockade. Before surgery, blood pressure should be consistently below 160/90 mmHg, with moderate orthostasis. Beta blockers (e.g., 10 mg propranolol three to four times per day) can be added after starting alpha blockers and increased as needed if tachycardia persists. Other antihypertensives, such as calcium channel blockers or angiotensin-converting enzyme inhibitors, have been used when blood pressure is difficult to control with phenoxybenzamine alone.

Surgery should be performed by teams of anesthesiologists and surgeons with experience in the management of pheochromocytomas. Blood pressure can be labile during surgery, particularly at the onset of intubation or when the tumor is manipulated. Nitroprusside infusion is useful for intraoperative hypertensive crises, and hypotension usually responds to volume infusion. Although laparotomy was the traditional surgical approach, endoscopic surgery, using either a transperitoneal or a retroperitoneal approach, is associated with fewer complications, a faster recovery, and optimal cosmetic results. Atraumatic endoscopic surgery has become the method of choice. It may be possible to preserve the normal adrenal cortex, particularly in hereditary disorders in which bilateral pheochromocytomas are more likely. Extra-adrenal abdominal as well as most thoracic pheochromocytomas also can be removed endoscopically. Postoperatively, catecholamine normalization should be documented. An adrenocorticotropic hormone test should be used to exclude cortisol deficiency when bilateral adrenal cortex–sparing surgery is performed.

MALIGNANT PHEOCHROMOCYTOMA

About 5–10% of pheochromocytomas and paragangliomas are malignant. The diagnosis of malignant pheochromocytoma is problematic. Typical histologic criteria of cellular atypia, presence of mitoses, and invasion of vessels or adjacent tissues do not reliably identify which tumors have the capacity to metastasize. Thus, the term *malignant pheochromocytoma* generally is restricted to tumors with distant metastases, most commonly found in lungs, bone, or liver, suggesting a vascular pathway of spread. Because hereditary syndromes are associated with multifocal tumor sites, these features should be anticipated in patients with germ-line mutations of *RET, VHL, SDHD, or SDHB*. However, distant metastases also occur in these syndromes, especially in carriers of *SDHB* mutations.

Treatment of malignant pheochromocytoma or paraganglioma is challenging. Options include tumor mass reduction, alpha blockers for symptoms, chemotherapy, and nuclear medicine radiotherapy. Averbuch's chemotherapy protocol includes dacarbazine (600 mg/m^2 days 1 and 2), cyclophosphamide (750 mg/m^2 day 1), and vincristine (1.4 mg/m^2 day 1), repeated every 21 days for three to six cycles. Palliation (stable disease to shrinkage) is achieved in about one-half of patients. Other chemotherapeutic protocols remain in the experimental stage. An alternative is ^{131}I-MIBG treatment using 200-mCi doses at monthly intervals over three to six cycles. The prognosis of metastatic pheochromocytoma or paraganglioma is variable, with a 5-year survival of 30–60%.

PHEOCHROMOCYTOMA IN PREGNANCY

Pheochromocytomas occasionally are diagnosed in pregnancy. Endoscopic removal, preferably in the forth to sixth month of gestation, is possible and can be followed by uneventful childbirth. Regular screening in families with inherited pheochromocytomas provides an opportunity to identify and remove asymptomatic tumors in women of reproductive age.

PHEOCHROMOCYTOMA-ASSOCIATED SYNDROMES

About 25–33% of patients with a pheochromocytoma or paraganglioma have an inherited syndrome. The mean age at diagnosis is about 15 years lower in patients with inherited syndromes compared with patients with sporadic tumors.

Neurofibromatosis type 1 (NF 1) was the first described pheochromocytoma-associated syndrome (Chap. 379). The *NF1* gene functions as a tumor suppressor by regulating the Ras signaling cascade. Classic features of neurofibromatosis include multiple neurofibromas, café au lait spots, axillary freckling of the skin, and Lisch nodules of the iris (Fig. 343-2). Pheochromocytomas occur in only about 1% of these patients and are located predominantly in the adrenals. Malignant pheochromocytoma is not uncommon.

The best-known pheochromocytoma-associated syndrome is the autosomal dominant disorder *multiple endocrine neoplasia type 2A and type 2B (MEN 2A, MEN 2B)* (Chap. 351). Both types of MEN 2 are caused by mutations in *RET* (*RE*arranged during *T*ransfection), which encodes a tyrosine kinase. The locations of RET mutations correlate with the severity of disease and the type of MEN 2 (Chap. 351). MEN 2A is characterized by medullary thyroid carcinoma (MTC), pheochromocytoma, and hyperparathyroidism; MEN 2B also includes MTC and pheochromocytoma, as well as multiple mucosal neuromas, marfanoid habitus, and other developmental disorders, though

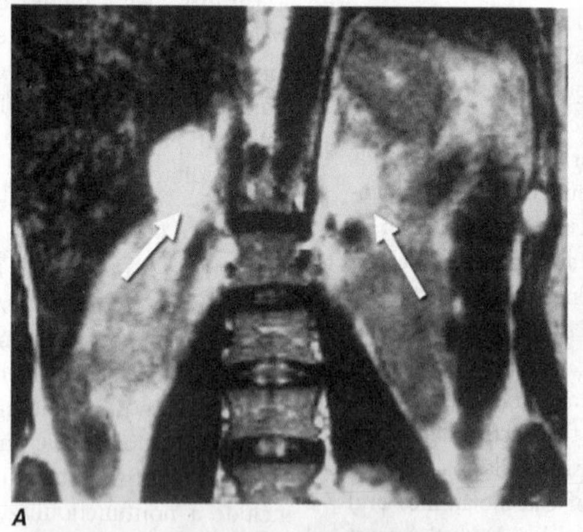

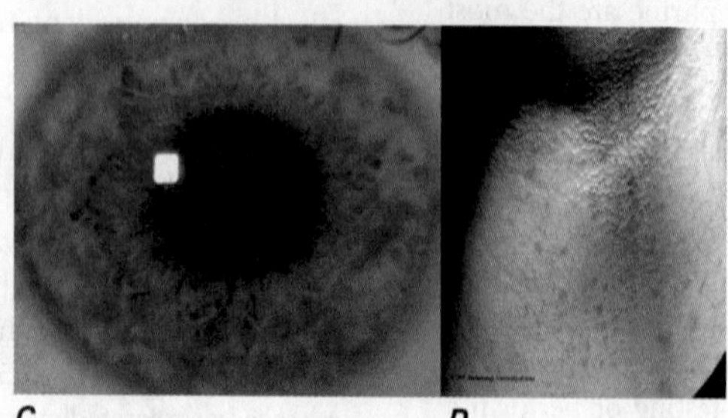

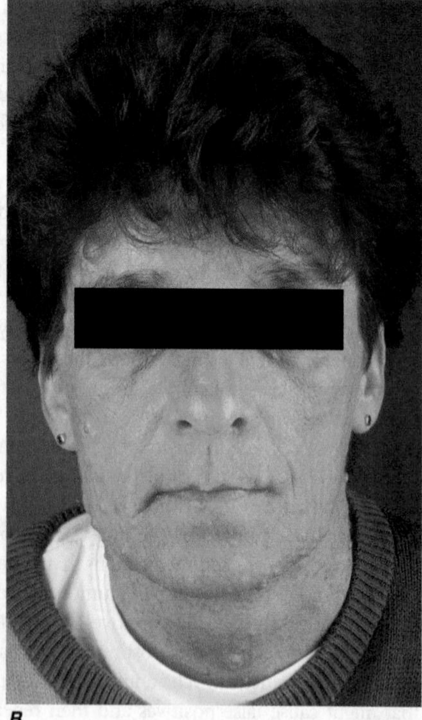

Figure 343-2 Neurofibromatosis. ***A.*** MRI of bilateral adrenal pheochromocytoma. ***B.*** Cutaneous neurofibromas. ***C.*** Lisch nodules of the iris. ***D.*** Axillary freckling. *(Part A from HPH Neumann et al: Keio J Med 54:15, 2005; with permission.)*

it typically lacks hyperparathyroidism. MTC is seen in virtually all patients with MEN 2, but pheochromocytoma occurs in only about 50% of these patients. Nearly all pheochromocytomas are benign and located in the adrenals, often bilateral (Fig. 343-3). Pheochromocytoma may be symptomatic before MTC. Prophylactic thyroidectomy is being performed in many carriers of *RET* mutations; pheochromocytomas should be excluded before any surgery in these patients.

Von Hippel-Lindau syndrome (VHL) is an autosomal dominant disorder that predisposes to retinal and cerebellar hemangioblastomas, which also occur in the brainstem and spinal cord (Fig. 343-4). Other important features of VHL are clear cell renal carcinomas, pancreatic islet cell tumors, endolymphatic sac tumors (ELSTs) of the inner ear, cystadenomas of the epididymis and broad ligament, and multiple pancreatic or renal cysts.

The *VHL* gene encodes an E3 ubiquitin ligase that regulates expression of hypoxia-inducible factor-1 (HIF-1), among other genes. Loss of *VHL* is associated with increased expression of vascular endothelial growth factor (VEGF) that induces angiogenesis. Although the *VHL* gene can be inactivated by all types of mutations, patients with pheochromocytoma predominantly have missense mutations. About 20–30% of patients with VHL have pheochromocytomas, but in some families the incidence can reach 90%. The recognition of pheochromocytoma as a VHL-associated feature provides an opportunity to diagnose retinal, central nervous system, renal, and pancreatic tumors at a stage when effective treatment may still be possible

The *paraganglioma syndromes (PGL)* have been classified by genetic analyses of families with head and neck paragangliomas. The susceptibility genes encode subunits of the enzyme succinate dehydrogenase (SDH), a component in the Krebs cycle and the mitochondrial electron transport chain. SDH is formed by four subunits (A–D). Mutations of *SDHB* (PGL4), *SDHC* (PGL3), *SDHD* (PGL1), and *SDHAF2* (PGL2) predispose to the paraganglioma syndromes. Mutations of SDHA do not predispose to paraganglioma tumors but instead cause Leigh's disease, a form of encephalopathy. The transmission of the disease in carriers of *SDHB, SDHC,* and *SDHAF2* germline mutations is autosomal dominant. In contrast, in SDHD families, only the progeny of affected fathers develop tumors if they inherit the mutation. In a small number of patients with familial pheochromocytoma, a mutation has not been identified. PGL1 is most common, followed by PGL4; PGL2 and PGL3 are rare. Adrenal, extra-adrenal abdominal, and thoracic pheochromocytomas that are components of PGL1 and PGL4, are rare in PGL3, but absent in PGL2 (Fig. 343-5). About one-third of the patients with PGL4 develop metastases.

Familial pheochromocytoma (FP) has been attributed to hereditary, exclusively adrenal tumors in patients with germline mutations in the *TMEM127* gene.

GUIDELINES FOR GENETIC SCREENING IN PATIENTS WITH PHEOCHROMOCYTOMA OR PARAGANGLIOMA

In addition to family history, general features suggesting an inherited syndrome include young age, multifocal tumors, extra-adrenal tumors, and malignant tumors (Fig. 343-6). Because of the relatively high prevalence of familial syndromes among patients who present with pheochromocytoma or paraganglioma, it is useful to identify germline mutations even in patients without a known family history. A first step is to search for clinical features of inherited syndromes and to perform an in-depth, multigenerational family history. Each of these syndromes exhibits autosomal dominant transmission with variable penetrance, but a proband with a mother affected by paraganglial tumors is not predisposed to PLG1 (*SDHD* mutation carrier). Cutaneous neurofibromas, café au lait spots, and axillary freckling suggest neurofibromatosis. Germ-line mutations in *NF1* have not been reported in patients with sporadic pheochromocytomas. Thus, *NF1* testing does not have to be performed in the absence of other clinical features of neurofibromatosis. A personal or family history of medullary thyroid cancer or elevation of serum calcitonin strongly suggest MEN 2 and should prompt testing for *RET* mutations. A history of visual impairment, or tumors of the cerebellum, kidney, brainstem, or spinal cord, suggests the possibility of VHL. A personal and/or family history for head and neck paraganglioma suggests PGL1 or PGL4.

A single adrenal pheochromocytoma in a patient with an otherwise unremarkable history may still be associated with mutations of *VHL, RET, SDHB,* or *SDHD* (in decreasing order of frequency). Two-thirds of extra-adrenal tumors are associated with one of these syndromes, and multifocal tumors occur with decreasing

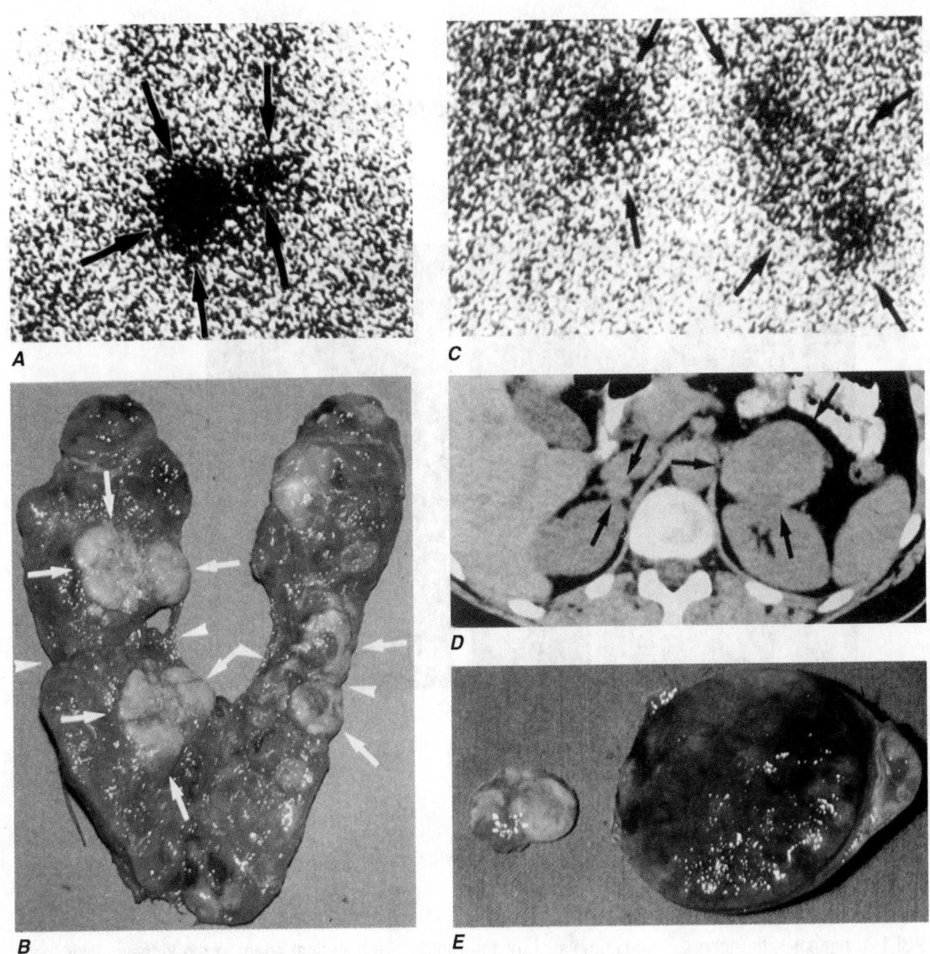

Figure 343-3 Multiple endocrine neoplasia type 2. Multifocal medullary thyroid carcinoma shown by (***A***) MIBG scintigraphy and (***B***) operative specimen Arrows demonstrate the tumors; arrowheads show the tissue bridge of the cut specimen. Bilateral adrenal pheochromocytoma shown by (***C***) MIBG scintigraphy, (***D***) CT imaging, and (***E***) operative specimens. *(From HPH Neumann et al: Keio J Med 54:15, 2005; with permission.)*

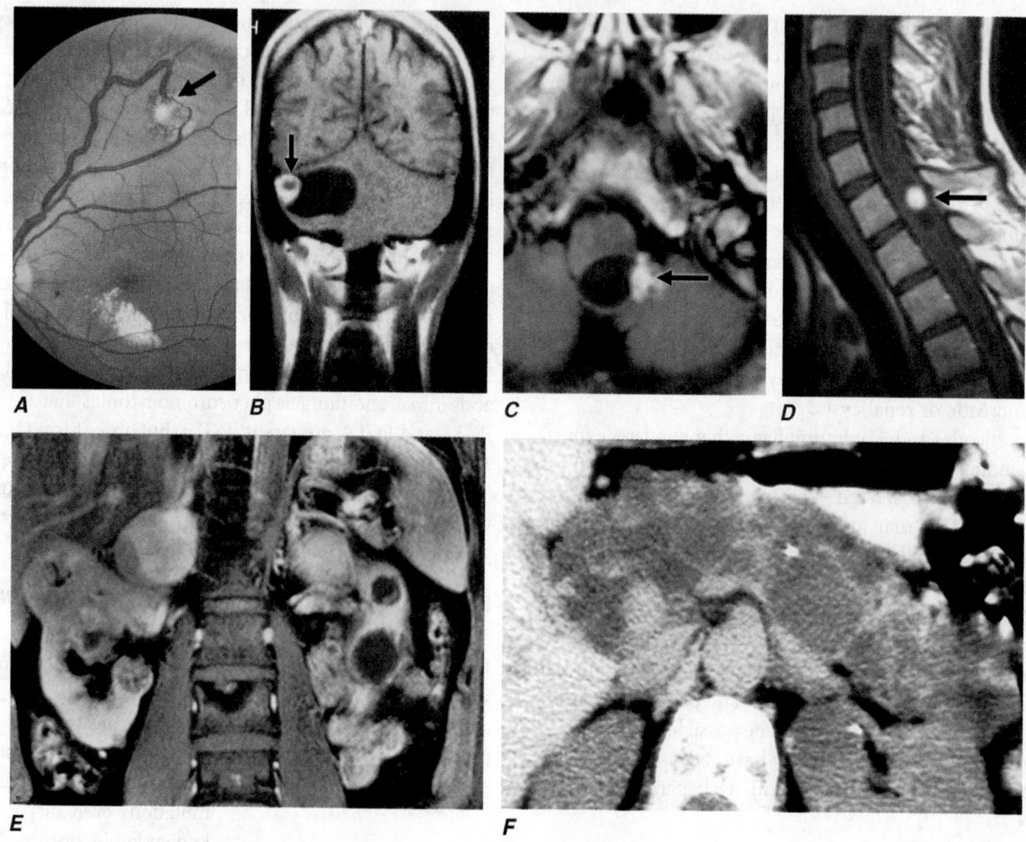

Figure 343-4 Von Hippel-Lindau disease. Retinal angioma (***A***); hemangioblastomas of cerebellum are shown by MRI in (***B***) brainstem; (***C*** and ***D***) spinal cord; (***E***) bilateral pheochromocytomas and bilateral renal clear cell carcinomas; and (***F***) multiple pancreatic cysts. *[Parts **A** and **D** from HPH Neumann et al: Adv Nephrol Necker Hosp 27:361, 1997. Copyright Elsevier. Part B from SH Morgan, J-P Grunfeld (eds): Inherited Disorders of the Kidney. Oxford, UK, Oxford University Press, 1998. Part **F** from HPH Neumann et al: Contrib Nephrol 136:193, 2001. Copyright S. Karger AG, Basel.]*

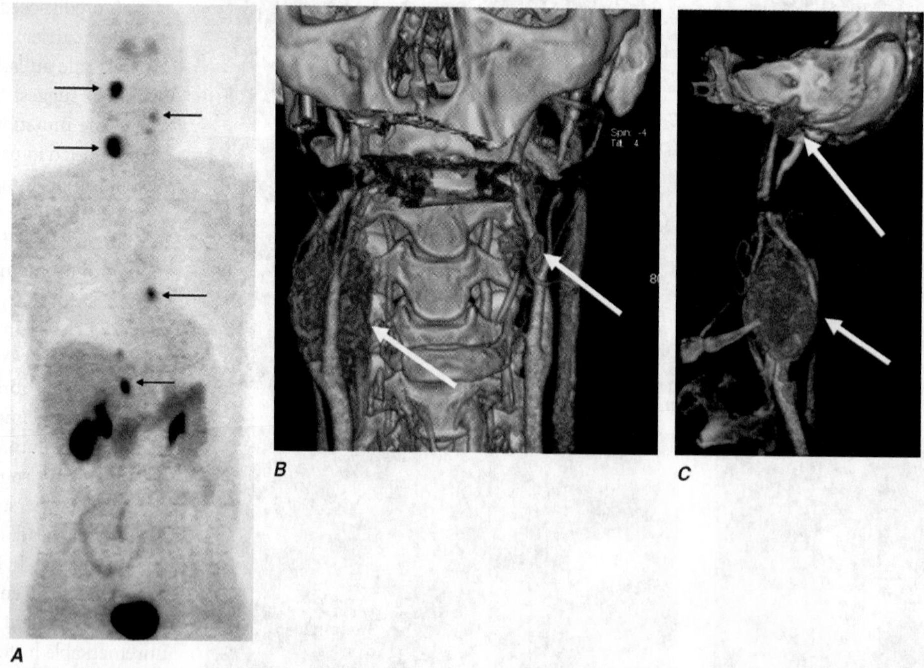

Figure 343-5 Paraganglioma syndrome. PGL1, a patient with incomplete resection of a left carotid body tumor and the SDHD W5X mutation. ***A***. ^{18}F-dopa positron emission tomography demonstrating tumor uptake in the right jugular glomus, the right carotid body, the left carotid body, the left coronary glomus, and the right adrenal gland. Note the physiologic accumulation of the radiopharmaceutical agent in the kidneys, liver, gallbladder, renal pelvis, and urinary bladder. ***B*** and ***C***. CT angiography with three-dimensional reconstruction. Arrows point to the paraganglial tumors. *(From S Hoegerle et al: Eur J Nucl Med Mol Imaging 30:689, 2003; with permission.)*

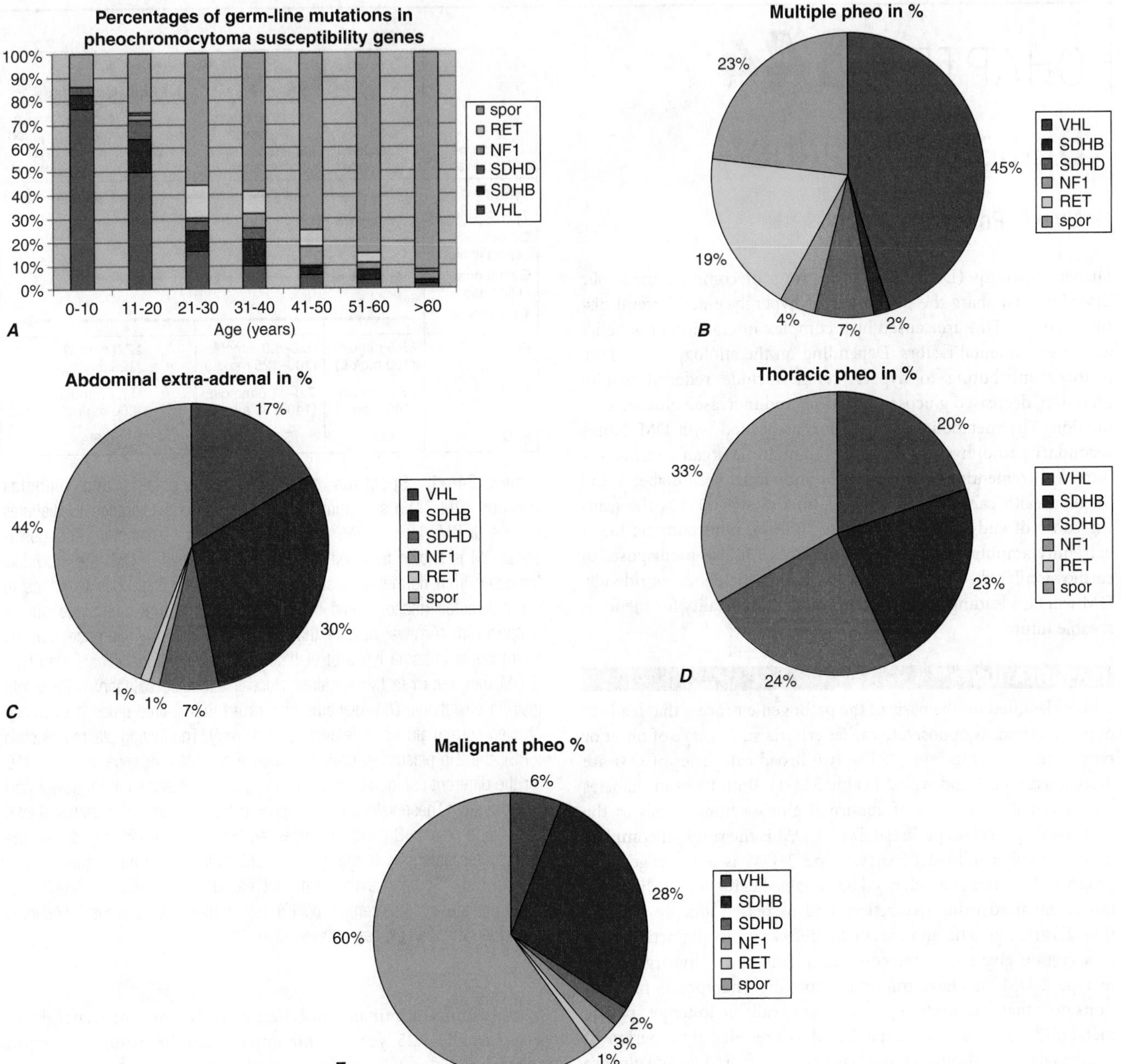

Figure 343-6 Mutation distribution in the *RET, VHL, NF1, SDHB,* and *SDHD* genes. *A.* Correlation with age. The bars depict the frequency of sporadic or various inherited forms of pheochromocytoma in different age groups. The inherited disorders are much more common among younger individuals presenting with pheochromocytoma. Germ-line mutations according to (***B***) multiple, (***C***) extraadrenal retroperitoneal, (***D***) thoracic, and (***E***) malignant pheochromocytomas *(Data from the Freiburg International Pheochromocytoma and Paraganglioma Registry in 2009.)*

frequency in carriers of *RET, SDHD, VHL,* and *SDHB* mutations. About 30% of head and neck paragangliomas are associated with germ-line mutations of one of the SDH subunit genes (particularly *SDHD*) and are rare in carriers of *VHL* and *RET* mutations.

Once the underlying syndrome is diagnosed, the benefit of genetic testing can be extended to relatives. For this purpose, it is necessary to identify the germ-line mutation in the proband and, after genetic counseling, perform DNA sequence analyses of the responsible gene in relatives to determine whether they are affected (Chap. 63). Other family members may benefit from biochemical screening for paraganglial tumors in individuals who carry a germ-line mutation.

FURTHER READINGS

Erlic Z et al: Clinical predictors and algorithm for the genetic diagnosis of pheochromocytoma patients. Clin Cancer Res 15:6378, 2009

Lenders JW et al: Phaeochromocytoma. Lancet 366:665, 2005

Neumann HP et al: Germ-line mutations in nonsyndromic pheochromocytoma. N Engl J Med 346:1459, 2002

———: Evidence of MEN-2 in the original description of classic pheochromocytoma. N Engl J Med 357:1311, 2007

Pacak K et al: Pheochromocytoma: Recommendations for clinical practice from the First International Symposium. Nat Clin Pract Endocrinol Metab 3:92, 2007

Tischler AS: Pheochromocytoma and extra-adrenal paraganglioma: Arch Pathol Lab Med 132:1272, 2008

Yao L et al: Spectrum and prevalence of FP/TMEM127 gene mutations in pheochromocytomas and paragangliomas. JAMA 304:2611, 2010

CHAPTER 344
Diabetes Mellitus

Alvin C. Powers

Diabetes mellitus (DM) refers to a group of common metabolic disorders that share the phenotype of hyperglycemia. Several distinct types of DM are caused by a complex interaction of genetics and environmental factors. Depending on the etiology of the DM, factors contributing to hyperglycemia include reduced insulin secretion, decreased glucose utilization, and increased glucose production. The metabolic dysregulation associated with DM causes secondary pathophysiologic changes in multiple organ systems that impose a tremendous burden on the individual with diabetes and on the health care system. In the United States, DM is the leading cause of end-stage renal disease (ESRD), nontraumatic lower extremity amputations, and adult blindness. It also predisposes to cardiovascular diseases. With an increasing incidence worldwide, DM will be a leading cause of morbidity and mortality for the foreseeable future.

CLASSIFICATION

DM is classified on the basis of the pathogenic process that leads to hyperglycemia, as opposed to earlier criteria such as age of onset or type of therapy (Fig. 344-1). The two broad categories of DM are designated type 1 and type 2 (Table 344-1). Both types of diabetes are preceded by a phase of abnormal glucose homeostasis as the pathogenic processes progress. Type 1 DM is the result of complete or near-total insulin deficiency. Type 2 DM is a heterogeneous group of disorders characterized by variable degrees of insulin resistance, impaired insulin secretion, and increased glucose production. Distinct genetic and metabolic defects in insulin action and/or secretion give rise to the common phenotype of hyperglycemia in type 2 DM and have important potential therapeutic implications now that pharmacologic agents are available to target specific metabolic derangements. Type 2 DM is preceded by a period of abnormal glucose homeostasis classified as impaired fasting glucose (IFG) or impaired glucose tolerance (IGT).

Two features of the current classification of DM diverge from previous classifications. First, the terms *insulin-dependent diabetes mellitus* (IDDM) and *non-insulin-dependent diabetes mellitus* (NIDDM) are obsolete. Since many individuals with type 2 DM eventually require insulin treatment for control of glycemia, the use of the term NIDDM generated considerable confusion. A second difference is that age is not a criterion in the classification system. Although type 1 DM most commonly develops before the age of 30, an autoimmune beta cell destructive process can develop at any age. It is estimated that between 5 and 10% of individuals who develop DM after age 30 years have type 1 DM. Although type 2 DM more typically develops with increasing age, it is now being diagnosed more frequently in children and young adults, particularly in obese adolescents.

OTHER TYPES OF DM

Other etiologies for DM include specific genetic defects in insulin secretion or action, metabolic abnormalities that impair insulin secretion, mitochondrial abnormalities, and a host of conditions that impair glucose tolerance (Table 344-1). *Maturity-onset diabetes of the young* (MODY) is a subtype of DM characterized by autosomal dominant inheritance, early onset of hyperglycemia (usually <25 years), and impairment in insulin secretion (discussed below). Mutations in the insulin receptor cause a group of rare disorders characterized by severe insulin resistance.

DM can result from pancreatic exocrine disease when the majority of pancreatic islets are destroyed. Cystic fibrosis-related DM is an important consideration in this patient population. Hormones that antagonize insulin action can also lead to DM. Thus, DM is often a feature of endocrinopathies such as acromegaly and Cushing's disease. Viral infections have been implicated in pancreatic islet destruction but are an extremely rare cause of DM. A form of acute onset of type 1 diabetes, termed *fulminant diabetes*, has been noted in Japan and may be related to viral infection of islets.

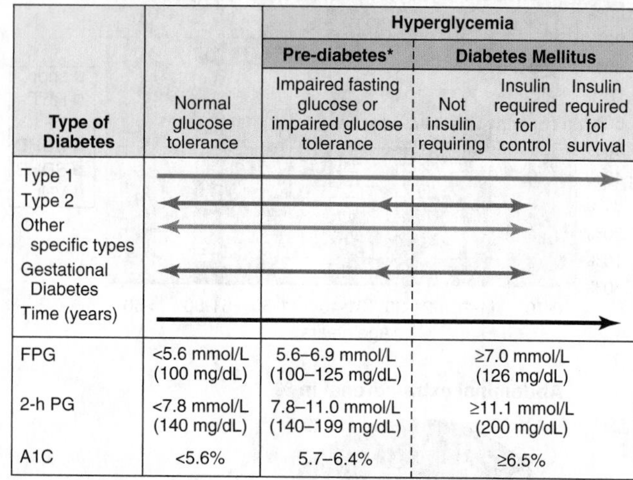

Figure 344-1 Spectrum of glucose homeostasis and diabetes mellitus (DM). The spectrum from normal glucose tolerance to diabetes in type 1 DM, type 2 DM, other specific types of diabetes, and gestational DM is shown from left to right. In most types of DM, the individual traverses from normal glucose tolerance to impaired glucose tolerance to overt diabetes (these should be viewed not as abrupt categories but as a spectrum). Arrows indicate that changes in glucose tolerance may be bidirectional in some types of diabetes. For example, individuals with type 2 DM may return to the impaired glucose tolerance category with weight loss; in gestational DM, diabetes may revert to impaired glucose tolerance or even normal glucose tolerance after delivery. The fasting plasma glucose (FPG), the 2-h plasma glucose (PG) after a glucose challenge, and the A1C for the different categories of glucose tolerance are shown at the lower part of the figure. These values do not apply to the diagnosis of gestational DM. The World Health Organization uses an FPG of 110–125 mg/dL for the prediabetes category. Some types of DM may or may not require insulin for survival. *Some use the term "increased risk for diabetes" (ADA) or "intermediate hyperglycemia" (WHO) rather than "prediabetes." *(Adapted from the American Diabetes Association, 2007.)*

GESTATIONAL DIABETES MELLITUS (GDM)

Glucose intolerance developing during pregnancy is classified as gestational diabetes. Insulin resistance is related to the metabolic changes of late pregnancy, and the increased insulin requirements may lead to IGT or diabetes. GDM occurs in ~7% (range 2–10%) of pregnancies in the United States; most women revert to normal glucose tolerance postpartum but have a substantial risk (35–60%) of developing DM in the next 10–20 years. The International Diabetes and Pregnancy Study Groups now recommends that diabetes diagnosed at the initial prenatal visit should be classified as "overt" diabetes rather than gestational diabetes.

TABLE 344-1 Etiologic Classification of Diabetes Mellitus

I. Type 1 diabetes (beta cell destruction, usually leading to absolute insulin deficiency)
    A. Immune-mediated
    B. Idiopathic
II. Type 2 diabetes (may range from predominantly insulin resistance with relative insulin deficiency to a predominantly insulin secretory defect with insulin resistance)
III. Other specific types of diabetes
    A. Genetic defects of beta cell function characterized by mutations in:
        1. Hepatocyte nuclear transcription factor (HNF) 4α (MODY 1)
        2. Glucokinase (MODY 2)
        3. HNF-1α (MODY 3)
        4. Insulin promoter factor-1 (IPF-1; MODY 4)
        5. HNF-1β (MODY 5)
        6. NeuroD1 (MODY 6)
        7. Mitochondrial DNA
        8. Subunits of ATP-sensitive potassium channel
        9. Proinsulin or insulin
    B. Genetic defects in insulin action
        1. Type A insulin resistance
        2. Leprechaunism
        3. Rabson-Mendenhall syndrome
        4. Lipodystrophy syndromes
    C. Diseases of the exocrine pancreas—pancreatitis, pancreatectomy, neoplasia, cystic fibrosis, hemochromatosis, fibrocalculous pancreatopathy, mutations in carboxyl ester lipase
    D. Endocrinopathies—acromegaly, Cushing's syndrome, glucagonoma, pheochromocytoma, hyperthyroidism, somatostatinoma, aldosteronoma
    E. Drug- or chemical-induced—glucocorticoids, vacor (a rodenticide), pentamidine, nicotinic acid, diazoxide, β-adrenergic agonists, thiazides, hydantoins, asparaginase, α-interferon, protease inhibitors, antipsychotics (atypicals and others), epinephrine
    F. Infections—congenital rubella, cytomegalovirus, coxsackievirus
    G. Uncommon forms of immune-mediated diabetes—"stiff-person" syndrome, anti-insulin receptor antibodies
    H. Other genetic syndromes sometimes associated with diabetes—Wolfram's syndrome, Down's syndrome, Klinefelter's syndrome, Turner's syndrome, Friedreich's ataxia, Huntington's chorea, Laurence-Moon-Biedl syndrome, myotonic dystrophy, porphyria, Prader-Willi syndrome
IV. Gestational diabetes mellitus (GDM)

Abbreviation: MODY, maturity-onset diabetes of the young.
Source: Adapted from American Diabetes Association, 2011.

EPIDEMIOLOGY

The worldwide prevalence of DM has risen dramatically over the past two decades, from an estimated 30 million cases in 1985 to 285 million in 2010. Based on current trends, the International Diabetes Federation projects that 438 million individuals will have diabetes by the year 2030 (Fig. 344-2). Although the prevalence of both type 1 and type 2 DM is increasing worldwide, the prevalence of type 2 DM is rising much more rapidly, presumably because of increasing obesity, reduced activity levels as countries become more industrialized, and the aging of the population. In 2010, the prevalence of diabetes ranged from 11.6 to 30.9% in the 10 countries with the highest prevalence (Naurua, United Arab Emigrates, Saudi Arabia, Mauritius, Bahrain, Reunion, Kuwait, Oman, Tonga, Malaysia—in descending prevalence; Fig. 344-2). In the most recent estimate for the United States (2010), the Centers for Disease Control and Prevention (CDC) estimated that 25.8 million persons, or 8.3% of the population, had diabetes (~27% of the individuals with diabetes were undiagnosed). Approximately 1.6 million individuals (>20 years) were newly diagnosed with diabetes in 2010. DM increases with aging. In 2010, the prevalence of DM in the United Sates was estimated to be 0.2% in individuals aged <20 years and 11.3% in individuals aged >20 years. In individuals aged >65 years, the prevalence of DM was 26.9%. The prevalence is similar in men and women throughout most age ranges (11.8% and 10.8%, respectively, in individuals aged >20 years). Worldwide estimates project that in 2030 the greatest number of individuals with diabetes will be aged 45–64 years.

There is considerable geographic variation in the incidence of both type 1 and type 2 DM. Scandinavia has the highest incidence of type 1 DM (e.g., in Finland, the incidence is 57.4/100,000 per year). The Pacific Rim has a much lower rate of type 1 DM (in Japan and China, the incidence is 0.6–2.4/100,000 per year); Northern Europe and the United States have an intermediate rate (8–20/100,000 per year). Much of the increased risk of type 1 DM is believed to reflect the frequency of high-risk human leukocyte antigen (HLA) alleles among ethnic groups in different geographic locations. The prevalence of type 2 DM and its harbinger, IGT, is highest in certain Pacific islands and the Middle East and intermediate in countries such as India and the United States. This variability is likely due to genetic, behavioral, and environmental factors. DM prevalence also varies among different ethnic populations within a given country. For example, the CDC estimated that the age-adjusted prevalence of DM in the United States (age > 20 years; 2007–2009) was 7.1% in non-Hispanic whites, 7.5% in Asian Americans, 11.8% in Hispanics, and 12.6% in non-Hispanic blacks. Comparable statistics for individuals belonging to American Indian, Alaska Native, or Pacific-Islander ethnic groups are not available, but the prevalence likely exceeds the rate in non-Hispanic whites. The onset of type 2 DM occurs, on average, at an earlier age in ethnic groups other than non-Hispanic whites. In Asia, the prevalence of diabetes is increasing rapidly and the diabetes phenotype appears to be different from that in the United States and Europe—onset at a lower BMI and younger age, greater visceral adiposity, and reduced insulin secretory capacity.

Diabetes is a major cause of mortality, but several studies indicate that diabetes is likely underreported as a cause of death. In the United States, diabetes was listed as the seventh leading cause of death in 2007; a recent estimate suggested that diabetes was the fifth leading cause of death worldwide and was responsible for almost 4 million deaths in 2010 (6.8% of deaths were attributed to diabetes worldwide).

DIAGNOSIS

Glucose tolerance is classified into three broad categories: normal glucose homeostasis, diabetes mellitus, and impaired glucose homeostasis. Glucose tolerance can be assessed using the fasting plasma glucose (FPG), the response to oral glucose challenge, or the hemoglobin A1C (A1C). An FPG <5.6 mmol/L (100 mg/dL), a plasma glucose <140 mg/dL (11.1 mmol/L) following an oral glucose challenge, and an A1C <5.6% are considered to define normal glucose tolerance. The International Expert Committee with members appointed by the American Diabetes Association, the European Association for the Study of Diabetes, and the International Diabetes Federation has issued diagnostic criteria

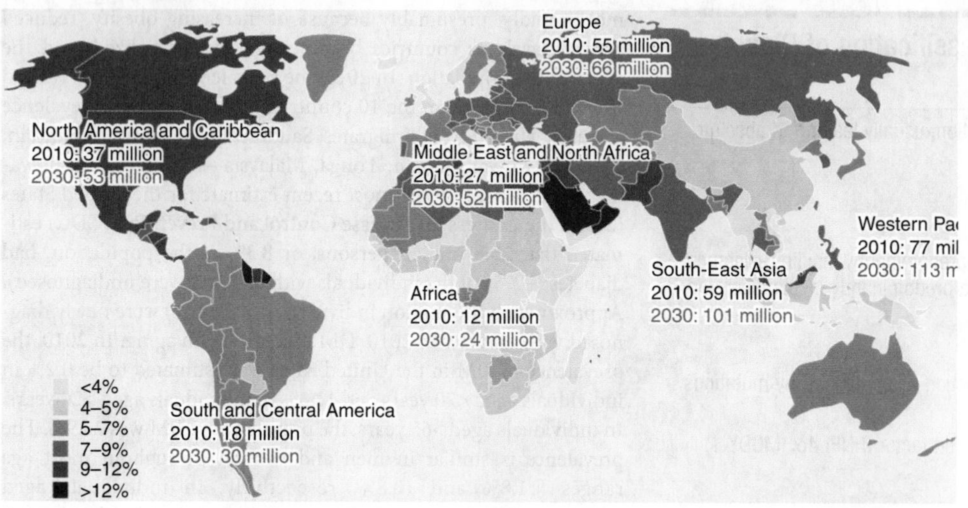

Figure 344-2 Worldwide prevalence of diabetes mellitus. Comparative prevalence (%) of estimates of diabetes (20–79 years), 2010. *(Used with permission from IDF Diabetes Atlas, the International Diabetes Federation, 2009.)*

glucose challenge, which is termed impaired glucose tolerance (IGT); or (3) A1C of 5.7–6.4%. An A1C of 5.7–6.4%, IFG, and IGT do not identify the same individuals, but individuals in all three groups are at greater risk of progressing to type 2 diabetes and have an increased risk of cardiovascular disease. Some use the term "prediabetes," "increased risk of diabetes" (ADA), or "intermediate hyperglycemia" (WHO) for this category. The current criteria for the diagnosis of DM emphasize that the A1C or the FPG as the most reliable and convenient tests for identifying DM in asymptomatic individuals. Oral glucose tolerance testing, although still a valid means for diagnosing DM, is not often used in routine clinical care.

for DM (Table 344-2) based on the following premises: (1) the FPG, the response to an oral glucose challenge (OGTT—oral glucose tolerance test), and A1C differ among individuals, and (2) DM is defined as the level of glycemia at which diabetes-specific complications occur rather than on deviations from a population-based mean. For example, the prevalence of retinopathy in Native Americans (Pima Indian population) begins to increase at an FPG >6.4 mmol/L (116 mg/dL) (Fig. 344-3).

An FPG ≥7.0 mmol/L (126 mg/dL), a glucose >11.1 mmol/L (200 mg/dL) 2 h after an oral glucose challenge, or an A1C ≥6.5% warrant the diagnosis of DM (Table 344-2). A random plasma glucose concentration ≥11.1 mmol/L (200 mg/dL) accompanied by classic symptoms of DM (polyuria, polydipsia, weight loss) also is sufficient for the diagnosis of DM (Table 344-2).

Abnormal glucose homeostasis (Fig. 344-1) is defined as (1) FPG = 5.6–6.9 mmol/L (100–125 mg/dL), which is defined as IFG (note that the World Health Organization uses an FPG of 6.1–6.9 mmol/L (110–125 mg/dL); (2) plasma glucose levels between 7.8 and 11 mmol/L (140 and 199 mg/dL) following an oral

TABLE 344-2 Criteria for the Diagnosis of Diabetes Mellitus

- Symptoms of diabetes plus random blood glucose concentration ≥11.1 mmol/L (200 mg/dL)[a] *or*
- Fasting plasma glucose ≥7.0 mmol/L (126 mg/dL)[b] *or*
- A1C > 6.5%[c] *or*
- Two-hour plasma glucose ≥11.1 mmol/L (200 mg/dL) during an oral glucose tolerance test[d]

[a]Random is defined as without regard to time since the last meal.
[b]Fasting is defined as no caloric intake for at least 8 h.
[c]The test should be performed in laboratory certified according to A1C standards of the Diabetes Control and Complications Trial.
[d]The test should be performed using a glucose load containing the equivalent of 75 g anhydrous glucose dissolved in water, not recommended for routine clinical use.
Note: In the absence of unequivocal hyperglycemia and acute metabolic decompensation, these criteria should be confirmed by repeat testing on a different day.
Source: American Diabetes Association, 2011.

The diagnosis of DM has profound implications for an individual from both a medical and a financial standpoint. Thus, abnormalities on screening tests for diabetes should be repeated before making a definitive diagnosis of DM, unless acute metabolic derangements or a markedly elevated plasma glucose are present (Table 344-2). These criteria also allow for the diagnosis of DM to be withdrawn in situations when the glucose intolerance reverts to normal.

■ SCREENING

Widespread use of the FPG or the A1C as a screening test for type 2 DM is recommended because (1) a large number of individuals who meet the current criteria for DM are asymptomatic and unaware

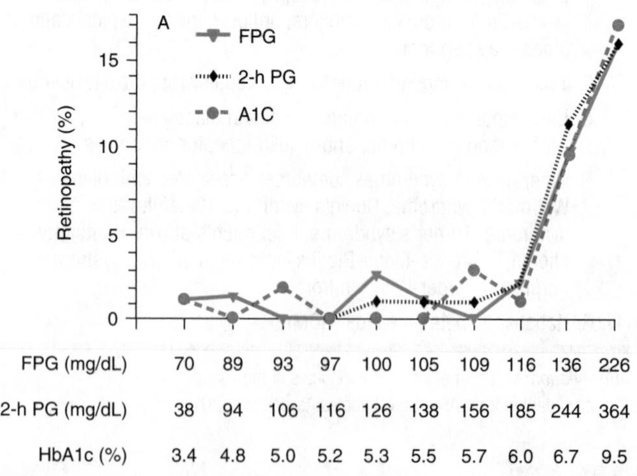

Figure 344-3 Relationship of diabetes-specific complication and glucose tolerance. This figure shows the incidence of retinopathy in Pima Indians as a function of the fasting plasma glucose (FPG), the 2-h plasma glucose after a 75-g oral glucose challenge (2-h PG), or the A1C. Note that the incidence of retinopathy greatly increases at a fasting plasma glucose >116 mg/dL, or a 2-h plasma glucose of 185 mg/dL, or an A1C > 6.5%. (Blood glucose values are shown in mg/dL; to convert to mmol/L, divide value by 18.) *(Copyright 2002, American Diabetes Association. From Diabetes Care 25(Suppl 1): S5–S20, 2002.)*

TABLE 344-3 Risk Factors for Type 2 Diabetes Mellitus

Family history of diabetes (i.e., parent or sibling with type 2 diabetes)
Obesity (BMI ≥25 kg/m^2)
Physical inactivity
Race/ethnicity (e.g., African American, Latino, Native American, Asian American, Pacific Islander)
Previously identified with IFG, IGT, or an A1C of 5.7–6.4%
History of GDM or delivery of baby >4 kg (9 lb)
Hypertension (blood pressure ≥140/90 mmHg)
HDL cholesterol level <35 mg/dL (0.90 mmol/L) and/or a triglyceride level >250 mg/dL (2.82 mmol/L)
Polycystic ovary syndrome or acanthosis nigricans
History of cardiovascular disease

Abbreviations: BMI, body mass index; GDM, gestational diabetes mellitus; HDL, high-density lipoprotein; IFG, impaired fasting glucose; IGT, impaired glucose tolerance.
Source: Adapted from American Diabetes Association, 2011.

that they have the disorder, (2) epidemiologic studies suggest that type 2 DM may be present for up to a decade before diagnosis, (3) some individuals with type 2 DM have one or more diabetes-specific complications at the time of their diagnosis, and (4) treatment of type 2 DM may favorably alter the natural history of DM. The ADA recommends screening all individuals >45 years every 3 years and screening individuals at an earlier age if they are overweight [body mass index (BMI) >25 kg/m^2] and have one additional risk factor for diabetes (Table 344-3). In contrast to type 2 DM, a long asymptomatic period of hyperglycemia is rare prior to the diagnosis of type 1 DM. A number of immunologic markers for type 1 DM are becoming available (discussed below), but their routine use is discouraged pending the identification of clinically beneficial interventions for individuals at high risk for developing type 1 DM.

INSULIN BIOSYNTHESIS, SECRETION, AND ACTION

BIOSYNTHESIS

Insulin is produced in the beta cells of the pancreatic islets. It is initially synthesized as a single-chain 86-amino-acid precursor polypeptide, preproinsulin. Subsequent proteolytic processing removes the amino-terminal signal peptide, giving rise to proinsulin. Proinsulin is structurally related to insulin-like growth factors I and II, which bind weakly to the insulin receptor. Cleavage of an internal 31-residue fragment from proinsulin generates the C peptide and the A (21 amino acids) and B (30 amino acids) chains of insulin, which are connected by disulfide bonds. The mature insulin molecule and C peptide are stored together and co-secreted from secretory granules in the beta cells. Because C peptide is cleared more slowly than insulin, it is a useful marker of insulin secretion and allows discrimination of endogenous and exogenous sources of insulin in the evaluation of hypoglycemia (Chaps. 345 and 350). Pancreatic beta cells co-secrete islet amyloid polypeptide (IAPP) or amylin, a 37-amino-acid peptide, along with insulin. The role of IAPP in normal physiology is incompletely defined, but it is the major component of the amyloid fibrils found in the islets of patients with type 2 diabetes, and an analogue is sometimes used in treating type 1 and type 2 DM. Human insulin is produced by recombinant DNA technology; structural alterations at one or more amino acid residues modify its physical and pharmacologic characteristics (see below).

SECRETION

Glucose is the key regulator of insulin secretion by the pancreatic beta cell, although amino acids, ketones, various nutrients, gastrointestinal peptides, and neurotransmitters also influence insulin secretion. Glucose levels >3.9 mmol/L (70 mg/dL) stimulate insulin synthesis, primarily by enhancing protein translation and processing. Glucose stimulation of insulin secretion begins with its transport into the beta cell by a facilitative glucose transporter (Fig. 344-4). Glucose phosphorylation by glucokinase is the rate-limiting step that controls glucose-regulated insulin secretion. Further metabolism of glucose-6-phosphate via glycolysis generates ATP, which inhibits the activity of an ATP-sensitive K^+ channel. This channel consists of two separate proteins: one is the binding site for certain oral hypoglycemics (e.g., sulfonylureas, meglitinides); the other is an inwardly rectifying K^+ channel protein (Kir6.2). Inhibition of this K^+ channel induces beta cell membrane depolarization, which opens voltage-dependent calcium channels (leading to an influx of calcium), and stimulates insulin secretion. Insulin secretory profiles reveal a pulsatile pattern of hormone release, with small secretory bursts occurring about every 10 min, superimposed upon greater amplitude oscillations of about 80–150 min. Incretins are released from neuroendocrine cells of the gastrointestinal tract following food ingestion and amplify glucose-stimulated insulin secretion and suppress glucagon secretion. Glucagon-like peptide 1 (GLP-1), the most potent incretin, is released from L cells in the small intestine and stimulates insulin secretion only when the blood glucose is above the fasting level. Incretin analogues, are used to enhance endogenous insulin secretion (see below).

ACTION

Once insulin is secreted into the portal venous system, ~50% is removed and degraded by the liver. Unextracted insulin enters

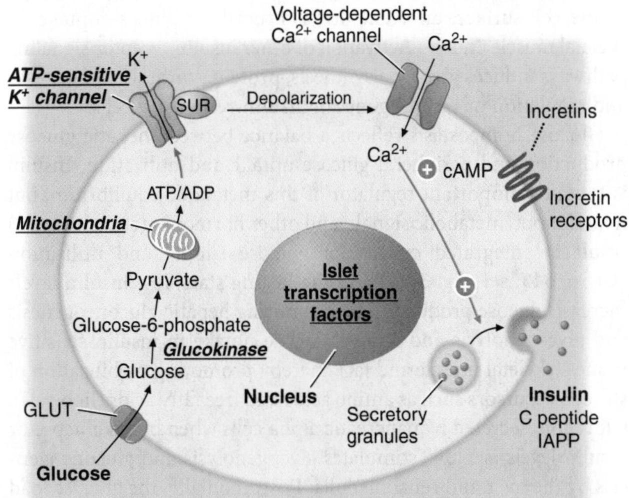

Figure 344-4 Mechanisms of glucose-stimulated insulin secretion and abnormalities in diabetes. Glucose and other nutrients regulate insulin secretion by the pancreatic beta cell. Glucose is transported by a glucose transporter (GLUT1 in humans, GLUT2 in rodents); subsequent glucose metabolism by the beta cell alters ion channel activity, leading to insulin secretion. The SUR receptor is the binding site for some drugs that act as insulin secretagogues. Mutations in the events or proteins underlined are a cause of maturity-onset diabetes of the young (MODY) or other forms of diabetes. SUR, sulfonylurea receptor; ATP, adenosine triphosphate; ADP, adenosine diphosphate, cAMP, cyclic adenosine monophosphate. IAPP, islet amyloid polypeptide or amylin.

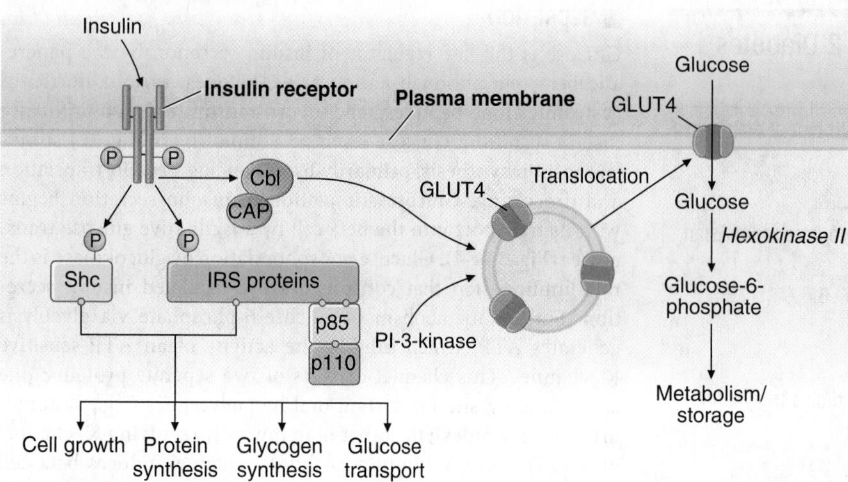

Figure 344-5 Insulin signal transduction pathway in skeletal muscle. The insulin receptor has intrinsic tyrosine kinase activity and interacts with insulin receptor substrates (IRS and Shc) proteins. A number of "docking" proteins bind to these cellular proteins and initiate the metabolic actions of insulin [GrB-2, SOS, SHP-2, p110, and phosphatidylinositol-3′-kinase (PI-3-kinase)]. Insulin increases glucose transport through PI-3-kinase and the Cbl pathway, which promotes the translocation of intracellular vesicles containing GLUT4 glucose transporter to the plasma membrane.

the systemic circulation where it binds to receptors in target sites. Insulin binding to its receptor stimulates intrinsic tyrosine kinase activity, leading to receptor autophosphorylation and the recruitment of intracellular signaling molecules, such as insulin receptor substrates (IRS) (Fig. 344-5). IRS and other adaptor proteins initiate a complex cascade of phosphorylation and dephosphorylation reactions, resulting in the widespread metabolic and mitogenic effects of insulin. As an example, activation of the phosphatidylinositol-3′-kinase (PI-3-kinase) pathway stimulates translocation of a facilitative glucose transporter (e.g., GLUT4) to the cell surface, an event that is crucial for glucose uptake by skeletal muscle and fat. Activation of other insulin receptor signaling pathways induces glycogen synthesis, protein synthesis, lipogenesis, and regulation of various genes in insulin-responsive cells.

Glucose homeostasis reflects a balance between hepatic glucose production and peripheral glucose uptake and utilization. Insulin is the most important regulator of this metabolic equilibrium, but neural input, metabolic signals, and other hormones (e.g., glucagon) result in integrated control of glucose supply and utilization (Chap. 345; see Fig. 345-1). In the fasting state, low insulin levels increase glucose production by promoting hepatic gluconeogenesis and glycogenolysis and reduce glucose uptake in insulin-sensitive tissues (skeletal muscle and fat), thereby promoting mobilization of stored precursors such as amino acids and free fatty acids (lipolysis). Glucagon, secreted by pancreatic alpha cells when blood glucose or insulin levels are low, stimulates glycogenolysis and gluconeogenesis by the liver and renal medulla. Postprandially, the glucose load elicits a rise in insulin and fall in glucagon, leading to a reversal of these processes. Insulin, an anabolic hormone, promotes the storage of carbohydrate and fat and protein synthesis. The major portion of postprandial glucose is utilized by skeletal muscle, an effect of insulin-stimulated glucose uptake. Other tissues, most notably the brain, utilize glucose in an insulin-independent fashion.

PATHOGENESIS

TYPE 1 DM

Type 1 DM is the result of interactions of genetic, environmental, and immunologic factors that ultimately lead to the destruction of the pancreatic beta cells and insulin deficiency. Type 1 DM results from autoimmune beta cell destruction, and most, but not all, individuals have evidence of islet-directed autoimmunity. Some individuals who have the clinical phenotype of type 1 DM lack immunologic markers indicative of an autoimmune process involving the beta cells and the genetic markers of type 1 diabetes. These individuals are thought to develop insulin deficiency by unknown, nonimmune mechanisms and are ketosis prone; many are African American or Asian in heritage. The temporal development of type 1 DM is shown schematically as a function of beta cell mass in Fig. 344-6. Individuals with a genetic susceptibility have normal beta cell mass at birth but begin to lose beta cells secondary to autoimmune destruction that occurs over months to years. This autoimmune process is thought to be triggered by an infectious or environmental stimulus and to be sustained by a beta cell–specific molecule. In the majority, immunologic markers appear after the triggering event but before diabetes becomes clinically overt. Beta cell mass then begins to decrease, and insulin secretion progressively declines, although normal glucose tolerance is maintained. The rate of decline in beta cell mass varies widely among individuals, with some patients progressing rapidly to clinical diabetes and others evolving more slowly. Features of diabetes do not become evident until a majority of beta cells are destroyed (70–80%). At this point, residual functional beta cells exist but are insufficient in number to maintain glucose tolerance. The events that trigger the transition

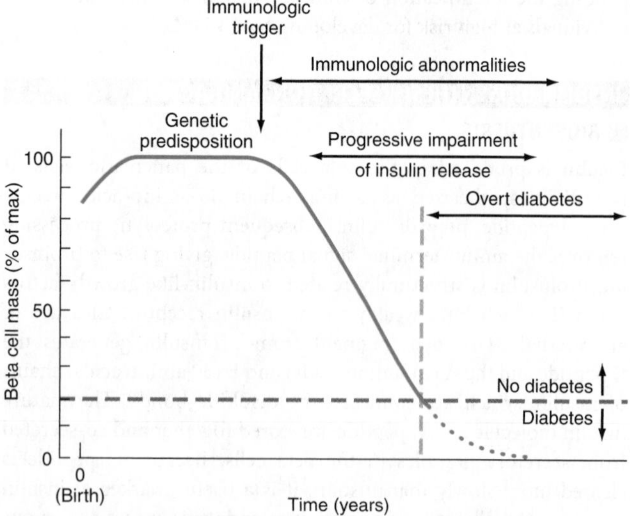

Figure 344-6 Temporal model for development of type 1 diabetes. Individuals with a genetic predisposition are exposed to an immunologic trigger that initiates an autoimmune process, resulting in a gradual decline in beta cell mass. The downward slope of the beta cell mass varies among individuals and may not be continuous. This progressive impairment in insulin release results in diabetes when ~80% of the beta cell mass is destroyed. A "honeymoon" phase may be seen in the first 1 or 2 years after the onset of diabetes and is associated with reduced insulin requirements. *[Adapted from Medical Management of Type 1 Diabetes, 3rd ed, JS Skyler (ed). American Diabetes Association, Alexandria, VA, 1998.]*

from glucose intolerance to frank diabetes are often associated with increased insulin requirements, as might occur during infections or puberty. After the initial clinical presentation of type 1 DM, a "honeymoon" phase may ensue during which time glycemic control is achieved with modest doses of insulin or, rarely, insulin is not needed. However, this fleeting phase of endogenous insulin production from residual beta cells disappears as the autoimmune process destroys remaining beta cells, and the individual becomes insulin deficient. Some individuals with long-standing type 1 diabetes produce a small amount of insulin (as reflected by C-peptide production) and some individuals have insulin-positive cells in the pancreas at autopsy.

GENETIC CONSIDERATIONS

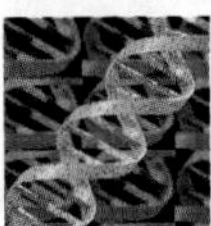

Susceptibility to type 1 DM involves multiple genes. The concordance of type 1 DM in identical twins ranges between 40 and 60%, indicating that additional modifying factors are likely involved in determining whether diabetes develops. The major susceptibility gene for type 1 DM is located in the HLA region on chromosome 6. Polymorphisms in the HLA complex account for 40–50% of the genetic risk of developing type 1 DM. This region contains genes that encode the class II major histocompatibility complex (MHC) molecules, which present antigen to helper T cells and thus are involved in initiating the immune response (Chap. 315). The ability of class II MHC molecules to present antigen is dependent on the amino acid composition of their antigen-binding sites. Amino acid substitutions may influence the specificity of the immune response by altering the binding affinity of different antigens for class II molecules.

Most individuals with type 1 DM have the HLA DR3 and/or DR4 haplotype. Refinements in genotyping of HLA loci have shown that the haplotypes DQA1*0301, DQB1*0302, and DQB1*0201 are most strongly associated with type 1 DM. These haplotypes are present in 40% of children with type 1 DM as compared to 2% of the normal U.S. population. However, most individuals with predisposing haplotypes do not develop diabetes.

In addition to MHC class II associations, genome association studies have identified at least 20 different genetic loci that contribute susceptibility to type 1 DM (polymorphisms in the promoter region of the insulin gene, the CTLA-4 gene, interleukin-2 receptor, *CTLA4*, and PTPN22, etc.). Genes that confer protection against the development of the disease also exist. The haplotype DQA1*0102, DQB1*0602 is extremely rare in individuals with type 1 DM (<1%) and appears to provide protection from type 1 DM.

Although the risk of developing type 1 DM is increased tenfold in relatives of individuals with the disease, the risk is relatively low: 3–4% if the parent has type 1 diabetes and 5–15% in a sibling (depending on which HLA haplotypes are shared). Hence, most individuals with type 1 DM do not have a first-degree relative with this disorder.

Pathophysiology

Although other islet cell types [alpha cells (glucagon-producing), delta cells (somatostatin-producing), or PP cells (pancreatic polypeptide-producing)] are functionally and embryologically similar to beta cells and express most of the same proteins as beta cells, they are spared from the autoimmune destruction. Pathologically, the pancreatic islets are infiltrated with lymphocytes (a process termed *insulitis*). After all beta cells are destroyed, the inflammatory process abates, the islets become atrophic, and most immunologic markers disappear. Studies of the autoimmune process in humans and in animal models of type 1 DM (NOD mouse and BB rat) have identified the following abnormalities in the humoral and cellular arms of the immune system: (1) islet cell autoantibodies; (2) activated lymphocytes in the islets, peripancreatic lymph nodes, and systemic circulation; (3) T lymphocytes that proliferate when stimulated with islet proteins; and (4) release of cytokines within the insulitis. Beta cells seem to be particularly susceptible to the toxic effect of some cytokines [tumor necrosis factor α (TNF-α), interferon γ, and interleukin 1 (IL-1)]. The precise mechanisms of beta cell death are not known but may involve formation of nitric oxide metabolites, apoptosis, and direct CD8+ T cell cytotoxicity. The islet destruction is mediated by T lymphocytes rather than islet autoantibodies, as these antibodies do not generally react with the cell surface of islet cells and are not capable of transferring DM to animals. Suppression of the autoimmune process at the time of diagnosis of diabetes slows the decline in beta cell destruction, but the safety of such interventions is unknown.

Pancreatic islet molecules targeted by the autoimmune process include insulin, glutamic acid decarboxylase (GAD, the biosynthetic enzyme for the neurotransmitter GABA), ICA-512/IA-2 (homology with tyrosine phosphatases), and a beta cell–specific zinc transporter (ZnT-8). Most of the autoantigens are not beta cell–specific, which raises the question of how the beta cells are selectively destroyed. Current theories favor initiation of an autoimmune process directed at one beta cell molecule, which then spreads to other islet molecules as the immune process destroys beta cells and creates a series of secondary autoantigens. The beta cells of individuals who develop type 1 DM do not differ from beta cells of normal individuals, since islets transplanted from a genetically identical twin are destroyed by a recurrence of the autoimmune process of type 1 DM.

Immunologic markers

Islet cell autoantibodies (ICAs) are a composite of several different antibodies directed at pancreatic islet molecules such as GAD, insulin, IA-2/ICA-512, and ZnT-8, and serve as a marker of the autoimmune process of type 1 DM. Assays for autoantibodies to GAD-65 are commercially available. Testing for ICAs can be useful in classifying the type of DM as type 1 and in identifying nondiabetic individuals at risk for developing type 1 DM. ICAs are present in the majority of individuals (>85%) diagnosed with new-onset type 1 DM, in a significant minority of individuals with newly diagnosed type 2 DM (5–10%), and occasionally in individuals with GDM (<5%). ICAs are present in 3–4% of first-degree relatives of individuals with type 1 DM. In combination with impaired insulin secretion after IV glucose tolerance testing, they predict a >50% risk of developing type 1 DM within 5 years. At present, the measurement of ICAs in nondiabetic individuals is a research tool because no treatments have been approved to prevent the occurrence or progression to type 1 DM. Clinical trials are testing interventions to slow the autoimmune beta cell destruction.

Environmental factors

Numerous environmental events have been proposed to trigger the autoimmune process in genetically susceptible individuals; however, none have been conclusively linked to diabetes. Identification of an environmental trigger has been difficult because the event may precede the onset of DM by several years (Fig. 344-6). Putative environmental triggers include viruses (coxsackie, rubella, enteroviruses most prominently), bovine milk proteins, and nitrosourea compounds.

Prevention of type 1 DM

A number of interventions have successfully delayed or prevented diabetes in animal models. Some interventions have targeted the immune system directly (immunosuppression, selective T cell subset deletion, induction of immunologic tolerance to islet proteins), whereas others have prevented islet cell death by blocking cytotoxic cytokines or increasing islet resistance to the destructive process. Though results in animal models are promising, these interventions have not been successful in preventing type 1 DM in humans. The Diabetes Prevention Trial—type 1 concluded that administering insulin (IV or PO) to individuals at high risk for developing type 1 DM did not prevent type 1 DM.

In patients with new-onset type 1 diabetes, treatment with anti-CD3 monoclonal antibodies, a GAD vaccine, and anti-B lymphocyte monoclonal antibody have been shown to slow the decline in C-peptide levels. This is an area of active clinical investigation.

■ TYPE 2 DM

Insulin resistance and abnormal insulin secretion are central to the development of type 2 DM. Although the primary defect is controversial, most studies support the view that insulin resistance precedes an insulin secretory defect but that diabetes develops only when insulin secretion becomes inadequate. Type 2 DM likely encompasses a range of disorders with common phenotype of hyperglycemia. Most of our current understanding (and the discussion below) of the pathophysiology and genetics is based on studies of individuals of European descent. It is becoming increasing apparent that DM in other ethnic groups (Asian, African, and Latin American) has a different, but yet undefined, pathophysiology. In these groups, DM that is ketosisprone (often obese) or ketosis-resistant (often lean) is commonly seen.

GENETIC CONSIDERATIONS

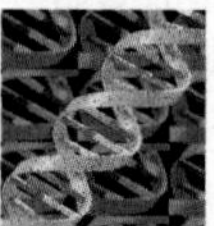

Type 2 DM has a strong genetic component. The concordance of type 2 DM in identical twins is between 70 and 90%. Individuals with a parent with type 2 DM have an increased risk of diabetes; if both parents have type 2 DM, the risk approaches 40%. Insulin resistance, as demonstrated by reduced glucose utilization in skeletal muscle, is present in many nondiabetic, first-degree relatives of individuals with type 2 DM. The disease is polygenic and multifactorial, since in addition to genetic susceptibility, environmental factors (such as obesity, nutrition, and physical activity) modulate the phenotype. The genes that predispose to type 2 DM are incompletely identified, but recent genome-wide association studies have identified a large number of genes that convey a relatively small risk for type 2 DM (>20 genes, each with a relative risk of 1.06–1.5). Most prominent is a variant of the transcription factor 7–like 2 gene that has been associated with type 2 diabetes in several populations and with impaired glucose tolerance in one population at high risk for diabetes. Genetic polymorphisms associated with type 2 diabetes have also been found in the genes encoding the peroxisome proliferators–activated receptor-γ, inward rectifying potassium channel, zinc transporter, IRS, and calpain 10. The mechanisms by which these genetic loci increase the susceptibility to type 2 diabetes are not clear, but most are predicted to alter islet function or development or insulin secretion. While the genetic susceptibility to type 2 diabetes is under active investigation (estimation that <10% of genetic risk is determined by loci identified thus far), it is currently not possible to use a combination of known genetic loci to predict type 2 diabetes.

Pathophysiology

Type 2 DM is characterized by impaired insulin secretion, insulin resistance, excessive hepatic glucose production, and abnormal fat metabolism. Obesity, particularly visceral or central (as evidenced by the hip-waist ratio), is very common in type 2 DM (80% or more are obese). In the early stages of the disorder, glucose tolerance remains near-normal, despite insulin resistance, because the pancreatic beta cells compensate by increasing insulin output (Fig. 344-7). As insulin resistance and compensatory hyperinsulinemia progress, the pancreatic islets in certain individuals are unable to sustain the hyperinsulinemic state. IGT, characterized by elevations in postprandial glucose, then

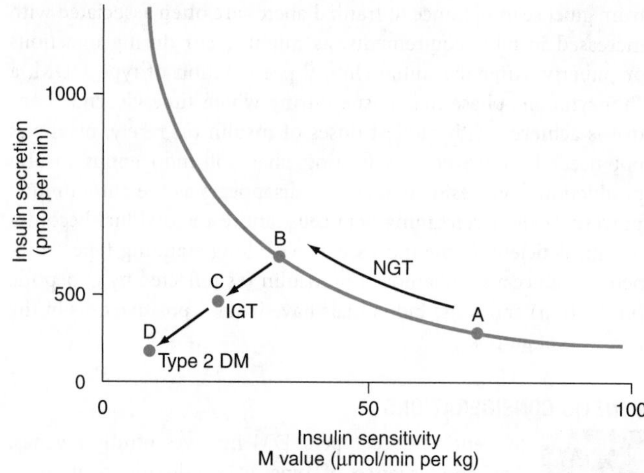

Figure 344-7 Metabolic changes during the development of type 2 diabetes mellitus (DM). Insulin secretion and insulin sensitivity are related, and as an individual becomes more insulin resistant (by moving from point A to point B), insulin secretion increases. A failure to compensate by increasing the insulin secretion results initially in impaired glucose tolerance (IGT; point C) and ultimately in type 2 DM (point D). *(Adapted from SE Kahn: J Clin Endocrinol Metab 86:4047, 2001; RN Bergman, M Ader: Trends Endocrinol Metab 11:351, 2000.)*

develops. A further decline in insulin secretion and an increase in hepatic glucose production lead to overt diabetes with fasting hyperglycemia. Ultimately, beta cell failure ensues.

Metabolic abnormalities

Abnormal muscle and fat metabolism Insulin resistance, the decreased ability of insulin to act effectively on target tissues (especially muscle, liver, and fat), is a prominent feature of type 2 DM and results from a combination of genetic susceptibility and obesity. Insulin resistance is relative, however, since supranormal levels of circulating insulin will normalize the plasma glucose. Insulin dose-response curves exhibit a rightward shift, indicating reduced sensitivity, and a reduced maximal response, indicating an overall decrease in maximum glucose utilization (30–60% lower than in normal individuals). Insulin resistance impairs glucose utilization by insulin-sensitive tissues and increases hepatic glucose output; both effects contribute to the hyperglycemia. Increased hepatic glucose output predominantly accounts for increased FPG levels, whereas decreased peripheral glucose usage results in postprandial hyperglycemia. In skeletal muscle, there is a greater impairment in nonoxidative glucose usage (glycogen formation) than in oxidative glucose metabolism through glycolysis. Glucose metabolism in insulin-independent tissues is not altered in type 2 DM.

The precise molecular mechanism leading to insulin resistance in type 2 DM has not been elucidated. Insulin receptor levels and tyrosine kinase activity in skeletal muscle are reduced, but these alterations are most likely secondary to hyperinsulinemia and are not a primary defect. Therefore, "postreceptor" defects in insulin-regulated phosphorylation/dephosphorylation appear to play the predominant role in insulin resistance (Fig. 344-5). For example, a PI-3-kinase signaling defect might reduce translocation of GLUT4 to the plasma membrane. Other abnormalities include the accumulation of lipid within skeletal myocytes, which may impair mitochondrial oxidative phosphorylation and reduce insulin-stimulated mitochondrial ATP production. Impaired fatty acid oxidation and lipid accumulation within skeletal myocytes also may generate reactive oxygen species such as lipid peroxides. Of note, not all insulin signal transduction pathways are resistant to the effects of insulin (e.g., those controlling cell growth and differentiation using the mitogenic-activated protein kinase pathway). Consequently, hyperinsulinemia may increase the insulin action through these pathways, potentially accelerating diabetes-related conditions such as atherosclerosis.

The obesity accompanying type 2 DM, particularly in a central or visceral location, is thought to be part of the pathogenic process. The increased adipocyte mass leads to increased levels of circulating free fatty acids and other fat cell products (Chap. 77). For example, adipocytes secrete a number of biologic products (nonesterified free fatty acids, retinol-binding protein 4, leptin, TNF-α, resistin, and adiponectin). In addition to regulating body weight, appetite, and energy expenditure, adipokines also modulate insulin sensitivity. The increased production of free fatty acids and some adipokines may cause insulin resistance in skeletal muscle and liver. For example, free fatty acids impair glucose utilization in skeletal muscle, promote glucose production by the liver, and impair beta cell function. In contrast, the production by adipocytes of adiponectin, an insulin-sensitizing peptide, is reduced in obesity, and this may contribute to hepatic insulin resistance. Adipocyte products and adipokines also produce an inflammatory state and may explain why markers of inflammation such as IL-6 and C-reactive protein are often elevated in type 2 DM. In addition, inflammatory cells have been found infiltrating adipose tissue. Inhibition of inflammatory signaling pathways such as the nuclear factor κB (NF-κB) pathway appears to reduce insulin resistance and improve hyperglycemia in animal models.

Impaired insulin secretion Insulin secretion and sensitivity are interrelated (Fig. 344-7). In type 2 DM, insulin secretion initially increases in response to insulin resistance to maintain normal glucose tolerance. Initially, the insulin secretory defect is mild and selectively involves glucose-stimulated insulin secretion. The response to other nonglucose secretagogues, such as arginine, is preserved. Abnormalities in proinsulin processing is reflected by increased secretion of proinsulin in type 2 diabetes. Eventually, the insulin secretory defect progresses to a state of inadequate insulin secretion.

The reason(s) for the decline in insulin secretory capacity in type 2 DM is unclear. The assumption is that a second genetic defect—superimposed upon insulin resistance—leads to beta cell failure. Beta cell mass is decreased by approximately 50% in individuals with long-standing type 2 diabetes. Islet amyloid polypeptide or amylin is co-secreted by the beta cell and forms the amyloid fibrillar deposit found in the islets of individuals with long-standing type 2 DM. Whether such islet amyloid deposits are a primary or secondary event is not known. The metabolic environment of diabetes may also negatively impact islet function. For example, chronic hyperglycemia paradoxically impairs islet function ("glucose toxicity") and leads to a worsening of hyperglycemia. Improvement in glycemic control is often associated with improved islet function. In addition, elevation of free fatty acid levels ("lipotoxicity") and dietary fat may also worsen islet function.

Increased hepatic glucose and lipid production In type 2 DM, insulin resistance in the liver reflects the failure of hyperinsulinemia to suppress gluconeogenesis, which results in fasting hyperglycemia and decreased glycogen storage by the liver in the postprandial state. Increased hepatic glucose production occurs early in the course of diabetes, though likely after the onset of insulin secretory abnormalities and insulin resistance in skeletal muscle. As a result of insulin resistance in adipose tissue, lipolysis and free fatty acid flux from adipocytes are increased, leading to increased lipid [very low density lipoprotein (VLDL) and triglyceride] synthesis in hepatocytes. This lipid storage or steatosis in the liver may lead to nonalcoholic fatty liver disease (Chap. 309) and abnormal liver function tests. This is also responsible for the dyslipidemia found in type 2 DM [elevated triglycerides, reduced high-density lipoprotein (HDL), and increased small dense low-density lipoprotein (LDL) particles].

Insulin resistance syndromes

The insulin resistance condition comprises a spectrum of disorders, with hyperglycemia representing one of the most readily diagnosed features. The *metabolic syndrome*, the *insulin resistance syndrome*, or *syndrome X* are terms used to describe a constellation of metabolic derangements that includes insulin resistance, hypertension, dyslipidemia (decreased HDL and elevated triglycerides), central or visceral obesity, type 2 diabetes or IGT/IFG, and accelerated cardiovascular disease. This syndrome is discussed in Chap. 242.

A number of relatively rare forms of severe insulin resistance include features of type 2 DM or IGT (Table 344-1). Mutations in the insulin receptor that interfere with binding or signal transduction are a rare cause of insulin resistance. Acanthosis nigricans and signs of hyperandrogenism (hirsutism, acne, and oligomenorrhea in women) are also common physical features. Two distinct syndromes of severe insulin resistance have been described in adults: (1) type A, which affects young women and is characterized by severe hyperinsulinemia, obesity, and features of hyperandrogenism; and (2) type B, which affects middle-aged women and is characterized by severe hyperinsulinemia, features of hyperandrogenism, and autoimmune disorders. Individuals with the type A insulin resistance syndrome have an undefined defect in the insulin-signaling pathway; individuals with the type B insulin resistance syndrome have autoantibodies directed at the insulin receptor. These receptor autoantibodies may block insulin binding or may stimulate the insulin receptor, leading to intermittent hypoglycemia.

Polycystic ovary syndrome (PCOS) is a common disorder that affects premenopausal women and is characterized by chronic anovulation and hyperandrogenism (Chap. 347). Insulin resistance is seen in a significant subset of women with PCOS, and the disorder substantially increases the risk for type 2 DM, independent of the effects of obesity.

Prevention

Type 2 DM is preceded by a period of IGT or IFG, and a number of lifestyle modifications and pharmacologic agents prevent or delay the onset of DM. The Diabetes Prevention Program (DPP) demonstrated that intensive changes in lifestyle (diet and exercise for 30 min/d five times/week) in individuals with IGT prevented or delayed the development of type 2 DM by 58% compared to placebo. This effect was seen in individuals regardless of age, sex, or ethnic group. In the same study, metformin prevented or delayed diabetes by 31% compared to placebo. The lifestyle intervention group lost 5–7% of their body weight during the 3 years of the study. Studies in Finnish and Chinese populations noted similar efficacy of diet and exercise in preventing or delaying type 2 DM; α-glucosidase inhibitors, metformin, thiazolidinediones, and orlistat prevent or delay type 2 DM but are not approved for this purpose. Individuals with a strong family history of type 2 DM and individuals with IFG or IGT should be strongly encouraged to maintain a normal BMI and engage in regular physical activity. Pharmacologic therapy for individuals with prediabetes is currently controversial because its cost-effectiveness and safety profile are not known. The ADA has suggested that metformin be considered in individuals with both IFG and IGT who are at very high risk for progression to diabetes (age <60 years, BMI ≥35 kg/m^2, family history of diabetes in first-degree relative, elevated triglycerides, reduced HDL, hypertension, or A1C >6.0%). Individuals with IFG, IGT, or an A1C of 5.7–6.4% should be monitored annually to determine if diagnostic criteria for diabetes are present.

GENETICALLY DEFINED, MONOGENIC FORMS OF DIABETES MELLITUS

Several monogenic forms of DM have been identified. Six different variants of MODY, caused by mutations in genes encoding islet-enriched transcription factors or glucokinase (Fig. 344-4; Table 344-1), are transmitted as autosomal dominant disorders. MODY 1, MODY 3, and MODY 5 are caused by mutations in the hepatocyte nuclear transcription factor (HNF) 4α, HNF-1α, and HNF-1β, respectively. As their names imply, these transcription factors are expressed in the liver but also in other tissues, including the pancreatic islets and kidney. These factors most likely affect islet development or the expression of genes important in glucose-stimulated insulin secretion or the maintenance of beta cell mass. For example, individuals with an HNF-1α mutation (MODY 3) have a progressive decline in glycemic control but may respond to sulfonylureas. In fact, some of these patients were initially thought to have type 1 DM but were later shown to respond to a sulfonylurea, and insulin was discontinued. Individuals with a HNF-1β mutation have progressive impairment of insulin secretion, hepatic insulin resistance, and require insulin treatment (minimal response to sulfonylureas). These individuals often have other abnormalities such as renal cysts, mild pancreatic exocrine insufficiency, and abnormal liver function tests. Individuals with MODY 2, the result of mutations in the glucokinase gene, have mild-to-moderate, stable hyperglycemia that does not respond to oral hypoglycemic agents. Glucokinase catalyzes the formation of glucose-6-phosphate from glucose, a reaction that is important for glucose sensing by the beta cells and for glucose utilization by the liver. As a result of glucokinase mutations, higher glucose levels are required to elicit insulin secretory responses, thus altering the set point for insulin secretion. MODY 4 is a rare variant caused by mutations in the insulin promoter factor (IPF) 1, which is a transcription factor that regulates pancreatic development and insulin gene transcription. Homozygous inactivating mutations cause pancreatic agenesis, whereas heterozygous mutations may result in DM. Studies of populations with type 2 DM suggest that mutations in MODY-associated genes are an uncommon (<5%) cause of type 2 DM.

Transient or permanent neonatal diabetes (onset <6 months of age) occurs. Permanent neonatal diabetes may be caused by several genetic mutations and usually requires treatment with insulin. Mutations in the ATP-sensitive potassium channel subunits (Kir6.2 and ABCC8) and the insulin gene (interfere with proinsulin folding and processing) (Fig. 344-4) are the major causes of permanent neonatal diabetes. Although these activating mutations in the ATP-sensitive potassium channel subunits impair glucose-stimulated insulin secretion, these individuals may respond to sulfonylureas and be treated with these agents. These mutations are associated with a spectrum of neurologic dysfunction. Homozygous glucokinase mutations cause a severe form of neonatal diabetes.

ACUTE COMPLICATIONS OF DM

Diabetic ketoacidosis (DKA) and hyperglycemic hyperosmolar state (HHS) are acute complications of diabetes. DKA was formerly considered a hallmark of type 1 DM, but also occurs in individuals who lack immunologic features of type 1 DM and who can sometimes subsequently be treated with oral glucose-lowering agents (these obese individuals with type 2 DM are often of Hispanic or African-American descent. The initial management of DKA is similar. HHS is primarily seen in individuals with type 2 DM. Both disorders are associated with absolute or relative insulin deficiency, volume depletion, and acid-base abnormalities. DKA and HHS exist along a continuum of hyperglycemia, with or without ketosis. The metabolic similarities and differences in DKA and HHS are highlighted in Table 344-4. Both disorders are associated with potentially serious complications if not promptly diagnosed and treated.

TABLE 344-4 Laboratory Values in Diabetic Ketoacidosis (DKA) and Hyperglycemic Hyperosmolar State (HHS) (Representative Ranges at Presentation)

	DKA	HHS
Glucose,[a] mmol/L (mg/dL)	13.9–33.3 (250–600)	33.3–66.6 (600–1200)
Sodium, meq/L	125–135	135–145
Potassium[a,b]	Normal to ↑	Normal
Magnesium[a]	Normal	Normal
Chloride[a]	Normal	Normal
Phosphate[a,b]	Normal	Normal
Creatinine	Slightly ↑	Moderately ↑
Osmolality (mOsm/mL)	300–320	330–380
Plasma ketones[a]	++++	+/–
Serum bicarbonate,[a] meq/L	<15 meq/L	Normal to slightly ↓
Arterial pH	6.8–7.3	>7.3
Arterial P_{CO_2},[a] mmHg	20–30	Normal
Anion gap[a] [Na – (Cl + HCO_3)]	↑	Normal to slightly ↑

[a]Large changes occur during treatment of DKA.
[b]Although plasma levels may be normal or high at presentation, total-body stores are usually depleted.

DIABETIC KETOACIDOSIS

Clinical features

The symptoms and physical signs of DKA are listed in Table 344-5 and usually develop over 24 h. DKA may be the initial symptom complex that leads to a diagnosis of type 1 DM, but more frequently

TABLE 344-5 Manifestations of Diabetic Ketoacidosis

Symptoms	Physical Findings
Nausea/vomiting	Tachycardia
Thirst/polyuria	Dehydration/hypotension
Abdominal pain	Tachypnea/Kussmaul respirations/respiratory distress
Shortness of breath	Abdominal tenderness (may resemble acute pancreatitis or surgical abdomen)
Precipitating events	Lethargy/obtundation/cerebral edema/possibly coma
Inadequate insulin administration	
Infection (pneumonia/UTI/gastroenteritis/sepsis)	
Infarction (cerebral, coronary, mesenteric, peripheral)	
Drugs (cocaine)	
Pregnancy	

Abbreviation: UTI, urinary tract infection.

it occurs in individuals with established diabetes. Nausea and vomiting are often prominent, and their presence in an individual with diabetes warrants laboratory evaluation for DKA. Abdominal pain may be severe and can resemble acute pancreatitis or ruptured viscus. Hyperglycemia leads to glucosuria, volume depletion, and tachycardia. Hypotension can occur because of volume depletion in combination with peripheral vasodilatation. Kussmaul respirations and a fruity odor on the patient's breath (secondary to metabolic acidosis and increased acetone) are classic signs of the disorder. Lethargy and central nervous system depression may evolve into coma with severe DKA but should also prompt evaluation for other reasons for altered mental status (infection, hypoxemia, etc.). Cerebral edema, an extremely serious complication of DKA, is seen most frequently in children. Signs of infection, which may precipitate DKA, should be sought on physical examination, even in the absence of fever. Tissue ischemia (heart, brain) can also be a precipitating factor. Omission of insulin because of an eating disorder may sometimes precipitate DKA.

Pathophysiology

DKA results from relative or absolute insulin deficiency combined with counterregulatory hormone excess (glucagon, catecholamines, cortisol, and growth hormone). Both insulin deficiency and glucagon excess, in particular, are necessary for DKA to develop. The decreased ratio of insulin to glucagon promotes gluconeogenesis, glycogenolysis, and ketone body formation in the liver, as well as increases in substrate delivery from fat and muscle (free fatty acids, amino acids) to the liver. Markers of inflammation (cytokines, C-reactive protein) are elevated in both DKA and HHS

The combination of insulin deficiency and hyperglycemia reduces the hepatic level of fructose-2,6-bisphosphate, which alters the activity of phosphofructokinase and fructose-1,6-bisphosphatase. Glucagon excess decreases the activity of pyruvate kinase, whereas insulin deficiency increases the activity of phosphoenolpyruvate carboxykinase. These changes shift the handling of pyruvate toward glucose synthesis and away from glycolysis. The increased levels of glucagon and catecholamines in the face of low insulin levels promote glycogenolysis. Insulin deficiency also reduces levels of the GLUT4 glucose transporter, which impairs glucose uptake into skeletal muscle and fat and reduces intracellular glucose metabolism (Fig. 344-5).

Ketosis results from a marked increase in free fatty acid release from adipocytes, with a resulting shift toward ketone body synthesis in the liver. Reduced insulin levels, in combination with elevations in catecholamines and growth hormone, increase lipolysis and the release of free fatty acids. Normally, these free fatty acids are converted to triglycerides or VLDL in the liver. However, in DKA, hyperglucagonemia alters hepatic metabolism to favor ketone body formation, through activation of the enzyme carnitine palmitoyltransferase I. This enzyme is crucial for regulating fatty acid transport into the mitochondria, where beta oxidation and conversion to ketone bodies occur. At physiologic pH, ketone bodies exist as ketoacids, which are neutralized by bicarbonate. As bicarbonate stores are depleted, metabolic acidosis ensues. Increased lactic acid production also contributes to the acidosis. The increased free fatty acids increase triglyceride and VLDL production. VLDL clearance is also reduced because the activity of insulin-sensitive lipoprotein lipase in muscle and fat is decreased. Hypertriglyceridemia may be severe enough to cause pancreatitis.

DKA is often precipitated by increased insulin requirements, as occurs during a concurrent illness (Table 344-5). Failure to augment insulin therapy often compounds the problem. Complete omission or inadequate administration of insulin by the patient or health care team (in a hospitalized patient with type 1 DM) may precipitate DKA. Patients using insulin infusion devices with short-acting insulin may develop DKA, since even a brief interruption in insulin delivery (e.g., mechanical malfunction) quickly leads to insulin deficiency.

Laboratory abnormalities and diagnosis

The timely diagnosis of DKA is crucial and allows for prompt initiation of therapy. DKA is characterized by hyperglycemia, ketosis, and metabolic acidosis (increased anion gap) along with a number of secondary metabolic derangements (Table 344-4). Occasionally, the serum glucose is only minimally elevated. Serum bicarbonate is frequently <10 mmol/L, and arterial pH ranges between 6.8 and 7.3, depending on the severity of the acidosis. Despite a total-body potassium deficit, the serum potassium at presentation may be mildly elevated, secondary to the acidosis. Total-body stores of sodium, chloride, phosphorus, and magnesium are reduced in DKA but are not accurately reflected by their levels in the serum because of dehydration and hyperglycemia. Elevated blood urea nitrogen (BUN) and serum creatinine levels reflect intravascular volume depletion. Interference from acetoacetate may falsely elevate the serum creatinine measurement. Leukocytosis, hypertriglyceridemia, and hyperlipoproteinemia are commonly found as well. Hyperamylasemia may suggest a diagnosis of pancreatitis, especially when accompanied by abdominal pain. However, in DKA the amylase is usually of salivary origin and thus is not diagnostic of pancreatitis. Serum lipase should be obtained if pancreatitis is suspected.

The measured serum sodium is reduced as a consequence of the hyperglycemia [1.6-mmol/L (1.6 meq) reduction in serum sodium for each 5.6-mmol/L (100 mg/dL) rise in the serum glucose]. A normal serum sodium in the setting of DKA indicates a more profound water deficit. In "conventional" units, the calculated serum osmolality [2 × (serum sodium + serum potassium) + plasma glucose (mg/dL)/18 + BUN/2.8] is mildly to moderately elevated, though to a lesser degree than that found in HHS (see below).

In DKA, the ketone body, β-hydroxybutyrate, is synthesized at a threefold greater rate than acetoacetate; however, acetoacetate is preferentially detected by a commonly used ketosis detection reagent (nitroprusside). Serum ketones are present at significant levels (usually positive at serum dilution of ≥1:8). The nitroprusside tablet, or stick, is often used to detect urine ketones; certain medications such as captopril or penicillamine may cause false-positive reactions. Serum or plasma assays for β-hydroxybutyrate are preferred since they more accurately reflect the true ketone body level.

The metabolic derangements of DKA exist along a spectrum, beginning with mild acidosis with moderate hyperglycemia evolving into more severe findings. The degree of acidosis and hyperglycemia do not necessarily correlate closely since a variety of factors determine the level of hyperglycemia (oral intake, urinary glucose loss). Ketonemia is a consistent finding in DKA and distinguishes it from simple hyperglycemia. The differential diagnosis of DKA includes starvation ketosis, alcoholic ketoacidosis (bicarbonate usually >15 meq/L) and other forms of increased anion-gap acidosis (Chap. 47).

TREATMENT Diabetic Ketoacidosis

The management of DKA is outlined in Table 344-6. After initiating IV fluid replacement and insulin therapy, the agent or event that precipitated the episode of DKA should be sought and aggressively treated. If the patient is vomiting or has altered mental status, a nasogastric tube should be inserted to prevent

TABLE 344-6 Management of Diabetic Ketoacidosis

1. Confirm diagnosis (↑plasma glucose, positive serum ketones, metabolic acidosis).
2. Admit to hospital; intensive-care setting may be necessary for frequent monitoring or if pH <7.00 or unconscious.
3. Assess:
   Serum electrolytes (K^+, Na^+, Mg^{2+}, Cl^-, bicarbonate, phosphate)
   Acid-base status—pH, HCO_3^-, P_{CO_2}, β-hydroxybutyrate
   Renal function (creatinine, urine output)
4. Replace fluids: 2–3 L of 0.9% saline over first 1–3 h (15–20 mL/kg per hour); subsequently, 0.45% saline at 250–500 mL/h; change to 5% glucose and 0.45% saline at 150–250 mL/h when plasma glucose reaches 200 mg/dL (11.2 mmol/L).
5. Administer short-acting insulin: IV (0.1 units/kg), then 0.1 units/kg per hour by continuous IV infusion; increase two- to threefold if no response by 2–4 h. If the initial serum potassium is <3.3 mmol/L (3.3 meq/L), do not administer insulin until the potassium is corrected. If the initial serum potassium is >5.2 mmol/L (5.2 meq/L), do not supplement K^+ until the potassium is corrected.
6. Assess patient: What precipitated the episode (noncompliance, infection, trauma, infarction, cocaine)? Initiate appropriate workup for precipitating event (cultures, CXR, ECG).
7. Measure capillary glucose every 1–2 h; measure electrolytes (especially K^+, bicarbonate, phosphate) and anion gap every 4 h for first 24 h.
8. Monitor blood pressure, pulse, respirations, mental status, fluid intake and output every 1–4 h.
9. Replace K^+: 10 meq/h when plasma K^+ < 5.0–5.2 meq/L (or 20–30 meq/L of infusion fluid), ECG normal, urine flow and normal creatinine documented; administer 40–80 meq/h when plasma K^+ < 3.5 meq/L or if bicarbonate is given. See text about bicarbonate or phosphate supplementation.
10. Continue above until patient is stable, glucose goal is 8.3–13.9 mmol/L (150–250 mg/dL), and acidosis is resolved. Insulin infusion may be decreased to 0.05–0.1 units/kg per hour.
11. Administer long-acting insulin as soon as patient is eating. Allow for overlap in insulin infusion and SC insulin injection.

Abbreviations: CXR, chest x-ray; ECG, electrocardiogram.
Source: Adapted from M Sperling, in *Therapy for Diabetes Mellitus and Related Disorders*, American Diabetes Association, Alexandria, VA, 1998; and AE Kitabchi et al: Diabetes Care 32:1335, 2009.

aspiration of gastric contents. Central to successful treatment of DKA is careful monitoring and frequent reassessment to ensure that the patient and the metabolic derangements are improving. A comprehensive flow sheet should record chronologic changes in vital signs, fluid intake and output, and laboratory values as a function of insulin administered.

After the initial bolus of normal saline, replacement of the sodium and free water deficit is carried out over the next 24 h (fluid deficit is often 3–5 L). When hemodynamic stability and adequate urine output are achieved, IV fluids should be switched to 0.45% saline depending on the calculated volume deficit. The change to 0.45% saline helps to reduce the trend toward hyperchloremia later in the course of DKA. Alternatively, initial use of lactated Ringer's IV solution may reduce the hyperchloremia that commonly occurs with normal saline.

A bolus of IV (0.1 units/kg) short-acting insulin should be administered immediately (Table 344-6), and subsequent treatment should provide continuous and adequate levels of circulating insulin. IV administration is preferred (0.1 units/kg of regular insulin per hour), because it ensures rapid distribution and allows adjustment of the infusion rate as the patient responds to therapy. In mild episodes of DKA, short-acting insulin analogues can be used SC. IV insulin should be continued until the acidosis resolves and the patient is metabolically stable. As the acidosis and insulin resistance associated with DKA resolve, the insulin infusion rate can be decreased (to 0.05–0.1 units/kg per hour). Long-acting insulin, in combination with SC short-acting insulin, should be administered as soon as the patient resumes eating, as this facilitates transition to an outpatient insulin regimen and reduces length of hospital stay. It is crucial to continue the insulin infusion until adequate insulin levels are achieved by administering long-acting insulin by the SC route. Even relatively brief periods of inadequate insulin administration in this transition phase may result in DKA relapse.

Hyperglycemia usually improves at a rate of 4.2–5.6 mmol/L (75–100 mg/dL) per hour as a result of insulin-mediated glucose disposal, reduced hepatic glucose release, and rehydration. The latter reduces catecholamines, increases urinary glucose loss, and expands the intravascular volume. The decline in the plasma glucose within the first 1–2 h may be more rapid and is mostly related to volume expansion. When the plasma glucose reaches 11.2 mmol/L (200 mg/dL), glucose should be added to the 0.45% saline infusion to maintain the plasma glucose in the 8.3–13.9 mmol/L (150–250 mg/dL) range, and the insulin infusion should be continued. Ketoacidosis begins to resolve as insulin reduces lipolysis, increases peripheral ketone body use, suppresses hepatic ketone body formation, and promotes bicarbonate regeneration. However, the acidosis and ketosis resolve more slowly than hyperglycemia. As ketoacidosis improves, β-hydroxybutyrate is converted to acetoacetate. Ketone body levels may appear to increase if measured by laboratory assays that use the nitroprusside reaction, which only detects acetoacetate and acetone. The improvement in acidosis and anion gap, a result of bicarbonate regeneration and decline in ketone bodies, is reflected by a rise in the serum bicarbonate level and the arterial pH. Depending on the rise of serum chloride, the anion gap (but not bicarbonate) will normalize. A hyperchloremic acidosis [serum bicarbonate of 15–18 mmol/L (15–18 meq/L)] often follows successful treatment and gradually resolves as the kidneys regenerate bicarbonate and excrete chloride.

Potassium stores are depleted in DKA [estimated deficit 3–5 mmol/kg (3–5 meq/kg)]. During treatment with insulin and fluids, various factors contribute to the development of hypokalemia. These include insulin-mediated potassium transport into cells, resolution of the acidosis (which also promotes potassium entry into cells), and urinary loss of potassium salts of organic acids. Thus, potassium repletion should commence as soon as adequate urine output and a normal serum potassium are documented. If the initial serum potassium level is elevated, then potassium repletion should be delayed until the potassium falls into the normal range. Inclusion of 20–40 meq of potassium in each liter of IV fluid is reasonable, but additional potassium supplements may also be required. To reduce the amount of chloride administered, potassium phosphate or acetate can be substituted for the chloride salt. The goal is to maintain the serum potassium at >3.5 mmol/L (3.5 meq/L).

Despite a bicarbonate deficit, bicarbonate replacement is not usually necessary. In fact, theoretical arguments suggest that bicarbonate administration and rapid reversal of acidosis may impair cardiac function, reduce tissue oxygenation, and promote hypokalemia. The results of most clinical trials do not support the routine use of bicarbonate replacement, and one study in children found that bicarbonate use was associated with an increased risk of cerebral edema. However, in the presence of severe acidosis (arterial pH <6.9), the ADA advises bicarbonate [50 mmol/L (meq/L) of sodium bicarbonate in 200 mL of sterile water with 10 meq/L KCl per hour for 2 h until the pH is >7.0]. Hypophosphatemia may result from increased glucose usage, but randomized clinical trials have not demonstrated that phosphate replacement is beneficial in DKA. If the serum phosphate < 0.32 mmol/L (1 mg/dL), then phosphate supplement should be considered and the serum calcium monitored. Hypomagnesemia may develop during DKA therapy and may also require supplementation.

With appropriate therapy, the mortality rate of DKA is low (<1%) and is related more to the underlying or precipitating event, such as infection or myocardial infarction. Venous thrombosis, upper gastrointestinal bleeding, and acute respiratory distress syndrome occasionally complicate DKA. The major nonmetabolic complication of DKA therapy is cerebral edema, which most often develops in children as DKA is resolving. The etiology of and optimal therapy for cerebral edema are not well established, but overreplacement of free water should be avoided.

Following treatment, the physician and patient should review the sequence of events that led to DKA to prevent future recurrences. Foremost is patient education about the symptoms of DKA, its precipitating factors, and the management of diabetes during a concurrent illness. During illness or when oral intake is compromised, patients should (1) frequently measure the capillary blood glucose; (2) measure urinary ketones when the serum glucose > 16.5 mmol/L (300 mg/dL); (3) drink fluids to maintain hydration; (4) continue or increase insulin; and (5) seek medical attention if dehydration, persistent vomiting, or uncontrolled hyperglycemia develop. Using these strategies, early DKA can be prevented or detected and treated appropriately on an outpatient basis.

HYPERGLYCEMIC HYPEROSMOLAR STATE

Clinical features

The prototypical patient with HHS is an elderly individual with type 2 DM, with a several-week history of polyuria, weight loss, and diminished oral intake that culminates in mental confusion, lethargy, or coma. The physical examination reflects profound dehydration and hyperosmolality and reveals hypotension, tachycardia, and altered mental status. Notably absent are symptoms of nausea, vomiting, and abdominal pain and the Kussmaul respirations characteristic of DKA. HHS is often precipitated by a serious, concurrent illness such as myocardial infarction or stroke. Sepsis, pneumonia, and other serious infections are frequent precipitants and should be sought. In addition, a debilitating condition (prior stroke or dementia) or social situation that compromises water intake usually contributes to the development of the disorder.

Pathophysiology

Relative insulin deficiency and inadequate fluid intake are the underlying causes of HHS. Insulin deficiency increases hepatic glucose production (through glycogenolysis and gluconeogenesis) and impairs glucose utilization in skeletal muscle (see above discussion of DKA). Hyperglycemia induces an osmotic diuresis that leads to intravascular volume depletion, which is exacerbated by inadequate fluid replacement. The absence of ketosis in HHS is not understood. Presumably, the insulin deficiency is only relative and less severe than in DKA. Lower levels of counterregulatory hormones and free fatty acids have been found in HHS than in DKA in some studies. It is also possible that the liver is less capable of ketone body synthesis or that the insulin/glucagon ratio does not favor ketogenesis.

Laboratory abnormalities and diagnosis

The laboratory features in HHS are summarized in Table 344-4. Most notable are the marked hyperglycemia [plasma glucose may be >55.5 mmol/L (1000 mg/dL)], hyperosmolality (>350 mosmol/L), and prerenal azotemia. The measured serum sodium may be normal or slightly low despite the marked hyperglycemia. The corrected serum sodium is usually increased [add 1.6 meq to measured sodium for each 5.6-mmol/L (100 mg/dL) rise in the serum glucose]. In contrast to DKA, acidosis and ketonemia are absent or mild. A small anion-gap metabolic acidosis may be present secondary to increased lactic acid. Moderate ketonuria, if present, is secondary to starvation.

TREATMENT Hyperglycemic Hyperosmolar State

Volume depletion and hyperglycemia are prominent features of both HHS and DKA. Consequently, therapy of these disorders shares several elements (Table 344-6). In both disorders, careful monitoring of the patient's fluid status, laboratory values, and insulin infusion rate is crucial. Underlying or precipitating problems should be aggressively sought and treated. In HHS, fluid losses and dehydration are usually more pronounced than in DKA due to the longer duration of the illness. The patient with HHS is usually older, more likely to have mental status changes, and more likely to have a life-threatening precipitating event with accompanying comorbidities. Even with proper treatment, HHS has a substantially higher mortality rate than DKA (up to 15% in some clinical series).

Fluid replacement should initially stabilize the hemodynamic status of the patient (1–3 L of 0.9% normal saline over the first 2–3 h). Because the fluid deficit in HHS is accumulated over a period of days to weeks, the rapidity of reversal of the hyperosmolar state must balance the need for free water repletion with the risk that too rapid a reversal may worsen neurologic function. If the serum sodium > 150 mmol/L (150 meq/L), 0.45% saline should be used. After hemodynamic stability is achieved, the IV fluid administration is directed at reversing the free water deficit using hypotonic fluids (0.45% saline initially, then 5% dextrose in water, D_5W). The calculated free water deficit (which averages 9–10 L) should be reversed over the next 1–2 days (infusion rates of 200–300 mL/h of hypotonic solution). Potassium repletion is usually necessary and should be dictated by repeated measurements of the serum potassium. In patients taking diuretics, the potassium deficit can be quite large and may be accompanied by magnesium deficiency. Hypophosphatemia may occur during therapy and can be improved by using KPO_4 and beginning nutrition.

As in DKA, rehydration and volume expansion lower the plasma glucose initially, but insulin is also required. A reasonable regimen for HHS begins with an IV insulin bolus of 0.1 units/kg followed by IV insulin at a constant infusion rate of 0.1 units/kg per hour. If the serum glucose does not fall, increase the insulin infusion rate by twofold. As in DKA, glucose should be added to IV fluid when the plasma glucose falls to 13.9–16.7 mmol/L (250–300 mg/dL), and the insulin infusion rate should be decreased to 0.05–0.1 units/kg per hour. The insulin infusion should be continued until the patient has resumed eating and can be transferred to a SC insulin regimen. The patient should be discharged from the hospital on insulin, though some patients can later switch to oral glucose-lowering agents.

CHRONIC COMPLICATIONS OF DM

The chronic complications of DM affect many organ systems and are responsible for the majority of morbidity and mortality associated with the disease. Chronic complications can be divided into vascular and nonvascular complications (Table 344-7). The vascular complications of DM are further subdivided into microvascular (retinopathy, neuropathy, nephropathy) and macrovascular complications [coronary heart disease (CHD), peripheral arterial disease (PAD), cerebrovascular disease]. Nonvascular complications include problems such as gastroparesis, infections, and skin changes. Long-standing diabetes may be associated with hearing loss. Whether type 2 DM in elderly individuals is associated with impaired mental function is not clear.

The risk of chronic complications increases as a function of the duration and degree of hyperglycemia; they usually do not become apparent until the second decade of hyperglycemia. Since type 2 DM often has a long asymptomatic period of hyperglycemia, many individuals with type 2 DM have complications at the time of diagnosis.

The microvascular complications of both type 1 and type 2 DM result from chronic hyperglycemia. Large, randomized clinical trials of individuals with type 1 or type 2 DM have conclusively demonstrated that a reduction in chronic hyperglycemia prevents or delays retinopathy, neuropathy, and nephropathy. Other incompletely defined factors may modulate the development of complications. For example, despite long-standing DM, some individuals never develop nephropathy or retinopathy. Many of these patients have glycemic control that is indistinguishable from those who develop microvascular complications, suggesting that there is a genetic susceptibility for developing particular complications.

Evidence implicating a causative role for chronic hyperglycemia in the development of macrovascular complications is less conclusive. However, coronary heart disease events and mortality rate are two to four times greater in patients with type 2 DM. These events correlate with fasting and postprandial plasma glucose levels as well as with the A1C. Other factors (dyslipidemia and hypertension) also play important roles in macrovascular complications.

TABLE 344-7 Chronic Complications of Diabetes Mellitus

Microvascular
Eye disease
Retinopathy (nonproliferative/proliferative)
Macular edema
Neuropathy
Sensory and motor (mono- and polyneuropathy)
Autonomic
Nephropathy
Macrovascular
Coronary heart disease
Peripheral arterial disease
Cerebrovascular disease
Other
Gastrointestinal (gastroparesis, diarrhea)
Genitourinary (uropathy/sexual dysfunction)
Dermatologic
Infectious
Cataracts
Glaucoma
Periodontal disease
Hearing loss

MECHANISMS OF COMPLICATIONS

Although chronic hyperglycemia is an important etiologic factor leading to complications of DM, the mechanism(s) by which it leads to such diverse cellular and organ dysfunction is unknown. At least four prominent theories, which are not mutually exclusive, have been proposed to explain how hyperglycemia might lead to the chronic complications of DM. An emerging hypothesis is that hyperglycemia leads to epigenetic changes in the affected cells.

One theory is that increased intracellular glucose leads to the formation of advanced glycosylation end products (AGEs), which bind to a cell surface receptor, via the nonenzymatic glycosylation of intra- and extracellular proteins. Nonenzymatic glycosylation results from the interaction of glucose with amino groups on proteins. AGEs have been shown to cross-link proteins (e.g., collagen, extracellular matrix proteins), accelerate atherosclerosis, promote glomerular dysfunction, reduce nitric oxide synthesis, induce endothelial dysfunction, and alter extracellular matrix composition and structure. The serum level of AGEs correlates with the level of glycemia, and these products accumulate as the glomerular filtration rate (GFR) declines.

A second theory is based on the observation that hyperglycemia increases glucose metabolism via the sorbitol pathway. Intracellular glucose is predominantly metabolized by phosphorylation and subsequent glycolysis, but when increased, some glucose is converted to sorbitol by the enzyme aldose reductase. Increased sorbitol concentration alters redox potential, increases cellular osmolality, generates reactive oxygen species, and likely leads to other types of cellular dysfunction. However, testing of this theory in humans, using aldose reductase inhibitors, has not demonstrated significant beneficial effects on clinical endpoints of retinopathy, neuropathy, or nephropathy.

A third hypothesis proposes that hyperglycemia increases the formation of diacylglycerol leading to activation of protein kinase C (PKC). Among other actions, PKC alters the transcription of genes for fibronectin, type IV collagen, contractile proteins, and extracellular matrix proteins in endothelial cells and neurons. Inhibitors of PKC are being studied in clinical trials.

A fourth theory proposes that hyperglycemia increases the flux through the hexosamine pathway, which generates fructose-6-phosphate, a substrate for O-linked glycosylation and proteoglycan production. The hexosamine pathway may alter function by glycosylation of proteins such as endothelial nitric oxide synthase or by changes in gene expression of transforming growth factor β (TGF-β) or plasminogen activator inhibitor-1 (PAI-1).

Growth factors appear to play an important role in some DM-related complications, and their production is increased by most of these proposed pathways. Vascular endothelial growth factor A (VEGF-A) is increased locally in diabetic proliferative retinopathy and decreases after laser photocoagulation. TGF-β is increased in diabetic nephropathy and stimulates basement membrane production of collagen and fibronectin by mesangial cells. Other growth factors, such as platelet-derived growth factor, epidermal growth factor, insulin-like growth factor I, growth hormone, basic fibroblast growth factor, and even insulin, have been suggested to play a role in DM-related complications. A possible unifying mechanism is that hyperglycemia leads to increased production of reactive oxygen species or superoxide in the mitochondria; these compounds may activate all four of the pathways described above. Although hyperglycemia serves as the initial trigger for complications of diabetes, it is still unknown whether the same pathophysiologic processes are operative in all complications or whether some pathways predominate in certain organs.

■ GLYCEMIC CONTROL AND COMPLICATIONS

The Diabetes Control and Complications Trial (DCCT) provided definitive proof that reduction in chronic hyperglycemia can prevent many of the early complications of type 1 DM. This large multicenter clinical trial randomized more than 1400 individuals with type 1 DM to either intensive or conventional diabetes management and prospectively evaluated the development of retinopathy, nephropathy, and neuropathy. Individuals in the intensive diabetes management group received multiple administrations of insulin each day along with extensive educational, psychological, and medical support. Individuals in the conventional diabetes management group received twice-daily insulin injections and quarterly nutritional, educational, and clinical evaluation. The goal in the former group was normoglycemia; the goal in the latter group was prevention of symptoms of diabetes. Individuals in the intensive diabetes management group achieved a substantially lower hemoglobin A1C (7.3%) than individuals in the conventional diabetes management group (9.1%).

The DCCT demonstrated that improvement of glycemic control reduced nonproliferative and proliferative retinopathy (47% reduction), microalbuminuria (39% reduction), clinical nephropathy (54% reduction), and neuropathy (60% reduction). Improved glycemic control also slowed the progression of early diabetic complications. There was a nonsignificant trend in reduction of macrovascular events during the trial (most individuals were young and had a low risk of cardiovascular disease). The results of the DCCT predicted that individuals in the intensive diabetes management group would gain 7.7 additional years of vision, 5.8 additional years free from ESRD, and 5.6 years free from lower extremity amputations. If all complications of DM were combined, individuals in the intensive diabetes management group would experience 15.3 more years of life without significant microvascular or neurologic complications of DM, compared to individuals who received standard therapy. This translates into an additional 5.1 years of life expectancy for individuals in the intensive diabetes management group. The long-term prognosis for type 1 diabetes continues to improve as shown by 30-year incidence data in the intensively treated group from the DCCT of retinopathy (21%), nephropathy (9%), and cardiovascular disease (9%). During this follow-up, fewer than 1% of the cohort had become blind, lost a limb to amputation, or required dialysis. The benefit of the improved glycemic control during the DCCT persisted even after the study concluded and glycemic control worsened. For example, individuals in the intensive diabetes management group for a mean of 6.5 years had a 42–57% reduction in cardiovascular events [nonfatal myocardial infarction (MI), stroke, or death from a cardiovascular event] at a mean follow-up of 17 years, even though their subsequent glycemic control was the same as those in the conventional diabetes management group from years 6.5–17 (discussed below).

The benefits of an improvement in glycemic control occurred over the entire range of A1C values (Fig. 344-8), suggesting that at any A1C level, an improvement in glycemic control is beneficial. The goal of therapy is to achieve an A1C level as close to normal as possible, without subjecting the patient to excessive risk of hypoglycemia.

The United Kingdom Prospective Diabetes Study (UKPDS) studied the course of >5000 individuals with type 2 DM for >10 years. This study utilized multiple treatment regimens and monitored the effect of intensive glycemic control and risk factor treatment on the development of diabetic complications. Newly diagnosed individuals with type 2 DM were randomized to (1) intensive management using various combinations of insulin, a sulfonylurea, or metformin or (2) conventional therapy using dietary modification and pharmacotherapy with the goal of symptom prevention. In addition, individuals were randomly assigned to different antihypertensive regimens. Individuals in the intensive treatment arm achieved an A1C of 7%, compared to a 7.9% A1C in the standard treatment group. The UKPDS demonstrated that each percentage point reduction in A1C was associated with a 35% reduction in microvascular complications. As in the DCCT, there was a continuous relationship between glycemic control and development of complications. Improved glycemic control did not conclusively reduce (nor worsen) cardiovascular mortality rate during the period of the trial, but was associated with improvement with lipoprotein risk profiles, such as reduced triglycerides and increased HDL.

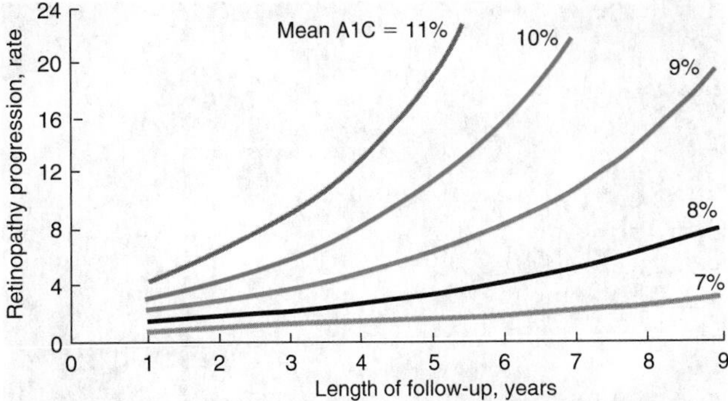

Figure 344-8 Relationship of glycemic control and diabetes duration to diabetic retinopathy. The progression of retinopathy in individuals in the Diabetes Control and Complications Trial is graphed as a function of the length of follow-up with different curves for different A1C values. *(Adapted from The Diabetes Control and Complications Trial Research Group: Diabetes 44:968, 1995.)*

One of the major findings of the UKPDS was that strict blood pressure control significantly reduced both macro- and microvascular complications. In fact, the beneficial effects of blood pressure control were greater than the beneficial effects of glycemic control. Lowering blood pressure to moderate goals (144/82 mmHg) reduced the risk of DM-related death, stroke, microvascular endpoints, retinopathy, and heart failure (risk reductions between 32 and 56%).

Similar reductions in the risks of retinopathy and nephropathy were also seen in a small trial of lean Japanese individuals with type 2 DM randomized to either intensive glycemic control or standard therapy with insulin (Kumamoto study). These results demonstrate the effectiveness of improved glycemic control in individuals of different ethnicity and, presumably, a different etiology of DM (i.e., phenotypically different from those in the DCCT and UKPDS).

The findings of the DCCT, UKPDS, and Kumamoto study strongly support the idea that chronic hyperglycemia plays a causative role in the pathogenesis of diabetic microvascular complications. These landmark studies prove the value of metabolic control and emphasize the importance of (1) intensive glycemic control in all forms of DM and (2) early diagnosis and strict blood pressure control in type 2 DM. Optimal targets for glycemic control and blood pressure are not entirely clear (see below).

■ OPHTHALMOLOGIC COMPLICATIONS OF DIABETES MELLITUS

DM is the leading cause of blindness between the ages of 20 and 74 in the United States. The gravity of this problem is highlighted by the finding that individuals with DM are 25 times more likely to become legally blind than individuals without DM. Blindness is primarily the result of progressive diabetic retinopathy and clinically significant macular edema. Diabetic retinopathy is classified into two stages: nonproliferative and proliferative. Nonproliferative diabetic retinopathy usually appears late in the first decade or early in the second decade of the disease and is marked by retinal

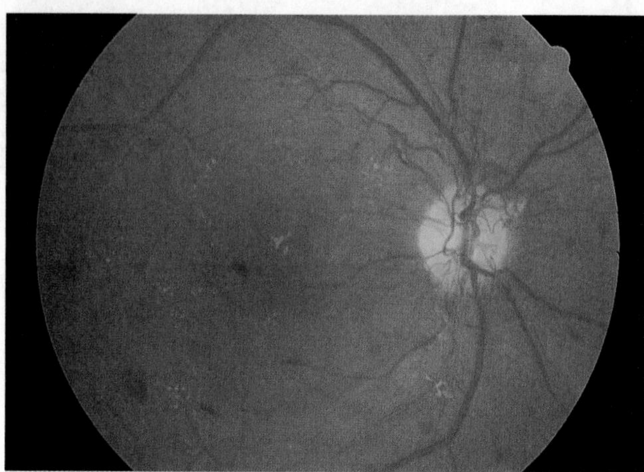

Figure 344-9 Diabetic retinopathy results in scattered hemorrhages, yellow exudates, and neovascularization. This patient has neovascular vessels proliferating from the optic disc, requiring urgent panretinal laser photocoagulation.

vascular microaneurysms, blot hemorrhages, and cotton-wool spots (Fig. 344-9). Mild nonproliferative retinopathy progresses to more extensive disease, characterized by changes in venous vessel caliber, intraretinal microvascular abnormalities, and more numerous microaneurysms and hemorrhages. The pathophysiologic mechanisms invoked in nonproliferative retinopathy include loss of retinal pericytes, increased retinal vascular permeability, alterations in retinal blood flow, and abnormal retinal microvasculature, all of which lead to retinal ischemia.

The appearance of neovascularization in response to retinal hypoxemia is the hallmark of proliferative diabetic retinopathy (Fig. 344-9). These newly formed vessels appear near the optic nerve and/or macula and rupture easily, leading to vitreous hemorrhage, fibrosis, and ultimately retinal detachment. Not all individuals with nonproliferative retinopathy develop proliferative retinopathy, but the more severe the nonproliferative disease, the greater the chance of evolution to proliferative retinopathy within 5 years. This creates an important opportunity for early detection and treatment of diabetic retinopathy. Clinically significant macular edema can occur when only nonproliferative retinopathy is present. Fluorescein angiography is useful to detect macular edema, which is associated with a 25% chance of moderate visual loss over the next 3 years.

Duration of DM and degree of glycemic control are the best predictors of the development of retinopathy; hypertension is also a risk factor. Nonproliferative retinopathy is found in many individuals who have had DM for >20 years (25% incidence with 5 years, and 80% incidence with 15 years of type 1 DM). Although there is genetic susceptibility for retinopathy, it confers less influence than either the duration of DM or the degree of glycemic control.

TREATMENT Diabetic Retinopathy

The most effective therapy for diabetic retinopathy is prevention. Intensive glycemic and blood pressure control will delay the development or slow the progression of retinopathy in individuals with either type 1 or type 2 DM. Paradoxically, during the first 6–12 months of improved glycemic control, established diabetic retinopathy may transiently worsen. Fortunately, this progression is temporary, and in the long term, improved glycemic control is associated with less diabetic retinopathy. Individuals with known retinopathy are candidates for prophylactic photocoagulation when initiating intensive therapy. Once advanced retinopathy is present, improved glycemic control imparts less benefit, though adequate ophthalmologic care can prevent most blindness.

Regular, comprehensive eye examinations are essential for all individuals with DM. Most diabetic eye disease can be successfully treated if detected early. Routine, nondilated eye examinations by the primary care provider or diabetes specialist are inadequate to detect diabetic eye disease, which requires an ophthalmologist for optimal care of these disorders. Laser photocoagulation is very successful in preserving vision. Proliferative retinopathy is usually treated with panretinal laser photocoagulation, whereas macular edema is treated with focal laser photocoagulation. Although exercise has not been conclusively shown to worsen proliferative diabetic retinopathy, most ophthalmologists advise individuals with advanced diabetic eye disease to limit physical activities associated with repeated Valsalva maneuvers. Aspirin therapy (650 mg/d) does not appear to influence the natural history of diabetic retinopathy.

RENAL COMPLICATIONS OF DIABETES MELLITUS

Diabetic nephropathy is the leading cause of ESRD in the United States and a leading cause of DM-related morbidity and mortality. Both microalbuminuria and macroalbuminuria in individuals with DM are associated with increased risk of cardiovascular disease. Individuals with diabetic nephropathy commonly have diabetic retinopathy.

Like other microvascular complications, the pathogenesis of diabetic nephropathy is related to chronic hyperglycemia. The mechanisms by which chronic hyperglycemia leads to ESRD, though incompletely defined, involve the effects of soluble factors (growth factors, angiotensin II, endothelin, AGEs), hemodynamic alterations in the renal microcirculation (glomerular hyperfiltration or hyperperfusion, increased glomerular capillary pressure), and structural changes in the glomerulus (increased extracellular matrix, basement membrane thickening, mesangial expansion, fibrosis). Some of these effects may be mediated through angiotensin II receptors. Smoking accelerates the decline in renal function. Because only 20–40% of patients with diabetes develop diabetic nephropathy, additional susceptibility factors remain unidentified. One known risk factor is a family history of diabetic nephropathy.

The natural history of diabetic nephropathy is characterized by a fairly predictable sequence of events that was initially defined for individuals with type 1 DM but appears to be similar in type 2 DM (Fig. 344-10). Glomerular hyperperfusion and renal hypertrophy occur in the first years after the onset of DM and are associated with an increase of the GFR. During the first 5 years of DM, thickening of the glomerular basement membrane, glomerular hypertrophy, and mesangial volume expansion occur as the GFR returns to normal. After 5–10 years of type 1 DM, ~40% of individuals begin to excrete small amounts of albumin in the urine. Microalbuminuria is defined as 30–299 mg/d in a 24-h collection or 30–299 μg/mg creatinine in a spot collection (preferred method). Although the appearance of microalbuminuria in type 1 DM is an important risk factor for progression to macroalbuminuria (>300 mg/d or > 300 μg/mg creatinine), only ~50% of individuals progress to macroalbuminuria over the next 10 years. In some individuals with type 1 diabetes and microalbuminuria of short duration, the microalbuminuria regresses. Microalbuminuria is a risk factor for cardiovascular disease. Once macroalbuminuria is present, there is a steady decline in GFR, and ~50% of individuals reach ESRD in 7–10 years. Once macroalbuminuria develops, blood pressure rises slightly and the pathologic changes are likely irreversible.

The nephropathy that develops in type 2 DM differs from that of type 1 DM in the following respects: (1) microalbuminuria or

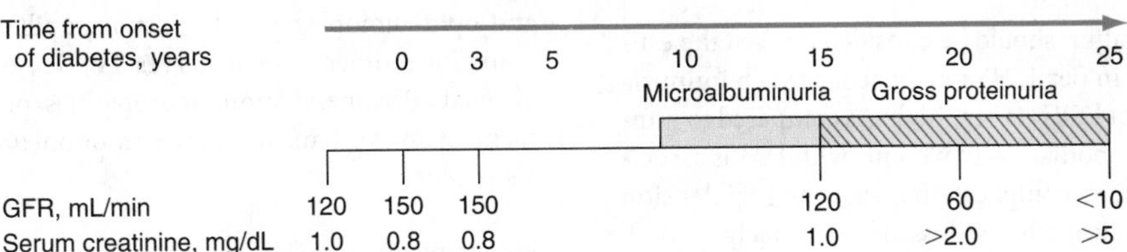

Figure 344-10 Time course of development of diabetic nephropathy. The relationship of time from onset of diabetes, the glomerular filtration rate (GFR), and the serum creatinine are shown. *(Adapted from RA DeFranzo, in Therapy for Diabetes Mellitus and Related Disorders, 3rd ed. American Diabetes Association, Alexandria, VA, 1998.)*

macroalbuminuria may be present when type 2 DM is diagnosed, reflecting its long asymptomatic period; (2) hypertension more commonly accompanies microalbuminuria or macroalbuminuria in type 2 DM; and (3) microalbuminuria may be less predictive of diabetic nephropathy and progression to macroalbuminuria in type 2 DM. Finally, it should be noted that albuminuria in type 2 DM may be secondary to factors unrelated to DM, such as hypertension, congestive heart failure (CHF), prostate disease, or infection. Diabetic nephropathy and ESRD secondary to DM develop more commonly in African Americans, Native Americans, and Hispanic individuals than in Caucasians with type 2 DM.

Type IV renal tubular acidosis (hyporeninemic hypoaldosteronism) may occur in type 1 or 2 DM. These individuals develop a propensity to hyperkalemia, which may be exacerbated by medications [especially angiotensin-converting enzyme (ACE) inhibitors and angiotensin receptor blockers (ARBs)]. Patients with DM are predisposed to radiocontrast-induced nephrotoxicity. Risk factors for radiocontrast-induced nephrotoxicity are preexisting nephropathy and volume depletion. Individuals with DM undergoing radiographic procedures with contrast dye should be well hydrated before and after dye exposure, and the serum creatinine should be monitored for 24–48 h following the procedure.

TREATMENT Diabetic Nephropathy

The optimal therapy for diabetic nephropathy is prevention by control of glycemia. As part of comprehensive diabetes care, microalbuminuria should be detected at an early stage when effective therapies can be instituted. The recommended strategy for detecting microalbuminuria is outlined in Fig. 344-11. Since some individuals with type 1 or type 2 DM have a decline in GFR in the absence of micro- or macroalbuminuria, annual measurement of the serum creatinine to estimate GFR should also be performed. Interventions effective in slowing progression from microalbuminuria to macroalbuminuria include (1) normalization of glycemia, (2) strict blood pressure control, and (3) administration of ACE inhibitors or ARBs. Dyslipidemia should also be treated.

Improved glycemic control reduces the rate at which microalbuminuria appears and progresses in type 1 and type 2 DM. However, once macroalbuminuria exists, it is unclear whether improved glycemic control will slow progression of renal disease. During the later phase of declining renal function, insulin requirements may fall as the kidney is a site of insulin degradation. Furthermore, many glucose-lowering medications (sulfonylureas and metformin) are contraindicated in advanced renal insufficiency.

Many individuals with type 1 or type 2 DM develop hypertension. Numerous studies in both type 1 and type 2 DM demonstrate the effectiveness of strict blood pressure control in reducing albumin excretion and slowing the decline in renal function. Blood pressure should be maintained at <130/80 mmHg in diabetic individuals.

Either ACE inhibitors or ARBs should be used to reduce the progression from microalbuminuria to macroalbuminuria and the associated decline in GFR that accompanies macroalbuminuria in individuals with type 1 or type 2 DM (see "Hypertension," below). Although direct comparisons of ACE inhibitors and ARBs are lacking, most experts believe that the two classes of drugs are equivalent in the patient with diabetes. ARBs can be used as an alternative in patients who develop ACE inhibitor–associated cough or angioedema. After 2–3 months of therapy in patients with microalbuminuria, the drug dose is increased until either the microalbuminuria disappears or the maximum dose is reached. If use of either ACE inhibitors or ARBs is not possible or the blood pressure is not controlled, then calcium channel blockers (non-dihydropyridine class), beta blockers, or diuretics should be used. However, their efficacy in slowing the fall in the GFR is not proven. Blood pressure control with any agent is extremely important, but a drug-specific benefit in diabetic nephropathy, independent of blood pressure control, has been shown only for ACE inhibitors and ARBs in patients with DM.

The ADA suggests modest restriction of protein intake in diabetic individuals with microalbuminuria (0.8–1.0 g/kg per day) or macroalbuminuria (<0.8 g/kg per day).

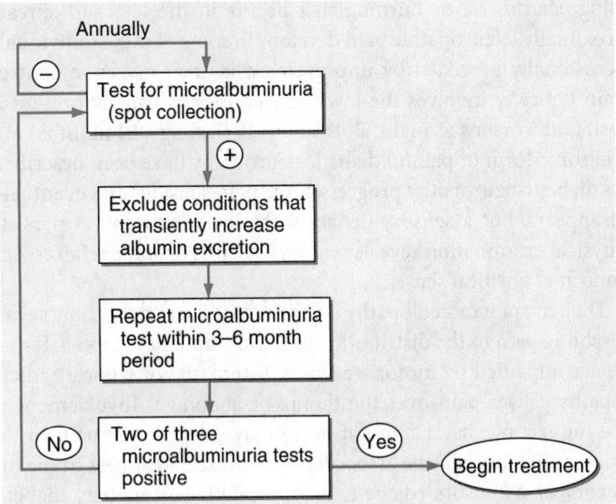

Figure 344-11 Screening for microalbuminuria should be performed in patients with type 1 diabetes for ≥5 years, in patients with type 2 diabetes, and during pregnancy. Non-diabetes-related conditions that might increase microalbuminuria are urinary tract infection, hematuria, heart failure, febrile illness, severe hyperglycemia, severe hypertension, and vigorous exercise. *(Adapted from RA DeFronzo, in Therapy for Diabetes Mellitus and Related Disorders, 3rd ed. American Diabetes Association, Alexandria, VA, 1998.)*

Nephrology consultation should be considered when the estimated GFR <60 mL/min per 1.743 m^2. Once macroalbuminuria ensues, the likelihood of ESRD is very high. As compared to nondiabetic individuals, hemodialysis in patients with DM is associated with more frequent complications, such as hypotension (due to autonomic neuropathy or loss of reflex tachycardia), more difficult vascular access, and accelerated progression of retinopathy. Survival after the onset of ESRD is shorter in the diabetic population compared to nondiabetics with similar clinical features. Atherosclerosis is the leading cause of death in diabetic individuals on dialysis, and hyperlipidemia should be treated aggressively. Renal transplantation from a living related donor is the preferred therapy but requires chronic immunosuppression. Combined pancreas-kidney transplant offers the promise of normoglycemia and freedom from dialysis.

NEUROPATHY AND DIABETES MELLITUS

Diabetic neuropathy occurs in ~50% of individuals with long-standing type 1 and type 2 DM. It may manifest as polyneuropathy, mononeuropathy, and/or autonomic neuropathy. As with other complications of DM, the development of neuropathy correlates with the duration of diabetes and glycemic control. Additional risk factors are BMI (the greater the BMI, the greater the risk of neuropathy) and smoking. The presence of cardiovascular disease, elevated triglycerides, and hypertension is also associated with diabetic peripheral neuropathy. Both myelinated and unmyelinated nerve fibers are lost. Because the clinical features of diabetic neuropathy are similar to those of other neuropathies, the diagnosis of diabetic neuropathy should be made only after other possible etiologies are excluded (Chap. 384).

Polyneuropathy/mononeuropathy

The most common form of diabetic neuropathy is distal symmetric polyneuropathy. It most frequently presents with distal sensory loss, but up to 50% of patients do not have symptoms of neuropathy. Hyperesthesia, paresthesia, and dysesthesia also may occur. Any combination of these symptoms may develop as neuropathy progresses. Symptoms may include a sensation of numbness, tingling, sharpness, or burning that begins in the feet and spreads proximally. Neuropathic pain develops in some of these individuals, occasionally preceded by improvement in their glycemic control. Pain typically involves the lower extremities, is usually present at rest, and worsens at night. Both an acute (lasting <12 months) and a chronic form of painful diabetic neuropathy have been described. As diabetic neuropathy progresses, the pain subsides and eventually disappears, but a sensory deficit in the lower extremities persists. Physical examination reveals sensory loss, loss of ankle reflexes, and abnormal position sense.

Diabetic polyradiculopathy is a syndrome characterized by severe disabling pain in the distribution of one or more nerve roots. It may be accompanied by motor weakness. Intercostal or truncal radiculopathy causes pain over the thorax or abdomen. Involvement of the lumbar plexus or femoral nerve may cause severe pain in the thigh or hip and may be associated with muscle weakness in the hip flexors or extensors (diabetic amyotrophy). Fortunately, diabetic polyradiculopathies are usually self-limited and resolve over 6–12 months.

Mononeuropathy (dysfunction of isolated cranial or peripheral nerves) is less common than polyneuropathy in DM and presents with pain and motor weakness in the distribution of a single nerve. A vascular etiology has been suggested, but the pathogenesis is unknown. Involvement of the third cranial nerve is most common and is heralded by diplopia. Physical examination reveals ptosis and ophthalmoplegia with normal pupillary constriction to light. Sometimes other cranial nerves IV, VI, or VII (Bell's palsy) are affected. Peripheral mononeuropathies or simultaneous involvement of more than one nerve (mononeuropathy multiplex) may also occur.

Autonomic neuropathy

Individuals with long-standing type 1 or 2 DM may develop signs of autonomic dysfunction involving the cholinergic, noradrenergic, and peptidergic (peptides such as pancreatic polypeptide, substance P, etc.) systems. DM-related autonomic neuropathy can involve multiple systems, including the cardiovascular, gastrointestinal, genitourinary, sudomotor, and metabolic systems. Autonomic neuropathies affecting the cardiovascular system cause a resting tachycardia and orthostatic hypotension. Reports of sudden death have also been attributed to autonomic neuropathy. Gastroparesis and bladder-emptying abnormalities are often caused by the autonomic neuropathy seen in DM (discussed below). Hyperhidrosis of the upper extremities and anhidrosis of the lower extremities result from sympathetic nervous system dysfunction. Anhidrosis of the feet can promote dry skin with cracking, which increases the risk of foot ulcers. Autonomic neuropathy may reduce counterregulatory hormone release (especially catecholamines), leading to an inability to sense hypoglycemia appropriately (hypoglycemia unawareness; Chap. 345), thereby subjecting the patient to the risk of severe hypoglycemia and complicating efforts to improve glycemic control.

TREATMENT Diabetic Neuropathy

Treatment of diabetic neuropathy is less than satisfactory. Improved glycemic control should be aggressively pursued and will improve nerve conduction velocity, but symptoms of diabetic neuropathy may not necessarily improve. Efforts to improve glycemic control may be confounded by autonomic neuropathy and hypoglycemia unawareness. Risk factors for neuropathy such as hypertension and hypertriglyceridemia should be treated. Avoidance of neurotoxins (alcohol) and smoking, supplementation with vitamins for possible deficiencies (B_{12}, folate; Chap. 74), and symptomatic treatment are the mainstays of therapy. Loss of sensation in the foot places the patient at risk for ulceration and its sequelae; consequently, prevention of such problems is of paramount importance. Patients with symptoms or signs of neuropathy (see "Physical Examination," below) should check their feet daily and take precautions (footwear) aimed at preventing calluses or ulcerations. If foot deformities are present, a podiatrist should be involved.

Chronic, painful diabetic neuropathy is difficult to treat but may respond to antidepressants (tricyclic antidepressants such as amitriptyline, desipramine, nortriptyline, imipramine or selective serotonin norepinephrine reuptake inhibitors such as duloxetine) or anticonvulsants (gabapentin, pregabalin, carbamazepine, lamotrigine). Two agents, duloxetine and pregabalin, have been approved by the U.S. Food and Drug Administration (FDA) for pain associated with diabetic neuropathy. However, pending further study, most recommend beginning with other agents such as a tricyclic antidepressant and switching if there is no response or if side effects develop. Referral to a pain management center may be necessary. Since the pain of acute diabetic neuropathy may resolve over time, medications may be discontinued as progressive neuronal damage from DM occurs.

Therapy of orthostatic hypotension secondary to autonomic neuropathy is also challenging. A variety of agents have limited success (fludrocortisone, midodrine, clonidine, octreotide, and yohimbine) but each has significant side effects. Nonpharmacologic maneuvers (adequate salt intake, avoidance of dehydration and diuretics, and lower extremity support hose) may offer some benefit.

GASTROINTESTINAL/GENITOURINARY DYSFUNCTION

Long-standing type 1 and 2 DM may affect the motility and function of gastrointestinal (GI) and genitourinary systems. The most prominent GI symptoms are delayed gastric emptying (gastroparesis) and altered small- and large-bowel motility (constipation or diarrhea). Gastroparesis may present with symptoms of anorexia, nausea, vomiting, early satiety, and abdominal bloating. Microvascular complications (retinopathy and neuropathy) are usually present. Nuclear medicine scintigraphy after ingestion of a radiolabeled meal may document delayed gastric emptying, but may not correlate well with the patient's symptoms. Noninvasive "breath tests" following ingestion of a radiolabeled meal are under development. Though parasympathetic dysfunction secondary to chronic hyperglycemia is important in the development of gastroparesis, hyperglycemia itself also impairs gastric emptying. Nocturnal diarrhea, alternating with constipation, is a feature of DM-related GI autonomic neuropathy. In type 1 DM, these symptoms should also prompt evaluation for celiac sprue because of its increased frequency. Esophageal dysfunction in long-standing DM may occur but is usually asymptomatic.

Diabetic autonomic neuropathy may lead to genitourinary dysfunction including cystopathy, erectile dysfunction, and female sexual dysfunction (reduced sexual desire, dyspareunia, reduced vaginal lubrication). Symptoms of diabetic cystopathy begin with an inability to sense a full bladder and a failure to void completely. As bladder contractility worsens, bladder capacity and the post-void residual increase, leading to symptoms of urinary hesitancy, decreased voiding frequency, incontinence, and recurrent urinary tract infections. Diagnostic evaluation includes cystometry and urodynamic studies.

Erectile dysfunction and retrograde ejaculation are very common in DM and may be one of the earliest signs of diabetic neuropathy (Chap. 48). Erectile dysfunction, which increases in frequency with the age of the patient and the duration of diabetes, may occur in the absence of other signs of diabetic autonomic neuropathy.

TREATMENT Gastrointestinal/Genitourinary Dysfunction

Current treatments for these complications of DM are inadequate. Improved glycemic control should be a primary goal, as some aspects (neuropathy, gastric function) may improve. Smaller, more frequent meals that are easier to digest (liquid) and low in fat and fiber may minimize symptoms of gastroparesis. Agents with some efficacy include dopamine antagonists metoclopramide, 5–10 mg, and domperidone, 10–20 mg, before each meal. Erythromycin interacts with the motilin receptor and may promote gastric emptying. Diabetic diarrhea in the absence of bacterial overgrowth is treated symptomatically with loperamide and may respond to octreotide (50–75 μg three times daily, SC). Treatment of bacterial overgrowth with antibiotics is sometimes useful (Chap. 294).

Diabetic cystopathy should be treated with timed voiding or self-catheterization, possibly with the addition of bethanechol. Drugs that inhibit type 5 phosphodiesterase are effective for erectile dysfunction, but their efficacy in individuals with DM is slightly lower than in the nondiabetic population (Chap. 48). Sexual dysfunction in women may be improved with use of vaginal lubricants, treatment of vaginal infections, and systemic or local estrogen replacement.

CARDIOVASCULAR MORBIDITY AND MORTALITY

Cardiovascular disease is increased in individuals with type 1 or type 2 DM. The Framingham Heart Study revealed a marked increase in PAD, CHF, CHD, MI, and sudden death (risk increase from one- to fivefold) in DM. The American Heart Association has designated DM as a "CHD risk equivalent." Type 2 diabetes patients without a prior MI have a similar risk for coronary artery–related events as nondiabetic individuals who have had a prior MI. Because of the extremely high prevalence of underlying cardiovascular disease in individuals with diabetes (especially in type 2 DM), evidence of atherosclerotic vascular disease (e.g., cardiac stress test) should be sought in an individual with diabetes who has symptoms suggestive of cardiac ischemia or peripheral or carotid arterial disease. The screening of asymptomatic individuals with diabetes for CHD is controversial, and recent studies have not shown a clinical benefit. The absence of chest pain ("silent ischemia") is common in individuals with diabetes, and a thorough cardiac evaluation should be considered in individuals undergoing major surgical procedures. The prognosis for individuals with diabetes who have CHD or MI is worse than for nondiabetics. CHD is more likely to involve multiple vessels in individuals with DM.

The increase in cardiovascular morbidity and mortality rates appears to relate to the synergism of hyperglycemia with other cardiovascular risk factors. For example, after controlling for all known cardiovascular risk factors, type 2 DM increases the cardiovascular death rate twofold in men and fourfold in women. Risk factors for macrovascular disease in diabetic individuals include dyslipidemia, hypertension, obesity, reduced physical activity, and cigarette smoking. Additional risk factors more prevalent in the diabetic population include microalbuminuria, macroalbuminuria, an elevation of serum creatinine, and abnormal platelet function. Insulin resistance, as reflected by elevated serum insulin levels, is associated with an increased risk of cardiovascular complications in individuals with and without DM. Individuals with insulin resistance and type 2 DM have elevated levels of plasminogen activator inhibitors (especially PAI-1) and fibrinogen, which enhances the coagulation process and impairs fibrinolysis, thus favoring the development of thrombosis. Diabetes is also associated with endothelial, vascular smooth-muscle, and platelet dysfunction.

Improved glycemic control started soon after the diagnosis of diabetes reduces cardiovascular complications in DM, but the glycemic goal for individuals with long-standing diabetes remains unclear. In both the DCCT (type 1 diabetes) and the UKPDS (type 2 diabetes), cardiovascular events were not reduced by intensive treatment during the trial but were reduced at follow-up 10–17 years later (this effect has been termed *legacy effect* or *metabolic memory*). During the DCCT, an improvement in the lipid profile of individuals in the intensive group (lower total and LDL cholesterol, lower triglycerides) during intensive diabetes management was noted. Trials to examine whether very aggressive glycemic targets (A1C near 6%) reduce cardiovascular events in type 2 diabetes did not show a survival benefit of reducing the A1C below 7% (and in one trial, the outcome was worse). Current recommendations do not suggest more aggressive glucose lowering in this patient population. The possibility of atherogenic potential of insulin is suggested by the data in nondiabetic individuals showing higher serum insulin levels (indicative of insulin resistance) in association with greater risk of cardiovascular morbidity and mortality. However, treatment with insulin and the sulfonylureas did not appear to increase the risk of cardiovascular disease in individuals with type 2 DM, refuting prior claims about the atherogenic potential of these agents.

In addition to CHD, cerebrovascular disease is increased in individuals with DM (threefold increase in stroke). Individuals with DM have an increased incidence of CHF. The etiology of this abnormality is probably multifactorial and includes factors such as myocardial ischemia from atherosclerosis, hypertension, and myocardial cell dysfunction secondary to chronic hyperglycemia.

TREATMENT Cardiovascular Disease

In general, the treatment of coronary disease is not different in the diabetic individual (Chap. 243). Revascularization procedures for CHD, including percutaneous coronary interventions (PCI) and coronary artery bypass grafting (CABG), may be less efficacious in the diabetic individual. Initial success rates of PCI in diabetic individuals are similar to those in the nondiabetic population, but diabetic patients have higher rates of restenosis and lower long-term patency and survival rates in older studies. More recently, the use of drug-eluting stents and a GPIIb/IIIa platelet inhibitor has improved the outcomes in diabetic patients, and whether there is a difference in efficacy of PCI in diabetic individuals is not clear. Although CABG may be preferred over PCI in diabetic individuals with multivessel coronary artery disease or recent Q-wave MI, PCI is preferred in patients with single-vessel coronary artery disease or two-vessel disease (no involvement of left anterior descending).

The ADA has emphasized the importance of glycemic control and aggressive cardiovascular risk modification in all individuals with DM (see below). Past trepidation about using beta blockers in individuals who have diabetes should not prevent use of these agents since they clearly benefit diabetic patients after MI. ACE inhibitors (or ARBs) may also be particularly beneficial and should be considered in individuals with type 2 DM and other risk factors (smoking, dyslipidemia, history of cardiovascular disease, microalbuminuria). Patients with atypical chest pain or an abnormal resting ECG should be considered for screening for CHD.

Antiplatelet therapy reduces cardiovascular events in individuals with DM who have CHD. Current recommendations by the ADA include the use of aspirin for secondary prevention of coronary events and the consideration of aspirin use in diabetic individuals with an increased cardiovascular risk (based on risk stratification using risk factors such as hypertension, smoking, family history, albuminuria, or dyslipidemia). Data demonstrating efficacy of aspirin in primary prevention of coronary events in individuals with DM and a low risk for CHD are lacking. The aspirin dose (75–162 mg) is the same as that in nondiabetic individuals. Aspirin therapy does not have detrimental effects on renal function or hypertension, nor does it influence the course of diabetic retinopathy.

Cardiovascular risk factors

Dyslipidemia Individuals with DM may have several forms of dyslipidemia (Chap. 356). Because of the additive cardiovascular risk of hyperglycemia and hyperlipidemia, lipid abnormalities should be assessed aggressively and treated as part of comprehensive diabetes care. The most common pattern of dyslipidemia is hypertriglyceridemia and reduced HDL cholesterol levels. DM itself does not increase levels of LDL, but the small dense LDL particles found in type 2 DM are more atherogenic because they are more easily glycated and susceptible to oxidation.

Almost all treatment studies of diabetic dyslipidemia have been performed in individuals with type 2 DM because of the greater frequency of dyslipidemia in this form of diabetes. Interventional studies have shown that the beneficial effects of LDL reduction are similar in the diabetic and nondiabetic populations. Large prospective trials of primary and secondary intervention for CHD have included some individuals with type 2 DM, and subset analyses have consistently found that reductions in LDL reduce cardiovascular events and morbidity in individuals with DM. No prospective studies have addressed similar questions in individuals with type 1 DM. Since the frequency of cardiovascular disease is low in children and young adults with diabetes, assessment of CV risk should be incorporated into the guidelines discussed below.

Based on the guidelines provided by the ADA and the American Heart Association, priorities in the treatment of dyslipidemia are as follows: (1) lower the LDL cholesterol, (2) raise the HDL cholesterol, and (3) decrease the triglycerides. A treatment strategy depends on the pattern of lipoprotein abnormalities. Initial therapy for all forms of dyslipidemia should include dietary changes, as well as the same lifestyle modifications recommended in the nondiabetic population (smoking cessation, blood pressure control, weight loss, increased physical activity). The dietary recommendations for individuals with DM are similar to those advocated by the National Cholesterol Education Program (Chap. 356) and include increased monounsaturated fat and carbohydrates and reduced saturated fats and cholesterol. Though viewed as important, the response to dietary alterations is often modest (<10% reduction in the LDL). Improvement in glycemic control will lower triglycerides and have a modest beneficial effect by raising HDL. HMG-CoA reductase inhibitors are the agents of choice for lowering the LDL. According to guidelines of the ADA and the American Heart Association, the target lipid values in diabetic individuals (age >40 years) without cardiovascular disease should be as follows: LDL < 2.6 mmol/L (100 mg/dL); HDL >1 mmol/L (40 mg/dL) in men and >1.3 mmol/L (50 mg/dL) in women; and triglycerides <1.7 mmol/L (150 mg/dL). In patients >40 years, the ADA recommends addition of a statin, regardless of the LDL level in patients with CHD and those without CHD, but who have CHD risk factors.

If the patient is known to have CHD, the ADA recommends an LDL goal of <1.8 mmol/L (70 mg/dL) as an "option" [in keeping with evidence that such a goal is beneficial in nondiabetic individuals with CHD (Chap. 356)]. Older studies with fibrates indicated efficacy, but recent trials have not shown a benefit of this class of agents. Combination therapy with an HMG-CoA reductase inhibitor and a fibrate or another lipid-lowering agent (ezetimibe, niacin) may be considered to reach LDL goals, but statin/fibrate combinations increase the possibility of side effects such as myositis. Nicotinic acid effectively raises HDL and can be used in patients with diabetes, but high doses (>2 g/d) may worsen glycemic control and increase insulin resistance. Bile acid–binding resins should not be used if hypertriglyceridemia is present.

Hypertension Hypertension can accelerate other complications of DM, particularly cardiovascular disease and nephropathy. In targeting a goal of BP <130/80 mmHg, therapy should first emphasize life-style modifications such as weight loss, exercise, stress management, and sodium restriction. Realizing that more than one agent is usually required to reach the blood pressure goal, the ADA recommends that all patients with diabetes and hypertension be treated with an ACE inhibitor or an ARB. Subsequently, agents that reduce cardiovascular risk (beta blockers, thiazide diuretics, and calcium channel blockers) should be incorporated into the regimen. While ACE inhibitors and ARBs are likely equivalent in most patients with diabetes and renal disease, the ADA notes (1) in patients with type 1 diabetes, hypertension, and micro- or macroalbuminuria, an ACE inhibitor slowed progression of nephropathy; (2) an ACE inhibitor or an ARB slowed the progression to macroalbuminuria in patients with type 2 diabetes, hypertension, and microalbuminuria; and (3) ARB slowed the decline in GFR in patients with type 2 diabetes, hypertension, macroalbuminuria, and renal insufficiency. Additional points of emphasis include the following:

1. ACE inhibitors are either glucose- and lipid-neutral or glucose- and lipid-beneficial and thus positively impact the cardiovascular risk profile. Calcium channel blockers, central adrenergic antagonists, and vasodilators are lipid- and glucose-neutral.
2. Beta blockers and thiazide diuretics can increase insulin resistance and negatively impact the lipid profile; beta blockers may slightly increase the risk of developing type 2 DM. Beta blockers are safe in patients with diabetes and reduce cardiovascular events.
3. Sympathetic inhibitors and α-adrenergic blockers may worsen orthostatic hypotension in the diabetic individual with autonomic neuropathy.
4. Equivalent reduction in blood pressure by different classes of agents may not translate into equivalent protection from cardiovascular and renal endpoints. Thiazides, beta blockers, ACE inhibitors, and ARBs positively impact cardiovascular endpoints (MI or stroke).
5. Serum potassium and renal function should be monitored.

Because of the high prevalence of atherosclerotic disease in individuals with type 2 DM, the possibility of renovascular hypertension should be considered when the blood pressure is not readily controlled.

LOWER EXTREMITY COMPLICATIONS

DM is the leading cause of nontraumatic lower extremity amputation in the United States. Foot ulcers and infections are also a major source of morbidity in individuals with DM. The reasons for the increased incidence of these disorders in DM involve the interaction of several pathogenic factors: neuropathy, abnormal foot biomechanics, PAD, and poor wound healing. The peripheral sensory neuropathy interferes with normal protective mechanisms and allows the patient to sustain major or repeated minor trauma to the foot, often without knowledge of the injury. Disordered proprioception causes abnormal weight bearing while walking and subsequent formation of callus or ulceration. Motor and sensory neuropathy lead to abnormal foot muscle mechanics and to structural changes in the foot (hammertoe, claw toe deformity, prominent metatarsal heads, Charcot joint). Autonomic neuropathy results in anhidrosis and altered superficial blood flow in the foot, which promote drying of the skin and fissure formation. PAD and poor wound healing impede resolution of minor breaks in the skin, allowing them to enlarge and to become infected.

Approximately 15% of individuals with type 2 DM develop a foot ulcer (great toe or MTP areas are most common), and a significant subset will ultimately undergo amputation (14–24% risk with that ulcer or subsequent ulceration). Risk factors for foot ulcers or amputation include: male sex, diabetes >10 years' duration, peripheral neuropathy, abnormal structure of foot (bony abnormalities, callus, thickened nails), peripheral arterial disease, smoking, history of previous ulcer or amputation, and poor glycemic control. Large calluses are often precursors to or overlie ulcerations.

TREATMENT Lower Extremity Complications

The optimal therapy for foot ulcers and amputations is prevention through identification of high-risk patients, education of the patient, and institution of measures to prevent ulceration. High-risk patients should be identified during the routine foot examination performed on all patients with DM (see "Ongoing Aspects of Comprehensive Diabetes Care," below). Patient education should emphasize (1) careful selection of footwear, (2) daily inspection of the feet to detect early signs of poor-fitting footwear or minor trauma, (3) daily foot hygiene to keep the skin clean and moist, (4) avoidance of self-treatment of foot abnormalities and high-risk behavior (e.g., walking barefoot), and (5) prompt consultation with a health care provider if an abnormality arises. Patients at high risk for ulceration or amputation may benefit from evaluation by a foot care specialist. Interventions directed at risk factor modification include orthotic shoes and devices, callus management, nail care, and prophylactic measures to reduce increased skin pressure from abnormal bony architecture. Attention to other risk factors for vascular disease (smoking, dyslipidemia, hypertension) and improved glycemic control are also important.

Despite preventive measures, foot ulceration and infection are common and represent a serious problem. Due to the multifactorial pathogenesis of lower extremity ulcers, management of these lesions is multidisciplinary and often demands expertise in orthopedics, vascular surgery, endocrinology, podiatry, and infectious diseases. The plantar surface of the foot is the most common site of ulceration. Ulcers may be primarily neuropathic (no accompanying infection) or may have surrounding cellulitis or osteomyelitis. Cellulitis without ulceration is also frequent and should be treated with antibiotics that provide broad-spectrum coverage, including anaerobes (see below).

An infected ulcer is a clinical diagnosis, since superficial culture of any ulceration will likely find multiple possible bacterial species. The infection surrounding the foot ulcer is often the result of multiple organisms (gram-positive and -negative organisms and anaerobes), and gas gangrene may develop in the absence of clostridial infection. Cultures taken from the surface of the ulcer are not helpful; a culture from the debrided ulcer base or from purulent drainage or aspiration of the wound is the most helpful. Wound depth should be determined by inspection and probing with a blunt-tipped sterile instrument. Plain radiographs of the foot should be performed to assess the possibility of osteomyelitis in chronic ulcers that have not responded to therapy. Nuclear medicine bone scans may be helpful, but overlying subcutaneous infection is often difficult to distinguish from osteomyelitis. Indium-labeled white cell studies are more useful in determining if the infection involves bony structures or only soft tissue, but they are technically demanding. MRI of the foot may be the most specific modality, although distinguishing bony destruction due to osteomyelitis from destruction secondary to Charcot arthropathy is difficult. If surgical debridement is necessary, bone biopsy and culture may provide the answer.

Osteomyelitis is best treated by a combination of prolonged antibiotics (IV, then oral) and possibly debridement of infected bone. The possible contribution of vascular insufficiency should be considered in all patients. Noninvasive blood-flow studies are often unreliable in DM, and angiography may be required, recognizing the risk of contrast-induced nephrotoxicity. Peripheral arterial bypass procedures are often effective in promoting wound healing and in decreasing the need for amputation of the ischemic limb.

A growing number of possible treatments for diabetic foot ulcers exist, but they have yet to demonstrate clear efficacy in prospective, controlled trials. A consensus statement from the ADA identified six interventions with demonstrated efficacy in diabetic foot wounds: (1) off-loading, (2) debridement, (3) wound dressings, (4) appropriate use of antibiotics, (5) revascularization, and (6) limited amputation. Off-loading is the complete avoidance of weight bearing on the ulcer, which removes the mechanical trauma that retards wound healing. Bed rest and a variety of orthotic devices or contact casting limit weight bearing on wounds or pressure points. Surgical debridement is important and effective, but clear efficacy of other modalities for wound cleaning (enzymes, soaking, whirlpools) is lacking. Dressings such as hydrocolloid dressings promote wound healing by creating a moist environment and protecting the wound. Antiseptic agents should be avoided. Topical antibiotics are of limited value. Referral for physical therapy, orthotic evaluation, and rehabilitation should occur once the infection is controlled.

Mild or non-limb-threatening infections can be treated with oral antibiotics (cephalosporin, clindamycin, amoxicillin/clavulanate, and fluoroquinolones), surgical debridement of necrotic tissue, local wound care (avoidance of weight bearing over the ulcer), and close surveillance for progression of infection. More severe ulcers may require IV antibiotics as well as bed rest and local wound care. Urgent surgical debridement may be required. Strict control of glycemia should be a goal (see below). IV antibiotics should provide broad-spectrum coverage directed toward *Staphylococcus aureus*, streptococci, gram-negative aerobes, and anaerobic bacteria. Initial antimicrobial regimens include ertapenem, piperacillin/tazobactam, cefotetan, ampicillin/sulbactam, linezolid, or the combination of clindamycin and a fluoroquinolone. Severe infections, or infections that do not improve after 48 h of antibiotic therapy, require expansion of antimicrobial therapy to treat methicillin-resistant *S. aureus* (e.g., vancomycin) and *Pseudomonas aeruginosa*. If the infection surrounding the ulcer is not improving with IV antibiotics, reassessment of antibiotic coverage and reconsideration of the need for surgical debridement or revascularization are indicated. With clinical improvement, oral antibiotics and local wound care can be continued on an outpatient basis with close follow-up.

New information about wound biology has led to a number of new technologies (e.g., living skin equivalents and growth factors) that may prove useful, especially in neuropathic ulcers. Hyperbaric oxygen has been used, but rigorous proof of efficacy is lacking. Negative wound pressure has been shown to accelerate wound healing of plantar wounds.

INFECTIONS

Individuals with DM have a greater frequency and severity of infection. The reasons for this include incompletely defined abnormalities in cell-mediated immunity and phagocyte function associated with hyperglycemia, as well as diminished vascularization. Hyperglycemia aids the colonization and growth of a variety of organisms (*Candida* and other fungal species). Many common infections are more frequent and severe in the diabetic population, whereas several rare infections are seen almost exclusively in the diabetic population. Examples of this latter category include rhinocerebral mucormycosis, emphysematous infections of the gall bladder and urinary tract, and "malignant" or invasive otitis externa. Invasive otitis externa is usually secondary to *P. aeruginosa* infection in the soft tissue surrounding the external auditory canal, usually begins with pain and discharge, and may rapidly progress to osteomyelitis and meningitis. These infections should be sought, in particular, in patients presenting with HHS.

Pneumonia, urinary tract infections, and skin and soft tissue infections are all more common in the diabetic population. In general, the organisms that cause pulmonary infections are similar to those found in the nondiabetic population; however, gram-negative organisms, *S. aureus*, and *Mycobacterium tuberculosis* are more frequent pathogens. Urinary tract infections (either lower tract or pyelonephritis) are the result of common bacterial agents such as *Escherichia coli*, though several yeast species (*Candida* and *Torulopsis glabrata*) are commonly observed. Complications of urinary tract infections include emphysematous pyelonephritis and emphysematous cystitis. Bacteriuria occurs frequently in individuals with diabetic cystopathy. Susceptibility to furunculosis, superficial candidal infections, and vulvovaginitis are increased. Poor glycemic control is a common denominator in individuals with these infections. Diabetic individuals have an increased rate of colonization of *S. aureus* in the skinfolds and nares. Diabetic patients also have a greater risk of postoperative wound infections. Strict glycemic control reduces postoperative infections in diabetic individuals undergoing CABG and should be the goal in all diabetic patients with an infection.

DERMATOLOGIC MANIFESTATIONS

The most common skin manifestations of DM are protracted wound healing and skin ulcerations. Diabetic dermopathy, sometimes termed *pigmented pretibial papules*, or "diabetic skin spots," begins as an erythematous area and evolves into an area of circular hyperpigmentation. These lesions result from minor mechanical trauma in the pretibial region and are more common in elderly men with DM. Bullous diseases, such as bullosa diabeticorum (shallow ulcerations or erosions in the pretibial region), are also seen. *Necrobiosis lipoidica diabeticorum* is a rare disorder of DM that predominantly affects young women with type 1 DM, neuropathy, and retinopathy. It usually begins in the pretibial region as an erythematous plaque or papules that gradually enlarge, darken, and develop irregular margins, with atrophic centers and central ulceration. They may be painful. Vitiligo occurs at increased frequency in individuals with type 1 diabetes. *Acanthosis nigricans* (hyperpigmented velvety plaques seen on the neck, axilla, or extensor surfaces) is sometimes a feature of severe insulin resistance and accompanying diabetes. Generalized or localized *granuloma annulare* (erythematous plaques on the extremities or trunk) and *scleredema* (areas of skin thickening on the back or neck at the site of previous superficial infections) are more common in the diabetic population. *Lipoatrophy* and *lipohypertrophy* can occur at insulin injection sites but are now unusual with the use of human insulin. Xerosis and pruritus are common and are relieved by skin moisturizers.

APPROACH TO THE PATIENT: Diabetes Mellitus

DM and its complications produce a wide range of symptoms and signs; those secondary to acute hyperglycemia may occur at any stage of the disease, whereas those related to chronic complications begin to appear during the second decade of hyperglycemia. Individuals with previously undetected type 2 DM may present with chronic complications of DM at the time of diagnosis. The history and physical examination should assess for symptoms or signs of acute hyperglycemia and should screen for the chronic complications and conditions associated with DM.

HISTORY A complete medical history should be obtained with special emphasis on DM-relevant aspects such as weight, family history of DM and its complications, risk factors for cardiovascular disease, exercise, smoking, and ethanol use. Symptoms of hyperglycemia include polyuria, polydipsia, weight loss, fatigue, weakness, blurry vision, frequent superficial infections (vaginitis, fungal skin infections), and slow healing of skin lesions after minor trauma. Metabolic derangements relate mostly to hyperglycemia (osmotic diuresis) and to the catabolic state of the patient (urinary loss of glucose and calories, muscle breakdown due to protein degradation and decreased protein synthesis). Blurred vision results from changes in the water content of the lens and resolves as the hyperglycemia is controlled.

In a patient with established DM, the initial assessment should also include special emphasis on prior diabetes care, including the type of therapy, prior A1C levels, self-monitoring blood glucose results, frequency of hypoglycemia, presence of DM-specific complications, and assessment of the patient's knowledge about diabetes, exercise, and nutrition. The chronic complications may afflict several organ systems, and an individual patient may exhibit some, all, or none of the symptoms related to the complications of DM (see above). In addition, the presence of DM-related comorbidities should be sought (cardiovascular disease, hypertension, dyslipidemia).

PHYSICAL EXAMINATION In addition to a complete physical examination, special attention should be given to DM-relevant aspects such as weight or BMI, retinal examination, orthostatic blood pressure, foot examination, peripheral pulses, and insulin injection sites. Blood pressure >130/80 mmHg is considered hypertension in individuals with diabetes. Careful examination of the lower extremities should seek evidence of peripheral arterial disease (pedal pulses), peripheral neuropathy, calluses, superficial fungal infections, nail disease, ankle reflexes, and foot deformities (such as hammertoes or claw toes and Charcot foot) in order to identify sites of potential skin ulceration. Vibratory sensation (128-MHz tuning fork at the base of the great toe), the ability to sense touch with a monofilament (5.07, 10-g monofilament), pinprick sensation, testing for ankle reflexes, and vibration perception threshold (using a biothesiometer) are used to detect moderately advanced diabetic neuropathy. Since periodontal disease is more frequent in DM, the teeth and gums should also be examined.

CLASSIFICATION OF DM IN AN INDIVIDUAL PATIENT The etiology of diabetes in an individual with new-onset disease can usually be assigned on the basis of clinical criteria. Individuals with type 1 DM tend to have the following characteristics: (1) onset of disease prior to age 30 years; (2) lean body habitus; (3) requirement of insulin as the initial therapy; (4) propensity to develop ketoacidosis; and (5) an increased risk of other autoimmune disorders such as autoimmune thyroid disease, adrenal insufficiency, pernicious anemia, celiac disease, and vitiligo. In contrast, individuals with type 2 DM often exhibit the following features: (1) develop diabetes after the age of 30 years; (2) are usually obese (80% are obese, but elderly individuals may be lean); (3) may not require insulin therapy initially; and (4) may have associated conditions such as insulin resistance, hypertension, cardiovascular disease, dyslipidemia, or PCOS. In type 2 DM, insulin resistance is often associated with abdominal obesity (as opposed to hip and thigh obesity) and hypertriglyceridemia. Although most individuals diagnosed with type 2 DM are older, the age of diagnosis is declining, and there is a marked increase among overweight children and adolescents. Some individuals with phenotypic type 2 DM present with DKA but lack autoimmune markers and may be later treated with oral glucose-lowering agents rather than insulin (this clinical picture is sometimes referred to as *ketosis-prone type 2 DM*). On the other hand, some individuals (5–10%) with the phenotypic appearance of type 2 DM do not have absolute insulin deficiency but have autoimmune markers (ICA, GAD autoantibodies) suggestive of type 1 DM (termed *latent autoimmune diabetes of the adult*). Such individuals are more likely to be <50 years of age, have a normal BMI, and have a personal or family history of other autoimmune disease. They are much more likely to require insulin treatment within 5 years. Monogenic forms of diabetes (discussed above) should be considered in those with diabetes onset <30 years of age, an autosomal pattern of diabetes inheritance, and the lack of nearly complete insulin deficiency. Despite recent advances in the understanding of the pathogenesis of diabetes, it remains difficult to categorize some patients unequivocally. Individuals who deviate from the clinical profile of type 1 and type 2 DM, or who have other associated defects such as deafness, pancreatic exocrine disease, and other endocrine disorders, should be classified accordingly (Table 344-1).

LABORATORY ASSESSMENT The laboratory assessment should first determine whether the patient meets the diagnostic criteria for DM (Table 344-2) and then assess the degree of glycemic control (A1C, discussed below). In addition to the standard laboratory evaluation, the patient should be screened for DM-associated conditions (e.g., microalbuminuria, dyslipidemia, thyroid dysfunction). Individuals at high risk for cardiovascular disease should be screened for asymptomatic CHD by appropriate cardiac stress testing, when indicated.

The classification of the type of DM may be facilitated by laboratory assessments. Serum insulin or C-peptide measurements do not always distinguish type 1 from type 2 DM, but a low C-peptide level confirms a patient's need for insulin. Many individuals with new-onset type 1 DM retain some C-peptide production. Measurement of islet cell antibodies at the time of diabetes onset may be useful if the type of DM is not clear based on the characteristics described above.

LONG-TERM TREATMENT

■ OVERALL PRINCIPLES

The goals of therapy for type 1 or type 2 DM are to (1) eliminate symptoms related to hyperglycemia, (2) reduce or eliminate the long-term microvascular and macrovascular complications of DM, and (3) allow the patient to achieve as normal a lifestyle as possible. To reach these goals, the physician should identify a target level of glycemic control for each patient, provide the patient with the educational and pharmacologic resources necessary to reach this level, and monitor/treat DM-related complications. Symptoms of diabetes usually resolve when the plasma glucose is <11.1 mmol/L (200 mg/dL), and thus most DM treatment focuses on achieving the second and third goals. The treatment goals for patients with diabetes are summarized in Table 344-8.

The care of an individual with either type 1 or type 2 DM requires a multidisciplinary team. Central to the success of this team are the patient's participation, input, and enthusiasm, all of which are essential for optimal diabetes management. Members of the health care team include the primary care provider and/or the endocrinologist or diabetologist, a certified diabetes educator, and a nutritionist. In addition, when the complications of DM arise, subspecialists (including neurologists, nephrologists, vascular surgeons, cardiologists, ophthalmologists, and podiatrists) with experience in DM-related complications are essential.

A number of names are sometimes applied to different approaches to diabetes care, such as intensive insulin therapy, intensive glycemic control, and "tight control." The current chapter, and other sources, use the term *comprehensive diabetes care* to emphasize the fact that optimal diabetes therapy involves more than plasma glucose management. Though glycemic control is central to optimal diabetes therapy, comprehensive diabetes care of both type 1 and type 2 DM should also detect and manage DM-specific complications and modify risk factors for

TABLE 344-8 Treatment Goals for Adults With Diabetes[a]

Index	Goal
Glycemic control[b]	
A1C	<7.0%[c]
Preprandial capillary plasma glucose	3.9–7.2 mmol/L (70–130 mg/dL)
Peak postprandial capillary plasma glucose [d]	<10.0 <1.7 mmol/L (<180 mg/dL)
Blood pressure	<130/80
Lipids[e]	
Low-density lipoprotein	<2.6 mmol/L (100 mg/dL)
High-density lipoprotein	>1 mmol/L (40 mg/dL) in men >1.3 mmol/L (50 mg/dL) in women
Triglycerides	<1.7 mmol/L (150 mg/dL)

[a]As recommended by the ADA; goals should be individualized for each patient (see text). Goals may be different for certain patient populations.
[b]A1C is primary goal.
[c]Normal range for A1C: 4.0–6.0% (DCCT-based assay).
[d]One–two hours after beginning of a meal.
[e]In decreasing order of priority.
Source: Adapted from American Diabetes Association, 2011.

DM-associated diseases. In addition to the physical aspects of DM, social, family, financial, cultural, and employment-related issues may impact diabetes care. The International Diabetes Federation (IDF), recognizing that resources available for diabetes care varies widely throughout the world, has issued guidelines for standard care (a well-developed service base and with health care funding systems consuming a significant part of their national wealth), minimal care (health care settings with very limited resources), and comprehensive care (health care settings with considerable resources). This chapter provides guidance for this comprehensive level of diabetes care.

PATIENT EDUCATION ABOUT DM, NUTRITION, AND EXERCISE

The patient with type 1 or type 2 DM should receive education about nutrition, exercise, care of diabetes during illness, and medications to lower the plasma glucose. Along with improved compliance, patient education allows individuals with DM to assume greater responsibility for their care. Patient education should be viewed as a continuing process with regular visits for reinforcement; it should not be a process that is completed after one or two visits to a nurse educator or nutritionist. The ADA refers to education about the individualized management plan for the patient as diabetes self-management education (DSME). More frequent contact between the patient and the diabetes management team (electronic, telephone, etc.) improves glycemic control.

Diabetes education

The diabetes educator is a health care professional (nurse, dietician, or pharmacist) with specialized patient education skills who is certified in diabetes education (e.g., American Association of Diabetes Educators). Education topics important for optimal diabetes care include self-monitoring of blood glucose; urine ketone monitoring (type 1 DM); insulin administration; guidelines for diabetes management during illnesses; prevention and management of hypoglycemia (Chap. 345); foot and skin care; diabetes management before, during, and after exercise; and risk factor-modifying activities.

Nutrition

Medical nutrition therapy (MNT) is a term used by the ADA to describe the optimal coordination of caloric intake with other aspects of diabetes therapy (insulin, exercise, weight loss). Primary prevention measures of MNT are directed at preventing or delaying the onset of type 2 DM in high-risk individuals (obese or with prediabetes) by promoting weight reduction. Medical treatment of obesity is a rapidly evolving area and is discussed in Chap. 78. Secondary prevention measures of MNT are directed at preventing or delaying diabetes-related complications in diabetic individuals by improving glycemic control. Tertiary prevention measures of MNT are directed at managing diabetes-related complications (cardiovascular disease, nephropathy) in diabetic individuals. For example, in individuals with diabetes and chronic kidney disease, protein intake should be limited to 0.8 g/kg of body weight per day. MNT in patients with diabetes and cardiovascular disease should incorporate dietary principles used in nondiabetic patients with cardiovascular disease. While the recommendations for all three types of MNT overlap, this chapter emphasizes secondary prevention measures of MNT. Pharmacologic approaches that facilitate weight loss and bariatric surgery should be considered in selected patients (Chap. 78).

In general, the components of optimal MNT are similar for individuals with type 1 or type 2 DM and similar to those for the general population (fruits, vegetables, fiber-containing foods, and low fat; Table 344-9). MNT education is an important component of comprehensive diabetes care and should be reinforced by regular patient education. Historically, nutrition education imposed restrictive, complicated regimens on the patient. Current practices have greatly changed, though many patients and health care providers still view the diabetic diet as monolithic and static. For example, MNT now

TABLE 344-9 Nutritional Recommendations for Adults With Diabetes[a]

Weight loss diet (in prediabetes and type 2 DM)
- Hypocaloric diet that is low-fat or low-carbohydrate

Fat in diet
- Minimal *trans* fat consumption

Carbohydrate in diet
- Monitor carbohydrate intake in regards to calories
- Sucrose-containing foods may be consumed with adjustments in insulin dose
- Amount of carbohydrate determined by estimating grams of carbohydrate in diet for (type 1 DM)
- Glycemic index reflects how consumption of a particular food affects the blood glucose

Protein in diet: as part of an optimal diet

Other components
- Nonnutrient sweeteners
- Routine supplements of vitamins, antioxidants, or trace elements not advised

[a]See text for differences for patients with type 1 or type 2 diabetes. As for the general population, a healthy diet includes fruits, vegetables, and fiber-containing foods.
Source: Adapted from American Diabetes Association, 2011.

includes foods with sucrose and seeks to modify other risk factors such as hyperlipidemia and hypertension rather than focusing exclusively on weight loss in individuals with type 2 DM. The *glycemic index* is an estimate of the postprandial rise in the blood glucose when a certain amount of that food is consumed. Consumption of foods with a low glycemic index appears to reduce postprandial glucose excursions and improve glycemic control. Reduced calorie and nonnutritive sweeteners are useful. Currently, evidence does not support supplementation of the diet with vitamins, antioxidants (vitamin C and E), or micronutrients (chromium) in patients with diabetes.

The goal of MNT in the individual with type 1 DM is to coordinate and match the caloric intake, both temporally and quantitatively, with the appropriate amount of insulin. MNT in type 1 DM and self-monitoring of blood glucose must be integrated to define the optimal insulin regimen. The ADA encourages patients and providers to utilize carbohydrate counting or exchange systems to estimate the nutrient content of a meal or snack. Based on the patient's estimate of the carbohydrate content of a meal, an insulin-to-carbohydrate ratio determines the bolus insulin dose for a meal or snack. MNT must be flexible enough to allow for exercise, and the insulin regimen must allow for deviations in caloric intake. An important component of MNT in type 1 DM is to minimize the weight gain often associated with intensive diabetes management.

The goals of MNT in type 2 DM should focus on weight loss and address the greatly increased prevalence of cardiovascular risk factors (hypertension, dyslipidemia, obesity) and disease in this population. The majority of these individuals are obese, and weight loss is strongly encouraged and should remain an important goal. Hypocaloric diets and modest weight loss (5–7%) often result in rapid and dramatic glucose lowering in individuals with new-onset type 2 DM. Nevertheless, numerous studies document that long-term weight loss is uncommon. MNT for type 2 DM should emphasize modest caloric reduction (low-carbohydrate or low-fat), reduced fat intake, and increased physical activity. Increased consumption of soluble, dietary fiber may improve glycemic control in individuals with type 2 DM. Weight loss and exercise improve insulin resistance.

Exercise

Exercise has multiple positive benefits including cardiovascular risk reduction, reduced blood pressure, maintenance of muscle mass, reduction in body fat, and weight loss. For individuals with type 1 or type 2 DM, exercise is also useful for lowering plasma glucose (during and following exercise) and increasing insulin sensitivity. In patients with diabetes, the ADA recommends 150 min/week (distributed over at least 3 days) of moderate aerobic physical activity. The exercise regimen should also include resistance training.

Despite its benefits, exercise presents challenges for individuals with DM because they lack the normal glucoregulatory mechanisms (normally, insulin falls and glucagon rises during exercise). Skeletal muscle is a major site for metabolic fuel consumption in the resting state, and the increased muscle activity during vigorous, aerobic exercise greatly increases fuel requirements. Individuals with type 1 DM are prone to either hyperglycemia or hypoglycemia during exercise, depending on the pre-exercise plasma glucose, the circulating insulin level, and the level of exercise-induced catecholamines. If the insulin level is too low, the rise in catecholamines may increase the plasma glucose excessively, promote ketone body formation, and possibly lead to ketoacidosis. Conversely, if the circulating insulin level is excessive, this relative hyperinsulinemia may reduce hepatic glucose production (decreased glycogenolysis, decreased gluconeogenesis) and increase glucose entry into muscle, leading to hypoglycemia.

To avoid exercise-related hyper- or hypoglycemia, individuals with type 1 DM should (1) monitor blood glucose before, during, and after exercise; (2) delay exercise if blood glucose is >14 mmol/L (250 mg/dL) and ketones are present; (3) if the blood glucose is <5.6 mmol/L (100 mg/dL), ingest carbohydrate before exercising; (3) monitor glucose during exercise and ingest carbohydrate to prevent hypoglycemia; (4) decrease insulin doses (based on previous experience) before exercise and inject insulin into a non-exercising area; and (5) learn individual glucose responses to different types of exercise and increase food intake for up to 24 h after exercise, depending on intensity and duration of exercise. In individuals with type 2 DM, exercise-related hypoglycemia is less common but can occur in individuals taking either insulin or insulin secretagogues.

Because asymptomatic cardiovascular disease appears at a younger age in both type 1 and type 2 DM, formal exercise tolerance testing may be warranted in diabetic individuals with any of the following: age >35 years, diabetes duration >15 years (type 1 DM) or >10 years (type 2 DM), microvascular complications of DM (retinopathy, microalbuminuria, or nephropathy), PAD, other risk factors of CHD, or autonomic neuropathy. Untreated proliferative retinopathy is a relative contraindication to vigorous exercise, as this may lead to vitreous hemorrhage or retinal detachment.

■ MONITORING THE LEVEL OF GLYCEMIC CONTROL

Optimal monitoring of glycemic control involves plasma glucose measurements by the patient and an assessment of long-term control by the physician (measurement of hemoglobin A1C and review of the patient's self-measurements of plasma glucose). These measurements are complementary: the patient's measurements provide a picture of short-term glycemic control, whereas the A1C reflects average glycemic control over the previous 2–3 months.

Self-monitoring of blood glucose

Self-monitoring of blood glucose (SMBG) is the standard of care in diabetes management and allows the patient to monitor his or her blood glucose at any time. In SMBG, a small drop of blood and an easily detectable enzymatic reaction allow measurement of the capillary plasma glucose. Many glucose monitors can rapidly and accurately measure glucose (calibrated to provide plasma glucose value even though blood glucose is measured) in small amounts of blood (3–10 μL) obtained from the fingertip; alternative testing sites (e.g., forearm) are less reliable, especially when the blood glucose is changing rapidly (postprandially). A large number of blood glucose monitors are available, and the certified diabetes educator is critical in helping the patient select the optimal device and learn to use it properly. By combining glucose measurements with diet history, medication changes, and exercise history, the diabetes management team and patient can improve the treatment program.

The frequency of SMBG measurements must be individualized and adapted to address the goals of diabetes care. Individuals with type 1 DM or individuals with type 2 DM taking multiple insulin injections each day should routinely measure their plasma glucose three or more times per day to estimate and select mealtime boluses of short-acting insulin and to modify long-acting insulin doses. Most individuals with type 2 DM require less frequent monitoring, though the optimal frequency of SMBG has not been clearly defined. Individuals with type 2 DM who are taking insulin should utilize SMBG more frequently than those on oral agents. Individuals with type 2 DM who are on oral medications should utilize SMBG as a means of assessing the efficacy of their medication and the impact of diet. Since plasma glucose levels fluctuate less in these individuals, one to two SMBG measurements per day (or fewer in patients who are on oral agents or are diet-controlled) may be sufficient. Most measurements in individuals with type 1 or type 2 DM should be performed prior to a meal and supplemented with postprandial measurements to assist in reaching postprandial glucose targets (Table 344-8).

Devices for continuous blood glucose monitoring (CGM) have been approved by the FDA, and others are in various stages of development. These devices do not replace the need for traditional glucose measurements. This rapidly evolving technology requires substantial expertise on the part of the diabetes management team and the patient. Current continuous glucose-monitoring systems measure the glucose in interstitial fluid, which is in equilibrium with the blood glucose. These devices provide useful short-term information about the patterns of glucose changes as well as an enhanced ability to detect hypoglycemic episodes. Alarms notify the patient if the blood glucose falls into the hypoglycemic range. Clinical experience with these devices is rapidly growing, and they are most useful in individuals with hypoglycemia unawareness, frequent hypoglycemia, or those who have not achieved glycemic targets despite major efforts. The utility of CGM in the ICU setting remains to be determined.

Ketones are an indicator of early diabetic ketoacidosis and should be measured in individuals with type 1 DM when the plasma glucose is consistently >16.7 mmol/L (300 mg/dL) during a concurrent illness or with symptoms such as nausea, vomiting, or abdominal pain. Blood measurement of β-hydroxybutyrate is preferred over urine testing with nitroprusside-based assays that measure only acetoacetate and acetone.

Assessment of long-term glycemic control

Measurement of glycated hemoglobin is the standard method for assessing long-term glycemic control. When plasma glucose is consistently elevated, there is an increase in nonenzymatic glycation of hemoglobin; this alteration reflects the glycemic history over the previous 2–3 months, since erythrocytes have an average life span of 120 days (glycemic level in the preceding month contributes about 50% to the A1C value). There are numerous laboratory methods for measuring the various forms of glycated hemoglobin, and these have significant interassay variations; assays that are calibrated against the DCCT A1C assay are essential. Depending on the assay methodology, hemoglobinopathies, anemias, reticulocytosis, transfusions, and uremia may interfere with the A1C result. Measurement of A1C at the "point of care" allows for more rapid feedback and may therefore assist in adjustment of therapy.

A1C should be measured in all individuals with DM during their initial evaluation and as part of their comprehensive diabetes care. As the primary predictor of long-term complications of DM, the A1C should mirror, to a certain extent, the short-term measurements of SMBG. These two measurements are complementary in that recent intercurrent illnesses may impact the SMBG measurements but not the A1C. Likewise, postprandial and nocturnal hyperglycemia may not be detected by the SMBG of fasting and preprandial capillary plasma glucose but will be reflected in the A1C. In standardized assays, the A1C approximates the following mean plasma glucose values: an A1C of 6% = 7.0 mmol/L (126 mg/dL), 7% = 8.6 mmol/L (154 mg/dL), 8% = 10.2 mmol/L (183 mg/dL), 9% = 11.8 mmol/L (212 mg/dL), 10% = 13.4 mmol/L (240 mg/dL), 11% = 14.9 mmol/L (269 mg/dL), and 12% = 16.5 mmol/L (298 mg/dL). In patients achieving their glycemic goal, the ADA recommends measurement of the A1C at least twice per year. More frequent testing (every 3 months) is warranted when glycemic control is inadequate or when therapy has changed. The degree of glycation of other proteins, such as albumin, can be used as an alternative indicator of glycemic control when the A1C is inaccurate (hemolytic anemia, hemoglobinopathies). The fructosamine assay (measuring glycated albumin) reflects the glycemic status over the prior 2 weeks. Alternative assays of glycemic control should not be routinely used since studies demonstrating that it accurately predicts the complications of DM are lacking.

TREATMENT Type 1 and Type 2 Diabetes Mellitus

ESTABLISHMENT OF TARGET LEVEL OF GLYCEMIC CONTROL Because the complications of DM are related to glycemic control, normoglycemia or near-normoglycemia is the desired, but often elusive, goal for most patients. However, normalization of the plasma glucose for long periods of time is extremely difficult, as demonstrated by the DCCT. Regardless of the level of hyperglycemia, improvement in glycemic control will lower the risk of diabetes complications (Fig. 344-8).

The target for glycemic control (as reflected by the A1C) must be individualized, and the goals of therapy should be developed in consultation with the patient after considering a number of medical, social, and lifestyle issues. Some important factors to consider include the patient's age, ability to understand and implement a complex treatment regimen, presence and severity of complications of diabetes, ability to recognize hypoglycemic symptoms, presence of other medical conditions or treatments that might alter the response to therapy, lifestyle and occupation (e.g., possible consequences of experiencing hypoglycemia on the job), and level of support available from family and friends.

The ADA suggests that the glycemic goal is to achieve an A1C as close to normal as possible without significant hypoglycemia. In general, the target A1C should be <7% (Table 344-8) with a more stringent target for some patients. A higher A1C goal may be appropriate for the very young or old or in individuals with limited life span or comorbid conditions. The major consideration is the frequency and severity of hypoglycemia, since this becomes more common with a more stringent A1C goal. More stringent glycemic control (A1C of 6% or less) is not beneficial, and may be determental, in type 2 DM and a high risk of CV disease.

TYPE 1 DIABETES MELLITUS

General Aspects The ADA recommendations for fasting and bedtime glycemic goals and A1C targets are summarized in Table 344-8. The goal is to design and implement insulin regimens that mimic physiologic insulin secretion. Because individuals with type 1 DM partially or completely lack endogenous insulin production, administration of basal insulin is essential for regulating glycogen breakdown, gluconeogenesis, lipolysis, and ketogenesis. Likewise, insulin replacement for meals should be appropriate for the carbohydrate intake and promote normal glucose utilization and storage.

Intensive Management Intensive diabetes management has the goal of achieving euglycemia or near-normal glycemia. This approach requires multiple resources, including thorough and continuing patient education, comprehensive recording of plasma glucose measurements and nutrition intake by the patient, and a variable insulin regimen that matches glucose intake and insulin dose. Insulin regimens usually include multiple-component insulin regimens, multiple daily injections (MDI), or insulin infusion devices (each discussed below).

The benefits of intensive diabetes management and improved glycemic control include a reduction in the microvascular complications of DM and a reduction in the macrovascular complications of DM, which persists after a period of near-normoglycemia. From a psychological standpoint, the patient experiences greater control over his or her diabetes and often notes an improved sense of well-being, greater flexibility in the timing and content of meals, and the capability to alter insulin dosing with exercise.

In addition, intensive diabetes management prior to and during pregnancy reduces the risk of fetal malformations and morbidity. Intensive diabetes management is strongly encouraged in newly diagnosed patients with type 1 DM because it may prolong the period of C-peptide production, which may result in better glycemic control and a reduced risk of serious hypoglycemia.

Although intensive management confers impressive benefits, it is also accompanied by significant personal and financial costs and is therefore not appropriate for all individuals.

Insulin Preparations Current insulin preparations are generated by recombinant DNA technology and consist of the amino acid sequence of human insulin or variations thereof. In the United States, most insulin is formulated as U-100 (100 units/mL). Regular insulin formulated as U-500 (500 units/mL) is available and sometimes useful in patients with severe insulin resistance. Human insulin has been formulated with distinctive pharmacokinetics or genetically modified to more closely mimic physiologic insulin secretion. Insulins can be classified as short-acting or long-acting (Table 344-10). For example, one short-acting insulin formulation, insulin lispro, is an insulin analogue in which the 28th and 29th amino acids (lysine and proline) on the insulin B chain have been reversed by recombinant DNA technology. Insulin aspart and insulin glulisine are other genetically modified insulin analogues with properties similar to lispro. These insulin analogues have full biologic activity but less tendency for self-aggregation, resulting in more rapid absorption and onset of action and a shorter duration of action. These characteristics are particularly advantageous for allowing entrainment of insulin injection and action to rising plasma glucose levels following meals. The shorter duration of action also appears to be associated with a decreased number of hypoglycemic episodes, primarily because the decay of insulin action corresponds to the decline in plasma glucose after a meal. Thus, insulin aspart, lispro, or glulisine is preferred over regular insulin for prandial coverage. Insulin glargine is a long-acting biosynthetic human insulin that differs from normal insulin in that asparagine is replaced by glycine at amino acid 21, and two arginine residues are added to the C terminus of the B chain. Compared to NPH insulin, the onset of insulin glargine action is later, the duration of action is longer (~24 h), and there is a less pronounced peak. A lower incidence of hypoglycemia, especially at night, has been reported with insulin glargine when compared to NPH insulin. The possible association between glargine and increased cancer risk is being investigated (FDA review underway) and is controversial. Insulin detemir has a fatty acid side chain that prolongs its action by slowing absorption and catabolism. Twice-daily injections of glargine of detemir are sometimes required to provide 24-h coverage. Regular and NPH insulin have the native insulin amino acid sequence.

Basal insulin requirements are provided by long-acting (NPH insulin, insulin glargine, or insulin detemir) insulin formulations. These are usually prescribed with short-acting insulin in an attempt to mimic physiologic insulin release with meals. Although mixing of NPH and short-acting insulin formulations is common practice, this mixing may alter the insulin absorption profile (especially the short-acting insulins). For example, lispro absorption is delayed by mixing with NPH. The alteration in insulin absorption when the patient mixes different insulin formulations should not discourage mixing insulins. However, the following guidelines should be followed: (1) Mix the different insulin formulations in the syringe immediately before injection (inject within 2 min after mixing); (2) do not store insulin as a mixture; (3) follow the same routine in terms of insulin mixing and administration to standardize the physiologic response to injected insulin; and (4) do not mix insulin glargine or detemir with other insulins. The miscibility of human regular and NPH insulin allows for the production of combination insulins that contain 70% NPH and 30% regular (70/30), or equal mixtures of NPH and regular (50/50). Other combination insulin formulations are insulin aspart (70/30) and insulin lispro (75/25 and 50/50). By including the insulin analogue mixed with protamine, these combinations have a short-acting and long-acting profile (Table 344-10). While more convenient for the patient (only two injections/day), combination insulin formulations do not allow independent adjustment of short-acting and long-acting activity. Several insulin formulations are available as insulin "pens," which may be more convenient for some patients. Insulin delivery by inhalation is no longer available but remains under investigation.

Insulin Regimens Representations of the various insulin regimens that may be utilized in type 1 DM are illustrated in Fig. 344-12. Although the insulin profiles are depicted as "smooth," symmetric curves, there is considerable patient-to-patient variation in the peak and duration. In all regimens, long-acting insulins (NPH, glargine, or detemir) supply basal insulin, whereas regular, insulin aspart, glulisine, or lispro insulin provides prandial insulin. Short-acting insulin analogues should be injected just before (<20 min) or just after a meal; regular insulin is given 30–45 min prior to a meal.

A shortcoming of current insulin regimens is that injected insulin immediately enters the systemic circulation, whereas endogenous insulin is secreted into the portal venous system.

TABLE 344-10 Properties of Insulin Preparations

Preparation	Time of Action		
	Onset, h	Peak, h	Effective Duration, h
Short-acting			
Aspart	<0.25	0.5–1.5	3–4
Glulisine	<0.25	0.5–1.5	3–4
Lispro	<0.25	0.5–1.5	3–4
Regular	0.5–1.0	2–3	4–6
Long-acting			
Detemir	1–4	—[a]	Up to 24
Glargine	1–4	—[a]	Up to 24
NPH	1–4	6–10	10–16
Insulin combinations			
75/25–75% protamine lispro, 25% lispro	<0.25	1.5 h	Up to 10–16
70/30–70% protamine aspart, 30% aspart	<0.25	1.5 h	Up to 10–16
50/50–50% protamine lispro, 50% lispro	<0.25	1.5 h	Up to 10–16
70/30–70% NPH, 30% regular	0.5–1	Dual[b]	10–16

[a]Glargine and detemir have minimal peak activity.

[b]Dual: two peaks—one at 2–3 h and the second one several hours later.

Source: Adapted from JS Skyler, Therapy for Diabetes Mellitus and Related Disorders, American Diabetes Association, Alexandria, VA, 2004.

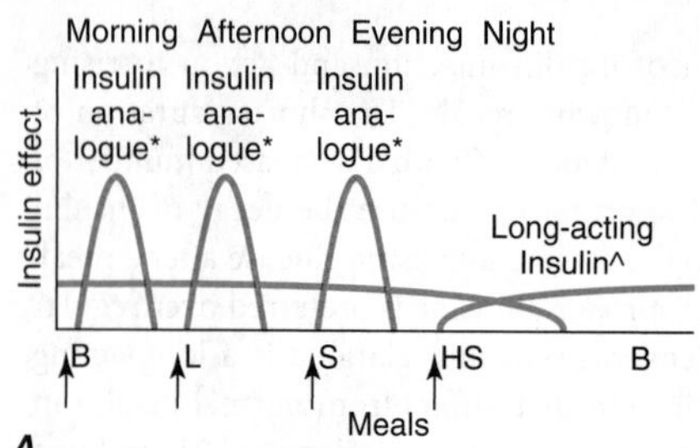

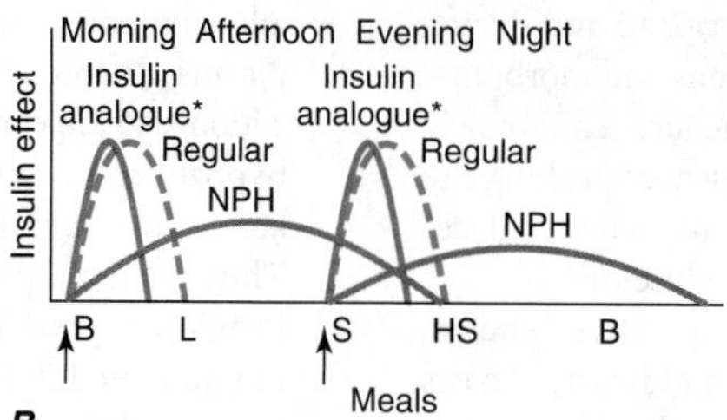

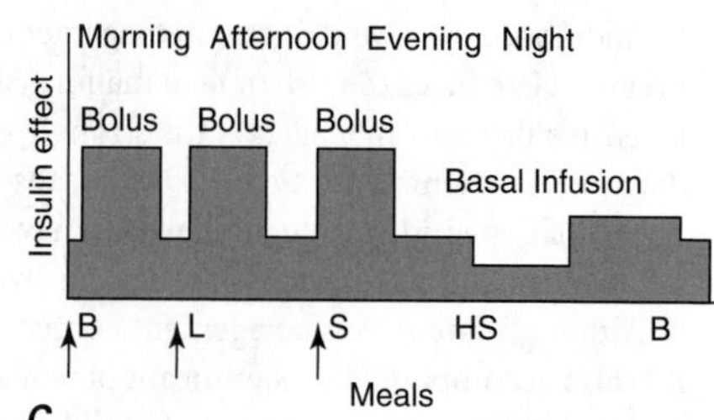

Figure 344-12 Representative insulin regimens for the treatment of diabetes. For each panel, the *y*-axis shows the amount of insulin effect and the *x*-axis shows the time of day. B, breakfast; L, lunch; S, supper; HS, bedtime; CSII, continuous subcutaneous insulin infusion. *Lispro, glulisine, or insulin aspart can be used. The time of insulin injection is shown with a vertical arrow. The type of insulin is noted above each insulin curve. ***A.*** A multiple-component insulin regimen consisting of long-acting insulin^ glargine or detemir may be required each day) to provide basal insulin coverage and three shots of glulisine, lispro, or insulin aspart to provide glycemic coverage for each meal. ***B.*** The injection of two shots of long-acting insulin (NPH) and short-acting insulin [glulisine, lispro, insulin aspart (solid red line), or regular (green dashed line)]. Only one formulation of short-acting insulin is used. ***C.*** Insulin administration by insulin infusion device is shown with the basal insulin and a bolus injection at each meal. The basal insulin rate is decreased during the evening and increased slightly prior to the patient awakening in the morning. Glulisine, lispro, or insulin aspart is used in the insulin pump. *[Adapted from H Lebovitz (ed): Therapy for Diabetes Mellitus. American Diabetes Association, Alexandria, VA, 2004.]*

Thus, exogenous insulin administration exposes the liver to subphysiologic insulin levels. No insulin regimen reproduces the precise insulin secretory pattern of the pancreatic islet. However, the most physiologic regimens entail more frequent insulin injections, greater reliance on short-acting insulin, and more frequent capillary plasma glucose measurements. In general, individuals with type 1 DM require 0.5–1 U/kg per day of insulin divided into multiple doses, with ~50% of the insulin given as basal insulin.

Multiple-component insulin regimens refer to the combination of basal insulin and bolus insulin (preprandial short-acting insulin). The timing and dose of short-acting, preprandial insulin are altered to accommodate the SMBG results, anticipated food intake, and physical activity. Such regimens offer the patient with type 1 diabetes more flexibility in terms of lifestyle and the best chance for achieving near normoglycemia. One such regimen, shown in Fig. 344-12*B*, consists of basal insulin with glargine or detemir and preprandial lispro, glulisine, or insulin aspart. The insulin aspart, glulisine, or lispro dose is based on individualized algorithms that integrate the preprandial glucose and the anticipated carbohydrate intake. To determine the meal component of the preprandial insulin dose, the patient uses an insulin-to-carbohydrate ratio (a common ratio for type 1 DM is 1–1.5 units/10 g of carbohydrate, but this must be determined for each individual). To this insulin dose is added the supplemental or correcting insulin based on the preprandial blood glucose [one formula uses 1 unit of insulin for every 2.7 mmol/L (50 mg/dL) over the preprandial glucose target; another formula uses (body weight in kg) × (blood glucose – desired glucose in mg/dL)/1700]. An alternative multiple-component insulin regimen consists of bedtime NPH insulin, a small dose of NPH insulin at breakfast (20–30% of bedtime dose), and preprandial short-acting insulin. Other variations of this regimen are in use but have the disadvantage that NPH has a significant peak, making hypoglycemia more common. Frequent SMBG (more than three times per day) is absolutely essential for these types of insulin regimens.

One commonly used regimen consists of twice-daily injections of NPH mixed with a short-acting insulin before the morning and evening meals (Fig. 344-12B). Such regimens usually prescribe two-thirds of the total daily insulin dose in the morning (with about two-thirds given as long-acting insulin and one-third as short-acting) and one-third before the evening meal (with approximately one-half given as long-acting insulin and one-half as short-acting). The drawback to such a regimen is that it enforces a rigid schedule on the patient, in terms of daily activity and the content and timing of meals. Although it is simple and effective at avoiding severe hyperglycemia, it does not generate near-normal glycemic control in individuals with type 1 DM. Moreover, if the patient's meal pattern or content varies or if physical activity is increased, hyperglycemia or hypoglycemia may result. Moving the long-acting insulin from before the evening meal to bedtime may avoid nocturnal hypoglycemia and provide more insulin as glucose levels rise in the early morning (so-called dawn phenomenon). The insulin dose in such regimens should be adjusted based on SMBG results with the following general assumptions: (1) the fasting glucose is primarily determined by the prior evening long-acting insulin; (2) the pre-lunch glucose is a function of the morning short-acting insulin; (3) the pre-supper glucose is a function of the morning long-acting insulin; and (4) the bedtime glucose is a function of the pre-supper, short-acting insulin. This is not an optimal regimen for the patient with type 1 DM, but is sometimes used for patients with type 2 diabetes.

Continuous SC insulin infusion (CSII) is a very effective insulin regimen for the patient with type 1 diabetes (Fig. 344-12*C*). To the basal insulin infusion, a preprandial insulin ("bolus") is delivered by the insulin infusion device based on instructions from the patient, who uses an individualized algorithm incorporating the preprandial plasma glucose and anticipated carbohydrate intake (see above). These sophisticated insulin infusion devices can accurately deliver small doses of insulin (microliters per hour) and have several advantages: (1) multiple basal infusion rates can be programmed to accommodate nocturnal versus daytime basal insulin requirement, (2) basal infusion rates can be altered during periods of exercise, (3) different waveforms of insulin infusion with meal-related bolus allow better matching of insulin depending on meal composition, and (4) programmed algorithms consider prior insulin administration and blood glucose values in calculating the insulin dose. These devices require instruction by a health professional with considerable experience with insulin infusion devices and very frequent patient interactions with the diabetes management team. Insulin infusion devices present unique challenges, such as infection at the infusion site, unexplained hyperglycemia because the infusion set becomes obstructed, or diabetic ketoacidosis if the pump becomes disconnected. Since most physicians use lispro, glulisine, or insulin aspart in CSII, the extremely short half-life of these insulins quickly lead to insulin deficiency if the delivery system is interrupted. Essential to the safe use of infusion devices is thorough patient education about pump function and frequent SMBG. Efforts to create a closed-loop system in which data from continuous glucose measurement regulates the insulin infusion rate continue.

Other Agents That Improve Glucose Control The role of amylin, a 37-amino-acid peptide co-secreted with insulin from pancreatic beta cells, in normal glucose homeostasis is uncertain. However, based on the rationale that patients who are insulin deficient are also amylin deficient, an analogue of amylin (pramlintide) was created and found to reduce postprandial glycemic excursions in type 1 and type 2 diabetic patients taking insulin. Pramlintide injected just before a meal slows gastric emptying and suppresses glucagon but does not alter insulin levels. Pramlintide is approved for insulin-treated patients with type 1 and type 2 DM. Addition of pramlintide produces a modest reduction in the A1C and seems to dampen meal-related glucose excursions. In type 1 diabetes, pramlintide is started as a 15-μg SC injection before each meal and titrated up to a maximum of 30–60 μg as tolerated. In type 2 DM, pramlintide is started as a 60-μg SC injection before each meal and may be titrated up to a maximum of 120 μg. The major side effects are nausea and vomiting, and dose escalations should be slow to limit these side effects. Because pramlintide slows gastric emptying, it may influence absorption of other medications and should not be used in combination with other drugs that slow GI motility. The short-acting insulin given before the meal should initially be reduced to avoid hypoglycemia and then titrated as the effects of the pramlintide become evident. α-Glucosidase inhibitors are another type of agent that is sometimes used in conjunction in patients with type 1 DM.

TYPE 2 DIABETES MELLITUS

General Aspects The goals of therapy for type 2 DM are similar to those in type 1. While glycemic control tends to dominate the management of type 1 DM, the care of individuals with type 2 DM must also include attention to the treatment of conditions associated with type 2 DM (obesity, hypertension, dyslipidemia, cardiovascular disease) and detection/management of DM-related complications (Fig. 344-13). DM-specific complications may be present in up to 20–50% of individuals with newly diagnosed type 2 DM. Reduction in cardiovascular risk is of paramount importance as this is the leading cause of mortality in these individuals. Efforts to achieve blood pressure and lipid goals (Table 344-8) should begin in concert with glucose-lowering interventions.

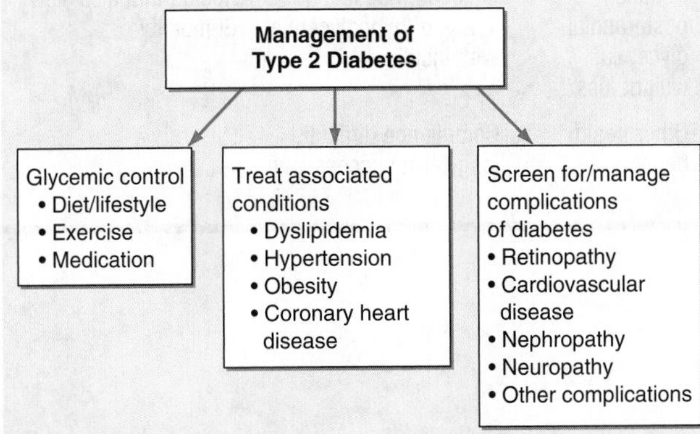

Figure 344-13 Essential elements in comprehensive diabetes care of type 2 diabetes.

Type 2 diabetes management should begin with MNT (discussed above). An exercise regimen to increase insulin sensitivity and promote weight loss should also be instituted. Pharmacologic approaches to the management of type 2 DM include oral glucose-lowering agents, insulin, and other agents that improve glucose control; most physicians and patients prefer oral glucose-lowering agents as the initial choice (discussed below) after review of various medications. Any therapy that improves glycemic control reduces "glucose toxicity" to the islet cells and improves endogenous insulin secretion. However, type 2 DM is a progressive disorder and ultimately requires multiple therapeutic agents and often insulin.

Glucose-Lowering Agents Advances in the therapy of type 2 DM have generated oral glucose-lowering agents that target different pathophysiologic processes in type 2 DM. Based on their mechanisms of action, glucose-lowering agents are subdivided into agents that increase insulin secretion, reduce glucose production, increase insulin sensitivity, and enhance GLP-1 action (Table 344-11). Glucose-lowering agents other than insulin (with the exception of amylin analogue and α-glucosidase inhibitors) are ineffective in type 1 DM and should not be used for glucose management of severely ill individuals with type 2 DM. Insulin is sometimes the initial glucose-lowering agent in type 2 diabetes.

Biguanides Metformin, representative of this class of agents, reduces hepatic glucose production and improves peripheral glucose utilization slightly (Table 344-11). Metformin activates AMP-dependent protein kinase and enters cells through organic cation transporters (polymorphisms of these may influence the response to metformin). Metformin reduces fasting plasma glucose and insulin levels, improves the lipid profile, and promotes modest weight loss. The initial starting dose of 500 mg once or twice a day can be increased to 1000 mg bid. An extended-release form is available and may have fewer gastrointestinal side effects (diarrhea, anorexia, nausea, metallic taste). Because of its relatively slow onset of action and gastrointestinal symptoms with higher doses, the dose should be escalated every 2–3 weeks based on SMBG measurements. Metformin is effective as monotherapy and can be used in combination with other oral agents or with insulin. The major toxicity of metformin, lactic acidosis is very rare and can be prevented by careful patient selection. Vitamin B_{12} levels are ~30% lower during metformin treatment. Metformin should not be used in patients with renal insufficiency [GFR < 60 mL/min], any form of acidosis, CHF, liver disease, or severe hypoxemia. Metformin should be discontinued in patients who are seriously ill, in patients who can take nothing orally, and in those receiving radiographic contrast material. Insulin should be used until metformin can be restarted.

Insulin Secretagogues—Agents That Affect the ATP-Sensitive K^+ Channel Insulin secretagogues stimulate insulin secretion by interacting with the ATP-sensitive potassium channel on the beta cell (Fig. 344-4). These drugs are most effective in individuals with type 2 DM of relatively recent onset (<5 years), who have residual endogenous insulin production. First-generation sulfonylureas (chlorpropamide, tolazamide, tolbutamide; not shown in Table 344-12) have a longer half-life, a greater incidence of hypoglycemia, more frequent drug interactions, and are now rarely used. Second-generation sulfonylureas have a more rapid onset of action and better coverage of the postprandial glucose

TABLE 344-11 Agents Used for Treatment of Type 1 and Type 2 Diabetes

	Mechanism of Action	Examples	A1C Reduction (%)[a]	Agent-Specific Advantages	Agent-Specific Disadvantages	Contraindications
Oral						
Biguanides[b]	↓ Hepatic glucose production	Metformin	1–2	Weight neutral, Do not cause hypoglycemia, inexpensive	Diarrhea, nausea, lactic acidosis	Serum creatinine >1.5 mg/dL (men) >1.4 mg/dL (women), CHF, radiographic contrast studies, seriously ill patients, acidosis
α-Glucosidase inhibitors[b]	↓ GI glucose absorption	Acarbose, Miglitol	0.5–0.8	Reduce postprandial glycemia	GI flatulence, liver function tests	Renal/liver disease
Dipeptidyl peptidase IV inhibitors[b]	Prolong endogenous GLP-1 action	Saxagliptin, Sitagliptin, Vildagliptin	0.5–0.8	Do not cause hypoglycemia		Reduce dose with renal disease
Insulin secretagogues: Sulfonylureas[b]	↑ Insulin secretion	See text and Table 344-12	1–2	Inexpensive	Hypoglycemia, weight gain	Renal/liver disease
Insulin secretagogues: Non-sulfonylureas[b]	↑ Insulin secretion	See text and Table 344-12	1–2	Short onset of action, lower postprandial glucose	Hypoglycemia	Renal/liver disease
Thiazolidinediones[b]	↓ Insulin resistance, ↑ glucose utilization	Rosiglitazone, Pioglitazone	0.5–1.4	Lower insulin requirements	Peripheral edema, CHF, weight gain, fractures, macular edema; rosiglitazone may increase cardiovascular risk	CHF, liver disease; see text about rosiglitazone
Bile acid sequestrants	Bind bile acids; mechanism of glucose lowering not known	Colesevelam	0.5		Constipation, dyspepsia, abdominal pain, nausea, ↑ triglycerides, interfere with absorption of other drugs, intestinal obstruction	Elevated plasma triglycerides
Parenteral						
Insulin[b,c]	↑ Glucose utilization, ↓ Hepatic glucose production, and other anabolic actions	See text and Table 344-10	Not limited	Known safety profile	Injection, weight gain, hypoglycemia	
GLP-1 receptor agonists[b]	↑ Insulin, ↓ glucagon, slow gastric emptying, satiety	Exenatide, liraglutide	0.5–1.0	Weight loss, do not cause hypoglycemia	Injection, nausea, ↑ risk of hypoglycemia with insulin secretagogues, pancreatitis, renal failure	Renal disease, agents that also slow GI motility; see text
Amylin agonists[b,c]	Slow gastric emptying, ↓ glucagon	Pramlintide	0.25–0.5	Reduce postprandial glycemia; weight loss	Injection, nausea, ↑ risk of hypoglycemia with insulin	Agents that also slow GI motility
Medical nutrition therapy and physical activity[b,c]	↓ Insulin resistance, ↑ insulin secretion	Low-calorie, low-fat diet, exercise	1–3	Other health benefits	Compliance difficult, long-term success low	

[a]A1C reduction (absolute) depends partly on starting A1C.
[b]Used for treatment of type 2 diabetes.
[c]Used in conjunction with insulin for treatment of type 1 diabetes.

TABLE 344-12 Properties of Insulin Secretagogues

Class/Generic Name	Daily Dosage, mg	Duration of Action, h
Sulfonylureas		
Glimepiride	1–8	24
Glipizide	5–40	12–18
Glipizide (extended release)	5–20	24
Glyburide	1.25–20	12–24
Glyburide (micronized)	0.75–12	12–24
Nonsulfonylureas (Meglitinides)		
Repaglinide	0.5–16	2–6
Nateglinide	180–360	2–4
GLP-1 agonist		
Exenatide	0.01–0.02	4–6
Liraglutide	0.6–1.8	12–24
Dipeptidyl Peptidase-4 Inhibitors		
Saxagliptin	2.5–5	12–16
Sitagliptin	100	12–16
Vildagliptin	50–100	12–24

Abbreviation: GLP-1, glucagon-like peptide 1.

rise, but the shorter half-life of some agents may require more than once-a-day dosing (Table 344-12). Sulfonylureas reduce both fasting and postprandial glucose and should be initiated at low doses and increased at 1- to 2-week intervals based on SMBG. In general, sulfonylureas increase insulin acutely and thus should be taken shortly before a meal; with chronic therapy, though, the insulin release is more sustained. Glimepiride and glipizide can be given in a single daily dose and are preferred over glyburide. Repaglinide and nateglinide are not sulfonylureas but also interact with the ATP-sensitive potassium channel. Because of their short half-life, these agents are given with each meal or immediately before to reduce meal-related glucose excursions.

These insulin secretagogues are generally well tolerated. These agents, especially the longer acting ones, have the potential to cause profound and persistent hypoglycemia, especially in elderly individuals. Hypoglycemia is usually related to delayed meals, increased physical activity, alcohol intake, or renal insufficiency. Individuals who ingest an overdose of some agents develop prolonged and serious hypoglycemia and should be monitored closely in the hospital (Chap. 345). Most sulfonylureas are metabolized in the liver to compounds (some of which are active) that are cleared by the kidney. Thus, their use in individuals with significant hepatic or renal dysfunction is not advisable. Weight gain, a common side effect of sulfonylurea therapy, results from the increased insulin levels and improvement in glycemic control. Some sulfonylureas have significant drug interactions with alcohol and some medications including warfarin, aspirin, ketoconazole, α-glucosidase inhibitors, and fluconazole. A related isoform of ATP-sensitive potassium channels is present in the myocardium and the brain. All of these agents except glyburide have a low affinity for this isoform. Despite concerns that this agent might affect the myocardial response to ischemia and observational studies suggesting that sulfonylureas increase cardiovascular risk, studies have not shown an increased cardiac mortality with glyburide.

Insulin Secretagogues—Agents That Enhance GLP-1 Receptor Signaling "Incretins" amplify glucose-stimulated insulin secretion (Fig. 344-4). Agents that either act as a GLP-1 agonist or enhance endogenous GLP-1 activity are approved for the treatment of type 2 diabetes (Table 344-12). Agents in this class do not cause hypoglycemia because of the glucose-dependent nature of incretin-stimulated insulin secretion (unless there is concomitant use of an agent that can lead to hypoglycemia—sulfonylureas, etc.). Exenatide, a synthetic version of a peptide initially identified in the saliva of the Gila monster (exendin-4), is an analogue of GLP-1. Unlike native GLP-1, which has a half-life of <5 min, differences in the exenatide amino acid sequence render it resistant to the enzyme that degrades GLP-1 (dipeptidyl peptidase IV, or DPP-IV). Thus, exenatide has prolonged GLP-1-like action and binds to GLP-1 receptors found in islets, the gastrointestinal tract, and the brain. Liraglutide, another GLP-1 receptor agonist, is almost identical to native GLP-1 except for an amino acid substitution and addition of a fatty acyl group (coupled with a γ-glutamic acid spacer) that promote binding to albumin and plasma proteins and prolong its half-life. GLP-1 receptor agonists increase glucose-stimulated insulin secretion, suppress glucagon, and slow gastric emptying. These agents do not promote weight gain; in fact, most patients experience modest weight loss and appetite suppression. Treatment with these agents should start at a low dose to minimize initial side effects (nausea being the limiting one). Exenatide is approved for monotherapy and for use as combination therapy with metformin, sulfonylureas, and thiazolidinediones. Some patients taking insulin secretagogues may require a reduction in those agents to prevent hypoglycemia. GLP-1 receptor agonists should not be used in patients taking insulin. The major side effects are nausea, vomiting, and diarrhea; pancreatitis and reduced renal function have been reported in surveillance data with exenatide. Liraglutide carries a black box warning from the FDA because of an increased risk of thyroid C-cell tumors in rodents and is contraindicated in individuals with medullary carcinoma of the thyroid and multiple endocrine neoplasia. Because GLP-1 receptor agonists slow gastric emptying, they may influence the absorption of other drugs. Whether GLP-1 receptor agonists enhance beta cell survival, promote beta cell proliferation, or alter the natural history of type 2 DM is not known. Other GLP-1 receptor agonists and formulations are under development.

DPP-IV inhibitors inhibit degradation of native GLP-1 and thus enhance the incretin effect. DPP-IV, which is widely expressed on the cell surface of endothelial cells and some lymphocytes, degrades a wide range of peptides (not GLP-1 specific). DPP-IV inhibitors promote insulin secretion in the absence of hypoglycemia or weight gain, and appear to have a preferential effect on postprandial blood glucose. DPP-IV inhibitors are used either alone or in combination with other oral agents in adults with type 2 DM. Reduced doses should be given to patients with renal insufficiency. These agents have relatively few side effects.

α-Glucosidase Inhibitors α-Glucosidase inhibitors (acarbose and miglitol) reduce postprandial hyperglycemia by delaying glucose absorption; they do not affect glucose utilization or insulin secretion (Table 344-11). Postprandial hyperglycemia, secondary to impaired hepatic and peripheral glucose disposal, contributes significantly to the hyperglycemic state in type 2 DM. These drugs, taken just before each meal, reduce glucose absorption by inhibiting the enzyme that cleaves oligosaccharides into simple sugars in the intestinal lumen. Therapy should be initiated at a low dose (25 mg of acarbose or miglitol) with the evening meal and may be increased to a maximal dose over weeks to months (50–100 mg for acarbose or 50 mg for miglitol with each meal). The major side effects (diarrhea, flatulence, abdominal distention) are related to increased delivery of oligosaccharides to the large bowel and can be reduced somewhat by gradual upward dose titration. α-Glucosidase inhibitors may increase levels of sulfonylureas and increase the incidence of hypoglycemia. Simultaneous treatment with bile acid resins and antacids should be avoided. These agents should not be used in individuals with inflammatory bowel disease, gastroparesis, or a serum creatinine >177 μmol/L (2 mg/dL). This class of agents is not as potent as other oral agents in lowering the A1C but is unique because it reduces the postprandial glucose rise even in individuals with type 1 DM. If hypoglycemia from other diabetes treatments occurs while taking these agents, the patient should consume glucose since the degradation and absorption of complex carbohydrates will be retarded.

Thiazolidinediones Thiazolidinediones reduce insulin resistance by binding to the PPAR-γ (peroxisome proliferator-activated receptor γ) nuclear receptor (which forms a heterodimer with the retinoid X receptor). The PPAR-γ receptor is found at highest levels in adipocytes but is expressed at lower levels in many other tissues. Agonists of this receptor regulate a large number of genes, promote adipocyte differentiation, reduce hepatic fat accumulation, and promote fatty acid storage (Table 344-11). Thiazolidinediones promote a redistribution of fat from central to peripheral locations. Circulating insulin levels decrease with use of the thiazolidinediones, indicating a reduction in insulin resistance. Although direct comparisons are not available, the two currently available thiazolidinediones appear to have similar efficacy; the therapeutic range for pioglitazone is 15–45 mg/d in a single daily dose, and for rosiglitazone the total daily dose is 2–8 mg/d administered either once daily or twice daily in divided doses. The prototype of this class of drugs, troglitazone, was withdrawn from the U.S. market after reports of hepatotoxicity and an association with an idiosyncratic liver reaction that sometimes led to hepatic failure. Although rosiglitazone and pioglitazone do not appear to induce the liver abnormalities seen with troglitazone, the FDA recommends measurement of liver function tests prior to initiating therapy with a thiazolidinedione and at regular intervals (every 2 months for the first year and then periodically).

Rosiglitazone raises LDL, HDL, and triglycerides slightly. Pioglitazone raises HDL to a greater degree and LDL a lesser degree but lowers triglycerides. The clinical significance of the lipid changes with these agents is not known and may be difficult to ascertain since most patients with type 2 diabetes are also treated with a statin.

Thiazolidinediones are associated with weight gain (2–3 kg), a small reduction in the hematocrit, and a mild increase in plasma volume. Peripheral edema and CHF are more common in individuals treated with these agents. These agents are contraindicated in patients with liver disease or CHF (class III or IV). The FDA has issued an alert that rare patients taking these agents may experience a worsening of diabetic macular edema. An increased risk of fractures has been noted in women taking these agents. Thiazolidinediones have been shown to induce ovulation in premenopausal women with PCOS. Women should be warned about the risk of pregnancy, since the safety of thiazolidinediones in pregnancy is not established.

Recent concerns about increased cardiovascular risk associated with rosiglitazone have led to considerable restrictions on its use. The FDA issued a "black box" warning for rosiglitazone in 2007. Under recent FDA guidelines (September 2010), new prescriptions for rosiglitazone in the United States must be written under a "risk evaluation and mitigation strategy" and only for patients with diabetes that cannot be controlled by other medications. The European Medicines Agency (2010) advised removal of rosiglitazone and formulations containing rosiglitazone from the European market. As a result of thesse rulings, rosiglitazone will be available in the United States on a limited basis, but will not be available in Europe.

Other Therapies for Type 2 Diabetes ***Bile acid–binding resins.*** Bile acid metabolism is abnormal type 2 diabetes. The bile acid–binding resin colesevelam has been approved for the treatment of type 2 diabetes (already approved for treatment of hypercholesterolemia). Emerging evidence indicates that bile acids, by signaling through nuclear receptors, may have a role in metabolism. Since bile acid–binding resins are minimally absorbed into the systemic circulation, how bile acid–binding resins lower blood glucose is not known. Colesevelam (available as a powder for oral solution and as 625-mg tablets) is prescribed as 3–6 tablets prior to meals. The most common side effects are gastrointestinal (constipation, abdominal pain, and nausea). Bile acid–binding resins can increase plasma triglycerides and should be used cautiously in patients with a tendency to hypertriglyceridemia. The role of this class of drugs in the treatment of type 2 diabetes is not yet defined.

Bromocriptine. A formulation of the dopamine receptor agonist bromocriptine (Cycloset), has been approved by the FDA for the treatment of type 2 diabetes (approved in 2009). However, this formulation is not available in the United States, and its role in the treatment of type 2 diabetes is uncertain.

Insulin Therapy in Type 2 DM Insulin should be considered as the initial therapy in type 2 DM, particularly in lean individuals or those with severe weight loss, in individuals with underlying renal or hepatic disease that precludes oral glucose-lowering agents, or in individuals who are hospitalized or acutely ill. Insulin therapy is ultimately required by a substantial number of individuals with type 2 DM because of the progressive nature of the disorder and the relative insulin deficiency that develops in patients with long-standing diabetes. Both physician and patient reluctance often delay the initiation of insulin therapy, but glucose control and patient well-being are improved by insulin therapy in patients who have not reached the glycemic target.

Because endogenous insulin secretion continues and is capable of providing some coverage of mealtime caloric intake, insulin is usually initiated in a single dose of long-acting insulin (0.3–0.4 U/kg per day), given either before breakfast and in the evening (NPH) or just before bedtime (NPH, glargine, detemir). Since fasting hyperglycemia and increased hepatic glucose production are prominent features of type 2 DM, bedtime insulin is more effective in clinical trials than a single dose of morning insulin. Glargine given at bedtime has less nocturnal hypoglycemia than NPH insulin. Some physicians prefer a relatively low, fixed starting dose of long-acting insulin (5–15 units) to reduce the chance of hypoglycemia in the initial treatment period. The insulin dose may then be adjusted in 10% increments as dictated by SMBG results. Both morning and bedtime long-acting insulin may be used in combination with oral glucose-lowering agents. Initially, basal insulin may be sufficient, but more often prandial insulin coverage with multiple insulin injections is needed as diabetes progresses (see insulin regimens used for type 1 diabetes). Other insulin formulations that have a combination of short-acting and long-acting insulin (Table 344-10) are sometimes used in patients with type 2 DM because of convenience but do not allow independent adjustment of short-acting and long-acting insulin dose and often do not achieve the same degree of glycemic control as basal/bolus regimens. In selected patients with type 2 DM (usually insulin deficient as defined by C-peptide level), insulin infusion devices may be considered.

Choice of Initial Glucose-Lowering Agent The level of hyperglycemia should influence the initial choice of therapy. Assuming maximal benefit of MNT and increased physical activity has been realized, patients with mild to moderate hyperglycemia [FPG <11.1–13.9 mmol/L (200–250 mg/dL)] often respond well to a single, oral glucose-lowering agent. Patients with more severe hyperglycemia [FPG >13.9 mmol/L (250 mg/dL)] may respond partially but are unlikely to achieve normoglycemia with oral monotherapy. A stepwise approach that starts with a single agent and adds a second agent to achieve the glycemic target can be used (see "Combination Therapy," below). Insulin can be used as initial therapy in individuals with severe hyperglycemia [FPG >13.9–16.7 mmol/L (250–300 mg/dL)] or in those who are symptomatic from the hyperglycemia. This approach is based on the rationale that more rapid glycemic control will reduce "glucose toxicity" to the islet cells, improve endogenous insulin secretion, and possibly allow oral glucose-lowering agents to be more effective. If this occurs, the insulin may be discontinued.

Insulin secretagogues, biguanides, α-glucosidase inhibitors, thiazolidinediones, GLP-1 receptor agonists, DPP-IV inhibitors, and insulin are approved for monotherapy of type 2 DM. Although each class of oral glucose-lowering agents has unique advantages and disadvantages, certain generalizations apply: (1) insulin secretagogues, biguanides, GLP-1 receptor agonists, and thiazolidinediones improve glycemic control to a similar degree (1–2% reduction in A1C) and are more effective than α-glucosidase inhibitors and DPP-IV inhibitors; (2) assuming a similar degree of glycemic improvement, no clinical advantage to one class of drugs has been demonstrated, and any therapy that improves glycemic control is likely beneficial; (3) insulin secretagogues, GLP-1 receptor agonists, DPP-IV inhibitors, and α-glucosidase inhibitors begin to lower the plasma glucose immediately, whereas the glucose-lowering effects of the biguanides and thiazolidinediones are delayed by several weeks; (4) not all agents are effective in all individuals with type 2 DM (primary failure); (5) biguanides, α-glucosidase inhibitors, GLP-1 receptor agonists, DPP-IV inhibitors, and thiazolidinediones do not directly cause hypoglycemia; and (6) most individuals will eventually require treatment with more than one class of oral glucose-lowering agents or insulin, reflecting the progressive nature of type 2 DM; (7) durability of glycemic control is slightly less for glyburide compared to metformin or rosiglitazone.

Considerable clinical experience exists with metformin and sulfonylureas because they have been available for several decades. It is assumed that the α-glucosidase inhibitors, GLP-1 agonists, DPP-IV inhibitors, and thiazolidinediones, which are newer classes of oral glucose-lowering drugs, will reduce DM-related complications by improving glycemic control, although long-term data are not yet available. The thiazolidinediones are theoretically attractive because they target a fundamental abnormality in type 2 DM, namely insulin resistance. However, all of these agents are currently more costly than metformin and sulfonylureas.

A reasonable treatment algorithm for initial therapy uses metformin as initial therapy because of its efficacy, known side-effect profile, and relatively low cost (Fig. 344-14). Metformin has the advantage that it promotes mild weight loss, lowers insulin levels, and improves the lipid profile slightly. Based on SMBG results and the A1C, the dose of metformin should be increased until the glycemic target is achieved or maximum dose is reached.

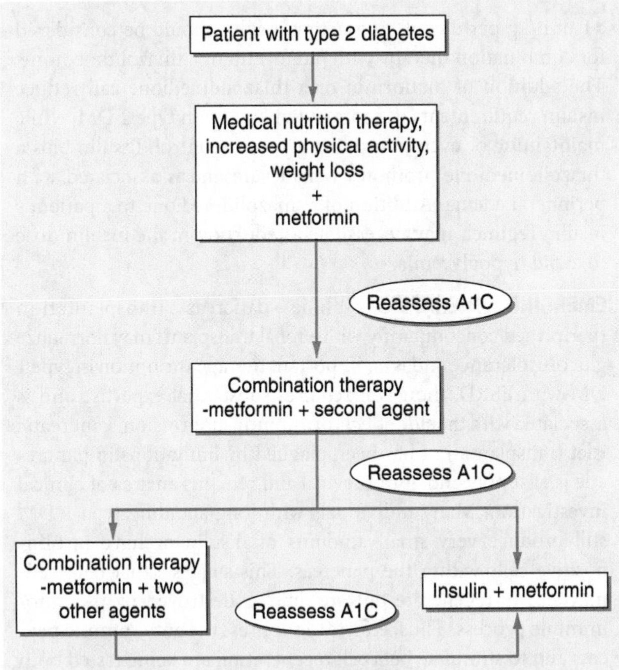

Figure 344-14 Glycemic management of type 2 diabetes. See text for discussion of treatment of severe hyperglycemia or symptomatic hyperglycemia. Agents that can be combined with metformin include insulin secretagogues, thiazolidinediones, α-glucosidase inhibitors, DPP-IV inhibitors, and GLP-1 receptor agonists. A1C, hemoglobin A1C.

Combination Therapy with Glucose-Lowering Agents A number of combinations of therapeutic agents are successful in type 2 DM, and the dosing of agents in combination is the same as when the agents are used alone. Because mechanisms of action of the first and second agents used are different, the effect on glycemic control is usually additive. Several fixed dose combinations of oral agents are available, but evidence that they are superior to titration of single agent to a maximum dose and then addition of a second agent is lacking. If adequate control is not achieved with the combination of two agents (based on reassessment of the A1C every 3 months), a third oral agent or basal insulin should be added (Fig. 344-14).

Treatment with insulin becomes necessary as type 2 DM enters the phase of relative insulin deficiency (as seen in long-standing DM) and is signaled by inadequate glycemic control with one or two oral glucose-lowering agents. Insulin alone or in combination should be used in patients who fail to reach the glycemic target. For example, a single dose of long-acting insulin at bedtime is effective in combination with metformin. As endogenous insulin production falls further, multiple injections of long-acting and short-acting insulin regimens are necessary to control postprandial glucose excursions. These insulin regimens are identical to the long-acting and short-acting combination regimens discussed above for type 1 DM. Since the hyperglycemia of type 2 DM tends to be more "stable," these regimens can be increased in 10% increments every 2–3 days using the FBG results. The daily insulin dose required can become quite large (1–2 units/kg per day) as endogenous insulin production falls and insulin resistance persists. Individuals who require

>1 unit/kg per day of long-acting insulin should be considered for combination therapy with metformin or a thiazolidinedione. The addition of metformin or a thiazolidinedione can reduce insulin requirements in some individuals with type 2 DM, while maintaining or even improving glycemic control. Insulin plus a thiazolidinedione promotes weight gain and is associated with peripheral edema. Addition of a thiazolidinedione to a patient's insulin regimen may necessitate a reduction in the insulin dose to avoid hypoglycemia.

EMERGING THERAPIES Whole pancreas transplantation (performed concomitantly with a renal transplant) may normalize glucose tolerance and is an important therapeutic option in type 1 DM with ESRD, though it requires substantial expertise and is associated with the side effects of immunosuppression. Pancreatic islet transplantation has been plagued by limitations in pancreatic islet supply and graft survival and remains an area of clinical investigation. Many individuals with long-standing type 1 DM still produce very small amounts of insulin or have insulin-positive cells within the pancreas. This suggests that beta cells may slowly regenerate but are quickly destroyed by the autoimmune process. Thus, efforts to suppress the autoimmune process and to stimulate beta cell regeneration are being tested both at the time of diagnosis and in years after the diagnosis of type 1 DM. Closed-loop pumps that infuse the appropriate amount of insulin in response to changing glucose levels are potentially feasible now that continuous glucose-monitoring technology has been developed. New therapies under development for type 2 diabetes include an inhibitor of the sodium-glucose co-transporter in the kidney, activators of glucokinase, an inhibitor of 11 β-hydroxysteroid dehydrogenase-1, and salsalate.

Bariatric surgery for markedly obese individuals with type 2 diabetes has shown considerable promise—sometimes with resolution of the diabetes or major reductions in the needed dose of glucose-lowering therapies (Chap. 78). The ADA clinical guidelines state that bariatric surgery should be considered in individuals with DM and a BMI >35 kg/m^2.

COMPLICATIONS OF THERAPY FOR DIABETES MELLITUS

As with any therapy, the benefits of efforts directed toward glycemic control must be balanced against the risks of treatment. Side effects of intensive treatment include an increased frequency of serious hypoglycemia, weight gain, increased economic costs, and greater demands on the patient. In the DCCT, quality of life was very similar in the intensive and standard therapy groups. The most serious complication of therapy for DM is hypoglycemia, and its treatment with oral glucose or glucagon injection is discussed in Chap. 345. Severe, recurrent hypoglycemia warrants examination of treatment regimen and glycemic goal for the individual patient. Weight gain occurs with most (insulin, insulin secretagogues, thiazolidinediones) but not all (metformin, α-glucosidase inhibitors, GLP-1 receptor agonists, DPP-IV inhibitors) therapies that improve glycemic control. The weight gain is partially due to the anabolic effects of insulin and the reduction in glucosuria. In the DCCT, individuals with the greatest weight gain exhibited increases in LDL cholesterol and triglycerides as well as increases in blood pressure (both systolic and diastolic) similar to those seen in individuals with type 2 DM and insulin resistance. These effects could increase the risk of cardiovascular disease. As discussed previously, transient worsening of diabetic retinopathy or neuropathy sometimes accompanies improved glycemic control. As a result of recent controversies about the optimal glycemic goal and concerns about safety, the FDA now requires information about the cardiovascular safety profile as part of its new evaluation for treatment of type 2 diabetes.

ONGOING ASPECTS OF COMPREHENSIVE DIABETES CARE

The morbidity and mortality rates of DM-related complications can be greatly reduced by timely and consistent surveillance procedures (Table 344-13). These screening procedures are indicated for all individuals with DM, but many individuals with diabetes do not receive comprehensive diabetes care. Screening for dyslipidemia and hypertension should be performed annually. In addition to routine health maintenance, individuals with diabetes should also receive the pneumococcal and tetanus vaccines (at recommended intervals) and the influenza vaccine (annually). As discussed above, aspirin therapy should be considered in many patients with diabetes (primary prevention in type 1 or type 2 DM men >50 years or women >60 years with one risk factor CV disease), but its role in primary prevention in low-risk individuals is uncertain and not recommended.

An annual comprehensive eye examination should be performed by a qualified optometrist or ophthalmologist. If abnormalities are detected, further evaluation and treatment require an ophthalmologist skilled in diabetes-related eye disease. Because many individuals with type 2 DM have had asymptomatic diabetes for several years before diagnosis, the ADA recommends the following ophthalmologic examination schedule: (1) individuals with type 1 DM should have an initial eye examination within 5 years of diagnosis, (2) individuals with type 2 DM should have an initial eye examination at the time of diabetes diagnosis, (3) women with DM who are pregnant or contemplating pregnancy should have an eye examination prior to conception and during the first trimester, and (4) if eye exam is normal, repeat examination in 2–3 years may be appropriate.

An annual foot examination should (1) assess blood flow, sensation (monofilament testing, pin prick, or tuning fork), ankle reflexes, and nail care; (2) look for the presence of foot deformities such as hammer or claw toes and Charcot foot; and (3) identify sites of potential ulceration. The ADA recommends annual screening for distal symmetric neuropathy beginning with the initial diagnosis of diabetes and annual screening for autonomic neuropathy 5 years after diagnosis of type 1 DM and at the time of diagnosis of type 2 DM. This includes testing for loss of protective sensation (LOPS) using monofilament testing plus one of the following tests: vibration, pinprick, ankle reflexes, or vibration perception threshold (using a biothesiometer). If the monofilament test or one of the other tests is abnormal, the patient is diagnosed with LOPS and counseled accordingly. Calluses and nail deformities should be treated by a podiatrist; the patient should be discouraged from self-care of even minor foot problems but should be strongly encouraged to check his or her feet daily for any early lesions. Providers should consider

TABLE 344-13 Guidelines for Ongoing Medical Care for Patients With Diabetes

- Self-monitoring of blood glucose (individualized frequency)
- A1C testing (2–4 times/year)
- Patient education in diabetes management (annual)
- Medical nutrition therapy and education (annual)
- Eye examination (annual)
- Foot examination (1–2 times/year by physician; daily by patient)
- Screening for diabetic nephropathy (annual; see Fig. 344-11)
- Blood pressure measurement (quarterly)
- Lipid profile and serum creatinine (estimate GFR) (annual)
- Influenza/pneumococcal immunizations
- Consider antiplatelet therapy (see text)

Abbreviation: A1C, hemoglobin A1C.

screening for asymptomatic peripheral arterial disease using ankle-brachial index testing in high-risk individuals.

An annual microalbuminuria measurement (albumin-to-creatinine ratio in spot urine) is advised in individuals with type 1 or type 2 DM (Fig. 344-10). The urine protein measurement in a routine urinalysis does not detect these low levels of albumin excretion (microalbuminuria). Screening for microalbuminuria should commence 5 years after the onset of type 1 DM and at the time of diagnosis of type 2 DM. Regardless of protein excretion results, the GFR should be estimated using the serum creatinine in all patients on an annual basis.

SPECIAL CONSIDERATIONS IN DIABETES MELLITUS

PSYCHOSOCIAL ASPECTS

Because the individual with DM can face challenges that affect many aspects of daily life, psychosocial assessment and treatment are a critical part of providing comprehensive diabetes care. The individual with DM must accept that he or she may develop complications related to DM. Even with considerable effort, normoglycemia can be an elusive goal, and solutions to worsening glycemic control may not be easily identifiable. The patient should view him- or herself as an essential member of the diabetes care team and not as someone who is cared for by the diabetes management team. Emotional stress may provoke a change in behavior so that individuals no longer adhere to a dietary, exercise, or therapeutic regimen. This can lead to the appearance of either hyper- or hypoglycemia. Eating disorders, including binge eating disorders, bulimia, and anorexia nervosa, appear to occur more frequently in individuals with type 1 or type 2 DM (Chap. 79).

MANAGEMENT IN THE HOSPITALIZED PATIENT

Virtually all medical and surgical subspecialties are involved in the care of hospitalized patients with diabetes. Hyperglycemia, whether in a patient with known diabetes or in someone without known diabetes, appears to be a predictor of poor outcome in hospitalized patients. General anesthesia, surgery, infection, or concurrent illness raises the levels of counterregulatory hormones (cortisol, growth hormone, catecholamines, and glucagon) and cytokines that may lead to transient insulin resistance and hyperglycemia. These factors increase insulin requirements by increasing glucose production and impairing glucose utilization and thus may worsen glycemic control. The concurrent illness or surgical procedure may lead to variable insulin absorption and also prevent the patient with DM from eating normally and, thus, may promote hypoglycemia. Glycemic control should be assessed on admission using the A1C. Electrolytes, renal function, and intravascular volume status should be assessed as well. The high prevalence of cardiovascular disease in individuals with DM (especially in type 2 DM) may require preoperative cardiovascular evaluation.

The goals of diabetes management during hospitalization are near-normoglycemia, avoidance of hypoglycemia, and transition back to the outpatient diabetes treatment regimen. Glycemic control appears to improve the clinical outcomes in a variety of settings, but optimal glycemic goals for the hospitalized patient are incompletely defined. In a number of cross-sectional studies of patients with diabetes, a greater degree of hyperglycemia was associated with worse cardiac, neurologic, and infectious outcomes. In some studies, patients who do not have preexisting diabetes but who develop modest blood glucose elevations during their hospitalization appear to benefit from achieving near-normoglycemia using insulin treatment. However, a large randomized clinical trial (NICE-SUGAR) of individuals in the intensive care unit (most of whom were receiving mechanical ventilation) found an increased mortality rate and a greater number of episodes of severe hypoglycemia with very strict glycemic control [target BG of 4.5–6 mmol/L or 81–108 mg/dL] compared to individuals with a more moderate glycemic goal (mean blood glucose of 8 mmol/L or 144 mg/dL). Currently, most data suggest that very strict blood glucose control in acutely ill patients likely worsens outcomes and increases the frequency of hypoglycemia. The ADA suggests these glycemic goals for hospitalized patients: (1) in critically ill patients: glucose of 7.8–10.0 mmol/L or 140–180 mg/dL; (2) in non–critically ill patients: pre-meal glucose <7.8 mmol/L (140 mg/dL) and at other times BG <10 mmol/L (180 mg/dL).

The physician caring for an individual with diabetes in the perioperative period, during times of infection or serious physical illness, or simply when the patient is fasting for a diagnostic procedure must monitor the plasma glucose vigilantly, adjust the diabetes treatment regimen, and provide glucose infusion as needed. Hypoglycemia is frequent in hospitalized patients, and many of these episodes are avoidable. Measures to reduce or prevent hypoglycemia include frequent glucose monitoring and anticipating potential modifications of insulin/glucose administration because of changes in the clinical situation or treatment (tapering of glucocorticoids, etc.) or interruption of enteral or parenteral infusions or PO intake.

Depending on the severity of the patient's illness and the hospital setting, the physician can use either an insulin infusion or SC insulin. Insulin infusions are preferred in the ICU or in a clinically unstable setting. The absorption of SC insulin may be variable in such situations. Insulin infusions can also effectively control plasma glucose in the perioperative period and when the patient is unable to take anything by mouth. Regular insulin is preferred over insulin analogues for IV insulin infusion since it is less expensive and equally effective. The physician must consider carefully the clinical setting in which an insulin infusion will be utilized, including whether adequate ancillary personnel are available to monitor the plasma glucose frequently and whether they can adjust the insulin infusion rate to maintain the plasma glucose within the optimal range. Insulin-infusion algorithms should integrate the insulin sensitivity of the patient, frequent blood glucose monitoring, and the trend of changes in the blood glucose to determine the insulin-infusion rate. Insulin-infusion algorithms jointly developed and implemented by nursing and physician staff are advised. Because of the short half-life of IV regular insulin, it is necessary to administer long-acting insulin prior to discontinuation of the insulin infusion (2–4 h) to avoid a period of insulin deficiency.

In patients who are not critically ill or not in the ICU, basal or "scheduled" insulin is provided by SC, long-acting insulin supplemented by prandial and/or "corrective" insulin using a short-acting insulin (insulin analogues preferred). The use of "sliding scale," short-acting insulin alone, where no insulin is given unless the blood glucose is elevated, is inadequate for in-patient glucose management and should not be used. The short-acting, preprandial insulin dose should include coverage for food consumption (based on anticipated carbohydrate intake) plus a corrective or supplemental insulin based on the patient's insulin sensitivity and the blood glucose. For example, if the patient is thin (and likely insulin-sensitive), a corrective insulin supplement might be 1 unit for each 2.7 mmol/L (50 mg/dL) over the glucose target. If the patient is obese and insulin-resistant, then the insulin supplement might be 2 units for each 2.7 mmol/L (50 mg/dL) over the glucose target. It is critical to individualize the regimen and adjust the basal or "scheduled" insulin dose frequently, based on the corrective insulin required. A "consistent carbohydrate diabetes meal plan" for hospitalized patients provides a predictable amount of carbohydrate for a particular meal each day (but not necessarily the same amount for breakfast, lunch, and supper). The hospital diet should be determined by a nutritionist; terms such as *ADA diet* or *low-sugar diet* are no longer used.

Individuals with type 1 DM who are undergoing general anesthesia and surgery, or who are seriously ill, should receive continuous insulin, either through an IV insulin infusion or by SC administration of a reduced dose of long-acting insulin. Short-acting insulin alone is insufficient. Prolongation of a surgical procedure or delay in the recovery room is not uncommon and may result in periods of insulin deficiency leading to DKA. Insulin infusion is the preferred method for managing patients with type 1 DM in the perioperative period or when serious concurrent illness is present (0.5–1.0 units/h of regular insulin). If the diagnostic or surgical procedure is brief and performed under local or regional anesthesia, a reduced dose of SC, long-acting insulin may suffice (30–50% reduction, with short-acting insulin withheld or reduced). This approach facilitates the transition back to long-acting insulin after the procedure. Glucose may be infused to prevent hypoglycemia. The blood glucose should be monitored frequently during the illness or in the perioperative period.

Individuals with type 2 DM can be managed with either an insulin infusion or SC long-acting insulin (25–50% reduction depending on clinical setting) plus preprandial, short-acting insulin. Oral glucose-lowering agents should be discontinued upon admission and are not useful in regulating the plasma glucose in clinical situations where the insulin requirements and glucose intake are changing rapidly. Moreover, these oral agents may be dangerous if the patient is fasting (e.g., hypoglycemia with sulfonylureas). Metformin should be withheld when radiographic contrast media will be given or if severe CHF, acidosis, or declining renal function is present.

Total parenteral nutrition

(See also Chap. 76.) Total parenteral nutrition (TPN) greatly increases insulin requirements. In addition, individuals not previously known to have DM may become hyperglycemic during TPN and require insulin treatment. IV insulin infusion is the preferred treatment for hyperglycemia, and rapid titration to the required insulin dose is done most efficiently using a separate insulin infusion. After the total insulin dose has been determined, insulin may be added directly to the TPN solution or, preferably, given as a separate infusion. Often, individuals receiving either TPN or enteral nutrition receive their caloric loads continuously and not at "meal times"; consequently, SC insulin regimens must be adjusted.

Glucocorticoids

Glucocorticoids increase insulin resistance, decrease glucose utilization, increase hepatic glucose production, and impair insulin secretion. These changes lead to a worsening of glycemic control in individuals with DM and may precipitate diabetes in other individuals ("steroid-induced diabetes"). The effects of glucocorticoids on glucose homeostasis are dose-related, usually reversible, and most pronounced in the postprandial period. If the FPG is near the normal range, oral diabetes agents (e.g., sulfonylureas, metformin) may be sufficient to reduce hyperglycemia. If the FPG >11.1 mmol/L (200 mg/dL), oral agents are usually not efficacious and insulin therapy is required. Short-acting insulin may be required to supplement long-acting insulin in order to control postprandial glucose excursions.

Reproductive issues

Reproductive capacity in either men or women with DM appears to be normal. Menstrual cycles may be associated with alterations in glycemic control in women with DM. Pregnancy is associated with marked insulin resistance; the increased insulin requirements often precipitate DM and lead to the diagnosis of GDM. Glucose, which at high levels is a teratogen to the developing fetus, readily crosses the placenta, but insulin does not. Thus, hyperglycemia from the maternal circulation may stimulate insulin secretion in the fetus. The anabolic and growth effects of insulin may result in macrosomia. GDM complicates ~7% of pregnancies in the United States. The incidence of GDM is greatly increased in certain ethnic groups, including African Americans and Latinas, consistent with a similar increased risk of type 2 DM. Current recommendations advise screening for glucose intolerance between weeks 24 and 28 of pregnancy in women with increased risk for GDM (≥25 years; obesity; family history of DM; member of an ethnic group such as Latina, Native American, Asian American, African American, or Pacific Islander). Therapy for GDM is similar to that for individuals with pregnancy-associated diabetes and involves MNT and insulin, if hyperglycemia persists. Oral glucose-lowering agents are not approved for use during pregnancy, but studies using metformin or glyburide have shown efficacy and have not found toxicity. However, most physicians use insulin to treat GDM. With current practices, the morbidity and mortality rates of the mother with GDM and the fetus are not different from those in the non-diabetic population. Individuals who develop GDM are at marked increased risk for developing type 2 DM in the future and should be screened periodically for DM. Most individuals with GDM revert to normal glucose tolerance after delivery, but some will continue to have overt diabetes or impairment of glucose tolerance after delivery. In addition, children of women with GDM appear to be at risk for obesity and glucose intolerance and have an increased risk of diabetes beginning in the later stages of adolescence.

Pregnancy in individuals with known DM requires meticulous planning and adherence to strict treatment regimens. Intensive diabetes management and normalization of the A1C are essential for individuals with existing DM who are planning pregnancy. The most crucial period of glycemic control is soon after fertilization. The risk of fetal malformations is increased 4–10 times in individuals with uncontrolled DM at the time of conception, and normal plasma glucose during the preconception period and throughout the periods of organ development in the fetus should be the goal.

■ LIPODYSTROPHIC DM

Lipodystrophy, or the loss of subcutaneous fat tissue, may be generalized in certain genetic conditions such as leprechaunism. Generalized lipodystrophy is associated with severe insulin resistance and is often accompanied by acanthosis nigricans and dyslipidemia. Localized lipodystrophy associated with insulin injections has been reduced considerably by the use of human insulin.

Protease inhibitors and lipodystrophy

Protease inhibitors used in the treatment of HIV disease (Chap. 189) have been associated with a centripetal accumulation of fat (visceral and abdominal area), accumulation of fat in the dorsocervical region, loss of extremity fat, decreased insulin sensitivity (elevations of the fasting insulin level and reduced glucose tolerance on IV glucose tolerance testing), and dyslipidemia. Although many aspects of the physical appearance of these individuals resemble Cushing's syndrome, increased cortisol levels do not account for this appearance. The possibility remains that this is related to HIV infection by some undefined mechanism, since some features of the syndrome were observed before the introduction of protease inhibitors. Therapy for HIV-related lipodystrophy is not well established.

FURTHER READINGS

American Diabetes Association: Standards of medical care in diabetes. Diabetes Care 34:S11, 2011

Chan JC et al: Diabetes in Asia: Epidemiology, risk factors, and pathophysiology. JAMA 301:2129, 2009

Grant RW et al: Genetic architecture of type 2 diabetes: Recent progress and clinical implications. Diabetes Care 32:1107, 2009

Holman RR et al: 10-year follow-up of intensive glucose control in type 2 diabetes. N Engl J Med 359:1577, 2008

Kahn SE et al: Glycemic durability of rosiglitazone, metformin, or glyburide monotherapy. N Engl J Med 355:2427, 2006

Kitabchi AE et al: Hyperglycemic crises in adult patients with diabetes. Diabetes Care 32:1335, 2009

Nathan DM et al: Modern-day clinical course of type 1 diabetes mellitus after 30 years' duration: The diabetes control and complications trial/epidemiology of diabetes interventions and complications and Pittsburgh epidemiology of diabetes complications experience (1983–2005). Arch Intern Med 169:1307, 2009

Vaxillaire M, Froguel P: Monogenic diabetes in the young, pharmacogenetics and relevance to multifactorial forms of type 2 diabetes. Endocr Rev 29:254, 2008

CHAPTER 345

Hypoglycemia

Philip E. Cryer
Stephen N. Davis

Hypoglycemia is most commonly caused by drugs used to treat diabetes mellitus or by exposure to other drugs, including alcohol. However, a number of other disorders, including critical organ failure, sepsis and inanition, hormone deficiencies, non–beta-cell tumors, insulinoma, and prior gastric surgery, may cause hypoglycemia (Table 345-1). Hypoglycemia is most convincingly documented by *Whipple's triad:* (1) symptoms consistent with hypoglycemia, (2) a low plasma glucose concentration measured with a precise method (not a glucose monitor), and (3) relief of those symptoms after the plasma glucose level is raised. The lower limit of the fasting plasma glucose concentration is normally approximately 70 mg/dL (3.9 mmol/L), but substantially lower venous glucose levels occur normally, late after a meal. Glucose levels <55 mg/dL (3.0 mmol/L) with symptoms that are relieved promptly after the glucose level is raised document hypoglycemia. Hypoglycemia can cause serious morbidity; if severe and prolonged, it can be fatal. It should be considered in any patient with episodes of confusion, an altered level of consciousness, or a seizure.

TABLE 345-1 Causes of Hypoglycemia in Adults

Ill or medicated individual
1. Drugs
Insulin or insulin secretagogue
Alcohol
Others
2. Critical illness
Hepatic, renal or cardiac failure
Sepsis
Inanition
3. Hormone deficiency
Cortisol
Glucagon and epinephrine (in insulin-deficient diabetes)
4. Non–islet cell tumor
Seemingly well individual
5. Endogenous hyperinsulinism
Insulinoma
Functional beta-cell disorders (nesidioblastosis)
Noninsulinoma pancreatogenous hypoglycemia
Post–gastric bypass hypoglycemia
Insulin autoimmune hypoglycemia
Antibody to insulin
Antibody to insulin receptor
Insulin secretagogue
Other
6. Accidental, surreptitious or malicious hypoglycemia

Source: From PE Cryer et al: J Clin Endocrinol Metab 94:709, 2009. © The Endocrine Society, 2009.

SYSTEMIC GLUCOSE BALANCE AND GLUCOSE COUNTERREGULATION

Glucose is an obligate metabolic fuel for the brain under physiologic conditions. The brain cannot synthesize glucose or store more than a few minutes' supply as glycogen and therefore requires a continuous supply of glucose from the arterial circulation. As the arterial plasma glucose concentration falls below the physiologic range, blood-to-brain glucose transport becomes insufficient to support brain energy metabolism and function. However, redundant glucose counterregulatory mechanisms normally prevent or rapidly correct hypoglycemia.

Plasma glucose concentrations are normally maintained within a relatively narrow range, roughly 70–110 mg/dL (3.9–6.1 mmol/L) in the fasting state with transient higher excursions after a meal, despite wide variations in exogenous glucose delivery from meals and in endogenous glucose utilization by, for example, exercising muscle. Between meals and during fasting, plasma glucose levels are maintained by endogenous glucose production, hepatic glycogenolysis, and hepatic (and renal) gluconeogenesis (Fig. 345-1). Although hepatic glycogen stores are usually sufficient to maintain plasma glucose levels for approximately 8 h, this time period can be shorter if glucose demand is increased by exercise or if glycogen stores are depleted by illness or starvation.

Gluconeogenesis normally requires low insulin levels and the presence of anti-insulin (counterregulatory) hormones, together with a coordinated supply of precursors from muscle and adipose tissue to the liver (and kidneys). Muscle provides lactate, pyruvate, alanine, glutamine, and other amino acids. Triglycerides in adipose tissue are broken down into fatty acids and glycerol, which is a gluconeogenic precursor. Fatty acids provide an alternative oxidative fuel to tissues other than the brain (which requires glucose).

Systemic glucose balance—maintenance of the normal plasma glucose concentration—is accomplished by a network of hormones, neural signals, and substrate effects that regulate endogenous glucose production and glucose utilization by tissues other than the brain (Chap. 344). Among the regulatory factors, insulin plays a

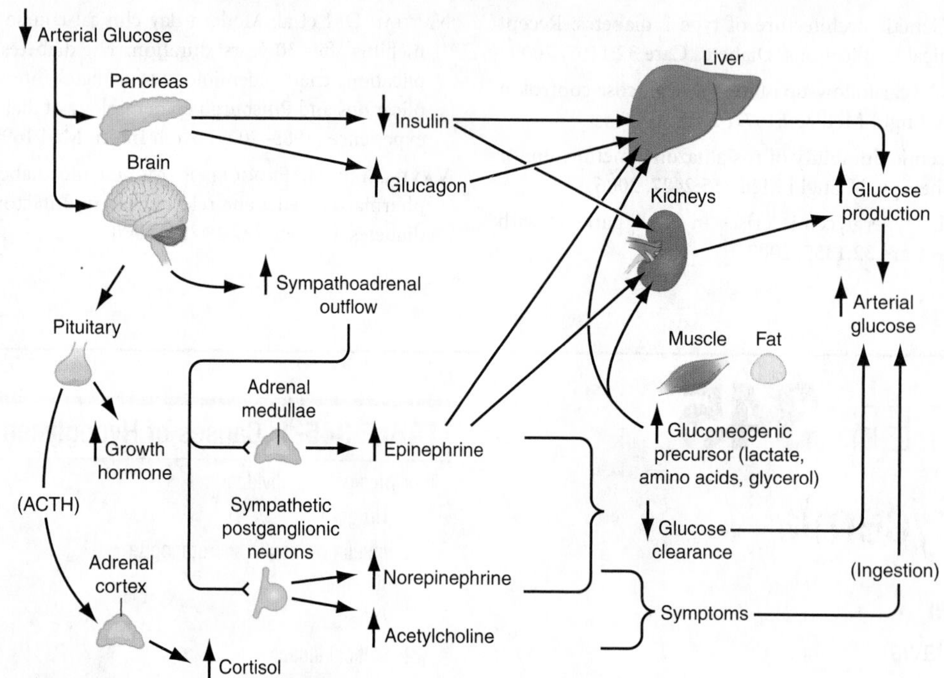

Figure 345-1 Physiology of glucose counterregulation—the mechanisms that normally prevent or rapidly correct hypoglycemia. In insulin-deficient diabetes, the key counterregulatory responses—suppression of insulin and increase of glucagon—are lost, and the stimulation of sympathoadrenal outflow is attenuated.

dominant role (Table 345-2; Fig. 345-1). As plasma glucose levels decline within the physiologic range in the fasting state, pancreatic beta-cell insulin secretion decreases, thereby increasing hepatic glycogenolysis and hepatic (and renal) gluconeogenesis. Low insulin levels also reduce glucose utilization in peripheral tissues, inducing lipolysis and proteolysis, thereby releasing gluconeogenic precursors. Thus, a decrease in insulin secretion is the first defense against hypoglycemia.

As plasma glucose levels decline just below the physiologic range, glucose counterregulatory (plasma glucose–raising) hormones are released (Table 345-2; Fig. 345-1). Among these, pancreatic α-cell glucagon, which stimulates hepatic glycogenolysis, plays a primary role. Glucagon is the second defense against hypoglycemia. Adrenomedullary epinephrine, which stimulates hepatic glycogenolysis and gluconeogenesis (and renal gluconeogenesis), is not normally critical. However, it becomes critical when glucagon is deficient. Epinephrine is the third defense against hypoglycemia. When hypoglycemia is prolonged beyond ~4 hours, cortisol and growth hormone also support glucose production and limit glucose utilization, albeit only ~20% of that of epinephrine.

As plasma glucose levels fall to lower levels, symptoms prompt the behavioral defense against hypoglycemia, including the ingestion of food (Table 345-2; Fig. 345-1).

The normal glycemic thresholds for these responses to decreasing plasma glucose concentrations are shown in Table 345-2. However, these thresholds are dynamic. They shift to higher-than-normal

TABLE 345-2 Physiologic Responses to Decreasing Plasma Glucose Concentrations

Response	Glycemic Threshold, mmol/L (mg/dL)	Physiologic Effects	Role in the Prevention or Correction of Hypoglycemia (Glucose Counterregulation)
↓ Insulin	4.4–4.7 (80–85)	↑ R_a (↓ R_d)	Primary glucose regulatory factor/first defense against hypoglycemia
↑ Glucagon	3.6–3.9 (65–70)	↑ R_a	Primary glucose counterregulatory factor/second defense against hypoglycemia
↑ Epinephrine	3.6–3.9 (65–70)	↑ R_a, ↓ R_c	Third defense against hypoglycemia, critical when glucagon is deficient
↑ Cortisol and growth hormone	3.6–3.9 (65–70)	↑ R_a, ↓ R_c	Involved in defense against prolonged hypoglycemia, not critical
Symptoms	2.8–3.1 (50–55)	Recognition of hypoglycemia	Prompt behavioral defense against hypoglycemia (food ingestion)
↓ Cognition	<2.8 (<50)	—	(Compromises behavioral defense against hypoglycemia)

Note: R_a, rate of glucose appearance, glucose production by the liver and kidneys; R_c, rate of glucose clearance, glucose utilization relative to the ambient plasma glucose concentration; R_d, rate of glucose disappearance, glucose utilization by the brain (which is unaltered by the glucoregulatory hormones) and by insulin-sensitive tissues such as skeletal muscle (which is regulated by insulin, epinephrine, cortisol, and growth hormone).

Source: From PE Cryer: Hypoglycemia, in *Williams Textbook of Endocrinology,* 11th ed, HM Kronenberg et al (eds). Philadelphia, Saunders, 2008.

glucose levels in people with poorly controlled diabetes who can experience symptoms of hypoglycemia when their glucose levels decline into the normal range. On the other hand, they shift to lower-than-normal glucose levels in people with recurrent hypoglycemia, e.g., those with aggressively treated diabetes or an insulinoma. Such patients have symptoms at glucose levels lower than those that cause symptoms in healthy individuals.

CLINICAL MANIFESTATIONS

Neuroglycopenic symptoms of hypoglycemia are the direct result of central nervous system (CNS) glucose deprivation. They include behavioral changes, confusion, fatigue, seizure, loss of consciousness, and, if hypoglycemia is severe and prolonged, death. Neurogenic (or autonomic) symptoms of hypoglycemia are the result of the perception of physiologic changes caused by the CNS-mediated sympathoadrenal discharge triggered by hypoglycemia. They include adrenergic symptoms (mediated largely by norepinephrine released from sympathetic postganglionic neurons but perhaps also by epinephrine released from the adrenal medullae) such as palpitations, tremor, and anxiety. They also include cholinergic symptoms (mediated by acetylcholine released from sympathetic postganglionic neurons) such as sweating, hunger, and paresthesias. Clearly, these are nonspecific symptoms. Their attribution to hypoglycemia requires a corresponding low plasma glucose concentration and their resolution after the glucose level is raised (Whipple's triad).

Common signs of hypoglycemia include diaphoresis and pallor. Heart rate and systolic blood pressure are typically increased but may not be raised in an individual who has experienced repeated, recent episodes of hypoglycemia. Neuroglycopenic manifestations are often observable. Transient focal neurologic deficits occur occasionally. Permanent neurologic deficits are rare.

ETIOLOGY AND PATHOPHYSIOLOGY

Hypoglycemia is most commonly a result of the treatment of diabetes. This topic is therefore addressed before considering other causes of hypoglycemia.

HYPOGLYCEMIA IN DIABETES

Impact and frequency

Hypoglycemia is the limiting factor in the glycemic management of diabetes. First, it causes recurrent morbidity in most people with type 1 diabetes (T1DM) and many with advanced type 2 diabetes (T2DM) and is sometimes fatal. Second, it precludes maintenance of euglycemia over a lifetime of diabetes and thus full realization of the well-established vascular benefits of glycemic control. Third, it causes a vicious cycle of recurrent hypoglycemia by producing hypoglycemia-associated autonomic failure—the clinical syndromes of defective glucose counterregulation and of hypoglycemia unawareness.

Hypoglycemia is a fact of life for people with T1DM. They suffer an average of two episodes of symptomatic hypoglycemia per week and at least one episode of severe, at least temporarily disabling, hypoglycemia each year. An estimated 6–10% of people with T1DM die as a result of hypoglycemia. Hypoglycemia occurs less frequently in T2DM. However, its prevalence in insulin-requiring T2DM is greater than commonly appreciated, Recent studies investigating insulin pump or multiple injection therapies have revealed a hypoglycemia prevalence approaching 70%. Metformin, thiazolidinediones, α-glucosidase inhibitors, glucagon-like peptide-1 (GLP-1) receptor agonists, and dipeptidyl peptidase-IV (DPP-IV) inhibitors should not cause hypoglycemia. However, they increase the risk when combined with an insulin secretagogue, such as one of the sulfonylureas or glinides, or with insulin. Notably, the frequency of hypoglycemia approaches that in T1DM as persons with T2DM develop absolute insulin deficiency and require more complex treatment with insulin.

Conventional risk factors

The conventional risk factors for hypoglycemia in diabetes are based on the premise that relative or absolute insulin excess is the sole determinant of risk. Relative or absolute insulin excess occurs when (1) insulin (or insulin secretagogue) doses are excessive, ill-timed, or of the wrong type; (2) the influx of exogenous glucose is reduced (e.g., during an overnight fast or following missed meals or snacks); (3) insulin-independent glucose utilization is increased (e.g., during exercise); (4) sensitivity to insulin is increased (e.g., with improved glycemic control, in the middle of the night, late after exercise, or with increased fitness or weight loss); (5) endogenous glucose production is reduced (e.g., following alcohol ingestion); and (6) insulin clearance is reduced (e.g., in renal failure). However, these conventional risk factors alone explain a minority of episodes; other factors are typically involved.

Hypoglycemia-associated autonomic failure

While marked insulin excess alone can cause hypoglycemia, iatrogenic hypoglycemia in diabetes is typically the result of the interplay of relative or absolute therapeutic insulin excess and compromised physiologic and behavioral defenses against falling plasma glucose concentrations (Table 345-2; Fig. 345-2). Defective glucose counterregulation compromises physiologic defense (particularly decrements in insulin and increments in glucagon and epinephrine), and hypoglycemia unawareness compromises behavioral defense (ingestion of carbohydrate).

Defective glucose counterregulation In the setting of absolute endogenous insulin deficiency, insulin levels do not decrease as plasma glucose levels fall; the first defense against hypoglycemia is lost. Furthermore, probably because the decrement in intraislet insulin is normally a signal to stimulate glucagon secretion, glucagon levels do not increase as plasma glucose levels fall further; the second defense against hypoglycemia is lost. Finally, the increase in epinephrine levels, the third defense against hypoglycemia, in response to a given level of hypoglycemia is typically attenuated. The glycemic threshold for the sympathoadrenal (adrenomedullary epinephrine and sympathetic neural norepinephrine) response is shifted to lower plasma glucose concentrations. That is typically the result of recent antecedent iatrogenic hypoglycemia. In the setting of absent decrements in insulin and of absent increments in glucagon, the attenuated increment in epinephrine causes the clinical syndrome of defective glucose counterregulation. Affected patients are at twenty-five-fold or greater increased risk of severe iatrogenic hypoglycemia during aggressive glycemic therapy of their diabetes compared with those with normal epinephrine responses. This functional, and reversible, disorder is distinct from classical diabetic autonomic neuropathy, a structural and irreversible disorder.

Hypoglycemia unawareness The attenuated sympathoadrenal response (largely the reduced sympathetic neural response) to hypoglycemia causes the clinical syndrome of hypoglycemia unawareness, i.e., loss of the warning adrenergic and cholinergic symptoms that previously allowed the patient to recognize developing hypoglycemia and therefore abort the episode by ingesting carbohydrates. Affected patients are at a sixfold increased risk of

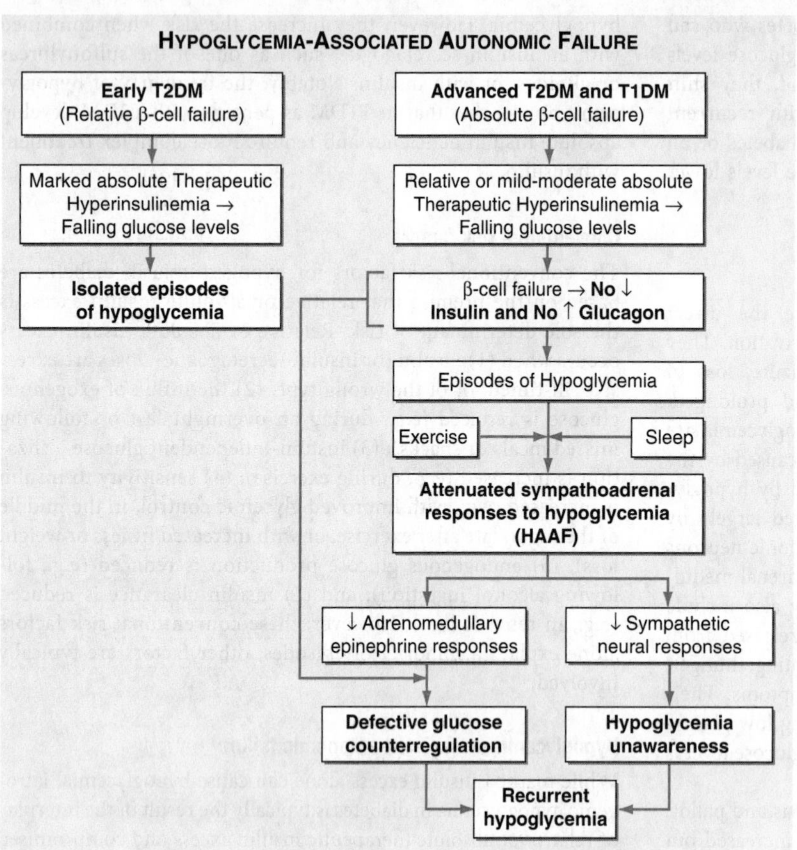

Figure 345-2 Hypoglycemia-associated autonomic failure in insulin-deficient diabetes.

severe iatrogenic hypoglycemia during aggressive glycemic therapy of their diabetes.

Hypoglycemia-associated autonomic failure The concept of hypoglycemia-associated autonomic failure (HAAF) in diabetes posits that recent antecedent iatrogenic hypoglycemia (or sleep or prior exercise) causes both defective glucose counterregulation (by reducing the epinephrine response to a given level of subsequent hypoglycemia in the setting of absent insulin and glucagon responses) and hypoglycemia unawareness (by reducing the sympathoadrenal response to a given level of subsequent hypoglycemia). These impaired responses create a vicious cycle of recurrent iatrogenic hypoglycemia (Fig. 345-2). Hypoglycemia unawareness, and to some extent the reduced epinephrine component of defective glucose counterregulation, is reversible by as little as 2–3 weeks of scrupulous avoidance of hypoglycemia in most affected patients.

Based on this pathophysiology, additional risk factors for hypoglycemia in diabetes include (1) absolute insulin deficiency that indicates that insulin levels will not decrease and glucagon levels will not increase as plasma glucose levels fall; (2) a history of severe hypoglycemia or of hypoglycemia unawareness, implying recent antecedent hypoglycemia, as well as prior exercise or sleep, that indicates that the sympathoadrenal response will be attenuated; and (3) lower HbA_{1C} levels or lower glycemic goals that, all other factors being equal, increase the probability of recent antecedent hypoglycemia.

Hypoglycemia risk factor reduction

Several recent multicenter randomized controlled trials investigating the potential benefits of tight glucose control in either inpatient or outpatient settings have reported a high prevalence of severe hypoglycemia. In the NICE-SUGAR study, attempts to control in-hospital plasma glucose values toward physiologic levels resulted in increased mortality. The ADVANCE, ACCORD, and VADT studies also reported a significant incidence of severe hypoglycemia in T2DM individuals. Somewhat surprisingly, all three studies found little or no benefit of intensive glucose control to reduce macrovascular events in T2DM. In fact, the ACCORD study was ended early due to increased mortality in the intensive glucose control arm. Whether iatrogenic hypoglycemia was the cause of the increased mortality is not known. In the light of the above findings, new recommendations and paradigms have been formulated. Whereas there is little debate regarding the need to reduce hyperglycemia in hospitalized patients, the glycemic maintenance goals have been modified to fall between 140 and 180 mg/dL. Thus, the benefits from insulin therapy and reduced hyperglycemia can be obtained while reducing the prevalence of hypoglycemia.

Similarly, evidence exists that intensive glucose control can reduce the prevalence of microvascular disease in both T1DM and T2DM. These benefits need to be weighed against the increased prevalence of hypoglycemia. The level of glucose control (HBA_{1C}) should be evaluated for each patient. Multicenter trials have demonstrated that patients with recently diagnosed T1DM or T2DM can have better glycemic control with less hypoglycemia. In addition, there is still long-term benefit in reducing HBA_{1C} from higher to lower levels, albeit still above recommended levels. Perhaps a reasonable therapeutic goal is the lowest HBA_{1C} that does not cause severe hypoglycemia and preserves awareness of hypoglycemia.

Pancreatic transplantation (both whole organ and islet cells) has been used as a treatment option for recurrent severe hypoglycemia. Generally, rates of hypoglycemia are reduced following transplantation. This appears to be due to more physiologic insulin and glucagon responses during hypoglycemia following whole organ transplant and resolution of insulin modulation following islet cell transplantation.

The use of continuous glucose monitors appears promising as a method of reducing hypoglycemia while improving HBA_{1C}. Other interventions to stimulate counterregulatory responses such as terbutaline, fluoxetine, thiazolidinediones or fructose remain experimental and have not been subjected to large-scale clinical trials.

Thus, intensive glycemic therapy (Chap. 344) needs to be applied in combination with patient education and empowerment; frequent self-monitoring of blood glucose; flexible insulin (and other drug) regimens including the use of insulin analogues (both short and longer acting); individualized glycemic goals; ongoing professional guidance and support; and consideration of both the conventional risk factors and those indicative of compromised glucose counterregulation. Given a history of hypoglycemia unawareness, a 2- to 3-week period of scrupulous avoidance of hypoglycemia is indicated.

■ HYPOGLYCEMIA WITHOUT DIABETES

There are many causes of hypoglycemia (Table 345-1). Because hypoglycemia is common in insulin- or insulin secretagogue–treated diabetes, it is often reasonable to assume that a clinically suspicious episode was the result of hypoglycemia. On the other hand, because hypoglycemia is rare in the absence of relevant drug-treated diabetes, it is reasonable to conclude that a hypoglycemic disorder is present only in patients in whom Whipple's triad can be demonstrated.

Particularly in patients who are ill or medicated, the initial diagnostic considerations should focus should on medications, and then critical illnesses, hormone deficiency, or nonislet cell tumor hypoglycemia. In the absence of any of these and in a seemingly well individual, the focus should shift to the possibilities of endogenous hyperinsulinism or accidental, surreptitious, or even malicious hypoglycemia.

Drugs

Insulin and insulin secretagogues suppress glucose production and stimulate glucose utilization. Ethanol blocks gluconeogenesis but not glycogenolysis. Thus, alcohol-induced hypoglycemia typically occurs after a several-day ethanol binge during which the person eats little food, thereby causing glycogen depletion. Ethanol is usually measurable in blood at the time of presentation, but its levels correlate poorly with plasma glucose concentrations. Because gluconeogenesis becomes the predominant route of glucose production during prolonged hypoglycemia, alcohol can contribute to the progression of hypoglycemia in patients with insulin-treated diabetes.

A large number of other drugs have been associated with hypoglycemia. These include commonly used drugs such as angiotensin-converting enzyme inhibitors and angiotensin receptor antagonists, β-adrenergic receptor antagonists, quinolone antibiotics, indomethacin, quinine, and sulfonamides among many others.

Critical illness

Among hospitalized patients, serious illnesses such as renal, hepatic, or cardiac failure, sepsis, and inanition are second only to drugs as causes of hypoglycemia.

Rapid and extensive hepatic destruction (e.g., toxic hepatitis) causes fasting hypoglycemia because the liver is the major site of endogenous glucose production. The mechanism of hypoglycemia in patients with cardiac failure is unknown. It may involve hepatic congestion and hypoxia. Although the kidneys are a source of glucose production, hypoglycemia in patients with renal failure is also caused by the reduced clearance of insulin and reduced mobilization of gluconeogenic precursors in renal failure.

Sepsis is a relatively common cause of hypoglycemia. Increased glucose utilization is induced by cytokine production in macrophage-rich tissues such as the liver, spleen, and lung. Hypoglycemia develops if glucose production fails to keep pace. Cytokine-induced inhibition of gluconeogenesis in the setting of nutritional glycogen depletion, in combination with hepatic and renal hypoperfusion, may also contribute to hypoglycemia.

Hypoglycemia can be seen with starvation, perhaps because of loss of whole-body fat stores and subsequent depletion of gluconeogenic precursors (e.g., amino acids), necessitating increased glucose utilization.

Hormone deficiencies

Neither cortisol nor growth hormone is critical to the prevention of hypoglycemia, at least in adults. Nonetheless, hypoglycemia can occur with prolonged fasting in patients with primary adrenocortical failure (Addison's disease) or hypopituitarism. Anorexia and weight loss are typical features of chronic cortisol deficiency and likely result in glycogen depletion. Cortisol deficiency is associated with impaired gluconeogenesis and low levels of gluconeogenic precursors, suggesting that substrate-limited gluconeogenesis, in the setting of glycogen depletion, is the cause of hypoglycemia. Growth hormone deficiency can cause hypoglycemia in young children. In addition to extended fasting, high rates of glucose utilization (e.g., during exercise or in pregnancy) or low rates of glucose production (e.g., following alcohol ingestion) can precipitate hypoglycemia in adults with previously unrecognized hypopituitarism.

Hypoglycemia is not a feature of the epinephrine-deficient state that results from bilateral adrenalectomy, when glucocorticoid replacement is adequate, nor does it occur during pharmacologic adrenergic blockade when other glucoregulatory systems are intact. Combined deficiencies of glucagon and epinephrine play a key role in the pathogenesis of iatrogenic hypoglycemia in people with insulin-deficient diabetes as discussed earlier. Otherwise, deficiencies of these hormones are not usually considered in the differential diagnosis of a hypoglycemic disorder.

Non–beta-cell tumors

Fasting hypoglycemia, often termed non–islet cell tumor hypoglycemia, occurs occasionally in patients with large mesenchymal or epithelial tumors (e.g., hepatomas, adrenocortical carcinomas, carcinoids). The glucose kinetic patterns resemble those of hyperinsulinism (see below), but insulin secretion is suppressed appropriately during hypoglycemia. In most instances, hypoglycemia is due to overproduction of an incompletely processed form of insulin-like growth factor II ("big IGF-II") that does not complex normally with circulating binding proteins and thus more readily gains access to target tissues. The tumors are usually apparent clinically, plasma IGF-II to IGF-I ratios are high and free IGF-II levels [and levels of pro-IGF-II (E1-21)] are elevated. Curative surgery is seldom possible, but reduction of tumor bulk may ameliorate hypoglycemia. Therapy with a glucocorticoid, growth hormone, or both has also been reported to alleviate hypoglycemia. Hypoglycemia attributed to ectopic IGF-I production has been reported but is rare.

Endogenous hyperinsulinism

Hypoglycemia due to endogenous hyperinsulinism can be caused by (1) a primary beta-cell disorder, typically a beta-cell tumor (insulinoma), sometimes multiple insulinomas, or a functional beta-cell disorder with beta-cell hypertrophy or hyperplasia; (2) an antibody to insulin or to the insulin receptor; (3) a beta-cell secretagogue such as a sulfonylurea; or (4) perhaps ectopic insulin secretion among other very rare mechanisms. None of these causes is common.

The fundamental pathophysiologic feature of endogenous hyperinsulinism caused by a primary beta-cell disorder or an insulin secretagogue is the failure of insulin secretion to fall to very low levels during hypoglycemia. This is assessed by measuring plasma insulin, C-peptide (the connecting peptide that is cleaved from proinsulin to produce insulin), proinsulin, and glucose concentrations during hypoglycemia. Insulin, C-peptide, and proinsulin levels need not be high relative to normal, euglycemic values; they are inappropriately high in the setting of a low plasma glucose concentration. Critical diagnostic findings are a plasma insulin concentration ≥3 μU/mL (≥18 pmol/L), a plasma C-peptide concentration ≥0.6 ng/mL (≥0.2 nmol/L) and a plasma proinsulin concentration ≥5.0 pmol/L when the plasma glucose concentration is <55 mg/dL (<3 mmol/L) with symptoms of hypoglycemia. A low plasma β-hydroxybutyrate concentration (≤2.7 mmol/L) and an increment in plasma glucose >25 mg/dL (1.4 mmol/L) following intravenous glucagon (1 mg) indicate increased insulin (or insulin-like growth factor) actions.

The diagnostic strategy is to obtain measurements of plasma glucose, insulin, C-peptide, proinsulin and β-hydroxybutyrate concentrations—and to screen for circulating oral hypoglycemic agents—during an episode of hypoglycemia and to assess symptoms during the episode and seek their resolution following correction of hypoglycemia by intravenous injection of glucagon (i.e., to document Whipple's triad). This approach is straightforward if the patient is hypoglycemic during evaluation. Since endogenous hyperinsulinemic disorders usually, but not invariably, cause fasting hypoglycemia, a diagnostic episode may develop after a relatively short outpatient fast. Serial sampling during an up to 72-h inpatient diagnostic fast or following a mixed meal is more problematic. An alternative is to give the patient a detailed list of the required measurements and ask them to present to an emergency room, with the list, during a symptomatic episode. Obviously, a normal plasma glucose concentration during a symptomatic episode indicates that the symptoms are not the result of hypoglycemia.

An insulinoma, an insulin-secreting pancreatic islet beta-cell tumor, is the prototypical cause of endogenous hyperinsulinism and, therefore, should be sought in patients with the clinical syndrome. However, insulinoma is not the only cause of endogenous hyperinsulinism. Some patients with fasting endogenous hyperinsulinemic hypoglycemia have diffuse islet involvement with beta-cell hypertrophy and sometimes hyperplasia. This pattern is commonly referred to as nesidioblastosis, although the finding of beta-cells budding from ducts is not invariably present. Other patients have a similar islet pattern but postprandial hypoglycemia, a disorder termed noninsulinoma pancreatogenous hypoglycemia. Post–gastric bypass postprandial hypoglycemia also involves diffuse islet involvement and endogenous hyperinsulinism. It most often follows Roux en Y gastric bypass. Some have suggested that exaggerated GLP-1 responses to meals may cause hyperinsulinemia and hypoglycemia, but the pathogenesis has not been clearly established. If medical treatments such as an α-glucosidase inhibitor or octreotide fail, partial pancreatectomy may be required. Autoimmune hypoglycemias include those caused by an antibody to insulin, which gradually disassociates, leading to late postprandial hypoglycemia. Alternatively, an insulin receptor antibody can function as an agonist. The presence of an insulin secretagogue, such as a sulfonylurea or a glinide, results in a clinical and biochemical pattern similar to that of an insulinoma but can be distinguished by the presence of the circulating secretagogue. Finally, very rare phenomena include ectopic insulin secretion, a gain of function insulin receptor mutation, and exercise-induced hyperinsulinemia.

Insulinomas are uncommon—the yearly incidence is estimated to be 1 in 250,000—but because more than 90% are benign, they are a treatable cause of potentially fatal hypoglycemia. The median age at presentation is 50 years in sporadic cases, but it usually presents in the third decade when it is a component of multiple endocrine neoplasia type 1 (Chap. 351). More than 99% of insulinomas are within the substance of the pancreas and they are usually small (90% <2.0 cm). Therefore, they come to clinical attention because of hypoglycemia rather than mass effects. CT or MRI detects approximately 70–80% of insulinomas. These methods detect metastases in the roughly 10% of patients with a malignant insulinoma. Transabdominal ultrasound will often identify insulinomas, and endoscopic ultrasound has a sensitivity of about 90%. Somatostatin receptor scintigraphy is thought to detect insulinomas in about half of patients. Selective pancreatic arterial calcium injections, with the endpoint of a sharp increase in hepatic venous insulin levels, regionalizes insulinomas with high sensitivity, but this invasive procedure is seldom necessary except to confirm endogenous hyperinsulinism in the diffuse islet disorders. Intraoperative pancreatic ultrasonography almost invariably localizes insulinomas that are not readily palpable by the surgeon. Surgical resection of a solitary insulinoma is generally curative. Diazoxide, which inhibits insulin secretion, or the somatostatin analogue octreotide can be used to treat hypoglycemia in patients with unresectable tumors; everolimus, an mTOR (mammalian target of rapamycin) inhibitor, is promising.

ACCIDENTAL, SURREPTITIOUS OR MALICIOUS HYPOGLYCEMIA

Accidental ingestion of an insulin secretagogue (e.g., the result of a pharmacy or other medical error), or administration of insulin, can occur. Factitious hypoglycemia, caused by surreptitious or even malicious administration of insulin or an insulin secretagogue, shares many clinical and laboratory features with insulinoma. It is most common among health care workers, patients with diabetes or their relatives, and people with a history of other factitious illnesses. However, it should be considered in all patients being evaluated for hypoglycemia of obscure cause. Ingestion of an insulin secretagogue causes hypoglycemia with increased C-peptide levels whereas exogenous insulin causes hypoglycemia with low C-peptide levels, reflecting suppression of insulin secretion.

Analytical error in the measurement of plasma glucose concentrations is rare. On the other hand, glucose monitors used to guide treatment of diabetes are not quantitative instruments, particularly at low glucose levels, and these should not be used for the definitive diagnosis of hypoglycemia. Even with a quantitative method, low measured glucose concentrations can be artifactual, e.g., the result of continued glucose metabolism by the formed elements of the blood ex vivo, particularly in the presence of leukocytosis, erythrocytosis, or thrombocytosis, or if separation of the serum from the formed elements is delayed (pseudohypoglycemia).

APPROACH TO THE PATIENT: Hypoglycemia

In addition to recognition and documentation of hypoglycemia, and often urgent treatment, diagnosis of the hypoglycemic mechanism is critical for choosing a treatment that prevents, or at least minimizes, recurrent hypoglycemia.

RECOGNITION AND DOCUMENTATION Hypoglycemia is suspected in patients with typical symptoms; in the presence of confusion, an altered level of consciousness, or a seizure; or in a clinical setting in which hypoglycemia is known to occur. Blood should be drawn, whenever possible, before the administration of glucose to allow documentation of a low plasma glucose concentration. Convincing documentation of hypoglycemia requires the fulfillment of Whipple's triad. Thus, the ideal time to measure the plasma glucose level is during a symptomatic episode. A normal glucose level excludes hypoglycemia as the cause of the symptoms. A low glucose level confirms that hypoglycemia is the cause of the symptoms, provided the latter resolve after the glucose level is raised. When the cause of the hypoglycemic episode is obscure, additional measurements, while the glucose level is low and before treatment, should include plasma insulin, C-peptide, proinsulin and β-hydroxybutyrate levels, as well as screening for circulating oral hypoglycemic agents, and symptoms should be assessed during and after the plasma glucose concentration is raised.

When the history suggests prior hypoglycemia, and a potential mechanism is not apparent, the diagnostic strategy is to measure these values, and assess for Whipple's triad, during and after an episode of hypoglycemia. On the other hand, while it cannot be ignored, a distinctly low plasma glucose concentration measured in a patient without corresponding symptoms raises the possibility of an artifact (pseudohypoglycemia).

DIAGNOSIS OF THE HYPOGLYCEMIC MECHANISM In a patient with documented hypoglycemia, a plausible hypoglycemic mechanism can often be deduced from the history, physical examination, and available laboratory data (Table 345-1). Drugs, particularly those used to treat diabetes or alcohol, should be the first consideration, even in the absence of known use of a relevant drug, given the possibility of surreptitious, accidental, or malicious drug administration. Other considerations include evidence of a relevant critical illness, less commonly hormone deficiencies, and rarely a non–beta-cell tumor that can be pursued diagnostically. Absent one of these mechanisms, in an otherwise seemingly well individual, one should consider endogenous hyperinsulinism and proceed with measurements and assessment of symptoms during spontaneous hypoglycemia or under conditions that might elicit hypoglycemia.

URGENT TREATMENT Oral treatment with glucose tablets or glucose-containing fluids, candy, or food is appropriate if the patient is able and willing to take these. A reasonable initial dose is 20 g of glucose. If the patient is unable or unwilling, because of neuroglycopenia, to take carbohydrates orally, parenteral therapy is necessary. Intravenous glucose (25 g) should be given and followed by a glucose infusion guided by serial plasma glucose measurements. If intravenous therapy is not practical, subcutaneous or intramuscular glucagon (1.0 mg in adults) can be used, particularly in patients with T1DM. Because it acts by stimulating glycogenolysis, glucagon is ineffective in glycogen-depleted individuals (e.g., those with alcohol-induced hypoglycemia). It also stimulates insulin secretion and is therefore less useful in T2DM. These treatments raise plasma glucose concentrations only transiently, and patients should therefore be urged to eat as soon as is practical to replete glycogen stores.

PREVENTION OF RECURRENT HYPOGLYCEMIA Prevention of recurrent hypoglycemia requires an understanding of the hypoglycemic mechanism. Offending drugs can be discontinued or their doses reduced. Hypoglycemia caused by a sulfonylurea can persist for hours, or even days. Underlying critical illnesses can often be treated. Cortisol and growth hormone can be replaced if they are deficient. Surgical, radiotherapeutic, or chemotherapeutic reduction of a non-islet cell tumor can alleviate hypoglycemia even if the tumor cannot be cured; glucocorticoid or growth hormone administration also may reduce hypoglycemic episodes in such patients. Surgical resection of an insulinoma is curative; medical therapy with diazoxide or octreotide can be used if resection is not possible and in patients with a nontumor beta-cell disorder. Partial pancreatectomy may be necessary in the latter patients. The treatment of autoimmune hypoglycemia (e.g., with a glucocorticoid or immunosuppressive drugs) is problematic, but the disorders are sometimes self-limited. Failing these treatments, frequent feedings and avoidance of fasting may be required. Administration of uncooked cornstarch at bedtime or even an overnight intragastric infusion of glucose may be necessary in some patients.

FURTHER READINGS

The Advance Collaborative Group: Intensive blood glucose control and vascular outcomes in patients with type 2 diabetes. N Engl J Med 358:2560, 2008

Cryer PE: *Hypoglycemia in Diabetes. Pathophysiology, Prevalence and Prevention*. Alexandria, VA, American Diabetes Association, 2009

——— et al: Evaluation and management of adult hypoglycemic disorders: An Endocrine Society clinical practice guideline. J Clin Endocrinol Metab 94:709, 2009

———: Hypoglycemia, in *Williams Textbook of Endocrinology*, 12th ed, S Melmed et al (eds). Philadelphia, Saunders, in press

Davis SN: Diabetes: Hypoglycemia—A new approach to an old problem. Nat Rev Endocrinol 5:243, 2009

——— et al: Effects of intensive therapy and antecedent hypoglycemia on counterregulatory responses to hypoglycemia in type 2 diabetes. Diabetes 58:701, 2009

Murad MH et al: Drug-induced hypoglycemia: A systematic review. J Clin Endocrinol Metab 94:741, 2009

The Nice-Sugar Study Investigators: Intensive versus conventional glucose control in critically ill patients. N Engl J Med 360:1283, 2009

CHAPTER **346**

Disorders of the Testes and Male Reproductive System

Shalender Bhasin
J. Larry Jameson

The male reproductive system regulates sex differentiation, virilization, and the hormonal changes that accompany puberty, ultimately leading to spermatogenesis and fertility. Under the control of the pituitary hormones—luteinizing hormone (LH) and follicle-stimulating hormone (FSH)—the Leydig cells of the testes produce testosterone and germ cells are nurtured by Sertoli cells to divide, differentiate, and mature into sperm. During embryonic development, testosterone and dihydrotestosterone (DHT) induce the wolffian duct and virilization of the external genitalia. During puberty, testosterone promotes somatic growth and the development of secondary sex characteristics. In adults, testosterone is necessary for spermatogenesis, stimulation of libido, normal sexual function, and maintenance of muscle and bone mass. This chapter focuses on the physiology of the testes and disorders associated with decreased androgen production, which may be caused by gonadotropin deficiency or primary testis dysfunction. A variety of testosterone formulations now allow more physiologic androgen replacement. Infertility occurs in ~5% of men and is increasingly amenable to treatment by hormone replacement or by using sperm transfer techniques. For further discussion of sexual dysfunction, disorders of the prostate, and testicular cancer, see Chaps. 48, 95, and 96, respectively.

DEVELOPMENT AND STRUCTURE OF THE TESTIS

The fetal testis develops from the undifferentiated gonad after expression of a genetic cascade that is initiated by the SRY (sex-related gene on the Y chromosome) (Chap. 349). SRY induces differentiation of Sertoli cells, which surround germ cells and, together with peritubular myoid cells, form testis cords that later develop into seminiferous tubules. Fetal Leydig cells and endothelial cells migrate into the gonad from the adjacent mesonephros but also may arise from interstitial cells that reside between testis cords. Leydig cells produce testosterone, which supports the growth and differentiation of wolffian duct structures that develop into the epididymis, vas deferens, and seminal vesicles. Testosterone is also converted to DHT (see below), which induces formation of the prostate and the external male genitalia, including the penis, urethra, and scrotum. Testicular descent through the inguinal canal is controlled in part by Leydig cell production of insulin-like factor 3 (INSL3), which acts via a receptor termed LGR8 (leucine-rich repeat-containing G protein–coupled receptor 8, also known as GREAT: *G* protein–coupled *re*ceptor *a*ffecting *t*estis descent). Sertoli cells produce müllerian inhibiting substance (MIS), which causes regression of the müllerian structures, including the fallopian tube, uterus, and upper segment of the vagina.

NORMAL MALE PUBERTAL DEVELOPMENT

Although *puberty* commonly refers to the maturation of the reproductive axis and the development of secondary sex characteristics, it involves a coordinated response of multiple hormonal systems

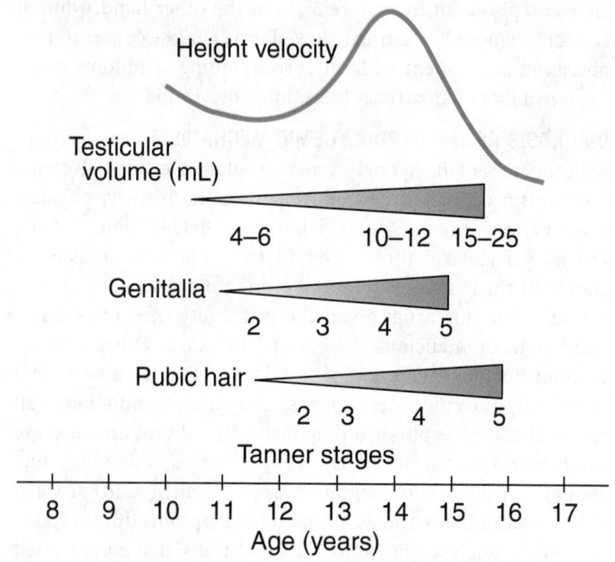

Figure 346-1 Pubertal events in males. Sexual maturity ratings for genitalia and pubic hair and divided into five stages. *(From WA Marshall, JM Tanner: Arch Dis Child 45:13, 1970.)*

that include the adrenal gland and the growth hormone (GH) axis (Fig. 346-1). The development of secondary sex characteristics is initiated by *adrenarche*, which usually occurs between 6 and 8 years of age when the adrenal gland begins to produce greater amounts of androgens from the zona reticularis, the principal site of dehydroepiandrosterone (DHEA) production. The sex maturation process is greatly accelerated by the activation of the hypothalamic-pituitary axis and the production of gonadotropin-releasing hormone (GnRH). The GnRH pulse generator in the hypothalamus is active during fetal life and early infancy but is restrained until the early stages of puberty by a neuroendocrine brake imposed by the inhibitory actions of glutamate, γ-amino butyric acid (GABA), and neuropeptide Y. Although the pathways that initiate reactivation of the GnRH pulse generator at the onset of puberty have been elusive, mounting evidence supports involvement of GPR54, a G protein–coupled receptor that binds an endogenous ligand, kisspeptin. Individuals with mutations of GPR54 fail to enter puberty, and experiments in primates demonstrate that infusion of kisspeptin is sufficient to induce premature puberty. Kisspeptin signaling plays an important role in mediating the feedback action of sex steroids on gonadotropin secretion and in regulating the tempo of sexual maturation at puberty. Leptin, a hormone produced by adipose cells, plays a permissive role in the resurgence of GnRH secretion at the onset of puberty, as leptin-deficient individuals also fail to enter puberty (Chap. 77).

The early stages of puberty are characterized by nocturnal surges of LH and FSH. Growth of the testes is usually the first sign of puberty, reflecting an increase in seminiferous tubule volume. Increasing levels of testosterone deepen the voice and increase muscle growth. Conversion of testosterone to DHT leads to growth of the external genitalia and pubic hair. DHT also stimulates prostate and facial hair growth and initiates recession of the temporal hairline. The growth spurt occurs at a testicular volume of about 10–12 mL. GH increases early in puberty and is stimulated in part by the rise in gonadal steroids. GH increases the level of insulin-like growth factor I (IGF-I), which enhances linear bone growth. The prolonged pubertal exposure to gonadal steroids (mainly estradiol) ultimately causes epiphyseal closure and limits further bone growth.

REGULATION OF TESTICULAR FUNCTION

REGULATION OF THE HYPOTHALAMIC-PITUITARY-TESTIS AXIS IN ADULT MEN

Hypothalamic GnRH regulates the production of the pituitary gonadotropins LH and FSH (Fig. 346-2). GnRH is released in discrete pulses approximately every 2 hours, resulting in corresponding pulses of LH and FSH. These dynamic hormone pulses account in part for the wide variations in LH and testosterone even within the same individual. LH acts primarily on the Leydig cell to stimulate testosterone synthesis. The regulatory control of androgen synthesis is mediated by testosterone and estrogen feedback on both the hypothalamus and the pituitary. FSH acts on the Sertoli cell to regulate spermatogenesis and the production of Sertoli products such as inhibin B, which acts to suppress pituitary FSH selectively. Despite these somewhat distinct Leydig and Sertoli cell–regulated pathways, testis function is integrated at several levels: GnRH regulates both gonadotropins; spermatogenesis requires high levels of testosterone; numerous paracrine interactions between Leydig and Sertoli cells are necessary for normal testis function.

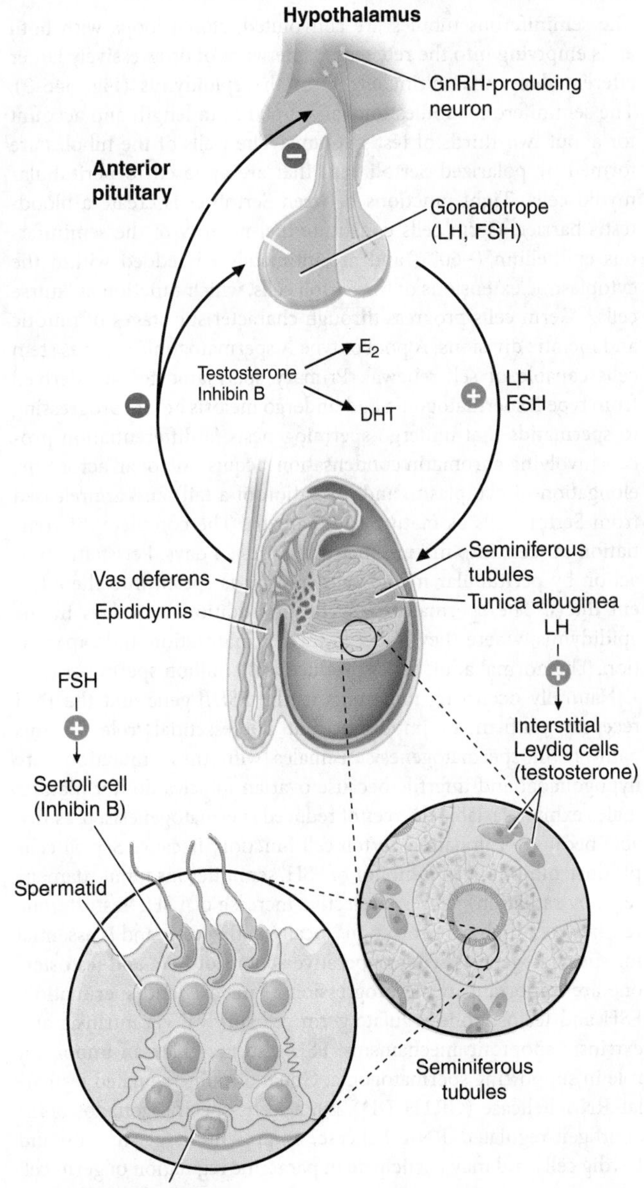

Figure 346-2 Human pituitary gonadotropin axis, structure of testis, seminiferous tubule. E_2, 17β–estradiol; DHT, dihydrotestosterone.

THE LEYDIG CELL: ANDROGEN SYNTHESIS

LH binds to its seven transmembrane, G protein–coupled receptor to activate the cyclic AMP pathway. Stimulation of the LH receptor induces *st*eroid *a*cute *r*egulatory (StAR) protein, along with several steroidogenic enzymes involved in androgen synthesis. LH receptor mutations cause Leydig cell hypoplasia or agenesis, underscoring the importance of this pathway for Leydig cell development and function. The rate-limiting process in testosterone synthesis is the delivery of cholesterol by the StAR protein to the inner mitochondrial membrane. Peripheral benzodiazepine receptor, a mitochondrial cholesterol-binding protein, is also an acute regulator of Leydig cell steroidogenesis. The five major enzymatic steps involved in testosterone synthesis are summarized in Fig. 346-3. After cholesterol transport into the mitochondrion, the formation of pregnenolone by CYP11A1 (side chain cleavage enzyme) is a limiting enzymatic step. The 17α-hydroxylase and the 17,20-lyase reactions are catalyzed by a single enzyme, CYP17; posttranslational modification (phosphorylation) of this enzyme and the presence of specific enzyme cofactors confer 17,20-lyase activity selectively in the testis and zona reticularis of the adrenal gland. Testosterone can be converted to the more potent DHT by 5α-reductase, or it can

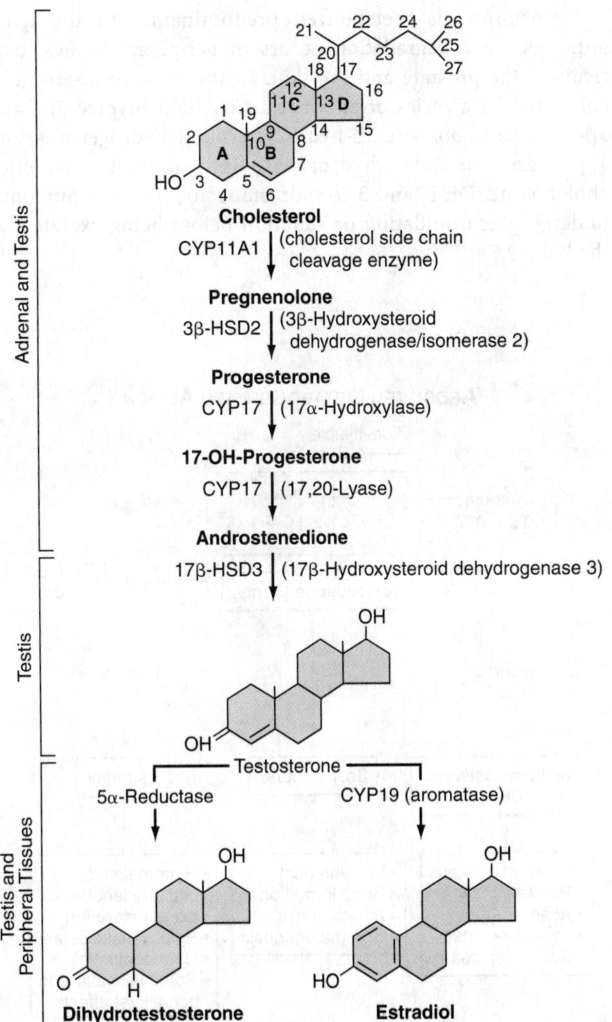

Figure 346-3 The biochemical pathway in the conversion of 27-carbon sterol cholesterol to androgens and estrogens.

be aromatized to estradiol by CYP19 (aromatase). Two isoforms of steroid 5α-reductase, SRD5A1 and SRD5A2, have been described; all known individuals with clinical features of 5α-reductase deficiency have mutations in SRD5A2, the predominant form in the prostate and the skin.

Testosterone transport and metabolism

In males, 95% of circulating testosterone is derived from testicular production (3–10 mg/d). Direct secretion of testosterone by the adrenal and peripheral conversion of androstenedione to testosterone collectively account for another 0.5 mg/d of testosterone. Only a small amount of DHT (70 μg/d) is secreted directly by the testis; most circulating DHT is derived from peripheral conversion of testosterone. Most of the daily production of estradiol (approximately 45 μg/d) in men is derived from aromatase-mediated peripheral conversion of testosterone and androstenedione.

Circulating testosterone is bound to two plasma proteins: sex hormone–binding globulin (SHBG) and albumin (Fig. 346-4). SHBG binds testosterone with much greater affinity than albumin. Only 0.5–3% of testosterone is unbound. According to the "free hormone" hypothesis, only the unbound fraction is biologically active; however, albumin-bound hormone dissociates readily in the capillaries and may be bioavailable. SHBG concentrations are decreased by androgens, obesity, diabetes mellitus, insulin, and nephrotic syndrome. Conversely, estrogen administration, hyperthyroidism, many chronic inflammatory illnesses, and aging are associated with high SHBG concentrations.

Testosterone is metabolized predominantly in the liver, although some degradation occurs in peripheral tissues, particularly the prostate and the skin. In the liver, testosterone is converted by a series of enzymatic steps that involve 5α- and 5β-reductases, 3α- and 3β-hydroxysteroid dehydrogenases, and 17β-hydroxysteroid dehydrogenase into androsterone, etiocholanolone, DHT, and 3-α-androstanediol. These compounds undergo glucuronidation or sulfation before being excreted by the kidneys.

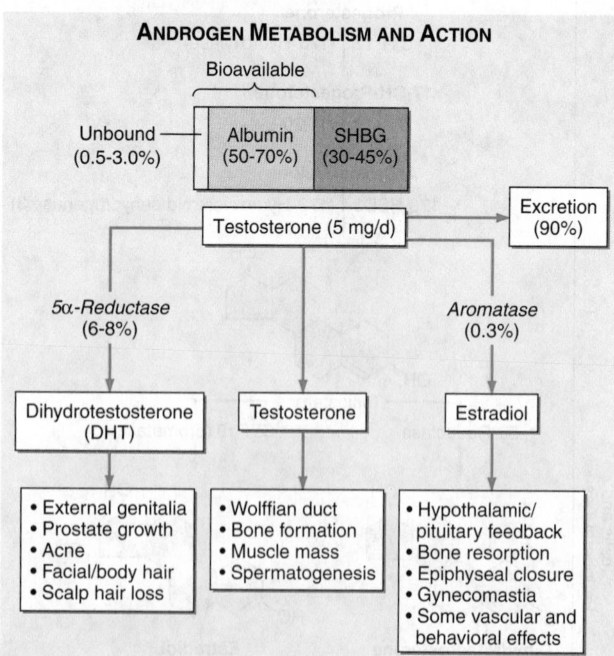

Figure 346-4 Androgen metabolism and actions. SHBG, sex hormone–binding globulin.

Mechanism of androgen action

The androgen receptor (AR) is structurally related to the nuclear receptors for estrogen, glucocorticoids, and progesterone (Chap. 338). The AR is encoded by a gene on the long arm of the X chromosome and has a molecular mass of about 110 kDa. A polymorphic region in the amino terminus of the receptor, which contains a variable number of glutamine repeats, modifies the transcriptional activity of the receptor. The AR protein is distributed in both the cytoplasm and the nucleus. Ligand binding to the AR induces conformational changes that allow the recruitment and assembly of tissue-specific cofactors and causes it to translocate into the nucleus, where it binds to DNA or other transcription factors already bound to DNA. Thus, the AR is a ligand-regulated transcription factor. Some androgen effects may be mediated by nongenomic AR signal transduction pathways. Testosterone binds to AR with one-half the affinity of DHT. The DHT-AR complex also has greater thermostability and a slower dissociation rate than the testosterone-AR complex. However, the molecular basis for selective testosterone versus DHT actions has not been explained completely.

THE SEMINIFEROUS TUBULES: SPERMATOGENESIS

The seminiferous tubules are convoluted, closed loops with both ends emptying into the rete testis, a network of progressively larger efferent ducts that ultimately form the epididymis (Fig. 346-2). The seminiferous tubules total about 600 m in length and account for about two-thirds of testis volume. The walls of the tubules are formed by polarized Sertoli cells that are apposed to peritubular myoid cells. Tight junctions between Sertoli cells create a blood-testis barrier. Germ cells constitute the majority of the seminiferous epithelium (~60%) and are intimately embedded within the cytoplasmic extensions of the Sertoli cells, which function as "nurse cells." Germ cells progress through characteristic stages of mitotic and meiotic divisions. A pool of type A spermatogonia serve as stem cells capable of self-renewal. Primary spermatocytes are derived from type B spermatogonia and undergo meiosis before progressing to spermatids that undergo spermiogenesis (a differentiation process involving chromatin condensation, acquisition of an acrosome, elongation of cytoplasm, and formation of a tail) and are released from Sertoli cells as mature spermatozoa. The complete differentiation process into mature sperm requires 74 days. Peristaltic-type action by peritubular myoid cells transports sperm into the efferent ducts. The spermatozoa spend an additional 21 days in the epididymis, where they undergo further maturation and capacitation. The normal adult testes produce >100 million sperm per day.

Naturally occurring mutations in the *FSHβ* gene and the FSH receptor confirm an important, but not essential, role for this pathway in spermatogenesis. Females with these mutations are hypogonadal and infertile because ovarian follicles do not mature; males exhibit variable degrees of reduced spermatogenesis, presumably because of impaired Sertoli cell function. Because Sertoli cells produce inhibin B, an inhibitor of FSH, seminiferous tubule damage (e.g., by radiation) causes a selective increase of FSH. Testosterone reaches very high concentrations locally in the testis and is essential for spermatogenesis. The cooperative actions of FSH and testosterone are important in the progression of meiosis and spermiation. FSH and testosterone regulate germ cell survival via intrinsic and extrinsic apoptotic mechanisms. FSH also may play an important role in supporting spermatogonia. Gonadotropin-regulated testicular RNA helicase (GRTH/DDX25), a testis-specific gonadotropin/androgen-regulated RNA helicase, is present in germ cells and Leydig cells and may participate in paracrine regulation of germ cell development.

A number of knockout mouse models exhibit impaired germ cell development or spermatogenesis, presaging possible mutations associated with male infertility. The human Y chromosome contains a small pseudoautosomal region that can recombine with homologous regions of the X chromosome. Most of the Y chromosome does not recombine with the X chromosome and is referred to as the male-specific region of the Y (MSY). The MSY contains 156 transcription units that encode for 26 proteins, including nine families of Y-specific multicopy genes; many of these Y-specific genes are also testis-specific and necessary for spermatogenesis. Microdeletions of several Y chromosome azoospermia factor (*AZF*) genes (e.g., RNA-binding motif, *RBM*; deleted in azoospermia, *DAZ*) are associated with oligospermia or azoospermia.

TREATMENT Male Factor Infertility

Treatment options for male factor infertility have expanded greatly in recent years. Secondary hypogonadism is highly amenable to treatment with gonadotropins (see below). Assisted reproductive technologies such as in vitro fertilization (IVF) and intracytoplasmic sperm injection (ICSI) have provided new opportunities for patients with male factor infertility primary testicular failure and disorders of sperm transport. Choice of initial treatment options depends on sperm concentration and motility. Expectant management should be attempted initially in men with mild male factor infertility (sperm count 15–20 × 10^6/mL and normal motility). Moderate male factor infertility (10–15 × 10^6/mL and 20–40% motility) should begin with intrauterine insemination alone or in combination with treatment of the female partner with clomiphene or gonadotropins, but it may require IVF with or without ICSI. For men with a severe defect (sperm count <10 × 10^6/mL, 10% motility), IVF with ICSI or donor sperm should be used.

CLINICAL AND LABORATORY EVALUATION OF MALE REPRODUCTIVE FUNCTION

HISTORY AND PHYSICAL EXAMINATION

The history should focus on developmental stages such as puberty and growth spurts, as well as androgen-dependent events such as early-morning erections, frequency and intensity of sexual thoughts, and frequency of masturbation or intercourse. Although libido and the overall frequency of sexual acts are decreased in androgen-deficient men, young hypogonadal men may achieve erections in response to visual erotic stimuli. Men with acquired androgen deficiency often report decreased energy and increased irritability.

The physical examination should focus on secondary sex characteristics such as hair growth, gynecomastia, testicular volume, prostate, and height and body proportions. *Eunuchoid proportions* are defined as an arm span >2 cm greater than height and suggest that androgen deficiency occurred before epiphyseal fusion. Hair growth on the face, axilla, chest, and pubic regions is androgen-dependent; however, changes may not be noticeable unless androgen deficiency is severe and prolonged. Ethnicity also influences the intensity of hair growth (Chap. 49). Testicular volume is best assessed by using a Prader orchidometer. Testes range from 3.5 to 5.5 cm in length, which corresponds to a volume of 12–25 mL. Advanced age does not influence testicular size, although the consistency becomes less firm. Asian men generally have smaller testes than Western Europeans, independent of differences in body size. Because of its possible role in infertility, the presence of varicocele should be sought by palpation while the patient is standing; it is more common on the left side. Patients with Klinefelter's syndrome have markedly reduced testicular volumes (1–2 mL). In congenital hypogonadotropic hypogonadism, testicular volumes provide a good index for the degree of gonadotropin deficiency and the likelihood of response to therapy.

GONADOTROPIN AND INHIBIN MEASUREMENTS

LH and FSH are measured by using two-site immunoradiometric, immunofluorometric, or chemiluminescent assays, which have very low cross-reactivity with other pituitary glycoprotein hormones and human chorionic gonadotropin (hCG) and have sufficient sensitivity to measure the low levels present in patients with hypogonadotropic hypogonadism. In men with a low testosterone level, an LH level can distinguish primary (high LH) from secondary (low or inappropriately normal LH) hypogonadism. An elevated LH level indicates a primary defect at the testicular level, whereas a low or inappropriately normal LH level suggests a defect at the hypothalamic-pituitary level. LH pulses occur about every 1–3 hours in normal men. Thus, gonadotropin levels fluctuate, and samples should be pooled or repeated when results are equivocal. FSH is less pulsatile than LH because it has a longer half-life. Selective increase in FSH suggests damage to the seminiferous tubules. Inhibin B, a Sertoli cell product that suppresses FSH, is reduced with seminiferous tubule damage. Inhibin B is a dimer with α-β_B subunits and is measured by two-site immunoassays.

GnRH stimulation testing

The GnRH test is performed by measuring LH and FSH concentrations at baseline and at 30 and 60 minutes after intravenous administration of 100 μg of GnRH. A minimally acceptable response is a twofold LH increase and a 50% FSH increase. In the prepubertal period or with severe GnRH deficiency, the gonadotrope may not respond to a single bolus of GnRH because it has not been primed by endogenous hypothalamic GnRH. With the advent of highly sensitive gonadotropin assays, this test is rarely used in practice.

TESTOSTERONE ASSAYS

Total testosterone

Total testosterone includes both unbound and protein-bound testosterone and is measured by radioimmunoassays, immunometric assays, or liquid chromatography tandem mass spectrometry (LC-MS/MS). LC-MS/MS involves extraction of serum by organic solvents, separation of testosterone from other steroids by high-performance liquid chromatography and mass spectrometry, and quantitation of unique testosterone fragments by mass spectrometry. LC-MS/MS provides accurate and sensitive measurements of testosterone levels even in the low range and is emerging as the method of choice for testosterone measurement. A single random sample provides a good approximation of the average testosterone concentration with the realization that testosterone levels fluctuate in response to pulsatile LH. Testosterone is generally lower in the late afternoon and is reduced by acute illness. The testosterone concentration in healthy young men ranges from 300 to 1000 ng/dL in most laboratories, although these reference ranges are not derived from population-based random samples. Alterations in SHBG levels due to aging, obesity, diabetes mellitus, hyperthyroidism, some types of medications, or chronic illness or on a congenital basis can affect total testosterone levels. Heritable factors contribute substantially to the population-level variation in testosterone levels. Genomewide association studies have revealed polymorphisms in the SHBG gene as important contributors to variation in testosterone levels.

Measurement of unbound testosterone levels

Most circulating testosterone is bound to SHBG and to albumin; only 0.5–3% of circulating testosterone is unbound, or "free." The unbound testosterone concentration can be measured by equilibrium dialysis or calculated from total testosterone, SHBG, and albumin concentrations by using published mass-action equations. Tracer analogue methods are relatively inexpensive and convenient but are inaccurate. *Bioavailable testosterone* refers to unbound testosterone plus testosterone that is loosely bound to albumin; it can be measured by the ammonium sulfate precipitation method.

hCG stimulation test

The hCG stimulation test is performed by administering a single injection of 1500–4000 IU of hCG intramuscularly and measuring testosterone levels at baseline and 24, 48, 72, and 120 hours after hCG injection. An alternative regimen involves three injections of 1500 units of hCG on successive days and measurement of testosterone levels 24 hours after the last dose. An acceptable response to hCG is a doubling of the testosterone concentration in adult men. In prepubertal boys, an increase in testosterone to >150 ng/dL indicates the presence of testicular tissue. No response may indicate an absence of testicular tissue or marked impairment of Leydig cell function. Measurement of MIS, a Sertoli cell product, is also used to detect the presence of testes in prepubertal boys with cryptorchidism.

SEMEN ANALYSIS

Semen analysis is the most important step in the evaluation of male infertility. Samples are collected by masturbation after a period of abstinence of 2–3 days. Semen volumes and sperm concentrations vary considerably among fertile men, and several samples may be needed before it is possible to conclude that the results are abnormal. Analysis should be performed within an hour of collection. The normal ejaculate volume is 2–6 mL and contains sperm counts >20 million/mL, with a motility of >50% and >15% normal morphology. Some men with low sperm counts are nevertheless fertile. A variety of tests for sperm function can be performed in specialized laboratories, but they add relatively little to the treatment options.

TESTICULAR BIOPSY

Testicular biopsy is useful in some patients with oligospermia or azoospermia as an aid in diagnosis and an indication for the feasibility of treatment. Using local anesthesia, fine-needle aspiration biopsy is performed to aspirate tissue for histology. Alternatively, open biopsies can be performed under local or general anesthesia when more tissue is required. A normal biopsy in an azoospermic man with a normal FSH level suggests obstruction of the vas deferens, which may be correctable surgically. Biopsies are also used to harvest sperm for ICSI and to classify disorders such as hypospermatogenesis (all stages present but in reduced numbers), germ cell arrest (usually at primary spermatocyte stage), and Sertoli cell–only syndrome (absent germ cells) or hyalinization (sclerosis with absent cellular elements).

DISORDERS OF SEXUAL DIFFERENTIATION

See Chap. 349.

DISORDERS OF PUBERTY

The onset and tempo of puberty vary greatly in the general population and are affected by genetic and environmental factors. Although some of the variance in the timing of puberty is explained by heritable factors, the genes involved, and their relative contributions to the timing of puberty are not known.

PRECOCIOUS PUBERTY

Puberty in boys before age 9 is considered precocious. *Isosexual precocity* refers to premature sexual development consistent with phenotypic sex and includes features such as the development of facial hair and phallic growth. Isosexual precocity is divided into gonadotropin-dependent and gonadotropin-independent causes of androgen excess (Table 346-1). *Heterosexual precocity* refers to the premature development of estrogenic features in boys such as breast development.

TABLE 346-1 Causes of Precocious or Delayed Puberty in Boys

I. Precocious puberty
- A. Gonadotropin-dependent
  - 1. Idiopathic
  - 2. Hypothalamic hamartoma or other lesions
  - 3. CNS tumor or inflammatory state
- B. Gonadotropin-independent
  - 1. Congenital adrenal hyperplasia
  - 2. hCG-secreting tumor
  - 3. McCune-Albright syndrome
  - 4. Activating LH receptor mutation
  - 5. Exogenous androgens

II. Delayed puberty
- A. Constitutional delay of growth and puberty
- B. Systemic disorders
  - 1. Chronic disease
  - 2. Malnutrition
  - 3. Anorexia nervosa
- C. CNS tumors and their treatment (radiotherapy and surgery)
- D. Hypothalamic-pituitary causes of pubertal failure (low gonadotropins)
  - 1. Congenital disorders (Table 346-2)
    - a. Hypothalamic syndromes (e.g., Prader-Willi)
    - b. Idiopathic hypogonadotropic hypogonadism
    - c. Congenital
    - d. PROP1 mutations and other mutations affecting pituitary development/function
  - 2. Acquired disorders
    - a. Pituitary tumors
    - b. Hyperprolactinemia
- E. Gonadal causes of pubertal failure (elevated gonadotropins)
  - 1. Klinefelter's syndrome
  - 2. Bilateral undescended testes
  - 3. Orchitis
  - 4. Chemotherapy or radiotherapy
  - 5. Anorchia
- F. Androgen insensitivity

Abbreviations: CNS, central nervous system; GnRH, gonadotropin-releasing hormone; hCG, human chronic gonadotropin; LH, luteinizing hormone.

Gonadotropin-dependent precocious puberty

This disorder, called *central precocious puberty* (CPP), is less common in boys than in girls. It is caused by premature activation of the GnRH pulse generator, sometimes because of central nervous system (CNS) lesions such as hypothalamic hamartomas, but it is often idiopathic. CPP is characterized by gonadotropin levels that are inappropriately elevated for age. Because pituitary priming has occurred, GnRH elicits LH and FSH responses typical of those seen in puberty or in adults. MRI should be performed to exclude a mass, structural defect, infection, or inflammatory process.

TABLE 346-2 Causes of Congenital Hypogonadotropic Hypogonadism

Gene	Locus	Inheritance	Associated Features
KAL1	Xp22	X-linked	Anosmia, renal agenesis, synkinesia, cleft lip/palate, oculomotor/visuospatial defects, gut malrotations
NELF	9q34.3	AR	Anosmia, hypogonadotropic hypogonadism
FGFR1	8p11-p12	AD	Anosmia, cleft lip/palate, synkinesia, syndactyly
PROK2	20p13	AR	Anosmia, hypogonadotropic hypogonadism
PROKR2	20p12.3	AR	Anosmia
LEP	7q31	AR	Obesity
LEPR	1p31	AR	Obesity
PC1	5q15-21	AR	Obesity, diabetes mellitus, ACTH deficiency
HESX1	3p21	AR	Septo-optic dysplasia, CPHD
		AD	Isolated GH insufficiency
LHX3	9q34	AR	CPHD (ACTH spared), cervical spine rigidity
PROP1	5q35	AR	CPHD (ACTH usually spared)
GPR54	19p13	AR	None
GnRHR	4q21	AR	None
FSHβ	11p13	AR	↑ LH
LHβ	19q13	AR	↑ FSH
SF1 (NR5A1)	9p33	AD/AR	Primary adrenal failure, XY sex reversal
DAX1 (NROB1)	Xp21	X-linked	Primary adrenal failure, impaired spermatogenesis
TAC3R	4q25	AR	None
TAC3	12q13-q21	AR	None

Abbreviations: ACTH, adrenocorticotropic hormone; AD, autosomal dominant; AR, autosomal recessive; CPHD, combined pituitary hormone deficiency; KAL1, Interval-1 gene; NELF, nasal embryonic LHRH factor; FGFR1, fibroblast growth factor receptor 1; PROKR2, prokineticin receptor 2; LEP, leptin; LEPR, leptin receptor; PC1, prohormone convertase 1; HESX1, homeobox gene expressed in embryonic stem cells 1; LHX3, LIM homeobox gene 3; PROP1, Prophet of Pit 1; GPR54, G protein–coupled receptor 54; GnRHR, gonadotropin-releasing hormone receptor; FSHβ, follicle-stimulating hormone β subunit; LHβ, luteinizing hormone β subunit; SF1, steroidogenic factor 1; DAX1, *d*osage-sensitive sex-reversal, *a*drenal hypoplasia congenita, *X*-chromosome.

Gonadotropin-independent precocious puberty

In these disorders, androgens from the testis or the adrenal are increased but gonadotropins are low. This group of disorders includes hCG-secreting tumors; congenital adrenal hyperplasia; sex steroid–producing tumors of the testis, adrenal, and ovary; accidental or deliberate exogenous sex steroid administration; hypothyroidism; and activating mutations of the LH receptor or $G_s\alpha$ subunit.

Familial male-limited precocious puberty Also called *testotoxicosis*, familial male-limited precocious puberty is an autosomal dominant disorder caused by activating mutations in the LH receptor, leading to constitutive stimulation of the cyclic AMP pathway and testosterone production. Clinical features include premature androgenization in boys, growth acceleration in early childhood, and advanced bone age followed by premature epiphyseal fusion. Testosterone is elevated, and LH is suppressed. Treatment options include inhibitors of testosterone synthesis (e.g., ketoconazole), androgen receptor antagonists (e.g., flutamide and bicalutamide), and aromatase inhibitors (e.g., anastrazole).

McCune-Albright syndrome This is a sporadic disorder caused by somatic (postzygotic) activating mutations in the $G_s\alpha$ subunit that links G protein–coupled receptors to intracellular signaling pathways (Chap. 355). The mutations impair the guanosine triphosphatase activity of the $G_s\alpha$ protein, leading to constitutive activation of adenylyl cyclase. Like activating LH receptor mutations, this stimulates testosterone production and causes gonadotropin-independent precocious puberty. In addition to sexual precocity, affected individuals may have autonomy in the adrenals, pituitary, and thyroid glands. Café au lait spots are characteristic skin lesions that reflect the onset of the somatic mutations in melanocytes during embryonic development. Polyostotic fibrous dysplasia is caused by activation of the parathyroid hormone receptor pathway in bone. Treatment is similar to that in patients with activating LH receptor mutations. Bisphosphonates have been used to treat bone lesions.

Congenital adrenal hyperplasia Boys with congenital adrenal hyperplasia (CAH) who are not well controlled with glucocorticoid suppression of adrenocorticotropic hormone (ACTH) can develop premature virilization because of excessive androgen production by the adrenal gland (Chaps. 342 and 349). LH is low, and the testes are small. Adrenal rests may develop within the testis of poorly controlled patients with CAH because of chronic ACTH stimulation; adrenal rests do not require surgical removal and regress with effective glucocorticoid therapy. Some children with CAH may develop gonadotropin-dependent precocious puberty with early maturation of the hypothalamic-pituitary-gonadal axis, elevated gonadotropins, and testicular growth.

Heterosexual sexual precocity

Breast enlargement in prepubertal boys can result from familial aromatase excess, estrogen-producing tumors in the adrenal gland, Sertoli cell tumors in the testis, marijuana smoking, or exogenous estrogens or androgens. Occasionally, germ cell tumors that secrete hCG can be associated with breast enlargement due to excessive stimulation of estrogen production (see "Gynecomastia," below).

APPROACH TO THE PATIENT Precocious Puberty

After verification of precocious development, serum LH and FSH levels should be measured to determine whether gonadotropins are increased in relation to chronologic age (gonadotropin-dependent) or whether sex steroid secretion is occurring independent of LH and FSH (gonadotropin-independent). In children with gonadotropin-dependent precocious puberty, CNS lesions should be excluded by history, neurologic examination, and MRI scan of the head. If organic causes are not found, one is left with the diagnosis of idiopathic central precocity. Patients with high testosterone but suppressed LH concentrations have gonadotropin-independent sexual precocity; in these patients, DHEA sulfate (DHEAS) and 17α-hydroxyprogesterone should be measured. High levels of testosterone and 17α-hydroxyprogesterone suggest the possibility of CAH due to 21α-hydroxylase or 11β-hydroxylase deficiency. If testosterone and DHEAS are elevated, adrenal tumors should be excluded by obtaining a CT scan of the adrenal glands. Patients with elevated testosterone but without increased 17α-hydroxyprogesterone or DHEAS should undergo careful evaluation of the testis by palpation and ultrasound to exclude a Leydig cell neoplasm. Activating mutations of the LH receptor should be considered in children with gonadotropin-independent precocious puberty in whom CAH, androgen abuse, and adrenal and testicular neoplasms have been excluded.

TREATMENT Precocious Puberty

In patients with a known cause (e.g., a CNS lesion or a testicular tumor), therapy should be directed toward the underlying disorder. In patients with idiopathic CPP, long-acting GnRH analogues can be used to suppress gonadotropins and decrease testosterone, halt early pubertal development, delay accelerated bone maturation, and prevent early epiphyseal closure, thus increasing final height and mitigating the psychosocial consequences of early pubertal development. The treatment is most effective for increasing final adult height if it is initiated before age 6. Puberty resumes after discontinuation of the GnRH analogue. Counseling is an important aspect of the overall treatment strategy.

In children with gonadotropin-independent precocious puberty, inhibitors of steroidogenesis such as ketoconazole, and AR antagonists have been used empirically. Long-term treatment with spironolactone (a weak androgen antagonist) and ketoconazole has been reported to normalize growth rate and bone maturation and to improve predicted height in small, nonrandomized trials in boys with familial male-limited precocious puberty. Aromatase inhibitors such as testolactone and letrozole have been used as an adjunct to antiandrogen and GnRH analogue therapy for children with familial male-limited precocious puberty, congenital adrenal hyperplasia, and McCune-Albright syndrome.

DELAYED PUBERTY

Puberty is delayed in boys if it has not ensued by age 14, an age that is 2–2.5 standard deviations above the mean for healthy children. Delayed puberty is more common in boys than in girls. There are four main categories of delayed puberty: (1) constitutional delay of growth and puberty (~60% of cases), (2) functional hypogonadotropic hypogonadism caused by systemic illness or malnutrition (~20% of cases), (3) hypogonadotropic hypogonadism caused by genetic or acquired defects in the hypothalamic-pituitary region (~10% of cases), and (4) hypergonadotropic hypogonadism secondary to primary gonadal failure (~15% of cases) (Table 346-1). Functional hypogonadotropic hypogonadism is more common in girls than in boys. Permanent causes of hypogonadotropic or hypergonadotropic hypogonadism are identified in <25% of boys with delayed puberty.

APPROACH TO THE PATIENT Delayed Puberty

Any history of systemic illness, eating disorders, excessive exercise, social and psychological problems, and abnormal patterns of linear growth during childhood should be verified. Boys with pubertal delay may have accompanying emotional and physical immaturity relative to their peers, which can be a source of anxiety. Physical examination should focus on height; arm span; weight; visual fields; and secondary sex characteristics, including hair growth, testicular volume, phallic size, and scrotal reddening and thinning. Testicular size >2.5 cm generally indicates that the child has entered puberty.

The main diagnostic challenge is to distinguish those with constitutional delay, who will progress through puberty at a later age, from those with an underlying pathologic process. Constitutional delay should be suspected when there is a family history and when there are delayed bone age and short stature. Pituitary priming by pulsatile GnRH is required before LH and FSH are synthesized and secreted normally. Thus, blunted responses to exogenous GnRH can be seen in patients with constitutional delay, GnRH deficiency, or pituitary disorders (see "GnRH Stimulation Testing," above). In contrast, low-normal basal gonadotropin levels or a normal response to exogenous GnRH is consistent with an early stage of puberty, which often is heralded by nocturnal GnRH secretion. Thus, constitutional delay is a diagnosis of exclusion that requires ongoing evaluation until the onset of puberty and the growth spurt.

TREATMENT Delayed Puberty

If therapy is considered appropriate, it can begin with 25–50 mg testosterone enanthate or testosterone cypionate every 2 weeks or by using a 2.5-mg testosterone patch or 25-mg testosterone gel. Because aromatization of testosterone to estrogen is obligatory for mediating androgen effects on epiphyseal fusion, concomitant treatment with aromatase inhibitors may allow attainment of greater final adult height. Testosterone treatment should be interrupted after 6 months to determine whether endogenous LH and FSH secretion has ensued. Other causes of delayed puberty should be considered when there are associated clinical features or when boys do not enter puberty spontaneously after a year of observation or treatment.

Reassurance without hormonal treatment is appropriate for many individuals with presumed constitutional delay of puberty. However, the impact of delayed growth and pubertal progression on a child's social relationships and school performance should be weighed. Also, boys with constitutional delay of puberty are less likely to achieve their full genetic height potential and have reduced total body bone mass as adults, mainly due to narrow limb bones and vertebrae as a result of impaired periosteal expansion during puberty. Administration of androgen therapy to boys with constitutional delay does not affect final height, and when administered with an aromatase inhibitor, it may improve final height.

DISORDERS OF THE MALE REPRODUCTIVE AXIS DURING ADULTHOOD

HYPOGONADOTROPIC HYPOGONADISM

Because LH and FSH are trophic hormones for the testes, impaired secretion of these pituitary gonadotropins results in secondary hypogonadism, which is characterized by low testosterone in the setting of low LH and FSH. Those with the most severe deficiency have complete absence of pubertal development, sexual infantilism, and, in some cases, hypospadias and undescended testes. Patients with partial gonadotropin deficiency have delayed or arrested sex development. The 24-hour LH secretory profiles are heterogeneous in patients with hypogonadotropic hypogonadism, reflecting variable abnormalities of LH pulse frequency or amplitude. In severe cases, basal LH is low and there are no LH pulses. A smaller subset of patients has low-amplitude LH pulses or markedly reduced pulse frequency. Occasionally, only sleep-entrained LH pulses occur, reminiscent of the pattern seen in the early stages of puberty. Hypogonadotropic hypogonadism can be classified into congenital and acquired disorders. Congenital disorders most commonly involve GnRH deficiency, which leads to gonadotropin deficiency. Acquired disorders are more common than congenital disorders and may result from a variety of sellar mass lesions or infiltrative diseases of the hypothalamus or pituitary.

Congenital disorders associated with gonadotropin deficiency

Most cases of congenital hypogonadotropic hypogonadism are idiopathic despite extensive endocrine testing and imaging studies of the sellar region. Among known causes, familial hypogonadotropic hypogonadism can be transmitted as an X-linked (20%), autosomal recessive (30%), or autosomal dominant (50%) trait. Some individuals with idiopathic hypogonadotropic hypogonadism (IHH) have sporadic mutations in the same genes that cause inherited forms of the disorder (Table 346-2). *Kallmann's syndrome* is an X-linked disorder caused by mutations in the *KAL1* gene, which encodes anosmin, a protein that mediates the migration of neural progenitors of the olfactory bulb and GnRH-producing neurons. These individuals have GnRH deficiency and variable combinations of anosmia or hyposmia, renal defects, and neurologic abnormalities, including mirror movements. Gonadotropin secretion and fertility can be restored by administration of pulsatile GnRH or gonadotropin replacement. Mutations in the *FGFR1* gene cause an autosomal dominant form of hypogonadotropic hypogonadism that clinically resembles Kallmann's syndrome; mutations in its putative ligand, the*FGF8* gene product, have also been associated with IHH. Prokineticin 2 (PROK2) also encodes a protein involved in migration and development of olfactory and GnRH neurons. Recessive mutations in PROK2 or in its receptor, PROKR2, have been associated with both anosmic and normosmic forms of hypogonadotropic hypogonadism. X-linked hypogonadotropic hypogonadism also occurs in *adrenal hypoplasia congenita*, a disorder caused by mutations in the *DAX1* gene, which encodes a nuclear receptor in the adrenal gland and reproductive axis. Adrenal hypoplasia congenita is characterized by absent development of the adult zone of the adrenal cortex, leading to neonatal adrenal insufficiency. Puberty usually does not occur or is arrested, reflecting variable degrees of gonadotropin deficiency. Although sexual differentiation is normal, some patients have testicular dysgenesis and impaired spermatogenesis despite gonadotropin replacement. Less commonly, adrenal hypoplasia congenita, sex reversal, and hypogonadotropic hypogonadism can be caused by mutations of steroidogenic factor 1 (SF1). *GnRH receptor mutations*, the most common identifiable cause of normosmic IHH, account for ~40% of autosomal recessive and 10% of sporadic cases of hypogonadotropic hypogonadism. These patients have decreased LH response to exogenous GnRH. Some receptor mutations alter GnRH binding affinity, allowing apparently normal responses to pharmacologic doses of exogenous GnRH, whereas other mutations may alter signal transduction downstream of hormone binding. Mutations of the *GnRH1* gene also have been reported in patients with hypogonadotropic hypogonadism, although they are rare. G protein–coupled receptor GPR54 and its cognate receptor, kisspeptin, are important regulators of sexual maturation. Recessive mutations in GPR54 cause gonadotropin deficiency without anosmia. Patients retain responsiveness to exogenous GnRH, suggesting an abnormality in the neural pathways that control GnRH release. The genes encoding neurokinin B (TAC3), which is involved in preferential activation of GnRH release in early development, and its receptor (TAC3R) have been implicated in some families with normosmic IHH. Mutations in more than one gene (digenicity) may contribute to clinical heterogeneity in IHH patients. Rarely, recessive mutations in the *LHβ* or *FSHβ* gene have been described in patients with selective deficiencies of these gonadotropins. In approximately 10% of men with IHH, reversal of gonadotropin deficiency may occur in adult life. Also, a small fraction of men with IHH may present with androgen deficiency and infertility in adult life after having gone through apparently normal pubertal development.

A number of homeodomain transcription factors are involved in the development and differentiation of the specialized hormone-producing cells within the pituitary gland (Table 346-2). Patients with mutations of *PROP1* have combined pituitary hormone deficiency that includes GH, prolactin (PRL), thyroid-stimulating hormone (TSH), LH, and FSH but not ACTH. *LHX3* mutations cause combined pituitary hormone deficiency in association with cervical spine rigidity. *HESX1* mutations cause septo-optic dysplasia and combined pituitary hormone deficiency.

Prader-Willi syndrome is characterized by obesity, hypotonic musculature, mental retardation, hypogonadism, short stature, and small hands and feet. Prader-Willi syndrome is a genomic imprinting disorder caused by deletions of the proximal portion of paternally derived chromosome 15q, uniparental disomy of the maternal alleles, or mutations of the genes/loci involved in imprinting (Chap. 62). *Laurence-Moon syndrome* is an autosomal recessive disorder characterized by obesity, hypogonadism, mental retardation, polydactyly, and retinitis pigmentosa. Recessive mutations of leptin, or its receptor, cause severe obesity and pubertal arrest, apparently because of hypothalamic GnRH deficiency (Chap. 77).

Acquired hypogonadotropic disorders

SEVERE ILLNESS, STRESS, MALNUTRITION, AND EXERCISE These factors may cause reversible gonadotropin deficiency. Although gonadotropin deficiency and reproductive dysfunction are well documented in these conditions in women, men exhibit similar but less pronounced responses. Unlike women, most male runners and other endurance athletes have normal gonadotropin and sex steroid levels despite low body fat and frequent intensive exercise. Testosterone levels fall at the onset of illness and recover during recuperation. The magnitude of gonadotropin suppression generally correlates with the severity of illness. Although hypogonadotropic hypogonadism is the most common cause of androgen deficiency in patients with acute illness, some have elevated levels of LH and FSH, which suggest primary gonadal dysfunction. The pathophysiology of reproductive dysfunction during acute illness is unknown but probably involves a combination of cytokine and/or glucocorticoid effects. There is a high frequency of low testosterone levels in patients with chronic illnesses such as HIV infection, end-stage renal disease, chronic obstructive lung disease, and many types of cancer and in patients receiving glucocorticoids. About 20% of HIV-infected men with low testosterone levels have elevated LH and FSH levels; these patients presumably have primary testicular dysfunction. The remaining 80% have either normal or low LH and FSH levels; these men have a central hypothalamic-pituitary defect or a dual defect involving both the testis and the hypothalamic-pituitary centers. Muscle wasting is common in chronic diseases associated with hypogonadism, which also leads to debility, poor quality of life, and adverse outcome of disease. There is great interest in exploring strategies that can reverse androgen deficiency or attenuate the sarcopenia associated with chronic illness.

Men using opioids for relief of cancer or noncancerous pain or because of addiction often have suppressed testosterone and LH levels; the degree of suppression is dose-related and particularly severe with long-acting opioids such as methadone. Opioids suppress GnRH secretion and alter the sensitivity to feedback inhibition by gonadal steroids. Men who are heavy users of marijuana have decreased testosterone secretion and sperm production. The mechanism of marijuana-induced hypogonadism is decreased GnRH secretion. Gynecomastia observed in marijuana users can also be caused by plant estrogens in crude preparations. Androgen deprivation therapy in men with prostate cancer has been associated with increased risk of bone fractures, diabetes mellitus, cardiovascular events, fatigue, sexual dysfunction, and poor quality of life.

Obesity In men with mild to moderate obesity, SHBG levels decrease in proportion to the degree of obesity, resulting in lower total testosterone levels. However, free testosterone levels usually remain within the normal range. The decrease in SHBG levels is caused by increased circulating insulin, which inhibits SHBG production. Estradiol levels are higher in obese men than in healthy, nonobese controls because of aromatization of testosterone to estradiol in adipose tissue. Weight loss is associated with reversal of these abnormalities, including an increase in total and free testosterone levels and a decrease in estradiol levels. A subset of massively obese men may have a defect in the hypothalamic-pituitary axis as suggested by low free testosterone in the absence of elevated gonadotropins. Weight gain in adult men can accelerate the rate of age-related decline in testosterone levels.

Hyperprolactinemia (See also Chap. 339.) Elevated PRL levels are associated with hypogonadotropic hypogonadism. PRL inhibits hypothalamic GnRH secretion either directly or through modulation of tuberoinfundibular dopaminergic pathways. A PRL-secreting tumor also may destroy the surrounding gonadotropes by invasion or compression of the pituitary stalk. Treatment with dopamine agonists reverses gonadotropin deficiency, although there may be a delay relative to PRL suppression.

Sellar mass lesions Neoplastic and nonneoplastic lesions in the hypothalamus or pituitary can affect gonadotrope function directly or indirectly. In adults, pituitary adenomas constitute the largest category of space-occupying lesions affecting gonadotropin and other pituitary hormone production. Pituitary adenomas that extend into the suprasellar region can impair GnRH secretion and mildly increase PRL secretion (usually <50 μg/L) because of impaired tonic inhibition by dopaminergic pathways. These tumors should be distinguished from prolactinomas, which typically secrete higher PRL levels. The presence of diabetes insipidus suggests the possibility of a craniopharyngioma, infiltrative disorder, or other hypothalamic lesions (Chap. 340).

Hemochromatosis (See also Chap. 357.) Both the pituitary and the testis can be affected by excessive iron deposition. However, the pituitary defect is the predominant lesion in most patients with hemochromatosis and hypogonadism. The diagnosis of hemochromatosis is suggested by the association of characteristic skin discoloration, hepatic enlargement or dysfunction, diabetes mellitus, arthritis, cardiac conduction defects, and hypogonadism.

■ PRIMARY TESTICULAR CAUSES OF HYPOGONADISM

Common causes of primary testicular dysfunction include Klinefelter's syndrome, uncorrected cryptorchidism, cancer chemotherapy, radiation to the testes, trauma, torsion, infectious orchitis, HIV infection, anorchia syndrome, and myotonic dystrophy. Primary testicular disorders may be associated with impaired spermatogenesis, decreased androgen production, or both. See Chap. 349 for disorders of testis development, androgen synthesis, and androgen action.

Klinefelter's syndrome

(See also Chap. 349.) Klinefelter's syndrome is the most common chromosomal disorder associated with testicular dysfunction and male infertility. It occurs in about 1 in 1000 live-born males. Azoospermia is the rule in men with Klinefelter's syndrome who have the 47,XXY karyotype; however, men with mosaicism may have germ cells, especially at a younger age. The clinical phenotype of Klinefelter's syndrome can be heterogeneous, possibly because of mosaicism, polymorphisms in androgen receptor gene, variable testosterone levels, or other genetic factors. Testicular histology shows hyalinization of seminiferous tubules and absence of spermatogenesis. Although their function is impaired, the number of Leydig cells appears to increase. Testosterone is decreased and estradiol is increased, leading to clinical features of undervirilization and gynecomastia. Men with Klinefelter's syndrome are at increased risk of systemic lupus erythematosus, breast cancer, non-Hodgkin's lymphoma, and lung cancer and reduced risk of prostate cancer. Periodic mammography for breast cancer surveillance is recommended for men with Klinefelter's syndrome. Fertility has been achieved by intracytoplasmic injection of sperm retrieved surgically from testicular biopsies of men with Klinefelter's syndrome, including some men with nonmosaic forms of Klinefelter's syndrome.

Cryptorchidism

Cryptorchidism occurs when there is incomplete descent of the testis from the abdominal cavity into the scrotum. About 3% of full-term and 30% of premature male infants have at least one undescended testis at birth, but descent is usually complete by the first few weeks of life. The incidence of cryptorchidism is <1% by 9 months of age. Androgens regulate both the transabdominal and inguinoscrotal descent of the testes through degeneration of the craniosuspensory ligament and a shortening of the gubernacula, respectively. Mutations in INSL3 and its receptor, which regulate the transabdominal portion of testicular descent, have been found in some patients with cryptorchidism.

Cryptorchidism is associated with increased risk of malignancy and infertility. Unilateral cryptorchidism, even when corrected before puberty, is associated with decreased sperm count, possibly reflecting unrecognized damage to the fully descended testis or other genetic factors. Epidemiologic, clinical, and molecular evidence supports the idea that cryptorchidism, hypospadias, impaired spermatogenesis, and testicular cancer may be causally related to common genetic and environment perturbations and are components of the testicular dysgenesis syndrome.

Acquired testicular defects

Viral orchitis may be caused by the mumps virus, echovirus, lymphocytic choriomeningitis virus, and group B arboviruses. Orchitis occurs in as many as one-fourth of adult men with mumps; the orchitis is unilateral in about two-thirds and bilateral in the remainder. Orchitis usually develops a few days after the onset of parotitis but may precede it. The testis may return to normal size and function or undergo atrophy. Semen analysis returns to normal for three-fourths of men with unilateral involvement but for only one-third of men with bilateral orchitis. *Trauma*, including testicular torsion, also can cause secondary atrophy of the testes. The exposed position of the testes in the scrotum renders them susceptible to both thermal and physical trauma, particularly in men with hazardous occupations.

The testes are sensitive to *radiation damage*. Doses >200 mGy (20 rad) are associated with increased FSH and LH levels and damage to the spermatogonia. After ~800 mGy (80 rad), oligospermia or azoospermia develops, and higher doses may obliterate the germinal epithelium. Permanent androgen deficiency in adult men is uncommon after therapeutic radiation; however, most boys given direct testicular radiation therapy for acute lymphoblastic leukemia have permanently low testosterone levels. Sperm banking should be considered before patients undergo radiation treatment or chemotherapy.

Drugs interfere with testicular function by several mechanisms, including inhibition of testosterone synthesis (e.g., ketoconazole), blockade of androgen action (e.g., spironolactone), increased estrogen (e.g., marijuana), or direct inhibition of spermatogenesis (e.g., chemotherapy).

Combination chemotherapy for acute leukemia, Hodgkin's disease, and testicular and other cancers may impair Leydig cell function and cause infertility. The degree of gonadal dysfunction depends on the type of chemotherapeutic agent and the dose and duration of therapy. Because of high response rates and the young age of these men, infertility and androgen deficiency have emerged as important long-term complications of cancer chemotherapy. Cyclophosphamide and combination regimens containing procarbazine are particularly toxic to germ cells. Thus, 90% of men with Hodgkin's lymphoma receiving MOPP (mechlorethamine, oncovin, procarbazine, prednisone) therapy develop azoospermia or extreme oligozoospermia; newer regimens that do not include procarbazine, such as ABVD (adriamycin, bleomycin, vinblastine, dacarbazine), are less toxic to germ cells.

Alcohol, when consumed in excess for prolonged periods, decreases testosterone, independent of liver disease or malnutrition. Elevated estradiol and decreased testosterone levels may occur in men taking digitalis.

The occupational and recreational history should be evaluated carefully in all men with infertility because of the toxic effects of many *chemical agents* on spermatogenesis. Known environmental hazards include microwaves and ultrasound and chemicals such as nematocide dibromochloropropane, cadmium, phthalates, and lead. In some populations, sperm density is said to have declined by as much as 40% in the last 50 years. Environmental estrogens or antiandrogens may be partly responsible.

Testicular failure also occurs as a part of *polyglandular autoimmune insufficiency* (Chap. 351). Sperm antibodies can cause isolated male infertility. In some instances, these antibodies are secondary phenomena resulting from duct obstruction or vasectomy. Granulomatous diseases can affect the testes, and testicular atrophy occurs in 10–20% of men with lepromatous leprosy because of direct tissue invasion by the mycobacteria. The tubules are involved initially, followed by endarteritis and destruction of Leydig cells.

Systemic disease can cause primary testis dysfunction in addition to suppressing gonadotropin production. In cirrhosis, a combined testicular and pituitary abnormality leads to decreased testosterone production independent of the direct toxic effects of ethanol. Impaired hepatic extraction of adrenal androstenedione leads to extraglandular conversion to estrone and estradiol, which partially suppresses LH. Testicular atrophy and gynecomastia are present in approximately one-half of men with cirrhosis. In chronic renal failure, androgen synthesis and sperm production decrease despite elevated gonadotropins. The elevated LH level is due to reduced clearance, but it does not restore normal testosterone production. About one-fourth of men with renal failure have hyperprolactinemia. Improvement in testosterone production with hemodialysis is incomplete, but successful renal transplantation may return testicular function to normal. Testicular atrophy is present in one-third of men with sickle cell anemia. The defect may be at either the testicular or the hypothalamic-pituitary level. Sperm density can decrease temporarily after acute febrile illness in the absence of a change in testosterone production. Infertility in men with celiac disease is associated with a hormonal pattern typical of androgen resistance, namely, elevated testosterone and LH levels.

Neurologic diseases associated with altered testicular function include myotonic dystrophy, spinobulbar muscular atrophy, and paraplegia. In myotonic dystrophy, small testes may be associated with impairment of both spermatogenesis and Leydig cell function. Spinobulbar muscular atrophy is caused by an expansion of the glutamine repeat sequences in the amino-terminal region of the AR; this expansion impairs function of the AR, but it is unclear how the alteration is related to the neurologic manifestations. Men with spinobulbar muscular atrophy often have undervirilization and infertility as a late manifestation. Spinal cord lesions that cause paraplegia can lead to a temporary decrease in testosterone levels and may cause persistent defects in spermatogenesis; some patients retain the capacity for penile erection and ejaculation.

ANDROGEN INSENSITIVITY SYNDROMES

Mutations in the AR cause resistance to the action of testosterone and DHT. These X-linked mutations are associated with variable degrees of defective male phenotypic development and undervirilization (Chap. 349). Although not technically hormone-insensitivity syndromes, two genetic disorders impair testosterone conversion to active sex steroids. Mutations in the *SRD5A2* gene, which encodes 5α-reductase type 2, prevent the conversion of testosterone to DHT, which is necessary for the normal development of the male external genitalia. Mutations in the *CYP19* gene, which encodes aromatase, prevent testosterone conversion to estradiol. Males with *CYP19* mutations have delayed epiphyseal fusion, tall stature, eunuchoid proportions, and osteoporosis, consistent with evidence from an estrogen receptor–deficient individual that these testosterone actions are mediated indirectly via estrogen.

GYNECOMASTIA

Gynecomastia refers to enlargement of the male breast. It is caused by excess estrogen action and is usually the result of an increased estrogen/androgen ratio. True gynecomastia is associated with glandular breast tissue that is >4 cm in diameter and often tender. Glandular tissue enlargement should be distinguished from excess adipose tissue: glandular tissue is firmer and contains fibrous-like cords. Gynecomastia occurs as a normal physiologic phenomenon in the newborn (due to transplacental transfer of maternal and placental estrogens), during puberty (high ratio of estrogen to androgen in early stages of puberty), and with aging (increased fat tissue and increased aromatase activity), but it also can result from pathologic conditions associated with androgen deficiency or estrogen excess. The prevalence of gynecomastia increases with age and body mass index (BMI), probably because of increased aromatase activity in adipose tissue. Medications that alter androgen metabolism or action may also cause gynecomastia. The relative risk of breast cancer is increased in men with gynecomastia, although the absolute risk is relatively small.

PATHOLOGIC GYNECOMASTIA

Any cause of *androgen deficiency* can lead to gynecomastia, reflecting an increased estrogen/androgen ratio, as estrogen synthesis still occurs by aromatization of residual adrenal and gonadal androgens. Gynecomastia is a characteristic feature of Klinefelter's syndrome (Chap. 349). *Androgen insensitivity* disorders also cause gynecomastia. *Excess estrogen production* may be caused by tumors, including Sertoli cell tumors in isolation or in association with Peutz-Jegher syndrome or Carney complex. Tumors that produce hCG, including some testicular tumors, stimulate Leydig cell estrogen synthesis. *Increased conversion of androgens to estrogens* can be a result of increased availability of substrate (androstenedione) for extraglandular estrogen formation (CAH, hyperthyroidism, and most feminizing adrenal tumors) or diminished catabolism of androstenedione (liver disease) so that androgen precursors are shunted to aromatase in peripheral sites. Obesity is associated with increased aromatization of androgen precursors to estrogens. Extraglandular aromatase activity can also be increased in tumors of the liver or adrenal gland or rarely as an inherited disorder. Several families with *increased peripheral aromatase activity* inherited as an autosomal dominant or an X-linked disorder have been described. In some families with this disorder, an inversion in chromosome 15q21.2-3 causes the *CYP19* gene to be activated by the regulatory elements of contiguous genes, resulting in excessive estrogen production in the fat and other extragonadal tissues. *Drugs* can cause gynecomastia by acting directly as estrogenic substances (e.g., oral contraceptives, phytoestrogens, digitalis), inhibiting androgen synthesis (e.g., ketoconazole), or action (e.g., spironolactone).

Because up to two-thirds of pubertal boys and one-half of hospitalized men have palpable glandular tissue that is benign, detailed investigation or intervention is not indicated in all men presenting with gynecomastia (Fig. 346-5). In addition to the extent of gynecomastia, recent onset, rapid growth, tender tissue, and occurrence in a lean subject should prompt more extensive evaluation. This should include a careful drug history, measurement and examination of the testes, assessment of virilization, evaluation of liver function, and hormonal measurements, including testosterone,

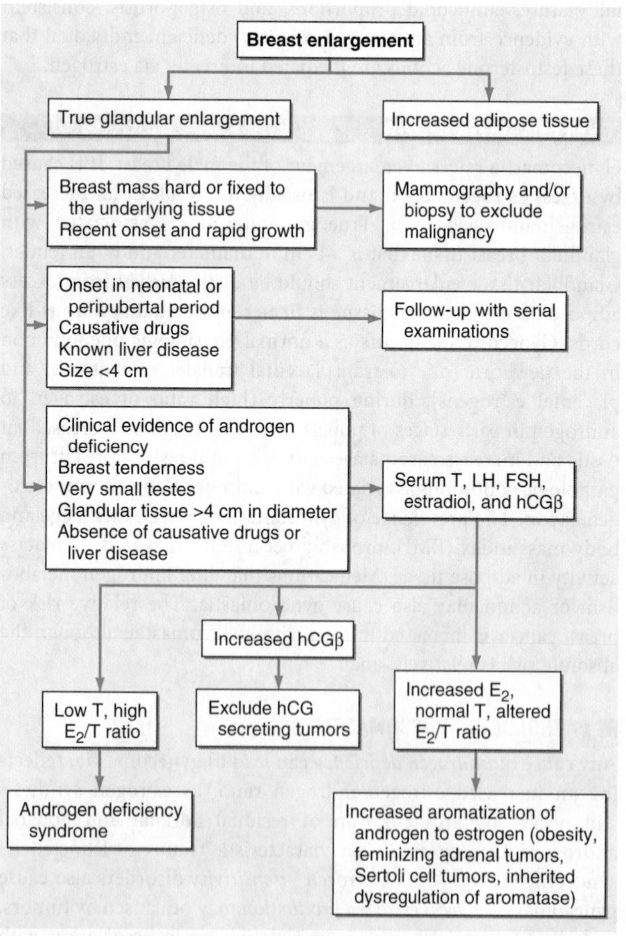

Breast enlargement

True glandular enlargement

Increased adipose tissue

Breast mass hard or fixed to the underlying tissue
Recent onset and rapid growth

Mammography and/or biopsy to exclude malignancy

Onset in neonatal or peripubertal period
Causative drugs
Known liver disease
Size <4 cm

Follow-up with serial examinations

Clinical evidence of androgen deficiency
Breast tenderness
Very small testes
Glandular tissue >4 cm in diameter
Absence of causative drugs or liver disease

Serum T, LH, FSH, estradiol, and hCGβ

Increased hCGβ

Low T, high E_2/T ratio

Exclude hCG secreting tumors

Increased E_2, normal T, altered E_2/T ratio

Androgen deficiency syndrome

Increased aromatization of androgen to estrogen (obesity, feminizing adrenal tumors, Sertoli cell tumors, inherited dysregulation of aromatase)

Figure 346-5 Evaluation of gynecomastia. T, testosterone; LH, luteinizing hormone; FSH, follicle-stimulating hormones; hCGβ, human chorionic gonadotropin β; E_2, 17β-estradiol.

estradiol, and androstenedione, LH, and hCG. A karyotype should be obtained in men with very small testes to exclude Klinefelter's syndrome. In spite of extensive evaluation, the etiology is established in fewer than one-half of patients.

TREATMENT Gynecomastia

When the primary cause can be identified and corrected, breast enlargement usually subsides over several months. However, if gynecomastia is of long duration, surgery is the most effective therapy. Indications for surgery include severe psychological and/or cosmetic problems, continued growth or tenderness, and suspected malignancy. In patients who have painful gynecomastia and in whom surgery cannot be performed, treatment with antiestrogens such as tamoxifen (20 mg/d) can reduce pain and breast tissue size in over one-half of the patients. The estrogen receptor antagonists tamoxifen and raloxifen have been reported in small trials to reduce breast size in men with pubertal gynecomastia, although complete regression of breast enlargement is unusual with the use of estrogen receptor antagonists. Aromatase inhibitors can be effective in the early proliferative phase of the disorder. However, in a randomized trial in men with established gynecomastia, anastrozole was no more effective than placebo in reducing breast size.

AGING-RELATED CHANGES IN MALE REPRODUCTIVE FUNCTION

A number of cross-sectional and longitudinal studies (e.g., the Baltimore Longitudinal Study of Aging, the Massachusetts Male Aging Study, and the European Male Aging Study) have established that testosterone concentrations decrease with advancing age. This age-related decline starts in the third decade of life and progresses slowly; the rate of decline in testosterone concentrations is greater in obese men, men with chronic illness, and those taking medications than in healthy older men. Because SHBG concentrations are higher in older men than in younger men, free or bioavailable testosterone concentrations decline with aging to a greater extent than do total testosterone concentrations. The age-related decline in testosterone is due to defects at all levels of the hypothalamic-pituitary-testicular axis: pulsatile GnRH secretion is attenuated, LH response to GnRH is reduced, and testicular response to LH is impaired. However, the gradual rise of LH with aging suggests that testis dysfunction is the main cause of declining androgen levels. The term *andropause* has been used to denote age-related decline in testosterone concentrations; this term is a misnomer because there is no discrete time when testosterone concentrations decline abruptly.

In epidemiologic surveys, low total and bioavailable testosterone concentrations have been associated with decreased appendicular skeletal muscle mass and strength, decreased self-reported physical function, higher visceral fat mass, insulin resistance, and increased risk of coronary artery disease and mortality. An analysis of signs and symptoms in older men in the European Male Aging Study revealed a syndromic association of sexual and physical symptoms with testosterone levels <320 ng/dL in community-dwelling older men. In systematic reviews of randomized controlled trials, testosterone therapy in healthy older men with low or low-normal testosterone levels was associated with greater increments in lean body mass, grip strength, and self-reported physical function than was the case with placebo. Testosterone therapy also induced greater improvement in vertebral but not femoral bone mineral density. Testosterone therapy in older men with sexual dysfunction and unequivocally low testosterone levels improves libido, but testosterone effects on erectile function and response to selective phosphodiesterase inhibitors have been inconsistent. Testosterone therapy has not been shown to improve depression scores, fracture risk, cognitive function, or clinical outcomes in older men. Furthermore, neither the long-term risks nor the clinical benefits of testosterone therapy in older men have been demonstrated in adequately powered trials. Although there is no evidence that testosterone causes prostate cancer, there is concern that testosterone therapy might induce the growth of subclinical prostate cancers or exacerbate cardiovascular disease. One randomized testosterone trial in older men with mobility limitation and a high burden of chronic conditions such as diabetes, heart disease, hypertension, and hyperlipidemia reported a greater number of cardiovascular events in men randomized to the testosterone arm of the study than in those randomized to the placebo arm. Population screening of all older men for low testosterone levels is not recommended, and testing should be restricted to men who have symptoms or physical features attributable to androgen deficiency. Testosterone therapy is not recommended for all older men with low testosterone levels. In older men with significant symptoms of androgen deficiency who have testosterone levels <200 ng/dL, testosterone therapy may be considered on an individualized basis and should be instituted after careful discussion of the risks and benefits (see "Testosterone Replacement," below).

Testicular morphology, semen production, and fertility are maintained up to a very old age in men. Although concern has been expressed about age-related increases in germ cell mutations and impairment of DNA repair mechanisms, the frequency of chromosomal aneuploidy or structural abnormalities does not increase in the sperm of older men. However, the incidence of autosomal dominant diseases such as achondroplasia, polyposis coli, Marfan's syndrome, and Apert's syndrome increases in the offspring of men who are advanced in age, consistent with transmission of sporadic missense mutations.

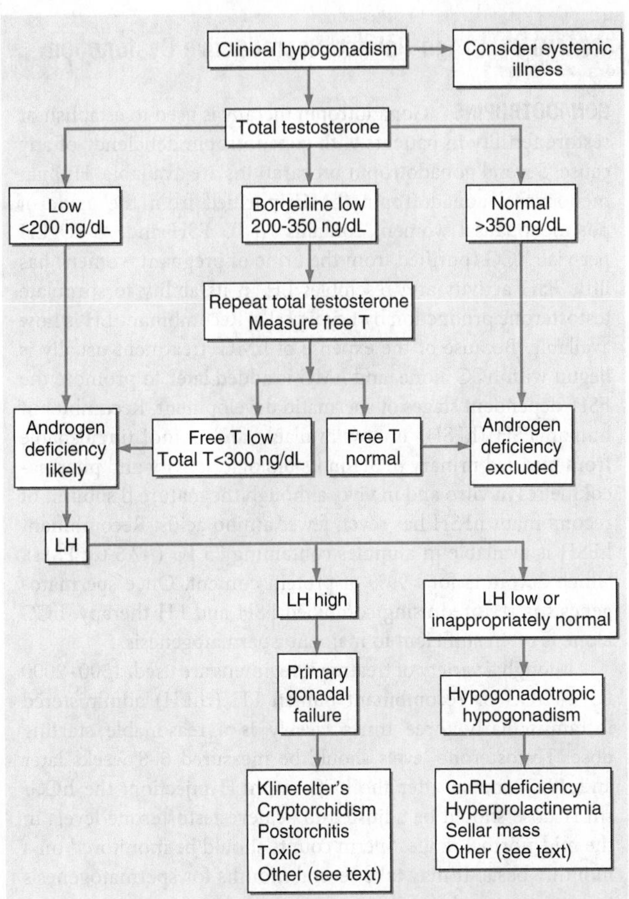

Figure 346-6 Evaluation of hypogonadism. GnRH, gonadotropin-releasing hormone; LH, luteinizing hormone; T, testosterone.

APPROACH TO THE PATIENT: Androgen Deficiency

Hypogonadism often is characterized by decreased sex drive, reduced frequency of sexual intercourse or inability to maintain erections, reduced beard growth, loss of muscle mass, decreased testicular size, and gynecomastia. Less than 10% of patients with erectile dysfunction alone have testosterone deficiency. Thus, it is useful to look for a constellation of symptoms and signs suggestive of androgen deficiency. Except when extreme, these clinical features may be difficult to distinguish from changes that occur with normal aging. Moreover, androgen deficiency may develop gradually. Although population studies such as the Massachusetts Male Aging Study and the Baltimore Longitudinal Study of Aging have reported a high prevalence of low testosterone levels in middle-aged and older men, the age-related decline in testosterone should be distinguished from classic hypogonadism due to diseases of the testes, the pituitary, or the hypothalamus.

When symptoms or clinical features suggest possible androgen deficiency, the laboratory evaluation is initiated by the measurement of total testosterone, preferably in the morning, using a reliable assay such as LC-MS/MS (Fig. 346-6). A consistently low total testosterone level <300 ng/dL measured by a reliable assay in association with symptoms provides evidence of testosterone deficiency. An early-morning testosterone level >350 ng/dL makes the diagnosis of androgen deficiency unlikely. In men with testosterone levels between 200 and 350 ng/dL, the total testosterone level should be repeated and a free testosterone level should be measured. In older men and in patients with other clinical states that are associated with alterations in SHBG levels, a direct measurement of free testosterone level by equilibrium dialysis can be useful in unmasking testosterone deficiency.

When androgen deficiency has been confirmed by low testosterone concentrations, LH should be measured to classify the patient as having primary (high LH) or secondary (low or inappropriately normal LH) hypogonadism. An elevated LH level indicates that the defect is at the testicular level. Common causes of primary testicular failure include Klinefelter's syndrome, HIV infection, uncorrected cryptorchidism, cancer chemotherapeutic agents, radiation, surgical orchiectomy, and prior infectious orchitis. Unless causes of primary testicular failure are known, a karyotype should be performed in men with low testosterone and elevated LH to exclude Klinefelter's syndrome. Men who have low testosterone but "inappropriately normal" or low LH levels have secondary hypogonadism; their defect resides at the hypothalamic-pituitary level. Common causes of acquired secondary hypogonadism include space-occupying lesions of the sella, hyperprolactinemia, chronic illness, hemochromatosis, excessive exercise, and substance abuse. Measurement of PRL and an MRI scan of the hypothalamic-pituitary region can help exclude the presence of a space-occupying lesion. Patients in whom known causes of hypogonadotropic hypogonadism have been excluded are classified as having IHH. It is not unusual for congenital causes of hypogonadotropic hypogonadism such as Kallmann's syndrome to be diagnosed in young adults.

TREATMENT Age-Related Reproductive Dysfunction

GONADOTROPINS Gonadotropin therapy is used to establish or restore fertility in patients with gonadotropin deficiency of any cause. Several gonadotropin preparations are available. Human menopausal gonadotropin (hMG; purified from the urine of postmenopausal women) contains 75 IU FSH and 75 IU LH per vial. hCG (purified from the urine of pregnant women) has little FSH activity and resembles LH in its ability to stimulate testosterone production by Leydig cells. Recombinant LH is now available. Because of the expense of hMG, treatment usually is begun with hCG alone, and hMG is added later to promote the FSH-dependent stages of spermatid development. Recombinant human FSH (hFSH) is now available and is indistinguishable from purified urinary hFSH in its biologic activity and pharmacokinetics in vitro and in vivo, although the mature β subunit of recombinant hFSH has seven fewer amino acids. Recombinant hFSH is available in ampules containing 75 IU (~7.5 μg FSH), which accounts for >99% of protein content. Once spermatogenesis is restored using combined FSH and LH therapy, hCG alone is often sufficient to maintain spermatogenesis.

Although a variety of treatment regimens are used, 1500–2000 IU of hCG or recombinant human LH (rhLH) administered intramuscularly three times weekly is a reasonable starting dose. Testosterone levels should be measured 6–8 weeks later and 48–72 hours after the hCG or rhLH injection; the hCG/rhLH dose should be adjusted to achieve testosterone levels in the mid-normal range. Sperm counts should be monitored on a monthly basis. It may take several months for spermatogenesis to be restored; therefore, it is important to forewarn patients about the potential length and expense of the treatment and to provide conservative estimates of success rates. If testosterone levels are in the mid-normal range but the sperm concentrations are low after 6 months of therapy with hCG alone, FSH should be added. This can be done by using hMG, highly purified urinary hFSH, or recombinant hFSH. The selection of the FSH dose is empirical. A common practice is to start with the addition of 75 IU FSH three times a week in conjunction with the hCG/rhLH injections. If sperm densities are still low after 3 months of combined treatment, the FSH dose should be increased to 150 IU. Occasionally, it may take ≥18–24 months for spermatogenesis to be restored.

The two best predictors of success using gonadotropin therapy in hypogonadotropic men are testicular volume at presentation and time of onset. In general, men with testicular volumes >8 mL have better response rates than those who have testicular volumes <4 mL. Patients who became hypogonadotropic after puberty experience higher success rates than those who have never undergone pubertal changes. Spermatogenesis usually can be reinitiated by hCG alone, with high rates of success for men with postpubertal onset of hypogonadotropism. The presence of a primary testicular abnormality such as cryptorchidism will attenuate testicular response to gonadotropin therapy. Prior androgen therapy does not preclude subsequent response to gonadotropin therapy, although some studies suggest that it may attenuate response to subsequent gonadotropin therapy.

TESTOSTERONE REPLACEMENT Androgen therapy is indicated to restore testosterone levels to normal to correct features of androgen deficiency. Testosterone replacement improves libido and overall sexual activity and increases energy, lean muscle mass, and bone density. The benefits of testosterone replacement therapy have been proved only in men who have documented androgen deficiency, as demonstrated by testosterone levels that are well below the lower limit of normal (<250 ng/dL).

Testosterone is available in a variety of formulations with distinct pharmacokinetics (Table 346-3). Testosterone serves as a prohormone and is converted to 17β-estradiol by aromatase and to 5α-dihydrotestosterone by 5α-reductase. Therefore, in evaluating testosterone formulations, it is important to consider whether the formulation being used can achieve physiologic estradiol and DHT concentrations in addition to normal testosterone concentrations. Although testosterone concentrations at the lower end of the normal male range can restore sexual function, it is not clear whether low-normal testosterone levels can maintain bone mineral density and muscle mass. The current recommendation is to restore testosterone levels to the mid-normal range.

Oral Derivatives of Testosterone Testosterone is well-absorbed after oral administration but is quickly degraded during the first pass through the liver. Therefore, it is difficult to achieve sustained blood levels of testosterone after oral administration of crystalline testosterone. 17α-Alkylated derivatives of testosterone (e.g., 17α-methyl testosterone, oxandrolone, fluoxymesterone) are relatively resistant to hepatic degradation and can be administered orally; however, because of the potential for hepatotoxicity, including cholestatic jaundice, peliosis, and hepatoma, these formulations should not be used for testosterone replacement. Hereditary angioedema due to C1 esterase deficiency is the only exception to this general recommendation; in this condition, oral 17α-alkylated androgens are useful because they stimulate hepatic synthesis of the C1 esterase inhibitor.

Injectable Forms of Testosterone The esterification of testosterone at the 17β-hydroxy position makes the molecule hydrophobic and extends its duration of action. The slow release of testosterone ester from an oily depot in the muscle accounts for its extended duration of action. The longer the side chain, the greater the hydrophobicity of the ester, and the longer the duration of action. Thus, testosterone enanthate, cypionate, and undecanoate with longer side chains have longer durations of action than does testosterone propionate. Within 24 hours after intramuscular administration of 200 mg testosterone enanthate or cypionate, testosterone levels rise into the high-normal or supraphysiologic range and then gradually decline into the hypogonadal range over the next 2 weeks. A bimonthly regimen of testosterone enanthate or cypionate therefore results in peaks and troughs in testosterone levels that are accompanied by changes in a patient's mood, sexual desire, and energy level. The kinetics of testosterone enanthate and cypionate are similar. Estradiol and DHT levels are normal if testosterone replacement is physiologic.

Transdermal Testosterone Patch Nongenital testosterone patches, when applied in an appropriate dose, can normalize testosterone, DHT, and estradiol levels 4–12 hours after application. Sexual function and well-being are restored in androgen-deficient men treated with the nongenital patch. One 5-mg patch may not be sufficient to increase testosterone into the mid-normal male range in all hypogonadal men; some patients may need two 5-mg patches daily to achieve the targeted testosterone concentrations. The use of testosterone patches may be associated with skin irritation in some individuals.

Testosterone Gel Two testosterone gels, Androgel and Testim, when applied topically to the skin in 5-, 7.5-, and 10-g doses, can maintain total and free testosterone concentrations in the mid- to high-normal range in hypogonadal men. The current recommendations are to begin with a 50-mg dose and adjust the dose on the

TABLE 346-3 Clinical Pharmacology of Some Testosterone Formulations

Formulation	Regimen	Pharmacokinetic profile	DHT and E2	Advantages	Disadvantages
Testosterone enanthate or cypionate	150–200 mg IM q 2 weeks or 75-100 mg/week	After a single IM injection, serum T levels rise into the supraphysiologic range, then decline gradually into the hypogonadal range by the end of the dosing interval	DHT and E_2 levels rise in proportion to the increase in T levels; T:DHT and T:E_2 ratios do not change	Corrects symptoms of androgen deficiency; relatively inexpensive if self-administered; flexibility of dosing	Requires IM injection; peaks and valleys in serum T levels
1% Testosterone gel	Available in sachets, tubes, and pumps 5–10 g T gel containing 50–100 mg T qid	Restores serum T and E_2 levels to physiologic male range	Serum DHT levels are higher and T:DHT ratios are lower in hypogonadal men treated with the T gel than in healthy eugonadal men	Corrects symptoms of androgen deficiency; provides flexibility of dosing, ease of application; good skin tolerability	Potential of transfer to a female partner or child by direct skin-to-skin contact; skin irritation in a small proportion of treated men; moderately high DHT levels
Transdermal testosterone patch	1 or 2 patches, designed to nominally deliver 5–10 mg T over 24 h applied qid on nonpressure areas	Restores serum T, DHT, and E_2 levels to physiologic male range	T:DHT and T:E_2 levels are in physiologic male range	Ease of application; corrects symptoms of androgen deficiency	Serum T levels in some androgen-deficient men may be in the low-normal range; these men may need application of 2 patches daily; skin irritation at the application site occurs frequently in many patients
Buccal, bioadhesive, T tablets	30-mg controlled-release, bioadhesive tablets bid	Absorbed from buccal mucosa	Normalizes serum T and DHT levels in hypogonadal men	Corrects symptoms of androgen deficiency in healthy, hypogonadal men	Gum-related adverse events in 16% of treated men.
Testosterone pellets	3–6 pellets implanted SC; dose and regimen vary with formulation	Serum T peaks at 1 month and then is sustained in normal range for 3–6 months, depending on formulation	T:DHT and T:E_2 ratios do not change	Corrects symptoms of androgen deficiency	Requires surgical incision for insertions; pellets may extrude spontaneously
17-α-methyl testosterone	This 17-α-alkylated compound should *not* be used because of potential for liver toxicity.	Orally active			Clinical responses are variable; potential for liver toxicity; should *not* be used for treatment of androgen deficiency
Oral testosterone undecanoate*	40–80 mg PO bid or tid with meals	When administered in oleic acid, T undecanoate is absorbed through lymphatics, bypassing portal system; considerable variability in the same individual on different days and among individuals	High DHT to T ratio	Convenience of oral administration	Not approved in the United States; variable clinical responses, variable serum T levels, high DHT:T ratio
Injectable long-acting testosterone undecanoate in oil*	European regimen 1000 mg IM, followed by 1000 mg at 6 weeks and 1000 mg q 10–14 weeks	When administered at a dose of 750–1000 mg IM, serum T levels are maintained in the normal range in a majority of treated men	DHT and E_2 levels rise in proportion to increase in T levels; T:DHT and T:E_2 ratios do not change	Corrects symptoms of androgen deficiency; requires infrequent administration.	Requires IM injection of a large volume (4 mL); cough reported immediately after injection in a very small number of men
Testosterone-inadhesive matrix patch*	2 × 60 cm^2 patches delivering approximately 4.8 mg of T/d	Restores serum T, DHT, and E_2 to physiologic range	T:DHT and T:E_2 are in physiologic range.	Lasts 2 d	Some skin irritation

*These formulations are not approved for clinical use in the United States but are available outside the United States in many countries. Physicians in countries where these formulations are available should follow the approved drug regimens.

Abbreviatons: DHT, dihydrotestosterone; E_2, estradiol; T, testosterone.

basis of testosterone levels. The advantages of the testosterone gel include ease of application and flexibility of dosing. A major concern is the potential for inadvertent transfer of the gel to a sexual partner or to children who may come in close contact with the patient. The ratio of DHT to testosterone concentrations is higher in men treated with the testosterone gel than in healthy men. Also, there is considerable intra- and interindividual variation in serum testosterone levels in men treated with the transdermal gel.

Buccal Adhesive Testosterone A buccal testosterone tablet that adheres to the buccal mucosa and releases testosterone as it is slowly dissolved has been approved. After twice-daily application of 30-mg tablets, serum testosterone levels are maintained within the normal male range in a majority of treated hypogonadal men. The adverse effects include buccal ulceration and gum problems in a few subjects. The effects of food and brushing on absorption have not been studied in detail.

Implants of crystalline testosterone can be inserted in the subcutaneous tissue by means of a trocar through a small skin incision. Testosterone is released by surface erosion of the implant and absorbed into the systemic circulation. Two to six 200-mg implants can maintain testosterone in the mid- to high-normal range for up to 6 months. Potential drawbacks include incising the skin for insertion and removal and spontaneous extrusions and fibrosis at the site of the implant.

Testosterone Formulations Not Available in the United States Testosterone undecanoate, when administered orally in oleic acid, is absorbed preferentially through the lymphatics into the systemic circulation and is spared first-pass degradation in the liver. Doses of 40–80 mg orally, two or three times daily, are typically used. However, the clinical responses are variable and suboptimal. Ratios of DHT to testosterone are higher in hypogonadal men treated with oral testosterone undecanoate compared with eugonadal men.

After initial priming, long-acting testosterone undecanoate in oil, when administered intramuscularly every 12 weeks, maintains serum testosterone, estradiol, and DHT in the normal male range and corrects symptoms of androgen deficiency in a majority of treated men. However, the large injection volume (4 mL) is a relative drawback.

Novel Androgen Formulations A number of androgen formulations with better pharmacokinetics or more selective activity profiles are under development. Two long-acting esters, testosterone buciclate and testosterone undecanoate, when injected intramuscularly, can maintain circulating testosterone concentrations in the male range for 7–12 weeks. Initial clinical trials have demonstrated the feasibility of administering testosterone by the sublingual or buccal route. 7α-Methyl-19-nortestosterone is an androgen that cannot be 5α-reduced; therefore, compared to testosterone, it has relatively greater agonist activity in muscle and gonadotropin suppression but lesser activity on the prostate.

Selective androgen receptor modulators (SARMs) are a class of androgen receptor ligands that bind the androgen receptor and display tissue-selective actions. A number of nonsteroidal SARMs that act as full agonists on the muscle and bone and spare the prostate to varying degrees have advanced to phase I and II human trials. Nonsteroidal SARMs do not serve as substrates for either the steroid 5α-reductase or the CYP19 aromatase. SARM binding to AR induces specific conformational changes in the AR protein, which then modulates protein-protein interactions between AR and its coregulators, resulting in tissue-specific regulation of gene expression.

Pharmacologic Uses of Androgens Androgens and SARMs are being evaluated as anabolic therapies for functional limitations associated with aging and chronic illness. Testosterone supplementation increases skeletal muscle mass, maximal voluntary strength, and muscle power in healthy men, hypogonadal men, older men with low testosterone levels, HIV-infected men with weight loss, and men receiving glucocorticoids. These anabolic effects of testosterone are related to testosterone dose and circulating concentrations. Systematic reviews have confirmed that testosterone therapy in HIV-infected men with weight loss promotes improvements in body weight, lean body mass, muscle strength, and depression indices, leading to the recommendation that testosterone be considered as an adjunctive therapy in HIV-infected men who are experiencing unexplained weight loss and have low testosterone levels. Similarly, in glucocorticoid-treated men, testosterone therapy should be considered to maintain muscle mass and strength and vertebral bone mineral density. It is not known whether testosterone therapy in older men with functional limitations is safe and effective in improving physical function and health-related quality of life and reducing disability. Concerns about potential adverse effects of testosterone on prostate and cardiovascular event rates have encouraged the development of selective androgen receptor modulators that are preferentially anabolic and spare the prostate.

Testosterone administration induces hypertrophy of both types 1 and 2 fibers and increases satellite cell (muscle progenitor cells) and myonuclear numbers. Androgens promote the differentiation of mesenchymal, multipotent progenitor cells into the myogenic lineage and inhibit their differentiation into the adipogenic lineage. Testosterone may have additional effects on satellite cell replication and muscle protein synthesis that may contribute to an increase in skeletal muscle mass.

Other indications for androgen therapy are in selected patients with anemia due to bone marrow failure (an indication largely supplanted by erythropoietin) and for hereditary angioedema.

Male Hormonal Contraception Based on Combined Administration of Testosterone and Gonadotropin Inhibitors Supraphysiologic doses of testosterone (200 mg testosterone enanthate weekly) suppress LH and FSH secretion and induce azoospermia in 50% of white men and >95% of Asian men. The World Health Organization (WHO)-supported multicenter efficacy trials have demonstrated that suppression of spermatogenesis to azoospermia or severe oligozoospermia (<3 million/mL) by administration of testosterone enanthate to men results in effective contraception. Because of concern about long-term adverse effects of supraphysiologic testosterone doses, regimens that combine other gonadotropin inhibitors such as GnRH antagonists and progestins, with replacement doses of testosterone are being investigated. Oral etonogestrel daily in combination with intramuscular testosterone decanoate every 4–6 weeks induced azoospermia or severe oligozoospermia (sperm density <1 million/mL) in 99% of treated men over a 1-year period. This regimen was associated with weight gain, deceased testicular volume, and decreased plasma high-density lipoprotein (HDL) cholesterol, and its long-term safety has not been demonstrated. Selective androgen receptor modulators that are more potent inhibitors of gonadotropins than testosterone and spare the prostate hold promise for their contraceptive potential.

Recommended Regimens for Androgen Replacement Testosterone esters are administered typically at doses of 75–100 mg intramuscularly every week or 150–200 mg every 2 weeks. One or two 5-mg nongenital testosterone patches can be applied daily over the skin of the back, thigh, or upper arm away from pressure areas. Testosterone gel typically is applied over a covered area of skin at a dose of 5–10 g daily; patients should wash their hands after gel application. Bioadhesive buccal testosterone tablets at a dose of 30 mg typically are applied twice daily on the buccal mucosa.

Establishing Efficacy of Testosterone Replacement Therapy Because a clinically useful marker of androgen action is not available, restoration of testosterone levels into the mid-normal range remains the goal of therapy. Measurements of LH and FSH are not useful in assessing the adequacy of testosterone replacement. Testosterone should be measured 3 months after initiating therapy to assess adequacy of therapy. There is substantial interindividual variability in serum testosterone levels, presumably due to genetic differences in testosterone clearance. In patients who are treated with testosterone enanthate or cypionate, testosterone levels should be 350–600 ng/dL 1 week after the injection. If testosterone levels are outside this range, adjustments should be made either in the dose or in the interval between injections. In men on transdermal patch or gel or buccal testosterone therapy, testosterone levels should be in the mid-normal range (500–700 ng/dL) 4–12 hours after application. If testosterone levels are outside this range, the dose should be adjusted.

Restoration of sexual function, secondary sex characteristics, energy, and well-being and maintenance of muscle and bone health are important objectives of testosterone replacement therapy. The patient should be asked about sexual desire and activity, the presence of early-morning erections, and the ability to achieve and maintain erections adequate for sexual intercourse. Some hypogonadal men continue to complain about sexual dysfunction even after testosterone replacement has been instituted; these patients may benefit from counseling. The hair growth in response to androgen replacement is variable and depends on ethnicity. Hypogonadal men with prepubertal onset of androgen deficiency who begin testosterone therapy in their late twenties or thirties may find it difficult to adjust to their newly found sexuality and may benefit from counseling. If the patient has a sexual partner, the partner should be included in counseling because of the dramatic physical and sexual changes that occur with androgen treatment.

Contraindications for Androgen Administration Testosterone administration is contraindicated in men with a history of prostate or breast cancer (Table 346-4). Testosterone therapy should not be administered without further urologic evaluation to men with a palpable prostate nodule or induration or prostate-specific antigen >4 ng/mL or >3 ng/mL in men at high risk for prostate cancer such as blacks or men with first-degree relatives with prostate cancer or with severe lower urinary tract symptoms (American Urological Association lower urinary tract symptom score >19). Testosterone replacement should not be administered to men with baseline hematocrit ≥50%, severe untreated obstructive sleep apnea, uncontrolled or poorly controlled congestive heart failure, or recent myocardial infarction or unstable angina.

TABLE 346-4 Conditions in Which Testosterone Administration is Associated With a Risk of Adverse Outcome

Conditions in Which Testosterone Administration is Associated with Very High Risk of Serious Adverse Outcomes:
Metastatic prostate cancer
Breast cancer
Conditions in Which Testosterone Administration is Associated with Moderate to High Risk of Adverse Outcomes:
Undiagnosed prostate nodule or induration
PSA >4 ng/mL (>3 ng/mL in individuals at high risk for prostate cancer, such as blacks and men with first-degree relatives who have prostate cancer)
Erythrocytosis (hematocrit >50%)
Severe lower urinary tract symptoms associated with benign prostatic hypertrophy as indicated by the American Urological Association/International prostate symptom score >19
Uncontrolled or poorly controlled congestive heart failure

Abbreviation: PSA, prostate-specific antigen.

Source: Reproduced from the Endocrine Society Guideline for Testosterone Therapy of Androgen Deficiency Syndromes in Men (Bhasin et al).

Monitoring Potential Adverse Experiences The clinical effectiveness and safety of testosterone replacement therapy should be assessed 3–6 months after initiating testosterone therapy and annually thereafter (Table 346-5). Potential adverse effects include acne, oiliness of skin, erythrocytosis, breast tenderness and enlargement, leg edema, induction and exacerbation of obstructive sleep apnea, and increased risk of detection of prostate disease. In addition, there may be formulation-specific adverse effects such as skin irritation with transdermal patches, risk of gel transfer to a sexual partner with testosterone gels, buccal ulceration and gum problems with buccal testosterone, and pain and mood fluctuation with injectable testosterone esters.

Hemoglobin Levels Administration of testosterone to androgen-deficient men typically is associated with a 3–5% increase in hemoglobin levels due to suppression of hepcidin and increased iron availability for erythropoiesis. The magnitude of hemoglobin increase during testosterone therapy is greater in older men than younger men and in men who have sleep apnea, a significant smoking history, or chronic obstructive lung disease. The frequency of erythrocytosis is higher in hypogonadal men treated with injectable testosterone esters than in those treated with transdermal formulations, presumably due to the higher testosterone dose delivered by the typical regimens of testosterone esters. Erythrocytosis is the most common adverse event reported in testosterone trials in middle-aged and older men and also the most common cause of treatment discontinuation in these trials. If hematocrit rises above 54%, testosterone therapy should be stopped until hematocrit has fallen to <50%. After evaluation of the patient for hypoxia and sleep apnea, testosterone therapy may be reinitiated at a lower dose.

Prostate and Serum PSA Levels Testosterone replacement therapy increases prostate volume to the size seen in age-matched controls but does not increase prostate volume beyond that expected for age. There is no evidence that testosterone therapy causes prostate cancer. However, androgen administration can exacerbate preexisting metastatic prostate cancer. Many older men harbor microscopic foci of cancer in their prostates. It is not known whether long-term testosterone administration will induce these microscopic foci to grow into clinically significant cancers.

Prostate-specific antigen (PSA) levels are lower in testosterone-deficient men and are restored to normal after testosterone replacement. There is considerable test-retest variability in PSA measurements. Increments in PSA levels after testosterone supplementation in androgen-deficient men are generally <0.5 ng/mL, and increments >1 ng/mL over a 3–6-month period are unusual. The 90% confidence interval for the change in PSA values in men with benign prostatic hypertrophy measured 3–6 months apart is 1.4 ng/mL. Therefore, the Endocrine Society expert panel suggests that an increase in PSA >1.4 ng/mL in any one year after starting testosterone therapy, if confirmed, should lead to urologic evaluation. PSA velocity criterion can be used for patients who have sequential PSA measurements for

TABLE 346-5 Monitoring Men Receiving Testosterone Therapy

1. Evaluate patient 3–6 months after treatment initiation and then annually to assess whether symptoms have responded to treatment and whether patient is experiencing any adverse effects.
2. Monitor testosterone level 3–6 months after initiation of testosterone therapy:
   - Therapy should aim to raise serum testosterone level into mid-normal range.
     - Injectable testosterone enanthate or cypionate: Measure serum testosterone level midway between injections. If testosterone is >700 ng/dL (24.5 nmol/L) or <400 ng/dL (14.1 nmol/L), adjust dose or frequency.
     - Transdermal patches: Assess testosterone level 3–12 h after application of the patch; adjust dose to achieve testosterone level in mid-normal range.
     - Buccal testosterone bioadhesive tablet: Assess level immediately before or after application of fresh system.
     - Transdermal gels: Assess testosterone level any time after patient has been on treatment for at least 1 week; adjust dose to achieve serum testosterone level in the mid-normal range.
     - Testosterone pellets: Measure testosterone levels at the end of dosing interval. Adjust number of pellets and/or dosing interval to achieve serum testosterone levels in normal range.
     - Oral testosterone undecanoate*: Monitor serum testosterone level 3 to 5 h after ingestion.
     - Injectable testosterone undecanoate: Measure serum testosterone level just before each subsequent injection and adjust dosing interval to maintain serum testosterone in mid-normal range.
3. Check hematocrit at baseline at 3–6 months and then annually. If hematocrit is >54%, stop therapy until hematocrit decreases to a safe level; evaluate patient for hypoxia and sleep apnea; reinitiate therapy with a reduced dose.
4. Measure bone mineral density of lumbar spine and/or femoral neck after 1–2 years of testosterone therapy in hypogonadal men with osteoporosis or low trauma fracture, consistent with regional standard of care.
5. In men 40 years of age or older with baseline PSA >0.6 ng/mL, perform digital rectal examination and check PSA level before initiating treatment at 3–6 months and then in accordance with guidelines for prostate cancer screening depending on age and race of patient.
6. Obtain urologic consultation if there is:
   - An increase in serum PSA concentration >1.4 ng/mL within any 12-month period of testosterone treatment.
   - A PSA velocity >0.4 ng/mL per year using PSA level after 6 months of testosterone administration as reference (applicable only if PSA data are available for a period exceeding 2 years).
   - Detection of a prostatic abnormality on digital rectal examination.
   - An AUA/IPSS prostate symptom score >19.
7. Evaluate formulation-specific adverse effects at each visit:
   - Buccal testosterone tablets: Inquire about alterations in taste and examine gums and oral mucosa for irritation.
   - Injectable testosterone esters (enanthate, cypionate, and undecanoate): Ask about fluctuations in mood or libido and, rarely, cough after injections.
   - Testosterone patches: Look for skin reaction at application site.
   - Testosterone gels: Advise patients to cover application sites with a shirt and wash skin with soap and water before having skin-to-skin contact because testosterone gels leave a testosterone residue on skin that can be transferred to a woman or child who comes in close contact. Serum testosterone levels are maintained when application site is washed 4–6 h after application of testosterone gel.
   - Testosterone pellets: Look for signs of infection, fibrosis, or pellet extrusion.

*Not approved for clinical use in the United States.

Abbreviations: AUA/IPSS, American Urological Association International Prostate Symptom Score; PSA, prostate-specific antigen.

Source: Reproduced with permission from the Endocrine Society Guideline for Testosterone Therapy of Androgen Deficiency Syndromes in Men (Bhasin et al).

>2 years; a change of >0.40 ng/mL per year merits closer urologic follow-up.

Cardiovascular Risk In epidemiologic studies, testosterone concentrations are negatively related to the risk of diabetes mellitus, heart disease, and all-cause and cardiovascular mortality. A recent testosterone trial in older men with mobility limitation was stopped early because of the higher rates of cardiovascular events in the testosterone arm than in the placebo arm of the trial. Meta-analyses of testosterone trials have found no statistically significant increase in cardiovascular event rates in men receiving testosterone therapy, although nonsignificant increases have been noted. Inferences about adverse events from previous trials included in these meta-analyses were limited by poor ascertainment, small numbers of events, and small numbers of participants. Adequately powered prospective studies are needed to determine the effect of testosterone replacement on cardiovascular risk.

Androgen Abuse by Athletes and Recreational Bodybuilders The illicit use of androgenic-anabolic steroids (AAS) to enhance athletic performance first surfaced in the 1950s among power lifters and spread rapidly to other sports, professional as well as high school athletes, and recreational bodybuilders. In the early 1980s, the use of AAS spread beyond the athletic community into the general population, and now as many as 2 million Americans, most of them men, probably have used these compounds. The most commonly used androgenic steroids include testosterone esters, nandrolone, stanozolol, methandienone, and methenolol. Athletes generally use increasing doses of multiple steroids in a practice known as stacking.

The adverse effects of long-term AAS abuse are poorly understood. Most of the information about the adverse effects of AAS has emerged from case reports, uncontrolled studies, or clinical trials that used replacement doses of testosterone. The adverse event data from clinical trials using physiologic replacement doses of testosterone have been extrapolated unjustifiably to AAS users who may administer 10–100 times the replacement doses of testosterone over many years and to support the claim that AAS use is safe. A substantial fraction of androgenic steroid users also use other drugs that are perceived to be muscle-building or performance-enhancing such as growth hormone; IGF-I; insulin; stimulants such as amphetamine, clenbuterol, cocaine, ephedrine, and thyroxine; and drugs perceived to reduce adverse effects such as hCG, aromatase inhibitors, and estrogen antagonists. The men who abuse androgenic steroids are more likely to engage in other high-risk behaviors than are nonusers. The adverse events associated with AAS use may be due to AAS themselves, concomitant use of other drugs, high-risk behaviors, and host characteristics that may render these individuals more susceptible to AAS use or other high-risk behaviors.

The high rates of mortality and morbidity observed in AAS users are alarming. One Finnish study reported 4.6 times the risk of death among elite power lifters than among age-matched men from the general population. The causes of death among power lifters included suicides, myocardial infarction, hepatic coma, and non-Hodgkin's lymphoma. A retrospective review of patient records in Sweden also reported higher standardized mortality ratios for AAS users than for nonusers.

Numerous reports of cardiac death among young AAS users raise concerns about the adverse cardiovascular effects of AAS. High doses of AAS may induce proatherogenic dyslipidemia, increase thrombosis risk via effects on clotting factors and platelets, and induce vasospasm through their effects on vascular nitric oxide. The finding of androgen receptors on myocardial cells suggests that AAS may be directly toxic to myocardial cells.

Replacement doses of testosterone, when administered parenterally, are associated with only a small decrease in HDL cholesterol and little or no effect on total cholesterol, low-density lipoprotein (LDL) cholesterol, and triglyceride levels. In contrast, supraphysiologic doses of testosterone and orally administered, 17α-alylated, nonaromatizable AAS are associated with marked reductions in HDL cholesterol and increases in LDL cholesterol.

Long-term AAS use suppresses LH and FSH secretion and inhibits endogenous testosterone production and spermatogenesis. Men who have used AAS for more than a few months experience suppression of the hypothalamic-pituitary-testicular (HPT) axis after stopping AAS that may be associated with sexual dysfunction, infertility, and depression; in some AAS users, gonadotropin suppression may last more than a year. The dysphoria caused by androgen withdrawal may cause some men to revert to using AAS, leading to continued use and AAS dependence. As many as 30% of AAS users develop a syndrome of AAS dependence that is characterized by long-term AAS use despite adverse medical and psychiatric effects.

Unsafe injection practices, high-risk behaviors, and increased rates of incarceration put AAS users at increased risk of HIV and hepatitis B and C. In one survey, nearly 1 in 10 gay men had injected AAS or other substances, and AAS users were more likely to report high-risk unprotected anal sex than were other men.

Some AAS users develop manic symptoms during AAS exposure (sometimes associated with violence) and major depression (sometimes associated with suicidality) during AAS withdrawal. Users also may engage in other forms of illicit drug use, which may be potentiated or exacerbated by AAS.

Elevated liver enzymes, cholestatic jaundice, hepatic neoplasms, and peliosis hepatis have been reported with oral 17α-alkylated AAS. AAS use may cause muscle hypertrophy without compensatory adaptations in tendons, ligaments, and joints, thus increasing the risk of tendon and joint injuries. AAS use is associated with acne and baldness, as well as increased body hair.

Accredited laboratories use gas chromatography–mass spectrometry or liquid chromatography–mass spectrometry to detect anabolic steroid abuse. In recent years, the availability of high-resolution mass spectrometry and tandem mass spectrometry has improved the sensitivity of detecting androgen abuse. Illicit testosterone use generally is detected by the application of the measurement of the ratio of urinary testosterone to epitestosterone and further confirmed by the use of the ^{13}C:^{12}C ratio in testosterone by the use of isotope ratio combustion mass spectrometry. Exogenous testosterone administration increases urinary testosterone glucuronide excretion and consequently the ratio of testosterone to epitestosterone. Ratios above 4 suggest exogenous testosterone use but can also reflect genetic variation. Synthetic testosterone has a lower ^{13}C:^{12}C ratio than endogenously produced testosterone, and these differences in the ^{13}C:^{12}C ratio can be detected by isotope ratio combustion mass spectrometry, which is used to confirm exogenous testosterone use in individuals with a high ratio of testosterone to epitestosterone.

FURTHER READINGS

Basaria S et al: Adverse events associated with testosterone administration. N Engl J Med 363:109, 2010

Bhasin S: An approach to infertile men. J Clin Endocrinol Metab 92:1995, 2007

——— et al: Testosterone therapy in men with androgen deficiency syndromes: An endocrine society clinical practice guideline. J Clin Endocrinol Metab 95:2536, 2010

Bolona ER et al: Testosterone use in men with sexual dysfunction: A systematic review and meta-analysis of randomized placebo-controlled trials. Mayo Clin Proc 82:20, 2007

Crowley WF Jr et al: New genes controlling human reproduction and how you find them. Trans Am Clin Climatol Assoc 119:29, 2008

Ferlin A et al: Molecular and clinical characterizations of Y chromosome microdeletions in infertile men: A 10-year experience in Italy. J Clin Endocrinol Metab 92:762, 2007

Fernández-Balsells MM et al: Clinical review: 1. Adverse effects of testosterone therapy in adult men: A systematic review and meta-analysis. J Clin Endocrinol Metab 95:2560, 2010

Kanayama G et al: Long-term psychiatric and medical consequences of anabolic-androgenic steroid abuse: A looming public health concern? Drug Alcohol Depend 98:1, 2008

Menke A et al: Sex steroid hormone concentrations and risk of death in US men. Am J Epidemiol 171:583, 2010

Sedlmeyer IL, Palmert MR: Delayed puberty: Analysis of a large case series from an academic center. J Clin Endocrinol Metab 87:1613, 2002

Srinivas-Shankar U et al: Effects of testosterone on muscle strength, physical function, body composition, and quality of life in intermediate-frail and frail elderly men: A randomized, double-blind, placebo-controlled study. J Clin Endocrinol Metab 95:639, 2010

Wu F et al: Identification of late-onset hypogonadism in middle-aged and elderly men. N Engl J Med 363:123, 2010

CHAPTER 347

The Female Reproductive System, Infertility, and Contraception

Janet E. Hall

The female reproductive system regulates the hormonal changes responsible for puberty and adult reproductive function. Normal reproductive function in women requires the dynamic integration of hormonal signals from the hypothalamus, pituitary, and ovary, resulting in repetitive cycles of follicle development, ovulation, and preparation of the endometrial lining of the uterus for implantation should conception occur.

For further discussion of related topics, see the following chapters: hyperandrogenic disorders (Chap. 49), menstrual cycle disorders (Chap. 50), gynecologic malignancies (Chap. 97), sexually transmitted diseases (Chap. 130), male hormonal contraception (Chap. 346), menopause (Chap. 348), and sexual differentiation (Chap. 349).

DEVELOPMENT OF THE OVARY AND EARLY FOLLICULAR GROWTH

The ovary orchestrates the development and release of a mature oocyte and also elaborates hormones (e.g., estrogen, progesterone, inhibin, relaxin) that are critical for pubertal development and preparation of the uterus for conception, implantation, and the early stages of pregnancy. To achieve these functions in repeated monthly cycles, the ovary undergoes some of the most dynamic changes of any organ in the body. Primordial germ cells can be identified by the third week of gestation and their migration to the genital ridge is complete by 6 weeks' gestation. Germ cells persist within the genital ridge, are then referred to as *oogonia*, and are essential for induction of ovarian development. Although one X chromosome undergoes X inactivation in somatic cells, it is reactivated in oogonia and genes on both X chromosomes are required for normal ovarian development. A streak ovary containing only stromal cells is found in patients with 45,X Turner's syndrome (Chap. 349).

The germ cell population expands, and starting at ~8 weeks' gestation, oogonia begin to enter prophase of the first meiotic division and become primary oocytes. This allows the oocyte to be surrounded by a single layer of flattened granulosa cells to form a primordial follicle (Fig. 347-1). Granulosa cells are derived from mesonephric cells that invade the ovary early in its development, pushing the germ cells to the periphery. Although recent studies have reopened the debate, the weight of evidence strongly supports the concept that the ovary contains a nonrenewable pool of germ

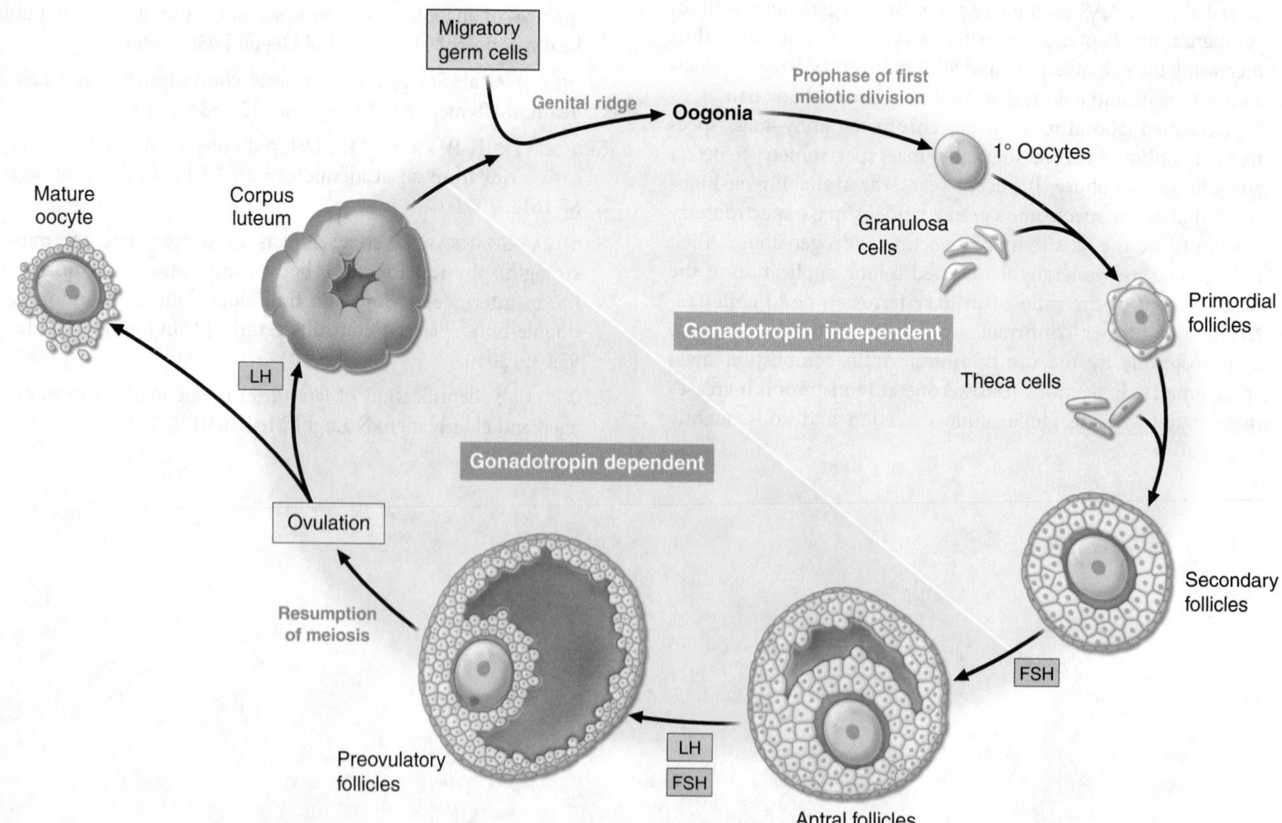

Figure 347-1 Stages of ovarian development from the arrival of the migratory germ cells at the genital ridge through gonadotropin-independent and gonadotropin-dependent phases that ultimately result in ovulation of a mature oocyte. FSH, follicle-stimulating hormone; LH, luteinizing hormone.

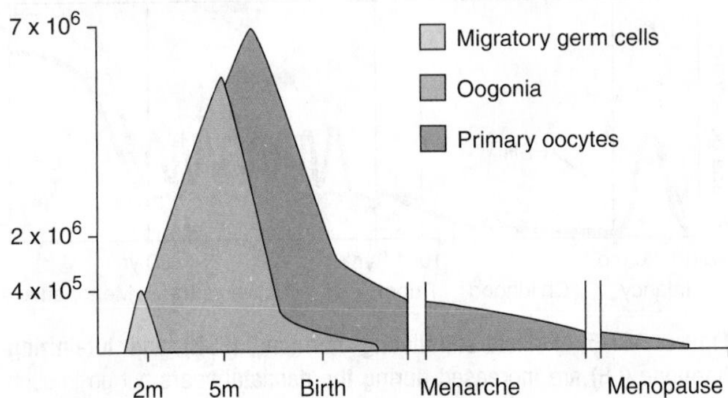

Figure 347-2 Ovarian germ cell number is maximal at mid-gestation, then decreases precipitously.

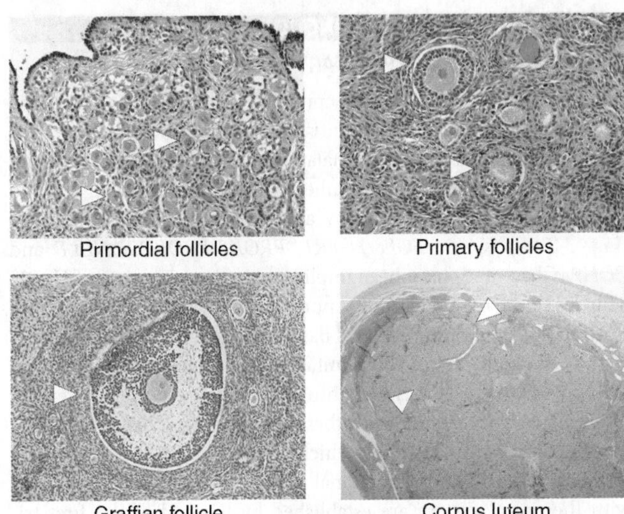

Figure 347-3 Development of ovarian follicles. The Graffian follicle is also known as a tertiary or preovulatory follicle. *(Courtesy of JH Eichhorn and D Roberts, Massachusetts General Hospital; with permission.)*

cells. Through the combined processes of mitosis, meiosis, and atresia, the population of oogonia reaches its maximum of 6–7 million by 20 weeks' gestation, after which there is a progressive loss of both oogonia and primordial follicles through the process of atresia. At birth, oogonia are no longer present in the ovary, and only 1–2 million germ cells remain in the form of primordial follicles (Fig. 347-2). The oocyte persists in prophase of the first meiotic division until just before ovulation, when meiosis resumes.

The quiescent primordial follicles are recruited to further growth and differentiation through a highly regulated process that limits the size of the developing cohort to ensure that folliculogenesis can continue throughout the reproductive life span. This initial recruitment of primordial follicles to form primary follicles (Fig. 347-1) is characterized by growth of the oocyte and the transition from squamous to cuboidal granulosa cells. The theca interna cells that surround the developing follicle begin to form as the primary follicle grows. Acquisition of a zona pellucida by the oocyte and the presence of several layers of surrounding cuboidal granulosa cells mark the development of secondary follicles. It is at this stage that granulosa cells develop follicle-stimulating hormone (FSH), estradiol, and androgen receptors and communicate with one another through the development of gap junctions.

Bidirectional signaling between the germ cells and the somatic cells in the ovary is a necessary component underlying the maturation of the oocyte and the capacity for hormone secretion. For example, the oocyte-derived factor in the germlineα(FIGα) is required for initial follicle formation. Anti-müllerian hormone [AMH, also known as mullerian inhibiting substance (MIS)] and activins derived from somatic cells induce the development of primary follicles from primordial follicles. Oocyte-derived growth differentiation factor 9 (GDF-9) is required for migration of pre-theca cells to the outer surface of the developing follicle. GDF-9 is also required for formation of secondary follicles, as are granulosa cell–derived KIT ligand (KITL) and the forkhead transcription factor (FOXL2). All of these genes are potential candidates for premature ovarian failure in women, and mutations in the human *FOXL2* gene have been shown to cause the syndrome of blepharophimosis/ptosis/epicanthus inversus, which is associated with ovarian failure.

DEVELOPMENT OF A MATURE FOLLICLE

The early stages of follicle growth are primarily driven by intraovarian factors and may take up to a year from the time of initial recruitment. Maturation to the state required for ovulation, including the resumption of meiosis in the oocyte, requires the combined stimulus of FSH and luteinizing hormone (LH) (Fig. 347-1) and can be accomplished within weeks. Recruitment of secondary follicles from the resting follicle pool requires the direct action of FSH. Accumulation of follicular fluid between the layers of granulosa cells creates an antrum that divides the granulosa cells into two functionally distinct groups: mural cells that line the follicle wall and cumulus cells that surround the oocyte (Fig. 347-3). Recent evidence suggests that, in addition to its role in normal development of the mullerian system, the WNT signaling pathway is required for normal antral follicle development and may also play a role in ovarian steroidogenesis. A single dominant follicle emerges from the growing follicle pool within the first 5–7 days after the onset of menses, and the majority of follicles fall off their growth trajectory and become atretic. Autocrine actions of activin and bone morphogenic protein 6 (BMP-6), derived from the granulosa cells, and paracrine actions of GDF-9, BMP-15, BMP-6, and Gpr149, derived from the oocyte, are involved in granulosa cell proliferation and modulation of FSH responsiveness. Differential exposure to these factors may explain why one follicle is selected for continued growth to the preovulatory stage. The dominant follicle can be distinguished by its size, evidence of granulosa cell proliferation, large number of FSH receptors, high aromatase activity, and elevated concentrations of estradiol and inhibin A in follicular fluid.

The dominant follicle undergoes rapid expansion during the 5–6 days prior to ovulation, reflecting granulosa cell proliferation and accumulation of follicular fluid. FSH induces LH receptors on the granulosa cells, and the preovulatory, or Graffian, follicle moves to the outer ovarian surface in preparation for ovulation. The LH surge triggers the resumption of meiosis, the suppression of granulosa cell proliferation, and the induction of cyclooxygenase 2 (COX-2), prostaglandins, and the progesterone receptor, each of which is required for ovulation. EGF-like factors are thought to mediate these follicular responses to LH. Ovulation also involves production of extracellular matrix leading to expansion of the cumulus cell population that surrounds the oocyte and the controlled expulsion of the egg and follicular fluid. Both progesterone and prostaglandins (induced by the ovulatory stimulus) are essential for this process. After ovulation, luteinization is induced by LH in conjunction with the acquisition of a rich vascular network in response to vascular endothelial growth factor (VEGF) and basic fibroblast growth factor (basic FGF). Traditional regulators of central reproductive control, gonadotropin-releasing hormone (GnRH) and its receptor (GnRHR), are also produced in the ovary and may be involved in corpus luteum function.

REGULATION OF OVARIAN FUNCTION

HYPOTHALAMIC AND PITUITARY SECRETION

GnRH neurons develop from epithelial cells outside the central nervous system and migrate, initially alongside the olfactory neurons, to the medial basal hypothalamus. Studies in GnRH-deficient patients who fail to undergo puberty have provided insights into genes that control the ontogeny and function of GnRH neurons (Fig. 347-4). *KAL1*, *FGF8/FGFR1*, *PROK2/PROKR2*, *NELF* and *CDH7* (Chap. 346) have been implicated in the migration of GnRH neurons to the hypothalamus. Approximately 7000 GnRH neurons, scattered throughout the medial basal hypothalamus, establish contacts with capillaries of the pituitary portal system in the median eminence. GnRH is secreted into the pituitary portal system in discrete pulses to stimulate synthesis and secretion of LH and FSH from pituitary gonadotropes, which comprise ~10% of cells in the pituitary (Chap. 339). Functional connections of GnRH neurons with the portal system are established by the end of the first trimester, coinciding with the production of pituitary gonadotropins. Thus, like the ovary, the hypothalamic and pituitary components of the reproductive system are present before birth. However, the high levels of estradiol and progesterone produced by the placenta suppress hypothalamic-pituitary stimulation of ovarian hormonal secretion in the fetus.

After birth and the loss of placenta-derived steroids, gonadotropin levels rise. FSH levels are much higher in girls than in boys. This rise in FSH results in ovarian activation (evident on ultrasound) and increased inhibin B and estradiol levels. Studies that have identified mutations in *TAC3*, which encodes neurokinin B, and its receptor, *TAC3R*, in patients with GnRH deficiency indicate that both are involved in control of GnRH secretion and may be particularly important at this early stage of development. By 12–20 months of age, the reproductive axis is again suppressed, and a period of relative quiescence persists until puberty (Fig. 347-5). At the onset of puberty, pulsatile GnRH secretion induces pituitary gonadotropin

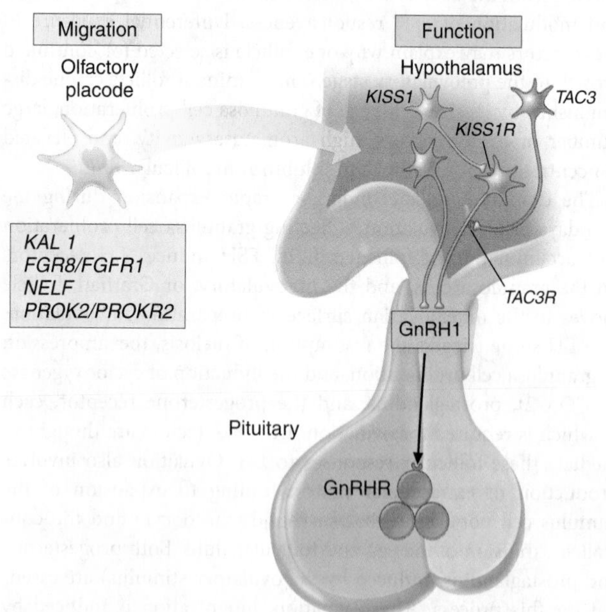

Figure 347-4 Establishment of a functional GnRH system requires the participation of a number of genes that are essential for development and migration of GnRH neurons from the olfactory placode to the hypothalamus in addition to genes involved in the functional control of GnRH secretion and action.

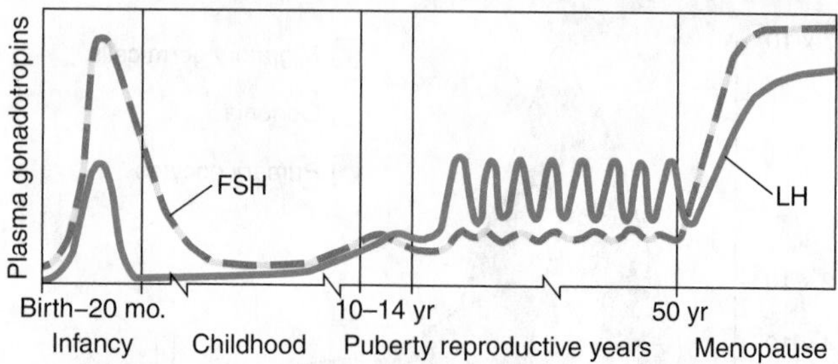

Figure 347-5 Follicle-stimulating hormone (FSH) and luteinizing hormone (LH) are increased during the neonatal years but go through a period of childhood quiescence before increasing again during puberty. Gonadotropin levels are cyclic during the reproductive years and increase dramatically with the loss of negative feedback that accompanies menopause.

production. In the early stages of puberty, LH and FSH secretion are apparent only during sleep, but as puberty develops, pulsatile gonadotropin secretion occurs throughout the day and night.

The mechanisms responsible for the childhood quiescence and pubertal reactivation of the reproductive axis remain incompletely understood. GnRH neurons in the hypothalamus respond to both excitatory and inhibitory factors. Increased sensitivity to the inhibitory influence of gonadal steroids has long been implicated in the inhibition of GnRH secretion during childhood but has not been definitively established in the human. Metabolic signals such as adipocyte-derived leptin, play a permissive role in reproductive function (Chap. 77). Studies of patients with isolated GnRH deficiency reveal that mutations in the G protein–coupled receptor 54 (*GPR54*) gene (now known as *KISS1R*) preclude the onset of puberty. The ligand for this receptor, metastin, is derived from the parent peptide, kisspeptin-1 (*KISS1*), and is a powerful stimulant for GnRH release. A potential role for kisspeptin in the onset of puberty has been suggested by upregulation of *KISS1* and *KISS1R* transcripts in the hypothalamus at the time of puberty. The KISS1/KISS1R system may also be involved in estrogen feedback regulation of GnRH secretion.

OVARIAN STEROIDS

Ovarian steroid-producing cells do not store hormones but produce them in response to LH and FSH during the normal menstrual cycle. The sequence of steps and the enzymes involved in the synthesis of steroid hormones are similar in the ovary, adrenal, and testis. However, the enzymes required to catalyze specific steps are compartmentalized and may not be abundant or even present in all cell types. Within the developing ovarian follicle, estrogen synthesis from cholesterol requires close integration between theca and granulosa cells—sometimes called the *two-cell model for steroidogenesis* (Fig. 347-6). FSH receptors are confined to the granulosa cells, whereas LH receptors are restricted to the theca cells until the late stages of follicular development, when they are also found on granulosa cells. The theca cells surrounding the follicle are highly vascularized and use cholesterol, derived primarily from circulating lipoproteins, as the starting point for the synthesis of androstenedione and testosterone under the control of LH. Androstenedione and testosterone are transferred across the basal lamina to the granulosa cells, which receive no direct blood supply. The mural granulosa cells are particularly rich in aromatase and, under the control of FSH, produce estradiol, the primary steroid secreted from the follicular phase ovary and the most potent estrogen. Theca cell–produced androstenedione and, to a lesser extent, testosterone are also secreted into peripheral blood, where they can be converted

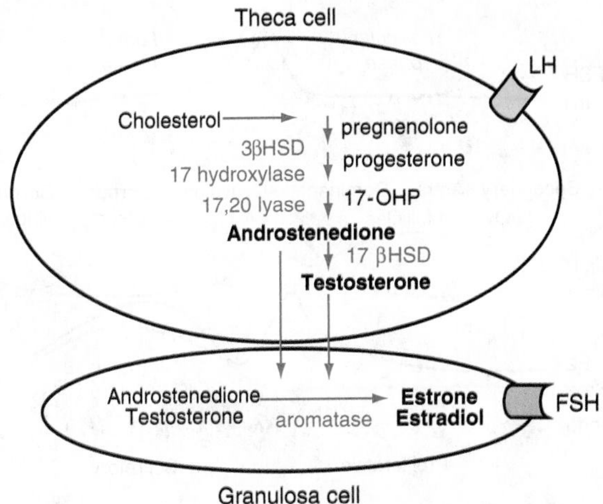

Figure 347-6 Estrogen production in the ovary requires the cooperative function of the theca and granulosa cells under the control of luteinizing hormone (LH) and follicle-stimulating hormone (FSH). HSD, hydroxysteroid dehydrogenase; OHP, hydroxyprogesterone.

to dihydrotestosterone in skin and to estrogens in adipose tissue. The hilar interstitial cells of the ovary are functionally similar to Leydig cells and are also capable of secreting androgens. Although stromal cells proliferate in response to androgens [as in polycystic ovarian syndrome (PCOS)], they do not secrete androgens.

Development of the rich capillary network following rupture of the follicle at the time of ovulation makes it possible for large molecules such as low-density lipoprotein (LDL) to reach the luteinized granulosa and theca lutein cells. As in the follicle, both cell types are required for steroidogenesis in the corpus luteum. The luteinized granulosa cells are the main source of progesterone production whereas the theca lutein cells produce 17-hydroxyprogesterone, a substrate for aromatization to estradiol by the luteinized granulosa cells. LH is critical for normal structure and function of the corpus luteum. Because LH and human chorionic gonadotropin (hCG) bind to a common receptor, the role of LH in support of the corpus luteum can be replaced by hCG in the first 10 weeks after conception, and hCG is commonly used for luteal phase support in the treatment of infertility.

Steroid hormone actions

Both estrogen and progesterone play critical roles in the expression of secondary sexual characteristics in women (Chap. 338). Estrogen promotes development of the ductule system in the breast, whereas progesterone is responsible for glandular development. In the reproductive tract, estrogens create a receptive environment for fertilization and support pregnancy and parturition through carefully coordinated changes in the endometrium, thickening of the vaginal mucosa, thinning of the cervical mucus, and uterine growth and contractions. Progesterone induces secretory activity in the estrogen-primed endometrium, increases the viscosity of cervical mucus, and inhibits uterine contractions. Both gonadal steroids play critical roles in the negative and positive feedback controls of gonadotropin secretion. Progesterone also increases basal body temperature and has therefore been used clinically as a marker of ovulation.

The vast majority of circulating estrogens and androgens are carried in the blood bound to carrier proteins, which restrain their free diffusion into cells and prolong their clearance, serving as a reservoir. High-affinity binding proteins include sex hormone–binding globulin (SHBG), which binds androgens with somewhat greater affinity than estrogens, and corticosteroid-binding globulin (CBG), which also binds progesterone. Modulations in binding protein levels by insulin, androgens, and estrogens contribute to high bioavailable testosterone levels in PCOS and to high circulating estrogen and progesterone levels during pregnancy.

Estrogens act primarily through binding to the nuclear receptors, estrogen receptor (ER) α and β. Transcriptional coactivators and co-repressors modulate ER action (Chap. 338). Both ER subtypes are present in the hypothalamus, pituitary, ovary, and reproductive tract. Although ERα and -β exhibit some functional redundancy, there is also a high degree of specificity, particularly in cell type expression. For example, ERα functions in the ovarian theca cells, whereas ERβ is critical for granulosa cell function. There is also evidence for membrane-initiated signaling by estrogen. Similar signaling mechanisms pertain for progesterone with evidence of transcriptional regulation through progesterone receptor (PR) A and B protein isoforms, as well as rapid membrane signaling.

■ OVARIAN PEPTIDES

Inhibin was initially isolated from gonadal fluids based on its ability to selectively inhibit FSH secretion from pituitary cells. Inhibin is a heterodimer composed of an α-subunit and a βA- or βB-subunit to form inhibin A or inhibin B, both of which are secreted from the ovary. Activin is a homodimer of inhibin β subunits with the capacity to stimulate the synthesis and secretion of FSH. Inhibins and activins are members of the transforming growth factor β (TGF-β) superfamily of growth and differentiation factors. During the purification of inhibin, follistatin, an unrelated monomeric protein that inhibits FSH secretion, was discovered. Within the pituitary, follistatin inhibits FSH secretion indirectly through binding and neutralizing activin.

Inhibin B is secreted from the granulosa cells of small antral follicles, whereas inhibin A is present in both granulosa and theca cells and is secreted by dominant follicles. Inhibin A is also present in luteinized granulosa cells and is a major secretory product of the corpus luteum. Inhibin B is constitutively secreted by granulosa cells and increases in serum in conjunction with cycle recruitment to the pool of actively growing follicles under the control of FSH. Inhibin B has been used clinically as a marker of ovarian reserve. Inhibin B is an important inhibitor of FSH, independent of estradiol, during the menstrual cycle. Although activin is also secreted from the ovary, the excess of follistatin in serum, combined with its nearly irreversible binding of activin, make it unlikely that ovarian activin plays an endocrine role in FSH regulation. However, there is evidence that activin plays an autocrine/paracrine role in the ovary, in addition to its intrapituitary role in modulation of FSH production.

AMH (also known as MIS) is important in ovarian biology in addition to the function from which it derived it name (i.e., promotion of the degeneration of the müllerian system during embryogenesis in the male). AMH is produced by granulosa cells and, like inhibin B, is a marker of ovarian reserve. AMH may also inhibit the recruitment of primordial follicles into the follicle pool and appears to inhibit the effect of FSH on aromatase expression.

Relaxin, which is produced by the theca lutein cells of the corpus luteum, is thought to play a role in decidualization of the endometrium and suppression of myometrial contractile activity, both of which are essential for the early establishment of pregnancy.

HORMONAL INTEGRATION OF THE NORMAL MENSTRUAL CYCLE

The sequence of changes responsible for mature reproductive function is coordinated through a series of negative and positive feedback loops that alter pulsatile GnRH secretion, the pituitary

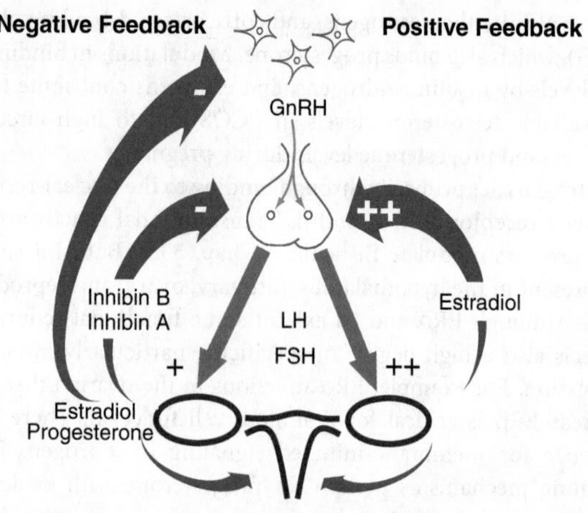

Figure 347-7 The reproductive system in women is critically dependent on both negative feedback of gonadal steroids and inhibin to modulate follicle-stimulating hormone (FSH) secretion and on estrogen positive feedback to generate the preovulatory luteinizing hormone (LH) surge. GnRH, gonadotropin-releasing hormone.

Figure 347-8 Relationship between gonadotropins, follicle development, gonadal secretion, and endometrial changes during the normal menstrual cycle. FSH, follicle-stimulating hormone; LH, luteinizing hormone; E_2, estradiol; Prog, progesterone; Endo, endometrium.

response to GnRH, and the relative secretion of LH and FSH from the gonadotrope. The frequency and amplitude of pulsatile GnRH secretion differentially modulate the synthesis and secretion of LH and FSH, with slow frequencies favoring FSH synthesis and increased amplitudes favoring LH synthesis. Activin is produced in both pituitary gonadotropes and folliculostellate cells and stimulates the synthesis and secretion of FSH. Inhibins function as potent antagonists of activins through sequestration of the activin receptors. Although inhibin is expressed in the pituitary, gonadal inhibin is the principal source of feedback inhibition of FSH.

For the majority of the cycle, the reproductive system functions in a classic endocrine negative feedback mode. Estradiol and progesterone inhibit GnRH secretion, and the inhibins act at the pituitary to selectively inhibit FSH synthesis and secretion (Fig. 347-7). This negative feedback control of FSH is critical for development of the single mature oocyte that characterizes normal reproductive function in women. In addition to these negative feedback controls, the menstrual cycle is uniquely dependent on estrogen-induced positive feedback to produce an LH surge that is essential for ovulation of a mature follicle. The neural signaling pathways that distinguish estrogen negative versus positive feedback are incompletely understood.

THE FOLLICULAR PHASE

The follicular phase is characterized by recruitment of a cohort of secondary follicles and the ultimate selection of a dominant preovulatory follicle (Fig. 347-8). The follicular phase begins, by convention, on the first day of menses. However, follicle recruitment is initiated by the rise in FSH that begins in the late luteal phase in conjunction with the loss of negative feedback of gonadal steroids and likely inhibin A. The fact that a 20–30% increase in FSH is adequate for follicular recruitment speaks to the marked sensitivity of the resting follicle pool to FSH. The resultant granulosa cell proliferation is responsible for increasing early follicular phase levels of inhibin B. Inhibin B in conjunction with rising levels of estradiol, and probably inhibin A, restrain FSH secretion during this critical period such that only a single follicle matures in the vast majority of cycles. The increased risk of multiple gestation associated with the increased levels of FSH characteristic of advanced maternal age, or with exogenous gonadotropin administration in the treatment of infertility, attest to the importance of the negative feedback regulation of FSH. With further growth of the dominant follicle, estradiol and inhibin A increase exponentially and the follicle acquires LH receptors. Increasing levels of estradiol are responsible for proliferative changes in the endometrium. The exponential rise in estradiol results in positive feedback on the pituitary, leading to the generation of an LH surge (and a smaller FSH surge), thereby triggering ovulation and luteinization of the granulosa cells.

THE LUTEAL PHASE

The luteal phase begins with the formation of the corpus luteum from the ruptured follicle. Progesterone and inhibin A are produced from the luteinized granulosa cells, which continue to aromatize theca-derived androgen precursors, producing estradiol. The combined actions of estrogen and progesterone are responsible for the secretory changes in the endometrium that are necessary for implantation. The corpus luteum is supported by LH but has a finite life span because of diminished sensitivity to LH. The demise of the corpus luteum results in a progressive decline in hormonal support of the endometrium. Inflammation or local hypoxia and ischemia result in vascular changes in the endometrium leading to the release of cytokines, cell death, and shedding of the endometrium.

If conception occurs, hCG produced by the trophoblast binds to LH receptors on the corpus luteum, maintaining steroid hormone production and preventing involution of the corpus luteum. The corpus luteum is essential for the hormonal maintenance of the endometrium during the first 6–10 weeks of pregnancy until this function is taken over by the placenta.

CLINICAL ASSESSMENT OF OVARIAN FUNCTION

Menstrual bleeding should become regular within 2 to 4 years of menarche, although anovulatory and irregular cycles are common before that. For the remainder of adult reproductive life, the cycle length counted from the first day of menses to the first day of subsequent menses, is ~28 days, with a range of 25–35 days. However, cycle-to-cycle variability for an individual woman is ±2 days. Luteal phase length is relatively constant between 12 and 14 days in normal cycles; thus, the major variability in cycle length is due to variations in the follicular phase. The duration of menstrual bleeding in ovulatory cycles varies between 4 and 6 days. There is a gradual shortening of cycle length with age such that women over the age of 35 have cycles that are shorter than during their younger reproductive years. Anovulatory cycles increase as women approach the menopause, and bleeding patterns may be erratic.

Women who report regular monthly bleeding with cycles that do not vary by >4 days generally have ovulatory cycles, but several other clinical signs can be used to assess the likelihood of ovulation. Some women experience *mittelschmerz*, described as midcycle pelvic discomfort that is thought to be caused by the rapid expansion of the dominant follicle at the time of ovulation. A constellation of premenstrual moliminal symptoms such as bloating, breast tenderness, and food cravings often occur several days before menses in ovulatory cycles, but their absence cannot be used as evidence of anovulation. Methods that can be used to determine whether ovulation is likely to include a serum progesterone level >5 ng/mL ~7 days before expected menses, an increase in basal body temperature of 0.24°C (>0.5°F) in the second half of the cycle due to the thermoregulatory effect of progesterone, or the detection of the urinary LH surge using ovulation predictor kits. Because ovulation occurs ~36 hours after the LH surge, urinary LH can be helpful in timing intercourse to coincide with ovulation.

Ultrasound can be used to detect the growth of the fluid-filled antrum of the developing follicle and to assess endometrial proliferation in response to increasing estradiol levels in the follicular phase, as well as the characteristic echogenicity of the secretory endometrium of the luteal phase.

PUBERTY

NORMAL PUBERTAL DEVELOPMENT IN GIRLS

The first menstrual period (*menarche*) occurs relatively late in the series of developmental milestones that characterize normal pubertal development (Table 347-1). Menarche is preceded by the appearance of pubic and then axillary hair as a result of maturation of the zona reticularis in the adrenal gland and increased adrenal androgen secretion, particularly dehydroepiandrosterone (DHEA). The triggers for adrenarche remain unknown but may involve increases in body mass index as well as in utero and neonatal factors. Menarche is also preceded by breast development (*thelarche*), which is exquisitely sensitive to the very low levels of estrogen that result from peripheral conversion of adrenal androgens and the low levels of estrogen secreted from the ovary early in pubertal maturation. Breast development precedes the appearance of pubic and axillary hair in ~60% of girls. The interval between the onset of breast development and menarche is ~2 years. There has been a gradual decline in the age of menarche over the past century, attributed in large part to improvement in nutrition, and there is a relationship between adiposity and earlier sexual maturation in girls. In the United States, menarche occurs at an average age of 12.5 years (Table 347-1). Much of the variation in the timing of puberty is due to genetic factors, with heritability estimates of 50–80%. Both adrenarche and breast development occur ~1 year earlier in black compared with white girls, although the timing of menarche differs by only 6 months between these ethnic groups.

Other important hormonal changes also occur in conjunction with puberty. Growth hormone (GH) levels increase early in puberty, stimulated in part by the pubertal increases in estrogen secretion. GH increases insulin-like growth factor-I (IGF-I), which enhances linear growth. The growth spurt is generally less pronounced in girls than in boys, with a peak growth velocity of ~7 cm/year. Linear growth is ultimately limited by closure of epiphyses in the long bones as a result of prolonged exposure to estrogen. Puberty is also associated with mild insulin resistance.

DISORDERS OF PUBERTY

The differential diagnosis of precocious and delayed puberty is similar in boys (Chap. 346) and girls. However, there are differences in the timing of normal puberty and differences in the relative frequency of specific disorders in girls compared with boys.

Precocious puberty

Traditionally, precocious puberty has been defined as the development of secondary sexual characteristics before the age of 8 in girls based on data from Marshall and Tanner in British girls studied in the 1960s. More recent studies led to recommendations that girls be evaluated for precocious puberty if breast development or pubic hair are present at <7 years of age for white girls or <6 years for black girls.

Precocious puberty is most often centrally mediated (Table 347-2), resulting from early activation of the hypothalamic-pituitary-ovarian axis. It is characterized by pulsatile LH secretion and an enhanced LH and FSH response to exogenous GnRH (two- to threefold stimulation) (Table 347-3). True precocity is marked by advancement in bone age of >2 SD, a recent history of growth acceleration, and progression of secondary sexual characteristics. In girls, centrally mediated precocious puberty is idiopathic in ~85% of cases; however, neurogenic causes must also be considered. GnRH agonists that induce pituitary desensitization are the mainstay of treatment to prevent premature epiphyseal closure and preserve adult height, as well as to manage psychosocial repercussions of precocious puberty.

Peripherally mediated precocious puberty does not involve activation of the hypothalamic-pituitary-ovarian axis and is characterized by suppressed gonadotropins in the presence of elevated estradiol. Management of peripheral precocious puberty involves treating the underlying disorder (Table 347-2) and limiting the effects of gonadal steroids using aromatase inhibitors, inhibitors of steroidogenesis, and estrogen receptor blockers. It is important to be aware that central precocious puberty can also develop in girls whose precocity was initially peripherally mediated, as in McCune-Albright syndrome and congenital adrenal hyperplasia.

Incomplete and intermittent forms of precocious puberty may also occur. For example, premature breast development may occur in girls before the age of 2 years, with no further progression and without significant advancement in bone age, androgen production, or compromised height. Premature adrenarche can also occur

TABLE 347-1 Mean Age (Years) of Pubertal Milestones in Girls

	Onset of Breast/Pubic Hair Development	Age of Peak Height Velocity	Menarche	Final Breast/Pubic Hair Development	Adult Height
White	10.2	11.9	12.6	14.3	17.1
Black	9.6	11.5	12	13.6	16.5

Source: From FM Biro et al: J Pediatr 148:234, 2006.

TABLE 347-2 Differential Diagnosis of Precocious Puberty

Central (GnRH Dependent)	Peripheral (GnRH Independent)
Idiopathic	Congenital adrenal hyperplasia
CNS tumors	Estrogen-producing tumors
Hamartomas	Adrenal tumors
Astrocytomas	Ovarian tumors
Adenomyomas	Gonadotropin/hCG-producing tumors
Gliomas	
Germinomas	Exogenous exposure to estrogen or androgen
CNS infection	
Head trauma	McCune-Albright syndrome
Iatrogenic	Aromatase excess syndrome
Radiation	
Chemotherapy	
Surgical	
CNS malformation	
Arachnoid or suprasellar cysts	
Septo-optic dysplasia	
Hydrocephalus	

Abbreviations: CNS, central nervous system; GnRH, gonadotropin-releasing hormone; hCG, human chorionic gonadotropin.

in the absence of progressive pubertal development, but it must be distinguished from late-onset congenital adrenal hyperplasia and androgen-secreting tumors, in which case it may be termed *heterosexual precocity.* Premature adrenarche may be associated with obesity, hyperinsulinemia, and the subsequent predisposition to PCOS.

Delayed puberty

Delayed puberty (Table 347-4) is defined as the absence of secondary sexual characteristics by age 13 in girls. The diagnostic considerations are very similar to those for primary amenorrhea (Chap. 50). Between 25 and 40% of delayed puberty in girls is of ovarian origin, with Turner's syndrome accounting for the majority of such patients. Functional hypogonadotropic hypogonadism encompasses diverse etiologies such as systemic illnesses, including celiac disease and chronic renal disease, and endocrinopathies such as diabetes and hypothyroidism. In addition, girls appear to be particularly susceptible to the adverse effects of abnormalities in energy balance that result from exercise, dieting, and/or eating disorders. Together these reversible conditions account for ~25% of delayed puberty in girls. Congenital hypogonadotropic hypogonadism in girls or boys can be caused by mutations in several different genes or combinations of genes (Fig. 347-4, Chap. 346, Table 346-2). Family studies suggest that genes identified in association with absent puberty may also cause delayed puberty, and recent reports have further suggested that a genetic susceptibility to environmental stresses such as diet and exercise may account for at least some cases of functional hypothalamic amenorrhea. Although neuroanatomic causes of delayed puberty are considerably less common in girls than in boys, it is always important to rule these out in the setting of hypogonadotropic hypogonadism.

TABLE 347-3 Evaluation of Precocious and Delayed Puberty

	Precocious	Delayed
Initial Screening Tests		
History and physical	×	×
Assessment of growth velocity	×	×
Bone age	×	×
LH, FSH	×	×
Estradiol, testosterone	×	×
DHEAS	×	×
17-Hydroxyprogesterone	×	
TSH, T_4	×	×
Complete blood count		×
Sedimentation rate, C-reactive protein		×
Electrolytes, renal function		×
Liver enzymes		×
IGF-I, IGFBP-3		×
Urinalysis		×
Secondary Tests		
Pelvic ultrasound	×	
Cranial MRI	×	×
β-hCG	×	
GnRH/agonist stimulation test	×	×
ACTH stimulation test	×	
Inflammatory bowel disease panel	×	×
Celiac disease panel	×	×
Prolactin		×
Karyotype		×

Abbreviations: LH, luteinizing hormone; FSH, follicle-stimulating hormone; DHEAS, dehydroepiandrosterone sulfate; TSH, thyroid-stimulating hormone; T_4, thyroxine; IGF-I, insulin-like growth factor-I; IGFBP-3, IGF-binding protein 3; hCG, human chorionic gonadotropin; ACTH, adrenocorticotropic hormone.

INFERTILITY

DEFINITION AND PREVALENCE

Infertility is defined as the inability to conceive after 12 months of unprotected sexual intercourse. In a study of 5574 English and American women who ultimately conceived, pregnancy occurred in 50% within 3 months, 72% within 6 months, and 85% within 12 months. These findings are consistent with predictions based on *fecundability*, the probability of achieving pregnancy in one menstrual cycle (approximately 20–25% in healthy young couples). Assuming a fecundability of 0.25, 98% of couples should conceive within 13 months. Based on this definition, the National Survey of Family Growth reports a 14% rate of infertility in the United States in married women aged 15–44. The infertility rate has remained relatively stable over the past 30 years, although the proportion of couples without children has risen, reflecting a trend to delay childbearing. This trend has important implications because of an

TABLE 347-4 Differential Diagnosis of Delayed Puberty

Hypergonadotropic
Ovarian
Turner's syndrome
Gonadal dysgenesis
Chemotherapy/radiation therapy
Galactosemia
Autoimmune oophoritis
Congenital lipoid hyperplasia
Steroidogenic enzyme abnormalities
17α-hydroxylase deficiency
Aromatase deficiency
Gonadotropin/receptor mutations
FSHβ, LHR, FSHR
Androgen resistance syndrome
Hypogonadotropic
Genetic
Hypothalamic syndromes
Leptin/leptin receptor
HESX1 (septo-optic dysplasia)
PC1 (prohormone convertase)
IHH and Kallmann syndrome
KAL1, FGF8, FGFR1, NELF, PROK2, PROKR2
KISS1, KISS1R, TAC3, TAC3R, GnRH1, GnRHR
Abnormalities of pituitary development/function
PROP1
CNS tumors/infiltrative disorders
Craniopharyngioma
Astrocytoma, germinoma, glioma
Prolactinomas, other pituitary tumors
Histiocytosis X
Chemotherapy/radiation
Functional
Chronic diseases
Malnutrition
Excessive exercise
Eating disorders

Abbreviations: CNS, central nervous system; FGF8, fibroblast growth factor 8; FGFR1, fibroblast growth factor 1 receptor; FSHβ, follicle-stimulating hormone β chain; FSHR, FSH receptor; GnRHR, gonadotropin-releasing hormone receptor; HESX1, homeobox, embryonic stem cell expressed 1; IHH, idiopathic hypogonadotropic hypogonadism; KAL, Kallmann; KISS1, kisspeptin 1; KISSR1, KISS1 receptor; LHR, luteinizing hormone receptor; NELF, nasal embryonic LHRH factor; PROK2, prokineticin 2; PROKR2 prokineticin receptor 2; PROP1, prophet of Pit1, paired-like homeodomain transcription factor.

age-related decrease in fecundability, which begins at age 35 and decreases markedly after age 40. It is estimated that ~8% of women in the United States have received medical assistance for infertility; of these, 74% received counseling, ~60% underwent infertility testing of the female and/or male partner, and ~46% used ovulation-inducing medication.

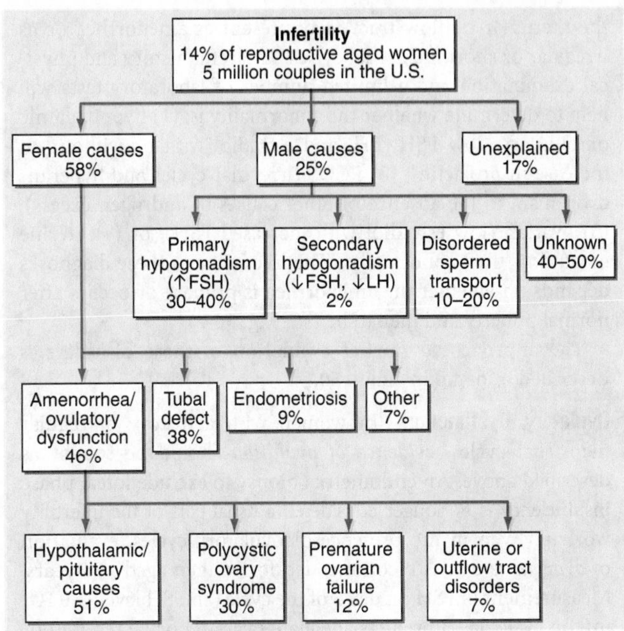

Figure 347-9 Causes of infertility. FSH, follicle-stimulating hormone; LH, luteinizing hormone.

CAUSES OF INFERTILITY

The spectrum of infertility ranges from reduced conception rates or the need for medical intervention to irreversible causes of infertility. Infertility can be attributed primarily to male factors in 25%, female factors in 58%, and is unexplained in about 17% of couples (Fig. 347-9). Not uncommonly, both male and female factors contribute to infertility.

APPROACH TO THE PATIENT Infertility

INITIAL EVALUATION In all couples presenting with infertility, the initial evaluation includes discussion of the appropriate timing of intercourse and discussion of modifiable risk factors such as smoking, alcohol, caffeine, and obesity. The range of required investigations should be reviewed as well as a brief description of infertility treatment options, including adoption. Initial investigations are focused on determining whether the primary cause of the infertility is male, female, or both. These investigations include a semen analysis in the male, confirmation of ovulation in the female, and, in the majority of situations, documentation of tubal patency in the female. In some cases, after an extensive workup excluding all male and female factors, a specific cause cannot be identified and infertility may ultimately be classified as unexplained.

PSYCHOLOGICAL ASPECTS OF INFERTILITY Infertility is invariably associated with psychological stress related not only to the diagnostic and therapeutic procedures themselves but also to repeated cycles of hope and loss associated with each new procedure or cycle of treatment that does not result in the birth of a child. These feelings are often combined with a sense of isolation from friends and family. Counseling and stress-management techniques should be introduced early in the evaluation of infertility. Importantly, infertility and its treatment do not appear to be associated with long-term psychological sequelae.

FEMALE CAUSES Abnormalities in menstrual function constitute the most common cause of female infertility. These disorders, which include ovulatory dysfunction and abnormalities of the uterus or outflow tract, may present as amenorrhea or as irregular or short menstrual cycles. A careful history and physical examination and a limited number of laboratory tests will help to determine whether the abnormality is: (1) hypothalamic or pituitary (low FSH, LH, and estradiol with or without an increase in prolactin), (2) PCOS (irregular cycles and hyperandrogenism in the absence of other causes of androgen excess), (3) ovarian (low estradiol with increased FSH), or (4) uterine or outflow tract abnormality. The frequency of these diagnoses depends on whether the amenorrhea is primary or occurs after normal puberty and menarche (see Fig. 50-2).

The approach to further evaluation of these disorders is described in detail in Chap. 50.

Ovulatory Dysfunction In women with a history of regular menstrual cycles, *evidence of ovulation* should be sought as described above. An endometrial biopsy to exclude luteal phase insufficiency is no longer considered a usual part of the infertility workup. Even in the presence of ovulatory cycles, evaluation of *ovarian reserve* is recommended for women aged >35 years. Measurement of FSH on day 3 of the cycle (an FSH level <10 IU/mL on cycle day 3 predicts adequate ovarian oocyte reserve) or in response to clomiphene (blocks estrogen negative feedback on FSH), antral follicle count and serum levels of inhibin B and AMH have all been used for this purpose.

Tubal Disease Tubal dysfunction may result from pelvic inflammatory disease (PID), appendicitis, endometriosis, pelvic adhesions, tubal surgery, previous use of an intrauterine device (IUD), and a previous ectopic pregnancy. However, a cause is not identified in up to 50% of patients with documented tubal factor infertility. Because of the high prevalence of tubal disease, evaluation of tubal patency by hysterosalpingogram (HSG) or laparoscopy should occur early in the majority of couples with infertility. Subclinical infections with *Chlamydia trachomatis* may be an underdiagnosed cause of tubal infertility and requires the treatment of both partners.

Endometriosis *Endometriosis* is defined as the presence of endometrial glands or stroma outside the endometrial cavity and uterine musculature. Its presence is suggested by a history of dyspareunia (painful intercourse), worsening dysmenorrhea that often begins before menses, or by a thickened rectovaginal septum or deviation of the cervix on pelvic examination. The pathogenesis of the infertility associated with endometriosis is unclear but may involve effects on fertilization, normal function of the endometrium, as well as adhesions. Endometriosis is often clinically silent, however, and can only be excluded definitively by laparoscopy.

MALE CAUSES (See also Chap. 346) Known causes of male infertility include primary testicular disease, disorders of sperm transport, and hypothalamic-pituitary disease resulting in secondary hypogonadism. However, the etiology is not ascertained in up to one-half of men with suspected male factor infertility. The key initial diagnostic test is a *semen analysis*. Testosterone levels should be measured if the sperm count is low on repeated examination or if there is clinical evidence of hypogonadism. Gonadotropin levels will help to determine a gonadal versus a central cause of hypogonadism.

TREATMENT Infertility

In addition to addressing the negative impact of smoking on fertility and pregnancy outcome, counseling about nutrition and weight is a critical part of infertility and pregnancy management. Both low and increased body mass index (BMI) are associated with infertility in women and with increased morbidity during pregnancy. Obesity has also been associated with infertility in men. The treatment of infertility should be tailored to the problems unique to each couple. In many situations, including unexplained infertility, mild-to-moderate endometriosis, and/or borderline semen parameters, a stepwise approach to infertility is optimal, beginning with low-risk interventions and moving to more invasive, higher risk interventions only if necessary. After determination of all infertility factors and their correction, if possible, this approach might include, in increasing order of complexity: (1) expectant management, (2) clomiphene citrate (see below) with or without intrauterine insemination (IUI), (3) gonadotropins with or without IUI, and (4) in vitro fertilization (IVF). The time used to complete the evaluation, correction, and expectant management can be longer in women aged <30 years, but this process should be advanced rapidly in women aged >35 years. In some situations, expectant management will not be appropriate.

OVULATORY DYSFUNCTION Treatment of ovulatory dysfunction should first be directed at identification of the etiology of the disorder to allow specific management when possible. Dopamine agonists, for example, may be indicated in patients with hyperprolactinemia (Chap. 339); lifestyle modification may be successful in women with obesity, low body weight, or a history of intensive exercise (Chap. 79).

Medications used for ovulation induction include clomiphene citrate, gonadotropins, and pulsatile GnRH. *Clomiphene citrate* is a nonsteroidal estrogen antagonist that increases FSH and LH levels by blocking estrogen negative feedback at the hypothalamus. The efficacy of clomiphene for ovulation induction is highly dependent on patient selection. It induces ovulation in ~60% of women with PCOS and is the initial treatment of choice. It may be combined with agents that modify insulin levels such as metformin. Clomiphene citrate is less successful in patients with hypogonadotropic hypogonadism. *Aromatase inhibitors* have also been investigated for the treatment of infertility. Initial studies are promising, but these medications have not been approved for this indication.

Gonadotropins are highly effective for ovulation induction in women with hypogonadotropic hypogonadism and PCOS and are used to induce the development of multiple follicles in unexplained infertility and in older reproductive-age women. Disadvantages include a significant risk of multiple gestation and the risk of ovarian hyperstimulation. Careful monitoring and a conservative approach to ovarian stimulation reduce these risks. Currently available gonadotropins include urinary preparations of LH and FSH, highly purified FSH, and recombinant FSH. Though FSH is the key component, there are growing data that the addition of some LH (or hCG) may improve results and this is particularly important in hypogonadotropic patients.

None of these methods are effective in women with premature ovarian failure in whom donor oocyte or adoption are the methods of choice.

TUBAL DISEASE If hysterosalpingography suggests a tubal or uterine cavity abnormality, or if a patient is aged ≥35 at the time of initial evaluation, laparoscopy with tubal lavage is recommended, often with a hysteroscopy. Although tubal reconstruction may be attempted if tubal disease is identified, it is generally being replaced by the use of IVF. These patients are at increased risk of developing an ectopic pregnancy.

ENDOMETRIOSIS Though 60% of women with minimal or mild endometriosis may conceive within 1 year without treatment, laparoscopic resection or ablation appears to improve conception rates. Medical management of advanced stages of endometriosis is widely used for symptom control but has not been shown to enhance fertility. In moderate-to-severe endometriosis, conservative surgery is associated with pregnancy rates of 50 and 39%, respectively, compared with rates of 25 and 5% with expectant management alone. In some patients, IVF may be the treatment of choice.

MALE FACTOR INFERTILITY The treatment options for male factor infertility have expanded greatly in recent years (Chap. 346). Secondary hypogonadism is highly amenable to treatment with pulsatile GnRH or gonadotropins. In vitro techniques have provided new opportunities for patients with primary testicular failure and disorders of sperm transport. Choice of initial treatment options depends on sperm concentration and motility. Expectant management should be attempted initially in men with mild male factor infertility (sperm count of 15 to 20 × 10^6/mL and normal motility). Moderate male factor infertility (10 to 15 × 10^6/mL and 20–40% motility) should begin with IUI alone or in combination with treatment of the female partner with clomiphene or gonadotropins, but it may require IVF with or without intracytoplasmic sperm injection (ICSI). For men with a severe defect (sperm count of <10 × 10^6/mL, 10% motility), IVF with ICSI or donor sperm should be used. If ICSI is performed because of azoospermia due to congenital bilateral absence of the vas deferens, genetic testing and counseling should be provided because of the risk of cystic fibrosis.

ASSISTED REPRODUCTIVE TECHNOLOGIES The development of assisted reproductive technologies (ARTs) has dramatically altered the treatment of male and female infertility. IVF is indicated for patients with many causes of infertility that have not been successfully managed with more conservative approaches. IVF or ICSI is often the treatment of choice in couples with a significant male factor or tubal disease, whereas IVF using donor oocytes is used in patients with premature ovarian failure and in women of advanced reproductive age. Success rates depend on the age of the woman and the cause of the infertility. The number of cycles canceled increases from approximately 10% in women aged <35 years to 24% in women aged >40 while the birth rate decreases from ~39% of cycles in which embryos were transferred in women aged <35 to 24% in women aged 38-40 and only 10% in women aged >40. Though often effective, IVF is expensive and requires careful monitoring of ovulation induction and invasive techniques, including the aspiration of multiple follicles. IVF is associated with a significant risk of multiple gestation, particularly in women aged <35, in whom it can be as high as 40%.

CONTRACEPTION

Only 15% of couples in the United States report having unprotected sexual intercourse in the past 3 months. However, despite the wide availability and widespread use of a variety of effective methods of contraception, approximately one-half of all births in the United States are the result of unintended pregnancy. Teenage pregnancies continue to represent a serious public health problem in the United States, with >1 million unintended pregnancies each year—a significantly greater incidence than in other industrialized nations.

Of the contraceptive methods available (Table 347-5), a reversible form of contraception is used by >50% of couples, while sterilization (male or female) has been employed as a permanent form of contraception by over one-third of couples. Pregnancy termination is relatively safe when directed by health care professionals, but is rarely the option of choice.

No single contraceptive method is ideal, although all are safer than carrying a pregnancy to term. The effectiveness of a given method of contraception does not just depend on the efficacy of the method itself. Discrepancies between theoretical and actual effectiveness emphasize the importance of patient education and compliance when considering various forms of contraception (Table 347-5). Knowledge of the advantages and disadvantages of each contraceptive is essential for counseling an individual about the methods that are safest and most consistent with his or her lifestyle. The World Health Organization (WHO) has extensive family planning resources for the physician and patient that can be accessed online. Similar resources for determining medical eligibility are available through the Centers for Disease Control and Prevention (CDC). Considerations for contraceptive use in obese patients and after bariatric surgery are discussed below.

BARRIER METHODS

Barrier contraceptives (such as condoms, diaphragms, and cervical caps) and spermicides are easily available, reversible, and have fewer side effects than hormonal methods. However, their effectiveness is highly dependent on adherence and proper use (Table 347-5). A major advantage of barrier contraceptives is the protection provided against sexually transmitted infections (STIs) (Chap. 130). Consistent use is associated with a decreased risk of HIV, gonorrhea, nongonococcal urethritis, and genital herpes, probably due in part to the concomitant use of spermicides. Natural membrane condoms may be less effective than latex condoms, and petroleum-based lubricants can degrade condoms and decrease their efficacy for preventing HIV infection. A highly effective female condom, which also provides protection against STIs, was approved in 1994 but has not achieved widespread use.

STERILIZATION

Sterilization is the method of birth control most frequently chosen by fertile men and multiparous women >30 (Table 347-5). Sterilization refers to a procedure that prevents fertilization by surgical interruption of the fallopian tubes in women or the vas deferens in men. Although tubal ligation and vasectomy are potentially reversible, these procedures should be considered permanent and should not be undertaken without patient counseling.

Several methods of *tubal ligation* have been developed, all of which are highly effective with a 10-year cumulative pregnancy rate of 1.85 per 100 women. However, when pregnancy does occur, the risk of ectopic pregnancy may be as high as 30%. The success rate of tubal reanastomosis depends on the method used, but even after successful reversal, the risk of ectopic pregnancy remains high. In addition to prevention of pregnancy, tubal ligation reduces the risk of ovarian cancer, possibly by limiting the upward migration of potential carcinogens.

Vasectomy is a highly effective outpatient surgical procedure that has little risk. The development of azoospermia may be delayed for 2–6 months, and other forms of contraception must be used until two sperm-free ejaculations provide proof of sterility. Reanastomosis may restore fertility in 30–50% of men, but the success rate declines with time after vasectomy and may be influenced by factors such as the development of antisperm antibodies.

INTRAUTERINE DEVICES

IUDs inhibit pregnancy primarily through a spermicidal effect caused by a sterile inflammatory reaction induced by the presence of a foreign body in the uterine cavity (copper IUDs) or by the release of progestins (Progestasert, Mirena). IUDs provide a high level of efficacy in the absence of systemic metabolic effects, and ongoing motivation is not required to ensure efficacy once the device has been placed. However, only 1% of women in the United States

TABLE 347-5 Effectiveness of Different Forms of Contraception

Method of Contraception	Theoretical[a] Effectiveness, %	Actual[a] Effectiveness, %	Percent Continuing Use at 1 Year[b]	Contraceptive Methods Used by U.S. Women[c]
Barrier methods				
Condoms	98	88	63	18
Diaphragm	94	82	58	2
Cervical cap	94	82	50	<1
Spermicides	97	79	43	1
Sterilization				
Male	99.9	99.9	100	9
Female	99.8	99.6	100	27
Intrauterine device				1
Copper T380	99	97	78	
Progestasert	98	97	81	
Mirena	99.9	99.8		
Hormonal contraceptives	99.7	92	72	31
Combination pill				
Progestin only pill				
Transdermal patch				
Vaginal ring				
Long-acting progestins				
Depo-Provera	99.7	99.7	70	9

[a]Adapted from J Trussel et al: Obstet Gynecol 76:558, 1990.
[b]Adapted from Contraceptive Technology Update. Contraceptive Technology, Feb. 1996, Vol 17, No 1, pp 13–24.
[c]Adapted from LJ Piccinino and WD Mosher: Fam Plan Perspective 30:4, 1998.

use this method compared to a utilization rate of 15–30% in much of Europe and Canada, despite evidence that the newer devices are not associated with increased rates of pelvic infection and infertility, as occurred with earlier devices. An IUD should not be used in women at high risk for development of STI or in women at high risk for bacterial endocarditis. The IUD may not be effective in women with uterine leiomyomas because they alter the size or shape of the uterine cavity. IUD use is associated with increased menstrual blood flow, although this is less pronounced with the progestin-releasing IUD, which is associated with a more frequent occurrence of spotting or amenorrhea.

HORMONAL METHODS

Oral contraceptive pills

Because of their ease of use and efficacy, oral contraceptive pills are the most widely used form of hormonal contraception. They act by suppressing ovulation, changing cervical mucus, and altering the endometrium. The current formulations are made from synthetic estrogens and progestins. The estrogen component of the pill consists of ethinyl estradiol or mestranol, which is metabolized to ethinyl estradiol. Multiple synthetic progestins are used. Norethindrone and its derivatives are used in many formulations. Low-dose norgestimate and the more recently developed progestins (desogestrel, gestodene, drospirenone) have a less androgenic profile; levonorgestrel appears to be the most androgenic of the progestins and should be avoided in patients with hyperandrogenic symptoms. The three major formulations of oral contraceptives are (1) fixed-dose estrogen-progestin combination, (2) phasic estrogen-progestin combination, and (3) progestin only. Each of these formulations is administered daily for 3 weeks followed by a week of no medication during which menstrual bleeding generally occurs. Two extended oral contraceptives are approved for use in the United States; Seasonale is a 3-month preparation with 84 days of active drug and 7 days of placebo, and Lybrel is a continuous preparation containing 90 μg of levonorgestrel and 10 μg of ethinyl estradiol. Current doses of ethinyl estradiol range from 20 to 50 μg. However, indications for the 50-μg dose are rare, and the majority of formulations contain 35 μg of ethinyl estradiol. The reduced estrogen and progestin content in the second- and third-generation pills has decreased both side effects and risks associated with oral contraceptive use (Table 347-6). At the currently used doses, patients must be cautioned not to miss pills due to the potential for ovulation. Side effects, including breakthrough bleeding, amenorrhea, breast tenderness, and weight gain, often respond to a change in formulation.

The microdose progestin-only minipill is less effective as a contraceptive, having a pregnancy rate of 2–7 per 100 women-years. However, it may be appropriate for women with cardiovascular disease or for women who cannot tolerate synthetic estrogens.

New methods

A *weekly contraceptive patch* (Ortho Evra) is available and has similar efficacy to oral contraceptives but may be associated with less breakthrough bleeding. Approximately 2% of patches fail to adhere, and a similar percentage of women have skin reactions. Efficacy is lower in women weighing >90 kg. The amount of estrogen delivered may be comparable to that of a 40-μg ethinyl estradiol oral contraceptive, raising

TABLE 347-6 Oral Contraceptives: Contraindications and Disease Risk

Contraindications
Absolute
Previous thromboembolic event or stroke
History of an estrogen-dependent tumor
Active liver disease
Pregnancy
Undiagnosed abnormal uterine bleeding
Hypertriglyceridemia
Women aged >35 years who smoke heavily
Relative
Hypertension
Women receiving anticonvulsant drug therapy
Women following bariatric surgery (malapsorptive procedure)
Disease Risks
Increased
Coronary heart disease—increased in smokers >35; no relation to progestin type
Hypertension—relative risk 1.8 (current users) and 1.2 (previous users)
Venous thrombosis—relative risk ~4; may be higher with third-generation progestin, drosperinone, and patch; compounded by obesity (tenfold increased risk compared with nonobese, no OCP); markedly increased with factor V Leiden or prothrombin-gene mutations (see Chap. 116)
Stroke—slight increase; unclear relation to migraine headache
Cerebral vein thrombosis—relative risk ~13–15; synergistic with prothrombin-gene mutation
Cervical cancer—relative risk 2–4
Breast cancer—may increase risk in carriers of BRCA1 and possible BRCA2
Decreased
Ovarian cancer—50% reduction in risk
Endometrial cancer—40% reduction in risk

Abbreviation: OCP, oral contraceptive pill.

the possibility of increased risk of venous thromboembolism, which must be balanced against potential benefits for women not able to successfully use other methods. A *monthly contraceptive estrogen/progestin injection* (Lunelle) is highly effective, with a first-year failure rate of <0.2%, but it may be less effective in obese women. Its use is associated with bleeding irregularities that diminish over time. Fertility returns rapidly after discontinuation. A *monthly vaginal ring* (NuvaRing) that is intended to be left in place during intercourse is also available for contraceptive use. It is highly effective, with a 12-month failure rate of 0.7%. Ovulation returns within the first recovery cycle after discontinuation.

Long-term contraceptives

Long-term progestin administration acts primarily by inhibiting ovulation and causing changes in the endometrium and cervical mucus that result in decreased implantation and sperm transport. Depot Medroxyprogesterone acetate (Depo Provera, DMPA), the only injectable form available in the United States, is effective for 3 months, but return of fertility after discontinuation may be delayed for up to 12–18 months. DMPA is now available for both SC and IM injection. Irregular bleeding, amenorrhea, and weight gain are the most common side effects. This form of contraception may be particularly good for women in whom an estrogen-containing contraceptive is contraindicated (e.g., migraine exacerbation, sickle-cell anemia, fibroids).

POSTCOITAL CONTRACEPTION

Postcoital contraceptive methods prevent implantation or cause regression of the corpus luteum and are highly efficacious if used appropriately. Unprotected intercourse without regard to the time of the month carries an 8% incidence of pregnancy, an incidence that can be reduced to 2% by the use of emergency contraceptives within 72 hours of unprotected intercourse. A notice published in 1997 by the U.S. Food and Drug Administration (FDA) indicated that certain oral contraceptive pills could be used within 72 hours of unprotected intercourse [Ovral (2 tablets, 12 hours apart) and Lo/Ovral (4 tablets, 12 hours apart)]. Preven (50 mg ethinyl estradiol and 0.25 mg levonorgestrel) and Plan B or Next Choice (0.75 mg levonorgestrel) are now approved for postcoital contraception and are available over the counter for women aged >17 years. Levonorgestrel is more effective and is associated with fewer side effects than the combination estrogen-progestin regimens. Ulipristal acetate is a progesterone antagonist that has been developed for emergency contraception. It is available in Europe and was approved by the FDA for prescription use in 2010. This medication is effective for up to 5 days after unprotected intercourse. Mifepristone is also a progesterone antagonist that is available for medical termination of intrauterine pregnancy but is not approved for emergency contraception in the United States. Insertion of a copper IUD within 5 days after unprotected intercourse is also a highly effective method.

IMPACT OF OBESITY ON CONTRACEPTIVE CHOICE

Approximately one-third of adults in the United States are obese. While obesity is associated with some reduction in fertility, the vast majority of obese women can conceive. The risk of pregnancy-associated complications is higher in obese women. Intrauterine contraception may be more effective than oral or transdermal methods for obese women. The WHO guidelines provide no restrictions (class 1) for the use of intrauterine contraception, DMPA, and progestin-only pills for obese women (BMI ≥30) in the absence of coexistent medical problems whereas methods that include estrogen (pill, patch, ring) are considered class 2 (advantages generally outweigh theoretical or proven risks) due to the increased risk of thromboembolic disease. There are no restrictions to the use of any contraceptive methods following restrictive bariatric surgery procedures, but both combined and progestin-only pills are relatively less effective following procedures associated with malabsorption.

FURTHER READINGS

Balasubramanian R et al: Human GnRH deficiency: A unique disease model to unravel the ontogeny of GnRH neurons. Neuroendocrinol 92:81, 2010

Boivin J et al: International estimates of infertility prevalence and treatment-seeking: Potential need and demand for infertility medical care. Hum Reprod 22:1506, 2007

Division of Reproductive Health et al: U S. medical eligibility criteria for contraceptive use, 2010: Adapted from the World Health Organization medical eligibility criteria for contraceptive use, 4th edition. MMWR Recomm Rep 59:1, 2010

Edson MA et al: The mammalian ovary from genesis to revelation. Endocr Rev 30:624, 2010

Gajdos ZK et al: Genetic determinants of pubertal timing in the general population. Mol Cell Endocrinol 324:21, 2010

CHAPTER 348

The Menopause Transition and Postmenopausal Hormone Therapy

JoAnn E. Manson
Shari S. Bassuk

Menopause is the permanent cessation of menstruation due to loss of ovarian follicular function. It is diagnosed retrospectively after 12 months of amenorrhea. The average age at menopause is 51 years among U.S. women. *Perimenopause* refers to the time period preceding menopause, when fertility wanes and menstrual cycle irregularity increases, until the first year after cessation of menses. The onset of perimenopause precedes the final menses by 2 to 8 years, with a mean duration of four years. Smoking accelerates the menopausal transition by 2 years.

Although the peri- and postmenopausal transitions share many symptoms, the physiology and clinical management differ. Low-dose oral contraceptives have become a therapeutic mainstay in perimenopause, whereas postmenopausal hormone therapy (HT) has been a common method of symptom alleviation after menstruation ceases.

PERIMENOPAUSE

PHYSIOLOGY

Ovarian mass and fertility decline sharply after age 35 and even more precipitously during perimenopause; depletion of primary follicles, a process that begins before birth, occurs steadily until menopause (Chap. 347). In perimenopause, intermenstrual intervals shorten significantly (typically by 3 days) due to an accelerated follicular phase. Follicle-stimulating hormone (FSH) levels rise due to altered folliculogenesis and reduced inhibin secretion. In contrast to the consistently high FSH and low estradiol levels seen in menopause, perimenopause is characterized by "irregularly irregular" hormone levels. The propensity for anovulatory cycles can produce a hyperestrogenic, hypoprogestagenic environment that may account for the increased incidence of endometrial hyperplasia or carcinoma, uterine polyps, and leiomyoma observed among women of perimenopausal age. Mean serum levels of selected ovarian and pituitary hormones during the menopausal transition are shown in Fig. 348-1. With transition into menopause, estradiol levels fall markedly, whereas estrone levels are relatively preserved, reflecting peripheral aromatization of adrenal and ovarian androgens. FSH levels increase more than those of luteinizing hormone (LH), presumably because of the loss of inhibin, as well as estrogen feedback.

DIAGNOSTIC TESTS

Because of their extreme intraindividual variability, FSH and estradiol levels are imperfect diagnostic indicators of perimenopause in menstruating women. However, a low FSH in the early follicular phase (days 2 through 5) of the menstrual cycle is inconsistent with a diagnosis of perimenopause. FSH measurement can also aid in assessing fertility; levels of <20 mIU/mL, 20 to <30 mIU/mL, and ≥30 mIU/mL measured on day 3 of the cycle indicate a good, fair, and poor likelihood of achieving pregnancy, respectively.

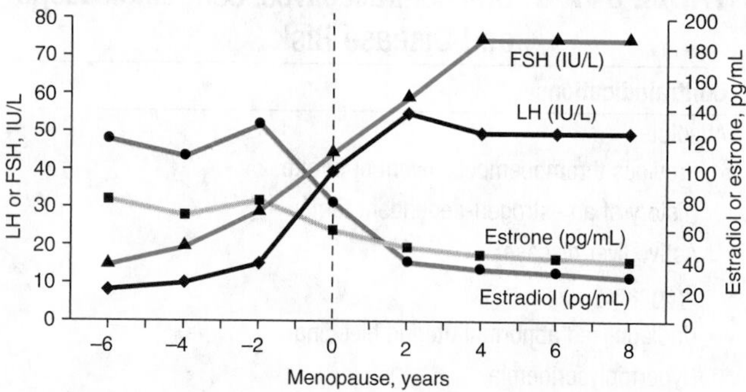

Figure 348-1 Mean serum levels of ovarian and pituitary hormones during the menopausal transition. FSH, follicle-stimulating hormone; LH, luteinizing hormone. *(From JL Shifren, I Schiff: J Womens Health Gend Based Med 9 Suppl 1:S3, 2000, with permission.)*

SYMPTOMS

Determining whether symptoms that develop in midlife are due to ovarian senescence or to other age-related changes is difficult. There is strong evidence that the menopausal transition can cause hot flashes, night sweats, irregular bleeding, and vaginal dryness, and moderate evidence that it can cause sleep disturbances in some women. There is inconclusive or insufficient evidence that ovarian aging is a major cause of mood swings, depression, impaired memory or concentration, somatic symptoms, urinary incontinence, or sexual dysfunction. In one U.S. study, nearly 60% of women reported hot flashes in the 2 years before their final menses. Symptom intensity, duration, frequency, and effects on quality of life are highly variable.

TREATMENT Perimenopause

For women with irregular or heavy menses or hormone-related symptoms that impair quality of life, low-dose combined oral contraceptives are a staple of therapy. Static doses of estrogen and progestin (e.g., 20 μg of ethinyl estradiol and 1 mg of norethindrone acetate daily for 21 days each month) can eliminate vasomotor symptoms and restore regular cyclicity. Oral contraceptives provide other benefits, including protection against ovarian and endometrial cancers and increased bone density, although it is not clear whether use during perimenopause decreases fracture risk later in life. Moreover, the contraceptive benefit is important, given that the unintentional pregnancy rate among women in their forties rivals that of adolescents. Contraindications to oral contraceptive use include cigarette smoking, liver disease, a history of thromboembolism or cardiovascular disease, breast cancer, or unexplained vaginal bleeding. Progestin-only formulations (e.g., 0.35 mg norethindrone daily) or medroxyprogesterone (Depo-Provera) injections (e.g., 150 mg IM every 3 months) may provide an alternative for the treatment of perimenopausal menorrhagia in women who smoke or have cardiovascular risk factors. Although progestins neither regularize cycles nor reduce the number of bleeding days, they reduce the volume of menstrual flow.

Nonhormonal strategies to reduce menstrual flow include use of nonsteroidal anti-inflammatory agents such as mefenamic acid (initial dose of 500 mg at start of menses, then 250 mg qid for 2–3 days) or, when medical approaches fail, endometrial ablation. It should be noted that menorrhagia requires an evaluation to rule out uterine disorders. Transvaginal ultrasound with saline enhancement is useful for detecting leiomyomata or polyps, and endometrial aspiration can identify hyperplastic changes.

TRANSITION TO MENOPAUSE For sexually active women using contraceptive hormones to alleviate perimenopausal symptoms, the question of when and if to switch to HT must be individualized. Doses of estrogen and progestogen (either synthetic progestins or natural forms of progesterone) in HT are lower than those in oral contraceptives and have not been documented to prevent pregnancy. Although a 1-year absence of spontaneous menses reliably indicates ovulation cessation, it is not possible to assess the natural menstrual pattern while a woman is taking an oral contraceptive. Women willing to switch to a barrier method of contraception should do so; if menses occur spontaneously, oral contraceptive use can be resumed. The average age of final menses among relatives can serve as a guide for when to initiate this process, which can be repeated yearly until menopause has occurred.

MENOPAUSE AND POSTMENOPAUSAL HORMONE THERAPY

One of the most complex health care decisions facing women is whether to use postmenopausal HT. Once prescribed primarily to relieve vasomotor symptoms, HT has been promoted as a strategy to forestall various disorders that accelerate after menopause, including osteoporosis and cardiovascular disease. In 2000, nearly 40% of postmenopausal women age 50–74 in the United States had used HT. This widespread use occurred despite the paucity of conclusive data, until recently, on the health consequences of such therapy. Although many women rely on their health care providers for a definitive answer to the question of whether to use postmenopausal hormones, balancing the benefits and risks for an individual patient is challenging.

Although observational studies suggest that HT prevents cardiovascular and other chronic diseases, the apparent benefits may result at least in part from differences between women who opt to take postmenopausal hormones and women who do not. Those choosing HT tend to be healthier, have greater access to medical care, are more compliant with prescribed treatments, and maintain a more health-promoting lifestyle. Randomized trials, which eliminate these confounding factors, have not consistently confirmed the benefits found in observational studies. Indeed, the largest HT trial to date, the Women's Health Initiative (WHI), which examined more than 27,000 postmenopausal women age 50–79 (mean age, 63) for an average of 5–7 years, was stopped early because of an overall unfavorable risk-benefit ratio in the estrogen-progestin arm and an excess risk of stroke that was not offset by a reduced risk of coronary heart disease (CHD) in the estrogen-only arm.

The following summary offers a decision-making guide based on a synthesis of currently available evidence. Prevention of cardiovascular disease is eliminated from the equation due to lack of evidence for such benefits in recent randomized clinical trials.

BENEFITS AND RISKS OF POSTMENOPAUSAL HORMONE THERAPY

(Table 348-1)

Definite benefits

Symptoms of menopause Compelling evidence, including data from randomized clinical trials, indicates that estrogen therapy is highly effective for controlling vasomotor and genitourinary symptoms. Alternative approaches, including the use of antidepressants (such as venlafaxine, 75–150 mg/d), gabapentin (300–900 mg/d), clonidine (0.1–0.2 mg/d), or vitamin E (400–800 IU/d), or the consumption of soy-based products or other phytoestrogens, may also alleviate vasomotor symptoms, although they are less effective than HT. For genitourinary symptoms, the efficacy of vaginal estrogen is similar to that of oral or transdermal estrogen.

Osteoporosis (See also Chap. 354)

Bone density By reducing bone turnover and resorption rates, estrogen slows the aging-related bone loss experienced by most postmenopausal women. More than 50 randomized trials have demonstrated that postmenopausal estrogen therapy, with or without a progestogen, rapidly increases bone mineral density at the spine by 4–6% and at the hip by 2–3%, and maintains those increases during treatment.

Fractures Data from observational studies indicate a 50–80% lower risk of vertebral fracture and a 25–30% lower risk of hip, wrist, and other peripheral fractures among current estrogen users; addition of a progestogen does not appear to modify this benefit. In the WHI, 5–7 years of either combined estrogen-progestin or estrogen-only therapy was associated with a 30–40% reduction in hip fracture and 20–30% fewer total fractures among a population unselected for osteoporosis. Bisphosphonates (such as alendronate, 10 mg/d or 70 mg once per week; risedronate, 5 mg/d or 35 mg once per week; or ibandronate, 2.5 mg/d or 150 mg once per month or 3 mg every 3 months IV) and raloxifene (60 mg/d), a selective estrogen receptor modulator (SERM), have been shown in randomized trials to increase bone mass density and decrease fracture rates. A recently available option for treatment of osteoporosis is parathyroid hormone (teriparatide, 20 μg/d SC). These agents, unlike estrogen, do not appear to have adverse effects on the endometrium or breast. Increased physical activity and adequate calcium (1000–1200 mg/d through diet or supplements in two to three divided doses) and vitamin D (600–1000 IU/d) intakes may also reduce the risk of osteoporosis-related fractures. (Blood levels of 25-hydroxyvitamin D of ≥75 nmol/L are optimal for bone-density maintenance and fracture prevention.) The Fracture Risk Assessment (FRAX®) score, an algorithm that combines an individual's bone-density score with age and other risk factors to predict her 10-year risk of hip and major osteoporotic fracture, may be of use in guiding decisions about pharmacologic treatment (see *http://www.shef.ac.uk/FRAX/index.htm*).

Definite risks

Endometrial cancer (with estrogen alone) A combined analysis of 30 observational studies found a tripling of endometrial cancer risk among short-term (1–5 years) users of unopposed estrogen and a nearly tenfold increased risk among users for 10 or more years. These findings are supported by results from the randomized Postmenopausal Estrogen/Progestin Interventions (PEPI) trial, in which 24% of women assigned to unopposed estrogen for 3 years developed atypical endometrial hyperplasia, a premalignant lesion, compared with only 1% of women assigned to placebo. Use of a progestogen, which opposes the effects of estrogen on the endometrium, eliminates these risks.

Venous thromboembolism A meta-analysis of 12 studies—8 case-control, 1 cohort, and 3 randomized trials—found that current estrogen use was associated with a doubling of venous thromboembolism risk in postmenopausal women. Relative risks of thromboembolic events were even greater (2.7–5.1) in the three trials included in the meta-analysis. Results from the WHI indicate a twofold increase in risk of venous and pulmonary thromboembolism

TABLE 348-1 Benefits and Risks of Postmenopausal Hormone Therapy (HT) in Primary Prevention Settings[a]

Outcome	Effect	Benefit or Risk: Relative — Observational Studies	Relative — WHI[b], Except Where Noted	Absolute — WHI[b], Except Where Noted
Definite Benefits				
Symptoms of menopause	Definite improvement	↓ 70–80% decreased risk	↓65–90% decreased risk[c]	
Osteoporosis	Definite increase in bone mineral density and decrease in fracture risk	↓ 20–50% decreased risk for fracture	E+P: ↓ 33% decreased risk for hip fracture E: ↓ 39% decreased risk for hip fracture	E+P: 50 fewer hip fractures (110 vs 160) per 100,000 woman-years E: 60 fewer hip fractures (110 vs 170) per 100,000 woman-years
Definite Risks				
Endometrial cancer	Definite increase in risk with estrogen alone; no increase in risk with estrogen-progestin	E+P: No increase in risk E: ↑ >300% increased risk (1–5 years); >600% increased risk (≥5 years)	E+P: No increase in risk E: Not applicable	E+P: No difference in risk E: 46 excess cases per 100,000 woman-years with unopposed estrogen (observational studies)[d]
Venous thromboembolism	Definite increase in risk	↑ 110% increased risk	E+P: ↑ 106% increased risk E: ↑ 32% increased risk	E+P: 180 excess cases (350 vs 170) per 100,000 woman-years E: 80 excess cases (300 vs 220) per 100,000 woman-years
Breast cancer	Increase in risk with long-term use (≥5 years) of estrogen-progestin	E+P: ↑ 63% increased risk (≥5 years) E: ↑ 20% increased risk (≥5 years)	E+P: ↑ 24% increased risk E: No increase in risk	10–30 excess cases per 10,000 women using HT for 5 years; 30–90 excess cases per 10,000 women after 10 years use; 50–200 excess cases per 10,000 women after 15 years' use (estimate derived from observational data and WHI E+P findings)
Gallbladder disease	Definite increase in risk	↑ 110% increased risk	E+P: ↑ 67% increased risk E: ↑ 93% increased risk	E+P: 180 excess cases (460 vs 280) per 100,000 woman-years E: 310 excess cases (650 vs 340) per 100,000 woman-years
Probable or Uncertain Risks and Benefits				
Coronary heart disease	Probable increase in risk among older women and women many years past menopause; possible decrease in risk or no effect in younger or recent menopausal women	E+P: ↓36% decreased risk E: ↓ 45% decreased risk	E+P: ↑ 24% increased risk E: No increase or decrease in risk	E+P: 60 excess cases (390 vs 330) per 100,000 woman-years E: No difference in risk
Stroke	Probable increase in risk	↑ 12% increased risk	E+P: ↑ 31% increased risk E: ↑ 39% increased risk	E+P: 70 excess cases (310 vs 240) per 100,000 woman-years E: 120 excess cases (440 vs 320) per 100,000 woman-years
Ovarian cancer	Probable increase in risk with long-term use (≥5 years)	E+P: No effect (<4 years use) E: ↑ 80% increased risk (≥10 years)	E+P: ↑ 58% increased risk[e] E: Not yet available	E+P: 10 excess cases (40 vs 30) per 100,000 woman-years[e]
Colorectal cancer	Probable decrease in risk with estrogen-progestin	↓ 34% decreased risk	E+P: ↓ 37% decreased risk E: No increase or decrease in risk	E+P: 70 fewer cases (90 vs 160) per 100,000 woman-years E: No difference in risk
Diabetes mellitus	Probable decrease in risk	↓ 20% decreased risk	E+P: ↓ 21% decreased risk E: ↓ 12% decreased risk[e]	E+P: 150 fewer cases (610 vs 760) per 100,000 woman-years E: 140 fewer cases (1160 vs 1300) per 100,000 woman-years[e]
Cognitive dysfunction	Unproven decrease in risk (inconsistent data from observational studies and randomized trials)	↓ 34% decreased risk	↑ 76% increased risk for dementia at age ≥65	120–230 excess cases of dementia per 100,000 woman-years

[a]E, estrogen alone; E+P, estrogen plus progestin. Most studies have assessed conjugated equine estrogen alone or in combination with medroxyprogesterone acetate.
[b]WHI, Women's Health Initiative. The estrogen–plus–progestin arm of the WHI assessed 5.6 years of conjugated equine estrogen (0.625 mg/d) plus medroxyprogesterone acetate (2.5 mg/d) versus placebo. The estrogen–alone arm of the WHI assessed 7.1 years of conjugated equine estrogen (0.625 mg/d) versus placebo.
[c]Data are from other randomized trials. The WHI was not designed to assess effect of HT on menopausal symptoms.
[d]JE Manson, KA Martin: N Engl J Med 345:34, 2001.
[e]Not statistically significant.

associated with estrogen-progestin and a one-third increase in this risk with estrogen-only therapy. Transdermal estrogen, taken alone or with certain progestogens (micronized progesterone or pregnane derivatives), appears to be a safer alternative with respect to thrombotic risk.

Breast cancer (with estrogen-progestin) An increased risk of breast cancer has been found among current or recent estrogen users in observational studies; this risk is directly related to duration of use. In a meta-analysis of 51 case-control and cohort studies, short-term use (<5 years) of postmenopausal HT did not appreciably elevate breast cancer incidence, whereas long-term use (≥5 years) was associated with a 35% increase in risk. In contrast to findings for endometrial cancer, combined estrogen-progestin regimens appear to increase breast cancer risk more than estrogen alone. Data from randomized trials also indicate that estrogen-progestin raises breast cancer risk. In the WHI, women assigned to receive combination hormones for an average of 5.6 years were 24% more likely to develop breast cancer than women assigned to placebo, but 7.1 years of estrogen-only therapy did not increase risk. Indeed, the WHI showed a trend toward a reduction in breast cancer risk with estrogen alone, although it is unclear whether this finding would pertain to formulations of estrogen other than conjugated equine estrogens or to treatment durations longer than 7 years. In the Heart and Estrogen/progestin Replacement Study (HERS), 4 years of combination therapy was associated with a 27% increase in breast cancer risk. Although the latter finding was not statistically significant, the totality of evidence strongly implicates estrogen-progestin therapy in breast carcinogenesis.

Gallbladder disease Large observational studies report a two- to threefold increased risk of gallstones or cholecystectomy among postmenopausal women taking oral estrogen. In the WHI, women randomized to estrogen-progestin or estrogen alone had a 67% and 93% greater risk, respectively, of undergoing cholecystectomy than those assigned to placebo. Increased risks were also observed in HERS. Transdermal HT might be a safer alternative, but further research is needed.

Probable or uncertain risks and benefits

Coronary heart disease/stroke Until recently, HT had been enthusiastically recommended as a possible cardioprotective agent. In the past 3 decades, multiple observational studies suggested, in the aggregate, that estrogen use leads to a 35–50% reduction in CHD incidence among postmenopausal women. The biologic plausibility of such an association is supported by data from randomized trials demonstrating that exogenous estrogen lowers plasma low-density lipoprotein (LDL) cholesterol and raises high-density lipoprotein (HDL) cholesterol levels by 10–15%. Administration of estrogen also favorably affects lipoprotein(a) levels, LDL oxidation, endothelial vascular function, fibrinogen, and plasminogen activator inhibitor-1. However, estrogen therapy also has unfavorable effects on other biomarkers of cardiovascular risk: it boosts triglyceride levels; promotes coagulation via factor VII, prothrombin fragments 1 and 2, and fibrinopeptide A elevations; and raises levels of the inflammatory marker C-reactive protein.

Randomized trials of estrogen or combined estrogen-progestin in women with preexisting cardiovascular disease (CVD) have not confirmed the benefits reported in observational studies. In HERS, a secondary prevention trial designed to test the efficacy and safety of estrogen-progestin therapy on clinical cardiovascular outcomes, the 4-year incidence of coronary mortality and nonfatal myocardial infarction was similar in the active treatment and placebo groups, and a 50% increase in risk of coronary events was noted during the first year of the study among participants assigned to the active treatment group. Although it is possible that progestin may mitigate estrogen's benefits, the Estrogen Replacement and Atherosclerosis (ERA) trial indicated that angiographically determined progression of coronary atherosclerosis was unaffected by either opposed or unopposed estrogen treatment. Moreover, the Papworth Hormone Replacement Therapy Atherosclerosis Study, a trial of transdermal estradiol with and without norethindrone; the Women's Estrogen for Stroke Trial (WEST), a trial of oral 17β-estradiol; and the EStrogen in the Prevention of ReInfarction Trial (ESPRIT), a trial of oral estradiol valerate, found no cardiovascular benefits of the regimens studied. Thus, in clinical trials, HT has not proved effective for the secondary prevention of CVD in postmenopausal women.

Primary prevention trials also suggest an early increase in cardiovascular risk and absence of cardioprotection with postmenopausal HT. Results from the WHI suggest a deleterious cardiovascular effect of HT. Women assigned to 5.6 years of estrogen-progestin therapy were 24% more likely to develop CHD and 31% more likely to suffer a stroke than those assigned to placebo. In the estrogen-only arm of the WHI, a similar increase in stroke and no effect on CHD were observed.

However, a closer look at available data suggests that timing of initiation of HT may critically influence the association between such therapy and CHD. Estrogen may slow early stages of atherosclerosis but have adverse effects on advanced atherosclerotic lesions. It has been hypothesized that the prothrombotic and proinflammatory effects of estrogen manifest themselves predominantly among women with subclinical lesions who initiate HT well after the menopausal transition, whereas women with less arterial damage who start HT early in menopause may derive cardiovascular benefit because they have not yet developed advanced lesions. Nonhuman primate data support this concept. Conjugated estrogens had no effect on the extent of coronary artery plaque in cynomolgus monkeys assigned to estrogen alone or combined with progestin starting 2 years (approximately 6 human years) after oophorectomy and well after the establishment of atherosclerosis. However, administration of exogenous hormones immediately after oophorectomy, during the early stages of atherosclerosis, reduced the extent of plaque by 70%.

Lending further credence to this hypothesis are results of subgroup analyses of observational and clinical trial data. For example, among women who entered the WHI trial with a better cholesterol profile, estrogen with or without progestin led to a 40% lower risk for incident CHD. Among women who entered with a worse cholesterol profile, therapy resulted in a 73% higher risk (p for interaction=0.02). Moreover, although there was no association between estrogen-only therapy and CHD in the WHI trial cohort as a whole, such therapy was associated with a CHD risk reduction of 37% among participants age 50–59. By contrast, a risk reduction of only 8% was observed among those age 60–69, and a risk increase of 11% was found among those age 70–79. Due to the relatively small number of cases of myocardial infarction or coronary death (the primary definition of CHD in the WHI), especially in the younger women, these intra- and inter-age group differences were not statistically significant. However, when the definition of CHD was widened to include coronary bypass surgery or percutaneous coronary interventions, estrogen-only therapy was associated with a significant 45% reduction in CHD among women in the youngest age group. Moreover, estrogen was associated with lower levels of coronary artery calcified plaque.

Although age did not have a similar effect in the estrogen-progestin arm of the WHI, CHD risks steadily increased with years since menopause. Estrogen-progestin was associated with an 11% risk reduction for women less than 10 years beyond menopause but was associated with a 22% increase in risk for women 10–19 years from menopause, and a 71% increase in risk for women 20 years or more from menopause (only the latter was statistically significant). In the large observational Nurses' Health Study, women who chose to start HT within 4 years of menopause experienced a lower risk of CHD than did nonusers, whereas those who began therapy 10 or more years after menopause appeared to receive little coronary benefit. Because observational studies include a high proportion of women who begin HT within 3–4 years of menopause and clinical trials include a high proportion of women 12 or more years past menopause, these findings help to reconcile some of the apparent discrepancies between the two types of studies.

Whether or not age at initiation of HT influences stroke risk is not well understood. In the WHI and the Nurses' Health Study, HT was associated with an excess risk of stroke in all age groups. Further research is needed on age, time since menopause, and other clinical characteristics as well as on biomarkers that predict increases or decreases in cardiovascular risk associated with exogenous HT. Furthermore, it remains uncertain whether different doses, formulations, or routes of administration of HT will produce different cardiovascular effects.

Colorectal cancer Observational studies have suggested that HT reduces risks of colon and rectal cancer, although the estimated magnitudes of the relative benefits ranged from 8 to 34% in various meta-analyses. In the WHI, the sole trial to examine the issue, estrogen-progestin was associated with a significant 44% reduction in colorectal cancer over a 5.6-year period, although no benefit was seen with 7 years of estrogen-only therapy.

Cognitive decline and dementia A meta-analysis of ten case-control and two cohort studies suggested that postmenopausal HT is associated with a 34% decreased risk of dementia. Subsequent randomized trials, including the WHI, however, have failed to demonstrate any benefit of estrogen or estrogen-progestin therapy on the progression of mild to moderate Alzheimer's disease and/or have indicated a potential adverse effect of HT on the incidence of dementia, at least in women age 65 and older. Determining whether timing of initiation of HT influences cognitive outcomes will require further study.

Ovarian cancer and other disorders On the basis of limited observational and randomized data, it has been hypothesized that HT increases the risk of ovarian cancer and reduces the risk of type 2 diabetes mellitus. Results from the WHI support these hypotheses. The WHI also found that estrogen-progestin use was associated with increased lung cancer mortality.

Changes in health status after discontinuation of hormone therapy In the WHI cohort as a whole, the elevated risks for CHD, stroke, and venous thromboembolism associated with active use of estrogen-progestin disappeared within 2.4 years after discontinuation of therapy, as did the benefits, including amelioration of hot flashes and protection against osteoporotic fractures and colorectal cancer. A slightly elevated risk for breast cancer persisted, and a suggestion of higher risks for lung cancer, total cancer, and total mortality emerged. Postintervention results stratified by age or time since menopause onset are not yet available.

APPROACH TO THE PATIENT: Postmenopausal Hormone Therapy

The rational use of postmenopausal HT requires balancing the potential benefits and risks. Figure 348-2 provides one approach to decision making. The clinician should first determine whether the patient has moderate to severe menopausal symptoms, the only indication for initiating systemic HT (urogenital symptoms in the absence of vasomotor symptoms may be treated with vaginal estrogen). The benefits and risks of such therapy should then be reviewed with the patient, giving more emphasis to absolute than to relative measures of effect, and pointing out uncertainties in clinical knowledge where relevant. Because chronic disease rates generally increase with age, absolute risks tend to be greater in older women, even when relative risks remain similar. Potential side effects—especially vaginal bleeding that may result from use of combined estrogen-progestogen formulations recommended for women with an intact uterus—should be noted. The patient's own preference regarding therapy should be elicited and factored into the decision. Contraindications to HT should be assessed routinely and include unexplained vaginal bleeding, active liver disease, venous thromboembolism, history of endometrial cancer (except stage 1 without deep invasion) or breast cancer, and history of CHD, stroke, transient ischemic attack, or diabetes. Relative contraindications include hypertriglyceridemia (>400 mg/dl) and active gallbladder disease; in such cases, transdermal estrogen may be an option. Primary prevention of heart disease should not be viewed as an expected benefit of HT, and an increase in stroke and a small early increase in coronary artery disease risk should be considered. Nevertheless, such therapy may be appropriate if the noncoronary benefits of treatment clearly outweigh risks. A woman who suffers an acute coronary event or stroke while on HT should stop therapy immediately.

Short-term use (<5 years) of HT is appropriate for relief of menopausal symptoms among women without contraindications to such use. However, such therapy should be avoided among women with an elevated baseline risk of future cardiovascular events. Women who have contraindications, or are opposed to HT, may derive benefit from the use of certain antidepressants (including venlafaxine, fluoxetine, or paroxetine), gabapentin, clonidine, soy, or black cohosh, and, for genitourinary symptoms, intravaginal estrogen creams or devices.

Long-term use (≥5 years) of HT, especially estrogen-progestogen, is more problematic because a heightened risk of breast cancer must be factored into the decision. Reasonable candidates for such use include a small percentage of postmenopausal women and comprise those who have persistent severe vasomotor symptoms along with an increased risk of osteoporosis (e.g., those with osteopenia, a personal or family history of nontraumatic fracture, or a weight below 125 lbs), who also have no personal or family history of breast cancer in a first-degree relative or other contraindications, and who have a strong personal preference for therapy. Poor candidates are women with elevated cardiovascular risk, those at increased risk of breast cancer (e.g., women who have a first-degree relative with breast cancer, susceptibility genes such as *BRCA1* or *BRCA2*, or a personal history of cellular atypia detected by breast biopsy), and those at low risk of osteoporosis. Even in reasonable candidates, strategies to minimize dose and duration of use should be employed. For example, women using HT to relieve intense vasomotor symptoms in early postmenopause should consider discontinuing therapy before 5 years, resuming it only if such symptoms persist. Because of the role of progestogens in increasing breast cancer risk, regimens that employ cyclic rather than continuous progestogen exposure should be considered if treatment is extended. For prevention of osteoporosis, alternative therapies such as bisphosphonates or SERMs should be considered. Research on androgen-containing preparations has been limited, particularly in terms of long-term safety. Additional research on the effects of these agents on CVD,

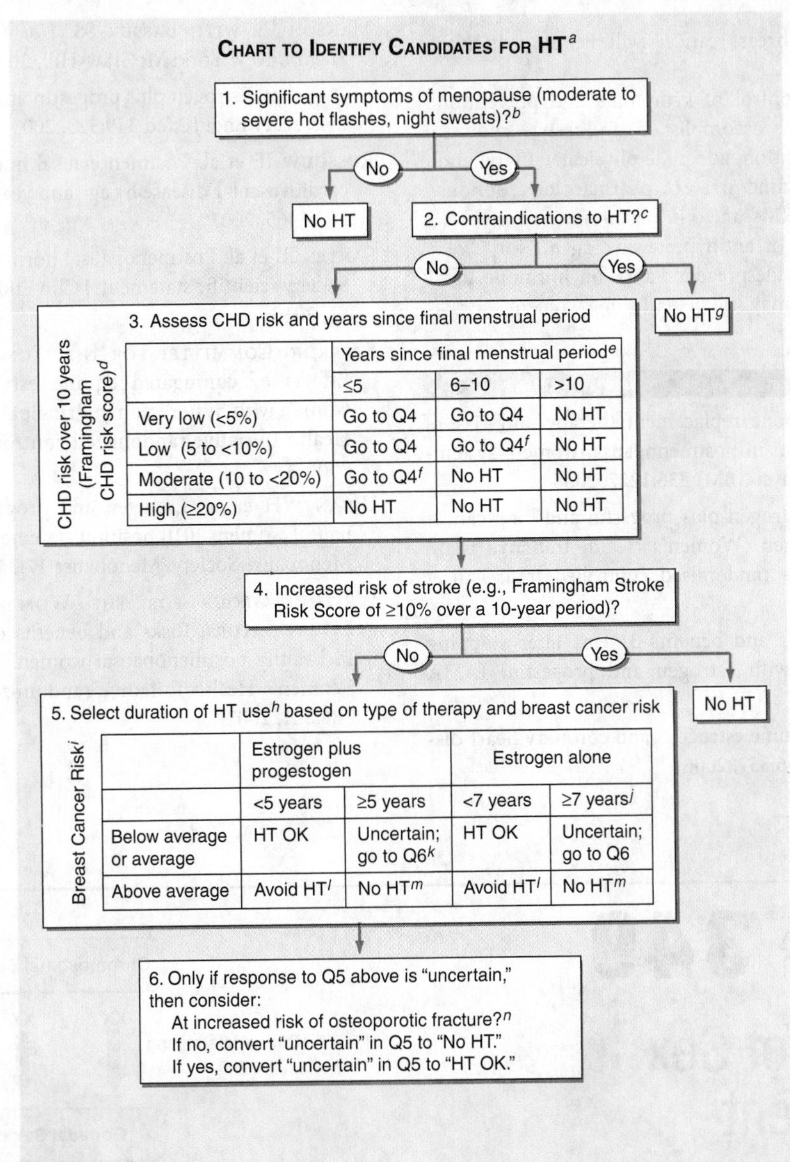

Figure 348-2 Chart for identifying appropriate candidates for postmenopausal hormone therapy (HT). CHD, coronary heart disease.

[a]Reassess each step at least once every 6–12 months (assuming patient's continued preference for HT).

[b]Women who have vaginal dryness without moderate to severe vasomotor symptoms may be candidates for vaginal estrogen.

[c]Traditional contraindications: unexplained vaginal bleeding; active liver disease; history of venous thromboembolism due to pregnancy, oral contraceptive use, or unknown etiology; blood clotting disorder; history of breast or endometrial cancer; history of CHD, stroke, transient ischemic attack, or diabetes. For other contraindications, including high triglycerides (>400 mg/dL); active gallbladder disease; and history of venous thromboembolism due to past immobility, surgery, or bone fracture; oral HT should be avoided but transdermal HT may be an option (see *f* below).

[d]10-year risk of CHD, based on Framingham Coronary Heart Disease Risk Score (Expert Panel on Detection, Evaluation, and Treatment of High Blood Cholesterol in Adults: JAMA 285:2486, 2001), as modified by JE Manson, with SS Bassuk: *Hot Flashes, Hormones & Your Health.* New York, McGraw-Hill, 2007.

[e]Women >10 years past menopause are not good candidates for starting (first use of) HT.

[f]Avoid oral HT. Transdermal HT may be an option because it has a less adverse effect on clotting factors, triglyceride levels, and inflammation factors than oral HT.

[g]Consider selective serotonin or serotonin-norepinephrine reuptake inhibitor, gabapentin, clonidine, soy, or alternative.

[h]HT should be continued only if moderate to severe menopausal symptoms persist. The recommended cutpoints for duration are based on results of the Women's Health Initiative estrogen-progestin and estrogen-alone trials, which lasted 5.6 and 7.1 years, respectively. For longer durations of HT use, balance of benefits and risks is not known.

[i]Above-average risk of breast cancer: one or more first-degree relatives with breast cancer; susceptibility genes such as *BRCA1* or *BRCA2*; or a personal history of breast biopsy demonstrating atypia.

[j]Women with premature surgical menopause may take HT until average age at menopause (age 51 in the United States) and then follow flowchart for subsequent decision making.

[k]If progestogen is taken daily, avoid extending duration. If progestogen is cyclical or infrequent, avoid extending duration more than 1–2 years.

[l]If menopausal symptoms are severe, estrogen plus progestin can be taken for 2–3 years maximum and estrogen alone for 4–5 years maximum.

[m]If at high risk of osteoporotic fracture (see Q6), consider bisphosphonate, raloxifene, or alternative.

[n]Increased risk of osteoporotic fracture: documented osteopenia, personal or family history of nontraumatic fracture, current smoking, or weight <125 lbs.

Source: Adapted from JE Manson with SS Bassuk: *Hot Flashes, Hormones & Your Health.* New York, McGraw-Hill, 2007.

glucose tolerance, and breast cancer will be of particular interest.

In addition to HT, control of symptoms and prevention of chronic disease can be accomplished by lifestyle choices, including smoking abstention, adequate physical activity, and a healthy diet. An expanding array of pharmacologic options (e.g., bisphosphonates, SERMs, and other agents for osteoporosis, and cholesterol-lowering or antihypertensive agents for CVD should also reduce the widespread reliance on hormone use. However, short-term HT may still benefit some women.

FURTHER READINGS

Canonico M et al: Hormone replacement therapy and risk of venous thromboembolism in postmenopausal women: systematic review and meta-analysis. BMJ 336:1227, 2008

Chlebowski RT et al: Oestrogen plus progestin and lung cancer in postmenopausal women (Women's Health Initiative trial): a post-hoc analysis of a randomised controlled trial. Lancet 374:1243, 2009

Heiss G et al: Health risks and benefits 3 years after stopping randomized treatment with estrogen and progestin. JAMA 299:1036, 2008

Hsia J et al: Conjugated equine estrogens and coronary heart disease. Arch Intern Med 166:357, 2006

Manson JE, with Bassuk SS: *Hot Flashes, Hormones & Your Health*. New York: McGraw-Hill, 2007

———, et al: Estrogen plus progestin and the risk of coronary heart disease. N Engl J Med 349:523, 2003

Rossouw JE et al: Postmenopausal hormone therapy and risk of cardiovascular disease by age and years since menopause. JAMA 297:1465, 2007

Santen RJ et al: Postmenopausal hormone therapy: An Endocrine Society scientific statement. J Clin Endocrinol Metab 95(Suppl 1): S1, 2010

Steering Committee for the Women's Health Initiative: Effects of conjugated equine estrogen in postmenopausal women with hysterectomy: Principal results from the Women's Health Initiative randomized controlled trial. JAMA 291:1701, 2004

Utian WH et al.: Estrogen and progestogen use in postmenopausal women: 2010 position statement of The North American Menopause Society. Menopause 17:242, 2010

Writing Group for the Women's Health Initiative Investigators: Risks and benefits of estrogen plus progestin in healthy postmenopausal women. Principal results from the Women's Health Initiative randomized controlled trial. JAMA 288:321, 2002

CHAPTER 349 Disorders of Sex Development

John C. Achermann
J. Larry Jameson

Sex development begins in utero but continues into young adulthood with the achievement of sexual maturity and reproductive capability. The major determinants of sex development can be divided into three major components: chromosomal sex, gonadal sex (sex determination), and phenotypic sex (sex differentiation) (Fig. 349-1). Abnormalities at each of these stages can result in disorders of sex development (DSDs) (Table 349-1). A child born with ambiguous genitalia requires urgent assessment, as some causes such as congenital adrenal hyperplasia (CAH), can be associated with life-threatening adrenal crises. Early gender assignment and clear communication with parents about the diagnosis and treatment options are essential. The involvement of an experienced multidisciplinary team is crucial for counseling, medical management, and surgical evaluation/intervention (if needed). Subtler forms of gonadal dysfunction [e.g., Klinefelter's syndrome (KS), Turner's syndrome (TS)] often are diagnosed later in life by internists. Because these conditions are associated with a variety of psychological, reproductive, and metabolic consequences, an open dialogue must be established between the patient and health care providers to ensure continuity and attention to these issues.

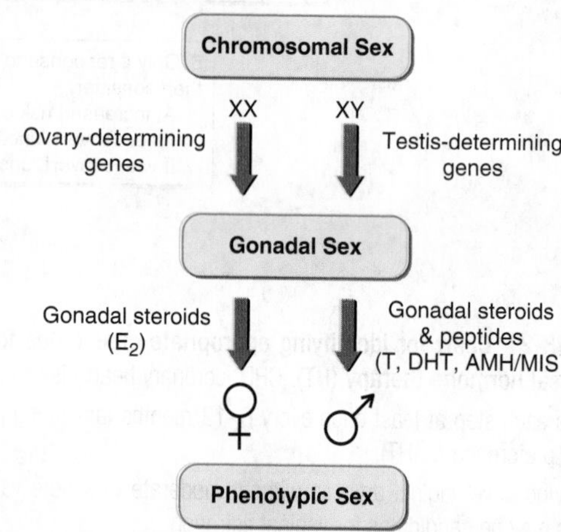

Figure 349-1 Sex development can be divided into three major components: chromosomal sex, gonadal sex, and phenotypic sex. T, testosterone; DHT, dihydrotestosterone; MIS, müllerian-inhibiting substance also known as anti-müllerian hormone, AMH.

SEX DEVELOPMENT

Chromosomal sex describes the X and/or Y chromosome complement (46,XY male; 46,XX female) that is established at the time of fertilization. The presence of a normal Y chromosome determines that testis development will occur even in the presence of multiple X chromosomes (e.g., 47,XXY or 48,XXXY). The loss of an X chromosome impairs gonad development (45,X or 45,X/46,XY mosaicism). Fetuses with no X chromosome (45,Y) are not viable.

Gonadal sex refers to the assignment of gonadal tissue as testis or ovary. The embryonic gonad is bipotential and can develop (from ~42 days gestation) into either a testis or an ovary, depending on which genes are expressed (Fig. 349-2). Testis development is

TABLE 349-1 Classification of Disorders of Sex Development (DSDs)

Sex Chromosome DSD	46,XY DSD	46,XX DSD
47,XXY (Klinefelter's syndrome and variants)	**Disorders of gonadal (testis) development**	**Disorders of gonadal (ovary) development**
45,X (Turner's syndrome and variants)	Complete or partial gonadal dysgenesis (e.g., *SRY, SOX9, SF1, WT1, DHH*)	Gonadal dysgenesis
45,X/46,XY mosaicism (mixed gonadal dysgenesis)	Impaired fetal Leydig cell function (e.g., *SF1/NR5A1, CXorf6/MAMLD1*)	Ovotesticular DSD
46,XX/46,XY (chimerism/mosaicism)	Ovotesticular DSD	Testicular DSD (e.g., *SRY+*, dup *SOX9, RSPO1*)
	Testis regression	
	Disorders in androgen synthesis or action (see Table 349-3)	**Androgen excess (see Table 349-4)**
	Disorders of androgen biosynthesis	Fetal
	LH receptor (*LHCGR*) mutations	3β-Hydroxysteroid dehydrogenase II (*HSD3β2*)
	Smith-Lemli-Opitz syndrome	21-Hydroxylase (*CYP21A2*)
	Steroidogenic acute regulatory (*STAR*) protein	P450 oxidoreductase (*POR*)
	Cholesterol side-chain cleavage (*CYP11A1*)	11β-Hydroxylase (*CYP11B1*)
	3β-Hydroxysteroid dehydrogenase II (*HSD3β2*)	Glucocorticoid receptor mutations
	17α-Hydroxylase/17,20-lyase (*CYP17A1*)	Fetoplacental
	P450 oxidoreductase (*POR*)	Aromatase deficiency (*CYP19*)
	17β-Hydroxysteroid dehydrogenase III (*HSD17β3*)	Oxidoreductase deficiency (*POR*)
	5α-Reductase II (*SRD5A2*)	Maternal
	Disorders of androgen action	Maternal virilizing tumors (e.g., luteomas)
	Androgen Insensitivity syndrome	Androgenic drugs
	Drugs and environmental modulators	
	Other	**Other**
	Syndromic associations of male genital development	Syndromic associations (e.g., cloacal anomalies)
	Persistent müllerian duct syndrome	Müllerian agenesis/hypoplasia (e.g., MRKH)
	Vanishing testis syndrome	Uterine abnormalities (e.g., MODY5)
	Isolated hypospadias	Vaginal atresia (e.g., McKusick-Kaufman)
	Congenital hypogonadotropic hypogonadism	Labial adhesions
	Cryptorchidism	
	Environmental influences	

Source: Modified from IA Hughes. Arch Dis Child 91:554, 2006.

initiated by expression of the Y chromosome gene *SRY* (sex-determining region on the Y chromosome) that encodes an HMG box transcription factor. *SRY* is expressed transiently in cells destined to become Sertoli cells and serves as a pivotal switch to establish the testis lineage. Mutation of *SRY* prevents testis development in chromosomal 46,XY males, whereas translocation of *SRY* in 46,XX females is sufficient to induce testis development and a male phenotype. Other genes are necessary to continue testis development. *SOX9* (*SRY*-related HMG-box gene 9) is upregulated by *SRY* in the developing male gonad but is suppressed in the female gonad. Transgenic expression of *SOX9* is sufficient to initiate testis formation in mice, and mutations that disrupt *SOX9* impair testis development. *WT1* (Wilms' tumor–related gene 1) acts early in the genetic pathway and regulates the transcription of several genes, including *SFI* (officially called *NRSA1*), *DAX1* (*NR0B1*), and *AMH* (encoding *MIS*, müllerian-inhibiting substance). *SF1* encodes steroidogenic factor 1, a nuclear receptor that functions in cooperation with other transcription factors to regulate a large array of adrenal and gonadal genes, including *SOX9* and many genes involved in steroidogenesis. Heterozygous *SF1* mutations account for ~10% of XY patients with gonadal dysgenesis and impaired androgenization, indicating the sensitivity of the testis to *SF1* gene dosage. The early expression pattern of *SF1* in the gonad parallels that of another orphan nuclear receptor, *DAX1* (dosage sensitive sex-reversal, adrenal hypoplasia congenita on the X chromosome, gene 1). Duplication of *DAX1* impairs testis development, whereas deletions or mutations of *DAX1* lead to disordered formation of testis cords, again revealing the exquisite sensitivity of the male sex-determining pathway to gene dosage effects. In addition to the genes mentioned above, studies of human and murine mutations indicate that at least 15 other genes are also involved in gonadal differentiation, gonadal development, and final positioning of the gonad (Fig. 349-2). These genes encode an array of signaling molecules and paracrine growth factors in addition to transcription factors.

Although ovarian development once was considered a "default" process, it is now clear that specific genes are expressed during the earliest stages of ovary development. Some of these factors may repress testis development (e.g., *WNT4*, R-spondin-1) (Fig. 349-2). Once the ovary has formed, additional genes are required for normal follicular development [e.g., follicle-stimulating hormone

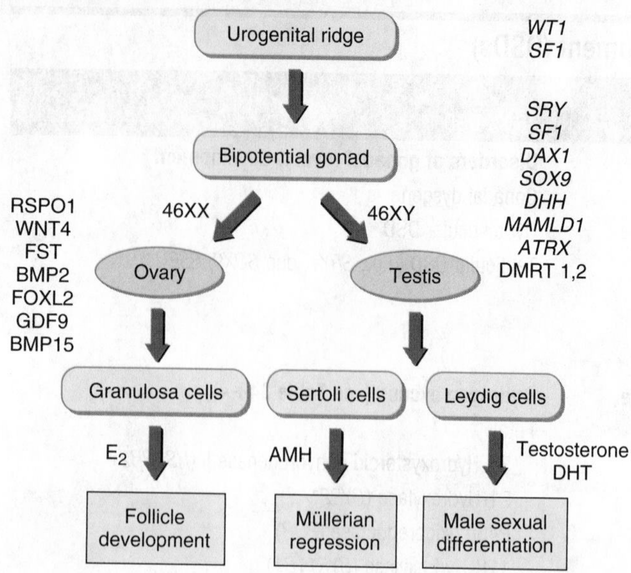

Figure 349-2 The genetic regulation of gonadal development. *WT1*, Wilms' tumor–related gene 1; *SF1*, steroidogenic factor 1 (also known as NR5A1); *SRY*, sex-determining region on the Y chromosome; *SOX9*, *SRY*-related HMG-box gene 9; *DHH*, desert hedgehog; *ATRX*, (α-thalassemia, mental retardation on the X); *DAX1*, dosage sensitive sex-reversal, adrenal hypoplasia congenita on the X chromosome, gene 1; DMRT 1,2, doublesex MAB3-related transcription factor 1,2; WNT4, wingless-type MMTV integration site 4; FST, follistatin; BMP2 and 15, bone morphogenic factors 2 and 15; FOXL2, forkhead transcription factor L2; GDF9, growth differentiation factor 9; AMH, anti-müllerian hormone (müllerian-inhibiting substance); DHT, dihydrotestosterone; RSPO1, R-spondin 1; *MAMLD1*, mastermind-like domain containing 1.

(FSH) receptor, *GDF9*]. Steroidogenesis in the ovary requires the development of follicles that contain granulosa cells and theca cells surrounding the oocytes (Chap. 347). Thus, there is relatively limited ovarian steroidogenesis until gonadotropins are produced at puberty.

Germ cells also develop in a sex dimorphic manner. In the developing ovary, primordial germ cells (PGCs) proliferate and enter meiosis, whereas they proliferate and then undergo mitotic arrest in the developing testis. PGC entry into meiosis is initiated by retinoic acid that activates *STRA8* (*stimulated by retinoic acid 8*) and other genes involved in meiosis. The developing testis produces high levels of CYP26B1, an enzyme that degrades retinoic acid, preventing PGC entry into meiosis. Approximately 7 million germ cells are present in the fetal ovary in the second trimester, and 1 million remain at birth. Only 400 are ovulated during a woman's reproductive life span (Chap. 347).

Phenotypic sex refers to the structures of the external and internal genitalia and secondary sex characteristics. The male phenotype requires the secretion of anti-müllerian hormone (AMH, also known as müllerian-inhibiting substance, *MIS*) from Sertoli cells and testosterone from testicular Leydig cells. AMH is a member of the transforming growth factor (TGF) β family and acts through specific receptors to cause regression of the müllerian structures (from 60–80 days' gestation). At ~60–140 days' gestation, testosterone supports the development of wolffian structures, including the epididymides, vasa deferentia, and seminal vesicles. Testosterone is the precursor for dihydrotestosterone (DHT), a potent androgen that promotes development of the external genitalia, including the penis and scrotum (65–100 days, and thereafter) (Fig. 349-3). The urogenital sinus develops into the prostate and prostatic urethra in the male and into the urethra and lower portion of the vagina in the female. The genital tubercle becomes the glans penis in the male and the clitoris in the female. The urogenital swellings form the scrotum or the labia majora, and the urethral folds fuse to form the shaft of the penis and the male urethra or the labia minora. In the female, wolffian ducts regress and the müllerian ducts form the fallopian tubes, uterus, and upper segment of the vagina. A female phenotype will develop in the absence of the gonad, but estrogen is needed for maturation of the uterus and breast at puberty.

DISORDERS OF CHROMOSOMAL SEX

Variations in sex chromosome number and structure can present as disorders of sex development (e.g., 45,X/46,XY). KS (47,XXY) and TS (45,X) do not usually present with genital ambiguity but are associated with gonadal dysfunction (Table 349-2).

KLINEFELTER'S SYNDROME (47,XXY)

Pathophysiology

The classic form of KS (47,XXY) occurs after meiotic nondisjunction of the sex chromosomes during gametogenesis (40% during spermatogenesis, 60% during oogenesis) (Chap. 62). Mosaic forms of KS (46,XY/47,XXY) are thought to result from chromosomal mitotic nondisjunction within the zygote and occur in at least 10% of individuals with this condition. Other chromosomal variants of KS (e.g., 48,XXYY, 48,XXXY) have been reported but are less common.

Clinical features

KS is characterized by small testes, infertility, gynecomastia, "eunuchoid" proportions, and incomplete virilization in phenotypic males. It has an incidence of at least 1 in 1000 men, but approximately 75% of cases are not diagnosed. In severe cases, individuals present prepubertally with small testes or with impaired androgenization and gynecomastia at the time of puberty. Developmental delay and learning disabilities may be a feature. Later in life, eunuchoid features or infertility lead to the diagnosis. Testes are small and firm [median length 2.5 cm (4 mL volume); almost always <3.5 cm (12 mL)] and typically seem inappropriately small for the degree of androgenization. Biopsies are not usually necessary but reveal seminiferous tubule hyalinization and azoospermia. Other clinical features of KS are listed in Table 349-2. Plasma concentrations of FSH and luteinizing hormone (LH) are increased in most patients with 47,XXY (90% and 80%, respectively), and plasma testosterone is decreased (50–75%), reflecting primary gonadal failure. Estradiol is often increased because of chronic Leydig cell stimulation by LH and because of aromatization of androstenedione by adipose tissue; the increased ratio of estradiol/testosterone results in gynecomastia. Patients with mosaic forms of KS have less severe clinical features, have larger testes, and sometimes achieve spontaneous fertility.

TREATMENT Klinefelter's Syndrome

Gynecomastia should be treated by surgical reduction if it causes concern (Chap. 346). Androgen supplementation improves virilization, libido, energy, hypofibrinolysis, and bone mineralization in underandrogenized men but may occasionally worsen gynecomastia (Chap. 346). Fertility has been achieved by using in vitro fertilization in men with oligospermia or with intracytoplasmic sperm injection (ICSI) after retrieval of spermatozoa by testicular sperm extraction techniques. In specialized centers, successful spermatozoa retrieval using this technique is possible in >50% of men with nonmosaic KS. After ICSI and embryo transfer, successful pregnancies can be achieved in ~50% of these cases. The risk of transmission of this

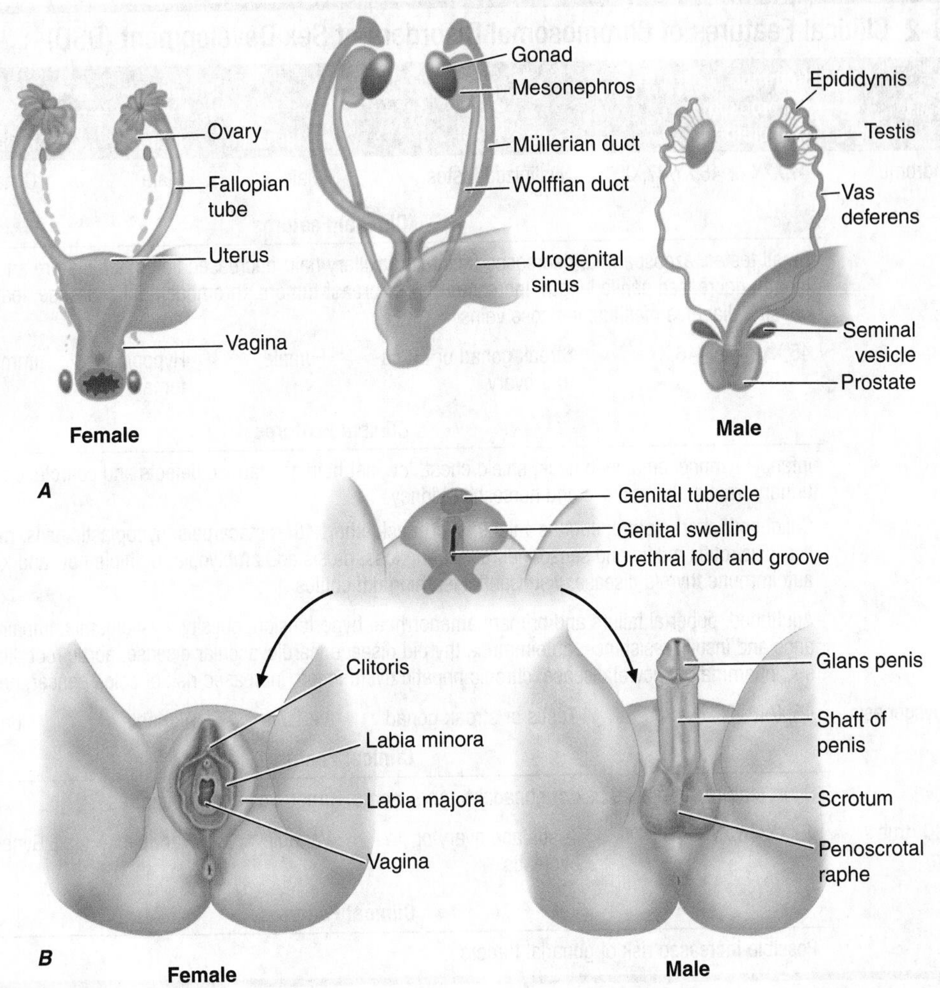

Figure 349-3 Sex development. ***A.*** Internal urogenital tract. ***B.*** External genitalia. *[After E Braunwald et al (eds): Harrison's Principles of Internal Medicine, 15th ed. New York, McGraw-Hill, 2001.]*

chromosomal abnormality needs to be considered, and preimplantation screening may be desired, although this outcome is much less common than originally predicted.

■ TURNER'S SYNDROME (GONADAL DYSGENESIS; 45,X)

Pathophysiology

Approximately one-half of individuals with Turner's syndrome have a 45,X karyotype, about 20% have 45,X/46,XX mosaicism, and the remainder have structural abnormalities of the X chromosome such as X fragments, isochromosomes, or rings. The clinical features of TS result from haploinsufficiency of multiple X chromosomal genes (e.g., short stature homeobox, *SHOX*). However, imprinted genes also may be affected when the inherited X has different parental origins.

Clinical features

TS is characterized by bilateral streak gonads, primary amenorrhea, short stature, and multiple congenital anomalies in phenotypic females. It affects ~1 in 2500 women and is diagnosed at different ages depending on the dominant clinical features (Table 349-2). Prenatally, a diagnosis of TS usually is made incidentally after chorionic villus sampling or amniocentesis for unrelated reasons such as advanced maternal age. Prenatal ultrasound findings include increased nuchal translucency. The postnatal diagnosis of TS should be considered in female neonates or infants with lymphedema, nuchal folds, low hairline, or left-sided cardiac defects and in girls with unexplained growth failure or pubertal delay. Although limited spontaneous pubertal development occurs in up to 30% of girls with TS (10%, 45,X; 30–40%, 45,X/46,XX) and ~2% reach menarche, the vast majority of women with TS develop complete ovarian failure. This diagnosis should be considered, therefore, in all women who present with primary or secondary amenorrhea and elevated gonadotropin levels.

TREATMENT Turner's Syndrome

The management of girls and women with TS requires a multidisciplinary approach because of the number of potentially involved organ systems. Detailed cardiac and renal evaluation should be performed at the time of diagnosis. Individuals with congenital heart defects (CHDs) (30%) (bicuspid aortic valve, 30–50%; coarctation of the aorta, 30%; aortic root dilation, 5%) require long-term follow-up by an experienced cardiologist, antibiotic prophylaxis for dental or surgical procedures, and serial imaging of aortic root dimensions, as progressive aortic root dilation is associated with increased risk of aortic dissection. Individuals found to have congenital renal and urinary tract malformations (30%) are at risk for urinary tract infections, hypertension, and nephrocalcinosis. Hypertension can occur

TABLE 349-2 Clinical Features of Chromosomal Disorders of Sex Development (DSD)

Disorder	Common Chromosomal Complement	Gonad	Genitalia		Breast Development
			External	Internal	
Klinefelter's syndrome	47,XXY or 46,XY/47,XXY	Hyalinized testes	Male	Male	Gynecomastia
	Clinical Features				
	Small testes, azoospermia, decreased facial and axillary hair, decreased libido, tall stature and increased leg length, decreased penile length, increased risk of breast tumors, thromboembolic disease, learning difficulties, obesity, diabetes mellitus, varicose veins				
Turner's syndrome	45,X or 45,X/46,XX	Streak gonad or immature ovary	Female	Hypoplastic female	Immature female
	Clinical Features				
	Infancy: lymphedema, web neck, shield chest, low-set hairline, cardiac defects and coarctation of the aorta, urinary tract malformations and horseshoe kidney Childhood: short stature, cubitus valgus, short neck, short 4th metacarpals, hypoplastic nails, micrognathia, scoliosis, otitis media and sensorineural hearing loss, ptosis and amblyopia, multiple nevi and keloid formation, autoimmune thyroid disease, visuospatial learning difficulties Adulthood: pubertal failure and primary amenorrhea, hypertension, obesity, dyslipidemia, impaired glucose tolerance and insulin resistance, autoimmune thyroid disease, cardiovascular disease, aortic root dilation, osteoporosis, inflammatory bowel disease, chronic hepatic dysfunction, increased risk of colon cancer, hearing loss				
Mixed gonadal dysgenesis	45,X/46,XY	Testis or streak gonad	Variable	Variable	Usually male
	Clinical Features				
	Short stature, increased risk of gonadal tumors, some Turner's syndrome features				
Ovotesticular DSD (true hermaphroditism)	46,XX/46,XY	Testis and ovary or ovotestis	Variable	Variable	Gynecomastia
	Clinical Features				
	Possible increased risk of gonadal tumors				

independently of cardiac and renal malformations and should be monitored and treated as in other patients with essential hypertension. Clitoral enlargement or other evidence of virilization suggests the presence of covert, translocated Y chromosomal material and is associated with increased risk of gonadoblastoma, apparently as a consequence of Y chromosomal genes distinct from *SRY*. Regular assessment of thyroid function, weight, dentition, hearing, speech, vision, and educational issues should be performed during childhood. Otitis media and middle-ear disease are prevalent in childhood (50–85%), and sensorineural hearing loss becomes progressively common with age (70–90%). Autoimmune hypothyroidism (15–30%) can occur in childhood but has a mean age of onset in the third decade. Counseling about long-term growth and fertility issues should be provided. Patient support groups are active throughout the world and can play an invaluable role.

The treatment of short stature in children with TS remains a challenge, as untreated final height rarely exceeds 150 cm in nonmosaic 45,X TS. High-dose recombinant growth hormone stimulates growth rate in children with TS and may be used alone or in combination with low doses of the nonaromatizable anabolic steroid oxandrolone (up to 0.05 mg/kg per d) in an older child (>9 years). However, final height increments are often modest (5–10 cm), and individualization of treatment response to regimens may be beneficial. Girls with evidence of gonadal failure require estrogen replacement to induce breast and uterine development, support growth, and maintain bone mineralization. Most physicians now choose to initiate low-dose estrogen therapy (one-tenth to one-eighth of the adult replacement dose) to induce puberty at an age-appropriate time (~12 years). Doses of estrogen are increased gradually to allow feminization over a 2–4 year period. Progestins are added later to regulate withdrawal bleeds, and some women with TS have achieved successful pregnancy after ovum donation and in vitro fertilization. Long-term follow-up of women with TS involves careful surveillance of sex hormone replacement and reproductive function, bone mineralization, cardiac function and aortic root dimensions, blood pressure, weight and glucose tolerance, hepatic and lipid profiles, thyroid function, and hearing. This service is provided by a dedicated TS clinic in some centers.

MIXED GONADAL DYSGENESIS (45,X/46,XY)

Mixed gonadal dysgenesis typically results from 45,X/46,XY mosaicism. The phenotype of patients with this condition varies considerably. Although some patients have a predominantly female phenotype with somatic features of TS, streak gonads, and müllerian structures, most 45,X/46,XY individuals have a male phenotype and testes, and the diagnosis is made incidentally after amniocentesis or during investigation of infertility. In practice, most children referred for assessment have ambiguous genitalia and variable somatic features. A female sex-of-rearing is often assigned (60%) if uterine structures are present, gonads are intraabdominal, and phallic development is poor. In such situations, gonadectomy usually is undertaken to prevent further androgen secretion and prevent development of gonadoblastoma (up to 25%). Individuals raised as males require reconstructive surgery for hypospadias and removal of dysgenetic gonads if the gonads cannot be brought down into the scrotum. Scrotal testes can be preserved but require regular examination for tumor development. Biopsy for carcinoma in situ is recommended in adolescence, and testosterone supplementation may be required to support androgenization in puberty. Height potential is usually attenuated.

■ OVOTESTICULAR DSD

Ovotesticular DSD (formerly called *true hermaphroditism*) occurs when both an ovary and a testis—or when an ovotestis—are found in one individual. For unclear reasons, gonadal asymmetry most often occurs with a testis on the right and an ovary on the left. Most individuals with this diagnosis have a 46,XX karyotype, especially in sub-Saharan Africa. A 46,XX/46,XY chimeric karyotype is less common and has a variable phenotype.

DISORDERS OF GONADAL AND PHENOTYPIC SEX

The clinical features of patients with disorders of gonadal and phenotypic sex are divided into the underandrogenization of 46,XY males (46,XY DSD) and the excess androgenization of 46,XX females (46,XX DSD) (Table 349-1). These disorders cover a spectrum of phenotypes ranging from "46,XY phenotypic females" or "46,XX males" to individuals with ambiguous genitalia.

■ 46,XY DSD (UNDERANDROGENIZED MALES)

Underandrogenization of the 46,XY fetus (formerly called *male pseudohermaphroditism*) reflects defects in androgen production or action. It can result from disorders of testis development, defects of androgen synthesis, or resistance to testosterone and DHT (Table 349-1).

Disorders of testis development

Testicular dysgenesis Patients with *pure* (or *complete*) *gonadal dysgenesis (Swyer syndrome)* have streak gonads, müllerian structures (due to insufficient AMH/MIS secretion), and a complete absence of androgenization. Serum AMH/MIS is low, and testosterone response to human chorionic gonadotropin (hCG) stimulation is impaired. Patients with *partial gonadal dysgenesis (dysgenetic testes)* may produce enough MIS to regress the uterus and, sometimes, sufficient testosterone for partial androgenization. Gonadal dysgenesis can result from mutations or deletions of testis-promoting genes (*WT1, SF1, SRY, SOX9, DHH, ATRX, ARX, DMRT*) or duplication of chromosomal loci containing "antitestis" genes (e.g., *WNT4/RSPO1, DAX1*) (Table 349-3). Among these, deletions or mutations of *SRY* and heterozygous mutations of *SF1 (NR5A1)* appear to be most common but still account collectively for <25% of cases. Associated clinical features may be present, reflecting additional functional roles for these genes. For example, renal dysfunction occurs in patients with specific *WT1* mutations (Denys-Drash and Fraser's syndromes), primary adrenal failure occurs in some patients with *SF1* mutations, and severe cartilage abnormalities (campomelic dysplasia) are the predominant clinical feature of *SOX9* mutations. A family history of DSD or premature ovarian insufficiency is important (e.g., *SF1/NR5A1*). Intraabdominal dysgenetic testes should be removed to prevent malignancy, and estrogens can be used to induce secondary sex characteristics in 46,XY individuals raised as females. *Absent (vanishing) testis syndrome (bilateral anorchia)* reflects regression of the testis during development. The etiology is unknown, but the absence of müllerian structures indicates adequate secretion of AMH in utero. Early testicular regression causes impaired androgenization in utero, and in most cases, androgenization of the external genitalia is either normal or slightly impaired (e.g., small penis, hypospadias). These individuals can be offered testicular prostheses and should receive androgen replacement in adolescence.

Disorders of androgen synthesis

Defects in the pathway that regulates androgen synthesis (Fig. 349-4) cause underandrogenization of the male fetus (Table 349-1). Müllerian regression is unaffected because Sertoli cell function is preserved.

LH receptor Mutations in the LH receptor (LHCGR) cause Leydig's cell hypoplasia and androgen deficiency. Defects of LH receptor synthesis or function preclude hCG stimulation of Leydig's cells in utero, as well as LH stimulation of Leydig's cells late in gestation and during the neonatal period. As a result, testosterone and DHT synthesis are insufficient for normal androgenization of the internal and external genitalia, causing a spectrum of phenotypes that range from complete underandrogenization to micropenis, depending on the severity of the mutation.

Steroidogenic enzyme pathways Mutations in *steroidogenic acute regulatory protein (StAR)* and *CYP11A1* affect both adrenal and gonadal steroidogenesis (Chap. 342). Affected individuals (46,XY) usually have severe early-onset salt-losing adrenal failure and a female phenotype, although later-onset milder variants have been reported. Defects in *3β-hydroxysteroid dehydrogenase type 2 (HSD3β2)* also cause adrenal insufficiency in severe cases, but the accumulation of dehydroepiandrosterone (DHEA) has a mild androgenizing effect, resulting in ambiguous genitalia or hypospadias. Patients with CAH due to *17α-hydroxylase (CYP17) deficiency* have variable underandrogenization and develop hypertension and hypokalemia due to the potent salt-retaining effects of corticosterone and 11-deoxycorticosterone. Patients with complete loss of 17α-hydroxylase function often present as phenotypic females who fail to enter puberty and are found to have inguinal testes and hypertension in adolescence. Some mutations in *CYP17* selectively impair 17,20 lyase activity without altering 17α-hydroxylase activity, leading to underandrogenization without mineralocorticoid excess and hypertension. Mutations in *P450 oxidoreductase (POR)* affect multiple steroidogenic enzymes, leading to impaired androgenization and a biochemical pattern of apparent combined 21-hydroxylase and 17α-hydroxylase deficiency, sometimes with skeletal abnormalities (Antley-Bixler craniosynostosis). Defects in *17β-hydroxysteroid dehydrogenase type 3 (HSD17β3)* and *5α-reductase type 2 (SRD5A2)* interfere with the synthesis of testosterone and DHT, respectively. These conditions are characterized by minimal or absent androgenization in utero, but some phallic development can occur during adolescence due to the action of other enzyme isoforms. Individuals with *5α-reductase type 2* deficiency have normal wolffian structures and usually do not develop breast tissue. At puberty, the increase in testosterone induces muscle mass and other virilizing features despite DHT deficiency. Some individuals change gender from female to male at puberty. Thus, the management of this disorder is challenging. DHT cream can improve prepubertal phallic growth in patients raised as male. Gonadectomy before adolescence and estrogen replacement at puberty can be considered in individuals raised as females.

Disorders of androgen action

Androgen insensitivity syndrome Mutations in the androgen receptor (AR) cause resistance to androgen (testosterone, DHT) action or the *androgen insensitivity syndrome (AIS)*. AIS is a spectrum of disorders that affects at least 1 in 100,000 46,XY individuals. Because the androgen receptor is X-linked, only 46,XY offspring are affected if the mother is a carrier of a mutation. XY individuals with *complete AIS* (formerly called *testicular feminization syndrome*)

TABLE 349-3 Selected Genetic Causes of Underandrogenization of Karyotypic Males (46,XY DSD)

Gene	Inheritance	Gonad	Uterus	External Genitalia	Associated Features
Disorders of Testis Development					
WT1	AD	Dysgenetic testis	+/–	Female or ambiguous	Wilms' tumor, renal abnormalities, gonadal tumors (WAGR, Denys-Drash and Fraser's syndromes)
CBX2	AD	Ovary	+	Female	
SF1	AR/AD	Dysgenetic testis/Leydig's dysfunction	+/–	Female or ambiguous	Primary adrenal failure; primary ovarian insufficiency in female (46,XX) relatives
SRY	Y	Dysgenetic testis or ovotestis	+/–	Female or ambiguous	
SOX9	AD	Dysgenetic testis or ovotestis	+/–	Female or ambiguous	Campomelic dysplasia
DHH	AR	Dysgenetic testis	+	Female	Minifascicular neuropathy
ATRX	X	Dysgenetic testis	–	Female or ambiguous	α Thalassemia, developmental delay
ARX	X	Dysgenetic testis	–	Male or ambiguous	Developmental delay; X-linked lissencephaly
MAMLD1	X	Dysgenetic testis/Leydig's dysfunction	–	Hypospadias	
DAX1	dupXp21	Dysgenetic testis	+/–	Female or ambiguous	
WNT4/ RSPO1	dup1p35	Dysgenetic testis	+	Ambiguous	
Disorders of Androgen Synthesis					
LHR	AR	Testis	–	Female, ambiguous or micropenis	Leydig's cell hypoplasia
DHCR7	AR	Testis	–	Variable	Smith-Lemli-Opitz syndrome: coarse facies, second-third toe syndactyly, failure to thrive, developmental delay, cardiac and visceral abnormalities
StAR	AR	Testis	–	Female or ambiguous	Congenital lipoid adrenal hyperplasia (primary adrenal failure)
CYP11A1	AR	Testis	–	Ambiguous	Primary adrenal failure
HSD3β2	AR	Testis	–	Ambiguous	CAH, primary adrenal failure ± salt loss, partial androgenization due to ↑ DHEA
CYP17	AR	Testis	–	Female or ambiguous	CAH, hypertension due to ↑ corticosterone and 11-deoxycorticosterone, except in isolated 17,20 lyase deficiency
POR	AR	Testis	–	Ambiguous or male	Mixed features of 21-hydroxylase deficiency and 17α-hydroxylase/17,20 lyase deficiency, sometimes associated with Antley-Bixler craniosynostosis
HSD17β3	AR	Testis	–	Female or ambiguous	Partial androgenization at puberty, ↑ androstenedione: testosterone ratio
SRD5A2	AR	Testis	–	Ambiguous or micropenis	Partial androgenization at puberty, ↑ testosterone: dihydrotestosterone ratio
Disorders of Androgen Action					
Androgen receptor	X	Testis	–	Female, ambiguous, micropenis or normal male	Phenotypic spectrum from complete androgen insensitivity syndrome (female external genitalia) and partial androgen insensitivity (ambiguous) to normal male genitalia and infertility

Abbreviations: AR, autosomal recessive; AD, autosomal dominant; CAH, congenital adrenal hyperplasia; *WT1*, Wilms' tumor–related gene 1; WAGR, Wilms' tumor, aniridia, genitourinary anomalies, and mental retardation; *SF1*, steroidogenic factor 1; *SRY*, sex-related gene on the Y chromosome; *SOX9*, *SRY*-related HMG-box gene 9; *DHH*, desert hedgehog; *ATRX*, (α-thalassemia, mental retardation on the X); *ARX*, aristaless related homeobox, X-linked; *DAX1*, dosage sensitive sex-reversal, adrenal hypoplasia congenita on the X chromosome, gene 1; *WNT4*, wingless-type mouse mammary tumor virus integration site, 4; *LHR*, LH receptor; *DHCR7*, sterol 7 δ reductase; *StAR*, steroidogenic acute regulatory protein; *CYP11A1*, P450 cholesterol side-chain cleavage; *HSD3β2*, 3β-hydroxysteroid dehydrogenase type 2; *CYP17*, 17α-hydroxylase and 17,20-lyase; *POR*, P450 oxidoreductase; *HSD17β3*, 17β-hydroxysteroid dehydrogenase type 3; *SRD5A2*, 5α-reductase type 2.

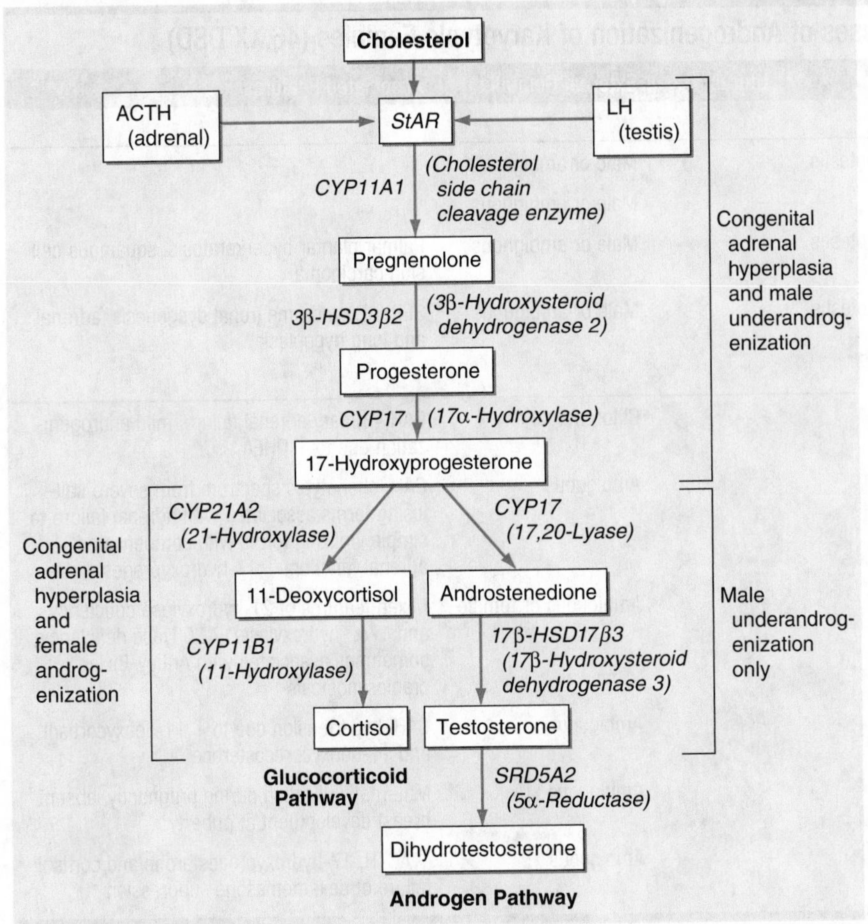

Figure 349-4 Simplified overview of glucocorticoid and androgen synthesis pathways. Defects in *CYP21A2* and *CYP11B1* shunt steroid precursors into the androgen pathway and cause androgenization of 46,XX females. Testosterone is synthesized in the testicular Leydig's cells and converted to dihydrotestosterone peripherally. Defects in enzymes involved in androgen synthesis result in underandrogenization of 46,XY males. *StAR*, steroidogenic acute regulatory protein. *[After E Braunwald et al (eds): Harrison's Principles of Internal Medicine, 15th ed. New York, McGraw-Hill, 2001.]*

have a female phenotype, normal breast development (due to aromatization of testosterone), a short vagina but no uterus (because MIS production is normal), scanty pubic and axillary hair, and a female psychosexual orientation. Gonadotropins and testosterone levels can be low, normal, or elevated, depending on the degree of androgen resistance and the contribution of estradiol to feedback inhibition of the hypothalamic-pituitary-gonadal axis. AMH/MIS levels in childhood are normal or high. Most patients present with inguinal hernias (containing testes) in childhood or with primary amenorrhea in adulthood. Gonadectomy sometimes is performed, as there is a low risk of malignancy, and estrogen replacement is prescribed. Alternatively, the gonads can be left in situ until breast development is complete. The use of graded dilators in adolescence is usually sufficient to dilate the vagina and permit sexual intercourse.

Partial AIS (Reifenstein's syndrome) results from less severe AR mutations. Patients often present in infancy with perineoscrotal hypospadias and small undescended testes and with gynecomastia at the time of puberty. Those individuals raised as males require hypospadias repair in childhood and breast reduction in adolescence. Supplemental testosterone rarely enhances androgenization significantly, as endogenous testosterone is already increased. More severely underandrogenized patients present with clitoral enlargement and labial fusion and may be raised as females. The surgical and psychosexual management of these patients is complex and requires active involvement of the parents and the patient during the appropriate stages of development. *Azoospermia* and male-factor infertility also have been described in association with mild loss-of-function mutations in the androgen receptor.

OTHER DISORDERS AFFECTING 46,XY MALES

Persistent müllerian duct syndrome is the presence of a uterus in an otherwise normal male. This condition can result from mutations in AMH or its receptor (AMHR2). The uterus may be removed, but damage to the vasa deferentia must be avoided. *Isolated hypospadias* occurs in ~1 in 200 males and is treated by surgical repair. Most cases are idiopathic, although evidence of penoscrotal hypospadias, poor phallic development, and/or bilateral cryptorchidism require investigation for an underlying disorder of sex development (e.g., partial gonadal dysgenesis, mild defect in testosterone action, or even severe forms of 46,XX CAH). Unilateral undescended testes (cryptorchidism) affects more than 3% of boys at birth. Orchidopexy should be considered if the testis has not descended by 6 to 9 months of age. Bilateral cryptorchidism occurs less frequently and should raise suspicion of gonadotropin deficiency or DSD. A small subset of patients with cryptorchidism may have mutations in the insulin-like 3 (*INSL3*) gene or its receptor LGR8 (also known as *GREAT*), which mediates normal testicular descent. Ascending testis is being recognized increasingly as a distinct condition for which management is currently unclear. *Syndromic associations* and *intrauterine growth retardation* also occur relatively frequently in association with impaired testicular function or target tissue responsiveness, but the underlying etiology of many of these conditions is unknown.

46,XX DSD (ANDROGENIZED FEMALES)

Inappropriate androgenization of females (formerly called *female pseudohermaphroditism*) occurs when the gonad (ovary) contains androgen-secreting testicular material or after increased androgen exposure, which is usually adrenal in origin (Table 349-1).

46,XX testicular/ovotesticular DSD

Testicular tissue can develop in 46,XX testicular DSD (46,XX males) after translocation of *SRY* or duplication of *SOX9* or defects in *RSPO1* (Table 349-4).

Increased androgen exposure

21-Hydroxylase deficiency (congenital adrenal hyperplasia) The *classic form* of 21-hydroxylase deficiency (21-OHD) is the most common cause of CAH (Chap. 342). It has an incidence between 1 in 10,000 and 1 in 15,000 and is the most common cause of androgenization in chromosomal 46,XX females (Table 349-4). Affected individuals are homozygous or compound heterozygous for severe mutations in the enzyme 21-hydroxylase (*CYP21A2*). This mutation causes a block in adrenal glucocorticoid and mineralocorticoid synthesis, increasing 17-hydroxyprogesterone and shunting steroid

TABLE 349-4 Selected Genetic Causes of Androgenization of Karyotypic Females (46,XX DSD)

Gene	Inheritance	Gonad	Uterus	External Genitalia	Associated Features
Testicular/Ovotesticular DSD					
SRY	Translocation	Testis or ovotestis	–	Male or ambiguous	
SOX9	dup17q24	Unknown	–	Male or ambiguous	
RSPO1	AR	Testis or ovotestis	±	Male or ambiguous	Palmar plantar hyperkeratosis, squamous cell skin carcinoma
WNT4	AR	Testis or ovotestis	–	Male or ambiguous	SERKAL syndrome (renal dysgenesis, adrenal and lung hypoplasia)
Increased Androgen Synthesis					
HSD3β2	AR	Ovary	+	Clitoromegaly	CAH, primary adrenal failure, mild androgenization due to ↑ DHEA
CYP21A2	AR	Ovary	+	Ambiguous	CAH, phenotypic spectrum from severe salt-losing forms associated with adrenal failure to simple virilizing forms with compensated adrenal function, ↑ 17-hydroxyprogesterone
POR	AR	Ovary	+	Ambiguous or female	Mixed features of 21-hydroxylase deficiency and 17α -hydroxylase/17,20 lyase deficiency, sometimes associated with Antley-Bixler craniosynostosis
CYP11B1	AR	Ovary	+	Ambiguous	CAH, hypertension due to ↑ 11-deoxycortisol and 11-deoxycorticosterone
CYP19	AR	Ovary	+	Ambiguous	Maternal virilization during pregnancy, absent breast development at puberty
Glucocorticoid receptor	AR	Ovary	+	Ambiguous	↑ ACTH, 17-hydroxyprogesterone and cortisol; failure of dexamethasone suppression

Abbreviations: DSD, disorders of sex development; AR, autosomal recessive; *SRY*, sex-related gene on the Y chromosome; *SOX9*, *SRY*-related HMG-box gene 9; CAH, congenital adrenal hyperplasia; *HSD3β2*, 3β-hydroxysteroid dehydrogenase type 2; *CYP21A2*, 21-hydroxylase; POR, P450 oxidoreductase; *CYP11B1*, 11β-hydroxylase; *CYP19*, aromatase; ACTH, adrenocorticotropin; *RSPO1*, R-spondin 1.

precursors into the androgen synthesis pathway (Fig. 349-4). Glucocorticoid insufficiency causes a compensatory elevation of adrenocorticotropin (ACTH), resulting in adrenal hyperplasia and additional synthesis of steroid precursors proximal to the enzymatic block. Increased androgen synthesis in utero causes androgenization of the female fetus in the first trimester. Ambiguous genitalia are seen at birth, with varying degrees of clitoral enlargement and labial fusion. Excess androgen production causes gonadotropin-independent precocious puberty in males with 21-OHD.

The *salt-wasting* form of 21-OHD results from severe combined glucocorticoid and mineralocorticoid deficiency. A salt-wasting crisis usually manifests between 7 and 21 days of life and is a potentially life-threatening event that requires urgent fluid resuscitation and steroid treatment. Thus, a diagnosis of 21-OHD should be considered in any baby with ambiguous genitalia with bilateral nonpalpable gonads. Males (46,XY) with 21-OHD have no genital abnormalities at birth but are equally susceptible to adrenal insufficiency and salt-losing crises.

Females with the *classic simple virilizing* form of 21-OHD also present with genital ambiguity. They have impaired cortisol biosynthesis but do not develop salt loss. Patients with *nonclassic 21-OHD* produce normal amounts of cortisol and aldosterone, but at the expense of producing excess androgens. Hirsutism (60%), oligomenorrhea (50%), and acne (30%) are the most common presenting features. This is one of the most common recessive disorders in humans, with an incidence as high as 1 in 100 to 500 in many populations and 1 in 27 in Ashkenazi Jews of Eastern European origin.

Biochemical features of acute salt-wasting 21-OHD are hyponatremia, hyperkalemia, hypoglycemia, low cortisol and aldosterone, and elevated 17-hydroxyprogesterone, ACTH, and plasma renin activity. Presymptomatic diagnosis of classic 21-OHD is now made by neonatal screening tests for increased 17-hydroxyprogesterone in many centers. In most cases, 17-hydroxyprogesterone is markedly increased. In adults, ACTH stimulation (0.25 mg cosyntropin IV) with assays for 17-hydroxyprogesterone at 0 and 30 min can be useful for detecting nonclassic 21-OHD and heterozygotes (Chap. 342).

TREATMENT Congenital Adrenal Hyperplasia

Acute salt-wasting crises require fluid resuscitation, IV hydrocortisone, and correction of hypoglycemia. Once the patient is stabilized, glucocorticoids must be given to correct the cortisol insufficiency and suppress ACTH stimulation, thereby preventing further virilization, rapid skeletal maturation, and the development of polycystic ovaries. Typically, hydrocortisone (10–15 mg/m^2 per day in three divided doses) is used in childhood with a goal of partially suppressing 17-hydroxyprogesterone (100–<1000 ng/dL). The aim of treatment is to use the lowest glucocorticoid dose that adequately suppresses adrenal androgen production without causing signs of glucocorticoid excess such as impaired growth and obesity. Salt-wasting conditions are treated with mineralocorticoid replacement. Infants usually need salt supplements up to the first year of life. Plasma renin activity and electrolytes are used to monitor mineralocorticoid replacement. Some patients with simple virilizing 21-OHD also benefit from mineralocorticoid supplements. Newer therapeutic approaches such as antiandrogens and aromatase inhibitors (to block premature epiphyseal closure) are under evaluation. Parents and patients should be aware of the need for increased doses of steroids during sickness, and patients should carry medic alert systems.

Older adolescents and adults often are treated with prednisolone or with dexamethasone at night to provide more complete ACTH suppression. Steroid doses should be adjusted to individual requirements as overtreatment results in weight gain and hypertension and can affect bone turnover. Androstenedione and testosterone may be useful measurements of long-term control, with less fluctuation than 17-hydroxyprogesterone. Mineralocorticoid requirements often decrease in adulthood, and doses should be reduced to avoid hypertension. In very severe cases, adrenalectomy has been advocated but incurs the risks of surgery and total adrenal insufficiency.

Girls with significant genital androgenization due to classic 21-OHD usually undergo vaginal reconstruction and clitoral reduction (maintaining the glans and nerve supply), but the optimal timing of these procedures is debated, as is the need for the individual to be able to consent. There is a higher threshold for undertaking clitoral surgery in some centers as long-term sensation and ability to achieve orgasm can be affected, but the long-term results of newer techniques are not yet known. If surgery is performed in infancy, surgical revision or regular vaginal dilatation may be needed in adolescence or adulthood, and long-term psychological support and psychosexual counseling may be appropriate. Women with 21-OHD frequently develop polycystic ovaries and have reduced fertility, especially when control is poor. Fecundity is achieved in up to 90% of women, but ovulation induction (or even adrenalectomy) is frequently required. Dexamethasone should be avoided in pregnancy. Men with poorly controlled 21-OHD may develop testicular adrenal rests and are at risk for reduced fertility. Prenatal treatment of 21-OHD by the administration of dexamethasone to mothers is still under evaluation. However, treatment of the mother and child must be started ideally before 6 to 7 weeks; long-term effects of prenatal dexamethasone exposure on fetal development are still under evaluation.

The treatment of other forms of CAH includes mineralocorticoid and glucocorticoid replacement for salt-losing conditions (e.g., *StAR, CYP11A1, HSD3β2*), suppression of ACTH drive with glucocorticoids in disorders associated with hypertension (e.g., *CYP17, CYP11B1*), and appropriate sex-hormone replacement in adolescence and adulthood, when necessary.

Other causes Increased androgen synthesis can also occur in CAH due to defects in *POR, 11β-hydroxylase (CYP11B1),* and *3β-hydroxysteroid dehydrogenase type 2 (HSD3β2)* and with mutations in the genes encoding *aromatase (CYP19)* and the glucocorticoid receptor. Increased androgen exposure in utero can occur with maternal virilizing tumors and with ingestion of androgenic compounds.

OTHER DISORDERS AFFECTING 46,XX FEMALES

Congenital absence of the vagina occurs in association with *müllerian agenesis* or *hypoplasia* as part of the Mayer-Rokitansky-Kuster-Hauser (MRKH) syndrome (rarely caused by *WNT4* mutations). This diagnosis should be considered in otherwise phenotypically normal females with primary amenorrhea. Associated features include renal (agenesis) and cervical spinal abnormalities.

GLOBAL CONSIDERATIONS

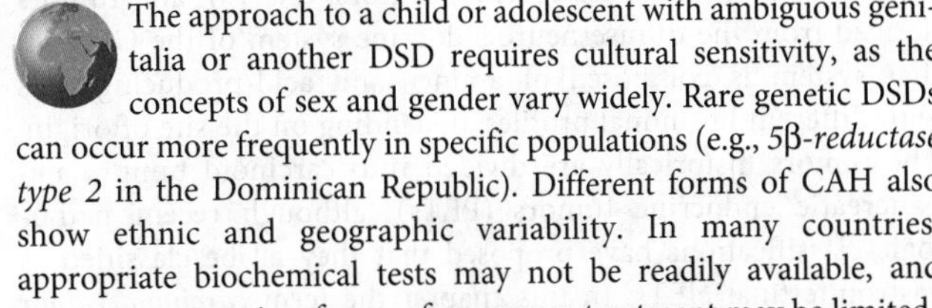

The approach to a child or adolescent with ambiguous genitalia or another DSD requires cultural sensitivity, as the concepts of sex and gender vary widely. Rare genetic DSDs can occur more frequently in specific populations (e.g., *5β-reductase type 2* in the Dominican Republic). Different forms of CAH also show ethnic and geographic variability. In many countries, appropriate biochemical tests may not be readily available, and access to appropriate forms of surgery or treatment may be limited.

FURTHER READINGS

Bojesen A, Gravholt CH: Klinefelter syndrome in clinical practice. Nat Clin Pract Urol 4:192, 2007

Bondy CA for the Turner Syndrome Study Group: Care of girls and women with Turner syndrome: A guideline of the Turner Syndrome Study Group. J Clin Endocrinol Metab 92:10, 2007

Brain CE et al: Holistic management of DSD. Best Pract Res Clin Endocrinol Metab 24:335, 2010

Cools M et al: Germ cell tumors in the intersex gonad: Old paths, new directions, moving frontiers. Endocrinol Rev 27:468, 2006

Lee PA et al: Consensus statement of management of intersex disorders. Pediatrics 118:e488, 2006

Mendonca BB et al: 46,XY disorders of sex development (DSD). Clin Endocrinol 70:173, 2009

Speiser PW et al: Congenital adrenal hyperplasia due to steroid 21-hydroxylase deficiency: An Endocrine Society clinical practice guideline. J Clin Endocrinol Metab 95:4133, 2010

Wilhelm D et al: Sex determination and gonadal development in mammals. Physiol Rev 87:1, 2007

CHAPTER 350

Endocrine Tumors of the Gastrointestinal Tract and Pancreas

Robert T. Jensen

GENERAL FEATURES OF GASTROINTESTINAL (GI) NEUROENDOCRINE TUMORS

Gastrointestinal neuroendocrine tumors (NETs) are tumors derived from the diffuse neuroendocrine system of the GI tract; that system is composed of amine- and acid-producing cells with different hormonal profiles, depending on the site of origin. The tumors historically are divided into carcinoid tumors and pancreatic endocrine tumors (PETs), although recent pathologic classifications have proposed that they all be classified as gastrointestinal NETs. In this chapter the term *carcinoid tumor* is retained because it is widely used. These tumors originally were classified as APUDomas (for *a*mine *p*recursor *u*ptake and *d*ecarboxylation), as were pheochromocytomas, melanomas, and medullary thyroid carcinomas, because they share certain cytochemical features as well as various pathologic, biologic, and molecular features (Table 350-1). It was originally proposed that APUDomas had a similar embryonic origin from neural crest cells, but it is now known the peptide-secreting cells are not of neuroectodermal origin. Nevertheless, the concept of APUDomas is useful because the tumors from the cells have important similarities as well as some differences (Table 350-1). In this section, the areas of similarity between PETs and carcinoids will be discussed together and areas in which there are important differences will be discussed separately.

CLASSIFICATION/PATHOLOGY/TUMOR BIOLOGY OF NETs

NETs generally are composed of monotonous sheets of small round cells with uniform nuclei, and mitoses are uncommon. They can be identified tentatively on routine histology; however, these tumors are now recognized principally by their histologic staining patterns due to shared cellular proteins. Historically, silver staining was used, and tumors were classified as showing an argentaffin reaction if they took up and reduced silver or as being argyrophilic if they did not reduce it. More recently immunocytochemical localization of chromogranins (A, B, C), neuron-specific enolase, and synaptophysin, which are all neuroendocrine cell markers, is used (Table 350-1). Chromogranin A is currently the most widely used.

Ultrastructurally, these tumors possess electron-dense neurosecretory granules and frequently contain small clear vesicles that correspond to synaptic vesicles of neurons. NETs synthesize numerous peptides, growth factors, and bioactive amines that may be ectopically secreted, giving rise to a specific clinical syndrome (Table 350-2). The diagnosis of the specific syndrome requires the clinical features of the disease (Table 350-2) and cannot be made

TABLE 350-1 General Characteristics of Gastrointestinal Neuroendocrine Tumors [Carcinoids, Pancreatic Endocrine Tumors (PETs)]

A. Share general neuroendocrine cell markers (identification used for diagnosis)
  1. Chromogranins (A, B, C) are acidic monomeric soluble proteins found in the large secretory granules. Chromogranin A is the most widely used.
  2. Neuron-specific enolase (NSE) is the γ-γ dimer of the enzyme enolase and is a cytosolic marker of neuroendocrine differentiation.
  3. Synaptophysin is an integral membrane glycoprotein of 38,000 molecular weight found in small vesicles of neurons and neuroendocrine tumors.

B. Pathologic similarities
  1. All are APUDomas showing *a*mine *p*recursor *u*ptake and *d*ecarboxylation.
  2. Ultrastructurally they have dense-core secretory granules (>80 nm).
  3. Histologically, generally appear similar with few mitoses and uniform nuclei.
  4. Frequently synthesize multiple peptides/amines, which can be detected immunocytochemically but may not be secreted.
  5. Presence or absence of clinical syndrome or type cannot be predicted by immunocytochemical studies.
  6. Histologic classifications increasingly predictive of biologic behavior. Only invasion or metastases establish malignancy

C. Similarities of biologic behavior
  1. Generally slow growing, but a proportion are aggressive.
  2. Secrete biologically active peptides/amines, which can cause clinical symptoms.
  3. Generally have high densities of somatostatin receptors, which are used for both localization and treatment.

D. Similarities/differences in molecular abnormalities
  1. Similarities
     a. Uncommon—alterations in common oncogenes (*ras, jun, fos*, etc).
     b. Uncommon—alterations in common tumor-suppressor genes (p53, retinoblastoma).
     c. Alterations at MEN 1 locus (11q13) and p16^{INK4a} (9p21) occur in a proportion (10–45%).
     d. Methylation of various genes occurs in 40–87% (*ras*-associated domain family I, p14, p16, O^6 methyl guanosine methyltransferases, retinoic acid receptor β)
  2. Differences
     a. PETs—loss of 1p (21%), 3p (8–47%), 3q (8–41%), 11q (21–62%), 6q (18–68%). Gains at 17q (10–55%), 7q (16–68%), 4q (33%).
     b. Carcinoids—loss of 18q (38–67%) >18p (33–43%) > 9p, 16q21(21–23%). Gains at 17q, 19p (57%), 4q (33%), 14q (20%).

Abbreviation: MEN 1, multiple endocrine neoplasia type 1.

TABLE 350-2 Gastrointestinal Neuroendocrine Tumor Syndrome

Name	Biologically Active Peptide(s) Secreted	Incidence (New Cases/10^6 Population/Year)	Tumor Location	Malignant, %	Associated with MEN 1, %	Main Symptoms/Signs
I. Established Specific Functional Syndrome						
A. Carcinoid tumor						
Carcinoid syndrome	Serotonin, possibly tachykinins, motilin, prostaglandins	0.5–2	Midgut (75–87%) Foregut (2–33%) Hindgut (1–8%) Unknown (2–15%)	95–100	Rare	Diarrhea (32–84%) Flushing (63–75%) Pain (10–34%) Asthma (4–18%) Heart disease (11–41%)
B. Pancreatic endocrine tumor						
Zollinger-Ellison syndrome	Gastrin	0.5–1.5	Duodenum (70%) Pancreas (25%) Other sites (5%)	60–90	20–25	Pain (79–100%) Diarrhea (30–75%) Esophageal symptoms (31–56%)
Insulinoma	Insulin	1–2	Pancreas (>99%)	<10	4–5	Hypoglycemic symptoms (100%)
VIPoma (Verner-Morrison syndrome, pancreatic cholera, WDHA)	Vasoactive intestinal peptide	0.05–0.2	Pancreas (90%, adult) Other (10%, neural,adrenal, periganglionic)	40–70	6	Diarrhea (90–100%) Hypokalemia (80–100%) Dehydration (83%)
Glucagonoma	Glucagon	0.01–0.1	Pancreas (100%)	50–80	1–20	Rash (67–90%) Glucose intolerance (38–87%) Weight loss (66–96%)
Somatostatinoma	Somatostatin	Rare	Pancreas (55%) Duodenum/jejunum (44%)	>70	45	Diabetes mellitus (63–90%) Cholelithiases (65–90%) Diarrhea (35–90%)
GRFoma	Growth hormone–releasing hormone	Unknown	Pancreas (30%) Lung (54%) Jejunum (7%) Other (13%)	>60	16	Acromegaly (100%)
ACTHoma	ACTH	Rare	Pancreas (4–16% all ectopic Cushing's)	>95	Rare	Cushing's syndrome (100%)
PET causing carcinoid syndrome	Serotonin, ?tachykinins	Rare (43 cases)	Pancreas (<1% all carcinoids)	60–88	Rare	Same as carcinoid syndrome above
PET causing hypercalcemia	PTHrP Others unknown	Rare	Pancreas (rare cause of hypercalcemia)	84	Rare	Abdominal pain due to hepatic metastases
II. Possible Specific Functional Syndrome						
PET secreting calcitonin	Calcitonin	Rare	Pancreas (rare cause of hypercalcitonemia)	>80	16	Diarrhea (50%)
PET secreting renin	Renin	Rare	Pancreas	Unknown	No	Hypertension
PET secreting luteinizing hormone	Luteinizing hormone	Rare	Pancreas	Unknown	No	Anovulation, virilization (female); reduced libido (male)
PET secreting erythropoietin	Erythropoietin	Rare	Pancreas	100	No	Polycythemia
PET secreting IF-II	Insulin-like growth factor II	Rare	Pancreas	Unknown	No	Hypoglycemia
III. No Functional Syndrome						
PPoma/nonfunctional	None	1–2	Pancreas (100%)	>60	18–44	Weight loss (30–90%) Abdominal mass (10–30%) Pain (30–95%)

Abbreviations: ACTH, adrenocorticotropic hormone; GRFoma, growth hormone-releasing factor secreting pancreatic endocrine tumor; IF-II, insulin-like growth factor 2; MEN, multiple endocrine neoplasia; PET, pancreatic endocrine tumor; PPoma, tumor secreting pancreatic polypeptide; PTHrP, parathyroid hormone–related peptide; VIPoma, tumor secreting vasoactive intestinal peptide; WDHA, *w*atery *d*iarrhea, *h*ypokalemia, and *a*chlorhydria syndrome.

from the immunocytochemistry results alone. The presence or absence of a specific clinical syndrome also cannot be predicted from the immunocytochemistry alone (Table 350-1). Furthermore, pathologists cannot distinguish between benign and malignant NETs unless metastases or invasion is present.

Carcinoid tumors frequently are classified according to their anatomic area of origin (i.e., foregut, midgut, hindgut) because tumors with similar areas of origin share functional manifestations, histochemistry, and secretory products (Table 350-3). Foregut tumors generally have a low serotonin (5-HT) content; are argentaffin-negative but argyrophilic; occasionally secrete adrenocorticotropic hormone (ACTH) or 5-hydroxytryptophan (5-HTP), causing an atypical carcinoid syndrome (Fig. 350-1); are often multihormonal; and may metastasize to bone. They uncommonly produce a clinical syndrome due to the secreted products. Midgut carcinoids are argentaffin-positive, have a high serotonin content, most frequently cause the typical carcinoid syndrome when they metastasize (Table 350-3, Fig. 350-1), release serotonin and tachykinins (substance P, neuropeptide K, substance K), rarely secrete 5-HTP or ACTH, and less commonly metastasize to bone. Hindgut carcinoids (rectum, transverse and descending colon) are argentaffin-negative, are often argyrophilic, rarely contain serotonin or cause the carcinoid syndrome (Fig. 350-1, Table 350-3), rarely secrete 5-HTP or ACTH, contain numerous peptides, and may metastasize to bone.

Pancreatic endocrine tumors can be classified into nine well-established specific functional syndromes (Table 350-2), five possible specific functional syndromes (PETs secreting calcitonin, renin, luteinizing hormone, erythropoietin, or insulin-like growth factor II) (Table 350-2), and nonfunctional PETs (pancreatic polypeptide-secreting tumors; PPomas). Other functional hormonal syndromes due to nonpancreatic tumors (usually intraabdominal in location) have been described only rarely and are not included in Table 350-2. They include secretion of glucagon-like peptide-2 (GLP-2) that causes intestinal villus hypertrophy (enteroglucagonomas), secretion of GLP-1 that causes hypoglycemia and delayed transit, and intestinal and ovarian tumors secreting peptide tyrosine tyrosine (PYY) that result in altered motility and constipation. Each of the functional syndromes listed in Table 350-2 is associated with symptoms due to the specific hormone released. In contrast, nonfunctional PETs release no products that cause a specific clinical syndrome. "Nonfunctional" is a misnomer in the strict sense because those tumors frequently ectopically secrete a number of peptides [pancreatic polypeptide (PP), chromogranin A, ghrelin, neurotensin, α subunits of human chorionic gonadotropin, neuron-specific enolase]; however, they cause no specific clinical syndrome. The symptoms caused by nonfunctional PETs are entirely due to the tumor per se.

Carcinoid tumors can occur in almost any GI tissue (Table 350-3); however, at present most (70%) have their origin in one of three sites: bronchus, jejunoileum, or colon/rectum. In the past, carcinoid tumors most frequently were reported in the appendix (i.e., 40%); however, the bronchus/lung, rectum, and small intestine are now the most common sites. Overall, the GI tract is the most common site for these tumors, accounting for 64%, with the respiratory tract a distant second at 28%. Both race and sex can

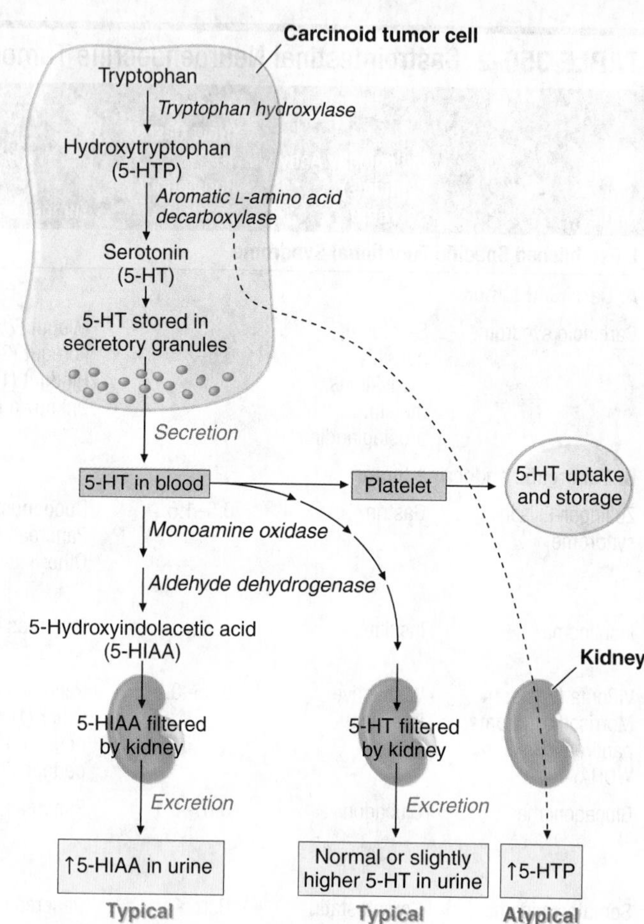

Figure 350-1 Synthesis, secretion, and metabolism of serotonin (5-HT) in patients with typical and atypical carcinoid syndromes. 5-HIAA, 5-hydroxyindolacetic acid.

TABLE 350-3 Carcinoid Tumor Location, Frequency of Metastases, and Association With the Carcinoid Syndrome

	Location (% of Total)	Incidence of Metastases	Incidence of Carcinoid Syndrome
Foregut			
Esophagus	<0.1	—	—
Stomach	4.6	10	9.5
Duodenum	2.0	—	3.4
Pancreas	0.7	71.9	20
Gallbladder	0.3	17.8	5
Bronchus, lung, trachea	27.9	5.7	13
Midgut			
Jejunum	1.8	{58.4	9
Ileum	14.9		9
Meckel's diverticulum	0.5	—	13
Appendix	4.8	38.8	<1
Colon	8.6	51	5
Liver	0.4	32.	—
Ovary	1.0	2 32	50
Testis	<0.1	—	50
Hindgut			
Rectum	13.6	3.9	—

Source: Location is from the PAN-SEER data (1973–1999), and incidence of metastases from the SEER data (1992–1999), reported by IM Modlin et al: Cancer 97:934, 2003. Incidence of carcinoid syndrome is from 4349 cases studied from 1950–1971, reported by JD Godwin: Cancer 36:560, 1975.

affect the frequency as well as the distribution of carcinoid tumors. African Americans have a high incidence of carcinoids, and rectal carcinoids are the most common. Females have a lower incidence of small-intestinal and pancreatic carcinoids.

The term *pancreatic endocrine tumor*, although widely used and therefore retained here, is also a misnomer, strictly speaking, because these tumors can occur either almost entirely in the pancreas (insulinomas, glucagonomas, nonfunctional PETs, PETs causing hypercalcemia) or at both pancreatic and extrapancreatic sites [gastrinomas, VIPomas (vasoactive intestinal peptide), somatostatinomas, GRFomas (growth hormone–releasing factor)]. PETs are also called islet cell tumors; however, the use of this term is discouraged because it is not established that they originate from the islets and many can occur at extrapancreatic sites.

A number of new classification systems have been proposed for both carcinoids and PETs. In the World Health Organization (WHO) classification it has been proposed that these tumors all be classified as GI neuroendocrine tumors (including carcinoids and PETs), which divides them into three general categories: (1a) well-differentiated NETs, (1b) well-differentiated neuroendocrine carcinomas that have low-grade malignancy, and (2) poorly differentiated neuroendocrine carcinomas that are usually small cell neuroendocrine carcinomas of high-grade malignancy. The term *carcinoid* is synonymous with *well-differentiated NETs* (1a). This classification is further divided on the basis of tumor location and biology. In addition, for the first time a standard TNM (tumor, node, metastasis) classification and grading system has been proposed for GI neuroendocrine tumors. The new WHO classification and the TNM classification and grading system were proposed to facilitate the comparison and evaluation of clinical, pathologic, and prognostic features and results of treatment in GI NETs from different studies. These classification systems may provide important prognostic information that can guide treatment (Table 350-4).

The exact incidence of carcinoid tumors or PETs varies according to whether only symptomatic tumors or all tumors are considered. The incidence of clinically significant carcinoids is

TABLE 350-4 Prognostic Factors in Neuroendocrine Tumors

I. Both carcinoid tumors and PETs	II. Carcinoid tumors
Presence of liver metastases ($p < .001$)	Presence of carcinoid syndrome
Extent of liver metastases ($p < .001$)	Laboratory results [urinary 5-HIAA levels ($p < .01$), plasma neuropeptide K ($p < .05$), serum chromogranin A ($p < .01$)]
Presence of lymph node metastases ($p < .001$)	Presence of a second malignancy
Depth of invasion ($p < .001$)	Male sex ($p < .001$)
Rapid rate of tumor growth	Mode of discovery (incidental > symptomatic)
Elevated serum alkaline phosphatase levels ($p = .003$)	Molecular findings [TGF-α expression ($p < .05$), chr 16q LOH or gain chr 4p ($p < .05$)]
Primary tumor site ($p < .001$)	WHO, TNM, and grading classification
Primary tumor size ($p < .005$)	Molecular findings [gain in chr 14, loss of 3p13 (ileal carcinoid), upregulation of Hoxc6]
Various histologic features	**III. PETs**
Tumor differentiation ($p < .001$)	Ha-*ras* oncogene or p53 overexpression
High growth indices (high $K_{i\text{-}67}$ index, PCNA expression)	Female gender
High mitotic counts ($p < .001$)	MEN 1 syndrome absent
Necrosis present	Presence of nonfunctional tumor (some studies, not all)
Presence of cytokeratin 19 ($p < .02$)	WHO, TNM, and grading classification
Vascular or perineural invasion	Laboratory findings (increased chromogranin A in some studies; gastrinomas—increased gastrin level)
Vessel density (low microvessel density, increased lymphatic density)	Molecular findings [increased HER2/*neu* expression ($p = .032$), chr 1q, 3p, 3q, or 6q LOH ($p = .0004$), EGF receptor overexpression ($p = .034$), gains in chr 7q, 17q, 17p, 20q; alterations in the VHL gene (deletion, methylation)]
High CD10 metalloproteinase expression (in series with all grades of NETs)	
Flow cytometric features (i.e., aneuploidy)	
High VEGF expression (in low-grade or well-differentiated NETs only)	
WHO, TNM, and grading classification	
Presence of a pancreatic NET rather than GI NET associated with poorer prognosis ($p = .0001$)	
Older age ($p < .01$)	

Abbreviations: 5-HIAA, 5-hydroxyindoleacetic acid; chr, chromosome; EGF, epidermal growth factor; Ki-67, proliferation-associated nuclear antigen recognized by Ki-67 monoclonal antibody; LOH, loss of heterozygosity; MEN, multiple endocrine neoplasia; NET, neuroendocrine tumors; PCNA, proliferating cell nuclear antigen; PET, pancreatic endocrine tumor; TGF-α, transforming growth factor α; TNM, tumor, node, metastasis; VEGF, vascular endothelial growth factor; WHO, World Health Organization.

7-13 cases/million population per year, whereas any malignant carcinoids at autopsy are reported in 21–84 cases/million population per year. The incidence of GI NETs is approximately 25–50 cases per million in the United States, which makes them less common than adenocarcinomas of the GI tract. However, their incidence has increased sixfold in the last 30 years. Clinically significant PETs have a prevalence of 10 cases/million population, with insulinomas, gastrinomas, and nonfunctional PETs having an incidence of 0.5–2 cases/million population per year (Table 350-2). VIPomas are two to eight times less common, glucagonomas are 17 to 30 times less common, and somatostatinomas are the least common. In autopsy studies 0.5–1.5% of all cases have a PET; however, in less than 1 in 1000 cases was a functional tumor thought to occur.

Both carcinoid tumors and PETs commonly show malignant behavior (Tables 350-2 and 350-3). With PETs, except for insulinomas in which <10% are malignant, 50–100% in different series are malignant. With carcinoid tumors the percentage showing malignant behavior varies in different locations. For the three most common sites of occurrence, the incidence of metastases varies greatly from jejunoileum (58%) > lung/bronchus (6%) > rectum (4%) (Table 350-3). With both carcinoid tumors and PETs, a number of factors, summarized in Table 350-4, are important prognostic factors in determining survival and the aggressiveness of the tumor. Patients with PETs (excluding insulinomas) generally have a poorer prognosis than do patients with GI NETs (carcinoids). The presence of liver metastases is the single most important prognostic factor in single and multivariate analyses for both carcinoid tumors and PETs. Particularly important in the development of liver metastases is the size of the primary tumor. For example, with small-intestinal carcinoids, which are the most common cause of the carcinoid syndrome due to metastatic disease in the liver (Table 350-2), metastases occur in 15–25% if the tumor diameter is <1 cm, 58–80% if it is 1–2 cm in diameter, and >75% if it is >2 cm in diameter. Similar data exist for gastrinomas and other PETs in which the size of the primary tumor is an independent predictor of the development of liver metastases. The presence of lymph node metastases; the depth of invasion; the rapid rate of growth; various histologic features [differentiation, mitotic rates, growth indices, vessel density, vascular endothelial growth factor (VEGF), and CD10 metalloproteinase expression]; necrosis; presence of cytokeratin; elevated serum alkaline phosphatase levels; older age; advanced stages in WHO, TNM, or grading classification systems; and flow cytometric results such as the presence of aneuploidy are all important prognostic factors for the development of metastatic disease (Table 350-4). For patients with carcinoid tumors, additional associations with a worse prognosis include the development of the carcinoid syndrome (especially the development of carcinoid heart disease), male sex, the presence of a symptomatic tumor or greater increases in a number of tumor markers [5-hydroxyindolacetic acid (5-HIAA), neuropeptide K, chromogranin A], and the presence of various molecular features. With PETs or gastrinomas, which have been the best studied PET long-term, a worse prognosis is associated with female sex, overexpression of the Ha-*ras* oncogene or p53, the absence of multiple endocrine neoplasia type 1 (MEN 1), higher levels of various tumor markers (i.e., chromogranin A, gastrin), and various molecular features (Table 350-4).

TABLE 350-5 Genetic Syndromes Associated With an Increased Incidence of Neuroendocrine Tumors (NETs) [Carcinoids or Pancreatic Endocrine Tumors (PETs)]

Syndrome	Location of Gene Mutation and Gene Product	NETs Seen/Frequency
Multiple endocrine neoplasia type 1 (MEN 1)	11q13 (encodes 610-amino-acid protein, menin)	80–100% develop PETs (microscopic), 20–80% (clinical): (nonfunctional > gastrinoma > insulinoma) Carcinoids: gastric (13–30%), bronchial/thymic (8%)
von Hippel–Lindau disease	3q25 (encodes 213-amino-acid protein)	12–17% develop PETs (almost always nonfunctional)
von Recklinghausen's disease [neurofibromatosis 1 (NF-1)]	17q11.2 (encodes 2485-amino-acid protein, neurofibromin)	0–10% develop PETs, primarily duodenal somatostatinomas (usually nonfunctional) Rarely insulinoma, gastrinoma
Tuberous sclerosis	9q34 (TSCI) encodes 1164-amino-acid protein, hamartin) 16p13 (TSC2) (encodes 1807-amino-acid protein, tuberin)	Uncommonly develop PETs [nonfunctional and functional (insulinoma, gastrinoma)]

A number of diseases due to various genetic disorders are associated with an increased incidence of neuroendocrine tumors (Table 350-5). Each one is caused by a loss of a possible tumor-suppressor gene. The most important is MEN 1, which is an autosomal dominant disorder due to a defect in a 10-exon gene on 11q13, which encodes for a 610-amino-acid nuclear protein, menin (Chap. 351). Patients with MEN 1 develop hyperparathyroidism due to parathyroid hyperplasia in 95–100% of cases, PETs in 80–100%, pituitary adenomas in 54–80%, adrenal adenomas in 27–36%, bronchial carcinoids in 8%, thymic carcinoids in 8%, gastric carcinoids in 13–30% of patients with Zollinger-Ellison syndrome, skin tumors [angiofibromas (88%), collagenomas (72%)], central nervous system (CNS) tumors [meningiomas (<8%)], and smooth-muscle tumors [leiomyomas, leiomyosarcomas (1–7%)]. Among patients with MEN 1, 80–100% develop nonfunctional PETs (most are microscopic with 0–13% large/symptomatic), functional PETs occur in 20–80% in different series with a mean of 54% developing Zollinger-Ellison syndrome, 18% insulinomas, 3% glucagonomas, 3% VIPomas, and <1% GRFomas or somatostatinomas. MEN 1 is present in 20–25% of all patients with Zollinger-Ellison syndrome, 4% of patients with insulinomas, and a low percentage (<5%) of patients with the other PETs.

Three phacomatoses associated with neuroendocrine tumors are von Hippel–Lindau disease (VHL), von Recklinghausen's disease [neurofibromatosis type 1 (NF-1)], and tuberous sclerosis (Bourneville's disease) (Table 350-5). VHL is an autosomal dominant disorder due to defects on chromosome 3p25, which encodes for a 213-amino-acid protein that interacts with the elongin family of proteins as a transcriptional regulator (Chaps. 284, 343, 351, 379). In addition to cerebellar hemangioblastomas, renal cancer, and pheochromocytomas, 10–17% develop a PET. Most are nonfunctional, although insulinomas and VIPomas have been reported. Patients with NF-1 (von Recklinghausen's disease) have defects in a gene on chromosome 17q11.2 that encodes for a 2845-amino-acid protein, neurofibromin, which functions in normal cells as a suppressor of the *ras* signaling cascade (Chap. 379). Up to 10% of these patients develop an upper GI carcinoid tumor, characteristically in the periampullary region (54%). Many are classified as somatostatinomas because they contain somatostatin immunocytochemically; however, they uncommonly secrete somatostatin and rarely produce a clinical somatostatinoma syndrome. NF-1 has rarely been associated with insulinomas and Zollinger-Ellison syndrome. NF-1 accounts for 48% of all duodenal somatostastinomas and 23% of all ampullary carcinoid tumors. Tuberous sclerosis is caused by mutations that alter either the 1164-amino-acid protein hamartin (TSC1) or the 1807-amino-acid protein tuberin (TSC2) (Chap. 379). Both hamartin and tuberin interact in a pathway related to phosphatidylinositol 3-kinases and mTor signaling cascades. A few cases including nonfunctional and functional PETs (insulinomas and gastrinomas) have been reported in these patients (Table 350-5).

In contrast to most common nonendocrine tumors, such as carcinoma of the breast, colon, lung, or stomach, in neither PETs nor carcinoid tumors have alterations in common oncogenes (*ras, myc, fos, src, jun*) or common tumor-suppressor genes (p53, retinoblastoma susceptibility gene) been found to be generally important in their molecular pathogenesis (Table 350-1). Alterations that may be important in their pathogenesis include changes in the *MEN 1* gene, p16/MTS1 tumor-suppressor gene, and *DPC 4/Smad 4* gene; amplification of the HER-2/*neu* protooncogene; alterations in transcription factors [Hoxc6 (GI carcinoids)], growth factors, and their receptor expression; methylation of a number of genes that probably results in their inactivation; and deletions of unknown tumor-suppressor genes as well as gains in other unknown genes (Table 350-1). Comparative genomic hybridization, genome-wide allelotyping studies, and genome-wide single-nucleotide polymorphism analyses have shown that chromosomal losses and gains are common in PETs and carcinoids, but they differ between these two NETs and some have prognostic significance (Table 350-4). Mutations in the *MEN 1* gene are probably particularly important. There is loss of heterozygosity at the MEN 1 locus on chromosome 11q13 in 93% of sporadic PETs (i.e., in patients without MEN 1) and in 26–75% of sporadic carcinoid tumors. Mutations in the *MEN 1* gene are reported in 31–34% of sporadic gastrinomas. The presence of a number of these molecular alterations (PET or carcinoid) correlates with tumor growth, tumor size, and disease extent or invasiveness and may have prognostic significance.

CARCINOID TUMORS AND CARCINOID SYNDROME

CHARACTERISTICS OF THE MOST COMMON GI CARCINOID TUMORS

Appendiceal carcinoids

Appendiceal carcinoids occur in 1 in every 200–300 appendectomies, usually in the appendiceal tip. Most (i.e., >90%) are <1 cm in diameter without metastases in older studies, but more recently 2–35% have had metastases (Table 350-3). In the SEER data of 1570 appendiceal carcinoids, 62% were localized, 27% had regional metastases, and 8% had distant metastases. Approximately 50% between 1 and 2 cm metastasized to lymph nodes. Their percentage of the total number of carcinoids decreased from 43.9% (1950–1969) to 2.4% (1992–1999).

Small-intestinal carcinoids

Small-intestinal carcinoids account for approximately one-third of all small-bowel tumors in various surgical series. These are frequently multiple; 70–80% are present in the ileum, and 70% within 6 cm (24 in.) of the ileocecal valve. Forty percent are <1 cm in diameter, 32% are 1–2 cm, and 29% are >2 cm. Between 35 and 70% are associated with metastases (Table 350-3). They characteristically cause a marked fibrotic reaction, which can lead to intestinal obstruction. Distant metastases occur to liver in 36–60%, to bone in 3%, and to lung in 4%. As discussed previously, tumor size is an important variable in the frequency of metastases. However, even a proportion of small carcinoid tumors of the small intestine (<1 cm) have metastases in 15–25% of cases, whereas the proportion increases to 58–100% for tumors 1–2 cm in diameter. Carcinoids also occur in the duodenum, with 31% having metastases. No duodenal tumor <1 cm in two series metastasized, whereas 33% of those >2 cm had metastases. Small-intestinal carcinoids are the most common cause (60–87%) of the carcinoid syndrome and are discussed in a later section (Table 350-6).

TABLE 350-6 Clinical Characteristics in Patients With Carcinoid Syndrome

	At Presentation	During Course of Disease
Symptoms/signs		
Diarrhea	32–73%	68–84%
Flushing	23–65%	63–74%
Pain	10%	34%
Asthma/wheezing	4–8%	3–18%
Pellagra	2%	5%
None	12%	22%
Carcinoid heart disease present	11%	14–41%
Demographics		
Male	46–59%	46–61%
Age		
Mean	57 yrs	52–54 yrs
Range	25–79 yrs	9–91 yrs
Tumor location		
Foregut	5–9%	2–33%
Midgut	78–87%	60–87%
Hindgut	1–5%	1–8%
Unknown	2–11%	2–15%

Rectal carcinoids

Rectal carcinoids represent 1–2% of all rectal tumors. They are found in approximately 1 in every 2500 proctoscopies. Nearly all occur between 4 and 13 cm above the dentate line. Most are small, with 66–80% being <1 cm in diameter, and rarely metastasize (5%). Tumors between 1 and 2 cm can metastasize in 5–30%, and those >2 cm, which are uncommon, in >70%.

Bronchial carcinoids

Bronchial carcinoids account for 1–2% of primary lung tumors. The frequency of bronchial carcinoids has increased more than fivefold over the last 30 years. A number of different classifications of bronchial carcinoid tumors have been proposed. In some studies, lung NETs are classified into four categories: typical carcinoid [also called bronchial carcinoid tumor, Kulchitsky cell carcinoma I (KCC-I)], atypical carcinoid [also called well-differentiated neuroendocrine carcinoma (KC-II)], intermediate small cell neuroendocrine carcinoma, and small cell neuroendocarcinoma (KC-III). Another proposed classification includes three categories of lung NETs: benign or low-grade malignant (typical carcinoid), low-grade malignant (atypical carcinoid), and high-grade malignant (poorly differentiated carcinoma of the large cell or small cell type). The WHO classification includes four general categories: typical carcinoid, atypical carcinoid, large cell neuroendocrine carcinoma, and small cell carcinoma. These different categories of lung NETs have different prognoses, varying from excellent for typical carcinoid to poor for small cell neuroendocrine carcinomas. The occurrence of large cell and small cell lung carcinoids, but not typical or atypical lung carcinoids, is related to tobacco use.

Gastric carcinoids

Gastric carcinoids account for 3 of every 1000 gastric neoplasms. Three different subtypes of gastric carcinoids are proposed to occur. Each originates from gastric enterochromaffin-like cells (ECL cells), one of the six types of gastric neuroendocrine cells, in the gastric mucosa. Two subtypes are associated with hypergastrinemic states, either chronic atrophic gastritis (type I) (80% of all gastric carcinoids) or Zollinger-Ellison syndrome, which is almost always a part of the MEN 1 syndrome (type II) (6% of all cases). These tumors generally pursue a benign course, with type 1 uncommonly (<10%) associated with metastases, whereas type II tumors are slightly more aggressive with 10–30% percentage associated with metastases. They are usually multiple and small and infiltrate only to the submucosa. The third subtype of gastric carcinoid (type III) (sporadic) occurs without hypergastrinemia (14–25% of all gastric carcinoids) and has an aggressive course, with 54–66% developing metastases. Sporadic carcinoids are usually single, large tumors; 50% have atypical histology, and they can be a cause of the carcinoid syndrome. Gastric carcinoids as a percentage of all carcinoids are increasing in frequency [1.96% (1969–1971), 3.6% (1973–1991), 5.8% (1991–1999)].

CARCINOID TUMORS WITHOUT THE CARCINOID SYNDROME

The age of patients at diagnosis ranges from 10 to 93 years, with a mean age of 63 years for the small intestine and 66 years for the rectum. The presentation is diverse and is related to the site of origin and the extent of malignant spread. In the appendix, carcinoid tumors usually are found incidentally during surgery for suspected appendicitis. Small-intestinal carcinoids in the jejunoileum present with periodic abdominal pain (51%), intestinal obstruction with ileus/invagination (31%), an abdominal tumor (17%), or GI bleeding (11%). Because of the vagueness of the symptoms, the diagnosis usually is delayed approximately 2 years from onset of the symptoms, with a range up to 20 years. Duodenal, gastric, and rectal carcinoids are most frequently found by chance at endoscopy. The most common symptoms of rectal carcinoids are melena/bleeding (39%), constipation (17%), and diarrhea (12%). Bronchial carcinoids frequently are discovered as a lesion on a chest radiograph, and 31% of the patients are asymptomatic. Thymic carcinoids present as anterior mediastinal masses, usually on chest radiograph or CT scan. Ovarian and testicular carcinoids usually present as masses discovered on physical examination or ultrasound. Metastatic carcinoid tumor in the liver frequently presents as hepatomegaly in a patient who may have minimal symptoms and nearly normal liver function test results.

CARCINOID TUMORS WITH SYSTEMIC SYMPTOMS DUE TO SECRETED PRODUCTS

Carcinoid tumors immunocytochemically can contain numerous GI peptides: gastrin, insulin, somatostatin, motilin, neurotensin, tachykinins (substance K, substance P, neuropeptide K), glucagon, gastrin-releasing peptide, vasoactive intestinal peptide (VIP), pancreatic polypeptide (PP), ghrelin, other biologically active peptides (ACTH, calcitonin, growth hormone), prostaglandins, and bioactive amines (serotonin). These substances may or may not be released in sufficient amounts to cause symptoms. In various studies of patients with carcinoid tumors, elevated serum levels of PP were found in 43%, motilin in 14%, gastrin in 15%, and VIP in 6%. Foregut carcinoids are more likely to produce various GI peptides than are midgut carcinoids. Ectopic ACTH production causing Cushing's syndrome is seen increasingly with foregut carcinoids (respiratory tract primarily) and in some series has been the most common cause of the ectopic ACTH syndrome, accounting for 64% of all cases. Acromegaly due to growth hormone–releasing factor release occurs with foregut carcinoids, as does the somatostatinoma syndrome, but rarely occurs with duodenal carcinoids. The most common systemic syndrome with carcinoid tumors is the carcinoid syndrome, which is discussed in detail in the next section.

CARCINOID SYNDROME

Clinical features

The cardinal features from a number of series at presentation as well as during the disease course are shown in Table 350-6. Flushing and diarrhea are the two most common symptoms, occurring in up to 73% initially and in up to 89% during the course of the disease. The characteristic flush is of sudden onset; it is a deep red or violaceous erythema of the upper body, especially the neck and face, often associated with a feeling of warmth and occasionally associated with pruritus, lacrimation, diarrhea, or facial edema. Flushes may be precipitated by stress; alcohol; exercise; certain foods, such as cheese; or certain agents, such as catecholamines, pentagastrin, and serotonin reuptake inhibitors. Flushing episodes may be brief, lasting 2 to 5 min, especially initially, or may last hours, especially later in the disease course. Flushing usually is associated with metastastic midgut carcinoids but can also occur with foregut carcinoids. With bronchial carcinoids the flushes frequently are prolonged for hours to days, reddish in color, and associated with salivation, lacrimation, diaphoresis, diarrhea, and hypotension. The flush associated with gastric carcinoids can also be reddish in color, but with a patchy distribution over the face and neck, although the classic flush seen with midgut carcinoids can also be seen with gastric carcinoids. It may be provoked by food and have accompanying pruritus.

Diarrhea is present in 32–73% initially and 68–84% at some time in the disease course. Diarrhea usually occurs with flushing (85% of cases). The diarrhea usually is described as watery, with 60% of patients having <1 L/d of diarrhea. Steatorrhea is present in 67%, and in 46% it is greater than 15 g/d (normal <7 g). Abdominal pain may be present with the diarrhea or independently in 10–34% of cases.

Cardiac manifestations occur in 11–20% initially of patients with carcinoid syndrome and in 17–56% (mean 40%) at some time in the disease course. The cardiac disease is due to the formation of fibrotic plaques (composed of smooth-muscle cells, myofibroblasts, and elastic tissue) involving the endocardium, primarily on the right side, although lesions on the left side also occur occasionally, especially if a patent foramen ovale exists. The dense fibrous deposits are most commonly on the ventricular aspect of the tricuspid valve and less commonly on the pulmonary valve cusps. They can result in constriction of the valves, and pulmonic stenosis is usually predominant, whereas the tricuspid valve is often fixed open, resulting in regurgitation predominating. Overall, in patients with carcinoid heart disease, 97% have tricuspid insufficiency, 59% tricuspid stenosis, 50% pulmonary insufficiency, 25% pulmonary stenosis, and 11% (0–25%) left-side lesions. Up to 80% of patients with cardiac lesions develop heart failure. Lesions on the left side are much less extensive, occur in 30% at autopsy, and most frequently affect the mitral valve.

Other clinical manifestations include wheezing or asthma-like symptoms (8–18%) and pellagra-like skin lesions (2–25%). A variety of noncardiac problems due to increased fibrous tissue have been reported, including retroperitoneal fibrosis causing urethral obstruction, Peyronie's disease of the penis, intraabdominal fibrosis, and occlusion of the mesenteric arteries or veins.

Pathobiology

Carcinoid syndrome occurred in 8% of 8876 patients with carcinoid tumors, with a rate of 1.4–18.4% in different studies. It occurs only when sufficient concentrations of products secreted by the tumor reach the systemic circulation. In 91% of cases this occurs after distant metastases to the liver. Rarely, primary gut carcinoids with nodal metastases with extensive retroperitoneal invasion, pancreatic carcinoids with retroperitoneal lymph nodes, or carcinoids of the lung or ovary with direct access to the systemic circulation can cause the carcinoid syndrome without hepatic metastases. All carcinoid tumors do not have the same propensity to metastasize and cause the carcinoid syndrome (Table 350-3). Midgut carcinoids account for 60–67% of cases of carcinoid syndrome, foregut tumors for 2–33%, hindgut for 1–8%, and an unknown primary location for 2–15%.

One of the main secretory products of carcinoid tumors involved in the carcinoid syndrome is serotonin [5-hydroxytryptamine (5-HT)] (Fig. 350-1), which is synthesized from tryptophan. Up to 50% of dietary tryptophan can be used in this synthetic pathway by tumor cells, and this can result in inadequate supplies for conversion to niacin; hence, some patients (2.5%) develop pellagra-like lesions. Serotonin has numerous biologic effects, including stimulating intestinal secretion with inhibition of absorption, stimulating increases in intestinal motility, and stimulating fibrogenesis. In various studies 56–88% of all carcinoid tumors were associated with serotonin overproduction; however, 12–26% of the patients did not have the carcinoid syndrome. In one study platelet serotonin was elevated in 96% of patients with midgut carcinoids, 43% with foregut tumors, and 0% with hindgut tumors. In 90–100% of patients with the carcinoid syndrome there is evidence of serotonin overproduction. Serotonin is thought to be predominantly responsible for the diarrhea because of its effects on gut motility and intestinal secretion, primarily through 5-HT_3 and, to a lesser degree, 5-HT_4 receptors. Serotonin receptor antagonists (especially 5-HT_3 antagonists) relieve the diarrhea in many, but not all, patients. Additional studies suggest that prostaglandin E_2 (PGE_2) and tachykinins may be important mediators of the diarrhea in some patients. In one study, plasma tachykinin levels correlated with symptoms of both flushing and diarrhea. Serotonin does not appear to be involved in the flushing because serotonin receptor antagonists do not relieve flushing. In patients with gastric carcinoids the characteristic red, patchy pruritic flush probably is due to histamine release because H_1 and H_2 receptor antagonists can prevent it. Numerous studies have shown that tachykinins are stored in carcinoid tumors and released during flushing. However, some studies have demonstrated that octreotide can relieve the flushing induced by pentagastrin in these patients without altering the stimulated increase in plasma substance P, suggesting that other mediators must be involved in the flushing. A correlation between plasma tachykinin levels, but not substance P levels, and flushing has been reported. Both histamine and serotonin may be responsible for the wheezing as well as the fibrotic reactions involving the heart, causing Peyronie's disease and intraabdominal fibrosis. The exact mechanism of the heart disease has remained unclear, although increasing evidence supports a central role for serotonin. The valvular heart disease caused by the appetite-suppressant drug dexfenfluramine is histologically indistinguishable from that observed in carcinoid disease. Furthermore, ergot-containing dopamine receptor agonists used for Parkinson's disease (pergolide, cabergoline) cause valvular heart disease that closely resembles that seen in the carcinoid syndrome. Metabolites of fenfluramine, as well as the dopamine receptor agonists, have high affinity for serotonin receptor subtype 5-HT_{2B} receptors, whose activation is known to cause fibroblast mitogenesis. Serotonin receptor subtypes $5\text{-HT}_{1B,1D,2A,2B}$ normally are expressed in human heart valve interstitial cells. High levels of 5-HT_{2B} receptors are known to occur in heart valves and occur in cardiac fibroblasts and cardiomyocytes. Studies of cultured interstitial cells from human cardiac valves have demonstrated that these valvulopathic drugs induce mitogenesis by activating 5-HT_{2B} receptors and stimulating upregulation of transforming growth factor β and collagen biosynthesis. These observations support the conclusion that serotonin overproduction by carcinoid tumors is important in mediating the valvular changes, possibly by activating 5-HT_{2B} receptors in the endocardium. Both the magnitude of serotonin overproduction and prior chemotherapy are important predictors of progression of the heart disease. Atrial natriuretic peptide (ANP) overproduction also has been reported in patients with cardiac disease, but its role in the pathogenesis is unknown. However, high plasma levels of ANP have a worse prognosis. Plasma connective tissue growth factor levels are elevated in many fibrotic conditions; elevated levels occur in patients with carcinoid heart disease and correlate with the presence of right-ventricular dysfunction and the extent of valvular regurgitation in patients with carcinoid tumors.

Patients may develop either a typical or, rarely, an atypical carcinoid syndrome. In patients with the typical form, which characteristically is caused by a midgut carcinoid tumor, the conversion of tryptophan to 5-HTP is the rate-limiting step (Fig. 350-1). Once 5-HTP is formed, it is rapidly converted to 5-HT and stored in secretory granules of the tumor or in platelets. A small amount remains in plasma and is converted to 5-HIAA, which appears in large amounts in the urine. These patients have an expanded serotonin pool size, increased blood and platelet serotonin, and increased urinary 5-hydroxyindolacetic acid (5-HIAA). Some carcinoid tumors cause an atypical carcinoid syndrome that is thought to be due to a deficiency in the enzyme dopa decarboxylase; thus, 5-HTP cannot be converted to 5-HT (serotonin), and 5-HTP is secreted into the bloodstream (Fig. 350-1). In these patients, plasma serotonin levels are normal but urinary levels may be increased because some 5-HTP is converted to 5-HT in the kidney. Characteristically, urinary 5-HTP and 5-HT are increased, but urinary 5-HIAA levels are only slightly elevated. Foregut carcinoids are the most likely to cause an atypical carcinoid syndrome.

One of the most immediate life-threatening complications of the carcinoid syndrome is the development of a carcinoid crisis. This is more common in patients who have intense symptoms or have greatly increased urinary 5-HIAA levels (i.e., >200 mg/d). The crises may occur spontaneously or be provoked by stress, anesthesia, chemotherapy, or a biopsy. Patients develop intense flushing, diarrhea, abdominal pain, cardiac abnormalities including tachycardia, hypertension, or hypotension. If not adequately treated, this can be a terminal event.

DIAGNOSIS OF THE CARCINOID SYNDROME AND CARCINOID TUMORS

The diagnosis of carcinoid syndrome relies on measurement of urinary or plasma serotonin or its metabolites in the urine. The measurement of 5-HIAA is used most frequently. False-positive elevations may occur if the patient is eating serotonin-rich foods such as bananas, pineapples, walnuts, pecans, avocados, or hickory nuts or is taking certain medications (cough syrup containing guaifenesin, acetaminophen, salicylates, serotonin reuptake inhibitors, or L-dopa). The normal range in daily urinary 5-HIAA excretion is 2–8 mg/d. Serotonin overproduction was noted in 92% of patients with carcinoid syndrome in one study, and in another study, 5-HIAA had 73% sensitivity and 100% specificity for carcinoid syndrome.

Most physicians use only the urinary 5-HIAA excretion rate; however, plasma and platelet serotonin levels, if available, may provide additional information. Platelet serotonin levels are more sensitive than urinary 5-HIAA but are not generally available.

Because patients with foregut carcinoids may produce an atypical carcinoid syndrome, if this syndrome is suspected and the urinary 5-HIAA is minimally elevated or normal, other urinary metabolites of tryptophan, such as 5-HTP and 5-HT, should be measured (Fig. 350-1).

Flushing occurs in a number of other diseases, including systemic mastocytosis, chronic myeloid leukemia with increased histamine release, menopause, reactions to alcohol or glutamate, side effects of chlorpropamide, calcium channel blockers, and nicotinic acid. None of these conditions cause increased urinary 5-HIAA.

The diagnosis of carcinoid tumor can be suggested by the carcinoid syndrome, recurrent abdominal symptoms in a healthy-appearing individual, or the discovery of hepatomegaly or hepatic metastases associated with minimal symptoms. Ileal carcinoids, which make up 25% of all clinically detected carcinoids, should be suspected in patients with bowel obstruction, abdominal pain, flushing, or diarrhea.

Serum chromogranin A levels are elevated in 56–100% of patients with carcinoid tumors, and the level correlates with tumor bulk. Serum chromogranin A levels are not specific for carcinoid tumors because they are also elevated in patients with PETs and other neuroendocrine tumors. Plasma neuron-specific enolase levels are also used as a marker of carcinoid tumors but are less sensitive than chromogranin A, being increased in only 17–47% of patients.

TREATMENT Carcinoid Syndrome and Nonmetastatic Carcinoid Tumors

CARCINOID SYNDROME Treatment includes avoiding conditions that precipitate flushing, dietary supplementation with nicotinamide, treatment of heart failure with diuretics, treatment of wheezing with oral bronchodilators, and control of the diarrhea with antidiarrheal agents such as loperamide and diphenoxylate. If patients still have symptoms, serotonin receptor antagonists or somatostatin analogues (Fig. 350-2) are the drugs of choice.

There are 14 subclasses of serotonin receptors, and antagonists for many are not available. The 5-HT_1 and 5-HT_2 receptor antagonists methylsergide, cyproheptadine, and ketanserin have all been used to control the diarrhea but usually do not decrease flushing. The use of methylsergide is limited because it can cause or enhance retroperitoneal fibrosis. Ketanserin diminishes diarrhea in 30–100% of patients. 5-HT_3 receptor antagonists (ondansetron, tropisetron, alosetron) can control diarrhea and nausea in up to 100% of patients and occasionally ameliorate the flushing. A combination of histamine H_1 and H_2 receptor antagonists (i.e., diphenhydramine and cimetidine or ranitidine) may control flushing in patients with foregut carcinoids.

Synthetic analogues of somatostatin (octreotide, lanreotide) are now the most widely used agents to control the symptoms of patients with carcinoid syndrome (Fig. 350-2). These drugs are effective at relieving symptoms and decreasing urinary 5-HIAA levels in patients with this syndrome. Octreotide-LAR and lanreotide-SR/autogel (Somatuline) control symptoms in 74% and 68%, respectively, of patients with carcinoid syndrome and show a biochemical response in 51% and 39%. Patients with mild to moderate symptoms usually are treated initially with octreotide 100 μg SC every 8 h and begun on long-acting monthly depot forms (octreotide-LAR or lanreotide-autogel). Forty percent of patients escape control after a median time of 4 months, and the depot dosage may have to be increased as well as supplemented with the shorter-acting formulation, SC octreotide.

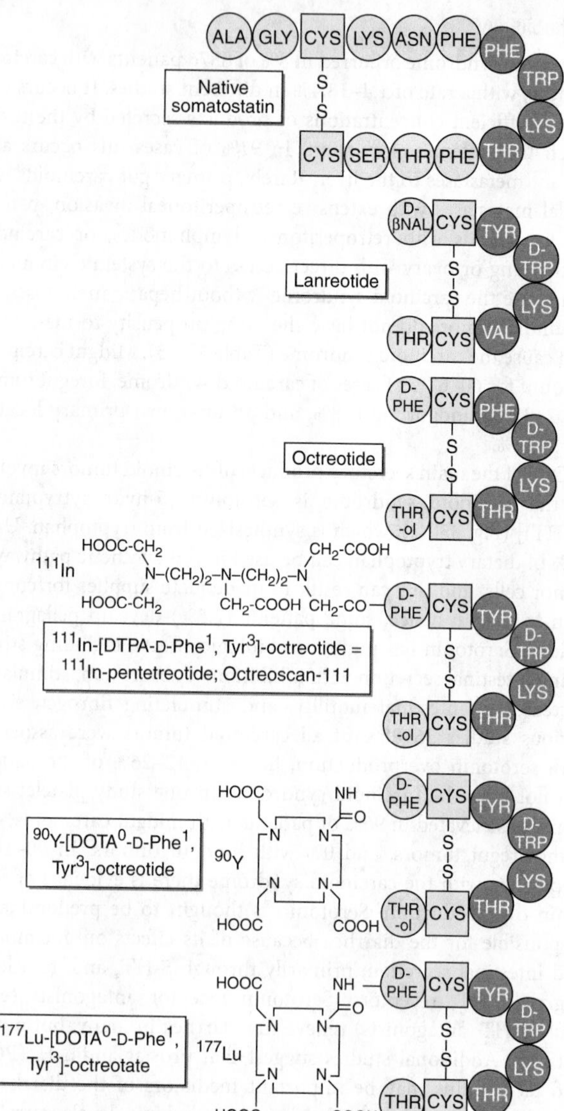

Figure 350-2 Structure of somatostatin and synthetic analogues used for diagnostic or therapeutic indications.

Carcinoid heart disease is associated with a decreased mean survival (3.8 years), and therefore it should be sought for and carefully assessed in all patients with carcinoid syndrome. Transthoracic echocardiography remains a key element in establishing the diagnosis of carcinoid heart disease and determining the extent and type of cardiac abnormalities. Treatment with diuretics and somatostatin analogues can reduce the negative hemodynamic effects and secondary heart failure. It remains unclear whether long-term treatment with these drugs will decrease the progression of carcinoid heart disease. Balloon valvuloplasty for stenotic valves or cardiac valve surgery may be required.

In patients with carcinoid crises, somatostatin analogues are effective at both treating the condition and preventing their development during known precipitating events such as surgery, anesthesia, chemotherapy, and stress. It is recommended that octreotide 150–250 μg SC every 6 to 8 h be used 24–48 h before anesthesia and then continued throughout the procedure.

Currently, sustained-release preparations of both octreotide [octreotide-LAR (long-acting release), 10, 20, 30 mg] and lanreotide [lanreotide-PR (prolonged release, lanreotide-autogel), 60, 90, 120 mg] are available and widely used because their use greatly facilitates long-term treatment. Octreotide-LAR (30 mg/month) gives a plasma level ≥1 ng/mL for 25 days, whereas this requires three to six injections a day of the non-sustained-release form. Lanreotide autogel (Somatuline) is given every 4–6 weeks.

Short-term side effects occur in up to one-half of patients. Pain at the injection site and side effects related to the GI tract (59% discomfort, 15% nausea, diarrhea) are the most common. They are usually short-lived and do not interrupt treatment. Important long-term side effects include gallstone formation, steatorrhea, and deterioration in glucose tolerance. The overall incidence of gallstones/biliary sludge in one study was 52%, with 7% having symptomatic disease that required surgical treatment.

Interferon α is reported to be effective in controlling symptoms of the carcinoid syndrome either alone or combined with hepatic artery embolization. With interferon α alone the response rate is 42%, and with interferon α with hepatic artery embolization, diarrhea was controlled for 1 year in 43% and flushing was controlled in 86%.

Hepatic artery embolization alone or with chemotherapy (chemoembolization) has been used to control the symptoms of carcinoid syndrome. Embolization alone is reported to control symptoms in up to 76% of patients, and chemoembolization (5-fluorouracil, doxorubicin, cisplatin, mitomycin) in 60–75% of patients. Hepatic artery embolization can have major side effects, including nausea, vomiting, pain, and fever. In two studies 5–7% of patients died from complications of hepatic artery occlusion.

Other drugs have been used successfully in small numbers of patients to control the symptoms of carcinoid syndrome. Parachlorophenylanine can inhibit tryptophan hydroxylase and therefore the conversion of tryptophan to 5-HTP. However, its severe side effects, including psychiatric disturbances, make it intolerable for long-term use. α-Methyldopa inhibits the conversion of 5-HTP to 5-HT, but its effects are only partial.

Peptide radioreceptor therapy (using radiotherapy with radiolabeled somatostatin analogues), the use of radiolabeled microspheres, and other methods for treatment of advanced metastatic disease may facilitate control of the carcinoid syndrome and are discussed in a later section dealing with treatment of advanced disease.

CARCINOID TUMORS (NONMETASTATIC) Surgery is the only potentially curative therapy. Because with most carcinoids the probability of metastatic disease increases with increasing size, the extent of surgical resection is determined accordingly. With appendiceal carcinoids <1 cm, simple appendectomy was curative in 103 patients followed for up to 35 years. With rectal carcinoids <1 cm, local resection is curative. With small-intestinal carcinoids <1 cm, there is not complete agreement. Because 15–69% of small-intestinal carcinoids this size have metastases in different studies, some recommend a wide resection with en bloc resection of the adjacent lymph-bearing mesentery. If the carcinoid tumor is >2 cm for rectal, appendiceal, or small-intestinal carcinomas, a full cancer operation should be done. This includes a right hemicolectomy for appendiceal carcinoid, an abdominoperineal resection or low anterior resection for rectal carcinoids, and an en bloc resection of adjacent lymph nodes for small-intestinal carcinoids. For carcinoids 1–2 cm in diameter for appendiceal tumors, a simple appendectomy is proposed by some, whereas others favor a formal right hemicolectomy. For rectal carcinoids 1–2 cm, it is recommended that a wide local full-thickness excision be performed.

With type I or II gastric carcinoids, which are usually <1 cm, endoscopic removal is recommended. In type I or II gastric carcinoids, if the tumor is >2 cm or if there is local invasion, some recommend total gastrectomy, whereas others recommend antrectomy in type I to reduce the hypergastrinemia, which led to regression of the carcinoids in a number of studies. For types I and II gastric carcinoids of 1–2 cm, there is no agreement, with some recommending endoscopic treatment followed by chronic somatostatin treatment and careful follow-up and others recommending surgical treatment. With type III gastric carcinoids >2 cm, excision and regional lymph node clearance are recommended. Most tumors <1 cm are treated endoscopically.

Resection of isolated or limited hepatic metastases may be beneficial and will be discussed in a later section on treatment of advanced disease.

PANCREATIC ENDOCRINE TUMORS

Functional PETs usually present clinically with symptoms due to the hormone-excess state. Only late in the course of the disease does the tumor per se cause prominent symptoms such as abdominal pain. In contrast, all the symptoms due to nonfunctional PETs are due to the tumor per se. The overall result of this is that some functional PETs may present with severe symptoms with a small or undetectable primary tumor, whereas nonfunctional tumors usually present late in the disease course with large tumors, which are frequently metastatic. The mean delay between onset of continuous symptoms and diagnosis of a functional PET syndrome is 4–7 years. Therefore, the diagnoses frequently are missed for extended periods.

TREATMENT Pancreatic Endocrine Tumor

Treatment of PETs requires two different strategies. First, treatment must be directed at the hormone-excess state such as the gastric acid hypersecretion in gastrinomas or the hypoglycemia in insulinomas. Ectopic hormone secretion usually causes the presenting symptoms and can cause life-threatening complications. Second, with all the tumors except insulinomas, >50% are malignant (Table 350-2); therefore, treatment must also be directed against the tumor per se. Because in many patients these tumors are not surgically curable due to the presence of advanced disease at diagnosis, surgical resection for cure, which addresses both treatment aspects, is often not possible.

■ GASTRINOMA (ZOLLINGER-ELLISON SYNDROME) (ZES)

A gastrinoma is a neuroendocrine tumor that secretes gastrin; the resultant hypergastrinemia causes gastric acid hypersecretion (Zollinger-Ellison syndrome). The chronic hypergastrinemia results in marked gastric acid hypersecretion and growth of the gastric mucosa with increased numbers of parietal cells and proliferation of gastric ECL cells. The gastric acid hypersecretion characteristically causes peptic ulcer disease, often refractory and severe, as well as diarrhea. The most common presenting symptoms are abdominal pain (70–100%), diarrhea (37–73%), and gastroesophageal reflux disease (GERD) (30–35%); 10–20% have diarrhea only. Although peptic ulcers may occur in unusual locations, most patients have a typical duodenal ulcer. Important observations that should suggest this diagnosis include peptic ulcer disease (PUD); with diarrhea; PUD in an unusual location or with multiple ulcers; PUD refractory to treatment or persistent; PUD associated with prominent gastric folds; PUD associated with findings suggestive of MEN 1 (endocrinopathy, family history of ulcer or endocrinopathy, nephrolithiases); and PUD without *Helicobacter pylori* present. *H. pylori* is present in >90% of idiopathic peptic ulcers but is present in <50% of patients with gastrinomas. Chronic unexplained diarrhea also should suggest gastrinoma.

Approximately 20–25% of patients with ZES have MEN 1, and in most cases hyperparathyroidism is present before the gastrinoma. These patients are treated differently from those without MEN 1; therefore, MEN 1 should be sought in all patients by family history and by measuring plasma ionized calcium and prolactin levels and plasma hormone levels (parathormone, growth hormone).

Most gastrinomas (50–70%) are present in the duodenum, followed by the pancreas (20–40%) and other intraabdominal sites (mesentery, lymph nodes, biliary tract, liver, stomach, ovary). Rarely, the tumor may involve extraabdominal sites. In MEN 1 the gastrinomas are also usually in the duodenum (70–90%), followed by the pancreas (10–30%), and are almost always multiple. About 60–90% of gastrinomas are malignant (Table 350-2) with metastatic spread to lymph nodes and liver. Distant metastases to bone occur in 12–30% of patients with liver metastases.

Diagnosis

The diagnosis of ZES requires the demonstration of inappropriate fasting hypergastrinemia, usually by demonstrating hypergastrinemia occurring with an increased basal gastric acid output (BAO) (hyperchlorhydria). More than 98% of patients with gastrinomas have fasting hypergastrinemia, although in 40–60% the level may be elevated less than tenfold. Therefore, when the diagnosis is suspected, a fasting gastrin should be determined first. It is important to remember that potent gastric acid suppressant drugs such as proton pump inhibitors (omeprazole, esomeprazole, pantoprazole, lansoprazole, rabeprazole) can suppress acid secretion sufficiently to cause hypergastrinemia; because of their prolonged duration of action, these drugs have to be discontinued for a week before the gastrin determination. Withdrawal of proton pump inhibitors (PPIs) should be performed carefully and is best done in consultation with GI units with experience in this area. The widespread use of PPIs can confound the diagnosis of ZES by raising a false-positive diagnosis by causing hypergastrinemia in a patient being treated with idiopathic peptic disease (without ZES) and lead to a false-negative diagnosis because at routine doses used to treat patients with idiopathic peptic disease, PPIs control symptoms in most ZES patients and thus mask the diagnosis. If ZES is suspected and the gastrin level is elevated, it is important to show that it is increased when gastric pH is ≤2.0 because physiologically hypergastrinemia secondary to achlorhydria (atrophic gastritis, pernicious anemia) is one of the most common causes of hypergastrinemia. Nearly all gastrinoma patients have a fasting pH ≤2 when off antisecretory drugs. If the fasting gastrin is >1000 pg/mL (increased tenfold) and the pH is ≤2.0, which occurs in 40–60% of patients with gastrinoma, the diagnosis of ZES is established after the possibility of retained antrum syndrome has been ruled out by history. In patients with hypergastrinemia with fasting gastrins <1000 pg/mL and gastric pH ≤2.0, other conditions, such as *H. pylori* infections, antral G-cell hyperplasia/hyperfunction, gastric outlet obstruction, and, rarely, renal failure, can masquerade as ZES. To establish the diagnosis in this group, a determination of BAO and a secretin provocative test should be done. In patients with ZES without previous gastric acid–reducing surgery, the BAO is usually (>90%) elevated (i.e., >15 meq/h). The secretin provocative test is usually positive, with the criterion of a >120-pg/mL increase over the basal level having the highest sensitivity (94%) and specificity (100%).

TREATMENT Gastrinomas

Gastric acid hypersecretion in patients with gastrinomas can be controlled in almost every case by oral gastric antisecretory drugs. Because of their long duration of action and potency, which allows dosing once or twice a day, the PPIs (H^+,K^+-ATPase inhibitors) are the drugs of choice. Histamine H_2-receptor antagonists are also effective, although more frequent dosing (q 4–8 h) and high doses are required. In patients with MEN 1 with hyperparathyroidism, correction of the hyperparathyroidism increases the sensitivity to gastric antisecretory drugs and decreases the basal acid output. Long-term treatment with PPIs (>15 years) has proved to be safe and effective, without development of tachyphylaxis. Although patients with ZES, especially those with MEN 1, more frequently develop gastric carcinoids, no data suggest that the long-term use of PPIs increases this risk in these patients. With long-term PPI use in ZES patients, vitamin B_{12} deficiency can develop; thus, vitamin B_{12} levels should be assessed during follow-up.

With the increased ability to control acid hypersecretion, more than 50% of patients who are not cured (>60% of patients) will die from tumor-related causes. At presentation, careful imaging studies are essential to localize the extent of the tumor. A third of patients present with hepatic metastases, and in <15% of those patients the disease is limited, so that surgical resection may be possible. Surgical short-term cure is possible in 60% of all patients without MEN 1 or liver metastases (40% of all patients) and in 30% of patients long-term. In patients with MEN 1, long-term surgical cure is rare because the tumors are multiple, frequently with lymph node metastases. Therefore, all patients with gastrinomas without MEN 1 or a medical condition that limits life expectancy should undergo surgery by a surgeon experienced in the treatment of these disorders.

INSULINOMAS

An insulinoma is an endocrine tumor of the pancreas that is thought to be derived from beta cells that ectopically secrete insulin, which results in hypoglycemia. The average age of occurrence is 40–50 years old. The most common clinical symptoms are due to the effect of the hypoglycemia on the CNS (neuroglycemic symptoms) and include confusion, headache, disorientation, visual difficulties, irrational behavior, and even coma. Also, most patients have symptoms due to excess catecholamine release secondary to the hypoglycemia, including sweating, tremor, and palpitations. Characteristically, these attacks are associated with fasting.

Insulinomas are generally small (>90% <2 cm) and usually not multiple (90%); only 5–15% are malignant, and they almost invariably occur only in the pancreas, distributed equally in the pancreatic head, body, and tail.

Insulinomas should be suspected in all patients with hypoglycemia, especially when there is a history suggesting that attacks are provoked by fasting, or with a family history of MEN 1. Insulin is synthesized as proinsulin, which consists of a 21-amino-acid α chain and a 30-amino-acid β chain connected by a 33-amino-acid connecting peptide (C peptide). In insulinomas, in addition to elevated plasma insulin levels, elevated plasma proinsulin levels are found, and C-peptide levels can be elevated.

Diagnosis

The diagnosis of insulinoma requires the demonstration of an elevated plasma insulin level at the time of hypoglycemia. A number of other conditions may cause fasting hypoglycemia, such as the inadvertent or surreptitious use of insulin or oral hypoglycemic agents, severe liver disease, alcoholism, poor nutrition, and other extrapancreatic tumors. Furthermore, postprandial hypoglycemia can be caused by a number of conditions that confuse the diagnosis of insulinoma. Particularly important here is the increased occurrence of hypoglycemia after gastric bypass surgery for obesity, which is now widely performed. The most reliable test to diagnose insulinoma is a fast up to 72 h with serum glucose, C-peptide, proinsulin, and insulin measurements every 4–8 h. If at any point the patient becomes symptomatic or glucose levels are persistently below <2.2 mmol/L (40 mg/dL), the test should be terminated and repeat samples for the above studies should be obtained before glucose is given. Some 70–80% of patients will develop hypoglycemia during the first 24 h, and 98% by 48 h. In nonobese normal subjects, serum insulin levels should decrease to <43 pmol/L (<6 μU/mL) when blood glucose decreases to <2.2 mmol/L (<40 mg/dL) and the ratio of insulin to glucose is <0.3 (in mg/dL). In addition to having an insulin level >6 μU/mL when blood glucose is <40 mg/dL, some investigators also require an elevated C-peptide and serum proinsulin level, an insulin/glucose ratio >0.3, and a decreased plasma β-hydroxybutyrate level for the diagnosis of insulinomas. Surreptitious use of insulin or hypoglycemic agents may be difficult to distinguish from insulinomas. The combination of proinsulin levels (normal in exogenous insulin/hypoglycemic agent users), C-peptide levels (low in exogenous insulin users), antibodies to insulin (positive in exogenous insulin users), and measurement of sulfonylurea levels in serum or plasma will allow the correct diagnosis to be made. The diagnosis of insulinoma has been complicated by the introduction of specific insulin assays that do not also interact with proinsulin, as do many of the older radioimmunoassays (RIAs), and therefore give lower plasma insulin levels. The increased use of these specific insulin assays has resulted in increased numbers of patients with insulinomas having lower plasma insulin values than the 6 μU/mL levels proposed to be characteristic of insulinomas by RIA. In these patients the assessment of proinsulin and C-peptide levels at the time of hypoglycemia is particularly helpful for establishing the correct diagnosis. An elevated proinsulin level when the fasting glucose level is <45 mg/dL is sensitive and specific.

TREATMENT Insulinomas

Only 5–15% of insulinomas are malignant; therefore, after appropriate imaging (see below), surgery should be performed. In different studies, 75–100% of patients are cured by surgery. Before surgery, the hypoglycemia can be controlled by frequent small meals and the use of diazoxide (150–800 mg/d). Diazoxide is a benzothiadiazide whose hyperglycemic effect is attributed to inhibition of insulin release. Its side effects are sodium retention and GI symptoms such as nausea. Approximately 50–60% of patients respond to diazoxide. Other agents effective in some patients to control the hypoglycemia include verapamil and diphenylhydantoin. Long-acting somatostatin analogues such as octreotide and lanreotide are acutely effective in 40% of patients. However, octreotide must be used with care because it inhibits growth hormone secretion and can alter plasma glucagon levels; therefore, in some patients it can worsen the hypoglycemia.

For the 5–15% of patients with malignant insulinomas, these drugs or somatostatin analogues are used initially. In a small number of patients with insulinomas, some with malignant tumors, mammalian target of rapamycin (mTor) inhibitors (everolimus, rapamycin) are reported to control the hypoglycemia. If they are not effective, various antitumor treatments such as hepatic arterial embolization, chemoembolization, chemotherapy, and peptide receptor radiotherapy have been used (see below).

Insulinomas, which are usually benign (>90%) and intrapancreatic in location, are increasingly resected using a laparoscopic approach, which has lower morbidity rates. This approach requires that the insulinoma be localized on preoperative imaging studies.

GLUCAGONOMAS

A glucagonoma is an endocrine tumor of the pancreas that secretes excessive amounts of glucagon, which causes a distinct syndrome characterized by dermatitis, glucose intolerance or diabetes, and weight loss. Glucagonomas principally occur between 45 and 70 years of age. The tumor is clinically heralded by a characteristic dermatitis (migratory necrolytic erythema) (67–90%), accompanied by glucose intolerance (40–90%), weight loss (66–96%), anemia (33–85%), diarrhea (15–29%), and thromboembolism (11–24%). The characteristic rash usually starts as an annular erythema at intertriginous and periorificial sites, especially in the groin or buttock. It subsequently becomes raised, and bullae form; when the bullae rupture, eroded areas form. The lesions can wax and wane. The development of a similar rash in patients receiving glucagon therapy suggests that the rash is a direct effect of the hyperglucagonemia. A characteristic laboratory finding is hypoaminoacidemia, which occurs in 26–100% of patients.

Glucagonomas are generally large tumors at diagnosis (5–10 cm). Some 50–80% occur in the pancreatic tail. From 50 to 82% have evidence of metastatic spread at presentation, usually to the liver. Glucagonomas are rarely extrapancreatic and usually occur singly.

Diagnosis

The diagnosis is confirmed by demonstrating an increased plasma glucagon level. Characteristically, plasma glucagon levels exceed 1000 pg/mL (normal is <150 pg/mL) in 90%; 7% are between 500 and 1000 pg/mL, and 3% are <500 pg/mL. A trend toward lower levels at diagnosis has been noted in the last decade. A plasma glucagon level >1000 pg/mL is considered diagnostic of glucagonoma. Other diseases causing increased plasma glucagon levels include renal insufficiency, acute pancreatitis, hypercorticism, hepatic insufficiency, severe stress, and prolonged fasting or familial hyperglucagonemia, as well as danazol treatment. With the exception of cirrhosis, these disorders do not increase plasma glucagon >500 pg/mL.

Necrolytic migratory erythema is not pathognomonic for glucagonoma and occurs in myeloproliferative disorders, hepatitis B infection, malnutrition, short-bowel syndrome, inflammatory bowel disease, and malabsorption disorders.

TREATMENT Glucagonomas

In 50–80% of patients, hepatic metastases are present, and so curative surgical resection is not possible. Surgical debulking in patients with advanced disease or other antitumor treatments may be beneficial (see below). Long-acting somatostatin analogues such as octreotide and lanreotide improve the skin rash in 75% of patients and may improve the weight loss, pain, and diarrhea but usually do not improve the glucose intolerance.

SOMATOSTATINOMA SYNDROME

The somatostatinoma syndrome is due to an NET that secretes excessive amounts of somatostatin, which causes a distinct syndrome

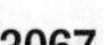

characterized by diabetes mellitus, gallbladder disease, diarrhea, and steatorrhea. There is no general distinction in the literature between a tumor that contains somatostatin-like immunoreactivity (somatostatinoma) and does (11–45%) or does not (55–90%) produce a clinical syndrome (somatostatinoma syndrome) by secreting somatostatin. In a review of 173 cases of somatostatinomas, only 11% were associated with the somatostatinoma syndrome. The mean age is 51 years. Somatostatinomas occur primarily in the pancreas and small intestine, and the frequency of the symptoms and occurrence of the somatostatinoma syndrome differ in each. Each of the usual symptoms is more common in pancreatic than in intestinal somatostatinomas: diabetes mellitus (95% vs. 21%), gallbladder disease (94% vs. 43%), diarrhea (92% vs. 38%), steatorrhea (83% vs. 12%), hypochlorhydria (86% vs. 12%), and weight loss (90% vs. 69%). The somatostatinoma syndrome occurs in 30–90% of pancreatic and 0–5% of small-intestinal somatostatinomas. In various series 43% of all duodenal NETs contain somatostatin; however, the somatostatinoma syndrome is rarely present (<2%). Somatostatinomas occur in the pancreas in 56–74% of cases, with the primary location being the pancreatic head. The tumors are usually solitary (90%) and large (mean size 4.5 cm). Liver metastases are common, being present in 69–84% of patients. Somatostatinomas are rare in patients with MEN 1, occurring in only 0.65%.

Somatostatin is a tetradecapeptide that is widely distributed in the CNS and GI tract, where it functions as a neurotransmitter or has paracrine and autocrine actions. It is a potent inhibitor of many processes, including release of almost all hormones, acid secretion, intestinal and pancreatic secretion, and intestinal absorption. Most of the clinical manifestations are directly related to these inhibitory actions.

Diagnosis

In most cases somatostatinomas have been found by accident either at the time of cholecystectomy or during endoscopy. The presence of psammoma bodies in a duodenal tumor should particularly raise suspicion. Duodenal somatostatin-containing tumors are increasingly associated with von Recklinghausen's disease. Most of these tumors (>98%) do not cause the somatostatinoma syndrome. The diagnosis of the somatostatinoma syndrome requires the demonstration of elevated plasma somatostatin levels.

TREATMENT Somatostatinomas

Pancreatic tumors are frequently (70–92%) metastatic at presentation, whereas 30–69% of small-intestinal somatostatinomas have metastases. Surgery is the treatment of choice for those without widespread hepatic metastases. Symptoms in patients with the somatostatinoma syndrome are also improved by octreotide treatment.

VIPOMAS

VIPomas are endocrine tumors that secrete excessive amounts of vasoactive intestinal peptide, which causes a distinct syndrome characterized by large-volume diarrhea, hypokalemia, and dehydration. This syndrome also is called Verner-Morrison syndrome, pancreatic cholera, and WDHA syndrome for *w*atery *d*iarrhea, *h*ypokalemia, and *a*chlorhydria, which some patients develop. The mean age of patients with this syndrome is 49 years; however, it can occur in children, and when it does, it is usually caused by a ganglioneuroma or ganglioneuroblastoma.

The principal symptoms are large-volume diarrhea (100%) severe enough to cause hypokalemia (80–100%), dehydration (83%), hypochlorhydria (54–76%), and flushing (20%). The diarrhea is secretory in nature, persisting during fasting, and is almost always >1 L/d and in 70% is >3 L/d. In a number of studies, the diarrhea was intermittent initially in up to half the patients. Most patients do not have accompanying steatorrhea (16%), and the increased stool volume is due to increased excretion of sodium and potassium, which, with the anions, accounts for the osmolality of the stool. Patients frequently have hyperglycemia (25–50%) and hypercalcemia (25–50%).

VIP is a 28-amino-acid peptide that is an important neurotransmitter, ubiquitously present in the CNS and GI tract. Its known actions include stimulation of small-intestinal chloride secretion as well as effects on smooth muscle contractility, inhibition of acid secretion, and vasodilatory effects, which explain most features of the clinical syndrome.

In adults 80–90% of VIPomas are pancreatic in location, with the rest due to VIP-secreting pheochromocytomas, intestinal carcinoids, and rarely ganglioneuromas. These tumors are usually solitary, 50–75% are in the pancreatic tail, and 37–68% have hepatic metastases at diagnosis. In children <10 years old, the syndrome is usually due to ganglioneuromas or ganglioblastomas and is less often malignant (10%).

Diagnosis

The diagnosis requires the demonstration of an elevated plasma VIP level and the presence of large-volume diarrhea. A stool volume <700 mL/d is proposed to exclude the diagnosis of VIPoma. When the patient fasts, a number of diseases can be excluded that can cause marked diarrhea. Other diseases that can produce a secretory large-volume diarrhea include gastrinomas, chronic laxative abuse, carcinoid syndrome, systemic mastocytosis, rarely medullary thyroid cancer, diabetic diarrhea, sprue, and AIDS. Among these conditions, only VIPomas caused a marked increase in plasma VIP. Chronic surreptitious use of laxatives/diuretics can be particularly difficult to detect clinically. Hence, in a patient with unexplained chronic diarrhea, screens for laxatives should be performed; they will detect many, but not all, laxative abusers.

TREATMENT Vasoactive Intestinal Peptidomas

The most important initial treatment in these patients is to correct their dehydration, hypokalemia, and electrolyte losses with fluid and electrolyte replacement. These patients may require 5 L/d of fluid and >350 meq/d of potassium. Because 37–68% of adults with VIPomas have metastatic disease in the liver at presentation, a significant number of patients cannot be cured surgically. In these patients long-acting somatostatin analogues such as octreotide and lanreotide are the drugs of choice.

Octreotide/lanreotide will control the diarrhea short- and long-term in 75–100% of patients. In nonresponsive patients the combination of glucocorticoids and octreotide/lanreotide has proved helpful in a small number of patients. Other drugs reported to be helpful in small numbers of patients include prednisone (60–100 mg/d), clonidine, indomethacin, phenothiazines, loperamide, lidamidine, lithium, propranolol, and metoclopramide. Treatment of advanced disease with embolization, chemoembolization, chemotherapy, radiotherapy, radiofrequency ablation, and peptide receptor radiotherapy may be helpful (see below).

NONFUNCTIONAL PANCREATIC ENDOCRINE TUMORS (NF-PETs)

NF-PETs are endocrine tumors that originate in the pancreas and secrete no products, or their products do not cause a specific clinical syndrome. The symptoms are due entirely to the tumor per se. NF-PETs secrete chromogranin A (90–100%), chromogranin B (90–100%), PP (58%), α-HCG (human chorionic gonadotropin) (40%), and β-HCG (20%). Because the symptoms are due to the tumor mass, patients with NF-PETs usually present late in the disease course with invasive tumors and hepatic metastases (64–92%) and the tumors are usually large (72% >5 cm). NF-PETs are usually solitary except in patients with MEN 1, in which case they are multiple. They occur primarily in the pancreatic head. Even though these tumors do not cause a functional syndrome, immunocytochemical studies show that they synthesize numerous peptides and cannot be distinguished from functional tumors by immunocytochemistry. In MEN 1, 80–100% of patients have microscopic NF-PETs, but they become large or symptomatic in only a minority (0–13%) of cases. In VHL 12–17% develop NF-PETs, and in 4% they are ≥3 cm in diameter.

The most common symptoms are abdominal pain (30–80%), jaundice (20–35%), and weight loss, fatigue, or bleeding; 10–30% are found incidentally. The average time from the beginning of symptoms to diagnosis is 5 years.

Diagnosis

The diagnosis is established by histologic confirmation in a patient without either the clinical symptoms or the elevated plasma hormone levels of one of the established syndromes. The principal difficulty in diagnosis is to distinguish an NF-PET from a nonendocrine pancreatic tumor, which is more common. Even though chromogranin A levels are elevated in almost every patient, this is not specific for this disease as it can be found in functional PETs, carcinoids, and other neuroendocrine disorders. Plasma pancreatic polypeptide is increased in 22–71% of patients and should strongly suggest the diagnosis in a patient with a pancreatic mass because it is usually normal in patients with pancreatic adenocarcinomas. Elevated plasma PP is not diagnostic of this tumor because it is elevated in a number of other conditions, such as chronic renal failure, old age, inflammatory conditions, and diabetes. A positive somatostatin receptor scan in a patient with a pancreatic mass should suggest the presence of PET/NF-PET rather than a nonendocrine tumor.

TREATMENT Nonfunctional Pancreatic Endocrine Tumors

Overall survival in patients with sporadic NF-PET is 30–63% at 5 years, with a median survival of 6 years. Unfortunately, surgical curative resection can be considered only in a minority of these patients because 64–92% present with metastatic disease. Treatment needs to be directed against the tumor per se using the various modalities discussed below for advanced disease. The treatment of NF-PETs in either MEN 1 patients or patients with VHL is controversial. Most recommend surgical resection for any tumor >2–3 cm in diameter; however, there is no consensus on smaller NF-PETs, with most recommending careful surveillance of these patients.

GRFOMAS

GRFomas are endocrine tumors that secrete excessive amounts of growth hormone–releasing factor (GRF) that cause acromegaly. GRF is a 44-amino-acid peptide, and 25–44% of PETs have GRF immunoreactivity, although it is uncommonly secreted. GRFomas are lung tumors in 47–54% of cases, PETs in 29–30%, and small-intestinal carcinoids in 8–10%; up to 12% occur at other sites. Patients have a mean age of 38 years, and the symptoms usually are due to either acromegaly or the tumor per se. The acromegaly caused by GRFomas is indistinguishable from classic acromegaly. The pancreatic tumors are usually large (>6 cm), and liver metastases are present in 39%. They should be suspected in any patient with acromegaly and an abdominal tumor, a patient with MEN 1 with acromegaly, or a patient without a pituitary adenoma with acromegaly or associated with hyperprolactinemia, which occurs in 70% of GRFomas. GRFomas are an uncommon cause of acromegaly. GRFomas occur in <1% of MEN 1 patients. The diagnosis is established by performing plasma assays for GRF and growth hormone. Most GRFomas have a plasma GRF level >300 pg/mL (normal <5 pg/mL men, <10 pg/mL women). Patients with GRFomas also have increased plasma levels of insulin-like growth factor type I (IGF-I) levels similar to those in classic acromegaly. Surgery is the treatment of choice if diffuse metastases are not present. Long-acting somatostatin analogues such as octreotide and lanreotide are the agents of choice, with 75–100% of patients responding.

OTHER RARE PANCREATIC ENDOCRINE TUMOR SYNDROMES

Cushing's syndrome (ACTHoma) due to a PET occurs in 4–16% of all ectopic Cushing's syndrome cases. It occurs in 5% of cases of sporadic gastrinomas, almost invariably in patients with hepatic metastases, and is an independent poor prognostic factor. Paraneoplastic hypercalcemia due to PETs releasing parathyroid hormone–related peptide (PTHrP), a PTH-like material, or unknown factor, is rarely reported. The tumors are usually large, and liver metastases are usually present. Most (88%) appear to be due to release of PTHrP. PETs occasionally can cause the carcinoid syndrome. PETs secreting calcitonin have been proposed as a specific clinical syndrome. One-half of the patients have diarrhea, which disappears with resection of the tumor. The proposal that this could be a discrete syndrome is supported by the finding that 25–42% of patients with medullary thyroid cancer with hypercalcitonemia develop diarrhea, probably secondary to a motility disorder. This is classified in Table 350-2 as a possible specific disorder because so few cases have been described. Similarly classified with only a few cases described are a renin-producing PET in a patient presenting with hypertension; PETs secreting luteinizing hormone, resulting in masculinization or decreased libido; a PET-secreting erythropoietin resulting in polycythemia; and PETs secreting insulin-like growth factor II causing hypoglycemia (Table 350-2). Ghrelin is a 28-amino-acid peptide with a number of metabolic functions. Even though it is detectable immunohistochemically in most PETs, no specific syndrome is associated with release of ghrelin by the PET.

TUMOR LOCALIZATION

Localization of the primary tumor and knowledge of the extent of the disease are essential to the proper management of all carcinoids and PETs. Without proper localization studies it is not possible to determine whether the patient is a candidate for curative resection or cytoreductive surgery or requires antitumor treatment or to predict the patient's prognosis reliably.

Numerous tumor localization methods are used in both types of NETs, including conventional imaging studies (computed tomographic scanning, magnetic resonance imaging, transabdominal ultrasound, selective angiography), somatostatin receptor scintigraphy (SRS), and positron emission tomographic scanning. In PETs, endoscopic ultrasound (EUS) and functional localization by measuring venous hormonal gradients are also reported to be useful. Bronchial carcinoids are usually detected by standard chest radiography and assessed by CT. Rectal, duodenal, colonic, and gastric carcinoids are usually detected by GI endoscopy.

PETs, as well as carcinoid tumors, frequently overexpress high-affinity somatostatin receptors in both their primary tumors and their metastases. Of the five types of somatostatin receptors (sst_{1-5}), radiolabeled octreotide binds with high affinity to sst_2 and sst_5, has a lower affinity for sst_3, and has a very low affinity for sst_1 and sst_4. Between 90 and 100% of carcinoid tumors and PETs possess sst_2, and many also have the other four sst subtypes. Interaction with these receptors can be used to localize NETs by using [^{111}In-DTPA-D-Phe^1]octreotide and radionuclide scanning (SRS) as well as for treatment of the hormone-excess state with octreotide or lanreotide, as discussed earlier. Because of its sensitivity and ability to localize tumor throughout the body, SRS is the initial imaging modality of choice for localizing both the primary and metastatic NETs. SRS localizes tumor in 73–89% of patients with carcinoids and in 56–100% of patients with PETs, except insulinomas. Insulinomas are usually small and have low densities of sst receptors, resulting in SRS being positive in only 12–50% of patients with insulinomas. Figure 350-3 shows an example of the increased sensitivity of SRS in a patient with a carcinoid tumor. The CT scan showed a single liver metastasis, whereas the SRS demonstrated three metastases in the liver in multiple locations. Occasional false-positive responses with SRS can occur (12% in one study) because numerous other normal tissues as well as diseases can have high densities of sst receptors, including granulomas (sarcoid, tuberculosis, etc.), thyroid diseases (goiter, thyroiditis), and activated lymphocytes (lymphomas, wound infections). For PETs in the pancreas, EUS is highly sensitive, localizing 77–100% of insulinomas, which occur almost exclusively within the pancreas. Endoscopic ultrasound is less sensitive for extrapancreatic tumors. It is increasingly used in patients with MEN 1 and to a lesser extent VHL to detect small PETs not seen with other modalities or for serial PET assessments to determine size changes or rapid growth in patients in whom surgery is deferred. EUS with cytologic evaluation also is used frequently to distinguish an NF-PET from a pancreatic adenocarcinoma or another nonendocrine pancreatic tumor.

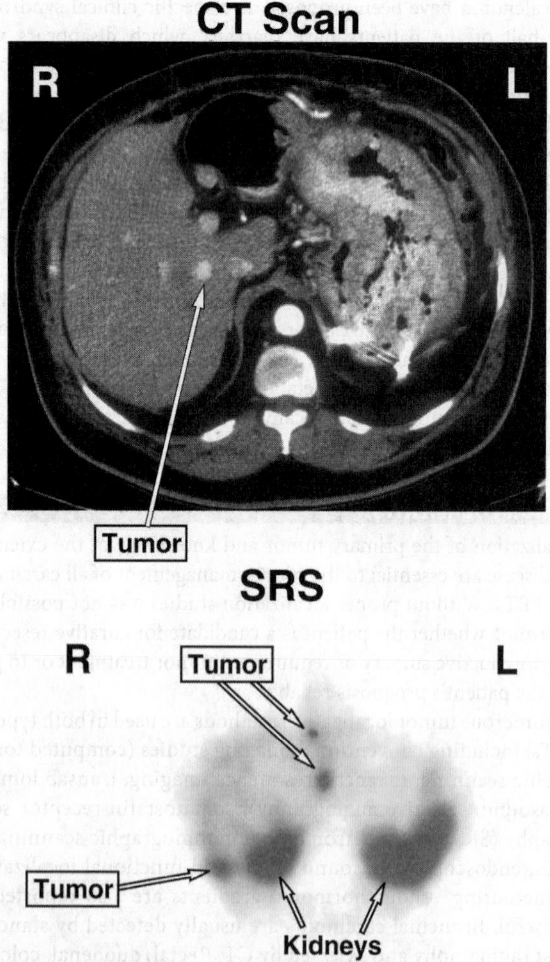

Figure 350-3 Ability of CT scanning (*top*) or somatostatin receptor scintigraphy (SRS) (*bottom*) to localize metastatic carcinoid in the liver.

Insulinomas overexpress receptors for GLP-1; a radiolabeled GLP-1 analogue can detect occult insulinomas not localized by other imaging modalities. Functional localization by measuring hormonal gradients is now uncommonly used with gastrinomas (after intraarterial secretin injections) but is still frequently used in insulinoma patients in whom other imaging studies are negative (assessing hepatic vein insulin concentrations post-intraarterial calcium injections). The intraarterial calcium test may also allow differentiation of the cause of the hypoglycemia and indicate whether it is due to an insulinoma or a nesidioblastosis. The latter entity is becoming increasingly important because hypoglycemia after gastric bypass surgery for obesity is increasing in frequency, and it is primarily due to nesidioblastosis, although it can occasionally be due to an insulinoma.

If liver metastases are identified by SRS, to plan the proper treatment either a CT or an MRI is recommended to assess the size and exact location of the metastases because SRS does not provide information on tumor size. Functional localization measuring hormone gradients after intraarterial calcium injections in insulinomas (insulin) or gastrin gradients after secretin injections in gastrinoma is a sensitive method, being positive in 80–100% of patients. However, this method provides only regional localization and therefore is reserved for cases in which the other imaging modalities are negative.

Two newer imaging modalities (positron emission tomography and use of hybrid scanners such as CT and SRS) may have increased sensitivity. Positron emission tomographic scanning with ^{18}F-fluoro-DOPA in patients with carcinoids or with ^{11}C-5-HTP or ^{68}gallium-labeled somatostatin analogues in patients with PETs or carcinoids has greater sensitivity than conventional imaging studies or SRS and probably will be used increasingly in the future. Positron emission tomographic scanning for GI NETs is not currently approved in the United States.

TREATMENT Advanced Disease (Diffuse Metastatic Disease)

The single most important prognostic factor for survival is the presence of liver metastases (Fig. 350-4). For patients with foregut carcinoids without hepatic metastases, the 5-year survival in one study was 95%, and with distant metastases, it was 20% (Fig. 350-4, bottom). With gastrinomas the 5-year survival without liver metastases is 98%; with limited metastases in one hepatic lobe, it is 78%; and with diffuse metastases, 16% (Fig. 350-4, top). In a large study of 156 patients (67 PETs, rest carcinoids) the overall 5-year survival rate was 77%; it was 96% without liver metastases, 73% with liver metastases, and 50% with distant disease. Therefore, treatment for advanced metastatic disease is an important challenge. A number of different modalities are reported to be effective, including cytoreductive surgery [surgically or by radio frequency ablation (RFA)], treatment with chemotherapy, somatostatin analogues, interferon α, hepatic embolization alone or with chemotherapy (chemoembolization), radiotherapy with radiolabeled beads/microspheres, peptide radio-receptor therapy, and liver transplantation.

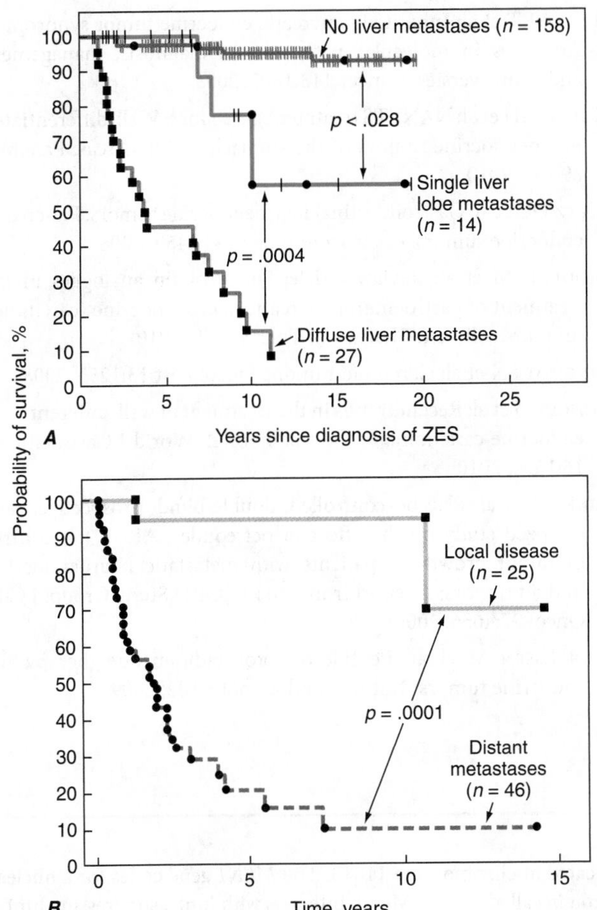

Figure 350-4 Effect of the presence and extent of liver metastases on survival in patients with gastrinomas **(A)** or carcinoid tumors **(B)**. ZES, Zollinger-Ellison syndrome. *(Top panel is drawn from data from 199 patients with gastrinomas modified from F Yu et al: J Clin Oncol 17:615, 1999. Bottom panel is drawn from data from 71 patients with foregut carcinoid tumors from EW McDermott et al: Br J Surg 81:1007, 1994.)*

SPECIFIC ANTITUMOR TREATMENTS Cytoreductive surgery, unfortunately, is possible in only 9–22% of patients who present with limited hepatic metastases. Although no randomized studies have proved that it extends life, results from a number of studies suggest that it probably increases survival; therefore, it is recommended, if possible. Radio frequency thermal ablation can be applied to GI NET liver metastases if they are limited in number (usually <5) and size (usually <3.5 cm in diameter). Response rates are >80%, the morbidity rate is low, and this procedure may be particularly helpful in patients with functional PETs that are difficult to control medically.

Chemotherapy for metastatic carcinoid tumors has generally been disappointing, with response rates of 0–40% with various two- and three-drug combinations. Chemotherapy for PETs has been more successful, with tumor shrinkage reported in 30–70% of patients. The current regimen of choice is streptozotocin and doxorubicin. In poorly differentiated PETs, chemotherapy with cisplatin, etoposide, or their derivatives is the recommended treatment, with response rates of 40–70%; however, responses are generally short-lived. Some newer combinations of chemotherapeutic agents show promise in small numbers of patients, including temozolomide (TMZ) alone, especially in PETs, which frequently have O^6-methylguanine DNA methyltransferase deficiency, which increases their TMZ sensitivity (34% response rate), and TMZ plus capecitabine (response rate 59–71%, retrospective studies).

Long-acting somatostatin analogues such as octreotide, lanreotide, and interferon α rarely decrease tumor size (i.e., 0–17%); however, these drugs have tumoristatic effects, stopping additional growth in 26–95% of patients with NETs. A randomized, double-blind study in patients with metastatic midgut carcinoids demonstrated a marked lengthening of time to progression (14.3 vs. 6 months, $p = .000072$) from the use of octreotide-LAR. This improvement was seen in patients with limited liver involvement. Whether this change will result in extended survival has not been proved. Somatostatin analogues can induce apoptosis in carcinoid tumors, and interferon α can decrease Bcl-2 protein expression, which probably contributes to its antiproliferative effects.

Hepatic embolization and chemoembolization (with dacarbazine, cisplatin, doxorubicin, 5-fluorouracil, or streptozotocin) have been reported to decrease tumor bulk and help control the symptoms of the hormone-excess state. These modalities generally are reserved for liver-directed therapy in cases in which treatment with somatostatin analogues, interferon (carcinoids), or chemotherapy (PETs) fails. Embolization, when combined with treatment with octreotide and interferon α, significantly reduces tumor progression ($p = .008$) compared with treatment with embolization and octreotide alone in patients with advanced midgut carcinoids.

Radiotherapy with radiolabeled somatostatin analogues that are internalized by the tumors is being investigated. Three different radionuclides are being used. High doses of [^{111}In-DTPA-D-Phe^1]octreotide, which emits γ-rays, internal conversion, and Auger electrons; yttrium-90, which emits high-energy β-particles coupled by a DOTA chelating group to octreotide or octreotate; and ^{177}lutetium-coupled analogues, which emit both, are all in clinical studies. ^{111}Indium-, ^{90}yttrium-, and ^{177}lutetium-labeled compounds caused tumor stabilization in 41–81%, 44–88%, and 23–40%, respectively, and a decrease in tumor size in 8–30%, 6–37%, and 38%, respectively, of patients with advanced metastatic NETs. Use of ^{177}Lu-labeled analogues to treat 504 patients with malignant NETs produced a reduction of tumor size of >50% in 30% of patients (2% complete) and tumor stabilization in 51%. An effect on survival has not been established. These results suggest that this novel therapy may be helpful, especially in patients with widespread metastatic disease.

Selective internal radiation therapy (SIRT) using ^{90}yttrium glass or resin microspheres is being evaluated in patients with unresectable NET liver metastases. The treatment requires careful evaluation for vascular shunting before treatment and generally is reserved for patients without extrahepatic metastatic disease and with adequate hepatic reserve. The ^{90}Y-microspheres are delivered to the liver by intraarterial injection from percutaneous placed catheters. In four studies involving metastatic NETs, the response rate varied from 50–61% (partial or complete), tumor stabilization occurred in 22–41%, and overall survival varied from 25–70 months. In the largest study (148 patients), no radiation-induced liver failure occurred and the most common side effect was fatigue (6.5%).

The use of liver transplantation has been abandoned for treatment of most metastatic tumors to the liver. However, for metastatic NETs, it is still a consideration. In a review of 103 cases of malignant NETs (48 PETs, 43 carcinoids) the 2- and 5-year survival rates were 60% and 47%, respectively. However, recurrence-free survival was low (<24%). For younger patients with metastatic NETs limited to the liver, liver transplantation may be justified.

Newer approaches show some promise in the treatment of advanced GI NETs. They include the use of growth factor inhibitors or inhibitors of their receptors (using tyrosine kinase inhibitors, monoclonal antibodies), inhibitors of mTor signaling (everolimus, temsirolimus), angiogenesis inhibitors, and VEGF or vascular endothelial growth factor receptor (VEGFR) tyrosine kinase inhibitors. A number of these agents, particularly sunitinib (tyrosine kinase inhibitor), various mTor inhibitors, and bevacizumub (monoclonal antibody against VEGF), show impressive activity. Additional value may result from selected combinations of agents.

FURTHER READINGS

Boudreaux JP et al: The NANETS consensus guideline for the diagnosis and management of neuroendocrine tumors: Well-differentiated neuroendocrine tumors of the jejunum, ileum, appendix, and cecum. Pancreas 2010 39:753, 2010

Capurso G et al: Molecular target therapy for gastroenteropancreatic endocrine tumours: Biological rationale and clinical perspectives. Crit Rev Oncol Hematol 72:110, 2009

Clark OH et al: NCCN Clinical Practice Guidelines in Oncology: Neuroendocrine tumors. J Natl Compr Canc Netw 7:712, 2009

Jensen RT et al: Inherited pancreatic endocrine tumor syndromes: Advances in molecular pathogenesis, diagnosis, management and controversies. Cancer 113:1807, 2008

Kulke MH et al: NANETS treatment guidelines: Well-differentiated neuroendocrine tumors of the stomach and pancreas. Pancreas 39:735, 2010

Metz DC et al: Gastrointestinal neuroendocrine tumors: Pancreatic endocrine tumors. Gastroenterology 135:1469, 2008

Modlin IM et al: Review article: Somatostatin analogues in the treatment of gastroenteropancreatic neuroendocrine (carcinoid) tumours. Aliment Pharmacol Ther 31:169, 2010

Pinchot SN et al: Carcinoid tumors. Oncologist 13:1255, 2008

Poncet G et al: Recent trends in the treatment of well-differentiated endocrine carcinoma of the small bowel. World J Gastroenterol 16:1696, 2010

Rinke A et al: Placebo-controlled, double-blind, prospective, randomized study on the effect of octreotide LAR in the control of tumor growth in patients with metastatic neuroendocrine midgut tumors: A report from the PROMID Study Group. J Clin Oncol 27:4656, 2009

Van Essen M et al: Peptide-receptor radionuclide therapy for endocrine tumors. Nat Rev Endocrinol 5:382, 2009

CHAPTER 351

Disorders Affecting Multiple Endocrine Systems

Camilo Jimenez Vasquez
Robert F. Gagel

NEOPLASTIC DISORDERS AFFECTING MULTIPLE ENDOCRINE ORGANS

Multiple endocrine neoplasia syndrome is defined as a disorder with neoplasms in two or more different hormonal tissues in several members of a family. Several distinct genetic disorders predispose to endocrine gland neoplasia and cause hormone excess syndromes (Table 351-1). DNA-based genetic testing is available for these disorders, but effective management requires an understanding of endocrine neoplasia and the range of clinical features that may be manifested in an individual patient.

MULTIPLE ENDOCRINE NEOPLASIA (MEN) TYPE 1

MEN 1, or Wermer's syndrome, is inherited as an autosomal dominant trait. This syndrome is characterized by neoplasia of the parathyroid glands, enteropancreatic tumors, anterior pituitary adenomas, and other neuroendocrine tumors with variable penetrance (Table 351-1). Although rare, MEN 1 is the most common multiple endocrine neoplasia syndrome, with an estimated prevalence of 2–20 per 100,000 in the general population. It is caused by inactivating mutations of the tumor-suppressor gene *MEN1* located at chromosome 11q13. The *MEN1* gene codes for a nuclear protein called Menin. Menin interacts with JunD, suppressing JunD-dependent transcriptional activation. It is unclear how this accounts for Menin growth regulatory activity, since JunD is associated with inhibition of cell growth. Each child born to an affected parent has a 50% probability of inheriting the gene. The variable penetrance of the several neoplastic components can make the differential diagnosis and treatment challenging.

Clinical manifestations

Primary hyperparathyroidism is the most common manifestation of MEN 1, with an estimated penetrance of 95–100%. Hypercalcemia may develop during the teenage years, and most individuals are affected by age 40 (Fig. 351-1). Hyperparathyroidism is the earliest manifestation of the syndrome in most MEN 1 patients. The neoplastic changes in hyperparathyroidism provide a specific example of one of the cardinal features of endocrine tumors in MEN 1: multicentricity. The neoplastic changes inevitably affect multiple parathyroid glands, making surgical cure difficult. Screening for hyperparathyroidism involves measurement of either an albumin-adjusted or an ionized serum calcium level. The diagnosis is established by demonstrating elevated levels of serum calcium and intact parathyroid hormone. Manifestations of hyperparathyroidism in MEN 1 do not differ substantially from those in sporadic hyperparathyroidism and include calcium-containing kidney stones, kidney failure, nephrocalcinosis, bone abnormalities (i.e., osteoporosis, osteitis fibrosa cystica), and gastrointestinal and musculoskeletal complaints. Management is challenging because of early onset, significant recurrence rates, and the multiplicity of parathyroid gland involvement. Differentiation of hyperparathyroidism of MEN 1 from other forms of familial primary hyperparathyroidism usually is based on family history, histologic features of resected parathyroid tissue, the presence of a *MEN1* mutation, and, sometimes, long-term observation to determine whether other manifestations of MEN 1 develop. Parathyroid hyperplasia is the most common cause of hyperparathyroidism in MEN 1, although single

TABLE 351-1 Disease Associations in the Multiple Endocrine Neoplasia (MEN) Syndromes

MEN 1	MEN 2	Mixed Syndromes
Parathyroid hyperplasia or adenoma	**MEN 2A**	**Von Hippel–Lindau syndrome**
Islet cell hyperplasia, adenoma, or carcinoma	MTC	Pheochromocytoma
Pituitary hyperplasia or adenoma	Pheochromocytoma	Islet cell tumor
Other, less common manifestations: foregut carcinoid, pheochromocytoma, subcutaneous or visceral lipomas	Parathyroid hyperplasia or adenoma	Renal cell carcinoma
	MEN 2A with cutaneous lichen amyloidosis	Hemangioblastoma of central nervous system
	MEN 2A with Hirschsprung disease	Retinal angiomas
	Familial MTC	**Neurofibromatosis with features of MEN 1 or 2**
	MEN 2B	**Carney complex**
	MTC	Myxomas of heart, skin, and breast
	Pheochromocytoma	Spotty cutaneous pigmentation
	Mucosal and gastrointestinal neuromas	Testicular, adrenal, and GH-producing pituitary tumors
	Marfanoid features	Peripheral nerve schwannomas
		Familial growth hormone or prolactin-producing pituitary tumors

Abbreviations: GH, growth hormone; MTC, medullary thyroid carcinoma.

and multiple adenomas have been described. Hyperplasia of one or more parathyroid glands is common in younger patients; adenomas usually are found in older patients or those with long-standing disease.

Enteropancreatic tumors are the second most common manifestation of MEN 1, with an estimated penetrance of 50%. They tend to occur in parallel with hyperparathyroidism (Fig. 351-1); 30% are malignant. Most of these tumors secrete peptide hormones that cause specific clinical syndromes. Those syndromes, however, may have an insidious onset and a slow progression, making their diagnosis difficult and in many cases delayed. Some enteropancreatic tumors do not secrete hormones. Those "silent" tumors usually are found during radiographic screening. Metastasis, most commonly to the liver, occurs in about a third of patients.

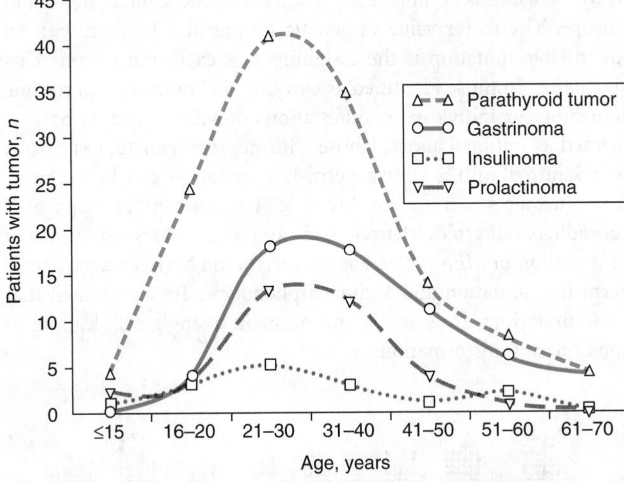

Figure 351-1 Age at onset of endocrine tumor expression in multiple endocrine neoplasia type 1 (MEN 1). Data derived from retrospective analysis for each endocrine organ hyperfunction in 130 cases of MEN 1. Age at onset is the age at first symptom or, with tumors not causing symptoms, age at the time of the first abnormal finding on a screening test. The rate of diagnosis of hyperparathyroidism increased sharply between ages 16 and 20 years. *(Reprinted with permission from S Marx et al: Ann Intern Med 129:484, 1998.)*

Gastrinomas are the most common enteropancreatic tumors observed in MEN 1 patients and result in the Zollinger-Ellison syndrome (ZES). ZES is caused by excessive gastrin production and occurs in more than one-half of MEN 1 patients with small carcinoid-like tumors in the duodenal wall or, less often, by pancreatic islet cell tumors. There may be more than one gastrin-producing tumor, making localization difficult. The robust acid production may cause esophagitis, duodenal ulcers throughout the duodenum, ulcers involving the proximal jejunum, and diarrhea. The ulcer diathesis is commonly refractory to conservative therapy such as antacids. The diagnosis is made by finding increased gastric acid secretion, elevated basal gastrin levels in the serum [generally >115 pmol/L (200 pg/mL)], and an exaggerated response of serum gastrin to either secretin or calcium. Other causes of elevated serum gastrin levels, such as achlorhydria, treatment with H_2 receptor antagonists or proton pump inhibitors, retained gastric antrum, small-bowel resection, gastric outlet obstruction, and hypercalcemia, should be excluded (Fig. 351-1). High-resolution, early-phase CT scanning, abdominal MRI with contrast, octreotide scan, and/or endoscopic ultrasound are the best preoperative techniques for identification of the primary and metastatic gastrinoma; intraoperative ultrasonography is the most sensitive method for detection of small tumors. Approximately one-fourth of all cases of ZES occur in the context of MEN 1.

Insulinomas are the second most common enteropancreatic tumors in patients who have MEN 1. Unlike gastrinomas, most insulinomas originate in the pancreas bed, becoming the most common pancreatic tumor in MEN 1. Hypoglycemia caused by insulinomas is observed in about one-third of MEN 1 patients with pancreatic islet cell tumors (Fig. 351-1). The tumors may be benign or malignant (25%). The diagnosis can be suggested by documenting hypoglycemia during a short fast with simultaneous inappropriate elevation of serum insulin and C-peptide levels. More commonly, it is necessary to subject the patient to a supervised 12- to 72-h fast to provoke hypoglycemia (Chap. 345). Large insulinomas may be identified by CT or MRI scanning; small tumors not detected by conventional radiographic techniques may be localized by endoscopic ultrasound or selective arteriographic injection of calcium into each of the arteries that supply the pancreas and sampling of the hepatic vein for insulin to determine the anatomic region containing the tumor. Intraoperative ultrasonography is used frequently to localize these tumors. The trend toward earlier diagnosis of, hence, smaller tumors has reduced the usefulness of octreotide scanning, which is positive in a minority of these patients.

Glucagonoma, which is seen occasionally in MEN 1, causes a syndrome of hyperglycemia, skin rash (necrolytic migratory erythema), anorexia, glossitis, anemia, depression, diarrhea, and venous thrombosis. In about half of these patients the plasma glucagon level is high, leading to its designation as the *glucagonoma syndrome*, although elevation of the plasma glucagon level in MEN 1 patients is not necessarily associated with these symptoms. Some patients with this syndrome also have elevated plasma ghrelin levels. The glucagonoma syndrome may represent a complex interaction between glucagon and ghrelin overproduction and the nutritional status of the patient.

The *Verner-Morrison*, or *watery diarrhea, syndrome* consists of watery diarrhea, hypokalemia, hypochlorhydria, and metabolic acidosis. The diarrhea can be voluminous and almost always is found in association with an islet cell tumor in the context of MEN 1, prompting use of the term *pancreatic cholera*. However, when not associated with MEN 1, the syndrome outside of MEN 1 is not restricted to pancreatic islet tumors and has been observed with carcinoids or other tumors. This syndrome is believed to be due to overproduction of vasoactive intestinal peptide (VIP), although plasma VIP levels may not be elevated. Hypercalcemia may be induced by the effects of VIP to stimulate osteoclastic bone resorption as well as by hyperparathyroidism. Other disorders that should be considered in the differential diagnosis of chronic diarrhea include infectious or parasitic diseases, inflammatory bowel disease, sprue, and other endocrine causes such as ZES, carcinoid, and medullary thyroid carcinoma.

The pancreatic neoplasms differ from the other components of MEN 1 in that approximately one-third of the tumors display malignant features, including hepatic metastases. The pancreatic neoplasms also can be used to highlight another characteristic of MEN 1: the specific impact of a hormone produced by one component of MEN 1 on another neoplastic component of this syndrome. Specific examples include the effects of either corticotropin-releasing hormone (CRH) or growth hormone–releasing hormone (GHRH) production by an islet cell tumor to cause a syndrome of excess adrenocorticotropin (ACTH) (Cushing's disease) or GH (acromegaly) production by the pituitary gland. These secondary interactions add complexity to the diagnosis and management of these tumor syndromes. Pancreatic islet cell tumors are diagnosed by identification of a characteristic clinical syndrome, hormonal assays with or without provocative stimuli, or radiographic techniques. One approach involves annual screening of individuals at risk with measurement of basal and meal-stimulated levels of pancreatic polypeptide to identify the tumors as early as possible; the rationale for this screening strategy is the concept that surgical removal of islet cell tumors at an early stage will be curative. Other approaches to screening include measurement of serum gastrin and pancreatic polypeptide levels every 2–3 years, with the rationale that pancreatic neoplasms will be detected at a later stage but can be managed medically, if possible, or by surgery. High-resolution, early-phase CT scanning or endoscopic ultrasound provides the best preoperative technique for identification of these tumors; intraoperative ultrasonography is the most sensitive method for detection of small tumors. Although fluorodeoxyglucose–positron emission tomography (FDG-PET) scanning detects ~50% of pancreatic islet cell tumors, most of these tumors are large; as most of these tumors can be identified by CT or ultrasound, the lack of sensitivity for small tumors makes FDG-PET scanning unhelpful for early diagnosis.

Pituitary tumors occur in 20–30% of patients with MEN 1 and tend to be multicentric. These tumors can exhibit aggressive behavior and local invasiveness that makes them difficult to resect (Chap. 339). Prolactinomas are the most common (Fig. 351-1) and are diagnosed by finding serum prolactin levels >200 μg/L with or without a pituitary mass evident on MRI. Values <200 μg/L may be due to a prolactin-secreting neoplasm or to compression of the pituitary stalk by a different type of pituitary tumor. Acromegaly due to excessive GH production is the second most common syndrome caused by pituitary tumors in MEN 1 and can rarely be due to production of GHRH by an islet cell tumor (see above). The possibility of hereditary growth hormone– or prolactin-secreting tumors (discussed below in "Other Genetic Endocrine Tumor Syndromes") should be considered in the differential diagnosis. Cushing's disease can be caused by ACTH-producing pituitary tumors or by ectopic production of ACTH or CRH by other components of the MEN 1 syndrome, including islet cell or carcinoid tumors or adrenal adenomas. Diagnosis of pituitary Cushing's disease is generally best accomplished by a high-dose dexamethasone suppression test or by petrosal venous sinus sampling for ACTH after IV injection of CRH. Differentiation of a primary pituitary tumor from an ectopic CRH-producing tumor may be difficult because the pituitary is the source of ACTH in both disorders; documentation of CRH production by a pancreatic islet or carcinoid tumor may be the only method of proving ectopic CRH production.

Adrenal cortical tumors are found in almost one-half of gene carriers but are rarely functional; malignancy in cortical adenomas is uncommon. Rare cases of pheochromocytoma have been described in the context of MEN 1. Due to their rarity, screening for these tumors is indicated only when there are suggestive symptoms.

Carcinoid tumors in MEN 1 are of the foregut type and are derived from thymus, lung, stomach, or duodenum; they may metastasize or be locally invasive. These tumors usually produce serotonin, calcitonin, or CRH; the typical carcinoid syndrome with flushing, diarrhea, and bronchospasm is rare (Chap. 350). Mediastinal carcinoid tumors (an upper mediastinal mass) are more common in men; bronchial carcinoid tumors are more common in women. Carcinoid tumors are a late manifestation of MEN 1; some reports have emphasized the importance of routine chest CT screening for mediastinal carcinoid tumors because of their high rate of malignant transformation and aggressive behavior.

Unusual manifestations of MEN 1 Subcutaneous or visceral lipomas and cutaneous leiomyomas also may be present but rarely undergo malignant transformation. Skin angiofibromas or collagenomas are seen in most patients with MEN 1 when carefully sought.

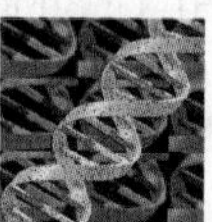

GENETIC CONSIDERATIONS

MEN1 gene mutations are found in >90% of families with the syndrome (Fig. 351-2). Genetic testing can be performed in individuals at risk for the development of MEN 1 and is commercially available in the United States and Europe. The major value of genetic testing in a kindred with an identifiable mutation is the assignment or exclusion of gene carrier status. In those identified as carrying the mutant gene, routine screening for individual manifestations of MEN 1 should be performed as outlined above. Those with negative genetic test results in a kindred with a known germ-line mutation can be excluded from further screening for MEN 1. A significant percentage of sporadic parathyroid, islet cell, and carcinoid tumors also have loss or mutation of *MEN1*. There is no correlation between a particular germ-line mutation and a clinical phenotype. It is presumed that these mutations are somatic and occur in a single cell, leading to subsequent transformation.

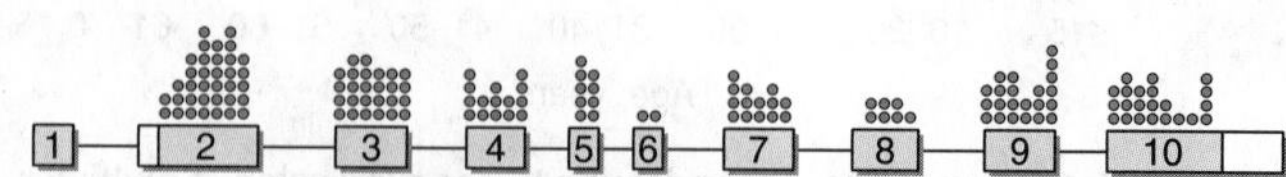

Figure 351-2 Schematic depiction of the MEN1 gene and the distribution of mutations. The shaded areas show coding sequence. The closed circles show the relative distribution of mutations, mostly inactivating, in each exon. Mutation data are derived from the Human Gene Mutation Database, from which more detailed information can be obtained at *www.uwcm.ac.uk/uwcm/mg/hgmd0.html. (From M Krawczak, DN Cooper: Trends Genet 13:1321, 1998.)*

TREATMENT Multiple Endocrine Neoplasia Type 1

Almost everyone who inherits a mutant *MEN1* gene develops at least one clinical manifestation of the syndrome. Most develop hyperparathyroidism, 80% develop pancreatic islet cell tumors, and more than half develop pituitary tumors. For most of these tumors, initial surgery is not curative and patients frequently require multiple surgical procedures and surgery on two or more endocrine glands during a lifetime. For this reason, it is essential to establish clear goals for management of these patients rather than to recommend surgery casually each time a tumor is discovered. Ranges for acceptable management are discussed below.

HYPERPARATHYROIDISM Individuals with serum calcium levels >3.0 mmol/L (12 mg/dL), evidence of calcium nephrolithiasis or renal dysfunction, neuropathic or muscular symptoms, or bone involvement (including osteopenia) and individuals <50 years of age should undergo parathyroid exploration. There is less agreement about the necessity for parathyroid exploration in individuals who do not meet these criteria, and observation may be appropriate in MEN 1 patients with asymptomatic hyperparathyroidism.

When parathyroid surgery is indicated in MEN 1, there are two approaches. In the first, all parathyroid tissue is identified and removed at the time of primary operation, and parathyroid tissue is implanted in the nondominant forearm. Thymectomy also should be performed because of the potential for later development of malignant carcinoid tumors. If reoperation for hyperparathyroidism is necessary at a later date, transplanted parathyroid tissue can be resected from the forearm with titration of tissue removal to lower the intact parathyroid hormone (PTH) to <50% of basal.

Another approach is to remove 3–3.5 parathyroid glands from the neck (leaving ~50 mg of parathyroid tissue), carefully marking the location of residual tissue so that the remaining tissue can be located easily during subsequent surgery. If this approach is used, intraoperative PTH measurements should be utilized to monitor adequacy of removal of parathyroid tissue with a goal of reducing postoperative serum intact PTH to ≤50% of basal values.

The use of high-resolution CT scanning (1 mm) and imaging during three phases of contrast flow has substantially improved the ability to identify aberrantly located parathyroid tissue. As this issue arises with some frequency in the context of parathyroid disease in MEN 1, this technique should be utilized to locate parathyroid tissue before reoperation for a failed exploration, and it may be useful before the initial operation.

PANCREATIC ISLET CELL TUMORS (See Chap. 350 for discussion of pancreatic islet cell tumors not associated with MEN 1.) Two features of pancreatic islet cell tumors in MEN 1 complicate management. First, the tumors are multicentric, are malignant about a third of the time, and cause death in 10–20% of patients. Second, performance of a total pancreatectomy to prevent malignancy causes diabetes mellitus, a disease with significant long-term complications that include neuropathy, retinopathy, and nephropathy. These features make it difficult to formulate clear-cut guidelines, but some general concepts appear to be valid. (1) Islet cell tumors producing insulin, glucagon, VIP, GHRH, or CRH should be resected because medical therapy for the hormonal effects of these tumors are generally ineffective. (2) Gastrin-producing islet cell tumors that cause ZES are frequently multicentric. Recent experience suggests that a high percentage of ZES in MEN 1 is caused by duodenal wall carcinoid tumors and that resection of these tumors improves the cure rate. Treatment with H_2 receptor antagonists (cimetidine or ranitidine) or proton pump inhibitors (omeprazole, lansoprazole, esomeprazole, etc.) provides an alternative, and some think preferable, therapy to surgery for control of ulcer disease in patients with multicentric tumors or hepatic metastases. (3) In families in which there is a high incidence of malignant islet cell tumors that cause death, total pancreatectomy at an early age may be considered to prevent malignancy, although it should be noted that this surgical intervention does not prevent the development of neuroendocrine tumors outside the pancreato-duodenal region.

Management of metastatic islet cell carcinoma is unsatisfactory. Hormonal abnormalities sometimes can be controlled. For example, ZES can be treated with H_2 receptor antagonists or proton pump inhibitors; the somatostatin analogues octreotide and lanreotide are useful in the management of carcinoid, glucagonoma, and the watery diarrhea syndrome. Bilateral adrenalectomy may be required for ectopic ACTH syndrome if medical therapy is ineffective (Chap. 342). Islet cell carcinomas frequently metastasize to the liver but may grow slowly. Hepatic artery embolization, radiofrequency ablation, or chemotherapy (5-fluorouracil, streptozocin, chlorozotocin, doxorubicin, or dacarbazine) may reduce tumor streptozotocin mass, control symptoms of hormone excess, and prolong life; however, these treatments are never curative. There is evolving evidence that everolimus, an inhibitor of mTor (mammalian target of rapamycin) causes regression of tumor size; 2 of 13 islet cell carcinomas and 2 of 12 carcinoid tumors had a >30% reduction in size and >60% had stable disease.

PITUITARY TUMORS Treatment of prolactinomas with dopamine agonists (bromocriptine, cabergoline, or quinagolide) usually returns the serum prolactin level to normal and prevents further tumor growth (Chap. 339). Surgical resection of a prolactinoma is rarely curative but may relieve mass effects. Transsphenoidal resection is appropriate for neoplasms that secrete ACTH, GH, or the α subunit of the pituitary glycoprotein hormones. Octreotide reduces tumor mass in one-third of GH-secreting tumors and reduces GH and insulin-like growth factor I levels in >75% of patients. Pegvisomant, a GH antagonist, rapidly lowers insulin-like growth factor levels in patients with acromegaly (Chap. 339). Radiation therapy may be useful for large or recurrent tumors.

Improvements in the management of MEN 1, particularly the earlier recognition of islet cell and pituitary tumors, have improved outcomes in these patients. As a result, other neoplastic manifestations that develop later in the course of this disorder, such as carcinoid syndrome, are now seen with increased frequency.

MULTIPLE ENDOCRINE NEOPLASIA TYPE 2

Clinical manifestations

Medullary thyroid carcinoma (MTC) and pheochromocytoma are associated in two major syndromes: MEN type 2A and MEN type 2B (Table 351-1). MEN 2A is the combination of MTC, hyperparathyroidism, and pheochromocytoma. Three subvariants of MEN 2A are familial medullary thyroid carcinoma (FMTC), MEN 2A with cutaneous lichen amyloidosis, and MEN 2A with Hirschsprung disease. MEN 2B is the combination of MTC, pheochromocytoma, mucosal neuromas, intestinal ganglioneuromatosis, and marfanoid features.

Multiple endocrine neoplasia type 2A MTC is the most common manifestation. This tumor usually develops in childhood, beginning as hyperplasia of the calcitonin-producing cells (C cells) of the thyroid. MTC typically is located at the junction of the upper one-third and lower two-thirds of each lobe of the thyroid, reflecting the high density of C cells in this location; tumors >1 cm in size frequently are associated with local or distant metastases.

Pheochromocytoma occurs in ~50% of patients with MEN 2A and causes palpitations, nervousness, headaches, and sometimes sweating (Chap. 343). About half of the tumors are bilateral, and >50% of patients who have had unilateral adrenalectomy develop a pheochromocytoma in the contralateral gland within a decade. A second feature of these tumors is a disproportionate increase in the secretion of epinephrine relative to norepinephrine. This characteristic differentiates the MEN 2 pheochromocytomas from sporadic pheochromocytoma and those associated with von Hippel–Lindau (VHL) syndrome, hereditary paraganglioma, or neurofibromatosis. Capsular invasion is common, but metastasis is uncommon. Finally, the pheochromocytomas almost always are found in the adrenal gland, differentiating the pheochromocytomas in MEN 2 from the extraadrenal tumors more commonly found in hereditary paraganglioma syndromes.

Hyperparathyroidism occurs in 15–20% of patients, with the peak incidence in the third or fourth decade. The manifestations of hyperparathyroidism do not differ from those in other forms of primary hyperparathyroidism (Chap. 353). Diagnosis is established by finding hypercalcemia, hypophosphatemia, hypercalciuria, and an inappropriately high serum level of intact PTH. Multiglandular parathyroid hyperplasia is the most common histologic finding, although with long-standing disease adenomatous changes may be superimposed on hyperplasia.

The most common subvariant of MEN 2A is familial MTC, an autosomal dominant syndrome in which MTC is the only manifestation (Table 351-1). The clinical diagnosis of FMTC is established by the identification of MTC in multiple generations without a pheochromocytoma. Since the penetrance of pheochromocytoma is 50% in MEN 2A, it is possible that MEN 2A could masquerade as FMTC in small kindreds. It is important to consider this possibility carefully before classifying a kindred as having FMTC; failure to do so could lead to death or serious morbidity from pheochromocytoma in an affected kindred member. The difficulty of differentiating MEN 2A and FMTC is discussed further below.

Multiple endocrine neoplasia type 2B The association of MTC, pheochromocytoma, mucosal neuromas, and a marfanoid habitus is designated MEN 2B. MTC in MEN 2B develops earlier and is more aggressive than in MEN 2A. Metastatic disease has been described before 1 year of age, and death may occur in the second or third decade of life. However, the prognosis is not invariably bad even in patients with metastatic disease, as evidenced by a number of multigenerational families with this disease.

Pheochromocytoma occurs in more than half of MEN 2B patients and does not differ from that in MEN 2A. Hypercalcemia is rare in MEN 2B, and there are no well-documented examples of hyperparathyroidism.

The mucosal neuromas and marfanoid body habitus are the most distinctive features and are recognizable in childhood. Neuromas are present on the tip of the tongue, under the eyelids, and throughout the gastrointestinal tract and are true neuromas, distinct from neurofibromas. The most common presentation in children relates to gastrointestinal symptomatology, including intermittent colic, pseudoobstruction, and diarrhea.

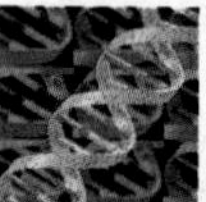

GENETIC CONSIDERATIONS

Mutations of the *RET* protooncogene have been identified in most patients with MEN 2 (Fig. 351-3). *RET* encodes a tyrosine kinase receptor that in combination with a co-receptor, GFRα, normally is activated by glial cell–derived neurotrophic factor (GDNF) or other members of this transforming growth factor β–like family of peptides, including artemin, persephin, and neurturin. In the C cell there is evidence that persephin normally activates the *RET*/GFRα-4 receptor complex and is partially responsible for migration of the C cells into the thyroid gland, whereas in the developing

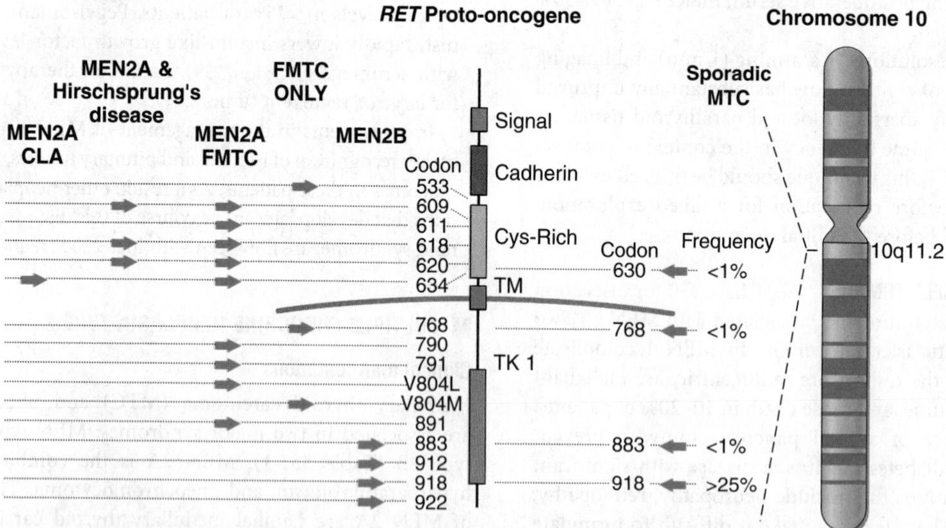

Figure 351-3 Schematic diagram of the *RET* protooncogene showing mutations found in MEN type 2 and sporadic medullary thyroid carcinoma (MTC). The *RET* protooncogene is located on the proximal arm of chromosome 10q (10q11.2). Activating mutations of two functional domains of RET tyrosine kinase receptor have been identified. The first affects a cysteine-rich (Cys-Rich) region in the extracellular portion of the receptor. Each germ-line mutation changes a cysteine at codons 609, 611, 618, 620, or 634 to another amino acid. The second region is the intracellular tyrosine kinase (TK) domain. Codon 634 mutations account for ~80% of all germ-line mutations. Mutations of codons 630, 768, 883, and 918 have been identified as somatic (non-germ-line) mutations that occur in a single parafollicular or C cell within the thyroid gland in sporadic MTC. A codon 918 mutation is the most common somatic mutation. MEN2, multiple endocrine neoplasia type 2; CLA, cutaneous lichen amyloidosis; FMTC, familial medullary thyroid carcinoma; Signal, the signal peptide; Cadherin, a cadherin-like region in the extracellular domain; TM, transmembrane domain; TK, tyrosine kinase domain.

neuronal system of the gastrointestinal tract, GDNF activates the *RET*/GFRα-1 complex. *RET* mutations induce constitutive activity of the receptor, explaining the autosomal dominant transmission of the disorder.

Naturally occurring mutations localize to two regions of the *RET* tyrosine kinase receptor. The first is a cysteine-rich extracellular domain; point mutations in the coding sequence for one of six cysteines (codons 609, 611, 618, 620, 630, and 634) cause amino acid substitutions that induce receptor dimerization and activation in the absence of its ligand. Codon 634 mutations occur in 80% of MEN 2A kindreds and are most commonly associated with classic MEN 2A features (Figs. 351-3 and 351-2); an arginine substitution at this codon accounts for half of all MEN 2A mutations. All reported families with MEN 2A and cutaneous lichen amyloidosis have a codon 634 mutation. Mutations of codon 609, 611, 618, or 620 occur in 10–15% of MEN 2A kindreds and are more commonly associated with FMTC (Fig. 351-3). Mutations in codons 609, 618, and 620 also have been identified in a variant of MEN 2A that includes Hirschsprung disease (Fig. 351-3). The second region of the *RET* tyrosine kinase that is mutated in MEN 2 is in the substrate recognition pocket at codon 918 (Fig. 351-3). This activating mutation is present in ~95% of patients with MEN 2B and accounts for 5% of all *RET* protooncogene mutations in MEN 2. Mutations of codon 883 and 922 also have been identified in a few patients with MEN 2B.

Uncommon mutations (<5% of the total) include those of codons 533 (exon 8), 666, 768, 777, 790, 791, 804, 891, and 912. Mutations associated with only FMTC include codons 533, 768, and 912. With greater experience, mutations that once were associated with FMTC only (666, 791, V804L, V804M, and 891) have been found in MEN 2A as there have been occasional descriptions of pheochromocytoma. At present it is reasonable to conclude that only kindreds with codon 533, 768, or 912 mutations are consistently associated with FMTC; in kindreds with all other *RET* mutations, pheochromocytoma is a possibility. The recognition that germ-line mutations occur in at least 6% of patients with apparently sporadic MTC has led to the firm recommendation that all patients with MTC should be screened for these mutations. The effort to screen patients with sporadic MTC, combined with the fact that new kindreds with classic MEN 2A are being recognized less frequently, has led to a shift in the mutation frequencies. These findings mirror results in other malignancies in which germ-line mutations of cancer-causing genes contribute to a greater percentage of apparently sporadic cancer than was considered previously. The recognition of new *RET* mutations suggests that more will be identified in the future.

Somatic mutations (found only in the tumor and not transmitted in the germ line) of the *RET* protooncogene have been identified in sporadic MTC; 25–60% of sporadic tumors have codon 918 mutations, and somatic mutations in codons 630, 768, and 804 have been identified (Fig. 351-3).

TREATMENT Multiple Endocrine Neoplasia Type 2

SCREENING FOR MULTIPLE ENDOCRINE NEOPLASIA TYPE 2

Death from MTC can be prevented by early thyroidectomy. The identification of *RET* protooncogene mutations and the application of DNA-based molecular diagnostic techniques to identify these mutations have simplified the screening process. During the initial evaluation of a kindred, a *RET* protooncogene analysis should be performed on an individual with proven MEN 2A. Establishment of the specific germ-line mutation facilitates the subsequent analysis of other family members. Each family member at risk should be tested twice for the presence of the specific mutation; the second analysis should be performed on a new DNA sample and, ideally, in a second laboratory to exclude sample mix-up or technical error (see *www.genetests.org* for an up-to-date list of laboratory testing sites). Both false-positive and false-negative analyses have been described. A false-negative test result is of the greatest concern because calcitonin testing is now rarely performed as a diagnostic backup study; if there is a genetic test error, a child may present in the second or third decade with metastatic MTC. Individuals in a kindred with a known mutation who have two normal analyses can be excluded from further screening.

There is a consensus that children with codon 883, 918, and 922 mutations, those associated with MEN 2B, should have a total thyroidectomy and central lymph node dissection (level VI) performed during the first months of life or soon after identification of the syndrome. If local metastasis is discovered, a more extensive lymph node dissection (levels II to V) is generally indicated. In children with codon 611, 618, 620, 630, 634, and 891 mutations, thyroidectomy should be performed before age 6 years because of reports of local metastatic disease in children this age. Finally, there are kindreds with codon 609, 768, 790, 791, 804, and 912 mutations in which the phenotype of MTC appears to be less aggressive. A clinician caring for children with one of these mutations faces a dilemma. In many kindreds there has never been a death from MTC caused by one of these mutations. However, in other kindreds there are examples of metastatic disease occurring early in life. For example, metastatic disease before age 6 years has been described with codon 609 and 804 mutations and before age 14 years in a patient with a codon 912 mutation. In kindreds with these mutations, two management approaches have been suggested: (1) perform a total thyroidectomy with or without central node dissection at some arbitrary age (perhaps 6–10 years of age) or (2) continue annual or biannual calcitonin provocative testing with performance of total thyroidectomy with or without central neck dissection when the test becomes abnormal. The pentagastrin test involves measurement of serum calcitonin basally and 2, 5, 10, and 15 min after a bolus injection of 5 μg pentagastrin per kilogram of body weight. Patients should be warned before pentagastrin injection of epigastric tightness, nausea, warmth, and tingling of extremities and reassured that the symptoms will last ~2 min. If pentagastrin is unavailable, an alternative is a short calcium infusion, performed by obtaining a baseline serum calcitonin and then infusing 150 mg calcium salt IV over 10 min with measurement of serum calcitonin at 5, 10, 15, 30 min after initiation of the infusion.

The *RET* protooncogene analysis should be performed in patients with suspected MEN 2B to detect codon 883, 918, and 922 mutations, especially in newborn children in whom the diagnosis is suspected but the clinical phenotype is not fully developed. Other family members at risk for MEN 2B also should be tested because the mucosal neuromas can be subtle. Most MEN 2B mutations represent de novo mutations derived from the paternal allele. In the rare families with proven germ-line transmission of MTC but no identifiable *RET* protooncogene mutation (sequencing of the entire *RET* gene should be performed), annual pentagastrin or calcium testing should be performed on members at risk.

Annual screening for pheochromocytoma in patients with germ-line *RET* mutations should be performed by measuring basal plasma or 24-h urine catecholamines and metanephrines. The goal is to identify a pheochromocytoma before it causes significant symptoms or is likely to cause sudden death, an event most commonly associated with large tumors. Although there are kindreds with FMTC and specific *RET* mutations in which no pheochromocytomas have been identified (Fig. 351-3), clinical experience is insufficient to exclude pheochromocytoma screening in these individuals. Radiographic studies such as MRI or CT scans generally are reserved for individuals with abnormal screening tests or symptoms suggestive of pheochromocytoma (Chap. 343). Women should be tested during pregnancy because undetected pheochromocytoma can cause maternal death during childbirth.

Measurement of serum calcium and parathyroid hormone levels every 2–3 years provides an adequate screen for hyperparathyroidism, except in families in which hyperparathyroidism is a prominent component, in which measurements should be made annually.

MEDULLARY THYROID CARCINOMA Hereditary MTC is a multicentric disorder. Total thyroidectomy with a central lymph node dissection should be performed in children who carry the mutant gene. Incomplete thyroidectomy leaves the possibility of later transformation of residual C cells. The goal of early therapy is cure, and a strategy that does not accomplish this goal is shortsighted. Long-term follow-up studies indicate an excellent outcome, with ~90% of children free of disease 15–20 years after surgery. In contrast, 15–25% of patients in whom the diagnosis is made on the basis of a palpable thyroid nodule die from the disease within 15–20 years.

In adults with MTC >1 cm in size, metastases to regional lymph nodes are common (>75%). Total thyroidectomy with central lymph node dissection and selective dissection of other regional chains provides the best chance for cure. In patients with extensive local metastatic disease in the neck, external radiation may prevent local recurrence or reduce tumor mass but is not curative. Chemotherapy with combinations of adriamycin, vincristine, cyclophosphamide, and dacarbazine may provide palliation. Clinical trials with small compounds (tyrosine kinase inhibitors) that interact with the ATP-binding pocket of the RET, vascular endothelial receptor, and type 2 and epidermal growth factor receptors and prevent phosphorylation have shown promise for treatment of hereditary and sporadic MTC. A phase I trial of vandetanib has shown that 45% of patients have a 30% or greater reduction of tumor size and prolongation of progression-free survival by at least 11 months. Similar phase II results have been observed for XL184, sunitinib, tipifarnib, and sorafenib, and phase II trials of E7080 and pazopanib are under way. It seems likely that one or more of these compounds will be approved for treatment of metastatic MTC within the next few years.

PHEOCHROMOCYTOMA The long-term goal for management of pheochromocytoma is to prevent death and cardiovascular complications. Improvements in radiographic imaging of the adrenals make direct examination of the apparently normal contralateral gland during surgery less important, and the rapid evolution of laparoscopic abdominal or retroperitoneal surgery has simplified management of early pheochromocytoma. The major question is whether to remove both adrenal glands or remove only the affected adrenal at the time of primary surgery. Issues to be considered in making this decision include the possibility of malignancy (<15 reported cases), the high probability of developing pheochromocytoma in the apparently unaffected gland over an 8- to 10-year period, and the risks of adrenal insufficiency caused by removal of both glands (at least two deaths related to adrenal insufficiency have occurred in MEN 2 patients). Most clinicians recommend removing only the affected gland. If both adrenals are removed, glucocorticoid and mineralocorticoid replacement is mandatory. An alternative approach is to perform a cortical-sparing adrenalectomy, removing the pheochromocytoma and adrenal medulla and leaving the adrenal cortex behind. This approach is usually successful and eliminates the necessity for steroid hormone replacement in most patients, although the pheochromocytoma recurs in a small percentage.

HYPERPARATHYROIDISM Hyperparathyroidism has been managed by one of two approaches. Removal of 3.5 glands with maintenance of the remaining half gland in the neck is the usual procedure. In families in which hyperparathyroidism is a prominent manifestation (almost always associated with a codon 634 *RET* mutation) and recurrence is common, total parathyroidectomy with transplantation of parathyroid tissue into the nondominant forearm is preferred. This approach is discussed above in the context of hyperparathyroidism associated with MEN 1.

OTHER GENETIC ENDOCRINE TUMOR SYNDROMES

A number of mixed syndromes exist in which the neoplastic associations differ from those in MEN 1 or 2 (Table 351-1).

The cause of VHL syndrome—the association of central nervous system tumors, renal cell carcinoma, pheochromocytoma, and islet cell neoplasms—is a mutation in the *VHL* tumor-suppressor gene. Germ-line-inactivating mutations of the *VHL* gene cause tumor formation when there is additional loss or somatic mutation of the normal *VHL* allele in brain, kidney, pancreatic islet, or adrenal medullary cells. Missense mutations been identified in >40% of VHL families with pheochromocytoma, suggesting that families with this type of mutation should be surveyed routinely for pheochromocytoma. A point that may be useful in differentiating VHL from MEN 1 (overlapping features include islet cell tumor and rare pheochromocytoma) or MEN 2 (overlapping feature is pheochromocytoma) is that hyperparathyroidism rarely occurs in VHL.

The molecular defect in type 1 neurofibromatosis inactivates neurofibromin, a cell membrane–associated protein that normally activates a GTPase. Inactivation of this protein impairs GTPase and causes continuous activation of p21 Ras and its downstream tyrosine kinase pathway. Endocrine tumors also form in less common neoplastic genetic syndromes. These include Cowden disease, Carney complex, familial growth hormone and prolactin tumors, and familial carcinoid syndrome. Carney complex includes myxomas of the heart, skin, and breast; peripheral nerve schwannomas; spotty skin pigmentation; and testicular, adrenal, and GH-secreting pituitary tumors. Linkage analysis has identified two loci: chromosome 2p in half of the families and 17q in the others. The 17q gene has been identified as the regulatory subunit (type IA) of protein kinase A (*PRKA1A*). Familial growth hormone– or prolactin-producing neoplasms without other manifestations of MEN 1 are caused by germ-line-inactivating mutation of the aryl hydrocarbon receptor interacting protein (AIP). It is transmitted in an autosomal dominant manner. Other types of endocrine tumors have not, to date, been associated with AIP mutations.

IMMUNOLOGIC SYNDROMES AFFECTING MULTIPLE ENDOCRINE ORGANS

When immune dysfunction affects two or more endocrine glands and other nonendocrine immune disorders are present, the *polyglandular autoimmune* (PGA) *syndromes* should be considered. The PGA syndromes are classified as two main types: the type I syndrome starts in childhood and is characterized by mucocutaneous candidiasis, hypoparathyroidism, and adrenal insufficiency; the type II, or Schmidt, syndrome is more likely to present in adults

TABLE 351-2 Features of Polyglandular Autoimmune (PGA) Syndromes

PGA I	PGA II
Epidemiology	
Autosomal recessive	Polygenic inheritance
Mutations in *APECED* gene	HLA-DR3 and HLA-DR4 associated
Childhood onset	Adult onset
Equal male:female ratio	Female predominance
Disease Associations	
Mucocutaneous candidiasis	Adrenal insufficiency
Hypoparathyroidism	Hypothyroidism
Adrenal insufficiency	Graves' disease
Hypogonadism	Type 1 diabetes
Alopecia	Hypogonadism
Hypothyroidism	Hypophysitis
Dental enamel hypoplasia	Myasthenia gravis
Malabsorption	Vitiligo
Chronic active hepatitis	Alopecia
Vitiligo	Pernicious anemia
Pernicious anemia	Celiac disease

Abbreviation: APECED, autoimmune polyendocrinopathy-candidiasis-ectodermal dystrophy.

and most commonly includes adrenal insufficiency, thyroiditis, or type 1 diabetes mellitus. Some authors have attempted to subdivide PGA II on the basis of association with some autoimmune disorders but not others (i.e., type II and type III). The type III syndrome is heterogeneous and may consist of autoimmune thyroid disease along with a variety of other autoimmune endocrine disorders (Table 351-2). However, little information is gained by making this subdivision in terms of understanding pathogenesis or prevention of future endocrine complications in individual patients or in the affected families.

POLYGLANDULAR AUTOIMMUNE SYNDROME TYPE I

PGA type I usually is recognized in the first decade of life and requires two of three components for diagnosis: mucocutaneous candidiasis, hypoparathyroidism, and adrenal insufficiency. Mucocutaneous candidiasis and hypoparathyroidism present with similar high frequency (100% and 79–96%, respectively). Adrenal insufficiency is observed in 60–72% of patients. Mineralocorticoids and glucocorticoids may be lost simultaneously or sequentially. PGA type 1 also is called *autoimmune polyendocrinopathy-candidiasis-ectodermal dystrophy* (APECED). Other endocrine defects can include gonadal failure (60% female, 14% male), hypothyroidism (5%), and destruction of the beta cells of the pancreatic islets and development of insulin-dependent (type 1) diabetes mellitus (14% lifetime risk). Additional features include hypoplasia of the dental enamel, nail dystrophy, tympanic membrane sclerosis, vitiligo, keratopathy, and gastric parietal cell dysfunction resulting in pernicious anemia (13%). Some patients develop autoimmune hepatitis (12%), malabsorption (variably attributed to intestinal lymphangiectasia, bacterial overgrowth, or hypoparathyroidism), asplenism, achalasia, and cholelithiasis (Table 351-2). At the outset, only one organ may be involved, but the number increases with time so that patients eventually manifest two to five components of the syndrome.

Most patients initially present with oral candidiasis in childhood; it is poorly responsive to treatment (Chap. 353) and relapses frequently. Chronic hypoparathyroidism usually occurs before adrenal insufficiency develops. More than 60% of postpubertal women develop premature hypogonadism. The endocrine components, including adrenal insufficiency and hypoparathyroidism, may not develop until the fourth decade, making continued surveillance necessary.

Type I PGA syndrome is not associated with a particular HLA type and usually is inherited as an autosomal recessive trait. It may occur sporadically. The responsible gene, designated as either *APECED* or *AIRE*, encodes a transcription factor that is expressed in thymus and lymph nodes; a variety of different mutations have been reported. The mechanism by which these mutations lead to the diverse manifestations of type I PGA is unknown.

POLYGLANDULAR AUTOIMMUNE SYNDROME TYPE II

PGA type II is characterized by two or more of the endocrinopathies listed in Table 351-2. Most often these endocrinopathies include primary adrenal insufficiency, Graves' disease or autoimmune hypothyroidism, type 1 diabetes mellitus, and primary hypogonadism. Because adrenal insufficiency is relatively rare, it is used frequently to define the presence of the syndrome. Among patients with adrenal insufficiency, type 1 diabetes mellitus coexists in 52% and autoimmune thyroid disease occurs in 69%. However, many patients with antimicrosomal and antithyroglobulin antibodies never develop abnormalities of thyroid function. Thus, increased antibody titers alone are poor predictors of future disease. Other associated conditions include hypophysitis, celiac disease (2–3%), atrophic gastritis, and pernicious anemia (13%). Vitiligo, which is caused by antibodies against the melanocyte, and alopecia are less common than in the type I syndrome. Mucocutaneous candidiasis does not occur. A few patients develop a late-onset, usually transient hypoparathyroidism caused by antibodies that compete with PTH for binding to the PTH receptor. Up to 25% of patients with myasthenia gravis and an even higher percentage who have myasthenia and a thymoma have PGA type II.

The type II syndrome is familial in nature, often transmitted as an autosomal dominant trait with incomplete penetrance. As in many of the individual autoimmune endocrinopathies, certain HL-DR3 and -DR4 alleles increase disease susceptibility; several different genes probably contribute to the expression of this syndrome.

A variety of autoantibodies are seen in PGA type II, including antibodies directed against (1) thyroid antigens such as thyroid peroxidase, thyroglobulin, and the thyroid-stimulating hormone (TSH) receptor; (2) adrenal side chain cleavage enzyme, steroid 21-hydroxylase, or ACTH receptor; and (3) pancreatic islet glutamic acid decarboxylase or the insulin receptor, among others. The roles of cytokines such as interferon and cell-mediated immunity are unclear.

DIAGNOSIS

The clinical manifestations of adrenal insufficiency often develop slowly, may be difficult to detect, and can be fatal if not diagnosed and treated appropriately. Thus, prospective screening should be performed routinely in all patients and family members at risk for PGA types I and II. The most effective screening test for adrenal disease is a cosyntropin stimulation test (Chap. 342). A fasting blood glucose level can be obtained to screen for hyperglycemia. Additional screening tests should include measurements of TSH, luteinizing hormone, follicle-stimulating hormone, and, in men, testosterone levels. In families with suspected type I PGA syndrome, calcium and phosphorus levels should be measured. These screening studies should be performed every 1–2 years up to about age 50 in families with PGA type II syndrome and until about age 40 in patients with type I syndrome. Screening measurements of autoantibodies against potentially affected endocrine organs are of uncertain prognostic value. The differential diagnosis of PGA syndrome should include the DiGeorge syndrome (hypoparathyroidism due to glandular agenesis and mucocutaneous candidiasis), Kearns-Sayre syndrome (hypoparathyroidism, primary hypogonadism, type 1 diabetes mellitus, and panhypopituitarism), Wolfram's syndrome (congenital diabetes insipidus and diabetes mellitus), IPEX syndrome (*i*mmunodysregulation, *p*olyendocrinopathy, and *e*nteropathy, *X*-linked), and congenital rubella (type 1 diabetes mellitus and hypothyroidism).

TREATMENT Polyglandular Autoimmune Syndrome

With the exception of Graves' disease, the management of each of the endocrine components of the disease involves hormone replacement and is covered in detail in the chapters on adrenal, thyroid, gonadal, and parathyroid disease (Chaps. 341, 342, 346, 347, and 353). Some aspects of therapy merit special emphasis. Primary hypothyroidism can mask adrenal insufficiency by prolonging the half-life of cortisol; consequently, administration of thyroid hormone to a patient with unsuspected adrenal insufficiency can precipitate adrenal crisis. Thus, all patients with hypothyroidism in the context of PGA syndrome should be screened for adrenal disease and, if it is present, treated with glucocorticoids before or concurrently with thyroid hormone therapy. Hypoglycemia or decreasing insulin requirements in a patient with diabetes mellitus type 1 may be the earliest symptom of adrenal insufficiency. Consequently, such patients should be screened for adrenal disease. Treatment of mucocutaneous candidiasis with ketoconazole may induce adrenal insufficiency. This drug also may elevate liver enzymes, making the diagnosis of autoimmune hepatitis more difficult. Hypocalcemia in PGA type II is more commonly due to malabsorption associated with celiac disease than to hypoparathyroidism.

OTHER AUTOIMMUNE ENDOCRINE SYNDROMES

Insulin resistance caused by antibodies

Rare insulin-resistance syndromes occur in patients who develop antibodies that block the interaction of insulin with its receptor. Conversely, other classes of anti-insulin receptor antibodies can activate the receptor and can cause hypoglycemia; this disorder should be considered in the differential diagnosis of fasting hypoglycemia (Chap. 345).

Patients with insulin receptor antibodies and acanthosis nigricans are often middle-aged women who acquire insulin resistance in association with other autoimmune disorders, such as systemic lupus erythematosus and Sjögren's syndrome. Vitiligo, alopecia, Raynaud's phenomenon, and arthritis also may be seen. Other autoimmune endocrine disorders, including thyrotoxicosis, hypothyroidism, and hypogonadism, occur rarely. Acanthosis nigricans, a velvety, hyperpigmented, thickened skin lesion, is prominent on the dorsum of the neck and other skinfold areas in the axillae or groin and often heralds the diagnosis in these patients. However, acanthosis nigricans also occurs in patients with obesity or polycystic ovarian syndrome, in which insulin resistance appears to be due to a postreceptor defect; thus, acanthosis nigricans itself is not diagnostic of the immunologic form of insulin resistance.

Some patients with acanthosis nigricans have mild glucose intolerance, with a compensatory increase in insulin secretion that is detected only when insulin levels are measured. Others have severe diabetes mellitus that requires massive doses of insulin (several thousand units per day) to lower the blood glucose levels. The nature of the antibodies determines the manifestations; though insulin resistance is more common, fasting hypoglycemia can result from insulinomimetic antibodies.

Insulin-resistant diabetes mellitus associated with anti-insulin antibodies occurs in patients with ataxia-telangiectasia. This is an autosomal recessive disorder caused by mutations in *ATM*, a gene involved in cellular responses to ionizing radiation and oxidative damage. This disorder is characterized by ataxia, telangiectasia, immune abnormalities, and an increased incidence of malignancies.

Autoimmune insulin syndrome with hypoglycemia

This disorder typically occurs in patients with other autoimmune disorders and is caused by polyclonal autoantibodies that bind to endogenously synthesized insulin. If the insulin dissociates from the antibodies several hours or more after a meal, hypoglycemia can result. Most cases of the syndrome have been described from Japan, and there may be a genetic component. In plasma cell dyscrasias such as multiple myeloma, the plasma cells may produce monoclonal antibodies against insulin and cause hypoglycemia by a similar mechanism.

Antithyroxine antibodies and hypothyroidism

Circulating autoantibodies against thyroid hormones in patients with both immune thyroid disease and plasma cell dyscrasias such as Waldenström's macroglobulinemia can bind thyroid hormones, decrease their biologic activity, and result in primary hypothyroidism. In other patients the antibodies simply interfere with thyroid hormone immunoassays and cause false elevations or decreases in measured hormone levels.

Crow-Fukase syndrome

The features of this syndrome are highlighted by an acronym that emphasizes its important features: *p*olyneuropathy, *o*rganomegaly, *e*ndocrinopathy, *M*-proteins, and *s*kin changes (POEMS). The most important feature is a severe, progressive sensorimotor polyneuropathy associated with a plasma cell dyscrasia. Localized collections of plasma cells (plasmacytomas) can cause sclerotic bone lesions and produce monoclonal IgG or IgA proteins. Endocrine manifestations in men or women include hyperprolactinemia, diabetes mellitus type 2, primary hypothyroidism, and adrenal insufficiency. Additional findings include ovarian failure and amenorrhea in women and testicular failure, impotence, and gynecomastia in men. Skin changes include hyperpigmentation, thickening of the dermis, hirsutism, and hyperhidrosis. Hepatomegaly and lymphadenopathy occur in about two-thirds of patients, and splenomegaly is seen in about one-third. Other manifestations include increased cerebrospinal fluid pressure with papilledema, peripheral edema, ascites, pleural effusions, glomerulonephritis, and fever. Median survival may be >10 years, though shorter in patients with extravascular volume overload or clubbing.

The systemic nature of the disorder may cause confusion with other connective tissue diseases. The endocrine manifestations suggest an autoimmune basis of the disorder, but circulating antibodies against endocrine cells have not been demonstrated. Increased serum and tissue levels of interleukin 6, interleukin 1β, vascular endothelial growth factor, matrix metalloproteins, and tumor necrosis factor α are present, but the pathophysiologic basis for the POEMS syndrome is uncertain. Therapy directed against the plasma cell dyscrasia such as local radiation of bony lesions, chemotherapy, thalidomide, plasmapheresis, bone marrow or stem cell transplantation, and treatment with all-*trans* retinoic acid may improve the endocrine manifestations.

FURTHER READINGS

Burgess J: How should the patient with multiple endocrine neoplasia type 1 (MEN 1) be followed? Clin Endocrinol (Oxf) 72:13, 2010

Falchetti A et al: Multiple endocrine neoplasia type 1 (MEN 1): Not only inherited endocrine tumors. Genet Med 11:825, 2009

Gracanin A et al: Tissue selectivity in multiple endocrine neoplasia type 1-associated tumorigenesis. Cancer Res 69:6371, 2009

Jensen RT et al: Inherited pancreatic endocrine tumor syndromes: Advances in molecular pathogenesis, diagnosis, management, and controversies. Cancer 113:1807, 2008

Jimenez C et al: Management of medullary thyroid carcinoma. Endocrinol Metab Clin North Am 37:481, 2008

Kahaly GJ: Polyglandular autoimmune syndromes. Eur J Endocrinol 161:11, 2009

Mathis D, Benoist C: Aire. Annu Rev Immunol 27:287, 2009

Vierimma O et al: Pituitary adenoma predisposition caused by germline mutations in the AIP gene. Science 312:1228, 2006

Ye L et al: The evolving field of tyrosine kinase inhibitors in the treatment of endocrine tumors. Endocrine Rev 31:578, 2010

CHAPTER 352

Bone and Mineral Metabolism in Health and Disease

F. Richard Bringhurst
Marie B. Demay
Stephen M. Krane
Henry M. Kronenberg

BONE STRUCTURE AND METABOLISM

Bone is a dynamic tissue that is remodeled constantly throughout life. The arrangement of compact and cancellous bone provides strength and density suitable for both mobility and protection. In addition, bone provides a reservoir for calcium, magnesium, phosphorus, sodium, and other ions necessary for homeostatic functions. Bone also hosts and regulates hematopoiesis by providing niches for hematopoietic cell proliferation and differentiation. The skeleton is highly vascular and receives about 10% of the cardiac output. Remodeling of bone is accomplished by two distinct cell types: osteoblasts produce bone matrix, and osteoclasts resorb the matrix.

The extracellular components of bone consist of a solid mineral phase in close association with an organic matrix, of which 90–95% is type I collagen (Chap. 363). The noncollagenous portion of the organic matrix is heterogeneous and contains serum proteins such as albumin as well as many locally produced proteins, whose functions are incompletely understood. Those proteins include cell attachment/signaling proteins such as thrombospondin, osteopontin, and fibronectin; calcium-binding proteins such as matrix gla protein and osteocalcin; and proteoglycans such as biglycan and decorin. Some of the proteins organize collagen fibrils; others influence mineralization and binding of the mineral phase to the matrix.

The mineral phase is made up of calcium and phosphate and is best characterized as a poorly crystalline hydroxyapatite. The mineral phase of bone is deposited initially in intimate relation to the collagen fibrils and is found in specific locations in the "holes" between the collagen fibrils. This architectural arrangement of mineral and matrix results in a two-phase material well suited to withstand mechanical stresses. The organization of collagen influences the amount and type of mineral phase formed in bone. Although the primary structures of type I collagen in skin and bone tissues are similar, there are differences in posttranslational modifications and distribution of intermolecular cross-links. The holes in the packing structure of the collagen are larger in mineralized collagen of bone and dentin than in unmineralized collagens such as those in tendon. Single amino acid substitutions in the helical portion of either the α1 (*COL1A1*) or α2 (*COL1A2*) chains of type I collagen disrupt the organization of bone in osteogenesis imperfecta. The severe skeletal fragility associated with this group of disorders highlights the importance of the fibrillar matrix in the structure of bone (Chap. 363).

Osteoblasts synthesize and secrete the organic matrix. They are derived from cells of mesenchymal origin (Fig. 352-1*A*). Active osteoblasts are found on the surface of newly forming bone. As an osteoblast secretes matrix, which then is mineralized, the cell becomes an *osteocyte*, still connected with its blood supply through a series of canaliculi. Osteocytes account for the vast majority of the cells in bone. They are thought to be the mechanosensors in bone that communicate signals to surface osteoblasts and their progenitors through the canalicular network and thereby serve as master regulators of bone formation and resorption. Remarkably, osteocytes also secrete fibroblast growth factor 23 (FGF23), a major regulator of phosphate metabolism (see below). Mineralization of the matrix, both in trabecular bone and in osteones of compact cortical bone (*Haversian systems*), begins soon after the matrix is secreted (primary mineralization) but is not completed for several weeks or even longer (secondary mineralization). Although this mineralization takes advantage of the high concentrations of calcium and phosphate, already near saturation in serum, mineralization is a carefully regulated process that is dependent on the activity of osteoblast-derived alkaline phosphatase, which probably works by hydrolyzing inhibitors of mineralization.

Genetic studies in humans and mice have identified several key genes that control osteoblast development. *Runx2* is a transcription factor expressed specifically in chondrocyte (cartilage cells) and osteoblast progenitors as well as in hypertrophic chondrocytes and mature osteoblasts. *Runx2* regulates the expression of several important osteoblast proteins, including osterix (another transcription factor needed for osteoblast maturation), osteopontin, bone sialoprotein, type I collagen, osteocalcin, and receptor-activator of NFκB (RANK) ligand. *Runx2* expression is regulated in part by bone morphogenic proteins (BMPs). *Runx2*-deficient mice are devoid of osteoblasts, whereas mice with a deletion of only one allele (*Runx2* +/–) exhibit a delay in formation of the clavicles and some cranial bones. The latter abnormalities are similar to those in the human disorder *cleidocranial dysplasia*, which is also caused by heterozygous inactivating mutations in *Runx2*.

The paracrine signaling molecule, Indian hedgehog (Ihh), also plays a critical role in osteoblast development, as evidenced by Ihh-deficient mice that lack osteoblasts in bone formed on a cartilage mold (endochondral ossification). Signals originating from members of the wnt (wingless-type mouse mammary tumor virus integration site) family of paracrine factors are also important for osteoblast proliferation and differentiation. Numerous other growth-regulatory factors affect osteoblast function, including the three closely related transforming growth factor βs, fibroblast growth factors (FGFs) 2 and 18, platelet-derived growth factor, and insulin-like growth factors (IGFs) I and II. Hormones such as parathyroid hormone (PTH) and 1,25-dihydroxyvitamin D [1,25$(OH)_2$D] activate receptors expressed by osteoblasts to assure mineral homeostasis and influence a variety of bone cell functions.

Resorption of bone is carried out mainly by *osteoclasts*, multinucleated cells that are formed by fusion of cells derived from the common precursor of macrophages and osteoclasts. Multiple factors that regulate osteoclast development have been identified (Fig. 352-1*B*). Factors produced by osteoblasts or marrow stromal

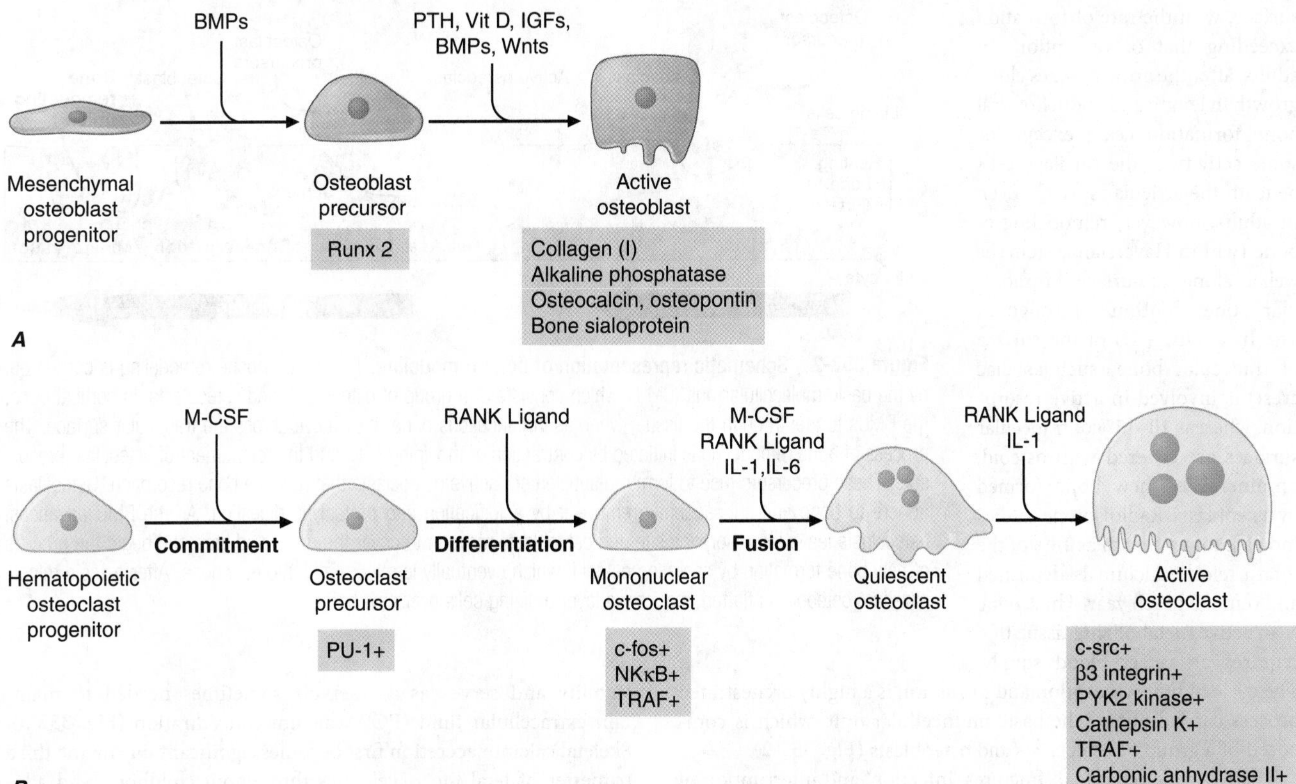

Figure 352-1 Pathways regulating development of *A.* osteoblasts and *B.* osteoclasts. Hormones, cytokines, and growth factors that control cell proliferation and differentiation are shown above the arrows. Transcription factors and other markers specific for various stages of development are depicted below the arrows. BMPs, bone morphogenic proteins; wnts, wingless-type mouse mammary tumor virus integration site; PTH, parathyroid hormone; Vit D, vitamin D; IGFs, insulin-like growth factors; Runx2, Runt-related transcription factor 2; M-CSF, macrophage colony-stimulating factor; PU-1, a monocyte- and B lymphocyte–specific ets family transcription factor; NFκB, nuclear factor κB; TRAF, tumor necrosis factor receptor–associated factors; RANK ligand, receptor activator of NFκB ligand; IL-1, interleukin 1; IL-6, interleukin 6. *(Modified from T Suda et al: Endocr Rev 20:345, 1999, with permission.)*

cells allow osteoblasts to control osteoclast development and activity. Macrophage colony-stimulating factor (M-CSF) plays a critical role during several steps in the pathway and ultimately leads to fusion of osteoclast progenitor cells to form multinucleated, active osteoclasts. RANK ligand, a member of the tumor necrosis factor (TNF) family, is expressed on the surface of osteoblast progenitors and stromal fibroblasts. In a process involving cell-cell interactions, RANK ligand binds to the RANK receptor on osteoclast progenitors, stimulating osteoclast differentiation and activation. Alternatively, a soluble decoy receptor, referred to as osteoprotegerin, can bind RANK ligand and inhibit osteoclast differentiation. Several growth factors and cytokines (including interleukins 1, 6, and 11; TNF; and interferon γ) modulate osteoclast differentiation and function. Most hormones that influence osteoclast function do not target these cells directly but instead influence M-CSF and RANK ligand signaling by osteoblasts. Both PTH and $1,25(OH)_2D$ increase osteoclast number and activity, whereas estrogen decreases osteoclast number and activity by this indirect mechanism. Calcitonin, in contrast, binds to its receptor on the basal surface of osteoclasts and directly inhibits osteoclast function.

Osteoclast-mediated resorption of bone takes place in scalloped spaces (*Howship's lacunae*) where the osteoclasts are attached through a specific $\alpha_v\beta_3$ integrin to components of the bone matrix such as osteopontin. The osteoclast forms a tight seal to the underlying matrix and secretes protons, chloride, and proteinases into a confined space that has been likened to an extracellular lysosome. The active osteoclast surface forms a ruffled border that contains a specialized proton-pump ATPase, which secretes acid and solubilizes the mineral phase. Carbonic anhydrase (type II isoenzyme) within the osteoclast generates the needed protons. The bone matrix is resorbed in the acid environment adjacent to the ruffled border by proteases that act at low pH such as cathepsin K.

In the embryo and the growing child, bone develops by remodeling and replacing previously calcified cartilage (endochondral bone formation) or is formed without a cartilage matrix (intramembranous bone formation). During endochondral bone formation, chondrocytes proliferate, secrete and mineralize a matrix, enlarge (hypertrophy), and then die, enlarging bone and providing the matrix and factors that stimulate endochondral bone formation. This program is regulated by both local factors such as IGF-I and -II, Ihh, parathyroid hormone–related peptide (PTHrP), and FGFs and by systemic hormones such as growth hormone, glucocorticoids, and estrogen.

New bone, whether formed in infants or in adults during repair, has a relatively high ratio of cells to matrix and is characterized by coarse fiber bundles of collagen that are interlaced and randomly dispersed (woven bone). In adults, the more mature bone is organized with fiber bundles regularly arranged in parallel or concentric sheets (lamellar bone). In long bones, deposition of lamellar bone in a concentric arrangement around blood vessels forms the Haversian systems. Growth in length of bones is dependent on proliferation of cartilage cells and the endochondral sequence at the growth plate. Growth in width and thickness is accomplished by formation of bone at the periosteal surface and by resorption at the endosteal surface, with the rate of formation exceeding that of resorption. In adults, after the growth plates close, growth in length and endochondral bone formation cease except for some activity in the cartilage cells beneath the articular surface. Even in adults, however, remodeling of bone (within Haversian systems as well as along the surfaces of trabecular bone) continues throughout life. In adults, ~4% of the surface of trabecular bone (such as iliac crest) is involved in active resorption, whereas 10–15% of trabecular surfaces are covered with osteoid, unmineralized new bone formed by osteoblasts. Radioisotope studies indicate that as much as 18% of the total skeletal calcium is deposited and removed each year. Thus, bone is an active metabolizing tissue that requires an intact blood supply. The cycle of bone resorption and formation is a highly orchestrated process carried out by the basic multicellular unit, which is composed of a group of osteoclasts and osteoblasts (Fig. 352-2).

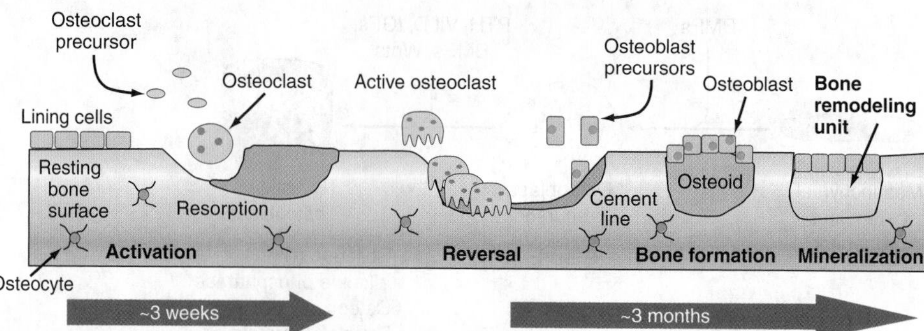

Figure 352-2 Schematic representation of bone remodeling. The cycle of bone remodeling is carried out by the basic multicellular unit (BMU), which consists of a group of osteoclasts and osteoblasts. In cortical bone, the BMUs tunnel through the tissue, whereas in cancellous bone, they move across the trabecular surface. The process of bone remodeling is initiated by contraction of the lining cells and the recruitment of osteoclast precursors. These precursors fuse to form multinucleated, active osteoclasts that mediate bone resorption. Osteoclasts adhere to bone and subsequently remove it by acidification and proteolytic digestion. As the BMU advances, osteoclasts leave the resorption site and osteoblasts move in to cover the excavated area and begin the process of new bone formation by secreting osteoid, which eventually is mineralized into new bone. After osteoid mineralization, osteoblasts flatten and form a layer of lining cells over new bone.

The response of bone to fractures, infection, and interruption of blood supply and to expanding lesions is relatively limited. Dead bone must be resorbed, and new bone must be formed, a process carried out in association with growth of new blood vessels into the involved area. In injuries that disrupt the organization of the tissue such as a fracture in which apposition of fragments is poor or when motion exists at the fracture site, the progenitor stromal cells recapitulate the endochondral bone formation of early development and form cartilage that is replaced by bone and, variably, fibrous tissue. When there is good apposition with fixation and little motion at the fracture site, repair occurs predominantly by formation of new bone without other mediating tissue.

Remodeling of bone occurs along lines of force generated by mechanical stress. The signals from these mechanical stresses are sensed by osteocytes, which transmit signals to osteoclasts and osteoblasts or their precursors. One such signal is sclerostin, an inhibitor of wnt signaling. Mechanical forces suppress sclerostin production and thus increase bone formation by osteoblasts. Expanding lesions in bone such as tumors induce resorption at the surface in contact with the tumor by producing ligands such as PTHrP that stimulate osteoclast differentiation and function. Even in a disorder as architecturally disruptive as Paget's disease, remodeling is dictated by mechanical forces. Thus, bone plasticity reflects the interaction of cells with each other and with the environment.

Measurement of the products of osteoblast and osteoclast activity can assist in the diagnosis and management of bone diseases. Osteoblast activity can be assessed by measuring serum bone-specific alkaline phosphatase. Similarly, osteocalcin, a protein secreted from osteoblasts, is made virtually only by osteoblasts. Osteoclast activity can be assessed by measurement of products of collagen degradation. Collagen molecules are covalently linked to each other in the extracellular matrix through the formation of hydroxypyridinium cross-links (Chap. 363). After digestion by osteoclasts, these cross-linked peptides can be measured both in urine and in blood.

CALCIUM METABOLISM

Over 99% of the 1–2 kg of calcium present normally in the adult human body resides in the skeleton, where it provides mechanical stability and serves as a reservoir sometimes needed to maintain extracellular fluid (ECF) calcium concentration (Fig. 352-3). Skeletal calcium accretion first becomes significant during the third trimester of fetal life, accelerates throughout childhood and adolescence, reaches a peak in early adulthood, and gradually declines thereafter at rates that rarely exceed 1–2% per year. These slow changes in total skeletal calcium content contrast with relatively high daily rates of closely matched fluxes of calcium into and out of bone (~250–500 mg each), a process mediated by coupled osteoblastic and osteoclastic activity. Another 0.5–1% of skeletal calcium is freely exchangeable (e.g., in chemical equilibrium) with that in the ECF.

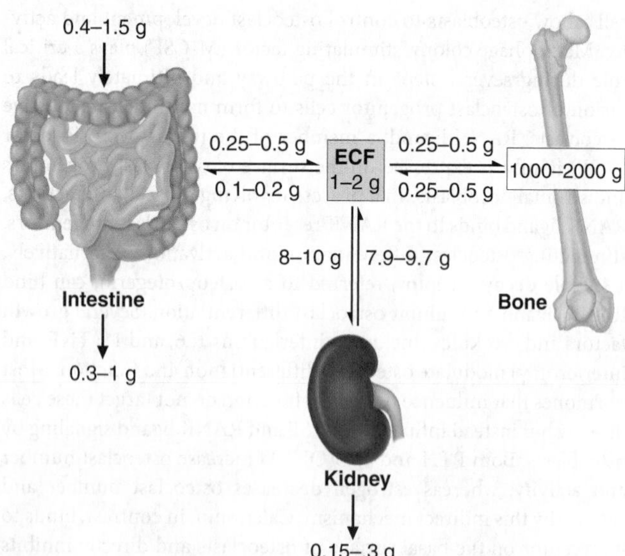

Figure 352-3 Calcium homeostasis. Schematic illustration of calcium content of extracellular fluid (ECF) and bone as well as of diet and feces; magnitude of calcium flux per day as calculated by various methods is shown at sites of transport in intestine, kidney, and bone. Ranges of values shown are approximate and were chosen to illustrate certain points discussed in the text. In conditions of calcium balance, rates of calcium release from and uptake into bone are equal.

The concentration of ionized calcium in the ECF must be maintained within a narrow range because of the critical role it plays in a wide array of cellular functions, especially those involved in neuromuscular activity, secretion, and signal transduction. Intracellular cytosolic free calcium levels are ~100 nmol/L and are 10,000-fold lower than ionized calcium concentration in the blood and ECF (1.1–1.3 mmol/L). Cytosolic calcium does not play the structural role played by extracellular calcium; instead, it serves a signaling function. The steep chemical gradient of calcium from outside to inside the cell promotes rapid calcium influx through various membrane calcium channels that can be activated by hormones, metabolites, or neurotransmitters, swiftly changing cellular function. In blood, total calcium concentration is normally 2.2–2.6 m*M* (8.5–10.5 mg/dL), of which ~50% is ionized. The remainder is bound ionically to negatively charged proteins (predominantly albumin and immunoglobulins) or loosely complexed with phosphate, citrate, sulfate, or other anions. Alterations in serum protein concentrations directly affect the total blood calcium concentration even if the ionized calcium concentration remains normal. An algorithm to correct for protein changes adjusts the total serum calcium (in mg/dL) upward by 0.8 times the deficit in serum albumin (g/dL) or by 0.5 times the deficit in serum immunoglobulin (in g/dL). Such corrections provide only rough approximations of actual free calcium concentrations, however, and may be misleading, particularly during acute illness. Acidosis also alters ionized calcium by reducing its association with proteins. The best practice is to measure blood ionized calcium directly by a method that employs calcium-selective electrodes in acute settings during which calcium abnormalities might occur.

Control of the ionized calcium concentration in the ECF ordinarily is accomplished by adjusting the rates of calcium movement across intestinal and renal epithelia. These adjustments are mediated mainly via changes in blood levels of the hormones PTH and 1,25(OH)$_2$D. Blood ionized calcium directly suppresses PTH secretion by activating parathyroid calcium-sensing receptors (CaSRs). Also, ionized calcium indirectly affects PTH secretion via effects on 1,25(OH)$_2$D production. This active vitamin D metabolite inhibits PTH production by an incompletely understood mechanism of negative feedback (Chap. 353).

Normal dietary calcium intake in the United States varies widely, ranging from 10–37 mmol/d (400–1500 mg/d). Many individuals, in an effort to prevent osteoporosis, routinely supplement this with oral calcium salts to a total intake of 37–50 mmol/d (1500–2000 mg/d). Intestinal absorption of ingested calcium involves both active (transcellular) and passive (paracellular) mechanisms. Passive calcium absorption is nonsaturable and approximates 5% of daily calcium intake, whereas active absorption involves apical calcium entry via specific ion channels (TRPV5 and TRPV6), whose expression is controlled principally by 1,25(OH)$_2$D, and normally ranges from 20 to 70%. Active calcium transport occurs mainly in the proximal small bowel (duodenum and proximal jejunum), although some active calcium absorption occurs in most segments of the small intestine. Optimal rates of calcium absorption require gastric acid. This is especially true for weakly dissociable calcium supplements such as calcium carbonate. In fact, large boluses of calcium carbonate are poorly absorbed because of their neutralizing effect on gastric acid. In achlorhydric subjects and for those taking drugs that inhibit gastric acid secretion, supplements should be taken with meals to optimize their absorption. Use of calcium citrate may be preferable in these circumstances. Calcium absorption may also be blunted in disease states such as pancreatic or biliary insufficiency, in which ingested calcium remains bound to unabsorbed fatty acids or other food constituents. At high levels of calcium intake, synthesis of 1,25(OH)$_2$D is reduced; this decreases the rate of active intestinal calcium absorption. The opposite occurs with dietary calcium restriction. Some calcium, ~2.5–5 mmol/d (100–200 mg/d), is excreted as an obligate component of intestinal secretions and is not regulated by calciotropic hormones.

The feedback-controlled hormonal regulation of intestinal absorptive efficiency results in a relatively constant daily net calcium absorption of ~5–7.5 mmol/d (200–400 mg/d) despite large changes in daily dietary calcium intake. This daily load of absorbed calcium is excreted by the kidneys in a manner that is also tightly regulated by the concentration of ionized calcium in the blood. Approximately 8–10 g/d of calcium is filtered by the glomeruli, of which only 2–3% appears in the urine. Most filtered calcium (65%) is reabsorbed in the proximal tubules via a passive, paracellular route that is coupled to concomitant NaCl reabsorption and not specifically regulated. The cortical thick ascending limb of Henle's loop (cTAL) reabsorbs roughly another 20% of filtered calcium, also via a paracellular mechanism. Calcium reabsorption in the cTAL requires a tight-junctional protein called paracellin-1 and is inhibited by increased blood concentrations of calcium or magnesium, acting via the CaSR, which is highly expressed on basolateral membranes in this nephron segment. Operation of the renal CaSR provides a mechanism, independent of those engaged directly by PTH or 1,25(OH)$_2$D, by which serum ionized calcium can control renal calcium reabsorption. Finally, ~10% of filtered calcium is reabsorbed in the distal convoluted tubules (DCTs) by a transcellular mechanism. Calcium enters the luminal surface of the cell through specific apical calcium channels (TRPV5), whose number is regulated. It then moves across the cell in association with a specific calcium-binding protein (calbindin-D28k) that buffers cytosolic calcium concentrations from the large mass of transported calcium. Ca^{2+}-ATPases and Na^+/Ca^{2+} exchangers actively extrude calcium across the basolateral surface and thereby maintain the transcellular calcium gradient. All these processes are stimulated directly or indirectly by PTH. The DCT is also the site of action of thiazide diuretics, which lower urinary calcium excretion by inducing sodium depletion and thereby augmenting proximal calcium reabsorption. Conversely, dietary sodium loads, or increased distal sodium delivery caused by loop diuretics or saline infusion, induce calciuresis.

The homeostatic mechanisms that normally maintain a constant serum ionized calcium concentration may fail at extremes of calcium intake or when the hormonal systems or organs involved are compromised. Thus, even with maximal activity of the vitamin D–dependent intestinal active transport system, sustained calcium intakes <5 mmol/d (<200 mg/d) cannot provide enough net calcium absorption to replace obligate losses via the intestine, the kidney, sweat, and other secretions. In this case, increased blood levels of PTH and 1,25(OH)$_2$D activate osteoclastic bone resorption to obtain needed calcium from bone, which leads to progressive bone loss and negative calcium balance. Increased PTH and 1,25(OH)$_2$D also enhance renal calcium reabsorption, and 1,25(OH)$_2$D enhances calcium absorption in the gut. At very high calcium intakes [>100 mmol/d (>4 g/d)], passive intestinal absorption continues to deliver calcium into the ECF despite maximally downregulated intestinal active transport and renal tubular calcium reabsorption. This can cause severe hypercalciuria, nephrocalcinosis, progressive renal failure, and hypercalcemia (e.g., "milk-alkali syndrome"). Deficiency or excess of PTH or vitamin D, intestinal disease, and renal failure represent other commonly encountered challenges to normal calcium homeostasis (Chap. 353).

PHOSPHORUS METABOLISM

Although 85% of the ~600 g of body phosphorus is present in bone mineral, phosphorus is also a major intracellular constituent both as the free anion(s) and as a component of numerous organophosphate compounds, including structural proteins, enzymes, transcription factors, carbohydrate and lipid intermediates, high-energy stores [ATP (adenosine triphosphate), creatine phosphate], and nucleic acids. Unlike calcium, phosphorus exists intracellularly at concentrations close to those present in ECF (e.g., 1–2 mmol/L). In cells and in the ECF, phosphorus exists in several forms, predominantly as $H_2PO_4^-$ or $NaHPO_4^-$, with perhaps 10% as HPO_4^{2-}. This mixture of anions will be referred to here as "phosphate." In serum, about 12% of phosphorus is bound to proteins. Concentrations of phosphates in blood and ECF generally are expressed in terms of elemental phosphorus, with the normal range in adults being 0.75–1.45 mmol/L (2.5–4.5 mg/dL). Because the volume of the intracellular fluid compartment is twice that of the ECF, measurements of ECF phosphate may not accurately reflect phosphate availability within cells that follows even modest shifts of phosphate from one compartment to the other.

Phosphate is widely available in foods and is absorbed efficiently (65%) by the small intestine even in the absence of vitamin D. However, phosphate absorptive efficiency may be enhanced (to 85–90%) via active transport mechanisms that are stimulated by $1,25(OH)_2D$. These mechanisms involve activation of Na^+/PO_4^{2-} co-transporters that move phosphate into intestinal cells against an unfavorable electrochemical gradient. Daily net intestinal phosphate absorption varies widely with the composition of the diet but is generally in the range of 500–1000 mg/d. Phosphate absorption can be inhibited by large doses of calcium salts or by sevelamer hydrochloride (Renagel), strategies commonly used to control levels of serum phosphate in renal failure. Aluminum hydroxide antacids also reduce phosphate absorption but are used less commonly because of the potential for aluminum toxicity. Low serum phosphate stimulates renal proximal tubular synthesis of $1,25(OH)_2D$, perhaps by suppressing blood levels of FGF23 (see below).

Serum phosphate levels vary by as much as 50% on a normal day. This reflects the effect of food intake but also an underlying circadian rhythm that produces a nadir between 7 and 10 A.M. Carbohydrate administration, especially as IV dextrose solutions in fasting subjects, can decrease serum phosphate by >0.7 mmol/L (2 mg/dL) due to rapid uptake into and utilization by cells. A similar response is observed in the treatment of diabetic ketoacidosis and during metabolic or respiratory alkalosis. Because of this wide variation in serum phosphate, it is best to perform measurements in the basal, fasting state.

Control of serum phosphate is determined mainly by the rate of renal tubular reabsorption of the filtered load, which is ~4–6 g/d. Because intestinal phosphate absorption is highly efficient, urinary excretion is not constant but varies directly with dietary intake. The fractional excretion of phosphate (ratio of phosphate to creatinine clearance) is generally in the range of 10–15%. The proximal tubule is the principal site at which renal phosphate reabsorption is regulated. This is accomplished by changes in the levels of apical expression and activity of specific Na^+/PO_4^{2-} co-transporters (NaPi-2 and NaPi-2c) in the proximal tubule. Levels of these transporters at the apical surface of these cells are reduced rapidly by PTH, the major known hormonal regulator of renal phosphate excretion. FGF23 can impair phosphate reabsorption dramatically by a similar mechnism. Activating *FGF23* mutations cause the rare disorder autosomal dominant hypophosphatemic rickets. In contrast to PTH, FGF23 also leads to reduced synthesis of $1,25(OH)_2D$, which may worsen the resulting hypophosphatemia by lowering intestinal phosphate absorption. Renal reabsorption of phosphate is responsive to changes in dietary intake such that experimental dietary phosphate restriction leads to a dramatic lowering of urinary phosphate within hours, preceding any decline in serum phosphate (e.g., filtered load). This physiologic renal adaptation to changes in dietary phosphate availability occurs independently of PTH and may be mediated in part by changes in levels of serum FGF23. Findings in *FGF23*-knockout mice suggest that FGF23 normally acts to lower blood phosphate and $1,25(OH)_2D$ levels. In turn, elevation of blood phosphate increases blood levels of FGF23.

Renal phosphate reabsorption is impaired by hypocalcemia, hypomagnesemia, and severe hypophosphatemia. Phosphate clearance is enhanced by ECF volume expansion and impaired by dehydration. Phosphate retention is an important pathophysiologic feature of renal insufficiency (Chap. 280).

HYPOPHOSPHATEMIA

Causes

Hypophosphatemia can occur by one or more of three primary mechanisms: (1) inadequate intestinal phosphate absorption, (2) excessive renal phosphate excretion, and (3) rapid redistribution of phosphate from the ECF into bone or soft tissue (Table 352-1). Because phosphate is so abundant in foods, inadequate intestinal absorption is almost never observed now that aluminum hydroxide antacids, which bind phosphate in the gut, are no longer used commonly. Fasting or starvation, however, may result in depletion of body phosphate and predispose to subsequent hypophosphatemia during refeeding, especially if this is accomplished with IV glucose alone.

Chronic hypophosphatemia usually signifies a persistent renal tubular phosphate-wasting disorder. Excessive activation of PTH/PTHrP receptors in the proximal tubule as a result of primary or secondary hyperparathyroidism or because of the PTHrP-mediated hypercalcemia syndrome in malignancy (Chap. 353) is among the more common causes of renal hypophosphatemia, especially because of the high prevalence of vitamin D deficiency in older Americans. Familial hypocalciuric hypercalcemia and Jansen's chondrodystrophy are rare examples of genetic disorders in this category (Chap. 353).

Several genetic and acquired diseases cause PTH/PTHrP-independent tubular phosphate wasting with associated rickets and osteomalacia. All these diseases manifest severe hypophosphatemia; renal phosphate wasting, sometimes accompanied by aminoaciduria; low blood levels of $1,25(OH)_2D$; low-normal serum levels of calcium; and evidence of impaired cartilage or bone mineralization. Analysis of these diseases has led to the discovery of the hormone FGF23, which is an important physiologic regulator of phosphate metabolism. FGF23 decreases phosphate reabsorption in the proximal tubule and also suppresses the 1α-hydroxylase responsible for synthesis of $1,25(OH)_2D$. FGF23 is synthesized by cells of the osteoblast lineage, primarily osteocytes. High-phosphate diets increase FGF23 levels, and low-phosphate diets decrease them. Autosomal dominant hypophosphatemic rickets (ADHR) was the first disease linked to abnormalities in FGF23. ADHR results from activating mutations in the gene that encodes FGF23. The most common inherited cause of hypophosphatemia is X-linked hypophosphatemic rickets (XLHR), which results from inactivating mutations in an endopeptidase termed *PHEX* (*p*hosphate-regulating gene with *h*omologies to *e*ndopeptidases on the *X* chromosome) that is expressed most abundantly on the surface of osteocytes and mature osteoblasts. Patients with XLH usually have high FGF23 levels, and ablation of the *FGF23* gene reverses the hypophosphatemia found in the mouse version of XLH. How inactivation of PHEX leads to increased levels of FGF23 has not been determined. A third hypophosphatemic disorder, tumor-induced osteomalacia (TIO), is an acquired disorder in which tumors, usually of mesenchymal origin and generally histologically benign, secrete molecules that induce renal phosphate wasting. The hypophosphatemic syndrome resolves completely within hours to days after successful resection of the responsible tumor. Such tumors express large amounts of FGF23 mRNA, and patients with TIO usually exhibit elevations of FGF23 in their blood.

TABLE 352-1 Causes of Hypophosphatemia

- I. Reduced renal tubular phosphate reabsorption
  - A. PTH/PTHrP-dependent
    - 1. Primary hyperparathyroidism
    - 2. Secondary hyperparathyroidism
      - a. Vitamin D deficiency/resistance
      - b. Calcium starvation/malabsorption
      - c. Bartter's syndrome
      - d. Autosomal recessive renal hypercalciuria with hypomagnesemia
    - 3. PTHrP-dependent hypercalcemia of malignancy
    - 4. Familial hypocalciuric hypercalcemia
  - B. PTH/PTHrP-independent
    - 1. Excess FGF23 or other "phosphatonins"
      - a. X-linked hypophosphatemic rickets (XLHR)
      - b. Autosomal recessive hypophosphatemia (ARHP)
      - c. Autosomal dominant hypophosphatemic rickets (ADHR)
      - d. Tumor-induced osteomalacia syndrome (TIO)
      - e. McCune-Albright syndrome (fibrous dysplasia)
      - f. Epidermal nevus syndrome
    - 2. Intrinsic renal disease
      - a. Fanconi's syndrome(s)
      - b. Cystinosis
      - c. Wilson's disease
      - d. NaPi-2a or NaPi-2c mutations
    - 3. Other systemic disorders
      - a. Poorly controlled diabetes mellitus
      - b. Alcoholism
      - c. Hyperaldosteronism
      - d. Hypomagnesemia
      - e. Amyloidosis
      - f. Hemolytic-uremic syndrome
      - g. Renal transplantation or partial liver resection
      - h. Rewarming or induced hyperthermia
    - 4. Drugs or toxins
      - a. Ethanol
      - b. Acetazolamide, other diuretics
      - c. High-dose estrogens or glucocorticoids
      - d. Heavy metals (lead, cadmium)
      - e. Toluene, *N*-methyl formamide
      - f. Cisplatin, ifosfamide, foscarnet, rapamycin
- II. Impaired intestinal phosphate absorption
  - A. Aluminum-containing antacids
  - B. Sevalamer
- III. Shifts of extracellular phosphate into cells
  - A. Intravenous glucose
  - B. Insulin therapy for prolonged hyperglycemia or diabetic ketoacidosis
  - C. Catecholamines (epinephrine, dopamine, albuterol)
  - D. Acute respiratory alkalosis
  - E. Gram-negative sepsis, toxic shock syndrome
  - F. Recovery from starvation or acidosis
  - G. Rapid cellular proliferation
    - 1. Leukemic blast crisis
    - 2. Intensive erythropoietin, other growth factor therapy
- IV. Accelerated net bone formation
  - A. After parathyroidectomy
  - B. Treatment of vitamin D deficiency, Paget's disease
  - C. Osteoblastic metastases

Dent's disease is an X-linked recessive disorder caused by inactivating mutations in CLCN5, a chloride transporter expressed in endosomes of the proximal tubule; features include hypercalciuria, hypophosphatemia, and recurrent kidney stones. Renal phosphate wasting is common among poorly controlled diabetic patients and alcoholics, who therefore are at risk for iatrogenic hypophosphatemia when treated with insulin or IV glucose, respectively. Diuretics and certain other drugs and toxins can cause defective renal tubular phosphate reabsorption (Table 352-1).

In hospitalized patients, hypophosphatemia is often attributable to massive redistribution of phosphate from the ECF into cells. Insulin therapy for diabetic ketoacidosis is a paradigm for this phenomenon, in which the severity of the hypophosphatemia is related to the extent of antecedent depletion of phosphate and other electrolytes (Chap. 344). The hypophosphatemia is usually greatest at a point many hours after initiation of insulin therapy and is difficult to predict from baseline measurements of serum phosphate at the time of presentation, when prerenal azotemia can obscure significant phosphate depletion. Other factors that may contribute to such acute redistributive hypophosphatemia include antecedent starvation or malnutrition, administration of IV glucose without other nutrients, elevated blood catecholamines (endogenous or exogenous), respiratory alkalosis, and recovery from metabolic acidosis.

Hypophosphatemia also can occur transiently (over weeks to months) during the phase of accelerated net bone formation that follows parathyroidectomy for severe primary hyperparathyroidism or during treatment of vitamin D deficiency or lytic Paget's disease. This is usually most prominent in patients who preoperatively have evidence of high bone turnover (e.g., high serum levels of alkaline phosphatase). Osteoblastic metastases can also lead to this syndrome.

Clinical and laboratory findings

The clinical manifestations of severe hypophosphatemia reflect a generalized defect in cellular energy metabolism because of ATP depletion, a shift from oxidative phosphorylation toward glycolysis, and associated tissue or organ dysfunction. Acute, severe hypophosphatemia occurs mainly or exclusively in hospitalized patients with underlying serious medical or surgical illness and preexisting phosphate depletion due to excessive urinary losses, severe malabsorption, or malnutrition. Chronic hypophosphatemia tends to be less severe, with a clinical presentation dominated by musculoskeletal complaints such as bone pain, osteomalacia, pseudofractures, and proximal muscle weakness or, in children, rickets and short stature.

Neuromuscular manifestations of severe hypophosphatemia are variable but may include muscle weakness, lethargy, confusion, disorientation, hallucinations, dysarthria, dysphagia, oculomotor palsies, anisocoria, nystagmus, ataxia, cerebellar tremor, ballismus, hyporeflexia, impaired sphincter control, distal sensory deficits, paresthesia, hyperesthesia, generalized or Guillain-Barré–like ascending paralysis, seizures, coma, and even death. Serious sequelae such as paralysis, confusion, and seizures are likely only at phosphate concentrations <0.25 mmol/L (<0.8 mg/dL). Rhabdomyolysis may develop during rapidly progressive hypophosphatemia. The diagnosis of hypophosphatemia-induced rhabdomyolysis may be overlooked, as up to 30% of patients with acute hypophosphatemia (<0.7 m*M*) have creatine phosphokinase elevations that peak one to two days after the nadir in serum phosphate, when the release of phosphate from injured myocytes may have led to a near normalization of circulating levels of phosphate.

Respiratory failure and cardiac dysfunction, which are reversible with phosphate treatment, may occur at serum phosphate levels of 0.5–0.8 mmol/L (1.5–2.5 mg/dL). Renal tubular defects, including tubular acidosis, glycosuria, and impaired reabsorption of sodium and calcium, may occur. Hematologic abnormalities correlate with reductions in intracellular ATP and 2,3-diphosphoglycerate and may include erythrocyte microspherocytosis and hemolysis; impaired oxyhemoglobin dissociation; defective leukocyte chemotaxis, phagocytosis, and bacterial killing; and platelet dysfunction with spontaneous gastrointestinal hemorrhage.

TREATMENT Hypophosphatemia

Severe hypophosphatemia [<0.75 mmol/L (<2 mg/dL)], particularly in the setting of underlying phosphate depletion, constitutes a dangerous electrolyte abnormality that should be corrected promptly. Unfortunately, the cumulative deficit in body phosphate cannot be predicted easily from knowledge of the circulating level of phosphate, and therapy must be approached empirically. The threshold for IV phosphate therapy and the dose administered should reflect consideration of renal function, the likely severity and duration of the underlying phosphate depletion, and the presence and severity of symptoms consistent with those of hypophosphatemia. In adults, phosphate may be safely administered IV as neutral mixtures of sodium and potassium phosphate salts at initial doses of 0.2–0.8 mmol/kg of elemental phosphorus over 6 hours (e.g., 10–50 mmol over 6 hours), with doses >20 mmol/6 hours reserved for those who have serum levels <0.5 mmol/L (1.5 mg/dL) and normal renal function. A suggested approach is presented in Table 352-2. Serum levels of phosphate and calcium must be monitored closely (every 6–12 hours) throughout treatment. It is necessary to avoid a serum calcium-phosphorus product >50 to reduce the risk of heterotopic calcification. Hypocalcemia, if present, should be corrected before administering IV phosphate. Less severe hypophosphatemia, in the range of 0.5–0.8 mmol/L (1.5–2.5 mg/dL), usually can be treated with oral phosphate in divided doses of 750–2000 mg/d as elemental phosphorus; higher doses can cause bloating and diarrhea.

Management of chronic hypophosphatemia requires knowledge of the cause(s) of the disorder. Hypophosphatemia related to the secondary hyperparathyroidism of vitamin D deficiency usually responds to treatment with vitamin D and calcium alone. XLHR, ADHR, TIO, and related renal tubular disorders usually are managed with divided oral doses of phosphate, often with calcium and $1,25(OH)_2D$ supplements to bypass the block in renal $1,25(OH)_2D$ synthesis and prevent secondary hyperparathyroidism caused by suppression of ECF calcium levels. Thiazide diuretics may be used to prevent nephrocalcinosis in patients who are managed this way. Complete normalization of hypophosphatemia is generally not possible in these conditions. Optimal therapy for TIO is extirpation of the responsible tumor, which may be localized by radiographic skeletal survey or bone scan (many are located in bone) or by radionuclide scanning using sestamibi or labeled octreotide. Successful treatment of TIO-induced hypophosphatemia with octreotide has been reported in a small number of patients.

HYPERPHOSPHATEMIA

Causes

When the filtered load of phosphate and glomerular filtration rate (GFR) are normal, control of serum phosphate levels is achieved by adjusting the rate at which phosphate is reabsorbed by the proximal tubular NaPi-2 co-transporters. The principal hormonal regulators of NaPi-2 activity are PTH and FGF23. Hyperphosphatemia, defined in adults as a fasting serum phosphate concentration >1.8 mmol/L (5.5 mg/dL), usually results from impaired glomerular filtration, hypoparathyroidism, excessive delivery of phosphate into the ECF (from bone, gut, or parenteral phosphate therapy), or a combination of these factors (Table 352-3). The upper limit

TABLE 352-2 Intravenous Therapy for Hypophosphatemia

Consider

Likely severity of underlying phosphate depletion

Concurrent parenteral glucose administration

Presence of neuromuscular, cardiopulmonary, or hematologic complications of hypophosphatemia

Renal function [reduce dose by 50% if serum creatinine >220 μmol/L (>2.5 mg/dL)]

Serum calcium level (correct hypocalcemia first; reduce dose by 50% in hypercalcemia)

Guidelines

Serum Phosphorus, m*M* (mg/dL)	Rate of Infusion, mmol/h	Duration, h	Total Administered, mmol
<0.8 (<2.5)	2	6	12
<0.5 (<1.5)	4	6	24
<0.3 (<1)	8	6	48

Rates shown are calculated for a 70-kg person; levels of serum calcium and phosphorus must be measured every 6 to 12 h during therapy; infusions can be repeated to achieve stable serum phosphorus levels >0.8 mmol/L (>2.5 mg/dL); most formulations available in the United States provide 3 mmol/mL of sodium or potassium phosphate.

TABLE 352-3 Causes of Hyperphosphatemia

I. Impaired renal phosphate excretion
  A. Renal insufficiency
  B. Hypoparathyroidism
    1. Developmental
    2. Autoimmune
    3. After neck surgery or radiation
    4. Activating mutations of the calcium-sensing receptor
  C. Parathyroid suppression
    1. Parathyroid-independent hypercalcemia
      a. Vitamin D or vitamin A intoxication
      b. Sarcoidosis, other granulomatous diseases
      c. Immobilization, osteolytic metastases
      d. Milk-alkali syndrome
    2. Severe hypermagnesemia or hypomagnesemia
  D. Pseudohypoparathyroidism
  E. Acromegaly
  F. Tumoral calcinosis
  G. Heparin therapy
II. Massive extracellular fluid phosphate loads
  A. Rapid administration of exogenous phosphate (intravenous, oral, rectal)
  B. Extensive cellular injury or necrosis
    1. Crush injuries
    2. Rhabdomyolysis
    3. Hyperthermia
    4. Fulminant hepatitis
    5. Cytotoxic therapy
    6. Severe hemolytic anemia
  C. Transcellular phosphate shifts
    1. Metabolic acidosis
    2. Respiratory acidosis

of normal serum phosphate concentrations is higher in children and neonates [2.4 mmol/L (7 mg/dL)]. It is useful to distinguish hyperphosphatemia caused by impaired renal phosphate excretion from that which results from excessive delivery of phosphate into the ECF (Table 352-3).

In chronic renal insufficiency, reduced GFR leads to phosphate retention. Hyperphosphatemia in turn further impairs renal synthesis of $1,25(OH)_2D$ and stimulates PTH secretion and hypertrophy both directly and indirectly (by lowering blood ionized calcium levels). Thus, hyperphosphatemia is a major cause of the secondary hyperparathyroidism of renal failure and must be addressed early in the course of the disease (Chaps. 280 and 353).

Hypoparathyroidism leads to hyperphosphatemia via increased expression of NaPi-2 co-transporters in the proximal tubule. Hypoparathyroidism, or parathyroid suppression, has multiple potential causes, including autoimmune disease; developmental, surgical, or radiation-induced absence of functional parathyroid tissue; vitamin D intoxication or other causes of PTH-independent hypercalcemia; cellular PTH resistance (pseudohypoparathyroidism or hypomagnesemia); infiltrative disorders such as Wilson's disease and hemochromatosis; and impaired PTH secretion caused by hypermagnesemia, severe hypomagnesemia, or activating mutations in the CaSR. Hypocalcemia may also contribute directly to impaired phosphate clearance, as calcium infusion can induce hyperphosphaturia in hypoparathyroid subjects. Increased tubular phosphate reabsorption also occurs in acromegaly, during heparin administration, and in tumoral calcinosis. Tumoral calcinosis is caused by a rare group of genetic disorders in which the *FGF23* gene is inactivated directly or FGF23 is processed in a way that leads to low levels of active FGF23 in the bloodstream. A similar syndrome results from FGF23 resistance due to inactivating mutations of the FGF23 co-receptor Klotho. These abnormalities cause elevated serum $1,25(OH)_2D$, parathyroid suppression, increased intestinal calcium absorption, and focal hyperostosis with large, lobulated periarticular heterotopic ossifications (especially at shoulders or hips) and are accompanied by hyperphosphatemia. In some forms of tumoral calcinosis serum phosphorus levels are normal.

When large amounts of phosphate are delivered rapidly into the ECF, hyperphosphatemia can occur despite normal renal function. Examples include overzealous IV phosphate therapy, oral or rectal administration of large amounts of phosphate-containing laxatives or enemas (especially in children), extensive soft tissue injury or necrosis (crush injuries, rhabdomyolysis, hyperthermia, fulminant hepatitis, cytotoxic chemotherapy), extensive hemolytic anemia, and transcellular phosphate shifts induced by severe metabolic or respiratory acidosis.

Clinical findings

The clinical consequences of acute, severe hyperphosphatemia are due mainly to the formation of widespread calcium phosphate precipitates and resulting hypocalcemia. Thus, tetany, seizures, accelerated nephrocalcinosis (with renal failure, hyperkalemia, hyperuricemia, and metabolic acidosis), and pulmonary or cardiac calcifications (including development of acute heart block) may occur. The severity of these complications relates to the elevation of serum phosphate levels, which can reach concentrations as high as 7 mmol/L (20 mg/dL) in instances of massive soft tissue injury or tumor lysis syndrome.

TREATMENT Hyperphosphatemia

Therapeutic options for management of severe hyperphosphatemia are limited. Volume expansion may enhance renal phosphate clearance. Aluminum hydroxide antacids or sevalamer may be helpful in chelating and limiting absorption of offending phosphate salts present in the intestine. Hemodialysis is the most effective therapeutic strategy and should be considered early in the course of severe hyperphosphatemia, especially in the setting of renal failure and symptomatic hypocalcemia.

MAGNESIUM METABOLISM

Magnesium is the major intracellular divalent cation. Normal concentrations of extracellular magnesium and calcium are crucial for normal neuromuscular activity. Intracellular magnesium forms a key complex with ATP and is an important cofactor for a wide range of enzymes, transporters, and nucleic acids required for normal cellular function, replication, and energy metabolism. The concentration of magnesium in serum is closely regulated within the range of 0.7–1 mmol/L (1.5–2 meq/L; 1.7–2.4 mg/dL), of which 30% is protein-bound and another 15% is loosely complexed to phosphate and other anions. One-half of the 25 g (1000 mmol) of total body magnesium is located in bone, only one-half of which is insoluble in the mineral phase. Almost all extraskeletal magnesium is present within cells, where the total concentration is 5 m*M*, 95% of which is bound to proteins and other macromolecules. Because only 1% of body magnesium resides in the ECF, measurements of serum magnesium levels may not accurately reflect the level of total body magnesium stores.

Dietary magnesium content normally ranges from 6 to 15 mmol/d (140–360 mg/d), of which 30–40% is absorbed, mainly in the jejunum and ileum. Intestinal magnesium absorptive efficiency is stimulated by $1,25(OH)_2D$ and can reach 70% during magnesium deprivation. Urinary magnesium excretion normally matches net intestinal absorption and is ~4 mmol/d (100 mg/d). Regulation of serum magnesium concentrations is achieved mainly by control of renal magnesium reabsorption. Only 20% of filtered magnesium is reabsorbed in the proximal tubule, whereas 60% is reclaimed in the cTAL and another 5–10% in the DCT. Magnesium reabsorption in the cTAL occurs via a paracellular route that requires both a lumen-positive potential, created by NaCl reabsorption, and tight-junction proteins encoded by members of the Claudin gene family. Magnesium reabsorption in the cTAL is increased by PTH but inhibited by hypercalcemia or hypermagnesemia, both of which activate the CaSR in this nephron segment.

HYPOMAGNESEMIA

Causes

Hypomagnesemia usually signifies substantial depletion of body magnesium stores (0.5–1 mmol/kg). Hypomagnesemia can result from intestinal malabsorption; protracted vomiting, diarrhea, or intestinal drainage; defective renal tubular magnesium reabsorption; or rapid shifts of magnesium from the ECF into cells, bone, or third spaces (Table 352-4). Dietary magnesium deficiency is unlikely except possibly in the setting of alcoholism. A rare genetic disorder that causes selective intestinal magnesium malabsorption has been described (primary infantile hypomagnesemia). Another rare inherited disorder (hypomagnesemia with secondary hypocalcemia) is caused by mutations in the gene encoding TRPM6, a protein that, along with TRPM7, forms a channel important for both intestinal and distal-tubular renal magnesium transport. Malabsorptive states, often compounded by vitamin D deficiency, can critically limit magnesium absorption and produce hypomagnesemia despite the compensatory effects of secondary hyperparathyroidism and of hypocalcemia and hypomagnesemia to enhance cTAL magnesium reabsorption. Diarrhea or surgical drainage fluid may contain ≥5 mmol/L of magnesium.

Several genetic magnesium-wasting syndromes have been described, including inactivating mutations of genes encoding the DCT NaCl co-transporter (Gitelman's syndrome), proteins required for cTAL Na-K-2Cl transport (Bartter's syndrome), paracellin-1 (autosomal recessive renal hypomagnesemia with hypercalciuria), a DCT Na^+,K^+-ATPase γ-subunit (autosomal dominant renal hypomagnesemia with hypocalciuria), and a mitochondrial DNA gene encoding a mitochondrial tRNA. ECF expansion, hypercalcemia, and severe phosphate depletion may impair magnesium reabsorption, as can various forms of renal injury, including those caused by drugs such as cisplatin, cyclosporine, aminoglycosides, and pentamidine as well as the EGF receptor inhibitory antibody cetuximab (Table 352-4). A rising blood concentration of ethanol directly impairs tubular magnesium reabsorption, and persistent glycosuria with osmotic diuresis leads to magnesium wasting and probably contributes to the high frequency of hypomagnesemia in poorly controlled diabetic patients. Magnesium depletion is aggravated by metabolic acidosis, which causes intracellular losses as well.

TABLE 352-4 Causes of Hypomagnesemia

I. Impaired intestinal absorption
   A. Hypomagnesemia with secondary hypocalcemia (TRPM6 mutations)
   B. Malabsorption syndromes
   C. Vitamin D deficiency
II. Increased intestinal losses
   A. Protracted vomiting/diarrhea
   B. Intestinal drainage, fistulas
III. Impaired renal tubular reabsorption
   A. Genetic magnesium-wasting syndromes
      1. Gitelman's syndrome
      2. Bartter's syndrome
      3. Claudin 16 or 19 mutations
      4. Na^+,K^+-ATPase γ-subunit mutations (FXYD2)
      5. Autosomal dominant, with low bone mass
   B. Acquired renal disease
      1. Tubulointerstitial disease
      2. Postobstruction, ATN (diuretic phase)
      3. Renal transplantation
   C. Drugs and toxins
      1. Ethanol
      2. Diuretics (loop, thiazide, osmotic)
      3. Cisplatin
      4. Pentamidine, foscarnet
      5. Cyclosporine
      6. Aminoglycosides, amphotericin B
      7. Cetuximab
   D. Other
      1. Extracellular fluid volume expansion
      2. Hyperaldosteronism
      3. SIADH
      4. Diabetes mellitus
      5. Hypercalcemia
      6. Phosphate depletion
      7. Metabolic acidosis
      8. Hyperthyroidism
IV. Rapid shifts from extracellular fluid
   A. Intracellular redistribution
      1. Recovery from diabetic ketoacidosis
      2. Refeeding syndrome
      3. Correction of respiratory acidosis
      4. Catecholamines
   B. Accelerated bone formation
      1. Post-parathyroidectomy
      2. Treatment of vitamin D deficiency
      3. Osteoblastic metastases
   C. Other
      1. Pancreatitis, burns, excessive sweating
      2. Pregnancy (third trimester) and lactation

Abbreviations: ATN, acute tubular necrosis; SIADH, syndrome of inappropriate antidiuretic hormone.

Hypomagnesemia due to rapid shifts of magnesium from ECF into the intracellular compartment can occur during recovery from diabetic ketoacidosis, starvation, or respiratory acidosis. Less acute shifts may be seen during rapid bone formation after parathyroidectomy, with treatment of vitamin D deficiency, or with osteoblastic metastases. Large amounts of magnesium may be lost with acute pancreatitis, extensive burns, and protracted and severe sweating and during pregnancy and lactation.

Clinical and laboratory findings

Hypomagnesemia may cause generalized alterations in neuromuscular function, including tetany, tremor, seizures, muscle weakness, ataxia, nystagmus, vertigo, apathy, depression, irritability, delirium, and psychosis. Patients are usually asymptomatic when serum magnesium concentrations are >0.5 mmol/L (1 meq/L; 1.2 mg/dL), although the severity of symptoms may not correlate with serum magnesium levels. Cardiac arrhythmias may occur, including sinus tachycardia, other supraventricular tachycardias, and ventricular arrhythmias. Electrocardiographic abnormalities may include prolonged PR or QT intervals, T-wave flattening or inversion, and ST straightening. Sensitivity to digitalis toxicity may be enhanced.

Other electrolyte abnormalities often seen with hypomagnesemia, including hypocalcemia (with hypocalciuria) and hypokalemia, may not be easily corrected unless magnesium is administered as well. The hypocalcemia may be a result of concurrent vitamin D deficiency, although hypomagnesemia can cause impaired synthesis of $1,25(OH)_2D$, cellular resistance to PTH, and, at very low serum magnesium [<0.4 mmol/L (<0.8 meq/L; <1 mg/dL)], a defect in PTH secretion; these abnormalities are reversible with therapy.

TREATMENT Hypomagnesemia

Mild, asymptomatic hypomagnesemia may be treated with oral magnesium salts [$MgCl_2$, MgO, $Mg(OH)_2$] in divided doses totaling 20–30 mmol/d (40–60 meq/d). Diarrhea may occur with larger doses. More severe hypomagnesemia should be treated parenterally, preferably with IV $MgCl_2$, which can be administered safely as a continuous infusion of 50 mmol/d (100 meq Mg^{2+}/d) if renal function is normal. If GFR is reduced, the infusion rate should be lowered by 50–75%. Use of IM $MgSO_4$ is discouraged; the injections are painful and provide relatively little magnesium (2 mL of 50% $MgSO_4$ supplies only 4 mmol). $MgSO_4$ may be given IV instead of $MgCl_2$, although the sulfate anions may bind calcium in serum and urine and aggravate hypocalcemia. Serum magnesium should be monitored at intervals of 12–24 hours during therapy, which may continue for several days because of impaired renal conservation of magnesium (only 50–70% of the daily IV magnesium dose is retained) and delayed repletion of intracellular deficits, which may be as high as 1–1.5 mmol/kg (2–3 meq/kg).

It is important to consider the need for calcium, potassium, and phosphate supplementation in patients with hypomagnesemia. Vitamin D deficiency frequently coexists and should be treated with oral or parenteral vitamin D or 25(OH)D [but not with $1,25(OH)_2D$, which may impair tubular magnesium reabsorption, possibly via PTH suppression]. In severely hypomagnesemic patients with concomitant hypocalcemia and hypophosphatemia, administration of IV magnesium alone may worsen hypophosphatemia, provoking neuromuscular symptoms or rhabdomyolysis, due to rapid stimulation of PTH secretion. This is avoided by administering both calcium and magnesium.

HYPERMAGNESEMIA

Causes

Hypermagnesemia is rarely seen in the absence of renal insufficiency, as normal kidneys can excrete large amounts (250 mmol/d) of magnesium. Mild hypermagnesemia due to excessive reabsorption in the cTAL occurs with calcium-sensing receptor mutations in familial hypocalciuric hypercalcemia and has been described in some patients with adrenal insufficiency, hypothyroidism, or hypothermia. Massive exogenous magnesium exposures, usually via the gastrointestinal tract, can overwhelm renal excretory capacity and cause life-threatening hypermagnesemia (Table 352-5). A notable example of this is prolonged retention of even normal amounts of magnesium-containing cathartics in patients with intestinal ileus, obstruction, or perforation. Extensive soft tissue injury or necrosis can also deliver large amounts of magnesium into the ECF in patients who have suffered trauma, shock, sepsis, cardiac arrest, or severe burns.

TABLE 352-5 Causes of Hypermagnesemia

I. Excessive magnesium intake
  A. Cathartics, urologic irrigants
  B. Parenteral magnesium administration
II. Rapid mobilization from soft tissues
  A. Trauma, shock, sepsis
  B. Cardiac arrest
  C. Burns
III. Impaired magnesium excretion
  A. Renal failure
  B. Familial hypocalciuric hypercalcemia
IV. Other
  A. Adrenal insufficiency
  B. Hypothyroidism
  C. Hypothermia
V. Excessive magnesium intake
  A. Cathartics, urologic irrigants
  B. Parenteral magnesium administration
VI. Rapid mobilization from soft tissues
  A. Trauma, shock, sepsis
  B. Cardiac arrest
  C. Burns
VII. Impaired magnesium excretion
  A. Renal failure
  B. Familial hypocalciuric hypercalcemia
VIII. Other
  A. Adrenal insufficiency
  B. Hypothyroidism
  C. Hypothermia

Clinical and laboratory findings

The most prominent clinical manifestations of hypermagnesemia are vasodilation and neuromuscular blockade, which may appear at serum magnesium concentrations >2 mmol/L (>4 meq/L; >4.8 mg/dL). Hypotension that is refractory to vasopressors or volume expansion may be an early sign. Nausea, lethargy, and weakness may progress to respiratory failure, paralysis, and coma, with hypoactive tendon reflexes, at serum magnesium levels >4 mmol/L. Other findings may include gastrointestinal hypomotility or ileus; facial flushing; pupillary dilation; paradoxical bradycardia; prolongation of PR, QRS, and QT intervals; heart block; and, at serum magnesium levels approaching 10 mmol/L, asystole.

Hypermagnesemia, acting via the CaSR, causes hypocalcemia and hypercalciuria due to both parathyroid suppression and impaired cTAL calcium reabsorption.

TREATMENT Hypermagnesemia

Successful treatment of hypermagnesemia generally involves identifying and interrupting the source of magnesium and employing measures to increase magnesium clearance from the ECF. Use of magnesium-free cathartics or enemas may be helpful in clearing ingested magnesium from the gastrointestinal tract. Vigorous IV hydration should be attempted, if appropriate. Hemodialysis is effective and may be required in patients with significant renal insufficiency. Calcium, administered IV in doses of 100–200 mg over 1–2 hours, has been reported to provide temporary improvement in signs and symptoms of hypermagnesemia.

VITAMIN D

SYNTHESIS AND METABOLISM

1,25-dihydroxyvitamin D [$1,25(OH)_2D$] is the major steroid hormone involved in mineral ion homeostasis regulation. Vitamin D and its metabolites are hormones and hormone precursors rather than vitamins, since in the proper biologic setting, they can be synthesized endogenously (Fig. 352-4). In response to ultraviolet radiation of the skin, a photochemical cleavage results in the formation of vitamin D from 7-dehydrocholesterol. Cutaneous production of vitamin D is decreased by melanin and high solar protection factor sunblocks, which effectively impair skin penetration by ultraviolet light. The increased use of sunblocks in North America and Western Europe and a reduction in the magnitude of solar exposure of the general population over the last several decades has led to an increased reliance on dietary sources of vitamin D. In the United States and Canada, these sources largely consist of fortified cereals and dairy products, in addition to fish oils and egg yolks. Vitamin D from plant sources is in the form of vitamin D_2, whereas that from animal sources is vitamin D_3. These two forms have equivalent biologic activity and are activated equally well by the vitamin D hydroxylases in humans. Vitamin D enters the circulation, whether absorbed from the intestine or synthesized cutaneously, bound to vitamin D–binding protein, an α-globulin synthesized in the liver. Vitamin D is subsequently 25-hydroxylated in the liver by cytochrome P450–like enzymes in the mitochondria and microsomes. The activity of this hydroxylase is not tightly regulated, and the resultant metabolite, 25-hydroxyvitamin D [25(OH)D], is the major circulating and storage form of vitamin D. Approximately 88% of 25(OH)D circulates bound to the vitamin D–binding protein, 0.03% is free, and the rest circulates bound to albumin. The half-life of 25(OH)D is approximately two to three weeks; however, it is shortened dramatically when vitamin D–binding protein levels are reduced, as can occur with increased urinary losses in the nephrotic syndrome.

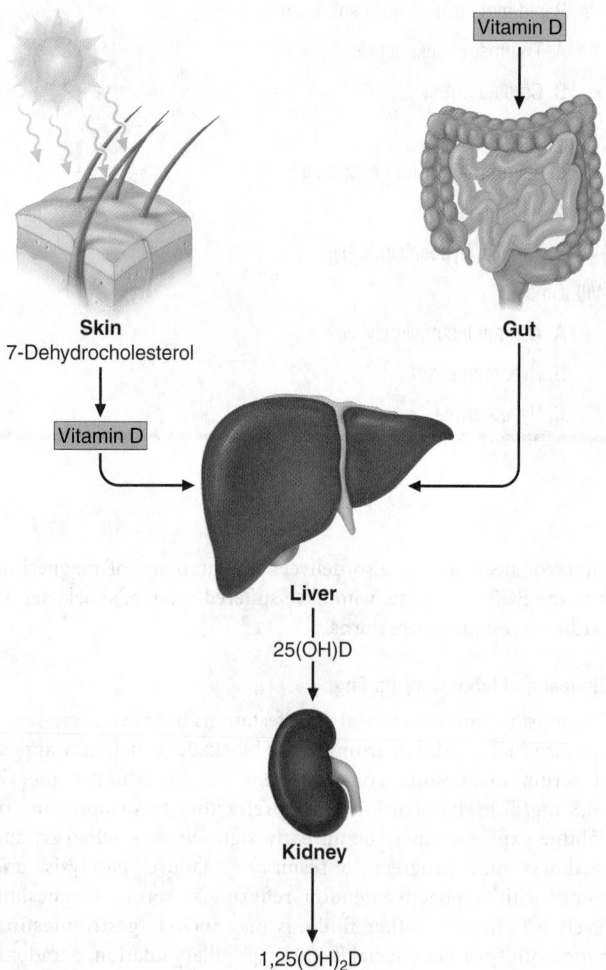

Figure 352-4 Vitamin D synthesis and activation. Vitamin D is synthesized in the skin in response to ultraviolet radiation and also is absorbed from the diet. It is then transported to the liver, where it undergoes 25-hydroxylation. This metabolite is the major circulating form of vitamin D. The final step in hormone activation, 1α-hydroxylation, occurs in the kidney.

The second hydroxylation, required for the formation of the mature hormone, occurs in the kidney (Fig. 352-5). The 25-hydroxyvitamin D-1α-hydroxylase is a tightly regulated cytochrome P450–like mixed-function oxidase expressed in the proximal convoluted tubule cells of the kidney. PTH and hypophosphatemia are the major inducers of this microsomal enzyme, whereas calcium, FGF23, and the enzyme's product, $1,25(OH)_2D$, repress it. The 25-hydroxyvitamin D-1α-hydroxylase is also present in epidermal keratinocytes, but keratinocyte production of $1,25(OH)_2D$ is not thought to contribute to circulating levels of this hormone. In addition to being present in the trophoblastic layer of the placenta, the 1α-hydroxylase is produced by macrophages associated with granulomas and lymphomas. In these latter pathologic states, the activity of the enzyme is induced by interferon γ and TNF-α but is not regulated by calcium or $1,25(OH)_2D$; therefore, hypercalcemia, associated with elevated levels of $1,25(OH)_2D$, may be observed. Treatment of sarcoidosis-associated hypercalcemia with glucocorticoids, ketoconazole, or chloroquine reduces $1,25(OH)_2D$ production and effectively lowers serum calcium. In contrast, chloroquine has not been shown to lower the elevated serum $1,25(OH)_2D$ levels in patients with lymphoma.

The major pathway for inactivation of vitamin D metabolites is an additional hydroxylation step by the vitamin D 24-hydroxylase, an enzyme that is expressed in most tissues. $1,25(OH)_2D$ is the major inducer of this enzyme; therefore, this hormone promotes its own inactivation, thereby limiting its biologic effects. Polar metabolites of $1,25(OH)_2D$ are secreted into the bile and reabsorbed via the enterohepatic circulation. Impairment of this recirculation, which is seen with diseases of the terminal ileum, leads to accelerated losses of vitamin D metabolites.

ACTIONS OF $1,25(OH)_2D$

$1,25(OH)_2D$ mediates its biologic effects by binding to a member of the nuclear receptor superfamily, the vitamin D receptor (VDR). This receptor belongs to the subfamily that includes the thyroid hormone receptors, the retinoid receptors, and the peroxisome proliferator–activated receptors; however, in contrast to the other members of this subfamily, only one VDR isoform

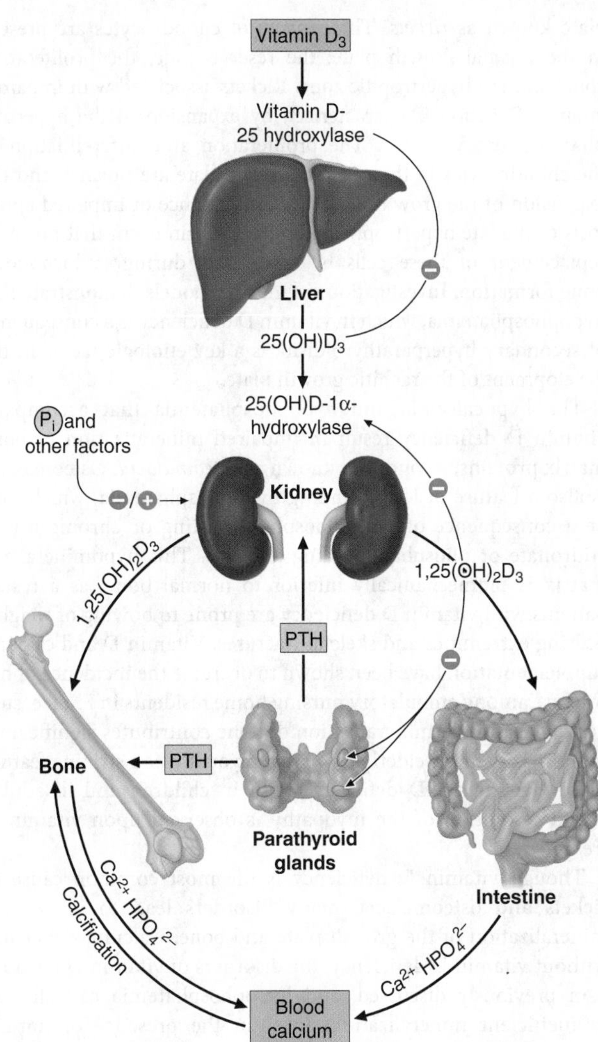

Figure 352-5 Schematic representation of the hormonal control loop for vitamin D metabolism and function. A reduction in the serum calcium below ~2.2 mmol/L (8.8 mg/dL) prompts a proportional increase in the secretion of parathyroid hormone (PTH) and so mobilizes additional calcium from the bone. PTH promotes the synthesis of $1,25(OH)_2D$ in the kidney, which in turn stimulates the mobilization of calcium from bone and intestine and regulates the synthesis of PTH by negative feedback.

has been isolated. The VDR binds to target DNA sequences as a heterodimer with the retinoid X receptor, recruiting a series of coactivators that modify chromatin and approximate the VDR to the basal transcriptional apparatus, resulting in the induction of target gene expression. The mechanism of transcriptional repression by the VDR varies with different target genes but has been shown to involve either interference with the action of activating transcription factors or the recruitment of novel proteins to the VDR complex, resulting in transcriptional repression.

The affinity of the VDR for $1,25(OH)_2D$ is approximately three orders of magnitude higher than that for other vitamin D metabolites. In normal physiologic circumstances, these other metabolites are not thought to stimulate receptor-dependent actions. However, in states of vitamin D toxicity, the markedly elevated levels of 25(OH)D may lead to hypercalcemia by interacting directly with the VDR and by displacing $1,25(OH)_2D$ from vitamin D–binding protein, resulting in increased bioavailability of the active hormone.

The VDR is expressed in a wide range of cells and tissues. The molecular actions of $1,25(OH)_2D$ have been studied most extensively in tissues involved in the regulation of mineral ion homeostasis. This hormone is a major inducer of calbindin 9K, a calcium-binding protein expressed in the intestine, which is thought to play an important role in the active transport of calcium across the enterocyte. The two major calcium transporters expressed by intestinal epithelia, TRPV5 and TRPV6 (transient receptor potential vanilloid), are also vitamin D responsive. By inducing the expression of these and other genes in the small intestine, $1,25(OH)_2D$ increases the efficiency of intestinal calcium absorption, and it also has been shown to have several important actions in the skeleton. The VDR is expressed in osteoblasts and regulates the expression of several genes in this cell. These genes include the bone matrix proteins osteocalcin and osteopontin, which are upregulated by $1,25(OH)_2D$, in addition to type I collagen, which is transcriptionally repressed by $1,25(OH)_2D$. Both $1,25(OH)_2D$ and PTH induce the expression of RANK ligand, which promotes osteoclast differentiation and increases osteoclast activity, by binding to RANK on osteoclast progenitors and mature osteoclasts. This is the mechanism by which $1,25(OH)_2D$ induces bone resorption. However, the skeletal features associated with VDR-knockout mice (rickets, osteomalacia) are largely corrected by increasing calcium and phosphorus intake, underscoring the importance of vitamin D action in the gut.

The VDR is expressed in the parathyroid gland, and $1,25(OH)_2D$ has been shown to have antiproliferative effects on parathyroid cells and to suppress the transcription of the parathyroid hormone gene. These effects of $1,25(OH)_2D$ on the parathyroid gland are an important part of the rationale for current therapies directed at preventing and treating hyperparathyroidism associated with renal insufficiency.

The VDR is also expressed in tissues and organs that do not play a role in mineral ion homeostasis. Notable in this respect is the observation that $1,25(OH)_2D$ has an antiproliferative effect on several cell types, including keratinocytes, breast cancer cells, and prostate cancer cells. The effects of $1,25(OH)_2D$ and the VDR on keratinocytes are particularly intriguing. Alopecia is seen in humans and mice with mutant VDRs but is not a feature of vitamin D deficiency; thus, the effects of the VDR on the hair follicle are ligand-independent.

VITAMIN D DEFICIENCY

The mounting concern about the relationship between solar exposure and the development of skin cancer has led to increased reliance on dietary sources of vitamin D. Although the prevalence of vitamin D deficiency varies, the third National Health and Nutrition Examination Survey (NHANES III) revealed that vitamin D deficiency is prevalent throughout the United States. The clinical syndrome of vitamin D deficiency can be a result of deficient production of vitamin D in the skin, lack of dietary intake, accelerated losses of vitamin D, impaired vitamin D activation, or resistance to the biologic effects of $1,25(OH)_2D$ (Table 352-6). The elderly and nursing home residents are particularly at risk for vitamin D deficiency, since both the efficiency of vitamin D synthesis in the skin and the absorption of vitamin D from the intestine decline with age. Similarly, intestinal malabsorption of dietary fats leads to vitamin D deficiency. This is further exacerbated in the presence of terminal ileal disease, which results in impaired enterohepatic circulation of vitamin D metabolites. In addition to intestinal diseases, accelerated inactivation of vitamin D metabolites can be seen with drugs that induce hepatic cytochrome P450 mixed-function oxidases such as barbiturates, phenytoin, and rifampin. Impaired 25-hydroxylation, associated with severe liver disease or isoniazid, is an uncommon cause of vitamin D deficiency. A mutation

TABLE 352-6 Causes of Impaired Vitamin D Action

Vitamin D deficiency	Impaired 1α-hydroxylation
Impaired cutaneous production	Hypoparathyroidism
Dietary absence	Renal failure
Malabsorption	Ketoconazole
Accelerated loss of vitamin D	1α-hydroxylase mutation
Increased metabolism (barbiturates, phenytoin, rifampin)	Oncogenic osteomalacia
Impaired enterohepatic circulation	X-linked hypophosphatemic rickets
Nephrotic syndrome	Target organ resistance
Impaired 25-hydroxylation	Vitamin D receptor mutation
Liver disease, isoniazid	Phenytoin

in the gene responsible for 25- hydroxylation has been identified in one kindred. Impaired 1α-hydroxylation is prevalent in the population with profound renal dysfunction due to an increase in circulating FGF23 levels and a decrease in functional renal mass. Thus, therapeutic interventions should be considered in patients whose creatinine clearance is <0.5 mL/s (30 mL/min). Mutations in the renal 1α-hydroxylase are the basis for the genetic disorder, pseudovitamin D–deficiency rickets. This autosomal recessive disorder presents with the syndrome of vitamin D deficiency in the first year of life. Patients present with growth retardation, rickets, and hypocalcemic seizures. Serum $1,25(OH)_2D$ levels are low despite normal 25(OH)D levels and elevated PTH levels. Treatment with vitamin D metabolites that do not require 1α-hydroxylation results in disease remission, although lifelong therapy is required. A second autosomal recessive disorder, hereditary vitamin D–resistant rickets, a consequence of vitamin D receptor mutations, is a greater therapeutic challenge. These patients present in a similar fashion during the first year of life, but alopecia often accompanies the disorder, demonstrating a functional role of the VDR in postnatal hair regeneration. Serum levels of $1,25(OH)_2D$ are dramatically elevated in these individuals both because of increased production due to stimulation of 1α-hydroxylase activity as a consequence of secondary hyperparathyroidism and because of impaired inactivation, since induction of the 24-hydroxylase by $1,25(OH)_2D$ requires an intact VDR. Since the receptor mutation results in hormone resistance, daily calcium and phosphorus infusions may be required to bypass the defect in intestinal mineral ion absorption.

Regardless of the cause, the clinical manifestations of vitamin D deficiency are largely a consequence of impaired intestinal calcium absorption. Mild to moderate vitamin D deficiency is asymptomatic, whereas long-standing vitamin D deficiency results in hypocalcemia accompanied by secondary hyperparathyroidism, impaired mineralization of the skeleton (osteopenia on x-ray or decreased bone mineral density), and proximal myopathy. Vitamin D deficiency also has been shown to be associated with an increase in overall mortality rates, including cardiovascular causes. In the absence of an intercurrent illness, the hypocalcemia associated with long-standing vitamin D deficiency rarely presents with acute symptoms of hypocalcemia such as numbness, tingling, and seizures. However, the concurrent development of hypomagnesemia, which impairs parathyroid function, or the administration of potent bisphosphonates, which impair bone resorption, can lead to acute symptomatic hypocalcemia in vitamin D–deficient individuals.

Rickets and osteomalacia

In children, before epiphyseal fusion, vitamin D deficiency results in growth retardation associated with an expansion of the growth plate known as *rickets*. Three layers of chondrocytes are present in the normal growth plate: the reserve zone, the proliferating zone, and the hypertrophic zone. Rickets associated with impaired vitamin D action is characterized by expansion of the hypertrophic chondrocyte layer. The proliferation and differentiation of the chondrocytes in the rachitic growth plate are normal, and the expansion of the growth plate is a consequence of impaired apoptosis of the late hypertrophic chondrocytes, an event that precedes replacement of these cells by osteoblasts during endochondral bone formation. Investigations in murine models demonstrate that hypophosphatemia, which in vitamin D deficiency is a consequence of secondary hyperparathyroidism, is a key etiologic factor in the development of the rachitic growth plate.

The hypocalcemia and hypophosphatemia that accompany vitamin D deficiency result in impaired mineralization of bone matrix proteins, a condition known as *osteomalacia*. Osteomalacia is also a feature of long-standing hypophosphatemia, which may be a consequence of renal phosphate wasting or chronic use of etidronate or phosphate-binding antacids. This hypomineralized matrix is biomechanically inferior to normal bone; as a result, patients with vitamin D deficiency are prone to bowing of weight-bearing extremities and skeletal fractures. Vitamin D and calcium supplementation have been shown to decrease the incidence of hip fracture among ambulatory nursing home residents in France, suggesting that undermineralization of bone contributes significantly to morbidity in the elderly. Proximal myopathy is a striking feature of severe vitamin D deficiency both in children and in adults. Rapid resolution of the myopathy is observed upon vitamin D treatment.

Though vitamin D deficiency is the most common cause of rickets and osteomalacia, many disorders lead to inadequate mineralization of the growth plate and bone. Calcium deficiency without vitamin D deficiency, the disorders of vitamin D metabolism previously discussed, and hypophosphatemia can all lead to inefficient mineralization. Even in the presence of normal calcium and phosphate levels, chronic acidosis and drugs such as bisphosphonates can lead to osteomalacia. The inorganic calcium/phosphate mineral phase of bone cannot form at low pH, and bisphosphonates bind to and prevent mineral crystal growth. Since alkaline phosphatase is necessary for normal mineral deposition, probably because the enzyme can hydrolyze inhibitors of mineralization such as inorganic pyrophosphate, genetic inactivation of the alkaline phosphatase gene (hereditary hypophosphatasia) also can lead to osteomalacia in the setting of normal calcium and phosphate levels.

Diagnosis of vitamin D deficiency, rickets, and osteomalacia

The most specific screening test for vitamin D deficiency in otherwise healthy individuals is a serum 25(OH)D level. Although the normal ranges vary, levels of 25(OH)D <37 nmol/L (<15 ng/mL) are associated with increasing PTH levels and lower bone density; optimal vitamin D levels are >80 nmol/L (>32 ng/mL). Vitamin D deficiency leads to impaired intestinal absorption of calcium, resulting in decreased serum total and ionized calcium values. This hypocalcemia results in secondary hyperparathyroidism, a homeostatic response that initially maintains serum calcium levels at the expense of the skeleton. Due to the PTH-induced increase in bone turnover, alkaline phosphatase levels are often increased. In addition to increasing bone resorption, PTH decreases urinary calcium excretion while promoting phosphaturia. This results in hypophosphatemia, which exacerbates the mineralization defect in the skeleton. With prolonged vitamin D deficiency resulting in osteomalacia, calcium stores in the skeleton become relatively inaccessible, since osteoclasts cannot resorb unmineralized osteoid, and frank hypocalcemia ensues. Since PTH is a major stimulus for the renal 25(OH)D 1α-hydroxylase, there is increased synthesis of the active hormone, $1,25(OH)_2D$. Paradoxically, levels of this hormone are often normal in severe vitamin D deficiency. Therefore, measurements of $1,25(OH)_2D$ are not accurate reflections of vitamin D stores and should not be used to diagnose vitamin D deficiency in patients with normal renal function.

Radiologic features of vitamin D deficiency in children include a widened, expanded growth plate that is characteristic of rickets. These findings not only are apparent in the long bones but also are present at the costochondral junction, where the expansion of the growth plate leads to swellings known as the "rachitic rosary." Impairment of intramembranous bone mineralization leads to delayed fusion of the calvarial sutures and a decrease in the radiopacity of cortical bone in the long bones. If vitamin D deficiency occurs after epiphyseal fusion, the main radiologic finding is a decrease in cortical thickness and relative radiolucency of the skeleton. A specific radiologic feature of osteomalacia, whether associated with phosphate wasting or vitamin D deficiency, is pseudofractures, or Looser's zones. These are radiolucent lines that occur where large arteries are in contact with the underlying skeletal elements; it is thought that the arterial pulsations lead to the radiolucencies. As a result, these pseudofractures are usually a few millimeters wide, are several centimeters long, and are seen particularly in the scapula, the pelvis, and the femoral neck.

TREATMENT Vitamin D Deficiency

Daily intake of a multivitamin (400 IU) is often insufficient to prevent vitamin D deficiency. Based on the observation that 800 IU of vitamin D, with calcium supplementation, decreases the risk of hip fractures in elderly women, this higher dose is thought to be an appropriate daily intake for prevention of vitamin D deficiency in adults. The safety margin for vitamin D is large, and vitamin D toxicity usually is observed only in patients taking doses in the range of 40,000 IU daily. Treatment of vitamin D deficiency should be directed at the underlying disorder, if possible, and also should be tailored to the severity of the condition. Vitamin D should always be repleted in conjunction with calcium supplementation since most of the consequences of vitamin D deficiency are a result of impaired mineral ion homeostasis. In patients in whom 1α-hydroxylation is impaired, metabolites that do not require this activation step are the treatment of choice. They include $1,25(OH)_2D_3$ [calcitriol (Rocaltrol), 0.25–0.5 μg/d] and 1α-hydroxyvitamin D_2 (Hectorol, 2.5–5 μg/d). If the pathway required for activation of vitamin D is intact, severe vitamin D deficiency can be treated with pharmacologic repletion initially (50,000 IU weekly for 3–12 weeks), followed by maintenance therapy (800 IU daily). Pharmacologic doses may be required for maintenance therapy in patients who are taking medications such as barbiturates or phenytoin, that accelerate metabolism of, or cause resistance to $1,25(OH)_2D$. Calcium supplementation should include 1.5–2 g/d of elemental calcium. Normocalcemia is usually observed within one week of the institution of therapy, although increases in PTH and alkaline phosphatase levels may persist for three to six months. The most efficacious methods to monitor treatment and resolution of vitamin D deficiency are serum and urinary calcium measurements. In patients who are vitamin D replete and are taking adequate calcium supplementation, the 24-hour urinary calcium excretion should be in the range of 100–250 mg/24 hours. Lower levels suggest problems with adherence to the treatment regimen or with absorption of calcium or vitamin D supplements. Levels >250 mg/24 hours predispose to nephrolithiasis and should lead to a reduction in vitamin D dosage and/or calcium supplementation.

FURTHER READINGS

Bouillon R et al: Vitamin D and human health: Lessons from the vitamin D receptor null mice. Endocr Rev 29:726, 2008

DeLuca HF: Overview of general physiologic features and functions of vitamin D. Am J Clin Nutr 80:1689S, 2004

Heaney RP: Bone health. Am J Clin Nutr 85:300S, 2007

Holick MF: Vitamin D deficiency. N Engl J Med 357:266, 2007

Karsenty G: The complexities of skeletal biology. Nature 423:316, 2003

Kobayashi T et al: Minireview: Transcriptional regulation in development of bone. Endocrinology 146:1012, 2005

Razzaque MS: The FGF23-Klotho axis: Endocrine regulation of phosphate homeostasis. Nat Rev Endocrinol 5:611, 2009.

Teitelbaum SL, Ross SP: Genetic regulation of osteoclast development and function. Nat Rev Genet 4:638, 2003

CHAPTER 353

Disorders of the Parathyroid Gland and Calcium Homeostasis

John T. Potts, Jr.
Harald Jüppner

The four parathyroid glands are located posterior to the thyroid gland. They produce parathyroid hormone (PTH), which is the primary regulator of calcium physiology. PTH acts directly on bone, where it induces calcium resorption, and on the kidney, where it enhances calcium reabsorption and synthesis of 1,25-dihydroxyvitamin D [1,25(OH)$_2$D], a hormone that increases gastrointestinal calcium absorption. Serum PTH levels are tightly regulated by a negative feedback loop. Calcium, acting through the calcium-sensing receptor, and vitamin D, acting through its nuclear receptor, reduce PTH release and synthesis. Additional evidence indicates that fibroblast growth factor 23 (FGF23), a phosphaturic hormone, can suppress PTH secretion. Understanding the hormonal pathways that regulate calcium levels and bone metabolism is essential for effective diagnosis and management of a wide array of hyper- and hypocalcemic disorders.

Hyperparathyroidism (HPT), characterized by excess production of PTH, is a common cause of hypercalcemia and is usually the result of autonomously functioning adenomas or hyperplasia. Surgery for this disorder is highly effective and has been shown to reverse some of the deleterious effects of long-standing PTH excess on bone density. Humoral hypercalcemia of malignancy is also common and is usually due to the overproduction of parathyroid hormone–related peptide (PTHrP) by cancer cells. The similarities in the biochemical characteristics of hyperparathyroidism and humoral hypercalcemia of malignancy, first noted by Albright in 1941, are now known to reflect the actions of PTH and PTHrP through the same G protein–coupled PTH/PTHrP receptor.

The genetic basis of multiple endocrine neoplasia (MEN) types 1 and 2, familial hypocalciuric hypercalcemia (FHH), different forms of pseudohypoparathyroidism (PHP), Jansen's syndrome, disorders of vitamin D synthesis and action, and the molecular events associated with parathyroid gland neoplasia have provided new insights into the regulation of calcium homeostasis. PTH and *possibly some* of its analogues are promising therapeutic agents for the treatment of postmenopausal or senile osteoporosis, and calcimimetic agents, which activate the calcium-sensing receptor, have provided new approaches for PTH suppression.

PARATHYROID HORMONE

PHYSIOLOGY

The primary function of PTH is to maintain the extracellular fluid (ECF) calcium concentration within a narrow normal range. The hormone acts directly on bone and kidney and indirectly on the intestine through its effects on synthesis of 1,25(OH)$_2$D to increase serum calcium concentrations; in turn, PTH production is closely regulated by the concentration of serum ionized calcium. This feedback system is the critical homeostatic mechanism for maintenance of ECF calcium. Any tendency toward hypocalcemia, as might be induced by calcium-deficient diets, is counteracted by an increased secretion of PTH. This in turn (1) increases the rate of dissolution of bone mineral, thereby increasing the flow of calcium from bone into blood; (2) reduces the renal clearance of calcium, returning more of the calcium filtered at the glomerulus into ECF; and (3) increases the efficiency of calcium absorption in the intestine by stimulating the production of 1,25(OH)$_2$D. Immediate control of blood calcium is due to PTH effects on bone and, to a lesser extent, on renal calcium clearance. Maintenance of steady-state calcium balance, on the other hand, probably results from the effects of 1,25(OH)$_2$D on calcium absorption (Chap. 352). The renal actions of the hormone are exerted at multiple sites and include inhibition of phosphate transport (proximal tubule), augmentation of calcium reabsorption (distal tubule), and stimulation of the renal 25(OH)D-1α-hydroxylase. As much as 12 mmol (500 mg) calcium is transferred between the ECF and bone each day (a large amount in relation to the total ECF calcium pool), and PTH has a major effect on this transfer. The homeostatic role of the hormone can preserve calcium concentration in blood at the cost of bone demineralization.

PTH has multiple actions on bone, some direct and some indirect. PTH-mediated changes in bone calcium release can be seen within minutes. The chronic effects of PTH are to increase the number of bone cells, both osteoblasts and osteoclasts, and to increase the remodeling of bone; these effects are apparent within hours after the hormone is given and persist for hours after PTH is withdrawn. Continuous exposure to elevated PTH (as in hyperparathyroidism or long-term infusions in animals) leads to increased osteoclast-mediated bone resorption. However, the intermittent administration of PTH, elevating hormone levels for 1–2 hours each day, leads to a net stimulation of bone formation rather than bone breakdown. Striking increases, especially in trabecular bone in the spine and hip, have been reported with the use of PTH in combination with estrogen. PTH(1-34) as monotherapy caused a highly significant reduction in fracture incidence in a worldwide placebo-controlled trial.

Osteoblasts (or stromal cell precursors), which have PTH/PTHrP receptors, are crucial to this bone-forming effect of PTH; osteoclasts, which mediate bone breakdown, lack such receptors. PTH-mediated stimulation of osteoclasts is indirect, acting in part, through cytokines released from osteoblasts to activate osteoclasts; in experimental studies of bone resorption in vitro, osteoblasts must be present for PTH to activate osteoclasts to resorb bone (Chap. 352).

STRUCTURE

PTH is an 84-amino-acid single-chain peptide. The amino-terminal portion, PTH(1–34), is highly conserved and is critical for the biologic actions of the molecule. Modified synthetic fragments of the amino-terminal sequence as small as PTH(1–11) are sufficient to activate the PTH/PTHrP receptor (see below). The carboxyl-terminal regions of the full-length PTH(1–84) molecule also can bind to a separate binding protein/receptor (cPTH-R), but this receptor has been incompletely characterized. Fragments shortened at the amino terminus possibly by binding to cPTH can inhibit some of the biologic actions of full-length PTH(1–84) and of PTH(1–34).

BIOSYNTHESIS, SECRETION, AND METABOLISM

Synthesis

Parathyroid cells have multiple methods of adapting to increased needs for PTH production. Most rapid (within minutes) is secretion of preformed hormone in response to hypocalcemia. Second, within hours, PTH mRNA expression is induced by sustained hypocalcemia. Finally, protracted challenge leads within days to cellular replication to increase gland mass.

PTH is initially synthesized as a larger molecule (preproparathyroid hormone, consisting of 115 amino acids). After a first cleavage step to remove the "pre" sequence of 25 amino acid residues, a second cleavage step removes the "pro" sequence of 6 amino acid residues before secretion of the mature peptide comprising 84 residues. In one kindred with hypoparathyroidism, a mutation in the preprotein region of the gene interferes with hormone transport and secretion.

Transcriptional suppression of the PTH gene by calcium is nearly maximal at physiologic calcium concentrations. Hypocalcemia increases transcriptional activity within hours. $1,25(OH)_2D_3$ strongly suppresses PTH gene transcription. In patients with renal failure, IV administration of supraphysiologic levels of $1,25(OH)_2D_3$ or analogues of this active metabolite can dramatically suppress PTH overproduction, which is sometimes difficult to control due to severe secondary HPT. Regulation of proteolytic destruction of preformed hormone (posttranslational regulation of hormone production) is an important mechanism for mediating rapid (minutes) changes in hormone availability. High calcium increases and low calcium inhibit the proteolytic destruction of hormone stores.

Regulation of PTH secretion

PTH secretion increases steeply to a maximum value of about five times the basal rate of secretion as calcium concentration falls from normal to the range of 1.9–2 mmol/L (7.5–8 mg/dL) (measured as total calcium). The ionized fraction of blood calcium is the important determinant of hormone secretion. Severe intracellular magnesium deficiency impairs PTH secretion (see below).

ECF calcium controls PTH secretion by interaction with a calcium sensor, a G protein–coupled receptor (GPCR) for which Ca^{2+} ions act as the primary ligand (see below). This receptor is a member of a distinctive subgroup of the GPCR superfamily that is characterized by a large extracellular domain suitable for "clamping" the small-molecule ligand. Stimulation of the receptor by high calcium levels suppresses PTH secretion. The receptor is present in parathyroid glands and the calcitonin-secreting cells of the thyroid (C cells), as well as in other sites such as brain and kidney. Genetic evidence has revealed a key biologic role for the calcium-sensing receptor in parathyroid gland responsiveness to calcium and in renal calcium clearance. Heterozygous point mutations associated with loss-of-function cause the syndrome of FHH, in which the blood calcium abnormality resembles that observed in hyperparathyroidism but with hypocalciuria. On the other hand, heterozygous gain-of-function mutations cause a form of hypocalcemia resembling hypoparathyroidism (see below).

Metabolism

The secreted form of PTH is indistinguishable by immunologic criteria and by molecular size from the 84-amino-acid peptide [PTH(1–84)] extracted from glands. However, much of the immunoreactive material found in the circulation is smaller than the extracted or secreted hormone. The principal circulating fragments of immunoreactive hormone lack a portion of the critical amino-terminal sequence required for biologic activity and, hence, are biologically inactive fragments (so-called middle and carboxyl-terminal fragments). Much of the proteolysis of hormone occurs in the liver and kidney. Peripheral metabolism of PTH does not appear to be regulated by physiologic states (high versus low calcium, etc.); hence, peripheral metabolism of hormone, although responsible for rapid clearance of secreted hormone, appears to be a high-capacity, metabolically invariant catabolic process.

The rate of clearance of the secreted 84-amino-acid peptide from blood is more rapid than the rate of clearance of the biologically inactive fragment(s) corresponding to the middle and carboxyl-terminal regions of PTH. Consequently, the interpretation of results obtained with earlier PTH radioimmunoassays is influenced by the nature of the peptide fragments detected by the antibodies.

Although the problems inherent in PTH measurements have been largely circumvented by use of double-antibody immunometric assays, it is now known that some of these assays detect, besides the intact molecule, large amino-terminally truncated forms of PTH, which are present in normal and uremic individuals in addition to PTH(1–84). The concentration of these fragments relative to that of intact PTH(1–84) is higher with induced hypercalcemia than in eucalcemic or hypocalcemic conditions and is higher in patients with renal failure. These fragments have limited portions of the amino-terminal portion of the hormone removed; PTH(7–84) has been identified as a major component of these amino-terminally truncated fragments. Growing evidence suggests that the PTH(7–84) (and probably related amino-terminally truncated fragments) can act, through yet undefined mechanisms, as an inhibitor of PTH action and may be of clinical significance, particularly in renal failure. In this group of patients, efforts to prevent secondary HPT by a variety of measures (vitamin D analogues, higher calcium intake, higher dialysate calcium, and phosphate-lowering strategies) may have led to oversuppression of biologically active, intact PTH since some amino-terminally truncated PTH fragments such as PTH(7–84), react in many immunometric PTH assays (now termed second-generation assays; see below under "Diagnosis"). Excessive parathyroid gland suppression due to overly aggressive treatment with vitamin D analogues and calcium-containing phosphate binders or inaccurate PTH measurements can lead to adynamic bone disease in renal failure (see below). Adynamic bone disease has been associated in children with further impaired growth and increased bone fracture rates in adults, and can furthermore lead to significant hypercalcemia. The measurement of PTH with newer third-generation immunometric assays, which use detection antibodies directed against extreme amino-terminal PTH epitopes and thus detect only full-length PTH(1–84), may provide some advantage to prevent bone disease in chronic kidney disease.

PARATHYROID HORMONE–RELATED PROTEIN (PTHrP)

PTHrP is responsible for most instances of hypercalcemia of malignancy (Chap. 100), a syndrome that resembles HPT but without elevated PTH levels. Most cell types produce PTHrP, including brain, pancreas, heart, lung, mammary tissue, placenta, endothelial cells, and smooth muscle. In fetal animals, PTHrP directs transplacental calcium transfer, and high concentrations of PTHrP are produced in mammary tissue and secreted into milk, but the biologic significance of the very high concentrations of this hormone in breast milk is unknown. PTHrP also plays an essential role in endochondral bone formation and in branching morphogenesis of the breast, and possibly in uterine contraction and other biologic functions.

PTH and PTHrP, although distinctive products of different genes, exhibit considerable functional and structural homology (Fig. 353-1) and have evolved from a shared ancestral gene. The structure of the gene for human PTHrP, however, is more complex than that of PTH, containing multiple additional exons, which can undergo alternate splicing patterns during formation of the mature mRNA. Protein products of 141, 139, and 173 amino acids are produced, and other molecular forms may result from tissue-specific degradation at accessible internal cleavage sites. The biologic roles of these various molecular species and the nature of the circulating forms of PTHrP are unclear. It is uncertain whether PTHrP circulates at any significant level in adults. As a paracrine factor, PTHrP may be produced, act, and be destroyed locally within tissues. In adults, PTHrP appears to have little influence on calcium

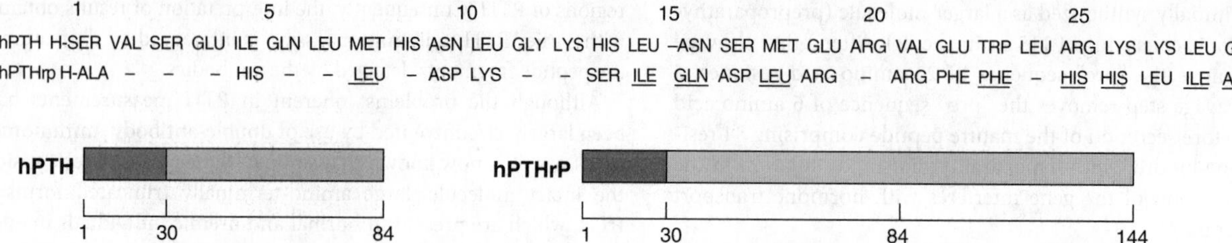

Figure 353-1 Schematic diagram to illustrate similarities and differences in structure of human parathyroid hormone (PTH) and human PTH-related peptide (PTHrP). Close structural (and functional) homology exists between the first 30 amino acids of hPTH and hPTHrP. The PTHrP sequence may be ≥144 amino acid residues in length. PTH is only 84 residues long; after residue 30, there is little structural homology between the two. Dashed lines in the PTHrP sequence indicate identity; underlined residues, although different from those of PTH, still represent conservative changes (charge or polarity preserved). Ten amino acids are identical, and a total of 20 of 30 are homologues.

homeostasis, except in disease states, when large tumors, especially of the squamous cell type as well as renal cell carcinomas, lead to massive overproduction of the hormone and hypercalcemia.

PTH AND PTHrP HORMONE ACTION

Both PTH and PTHrP bind to and activate the PTH/PTHrP receptor. The PTH/PTHrP receptor (also known as the PTH-1 receptor, PTH1R) belongs to a subfamily of GPCRs that includes the receptors for calcitonin, glucagon, secretin, vasoactive intestinal peptide, and other peptides. Although both ligands activate the PTH1R, the two peptides induce distinct responses in the receptor, which explains how a single receptor without isoforms can serve two biologic roles. The extracellular regions of the receptor are involved in hormone binding, and the intracellular domains, after hormone activation, bind G protein subunits to transduce hormone signaling into cellular responses through the stimulation of second messenger formation. A second receptor that binds PTH, originally termed the *PTH-2 receptor* (PTH2R), is primarily expressed in brain, pancreas, and testis. Different mammalian PTH1Rs respond equivalently to PTH and PTHrP, whereas only the human PTH2R responds efficiently to PTH (but not to PTHrP), PTH2Rs from other species show little or no stimulation of second-messenger formation in response to PTH or PTHrP. The endogenous ligand of the PTH2R was shown to be a hypothalamic peptide referred to as *tubular infundibular peptide of 39 residues*, TIP39, that is distantly related to PTH. The PTH1R and the PTH2R can be traced backward in evolutionary time to fish; in fact, the zebrafish genome contains, in addition to the PTH1R and the PTH2R orthologs, a third receptor, the PTH3R, that is more closely related to the fish PTH1R than the fish PTH2R. The evolutionary conservation of structure and function suggests important biologic roles for these receptors, even in fish, which lack discrete parathyroid glands but produce two molecules that are closely related to mammalian PTH.

Studies using the cloned PTH1R confirm that it can be coupled to more than one G protein and second-messenger pathway, apparently explaining the multiplicity of pathways stimulated by PTH. Stimulation of protein kinases (A and C) and calcium transport channels is associated with a variety of hormone-specific tissue responses. These responses include inhibition of phosphate and bicarbonate transport, stimulation of calcium transport, and activation of renal 1α-hydroxylase in the kidney. The responses in bone include effects on collagen synthesis, alkaline phosphatase, ornithine decarboxylase, citrate decarboxylase, and glucose-6-phosphate dehydrogenase activities, phospholipid synthesis, as well as calcium and phosphate transport. Ultimately, these biochemical events lead to an integrated hormonal response in bone turnover and calcium homeostasis. PTH also activates Na^+/Ca^{2+} exchangers at renal distal tubular sites and stimulates translocation of preformed calcium transport channels, moving them from the interior to the apical surface to increase tubular uptake of calcium. PTH-dependent stimulation of phosphate excretion (reducing reabsorption—the opposite effect from actions on calcium in the kidney) involves the down regulation of two sodium-dependent phosphate co-transporters, NPT2a and NPT2c, and expression at the apical membrane, thereby reducing phosphate reabsorption. Similar mechanisms may be involved in other renal tubular transporters that are influenced by PTH.

PTHrP exerts important developmental influences on fetal bone development and in adult physiology. A homozygous ablation of the gene encoding PTHrP (or disruption of the gene encoding the PTH/PTHrP receptor) in mice causes a lethal phenotype in which animals are born with pronounced acceleration of chondrocyte maturation that resembles a lethal form of chondrodysplasia in humans (Fig. 353-2). Mice that are heterozygous for ablation of the PTHrP gene display reduced mineral density consistent with osteoporosis. Experiments with these mouse models point to a hitherto unappreciated role of PTHrP as a paracrine/autocrine factor that modulates bone metabolism in adults as well as during bone development.

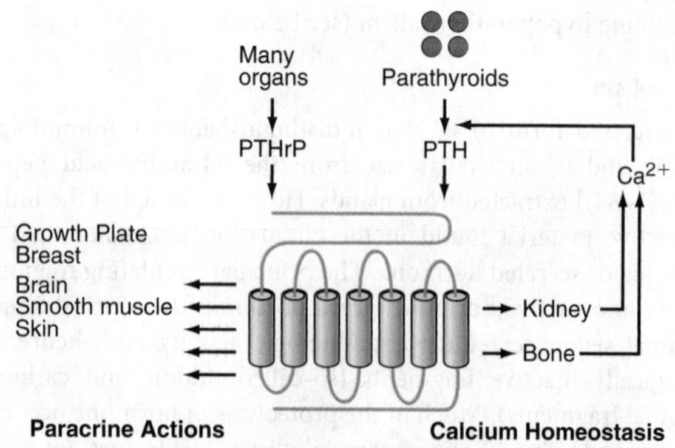

Figure 353-2 Dual role for the actions of the PTH/PTHrP receptor (PTH1R). Parathyroid hormone (PTH; endocrine-calcium homeostasis) and PTH-related peptide (PTHrP; paracrine–multiple tissue actions including growth plate cartilage in developing bone) use the single receptor for their disparate functions mediated by the amino-terminal 30 residues of either peptide. Other regions of both ligands interact with other receptors (not shown).

CALCITONIN

(See also Chap. 351) Calcitonin is a hypocalcemic peptide hormone that in several mammalian species acts as an antagonist to PTH. Calcitonin seems to be of limited physiologic significance in humans, at least with regard to calcium homeostasis. It is of medical significance because of its role as a tumor marker in sporadic and hereditary cases of medullary carcinoma and its medical use as an adjunctive treatment in severe hypercalcemia and in Paget's disease of bone.

The hypocalcemic activity of calcitonin is accounted for primarily by inhibition of osteoclast-mediated bone resorption and secondarily by stimulation of renal calcium clearance. These effects are mediated by receptors on osteoclasts and renal tubular cells. Calcitonin exerts additional effects through receptors present in the brain, the gastrointestinal tract, and the immune system. The hormone, for example, exerts analgesic effects directly on cells in the hypothalamus and related structures, possibly by interacting with receptors for related peptide hormones such as calcitonin gene–related peptide (CGRP) or amylin. The latter ligands have specific high-affinity receptors and can also bind to and trigger calcitonin receptors. The calcitonin receptor shares considerable structural similarity with the PTH1R.

The thyroid is the major source of the hormone, and the cells involved in calcitonin synthesis arise from neural crest tissue. During embryogenesis, these cells migrate into the ultimobranchial body, derived from the last branchial pouch. In submammalian vertebrates, the ultimobranchial body constitutes a discrete organ, anatomically separate from the thyroid gland; in mammals, the ultimobranchial gland fuses with and is incorporated into the thyroid gland.

The naturally occurring calcitonins consist of a peptide chain of 32 amino acids. There is considerable sequence variability among species. Calcitonin from salmon, which is used therapeutically, is 10–100 times more potent than mammalian forms in lowering serum calcium.

There are two calcitonin genes, α and β; the transcriptional control of these genes is complex. Two different mRNA molecules are transcribed from the α gene; one is translated into the precursor for calcitonin, and the other message is translated into an alternative product, CGRP. CGRP is synthesized wherever the calcitonin mRNA is expressed (e.g., in medullary carcinoma of the thyroid). The β, or CGRP-2, gene is transcribed into the mRNA for CGRP in the central nervous system (CNS); this gene does not produce calcitonin, however. CGRP has cardiovascular actions and may serve as a neurotransmitter or play a developmental role in the CNS.

The circulating level of calcitonin in humans is lower than that in many other species. In humans, even extreme variations in calcitonin production do not change calcium and phosphate metabolism; no definite effects are attributable to calcitonin deficiency (totally thyroidectomized patients receiving only replacement thyroxine) or excess (patients with medullary carcinoma of the thyroid, a calcitonin-secreting tumor) (Chap. 351). Calcitonin has been a useful pharmacologic agent to suppress bone resorption in Paget's disease (Chap. 355) and osteoporosis (Chap. 354) and in the treatment of hypercalcemia of malignancy (see below). However, the physiologic role, if any, of calcitonin in humans is uncertain. On the other hand, a knockout of the calcitonin gene in mice leads to reduced bone mineral density, suggesting that its biologic role in mammals is still not fully understood.

HYPERCALCEMIA

(See also Chap. 46) Hypercalcemia can be a manifestation of a serious illness such as malignancy or can be detected coincidentally by laboratory testing in a patient with no obvious illness. The number of patients recognized with asymptomatic hypercalcemia, usually hyperparathyroidism, increased in the late twentieth century.

Whenever hypercalcemia is confirmed, a definitive diagnosis must be established. Although hyperparathyroidism, a frequent cause of asymptomatic hypercalcemia, is a chronic disorder in which manifestations, if any, may be expressed only after months or years, hypercalcemia can also be the earliest manifestation of malignancy, the second most common cause of hypercalcemia in the adult. The causes of hypercalcemia are numerous (Table 353-1), but hyperparathyroidism and cancer account for 90% of all cases.

Before undertaking a diagnostic workup, it is essential to be sure that true hypercalcemia, not a false-positive laboratory test, is present. A false-positive diagnosis of hypercalcemia is usually the result of inadvertent hemoconcentration during blood collection or elevation in serum proteins such as albumin. Hypercalcemia is a chronic problem, and it is cost-effective to obtain several serum calcium measurements; these tests need not be in the fasting state.

Clinical features are helpful in differential diagnosis. Hypercalcemia in an adult who is asymptomatic is usually due to primary hyperparathyroidism. In malignancy-associated hypercalcemia, the disease is usually not occult; rather, symptoms of malignancy bring the patient to the physician, and hypercalcemia is discovered during the evaluation. In such patients, the interval

TABLE 353-1 Classification of Causes of Hypercalcemia

I. Parathyroid-Related
- A. Primary hyperparathyroidism
  - 1. Adenoma(s)
  - 2. Multiple endocrine neoplasia
  - 3. Carcinoma
- B. Lithium therapy
- C. Familial hypocalciuric hypercalcemia

II. Malignancy-Related
- A. Solid tumor with metastases (breast)
- B. Solid tumor with humoral mediation of hypercalcemia (lung, kidney)
- C. Hematologic malignancies (multiple myeloma, lymphoma, leukemia)

III. Vitamin D–Related
- A. Vitamin D intoxication
- B. ↑ $1,25(OH)_2D$; sarcoidosis and other granulomatous diseases
- C. Idiopathic hypercalcemia of infancy

IV. Associated with High Bone Turnover
- A. Hyperthyroidism
- B. Immobilization
- C. Thiazides
- D. Vitamin A intoxication

V. Associated with Renal Failure
- A. Severe secondary hyperparathyroidism
- B. Aluminum intoxication
- C. Milk-alkali syndrome

between detection of hypercalcemia and death, especially without vigorous treatment, is often <6 months. Accordingly, if an asymptomatic individual has had hypercalcemia or some manifestation of hypercalcemia such as kidney stones for >1 or 2 years, it is unlikely that malignancy is the cause. Nevertheless, differentiating primary hyperparathyroidism from *occult* malignancy can occasionally be difficult, and careful evaluation is required, particularly when the duration of the hypercalcemia is unknown. Hypercalcemia not due to hyperparathyroidism or malignancy can result from excessive vitamin D action, high bone turnover from any of several causes, or from renal failure (Table 353-1). Dietary history and a history of ingestion of vitamins or drugs are often helpful in diagnosing some of the less frequent causes. Immunometric PTH assays serve as the principal laboratory test in establishing the diagnosis.

Hypercalcemia from any cause can result in fatigue, depression, mental confusion, anorexia, nausea, vomiting, constipation, reversible renal tubular defects, increased urination, a short QT interval in the electrocardiogram, and, in some patients, cardiac arrhythmias. There is a variable relation from one patient to the next between the severity of hypercalcemia and the symptoms. Generally, symptoms are more common at calcium levels >2.9–3 mmol/L (11.5–12 mg/dL), but some patients, even at this level, are asymptomatic. When the calcium level is >3.2 mmol/L (13 mg/dL), calcification in kidneys, skin, vessels, lungs, heart, and stomach occurs and renal insufficiency may develop, particularly if blood phosphate levels are normal or elevated due to impaired renal function. Severe hypercalcemia, usually defined as ≥3.7–4.5 mmol/L (15–18 mg/dL), can be a medical emergency; coma and cardiac arrest can occur.

Acute management of the hypercalcemia is usually successful. The type of treatment is based on the severity of the hypercalcemia and the nature of associated symptoms, as outlined below.

■ PRIMARY HYPERPARATHYROIDISM

Natural history and incidence

Primary hyperparathyroidism is a generalized disorder of calcium, phosphate, and bone metabolism due to an increased secretion of PTH. The elevation of circulating hormone usually leads to hypercalcemia and hypophosphatemia. There is great variation in the manifestations. Patients may present with multiple signs and symptoms, including recurrent nephrolithiasis, peptic ulcers, mental changes, and, less frequently, extensive bone resorption. However, with greater awareness of the disease and wider use of multiphasic screening tests, including measurements of blood calcium, the diagnosis is frequently made in patients who have no symptoms and minimal, if any, signs of the disease other than hypercalcemia and elevated levels of PTH. The manifestations may be subtle, and the disease may have a benign course for many years or a lifetime. This milder form of the disease is usually termed *asymptomatic HPT*. Rarely, hyperparathyroidism develops or worsens abruptly and causes severe complications such as marked dehydration and coma, so-called hypercalcemic parathyroid crisis.

The annual incidence of the disease is calculated to be as high as 0.2% in patients >60, with an estimated prevalence, including undiscovered asymptomatic patients, of ≥1%; some reports suggest the incidence may be declining. If confirmed, these changing estimates may reflect less frequent routine testing of serum calcium in recent years, earlier overestimates in incidence, or unknown factors. The disease has a peak incidence between the third and fifth decades but occurs in young children and in the elderly.

Etiology

Parathyroid tumors are most often encountered as isolated adenomas without other endocrinopathy. They may also arise in hereditary syndromes such as MEN syndromes. Parathyroid tumors may also arise as secondary to underlying disease (excessive stimulation in secondary hyperparathyroidism, especially chronic renal failure), or after other forms of excessive stimulation such as lithium therapy. These etiologies are discussed below.

Solitary adenomas A single abnormal gland is the cause in ~80% of patients; the abnormality in the gland is usually a benign neoplasm or adenoma and rarely a parathyroid carcinoma. Some surgeons and pathologists report that the enlargement of multiple glands is common; double adenomas are reported. In ~15% of patients, all glands are hyperfunctioning; *chief cell parathyroid hyperplasia* is usually hereditary and frequently associated with other endocrine abnormalities.

Hereditary syndromes and multiple parathyroid tumors Hereditary hyperparathyroidism can occur without other endocrine abnormalities but is usually part of a *multiple endocrine neoplasia* syndrome (Chap. 351). MEN 1 (Wermer's syndrome) consists of hyperparathyroidism and tumors of the pituitary and pancreas, often associated with gastric hypersecretion and peptic ulcer disease (Zollinger-Ellison syndrome). MEN 2A is characterized by pheochromocytoma and medullary carcinoma of the thyroid, as well as hyperparathyroidism; MEN 2B has additional associated features such as multiple neuromas but usually lacks hyperparathyroidism. Each of these MEN syndromes is transmitted in an apparent autosomal dominant manner, although, as noted below, the genetic basis of MEN 1 involves biallelic loss of a tumor suppressor.

The *hyperparathyroidism jaw tumor* (HPT-JT) syndrome occurs in families with parathyroid tumors (sometimes carcinomas) in association with benign jaw tumors. Some kindreds exhibit hereditary hyperparathyroidism without other endocrinopathies. This disorder is often termed *nonsyndromic familial isolated hyperparathyroidism* (FIHP). There is speculation that these families may be examples of variable expression of the other syndromes such as MEN 1, MEN 2, or the HPT-JT syndrome, but they may also have distinctive, still unidentified genetic causes.

Pathology

Adenomas are most often located in the inferior parathyroid glands, but in 6–10% of patients, parathyroid adenomas may be located in the thymus, the thyroid, the pericardium, or behind the esophagus. Adenomas are usually 0.5–5 g in size but may be as large as 10–20 g (normal glands weigh 25 mg on average). Chief cells are predominant in both hyperplasia and adenoma. With chief cell hyperplasia, the enlargement may be so asymmetric that some involved glands appear grossly normal. If generalized hyperplasia is present, however, histologic examination reveals a uniform pattern of chief cells and disappearance of fat even in the absence of an increase in gland weight. Thus, microscopic examination of biopsy specimens of several glands is essential to interpret findings at surgery.

Parathyroid carcinoma is often not aggressive. Long-term survival without recurrence is common if at initial surgery the entire gland is removed without rupture of the capsule. Recurrent parathyroid carcinoma is usually slow-growing with local spread in the neck, and surgical correction of recurrent disease may be feasible. Occasionally, however, parathyroid carcinoma is more aggressive, with distant metastases (lung, liver, and bone) found at the time of initial operation. It may be difficult to appreciate initially that a primary tumor is carcinoma; increased numbers of mitotic figures and increased fibrosis of the gland stroma may precede invasion. The diagnosis of carcinoma is often made in retrospect. Hyperparathyroidism from a parathyroid carcinoma may be indistinguishable from other forms of primary hyperparathyroidism but is usually more severe clinically. A potential clue to the diagnosis is offered by the degree of calcium elevation. Calcium values of 3.5–3.7 mmol/L (14–15 mg/dL) are frequent with carcinoma and may alert the surgeon to remove the abnormal gland with care to avoid capsular rupture. Recent findings concerning the genetic basis of parathyroid carcinoma (distinct from that of benign adenomas) indicate the need, in these kindreds, for family screening (see below).

GENETIC DEFECTS ASSOCIATED WITH HYPERPARATHYROIDISM

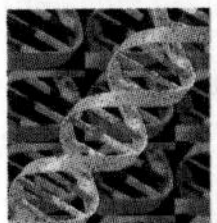

As in many other types of neoplasia, two fundamental types of genetic defects have been identified in parathyroid gland tumors: (1) overactivity of protooncogenes and (2) loss of function of tumor-suppressor genes. The former, by definition, can lead to uncontrolled cellular growth and function by activation (gain-of-function mutation) of a single allele of the responsible gene, whereas the latter requires loss of function of both allelic copies. Biallelic loss of function of a tumor-suppressor gene is usually characterized by a germ-line defect (all cells) and an additional somatic deletion/mutation in the tumor (Fig. 353-3).

Mutations in the *MEN1* gene locus, encoding the protein MENIN, on chromosome 11q13 are responsible for causing MEN 1; the normal allele of this gene fits the definition of a tumor-suppressor gene. Inheritance of one mutated allele in this hereditary syndrome, followed by loss of the other allele via somatic cell mutation, leads to monoclonal expansion and tumor development. Also, in ~15–20% of sporadic parathyroid adenomas, both alleles of the *MEN1* locus on chromosome 11 are somatically deleted, implying that the same defect responsible for MEN 1 can also cause the sporadic disease (Fig. 353-3A). Consistent with the Knudson hypothesis for two-step neoplasia in certain inherited cancer syndromes (Chap. 83), the earlier onset of hyperparathyroidism in the hereditary syndromes reflects the need for only one mutational event to trigger the monoclonal outgrowth. In sporadic adenomas, typically occurring later in life, two different somatic events must occur before the *MEN1* gene is silenced.

Other presumptive anti-oncogenes involved in hyperparathyroidism include a still unidentified gene mapped to chromosome 1p seen in 40% of sporadic parathyroid adenomas and a gene mapped to chromosome Xp11 in patients with secondary hyperparathyroidism and renal failure, who progressed to "tertiary" hyperparathyroidism, now known to reflect monoclonal outgrowths within previously hyperplastic glands.

A more complex pattern, still incompletely resolved, arises with genetic defects and carcinoma of the parathyroids. This appears to be due to biallelic loss of a functioning copy of a gene, *HRPT2* (or CDC73), originally identified as the cause of the HPT-JT syndrome. Several inactivating mutations have been identified in *HRPT2* (located on chromosome 1q21-31), which encodes a 531-amino-acid protein called parafibromin. The responsible genetic mutations in *HRPT2* appear to be necessary, but not sufficient, for parathyroid cancer.

In general, the detection of additional genetic defects in these parathyroid tumor–related syndromes and the variations seen in phenotypic expression/penetrance indicate the multiplicity of the genetic factors responsible. Nonetheless, the ability to detect the presence of the major genetic contributors has greatly aided a more informed management of family members of patients identified in the hereditary syndromes such as MEN 1, MEN 2, and HPT-JT.

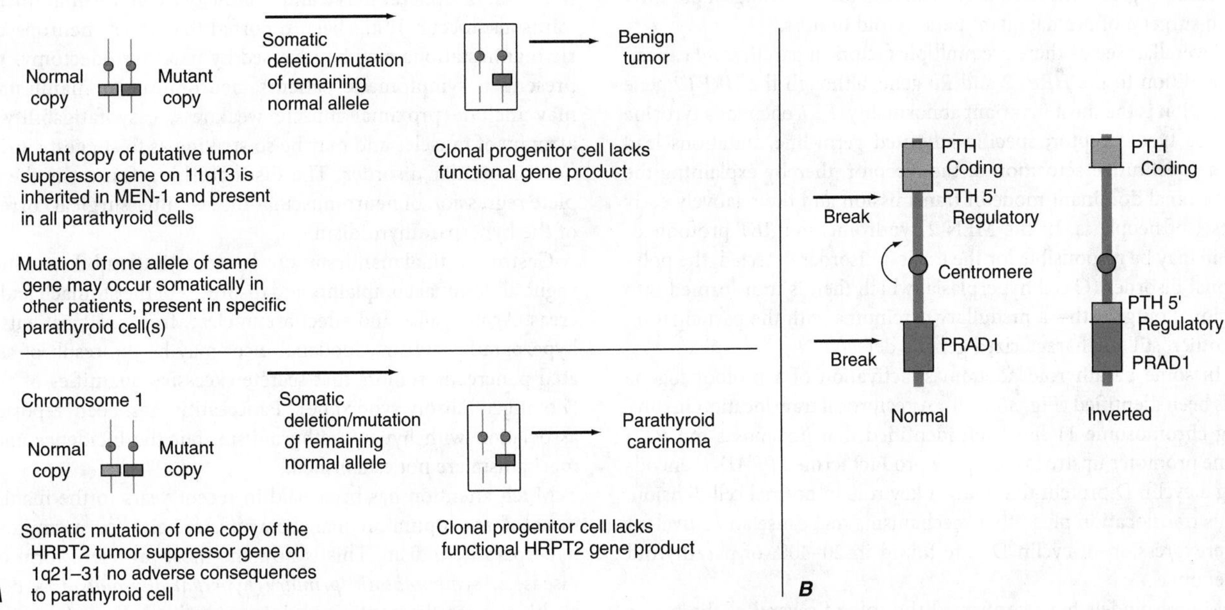

Figure 353-3 ***A.*** **Schematic diagram indicating molecular events** in tumor susceptibility. The patient with the hereditary abnormality (multiple endocrine neoplasia, or MEN) is envisioned as having one defective gene inherited from the affected parent on chromosome 11, but one copy of the normal gene is present from the other parent. In the monoclonal tumor (benign tumor), a somatic event, here partial chromosomal deletion, removes the remaining normal gene from a cell. In nonhereditary tumors, two successive somatic mutations must occur, a process that takes a longer time. By either pathway, the cell, deprived of growth-regulating influence from this gene, has unregulated growth and becomes a tumor. A different genetic locus also involving loss of a tumor-suppressor gene termed HRPT2 is involved in the pathogenesis of parathyroid carcinoma. *(From A Arnold: J Clin Endocrine Metab 77:1108, 1993. Copyright 1993, The Endocrine Society.)* ***B.*** **Schematic illustration of the mechanism and consequences of gene rearrangement** and overexpression of the PRAD 1 protooncogene (pericentromeric inversion of chromosome 11) in parathyroid adenomas. The excessive expression of PRAD 1 (a cell cycle control protein, cyclin D_1) by the highly active PTH gene promoter in the parathyroid cell contributes to excess cellular proliferation. *[From J Habener et al, in L DeGroot, JL Jameson (eds): Endocrinology, 4th ed. Philadelphia, Saunders, 2001; with permission.]*

An important contribution from studies on the genetic origin of parathyroid carcinoma has been the realization that the mutations involve a different pathway than that involved with the benign gland enlargements. Unlike the pathogenesis of genetic alterations seen in colon cancer, where lesions evolve from benign adenomas to malignant disease by progressive genetic changes, the alterations commonly seen in most parathyroid cancers (*HRPT2* mutations) are infrequently seen in sporadic parathyroid adenomas.

Abnormalities at the *Rb* gene were the first to be noted in parathyroid cancer. The *Rb* gene, a tumor-suppressor gene located on chromosome 13q14, was initially associated with retinoblastoma but has since been implicated in other neoplasias, including parathyroid carcinoma. Early studies implicated allelic deletions of the *Rb* gene in many parathyroid carcinomas and decreased or absent expression of the Rb protein. However, because there are often large deletions in chromosome 13 that include many genes in addition to the *Rb* locus (with similar findings in some pituitary carcinomas), it remains possible that other tumor-suppressor genes on chromosome 13 may be playing a role in parathyroid carcinoma.

Study of the parathyroid cancers found in some patients with the HPT-JT syndrome has led to identification of a much larger role for mutations in the *HRPT2* gene in most parathyroid carcinomas, including those that arise sporadically, without apparent association with the HPT-JT syndrome. Mutations in the coding region have been identified in 75–80% of all parathyroid cancers analyzed, leading to the conclusion that, with addition of presumed mutations in the noncoding regions, this genetic defect may be seen in essentially all parathyroid carcinomas. Of special importance was the discovery that, in some sporadic parathyroid cancers, germ-line mutations have been found; this, in turn, has led to careful investigation of the families of these patients and a new clinical indication for genetic testing in this setting.

Hypercalcemia occurring in family members (who are also found to have the germ-line mutations) can lead to the finding, at parathyroid surgery, of premalignant parathyroid tumors.

Overall, it seems there are multiple factors in parathyroid cancer, in addition to the *HRPT2* and *Rb* gene, although the *HRPT2* gene mutation is the most invariant abnormality. *RET* encodes a tyrosine kinase type receptor; specific inherited germ-line mutations lead to a constitutive activation of the receptor, thereby explaining the autosomal dominant mode of transmission and the relatively early onset of neoplasia. In the MEN 2 syndrome, the *RET* protooncogene may be responsible for the earliest disorder detected, the polyclonal disorder (C cell hyperplasia, which then is transformed into a clonal outgrowth—a medullary carcinoma with the participation of other, still uncharacterized genetic defects).

In some parathyroid adenomas, activation of a protooncogene has been identified (Fig. 353-3*B*). A reciprocal translocation involving chromosome 11 has been identified that juxtaposes the *PTH* gene promoter upstream of a gene product termed *PRAD-1*, encoding a cyclin D protein that plays a key role in normal cell division. This translocation plus other mechanisms that cause an equivalent overexpression of cyclin D1 are found in 20–40% of parathyroid adenomas.

Mouse models have confirmed the role of several of the major identified genetic defects in parathyroid disease and the MEN syndromes. Loss of the *MEN1* gene locus or overexpression of the *PRAD-1* protooncogene or the mutated *RET* protooncogene have been analyzed by genetic manipulation in mice, with the expected onset of parathyroid tumors or medullary carcinoma, respectively.

Signs and symptoms

One-half or more of patients with hyperparathyroidism are asymptomatic. In series in which patients are followed without operation, as many as 80% are classified as without symptoms. Manifestations of hyperparathyroidism involve primarily the kidneys and the skeletal system. Kidney involvement, due either to deposition of calcium in the renal parenchyma or to recurrent nephrolithiasis, was present in 60–70% of patients prior to 1970. With earlier detection, renal complications occur in <20% of patients in many large series. Renal stones are usually composed of either calcium oxalate or calcium phosphate. In occasional patients, repeated episodes of nephrolithiasis or the formation of large calculi may lead to urinary tract obstruction, infection, and loss of renal function. Nephrocalcinosis may also cause decreased renal function and phosphate retention.

The distinctive bone manifestation of hyperparathyroidism is *osteitis fibrosa cystica*, which occurred in 10–25% of patients in series reported 50 years ago. Histologically, the pathognomonic features are an increase in the giant multinucleated osteoclasts in scalloped areas on the surface of the bone (Howship's lacunae) and a replacement of the normal cellular and marrow elements by fibrous tissue. X-ray changes include resorption of the phalangeal tufts and replacement of the usually sharp cortical outline of the bone in the digits by an irregular outline (subperiosteal resorption). In recent years, osteitis fibrosa cystica is very rare in primary hyperparathyroidism, probably due to the earlier detection of the disease.

Dual-energy x-ray absorptiometry (DEXA) of the spine provides reproducible quantitative estimates (within a few percent) of spinal bone density. Similarly, bone density in the extremities can be quantified by densitometry of the hip or of the distal radius at a site chosen to be primarily cortical. CT is a very sensitive technique for estimating spinal bone density, but reproducibility of standard CT is no better than 5%. Newer CT techniques (spiral, "extreme" CT) are more reproducible but are currently available in a limited number of medical centers. Cortical bone density is reduced while cancellous bone density, especially in the spine, is relatively preserved. In symptomatic patients, dysfunctions of the CNS, peripheral nerve and muscle, gastrointestinal tract, and joints also occur. It has been reported that severe neuropsychiatric manifestations may be reversed by parathyroidectomy. When present in symptomatic patients, neuromuscular manifestations may include proximal muscle weakness, easy fatigability, and atrophy of muscles and may be so striking as to suggest a primary neuromuscular disorder. The distinguishing feature is the complete regression of neuromuscular disease after surgical correction of the hyperparathyroidism.

Gastrointestinal manifestations are sometimes subtle and include vague abdominal complaints and disorders of the stomach and pancreas. Again, cause and effect are unclear. In MEN 1 patients with hyperparathyroidism, duodenal ulcer may be the result of associated pancreatic tumors that secrete excessive quantities of gastrin (Zollinger-Ellison syndrome). Pancreatitis has been reported in association with hyperparathyroidism, but the incidence and the mechanism are not established.

Much attention has been paid in recent years to the manifestations of and optimum management strategies for asymptomatic hyperparathyroidism. This is now the most prevalent form of the disease. *Asympomatatic primary hyperparathyroidism* is defined as biochemically confirmed hyperparathyroidism (elevated or inappropriately normal PTH levels despite hypercalcemia) with the absence of signs and symptoms typically associated with more severe hyperparathyroidism such as features of renal or bone disease.

Three conferences on the topic have been held in the United States over the past two decades, with the most recent in 2008. The published proceedings include discussion of more subtle manifestations of disease, its natural history (without parathyroidectomy), and guidelines both for indications for surgery and medical monitoring in nonoperated patients.

TABLE 353-2 Guidelines for Surgery in Asymptomatic Primary Hyperparathyroidism[a]

Parameter	Guideline
Serum calcium (above normal)	>1 mg/dL
24-h urinary Ca	No indication
Creatinine clearance (calculated)	If <60 mL/min
Bone density	*T* score <–2.5 at Any of 3 sites[b]
Age	<50

[a]Bilezikian et al.
[b]Spine, distal radius, hip.

Issues of concern include the potential for cardiovascular deterioration, the presence of subtle neuropsychiatric symptoms, and the longer-term status of skeletal integrity in patients not treated surgically. The current consensus is that medical monitoring rather than surgical correction of hyperparathyroidism may be justified in certain patients. The current recommendation is that patients who show mild disease, as defined by specific criteria (Table 353-2), can be safely followed under management guidelines (Table 353-3). There is, however, growing uncertainty about subtle disease manifestations and whether surgery is therefore indicated in most patients. Among the issues is the evidence of eventual (>8 years) deterioration in bone mineral density after a decade of relative stability. There is concern that this late-onset deterioration in bone density in nonoperated patients could contribute significantly to the well-known age-dependent fracture risk (osteoporosis). One study reported significant and sustained improvements in bone mineral density after successful parathyroidectomy, again raising the issue regarding benefits of surgery. Other randomized studies, however, did not report major gains post-surgery.

Cardiovascular disease including left ventricular hypertrophy, cardiac functional defects, and endothelial dysfunction have been reported as reversible in European patients with more severe symptomatic disease after surgery, leading to numerous studies of these cardiovascular features in those with milder disease. There are reports of endothelial dysfunction in patients with mild asymptomatic hyperparathyroidism, but more observation is needed the expert panels concluded, especially whether there is reversibility with surgery.

A topic of considerable interest and some debate is assessment of neuropsychiatric status and health-related quality of life (QOL) status in hyperparathyroid patients both before surgery and in response to parathyroidectomy. Several observational studies suggest considerable improvements in symptom score after surgery. Randomized studies of surgery versus observation, however, have yielded inconclusive results, especially regarding benefits of surgery. Most studies report that hyperparathyroidism is associated with increased neuropsychiatric symptoms, so the issue remains a significant factor in decisions regarding the impact of surgery in this disease.

TABLE 353-3 Guidelines for Monitoring in Asymptomatic Primary Hyperparathyroidism[a]

Parameter	Guideline
Serum calcium	Annually
24-h urinary calcium	Not recommended
Creatinine clearance	Not recommended
Serum creatinine[b]	Annually
Bone density	Annually (3 sites)[a]

[a]Updates guidelines (Bilezikian et al).
[b]Creatinine clearance calculated by Cockcroft-Gault equation or MDRD equation.

DIAGNOSIS

The diagnosis is typically made by detecting an elevated immunoreactive PTH level in a patient with asymptomatic hypercalcemia (see "Differential Diagnosis: Special Tests," below). Serum phosphate is usually low but may be normal, especially if renal failure has developed.

Several modifications in PTH assays have been introduced in efforts to improve their utility in light of information about metabolism of PTH (as discussed above). First-generation assays were based on displacement of radiolabeled PTH from antibodies that reacted with PTH (often also PTH fragments). Double-antibody or immunometric assays (one antibody that is usually directed against the carboxyl-terminal portion of intact PTH to capture the hormone and a second radio- or enzyme-labeled antibody that is usually directed against the amino-terminal portion of intact PTH) greatly improved the diagnostic discrimination of the tests by eliminating interference from circulating biologically inactive fragments, detected by the original first-generation assays. Double-antibody assays are now referred to as second-generation. Such PTH assays have in some centers and testing laboratories been replaced by third-generation assays after it was discovered that large PTH fragments, devoid of only the extreme amino-terminal portion of the PTH molecule, are also present in blood and are detected, incorrectly as intact PTH. These amino-terminally truncated PTH fragments were prevented from registering in the newer third-generation assays by use of a detection antibody directed against the extreme amino-terminal epitope. These assays may be useful for clinical research studies as in management of chronic renal disease, but the consensus is that either second- or third-generation assays are useful in the diagnosis of primary hyperparathyroidism and for the diagnosis of high-turnover bone disease in chronic kidney disease.

Many tests based on renal responses to excess PTH (renal calcium and phosphate clearance; blood phosphate, chloride, magnesium; urinary or nephrogenous cyclic AMP) were used in earlier decades. These tests have low specificity for hyperparathyroidism and are therefore not cost-effective; they have been replaced by PTH immunometric assays combined with simultaneous blood calcium measurements (Fig. 353-4).

TREATMENT Hyperparathyroidism

Surgical excision of the abnormal parathyroid tissue is the definitive therapy for this disease. As noted above, medical surveillance without operation for patients with mild, asymptomatic disease is, however, still preferred by some physicians and patients, particularly when the patients are more elderly. Evidence favoring surgery, if medically feasible, is growing

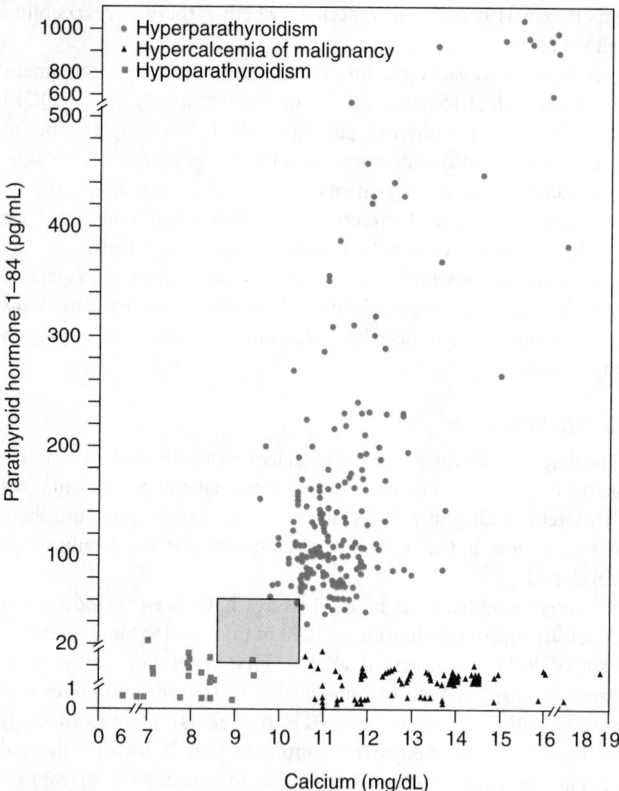

Figure 353-4 Levels of immunoreactive parathyroid hormone (PTH) detected in patients with primary hyperparathyroidism, hypercalcemia of malignancy, and hypoparathyroidism. Boxed area represents the upper and normal limits of blood calcium and/or immunoreactive PTH. *[From SR Nussbaum, JT Potts, Jr, in L DeGroot, JL Jameson (eds): Endocrinology, 4th ed. Philadelphia, Saunders, 2001; with permission.]*

because of concerns about skeletal, cardiovascular, and neuropsychiatric disease, even in mild hyperparathyroidism.

Two surgical approaches are generally practiced. The conventional parathyroidectomy procedure was neck exploration with general anesthesia; this procedure is being replaced in many centers, whenever feasible, by an outpatient procedure with local anesthesia, termed *minimally invasive parathyroidectomy.*

Parathyroid exploration is challenging and should be undertaken by an experienced surgeon. Certain features help in predicting the pathology (e.g., multiple abnormal glands in familial cases). However, some critical decisions regarding management can be made only during the operation.

With conventional surgery, one approach is still based on the view that typically only one gland (the adenoma) is abnormal. If an enlarged gland is found, a normal gland should be sought. In this view, if a biopsy of a normal-sized second gland confirms its histologic (and presumed functional) normality, no further exploration, biopsy, or excision is needed. At the other extreme is the minority viewpoint that all four glands be sought and that most of the total parathyroid tissue mass be removed. The concern with the former approach is that the recurrence rate of hyperparathyroidism may be high if a second abnormal gland is missed; the latter approach could involve unnecessary surgery and an unacceptable rate of hypoparathyroidism. When normal glands are found in association with one enlarged gland, excision of the single adenoma usually leads to cure or at least years free of symptoms. Long-term follow-up studies to establish true rates of recurrence are limited.

Recently, there has been growing experience with new surgical strategies that feature a minimally invasive approach guided by improved preoperative localization and intraoperative monitoring by PTH assays. Preoperative ^{99m}Tc sestamibi scans with single-photon emission CT (SPECT) are used to predict the location of an abnormal gland and intraoperative sampling of PTH before and at 5-minute intervals after removal of a suspected adenoma to confirm a rapid fall (>50%) to normal levels of PTH. In several centers, a combination of preoperative sestamibi imaging, cervical block anesthesia, minimal surgical incision, and intraoperative PTH measurements has allowed successful outpatient surgical management with a clear-cut cost benefit compared to general anesthesia and more extensive neck surgery. The use of these minimally invasive approaches requires clinical judgment to select patients unlikely to have multiple gland disease (e.g., MEN or secondary hyperparathyroidism). The growing acceptance of the technique and its relative ease for the patient has lowered the threshold for surgery.

Usually the severity of the hypercalcemia provides a preoperative clue to parathyroid carcinoma. In such cases, when neck exploration is undertaken, the tissue should be widely excised; care is taken to avoid rupture of the capsule to prevent local seeding of tumor cells.

Multiple-gland hyperplasia, as predicted in familial cases, poses more difficult questions of surgical management. Once a diagnosis of hyperplasia is established, all the glands must be identified. Two schemes have been proposed for surgical management. One is to totally remove three glands with partial excision of the fourth gland; care is taken to leave a good blood supply for the remaining gland. Other surgeons advocate total parathyroidectomy with immediate transplantation of a portion of a removed, minced parathyroid gland into the muscles of the forearm, with the view that surgical excision is easier from the ectopic site in the arm if there is recurrent hyperfunction.

In a minority of cases, if no abnormal parathyroid glands are found in the neck, the issue of further exploration must be decided. There are documented cases of five or six parathyroid glands and of unusual locations for adenomas such as in the mediastinum.

When a second parathyroid exploration is indicated, the minimally invasive techniques for preoperative localization such as ultrasound, CT scan, and isotope scanning are combined with venous sampling and/or selective digital arteriography in one of the centers specializing in these procedures. Intraoperative monitoring of PTH levels by rapid PTH immunoassays may be useful in guiding the surgery. At one center, long-term cures have been achieved with selective embolization or injection of large amounts of contrast material into the end-arterial circulation feeding the parathyroid tumor.

A decline in serum calcium occurs within 24 hours after successful surgery; usually blood calcium falls to low-normal values for 3–5 days until the remaining parathyroid tissue resumes full hormone secretion. Acute postoperative hypocalcemia is likely only if severe bone mineral deficits are present or if injury to all the normal parathyroid glands occurs during surgery. In general, there are few problems encountered in patients with uncomplicated disease such as a single adenoma (the clear majority), who do not have symptomatic bone disease nor a large deficit in bone mineral, who are vitamin D and magnesium sufficient, and who have good renal and gastrointestinal function. The extent of postoperative hypocalcemia varies with the surgical approach. If all glands are biopsied, hypocalcemia may be transiently symptomatic and more prolonged. Hypocalcemia is more likely to be symptomatic after second parathyroid explorations, particularly when normal parathyroid tissue was removed at the initial operation and when the manipulation and/or biopsy of the remaining normal glands are more extensive in the search for the missing adenoma.

Patients with hyperparathyroidism have efficient intestinal calcium absorption due to the increased levels of $1,25(OH)_2D$ stimulated by PTH excess. Once hypocalcemia signifies successful surgery, patients can be put on a high-calcium intake or be given oral calcium supplements. Despite mild hypocalcemia, most patients do not require parenteral therapy. If the serum calcium falls to <2 mmol/L (8 mg/dL), *and if the phosphate level rises simultaneously*, the possibility that surgery has caused hypoparathyroidism must be considered. With unexpected hypocalcemia, coexistent hypomagnesemia should be considered, as it interferes with PTH secretion and causes functional hypoparathyroidism (Chap. 352).

Signs of hypocalcemia include symptoms such as muscle twitching, a general sense of anxiety, and positive Chvostek's and Trousseau's signs coupled with serum calcium consistently <2 mmol/L (8 mg/dL). Parenteral calcium replacement at a low level should be instituted when hypocalcemia is symptomatic. The rate and duration of IV therapy are determined by the severity of the symptoms and the response of the serum calcium to treatment. An infusion of 0.5–2 mg/kg per hour or 30–100 mL/h of a 1-mg/mL solution usually suffices to relieve symptoms. Usually, parenteral therapy is required for only a few days. If symptoms worsen or if parenteral calcium is needed for >2–3 days, therapy with a vitamin D analogue and/or oral calcium (2–4 g/d) should be started (see below). It is cost-effective to use calcitriol (doses of 0.5–1 μg/d) because of the rapidity of onset of effect and prompt cessation of action when stopped, in comparison to other forms of vitamin D. A rise in blood calcium after several months of vitamin D replacement may indicate restoration of parathyroid function to normal. It is also appropriate to monitor serum PTH serially to estimate gland function in such patients.

If magnesium deficiency was present, it can complicate the postoperative course since magnesium deficiency impairs the secretion of PTH. Hypomagnesemia should be corrected whenever detected. Magnesium replacement can be effective orally (e.g., $MgCl_2$, $MgOH_2$), but parenteral repletion is usual to ensure postoperative recovery, if magnesium deficiency is suspected due to low blood magnesium levels. Because the depressant effect of magnesium on central and peripheral nerve functions does not occur at levels <2 mmol/L (normal range 0.8–1.2 mmol/L), parenteral replacement can be given rapidly. A cumulative dose as great as 0.5–1 mmol/kg of body weight can be administered if severe hypomagnesemia is present; often, however, total doses of 20–40 mmol are sufficient.

MEDICAL MANAGEMENT The guidelines for recommending surgical intervention, if feasible (Table 353-2), as well as for monitoring patients with asymptomatic hyperparathyroidism who elect not to undergo parathyroidectomy (Table 353-3), reflect the changes over time since the first conference on the topic in 1990. Medical monitoring rather than corrective surgery is still acceptable, but it is clear that surgical intervention is the more frequently recommended option for the reasons noted above. Tightened guidelines favoring surgery include lowering the recommended level of serum calcium elevation, more careful attention to skeletal integrity through reference to peak skeletal mass at baseline (T scores) rather than age-adjusted bone density (*Z* scores), as well as the presence of any fragility fracture. The other changes noted in the two guidelines (Tables 353-2 and 353-3) reflect accumulated experience and practical consideration, such as a difficulty in quantity of urine collections. Despite the usefulness of the guidelines, the importance of individual patient and physician judgment and preference are clear in all recommendations.

When surgery is not selected, or not medically feasible, there is interest in the potential value of specific medical therapies. There is no long-term experience regarding specific clinical outcomes such as fracture prevention, but it has been established that bisphosphonates increase bone mineral density significantly without changing serum calcium (as does estrogen, but the latter is not favored because of reported adverse effects in other organ systems). Calcimimetics that lower PTH secretion lower calcium but do not affect bone mass density (BMD).

■ OTHER PARATHYROID-RELATED CAUSES OF HYPERCALCEMIA

Lithium therapy

Lithium, used in the management of bipolar depression and other psychiatric disorders, causes hypercalcemia in ~10% of treated patients. The hypercalcemia is dependent on continued lithium treatment, remitting and recurring when lithium is stopped and restarted. The parathyroid adenomas reported in some hypercalcemic patients with lithium therapy may reflect the presence of an independently occurring parathyroid tumor; a permanent effect of lithium on parathyroid gland growth need not be implicated as most patients have complete reversal of hypercalcemia when lithium is stopped. However, long-standing stimulation of parathyroid cell replication by lithium may predispose to development of adenomas (as is documented in secondary hyperparathyroidism and renal failure).

At the levels achieved in blood in treated patients, lithium can be shown in vitro to shift the PTH secretion curve to the right in response to calcium; i.e., higher calcium levels are required to lower PTH secretion, probably acting at the calcium sensor (see below). This effect can cause elevated PTH levels and consequent hypercalcemia in otherwise normal individuals. Fortunately, there are usually alternative medications for the underlying psychiatric illness. Parathyroid surgery should not be recommended unless hypercalcemia and elevated PTH levels persist after lithium is discontinued.

■ GENETIC DISORDERS CAUSING HYPERPARATHYROID-LIKE SYNDROMES

Familial hypocalciuric hypercalcemia

FHH (also called *familial benign hypercalcemia*) is inherited as an autosomal dominant trait. Affected individuals are discovered because of asymptomatic hypercalcemia. FHH, which is caused by an inactivating mutation in a single allele of the calcium sensing receptor (see below), involves inappropriately normal or even increased secretion of PTH, whereas another hypercalcemic disorder, namely the exceedingly rare Jansen's disease, is caused by a constitutively active PTH/PTHrP receptor in target tissues. Neither FHH nor Jansen's disease, however, is a growth disorder of the parathyroids.

The pathophysiology of FHH is now understood. The primary defect is abnormal sensing of the blood calcium by the parathyroid gland and renal tubule, causing inappropriate secretion of PTH and excessive renal reabsorption of calcium. The calcium-sensing receptor is a member of the third family of GPCRs (type C, or III). The receptor responds to increased ECF calcium concentration by suppressing PTH secretion through second-messenger signaling, thereby providing negative-feedback regulation of PTH secretion. Many different inactivating mutations in the calcium-sensing receptor have been identified in patients with FHH. These mutations lower the capacity of the sensor to bind calcium, and the mutant receptors function as though blood calcium levels were low; excessive secretion of PTH occurs from an otherwise normal gland. Approximately two-thirds of patients with FHH have mutations within the protein-coding region of the gene. The remaining one-third of kindreds may have mutations in the gene promoter or may involve still unknown mechanisms in other regions of the genome identified through mapping studies (e.g., chromosome 19p and 19q).

Even before elucidation of the pathophysiology of FHH, abundant clinical evidence served to separate the disorder from primary hyperparathyroidism; these clinical features are still useful in differential diagnosis. Patients with primary hyperparathyroidism have <99% renal calcium reabsorption, whereas most patients with FHH have >99% reabsorption. The hypercalcemia in FHH is often detectable in affected members of the kindreds in the first decade of life, whereas hypercalcemia rarely occurs in patients with primary hyperparathyroidism or the MEN syndromes who are aged <10 years. PTH may be elevated in FHH, but the values are usually normal or lower for the same degree of calcium elevation that is observed in patients with primary hyperparathyroidism. Parathyroid surgery performed in a few patients with FHH before the nature of the syndrome was understood led to permanent hypoparathyroidism; nevertheless, hypocalciuria persisted, establishing that hypocalciuria is not PTH-dependent (now known to be due to the abnormal calcium-sensing receptor in the kidney).

Few clinical signs or symptoms are present in patients with FHH, and other endocrine abnormalities are not present. Most patients are detected as a result of family screening after hypercalcemia is detected in a proband. In those patients inadvertently operated upon, the parathyroids appeared normal or moderately hyperplastic. Parathyroid surgery is not appropriate, nor, in view of the lack of symptoms, does medical treatment seem needed to lower the calcium. One striking exception to the rule against parathyroid surgery in this syndrome is the occurrence, usually in consanguineous marriages (due to the rarity of the gene mutation), of a homozygous or compound heterozygote state, resulting in severe impairment of calcium-sensing receptor function. In this condition, neonatal severe hypercalcemia, total parathyroidectomy is mandatory. Rare but well-documented cases of acquired hypocalciuric hypercalcemia are reported due to antibodies against the calcium-sensing receptor. They appear to be a complication of an underlying autoimmune disorder and respond to therapies directed against the underlying disorder.

Jansen's disease

Activating mutations in the PTH/PTHrP receptor (PTH1R) have been identified as the cause of this rare autosomal dominant syndrome. Because the mutations lead to constitutive receptor function, one abnormal copy of the mutant receptor is sufficient to cause the disease, thereby accounting for its dominant mode of transmission. The disorder leads to short-limbed dwarfism due to abnormal regulation of chondrocyte maturation in the growth plates of the bone that are formed through an endochondral process. In adult life, there are numerous abnormalities in bone, including multiple cystic resorptive areas resembling those seen in severe hyperparathyroidism. Hypercalcemia and hypophosphatemia with undetectable or low PTH levels are typically seen. The pathogenesis of the growth plate abnormalities in Jansen's disease has been confirmed by transgenic experiments in which targeted expression of the mutant PTH/PTHrP receptor to the proliferating chondrocyte layer of growth plate emulated several features of the human disorder. Figure 353-5 illustrates some of these genetic mutations in the parathyroid gland or PTH target cells that affect Ca^{2+} metabolism.

MALIGNANCY-RELATED HYPERCALCEMIA

Clinical syndromes and mechanisms of hypercalcemia

Hypercalcemia due to malignancy is common (occurring in as many as 20% of cancer patients, especially with certain types of tumor such as lung carcinoma), often severe and difficult to manage, and, on rare occasions, difficult to distinguish from primary hyperparathyroidism. Although malignancy is often clinically obvious or readily detectable by medical history, hypercalcemia can occasionally be due to an occult tumor. Previously, hypercalcemia associated with malignancy was thought to be due to local invasion and destruction of bone by tumor cells; many cases are now known to result from the elaboration by the malignant cells of humoral mediators of hypercalcemia. PTHrP is the responsible humoral agent in most solid tumors that cause hypercalcemia.

The histologic character of the tumor is more important than the extent of skeletal metastases in predicting hypercalcemia. Small cell carcinoma (oat cell) and adenocarcinoma of the lung, though the most common lung tumors associated with skeletal metastases, rarely cause hypercalcemia. By contrast, many patients with squamous cell carcinoma of the lung develop hypercalcemia. Histologic studies of bone in patients with squamous cell or epidermoid carcinoma of the lung, in sites invaded by tumor as well as areas remote from tumor invasion, reveal increased bone resorption.

Two main mechanisms of hypercalcemia are operative in cancer hypercalcemia. Many solid tumors associated with hypercalcemia, particularly squamous cell and renal tumors, produce and secrete PTHrP that causes increased bone resorption and mediate the hypercalcemia through systemic actions on the skeleton. Alternatively, direct bone marrow invasion occurs with hematologic malignancies such as leukemia, lymphoma, and multiple myeloma. Lymphokines and cytokines (including PTHrP) produced by cells involved in the marrow response to the tumors promote resorption of bone through local destruction. Several hormones, hormone analogues, cytokines, and growth factors have been implicated as the result of clinical assays, in vitro tests, or chemical isolation. The etiologic factor produced by activated normal lymphocytes and by myeloma and lymphoma cells, originally termed *osteoclast activation factor*, now appears to represent the biologic action of several different cytokines, probably interleukin 1 and lymphotoxin or tumor necrosis factor (TNF). In some lymphomas, there is a third mechanism, caused by an increased blood level of $1,25(OH)_2D$, produced by the abnormal lymphocytes.

In the more common mechanism, usually termed *humoral hypercalcemia of malignancy*, solid tumors (cancers of the lung and kidney, in particular), in which bone metastases are absent, minimal, or not detectable clinically, secrete PTHrP measurable by immunoassay. Secretion by the tumors of the PTH-like factor, PTHrP, activates the PTH1R, resulting in a pathophysiology closely resembling hyperparathyroidism. The clinical picture resembles primary hyperparathyroidism (hypophosphatemia accompanies hypercalcemia), and elimination or regression of the primary tumor leads to disappearance of the hypercalcemia.

As in hyperparathyroidism, patients with the humoral hypercalcemia of malignancy have elevated urinary nephrogenous cyclic AMP excretion, hypophosphatemia, and increased urinary phosphate clearance. However, in humoral hypercalcemia of malignancy, immunoreactive PTH is undetectable or suppressed, making the differential diagnosis easier. Other features of the disorder differ from those of true hyperparathyroidism. Although

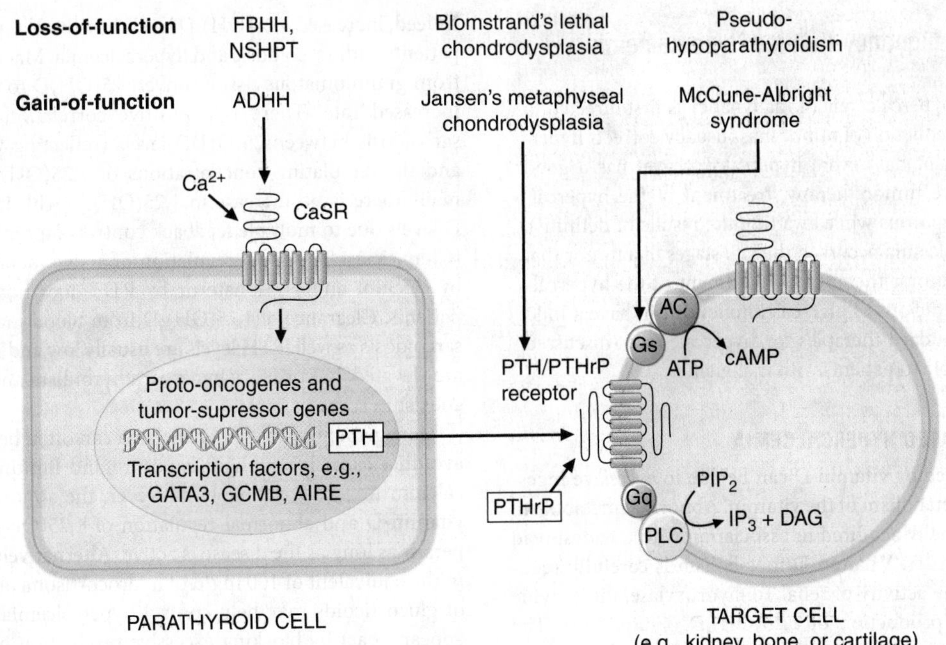

Figure 353-5 Illustration of some genetic mutations that alter calcium metabolism by effects on the parathyroid cell or target cells of PTH action. Alterations in PTH production by the parathyroid cell can be caused by changes in the response to extracellular fluid calcium (Ca^{2+}) that are detected by the calcium-sensing receptor (CaSR). Furthermore, PTH (or PTHrP) can show altered efficacy in target cells such as in proximal tubular cells, by altered function of its receptor (PTH/PTHrP receptor) or the signal transduction proteins, G proteins such as $G_s\alpha$ that is linked to adenylate cyclase (AC), the enzyme responsible for producing cyclic AMP (cAMP) [also illustrated is Gq, which activates an alternate pathway of receptor signal transmission involving the generation of inositol triphosphate (IP_3) or diacylglycerol (DAG)]. Heterozygous loss-of-function mutations in the CaSR cause familial benign hypocalciuric hypercalcemia (FBHH) and homozygous mutations (both alleles mutated) and severe neonatal hyperparathyroidism (NSHPT); heterozygous gain-of-functions causes autosomal dominant hypercalciuric hypocalcemia (ADHH). Other defects in parathyroid cell function that occur at the level of gene regulation (oncogenes or tumor suppressor genes) or transcription factors are discussed in the text. Blomstrand's lethal chondrodysplasia is due to homozygous or compound heterozygous loss-of-function mutations in the PTH/PTHrP receptor, a neonatally lethal disorder, while pseudohypoparathyroidism involves inactivation at the level of the G proteins, specifically mutations that eliminate or reduce $G_s\alpha$ activity in the kidney (see text for details). Jansen's metaphyseal chondrodysplasia and McCune-Albright syndrome represent gain-of-function mutations in the PTH/PTHrP receptor and $G_s\alpha$ protein, respectively.

the biologic actions of PTH and PTHrP are exerted through the same receptor, subtle differences in receptor activation by the two ligands must account for some of the discordance in pathophysiology, when an excess of one or the other peptide occurs. Other cytokines elaborated by the malignancy may contribute to the variations from hyperparathyroidism in these patients as well. Patients with humoral hypercalcemia of malignancy may have low to normal levels of $1,25(OH)_2D$ instead of elevated levels as in true hyperparathyroidism. In some patients with the humoral hypercalcemia of malignancy, osteoclastic resorption is unaccompanied by an osteoblastic or bone-forming response, implying inhibition of the normal coupling of bone formation and resorption.

Several different assays (single- or double-antibody, different epitopes) have been developed to detect PTHrP. Most data indicate that circulating PTHrP levels are undetectable (or low) in normal individuals except perhaps in pregnancy (high in human milk) and elevated in most cancer patients with the humoral syndrome. The etiologic mechanisms in cancer hypercalcemia may be multiple in the same patient. For example, in breast carcinoma (metastatic to bone) and in a distinctive type of T cell lymphoma/leukemia initiated by human T cell lymphotropic virus I, hypercalcemia is caused by direct local lysis of bone as well as by a humoral mechanism involving excess production of PTHrP. Hyperparathyroidism has been reported to coexist with the humoral cancer syndrome and, rarely, ectopic hyperparathyroidism due to tumor elaboration of true PTH is reported.

Diagnostic issues

Levels of PTH measured by the double-antibody technique are undetectable or extremely low in tumor hypercalcemia, as would be expected with the mediation of the hypercalcemia by a factor other than PTH (the hypercalcemia suppresses the normal parathyroid glands). In a patient with minimal symptoms referred for hypercalcemia, low or undetectable PTH levels would focus attention on a possible occult malignancy (except for very rare cases of ectopic hyperparathyroidism).

Ordinarily, the diagnosis of cancer hypercalcemia is not difficult because tumor symptoms are prominent when hypercalcemia is detected. Indeed, hypercalcemia may be noted incidentally during the workup of a patient with known or suspected malignancy. Clinical suspicion that malignancy is the cause of the hypercalcemia is heightened when there are other signs or symptoms of a paraneoplastic process such as weight loss, fatigue, muscle weakness, or unexplained skin rash, or when symptoms specific for a particular tumor are present. Squamous cell tumors are most frequently associated with hypercalcemia, particularly tumors of the lung, kidney, head and neck, and urogenital tract. Radiologic examinations can focus on these areas when clinical evidence is unclear. Bone scans with technetium-labeled bisphosphonate are useful for detection of osteolytic metastases; the sensitivity is high, but specificity is low; results must be confirmed by conventional x-rays to be certain that areas of increased uptake are due to osteolytic metastases per se. Bone marrow biopsies are helpful in patients with anemia or abnormal peripheral blood smears.

TREATMENT Malignancy-Related Hypercalcemia

Treatment of the hypercalcemia of malignancy is first directed to control of tumor; reduction of tumor mass usually corrects hypercalcemia. If a patient has severe hypercalcemia yet has a good chance for effective tumor therapy, treatment of the hypercalcemia should be vigorous while awaiting the results of definitive therapy. If hypercalcemia occurs in the late stages of a tumor that is resistant to antitumor therapy, the treatment of the hypercalcemia should be judicious as high calcium levels can have a mild sedating effect. Standard therapies for hypercalcemia (discussed below) are applicable to patients with malignancy.

VITAMIN D–RELATED HYPERCALCEMIA

Hypercalcemia caused by vitamin D can be due to excessive ingestion or abnormal metabolism of the vitamin. Abnormal metabolism of the vitamin is usually acquired in association with a widespread granulomatous disorder. Vitamin D metabolism is carefully regulated, particularly the activity of renal 1α-hydroxylase, the enzyme responsible for the production of $1,25(OH)_2D$ (Chap. 352). The regulation of 1α-hydroxylase and the normal feedback suppression by $1,25(OH)_2D$ seem to work less well in infants than in adults and to operate poorly, if at all, in sites other than the renal tubule; these phenomena may explain the occurrence of hypercalcemia secondary to excessive $1,25(OH)_2D_3$ production in infants with Williams' syndrome (see below) and in adults with sarcoidosis or lymphoma.

Vitamin D intoxication

Chronic ingestion of 40–100 times the normal physiologic requirement of vitamin D (amounts >40,000–100,000 U/d) is usually required to produce significant hypercalcemia in normal individuals. The stated upper limit of safe dietary intake is 2000 U/d (50 μg/d) in adults because of concerns about potential toxic effects of cumulative supraphysiologic doses. These recommendations are now regarded as too restrictive, since some estimates are that in elderly individuals in northern latitudes, 2000 U/daily or more may be necessary to avoid vitamin D insufficiency.

Hypercalcemia in vitamin D intoxication is due to an excessive biologic action of the vitamin, perhaps the consequence of increased levels of 25(OH)D rather than merely increased levels of the active metabolite $1,25(OH)_2D$ (the latter may not be elevated in vitamin D intoxication). 25(OH)D has definite, if low, biologic activity in the intestine and bone. The production of 25(OH)D is less tightly regulated than is the production of $1,25(OH)_2D$. Hence concentrations of 25(OH)D are elevated severalfold in patients with excess vitamin D intake.

The diagnosis is substantiated by documenting elevated levels of 25(OH)D >100 mg/mL. Hypercalcemia is usually controlled by restriction of dietary calcium intake and appropriate attention to hydration. These measures, plus discontinuation of vitamin D, usually lead to resolution of hypercalcemia. However, vitamin D stores in fat may be substantial, and vitamin D intoxication may persist for weeks after vitamin D ingestion is terminated. Such patients are responsive to glucocorticoids, which in doses of 100 mg/d of hydrocortisone or its equivalent usually return serum calcium levels to normal over several days; severe intoxication may require intensive therapy.

Sarcoidosis and other granulomatous diseases

In patients with sarcoidosis and other granulomatous diseases, such as tuberculosis and fungal infections, excess $1,25(OH)_2D$ is synthesized in macrophages or other cells in the granulomas. Indeed, increased $1,25(OH)_2D$ levels have been reported in anephric patients with sarcoidosis and hypercalcemia. Macrophages obtained from granulomatous tissue convert 25(OH)D to $1,25(OH)_2D$ at an increased rate. There is a positive correlation in patients with sarcoidosis between 25(OH)D levels (reflecting vitamin D intake) and the circulating concentrations of $1,25(OH)_2D$, whereas normally there is no increase in $1,25(OH)_2D$ with increasing 25(OH) D levels due to multiple feedback controls on renal 1α-hydroxylase (Chap. 352). The usual regulation of active metabolite production by calcium and phosphate or by PTH does not operate in these patients. Clearance of $1,25(OH)_2D$ from blood may be decreased in sarcoidosis as well. PTH levels are usually low and $1,25(OH)_2D$ levels are elevated, but primary hyperparathyroidism and sarcoidosis may coexist in some patients.

Management of the hypercalcemia can often be accomplished by avoiding excessive sunlight exposure and limiting vitamin D and calcium intake. Presumably, however, the abnormal sensitivity to vitamin D and abnormal regulation of $1,25(OH)_2D$ synthesis will persist as long as the disease is active. Alternatively, glucocorticoids in the equivalent of 100 mg/d of hydrocortisone or equivalent doses of glucorticoids may help control hypercalcemia. Glucocorticoids appear to act by blocking excessive production of $1,25(OH)_2D$, as well as the response to it in target organs.

Idiopathic hypercalcemia of infancy

This rare disorder, usually referred to as *Williams' syndrome*, is an autosomal dominant disorder characterized by multiple congenital development defects, including supravalvular aortic stenosis, mental retardation, and an elfin facies, in association with hypercalcemia due to abnormal sensitivity to vitamin D. The hypercalcemia associated with the syndrome was first recognized in England after fortification of milk with vitamin D. The cardiac and developmental abnormalities were independently described, but the connection between these defects and hypercalcemia were not described until later. Levels of $1,25(OH)_2D$ can be elevated, ranging from 46 to 120 nmol/L (150–500 pg/mL). The mechanism of the abnormal sensitivity to vitamin D and of the increased circulating levels of $1,25(OH)_2D$ is still unclear. Studies suggest that genetic mutations involving microdeletions at the elastin locus and perhaps other genes on chromosome 7 may play a role in the pathogenesis.

HYPERCALCEMIA ASSOCIATED WITH HIGH BONE TURNOVER

Hyperthyroidism

As many as 20% of hyperthyroid patients have high-normal or mildly elevated serum calcium concentrations; hypercalciuria is even more common. The hypercalcemia is due to increased bone turnover, with bone resorption exceeding bone formation. Severe calcium elevations are not typical, and the presence of such suggests a concomitant disease such as hyperparathyroidism. Usually, the diagnosis is obvious, but signs of hyperthyroidism may occasionally be occult, particularly in the elderly (Chap. 341). Hypercalcemia is managed by treatment of the hyperthyroidism. Reports that thyroid-stimulating hormone (TSH) itself normally has a bone-protective effect suggest that suppressed TSH levels also play a role in hypercalcemia.

Immobilization

Immobilization is a rare cause of hypercalcemia in adults in the absence of an associated disease but may cause hypercalcemia in children and adolescents, particularly after spinal cord injury and paraplegia or quadriplegia. With resumption of ambulation, the hypercalcemia in children usually returns to normal.

The mechanism appears to involve a disproportion between bone formation and bone resorption; the former decreased and the latter increased. Hypercalciuria and increased mobilization of skeletal calcium can develop in normal volunteers subjected to extensive bed rest, although hypercalcemia is unusual. Immobilization of an adult with a disease associated with high bone turnover, however, such as Paget's disease, may cause hypercalcemia.

Thiazides

Administration of benzothiadiazines (thiazides) can cause hypercalcemia in patients with high rates of bone turnover such as patients with hypoparathyroidism treated with high doses of vitamin D. Traditionally, thiazides are associated with aggravation of hypercalcemia in primary hyperparathyroidism, but this effect can be seen in other high-bone-turnover states as well. The mechanism of thiazide action is complex. Chronic thiazide administration leads to reduction in urinary calcium; the hypocalciuric effect appears to reflect the enhancement of proximal tubular resorption of sodium and calcium in response to sodium depletion. Some of this renal effect is due to augmentation of PTH action and is more pronounced in individuals with intact PTH secretion. However, thiazides cause hypocalciuria in hypoparathyroid patients on high-dose vitamin D and oral calcium replacement if sodium intake is restricted. This finding is the rationale for the use of thiazides as an adjunct to therapy in hypoparathyroid patients, as discussed below. Thiazide administration to normal individuals causes a transient increase in blood calcium (usually within the high-normal range) that reverts to preexisting levels after a week or more of continued administration. If hormonal function and calcium and bone metabolism are normal, homeostatic controls are reset to counteract the calcium-elevating effect of the thiazides. In the presence of hyperparathyroidism or increased bone turnover from another cause, homeostatic mechanisms are ineffective. The abnormal effects of the thiazide on calcium metabolism disappear within days of cessation of the drug.

Vitamin A intoxication

Vitamin A intoxication is a rare cause of hypercalcemia and is most commonly a side effect of dietary faddism (Chap. 74). Calcium levels can be elevated into the 3–3.5-mmol/L (12–14 mg/dL) range after the ingestion of 50,000–100,000 units of vitamin A daily (10–20 times the minimum daily requirement). Typical features of severe hypercalcemia include fatigue, anorexia, and, in some, severe muscle and bone pain. Excess vitamin A intake is presumed to increase bone resorption.

The diagnosis can be established by history and by measurement of vitamin A levels in serum. Occasionally, skeletal x-rays reveal periosteal calcifications, particularly in the hands. Withdrawal of the vitamin is usually associated with prompt disappearance of the hypercalcemia and reversal of the skeletal changes. As in vitamin D intoxication, administration of 100 mg/d hydrocortisone or its equivalent leads to a rapid return of the serum calcium to normal.

HYPERCALCEMIA ASSOCIATED WITH RENAL FAILURE

Severe secondary hyperparathyroidism

The pathogenesis of secondary hyperparathyroidism in chronic kidney disease is incompletely understood. Resistance to the normal level of PTH is a major factor contributing to the development of hypocalcemia, which, in turn, is a stimulus to parathyroid gland enlargement. However, recent findings have indicated that an increase of FGF23 production by osteocytes (and possibly osteoblasts) in bone occurs well before an elevation in PTH is detected. FGF23 is a potent inhibitor of the renal 1-alpha hydroxylase, and the FGF23-dependent reduction in $1,25(OH)_2$ vitamin D may be an important stimulus for the development of secondary hyperparathyroidism.

Secondary hyperparathyroidism occurs not only in patients with renal failure but also in those with osteomalacia due to multiple causes (Chap. 352), including deficiency of vitamin D action and PHP (deficient response to PTH at the level of the receptor). For both disorders, hypocalcemia seems to be the common denominator in initiating the development of secondary hyperparathyroidism. Primary (1°) and secondary (2°) hyperparathyroidism can be distinguished conceptually by the autonomous growth of the parathyroid glands in primary hyperparathyroidism (presumably irreversible) and the adaptive response of the parathyroids in secondary hyperparathyroidism (typically reversible). In fact, reversal over weeks from an abnormal pattern of secretion, presumably accompanied by involution of parathyroid gland mass to normal, occurs in patients with osteomalacia who have been treated effectively with calcium and vitamin D. However, it is now recognized that a true clonal outgrowth (irreversible) can arise in long-standing, inadequately treated chronic renal failure [e.g., tertiary (3°) hyperparathyroidism; see below].

Patients with secondary hyperparathyroidism may develop bone pain, ectopic calcification, and pruritus. The bone disease seen in patients with secondary hyperparathyroidism and chronic kidney disease is termed *renal osteodystrophy* and affects primarily bone turnover. However, osteomalacia is frequently encountered as well and may be related to the circulating levels of FGF23.

Two other skeletal disorders have been frequently associated in the past with CKD patients treated by long-term dialysis who received aluminum-containing phosphate binders. Aluminum deposition in bone (see below) leads to an osteomalacia-like picture. The other entity is a low-bone-turnover state termed "aplastic" or "adynamic" bone disease; PTH levels are lower than typically observed in CKD patients with secondary hyperparathyroidism. It is believed that the condition is caused, at least in part, by excessive PTH suppression, which may be even greater than previously appreciated in light of evidence that some of the immunoreactive PTH detected by most commercially available PTH assays is not the full-length biologically active molecule (as discussed above) but may consist of amino-terminally truncated fragments that do not activate the PTH1R.

TREATMENT Secondary Hyperparathyroidism

Medical therapy to reverse secondary hyperparathyroidism in CKD includes reduction of excessive blood phosphate by restriction of dietary phosphate, the use of nonabsorbable antacids, and careful, selective addition of calcitriol (0.25–2 μg/d) or related analogues. Calcium carbonate became preferred over aluminum-containing antacids to prevent aluminum-induced bone disease. However, synthetic gels that also bind phosphate (such as sevelamer; Chap. 280) are now widely used, with the advantage of avoiding not only aluminum retention but excess calcium elevation. Intravenous calcitriol (or related analogues), administered as several pulses each week, helps control secondary hyperparathyroidism. Aggressive but carefully administered medical therapy can often, but not always, reverse hyperparathyroidism and its symptoms and manifestations.

Occasional patients develop severe manifestations of secondary hyperparathyroidism, including hypercalcemia, pruritus, extraskeletal calcifications, and painful bones, despite aggressive medical efforts to suppress the hyperparathyroidism. PTH hypersecretion no longer responsive to medical therapy, a state of severe hyperparathyroidism in patients with renal failure that requires surgery, has been referred to as *tertiary hyperparathyroidism*. Parathyroid surgery is necessary to control this condition. Based on genetic evidence from examination of tumor samples in these patients, the emergence of autonomous parathyroid function is due to a monoclonal outgrowth of one or more previously hyperplastic parathyroid glands. The adaptive response has become an independent contributor to disease; this finding seems to emphasize the importance of optimal medical management to reduce the proliferative response of the parathyroid cells that enables the irreversible genetic change.

Aluminum intoxication

Aluminum intoxication (and often hypercalcemia as a complication of medical treatment) in the past occurred in patients on chronic dialysis; manifestations included acute dementia and unresponsive and severe osteomalacia. Bone pain, multiple nonhealing fractures, particularly of the ribs and pelvis, and a proximal myopathy occur. Hypercalcemia develops when these patients are treated with vitamin D or calcitriol because of impaired skeletal responsiveness. Aluminum is present at the site of osteoid mineralization, osteoblastic activity is minimal, and calcium incorporation into the skeleton is impaired. The disorder is now rare because of the avoidance of aluminum-containing antacids or aluminum excess in the dialysis regimen (Chap. 360).

Milk-alkali syndrome

The milk-alkali syndrome is due to excessive ingestion of calcium and absorbable antacids such as milk or calcium carbonate. It is much less frequent since proton-pump inhibitors and other treatments became available for peptic ulcer disease. For a time, the increased use of calcium carbonate in the management of secondary hyperparathyroidism led to reappearance of the syndrome. Several clinical presentations—acute, subacute, and chronic—have been described, all of which feature hypercalcemia, alkalosis, and renal failure. The chronic form of the disease, termed *Burnett's syndrome*, is associated with irreversible renal damage. The acute syndromes reverse if the excess calcium and absorbable alkali are stopped.

Individual susceptibility is important in the pathogenesis, as some patients are treated with calcium carbonate and alkali regimens without developing the syndrome. One variable is the fractional calcium absorption as a function of calcium intake. Some individuals absorb a high fraction of calcium, even with intakes ≥2 g of elemental calcium per day, instead of reducing calcium absorption with high intake, as occurs in most normal individuals. Resultant mild hypercalcemia after meals in such patients is postulated to contribute to the generation of alkalosis. Development of hypercalcemia causes increased sodium excretion and some depletion of total-body water. These phenomena and perhaps some suppression of endogenous PTH secretion due to mild hypercalcemia lead to increased bicarbonate resorption and to alkalosis in the face of continued calcium carbonate ingestion. Alkalosis per se selectively enhances calcium resorption in the distal nephron, thus aggravating the hypercalcemia. The cycle of mild hypercalcemia → bicarbonate retention → alkalosis → renal calcium retention → severe hypercalcemia perpetuates and aggravates hypercalcemia and alkalosis as long as calcium and absorbable alkali are ingested.

DIFFERENTIAL DIAGNOSIS: SPECIAL TESTS

Differential diagnosis of hypercalcemia is best achieved by using clinical criteria, but immunometric assays to measure PTH is especially useful in distinguishing among major causes (Fig. 353-6). The clinical features that deserve emphasis are the presence or absence of symptoms or signs of disease and evidence of chronicity. If one discounts fatigue or depression, >90% of patients with primary hyperparathyroidism have *asymptomatic hypercalcemia*; symptoms of malignancy are usually present in cancer-associated hypercalcemia. Disorders other than hyperparathyroidism and malignancy cause <10% of cases of hypercalcemia, and some of the nonparathyroid causes are associated with clear-cut manifestations such as renal failure.

Hyperparathyroidism is the likely diagnosis in patients with *chronic hypercalcemia*. If hypercalcemia has been manifest for >1 year, malignancy can usually be excluded as the cause. A striking feature of malignancy-associated hypercalcemia is the rapidity of the course, whereby signs and symptoms of the underlying malignancy are evident within months of the detection of hypercalcemia. Although clinical considerations are helpful in arriving at the correct diagnosis of the cause of hypercalcemia, appropriate laboratory testing is essential for definitive diagnosis. The immunoassay for PTH usually separates hyperparathyroidism from all other causes of hypercalcemia. There are very rare reports of ectopic production of excess PTH by nonparathyroid tumors. Patients with hyperparathyroidism have elevated PTH levels despite hypercalcemia, whereas patients with malignancy and the other causes of hypercalcemia (except for disorders mediated by PTH such as lithium-induced hypercalcemia) have levels of hormone below normal or undetectable. Assays based on the double-antibody method for PTH exhibit very high sensitivity (especially if serum calcium is simultaneously

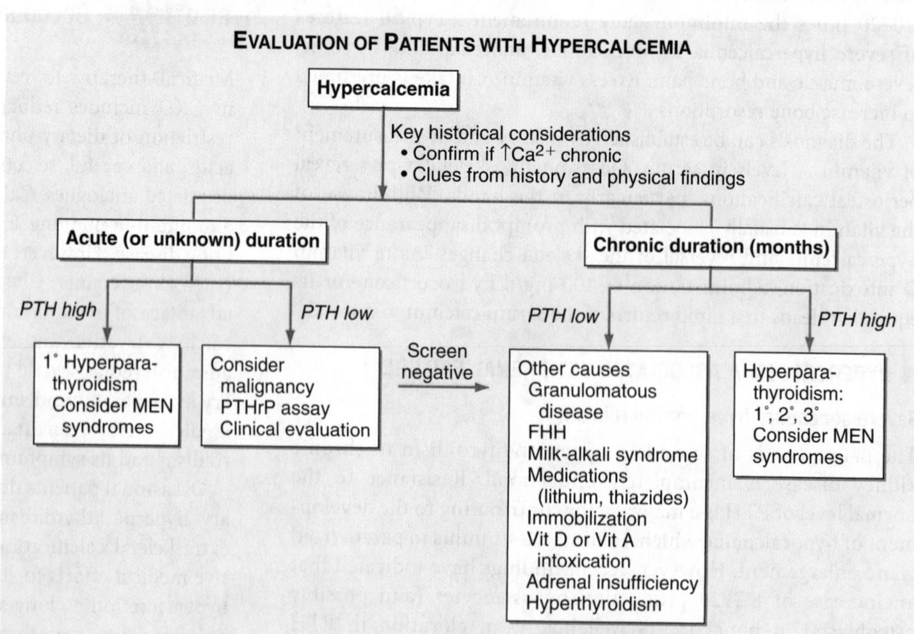

Figure 353-6 Algorithm for the evaluation of patients with hypercalcemia. See text for details. FHH, familial hypocalciuric hypercalcemia; MEN, multiple endocrine neoplasia; PTH, parathyroid hormone; PTHrP, parathyroid hormone–related peptide.

evaluated) and specificity for the diagnosis of primary hyperparathyroidism (Fig. 353-4).

In summary, PTH values are elevated in >90% of parathyroid-related causes of hypercalcemia, undetectable or low in malignancy-related hypercalcemia, and undetectable or normal in vitamin D–related and high-bone-turnover causes of hypercalcemia. In view of the specificity of the PTH immunoassay and the high frequency of hyperparathyroidism in hypercalcemic patients, it is cost-effective to measure the PTH level in all hypercalcemic patients unless malignancy or a specific nonparathyroid disease is obvious. False-positive PTH assay results are rare. Immunoassays for PTHrP are helpful in diagnosing certain types of malignancy-associated hypercalcemia. Although FHH is parathyroid-related, the disease should be managed distinctively from hyperparathyroidism. Clinical features and the low urinary calcium excretion can help make the distinction. Because the incidence of malignancy and hyperparathyroidism both increase with age, they can coexist as two independent causes of hypercalcemia.

$1,25(OH)_2D$ levels are elevated in many (but not all) patients with primary hyperparathyroidism. In other disorders associated with hypercalcemia, concentrations of $1,25(OH)_2D$ are low or, at the most, normal. However, this test is of low specificity and is not cost-effective, as not all patients with hyperparathyroidism have elevated $1,25(OH)_2D$ levels and not all nonparathyroid hypercalcemic patients have suppressed $1,25(OH)_2D$. Measurement of $1,25(OH)_2D$ is, however, critically valuable in establishing the cause of hypercalcemia in sarcoidosis and certain lymphomas.

A useful general approach is outlined in Fig. 353-6. If the patient is *asymptomatic* and there is evidence of *chronicity* to the hypercalcemia, hyperparathyroidism is almost certainly the cause. If PTH levels (usually measured at least twice) are elevated, the clinical impression is confirmed and little additional evaluation is necessary. If there is only a short history or no data as to the duration of the hypercalcemia, *occult malignancy* must be considered; if the PTH levels are not elevated, then a thorough workup must be undertaken for malignancy, including chest x-ray, CT of chest and abdomen, and bone scan. Immunoassays for PTHrP may be especially useful in such situations. Attention should also be paid to clues for underlying hematologic disorders such as anemia, increased plasma globulin, and abnormal serum immunoelectrophoresis; bone scans can be negative in some patients with metastases such as in multiple myeloma. Finally, if a patient with chronic hypercalcemia is asymptomatic and malignancy therefore seems unlikely on clinical grounds, but PTH values are not elevated, it is useful to search for other chronic causes of hypercalcemia such as occult sarcoidosis. A careful history of dietary supplements and drug use may suggest intoxication with vitamin D or vitamin A or the use of thiazides.

TREATMENT Hypercalcemic States

The approach to medical treatment of hypercalcemia varies with its severity (Table 353-4). Mild hypercalcemia, <3 mmol/L (12 mg/dL), can be managed by hydration. More severe hypercalcemia [levels of 3.2–3.7 mmol/L (13–15 mg/dL)] must be managed aggressively; above that level, hypercalcemia can be life-threatening and requires emergency measures. By using a

TABLE 353-4 Therapies for Severe Hypercalcemia

Treatment	Onset of Action	Duration of Action	Advantages	Disadvantages
Most Useful Therapies				
Hydration with saline	Hours	During infusion	Rehydration invariably needed	Volume overload
Forced diuresis; saline plus loop diuretic	Hours	During treatment	Rapid action	Volume overload, cardiac decompensation, intensive monitoring, electrolyte disturbance, inconvenience
Bisphosphonates				
Pamidronate	1–2 days	10–14 days to weeks	High potency; intermediate onset of action	Fever in 20%, hypophosphatemia, hypocalcemia, hypomagnesemia, rarely jaw necrosis
Zolendronate	1–2 days	>3 weeks	Same as for pamidronate (may last longer)	Same as pamidronate above
Calcitonin	Hours	1–2 days	Rapid onset of action; useful as adjunct in severe hypercalcemia	Rapid tachyphylaxis
Special Use Therapies				
Phosphate Oral	24 h	During use	Chronic management (with hypophosphatemia); low toxicity if P <4 mg/dL	Limited use except as adjuvant or chronic therapy
Glucocorticoids	Days	Days, weeks	Oral therapy, antitumor agent	Active only in certain malignancies, vitamin D excess and sarcoidosis; glucocorticoid side effects
Dialysis	Hours	During use and 24–48 h afterward	Useful in renal failure; onset of effect in hours; can immediately reverse life-threatening hypercalcemia	Complex procedure, reserved for extreme or special circumstances

combination of approaches in severe hypercalcemia, the serum calcium concentration can be decreased by 0.7–2.2 mmol/L (3–9 mg/dL) within 24–48 hours in most patients, enough to relieve acute symptoms, prevent death from hypercalcemic crisis, and permit diagnostic evaluation. Therapy can then be directed at the underlying disorder—the second priority.

Hypercalcemia develops because of excessive skeletal calcium release, increased intestinal calcium absorption, or inadequate renal calcium excretion. Understanding the particular pathogenesis helps guide therapy. For example, hypercalcemia in patients with malignancy is primarily due to excessive skeletal calcium release and is, therefore, minimally improved by restriction of dietary calcium. On the other hand, patients with vitamin D hypersensitivity or vitamin D intoxication have excessive intestinal calcium absorption, and restriction of dietary calcium is beneficial. Decreased renal function or ECF depletion decreases urinary calcium excretion. In such situations, rehydration may rapidly reduce or reverse the hypercalcemia, even though increased bone resorption persists. As outlined below, the more severe the hypercalcemia, the greater the number of combined therapies that should be used. Rapid acting (hours) approaches—rehydration, forced diuresis, and calcitonin—can be used with the most effective antiresorptive agents such as bisphosphonates (since severe hypercalcemia usually involves excessive bone resorption).

HYDRATION, INCREASED SALT INTAKE, MILD AND FORCED DIURESIS The first principle of treatment is to restore normal hydration. Many hypercalcemic patients are dehydrated because of vomiting, inanition, and/or hypercalcemia-induced defects in urinary concentrating ability. The resultant drop in glomerular filtration rate is accompanied by an additional decrease in renal tubular sodium and calcium clearance. Restoring a normal ECF volume corrects these abnormalities and increases urine calcium excretion by 2.5–7.5 mmol/d (100–300 mg/d). Increasing urinary sodium excretion to 400–500 mmol/d increases urinary calcium excretion even further than simple rehydration. After rehydration has been achieved, saline can be administered or furosemide or ethacrynic acid can be given twice daily to depress the tubular reabsorptive mechanism for calcium (care must be taken to prevent dehydration). The combined use of these therapies can increase urinary calcium excretion to ≥12.5 mmol/d (500 mg/d) in most hypercalcemic patients. Since this is a substantial percentage of the exchangeable calcium pool, the serum calcium concentration usually falls 0.25–0.75 mmol/L (1–3 mg/dL) within 24 hours. Precautions should be taken to prevent potassium and magnesium depletion; calcium-containing renal calculi are a potential complication.

Under life-threatening circumstances, the preceding approach can be pursued more aggressively, but the availability of effective agents to block bone resorption (such as bisphosphonates) has reduced the need for extreme diuresis regimens (Table 353-5). Depletion of potassium and magnesium is inevitable unless replacements are given; pulmonary edema can be precipitated. The potential complications can be reduced by careful monitoring of central venous pressure and plasma or urine electrolytes; catheterization of the bladder may be necessary. Dialysis treatment may be needed when renal function is compromised.

BISPHOSPHONATES The bisphosphonates are analogues of pyrophosphate, with high affinity for bone, especially in areas of increased bone turnover, where they are powerful inhibitors of bone resorption. These bone-seeking compounds are stable in vivo because phosphatase enzymes cannot hydrolyze the central carbon-phosphorus-carbon bond. The bisphosphonates are concentrated in areas of high bone turnover and are taken up by

TABLE 353-5 Functional Classification of Hypocalcemia (Excluding Neonatal Conditions)

PTH Absent	
Hereditary hypoparathyroidism	Hypomagnesemia
Acquired hypoparathyroidism	
PTH Ineffective	
Chronic renal failure	Active vitamin D ineffective
Active vitamin D lacking	Intestinal malabsorption
↓ Dietary intake or sunlight	Vitamin D–dependent rickets type II
Defective metabolism:	
Anticonvulsant therapy	Pseudohypoparathyroidism
Vitamin D–dependent rickets type I	
PTH Overwhelmed	
Severe, acute hyperphosphatemia	Osteitis fibrosa after parathyroidectomy
Tumor lysis	
Acute renal failure	
Rhabdomyolysis	

Abbreviation: PTH, parathyroid hormone.

and inhibit osteoclast action; the mechanism of action is complex. The bisphosphonate molecules that contain amino groups in the side chain structure (see below) interfere with prenylation of proteins and can lead to cellular apoptosis. The highly active nonamino group–containing bisphosphonates are also metabolized to cytotoxic products.

The initial bisphosphonate widely used in clinical practice, etidronate, was effective but had several disadvantages, including the capacity to inhibit bone formation as well as blocking resorption. Subsequently, a number of second- or third-generation compounds have become the mainstays of antiresorptive therapy for treatment of hypercalcemia and osteoporosis. The newer bisphosphonates have a highly favorable ratio of blocking resorption versus inhibiting bone formation; they inhibit osteoclast-mediated skeletal resorption yet do not cause mineralization defects at ordinary doses. Though the bisphosphonates have similar structures, the routes of administration, efficacy, toxicity, and side effects vary. The potency of the compounds for inhibition of bone resorption varies more than 10,000-fold, increasing in the order of etidronate, tiludronate, pamidronate, alendronate, risedronate, and zolendronate. The IV use of pamidronate and zolendronate is approved for the treatment of hypercalcemia; between 30 and 90 mg pamidronate, given as a single IV dose over a few hours, returns serum calcium to normal within 24–48 hours with an effect that lasts for weeks in 80–100% of patients. Zolendronate given in doses of 4 or 8 mg/5-minute infusion has a more rapid and more sustained effect than pamidronate in direct comparison.

These drugs are used extensively in cancer patients. Absolute survival improvements are noted with pamidronate and zolendronate in multiple myeloma, for example. However, though still rare, there are increasing reports of jaw necrosis, especially after dental surgery, mainly in cancer patients treated with multiple doses of the more potent bisphosphonates.

CALCITONIN Calcitonin acts within a few hours of its administration, principally through receptors on osteoclasts, to block bone resorption. Calcitonin, after 24 hours of use, is no longer effective in lowering calcium. Tachyphylaxis, a known phenomenon with this drug, seems to explain the results, since the drug is often effective in the first 24 hours of use. Therefore, in life-threatening hypercalcemia, calcitonin can be used effectively within the first 24 hours in combination with rehydration and saline diuresis while waiting for more sustained effects from a simultaneously administered bisphosphonate such as pamidronate. Usual doses of calcitonin are 2–8 U/kg of body weight IV, SC, or IM every 6–12 hours.

OTHER THERAPIES *Plicamycin* (formerly mithramycin), which inhibits bone resorption, has been a useful therapeutic agent but is now seldom used because of its toxicity and the effectiveness of bisphosphonates. Plicamycin must be given IV, either as a bolus or by slow infusion; the usual dose is 25 μg/kg body weight. *Gallium nitrate* exerts a hypocalcemic action by inhibiting bone resorption and altering the structure of bone crystals. It is not often used now because of superior alternatives.

Glucocorticoids have utility, especially in hypercalcemia complicating certain malignancies. They increase urinary calcium excretion and decrease intestinal calcium absorption when given in pharmacologic doses, but they also cause negative skeletal calcium balance. In normal individuals and in patients with primary hyperparathyroidism, glucocorticoids neither increase nor decrease the serum calcium concentration. In patients with hypercalcemia due to certain osteolytic malignancies, however, glucocorticoids may be effective as a result of antitumor effects. The malignancies in which hypercalcemia responds to glucocorticoids include multiple myeloma, leukemia, Hodgkin's disease, other lymphomas, and carcinoma of the breast, at least early in the course of the disease. Glucocorticoids are also effective in treating hypercalcemia due to vitamin D intoxication and sarcoidosis. Glucocorticoids are also useful in the rare form of hypercalcemia, now recognized in certain autoimmune disorders in which inactivating antibodies against the receptor imitate FHH. Elevated PTH and calcium levels are effectively lowered by the glucocorticoids. In all the preceding situations, the hypocalcemic effect develops over several days, and the usual glucocorticoid dosage is 40–100 mg prednisone (or its equivalent) daily in four divided doses. The side effects of chronic glucocorticoid therapy may be acceptable in some circumstances.

Dialysis is often the treatment of choice for severe hypercalcemia complicated by renal failure, which is difficult to manage medically. Peritoneal dialysis with calcium-free dialysis fluid can remove 5–12.5 mmol (200–500 mg) of calcium in 24–48 hours and lower the serum calcium concentration by 0.7–3 mmol/L (3–12 mg/dL). Large quantities of phosphate are lost during dialysis, and serum inorganic phosphate concentration usually falls, potentially aggravating hypercalcemia. Therefore, the serum inorganic phosphate concentration should be measured after dialysis, and phosphate supplements should be added to the diet or to dialysis fluids if necessary.

Phosphate therapy, PO or IV, has a limited role in certain circumstances (Chap. 352). Correcting hypophosphatemia lowers the serum calcium concentration by several mechanisms, including bone/calcium exchange. The usual oral treatment is 1–1.5 g phosphorus per day for several days, given in divided doses. It is generally believed, but not established, that toxicity does not occur if therapy is limited to restoring serum inorganic phosphate concentrations to normal.

Raising the serum inorganic phosphate concentration above normal decreases serum calcium levels, sometimes strikingly. Intravenous phosphate is one of the most dramatically effective treatments available for severe hypercalcemia but is toxic and even dangerous (fatal hypocalcemia). For these reasons, it is used rarely and only in severely hypercalcemic patients with cardiac or renal failure where dialysis, the preferable alternative, is not feasible or is unavailable.

SUMMARY The various therapies for hypercalcemia are listed in Table 353-4. The choice depends on the underlying disease, the severity of the hypercalcemia, the serum inorganic phosphate level, and the renal, hepatic, and bone marrow function. Mild hypercalcemia [≤3 mmol/L (12 mg/dL)] can usually be managed by hydration. Severe hypercalcemia [≥3.7 mmol/L (15 mg/dL)] requires rapid correction. Calcitonin should be given for its rapid, albeit short-lived, blockade of bone resorption, and IV pamidronate or zolendronate should be administered, although its onset of action is delayed for 1–2 days. In addition, for the first 24–48 hours, aggressive sodium-calcium diuresis with IV saline should be given and, following rehydration, large doses of furosemide or ethacrynic acid, but only if appropriate monitoring is available and cardiac and renal function are adequate. Otherwise, dialysis may be necessary. Intermediate degrees of hypercalcemia between 3 and 3.7 mmol/L (12 and 15 mg/dL) should be approached with vigorous hydration and then the most appropriate selection for the patient of the combinations used with severe hypercalcemia.

HYPOCALCEMIA

(See also Chap. 46)

PATHOPHYSIOLOGY OF HYPOCALCEMIA: CLASSIFICATION BASED ON MECHANISM

Chronic hypocalcemia is less common than hypercalcemia; causes include chronic renal failure, hereditary and acquired hypoparathyroidism, vitamin D deficiency, PHP, and hypomagnesemia.

Acute rather than chronic hypocalcemia is seen in critically ill patients or as a consequence of certain medications and often does not require specific treatment. Transient hypocalcemia is seen with severe sepsis, burns, acute renal failure, and extensive transfusions with citrated blood. Although as many as one-half of patients in an intensive care setting are reported to have calcium concentrations <2.1 mmol/L (8.5 mg/dL), most do not have a reduction in ionized calcium. Patients with severe sepsis may have a decrease in ionized calcium (true hypocalcemia), but in other severely ill individuals, hypoalbuminemia is the primary cause of the reduced total calcium concentration. Alkalosis increases calcium binding to proteins, and in this setting direct measurements of ionized calcium should be made.

Medications such as protamine, heparin, and glucagon may cause transient hypocalcemia. These forms of hypocalcemia are usually not associated with tetany and resolve with improvement in the overall medical condition. The hypocalcemia after repeated transfusions of citrated blood usually resolves quickly.

Patients with *acute pancreatitis* have hypocalcemia that persists during the acute inflammation and varies in degree with the severity of the pancreatitis. The cause of hypocalcemia remains unclear. PTH values are reported to be low, normal, or elevated, and both resistance to PTH and impaired PTH secretion have been postulated. Occasionally, a chronic low total calcium and low ionized calcium concentration are detected in an elderly patient without obvious cause and with a paucity of symptoms; the pathogenesis is unclear.

Chronic hypocalcemia, however, is usually symptomatic and requires treatment. Neuromuscular and neurologic manifestations of chronic hypocalcemia include muscle spasms, carpopedal spasm, facial grimacing, and, in extreme cases, laryngeal spasm and convulsions. Respiratory arrest may occur. Increased intracranial pressure occurs in some patients with long-standing hypocalcemia, often in association with papilledema. Mental changes include irritability, depression, and psychosis. The QT interval on the electrocardiogram is prolonged, in contrast to its shortening with hypercalcemia. Arrhythmias occur, and digitalis effectiveness may be reduced. Intestinal cramps and chronic malabsorption may occur. Chvostek's or Trousseau's sign can be used to confirm latent tetany.

The classification of hypocalcemia shown in Table 353-5 is based on an organizationally useful premise that PTH is responsible for minute-to-minute regulation of plasma calcium concentration and, therefore, that the occurrence of hypocalcemia must mean a failure of the homeostatic action of PTH. Failure of the PTH response can occur if there is hereditary or acquired parathyroid gland failure, if PTH is ineffective in target organs, or if the action of the hormone is overwhelmed by the loss of calcium from the ECF at a rate faster than it can be replaced.

■ PTH ABSENT

Whether hereditary or acquired, hypoparathyroidism has a number of common components. Symptoms of untreated hypocalcemia are shared by both types of hypoparathyroidism, although the onset of hereditary hypoparathyroidism is more gradual and is often associated with other developmental defects. Basal ganglia calcification and extrapyramidal syndromes are more common and earlier in onset in hereditary hypoparathyroidism. In earlier decades, acquired hypoparathyroidism secondary to surgery in the neck was more common than hereditary hypoparathyroidism, but the frequency of surgically induced parathyroid failure has diminished as a result of improved surgical techniques that spare the parathyroid glands and increased use of nonsurgical therapy for hyperthyroidism. PHP, an example of ineffective PTH action rather than a failure of parathyroid gland production, may share several features with hypoparathyroidism, including extraosseous calcification and extrapyramidal manifestations such as choreoathetotic movements and dystonia.

Papilledema and raised intracranial pressure may occur in both hereditary and acquired hypoparathyroidism, as do chronic changes in fingernails and hair and lenticular cataracts, the latter usually reversible with treatment of hypocalcemia. Certain skin manifestations, including alopecia and candidiasis, are characteristic of hereditary hypoparathyroidism associated with autoimmune polyglandular failure (Chap. 351).

Hypocalcemia associated with hypomagnesemia is associated with both deficient PTH release and impaired responsiveness to the hormone. Patients with hypocalcemia secondary to hypomagnesemia have absent or low levels of circulating PTH, indicative of diminished hormone release despite a maximum physiologic stimulus by hypocalcemia. Plasma PTH levels return to normal with correction of the hypomagnesemia. Thus hypoparathyroidism with low levels of PTH in blood can be due to hereditary gland failure, acquired gland failure, or acute but reversible gland dysfunction (hypomagnesemia).

Genetic abnormalities and hereditary hypoparathyroidism

Hereditary hypoparathyroidism can occur as an isolated entity without other endocrine or dermatologic manifestations. More typically, it occurs in association with other abnormalities such as defective development of the thymus or failure of other endocrine organs such as the adrenal, thyroid, or ovary (Chap. 351). Hereditary hypoparathyroidism is often manifest within the first decade but may appear later.

Genetic defects associated with hypoparathyroidism serve to illuminate the complexity of organ development, hormonal biosynthesis and secretion, and tissue-specific patterns of endocrine effector function (Fig. 353-5). Often, hypoparathyroidism is isolated, signifying a highly specific functional disturbance. When hypoparathyroidism is associated with other developmental or organ defects, treatment of the hypocalcemia can still be effective.

A rare form of hypoparathyroidism associated with defective development of both the thymus and the parathyroid glands is termed the *DiGeorge syndrome*, or the *velocardiofacial syndrome*. Congenital cardiovascular, facial, and other developmental defects are present, and patients may die in early childhood with severe infections, hypocalcemia and seizures, or cardiovascular complications. Patients can survive into adulthood, and milder, incomplete forms occur. Most cases are sporadic, but an autosomal dominant form involving microdeletions of chromosome 22q11.2 has been described. Smaller deletions in chromosome 22 are seen in incomplete forms of the DiGeorge syndrome, appearing in childhood or adolescence, that are manifest primarily by parathyroid gland failure. The chromosome 22 defect is now termed *DSG1*; more recently, a defect in chromosome 10p is also recognized—now called *DSG2*. The phenotypes seem similar. Studies on the chromosome 22 defect have pinpointed a transcription factor, TBX1. Deletions of the orthologous mouse gene show a phenotype similar to the human syndrome.

Another autosomal dominant developmental defect, featuring hypoparathyroidism, deafness, and renal dysplasia (HDR) has been studied at a genetic level. Cytogenic abnormalities in some, but not all kindred, point to translocation defects on chromosome 10, as in DiGeorge syndrome. However, the lack of immunodeficiency and heart defects distinguishes the two syndromes. Mouse models, as well as deletional analysis in some HDR patients, has pointed to transcription factor GATA3, which is important in embryonic development and is expressed in developing kidney, ear structures, and the parathyroids.

Another pair of linked developmental disorders involving the parathyroids is recognized. *Kenney-Caffey syndrome* features hypoparathyroidism, short stature, osteosclerosis, and thick cortical bones. A defect seen in Middle Eastern patients, particularly in Saudi Arabia, termed *Sanjad-Sakati syndrome*, also exhibits growth failure and other dysmorphic features. This syndrome, which is clearly autosomal recessive, involves a gene on chromosome 1q42-q43. Both syndromes apparently involve a chaperone protein, called *TBCE*, relevant to tubulin function.

Hypoparathyroidism can occur in association with a complex hereditary autoimmune syndrome involving failure of the adrenals, the ovaries, the immune system, and the parathyroids in association with recurrent mucocutaneous candidiasis, alopecia, vitiligo, and pernicious anemia (Chap. 351). The responsible gene on chromosome 21q22.3 has been identified. The protein product, which resembles a transcription factor, has been termed the *autoimmune regulator*, or AIRE. A stop codon mutation occurs in many Finnish families with the disorder, commonly referred to as *polyglandular autoimmune type 1 deficiency*.

Hypoparathyroidism is seen in two disorders associated with mitochondrial dysfunction and myopathy, one termed the *Kearns-Sayre syndrome* (KSS), with ophthalmoplegia and pigmentary retinopathy, and the other termed the *MELAS syndrome*, mitochondrial encephalopathy, lactic acidosis, and stroke-like episodes. Mutations or deletions in mitochondrial genes have been identified.

Several forms of hypoparathyroidism, each rare in frequency, are seen as isolated defects; the genetic mechanisms are varied. The inheritance includes autosomal dominant, autosomal recessive, and

X-linked modes. Three separate autosomal defects involving the parathyroid gene have been recognized: one is dominant and the other two are recessive. The dominant form has a point mutation in the signal sequence, a critical region involved in intracellular transport of the hormone precursor. An Arg for Cys mutation interferes with processing of the precursor and is believed to trigger an apoptotic cellular response, hence acting as a dominant negative. The other two forms are recessive. One point mutation also blocks cleavage of the PTH precursor but requires both alleles to cause hypoparathyroidism. The third involves a single-nucleotide base change that results in an exon splicing defect; the lost exon contains the promoter—hence, the gene is silenced. An X-linked recessive form of hypoparathyroidism has been described in males and the defect has been localized to chromosome Xq26-q27, perhaps involving the *SOX3* gene.

Abnormalities in the calcium-sensing receptor (CaSR) are detected in three distinctive hypocalcemic disorders. All are rare but more than 10 different gain-of-function mutations have been found in one form of hypocalcemia termed *autosomal dominant hypocalcemic hypercalciuria (ADHH)*. The receptor senses the ambient calcium level as excessive and suppresses PTH secretion, leading to hypocalcemia. The hypocalcemia is aggravated by constitutive receptor activity in the renal tubule causing excretion of inappropriate amounts of calcium. Recognition of the syndrome is important because efforts to treat the hypocalcemia with vitamin D analogues and increased oral calcium exacerbate the already excessive urinary calcium excretion (several grams or more per 24 hours), leading to irreversible renal damage from stones and ectopic calcification.

Other causes of isolated hypoparathyroidism include homozygous, inactivating mutations in the parathyroid-specific transcription factor GCMB, which lead to an autosomal recessive form of the disease, or heterozygous point mutations in GCMB, which have a dominant negative effect on the wild-type protein and thus lead to an autosomal dominant form of hypoparathyroidism.

The *Bartter syndrome* is a group of disorders associated with disturbances in electrolyte and acid/base balance, sometimes with nephrocalcinosis and other features. Several types of ion channels or transporters are involved. Curiously, *Bartter syndrome type V* has the electrolyte and pH disturbances seen in the other syndromes but appears to be due to a gain of function in the CaSR. The defect may be more severe than in ADHH and explains the additional features seen beyond hypocalcemia and hypercalciuria.

As with autoimmune disorders that block the CaSR (discussed above under hypercalcemic conditions), there are autoantibodies that at least transiently activate the CaSR, leading to suppressed PTH secretion and hypocalcemia. This disorder, which may wax and wane, could be classified as an acquired form of hypoparathyroidism but is listed here with other disorders involving the CaSR.

Acquired hypoparathyroidism

Acquired chronic hypoparathyroidism is usually the result of inadvertent surgical removal of all the parathyroid glands; in some instances, not all the tissue is removed, but the remainder undergoes vascular supply compromise secondary to fibrotic changes in the neck after surgery. In the past, the most frequent cause of acquired hypoparathyroidism was surgery for hyperthyroidism. Hypoparathyroidism now usually occurs after surgery for hyperparathyroidism when the surgeon, facing the dilemma of removing too little tissue and thus not curing the hyperparathyroidism, removes too much. Parathyroid function may not be totally absent in all patients with postoperative hypoparathyroidism.

Even rarer causes of acquired chronic hypoparathyroidism include radiation-induced damage subsequent to radioiodine therapy of hyperthyroidism and glandular damage in patients with hemochromatosis or hemosiderosis after repeated blood transfusions. Infection may involve one or more of the parathyroids but usually does not cause hypoparathyroidism because all four glands are rarely involved.

Transient hypoparathyroidism is frequent following surgery for hyperparathyroidism. After a variable period of hypoparathyroidism, normal parathyroid function may return due to hyperplasia or recovery of remaining tissue. Occasionally, recovery occurs months after surgery.

TREATMENT Acquired and Hereditary Hypoparathyroidism

Treatment involves replacement with vitamin D or $1,25(OH)_2D_3$ (calcitriol) combined with a high oral calcium intake. In most patients, blood calcium and phosphate levels are satisfactorily regulated, but some patients show resistance and a brittleness, with a tendency to alternate between hypocalcemia and hypercalcemia. For many patients, vitamin D in doses of 40,000–120,000 U/d (1–3 mg/d) combined with ≥1 g elemental calcium is satisfactory. The wide dosage range reflects the variation encountered from patient to patient; precise regulation of each patient is required. Compared to typical daily requirements in euparathyroid patients of 200 U/d (or in older patients as high as 800 U/d), the high dose of vitamin D (as much as 100-fold higher) reflects the reduced conversion of vitamin D to $1,25(OH)_2D$. Many physicians now use 0.5–1 μg of calcitriol in management of such patients, especially if they are difficult to control. Because of its storage in fat, when vitamin D is withdrawn, weeks are required for the disappearance of the biologic effects, compared with a few days for calcitriol, which has a rapid turnover.

Oral calcium and vitamin D restore the overall calcium-phosphate balance but do not reverse the lowered urinary calcium reabsorption typical of hypoparathyroidism. Therefore, care must be taken to avoid excessive urinary calcium excretion after vitamin D and calcium replacement therapy; otherwise, kidney stones can develop. Thiazide diuretics lower urine calcium by as much as 100 mg/d in hypoparathyroid patients on vitamin D, provided they are maintained on a low-sodium diet. Use of thiazides seems to be of benefit in mitigating hypercalciuria and easing the daily management of these patients.

There are now trials of parenterally administered PTH [either PTH(1–34) or PTH(1–84)] in patients with hypoparathyroidism providing greater ease of maintaining serum calcium and reducing urinary calcium excretion (desirable to protect any renal damage). However, PTH therapy is not approved as of yet.

Hypomagnesemia

Severe hypomagnesemia (<0.4 mmol/L; <0.8 meq/L) is associated with hypocalcemia (Chap. 352). Restoration of the total-body magnesium deficit leads to rapid reversal of hypocalcemia. There are at least two causes of the hypocalcemia—impaired PTH secretion and reduced responsiveness to PTH. For further discussion of causes and treatment of hypomagnesemia, see Chap. 352.

The effects of magnesium on PTH secretion are similar to those of calcium; hypermagnesemia suppresses and hypomagnesemia stimulates PTH secretion. The effects of magnesium on PTH secretion are normally of little significance, however, because the calcium effects dominate. Greater change in magnesium than in calcium is needed to influence hormone secretion. Nonetheless, hypomagnesemia might be expected to increase hormone secretion. It is therefore surprising to find that severe hypomagnesemia is associated with blunted secretion of PTH. The explanation for the paradox is that severe, chronic hypomagnesemia leads to intracellular magnesium deficiency, which interferes with secretion and peripheral responses to PTH. The mechanism of the cellular abnormalities caused by hypomagnesemia is unknown, although effects on adenylate cyclase (for which magnesium is a cofactor) have been proposed.

PTH levels are undetectable or inappropriately low in severe hypomagnesemia despite the stimulus of severe hypocalcemia, and acute repletion of magnesium leads to a rapid increase in PTH level. Serum phosphate levels are often not elevated, in contrast to the situation with acquired or idiopathic hypoparathyroidism, probably because phosphate deficiency is often seen in hypomagnesmia (see Chap. 331).

Diminished peripheral responsiveness to PTH also occurs in some patients, as documented by subnormal response in urinary phosphorus and urinary cyclic AMP excretion after administration of exogenous PTH to patients who are hypocalcemic and hypomagnesemic. Both blunted PTH secretion and lack of renal response to administered PTH can occur in the same patient. When acute magnesium repletion is undertaken, the restoration of PTH levels to normal or supranormal may precede restoration of normal serum calcium by several days.

TREATMENT Hypomagnesemia

Repletion of magnesium cures the condition. Repletion should be parenteral. Attention must be given to restoring the intracellular deficit, which may be considerable. After IV magnesium administration, serum magnesium may return transiently to the normal range, but unless replacement therapy is adequate, serum magnesium will again fall. If the cause of the hypomagnesemia is renal magnesium wasting, magnesium may have to be given long-term to prevent recurrence (Chap. 352).

PTH INEFFECTIVE

PTH is ineffective when the PTH/PTHrP receptor–guanyl nucleotide–binding protein complex is defective (PHP, discussed below), when PTH action to promote calcium absorption from the diet is impaired because of vitamin D deficiency or because vitamin D is ineffective (defects in vitamin D receptor or vitamin D synthesis), or in chronic renal failure in which the calcium-elevating action of PTH is impaired.

Typically, hypophosphatemia is more severe than hypocalcemia in vitamin D deficiency states because of the increased secretion of PTH, which, although only partly effective in elevating blood calcium, is capable of promoting phosphaturia.

PHP, on the other hand, has a pathophysiology different from the other disorders of ineffective PTH action. PHP resembles hypoparathyroidism (in which PTH synthesis is deficient) and is manifested by hypocalcemia and hyperphosphatemia, yet elevated PTH levels. The cause of the disorder is defective PTH-dependent activation of guanyl nucleotide–binding proteins, resulting in failure of PTH to increase intracellular cyclic AMP (see below).

Chronic renal failure

Improved medical management of chronic kidney disease now allows many patients to survive for decades and hence time enough to develop features of renal osteodystrophy, which must be controlled to avoid additional morbidity. Impaired production of $1,25(OH)_2D$ is now thought to be the principal factor that causes calcium deficiency, secondary hyperparathyroidism, and bone disease; hyperphosphatemia typically occurs only in the later stages of CKD. Low levels of $1,25(OH)_2D$ due to increased FGF23 production in bone are critical in the development of hypocalcemia. The uremic state also causes impairment of intestinal absorption by mechanisms other than defects in vitamin D metabolism. Nonetheless, treatment with supraphysiologic amounts of vitamin D or calcitriol corrects the impaired calcium absorption. Since increased FGF23 levels are seen even in early stages of renal failure in some patients, and have been reported to correlate with increased mortality, there is current interest in methods (lowering phosphate absorption) to lower FGF23 levels and concern as to whether vitamin D supplementation (known physiologically to increase FGF23) increases FGF23 in CKD.

Hyperphosphatemia in renal failure lowers blood calcium levels by several mechanisms, including extraosseous deposition of calcium and phosphate, impairment of the bone-resorbing action of PTH, and reduction in $1,25(OH)_2D$ production by remaining renal tissue.

TREATMENT Chronic Renal Failure

Therapy of chronic renal failure (Chap. 280) involves appropriate management of patients prior to dialysis and adjustment of regimens once dialysis is initiated. Attention should be paid to restriction of phosphate in the diet; avoidance of aluminum-containing phosphate-binding antacids to prevent the problem of aluminum intoxication; provision of an adequate calcium intake by mouth, usually 1–2 g/d; and supplementation with 0.25–1 μg/d calcitriol. Each patient must be monitored closely. The aim of therapy is to restore normal calcium balance to prevent osteomalacia and severe secondary hyperparathyroidism (it is usually recommended to maintain PTH levels between 100 and 300 pg/mL) and, in light of evidence of genetic changes and monoclonal outgrowths of parathyroid glands in CKD patients, to prevent secondary from becoming autonomous hyperparathyroidism. Reduction of hyperphosphatemia and restoration of normal intestinal calcium absorption by calcitriol can improve blood calcium levels and reduce the manifestations of secondary hyperparathyroidism. Since adynamic bone disease can occur in association with low PTH levels, it is important to avoid excessive suppression of the parathyroid glands while recognizing the beneficial effects of controlling the secondary hyperparathyroidism. These patients should probably be closely monitored with PTH assays that detect only the full-length PTH(1–84) to ensure that biologically active PTH and not inactive, inhibitory PTH fragments are measured. Use of phosphate-binding agents such as sevelamer are approved for payment only in end-stage renal disease (ESRD).

Vitamin D deficiency due to inadequate diet and/or sunlight

Vitamin D deficiency due to inadequate intake of dairy products enriched with vitamin D, lack of vitamin supplementation, and reduced sunlight exposure in the elderly, particularly during winter in northern latitudes, is more common in the United States than previously recognized. Biopsies of bone in elderly patients with hip fracture (documenting osteomalacia) and abnormal levels of vitamin D metabolites, PTH, calcium, and phosphate indicate that vitamin D deficiency may occur in as many as 25% of elderly patients, particularly in northern latitudes in the United States. Concentrations of 25(OH)D are low or low-normal in these patients. Quantitative histomorphometry of bone biopsy specimens reveals widened osteoid seams consistent with osteomalacia (Chap. 352). PTH hypersecretion compensates for the tendency for the blood calcium to fall but also induces renal phosphate wasting and results in osteomalacia.

Treatment involves adequate replacement with vitamin D and calcium until the deficiencies are corrected. Severe hypocalcemia rarely occurs in moderately severe vitamin D deficiency of the elderly, but vitamin D deficiency must be considered in the differential diagnosis of mild hypocalcemia.

Mild hypocalcemia, secondary hyperparathyroidism, severe hypophosphatemia, and a variety of nutritional deficiencies occur with gastrointestinal diseases. Hepatocellular dysfunction can lead to reduction in 25(OH)D levels, as in portal or biliary cirrhosis of the liver, and malabsorption of vitamin D and its metabolites, including $1,25(OH)_2D$, may occur in a variety of bowel diseases, hereditary or acquired. Hypocalcemia itself can lead to steatorrhea, due to deficient production of pancreatic enzymes and bile salts. Depending on the disorder, vitamin D or its metabolites can be given parenterally, guaranteeing adequate blood levels of active metabolites.

TABLE 353-6 Classification of Pseudohypoparathyroidism (PHP) and Pseudopseudohypoparathyroidism (PPHP)

Type	Hypocalcemia, Hyperphosphatemia	Response of Urinary cAMP to PTH	Serum PTH	$G_s\alpha$ Subunit Deficiency	AHO	Resistance to Hormones in Addition to PTH
PHP-Ia	Yes	↓	↑	Yes	Yes	Yes
PHP-Ib	Yes	↓	↑	No	No	Yes (in some patients)
PHP-II	Yes	Normal	↑	No	No	No
PPHP	No	Normal	Normal	Yes	Yes	No

Abbreviations: ↓, decreased; ↑, increased; AHO, Albright's hereditary osteodystrophy; PTH, parathyroid hormone.

Defective vitamin D metabolism

Anticonvulsant therapy Anticonvulsant therapy with any of several agents induces acquired vitamin D deficiency by increasing the conversion of vitamin D to inactive compounds and/or causing resistance to its action. The more marginal the vitamin D intake in the diet, the more likely that anticonvulsant therapy will lead to abnormal mineral and bone metabolism.

Vitamin D–dependent rickets type I Rickets can be due to *resistance to the action* of vitamin D as well as to vitamin D deficiency. Vitamin D–dependent rickets type I, previously termed *pseudovitamin D–resistant rickets*, differs from true vitamin D–resistant rickets (vitamin D–dependent rickets type II, see below) in that it is less severe and the biochemical and radiographic abnormalities can be reversed with appropriate doses of the vitamin's active metabolite, $1,25(OH)_2D_3$. Physiologic amounts of calcitriol cure the disease (Chap. 352). This finding fits with the pathophysiology of the disorder, which is autosomal recessive, and is now known to be caused by mutations in the gene encoding 25(OH)D-1α-hydroxylase. Both alleles are inactivated in all patients, and compound heterozygotes, harboring distinct mutations, are common.

Clinical features include hypocalcemia, often with tetany or convulsions, hypophosphatemia, secondary hyperparathyroidism, and osteomalacia, often associated with skeletal deformities and increased alkaline phosphatase. Treatment involves physiologic replacement doses of $1,25(OH)_2D_3$ (Chap. 352).

Vitamin D–dependent rickets type II Vitamin D–dependent rickets type II results from end-organ resistance to the active metabolite $1,25(OH)_2D_3$. The clinical features resemble those of the type I disorder and include hypocalcemia, hypophosphatemia, secondary hyperparathyroidism, and rickets but also partial or total alopecia. Plasma levels of $1,25(OH)_2D$ are elevated, in keeping with the refractoriness of the end organs. This disorder is caused by mutations in the gene encoding the vitamin D receptor; treatment is difficult and requires regular, usually nocturnal calcium infusions (Chap. 352).

Pseudohypoparathyroidism

PHP refers to a group of distinct inherited disorders. Patients are characterized by symptoms and signs of hypocalcemia in association with distinctive skeletal and developmental defects. The hypocalcemia is due to a deficient response to PTH, which is probably restricted to the proximal renal tubules. Hyperplasia of the parathyroids, a response to hormone-resistant hypocalcemia, causes elevation of PTH levels. Studies, both clinical and basic, have clarified some aspects of these disorders, including the variable clinical spectrum, the pathophysiology, the genetic defects, and their mode of inheritance.

A working classification of the various forms of PHP is given in Table 353-6. The classification scheme is based on the signs of ineffective PTH action (low calcium and high phosphate), urinary cyclic AMP response to exogenous PTH, the presence or absence of *Albright's hereditary osteodystrophy* (AHO), and assays to measure the concentration of the $G_s\alpha$ subunit of the adenylate cyclase enzyme. Using these criteria, there are four types: PHP types Ia and Ib; pseudopseudohypoparathyroidism (PPHP), and the related disorder POH, and PHP-II.

PHP-Ia and PHP-Ib Individuals with PHP-I, the most common of the disorders, show a deficient urinary cyclic AMP response to administration of exogenous PTH. Patients with PHP-I are divided into type Ia and type Ib. Patients with PHP-Ia show evidence for AHO and reduced amounts of $G_s\alpha$ protein/activity in readily accessible tissues, such as erythrocytes, lymphocytes, and fibroblasts. Patients with PHP-Ib typically lack evidence for AHO and they have normal $G_s\alpha$ activity. PHP-Ic, sometimes listed as a third form of PHP, is really a variant of PHP-Ia, since the mutant $G_s\alpha$ shows normal activity in certain in vitro assays.

Most patients who have PHP-Ia reveal characteristic features of AHO, consisting of short stature, round face, skeletal anomalies (brachydactyly), and/or heterotopic calcification. Patients have low calcium and high phosphate levels, as with true hypoparathyroidism. PTH levels, however, are elevated, reflecting resistance to hormone action.

Amorphous deposits of calcium and phosphate are found in the basal ganglia in about one-half of patients. The defects in metacarpal and metatarsal bones are sometimes accompanied by short phalanges as well, possibly reflecting premature closing of the epiphyses. The typical findings are short fourth and fifth metacarpals and metatarsals. The defects are usually bilateral. Exostoses and radius curvus are frequent. Impairments in olfaction and taste and unusual dermatoglyphic abnormalities have been reported.

Inheritance and genetic patterns

Multiple defects at the *GNAS* locus have now been identified in PHP-Ia, PHP-Ib, and PPHP patients. This gene, which is located

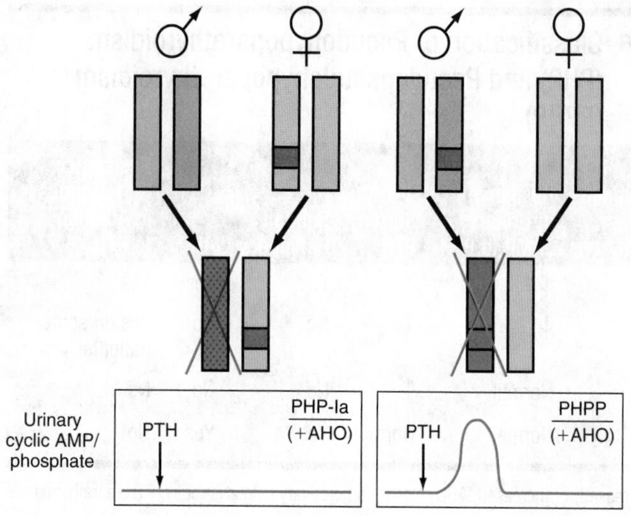

Figure 353-7 Paternal imprinting of renal parathyroid hormone (PTH) resistance (*GNAS-1* gene for $G_s\alpha$ subunit) in pseudohypoparathyroidism (PHPIa). An impaired excretion of urinary cyclic AMP and phosphate is observed in patients with PHP. In the renal cortex, there is selective silencing of the paternal $G_s\alpha$ gene mRNA. The disease becomes manifest only in patients who inherit the defective gene from an obligate female carrier (*left*). If the genetic defect is inherited from an obligate male gene carrier, there is no biochemical abnormality; administration of PTH causes an appropriate increase in the urinary cyclic AMP and phosphate concentration [pseudo-PHP (PPHP); *right*]. Both patterns of inheritance lead to Albright's hereditary osteodystrophy (AHO), perhaps because of haplotype insufficiency—i.e., both copies of $G_s\alpha$ must be active in the fetus for normal bone development.

on chromosome 20q13.3, encodes the α-subunit of the stimulatory G-protein ($G_s\alpha$), among other products (see below). Mutations include abnormalities in splice junctions associated with deficient mRNA production, point mutations, insertions, and/or deletion that all result in a protein with defective function, i.e. a 50% reduction in $G_s\alpha$ activity in erythrocytes or other cells.

Detailed analyses of disease transmission in affected kindreds have clarified many features of PHP-Ia, PPHP, and PHP-Ib (Fig. 353-7). The former two entities, traced through multiple kindreds, have an inheritance pattern consistent with gene imprinting—only females, not males, can transmit the full disease with hypocalcemia—and PHP-Ia and PPHP do not coexist in the same generation. The phenomenon of gene imprinting, involving methylation of gene loci, independent of any mutation, involves selective inactivation of either the maternal or the paternal allele (Chap. 61). In the case of the $G_s\alpha$ transcript, it is paternally imprinted (silenced) in the renal cortex (where the disease manifestation is expressed), so that the disease PHP-Ia can never be inherited from the father carrying the defective allele but only from a mother whose allelic product is critical for the PTH-dependent function in the proximal tubules of the kidney. In the renal cortex, it is postulated that only the maternal allele is normally active (independent of any mutation), such that lack of activity from a defective paternal allele is not of consequence. This explains the occurrence in PHP-Ia of hypocalcemia, hyperphosphatemia, and resistance to PTH and often to other hormones that mediate their actions through a G protein–coupled receptor in tissues where imprinting also occurs. Strong additional evidence favoring this overall hypothesis comes from gene knockout studies in the mouse (ablating exon 2 of the gene responsible for $G_s\alpha$ synthesis). Mice inheriting the mutant allele from the female had undetectable $G_s\alpha$ protein in renal cortex and were hypocalcemic and resistant to renal actions of PTH. Offspring inheriting the mutant allele from the male showed no evidence of PTH resistance or hypocalcemia.

Imprinting is tissue selective. Paternal $G_s\alpha$ expression is not silenced in most tissues. It seems likely, therefore, that the AHO phenotype recognized in PPHP as well as PHP-Ia reflects $G_s\alpha$ haploinsufficiency during embryonic or postnatal development.

The complex mechanisms that control the *GNAS* gene contribute to challenges involved in unraveling the pathogenesis of these disorders, especially that of PHP-Ib. Much intensive work with families in which multiple members are affected by PHP-Ib, as well as studies of the complex regulation of the *GNAS* gene locus, have now shown that PHP-Ib is caused by microdeletions within or up-stream of the *GNAS* locus, which are associated with a loss of DNA methylation at one or several loci of the maternal allele (Table 353-6). These abnormalities in methylation silence the expression of the gene. This leads in the renal cortex—where $G_s\alpha$ appears to be expressed exclusively from the maternal allele—to PTH resistance. In other tissues, $G_s\alpha$ expression is not imprinted; hence erythrocytes show normal levels of $G_s\alpha$.

PHP-Ib, lacking the AHO phenotype in most instances, shares with PHP-Ia the hypocalcemia and hyperphosphatemia caused by PTH resistance, and thus the blunted urinary cyclic AMP response to administered PTH, a standard test to assess the presence or absence of hormone resistance (Table 353-6). Furthermore, these endocrine abnormalities become apparent only if the disease-causing mutation is inherited maternally. Bone responsiveness may be excessive rather than blunted in PHP-Ib (and in PHP-Ia) patients, based on case reports that have emphasized an osteitis fibrosa–like pattern in several PHP-Ib patients.

PHP-II refers to patients with hypocalcemia and hyperphosphatemia who have a normal urinary cyclic AMP, but an impaired urinary phosphaturic response to PTH. These patients are assumed to have a defect in the response to PTH at a locus distal to cyclic AMP production. It remains unclear why the PTH resistance in some patients, labeled as PHP-II, can be treated with vitamin D supplements.

The diagnosis of these hormone-resistant states can usually be made without difficulty when there is a positive family history for features of AHO, in association with the signs and symptoms of hypocalcemia. In both categories—PHP-Ia and PHP-Ib—serum PTH levels are elevated, particularly when patients are hypocalcemic. However, patients with PHP-Ib or PHP-II usually do not have phenotypic abnormalities, only hypocalcemia with high PTH levels, as evidence for hormone resistance. In PHP-Ib, the response of urinary cyclic AMP to the administration of exogenous PTH is blunted. The diagnosis of PHP-II is more complex, in that cyclic AMP responses in urine are, by definition, normal. Vitamin D deficiency must be excluded before the diagnosis of PHP-II can be entertained.

TREATMENT Pseudohypoparathyroidism

Treatment of PHP is similar to that of hypoparathyroidism, except that calcium and vitamin D doses are usually lower. Patients with PHP show no PTH resistance in the distal tubules—hence, urinary calcium clearance is not affected and they are at less risk of developing nephrocalcinosis than in patients with true hypoparathyroidism. Variability in response makes it necessary to establish the optimal regimen for each patient, based on maintaining the appropriate blood calcium level and urinary calcium excretion.

PTH OVERWHELMED

Occasionally, loss of calcium from the ECF is so severe that PTH cannot compensate. Such situations include acute pancreatitis and severe, acute hyperphosphatemia, often in association with renal failure, conditions in which there is rapid efflux of calcium from the ECF. Severe hypocalcemia can occur quickly; PTH rises in response to hypocalcemia but does not return blood calcium to normal.

Severe, acute hyperphosphatemia

Severe hyperphosphatemia is associated with extensive tissue damage or cell destruction (Chap. 352). The combination of increased release of phosphate from muscle and impaired ability to excrete phosphorus because of renal failure causes moderate to severe hyperphosphatemia, the latter causing calcium loss from the blood and mild to moderate hypocalcemia. Hypocalcemia is usually reversed with tissue repair and restoration of renal function as phosphorus and creatinine values return to normal. There may even be a mild hypercalcemic period in the oliguric phase of renal function recovery. This sequence, severe hypocalcemia followed by mild hypercalcemia, reflects widespread deposition of calcium in muscle and subsequent redistribution of some of the calcium to the ECF after phosphate levels return to normal.

Other causes of hyperphosphatemia include hypothermia, massive hepatic failure, and hematologic malignancies, either because of high cell turnover of malignancy or because of cell destruction by chemotherapy.

TREATMENT Severe, Acute Hyperphosphatemia

Treatment is directed toward lowering of blood phosphate by the administration of phosphate-binding antacids or dialysis, often needed for the management of renal failure. Although calcium replacement may be necessary if hypocalcemia is severe and symptomatic, calcium administration during the hyperphosphatemic period tends to increase extraosseous calcium deposition and aggravate tissue damage. The levels of $1,25(OH)_2D$ may be low during the hyperphosphatemic phase and return to normal during the oliguric phase of recovery.

Osteitis fibrosa after parathyroidectomy

Severe hypocalcemia after parathyroid surgery is rare now that osteitis fibrosa cystica is an infrequent manifestation of hyperparathyroidism. When osteitis fibrosa cystica is severe, however, bone mineral deficits can be large. After parathyroidectomy, hypocalcemia can persist for days if calcium replacement is inadequate. Treatment may require parenteral administration of calcium; addition of calcitriol and oral calcium supplementation is sometimes needed for weeks to a month or two until bone defects are filled (which, of course, is of therapeutic benefit in the skeleton), making it possible to discontinue parenteral calcium and/or reduce the amount.

DIFFERENTIAL DIAGNOSIS OF HYPOCALCEMIA

Care must be taken to ensure that true hypocalcemia is present; in addition, acute transient hypocalcemia can be a manifestation of a variety of severe, acute illnesses, as discussed above. *Chronic hypocalcemia*, however, can usually be ascribed to a few disorders associated with absent or ineffective PTH. Important clinical criteria include the duration of the illness, signs or symptoms of associated disorders, and the presence of features that suggest a hereditary abnormality. A nutritional history can be helpful in recognizing a low intake of vitamin D and calcium in the elderly, and a history of excessive alcohol intake may suggest magnesium deficiency.

Hypoparathyroidism and PHP are typically lifelong illnesses, usually (but not always) appearing by adolescence; hence, a recent onset of hypocalcemia in an adult is more likely due to nutritional deficiencies, renal failure, or intestinal disorders that result in deficient or ineffective vitamin D. Neck surgery, even long past, however, can be associated with a delayed onset of postoperative hypoparathyroidism. A history of seizure disorder raises the issue of anticonvulsive medication. Developmental defects may point to the diagnosis of PHP. Rickets and a variety of neuromuscular syndromes and deformities may indicate ineffective vitamin D action, either due to defects in vitamin D metabolism or to vitamin D deficiency.

A pattern of *low calcium with high phosphorus* in the absence of renal failure or massive tissue destruction almost invariably means hypoparathyroidism or PHP. A *low calcium and low phosphorus* pattern points to absent or ineffective vitamin D, thereby impairing the action of PTH on calcium metabolism (but not phosphate clearance). The relative ineffectiveness of PTH in calcium homeostasis in vitamin D deficiency, anticonvulsant therapy, gastrointestinal disorders, and hereditary defects in vitamin D metabolism leads to secondary hyperparathyroidism as a compensation. The excess PTH on renal tubule phosphate transport accounts for renal phosphate wasting and hypophosphatemia.

Exceptions to these patterns may occur. Most forms of hypomagnesemia are due to long-standing nutritional deficiency as seen in chronic alcoholics. Despite the fact that the hypocalcemia is principally due to an acute absence of PTH, phosphate levels are usually low, rather than elevated, as in hypoparathyroidism. Chronic renal failure is often associated with hypocalcemia and hyperphosphatemia, despite secondary hyperparathyroidism.

Diagnosis is usually established by application of the PTH immunoassay, tests for vitamin D metabolites, and measurements of the urinary cyclic AMP response to exogenous PTH. In hereditary and acquired hypoparathyroidism and in severe hypomagnesemia, PTH is either undetectable or in the normal range (Fig. 353-4). This finding in a hypocalcemic patient is supportive of hypoparathyroidism, as distinct from ineffective PTH action, in which even mild hypocalcemia is associated with elevated PTH levels. Hence a failure to detect elevated PTH levels establishes the diagnosis of hypoparathyroidism; elevated levels suggest the presence of secondary hyperparathyroidism, as found in many of the situations in which the hormone is ineffective due to associated abnormalities in vitamin D action. Assays for 25(OH)D can be helpful. Low or low-normal 25(OH)D indicates vitamin D deficiency due to lack of sunlight, inadequate vitamin D intake, or intestinal malabsorption. Recognition that mild hypocalcemia, rickets, and hypophosphatemia are due to anticonvulsant therapy is made by history.

TREATMENT Hypocalcemic States

The management of hypoparathyroidism, PHP, chronic renal failure, and hereditary defects in vitamin D metabolism involves the use of vitamin D or vitamin D metabolites and calcium supplementation. Vitamin D itself is the least expensive form of vitamin D replacement and is frequently used in the management of uncomplicated hypoparathyroidism and some disorders associated with ineffective vitamin D action. When vitamin D is used prophylactically, as in the elderly or in those with chronic anticonvulsant therapy, there is a wider margin of safety than with the more potent metabolites. However, most of the conditions in which vitamin D is administered chronically for hypocalcemia require amounts 50–100 times the daily replacement dose because the formation of $1,25(OH)_2D$ is deficient. In such situations, vitamin D is no safer than the active metabolite because intoxication can occur with high-dose therapy (because of storage in fat). Calcitriol is more rapid in onset of action and also has a short biologic half-life.

Vitamin D [at least 1000 U/d (2–3 μg/d) (higher levels required in older persons)] or calcitriol (0.25–1 μg/d) is required to prevent rickets in normal individuals. In contrast, 40,000–120,000 U (1–3 mg) of vitamin D_2 or D_3 is typically required in hypoparathyroidism. The dose of calcitriol is unchanged in hypoparathyroidism, since the defect is in hydroxylation by the 25(OH)D-1α-hydroxylase. Calcitriol is also used in disorders of 25(OH)D-1α-hydroxylase; vitamin D receptor defects are much more difficult to treat.

Patients with hypoparathyroidism should be given 2–3 g elemental calcium PO each day. The two agents, vitamin D or calcitriol and oral calcium, can be varied independently. Urinary calcium excretion needs to be monitored carefully. If hypocalcemia alternates with episodes of hypercalcemia in high-brittleness patients with hypoparathyroidism, administration of calcitriol and use of thiazides, as discussed above, may make management easier.

FURTHER READINGS

BASTEPE M, JÜPPNER H: Pseudohypoparathyroidism, Albright's hereditary osteodystrophy, and progressive osseous heteroplasia: Disorders caused by inactivating GNAS mutations, in *Endocrinology*, 6th ed, in *Endocrinology*, JL Jameson, LJ DeGroot (eds), Philadelphia, W.B. Saunders Company, 2011

BILEZIKIAN JP et al: Guidelines for the management of asymptomatic primary hyperparathyroidism: Summary statement from the third international workshop. J Clin Endocrinol Metab 94:335, 2009

THAKKER RV et al: Genetic disorders of calcium homeostasis caused by abnormal regulation of parathyroid hormone secretion or responsiveness, in *Endocrinology*, 6th ed, in *Endocrinology*, JL Jameson, LJ DeGroot (eds), Philadelphia, W.B. Saunders Company, 2011

CHAPTER 354

Osteoporosis

Robert Lindsay
Felicia Cosman

Osteoporosis, a condition characterized by decreased bone strength, is prevalent among postmenopausal women but also occurs in men and women with underlying conditions or major risk factors associated with bone demineralization. Its chief clinical manifestations are vertebral and hip fractures, although fractures can occur at any skeletal site. Osteoporosis affects >10 million individuals in the United States, but only a small proportion are diagnosed and treated.

DEFINITION

Osteoporosis is defined as a reduction in the strength of bone that leads to an increased risk of fractures. Loss of bone tissue is associated with deterioration in skeletal microarchitecture. The World Health Organization (WHO) operationally defines osteoporosis as a bone density that falls 2.5 standard deviations (SD) below the mean for young healthy adults of the same sex—also referred to as a *T-score* of −2.5. Postmenopausal women who fall at the lower end of the young normal range (a T-score <−1.0) are defined as having low bone density and are also at increased risk of osteoporosis. More than 50% of fractures among postmenopausal women, including hip fractures, occur in this group with low bone density.

EPIDEMIOLOGY

In the United States, as many as 8 million women and 2 million men have osteoporosis (T-score <−2.5), and an additional 18 million individuals have bone mass levels that put them at increased risk of developing osteoporosis (e.g., bone mass T-score <−1.0). Osteoporosis occurs more frequently with increasing age as bone tissue is lost progressively. In women, the loss of ovarian function at menopause (typically about age 50) precipitates rapid bone loss so that most women meet the diagnostic criterion for osteoporosis by age 70–80.

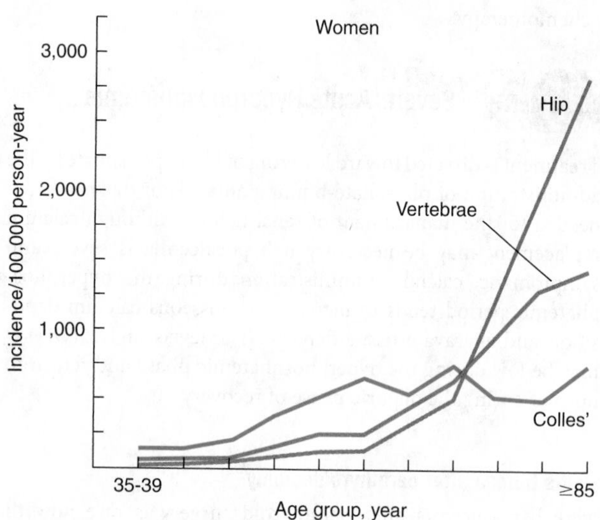

Figure 354-1 Epidemiology of vertebral, hip, and Colles' fractures with age. *(Adapted from C Cooper, LJ Melton III: Trends Endocrinol Metab 3:224, 1992; with permission.)*

The epidemiology of fractures follows the trend for loss of bone density. Fractures of the distal radius increase in frequency before age 50 and plateau by age 60, with only a modest age-related increase thereafter. In contrast, incidence rates for hip fractures double every 5 years after age 70 (Fig. 354-1). This distinct epidemiology may be related to the way people fall as they age, with fewer falls on an outstretched hand and more falls directly on the hip. At least 1.5 million fractures occur each year in the United States as a consequence of osteoporosis. As the population continues to age, the total number of fractures will continue to escalate.

About 300,000 hip fractures occur each year in the United States, most of which require hospital admission and surgical intervention. The probability that a 50-year-old white individual will have a hip fracture during his or her lifetime is 14% for women and 5% for men; the risk for blacks is lower (about one-half those rates). Hip fractures are associated with a high incidence of deep vein thrombosis and pulmonary embolism (20–50%) and a mortality rate between 5 and 20% during the year after surgery.

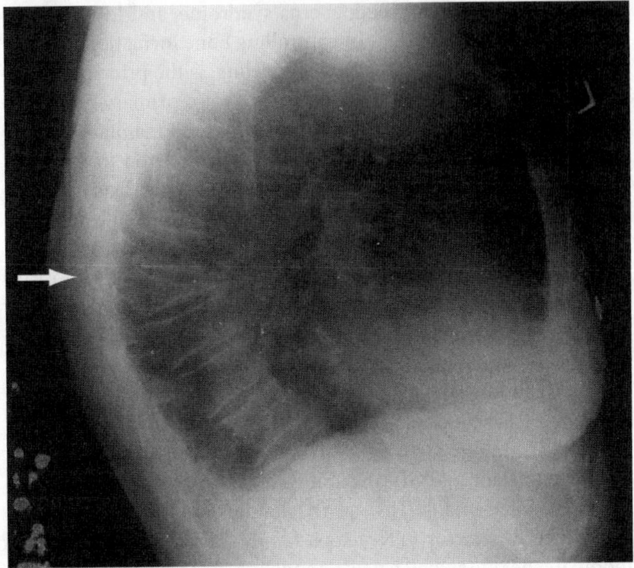

Figure 354-2 **Lateral spine x-ray** showing severe osteopenia and a severe wedge-type deformity (severe anterior compression).

There are about 700,000 vertebral crush fractures per year in the United States. Only a fraction of them are recognized clinically, since many are relatively asymptomatic and are identified incidentally during radiography for other purposes (Fig. 354-2). Vertebral fractures rarely require hospitalization but are associated with long-term morbidity and a slight increase in mortality rates, primarily related to pulmonary disease. Multiple vertebral fractures lead to height loss (often of several inches), kyphosis, and secondary pain and discomfort related to altered biomechanics of the back. Thoracic fractures can be associated with restrictive lung disease, whereas lumbar fractures are associated with abdominal symptoms that include distention, early satiety, and constipation.

Approximately 250,000 wrist fractures occur in the United States each year. Fractures of other bones (estimated to be ~300,000 per year) also occur with osteoporosis; this is not surprising in light of the fact that bone loss is a systemic phenomenon. Fractures of the pelvis and proximal humerus clearly are associated with osteoporosis. Although some fractures result from major trauma, the threshold for fracture is reduced for an osteoporotic bone (Fig. 354-3). In addition to bone density, there are a number of risk factors for fracture; the common ones are summarized in Table 354-1. Age, prior fractures, a family history of osteoporosis-related fractures, low body weight, cigarette consumption, and excessive alcohol use are all independent predictors of fracture. Chronic diseases with inflammatory components that increase skeletal remodeling such as rheumatoid arthritis, increase the risk of osteoporosis, as do diseases associated with malabsorption. Chronic diseases that increase the risk of falling or frailty, including dementia, Parkinson's disease, and multiple sclerosis, also increase fracture risk.

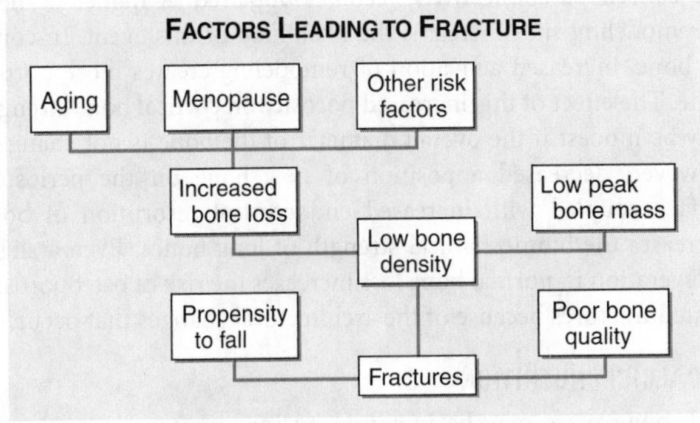

Figure 354-3 **Factors leading to osteoporotic fractures.**

TABLE 354-1 Risk Factors for Osteoporosis Fracture

Nonmodifiable	Estrogen deficiency
Personal history of fracture as an adult	Early menopause (<45 years) or bilateral ovariectomy
History of fracture in first-degree relative	Prolonged premenstrual amenorrhea (>1 year)
Female sex	Low calcium intake
Advanced age	Alcoholism
White race	Impaired eyesight despite adequate correction
Dementia	
Potentially modifiable	Recurrent falls
Current cigarette smoking	Inadequate physical activity
Low body weight [<58 kg (127 lb)]	Poor health/frailty

In the United States and Europe, osteoporosis-related fractures are more common among women than men, presumably due to a lower peak bone mass as well as postmenopausal bone loss in women. However, this sex difference in bone density and age-related increase in hip fractures is not as apparent in some other cultures, possibly due to genetics, physical activity level, or diet.

Fractures are themselves risk factors for future fractures (Table 354-1). Vertebral fractures increase the risk of other vertebral fractures as well as fractures of the peripheral skeleton such as the hip and wrist. Wrist fractures also increase the risk of vertebral and hip fractures. Consequently, among individuals over age 50, any fracture should be considered as potentially related to osteoporosis regardless of the circumstances of the fracture. Osteoporotic bone is more likely to fracture than is normal bone at any level of trauma, and a fracture in a person over 50 should trigger evaluation for osteoporosis.

PATHOPHYSIOLOGY

BONE REMODELING

Osteoporosis results from bone loss due to age-related changes in bone remodeling as well as extrinsic and intrinsic factors that exaggerate this process. These changes may be superimposed on a low peak bone mass. Consequently, understanding the bone remodeling process is fundamental to understanding the pathophysiology of osteoporosis (Chap. 352). During growth, the skeleton increases in size by linear growth and by apposition of new bone tissue on the outer surfaces of the cortex (Fig. 354-4). The latter process is called *modeling*, a process that also allows the long bones to adapt in shape to the stresses placed on them. Increased sex hormone production at puberty is required for skeletal maturation, which reaches maximum mass and density in early adulthood. It is around puberty that the sexual dimorphism in skeletal size becomes obvious, although true bone density remains similar between the sexes. Nutrition and lifestyle also play an important role in growth, though genetic factors primarily determine peak skeletal mass and density. Numerous genes control skeletal growth, peak bone mass, and body size, as well as skeletal structure and density. Heritability estimates of 50–80% for bone density and size have been derived on the basis of twin

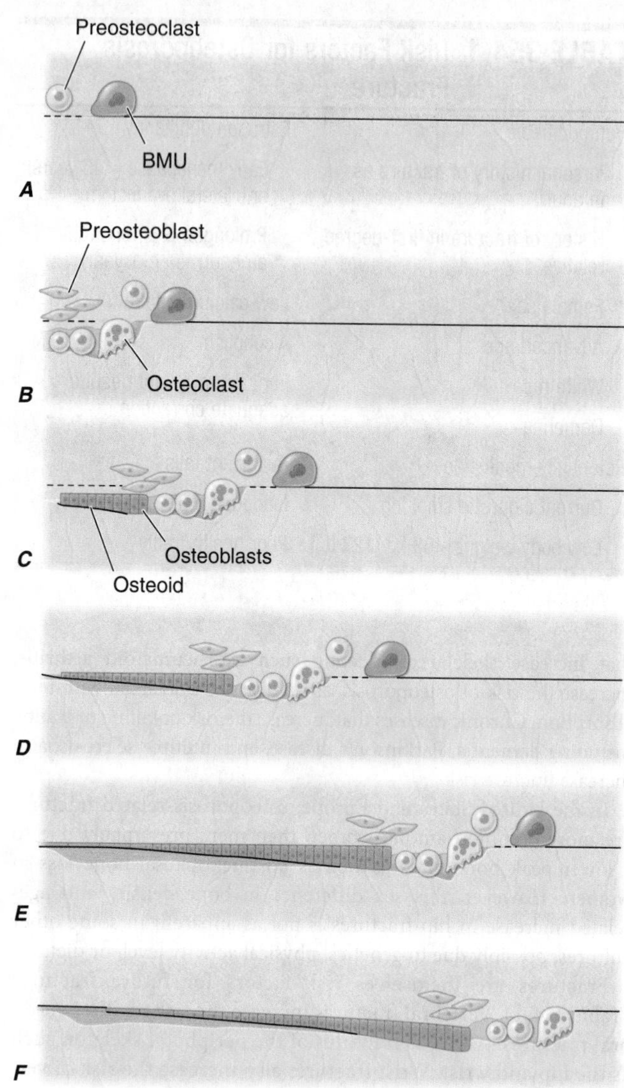

Figure 354-4 Mechanism of bone remodeling. The basic molecular unit (BMU) moves along the trabecular surface at a rate of about 10 μm/d. The figure depicts remodeling over ~120 days. ***A.*** Origination of BMU-lining cells contracts to expose collagen and attract preosteoclasts. ***B.*** Osteoclasts fuse into multinucleated cells that resorb a cavity. Mononuclear cells continue resorption, and preosteoblasts are stimulated to proliferate. ***C.*** Osteoblasts align at bottom of cavity and start forming osteoid (black). ***D.*** Osteoblasts continue formation and mineralization. Previous osteoid starts to mineralize (horizontal lines). ***E.*** Osteoblasts begin to flatten. ***F.*** Osteoblasts turn into lining cells; bone remodeling at initial surface (left of drawing) is now complete, but BMU is still advancing (to the right). *[Adapted from SM Ott, in JP Bilezikian et al (eds): Principles of Bone Biology, vol. 18. San Diego, Academic Press, 1996, pp 231–241.]*

studies. Though peak bone mass is often lower among individuals with a family history of osteoporosis, association studies of candidate genes [vitamin D receptor; type I collagen, the estrogen receptor (ER), and interleukin 6 (IL-6); and insulin-like growth factor I (IGF-I)] and bone mass, bone turnover, and fracture prevalence have been inconsistent. Linkage studies suggest that a genetic locus on chromosome 11 is associated with high bone mass. Families with high bone mass and without much apparent age-related bone loss have been shown to have a point mutation in LRP5, a low-density lipoprotein receptor–related protein. The role of this gene in the general population is not clear, although a nonfunctional mutation results in osteoporosis-pseudoglioma syndrome, and LRP5 signaling appears to be important in controlling bone formation.

In adults, bone remodeling, not modeling, is the principal metabolic skeletal process. Bone remodeling has two primary functions: (1) to repair microdamage within the skeleton to maintain skeletal strength and (2) to supply calcium from the skeleton to maintain serum calcium. Remodeling may be activated by microdamage to bone as a result of excessive or accumulated stress. Acute demands for calcium involve osteoclast-mediated resorption as well as calcium transport by osteocytes. Chronic demands for calcium result in secondary hyperparathyroidism, increased bone remodeling, and overall loss of bone tissue.

Bone remodeling also is regulated by several circulating hormones, including estrogens, androgens, vitamin D, and parathyroid hormone (PTH), as well as locally produced growth factors such as IGF-I and immunoreactive growth hormone II (IGH-II), transforming growth factor β (TGF-β), parathyroid hormone–related peptide (PTHrP), interleukins (ILs), prostaglandins, and members of the tumor necrosis factor (TNF) superfamily. These factors primarily modulate the rate at which new remodeling sites are activated, a process that results initially in bone resorption by osteoclasts, followed by a period of repair during which new bone tissue is synthesized by osteoblasts. The cytokine responsible for communication between the osteoblasts, other marrow cells, and osteoclasts has been identified as RANK ligand (RANKL) [receptor activator of nuclear factor-kappa-B (NFκB); RANKL]. RANKL, a member of the TNF family, is secreted by osteoblasts and certain cells of the immune system (Chap. 352). The osteoclast receptor for this protein is referred to as *RANK*. Activation of RANK by RANKL is a final common path in osteoclast development and activation. A humoral decoy for RANKL, also secreted by osteoblasts, is referred to as *osteoprotegerin* (Fig. 354-5). Modulation of osteoclast recruitment and activity appears to be related to the interplay among these three factors. Additional influences include nutrition (particularly calcium intake) and physical activity level.

In young adults resorbed bone is replaced by an equal amount of new bone tissue. Thus, the mass of the skeleton remains constant after peak bone mass is achieved in adulthood. After age 30–45, however, the resorption and formation processes become imbalanced, and resorption exceeds formation. This imbalance may begin at different ages and varies at different skeletal sites; it becomes exaggerated in women after menopause. Excessive bone loss can be due to an increase in osteoclastic activity and/or a decrease in osteoblastic activity. In addition, an increase in remodeling activation frequency, and thus the number of remodeling sites, can magnify the small imbalance seen at each remodeling unit. Increased recruitment of bone remodeling sites produces a reversible reduction in bone tissue but also can result in permanent loss of tissue and disrupted skeletal architecture. In trabecular bone, if the osteoclasts penetrate trabeculae, they leave no template for new bone formation to occur, and, consequently, rapid bone loss ensues and cancellous connectivity becomes impaired. A higher number of remodeling sites increases the likelihood of this event. In cortical bone, increased activation of remodeling creates more porous bone. The effect of this increased porosity on cortical bone strength may be modest if the overall diameter of the bone is not changed. However, decreased apposition of new bone on the periosteal surface coupled with increased endocortical resorption of bone decreases the biomechanical strength of long bones. Even a slight exaggeration in normal bone loss increases the risk of osteoporosis-related fractures because of the architectural changes that occur.

CALCIUM NUTRITION

Peak bone mass may be impaired by inadequate calcium intake during growth among other nutritional factors (calories, protein,

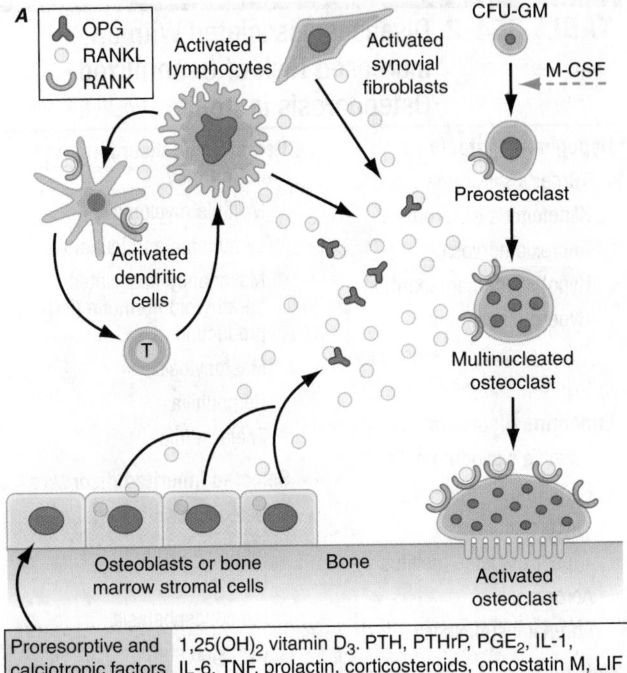

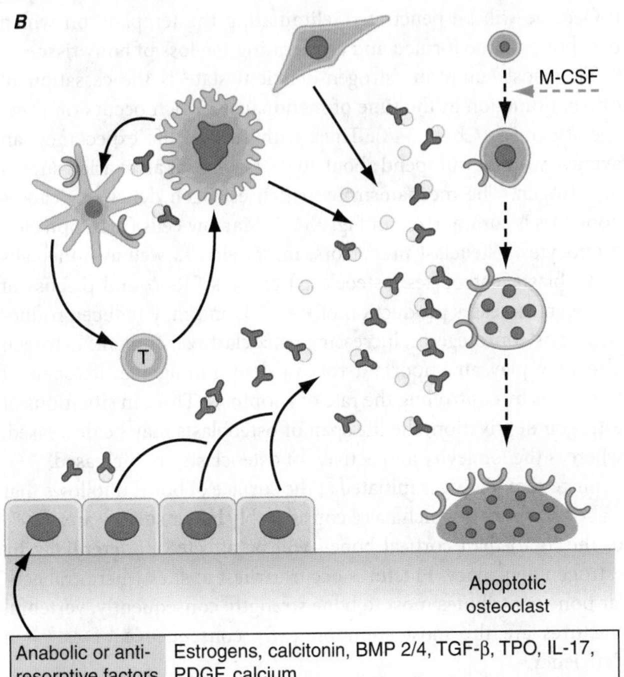

Figure 354-5 Hormonal control of bone resorption. ***A.*** Proresorptive and calciotropic factors. ***B.*** Anabolic and antiosteoclastic factors. RANKL expression is induced in osteoblasts, activated T cells, synovial fibroblasts, and bone marrow stromal cells. It binds to membrane-bound receptor RANK to promote osteoclast differentiation, activation, and survival. Conversely, osteoprotegerin (OPG) expression is induced by factors that block bone catabolism and promote anabolic effects. OPG binds and neutralizes RANKL, leading to a block in osteoclastogenesis and decreased survival of preexisting osteoclasts. CFU-GM, colony-forming units, granulocyte macrophage; M-CSF, macrophage colony-stimulating factor; RANKL, receptor activator of nuclear factor NFκB; PTH, parathyroid hormone; PGE_2, prostaglandin E_2; TNF, tumor necrosis factor; LIF, leukemia inhibitory factor; TPO, thrombospondin; PDGF, platelet-derived growth factor; OPG-L, osteoprotegerin-ligand; IL, interleukin; TGF-β, transforming growth factor β. *(From WJ Boyle et al: Nature 423: 337, 2003.)*

and other minerals), leading to increased risk of osteoporosis later in life. During the adult phase of life, insufficient calcium intake contributes to relative secondary hyperparathyroidism and an increase in the rate of bone remodeling to maintain normal serum calcium levels. PTH stimulates the hydroxylation of vitamin D in the kidney, leading to increased levels of 1,25-dihydroxyvitamin D [$1,25(OH)_2D$] and enhanced gastrointestinal calcium absorption. PTH also reduces renal calcium loss. Although these are all appropriate compensatory homeostatic responses for adjusting calcium economy, the long-term effects are detrimental to the skeleton because the increased remodeling rates and the ongoing imbalance between resorption and formation at remodeling sites combine to accelerate loss of bone tissue.

Total daily calcium intakes <400 mg are detrimental to the skeleton, and intakes in the range of 600–800 mg, which is about the average intake among adults in the United States, are also probably suboptimal. The recommended daily required intake of 1000–1200 mg for adults accommodates population heterogeneity in controlling calcium balance (Chap. 73).

■ VITAMIN D

(See also Chap. 352) Severe vitamin D deficiency causes rickets in children and osteomalacia in adults. However, there is accumulating evidence that vitamin D insufficiency may be more prevalent than previously thought, particularly among individuals at increased risk such as the elderly; those living in northern latitudes; and individuals with poor nutrition, malabsorption, or chronic liver or renal disease. Dark-skinned individuals are also at high risk of vitamin D deficiency. An expert consensus panel has suggested that the accepted levels for serum 25-hydroxyvitamin D [25(OH)D] have been set too low and that optimal targets for serum 25(OH)D are >75 nmol/L (30 ng/mL). To achieve this level for most adults requires an intake of 800–1000 units/d, particularly in individuals who avoid sunlight or routinely use ultraviolet-blocking lotions. Vitamin D insufficiency leads to compensatory secondary hyperparathyroidism and is an important risk factor for osteoporosis and fractures. Some studies have shown that >50% of inpatients on a general medical service exhibit biochemical features of vitamin D deficiency, including increased levels of PTH and alkaline phosphatase and lower levels of ionized calcium. In women living in northern latitudes, vitamin D levels decline during the winter months. This is associated with seasonal bone loss, reflecting increased bone turnover. Even among healthy ambulatory individuals, mild vitamin D deficiency is increasing in prevalence. Treatment with vitamin D can return levels to normal [>75 μmol/L (30 ng/mL)] and prevent the associated increase in bone remodeling, bone loss, and fractures. Reduced fracture rates also have been documented among individuals in northern latitudes who have greater vitamin D intake and have higher 25(OH)D levels (see below). Vitamin D adequacy also may affect risk and/or severity of other diseases, including cancers (colorectal, prostate, and breast), autoimmune diseases, and diabetes.

■ ESTROGEN STATUS

Estrogen deficiency probably causes bone loss by two distinct but interrelated mechanisms: (1) activation of new bone remodeling sites and (2) exaggeration of the imbalance between bone formation and resorption. The change in activation frequency causes a transient bone loss until a new steady state between resorption and formation is achieved. The remodeling imbalance, however, results in a permanent decrement in mass. In addition, the very presence of more remodeling sites in the skeleton increases the probability that trabeculae will be penetrated, eliminating the template on which new bone can be formed and accelerating the loss of bony tissue.

The most common estrogen-deficient state is the cessation of ovarian function at the time of menopause, which occurs on average at age 51 (Chap. 348). Thus, with current life expectancy, an average woman will spend about 30 years without an ovarian supply of estrogen. The mechanism by which estrogen deficiency causes bone loss is summarized in Fig. 354-5. Marrow cells (macrophages, monocytes, osteoclast precursors, mast cells) as well as bone cells (osteoblasts, osteocytes, osteoclasts) express ERs α and β. Loss of estrogen increases production of RANKL and may reduce production of osteoprotegerin, increasing osteoclast recruitment. Estrogen also may play an important role in determining the life span of bone cells by controlling the rate of apoptosis. Thus, in situations of estrogen deprivation, the life span of osteoblasts may be decreased, whereas the longevity and activity of osteoclasts are increased.

Since remodeling is initiated at the surface of bone, it follows that trabecular bone—which has a considerably larger surface area (80% of the total) than cortical bone—will be affected preferentially by estrogen deficiency. Fractures occur earliest at sites where trabecular bone contributes most to bone strength; consequently, vertebral fractures are the most common early consequence of estrogen deficiency.

■ PHYSICAL ACTIVITY

Inactivity such as prolonged bed rest or paralysis, results in significant bone loss. Concordantly, athletes have higher bone mass than does the general population. These changes in skeletal mass are most marked when the stimulus begins during growth and before the age of puberty. Adults are less capable than children of increasing bone mass after restoration of physical activity. Epidemiologic data support the beneficial effects on the skeleton of chronic high levels of physical activity. Fracture risk is lower in rural communities and in countries where physical activity is maintained into old age. However, when exercise is initiated during adult life, the effects of moderate exercise on the skeleton are modest, with a bone mass increase of 1–2% in short-term studies of <2 years' duration. It is argued that more active individuals are less likely to fall and are more capable of protecting themselves upon falling, thereby reducing fracture risk.

■ CHRONIC DISEASE

Various genetic and acquired diseases are associated with an increase in the risk of osteoporosis (Table 354-2). Mechanisms that contribute to bone loss are unique for each disease and typically result from multiple factors, including nutrition, reduced physical activity levels, and factors that affect rates of bone remodeling. In most, but not all, circumstances the primary diagnosis is made before osteoporosis presents clinically.

■ MEDICATIONS

A large number of medications used in clinical practice have potentially detrimental effects on the skeleton (Table 354-3). *Glucocorticoids* are the most common cause of medication-induced osteoporosis. It is often not possible to determine the extent to which osteoporosis is related to glucocorticoid or to other factors, as treatment is superimposed on the effects of the primary disease, which in itself may be associated with bone loss (e.g., rheumatoid arthritis). Excessive doses of thyroid hormone can accelerate bone remodeling and result in bone loss.

Other medications have less detrimental effects on the skeleton than pharmacologic doses of glucocorticoids. *Anticonvulsants* are thought to increase the risk of osteoporosis, although many affected individuals have concomitant insufficiency of 1,25(OH)2D, as some anticonvulsants induce the cytochrome P450 system and vitamin D metabolism. Patients undergoing transplantation are at high risk for rapid bone loss and fracture not only from glucocorticoids but also from treatment with other *immunosuppressants* such as cyclosporine and tacrolimus (FK506). In addition these patients often have underlying metabolic abnormalities such as hepatic or renal failure, that predispose to bone loss.

TABLE 354-2 Diseases Associated With an Increased Risk of Generalized Osteoporosis in Adults

Hypogonadal states	**Hematologic disorders/malignancy**
Turner's syndrome	Multiple myeloma
Klinefelter's syndrome	Lymphoma and leukemia
Anorexia nervosa	Malignancy-associated parathyroid hormone (PTHrP) production
Hypothalamic amenorrhea	Mastocytosis
Hyperprolactinemia	Hemophilia
Other primary or secondary hypogonadal states	Thalassemia
Endocrine disorders	**Selected inherited disorders**
Cushing's syndrome	Osteogenesis imperfecta
Hyperparathyroidism	Marfan's syndrome
Thyrotoxicosis	Hemochromatosis
Type 1 diabetes mellitus	Hypophosphatasia
Acromegaly	Glycogen storage diseases
Adrenal insufficiency	Homocystinuria
Nutritional and gastrointestinal disorders	Ehlers-Danlos syndrome
Malnutrition	Porphyria
Parenteral nutrition	Menkes' syndrome
Malabsorption syndromes	Epidermolysis bullosa
Gastrectomy	**Other disorders**
Severe liver disease, especially biliary cirrhosis	Immobilization
Pernicious anemia	Chronic obstructive pulmonary disease
Rheumatologic disorders	Pregnancy and lactation
Rheumatoid arthritis	Scoliosis
Ankylosing spondylitis	Multiple sclerosis
	Sarcoidosis
	Amyloidosis

TABLE 354-3 Drugs Associated With an Increased Risk of Generalized Osteoporosis in Adults

Glucocorticoids	Excessive thyroxine
Cyclosporine	Aluminum
Cytotoxic drugs	Gonadotropin-releasing hormone agonists
Anticonvulsants	Heparin
Excessive alcohol	Lithium
Aromatase inhibitors	

Aromatase inhibitors, which potently block the aromatase enzyme that converts androgens and other adrenal precursors to estrogen, reduce circulating postmenopausal estrogen levels dramatically. These agents, which are used in various stages for breast cancer treatment, also have been shown to have a detrimental effect on bone density and risk of fracture.

CIGARETTE CONSUMPTION

The use of cigarettes over a long period has detrimental effects on bone mass. These effects may be mediated directly by toxic effects on osteoblasts or indirectly by modifying estrogen metabolism. On average, cigarette smokers reach menopause 1–2 years earlier than the general population. Cigarette smoking also produces secondary effects that can modulate skeletal status, including intercurrent respiratory and other illnesses, frailty, decreased exercise, poor nutrition, and the need for additional medications (e.g., glucocorticoids for lung disease).

MEASUREMENT OF BONE MASS

Several noninvasive techniques are available for estimating skeletal mass or density. They include dual-energy x-ray absorptiometry (DXA), single-energy x-ray absorptiometry (SXA), quantitative CT, and ultrasound (US).

DXA is a highly accurate x-ray technique that has become the standard for measuring bone density in most centers. Though it can be used for measurement in any skeletal site, clinical determinations usually are made of the lumbar spine and hip. Portable DXA machines have been developed that measure the heel (calcaneus), forearm (radius and ulna), or finger (phalanges). DXA also can be used to measure body composition. In the DXA technique, two x-ray energies are used to estimate the area of mineralized tissue, and the mineral content is divided by the area, which partially corrects for body size. However, this correction is only partial since DXA is a two-dimensional scanning technique and cannot estimate the depth or posteroanterior length of the bone. Thus, small people tend to have lower than average bone mineral density (BMD). Bone spurs, which are common in osteoarthritis, tend to falsely increase bone density of the spine and are a particular problem in measuring the spine in older individuals. Because DXA instrumentation is provided by several different manufacturers, the output varies in absolute terms. Consequently, it has become standard practice to relate the results to "normal" values by using T-scores, which compare individual results to those in a young population that is matched for race and sex. Z-scores compare individual results to those of an age-matched population that also is matched for race and sex. Thus, a 60-year-old woman with a Z-score of –1 (1 SD below mean for age) has a T-score of –2.5 (2.5 SD below mean for a young control group) (Fig. 354-6). A T-score below –2.5 in the lumbar spine, femoral neck, or total hip is taken as a diagnosis of osteoporosis.

CT is used primarily to measure the spine and, more recently, the hip. Peripheral CT is used to measure bone in the forearm or tibia. The results obtained from CT are different from all others currently available since this technique is three-dimensional and can provide a true density (mass of bone tissue per unit volume). CT also can specifically analyze trabecular bone and cortical bone content and volume separately. However, CT remains expensive, involves greater radiation exposure, and is less reproducible than DXA. A new technique employing high-resolution CT scanning called *Xtreme CT* also can provide information on skeletal architecture, including cancellous connectivity.

US is used to measure bone mass by calculating the attenuation of the signal as it passes through bone or the speed with which it traverses the bone. It is unclear whether US assesses properties of bone other than mass (e.g., quality), but this is a potential advantage of the technique. Because of its relatively low cost and mobility, US is amenable for use as a screening procedure.

All these techniques for measuring BMD have been approved by the U.S. Food and Drug Administration (FDA) on the basis of their capacity to predict fracture risk. The hip is the preferred site of measurement in most individuals, since it predicts the risk of hip fracture, the most important consequence of osteoporosis, better than any other bone density measurement site. When hip measurements are performed by DXA, the spine can be measured at the same time. In younger individuals such as perimenopausal or early postmenopausal women, spine measurements may be the most sensitive indicator of bone loss.

WHEN TO MEASURE BONE MASS

Clinical guidelines have been developed for the use of bone densitometry in clinical practice. The original National Osteoporosis Foundation guidelines recommend bone mass measurements in postmenopausal women, assuming they have one or more risk factors for osteoporosis in addition to age, sex, and estrogen deficiency. The guidelines further recommend that bone mass measurement be considered in *all* women by age 65, a position ratified by the U.S. Preventive Health Services Task Force. Criteria approved for Medicare reimbursement of BMD are summarized in Table 354-4.

WHEN TO TREAT BASED ON BONE MASS RESULTS

Most guidelines suggest that patients be considered for treatment when BMD is >2.5 SD below the mean value for young adults (T-score ≤–2.5), a level consistent with the diagnosis of osteoporosis. Treatment also should also be considered in postmenopausal

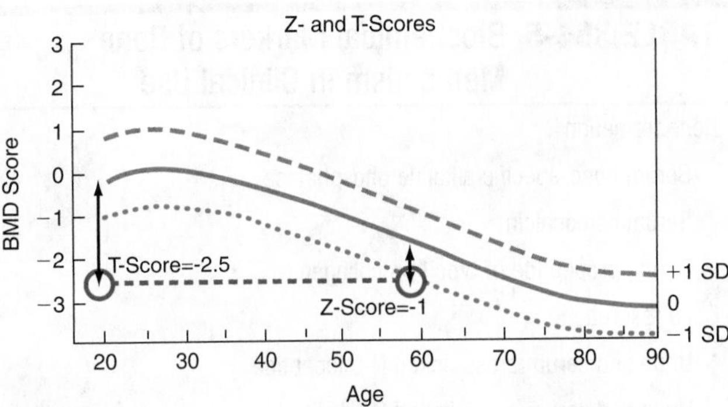

Figure 354-6 Relationship between Z-scores and T-scores in a 60-year-old woman. BMD, bone mineral density; SD, standard deviation.

TABLE 354-4 FDA-Approved Indications for BMD Tests*

Estrogen-deficient women at clinical risk of osteoporosis
Vertebral abnormalities on x-ray suggestive of osteoporosis (osteopenia, vertebral fracture)
Glucocorticoid treatment equivalent to ≥7.5 mg of prednisone or duration of therapy >3 months
Primary hyperparathyroidism
Monitoring response to an FDA-approved medication for osteoporosis
Repeat BMD evaluations at >23-month intervals or more frequently if medically justified

*Criteria adapted from the 1998 Bone Mass Measurement Act.

Abbreviations: BMD, bone mineral density; FDA, U.S. Food and Drug Administration.

women with fracture risk factors even if BMD is not in the osteoporosis range. Risk factors (age, prior fracture, family history of hip fracture, low body weight, cigarette consumption, excessive alcohol use, steroid use, and rheumatoid arthritis) can be combined with BMD to assess the likelihood of a fracture over a 5- or 10-year period. Treatment thresholds depend on cost-effectiveness analyses but probably is ~1% per year of risk in the United States.

APPROACH TO THE PATIENT: Osteoporosis

The perimenopausal transition is a good opportunity to initiate a discussion about risk factors for osteoporosis and consideration of indications for a BMD test. A careful history and physical examination should be performed to identify risk factors for osteoporosis. A low Z-score increases the suspicion of a secondary disease. Height loss >2.5–3.8 cm (>1–1.5 in.) is an indication for radiography or vertebral fracture assessment by DXA to rule out asymptomatic vertebral fractures, as is the presence of significant kyphosis or back pain, particularly if it began after menopause. For patients who present with fractures, it is important to ensure that the fractures are not caused by an underlying malignancy. Usually this is clear on routine radiography, but on occasion, CT, MRI, or radionuclide scans may be necessary.

ROUTINE LABORATORY EVALUATION There is no established algorithm for the evaluation of women who present with osteoporosis. A general evaluation that includes complete blood count, serum and 24-h urine calcium, and renal and hepatic function tests is useful for identifying selected secondary causes of low bone mass, particularly for women with fractures or very low Z-scores. An elevated serum calcium level suggests hyperparathyroidism or malignancy, whereas a reduced serum calcium level may reflect malnutrition and osteomalacia. In the presence of hypercalcemia, a serum PTH level differentiates between hyperparathyroidism (PTH↑) and malignancy (PTH↓), and a high PTHrP level can help document the presence of humoral hypercalcemia of malignancy (Chap. 353). A low urine calcium (<50 mg/24 h) suggests osteomalacia, malnutrition, or malabsorption; a high urine calcium (>300 mg/24 h) is indicative of hypercalciuria and must be investigated further. Hypercalciuria occurs primarily in three situations: (1) a renal calcium leak, which is more common in males with osteoporosis; (2) absorptive hypercalciuria, which can be idiopathic or associated with increased 1,25$(OH)_2$D in granulomatous disease; or (3) hematologic malignancies or conditions associated with excessive bone turnover such as Paget's disease, hyperparathyroidism, and hyperthyroidism.

Individuals who have osteoporosis-related fractures or bone density in the osteoporotic range should have a measurement of serum 25(OH)D level, since the intake of vitamin D required to achieve a target level >32 ng/mL is highly variable. Vitamin D levels should be optimized in all individuals being treated for osteoporosis. Hyperthyroidism should be evaluated by measuring thyroid-stimulating hormone (TSH).

When there is clinical suspicion of Cushing's syndrome, urinary free cortisol levels or a fasting serum cortisol should be measured after overnight dexamethasone. When bowel disease, malabsorption, or malnutrition is suspected, serum albumin, cholesterol, and a complete blood count should be checked. Asymptomatic malabsorption may be heralded by anemia (macrocytic—vitamin B_{12} or folate deficiency; microcytic—iron deficiency) or low serum cholesterol or urinary calcium levels. If these or other features suggest malabsorption, further evaluation is required. Asymptomatic celiac disease with selective malabsorption is being found with increasing frequency; the diagnosis can be made by testing for antigliadin, antiendomysial, or transglutaminase antibodies but may require endoscopic biopsy. A trial of a gluten-free diet can be confirmatory (Chap. 294). When osteoporosis is found associated with symptoms of rash, multiple allergies, diarrhea, or flushing, mastocytosis should be excluded by using 24-h urine histamine collection or serum tryptase.

Myeloma can masquerade as generalized osteoporosis, although it more commonly presents with bone pain and characteristic "punched-out" lesions on radiography. Serum and urine electrophoresis and evaluation for light chains in urine are required to exclude this diagnosis. A bone marrow biopsy may be required to rule out myeloma (in patients with equivocal electrophoretic results) and also can be used to exclude mastocytosis, leukemia, and other marrow infiltrative disorders such as Gaucher's disease.

BONE BIOPSY Tetracycline labeling of the skeleton allows determination of the rate of remodeling as well as evaluation for other metabolic bone diseases. The current use of BMD tests, in combination with hormonal evaluation and biochemical markers of bone remodeling, has largely replaced the clinical use of bone biopsy, although it remains an important tool in clinical research.

BIOCHEMICAL MARKERS Several biochemical tests are available that provide an index of the overall rate of bone remodeling (Table 354-5). Biochemical markers usually are characterized as those related primarily to *bone formation* or *bone resorption*. These tests measure the overall state of bone remodeling at a single point in time. Clinical use of these tests has been hampered by biologic variability (in part related to circadian rhythm) as well as analytic variability, although the latter is improving.

For the most part, remodeling markers do not predict rates of bone loss well enough for this information to be used clinically. However, markers of bone resorption may help in the prediction of fracture risk, independently of bone density, particularly in older individuals. In women ≥65 years, when bone density results are greater than the usual treatment thresholds noted above, a high level of bone resorption should prompt consideration of treatment. The primary use of biochemical markers is for monitoring the response to treatment. With the introduction of antiresorptive therapeutic agents, bone remodeling declines rapidly, with the fall in resorption occurring earlier than the fall in formation. Inhibition of bone resorption is maximal within 3–6 months. Thus, measurement of bone

TABLE 354-5 Biochemical Markers of Bone Metabolism in Clinical Use

Bone formation
Serum bone-specific alkaline phosphatase
Serum osteocalcin
Serum propeptide of type I procollagen
Bone resorption
Urine and serum cross-linked N-telopeptide
Urine and serum cross-linked C-telopeptide
Urine total free deoxypyridinoline

resorption before initiating therapy and 4–6 months after starting therapy provides an earlier estimate of patient response than does bone densitometry. A decline in resorptive markers can be ascertained after treatment with bisphosphonates or estrogen; this effect is less marked after treatment with either raloxifene or intranasal calcitonin. A biochemical marker response to therapy is particularly useful for asymptomatic patients and may help ensure long-term adherence to treatment. Bone turnover markers are also useful in monitoring the effects of 1-34hPTH, or teriparatide, which rapidly increases bone formation and later bone resorption.

TREATMENT Osteoporosis

MANAGEMENT OF OSTEOPOROTIC FRACTURES Treatment of a patient with osteoporosis frequently involves management of acute fractures as well as treatment of the underlying disease. Hip fractures almost always require surgical repair if the patient is to become ambulatory again. Depending on the location and severity of the fracture, condition of the neighboring joint, and general status of the patient, procedures may include open reduction and internal fixation with pins and plates, hemiarthroplasties, and total arthroplasties. These surgical procedures are followed by intense rehabilitation in an attempt to return patients to their prefracture functional level. Long bone fractures often require either external or internal fixation. Other fractures (e.g., vertebral, rib, and pelvic fractures) usually are managed with supportive care, requiring no specific orthopedic treatment.

Only ~25–30% of vertebral compression fractures present with sudden-onset back pain. For acutely symptomatic fractures, treatment with analgesics is required, including nonsteroidal anti-inflammatory agents and/or acetaminophen, sometimes with the addition of a narcotic agent (codeine or oxycodone). A few small, randomized clinical trials suggest that calcitonin may reduce pain related to acute vertebral compression fracture. A recently developed technique involves percutaneous injection of artificial cement (polymethylmethacrylate) into the vertebral body (vertebroplasty or kyphoplasty); this offers significant immediate pain relief in the majority of patients. Long-term effects are unknown, and conclusions are based on observational studies in patients with severe persistent back pain from acute or subacute vertebral fractures. There have been no long-term randomized controlled trials of either vertebroplasty or kyphoplasty to date. Short periods of bed rest may be helpful for pain management, but in general, early mobilization is recommended as it helps prevent further bone loss associated with immobilization. Occasionally, use of a soft elastic-style brace may facilitate earlier mobilization. Muscle spasms often occur with acute compression fractures and can be treated with muscle relaxants and heat treatments.

Severe pain usually resolves within 6–10 weeks. Chronic pain is probably not bony in origin; instead, it is related to abnormal strain on muscles, ligaments, and tendons and to secondary facet-joint arthritis associated with alterations in thoracic and/or abdominal shape. Chronic pain is difficult to treat effectively and may require analgesics, sometimes including narcotic analgesics. Frequent intermittent rest in a supine or semireclining position is often required to allow the soft tissues, which are under tension, to relax. Back-strengthening exercises (paraspinal) may be beneficial. Heat treatments help relax muscles and reduce the muscular component of discomfort. Various physical modalities, such as US and transcutaneous nerve stimulation, may be beneficial in some patients. Pain also occurs in the neck region, not as a result of compression fractures (which almost never occur in the cervical spine as a result of osteoporosis) but because of chronic strain associated with trying to elevate the head in a person with a severe thoracic kyphosis.

Multiple vertebral fractures often are associated with psychological symptoms; this is not always appreciated. The changes in body configuration and back pain can lead to marked loss of self-image and a secondary depression. Altered balance, precipitated by the kyphosis and the anterior movement of the body's center of gravity, leads to a fear of falling, a consequent tendency to remain indoors, and the onset of social isolation. These symptoms sometimes can be alleviated by family support and/or psychotherapy. Medication may be necessary when depressive features are present.

MANAGEMENT OF THE UNDERLYING DISEASE

Risk Factor Reduction Assessment of fracture risk can be estimated by using FRAX calculators that are available online (*http://www.shef.ac.uk/FRAX/tool.jsp?locationValue=9*) (Fig. 354-7). Patients should be thoroughly educated to reduce the impact of modifiable risk factors associated with bone loss and falling. Medications should be reviewed to ensure that all are necessary. Glucocorticoid medication, if present, should be evaluated to determine that it is truly indicated and is being given in doses that are as low as possible. For those on thyroid hormone replacement, TSH testing should be performed to determine that an excessive dose is not being used, as thyrotoxicosis can be associated with increased bone loss. In patients who smoke, efforts should be made to facilitate smoking cessation. Reducing risk factors for falling also include alcohol abuse treatment and a review of the medical regimen for any drugs that might be associated with orthostatic hypotension and/or sedation, including hypnotics and anxiolytics. If nocturia occurs, the frequency should be reduced, if possible (e.g., by decreasing or modifying diuretic use), as arising in the middle of sleep is a common precipitant of a fall. Patients should be instructed about environmental safety with regard to eliminating exposed wires, curtain strings, slippery rugs, and mobile tables. Avoiding stocking feet on wood floors, checking carpet condition (particularly on stairs), and providing good light in paths to bathrooms and outside the home are important preventive measures. Treatment for impaired vision is recommended, particularly a problem with depth perception, which is specifically associated with increased falling risk. Elderly patients with neurologic impairment (e.g., stroke, Parkinson's disease, Alzheimer's disease) are particularly at risk of falling and require specialized supervision and care.

Nutritional Recommendations

Calcium A large body of data indicates that optimal calcium intake reduces bone loss and suppresses bone turnover. Recommended intakes from an Institute of Medicine report are shown in Table 354-6. The National Health and Nutritional Evaluation Studies (NHANES) have consistently documented that average calcium intakes fall considerably short of these recommendations. The preferred source of calcium is dairy products and other foods, but many patients require calcium supplementation. Food sources of calcium are dairy products (milk, yogurt, and cheese) and fortified foods such as certain cereals, waffles, snacks, juices, and crackers. Some of these fortified foods contain as much calcium per serving as milk.

If a calcium supplement is required, it should be taken in doses ≤600 mg at a time, as the calcium absorption fraction

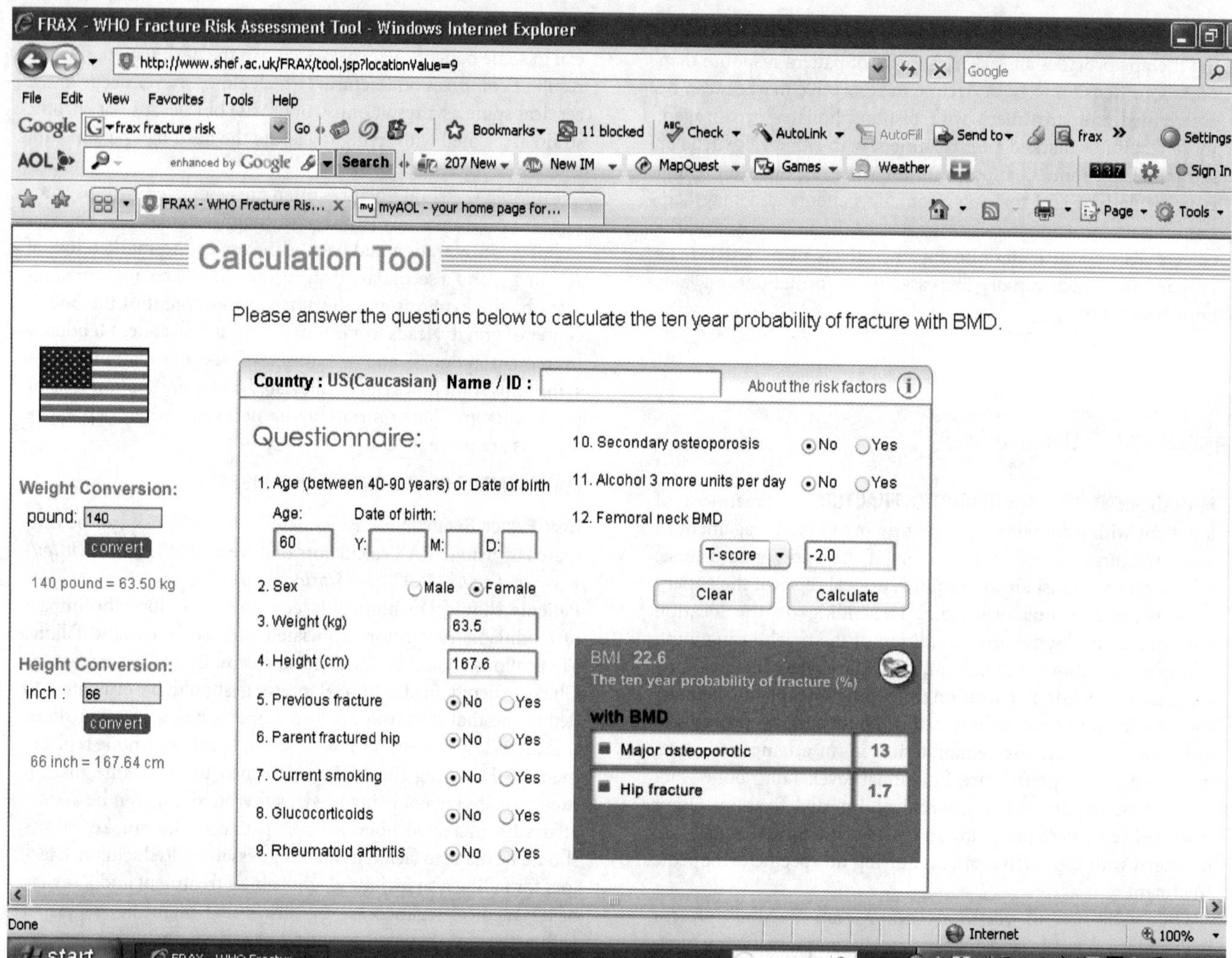

Figure 354-7 FRAX calculation tool. When the answers to the indicated questions are filled in, the calculator can be used to assess the 10-year probability of fracture. The calculator (available online at *http://www.shef.ac.uk/FRAX/tool.jsp?locationValue=9)* also can risk adjust for various ethnic groups.

decreases at higher doses. Calcium supplements should be calculated on the basis of the elemental calcium content of the supplement, not the weight of the calcium salt (Table 354-7). Calcium supplements containing carbonate are best taken with food since they require acid for solubility. Calcium citrate supplements can be taken at any time. To confirm bioavailability, calcium supplements can be placed in distilled vinegar. They should dissolve within 30 min.

Several controlled clinical trials of calcium plus vitamin D have confirmed reductions in clinical fractures, including fractures of the hip (~20–30% risk reduction). All recent studies of pharmacologic agents have been conducted in the context of

TABLE 354-6 Adequate Calcium Intake

Life Stage Group	Estimated Adequate Daily Calcium Intake, mg/d
Young children (1–3 years)	500
Older children (4–8 years)	800
Adolescents and young adults (9–18 years)	1300
Men and women (19–50 years)	1000
Men and women (51 and older)	1200

Note: Pregnancy and lactation needs are the same as for nonpregnant women (e.g., 1300 mg/d for adolescents/young adults and 1000 mg/d for ≥19 years).

Source: Adapted from the Standing Committee on the Scientific Evaluation of Dietary Reference Intakes. Food and Nutrition Board. Institute of Medicine. Washington, DC, 1997, National Academy Press.

TABLE 354-7 Elemental Calcium Content of Various Oral Calcium Preparations

Calcium Preparation	Elemental Calcium Content
Calcium citrate	60 mg/300 mg
Calcium lactate	80 mg/600 mg
Calcium gluconate	40 mg/500 mg
Calcium carbonate	400 mg/g
Calcium carbonate + 5 μg vitamin D_2 (OsCal 250)	250 mg/tablet
Calcium carbonate (Tums 500)	500 mg/tablet

Source: Adapted from SM Krane, MF Holick, Chap. 355, in *Harrison's Principles of Internal Medicine,* 14th ed. New York, McGraw-Hill, 1998.

calcium replacement (± vitamin D). Thus, it is standard practice to ensure an adequate calcium and vitamin D intake in patients with osteoporosis whether they are receiving additional pharmacologic therapy or not. A systematic review confirmed a greater BMD response to antiresorptive therapy when calcium intake was adequate.

Although side effects from supplemental calcium are minimal (eructation and constipation mostly with carbonate salts), individuals with a history of kidney stones should have a 24-h urine calcium determination before starting increased calcium to avoid significant hypercalciuria.

Vitamin D Vitamin D is synthesized in skin under the influence of heat and ultraviolet light (Chap. 352). However, large segments of the population do not obtain sufficient vitamin D to maintain what is now considered an adequate supply [serum 25(OH)D consistently >75 μmol/L (30 ng/mL)]. Since vitamin D supplementation at doses that would achieve these serum levels is safe and inexpensive, the Institute of Medicine recommends daily intakes of 200 IU for adults <50 years of age, 400 IU for those 50–70 years, and 600 IU for those >70 years. Multivitamin tablets usually contain 400 IU, and many calcium supplements also contain vitamin D. Some data suggest that higher doses (≥1000 IU) may be required in the elderly and chronically ill.

Other Nutrients Other nutrients such as salt, high animal protein intakes, and caffeine may have modest effects on calcium excretion or absorption. Adequate vitamin K status is required for optimal carboxylation of osteocalcin. States in which vitamin K nutrition or metabolism is impaired, such as with long-term warfarin therapy, have been associated with reduced bone mass. Research concerning cola intake is controversial but suggests a possible link to reduced bone mass through factors that are independent of caffeine.

Magnesium is abundant in foods, and magnesium deficiency is quite rare in the absence of a serious chronic disease. Magnesium supplementation may be warranted in patients with inflammatory bowel disease, celiac disease, chemotherapy, severe diarrhea, malnutrition, or alcoholism. Dietary phytoestrogens, which are derived primarily from soy products and legumes [e.g., garbanzo beans (chickpeas) and lentils], exert some estrogenic activity but are insufficiently potent to justify their use in place of a pharmacologic agent in the treatment of osteoporosis.

Patients with hip fractures are often frail and relatively malnourished. Some data suggest an improved outcome in such patients when they are provided calorie and protein supplementation. Excessive protein intake can increase renal calcium excretion, but this can be corrected by an adequate calcium intake.

Exercise Exercise in young individuals increases the likelihood that they will attain the maximal genetically determined peak bone mass. Meta-analyses of studies performed in postmenopausal women indicate that weight-bearing exercise prevents bone loss but does not appear to result in substantial gain of bone mass. This beneficial effect wanes if exercise is discontinued. Most of the studies are short term, and a more substantial effect on bone mass is likely if exercise is continued over a long period. Exercise also has beneficial effects on neuromuscular function, and it improves coordination, balance, and strength, thereby reducing the risk of falling. A walking program is a practical way to start. Other activities such as dancing, racquet sports, cross-country skiing, and use of gym equipment, are also recommended, depending on the patient's personal preference and general condition. Even women who cannot walk benefit from swimming or water exercises, not so much for the effects on bone, which are quite minimal, but because of effects on muscle. Exercise habits should be consistent, optimally at least three times a week.

PHARMACOLOGIC THERAPIES Until fairly recently, estrogen treatment, either by itself or in concert with a progestin, was the primary therapeutic agent for prevention or treatment of osteoporosis. However, a number of new drugs have appeared, and more are expected in the near future. Some are agents that specifically treat osteoporosis (bisphosphonates, calcitonin, PTH); others such as selective estrogen response modulators (SERMs), have broader effects. The availability of these drugs allows therapy to be tailored to the needs of an individual patient.

Estrogens A large body of clinical trial data indicates that various types of estrogens (conjugated equine estrogens, estradiol, estrone, esterified estrogens, ethinyl estradiol, and mestranol) reduce bone turnover, prevent bone loss, and induce small increases in bone mass of the spine, hip, and total body. The effects of estrogen are seen in women with natural or surgical menopause and in late postmenopausal women with or without established osteoporosis. Estrogens are efficacious when administered orally or transdermally. For both oral and transdermal routes of administration, combined estrogen/progestin preparations are now available in many countries, obviating the problem of taking two tablets or using a patch and oral progestin. One large study, referred to as PEPI (Postmenopausal Estrogen/Progestin Intervention Trial), indicated that C-21 progestins alone do not augment the effect of standard estrogen doses on bone mass.

Dose of Estrogen For oral estrogens, the standard recommended doses have been 0.3 mg/d for esterified estrogens, 0.625 mg/d for conjugated equine estrogens, and 5 μg/d for ethinyl estradiol. For transdermal estrogen, the commonly used dose supplies 50 μg estradiol per day, but a lower dose may be appropriate for some individuals. Dose-response data for conjugated equine estrogens indicate that lower doses (0.3 and 0.45 mg/d) are effective. Doses even lower have been associated with bone mass protection.

Fracture Data Epidemiologic databases indicate that women who take estrogen replacement have a 50% reduction, on average, of osteoporotic fractures, including hip fractures. The beneficial effect of estrogen is greatest among those who start replacement early and continue the treatment; the benefit declines after discontinuation to the extent that there is no residual protective effect against fracture by 10 years after discontinuation. The first clinical trial evaluating fractures as secondary outcomes, the Heart and Estrogen-Progestin Replacement Study (HERS) trial, showed no effect of hormone therapy on hip or other clinical fractures in women with established coronary artery disease. These data made the results of the Women's Health Initiative (WHI) exceedingly important (Chap. 348). The estrogen-progestin arm of the WHI in >16,000 postmenopausal healthy women indicated that hormone therapy reduces the risk of hip and clinical spine fracture by 34% and that of all clinical fractures by 24%.

A few smaller clinical trials have evaluated spine fracture occurrence as an outcome with estrogen therapy. They have consistently shown that estrogen treatment reduces the incidence of vertebral compression fracture.

The WHI has provided a vast amount of data on the multisystemic effects of hormone therapy. Although earlier observational studies suggested that estrogen replacement might reduce heart disease, the WHI showed that combined estrogen-progestin treatment increased risk of fatal and nonfatal myocardial infarction by ~29%, confirming data from the HERS study. Other important

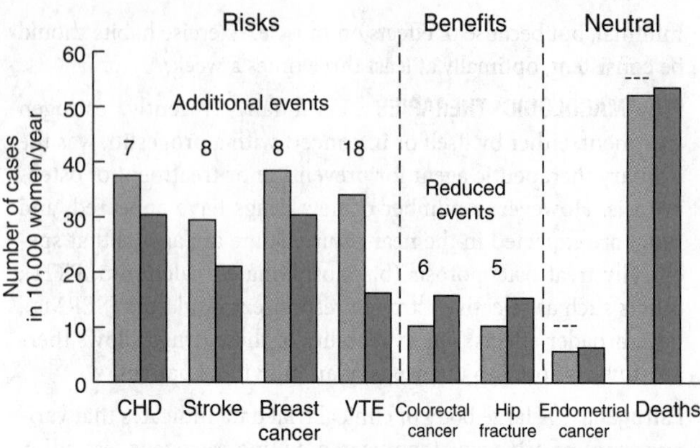

Figure 354-8 Effects of hormone therapy on event rates: green, placebo; purple, estrogen and progestin. CHD, coronary heart disease; VTE, venous thromboembolic events. *(Adapted from Women's Health Initiative. WHI HRT Update. Available at http://www.nhlbi.nih.gov/health/women/upd2002.htm.)*

relative risks included a 40% increase in stroke, a 100% increase in venous thromboembolic disease, and a 26% increase in risk of breast cancer. Subsequent analyses have confirmed the increased risk of stroke and shown a twofold increase in dementia. Benefits other than the fracture reductions noted above included a 37% reduction in the risk of colon cancer. These relative risks have to be interpreted in light of absolute risk (Fig. 354-8). For example, out of 10,000 women treated with estrogen-progestin for 1 year, there will be 8 excess heart attacks, 8 excess breast cancers, 18 excess venous thromboembolic events, 5 fewer hip fractures, 44 fewer clinical fractures, and 6 fewer colorectal cancers. These numbers must be multiplied by years of hormone treatment. There was no effect of hormone treatment on the risk of uterine cancer or total mortality.

It is important to note that these WHI findings apply specifically to hormone treatment in the form of conjugated equine estrogen plus medroxyprogesterone acetate. The relative benefits and risks of unopposed estrogen in women who had hysterectomies vary somewhat. They still show benefits against fracture occurrence and increased risk of venous thrombosis and stroke, similar in magnitude to the risks for combined hormone therapy. In contrast, though, the estrogen-only arm of WHI indicated no increased risk of heart attack or breast cancer. The data suggest that at least some of the detrimental effects of combined therapy are related to the progestin component.

Mode of Action Two subtypes of ERs, α and β, have been identified in bone and other tissues. Cells of monocyte lineage express both ERα and ERβ, as do osteoblasts. Estrogen-mediated effects vary with the receptor type. Using ER knockout mouse models, elimination of ERα produces a modest reduction in bone mass, whereas mutation of ERβ has less of an effect on bone. A male patient with a homozygous mutation of ERα had markedly decreased bone density as well as abnormalities in epiphyseal closure, confirming the important role of ERα in bone biology. The mechanism of estrogen action in bone is an area of active investigation (Fig. 354-5). Although data are conflicting, estrogens may inhibit osteoclasts directly. However, the majority of estrogen (and androgen) effects on bone resorption are mediated indirectly through paracrine factors produced by osteoblasts. These actions include (1) increasing IGF-I and TGF-β and (2) suppressing IL-1 (α and β), IL-6, TNF-α, and osteocalcin synthesis. The indirect estrogen actions primarily decrease bone resorption.

Progestins In women with a uterus, daily progestin or cyclical progestins at least 12 days per month are prescribed in combination with estrogens to reduce the risk of uterine cancer. Medroxyprogesterone acetate and norethindrone acetate blunt the high-density lipoprotein response to estrogen, but micronized progesterone does not. Neither medroxyprogesterone acetate nor micronized progesterone appears to have an independent effect on bone; at lower doses of estrogen, norethindrone acetate may have an additive benefit. On breast tissue, progestins may increase the risk of breast cancer.

SERMs Two SERMs are used currently in postmenopausal women: raloxifene, which is approved for the prevention and treatment of osteoporosis, and tamoxifen, which is approved for the prevention and treatment of breast cancer.

Tamoxifen reduces bone turnover and bone loss in postmenopausal women compared with placebo groups. These findings support the concept that tamoxifen acts as an estrogenic agent in bone. There are limited data on the effect of tamoxifen on fracture risk, but the Breast Cancer Prevention study indicated a possible reduction in clinical vertebral, hip, and Colles' fractures. The major benefit of tamoxifen is on breast cancer occurrence. The breast cancer prevention trial indicated that tamoxifen administration over 4–5 years reduced the incidence of new invasive and noninvasive breast cancer by ~45% in women at increased risk of breast cancer. The incidence of ER-positive breast cancers was reduced by 65%. Tamoxifen increases the risk of uterine cancer in postmenopausal women, limiting its use for breast cancer prevention in women at low or moderate risk.

Raloxifene (60 mg/d) has effects on bone turnover and bone mass that are very similar to those of tamoxifen, indicating that this agent is also estrogenic on the skeleton. The effect of raloxifene on bone density (+1.4–2.8% versus placebo in the spine, hip, and total body) is somewhat less than that seen with standard doses of estrogens. Raloxifene reduces the occurrence of vertebral fracture by 30–50%, depending on the population; however, there are no data confirming that raloxifene can reduce the risk of nonvertebral fractures over 8 years of observation.

Raloxifene, like tamoxifen and estrogen, has effects in other organ systems. The most beneficial effect appears to be a reduction in invasive breast cancer (mainly decreased ER-positive) occurrence of ~65% in women who take raloxifene compared to placebo. In a head-to-head study raloxifene was as effective as tamoxifen in preventing breast cancer in high-risk women, but in a separate study it had no effect on heart disease in women with increased risk for this outcome. In contrast to tamoxifen, raloxifene is not associated with an increase in the risk of uterine cancer or benign uterine disease. Raloxifene increases the occurrence of hot flashes but reduces serum total and low-density lipoprotein cholesterol, lipoprotein(a), and fibrinogen.

Mode of Action of SERMs All SERMs bind to the ER, but each agent produces a unique receptor-drug conformation. As a result, specific coactivator or co-repressor proteins are bound to the receptor (Chap. 338), resulting in differential effects on gene transcription that vary depending on other transcription factors present in the cell. Another aspect of selectivity is the affinity of each SERM for the different ERα and ERβ subtypes, which are expressed differentially in various tissues. These tissue-selective effects of SERMs offer the possibility of tailoring estrogen therapy to best meet the needs and risk factor profile of an individual patient.

Bisphosphonates Alendronate, risedronate, and ibandronate are approved for the prevention and treatment of postmenopausal osteoporosis. Risedronate and alendronate are approved for the treatment of steroid-induced osteoporosis, and risedronate also is approved for prevention of steroid-induced osteoporosis. Both alendronate and risedronate are approved for treatment of osteoporosis in men.

Alendronate has been shown to decrease bone turnover and increase bone mass in the spine by up to 8% versus placebo and by 6% versus placebo in the hip. Multiple trials have evaluated its effect on fracture occurrence. The Fracture Intervention Trial provided evidence in >2000 women with prevalent vertebral fractures that daily alendronate treatment (5 mg/d for 2 years and 10 mg/d for 9 months afterward) reduces vertebral fracture risk by about 50%, multiple vertebral fractures by up to 90%, and hip fractures by up to 50%. Several subsequent trials have confirmed these findings (Figs. 354-9 and 354-10). For example, in a study of >1900 women with low bone mass treated with alendronate (10 mg/d) versus placebo, the incidence of all nonvertebral fractures was reduced by ~47% after only 1 year.

Trials comparing once-weekly alendronate, 70 mg, with daily 10-mg dosing have shown equivalence with regard to bone mass and bone turnover responses. Consequently, once-weekly therapy generally is preferred because of the low incidence of gastrointestinal side effects and ease of administration. Alendronate should be given with a full glass of water before breakfast, as bisphosphonates are poorly absorbed. Because of the potential for esophageal irritation, alendronate is contraindicated in patients who have stricture or inadequate emptying of the esophagus. It is recommended that patients remain upright for at least 30 min after taking the medication to avoid esophageal irritation. Cases of esophagitis, esophageal ulcer, and esophageal stricture have been described, but the incidence appears to be low. In clinical trials, overall gastrointestinal symptomatology was no different with alendronate than with placebo. Alendronate is also available in a preparation that contains vitamin D.

Risedronate also reduces bone turnover and increases bone mass. Controlled clinical trials have demonstrated 40–50% reduction in vertebral fracture risk over 3 years, accompanied by a 40% reduction in clinical nonspine fractures. The only clinical trial specifically designed to evaluate hip fracture outcome (HIP) indicated that risedronate reduced hip fracture risk in women in their seventies with confirmed osteoporosis by 40%. In contrast, risedronate was not effective at reducing hip fracture occurrence in older women (80+ years) without proven osteoporosis. Studies have shown that 35 mg of risedronate administered once weekly is therapeutically equivalent to 5 mg/d. Patients should take risedronate with a full glass of plain water to facilitate delivery to the stomach and should not lie down for 30 min after taking the drug. The incidence of gastrointestinal side effects in trials with risedronate was similar to that of placebo.

Etidronate was the first bisphosphonate to be approved, initially for use in Paget's disease and hypercalcemia. This agent has also been used in osteoporosis trials of smaller magnitude than those performed for alendronate and risedronate but is not approved by the FDA for treatment of osteoporosis. Etidronate probably has some efficacy against vertebral fracture when given as an intermittent cyclical regimen (2 weeks on, 2.5 months off). Its effectiveness against nonvertebral fractures has not been studied.

Ibandronate is the third amino-bisphosphonate approved in the United States. Ibandronate (2.5 mg/d) has been shown in clinical trials to reduce vertebral fracture risk by ~40% but with no overall effect on nonvertebral fractures. In a post hoc analysis of subjects with a femoral neck T-score of –3 or below, ibandronate reduced the risk of nonvertebral fractures by ~60%. In clinical trials, ibandronate doses of 150 mg/month PO or 3 mg every 3 months IV had greater effects on turnover and bone mass than did 2.5 mg/d. Patients should take oral ibandronate in the same way as other bisphosphonates, but with 1 h elapsing before other food or drink (other than plain water).

Zoledronic acid is a potent bisphosphonate with unique administration regimens (once yearly IV). Although it has not been approved for use in osteoporosis, the data suggest that it is highly effective in fracture risk reduction. In a study of >7000 women followed for 3 years, zoledronic acid (5 mg as a single IV infusion annually) reduced the risk of vertebral fractures by 70%, nonvertebral fractures by 25%, and hip fractures by 40%. These results were associated with less height loss and disability. In the treated population, there was an increased risk of atrial fibrillation (2%) and arthralgia and a 15% risk of fever in comparison to placebo.

Mode of Action Bisphosphonates are structurally related to pyrophosphates, compounds that are incorporated into bone matrix. Bisphosphonates specifically impair osteoclast function and reduce osteoclast number, in part by inducing apoptosis. Recent evidence suggests that the nitrogen-containing bisphosphonates also inhibit protein prenylation, one of the end products in the mevalonic acid pathway, by inhibiting the enzyme farnesyl pyrophosphate synthase. This effect disrupts intracellular protein trafficking and ultimately may lead to apoptosis. Some bisphosphonates have very long retention in the skeleton and may exert long-term effects. The consequences of this, if any, are unknown. A phenomenon that has been called *osteonecrosis of the jaw* (ONJ) has been described, mostly in patients with cancer who are given high doses of zoledronic acid or pamidronate. A few cases have been described in patients with osteoporosis treated with oral bisphosphonates. The background incidence of ONJ in this population is not known, and thus the attributable risk for bisphosphonates is not clear, although it appears to be relatively low.

Calcitonin Calcitonin is a polypeptide hormone produced by the thyroid gland (Chap. 353). Its physiologic role is unclear as no skeletal disease has been described in association with calcitonin deficiency or excess. Calcitonin preparations are approved by the FDA for Paget's disease, hypercalcemia, and osteoporosis in women >5 years past menopause.

Injectable calcitonin produces small increments in bone mass of the lumbar spine. However, difficulty of administration and frequent reactions, including nausea and facial flushing, make general use limited. A nasal spray containing calcitonin (200 IU/d) is available for treatment of osteoporosis in postmenopausal women. One study suggests that nasal calcitonin produces small increments in bone mass and a small reduction in new vertebral fractures in calcitonin-treated patients versus those on calcium alone. There has been no proven effectiveness against nonvertebral fractures. An oral preparation of calcitonin recently was approved for use in osteoporosis.

Calcitonin is not indicated for prevention of osteoporosis and is not sufficiently potent to prevent bone loss in early postmenopausal women. Calcitonin might have an analgesic effect on bone pain, both in the subcutaneous and possibly in the nasal form.

Mode of Action Calcitonin suppresses osteoclast activity by direct action on the osteoclast calcitonin receptor. Osteoclasts exposed to calcitonin cannot maintain their active ruffled border, which normally maintains close contact with underlying bone.

Denosumab A novel agent that was given twice yearly by SC administration in a randomized controlled trial in postmenopausal women with osteoporosis has been shown to increase BMD in the spine, hip, and forearm and reduce vertebral, hip, and nonvertebral fractures over a 3-year period by 70, 40, and

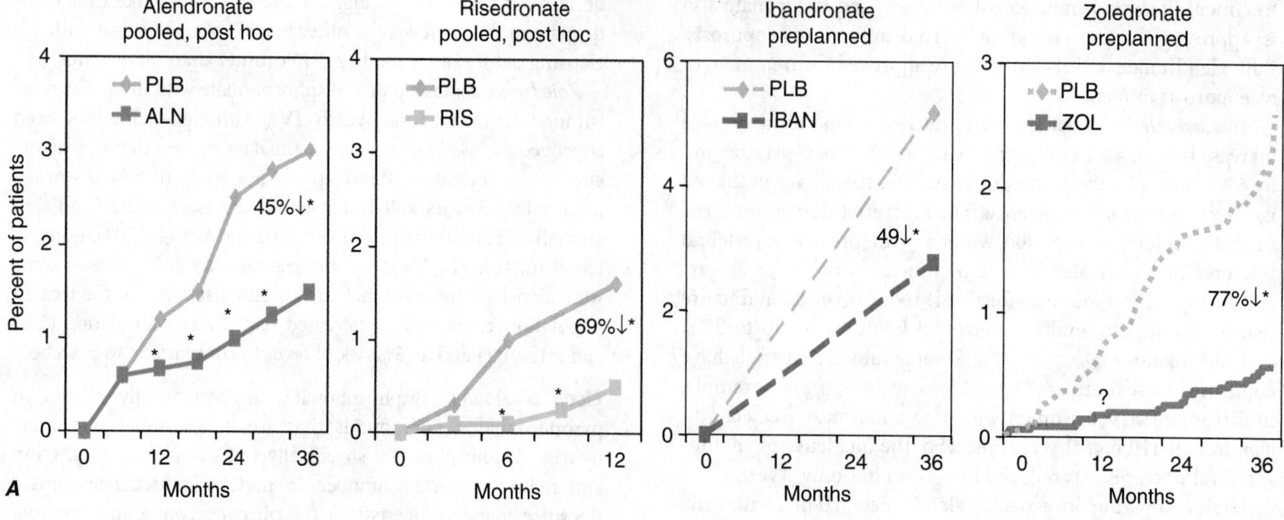

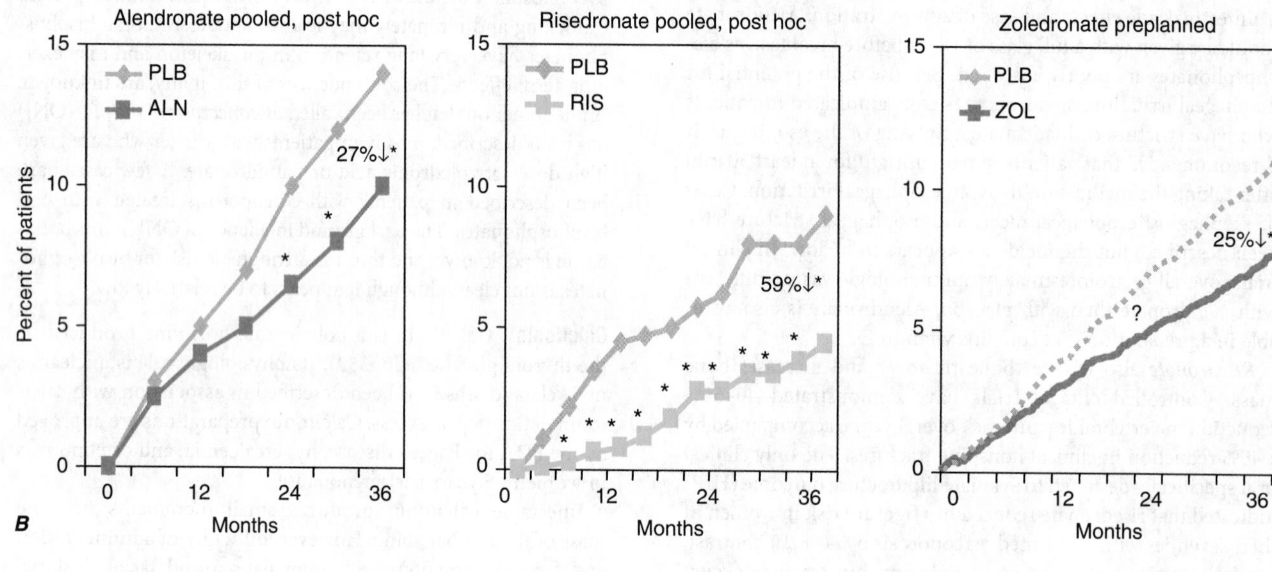

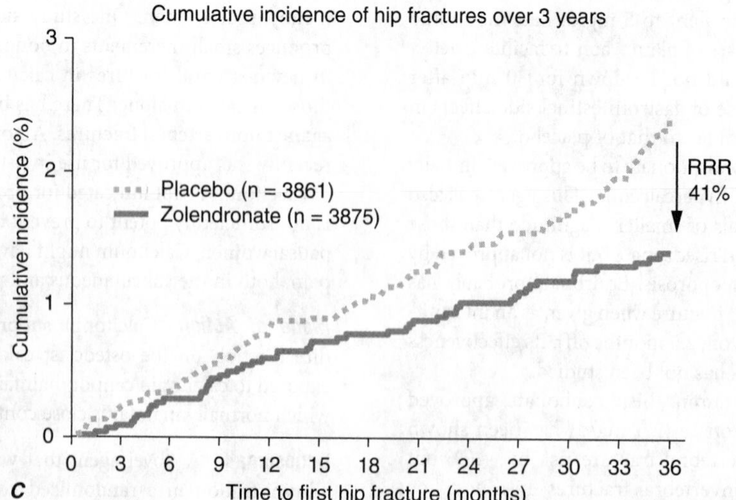

Figure 354-9 Effects of various bisphosphonates on clinical vertebral fractures **A.**, nonvertebral fractures **B.**, and hip fractures **C.** Plb, placebo; RRR, relative rish reduction. (*After DM Black et al: J Clin Endocrinol Metab 85:4118, 2000; C Roux et al: Curr Med Res Opin 4:433, 2004; CH Chesnut et al: J Bone Miner Res 19: 1241, 2004; DM Black et al: N Engl J Med 356:1809, 2007; JT Harrington et al: Calcif Tissue Int 74:129, 2003.*)

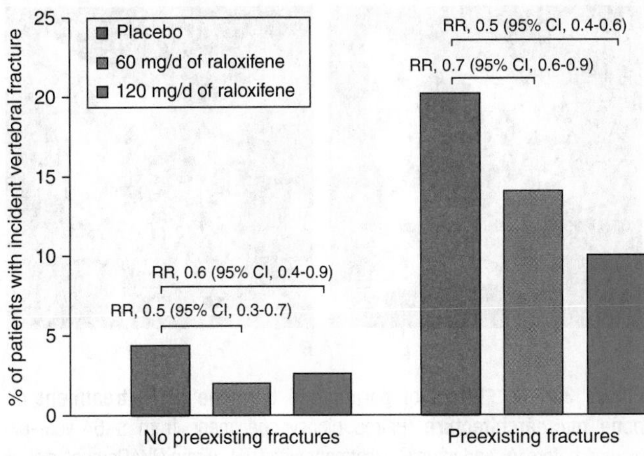

Figure 354-10 Effects of two doses of raloxifene on incident vertebral fractures in the MORE trial. *(After B Ettinger et al: JAMA:282:637, 1999.)*

20%, respectively (Fig. 354-11). Other clinical trials indicate ability to increase bone mass in postmenopausal women with low bone mass (above osteoporosis range) and in postmenopausal women with breast cancer treated with hormonal agents. Furthermore, a study of men with prostate cancer treated with gonadotropin-releasing hormone (GnRH) agonist therapy indicated the ability of denosumab to improve bone mass and reduce vertebral fracture occurrence. Denosumab was approved by the FDA in 2010 for the treatment of postmenopausal women who have a high risk for osteoporotic fractures, including those with a history of fracture or multiple risk factors for fracture, and those who have failed or are intolerant to other osteoporosis therapy.

Mode of Action Denosumab is a fully human monoclonal antibody to RANKL, the final common effector of osteoclast formation, activity, and survival. Denosumab binds to RANKL, inhibiting its ability to initiate formation of mature osteoclasts from osteoclast precursors and to bring mature osteoclasts to the bone surface and initiate bone resorption. Denosumab also plays a role in reducing the survival of the osteoclast. Through these actions on the osteoclast, denosumab induces potent antiresorptive action, as assessed biochemically and histomorphometrically, and may contribute to the occurrence of ONJ. Serious adverse reactions include hypocalcemia, infections, and dermatologic reactions such as dermatitis, rashes, and eczema.

Parathyroid Hormone Endogenous PTH is an 84-amino-acid peptide that is largely responsible for calcium homeostasis (Chap. 353). Although chronic elevation of PTH, as occurs in hyperparathyroidism, is associated with bone loss (particularly cortical bone), PTH also can exert anabolic effects on bone. Consistent with this, some observational studies have indicated that mild elevations in PTH are associated with maintenance of trabecular bone mass. On the basis of these findings, several clinical trials have been performed using an exogenous PTH analogue (1-34hPTH; teriparatide) that has been approved for the treatment of established osteoporosis in both men and women. The first randomized controlled trial in postmenopausal women showed that PTH, when superimposed on ongoing estrogen therapy, produced substantial increments in bone mass (13% over a 3-year period compared with estrogen alone) and reduced the risk of vertebral compression deformity. In the pivotal study (median, 19 months' duration), 20 μg PTH(1–34) daily by SC injection reduced vertebral fractures by 65% and nonvertebral fractures by 45% (Fig. 354-12). Treatment is administered as a single daily injection given for a maximum of 2 years. Teriparatide

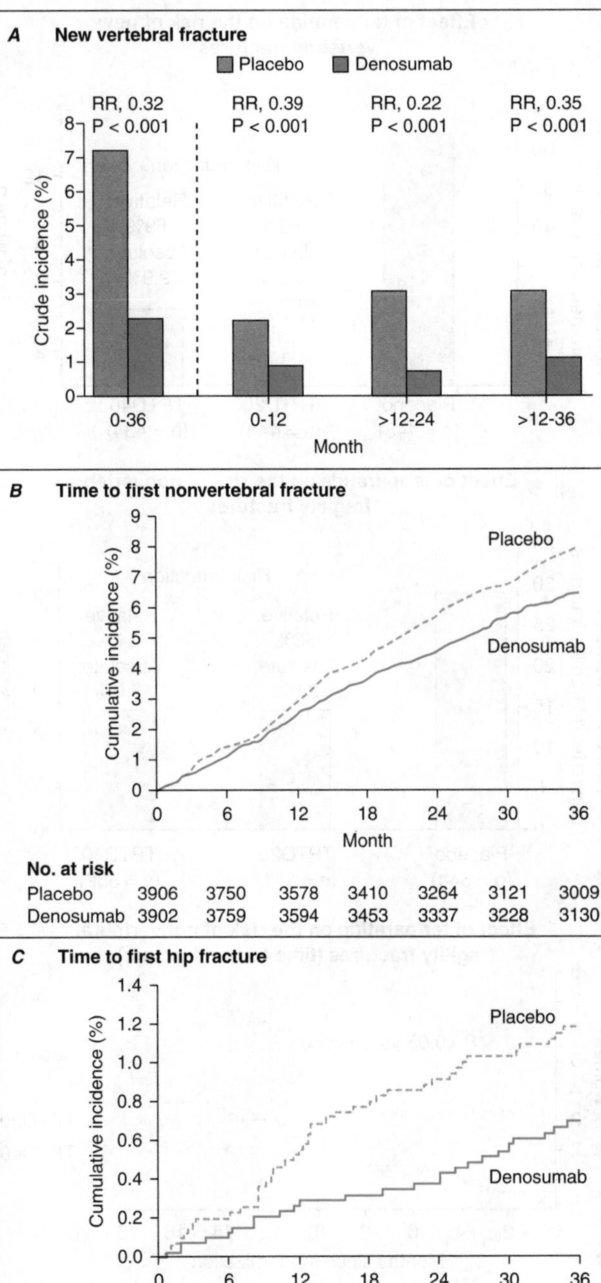

Figure 354-11 Effects of denosumab on new vertebral fractures ***A.*** and times to nonvertebral and hip fracture ***B.*** and ***C.*** *(After SR Cummings et al: N Engl J Med:361:756, 2009.)*

produces increases in bone mass and mediates architectural improvements in skeletal structure. These effects are lower when patients have been exposed previously to bisphosphonates, possibly in proportion to the potency of the antiresorptive effect. When 1–34hPTH is being considered for treatment-naive patients, it is best administered as monotherapy and followed by an antiresorptive agent such as a bisphosphonate.

Side effects of teriparatide are generally mild and can include muscle pain, weakness, dizziness, headache, and nausea. Rodents given prolonged treatment with PTH in relatively high doses developed osteogenic sarcomas. One case of osteosarcoma has

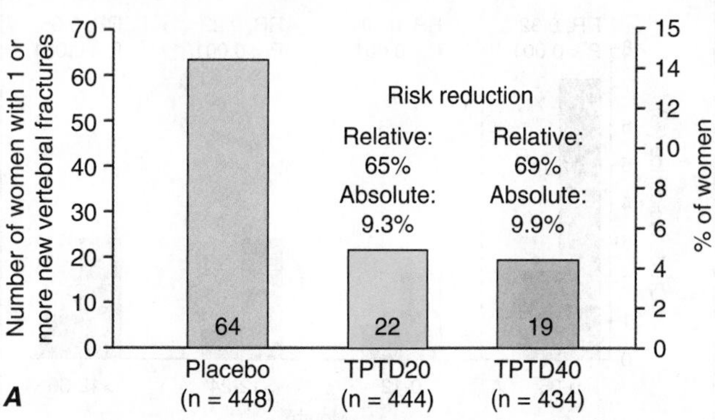

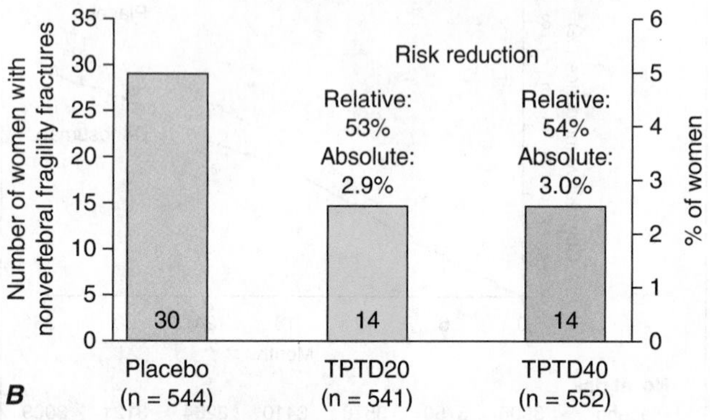

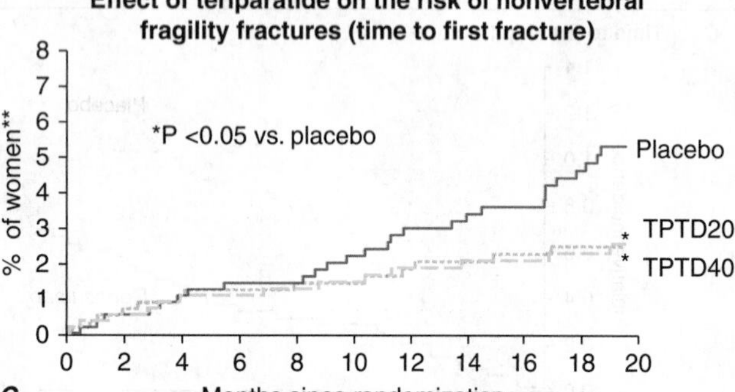

Figure 354-12 Effects of teriparatide on new vertebral fractures ***A.*** and nonvertebral fragility fractures ***B.*** and ***C.*** *(After RM Neer et al: N Engl J Med 344:1434, 2001.)*

been described in a patient treated with teriparatide. At present this seems to equate to the background incidence of osteosarcoma in this population.

PTH use may be limited by its mode of administration; alternative modes of delivery are being investigated. The optimal frequency of administration also remains to be established, and it is possible that PTH might be effective when used intermittently. Cost also may be a limiting factor.

Mode of Action Exogenously administered PTH appears to have direct actions on osteoblast activity, with biochemical and histomorphometric evidence of de novo bone formation early in response to PTH, before activation of bone resorption. Subsequently, PTH activates bone remodeling but still appears to favor bone formation over bone resorption. PTH stimulates IGF-I and collagen production and appears to increase osteoblast number by stimulating replication, enhancing osteoblast recruitment, and inhibiting apoptosis. Unlike all other treatments, PTH produces a true increase in bone tissue and an apparent restoration of bone microarchitecture (Fig. 354-13).

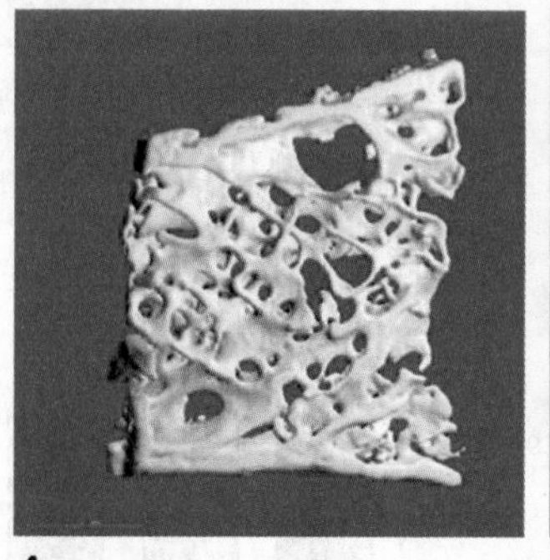

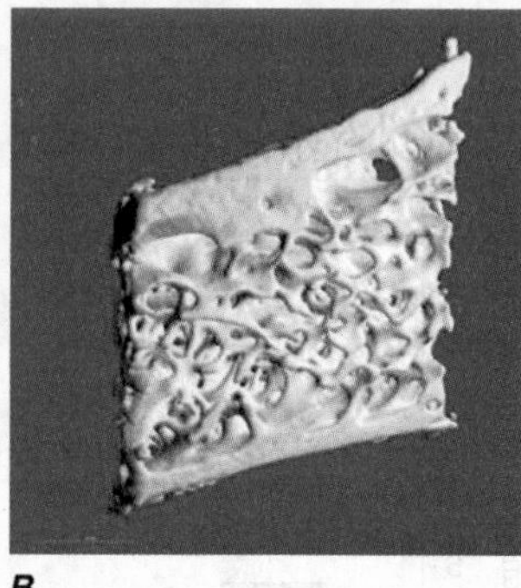

Figure 354-13 Effect of parathyroid hormone (PTH) treatment on bone microarchitecture. Paired biopsy specimens from a 64-year-old woman before ***A.*** and after ***B.*** treatment with PTH. *(From DW Dempster et al: J Bone Miner Res 16:1846, 2001.)*

Fluoride Fluoride has been available for many years and is a potent stimulator of osteoprogenitor cells when studied in vitro. It has been used in multiple osteoporosis studies with conflicting results, in part because of the use of varying doses and preparations. Despite increments in bone mass of up to 10%, there are no consistent effects of fluoride on vertebral or nonvertebral fracture; the latter may actually increase when high doses of fluoride are used. Fluoride remains an experimental agent despite its long history and multiple studies.

Strontium Ranelate Strontium ranelate is approved in several European countries for the treatment of osteoporosis. It increases bone mass throughout the skeleton; in clinical trials, the drug reduced the risk of vertebral fractures by 37% and that of nonvertebral fractures by 14%. It appears to be modestly antiresorptive while at the same time not causing as much of a decrease in bone formation (measured biochemically). Strontium is incorporated into hydroxyapatite, replacing calcium, a feature that might explain some of its fracture benefits. Small increased risks of venous thrombosis, seizures, and abnormal cognition have been seen and require further study.

Other Potential Anabolic Agents Several small studies of growth hormone (GH), alone or in combination with other agents, have not shown consistent or substantial positive effects on skeletal mass. Many of these studies have been relatively short term, and the effects of GH, growth hormone–releasing hormone, and the IGFs are still under investigation. Anabolic steroids, mostly derivatives of testosterone, act primarily as antiresorptive agents to reduce bone turnover but also may stimulate osteoblastic activity. Effects on bone mass remain unclear but appear weak in general, and use is limited by masculinizing side effects. Several recent observational studies suggest that the statin drugs, which currently are used to treat hypercholesterolemia, may be associated with increased bone mass and reduced fractures, but conclusions from clinical trials are mixed.

NONPHARMACOLOGIC APPROACHES Protective pads worn around the outer thigh, which cover the trochanteric region of the hip, can prevent hip fractures in elderly residents in nursing homes. The use of hip protectors is limited largely by issues of compliance and comfort, but new devices are being developed that may circumvent these problems and provide adjunctive treatments.

Kyphoplasty and *vertebroplasty* are also useful nonpharmacologic approaches for the treatment of painful vertebral fractures. However, no long-term data are available.

TREATMENT MONITORING There are currently no well-accepted guidelines for monitoring treatment of osteoporosis. Because most osteoporosis treatments produce small or moderate bone mass increments on average, it is reasonable to consider BMD as a monitoring tool. Changes must exceed ~4% in the spine and 6% in the hip to be considered significant in any individual. The hip is the preferred site due to larger surface area and greater reproducibility. Medication-induced increments may require several years to produce changes of this magnitude (if they do at all). Consequently, it can be argued that BMD should be repeated at intervals >2 years. Only significant BMD reductions should prompt a change in medical regimen, as it is expected that many individuals will not show responses greater than the detection limits of the current measurement techniques.

Biochemical markers of bone turnover may prove useful for treatment monitoring, but little hard evidence currently supports this concept; it remains unclear which endpoint is most useful. If bone turnover markers are used, a determination should be made before therapy is started and repeated ≥4 months after therapy is initiated. In general, a change in bone turnover markers must be 30–40% lower than the baseline to be significant because of the biologic and technical variability in these tests. A positive change in biochemical markers and/or bone density can be useful to help patients adhere to treatment regimens.

GLUCOCORTICOID-INDUCED OSTEOPOROSIS

Osteoporotic fractures are a well-characterized consequence of the hypercortisolism associated with Cushing's syndrome. However, the therapeutic use of glucocorticoids is by far the most common form of glucocorticoid-induced osteoporosis. Glucocorticoids are used widely in the treatment of a variety of disorders, including chronic lung disorders, rheumatoid arthritis, and other connective tissue diseases, inflammatory bowel disease, and after transplantation. Osteoporosis and related fractures are serious side effects of chronic glucocorticoid therapy. Because the effects of glucocorticoids on the skeleton are often superimposed on the consequences of aging and menopause, it is not surprising that women and the elderly are most frequently affected. The skeletal response to steroids is remarkably heterogeneous, however, and even young, growing individuals treated with glucocorticoids can present with fractures.

The risk of fractures depends on the dose and duration of glucocorticoid therapy, although recent data suggest that there may be no completely safe dose. Bone loss is more rapid during the early months of treatment, and trabecular bone is affected more severely than cortical bone. As a result, fractures have been shown to increase within 3 months of steroid treatment. There is an increase in fracture risk in both the axial skeleton and the appendicular skeleton, including risk of hip fracture. Bone loss can occur with any route of steroid administration, including high-dose inhaled glucocorticoids and intraarticular injections. Alternate-day delivery does not appear to ameliorate the skeletal effects of glucocorticoids.

PATHOPHYSIOLOGY

Glucocorticoids increase bone loss by multiple mechanisms, including (1) inhibition of osteoblast function and an increase in osteoblast apoptosis, resulting in impaired synthesis of new bone; (2) stimulation of bone resorption, probably as a secondary effect; (3) impairment of the absorption of calcium across the intestine, probably by a vitamin D–independent effect; (4) increase of urinary calcium loss and perhaps induction of some degree of secondary hyperparathyroidism; (5) reduction of adrenal androgens and suppression of ovarian and testicular secretion of estrogens and androgens; and (6) induction of glucocorticoid myopathy, which may exacerbate effects on skeletal and calcium homeostasis as well as increase the risk of falls.

EVALUATION OF THE PATIENT

Because of the prevalence of glucocorticoid-induced bone loss, it is important to evaluate the status of the skeleton in all patients starting or already receiving long-term glucocorticoid therapy. Modifiable risk factors should be identified, including those for falls. Examination should include testing of height and muscle strength. Laboratory evaluation should include an assessment of 24-h urinary calcium. All patients on long-term (>3 months) glucocorticoids should have measurement of bone mass at both the spine and the hip using DXA. If only one skeletal site can be measured, it is best to assess the spine in individuals <60 years and the hip in those >60 years.

PREVENTION

Bone loss caused by glucocorticoids can be prevented, and the risk of fractures significantly reduced. Strategies must include using the lowest dose of glucocorticoid for disease management. Topical and inhaled routes of administration are preferred, where appropriate. Risk factor reduction is important, including smoking cessation, limitation of alcohol consumption, and participation in weight-bearing exercise, when appropriate. All patients should receive an adequate calcium and vitamin D intake from the diet or from supplements.

TREATMENT Glucocorticoid-Induced Osteoporosis

Only bisphosphonates have been demonstrated in large clinical trials to reduce the risk of fractures in patients being treated with glucocorticoids. Risedronate prevents bone loss and reduces vertebral fracture risk by ~70%. Similar beneficial effects are observed in studies of alendronate. Controlled trials of hormone therapy have shown bone-sparing effects, and calcitonin also has some protective effect in the spine. Thiazides reduce urine calcium loss, but their role in prevention of fractures is unclear. PTH has been studied in a small group of women with glucocorticoid-induced osteoporosis, among whom bone mass increased substantially, and teriparatide is being investigated in a larger multicenter trial.

FURTHER READINGS

Bischoff-Ferrari HA et al: Benefit-risk assessment of vitamin D supplementation. Osteoporos Int 21:1121, 2010

Bolognese MA: SERMS and SERMS with estrogens for postmenopausal osteoporosis. Rev Endocr Metab Disord 11:253, 2010

Cosman F: Parathyroid hormone treatment for osteoporosis. Curr Opin Endocrinol Diabetes Obes 15:495, 2008

Cummings SR et al: FREEDOM Trial: Denosumab for prevention of fractures in postmenopausal women with osteoporosis. N Engl J Med 361:756, 2009

Ettinger B et al: Updated fracture incidence rates for the US version of FRAX. Osteoporos Int 2010 21:25, 2009

Khosla S: Update on estrogens and the skeleton. J Clin Endocrinol Metab 95:3569, 2010

Lyles KW et al: Zolendroic acid and clinical fractures and mortality after hip fracture. N Engl J Med 357:1799, 2007

Tucker KL: Osteoporosis prevention and nutrition. Current Curr Osteoporos Rep 7:111, 2009

CHAPTER 355

Paget's Disease and Other Dysplasias of Bone

Murray J. Favus
Tamara J. Vokes

PAGET'S DISEASE OF BONE

Paget's disease is a localized bone-remodeling disorder that affects widespread, noncontiguous areas of the skeleton. The pathologic process is initiated by overactive osteoclastic bone resorption followed by a compensatory increase in osteoblastic new bone formation, resulting in a structurally disorganized mosaic of woven and lamellar bone. Pagetic bone is expanded, less compact, and more vascular; thus, it is more susceptible to deformities and fractures. Although most patients are asymptomatic, symptoms resulting directly from bony involvement (bone pain, secondary arthritis, fractures) or secondarily from the expansion of bone causing compression of surrounding neural tissue are not uncommon.

Epidemiology

There is a marked geographic variation in the frequency of Paget's disease, with high prevalence in Western Europe (Great Britain, France, and Germany, but not Switzerland or Scandinavia) and among those who have immigrated to Australia, New Zealand, South Africa, and North and South America. The disease is rare in native populations of the Americas, Africa, Asia, and the Middle East; when it does occur, the affected subjects usually have evidence of European ancestry, supporting the migration theory. For unclear reasons, the prevalence and severity of Paget's disease are decreasing, and the age of diagnosis is increasing.

The prevalence is greater in males and increases with age. Autopsy series reveal Paget's disease in about 3% of those over age 40. Prevalence of positive skeletal radiographs in patients over age 55 is 2.5% for men and 1.6% for women. Elevated alkaline phosphatase (ALP) levels in asymptomatic patients have an age-adjusted incidence of 12.7 and 7 per 100,000 person-years in men and women, respectively.

Etiology

The etiology of Paget's disease of bone remains unknown, but evidence supports both genetic and viral etiologies. A positive family history is found in 15–25% of patients and, when present, raises the prevalence of the disease seven- to tenfold among first-degree relatives.

A clear genetic basis has been established for several rare familial bone disorders that clinically and radiographically resemble Paget's disease but have more severe presentation and earlier onset. A homozygous deletion of the *TNFRSF11B* gene, which encodes osteoprotegrin (Fig. 355-1), causes *juvenile Paget's disease,* also known as *familial idiopathic hypophosphatasia*, a disorder characterized by uncontrolled osteoclastic differentiation and resorption. Familial patterns of disease in several large kindred are consistent with an autosomal-dominant pattern of inheritance with variable

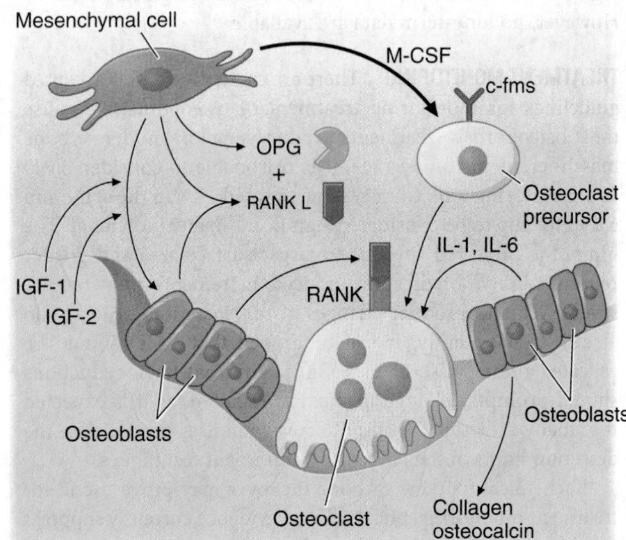

Figure 355-1 Diagram illustrating factors that promote differentiation and function of osteoclasts and osteoblasts and the role of the RANK pathway. Stromal bone marrow (mesenchymal) cells and differentiated osteoblasts produce multiple growth factors and cytokines, including macrophage colony-stimulating factor (M-CSF), to modulate osteoclastogenesis. RANKL (receptor activator of NFκB ligand) is produced by osteoblast progenitors and mature osteoblasts and can bind to a soluble decoy receptor known as OPG (osteoprotegerin) to inhibit RANKL action. Alternatively, a cell-cell interaction between osteoblast and osteoclast progenitors allows RANKL to bind to its membrane-bound receptor, RANK, thereby stimulating osteoclast differentiation and function. RANK binds intracellular proteins called TRAFs (tumor necrosis factor receptor–associated factors) that mediate receptor signaling through transcription factors such as NFκB. M-CSF binds to its receptor, c-fms, which is the cellular homologue of the *fms* oncogene. See text for the potential role of these pathways in disorders of osteoclast function such as Paget's disease and osteopetrosis.

penetrance. *Familial expansile osteolysis, expansile skeletal hyperphosphatasia, and early-onset Paget's disease* are associated with mutations in *TNFRSF11A* gene, which encodes RANK (receptor activator of nuclear factor-κB), a member of the tumor-necrosis factor superfamily critical for osteoclast differentiation (Fig. 355-1). Finally, mutations in the gene for valosin-containing protein cause a rare syndrome with autosomal-dominant inheritance and variable penetrance known as *inclusion body myopathy with Paget's disease and frontotemporal dementia (IBMPFD).* The role of genetic factors is less clear in the more common form of late-onset Paget's disease. Although a few families with mutations in the gene encoding RANK have been reported, the most common mutations identified in familial and sporadic cases of Paget's disease have been in the *SQSTM1* gene (sequestasome-1 or p62 protein) in the C-terminal ubiquitin-binding domain. The p62 protein is involved in NF-κB signaling and regulates osteoclastic differentiation. The phenotypic variability in patients with *SQSTM1* mutations suggests that additional factors, such as other genetic influences or viral infection, may influence clinical expression of the disease.

Several lines of evidence suggest that a viral infection may contribute to the clinical manifestations of Paget disease, including (1) the presence of cytoplasmic and nuclear inclusions resembling paramyxoviruses (measles and respiratory syncytial virus) in pagetic osteoclasts and (2) viral mRNA in precursor and mature osteoclasts. The viral etiology is further supported by conversion of osteoclast precursors to pagetic-like osteoclasts by vectors containing the measles virus nucleocapsid or matrix genes. However, the viral etiology has been questioned by the inability to culture a live virus from pagetic bone and by failure to clone the full-length viral genes from material obtained from patients with Paget's disease.

Pathophysiology

The principal abnormality in Paget's disease is the increased number and activity of osteoclasts. Pagetic osteoclasts are large, increased 10- to 100-fold in number and have a greater number of nuclei (as many as 100 compared to 3–5 nuclei in the normal osteoclast). The overactive osteoclasts may create a sevenfold increase in resorptive surfaces and an erosion rate of 9 μg/day (normal is 1 μg/day). Several causes for the increased number and activity of pagetic osteoclasts have been identified: (1) osteoclastic precursors are hypersensitive to $1,25(OH)_2D_3$; (2) osteoclasts are hyperresponsive to RANK ligand (RANKL), the osteoclast stimulatory factor that mediates the effects of most osteotropic factors on osteoclast formation; (3) marrow stromal cells from pagetic lesions have increased RANKL expression; (4) osteoclast precursor recruitment is increased by interleukin (IL) 6, which is increased in the blood of patients with active Paget disease and is overexpressed in pagetic osteoclasts; (5) expression of the proto-oncogene *c-fos*, which increases osteoclastic activity, is increased; and (6) the antiapoptotic oncogene *Bcl-2* in pagetic bone is overexpressed. Numerous osteoblasts are recruited to active resorption sites and produce large amounts of new bone matrix. As a result, bone turnover is high, and bone mass is normal or increased, not reduced, unless there is concomitant deficiency of calcium and/or vitamin D.

The characteristic feature of Paget's disease is increased bone resorption accompanied by accelerated bone formation. An initial osteolytic phase involves prominent bone resorption and marked hypervascularization. Radiographically, this manifests as an advancing lytic wedge, or "blade of grass" lesion. The second phase is a period of very active bone formation and resorption that replaces normal lamellar bone with haphazard (woven) bone. Fibrous connective tissue may replace normal bone marrow. In the final sclerotic phase, bone resorption declines progressively and leads to a hard, dense, less vascular pagetic or mosaic bone, which represents the so-called burned-out phase of Paget's disease. All three phases may be present at the same time at different skeletal sites.

Clinical manifestations

Diagnosis is often made in asymptomatic patients because they have elevated ALP levels on routine blood chemistry testing or an abnormality on a skeletal radiograph obtained for another indication. The skeletal sites most commonly involved are the pelvis, vertebral bodies, skull, femur, and tibia. Familial cases with an early presentation often have numerous active sites of skeletal involvement.

The most common presenting symptom is pain, which may result from increased bony vascularity, expanding lytic lesions, fractures, bowing, or other deformities. Bowing of the femur or tibia causes gait abnormalities and abnormal mechanical stresses with secondary osteoarthritis of the hip or knee joints. Long bone bowing also causes extremity pain by stretching the muscles attached to the bone softened by the pagetic process. Back pain results from enlarged pagetic vertebrae, vertebral compression fractures, spinal stenosis, degenerative changes of the joints, and altered body mechanics with kyphosis and forward tilt of the upper back. Rarely, spinal cord compression may result from bone enlargement or from the vascular steal syndrome. Skull involvement may cause headaches, symmetric or asymmetric enlargement of the parietal or frontal bones (frontal bossing), and increased head size. Cranial expansion may narrow cranial foramens and cause neurologic complications including hearing loss from cochlear nerve damage from temporal bone involvement, cranial nerve palsies, and softening of the base of the skull (*platybasia*) with the risk of brainstem compression. Pagetic involvement of the facial bones may cause facial deformity; loss of teeth and other dental conditions; and, rarely, airway compression.

Fractures are serious complications of Paget's disease and usually occur in long bones at areas of active or advancing lytic lesions. Common fracture sites are the femoral shaft and subtrochanteric regions. Neoplasms arising from pagetic bone are rare. The incidence of sarcoma appears to be decreasing, possibly because of earlier, more effective treatment with potent antiresorptive agents. The majority of tumors are osteosarcomas, which usually present with new pain in a long-standing pagetic lesion. Osteoclast-rich benign giant cell tumors may arise in areas adjacent to pagetic bone, and they respond to glucocorticoid therapy.

Cardiovascular complications may occur in patients with involvement of large (15–35%) portions of the skeleton and a high degree of disease activity (ALP four times above normal). The extensive arteriovenous shunting and marked increases in blood flow through the vascular pagetic bone lead to a high-output state and cardiac enlargement. However, high-output heart failure is relatively rare and usually develops in patients with concomitant cardiac pathology. In addition, calcific aortic stenosis and diffuse vascular calcifications have been associated with Paget's disease.

Diagnosis

The diagnosis may be suggested on clinical examination by the presence of an enlarged skull with frontal bossing, bowing of an extremity, or short stature with simian posturing. An extremity with an area of warmth and tenderness to palpation may suggest an underlying pagetic lesion. Other findings include bony deformity of the pelvis, skull, spine, and extremities; arthritic involvement of the joints adjacent to lesions; and leg-length discrepancy resulting from deformities of the long bones.

Paget's disease is usually diagnosed from radiologic and biochemical abnormalities. Radiographic findings typical of Paget's disease include enlargement or expansion of an entire bone or area of a long bone, cortical thickening, coarsening of trabecular markings, and typical lytic and sclerotic changes. Skull radiographs (Fig. 355-2) reveal regions of "cotton wool," or osteoporosis circumscripta, thickening of diploic areas, and enlargement and sclerosis of a portion or all of one or more skull bones. Vertebral cortical thickening of the superior and inferior end plates creates a "picture frame" vertebra. Diffuse radiodense enlargement of a vertebra is referred to as "ivory vertebra." Pelvic radiographs may demonstrate disruption or fusion of the sacroiliac joints; porotic and radiodense lesions of the ilium with whorls of coarse trabeculation; thickened and sclerotic iliopectineal line (brim sign); and softening with protrusio acetabuli, with axial migration of the hips and functional flexion contracture. Radiographs of long bones reveal bowing deformity and typical pagetic changes of cortical thickening and expansion and areas of lucency and sclerosis (Fig. 355-3). Radionuclide ^{99m}Tc bone scans are less specific but are more sensitive than standard radiographs for identifying sites of active skeletal lesions. Although CT and MRI studies are not necessary in most cases, CT may be useful for the assessment of possible fracture and MRI is necessary to assess the possibility of sarcoma, giant cell tumor, or metastatic disease in pagetic bone. Definitive diagnosis of malignancy often requires bone biopsy.

Biochemical evaluation is useful in the diagnosis and management of Paget disease. The marked increase in bone turnover can be monitored using biochemical markers of bone formation and resorption. The parallel rise in markers of bone formation and resorption confirms the coupling of bone formation and resorption in Paget's

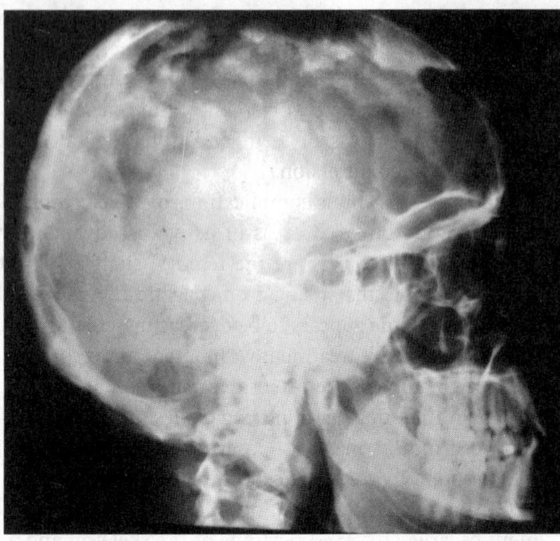

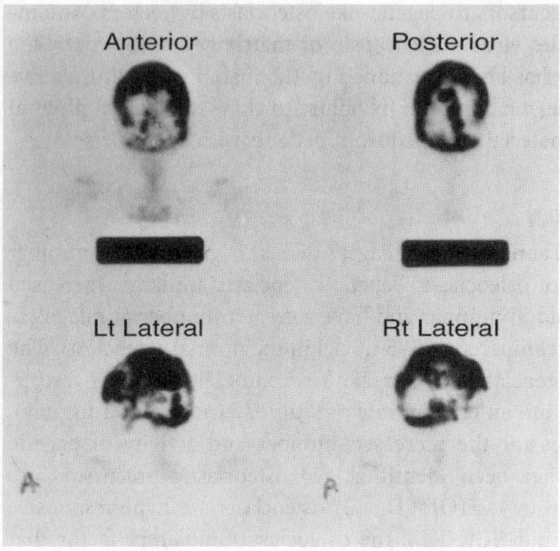

Figure 355-2 A 48-year-old woman with Paget's disease of the skull. ***Left.*** Lateral radiograph showing areas of both bone resorption and sclerosis. ***Right.*** ^{99m}Tc HDP bone scan with anterior, posterior, and lateral views of the skull showing diffuse isotope uptake by the frontal, parietal, occipital, and petrous bones.

disease. The degree of bone-marker elevation reflects the extent and severity of the disease. Patients with the highest elevation of ALP (10 times the upper limit of normal) typically have involvement of the skull and at least one other skeletal site. Lower values suggest less extensive involvement or a quiescent phase of the disease. For most patients, serum total ALP remains the test of choice both for diagnosis and assessing response to therapy. Occasionally, a symptomatic patient with evidence of progression at a single site may have a normal total ALP level but increased bone-specific ALP. For unclear reasons, serum osteocalcin, another marker of bone formation, is not always elevated and is not recommended for use in diagnosis or management of Paget's disease. Bone-resorption markers (serum or urine N-telopeptide or C-telopeptide measured in the blood or urine) are also elevated in active Paget's disease and decrease more rapidly in response to therapy than does ALP.

Serum calcium and phosphate levels are normal in Paget's disease. Immobilization of a patient with active Paget's disease may rarely cause hypercalcemia and hypercalciuria and increase the risk for nephrolithiasis. However, the discovery of hypercalcemia, even in the presence of immobilization, should prompt a search for another cause of hypercalcemia. In contrast, hypocalcemia or mild secondary hyperparathyroidism may develop in Paget patients with very active bone formation and insufficient dietary calcium intake, particularly during bisphosphonate therapy when bone resorption is rapidly suppressed and active bone formation continues. Therefore, adequate calcium and vitamin D intake should be instituted prior to administration of bisphosphonates.

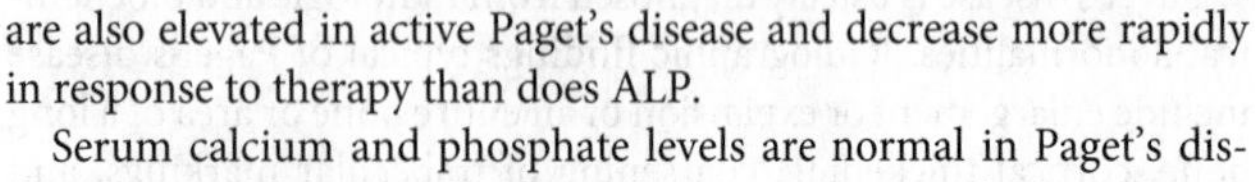

Figure 355-3 Radiograph of a 73-year-old man with Paget's disease of the right proximal femur. Note the coarsening of the trabecular pattern with marked cortical thickening and narrowing of the joint space consistent with osteoarthritis secondary to pagetic deformity of the right femur.

TREATMENT Paget's Disease of Bone

The development of effective and potent pharmacologic agents (Table 355-1) has changed the treatment philosophy from treating only symptomatic patients to treating asymptomatic patients who are at risk for complications. Pharmacologic therapy is indicated in the following circumstances: to control symptoms caused by metabolically active Paget's disease such as bone pain, fracture, headache, pain from pagetic radiculopathy or arthropathy, or neurologic complications; to decrease local blood flow and minimize operative blood loss in patients who need surgery at an active pagetic site; to reduce hypercalciuria that may occur during immobilization; and to decrease the risk of complications when disease activity is high (elevated ALP) and when the site of involvement involves weight-bearing bones, areas adjacent to major joints, vertebral bodies, and the skull. Whether or not early therapy prevents late complications remains to be determined. A recent randomized study of over 1200 patients from the UK showed no difference in bone pain, fracture rates, quality of life, and hearing loss between patients who received pharmacologic therapy to control symptoms (bone pain) and those receiving bisphosphonates to normalize serum ALP. However, the most potent agent (zoledronic acid) was not used and the duration of observation (mean of 3 years with a range of 2 to 5 years) may not be long enough to assess the impact of treatment on long-term outcomes. It seems likely that the restoration of normal bone architecture following suppression of pagetic activity will prevent further deformities and complications.

Agents approved for treatment of Paget's disease suppress the very high rates of bone resorption and secondarily decrease

TABLE 355-1 Pharmacologic Agents Approved for Treatment of Paget's Disease

Name (Brand)	Dose and Mode of Delivery	Normalization of ALP
Zoledronate (Zometa)	5 mg IV over 15 min	90% of patients at 6 mo
Pamidronate (Aredia)	30 mg IV/d over 4 h on 3 days	~50% of patients
Risedronate (Actonel)	30 mg PO/d for 2 mo	73% of patients
Alendronate (Fosamax)	40 mg PO/d for 6 mo	63% of patients
Tiludronate (Skelid)	800 mg PO daily for 3 mo	35% of patients
Etidronate (Didronel)	200–400 mg PO/d x 6 mo	15% of patients
Calcitonin (Miacalcin)	100 U SC daily for 6–18 mo (may reduce to 50 U 3 times per wk)	(Reduction of ALP by to 50%)

the high rates of bone formation (Table 355-1). As a result of decreasing bone turnover, pagetic structural patterns, including areas of poorly mineralized woven bone, are replaced by more normal cancellous or lamellar bone. Reduced bone turnover can be documented by a decline in serum ALP and urine or serum resorption markers (N-telopeptide, C-telopeptide).

The first clinically useful agent, etidronate, is now rarely used because the doses required to suppress bone resorption may impair mineralization, necessitating that the drug be given for a maximum of 6 months followed by a 6-month drug-free period. The second-generation oral bisphosphonates—tiludronate, alendronate, and risedronate—are more potent than etidronate in controlling bone turnover and, thus, induce a longer remission at a lower dose. The lower doses reduce the risks of impaired mineralization and osteomalacia. Oral bisphosphonates should be taken first thing in the morning on an empty stomach, followed by maintenance of upright posture with no food, drink, or other medications for 30–60 minutes. The efficacy of different agents, based on their ability to normalize or decrease ALP levels, is summarized in Table 355-1, although the response rates are not comparable because they are obtained from different studies.

Intravenous bisphosphonates approved for Paget's disease include pamidronate and zoledronic acid. Although the recommended dose for pamidronate is 30 mg dissolved in 500 mL of normal saline or dextrose IV over 4 h on three consecutive days, a more commonly used simpler regimen is a single infusion of 60–90 mg in patients with mild elevation of serum ALP and multiple 90-mg infusions in those with higher levels of ALP. In many patients, particularly those who have severe disease or need rapid normalization of bone turnover (neurologic symptoms, severe bone pain due to a lytic lesion, risk of an impending fracture, or pretreatment prior to elective surgery in an area of active disease), treatment with zoledronic acid is the first choice. It normalizes ALP in about 90% of patients by 6 months, and the therapeutic effect persists for at least 6 more months in most patients. About 10–20% of patients experience a flulike syndrome after the first infusion, which can be partly ameliorated by pretreatment with acetaminophen or NSAIDs. In patients with high bone turnover, vitamin D (400–800 IU daily) and calcium (500 mg three times daily) should be provided to prevent hypocalcemia and secondary hyperparathyroidism. Remission following treatment with IV bisphosphonates, particularly zoledronic acid, may persist for well over 1 year. Bisphosphonates should not be used in patients with renal insufficiency (glomerular filtration rate <35ml/min).

The subcutaneous injectable form of salmon calcitonin is approved for the treatment of Paget's disease. Intranasal calcitonin spray is approved for osteoporosis at a dose of 200 U/d; however, the efficacy of this dose in Paget's disease has not been thoroughly studied. The usual starting dose of injectable calcitonin (100 U/d) reduces ALP by 50% and may relieve skeletal symptoms. The dose may be reduced to 50 U/d three times weekly after an initial favorable response to 100 U daily; however, the lower dose may require long-term use to sustain efficacy. The common side effects of calcitonin therapy are nausea and facial flushing. Secondary resistance after prolonged use may be due to either the formation of anticalcitonin antibodies or downregulation of osteoclastic cell–surface calcitonin receptors. The lower potency and injectable mode of delivery make this agent a less-attractive treatment option that should be reserved for patients who either do not tolerate bisphosphonates or have a contraindication to their use.

SCLEROSING BONE DISORDERS

OSTEOPETROSIS

Osteopetrosis refers to a group of disorders caused by severe impairment of osteoclast-mediated bone resorption. Other terms that are often used include marble bone disease, which captures the solid x-ray appearance of the involved skeleton, and Albers-Schonberg disease, which refers to the milder, adult form of osteopetrosis also known as autosomal-dominant osteopetrosis type II. The major types of osteopetrosis include malignant (severe, infantile, autosomal recessive) osteopetrosis and benign (adult, autosomal dominant) osteopetrosis types I and II. A rare autosomal recessive intermediate form has a more benign prognosis. Autosomal recessive carbonic anhydrase (CA) II deficiency produces osteopetrosis of intermediate severity associated with renal tubular acidosis and cerebral calcification.

Etiology and genetics

Naturally occurring and gene-knockout animal models with phenotypes similar to those of the human disorders have been used to explore the genetic basis of osteopetrosis. The primary defect in osteopetrosis is the loss of osteoclastic bone resorption and preservation of normal osteoblastic bone formation. Osteoprotegerin (OPG) is a soluble decoy receptor that binds osteoblast-derived RANK ligand, which mediates osteoclast differentiation and activation (Fig. 355-1). Transgenic mice that overexpress OPG develop osteopetrosis, presumably by blocking RANK ligand. Mice deficient in RANK lack osteoclasts and develop severe osteopetrosis.

Recessive mutations of CA II prevent osteoclasts from generating an acid environment in the clear zone between its ruffled border and the adjacent mineral surface. Absence of CA II, therefore, impairs osteoclastic bone resorption. Other forms of human disease have less clear genetic defects. About one-half of the patients with malignant infantile osteopetrosis have a mutation in the *TCIRG1* gene encoding the osteoclast-specific subunit of the vacuolar proton pump, which mediates the acidification of the interface between bone mineral and the osteoclast ruffled border. Mutations in the *CICN7* chloride channel gene cause autosomal-dominant osteopetrosis type II.

Clinical presentation

The incidence of autosomal-recessive severe (malignant) osteopetrosis ranges from 1 in 200,000 to 1 in 500,000 live births. As bone and cartilage fail to undergo modeling, paralysis of one or more cranial nerves may occur due to narrowing of the cranial foramens. Failure of skeletal modeling also results in inadequate marrow space, leading to extramedullary hematopoiesis with hypersplenism and pancytopenia. Hypocalcemia due to lack of osteoclastic bone resorption may occur in infants and young children. The untreated infantile disease is fatal, often before age five.

Adult (benign) osteopetrosis is an autosomal-dominant disease that is usually diagnosed by the discovery of typical skeletal changes in young adults who undergo radiologic evaluation of a fracture. The prevalence is 1 in 100,000 to 1 in 500,000 adults. The course is not always benign, because fractures may be accompanied by loss of vision, deafness, psychomotor delay, mandibular osteomyelitis, and other complications usually associated with the juvenile form. In some kindred, nonpenetrance results in skip generations, while in other families, severely affected children are born into families with benign disease. The milder form of the disease does not usually require treatment.

Radiography

Typically, there are generalized symmetric increases in bone mass with thickening of both cortical and trabecular bone. Diaphyses and metaphyses are broadened, and alternating sclerotic and lucent bands may be seen in the iliac crests, at the ends of long bones, and in vertebral bodies. The cranium is usually thickened, particularly at the base of the skull, and the paranasal and mastoid sinuses are underpneumatized.

Laboratory findings

The only significant laboratory findings are elevated serum levels of osteoclast-derived tartrate-resistant acid phosphatase (TRAP) and the brain isoenzyme of creatine kinase. Serum calcium may be low in severe disease, and parathyroid hormone and 1,25-dihydroxyvitamin D levels may be elevated in response to hypocalcemia.

TREATMENT Osteopetrosis

Allogeneic HLA-identical bone marrow transplantation has been successful in some children. Following transplantation, the marrow contains progenitor cells and normally functioning osteoclasts. A cure is most likely when children are transplanted before age four. Marrow transplantation from nonidentical HLA-matched donors has a much higher failure rate. Limited studies in small numbers of patients have suggested variable benefits following treatment with interferon γ-1β, 1,25-dihydroxyvitamin D (which stimulates osteoclasts directly), methylprednisolone, and a low-calcium/high-phosphate diet.

Surgical intervention is indicated to decompress optic or auditory nerve compression. Orthopedic management is required for the surgical treatment of fractures and their complications including malunion and postfracture deformity.

PYKNODYSOSTOSIS

This is an autosomal-recessive form of osteosclerosis that is believed to have affected the French impressionist painter Henri de Toulouse-Lautrec. The molecular basis involves mutations in the gene that encodes cathepsin K, a lysosomal metalloproteinase highly expressed in osteoclasts and important for bone-matrix degradation. Osteoclasts are present but do not function normally. Pyknodysostosis is a form of short-limb dwarfism that presents with frequent fractures but usually a normal life span. Clinical features include short stature; kyphoscoliosis and deformities of the chest; high arched palate; proptosis; blue sclerae; dysmorphic features including small face and chin, frontooccipital prominence, pointed beaked nose, large cranium, and obtuse mandibular angle; and small, square hands with hypoplastic nails. Radiographs demonstrate a generalized increase in bone density, but in contrast to osteopetrosis, the long bones are normally shaped. Separated cranial sutures, including the persistent patency of the anterior fontanel, are characteristic of the disorder. There may also be hypoplasia of the sinuses, mandible, distal clavicles, and terminal phalanges. Persistence of deciduous teeth and sclerosis of the calvarium and base of the skull are also common. Histologic evaluation shows normal cortical bone architecture with decreased osteoblastic and osteoclastic activities. Serum chemistries are normal, and, unlike osteopetrosis, there is no anemia. There is no known treatment for this condition, and there are no reports of attempted bone marrow transplant.

PROGRESSIVE DIAPHYSEAL DYSPLASIA

Also known as *Camurati-Engelmann disease*, progressive diaphyseal dysplasia is an autosomal-dominant disorder that is characterized radiographically by diaphyseal hyperostosis and a symmetric thickening and increased diameter of the endosteal and periosteal surfaces of the diaphyses of the long bones, particularly the femur and tibia, and, less often, the fibula, radius, and ulna. The genetic defect responsible for the disease has been localized to the area of chromosome 19q13.2 encoding tumor growth factor (TGF)-β1. The mutation promotes activation of TGF-β1. The clinical severity is variable. The most common presenting symptoms are pain and tenderness of the involved areas, fatigue, muscle wasting, and gait disturbance. The weakness may be mistaken for muscular dystrophy. Characteristic body habitus includes thin limbs with little muscle mass yet prominent and palpable bones and, when the skull is involved, large head with prominent forehead and proptosis. Patients may also display signs of cranial nerve palsies, hydrocephalus, central hypogonadism, and Raynaud's phenomenon. Radiographically, patchy progressive endosteal and periosteal new bone formation is observed along the diaphyses of the long bones. Bone scintigraphy shows increased radiotracer uptake in involved areas.

Treatment with low-dose glucocorticoids relieves bone pain and may reverse the abnormal bone formation. Intermittent bisphosphonate therapy has produced clinical improvement in a limited number of patients.

HYPEROSTOSIS CORTICALIS GENERALISATA

This is also known as *van Buchem's disease*; it is an autosomal-recessive disorder characterized by endosteal hyperostosis in which osteosclerosis involves the skull, mandible, clavicles, and ribs. The major manifestations are due to narrowed cranial foramens with neural compressions that may result in optic atrophy, facial paralysis, and deafness. Adults may have an enlarged mandible. Serum ALP levels may be elevated, which reflect the uncoupled bone remodeling with high osteoblastic formation rates and low osteoclastic resorption. As a result, there is increased accumulation of normal bone. Endosteal hyperostosis with syndactyly, known as *sclerosteosis*, is a more severe form. The genetic defects for both sclerosteosis and van Buchem's disease have been assigned to the same region of the chromosome 17q12-q21. It is possible that both conditions may have deactivating mutations in the *BEER* (bone-expressed equilibrium regulator) gene.

MELORHEOSTOSIS

Melorheostosis (Greek, "flowing hyperostosis") may occur sporadically or follow a pattern consistent with an autosomal-recessive disorder. The major manifestation is progressive linear hyperostosis in one or more bones of one limb, usually a lower extremity. The name comes from the radiographic appearance of the involved bone, which resembles melted wax that has dripped down a candle. Symptoms appear during childhood as pain or stiffness in the area of sclerotic bone. There may be associated ectopic soft tissue masses, composed of cartilage or osseous tissue, and skin changes overlying the involved bone, consisting of scleroderma-like areas and hypertrichosis. The disease does not progress in adults, but pain and stiffness may persist. Laboratory tests are unremarkable. No specific etiology is known. There is no specific treatment. Surgical interventions to correct contractures are often unsuccessful.

OSTEOPOIKILOSIS

The literal translation of osteopoikilosis is "spotted bones"; it is a benign autosomal-dominant condition in which numerous small, variably shaped (usually round or oval) foci of bony sclerosis are seen in the epiphyses and adjacent metaphyses. The lesions may involve any bone except the skull, ribs, and vertebrae. They may be misidentified as metastatic lesions. The main differentiating points are that bony lesions of osteopoikilosis are stable over time and do not accumulate radionucleotide on bone scanning. In some kindred, osteopoikilosis is associated with connective tissue nevi known as *dermatofibrosis lenticularis disseminata*, also known as *Buschke-Ollendorff syndrome*. Histologic inspection reveals thickened but otherwise normal trabeculae and islands of normal cortical bone. No treatment is indicated.

HEPATITIS C–ASSOCIATED OSTEOSCLEROSIS

Hepatitis C–associated osteosclerosis (HCAO) is a rare acquired diffuse osteosclerosis in adults with prior hepatitis C infection. After a latent period of several years, patients develop diffuse appendicular bone pain and a generalized increase in bone mass with elevated serum ALP. Bone biopsy and histomorphometry reveal increased rates of bone formation, decreased bone resorption with a marked decrease in osteoclasts, and dense lamellar bone. One patient had increased serum OPG levels, and bone biopsy showed large numbers of osteoblasts positive for OPG and reduced osteoclast number. Empirical therapy includes pain control, and there may be beneficial response to either calcitonin or bisphosphonate.

DISORDERS ASSOCIATED WITH DEFECTIVE MINERALIZATION

HYPOPHOSPHATASIA

This is a rare inherited disorder that presents as rickets in infants and children or osteomalacia in adults with paradoxically low serum levels of ALP. The frequency of the severe neonatal and infantile forms is about 1 in 100,000 live births in Canada, where the disease is most common because of its high prevalence among Mennonites and Hutterites. It is rare in African Americans. The severity of the disease is remarkably variable, ranging from intrauterine death associated with profound skeletal hypomineralization at one extreme to premature tooth loss as the only manifestation in some adults. Severe cases are inherited in an autosomal-recessive manner, but the genetic patterns are less clear for the milder forms. The disease is caused by a deficiency of tissue nonspecific (bone/liver/kidney) ALP (TNSALP), which, although ubiquitous, results only in bone abnormalities. Protein levels and functions of the other ALP isozymes (germ cell, intestinal, placental) are normal. Defective ALP permits accumulation of its major naturally occurring substrates including phosphoethanolamine (PEA), inorganic pyrophosphate (PPi), and pyridoxal 5′-phosphate (PLP). The accumulation of PPi interferes with mineralization through its action as a potent inhibitor of hydroxyapatite crystal growth.

Perinatal hypophosphatasia becomes manifest during pregnancy and is often complicated by polyhydramnios and intrauterine death. The infantile form becomes clinically apparent before the age of 6 months with failure to thrive, rachitic deformities, functional craniosynostosis despite widely open fontanels (which are actually hypomineralized areas of the calvarium), raised intracranial pressure, and flail chest and predisposition to pneumonia. Hypercalcemia and hypercalciuria are common. This form has a mortality rate of about 50%. Prognosis seems to improve for the children who survive infancy. Childhood hypophosphatasia has variable clinical presentation. Premature loss of deciduous teeth (before age five) is the hallmark of the disease. Rickets causes delayed walking with waddling gait, short stature, and dolichocephalic skull with frontal bossing. The disease often improves during puberty but may recur in adult life. Adult hypophosphatasia presents during middle age with painful, poorly healing metatarsal stress fractures or thigh pain due to femoral pseudofractures.

Laboratory investigation reveals low ALP levels and normal or elevated levels of serum calcium and phosphorus despite clinical and radiologic evidence of rickets or osteomalacia. Serum parathyroid hormone, 25-hydroxyvitamin D, and 1,25-dihydroxyvitamin D levels are normal. The elevation of PLP is specific for the disease and may even be present in asymptomatic parents of severely affected children. Because vitamin B_6 increases PLP levels, vitamin B_6 supplements should be discontinued one week before testing.

There is no established medical therapy. In contrast to other forms of rickets and osteomalacia, calcium and vitamin D supplementation should be avoided because they may aggravate hypercalcemia and hypercalciuria. A low-calcium diet, glucocorticoids, and calcitonin have been used in a small number of patients with variable responses. Because fracture healing is poor, placement of intramedullary rods is best for acute fracture repair and for prophylactic prevention of fractures.

AXIAL OSTEOMALACIA

This is a rare disorder characterized by defective skeletal mineralization despite normal serum calcium and phosphate levels. Clinically, the disorder presents in middle-aged or elderly men with chronic axial skeletal discomfort. Cervical spine pain may also be present. Radiographic findings are mainly osteosclerosis due to coarsened trabecular patterns typical of osteomalacia. Spine, pelvis, and ribs are most commonly affected. Histologic changes show defective mineralization and flat, inactive osteoblasts. The primary defect appears to be an acquired defect in osteoblast function. The course is benign, and there is no established treatment. Calcium and vitamin D therapies are not effective.

FIBROGENESIS IMPERFECTA OSSIUM

This is a rare condition of unknown etiology. It presents in both sexes; in middle age or later; with progressive, intractable skeletal pain and fractures; worsening immobilization; and a debilitating course. Radiographic evaluation reveals generalized osteomalacia, osteopenia, and occasional pseudofractures. Histologic features include a tangled pattern of collagen fibrils with abundant osteoblasts and osteoclasts. There is no effective treatment. Spontaneous remission has been reported in a small number of patients. Calcium and vitamin D have not been beneficial.

FIBROUS DYSPLASIA AND McCUNE-ALBRIGHT SYNDROME

Fibrous dysplasia is a sporadic disorder characterized by the presence of one (monostotic) or more (polyostotic) expanding fibrous skeletal lesions composed of bone-forming mesenchyme. The association of the polyostotic form with café-au-lait spots and hyperfunction of an endocrine system such as pseudo-precocious puberty of ovarian origin is known as *McCune-Albright syndrome* (MAS). A spectrum of the phenotypes is caused by activating mutations in the *GNAS1* gene, which encodes the α subunit of the stimulatory G protein ($G_s\alpha$). As the postzygotic mutations occur at different stages of early development, the extent and type of tissue affected are variable and explain the mosaic pattern of skin and bone changes. GTP binding activates the $G_s\alpha$ regulatory protein and mutations in regions of $G_s\alpha$ that selectively inhibit GTPase activity, which results in constitutive stimulation of the cyclic AMP–protein kinase A signal transduction pathway. Such mutations of the $G_s\alpha$ protein–coupled receptor may cause autonomous function in bone (parathyroid hormone receptor); skin (melanocyte-stimulating hormone receptor); and various endocrine glands including ovary (follicle-stimulating hormone receptor), thyroid (thyroid-stimulating hormone receptor), adrenal (adrenocorticotropic hormone receptor), and pituitary (growth hormone–releasing hormone receptor). The skeletal lesions are composed largely of mesenchymal cells that do not differentiate into osteoblasts, resulting in the formation of imperfect bone. In some areas of bone, fibroblast-like cells develop features of osteoblasts in that they produce extracellular matrix that organizes into woven bone. Calcification may occur in some areas. In other areas, cells have features of chondrocytes and produce cartilage-like extracellular matrix.

Clinical presentation

Fibrous dysplasia occurs with equal frequency in both sexes, whereas MAS with precocious puberty is more common (10:1) in girls. The monostotic form is the most common and is usually diagnosed in patients between 20 and 30 years of age without associated skin lesions. The polyostotic form typically manifests in children <10 years old and may progress with age. Early-onset disease is generally more severe. Lesions may become quiescent in puberty and progress during pregnancy or with estrogen therapy. In polyostotic fibrous dysplasia, the lesions most commonly involve the maxilla and other craniofacial bones, ribs, and metaphyseal or diaphyseal portions of the proximal femur or tibia. Expanding bone lesions may cause pain, deformity, fractures, and nerve entrapment. Sarcomatous degeneration involving the facial bones or femur is infrequent (<1%). The risk of malignant transformation is increased by radiation, which has proven to be ineffective treatment. In rare patients with widespread lesions, renal phosphate wasting and hypophosphatemia may cause rickets or osteomalacia. Hypophosphatemia may be due to production of a phosphaturic factor by the abnormal fibrous tissue.

MAS patients may have café-au-lait spots, which are flat, hyperpigmented skin lesions that have rough borders ("coast of Maine") in contrast to the café-au-lait lesions of neurofibromatosis that have smooth borders ("coast of California"). The most common endocrinopathy is isosexual pseudoprecocious puberty in girls. Other less common endocrine disorders include thyrotoxicosis, Cushing's syndrome, acromegaly, hyperparathyroidism, hyperprolactinemia, and pseudoprecocious puberty in boys.

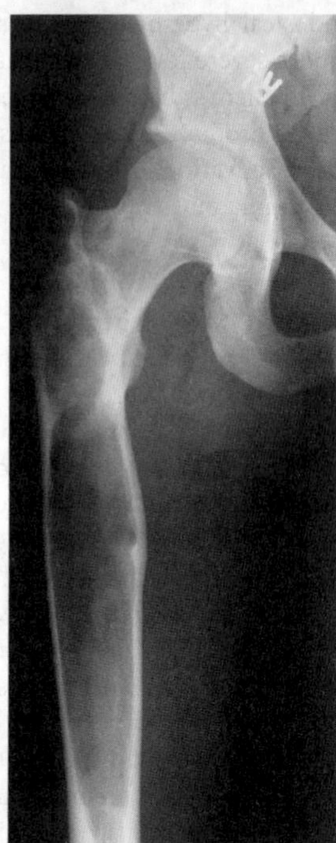

Figure 355-4 Radiograph of a 16-year-old male with fibrous dysplasia of the right proximal femur. Note the multiple cystic lesions, including the large lucent lesion in the proximal midshaft with scalloping of the interior surface. The femoral neck contains two lucent cystic lesions.

Radiographic findings

In long bones, the fibrous dysplastic lesions are typically well-defined, radiolucent areas with thin cortices and a ground-glass appearance. Lesions may be lobulated with trabeculated areas of radiolucency (Fig. 355-4). Involvement of facial bones usually presents as radiodense lesions, which may create a leonine appearance (leontiasis osea). Expansile cranial lesions may narrow foramens and cause optic lesions, reduce hearing, and create other manifestations of cranial nerve compression.

LABORATORY RESULTS

Serum ALP is occasionally elevated but calcium, parathyroid hormone, 25-hydroxyvitamin D, and 1,25-dihydroxyvitamin D levels are normal. Patients with extensive polyostotic lesions may have hypophosphatemia, hyperphosphaturia, and osteomalacia. The hypophosphatemia and phosphaturia are directly related to the levels of fibroblast growth factor 23 (FGF23). Biochemical markers of bone turnover may be elevated.

TREATMENT Fibrous Dysplasia and McCune-Albright Syndrome

Spontaneous healing of the lesions does not occur, and there is no established effective treatment. Improvement in bone pain and partial or complete resolution of radiographic lesions have been reported after IV bisphosphonate therapy. Surgical stabilization is used to prevent pathologic fracture or destruction of a major joint space and to relieve nerve root or cranial nerve compression or sinus obstruction.

OTHER DYSPLASIAS OF BONE AND CARTILAGE

PACHYDERMOPERIOSTOSIS

Pachydermoperiostosis, or hypertrophic osteoarthropathy (primary or idiopathic), is an autosomal-dominant disorder characterized by periosteal new bone formation that involves the distal extremities.

The lesions present as clubbing of the digits and hyperhydrosis and thickening of the skin, primarily of the face and forehead. The changes usually appear during adolescence, progress over the next decade, and then become quiescent. During the active phase, progressive enlargement of the hands and feet produces a pawlike appearance, which may be mistaken for acromegaly. Arthralgias, pseudogout, and limited mobility may also occur. The disorder must be differentiated from secondary hypertrophic osteopathy that develops during the course of serious pulmonary disorders. The two conditions can be differentiated by standard radiography of the digits in which secondary pachydermoperiostosis has exuberant periosteal new bone formation and a smooth and undulating surface. In contrast, primary hypertrophic osteopathy has an irregular periosteal surface.

There are no diagnostic blood or urine tests. Synovial fluid does not have an inflammatory profile. There is no specific therapy, although a limited experience with colchicine suggests some benefit in controlling the arthralgias.

OSTEOCHONDRODYSPLASIAS

These include several hundred heritable disorders of connective tissue. These primary abnormalities of cartilage manifest as disturbances in cartilage and bone growth. Selected growth-plate chondrodysplasias are described here. For discussion of chondrodysplasias, see Chap. 363.

Achondrodysplasia

This is a relatively common form of short-limb dwarfism that occurs in 1 in 15,000 to 1 in 40,000 live births. The disease is caused by a mutation of the fibroblast growth factor receptor 3 (*FGFR3*) gene that results in a gain-of-function state. Most cases are sporadic mutations. However, when the disorder appears in families, the inheritance pattern is consistent with an autosomal-dominant disorder. The primary defect is abnormal chondrocyte proliferation at the growth plate that causes development of short, but proportionately thick, long bones. Other regions of the long bones may be relatively unaffected. The disorder is manifest by the presence of short limbs (particularly the proximal portions), normal trunk, large head, saddle nose, and an exaggerated lumbar lordosis. Severe spinal deformity may lead to cord compression. The homozygous disorder is more serious than the sporadic form and may cause neonatal death. Pseudoachondroplasia clinically resembles achondrodysplasia but has no skull abnormalities.

Enchondromatosis

This is also called *dyschondroplasia* or *Ollier's disease*; it is also a disorder of the growth plate in which the primary cartilage is not resorbed. Cartilage ossification proceeds normally, but it is not resorbed normally, leading to cartilage accumulation. The changes are most marked at the ends of long bones, where the highest growth rates occur. Chondrosarcoma develops infrequently. The association of enchondromatosis and cavernous hemangiomas of the skin and soft tissues is known as *Maffucci syndrome*. Both Ollier's disease and Maffucci syndrome are associated with various malignancies, including granulosa cell tumor of the ovary and cerebral glioma.

Multiple exostoses

This is also called *diaphyseal aclasis* or *osteochondromatosis*; it is a genetic disorder that follows an autosomal-dominant pattern of inheritance. In this condition, areas of growth plates become displaced, presumably by growing through a defect in the perichondrium. The lesion begins with vascular invasion of the growth-plate cartilage, resulting in a characteristic radiographic finding of a mass that is in direct communication with the marrow cavity of the parent bone. The underlying cortex is resorbed. The disease is caused by inactivating mutations of the *EXT1* and *EXT2* genes, whose products normally regulate processing of chondrocyte cytoskeletal proteins. The products of the *EXT* gene likely function as tumor suppressors, with the loss-of-function mutation resulting in abnormal proliferation of growth-plate cartilage. Solitary or multiple lesions are located in the metaphyses of long bones. Although usually asymptomatic, the lesions may interfere with joint or tendon function or compress peripheral nerves. The lesions stop growing when growth ceases but may recur during pregnancy. There is a small risk for malignant transformation into chondrosarcoma.

EXTRASKELETAL (ECTOPIC) CALCIFICATION AND OSSIFICATION

Deposition of calcium phosphate crystals (*calcification*) or formation of true bone (*ossification*) in nonosseous soft tissue may occur by one of three mechanisms: (1) metastatic calcification due to a supranormal calcium × phosphate concentration product in extracellular fluid; (2) dystrophic calcification due to mineral deposition into metabolically impaired or dead tissue despite normal serum levels of calcium and phosphate; and (3) ectopic ossification, or true bone formation. Disorders that may cause extraskeletal calcification or ossification are listed in Table 355-2.

METASTATIC CALCIFICATION

Soft tissue calcification may complicate diseases associated with significant hypercalcemia, hyperphosphatemia, or both. In addition, vitamin D and phosphate treatments or calcium administration in the presence of mild hyperphosphatemia, such as during hemodialysis, may induce ectopic calcification. Calcium phosphate precipitation may complicate any disorder when the serum calcium × phosphate concentration product is >75. The initial calcium phosphate deposition is in the form of small, poorly organized crystals, which subsequently organize into hydroxyapatite crystals. Calcifications that occur in hypercalcemic states with normal or low phosphate have a predilection for kidney, lungs, and gastric mucosa. Hyperphosphatemia with normal or low serum calcium may promote soft tissue calcification with predilection for the kidney and arteries. The disturbances of calcium and phosphate in renal failure and hemodialysis are common causes of soft tissue (metastatic) calcification.

TABLE 355-2 Diseases and Conditions Associated With Ectopic Calcification and Ossification

Metastatic calcification	Dystrophic calcification
Hypercalcemic states	Inflammatory disorders
Primary hyperparathyroidism	Scleroderma
Sarcoidosis	Dermatomyositis
Vitamin D intoxication	Systemic lupus erythematosus
Milk-alkali syndrome	Trauma-induced
Renal failure	Ectopic ossification
Hyperphosphatemia	Myositis ossificans
Tumoral calcinosis	Postsurgery
Secondary hyperparathyroidism	Burns
Pseudohypoparathyroidism	Neurologic injury
Renal failure	Other trauma
Hemodialysis	Fibrodysplasia ossificans progressiva
Cell lysis following chemotherapy	
Therapy with vitamin D and phosphate	

TUMORAL CALCINOSIS

This is a rare genetic disorder characterized by masses of metastatic calcifications in soft tissues around major joints, most often shoulders, hips, and ankles. Tumoral calcinosis differs from other disorders in that the periarticular masses contain hydroxyapatite crystals or amorphous calcium phosphate complexes, while in fibrodysplasia ossificans progressiva (below), true bone is formed in soft tissues. About one-third of tumoral calcinosis cases are familial, with both autosomal-recessive and autosomal-dominant modes of inheritance reported. The disease is also associated with a variably expressed abnormality of dentition marked by short bulbous roots, pulp calcification, and radicular dentin deposited in swirls. The primary defect responsible for the metastatic calcification appears to be hyperphosphatemia resulting from the increased capacity of the renal tubule to reabsorb filtered phosphate. Spontaneous soft tissue calcification is related to the elevated serum phosphate, which, along with normal serum calcium, exceeds the concentration product of 75.

All of the North American patients reported have been African American. The disease usually presents in childhood and continues throughout the patient's life. The calcific masses are typically painless and grow at variable rates, sometimes becoming large and bulky. The masses are often located near major joints but remain extracapsular. Joint range of motion is not usually restricted unless the tumors are very large. Complications include compression of neural structures and ulceration of the overlying skin with drainage of chalky fluid and risk of secondary infection. Small deposits not detected by standard radiographs may be detected by ^{99m}Tc bone scanning. The most common laboratory findings are hyperphosphatemia and elevated serum 1,25-dihydroxyvitamin D levels. Serum calcium, parathyroid hormone, and ALP levels are usually normal. Renal function is also usually normal. Urine calcium and phosphate excretions are low, and calcium and phosphate balances are positive.

An acquired form of the disease may occur with other causes of hyperphosphatemia, such as secondary hyperparathyroidism associated with hemodialysis, hypoparathyroidism, pseudohypoparathyroidism, and massive cell lysis following chemotherapy for leukemia. Tissue trauma from joint movement may contribute to the periarticular calcifications. Metastatic calcifications are also seen in conditions associated with hypercalcemia, such as in sarcoidosis, vitamin D intoxication, milk-alkali syndrome, and primary hyperparathyroidism. In these conditions, however, mineral deposits are more likely to occur in proton-transporting organs such as kidney, lungs, and gastric mucosa in which an alkaline milieu is generated by the proton pumps.

TREATMENT Tumoral Calcinosis

Therapeutic successes have been achieved with surgical removal of subcutaneous calcified masses, which tend not to recur if all calcification is removed from the site. Reduction of serum phosphate by chronic phosphorus restriction may be accomplished using low dietary phosphorus intake alone or in combination with oral phosphate binders. The addition of the phosphaturic agent acetazolamide may be useful. Limited experience using the phosphaturic action of calcitonin deserves further testing.

DYSTROPHIC CALCIFICATION

Posttraumatic calcification may occur with normal serum calcium and phosphate levels and normal ion-solubility product. The deposited mineral is either in the form of amorphous calcium phosphate or hydroxyapatite crystals. Soft tissue calcification complicating connective tissue disorders such as scleroderma, dermatomyositis, and systemic lupus erythematosus may involve localized areas of the skin or deeper subcutaneous tissue and is referred to as *calcinosis circumscripta*. Mineral deposition at sites of deeper tissue injury including periarticular sites is called *calcinosis universalis*.

ECTOPIC OSSIFICATION

True extraskeletal bone formation that begins in areas of fasciitis following surgery, trauma, burns, or neurologic injury is referred to as *myositis ossificans*. The bone formed is organized as lamellar or trabecular, with normal osteoblasts and osteoclasts conducting active remodeling. Well-developed haversian systems and marrow elements may be present. A second cause of ectopic bone formation occurs in an inherited disorder, *fibrodysplasia ossificans progressiva*.

FIBRODYSPLASIA OSSIFICANS PROGRESSIVA

This is also called *myositis ossificans progressiva*; it is a rare autosomal-dominant disorder characterized by congenital deformities of the hands and feet and episodic soft tissue swellings that ossify. Ectopic bone formation occurs in fascia, tendons, ligaments, and connective tissue within voluntary muscles. Tender, rubbery induration, sometimes precipitated by trauma, develops in the soft tissue and gradually calcifies. Eventually, heterotopic bone forms at these sites of soft tissue trauma. Morbidity results from heterotopic bone interfering with normal movement and function of muscle and other soft tissues. Mortality is usually related to restrictive lung disease caused by an inability of the chest to expand. Laboratory tests are unremarkable.

There is no effective medical therapy. Bisphosphonates, glucocorticoids, and a low-calcium diet have largely been ineffective in halting progression of the ossification. Surgical removal of ectopic bone is not recommended, because the trauma of surgery may precipitate formation of new areas of heterotopic bone. Dental complications including frozen jaw may occur following injection of local anesthetics. Thus, CT imaging of the mandible should be undertaken to detect early sites of soft tissue ossification before they are appreciated by standard radiography.

FURTHER READINGS

Albagha OM et al: Genome-wide association study identifies variants at CSF1, OPTN and TNFRSF11A as genetic risk factors for Paget's disease of bone. Nat Genet 42:520, 2010

Avramidis A et al: Scintigraphic, biochemical, and clinical response to zoledronic acid treatment in patients with Paget's disease of bone. J Bone Miner Metab 26:635, 2008

Goode A, Layfield R: Recent advances in understanding the molecular basis of Paget's disease of bone. J Clin Pathol 63:199, 2010

Hiruma Y et al: A SQSTM1/p62 mutation linked to Paget's disease increases the osteoclastogenic potential of the bone microenvironment. Hum Mol Genet 17:3708, 2008

Hosking D et al: Long-term control of bone turnover in Paget's disease with zoledronic acid and risedronate. J Bone Miner Res 22:142, 2007

Langston AL et al: Randomized trial of intensive bisphosphonate treatment versus symptomatic management in Paget's disease of bone. J Bone Miner Res 25:20, 2010

Ralston SH et al: Pathogenesis and management of Paget's disease of bone. Lancet 372:155, 2008

Reid IR et al: Comparison of a single infusion of zoledronic acid with risedronate for Paget's disease. N Engl J Med 353:898,2005

Roodman GE et al: Paget's disease of bone. J Clin Invest 115: 200, 2005

Whyte MP: Paget's disease of bone. N Engl J Med 355:593, 2006

CHAPTER 356
Disorders of Lipoprotein Metabolism

Daniel J. Rader
Helen H. Hobbs

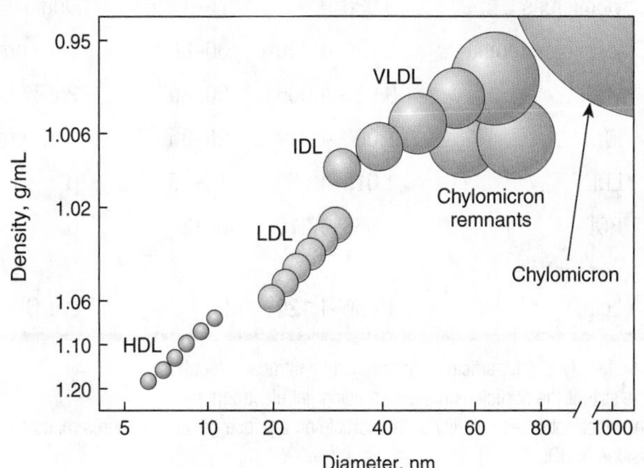

Figure 356-1 The density and size-distribution of the major classes of lipoprotein particles. Lipoproteins are classified by density and size, which are inversely related. VLDL, very low-density lipoprotein; IDL, intermediate-density lipoprotein; LDL, low-density lipoprotein; HDL, high-density lipoprotein.

Lipoproteins are complexes of lipids and proteins that are essential for the transport of cholesterol, triglycerides, and fat-soluble vitamins. Previously, lipoprotein disorders were the purview of specialized lipidologists, but the demonstration that lipid-lowering therapy significantly reduces the clinical complications of atherosclerotic cardiovascular disease (ASCVD) has brought the diagnosis and treatment of these disorders into the domain of the internist. The number of individuals who are candidates for lipid-lowering therapy has continued to increase. The development of safe, effective, and well-tolerated pharmacologic agents has greatly expanded the therapeutic armamentarium available to the physician to treat disorders of lipid metabolism. Therefore, the appropriate diagnosis and management of lipoprotein disorders is of critical importance in the practice of medicine. This chapter will review normal lipoprotein physiology, the pathophysiology of primary (inherited) disorders of lipoprotein metabolism, the diseases and environmental factors that cause secondary disorders of lipoprotein metabolism, and the practical approaches to their diagnosis and management.

LIPOPROTEIN METABOLISM

LIPOPROTEIN CLASSIFICATION AND COMPOSITION

Lipoproteins are large macromolecular complexes that transport hydrophobic lipids (primarily triglycerides, cholesterol, and fat-soluble vitamins) through body fluids (plasma, interstitial fluid, and lymph) to and from tissues. Lipoproteins play an essential role in the absorption of dietary cholesterol, long-chain fatty acids, and fat-soluble vitamins; the transport of triglycerides, cholesterol, and fat-soluble vitamins from the liver to peripheral tissues; and the transport of cholesterol from peripheral tissues to the liver.

Lipoproteins contain a core of hydrophobic lipids (triglycerides and cholesteryl esters) surrounded by hydrophilic lipids (phospholipids, unesterified cholesterol) and proteins that interact with body fluids. The plasma lipoproteins are divided into five major classes based on their relative density (Fig. 356-1 and Table 356-1): chylomicrons, very low-density lipoproteins (VLDLs), intermediate-density lipoproteins (IDLs), low-density lipoproteins (LDLs), and high-density lipoproteins (HDLs). Each lipoprotein class comprises a family of particles that vary slightly in density, size and protein composition. The density of a lipoprotein is determined by the amount of lipid per particle. HDL is the smallest and most dense lipoprotein, whereas chylomicrons and VLDLs are the largest and least dense lipoprotein particles. Most plasma triglyceride is transported in chylomicrons or VLDLs, and most plasma cholesterol is carried as cholesteryl esters in LDLs and HDLs.

The proteins associated with lipoproteins, called *apolipoproteins* (Table 356-2), are required for the assembly, structure, and function of lipoproteins. Apolipoproteins activate enzymes important in lipoprotein metabolism and act as ligands for cell surface receptors. ApoA-I, which is synthesized in the liver and intestine, is found on virtually all HDL particles. ApoA-II is the second most abundant HDL apolipoprotein and is on approximately two-thirds of the HDL particles. ApoB is the major structural protein of chylomicrons, VLDLs, IDLs, and LDLs; one molecule of apoB, either apoB-48 (chylomicron) or apoB-100 (VLDL, IDL or LDL), is present on each lipoprotein particle. The human liver synthesizes apoB-100, and the intestine makes apoB-48, which is derived from the same gene by mRNA editing. ApoE is present in multiple copies on chylomicrons, VLDL, and IDL, and it plays a critical role in the metabolism and clearance of triglyceride-rich particles. Three apolipoproteins of the C-series (apoC-I, apoC-II, and apoC-III) also participate in the metabolism of triglyceride-rich lipoproteins. ApoB is the only major apolipoprotein that does not transfer between lipoprotein particles. Some of the minor apolipoproteins are listed in Table 356-2.

TRANSPORT OF DIETARY LIPIDS (EXOGENOUS PATHWAY)

The exogenous pathway of lipoprotein metabolism permits efficient transport of dietary lipids (Fig. 356-2). Dietary triglycerides are hydrolyzed by lipases within the intestinal lumen and emulsified with bile acids to form micelles. Dietary cholesterol, fatty acids, and fat-soluble vitamins are absorbed in the proximal small intestine. Cholesterol and retinol are esterified (by the addition of a fatty acid) in the enterocyte to form cholesteryl esters and retinyl esters, respectively. Longer-chain fatty acids (>12 carbons) are incorporated into triglycerides and packaged with apoB-48, cholesteryl esters, retinyl esters, phospholipids, and cholesterol to form chylomicrons. Nascent chylomicrons are secreted into the intestinal lymph and delivered via the thoracic duct directly to the systemic circulation, where they are extensively processed by peripheral tissues before reaching the liver. The particles encounter

TABLE 356-1 Major Lipoprotein Classes

Lipoprotein	Density, g/mL[a]	Size, nm[b]	Electrophoretic Mobility[c]	Apolipoproteins		Other Constituents
				Major	Other	
Chylomicrons	0.930	75–1200	Origin	ApoB-48	A-I, A-IV, C-I, C-II, C-III, E	Retinyl esters
Chylomicron remnants	0.930–1.006	30–80	Slow pre-β	ApoB-48	A-I, A-IV, C-I, C-II, C-III, E	Retinyl esters
VLDL	0.930–1.006	30–80	Pre-β	ApoB-100	A-I, A-II, A-V, C-I, C-II, C-III, E	Vitamin E
IDL	1.006–1.019	25–35	Slow pre-β	ApoB-100	C-I, C-II, C-III, E	Vitamin E
LDL	1.019–1.063	18–25	β	ApoB-100		Vitamin E
HDL	1.063–1.210	5–12	α	ApoA-I	A-II, A-IV, A-V, C-III, E	LCAT, CETP paroxonase
Lp(a)	1.050–1.120	25	Pre-β	ApoB-100	Apo(a)	

[a]The density of the particle is determined by ultracentrifugation.
[b]The size of the particle is measured using gel electrophoresis.
[c]The electrophoretic mobility of the particle on agarose gel electrophores reflects the size and surface charge of the particle, with β being the position of LDL and α being the position of HDL.
Note: All of the lipoprotein classes contain phospholipids, esterified and unesterified cholesterol, and triglycerides to varying degrees.
Abbreviations: CETP, cholesteryl ester transfer protein; HDL, high-density lipoprotein; IDL, intermediate-density lipoprotein; LCAT, lecithin-cholesterol acyltransferase; LDL, low-density lipoprotein; Lp(a), lipoprotein A; VLDL, very low-density lipoprotein.

TABLE 356-2 Major Apolipoproteins

Apolipoprotein	Primary Source	Lipoprotein Association	Function
ApoA-I	Intestine, liver	HDL, chylomicrons	Structural protein for HDL Activates LCAT
ApoA-II	Liver	HDL, chylomicrons	Structural protein for HDL
ApoA-IV	Intestine	HDL, chylomicrons	Unknown
ApoA-V	Liver	VLDL, chylomicrons	Promotes LPL-mediated triglyceride lipolysis
Apo(a)	Liver	Lp(a)	Unknown
ApoB-48	Intestine	Chylomicrons	Structural protein for chylomicrons
ApoB-100	Liver	VLDL, IDL, LDL, Lp(a)	Structural protein for VLDL, LDL, IDL, Lp(a) Ligand for binding to LDL receptor
ApoC-I	Liver	Chylomicrons, VLDL, HDL	Unknown
ApoC-II	Liver	Chylomicrons, VLDL, HDL	Cofactor for LPL
ApoC-III	Liver	Chylomicrons, VLDL, HDL	Inhibits lipoprotein binding to receptors
ApoE	Liver	Chylomicron remnants, IDL, HDL	Ligand for binding to LDL receptor
ApoH	Liver	Chylomicrons, VLDL, LDL, HDL	B_2 glycoprotein I
ApoJ	Liver	HDL	Unknown
ApoL	Unknown	HDL	Unknown
ApoM	Liver	HDL	Unknown

Abbreviations: HDL, high-density lipoprotein; IDL, intermediate-density lipoprotein; LCAT, lecithin-cholesterol acyltransferase; LDL, low-density lipoprotein; Lp(a), lipoprotein A; LPL, lipoprotein lipase; VLDL, very low-density lipoprotein.

lipoprotein lipase (LPL), which is anchored to a glycosylphosphatidylinositol-anchored protein, GPIHBP1, that is attached to the endothelial surfaces of capillaries in adipose tissue, heart, and skeletal muscle (Fig. 356-2). The triglycerides of chylomicrons are hydrolyzed by LPL, and free fatty acids are released. ApoC-II, which is transferred to circulating chylomicrons from HDL, acts as a required cofactor for LPL in this reaction. The released free fatty acids are taken up by adjacent myocytes or adipocytes and either oxidized to generate energy or reesterified and stored as triglyceride. Some of the released free fatty acids bind albumin before entering cells and are transported to other tissues, especially the liver. The chylomicron particle progressively shrinks in size as the hydrophobic core is hydrolyzed and the hydrophilic lipids (cholesterol and phospholipids) and apolipoproteins on the particle surface are transferred to HDL, creating chylomicron remnants. Chylomicron remnants are rapidly removed from the circulation by the liver through a process that requires apoE as a ligand for receptors in the liver. Consequently, few, if any, chylomicrons or chylomicron remnants are present in the blood after a 12-hour fast, except in patients with disorders of chylomicron metabolism.

■ TRANSPORT OF HEPATIC LIPIDS (ENDOGENOUS PATHWAY)

The endogenous pathway of lipoprotein metabolism refers to the secretion of apoB-containing lipoproteins from the liver and the metabolism of these triglyceride-rich particles in peripheral tissues (Fig. 356-2). VLDL

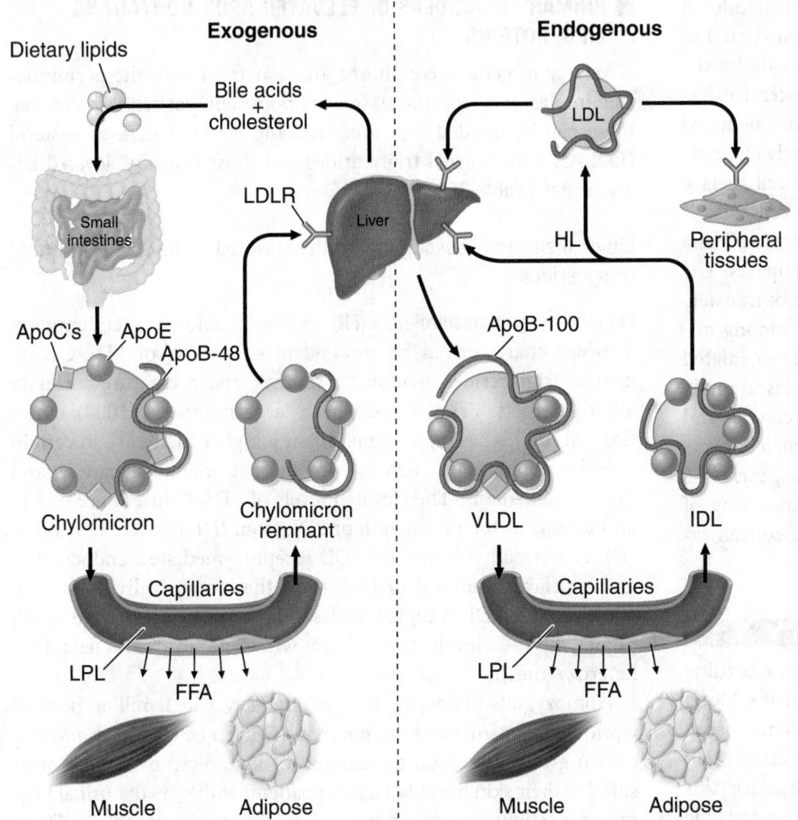

Figure 356-2 The exogenous and endogenous lipoprotein metabolic pathways. The exogenous pathway transports dietary lipids to the periphery and the liver. The endogenous pathway transports hepatic lipids to the periphery. LPL, lipoprotein lipase; FFA, free fatty acid; VLDL, very low density lipoprotein; IDL, intermediate-density lipoprotein; LDL, low-density lipoprotein; LDLR, low-density lipoprotein receptor; HL, hepatic lipase.

particles resemble chylomicrons in protein composition but contain apoB-100 rather than apoB-48 and have a higher ratio of cholesterol to triglyceride (~1 mg of cholesterol for every 5 mg of triglyceride). The triglycerides of VLDL are derived predominantly from the esterification of long-chain fatty acids in the liver. The packaging of hepatic triglycerides with the other major components of the nascent VLDL particle (apoB-100, cholesteryl esters, phospholipids, and vitamin E) requires the action of the enzyme microsomal triglyceride transfer protein (MTP). After secretion into the plasma, VLDL acquires multiple copies of apoE and apolipoproteins of the C series by transfer from HDL. As with chylomicrons, the triglycerides of VLDL are hydrolyzed by LPL, especially in muscle, heart, and adipose tissue. After the VLDL remnants dissociate from LPL, they are referred to as IDLs, which contain roughly similar amounts of cholesterol and triglyceride. The liver removes approximately 40–60% of IDL by LDL receptor–mediated endocytosis via binding to apoE. The remainder of IDL is remodeled by hepatic lipase (HL) to form LDL. During this process, most of the triglyceride in the particle hydrolyzed, and all apolipoproteins except apoB-100 are transferred to other lipoproteins. The cholesterol in LDL accounts for more than one-half of the plasma cholesterol in most individuals. Approximately 70% of circulating LDL is cleared by LDL receptor–mediated endocytosis in the liver. *Lipoprotein(a)* [Lp(a)] is a lipoprotein similar to LDL in lipid and protein composition, but it contains an additional protein called *apolipoprotein(a)* [apo(a)]. Apo(a) is synthesized in the liver and attached to apoB-100 by a disulfide linkage. The major site of clearance of Lp(a) is the liver, but the uptake pathway is not known.

HDL METABOLISM AND REVERSE CHOLESTEROL TRANSPORT

All nucleated cells synthesize cholesterol, but only hepatocytes and enterocytes can effectively excrete cholesterol from the body, into either the bile or the gut lumen. In the liver, cholesterol is secreted into the bile, either directly or after conversion to bile acids. Cholesterol in peripheral cells is transported from the plasma membranes of peripheral cells to the liver and intestine by a process termed "reverse cholesterol transport" that is facilitated by HDL (Fig. 356-3).

Nascent HDL particles are synthesized by the intestine and the liver. Newly secreted apoA-I rapidly acquires phospholipids and unesterified cholesterol from its site of synthesis (intestine or liver) via efflux promoted by the membrane protein ATP-binding cassette protein A1 (ABCA1). This process results in the formation of discoidal HDL particles, which then recruit additional unesterified cholesterol from the periphery. Within the HDL particle, the cholesterol is esterified by lecithin-cholesterol acyltransferase (LCAT), a plasma enzyme associated with HDL, and the more hydrophobic cholesteryl ester moves to the core of the HDL particle. As HDL acquires more cholesteryl ester it becomes spherical, and additional apolipoproteins and lipids are transferred to the particles from the surfaces of chylomicrons and VLDLs during lipolysis.

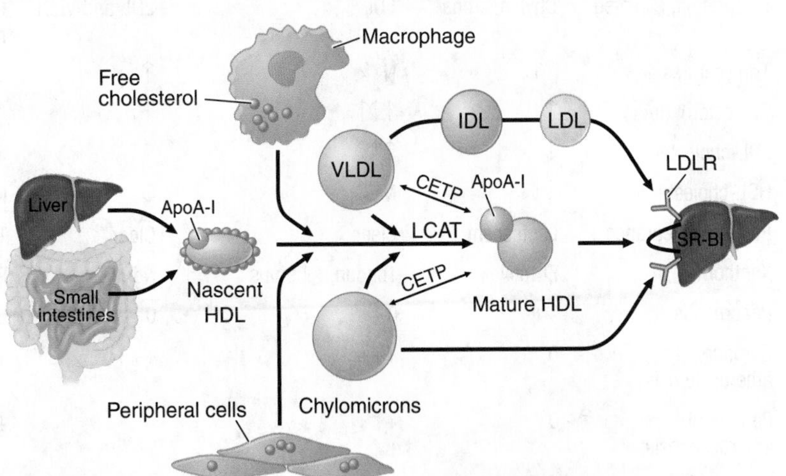

Figure 356-3 HDL metabolism and reverse cholesterol transport. This pathway transports excess cholesterol from the periphery back to the liver for excretion in the bile. The liver and the intestine produce nascent HDLs. Free cholesterol is acquired from macrophages and other peripheral cells and esterified by LCAT, forming mature HDLs. HDL cholesterol can be selectively taken up by the liver via SR-BI (scavenger receptor class BI). Alternatively, HDL cholesteryl ester can be transferred by CETP from HDLs to VLDLs and chylomicrons, which can then be taken up by the liver. LCAT, lecithin-cholesterol acyltransferase; CETP, cholesteryl ester transfer protein; VLDL, very low-density lipoprotein; IDL, intermediate-density lipoprotein; LDL, low-density lipoprotein; HDL, high-density lipoprotein; LDLR, low-density lipoprotein receptor.

HDL cholesterol is transported to hepatocytes by both an indirect and a direct pathway. HDL cholesteryl esters can be transferred to apoB-containing lipoproteins in exchange for triglyceride by the cholesteryl ester transfer protein (CETP). The cholesteryl esters are then removed from the circulation by LDL receptor–mediated endocytosis. HDL cholesterol can also be taken up directly by hepatocytes via the scavenger receptor class B1 (SR-B1), a cell surface receptor that mediates the selective transfer of lipids to cells.

HDL particles undergo extensive remodeling within the plasma compartment by a variety of lipid transfer proteins and lipases. The phospholipid transfer protein (PLTP) has the net effect of transferring phospholipids from other lipoproteins to HDL or among different classes of HDL particles. After CETP- and PLTP-mediated lipid exchange, the triglyceride-enriched HDL becomes a much better substrate for HL, which hydrolyzes the triglycerides and phospholipids to generate smaller HDL particles. A related enzyme called *endothelial lipase* hydrolyzes HDL phospholipids, generating smaller HDL particles that are catabolized faster. Remodeling of HDL influences the metabolism, function, and plasma concentrations of HDL.

DISORDERS OF LIPOPROTEIN METABOLISM

Fredrickson and Levy classified hyperlipoproteinemias according to the type of lipoprotein particles that accumulate in the blood (Type I to Type V) (Table 356-3). A classification scheme based on the molecular etiology and pathophysiology of the lipoprotein disorders complements this system and forms the basis for this chapter. The identification and characterization of genes responsible for the genetic forms of hyperlipidemia have provided important molecular insights into the critical roles of structural apolipoproteins, enzymes, and receptors in lipid metabolism (Table 356-4).

PRIMARY DISORDERS OF ELEVATED APOB-CONTAINING LIPOPROTEINS

A variety of genetic conditions are associated with the accumulation in plasma of specific classes of lipoprotein particles. In general, these can be divided into those causing elevated LDL-cholesterol (LDL-C) with normal triglycerides and those causing elevated triglycerides (Table 356-4).

Lipid disorders associated with elevated LDL-C and normal triglycerides

Familial hypercholesterolemia (FH) FH is an autosomal codominant disorder characterized by elevated plasma levels of LDL-C with normal triglycerides, tendon xanthomas, and premature coronary atherosclerosis. FH is caused by a large number (>1000) mutations in the LDL receptor gene. It has a higher incidence in certain founder populations, such as Afrikaners, Christian Lebanese, and French Canadians. The elevated levels of LDL-C in FH are due to an increase in the production of LDL from IDL (since a portion of IDL is normally cleared by LDL receptor–mediated endocytosis) and a delayed removal of LDL from the blood. Individuals with two mutated LDL receptor alleles (FH homozygotes) have much higher LDL-C levels than those with one mutant allele (FH heterozygotes).

Homozygous FH occurs in approximately 1 in 1 million persons worldwide. Patients with homozygous FH can be classified into one of two groups based on the amount of LDL receptor activity measured in their skin fibroblasts: those patients with <2% of normal LDL receptor activity (receptor negative) and those patients with 2–25% of normal LDL receptor activity (receptor defective). Most patients with homozygous FH present in childhood with cutaneous xanthomas on the hands, wrists, elbows, knees, heels, or buttocks. Total cholesterol

TABLE 356-3 Fredrickson Classification of Hyperlipoproteinemias

Phenotype	I	IIa	IIb	III	IV	V
Lipoprotein, elevated	Chylomicrons	LDL	LDL and VLDL	Chylomicron and VLDL remnants	VLDL	Chylomicrons and VLDL
Triglycerides	↑↑↑	N	↑	↑↑	↑↑	↑↑↑
Cholesterol (total)	↑	↑↑↑	↑↑	↑↑	N/↑	↑↑
LDL-cholesterol	↓	↑↑↑	↑↑	↓	↓	↓
HDL-cholesterol	↓↓↓	N/↓	↓	N	↓↓	↓↓↓
Plasma appearance	Lactescent	Clear	Clear	Turbid	Turbid	Lactescent
Xanthomas	Eruptive	Tendon, tuberous	None	Palmar, tuberoeruptive	None	Eruptive
Pancreatitis	+++	0	0	0	0	+++
Coronary atherosclerosis	0	+++	+++	+++	+/–	+/–
Peripheral atherosclerosis	0	+	+	++	+/–	+/–
Molecular defects	LPL and ApoC-II	LDL receptor, ApoB-100, PCSK9, LDLRAP, ABCG5 and ABCG8		ApoE	ApoA-V	ApoA-V and GPIHBP1
Genetic nomenclature	FCS	FH, FDB, ADH, ARH, sitosterolemia	FCHL	FDBL	FHTG	FHTG

Abbreviations: ADH, autosomal dominant hypercholesterolemia; Apo, apolipoprotein; ARH, autosomal recessive hypercholesterolemia; FCHL, familial combined hyperlipidemia; FCS, familial chylomicronemia syndrome; FDB, familial defective ApoB; FDBL, familial dysbetalipoproteinemia; FH, familial hypercholesterolemia; FHTG, familial hypertriglyceridemia; LPL, lipoprotein lipase; LDLRAP, LDL receptor associated protein; GPIHBP1, glycosylphosphatidylinositol-anchored high density lipoprotein binding protein1; N, normal

TABLE 356-4 Primary Hyperlipoproteinemias Caused by Known Single Gene Mutations

Genetic Disorder	Protein (Gene) Defect	Lipoproteins Elevated	Clinical Findings	Genetic Transmission	Estimated Incidence
Lipoprotein lipase deficiency	LPL (*LPL*)	Chylomicrons	Eruptive xanthomas, hepatosplenomegaly, pancreatitis	AR	1/1,000,000
Familial apolipoprotein C-II deficiency	ApoC-II (*APOC2*)	Chylomicrons	Eruptive xanthomas, hepatosplenomegaly, pancreatitis	AR	<1/1,000,000
ApoA-V deficiency	ApoA-V (*APOA5*)	Chylomicrons, VLDL	Eruptive xanthomas, hepatosplenomegaly, pancreatitis	AD	<1/1,000,000
GPIHBP1 deficiency	*GDIHBP1*	Chylomicrons	Eruptive xanthomas, pancreatitis	AD	<1/1,000,000
Familial hepatic lipase deficiency	Hepatic lipase (*LIPC*)	VLDL remnants	Pancreatitis, CHD	AR	<1/1,000,000
Familial dysbetalipoproteinemia	ApoE (*APOE*)	Chylomicron and VLDL remnants	Palmar and tuberoeruptive xanthomas, CHD, PVD	AR AD	1/10,000
Familial hypercholesterolemia	LDL receptor (*LDLR*)	LDL	Tendon xanthomas, CHD	AD	1/500
Familial defective apoB-100	ApoB-100 (*APOB*)	LDL	Tendon xanthomas, CHD	AD	<1/1000
Autosomal dominant hypercholesterolemia	PCSK9 (*PCSK9*)	LDL	Tendon xanthomas, CHD	AD	<1/1,000,000
Autosomal recessive hypercholesterolemia	*LDLRAP*	LDL	Tendon xanthomas, CHD	AR	<1/1,000,000
Sitosterolemia	*ABCG5* or *ABCG8*	LDL	Tendon xanthomas, CHD	AR	<1/1,000,000

Abbreviations: AD, autosomal dominant; AR, autosomal recessive; ARH, autosomal recessive hypercholesterolemia; CHD, coronary heart disease; LDL, low-density lipoprotein; LPL, lipoprotein lipase; PVD, peripheral vascular disease; VLDL, very-low density lipoprotein.

levels are usually >500 mg/dL and can be higher than 1000 mg/dL. The devastating complication of homozygous FH is accelerated atherosclerosis, which can result in disability and death in childhood. Atherosclerosis often develops first in the aortic root, where it can cause aortic valvular or supravalvular stenosis, and typically extends into the coronary ostia, which become stenotic. Children with homozygous FH often develop symptomatic coronary atherosclerosis before puberty; symptoms can be atypical, and sudden death is not uncommon. Untreated, receptor-negative patients with homozygous FH rarely survive beyond the second decade; patients with receptor-defective LDL receptor defects have a better prognosis but almost invariably develop clinically apparent atherosclerotic vascular disease by age 30, and often much sooner. Carotid and femoral disease develops later in life and is usually not clinically significant.

A careful family history should be taken, and plasma lipid levels should be measured in the parents and other first-degree relatives of patients with homozygous FH. The disease has >90% penetrance so both parents of FH homozygotes usually have hypercholesterolemia. The diagnosis of homozygous FH can be confirmed by obtaining a skin biopsy and measuring LDL receptor activity in cultured skin fibroblasts, or by quantifying the number of LDL receptors on the surfaces of lymphocytes using cell sorting technology. Molecular assays are also available to define the mutations in the LDL receptor by DNA sequencing. In selected populations where particular mutations predominate (e.g., Africaners and French Canadians), the common mutations can be screened for directly. Alternatively, the entire coding region needs to be sequenced for mutation detection because a large number of different LDL receptor mutations can cause disease. Ten to 15% of LDL receptor mutations are large deletions or insertions, which may be missed by routine DNA sequencing.

Combination therapy with an HMG-CoA reductase inhibitor and a second drug (cholesterol absorption inhibitor or bile acid sequestrant) sometimes reduces plasma LDL-C in those FH homozygotes who have residual LDL receptor activity, but patients with homozygous FH invariably require additional lipid-lowering therapy. Since the liver is quantitatively the most important tissue for removing circulating LDLs via the LDL receptor, liver transplantation is effective in decreasing plasma LDL-C levels in this disorder. Liver transplantation, however, is associated with substantial risks, including the requirement for long-term immunosuppression. The current treatment of choice for homozygous FH is LDL apheresis (a process by which the LDL particles are selectively removed from the circulation), which can promote regression of xanthomas and may slow the progression of atherosclerosis. Initiation of LDL apheresis should generally be delayed until approximately 5 years of age, except when evidence of atherosclerotic vascular disease is present.

Heterozygous FH is caused by the inheritance of one mutant LDL receptor allele and occurs in approximately 1 in 500 persons worldwide, making it one of the most common single-gene disorders. It is characterized by elevated plasma levels of LDL-C (usually 200–400 mg/dL) and normal levels of triglyceride. Patients with heterozygous FH have hypercholesterolemia from birth, and disease recognition is usually based on detection of hypercholesterolemia on routine screening, the appearance of tendon xanthomas, or the development of symptomatic ASCVD. Since the disease is codominant in inheritance, one parent and ~50% of the patient's siblings usually also have hypercholesterolemia. The family history is frequently positive for premature ASCVD on one side of the family. Corneal arcus is common, and tendon xanthomas involving the dorsum of the hands, elbows, knees, and especially the Achilles tendons are present in ~75% of patients. The age of onset of ASCVD is highly variable and depends in part on the molecular defect in the LDL receptor gene and also on coexisting cardiac risk factors. FH heterozygotes with elevated plasma levels of Lp(a) appear to be at greater risk for cardiovascular complications. Untreated men with heterozygous FH have an ~50% chance of having a myocardial infarction before age 60 years. Although the age of onset of atherosclerotic heart disease is later in women with FH, coronary heart disease (CHD) is significantly more common in women with FH than in the general female population.

No definitive diagnostic test for heterozygous FH is available. Although FH heterozygotes tend to have reduced levels of LDL receptor function in skin fibroblasts, significant overlap with the LDL receptor activity levels in normal fibroblasts exists. Molecular assays are now available to identify mutations in the LDL receptor gene by DNA sequencing, but the clinical utility of pinpointing the mutation has not been demonstrated. The clinical diagnosis is usually not problematic, but it is critical that hypothyroidism, nephrotic syndrome, and obstructive liver disease be excluded before initiating therapy.

FH patients should be aggressively treated to lower plasma levels of LDL-C. Initiation of a low-cholesterol, low-fat diet is recommended, but heterozygous FH patients require lipid-lowering drug therapy. Statins are effective in heterozygous FH, but combination drug therapy with the addition of a cholesterol absorption inhibitor and/or bile acid sequestrant is frequently required, and the addition of nicotinic acid is sometimes needed. Heterozygous FH patients who cannot be adequately controlled on combination drug therapy are candidates for LDL apheresis.

Familial defective ApoB-100 (FDB)

FDB is a dominantly inherited disorder that clinically resembles heterozygous FH. The disease is rare in most populations except individuals of German descent, where the frequency can be as high as 1 in 1000. FDB is characterized by elevated plasma LDL-C levels with normal triglycerides, tendon xanthomas, and an increased incidence of premature ASCVD. FDB is caused by mutations in the LDL receptor–binding domain of apoB-100, most commonly due to a substitution of glutamine for arginine at position 3500. As a consequence of the mutation in apoB-100, LDL binds the LDL receptor with reduced affinity, and LDL is removed from the circulation at a reduced rate. Patients with FDB cannot be clinically distinguished from patients with heterozygous FH, although patients with FDB tend to have lower plasma levels of LDL-C than FH heterozygotes. The apoB-100 gene mutation can be detected directly, but genetic diagnosis is not currently encouraged since the recommended management of FDB and heterozygous FH is identical.

Autosomal dominant hypercholesterolemia due to mutations in PCSK9 (ADH-PCSK9 or ADH3) ADH-PCSK9 is a rare autosomal dominant disorder caused by gain-of-function mutations in proprotein convertase subtilisin/kexin type 9 (PCSK9). PCSK9 is a secreted protein that binds to the LDL receptor, resulting in its degradation. Normally, after LDL binds to the receptor it is internalized along with the receptor. In the low pH of the endosome, LDL dissociates from the receptor and returns to the cell surface. The LDL is delivered to the lysosome. When PCSK9 binds the receptor, the complex is internalized and the receptor is redirected to the lysosome rather than to the cell surface. The missense mutations in PCSK9 that cause hypercholesterolemia enhance the activity of PCSK9. As a consequence, the number of hepatic LDL receptors is reduced. Patients with ADH-PCSK9 are indistinguishable clinically from patients with FH. Interestingly, loss-of-function mutations in PCSK9 cause low LDL-C levels (see below).

Autosomal recessive hypercholesterolemia (ARH) ARH is a rare disorder (except in Sardinia, Italy) due to mutations in a protein (ARH, also called LDLR adaptor protein, LDLRAP) involved in LDL receptor–mediated endocytosis in the liver. In the absence of LDLRAP, LDL binds to the LDL receptor but the lipoprotein-receptor complex fails to be internalized. ARH, like homozygous FH, is characterized by hypercholesterolemia, tendon xanthomas, and premature coronary artery disease (CAD). The levels of plasma LDL-C tend to be intermediate between the levels present in FH homozygotes and FH heterozygotes, and CAD is not usually symptomatic until at least the third decade. LDL receptor function in cultured fibroblasts is normal or only modestly reduced in ARH, whereas LDL receptor function in lymphocytes and the liver is negligible. Unlike FH homozygotes, the hyperlipidemia responds partially to treatment with HMG-CoA reductase inhibitors, but these patients usually require LDL apheresis to lower plasma LDL-C to recommended levels.

Sitosterolemia Sitosterolemia is another rare autosomal recessive disease that can result in severe hypercholesterolemia, tendon xanthomas, and premature ASCVD. Sitosterolemia is caused by mutations in either of two members of the ATP-binding cassette (ABC) half transporter family, ABCG5 and ABCG8. These genes are expressed in enterocytes and hepatocytes. The proteins heterodimerize to form a functional complex that pumps plant sterols such as sitosterol and campesterol, and animal sterols, predominantly cholesterol, into the gut lumen and into the bile. In normal individuals, <5% of dietary plant sterols are absorbed by the proximal small intestine and delivered to the liver. Absorbed plant sterols are preferentially secreted into the bile and are maintained at very low levels. In sitosterolemia, the intestinal absorption of sterols is increased and biliary excretion of the sterols is reduced, resulting in increased plasma and tissue levels of both plant sterols and cholesterol.

Incorporation of plant sterols into cell membranes results in misshapen red blood cells and megathrombocytes that are visible on blood smear. Episodes of hemolysis are a distinctive clinical feature of this disease compared to other genetic forms of hypercholesterolemia.

Sitosterolemia is diagnosed by demonstrating an increase in the plasma level of sitosterol using gas chromatography. The hypercholesterolemia is unusually responsive to reductions in dietary cholesterol content and should be suspected in individuals who have a >40% reduction in plasma cholesterol level on a low-cholesterol diet. The hypercholesterolemia does not respond to HMG-CoA reductase inhibitors, whereas bile acid sequestrants and cholesterol-absorption inhibitors such as ezetimibe, are effective in reducing plasma sterol levels in these patients.

Polygenic hypercholesterolemia This condition is characterized by hypercholesterolemia due to elevated LDL-C with a normal plasma level of triglyceride in the absence of secondary causes of hypercholesterolemia. Plasma LDL-C levels are generally not as elevated as they are in FH and FDB. Family studies are useful to differentiate polygenic hypercholesterolemia from the single-gene disorders described above; one-half of the first-degree relatives of patients with FH and FDB are hypercholesterolemic, whereas <10% of first-degree relatives of patients with polygenic hypercholesterolemia have hypercholesterolemia. Treatment of polygenic hypercholesterolemia is identical to that of other forms of hypercholesterolemia.

Elevated plasma levels of lipoprotein(a)

Unlike the other major classes of lipoproteins, that have a normal distribution in the population, plasma levels of Lp(a) have a highly skewed distribution with levels varying over a 1000-fold range. Levels are strongly influenced by genetic factors, with individuals of African and South Asian descent having higher levels than those of European descent. Although it has been well documented that elevated levels of Lp(a) are associated with an increase in ASCVD, lowering plasma levels of Lp(a) has not been demonstrated to reduce cardiovascular risk.

Lipid disorders associated with elevated triglycerides

Familial chylomicronemia syndrome (Type I hyperlipoproteinemia; lipoprotein lipase and ApoC-II Deficiency) As noted above, LPL is required for the hydrolysis of triglycerides in chylomicrons and VLDLs, and apoC-II is a cofactor for LPL (Fig. 356-2). Genetic deficiency or inactivity of either protein results in impaired lipolysis and profound elevations in plasma chylomicrons. These patients can also have elevated plasma levels of VLDL, but chylomicronemia predominates. The fasting plasma is turbid, and if left at 4°C (39.2°F) for a few hours, the chylomicrons float to the top and form a creamy supernatant. In these disorders, called *familial chylomicronemia syndromes*, fasting triglyceride levels are almost invariably >1000 mg/dL. Fasting cholesterol levels are also elevated but to a lesser degree.

LPL deficiency has autosomal recessive inheritance and has a frequency of approximately 1 in 1 million in the population. *ApoC-II deficiency* is also recessive in inheritance pattern and is even less common than LPL deficiency. Multiple different mutations in the LPL and apoC-II genes cause these diseases. Obligate LPL heterozygotes have normal or mild-to-moderate elevations in plasma triglyceride levels, whereas individuals heterozygous for mutation in apoC-II do not have hypertriglyceridemia.

Both LPL and apoC-II deficiency usually present in childhood with recurrent episodes of severe abdominal pain due to acute pancreatitis. On funduscopic examination, the retinal blood vessels are opalescent (lipemia retinalis). Eruptive xanthomas, which are small, yellowish-white papules, often appear in clusters on the back, buttocks, and extensor surfaces of the arms and legs. These typically painless skin lesions may become puritic. Hepatosplenomegaly results from the uptake of circulating chylomicrons by reticuloendothelial cells in the liver and spleen. For unknown reasons, some patients with persistent and pronounced chylomicronemia never develop pancreatitis, eruptive xanthomas, or hepatosplenomegaly. Premature CHD is not generally a feature of familial chylomicronemia syndromes.

The diagnoses of LPL and apoC-II deficiency are established enzymatically in specialized laboratories by assaying triglyceride lipolytic activity in postheparin plasma. Blood is sampled after an IV heparin injection to release the endothelial-bound LPL. LPL activity is profoundly reduced in both LPL and apoC-II deficiency; in patients with apoC-II deficiency, it normalizes after the addition of normal plasma (providing a source of apoC-II). Molecular sequencing of the genes can be used to confirm the diagnosis.

The major therapeutic intervention in familial chylomicronemia syndromes is dietary fat restriction (to as little as 15 g/d) with fat-soluble vitamin supplementation. Consultation with a registered dietician familiar with this disorder is essential. Caloric supplementation with medium-chain triglycerides, which are absorbed directly into the portal circulation, can be useful but may be associated with hepatic fibrosis if used for prolonged periods. If dietary fat restriction alone is not successful in resolving the chylomicronemia, fish oils have been effective in some patients. In patients with apoC-II deficiency, apoC-II can be provided by infusing fresh-frozen plasma to resolve the chylomicronemia in the acute setting. Management of patients with familial chylomicronemia syndrome is particularly challenging during pregnancy when VLDL production is increased and may require plasmapheresis to remove the circulating chylomicrons.

ApoA-V deficiency Another apolipoprotein, ApoA-V, circulates at much lower concentrations than the other major apolipoproteins. Individuals harboring mutations in both ApoA-V alleles can present as adults with chylomicronemia. The exact mechanism of action of ApoA-V is not known, but it appears to be required for the association of VLDL and chylomicrons with LPL.

GPIHBP1 deficiency After LPL is synthesized in adipocytes, myocytes or other cells, it is transported across the vascular endothelium and is attached to a protein on the endothelial surface of capillaries called GPIHBP1. Homozygosity for mutations that interfere with GPIHBP1 synthesis or folding cause severe hypertriglyceridemia. The frequency of chylomicronemia due to mutations in GHIHBP1 has not been established but appears to be very rare.

Hepatic lipase deficiency HL is a member of the same gene family as LPL and hydrolyzes triglycerides and phospholipids in remnant lipoproteins and HDLs. HL deficiency is a very rare autosomal recessive disorder characterized by elevated plasma levels of cholesterol and triglycerides (mixed hyperlipidemia) due to the accumulation of circulating lipoprotein remnants and either a normal or elevated plasma level of HDL-C. The diagnosis is confirmed by measuring HL activity in postheparin plasma. Due to the small number of patients with HL deficiency, the association of this genetic defect with ASCVD is not clearly known, but lipid-lowering therapy is recommended.

Familial dysbetalipoproteinemia (Type III hyperlipoproteinemia) Like HL deficiency, familial dysbetalipoproteinemia (FDBL) (also known as *type III hyperlipoproteinemia* or *familial broad* β *disease*) is characterized by a mixed hyperlipidemia due to the accumulation of remnant lipoprotein particles. ApoE is present in multiple copies on chylomicron and VLDL remnants and mediates their removal via hepatic lipoprotein receptors (Fig. 356-2). FDBL is due to genetic variations in apoE that interfere with its ability to bind lipoprotein receptors. The *APOE* gene is polymorphic in sequence, resulting in the expression of three common isoforms: apoE3, which is the most common; and apoE2 and apoE4, which both differ from apoE3 by a single amino acid. Although associated with slightly higher LDL-C levels and increased CHD risk, the apoE4 allele is not associated with FDBL. Patients with apoE4 have an increased incidence of late-onset Alzheimer's disease. ApoE2 has a lower affinity for the LDL receptor; therefore, chylomicron and VLDL remnants containing apoE2 are removed from plasma at a slower rate. Individuals who are homozygous for the E2 allele (the E2/E2 genotype) comprise the most common subset of patients with FDBL.

Approximately 0.5% of the general population are apoE2/E2 homozygotes, but only a small minority of these individuals develop FDBL. In most cases, an additional, identifiable factor precipitates the development of hyperlipoproteinemia. The most common precipitating factors are a high-fat diet, diabetes mellitus, obesity, hypothyroidism, renal disease, HIV infection, estrogen deficiency, alcohol use, or certain drugs. Other mutations in apoE can cause a dominant form of FDBL where the hyperlipidemia is fully manifest in the heterozygous state, but these mutations are rare.

Patients with FDBL usually present in adulthood with incidental hyperlipidemia, xanthomas, premature coronary disease, or peripheral vascular disease. The disease seldom presents in women before menopause. Two distinctive types of xanthomas, tuberoeruptive and palmar, are seen in FDBL patients. Tuberoeruptive xanthomas begin as clusters of small papules on the elbows, knees, or buttocks and can grow to the size of small grapes. Palmar xanthomas (alternatively called *xanthomata striata palmaris*) are orange-yellow discolorations of the creases in the palms and wrists. In FDBL, in contrast to other disorders of elevated triglycerides, the plasma levels of cholesterol and triglyceride are often elevated to a similar degree and the level of HDL-C is usually normal rather than being low.

The traditional approaches to diagnosis of this disorder are lipoprotein electrophoresis (broad β band) or ultracentrifugation (ratio of VLDL-C to total plasma triglyceride >0.30). Protein methods (apoE phenotyping) or DNA-based methods (apoE genotyping) can be performed to confirm homozygosity for apoE2. However, absence of the apoE2/E2 genotype does not rule out the diagnosis of FDBL, since other mutations in apoE can cause this condition.

Since FDBL is associated with increased risk of premature ASCVD, it should be treated aggressively. Subjects with FDBL tend to have more peripheral vascular disease than is typically seen in FH. Other metabolic conditions that can worsen the hyperlipidemia (see above) should be aggressively treated. Patients with FDBL are typically very diet-responsive and can respond favorably to weight reduction and to low-cholesterol, low-fat diets. Alcohol intake should be curtailed. HMG-CoA reductase inhibitors, fibrates, and niacin are all generally effective in the treatment of FDBL, and sometimes combination drug therapy is required.

Familial hypertriglyceridemia (FHTG) FHTG is a relatively common (~1 in 500) autosomal dominant disorder of unknown etiology characterized by moderately elevated plasma triglycerides accompanied by more modest elevations in cholesterol. Since the major class of lipoproteins elevated in this disorder is VLDL, patients with this disorder are often referred to as having *Type IV hyperlipoproteinemia* (Fredrickson classification, Table 356-3). The elevated plasma levels of VLDL are due to increased production of VLDL, impaired catabolism of VLDL, or a combination of these mechanisms. Some patients with FHTG have a more severe form of hyperlipidemia in which both VLDLs and chylomicrons are elevated (*Type V hyperlipidemia*), since these two classes of lipoproteins compete for the same lipolytic pathway. Increased intake of simple carbohydrates, obesity, insulin resistance, alcohol use, and estrogen treatment, all of which increase VLDL synthesis, can exacerbate this syndrome. FHTG appears not to be associated with increased risk of ASCVD in many families.

The diagnosis of FHTG is suggested by the triad of elevated levels of plasma triglycerides (250–1000 mg/dL), normal or only mildly increased cholesterol levels (<250 mg/dL), and reduced plasma levels of HDL-C. Plasma LDL-C levels are generally not increased and are often reduced due to defective metabolism of the triglyceride-rich particles, The identification of other first-degree relatives with hypertriglyceridemia is useful in making the diagnosis. FDBL and familial combined hyperlipidemia (FCHL) should also be ruled out since these two conditions are associated with a significantly increased risk of ASCVD. The plasma apoB levels are lower and the ratio of plasma triglyceride to cholesterol is higher in FHTG than in either FDBL or FCHL.

It is important to consider and rule out secondary causes of the hypertriglyceridemia (Table 356-5) before making the diagnosis of FHTG. Lipid-lowering drug therapy can frequently be avoided with appropriate dietary and lifestyle changes. Patients with plasma triglyceride levels >500 mg/dL after a trial of diet and exercise should be considered for drug therapy to avoid the development of chylomicronemia and pancreatitis. Fibrate drugs or fish oils (omega 3 fatty acids) are reasonable first-line approaches for FHTG, and niacin can also be considered in this condition. For more moderate elevations in triglyceride levels (250-500 mg/dL), statins are effective at lowering triglyceride levels.

TABLE 356-5 Secondary Forms of Hyperlipidemia

LDL		HDL					
Elevated	Reduced	Elevated	Reduced	VLDL Elevated	IDL Elevated	Chylomicrons Elevated	Lp(a) Elevated
Hypothyroidism	Severe liver disease	Alcohol	Smoking	Obesity	Multiple myeloma	Autoimmune disease	Renal insufficiency
Nephrotic syndrome	Malabsorption	Exercise	DM type 2	DM type 2			
	Malnutrition	Exposure to chlorinated hydrocarbons	Obesity	Glycogen storage disease	Monoclonal gammopathy	DM type 2	Inflammation
Cholestasis	Gaucher's disease		Malnutrition				Menopause
Acute intermittent porphyria	Chronic infectious disease	Drugs: estrogen	Gaucher's disease	Hepatitis	Autoimmune disease		Orchidectomy
				Alcohol			
Anorexia nervosa	Hyperthyroidism		Drugs: anabolic steroids, beta blockers	Renal failure	Hypothyroidism		Hypothyroidism
Hepatoma	Drugs: niacin toxicity			Sepsis			Acromegaly
Drugs: thiazides, cyclosporin, tegretol				Stress			Nephrosis
				Cushing's syndrome			Drugs: growth hormone, isotretinoin
				Pregnancy			
				Acromegaly			
				Lipodystrophy			
				Drugs: estrogen, beta blockers, glucocorticoids, bile acid binding resins, retinoic acid			

Abbreviations: DM, diabetes mellitus; HDL, high-density lipoprotein; IDL, intermediate-density lipoprotein; LDL, low-density lipoprotein; Lp(a), lipoprotein A; VLDL, very low-density lipoprotein.

Familial combined hyperlipidemia (FCHL) FCHL is generally characterized by moderate elevations in plasma levels of triglycerides (VLDL) and cholesterol (LDL) and reduced plasma levels of HDL-C. Approximately 20% of patients who develop CHD under age 60 have FCHL. The disease appears to be autosomal dominant with incomplete penetrance and affected family members typically have one of three possible phenotypes: (1) elevated plasma levels of LDL-C, (2) elevated plasma levels of triglycerides due to elevation in VLDL, or (3) elevated plasma levels of both LDL-C and triglyceride. A classic feature of FCHL is that the lipoprotein profile can switch among these three phenotypes in the same individual over time and may depend on factors such as diet, exercise, and weight. FCHL can manifest in childhood but is usually not fully expressed until adulthood. A cluster of other metabolic risk factors are often found in association with this hyperlipidemia, including obesity, glucose intolerance, insulin resistance, and hypertension (the so-called metabolic syndrome, Chap. 242). These patients do not develop xanthomas.

Patients with FCHL almost always have significantly elevated plasma levels of apoB. The levels of apoB are disproportionately high relative to the plasma LDL-C concentration, indicating the presence of small, dense LDL particles, which are characteristic of this syndrome. *Hyperapobetalipoproteinemia*, which has been used to describe the state of elevated plasma levels of apoB with normal plasma LDL-C levels, is probably a form of FCHL. Individuals with FCHL generally share the same metabolic defect, which is overproduction of VLDL by the liver. The molecular etiology of FCHL remains poorly understood, and it is likely that defects in several different genes can cause the phenotype of FCHL.

The presence of a mixed dyslipidemia (plasma triglyceride levels between 200 and 800 mg/dL and total cholesterol levels between 200 and 400 mg/dL, usually with HDL-C levels <40 mg/dL in men and <50 mg/dL in women) and a family history of hyperlipidemia and/or premature CHD strongly suggests the diagnosis of FCHL.

Individuals with FCHL should be treated aggressively due to significantly increased risk of premature CHD. Decreased dietary intake of saturated fat and simple carbohydrates, aerobic exercise, and weight loss can all have beneficial effects on the lipid profile. Patients with diabetes should be aggressively treated to maintain good glucose control. Most patients with FCHL require lipid-lowering drug therapy to reduce lipoprotein levels to the recommended range and reduce the high risk of ASCVD. Statins are effective in this condition, but many patients will require a second drug (cholesterol absorption inhibitor, niacin, fibrate, or fish oils) for optimal control of lipoprotein levels.

■ INHERITED CAUSES OF LOW LEVELS OF ApoB-CONTAINING LIPOPROTEINS

Familial hypobetalipoproteinemia (FHB)

Low plasma levels of LDL-C (the "β-lipoprotein") with a genetic or inherited basis are referred to generically as *familial hypobetalipoproteinemia*. Traditionally this term has been used to refer to the condition of low total cholesterol and LDL-C due to mutations in apoB, which represents the most common inherited form of hypocholesterolemia. Most of the mutations causing FHB interfere with the production of apoB, resulting in reduced secretion and/or accelerated catabolism of the protein. Individuals heterozygous for these mutations usually have LDL-C levels <80 mg/dL and may enjoy protection from ASCVD, though this has not been rigorously demonstrated. Some heterozygotes have elevated levels of hepatic triglycerides.

Mutations in both apoB alleles cause homozygous FHB, a disorder resembling abetalipoproteinemia (see below), although the neurologic findings tend to be less severe. Patients with homozygous hypobetalipoproteinemia can be distinguished from individuals with abetalipoproteinemia by measuring the levels of LDL-C in the parents, which are low in hypobetalipoproteinemia and normal in abetalipoproteinemia.

PCSK9 deficiency

A phenocopy of FHB results from loss-of-function mutations in PCSK9. As reviewed previously, PCSK9 normally promotes the degradation of the LDL receptor. Mutations that interfere with the synthesis of PCSK9, which are more common in individuals of African descent, result in increased LDL receptor activity and ~40% reduction in plasma level of LDL-C. A sequence variation of higher frequency (R46L) is found predominantly in individuals of European descent and is associated with a 15% reduction in LDL-C. Individuals with inactivating mutations are protected from developing CHD relative to those without these sequence variations, presumably due to having lower plasma cholesterol levels since birth.

Abetalipoproteinemia

The synthesis and secretion of apoB-containing lipoproteins in the enterocytes of the proximal small bowel and in the hepatocytes of the liver involve a complex series of events that coordinate the coupling of various lipids with apoB-48 and apoB-100, respectively. Abetalipoproteinemia is a rare autosomal recessive disease caused by loss-of-function mutations in the gene encoding microsomal triglyceride transfer protein (MTP), a protein that transfers lipids to nascent chylomicrons and VLDLs in the intestine and liver, respectively. Plasma levels of cholesterol and triglyceride are extremely low in this disorder, and chylomicrons, VLDLs, LDLs, and apoB are undetectable in plasma. The parents of patients with abetalipoproteinemia (obligate heterozygotes) have normal plasma lipid and apoB levels. Abetalipoproteinemia usually presents in early childhood with diarrhea and failure to thrive due to fat malabsorption. The initial neurologic manifestations are loss of deep-tendon reflexes, followed by decreased distal lower extremity vibratory and proprioceptive sense, dysmetria, ataxia, and the development of a spastic gait, often by the third or fourth decade. Patients with abetalipoproteinemia also develop a progressive pigmented retinopathy presenting with decreased night and color vision, followed by reductions in daytime visual acuity and ultimately progressing to near-blindness. The presence of spinocerebellar degeneration and pigmented retinopathy in this disease has resulted in some patients with abetalipoproteinemia being misdiagnosed as having Friedreich's ataxia.

Most clinical manifestations of abetalipoproteinemia result from defects in the absorption and transport of fat-soluble vitamins. Vitamin E and retinyl esters are normally transported from enterocytes to the liver by chylomicrons, and vitamin E is dependent on VLDL for transport out of the liver and into the circulation. As a consequence of the inability of these patients to secrete apoB-containing particles, patients with abetalipoproteinemia are markedly deficient in vitamin E and are also mildly to moderately deficient in vitamins A and K. Patients with abetalipoproteinemia should be referred to specialized centers for confirmation of the diagnosis and appropriate therapy. Treatment consists of a low-fat, high-caloric, vitamin-enriched diet accompanied by large supplemental doses of vitamin E. It is imperative that treatment be initiated as soon as possible to help forestall development of neurologic sequelae, which can progress even with appropriate therapy. New therapies for this serious disease are needed.

■ GENETIC DISORDERS OF HDL METABOLISM

Mutations in genes encoding proteins that play critical roles in HDL synthesis and catabolism can result in both reductions and elevations in plasma levels of HDL-C. Unlike the genetic forms of hypercholesterolemia, which are invariably associated with premature coronary atherosclerosis, genetic forms of hypoalphalipoproteinemia (low HDL-C) are not always associated with accelerated atherosclerosis.

INHERITED CAUSES OF LOW LEVELS OF HDL-C

Gene deletions in the ApoAV-AI-CIII-AIV locus and coding mutations in ApoA-I

Complete genetic deficiency of apoA-I due to deletion of the apoA-I gene results in the virtual absence of HDL from the plasma. The genes encoding apoA-I, apoC-III, apoA-IV, and apoA-V are clustered together on chromosome 11, and some patients with no apoA-I have genomic deletions that include other genes in the cluster. ApoA-I is required for LCAT activity. In the absence of LCAT, free cholesterol levels increase in both HDL and in tissues. The free cholesterol can form deposits in the cornea and in the skin, resulting in corneal opacities and planar xanthomas. Premature CHD is a common feature of apoA-I deficiency, especially when additional genes in the complex are also deleted.

Missense and nonsense mutations in the apoA-I gene have been identified in some patients with low plasma levels of HDL-C (usually 15–30 mg/dL), but these are very rare causes of low HDL-C levels. Patients heterozygous for an Arg173Cys substitution in APOAI (so-called apoA-I_{Milano}) have very low plasma levels of HDL due to impaired LCAT activation and rapid catabolism of the mutant apolipoprotein and yet have no increased risk of premature CHD. Most other individuals with low plasma HDL-C levels due to missense mutations in apoA-I do not appear to have premature CHD. A few selected missense mutations in apoA-I and apoA-II promote the formation of amyloid fibrils causing systemic amyloidosis.

Tangier disease (ABCA1 deficiency)

Tangier disease is a very rare autosomal codominant form of extremely low plasma HDL-C caused by mutations in the gene encoding ABCA1, a cellular transporter that facilitates efflux of unesterified cholesterol and phospholipids from cells to apoA-I (Fig. 356-3). ABCA1 in the liver and intestine rapidly lipidates the apoA-I secreted from these tissues. In the absence of ABCA1, the nascent, poorly lipidated apoA-I is immediately cleared from the circulation. Thus, patients with Tangier disease have extremely low circulating plasma levels of HDL-C (<5 mg/dL) and apoA-I (<5 mg/dL). Cholesterol accumulates in the reticuloendothelial system of these patients, resulting in hepatosplenomegaly and pathognomonic enlarged, grayish yellow or orange tonsils. An intermittent peripheral neuropathy (mononeuritis multiplex) or a sphingomyelia-like neurologic disorder can also be seen in this disorder. Tangier disease is probably associated with some increased risk of premature atherosclerotic disease, although the association is not as robust as might be anticipated, given the very low levels of HDL-C and apoA-I in these patients. Patients with Tangier disease also have low plasma levels of LDL-C, which may attenuate the atherosclerotic risk. Obligate heterozygotes for ABCA1 mutations have moderately reduced plasma HDL-C levels (15–30 mg/dL) but their risk of premature CHD remains uncertain. ABCA1 mutations appear to be the cause of low HDL-C in a minority of individuals.

LCAT deficiency

This very rare autosomal recessive disorder is caused by mutations in LCAT, an enzyme synthesized in the liver and secreted into the plasma, where it circulates associated with lipoproteins (Fig. 356-3). As reviewed previously, the enzyme is activated by apoA-I and mediates the esterification of cholesterol to form cholesteryl esters. Consequently, in LCAT deficiency the proportion of free cholesterol in circulating lipoproteins is greatly increased (from ~25% to >70% of total plasma cholesterol). Lack of normal cholesterol esterification impairs formation of mature HDL particles, resulting in the rapid catabolism of circulating apoA-I. Two genetic forms of LCAT deficiency have been described in humans: complete deficiency (also called *classic LCAT deficiency*) and partial deficiency (also called *fish-eye disease*). Progressive corneal opacification due to the deposition of free cholesterol in the cornea, very low plasma levels of HDL-C (usually <10 mg/dL), and variable hypertriglyceridemia are characteristic of both disorders. In partial LCAT deficiency, there are no other known clinical sequelae. In contrast, patients with complete LCAT deficiency have hemolytic anemia and progressive renal insufficiency that eventually leads to end-stage renal disease (ESRD). Remarkably, despite the extremely low plasma levels of HDL-C and apoA-I, premature ASCVD is not a consistent feature of either LCAT deficiency or fish eye disease. The diagnosis can be confirmed in a specialized laboratory by assaying plasma LCAT activity or by sequencing the LCAT gene.

Primary hypoalphalipoproteinemia

Low plasma levels of HDL-C (the "alpha lipoprotein") is referred to as *hypoalphalipoproteinemia*. Primary hypoalphalipoproteinemia is defined as a plasma HDL-C level below the tenth percentile in the setting of relatively normal cholesterol and triglyceride levels, no apparent secondary causes of low plasma HDL-C, and no clinical signs of LCAT deficiency or Tangier disease. This syndrome is often referred to as *isolated low HDL*. A family history of low HDL-C facilitates the diagnosis of an inherited condition, which usually follows an autosomal dominant pattern. The metabolic etiology of this disease appears to be primarily accelerated catabolism of HDL and its apolipoproteins. Some of these patients may have ABCA1 mutations and therefore technically have heterozygous Tangier disease. Several kindreds with primary hypoalphalipoproteinemia have been described in association with an increased incidence of premature CHD, although this is not an invariant association. Association of hypoalphalipoproteinemia with premature CHD may depend on the specific nature of the gene defect or the underlying metabolic defect responsible for the low plasma HDL-C level.

INHERITED CAUSES OF HIGH LEVELS OF HDL-C

CETP deficiency

Loss-of-function mutations in both alleles of the gene encoding CETP cause substantially elevated HDL-C levels (usually >150 mg/dL). As noted above, CETP facilitates the transfer of cholesteryl esters from HDL to apoB-containing lipoproteins (Fig. 356-3). The absence of this transfer results in an increase in the cholesteryl ester content of HDL and a reduction in plasma levels of LDL-C. The large, cholesterol-rich HDL particles circulating in these patients are cleared at a reduced rate. CETP deficiency was first diagnosed in Japanese persons and is rare outside of Japan. The relationship of CETP deficiency to ASCVD remains unresolved. Heterozygotes for CETP deficiency have only modestly elevated HDL-C levels. Based on the phenotype of high HDL-C in CETP deficiency, pharmacologic inhibition of CETP is under development as a new therapeutic approach to both raise HDL-C levels and lower LDL-C levels, but whether it will reduce risk of ASCVD remains to be determined.

Familial hyperalphalipoproteinemia

The condition of high plasma levels of HDL-C is referred to as *hyperalphalipoproteinemia* and is defined as a plasma HDL-C level above the ninetieth percentile. This trait runs in families, and outside of Japan it is unlikely to be due to CETP deficiency. Most, but not all, persons with this condition appear to have a reduced risk of CHD and increased longevity. Recent evidence is consistent with mutations in endothelial lipase contributing to this phenotype in some cases.

SECONDARY DISORDERS OF LIPOPROTEIN METABOLISM

Significant changes in plasma levels of lipoproteins are seen in a variety of diseases. It is crucial that secondary causes of dyslipidemias (Table 356-5) are considered prior to initiation of lipid-lowering therapy.

Obesity

(See also Chaps. 77 and 78) Obesity is frequently accompanied by dyslipidemia. The increase in adipocyte mass and accompanying decreased insulin sensitivity associated with obesity has multiple effects on lipid metabolism. More free fatty acids are delivered from the expanded adipose tissue to the liver, where they are reesterified in hepatocytes to form triglycerides, which are packaged into VLDLs for secretion into the circulation. The increased insulin levels promote fatty acid synthesis in the liver. Increased dietary intake of simple carbohydrates also drives hepatic production of VLDLs, resulting in elevations in VLDL and/or LDL in some obese subjects. Plasma levels of HDL-C tend to be low in obesity, due in part to reduced lipolysis. Weight loss is often associated with reductions in plasma levels of circulating apoB-containing lipoproteins and increases in the plasma levels of HDL-C.

Diabetes mellitus

(See also Chap. 344) Patients with type I diabetes mellitus generally do not have hyperlipidemia if they remain under good glycemic control. Diabetic ketoacidosis is frequently accompanied by hypertriglyceridemia due to an increased hepatic influx of free fatty acids from adipose tissue. Patients with type II diabetes mellitus are usually dyslipidemic, even when under relatively good glycemic control. The high levels of insulin and insulin resistance associated with type II diabetes has multiple effects on fat metabolism: (1) a decrease in LPL activity resulting in reduced catabolism of chylomicrons and VLDLs, (2) an increase in the release of free fatty acid from the adipose tissue, (3) an increase in fatty acid synthesis in the liver, and (4) an increase in hepatic VLDL production. Patients with type II diabetes mellitus have several lipid abnormalities, including elevated plasma triglycerides (due to increased VLDL and lipoprotein remnants), elevated levels of dense LDL, and decreased plasma levels of HDL-C. In some diabetic patients, especially those with a genetic defect in lipid metabolism, the triglycerides can be extremely elevated, resulting in the development of pancreatitis. Elevated plasma LDL-C levels usually are not a feature of diabetes mellitus and suggest the presence of an underlying lipoprotein abnormality or may indicate the development of diabetic nephropathy.

Lipodystrophy is associated with profound insulin resistance and elevated plasma levels of VLDL and chylomicrons that can be especially difficult to control. Those with congenital generalized lipodystrophy have absence of subcutaneous fat associated with muscle hypertrophy and hepatic steatosis; some of these patients have been treated successfully with leptin. Partial lipodystropy can present with dyslipidemia and the diagnosis should be entertained in patients with variations in body fat distribution, particularly increased truncal fat accompanied by reduced fat in the buttocks and extremities.

Thyroid disease

(See also Chap. 341) Hypothyroidism is associated with elevated plasma LDL-C levels due primarily to a reduction in hepatic LDL receptor function and delayed clearance of LDL. Conversely, plasma levels of LDL-C are often reduced in the hyperthyroid patient. Hypothyroid patients also frequently have increased levels of circulating IDL, and some patients with hypothyroidism also have mild hypertriglyceridemia. Because hypothyroidism is often subtle and therefore easily overlooked, all patients presenting with elevated plasma levels of LDL-C, IDL or triglycerides should be screened for hypothyroidism. Thyroid replacement therapy usually ameliorates the hypercholesterolemia; if not, the patient probably has a primary lipoprotein disorder and may require lipid-lowering drug therapy.

Renal disorders

(See also Chap. 280) Nephrotic syndrome is often associated with pronounced hyperlipoproteinemia, which is usually mixed but can manifest as hypercholesterolemia or hypertriglyceridemia. The hyperlipidemia of nephrotic syndrome appears to be due to a combination of increased hepatic production and decreased clearance of VLDLs, with increased LDL production. Effective treatment of the underlying renal disease normalizes the lipid profile, but most patients with chronic nephrotic syndrome require lipid-lowering drug therapy.

ESRD is often associated with mild hypertriglyceridemia (<300 mg/dL) due to the accumulation of VLDLs and remnant lipoproteins in the circulation. Triglyceride lipolysis and remnant clearance are both reduced in patients with renal failure. Because the risk of ASCVD is increased in ESRD subjects with hyperlipidemia, they should probably be aggressively treated with lipid-lowering agents, even though there is inadequate data at present to indicate that this population benefits from LDL-lowering therapy.

Patients with renal transplants usually have increased lipid levels due to the effect of the drugs required for immunosuppression (cyclosporine and glucocorticoids) and present a difficult management problem since HMG-CoA reductase inhibitors must be used cautiously in these patients.

Liver disorders

(See also Chap. 301) Because the liver is the principal site of formation and clearance of lipoproteins, it is not surprising that liver diseases can affect plasma lipid levels in a variety of ways. Hepatitis due to infection, drugs, or alcohol is often associated with increased VLDL synthesis and mild to moderate hypertriglyceridemia. Severe hepatitis and liver failure are associated with dramatic reductions in plasma cholesterol and triglycerides due to reduced lipoprotein biosynthetic capacity. Cholestasis is associated with hypercholesterolemia, which can be very severe. A major pathway by which cholesterol is excreted from the body is via secretion into bile, either directly or after conversion to bile acids, and cholestasis blocks this critical excretory pathway. In cholestasis, free cholesterol, coupled with phospholipids, is secreted into the plasma as a constituent of a lamellar particle called *LP-X*. The particles can deposit in skinfolds, producing lesions resembling those seen in patients with FDBL (xanthomata strata palmaris). Planar and eruptive xanthomas can also be seen in patients with cholestasis.

Alcohol

Regular alcohol consumption has a variable effect on plasma lipid levels. The most common effect of alcohol is to increase plasma triglyceride levels. Alcohol consumption stimulates hepatic secretion of VLDL, possibly by inhibiting the hepatic oxidation of free fatty acids, which then promote hepatic triglyceride synthesis and VLDL secretion. The usual lipoprotein pattern seen with alcohol consumption is Type IV (increased VLDLs), but persons with an underlying primary lipid disorder may develop severe hypertriglyceridemia (Type V) if they drink alcohol. Regular alcohol use also raises plasma levels of HDL-C.

Estrogen

Estrogen administration is associated with increased VLDL and HDL synthesis, resulting in elevated plasma levels of both triglycerides and HDL-C. This lipoprotein pattern is distinctive since the levels of plasma triglyceride and HDL-C are typically inversely related. Plasma triglyceride levels should be monitored when birth control pills or postmenopausal estrogen therapy is initiated to ensure that the increase in VLDL production does not lead to severe hypertriglyceridemia. Use of low-dose preparations of estrogen or the estrogen patch can minimize the effect of exogenous estrogen on lipids.

Lysosomal storage diseases

(See also Chap. 361) Cholesteryl ester storage disease (due to deficiency in lysosomal acid lipase) and glycogen storage diseases such as von Gierke's disease (caused by mutations in glucose-6-phosphatase) are rare causes of secondary hyperlipidemias.

Cushing's syndrome

(See also Chap. 342) Glucocorticoid excess is associated with increased VLDL synthesis and hypertriglyceridemia. Patients with Cushing's syndrome can also have mild elevations in plasma levels of LDL-C.

Drugs

Many drugs have an impact on lipid metabolism and can result in significant alterations in the lipoprotein profile (Table 356-5).

■ SCREENING

(See also Chaps. 225 and 242) Guidelines for the screening and management of lipid disorders have been provided by an expert Adult Treatment Panel (ATP) convened by the National Cholesterol Education Program (NCEP) of the National Heart, Lung, and Blood Institute. The NCEP ATPIII guidelines published in 2001 recommend that all adults older than age 20 years should have plasma levels of cholesterol, triglyceride, LDL-C, and HDL-C measured after a 12-hour overnight fast. In most clinical laboratories, the total cholesterol and triglycerides in the plasma are measured enzymatically, and then the cholesterol in the supernatant is measured after precipitation of apoB-containing lipoproteins to determine the HDL-C. The LDL-C is estimated using the following equation:

$$LDL\text{-}C = total\ cholesterol - (triglycerides/5) - HDL\text{-}C.$$

(The VLDL-C is estimated by dividing the plasma triglyceride by 5, reflecting the ratio of cholesterol to triglyceride in VLDL particles.) This formula is reasonably accurate if test results are obtained on fasting plasma and if the triglyceride level does not exceed ~200 mg/dL; by convention it cannot be used if the triglyceride level is >400 mg/dL. The accurate determination of LDL-C levels in patients with triglyceride levels >200 mg/dL requires application of ultracentrifugation techniques or other direct assays for LDL-C. If the triglyceride level is >200 mg/dL, the guidelines recommend that the "non-HDL-C" be calculated by simple subtraction of HDL-C from the total cholesterol and that this be considered a secondary target of therapy. Further evaluation and treatment is based primarily on the plasma LDL-C and non-HDL-C levels as well as assessment of overall cardiovascular risk.

■ DIAGNOSIS

The critical first step in managing a lipid disorder is to determine the class or classes of lipoproteins that are increased or decreased in the patient. The Fredrickson classification scheme for hyperlipoproteinemias (Table 356-3), though less commonly used now than in the past, can be helpful in this regard. Once the hyperlipidemia is accurately classified, efforts should be directed to rule out any possible secondary causes of the hyperlipidemia (Table 356-5). Although many patients with hyperlipidemia have a primary or genetic cause of their lipid disorder, secondary factors frequently contribute to the hyperlipidemia. A fasting glucose should be obtained in the initial workup of all subjects with an elevated triglyceride level. Nephrotic syndrome and chronic renal insufficiency should be excluded by obtaining urine protein and serum creatinine. Liver function tests should be performed to rule out hepatitis and cholestasis. Hypothyroidism should be ruled out by measuring serum TSH. Patients with hyperlipidemia, especially hypertriglyceridemia, who drink alcohol should be encouraged to decrease their intake. Sedentary lifestyle, obesity, and smoking are all associated with low HDL-C levels, and patients should be counseled about these issues.

Once secondary causes for the elevated lipoprotein levels have been ruled out, attempts should be made to diagnose the primary lipid disorder since the underlying etiology has a significant effect on the risk of developing CHD, on the response to drug therapy, and on the management of other family members. Often, determining the correct diagnosis requires a detailed family medical history and, in some cases, lipid analyses in family members.

If the fasting plasma triglyceride level is >1000 mg/dL, the patient almost always has chylomicronemia and either has Type I or Type V hyperlipoproteinemia (Table 356-3). The plasma triglyceride to cholesterol ratio helps distinguish between these two possibilities and is higher in Type I than Type V hyperlipoproteinemia. If the patient has Type I hyperlipoproteinemia, a postheparin lipolytic assay should be performed to determine if the patient has LPL or apoC-II deficiency. Type V is a much more frequent form of chylomicronemia in the adult patient. Often treatment of secondary factors contributing to the hyperlipidemia (diet, obesity, glucose intolerance, alcohol ingestion, estrogen therapy) will change a Type V into a Type IV pattern, reducing the risk of developing acute pancreatitis.

If the levels of LDL-C are very high (greater than a ninety-fifth percentile), it is likely the patient has a genetic form of hyperlipidemia. The presence of severe hypercholesterolemia, tendon xanthomas, and an autosomal dominant pattern of inheritance are consistent with the diagnosis of either FH, FDB, or ADH-PCSK9. At the present time, there is no compelling reason to perform molecular studies to further refine the molecular diagnosis, since the treatment of FH and FDB is identical. Recessive forms of severe hypercholesterolemia are rare and if the patient with severe hypercholesterolemia has parents with normal cholesterol levels, sitosterolemia should be considered; a clue to the diagnosis of sitosterolemia is the greater than expected response of the hypercholesterolemia to reductions in dietary cholesterol content or to treatment with either a cholesterol absorption inhibitor (ezetimibe) or to bile acid resins. Patients with more moderate hypercholesterolemia that does not segregate in families as a monogenic trait are likely to have polygenic hypercholesterolemia.

The most common error in the diagnosis and treatment of lipid disorders is in patients with a mixed hyperlipidemia without chylomicronemia. Elevations in the plasma levels of both cholesterol and triglycerides are seen in patients with increased plasma levels of IDL (Type III) and of LDL and VLDL (Type IIB) and in patients with increased levels of VLDL (Type IV). The ratio of triglyceride to cholesterol is higher in Type IV than the other two disorders. The plasma levels of apoB are highest in Type IIB. A beta quantification to determine the VLDL-C/triglyceride ratio in plasma (see discussion of FDBL) or a direct measurement of the plasma LDL-C should be performed at least once prior to initiation of lipid-lowering therapy to determine if the hyperlipidemia is due to the accumulation of remnants or to an increase in both LDL and VLDL.

TREATMENT **Lipoprotein Disorders**

CLINICAL EVIDENCE THAT TREATMENT OF DYSLIPIDEMIA REDUCES RISK OF CHD

Observational Data Multiple epidemiologic studies have demonstrated a strong relationship between plasma levels of LDL-C and CHD. A direct connection between plasma cholesterol levels and the atherosclerotic process was made in humans when aortic fatty streaks in young persons were shown to be strongly correlated with serum cholesterol levels. The elucidation of homozygous familial hypercholesterolemia was proof that high plasma levels of LDL-C alone are sufficient to cause CAD. Moreover, PCSK9 deficiency proves that having a lifelong reduction in plasma level of LDL-C is associated with a marked reduction in cardiovascular risk.

Clinical Trials: LDL-C Reduction Early clinical trials of cholesterol (mostly LDL-C) reduction utilized niacin, bile acid sequestrants, and even the surgical approach of partial ileal bypass to reduce serum cholesterol levels. Although most of these early studies found a small but significant reduction in cardiac events, no decrease in total mortality was seen. The discovery of more potent and well-tolerated cholesterol-lowering agents, namely HMG-CoA reductase inhibitors (statins), ushered in a series of large cholesterol reduction trials that unequivocally established the benefit of cholesterol reduction. The first of these studies was the Scandinavian Simvastatin Survival Study (4S) in which hypercholesterolemic men with CHD who were treated with simvastatin had a reduction in major coronary events of 44% and a reduction in total mortality of 30%. These impressive results were followed by additional studies using statins. The consistency of results of these studies is remarkable. They demonstrated statins to be effective in primary as well as secondary prevention, in women as well as men, in elderly as well as middle-aged individuals, and in patients with only modestly elevated LDL-C levels as well as those with severe hypercholesterolemia. In general, these studies demonstrated that a 1% reduction in LDL-C level is associated with a reduction in coronary events of a similar magnitude, and an ~40 mg/dL reduction in LDL-C is associated with an ~22% reduction in coronary events.

More recent studies have enrolled subjects with average or subaverage plasma LDL-C levels and have involved targeting the on-treatment LDL-C to even lower levels. For example, the Heart Protection Study (HPS) included 20,536 men and women, ages 40–80 years, who had either established ASCVD or were at high risk for the development of CHD (primarily diabetes); the only lipid entry criterion was a total plasma cholesterol level of >135 mg/dL. Treatment with simvastatin for an average of 5 years resulted in a 24% reduction in major coronary events and a highly significant 13% reduction in all-cause mortality. Importantly, the relative benefit of statin therapy was similar across tertiles of baseline LDL-C, and even the large subgroup of individuals with an LDL-C <100 mg/dL at baseline experienced significant benefit from therapy. This study demonstrated that statin therapy is beneficial in high-risk subjects, even if the baseline LDL-C level is below the currently recommended targeted goal; it also helped to shift the emphasis from simply treating elevated cholesterol to treating patients at high risk of CHD. Additional large-scale clinical trials have expanded on these findings and confirmed that individuals with other cardiovascular risk factors (hypertension, diabetes) benefit from LDL-lowering therapy even when the initial LDL-C level is only modestly elevated. The JUPITER trial was a primary prevention trial in subjects without CHD and with LDL-C <130 mg/dL but with an elevated plasma level of C-reactive protein (CRP). Treatment with rosuvastatin reduced LDL-C by an average of 50% and significantly reduced cardiovascular events, further extending the indication for statin therapy in primary prevention.

Further studies have compared different statin regimens to show that greater reductions in LDL-C levels with treatment are associated with a greater reduction in major cardiovascular events. Based on several of these studies, a white paper was issued by the NCEP in 2004 establishing an "optional" LDL-C goal of <70 mg/dL in high-risk patients with CHD and of <100 mg/dL in very-high-risk patients without known CHD. These optional targets have been widely embraced, and clinical practice is clearly evolving to treating CHD and high-risk patients more aggressively for LDL reduction.

Clinical Trials: The Triglyceride-HDL Axis Abnormalities of the triglyceride high-density lipoprotein (TG-HDL) axis are common in patients with CHD, although data supporting pharmacologic intervention in the TG-HDL axis is less compelling than data supporting LDL-C reduction. Fibric acid derivatives (fibrates), nicotinic acid (niacin), and omega 3 fatty acids (fish oils) are the primary agents currently available to lower plasma triglyceride levels and increase plasma levels of HDL-C. Fibrates have been used as lipid-lowering drugs for several decades and are more effective in reducing plasma triglyceride levels and relatively less effective in increasing plasma HDL-C levels. The results of clinical trials using fibrates have been mixed. Some studies such as the Helsinki Heart Study (HHS) and the Veteran Affairs High-Density Lipoprotein Cholesterol Intervention Trial (VA-HIT) demonstrated a significant reduction in nonfatal myocardial infarction and coronary death with gemfibrozil therapy. However, the Bezafibrate Infarction Prevention (BIP) trial of bezafibrate vs placebo in CHD patients with low HDL-C failed to demonstrate a statistically significant reduction in coronary events, the Fenofibrate Intervention and Event Lowering in Diabetes (FIELD) trial of fenofibrate in patients with type 2 diabetes failed to show a significant reduction in its primary endpoint of nonfatal myocardial infarction and coronary death, and the Action to Control Cardiovascular Risk in Diabetes (ACCORD) study of fenofibrate vs. placebo added to simvastatin in patients with type 2 diabetes failed to show a significant reduction in its primary end point of major acute cardiovascular events. In each of these studies, the subgroup with elevated baseline triglycerides suggested benefit.

While niacin is the most effective HDL-raising drug currently available, it has not been tested for its ability to reduce cardiovascular risk in subjects with low plasma levels of HDL-C. The AIM-HIGH and HPS2-THRIVE trials are ongoing studies of the effect of niacin added to baseline statin therapy in patients with CHD and low HDL-C. Finally, while low-dose fish oils have been shown to reduce cardiovascular events, higher doses that reduce triglyceride levels have not been tested for their ability to reduce cardiovascular events. Definitive proof that treating the TG-HDL axis reduces cardiovascular events is likely to come from new therapies that are more effective at specifically targeting VLDL and/or HDL particles.

CLINICAL APPROACH TO LIPID-MODIFYING THERAPY The major goal of lipid-modifying therapy in most patients with disorders of lipid metabolism is to prevent ASCVD and its complications. Management of lipid disorders should be based on clinical trial data demonstrating that treatment reduces cardiovascular morbidity and mortality, although reasonable extrapolation of these data to specific subgroups is sometimes required. Clearly, elevated plasma levels of LDL-C are strongly associated with increased risk of ASCVD, and treatment to lower the levels of plasma LDL-C decreases the risk of clinical cardiovascular events in both secondary and primary prevention. Although the proportional benefit accrued from reducing plasma LDL-C appears to be similar over the entire range of LDL-C values, the absolute risk reduction depends on the baseline level of cardiovascular risk. The treatment guidelines developed by NCEP ATPIII and the 2004 white paper incorporate these principles. As noted above, abnormalities in the TG-HDL axis (elevated triglyceride, low HDL-C, or both) are commonly seen in patients with CHD or who are at high risk for developing it, but clinical trial data supporting the treatment of these abnormalities is much less compelling, and the pharmacologic tools for their management are more limited. Importantly, the NCEP ATPIII guidelines promote the use of the "non-HDL-C" as a secondary target of therapy in patients with triglyceride levels >200 mg/dL. The goals for non-HDL-C are 30 mg/dL higher than the goals for LDL-C. Thus, many patients with abnormalities of the TG-HDL axis require additional therapy for reduction of non-HDL-C to recommended goals.

NONPHARMACOLOGIC TREATMENT

Diet Dietary modification is an important component in the management of dyslipidemia. The physician should assess the content of the patient's diet and provide suggestions for dietary modifications. In the patient with elevated LDL-C, dietary saturated fat and cholesterol should be restricted. For individuals with hypertriglyceridemia, the intake of simple carbohydrates should be curtailed. For severe hypertriglyceridemia (>1000 mg/dL), restriction of total fat intake is critical. The most widely used diet to lower the LDL-C level is the "Step I diet" developed by the American Heart Association. Most patients have a relatively modest (<10%) decrease in plasma levels of LDL-C on a Step I diet in the absence of any associated weight loss. Almost all persons experience a decrease in plasma HDL-C levels with a reduction in the amount of total and saturated fat in their diet.

Foods and Additives Certain foods and dietary additives are associated with modest reductions in plasma cholesterol levels. Plant stanol and sterol esters are available in a variety of foods, such as spreads, salad dressings, and snack bars. Plant sterol and sterol esters interfere with cholesterol absorption and reduce plasma LDL-C levels by ~10% when taken three times per day. The addition to the diet of psyllium, soy protein, or Chinese red yeast rice (which contains lovastatin) can have modest cholesterol-lowering effects. No controlled studies have been performed in which several of these nonpharmacologic options have been combined to address their additive or synergistic effects.

Weight Loss and Exercise The treatment of obesity, if present, can have a favorable impact on plasma lipid levels and should be actively encouraged. Plasma triglyceride and LDL-C levels tend to fall and HDL-C levels tend to increase in obese subjects after weight reduction. Regular aerobic exercise can also have a positive effect on lipids, in large measure due to the associated weight reduction. Aerobic exercise has a very modest elevating effect on plasma levels of HDL-C in most individuals but also has cardiovascular benefits that extend beyond the effects on plasma lipid levels.

PHARMACOLOGIC TREATMENT The decision to use drug therapy depends on the level of cardiovascular risk. Drug therapy for hypercholesterolemia in patients with established CHD is well supported by clinical trial data, as reviewed above. Even patients with CHD or risk factors who have "average" LDL-C levels benefit from treatment. Drug treatment to lower LDL-C levels in patients with CHD is also highly cost-effective. Patients with diabetes mellitus without known CHD have similar cardiovascular risk to those without diabetes but with preexisting CHD. The NCEP ATPIII guidelines recommended estimating absolute risk of a cardiovascular event over 10 years using a scoring system based on the Framingham Heart Study database. Patients with a 10-year absolute CHD risk of >20% are considered "CHD risk equivalents" to be treated as aggressively as patients with existing CHD. Current NCEP ATPIII guidelines call for drug therapy to reduce LDL-C to <100 mg/dL in patients with established CHD, other ASCVD (aortic aneurysm, peripheral vascular disease, or cerebrovascular disease), diabetes mellitus, or CHD risk equivalents; and "optionally" to reduce LDL-C to <70 mg/dL in high-risk CHD patients. Based on these guidelines, virtually all CHD and CHD risk-equivalent patients require cholesterol-lowering drug therapy. Moderate-risk patients with two or more risk factors and a 10-year absolute risk of 10–20% should be treated to a goal LDL-C of <130 mg/dL or "optionally" to LDL-C <100 mg/dL.

Although helpful to consider 10-year absolute risk in making clinical decisions about lipid-altering drug therapy, there are situations where 10-year risk is low but lifetime risk is very high and therefore treatment is indicated. A typical example would be a young adult with heterozygous FH and an LDL-C >220 mg/dL. Despite a very low 10-year absolute risk, every such patient should be treated with drug therapy to reduce lifetime risk. Indeed, all patients with markedly elevated plasma levels of LDL-C levels (>190 mg/dL) should be strongly considered for drug therapy even if their 10-year absolute CHD risk is not elevated. The decision of whether to initiate drug treatment in individuals with plasma LDL-C levels between 130 and 190 mg/dL remains controversial and depends on both 10-year and lifetime risk. Although it is desirable to avoid drug treatment in patients who are unlikely to develop CHD, a high proportion of patients who eventually develop CHD have plasma LDL-C levels within this range. The presence of other risk factors such as a low plasma level of HDL-C (<40 mg/dL) or the diagnosis of the metabolic syndrome would argue in favor of drug therapy (Chap. 242). Other laboratory tests such as an elevated plasma level of apoB, Lp(a), or high-sensitivity C-reactive protein, may assist in the identification of high-risk individuals who should be considered for drug therapy when their LDL-C is in a "gray zone."

Drug treatment is also indicated in patients with triglycerides >500 mg/dL who have been screened and treated for secondary causes of hypertriglyceridemia. The goal is to reduce fasting plasma triglycerides to below 500 mg/dL to prevent the risk of acute pancreatitis. When triglycerides are 200–500 mg/dL, the decision to use drug therapy depends on the risk of the patient developing chylomicronemia and an assessment of cardiovascular risk. Most major clinical endpoint trials with statins have excluded persons with triglyceride levels >350–450 mg/dL, and there are therefore few data regarding the effectiveness of statins in reducing cardiovascular risk in persons with hypertriglyceridemia. More data are needed regarding the relative effectiveness of statins, fibrates, niacin, and fish oils for reducing cardiovascular risk in this setting. Combination therapy is often required for optimal control of mixed dyslipidemia.

HMG-CoA Reductase Inhibitors (Statins) HMG-CoA reductase is a key enzyme in cholesterol biosynthesis, and inhibition of this enzyme decreases cholesterol synthesis. By inhibiting cholesterol biosynthesis, statins lead to increased hepatic LDL receptor activity as a counterregulatory mechanism and thus accelerated clearance of circulating LDL, resulting in a dose-dependent reduction in plasma levels of LDL-C. The magnitude of LDL lowering associated with statin treatment varies widely among individuals, but once a patient is on a statin, the doubling of the statin dose produces an ~6% further reduction in the level of plasma

TABLE 356-6 Summary of the Major Drugs Used for the Treatment of Hyperlipidemia

Drug	Major Indications	Starting Dose	Maximal Dose	Mechanism	Common Side Effects
HMG-CoA reductase inhibitors (statins)	Elevated LDL-C			↓ Cholesterol synthesis, ↑ hepatic LDL receptors, ↓ VLDL production	Myalgias, arthralgias, elevated transaminases, dyspepsia
Lovastatin		20 mg daily	80 mg daily		
Pravastatin		40 mg qhs	80 mg qhs		
Simvastatin		20 mg qhs	80 mg qhs		
Fluvastatin		20 mg qhs	80 mg qhs		
Atorvastatin		10 mg qhs	80 mg qhs		
Rosuvastatin		10 mg qhs	40 mg qhs		
Cholesterol absorption inhibitors				↓ Intestinal cholesterol absorption	Elevated transaminases
Ezetimibe	Elevated LDL-C	10 mg daily	10 mg daily	LDL receptors	
Bile acid sequestrants	Elevated LDL-C			↑ Bile acid excretion and ↑ LDL receptors	Bloating, constipation, elevated triglycerides
Cholestyramine		4 g daily	32 g daily		
Colestipol		5 g daily	40 g daily		
Colesevelam		3750 mg daily	4375 mg daily		
Nicotinic acid	Elevated LDL-C, low HDL-C, elevated TG			↓ VLDL production	Cutaneous flushing, GI upset, elevated glucose, uric acid, and liver function tests
Immediate-release		100 mg tid	1 g tid		
Sustained-release		250 mg bid	1.5 g bid		
Extended-release		500 mg qhs	2 g qhs		
Fibric acid derivatives	Elevated TG, elevated remnants			↑ LPL, ↓ VLDL synthesis	Dyspepsia, myalgia, gallstones, elevated transaminases
Gemfibrozil		600 mg bid	600 mg bid		
Fenofibrate		145 mg qd	145 mg qd		
Omega 3 fatty acids	Elevated TG	3 g daily	6 g daily	↑ TG catabolism	Dyspepsia, diarrhea, fishy odor to breath

Abbreviations: GI, gastrointestinal; HDL-C, HDL-cholesterol; LDL, low-density lipoprotein; LDL-C, LDL-cholesterol; LPL, lipoprotein lipase; TG, triglyceride; VLDL, very low-density lipoprotein.

LDL-C. The statins currently available differ in their LDL-C reducing potency (Table 356-6). Currently, there is no convincing evidence that any of the different statins confer an advantage that is independent of the effect on LDL-C. Statins also reduce plasma triglycerides in a dose-dependent fashion, which is roughly proportional to their LDL-C–lowering effects (if the triglycerides are <400 mg/dL). Statins have a modest HDL-raising effect (5–10%) that is not generally dose-dependent.

Statins are well tolerated and can be taken in tablet form once a day. Potential side effects include dyspepsia, headaches, fatigue, and muscle or joint pains. Severe myopathy and even rhabdomyolysis occur rarely with statin treatment. The risk of statin-associated myopathy is increased by the presence of older age, frailty, renal insufficiency, and coadministration of drugs that interfere with the metabolism of statins such as erythromycin and related antibiotics, antifungal agents, immunosuppressive drugs, and fibric acid derivatives (particularly gemfibrozil). Severe myopathy can usually be avoided by careful patient selection, avoidance of interacting drugs, and instructing the patient to contact the physician immediately in the event of unexplained muscle pain. In the event of muscle symptoms, the plasma creatine kinase (CK) level should be obtained to document the myopathy. Serum CK levels need not be monitored on a routine basis in patients taking statins, as an elevated CK in the absence of symptoms does not predict the development of myopathy and does not necessarily suggest the need for discontinuing the drug.

Another consequence of statin therapy can be elevation in liver transaminases [alanine (ALT) and aspartate (AST)]. They should be checked before starting therapy, at 2–3 months, and then annually. Substantial (greater than three times the upper limit of normal) elevation in transaminases is relatively rare and mild-to-moderate (one to three times normal) elevation in transaminases in the absence of symptoms need not mandate discontinuing the medication. Severe clinical hepatitis associated with statins is exceedingly rare, and the trend is toward less frequent monitoring of transaminases in patients taking statins. The statin-associated elevation in liver enzymes resolves upon discontinuation of the medication.

Statins appear to be remarkably safe. Meta-analyses of large randomized controlled clinical trials with statins do not suggest an increase in any major noncardiac diseases. Statins are the drug class of choice for LDL-C reduction and are by far the most widely used class of lipid-lowering drugs.

Cholesterol Absorption Inhibitors Cholesterol within the lumen of the small intestine is derived from the diet (about one-third) and the bile (about two-thirds) and is actively absorbed by the enterocyte through a process that involves the protein NPC1L1.

Ezetimibe (Table 356-6) is a cholesterol absorption inhibitor that binds directly to and inhibits NPC1L1 and blocks the intestinal absorption of cholesterol. Ezetimibe (10 mg) inhibits cholesterol absorption by almost 60%, resulting in a reduction in delivery of dietary sterols in the liver and an increase in hepatic LDL receptor expression. The mean reduction in plasma LDL-C on ezetimibe (10 mg) is 18%, and the effect is additive when used in combination with a statin. Effects on triglyceride and HDL-C levels are negligible, and no cardiovascular outcome data have been reported. When used in combination with a statin, monitoring of liver transaminases is recommended. The only role for ezetimibe in monotherapy is in patients who do not tolerate statins; the drug is often added to a statin in patients who require further LDL-C reduction.

Bile Acid Sequestrants (Resins) Bile acid sequestrants bind bile acids in the intestine and promote their excretion rather than reabsorption in the ileum. To maintain the bile acid pool size, the liver diverts cholesterol to bile acid synthesis. The decreased hepatic intracellular cholesterol content results in upregulation of the LDL receptor and enhanced LDL clearance from the plasma. Bile acid sequestrants, including cholestyramine, colestipol, and colesevelam (Table 356-6), primarily reduce plasma LDL-C levels but can cause an increase in plasma triglycerides. Therefore, patients with hypertriglyceridemia should not be treated with bile acid–binding resins. Cholestyramine and colestipol are insoluble resins that must be suspended in liquids. Colesevelam is available as tablets but generally requires up to six to seven tablets per day for effective LDL-C lowering. Most side effects of resins are limited to the gastrointestinal tract and include bloating and constipation. Since bile acid sequestrants are not systemically absorbed, they are very safe and the cholesterol-lowering drug of choice in children and in women of childbearing age who are lactating, pregnant, or could become pregnant. They are effective in combination with statins as well as in combination with ezetimibe and are particularly useful with one or both of these drugs for difficult-to-treat patients or those with statin intolerance.

Nicotinic Acid (Niacin) Nicotinic acid, or niacin, is a B-complex vitamin that has been used as a lipid-modifying agent for more than five decades. Niacin reduces the flux of nonesterified fatty acids (NEFAs) to the liver, which is thought to be the mechanism for reduced hepatic triglyceride synthesis and VLDL secretion. Recently, a nicotinic acid receptor (GPR109A) was discovered that suppresses release of NEFA by adipose tissue, thus mediating the effect of niacin on NEFA suppression. Niacin reduces plasma triglyceride and LDL-C levels and raises the plasma concentration of HDL-C (Table 356-6), but it appears that these effects may not be mediated solely by GPR109A. Niacin is also the only currently available lipid-lowering drug that significantly reduces plasma levels of Lp(a) (up to 40%). If properly prescribed and monitored, niacin is a safe and effective lipid-lowering agent.

The most frequent side effect of niacin is cutaneous flushing, which is mediated by activating GPR109A in the skin, leading to local generation of prostaglandin D2 (PGD2) and prostaglandin E2. Flushing can be reduced by formulations that slow the absorption and by taking aspirin prior to dosing. A product is available in Europe that blocks the receptor for PGD2 and attenuates flushing. There is rapid tachyphylaxis to the flushing. Niacin therapy is generally started at lower doses and gradually titrated up to higher doses. Immediate-release crystalline niacin is generally administered three times per day, over-the-counter sustained-release niacin is taken twice a day, and a prescription form of extended-release niacin is taken once a day. Mild elevations in transaminases occur in up to 15% of patients treated with any form of niacin, and on occasion these elevations may require stopping the medication. Niacin potentiates the effect of warfarin, and these two drugs should be prescribed together with caution. Acanthosis nigricans, a dark-colored coarse skin lesion, and maculopathy are infrequent side effects of niacin. Niacin is contraindicated in patients with peptic ulcer disease and can exacerbate the symptoms of esophageal reflux. It can also raise plasma levels of uric acid and precipitate gouty attacks in susceptible patients.

Niacin can raise fasting plasma glucose levels. A study in type 2 diabetics found only a slight increase in fasting glucose and no significant change in HbA1c level with niacin treatment. Low-dose niacin can be used effectively to reduce plasma triglyceride levels and increase HDL-C without adversely impacting on glycemic control. Thus, niacin can be used in diabetic patients, but every effort should be made to optimize the diabetes management before initiating niacin. Glucose should be carefully monitored in nondiabetic patients with impaired fasting glucose after initiation of niacin therapy.

Successful therapy with niacin requires careful education and motivation on the part of the patient. Its advantages are its low cost and long-term safety. It is the most effective drug currently available for raising HDL-C levels. It is particularly useful in patients with combined hyperlipidemia and low plasma levels of HDL-C and is effective in combination with statins. Outcome data are somewhat limited with niacin, but two clinical trials assessing the benefits of adding niacin to a statin in high-risk patients with low HDL-C are currently ongoing.

Fibric Acid Derivatives (Fibrates) Fibric acid derivatives are agonists of PPARα, a nuclear receptor involved in the regulation of lipid metabolism. Fibrates stimulate LPL activity (enhancing triglyceride hydrolysis), reduce apoC-III synthesis (enhancing lipoprotein remnant clearance), promote beta-oxidation of fatty acids, and may reduce VLDL triglyceride production. Fibrates are the most effective drugs available for reducing triglyceride levels and also raise HDL-C levels modestly (Table 356-6). They have variable effects on LDL-C and in hypertriglyceridemic patients can sometimes be associated with increases in plasma LDL-C levels.

Fibrates are generally very well tolerated. The most common side effect is dyspepsia. Myopathy and hepatitis occur rarely in the absence of other lipid-lowering agents. Fibrates promote cholesterol secretion into bile and are associated with an increased risk of gallstones. Fibrates can raise creatinine and should be used with caution in patients with chronic kidney disease. Importantly, fibrates can potentiate the effect of warfarin and certain oral hypoglycemic agents, so the anticoagulation status and plasma glucose levels should be closely monitored in patients on these agents.

Fibrates are useful and are a reasonable consideration for first-line therapy in patients with severe hypertriglyceridemia (>500 mg/dL) to prevent pancreatitis. Their role in patients with moderate hypertriglyceridemia (200–500 mg/dL) is to promote reduction in non-HDL-C levels, but outcome data regarding their effects on coronary events in this setting remains mixed. In patients with a triglyceride level <500 mg/dL, the role of fibrates is primarily in combination with statins in selected patients with mixed dyslipidemia. In this setting, the risk of myopathy can be minimized with appropriate patient and drug selection and must be carefully weighed against the clinical benefit of the therapy.

Omega 3 Fatty Acids (Fish Oils) N-3 polyunsaturated fatty acids (n-3 PUFAs) are present in high concentration in fish and in flaxseeds. The most widely used n-3 PUFAs for the treatment of hyperlipidemias are the two active molecules in fish oil: eicosapentaenoic acid (EPA) and decohexanoic acid (DHA).

N-3 PUFAs have been concentrated into tablets and in doses of 3–4 g/d are effective at lowering fasting triglyceride levels. Fish oils can cause an increase in plasma LDL-C levels in some patients. Fish oil supplements can be used in combination with fibrates, niacin, or statins to treat hypertriglyceridemia. In general, fish oils are well tolerated and appear to be safe, at least at doses up to 3–4 g. Although fish oil administration is associated with a prolongation in the bleeding time, no increase in bleeding has been seen in clinical trials. A lower dose of omega 3 (about 1 g) has been associated with reduction in cardiovascular events in CHD patients and is used by some clinicians for this purpose.

Combination Drug Therapy Combination drug therapy is frequently used for (1) patients unable to reach LDL-C and non-HDL-C goals on statin monotherapy, (2) patients with combined elevated LDL-C and abnormalities of the TG-HDL axis, and (3) patients with severe hypertriglyceridemia who do not achieve non-HDL-C goal on a fibrate or on fish oils alone. When LDL-C and non-HDL-C goals are not achieved on statin monotherapy, a cholesterol absorption inhibitor or bile acid sequestrant can be added to the drug regimen. Combination of niacin with a statin is an attractive option for high-risk patients who do not attain their target LDL-C level on statin monotherapy and have a low HDL-C level. Conversely, in high-risk patients on statin therapy who have an elevated plasma triglyceride level, addition of a fibrate or fish oils is a reasonable consideration.

Severely hypertriglyceridemic patients treated first with a fibrate often fail to reach LDL-C and non-HDL-C goals and are therefore candidates for addition of a statin. Coadministration of statins and fibrates has obvious appeal in patients with combined hyperlipidemia, but no clinical trial has assessed the effectiveness of a statin-fibrate combination compared with either a statin or a fibrate alone in reducing cardiovascular events. The long-term safety of the statin-fibrate combination is not known. Since coadministration of statins and fibrates is associated with an increased incidence of severe myopathy and rhabdomyolysis, patients treated with this combination must be carefully counseled and monitored. This combination of drugs should be used cautiously in patients with underlying renal or hepatic insufficiency; in the elderly, frail, and chronically ill; and in those on multiple medications.

OTHER APPROACHES Occasionally, patients cannot tolerate any of the existing lipid-lowering drugs at doses required for adequate control of their lipid levels. A larger group of patients, most of whom have genetic lipid disorders, remain significantly hypercholesterolemic despite combination drug therapy. These patients are at high risk for the development or progression of CHD and clinical CHD events. The preferred option for management of patients with severe refractory hypercholesterolemia is LDL apheresis. In this process, the patient's plasma is passed over a column that selectively removes the LDL, and the LDL-depleted plasma is returned to the patient. Patients on maximally tolerated combination drug therapy who have CHD and a plasma LDL-C level >200 mg/dL or no CHD and a plasma LDL-C level >300 mg/dL are candidates for every-other-week LDL apheresis and should be referred to a specialized lipid center.

MANAGEMENT OF LOW HDL-C Severely reduced plasma levels of HDL-C (<20 mg/dL) accompanied by triglycerides <400 mg/dL usually indicate the presence of a genetic disorder such as a mutation in apoA-I, LCAT deficiency, or Tangier disease. HDL-C levels <20 mg/dL are common in the setting of severe hypertriglyceridemia, in which case the primary focus should be on the management of the triglycerides. HDL-C levels <20 mg/dL also occur in individuals using anabolic steroids. Secondary causes of more moderate reductions in plasma HDL (20–40 mg/dL) should be considered (Table 356-5). Smoking should be discontinued, obese persons should be encouraged to lose weight, sedentary persons should be encouraged to exercise, and diabetes should be optimally controlled. When possible, medications associated with reduced plasma levels of HDL-C should be discontinued. The presence of an isolated low plasma level of HDL-C in a patient with a borderline plasma level of LDL-C should prompt consideration of LDL-lowering drug therapy in high-risk individuals. Statins increase plasma levels of HDL-C only modestly (~5–10%). Fibrates also have only a modest effect on plasma HDL-C levels (increasing levels ~5–15%), except in patients with coexisting hypertriglyceridemia, where the effect on HDL levels can be greater. Niacin is the most effective HDL-C–raising therapeutic agent available and can increase plasma HDL-C by up to ~30%, although some patients fail to achieve clinically important increases in HDL-C levels from niacin therapy.

The issue of whether pharmacologic intervention should be used to specifically raise HDL-C levels has not been adequately addressed in clinical trials. In persons with established CHD and low HDL-C levels whose plasma LDL-C levels are at or below the goal, it may be reasonable to initiate therapy (with a fibrate or niacin) directed specifically at reducing plasma triglyceride levels and raising the level of plasma HDL-C. More data are required before broad recommendations are made to use drug therapy to specifically raise HDL-C levels to prevent cardiovascular events. New HDL-raising approaches are under development that may help to address this important issue.

Management of Elevated Levels of Lp(a) High levels of Lp(a) are associated with increased risk of ASCVD. Genetic studies suggest that this association is causal, but there is no evidence that reducing plasma Lp(a) levels reduces cardiovascular risk. Until such studies are performed, the major therapeutic approach to patients with high plasma levels of Lp(a) and established CAD is to aggressively lower plasma levels of LDL-C. Niacin is the only drug currently available that lowers Lp(a), and might be considered as an addition to a statin in a very-high-risk patient with elevated Lp(a).

FURTHER READINGS

Ashen MD, Blumenthal RS: Clinical practice: Low HDL cholesterol levels. N Engl J Med 353:1252, 2005

Baigent C et al: Efficacy and safety of cholesterol-lowering treatment: Prospective meta-analysis of data from 90,056 participants in 14 randomised trials of statins. Lancet 366:1267, 2005

Brunzell JD: Clinical practice. Hypertriglyceridemia. N Engl J Med 357:1009, 2007

Grundy SM: The issue of statin safety: Where do we stand? Circulation 111:3016, 2005

——— et al: Implications of recent clinical trials for the National Cholesterol Education Program Adult Treatment Panel III guidelines. Circulation 110:227, 2004

National Cholesterol Education Program: Executive summary of the third report of the National Cholesterol Education Program (NCEP) Expert Panel on Detection, Evaluation, and Treatment of High Blood Cholesterol in Adults (Adult Treatment Panel III). JAMA 285:2486, 2001

Rader DJ et al: Monogenic hypercholesterolemia: New insights in pathogenesis and treatment. J Clin Invest 111:1795, 2003

Ridker PM et al: Rosuvastatin to prevent vascular events in men and women with elevated C-reactive protein. N Engl J Med 359:2195, 2008

CHAPTER 357
Hemochromatosis

Lawrie W. Powell

DEFINITION

Hemochromatosis is a common inherited disorder of iron metabolism in which dysregulation of intestinal iron absorption results in deposition of excessive amounts of iron in parenchymal cells with eventual tissue damage and impaired function in a wide range of organs. The iron-storage pigment in tissues is called *hemosiderin* because it is believed to be derived from the blood. The term *hemosiderosis* is used to describe the presence of stainable iron in tissues, but tissue iron must be quantified to assess body-iron status accurately (see below and Chap. 103). *Hemochromatosis* refers to a group of genetic diseases that predispose to iron overload, potentially leading to fibrosis and organ failure. Cirrhosis of the liver, diabetes mellitus, arthritis, cardiomyopathy, and hypogonadotropic hypogonadism are the major clinical manifestations.

Although there is debate about definitions, the following terminology is widely accepted.

1. *Hereditary hemochromatosis* is most often caused by a mutant gene, termed *HFE*, which is tightly linked to the HLA-A locus on chromosome 6p (see "Genetic Basis," below). Persons who are homozygous for the mutation are at increased risk of iron overload and account for 80 to 90% of clinical hereditary hemochromatosis in persons of northern European descent. In such subjects, the presence of hepatic fibrosis, cirrhosis, arthropathy, or hepatocellular carcinoma constitutes iron overload–related disease. Rarer forms of non-*HFE* hemochromatosis are caused by mutations in other genes involved in iron metabolism (Table 357-1). The disease can be recognized during its early stages when iron overload and organ damage are minimal. At this stage, the disease is best referred to as *early hemochromatosis* or *precirrhotic hemochromatosis*.
2. *Secondary iron overload* occurs as a result of an iron-loading anemia, such as thalassemia or sideroblastic anemia, in which erythropoiesis is increased but ineffective. In the acquired iron-loading disorders, massive iron deposits in parenchymal tissues can lead to the same clinical and pathologic features as in hemochromatosis.

PREVALENCE

HFE-associated hemochromatosis mutations are among the most common inherited disease alleles, although the prevalence varies in different ethnic groups. It is most common in populations of northern European extraction in whom approximately 1 in 10 persons are heterozygous carriers and 0.3–0.5% are homozygotes. However, expression of the disease is variable and modified by several factors, especially alcohol consumption and dietary iron intake, blood loss associated with menstruation and pregnancy, and blood donation. Recent population studies indicate that approximately 30% of homozygous men develop iron overload–related disease and about 6% develop hepatic cirrhosis; for women, the figure is closer to 1%. Nearly 70% of patients develop the first symptoms between ages 40 and 60. The disease is rarely evident before age 20, although with family screening (see "Screening for Hemochromatosis," below) and periodic health examinations, asymptomatic subjects with iron overload can be identified, including young menstruating women.

In contrast to *HFE*-associated hemochromatosis, the non-*HFE*-associated forms of hemochromatosis (Table 357-1) are rare, but they affect all races and young people (juvenile hemochromatosis).

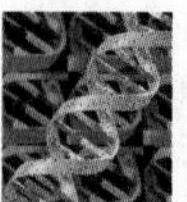

GENETIC BASIS

The *HFE* gene responsible for the most common form of hemochromatosis was identified in 1996. A homozygous G to A mutation resulting in a cysteine to tyrosine substitution at position 282 (C282Y) is the most common mutation. It is identified in 85–90% of patients with hereditary hemochromatosis in populations of northern European descent but is found in only 60% of cases from Mediterranean populations (e.g., southern Italy). A second, relatively common *HFE* mutation (H63D) results in a substitution of histidine to aspartic acid at codon 63. Homozygosity for H63D is not associated with clinically significant iron overload. Some compound heterozygotes (e.g., one copy each of C282Y and H63D) have mild to moderately increased body-iron stores but develop clinical disease only in association with cofactors such as heavy alcohol intake or hepatic steatosis. Thus, *HFE*-associated hemochromatosis is inherited as an autosomal recessive trait; heterozygotes have no, or minimal, increase in iron stores. However, this slight increase in hepatic iron can act as a cofactor that may modify the expression of other diseases such as porphyria cutanea tarda (PCT) or nonalcoholic steatohepatitis.

Mutations in other genes involved in iron metabolism are responsible for non-*HFE*-associated hemochromatosis, including juvenile hemochromatosis, which affects persons in the second and third decades of life (Table 357-1). Mutations in the genes encoding hepcidin, transferrin receptor 2 (TfR2), and hemojuvelin (Fig. 357-1) result in clinicopathologic features that are indistinguishable from

TABLE 357-1 Classification of Iron Overload States

Hereditary Hemochromatosis	
Hemochromatosis, *HFE*-related (type 1)	
C282Y homozygosity	
C282Y/H63D compound heterozygosity	
Hemochromatosis, non-*HFE*-related	
Juvenile hemochromatosis (type 2A) (hemojuvelin mutations)	
Juvenile hemochromatosis (type 2B) (hepcidin mutation)	
Mutated transferrin receptor 2 *TFR2* (type 3)	
Mutated ferroportin 1 gene, *SLC11A3* (type 4)	
Acquired Iron Overload	
Iron-loading anemias	Chronic liver disease
Thalassemia major	Hepatitis C
Sideroblastic anemia	Alcoholic cirrhosis, especially when advanced
Chronic hemolytic anemias	Nonalcoholic steatohepatitis
Transfusional and parenteral iron overload	Porphyria cutanea tarda
Dietary iron overload	Dysmetabolic iron overload syndrome
	Post-portacaval shunting
Miscellaneous	
Iron overload in sub-Saharan Africa	
Neonatal iron overload	
Aceruloplasminemia	
Congenital atransferrinemia	

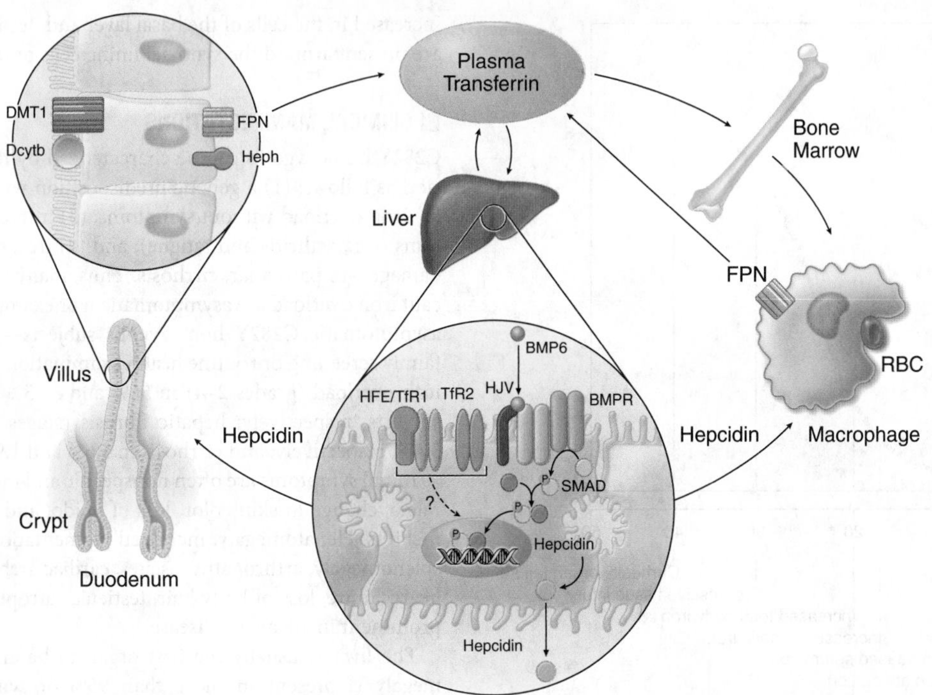

Figure 357-1 Pathways of normal iron homeostasis. Dietary inorganic iron traverses the brush border membrane of duodenal enterocytes via DMT1 after reduction of ferric (Fe^{3+}) iron to the ferrous (Fe^{2+}) state by duodenal cytochrome B (DcytB). Iron then moves from the enterocyte to the circulation via a process requiring the basolateral iron exporter ferroportin (FPN) and the iron oxidase hephaestin (Heph). In the circulation, iron binds to plasma transferrin and is thereby distributed to sites of iron utilization and storage. Much of the diferric transferrin supplies iron to immature erythrocyte cells in the bone marrow for hemoglobin synthesis. At the end of their life, senescent red blood cells (RBC) are phagocytosed by macrophages and iron is returned to the circulation after export through ferroportin. The liver-derived peptide hepcidin represses basolateral iron transport in the gut as well as iron released from macrophages and other cells and serves as a central regulator of body-iron traffic. Hepcidin responds to changes in body-iron requirements by signals mediated by diferric transferrin through two mechanisms. One involves HFE and TfR2, while the other involves hemojuvelin (HJV) and the Bone Morphogenetic Protein (BMP)/SMAD pathway. Heme is metabolized by heme oxygenase within the enterocytes and the released iron then follows the same pathway.

Mutations in the genes encoding HFE, TfR2, hemojuvelin and hepcidin all lead to decreased hepcidin release and increased iron absorption, resulting in hemochromatosis (Table 357-1).

HFE-associated hemochromatosis. However, mutations in ferroportin, responsible for the efflux of iron from enterocytes and most other cell types, result in iron loading of reticuloendothelial cells and macrophages as well as parenchymal cells.

PATHOPHYSIOLOGY

Normally, the body-iron content of 3–4 g is maintained such that intestinal mucosal absorption of iron is equal to iron loss. This amount is approximately 1 mg/d in men and 1.5 mg/d in menstruating women. In hemochromatosis, mucosal absorption is greater than body requirements and amounts to 4 mg/d or more. The progressive accumulation of iron increases plasma iron, saturation of transferrin, and results in a progressive increase of plasma ferritin (Fig. 357-2). A liver-derived peptide, hepcidin, represses basolateral iron transport in the intestine and iron release from macrophages and other cells by binding to ferroportin. Hepcidin, in turn, responds to signals in the liver mediated by HFE, TfR2, and hemojuvelin (Fig. 357-1). Thus, hepcidin is a crucial molecule in iron metabolism, linking body stores with intestinal iron absorption.

The *HFE* gene encodes a 343-amino-acid protein that is structurally related to MHC class I proteins. The basic defect in *HFE*-associated hemochromatosis is a lack of cell surface expression of HFE (due to the C282Y mutation). The normal (wild-type) HFE protein forms a complex with β_2-microglobulin and transferrin receptor 1 (TfR1). The C282Y mutation completely abrogates this interaction. As a result, the mutant HFE protein remains trapped intracellularly, reducing TfR1-mediated iron uptake by the intestinal crypt cell. This impaired TfR1-mediated iron uptake leads to upregulation of the divalent metal transporter (DMT1) on the brush border of the villus cells, causing inappropriately increased intestinal iron absorption (Fig. 357-1). In advanced disease, the body may contain 20 g or more of iron that is deposited mainly in parenchymal cells of the liver, pancreas, and heart. Iron may be increased 50- to 100-fold in the liver and pancreas and 5- to 25-fold in the heart. Iron deposition in the pituitary causes hypogonadotropic hypogonadism in both men and women. Tissue injury may result from disruption of iron-laden lysosomes, from lipid peroxidation of subcellular organelles by excess iron, or from stimulation of collagen synthesis by activated stellate cells.

Secondary iron overload with deposition in parenchymal cells occurs in chronic disorders of erythropoiesis, particularly in those due to defects in hemoglobin synthesis or ineffective erythropoiesis such as sideroblastic anemia and thalassemia (Chap. 104). In these disorders, iron absorption is increased. Moreover, these patients require blood transfusions and are frequently treated inappropriately with iron. PCT, a disorder characterized by a defect in porphyrin biosynthesis (Chap. 358), can also be associated with excessive parenchymal iron deposits. The magnitude of the iron load in PCT is usually insufficient to produce tissue damage. However, some patients with PCT also have mutations in the *HFE* gene, and some

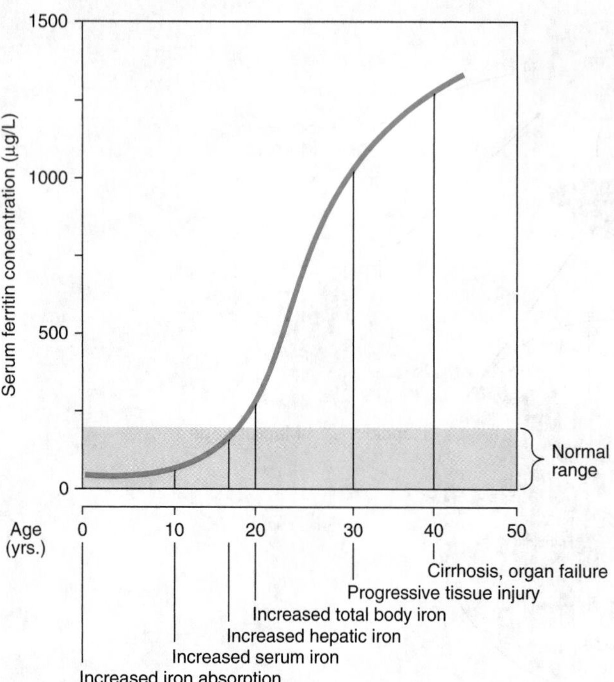

Figure 357-2 Sequence of events in genetic hemochromatosis and their correlation with the serum ferritin concentration. Increased iron absorption is present throughout life. Overt, symptomatic disease usually develops between ages 40 and 60, but latent disease can be detected long before this.

have associated hepatitis C virus (HCV) infection. Although the relationship between these disorders remains to be clarified, iron overload accentuates the inherited enzyme deficiency in PCT and should be avoided along with other agents (alcohol, estrogens, haloaromatic compounds) that may exacerbate PCT. Another cause of hepatic parenchymal iron overload is hereditary aceruloplasminemia. In this disorder, impairment of iron mobilization due to deficiency of ceruloplasmin (a ferroxidase) causes iron overload in hepatocytes.

Excessive iron ingestion over many years rarely results in hemochromatosis. An important exception has been reported in South Africa among groups who brew fermented beverages in vessels made of iron. Hemochromatosis has been described in apparently normal persons who have taken medicinal iron over many years, but such individuals probably had genetic disorders.

The common denominator in all patients with hemochromatosis is *excessive amounts of iron in parenchymal tissues.* Parenteral administration of iron in the form of blood transfusions or iron preparations results predominantly in reticuloendothelial cell iron overload. This appears to lead to less tissue damage than iron loading of parenchymal cells.

In the liver, parenchymal iron is in the form of ferritin and hemosiderin. In the early stages, these deposits are seen in the periportal parenchymal cells, especially within lysosomes in the pericanalicular cytoplasm of the hepatocytes. This stage progresses to perilobular fibrosis and eventually to deposition of iron in bile-duct epithelium, Kupffer cells, and fibrous septa due to activation of stellate cells. In the advanced stage, a macronodular or mixed macro- and micronodular cirrhosis develops. Hepatic fibrosis and cirrhosis correlate significantly with hepatic iron concentration.

At autopsy, the enlarged nodular liver and pancreas are rusty in color. Histologically, iron is increased in many organs, particularly in the liver, heart, and pancreas, and, to a lesser extent, in the endocrine glands. The epidermis of the skin is thin, and melanin is increased in the cells of the basal layer and dermis. Deposits of iron are present around the synovial lining cells of the joints.

CLINICAL MANIFESTATIONS

C282Y homozygotes can be characterized by the stage of progression as follows: (1) a genetic predisposition without abnormalities; (2) iron overload without symptoms; (3) iron overload with symptoms (e.g., arthritis and fatigue); and (4) iron overload with organ damage—in particular, cirrhosis. Thus, many subjects with significant iron overload are asymptomatic. For example, in a study of 672 asymptomatic C282Y homozygous subjects—identified by either family screening or routine health examinations—there was hepatic iron overload (grades 2–4) in 56% and 34.5% of male and female subjects, respectively; hepatic fibrosis (stages 2–4) in 18.4% and 5.4%, respectively; and cirrhosis in 5.6% and 1.9%, respectively.

Initial symptoms are often nonspecific and include lethargy, arthralgia, change in skin color, loss of libido, and features of diabetes mellitus. Hepatomegaly, increased pigmentation, spider angiomas, splenomegaly, arthropathy, ascites, cardiac arrhythmias, congestive heart failure, loss of body hair, testicular atrophy, and jaundice are prominent in advanced disease.

The *liver* is usually the first organ to be affected, and hepatomegaly is present in more than 95% of symptomatic patients. Hepatic enlargement may exist in the absence of symptoms or of abnormal liver-function tests. Manifestations of portal hypertension and esophageal varices occur less commonly than in cirrhosis from other causes. Hepatocellular carcinoma develops in about 30% of patients with cirrhosis, and it is the most common cause of death in treated patients—hence the importance of early diagnosis and therapy. The incidence increases with age, it is more common in men, and it occurs almost exclusively in cirrhotic patients.

Excessive skin pigmentation is present in patients with advanced disease. The characteristic metallic or slate-gray hue is sometimes referred to as *bronzing* and results from increased melanin and iron in the dermis. Pigmentation usually is diffuse and generalized, but it may be more pronounced on the face, neck, extensor aspects of the lower forearms, dorsa of the hands, lower legs, and genital regions, as well as in scars.

Diabetes mellitus occurs in about 65% of patients with advanced disease and is more likely to develop in those with a family history of diabetes, suggesting that direct damage to the pancreatic islets by iron deposition occurs in combination with other risk factors. The management is similar to that of other forms of diabetes, although insulin resistance is more common in association with hemochromatosis. Late complications are the same as seen in other causes of diabetes mellitus.

Arthropathy develops in 25–50% of symptomatic patients. It usually occurs after age 50 but may occur as a first manifestation, or long after therapy. The joints of the hands, especially the second and third metacarpophalangeal joints, are usually the first joints involved, a feature that helps to distinguish the chondrocalcinosis associated with hemochromatosis from the idiopathic form (Chap. 333). A progressive polyarthritis involving wrists, hips, ankles, and knees may also ensue. Acute brief attacks of synovitis may be associated with deposition of calcium pyrophosphate (chondrocalcinosis or pseudogout), mainly in the knees. Radiologic manifestations include cystic changes of the subchondral bones, loss of articular cartilage with narrowing of the joint space, diffuse demineralization, hypertrophic bone proliferation, and calcification of the synovium. The arthropathy tends to progress despite removal of iron by phlebotomy. Although the relation of these abnormalities to iron metabolism is not known, the fact that similar changes occur in other forms of iron overload suggests that iron is directly involved.

TABLE 357-2 Representative Iron Values in Normal Subjects, Patients With Hemochromatosis, and Patients With Alcoholic Liver Disease

Determination	Normal	Symptomatic Hemochromatosis	Homozygotes with Early, Asymptomatic Hemochromatosis	Heterozygotes	Alcoholic Liver Disease
Plasma iron, μmol/L (μg/dL)	9–27 (50–150)	32–54 (180–300)	Usually elevated	Elevated or normal	Often elevated
Total iron-binding capacity, μmol/L (μg/dL)	45–66 (250–370)	36–54 (200–300)	36–54 (200–300)	Elevated or normal	45–66 (250–370)
Transferrin saturation, percent	22–46	50–100	50–100	Normal or elevated	27–60
Serum ferritin, μg/L		900–6000	200–500	Usually <500	10–500
Men	20–250				
Women	15–150				
Liver iron, μg/g dry wt	300–1400	6000–18,000	2000–4000	300–3000	300–2000
Hepatic iron index	<1.0	>2	1.5–2	<2	<2

Cardiac involvement is the presenting manifestation in about 15% of symptomatic patients. The most common manifestation is congestive heart failure, which occurs in about 10% of young adults with the disease, especially those with juvenile hemochromatosis. Symptoms of congestive heart failure may develop suddenly, with rapid progression to death if untreated. The heart is diffusely enlarged; this may be misdiagnosed as idiopathic cardiomyopathy if other overt manifestations are absent. Cardiac arrhythmias include premature supraventricular beats, paroxysmal tachyarrhythmias, atrial flutter, atrial fibrillation, and varying degrees of atrioventricular block.

Hypogonadism occurs in both sexes and may antedate other clinical features. Manifestations include loss of libido, impotence, amenorrhea, testicular atrophy, gynecomastia, and sparse body hair. These changes are primarily the result of decreased production of gonadotropins due to impairment of hypothalamic-pituitary function by iron deposition. Adrenal insufficiency, hypothyroidism, and hypoparathyroidism are rare manifestations.

DIAGNOSIS

The association of (1) hepatomegaly, (2) skin pigmentation, (3) diabetes mellitus, (4) heart disease, (5) arthritis, and (6) hypogonadism should suggest the diagnosis. However, as stated above, significant iron overload may exist with none or only some of these manifestations. Therefore, a high index of suspicion is needed to make the diagnosis early. Treatment before permanent organ damage occurs can reverse the iron toxicity and restore life expectancy to normal.

The history should be particularly detailed in regard to disease in other family members; alcohol ingestion; iron intake; and ingestion of large doses of ascorbic acid, which promotes iron absorption (Chap. 74). Appropriate tests should be performed to exclude iron deposition due to hematologic disease. The presence of liver, pancreatic, cardiac, and joint disease should be confirmed by physical examination, radiography, and standard function tests of these organs.

The degree of increase in total body–iron stores can be assessed by (1) measurement of serum iron and the percent saturation of transferrin (or the unsaturated iron-binding capacity), (2) measurement of serum ferritin concentration, (3) liver biopsy with measurement of the iron concentration and calculation of the hepatic iron index (Table 357-2), and (4) MRI of the liver. In addition, a retrospective assessment of body-iron storage is also provided by performing weekly phlebotomy and calculating the amount of iron removed before iron stores are exhausted (1 mL blood = approximately 0.5 mg iron).

Each of these methods for assessing iron stores has advantages and limitations. The serum iron level and percent saturation of transferrin are elevated early in the course, but their specificity is reduced by significant false-positive and false-negative rates. For example, serum iron concentration may be increased in patients with alcoholic liver disease without iron overload; in this situation, however, the hepatic iron index is usually not increased as in hemochromatosis (Table 357-1). In otherwise healthy persons, a fasting serum transferrin saturation greater than 50% is abnormal and suggests homozygosity for hemochromatosis.

The serum ferritin concentration is usually a good index of body-iron stores, whether decreased or increased. In fact, an increase of 1 μg/L in serum ferritin level reflects an increase of about 5 mg in body stores. In most untreated patients with hemochromatosis, the serum ferritin level is significantly increased (Fig. 357-2 and Table 357-1), and a serum ferritin level >1000 μg/L is the strongest predictor of disease expression among individuals homozygous for the C282Y mutation. However, in patients with inflammation and hepatocellular necrosis, serum ferritin levels may be elevated out of proportion to body-iron stores due to increased release from tissues. Therefore, a repeat determination of serum ferritin should be carried out after acute hepatocellular damage has subsided (e.g., in alcoholic liver disease). Ordinarily, the combined measurements of the percent transferrin saturation and serum ferritin level provide a simple and reliable screening test for hemochromatosis, including the precirrhotic phase of the disease. If either of these tests is abnormal, genetic testing for hemochromatosis should be performed (Fig. 357-3).

The role of liver biopsy in the diagnosis and management of hemochromatosis has been reassessed as a result of the widespread availability of genetic testing for the C282Y mutation. The absence of severe fibrosis can be accurately predicted in most patients using clinical and biochemical variables. Thus, there is virtually no risk of severe fibrosis in a C282Y homozygous subject with (1) serum ferritin level less than 1000 μg/L, (2) normal serum alanine amino transaminase values, (3) no hepatomegaly, and (4) no excess alcohol intake. However, it should be emphasized that liver biopsy is the only reliable method for establishing or excluding the presence of hepatic cirrhosis, which is the critical factor determining prognosis and the risk of developing hepatocellular carcinoma. Biopsy also permits histochemical estimation of tissue iron and measurement

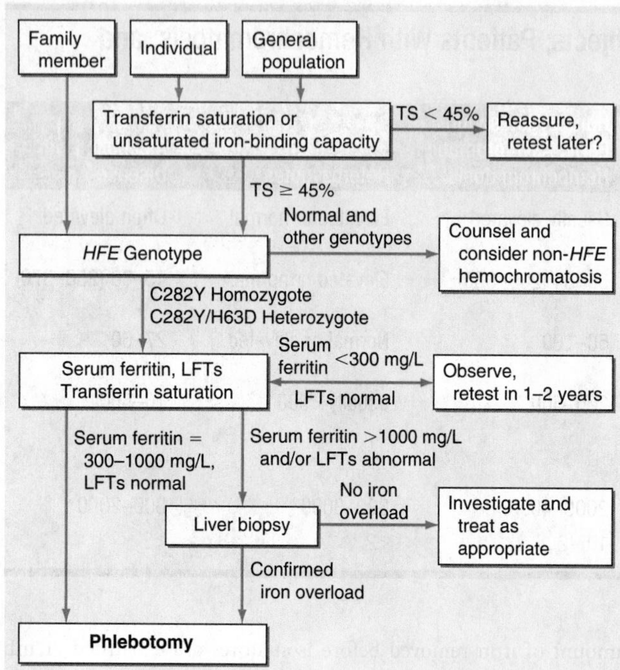

Figure 357-3 Algorithm for screening for *HFE*-associated hemochromatosis. LFT, liver function test; TS, transferrin saturation. *(From EJ Eijkelkamp et al: Can J Gastroenterol 14:121, 2000; with permission.)*

of hepatic iron concentration. Increased density of the liver due to iron deposition can be demonstrated by CT or MRI, and, with improved technology, MRI has become more accurate in determining hepatic iron concentration.

SCREENING FOR HEMOCHROMATOSIS

When the diagnosis of hemochromatosis is established, it is important to counsel and screen other family members (Chap. 63). Asymptomatic as well as symptomatic family members with the disease usually have an increased saturation of transferrin and an increased serum-ferritin concentration. These changes occur even before the iron stores are greatly increased (Fig. 357-2). All adult first-degree relatives of patients with hemochromatosis should be tested for the C282Y and H63D mutations and counseled appropriately (Fig. 357-3). In affected individuals, it is important to confirm or exclude the presence of cirrhosis and begin therapy as early as possible. When children of a proband are affected, a homozygote-heterozygote mating is most likely. For practical purposes, children need not be checked before they are 18 years old.

The role of population screening for hemochromatosis is controversial. Recent studies indicate that it is highly effective for primary care physicians to screen subjects using serum iron, transferrin saturation, and serum ferritin levels. Such screening also detects iron deficiency. Genetic screening of the normal population is feasible, but its cost-effectiveness has not been established.

TREATMENT Hemochromatosis

The therapy of hemochromatosis involves removal of the excess body iron and supportive treatment of damaged organs. Iron removal is best accomplished by weekly or twice-weekly phlebotomy of 500 mL. Although there is an initial modest decline in the volume of packed red blood cells to about 35 mL/dL, the level stabilizes after several weeks. The plasma transferrin saturation remains increased until the available iron stores are depleted. In contrast, the plasma ferritin concentration falls progressively, reflecting the gradual decrease in body-iron stores. One 500 mL unit of blood contains 200–250 mg iron, and up to 25 g iron or more may have to be removed. Therefore, in patients with advanced disease, weekly phlebotomy may be required for 1–2 years, and it should be continued until the serum ferritin level is under 50 μg/L. Thereafter, phlebotomies are performed at appropriate intervals to maintain ferritin levels between 50 and 100 μg/L. Usually one phlebotomy every three months will suffice.

Chelating agents such as deferoxamine, when given parenterally, remove 10–20 mg iron per day, which is much less than that mobilized by once-weekly phlebotomy. Phlebotomy is also less expensive, more convenient, and safer for most patients. However, chelating agents are indicated when anemia or hypoproteinemia is severe enough to preclude phlebotomy. Subcutaneous infusion of deferoxamine using a portable pump is the most effective means of its administration.

An effective oral iron chelating agent, deferasirox (Exjade), has recently become available but is still in clinical trials. This agent is effective in thalassemia and secondary iron overload, but its role in primary iron overload has yet to be established.

Alcohol consumption should be severely curtailed or eliminated because it increases the risk of cirrhosis in hereditary hemochromatosis nearly tenfold. The management of hepatic failure, cardiac failure, and diabetes mellitus is similar to conventional therapy for these conditions. Loss of libido and change in secondary sex characteristics are managed with testosterone replacement or gonadotropin therapy (Chap. 346).

End-stage liver disease may be an indication for liver transplantation, although results are improved if the excess iron can be removed beforehand. The available evidence indicates that the fundamental metabolic abnormality in hemochromatosis is reversed by successful liver transplantation.

PROGNOSIS

The principal causes of death are cardiac failure, hepatocellular failure or portal hypertension, and hepatocellular carcinoma.

Life expectancy is improved by removal of the excessive stores of iron and maintenance of these stores at near-normal levels. The 5-year survival rate with therapy increases from 33 to 89%. With repeated phlebotomy, the liver decreases in size, liver function improves, pigmentation of skin decreases, and cardiac failure may be reversed. Diabetes improves in about 40% of patients, but removal of excess iron has little effect on hypogonadism or arthropathy. Hepatic fibrosis may decrease, but established cirrhosis is irreversible. Hepatocellular carcinoma occurs as a late sequela in patients who are cirrhotic at presentation. The apparent increase in its incidence in treated patients is probably related to their increased life span. Hepatocellular carcinoma rarely develops if the disease is treated in the precirrhotic stage. Indeed, the life expectancy of homozygotes treated before the development of cirrhosis is normal.

The importance of family screening and early diagnosis and treatment cannot be overemphasized. Asymptomatic individuals detected by family studies should have phlebotomy therapy if iron stores are moderately to severely increased. Assessment of iron stores at appropriate intervals is also important. With this management approach, most manifestations of the disease can be prevented.

ROLE OF *HFE* MUTATIONS IN OTHER LIVER DISEASES

There is considerable interest in the role of *HFE* mutations and hepatic iron in several other liver diseases. Several studies have shown an increased prevalence of *HFE* mutations in PCT patients. Iron accentuates the inherited enzyme deficiency in PCT and clinical manifestations of PCT. The situation in nonalcoholic steatosis (NASH) is less clear, but some studies have shown an increased prevalence of *HFE* mutations in NASH patients. The role of phlebotomy therapy, however, is unproven. In chronic HCV infection, *HFE* mutations are not more common, but some subjects have increased hepatic iron. Before initiating antiviral therapy in these patients, it is reasonable to perform phlebotomy therapy to remove excess iron stores, because this reduces liver enzyme levels.

HFE mutations are not increased in frequency in alcoholic liver disease. Hemochromatosis in a heavy drinker can be distinguished from alcoholic liver disease by the presence of the C282Y mutation.

End-stage liver disease may also be associated with iron overload of the degree seen in hemochromatosis. The mechanism is uncertain, although recent evidence suggests that alcohol suppresses hepatic hepcidin secretion. Hemolysis also plays a role. *HFE* mutations are uncommon.

A recent large population study has shown that subjects homozygous for C282Y are at increased risk of breast and colorectal cancer.

FURTHER READINGS

Adams PC et al: Hemochromatosis and iron-overload screening in a racially diverse population. N Engl J Med 352:1769, 2005

Allen KJ et al: Iron-overload-related disease in *HFE* hereditary hemochromatosis. New Engl J Med 358:221, 2008

Crawford DH et al: Serum hyaluronic acid with serum ferritin accurately predicts cirrhosis and reduces the need for liver biopsy in C282Y hemochromatosis. Hepatology 49:418, 2009

Gurrin LC et al: HFE C282Y/H63D compound heterozygotes are at low risk of hemochromatosis-related morbidity. Hepatology 50:94, 2009

Osborne NJ et al: HFE C282Y homozygotes are at increased risk of breast and colorectal cancer. Hepatology 51:1311, 2010

Pietrangelo A: Non-HFE-linked hemochromatosis. Semin Liver Dis 25:450, 2005

Powell LW et al: Screening for hemochromatosis in asymptomatic subjects with or without a family history. Arch Intern Med 166:294, 2006

CHAPTER 358

The Porphyrias

Robert J. Desnick
Manisha Balwani

The porphyrias are metabolic disorders, each resulting from the deficiency of a specific enzyme in the heme biosynthetic pathway (Fig. 358-1 and Table 358-1). These enzyme deficiencies are inherited as autosomal dominant, autosomal recessive, or X-linked traits, with the exception of porphyria cutanea tarda (PCT), which usually is sporadic (Table 358-1). The porphyrias are classified as either *hepatic* or *erythropoietic*, depending on the primary site of overproduction and accumulation of their respective porphyrin precursors or porphyrins (Tables 358-1 and 358-2), although some have overlapping features. For example, PCT, the most common porphyria, is hepatic and presents with blistering cutaneous photosensitivity, which is usually a manifestation of the erythropoietic porphyrias. The major manifestations of the acute hepatic porphyrias are neurologic, including neuropathic abdominal pain, peripheral motor neuropathy, and mental disturbances, with attacks often precipitated by steroid hormones, certain drugs, and nutritional changes such as dieting. While hepatic porphyrias are symptomatic primarily in adults, rare homozygous variants of the autosomal dominant hepatic porphyrias usually manifest clinically prior to puberty.

In contrast, the erythropoietic porphyrias usually present with cutaneous photosensitivity at birth or in early childhood, or in the case of congenital erythropoietic porphyria (CEP), even in utero as nonimmune hydrops fetalis. Cutaneous sensitivity to sunlight results from excitation of excess porphyrins in the skin by long-wave ultraviolet light, leading to cell damage, scarring, and disfigurement. Thus, the porphyrias are metabolic disorders in which genetic, physiologic, and environmental factors interact to cause disease.

Because many symptoms of the porphyrias are nonspecific, diagnosis is often delayed. Laboratory measurement of porphyrin precursors [5′-aminolevulinic acid (ALA) and porphobilinogen (PBG)] or porphyrins in urine, plasma, erythrocytes, or feces is required to confirm or exclude the various types of porphyria (see below). However, a definite diagnosis requires demonstration of the specific enzyme deficiency or gene defect (Table 358-3). The isolation and characterization of the genes encoding all the heme biosynthetic enzymes has permitted identification of the mutations causing each porphyria (Table 358-2). Molecular genetic analyses now make it possible to provide precise heterozygote or homozygote identification and prenatal diagnoses in families with known mutations.

In addition to recent reviews of the porphyrias (see Further Readings), informative and up-to-date websites are sponsored by the American Porphyria Foundation (*www.porphyriafoundation.com*) and the European Porphyria Initiative (*www.porphyria-europe.org*). An extensive list of unsafe and safe drugs for individuals with acute porphyrias is provided at the Drug Database for Acute Porphyrias (*www.drugs-porphyria.com*).

HEME BIOSYNTHESIS

Heme biosynthesis involves eight enzymatic steps in the conversion of glycine and succinyl-CoA to heme (Fig. 358-2 and Table 358-2). These eight enzymes are encoded by nine genes, as the first enzyme in the pathway, 5′-aminolevulinate synthase (ALA-synthase), has two genes that encode unique housekeeping (ALAS1) and erythroid-specific (ALAS2) isozymes. The first and last three enzymes in the pathway are located in the mitochondrion, whereas the other four are in the cytosol. Heme is required for a variety of hemoproteins such as hemoglobin, myoglobin, respiratory cytochromes, and the cytochrome P450 enzymes (CYPs). Hemoglobin synthesis in erythroid precursor cells accounts for approximately 85% of daily heme synthesis in humans. Hepatocytes account for most of the rest, primarily for the synthesis of CYPs, which are especially abundant in the liver endoplasmic reticulum, and turn over more rapidly than many other hemoproteins, such as the mitochondrial respiratory

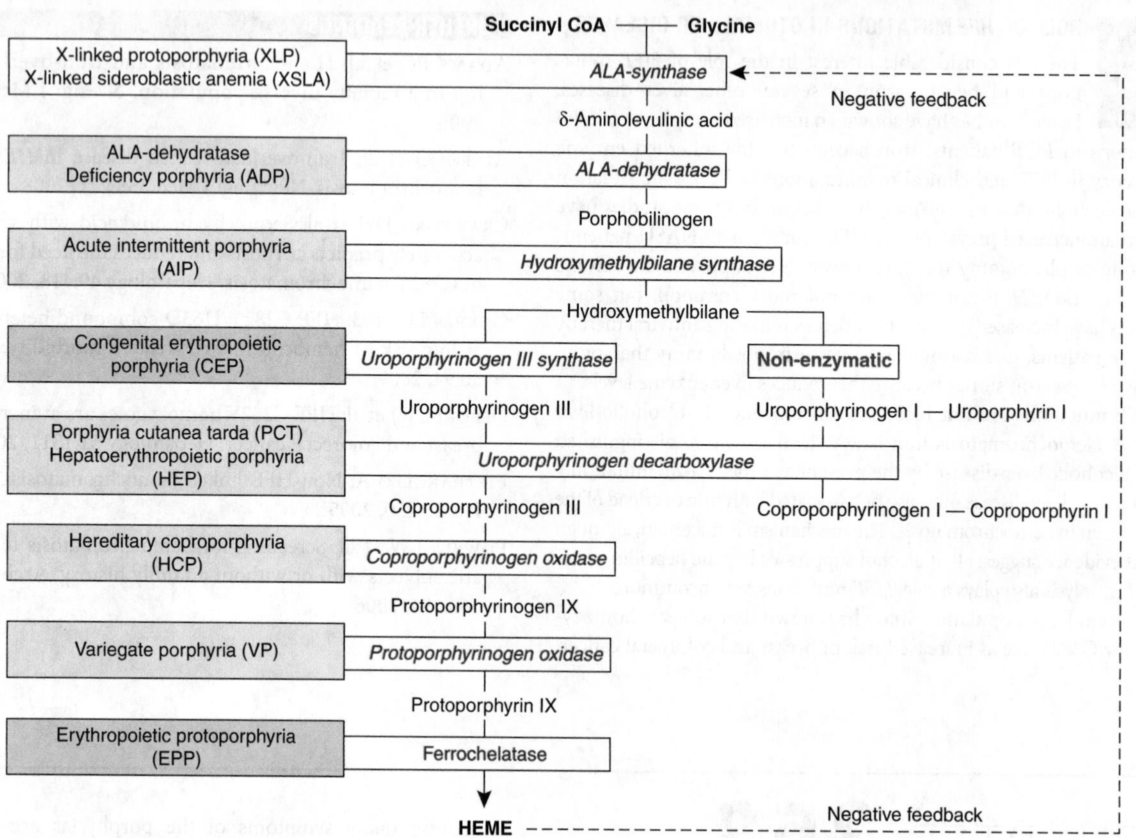

Figure 358-1 **The human heme biosynthetic pathway** indicating in linked boxes the enzyme that, when deficient, causes the respective porphyria. Hepatic porphyrias are shown in yellow boxes and erythropoietic porphyrias in pink boxes.

TABLE 358-1 Human Porphyrias: Major Clinical and Laboratory Features

Porphyria	Deficient Enzyme	Inheritance	Principal Symptoms NV or CP+	Enzyme Activity % of Normal	Increased Porphyrin Precursors and/or Porphyrins: Erythrocytes	Urine	Stool
Hepatic porphyrias							
5-ALA dehydratase-deficient porphyria (ADP)	ALA-dehydratase	AR	NV	~5	Zn-Protoporphyrin	ALA, Coproporphyrin III	—
Acute intermittent porphyria (AIP)	HMB-synthase	AD	NV	~50	—	ALA[a], PBG, Uroporphyrin	—
Porphyria cutanea tarda (PCT)	URO-decarboxylase	AD	CP	~20	—	Uroporphyrin, 7-carboxylate porphyrin	Isocoproporphyrin
Hereditary coproporphyria (HCP)	COPRO-oxidase	AD	NV & CP	~50	—	ALA, PBG, Coproporphyrin III	Coproporphyrin III
Variegate porphyria (VP)	PROTO-oxidase	AD	NV & CP	~50	—	ALA, PBG, Coproporphyrin III	Coproporphyrin III Protoporphyrin
Erythropoietic porphyrias							
Congenital erythropoietic porphyria (CEP)	URO-synthase	AR	CP	1–5	Uroporphyrin I Coproporphyrin I	Uroporphyrin I[b] Coproporphyrin I[b]	Coproporphyrin I
Erythropoietic protoporphyria (EPP)	Ferrochelatase	AR[a]	CP	~20–30	Protoporphyrin	—	Protoporphyrin
X-linked protoporphyria (XLP)	ALA-synthase 2	XL	CP	>100[c]	Protoporphyrin	—	Protoporphyrin

[a]Polymorphism in intron 3 of wild-type allele affects level of enzyme activity and clinical expression.
[b]Type I isomers.
[c]Increased activity due to "gain-of-function" mutations in ALAS2 exon 11.
Abbreviations: AD, autosomal dominant; ALA, 5-aminolevulinic acid; AR, autosomal recessive; COPRO I, coproporphyrin I; COPRO III, coproporphyirn III; CP, cutaneous photosensitivity; ISOCOPRO, isocoproporphyrin; + Nv, neurovisceral; PBG, porphobilinogen; PROTO, protoporphyrin IX; URO I, uroporphyrin I; URO III, uroporphyrin III; XL, X-linked.

TABLE 358-2 Human Heme Biosynthetic Enzymes and Genes

Enzyme	Gene Symbol	Chromosomal Location	cDNA (bp)	Gene: Size (kb)	Gene: Exons[a]	Protein (aa)	Subcellular Location	Known Mutations[b]	3D Structure[c]
ALA-synthase Housekeeping	ALAS1	3p21.1	2199	17	11	640	M	—	
Erythroid-specific	ALAS2	Xp11.2	1937	22	11	587	M	>30	—
ALA-dehydratase Housekeeping	ALAD	9q32	1149	15.9	12 (1A + 2 – 12)	330	C	12	Y
Erythroid-specific	ALAD	9q32	1154	15.9	12 (1B + 2 – 12)	330	C	—	
HMB-synthase Housekeeping	HMBS	11q23.3	1086	11	15 (1 + 3 – 15)	361	C	>315	E
Erythroid-specific	HMBS	11q23.3	1035	11	15 (2 – 15)	344	C	10	
URO-synthase Housekeeping	UROS	10q26.2	1296	34	10 (1 + 2B – 10)	265	C	39	H
Erythroid-specific	UROS	10q26.2	1216	34	10 (2A + 2B – 10)	265	C	4	
URO-decarboxylase	UROD	1p34.1	1104	3	10	367	C	108	H
COPRO-oxidase	CPOX	3q12.1	1062	14	7	354	M	51	H
PROTO-oxidase	PPOX	1q23.3	1431	5.5	13	477	M	129	—
Ferrochelatase	FECH	18q21.31	1269	45	11	423	M	125	B

[a]Number of exons and those encoding separate housekeeping and erythroid-specific forms indicated in parentheses.
[b]Number of known mutations from the Human Gene Mutation Database (*www.hgmd.org*).
[c]Crystallized from human (H), murine (M), *Escherichia coli* (E), *Bacillus subtilis* (B), or yeast (Y) purified enzyme; references in Protein Data Bank (*www.rcsb.org*).
Abbreviations: C, cytoplasm; M, mitochondria.
Source: From Anderson et al.

cytochromes. As shown in Fig. 358-2, pathway intermediates are the porphyrin precursors, ALA and PBG, and porphyrins (mostly in their reduced forms, known as *porphyrinogens*). At least in humans, these intermediates do not accumulate in significant amounts under normal conditions or have important physiologic functions.

The first enzyme, ALA-synthase, catalyzes the condensation of glycine, activated by pyridoxal phosphate and succinyl coenzyme A, to form ALA. In the liver, this rate-limiting enzyme can be induced by a variety of drugs, steroids, and other chemicals. Distinct nonerythroid (e.g., housekeeping) and erythroid-specific forms of ALA-synthase are encoded by separate genes located on chromosomes 3p21.1 (ALAS1) and Xp11.2 (ALAS2), respectively. Defects in the erythroid gene ALAS2 that decrease its activity cause X-linked sideroblastic anemia (XLSA). Recently, gain of function mutations in exon 11 of ALAS2 that increase its activity have been shown to cause an X-linked form of erythropoietic protoporphyria (EPP), known as X-linked protoporphyria (XLP).

The second enzyme, 5′-aminolevulinate dehydratase (ALA-dehydratase), catalyzes the condensation of two molecules of ALA to form PBG. Hydroxymethylbilane synthase (HMB-synthase; also known as PBG-deaminase) catalyzes the head-to-tail condensation of four PBG molecules by a series of deaminations to form the linear tetrapyrrole, HMB. Uroporphyrinogen III synthase (URO-synthase) catalyzes the rearrangement and rapid cyclization of HMB to form the asymmetric, physiologic, octacarboxylate porphyrinogen uroporphyrinogen (URO'gen) III.

The fifth enzyme in the pathway, uroporphyrinogen decarboxylase (URO-decarboxylase), catalyzes the sequential removal of the four carboxyl groups from the acetic acid side chains of URO'gen III to form coproporphyrinogen (COPRO'gen) III, a tetracarboxylate porphyrinogen. This compound then enters the mitochondrion via a specific transporter, ABCB6, where COPRO-oxidase, the sixth enzyme, catalyzes the decarboxylation of two of the four propionic acid groups to form the two vinyl groups of protoporphyrinogen (PROTO'gen) IX, a decarboxylate porphyrinogen. Next, PROTO-oxidase oxidizes PROTO IX'gen to protoporphyrin IX by the removal of six hydrogen atoms. The product of the reaction is a porphyrin (oxidized form), in contrast to the preceding tetrapyrrole intermediates, which are porphyrinogens (reduced forms). Finally, ferrous iron is inserted into protoporphyrin IX to form heme, a reaction catalyzed by the eighth enzyme in the pathway, ferrochelatase (also known as heme synthetase or protoheme ferrolyase).

■ REGULATION OF HEME BIOSYNTHESIS

Regulation of heme synthesis differs in the two major heme-forming tissues, the liver and erythron. In the liver, the concentration of "free" heme regulates the synthesis and mitochondrial translocation of the housekeeping form of ALA-synthase 1. Heme represses the synthesis of the ALA-synthase 1 mRNA and interferes with the transport of the enzyme from the cytosol into mitochondria. Hepatic ALA-synthase 1 is increased by many of the same chemicals that induce the cytochrome P450 enzymes in the endoplasmic reticulum of the liver. Because most of the heme in the liver is used for the synthesis of cytochrome P450 enzymes, hepatic ALA-synthase 1 and the cytochrome P450s are regulated in a coordinated fashion, and many drugs that induce hepatic ALA-synthase 1 also induce the CYPs. The other hepatic heme biosynthetic enzymes are presumably expressed at constant levels, although their relative activities and kinetic properties differ. For example, normal individuals have high activities of ALA-dehydratase, but low activities of HMB-synthase, the latter being the second rate-limiting step in the pathway.

In the erythron, novel regulatory mechanisms allow for the production of the very large amounts of heme needed for hemoglobin synthesis. The response to stimuli for hemoglobin synthesis occurs during cell differentiation, leading to an increase in cell number. The erythroid-specific ALA-synthase 2 is expressed at higher levels than the housekeeping enzyme, and erythroid-specific control mechanisms

TABLE 358-3 Diagnosis of Acute and Cutaneous Porphyrias

Symptoms	First-Line Test: Abnormality	Possible Porphyria:	Second-Line Testing if First-Line Testing Is Positive: To include: urine (U), plasma (P), and fecal (F) porphyrins; for acute porphyrias add red blood cell (RBC) HMB-synthase; for blistering skin lesions add P & RBC porphyrins	Confirmatory Test: Enzyme Assay and/or Mutation Analysis
Neurovisceral	**Spot U:** ↑↑ ALA & normal PBG	ADP	**U porphyrins:** ↑↑, mostly COPRO III **P & F porphyrins:** normal or slightly ↑ **RBC HMB-synthase:** normal	Rule out other causes of elevated ALA; ↓↓ RBC ALA-dehydratase activity (<10%); ALA-dehydratase mutation analysis
	Spot U: ↑↑ PBG	AIP	**U porphyrins:** ↑↑, mostly URO & COPRO **P & F porphyrins:** normal or slightly ↑ **RBC HMB-synthase:** usually ↓	HMB-synthase mutation analysis
	"	HCP	**U porphyrins:** ↑↑, mostly COPRO III **P porphyrins:** normal or slightly ↑ (↑ if skin lesions present) **F porphyrins:** ↑↑, mostly COPRO III	Measure RBC HMB-synthase: normal activity COPRO-oxidase mutation analysis
	"	VP	**U porphyrins:** ↑↑, mostly COPRO III **P porphyrins:** ↑↑ (characteristic fluorescence peak at neutral pH) **F porphyrins:** ↑↑, mostly COPRO & PROTO	Measure RBC HMB-synthase: normal activity PROTO-oxidase mutation analysis
Blistering Skin Lesions	**P:** ↑ porphyrins	PCT & HEP	**U porphyrins:** ↑↑, mostly URO & heptacarboxylate porphyrin **P porphyrins:** ↑↑ **F porphyrins:** ↑↑, including increased isocoproporphyrin **RBC porphyrins:** ↑↑ zinc PROTO in HEP[a]	RBC URO-decarboxylase activity: half-normal in familial PCT (~20% of all PCT cases); substantially deficient in HEP URO-decarboxylase mutation analysis: mutation(s) present in familial PCT (heterozygous) &HEP (homozygous)
	"	HCP & VP	See HCP &VP above. Also, U ALA & PBG: may be ↑	
	"	CEP	**RBC & U porphyrins:** ↑↑, mostly URO I and COPRO I **F porphyrins:** ↑↑; mostly COPRO I	↓↓RBC URO-synthase activity (<15%) URO-synthase mutation analysis
Nonblistering Photosensitivity	**P:** porphyrins usually ↑	EPP	**RBC porphyrins:** ↑↑, mostly free PROTO **U porphyrins:** normal **F porphyrins:** normal or ↑, mostly PROTO	FECH mutation analysis
	P: porphyrins usually ↑	XLP	**RBC porphyrins:** ↑↑, approx equal free and zinc PROTO **U porphyrins:** normal **F porphyrins:** normal or ↑, mostly PROTO	ALA S2 mutation analysis

[a]Nonspecific increases in zinc protoporphyrins are common in other porphyrias

Abbreviations: ALA, 5-aminolevulinic acid; COPRO I, coproporphyrin I; COPRO III, coproporphyrin III; ISOCOPRO, isocoproporphyrin; F, fecal; P, plasma; PBG, porphobilinogen; PROTO, protoporphyrin IX; RBC, erythrocytes; U, urine; URO I, uroporphyrin I; URO III, uroporphyrin III.

Source: Based on KE Anderson et al: Ann Intern Med 142:439, 2005.

regulate other pathway enzymes as well as iron transport into erythroid cells. Separate erythroid-specific and nonerythroid or "housekeeping" transcripts are known for the first four enzymes in the pathway. As noted above, housekeeping and erythroid-specific ALA-synthases are encoded by genes on different chromosomes, but for each of the next three genes in the pathway, both erythroid and nonerythroid transcripts are transcribed by alternative promoters from their single respective genes (Table 358-2).

■ CLASSIFICATION OF THE PORPHYRIAS

As mentioned above, the porphyrias can be classified as either *hepatic* or *erythropoietic*, depending on whether the heme biosynthetic intermediates that accumulate arise initially from the liver or developing erythrocytes, or as *acute* or *cutaneous*, based on their clinical manifestations. Table 358-1 lists the porphyrias, their principal symptoms, and major biochemical abnormalities. Four of the five hepatic porphyrias—acute intermittent porphyria (AIP), hereditary coproporphyria (HCP), variegate porphyria (VP), and ALA-dehydratase porphyria (ADP)—present during adult life with acute attacks of neurologic manifestations and elevated levels of one or both of the porphyrin precursors, ALA and PBG, and are thus classified as *acute porphyrias*. Patients with ADP have also presented in infancy and adolescence. The fifth hepatic disorder, porphyria cutanea tarda (PCT), presents with blistering skin lesions. HCP and VP also may have cutaneous manifestations similar to PCT.

The erythropoietic porphyrias—congenital erythropoietic porphyria (CEP) and erythropoietic protoporphyria (EPP), including the recently described X-linked form, XLP—are characterized by elevations of porphyrins in bone marrow and erythrocytes and present with cutaneous photosensitivity. The skin lesions in CEP resemble PCT but are usually much more severe, whereas EPP and XLP cause a more immediate, painful, and nonblistering type of photosensitivity. EPP is the most common porphyria to cause symptoms before puberty. About 20% of EPP patients develop minor abnormalities of liver function, with up to about 5% developing hepatic complications that can become life-threatening. XLP has a clinical presentation similar to EPP causing photosensitivity and liver disease.

DIAGNOSIS OF PORPHYRIA

A few specific and sensitive first-line laboratory tests should be used whenever symptoms or signs suggest the diagnosis of porphyria (Table 358-3). If a first-line test is significantly abnormal, more comprehensive testing should follow to establish the type of porphyria, and finally the specific causative gene mutation.

Acute porphyrias

An acute porphyria should be suspected in patients with neurovisceral symptoms after puberty, such as abdominal pain, and when the initial clinical evaluation does not suggest another cause, the urinary porphyrin precursors (ALA and PBG) should be measured (Fig. 358-2). Urinary PBG is virtually always increased

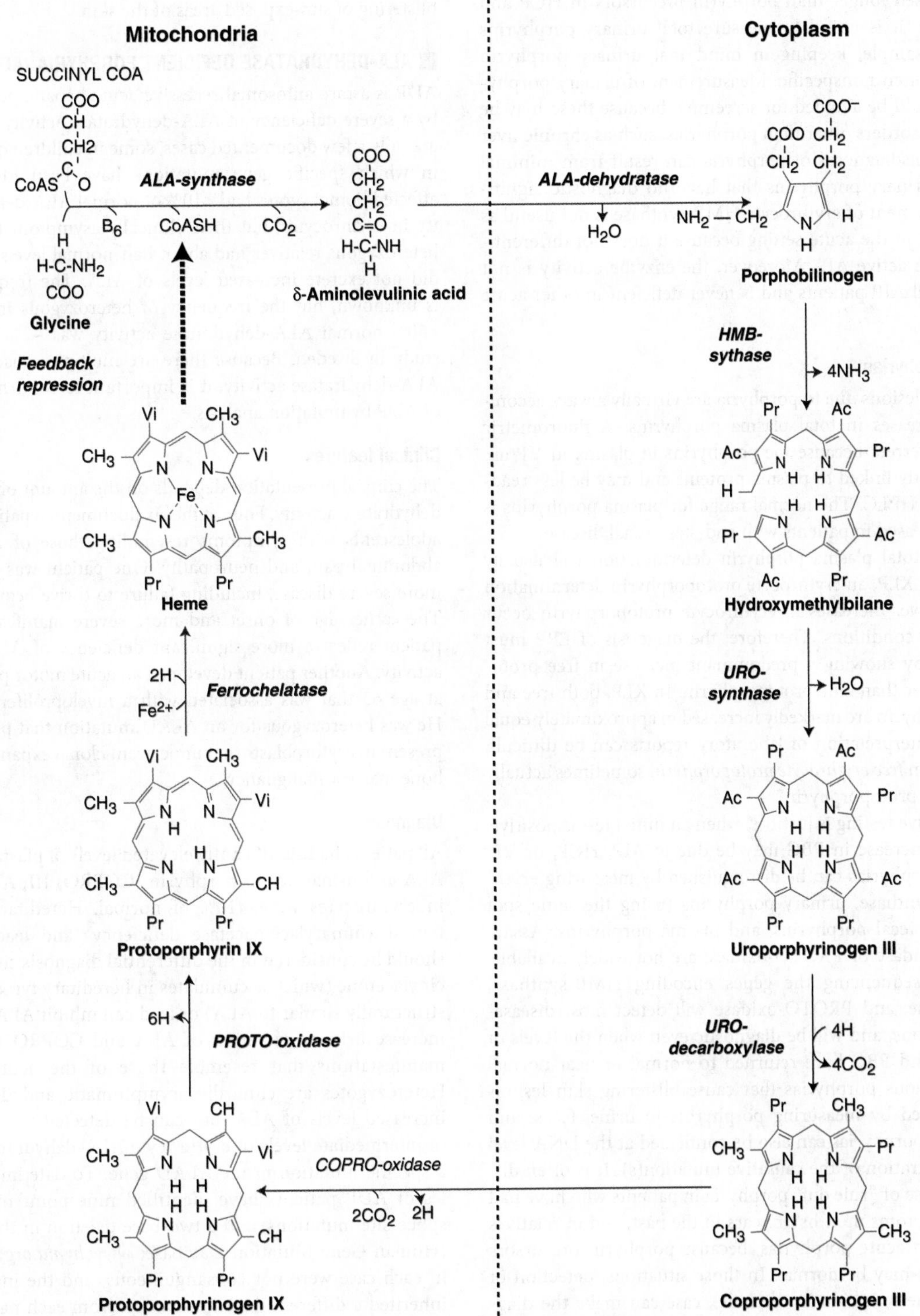

Figure 358-2 The heme biosynthetic pathway showing the eight enzymes and their substrates and products. Four of the enzymes are localized in the mitochondria and four in the cytosol.

during acute attacks of AIP, HCP, and VP and is not substantially increased in any other medical condition. Therefore, this measurement is both sensitive and specific. A method for rapid, in-house testing for urinary PBG, such as the Trace PBG kit (Trace America/Trace Diagnostics, Louisville, Colorado), can be used. Results from spot (single void) urine specimens are highly informative because very substantial increases in PBG are expected during acute attacks of porphyria. A 24-h collection can unnecessarily delay diagnosis. The same spot urine specimen should be saved for quantitative determination of ALA, PBG, and creatinine, in order to confirm the qualitative PBG result and also to detect patients with ALAD-deficient porphyria (ADP). Urinary porphyrins may remain increased longer than porphyrin precursors in HCP and VP. Therefore, it is useful to measure total urinary porphyrins in the same sample, keeping in mind that urinary porphyrin increases are often nonspecific. Measurement of urinary porphyrins alone should be avoided for screening, because these may be increased in disorders other than porphyrias, such as chronic liver disease, and misdiagnoses of porphyria can result from minimal increases in urinary porphyrins that have no diagnostic significance. Measurement of erythrocyte HMB-synthase is not useful as a first-line test in the acute setting because it does not differentiate latent from active AIP. Moreover, the enzyme activity is not decreased in all AIP patients and is never deficient in other acute porphyrias.

Cutaneous porphyrias

Blistering skin lesions due to porphyria are virtually always accompanied by increases in total plasma porphyrins. A fluorometric method is preferred, because the porphyrins in plasma in VP are mostly covalently linked to plasma proteins and may be less readily detected by HPLC. The normal range for plasma porphyrins is somewhat increased in patients with end-stage renal disease.

Although a total plasma porphyrin determination will usually detect EPP and XLP, an erythrocyte protoporphyrin determination is more sensitive. Increases in erythrocyte protoporphyrin occur in many other conditions. Therefore, the diagnosis of EPP must be confirmed by showing a predominant increase in free protoporphyrin rather than zinc protoporphyrin. In XLP, both free and zinc protoporphyrin are markedly increased in approximately equal proportions. Interpretation of laboratory reports can be difficult, because the term *free erythrocyte protoporphyrin* sometimes actually represents zinc protoporphyrin.

More extensive testing is justified when an initial test is positive. A substantial increase in PBG may be due to AIP, HCP, or VP. These acute porphyrias can be distinguished by measuring erythrocyte HMB-synthase, urinary porphyrins (using the same spot urine sample), fecal porphyrins, and plasma porphyrins. Assays for COPRO-oxidase or PROTO-oxidase are not widely available. Alternatively, sequencing the genes encoding HMB-synthase, COPRO-oxidase, and PROTO-oxidase will detect most disease-causing mutations, and will be diagnostic even when the levels of urinary ALA and PBG have returned to normal or near-normal levels. The various porphyrias that cause blistering skin lesions are differentiated by measuring porphyrins in urine, feces, and plasma. These porphyrias can also be confirmed at the DNA level by the demonstration of the causative mutation(s). It is often difficult to diagnose or "rule out" porphyria in patients who have had suggestive symptoms months or years in the past, and in relatives of patients with acute porphyrias, because porphyrin precursors and porphyrins may be normal. In those situations, detection of the specific gene mutation in the index case can make the diagnosis. Consultation with a specialist laboratory and physician is useful for selecting which heme biosynthetic gene or genes to be sequenced. Before evaluating relatives, the gene-based diagnosis of porphyria should be established in an index case. Once a specific mutation is identified in an affected member, other at-risk relatives can be offered genetic counseling and testing for that mutation. Further details are provided in the sections below on each type of porphyria.

THE HEPATIC PORPHYRIAS

Markedly elevated plasma and urinary concentrations of the porphyrin precursors ALA or PBG, which originate from the liver, are especially evident during attacks of neurologic manifestations of the four acute porphyrias, ADP, AIP, HCP, and VP. In PCT, excess porphyrins also accumulate initially in the liver and cause chronic blistering of sun-exposed areas of the skin.

ALA-DEHYDRATASE DEFICIENT PORPHYRIA (ADP)

ADP is a rare autosomal recessive acute hepatic porphyria caused by a severe deficiency of ALA-dehydratase activity. To date, there are only a few documented cases, some in children or young adults, in which specific gene mutations have been identified. These affected homozygotes had <10% of normal ALA-dehydratase activity in erythrocytes, but their clinically asymptomatic parents and heterozygous relatives had about half-normal levels of activity and did not excrete increased levels of ALA. The frequency of ADP is unknown, but the frequency of heterozygous individuals with <50% normal ALA-dehydratase activity was ~2% in a screening study in Sweden. Because there are multiple causes for deficient ALA-dehydratase activity, it is important to confirm the diagnosis of ADP by mutation analysis.

Clinical features

The clinical presentation depends on the amount of residual ALA-dehydratase activity. Four of the six documented patients were male adolescents with symptoms resembling those of AIP, including abdominal pain and neuropathy. One patient was an infant with more severe disease, including failure to thrive beginning at birth. The earlier age of onset and more severe manifestations in this patient reflect a more significant deficiency of ALA-dehydratase activity. Another patient developed an acute motor polyneuropathy at age 63 that was associated with a myeloproliferative disorder. He was heterozygous for an ALAD mutation that presumably was present in erythroblasts that underwent clonal expansion due to the bone marrow malignancy.

Diagnosis

All patients had significantly elevated levels of plasma and urinary ALA and urinary coproporphyrin (COPRO) III; ALAD activities in erythrocytes were <10% of normal. Hereditary tyrosinemia type 1 (fumarylacetoacetase deficiency) and lead intoxication should be considered in the differential diagnosis since either succinylacetone (which accumulates in hereditary tyrosinemia and is structurally similar to ALA) or lead can inhibit ALA-dehydratase, increase urinary excretion of ALA and COPRO III, and cause manifestations that resemble those of the acute porphyrias. Heterozygotes are clinically asymptomatic and do not excrete increased levels of ALA, but can be detected by demonstration of intermediate levels of erythrocyte ALA-dehydratase activity or a specific mutation in the ALAD gene. To date, molecular studies of ADP patients have identified nine point mutations, two splice-site mutations, and a two-base deletion in the ALAD gene (Human Gene Mutation Database; *www.hgmd.org*). The parents in each case were not consanguineous, and the index cases had inherited a different ALAD mutation from each parent. Prenatal diagnosis of this disorder is possible by determination of ALA-dehydratase activity and/or gene mutation in cultured chorionic villi or amniocytes.

TREATMENT ALA-Dehydratase Deficient Porphyria

The treatment of ADP acute attacks is similar to that of AIP (see below). The severely affected infant referred to above was supported by hyperalimentation and periodic blood transfusions, but did not respond to intravenous hemin and died after liver transplantation.

ACUTE INTERMITTENT PORPHYRIA (AIP)

This hepatic porphyria is an autosomal dominant condition resulting from the half-normal level of HMB-synthase activity. The disease is widespread but is especially common in Scandinavia and Great Britain. Clinical expression is highly variable, and activation of the disease is often related to environmental or hormonal factors, such as drugs, diet, and steroid hormones. Attacks can be prevented by avoiding known precipitating factors. Rare homozygous dominant AIP also has been described in children (see below).

Clinical features

Induction of the rate-limiting hepatic enzyme ALA-synthase in AIP heterozygotes with half-normal HMB-synthase activity is thought to underlie the acute attacks in AIP and other acute porphyrias. The disorder remains latent (or asymptomatic) in the great majority of those who are heterozygous for HMB-synthase mutations, and this is almost always the case prior to puberty. In patients with no history of acute symptoms, porphyrin precursor excretion is usually normal, suggesting that half-normal hepatic HMB-synthase activity is sufficient, and that hepatic ALA-synthase activity is not increased. However, under conditions where heme synthesis is increased in the liver, half-normal HMB-synthase activity may become limiting, and ALA, PBG, and other heme pathway intermediates may accumulate and be excreted in the urine. Common precipitating factors include endogenous and exogenous steroids, porphyrinogenic drugs, alcohol ingestion, and low-calorie diets, usually instituted for weight loss.

The fact that AIP is almost always latent before puberty suggests that adult levels of steroid hormones are important for clinical expression. Symptoms are more common in women, suggesting a role for estrogens or progestins. Premenstrual attacks are probably due to endogenous progesterone. Acute porphyrias are sometimes exacerbated by exogenous steroids, including oral contraceptive preparations containing progestins. Surprisingly, pregnancy is usually well tolerated, suggesting that beneficial metabolic changes may ameliorate the effects of high levels of progesterone. Table 358-4 provides a partial list of the major drugs that are harmful in AIP (and also in HCP and VP). Extensive lists of unsafe and safe drugs are available on websites sponsored by the American Porphyria Foundation (*www.porphyriafoundation.com*), the European Porphyria Initiative (*www.porphyria-europe.org*), and at the Drug Database for Acute Porphyrias website (*www.drugs-porphyria.com*). Reduced intake of calories and carbohydrate, as may occur with illness or attempts to lose weight, can also increase porphyrin precursor excretion and induce attacks of porphyria. Increased carbohydrate intake can ameliorate attacks. Studies in a knockout AIP mouse model indicate that the hepatic ALAS1 gene is regulated by the peroxisome proliferator–activated receptor γ coactivator 1α (PGC-1α). Hepatic PGC-1α is induced by fasting, which in turn activates ALAS1 transcription, resulting in increased heme biosynthesis. This finding suggests an important link between nutritional status and the attacks in acute porphyrias. Attacks also can be provoked by infections, surgery, and ethanol.

Because the neurovisceral symptoms rarely occur before puberty and are often nonspecific, a high index of suspicion is required to make the diagnosis. The disease can be disabling but is rarely fatal. Abdominal pain, the most common symptom, is usually steady and poorly localized but may be cramping. Ileus, abdominal distention, and decreased bowel sounds are common. However, increased bowel sounds and diarrhea may occur. Abdominal tenderness, fever, and leukocytosis are usually absent or mild because the symptoms are neurologic rather than inflammatory. Nausea; vomiting; constipation; tachycardia; hypertension; mental symptoms; pain in the limbs, head, neck, or chest; muscle weakness; sensory loss; dysuria; and urinary retention are characteristic. Tachycardia, hypertension, restlessness, tremors, and excess sweating are due to sympathetic overactivity.

The peripheral neuropathy is due to axonal degeneration (rather than demyelinization) and primarily affects motor neurons. Significant neuropathy does not occur with all acute attacks; abdominal symptoms are usually more prominent. Motor neuropathy affects the proximal muscles initially, more often in the shoulders and arms. The course and degree of involvement are variable and sometimes may be focal and involve cranial nerves. Deep tendon reflexes initially may be normal or hyperactive but become decreased or absent as the neuropathy advances. Sensory changes such as paresthesia and loss of sensation are less prominent. Progression to respiratory and bulbar paralysis and death occurs especially when the diagnosis and treatment are delayed. Sudden death may result from sympathetic overactivity and cardiac arrhythmia.

Mental symptoms such as anxiety, insomnia, depression, disorientation, hallucinations, and paranoia can occur in acute attacks. Seizures can be due to neurologic effects or to hyponatremia. Treatment of seizures is difficult because most antiseizure drugs can exacerbate AIP (clonazepam may be safer than phenytoin or barbiturates). Hyponatremia results from hypothalamic involvement and inappropriate vasopressin secretion or from electrolyte depletion due to vomiting, diarrhea, poor intake, or excess renal sodium loss. Persistent hypertension and impaired renal function may occur. When an attack resolves, abdominal pain may disappear within hours, and paresis begins to improve within days and may continue to improve over several years.

Homozygous dominant AIP is a rare form of AIP in which patients inherit HMBS mutations from each of their heterozygous parents and, therefore, have very low (<2%) enzyme activity. The disease has been described in a Dutch girl, two young British siblings, and a Spanish boy. In these homozygous affected patients, the disease presented in infancy with failure to thrive, developmental delay, bilateral cataracts, and/or hepatosplenomegaly. Urinary ALA and PBG concentrations were markedly elevated. All of these patients' HMBS mutations (R167W, R167Q, and R172Q) were in exon 10 within five bases of each other. Studies of the brain MRIs of children with homozygous AIP have suggested damage primarily in white matter that was myelinated postnatally, while tracks that myelinated prenatally were normal. Most children with homozygous AIP die at an early age.

Diagnosis

ALA and PBG levels are substantially increased in plasma and urine, especially during acute attacks, and become normal only after prolonged latency. For example, urinary PBG excretion during an attack is usually 50–200 mg/24 h (220–880 μmol/24 h) [normal, 0–4 mg/24 h (0–18 μmol/24 h)], and urinary ALA excretion is 20–100 mg/24 h (150–760 μmol/24 h) [normal, 1–7 mg/24 h (8–53 μmol/24 h)]. Because levels often remain high after symptoms resolve, the diagnosis of an acute attack in a patient with biochemically proven AIP is based primarily on clinical features. Excretion of ALA and

TABLE 358-4 Unsafe Drugs in Porphyria

Documented Porphyrinogenic	Probably Porphyrinogenic	Possibly Porphyrinogenic	
Carbamazepine	Altretamine	Aceclofenac	Parecoxib
Carisoprodol	Aminophylline	Acitretin	Pentifylline
Chloramphenicol	Amiodarone	Acrivastine	Pentoxyverine
Clindamycin	Amitriptyline	Alfuzosin	Phenylpropanolamine
Dextropropoxyphene	Amlodipine	Anastrozole	+ Cinnarizine
Dihydralazine	Amprenavir	Auranofin	Pizotifen
Dihydroergotamine	Aprepitant	Azelastine	Polidocanol
Drospirenone + estrogen	Atorvastatin	Benztropine	Polyestradiol
Dydrogesterone	Azathioprine	Benzydamine	Phosphate
Etonogestrel	Bosentan	Betaxolol	Potassium canrenoate
Fosphenytoin sodium	Bromocriptine	Bicalutamide	Pravastatin
Hydralazine	Buspirone	Biperiden	Prednisolone
Hydroxyzine	Busulfan	Bupropion	Prilocaine
Indinavir	Butylscopolamine	Carvedilol	Proguanil
Ketamine	Cabergoline	Chlorambucil	Propafenone
Ketoconazole	Ceftriaxone +	Chlorcyclizine +	Pseudoephedrine +
Lidocaine	Lidocaine	Guaifenesin	Dexbrompheniramine
Lynestrenol	Cerivastatin	Chloroquine	Quillaia extract
Lynestrenol + estrogen	Cetirizine	Chlorprothixene	Quinagolide
Mecillinam	Cholinetheophyllinate	Chlorzoxazone	Quinine
Medroxyprogesterone	Clarithromycin	Chorionic	Quinupristin +
Megestrol	Clemastine	Gonadotrophin	Dalfopristin
Methylergometrine	Clonidine	Ciclosporin	Reboxetine
Methyldopa	Cyclizine	Cisapride	Repaglinide
Mifepristone	Cyproterone	Citalopram	Rizatriptan
Nicotinic	Danazol	Clomethiazole	Rofecoxib
Acid/meclozine/hydroxyzine	Delavirdine	Clomiphene	Ropinirole
Nitrofurantoin	Desogestrel + estrogen	Clomipramine	Ropivacaine
Norethisterone	Diazepam	Clopidogrel	Roxithromycin
Norgestimate + estrogen	Dienogest + estrogen	Clotrimazole	Sertraline
Orphenadrine	Diclofenac	Cortisone	Sevoflurane
Phenobarbital	Diltiazem	Cyclandelate	Sibutramine
Phenytoin	Diphenhydramine	Cyclophosphamide	Sildenafil
Pivampicillin	Disopyramide	Cyproheptadine	Sirolimus
Pivmecillinam	Disulfiram	Dacarbazine	Sodium
Primidone	Drospirenone +	Daunorubicin	Aurothiomalate
Rifampicin	Estrogen	Desogestrel	Sodium oleate +
Ritonavir	Dydrogesterone	Dichlorobenzyl	Chlorocymol
Spironolactone	Ergoloid mesylate	Alcohol	Stavudine
Sulfadiazine +	Erythromycin	Dithranol	Sulindac
Trimethoprim	Estramustine	Docetaxel	Sumatriptan
Tamoxifen	Ethosuximide	Donepezil	Tacrolimus
Testosterone, injection	Etoposide	Doxycycline	Tadalafil
Thiopental	Exemestane	Ebastine	Tegafur + uracil
Trimethoprim	Felbamate	Econazole	Telmisartan
Valproic acid	Felodipine	Efavirenz	Thioridazine
Venlafaxine	Fluconazole	Escitalopram	Tioguanine
Vinblastine	Flunitrazepam	Esomeprazole	Tolfenamic acid
Vincristine	FLuvastatin	Estradiol/tablets	Tolterodine
Vindesine	Glibenclamide	Estriol/tablets	Torsemide
Vinorelbine	Halothane	Estrio/vainal crème, tablet	Triamcinolone

(continued)

TABLE 358-4 Unsafe Drugs in Porphyria (*Continued*)

Documented Porphyrinogenic	Probably Porphyrinogenic	Possibly Porphyrinogenic	
Xylometazoline	Hyoscyamine		Trihexyphenidyl
Zaleplon	Ifosfamide	Estrogen, Conjugate	Trimipramine
Ziprasidone	Imipramine	Finasteride	Valerian
Zolmitriptan	Irinotecan	Flecainide	Venlafaxine
Zolpidem	Isoniazid	Flucloxacillin	Vinblastine
Zuclopenthixol	Isradipine	Fluoxetine	Vincristine
	Itraconazole	Flupentixol	Vindesine
	Lamivudine	Flutamide	Vinorelbine
	+Zidovudine	Fluvoxamine	Xylometazoline
	Lansoprazole	Follitropin alfa and	Zaleplon
	Lercanidipine	Beta	Ziprasidone
	Levonorgestrel	Galantamine	ZolmitriPtan
	Lidocaine,	Glimepiride	Zolpidem
	Lopinavir	Glipizide	Zuclopenthixol
	Lutropin alfa	Gonadorelin	
	Lymecycline	Gramicidin	
	Meclozine	Guaifenesin	
	Medroxyprogesterone	Hydrocortisone	
	+ Estrogen	Hydroxycarbamide	
	Metoclopramide	Hydroxychloroquine	
	Metronidazole	Ibutilide	
	Metyrapone	Imatinib	
	Moxonidine	Indomethacin	
	Nandrolone	Ketobemidone +	
	Nefazodone	Ddba	
	Nelfinavir	Ketoconazole	
	Nevirapine	Ketorolac	
	Nifedipine	Lamotrigine	
	Nimodipine	Letrozole	
	Nitrazepam	Levodopa +	
	Norethisterone	Benserazide	
	Nortriptyline	Levonorgestrel	
	Oxcarbazepine	Intrauterine	
	Oxytetracycline	Levosimendan	
	Paclitaxel	Lidocaine	
	Paroxetine	Linezolid	
	Phenazone + caffeine	Lofepramine	
	Pioglitazone	Lomustine	
	Probenecid	Malathion	
	Progesterone, vaginal	Maprotiline	
	Gel	Mebendazole	
	Quinidine	Mefloquine	
	Rabeprazole	Melperone	
	Raloxifene	Melphalan	
	Rifabutin	Mepenzolate	
	Riluzole	Mepivacaine	
	Risperidone	Mercaptopurine	
	Rosiglitazone	Methadone	
	Saquinavir	Methylprednisolone	
	Selegiline	Methixene	
	Simvastatin	Metolazone	

(*continued*)

TABLE 358-4 Unsafe Drugs in Porphyria (*Continued*)

Documented Porphyrinogenic	Probably Porphyrinogenic	Possibly Porphyrinogenic
	Sulfasalazine	Metronidazole
	Telithromycin	Mexiletine
	Terbinafine	Mianserin
	Terfenadine	Midazolam
	Testosterone,	Minoxidil
	Transdermal patch	Mirtazapine
	Tetracycline	Mitomycin
	Theophylline	Mitoxantrone
	Thiamazole	Moclobemide
	Tibolone	Montelukast
	Ticlopidine	Morphine +
	Tinidazole	Scopolamine
	Thiotepa	Multivitamins
	Topiramate	Mupirocin
	Topotecan	Nabumetone
	Toremifene	Nafarelin
	Tramadol	Naltrexone
	Trimegestone +	Nateglinide
	Estrogen	Nilutamide
	Verapamil	Noscapine
	Voriconazole	Omeprazole
	Zidovudine/azt	Oxybutynin
		Oxycodone
		Pantoprazole
		Papaverine

Note: Based on list in "Patient's and Doctor's Guide to Medication in Acute Porphyria," Swedish Porphyria Association and Porphyria Centre Sweden. Also see the website Drug Database for Acute Porphyrias (*www.drugs-porphyria.com*) for a searchable list of safe and unsafe drugs.

PBG decrease dramatically after intravenous hemin. A normal urinary PBG level before hemin effectively excludes AIP as a cause for current symptoms. Fecal porphyrins are usually normal or minimally increased in AIP, in contrast to HCP and VP. Most heterozygotes with HMB-synthase deficiency with no history of symptoms have normal urinary excretion of ALA and PBG. Therefore, measurement of HMB-synthase in erythrocytes or, better, the detection of the family's HMBS mutation will diagnose asymptomatic family members.

The enzyme deficiency is detectable in erythrocytes from most AIP heterozygotes. Because the activity is higher in young erythrocytes, it may increase into the normal range if erythropoiesis is increased due to a concurrent condition. Furthermore, patients with HMBS mutations in the initiation of translation codon in exon 1 and in the intron 1 5′-splice donor site have normal enzyme levels in erythrocytes and deficient activity only in nonerythroid tissues. This occurs because the erythroid and housekeeping forms of HMB-synthase are encoded by a single gene, which has two promoters. More than 315 HMBS mutations have been identified in AIP, including missense, nonsense, and splicing mutations and insertions and deletions, with most mutations found in only one or a few families (Human Gene Mutation Database, *www.hgmd.org*). The prenatal diagnosis of a fetus at risk can be made with cultured amniotic cells or chorionic villi. However, this is seldom done, because the prognosis of individuals with HMBS mutations is generally favorable.

TREATMENT Acute Intermittent Porphyria

During acute attacks, narcotic analgesics may be required for abdominal pain, and phenothiazines are useful for nausea, vomiting, anxiety, and restlessness. Chloral hydrate can be given for insomnia, and benzodiazepines are probably safe in low doses if a minor tranquilizer is required. Carbohydrate loading, usually with intravenous glucose (at least 300 g/dL of 10% dextrose in water daily), may be effective in milder acute attacks of porphyria (without paresis, hyponatremia, etc.). Because intravenous hemin is more effective and the response slower if treatment is delayed, it is no longer recommended that hemin therapy for a severe attack be started only after an unsuccessful trial of intravenous glucose for several days. Hemin should be used initially for severe attacks and for mild attacks that do not respond to carbohydrate loading within 1–2 days. The standard regimen is 3–4 mg/kg of heme, in the form of lyophilized hematin (Lundbeck Pharmaceuticals), heme albumin (hematin reconstituted with human albumin), or heme arginate (Orphan Europe), infused daily for 4 days. Heme arginate and heme albumin are chemically stable and are less likely than hematin to produce phlebitis or an anticoagulant effect. Recovery depends on the degree of neuronal damage and usually is rapid if therapy is started early. Recovery from severe motor neuropathy may require months or years. Identification and avoidance of inciting factors can hasten recovery from an attack and prevent future attacks. Inciting factors are usually multiple, and removal of one or more hastens recovery and helps prevent future attacks. Frequent attacks that occur during the luteal phase of the menstrual cycle may be prevented with a gonadotropin-releasing hormone analogue, which prevents ovulation and progesterone production, or by preventive monthly hematin administration.

The long-term risk of hypertension and chronic renal disease is increased in AIP; a number of patients have undergone successful renal transplantation. Chronic, low-grade abnormalities in liver function tests are common, and the risk of hepatocellular carcinoma is increased. Hepatic imaging is recommended at least yearly for early detection of these tumors.

An allogeneic liver transplant was performed on a 19-year-old female AIP heterozygote who had 37 acute attacks in the 29 months prior to transplantation. Post-transplantation, her elevated urinary ALA and BPG levels returned to normal in 24 h, and she did not experience acute neurologic, attacks for more than 3 years post-transplant. Two AIP patients had combined liver and kidney transplants secondary to uncontrolled acute porphyria attacks, chronic peripheral neuropathy, and renal failure requiring dialysis. Both patients had a marked improvement with no attacks and normal urinary PBG levels post-transplantation, as well as improvement of their neuropathic manifestations. To date, a number of women with AIP have had successful liver transplants for severe recurrent neurologic attacks and secondary organ damage with amelioration of their neurologic attacks and normalization of their heme precursors. However, liver transplantation is a high-risk procedure and should be considered as a last resort in patients with severe recurrent attacks. Recently, liver-directed gene therapy has been successful in the prevention of drug-induced biochemical attacks in a murine model of human AIP.

PORPHYRIA CUTANEA TARDA (PCT)

PCT, the most common of the porphyrias, can be either sporadic (type 1) or familial (type 2) and can also develop after exposure to halogenated aromatic hydrocarbons. Hepatic URO-decarboxylase is deficient in all types of PCT, and for clinical symptoms to manifest, this enzyme deficiency must be substantial (~20% of normal activity or less); it is currently attributed to generation of an URO-decarboxylase inhibitor in the liver in the presence of iron and under conditions of oxidative stress, although it remains to be isolated and characterized.

The majority of PCT patients (~80%) have no UROD mutations and are said to have sporadic (type 1) disease. PCT patients heterozygous for UROD mutations have familial (type 2) PCT. In these patients, inheritance of a UROD mutation from one parent results in half-normal enzyme activity in liver and all other tissues, which is a significant predisposing factor, but is insufficient by itself to cause symptomatic PCT. As discussed below, other genetic and environmental factors contribute to susceptibility for both types of PCT. Because penetrance of the genetic trait is low, many patients with familial (type 2) PCT have no family history of the disease. Hepatoerythropoietic porphyria (HEP) is an autosomal recessive form of porphyria that results from the marked systemic deficiency of URO-decarboxylase activity with clinical symptoms in childhood.

Clinical features

Blistering skin lesions that appear most commonly on the backs of the hands are the major clinical feature (Fig. 358-3). These rupture and crust over, leaving areas of atrophy and scarring. Lesions may also occur on the forearms, face, legs, and feet. Skin friability and small white papules termed milia are common, especially on the backs of the hands and fingers. Hypertrichosis and hyperpigmentation, especially of the face, are especially troublesome in women. Occasionally, the skin over sun-exposed areas becomes severely thickened, with scarring and calcification that resembles systemic sclerosis. Neurologic features are absent.

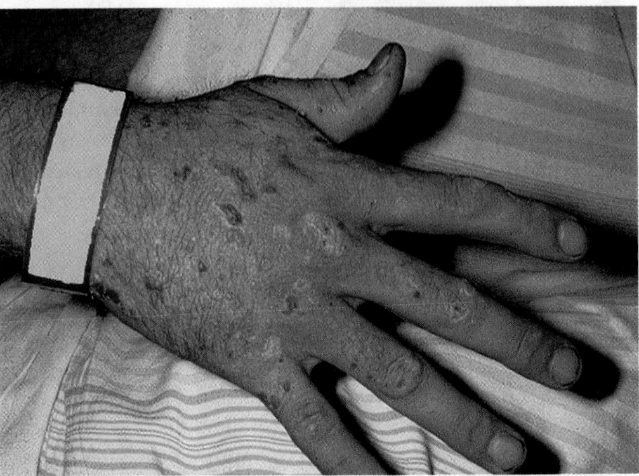

Figure 358-3 Typical cutaneous lesions in a patient with porphyria cutanea tarda. Chronic, crusted lesions resulting from blistering due to photosensitivity on the dorsum of the hand of a PCT patient. *(Courtesy of Dr. Karl E. Anderson; with permission.)*

A number of susceptibility factors, in addition to inherited UROD mutations in type 2 PCT, can be recognized clinically and can affect management. These include hepatitis C, HIV, excess alcohol, elevated iron levels, and estrogens. The importance of excess hepatic iron as a precipitating factor is underscored by the finding that the incidence of the common hemochromatosis-causing mutations, hemochromatosis gene (HFE) mutations C282Y and H63D, is increased in patients with types 1 and 2 PCT (Chap. 357). Excess alcohol is a long-recognized contributor, as is estrogen use in women. HIV is probably an independent but less common risk factor that, like hepatitis C, does not cause PCT in isolation. Multiple susceptibility factors that appear to act synergistically can be identified in the individual PCT patient. Patients with PCT characteristically have chronic liver disease and sometimes cirrhosis and are at risk for hepatocellular carcinoma. Various chemicals can also induce PCT; an epidemic of PCT occurred in eastern Turkey in the 1950s as a consequence of wheat contaminated with the fungicide hexachlorobenzene. PCT also occurs after exposure to other chemicals, including di- and trichlorophenols and 2,3,7,8-tetrachlorodibenzo-(*p*)-dioxin (TCDD, dioxin).

Diagnosis

Porphyrins are increased in the liver, plasma, urine, and stool. The urinary ALA level may be slightly increased, but the PBG level is normal. Urinary porphyrins consist mostly of URO and heptacarboxylate porphyrin, with lesser amounts of COPRO and hexa- and pentacarboxylate porphyrins. Plasma porphyrins are also increased, and fluorometric scanning of diluted plasma at neutral pH can rapidly distinguish VP and PCT (Table 358-3). Isocoproporphyrins, which are increased in feces and sometimes in plasma and urine, are diagnostic for hepatic URO-decarboxylase deficiency.

Type 2 PCT and HEP can be distinguished from type 1 by finding decreased URO-decarboxylase in erythrocytes. URO-decarboxylase activity in liver, erythrocytes, and cultured skin fibroblasts in type 2

PCT is approximately 50% of normal in affected individuals and in family members with latent disease. In HEP, the URO-decarboxylase activity is markedly deficient, with typical levels of 3–10% of normal. More than 105 mutations have been identified in the UROD gene (Human Gene Mutation Database; *www.hgmd.org*). Of the mutations listed in the database, ~65% are missense or nonsense and ~10% are splice-site mutations. Most UROD mutations have been identified in only one or two families.

TREATMENT Porphyria Cutanea Tarda

Alcohol, estrogens, iron supplements, and, if possible, any drugs that may exacerbate the disease should be discontinued, but this step does not always lead to improvement. A complete response can almost always be achieved by the standard therapy, repeated phlebotomy, to reduce hepatic iron. A unit (450 mL) of blood can be removed every 1–2 weeks. The aim is to gradually reduce excess hepatic iron until the serum ferritin reaches the lower limits of normal. Because iron overload is not marked in most cases, remission may occur after only five or six phlebotomies; however, PCT patients with hemochromatosis may require more treatments to bring their iron levels down to the normal range. To document improvement in PCT, it is most convenient to follow the total plasma porphyrin concentration, which becomes normal some time after the target ferritin level is reached. Hemoglobin levels or hematocrits and serum ferritin should be followed closely to prevent development of iron deficiency and anemia. After remission, continued phlebotomy may not be needed. Plasma porphyrin levels are followed at 6–12-month intervals for early detection of recurrences, which are treated by additional phlebotomy.

An alternative when phlebotomy is contraindicated or poorly tolerated is a low-dose regimen of chloroquine or hydroxychloroquine, both of which complex with the excess porphyrins and promote their excretion. Small doses (e.g., 125 mg chloroquine phosphate twice weekly) should be given, because standard doses can induce transient, sometimes marked increases in photosensitivity and hepatocellular damage. Hepatic imaging can diagnose or exclude complicating hepatocellular carcinoma. Treatment of PCT in patients with end-stage renal disease is facilitated by administration of erythropoietin.

HEREDITARY COPROPORPHYRIA (HCP)

HCP is an autosomal dominant hepatic porphyria that results from the half-normal activity of COPRO-oxidase. The disease presents with acute attacks, as in AIP. Cutaneous photosensitivity also may occur, but much less commonly than in VP. HCP patients may have acute attacks and cutaneous photosensitivity together or separately. HCP is less common than AIP and VP. Homozygous dominant HCP and harderoporphyria, a biochemically distinguishable variant of HCP, present with clinical symptoms in children (see below).

Clinical features

HCP is influenced by the same factors that cause attacks in AIP. The disease is latent before puberty, and symptoms, which are virtually identical to those of AIP, are more common in women. HCP is generally less severe than AIP. Blistering skin lesions are identical to PCT and VP and begin in childhood in rare homozygous cases.

Diagnosis

COPRO III is markedly increased in the urine and feces in symptomatic disease and often persists, especially in feces, when there are no symptoms. Urinary ALA and PBG levels are increased (but less than in AIP) during acute attacks, but may revert to normal more quickly than in AIP when symptoms resolve. Plasma porphyrins are usually normal or only slightly increased, but they may be higher in cases with skin lesions. The diagnosis of HCP is readily confirmed by increased fecal porphyrins consisting almost entirely of COPRO III, which distinguishes it from other porphyrias.

Although the diagnosis can be confirmed by measuring COPRO-oxidase activity, the assays for this mitochondrial enzyme are not widely available and require cells other than erythrocytes. The CPOX gene has been cloned and more than 50 mutations, 70% of which are missense or nonsense, have been identified in unrelated patients (Human Gene Mutation Database; *www.hgmd.org*). Detection of a CPOX mutation in a symptomatic individual permits the identification of asymptomatic family members.

TREATMENT Hereditary Coproporphyria

Neurologic symptoms are treated as in AIP (see above). Phlebotomy and chloroquine are ineffective when cutaneous lesions are present.

VARIEGATE PORPHYRIA (VP)

VP is an autosomal dominant hepatic porphyria that results from the deficient activity of PROTO-oxidase, the seventh enzyme in the heme biosynthetic pathway, and can present with neurologic symptoms, photosensitivity, or both. VP is particularly common in South Africa, where 3 of every 1000 whites have the disorder. Most are descendants of a couple who emigrated from Holland to South Africa in 1688. In other countries, VP is less common than AIP. Rare cases of homozygous dominant VP, presenting in childhood with cutaneous symptoms, also have been reported.

Clinical features

VP can present with skin photosensitivity, acute neurovisceral crises, or both. In two large studies of VP patients, 59% had only skin lesions, 20% had only acute attacks, and 22% had both. Acute attacks are identical to those in AIP and are precipitated by the same factors as AIP (see above). Blistering skin manifestations are similar to those in PCT, but are more difficult to treat and usually are of longer duration. Homozygous VP is associated with photosensitivity, neurologic symptoms, and developmental disturbances, including growth retardation, in infancy or childhood; all cases had increased erythrocyte levels of zinc protoporphyrin, a characteristic finding in all homozygous porphyrias so far described.

Diagnosis

Urinary ALA and PBG levels are increased during acute attacks but may return to normal more quickly than in AIP. Increases in fecal protoporphyrin and COPRO III and in urinary COPRO III are more persistent. Plasma porphyrin levels also are increased, particularly when there are cutaneous lesions. VP can be distinguished rapidly from all other porphyrias by examining the fluorescence emission spectrum of porphyrins in plasma at neutral pH since VP has a unique fluorescence peak at neutral pH.

Assays of PROTO-oxidase activity in cultured fibroblasts or lymphocytes are not widely available. More than 145 mutations have been identified in the PPOX gene from unrelated VP patients (Human Gene Mutation Database; *www.hgmd.org*). The missense mutation R59W is the common mutation in most South Africans with VP of Dutch descent. Five missense mutations were common in English and French VP patients; however, most mutations have been found in only one or two families.

TREATMENT Variegate Porphyria

Acute attacks are treated as in AIP, and hemin should be started early in most cases. Other than avoiding sun exposure, there are few effective measures for treating the skin lesions. β-Carotene, phlebotomy, and chloroquine are not helpful.

THE ERYTHROPOIETIC PORPHYRIAS

In the erythropoietic porphyrias, excess porphyrins from bone marrow erythrocyte precursors are transported via the plasma to the skin and lead to cutaneous photosensitivity.

X-LINKED SIDEROBLASTIC ANEMIA (XLSA)

XLSA results from the deficient activity of the erythroid form of ALA-synthase and is associated with ineffective erythropoiesis, weakness, and pallor.

Clinical features

Typically, males with XLSA develop refractory hemolytic anemia, pallor, and weakness during infancy. They have secondary hypersplenism, become iron overloaded, and can develop hemosiderosis. The severity depends on the level of residual erythroid ALA-synthase activity and on the responsiveness of the specific mutation to pyridoxal 5′-phosphate supplementation (see below). Peripheral blood smears reveal a hypochromic, microcytic anemia with striking anisocytosis, poikilocytosis, and polychromasia; the leukocytes and platelets appear normal. Hemoglobin content is reduced, and the mean corpuscular volume and mean corpuscular hemoglobin concentration are decreased. Patients with milder, late-onset disease have been reported recently.

Diagnosis

Bone marrow examination reveals hypercellularity with a left shift and megaloblastic erythropoiesis with an abnormal maturation. A variety of Prussian blue–staining sideroblasts are observed. Levels of urinary porphyrin precursors and of both urinary and fecal porphyrins are normal. The level of erythroid ALA-synthase is decreased in bone marrow, but this enzyme is difficult to measure in the presence of the normal ALA-synthase housekeeping enzyme. Definitive diagnosis requires the demonstration of mutations in the erythroid ALAS2 gene.

TREATMENT X-Linked Sideroblastic Anemia

The severe anemia may respond to pyridoxine supplementation. This cofactor is essential for ALA-synthase activity, and mutations in the pyridoxine-binding site of the enzyme have been found in several responsive patients. Cofactor supplementation may make it possible to eliminate or reduce the frequency of transfusion. Unresponsive patients may be transfusion-dependent and require chelation therapy.

CONGENITAL ERYTHROPOIETIC PORPHYRIA (CEP)

CEP, also known as Günther disease, is an autosomal recessive disorder. It is due to the markedly deficient, but not absent, activity of URO-synthase and the resultant accumulation of URO I and COPRO I isomers. CEP is associated with hemolytic anemia and cutaneous lesions.

Clinical features

Severe cutaneous photosensitivity begins in early infancy. The skin over light-exposed areas is friable, and bullae and vesicles are prone to rupture and infection. Skin thickening, focal hypo- and hyperpigmentation, and hypertrichosis of the face and extremities are characteristic. Secondary infection of the cutaneous lesions can lead to disfigurement of the face and hands. Porphyrins are deposited in teeth and in bones. As a result, the teeth are reddish-brown and fluoresce on exposure to long-wave ultraviolet light. Hemolysis is probably due to the marked increase in erythrocyte porphyrins and leads to splenomegaly. Adults with a milder form of the disease also have been described.

Diagnosis

URO and COPRO (mostly type I isomers) accumulate in the bone marrow, erythrocytes, plasma, urine, and feces. The predominant porphyrin in feces is COPRO I. The diagnosis of CEP can be confirmed by demonstration of markedly deficient URO-synthase activity and/or the identification of specific mutations in the UROS gene. The disease can be detected in utero by measuring porphyrins in amniotic fluid and URO-synthase activity in cultured amniotic cells or chorionic villi, or by the detection of the family's specific gene mutations. Molecular analyses of the mutant alleles from more than 50 unrelated patients have revealed the presence of more than 35 mutations in the UROS gene, including four in the erythroid-specific promoter of the UROS gene. Genotype/phenotype correlations can predict the severity of the disease.

TREATMENT Congenital Erythropoietic Porphyria

Severe cases often require transfusions for anemia. Chronic transfusions of sufficient blood to suppress erythropoiesis are effective in reducing porphyrin production, but results in iron overload. Splenectomy may reduce hemolysis and decrease transfusion requirements. Protection from sunlight and from minor skin trauma is important. β-Carotene may be of some value. Complicating bacterial infections should be treated promptly. Recently, bone marrow and cord blood transplantation has proven curative in several transfusion-dependent children, providing the rationale for stem-cell gene therapy.

ERYTHROPOIETIC PROTOPORPHYRIA (EPP)

EPP is an inherited disorder resulting from the deficient activity of ferrochelatase, the last enzyme in the heme biosynthetic pathway. EPP is the most common erythropoietic porphyria in children and, after PCT, the second most common porphyria in adults. EPP patients have ferrochelatase activities as low as 15–25% in lymphocytes and cultured fibroblasts. Protoporphyrin accumulates in bone marrow reticulocytes and then appears in plasma, is taken up in the liver, and excreted in bile and feces. Protoporphyrin transported to the skin causes nonblistering photosensitivity. In most symptomatic patients (~90%) with this autosomal recessive disorder, a mutation in one FECH allele is inherited with a relatively common (~10% normal whites) intronic 3 (IVS3) alteration (IVS3-48T>C) that results in the low expression of the normal enzyme. In about 10% of EPP families, two FECH mutations have been found. Recently, deletion mutations in exon 11 of the ALAS2 gene have been described, which cause an X-linked protoporphyria (XLP) that is clinically indistinguishable from EPP. The deletion of the carboxy-terminal amino acid of ALAS2 results in increased ALA-synthase 2 activity and the accumulation of protoporphyrin. XLP accounts for approximately 2% of cases with the EPP phenotype.

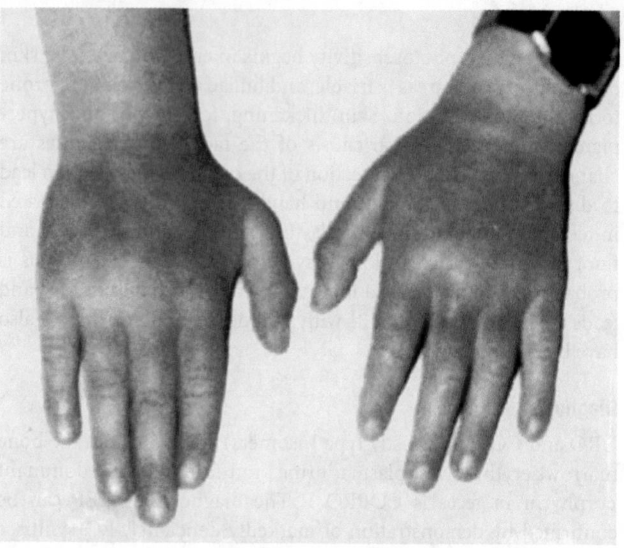

Figure 358-4 Erythema and edema of the hands due to acute photosensitivity in a 10-year-old boy with erythropoietic protoporphyria. *(From P. Poblette-Gutierrez et al.)*

Clinical features

Skin photosensitivity, which differs from that in other porphyrias, usually begins in childhood and consists of pain, redness, and itching occurring within minutes of sunlight exposure (Fig. 358-4). Photosensitivity is associated with substantial elevations in erythrocyte protoporphyrin and occurs only in patients with genotypes that result in ferrochelatase activities lower than ~35% of normal. Vesicular lesions are uncommon. Redness, swelling, burning, and itching can develop shortly after sun exposure and resemble angioedema. Symptoms may seem out of proportion to the visible skin lesions. Sparse vesicles and bullae occur in 10% of cases. Chronic skin changes may include lichenification, leathery pseudovesicles, labial grooving, and nail changes. Severe scarring is rare, as are pigment changes, friability, and hirsutism. Unless hepatic or other complications develop, protoporphyrin levels and symptoms of photosensitivity remain remarkably stable over many years in most patients. Factors that exacerbate the hepatic porphyrias play little or no role in EPP.

The primary source of excess protoporphyrin is the bone marrow reticulocytes. Erythrocyte protoporphyrin is free (not complexed with zinc) and is mostly bound to hemoglobin. In plasma, protoporphyrin is bound to albumin. Hemolysis and anemia are usually absent or mild.

Although EPP is an erythropoietic porphyria, up to 20% of EPP patients may have minor abnormalities of liver function, and in about 5% of these patients the accumulation of protoporphyrins causes chronic liver disease that can progress to liver failure and death. Protoporphyrin is insoluble, and excess amounts form crystalline structures in liver cells (Fig. 358-4) and can decrease hepatic bile flow. Studies in the mouse model of EPP have shown that the bile duct epithelium may be damaged by toxic bile, leading to biliary fibrosis. Thus, rapidly progressive liver disease appears to be related to the cholestatic effects of protoporphyrins and is associated with increasing hepatic protoporphyrin levels due to impaired hepatobiliary excretion and increased photosensitivity. The hepatic complications also are often characterized by increasing levels of protoporphyrins in erythrocytes and plasma as well as severe abdominal and back pains, especially in the right upper quadrant. Gallstones composed at least in part of protoporphyrin occur in some patients. Hepatic complications appear to be higher in autosomal recessive EPP due to two FECH mutations and in XLP.

Diagnosis

A substantial increase in erythrocyte protoporphyrin, which is predominantly free and not complexed with zinc, is the hallmark of EPP. Protoporphyrin levels are also variably increased in bone marrow, plasma, bile, and feces. Erythrocyte protoporphyrin concentrations are increased in other conditions such as lead poisoning, iron deficiency, various hemolytic disorders, all homozygous forms of other porphyrias, and sometimes even in acute porphyrias. In all these conditions, however, in contrast to EPP, protoporphyrin is complexed with zinc. Therefore, after an increase in erythrocyte protoporphyrin is found in a suspected EPP patient, it is important to confirm the diagnosis by an assay that distinguishes free and zinc-complexed protoporphyrin. Erythrocytes in EPP also exhibit red fluorescence under a fluorescence microscopy at 620 nm. Urinary levels of porphyrins and porphyrin precursors are normal. Ferrochelatase activity in cultured lymphocytes or fibroblasts is decreased. DNA diagnosis by mutation analysis is recommended to detect the causative FECH mutation(s) and/or the presence of the IVS3-48T>C hypo-expression allele. To date, 125 mutations have been identified in the FECH gene, many of which result in an unstable or absent enzyme protein (null alleles) (Human Gene Mutation Database; *www.hgmd.org*). Studies suggest that EPP patients with a null allele (and the IVS3-48T>C hypo-expression allele) have a great risk for developing severe liver complications. In XLP, the erythrocyte protoporphyrin levels appear to be higher than other forms of EPP and the proportions of free and zinc protoporphyrins are approximately equivalent. To date, two ALAS2 mutations, all deletions of 1 to 4 bases, have been described, which markedly increase ALAS2 activity and cause XLP.

TREATMENT Erythropoietic Protoporphyria

Avoiding sunlight exposure and wearing clothing designed to provide protection for conditions with chronic photosensitivity are essential. Oral β-carotene (120–180 mg/dL) improves tolerance to sunlight in some patients. The beneficial effects of β-carotene may involve quenching of singlet oxygen or free radicals. The dosage may need to be adjusted to maintain serum carotene levels in the recommended range of 10–15 mmol/L (600–800 mg/dL). Mild skin discoloration due to carotenemia is the only significant side effect.

Treatment of hepatic complications, which may be accompanied by motor neuropathy, is difficult. Cholestyramine and other porphyrin absorbents such as activated charcoal may interrupt the enterohepatic circulation of protoporphyrin and promote its fecal excretion, leading to some improvement. Splenectomy may be helpful when the disease is accompanied by hemolysis and significant splenomegaly. Plasmapheresis and intravenous hemin are sometimes beneficial.

Liver transplantation has been carried out in some EPP and XLP patients with severe liver complications and is often successful in the short term. However, disease often recurs in the transplanted liver due to continued bone marrow production of excess protoporphyrin. In a retrospective study of 17 liver-transplanted EPP patients, 11 (65%) had recurrent EPP liver disease. Posttransplantation treatment with hematin and plasmapheresis should be considered to prevent the recurrence of liver disease. Bone marrow transplantation, which has been successful in human EPP and prevents liver disease in a mouse model, should be considered after the liver transplantation, if a suitable donor can be found.

ACKNOWLEDGMENT

The authors thank Dr. Karl E. Anderson for his review of the manuscript and helpful comments and suggestions.

FURTHER READINGS

Anderson KE et al: Disorders of heme biosynthesis: X-linked sideroblastic anemia and the porphyrias, in *The Metabolic and Molecular Bases of Inherited Diseases*, CR Scriver et al (eds). New York, McGraw-Hill, 2001, pp 2991–3062

Handschin C et al: Nutritional regulation of hepatic heme biosynthesis and porphyria through PCG-1α. Cell 122:505, 2005

Herve P et al: Porphyrias. Lancet 375:924, 2010

Lambrecht RW et al: Genetic aspects of porphyria cutanea tarda. Semin Liver Dis 27:99, 2007

Poblete-Gutierrez P et al: The porphyrias: Clinical diagnosis and treatment. Eur J Dermatol 16:230, 2006

Soonawalla ZF et al: Liver transplantation as a cure for acute intermittent porphyria. Lancet 363:705, 2004

Whatley SD et al: Molecular epidemiology of erythropoietic protoporphyria in the U.K. Br J Dermatol 162:642, 2010

Yasuda M et al: AAV8-mediated gene therapy prevents induced biochemical attacks of intermittent porphyria and improves neuromotor function. Mol Ther 18:17, 2010

CHAPTER 359 Disorders of Purine and Pyrimidine Metabolism

Christopher M. Burns
Robert L. Wortmann

Purines (adenine and guanine) and pyrimidines (cytosine, thymine, uracil) serve fundamental roles in the replication of genetic material, gene transcription, protein synthesis, and cellular metabolism. Disorders that involve abnormalities of nucleotide metabolism range from relatively common diseases such as hyperuricemia and gout, in which there is increased production or impaired excretion of a metabolic end product of purine metabolism (uric acid), to rare enzyme deficiencies that affect purine and pyrimidine synthesis or degradation. Understanding these biochemical pathways has led, in some instances, to the development of specific forms of treatment, such as the use of allopurinol, to reduce uric acid production.

URIC ACID METABOLISM

Uric acid is the final breakdown product of purine degradation in humans. It is a weak acid with pK_as of 5.75 and 10.3. Urates, the ionized forms of uric acid, predominate in plasma extracellular fluid and synovial fluid, with ~98% existing as monosodium urate at pH 7.4.

Plasma is saturated with monosodium urate at a concentration of 405 μmol/L (6.8 mg/dL) at 37°C. At higher concentrations, plasma is therefore supersaturated, creating the potential for urate crystal precipitation. However, plasma urate concentrations can reach 4800 μmol/L (80 mg/dL) without precipitation, perhaps because of the presence of solubilizing substances.

The pH of urine greatly influences the solubility of uric acid. At pH 5.0, urine is saturated with uric acid at concentrations ranging from 360 to 900 μmol/L (6–15 mg/dL). At pH 7, saturation is reached at concentrations between 9480 and 12,000 μmol/L (158 and 200 mg/dL). Ionized forms of uric acid in urine include mono- and disodium, potassium, ammonium, and calcium urates.

Although purine nucleotides are synthesized and degraded in all tissues, urate is produced only in tissues that contain xanthine oxidase, primarily the liver and small intestine. Urate production varies with the purine content of the diet and the rates of purine biosynthesis, degradation, and salvage (Fig. 359-1). Normally, two-thirds to three-fourths of urate is excreted by the kidneys, and most of the remainder is eliminated through the intestines.

The kidneys clear urate from the plasma and maintain physiologic balance by utilizing specific organic anion transporters (OATs), including urate transporter 1 (URAT1) and human uric acid transporter (hUAT) (Fig. 359-2). URAT1 and other OATs carry urate into the tubular cells from the apical side of the lumen. Once inside the cell, urate must pass to the basolateral side of the lumen in a process controlled by the voltage-dependent carrier hUAT. Until recently, a four-component model has been used to describe the renal handling of urate/uric acid: (1) glomerular filtration, (2) tubular reabsorption, (3) secretion, and (4) postsecretory reabsorption. Although these processes have been considered sequential, it is now apparent that they are carried out in parallel by these transporters. URAT1 is a novel transporter expressed at the apical brush border of the proximal nephron. Uricosuric compounds (Table 359-1) directly inhibit URAT1 on the apical side of the tubular cell (so-called *cis*-inhibition). In contrast, antiuricosuric compounds (those that promote hyperuricemia), such as nicotinate, pyrazinoate, lactate, and other aromatic organic acids, serve

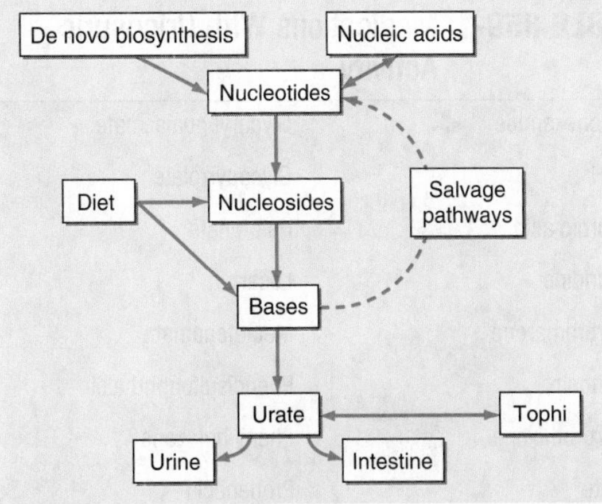

Figure 359-1 The total-body urate pool is the net result between urate production and excretion. Urate production is influenced by dietary intake of purines and the rates of de novo biosynthesis of purines from nonpurine precursors, nucleic acid turnover, and salvage by phosphoribosyltransferase activities. The formed urate is normally excreted by urinary and intestinal routes. Hyperuricemia can result from increased production, decreased excretion, or a combination of both mechanisms. When hyperuricemia exists, urate can precipitate and deposit in tissues as tophi.

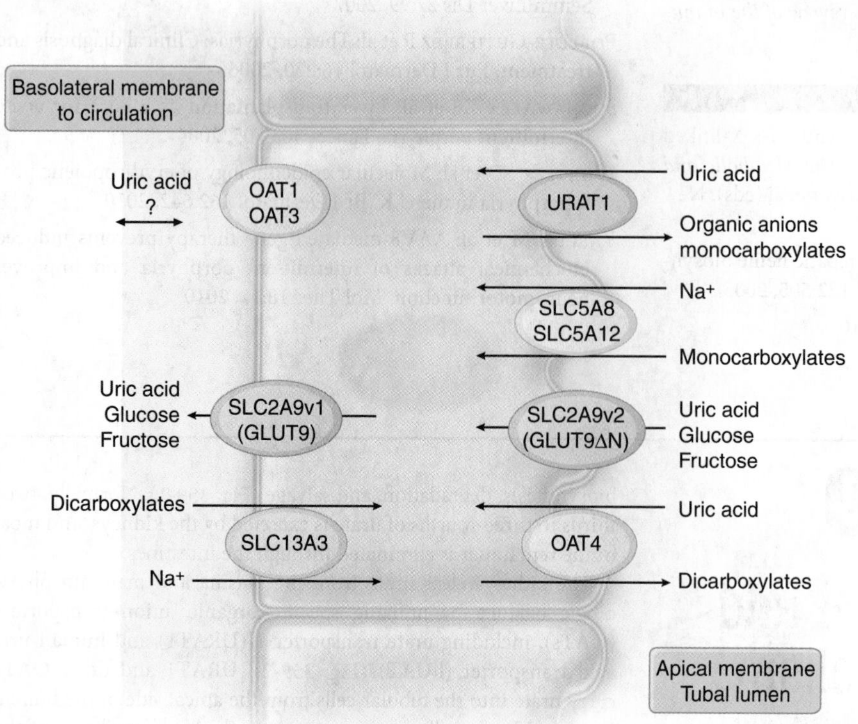

Figure 359-2 Schematic for handling of uric acid by the kidney. A complex interplay of transporters on both the apical and basolateral aspects of the renal tubule epithelial cell is involved in the reabsorption of uric acid. Please see text for details. Most uricosuric compounds inhibit URAT1 on the apical side, as well as OAT1, OAT3, and GLUT9 on the basolateral side.

as the exchange anion inside the cell, thereby stimulating anion exchange and urate reabsorption (*trans*-stimulation). The activities of URAT1, other OATs, and sodium anion transporter result in 8–12% of the filtered urate being excreted as uric acid.

Most children have serum urate concentrations of 180–240 μmol/L (3–4 mg/dL). Levels begin to rise in males during puberty but remain low in females until menopause. Mean serum urate values of adult men and premenopausal women are 415 and 360 μmol/L (6.8 and 6 mg/dL), respectively. After menopause, values for women increase to approximate those of men. In adulthood, concentrations rise steadily over time and vary with height, body weight, blood pressure, renal function, and alcohol intake.

HYPERURICEMIA

Hyperuricemia can result from increased production or decreased excretion of uric acid or from a combination of the two processes. Sustained hyperuricemia predisposes some individuals to develop clinical manifestations including gouty arthritis (Chap. 333), urolithiasis, and renal dysfunction (see below).

Hyperuricemia is defined as a plasma (or serum) urate concentration >405 μmol/L (6.8 mg/dL). The risk of developing gouty arthritis or urolithiasis increases with higher urate levels and escalates in proportion to the degree of elevation. Hyperuricemia is present in between 2 and 13.2% of ambulatory adults and is even more frequent in hospitalized individuals.

■ CAUSES OF HYPERURICEMIA

Hyperuricemia may be classified as primary or secondary depending on whether the cause is innate or is the result of an acquired disorder. However, it is more useful to classify hyperuricemia in relation to the underlying pathophysiology, i.e., whether it results from increased production, decreased excretion, or a combination of the two (Fig. 359-1, Table 359-2).

Increased urate production

Diet contributes to the serum urate in proportion to its purine content. Strict restriction of purine intake reduces the mean serum urate level by about 60 μmol/L (1 mg/dL) and urinary uric acid excretion by ~1.2 mmol/d (200 mg/d). Foods high in nucleic acid content include liver, "sweetbreads" (i.e., thymus and pancreas), kidney, and anchovy.

Endogenous sources of purine production also influence the serum urate level (Fig. 359-3). De novo purine biosynthesis is an 11-step process that forms inosine monophosphate (IMP). The rates of purine biosynthesis and urate production are determined, for the most part, by amidophosphoribosyltransferase (amidoPRT), which combines phosphoribosylpyrophosphate (PRPP) and glutamine. A secondary regulatory pathway is the salvage of purine bases by hypoxanthine phosphoribosyltransferase (HPRT). HPRT catalyzes the combination of the purine bases hypoxanthine and guanine with PRPP to form the respective ribonucleotides IMP and guanosine monophosphate (GMP).

Serum urate levels are closely coupled to the rates of de novo purine biosynthesis, which is driven in part by the level of PRPP, as evidenced by two X-linked inborn errors of purine metabolism. Both increased PRPP synthetase activity and HPRT deficiency are associated with overproduction of purines, hyperuricemia, and hyperuricaciduria (see below for clinical descriptions).

Accelerated purine nucleotide degradation can also cause hyperuricemia, i.e., with conditions of rapid cell turnover, proliferation,

TABLE 359-1 Medications With Uricosuric Activity

Acetohexamide	Glyceryl guaiacolate
ACTH	Glycopyrrolate
Ascorbic acid	Halofenate
Azauridine	Losartan
Benzbromarone	Meclofenamate
Calcitonin	Phenolsulfonphthalein
Chlorprothixene	Phenylbutazone
Citrate	Probenecid
Dicumarol	Radiographic contrast agents
Diflunisal	Salicylates (>2 g/d)
Estrogens	Sulfinpyrazone
Fenofibrate	Tetracycline that is outdated
Glucocorticoids	Zoxazolamine

TABLE 359-2 Classification of Hyperuricemia by Pathophysiology

Urate Overproduction		
Primary idiopathic	Myeloproliferative diseases	Rhabdomyolysis
HPRT deficiency	Polycythemia vera	Exercise
PRPP synthetase overactivity	Psoriasis	Alcohol
Hemolytic processes	Paget's disease	Obesity
Lymphoproliferative diseases	Glycogenosis III, V, and VII	Purine-rich diet
Decreased Uric Acid Excretion		
Primary idiopathic	Starvation ketosis	Drug ingestion
Renal insufficiency	Berylliosis	Salicylates (>2 g/d)
Polycystic kidney disease	Sarcoidosis	Diuretics
Diabetes insipidus	Lead intoxication	Alcohol
Hypertension	Hyperparathyroidism	Levodopa
Acidosis	Hypothyroidism	Ethambutol
Lactic acidosis	Toxemia of pregnancy	Pyrazinamide
Diabetic ketoacidosis	Bartter's syndrome	Nicotinic acid
	Down syndrome	Cyclosporine
Combined Mechanism		
Glucose-6-phosphatase deficiency	Fructose-1-phosphate aldolase deficiency	Alcohol
		Shock

Abbreviations: HPRT, hypoxanthine phosphoribosyltransferase; PRPP, phosphoribosylpyrophosphate.

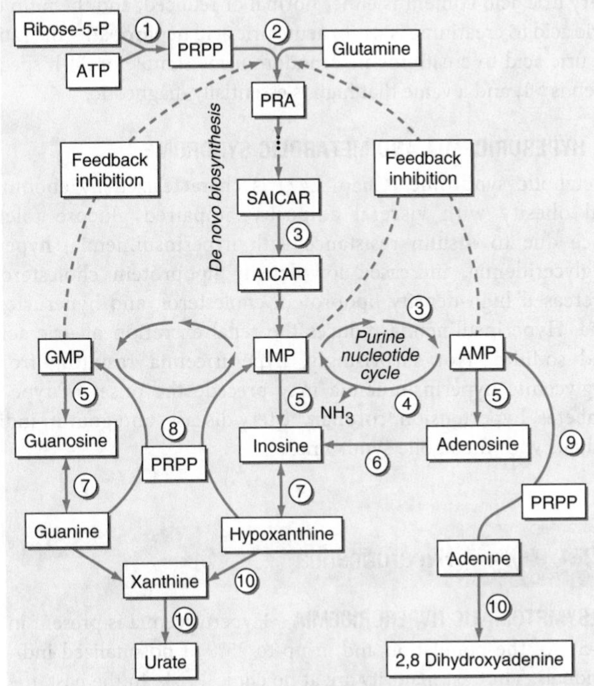

Figure 359-3 Abbreviated scheme of purine metabolism. (1) Phosphoribosylpyrophosphate (PRPP) synthetase, (2) amidophosphoribosyltransferase (amidoPRT), (3) adenylosuccinate lyase, (4) (myo-)adenylate (AMP) deaminase, (5) 5′-nucleotidase, (6) adenosine deaminase, (7) purine nucleoside phosphorylase, (8) hypoxanthine phosphoribosyltransferase (HPRT), (9) adenine phosphoribosyltransferase (APRT), and (10) xanthine oxidase. PRA, phosphoribosylamine; SAICAR, succinylaminoimidazole carboxamide ribotide; AICAR, aminoimidazole carboxamide ribotide; GMP, guanylate; IMP, inosine monophosphate; ATP, adenosine triphosphate.

or cell death, as in leukemic blast crises, cytotoxic therapy for malignancy, hemolysis, or rhabdomyolysis. Hyperuricemia can result from excessive degradation of skeletal muscle ATP after strenuous physical exercise or status epilepticus and in glycogen storage diseases types III, V, and VII (Chap. 362). The hyperuricemia of myocardial infarction, smoke inhalation, and acute respiratory failure may also be related to accelerated breakdown of ATP.

Decreased uric acid excretion

More than 90% of individuals with sustained hyperuricemia have a defect in the renal handling of uric acid. Gouty individuals excrete ~40% less uric acid than nongouty individuals for any given plasma urate concentration. Uric acid excretion increases in gouty and nongouty individuals when plasma urate levels are raised by purine ingestion or infusion, but in those with gout, plasma urate concentrations must be 60–120 μmol/L (1–2 mg/dL) higher than normal to achieve equivalent uric acid excretion rates.

Altered uric acid excretion could theoretically result from decreased glomerular filtration, decreased tubular secretion, or enhanced tubular reabsorption. Decreased urate filtration does not appear to cause primary hyperuricemia but does contribute to the hyperuricemia of renal insufficiency. Although hyperuricemia is invariably present in chronic renal disease, the correlation between serum creatinine, urea nitrogen, and urate concentration is poor. Uric acid excretion per unit of glomerular filtration rate increases progressively with chronic renal insufficiency, but tubular secretory capacity tends to be preserved, tubular reabsorptive capacity is reduced, and extrarenal clearance of uric acid increases as renal damage becomes more severe.

Many agents that cause hyperuricemia exert their effects by stimulating reabsorption rather than inhibiting secretion. This appears to occur through a process of "priming" renal urate reabsorption through the sodium-dependent loading of proximal tubular epithelial cells with anions capable of *trans*-stimulating urate reabsorption. The sodium-coupled monocarboxyl transporters SMCT1 and 2 (SLC5A8, SLC5A12) in the brush border of the proximal tubular cells mediate sodium-dependent loading of these cells with monocarboxylates. A similar transporter, SLC13A3, mediates sodium-dependent influx of dicarboxylates into the epithelial cell from the basolateral membrane. Some of these carboxylates are well known to cause hyperuricemia, including pyrazinoate (from pyrazinamide treatment), nicotinate (from niacin therapy), and the organic acids lactate, β-hydroxybutyrate, and acetoacetate. The mono- and divalent anions then become substrates for URAT1 and organic anion transporter (OAT4), respectively, and are exchanged for uric acid from the proximal tubule. Increased blood levels of these anions result in their increased glomerular filtration and greater reabsorption by proximal tubular cells. The increased intraepithelial cell concentrations lead to increased uric acid reabsorption by promoting URAT1- and OAT4-dependent anion exchange. Low doses of salicylates also promote hyperuricemia by this mechanism. Sodium loading of proximal tubular cells also provokes urate retention by reducing extracellular fluid volume and increasing angiotensin II, insulin, and parathyroid hormone release. Additional organic anion transporters OAT1 and OAT3 are involved in the movement of uric acid through the basolateral membrane, although the detailed mechanisms are still being elucidated.

Glucose transporter 9 (GLUT9, SLC2A9) is an electrogenic hexose transporter with splicing variants that mediate co-reabsorption of uric acid along with glucose and fructose at the apical membrane (GLUT9ΔN/SLC2A9v2), as well as through the basolateral membrane, and thus into the circulation (SLC2A9v1). This might be a mechanism for the observed association of the consumption of fructose-sweetened soft drinks with an increased risk of hyperuricemia and gout. Genomewide association scanning (GWAS) suggests that polymorphisms in SLC2A9 may play an important role in susceptibility to gout in the white population. The presence of one predisposing variant allele increases the relative risk of developing gout by 30–70%, most likely by increasing expression of the shorter isoform, SLC2A9v2 (GLUT9ΔN). Notably, these polymorphisms explain <5% of the variation in serum uric acid levels in whites.

Alcohol promotes hyperuricemia because of increased urate production and decreased uric acid excretion. Excessive alcohol consumption accelerates hepatic breakdown of ATP to increase urate production. Alcohol consumption can also induce hyperlacticacidemia, which blocks uric acid secretion. The higher purine content in some alcoholic beverages such as beer may also be a factor.

EVALUATION

Hyperuricemia does not necessarily represent a disease, nor is it a specific indication for therapy. The decision to treat depends on the cause and the potential consequences of the hyperuricemia in each individual.

Quantification of uric acid excretion can be used to determine whether hyperuricemia is caused by overproduction or decreased excretion. On a purine-free diet, men with normal renal function excrete <3.6 mmol/d (600 mg/d). Thus, the hyperuricemia of individuals who excrete uric acid above this level while on a purine-free diet is due to purine overproduction; for those who excrete lower amounts on the purine-free diet, it is due to decreased excretion. If the assessment is performed while the patient is on a regular diet, the level of 4.2 mmol/d (800 mg/d) can be used as the discriminating value.

COMPLICATIONS

The most recognized complication of hyperuricemia is *gouty arthritis*. In the general population, the prevalence of hyperuricemia ranges between 2.0 and 13.2%, and the prevalence of gout is between 1.3 and 3.7%. The higher the serum urate level, the more likely an individual is to develop gout. In one study, the incidence of gout was 4.9% for individuals with serum urate concentrations >540 μmol/L (9.0 mg/dL) compared with 0.5% for those with values between 415 and 535 μmol/L (7.0 and 8.9 mg/dL). The complications of gout correlate with both the duration and severity of hyperuricemia. For further discussion of gout, see Chap. 333.

Hyperuricemia also causes several renal problems: (1) nephrolithiasis; (2) urate nephropathy, a rare cause of renal insufficiency attributed to monosodium urate crystal deposition in the renal interstitium; and (3) uric acid nephropathy, a reversible cause of acute renal failure resulting from deposition of large amounts of uric acid crystals in the renal collecting ducts, pelvis, and ureters.

NEPHROLITHIASIS

Uric acid nephrolithiasis occurs most commonly, but not exclusively, in individuals with gout. In gout, the prevalence of nephrolithiasis correlates with the serum and urinary uric acid levels, reaching ~50% with serum urate levels of 770 μmol/L (13 mg/dL) or urinary uric acid excretion >6.5 mmol/d (1100 mg/d).

Uric acid stones can develop in individuals with no evidence of arthritis, only 20% of whom are hyperuricemic. Uric acid can also play a role in other types of kidney stones. Some nongouty individuals with calcium oxalate or calcium phosphate stones have hyperuricemia or hyperuricaciduria. Uric acid may act as a nidus on which calcium oxalate can precipitate or lower the formation product for calcium oxalate crystallization.

Urate nephropathy

Urate nephropathy, sometimes referred to as *urate nephrosis*, is a late manifestation of severe gout and is characterized histologically by deposits of monosodium urate crystals surrounded by a giant cell inflammatory reaction in the medullary interstitium and pyramids. The disorder is now rare and cannot be diagnosed in the absence of gouty arthritis. The lesions may be clinically silent or cause proteinuria, hypertension, and renal insufficiency.

Uric acid nephropathy

This reversible cause of acute renal failure is due to precipitation of uric acid in renal tubules and collecting ducts that causes obstruction to urine flow. Uric acid nephropathy develops following sudden urate overproduction and marked hyperuricaciduria. Factors that favor uric acid crystal formation include dehydration and acidosis. This form of acute renal failure occurs most often during an aggressive "blastic" phase of leukemia or lymphoma prior to or coincident with cytolytic therapy but has also been observed in individuals with other neoplasms, following epileptic seizures, and after vigorous exercise with heat stress. Autopsy studies have demonstrated intraluminal precipitates of uric acid, dilated proximal tubules, and normal glomeruli. The initial pathogenic events are believed to include obstruction of collecting ducts with uric acid and obstruction of distal renal vasculature.

If recognized, uric acid nephropathy is potentially reversible. Appropriate therapy has reduced the mortality from about 50% to practically nil. Serum levels cannot be relied on for diagnosis because this condition has developed in the presence of urate concentrations varying from 720 to 4800 μmol/L (12–80 mg/dL). The distinctive feature is the urinary uric acid concentration. In most forms of acute renal failure with decreased urine output, urinary uric acid content is either normal or reduced, and the ratio of uric acid to creatinine is <1. In acute uric acid nephropathy the ratio of uric acid to creatinine in a random urine sample or 24-h specimen is >1, and a value that high is essentially diagnostic.

HYPERURICEMIA AND METABOLIC SYNDROME

Metabolic syndrome (Chap. 242) is characterized by abdominal obesity with visceral adiposity, impaired glucose tolerance due to insulin resistance with hyperinsulinemia, hypertriglyceridemia, increased low-density lipoprotein cholesterol, decreased high-density lipoprotein cholesterol, and hyperuricemia. Hyperinsulinemia reduces the renal excretion of uric acid and sodium. Not surprisingly, hyperuricemia resulting from euglycemic hyperinsulinemia may precede the onset of type 2 diabetes, hypertension, coronary artery disease, and gout in individuals with metabolic syndrome.

TREATMENT Hyperuricemia

ASYMPTOMATIC HYPERURICEMIA Hyperuricemia is present in ~5% of the population and in up to 25% of hospitalized individuals. The vast majority are at no clinical risk. In the past, the association of hyperuricemia with cardiovascular disease and renal failure led to the use of urate-lowering agents for patients with asymptomatic hyperuricemia. This practice is no longer recommended except for individuals receiving cytolytic therapy for neoplastic disease, in which treatment is given in an effort to prevent uric acid nephropathy. Because hyperuricemia can be a component of the metabolic syndrome, its presence is an indication to screen for and aggressively treat any accompanying obesity, hyperlipidemia, diabetes mellitus, or hypertension.

Hyperuricemic individuals are at risk to develop gouty arthritis, especially those with higher serum urate levels. However, most hyperuricemic persons never develop gout, and prophylactic treatment is not indicated. Furthermore, neither structural kidney damage nor tophi are identifiable before the first attack. Reduced renal function cannot be attributed to asymptomatic hyperuricemia, and treatment of asymptomatic hyperuricemia does not alter the progression of renal dysfunction in patients with renal disease. Increased risk of stone formation in those with asymptomatic hyperuricemia is not established.

Thus, because treatment with specific antihyperuricemic agents entails inconvenience, cost, and potential toxicity, routine treatment of asymptomatic hyperuricemia cannot be justified other than for prevention of acute uric acid nephropathy. In addition, routine screening for asymptomatic hyperuricemia is not recommended. If hyperuricemia is diagnosed, however, the cause should be determined. Causal factors should be corrected if the condition is secondary, and associated problems such as hypertension, hypercholesterolemia, diabetes mellitus, and obesity should be treated.

SYMPTOMATIC HYPERURICEMIA Nephrolithiasis (See Chap. 333 for treatment of gout.) Antihyperuricemic therapy is recommended for the individual who has both gouty arthritis and either uric acid– or calcium-containing stones, both of which may occur in association with hyperuricaciduria. Regardless of the nature of the calculi, fluid ingestion should be sufficient to produce a daily urine volume >2 L. Alkalinization of the urine with sodium bicarbonate or acetazolamide may be justified to increase the solubility of uric acid. Specific treatment of uric acid calculi requires reducing the urine uric acid concentration with a xanthine oxidase inhibitor, such as allopurinol or febuxostat. These agents decrease the serum urate concentration and the urinary excretion of uric acid in the first 24 h, with a maximum reduction occurring within 2 weeks. The average effective dose of allopurinol is 300–400 mg/d. Allopurinol can be given once a day because of the long half-life (18 h) of its active metabolite, oxypurinol. The drug is effective in patients with renal insufficiency, but the dose should be reduced. Allopurinol is also useful in reducing the recurrence of calcium oxalate stones in gouty patients and in nongouty individuals with hyperuricemia or hyperuricaciduria. Febuxostat (40–80 mg/d) is also taken once daily, and doses do not need to be adjusted in the presence of mild to moderate renal dysfunction. Potassium citrate (30–80 mmol/d orally in divided doses) is an alternative therapy for patients with uric acid stones alone or mixed calcium/uric acid stones. A xanthine oxidase inhibitor is also indicated for the treatment of 2,8-dihydroxyadenine kidney stones.

Uric Acid Nephropathy Uric acid nephropathy is often preventable, and immediate, appropriate therapy has greatly reduced the mortality rate. Vigorous IV hydration and diuresis with furosemide dilute the uric acid in the tubules and promote urine flow to ≥100 mL/h. The administration of acetazolamide, 240–500 mg every 6–8 h, and sodium bicarbonate, 89 mmol/L, IV enhances urine alkalinity and thereby solubilizes more uric acid. It is important to ensure that the urine pH remains >7.0 and to watch for circulatory overload. In addition, antihyperuricemic therapy in the form of allopurinol in a single dose of 8 mg/kg is administered to reduce the amount of urate that reaches the kidney. If renal insufficiency persists, subsequent daily doses should be reduced to 100–200 mg because oxypurinol, the active metabolite of allopurinol, accumulates in renal failure. Despite these measures, hemodialysis may be required. Urate oxidase (Rasburicase) can also be administered IV to prevent or to treat tumor lysis syndrome.

HYPOURICEMIA

Hypouricemia, defined as a serum urate concentration <120 μmol/L (2.0 mg/dL) can result from decreased production of urate, increased excretion of uric acid, or a combination of both mechanisms. It occurs in <0.2% of the general population and <0.8% of hospitalized individuals. Hypouricemia causes no symptoms or pathology and therefore requires no therapy.

Most hypouricemia results from increased renal uric acid excretion. The finding of normal amounts of uric acid in a 24-h urine collection in an individual with hypouricemia is evidence for a renal cause. Medications with uricosuric properties (Table 359-1) include aspirin (at doses >2.0 g/d), losartan, fenofibrate, x-ray contrast materials, and glyceryl guaiacolate. Total parenteral hyperalimentation can also cause hypouricemia, possibly a result of the high glycine content of the infusion formula. Other causes of increased urate clearance include conditions such as neoplastic disease, hepatic cirrhosis, diabetes mellitus, and inappropriate secretion of vasopressin; defects in renal tubular transport such as primary Fanconi syndrome and Fanconi syndromes caused by Wilson's disease, cystinosis, multiple myeloma, and heavy metal toxicity; and isolated congenital defects in the bidirectional transport of uric acid. Hypouricemia can be familial, generally inherited in an autosomal recessive manner. Most cases are caused by a loss of function mutation in *SLC12A12*, the gene that encodes URAT-1, resulting in increased renal urate clearance. Individuals with normal *SLC12A12* most likely have a defect in other urate transporters. Although usually asymptomatic, some patients suffer from urate nephrolithiasis or exercise-induced renal failure.

SELECTED INBORN ERRORS OF PURINE METABOLISM

(See also Table 359-3, Fig. 359-3.) More than 30 defects in human purine and pyrimidine metabolic pathways have been identified thus far. Many are benign, but about half are associated with clinical manifestations, some causing major morbidity and mortality. Advances in genetics, as well as high-performance liquid chromatography and tandem mass spectrometry, have allowed for better diagnosis.

PURINE DISORDERS

HPRT DEFICIENCY

The HPRT gene is located on the X chromosome. Affected males are hemizygous for the mutant gene; carrier females are asymptomatic. A complete deficiency of HPRT, the Lesch-Nyhan syndrome, is characterized by hyperuricemia, self-mutilative behavior, choreoathetosis, spasticity, and mental retardation. A partial deficiency of HPRT, the Kelley-Seegmiller syndrome, is associated with hyperuricemia but no central nervous system manifestations. In both disorders, the hyperuricemia results from urate overproduction and can cause uric acid crystalluria, nephrolithiasis, obstructive uropathy, and gouty arthritis. Early diagnosis and appropriate therapy with allopurinol can prevent or eliminate all the problems attributable to hyperuricemia but have no effect on the behavioral or neurologic abnormalities.

INCREASED PRPP SYNTHETASE ACTIVITY

Like the HPRT deficiency states, PRPP synthetase overactivity is X-linked and results in gouty arthritis and uric acid nephrolithiasis. Nerve deafness occurs in some families.

ADENINE PHOSPHORIBOSYLTRANSFERASE (APRT) DEFICIENCY

APRT deficiency is inherited as an autosomal recessive trait. Affected individuals develop kidney stones composed of 2,8-dihydroxyadenine. Whites with the disorder have a complete

TABLE 359-3 Inborn Errors of Purine Metabolism

Enzyme	Activity	Inheritance	Clinical Features	Laboratory Features
Hypoxanthine phosphoribosyltransferase	Complete deficiency	X-linked	Self-mutilation, choreoathetosis, gout, and uric acid lithiasis	Hyperuricemia, hyperuricosuria
	Partial deficiency	X-linked	Gout, and uric acid lithiasis	Hyperuricemia, hyperuricosuria
Phosphoribosylpyrophosphate synthetase	Overactivity	X-linked	Gout, uric acid lithiasis, and deafness	Hyperuricemia, hyperuricosuria
Adenine phosphoribosyltransferase	Deficiency	Autosomal recessive	2,8-Dihydroxyadenine lithiasis	—
Xanthine oxidase	Deficiency	Autosomal recessive	Xanthinuria and xanthine lithiasis	Hypouricemia, hypouricosuria
Adenylosuccinate lyase	Deficiency	Autosomal recessive	Autism and psychomotor retardation	—
Myoadenylate deaminase	Deficiency	Autosomal recessive	Myopathy with exercise intolerance or asymptomatic	—
Adenosine deaminase	Deficiency	Autosomal recessive	Severe combined immunodeficiency disease and chondroosseous dysplasia	—
Purine nucleoside phosphorylase	Deficiency	Autosomal recessive	T cell–mediated immunodeficiency	—

deficiency (type I), whereas Japanese subjects have some measurable enzyme activity (type II). Expression of the defect is similar in the two populations, as is the frequency of the heterozygous state (0.4–1.1 per 100). Allopurinol treatment prevents stone formation.

HEREDITARY XANTHINURIA

A deficiency of xanthine oxidase causes all purine in the urine to occur in the form of hypoxanthine and xanthine. About two-thirds of deficient individuals are asymptomatic. The remainder develop kidney stones composed of xanthine.

MYOADENYLATE DEAMINASE DEFICIENCY

Primary (inherited) and secondary (acquired) forms of myoadenylate deaminase deficiency have been described. The primary form is inherited as an autosomal recessive trait. Clinically, some may have relatively mild myopathic symptoms with exercise or other triggers, but most individuals with this defect are asymptomatic. Therefore, another explanation for the myopathy should be sought in symptomatic patients with this deficiency. The acquired deficiency occurs in association with a wide variety of neuromuscular disease, including muscular dystrophies, neuropathies, inflammatory myopathies, and collagen vascular diseases.

ADENYLOSUCCINATE LYASE DEFICIENCY

Deficiency of this enzyme is due to an autosomal recessive trait and causes profound psychomotor retardation, seizures, and other movement disorders. All individuals with this deficiency are mentally retarded, and most are autistic.

ADENOSINE DEAMINASE DEFICIENCY AND PURINE NUCLEOSIDE PHOSPHORYLASE DEFICIENCY

See Chap. 316.

PYRIMIDINE DISORDERS

The pyrimidine cytidine is found in both DNA and RNA; it is a complementary base pair for guanine. Thymidine is found only in DNA, where it is paired with adenine. Uridine is found only in RNA and can pair with either adenine or guanine in RNA secondary structures. Pyrimidines can be synthesized by a de novo pathway (Fig. 359-4) or reused in a salvage pathway. Although >25 different enzymes are involved in pyrimidine metabolism, disorders of these pathways are rare. Seven disorders of pyrimidine metabolism have been discovered (Table 359-4), three of which are discussed below.

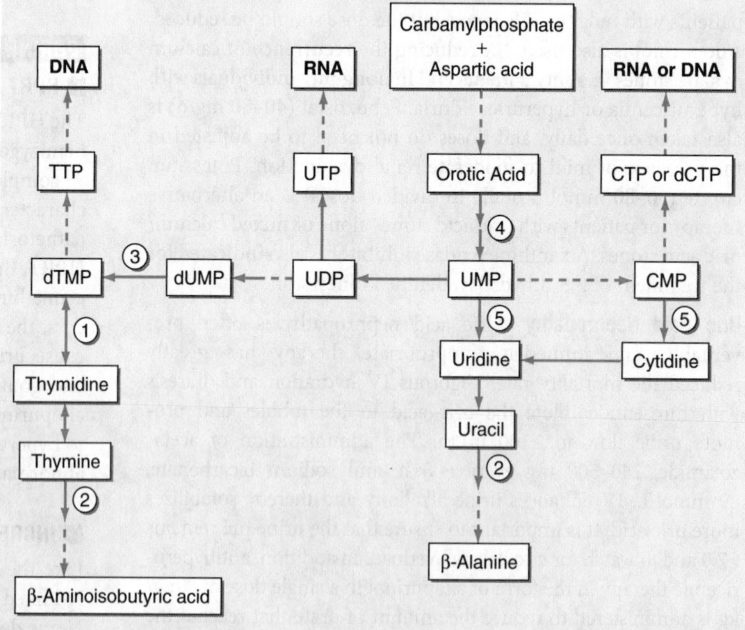

Figure 359-4 Abbreviated scheme of pyrimidine metabolism. (1) thymidine kinase, (2) dihydropyrimidine dehydrogenase, (3) thymidylate synthase, (4) UMP synthase, (5) 5′-nucleotidase. CMP, cytidine-5′-monophosphate; UMP, uridine-5′-monophosphate; UDP, uridine-5′-diphosphate; dUMP, deoxyuridine-5′-monophosphate; dTMP, deoxythymidine-5′-monophosphate; TTP, thymidine triphosphate; UTP, uridine triphosphate.

TABLE 359-4 Inborn Errors of Pyrimidine Metabolism

Enzyme	Activity	Inheritance	Clinical Features	Laboratory Features
Uridine-5′-monophosphate synthetase	Deficiency	Autosomal recessive	Orotic acid crystalluria; obstructive uropathy, hypochromic megaloblastic anemia	Orotic aciduria
Pyrimidine 5′-nucleotidase	Deficiency	Autosomal recessive	Hemolytic anemia	Basophilic stippling of erythrocytes; high levels of cytidine and uridine ribonucleotides
Pyrimidine 5′-nucleotidase	Superactivity	Uncertain	Developmental delay, seizures, ataxia, language deficit	Hypouricosuria
Thymidine phosphorylase	Deficiency	Autosomal recessive	Mitochondrial neurogastrointestinal encephalopathy	Hypouricosuria
Dihydropyrimidine dehydrogenase	Deficiency	Autosomal recessive	Seizures, motor and mental retardation	High levels of uracil, thymine, and 5-hydroxymethyluracil and low levels of dihydropyrimidines in urine
Dihydropyrimidinase	Deficiency	Uncertain	Seizures, mental retardation	Dihydropyrimidinuria
Ureidopropionase	Deficiency	Uncertain	Hypotonia, dystonia, developmental delay	High urinary excretion of *N*-carbamyl-β-alanine and *N*-carbamyl β-aminoisobutyric acid

OROTIC ACIDURIA

Hereditary orotic aciduria is caused by mutations in a bifunctional enzyme, uridine-5′-monophosphate (UMP) synthase, which converts orotic acid to UMP in the de novo synthesis pathway (Fig. 359-4). The disorder is characterized by hypochromic megaloblastic anemia that is unresponsive to vitamin B_{12} and folic acid, growth retardation, and neurologic abnormalities. Increased excretion of orotic acid causes crystalluria and obstructive uropathy. Replacement of uridine (100–200 mg/kg per day) corrects the anemia, reduces orotic acid excretion, and improves the other sequelae of the disorder.

PYRIMIDINE 5′-NUCLEOTIDASE DEFICIENCY

Pyrimidine 5′-nucleotidase catalyzes the removal of the phosphate group from pyrimidine ribonucleoside monophosphates (cytidine-5′-monophosphate or UMP) (Fig. 359-4). An inherited deficiency of this enzyme causes hemolytic anemia with prominent basophilic stippling of erythrocytes. The accumulation of pyrimidines or cytidine diphosphate choline (CDPC) is thought to induce hemolysis. There is no specific treatment. Acquired pyrimidine 5′-nucleotidase deficiency has been reported in lead poisoning and in thalassemia.

DIHYDROPYRIMIDINE DEHYDROGENASE DEFICIENCY

Dihydropyrimidine dehydrogenase (DPD) is the rate-limiting enzyme in the pathway of uracil and thymine degradation (Fig. 359-4). Deficiency of this enzyme causes excessive urinary excretion of uracil and thymine. DPD deficiency causes nonspecific cerebral dysfunction with convulsive disorders, motor retardation, and mental retardation. No specific treatment is available.

MEDICATION EFFECTS ON PYRIMIDINE METABOLISM

A variety of medications can influence pyrimidine metabolism. The anticancer agents fluorodeoxyuridine and 5-fluorouracil (5-FU) and the antimicrobial agent fluorocytosine cause cytotoxicity when converted to fluorodeoxyuridylate (FdUMP), a specific suicide inhibitor of thymidylate synthase. Fluorocytosine must be converted to 5-FU to be effective. This conversion is catalyzed by cytosine deaminase activity. Fluorocytosine's action is selective because cytosine deaminase is present in bacteria and fungi but not in human cells. DPD is involved in the degradation of 5-FU. Consequently, deficiency of this enzyme is associated with 5-FU neurotoxicity.

Leflunomide, which is used to treat rheumatoid arthritis, inhibits de novo pyrimidine synthesis by inhibiting dihydroorotate dehydrogenase, resulting in an antiproliferative effect on T cells. Allopurinol, which is used to block xanthine oxidase and purine synthesis, also inhibits orotidine-5′-phosphate decarboxylase, a step in UMP synthesis. Consequently, allopurinol use is associated with increased excretion of orotidine and orotic acid; there are no known clinical effects of this inhibition.

FURTHER READINGS

Burns CM, Wortmann RL: Gout therapeutics: New drugs for an old disease. Lancet 377:165, 2011

Dalbeth N, Merriman T: Crystal ball gazing: New therapeutic targets for hyperuricaemia and gout. Rheumatol 48:222, 2009

Van Gennip AH et al: Inborn errors of purine and pyrimidine metabolism, in *Physician's Guide to the Treatment and Follow-up of Metabolic Diseases*, N Blau et al (eds). New York, Springer-Verlag, 2005, pp 245–254

Wortmann RL: Gout and hyperuricemia, in *Kelly's Textbook of Rheumatology*, 8th ed, GS Firestein et al (eds). Philadelphia, Saunders, 2009, pp 1481–1506

——— et al (eds): *Crystal-Induced Arthropathies*. New York, Informa Healthcare, 2006, pp 189–212, 255–276, 369–400

CHAPTER 360
Wilson's Disease

George J. Brewer

Wilson's disease is an autosomal recessive disorder caused by mutations in the *ATP7B* gene, a membrane-bound, copper-transporting ATPase. Clinical manifestations are caused by copper toxicity and primarily involve the liver and the brain. Because effective treatment is available, it is important to make this diagnosis early.

The frequency of Wilson's disease in most populations is about 1 in 30,000–40,000, and the frequency of carriers of *ATP7B* mutations is ~1%. Siblings of a diagnosed patient have a 1 in 4 risk of Wilson's disease, whereas children of an affected patient have about a 1 in 200 risk. Because a large number of inactivating mutations have been reported in the *ATP7B* gene, mutation screening for diagnosis is not routine, although this may be practical in the future. DNA haplotype analysis can be used to genotype siblings of an affected patient.

PATHOGENESIS

ATP7B protein deficiency impairs biliary copper excretion, resulting in positive copper balance, hepatic copper accumulation, and copper toxicity from oxidant damage. Excess hepatic copper is initially bound to metallothionein, but as this storage capacity is exceeded, liver damage begins as early as three years of age. Defective copper incorporation into apoceruloplasmin leads to excess catabolism and low blood levels of ceruloplasmin. Serum copper levels are usually lower than normal because of low blood ceruloplasmin, which normally binds >90% of serum copper. As the disease progresses, nonceruloplasmin serum copper ("free" copper) levels increase, resulting in copper buildup in other parts of the body, such as the brain, leading to neurologic and psychiatric disease.

CLINICAL PRESENTATION

Hepatic

Wilson's disease may present as hepatitis, cirrhosis, or as hepatic decompensation, typically in the mid to late teenage years in western countries, although the age of presentation is quite broad and extends into the fifth decade of life.

An episode of hepatitis may occur, with elevated blood transaminase enzymes, with or without jaundice, and then spontaneously regress. Hepatitis often reoccurs, and most of these patients eventually develop cirrhosis.

Hepatic decompensation is associated with elevated serum bilirubin, reduced serum albumin and coagulation factors, ascites, peripheral edema, and hepatic encephalopathy. In severe hepatic failure, hemolytic anemia may occur because large amounts of copper derived from hepatocellular necrosis are released into the bloodstream. The association of hemolysis and liver disease makes Wilson's disease a likely diagnosis.

Neurologic

The neurologic manifestations of Wilson's disease typically occur in patients in their early twenties, although the age of onset extends into the sixth decade of life. MRI and CT scans reveal damage in the basal ganglia and occasionally in the pons, medulla, thalamus, cerebellum, and subcortical areas. The three main movement disorders include dystonia, incoordination, and tremor. Dysarthria and dysphagia are common. In some patients, the clinical picture closely resembles that of Parkinson's disease. Dystonia can involve any part of the body and eventually leads to grotesque positions of the limbs, neck, and trunk. Autonomic disturbances may include orthostatic hypotension and sweating abnormalities as well as bowel, bladder, and sexual dysfunction. Memory loss, migraine-type headaches, and seizures may occur. Patients have difficulties focusing on tasks, but cognition is not usually grossly impaired. Sensory abnormalities and muscular weakness are not features of the disease.

Psychiatric

A history of behavioral disturbances, with onset in the five years before diagnosis, is present in half of patients with neurologic disease. The features are diverse and may include loss of emotional control (temper tantrums, crying bouts), depression, hyperactivity, or loss of sexual inhibition.

Other manifestations

Some female patients have repeated spontaneous abortions, and most become amenorrheic prior to diagnosis. Cholelithiasis and nephrolithiasis occur with increased frequency. Some patients have osteoarthritis, particularly of the knee. Microscopic hematuria is common, and increased urinary excretion of phosphates, amino acids, glucose, or urates may occur; however, a full-blown Fanconi syndrome is rare. Sunflower cataracts and Kayser-Fleischer rings (copper deposits in the outer rim of the cornea) may be seen. Electrocardiographic and other cardiac abnormalities have been reported but are not common.

DIAGNOSIS

Diagnostic tests for Wilson's disease are listed in Table 360-1. Serum ceruloplasmin levels should not be used for definitive diagnosis, because they are normal in up to 10% of affected patients and are reduced in 20% of carriers. Kayser-Fleischer rings (Fig. 360-1) can only be diagnosed definitively by an ophthalmologist using a slit lamp. They are present in >99% of patients with neurologic/psychiatric forms of the disease and have been described very rarely in the absence of Wilson's disease. Kayser-Fleischer rings are present in only ~30–50% of patients diagnosed in the hepatic or presymptomatic state; thus, the absence of rings does not exclude the diagnosis.

Urine copper is an important diagnostic tool, but it must be collected carefully to avoid contamination. Symptomatic patients invariably have urine copper levels > 1.6 μmol (>100 μg) per 24 h. Heterozygotes have values < 1.3 μmol (<80 μg) per 24 h. About half of presymptomatic patients who are ultimately affected have diagnostically elevated urine copper values, but the other half are in an intermediate range between 0.9 and 1.6 μmol (60 and 100 μg) per 24 h. Because heterozygotes may have values up to 1.3 μmol (80 μg) per 24 h, patients in this range may require a liver biopsy for definitive diagnosis.

The gold standard for diagnosis remains liver biopsy with quantitative copper assays. Affected patients have values > 3.1 μmol/g (> 200 μg/g dry weight of liver). Copper stains are not reliable. False-positive results can occur with long-standing obstructive liver disease, which can elevate hepatic and urine copper and rarely causes Kayser-Fleischer rings.

TREATMENT Wilson's disease

Recommended anticopper treatments are listed in Table 360-2. Penicillamine was previously the primary anticopper treatment but now plays a minor role because of its toxicity and because it often worsens existing neurologic disease if used as initial therapy.

TABLE 360-1 Useful Tests for Wilson's disease

Test	Usefulness[a]	Normal Value	Heterozygous Carriers	Wilson's disease
Serum ceruloplasmin	+	180–350 mg/L (18–35 mg/dL)	Low in 20%	Low in 90%
KF rings	++	Absent	Absent	Present in 99% + if neurologic or psychiatric symptoms present Present in 30–50% in hepatic presentation and presymptomatic state
24-h urine Cu	+++	0.3–0.8 μmol (20–50 μg)	Normal to 1.3 μmol (80 μg)	>1.6 μmol (>100 μg) in symptomatic patients 0.9 to >1.6 μmol (60 to >100 μg) in presymptomatic patients
Liver Cu	++++	0.3–0.8 μmol/g (20–50 μg per g tissue)	Normal to 2.0 μmol (125 μg)	>3.1 μmol (>200 μg) (obstructive liver disease can cause false-positive results)
Haplotype analysis	++++ (Siblings only)	0 Matches	1 Match	2 Matches

[a]Usefulness: +, somewhat useful, to ++++, very useful.
Abbreviations: Cu, copper; KF, Kayser-Fleischer.

If penicillamine is given, it should always be accompanied by 25 mg/d of pyridoxine. Trientine is a less toxic chelator and is supplanting penicillamine when a chelator is indicated.

For patients with hepatitis or cirrhosis, but without evidence of hepatic decompensation or neurologic/psychiatric symptoms, zinc is the therapy of choice, although some advocate therapy with trientine. Zinc has proven efficacy in Wilson's disease and is essentially nontoxic. It produces a negative copper balance by blocking intestinal absorption of copper, and it induces hepatic metallothionein synthesis, which sequesters additional toxic copper. All presymptomatic patients should be treated prophylactically, because the disease is close to 100% penetrant.

The first step in evaluating patients presenting with hepatic decompensation is to establish disease severity, which can be estimated using the Nazer prognostic index (Table 360-3). Patients with scores < 7 can usually be managed with medical therapy. Patients with scores > 9 should be considered immediately for liver transplantation, and those with scores between 7 and 9 require clinical judgment as to whether to recommend transplantation or medical therapy. A combination of trientine and zinc has been used to treat patients with Nazer scores as high as 9, but such patients should be watched carefully for indications of hepatic deterioration, which mandates transplantation.

For initial medical therapy of patients with hepatic decompensation, a chelator (trientine is preferred) plus zinc is recommended (Table 360-2). Zinc should not, however, be ingested

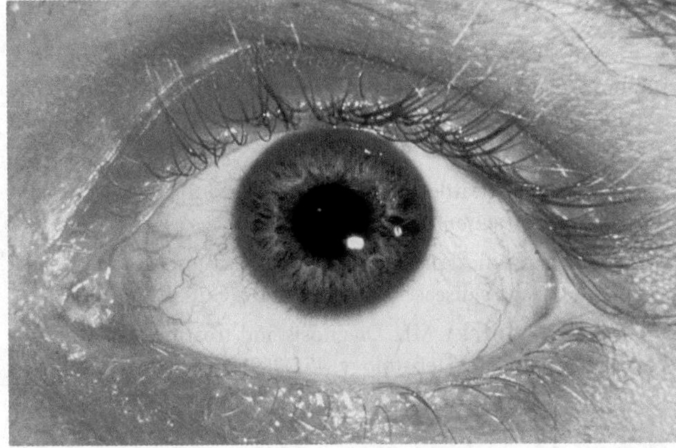

Figure 360-1 A Kayser-Fleischer ring. Although in this case, the brownish ring rimming the cornea is clearly visible to the naked eye, confirmation is usually by slit-lamp examination.

TABLE 360-2 Recommended Anticopper Drugs for Wilson's Disease

Disease Status	First Choice	Second Choice
Initial hepatic		
Hepatitis or cirrhosis without decompensation	Zinc[a]	Trientine
Hepatic decompensation		
Mild	Trientine[b] and zinc	Penicillamine[b] and zinc
Moderate	Trientine and zinc	Hepatic transplantation
Severe	Hepatic transplantation	Trientine and zinc
Initial neurologic/psychiatric	Tetrathiomolybdate[c] and zinc	Zinc
Maintenance	Zinc	Trientine
Presymptomatic	Zinc	Trientine
Pediatric	Zinc	Trientine
Pregnant	Zinc	Trientine

[a]Zinc acetate is supplied as Galzin, manufactured by Gate Pharmaceutical. Recommended adult dose for all the above indications is 50 mg of elemental zinc three times daily, each dose separated from food and beverages other than water by at least 1 h, and separated from trientine or penicillamine doses by at least 1 h.

[b]Trientine is supplied as Syprine and penicillamine as Cuprimine, both manufactured by Merck. Recommended adult dosage for both drugs is 500 mg twice daily, each dose at least 1/2 h before or 2 h after meals.

[c]Tetrathiomolybdate is being studied in clinical trials.

TABLE 360-3 Prognostic Index of Nazer

Laboratory Measurement	Normal Value	Score (in Points) 0	1	2	3	4
Serum bilirubin[a]	0.2–1.2 mg/dL	<5.8	5.8–8.8	8.8–11.7	11.7–17.5	>17.5
Serum aspartate transferase (AST)	10–35 IU/L	<100	100–150	151–200	201–300	>300
Prolongation of prothrombin time (seconds)	—	<4	4–8	9–12	13–20	>20

[a]If hemolysis is present, the serum bilirubin cannot be used as a measure of liver function until the hemolysis subsides.

Source: Modified from H Nazer et al: Gut 27:1377, 1986; with permission from BMJ Publishing Group.

simultaneously with trientine, because it will chelate zinc and form therapeutically ineffective complexes; administration of the two drugs should be separated by at least one hour.

For initial neurologic therapy, tetrathiomolybdate is emerging as the drug of choice because of its rapid control of free copper, preservation of neurologic function, and low toxicity. Penicillamine and trientine should be avoided because they each have a high risk of worsening the neurologic condition. Until tetrathiomolybdate is commercially available, zinc therapy is recommended. Although it is relatively slow-acting, zinc itself does not cause neurologic worsening. Although hepatic transplantation may improve neurologic symptoms, it does so only by removing copper, which can be done more safely and inexpensively with anticopper drugs. Pregnant patients should be treated with zinc or trientine throughout pregnancy, but without tight copper control, because copper deficiency can be teratogenic.

Anticopper therapy must be lifelong. With treatment, liver function usually recovers after about a year, although residual liver damage is usually present. Neurologic and psychiatric symptoms usually improve after 6 to 24 months of treatment.

Monitoring anticopper therapy When first using trientine or penicillamine, it is necessary to monitor for drug toxicity—particularly bone marrow suppression and proteinuria. Complete blood counts, standard biochemical profiles, and a urinalysis should be performed at weekly intervals for a month, then at twice-weekly intervals for two to three months, then at monthly intervals for three or four months, and at four- to six-month intervals thereafter.

The anticopper effects of trientine and penicillamine can be monitored by following 24-h "free" serum copper. Changes in urine copper are more difficult to interpret because excretion reflects the effect of the drug, as well as body loading with copper. Free serum copper is calculated by subtracting the ceruloplasmin copper from the total serum copper. Each 10 mg/L (mg/dL) of ceruloplasmin contributes 0.5 μmol/L (3 μg/dL) of serum copper. The normal free copper value is 1.6–2.4 μmol/L (10–15 μg/dL), and it is often as high as 7.9 μmol/L (50 μg/dL) in untreated Wilson's disease. With treatment, free copper should be <3.9 μmol/L (<25 μg/dL).

Zinc treatment does not require blood or urine monitoring for toxicity. Its only significant side effect is gastric burning or nausea in ~10% of patients, usually with the first morning dose. This can be mitigated by taking the first dose an hour after breakfast or taking the zinc with a small amount of protein. Because zinc mainly affects stool copper, 24-h urine copper can be used to reflect body loading. The typical value in untreated symptomatic patients is >3.1 μmol (>200 μg) per 24 h. This level should decrease during the first 1–2 years of therapy to <2.0 μmol (<125 μg) per 24 h. A normal value [0.3 to 0.8 μmol (20 to 50 μg)] is rarely reached during the first decade of therapy and should raise concern about overtreatment (copper deficiency), the first sign of which is anemia and/or leukopenia.

GLOBAL CONSIDERATIONS

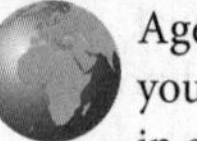

Age of onset of clinical disease may be considerably younger in India and far Eastern countries, often occurring in children only five or six years of age. The incidence of the disease may be increased in certain populations due to founder effects. For example, in Sardinia, the incidence may be 1 in 3000. In countries where penicillamine, trientine, and zinc acetate (as Galzin) are not available or cannot be afforded, zinc salts such as the gluconate or sulfate provide an alternative treatment option.

FURTHER READINGS

Askari FK et al: Treatment of Wilson's disease with zinc XVIII. Initial treatment of the hepatic decompensation presentation with trientine and zinc. J Lab Clin Med 142:385, 2003

Brewer GJ, Askari FK: Wilson's disease: Clinical management and therapy. J Hepatol 42:S13, 2005

——— et al: Treatment of Wilson's disease with ammonium tetrathiomolybdate: V. Control of free copper by tetrathiomolybdate and a comparison with trientine. Transl Res. 154:70, 2009

Cox DW, Roberts EA: Wilson's disease. GeneClinics, University of Washington, Seattle. Online. Available at *http://www.geneclinics.org/profiles/wilson/details.html*

Merle U et al: Clinical presentation, diagnosis, and long-term outcome of Wilson's disease: A cohort study. Gut 56:115, 2007

Roberts EA, Schilsky ML: Diagnosis and treatment of Wilson's disease: An update. Hepatology. 47:2089, 2008

CHAPTER 361

Lysosomal Storage Diseases

Robert Hopkin
Gregory A. Grabowski

Lysosomes are heterogeneous subcellular organelles containing specific hydrolyses that allow selective processing or degradation of proteins, nucleic acids, carbohydrates, and lipids. There are >40 different lysosomal storage diseases, classified based on the nature of the stored material (Table 361-1). Several of the most prevalent disorders are reviewed here, including Tay-Sachs disease, Fabry's disease, Gaucher's disease, Niemann-Pick disease, the mucopolysaccharidosis, and Pompe's disease. Lysosomal storage diseases should be considered in the differential diagnosis of patients with neurologic, renal, or muscular degeneration and/or unexplained hepatomegaly, splenomegaly, cardiomyopathy, or skeletal dysplasias and deformations. Physical findings are disease-specific, and enzyme assays or genetic testing can be used to make a definitive diagnosis. Although the nosology of these diseases segregates the variants into distinct phenotypes, these are heuristic and, in the clinic, each disease exhibits, more or less, a continuous spectrum of manifestations from severe to attenuated variants.

PATHOGENESIS OF LYSOSOMAL STORAGE DISEASES

Lysosomal biogenesis involves ongoing synthesis of lysosomal hydrolases, membrane constitutive proteins, and new membranes. Lysosomes originate from the fusion of trans-Golgi network (TGN) vesicles with late endosomes. Progressive vesicular acidification accompanies the maturation of TGN vesicles, and this gradient facilitates the pH-dependent dissociation of receptors and ligands, as well as activating lysosomal hydrolases.

Abnormalities at any biosynthetic step can impair enzyme activation and lead to a lysosomal storage disorder. Following leader sequence clipping, complex oligosaccharide modifications occur during transit through the Golgi, including the lysosomal targeting ligand, mannose-6-phosphate, and modification of high-mannose oligosaccharide chains of many soluble lysosomal hydrolases. Lysosomal integral or associated membrane proteins are sorted to the membrane or interior of the lysosome by several different peptide signals. Phosphorylation, sulfation, additional proteolytic processing, and macromolecular assembly of heteromers occur concurrently. Such posttranslational modifications are critical to enzyme function, and defects can result in multiple enzyme/protein deficiencies.

The final common pathway for lysosomal storage diseases is the accumulation of specific macromolecules within tissues and cells that normally have a high flux of these substrates. The majority of lysosomal enzyme deficiencies result from point mutations or genetic rearrangements at a locus that encodes a single lysosomal hydrolase. However, some mutations cause deficiencies of several different lysosomal hydrolases by altering the enzymes/proteins involved in targeting, active site modifications, or macromolecular association or trafficking. All are inherited as autosomal recessive disorders, except Hunter's (mucopolysaccharidosis type II) and Fabry's diseases, which are X-linked. Substrate accumulation leads to lysosomal distortion, which has significant pathologic consequences. In addition, abnormal amounts of metabolites may also have pharmacologic effects important to disease pathophysiology and propagation.

For many lysosomal diseases, the accumulated substrates are endogenously synthesized within particular tissue sites of pathology. Other diseases have greater exogenous substrate supplies. For example, they are delivered by low-density lipoprotein receptor–mediated uptake in Fabry's and cholesteryl ester storage diseases or by phagocytosis in Gaucher's disease type 1. The threshold hypothesis refers to a level of enzyme activity below which disease develops. Consequently, small changes in enzyme activity near the threshold can lead to or prevent disease. A critical element of this model is that enzymatic activity can be challenged by changes in substrate flux based on genetic background, cell turnover, recycling, or metabolic demands. Thus, a set level of residual enzyme may be adequate for substrate in some tissues or cells, but not in others. In addition, several variants of each lysosomal storage disease exist at a clinical level. These disorders, therefore, represent a continuum of manifestations that are not easily dissociated into discrete entities. The bases for such variations have not been elucidated in any detail.

SELECTED DISORDERS

TAY-SACHS DISEASE

About 1 in 30 Ashkenazi Jews is a carrier for Tay-Sachs disease, which is caused by total hexosaminidase A (Hex A) deficiency—defective α-chains. The infantile form is a fatal neurodegenerative disease with macrocephaly, loss of motor skills, increased startle reaction, and a macular cherry red spot. The juvenile-onset form presents with ataxia and dementia, with death by age 10–15 years. The adult-onset disorder is characterized by clumsiness in childhood; progressive motor weakness in adolescence; and additional spinocerebellar, lower motor neuron symptoms, and dysarthria in adulthood. Intelligence declines slowly, and psychosis is common. Screening for Tay-Sachs disease carriers is recommended in the Ashkenazi Jewish population. Sandhoff's disease, defective β-chains, is phenotypically similar to Tay-Sachs disease, but hepatosplenomegaly and bony dysplasias are also present.

FABRY'S DISEASE

Fabry's disease is an X-linked disorder that results from mutations in the α-galactosidase gene. The estimated prevalence of hemizygous males is 1/40,000 to 1/3500 in selected populations. Clinically, the disease manifests with angiokeratomas (telangiectatic skin lesions), hypohidrosis, corneal and lenticular opacities, acroparesthesia; and small-vessel disease of the kidney, heart, and brain.

The angiokeratomas and acroparesthesia may appear in childhood and lead to early diagnosis, if suspected. Angiokeratomas are punctate, dark red to blue-black, flat or slightly raised, and usually symmetric; they do not blanch with pressure. They range from barely visible to several millimeters in diameter and have a tendency to increase in size and number with age. They usually are most dense between the umbilicus and knees—the "bathing suit area"—but may occur anywhere, including the mucosal surfaces. Angiokeratomas also occur in Fordyce scrotal angiokeratoma and several other very rare lysosomal storage diseases. Corneal and lenticular lesions, detectable on slit-lamp examination, may help in establishing a diagnosis of Fabry's disease. Debilitating episodic burning pain of the hands, feet, and proximal extremities (acroparesthesia) can last from minutes to days and can be precipitated by changes in temperature, exercise, fatigue, or fever. Abdominal pain can resemble that from appendicitis or renal colic. Proteinuria, isosthenuria, and progressive renal dysfunction occur in the second

TABLE 361-1 Selected Lysosomal Storage Diseases

Disorder[a]	Enzyme Deficiency [Specific Therapy]	Stored Material	Clinical Types (Onset)	Inheritance	Clinical Features: Neurologic	Liver Spleen Enlargement	Skeletal Dysplasia	Ophthalmologic	Hematologic	Unique Features
Mucopolysaccharidoses (MPS)										
MPS I H, Hurler (136) MPS I H/S, Hurler/Scheie MPS I S, Scheie	α-L-Iduronidase [ET, BMT]	Dermatan sulfate Heparan sulfate	Infantile Intermediate Adult	AR	Mental retardation Mental retardation None	+++	++++	Corneal clouding	Vacuolated lymphocytes	Coarse facies; cardiovascular involvement; joint stiffness
MPS II, Hunter (136)	Iduronate sulfatase [ET]	Dermatan sulfate Heparan sulfate	Severe infantile Mild juvenile	X-linked	Mental retardation, less in mild form	+++	++++	Retinal degeneration, no corneal clouding	Granulated lymphocytes	Coarse facies; cardiovascular involvement; joint stiffness; distinctive pebbly skin lesions
MPS III A, Sanfilippo A (136)	Heparan-*N*-sulfatase	Heparan sulfate	Late infantile	AR	Severe mental retardation	+	+	None	Granulated lymphocytes	Mild coarse facies
MPS III B, Sanfilippo B	*N*-Acetyl-α-glucosaminidase	Heparan sulfate	Late infantile	AR	Severe mental retardation	+	+	None	Granulated lymphocytes	Mild coarse facies
MPS III C, Sanfilippo C	Acetyl-CoA: α-glucosaminide *N*-acetyltransferase	Heparan sulfate	Late infantile	AR	Severe mental retardation	+	+	None	Granulated lymphocytes	Mild coarse facies
MPS III D, Sanfilippo D	*N*-Acetylglucosamine-6-sulfate sulfatase	Heparan sulfate	Late infantile	AR	Severe mental retardation	+	+	None	Granulated lymphocytes	Mild coarse facies
MPS IV A, Morquio (136)	*N*-Acetylgalactosamine-6-sulfate sulfatase	Keratan sulfate Chondroitin-6 sulfate	Childhood	AR	None	+	++++	Corneal clouding	Granulated neutrophils	Distinctive skeletal deformity; odontoid hypoplasia; aortic valve disease
MPS VI B, Morquio (136)	β-Galactosidase		Childhood	AR	None	±	++++			
MPS VI, Maroteaux-Lamy (136)	Arylsulfatase B [ET, BMT]	Dermatan sulfate	Late infantile	AR	None	++	++++	Corneal clouding	Granulated neutrophils and lymphocytes	Coarse facies; valvular heart disease

MPS VII (136)	β-Glucuronidase	Dermatan sulfate Heparan sulfate	Neonatal Infantile Adult	AR	Mental retardation, absent in some adults	+++	+++	Corneal clouding	Granulated neutrophils	Coarse facies; vascular involvement; hydrops fetalis in neonatal form
GM_2 Gangliosidoses										
Tay-Sachs disease (153)	β-Hexosaminidase A	GM_2 gangliosides	Infantile Juvenile	AR	Mental retardation; seizures; later juvenile form	None	None	Cherry red spot in infantile form	None	Macrocephaly; hyperacusis in infantile form
Sandhoff's disease (153)	β-Hexosaminidases A and B	GM_2 gangliosides	Infantile	AR	Mental retardation; seizures	++	±	Cherry red spot	None	Macrocephaly; hyperacusis
Neutral Glycosphingolipidoses										
Fabry's disease (150)	α-Galactosidase A [ET]	Globotriaosylceramide	Childhood	X-linked	Painful acroparesthesias	None	None	Corneal dystrophy, vascular lesions	None	Cutaneous angiokeratomas; hypohydrosis
Gaucher's disease (146)	Acid β-glucosidase [ET, SRT]	Glucosylceramide	Type 1 Type 2 Type 3	AR	None ++++ ++	++++ +++ ++++	++++ + ++++	None Eye movements Eye movements	Gaucher's cells in bone marrow; cytopenias	Adult form highly variable
Niemann-Pick disease (144) A and B	Sphingomyelinase	Sphingomyelin	Neuronopathic, type A Nonneuronopathic, type B	AR	Mental retardation; seizures	++++	None Osteoporosis	Macular degeneration	Foam cells in bone marrow	Pulmonary infiltrates Lung failure
Glycoproteinoses										
Fucosidosis (140)	α-Fucosidase	Glycopeptides; oligosaccharides	Infantile Juvenile	AR	Mental retardation	++	++	None	Vacuolated lymphocytes; foam cells	Coarse facies; angiokeratomas in juvenile form
α-Mannosidosis (140)	α-Mannosidase	Oligosaccharides	Infantile Milder variant	AR	Mental retardation	+++	++	Cataracts, corneal clouding	Vacuolated lymphocytes, granulated neutrophils	Coarse facies; enlarged tongue

(*continued*)

TABLE 361-1 Selected Lysosomal Storage Diseases (*Continued*)

					Clinical Features					
Disorder[a]	Enzyme Deficiency [Specific Therapy]	Stored Material	Clinical Types (Onset)	Inheritance	Neurologic	Liver Spleen Enlargement	Skeletal Dysplasia	Ophthalmologic	Hematologic	Unique Features
β-Mannosidosis (140)	β-Mannosidase	Oligosaccharides		AR	Seizures; mental retardation		++	None	Vacuolated lymphocytes, foam cells	Angiokeratomas
Aspartylglucosaminuria (140)	Aspartylglucosaminidase	Aspartylglucosamine; glycopeptides	Young adult onset	AR	Mental retardation	±	++	None	Vacuolated lymphocytes, foam cells	Coarse facies
Sialidosis (140)	Neuraminidase	Sialyloligosaccharides	Type I, congenital Type II, infantile and juvenile forms	AR	Myoclonus; mental retardation	++, less in type I	++ less in type I	Cherry red spot	Vacuolated lymphocytes	MPS phenotype in type II
Mucolipidoses (ML)										
ML-II, I-cell disease (138)	UDP-*N*-Acetylglucosamine-1-phosphotransferase	Glycoprotein; glycolipids	Infantile	AR	Mental retardation	±	++++	Corneal clouding	Vacuolated and granulated neutrophils	Coarse facies; absence of mucopolysacchariduria; gingival hypoplasia
ML-III, pseudo-Hurler polydystrophy (138)	UDP-*N*-Acetylglucosamine-1-phosphotransferase	Glycoprotein; glycolipids	Late infantile	AR	Mild mental retardation	None	+++	Corneal clouding, mild retinopathy, hyperopic astigmatism		Coarse facies; stiffness of hands and shoulders
Leukodystrophies										
Krabbe's disease (147)	Galactosylceramidase [BMT]	Galactosylceramide Galactosylsphingosine	Infantile	AR	Mental retardation	None	None	None	None	White matter globoid cells
Metachromatic leukodystrophy (148)	Arylsulfatase A	Cerebroside sulfate	Infantile Juvenile Adult	AR	Mental retardation; dementia; and psychosis in adult	None	None	Optic atrophy	None	Gait abnormalities in late infantile form
Multiple sulfatase deficiency (149)	Active site cysteine to C_{α}-formylglycine-converting enzyme	Sulfatides; mucopolysaccharides	Late infantile	AR	Mental retardation	+	++	Retinal degeneration	Vacuolated and granulated cells	Absent activity of all known cellular sulfatases

Disorders of Neutral Lipids										
Wolman's disease (142)	Acid lysosomal lipase [BMT]	Cholesteryl esters; triglycerides	Infantile	AR	Mild mental retardation	+++	None	None	None	Adrenal calcification
Cholesteryl ester storage disease (142)	Acid lysosomal lipase	Cholesteryl esters	Childhood	AR	None	Hepatomegaly	None	None	None	Fatty liver disease; cirrhosis
Farber's disease (142)	Acid ceramidase	Ceramide	Infantile Juvenile	AR	Occasional mental retardation	+/–	None	Macular degeneration	None	Arthropathy, subcutaneous nodules
Disorders of Glycogen										
Pompe's disease (135)	Acid α-glucosidase [ET]	Glycogen	Infantile late onset	AR	Neuromuscular	+/–	None	None	None	Myocardiopathy
Late onset GAA deficiency (135)	Acid α-glucosidase [ET]	Glycogen	Variable–juvenile to adulthood	AR	Neuromuscular	None	None	None	None	Respiratory insufficiency; neuromuscular disease
Danon's disease	LAMP-2 (lysosomal associated membrane protein-2)	Glycogen	Variable–childhood to adulthood	X-linked (?Dominant)	Cardiomyopathy Neuromuscular Inconsistent mental retardation	None	None	None	None	Myocardial vacuolar degeneration

[a]Numbers in parentheses refer to the chapters in Scriver et al, 8th ed, for comprehensive reviews.

Abbreviations: AR, autosomal recessive; ET, enzyme therapy; SRT, substrate reduction therapy; BMT, bone marrow (or stem cell) transplantation.

to fourth decades; about 5% of idiopathic renal failure males have α-galactosidase mutations. Hypertension, left ventricular hypertrophy, anginal chest pain with or without myocardial ischemia or infarction, and congestive heart failure can occur in the third to fourth decades. About 1–3% of patients with idiopathic hypertrophic myocardiopathy were found to have Fabry's disease. Similarly, ~3–5% of idiopathic stroke in males (35–50 years) have α-galactosidase mutations. Leg lymphedema without hypoproteinemia and episodic diarrhea also occur. Death is due to renal failure or cardiovascular or cerebrovascular disease in untreated patients. Variants with residual α-galactosidase activity may have late-onset manifestations limited to the cardiovascular system that resemble hypertrophic cardiomyopathy. Variants with predominant cardiac, renal, or central nervous system (CNS) manifestations are becoming better defined. Up to 70% of heterozygous females may exhibit clinical manifestations, including acroparesthesia and CNS, cardiac, and renal disease.

Phenytoin and carbamazepine diminish the chronic and episodic acroparesthesia. Chronic hemodialysis or kidney transplantation can be lifesaving in patients with renal failure. Enzyme therapy clears stored lipids from a variety of cells, particularly those of the renal, cardiac, and skin vascular endothelium. Renal insufficiency appears irreversible. Early institution of enzyme therapy may prevent or slow the progression of the life-threatening complications.

GAUCHER'S DISEASE

Gaucher's disease is an autosomal recessive disorder that results from defective activity of acid β-glucosidase; >400 mutations have been described at the *GBA* locus of such patients. Disease variants are classified based on the absence or presence and progression of neuronopathic involvement.

Gaucher's disease type 1 is a nonneuronopathic disease that can present in childhood to adulthood with slowly to rapidly progressive visceral disease. About 55–60% of such patients are diagnosed at <20 years in white populations and even younger in other groups. This pattern of presentation is distinctly bimodal, with peaks at <10 to 15 years and at ~25 years. Younger patients tend to have a greater degree of hepatosplenomegaly and accompanying blood cytopenias. In contrast, the older group has a greater tendency for chronic bone disease. Hepatosplenomegaly occurs in virtually all symptomatic patients and can be minor or massive. Accompanying anemia and thrombocytopenia are variable and are not directly related to liver or spleen volumes. Severe liver dysfunction is unusual. Splenic infarctions can resemble an acute abdomen. Pulmonary hypertension and alveolar Gaucher's cell accumulation are uncommon, but life threatening, and can occur at any age. *GBA* mutations in the hetero- or homozygous states are a significant risk factor for early onset or more progressive Parkinson's disease.

All patients with Gaucher's disease have nonuniform infiltration of bone marrow by lipid-laden macrophages termed Gaucher's cells. This can lead to marrow packing with subsequent infarction, ischemia, necrosis, and cortical bone destruction. Bone marrow involvement spreads from proximal to distal in the limbs and can involve the axial skeleton extensively, causing vertebral collapse. In addition to bone marrow involvement, bone remodeling is defective, with loss of total bone calcium leading to osteopenia, osteonecrosis, avascular infarction, and vertebral compression fractures and spinal cord involvement. Aseptic necrosis of the femoral head is common, as is fracture of the femoral neck. The mechanism by which diseased bone marrow macrophages interact with osteoclasts and/or osteoblasts to cause bone disease is not well understood. Chronic, ill-defined bone pain can be debilitating and poorly correlated with radiographic findings. "Bone crises" are associated with localized, excruciating pain, and, on occasion, local erythema, fever, and leukocytosis. Some patients have frequent crises, whereas other patients experience only one. These crises represent acute infarctions of bone, as evidenced in nuclear scans by localized absent uptake of pyrophosphate agents. Osteomyelitis should be excluded by appropriate cultures.

Decreased acid β-glucosidase activity (0–20% of normal) in nucleated cells makes the diagnosis. The enzyme is not present in bodily fluids. The sensitivity of enzyme testing is poor for heterozygote detection; molecular testing is preferred when the mutations are known. The disease frequency varies from about 1 in 1000 in Ashkenazi Jews to <1 in 100,000 in other populations. About 1 in 12–15 Ashkenazi Jews carries a Gaucher's disease allele. Four common mutations account for ~85% of the mutations in that population of affected patients: N370S (1226G), 84GG (a G insertion at cDNA position 84), L444P (1448C), and IVS-2 (an intron 2 splice junction mutation).

Genotype/phenotype studies indicate a significant correlation, though not absolute, between disease type and severity and the acid β-glucosidase genotype. The most common mutation in the Ashkenazi Jewish population (N370S) shares a 100% association with nonneuronopathic or type 1 Gaucher's disease. The N370S/N370S and N370S/other mutant allele genotypes are associated with later onset/less severe disease and with earlier onset/severe disease, respectively. As many as 50–60% of individuals with the N370S/N370S genotype are asymptomatic. Other alleles include L444P (very low activity), 84GG (null), or IVS-2 (null), and rare/private or uncharacterized alleles. The L444P/L444P patients almost always have life-threatening to very severe/early-onset disease, and many, though not all, develop CNS involvement in the first 2 decades of life.

Symptomatic management of the blood cytopenias and joint replacement surgeries continue to have important roles in management. However, regular, intravenous enzyme therapy is currently the treatment of choice in significantly affected patients and is highly efficacious and safe in diminishing the hepatosplenomegaly and improving bone marrow involvement and hematologic findings. The bone disease is decreased but not eliminated by enzyme therapy. Adult patients may benefit from adjunctive treatment with bisphosphonates to improve bone density. Patients who cannot be treated with enzyme, either because it is not effective or because they have an allergy or other hypersensitivities, may be treated with medications that decrease the production of the complex lipid molecules that are broken down by acid β-glucosidase (so-called, substrate reduction therapy). Other approaches to stabilize the abnormal enzyme produced by mutant alleles allowing improved enzyme function (referred to as *pharmacologic chaperone therapy*) are under investigation as alternative treatments for Gaucher's disease, Fabry's disease, and other lysosomal diseases.

Gaucher's disease type 2 is a rare, severe CNS disease that leads to death by 2 years of age. Type 3 Gaucher's disease has highly variable manifestations in the CNS and viscera. It can present in early childhood with rapidly progressive, massive visceral disease and slowly progresses to static CNS involvement; in adolescence with dementia; or in early adulthood with rapidly progressive, uncontrollable myoclonic seizures and mild visceral disease. Visceral disease in type 3 is nearly identical to that in type 1 but is generally more severe. Early CNS findings may be limited to defects in lateral gaze tracking, which may remain static for decades. Mental retardation can be slowly progressive or static. This variant is most frequent among individuals of Swedish descent. The visceral, but not the CNS, involvement responds to enzyme therapy.

NIEMANN-PICK DISEASE

This is an autosomal recessive disorder that results from defects in acid sphingomyelinase. Types A and B are distinguished by an early age of onset and progressive CNS disease in type A. Type A typically has onset in the first 6 months, with rapidly progressive CNS deterioration, spasticity, failure to thrive, and massive hepatosplenomegaly. In contrast, type B has a later, more variable onset and progression of hepatosplenomegaly, with eventual development of cirrhosis and hepatic replacement by foam cells. Affected patients develop progressive pulmonary disease with dyspnea, hypoxemia, and a reticular infiltrative pattern on chest x-ray. Foam cells are present in alveoli, lymphatic vessels, and pulmonary arteries. Progressive hepatic or lung disease leads to demise in adolescence to early adulthood.

The diagnosis is established by markedly decreased (1–10% of normal) sphingomyelinase activity in nucleated cells. There is no specific treatment for Niemann-Pick disease. The efficacy of hepatic or bone marrow transplantation has not been clearly established. Clinical trials using enzyme therapy are anticipated in the near future.

MUCOPOLYSACCHARIDOSES

Mucopolysaccharidosis type I (MPS I) is an autosomal recessive disorder caused by deficiency of α-L-iduronidase. The continuum of involvement traditionally has been divided into three categories: (1) Hurler's disease (MPS I H) for severe deficiency with neurodegeneration, (2) Scheie's disease (MPS I S) for later-onset disease without neurologic involvement and with relatively less severe disease in other organ systems, and (3) Hurler-Scheie syndrome (MPS I H/S) for patients intermediate between these extremes. MPS I H/S is characterized by severe somatic disease and usually without overt neurologic deterioration.

MPS I often presents in infancy or early childhood with chronic rhinitis, clouding of the corneas, and hepatosplenomegaly. As the disease progresses, nearly every organ system can be affected. For the more severe forms, cardiac and respiratory diseases become life threatening in childhood. Skeletal disease can be quite severe, resulting in very limited mobility.

There are two current treatments for the MPS I diseases. Stem cell transplantation is the standard treatment for patients presenting in infancy who appear to have or are at risk for neurologic degeneration. Stem cell engraftment results in stabilization of the CNS disease and reverses the hepatosplenomegaly. It also improves the cardiac and respiratory disease. Stem cell transplantation does not eliminate the corneal disease or resolve the progressive skeletal disease. Intravenous enzyme therapy effectively addresses the hepatosplenomegaly and improves cardiac and respiratory disease. The enzyme does not effectively penetrate the CNS and does not directly alter the CNS disease. Enzyme therapy and stem cell transplant appear to have similar effects for signs and symptoms outside the CNS. Enzyme therapy has a lower risk for life-threatening complications and may, therefore, have advantages for patients without CNS degeneration. A combination of enzyme therapy and stem cell transplantation has been used with enzyme therapy started prior to transplantation in an attempt to decrease the disease burden prior to transplantation. The experience with this approach is not well documented, but it appears to have advantages over stem cell therapy alone.

Enzyme therapy for Maroteaux-Lamy disease (MPS VI) has received U.S. Food and Drug Administration (FDA) approval for treatment. This very rare autosomal recessive disorder is characterized by hepatosplenomegaly, bone disease, heart disease, and respiratory compromise similar to those seen in MPS I, but it is due to deficiency of arylsulfatase B and is not associated with neurologic degeneration.

Hunter's disease (MPS II) is an X-linked disorder due to deficiency in iduronate sulfate sulfatase; it has manifestations similar to MPS I, including neurologic degeneration, but there is no corneal clouding or other eye disease. Like MPS I, MPS II is clinically variable with CNS and non-CNS variants. Stem cell transplantation has not been successful in treating the CNS disease associated with MPS II. The FDA and the European Agency for the Evaluation of Medicinal Products (EMEA) have approved enzyme replacement for treatment of the visceral manifestations of MPS II.

POMPE'S DISEASE

Acid maltase (acid α-glucosidase's GAA) deficiency, also called Pompe's disease, is the only glycogen lysosomal storage disease. The classic severe infantile form presents with hypotonia, myocardiopathy, and hepatosplenomegaly. This variant is rapidly progressive and generally results in death in the first year of life. However, as with other lysosomal diseases, there are early- and late-onset forms of this disorder. The late-onset variants may be as common as 1/40,000. The late-onset patients typically present with a slowly progressive myopathy that may resemble a limb-girdle muscular dystrophy. Respiratory insufficiency may be the presenting sign or it may develop with advancing disease. In late stages of the disease, patients may require mechanical ventilation, report swallowing difficulties, and experience loss of bowel and bladder control. Myocardiopathy is not usually seen in late-onset variants of Pompe's disease.

The FDA has approved enzyme infusion therapy for Pompe's disease. This is clearly life-prolonging for the infantile form, consistently resulting in improved cardiac function. Improved respiratory function is seen in most treated infants. Some infants demonstrated marked improvement in motor functions while others had minor changes in muscle tone or strength. Prevention of deterioration has been shown with GAA enzyme therapy in the late-onset forms. Early intervention with GAA enzyme therapy in such patients may limit or prevent the deterioration, but very advanced disease will have significant irreversible components.

FURTHER READINGS

GRABOWSKI GA et al: Dose-response relationships for enzyme replacement therapy with imiglucerase/alglucerase in patients with Gaucher disease type 1. Genet Med 11:92, 2009

MARTINS AM et al: Guidelines for the management of mucopolysaccharidosis type I. J Pediatr 155:S32, 2009

MUENZER J et al: Multidisciplinary management of Hunter syndrome. Pediatrics 124:e1228, 2009

SCRIVER CR et al (eds): *The Metabolic and Molecular Bases of Inherited Disease,* 8th ed. New York, McGraw-Hill, 2001; *ommbid.com,* 2006

VAN DER PLOEG AT, REUSER AJ: Pompe's disease. Lancet 372:1342, 2008

WEINREB NJ et al:. 2009. A validated disease severity scoring system for adults with type 1 Gaucher disease. Genet Med 12:44, 2010

ZARATE YA, HOPKIN, RJ: Fabry's disease. Lancet 372:1427, 2008

CHAPTER 362

Glycogen Storage Diseases and Other Inherited Disorders of Carbohydrate Metabolism

Priya S. Kishnani
Yuan-Tsong Chen

Carbohydrate metabolism plays a vital role in cellular function by providing the energy required for most metabolic processes. The relevant biochemical pathways involved in the metabolism of these carbohydrates are shown in Fig. 362-1. Glucose is the principle substrate of energy metabolism in humans. Metabolism of glucose generates ATP through glycolysis and mitochondrial oxidative phosphorylation. The body obtains glucose through the ingestion of polysaccharides, primarily starch, and disaccharides including lactose, maltose, and sucrose. Galactose and fructose are two other monosaccharides that serve as sources of fuel for cellular metabolism; however, their role as fuel sources is much less significant than that of glucose. Galactose is derived from lactose (galactose + glucose), which is found in milk products, and is an important component for certain glycolipids, glycoproteins, and glycosaminoglycans. Fructose is found in fruits, vegetables, and honey. Sucrose (fructose + glucose) is another dietary source of fructose and is a commonly used sweetener.

Glycogen, the storage form of glucose in animal cells, is composed of glucose residues joined in straight chains by α1-4 linkages and branched at intervals of 4–10 residues by α1-6 linkages. Glycogen forms a treelike molecule and can have a molecular weight of many millions. Glycogen may aggregate to form structures recognizable by electron microscopy. With the exception of glycogen storage disease (GSD) type 0, defects in glycogen metabolism typically cause an accumulation of glycogen in the tissues, hence the name *glycogen storage diseases*. The stored glycogen could be normal or abnormal in structure in the various disorders. The defects in gluconeogenesis or glycolytic pathways, including galactose and fructose metabolism, do not usually result in glycogen accumulation.

Clinical manifestations of the various disorders of carbohydrate metabolism differ markedly. The symptoms range from harmless to lethal. Unlike disorders of lipid metabolism, mucopolysaccharidoses, or other storage diseases, dietary therapy has been effective in many of the carbohydrate disorders. All of the genes responsible for the inherited defects of carbohydrate metabolism have been cloned, and mutations have been identified. Advances in our understanding of the molecular basis of these diseases are being used to improve diagnosis and management. Some of these disorders are candidates for enzyme replacement, substrate reduction, and early trials of gene therapy.

Historically, the glycogen storage diseases were categorized numerically in the order in which the enzymatic defects were identified. They are also classified by the organs involved and clinical manifestations. This is the system followed in this chapter (Table 362-1). The overall frequency of all forms of glycogen storage disease is approximately 1 in 20,000 live births. Most are inherited as autosomal recessive traits; however, phosphoglycerate kinase deficiency and one form of phosphorylase kinase deficiency are X-linked disorders. The most

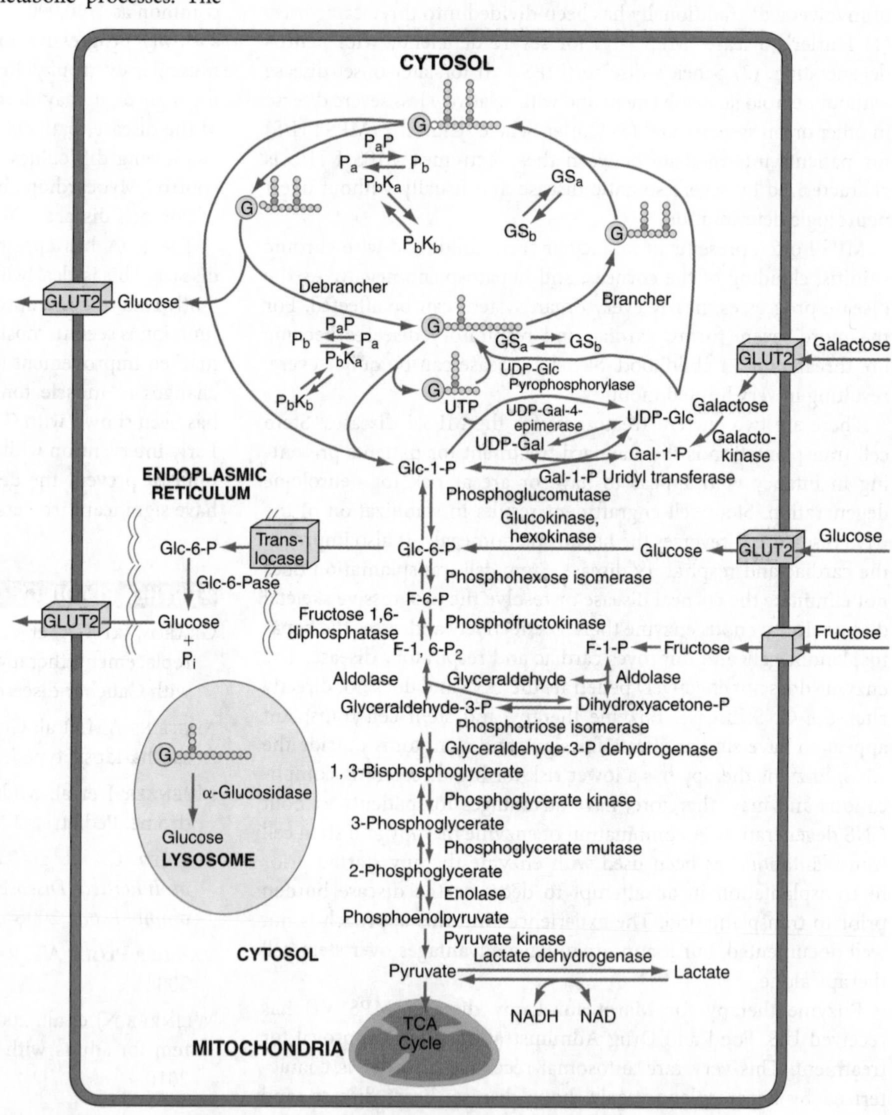

Figure 362-1 Metabolic pathways related to glycogen storage diseases and galactose and fructose disorders. Nonstandard abbreviations are as follows: GS_a, active glycogen synthase; GS_b, inactive glycogen synthase; P_a, active phosphorylase; P_b, inactive phosphorylase; P_aP, phosphorylase *a* phosphatase; P_bK_a, active phosphorylase *b* kinase; P_bK_b, inactive phosphorylase *b* kinase; G, glycogenin, the primer protein for glycogen synthesis. [*Modified from AR Beaudet, in KJ Isselbacher et al (eds): Harrison's Principles of Internal Medicine, 13th ed., New York, McGraw-Hill, 1994, p 1855.*]

TABLE 362-1 Features of Glycogen Storage Diseases and Galactose and Fructose Disorders

Type/Common Name	Basic Defect	Clinical Features	Comments
Liver Glycogenoses			
Disorders with hepatomegaly and hypoglycemia			
Ia/von Gierke	Glucose-6-phosphatase	Growth retardation, enlarged liver and kidney, hypoglycemia, elevated blood lactate, cholesterol, triglycerides, and uric acid	Common, severe hypoglycemia Complications in adulthood include hepatic adenomas, hepatic carcinoma, renal failure
Ib	Glucose-6-phosphate translocase	As for Ia, with additional findings of neutropenia and neutrophil dysfunction	~10% of type I
IIIa/Cori or Forbes	Liver and muscle debranching enzyme	Childhood: Hepatomegaly, growth retardation, muscle weakness, hypoglycemia, hyperlipidemia, elevated liver transaminases; liver symptoms improve with age Adulthood: muscle atrophy and weakness; onset: third to fourth decades; variable cardiomyopathy	Common, intermediate severity of hypoglycemia; hepatic adenomas, liver cirrhosis, and hepatic carcinoma can occur
IIIb	Liver debranching enzyme (normal muscle debrancher activity)	Liver symptoms same as in type IIIa; no muscle symptoms	~15% of type III
VI/Hers	Liver phosphorylase	Hepatomegaly, variable hypoglycemia, hyperlipidemia and ketosis; symptoms may improve with age	Rare, often a "benign" glycogenosis, severe cases being recognized
IX/phosphorylase kinase deficiency	Liver phosphorylase kinase a subunit	As for VI	Common, X-linked, typically less severe than autosomal forms; clinical variability within and between subtypes; severe cases being recognized
0/glycogen synthase deficiency	Glycogen synthase	Fasting hypoglycemia and ketosis, elevated lactic acid and hyperglycemia after glucose load	Decreased glycogen stores
XI/Fanconi-Bickel	Glucose transporter-2	Failure to thrive, rickets, hepatomegaly, proximal renal tubular dysfunction, impaired glucose and galactose utilization	Rare, consanguinity in 70%
Disorders with liver cirrhosis			
IV/Andersen	Branching enzyme	Failure to thrive, hypotonia, hepatomegaly, splenomegaly, progressive liver cirrhosis and failure (death usually before fifth year); some without progression	One of the rarer glycogenoses; other neuromuscular variants exist
Muscle Glycogenoses			
Disorders with muscle-energy impairment V/McArdle	Muscle phosphorylase	Exercise intolerance, muscle cramps, myoglobinuria on strenuous exercise, increased CK	Common, male predominance
VII/Tarui	Phosphofructokinase—M subunit	As for type V, with additional findings of a compensated hemolysis	Prevalent in Ashkenazi Jews and Japanese
Phosphoglycerate kinase deficiency	Phosphoglycerate kinase	As for type V, with additional findings of a hemolytic anemia and CNS dysfunction	Rare, X-linked
Phosphoglycerate mutase deficiency	Phosphoglycerate mutase—M subunit	As for type V	Rare; most patients are African American
Lactate dehydrogenase deficiency	Lactic acid dehydrogenase—M subunit	As for type V, with additional findings of erythematous skin eruption and uterine stiffness resulting in childbirth difficulty in female	Rare
Fructose 1,6-bisphosphate aldolase A deficiency	Fructose 1,6-bisphosphate aldolase A	As for type V, with additional finding of hemolytic anemia	Rare
Pyruvate kinase deficiency	Pyruvate kinase—muscle isozyme	Muscle cramps and/or fixed muscle weakness	Rare
Muscle phosphorylase kinase deficiency	Muscle-specific phosphorylase kinase	As for type V, some patients may have muscle weakness and atrophy	Rare, autosomal recessive

(*continued*)

TABLE 362-1 Features of Glycogen Storage Diseases and Galactose and Fructose Disorders (*Continued*)

Type/Common Name	Basic Defect	Clinical Features	Comments
b-enolase deficiency	Muscle b-enolase	Exercise intolerance	Rare
Disorders with progressive skeletal myopathy and/or cardiomyopathy			
II/Pompe	Lysosomal acid a-glucosidase	Infantile: hypotonia, muscle weakness, cardiac enlargement and failure, fatal early; Juvenile and adult: progressive skeletal muscle weakness and atrophy, proximal muscle and respiratory muscle are seriously affected	Common, undetectable, or very low level of enzyme activity in infantile form; residual enzyme activity in late-onset
Cardiac phosphorylase kinase deficiency	Cardiac-specific phosphorylase kinase	Severe cardiomyopathy and early heart failure	Very rare
Galactose Disorders			
Galactosemia with uridyl transferase deficiency	Galactose 1-phosphate uridyl transferase	Vomiting, hepatomegaly, jaundice, cataracts, amino aciduria, failure to thrive	Long-term complications exist despite early diagnosis and treatment
Galactokinase deficiency	Galactokinase	Cataracts	Benign
Uridine diphosphate galactose 4-epimerase deficiency	Uridine diphosphate galactose 4-epimerase	Similar to transferase deficiency with additional findings of hypotonia and nerve deafness	Benign variant exists
Fructose Disorders			
Essential fructosuria	Fructokinase	Asymptomatic, positive urine reducing substance	Benign
Hereditary fructose intolerance	Fructose 1-6 bisphosphate aldolase B	Vomiting, lethargy, failure to thrive, hepatic failure	Prognosis good with early diagnosis and fructose restriction
Fructose 1,6-diphosphatase deficiency	Fructose 1,6-diphosphatase	Episodic hypoglycemia and lactic acidosis	Avoid fasting, good prognosis

Abbreviations: CK, creatine kinase; CNS, central nervous system; M, muscle.

common childhood disorders are glucose-6-phosphatase deficiency (type I), lysosomal acid α-glucosidase deficiency (type II), debrancher deficiency (type III), and liver phosphorylase kinase deficiency (type IX). The most common adult disorder is myophosphorylase deficiency (type V, or McArdle disease).

SELECTED LIVER GLYCOGENOSES

DISORDERS WITH HEPATOMEGALY AND HYPOGLYCEMIA

Type I glycogen storage disease (glucose-6-phosphatase or translocase deficiency, von Gierke's disease)

Type I glycogen storage disease is an autosomal recessive disorder caused by glucose-6-phosphatase deficiency in liver, kidney, and intestinal mucosa. There are two subtypes of GSD I: type Ia, in which the glucose-6-phosphatase enzyme is defective, and type Ib, in which the translocase that transports glucose-6-phosphate across the microsomal membrane is defective. The defects in both subtypes lead to inadequate conversion in the liver of glucose-6-phosphate to glucose and thus make affected individuals susceptible to fasting hypoglycemia.

Clinical and laboratory findings Persons with type I disease may develop hypoglycemia and lactic acidosis during the neonatal period; however, more commonly, they exhibit hepatomegaly at 3–4 months of age. Hypoglycemia and lactic acidosis can develop after a short fast. These children usually have doll-like faces with fat cheeks, relatively thin extremities, short stature, and a protuberant abdomen that is due to massive hepatomegaly. The kidneys are enlarged, but the spleen and heart are of normal size. The hepatocytes are distended by glycogen and fat with large and prominent lipid vacuoles. Despite hepatomegaly, liver enzymes are usually normal or near normal. Easy bruising and epistaxis are associated with a prolonged bleeding time as a result of impaired platelet aggregation/adhesion. Hyperuricemia is present. Hyperlipidemia includes elevation of triglycerides, cholesterol, and phospholipids. Type Ib patients have additional findings of neutropenia and impaired neutrophil function, resulting in recurrent bacterial infections and oral and intestinal mucosal ulceration. GSD I patients may experience intermittent diarrhea, which can worsen with age. In GSD Ib, it is largely due to loss of mucosal barrier function caused by inflammation.

Long-term complications Gout usually becomes symptomatic at puberty as a result of the long-term hyperuricemia. Puberty is often delayed. Nearly all females have ultrasound findings consistent with polycystic ovaries; however, the other clinical features of polycystic ovary syndrome, such as acne and hirsutism, are not seen. Several reports of successful pregnancy in women with GSD I suggest fertility is not affected. Increased bleeding during menstrual cycles, including life-threatening menorrhagia, has been reported. Secondary to the lipid abnormalities, there is an increased risk of pancreatitis. Patients with GSD I may be at an increased risk for cardiovascular disease. Frequent fractures and radiographic evidence of osteopenia/osteoporosis can be observed in adult patients, and radial bone mineral content is significantly reduced in prepubertal patients. Pulmonary hypertension, although rare, has been reported. By the second or third decade, most patients with type I glycogen storage disease develop hepatic adenomas that can hemorrhage and, in some cases, become malignant. Renal disease is a serious late complication. Almost all patients older than 20 years have proteinuria, and many have hypertension, kidney stones, nephrocalcinosis, and altered creatinine clearance. In some patients, renal function deteriorates and progresses to complete failure, requiring dialysis or transplantation.

Diagnosis Clinical presentation and abnormal plasma lactate and lipid values suggest that a patient may have GSD I, but gene-based mutation analysis provides a noninvasive means of reaching a definitive diagnosis for most patients with types Ia and Ib disease. Before the glucose-6-phosphatase and glucose-6-phosphate translocase genes were cloned, a definitive diagnosis required a liver biopsy to demonstrate a deficiency.

TREATMENT Type I Glycogen Storage Disease

Treatment involves the maintenance of normal blood glucose levels through continuous infusion of glucose via feeding tube or oral administration of uncooked cornstarch. Uncooked cornstarch serves as a slow-release form of glucose and can be given at a dose of 1.6 g/kg every 4 h for infants younger than 2 years. As the child grows older, the cornstarch regimen can be changed to every 6 h at a dose of 1.75–2.5 g/kg of body weight. Newer starch products may be longer acting, better tolerated, and more palatable. Since fructose and galactose cannot be converted to free glucose, their dietary intake should be restricted. Dietary supplements of multivitamins, calcium, and Vitamin D are often required. Allopurinol is given to lower uric acid levels, if levels remain elevated despite diet and metabolic control. The hyperlipidemia can be reduced with dietary control, use of medium chain triglycerides, fish oil and lipid-lowering drugs such as statins and fibric acids. Angiotensin-converting enzyme (ACE) inhibitors are beneficial for treating microalbuminuria, an early indicator of renal dysfunction in these patients. Citrate supplementation may be beneficial in preventing or ameliorating nephrocalcinosis and development of urinary calculi. Orthotropic liver transplantation is a treatment usually reserved for GSD I patients with liver malignancy, multiple liver adenomas, metabolic derangements refractory to medical management, and/or liver failure.

Type III glycogen storage disease (debrancher deficiency, limit dextrinosis)

Type III GSD is an autosomal recessive disorder caused by a deficiency of glycogen debranching enzyme. Debranching and phosphorylase enzyme are responsible for complete degradation of glycogen. When the debranching enzyme is defective, glycogen breakdown is incomplete. Abnormal glycogen accumulates with short outer chains and resembles dextrin.

Clinical and laboratory findings Deficiency of glycogen debranching enzyme causes hepatomegaly, hypoglycemia, short stature, variable skeletal myopathy, and cardiomyopathy. The disorder usually involves both liver and muscle and is termed *type IIIa* glycogen storage disease. However, in about 15% of patients, the disease appears to involve only the liver and is classified as *type IIIb*. Hypoglycemia, hyperlipidemia, and elevated liver transaminases occur in children. In contrast to type I disease, fasting ketosis can be prominent, transaminases are elevated, and blood lactate and uric acid concentrations are usually normal. Serum creatine kinase (CK) levels can sometimes be used to identify patients with muscle involvement, but normal levels do not rule out muscle enzyme deficiency. In most patients with type III disease, hepatomegaly improves with age; however, liver cirrhosis and hepatocellular carcinoma may occur in late adulthood. Hepatic adenomas may occur although less common than in GSOI. Left ventricular hypertrophy and life-threatening arrhythmias have been reported. Those with type IIIa may experience muscle weakness in childhood that can become severe after the third or fourth decade of life. Polycystic ovaries are common in GSD III, and some patients develop features of polycystic ovarian syndrome, such as hirsutism and irregular menstrual cycles. Reports of successful pregnancy in women with GSD III suggest fertility is normal.

Diagnosis In type IIIa glycogen storage disease, deficient debranching enzyme activity can be demonstrated in liver, skeletal muscle, and heart. In contrast, patients with type IIIb have debranching enzyme deficiency in the liver but not in muscle. In the past, definitive assignment of subtype required enzyme assays in both liver and muscle. DNA-based analyses now provide a noninvasive way of subtyping these disorders in most patients. However, the large size of the gene and the distribution of private mutations across it pose challenges in DNA based analysis.

TREATMENT Type III Glycogen Storage Disease

Dietary management of type III disease is less demanding than that of type I. Frequent high-carbohydrate meals with cornstarch supplements or nocturnal gastric drip feedings are usually effective in treating hypoglycemia. A high-protein diet is recommended as neoglucogenesis is intact in GSD III thus providing a source for glucose.

Type IX glycogen storage disease (liver phosphorylase kinase deficiency)

Defects of phosphorylase kinase cause a heterogeneous group of glycogenoses. The phosphorylase kinase enzyme complex consists of four subunits (α, β, γ, and δ). Each is encoded by different genes (X chromosome as well as autosomes) that are differentially expressed in various tissues. Phosphorylase kinase deficiency can be divided into several subtypes on the basis of the gene/subunit involved, the tissues primarily affected, and the mode of inheritance. The most common subtype is X-linked liver phosphorylase kinase deficiency, which is one of the most common liver glycogenoses. Phosphorylase kinase activity may also be deficient in erythrocytes and leukocytes but is normal in muscle. Typically, a child between the ages of 1 and 5 years presents with growth retardation and hepatomegaly. Levels of cholesterol, triglycerides, and liver enzymes are mildly elevated. Fasting ketosis is another feature of the disease. Lactic and uric acid levels are usually normal. Hypoglycemia is typically mild, in the X-linked form of the disease. Phenotypic variability is being increasingly recognized in the X-linked form. The accumulated glycogen in liver (β particles, rosette form) has a frayed or burst appearance and is less compact than the glycogen seen in type I or type III GSD. Hepatomegaly and abnormal blood chemistries gradually return to normal with age. Most adults reach a normal final height and are practically asymptomatic, despite a persistent phosphorylase kinase deficiency. Prognosis is usually good, and adult patients have normal stature and minimal hepatomegaly. "With further study, long term issues will be better understood."

Treatment is symptomatic. A high-carbohydrate diet and frequent feedings are effective in preventing hypoglycemia. Some patients require no specific treatment.

Other subtypes of type IX include an autosomal recessive form of liver and muscle phosphorylase kinase deficiency, an autosomal recessive form of liver phosphorylase kinase deficiency that often develops into liver cirrhosis, a muscle-specific phosphorylase kinase deficiency that causes cramps and myoglobinuria with exercise, and a cardiac-specific phosphorylase kinase deficiency that is lethal during infancy because of massive glycogen deposition in the myocardium. The finding of PK deficiency maybe a secondary phenomena as a subset of these patients have been found to have mutations in PRKAG2.

Other Liver Glycogenoses with Hepatomegaly and Hypoglycemia

These disorders include glycogen synthase deficiency (type 0) and hepatic glycogenosis with renal Fanconi syndrome (type XI). The latter is caused by defects in the facilitative glucose transporter 2 (GLUT-2), which transports glucose in and out of hepatocytes, pancreatic cells, and the basolateral membranes of intestinal and renal epithelial cells. The disease is characterized by proximal renal tubular dysfunction, impaired glucose and galactose utilization, and accumulation of glycogen in liver and kidney.

SELECTED MUSCLE GLYCOGENOSES

■ DISORDERS WITH MUSCLE-ENERGY IMPAIRMENT

Type V glycogen storage disease (muscle phosphorylase deficiency, McArdle disease)

Type V glycogen storage disease is an autosomal recessive disorder caused by deficiency of muscle phosphorylase. McArdle disease is a prototypical muscle energy disorder as the enzyme deficiency limits ATP generation by glycogenolysis and results in glycogen accumulation.

Clinical and laboratory findings Symptoms usually first develop in adulthood and involve exercise intolerance with muscle cramps. Two types of activity tend to cause symptoms: (1) brief exercise of great intensity, such as sprinting or carrying heavy loads; and (2) less-intense but sustained activity, such as climbing stairs or walking uphill. Most patients can engage in moderate exercise, such as walking on level ground, for long periods. Although most patients experience episodic muscle pain and cramping as a result of exercise, 35% report permanent pain that seriously affects sleep and other activities. About half of patients report burgundy-colored urine after exercise, resulting from myoglobinuria secondary to rhabdomyolysis. Intense myoglobinuria after vigorous exercise can lead to renal failure. Clinical heterogeneity is uncommon, however there are cases with symptom onset as late as the eighth decade and cases that present early with hypotonia, generalized muscle weakness, and progressive respiratory insufficiency, which is often fatal.

In rare cases, electromyography (EMG) findings may suggest an inflammatory myopathy, a diagnosis that may be confused with polymyositis. These patients may be at risk for a statin-induced myopathy and rhabdomyolysis.

During rest, the serum CK level is usually elevated; after exercise, the CK level increases even more. Exercise also increases the levels of blood ammonia, inosine, hypoxanthine, and uric acid. The latter abnormalities are caused by accelerated recycling of muscle purine nucleotides in the face of insufficient ATP production.

Diagnosis Lack of an increase in blood lactate and exaggerated blood ammonia elevations after an ischemic exercise test are indicative of a muscle glycogenosis and suggest a defect in the conversion of glycogen or glucose to lactate. The abnormal exercise response, however, can also occur with other defects in glycogenolysis or glycolysis, such as deficiencies of muscle phosphofructokinase or debranching enzyme (when the test is done after fasting). Definitive diagnosis is made by enzymatic assay in muscle tissue or by mutation analysis of the myophosphorylase gene.

TREATMENT Type V Glycogen Storage Disease

In general, avoidance of strenuous exercise can prevent major episodes of rhabdomyolysis; however, regular and moderate exercise is recommended to improve exercise capacity. Sucrose administered before exercise can markedly improve tolerance in these patients. A high-protein diet may increase exercise endurance. Creatine and vitamin B6 supplementation have also been shown to improve muscle function in some patients. In general, longevity does not appear to be affected.

■ DISORDERS WITH PROGRESSIVE SKELETAL MUSCLE MYOPATHY AND/OR CARDIOMYOPATHY

Pompe disease, type II glycogen storage disease (acid α-1,4 glucosidase deficiency)

Pompe disease is an autosomal recessive disorder caused by a deficiency of lysosomal acid α-1,4 glucosidase (acid maltase), an enzyme responsible for the degradation of glycogen in the lysosomes. It is characterized by the accumulation of glycogen in the lysosomes as opposed to accumulation in cytoplasm as in the other glycogenoses.

Clinical and laboratory findings The disorder encompasses a range of phenotypes. Each includes myopathy but differs in the age of onset, organ involvement, and clinical severity. The most severe is the infantile form with cardiomegaly, hypotonia, and death before age 1. Infants may appear normal at birth but soon develop generalized muscle weakness with feeding difficulties, macroglossia, hepatomegaly, and congestive heart failure due to a hypertrophic cardiomyopathy.

The late onset form (juvenile, or late-childhood, or adult form) is characterized by skeletal muscle manifestations, usually without or with minimal cardiac involvement, and a more slowly progressive course. The juvenile form typically presents as delayed motor milestones (if age of onset is early enough) and difficulty in walking. With disease progression, patients often develop swallowing difficulties, proximal muscle weakness, and respiratory muscle involvement. Death may occur before the end of the second decade.

The adult form presents as a slowly progressive myopathy without overt cardiac involvement and typically has its onset between the second and seventh decades. The clinical picture is dominated by slowly progressive proximal muscle weakness with truncal involvement. The pelvic girdle, paraspinal muscles, and diaphragm are most seriously affected. Respiratory symptoms include somnolence, morning headache, orthopnea, and exertional dyspnea. In rare instances patients present with respiratory insufficiency as the initial symptom.

Laboratory findings include elevated levels of serum CK, aspartate transaminase, and lactate dehydrogenase. In infants, chest x-ray shows massive cardiomegaly and electrocardiographic findings include a high-voltage QRS complex and a shortened PR interval. Muscle biopsy shows the presence of vacuoles that stain positively for glycogen; muscle acid phosphatase is increased, presumably from a compensatory increase of lysosomal enzymes. EMG reveals myopathic features with irritability of muscle fibers and pseudomyotonic discharges. Serum CK is not always elevated in adults, and depending on the muscle biopsied or tested, muscle histology or EMG may not be abnormal. The affected muscle should be examined.

Diagnosis The confirmatory step for a diagnosis of Pompe disease is enzyme assay demonstrating deficient acid α-glucosidase or gene sequence showing 2 pathogenic mutations in the GAA gene. Enzyme activity can be measured in muscle, cultured skin fibroblasts, or blood. Deficiency is usually more severe in the infantile form than in the juvenile and adult disorders.

TREATMENT Type II Glycogen Storage Disease

Nocturnal ventilatory support in late-onset patients improves the quality of life and is beneficial during a period of respiratory decompensation. A definitive therapy is now available using aglucosidase alfa (Myozyme), a recombinant human acid α-glucosidase at 20 mg/kg body weight every 2 weeks as an intravenous infusion. In the clinical trials, aglucosidase alfa has been shown to improve ventilator-free survival and motor function in patients with infantile-onset Pompe disease as compared to untreated controls. A randomized placebo-controlled trial in adults demonstrated stabilization of musculoskeletal outcomes and respiratory parameters.

GLYCOGEN STORAGE DISEASE MIMICKING HYPERTROPHIC CARDIOMYOPATHY

Deficiencies of lysosomal-associated membrane protein 2 (LAMP2, also called Danon's disease) and protein kinase, adenosine monophosphate (AMP)-activated gamma 2 noncatalytic subunit (PRKAG2) result in the accumulation of glycogen in the heart and skeletal muscle. Clinically, these patients present primarily as hypertrophic cardiomyopathy. Their electrophysiologic abnormalities, particularly ventricular preexcitation and conduction defects, can distinguish them from patients with hypertrophic cardiomyopathy resulting from defects in sarcomere-protein genes. In patients with LAMP2 deficiency, the onset of cardiac symptoms, including chest pain, palpitation, syncope, and cardiac arrest, can occur between the ages of 8 and 15 years, which is younger than the average age of 33 years for patients with PRKAG2 deficiency. The prognosis for LAMP2 deficiency is poor, with progressive end-stage heart failure early in adulthood. By contrast, long-term survival is possible for patients with cardiomyopathy due to PRKAG2 mutations, although some patients may require the implantation of a pacemaker and aggressive control of arrhythmias. There is a congenital form of PRKAG2 that presents in early infancy with severe hypertrophic cardiomyopathy and a rapidly fatal course. In these patients, levels of phosphorylase kinase have been found to be low.

SELECTED DISORDERS OF GALACTOSE METABOLISM

"Classic" *galactosemia* is caused by galactose 1-phosphate uridyl transferase deficiency. It is a serious disease with an incidence of 1 in 60,000 and an early onset of symptoms. The newborn infant normally receives up to 20% of caloric intake as lactose, which consists of glucose and galactose. Without the transferase, the infant is unable to metabolize galactose 1-phosphate (Fig. 362-1), which accumulates, resulting in injury to parenchymal cells of the kidney, liver, and brain. Patients with galactosemia are at increased risk for *Escherichia coli* neonatal sepsis; the onset of sepsis often precedes the diagnosis of galactosemia.

Widespread newborn screening for galactosemia has identified these infants early and allowed them to be placed on dietary restriction. Elimination of galactose from the diet reverses growth failure and renal and hepatic dysfunction, improving the prognosis. However, on long-term follow-up, some patients still have ovarian failure manifest as primary or secondary amenorrhea, as well as developmental delays and learning disabilities, which increase in severity with age. Eighty to over ninety percent of women with classic galactosemia report hypergonadotropic hypogonadism. While most female patients are infertile when they reach childbearing age, a small number have given birth. There are several mutations that appear protective, particularly the S135L mutation, which is more common in the African American population. In addition, most patients have speech disorders, and a smaller number demonstrate poor growth and impaired motor function and balance (with or without overt ataxia). The treatment of galactosemia to prevent long-term complications remains a challenge.

Deficiency of *galactokinase* (Fig. 362-1) causes cataracts. Deficiency of *uridine diphosphate galactose 4-epimerase* can be benign when the enzyme deficiency is limited to blood cells but can be as severe as classic galactosemia when the enzyme deficiency is generalized.

SELECTED DISORDERS OF FRUCTOSE METABOLISM

Fructokinase deficiency (Fig. 362-1) causes a benign condition that is usually an incidental finding made through the detection of fructose as a reducing substance in the urine.

Deficiency of *fructose 1-6 bisphosphate aldolase* (aldolase B, hereditary fructose intolerance) is a serious disease in infants. These patients are healthy and asymptomatic until fructose or sucrose (table sugar) is ingested (usually from fruit, sweetened cereal, or sucrose-containing formula). Clinical manifestations may include jaundice, hepatomegaly, vomiting, lethargy, irritability, and convulsions. There is a higher incidence of celiac disease in patients with hereditary fructose intolerance (>10%) than in the general population (1–3%). Laboratory findings show a prolonged clotting time, hypoalbuminemia, elevation of bilirubin and transaminases, and proximal renal tubular dysfunction. If the disease is not diagnosed and intake of the noxious sugar continues, hypoglycemic episodes recur, and liver and kidney failure progresses, eventually leading to death. Treatment requires the elimination of all sources of sucrose, fructose, and sorbitol from the diet. Through this treatment, liver and kidney dysfunction improve, and catch-up growth is common; intellectual development is usually unimpaired. Over time, the patient's symptoms become milder, even after fructose ingestion, and the long-term prognosis is good.

Fructose 1,6-diphosphatase deficiency is characterized by childhood life-threatening episodes of acidosis, hypoglycemia, hyperventilation, convulsions, and coma. These episodes are triggered by febrile infections and gastroenteritis when oral food intake decreases. Laboratory findings show low blood glucose, high lactate and uric acid levels, and metabolic acidosis. Unlike hereditary fructose intolerance, there is usually no aversion to sweets, and renal tubular and liver functions are normal. Treatment of acute attacks requires the correction of hypoglycemia and acidosis by intravenous infusion. Later, avoidance of fasting and elimination of fructose and sucrose from the diet prevent further episodes. A slowly released carbohydrate such as cornstarch is useful for the long-term prevention of hypoglycemia. Prognosis is good as patients who survive childhood develop normally.

GLOBAL CONSIDERATIONS

The glycogen storage diseases and other inherited disorders of carbohydrate metabolism although rare, have been reported in most ethnic populations. The prevalent genetic mutations for each disease may vary in different ethnic populations but clinical symptoms are remarkably similar and treatment guidelines apply to all populations.

FURTHER READINGS

ARAD M et al: Glycogen storage diseases presenting as hypertrophic cardiomyopathy. N Engl J Med 352:362, 2005

BEAUCHAMP NJ et al: Glycogen storage disease type IX: High variability in clinical phenotype. Mol Genet Metab 92: 88, 2007

KISHNANI PS et al: Glycogen storage diseases, in *The Online Metabolic and Molecular Bases of Inherited Disease,* CR Scriver et al (eds). New York, McGraw-Hill, 2009, pp 1–85

———: Recombinant human acid α-glucosidase: Major clinical benefits in patients with infantile-onset Pompe disease. Neurology 68:99, 2007

KOERBERL DD et al: Glycogen storage disease types I and II: Treatment updates. J Inherit Metab Dis 30:159, 2007

———: Emerging therapies for glycogen storage disease type 1. Trends Endocrinol Metab 20: 252, 2009

CHAPTER 363

Heritable Disorders of Connective Tissue

Darwin J. Prockop
John F. Bateman

Some of the most common heritable disorders involve the major connective tissues of the body such as bone, skin, cartilage, blood vessels, and basement membranes. Identification of the causes of these disorders has underscored the important structural role of connective tissue proteins, such as the collagens, fibrillin, and elastin. However, these studies have also uncovered unanticipated defects in other proteins and enzymes involved in cell signaling and protein processing. The literature on connective tissue disorders is vast. Consequently, this chapter will focus on the classification and pathophysiology of these disorders and summarize the clinical features and management of the more common disorders.

CLASSIFICATION OF CONNECTIVE TISSUE DISORDERS

The original classification of connective tissue diseases was based on the pattern of inheritance, the cluster of signs and symptoms, as well as radiologic and histologic features. Identification of the mutations causing the diseases has provided a rational framework for understanding the multiple manifestations of the diseases and has led to revisions in the classifications. Also, it has provided tests for prenatal diagnosis and important information for genetic counseling. The usefulness of these tests is likely to increase with the capability to analyze the complete genomes of patients. At the same time, the identification of mutations has thus far provided few new therapies. Also, as with many genetic diseases, the mutations are not always reliable predictors of clinical outcomes. For example, identical collagen I mutations in patients with osteogenesis imperfecta (OI) can be associated with clinical mild or lethal phenotypes for reasons that are not apparent. Also, the current classifications tend to overemphasize the etiologic differences between genetic diseases that are apparent in infants versus similar diseases that appear later in life. For example, small subsets of patients with initial diagnoses of postmenopausal osteoporosis, familial aortic aneurysms, or osteoarthritis have mutations in collagen genes similar to the mutations that are found in patients with OI or chondrodysplasia (CD).

COMPOSITION OF CONNECTIVE TISSUES

Connective tissues contain a large number of complex macromolecules (Table 363-1). The most abundant components are three similar fibrillar collagens (types I, II, and III). They have about the same tensile strength as steel wires. The three fibrillar collagens are distributed in a tissue-specific manner: Type I collagen accounts for most of the protein of dermis, ligaments, tendons, and demineralized bone; type I and type III are the most abundant proteins of large blood vessels; and type II is the most abundant protein of cartilage.

BIOSYNTHESIS AND TURNOVER OF CONNECTIVE TISSUES

Connective tissues are among the most stable components in living organisms, but they are not inert. During embryonic development, connective tissue membranes appear as early as the four-cell blastocyst to provide strength and a structural scaffold for the developing embryo. With the development of blood vessels and skeleton, there is a rapid increase in the synthesis, degradation, and resynthesis of connective tissues. The turnover continues at a slower but still rapid pace throughout postnatal development and then spikes during the growth spurt of puberty. During adulthood, the metabolic turnover of most connective tissues is slow, but it continues at a moderate pace in bone. With age, malnutrition, physical inactivity, and low gravitational stress, the rate of degradation of most connective tissues, especially bone and skin, begins to exceed the rate of synthesis and the tissues shrink. In starvation, a large fraction of the collagen in skin and other connective tissues is degraded and provides amino acids for gluconeogenesis (Chap. 75). In both osteoarthritis and rheumatoid arthritis, there is extensive degradation of articular cartilage collagen. Glucocorticoids weaken most tissues by decreasing collagen synthesis. In many pathologic states, however, collagen is deposited in excess. With most injuries to tissues, inflammatory and immune responses stimulate the deposition of collagen fibrils in the form of fibrotic scars. The deposition of the fibrils is largely irreversible and prevents regeneration of normal tissues in hepatic cirrhosis, pulmonary fibrosis, atherosclerosis, and nephrosclerosis.

Structure and biosynthesis of fibrillar collagens

The tensile strength of collagen fibers derives primarily from the self-assembly of protein monomers into large fibril structures in a process that resembles crystallization. The self-assembly requires monomers of highly uniform and rigid structure. It also requires a complex series of posttranslational processing steps that maintain the solubility of the monomers until they are transported to the appropriate extracellular sites for fibril assembly. Because of the stringent requirements for correct self-assembly, it is not surprising that mutations in genes for fibrillar collagens cause many of the diseases of connective tissues.

The monomers of the three fibrillar collagens are formed from three polypeptide chains, called *α chains*, that are wrapped around each other into a ropelike triple-helical conformation. The triple helix is a unique structure among proteins, and it provides rigidity to the molecule. It also orients the side chains of amino acids in an "inside out" manner relative to most other proteins so that the charged and hydrophobic residues on the surface can direct self-assembly of the monomers into fibrils. The triple-helical conformation of the monomer is generated because each of the α chains has a repetitive amino acid sequence in which glycine (Gly) appears as every third amino acid. Each α chain contains about 1000 amino acids. Therefore, the sequence of each α chain can be designated as $(\text{-Gly-X-Y-})_n$, where X and Y represent amino acids other than glycine and n is >338. The presence of glycine, the smallest amino acid, in every third position in the sequence is critical because this residue must fit in a sterically restricted space in the middle of the helix where the three chains come together. The requirement for a glycine residue at every third position explains the severe effects of mutations that convert any of the glycine residues to an amino acid with a bulkier side chain (see below). Many of the X- and Y-position amino acids are proline and hydroxyproline, which, because of their ring structures, provide additional rigidity to the triple helix. Other X- and Y-positions are occupied by charged or hydrophobic amino acids that precisely direct lateral and longitudinal assembly of the monomers into highly ordered thin fibrils. Mutations that substitute amino acids in some X- and Y-positions can, in rare instances, also produce genetic diseases.

The fibers formed by the three fibrillar collagens differ in thickness and length, but they have a similar fine structure. As viewed by electron microscopy, they all have a characteristic pattern

TABLE 363-1 Constituents of Connective Tissues in Various Tissues

Connective Tissue	Major Constituents	Approximate Amounts, % dry wt	Characteristics or Functions
Dermis, ligaments, tendons	Type I collagen	80	Large bundles of fibrils
	Type III collagen	5–15	Thin fibrils
	Type IV collagen, laminins, and nidogen	<5	Form basal laminae under epithelium
	Types V, VI, and VII collagens	<5	V modifies type I fibrils; VI forms pericellular hexagonal network; VII forms anchoring fibrils for epidermis
	Fibrillin aggregates/elastin	<5	Provide elasticity
	Fibronectin	<5	Associated with collagen fibers and cell surfaces
	Proteoglycans[a]/ hyaluronan	<0.5	Provide resiliency
Bone (demineralized)	Type I collagen	90	Complex fibril network
	Type VI collagen	1–2	Pericellular hexagonal network
	Proteoglycans[a]/ hyaluronan	1	Function unclear
	Osteonectin, osteopontin, osteocalcin, α2-glycoprotein, and sialoproteins	1–5	May regulate mineralization
Aorta	Type I collagen	20–40	Fibril network
	Type III collagen	20–40	Thin fibrils
	Fibrillin aggregates/elastin	20–40	Provide elasticity
	Type IV collagen, laminins, and nidogen	<5	Form basal lamina under endothelial cells
	Types V and VI collagens	<2	V modifies type I fibrils; VI forms pericellular hexagonal network
	Proteoglycans[a]/ hyaluronan	<3	Provide resiliency
Cartilage	Type II collagen	40–50	Arcades of thin fibrils
	Type IX collagen	5–10	Links type II fibrils and other components
	Type X collagen	5–10	Surrounds hypertrophic cells
	Type XI collagen	<10	Incorporated into some type II fibrils
	Proteoglycans[a]/hyaluronan	15–50	Provide resiliency
	Small leucine-rich repeat proteins (SLRPs; >6 kinds)	<5	Multiple functions in assembly and function of the tissue

[a]Over 30 proteoglycans have now been identified. They differ in the structures of their core proteins and their contents of glycosaminoglycan side chains of chondroitin-4-sulfate, chondroitin-6-sulfate, dermatan sulfate, and keratin sulfate. Basal lamina contains a proteoglycan with a side chain of heparan sulfate that resembles heparin.

of cross-striations that are about one-quarter the length of the monomers and reflect the precise packing into fibrils. The three fibrillar collagens, however, differ in sequences found in the X- and Y-positions of the α chains and therefore in some of their physical properties. Type I collagen is composed of two identical α1(I) chains and a third α2(I) chain that differs slightly in its amino acid sequence. Type II collagen is composed of three identical α(II) chains. Type III collagen is composed of three identical α1(III) chains.

To deliver a monomer of the correct structure to the appropriate site of fibril assembly, the biosynthesis of fibrillar collagens involves a large number of unique processing steps (Fig. 363-1). The monomer, first synthesized as a soluble precursor called *procollagen,* contains an additional globular domain at each end. As the proα chains of procollagen are synthesized on ribosomes, the free N-terminal ends move into the cisternae of the rough endoplasmic reticulum. Signal peptides at the N termini are cleaved, and additional post-translational reactions begin. Proline residues in the Y-position of the repeating -Gly-X-Y- sequences are converted to hydroxyproline by the enzyme prolyl hydroxylase. The hydroxylation of prolyl residues is essential for the three α chains of the monomer to fold into a triple helix at body temperature. The enzyme requires ascorbic acid as one of its essential cofactors, an observation that explains why wounds fail to heal in scurvy (Chap. 74).

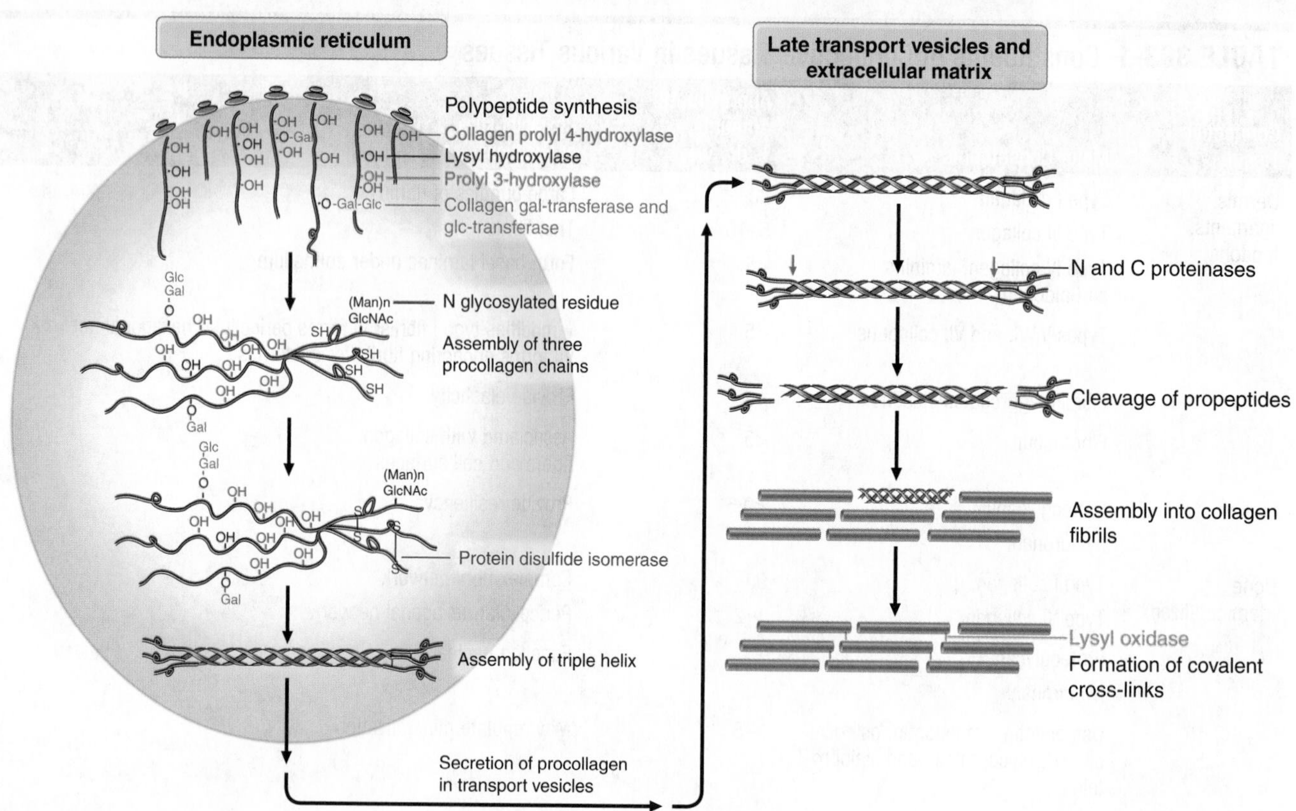

Figure 363-1 Schematic summary of biosynthesis of fibrillar collagens. *(Modified and reproduced with permission from J Myllyharju, KI Kivirikko: Trends in Genetics 20:33, 2004.)*

In scurvy, some of the underhydroxylated and unfolded protein accumulates in the cisternae of the rough endoplasmic reticulum and is slowly degraded. Lysine residues in the Y-position are also hydroxylated to hydroxylysine by a separate lysyl hydroxylase. Many of the hydroxylysine residues are glycosylated with galactose or with galactose and glucose. A large mannose-rich oligosaccharide is assembled on the C-terminal propeptide of each chain. The proα chains are assembled by interactions among these C-terminal propeptides that control the selection of the appropriate partner chains to form hetero- or homotrimers and provide the correct chain registration required for subsequent formation of the collagen triple helix. After the C-terminal propeptides assemble three proα chains, a nucleus of triple helix is formed near the C terminus, and the helical conformation is propagated toward the N terminus in a zipper-like manner that resembles crystallization. The folding into the triple helix is spontaneous in solution, but as discussed below, identification of rare mutations causing OI demonstrated that the folding *in cellulo* is assisted by ancillary proteins. The fully folded protein is then secreted. After secretion, procollagen is processed to collagen by cleavage of the N propeptides and C propeptides by two specific proteinases. The release of the propeptides decreases the solubility of the protein about 1000-fold. The entropic energy that is released drives the self-assembly of the collagen into fibrils. Self-assembled collagen fibers have considerable tensile strength, but their strength is increased further by cross-linking reactions that form covalent bonds between α chains in one molecule and α chains in adjacent molecules.

Although the assembly of collagen monomers into fibers is a spontaneous reaction, the process in tissues is modulated by the presence of less abundant collagens (type V with type I, and type XI with type II) and by other components such as a series of small leucine-rich proteins (SLRPs). Some of the less abundant components alter the rate of fibril assembly, whereas others change the morphology of the fibers or their interactions with cells and other molecules.

Collagen fibers are resistant to most proteases, but during degradation of connective tissues, they are cleaved by specific matrix metalloproteinases (collagenases) that cause partial unfolding of the triple helices into gelatin-like structures that are further degraded by less specific proteinases.

OTHER COLLAGENS AND RELATED MOLECULES

The unique properties of the triple helix are used to define a family of at least 29 collagens that contain repetitive -Gly-X-Y- sequences and form triple helices of varying length and complexity. The proteins are heterogeneous both in structure and function, and many are the sites of mutations causing genetic diseases. For example, the type IV collagen found in basement membranes is composed of three α chains synthesized from any of six different genes. Mutations in any of the six genes can cause Alport syndrome.

Fibrillin aggregates and elastin

In addition to tensile strength, many tissues such as the lung, large blood vessels, and ligaments require elasticity. The elasticity was originally ascribed to an amorphous rubber-like protein named *elastin*. Subsequent analyses, largely sparked by discoveries of mutations causing the Marfan syndrome (MFS), demonstrated that the elasticity resided in thin fibrils composed primarily of large glycoproteins named *fibrillins*. The fibrillins contain large numbers of epidermal growth factor–like domains interspersed with characteristic cysteine-rich domains that are also found in latent transforming growth factor β (TGF-β) binding proteins. The fibrillins assemble into long beadlike strands that also contain numerous other components including small and variable amounts of elastin, bone morphogenic proteins (BMPs), and microfibril-associated glycoproteins (MAGPs). The principles whereby the fibrils provide elasticity to tissue and their biosynthetic assembly are still under investigation.

Proteoglycans

The resiliency to compression of connective tissues such as cartilage or the aorta is largely explained by the presence of proteoglycans. Proteoglycans are composed of a core protein to which are attached a large series of negatively charged polymers of disaccharides (largely chondroitin sulfates). At least 30 proteoglycans have been identified. They vary in their binding to collagens and other components of matrix, but specific functions have not been assigned to most. The major proteoglycan of cartilage, called *aggrecan*, has a core 2000-amino-acid protein that is decorated with about 100 side chains of chondroitin sulfate and keratin sulfate. The core protein, in turn, binds to long chains of the polymeric disaccharide hyaluronan to form proteoglycan aggregates, one of the largest soluble macromolecular structures in nature. Because of its highly negative charge and extended structure, the proteoglycan aggregate binds large amounts of water and small ions to distend the three-dimensional arcade of collagen fibers found in the same tissues. They thereby make the cartilage resilient to pressure.

SPECIFIC DISORDERS

OSTEOGENESIS IMPERFECTA (OI)

The central feature of OI is a severe decrease in bone mass that makes bones brittle. The disorder is frequently associated with blue sclerae, dental abnormalities (dentinogenesis imperfecta), progressive hearing loss, and a positive family history.

Classification

An extensive classification for OI has recently been revised (Table 363-2). Type I is the mildest subtype and can produce either mild or no apparent deformities of the skeleton. Most patients have distinctly blue sclerae. Type II produces bone so brittle that it is lethal in utero or shortly after birth; it is subclassified into types II A, B, and C, depending on radiologic findings. Of the severe nonlethal forms, type III is severely deforming, and type IV is moderately deforming. The rarer types V to VIII of OI are moderately to severely deforming (Table 363-2).

The initial classifications of patients by types of OI do not always predict the clinical course of the disease. Some patients appear normal at birth and become progressively worse; others have multiple fractures in infancy and childhood, improve after puberty, and fracture more frequently later in life. Women are particularly prone to fracture during pregnancy and after menopause. A few women from families with mild variants of OI do not develop fractures until after menopause, and their disease may be difficult to distinguish from postmenopausal osteoporosis.

Incidence

Type I OI has a frequency of about 1 in 30,000 births. Type II OI has a reported incidence of about 1 in 60,000, but the combined incidence of the three severe forms that are recognizable at birth (types II, III, and IV) may be much higher. Only a few patients with types V, VI, VII, and VIII have been reported.

Skeletal effects

In type I OI, the fragility of bones may be severe enough to limit physical activity or be so mild that individuals are unaware of any disability. Radiographs of the skull in patients with mild disease may show a mottled appearance because of small islands of irregular ossification. In type II OI, ossification of many bones is frequently incomplete. Continuously beaded or broken ribs and crumpled long bones (accordina femora) may be present. For reasons that are not apparent, the long bones may be either thick or thin. In types III and IV, multiple fractures from minor physical stress can produce severe deformities. Kyphoscoliosis can impair respiration, cause cor pulmonale, and predispose to pulmonary infections. The appearance of "popcorn-like" deposits of mineral in x-rays of the ends of long bones is an ominous sign. Progressive neurologic symptoms may result from basilar compression and communicating hydrocephalus. Type V OI is recognized by the presence of dislocated radial heads and hyperplastic callus formation. Rhizomelia and coxa vara are observed in patients with type VII. Type VIII is characterized by severe growth deficiency, skeletal undermineralization, and bulbous metaphyses.

In all forms of OI, bone mineral density is decreased. However, the degree of osteopenia may be difficult to evaluate because

TABLE 363-2 Expanded Classification of Osteogenesis Imperfecta (OI)

Type	Bone Fragility	Blue Sclerae	Abnormal Dentition	Hearing Loss	Inheritance
I	Mild	Present	Present in some	Present in most	AD
II	Extreme	Present	Present in some	Unknown	S, rarely AR
III	Severe	Bluish at birth	Present in some	High incidence	AD, rarely AR
IV	Variable	Absent	Absent in IVA, present in IVB	High incidence	AD
V	Moderate to severe	Absent	Absent		AD
VI	Moderate to severe	Absent	Absent		Unknown
VII	Moderate	Absent	Absent	Absent	AR

Abbreviations: AD, autosomal dominant; AR, autosomal recessive; S, sporadic.

recurrent fractures limit exercise and thereby diminish bone mass. Surprisingly, fractures appear to heal normally.

Ocular features

The sclerae can be normal, slightly bluish, or bright blue. The color is probably caused by a thinness of the collagen layers of the sclerae that allows the choroid layers to be seen. Blue sclerae, however, are an inherited trait in some families who do not have increased bone fragility.

Dentinogenesis

The teeth may be normal, moderately discolored, or grossly abnormal. The enamel generally appears normal, but the teeth may have a characteristic amber, yellowish brown, or translucent bluish gray color because of a deficiency of dentin that is rich in type I collagen. The deciduous teeth are usually smaller than normal, whereas permanent teeth are frequently bell-shaped and restricted at the base. In some patients, the teeth readily fracture and need to be extracted. Similar tooth defects, however, can be inherited without any evidence of OI.

Hearing loss

Hearing loss usually begins during the second decade of life and occurs in more than 50% of individuals over age 30. The loss can be conductive, sensorineural, or mixed, and it varies in severity. The middle ear usually exhibits maldevelopment, deficient ossification, persistence of cartilage in areas that are normally ossified, and abnormal calcium deposits.

Other features

Changes in other connective tissues can include thin skin that scars extensively, joint laxity with permanent dislocations indistinguishable from those of Ehlers-Danlos syndrome (EDS), and occasionally, cardiovascular manifestations such as aortic regurgitation, floppy mitral valves, mitral incompetence, and fragility of large blood vessels. For unknown reasons, some patients develop bouts of a hypermetabolic state with elevated serum thyroxine levels, hyperthermia, and excessive sweating.

Molecular defects

Most patients who meet the clinical criteria for OI are heterozygous for mutations in either the proα1 chain gene or the proα2 chain gene of type I procollagen (the *COL1A1* and *COL1A2* genes). Over 90% of patients with type I OI and blue sclerae have mutations that reduce the synthesis of pro α1chains to about one half. Mutations that reduce the synthesis of proα2 chains produce slightly more severe phenotypes and skin defects similar to EDS.

In contrast to the null mutations found in type I OI, most of the severe variants (types II, III, and IV) are caused by mutations that produce structurally abnormal proα chains that have compromised assembly or abnormal folding of the triple helix. As with collagen mutations in other connective tissue diseases, these structural mutations generally fall into two functional categories. Firstly, the relatively rare mutations in the C-propeptide domain can prevent or seriously impair initial assembly of the procollagen trimers. These misfolded chains are retained in the endoplasmic reticulum (ER) and targeted for degradation by the ER-associated proteasomal pathway. Because these mutations induce an ER-stress response, the unfolded protein response (UPR) may have many downstream effects on cells. ER stress is a new concept in the pathophysiology of connective tissue disease and has been best characterized for chondrodysplasias (see below).

The most common type I collagen mutations, however, are single base substitutions that introduce an amino acid with a bulky side chain for one of the glycine residues that appear as every third amino acid in the triple helix. In effect, any of the 338 glycine residues in either the proα1 or proα2 chain of type I procollagen is a potential site for a disease-producing mutation. These mutations compromise the structural integrity of the triple helix, causing disruption to helix folding, retention of the mutant trimers in the ER, and increased posttranslational hydroxylation and glycosylation of lysines. Collagen-containing helix mutations can form insoluble aggregates in the ER that are degraded by the autophagosome-endosome system, rather than the proteasomes.

A similar sequence of events occurs with less common mutations that produce partial gene deletions, partial gene duplications, and splicing mutations. The search for mutations causing the very rare recessive types of OI (VII and VIII) identified mutations in genes for a series of chaperone proteins that are essential for the timely folding of the procollagen monomer: cartilage-associated protein (CRTAP), prolyl-3-hydroxylase (LEPRE1/P3H1), cyclophilin B (PPIB), collagen chaperone-like protein HSP47 (SERPINH1), and the procollagen chaperone protein FKBP65 (FKBP10).

In addition to their intracellular effects, the structurally abnormal mutant-containing collagen that is secreted by the cell can also have important extracellular affects. For example, the presence of one abnormal proα chain in a procollagen molecule can interfere with cleavage of the N propeptide from the protein. The persistence of the N propeptide on a fraction of the molecules interferes with the self-assembly of normal collagen so that thin and irregular collagen fibrils are formed. Furthermore, if structurally abnormal collagens are incorporated into fibrils, they may have a destabilizing effect and be selectively degraded, or they may alter the interactions of collagen with other connective tissue components, disturbing architecture and stability.

Several generalizations can be made about mutations in type I collagen genes. One is that unrelated patients rarely have the same mutation in the same gene. Over 900 such "private" mutations have been identified. Glycine substitutions in the N-terminal region of the triple helix tend to produce milder phenotypes, apparently because they have less effect on the zipper-like propagation of the triple-helical conformation from the C terminus. Rare substitutions of charged amino acids (Asp, Arg) or a branched amino acid (Val) in X- or Y-positions produce lethal phenotypes, apparently because they are located at sites for lateral assembly of the monomers or binding of other components of matrix.

Inheritance and mosaicism in germ-line cells and in somatic cells

Type I OI is usually inherited as an autosomal dominant trait. However, some patients with type I OI appear to represent sporadic new mutations or a diagnosis that was missed in earlier generations. Most lethal OI is the result of sporadic mutations that occur in the germ line in one of the parents. Because of the possibility for germ-line mosaicism for newly generated mutations, there is about a 7% probability that a second child could inherit a severe variant of OI.

Diagnosis

OI is usually diagnosed on the basis of clinical criteria. The presence of fractures together with blue sclerae, dentinogenesis imperfecta, or family history of the disease is usually sufficient to make the diagnosis. Other causes of pathologic fractures must be excluded, including battered child syndrome, nutritional deficiencies, malignancies, and other inherited disorders such as CDs and hypophosphatasia, that can have overlapping presentations. The absence of superficial bruises can be helpful in distinguishing OI from battered child syndrome. X-rays usually reveal a decrease in bone density that can be verified by photon or x-ray absorptiometry. Bone microscopy can be helpful in the diagnosis. A molecular defect in type I procollagen can be demonstrated in over two-thirds of patients by incubating skin fibroblasts with radioactive amino acids and then analyzing the proα chains by polyacrylamide gel electrophoresis. The mutations themselves can be defined in most patients by the sequencing of genomic DNA with tests that are currently available from specialized laboratories.

TREATMENT Osteogenesis Imperfecta

Many patients with OI lead productive and successful lives despite severe deformities. Those with mild disorder may need little treatment when fractures decrease after puberty, but women require special attention during pregnancy and after menopause, when fractures again increase. More severely affected children require a comprehensive program of physical therapy and surgical management of fractures and skeletal deformities.

Many fractures are only slightly displaced and have little soft tissue swelling. Therefore, they can be treated with minimal support or traction for a week or two followed by a light cast. If fractures are relatively painless, physical therapy can be initiated early. A judicious amount of exercise prevents loss of bone mass secondary to physical inactivity. Some physicians advocate insertion of steel rods into long bones to correct limb deformities; the risk/benefits and cost/benefits of such procedures are difficult to evaluate. Aggressive conventional intervention is usually warranted for pneumonia and cor pulmonale. For severe hearing loss, stapedectomy or replacement of the stapes with a prosthesis may be successful. Moderately to severely affected patients should be evaluated periodically to anticipate possible neurologic problems. About half of children have a substantial increase in growth when given growth hormone. Treatment with bisphosphonates to decrease bone loss has been introduced for moderate to severe forms of OI. Initial responses were promising, particularly in decreasing bone pain. However the long-term effects of the drugs are still unknown. Also, a clinical trial was performed in which patients were treated by intravenous infusion of cells from bone marrow referred to as mesenchymal stem cells, or multipotential stromal cells (MSCs; see Chap. 67). Promising results were obtained, but the trial required a prior bone marrow transplant with marrow from a normal donor who subsequently was used as a source of normal MSCs. As a result, the procedure has not been widely adopted. However, the results raise the possibility that it may be possible in the future to develop effective stem cell therapies for OI.

Counseling and emotional support are important for patients and their parents; lay organizations in some countries provide help in these areas. Prenatal ultrasonography will detect severely affected fetuses at about 16 weeks of pregnancy. Diagnosis by demonstrating synthesis of abnormal proα chains or by DNA sequencing can be carried out in chorionic villus biopsies at 8–12 weeks of pregnancy.

EHLERS-DANLOS SYNDROME

EDS is characterized by hyperelasticity of the skin and hypermobile joints.

Classification

Several types of EDS have been defined, based on the extent to which the skin, joints, and other tissues are involved, mode of inheritance, and by molecular and biochemical analysis (Table 363-3). Classical EDS includes a severe form of the disease (type I) and a milder form (type II), both characterized by joint hypermobility and skin that is velvety in texture, hyperextensible, and easily scarred. In hypermobile EDS (type III), joint hypermobility is more prominent than skin changes. In vascular-type EDS (type IV), the skin changes are more prominent than joint changes, and the patients are predisposed to sudden death from rupture of large blood vessels or other hollow organs. EDS V is similar to EDS II but is inherited as an X-linked trait. The ocular-scoliotic type of EDS (type VI) is characterized by scoliosis, ocular fragility, and a cone-shaped deformity of the cornea (keratoconus). The arthrochalasic type of EDS (type VII A and B) is characterized by marked joint hypermobility that is difficult to distinguish from EDS III except by the specific molecular defects in the processing of type I procollagen to collagen. The periodontotic-type EDS (type VIII) is distinguished by prominent periodontal changes. EDS IX, X, and XI were defined on the basis of preliminary biochemical and clinical data. EDS due to tenascin X deficiency has not been assigned a type; it is an autosomal recessive form of the syndrome similar to EDS II. The cardiac valvular form of EDS has similar features to EDS II but also involves severe changes to the aorta. The progeroid form of EDS displays features of both EDS and progeria. Because of overlapping signs and symptoms, many patients and families with some of the features of EDS cannot be assigned to any of the defined types.

Incidence

The overall incidence of EDS is about 1 in 5000 births, with a higher rate for blacks. Classical and hypermobile types of EDS are the most common. Patients with milder forms frequently do not seek medical attention.

Skin

Skin changes vary from thin and velvety to skin that is either dramatically hyperextensible ("rubber person" syndrome) or easily torn or scarred. Patients with classical EDS develop characteristic "cigarette-paper" scars. In vascular-type EDS, extensive scars and hyperpigmentation develop over bony prominences, and the skin may be so thin that subcutaneous blood vessels are visible. In the periodontotic type of EDS, the skin is more fragile than hyperextensible, and it heals with atrophic, pigmented scars. Easy bruisability occurs in several types of EDS.

Ligament and joint changes

Laxity and hypermobility of joints vary from mild to unreducible dislocations of hips and other large joints. In mild forms, patients learn to avoid dislocations by limiting physical activity. In more severe forms, surgical repair may be required. Some patients have progressive difficulty with age.

Other features

Mitral valve prolapse and hernias occur, particularly with type I. Pes planus and mild to moderate scoliosis are common. Extreme joint laxity and repeated dislocations may lead to degenerative arthritis. In the ocular-scoliotic type of EDS, the eye may rupture with minimal trauma, and kyphoscoliosis can cause respiratory impairment. Also, sclerae may be blue.

Molecular defects

Subsets of patients with different types of EDS have mutations in the structural genes for collagens (Table 363-3). These include mutations in the *COL1A1* gene in a few patients with moderately severe classical EDS (type I); mutations in *COL1A2* in rare patients with an aortic valvular form of EDS; mutations in two of the three

TABLE 363-3 Different Forms of Ehlers-Danlos Syndrome

Type	Typical Features	Inheritance	Gene Defect	Protein Defect
Classic (EDS I—severe and EDS II—mild)	Skin hyperextensibility and fragility, joint hypermobility, tissue fragility manifested by widened atrophic scarring	AD	*COL5A1* *COL5A2*	Collagen V
		AD AD, AR	*COL1A1* *COL1A2*	Proα1 (I) and proα2 (I) chains of procollagen I
Hypermobile (EDS III)	Joint hypermobility, moderate skin involvement, absence of tissue fragility	AD	*TNXB*	Tenascin X
Vascular (EDS IV)	Markedly reduced life span due to spontaneous rupture of internal organs such as arteries and intestines; skin is thin, translucent, and fragile, with extensive bruising; hypermobile minor joints; characteristic facial appearance	AD	*COL3A1*	Collagen III
X-linked EDS (EDS V)	Similar to classic type	X-linked recessive	Unknown	Unknown
Ocular-scoliotic EDS VI (EDS VIA and EDS VIB)	Features of classic EDS as well as severe muscular hypotonia after birth, progressive kyphoscoliosis, a Marfanoid habitus, osteopenia, occasionally rupture of the eye globe and great arteries	AR	*PLOD1*	Deficiency of procollagen-lysine 5-dioxygenase activity (EDS VIA)
			Unknown for EDS VIB	Unknown for EDS VIB
Arthrochalasic EDS VII (EDS VIIA and EDS VIIB)	Congenital bilateral hip dislocation, hypermobile joints, moderate skin involvement, osteopenia	AD	*COL1A1* *COL1A2*	Mutations that prevent cleavage of the N propeptides
Dermatosparactic EDS VII C	Redundant and fragile skin, prominent hernias, joint laxity, dysmorphic features	AR	*ADAMTS2*	Deficiency of procollagen I N-terminal proteinase
Periodontotic EDS VIII	Absorptive periodontosis with premature loss of permanent teeth, fragility of the skin, skin lesions	AD	Unknown	Unknown
EDS due to tenascin X deficiency	Similar to EDS II	AR	*TNXB*	Tenascin X
EDS, progeroid form		AR?	*B4GALT7*	Deficiency of galactosyltransferase 7 (defective synthesis of dermatan sulfate proteoglycans)

Abbreviations: AD, autosomal dominant; AR, autosomal recessive.

genes (*COL5A1* and *COL5A2*) for type V collagen, a minor collagen found in association with type I collagen, in about half the patients with classical EDS (types I and II); mutations in the *COL3A1* gene for type III collagen that is abundant in the aorta in patients with the frequently lethal vascular EDS (type IV).

Some of the type I collagen-related mutations alter processing of the protein or genes for the processing enzymes. Arthrochalasic EDS (type VII) is caused by mutations in amino acid sequence that make type I procollagen resistant to cleavage by procollagen N-proteinase or by mutations that decrease the activity of the enzyme. The persistence of the N propeptide causes the formation of collagen fibrils that are thin and irregular. Some of the patients have fragile bones and therefore a phenotype that overlaps with OI. The ocular-scoliotic type of EDS (type VI) is caused by homozygous or compound heterozygous mutations in the *PLOD 1* gene, which encodes procollagen-lysine 5-dioxygenase (lysyl hydroxylase 1), an enzyme required for formation of stable cross-links in collagen fibers.

Some patients with the hypermobile EDS (type III) and a few with mild EDS (type II) have mutations in the *TNXB* gene, which encodes tenascin X, another minor component of connective tissue that appears to regulate the assembly of collagen fibers. Mutations in proteoglycans have been found in a few patients. The progeroid form of EDS results from autosomal recessive mutations in *B4GALT7*, the gene for β-1,4-galactosyltransferase 7, a key enzyme in the addition of glycosaminoglycan chains to proteoglycans.

Diagnosis

The diagnosis is based on clinical criteria. Biochemical assays and gene analyses for known molecular defects in EDS are difficult and time-consuming, but tests are sometimes available from specialized laboratories. Correlations between genotype and phenotype are challenging, but the tests are particularly useful for the diagnosis of vascular-type IV EDS with its dire prognosis.

As with other heritable diseases of connective tissue, there is a large degree of variability among members of the same family carrying the same mutation. Some patients have increased fractures and are difficult to distinguish from OI. A few families with heritable aortic aneurysms have mutations in the gene for type III collagen without any evidence of EDS or OI.

TREATMENT Ehlers-Danlos Syndrome

Surgical repair and tightening of joint ligaments require careful evaluation of individual patients, as the ligaments frequently do not hold sutures. Patients with easy bruisability should be evaluated for bleeding disorders. Patients with type IV EDS and members of their families should be evaluated at regular intervals for early detection of aneurysms, but surgical repair may be difficult because of friable tissues. Also, women with type IV EDS should be counseled about the increased risk of uterine rupture, bleeding, and other complications of pregnancy.

CHONDRODYSPLASIAS

(See also Chap. 355) Chondrodysplasias (CDs), also referred to as skeletal dysplasias, are heritable skeletal disorders that are characterized by dwarfism and abnormal body proportions. The category also includes some individuals with normal stature and body proportions who have features such as ocular changes or cleft palate, which are common in more severe CDs. Many patients develop degenerative joint changes, and mild CD in adults may be difficult to differentiate from primary generalized osteoarthritis.

Classification

Over 200 distinct types and subtypes have been defined based on criteria such as "bringing death" (thanatophoric), causing "twisted" bones (diastrophic), affecting metaphyses (metaphyseal), affecting epiphyses (epiphyseal), affecting spine (spondylo-), and producing histologic changes such as an apparent increase in the fibrous material in the epiphyses (fibrochondrogenesis). Also, a number of eponyms are based on the first or most comprehensive case reports. Severe forms of the diseases produce dwarfism with gross distortions of most cartilaginous structures and of other structures including the eye. Mild forms are more difficult to classify. Among the features are cataracts, degeneration of the vitreous, and retinal detachment high forehead hypoplastic facies cleft palate short extremities and gross distortions of the epiphyses, metaphyses, and joint surfaces. Patients with Stickler syndrome (hereditary arthro-ophthalmopathy) have been classified into three types based on a combination of the ocular phenotype and mutated genes.

Incidence

The overall incidence of all forms of CD ranges from 1 per 2500 to 1 per 4000 births. Data on the frequency of individual CDs are incomplete, but the incidence of the Stickler syndrome is 1 in 10,000. Therefore, the disease is probably among the more common heritable disorders of connective tissue.

Molecular defects

Mutations in the *COL2A1* gene for the type II collagen of cartilage are found in a fraction of patients with both mild and severe CDs. For example, a mutation in the gene substituting a cysteine residue for an arginine was found in three unrelated families with spondyloepiphyseal dysplasia (SED) and precocious generalized osteoarthritis (OA). Mutations in the gene were also found in some lethal CDs characterized by gross deformities of bones and cartilage, such as those found in spondyloepiphyseal dysplasia congenita, spondyloepimetaphyseal dysplasia congenita, hypochondrogenesis/achondrogenesis type II, and Kniest syndrome. The highest incidence of *COL2A1* mutations, however, occurs in patients with the distinctive features of the Stickler syndrome, which is characterized by skeletal changes, orofacial abnormalities, and auditory abnormalities. Most of the mutations in *COL2A1* are premature stop codons that produce haploinsufficiency. In addition, some of the patients with the Stickler syndrome or a closely related syndrome have mutations in two genes specific for type XI collagen, which is an unusual heterotrimer formed from α chains encoded by the gene for type II collagen (*COL2A1*) and two distinctive genes for type XI collagen (*COL11A1* and *COL11A2*). Mutations in the *COL11A1* gene are also found in patients with Marshall syndrome, which is similar to classic Stickler syndrome but with more severe hearing loss and dysmorphic features, such as a flat or retracted midface with flat nasal bridge, short nose, anteverted nostrils, long philtrum, and large-appearing eyes.

CDs are also caused by mutations in the less abundant collagens found in cartilage. For example, patients with Schmid metaphyseal CD have mutations in the gene for type X collagen, a short, network-forming collagen found in the hypertrophic zone of endochondral cartilage. The syndrome is characterized by short stature, coxa vara, flaring metaphyses, and waddling gait. As with other collagen genes, the most common mutations are of two types: Nonsense mutations that lead to haploinsufficiency and structural mutations that compromise collagen assembly. In type X collagen all the structural mutations detected occur in the C-terminal NC1 domain that coordinates the formation of the trimers. This NC1 domain is functionally equivalent to the C propeptide of the fibrillar collagens. These mutations disturb the structure of the NC1 domain, leading to misfolding and initiation of cellular ER stress via the unfolded protein response (UPR). While the UPR evolved to allow cells to adjust their ER folding capacity to differing protein folding loads, it is deployed by cells when mutant misfolded proteins accumulate in the ER. Activation of the UPR attenuates protein translation and activates mutant protein degradation pathways such as ER-associated degradation. If these strategies do not sufficiently reduce the stress response, cell death may occur. In Schmid metaphyseal CD, mutant misfolded type X collagen induces the UPR, resulting in downstream consequences that contribute to the pathophysiology.

Some patients have mutations in genes for proteins that interact with collagens. Patients with pseudoachondroplasia, or autosomal dominant multiple epiphyseal dysplasia, have mutations in the gene for the cartilage oligomeric matrix protein (*COMP*), a protein that interacts with both collagens and proteoglycans in cartilage. However, some families with multiple epiphyseal dysplasia have a defect in one of the three genes for type IX collagen (*COL9A1*, *COL9A2*, and *COL9A3*) or in matrilin-3, another extracellular protein found in cartilage. With misfolding mutations in COMP and matrilin-3, the activation of the UPR has been described, providing further evidence that the UPR is a component of pathology of these conditions.

Some CDs are caused by mutations in genes that affect early development of cartilage and related structures. The most common form of short-limbed dwarfism, achondroplasia, is caused by mutations in the gene for a receptor for a fibroblastic growth factor (*FGFR3*). The mutations in the *FGFR3* gene causing achondroplasias are unusual in several respects. The same single-base mutation in the gene that converts glycine to arginine at position 380 in the *FGFR3* gene is present in over 90% of patients. Most patients harbor sporadic new mutations, and therefore this nucleotide change must be one of the most common recurring mutations in the human genome. The mutation causes unregulated signal transduction through the receptor and inappropriate development of cartilage. Mutations that alter other domains of *FGFR3* have been found in patients with the more severe disorders of hypochondroplasia and thanatophoric dysplasia and in a few families with a variant of craniosynostosis. However, most patients with craniosynostosis appear to have mutations in the related *FGFR2* gene. The similarities between the phenotypes produced by mutations in genes for FGF receptors and mutations in structural proteins of cartilage are probably explained by the observation that the activity of FGFs is regulated in part by binding of FGFs to proteins sequestered in the extracellular matrix. Therefore, the situation parallels the interactions between transforming growth factors (TGFs) and fibrillin in MFS (see below).

Rare mutations involve the proteoglycans of cartilage. Patients with an autosomal recessive form of multiple epiphyseal dysplasia have mutations in a gene encoding a sulfate transporter protein (*DTDST*) required for synthesis of chondroitin sulfates and proteoglycans.

Diagnosis

The diagnosis of CDs is made on the basis of the physical appearance, slit-lamp eye examinations, x-ray findings, histologic changes, and clinical course. Evaluation of patients by specialists in the field is usually required for a diagnosis. DNA tests for mutations in some of the genes are available from specialized laboratories. For Stickler syndrome, more precise diagnostic criteria have made it possible to identify type I variants with mutations in the *COL2A1* gene with a high degree of accuracy. It has been suggested that the type II variant with mutations in the *COL11A1* gene can be identified on the basis of a "beaded" vitreous phenotype, and the type III variant with mutations in the *COL11A2* gene can be identified on the basis of the characteristic systemic features without the ocular involvement. Prenatal diagnosis based on analysis of DNA obtained from chorionic villus or amniotic fluid is possible.

TREATMENT Chondrodysplasias

The treatment is symptomatic and is directed to secondary features such as degenerative arthritis. Many patients require joint replacement surgery and corrective surgery for cleft palate. The eyes should be monitored carefully for the development of cataracts and the need for laser therapy to prevent retinal detachment. Patients should be advised to avoid obesity and contact sports. Counseling for the psychological problems of short stature is critical, and support groups have formed in many countries.

■ MARFAN SYNDROME (MFS)

MFS includes features that primarily affect the skeleton, the cardiovascular system, and the eyes.

Classification

MFS was initially characterized by a triad of features: (1) skeletal changes that include long, thin extremities, frequently associated with loose joints; (2) reduced vision as the result of dislocations of the lenses (ectopia lentis); and (3) aortic aneurysms. An international panel has developed a series of "Ghent criteria" that are useful in classifying patients.

Incidence and inheritance

The incidence of MFS is among the highest of any heritable disorder: about 1 in 3000/5000 births in most racial and ethnic groups. The related syndromes are less common. Mutations are generally inherited as autosomal dominant traits, but about one-fourth of patients have sporadic new mutations.

Skeletal effects

Patients have long limbs and are usually tall compared to other members of the same family. The ratio of the upper segment (top of the head to the top of the pubic ramus) to the lower segment (top of the pubic ramus to the floor) is usually 2 SDs below mean for age, race, and sex. The fingers and hands are long and slender and have a spider-like appearance (arachnodactyly). Many patients have severe chest deformities, including depression (pectus excavatum), protrusion (pectus carinatum), or asymmetry. Scoliosis is frequent and usually accompanied by kyphosis. CT or MRI examinations of the lumbar sacral region frequently reveals enlargement of the neural canal, thinning of the pedicles and laminae, widening of the foramins, or anterior meningocele (dural ectasia). High-arched palate and high pedal arches or pes planus are common. A few patients have severe joint hypermobility similar to EDS.

Cardiovascular features

Cardiovascular abnormalities are the major source of morbidity and mortality (Chap. 248). Mitral valve prolapse develops early in life and progresses to mitral valve regurgitation of increasing severity in about one-quarter of patients. Dilation of the root of the aorta and the sinuses of Valsalva are characteristic and ominous features of the disease that can develop at any age. The rate of dilation is unpredictable, but it can lead to aortic regurgitation, dissection of the aorta, and rupture. Dilation is probably accelerated by physical and emotional stress, as well as by pregnancy. Patients with familial aortic aneurysms tend to develop aneurysms at the base of the abdominal aorta. The location of the aneurysms, however, is somewhat variable, and the high incidence of aortic aneurysms in the general population (1 in 100) makes the differential diagnosis difficult unless other features of MFS are clearly present.

Ocular features

Upward displacement of the lens is common. It is usually not progressive but may contribute to the formation of cataracts. The ocular globe is frequently elongated, and most patients are myopic but with adequate vision. Retinal detachment can occur.

Other features

Striae may occur over the shoulders and buttocks. A number of patients develop spontaneous pneumothorax. Inguinal and incisional hernias are common. Patients are typically thin with little subcutaneous fat, but adults may develop centripetal obesity.

Molecular defects

More than 90% of patients clinically classified as having MFS by the "Ghent criteria" have a mutation in the gene for fibrillin-1 (*FBN1*). Mutations in the same gene are found in a few patients who do not meet the Ghent criteria. Also, a few MFS patients without mutations in the *FBN1* gene have mutations in the gene for TGF-β receptor 2 (*TGFBR2*). In addition, mutations in either *TGFBR2* or *TGFBR1* are found in the related Loeys-Dietz syndrome (LDS), which is characterized by aortic aneurysms, cleft palate, and hypertelorism. Mutations in the *FBN2* gene, which is structurally similar to the *FBN1* gene, which, are found in patients with MFS-like syndrome of congenital contractual arachnodactyly (CCA).

Over 550 different mutations have been found in the *FBN1* gene, scattered throughout its 65 coding exons. Most are private mutations, but about 10% are recurrent new mutations that are largely located in CpG sequences known to be "hot spots." Most severe mutations are located in the central codons (24–32). About one-third of the mutations introduce premature termination codons, and about two-thirds are missense mutations that alter calcium-binding domains in the repetitive epidermal growth factor–like domains of the protein. Rarer mutations alter the processing of the protein. As in many genetic diseases, the severity of the phenotype cannot be predicted from the nature of the mutation.

The discovery that syndromes similar to MFS are caused by mutations in *TGFBR1* and *TGFBR2* refocused attention on structural similarity between fibrillin-1 and TGF-β binding proteins that sequester TGF-β in the extracellular matrix. As a result, some of the manifestations of MFS have been shown to arise from alterations in binding sites that modulate the activity of TGF-β during early development of the skeleton and other tissues.

Diagnosis

All patients with a suspected diagnosis of MFS should have a slit-lamp examination and an echocardiogram. Also, homocystinuria should be ruled out by amino acid analysis of plasma (Chap. 364). The diagnosis of MFS according to the international Ghent standards places emphasis on major criteria that include presence of at least four skeletal abnormalities: ectopia lentis; dilation of the ascending aorta with or without dissection; dural ectasia; and a blood relative who meets the same criteria, with or without a DNA diagnosis. A final diagnosis is based on a balanced assessment of the major criteria together with several minor criteria. The absence of ocular changes suggests LDS, and the presence of contractures with some of the signs of OI suggests CCA.

Diagnostic tests based on detection of protein defects in fibrillin-1 in cultured skin fibroblasts or DNA analyses of most of the gene are now available from several laboratories. The results are unlikely to alter the treatment or prognosis, but are helpful to inform the patients and families and to rapidly exclude the diagnosis in unaffected family members.

TREATMENT Marfan Syndrome

Propranolol or other β-adrenergic blocking agents are used to lower blood pressure and thereby delay or prevent aortic dilation. Surgical correction of the aorta, aortic valve, and mitral valve has been successful in many patients, but tissues are frequently friable. Patients should be advised of the risks of severe physical and emotional stress and of pregnancy.

The scoliosis tends to be progressive and should be treated by mechanical bracing and physical therapy if >20° or by surgery if it progresses to >45°. Dislocated lenses rarely require surgical removal, but patients should be followed closely for retinal detachment. The finding that MFS pathophysiology involves alterations in TGF-β signaling has raised the possibility of new therapeutic strategies. Attenuation of TGF-β signaling with agents such as angiotensin II receptor blockers (e.g., Losartan) appears promising based on studies in animal models and is undergoing clinical trials.

■ ELASTIN-RELATED DISEASES

Mutations in the elastin gene (*ELN*) have been found in patients with supravalvular aortic stenosis and cutis laxa.

■ EPIDERMOLYSIS BULLOSA (EB)

EB is of a group of similar disorders in which the skin and related epithelial tissues break and blister as the result of minor trauma.

Classification and incidence

Four types of EB are defined on the basis of the level at which blistering occurs: (1) EB simplex for blistering in the epidermis, (2) EB hemidesmosomal for fissures between keratinocytes and the basal lamina, (3) EB junctional for blistering in the dermal-epidermal junction, and (4) EB dystrophica for blistering in the dermis.

The incidence of EB in the United States is about 1 in 50,000.

Molecular defects

The distinctive anatomic features of skin have made it possible to relate the clinical features of subtypes of EB to mutations for specific components. Mutations in the genes for the major keratins of basal epithelial cells (keratins 14 and 15) are found in patients with the blistering skin of EB simplex. Patients with the related syndrome, epidermolytic ichthyosis, have mutations in keratin 1 and keratin 10. Mutations in a large number of genes for the complex structure of hemidesmosomes are found in EB hemidesmosomal. Hemidesmosomal mutations occur in genes for type XVII collagen, lamin 3, α6 integrin, α4 integrin, and plectin. Mutations in the genes for components of the dermal-epidermal junction are found in EB junctional and include: three lamin genes (*A3, B3,* and *C2*) and type XVII collagen. Mutations in the gene that codes for type VII collagen that forms long anchoring fibrils for the basement membrane are found in the severe syndrome of EB dystrophica.

Diagnosis and treatment

The diagnosis is based on skin that readily breaks and forms blisters. EB simplex and EB hemidesmosomal are generally milder than EB junctional or EB dystrophica. EB dystrophica variants usually cause large and prominent scars. Precise classification within subtypes usually requires electron microscopy. DNA diagnostic tests are also available. The treatment is symptomatic.

■ ALPORT SYNDROME (AS)

AS is an inherited disorder characterized by hematuria and several associated features. Four forms of the disease are now recognized: (1) classic AS, which is inherited as an X-linked disorder with hematuria, sensorineural deafness, and conical deformation of the anterior surface of the lens (lenticonus); (2) a subtype of the X-linked form associated with diffuse leiomyomatosis; (3) an autosomal recessive form; and (4) an autosomal dominant form. Both autosomal recessive and dominant forms can cause renal disease without deafness or lenticonus.

Incidence

The incidence of AS is about 1 in 10,000 births in the general population and as high as 1 in 5000 in some ethnic groups. About 80% of AS patients have the classical X-linked variant.

Molecular defects

Most patients have mutations in four of the six genes for the chains of type IV collagen (*COL4A3, COL4A4, COL4A5,* and *COL4A6*). The genes for the proteins are arranged in tandem pairs on different chromosomes in an unusual head-to-head orientation and with overlapping promoters; i.e., the *COL4A1* and *COL4A2* genes are head-to-head on chromosome 13q34, the *COL4A3* and *COL4A4* genes are on chromosome 2q35–37, and the *COL4A5* and *COL4A6* genes are on chromosome Xq22. The X-linked variants are caused by either mutations in the COL4A5 gene or by partial deletions of both of the adjacent *COL4A4* and *COL4A5* genes. The autosomal recessive variants are caused by mutations in either the *COL4A3* or *COL4A4* genes. The mutations responsible for the autosomal dominant variants are still unknown, but they have been mapped to the same locus as the *COL4A3* and *COL4A4* genes.

Diagnosis

The diagnosis of classic AS is based on X-linked inheritance of hematuria, sensorineural deafness, and lenticonus. The lenticonus together with hematuria is pathognomonic of classic AS. The sensorineural deafness is primarily in the high-tone range. It can frequently be detected only by an audiogram and is usually not progressive. Because of the X-linked transmission, women are generally underdiagnosed and are usually less severely affected than men. The hematuria usually progresses to nephritis and may cause renal failure in late adolescence in affected males and at older ages in some women. Renal transplantation is usually successful.

ACKNOWLEDGMENTS

The authors acknowledge the contributions of Helena Kuivaniemi, Gerard Tromp, Leena Ala-Kokko, and Malwina Czarny-Ratajcak to this chapter in previous editions of Harrison's.

FURTHER READINGS

BATEMAN JF et al: Genetic diseases of connective tissues: Cellular and extracellular effects of ECM mutations. Nat Rev Genet 10:173, 2009

BOILEAU C et al: Molecular genetics of Marfan syndrome. Curr Opin Cardiol 20:194, 2005

CABRAL WA et al: Prolyl 3-hydroxylase 1 deficiency causes a recessive metabolic bone disorder resembling lethal/severe osteogenesis imperfecta. Nat Genet 39:359, 2007

CALLEWAERT B et al: Ehlers-Danlos and Marfan syndrome. Best Pract Res Clin Rheumatol 22:1521, 2008

HEINEGARD D: Proteoglycans and more—from molecules to biology. Int J Exp Pathol 90:575, 2009

ISHIDA Y et al: Autophagic elimination of misfolded procollagen aggregates in the endoplasmic reticulum as a means of cell protection. Mol Cell Biol 284:12020, 2009

MARINI JC et al: Consortium for osteogenesis imperfecta mutations in the helical domain of type I collagen: Regions rich in lethal mutations align with collagen binding sites for integrins and proteoglycans. Hum Mutat 28:209, 2009

RAMIREZ F, DIETZ HC: Marfan's syndrome: From molecular pathogenesis to clinical treatment. Curr Opin Genet Dev 17:252, 2007

——— SAKAI LY: Biogenesis and function of fibrillin assemblies. Cell Tissue Res 339:71, 2010

CHAPTER 364

Inherited Disorders of Amino Acid Metabolism in Adults

Nicola Longo

Amino acids are not only the building blocks of proteins but also serve as neurotransmitters (glycine, glutamate, γ-aminobutyric acid) or as precursors of hormones, coenzymes, pigments, purines, or pyrimidines. Eight amino acids, referred to as *essential*, cannot be synthesized by humans and must be obtained from dietary sources. The others are formed endogenously. Each amino acid has a unique degradative pathway by which its nitrogen and carbon components are used for the synthesis of other amino acids, carbohydrates, and lipids. Disorders of amino acid metabolism and transport (Chap. 365) are individually rare—the incidences range from 1 in 10,000 for cystinuria or phenylketonuria to 1 in 200,000 for homocystinuria or alkaptonuria—but collectively they affect perhaps 1 in 1,000 newborns. Almost all are transmitted as autosomal recessive traits.

The features of inherited disorders of amino acid catabolism are summarized in Table 364-1. In general, these disorders are named for the compound that accumulates to highest concentration in blood (*-emias*) or urine (*-urias*). For many conditions (often called *aminoacidopathies*), the parent amino acid is found in excess; for others, generally referred to as *organic acidemias*, products in the catabolic pathway accumulate. Which compound(s) accumulates depends on the site of the enzymatic block, the reversibility of the reactions proximal to the lesion, and the availability of alternative pathways of metabolic "runoff." Biochemical and genetic heterogeneity are common. Five distinct forms of hyperphenylalaninemia, seven forms of homocystinuria, and seven types of methylmalonic acidemia are recognized. Such heterogeneity reflects the presence of an even larger array of molecular defects.

The manifestations of these conditions differ widely (Table 364-1). Some, such as sarcosinemia, produce no clinical consequences. At the other extreme, complete deficiency of ornithine transcarbamylase is lethal in the untreated neonate. Central nervous system (CNS) dysfunction, in the form of developmental retardation, seizures, alterations in sensorium, or behavioral disturbances, is present in more than half the disorders. Protein-induced vomiting, neurologic dysfunction, and hyperammonemia occur in many disorders of urea cycle intermediates. Metabolic ketoacidosis, often accompanied by hyperammonemia, is a frequent presenting finding in disorders of branched-chain amino acid metabolism. Some disorders produce focal tissue or organ involvement such as liver disease, renal failure, cutaneous abnormalities, or ocular lesions.

The analysis of plasma amino acids (by ion-exchange chromatography), urine organic acids (by gas chromatography/mass spectrometry), and plasma acylcarnitines (by tandem mass spectrometry) is commonly used to diagnose and monitor most of these disorders. The diagnosis is confirmed by enzyme assay on cells or tissues from the patients or by DNA testing. The clinical manifestations in many of these conditions can be prevented or mitigated if a diagnosis is achieved early and appropriate treatment (e.g., dietary protein or amino acid restriction or vitamin supplementation) is instituted promptly. For this reason, newborn screening programs seek to identify several of these disorders. Infants with a positive screening test need additional metabolic testing (usually suggested by the newborn screening program) to confirm or exclude the diagnosis. Confirmed cases should be referred to a metabolic center for initiation of therapy. The parents need to be counseled about the recurrence risk of the disease in future pregnancies. In some cases, parents need testing to exclude metabolic alterations seen in carriers for some of these disorders (such as some forms of homocystinuria) or because they might have a disorder themselves (such as methylcrotonyl CoA carboxylase deficiency, glutaric acidemia type 1, primary carnitine deficiency, or fatty acid oxidation defects). Some metabolic disorders can remain asymptomatic until adult age, presenting only when fasting or severe stress require full activity of affected metabolic pathways to provide energy.

Selected disorders that illustrate the principles, properties, and problems presented by the disorders of amino acid metabolism are discussed in this chapter.

TABLE 364-1 Inherited Disorders of Amino Acid Metabolism

Amino acid(s)	Condition	Enzyme Defect	Clinical Findings	Inheritance
Phenylalanine	Phenylketonuria	Phenylalanine hydroxylase	Mental retardation, microcephaly, hypopigmented skin and hairs, eczema, "mousy" odor	AR
	DHPR deficiency hyperphenylalaninemia	Dihydropteridine reductase	Mental retardation, hypotonia, spasticity, myoclonus	AR
	PTS deficiency hyperphenylalaninemia	6-Pyruvoyl-tetrahydropterin synthase	Dystonia, neurologic deterioration, seizures, mental retardation	AR
	GCH1 deficiency hyperphenylalaninemia	GTP cyclohydrolase I	Mental retardation, seizures, dystonia, temperature instability	AR
	Carbinolamine dehydratase deficiency	Pterin-4α-carbinolamine dehydratase	Transient hyperphenylalaninemia (benign)	AR
Tyrosine	Tyrosinemia type I (hepatorenal)	Fumarylacetoacetate hydrolase	Liver failure, cirrhosis, rickets, failure to thrive, peripheral neuropathy, "boiled cabbage" odor	AR
	Tyrosinemia type II (oculocutaneous)	Tyrosine transaminase	Palmoplantar keratosis, painful corneal erosions with photophobia, mental retardation (?)	AR
	Tyrosinemia type III	4-Hydroxyphenylpyruvate dioxygenase	Hypertyrosinemia with normal liver function, occasional mental delay	AR
	Hawkinsinuria	4-Hydroxyphenylpyruvate dioxygenase	Transient failure to thrive, metabolic acidosis in infancy	AD
	Alkaptonuria	Homogentisic acid oxidase	Ochronosis, arthritis, cardiac valve involvement, coronary artery calcification	AR
	Albinism (oculocutaneous)	Tyrosinase	Hypopigmentation of hair, skin, and optic fundus; visual loss; photophobia	AR
	Albinism (ocular)	Different enzymes or transporters	Hypopigmentation of optic fundus, visual loss	AR, XL
	DOPA-responsive dystonia	Tyrosine hydroxylase	Rigidity, truncal hypotonia, tremor, mental retardation	AR
GABA	4-Hydroxybutyric aciduria	Succinic semialdehyde dehydrogenase	Seizures, mental retardation, ataxia	AR
Tryptophan	Kynurenic aciduria	Kynurenine-3-monooxygenase	Niacin deficiency, pellagra, colitis	AR
	Hydroxykynureninuria (xanthurenic aciduria)	Kynureninase	Niacin deficiency, mental retardation, spasticity	AR
Histidine	Histidinemia	Histidine-ammonia lyase	Benign	AR
	Urocanic aciduria	Urocanase	Benign	AR
	Formiminoglutamic aciduria	Formiminotransferase	Occasional mental retardation	AR
Glycine	Glycine encephalopathy	Glycine cleavage (4 enzymes)	Infantile seizures, lethargy, apnea, profound mental retardation	AR
	Sarcosinemia	Sarcosine dehydrogenase	Benign	AR
	Hyperoxaluria type I	Alanine:glyoxylate aminotransferase	Calcium oxalate nephrolithiasis, renal failure	AR
	Hyperoxaluria type II	D-Glyceric acid dehydrogenase/glyoxylate reductase	Calcium oxalate nephrolithiasis, renal failure	AR
Serine	Phosphoglycerate dehydrogenase deficiency	Phosphoglycerate dehydrogenase	Seizures, microcephaly, mental retardation	AR
Proline	Hyperprolinemia type I	Proline oxidase	Benign	AR
	Hyperprolinemia type II	Δ^1-Pyrroline-5-carboxylate dehydrogenase	Febrile seizures, mental retardation	AR
	Hyperhydroxyprolinemia	Hydroxyproline oxidase	Benign	AR
	Prolidase deficiency	Prolidase	Mild mental retardation, chronic dermatitis	AR

(continued)

TABLE 364-1 Inherited Disorders of Amino Acid Metabolism (*Continued*)

Amino acid(s)	Condition	Enzyme Defect	Clinical Findings	Inheritance
Methionine	Hypermethioninemia	Methionine adenosyltransferase	Usually benign	AR
	S-Adenosylhomocysteine hydrolase deficiency	S-Adenosylhomocysteine hydrolase	Hypotonia, mental retardation, absent tendon reflexes, delayed myelination	AR
	Glycine N-methyltransferase deficiency	Glycine N-methyltransferase	Elevated liver transaminases	AR
Homocystine	Homocystinuria	Cystathionine β-synthase	Lens dislocation, thrombotic vascular disease, mental retardation, osteoporosis	AR
	Homocystinuria	5,10-Methylenetetrahydrofolate reductase	Mental retardation, gait and psychiatric abnormalities, recurrent strokes	AR
	Homocystinuria	Methionine synthase (cblE, -G)	Mental retardation, hypotonia, seizures, megaloblastic anemia	AR
	Homocystinuria and methylmalonic acidemia	Vitamin B_{12} lysosomal efflux and metabolism (cbl C, -D, -F)	Mental retardation, lethargy, failure to thrive, hypotonia, seizures, megaloblastic anemia	AR
Cystathionine	Cystathioninuria	β-Cystathionase	Benign	AR
Cystine	Cystinosis	Cystinosin CTNS (lysosomal efflux)	Renal Fanconi syndrome, rickets, photophobia, hypotonia, renal failure	AR
S-Sulfo-L-cysteine	Sulfocysteinuria	Sulfate oxidase or molybdenum cofactor deficiency	Seizures, mental retardation, dislocated lenses	AR
Lysine	Hyperlysinemia, saccharopinuria	α-Aminoadipic semialdehyde synthase	Benign	AR
	Pyridoxine-dependent seizures	L-Δ^1-Piperideine-6-carboxilate dehydrogenase	Seizures	AR
Lysine, tryptophan	α-Ketoadipic acidemia	α-Ketoadipic acid dehydrogenase	Benign	?
	Glutaric acidemia type I	Glutaryl-CoA dehydrogenase	Severe dystonia and athetosis, mild mental retardation	AR
	Glutaric acidemia type II	Electron transfer flavoprotein (ETF) or ETF:ubiquinone oxidoreductase	Hypoglycemia, metabolic acidosis, "sweaty feet" odor, hypotonia, cardiomyopathy, exercise-induced myopathy	AR
Ornithine	Gyrate atrophy of the choroid and retina	Ornithine-δ-aminotransferase	Myopia, night blindness, loss of peripheral vision, cataracts, chorioretinal degeneration	AR
Urea cycle	Carbamoylphosphate synthase-1 deficiency	Carbamoylphosphate synthase-1	Lethargy progressing to coma, protein aversion, mental retardation, hyperammonemia	AR
	N-Acetylglutamate synthase deficiency	*N*-Acetylglutamate synthase	Lethargy progressing to coma, protein aversion, mental retardation, hyperammonemia	AR
	Ornithine transcarbamylase deficiency	Ornithine transcarbamylase	Lethargy progressing to coma, protein aversion, mental retardation, hyperammonemia	XL
	Citrullinemia type I	Argininosuccinate synthase	Lethargy progressing to coma, protein aversion, mental retardation, hyperammonemia	AR
	Argininosuccinic acidemia	Argininosuccinate lyase	Lethargy progressing to coma, protein aversion, mental retardation, hyperammonemia, trichorrhexis nodosa	AR
	Arginase deficiency	Arginase	Spastic tetraparesis, mental retardation, mild hyperammonemia	AR
	Hyperornithinemia, hyperammonemia, homocitrullinuria	Mitochondrial ornithine carrier ORNT1	Vomiting, lethargy, failure to thrive, mental retardation, episodic confusion, hyperammonemia, protein intolerance	AR
	Citrullinemia type 2	Mitochondrial aspartate/glutamate carrier CTLN2	Neonatal intrahepatic cholestasis, adult presentation with sudden behavioral changes and stupor, coma, hyperammonemia	AR

(continued)

TABLE 364-1 Inherited Disorders of Amino Acid Metabolism (*Continued*)

Amino acid(s)	Condition	Enzyme Defect	Clinical Findings	Inheritance
Proline, ornithine, arginine	Δ^1-pyrroline-5-carboxylate synthase deficiency	Δ^1-pyrroline-5-carboxylate synthase	Hypotonia, seizures, hyperammonemia, neurodegeneration	AR
Glutamine	Glutamine synthase deficiency	Glutamine synthase	Brain malformations, pachygyria, seizures, hypotonia, dysmorphic features	AR
Valine	Isobutyryl-CoA dehydrogenase deficiency	Isobutyryl-CoA dehydrogenase	Failure to thrive, anemia, and dilated cardiomyopathy(?)	AR
Valine, leucine, isoleucine	Maple syrup urine disease (defective E1α, E1β, E2, E3)	Branched chain ketoacid dehydrogenase	Lethargy, vomiting, encephalopathy, seizures, mental retardation, "maple syrup" odor, protein intolerance	AR
Leucine	Isovaleric acidemia	Isovaleryl-CoA dehydrogenase	Acidosis, ketosis, vomiting, coma, hyperammonemia, "sweaty feet" odor, protein intolerance	AR
	3-Methylcrotonyl glycinuria	3-Methylcrotonyl-CoA carboxylase	Stress-induced metabolic acidosis, hypotonia, hypoglycemia, "cat's urine" odor	AR
	3-Methylglutaconic aciduria type I	3-Methylglutaconyl-CoA hydratase deficiency	Stress-induced acidosis, leukoencephalopathy	AR
	3-Hydroxy-3-methylglutaric aciduria	3-Hydroxy-3-methylglutaryl-CoA lyase	Stress-induced hypoketotic hypoglycemia and acidosis, encephalopathy, hyperammonemia	AR
Isoleucine	2-Methylbutyryl-glycinuria	2-Methylbutyryl-CoA dehydrogenase	Fasting-induced metabolic acidosis/ hypoglycemia	AR
	2-Methyl-3-hydroxybutyryl-CoA dehydrogenase deficiency	2-Methyl-3-hydroxybutyryl-CoA dehydrogenase	Developmental regression, seizures, and rigidity sometimes triggered by illnesses	XL
	3-Oxothiolase deficiency	3-Oxothiolase	Fasting-induced acidosis and ketosis, vomiting, lethargy	AR
Valine, isoleucine, methionine, threonine	Propionic acidemia (pccA,-B,-C)	Propionyl-CoA carboxylase	Metabolic ketoacidosis, hyperammonemia, hypotonia, lethargy, coma, protein intolerance, mental retardation, hyperglycinemia	AR
	Multiple carboxylase/ biotinidase deficiency	Holocarboxylase synthase or biotinidase	Metabolic ketoacidosis, diffuse rash, alopecia, seizures, mental retardation	AR
	Methylmalonic acidemia (mutase, racemase, CblA, -B, -D)	Methylmalonyl-CoA mutase/ racemase or cobalamin reductase/adenosyltransferase	Metabolic ketoacidosis, hyperammonemia, hypertonia, lethargy, coma, protein intolerance, mental retardation, hyperglycinemia	AR

Abbreviations: AD, autosomal dominant; AR, autosomal recessive; Cbl, cobalamin; DHPR, dihydropteridine reductase; DOPA, dihydroxyphenylalanine; GABA, g-aminobutyric acid; GTP, guanosine 5′-triphosphate; XL, X-linked.

THE HYPERPHENYLALANINEMIAS

The hyperphenylalaninemias (Table 364-1) result from impaired conversion of phenylalanine to tyrosine. The most common and clinically important is *phenylketonuria* (frequency 1:10,000), which is an autosomal recessive disorder characterized by an increased concentration of phenylalanine and its by-products in body fluids and by severe mental retardation if untreated in infancy. It results from reduced activity of phenylalanine hydroxylase (PAH deficiency phenylketonuria). The accumulation of phenylalanine inhibits the transport of other amino acids required for protein or neurotransmitter synthesis, reduces synthesis and increases degradation of myelin, and leads to inadequate formation of norepinephrine and serotonin. Phenylalanine is a competitive inhibitor of tyrosinase, a key enzyme in the pathway of melanin synthesis, and accounts for the hypopigmentation of hair and skin. Untreated children with classic phenylketonuria are normal at birth but fail to attain early developmental milestones, develop microcephaly, and demonstrate progressive impairment of cerebral function. Hyperactivity, seizures, and severe mental retardation are major clinical problems later in life. Electroencephalographic abnormalities; "mousy" odor of skin, hair, and urine (due to phenylacetate accumulation); and a tendency to hypopigmentation and eczema complete the devastating clinical picture. In contrast, affected children who are detected and treated at birth show none of these abnormalities.

TREATMENT Phenylketonuria

To prevent mental retardation, diagnosis and initiation of dietary treatment of classic phenylketonuria must occur before the child is 3 weeks of age. For this reason, most newborns in North America, Australia, and Europe are screened by determinations of blood phenylalanine levels. Abnormal values are confirmed using quantitative analysis of plasma amino acids. Dietary phenylalanine restriction is usually instituted if blood phenylalanine levels are >300 μmol/L (5 mg/dL). Treatment consists of a special diet low in phenylalanine and supplemented with tyrosine, since tyrosine becomes an essential amino acid in phenylalanine hydroxylase deficiency. With therapy, plasma phenylalanine concentrations should be maintained between 60 and 360 μmol/L (1 and 6 mg/dL). Dietary restriction should be continued and monitored indefinitely. About one-third of all patients with phenylketonuria and the majority of those with milder forms (phenylalanine <1200 μmol/L at presentation) show increased tolerance to dietary proteins and improved metabolic control when treated with tetrahydrobiopterin (5–20 mg/kg per day), an essential cofactor of phenylalanine hydroxylase. This drug should be used in addition to dietary therapy.

Women with phenylketonuria, who have been treated since infancy, reach adulthood and can become pregnant. If maternal phenylalanine levels are not strictly controlled before and during pregnancy, their offspring are at increased risk for congenital defects and microcephaly (*maternal phenylketonuria*). After birth, these children have severe mental and growth retardation. Pregnancy risks can be minimized by continuing lifelong phenylalanine-restricted diets and assuring strict phenylalanine restriction 2 months prior to conception and throughout gestation.

THE HOMOCYSTINURIAS (HYPERHOMOCYSTEINEMIAS)

The homocystinurias are seven biochemically and clinically distinct disorders (Table 364-1) characterized by increased concentration of the sulfur-containing amino acid homocystine in blood and urine.

Classic homocystinuria, the most common (frequency 1:200,000), results from reduced activity of cystathionine β-synthase (Fig. 364-1), the pyridoxal phosphate–dependent enzyme that condenses homocysteine with serine to form cystathionine. Most patients present between 3 and 5 years of age with dislocated optic lenses and mental retardation (in about half of cases). Some patients develop a marfanoid habitus and radiologic evidence of osteoporosis.

Life-threatening vascular complications (affecting coronary, renal, and cerebral arteries) can occur during the first decade of life and are the major cause of morbidity and mortality. Classic homocystinuria can be diagnosed with analysis of plasma amino acids, showing elevated methionine and presence of free homocystine. Total plasma homocysteine is also extremely elevated (usually >100 μ*M*). Treatment consists of a special diet restricted in protein and methionine and supplemented with cystine. In approximately half of patients, oral pyridoxine (25–500 mg/d) produces a decrease in plasma methionine and homocystine concentration in body fluids. Folate and vitamin B_{12} deficiency should be prevented by adequate supplementation. Betaine is also effective in reducing homocystine levels.

The other forms of homocystinuria are the result of impaired remethylation of homocysteine to methionine. This can be caused by defective methionine synthase or reduced availability of two essential cofactors, 5-methyltetrahydrofolate and methylcobalamin (methyl-vitamin B_{12}).

Hyperhomocysteinemia refers to increased total plasma concentration of homocysteine with or without an increase in free homocystine (disulfide form). Hyperhomocysteinemia, in the absence of significant homocystinuria, is found in some heterozygotes for the genetic defects noted above or in homozygotes for milder variants. Changes of homocysteine levels are also observed with increasing age; with smoking; in postmenopausal women; in patients with renal failure, hypothyroidism, leukemias, inflammatory bowel disease, or psoriasis; and during therapy with drugs such as methotrexate, nitrous oxide, isoniazid, and some antiepileptic agents. Homocysteine acts as an atherogenic and thrombophilic agent. An increase in total plasma homocysteine represents an independent risk factor for coronary, cerebrovascular, and peripheral arterial disease as well as for deep-vein thrombosis (Chap. 241). Homocysteine is synergistic with hypertension and smoking, and it is additive with other risk factors that predispose to peripheral

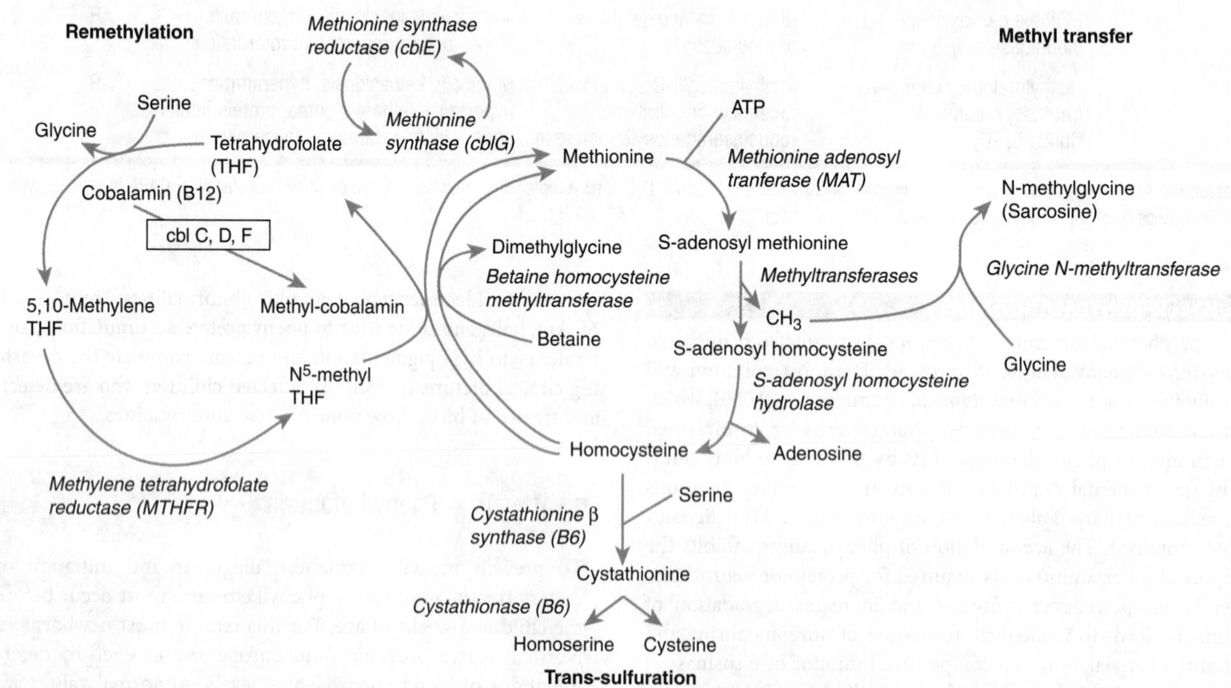

Figure 364-1 Pathways, enzymes, and coenzymes involved in the homocystinurias. Methionine transfers a methyl group during its conversion to homocysteine. Defects in methyl transfer or in the subsequent metabolism of homocysteine by the pyridoxal phosphate (vitamin B_6)-dependent cystathionine β-synthase increase plasma methionine levels. Homocysteine is transformed into methionine via remethylation. This occurs through methionine synthase, a reaction requiring methylcobalamin and folic acid. Deficiencies in these enzymes or lack of cofactors is associated with decreased or normal methionine levels. In an alternative pathway, homocysteine can be remethylated by betaine:homocysteine methyl transferase.

arterial disease. In addition, hyperhomocysteinemia and folate and vitamin B_{12} deficiency have been associated with an increased risk of neural tube defects in pregnant women. Vitamin supplements are effective in reducing plasma homocysteine levels in these cases, although the risk reduction for cardiovascular disease and stroke has been inconsistent among different studies.

ALKAPTONURIA

Alkaptonuria is a rare (frequency 1:200,000) disorder of tyrosine catabolism in which deficiency of homogentisate 1,2-dioxygenase (also known as *homogentisic acid oxidase*) leads to excretion of large amounts of homogentisic acid in urine and accumulation of oxidized homogentisic acid pigment in connective tissues (*ochronosis*). Alkaptonuria may go unrecognized until middle life, when degenerative joint disease develops. Prior to this time, about half of patients might be diagnosed for the presence of dark urine. Foci of gray-brown scleral pigment and generalized darkening of the concha, anthelix, and, finally, helix of the ear usually develop after age 30. Low back pain usually starts between 30 and 40 years of age. *Ochronotic arthritis* is heralded by pain, stiffness, and some limitation of motion of the hips, knees, and shoulders. Acute arthritis may resemble rheumatoid arthritis, but small joints are usually spared. Pigmentation of heart valves, larynx, tympanic membranes, and skin occurs, and occasional patients develop pigmented renal or prostatic calculi. Degenerative cardiovascular disease is increased in older patients. The diagnosis should be suspected in a patient whose urine darkens to blackness. Homogentisic acid in urine is identified by urine organic acid analysis or by a specific colorimetric test. Ochronotic arthritis is treated symptomatically (Chap. 332). Nitisinone [2-(2-nitro-4-trifluoromethylbenzoyl)-1,3-cyclohexanedione], a drug used in tyrosinemia type I, reduces urinary excretion of homogentisic acid, but it is still unclear whether it can prevent the long-term complications of alkaptonuria.

UREA CYCLE DEFECTS

Excess ammonia generated from protein nitrogen is removed by the urea cycle, a process mediated by several enzymes and transporters (Table 364-1). Complete absence of any of these enzymes usually causes severe hyperammonemia in newborns, while milder variants can be seen in adults. The accumulation of ammonia and glutamine leads to brain edema and direct neuronal toxicity. Deficiencies in urea cycle enzymes are individually rare, but as a group they affect about 1:25,000 individuals. They are all transmitted as autosomal recessive traits, with the exception of ornithine transcarbamylase deficiency, which is X-linked. Hepatocytes of females with ornithine transcarbamylase deficiency express either the normal or the mutant allele due to random X-inactivation and may be unable to remove excess ammonia if mutant cells are predominant.

Infants with classic urea cycle defects present at 1–4 days of life with refusal to eat and lethargy progressing to coma and death. Milder enzyme deficiencies present with protein avoidance, recurrent vomiting, migraine, mood swings, chronic fatigue, irritability, and disorientation that can progress to coma. Acute liver failure can also be observed in adults. Females with ornithine transcarbamylase deficiency or milder forms of other urea cycle defects can present at time of childbirth due to the combination of involuntary fasting and stress that favor catabolism. The diagnosis requires measurement of plasma ammonia, plasma amino acids, and urine orotic acid, useful for differentiating ornithine transcarbamylase deficiency from carbamyl phosphate synthase-1 and *N*-acetylglutamate synthase deficiency. Hyperammonemia can also be caused by liver disease from any cause and several organic acidemias and fatty acid oxidation defects (the latter two excluded by the analysis of urine organic acids and plasma acylcarnitine profile).

TREATMENT Urea Cycle Defects

Therapy is aimed at stopping catabolism and ammonia production by providing adequate calories (as intravenous glucose and lipids in the comatose patient) and, if needed, insulin. Excess nitrogen is removed by intravenous phenylacetate and benzoate (0.25 g/kg for the priming dose and subsequently as an infusion over 24 h) that conjugate with glutamine and glycine, respectively, to form phenylacetylglutamine and hippuric acid, water-soluble molecules efficiently excreted in urine. Arginine (200 mg/kg/d) becomes an essential amino acid (except in arginase deficiency) and should be provided intravenously to resume protein synthesis. Standard therapy of brain edema with mannitol and hypertonic saline should also be instituted in the comatose patient. If these measures fail to reduce ammonia, hemodialysis should be initiated promptly. Chronic therapy consists of a protein-restricted diet, phenylbutyrate (a more palatable precursor of phenylacetate), arginine or citrulline supplements, depending on the specific diagnosis. Liver transplantation should be considered in patients with severe urea cycle defects that are difficult to control medically.

Hyperammonemia due to a functional deficiency of glutamine synthase can occur in patients receiving chemotherapy for different malignancies or undergoing solid organ transplants. Several of these patients have been successfully rescued from hyperammonemia using the protocol described above for urea cycle defects.

FURTHER READINGS

Burgard P et al: Phenylketonuria, in *Pediatric Endocrinology and Inborn Errors of Metabolism*, K Sarafoglou et al (eds). New York, McGraw-Hill, 2009, pp 163–168

Maron BA, Loscalzo J: The treatment of hyperhomocysteinemia. Annu Rev Med 60:394, 2009

Mudd SH: Hypermethioninemias of genetic and non-genetic origin: A review. Am J Med Genet C Semin Med Genet 157:3, 2011

Salek J et al: Recurrent liver failure in a 25-year-old female. Liver Transpl 16:1049, 2010

Trefz FK et al: Efficacy of sapropterin dihydrochloride in increasing phenylalanine tolerance in children with phenylketonuria: A phase III, randomized, double-blind, placebo-controlled study. J Pediatr 154:700, 2009.

Vilboux T et al: Mutation spectrum of homogentisic acid oxidase (HGD) in alkaptonuria. Hum Mutat 30:1611, 2009

CHAPTER 365
Inherited Defects of Membrane Transport

Nicola Longo

Specific membrane transporters mediate the passage of a wide variety of substances across cellular membranes. Classes of substrates include amino acids, sugars, cations, anions, vitamins, and water. The number of inherited disorders of membrane transport continues to increase with the identification of new transporters and the clarification of the molecular basis of diseases with previously unknown pathophysiology. The first transport disorders identified affected the gut or the kidney, but transport processes are essential for the normal function of every organ. Mutations in transporter molecules cause disorders of the heart, muscle, brain, and endocrine and sensory organs (Table 365-1). Inherited defects impairing the transport of selected amino acids that can present in adults are discussed here as examples of the abnormalities encountered; others are considered elsewhere in this text.

CYSTINURIA

Cystinuria (frequency of 1 in 10,000 to 1 in 15,000) is an autosomal recessive disorder caused by defective transporters in the apical brush border of proximal renal tubule and small intestinal cells. It is characterized by impaired reabsorption and excessive urinary excretion of the dibasic amino acids lysine, arginine, ornithine, and cystine. Because cystine is poorly soluble, its excess excretion predisposes to the formation of renal, ureteral, and bladder stones. Such stones are responsible for the signs and symptoms of the disorder.

There are two variants of cystinuria. Homozygotes for both variants have high urinary excretion of cystine, lysine, arginine, and ornithine. Type I heterozygotes usually have normal urinary amino acids, whereas most non-type I (formerly type II and type III) heterozygotes have moderately increased urinary excretion of each of the four amino acids. The gene for type I cystinuria (*SLC3A1*, chromosome 2p16.3) encodes a membrane glycoprotein. Non-type I cystinuria is caused by mutations in *SLC7A9* (chromosome 19q13) that encodes the $b^{0,+}$ amino acid transporter. The glycoprotein encoded by *SLC3A1* favors the correct processing of the $b^{0,+}$ membrane transporter, and explains why mutations in two different genes cause a similar disease.

Cystine stones account for 1–2% of all urinary tract calculi but are the most common cause of stones in children. Cystinuria homozygotes regularly excrete 2400–7200 μmol (600–1800 mg) of cystine daily. Since the maximum solubility of cystine in the physiologic urinary pH range of 4.5–7.0 is about 1200 μmol/L (300 mg/L), cystine needs to be diluted to 2.5–7 L of water to prevent crystalluria. Stone formation usually manifests in the second or third decade but may occur in the first year of life. Symptoms and signs are those typical of urolithiasis: hematuria, flank pain, renal colic, obstructive uropathy, and infection (Chap. 287). Recurrent urolithiasis may lead to progressive renal insufficiency.

Cystinuria is suspected after observing typical hexagonal crystals in the sediment of acidified, concentrated, chilled urine or after performing a urinary nitroprusside test. Quantitative urine amino acid analysis confirms the diagnosis of cystinuria by showing selective over excretion of cystine, lysine, arginine, and ornithine. Quantitative measurements are important for differentiating heterozygotes from homozygotes and for following free cystine excretion during therapy.

Management is aimed at preventing cystine crystal formation by increasing urinary volume and by maintaining an alkaline urine pH. Fluid ingestion in excess of 4 L/d is essential, and 5–7 L/d is optimal. Urinary cystine concentration should be <1000 μmol/L (250 mg/L). The daily fluid ingestion necessary to maintain this dilution of excreted cystine should be spaced over 24 h, with one-third of the total volume ingested between bedtime and 3 A.M. Cystine solubility rises sharply above pH 7.5, and urinary alkalinization (with potassium citrate) can be therapeutic. Penicillamine (1–3 g/d) and tiopronin (α-mercaptopropionylglycine, 800–1200 mg/d in four divided doses) undergo sulfhydryl-disulfide exchange with cystine to form mixed disulfides. Since these disulfides are much more soluble than cystine, pharmacologic therapy can prevent and promote dissolution of calculi. Penicillamine can have significant side effects and should be reserved for patients who fail to respond to hydration alone or who are in a high-risk category (one remaining kidney, renal insufficiency). The dose of penicillamine should be increased gradually to limit side-effects. When medical management fails, shock wave lithotripsy, ureteroscopy, and percutaneous nephrolithotomy are effective for most stones. Open urologic surgery is considered for complex staghorn stones or when the patient has concomitant renal or ureteral abnormalities. Occasional patients progress to renal failure and require kidney transplantation.

DIBASIC AMINOACIDURIA

This disorder is characterized by a defect in renal tubular reabsorption of the three dibasic amino acids lysine, arginine, and ornithine but *not* cystine. There are two variants, transmitted as autosomal recessive traits. In the common form of dibasic aminoaciduria (type II), also known as *lysinuric protein intolerance*, homozygotes show defective intestinal transport of dibasic amino acids as well as exaggerated renal losses. It is most common in Finland (1 in 60,000), Southern Italy, and Japan, but is rare elsewhere. The transport defect affects basolateral rather than luminal membrane transport and is associated with impairment of the urea cycle. The defective gene (*SLC7A7*, chromosome 14q11.2) encodes the membrane transporter, y^+LAT, which associates with the cell-surface glycoprotein 4F2 heavy chain to form the complete sodium-independent transporter y^+L.

Manifestations are related to the losses of ornithine, arginine, and lysine. Affected patients can present in childhood with hepatosplenomegaly, protein intolerance, and episodic ammonia intoxication. Older patients may present with severe osteoporosis, impairment of kidney function, or interstitial changes in the lungs. Plasma concentrations of lysine, arginine, and ornithine can be reduced, whereas urinary excretion of lysine and orotic acid are increased. Hyperammonemia may develop after the ingestion of protein loads or with infections, probably because of insufficient amounts of arginine and ornithine to maintain proper function of the urea cycle. The clinical features have been attributed to the hyperammonemia, to insufficient amounts of lysine to support protein synthesis during growth, and to decreased production of nitric oxide caused by arginine deficiency.

Therapy consists of dietary protein restriction and supplementation of citrulline (2–8 g/d), a neutral amino acid that fuels the urea cycle when metabolized to arginine and ornithine. Pulmonary disease responds to glucocorticoids or bronchoalveolar lavage in some patients. Women with lysinuric protein intolerance, who become pregnant, have an increased risk of anemia, toxemia, and

TABLE 365-1 Genetic Disorders of Membrane Transport (Selected Examples)

Class of Substance and Disorder	Individual Substrates	Tissues Manifesting Transport Defect	Molecular Defect	Major Clinical Manifestations	Inheritance
Amino Acids					
Cystinuria	Cystine, lysine, arginine, ornithine	Proximal renal tubule, jejunal mucosa	Shared dibasic-cystine transporter SLC3A1, SLC7A9	Cystine nephrolithiasis	AR
Dibasic aminoaciduria	Lysine, arginine, ornithine	Proximal renal tubule, jejunal mucosa	Dibasic transporter SLC7A7	Type I: Benign Type II: Protein intolerance, hyperammonemia, mental retardation	AR
Hartnup disease	Neutral amino acids	Proximal renal tubule, jejunal mucosa	Neutral amino acid transporter SLC6A19	Constant neutral aminoaciduria, intermittent symptoms of pellagra	AR
Methionine malabsorption	Methionine	Jejunal mucosa	Methionine transporter	White hair, mental retardation, convulsions, hyperpneic attacks, edema	Probable AR
Histidinuria	Histidine	Proximal renal tubule, jejunal mucosa	Histidine transporter	Mental retardation	AR
Iminoglycinuria	Glycine, proline, hydroxyproline	Proximal renal tubule, jejunal mucosa	Shared glycine–imino acid transporter	None	AR
Dicarboxylic aminoaciduria	Glutamic acid, aspartic acid	Proximal renal tubule, jejunal mucosa	Shared dicarboxylic amino acid transporter	None	Probable AR
Cystinosis	Cystine	Lysosomal membranes	Lysosomal cystine transporter CTNS	Renal failure, hypothyroidism, blindness	AR
Hexoses					
Glucose-galactose malabsorption	D-Glucose D-Galactose	Proximal renal tubule, jejunal mucosa	Sodium-dependent glucose/galactose transporter SGLT1	Watery diarrhea on feeding glucose, lactose, sucrose, or galactose	AR
Glucose-transport defect	D-Glucose	Ubiquitous blood brain barrier	Facilitative glucose transporter GLUT1	Seizures, mental retardation	AD
Fanconi-Bickel syndrome	D-Glucose	Liver, kidney, pancreas, intestine	Facilitative glucose transporter GLUT2	Growth retardation, rickets, hepatorenal glycogenosis, hypo- and hyperglycemia	AR
Urate					
Hypouricemia	Uric acid	Proximal renal tubule	Urate transporter SLC22A12	Hypouricemia, uric acid urolithiasis	AR
Anions					
Congenital chloridorrhea	Chloride, sulfate	Ileal and colonic mucosa	Cl-/HCO3- exchanger (DRA)	Hydramnios, watery diarrhea, elevated fecal chloride, metabolic alkalosis with volume depletion, hyperaldosteronism	AR
Dent disease, X-linked recessive hypophosphatemic rickets and nephrocalcinosis	Chloride, phosphate	Proximal renal tubule	Voltage-gated Cl-channel CLCN5	Proteinuria, hypercalciuria, nephrocalcinosis, nephrolithiasis, rickets	XL
Cations					
Hyperinsulinemic hypoglycemia	Potassium	Pancreatic β cell	Sulfonylurea receptor SUR1, K^+ channel KCNJ11	Neonatal hypoglycemia, hyperinsulinemia	AR

(continued)

TABLE 365-1 Genetic Disorders of Membrane Transport (Selected Examples) (*Continued*)

Class of Substance and Disorder	Individual Substrates	Tissues Manifesting Transport Defect	Molecular Defect	Major Clinical Manifestations	Inheritance
Benign familial neonatal epilepsy	Potassium	Brain	Voltage-gated K+ channels KCNQ2, KCNQ3	Neonatal seizures, normal development	AD
Water					
Nephrogenic diabetes insipidus type 2	Water	Renal collecting tubule	Aquaporin 2 (water channel)	Polyuria, dehydration, hyposthenuria	AR
Vitamins					
Thiamine-responsive megaloblastic anemia	Thiamine	Ubiquitous	Thiamine transporter SLC19A2	Megaloblastic anemia, deafness, diabetes mellitus	AR
Other					
Carnitine deficiency	Carnitine	Kidney, muscle, heart	Carnitine transporter OCTN2	Hypoketotic hypoglycemia, cardiomyopathy, hypotonia	AR
Creatine deficiency	Creatine	Brain	Creatine transporter SLC6A8	Mental retardation, seizures, hypotonia	XL

Abbreviations: AD, autosomal dominant; AR, autosomal recessive; XL, X-linked recessive.

bleeding complications during delivery. These can be minimized by aggressive nutritional therapy and control of blood pressure. Their infants can have intrauterine growth restriction but have normal neurologic function.

HARTNUP DISEASE

Hartnup disease (frequency 1 in 24,000) is an autosomal recessive disorder characterized by pellagra-like skin lesions, variable neurologic manifestations, and neutral and aromatic aminoaciduria. Alanine, serine, threonine, valine, leucine, isoleucine, phenylalanine, tyrosine, tryptophan, glutamine, asparagine, and histidine are excreted in urine in quantities 5–10 times greater than normal, and intestinal transport of these same amino acids is defective. The defective neutral amino acid transporter, B^0AT1 encoded by the *SLC6A19* gene on chromosome 5p15, localizes to the apical membrane in renal tubular and intestinal cells.

The clinical manifestations result from nutritional deficiency of the essential amino acid tryptophan, caused by its intestinal and renal malabsorption, and of niacin, which derives in part from tryptophan metabolism. Only a small fraction of patients with the chemical findings of this disorder develop a pellagra-like syndrome, implying that manifestations depend on other factors in addition to the transport defect. The diagnosis of Hartnup disease should be suspected in any patient with clinical features of pellagra who does not have a history of dietary niacin deficiency (Chap. 74). The neurologic and psychiatric manifestations range from attacks of cerebellar ataxia to mild emotional lability to frank delirium, and they are usually accompanied by exacerbations of the erythematous, eczematoid skin rash. Fever, sunlight, stress, and sulfonamide therapy provoke clinical relapses. Diagnosis is made by detection of the neutral aminoaciduria, which does not occur in dietary niacin deficiency. Treatment is directed at niacin repletion and includes a high-protein diet and daily nicotinamide supplementation (50–250 mg).

FURTHER READINGS

Broer S: Amino acid transport across mammalian intestinal and renal epithelia. Physiol Rev 88: 249, 2008

Camargo SM et al: Aminoacidurias: Clinical and molecular aspects. Kidney Int 73:918, 2008

Kleta R et al: Mutations in SLC6A19, encoding B^0AT1, cause Hartnup disorder. Nat Genet 36:999, 2004

Palacin M et al: The genetics of heteromeric amino acid transporters. Physiology (Bethesda) 20:112, 2005

Sebastio G et al: Lysinuric protein intolerance: Reviewing concepts on a multisystem disease. Am J Med Genet C Semin Med Genet 157:54, 2011

PART 17

Neurologic Disorders

CHAPTER 366 Biology of Neurologic Diseases

Stephen L. Hauser
M. Flint Beal

The human nervous system is the organ of consciousness, cognition, ethics, and behavior; as such, it is the most intricate structure known to exist. More than one-third of the 23,000 genes encoded in the human genome are expressed in the nervous system. Each mature brain is composed of 100 billion neurons, several million miles of axons and dendrites, and $>10^{15}$ synapses. Neurons exist within a dense parenchyma of multifunctional glial cells that synthesize myelin, preserve homeostasis, and regulate immune responses. Measured against this background of complexity, the achievements of molecular neuroscience have been extraordinary. This chapter reviews selected themes in neuroscience that provide a context for understanding fundamental mechanisms that underlie neurologic disorders.

NEUROGENETICS

The landscape of neurology has been transformed by modern molecular genetics. More than 350 different disease-causing genes have been identified, and >1000 neurologic disorders have been genetically mapped to various chromosomal locations. Several hundred neurologic and psychiatric disorders now can be diagnosed through genetic testing (*http://www.ncbi.nlm.nih.gov/sites/GeneTests/?db=GeneTests*). The vast majority of these disorders represent highly penetrant mutations that cause rare neurologic disorders; alternatively, they represent rare monogenic causes of common phenotypes. Examples of the latter include mutations of the amyloid precursor protein in familial Alzheimer's disease, the microtubule-associated protein tau (MAPT) in frontotemporal dementia, and α-synuclein in Parkinson's disease. These discoveries have been profoundly important because the mutated gene in a familial disorder often encodes a protein that is also pathogenetically involved (although not mutated) in the typical, sporadic form. The common mechanism involves disordered processing and, ultimately, aggregation of the protein, leading to cell death (see "Protein Aggregation and Neurodegeneration," below).

There is great optimism that complex genetic disorders that are caused by combinations of genetic and environmental factors have become tractable problems. Genome-wide association studies (GWAS) have been carried out in many complex neurologic disorders, with many hundreds of variants identified, nearly all of which confer only a small increment in disease risk (1.15–1.5 fold). GWAS are rooted in the "common disease, common variant" hypothesis, as they examine potential risk alleles that are relatively common (e.g. >5%) in the general population. More than 1000 GWAS have been carried out to date, with notable successes such as the identification of >50 risk alleles for multiple sclerosis. Furthermore, when bioinformatics tools are used, risk variants can be aligned in functional biologic pathways to identify novel pathogenic mechanisms as well as to reveal heterogeneity (e.g., different pathways in different individuals). Despite these successes, many experienced geneticists question the value of common disease-associated variants, particularly whether they are actually causative or merely mark the approximate locations of more important—truly causative—rare mutations.

This debate has set the stage for the next revolution in human genetics, made possible by the development of increasingly efficient and cost-effective high-throughput sequencing methodologies. It is currently possible to sequence an entire human genome in approximately an hour, at a cost of only $4000 for the entire coding sequence ("whole-exome") or $10,000 for the entire genome; it is certain that these costs will continue to decline. This makes it feasible to look for disease-causing sequence variations in individual patients with the possibility of identifying rare variants that cause disease. The utility of this approach was demonstrated by whole-genome sequencing in a patient with Charcot-Marie-Tooth neuropathy in which compound heterozygous mutations were identified in the *SH3TC2* gene that then were shown to co-segregate with the disease in other members of the family.

It is also increasingly recognized that not all genetic diseases or predispositions are caused by simple changes in the linear nucleotide sequence of genes. As the complex architecture of the human genome becomes better defined, many disorders that result from alterations in copy numbers of genes ("gene-dosage" effects) resulting from unequal crossing-over are likely to be identified. As much as 5–10% of the human genome consists of nonhomologous duplications and deletions, and these appear to occur with a much higher mutational rate than is the case for single base pair mutations. The first copy-number disorders to be recognized were Charcot-Marie-Tooth disease type 1A (CMT1A), caused by a duplication in the gene encoding the myelin protein PMP22, and the reciprocal deletion of the gene causing hereditary liability to pressure palsies (HNPP) (Chap. 384). Gene-dosage effects are causative in some cases of Parkinson's disease (α-synuclein), Alzheimer's disease (amyloid precursor protein), spinal muscular atrophy (survival motor neuron 2), the dysmyelinating disorder Pelizaeus-Merzbacher syndrome (proteolipid protein 1), late-onset leukodystrophy (lamin B1), and a variety of developmental neurologic disorders. It is now evident that copy-number variations contribute substantially to normal human genomic variation for numerous genes involved in neurologic function, regulation of cell growth, and regulation of metabolism. It is also already clear that gene-dosage effects will influence many behavioral phenotypes, learning disorders, and autism spectrum disorders. Deletions at ch1q and ch15q have been associated with schizophrenia, and deletions at 15q and 16p with autism. Interestingly, the 16p deletion also is associated with epilepsy. Duplications of the X-linked *MeCP2* gene cause autism in males and psychiatric disorders with anxiety in females, whereas point mutations in this gene produce the neurodevelopmental disorder Rett syndrome. The understanding of the role of copy-number variation in human disease is still in its infancy.

The role of splicing variation as a contributor to neurologic disease is another area of active investigation. *Alternative splicing* refers to the inclusion of different combinations of exons in mature mRNA, resulting in the potential for many different protein products encoded by a single gene. Alternative splicing represents a powerful mechanism for generation of complexity and variation, and this mechanism appears to be highly prevalent in the nervous system, affecting key processes such as neurotransmitter receptors and ion channels. Numerous diseases are known to result from abnormalities in alternative splicing. Increased inclusion of exon 10–containing transcripts of *MAPT* can cause frontotemporal dementia. Aberrant splicing also contributes to the pathogenesis of Duchenne's, myotonic, and fascioscapulohumeral muscular dystrophies; ataxia-telangiectasia; neurofibromatosis; some inherited ataxias; and fragile X syndrome, among other disorders. It is also likely that subtle variations of splicing will influence many genetically complex disorders. For example, a splicing variant of the interleukin 7 receptor α chain, resulting in production of more soluble and less membrane-bound receptor, was found to be associated with susceptibility to multiple sclerosis (MS) in multiple different populations.

Epigenetics refers to the mechanisms by which levels of gene expression can be exquisitely modulated not by variations in the primary genetic sequence of DNA but rather by postgenomic alterations in DNA and chromatin structure, which influence how, when, and where genes are expressed. DNA methylation and the methylation and acetylation of histone proteins that interact with nuclear DNA to form chromatin are key mediators of these events. Epigenetic processes appear to be dynamically active even in postmitotic neurons. *Imprinting* refers to an epigenetic feature, present for a subset of genes, in which the predominant expression of one allele is determined by its parent of origin. The distinctive neurodevelopmental disorders Prader-Willi syndrome (mild mental retardation and endocrine abnormalities) and Angelman syndrome (cortical atrophy, cerebellar dysmyelination, Purkinje cell loss) are classic examples of imprinting disorders whose distinctive features are determined by whether the paternal or maternal copy of chromosome of the critical genetic region 15q11-13 was responsible. In a study of discordant monozygotic twins for MS in which the entire DNA sequence, transcriptome (e.g., mRNA levels), and methylome were assessed genomewide, tantalizing allelic differences in the use of the paternal, compared to maternal, copy for a group of genes were identified. Preferential allelic expression, whether due to imprinting, resistance to X inactivation, or other mechanisms, is likely to play a major role in determining complex behaviors and susceptibility to many neurologic and psychiatric disorders.

Another advance is the development of transgenic mouse models of neurologic diseases, which has been particularly fruitful in producing models relevant to Alzheimer's disease, Parkinson's disease, Huntington's disease, and amyotrophic lateral sclerosis. These models are useful in both studying disease pathogenesis and developing and testing new therapies. Models in both *Caenorhabditis elegans* and *Drosophila* have also been extremely useful, particularly in studying genetic modifiers as well as therapeutic interventions.

ION CHANNELS AND CHANNELOPATHIES

The resting potential of neurons and the action potentials responsible for impulse conduction are generated by ion currents and ion channels. Most ion channels are gated, meaning that they can transition between conformations that are open or closed to ion conductance. Individual ion channels are distinguished by the specific ions they conduct; their kinetics; and whether they directly sense voltage, are linked to receptors for neurotransmitters or other ligands such as neurotrophins, or are activated by second messengers. The diverse characteristics of different ion channels provide a means by which neuronal excitability can be modulated exquisitely at both the cellular and subcellular levels. Disorders of ion channels—channelopathies—are responsible for a growing list of human neurologic diseases (Table 366-1). Most are caused by mutations in ion channel genes or by autoantibodies against ion channel proteins. One example is epilepsy, a syndrome of diverse causes characterized by repetitive, synchronous firing of neuronal action potentials. Action potentials normally are generated by the opening of sodium channels and the inward movement of sodium ions down the intracellular concentration gradient. Depolarization of the neuronal membrane opens potassium channels, resulting in outward movement of potassium ions, repolarization, closure of the sodium channel, and hyperpolarization. Sodium or potassium channel subunit genes have long been considered candidate disease genes in inherited epilepsy syndromes, and recently such mutations were identified. These mutations appear to alter the normal gating function of these channels, increasing the

TABLE 366-1 Examples of Neurologic Channelopathies

Category	Disorder	Channel Type	Mutated Gene	Chap. Ref.
Genetic				
Ataxias	Episodic ataxia-1	K	*KCNA1*	373
	Episodic ataxia-2	Ca	*CACNL1A*	
	Spinocerebellar ataxia-6	Ca	*CACNL1A*	
Migraine	Familial hemiplegic migraine 1	Ca	*CACNL1A*	14
	Familial hemiplegic migraine 3	Na	*SCN1A*	
Epilepsy	Benign neonatal familial convulsions	K	*KCNQ2, KCNQ3*	369
	Generalized epilepsy with febrile convulsions plus	Na	*SCN1B*	
Periodic paralysis	Hyperkalemic periodic paralysis	Na	*SCN4A*	387
	Hypokalemic periodic paralysis	Ca	*CACNL1A3*	
Myotonia	Myotonia congenita	Cl	*CLCN1*	387
	Paramyotonia congenita	Na	*SCN4A*	
Deafness	Jervell and Lange-Nielsen syndrome (deafness, prolonged QT interval, and arrhythmia)	K	*KCNQ1, KCNE1*	30
	Autosomal dominant progressive deafness	K	*KCNQ4*	
Autoimmune				
Paraneoplastic	Limbic encephalitis	Kv1	—	101
	Acquired neuromyotonia	Kv1	—	101
	Cerebellar ataxia	Ca (P/Q type)		101
	Lambert-Eaton syndrome	Ca (P/Q type)	—	101

inherent excitability of neuronal membranes in regions where the abnormal channels are expressed.

Whereas the specific clinical manifestations of channelopathies are quite variable, one common feature is that manifestations tend to be intermittent or paroxysmal, as occurs in epilepsy, migraine, ataxia, myotonia, or periodic paralysis. Exceptions are clinically progressive channel disorders such as autosomal dominant hearing impairment. The genetic channelopathies identified to date are all uncommon disorders caused by obvious mutations in channel genes. As the full repertoire of human ion channels and related proteins is identified, it is likely that additional channelopathies will be discovered. In addition to rare disorders that result from obvious mutations, it is likely that less penetrant allelic variations in channel genes or their pattern of expression might underlie susceptibility to some apparently sporadic forms of epilepsy, migraine, or other disorders. For example, mutations in the potassium channel gene Kir2.6 have been found in many individuals with thyrotoxic hypokalemic periodic paralysis, a disorder similar to hypokalemic periodic paralysis but precipitated by stress from thyrotoxicosis or carbohydrate loading.

NEUROTRANSMITTERS AND NEUROTRANSMITTER RECEPTORS

Synaptic neurotransmission is the predominant means by which neurons communicate with each other. Classic neurotransmitters are synthesized in the presynaptic region of the nerve terminal; stored in vesicles; and released into the synaptic cleft, where they bind to receptors on the postsynaptic cell. Secreted neurotransmitters are eliminated by reuptake into the presynaptic neuron (or glia), diffusion away from the synaptic cleft, and/or specific inactivation. In addition to the classic neurotransmitters, many neuropeptides have been identified as definite or probable neurotransmitters; they include substance P, neurotensin, enkephalins, β-endorphin, histamine, vasoactive intestinal polypeptide, cholecystokinin, neuropeptide Y, and somatostatin. Peptide neurotransmitters are synthesized in the cell body rather than the nerve terminal and may colocalize with classic neurotransmitters in single neurons. A number of neuropeptides are important in pain modulation, including substance P and calcitonin gene-related peptide (CGRP), which causes migraine-like headaches in patients. As a consequence, CGRP receptor antagonists have been developed and shown to be effective in treating migraine headaches. Nitric oxide and carbon monoxide are gases that appear also to function as neurotransmitters, in part by signaling in a retrograde fashion from the postsynaptic to the presynaptic cell.

Neurotransmitters modulate the function of postsynaptic cells by binding to specific neurotransmitter receptors, of which there are two major types. *Ionotropic receptors* are direct ion channels that open after engagement by the neurotransmitter. *Metabotropic receptors* interact with G proteins, stimulating production of second messengers and activating protein kinases, which modulate a variety of cellular events. Ionotropic receptors are multiple-subunit structures, whereas metabotropic receptors are composed of single subunits only. One important difference between ionotropic and metabotropic receptors is that the kinetics of ionotropic receptor effects are fast (generally <1 ms) because neurotransmitter binding directly alters the electrical properties of the postsynaptic cell, whereas metabotropic receptors function over longer periods. These different properties contribute to the potential for selective and finely modulated signaling by neurotransmitters.

Neurotransmitter systems are perturbed in a large number of clinical disorders, examples of which are highlighted in Table 366-2. One example is the involvement of dopaminergic neurons originating in the substantia nigra of the midbrain and projecting to the striatum (nigrostriatal pathway) in Parkinson's disease and in heroin addicts after the ingestion of the toxin MPTP (1-methyl-4-phenyl-1,2,5,6-tetrahydropyridine).

A second important dopaminergic system arising in the midbrain is the mediocorticolimbic pathway, which is implicated in the pathogenesis of addictive behaviors including drug reward. Its key components include the midbrain ventral tegmental area (VTA), median forebrain bundle, and nucleus accumbens (see Fig. 390-1). The cholinergic pathway originating in the nucleus basalis of Meynert plays a role in memory function in Alzheimer's disease.

Addictive drugs share the property of increasing dopamine release in the nucleus accumbens. Amphetamine increases intracellular release of dopamine from vesicles and reverses transport of dopamine through the dopamine transporters. Patients prone to addiction show increased activation of the nucleus accumbens after administration of amphetamine. Cocaine binds to dopamine transporters and inhibits dopamine reuptake. Ethanol inhibits inhibitory neurons in the VTA, leading to increased dopamine release in the nucleus accumbens. Opioids also disinhibit these dopaminergic neurons by binding to μ receptors expressed by γ-aminobutyric acid (GABA)-containing interneurons in the VTA. Nicotine increases dopamine release by activating nicotinic acetylcholine receptors on cell bodies and nerve terminals of dopaminergic VTA neurons. Tetrahydrocannabinol, the active ingredient of cannabis, also increases dopamine levels in the nucleus accumbens. Blockade of dopamine in the nucleus accumbens can terminate the rewarding effects of addictive drugs.

Not all cell-to-cell communication in the nervous system occurs via neurotransmission. Gap junctions provide for direct neuron-neuron electrical conduction and also create openings for the diffusion of ions and metabolites between cells. In addition to neurons, gap junctions are widespread in glia, creating a syncytium that protects neurons by removing glutamate and potassium from the extracellular environment. Gap junctions consist of membrane-spanning proteins, termed *connexins,* that pair across adjacent cells. Mechanisms that involve gap junctions have been related to a variety of neurologic disorders. Mutations in connexin 32, a gap junction protein expressed by Schwann cells, are responsible for the X-linked form of CMT disease. Mutations in either of two gap junction proteins expressed in the inner ear—connexin 26 and connexin 31—result in autosomal dominant progressive hearing loss (Chap. 30). Glial calcium waves mediated through gap junctions also appear to explain the phenomenon of spreading depression associated with migraine auras and the march of epileptic discharges. Spreading depression is a neural response that follows a variety of different stimuli and is characterized by a circumferentially expanding negative potential that propagates at a characteristic speed of 20 m/s and is associated with an increase in extracellular potassium.

SIGNALING PATHWAYS AND GENE TRANSCRIPTION

The fundamental issue of how memory, learning, and thinking are encoded in the nervous system is likely to be clarified by identification of the signaling pathways involved in neuronal differentiation, axon guidance, and synapse formation and by an understanding of how these pathways are modulated by experience. Many families of transcription factors, each consisting of multiple individual components, are expressed in the nervous system. Elucidation of these signaling pathways has begun to provide insights into the causes of a variety of neurologic disorders, including inherited disorders of cognition such as X-linked mental retardation. This problem affects ~1 in 500 males, and linkage studies in different families suggest that as many as 60 different X-chromosome-encoded genes may be responsible. Rett syndrome,

TABLE 366-2 Principal Classic Neurotransmitters

Neurotransmitter	Anatomy	Clinical Aspects
Acetylcholine (ACh) $CH_3—C(=O)—O—CH_2—N—(CH_3)_3$	Motor neurons in spinal cord → neuromuscular junction	Acetylcholinesterases (nerve gases) Myasthenia gravis (antibodies to ACh receptor) Congenital myasthenic syndromes (mutations in ACh receptor subunits) Lambert-Eaton syndrome (antibodies to Ca channels impair ACh release) Botulism (toxin disrupts ACh release by exocytosis)
	Basal forebrain → widespread cortex	Alzheimer's disease (selective cell death) Autosomal dominant frontal lobe epilepsy (mutations in CNS ACh receptor)
	Interneurons in striatum	Parkinson's disease (tremor)
	Autonomic nervous system (preganglionic and postganglionic parasympathetic; preganglionic sympathetic)	
Dopamine 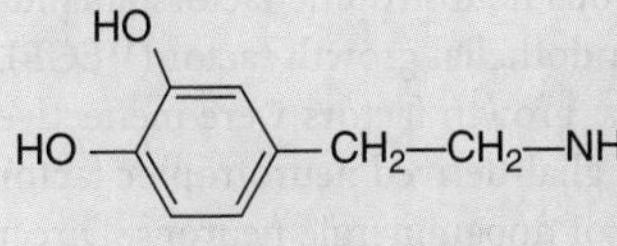 HO, HO —(benzene ring)— $CH_2—CH_2—NH_3$	Substantia nigra → striatum (nigrostriatal pathway)	Parkinson's disease (selective cell death) MPTP parkinsonism (toxin transported into neurons)
	Substantia nigra → limbic system and widespread cortex	Addiction, behavioral disorders
	Arcuate nucleus of hypothalamus → anterior pituitary (via portal veins)	Inhibits prolactin secretion
Norepinephrine (NE) 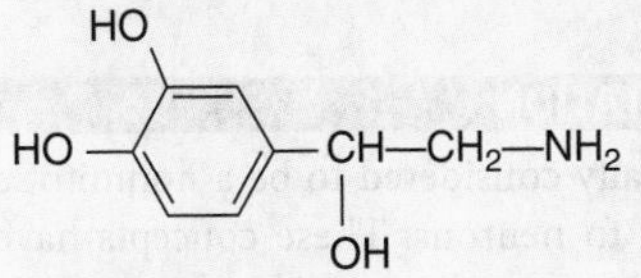 HO, HO —(benzene ring)— $CH(OH)—CH_2—NH_2$	Locus coeruleus (pons) → limbic system, hypothalamus, cortex	Mood disorders (MAOA inhibitors and tricyclics increase NE and improve depression)
	Medulla → locus coeruleus, spinal cord	Anxiety
	Postganglionic neurons of sympathetic nervous system	Orthostatic tachycardia syndrome (mutations in NE transporter)
Serotonin 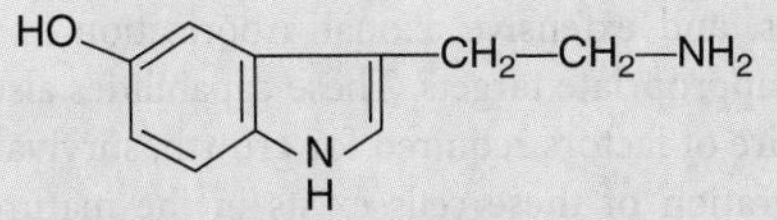 HO —(indole ring, N–H)— $CH_2—CH_2—NH_2$	Pontine raphe nuclei → widespread projections	Mood disorders (SSRIs improve depression) Migraine pain pathway
	Medulla/pons → dorsal horn of spinal cord	Pain pathway
γ-Aminobutyric acid (GABA) $H_2N—CH_2—CH_2—CH_2—COOH$	Major inhibitory neurotransmitter in brain; widespread cortical interneurons and long projection pathways	Stiff-person syndrome (antibodies to glutamic acid decarboxylase, the biosynthetic enzyme for GABA) Epilepsy (gabapentin and valproic acid increase GABA)
Glycine $H_2N—CH_2—COOH$	Major inhibitory neurotransmitter in spinal cord	Spasticity Hyperekplexia (myoclonic startle syndrome) due to mutations in glycine receptor
Glutamate $H_2N—CH(COOH)—CH_2—CH_2—COOH$	Major excitatory neurotransmitter; located throughout CNS, including cortical pyramidal cells	Seizures due to ingestion of domoic acid (a glutamate analogue) Rasmussen's encephalitis (antibody against glutamate receptor 3) Excitotoxic cell death

Abbreviations: CNS, central nervous system; MAOA, monoamine oxidase A; MPTP, 1-methyl-4-phenyl-1,2,3,6-tetrahydropyridine; SSRI, selective serotonin reuptake inhibitor.

a common cause of (dominant) X-linked progressive mental retardation in females, is due to a mutation in a gene (*MECP2*) that encodes a DNA-binding protein involved in transcriptional repression. As the X chromosome accounts for only ~3% of germ-line DNA, by extrapolation, the number of genes that potentially contribute to clinical disorders affecting intelligence in humans must be potentially very large. As discussed below, there is increasing evidence that abnormal gene transcription may play a role in neurodegenerative diseases such as Huntington's disease, in which proteins with polyglutamine expansions bind to and sequester transcription factors. A critical transcription factor for neuronal survival is CREB (cyclic adenosine monophosphate responsive element-binding) protein, which also plays an important role in memory in the hippocampus.

MYELIN

Myelin is the multilayered insulating substance that surrounds axons and speeds impulse conduction by permitting action potentials to jump between naked regions of axons (nodes of Ranvier) and across myelinated segments. Molecular interactions between the myelin membrane and the axon are required to maintain the stability, function, and normal life span of both structures. A single oligodendrocyte usually ensheathes multiple axons in the central nervous system (CNS), whereas in the peripheral nervous system (PNS) each Schwann cell typically myelinates a single axon. Myelin is a lipid-rich material formed by a spiraling process of the membrane of the myelinating cell around the axon, creating multiple membrane bilayers that are tightly apposed (compact myelin) by charged protein interactions. Several inhibitors of axon growth are expressed on the innermost (periaxonal) lamellae of the myelin membrane (see "Stem Cells and Transplantation," below). A number of clinically important neurologic disorders are caused by inherited mutations in myelin proteins of the CNS or PNS (Fig. 366-1). Constituents of myelin also have a propensity to be targeted as autoantigens in autoimmune demyelinating disorders (Fig. 366-2). Specification to oligodendrocyte precursor cells (OPCs) is transcriptionally regulated by the *Olig 2* and *Yin Yang 1* genes, whereas myelination mediated by postmitotic oligodendrocytes depends on a different transcription factor, *myelin gene regulatory factor (MRF).* It is noteworthy that in the normal adult brain large numbers of OPCs [expressing platelet-derived growth factor receptor alpha (PDGFR-α) and NG2] are widely distributed but do not myelinate axons, even in demyelinating environments such as lesions of MS. The characterization of these cells, including an understanding of their transcriptional regulation and functional roles, could result in novel approaches to remyelination and brain repair.

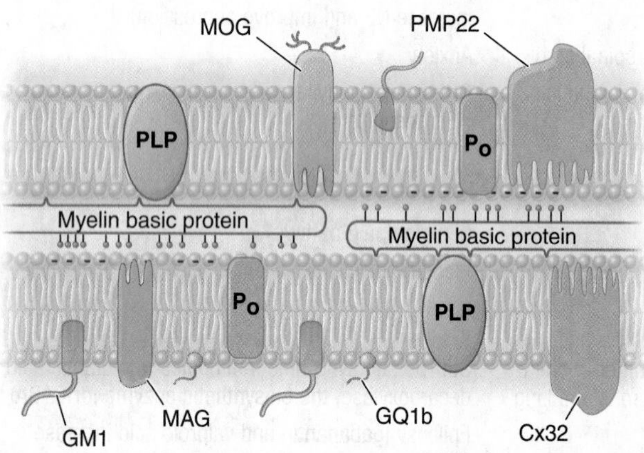

Figure 366-1 The molecular architecture of the myelin sheath illustrating the most important disease-related proteins. The illustration represents a composite of CNS and PNS myelin. Proteins restricted to CNS myelin are shown in green, proteins of PNS myelin are lavender, and proteins present in both CNS and PNS are red. In the CNS, the X-linked allelic disorders Pelizaeus-Merzbacher disease and one variant of familial spastic paraplegia are caused by mutations in the gene for proteolipid protein (PLP) that normally promotes extracellular compaction between adjacent myelin lamellae. The homologue of PLP in the PNS is the P_0 protein, mutations in which cause the neuropathy Charcot-Marie-Tooth disease (CMT) type 1B. The most common form of CMT is the 1A subtype caused by a duplication of the *PMP22* gene; deletions in *PMP22* are responsible for another inherited neuropathy termed *hereditary liability to pressure palsies* (Chap. 384).

In multiple sclerosis (MS), myelin basic protein (MBP) and the quantitatively minor CNS protein myelin oligodendrocyte glycoprotein (MOG) are probably T cell and B cell antigens, respectively (Chap. 380). The location of MOG at the outermost lamella of the CNS myelin membrane may facilitate its targeting by autoantibodies. In the PNS, autoantibodies against myelin gangliosides are implicated in a variety of disorders, including GQ1b in the Fisher variant of Guillain-Barré syndrome, GM1 in multifocal motor neuropathy, and sulfatide constituents of myelin-associated glycoprotein (MAG) in peripheral neuropathies associated with monoclonal gammopathies (Chap. 385).

NEUROTROPHIC FACTORS

Neurotrophic factors (Table 366-3) are secreted proteins that modulate neuronal growth, differentiation, repair, and survival; some have additional functions, including roles in neurotransmission and in the synaptic reorganization involved in learning and memory. The neurotrophin (NT) family contains nerve growth factor (NGF), brain-derived neurotrophic factor (BDNF), NT3, and NT4/5. The neurotrophins act at TrK and p75 receptors to promote survival of neurons. Because of their survival-promoting and antiapoptotic effects, neurotrophic factors are in theory outstanding candidates for therapy for disorders characterized by premature death of neurons as occurs in amyotrophic lateral sclerosis (ALS) and other degenerative motor neuron disorders. Knockout mice lacking receptors for ciliary neurotrophic factor (CNTF) or BDNF show loss of motor neurons, and experimental motor neuron death can be rescued by treatment with various neurotrophic factors, including CNTF, BDNF, and vascular endothelial growth factor (VEGF). However, in phase 3 clinical trials, growth factors were ineffective in human ALS. The growth factor glial-derived neurotrophic factor (GDNF) is important for survival of dopaminergic neurons. Direct infusions of GDNF showed initial promise in Parkinson's disease (PD), but the benefits were not replicated in a larger clinical trial.

STEM CELLS AND TRANSPLANTATION

The nervous system is traditionally considered to be a nonmitotic organ, particularly with respect to neurons. These concepts have been challenged by the finding that neural progenitor or stem cells exist in the adult CNS that are capable of differentiation, migration over long distances, and extensive axonal arborization and synapse formation with appropriate targets. These capabilities also indicate that the repertoire of factors required for growth, survival, differentiation, and migration of these cells exists in the mature nervous system. In rodents, neural stem cells, defined as progenitor cells capable of differentiating into mature cells of neural or glial lineage, have been experimentally propagated from fetal CNS and neuroectodermal tissues and also from adult germinal matrix and ependyma regions. Human fetal CNS tissue is also capable of differentiation into cells with neuronal, astrocyte, and oligodendrocyte morphology when cultured in the presence of growth factors.

Once the repertoire of signals required for cell type specification is better understood, differentiation into specific neural or glial subpopulations could be directed in vitro; such cells also could be engineered to express therapeutic molecules. Another promising approach is to utilize growth factors such as BDNF to stimulate endogenous stem cells to proliferate and migrate to areas of neuronal damage. Administration of epidermal growth factor with fibroblast growth factor replenished up to 50% of hippocampal CA1 neurons a month after global ischemia in rats. The new neurons made connections and improved performance in a memory task.

A major advance has been the development of induced pluripotent stem cells. Using this technique, adult somatic cells such as skin fibroblasts are treated with four pluripotency factors (SOX2, KLF4, cMYC, and Oct4), and this generates induced pluripotent stem cells (iPSCs). These adult-derived stem cells sidestep the ethical issues of utilizing stem cells derived from human embryos. The development of these cells has tremendous promise for both studying disease mechanisms and testing therapeutics. There is no consensus on the best way to generate and differentiate iPSCs; however, techniques to

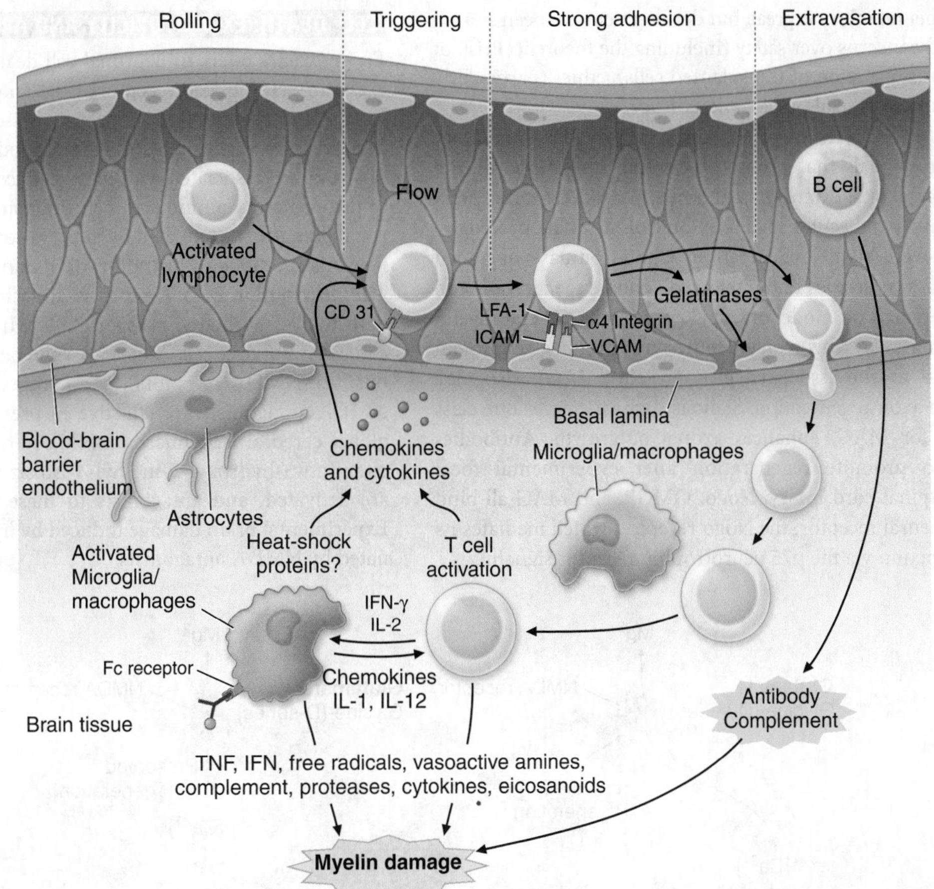

Figure 366-2 A model for experimental allergic encephalomyelitis (EAE). Crucial steps for disease initiation and progression include peripheral activation of preexisting autoreactive T cells; homing to the CNS and extravasation across the blood-brain barrier; reactivation of T cells by exposed autoantigens; secretion of cytokines; activation of microglia and astrocytes and recruitment of a secondary inflammatory wave; and immune-mediated myelin destruction. ICAM, intercellular adhesion molecule; LFA-1, lymphocyte function-associated antigen-1; VCAM, vascular cell adhesion molecule; IFN, interferon; IL, interleukin; TNF, tumor necrosis factor.

avoid using viral vectors and the use of Cre-lox systems to remove reprogramming factors result in a better match of gene expression profiles with those of embryonic stem cells. Thus far, iPSC cells have been made from patients with all the major human neurodegenerative diseases, and studies utilizing them are under way.

TABLE 366-3 Neurotrophic Factors

Neurotrophin family	Transforming growth factor β family
Nerve growth factor	Glial-derived neurotrophic family
Brain-derived neurotrophic factor	Neurturin
	Persephin
Neurotrophin-3	Fibroblast growth factor family
Neurotrophin-4	Hepatocyte growth factor
Neurotrophin-6	Insulin-like growth factor (IGF) family
Cytokine family	IGF-1
Ciliary neurotrophic factor	IGF-2
Leukemia inhibitory factor	
Interleukin 6	
Cardiotrophin-1	

Although stem cells hold tremendous promise for the treatment of debilitating neurologic diseases such as Parkinson's disease and spinal cord injury, it should be emphasized that medical application is in its infancy. Major obstacles are the generation of position- and neurotransmitter-defined subtypes of neurons and their isolation as pure populations of the desired cells. This is crucial to avoid persistence of undifferentiated embryonic stem (ES) cells, which can generate tumors. The establishment of appropriate neural connections and afferent control is also critical. For instance, human ES motor neurons will have to be introduced at multiple segments in the neuraxis, and then their axons will have to regenerate from the spinal cord to distal musculature.

Experimental transplantation of human fetal dopaminergic neurons in patients with Parkinson's disease has shown that these transplanted cells can survive within the host striatum; however, some patients developed disabling dyskinesias, and this approach is no longer in clinical development. Human ES cells can be differentiated into dopaminergic neurons, which reverse symptoms of Parkinson's disease in experimental animal models. Studies of transplantation for patients with Huntington's disease have reported encouraging, although very preliminary, results. Oligodendrocyte precursor cells transplanted into mice with a dysmyelinating disorder effectively migrated in the new environment, interacted with axons, and mediated myelination; such experiments raise hope that similar transplantation strategies may be feasible in human disorders of myelin such as MS. The promise of stem cells for treatment of both neurodegenerative diseases and neural injury is great, but development has been slowed by unresolved concerns over safety (including the theoretical risk of malignant transformation of transplanted cells), ethics (particularly with respect to use of fetal tissue), and efficacy.

In developing brain, the extracellular matrix provides stimulatory and inhibitory signals that promote neuronal migration, neurite outgrowth, and axonal extension. After neuronal damage, reexpression of inhibitory molecules such as chondroitin sulfate proteoglycans may prevent tissue regeneration. Chondroitinase degraded these inhibitory molecules and enhanced axonal regeneration and motor recovery in a rat model of spinal cord injury. Several myelin proteins, specifically Nogo, oligodendrocyte myelin glycoprotein (OMGP), and myelin-associated glycoprotein (MAG), also may interfere with axon regeneration. Sialidase, which cleaves one class of receptors for MAG, enhances axonal outgrowth. Antibodies against Nogo promote regeneration after experimental focal ischemia or spinal cord injury. Nogo, OMGP, and MAG all bind to the same neural receptor, the Nogo receptor, which mediates its inhibitory function via the p75 neurotrophin receptor signaling.

CELL DEATH: EXCITOTOXICITY AND APOPTOSIS

Excitotoxicity refers to neuronal cell death caused by activation of excitatory amino acid receptors (Fig. 366-3). Compelling evidence for a role of excitotoxicity, especially in ischemic neuronal injury, is derived from experiments in animal models. Experimental models of stroke are associated with increased extracellular concentrations of the excitatory amino acid neurotransmitter glutamate, and neuronal damage is attenuated by denervation of glutamate-containing neurons or the administration of glutamate receptor antagonists. The distribution of cells sensitive to ischemia corresponds closely with that of *N*-methyl-D-aspartate (NMDA) receptors (except for cerebellar Purkinje cells, which are vulnerable to hypoxemia-ischemia but lack NMDA receptors), and competitive and noncompetitive NMDA antagonists are effective in preventing focal ischemia. In global cerebral ischemia, non-NMDA receptors [kainic acid and α-amino-3-hydroxyl-5-methyl-4-isoxazole-propionate (AMPA)] are activated, and antagonists to these receptors are protective. Experimental brain damage induced by hypoglycemia also is attenuated by NMDA antagonists.

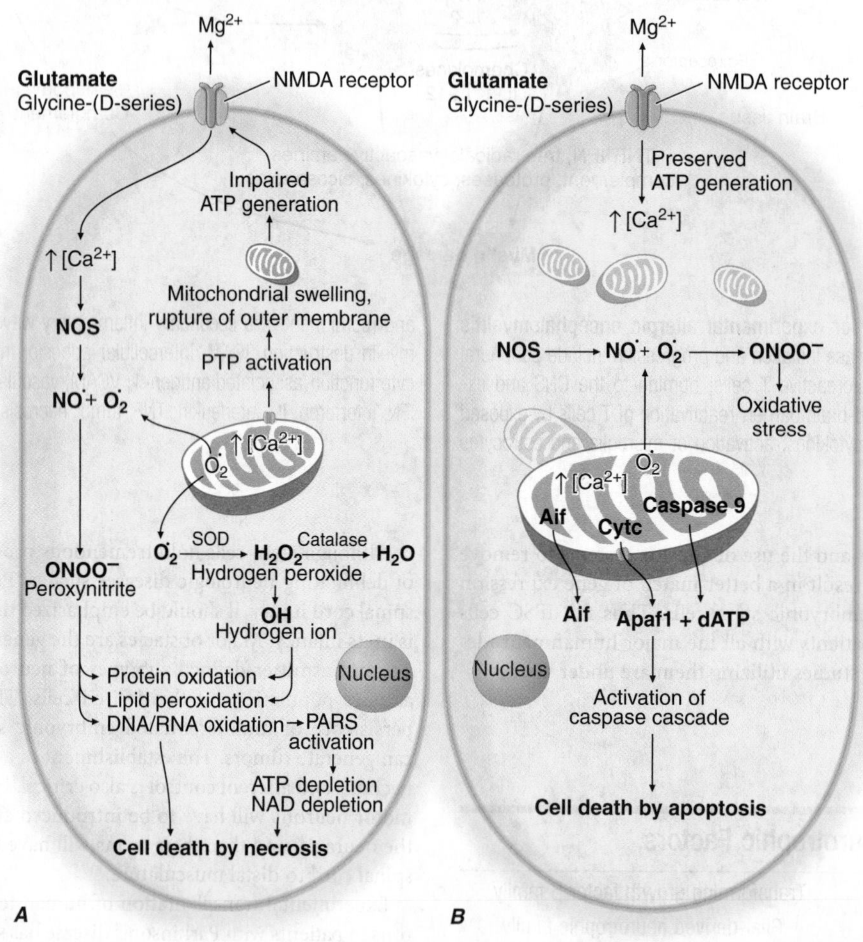

Figure 366-3 Involvement of mitochondria in cell death. A severe excitotoxic insult (***A***) results in cell death by necrosis, whereas a mild excitotoxic insult (***B***) results in apoptosis. After a severe insult (such as ischemia), there is a large increase in glutamate activation of NMDA receptors, an increase in intracellular Ca^{2+} concentrations, activation of nitric oxide synthase (NOS), and increased mitochondrial Ca^{2+} and superoxide generation followed by the formation of $ONOO^-$. This sequence results in damage to cellular macromolecules including DNA, leading to activation of poly-ADP-ribose polymerase (PARS). Both mitochondrial accumulation of Ca^{2+} and oxidative damage lead to activation of the permeability transition pore (PTP) that is linked to excitotoxic cell death. A mild excitotoxic insult can occur due either to an abnormality in an excitotoxicity amino acid receptor, allowing more Ca^{2+} flux, or to impaired functioning of other ionic channels or of energy production, which may allow the voltage-dependent NMDA receptor to be activated by ambient concentrations of glutamate. This event can then lead to increased mitochondrial Ca^{2+} and free radical production, yet relatively preserved ATP generation. The mitochondria may then release cytochrome *c* (Cytc), caspase 9, apoptosis-inducing factor (Aif), and perhaps other mediators that lead to apoptosis. The precise role of the PTP in this mode of cell death is still being clarified, but there does appear to be involvement of the adenine nucleotide transporter that is a key component of the PTP.

Excitotoxicity is not a single event but rather a cascade of cell injury. Excitotoxicity causes influx of calcium into cells, and much of the calcium is sequestered in mitochondria rather than in the cytoplasm. Increased cytoplasmic calcium causes metabolic dysfunction and free radical generation; activates protein kinases, phospholipases, nitric oxide synthase, proteases, and endonucleases; and inhibits protein synthesis. Activation of nitric oxide synthase generates nitric oxide (NO•), which can react with superoxide ($O^{\bullet}_2$) to generate peroxynitrite ($ONOO^-$), which may play a direct role in neuronal injury. Another critical pathway is activation of poly-ADP-ribose polymerase, which occurs in response to free radical–mediated DNA damage. Experimentally, mice with knockout mutations of neuronal nitric oxide synthase or poly-ADP-ribose polymerase, or those which overexpress superoxide dismutase, are resistant to focal ischemia.

Another aspect of excitotoxicity is that it has been demonstrated that stimulation of extrasynaptic NMDA receptors mediates cell death, whereas stimulation of synaptic receptors is protective. This has been shown to play a role in excitotoxicity in transgenic mouse models of Huntington's disease, in which the use of low-dose memantine to selectively block the extrasynaptic receptors is beneficial.

Although excitotoxicity is clearly implicated in the pathogenesis of cell death in stroke, to date treatment with NMDA antagonists has not proved clinically useful. Transient receptor potentials (TRPs) are calcium channels that are activated by oxidative stress in parallel with excitotoxic signal pathways. In addition, glutamate-independent pathways of calcium influx via acid-sensing ion channels have been identified. These channels transport calcium in the setting of acidosis and substrate depletion, and pharmacologic blockade of these channels markedly attenuates stroke injury. These channels offer a potential new therapeutic target for stroke.

Apoptosis, or programmed cell death, plays an important role in both physiologic and pathologic conditions. During embryogenesis, apoptotic pathways operate to destroy neurons that fail to differentiate appropriately or reach their intended targets. There is mounting evidence for an increased rate of apoptotic cell death in a variety of acute and chronic neurologic diseases. Apoptosis is characterized by neuronal shrinkage, chromatin condensation, and DNA fragmentation, whereas necrotic cell death is associated with cytoplasmic and mitochondrial swelling followed by dissolution of the cell membrane. Apoptotic death and necrotic cell death can coexist or be sequential events, depending on the severity of the initiating insult. Cellular energy reserves appear to have an important role in these two forms of cell death, with apoptosis favored under conditions in which ATP levels are preserved. Evidence of DNA fragmentation has been found in a number of degenerative neurologic disorders, including Alzheimer's disease, Huntington's disease, and ALS. The best characterized genetic neurologic disorder related to apoptosis is infantile spinal muscular atrophy (Werdnig-Hoffmann disease), in which two genes thought to be involved in the apoptosis pathways are causative.

Mitochondria are essential in controlling specific apoptosis pathways. The redistribution of cytochrome *c*, as well as apoptosis-inducing factor (AIF), from mitochondria during apoptosis leads to the activation of a cascade of intracellular proteases known as *caspases*. Caspase-independent apoptosis occurs after DNA damage, activation of poly-ADP-ribose polymerase, and translocation of AIF into the nucleus. Redistribution of cytochrome *c* is prevented by overproduction of the apoptotic protein BCL2 and is promoted by the proapoptotic protein BAX. These pathways may be triggered by activation of a large pore in the mitochondrial inner membrane known as the *permeability transition pore*, although in other circumstances they occur independently. Recent studies suggest that blocking the mitochondrial pore reduces both hypoglycemic and ischemic cell death. Mice deficient in cyclophilin D, a key protein involved in opening the permeability transition pore, are resistant to necrosis produced by focal cerebral ischemia.

PROTEIN AGGREGATION AND NEURODEGENERATION

The possibility that protein aggregation plays a role in the pathogenesis of neurodegenerative diseases is a major focus of current research. Protein aggregation is a major histopathologic hallmark of neurodegenerative diseases. Deposition of β-amyloid is strongly implicated in the pathogenesis of Alzheimer's disease. Genetic mutations in familial Alzheimer's disease cause increased production of β-amyloid with 42 amino acids, which has an increased propensity to aggregate, compared with β-amyloid with 40 amino acids. Mutations in genes encoding the MAPT lead to altered splicing of tau and the production of neurofibrillary tangles in frontotemporal dementia and progressive supranuclear palsy. Familial Parkinson's disease is associated with mutations in *leucine-rich repeat kinase 2 (LRRK2), α-synuclein, parkin, PINK1,* and *DJ-1.* PINK1 is a mitochondrial kinase (see below), and DJ-1 is a protein involved in protection from oxidative stress. Parkin, which causes autosomal recessive early-onset Parkinson's disease, is a ubiquitin ligase. The characteristic histopathologic feature of Parkinson's disease is the Lewy body, an eosinophilic cytoplasmic inclusion that contains both neurofilaments and α-synuclein. Huntington's disease and cerebellar degenerations are associated with expansions of polyglutamine repeats in proteins, which aggregate to produce neuronal intranuclear inclusions. Familial ALS is associated with superoxide dismutase mutations and cytoplasmic inclusions that contain superoxide dismutase. An important finding was the discovery that the ubiquinated inclusions observed in most cases of ALS and the most common form of frontotemporal dementia are composed of TAR DNA binding protein 43 (TDP-43). Subsequently, mutations in the TDP-43 gene and in the fused in sarcoma gene (FUS) were found in familial ALS. These two proteins are involved in transcription regulation as well as RNA metabolism. In autosomal dominant neurohypophyseal diabetes insipidus, mutations in vasopressin result in abnormal protein processing, accumulation in the endoplasmic reticulum, and cell death.

Another key mechanism linked to cell death is mitochondrial dynamics, which refer to the processes involved in movement of mitochondria, as well as in mitochondrial fission and fusion, which play a critical role in mitochondrial turnover and in replenishment of damaged mitochondria. Mitochondrial dysfunction is strongly linked to the pathogenesis of a number of neurodegenerative diseases, such as Friedreich's ataxia, which is caused by mutations in an iron-binding protein that plays an important role in transferring iron to iron-sulfur clusters in aconitase and complex I and II of the electron transport chain. Mitochondrial fission is dependent on the dynamin-related proteins (Drp1), which bind to its receptor Fis, whereas mitofuscins 1 and 2 (MF 1/ 2) and optic atrophy protein 1(Opa1) are responsible for fusion of the outer and inner mitochondrial membrane, respectively. Mutations in Mfn2 cause Charcot-Marie-Tooth neuropathy type 2A, and mutations in Opa1 cause autosomal dominant optic atrophy. Both β-amyloid and mutant huntingtin protein induce mitochondrial fragmentation and neuronal cell death associated with increased activity of Drp1. In addition, mutations in genes causing autosomal recessive Parkinson's disease, *parkin* and *PINK1*, cause abnormal mitochondrial morphology and result in impairment of the ability of the cell to remove damaged mitochondria by autophagy.

The current major scientific question is whether protein aggregates contribute to neuronal death or whether they are merely secondary bystanders. A major focus in all the neurodegenerative diseases is now on small protein aggregates termed *oligomers*. These aggregates may be the toxic species of β-amyloid, α-synuclein, and proteins with expanded polyglutamines such as those that are associated with Huntington's disease. Protein aggregates are usually ubiquinated, which targets them for degradation by the 26S component of the proteasome. An inability to degrade protein aggregates could lead to cellular dysfunction, impaired axonal transport, and cell death by apoptotic mechanisms.

Autophagy is the degradation of cystolic components in lysosomes. There is increasing evidence that autophagy plays an important role in degradation of protein aggregates in the neurodegenerative diseases, and it is impaired in Alzheimer's disease (AD), Parkinson's disease, and Huntington's disease (HD). Autophagy is particularly important to the health of neurons, and failure of autophagy contributes to cell death. In Huntington's disease, a failure of cargo recognition occurs, contributing to protein aggregates and cell death. Rapamycin, which induces autophagy, exerts beneficial therapeutic effects in transgenic mouse models of AD, PD, and HD.

In experimental models of Huntington's disease and cerebellar degeneration, protein aggregates are not well correlated with neuronal death and may be protective. A substantial body of evidence suggests that the mutant proteins with polyglutamine expansions in these diseases bind to transcription factors and that this contributes to disease pathogenesis. In Huntington's disease there is dysfunction of the transcriptional co-regulator PGC-1α, a key regulator of mitochondrial biogenesis. There is evidence that impaired function of PGC-1α is also important in both Parkinson's disease and Alzheimer's disease, making it an attractive target for treatments. Agents that upregulate gene transcription are neuroprotective in animal models of these diseases. A number of compounds have been developed to block β-amyloid production and/or aggregation, and these agents are being studied in early clinical trials in humans. Another approach under investigation is immunotherapy with antibodies that bind β-amyloid, tau, or α-synuclein.

Another emerging theme is the role of chronic inflammation, and in particular of activated microglia and innate immunity (Chap 314), in the pathogenesis of many neurodegenerative diseases. Activation of Toll-like receptors (TLR) in response to pattern-recognition signals from damaged or aging cells, including those mediated by heat shock proteins or aggregated proteins, can trigger or amplify pro-inflammatory responses. Familial frontotemporal degeneration (Chap. 371) is caused by mutations in the gene encoding progranulin, a growth factor that regulates inflammation via binding to tumor necrosis factor (TNF) receptors.

SYSTEMS NEUROSCIENCE

Systems neuroscience refers to study of the functions of neurocircuits and the way they relate to brain function, behavior, motor activity, and cognition. Brain imaging techniques, primarily functional MRI (fMRI) and positron emission tomography (PET), have made it possible to investigate cognitive processes such as perception, making judgments, paying attention, and thinking. This has allowed insights into how networks of neurons operate to produce behavior. Many of these studies at present are based on determining the connectivity of neural circuits and how they operate and how this can be modeled to produce improved understanding of physiologic processes. fMRI uses contrast mechanisms related to physiologic changes in tissue, and brain perfusion can be studied by observing the time course of changes in brain water signal as a bolus of injected paramagnetic gadolinium contrast moves through the brain. More recently, to study intrinsic contrast-related local changes in blood oxygenation with brain activity, blood-oxygen-level-dependent (BOLD) contrast has been used to provide a rapid noninvasive approach for functional assessment. These techniques have been used reliably in both behavioral and cognitive sciences. One example is the use of fMRI to demonstrate mirror neuron systems, imitative pathways activated when observing actions of others (Fig. 366-4). Mirror neurons are thought to be important for social conditioning and for many forms of learning, and abnormalities in mirror neurons may underlie some autism disorders. Data also suggest that enhancement of mirror neuron pathways might have potential for rehabilitation after stroke. Other examples of the use of fMRI include the study of memory. Recent studies have shown that not only is hippocampal activity correlated with declarative memory consolidation, it also involves activation in the ventral medial prefrontal cortex. Consolidation of memory over time results in decreased activity of the hippocampus and progressively stronger activation in the ventral medial prefrontal region associated with retrieval of consolidated memories. fMRI also has been utilized to identify sequences of brain activation involved in normal movements and alterations in their activation associated with both injury and recovery and to plan neurosurgical operations. Diffusion tensor imaging is a recently developed MRI technique that can measure macroscopic axonal organization in nervous system tissues; it appears to be useful in assessing myelin and axonal injuries as well as brain development. Advances in understanding neural processing have led to the development of the ability to demonstrate that humans have on-line voluntary control of human temporal lobe neurons.

A further advance that has far-reaching implications for the development of novel interventions for neurologic, including behavioral, conditions has been the development of deep-brain stimulation as a highly effective therapeutic intervention for treating excessively firing neurons in the subthalamic nucleus of patients with Parkinson's disease and the precingulate cortex in patients with depression.

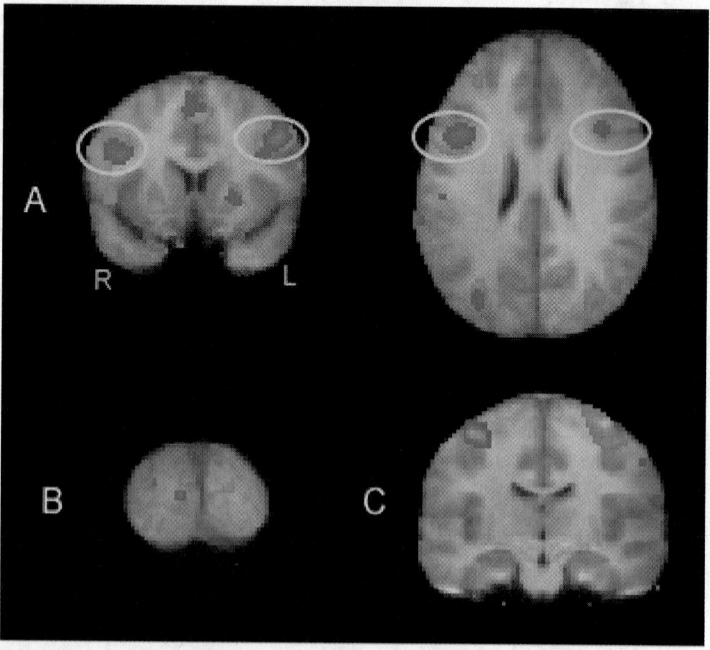

Figure 366-4 Mirror neuron systems are bilaterally activated during imitation. ***A.*** Bilateral activations (circled in yellow) in inferior frontal mirror neuron areas during imitation, as measured by BOLD fMRI signal changes. In red, activation during right hand imitation. In blue, activation during left hand imitation. ***B.*** In contrast, there is lateralized (contralateral) primary visual activation of the primary visual cortex for imitated actions presented to the right visual field (in red, left visual cortex) and to the left visual field (in blue, right visual cortex). ***C.*** Lateralized primary motor activation for hand actions imitated with the right hand (in red, left motor cortex) and with the left hand (in blue, right motor cortex). *(From L Aziz-Zadeh et al: J Neurosci 26:2964, 2006.)*

FURTHER READINGS

Amor S et al: Inflammation in neurodegenerative diseases. Immunology 129:154, 2010

Baranzini SE et al: Genome, epigenome, and RNA sequences of monozygotic twins discordant for multiple sclerosis. Nature 464:1391, 2010

Bilguvar K et al: Whole-exome sequencing identifies recessive WDR62 mutations in severe brain malformations. Nature 467:207, 2010

Catteneo L, Rizzolatti G: The mirror neuron system. Arch Neurol 66:557, 2009

Cerf M et al: Genetic diagnosis by whole exome capture and massively parallel DNA sequencing. Proc Natl Acad Sci USA 106:19096, 2009

Chong SYC, Chan JR: Tapping into the glial reservoir: Cells committed to remaining uncommitted. J Cell Biol 188:305, 2010

Doyle KP et al: Mechanisms of ischemic brain damage. Neuropharmacology 55:310, 2008

Emery B et al: Myelin gene regulatory factor is a critical transcriptional regulator required for CNS myelination. Cell 138:172, 2009

Ercan-Sencicek AG et al: L-histidine decarboxylase and Tourette's syndrome. N Engl J Med 362:1901, 2010

Kriegstein A, Alvarez-Buylla A: The glial nature of embryonic and adult neural stem cells. Annu Rev Neurosci 32:149, 2009

Lukong KE et al: RNA-binding proteins in human genetic disease. Trends Genet. 24:416, 2008

Lupski JR et al: Whole-genome sequencing in a patient with Charcot-Marie-Tooth neuropathy. N Engl J Med 362:1181, 2010

Mackenzie IRA et al: TDP-43 and FUS in amyotrophic lateral sclerosis and frontotemporal dementia. Lancet Neurol 9:995, 2010

Mehler MF: Epigenetics and the nervous system. Ann Neurol 64:602, 2008

Ramocki MB et al: Autism and other neuropsychiatric symptoms are prevalent in individuals with MeCP2 duplication syndrome. Ann Neurol 66:771, 2009

Rosenzweig A: Illuminating the potential of pluripotent stem cells. N Engl J Med 363:1471, 2010

Ryan DP et al: Mutations in potassium channel Kir2.6 cause susceptibility to thyrotoxic hypokalemic periodic paralysis. Cell 140:88, 2010

Tang W et al: The growth factor progranulin binds to TNF receptors and is therapeutic against inflammatory arthritis in mice. Science epub 10 March 2010

Wong E, Cuervo AM: Autophagy gone awry in neurodegenerative diseases. Nat Neurosci 13:805, 2010

Zoghbi HY, Warren ST: Neurogenetics: Advancing the "next-generation" of brain research. Neuron 68:165, 2010

CHAPTER 367

Approach to the Patient With Neurologic Disease

Daniel H. Lowenstein

Joseph B. Martin

Stephen L. Hauser

Neurologic diseases are common and costly. According to recent estimates by the World Health Organization, neurologic disorders affect over 1 billion people worldwide (Table 367-1), constitute 6.3% of the global burden of disease, and cause 12% of global deaths. Most patients with neurologic symptoms seek care from internists and other generalists rather than from neurologists.

TABLE 367-1 Prevalence of Neurologic and Psychiatric Diseases Worldwide

Disorder	Patients, Millions
Nutritional disorders and neuropathies	352
Migraine	326
Trauma	170
Cerebrovascular diseases	61
Epilepsy	50
Dementia	24
Neurologic infections	18

Source: World Health Organization estimates, 2002–2005.

Because therapies now exist for many neurologic disorders, a skillful approach to diagnosis is essential. Errors commonly result from an overreliance on costly neuroimaging procedures and laboratory tests, which, while useful, do not substitute for an adequate history and examination. The proper approach to the patient with a neurologic illness begins with the patient and focuses the clinical problem first in anatomic and then in pathophysiologic terms; only then should a specific diagnosis be entertained. This method ensures that technology is judiciously applied, a correct diagnosis is established in an efficient manner, and treatment is promptly initiated.

THE NEUROLOGIC METHOD

■ LOCATE THE LESION(S)

The first priority is to identify the region of the nervous system that is likely to be responsible for the symptoms. Can the disorder be mapped to one specific location, is it multifocal, or is a diffuse process present? Are the symptoms restricted to the nervous system, or do they arise in the context of a systemic illness? Is the problem in the central nervous system (CNS), the peripheral nervous system (PNS), or both? If in the CNS, is the cerebral cortex, basal ganglia, brainstem, cerebellum, or spinal cord responsible? Are the pain-sensitive meninges involved? If in the PNS, could the disorder be located in peripheral nerves and, if so, are motor or sensory nerves primarily affected, or is a lesion in the neuromuscular junction or muscle more likely?

The first clues to defining the anatomic area of involvement appear in the history, and the examination is then directed to confirm or rule out these impressions and to clarify uncertainties. A more detailed examination of a particular region of the CNS or PNS is often indicated. For example, the examination of a patient who presents with a history of ascending paresthesias and weakness should be directed toward deciding, among other things, if the location of the lesion is in the spinal cord or peripheral nerves. Focal back pain, a spinal cord sensory level, and incontinence suggest a spinal cord origin, whereas a stocking-glove pattern of sensory loss suggests peripheral nerve disease; areflexia usually indicates peripheral neuropathy but may also be present with spinal shock in acute spinal cord disorders.

Deciding "where the lesion is" accomplishes the task of limiting the possible etiologies to a manageable, finite number. In addition, this strategy safeguards against making serious errors. Symptoms of recurrent vertigo, diplopia, and nystagmus should not trigger "multiple sclerosis" as an answer (etiology) but "brainstem" or "pons" (location); then a diagnosis of brainstem arteriovenous malformation will not be missed for lack of consideration. Similarly, the combination of optic neuritis and spastic ataxic paraparesis should initially suggest optic nerve and spinal cord disease; multiple sclerosis (MS), CNS syphilis, and vitamin B_{12} deficiency are treatable disorders that can produce this syndrome. Once the question, "Where is the lesion?" is answered, then the question, "What is the lesion?" can be addressed.

DEFINE THE PATHOPHYSIOLOGY

Clues to the pathophysiology of the disease process may also be present in the history. Primary neuronal (gray matter) disorders may present as early cognitive disturbances, movement disorders, or seizures, whereas white matter involvement produces predominantly "long tract" disorders of motor, sensory, visual, and cerebellar pathways. Progressive and symmetric symptoms often have a metabolic or degenerative origin; in such cases lesions are usually not sharply circumscribed. Thus, a patient with paraparesis and a clear spinal cord sensory level is unlikely to have vitamin B_{12} deficiency as the explanation. A Lhermitte symptom (electric shock–like sensations evoked by neck flexion) is due to ectopic impulse generation in white matter pathways and occurs with demyelination in the cervical spinal cord; among many possible causes, this symptom may indicate MS in a young adult or compressive cervical spondylosis in an older person. Symptoms that worsen after exposure to heat or exercise may indicate conduction block in demyelinated axons, as occurs in MS. A patient with recurrent episodes of diplopia and dysarthria associated with exercise or fatigue may have a disorder of neuromuscular transmission such as myasthenia gravis. Slowly advancing visual scotoma with luminous edges, termed *fortification spectra*, indicates spreading cortical depression, typically with migraine.

THE NEUROLOGIC HISTORY

Attention to the description of the symptoms experienced by the patient and substantiated by family members and others often permits an accurate localization and determination of the probable cause of the complaints, even before the neurologic examination is performed. The history also helps to bring a focus to the neurologic examination that follows. Each complaint should be pursued as far as possible to elucidate the location of the lesion, the likely underlying pathophysiology, and potential etiologies. For example, a patient complains of weakness of the right arm. What are the associated features? Does the patient have difficulty with brushing hair or reaching upward (proximal) or buttoning buttons or opening a twist-top bottle (distal)? Negative associations may also be crucial. A patient with a right hemiparesis without a language deficit likely has a lesion (internal capsule, brainstem, or spinal cord) different from that of a patient with a right hemiparesis and aphasia (left hemisphere). Other pertinent features of the history include the following:

1. *Temporal course of the illness.* It is important to determine the precise time of appearance and rate of progression of the symptoms experienced by the patient. The rapid onset of a neurologic complaint, occurring within seconds or minutes, usually indicates a vascular event, a seizure, or migraine. The onset of sensory symptoms located in one extremity that spread over a few seconds to adjacent portions of that extremity and then to the other regions of the body suggests a seizure. A more gradual onset and less well-localized symptoms point to the possibility of a transient ischemic attack (TIA). A similar but slower temporal march of symptoms accompanied by headache, nausea, or visual disturbance suggests migraine. The presence of "positive" sensory symptoms (e.g., tingling or sensations that are difficult to describe) or involuntary motor movements suggests a seizure; in contrast, transient loss of function (negative symptoms) suggests a TIA. A stuttering onset where symptoms appear, stabilize, and then progress over hours or days also suggests cerebrovascular disease; an additional history of transient remission or regression indicates that the process is more likely due to ischemia rather than hemorrhage. A gradual evolution of symptoms over hours or days suggests a toxic, metabolic, infectious, or inflammatory process. Progressing symptoms associated with the systemic manifestations of fever, stiff neck, and altered level of consciousness imply an infectious process. Relapsing and remitting symptoms involving different levels of the nervous system suggest MS or other inflammatory processes. Slowly progressive symptoms without remissions are characteristic of neurodegenerative disorders, chronic infections, gradual intoxications, and neoplasms.
2. *Patients' descriptions of the complaint.* The same words often mean different things to different patients. "Dizziness" may imply impending syncope, a sense of disequilibrium, or true spinning vertigo. "Numbness" may mean a complete loss of feeling, a positive sensation such as tingling, or even weakness. "Blurred vision" may be used to describe unilateral visual loss, as in transient monocular blindness, or diplopia. The interpretation of the true meaning of the words used by patients to describe symptoms obviously becomes even more complex when there are differences in primary languages and cultures.
3. *Corroboration of the history by others.* It is almost always helpful to obtain additional information from family, friends, or other observers to corroborate or expand the patient's description. Memory loss, aphasia, loss of insight, intoxication, and other factors may impair the patient's capacity to communicate normally with the examiner or prevent openness about factors that have contributed to the illness. Episodes of loss of consciousness necessitate that details be sought from observers to ascertain precisely what has happened during the event.
4. *Family history.* Many neurologic disorders have an underlying genetic component. The presence of a Mendelian disorder, such as Huntington's disease or Charcot-Marie-Tooth neuropathy, is often obvious if family data are available. More detailed questions about family history are often necessary in polygenic disorders such as MS, migraine, and many types of epilepsy. It is important to elicit family history about all illnesses, in addition to neurologic and psychiatric disorders. A familial propensity to hypertension or heart disease is relevant in a patient who presents with a stroke. There are numerous inherited neurologic diseases that are associated with multisystem manifestations that may provide clues to the correct diagnosis (e.g., neurofibromatosis, Wilson's disease, neuro-ophthalmic syndromes).
5. *Medical illnesses.* Many neurologic diseases occur in the context of systemic disorders. Diabetes mellitus, hypertension, and abnormalities of blood lipids predispose to cerebrovascular disease. A solitary mass lesion in the brain may be an abscess in a patient with valvular heart disease, a primary hemorrhage in a patient with a coagulopathy, a lymphoma or toxoplasmosis in a patient with AIDS, or a metastasis in a patient with underlying cancer. Patients with malignancy may also present with a neurologic paraneoplastic syndrome (Chap. 101) or complications from chemotherapy or radiotherapy. Marfan's syndrome and related collagen disorders predispose to dissection of the cranial arteries and aneurysmal subarachnoid hemorrhage; the

latter may also occur with polycystic kidney disease. Various neurologic disorders occur with dysthyroid states or other endocrinopathies. It is especially important to look for the presence of systemic diseases in patients with peripheral neuropathy. Most patients with coma in a hospital setting have a metabolic, toxic, or infectious cause.

6. *Drug use and abuse and toxin exposure.* It is essential to inquire about the history of drug use, both prescribed and illicit. Sedatives, antidepressants, and other psychoactive medications are frequently associated with acute confusional states in the elderly. Aminoglycoside antibiotics may exacerbate symptoms of weakness in patients with disorders of neuromuscular transmission, such as myasthenia gravis, and may cause dizziness secondary to ototoxicity. Vincristine and other antineoplastic drugs can cause peripheral neuropathy, and immunosuppressive agents such as cyclosporine can produce encephalopathy. Excessive vitamin ingestion can lead to disease; for example vitamin A and pseudotumor cerebri, or pyridoxine and peripheral neuropathy. Many patients are unaware that over-the-counter sleeping pills, cold preparations, and diet pills are actually drugs. Alcohol, the most prevalent neurotoxin, is often not recognized as such by patients, and other drugs of abuse such as cocaine and heroin can cause a wide range of neurologic abnormalities. A history of environmental or industrial exposure to neurotoxins may provide an essential clue; consultation with the patient's coworkers or employer may be required.
7. *Formulating an impression of the patient.* Use the opportunity while taking the history to form an impression of the patient. Is the information forthcoming, or does it take a circuitous course? Is there evidence of anxiety, depression, hypochondriasis? Are there any clues to defects in language, memory, insight, or inappropriate behavior? The neurologic assessment begins as soon as the patient comes into the room and the first introduction is made.

THE NEUROLOGIC EXAMINATION

The neurologic examination is challenging and complex; it has many components and includes a number of skills that can be mastered only through repeated use of the same techniques on a large number of individuals with and without neurologic disease. Mastery of the complete neurologic examination is usually important only for physicians in neurology and associated specialties. However, knowledge of the basics of the examination, especially those components that are effective in screening for neurologic dysfunction, is essential for all clinicians, especially generalists.

There is no single, universally accepted sequence of the examination that must be followed, but most clinicians begin with assessment of mental status followed by the cranial nerves, motor system, sensory system, coordination, and gait. Whether the examination is basic or comprehensive, it is essential that it be performed in an orderly and systematic fashion to avoid errors and serious omissions. Thus, the best way to learn and gain expertise in the examination is to choose one's own approach and practice it frequently and do it in the same exact sequence each time.

The detailed description of the neurologic examination that follows describes the more commonly used parts of the examination, with a particular emphasis on the components that are considered most helpful for the assessment of common neurologic problems. Each section also includes a brief description of the minimal examination necessary for adequate screening for abnormalities in a patient who has no symptoms suggesting neurologic dysfunction. A screening examination done in this way can be completed in 3–5 min.

Several additional points about the examination are worth noting. First, in recording observations, it is important to describe what is found rather than to apply a poorly defined medical term (e.g., "patient groans to sternal rub" rather than "obtunded"). Second, subtle CNS abnormalities are best detected by carefully comparing a patient's performance on tasks that require simultaneous activation of both cerebral hemispheres (e.g., eliciting a pronator drift of an outstretched arm with the eyes closed; extinction on one side of bilaterally applied light touch, also with eyes closed; or decreased arm swing or a slight asymmetry when walking). Third, if the patient's complaint is brought on by some activity, reproduce the activity in the office. If the complaint is of dizziness when the head is turned in one direction, have the patient do this and also look for associated signs on examination (e.g., nystagmus or dysmetria). If pain occurs after walking two blocks, have the patient leave the office and walk this distance and immediately return, and repeat the relevant parts of the examination. Finally, the use of tests that are individually tailored to the patient's problem can be of value in assessing changes over time. Tests of walking a 7.5-m (25-ft) distance (normal, 5–6 s; note assistance, if any), repetitive finger or toe tapping (normal, 20–25 taps in 5 s), or handwriting are examples.

MENTAL STATUS EXAMINATION

- *The bare minimum: During the interview, look for difficulties with communication and determine whether the patient has recall and insight into recent and past events.*

The mental status examination is underway as soon as the physician begins observing and talking with the patient. If the history raises any concern for abnormalities of higher cortical function or if cognitive problems are observed during the interview, then detailed testing of the mental status is indicated. The patient's ability to understand the language used for the examination, cultural background, educational experience, sensory or motor problems, or comorbid conditions need to be factored into the applicability of the tests and interpretation of results.

The Folstein mini-mental status examination (MMSE) (Table 371-5) is a standardized screening examination of cognitive function that is extremely easy to administer and takes <10 min to complete. Using age-adjusted values for defining normal performance, the test is ~85% sensitive and 85% specific for making the diagnosis of dementia that is moderate or severe, especially in educated patients. When there is sufficient time available, the MMSE is one of the best methods for documenting the current mental status of the patient, and this is especially useful as a baseline assessment to which future scores of the MMSE can be compared.

Individual elements of the mental status examination can be subdivided into level of consciousness, orientation, speech and language, memory, fund of information, insight and judgment, abstract thought, and calculations.

Level of consciousness is the patient's relative state of awareness of the self and the environment, and ranges from fully awake to comatose. When the patient is not fully awake, the examiner should describe the responses to the minimum stimulus necessary to elicit a reaction, ranging from verbal commands to a brief, painful stimulus such as a squeeze of the trapezius muscle. Responses that are directed toward the stimulus and signify some degree of intact cerebral function (e.g., opening the eyes and looking at the examiner or reaching to push away a painful stimulus) must be distinguished from reflex responses of a spinal origin (e.g., triple flexion response—flexion at the ankle, knee, and hip in response to a painful stimulus to the foot).

Orientation is tested by asking the person to state his or her name, location, and time (day of the week and date); time is usually the first to be affected in a variety of conditions.

Speech is assessed by observing articulation, rate, rhythm, and prosody (i.e., the changes in pitch and accentuation of syllable and words).

Language is assessed by observing the content of the patient's verbal and written output, response to spoken commands, and ability to read. A typical testing sequence is to ask the patient to name successively more detailed components of clothing, a watch or a pen; repeat the phrase "No ifs, ands, or buts"; follow a three-step, verbal command; write a sentence; and read and respond to a written command.

Memory should be analyzed according to three main time scales: (1) immediate memory is assessed by saying a list of three items and having the patient repeat the list immediately, (2) short-term memory is tested by asking the patient to recall the same three items 5 and 15 min later, and (3) long-term memory is evaluated by determining how well the patient is able to provide a coherent chronologic history of his or her illness or personal events.

Fund of information is assessed by asking questions about major historic or current events, with special attention to educational level and life experiences.

Abnormalities of *insight and judgment* are usually detected during the patient interview; a more detailed assessment can be elicited by asking the patient to describe how he or she would respond to situations having a variety of potential outcomes (e.g., "What would you do if you found a wallet on the sidewalk?").

Abstract thought can be tested by asking the patient to describe similarities between various objects or concepts (e.g., apple and orange, desk and chair, poetry and sculpture) or to list items having the same attributes (e.g., a list of four-legged animals).

Calculation ability is assessed by having the patient carry out a computation that is appropriate to the patient's age and education (e.g., serial subtraction of 7 from 100 or 3 from 20; or word problems involving simple arithmetic).

CRANIAL NERVE EXAMINATION

- *The bare minimum: Check the fundi, visual fields, pupil size and reactivity, extraocular movements, and facial movements.*

The cranial nerves (CN) are best examined in numerical order, except for grouping together CN III, IV, and VI because of their similar function.

CN I (olfactory)

Testing is usually omitted unless there is suspicion for inferior frontal lobe disease (e.g., meningioma). With eyes closed, ask the patient to sniff a mild stimulus such as toothpaste or coffee and identify the odorant.

CN II (optic)

Check visual acuity (with eyeglasses or contact lens correction) using a Snellen chart or similar tool. Test the visual fields by confrontation, i.e., by comparing the patient's visual fields to your own. As a screening test, it is usually sufficient to examine the visual fields of both eyes simultaneously; individual eye fields should be tested if there is any reason to suspect a problem of vision by the history or other elements of the examination, or if the screening test reveals an abnormality. Face the patient at a distance of approximately 0.6–1.0 m (2–3 ft) and place your hands at the periphery of your visual fields in the plane that is equidistant between you and the patient. Instruct the patient to look directly at the center of your face and to indicate when and where he or she sees one of your fingers moving. Beginning with the two inferior quadrants and then the two superior quadrants, move your index finger of the right hand, left hand, or both hands simultaneously and observe whether the patient detects the movements. A single small-amplitude movement of the finger is sufficient for a normal response. Focal perimetry and tangent screen examinations should be used to map out visual field defects fully or to search for subtle abnormalities. Optic fundi should be examined with an ophthalmoscope, and the color, size, and degree of swelling or elevation of the optic disc noted, as well as the color and texture of the retina. The retinal vessels should be checked for size, regularity, arterial-venous nicking at crossing points, hemorrhage, exudates, etc.

CN III, IV, VI (oculomotor, trochlear, abducens)

Describe the size and shape of pupils and reaction to light and accommodation (i.e., as the eyes converge while following your finger as it moves toward the bridge of the nose). To check extraocular movements, ask the patient to keep his or her head still while tracking the movement of the tip of your finger. Move the target slowly in the horizontal and vertical planes; observe any paresis, nystagmus, or abnormalities of smooth pursuit (saccades, oculomotor ataxia, etc.). If necessary, the relative position of the two eyes, both in primary and multidirectional gaze, can be assessed by comparing the reflections of a bright light off both pupils. However, in practice it is typically more useful to determine whether the patient describes diplopia in any direction of gaze; true diplopia should almost always resolve with one eye closed. Horizontal nystagmus is best assessed at 45° and not at extreme lateral gaze (which is uncomfortable for the patient); the target must often be held at the lateral position for at least a few seconds to detect an abnormality.

CN V (trigeminal)

Examine sensation within the three territories of the branches of the trigeminal nerve (ophthalmic, maxillary, and mandibular) on each side of the face. As with other parts of the sensory examination, testing of two sensory modalities derived from different anatomic pathways (e.g., light touch and temperature) is sufficient for a screening examination. Testing of other modalities, the corneal reflex, and the motor component of CN V (jaw clench—masseter muscle) is indicated when suggested by the history.

CN VII (facial)

Look for facial asymmetry at rest and with spontaneous movements. Test eyebrow elevation, forehead wrinkling, eye closure, smiling, and cheek puff. Look in particular for differences in the lower versus upper facial muscles; weakness of the lower two-thirds of the face with preservation of the upper third suggests an upper motor neuron lesion, whereas weakness of an entire side suggests a lower motor neuron lesion.

CN VIII (vestibulocochlear)

Check the patient's ability to hear a finger rub or whispered voice with each ear. Further testing for air versus mastoid bone conduction (Rinne) and lateralization of a 512-Hz tuning fork placed at the center of the forehead (Weber) should be done if an abnormality is detected by history or examination. Any suspected problem should be followed up with formal audiometry. For further discussion of assessing vestibular nerve function in the setting of dizziness, hearing loss, or coma, see Chaps. 21, 30, and 274, respectively.

CN IX, X (Glossopharyngeal, Vagus)

Observe the position and symmetry of the palate and uvula at rest and with phonation ("aah"). The pharyngeal ("gag") reflex is evaluated by stimulating the posterior pharyngeal wall on each side with a sterile, blunt object (e.g., tongue blade), but the reflex is often absent in normal individuals.

CN XI (spinal accessory)

Check shoulder shrug (trapezius muscle) and head rotation to each side (sternocleidomastoid) against resistance.

CN XII (hypoglossal)

Inspect the tongue for atrophy or fasciculations, position with protrusion, and strength when extended against the inner surface of the cheeks on each side.

MOTOR EXAMINATION

- *The bare minimum: Look for muscle atrophy and check extremity tone. Assess upper extremity strength by checking for pronator drift and strength of wrist or finger extensors. Tap the biceps, patellar, and Achilles reflexes. Test for lower extremity strength by having the patient walk normally and on heels and toes.*

The motor examination includes observations of muscle appearance, tone, strength, and reflexes. Although gait is in part a test of motor function, it is usually evaluated separately at the end of the examination.

Appearance

Inspect and palpate muscle groups under good light and with the patient in a comfortable and symmetric position. Check for muscle fasciculations, tenderness, and atrophy or hypertrophy. Involuntary movements may be present at rest (e.g., tics, myoclonus, choreoathetosis), during maintained posture (pill-rolling tremor of Parkinson's disease), or with voluntary movements (intention tremor of cerebellar disease or familial tremor).

Tone

Muscle tone is tested by measuring the resistance to passive movement of a relaxed limb. Patients often have difficulty relaxing during this procedure, so it is useful to distract the patient to minimize active movements. In the upper limbs, tone is assessed by rapid pronation and supination of the forearm and flexion and extension at the wrist. In the lower limbs, while the patient is supine the examiner's hands are placed behind the knees and rapidly raised; with normal tone the ankles drag along the table surface for a variable distance before rising, whereas increased tone results in an immediate lift of the heel off the surface. Decreased tone is most commonly due to lower motor neuron or peripheral nerve disorders. Increased tone may be evident as spasticity (resistance determined by the angle and velocity of motion; corticospinal tract disease), rigidity (similar resistance in all angles of motion; extrapyramidal disease), or paratonia (fluctuating changes in resistance; frontal lobe pathways or normal difficulty in relaxing). Cogwheel rigidity, in which passive motion elicits jerky interruptions in resistance, is seen in parkinsonism.

Strength

Testing for pronator drift is an extremely useful method for screening upper limb weakness. The patient is asked to hold both arms fully extended and parallel to the ground with eyes closed. This position should be maintained for ~10 s; any flexion at the elbow or fingers or pronation of the forearm, especially if asymmetric, is a sign of potential weakness. Muscle strength is further assessed by having the patient exert maximal effort for the particular muscle or muscle group being tested. It is important to isolate the muscles as much as possible, i.e., hold the limb so that only the muscles of interest are active. It is also helpful to palpate accessible muscles as they contract. Grading muscle strength and evaluating the patient's effort is an art that takes time and practice. Muscle strength is traditionally graded using the following scale:

0 = no movement
1 = flicker or trace of contraction but no associated movement at a joint
2 = movement with gravity eliminated
3 = movement against gravity but not against resistance
4– = movement against a mild degree of resistance
4 = movement against moderate resistance
4+ = movement against strong resistance
5 = full power

However, in many cases it is more practical to use the following terms:

Paralysis = no movement
Severe weakness = movement with gravity eliminated
Moderate weakness = movement against gravity but not against mild resistance
Mild weakness = movement against moderate resistance
Full strength

Noting the pattern of weakness is as important as assessing the magnitude of weakness. Unilateral or bilateral weakness of the upper limb extensors and lower limb flexors ("pyramidal weakness") suggests a lesion of the pyramidal tract, bilateral proximal weakness suggests myopathy, and bilateral distal weakness suggests peripheral neuropathy.

Reflexes

Muscle stretch reflexes Those that are typically assessed include the biceps (C5, C6), brachioradialis (C5, C6), and triceps (C7, C8) reflexes in the upper limbs and the patellar or quadriceps (L3, L4) and Achilles (S1, S2) reflexes in the lower limbs. The patient should be relaxed and the muscle positioned midway between full contraction and extension. Reflexes may be enhanced by asking the patient to voluntarily contract other, distant muscle groups (Jendrassik maneuver). For example, upper limb reflexes may be reinforced by voluntary teeth-clenching, and the Achilles reflex by hooking the flexed fingers of the two hands together and attempting to pull them apart. For each reflex tested, the two sides should be tested sequentially, and it is important to determine the smallest stimulus required to elicit a reflex rather than the maximum response. Reflexes are graded according to the following scale:

0 = absent
1 = present but diminished
2 = normoactive
3 = exaggerated
4 = clonus

Cutaneous reflexes The plantar reflex is elicited by stroking, with a noxious stimulus such as a tongue blade, the lateral surface of the sole of the foot beginning near the heel and moving across the ball of the foot to the great toe. The normal reflex consists of plantar flexion of the toes. With upper motor neuron lesions above the S1 level of the spinal cord, a paradoxical extension of the toe is observed, associated with fanning and extension of the other toes (termed an *extensor plantar response*, or *Babinski sign*). However, despite its popularity, the reliability and validity of the Babinski sign for identifying upper motor neuron weakness is limited—it is far more useful to rely on tests of tone, strength, stretch reflexes, and coordination. Superficial abdominal reflexes are elicited by gently stroking the abdominal surface near the umbilicus in a diagonal fashion with a sharp object (e.g., the wooden end of a cotton-tipped swab) and observing the movement of the umbilicus. Normally, the umbilicus will pull toward the stimulated quadrant. With upper motor neuron lesions, these reflexes are absent. They are most helpful when there is preservation of the upper (spinal cord level T9) but not lower (T12) abdominal reflexes, indicating a spinal lesion between T9 and T12, or when the response is asymmetric. Other useful cutaneous reflexes include the cremasteric (ipsilateral elevation of the testicle following stroking of the medial thigh; mediated by L1 and L2) and anal (contraction of the anal sphincter when the perianal skin is scratched; mediated by S2, S3, S4) reflexes. It is particularly important to test for these reflexes in any patient with suspected injury to the spinal cord or lumbosacral roots.

Primitive reflexes With disease of the frontal lobe pathways, several primitive reflexes not normally present in the adult may appear. The suck response is elicited by lightly touching the center of the lips, and the root response the corner of the lips, with a tongue blade; the patient will move the lips to suck or root in the direction of the stimulus. The grasp reflex is elicited by touching the palm between the thumb and index finger with the examiner's fingers; a positive response is a forced grasp of the examiner's hand. In many instances stroking the back of the hand will lead to its release. The palmomental response is contraction of the mentalis muscle (chin) ipsilateral to a scratch stimulus diagonally applied to the palm.

Sensory examination

- *The bare minimum: Ask whether the patient can feel light touch and the temperature of a cool object in each distal extremity. Check double simultaneous stimulation using light touch on the hands.*

Evaluating sensation is usually the most unreliable part of the examination, because it is subjective and is difficult to quantify. In the compliant and discerning patient, the sensory examination can be extremely helpful for the precise localization of a lesion. With patients who are uncooperative or lack an understanding of the tests, it may be useless. The examination should be focused on the suspected lesion. For example, in spinal cord, spinal root, or peripheral nerve abnormalities, all major sensory modalities should be tested while looking for a pattern consistent with a spinal level and dermatomal or nerve distribution. In patients with lesions at or above the brainstem, screening the primary sensory modalities in the distal extremities along with tests of "cortical" sensation is usually sufficient.

The five primary sensory modalities—light touch, pain, temperature, vibration, and joint position—are tested in each limb. Light touch is assessed by stimulating the skin with single, very gentle touches of the examiner's finger or a wisp of cotton. Pain is tested using a new pin, and temperature is assessed using a metal object (e.g., tuning fork) that has been immersed in cold and warm water. Vibration is tested using a 128-Hz tuning fork applied to the distal phalanx of the great toe or index finger just below the nail bed. By placing a finger on the opposite side of the joint being tested, the examiner compares the patient's threshold of vibration perception with his or her own. For joint position testing, the examiner grasps the digit or limb laterally and distal to the joint being assessed; small 1- to 2-mm excursions can usually be sensed. The Romberg maneuver is primarily a test of proprioception. The patient is asked to stand with the feet as close together as necessary to maintain balance while the eyes are open, and the eyes are then closed. A loss of balance with the eyes closed is an abnormal response.

"Cortical" sensation is mediated by the parietal lobes and represents an integration of the primary sensory modalities; testing cortical sensation is only meaningful when primary sensation is intact. Double simultaneous stimulation is especially useful as a screening test for cortical function; with the patient's eyes closed, the examiner lightly touches one or both hands and asks the patient to identify the stimuli. With a parietal lobe lesion, the patient may be unable to identify the stimulus on the contralateral side when both hands are touched. Other modalities relying on the parietal cortex include the discrimination of two closely placed stimuli as separate (two-point discrimination), identification of an object by touch and manipulation alone (stereognosis), and the identification of numbers or letters written on the skin surface (graphesthesia).

COORDINATION EXAMINATION

- *The bare minimum: Test rapid alternating movements of the hands and the finger-to-nose and heel-knee-shin maneuvers.*

Coordination refers to the orchestration and fluidity of movements. Even simple acts require cooperation of agonist and antagonist muscles, maintenance of posture, and complex servomechanisms to control the rate and range of movements. Part of this integration relies on normal function of the cerebellar and basal ganglia systems. However, coordination also requires intact muscle strength and kinesthetic and proprioceptive information. Thus, if the examination has disclosed abnormalities of the motor or sensory systems, the patient's coordination should be assessed with these limitations in mind.

Rapid alternating movements in the upper limbs are tested separately on each side by having the patient make a fist, partially extend the index finger, and then tap the index finger on the distal thumb as quickly as possible. In the lower limb, the patient rapidly taps the foot against the floor or the examiner's hand. Finger-to-nose testing is primarily a test of cerebellar function; the patient is asked to touch his or her index finger repetitively to the nose and then to the examiner's outstretched finger, which moves with each repetition. A similar test in the lower extremity is to have the patient raise the leg and touch the examiner's finger with the great toe. Another cerebellar test in the lower limbs is the heel-knee-shin maneuver; in the supine position the patient is asked to slide the heel of each foot from the knee down the shin of the other leg. For all these movements, the accuracy, speed, and rhythm are noted.

GAIT EXAMINATION

- *The bare minimum: Observe the patient while walking normally, on the heels and toes, and along a straight line.*

Watching the patient walk is the most important part of the neurologic examination. Normal gait requires that multiple systems—including strength, sensation, and coordination—function in a highly integrated fashion. Unexpected abnormalities may be detected that prompt the examiner to return in more detail to other aspects of the examination. The patient should be observed while walking and turning normally, walking on the heels, walking on the toes, and walking heel-to-toe along a straight line. The examination may reveal decreased arm swing on one side (corticospinal tract disease), a stooped posture and short-stepped gait (parkinsonism), a broad-based unstable gait (ataxia), scissoring (spasticity), or a high-stepped, slapping gait (posterior column or peripheral nerve disease), or the patient may appear to be stuck in place (apraxia with frontal lobe disease).

NEUROLOGIC DIAGNOSIS

The clinical data obtained from the history and examination are interpreted to arrive at an anatomic localization that best explains the clinical findings (Table 367-2), to narrow the list of diagnostic

TABLE 367-2 Findings Helpful for Localization Within the Nervous System

	Signs
Cerebrum	Abnormal mental status or cognitive impairment
	Seizures
	Unilateral weakness[a] and sensory abnormalities including head and limbs
	Visual field abnormalities
	Movement abnormalities (e.g., diffuse incoordination, tremor, chorea)
Brainstem	Isolated cranial nerve abnormalities (single or multiple)
	"Crossed" weakness[a] and sensory abnormalities of head and limbs, e.g., weakness of right face and left arm and leg
Spinal cord	Back pain or tenderness
	Weakness[a] and sensory abnormalities sparing the head
	Mixed upper and lower motor neuron findings
	Sensory level
	Sphincter dysfunction
Spinal roots	Radiating limb pain
	Weakness[b] or sensory abnormalities following root distribution (see Figs. 23-2 and 23-3)
	Loss of reflexes
Peripheral nerve	Mid or distal limb pain
	Weakness[b] or sensory abnormalities following nerve distribution (see Figs. 23-2 and 23-3)
	"Stocking or glove" distribution of sensory loss
	Loss of reflexes
Neuromuscular junction	Bilateral weakness including face (ptosis, diplopia, dysphagia) and proximal limbs
	Increasing weakness with exertion
	Sparing of sensation
Muscle	Bilateral proximal or distal weakness
	Sparing of sensation

[a]Weakness along with other abnormalities having an "upper motor neuron" pattern, i.e., spasticity, weakness of extensors > flexors in the upper extremity and flexors > extensors in the lower extremity, hyperreflexia.
[b]Weakness along with other abnormalities having a "lower motor neuron" pattern, i.e., flaccidity and hyporeflexia.

possibilities, and to select the laboratory tests most likely to be informative. The laboratory assessment may include (1) serum electrolytes; complete blood count; and renal, hepatic, endocrine, and immune studies; (2) cerebrospinal fluid examination; (3) focused neuroimaging studies (Chap. 368); or (4) electrophysiologic studies (Chap. e45). The anatomic localization, mode of onset and course of illness, other medical data, and laboratory findings are then integrated to establish an etiologic diagnosis.

The neurologic examination may be normal even in patients with a serious neurologic disease, such as seizures, chronic meningitis, or a TIA. A comatose patient may arrive with no available history, and in such cases the approach is as described in Chap. 274. In other patients, an inadequate history may be overcome by a succession of examinations from which the course of the illness can be inferred. In perplexing cases it is useful to remember that uncommon presentations of common diseases are more likely than rare etiologies. Thus, even in tertiary care settings, multiple strokes are usually due to emboli and not vasculitis, and dementia with myoclonus is usually Alzheimer's disease and not due to a prion disorder or a paraneoplastic cause. Finally, the most important task of a primary care physician faced with a patient who has a new neurologic complaint is to assess the urgency of referral to a specialist. Here, the imperative is to rapidly identify patients likely to have nervous system infections, acute strokes, and spinal cord compression or other treatable mass lesions and arrange for immediate care.

FURTHER READINGS

Blumenthal H: *Neuroanatomy Through Clinical Cases,* 2nd ed. Sunderland, MA, Sinauer, 2010

Campbell WW: *DeJong's The Neurological Examination,* 6th ed. Philadelphia, Lippincott Williams & Wilkins, 2005

Ropper AH, Samuels M: *Adams and Victor's Principles of Neurology,* 9th ed. New York, McGraw-Hill, 2009

CHAPTER 368 Neuroimaging in Neurologic Disorders

William P. Dillon

The clinician caring for patients with neurologic symptoms is faced with myriad imaging options, including computed tomography (CT), CT angiography (CTA), perfusion CT (pCT), magnetic resonance imaging (MRI), MR angiography (MRA), functional MRI (fMRI), MR spectroscopy (MRS), MR neurography (MRN), diffusion and diffusion track imaging (DTI), susceptibility weighted MR imaging (SWI), and perfusion MRI (pMRI). In addition, an increasing number of interventional neuroradiologic techniques are available, including angiography catheter embolization, coiling, and stenting of vascular structures; and spine diagnostic and interventional techniques such as diskography, transforaminal and translaminar epidural and nerve root injections and blood patches. Recent developments such as multidetector CTA (MDCTA) and gadolinium-enhanced MRA, have narrowed the indications for conventional angiography, which is now reserved for patients in whom small-vessel detail is essential for diagnosis or for whom concurrent interventional therapy is planned (Table 368-1).

In general, MRI is more sensitive than CT for the detection of lesions affecting the central nervous system (CNS), particularly those of the spinal cord, cranial nerves, and posterior fossa structures. Diffusion MR, a sequence sensitive to the microscopic motion of water, is the most sensitive technique for detecting acute ischemic stroke of the brain or spinal cord, and it is also useful in the detection of encephalitis, abscesses, and prion diseases. CT, however, is quickly acquired and is widely available, making it a pragmatic choice for the initial evaluation of patients with acute changes in mental status, suspected acute stroke, hemorrhage, and intracranial or spinal trauma. CT is also more sensitive than MRI for visualizing fine osseous detail and is indicated in the initial evaluation of conductive hearing loss as well as lesions affecting the skull base and calvarium. MR may, however, add important diagnostic information regarding bone marrow infiltrative processes that are difficult to detect on CT.

COMPUTED TOMOGRAPHY

TECHNIQUE

The CT image is a cross-sectional representation of anatomy created by a computer-generated analysis of the attenuation of x-ray beams passed through a section of the body. As the x-ray beam, collimated to the desired slice width, rotates around the patient, it passes through selected regions in the body. X-rays that are not attenuated by body structures are detected by sensitive x-ray detectors aligned 180° from the x-ray tube. A computer calculates a "back projection" image from the 360° x-ray attenuation profile. Greater x-ray attenuation (e.g., as caused by bone), results in areas of high "density," while soft tissue structures that have poor attenuation of x-rays such as organs and air-filled cavities, are lower in density. The resolution of an image depends on the radiation dose, the detector size, collimation (slice thickness), the field of view, and the matrix size of the display. A modern CT scanner is capable of

TABLE 368-1 Guidelines for the Use of CT, Ultrasound, and MRI

Condition	Recommended Technique
Hemorrhage	
Acute parenchymal	CT, MR
Subacute/chronic	MRI
Subarachnoid hemorrhage	CT, CTA, lumbar puncture → angiography
Aneurysm	Angiography > CTA, MRA
Ischemic infarction	
Hemorrhagic infarction	CT or MRI
Bland infarction	MRI > CT, CTA, angiography
Carotid or vertebral dissection	MRI/MRA
Vertebral basilar insufficiency	CTA, MRI/MRA
Carotid stenosis	CTA > Doppler ultrasound, MRA
Suspected mass lesion	
Neoplasm, primary or metastatic	MRI + contrast
Infection/abscess	MRI + contrast
Immunosuppressed with focal findings	MRI + contrast
Vascular malformation	MRI ± angiography
White matter disorders	MRI
Demyelinating disease	MRI ± contrast
Dementia	MRI > CT
Trauma	
Acute trauma	CT (noncontrast)
Shear injury/chronic hemorrhage	MRI + gradient echo imaging
Headache/migraine	CT (noncontrast) / MRI
Seizure	
First time, no focal neurologic deficits	?CT as screen ± contrast
Partial complex/refractory	MRI with coronal T2W imaging
Cranial neuropathy	MRI with contrast
Meningeal disease	MRI with contrast
Spine	
Low back pain	
No neurologic deficits	MRI or CT after 4 weeks
With focal deficits	MRI > CT
Spinal stenosis	MRI or CT
Cervical spondylosis	MRI or CT myelography
Infection	MRI + contrast, CT
Myelopathy	MRI + contrast
Arteriovenous malformation	MRI, angiography

Abbreviations: CT, computed tomography; CTA, CT angiography; MRA, MR angiography; MRI, magnetic resonance imaging; T2W, T2-weighted.

obtaining sections as thin as 0.5–1 mm with submillimeter resolution at a speed of 0.3–1 s per rotation; complete studies of the brain can be completed in 2–10 s.

Multidetector CT (MDCT) is now standard in most radiology departments. Single or multiple (from 4 to 256) detectors positioned 180° to the x-ray source result in multiple slices per revolution of the beam around the patient. The table moves continuously through the rotating x-ray beam, generating a continuous "helix" of information that can be reformatted into various slice thicknesses and planes. Advantages of MDCT include shorter scan times, reduced patient and organ motion, and the ability to acquire images dynamically during the infusion of intravenous contrast that can be used to construct CT angiograms of vascular structures and CT perfusion images (Fig. 368-1*B* and *C*). CTA images are post-processed for display in three dimensions to yield angiogram-like images (Fig. 368-1*C*, 368-2 *E* and *F*, and see Fig. 370-4). CTA has proved useful in assessing the cervical and intracranial arterial and venous anatomy.

Intravenous iodinated contrast is often administered prior to or during a CT study to identify vascular structures and to detect defects in the blood-brain barrier (BBB) that are associated with disorders such as tumors, infarcts, and infections. In the normal CNS, only vessels and structures lacking a BBB (e.g., the pituitary gland, choroid plexus, and dura) enhance after contrast administration. The use of iodinated contrast agents carries a small risk of allergic reaction and adds additional expense. While helpful in characterizing mass lesions as well as essential for the acquisition of CTA studies, the decision to use contrast material should always be considered carefully.

INDICATIONS

CT is the primary study of choice in the evaluation of an acute change in mental status, focal neurologic findings, acute trauma to the brain and spine, suspected subarachnoid hemorrhage, and conductive hearing loss (Table 368-1). CT is complementary to MR in the evaluation of the skull base, orbit, and osseous structures of the spine. In the spine, CT is useful in evaluating patients with osseous spinal stenosis and spondylosis, but MRI is often preferred in those with neurologic deficits. CT can also be obtained following intrathecal contrast injection to evaluate the intracranial cisterns (*CT cisternography*) for cerebrospinal fluid (CSF) fistula, as well as the spinal subarachnoid space (*CT myelography*).

COMPLICATIONS

CT is safe, fast, and reliable. Radiation exposure depends on the dose used but is normally between 2 and 5 mSv (millisievert) for a routine brain CT study. Care must be taken to reduce exposure when imaging children. With the advent of MDCT, CTA, and CT perfusion, care must be taken to appropriately minimize radiation dose whenever possible. Advanced software that permits noise reduction may permit lower radiation doses. The most frequent complications are associated with use of intravenous contrast agents. Two broad categories of contrast media, ionic and nonionic, are in use. Although ionic agents are relatively safe and inexpensive, they are associated with a higher incidence of reactions and side effects. As a result, ionic agents have been largely replaced by safer nonionic compounds.

Contrast nephropathy may result from hemodynamic changes, renal tubular obstruction and cell damage, or immunologic reactions to contrast agents. A rise in serum creatinine of at least 85 μmol/L (1 mg/dL) within 48 hours of contrast administration is often used as a definition of contrast nephropathy, although other causes of acute renal failure must be excluded. The prognosis is usually favorable, with serum creatinine levels returning to baseline within 1–2 weeks. Risk factors for contrast nephropathy include advanced age (>80 years), preexisting renal disease (serum creatinine exceeding 2 mg/dL), solitary kidney, diabetes mellitus, dehydration, paraproteinemia, concurrent use of nephrotoxic medication or chemotherapeutic agents, and high contrast dose. Patients with diabetes and those with mild renal failure should be well hydrated prior to the administration of contrast agents, although careful consideration should be given to alternative imaging techniques such as MR imaging or noncontrast CT or ultrasound (US) examinations. Nonionic, low-osmolar media produce fewer abnormalities in renal blood flow and less endothelial cell damage but should still be used carefully in patients at risk for allergic reaction. Estimated glomerular filtration rate (eGFR)

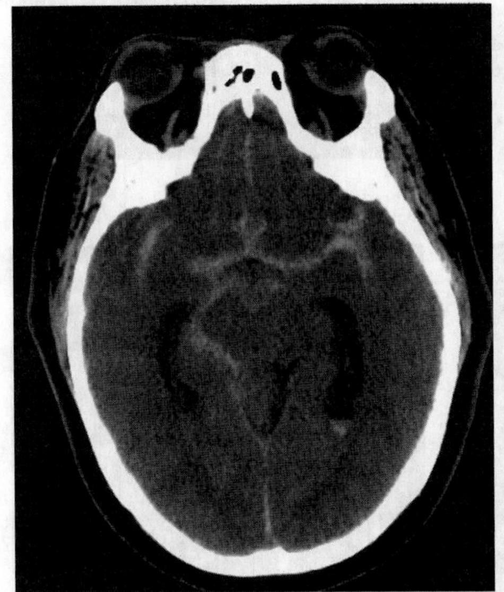

A

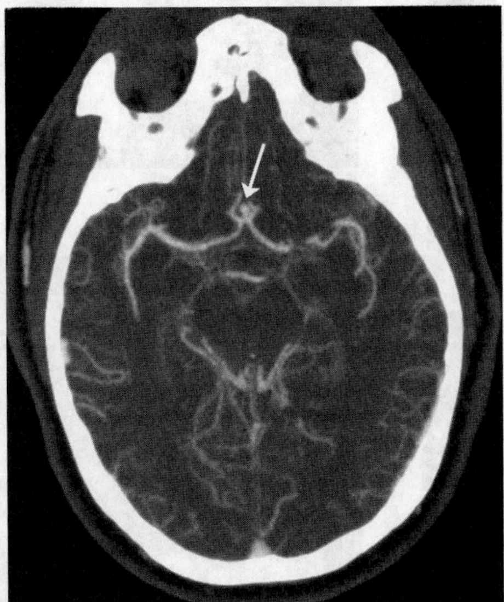

B

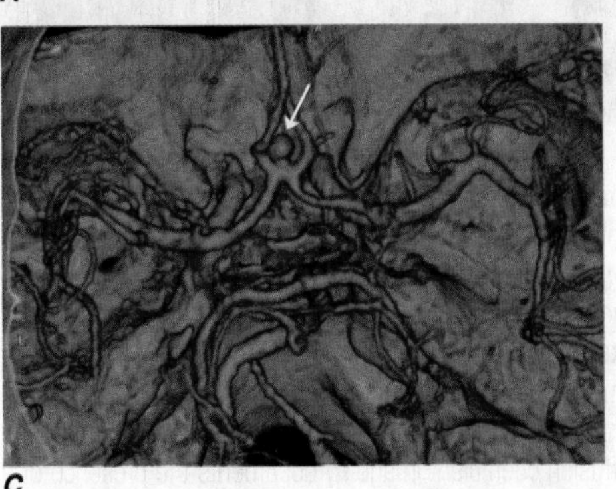

C

Figure 368-1 CT angiography (CTA) of ruptured anterior cerebral artery aneurysm in a patient presenting with acute headache. ***A.*** Noncontrast CT demonstrates subarachnoid hemorrhage and mild obstructive hydrocephalus. ***B.*** Axial maximum-intensity projection from CT angiography demonstrates enlargement of the anterior cerebral artery (*arrow*). ***C.*** 3D surface reconstruction using a workstation confirms the anterior cerebral aneurysm and demonstrates its orientation and relationship to nearby vessels (*arrow*). CTA image is produced by 0.5- 1-mm helical CT scans performed during a rapid bolus infusion of intravenous contrast medium.

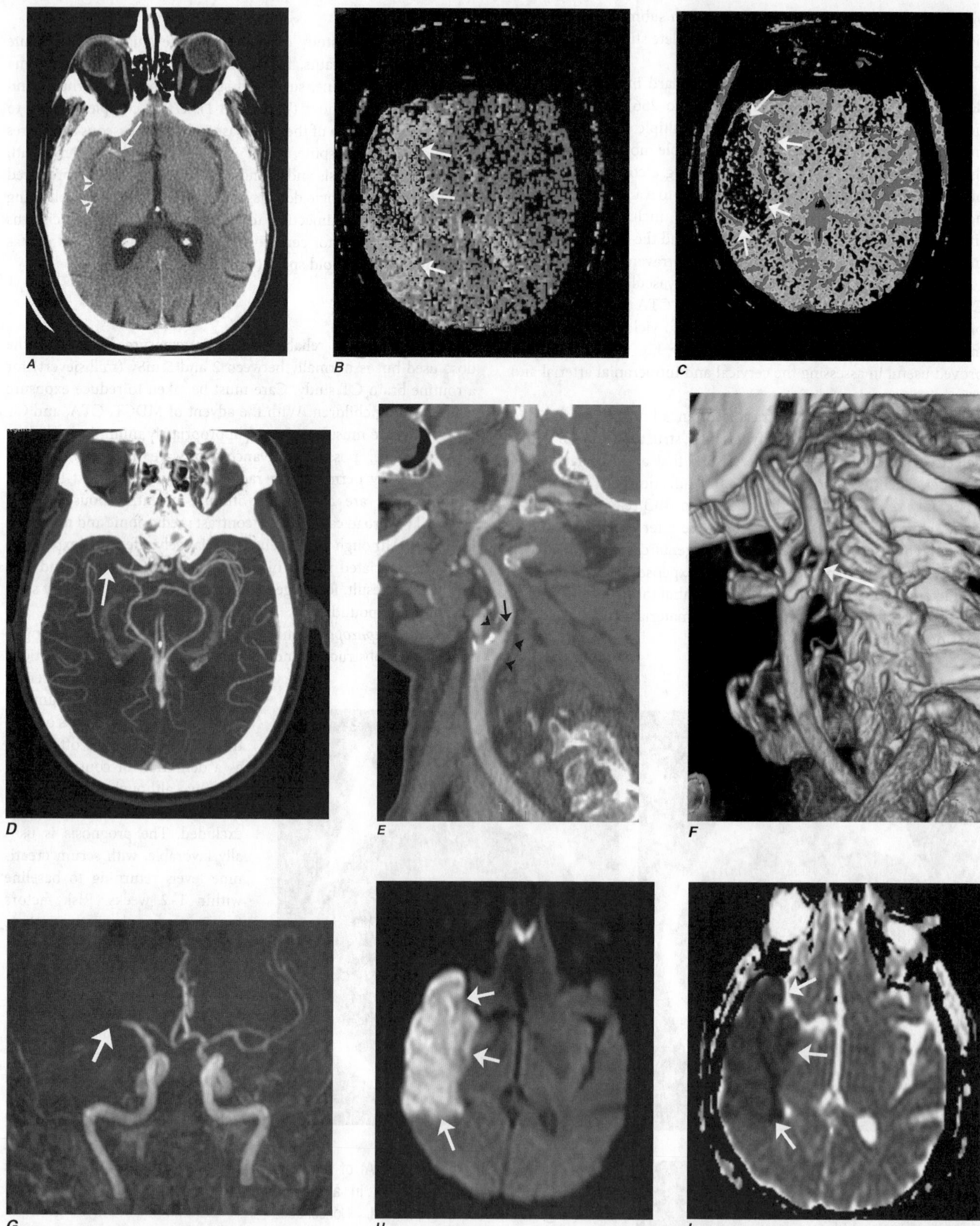

Figure 368-2 Acute left hemiparesis due to middle cerebral artery occlusion. ***A***. Axial noncontrast CT scan demonstrates high density within the right middle cerebral artery (*arrow*) associated with subtle low density involving the right putamen (*arrowheads*). ***B***. Mean transit time CT perfusion parametric map indicating prolonged mean transit time involving the right middle cerebral territory (*arrows*). ***C***. Cerebral blood volume map shows reduced CBV involving an area within the defect shown in ***B***, indicating a high likelihood of infarction (*arrows*). ***D***. Axial maximum-intensity projection from a CTA study through the circle of Willis demonstrates an abrupt occlusion of the proximal right middle cerebral artery (*arrow*). ***E***. Sagittal reformation through the right internal carotid artery demonstrates a low-density lipid-laden plaque (*arrowheads*) narrowing the lumen (*black arrow*) ***F***. 3D surface-rendered CTA image demonstrates calcification and narrowing of the right internal carotid artery (*arrow*), consistent with atherosclerotic disease. ***G***. Coronal maximum-intensity projection from MRA shows right middle cerebral artery (MCA) occlusion (*arrow*). ***H***. and ***I***. Axial diffusion-weighted image (***H***) and apparent diffusion coefficient image (***I***) documents the presence of a right middle cerebral artery infarction.

TABLE 368-2 Guidelines for Premedication of Patients With Prior Contrast Allergy

12 h prior to examination:

Prednisone, 50 mg PO *or* methylprednisolone, 32 mg PO

2 h prior to examination:

Prednisone, 50 mg PO *or* methylprednisolone, 32 mg PO *and*

Cimetidine, 300 mg PO *or* ranitidine, 150 mg PO

Immediately prior to examination:

Benadryl, 50 mg IV (alternatively, can be given PO 2 h prior to exam)

is a more reliable indicator of renal function compared to creatinine alone as it takes into account age, race and sex. In one study, 15% of outpatients with a normal serum creatinine had an estimated creatinine clearance of 50 mL/min/1.73 m^2 or less (normal is 90 mL/min/1.73 m^2 or more). The exact eGFR threshold, below which withholding intravenous contrast should be considered, is controversial. The risk of contrast nephropathy increases in patients with an eGFR <60 mL/min/1.73^2; however the majority of these patients will only have a temporary rise in creatinine. The risk of dialysis after receiving contrast significantly increases in patients with eGFR <30 mL/min/1.73^2. Thus, an eGFR threshold between 60 and 30 mL/min/1.73^2 is appropriate; however the exact number is somewhat arbitrary. A creatinine of 1.6 in a 70-year-old, non-African-American male corresponds to an eGFR of approximately 45 mL/min/1.73^2. The American College of Radiology suggests using an eGFR of 45 as a threshold below which iodinated contrast should not be given without serious consideration of the potential for contrast nephropathy. If contrast must be administered to a patient with an eGRF below 45, the patient should be well hydrated, and a reduction in the dose of contrast should be considered. Use of other agents such as bicarbonate and acetylcysteine may reduce the incidence of contrast nephropathy. Other side effects of CT scanning are rare but include a sensation of warmth throughout the body and a metallic taste during intravenous administration of iodinated contrast media. The most serious side effects are anaphylactic reactions, which range from mild hives to bronchospasm, acute anaphylaxis, and death. The pathogenesis of these allergic reactions is not fully understood but is thought to include the release of mediators such as histamine, antibody-antigen reactions, and complement activation. Severe allergic reactions occur in ~0.04% of patients receiving nonionic media, sixfold lower than with ionic media. Risk factors include a history of prior contrast reaction, food allergies to shellfish, and atopy (asthma and hay fever). In such patients, a noncontrast CT or MRI procedure should be considered as an alternative to contrast administration. If iodinated contrast is absolutely required, a nonionic agent should be used in conjunction with pretreatment with glucocorticoids and antihistamines (Table 368-2). Patients with allergic reactions to iodinated contrast material do not usually react to gadolinium-based MR contrast material, although such reactions can occur. It would be wise to pretreat patients with a prior allergic history to MR contrast administration in a similar fashion.

MAGNETIC RESONANCE IMAGING

TECHNIQUE

MRI is a complex interaction between hydrogen protons in biologic tissues, a static magnetic field (the magnet), and energy in the form of radiofrequency (Rf) waves of a specific frequency introduced by coils placed next to the body part of interest. Images are made by computerized processing of resonance information received from protons in the body. Field strength of the magnet is directly related to signal-to-noise ratio. While 1.5-Telsa magnets have become the standard high-field MRI units, 3T–8T magnets are now available and have distinct advantages in the brain and musculoskeletal systems. Spatial localization is achieved by magnetic gradients surrounding the main magnet, which impart slight changes in magnetic field throughout the imaging volume. Rf pulses transiently excite the energy state of the hydrogen protons in the body. Rf is administered at a frequency specific for the field strength of the magnet. The subsequent return to equilibrium energy state (*relaxation*) of the hydrogen protons results in a release of Rf energy (the *echo*), which is detected by the coils that delivered the Rf pulses. The echo is transformed by Fourier analysis into the information used to form an MR image. The MR image thus consists of a map of the distribution of hydrogen protons, with signal intensity imparted by both density of hydrogen protons as well as differences in the relaxation times (see below) of hydrogen protons on different molecules. While clinical MRI currently makes use of the ubiquitous hydrogen proton, research into sodium and carbon imaging appears promising.

T1 and T2 relaxation times

The rate of return to equilibrium of perturbed protons is called the *relaxation rate*. The relaxation rate varies among normal and pathologic tissues. The relaxation rate of a hydrogen proton in a tissue is influenced by local interactions with surrounding molecules and atomic neighbors. Two relaxation rates, T1 and T2, influence the signal intensity of the image. The T1 relaxation time is the time, measured in milliseconds, for 63% of the hydrogen protons to return to their normal equilibrium state, while the T2 relaxation is the time for 63% of the protons to become dephased owing to interactions among nearby protons. The intensity of the signal within various tissues and image contrast can be modulated by altering acquisition parameters such as the interval between Rf pulses (TR) and the time between the Rf pulse and the signal reception (TE). So-called T1-weighted (T1W) images are produced by keeping the TR and TE relatively short. T2-weighted (T2W) images are produced by using longer TR and TE times. Fat and subacute hemorrhage have relatively shorter T1 relaxation rates and thus higher signal intensity than brain on T1W images. Structures containing more water such as CSF and edema, have long T1 and T2 relaxation rates, resulting in relatively lower signal intensity on T1W images and a higher signal intensity on T2W images (Table 368-3). Gray matter contains 10–15% more water than white matter, which accounts for much of the intrinsic contrast between the two on MRI (Fig. 368-6B). T2W images are more sensitive than T1W images to

TABLE 368-3 Some Common Intensities on T1- and T2-Weighted MRI Sequences

			Signal Intensity			
Image	TR	TE	CSF	Fat	Brain	Edema
T1W	Short	Short	Low	High	Low	Low
T2W	Long	Long	High	Low	High	High
FLAIR (T2)	Long	Long	Low	Medium	High	High

Abbreviations: CSF, cerebrospinal fluid; TE, interval between Rf pulse and signal reception; TR, interval between radiofrequency (Rf) pulses; T1W and T2W, T1- and T2-weighted.

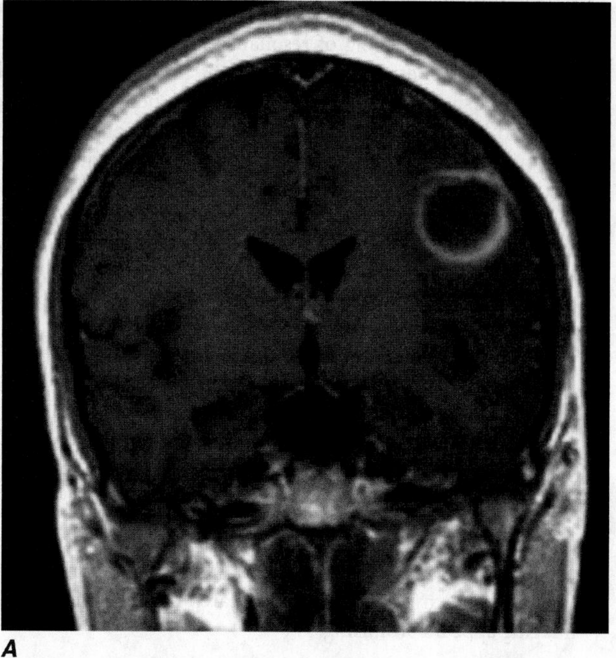

A

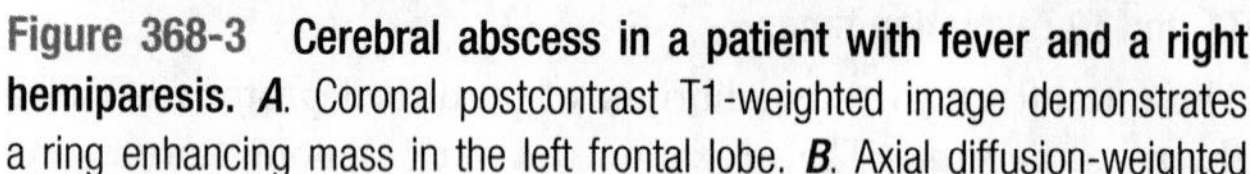

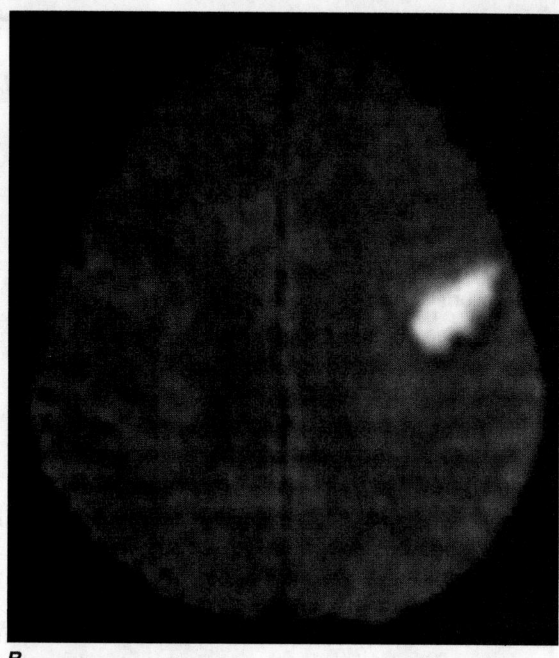

B

Figure 368-3 Cerebral abscess in a patient with fever and a right hemiparesis. ***A.*** Coronal postcontrast T1-weighted image demonstrates a ring enhancing mass in the left frontal lobe. ***B.*** Axial diffusion-weighted image demonstrates restricted diffusion (high signal intensity) within the lesion, which in this setting is highly suggestive of cerebral abscess.

edema, demyelination, infarction, and chronic hemorrhage, while T1W imaging is more sensitive to subacute hemorrhage and fat-containing structures.

Many different MR pulse sequences exist, and each can be obtained in various planes (Figs. 368-2, 368-3, 368-4). The selection of a proper protocol that will best answer a clinical question depends on an accurate clinical history and indication for the examination. Fluid-attenuated inversion recovery (FLAIR) is a useful pulse sequence that produces T2W images in which the normally high signal intensity of CSF is suppressed (Fig. 368-6*B*). FLAIR images are more sensitive than standard spin echo images for any water-containing lesions or edema. Susceptibility weighted imaging such as gradient echo imaging, is most sensitive to magnetic susceptibility generated by blood, calcium, and air and is indicated in patients suspected of pathology that might result in microhemorrhages (Fig. 368-5*C*). MR images can be generated in any plane without changing the patient's position. Each sequence, however, must be obtained separately and takes 1–10 minutes on average to complete. Three-dimensional volumetric imaging is also possible with MRI, resulting in a 3D volume of data that can be reformatted in any orientation to highlight certain disease processes.

MR contrast material

The heavy-metal element gadolinium forms the basis of all currently approved intravenous MR contrast agents. Gadolinium is a paramagnetic substance, which means that it reduces the T1 and T2 relaxation times of nearby water protons, resulting in a high signal on T1W images and a low signal on T2W images (the latter requires a sufficient local concentration, usually in the form of an intravenous bolus). Unlike iodinated contrast agents, the effect of MR contrast agents depends on the presence of local hydrogen protons on which it must act to achieve the desired effect. Gadolinium is chelated to DTPA (diethylenetriaminepentaacetic acid), which allows safe renal excretion. Approximately 0.2 mL/kg body weight is administered intravenously; the cost is ~$60 per dose. Gadolinium-DTPA does not normally cross the intact BBB immediately but will enhance lesions lacking a BBB (Fig. 368-3*A*) and areas of the brain that normally are devoid of the BBB (pituitary, choroid plexus). However, gadolinium contrast has been noted to slowly cross an intact BBB if given over time and especially in the setting of reduced renal clearance. The agents are generally well tolerated; severe allergic reactions are rare but have been reported. The adverse reaction rate in patients with a prior history of atopy or asthma is 3.7%; however, the reaction rate increases to 6.3% in those patients with a prior history of unspecified allergic reaction to iodinated contrast agents. Gadolinium contrast material can be administered safely to children as well as adults, although these agents are generally avoided in those under 6 months of age. Renal failure does not occur.

A rare complication, nephrogenic systemic fibrosis (NSF), has recently been reported in patients with renal insufficiency who have been exposed to gadolinium contrast agents. The onset of NSF has been reported between 5 and 75 days following exposure; histologic features include thickened collagen bundles with surrounding clefts, mucin deposition, and increased numbers of fibrocytes and elastic fibers in skin. In addition to dermatologic symptoms, other manifestations include widespread fibrosis of the skeletal muscle, bone, lungs, pleura, pericardium, myocardium, kidney, muscle, bone, testes, and dura. For this reason, the American College of Radiology recommends that prior to elective gadolinium-based MR contrast agent (GBMCA) administration, a recent (e.g., past 6 weeks') glomerular filtration rate (GFR) assessment be obtained in patients with a history of:

1. Renal disease (including solitary kidney, renal transplant, renal tumor)
2. Age >60 years
3. History of hypertension
4. History of diabetes
5. History of severe hepatic disease/liver transplant/pending liver transplant: for these patients it is recommended that the patient's GFR assessment be nearly contemporaneous with the MR examination.

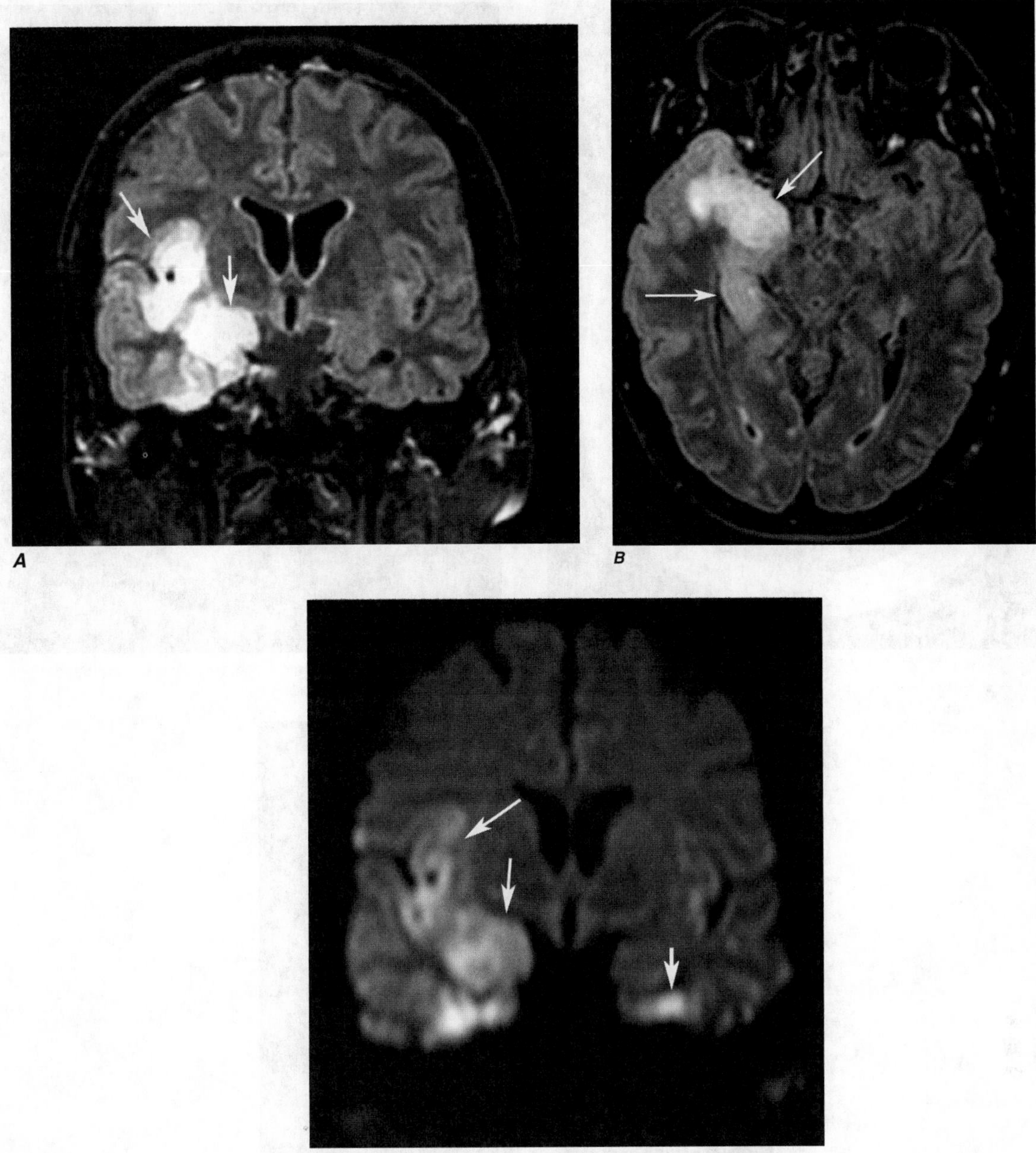

Figure 368-4 Herpes simplex encephalitis in a patient presenting with altered mental status and fever. ***A*****.** and ***B*****.** Coronal ***(A)*** and axial ***(B)*** T2-weighted FLAIR images demonstrates expansion and high signal intensity involving the right medial temporal lobe and insular cortex (*arrows*). ***C*****.** Coronal diffusion-weighted image demonstrates high signal intensity indicating restricted diffusion involving the right medial temporal lobe and hippocampus (*arrows*) as well as subtle involvement of the left inferior temporal lobe (*arrowhead*). This is most consistent with neuronal death and can be seen in acute infarction as well as encephalitis and other inflammatory conditions. The suspected diagnosis of herpes simplex encephalitis was confirmed by CSF PCR analysis.

The incidence of NSF in patients with severe renal dysfunction (GFR <30) varies from 0.19 to 4%. A recent meta-analysis reported an odds ratio of 26.7 (95% CI = 10.3–69.4) for development of NSF after gadolinium administration in patients with impaired renal function (GFR <30 mL/min/1.72 m). Thus, it is not recommended to administer gadolinium to any patient with a GRF below 30. Caution is advised for patients with a GRF below 45.

COMPLICATIONS AND CONTRAINDICATIONS

From the patient's perspective, an MRI examination can be intimidating, and a higher level of cooperation is required than with CT. The patient lies on a table that is moved into a long, narrow gap within the magnet. Approximately 5% of the population experiences severe claustrophobia in the MR environment. This can be reduced by mild sedation but remains a problem for some. Unlike CT, movement of the patient during an MR sequence distorts all the images; therefore, uncooperative patients should either be sedated for the MR study or scanned with CT. Generally, children under the age of 10 years usually require conscious sedation in order to complete the MR examination without motion degradation.

MRI is considered safe for patients, even at very high field strengths (>3–4 T). Serious injuries have been caused, however, by

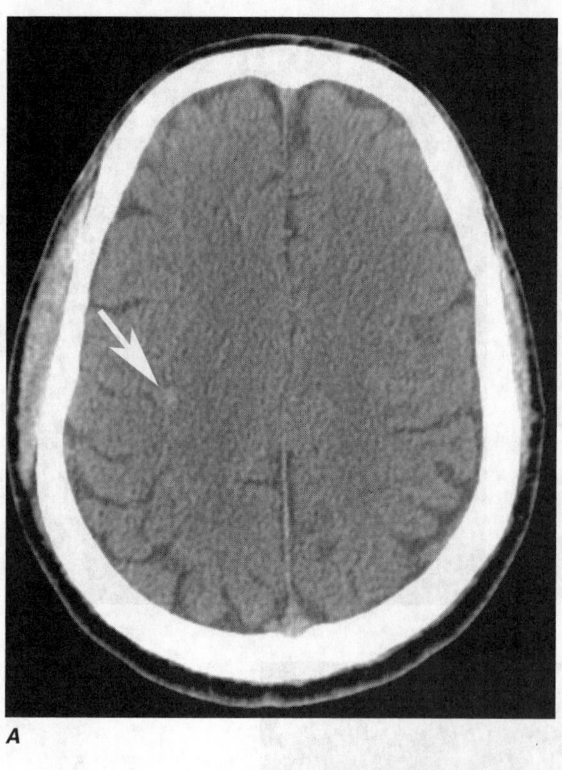

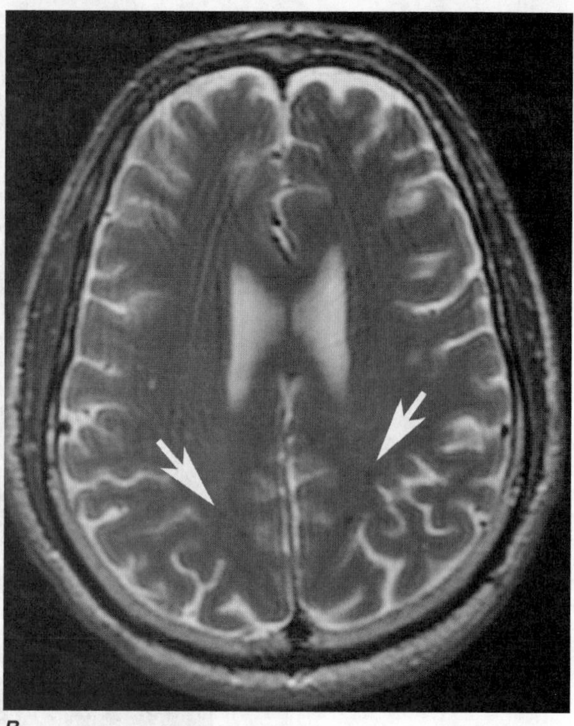

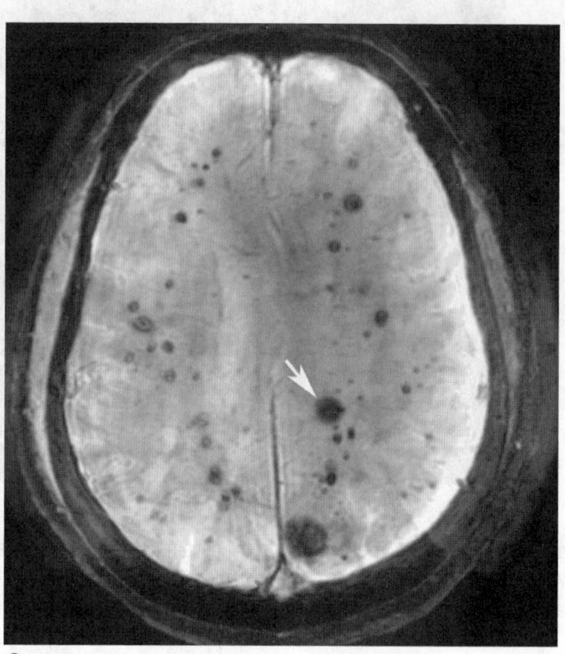

Figure 368-5 Susceptibility weighted imaging in a patient with familial cavernous malformations. ***A.*** Noncontrast CT scan shows one hyperdense lesion in the right hemisphere (*arrow*). ***B.*** T2-weighted fast spin echo image shows subtle low-intensity lesions (*arrows*). ***C.*** Susceptibility weighted image shows numerous low-intensity lesions consistent with hemosiderin-laden cavernous malformations (*arrow*).

attraction of ferromagnetic objects into the magnet, which act as missiles if brought too close to the magnet. Likewise, ferromagnetic implants such as aneurysm clips, may torque within the magnet, causing damage to vessels and even death. Metallic foreign bodies in the eye have moved and caused intraocular hemorrhage; screening for ocular metallic fragments is indicated in those with a history of metal work or ocular metallic foreign bodies. Implanted cardiac pacemakers are generally a contraindication to MRI owing to the risk of induced arrhythmias; however, some newer pacemakers have been shown to be safe. All health care personnel and patients must be screened and educated thoroughly to prevent such disasters as the magnet is always "on." Table 368-4 lists common contraindications for MRI.

MAGNETIC RESONANCE ANGIOGRAPHY

MR angiography is a general term describing several MR techniques that result in vascular-weighted images. These provide a vascular flow map rather than the anatomic map shown by conventional angiography. On routine spin echo MR sequences, moving protons (e.g., flowing blood, CSF) exhibit complex MR signals that range from high- to low-signal intensity relative to background stationary tissue. Fast-flowing blood returns no signal (flow void) on routine T1W or

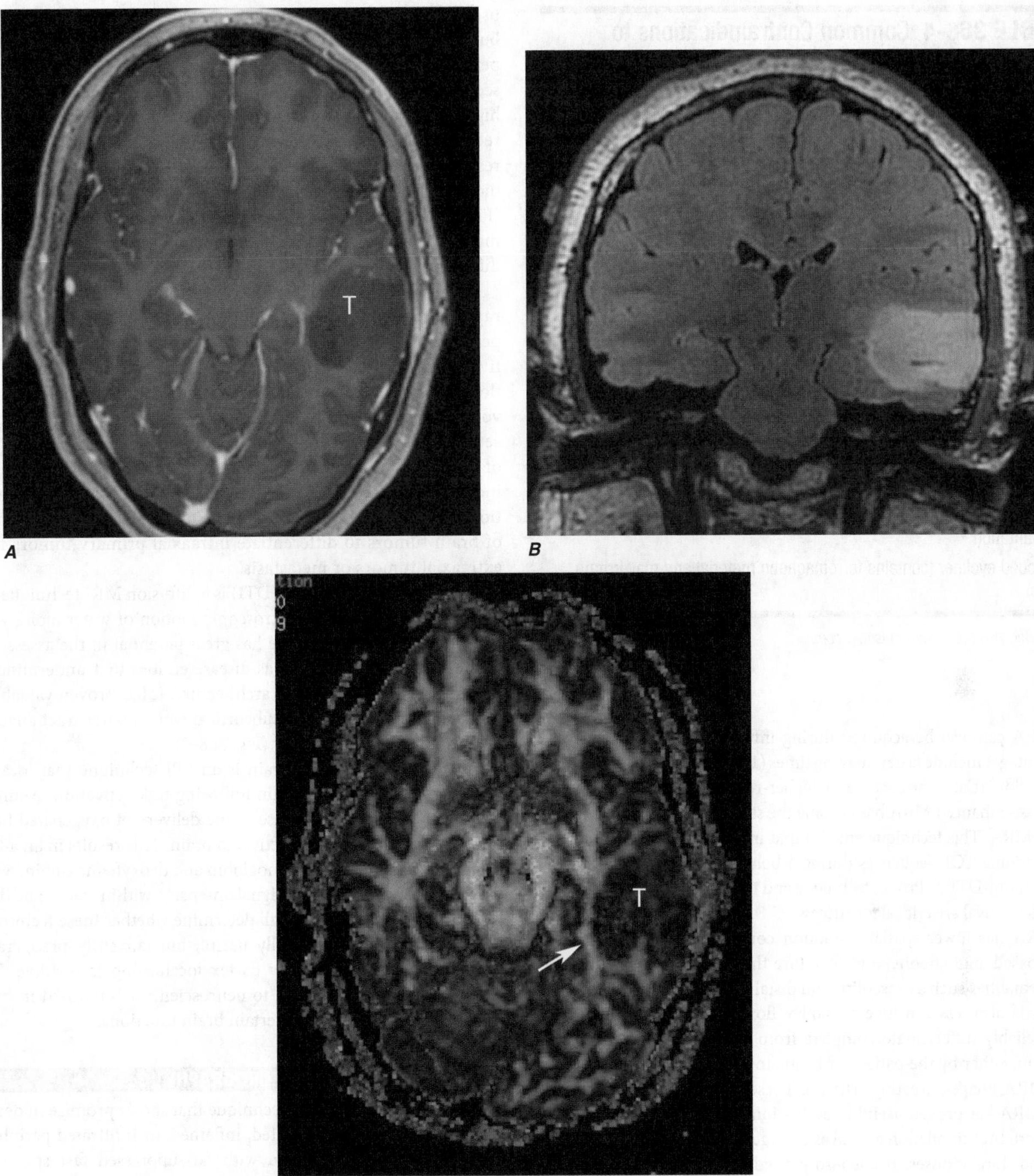

Figure 368-6 Diffusion tractography in cerebral glioma. ***A.*** An axial postcontrast T1-weighted image shows a nonenhancing glioma (T) of the left temporal lobe cortex lateral to the fibers of the internal capsule. ***B.*** Coronal T2 FLAIR image demonstrates high signal glioma in left temporal lobe. ***C.*** Axial diffusion fractional anisotropy image shows the position of the deep white matter fibers (*arrow*) relative to the enhancing tumor (T).

T2W spin echo MR images. Slower-flowing blood, as occurs in veins or distal to arterial stenosis, may appear high in signal. However, using special pulse sequences called *gradient echo sequences*, it is possible to increase the signal intensity of moving protons in contrast to the low signal background intensity of stationary tissue. This creates angiography-like images, which can be manipulated in three dimensions to highlight vascular anatomy and relationships.

Time-of-flight (TOF) imaging, currently the technique used most frequently, relies on the suppression of nonmoving tissue to provide a low-intensity background for the high signal intensity of flowing blood entering the section; arterial or venous structures may be highlighted. A typical TOF angiography sequence results in a series of contiguous, thin MR sections (0.6–0.9 mm thick), which can be viewed as a stack and manipulated to create an angiographic image data set that can be reformatted and viewed in various planes and angles, much like that seen with conventional angiography (Fig. 368-2G).

Phase-contrast MRA has a longer acquisition time than TOF MRA, but in addition to providing anatomic information similar to that of TOF imaging, it can be used to reveal the velocity and direction of blood flow in a given vessel. Through the selection of different imaging parameters, differing blood velocities can be highlighted; selective venous and arterial MRA images can thus be obtained. One advantage of phase-contrast MRA is the excellent suppression of high-signal-intensity background structures.

TABLE 368-4 Common Contraindications to MR Imaging

Cardiac pacemaker or permanent pacemaker leads
Internal defibrillatory device
Cochlear prostheses
Bone growth stimulators
Spinal cord stimulators
Electronic infusion devices
Intracranial aneurysm clips (some but not all)
Ocular implants (some) or ocular metallic foreign body
McGee stapedectomy piston prosthesis
Duraphase penile implant
Swan-Ganz catheter
Magnetic stoma plugs
Magnetic dental implants
Magnetic sphincters
Ferromagnetic IVC filters, coils, stents—safe 6 weeks after implantation
Tattooed eyeliner (contains ferromagnetic material and may irritate eyes)

Note: See also *http://www.mrisafety.com.*

MRA can also be acquired during infusion of contrast material. Advantages include faster imaging times (1–2 minutes vs. 10 minutes), fewer flow-related artifacts, and higher-resolution images. Recently, contrast-enhanced MRA has become the standard for extracranial vascular MRA. This technique entails rapid imaging using coronal three-dimensional TOF sequences during a bolus infusion of 15–20 mL of gadolinium-DTPA. Proper technique and timing of acquisition relative to bolus arrival are critical for success.

MRA has lower spatial resolution compared with conventional film-based angiography, and therefore the detection of small-vessel abnormalities such as vasculitis and distal vasospasm, is problematic. MRA is also less sensitive to slowly flowing blood and thus may not reliably differentiate complete from near-complete occlusions. Motion, either by the patient or by anatomic structures, may distort the MRA images, creating artifacts. These limitations notwithstanding, MRA has proved useful in evaluation of the extracranial carotid and vertebral circulation as well as of larger-caliber intracranial arteries and dural sinuses. It has also proved useful in the noninvasive detection of intracranial aneurysms and vascular malformations.

ECHO-PLANAR MR IMAGING

Recent improvements in gradients, software, and high-speed computer processors now permit extremely rapid MRI of the brain. With echo-planar MRI (EPI), fast gradients are switched on and off at high speeds to create the information used to form an image. In routine spin echo imaging, images of the brain can be obtained in 5–10 minutes. With EPI, all of the information required for processing an image is accumulated in 50–150 milliseconds, and the information for the entire brain is obtained in 1–2 minutes, depending on the degree of resolution required or desired. Fast MRI reduces patient and organ motion, permitting diffusion imaging and tractography (Figs. 368-2*H*, 368-3, 368-4*C*, 368-6; and see Fig. 370-16), perfusion imaging during contrast infusion, fMRI, and kinematic motion studies.

Perfusion and diffusion imaging are EPI techniques that are useful in early detection of ischemic injury of the brain and may be useful together to demonstrate infarcted tissue as well as ischemic but potentially viable tissue at risk of infarction (e.g., the ischemic penumbra). Diffusion-weighted imaging (DWI) assesses microscopic motion of water; restriction of motion appears as relative high-signal intensity on diffusion-weighted images. Infarcted tissue reduces the water motion within cells and in the interstitial tissues, resulting in high signal on DWI. DWI is the most sensitive technique for detection of acute cerebral infarction of <7 days' duration (Fig. 368-2*H*) and is also sensitive to encephalitis and abscess formation, which have reduced diffusion and result in high signal on diffusion-weighted images (Fig. 368-3*B*).

Perfusion MRI involves the acquisition of EPI images during a rapid intravenous bolus of gadolinium contrast material. Relative perfusion abnormalities can be identified on images of the relative cerebral blood volume, mean transit time, and cerebral blood flow. Delay in mean transit time and reduction in cerebral blood volume and cerebral blood flow are typical of infarction. In the setting of reduced blood flow, a prolonged mean transit time of contrast but normal or elevated cerebral blood volume may indicate tissue supplied by collateral flow that is at risk of infarction. Perfusion MRI imaging can also be used in the assessment of brain tumors to differentiate intraaxial primary tumors from extraaxial tumors or metastasis.

Diffusion tensor imaging (DTI) is a diffusion MRI technique that assesses the direction of microscopic motion of water along white matter tracts. This technique has great potential in the assessment of brain maturation as well as disease entities that undermine the integrity of the white matter architecture. It has proven valuable in preoperative assessment of subcortical white matter tract anatomy prior to brain tumor surgery (Fig. 368-6).

Functional MRI of the brain is an EPI technique that localizes regions of activity in the brain following task activation. Neuronal activity elicits a slight increase in the delivery of oxygenated blood flow to a specific region of activated brain. This results in an alteration in the balance of oxyhemoglobin and deoxyhemoglobin, which yields a 2–3% increase in signal intensity within veins and local capillaries. Further studies will determine whether these techniques are cost-effective or clinically useful, but currently preoperative somatosensory and auditory cortex localization is possible. This technique has proved useful to neuroscientists interested in interrogating the localization of certain brain functions.

MAGNETIC RESONANCE NEUROGRAPHY

MRN is a T2 weighted MR technique that shows promise in detecting increased signal in irritated, inflamed, or infiltrated peripheral nerves. Images are obtained with fat-suppressed fast spin echo imaging or short inversion recovery sequences. Irritated or infiltrated nerves will demonstrate high signal on T2W imaging. This is indicated in patients with radiculopathy whose conventional MR studies of the spine are normal, or in those suspected of peripheral nerve entrapment or trauma.

POSITRON EMISSION TOMOGRAPHY (PET)

PET relies on the detection of positrons emitted during the decay of a radionuclide that has been injected into a patient. The most frequently used moiety is 2-[^{18}F]fluoro-2-deoxy-D-glucose (FDG), which is an analogue of glucose and is taken up by cells competitively with 2-deoxyglucose. Multiple images of glucose uptake activity are formed after 45–60 minutes. Images reveal differences in regional glucose activity among normal and pathologic brain structures. A lower activity of FDG in the parietal lobes has been associated with Alzheimer's disease. FDG PET is used primarily for the detection of extracranial metastatic disease. Combination PET-CT scanners, in which both CT and PET are obtained at one sitting, are replacing

PET scans alone for most clinical indications. Functional images superimposed on high-resolution CT scans result in more precise anatomic diagnoses.

MYELOGRAPHY

TECHNIQUE

Myelography involves the intrathecal instillation of specially formulated water-soluble iodinated contrast medium into the lumbar or cervical subarachnoid space. CT scanning is usually performed after myelography (*CT myelography*) to better demonstrate the spinal cord and roots, which appear as filling defects in the opacified subarachnoid space. *Low-dose CT myelography*, in which CT is performed after the subarachnoid injection of a small amount of relatively dilute contrast material, has replaced conventional myelography for many indications, thereby reducing exposure to radiation and contrast media. Newer multidetector scanners now obtain CT studies quickly so that reformations in sagittal and coronal planes, equivalent to traditional myelography projections, are now routine.

INDICATIONS

Myelography has been largely replaced by CT myelography and MRI for diagnosis of diseases of the spinal canal and cord (Table 368-1). Remaining indications for conventional plain-film myelography include the evaluation of suspected meningeal or arachnoid cysts and the localization of spinal dural arteriovenous or CSF fistulas. Conventional myelography and CT myelography provide the most precise information in patients with prior spinal fusion and spinal fixation hardware.

CONTRAINDICATIONS

Myelography is relatively safe; however, it should be performed with caution in any patient with elevated intracranial pressure, evidence of a spinal block, or a history of allergic reaction to intrathecal contrast media. In patients with a suspected spinal block, MR is the preferred technique. If myelography is necessary, only a small amount of contrast medium should be instilled below the lesion in order to minimize the risk of neurologic deterioration. Lumbar puncture is to be avoided in patients with bleeding disorders, including patients receiving anticoagulant therapy, as well as in those with infections of the overlying soft tissues.

COMPLICATIONS

Headache, nausea, and vomiting are the most frequent complications of myelography and are reported to occur in up to 38% of patients. These symptoms result from either neurotoxic effects of the contrast agent, persistent leakage of CSF at the puncture site, or psychological reactions to the procedure. Vasovagal syncope may occur during lumbar puncture; it is accentuated by the upright position used during lumbar myelography. Adequate hydration before and after myelography will reduce the incidence of this complication. Postural headache (post–lumbar puncture headache) is generally due to leakage of CSF from the puncture site, resulting in CSF hypotension. Management of postlumbar-puncture headache is discussed in Chap. 14.

If significant headache persists for longer than 48 hours, placement of an epidural blood patch should be considered. Hearing loss is a rare complication of myelography. It may result from a direct toxic effect of the contrast medium or from an alteration of the pressure equilibrium between CSF and perilymph in the inner ear. Puncture of the spinal cord is a rare but serious complication of cervical (C1–2) or high lumbar puncture. The risk of cord puncture is greatest in patients with spinal stenosis, Chiari malformations, or conditions that reduce CSF volume. In these settings, a low-dose lumbar injection followed by thin-section CT or MRI is a safer alternative to cervical puncture. Intrathecal contrast reactions are rare, but aseptic meningitis and encephalopathy may occur. The latter is usually dose related and associated with contrast entering the intracranial subarachnoid space. Seizures occur following myelography in 0.1–0.3% of patients. Risk factors include a preexisting seizure disorder and the use of a total iodine dose of >4500 mg. Other reported complications include hyperthermia, hallucinations, depression, and anxiety states. These side effects have been reduced by the development of nonionic, water-soluble contrast agents as well as by head elevation and generous hydration following myelography.

SPINE INTERVENTIONS

DISKOGRAPHY

The evaluation of back pain and radiculopathy may require diagnostic procedures that attempt either to reproduce the patient's pain or relieve it, indicating its correct source prior to lumbar fusion. Diskography is performed by fluoroscopic placement of a 22- to 25-gauge needle into the intervertebral disk and subsequent injection of 1–3 mL of contrast media. The intradiskal pressure is recorded, as is an assessment of the patient's response to the injection of contrast material. Typically little or no pain is felt during injection of a normal disk, which does not accept much more than 1 mL of contrast material, even at pressures as high as 415–690 kPa (60–100 lb/in^2). CT and plain films are obtained following the procedure. Concerns have been raised that diskography may contribute to an accelerated rate of disk degeneration.

SELECTIVE NERVE ROOT AND EPIDURAL SPINAL INJECTIONS

Percutaneous selective nerve root and epidural blocks with glucocorticoid and anesthetic mixtures may be both therapeutic as well as diagnostic, especially if a patient's pain is relieved. Typically, 1–2 mL of an equal mixture of a long-acting glucocorticoid such as betamethasone and a long-acting anesthetic such as bupivacaine 0.75% is instilled under CT or fluoroscopic guidance in the intraspinal epidural space or adjacent to an existing nerve root.

ANGIOGRAPHY

Catheter angiography is indicated for evaluating intracranial small-vessel pathology (such as vasculitis), for assessing vascular malformations and aneurysms, and in endovascular therapeutic procedures (Table 368-1). Angiography has been replaced for many indications by CT/CTA or MRI/MRA.

Angiography carries the greatest risk of morbidity of all diagnostic imaging procedures, owing to the necessity of inserting a catheter into a blood vessel, directing the catheter to the required location, injecting contrast material to visualize the vessel, and removing the catheter while maintaining hemostasis. Therapeutic transcatheter procedures (see below) have become important options for the treatment of some cerebrovascular diseases. The decision to undertake a diagnostic or therapeutic angiographic procedure requires careful assessment of the goals of the investigation and its attendant risks.

To improve tolerance to contrast agents, patients undergoing angiography should be well hydrated before and after the procedure. Since the femoral route is used most commonly, the femoral artery must be compressed after the procedure to prevent a hematoma from developing. The puncture site and distal pulses should be evaluated carefully after the procedure; complications can include thigh hematoma or lower extremity emboli.

■ COMPLICATIONS

A common femoral arterial puncture provides retrograde access via the aorta to the aortic arch and great vessels. The most feared complication of cerebral angiography is stroke. Thrombus can form on or inside the tip of the catheter, and atherosclerotic thrombus or plaque can be dislodged by the catheter or guidewire or by the force of injection and can embolize distally in the cerebral circulation. Risk factors for ischemic complications include limited experience on the part of the angiographer, atherosclerosis, vasospasm, low cardiac output, decreased oxygen-carrying capacity, advanced age, and prior history of migraine. The risk of a neurologic complication varies but is ~4% for transient ischemic attack and stroke, 1% for permanent deficit, and <0.1% for death.

Ionic contrast material injected into the cerebral vasculature can be neurotoxic if the BBB is breached, either by an underlying disease or by the injection of hyperosmolar contrast agent. Ionic contrast media are less well tolerated than nonionic media, probably because they can induce changes in cell membrane electrical potentials. Patients with dolichoectasia of the basilar artery can suffer reversible brainstem dysfunction and acute short-term memory loss during angiography, owing to the slow percolation of the contrast material and the consequent prolonged exposure of the brain. Rarely, an intracranial aneurysm ruptures during an angiographic contrast injection, causing subarachnoid hemorrhage, perhaps as a result of injection under high pressure.

■ SPINAL ANGIOGRAPHY

Spinal angiography may be indicated to evaluate vascular malformations and tumors and to identify the artery of Adamkiewicz (Chap. 377) prior to aortic aneurysm repair. The procedure is lengthy and requires the use of relatively large volumes of contrast; the incidence of serious complications, including paraparesis, subjective visual blurring, and altered speech, is ~2%. Gadolinium-enhanced MRA has been used successfully in this setting, as has iodinated contrast CTA, which has promise for replacing diagnostic spinal angiography for some indications.

INTERVENTIONAL NEURORADIOLOGY

This rapidly developing field is providing new therapeutic options for patients with challenging neurovascular problems. Available procedures include detachable coil therapy for aneurysms, particulate or liquid adhesive embolization of arteriovenous malformations, balloon angioplasty and stenting of arterial stenosis or vasospasm, transarterial or transvenous embolization of dural arteriovenous fistulas, balloon occlusion of carotid-cavernous and vertebral fistulas, endovascular treatment of vein-of-Galen malformations, preoperative embolization of tumors, and thrombolysis of acute arterial or venous thrombosis. Many of these disorders place the patient at high risk of cerebral hemorrhage, stroke, or death.

The highest complication rates are found with the therapies designed to treat the highest-risk diseases. The advent of electrolytically detachable coils has ushered in a new era in the treatment of cerebral aneurysms. One randomized trial found a 28% reduction of morbidity and mortality at 1 year among those treated for anterior circulation aneurysm with detachable coils compared with neurosurgical clipping. It remains to be determined what the role of coils will be relative to surgical options, but in many centers, coiling has become standard therapy for many aneurysms.

FURTHER READINGS

AGARWAL R et al: Gadolinium-based contrast agents and nephrogenic systemic fibrosis: A systematic review and meta-analysis. Nephrol Dial Transplant 24:856, 2009

BERMAN JI et al: Diffusion-tensor imaging-guided tracking of fibers of the pyramidal tract combined with intraoperative cortical stimulation mapping in patients with gliomas. J Neurosurg 101:66, 2004

CARRAGEE EJ et al: 2009 ISSLS Prize Winner: Does discography cause accelerated progression of degeneration changes in the lumbar disc: A ten-year matched cohort study. Spine 34:2338, 2009

GONZALEZ RG: Imaging-guided acute ischemic stroke therapy: From "time is brain" to "physiology is brain." Am J Neuroradiol 27:728, 2006

SCHAEFER PW: Diffusion-weighted imaging in acute stroke. Magn Reson Imaging Clin N Am 14:141, 2006

CHAPTER 369 Seizures and Epilepsy

Daniel H. Lowenstein

A *seizure* (from the Latin *sacire*, "to take possession of") is a paroxysmal event due to abnormal excessive or synchronous neuronal activity in the brain. Depending on the distribution of discharges, this abnormal brain activity can have various manifestations, ranging from dramatic convulsive activity to experiential phenomena not readily discernible by an observer. Although a variety of factors influence the incidence and prevalence of seizures, ~5–10% of the population will have at least one seizure, with the highest incidence occurring in early childhood and late adulthood.

The meaning of the term *seizure* needs to be carefully distinguished from that of epilepsy. *Epilepsy* describes a condition in which a person has *recurrent* seizures due to a chronic, underlying process. This definition implies that a person with a single seizure, or recurrent seizures due to correctable or avoidable circumstances, does not necessarily have epilepsy. Epilepsy refers to a clinical phenomenon rather than a single disease entity, since there are many forms and causes of epilepsy. However, among the many causes of epilepsy there are various *epilepsy syndromes* in which the clinical and pathologic characteristics are distinctive and suggest a specific underlying etiology.

Using the definition of epilepsy as two or more unprovoked seizures, the incidence of epilepsy is ~0.3–0.5% in different populations throughout the world, and the prevalence of epilepsy has been estimated at 5–10 persons per 1000.

CLASSIFICATION OF SEIZURES

Determining the type of seizure that has occurred is essential for focusing the diagnostic approach on particular etiologies, selecting the appropriate therapy, and providing potentially vital information regarding prognosis. The International League against Epilepsy (ILAE) Commission on Classification and Terminology, 2005–2009 has provided an updated approach to classification of seizures (Table 369-1). This system is based on the clinical features of seizures and associated electroencephalographic findings. Other potentially distinctive features such as etiology or cellular substrate are not considered in this classification system, although this will undoubtedly change in the future as more is learned about the pathophysiologic mechanisms that underlie specific seizure types.

A fundamental principle is that seizures may be either focal or generalized. *Focal seizures* originate within networks limited to one cerebral hemisphere (note that the term *partial seizures* is no longer used). *Generalized seizures* arise within and rapidly engage networks distributed across both cerebral hemispheres. Focal seizures are usually associated with structural abnormalities of the brain. In contrast, generalized seizures may result from cellular, biochemical, or structural abnormalities that have a more widespread distribution. There are clear exceptions in both cases, however.

TABLE 369-1 Classification of Seizures

1. Focal seizures
   (Can be further described as having motor, sensory, autonomic, cognitive, or other features)
2. Generalized seizures
   a. Absence
      Typical
      Atypical
   b. Tonic clonic
   c. Clonic
   d. Tonic
   e. Atonic
   f. Myoclonic
3. May be focal, generalized, or unclear
   Epileptic spasms

FOCAL SEIZURES

Focal seizures arise from a neuronal network either discretely localized within one cerebral hemisphere or more broadly distributed but still within the hemisphere. With the new classification system, the subcategories of "simple focal seizures" and "complex focal seizures" have been eliminated. Instead, depending on the presence of cognitive impairment, they can be described as focal seizures with or without dyscognitive features. Focal seizures can also evolve into generalized seizures. In the past this was referred to as *focal seizures with secondary generalization*, but the new system relies on specific descriptions of the type of generalized seizures that evolve from the focal seizure.

The routine interictal (i.e., between seizures) electroencephalogram (EEG) in patients with focal seizures is often normal or may show brief discharges termed *epileptiform spikes*, or *sharp waves*. Since focal seizures can arise from the medial temporal lobe or inferior frontal lobe (i.e., regions distant from the scalp), the EEG recorded during the seizure may be nonlocalizing. However, the seizure focus is often detected using sphenoidal or surgically placed intracranial electrodes.

Focal seizures without dyscognitive features

Focal seizures can cause motor, sensory, autonomic, or psychic symptoms without impairment of cognition. For example, a patient having a focal motor seizure arising from the right primary motor cortex near the area controlling hand movement will note the onset of involuntary movements of the contralateral, left hand. These movements are typically clonic (i.e., repetitive, flexion/extension movements) at a frequency of ~2–3 Hz; pure tonic posturing may be seen as well. Since the cortical region controlling hand movement is immediately adjacent to the region for facial expression, the seizure may also cause abnormal movements of the face synchronous with the movements of the hand. The EEG recorded with scalp electrodes during the seizure (i.e., an ictal EEG) may show abnormal discharges in a very limited region over the appropriate area of cerebral cortex if the seizure focus involves the cerebral convexity. Seizure activity occurring within deeper brain structures is often not recorded by the standard EEG, however, and may require intracranial electrodes for its detection.

Three additional features of focal motor seizures are worth noting. First, in some patients the abnormal motor movements may begin in a very restricted region such as the fingers and gradually progress (over seconds to minutes) to include a larger portion of the extremity. This phenomenon, described by Hughlings Jackson and known as a "Jacksonian march," represents the spread of seizure activity over a progressively larger region of motor cortex. Second, patients may experience a localized paresis (Todd's paralysis) for minutes to many hours in the involved region following the seizure. Third, in rare instances the seizure may continue for hours or days. This condition, termed *epilepsia partialis continua*, is often refractory to medical therapy.

Focal seizures may also manifest as changes in somatic sensation (e.g., paresthesias), vision (flashing lights or formed hallucinations), equilibrium (sensation of falling or vertigo), or autonomic function (flushing, sweating, piloerection). Focal seizures arising from the temporal or frontal cortex may also cause alterations in hearing, olfaction, or higher cortical function (psychic symptoms). This includes the sensation of unusual, intense odors (e.g., burning rubber or kerosene) or sounds (crude or highly complex sounds), or an epigastric sensation that rises from the stomach or chest to the head. Some patients describe odd, internal feelings such as fear, a sense of impending change, detachment, depersonalization, déjá vu, or illusions that objects are growing smaller (micropsia) or larger (macropsia). These subjective, "internal" events that are not directly observable by someone else are referred to as *auras*.

Focal seizures with dyscognitive features

Focal seizures may also be accompanied by a transient impairment of the patient's ability to maintain normal contact with the environment. The patient is unable to respond appropriately to visual or verbal commands during the seizure and has impaired recollection or awareness of the ictal phase. The seizures frequently begin with an aura (i.e., a focal seizure without cognitive disturbance) that is stereotypic for the patient. The start of the ictal phase is often a sudden behavioral arrest or motionless stare, which marks the onset of the period of impaired awareness. The behavioral arrest is usually accompanied by *automatisms*, which are involuntary, automatic behaviors that have a wide range of manifestations. Automatisms may consist of very basic behaviors such as chewing, lip smacking, swallowing, or "picking" movements of the hands, or more elaborate behaviors such as a display of emotion or running. The patient is typically confused following the seizure, and the transition to full recovery of consciousness may range from seconds up to an hour. Examination immediately following the seizure may show an anterograde amnesia or, in cases involving the dominant hemisphere, a postictal aphasia.

The range of potential clinical behaviors linked to focal seizures is so broad that extreme caution is advised before concluding that stereotypic episodes of bizarre or atypical behavior are not due to seizure activity. In such cases additional, detailed EEG studies may be helpful.

EVOLUTION OF FOCAL SEIZURES TO GENERALIZED SEIZURES

Focal seizures can spread to involve both cerebral hemispheres and produce a generalized seizure, usually of the tonic-clonic variety (discussed below). This evolution is observed frequently following focal seizures arising from a focus in the frontal lobe, but may also be associated with focal seizures occurring elsewhere in the brain. A focal seizure that evolves into a generalized seizure is often difficult to distinguish from a primary generalized-onset tonic-clonic seizure, since bystanders tend to emphasize the more dramatic, generalized convulsive phase of the seizure and overlook the more subtle, focal symptoms present at onset. In some cases, the focal onset of the seizure becomes apparent only when a careful history identifies a preceding aura. Often, however, the focal onset is not clinically evident and may be established only through careful EEG analysis. Nonetheless, distinguishing between these two entities is extremely important, as there may be substantial differences in the evaluation and treatment of epilepsies associated with focal versus generalized seizures.

GENERALIZED SEIZURES

Generalized seizures are thought to arise at some point in the brain but immediately and rapidly engage neuronal networks in both cerebral hemispheres. Several types of generalized seizures have features that place them in distinctive categories and facilitate clinical diagnosis.

Typical absence seizures

Typical absence seizures are characterized by sudden, brief lapses of consciousness without loss of postural control. The seizure typically lasts for only seconds, consciousness returns as suddenly as it was lost, and there is no postictal confusion. Although the brief loss of consciousness may be clinically inapparent or the sole manifestation of the seizure discharge, absence seizures are usually accompanied by subtle, bilateral motor signs such as rapid blinking of the eyelids, chewing movements, or small-amplitude, clonic movements of the hands.

Typical absence seizures are associated with a group of genetically determined epilepsies with onset usually in childhood (ages 4–8 years) or early adolescence and are the main seizure type in 15–20% of children with epilepsy. The seizures can occur hundreds of times per day, but the child may be unaware of or unable to convey their existence. Since the clinical signs of the seizures are subtle, especially to parents who may not have had previous experience with seizures, it is not surprising that the first clue to absence epilepsy is often unexplained "daydreaming" and a decline in school performance recognized by a teacher.

The electrophysiologic hallmark of typical absence seizures is a generalized, symmetric, 3-Hz spike-and-wave discharge that begins and ends suddenly, superimposed on a normal EEG background. Periods of spike-and-wave discharges lasting more than a few seconds usually correlate with clinical signs, but the EEG often shows many more brief bursts of abnormal cortical activity than were suspected clinically. Hyperventilation tends to provoke these electrographic discharges and even the seizures themselves and is routinely used when recording the EEG.

Atypical absence seizures

Atypical absence seizures have features that deviate both clinically and electrophysiologically from typical absence seizures. For example, the lapse of consciousness is usually of longer duration and less abrupt in onset and cessation, and the seizure is accompanied by more obvious motor signs that may include focal or lateralizing features. The EEG shows a generalized, slow spike-and-wave pattern with a frequency of ≤2.5 per second, as well as other abnormal activity. Atypical absence seizures are usually associated with diffuse or multifocal structural abnormalities of the brain and therefore may accompany other signs of neurologic dysfunction such as mental retardation. Furthermore, the seizures are less responsive to anticonvulsants compared to typical absence seizures.

Generalized, tonic-clonic seizures

Generalized-onset tonic-clonic seizures are the main seizure type in ~10% of all persons with epilepsy. They are also the most common seizure type resulting from metabolic derangements and are therefore frequently encountered in many different clinical settings. The seizure usually begins abruptly without warning, although some patients describe vague premonitory symptoms in the hours leading up to the seizure. This prodrome is distinct from the stereotypic auras associated with focal seizures that generalize. The initial phase of the seizure is usually tonic contraction of muscles throughout the body, accounting for a number of the classic features of the event. Tonic contraction of the muscles of expiration and the larynx at the onset will produce a loud moan or "ictal cry." Respirations are impaired, secretions pool in the oropharynx, and cyanosis develops. Contraction of the jaw muscles may cause biting of the tongue. A marked enhancement of sympathetic tone leads to increases in heart rate, blood pressure, and pupillary size. After 10–20 seconds, the tonic phase of the seizure typically evolves into the clonic phase, produced by the superimposition of periods of muscle relaxation on the tonic muscle contraction. The periods of relaxation progressively increase until the end of the ictal phase, which usually lasts no more than 1 minute. The postictal phase is characterized by unresponsiveness, muscular flaccidity, and excessive salivation that can cause stridorous breathing and partial airway obstruction. Bladder or bowel incontinence may occur at this point. Patients gradually regain consciousness over minutes to hours, and during this transition there is typically a period of postictal confusion. Patients subsequently complain of headache, fatigue, and muscle ache that can last for many hours. The duration of impaired consciousness in the postictal phase can be extremely long (i.e., many hours) in patients with prolonged seizures or underlying central nervous system (CNS) diseases such as alcoholic cerebral atrophy.

The EEG during the tonic phase of the seizure shows a progressive increase in generalized low-voltage fast activity, followed by generalized high-amplitude, polyspike discharges. In the clonic phase, the high-amplitude activity is typically interrupted by slow waves to create a spike-and-wave pattern. The postictal EEG shows diffuse slowing that gradually recovers as the patient awakens.

There are a number of variants of the generalized tonic-clonic seizure, including pure tonic and pure clonic seizures. Brief tonic seizures lasting only a few seconds are especially noteworthy since they are usually associated with specific epileptic syndromes having mixed seizure phenotypes, such as the Lennox-Gastaut syndrome (discussed below).

Atonic seizures

Atonic seizures are characterized by sudden loss of postural muscle tone lasting 1–2 seconds. Consciousness is briefly impaired, but there is usually no postictal confusion. A very brief seizure may cause only a quick head drop or nodding movement, while a longer seizure will cause the patient to collapse. This can be extremely dangerous, since there is a substantial risk of direct head injury with the fall. The EEG shows brief, generalized spike-and-wave discharges followed immediately by diffuse slow waves that correlate with the loss of muscle tone. Similar to pure tonic seizures, atonic seizures are usually seen in association with known epilepsy syndromes.

Myoclonic seizures

Myoclonus is a sudden and brief muscle contraction that may involve one part of the body or the entire body. A normal, common physiologic form of myoclonus is the sudden jerking movement observed while falling asleep. Pathologic myoclonus is most commonly seen in association with metabolic disorders, degenerative CNS diseases, or anoxic brain injury (Chap. 275). Although the distinction from other forms of myoclonus is imprecise, myoclonic seizures are considered to be true epileptic events since they are caused by cortical (versus subcortical or spinal) dysfunction. The EEG may show bilaterally synchronous spike-and-wave discharges synchronized with the myoclonus, although these can be obscured by movement artifact. Myoclonic seizures usually coexist with other forms of generalized seizures but are the predominant feature of juvenile myoclonic epilepsy (discussed below).

CURRENTLY UNCLASSIFIABLE SEIZURES

Not all seizure types can be designated as focal or generalized, and they should therefore be labeled as "unclassifiable" until additional evidence allows a valid classification. *Epileptic spasms* are such an example. These are characterized by a briefly sustained flexion or extension of predominantly proximal muscles, including truncal muscles. The EEG in these patients usually shows hypsarrhythmias, which consist of diffuse, giant slow waves with a chaotic background of irregular, multifocal spikes and sharp waves. During the clinical spasm, there is a marked suppression of the EEG background (the "electrodecremental response"). The electromyogram (EMG) also reveals a characteristic rhomboid pattern that may help distinguish spasms from brief tonic and myoclonic seizures. Epileptic spasms occur predominantly in infants and likely result from differences in neuronal function and connectivity in the immature versus mature CNS.

EPILEPSY SYNDROMES

Epilepsy syndromes are disorders in which epilepsy is a predominant feature, and there is sufficient evidence (e.g., through clinical, EEG, radiologic, or genetic observations) to suggest a common underlying mechanism. Three important epilepsy syndromes are listed below; additional examples with a known genetic basis are shown in Table 369-2.

JUVENILE MYOCLONIC EPILEPSY

Juvenile myoclonic epilepsy (JME) is a generalized seizure disorder of unknown cause that appears in early adolescence and is usually characterized by bilateral myoclonic jerks that may be single or repetitive. The myoclonic seizures are most frequent in the morning after awakening and can be provoked by sleep deprivation. Consciousness is preserved unless the myoclonus is especially severe. Many patients also experience generalized tonic-clonic seizures, and up to one-third have absence seizures. Although complete remission is relatively uncommon, the seizures respond well to appropriate anticonvulsant medication. There is often a family history of epilepsy, and genetic linkage studies suggest a polygenic cause.

LENNOX-GASTAUT SYNDROME

Lennox-Gastaut syndrome occurs in children and is defined by the following triad: (1) multiple seizure types (usually including generalized tonic-clonic, atonic, and atypical absence seizures); (2) an EEG showing slow (<3 Hz) spike-and-wave discharges and a variety of other abnormalities; and (3) impaired cognitive function in most but not all cases. Lennox-Gastaut syndrome is associated with CNS disease or dysfunction from a variety of causes, including developmental abnormalities, perinatal hypoxia/ischemia, trauma, infection, and other acquired lesions. The multifactorial nature of this syndrome suggests that it is a nonspecific response of the brain to diffuse neural injury. Unfortunately, many patients have a poor prognosis due to the underlying CNS disease and the physical and psychosocial consequences of severe, poorly controlled epilepsy.

MESIAL TEMPORAL LOBE EPILEPSY SYNDROME

Mesial temporal lobe epilepsy (MTLE) is the most common syndrome associated with focal seizures with dyscognitive features and is an example of an epilepsy syndrome with distinctive clinical, electroencephalographic, and pathologic features (Table 369-3). High-resolution MRI can detect the characteristic hippocampal sclerosis that appears to be essential in the pathophysiology of MTLE for many patients (Fig. 369-1). Recognition of this syndrome is especially important because it tends to be refractory to treatment with anticonvulsants but responds extremely well to surgical

TABLE 369-2 Examples of Genes Associated With Epilepsy Syndromes[a]

Gene (Locus)	Function of Gene	Clinical Syndrome	Comments
CHRNA4 (20q13.2)	Nicotinic acetylcholine receptor subunit; mutations cause alterations in Ca^{2+} flux through the receptor; this may reduce amount of GABA release in presynaptic terminals	Autosomal dominant nocturnal frontal lobe epilepsy (ADNFLE); childhood onset; brief, nighttime seizures with prominent motor movements; often misdiagnosed as primary sleep disorder	Rare; first identified in a large Australian family; other families found to have mutations in CHRNA2 or CHRNB2, and some families appear to have mutations at other loci
KCNQ2 (20q13.3)	Voltage-gated potassium channel subunits; mutation in pore regions may cause a 20–40% reduction of potassium currents, which will lead to impaired repolarization	Benign familial neonatal convulsions (BFNC); autosomal dominant inheritance; onset in 1st week of life in infants who are otherwise normal; remission usually within weeks to months; long-term epilepsy in 10–15%	Rare; other families found to have mutations in KCNQ3; sequence and functional homology to KCNQ1, mutations of which cause long QT syndrome and a cardiac-auditory syndrome
SCN1B (19q12.1)	β-subunit of a voltage-gated sodium channel; mutation disrupts disulfide bridge that is crucial for structure of extracellular domain; mutated β-subunit leads to slower sodium channel inactivation	Generalized epilepsy with febrile seizures plus (GEFS+); autosomal dominant inheritance; presents with febrile seizures at median 1 year, which may persist >6 years, then variable seizure types not associated with fever	Incidence uncertain; GEFS+ identified in other families with mutations in other sodium channel subunits (SCN1A and SCN2A) and $GABA_A$ receptor subunit (GABRG2 and GABRA1); significant phenotypic heterogeneity within same family, including members with febrile seizures only
LGI1 (10q24)	Leucine-rich glioma-inactivated 1 gene; previous evidence for role in glial tumor progression; protein homology suggests a possible role in nervous system development	Autosomal dominant partial epilepsy with auditory features (ADPEAF); a form of idiopathic lateral temporal lobe epilepsy with auditory symptoms or aphasia as a major simple partial seizure manifestation; age of onset usually between 10 and 25 years	Mutations found in approximately 50% of families containing two or more subjects with idiopathic localization-related epilepsy with ictal auditory symptoms, suggesting that at least one other gene may underlie this syndrome. *LGI1* is the only gene identified so far in temporal lobe epilepsy
CSTB (21q22.3)	Cystatin B, a noncaspase cysteine protease inhibitor; normal protein may block neuronal apoptosis by inhibiting caspases directly or indirectly (via cathepsins), or controlling proteolysis	Progressive myoclonus epilepsy (PME) (Unverricht-Lundborg disease); autosomal recessive inheritance; age of onset between 6 and 15 years, myoclonic seizures, ataxia, and progressive cognitive decline; brain shows neuronal degeneration	Overall rare, but relatively common in Finland and Western Mediterranean (>1 in 20,000); precise role of cystatin B in human disease unknown, although mice with null mutations of cystatin B have similar syndrome
EPM2A (6q24)	Laforin, a protein tyrosine phosphatase (PTP); involved in glycogen metabolism and may have antiapoptotic activity	Progressive myoclonus epilepsy (Lafora's disease); autosomal recessive inheritance; onset age 6–19 years, death within 10 years; brain degeneration associated with polyglucosan intracellular inclusion bodies in numerous organs	Most common PME in Southern Europe, Middle East, Northern Africa, and Indian subcontinent; genetic heterogeneity; unknown whether seizure phenotype due to degeneration or direct effects of abnormal laforin expression
Doublecortin (Xq21-24)	Doublecortin, expressed primarily in frontal lobes; directly regulates microtubule polymerization and bundling	Classic lissencephaly associated with severe mental retardation and seizures in males; subcortical band heterotopia with more subtle findings in females (presumably due to random X-inactivation); X-linked dominant	Relatively rare but of uncertain incidence, recent increased ascertainment due to improved imaging techniques; relationship between migration defect and seizure phenotype unknown

[a]The first four syndromes listed in the table (ADNFLE, BFNC, GEFS+, and ADPEAF) are examples of idiopathic epilepsies associated with identified gene mutations. The last three syndromes are examples of the numerous Mendelian disorders in which seizures are one part of the phenotype.

Abbreviations: GABA, γ-aminobutyric acid; PME, progressive myoclonus epilepsy.

intervention. Advances in the understanding of basic mechanisms of epilepsy have come through studies of experimental models of MTLE, discussed below.

THE CAUSES OF SEIZURES AND EPILEPSY

Seizures are a result of a shift in the normal balance of excitation and inhibition within the CNS. Given the numerous properties that control neuronal excitability, it is not surprising that there are many different ways to perturb this normal balance, and therefore many different causes of both seizures and epilepsy. Three clinical observations emphasize how a variety of factors determine why certain conditions may cause seizures or epilepsy in a given patient.

1. *The normal brain is capable of having a seizure under the appropriate circumstances, and there are differences between individuals in the susceptibility or threshold for seizures.* For example, seizures may be induced by high fevers in children who are otherwise normal and who never develop other neurologic problems, including epilepsy. However, febrile seizures occur only in a relatively small proportion of children. This implies there are various underlying

TABLE 369-3 Characteristics of the Mesial Temporal Lobe Epilepsy Syndrome

History	
History of febrile seizures	Rare generalized seizures
Family history of epilepsy	Seizures may remit and reappear
Early onset	Seizures often intractable
Clinical Observations	
Aura common	Postictal disorientation
Behavioral arrest/stare	Memory loss
Complex automatisms	Dysphasia (with focus in dominant hemisphere)
Unilateral posturing	
Laboratory Studies	
Unilateral or bilateral anterior temporal spikes on EEG	
Hypometabolism on interictal PET	
Hypoperfusion on interictal SPECT	
Material-specific memory deficits on intracranial amobarbital (Wada) test	
MRI Findings	
Small hippocampus with increased signal on T2-weighted sequences	
Small temporal lobe	
Enlarged temporal horn	
Pathologic Findings	
Highly selective loss of specific cell populations within hippocampus in most cases	

Abbreviations: EEG, electroencephalogram; PET, positron emission tomography; SPECT, single photon emission computed tomography.

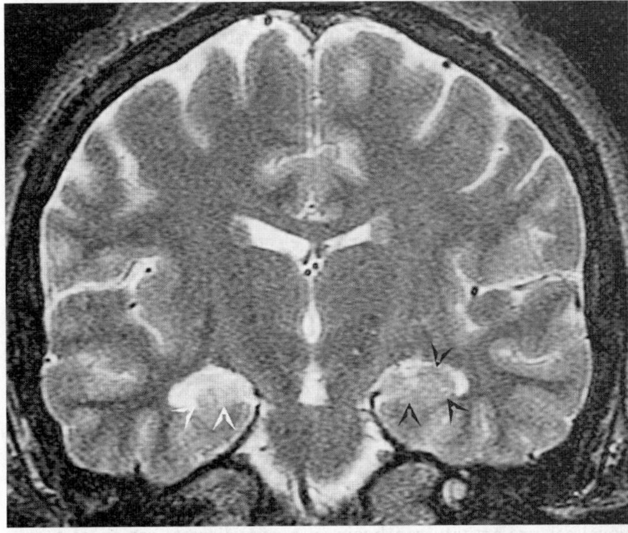

Figure 369-1 Mesial temporal lobe epilepsy. The EEG suggested a right temporal lobe focus. Coronal high-resolution T2-weighted fast spin echo magnetic resonance image obtained through the body of the hippocampus demonstrates abnormal high-signal intensity in the right hippocampus (*white arrows*; compare with the normal hippocampus on the left, *black arrows*) consistent with mesial temporal sclerosis.

endogenous factors that influence the threshold for having a seizure. Some of these factors are clearly genetic, as it has been shown that a family history of epilepsy will influence the likelihood of seizures occurring in otherwise normal individuals. Normal development also plays an important role, since the brain appears to have different seizure thresholds at different maturational stages.

2. *There are a variety of conditions that have an extremely high likelihood of resulting in a chronic seizure disorder.* One of the best examples of this is severe, penetrating head trauma, which is associated with up to a 45% risk of subsequent epilepsy. The high propensity for severe traumatic brain injury to lead to epilepsy suggests that the injury results in a long-lasting pathologic change in the CNS that transforms a presumably normal neural network into one that is abnormally hyperexcitable. This process is known as *epileptogenesis,* and the specific changes that result in a lowered seizure threshold can be considered *epileptogenic factors.* Other processes associated with epileptogenesis include stroke, infections, and abnormalities of CNS development. Likewise, the genetic abnormalities associated with epilepsy likely involve processes that trigger the appearance of specific sets of epileptogenic factors.
3. *Seizures are episodic.* Patients with epilepsy have seizures intermittently and, depending on the underlying cause, many patients are completely normal for months or even years between seizures. This implies there are important provocative or *precipitating factors* that induce seizures in patients with epilepsy. Similarly, precipitating factors are responsible for causing the single seizure in someone without epilepsy. Precipitants include those due to intrinsic physiologic processes such as psychological or physical stress, sleep deprivation, or hormonal changes associated with the menstrual cycle. They also include exogenous factors such as exposure to toxic substances and certain medications.

These observations emphasize the concept that the many causes of seizures and epilepsy result from a dynamic interplay between endogenous factors, epileptogenic factors, and precipitating factors. The potential role of each needs to be carefully considered when determining the appropriate management of a patient with seizures. For example, the identification of predisposing factors (e.g., family history of epilepsy) in a patient with febrile seizures may increase the necessity for closer follow-up and a more aggressive diagnostic evaluation. Finding an epileptogenic lesion may help in the estimation of seizure recurrence and duration of therapy. Finally, removal or modification of a precipitating factor may be an effective and safer method for preventing further seizures than the prophylactic use of anticonvulsant drugs.

CAUSES ACCORDING TO AGE

In practice, it is useful to consider the etiologies of seizures based on the age of the patient, as age is one of the most important factors determining both the incidence and the likely causes of seizures or epilepsy (Table 369-4). During the *neonatal period and early infancy,* potential causes include hypoxic-ischemic encephalopathy, trauma, CNS infection, congenital CNS abnormalities, and metabolic disorders. Babies born to mothers using neurotoxic drugs such as cocaine, heroin, or ethanol are susceptible to drug-withdrawal seizures in the first few days after delivery. Hypoglycemia and hypocalcemia, which can occur as secondary complications of perinatal injury, are also causes of seizures early after delivery. Seizures due to inborn errors of metabolism usually present once regular feeding begins, typically 2–3 days after birth. Pyridoxine (vitamin B_6) deficiency, an important cause of neonatal seizures, can be effectively treated with pyridoxine replacement. The idiopathic or inherited forms of benign neonatal convulsions are also seen during this time period.

TABLE 369-4 Causes of Seizures

Neonates (<1 month)	Perinatal hypoxia and ischemia Intracranial hemorrhage and trauma Acute CNS infection Metabolic disturbances (hypoglycemia, hypocalcemia, hypomagnesemia, pyridoxine deficiency) Drug withdrawal Developmental disorders Genetic disorders
Infants and children (>1 month and <12 years)	Febrile seizures Genetic disorders (metabolic, degenerative, primary epilepsy syndromes) CNS infection Developmental disorders Trauma Idiopathic
Adolescents (12–18 years)	Trauma Genetic disorders Infection Brain tumor Illicit drug use Idiopathic
Young adults (18–35 years)	Trauma Alcohol withdrawal Illicit drug use Brain tumor Idiopathic
Older adults (>35 years)	Cerebrovascular disease Brain tumor Alcohol withdrawal Metabolic disorders (uremia, hepatic failure, electrolyte abnormalities, hypoglycemia, hyperglycemia) Alzheimer's disease and other degenerative CNS diseases Idiopathic

Abbreviation: CNS, central nervous system.

The most common seizures arising in *late infancy and early childhood* are febrile seizures, which are seizures associated with fevers but without evidence of CNS infection or other defined causes. The overall prevalence is 3–5% and even higher in some parts of the world such as Asia. Patients often have a family history of febrile seizures or epilepsy. Febrile seizures usually occur between 3 months and 5 years of age and have a peak incidence between 18 and 24 months. The typical scenario is a child who has a generalized, tonic-clonic seizure during a febrile illness in the setting of a common childhood infection such as otitis media, respiratory infection, or gastroenteritis. The seizure is likely to occur during the rising phase of the temperature curve (i.e., during the first day) rather than well into the course of the illness. A *simple* febrile seizure is a single, isolated event, brief, and symmetric in appearance. *Complex* febrile seizures are characterized by repeated seizure activity, duration >15 minutes, or by focal features. Approximately one-third of patients with febrile seizures will have a recurrence, but <10% have three or more episodes. Recurrences are much more likely when the febrile seizure occurs in the first year of life. Simple febrile seizures are not associated with an increase in the risk of developing epilepsy, while complex febrile seizures have a risk of 2–5%; other risk factors include the presence of preexisting neurologic deficits and a family history of nonfebrile seizures.

Childhood marks the age at which many of the well-defined epilepsy syndromes present. Some children who are otherwise normal develop idiopathic, generalized tonic-clonic seizures without other features that fit into specific syndromes. Temporal lobe epilepsy usually presents in childhood and may be related to mesial temporal lobe sclerosis (as part of the MTLE syndrome) or other focal abnormalities such as cortical dysgenesis. Other types of focal seizures, including those that evolve into generalized seizures, may be the relatively late manifestation of a developmental disorder, an acquired lesion such as head trauma, CNS infection (especially viral encephalitis), or very rarely a CNS tumor.

The period of *adolescence and early adulthood* is one of transition during which the idiopathic or genetically based epilepsy syndromes, including JME and juvenile absence epilepsy, become less common, while epilepsies secondary to acquired CNS lesions begin to predominate. Seizures that begin in patients in this age range may be associated with head trauma, CNS infections (including parasitic infections such as cysticercosis), brain tumors, congenital CNS abnormalities, illicit drug use, or alcohol withdrawal.

Head trauma is a common cause of epilepsy in adolescents and adults. The head injury can be caused by a variety of mechanisms, and the likelihood of developing epilepsy is strongly correlated with the severity of the injury. A patient with a penetrating head wound, depressed skull fracture, intracranial hemorrhage, or prolonged posttraumatic coma or amnesia has a 40–50% risk of developing epilepsy, while a patient with a closed head injury and cerebral contusion has a 5–25% risk. Recurrent seizures usually develop within 1 year after head trauma, although intervals of ≥10 years are well known. In controlled studies, mild head injury, defined as a concussion with amnesia or loss of consciousness of <30 minutes, was found to be associated with only a slightly increased likelihood of epilepsy. Nonetheless, most epileptologists know of patients who have focal seizures within hours or days of a mild head injury and subsequently develop chronic seizures of the same type; such cases may represent rare examples of chronic epilepsy resulting from mild head injury.

The causes of seizures in *older adults* include cerebrovascular disease, trauma (including subdural hematoma), CNS tumors, and degenerative diseases. Cerebrovascular disease may account for ~50% of new cases of epilepsy in patients older than age 65. Acute seizures (i.e., occurring at the time of the stroke) are seen more often with embolic rather than hemorrhagic or thrombotic stroke. Chronic seizures typically appear months to years after the initial event and are associated with all forms of stroke.

Metabolic disturbances such as electrolyte imbalance, hypo- or hyperglycemia, renal failure, and hepatic failure may cause seizures at any age. Similarly, endocrine disorders, hematologic disorders, vasculitides, and many other systemic diseases may cause seizures over a broad age range. A wide variety of medications and abused substances are known to precipitate seizures as well (Table 369-5).

BASIC MECHANISMS

MECHANISMS OF SEIZURE INITIATION AND PROPAGATION

Focal seizure activity can begin in a very discrete region of cortex and then spread to neighboring regions, i.e., there is a *seizure initiation* phase and a *seizure propagation* phase. The initiation phase is characterized by two concurrent events in an aggregate of neurons: (1) high-frequency bursts of action potentials and (2) hypersynchronization. The bursting activity is caused by a relatively long-lasting depolarization of the neuronal membrane due to influx of

TABLE 369-5 Drugs and Other Substances That Can Cause Seizures

Alkylating agents (e.g., busulfan, chlorambucil)	**Psychotropics**
Antimalarials (chloroquine, mefloquine)	Antidepressants
Antimicrobials/antivirals	Antipsychotics
β-lactam and related compounds	Lithium
Quinolones	**Radiographic contrast agents**
Acyclovir	**Theophylline**
Isoniazid	**Sedative-hypnotic drug withdrawal**
Ganciclovir	Alcohol
Anesthetics and analgesics	Barbiturates (short-acting)
Meperidine	Benzodiazepines (short-acting)
Tramadol	**Drugs of abuse**
Local anesthetics	Amphetamine
Dietary supplements	Cocaine
Ephedra (ma huang)	Phencyclidine
Gingko	Methylphenidate
Immunomodulatory drugs	**Flumazenil**[a]
Cyclosporine	
OKT3 (monoclonal antibodies to T cells)	
Tacrolimus	
Interferons	

[a]In benzodiazepine-dependent patients.

extracellular calcium (Ca^{2+}), which leads to the opening of voltage-dependent sodium (Na^+) channels, influx of Na^+, and generation of repetitive action potentials. This is followed by a hyperpolarizing afterpotential mediated by γ-aminobutyric acid (GABA) receptors or potassium (K^+) channels, depending on the cell type. The synchronized bursts from a sufficient number of neurons result in a so-called spike discharge on the EEG.

Normally, the spread of bursting activity is prevented by intact hyperpolarization and a region of "surround" inhibition created by inhibitory neurons. With sufficient activation there is a recruitment of surrounding neurons via a number of synaptic and nonsynaptic mechanisms, including: (1) an increase in extracellular K^+, which blunts hyperpolarization and depolarizes neighboring neurons; (2) accumulation of Ca^{2+} in presynaptic terminals, leading to enhanced neurotransmitter release; and (3) depolarization-induced activation of the *N*-methyl-D-aspartate (NMDA) subtype of the excitatory amino acid receptor, which causes additional Ca^{2+} influx and neuronal activation; and (4) ephaptic interactions related to changes in tissue osmolarity and cell swelling. The recruitment of a sufficient number of neurons leads to the propagation of seizure activity into contiguous areas via local cortical connections, and to more distant areas via long commissural pathways such as the corpus callosum.

Many factors control neuronal excitability, and thus there are many potential mechanisms for altering a neuron's propensity to have bursting activity. Mechanisms *intrinsic* to the neuron include changes in the conductance of ion channels, response characteristics of membrane receptors, cytoplasmic buffering, second-messenger systems, and protein expression as determined by gene transcription, translation, and posttranslational modification. Mechanisms *extrinsic* to the neuron include changes in the amount or type of neurotransmitters present at the synapse, modulation of receptors by extracellular ions and other molecules, and temporal and spatial properties of synaptic and nonsynaptic input. Nonneural cells such as astrocytes and oligodendrocytes, have an important role in many of these mechanisms as well.

Certain recognized causes of seizures are explained by these mechanisms. For example, accidental ingestion of domoic acid, which is an analogue of glutamate (the principal excitatory neurotransmitter in the brain), causes profound seizures via direct activation of excitatory amino acid receptors throughout the CNS. Penicillin, which can lower the seizure threshold in humans and is a potent convulsant in experimental models, reduces inhibition by antagonizing the effects of GABA at its receptor. The basic mechanisms of other precipitating factors of seizures such as sleep deprivation, fever, alcohol withdrawal, hypoxia, and infection, are not as well understood but presumably involve analogous perturbations in neuronal excitability. Similarly, the endogenous factors that determine an individual's seizure threshold may relate to these properties as well.

Knowledge of the mechanisms responsible for initiation and propagation of most generalized seizures (including tonic-clonic, myoclonic, and atonic types) remains rudimentary and reflects the limited understanding of the connectivity of the brain at a systems level. Much more is understood about the origin of generalized spike-and-wave discharges in absence seizures. These appear to be related to oscillatory rhythms normally generated during sleep by circuits connecting the thalamus and cortex. This oscillatory behavior involves an interaction between $GABA_B$ receptors, T-type Ca^{2+} channels, and K^+ channels located within the thalamus. Pharmacologic studies indicate that modulation of these receptors and channels can induce absence seizures, and there is good evidence that the genetic forms of absence epilepsy may be associated with mutations of components of this system.

MECHANISMS OF EPILEPTOGENESIS

Epileptogenesis refers to the transformation of a normal neuronal network into one that is chronically hyperexcitable. There is often a delay of months to years between an initial CNS injury such as trauma, stroke, or infection and the first seizure. The injury appears to initiate a process that gradually lowers the seizure threshold in the affected region until a spontaneous seizure occurs. In many genetic and idiopathic forms of epilepsy, epileptogenesis is presumably determined by developmentally regulated events.

Pathologic studies of the hippocampus from patients with temporal lobe epilepsy have led to the suggestion that some forms of epileptogenesis are related to *structural changes in neuronal networks*. For example, many patients with MTLE have a highly selective loss of neurons that may contribute to inhibition of the main excitatory neurons within the dentate gyrus. There is also evidence that, in response to the loss of neurons, there is reorganization or "sprouting" of surviving neurons in a way that affects the excitability of the network. Some of these changes can be seen in experimental models of prolonged electrical seizures or traumatic brain injury. Thus, an initial injury such as head injury may lead to a very focal, confined region of structural change that causes local hyperexcitability. The local hyperexcitability leads to further structural changes that evolve over time until the focal lesion produces clinically evident seizures. Similar models have provided strong evidence for long-term alterations in *intrinsic, biochemical properties of cells* within the network such as chronic changes in glutamate or GABA receptor function. Recent work has suggested that induction of inflammatory cascades may be a critical factor in these processes as well.

GENETIC CAUSES OF EPILEPSY

The most important recent progress in epilepsy research has been the identification of genetic mutations associated with a variety of epilepsy syndromes (Table 369-2). Although all of the mutations identified to date cause rare forms of epilepsy, their discovery has led to extremely important conceptual advances. For example, it appears that many of the inherited, idiopathic epilepsies (i.e., the relatively "pure" forms of epilepsy in which seizures are the phenotypic abnormality and brain structure and function are otherwise normal) are due to mutations affecting ion channel function. These syndromes are therefore part of the larger group of channelopathies causing paroxysmal disorders such as cardiac arrhythmias, episodic ataxia, periodic weakness, and familial hemiplegic migraine. In contrast, gene mutations observed in symptomatic epilepsies (i.e., disorders in which other neurologic abnormalities such as cognitive impairment, coexist with seizures) are proving to be associated with pathways influencing CNS development or neuronal homeostasis. A current challenge is to identify the multiple susceptibility genes that underlie the more common forms of idiopathic epilepsies. Recent studies suggest that ion channel mutations and chromosomal microdeletions may be the cause of epilepsy in a subset of these patients.

MECHANISMS OF ACTION OF ANTIEPILEPTIC DRUGS

Antiepileptic drugs appear to act primarily by blocking the initiation or spread of seizures. This occurs through a variety of mechanisms that modify the activity of ion channels or neurotransmitters, and in most cases the drugs have pleiotropic effects. The mechanisms include inhibition of Na^+-dependent action potentials in a frequency-dependent manner (e.g., phenytoin, carbamazepine, lamotrigine, topiramate, zonisamide, lacosamide, rufinamide), inhibition of voltage-gated Ca^{2+} channels (phenytoin, gabapentin, pregabalin), attenuation of glutamate activity (lamotrigine, topiramate, felbamate), potentiation of GABA receptor function (benzodiazepines and barbiturates), increase in the availability of GABA (valproic acid, gabapentin, tiagabine), and modulation of release of synaptic vesicles (levetiracetam). The two most effective drugs for absence seizures, ethosuximide and valproic acid, probably act by inhibiting T-type Ca^{2+} channels in thalamic neurons.

In contrast to the relatively large number of antiepileptic drugs that can attenuate seizure activity, there are currently no drugs known to prevent the formation of a seizure focus following CNS injury. The eventual development of such "antiepileptogenic" drugs will provide an important means of preventing the emergence of epilepsy following injuries such as head trauma, stroke, and CNS infection.

APPROACH TO THE PATIENT Seizure

When a patient presents shortly after a seizure, the first priorities are attention to vital signs, respiratory and cardiovascular support, and treatment of seizures if they resume (see "Treatment: Seizures and Epilepsy"). Life-threatening conditions such as CNS infection, metabolic derangement, or drug toxicity must be recognized and managed appropriately.

When the patient is not acutely ill, the evaluation will initially focus on whether there is a history of earlier seizures (Fig. 369-2). If this is the first seizure, then the emphasis will be to: (1) establish whether the reported episode was a seizure rather than another paroxysmal event, (2) determine the cause of the seizure by identifying risk factors and precipitating events, and (3) decide whether anticonvulsant therapy is required in addition to treatment for any underlying illness.

In the patient with prior seizures or a known history of epilepsy, the evaluation is directed toward (1) identification of the underlying cause and precipitating factors, and (2) determination of the adequacy of the patient's current therapy.

HISTORY AND EXAMINATION

The first goal is to determine whether the event was truly a seizure. An in-depth history is essential, for *in many cases the diagnosis of a seizure is based solely on clinical grounds—the examination and laboratory studies are often normal.* Questions should focus on the symptoms before, during, and after the episode in order to differentiate a seizure from other paroxysmal events (see "Differential Diagnosis of Seizures" below). Seizures frequently occur out-of-hospital, and the patient may be unaware of the ictal and immediate postictal phases; thus, witnesses to the event should be interviewed carefully.

The history should also focus on risk factors and predisposing events. Clues for a predisposition to seizures include a history of febrile seizures, earlier auras or brief seizures not recognized as such, and a family history of seizures. Epileptogenic factors such as prior head trauma, stroke, tumor, or infection of the nervous system should be identified. In children, a careful assessment of developmental milestones may provide evidence for underlying CNS disease. Precipitating factors such as sleep deprivation, systemic diseases, electrolyte or metabolic derangements, acute infection, drugs that lower the seizure threshold (Table 369-5), or alcohol or illicit drug use should also be identified.

The general physical examination includes a search for signs of infection or systemic illness. Careful examination of the skin may reveal signs of neurocutaneous disorders such as tuberous sclerosis or neurofibromatosis, or chronic liver or renal disease. A finding of organomegaly may indicate a metabolic storage disease, and limb asymmetry may provide a clue to brain injury early in development. Signs of head trauma and use of alcohol or illicit drugs should be sought. Auscultation of the heart and carotid arteries may identify an abnormality that predisposes to cerebrovascular disease.

All patients require a complete neurologic examination, with particular emphasis on eliciting signs of cerebral hemispheric disease (Chap. 367). Careful assessment of mental status (including memory, language function, and abstract thinking) may suggest lesions in the anterior frontal, parietal, or temporal lobes. Testing of visual fields will help screen for lesions in the optic pathways and occipital lobes. Screening tests of motor function such as pronator drift, deep tendon reflexes, gait, and coordination may suggest lesions in motor (frontal) cortex, and cortical sensory testing (e.g., double simultaneous stimulation) may detect lesions in the parietal cortex.

LABORATORY STUDIES

Routine blood studies are indicated to identify the more common metabolic causes of seizures such as abnormalities in electrolytes, glucose, calcium, or magnesium, and hepatic or renal disease. A screen for toxins in blood and urine should also be obtained from all patients in appropriate risk groups, especially when no clear precipitating factor has been identified. A lumbar puncture is indicated if there is any suspicion of meningitis or encephalitis, and it is mandatory in all patients infected with HIV, even in the absence of symptoms or signs suggesting infection.

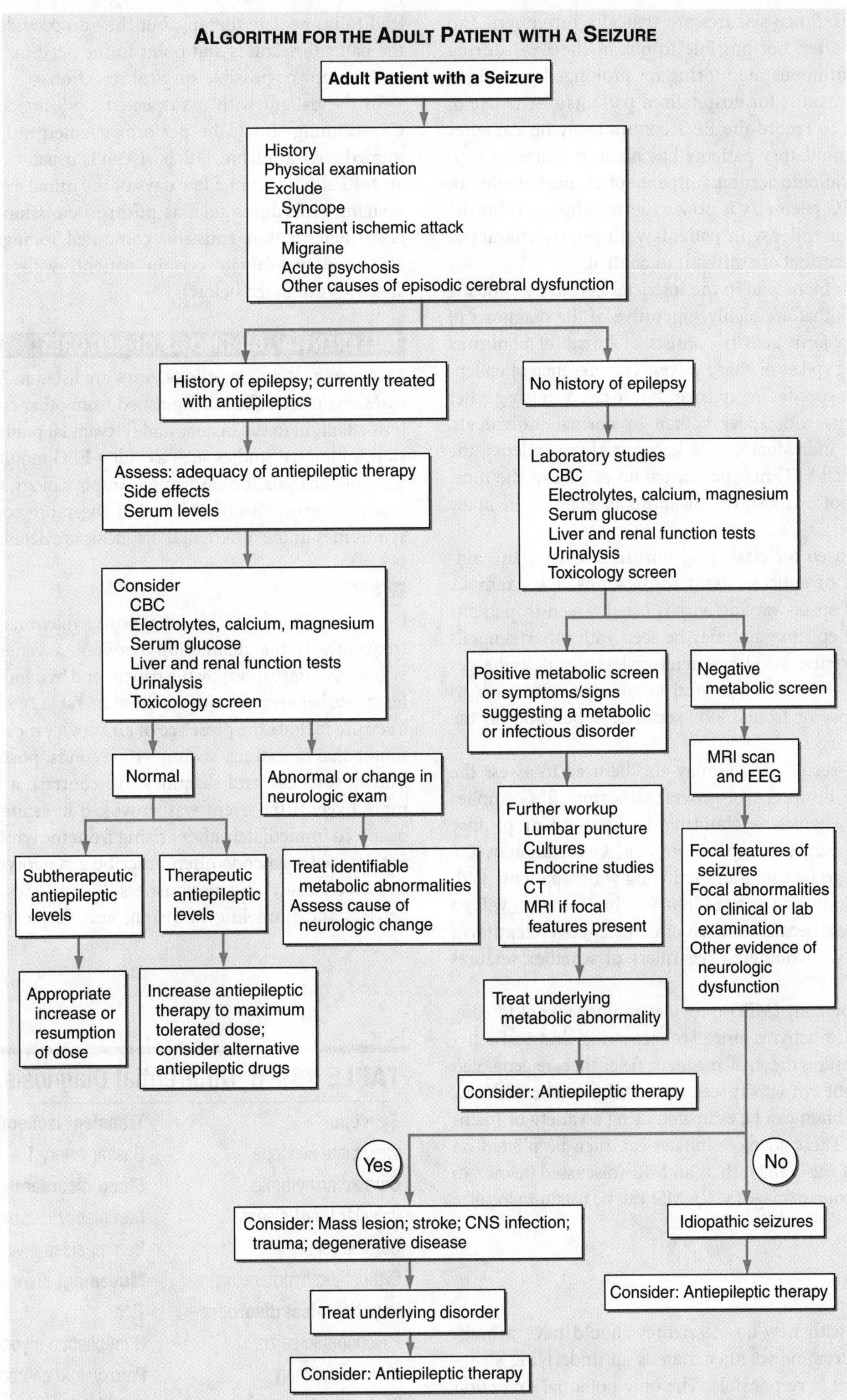

Figure 369-2 Evaluation of the adult patient with a seizure. CBC, complete blood count; CNS, central nervous system; CT, computed tomography; EEG, electroencephalogram; MRI, magnetic resonance imaging.

■ ELECTROPHYSIOLOGIC STUDIES

All patients who have a possible seizure disorder should be evaluated with an EEG as soon as possible. Details about the EEG are covered in Chap. e45.

In the evaluation of a patient with suspected epilepsy, the presence of *electrographic seizure activity* during the clinically evident event (i.e., abnormal, repetitive, rhythmic activity having a discrete onset and termination) clearly establishes the diagnosis. The absence of electrographic seizure activity does not exclude a seizure disorder, however, because focal seizures may originate from a region of the cortex that cannot be detected by standard scalp electrodes. The EEG is always abnormal during generalized tonic-clonic seizures. Since seizures are typically infrequent and unpredictable, it is often not possible to obtain the EEG during a clinical event. Continuous monitoring for prolonged periods in video-EEG telemetry units for hospitalized patients or the use of portable equipment to record the EEG continuously on cassettes for ≥24 hours in ambulatory patients has made it easier to capture the electrophysiologic accompaniments of clinical events. In particular, video-EEG telemetry is now a routine approach for the accurate diagnosis of epilepsy in patients with poorly characterized events or seizures that are difficult to control.

The EEG may also be helpful in the interictal period by showing certain abnormalities that are highly supportive of the diagnosis of epilepsy. Such *epileptiform activity* consists of bursts of abnormal discharges containing spikes or sharp waves. The presence of epileptiform activity is not specific for epilepsy, but it has a much greater prevalence in patients with epilepsy than in normal individuals. However, even in an individual who is known to have epilepsy, the initial routine interictal EEG may be normal up to 60% of the time. Thus, the EEG cannot establish the diagnosis of epilepsy in many cases.

The EEG is also used for classifying seizure disorders and aiding in the selection of anticonvulsant medications. For example, episodic generalized spike-wave activity is usually seen in patients with typical absence epilepsy and may be seen with other generalized epilepsy syndromes. Focal interictal epileptiform discharges would support the diagnosis of a focal seizure disorder such as temporal lobe epilepsy or frontal lobe seizures, depending on the location of the discharges.

The routine scalp-recorded EEG may also be used to assess the prognosis of seizure disorders; in general, a normal EEG implies a better prognosis, whereas an abnormal background or profuse epileptiform activity suggests a poor outlook. Unfortunately, the EEG has not proved to be useful in predicting which patients with predisposing conditions such as head injury or brain tumor, will go on to develop epilepsy, because in such circumstances epileptiform activity is commonly encountered regardless of whether seizures occur.

Magnetoencephalography (MEG) provides another way of looking noninvasively at cortical activity. Instead of measuring electrical activity of the brain, it measures the small magnetic fields that are generated by this activity. Epileptiform activity seen on the MEG can be analyzed, and its source in the brain can be estimated using a variety of mathematical techniques. These source estimates can then be plotted on an anatomic image of the brain such as an MRI (discussed below), to generate a magnetic source image (MSI). MSI can be useful to localize potential seizure foci.

■ BRAIN IMAGING

Almost all patients with new-onset seizures should have a brain imaging study to determine whether there is an underlying structural abnormality that is responsible. The only potential exception to this rule is children who have an unambiguous history and examination suggestive of a benign, generalized seizure disorder such as absence epilepsy. MRI has been shown to be superior to CT for the detection of cerebral lesions associated with epilepsy. In some cases MRI will identify lesions such as tumors, vascular malformations, or other pathologies that need immediate therapy. The use of newer MRI methods such as 3-Tesla scanners, multichannel head coils, three-dimensional structural imaging at submillimeter resolution, and new pulse sequences including fluid-attenuated inversion recovery (FLAIR), has increased the sensitivity for detection of abnormalities of cortical architecture, including hippocampal atrophy associated with mesial temporal sclerosis, as well as abnormalities of cortical neuronal migration. In such cases the findings may not lead to immediate therapy, but they do provide an explanation for the patient's seizures and point to the need for chronic anticonvulsant therapy or possible surgical resection.

In the patient with a suspected CNS infection or mass lesion, CT scanning should be performed emergently when MRI is not immediately available. Otherwise, it is usually appropriate to obtain an MRI study within a few days of the initial evaluation. Functional imaging procedures such as positron emission tomography (PET) and single-photon emission computed tomography (SPECT) are also used to evaluate certain patients with medically refractory seizures (discussed below).

DIFFERENTIAL DIAGNOSIS OF SEIZURES

Disorders that may mimic seizures are listed in Table 369-6. In most cases seizures can be distinguished from other conditions by meticulous attention to the history and relevant laboratory studies. On occasion, additional studies such as video-EEG monitoring, sleep studies, tilt-table analysis, or cardiac electrophysiology, may be required to reach a correct diagnosis. Two of the more common nonepileptic syndromes in the differential diagnosis are detailed below.

■ SYNCOPE

(See also Chap. 20) The diagnostic dilemma encountered most frequently is the distinction between a generalized seizure and syncope. Observations by the patient and bystanders that can help differentiate between the two are listed in Table 369-7. Characteristics of a seizure include the presence of an aura, cyanosis, unconsciousness, motor manifestations lasting >15 seconds, postictal disorientation, muscle soreness, and sleepiness. In contrast, a syncopal episode is more likely if the event was provoked by acute pain or anxiety or occurred immediately after arising from the lying or sitting position. Patients with syncope often describe a stereotyped transition from consciousness to unconsciousness that includes tiredness, sweating, nausea, and tunneling of vision, and they experience a relatively

TABLE 369-6 Differential Diagnosis of Seizures

Syncope	**Transient ischemic attack (TIA)**
Vasovagal syncope	Basilar artery TIA
Cardiac arrhythmia	**Sleep disorders**
Valvular heart disease	Narcolepsy/cataplexy
Cardiac failure	Benign sleep myoclonus
Orthostatic hypotension	**Movement disorders**
Psychological disorders	Tics
Psychogenic seizure	Nonepileptic myoclonus
Hyperventilation	Paroxysmal choreoathetosis
Panic attack	**Special considerations in children**
Metabolic disturbances	Breath-holding spells
Alcoholic blackouts	Migraine with recurrent abdominal pain and cyclic vomiting
Delirium tremens	Benign paroxysmal vertigo
Hypoglycemia	Apnea
Hypoxia	Night terrors
Psychoactive drugs (e.g., hallucinogens)	Sleepwalking
Migraine	
Confusional migraine	
Basilar migraine	

TABLE 369-7 Features That Distinguish Generalized Tonic-Clonic Seizure From Syncope

Features	Seizure	Syncope
Immediate precipitating factors	Usually none	Emotional stress, Valsalva, orthostatic hypotension, cardiac etiologies
Premonitory symptoms	None or aura (e.g., odd odor)	Tiredness, nausea, diaphoresis, tunneling of vision
Posture at onset	Variable	Usually erect
Transition to unconsciousness	Often immediate	Gradual over seconds[a]
Duration of unconsciousness	Minutes	Seconds
Duration of tonic or clonic movements	30–60 s	Never more than 15 s
Facial appearance during event	Cyanosis, frothing at mouth	Pallor
Disorientation and sleepiness after event	Many minutes to hours	<5 min
Aching of muscles after event	Often	Sometimes
Biting of tongue	Sometimes	Rarely
Incontinence	Sometimes	Sometimes
Headache	Sometimes	Rarely

[a]May be sudden with certain cardiac arrhythmias.

brief loss of consciousness. Headache or incontinence usually suggests a seizure but may on occasion also occur with syncope. A brief period (i.e., 1–10 seconds) of convulsive motor activity is frequently seen immediately at the onset of a syncopal episode, especially if the patient remains in an upright posture after fainting (e.g., in a dentist's chair) and therefore has a sustained decrease in cerebral perfusion. Rarely, a syncopal episode can induce a full tonic-clonic seizure. In such cases the evaluation must focus on both the cause of the syncopal event as well as the possibility that the patient has a propensity for recurrent seizures.

PSYCHOGENIC SEIZURES

Psychogenic seizures are nonepileptic behaviors that resemble seizures. They are often part of a conversion reaction precipitated by underlying psychological distress. Certain behaviors such as side-to-side turning of the head, asymmetric and large-amplitude shaking movements of the limbs, twitching of all four extremities without loss of consciousness, and pelvic thrusting are more commonly associated with psychogenic rather than epileptic seizures. Psychogenic seizures often last longer than epileptic seizures and may wax and wane over minutes to hours. However, the distinction is sometimes difficult on clinical grounds alone, and there are many examples of diagnostic errors made by experienced epileptologists. This is especially true for psychogenic seizures that resemble focal seizures with dyscognitive features, since the behavioral manifestations of focal seizures (especially of frontal lobe origin) can be extremely unusual, and in both cases the routine surface EEG may be normal. Video-EEG monitoring is very useful when historic features are nondiagnostic. Generalized tonic-clonic seizures always produce marked EEG abnormalities during and after the seizure. For suspected focal seizures of temporal lobe origin, the use of additional electrodes beyond the standard scalp locations (e.g., sphenoidal electrodes) may be required to localize a seizure focus. Measurement of serum prolactin levels may also help to distinguish between organic and psychogenic seizures, since most generalized seizures and some focal seizures are accompanied by rises in serum prolactin (during the immediate 30-minute postictal period), whereas psychogenic seizures are not. The diagnosis of psychogenic seizures does not exclude a concurrent diagnosis of epilepsy, since the two often coexist.

TREATMENT Seizures and Epilepsy

Therapy for a patient with a seizure disorder is almost always multimodal and includes treatment of underlying conditions that cause or contribute to the seizures, avoidance of precipitating factors, suppression of recurrent seizures by prophylactic therapy with antiepileptic medications or surgery, and addressing a variety of psychological and social issues. Treatment plans must be individualized, given the many different types and causes of seizures as well as the differences in efficacy and toxicity of antiepileptic medications for each patient. In almost all cases a neurologist with experience in the treatment of epilepsy should design and oversee implementation of the treatment strategy. Furthermore, patients with refractory epilepsy or those who require polypharmacy with antiepileptic drugs should remain under the regular care of a neurologist.

TREATMENT OF UNDERLYING CONDITIONS If the sole cause of a seizure is a metabolic disturbance such as an abnormality of serum electrolytes or glucose, then treatment is aimed at reversing the metabolic problem and preventing its recurrence. Therapy with antiepileptic drugs is usually unnecessary unless the metabolic disorder cannot be corrected promptly and the patient is at risk of having further seizures. If the apparent cause of a seizure was a medication (e.g., theophylline) or illicit drug use (e.g., cocaine), then appropriate therapy is avoidance of the drug; there is usually no need for antiepileptic medications unless subsequent seizures occur in the absence of these precipitants.

Seizures caused by a structural CNS lesion such as a brain tumor, vascular malformation, or brain abscess may not recur after appropriate treatment of the underlying lesion. However, despite removal of the structural lesion, there is a risk that the seizure focus will remain in the surrounding tissue or develop de novo as a result of gliosis and other processes induced by surgery, radiation, or other therapies. Most patients are therefore maintained on an antiepileptic medication for at least 1 year, and an attempt is made to withdraw medications only if the patient has been completely seizure free. If seizures are refractory to medication, the patient may benefit from surgical removal of the epileptic brain region (see below).

AVOIDANCE OF PRECIPITATING FACTORS Unfortunately, little is known about the specific factors that determine precisely when a seizure will occur in a patient with epilepsy. Some patients can identify particular situations that appear to lower their seizure threshold; these situations should be avoided. For example, a patient who has seizures in the setting of sleep deprivation should obviously be advised to maintain a normal sleep schedule. Many patients note an association between alcohol intake and seizures, and they should be encouraged to modify their drinking habits accordingly. There are also relatively rare cases of patients with seizures that are induced by highly specific stimuli such as a video game monitor, music, or an individual's voice ("reflex epilepsy"). If there is an association between stress and seizures, stress reduction techniques such as physical exercise, meditation, or counseling may be helpful.

ANTIEPILEPTIC DRUG THERAPY Antiepileptic drug therapy is the mainstay of treatment for most patients with epilepsy. The overall goal is to completely prevent seizures without causing any untoward side effects, preferably with a single medication and a dosing schedule that is easy for the patient to follow. Seizure classification is an important element in designing the treatment plan, since some antiepileptic drugs have different activities against various seizure types. However, there is considerable overlap between many antiepileptic drugs such that the choice of therapy is often determined more by the patient's specific needs, especially his or her assessment of side effects.

When to Initiate Antiepileptic Drug Therapy Antiepileptic drug therapy should be started in any patient with recurrent seizures of unknown etiology or a known cause that cannot be reversed. Whether to initiate therapy in a patient with a single seizure is controversial. Patients with a single seizure due to an identified lesion such as a CNS tumor, infection, or trauma, in which there is strong evidence that the lesion is epileptogenic, should be treated. The risk of seizure recurrence in a patient with an apparently unprovoked or idiopathic seizure is uncertain, with estimates ranging from 31 to 71% in the first 12 months after the initial seizure. This uncertainty arises from differences in the underlying seizure types and etiologies in various published epidemiologic studies. Generally accepted risk factors associated with recurrent seizures include the following: (1) an abnormal neurologic examination, (2) seizures presenting as status epilepticus, (3) postictal Todd's paralysis, (4) a strong family history of seizures, or (5) an abnormal EEG. Most patients with one or more of these risk factors should be treated. Issues such as employment or driving may influence the decision whether to start medications as well. For example, a patient with a single, idiopathic seizure whose job depends on driving may prefer taking antiepileptic drugs rather than risk a seizure recurrence and the potential loss of driving privileges.

Selection of Antiepileptic Drugs Antiepileptic drugs available in the United States are shown in Table 369-8, and the main pharmacologic characteristics of commonly used drugs are listed in Table 369-9. Worldwide, older medications such as phenytoin, valproic acid, carbamazepine, phenobarbital, and ethosuximide are generally used as first-line therapy for most seizure disorders since, overall, they are as effective as recently marketed drugs and significantly less expensive. Most of the new drugs that have become available in the past decade are used as add-on or alternative therapy, although some are now being used as first-line monotherapy.

In addition to efficacy, factors influencing the choice of an initial medication include the convenience of dosing (e.g., once daily versus three or four times daily) and potential side effects. In this regard, a number of the newer drugs have the advantage of a relative lack of drug-drug interactions and easier dosing. Almost all of the commonly used antiepileptic drugs can cause similar, dose-related side effects such as sedation, ataxia, and diplopia. Long-term use of some agents in adults, especially the elderly, can lead to osteoporosis. Close follow-up is required to ensure these side effects are promptly recognized and reversed. Most of the older drugs and some of the newer ones can also cause

TABLE 369-8 Selection of Antiepileptic Drugs

Generalized-onset Tonic-Clonic	Focal	Typical Absence	Atypical Absence, Myoclonic, Atonic
First-Line			
Valproic acid	Lamotrigine	Valproic acid	Valproic acid
Lamotrigine	Carbamazepine	Ethosuximide	Lamotrigine
Topiramate	Oxcarbazepine		Topiramate
	Phenytoin		
	Levetiracetam		
Alternatives			
Zonisamide[a]	Topiramate	Lamotrigine	Clonazepam
Phenytoin	Zonisamide[a]	Clonazepam	Felbamate
Carbamazepine	Valproic acid		
Oxcarbazepine	Tiagabine[a]		
Phenobarbital	Gabapentin[a]		
Primidone	Lacosamide[a]		
Felbamate	Phenobarbital		
	Primidone		
	Felbamate		

[a]As adjunctive therapy.

idiosyncratic toxicity such as rash, bone marrow suppression, or hepatotoxicity. Although rare, these side effects should be considered during drug selection, and patients must be instructed about symptoms or signs that should signal the need to alert their health care provider. For some drugs, laboratory tests (e.g., complete blood count and liver function tests) are recommended prior to the institution of therapy (to establish baseline values) and during initial dosing and titration of the agent. Importantly, recent studies have shown that Asian individuals carrying the human leukocyte antigen allele, HLA-B*1502, are at particularly high risk of developing serious skin reactions from carbamazepine and phenytoin, so racial background and genotype are additional factors to consider in drug selection.

Antiepileptic Drug Selection for Focal Seizures Carbamazepine (or a related drug, oxcarbazepine), lamotrigine and phenytoin are currently the drugs of choice approved for the initial treatment of focal seizures, including those that evolve into generalized seizures. Overall they have very similar efficacy, but differences in pharmacokinetics and toxicity are the main determinants for use in a given patient. For example, an advantage of carbamazepine (which is also available in an extended-release form) is that its metabolism follows first-order pharmacokinetics, and the relationship between drug dose, serum levels, and toxicity is linear. Carbamazepine can cause leukopenia, aplastic anemia, or hepatotoxicity and would therefore be contraindicated in patients with predispositions to these problems. Oxcarbazepine has the advantage of being metabolized in a way that avoids an intermediate metabolite associated with some of the side effects of carbamazepine. Oxcarbazepine also has fewer drug interactions than carbamazepine. Lamotrigine tends to be well tolerated in terms of side effects. However, patients need to be particularly vigilant about the possibility of a skin rash during the initiation of therapy. This can be extremely severe and lead to Stevens-Johnson syndrome if unrecognized and if the medication is not

TABLE 369-9 Dosage and Adverse Effects of Commonly Used Antiepileptic Drugs

Generic Name	Trade Name	Principal Uses	Typical Dose; Dose Interval	Half-Life	Therapeutic Range	Adverse Effects: Neurologic	Adverse Effects: Systemic	Drug Interactions
Phenytoin (diphenyl-hydantoin	Dilantin	Tonic-clonic Focal-onset	300–400 mg/d (3–6 mg/kg, adult; 4–8 mg/kg, child); qd-bid	24 h (wide variation, dose-dependent)	10–20 μg/mL	Dizziness Diplopia Ataxia Incoordination Confusion	Gum hyperplasia Lymphadenopathy Hirsutism Osteomalacia Facial coarsening Skin rash	Level increased by isoniazid, sulfonamides, fluoxetine Level decreased by enzyme-inducing drugs[a] Altered folate metabolism
Carbamazepine	Tegretol[b] Carbatrol	Tonic-clonic Focal-onset	600–1800 mg/d (15–35 mg/kg, child); bid-qid	10–17 h	6–12 μg/mL	Ataxia Dizziness Diplopia Vertigo	Aplastic anemia Leukopenia Gastrointestinal irritation Hepatotoxicity Hyponatremia	Level decreased by enzyme-inducing drugs[a] Level increased by erythromycin, propoxyphene, isoniazid, cimetidine, fluoxetine
Valproic acid	Depakene Depakote[b]	Tonic-clonic Absence Atypical absence Myoclonic Focal-onset Atonic	750–2000 mg/d (20–60 mg/kg); bid-qid	15 h	50–125 μg/mL	Ataxia Sedation Tremor	Hepatotoxicity Thrombocytopenia Gastrointestinal irritation Weight gain Transient alopecia Hyperammonemia	Level decreased by enzyme-inducing drugs[a]
Lamotrigine	Lamictal[b]	Focal-onset Tonic-clonic Atypical absence Myoclonic Lennox-Gastaut syndrome	150–500 mg/d; bid	25 h 14 h (with enzyme-inducers) 59 h (with valproic acid)	Not established	Dizziness Diplopia Sedation Ataxia Headache	Skin rash Stevens-Johnson syndrome	Level decreased by enzyme-inducing drugs[a] and oral contraceptives Level increased by valproic acid
Ethosuximide	Zarontin	Absence	750–1250 mg/d (20-40 mg/kg); qd-bid	60 h, adult 30 h, child	40–100 μg/mL	Ataxia Lethargy Headache	Gastrointestinal irritation Skin rash Bone marrow suppression	Level decreased by enzyme-inducing drugs[a] Level increased by valproic acid
Gabapentin	Neurontin	Focal-onset	900–2400 mg/d; tid-qid	5–9 h	Not established	Sedation Dizziness Ataxia Fatigue	Gastrointestinal irritation Weight gain Edema	No known significant interactions

(continued)

TABLE 369-9 Dosage and Adverse Effects of Commonly Used Antiepileptic Drugs (*Continued*)

Generic Name	Trade Name	Principal Uses	Typical Dose; Dose Interval	Half-Life	Therapeutic Range	Adverse Effects		Drug Interactions
						Neurologic	Systemic	
Topiramate	Topamax	Focal-onset Tonic-clonic Lennox-Gastaut syndrome	200–400 mg/d; bid	20–30 h	Not established	Psychomotor slowing Sedation Speech or language problems Fatigue Paresthesias	Renal stones (avoid use with other carbonic anhydrase inhibitors) Glaucoma Weight loss Hypohidrosis	Level decreased by enzyme-inducing drugs[a]
Tiagabine	Gabitril	Focal-onset	32–56 mg/d; bid-qid	7–9 h	Not established	Confusion Sedation Depression Dizziness Speech or language problems Paresthesias Psychosis	Gastrointestinal irritation	Level decreased by enzyme-inducing drugs[a]
Phenobarbital	Luminol	Tonic-clonic Focal-onset	60–180 mg/d; qd	90 h	10–40 μg/mL	Sedation Ataxia Confusion Dizziness Decreased libido Depression	Skin rash	Level increased by valproic acid, phenytoin
Primidone	Mysoline	Tonic-clonic Focal-onset	750–1000 mg/d; bid-tid	Primidone, 8–15 h Phenobarbital, 90 h	Primidone, 4–12 μg/mL Phenobarbital, 10–40 μg/mL	Same as phenobarbital		Level increased by valproic acid, phenytoin
Clonazepam	Klonopin	Absence Atypical absence Myoclonic	1–12 mg/d; qd-tid	24–48 h	10–70 ng/mL	Ataxia Sedation Lethargy	Anorexia	Level decreased by enzyme-inducing drugs[a]
Felbamate	Felbatol	Focal-onset Lennox-Gastaut syndrome Tonic-clonic	2400–3600 mg/d, tid-qid	16–22 h	Not established	Insomnia Dizziness Sedation Headache	Aplastic anemia Hepatic failure Weight loss Gastrointestinal irritation	Increases phenytoin, valproic acid, active carbamazepine metabolite

Levetiracetam	Keppra[b]	Focal-onset	1000–3000 mg/d; qd-bid	6–8 h	Not established	Sedation Fatigue Incoordination Mood changes	Anemia Leukopenia	No known significant interactions
Zonisamide	Zonegran	Focal-onset Tonic-clonic	200–400 mg/d; qd-bid	50–68 h	Not established	Sedation Dizziness Confusion Headache Psychosis	Anorexia Renal stones Hypohidrosis	Level decreased by enzyme-inducing drugs[a]
Oxcarbazepine	Trileptal	Focal-onset Tonic-clonic	900–2400 mg/d (30–45 mg/kg, child); bid	10–17 h (for active metabolite)	Not established	Fatigue Ataxia Dizziness Diplopia Vertigo Headache	See carbamazepine	Level decreased by enzyme-inducing drugs[a] May increase phenytoin
Lacosamide	Vimpat	Focal-onset	200-400 mg/d; bid	13 h	Not established	Dizziness Ataxia Diplopia Vertigo	GI irritation Cardiac conduction (PR interval prolongation)	Level decreased by enzyme-inducing drugs[a]
Rufinamide	Banzel	Lennox-Gastaut syndrome	3200 mg/d (45 mg/kg, child); bid	6-10 h	Not established	Sedation Fatigue Dizziness Ataxia Headache Diplopia	GI irritation Leukopenia Cardiac conduction (QT interval prolongation)	Level decreased by enzyme-inducing drugs[a] Level increased by valproic acid May increase phenytoin

[a]Phenytoin, carbamazepine, phenobarbital.
[b]Extended-release product available.

discontinued immediately. This risk can be reduced by slow introduction and titration. Lamotrigine must be started slowly when used as add-on therapy with valproic acid, since valproic acid inhibits lamotrigine metabolism, thereby substantially prolonging its half-life. Phenytoin has a relatively long half-life and offers the advantage of once or twice daily dosing compared to two or three times daily dosing for many of the other drugs. However, phenytoin shows properties of saturation kinetics, such that small increases in phenytoin doses above a standard maintenance dose can precipitate marked side effects. This is one of the main causes of acute phenytoin toxicity. Long-term use of phenytoin is associated with untoward cosmetic effects (e.g., hirsutism, coarsening of facial features, and gingival hypertrophy), and effects on bone metabolism, so it is often avoided in young patients who are likely to require the drug for many years. Topiramate can be used for both focal and generalized seizures. Similar to some of the other antiepileptic drugs, topiramate can cause significant psychomotor slowing and other cognitive problems, and it should not be used in patients at risk for the development of glaucoma or renal stones.

Valproic acid is an effective alternative for some patients with focal seizures, especially when the seizures generalize. Gastrointestinal side effects are fewer when using the valproate semisodium formulation (Depakote). Valproic acid also rarely causes reversible bone marrow suppression and hepatotoxicity, and laboratory testing is required to monitor toxicity. This drug should generally be avoided in patients with preexisting bone marrow or liver disease. Irreversible, fatal hepatic failure appearing as an idiosyncratic rather than dose-related side effect is a relatively rare complication; its risk is highest in children <2 years old, especially those taking other antiepileptic drugs or with inborn errors of metabolism.

Levetiracetam, zonisamide, tiagabine, gabapentin, and lacosamide are additional drugs currently used for the treatment of focal seizures with or without evolution into generalized seizures. Phenobarbital and other barbiturate compounds were commonly used in the past as first-line therapy for many forms of epilepsy. However, the barbiturates frequently cause sedation in adults, hyperactivity in children, and other more subtle cognitive changes; thus, their use should be limited to situations in which no other suitable treatment alternatives exist.

Antiepileptic Drug Selection for Generalized Seizures Valproic acid and lamotrigine are currently considered the best initial choice for the treatment of primary generalized, tonic-clonic seizures. Topiramate, zonisamide, phenytoin, and carbamazepine are suitable alternatives. Valproic acid is also particularly effective in absence, myoclonic, and atonic seizures and is therefore the drug of choice in patients with generalized epilepsy syndromes having mixed seizure types. Importantly, carbamazepine, oxcarbazepine, and phenytoin can worsen certain types of generalized seizures, including absence, myoclonic, tonic, and atonic seizures. Ethosuximide is a particularly effective drug for the treatment of uncomplicated absence seizures, but it is not useful for tonic-clonic or focal seizures. Ethosuximide rarely causes bone marrow suppression, so that periodic monitoring of blood cell counts is required. Lamotrigine appears to be particularly effective in epilepsy syndromes with mixed, generalized seizure types such as JME and Lennox-Gastaut syndrome. Topiramate, zonisamide, and felbamate may have similar broad efficacy.

Initiation and Monitoring of Therapy Because the response to any antiepileptic drug is unpredictable, patients should be carefully educated about the approach to therapy. The goal is to prevent seizures and minimize the side effects of therapy; determination of the optimal dose is often a matter of trial and error. This process may take months or longer if the baseline seizure frequency is low. Most anticonvulsant drugs need to be introduced relatively slowly to minimize side effects, and patients should expect that minor side effects such as mild sedation, slight changes in cognition, or imbalance will typically resolve within a few days. Starting doses are usually the lowest value listed under the dosage column in Table 369-9. Subsequent increases should be made only after achieving a steady state with the previous dose (i.e., after an interval of five or more half-lives).

Monitoring of serum antiepileptic drug levels can be very useful for establishing the initial dosing schedule. However, the published therapeutic ranges of serum drug concentrations are only an approximate guide for determining the proper dose for a given patient. The key determinants are the clinical measures of seizure frequency and presence of side effects, not the laboratory values. Conventional assays of serum drug levels measure the total drug (i.e., both free and protein bound). However, it is the concentration of free drug that reflects extracellular levels in the brain and correlates best with efficacy. Thus, patients with decreased levels of serum proteins (e.g., decreased serum albumin due to impaired liver or renal function) may have an increased ratio of free to bound drug, yet the concentration of free drug may be adequate for seizure control. These patients may have a "subtherapeutic" drug level, but the dose should be changed only if seizures remain uncontrolled, not just to achieve a "therapeutic" level. It is also useful to monitor free drug levels in such patients. In practice, other than during the initiation or modification of therapy, monitoring of antiepileptic drug levels is most useful for documenting compliance.

If seizures continue despite gradual increases to the maximum tolerated dose and documented compliance, then it becomes necessary to switch to another antiepileptic drug. This is usually done by maintaining the patient on the first drug while a second drug is added. The dose of the second drug should be adjusted to decrease seizure frequency without causing toxicity. Once this is achieved, the first drug can be gradually withdrawn (usually over weeks unless there is significant toxicity). The dose of the second drug is then further optimized based on seizure response and side effects. Monotherapy should be the goal whenever possible.

When to Discontinue Therapy Overall, about 70% of children and 60% of adults who have their seizures completely controlled with antiepileptic drugs can eventually discontinue therapy. The following patient profile yields the greatest chance of remaining seizure free after drug withdrawal: (1) complete medical control of seizures for 1–5 years; (2) single seizure type, either focal or generalized; (3) normal neurologic examination, including intelligence; and (4) normal EEG. The appropriate seizure-free interval is unknown and undoubtedly varies for different forms of epilepsy. However, it seems reasonable to attempt withdrawal of therapy after 2 years in a patient who meets all of the above criteria, is motivated to discontinue the medication, and clearly understands the potential risks and benefits. In most cases it is preferable to reduce the dose of the drug gradually over 2–3 months. Most recurrences occur in the first 3 months after discontinuing therapy, and patients should be advised to avoid potentially dangerous situations such as driving or swimming during this period.

Treatment of Refractory Epilepsy Approximately one-third of patients with epilepsy do not respond to treatment with a single antiepileptic drug, and it becomes necessary to try a combination of drugs to control seizures. Patients who have focal epilepsy related to an underlying structural lesion or those with multiple seizure types and developmental delay are particularly likely to require multiple drugs. There are currently no clear guidelines for rational polypharmacy, although in theory a combination of drugs with different mechanisms of action may be most useful. In most cases the initial combination therapy combines first-line drugs (i.e., carbamazepine, oxcarbazepine, lamotrigine, valproic acid, and phenytoin). If these drugs are unsuccessful, then the addition of a newer drug such as levetiracetam, topiramate, and zonisamide is indicated. Patients with myoclonic seizures resistant to valproic acid may benefit from the addition of clonazepam, and those with absence seizures may respond to a combination of valproic acid and ethosuximide. The same principles concerning the monitoring of therapeutic response, toxicity, and serum levels for monotherapy apply to polypharmacy, and potential drug interactions need to be recognized. If there is no improvement, a third drug can be added while the first two are maintained. If there is a response, the less effective or less well tolerated of the first two drugs should be gradually withdrawn.

SURGICAL TREATMENT OF REFRACTORY EPILEPSY

Approximately 20–30% of patients with epilepsy continue to have seizures despite efforts to find an effective combination of antiepileptic drugs. For some, surgery can be extremely effective in substantially reducing seizure frequency and even providing complete seizure control. Understanding the potential value of surgery is especially important when a patient's seizures are not controlled with initial treatment, as such patients often fail to respond to subsequent medication trials. Rather than submitting the patient to years of unsuccessful medical therapy and the psychosocial trauma and increased mortality associated with ongoing seizures, the patient should have an efficient but relatively brief attempt at medical therapy and then be referred for surgical evaluation.

The most common surgical procedure for patients with temporal lobe epilepsy involves resection of the anteromedial temporal lobe (temporal lobectomy) or a more limited removal of the underlying hippocampus and amygdala (amygdalohippocampectomy). Focal seizures arising from extratemporal regions may be abolished by a focal neocortical resection with precise removal of an identified lesion (lesionectomy). When the cortical region cannot be removed, multiple subpial transection, which disrupts intracortical connections, is sometimes used to prevent seizure spread. Hemispherectomy or multilobar resection is useful for some patients with severe seizures due to hemispheric abnormalities such as hemimegalencephaly or other dysplastic abnormalities, and corpus callosotomy has been shown to be effective for disabling tonic or atonic seizures, usually when they are part of a mixed-seizure syndrome (e.g., Lennox-Gastaut syndrome).

Presurgical evaluation is designed to identify the functional and structural basis of the patient's seizure disorder. Inpatient video-EEG monitoring is used to define the anatomic location of the seizure focus and to correlate the abnormal electrophysiologic activity with behavioral manifestations of the seizure. Routine scalp or scalp-sphenoidal recordings are usually sufficient for localization, and advances in neuroimaging have made the use of invasive electrophysiologic monitoring such as implanted depth electrodes or subdural electrodes less common. A high-resolution MRI scan is routinely used to identify structural lesions, and this is sometimes augmented with MEG. Functional imaging studies such as SPECT and PET are adjunctive tests that may help verify the localization of an apparent epileptogenic region. Once the presumed location of the seizure onset is identified, additional studies, including neuropsychological testing and the intracarotid amobarbital test (Wada test) may be used to assess language and memory localization and to determine the possible functional consequences of surgical removal of the epileptogenic region. In some cases, the exact extent of the resection to be undertaken is determined by performing cortical mapping at the time of the surgical procedure, allowing for a tailored resection. This involves electrocorticographic recordings made with electrodes on the surface of the brain to identify the extent of epileptiform disturbances. If the region to be resected is within or near brain regions suspected of having sensorimotor or language function, electrical cortical stimulation mapping is performed on the awake patient to determine the function of cortical regions in question in order to avoid resection of so-called eloquent cortex and thereby minimize postsurgical deficits.

Advances in presurgical evaluation and microsurgical techniques have led to a steady increase in the success of epilepsy surgery. Clinically significant complications of surgery are <5%, and the use of functional mapping procedures has markedly reduced the neurologic sequelae due to removal or sectioning of brain tissue. For example, about 70% of patients treated with temporal lobectomy will become seizure free, and another 15–25% will have at least a 90% reduction in seizure frequency. Marked improvement is also usually seen in patients treated with hemispherectomy for catastrophic seizure disorders due to large hemispheric abnormalities. Postoperatively, patients generally need to remain on antiepileptic drug therapy, but the marked reduction of seizures following resective surgery can have a very beneficial effect on quality of life.

Not all medically refractory patients are suitable candidates for resective surgery. For example, some patients have seizures arising from more than one site, making the risk of ongoing seizures or potential harm from the surgery unacceptably high. Vagus nerve stimulation (VNS) may be useful in some of these cases, although the benefit for most patients seems to be very limited (i.e., the efficacy of VNS appears to be no greater than trying another drug, which rarely works if a patient has proved to be refractory to the first two to three drugs). The precise mechanism of action of VNS is unknown, although experimental studies have shown that stimulation of vagal nuclei leads to widespread activation of cortical and subcortical pathways and an associated increased seizure threshold. Adverse effects of the surgery are rare, and stimulation-induced side effects, including transient hoarseness, cough, and dyspnea, are usually mild.

Although still in development, there are some additional therapies that will likely be of benefit to patients with medically refractory epilepsy. Preliminary studies suggest that stereotactic radiosurgery may be effective in certain focal seizure disorders. There has also been great interest in the development of implantable devices that can detect the onset of a seizure (in some instances, before the seizure becomes clinically apparent) and deliver either an electrical stimulation or drug directly to the seizure focus to abort the event.

■ STATUS EPILEPTICUS

Status epilepticus refers to continuous seizures or repetitive, discrete seizures with impaired consciousness in the interictal period. Status epilepticus has numerous subtypes, including generalized convulsive status epilepticus (GCSE) (e.g., persistent, generalized electrographic seizures, coma, and tonic-clonic movements), and nonconvulsive status epilepticus (e.g., persistent absence seizures or focal seizures, confusion or partially impaired consciousness, and minimal motor abnormalities). The duration of seizure activity sufficient to meet the definition of status epilepticus has traditionally been specified as 15–30 minutes. However, a more practical definition is to consider status epilepticus as a situation in which the duration of seizures prompts the acute use of anticonvulsant therapy. For GCSE, this is typically when seizures last beyond 5 minutes.

GCSE is an emergency and must be treated immediately, since cardiorespiratory dysfunction, hyperthermia, and metabolic derangements can develop as a consequence of prolonged seizures, and these can lead to irreversible neuronal injury. Furthermore, CNS injury can occur even when the patient is paralyzed with neuromuscular blockade but continues to have electrographic seizures. The most common causes of GCSE are anticonvulsant withdrawal or noncompliance, metabolic disturbances, drug toxicity, CNS infection, CNS tumors, refractory epilepsy, and head trauma.

GCSE is obvious when the patient is having overt convulsions. However, after 30–45 minutes of uninterrupted seizures, the signs may become increasingly subtle. Patients may have mild clonic movements of only the fingers or fine, rapid movements of the eyes. There may be paroxysmal episodes of tachycardia, hypertension, and pupillary dilation. In such cases, the EEG may be the only method of establishing the diagnosis. Thus, if the patient stops having overt seizures, yet remains comatose, an EEG should be performed to rule out ongoing status epilepticus. This is obviously also essential when a patient with GCSE has been paralyzed with neuromuscular blockade in the process of protecting the airway.

The first steps in the management of a patient in GCSE are to attend to any acute cardiorespiratory problems or hyperthermia, perform a brief medical and neurologic examination, establish venous access, and send samples for laboratory studies to identify metabolic abnormalities. Anticonvulsant therapy should then begin without delay; a treatment approach is shown in Fig. 369-3.

The treatment of nonconvulsive status epilepticus is thought to be less urgent than GCSE, since the ongoing seizures are not accompanied by the severe metabolic disturbances seen with GCSE. However, evidence suggests that nonconvulsive status epilepticus, especially that caused by ongoing, focal seizure activity, is associated with cellular injury in the region of the seizure focus; therefore this condition should be treated as promptly as possible using the general approach described for GCSE.

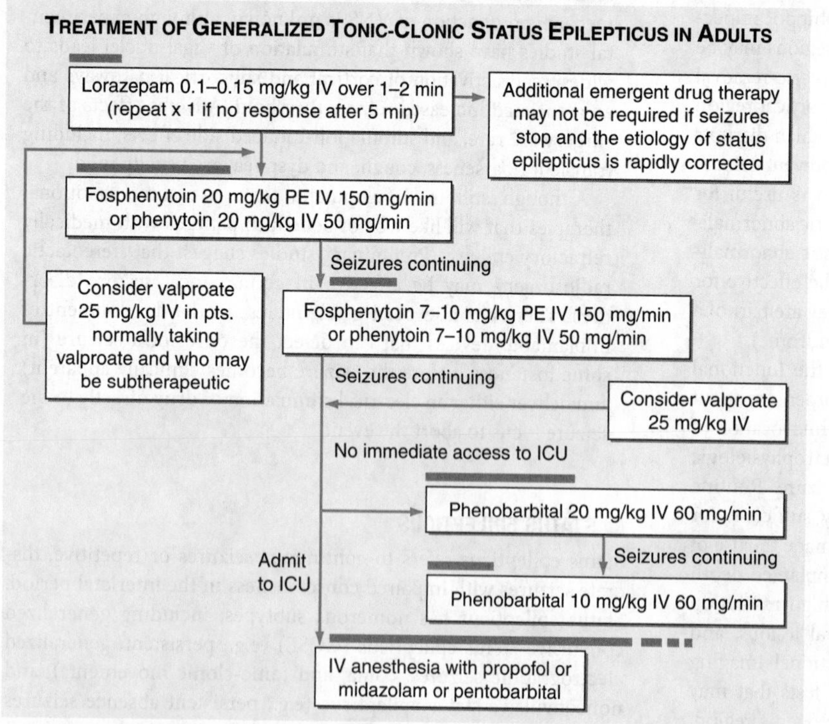

Treatment of Generalized Tonic-Clonic Status Epilepticus in Adults

Lorazepam 0.1–0.15 mg/kg IV over 1–2 min (repeat x 1 if no response after 5 min)
Additional emergent drug therapy may not be required if seizures stop and the etiology of status epilepticus is rapidly corrected
Fosphenytoin 20 mg/kg PE IV 150 mg/min or phenytoin 20 mg/kg IV 50 mg/min
Seizures continuing
Consider valproate 25 mg/kg IV in pts. normally taking valproate and who may be subtherapeutic
Fosphenytoin 7–10 mg/kg PE IV 150 mg/min or phenytoin 7–10 mg/kg IV 50 mg/min
Seizures continuing
Consider valproate 25 mg/kg IV
No immediate access to ICU
Phenobarbital 20 mg/kg IV 60 mg/min
Seizures continuing
Admit to ICU
Phenobarbital 10 mg/kg IV 60 mg/min
IV anesthesia with propofol or midazolam or pentobarbital

Figure 369-3 Pharmacologic treatment of generalized tonic-clonic status epilepticus in adults. The horizontal bars indicate the approximate duration of drug infusions. IV, intravenous; PE, phenytoin equivalents.

BEYOND SEIZURES: OTHER MANAGEMENT ISSUES

INTERICTAL BEHAVIOR

The adverse effects of epilepsy often go beyond the occurrence of clinical seizures, and the extent of these effects largely depends on the etiology of the seizure disorder, the degree to which the seizures are controlled, and the presence of side effects from antiepileptic therapy. Many patients with epilepsy are completely normal between seizures and able to live highly successful and productive lives. In contrast, patients with seizures secondary to developmental abnormalities or acquired brain injury may have impaired cognitive function and other neurologic deficits. Frequent interictal EEG abnormalities have been shown to be associated with subtle dysfunction of memory and attention. Patients with many seizures, especially those emanating from the temporal lobe, often note an impairment of short-term memory that may progress over time.

Patients with epilepsy are at risk of developing a variety of psychiatric problems, including depression, anxiety, and psychosis. This risk varies considerably depending on many factors, including the etiology, frequency, and severity of seizures and the patient's age and previous history. Depression occurs in ~20% of patients, and the incidence of suicide is higher in epileptic patients than in the general population. Depression should be treated through counseling or medication. The selective serotonin reuptake inhibitors (SSRIs) typically have no effect on seizures, while high doses of tricyclic antidepressants may lower the seizure threshold. Anxiety can appear as a manifestation of a seizure, and anxious or psychotic behavior can sometimes be observed as part of a postictal delirium. Postictal psychosis is a rare phenomenon that typically occurs after a period of increased seizure frequency. There is usually a brief lucid interval lasting up to a week, followed by days to weeks of agitated, psychotic behavior. The psychosis will usually resolve spontaneously but frequently will require short-term treatment with antipsychotic or anxiolytic medications.

There is ongoing controversy as to whether some patients with epilepsy (especially temporal lobe epilepsy) have a stereotypical "interictal personality." The predominant view is that the unusual or abnormal personality traits observed in such patients are, in most cases, not due to epilepsy but result from an underlying structural brain lesion, the effects of antiepileptic drugs, or psychosocial factors related to suffering from a chronic disease.

MORTALITY OF EPILEPSY

Patients with epilepsy have a risk of death that is roughly two to three times greater than expected in a matched population without epilepsy. Most of the increased mortality is due to the underlying etiology of epilepsy (e.g., tumors or strokes in older adults). However, a significant number of patients die from accidents, status epilepticus, and a syndrome known as *sudden unexpected death in epileptic patients* (SUDEP), which usually affects young people with convulsive seizures and tends to occur at night. The cause of SUDEP is unknown; it may result from brainstem-mediated effects of seizures on cardiac rhythms or pulmonary function.

PSYCHOSOCIAL ISSUES

There continues to be a cultural stigma about epilepsy, although it is slowly declining in societies with effective health education programs. Many patients with epilepsy harbor fears such as the fear of becoming mentally retarded or dying during a seizure. These issues need to be carefully addressed by educating the patient about epilepsy and by ensuring that family members, teachers, fellow employees, and other associates are equally well informed. The Epilepsy Foundation of America (*www.epilepsyfoundation.org*) is a patient advocacy organization and a useful source of educational material as is the Web site *www.epilepsy.com.*

EMPLOYMENT, DRIVING, AND OTHER ACTIVITIES

Many patients with epilepsy face difficulty in obtaining or maintaining employment, even when their seizures are well controlled. Federal and state legislation is designed to prevent employers from discriminating against patients with epilepsy, and patients should be encouraged to understand and claim their legal rights. Patients in these circumstances also benefit greatly from the assistance of health providers who act as strong patient advocates.

Loss of driving privileges is one of the most disruptive social consequences of epilepsy. Physicians should be very clear about local regulations concerning driving and epilepsy, since the laws vary considerably among states and countries. In all cases, it is the physician's responsibility to warn patients of the danger imposed on themselves and others while driving if their seizures are uncontrolled (unless the seizures are not associated with impairment of consciousness or motor control). In general, most states allow patients to drive after a seizure-free interval (on or off medications) of between 3 months and 2 years.

Patients with incompletely controlled seizures must also contend with the risk of being in situations where an impairment of consciousness or loss of motor control could lead to major injury or death. Thus, depending on the type and frequency of seizures, many patients need to be instructed to avoid working at heights or with machinery, or to have someone close by for activities such as bathing and swimming.

SPECIAL ISSUES RELATED TO WOMEN AND EPILEPSY

CATAMENIAL EPILEPSY

Some women experience a marked increase in seizure frequency around the time of menses. This is believed to be mediated by either the effects of estrogen and progesterone on neuronal excitability or changes in antiepileptic drug levels due to altered protein binding or metabolism. Some patients may benefit from increases in antiepileptic drug dosages during menses. Natural progestins or intramuscular medroxyprogesterone may be of benefit to a subset of women.

PREGNANCY

Most women with epilepsy who become pregnant will have an uncomplicated gestation and deliver a normal baby. However, epilepsy poses some important risks to a pregnancy. Seizure frequency during pregnancy will remain unchanged in ~50% of women, increase in 30%, and decrease in 20%. Changes in seizure frequency are attributed to endocrine effects on the CNS, variations in antiepileptic drug pharmacokinetics (such as acceleration of hepatic drug metabolism or effects on plasma protein binding), and changes in medication compliance. It is useful to see patients at frequent intervals during pregnancy and monitor serum antiepileptic drug levels. Measurement of the unbound drug concentrations may be useful if there is an increase in seizure frequency or worsening of side effects of antiepileptic drugs.

The overall incidence of fetal abnormalities in children born to mothers with epilepsy is 5–6%, compared to 2–3% in healthy women. Part of the higher incidence is due to teratogenic effects of antiepileptic drugs, and the risk increases with the number of medications used (e.g., 10–20% risk of malformations with three drugs) and possibly with higher doses. A recent meta-analysis of published pregnancy registries and cohorts found that the most common malformations were defects in the cardiovascular and musculoskeletal system (1.4–1.8%). Valproic acid is strongly associated with an increased risk of adverse fetal outcomes (7–20%). Little is currently known about the safety of newer drugs, although reports suggest a higher than expected incidence of cleft lip or palate with the use of lamotrigine during pregnancy.

Since the potential harm of uncontrolled convulsive seizures on the mother and fetus is considered greater than the teratogenic effects of antiepileptic drugs, it is currently recommended that pregnant women be maintained on effective drug therapy. When possible, it seems prudent to have the patient on monotherapy at the lowest effective dose, especially during the first trimester. For some women, however, the type and frequency of their seizures may allow for them to safely wean off antiepileptic drugs prior to conception. Patients should also take folate (1–4 mg/d), since the antifolate effects of anticonvulsants are thought to play a role in the development of neural tube defects, although the benefits of this treatment remain unproved in this setting.

Enzyme-inducing drugs such as phenytoin, carbamazepine, oxcarbazepine, topiramate, phenobarbital, and primidone cause a transient and reversible deficiency of vitamin K–dependent clotting factors in ~50% of newborn infants. Although neonatal hemorrhage is uncommon, the mother should be treated with oral vitamin K (20 mg/d, phylloquinone) in the last 2 weeks of pregnancy, and the infant should receive intramuscular vitamin K (1 mg) at birth.

CONTRACEPTION

Special care should be taken when prescribing antiepileptic medications for women who are taking oral contraceptive agents. Drugs such as carbamazepine, phenytoin, phenobarbital, and topiramate can significantly decrease the efficacy of oral contraceptives via enzyme induction and other mechanisms. Patients should be advised to consider alternative forms of contraception, or their contraceptive medications should be modified to offset the effects of the antiepileptic medications.

BREAST-FEEDING

Antiepileptic medications are excreted into breast milk to a variable degree. The ratio of drug concentration in breast milk relative to serum ranges from ~5% (valproic acid) to 300% (levetiracetam). Given the overall benefits of breast-feeding and the lack of evidence for long-term harm to the infant by being exposed to antiepileptic drugs, mothers with epilepsy can be encouraged to breast-feed. This should be reconsidered, however, if there is any evidence of drug effects on the infant such as lethargy or poor feeding.

FURTHER READINGS

Baulac S, Baulac M: Advances on the genetics of mendelian idiopathic epilepsies. Neurol Clin 27:1041, 2009

Bonnett LJ et al: Risk of recurrence after a first seizure and implications for driving: Further analysis of the Multicentre study of early Epilepsy and Single Seizures. BMJ 341:6477, 2010

Brodie MJ et al: Epilepsy in later life. Lancet Neurol 8:1019, 2009

French JA, Pedley TA: Clinical practice. Initial management of epilepsy. N Engl J Med 359:166, 2008.

——— et al: Efficacy and tolerability of the new antiepileptic drugs I: Treatment of new onset epilepsy: Report of the Therapeutics and Technology Assessment Subcommittee and Quality Standards Subcommittee of the American Academy of Neurology and the American Epilepsy Society. Neurology 62:1252, 2004

———: Efficacy and tolerability of the new antiepileptic drugs II: Treatment of refractory epilepsy: Report of the Therapeutics and Technology Assessment Subcommittee and Quality Standards Subcommittee of the American Academy of Neurology and the American Epilepsy Society. Neurology 62:1261, 2004

Millikan D et al: Emergency treatment of status epilepticus: Current thinking. Emerg Med Clin North Am 27:101, 2009

Pitkänen A, Lukasiuk K: Molecular and cellular basis of epileptogenesis in symptomatic epilepsy. Epilepsy Behav 14:16, 2009

Rakhade SN, Jensen FE. Epileptogenesis in the immature brain: emerging mechanisms. Nat Rev Neurol 5:380, 2009

Schuele SU, Lüders HO: Intractable epilepsy: management and therapeutic alternatives. Lancet Neurol 7:514, 2008

Tomson T et al: Sudden unexpected death in epilepsy: current knowledge and future directions. Lancet Neurol 7:1021, 2008

Walker SP et al: The management of epilepsy in pregnancy. BJOG 116:758, 2009

CHAPTER 370

Cerebrovascular Diseases

Wade S. Smith
Joey D. English
S. Claiborne Johnston

Cerebrovascular diseases include some of the most common and devastating disorders: ischemic stroke, hemorrhagic stroke, and cerebrovascular anomalies such as intracranial aneurysms and arteriovenous malformations (AVMs). They cause ~200,000 deaths each year in the United States and are a major cause of disability. The incidence of cerebrovascular diseases increases with age, and the number of strokes is projected to increase as the elderly population grows, with a doubling in stroke deaths in the United States by 2030. Most cerebrovascular diseases are manifest by the abrupt onset of a focal neurologic deficit, as if the patient was "struck by the hand of God." A stroke, or cerebrovascular accident, is defined by this abrupt onset of a neurologic deficit that is attributable to a focal vascular cause. Thus, the definition of stroke is clinical, and laboratory studies including brain imaging are used to support the diagnosis. The clinical manifestations of stroke are highly variable because of the complex anatomy of the brain and its vasculature. *Cerebral ischemia* is caused by a reduction in blood flow that lasts longer than several seconds. Neurologic symptoms are manifest within seconds because neurons lack glycogen, so energy failure is rapid. If the cessation of flow lasts for more than a few minutes, *infarction* or death of brain tissue results. When blood flow is quickly restored, brain tissue can recover fully and the patient's symptoms are only transient: This is called a *transient ischemic attack* (TIA). The standard definition of TIA requires that all neurologic signs and symptoms resolve within 24 hours regardless of whether there is imaging evidence of new permanent brain injury; stroke has occurred if the neurologic signs and symptoms last for >24 hours. However, a newly proposed definition classifies those with new brain infarction as ischemic strokes regardless of whether symptoms persist. A generalized reduction in cerebral blood flow due to systemic hypotension (e.g., cardiac arrhythmia, myocardial infarction, or hemorrhagic shock) usually produces syncope (Chap. 20). If low cerebral blood flow persists for a longer duration, then infarction in the border zones between the major cerebral artery distributions may develop. In more severe instances, *global hypoxia-ischemia* causes widespread brain injury; the constellation of cognitive sequelae that ensues is called *hypoxic-ischemic encephalopathy* (Chap. 275). *Focal ischemia* or infarction, conversely, is usually caused by thrombosis of the cerebral vessels themselves or by emboli from a proximal arterial source or the heart. *Intracranial hemorrhage* is caused by bleeding directly into or around the brain; it produces neurologic symptoms by producing a mass effect on neural structures, from the toxic effects of blood itself, or by increasing intracranial pressure.

APPROACH TO THE PATIENT Cerebrovascular Disease

Rapid evaluation is essential for use of time-sensitive treatments such as thrombolysis. However, patients with acute stroke often do not seek medical assistance on their own, both because they are rarely in pain, as well as because they may lose the appreciation that something is wrong (anosognosia); it is often a family member or a bystander who calls for help. Therefore, patients and their family members should be counseled to call emergency medical services immediately if they experience or witness the sudden onset of any of the following: loss of sensory and/or motor function on one side of the body (nearly 85% of ischemic stroke patients have hemiparesis); change in vision, gait, or ability to speak or understand; or if they experience a sudden, severe headache.

There are several common causes of sudden-onset neurologic symptoms that may mimic stroke, including seizure, intracranial tumor, migraine, and metabolic encephalopathy. An adequate history from an observer that no convulsive activity occurred at the onset reasonably excludes seizure; however, ongoing complex partial seizures without tonic-clonic activity may mimic stroke. Tumors may present with acute neurologic symptoms due to hemorrhage, seizure, or hydrocephalus. Surprisingly, migraine can mimic stroke, even in patients without a significant migraine history. When it develops without head pain (*acephalgic migraine*), the diagnosis may remain elusive. Patients without any prior history of migraine may develop acephalgic migraine even after age 65. A sensory disturbance is often prominent, and the sensory deficit, as well as any motor deficits, tends to migrate slowly across a limb over minutes rather than seconds as with stroke. The diagnosis of migraine becomes more secure as the cortical disturbance begins to cross vascular boundaries or if typical visual symptoms are present such as scintillating scotomata (Chap. 14). At times it may be difficult to make the diagnosis until multiple episodes have occurred leaving behind no residual symptoms and with a normal MRI study of the brain. Classically, metabolic encephalopathies produce fluctuating mental status

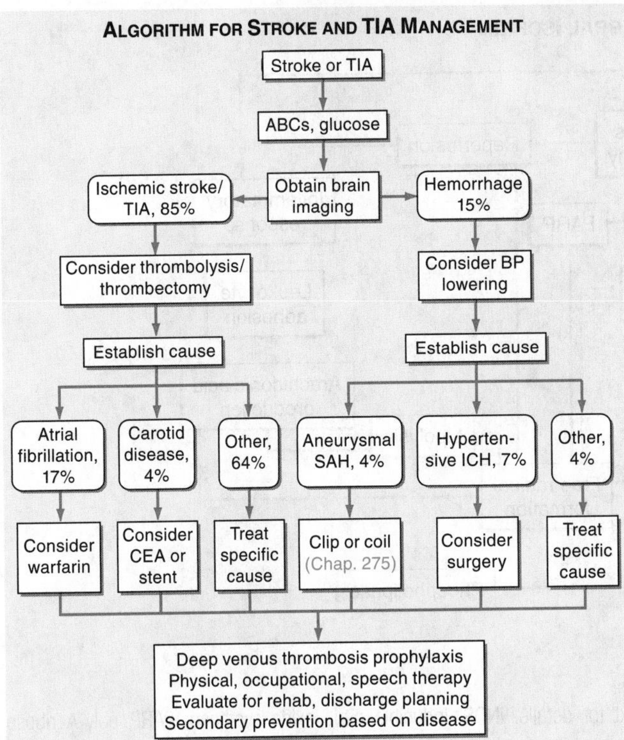

Figure 370-1 Medical management of stroke and TIA. Rounded boxes are diagnoses; rectangles are interventions. Numbers are percentages of stroke overall. ABCs, airway, breathing, circulation; BP, blood pressure; CEA, carotid endarterectomy; ICH, intracerebral hemorrhage; SAH, subarachnoid hemorrhage; TIA, transient ischemic attack.

without focal neurologic findings. However, in the setting of prior stroke or brain injury, a patient with fever or sepsis may manifest hemiparesis, which clears rapidly when the infection is remedied. The metabolic process serves to "unmask" a prior deficit.

Once the diagnosis of stroke is made, a brain imaging study is necessary to determine if the cause of stroke is ischemia or hemorrhage (Fig. 370-1). CT imaging of the brain is the standard imaging modality to detect the presence or absence of intracranial hemorrhage (see "Imaging Studies," below). If the stroke is ischemic, administration of recombinant tissue plasminogen activator (rtPA) or endovascular mechanical thrombectomy may be beneficial in restoring cerebral perfusion (see "Treatment: Acute Ischemic Stroke"). Medical management to reduce the risk of complications becomes the next priority, followed by plans for secondary prevention. For ischemic stroke, several strategies can reduce the risk of subsequent stroke in all patients, while other strategies are effective for patients with specific causes of stroke such as cardiac embolus and carotid atherosclerosis. For hemorrhagic stroke, aneurysmal subarachnoid hemorrhage (SAH) and hypertensive intracranial hemorrhage are two important causes. The treatment and prevention of hypertensive intracranial hemorrhage are discussed later in this chapter. SAH is discussed in Chap. 275.

ISCHEMIC STROKE

PATHOPHYSIOLOGY OF ISCHEMIC STROKE

Acute occlusion of an intracranial vessel causes reduction in blood flow to the brain region it supplies. The magnitude of flow reduction is a function of collateral blood flow and this depends on individual vascular anatomy, the site of occlusion, and likely systemic blood pressure. A decrease in cerebral blood flow to zero causes death of brain tissue within 4–10 minutes; values <16–18 mL/100 g tissue per minute cause infarction within an hour; and values <20 mL/100 g tissue per minute cause ischemia without infarction unless prolonged for several hours or days. If blood flow is restored prior to a significant amount of cell death, the patient may experience only transient symptoms, and the clinical syndrome is called a TIA. Tissue surrounding the core region of infarction is ischemic but reversibly dysfunctional and is referred to as the *ischemic penumbra*. The penumbra may be imaged by using perfusion-diffusion imaging with MRI or CT (see below and Figs. 370-15 and 370-16). The ischemic penumbra will eventually infarct if no change in flow occurs, and hence saving the ischemic penumbra is the goal of revascularization therapies.

Focal cerebral infarction occurs via two distinct pathways (Fig. 370-2): (1) a necrotic pathway in which cellular cytoskeletal breakdown is rapid, due principally to energy failure of the cell; and (2) an apoptotic pathway in which cells become programmed to die. Ischemia produces necrosis by starving neurons of glucose and oxygen, which in turn results in failure of mitochondria to produce ATP. Without ATP, membrane ion pumps stop functioning and neurons depolarize, allowing intracellular calcium to rise. Cellular depolarization also causes glutamate release from synaptic terminals; excess extracellular glutamate produces neurotoxicity by activating postsynaptic glutamate receptors that increase neuronal calcium influx. Free radicals are produced by membrane lipid degradation and mitochondrial dysfunction. Free radicals cause catalytic destruction of membranes and likely damage other vital functions of cells. Lesser degrees of ischemia, as are seen within the ischemic penumbra, favor apoptotic cellular death causing cells to die days to weeks later. Fever dramatically worsens brain injury during ischemia, as does hyperglycemia [glucose >11.1 mmol/L (200 mg/dL)], so it is reasonable to suppress fever and prevent hyperglycemia as much as possible. Induced moderate hypothermia to mitigate stroke is the subject of continuing clinical research.

TREATMENT Acute Ischemic Stroke

After the clinical diagnosis of stroke is made, an orderly process of evaluation and treatment should follow (Fig. 370-1). The first goal is to prevent or reverse brain injury. Attend to the patient's airway, breathing, circulation (ABC's), and treat hypoglycemia or hyperglycemia if identified. Perform an emergency noncontrast head CT scan to differentiate between ischemic stroke and hemorrhagic stroke; there are no reliable clinical findings that conclusively separate ischemia from hemorrhage, although a more depressed level of consciousness, higher initial blood pressure, or worsening of symptoms after onset favor hemorrhage, and a deficit that is maximal at onset, or remits, suggests ischemia. Treatments designed to reverse or lessen the amount of tissue infarction and improve clinical outcome fall within six categories: (1) medical support (2) IV thrombolysis, (3) endovascular techniques, (4) antithrombotic treatment, (5) neuroprotection, and (6) stroke centers and rehabilitation.

MEDICAL SUPPORT When ischemic stroke occurs, the immediate goal is to optimize cerebral perfusion in the surrounding ischemic penumbra. Attention is also directed toward preventing the common complications of bedridden patients—infections (pneumonia, urinary, and skin) and deep venous thrombosis (DVT) with pulmonary embolism. Many physicians use pneumatic

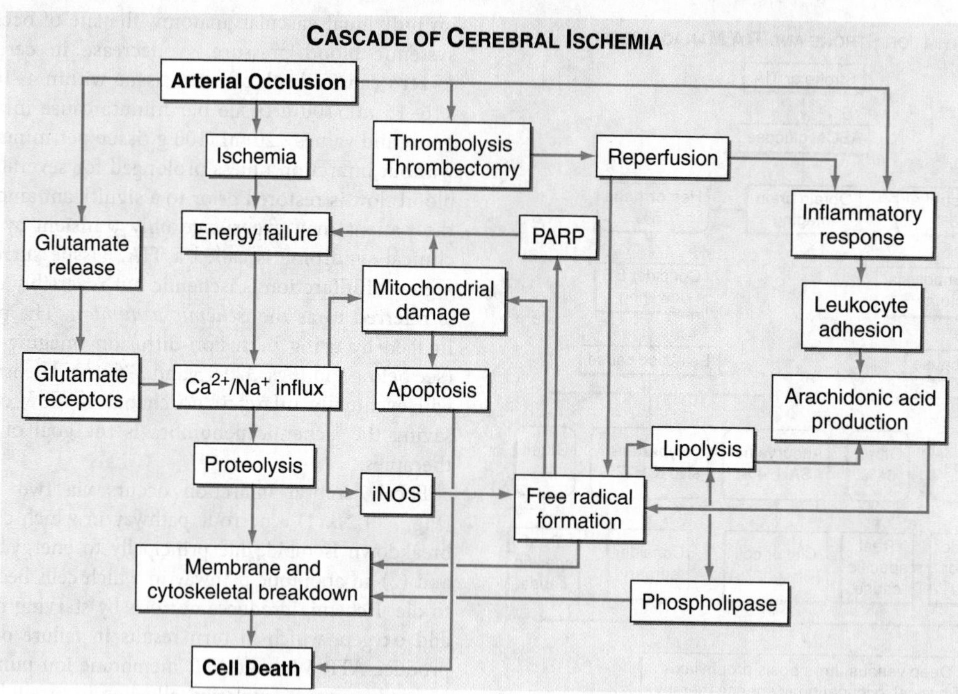

Figure 370-2 Major steps in the cascade of cerebral ischemia. See text for details. iNOS, inducible nitric oxide synthase; PARP, poly-A ribose polymerase.

compression stockings to prevent DVT; subcutaneous heparin (unfractionated and low-molecular weight) is safe and more effective and can be used concomitantly.

Because collateral blood flow within the ischemic brain is blood pressure dependent, there is controversy about whether blood pressure should be lowered acutely. Blood pressure should be lowered if there is malignant hypertension (Chap. 247) or concomitant myocardial ischemia or if blood pressure is >185/110 mm Hg and thrombolytic therapy is anticipated. When faced with the competing demands of myocardium and brain, lowering the heart rate with a β_1-adrenergic blocker (such as esmolol) can be a first step to decrease cardiac work and maintain blood pressure. Fever is detrimental and should be treated with antipyretics and surface cooling. Serum glucose should be monitored and kept at <6.1 mmol/L (110 mg/dL) using an insulin infusion if necessary.

Between 5 and 10% of patients develop enough cerebral edema to cause obtundation or brain herniation. Edema peaks on the second or third day but can cause mass effect for ~10 days. The larger the infarct, the greater the likelihood that clinically significant edema will develop. Water restriction and IV mannitol may be used to raise the serum osmolarity, but hypovolemia should be avoided as this may contribute to hypotension and worsening infarction. Combined analysis of three randomized European trials of hemicraniectomy (craniotomy and temporary removal of part of the skull) shows that hemicraniectomy markedly reduces mortality, and the clinical outcomes of survivors are acceptable.

Special vigilance is warranted for patients with cerebellar infarction. Such strokes may mimic labyrinthitis because of prominent vertigo and vomiting; the presence of head or neck pain should alert the physician to consider cerebellar stroke from vertebral artery dissection. Even small amounts of cerebellar edema can acutely increase intracranial pressure (ICP) or directly compress the brainstem. The resulting brainstem compression can result in coma and respiratory arrest and require emergency surgical decompression. Prophylactic suboccipital decompression of large cerebellar infarcts before brainstem compression, although not tested rigorously in a clinical trial, is practiced at most stroke centers.

INTRAVENOUS THROMBOLYSIS The National Institute of Neurological Disorders and Stroke (NINDS) recombinant tPA (rtPA) Stroke Study showed a clear benefit for IV rtPA in selected patients with acute stroke. The NINDS study used IV rtPA (0.9 mg/kg to a 90-mg max; 10% as a bolus, then the remainder over 60 minutes) versus placebo in patients with ischemic stroke within 3 hours of onset. One-half of the patients were treated within 90 minutes. Symptomatic intracerebral hemorrhage occurred in 6.4% of patients on rtPA and 0.6% on placebo. There was a nonsignificant 4% reduction in mortality in patients on rtPA (21% on placebo and 17% on rtPA); there was a significant 12% absolute increase in the number of patients with only minimal disability (32% on placebo and 44% on rtPA.) Thus, despite an increased incidence of symptomatic intracerebral hemorrhage, treatment with IV rtPA within 3 hours of the onset of ischemic stroke improved clinical outcome.

Three subsequent trials of IV rtPA did not confirm this benefit, perhaps because of the dose of rtPA used, the timing of its delivery, and small sample size. When data from all randomized IV rtPA trails were combined, however, efficacy was confirmed in the <3-hour time window, and efficacy likely extended to 4.5 hours if not 6 hours. Based on these combined results, the European Cooperative Acute Stroke Study (ECASS) III study explored the safety and efficacy of rtPA in the 3- to 4.5-hour time window. Unlike the NINDS study, patients older than 85 years of age, and diabetic patients were excluded. In this 821-patient, randomized study efficacy was again confirmed although less robust than in the 0–3 hour time window. In the rtPA group, 52.4% achieved a good outcome while 45.2% of the placebo group had a good outcome at 90 days (OR 1.34, $p = 0.04$). The symptomatic intracranial hemorrhage rate was 2.4% in the rtPA group and 0.2% in the placebo group ($p = 0.008$).

Based on these data, rtPA is being reviewed for approval in the 3–4.5-hour window in Europe, but is only approved for 0–3 hours in the United States and Canada. Use of IV tPA is now considered a central component of primary stroke centers (see below) as the first treatment proven to improve clinical outcomes in ischemic stroke and is cost-effective and cost-saving. One may be able to select patients beyond the 4.5-hour window, who will benefit from thrombolysis using advanced neuroimaging (see neuroimaging section below), but this is currently investigational. The time of stroke onset is defined as the time the patient's symptoms began or the time the patient was last seen as normal. Patients who awaken with stroke have the onset defined as when they went to bed. Table 370-1 summarizes eligibility criteria and instructions for administration of IV rtPA.

TABLE 370-1 Administration of Intravenous Recombinant Tissue Plasminogen Activator (rtPA) for Acute Ischemic Stroke (AIS)[a]

Indication	Contraindication
Clinical diagnosis of stroke	Sustained BP >185/110 mm Hg despite treatment
Onset of symptoms to time of drug administration ≤3 h	Platelets <100,000; HCT <25%; glucose <50 or >400 mg/dL
CT scan showing no hemorrhage or edema of >1/3 of the MCA territory	Use of heparin within 48 h and prolonged PTT, or elevated INR
Age ≥18 years	Rapidly improving symptoms
Consent by patient or surrogate	Prior stroke or head injury within 3 months; prior intracranial hemorrhage
	Major surgery in preceding 14 days
	Minor stroke symptoms
	Gastrointestinal bleeding in preceding 21 days
	Recent myocardial infarction
	Coma or stupor

Administration of rtPA

- Intravenous access with two peripheral IV lines (avoid arterial or central line placement)
- Review eligibility for rtPA
- Administer 0.9 mg/kg IV (maximum 90 mg) IV as 10% of total dose by bolus, followed by remainder of total dose over 1 h
- Frequent cuff blood pressure monitoring
- No other antithrombotic treatment for 24 h
- For decline in neurologic status or uncontrolled blood pressure, stop infusion, give cryoprecipitate, and reimage brain emergently
- Avoid urethral catheterization for ≥2 h

[a]See Activase (tissue plasminogen activator) package insert for complete list of contraindications and dosing.

Abbreviations: BP, blood pressure; HCT, hematocrit; INR, international normalized ratio; MCA, middle cerebral artery; PTT, partial thromboplastin time.

ENDOVASCULAR TECHNIQUES Ischemic stroke from large-vessel intracranial occlusion results in high rates of mortality and morbidity. Occlusions in such large vessels [middle cerebral artery (MCA), internal carotid artery, and the basilar artery] generally involve a large clot volume and often fail to open with IV rtPA alone. Therefore, there is growing interest in using thrombolytics via an intraarterial route to increase the concentration of drug at the clot and minimize systemic bleeding complications. The Prolyse in Acute Cerebral Thromboembolism (PROACT) II trial found benefit for intraarterial pro urokinase for acute MCA occlusions up to the sixth hour following onset of stroke. Intraarterial treatment of basilar artery occlusions may also be beneficial for selected patients. Intraarterial administration of a thrombolytic agent for acute ischemic stroke (AIS) is not approved by the U.S. Food and Drug Administration (FDA); however, many stroke centers offer this treatment based on these data.

Endovascular mechanical thrombectomy has recently shown promise as an alternative or adjunctive treatment of acute stroke in patients who are ineligible for, or have contraindications to, thrombolytics or in those who have failed to have vascular recanalization with IV thrombolytics (see Fig. 370-15). The Mechanical Embolus Removal in Cerebral Ischemia (MERCI) and multi-MERCI single-arm trials investigated the ability of a novel endovascular thrombectomy device to restore patency of occluded intracranial vessels within 8 hours of ischemic stroke symptoms. Recanalization of the target vessel occurred in 48–58% of treated patients and in 60–69% following use of adjuvant endovascular methods, and successful recanalization at 90 days correlated well with favorable outcomes. Based upon these nonrandomized data, the FDA approved this device as the first device for revascularization of occluded vessels in acute ischemic stroke even if the patient has been given rtPA and that therapy has failed. The Penumbra Pivotal Stroke trial tested another mechanical device that showed even higher rates of recanalization and led to FDA clearance of the tested device as well. Because use of endovascular devices in combination with rtPA appears safe, primary stroke centers may administer rtPA to eligible patients, and then rapidly refer such patients to comprehensive stroke centers that have endovascular capability for further intervention. Such a design allows centralization of resource-intensive endovascular centers in order to serve larger populations of patients. Use of mechanical techniques to restore blood flow have not as yet been studied in a randomized trial so the clinical efficacy of these treatments remain unproven and the focus of active investigation.

ANTITHROMBOTIC TREATMENT

Platelet Inhibition Aspirin is the only antiplatelet agent that has been proven effective for the acute treatment of ischemic stroke; there are several antiplatelet agents proven for the secondary prevention of stroke (see below). Two large trials, the International Stroke Trial (IST) and the Chinese Acute Stroke Trial (CAST), found that the use of aspirin within 48 hours of stroke onset reduced both stroke recurrence risk and mortality minimally. Among 19,435 patients in IST, those allocated to aspirin, 300 mg/d, had slightly fewer deaths within 14 days (9.0 versus 9.4%), significantly fewer recurrent ischemic strokes (2.8 versus 3.9%), no excess of hemorrhagic strokes (0.9 versus 0.8%), and a trend toward a reduction in death or dependence at 6 months (61.2 versus 63.5%). In CAST, 21,106 patients with ischemic stroke received 160 mg/d of aspirin or a placebo for up to 4 weeks. There were very small reductions in the aspirin group in early mortality (3.3 versus 3.9%), recurrent ischemic strokes (1.6 versus 2.1%), and dependency at discharge or death (30.5 versus 31.6%). These trials demonstrate that the use of aspirin in the treatment of AIS is safe and produces a small net benefit. For every 1000 acute strokes treated with aspirin, about 9 deaths or nonfatal stroke recurrences will be prevented in the first few weeks and ~13 fewer patients will be dead or dependent at 6 months.

The glycoprotein IIb/IIIa receptor inhibitor abciximab was found to cause excess intracranial hemorrhage and should be avoided in acute stroke. Clopidogrel is being tested as a way to prevent stroke following TIA and minor ischemic stroke.

Anticoagulation Numerous clinical trials have failed to demonstrate any benefit of anticoagulation in the primary treatment of atherothrombotic cerebral ischemia. Several trials have investigated antiplatelet versus anticoagulant medications given within 12–24 hours of the initial event. The U.S. Trial of Organon 10172 in Acute Stroke Treatment (TOAST), an investigational low-molecular-weight heparin (LMWH), failed to show any benefit over aspirin. Use of SC unfractionated heparin versus aspirin was tested in IST. Heparin given SC afforded no additional benefit over aspirin and increased bleeding rates. Several trials of LMWHs have also shown no consistent benefit in AIS. Furthermore, trials generally have shown an excess risk of brain and systemic hemorrhage with acute anticoagulation. Therefore, trials do not support the routine use of heparin or other anticoagulants for patients with atherothrombotic stroke.

NEUROPROTECTION Neuroprotection is the concept of providing a treatment that prolongs the brain's tolerance to ischemia. Drugs that block the excitatory amino acid pathways have been shown to protect neurons and glia in animals, but despite multiple human trials, they have not yet been proven to be beneficial. Hypothermia is a powerful neuroprotective treatment in patients with cardiac arrest (Chap. 275) and is neuroprotective in animal models of stroke, but it has not been adequately studied in patients with ischemic stroke.

STROKE CENTERS AND REHABILITATION Patient care in comprehensive stroke units followed by rehabilitation services improves neurologic outcomes and reduces mortality. Use of clinical pathways and staff dedicated to the stroke patient can improve care. Stroke teams that provide emergency 24-hour evaluation of acute stroke patients for acute medical management and consideration of thrombolysis or endovascular treatments are essential components of primary and comprehensive stroke centers, respectively.

Proper rehabilitation of the stroke patient includes early physical, occupational, and speech therapy. It is directed toward educating the patient and family about the patient's neurologic deficit, preventing the complications of immobility (e.g., pneumonia, DVT and pulmonary embolism, pressure sores of the skin, and muscle contractures), and providing encouragement and instruction in overcoming the deficit. The goal of rehabilitation is to return the patient to home and to maximize recovery by providing a safe, progressive regimen suited to the individual patient. Additionally, the use of restraint therapy (immobilizing the unaffected side) has been shown to improve hemiparesis following stroke, even years following the stroke, suggesting that physical therapy can recruit unused neural pathways. This finding suggests that the human nervous system is more adaptable than originally thought and has stimulated active research into physical and pharmacologic strategies that can enhance long-term neural recovery.

ETIOLOGY OF ISCHEMIC STROKE

(Figs. 370-1 and 370-3 and Table 370-2) Although the initial management of AIS often does not depend on the etiology, establishing a cause is essential in reducing the risk of recurrence. Particular focus should be on atrial fibrillation and carotid atherosclerosis, as these etiologies have proven secondary prevention strategies. The clinical presentation and examination findings often establish the cause of stroke or narrow the possibilities to a few. Judicious use of laboratory testing and imaging studies completes the initial evaluation. Nevertheless, nearly 30% of strokes remain unexplained despite extensive evaluation.

Clinical examination should focus on the peripheral and cervical vascular system (carotid auscultation for bruits, blood pressure, and pressure comparison between arms), the heart (dysrhythmia, murmurs), extremities (peripheral emboli), and retina [effects of hypertension and cholesterol emboli (Hollenhorst plaques)]. A complete neurologic examination is performed to localize the site of stroke. An imaging study of the brain is nearly always indicated and is required for patients being considered for thrombolysis; it may be combined with CT- or MRI-based angiography to interrogate the neck and intracranial vessels (see "Imaging Studies," below). A chest x-ray, electrocardiogram (ECG), urinalysis, complete blood count, erythrocyte sedimentation rate (ESR), serum electrolytes, blood urea nitrogen (BUN), creatinine, blood sugar, serologic test for syphilis, serum lipid profile, prothrombin time (PT), and partial thromboplastin time (PTT) are often useful and should be considered in all patients. An ECG may demonstrate arrhythmias or reveal evidence of recent myocardial infarction (MI).

Cardioembolic stroke

Cardioembolism is responsible for ~20% of all ischemic strokes. Stroke caused by heart disease is primarily due to embolism of thrombotic material forming on the atrial or ventricular wall or the left heart valves. These thrombi then detach and embolize into the arterial circulation. The thrombus may fragment or lyse quickly, producing only a TIA. Alternatively, the arterial occlusion may last longer, producing stroke. Embolic strokes tend to be sudden in onset, with maximum neurologic deficit at once. With reperfusion following more prolonged ischemia, petechial hemorrhage can occur within the ischemic territory. This is usually of no clinical significance and should be distinguished from frank intracranial hemorrhage into a region of ischemic stroke where the mass effect from the hemorrhage can cause a decline in neurologic function.

Emboli from the heart most often lodge in the MCA, the posterior cerebral artery (PCA), or one of their branches; infrequently, the anterior cerebral artery (ACA) territory is involved. Emboli large enough to occlude the stem of the MCA (3–4 mm) lead to large infarcts that involve both deep gray and white matter and some portions of the cortical surface and its underlying white matter. A smaller embolus may occlude a small cortical or penetrating arterial branch. The location and size of an infarct within a vascular territory depend on the extent of the collateral circulation.

The most significant causes of cardioembolic stroke in most of the world are nonrheumatic (often called nonvalvular) atrial fibrillation, MI, prosthetic valves, rheumatic heart disease, and ischemic cardiomyopathy (Table 370-2). Cardiac disorders causing brain embolism are discussed in the respective chapters on heart diseases. A few pertinent aspects are highlighted here.

Nonrheumatic atrial fibrillation is the most common cause of cerebral embolism overall. The presumed stroke mechanism is thrombus formation in the fibrillating atrium or atrial appendage, with subsequent embolization. Patients with atrial fibrillation have an average annual risk of stroke of ~5%. The risk of stroke can be estimated by calculating the CHADS2 score (see Table 370-3)

Left atrial enlargement is an additional risk factor for formation of atrial thrombi. Rheumatic heart disease usually causes ischemic stroke when there is prominent mitral stenosis or atrial fibrillation. Recent MI may be a source of emboli, especially when transmural and involving the anteroapical ventricular wall, and prophylactic anticoagulation following MI has been shown to reduce stroke risk. Mitral valve prolapse is not usually a source of emboli unless the prolapse is severe.

Paradoxical embolization occurs when venous thrombi migrate to the arterial circulation, usually via a patent foramen ovale or atrial septal defect. Bubble-contrast echocardiography (IV injection of agitated saline coupled with either transthoracic or transesophageal echocardiography) can demonstrate a right-to-left cardiac shunt, revealing the conduit for paradoxical embolization. Alternatively, a right-to-left shunt is implied if immediately following IV injection of agitated saline, the ultrasound signature of bubbles is observed during transcranial Doppler insonation of the MCA; pulmonary AVMs should be considered if this test is positive yet an echocardiogram fails to reveal an intracardiac shunt. Both techniques are highly sensitive for detection of right-to-left shunts. Besides venous clot, fat and tumor emboli, bacterial endocarditis, IV air, and amniotic fluid emboli at childbirth may occasionally be responsible for paradoxical embolization. The importance of right-to-left shunt as a cause of stroke is debated, particularly because such shunts are present in ~15% of the general population. Some studies have suggested that the risk is only elevated in the presence of a coexisting atrial septal aneurysm. The presence of a venous source of embolus, most commonly a deep venous thrombus, may provide confirmation of the importance of a right-to-left shunt in a particular case.

Bacterial endocarditis can cause valvular vegetations that can give rise to septic emboli. The appearance of multifocal symptoms and signs in a patient with stroke makes bacterial endocarditis more likely. Infarcts of microscopic size occur, and large septic infarcts may evolve into brain abscesses or cause hemorrhage into the infarct, which generally precludes use of anticoagulation or thrombolytics. Mycotic aneurysms caused by septic emboli give rise to SAH or intracerebral hemorrhage.

Artery-to-artery embolic stroke

Thrombus formation on atherosclerotic plaques may embolize to intracranial arteries producing an artery-to-artery embolic stroke. Less commonly, a diseased vessel may acutely thrombose. Unlike the myocardial vessels, artery-to-artery embolism, rather than local thrombosis, appears to be the dominant vascular mechanism causing brain ischemia. Any diseased vessel may be an embolic source, including the aortic arch, common carotid, internal carotid, vertebral, and basilar arteries. Carotid bifurcation atherosclerosis is the most common source of artery-to-artery embolus, and specific treatments have proven efficacy in reducing risk.

Carotid Atherosclerosis Atherosclerosis within the carotid artery occurs most frequently within the common carotid bifurcation and proximal internal carotid artery. Additionally, the carotid siphon (portion within the cavernous sinus) is also vulnerable to atherosclerosis. Male gender, older age, smoking, hypertension, diabetes, and hypercholesterolemia are risk factors for carotid disease, as they are for stroke in general (Table 370-4). Carotid atherosclerosis produces an estimated 10% of ischemic stroke. **For further discussion of the pathogenesis of atherosclerosis, see Chap. 241.**

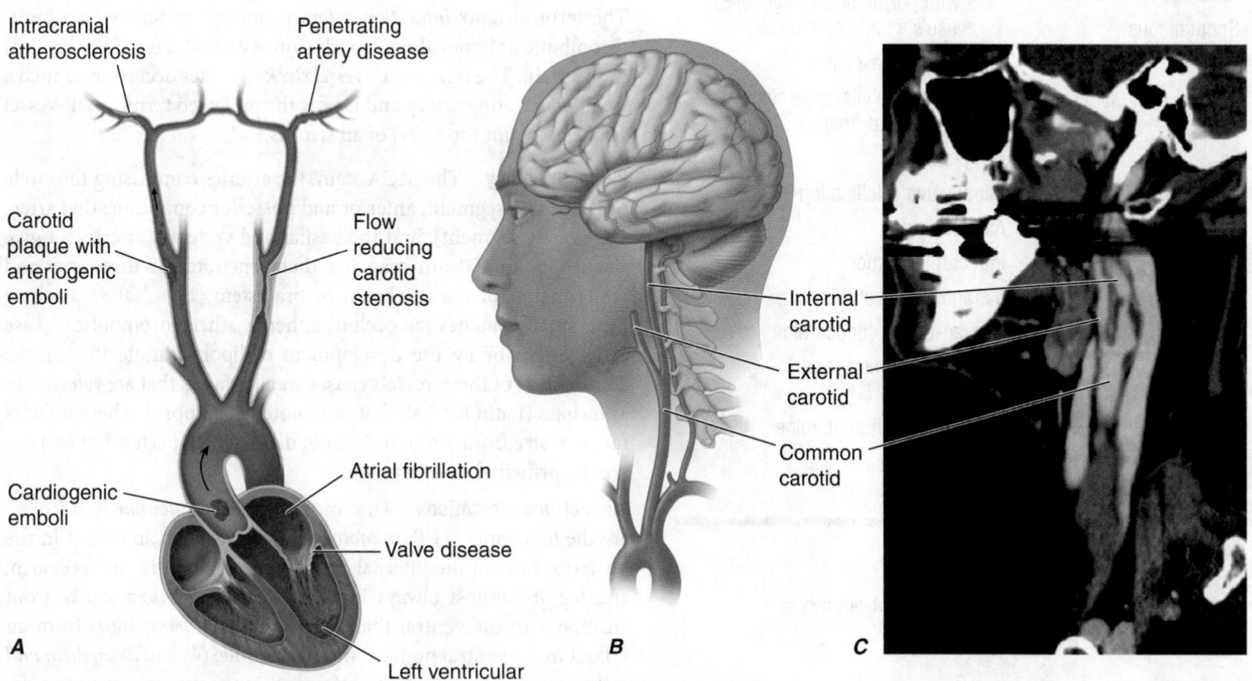

Figure 370-3 Pathophysiology of ischemic stroke. ***A.*** Diagram illustrating the three major mechanisms that underlie ischemic stroke: (1) occlusion of an intracranial vessel by an embolus that arises at a distant site (e.g., cardiogenic sources such as atrial fibrillation or artery-to-artery emboli from carotid atherosclerotic plaque), often affecting the large intracranial vessels; (2) in situ thrombosis of an intracranial vessel, typically affecting the small penetrating arteries that arise from the major intracranial arteries; (3) hypoperfusion caused by flow-limiting stenosis of a major extracranial (e.g., internal carotid) or intracranial vessel, often producing "watershed" ischemia. ***B*** and ***C.*** Diagram and reformatted CT angiogram of the common, internal, and external carotid arteries. High-grade stenosis of the internal carotid artery, which may be associated with either cerebral emboli or flow-limiting ischemia, was identified in this patient.

TABLE 370-2 Causes of Ischemic Stroke

Common Causes	Uncommon Causes
Thrombosis	Hypercoagulable disorders
Lacunar stroke (small vessel)	Protein C deficiency
Large vessel thrombosis	Protein S deficiency
Dehydration	Antithrombin III deficiency
Embolic occlusion	Antiphospholipid syndrome
Artery-to-artery	Factor V Leiden mutation[a]
Carotid bifurcation	Prothrombin G20210 mutation[a]
Aortic arch	Systemic malignancy
Arterial dissection	Sickle cell anemia
Cardioembolic	β-Thalassemia
Atrial fibrillation	Polycythemia vera
Mural thrombus	Systemic lupus erythematosus
Myocardial infarction	Homocysteinemia
Dilated cardiomyopathy	Thrombotic thrombocytopenic purpura
Valvular lesions	Disseminated intravascular coagulation
Mitral stenosis	Dysproteinemias
Mechanical valve	Nephrotic syndrome
Bacterial endocarditis	Inflammatory bowel disease
Paradoxical embolus	Oral contraceptives
Atrial septal defect	Venous sinus thrombosis[b]
Patent foramen ovale	Fibromuscular dysplasia
Atrial septal aneurysm	Vasculitis
Spontaneous echo contrast	Systemic vasculitis [PAN, granulomatosis with polyangiitis (Wegener's), Takayasu's, giant cell arteritis]
	Primary CNS vasculitis
	Meningitis (syphilis, tuberculosis, fungal, bacterial, zoster)
	Cardiogenic
	Mitral valve calcification
	Atrial myxoma
	Intracardiac tumor
	Marantic endocarditis
	Libman-Sacks endocarditis
	Subarachnoid hemorrhage vasospasm
	Drugs: cocaine, amphetamine
	Moyamoya disease
	Eclampsia

[a]Chiefly cause venous sinus thrombosis.
[b]May be associated with any hypercoagulable disorder.
Abbreviations: CNS, central nervous system; PAN, polyarteritis nodosa.

Carotid disease can be classified by whether the stenosis is symptomatic or asymptomatic and by the degree of stenosis (percent narrowing of the narrowest segment compared to a more distal internal carotid segment). Symptomatic carotid disease implies that the patient has experienced a stroke or TIA within the vascular distribution of the artery, and it is associated with a greater risk of subsequent stroke than asymptomatic stenosis, in which the patient is symptom free and the stenosis is detected through screening. Greater degrees of arterial narrowing are generally associated with a greater risk of stroke, except that those with near occlusions are at lower risk of stroke.

Other causes of artery-to-artery embolic stroke *Intracranial atherosclerosis* produces stroke either by an embolic mechanism or by in situ thrombosis of a diseased vessel. It is more common in patients of Asian and African-American descent. Recurrent stroke risk is ~15% per year, similar to symptomatic untreated carotid atherosclerosis.

Dissection of the internal carotid or vertebral arteries or even vessels beyond the circle of Willis is a common source of embolic stroke in young (age <60 years) patients. The dissection is usually painful and precedes the stroke by several hours or days. Extracranial dissections do not cause hemorrhage because of the tough adventitia of these vessels. Intracranial dissections, conversely, may produce SAH because the adventitia of intracranial vessels is thin and pseudoaneurysms may form, requiring urgent treatment to prevent rerupture. Treating asymptomatic pseudoaneurysms following dissection is controversial. The cause of dissection is usually unknown and recurrence is rare. Ehlers-Danlos type IV, Marfan's disease, cystic medial necrosis, and fibromuscular dysplasia are associated with dissections. Trauma (usually a motor vehicle accident or a sports injury) can cause carotid and vertebral artery dissections. Spinal manipulative therapy is independently associated with vertebral artery dissection and stroke. Most dissections heal spontaneously, and stroke or TIA is uncommon beyond 2 weeks. Although there are no trials comparing anticoagulation to antiplatelet agents, many physicians treat acutely with anticoagulants then convert to antiplatelet therapy after demonstration of satisfactory vascular recanalization.

SMALL-VESSEL STROKE

The term *lacunar infarction* refers to infarction following atherothrombotic or lipohyalinotic occlusion of a small artery (30–300 μm) in the brain. The term *small-vessel stroke* denotes occlusion of such a small penetrating artery and is now the preferred term. Small-vessel strokes account for ~20% of all strokes.

Pathophysiology The MCA stem, the arteries comprising the circle of Willis (A1 segment, anterior and posterior communicating arteries, and P1 segment), and the basilar and vertebral arteries all give rise to 30- to 300-μm branches that penetrate the deep gray and white matter of the cerebrum or brainstem (Fig. 370-4). Each of these small branches can occlude either by atherothrombotic disease at its origin or by the development of lipohyalinotic thickening. Thrombosis of these vessels causes small infarcts that are referred to as *lacunes* (Latin for "lake" of fluid noted at autopsy). These infarcts range in size from 3 mm to 2 cm in diameter. Hypertension and age are the principal risk factors.

Clinical manifestations The most common *lacunar syndromes* are the following: (1) *Pure motor hemiparesis* from an infarct in the posterior limb of the internal capsule or basis pontis; the face, arm, and leg are almost always involved; (2) *pure sensory stroke* from an infarct in the ventral thalamus; (3) *ataxic hemiparesis* from an infarct in the ventral pons or internal capsule; (4) and *dysarthria and a clumsy hand* or arm due to infarction in the ventral pons or in the genu of the internal capsule.

Transient symptoms (small vessel TIAs) may herald a small-vessel infarct; they may occur several times a day and last only a few minutes. Recovery from small-vessel strokes tends to be more rapid and complete than recovery from large-vessel strokes; in some cases, however, there is severe permanent disability. Often, institution of combined antithrombotic treatments does not prevent eventual stroke in "stuttering lacunes."

TABLE 370-3 Recommendations on Chronic Use of Antithrombotics for Various Cardiac Conditions

Condition	Recommendation
Nonvalvular atrial fibrillation	Calculate CHADS2[a] score
• CHADS2 score 0	Aspirin or no antithrombotic
• CHADS2 score 1	Aspirin or VKA
• CHADS2 score >1	VKA
Rheumatic mitral valve disease	
• With atrial fibrillation, previous embolization, or atrial appendage thrombus, or left atrial diameter >55 mm	VKA
• Embolization or appendage clot despite INR 2–3	VKA plus aspirin
Mitral valve prolapse	
• Asymptomatic	No therapy
• With otherwise cryptogenic stroke or TIA	Aspirin
• Atrial fibrillation	VKA
Mitral annular calcification	
• Without atrial fibrillation but systemic embolization, or otherwise cryptogenic stroke or TIA	Aspirin
• Recurrent embolization despite aspirin	VKA
• With atrial fibrillation	VKA
Aortic valve calcification	
• Asymptomatic	No therapy
• Otherwise cryptogenic stroke or TIA	Aspirin
Aortic arch mobile atheroma	
• Otherwise cryptogenic stroke or TIA	Aspirin or VKA
Patent foramen ovale	
• Otherwise cryptogenic ischemic stroke or TIA	Aspirin
• Indication for VKA (deep venous thrombosis or hypercoagulable state)	VKA
Mechanical heart value	
• Aortic position, bileaflet or Medtronic Hall tilting disk with normal left atrial size and sinus rhythm	VKA INR 2.5, range 2–3
• Mitral position tilting disk or bileaflet valve	VKA INR 3.0, range 2.5–3.5
• Mitral or aortic position, anterior-apical myocardial infarct or left atrial enlargement	VKA INR 3.0 , range 2.5–3.5
• Mitral or aortic position, with atrial fibrillation, or hypercoagulable state, or low ejection fraction, or atherosclerotic vascular disease	Aspirin plus VKA INR 3.0, range 2.5–3.5
• Systemic embolization despite target INR	Add aspirin and/or increase INR: prior target was 2.5 increase to 3.0, range 2.5–3.5; prior target was 3.0 increase to 3.5, range 3–4
Bioprosthetic valve	
• No other indication for VKA therapy	Aspirin
Infective endocarditis	Avoid antithrombotic agents
Nonbacterial thrombotic endocarditis	
• With systemic embolization	Full dose unfractionated heparin or SC LMWH

[a]CHADS2 score calculated as follows: 1 point for age >75 years, 1 point for hypertension, 1 point for congestive heart failure, 1 point for diabetes, and 2 points for stroke or TIA; sum of points is the total CHADS2 score.

Abbreviations: Dose of aspirin is 50–325 mg/d; target INR for VKA is 2.5 unless otherwise specified. INR, international normalized ratio; LMWH, low-molecular-weight heparin; TIA, transient ischemic attack; VKA, vitamin K antagonist.

Sources: Modified from DE Singer et al: Chest 133:546S, 2008; DN Salem et al: Chest 133:593S, 2008.

A large-vessel source (either thrombosis or embolism) may manifest initially as a lacunar syndrome with small-vessel infarction. Therefore, the search for embolic sources (carotid and heart) should not be completely abandoned in the evaluation of these patients. Secondary prevention of lacunar stroke involves risk factor modification, specifically reduction in blood pressure (see "Primary and Secondary Prevention of Stroke and TIA," below).

■ LESS COMMON CAUSES OF STROKE

(**Table 370-2**) *Hypercoagulable disorders* (Chap. 58) primarily cause increased risk of venous thrombosis and therefore may cause venous sinus thrombosis. Protein S deficiency and homocysteinemia may cause arterial thromboses as well. Systemic lupus erythematosus with Libman-Sacks endocarditis can be a cause of embolic stroke. These conditions overlap with the antiphospholipid syndrome, which probably requires long-term anticoagulation to prevent further stroke.

Venous sinus thrombosis of the lateral or sagittal sinus or of small cortical veins (cortical vein thrombosis) occurs as a complication of oral contraceptive use, pregnancy and the postpartum period, inflammatory bowel disease, intracranial infections (meningitis), and dehydration. It is also seen with increased incidence in patients with laboratory-confirmed thrombophilia (**Table 370-2**) including polycythemia, sickle cell anemia, deficiencies of proteins C and S, factor V Leiden mutation (resistance to activated protein C), antithrombin III deficiency, homocysteinemia, and the prothrombin G20210 mutation. Women who take oral contraceptives and have the prothrombin G20210 mutation may be at particularly high risk for sinus thrombosis. Patients present with headache and may also have focal neurologic signs (especially paraparesis) and seizures. Often, CT imaging is normal unless an intracranial venous hemorrhage has occurred, but the venous sinus occlusion is readily visualized using MR- or CT-venography or conventional x-ray angiography. With greater degrees of sinus thrombosis, the patient may develop signs of increased ICP and coma. Intravenous heparin, regardless of the presence of intracranial hemorrhage, has been shown to reduce morbidity and mortality, and the long-term outcome is generally good. Heparin prevents further thrombosis and reduces venous hypertension and ischemia. If an underlying hypercoagulable state is not found, many physicians treat with vitamin K antagonists (VKAs) for 3–6 months then convert to aspirin, depending on the degree of resolution of the venous sinus thrombus. Anticoagulation is often continued indefinitely if thrombophilia is diagnosed.

Sickle cell anemia (SS disease) is a common cause of stroke in children. A subset of homozygous carriers of this hemoglobin mutation develop stroke in childhood and this may be predicted by documenting high-velocity blood flow within the MCAs using transcranial Doppler ultrasonography. In children who are identified to have high velocities, treatment with aggressive exchange transfusion dramatically reduces risk of stroke, and if exchange transfusion is ceased, their stroke rate increases again along with MCA velocities.

Fibromuscular dysplasia affects the cervical arteries and occurs mainly in women. The carotid or vertebral arteries show multiple rings of segmental narrowing alternating with dilatation. Occlusion is usually incomplete. The process is often asymptomatic but occasionally is associated with an audible bruit, TIAs, or stroke. Involvement of the renal arteries is common and may cause hypertension. The cause and natural history of fibromuscular dysplasia are unknown (Chap. 249). TIA or stroke generally occurs only when the artery is severely narrowed or dissects. Anticoagulation or antiplatelet therapy may be helpful.

Temporal (giant cell) arteritis (Chap. 326) is a relatively common affliction of elderly persons in which the external carotid system, particularly the temporal arteries, undergo subacute granulomatous inflammation with giant cells. Occlusion of posterior ciliary arteries derived from the ophthalmic artery results in blindness in one or both eyes and can be prevented with glucocorticoids. It rarely causes stroke as the internal carotid artery is usually not inflamed. Idiopathic giant cell arteritis involving the great vessels arising from the aortic arch (*Takayasu's arteritis*) may cause carotid or vertebral thrombosis; it is rare in the Western hemisphere.

Necrotizing (or granulomatous) arteritis, occurring alone or in association with generalized polyarteritis nodosa or granulomatosis with polyangiitis (Wegener's), involves the distal small branches (<2 mm diameter) of the main intracranial arteries and produces small ischemic infarcts in the brain, optic nerve, and spinal cord. The cerebrospinal fluid (CSF) often shows pleocytosis, and the protein level is elevated. *Primary central nervous system vasculitis* is rare; small or medium-sized vessels are usually affected, without apparent systemic vasculitis. The differential diagnosis includes other inflammatory causes of vascular caliber change including infection (tubercular, fungal), sarcoidosis, angiocentric lymphoma, carcinomatous meningitis, as well as noninflammatory causes such as atherosclerosis, emboli, connective tissue disease, vasospasm, migraine-associated vasculopathy, and drug-associated causes. Some cases follow the postpartum period and are self-limited.

Patients with any form of vasculopathy may present with insidious progression of combined white and gray matter infarctions, prominent headache, and cognitive decline. Brain biopsy or high-resolution conventional x-ray angiography is usually

TABLE 370-4 Risk Factors for Stroke

Risk Factor	Relative Risk	Relative Risk Reduction with Treatment	Number Needed to Treat[a] Primary Prevention	Number Needed to Treat[a] Secondary Prevention
Hypertension	2–5	38%	100–300	50–100
Atrial fibrillation	1.8–2.9	68% warfarin, 21% aspirin	20–83	13
Diabetes	1.8–6	No proven effect		
Smoking	1.8	50% at 1 year, baseline risk at 5 years' postcessation		
Hyperlipidemia	1.8–2.6	16–30%	560	230
Asymptomatic carotid stenosis	2.0	53%	85	N/A
Symptomatic carotid stenosis (70–99%)		65% at 2 years	N/A	12
Symptomatic carotid stenosis (50–69%)		29% at 5 years	N/A	77

[a]Number needed to treat to prevent one stroke annually. Prevention of other cardiovascular outcomes is not considered here.
Abbreviation: N/A, not applicable.

Anterior cerebral a.
Deep branches of the middle cerebral a.
Internal carotid a.
Middle cerebral a.

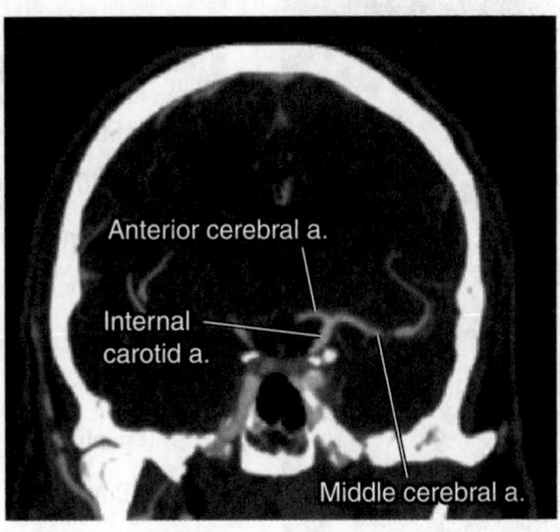

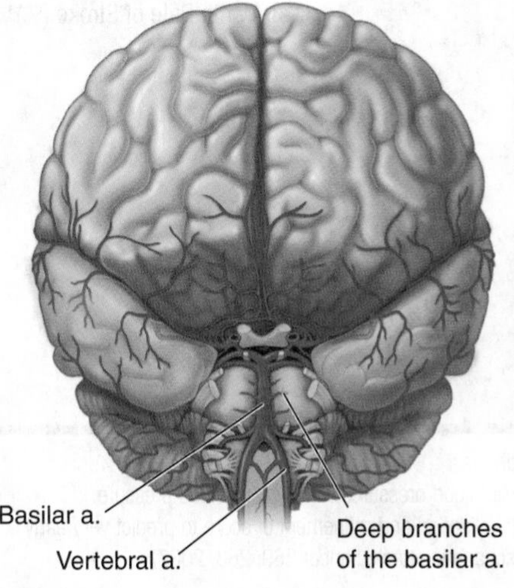

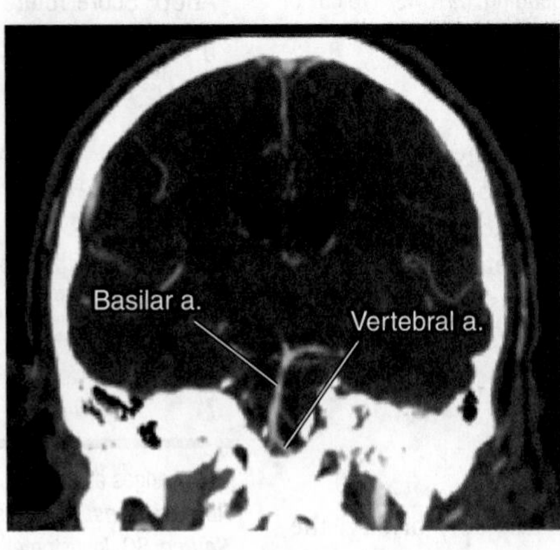

Figure 370-4 Diagrams and reformatted CT angiograms in the coronal section illustrating the deep penetrating arteries involved in small-vessel strokes. In the anterior circulation, small penetrating arteries called *lenticulostriates* arise from the proximal portion of the anterior and middle cerebral arteries and supply deep subcortical structures (***upper panels***). In the posterior circulation, similar arteries arise directly from the vertebral and basilar arteries to supply the brainstem (***lower panels***). Occlusion of a single penetrating artery gives rise to a discrete area of infarct (pathologically termed a "lacune," or lake). Note that these vessels are too small to be visualized on CT angiography.

required to make the diagnosis (Fig. 370-5). An inflammatory profile found on lumbar puncture favors an inflammatory cause. In cases where inflammation is confirmed, aggressive immunosuppression with glucocorticoids, and often cyclophosphamide, is usually necessary to prevent progression; a diligent investigation for infectious causes such as tuberculosis is essential prior to immunosuppression. With prompt recognition and treatment, many patients can make an excellent recovery.

Drugs, in particular amphetamines and perhaps cocaine, may cause stroke on the basis of acute hypertension or drug-induced vasculopathy. No data exist on the value of any treatment. Phenylpropanolamine has been linked with intracranial hemorrhage, as has cocaine and methamphetamine, perhaps related to a drug-induced vasculopathy. *Moyamoya disease* is a poorly understood occlusive disease involving large intracranial arteries, especially the distal internal carotid artery and the stem of the MCA and ACA. Vascular inflammation is absent. The lenticulostriate arteries develop a rich collateral circulation around the occlusive lesion, which gives the impression of a "puff of smoke" (*moyamoya* in Japanese) on conventional x-ray angiography. Other collaterals include transdural anastomoses between the cortical surface branches of the meningeal and scalp arteries. The disease occurs mainly in Asian children or young adults, but the appearance may be identical in adults who have atherosclerosis, particularly in association with diabetes. Because of the occurrence of intracranial hemorrhage from rupture of the transdural and pial anastomotic channels, anticoagulation is risky. Breakdown of dilated lenticulostriate arteries may produce parenchymal hemorrhage, and progressive occlusion of large surface arteries can occur, producing large-artery distribution strokes. Surgical bypass of extracranial carotid arteries to the dura or MCAs may prevent stroke and hemorrhage.

Reversible posterior leukoencephalopathy can occur in head injury, seizure, migraine, sympathomimetic drug use, eclampsia, and the postpartum period. The pathophysiology is uncertain but likely involves widespread cerebral segmental vasoconstriction and cerebral edema. Patients complain of headache and manifest fluctuating neurologic symptoms and signs, especially visual symptoms. Sometimes cerebral infarction ensues, but typically the clinical and imaging findings suggest that ischemia reverses completely. MRI findings are characteristic, and conventional x-ray angiography may also be helpful in establishing the diagnosis.

Leukoaraiosis, or *periventricular white matter disease,* is the result of multiple small-vessel infarcts within the subcortical white matter. It is readily seen on CT or MRI scans as areas of white matter injury surrounding the ventricles and within the corona radiata. Areas of lacunar infarction are often seen also. The pathophysiologic basis of the disease is lipohyalinosis of small penetrating arteries within the white matter, likely produced by chronic hypertension. Patients with periventricular white matter disease may develop a subcortical dementia syndrome, depending on the amount of white matter infarction, and it is likely that this common form of dementia may be delayed or prevented with antihypertensive medications (Chap. 371).

CADASIL (cerebral autosomal dominant arteriopathy with subcortical infarcts and leukoencephalopathy) is an inherited disorder that presents as small-vessel strokes, progressive dementia, and extensive symmetric white matter changes visualized by MRI. Approximately 40% of patients have migraine with aura, often manifest as transient motor or sensory deficits. Onset is usually in the fourth or fifth decade of life. This autosomal dominant condition is caused by one of several mutations in Notch-3, a member of a highly conserved gene family characterized by epidermal growth

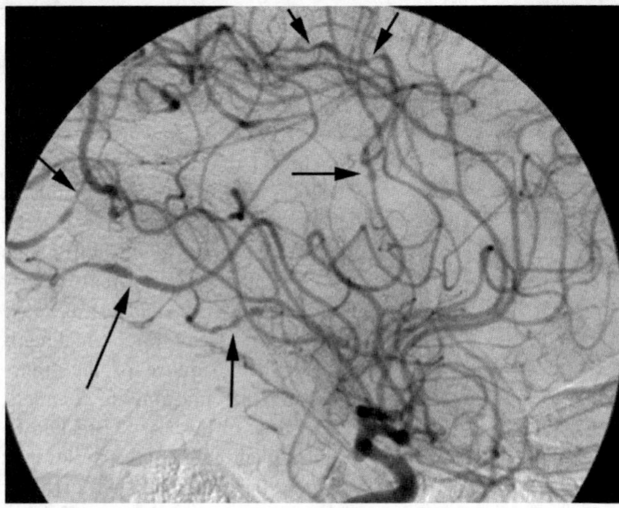

Figure 370-5 Cerebral angiogram from a 32-year-old male with central nervous system vasculopathy. Dramatic beading (*arrows*) typical of vasculopathy is seen.

factor repeats in its extracellular domain. Other monogenic ischemic stroke syndromes include cerebral autosomal recessive arteriopathy with subcortical infarcts and leukoencephalopathy (CARASIL) and hereditary endotheliopathy, retinopathy, nephropathy, and stroke (HERNS). Fabry's disease also produces both large-vessel arteriopathy and small-vessel infarcts by an unknown mechanism.

TRANSIENT ISCHEMIC ATTACKS

TIAs are episodes of stroke symptoms that last only briefly; the standard definition of duration is <24 hours, but most TIAs last <1 hour. The causes of TIA are similar to the causes of ischemic stroke, but because TIAs may herald stroke they are an important risk factor that should be considered separately. TIAs may arise from emboli to the brain or from in situ thrombosis of an intracranial vessel. With a TIA, the occluded blood vessel reopens and neurologic function is restored. However, infarcts of the brain do occur in 15–50% of TIAs even though neurologic signs and symptoms are absent. Newer definitions of TIA categorize those with new infarct as having ischemic stroke rather than TIA regardless of symptom duration, but the vast majority of studies have used the standard, time-based definition.

In addition to the stroke syndromes discussed below, one specific TIA symptom should receive special notice. *Amaurosis fugax*, or transient monocular blindness, occurs from emboli to the central retinal artery of one eye. This may indicate carotid stenosis as the cause or local ophthalmic artery disease.

The risk of stroke after a TIA is ~10–15% in the first 3 months, with most events occurring in the first 2 days. This risk can be directly estimated using the well validated ABCD² method (Table 370-5). Therefore, urgent evaluation and treatment are justified. Since etiologies for stroke and TIA are identical, evaluation for TIA should parallel that of stroke (Figs. 370-1 and 370-3). The improvement characteristic of TIA is a contraindication to thrombolysis. However, since the risk of subsequent stroke in the first few days after a TIA is high, the opportunity to give rtPA rapidly if a stroke occurs probably justifies hospital admission for most patients. Acute antiplatelet therapy has not been tested specifically after TIA but is likely to be effective and is recommended. A large-scale trial of acute antithrombotic treatment to prevent stroke following TIA is ongoing.

TABLE 370-5 Risk of Stroke Following TIA: The ABCD² Score

Clinical Factor	Score
A: Age ≥60 years	1
B: SBP >140 mm Hg or DBP >90 mm Hg	1
C: Clinical symptoms	
Unilateral weakness	2
Speech disturbance without weakness	1
D: Duration	
>60 minutes	2
10–59 minutes	1
D: Diabetes (oral medications or insulin)	1
Total Score	**Sum Each Category**
ABCD² Score Total	3-Month Rate of Stroke (%)[a]
0	0
1	2
2	3
3	3
4	8
5	12
6	17
7	22

[a]Data ranges are from 5 cohorts.

Abbreviations: DBP, diastolic blood pressure; SBP, systolic blood pressure.

Source: SC Johnston et al: Validation and refinement of score to predict very early stroke risk after transient ischaemic attack, Lancet 369: 283, 2007.

TREATMENT Primary and Secondary Prevention of Stroke and TIA

GENERAL PRINCIPLES A number of medical and surgical interventions, as well as lifestyle modifications, are available for preventing stroke. Some of these can be widely applied because of their low cost and minimal risk; others are expensive and carry substantial risk but may be valuable for selected high-risk patients. Identification and control of modifiable risk factors is the best strategy to reduce the burden of stroke, and the total number of strokes could be reduced substantially by these means (Table 370-4).

ATHEROSCLEROSIS RISK FACTORS The relationship of various factors to the risk of atherosclerosis is described in Chap. 241. Older age, family history of thrombotic stroke, diabetes mellitus, hypertension, tobacco smoking, abnormal blood cholesterol [particularly, low high-density lipoprotein (HDL) and/or high low-density lipoprotein (LDL)], and other factors are either proven or probable risk factors for ischemic stroke, largely by their link to atherosclerosis. Risk of stroke is much greater in those with prior stroke or TIA. Many cardiac conditions predispose to stroke, including atrial fibrillation and recent MI. Oral contraceptives and hormone replacement therapy increase stroke risk, and certain inherited and acquired hypercoagulable states predispose to stroke.

Hypertension is the most significant of the risk factors; in general, all hypertension should be treated. The presence of known cerebrovascular disease is not a contraindication to treatment aimed at achieving normotension. Also, the value of treating systolic hypertension in older patients has been clearly established. Lowering blood pressure to levels below those traditionally defining hypertension appears to reduce the risk of stroke even further. Data are particularly strong in support of thiazide diuretics and angiotensin-converting enzyme inhibitors.

Several trials have confirmed that statin drugs reduce the risk of stroke even in patients without elevated LDL or low HDL. The Stroke Prevention by Aggressive Reduction in Cholesterol Levels (SPARCL) trial showed benefit in secondary stroke reduction for patients with recent stroke or TIA, who were prescribed atorvastatin, 80 mg/d. The primary prevention trial, Justification for the Use of Statins in Prevention: An Intervention Trial Evaluating Rosuvastatin (JUPITER), found that patients with low LDL (<130 mg/dL) caused by elevated C-reactive protein benefitted by daily use of this statin. Primary stroke occurrence was reduced by 51% (hazard ratio 0.49, $p = 0.004$) and there was no increase in the rates of intracranial hemorrhage. Therefore, a statin should be considered in all patients with prior ischemic stroke. Tobacco smoking should be discouraged in all patients (Chap. 395). Tight control of blood sugar in patients with type II diabetes lowers stroke risk MI and death of any cause, but no trial sufficiently powered to detect a significant reduction in stroke has yet been performed. Statins, more aggressive blood pressure control, and pioglitazone (an agonist of peroxisome proliferator-activated receptor gamma) are effective.

ANTIPLATELET AGENTS *Platelet antiaggregation agents* can prevent atherothrombotic events, including TIA and stroke, by inhibiting the formation of intraarterial platelet aggregates. These can form on diseased arteries, induce thrombus formation, and occlude the artery or embolize into the distal circulation. Aspirin, clopidogrel, and the combination of aspirin plus extended-release dipyridamole are the antiplatelet agents most commonly used for this purpose. Ticlopidine has been largely abandoned because of its adverse effects but may be used as an alternative to clopidogrel.

Aspirin is the most widely studied antiplatelet agent. Aspirin acetylates platelet cyclooxygenase, which irreversibly inhibits the formation in platelets of thromboxane A_2, a platelet aggregating and vasoconstricting prostaglandin. This effect is permanent and lasts for the usual 8-day life of the platelet. Paradoxically, aspirin also inhibits the formation in endothelial cells of prostacyclin, an antiaggregating and vasodilating prostaglandin. This effect is transient. As soon as aspirin is cleared from the blood, the nucleated endothelial cells again produce prostacyclin. Aspirin in low doses given once daily inhibits the production of thromboxane A_2 in platelets without substantially inhibiting prostacyclin formation. Higher doses of aspirin have not been proven to be more effective than lower doses, and 50–325 mg/d of aspirin is generally recommended for stroke prevention.

Ticlopidine and clopidogrel block the adenosine diphosphate (ADP) receptor on platelets and thus prevent the cascade resulting in activation of the glycoprotein IIb/IIIa receptor that leads to fibrinogen binding to the platelet and consequent platelet aggregation. Ticlopidine is more effective than aspirin; however, it has the disadvantage of causing diarrhea, skin rash, and, in rare instances, neutropenia and thrombotic thrombocytopenic purpura (TTP). Clopidogrel rarely causes TTP but does not cause neutropenia. The Clopidogrel versus Aspirin in Patients at Risk of Ischemic Events (CAPRIE) trial, which led to FDA approval, found that it was only marginally more effective than aspirin in reducing risk of stroke. The Management of Atherothrombosis with Clopidogrel in High-Risk Patients (MATCH) trial was a large multicenter, randomized double-blind study that compared clopidogrel in combination with aspirin to clopidogrel alone in the secondary prevention of TIA or stroke. The MATCH trial found no difference in TIA or stroke prevention with this combination, but did show a small but significant increase in major bleeding complications (3% versus 1%). In the Clopidogrel for High Atherothrombotic Risk and Ischemic Stabilization, Management, and Avoidance (CHARISMA) trial, which included a subgroup of patients with prior stroke or TIA along with other groups at high risk of cardiovascular events, there was no benefit of clopidogrel combined with aspirin compared to aspirin alone. Thus, the use of clopidogrel in combination with aspirin is not recommended for stroke prevention. However, these trials did not enroll patients immediately after the stroke or TIA, and the benefits of combination therapy were greater among those treated earlier, so it is possible that clopidogrel combined with aspirin may be beneficial in this acute period. Ongoing studies are currently addressing this question.

Dipyridamole is an antiplatelet agent that inhibits the uptake of adenosine by a variety of cells, including those of the vascular endothelium. The accumulated adenosine is an inhibitor of aggregation. At least in part through its effects on platelet and vessel wall phosphodiesterases, dipyridamole also potentiates the antiaggregatory effects of prostacyclin and nitric oxide produced by the endothelium and acts by inhibiting platelet phosphodiesterase, which is responsible for the breakdown of cyclic AMP. The resulting elevation in cyclic AMP inhibits aggregation of platelets. Dipyridamole is erratically absorbed depending on stomach pH, but a newer formulation combines timed-release dipyridamole, 200 mg, with aspirin, 25 mg, and has better oral bioavailability. This combination drug was studied in three trials. The European Stroke Prevention Study (ESPS) II showed efficacy of both 50 mg/d of aspirin and extended-release dipyridamole in preventing stroke, and a significantly better risk reduction when the two agents were combined. The ESPRIT (European/Australasian Stroke Prevention in Reversible Ischaemia Trial) trial confirmed the ESPS-II results. This was an open-label, academic trial in which 2,739 patients with stroke or TIA treated with aspirin were randomized to dipyridamole, 200 mg twice daily, or no dipyridamole. Primary outcome was the composite of death from all vascular causes, nonfatal stroke, nonfatal MI, or major bleeding complication. After 3.5 years of follow-up, 13% of patients on aspirin and dipyridamole and 16% on aspirin alone [hazard ratio 0.80, 95% confidence index (CI) 0.66–0.98] met the primary outcome. In the Prevention Regimen for Effectively Avoiding Second Strokes (PRoFESS) trial, the combination of extended-release dipyridamole and aspirin was compared directly with clopidogrel with and without the angiotensin receptor blocker telmisartan in a study of 20,332 patients. There were no differences in the rates of second stroke (9% each) or degree of disability in patients with median follow-up of 2.4 years. Telmisartan also had no effect on these outcomes. This suggests that these antiplatelet regimens are similar, and also raises questions about default prescription of agents to block the angiotensin pathway in all stroke patients. The principal side effect of dipyridamole is headache. The combination capsule of extended-release dipyridamole and aspirin is approved for prevention of stroke.

Many large clinical trials have demonstrated clearly that most antiplatelet agents reduce the risk of all important vascular atherothrombotic events (i.e., ischemic stroke, MI, and death due to all vascular causes) in patients at risk for these events. The overall *relative* reduction in risk of nonfatal stroke is about 25–30% and of all vascular events is about 25%. The *absolute* reduction varies considerably, depending on the particular patient's risk. Individuals at very low risk for stroke seem to experience the same relative reduction, but their risks may be so low that the "benefit" is meaningless. Conversely, individuals with a 10–15% risk of vascular events per year experience a reduction to about 7.5–11%.

Aspirin is inexpensive, can be given in low doses, and could be recommended for all adults to prevent both stroke and MI. However, it causes epigastric discomfort, gastric ulceration, and gastrointestinal hemorrhage, which may be asymptomatic or life threatening. Consequently, not every 40- or 50-year-old should be advised to take aspirin regularly because the risk of atherothrombotic stroke is extremely low and is outweighed by the risk of adverse side effects. Conversely, every patient who has experienced an atherothrombotic stroke or TIA and has no contraindication should be taking an antiplatelet agent regularly because the average annual risk of another stroke is 8–10%; another few percent will experience an MI or vascular death. Clearly, the likelihood of benefit far outweighs the risks of treatment.

The choice of antiplatelet agent and dose must balance the risk of stroke, the expected benefit, and the risk and cost of treatment. However, there are no definitive data, and opinions vary. Many authorities believe low-dose (30–75 mg/d) and high-dose (650–1300 mg/d) aspirin are about equally effective. Some advocate very low doses to avoid adverse effects, and still others advocate very high doses to be sure the benefit is maximal. Most physicians in North America recommend 81–325 mg/d, while most Europeans recommend 50–100 mg. Clopidogrel or extended-release dipyridamole plus aspirin are being increasingly recommended as first-line drugs for secondary prevention. Similarly, the choice of aspirin, clopidogrel, or dipyridamole plus aspirin must balance the fact that the latter are more effective than aspirin but the cost is higher, and this is likely to affect long-term patient adherence. The use of platelet aggregation studies in individual patients taking aspirin is controversial because of limited data.

ANTICOAGULATION THERAPY AND EMBOLIC STROKE Several trials have shown that anticoagulation (INR range, 2–3) in patients with chronic nonvalvular (nonrheumatic) atrial fibrillation prevents cerebral embolism and is safe. For primary prevention and for patients who have experienced stroke or TIA, anticoagulation with a VKA reduces the risk by about 67%, which clearly outweighs the 1–3% risk per year of a major bleeding complication. A recent randomized trial compared the new oral thrombin inhibitor dabigatran to VKAs in a noninferiority trial to prevent stroke or systemic embolization in nonvalvular atrial fibrillation. Two doses of dabigatran were used: 110 mg/d and 150 mg/d. Both dose tiers of dabigatran were noninferior to VKAs in preventing second stroke and systemic embolization, and the higher dose tier was superior (relative risk 0.66; 95% CI, 0.53 to 0.82; $P < 0.001$) and the rate of major bleeding was lower in the lower dose tier of dabigatran compared to VKAs. This drug is likely more convenient to take as no blood monitoring is required to titrate the dose and its effect is independent of oral intake of vitamin K. For patients who cannot take anticoagulant medications, clopidogrel plus aspirin was compared to aspirin alone in the Atrial Fibrillation Clopidogrel Trial with Irbesartan for Prevention of Vascular Events (ACTIVE-A). Clopidogrel combined with aspirin was more effective than aspirin alone in preventing vascular events, principally stroke, but increases the risk of major bleeding (relative risk 1.57, $P < 0.001$).

The decision to use anticoagulation for primary prevention is based primarily on risk factors (Table 370-3). The history of a TIA or stroke tips the balance in favor of anticoagulation regardless of other risk factors. Since this risk factor is so important, many clinicians are performing extended ambulatory monitoring to detect intermittent atrial fibrillation in otherwise cryptogenic stroke since its detection would shift toward prescription of oral anticoagulation long term.

Because of the high annual stroke risk in untreated rheumatic heart disease with atrial fibrillation, primary prophylaxis against stroke has not been studied in a double-blind fashion. These patients generally should receive long-term anticoagulation.

Anticoagulation also reduces the risk of embolism in acute MI. Most clinicians recommend a 3-month course of anticoagulation when there is anterior Q-wave infarction, substantial left ventricular dysfunction, congestive heart failure, mural thrombosis, or atrial fibrillation. VKAs are recommended long-term if atrial fibrillation persists.

Stroke secondary to thromboembolism is one of the most serious complications of prosthetic heart valve implantation. The intensity of anticoagulation and/or antiplatelet therapy is dictated by the type of prosthetic valve and its location.

If the embolic source cannot be eliminated, anticoagulation should in most cases be continued indefinitely. Many neurologists recommend combining antiplatelet agents with anticoagulants for patients who "fail" anticoagulation (i.e., have another stroke or TIA).

ANTICOAGULATION THERAPY AND NONCARDIOGENIC STROKE Data do not support the use of long-term VKAs for preventing atherothrombotic stroke for either intracranial or extracranial cerebrovascular disease. The Warfarin-Aspirin Reinfarction Stroke Study (WARSS) study found no benefit of warfarin sodium (INR, 1.4–2.8) over aspirin, 325 mg, for secondary prevention of stroke but did find a slightly higher bleeding rate in the warfarin group. A recent European study confirmed this finding. The Warfarin-Aspirin Symptomatic Intracranial Disease (WASID) study (see below) demonstrated no benefit of warfarin (INR, 2–3) over aspirin in patients with symptomatic intracranial atherosclerosis, and also found higher bleeding complications.

TREATMENT Carotid Atherosclerosis

Carotid atherosclerosis can be removed surgically (endarterectomy) or mitigated with endovascular stenting with or without balloon angioplasty. Anticoagulation has not been directly compared with antiplatelet therapy for carotid disease.

SURGICAL THERAPY *Symptomatic carotid stenosis* was studied in the North American Symptomatic Carotid Endarterectomy Trial (NASCET) and the European Carotid Surgery Trial (ECST). Both showed a substantial benefit for surgery in patients with a stenosis of ≥70%. In NASCET, the average cumulative ipsilateral stroke risk at 2 years was 26% for patients treated medically and 9% for those receiving the same medical treatment plus a carotid endarterectomy. This 17% *absolute* reduction in the surgical group is a 65% *relative* risk reduction favoring surgery (Table 370-4). NASCET also showed a significant, although less robust, benefit for patients with 50–70% stenosis. ECST found harm for patients with stenosis <30% treated surgically.

A patient's risk of stroke and possible benefit from surgery are related to the presence of retinal versus hemispheric symptoms, degree of arterial stenosis, extent of associated medical conditions (of note, NASCET and ECST excluded "high-risk" patients with significant cardiac, pulmonary, or renal disease), institutional surgical morbidity and mortality, timing of surgery relative to symptoms, and other factors. A recent meta-analysis of the NASCET and ECST trials demonstrated that endarterectomy is most beneficial when performed within 2 weeks of symptom onset. In addition, benefit is more pronounced in patients >75 years, and men appear to benefit more than women.

In summary, a patient with recent symptomatic hemispheric ischemia, high-grade stenosis in the appropriate internal carotid artery, and an institutional perioperative morbidity and mortality rate of ≤6% generally should undergo carotid endarterectomy. If the perioperative stroke rate is >6% for any particular surgeon, however, the benefits of carotid endarterectomy are questionable.

The indications for surgical treatment of *asymptomatic carotid disease* have been clarified by the results of the Asymptomatic Carotid Atherosclerosis Study (ACAS) and the Asymptomatic Carotid Surgery Trial (ACST). ACAS randomized asymptomatic patients with ≥60% stenosis to medical treatment with aspirin or the same medical treatment plus carotid endarterectomy. The surgical group had a risk over 5 years for ipsilateral stroke (and any perioperative stroke or death) of 5.1%, compared to a risk in the medical group of 11%. While this demonstrates a 53% *relative* risk reduction, the *absolute* risk reduction is only 5.9% over 5 years, or 1.2% annually (Table 370-4). Nearly one-half of the strokes in the surgery group were caused by preoperative angiograms. The recently published ACST randomized 3120 asymptomatic patients with >60% carotid stenosis to endarterectomy or medical therapy. The 5-year risk of stroke in the surgical group (including perioperative stroke or death) was 6.4%, compared to 11.8% in the medically treated group (46% relative risk reduction and 5.4% absolute risk reduction).

In both ACAS and ACST, the perioperative complication rate was higher in women, perhaps negating any benefit in the reduction of stroke risk within 5 years. It is possible that with longer follow-up, a clear benefit in women will emerge. At present, carotid endarterectomy in asymptomatic women remains particularly controversial.

In summary, the natural history of asymptomatic stenosis is a ~2% per year stroke rate, while symptomatic patients experience a 13% per year risk of stroke. Whether to recommend carotid revascularization for an asymptomatic patient is somewhat controversial and depends on many factors, including patient preference, degree of stenosis, age, gender, and comorbidities. Medical therapy for reduction of atherosclerosis risk factors, including cholesterol-lowering agents and antiplatelet medications, is generally recommended for patients with asymptomatic carotid stenosis. As with atrial fibrillation, it is imperative to counsel the patient about TIAs so that therapy can be revised if symptoms develop.

ENDOVASCULAR THERAPY Balloon angioplasty coupled with stenting is being used with increasing frequency to open stenotic carotid arteries and maintain their patency. These techniques can treat carotid stenosis not only at the bifurcation but also near the skull base and in the intracranial segments. The Stenting and Angioplasty with Protection in Patients at High Risk for Endarterectomy (SAPPHIRE) trial randomized high-risk patients (defined as patients with clinically significant coronary or pulmonary disease, contralateral carotid occlusion, restenosis after endarterectomy, contralateral laryngeal-nerve palsy, prior radical neck surgery or radiation, or age >80) with symptomatic carotid stenosis >50% or asymptomatic stenosis >80% to either stenting combined with a distal emboli-protection device or endarterectomy. The risk of death, stroke, or MI within 30 days and ipsilateral stroke or death within 1 year was 12.2% in the stenting group and 20.1% in the endarterectomy group (p = .055), suggesting that stenting is at the very least comparable to endarterectomy as a treatment option for this patient group at high risk of surgery. However, the outcomes with both interventions may not have been better than leaving the carotid stenoses untreated, particularly for the asymptomatic patients, and much of the benefit seen in the stenting group was due to a reduction in periprocedure MI. In 2010, the results of two randomized trials comparing stents to endarterectomy in low-risk patients were published. The Carotid Revascularization Endarterectomy versus Stenting Trial (CREST) enrolled 2,502 patients with either asymptomatic or symptomatic stenosis. The 30-day risk of stroke was 4.1% in the stent group and 2.3% in the surgical group, but the 30-day risk of MI was 1.1% in the stent group and 2.3% in the surgery group, suggesting relative equivalence of risk between the procedures. At median follow-up of 2.5 years, the combined endpoint of stroke, MI, and death was the same (7.2% stent versus 6.8% surgery). The International Carotid Stenting (ICSS) trial randomized 1,713 symptomatic patients to stents versus endarterectomy and found a different result: At 120 days, the incidence of stroke, MI, or death was 8.5% in the stenting group versus 5.2% in the endarterectomy group (p = 0.006) and longer term follow-up is currently under way. Differences between trial designs, selection of stent, and operator experience may explain these important differences. Until more data are available on both trials, there remains controversy as to who should receive a stent or have endarterectomy; it is likely that the procedures carry similar risks if performed by experienced physicians.

BYPASS SURGERY Extracranial-to-intracranial (EC-IC) bypass surgery has been proven ineffective for atherosclerotic stenoses that are inaccessible to conventional carotid endarterectomy. However, a trial is under way to evaluate whether patients with decreased brain perfusion based on positron emission tomography (PET) imaging will benefit from EC-IC bypass.

INTRACRANIAL ATHEROSCLEROSIS The WASID trial randomized patients with symptomatic stenosis (50–99%) of a major intracranial vessel to either high-dose aspirin (1300 mg/d) or warfarin (target INR, 2.0–3.0), with a combined primary endpoint of ischemic stroke, brain hemorrhage, or death from vascular cause other than stroke. The trial was terminated early because of an increased risk of adverse events related to warfarin anticoagulation. With a mean follow-up of 1.8 years, the primary endpoint was seen in 22.1% in the aspirin group and 21.8% of the warfarin group. Death from any cause was seen in 4.3% of the aspirin group and 9.7% of the warfarin group; 3.2% of patients on aspirin experienced major hemorrhage, compared to 8.3% of patients taking warfarin.

Given the worrisome natural history of symptomatic intracranial atherosclerosis (in the aspirin arm of the WASID trial, 15% of patients experienced a stroke within the first year, despite current standard aggressive medical therapy), some centers treat symptomatic lesions with intracranial angioplasty and stenting. This intervention is currently being compared to aspirin therapy in a prospective, randomized trial. It is unclear whether EC-IC bypass, or other grafting procedures of extracranial blood supply to the pial arteries, are of value in such patients.

Dural Sinus Thrombosis Limited evidence exists to support short-term usage of anticoagulants, regardless of the presence of intracranial hemorrhage, for venous infarction following sinus thrombosis.

STROKE SYNDROMES

A careful history and neurologic examination can often localize the region of brain dysfunction; if this region corresponds to a particular arterial distribution, the possible causes responsible for the syndrome can be narrowed. This is of particular importance when the patient presents with a TIA and a normal examination. For example, if a patient develops language loss and a right homonymous hemianopia, a search for causes of left middle cerebral emboli should be performed. A finding of an isolated stenosis of the right internal carotid artery in that patient, for example, suggests an asymptomatic carotid stenosis, and the search for other causes of stroke should continue. The following sections describe the clinical findings of cerebral ischemia associated with cerebral vascular territories depicted in Figs. 370-4, and 370-6 through 370-14. Stroke syndromes are divided into: (1) large-vessel stroke within the anterior circulation, (2) large-vessel stroke within the posterior circulation, and (3) small-vessel disease of either vascular bed.

Stroke within the anterior circulation

The internal carotid artery and its branches comprise the anterior circulation of the brain. These vessels can be occluded by intrinsic disease of the vessel (e.g., atherosclerosis or dissection) or by embolic occlusion from a proximal source as discussed above. Occlusion of each major intracranial vessel has distinct clinical manifestations.

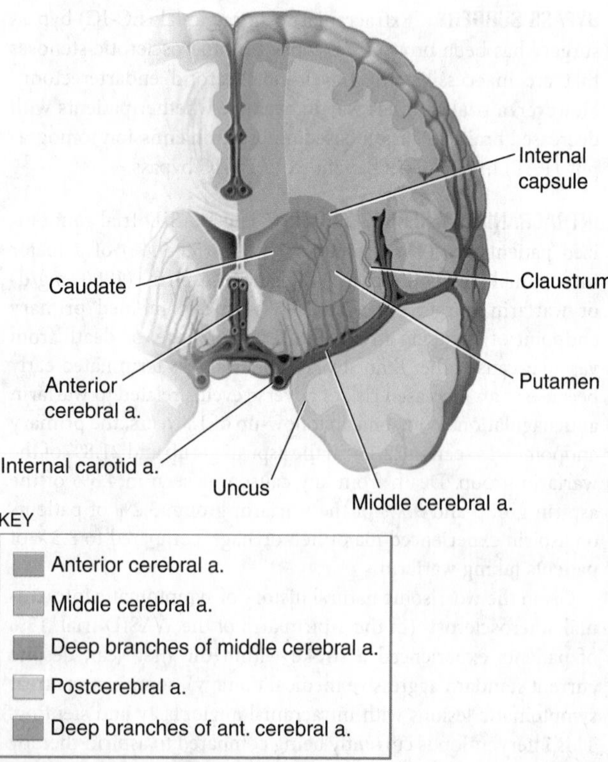

Figure 370-6 Diagram of a cerebral hemisphere in coronal section showing the territories of the major cerebral vessels that branch from the internal carotid arteries.

Middle cerebral artery Occlusion of the proximal MCA or one of its major branches is most often due to an embolus (artery-to-artery, cardiac, or of unknown source) rather than intracranial atherothrombosis. Atherosclerosis of the proximal MCA may cause distal emboli to the middle cerebral territory or, less commonly, may produce low-flow TIAs. Collateral formation via leptomeningeal vessels often prevents MCA stenosis from becoming symptomatic.

The cortical branches of the MCA supply the lateral surface of the hemisphere except for (1) the frontal pole and a strip along the superomedial border of the frontal and parietal lobes supplied by the ACA, and (2) the lower temporal and occipital pole convolutions supplied by the PCA (Figs. 370-6, 370-7, 370-8, and 370-9).

The proximal MCA (M1 segment) gives rise to penetrating branches (termed *lenticulostriate arteries*) that supply the putamen, outer globus pallidus, posterior limb of the internal capsule, the adjacent corona radiata, and most of the caudate nucleus (Fig. 370-6). In the sylvian fissure, the MCA in most patients divides into *superior* and *inferior* divisions (M2 branches). Branches of the inferior division supply the inferior parietal and temporal cortex, and those from the superior division supply the frontal and superior parietal cortex (Fig. 370-7).

If the entire MCA is occluded at its origin (blocking both its penetrating and cortical branches) and the distal collaterals are limited, the clinical findings are contralateral hemiplegia, hemianesthesia, homonymous hemianopia, and a day or two of gaze preference to the ipsilateral side. Dysarthria is common because of facial weakness. When the dominant hemisphere is involved, global aphasia is present also, and when the nondominant hemisphere is affected, anosognosia, constructional apraxia, and neglect are found (Chap. 26).

Complete MCA syndromes occur most often when an embolus occludes the stem of the artery. Cortical collateral blood flow and differing arterial configurations are probably responsible for the development of many partial syndromes. Partial syndromes may also be due to emboli that enter the proximal MCA without complete occlusion, occlude distal MCA branches, or fragment and move distally.

Partial syndromes due to embolic occlusion of a single branch include hand, or arm and hand, weakness alone (brachial syndrome) or facial weakness with nonfluent (Broca) aphasia (Chap. 26), with or without arm weakness (frontal opercular syndrome). A combination of sensory disturbance, motor weakness, and nonfluent aphasia suggests that an embolus has occluded the proximal superior division and infarcted large portions of the frontal and parietal cortices (Fig. 370-7). If a fluent (Wernicke's) aphasia occurs without weakness, the inferior division of the MCA supplying the posterior part (temporal cortex) of the dominant hemisphere is probably involved. Jargon speech and an inability to comprehend written and spoken language are prominent features, often accompanied by a contralateral, homonymous superior quadrantanopia. Hemineglect or spatial agnosia without weakness indicates that the inferior division of the MCA in the nondominant hemisphere is involved.

Occlusion of a lenticulostriate vessel produces small-vessel (lacunar) stroke within the internal capsule (Fig. 370-6). This produces pure motor stroke or sensory-motor stroke contralateral to the lesion. Ischemia within the genu of the internal capsule causes primarily facial weakness followed by arm then leg weakness as the ischemia moves posterior within the capsule. Alternatively, the contralateral hand may become ataxic and dysarthria will be prominent (clumsy hand, dysarthria lacunar syndrome). Lacunar infarction affecting the globus pallidus and putamen often has few clinical signs, but parkinsonism and hemiballismus have been reported.

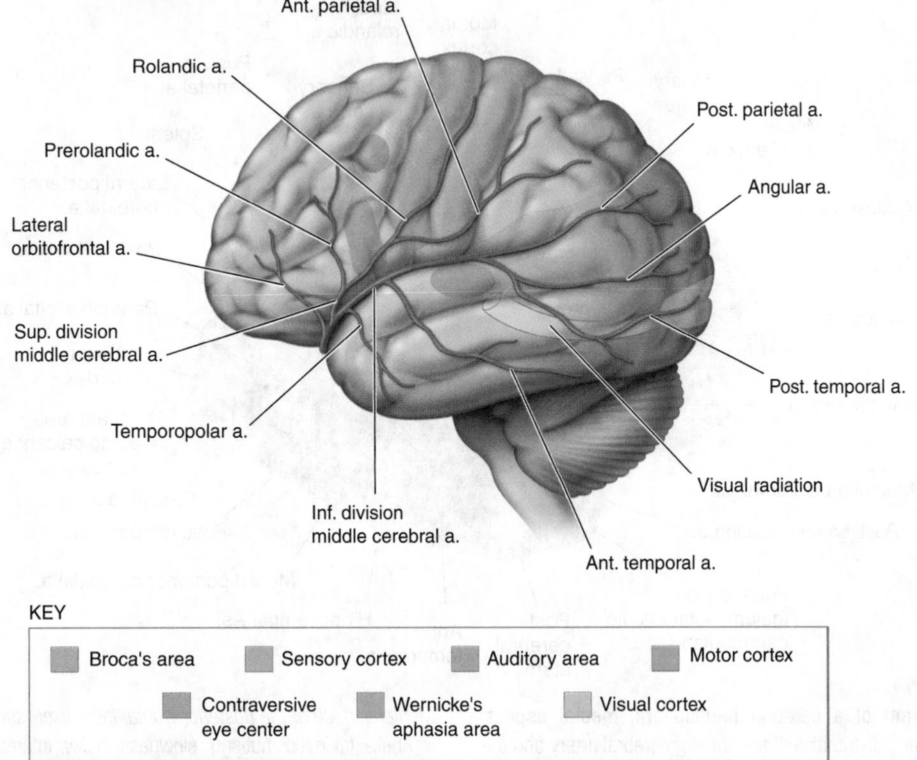

Figure 370-7 Diagram of a cerebral hemisphere, lateral aspect, showing the branches and distribution of the middle cerebral artery and the principal regions of cerebral localization. Note the bifurcation of the middle cerebral artery into a superior and inferior division.

Signs and symptoms: *Structures involved*

Paralysis of the contralateral face, arm, and leg; sensory impairment over the same area (pinprick, cotton touch, vibration, position, two-point discrimination, stereognosis, tactile localization, barognosis, cutaneographia): *Somatic motor area for face and arm and the fibers descending from the leg area to enter the corona radiata and corresponding somatic sensory system*

Motor aphasia: *Motor speech area of the dominant hemisphere*

Central aphasia, word deafness, anomia, jargon speech, sensory agraphia, acalculia, alexia, finger agnosia, right-left confusion (the last four comprise the Gerstmann syndrome): *Central, suprasylvian speech area and parietooccipital cortex of the dominant hemisphere*

Conduction aphasia: *Central speech area (parietal operculum)*

Apractagnosia of the nondominant hemisphere, anosognosia, hemiasomatognosia, unilateral neglect, agnosia for the left half of external space, dressing "apraxia," constructional "apraxia," distortion of visual coordinates, inaccurate localization in the half field, impaired ability to judge distance, upside-down reading, visual illusions (e.g., it may appear that another person walks through a table): *Nondominant parietal lobe (area corresponding to speech area in dominant hemisphere); loss of topographic memory is usually due to a nondominant lesion, occasionally to a dominant one*

Homonymous hemianopia (often homonymous inferior quadrantanopia): *Optic radiation deep to second temporal convolution*

Paralysis of conjugate gaze to the opposite side: *Frontal contraversive eye field or projecting fibers*

Anterior cerebral artery The ACA is divided into two segments: the precommunal (A1) circle of Willis, or stem, which connects the internal carotid artery to the anterior communicating artery, and the postcommunal (A2) segment distal to the anterior communicating artery (Figs. 370-4, 370-6, and 370-8). The A1 segment gives rise to several deep penetrating branches that supply the anterior limb of the internal capsule, the anterior perforate substance, amygdala, anterior hypothalamus, and the inferior part of the head of the caudate nucleus (Fig. 370-6).

Occlusion of the proximal ACA is usually well tolerated because of collateral flow through the anterior communicating artery and collaterals through the MCA and PCA. Occlusion of a single A2 segment results in the contralateral symptoms noted in Fig. 370-8. If both A2 segments arise from a single anterior cerebral stem (contralateral A1 segment atresia), the occlusion may affect both hemispheres. Profound abulia (a delay in verbal and motor response) and bilateral pyramidal signs with paraparesis or quadriparesis and urinary incontinence result.

Anterior choroidal artery This artery arises from the internal carotid artery and supplies the posterior limb of the internal capsule and the white matter posterolateral to it, through which pass some of the geniculocalcarine fibers (Fig. 370-9). The complete syndrome of anterior choroidal artery occlusion consists of contralateral hemiplegia, hemianesthesia (hypesthesia), and homonymous hemianopia. However, because this territory is also supplied by penetrating vessels of the proximal MCA and the posterior communicating and posterior choroidal arteries, minimal deficits may occur, and patients frequently recover substantially. Anterior choroidal strokes are usually the result of in situ thrombosis of the vessel, and the vessel is particularly vulnerable to iatrogenic occlusion during surgical clipping of aneurysms arising from the internal carotid artery.

Internal carotid artery The clinical picture of internal carotid occlusion varies depending on whether the cause of ischemia is propagated thrombus, embolism, or low flow. The cortex supplied by the MCA territory is affected most often. With a competent circle of

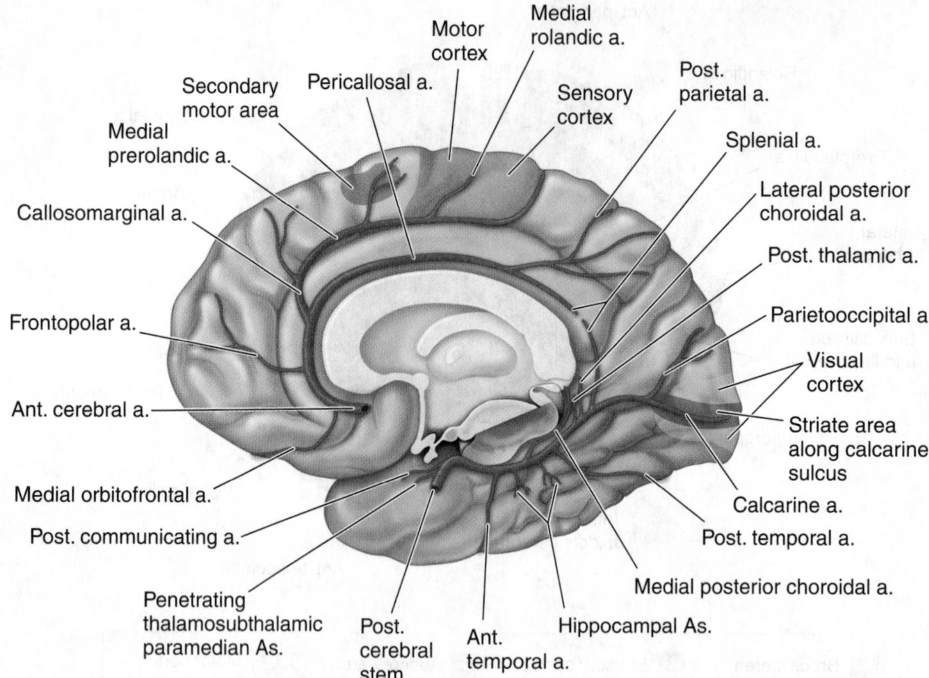

Figure 370-8 Diagram of a cerebral hemisphere, medial aspect, showing the branches and distribution of the anterior cerebral artery and the principal regions of cerebral localization.

Signs and symptoms: *Structures involved*

Paralysis of opposite foot and leg: *Motor leg area*

A lesser degree of paresis of opposite arm: *Arm area of cortex or fibers descending to corona radiata*

Cortical sensory loss over toes, foot, and leg: *Sensory area for foot and leg*

Urinary incontinence: *Sensorimotor area in paracentral lobule*

Contralateral grasp reflex, sucking reflex, gegenhalten (paratonic rigidity): *Medial surface of the posterior frontal lobe; likely supplemental motor area*

Abulia (akinetic mutism), slowness, delay, intermittent interruption, lack of spontaneity, whispering, reflex distraction to sights and sounds: *Uncertain localization—probably cingulate gyrus and medial inferior portion of frontal, parietal, and temporal lobes*

Impairment of gait and stance (gait apraxia): *Frontal cortex near leg motor area*

Dyspraxia of left limbs, tactile aphasia in left limbs: *Corpus callosum*

Willis, occlusion may go unnoticed. If the thrombus propagates up the internal carotid artery into the MCA or embolizes it, symptoms are identical to proximal MCA occlusion (see above). Sometimes there is massive infarction of the entire deep white matter and cortical surface. When the origins of both the ACA and MCA are occluded at the top of the carotid artery, abulia or stupor occurs with hemiplegia, hemianesthesia, and aphasia or anosognosia. When the PCA arises from the internal carotid artery (a configuration called a *fetal posterior cerebral artery*), it may also become occluded and give rise to symptoms referable to its peripheral territory (Figs. 370-8 and 370-9).

In addition to supplying the ipsilateral brain, the internal carotid artery perfuses the optic nerve and retina via the ophthalmic artery. In ~25% of symptomatic internal carotid disease, recurrent transient monocular blindness (amaurosis fugax) warns of the lesion. Patients typically describe a horizontal shade that sweeps down or up across the field of vision. They may also complain that their vision was blurred in that eye or that the upper or lower half of vision disappeared. In most cases, these symptoms last only a few minutes. Rarely, ischemia or infarction of the ophthalmic artery or central retinal arteries occurs at the time of cerebral TIA or infarction.

A high-pitched prolonged carotid bruit fading into diastole is often associated with tightly stenotic lesions. As the stenosis grows tighter and flow distal to the stenosis becomes reduced, the bruit becomes fainter and may disappear when occlusion is imminent.

Common carotid artery All symptoms and signs of internal carotid occlusion may also be present with occlusion of the common carotid artery. Jaw claudication may result from low flow in the external carotid branches. Bilateral common carotid artery occlusions at their origin may occur in Takayasu's arteritis (Chap. 326).

Stroke within the posterior circulation

The posterior circulation is composed of the paired vertebral arteries, the basilar artery, and the paired posterior cerebral arteries. The vertebral arteries join to form the basilar artery at the pontomedullary junction. The basilar artery divides into two posterior cerebral arteries in the interpeduncular fossa (Figs. 370-4, 370-8, and 370-9). These major arteries give rise to long and short circumferential branches and to smaller deep penetrating branches that supply the cerebellum, medulla, pons, midbrain, subthalamus, thalamus, hippocampus, and medial temporal and occipital lobes. Occlusion of each vessel produces its own distinctive syndrome.

Posterior cerebral artery In 75% of cases, both PCAs arise from the bifurcation of the basilar artery; in 20%, one has its origin from the ipsilateral internal carotid artery via the posterior communicating artery; in 5%, both originate from the respective ipsilateral internal carotid arteries (Figs. 370-8 and 370-9). The precommunal, or P1, segment of the true posterior cerebral artery is atretic in such cases.

PCA syndromes usually result from atheroma formation or emboli that lodge at the top of the basilar artery; posterior

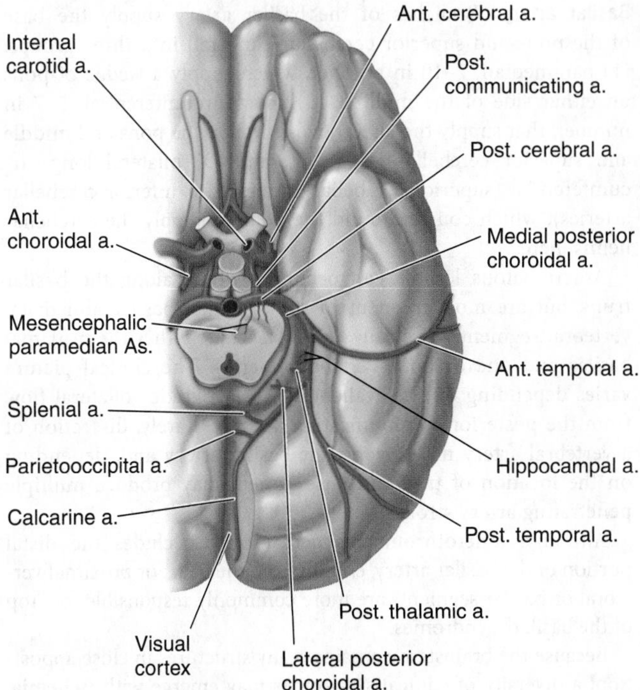

Figure 370-9 Inferior aspect of the brain with the branches and distribution of the posterior cerebral artery and the principal anatomic structures shown.

Signs and symptoms: *Structures involved*

Peripheral territory (see also Fig. 370-12). Homonymous hemianopia (often upper quadrantic): *Calcarine cortex or optic radiation nearby.* Bilateral homonymous hemianopia, cortical blindness, awareness or denial of blindness; tactile naming, achromatopia (color blindness), failure to see to-and-fro movements, inability to perceive objects not centrally located, apraxia of ocular movements, inability to count or enumerate objects, tendency to run into things that the patient sees and tries to avoid: *Bilateral occipital lobe with possibly the parietal lobe involved.* Verbal dyslexia without agraphia, color anomia: *Dominant calcarine lesion and posterior part of corpus callosum.* Memory defect: *Hippocampal lesion bilaterally or on the dominant side only.* Topographic disorientation and prosopagnosia: *Usually with lesions of nondominant, calcarine, and lingual gyrus.* Simultanagnosia, hemivisual neglect: *Dominant visual cortex, contralateral hemisphere.* Unformed visual hallucinations, peduncular hallucinosis, metamorphopsia, teleopsia, illusory visual spread, palinopsia, distortion of outlines, central photophobia: *Calcarine cortex.* Complex hallucinations: *Usually nondominant hemisphere.*

Central territory. Thalamic syndrome: sensory loss (all modalities), spontaneous pain and dysesthesias, choreoathetosis, intention tremor, spasms of hand, mild hemiparesis: *Posteroventral nucleus of thalamus; involvement of the adjacent subthalamus body or its afferent tracts.* Thalamoperforate syndrome: crossed cerebellar ataxia with ipsilateral third nerve palsy (Claude's syndrome): *Dentatothalamic tract and issuing third nerve.* Weber's syndrome: third nerve palsy and contralateral hemiplegia: *Third nerve and cerebral peduncle.* Contralateral hemiplegia: *Cerebral peduncle.* Paralysis or paresis of vertical eye movement, skew deviation, sluggish pupillary responses to light, slight miosis and ptosis (retraction nystagmus and "tucking" of the eyelids may be associated): *Supranuclear fibers to third nerve, interstitial nucleus of Cajal, nucleus of Darkschewitsch, and posterior commissure.* Contralateral rhythmic, ataxic action tremor; rhythmic postural or "holding" tremor (rubral tremor): *Dentatothalamic tract.*

circulation disease may also be caused by dissection of either vertebral artery and fibromuscular dysplasia.

Two clinical syndromes are commonly observed with occlusion of the PCA: (1) *P1 syndrome*: midbrain, subthalamic, and thalamic signs, which are due to disease of the proximal P1 segment of the PCA or its penetrating branches (thalamogeniculate, Percheron, and posterior choroidal arteries); and (2) *P2 syndrome*: cortical temporal and occipital lobe signs, due to occlusion of the P2 segment distal to the junction of the PCA with the posterior communicating artery.

P1 syndromes Infarction usually occurs in the ipsilateral subthalamus and medial thalamus and in the ipsilateral cerebral peduncle and midbrain (Figs. 370-9 and 370-14). A third nerve palsy with contralateral ataxia (Claude's syndrome) or with contralateral hemiplegia (Weber's syndrome) may result. The ataxia indicates involvement of the red nucleus or dentatorubrothalamic tract; the hemiplegia is localized to the cerebral peduncle (Fig. 370-14). If the subthalamic nucleus is involved, contralateral hemiballismus may occur. Occlusion of the artery of Percheron produces paresis of upward gaze and drowsiness, and often abulia. Extensive infarction in the midbrain and subthalamus occurring with bilateral proximal PCA occlusion presents as coma, unreactive pupils, bilateral pyramidal signs, and decerebrate rigidity.

Occlusion of the penetrating branches of thalamic and thalamogeniculate arteries produces less extensive thalamic and thalamocapsular lacunar syndromes. The *thalamic Déjérine-Roussy syndrome* consists of contralateral hemisensory loss followed later by an agonizing, searing or burning pain in the affected areas. It is persistent and responds poorly to analgesics. Anticonvulsants (carbamazepine or gabapentin) or tricyclic antidepressants may be beneficial.

P2 syndromes (See also Figs. 370-8 and 370-9.) Occlusion of the distal PCA causes infarction of the medial temporal and occipital lobes. Contralateral homonymous hemianopia with macula sparing is the usual manifestation. Occasionally, only the upper quadrant of visual field is involved. If the visual association areas are spared and only the calcarine cortex is involved, the patient may be aware of visual defects. Medial temporal lobe and hippocampal involvement may cause an acute disturbance in memory, particularly if it occurs in the dominant hemisphere. The defect usually clears because memory has bilateral representation. If the dominant hemisphere is affected and the infarct extends to involve the splenium of the corpus callosum, the patient may demonstrate alexia without agraphia. Visual agnosia for faces, objects, mathematical symbols, and colors and anomia with paraphasic errors (amnestic aphasia) may also occur in this setting, even without callosal involvement. Occlusion of the posterior cerebral artery can produce *peduncular hallucinosis* (visual hallucinations of brightly colored scenes and objects).

Bilateral infarction in the distal PCAs produces cortical blindness (blindness with preserved pupillary light reaction). The patient is often unaware of the blindness or may even deny it (*Anton's syndrome*). Tiny islands of vision may persist, and the patient may report that vision fluctuates as images are captured in the preserved portions. Rarely, only peripheral vision is lost and central vision is spared, resulting in "gun-barrel" vision. Bilateral visual association area lesions may result in *Balint's syndrome*, a disorder of the orderly visual scanning of the environment (Chap. 26), usually resulting from infarctions secondary to low flow in the "watershed" between the distal PCA and MCA territories, as occurs after cardiac arrest. Patients may experience persistence of a visual image for several minutes despite gazing at another scene (*palinopsia*) or an inability to synthesize the whole of an image (*asimultanagnosia*). Embolic occlusion of the top of the basilar artery can produce any or all of the central or peripheral territory symptoms. The hallmark is the sudden onset of bilateral signs, including ptosis, pupillary asymmetry or lack of reaction to light, and somnolence.

Vertebral and posterior inferior cerebellar arteries The vertebral artery, which arises from the innominate artery on the right and the subclavian artery on the left, consists of four segments. The first (V1) extends from its origin to its entrance into the sixth or fifth transverse vertebral foramen. The second segment (V2) traverses the vertebral foramina from C6 to C2. The third (V3) passes through the transverse foramen and circles around the arch of the atlas to pierce the dura at the foramen magnum. The fourth (V4) segment courses upward to join the other vertebral artery to form the basilar artery; only the fourth segment gives rise to branches that supply the brainstem and cerebellum. The posterior inferior cerebellar artery (PICA) in its proximal segment supplies the lateral medulla and, in its distal branches, the inferior surface of the cerebellum.

Atherothrombotic lesions have a predilection for V1 and V4 segments of the vertebral artery. The first segment may become diseased at the origin of the vessel and may produce posterior circulation emboli; collateral flow from the contralateral vertebral artery or the ascending cervical, thyrocervical, or occipital arteries is usually sufficient to prevent low-flow TIAs or stroke. When one vertebral artery is atretic and an atherothrombotic lesion threatens the origin of the other, the collateral circulation, which may also include retrograde flow down the basilar artery, is often insufficient (Figs. 370-4 and 370-9). In this setting, low-flow TIAs may occur, consisting of syncope, vertigo, and alternating hemiplegia; this state also sets the stage for thrombosis. Disease of the distal fourth segment of the vertebral artery can promote thrombus formation manifest as embolism or with propagation as basilar artery thrombosis. Stenosis proximal to the origin of the PICA can threaten the lateral medulla and posterior inferior surface of the cerebellum.

If the subclavian artery is occluded proximal to the origin of the vertebral artery, there is a reversal in the direction of blood flow in the ipsilateral vertebral artery. Exercise of the ipsilateral arm may increase demand on vertebral flow, producing posterior circulation TIAs, or "subclavian steal."

Although atheromatous disease rarely narrows the second and third segments of the vertebral artery, this region is subject to dissection, fibromuscular dysplasia, and, rarely, encroachment by osteophytic spurs within the vertebral foramina.

Embolic occlusion or thrombosis of a V4 segment causes ischemia of the lateral medulla. The constellation of vertigo, numbness of the ipsilateral face and contralateral limbs, diplopia, hoarseness, dysarthria, dysphagia, and ipsilateral Horner's syndrome is called the *lateral medullary (or Wallenberg's) syndrome* (Fig. 370-10). Most cases result from ipsilateral vertebral artery occlusion; in the remainder, PICA occlusion is responsible. Occlusion of the medullary penetrating branches of the vertebral artery or PICA results in partial syndromes. *Hemiparesis is not a feature of vertebral artery occlusion, however, quadriparesis may result from occlusion of the anterior spinal artery.*

Rarely, a *medial medullary syndrome* occurs with infarction of the pyramid and contralateral hemiparesis of the arm and leg, sparing the face. If the medial lemniscus and emerging hypoglossal nerve fibers are involved, contralateral loss of joint position sense and ipsilateral tongue weakness occur.

Cerebellar infarction with edema can lead to *sudden respiratory arrest* due to raised ICP in the posterior fossa. Drowsiness, Babinski signs, dysarthria, and bifacial weakness may be absent, or present only briefly, before respiratory arrest ensues. Gait unsteadiness, headache, dizziness, nausea, and vomiting may be the only early symptoms and signs and should arouse suspicion of this impending complication, which may require neurosurgical decompression, often with an excellent outcome. Separating these symptoms from those of viral labyrinthitis can be a challenge, but headache, neck stiffness, and unilateral dysmetria favor stroke.

Basilar artery Branches of the basilar artery supply the base of the pons and superior cerebellum and fall into three groups: (1) paramedian, 7–10 in number, which supply a wedge of pons on either side of the midline; (2) short circumferential, 5–7 in number, that supply the lateral two-thirds of the pons and middle and superior cerebellar peduncles; and (3) bilateral long circumferential (superior cerebellar and anterior inferior cerebellar arteries), which course around the pons to supply the cerebellar hemispheres.

Atheromatous lesions can occur anywhere along the basilar trunk but are most frequent in the proximal basilar and distal vertebral segments. Typically, lesions occlude either the proximal basilar and one or both vertebral arteries. The clinical picture varies depending on the availability of retrograde collateral flow from the posterior communicating arteries. Rarely, dissection of a vertebral artery may involve the basilar artery and, depending on the location of true and false lumen, may produce multiple penetrating artery strokes.

Although atherothrombosis occasionally occludes the distal portion of the basilar artery, emboli from the heart or proximal vertebral or basilar segments are more commonly responsible for "top of the basilar" syndromes.

Because the brainstem contains many structures in close apposition, a diversity of clinical syndromes may emerge with ischemia, reflecting involvement of the corticospinal and corticobulbar tracts, ascending sensory tracts, and cranial nerve nuclei (Figs. 370-11, 370-12, 370-13, and 370-14).

The symptoms of transient ischemia or infarction in the territory of the basilar artery often do not indicate whether the basilar artery itself or one of its branches is diseased, yet this distinction has important implications for therapy. *The picture of complete basilar occlusion, however, is easy to recognize as a constellation of bilateral long tract signs (sensory and motor) with signs of cranial nerve and cerebellar dysfunction.* A "locked-in" state of preserved consciousness with quadriplegia and cranial nerve signs suggests complete pontine and lower midbrain infarction. The therapeutic goal is to identify *impending* basilar occlusion before devastating infarction occurs. A series of TIAs and a slowly progressive, fluctuating stroke are extremely significant, as they often herald an atherothrombotic occlusion of the distal vertebral or proximal basilar artery.

TIAs in the proximal basilar distribution may produce vertigo (often described by patients as "swimming," "swaying," "moving," "unsteadiness," or "light-headedness"). Other symptoms that warn of basilar thrombosis include diplopia, dysarthria, facial or circumoral numbness, and hemisensory symptoms. In general, symptoms of basilar branch TIAs affect one side of the brainstem, whereas symptoms of basilar artery TIAs usually affect both sides, although a "herald" hemiparesis has been emphasized as an initial symptom of basilar occlusion. Most often TIAs, whether due to impending occlusion of the basilar artery or a basilar branch, are short lived (5–30 minutes) and repetitive, occurring several times a day. The pattern suggests intermittent reduction of flow. Many neurologists treat with heparin to prevent clot propagation.

Atherothrombotic occlusion of the basilar artery with infarction usually causes *bilateral* brainstem signs. A gaze paresis or internuclear ophthalmoplegia associated with ipsilateral hemiparesis may be the only manifestation of bilateral brainstem ischemia. More often, unequivocal signs of bilateral pontine disease are present. Complete basilar thrombosis carries a high mortality.

Occlusion of a branch of the basilar artery usually causes *unilateral* symptoms and signs involving motor, sensory, and cranial nerves. As long as symptoms remain unilateral, concern over pending basilar occlusion should be reduced.

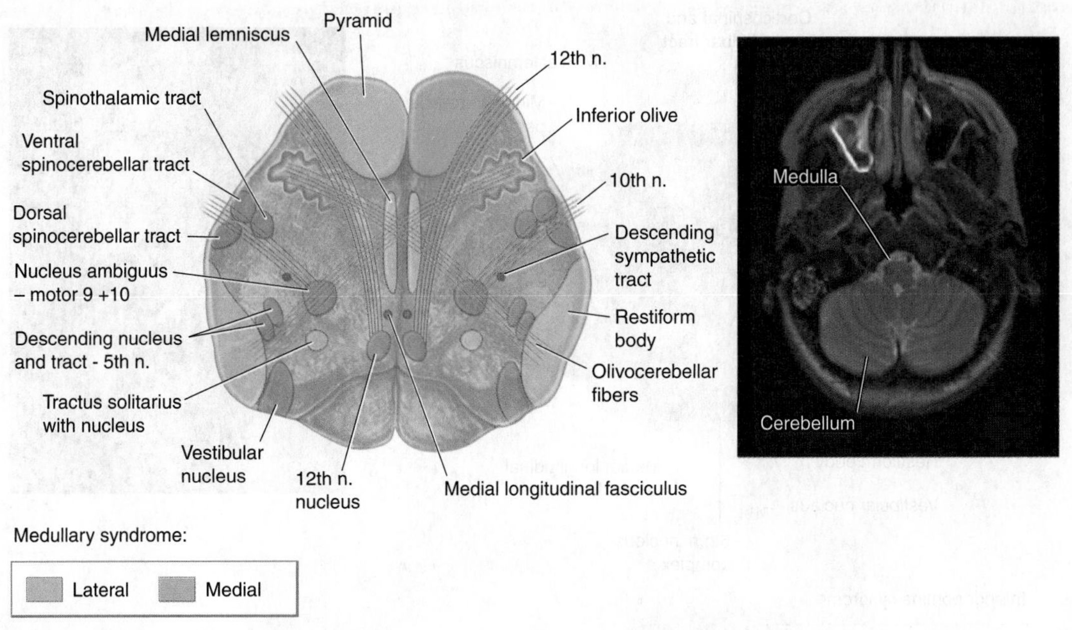

Figure 370-10 Axial section at the level of the medulla, depicted schematically on the left, with a corresponding MR image on the right. Note that in Figs. 370-10 through 370-14, all drawings are oriented with the dorsal surface at the bottom, matching the orientation of the brainstem that is commonly seen in all modern neuroimaging studies. Approximate regions involved in medial and lateral medullary stroke syndromes are shown.

Signs and symptoms: *Structures involved*

1. Medial medullary syndrome (occlusion of vertebral artery or of branch of vertebral or lower basilar artery)
   On side of lesion
   Paralysis with atrophy of one-half half the tongue: *Ipsilateral twelfth nerve*
   On side opposite lesion
   Paralysis of arm and leg, sparing face; impaired tactile and proprioceptive sense over one-half the body: *Contralateral pyramidal tract and medial lemniscus*
2. Lateral medullary syndrome (occlusion of any of five vessels may be responsible—vertebral, posterior inferior cerebellar, superior, middle, or inferior lateral medullary arteries)
   On side of lesion
   Pain, numbness, impaired sensation over one-half the face: *Descending tract and nucleus fifth nerve*
   Ataxia of limbs, falling to side of lesion: *Uncertain—restiform body, cerebellar hemisphere, cerebellar fibers, spinocerebellar tract (?)*
   Nystagmus, diplopia, oscillopsia, vertigo, nausea, vomiting: *Vestibular nucleus*
   Horner's syndrome (miosis, ptosis, decreased sweating): *Descending sympathetic tract*
   Dysphagia, hoarseness, paralysis of palate, paralysis of vocal cord, diminished gag reflex: *Issuing fibers ninth and tenth nerves*
   Loss of taste: *Nucleus and tractus solitarius*
   Numbness of ipsilateral arm, trunk, or leg: *Cuneate and gracile nuclei*
   Weakness of lower face: *Genuflected upper motor neuron fibers to ipsilateral facial nucleus*
   On side opposite lesion
   Impaired pain and thermal sense over half the body, sometimes face: *Spinothalamic tract*
3. Total unilateral medullary syndrome (occlusion of vertebral artery): Combination of medial and lateral syndromes
4. Lateral pontomedullary syndrome (occlusion of vertebral artery): Combination of lateral medullary and lateral inferior pontine syndrome
5. Basilar artery syndrome (the syndrome of the lone vertebral artery is equivalent): A combination of the various brainstem syndromes plus those arising in the posterior cerebral artery distribution.
   Bilateral long tract signs (sensory and motor; cerebellar and peripheral cranial nerve abnormalities): *Bilateral long tract; cerebellar and peripheral cranial nerves*
   Paralysis or weakness of all extremities, plus all bulbar musculature: *Corticobulbar and corticospinal tracts bilaterally*

Occlusion of the superior cerebellar artery results in severe ipsilateral cerebellar ataxia, nausea and vomiting, dysarthria, and contralateral loss of pain and temperature sensation over the extremities, body, and face (spino- and trigeminothalamic tract). Partial deafness, ataxic tremor of the ipsilateral upper extremity, Horner's syndrome, and palatal myoclonus may occur rarely. Partial syndromes occur frequently (Fig. 370-13). With large strokes, swelling and mass effects may compress the midbrain or produce hydrocephalus; these symptoms may evolve rapidly. Neurosurgical intervention may be lifesaving in such cases.

Occlusion of the anterior inferior cerebellar artery produces variable degrees of infarction because the size of this artery and the territory it supplies vary inversely with those of the PICA. The principal symptoms include: (1) ipsilateral deafness, facial weakness, vertigo, nausea and vomiting, nystagmus, tinnitus, cerebellar ataxia, Horner's syndrome, and paresis of conjugate lateral gaze; and (2) contralateral loss of pain and temperature sensation. An occlusion close to the origin of the artery may cause corticospinal tract signs (Fig. 370-11).

Occlusion of one of the short circumferential branches of the basilar artery affects the lateral two-thirds of the pons and middle or superior cerebellar peduncle, whereas occlusion of one of the paramedian branches affects a wedge-shaped area on either side of the medial pons (Figs. 370-11 through 370-13).

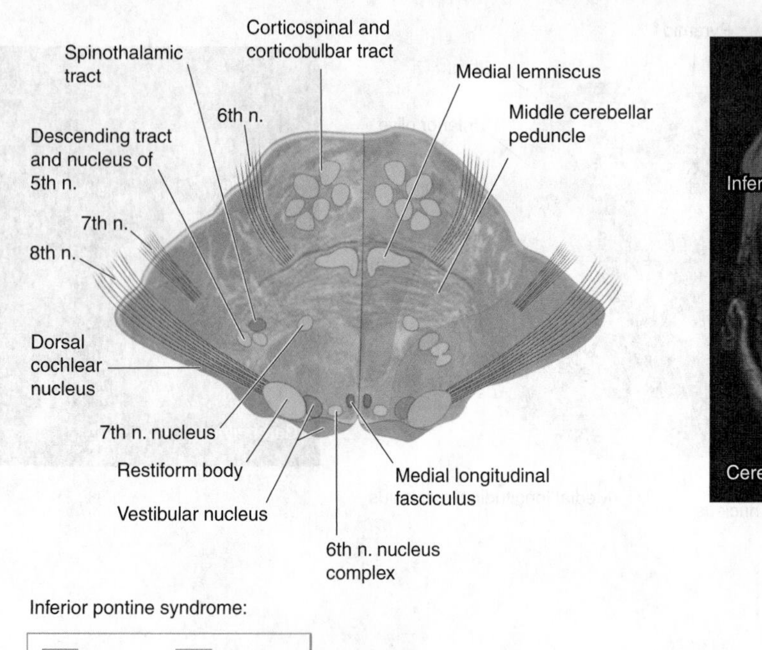

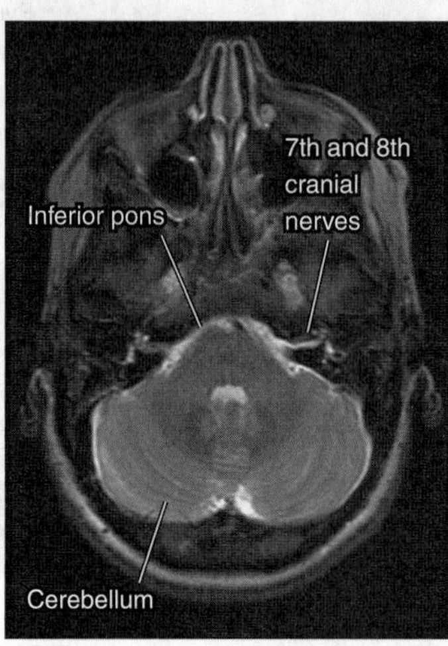

Figure 370-11 Axial section at the level of the inferior pons, depicted schematically on the left, with a corresponding MR image on the right. Approximate regions involved in medial and lateral inferior pontine stroke syndromes are shown.

Signs and symptoms: *Structures involved*

1. Medial inferior pontine syndrome (occlusion of paramedian branch of basilar artery)
   On side of lesion
   - Paralysis of conjugate gaze to side of lesion (preservation of convergence): *Center for conjugate lateral gaze*
   - Nystagmus: *Vestibular nucleus*
   - Ataxia of limbs and gait: Likely *middle cerebellar peduncle*
   - Diplopia on lateral gaze: *Abducens nerve*

   On side opposite lesion
   - Paralysis of face, arm, and leg: *Corticobulbar and corticospinal tract in lower pons*
   - Impaired tactile and proprioceptive sense over one-half of the body: *Medial lemniscus*
2. Lateral inferior pontine syndrome (occlusion of anterior inferior cerebellar artery)
   On side of lesion
   - Horizontal and vertical nystagmus, vertigo, nausea, vomiting, oscillopsia: *Vestibular nerve or nucleus*
   - Facial paralysis: *Seventh nerve*
   - Paralysis of conjugate gaze to side of lesion: *Center for conjugate lateral gaze*
   - Deafness, tinnitus: *Auditory nerve or cochlear nucleus*
   - Ataxia: *Middle cerebellar peduncle and cerebellar hemisphere*
   - Impaired sensation over face: *Descending tract and nucleus fifth nerve*

   On side opposite lesion
   - Impaired pain and thermal sense over one-half the body (may include face): *Spinothalamic tract*

IMAGING STUDIES

See also Chap. 368.

CT scans

CT radiographic images identify or exclude hemorrhage as the cause of stroke, and they identify extraparenchymal hemorrhages, neoplasms, abscesses, and other conditions masquerading as stroke. Brain CT scans obtained in the first several hours after an infarction generally show no abnormality, and the infarct may not be seen reliably for 24–48 hours. CT may fail to show small ischemic strokes in the posterior fossa because of bone artifact; small infarcts on the cortical surface may also be missed.

Contrast-enhanced CT scans add specificity by showing contrast enhancement of subacute infarcts and allow visualization of venous structures. Coupled with newer generation multidetector scanners, CT angiography (CTA) can be performed with administration of IV iodinated contrast allowing visualization of the cervical and intracranial arteries, intracranial veins, aortic arch, and even the coronary arteries in one imaging session. Carotid disease and intracranial vascular occlusions are readily identified with this method (Fig. 370-3). After an IV bolus of contrast, deficits in brain perfusion produced by vascular occlusion can also be demonstrated (Fig. 370-15) and used to predict the region of infarcted brain and the brain at risk of further infarction (i.e., the ischemic penumbra, see "Pathophysiology of Ischemic Stroke" above). CT imaging is also sensitive for detecting SAH (though by itself does not rule it out), and CTA can readily identify intracranial aneurysms (Chap. 275). Because of its speed and wide availability, noncontrast head CT is the imaging modality of choice in patients with acute stroke (Fig. 370-1), and CTA and CT perfusion imaging may also be useful and convenient adjuncts.

MRI

MRI reliably documents the extent and location of infarction in all areas of the brain, including the posterior fossa and cortical surface. It also identifies intracranial hemorrhage and other abnormalities but is less sensitive than CT for detecting acute blood. MRI scanners with magnets of higher field strength produce more reliable and precise images. Diffusion-weighted imaging is more sensitive for early brain infarction than standard

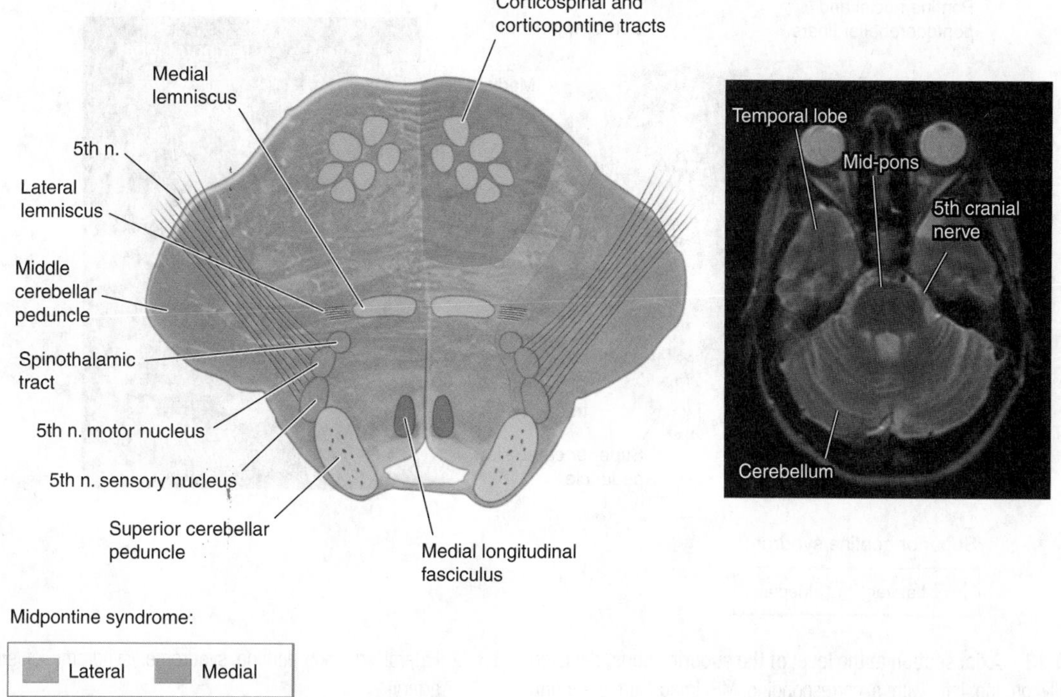

Figure 370-12 Axial section at the level of the midpons, depicted schematically on the left, with a corresponding MR image on the right. Approximate regions involved in medial and lateral midpontine stroke syndromes are shown.

Signs and symptoms: *Structures involved*

1. Medial midpontine syndrome (paramedian branch of midbasilar artery)
   On side of lesion
   Ataxia of limbs and gait (more prominent in bilateral involvement): *Pontine nuclei*
   On side opposite lesion
   Paralysis of face, arm, and leg: *Corticobulbar and corticospinal tract*
   Variable impaired touch and proprioception when lesion extends posteriorly: *Medial lemniscus*
2. Lateral midpontine syndrome (short circumferential artery)
   On side of lesion
   Ataxia of limbs: *Middle cerebellar peduncle*
   Paralysis of muscles of mastication: *Motor fibers or nucleus of fifth nerve*
   Impaired sensation over side of face: *Sensory fibers or nucleus of fifth nerve*
   On side opposite lesion
   Impaired pain and thermal sense on limbs and trunk: *Spinothalamic tract*

MR sequences or CT (Fig. 370-16), as is fluid-attenuated inversion recovery (FLAIR) imaging (Chap. 368). Using IV administration of gadolinium contrast, MR perfusion studies can be performed. Brain regions showing poor perfusion but no abnormality on diffusion are equivalent measure of the ischemic penumbra (see "Pathophysiology of Ischemic Stroke," above and Fig. 370-16), and patients showing large regions of mismatch may be better candidates for acute revascularization. MR angiography is highly sensitive for stenosis of extracranial internal carotid arteries and of large intracranial vessels. With higher degrees of stenosis, MR angiography tends to overestimate the degree of stenosis when compared to conventional x-ray angiography. MRI with fat saturation is an imaging sequence used to visualize extra or intracranial arterial dissection. This sensitive technique images clotted blood within the dissected vessel wall.

MRI is less sensitive for acute blood products than CT and is more expensive and time consuming and less readily available. Claustrophobia also limits its application. Most acute stroke protocols use CT because of these limitations. However, MRI is useful outside the acute period by more clearly defining the extent of tissue injury and discriminating new from old regions of brain infarction. MRI may have particular utility in patients with TIA: It is also more likely to identify new infarction, which is a strong predictor of subsequent stroke.

Cerebral angiography

Conventional x-ray cerebral angiography is the gold standard for identifying and quantifying atherosclerotic stenoses of the cerebral arteries and for identifying and characterizing other pathologies, including aneurysms, vasospasm, intraluminal thrombi, fibromuscular dysplasia, arteriovenous fistula, vasculitis, and collateral channels of blood flow. Endovascular techniques, which are evolving rapidly, can be used to deploy stents within delicate intracranial vessels, to perform balloon angioplasty of stenotic lesions, to treat intracranial aneurysms by embolization, and to open occluded vessels in acute stroke with mechanical thrombectomy devices. Randomized trials support use of thrombolytic agents delivered intraarterially in patients with acute MCA stroke by showing that vessels are effectively recanalized and clinical outcomes are improved at 90 days. Cerebral angiography coupled with endovascular techniques for cerebral revascularization are becoming routine in the United States and Europe and likely soon in Japan. Centers capable of these techniques are termed *comprehensive stroke centers* to distinguish them from primary stroke centers that can administer IV rtPA but not perform endovascular therapy. Conventional angiography carries risks of arterial damage, groin hemorrhage, embolic stroke, and renal failure from contrast nephropathy, so it should be reserved for situations where less invasive means are inadequate.

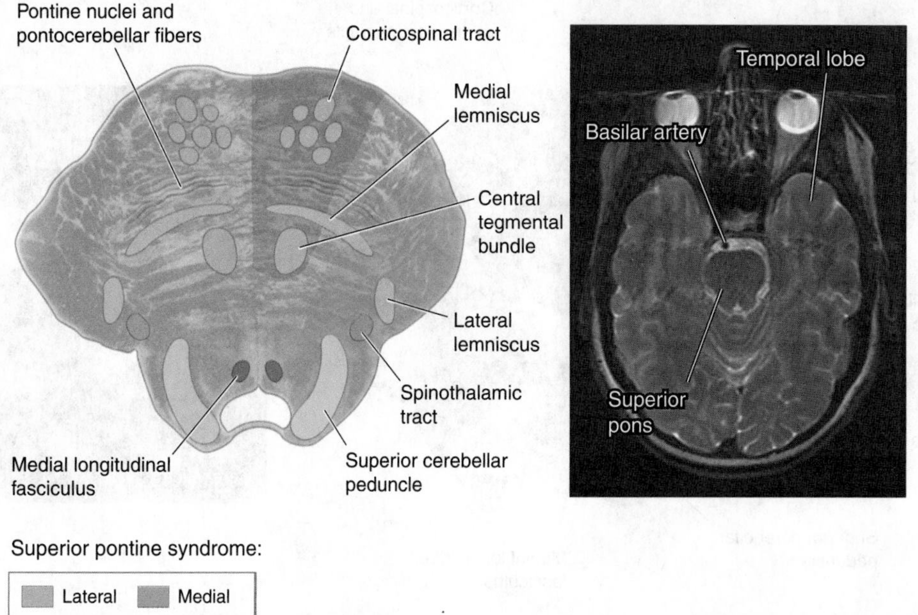

Figure 370-13 Axial section at the level of the superior pons, depicted schematically on the left, with a corresponding MR image on the right. Approximate regions involved in medial and lateral superior pontine stroke syndromes are shown.

Signs and symptoms: *Structures involved*

1. Medial superior pontine syndrome (paramedian branches of upper basilar artery)
   On side of lesion
   Cerebellar ataxia (probably): *Superior and/or middle cerebellar peduncle*
   Internuclear ophthalmoplegia: *Medial longitudinal fasciculus*
   Myoclonic syndrome, palate, pharynx, vocal cords, respiratory apparatus, face, oculomotor apparatus, etc.: *Localization uncertain—central tegmental bundle, dentate projection, inferior olivary nucleus*
   On side opposite lesion
   Paralysis of face, arm, and leg: *Corticobulbar and corticospinal tract*
   Rarely touch, vibration, and position are affected: *Medial lemniscus*
2. Lateral superior pontine syndrome (syndrome of superior cerebellar artery)
   On side of lesion
   Ataxia of limbs and gait, falling to side of lesion: *Middle and superior cerebellar peduncles, superior surface of cerebellum, dentate nucleus*
   Dizziness, nausea, vomiting; horizontal nystagmus: *Vestibular nucleus*
   Paresis of conjugate gaze (ipsilateral): *Pontine contralateral gaze*
   Skew deviation: *Uncertain*
   Miosis, ptosis, decreased sweating over face (Horner's syndrome): *Descending sympathetic fibers*
   Tremor: Localization unclear—*Dentate nucleus, superior cerebellar peduncle*
   On side opposite lesion
   Impaired pain and thermal sense on face, limbs, and trunk: *Spinothalamic tract*
   Impaired touch, vibration, and position sense, more in leg than arm (there is a tendency to incongruity of pain and touch deficits): *Medial lemniscus (lateral portion)*

Ultrasound techniques

Stenosis at the origin of the internal carotid artery can be identified and quantified reliably by ultrasonography that combines a B-mode ultrasound image with a Doppler ultrasound assessment of flow velocity ("duplex" ultrasound). Transcranial Doppler (TCD) assessment of MCA, ACA, and PCA flow and of vertebrobasilar flow is also useful. This latter technique can detect stenotic lesions in the large intracranial arteries because such lesions increase systolic flow velocity. Furthermore, TCD can assist thrombolysis and improve large artery recanalization following rtPA administration; the potential clinical benefit of this treatment is the subject of ongoing study. In many cases, MR angiography combined with carotid and transcranial ultrasound studies eliminates the need for conventional x-ray angiography in evaluating vascular stenosis. Alternatively, CT angiography of the entire head and neck can be performed during the initial imaging of acute stroke. Because this images the entire arterial system relevant to stroke, with the exception of the heart, much of the clinician's stroke workup can be completed with this single imaging study.

Perfusion techniques

Both xenon techniques (principally xenon-CT) and PET can quantify cerebral blood flow. These tools are generally used for research (Chap. 368) but can be useful for determining the significance of arterial stenosis and planning for revascularization surgery. Single-photon emission computed tomography (SPECT) and MR perfusion techniques report relative cerebral blood flow. Since CT imaging is used as the initial imaging modality for acute stroke, some centers combine both CT angiography and CT perfusion imaging together with the noncontrast CT scan. CT perfusion imaging increases the sensitivity for detecting ischemia, and can measure the ischemic penumbra (Fig. 370-15). Alternatively, MR perfusion can be combined with MR diffusion imaging to identify the ischemic penumbra as the mismatch between these two imaging sequences (Fig. 370-16). The ability to image the ischemic penumbra allows more judicious selection of patients who may or may not benefit from acute interventions such as thrombolysis, thrombectomy, or investigational neuroprotective strategies.

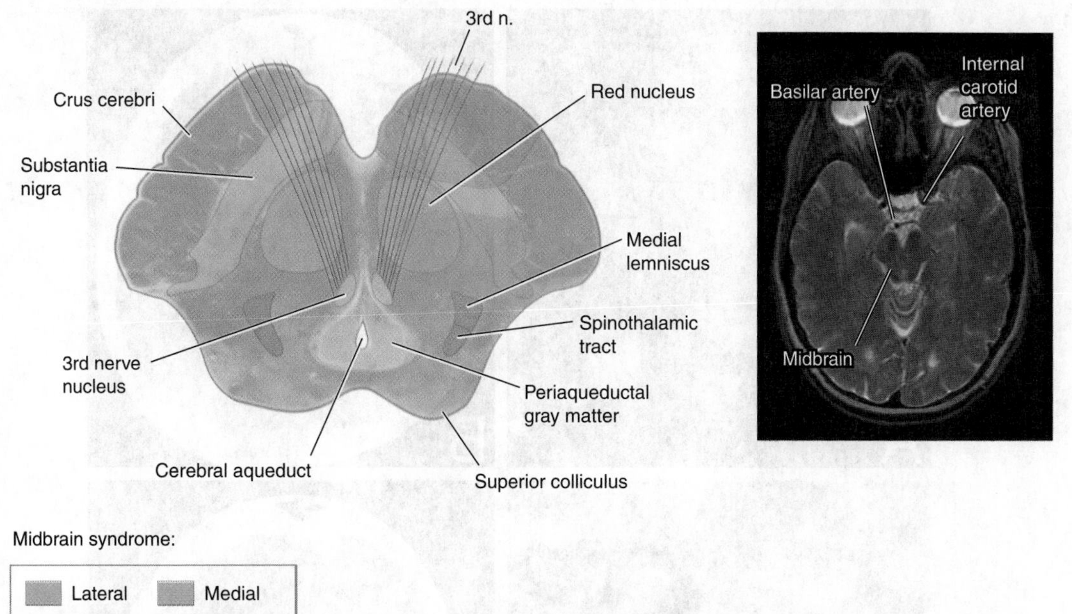

Figure 370-14 Axial section at the level of the midbrain, depicted schematically on the left, with a corresponding MR image on the right. Approximate regions involved in medial and lateral midbrain stroke syndromes are shown.

Signs and symptoms: *Structures involved*

1. Medial midbrain syndrome (paramedian branches of upper basilar and proximal posterior cerebral arteries)
   On side of lesion
      Eye "down and out" secondary to unopposed action of fourth and sixth cranial nerves, with dilated and unresponsive pupil: *Third nerve fibers*
   On side opposite lesion
      Paralysis of face, arm, and leg: *Corticobulbar and corticospinal tract descending in crus cerebri*
2. Lateral midbrain syndrome (syndrome of small penetrating arteries arising from posterior cerebral artery)
   On side of lesion
      Eye "down and out" secondary to unopposed action of fourth and sixth cranial nerves, with dilated and unresponsive pupil: *Third nerve fibers and/or third nerve nucleus*
   On side opposite lesion
      Hemiataxia, hyperkinesias, tremor: *Red nucleus, dentatorubrothalamic pathway*

INTRACRANIAL HEMORRHAGE

Hemorrhages are classified by their location and the underlying vascular pathology. Bleeding into subdural and epidural spaces is principally produced by trauma. SAHs are produced by trauma and rupture of intracranial aneurysms (Chap. 275). Intraparenchymal and intraventricular hemorrhage will be considered here.

DIAGNOSIS

Intracranial hemorrhage is often discovered on noncontrast CT imaging of the brain during the acute evaluation of stroke. Since CT is more sensitive than routine MRI for acute blood, CT imaging is the preferred method for acute stroke evaluation (Fig. 370-1). The location of the hemorrhage narrows the differential diagnosis to a few entities. Table 370-6 lists the causes and anatomic spaces involved in hemorrhages.

EMERGENCY MANAGEMENT

Close attention should be paid to airway management since a reduction in the level of consciousness is common and often progressive. The initial blood pressure should be maintained until the results of the CT scan are reviewed. Expansion of hemorrhage volume is associated with elevated blood pressure, but it remains unclear if lowering of blood pressure reduces hematoma growth. A recent feasibility trial of 60 patients showed that blood pressure could be safely lowered in acute spontaneous intraparenchymal (intracerebral) hemorrhage (ICH) using nicardipine and forms the basis for a planned pivotal trial powered for detecting improved clinical outcome. Another trial [Intensive Blood Pressure Reduction in Acute Cerebral Hemorrhage Trial (INTERACT)] randomized hypertensive, spontaneous ICH patients to maintain systolic blood pressure (SBP) <180 mm Hg versus SBP <140 mm Hg using IV antihypertensives. There was a statistical decrease in hematoma growth and a reduction in perihematoma edema in the patients assigned to the lower blood pressure goal. Whether these reductions in hematoma growth will translate to clinical benefit is unclear. Until more results are available it is recommended to keep mean arterial pressure (MAP) <130 mm Hg, unless an increase in ICP is suspected. In patients who have ICP monitors in place, current recommendations are to keep the cerebral perfusion pressure (MAP-ICP) above 60 mm Hg (i.e., one should lower MAP to this target if blood pressure is elevated). Blood pressure should be lowered with nonvasodilating IV drugs such as nicardipine, labetalol, or esmolol. Patients with cerebellar hemorrhages or with depressed mental status and radiographic evidence of hydrocephalus should undergo urgent neurosurgical evaluation. Based on the clinical examination and CT findings, further imaging studies may be necessary, including MRI or conventional x-ray angiography. Stuporous or comatose patients generally are treated presumptively for elevated ICP, with tracheal intubation and hyperventilation, mannitol administration, and elevation of the head of the bed while surgical consultation is obtained (Chap. 275).

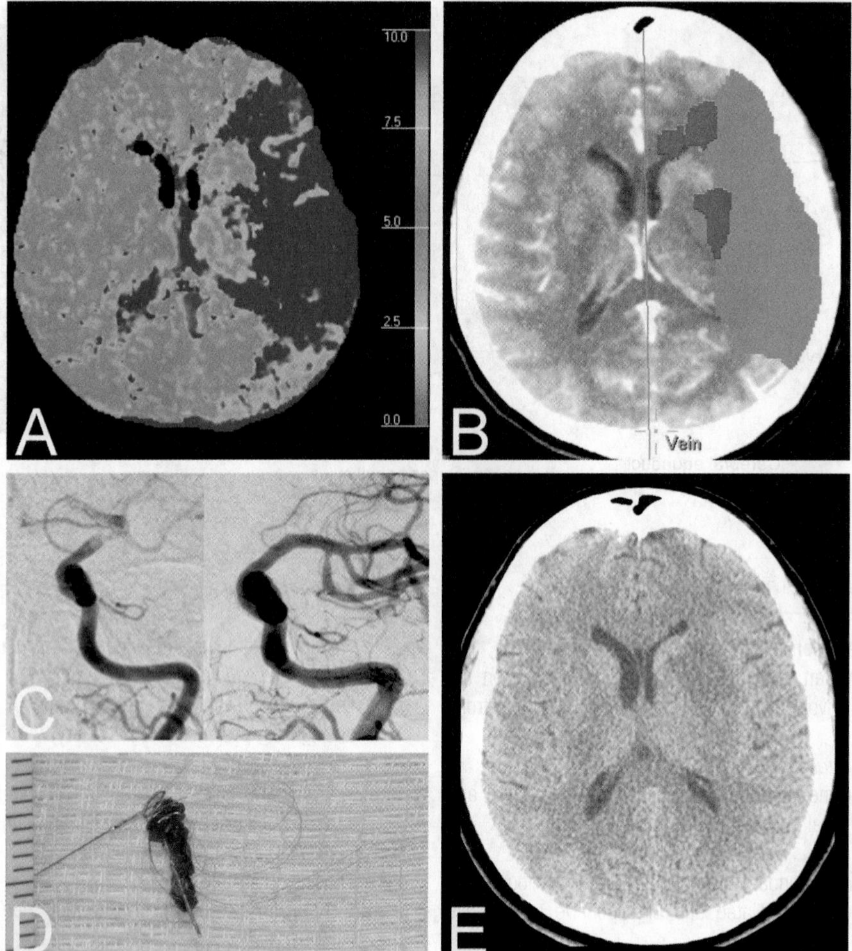

Figure 370-15 Acute left middle cerebral artery (MCA) stroke with right hemiplegia but preserved language. ***A.*** CT perfusion mean-transit time map showing delayed perfusion of the left MCA distribution (blue). ***B.*** Predicted region of infarct (*red*) and penumbra (*green*) based on CT perfusion data. ***C.*** Conventional angiogram showing occlusion of the left internal carotid–MCA bifurcation (*left panel*), and revascularization of the vessels following successful thrombectomy 8 hours after stroke symptom onset (*right panel*). ***D.*** The clot removed with a thrombectomy device (L5, Concentric Medical, Inc.). ***E.*** CT scan of the brain 2 days later; note infarction in the region predicted in ***B*** but preservation of the penumbral region by successful revascularization.

INTRAPARENCHYMAL HEMORRHAGE

ICH is the most common type of intracranial hemorrhage. It accounts for ~10% of all strokes and is associated with a 50% case fatality rate. Incidence rates are particularly high in Asians and blacks. Hypertension, trauma, and cerebral amyloid angiopathy cause the majority of these hemorrhages. Advanced age and heavy alcohol consumption increase the risk, and cocaine and methamphetamine use is one of the most important causes in the young.

Hypertensive intraparenchymal hemorrhage

Pathophysiology Hypertensive intraparenchymal hemorrhage (hypertensive hemorrhage or hypertensive intracerebral hemorrhage) usually results from spontaneous rupture of a small penetrating artery deep in the brain. The most common sites are the basal ganglia (especially the putamen), thalamus, cerebellum, and pons. When hemorrhages occur in other brain areas or in nonhypertensive patients, greater consideration should be given to hemorrhagic disorders, neoplasms, vascular malformations, and other causes. The small arteries in these areas seem most prone to hypertension-induced vascular injury. The hemorrhage may be small or a large clot may form and compress adjacent tissue, causing herniation and death. Blood may dissect into the ventricular space, which substantially increases morbidity and may cause hydrocephalus.

Most hypertensive intraparenchymal hemorrhages develop over 30–90 minutes, whereas those associated with anticoagulant therapy may evolve for as long as 24–48 hours. Within 48 hours macrophages begin to phagocytize the hemorrhage at its outer surface. After 1–6 months, the hemorrhage is generally resolved to a slitlike orange cavity lined with glial scar and hemosiderin-laden macrophages.

Clinical manifestations Although not particularly associated with exertion, ICHs almost always occur while the patient is awake and sometimes when stressed. The hemorrhage generally presents as the abrupt onset of focal neurologic deficit. Seizures are uncommon. The focal deficit typically worsens steadily over 30–90 minutes and is associated with a diminishing level of consciousness and signs of increased ICP such as headache and vomiting.

The putamen is the most common site for hypertensive hemorrhage, and the adjacent internal capsule is usually damaged (Fig. 370-17). Contralateral hemiparesis is therefore the sentinel sign. When mild, the face sags on one side over 5–30 minutes,

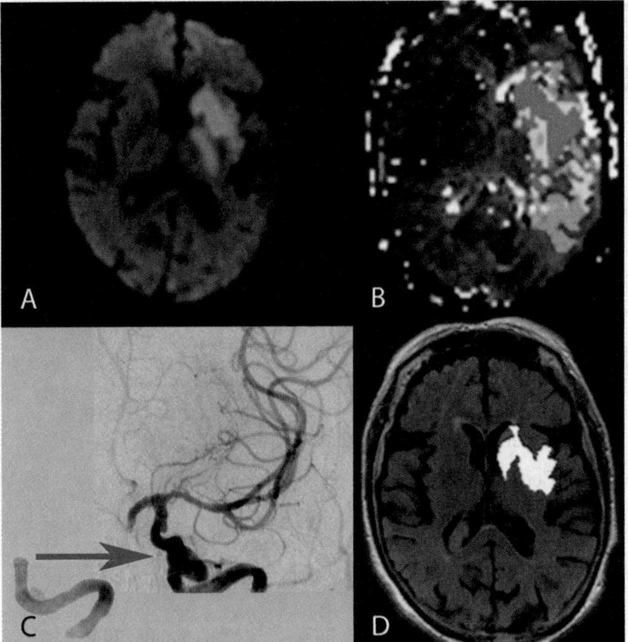

Figure 370-16 MRI of acute stroke. ***A.*** MRI diffusion-weighted image (DWI) of an 82-year-old woman 2.5 hours after onset of right-sided weakness and aphasia reveals restricted diffusion within the left basal ganglia and internal capsule (*colored regions.*) ***B.*** Perfusion defect within the left hemisphere (*colored signal*) imaged after administration of an IV bolus of gadolinium contrast. The discrepancy between the region of poor perfusion shown in ***B*** and the diffusion deficit shown in ***A*** is called *diffusion-perfusion mismatch* and provides an estimate of the ischemic penumbra. Without specific therapy the region of infarction will expand into much or all of the perfusion deficit. ***C.*** Cerebral angiogram of the left internal carotid artery in this patient before (*left*) and after (*right*) successful endovascular embolectomy. The occlusion is within the carotid terminus. ***D.*** FLAIR image obtained 3 days later showing a region of infarction (*coded as white*) that corresponds to the initial DWI image in ***A***, but not the entire area at risk shown in ***B***, suggesting that successful embolectomy saved a large region of brain tissue from infarction. *(Courtesy of Gregory Albers, MD, Stanford University; with permission.)*

speech becomes slurred, the arm and leg gradually weaken, and the eyes deviate away from the side of the hemiparesis. The paralysis may worsen until the affected limbs become flaccid or extend rigidly. When hemorrhages are large, drowsiness gives way to stupor as signs of upper brainstem compression appear. Coma ensues, accompanied by deep, irregular, or intermittent respiration, a dilated and fixed ipsilateral pupil, and decerebrate rigidity. In milder cases, edema in adjacent brain tissue may cause progressive deterioration over 12–72 hours.

Thalamic hemorrhages also produce a contralateral hemiplegia or hemiparesis from pressure on, or dissection into, the adjacent internal capsule. A prominent sensory deficit involving all modalities is usually present. Aphasia, often with preserved verbal repetition, may occur after hemorrhage into the dominant thalamus, and constructional apraxia or mutism occurs in some cases of nondominant hemorrhage. There may also be a homonymous visual field defect. Thalamic hemorrhages cause several typical ocular disturbances by virtue of extension inferiorly into the upper midbrain. These include deviation of the eyes downward and inward so that they appear to be looking at the nose, unequal pupils with absence of light reaction, skew deviation with the eye opposite the hemorrhage displaced downward and medially, ipsilateral Horner's syndrome, absence of convergence, paralysis of vertical gaze, and retraction nystagmus. Patients may later develop a chronic, contralateral pain syndrome (Déjérine-Roussy syndrome).

In pontine hemorrhages, deep coma with quadriplegia usually occurs over a few minutes. There is often prominent decerebrate rigidity and "pinpoint" (1 mm) pupils that react to light. There is impairment of reflex horizontal eye movements evoked by head turning (doll's-head or oculocephalic maneuver) or by irrigation of the ears with ice water (Chap. 274). Hyperpnea, severe hypertension, and hyperhidrosis are common. Death often occurs within a few hours, but small hemorrhages are compatible with survival.

Cerebellar hemorrhages usually develop over several hours and are characterized by occipital headache, repeated vomiting, and ataxia of gait. In mild cases there may be no other neurologic signs other than gait ataxia. Dizziness or vertigo may be prominent. There is often paresis of conjugate lateral gaze toward the side of the hemorrhage, forced deviation of the eyes to the opposite side, or an ipsilateral sixth nerve palsy. Less frequent ocular signs include blepharospasm, involuntary closure of one eye, ocular bobbing, and skew deviation. Dysarthria and dysphagia may occur. As the hours pass, the patient often becomes stuporous and then comatose from brainstem compression or obstructive hydrocephalus; immediate surgical evacuation before brainstem compression occurs may be lifesaving. Hydrocephalus from fourth ventricle compression can be relieved by external ventricular drainage, but definitive hematoma evacuation is essential for survival. If the deep cerebellar nuclei are spared, full recovery is common.

Lobar hemorrhage

Symptoms and signs appear over several minutes. Most lobar hemorrhages are small and cause a restricted clinical syndrome that simulates an embolus to an artery supplying one lobe. For example, the major neurologic deficit with an occipital hemorrhage is hemianopia; with a left temporal hemorrhage, aphasia and delirium; with a parietal hemorrhage, hemisensory loss; and with frontal hemorrhage, arm weakness. Large hemorrhages may be associated with stupor or coma if they compress the thalamus or midbrain. Most patients with lobar hemorrhages have focal headaches, and more than one-half vomit or are drowsy. Stiff neck and seizures are uncommon.

Other causes of intracerebral hemorrhage

Cerebral amyloid angiopathy is a disease of the elderly in which arteriolar degeneration occurs and amyloid is deposited in the walls of the cerebral arteries. Amyloid angiopathy causes both single and recurrent lobar hemorrhages and is probably the most common cause of lobar hemorrhage in the elderly. It accounts for some intracranial hemorrhages associated with IV thrombolysis given for MI. This disorder can be suspected in patients who present with multiple hemorrhages (and infarcts) over several months or years, or in patients with "micro-bleeds" seen on brain MRI sequences sensitive for hemosiderin, but it is definitively diagnosed by pathologic demonstration of Congo red staining of amyloid in cerebral vessels. The ε2 and ε4 allelic variations of the apolipoprotein E gene are associated with increased risk of recurrent lobar hemorrhage and may therefore be markers of amyloid angiopathy. Currently, there is no specific therapy, although antiplatelet and anticoagulating agents are typically avoided.

Cocaine and methamphetamine are frequent causes of stroke in young (age <45 years) patients. ICH, ischemic stroke, and SAH are all associated with stimulant use. Angiographic

TABLE 370-6 Causes of Intracranial Hemorrhage

Cause	Location	Comments
Head trauma	Intraparenchymal: frontal lobes, anterior temporal lobes; subarachnoid	Coup and contrecoup injury during brain deceleration
Hypertensive hemorrhage	Putamen, globus pallidus, thalamus, cerebellar hemisphere, pons	Chronic hypertension produces hemorrhage from small (~100 μm) vessels in these regions
Transformation of prior ischemic infarction	Basal ganglion, subcortical regions, lobar	Occurs in 1–6% of ischemic strokes with predilection for large hemispheric infarctions
Metastatic brain tumor	Lobar	Lung, choriocarcinoma, melanoma, renal cell carcinoma, thyroid, atrial myxoma
Coagulopathy	Any	Uncommon cause; often associated with prior stroke or underlying vascular anomaly
Drug	Lobar, subarachnoid	Cocaine, amphetamine, phenylpropanolamine
Arteriovenous malformation	Lobar, intraventricular, subarachnoid	Risk is ~2–4% per year for bleeding
Aneurysm	Subarachnoid, intraparenchymal, rarely subdural	Mycotic and nonmycotic forms of aneurysms
Amyloid angiopathy	Lobar	Degenerative disease of intracranial vessels; linkage to Alzheimer's disease, rare in patients <60 years
Cavernous angioma	Intraparenchymal	Multiple cavernous angiomas linked to mutations in KRIT1, CCM2, and PDCD10 genes
Dural arteriovenous fistula	Lobar, subarachnoid	Produces bleeding by venous hypertension
Capillary telangiectasias	Usually brainstem	Rare cause of hemorrhage

findings vary from completely normal arteries to large-vessel occlusion or stenosis, vasospasm, or changes consistent with vasculopathy. The mechanism of sympathomimetic-related stroke is not known, but cocaine enhances sympathetic activity causing acute, sometimes severe, hypertension, and this may lead to hemorrhage. Slightly more than one-half of stimulant-related intracranial hemorrhages are intracerebral, and the rest are subarachnoid. In cases of SAH, a saccular aneurysm is usually identified. Presumably, acute hypertension causes aneurysmal rupture.

Head injury often causes intracranial bleeding. The common sites are intracerebral (especially temporal and inferior frontal lobes) and into the subarachnoid, subdural, and epidural spaces. Trauma must be considered in any patient with an unexplained acute neurologic deficit (hemiparesis, stupor, or confusion), particularly if the deficit occurred in the context of a fall (Chap. 378).

Intracranial hemorrhages associated with *anticoagulant therapy* can occur at any location; they are often lobar or subdural. Anticoagulant-related ICHs may evolve slowly, over 24–48 hours. Coagulopathy and thrombocytopenia should be reversed rapidly, as discussed below. ICH associated with *hematologic disorders* (leukemia, aplastic anemia, thrombocytopenic purpura) can occur at any site and may present as multiple ICHs. Skin and mucous membrane bleeding is usually evident and offers a diagnostic clue.

Hemorrhage into a *brain tumor* may be the first manifestation of neoplasm. Choriocarcinoma, malignant melanoma, renal cell carcinoma, and bronchogenic carcinoma are among the most common metastatic tumors associated with ICH. Glioblastoma multiforme in adults and medulloblastoma in children may also have areas of ICH.

Hypertensive encephalopathy is a complication of malignant hypertension. In this acute syndrome, severe hypertension is associated with headache, nausea, vomiting, convulsions, confusion, stupor, and coma. Focal or lateralizing neurologic signs, either transitory or permanent, may occur but are infrequent and therefore suggest some other vascular disease (hemorrhage, embolism, or atherosclerotic thrombosis). There are retinal hemorrhages, exudates, papilledema (hypertensive retinopathy), and evidence of renal and cardiac disease. In most cases ICP and CSF protein levels are elevated. MRI brain imaging shows a pattern of typically posterior (occipital > frontal) brain edema that is reversible and termed *reversible posterior leukoencephalopathy*. The hypertension may be essential or due to chronic renal disease, acute glomerulonephritis, acute toxemia of pregnancy, pheochromocytoma, or other causes. Lowering the blood pressure reverses the process, but stroke can occur, especially if blood pressure is lowered too rapidly. Neuropathologic examination reveals multifocal to diffuse cerebral edema and hemorrhages of various sizes from petechial to massive. Microscopically, there are necrosis of arterioles, minute cerebral infarcts, and hemorrhages. The term *hypertensive encephalopathy* should be reserved for this syndrome and not for chronic recurrent headaches, dizziness, recurrent TIAs, or small strokes that often occur in association with high blood pressure.

Primary intraventricular hemorrhage is rare. It usually begins within the substance of the brain and dissects into the ventricular system without leaving signs of intraparenchymal hemorrhage. Alternatively, bleeding can arise from periependymal veins. Vasculitis, usually polyarteritis nodosa or lupus erythematosus, can produce hemorrhage in any region of the central nervous system; most hemorrhages are associated with hypertension, but

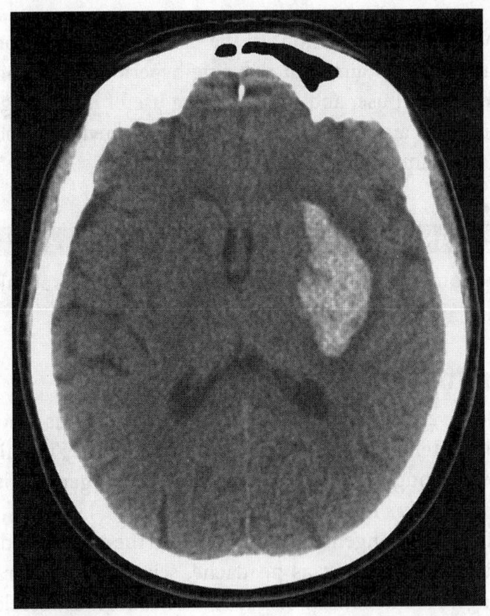

Figure 370-17 Hypertensive hemorrhage. Transaxial noncontrast CT scan through the region of the basal ganglia reveals a hematoma involving the left putamen in a patient with rapidly progressive onset of right hemiparesis.

the arteritis itself may cause bleeding by disrupting the vessel wall. Nearly one-half of patients with primary intraventricular hemorrhage have identifiable bleeding sources seen using conventional angiography. *Sepsis* can cause small petechial hemorrhages throughout the cerebral white matter. *Moyamoya disease*, mainly an occlusive arterial disease that causes ischemic symptoms, may on occasion produce intraparenchymal hemorrhage, particularly in the young. Hemorrhages into the spinal cord are usually the result of an AVM, cavernous malformation, or metastatic tumor. *Epidural spinal hemorrhage* produces a rapidly evolving syndrome of spinal cord or nerve root compression (Chap. 377). Spinal hemorrhages usually present with sudden back pain and some manifestation of myelopathy.

Laboratory and imaging evaluation

Patients should have routine blood chemistries and hematologic studies. Specific attention to the platelet count and PT/PTT are important to identify coagulopathy. CT imaging reliably detects acute focal hemorrhages in the supratentorial space. Small pontine hemorrhages may not be identified because of motion and bone-induced artifact that obscure structures in the posterior fossa. After the first 2 weeks, x-ray attenuation values of clotted blood diminish until they become isodense with surrounding brain. Mass effect and edema may remain. In some cases, a surrounding rim of contrast enhancement appears after 2–4 weeks and may persist for months. MRI, although more sensitive for delineating posterior fossa lesions, is generally not necessary in most instances. Images of flowing blood on MRI scan may identify AVMs as the cause of the hemorrhage. MRI, CT angiography, and conventional x-ray angiography are used when the cause of intracranial hemorrhage is uncertain, particularly if the patient is young or not hypertensive and the hematoma is not in one of the four usual sites for hypertensive hemorrhage. Postcontrast CT imaging may reveal acute hematoma enhancement signifying bleeding at the time of imaging; this "dot-sign" portends increased mortality. Some centers routinely perform CT and CT angiography with postcontrast CT imaging in one sitting to rapidly identify any macrovascular etiology of the hemorrhage and provide prognostic information at the same time. Since patients typically have focal neurologic signs and obtundation, and often show signs of increased ICP, a lumbar puncture should be avoided as it may induce cerebral herniation.

TREATMENT Intracerebral Hemorrhage

ACUTE MANAGEMENT Nearly 50% of patients with a hypertensive ICH die, but others have a good to complete recovery if they survive the initial hemorrhage. The ICH scoring system (Table 370-7) is a validated metric that is useful for prediction of mortality and clinical outcomes. Any identified coagulopathy

TABLE 370-7 Prognosis and Clinical Outcomes in Intracerebral Hemorrhage

Clinical or Imaging Factor	Point Score	
Age		
<80 years	0	
≥80 years	1	
Hematoma Volume		
<30 cc	0	
≥30 cc	1	
Intraventricular Hemorrhage Present		
No	0	
Yes	1	
Infratentorial Origin of Hemorrhage		
No	0	
Yes	1	
Glasgow Coma Scale Score		
13–15	0	
5–12	1	
3–4	2	
Total Score	Sum of each category above	
ICH Score Total	**Observed Mortality at 30 days (%)**	**Walk Independently at 12 months (%)**
0	0	70
1	13	60
2	26	33
3	72	3
4	97	8
5	100	None

Although a score of 6 is possible with the scale, no patient was observed to present with this combination of findings, and it is considered highly likely to be fatal.
Abbreviation: ICH, intracerebral hemorrhage.
Sources: JC Hemphill et al: Stroke 32:891, 2001; JC Hemphill et al: Neurology 73:1088, 2009.

should be reversed as soon as possible. For patients taking VKAs, rapid reversal of coagulopathy can be achieved by infusing prothrombin complex concentrates which can be administered quickly, followed by fresh-frozen plasma and vitamin K. When ICH is associated with thrombocytopenia (platelet count <50,000/μL), transfusion of fresh platelets is indicated. The role of urgent platelet inhibition assays in the decision to transfuse platelets remains unclear.

At present, little can be done about the hemorrhage itself. Hematomas may expand for several hours following the initial hemorrhage, so treating severe hypertension seems reasonable to prevent hematoma progression. A phase 3 trial of treatment with recombinant factor VIIa reduced hematoma expansion; however, clinical outcomes were not improved, so use of this drug cannot be advocated at present.

Evacuation of supratentorial hematomas does not appear to improve outcome. The International Surgical Trial in Intracerebral Haemorrhage (STICH) randomized 1,033 patients with supratentorial ICH to either early surgical evacuation or initial medical management. No benefit was found in the early surgery arm, although analysis was complicated by the fact that 26% of patients in the initial medical management group ultimately had surgery for neurologic deterioration. Overall, these data do not support routine surgical evacuation of supratentorial hemorrhages; however, many centers operate on patients with progressive neurologic deterioration. Surgical techniques continue to evolve, and minimally invasive endoscopic hematoma evacuation may prove beneficial in future trials.

For cerebellar hemorrhages, a neurosurgeon should be consulted immediately to assist with the evaluation; most cerebellar hematomas >3 cm in diameter will require surgical evacuation. If the patient is alert without focal brainstem signs and if the hematoma is <1 cm in diameter, surgical removal is usually unnecessary. Patients with hematomas between 1 and 3 cm require careful observation for signs of impaired consciousness and precipitous respiratory failure.

Tissue surrounding hematomas is displaced and compressed but not necessarily infarcted. Hence, in survivors, major improvement commonly occurs as the hematoma is reabsorbed and the adjacent tissue regains its function. Careful management of the patient during the acute phase of the hemorrhage can lead to considerable recovery.

Surprisingly, ICP is often normal even with large intraparenchymal hemorrhages. However, if the hematoma causes marked midline shift of structures with consequent obtundation, coma, or hydrocephalus, osmotic agents coupled with induced hyperventilation can be instituted to lower ICP (Chap. 275). These maneuvers will provide enough time to place a ventriculostomy or ICP monitor. Once ICP is recorded, further hyperventilation and osmotic therapy can be tailored to the individual patient to keep cerebral perfusion pressure (MAP-ICP) above 60 mm Hg. For example, if ICP is found to be high, CSF can be drained from the ventricular space and osmotic therapy continued; persistent or progressive elevation in ICP may prompt surgical evacuation of the clot or withdrawal of support. Alternately, if ICP is normal or only mildly elevated, induced hyperventilation can be reversed and osmotic therapy tapered. Since hyperventilation may actually produce ischemia by cerebral vasoconstriction, induced hyperventilation should be limited to acute resuscitation of the patient with presumptive high ICP and eliminated once other treatments (osmotic therapy or surgical treatments) have been instituted. Glucocorticoids are not helpful for the edema from intracerebral hematoma.

PREVENTION Hypertension is the leading cause of primary ICH. Prevention is aimed at reducing hypertension, eliminating excessive alcohol use, and discontinuing use of illicit drugs such as cocaine and amphetamines. Patients with amyloid angiopathy should avoid antithrombotic agents.

VASCULAR ANOMALIES

Vascular anomalies can be divided into congenital vascular malformations and acquired vascular lesions.

CONGENITAL VASCULAR MALFORMATIONS

True *arteriovenous malformations* (AVMs), venous anomalies, and capillary telangiectasias are lesions that usually remain clinically silent through life. AVMs are probably congenital but cases of acquired lesions have been reported.

True AVMs are congenital shunts between the arterial and venous systems that may present as headache, seizures, and intracranial hemorrhage. AVMs consist of a tangle of abnormal vessels across the cortical surface or deep within the brain substance. AVMs vary in size from a small blemish a few millimeters in diameter to a large mass of tortuous channels composing an arteriovenous shunt of sufficient magnitude to raise cardiac output and precipitate heart failure. Blood vessels forming the tangle interposed between arteries and veins are usually abnormally thin and histologically resemble both arteries and veins. AVMs occur in all parts of the cerebral hemispheres, brainstem, and spinal cord, but the largest ones are most frequently in the posterior half of the hemispheres, commonly forming a wedge-shaped lesion extending from the cortex to the ventricle.

Bleeding, headache, or seizures are most common between the ages of 10 and 30, occasionally as late as the fifties. AVMs are more frequent in men, and rare familial cases have been described. Familial AVM may be a part of the autosomal dominant syndrome of hereditary hemorrhagic telangiectasia (Osler-Rendu-Weber) syndrome due to mutations in endoglin (chromosome 9) or activin receptor-like kinase 1 (chromosome 12).

Headache (without bleeding) may be hemicranial and throbbing, like migraine, or diffuse. Focal seizures, with or without generalization, occur in ~30% of cases. one-half of AVMs become evident as ICHs. In most, the hemorrhage is mainly intraparenchymal with extension into the subarachnoid space in some cases. Blood is usually not deposited in the basal cisterns, and symptomatic cerebral vasospasm is rare. The risk of rerupture is ~2–4% per year and is particularly high in the first few weeks. Hemorrhages may be massive, leading to death, or may be as small as 1 cm in diameter, leading to minor focal symptoms or no deficit. The AVM may be large enough to steal blood away from adjacent normal brain tissue or to increase venous pressure significantly to produce venous ischemia locally and in remote areas of the brain. This is seen most often with large AVMs in the territory of the MCA.

Large AVMs of the anterior circulation may be associated with a systolic and diastolic bruit (sometimes self-audible) over the eye, forehead, or neck and a bounding carotid pulse. Headache at the onset of AVM rupture is not generally as explosive as with aneurysmal rupture. MRI is better than CT for diagnosis, although noncontrast CT scanning sometimes detects calcification of the AVM and contrast may demonstrate the abnormal blood vessels. Once identified, conventional x-ray angiography is the gold standard for evaluating the precise anatomy of the AVM.

Surgical treatment of symptomatic AVMs, often with preoperative embolization to reduce operative bleeding, is usually indicated for accessible lesions. Stereotaxic radiation, an alternative to surgery, can produce a slow sclerosis of the AVM over 2–3 years.

Patients with asymptomatic AVMs have about an ~2–4% per year risk for hemorrhage. Several angiographic features can be used to help predict future bleeding risk. Paradoxically, smaller lesions seem to have a higher hemorrhage rate. The impact of recurrent hemorrhage on disability is relatively modest, so the indication for surgery in asymptomatic AVMs is debated. A large-scale randomized trial is currently addressing this question.

Venous anomalies are the result of development of anomalous cerebral, cerebellar, or brainstem venous drainage. These structures, unlike AVMs, are functional venous channels. They are of little clinical significance and should be ignored if found incidentally on brain imaging studies. Surgical resection of these anomalies may result in venous infarction and hemorrhage. Venous anomalies may be associated with cavernous malformations (see below), which do carry some bleeding risk. If resection of a cavernous malformation is attempted, the venous anomaly should not be disturbed.

Capillary telangiectasias are true capillary malformations that often form extensive vascular networks through an otherwise normal brain structure. The pons and deep cerebral white matter are typical locations, and these capillary malformations can be seen in patients with hereditary hemorrhagic telangiectasia (Osler-Rendu-Weber) syndrome. If bleeding does occur, it rarely produces mass effect or significant symptoms. No treatment options exist.

ACQUIRED VASCULAR LESIONS

Cavernous angiomas are tufts of capillary sinusoids that form within the deep hemispheric white matter and brainstem with no normal intervening neural structures. The pathogenesis is unclear. Familial cavernous angiomas have been mapped to several different chromosomal loci: KRIT1 (7q21-q22), CCM2 (7p13), and PDCD10 (3q26.1). Both KRIT1 and CCM2 have roles in blood vessel formation while PDCD10 is an apoptotic gene. Cavernous angiomas are typically <1 cm in diameter and are often associated with a venous anomaly. Bleeding is usually of small volume, causing slight mass effect only. The bleeding risk for single cavernous malformations is 0.7–1.5% per year and may be higher for patients with prior clinical hemorrhage or multiple malformations. Seizures may occur if the malformation is located near the cerebral cortex. Surgical resection eliminates bleeding risk and may reduce seizure risk, but it is reserved for those malformations that form near the brain surface. Radiation treatment has not been shown to be of benefit.

Dural arteriovenous fistulas are acquired connections usually from a dural artery to a dural sinus. Patients may complain of a pulse-synchronous cephalic bruit ("pulsatile tinnitus") and headache. Depending on the magnitude of the shunt, venous pressures may rise high enough to cause cortical ischemia or venous hypertension and hemorrhage, particularly subarachnoid hemorrhage. Surgical and endovascular techniques are usually curative. These fistulas may form because of trauma, but most are idiopathic. There is an association between fistulas and dural sinus thrombosis. Fistulas have been observed to appear months to years following venous sinus thrombosis, suggesting that angiogenesis factors elaborated from the thrombotic process may cause these anomalous connections to form. Alternatively, dural arteriovenous fistulas can produce venous sinus occlusion over time, perhaps from the high pressure and high flow through a venous structure.

FURTHER READINGS

Adams HP Jr. et al: Guidelines for the Early Management of Adults with Ischemic Stroke. Stroke 38:1655, 2007

———: Update to the AHA/ASA recommendations for the prevention of stroke in patients with stroke and transient ischemic attack. Stroke 39:1647, 2008

Albers GW et al: Antithrombotic and thrombolytic therapy for ischemic stroke: American College of Chest Physicians Evidence-Based Clinical Practice Guidelines, 8th ed. Chest 133:630S, 2008

Alberts MJ et al: Recommendations for the establishment of primary stroke centers. Brain Attack Coalition. JAMA 238:3102, 2000

———: Recommendations for comprehensive stroke centers: A consensus statement from the Brain Attack Coalition. Stroke 36:1597, 2005

Choi JH, Mohr JP: Brain arteriovenous malformations in adults. Lancet Neurol 4:299, 2005

Del Zoppo, GJ et al: Expansion of the time window for treatment of acute ischemic stroke with intravenous tissue plasminogen activator: a science advisory from the American Heart Association/American Stroke Association. Stroke 40:2945, 2009

Easton JD et al: Definition and evaluation of transient ischemic attack. Stroke 40: 2276, 2009

Goldstein LB et al: Primary prevention of ischemic stroke. Stroke 37:1583, 2006

Morgenstern LB et al: Guidelines for the management of spontaneous intracerebral hemorrhage. Stroke 42:e23, 2011

CHAPTER 371 Dementia

William W. Seeley
Bruce L. Miller

Dementia, a syndrome with many causes, affects >4 million Americans and results in a total health care cost of >$100 billion annually. It is defined as an acquired deterioration in cognitive abilities that impairs the successful performance of activities of daily living. Memory is the most common cognitive ability lost with dementia; 10% of persons >70 and 20–40% of individuals >85 have clinically identifiable memory loss. In addition to memory, other mental faculties may be affected; these include language, visuospatial ability, calculation, judgment, and problem solving. Neuropsychiatric and social deficits also arise in many dementia syndromes, resulting in depression, apathy, hallucinations, delusions, agitation, insomnia, and disinhibition. The most common forms of dementia are progressive, but some are static and unchanging or fluctuate from day to day or even minute to minute. Most patients with Alzheimer's disease (AD), the most prevalent form of dementia, begin with memory impairment, although in other dementias, such as frontotemporal dementia, memory loss is not a presenting feature. Focal cerebral disorders are discussed in Chap. 26 and illustrated in a video library in Chap. e10; memory loss is discussed in Chap. e9.

FUNCTIONAL ANATOMY OF THE DEMENTIAS

Dementia syndromes result from the disruption of specific large-scale neuronal networks; the location and severity of synaptic and neuronal loss combine to produce the clinical features (Chap. 26). Behavior and mood are modulated by noradrenergic, serotonergic, and dopaminergic pathways, whereas cholinergic signaling is critical for attention and memory functions. The dementias differ in the relative neurotransmitter deficit profiles; accordingly, accurate diagnosis guides effective pharmacotherapy.

AD begins in the transentorhinal region, spreads to the hippocampus, and then moves to lateral and posterior temporal and parietal neocortex, eventually causing a more widespread degeneration. *Vascular dementia* is associated with focal damage in a random patchwork of cortical and subcortical regions or white matter tracts that disconnect nodes within distributed networks. In keeping with the anatomy, AD typically presents with memory loss accompanied later by aphasia or navigational problems. In contrast, patients with dementias that begin in frontal or subcortical regions such as *frontotemporal dementia* (FTD) or *Huntington's disease* (HD) are less likely to begin with memory problems and more likely to have difficulties with judgment, mood, and behavior.

Lesions of cortical-striatal pathways produce specific effects on behavior. The dorsolateral prefrontal cortex bears connections with a central band of the caudate. Lesions of either node or connecting white matter pathways result in poor organization and planning, decreased cognitive flexibility, and impaired working memory. The lateral orbital frontal cortex connects with the ventromedial caudate. Lesions of this system cause impulsiveness, distractibility, and disinhibition. The anterior cingulate cortex projects to the nucleus accumbens, and interruption of these connections produces apathy, poverty of speech, or even akinetic mutism. All corticostriatal systems also include topographically organized projections through the pallidum and thalamus, and damage to these nodes can likewise reproduce the clinical syndrome of corticostriatal damage.

THE CAUSES OF DEMENTIA

The single strongest risk factor for dementia is increasing age. The prevalence of disabling memory loss increases with each decade over age 50 and is usually associated with the microscopic changes of AD at autopsy. Yet some centenarians have intact memory function and no evidence of clinically significant dementia. Whether dementia is an inevitable consequence of normal human aging remains controversial.

The many causes of dementia are listed in Table 371-1. The frequency of each condition depends on the age group under study, the access of the group to medical care, the country of origin, and perhaps racial or ethnic background. AD is the most common cause of dementia in Western countries, accounting for more than half of all patients. Vascular disease is considered the second most frequent cause for dementia and is particularly common in elderly patients or populations with limited access to medical care, where vascular risk factors are undertreated. Often, vascular disease is mixed with other neurodegenerative disorders, making it difficult, even for the neuropathologist, to estimate the contribution of cerebrovascular disease to the cognitive disorder in an individual patient. Dementias related to Parkinson's disease (PD) are extremely common, and temporally can follow a parkinsonian disorder as seen with PD-related dementia (PDD) or can occur concurrently with or preceding the motor syndrome as with dementia with Lewy bodies (DLB). In patients under the age of 65, FTD rivals AD as the most common cause of dementia. Chronic intoxications, including those resulting from alcohol and prescription drugs, are an important and often treatable cause of dementia. Other disorders listed in the table are uncommon but important because many are reversible. The classification of dementing illnesses into reversible and irreversible disorders is a useful approach to differential diagnosis. When effective treatments for the neurodegenerative conditions emerge, this dichotomy will become obsolete.

In a study of 1000 persons attending a memory disorders clinic, 19% had a potentially reversible cause of the cognitive impairment and 23% had a potentially reversible concomitant condition. The three most common potentially reversible diagnoses were depression, hydrocephalus, and alcohol dependence (Table 371-1).

Subtle cumulative decline in episodic memory is a natural part of aging. This frustrating experience, often the source of jokes and humor, is referred to as *benign forgetfulness of the elderly. Benign* means that it is not so progressive or serious that it impairs reasonably successful and productive daily functioning, although the distinction between benign and more significant memory loss can be difficult to make. At age 85, the average person is able to learn and recall approximately one-half the number of items (e.g., words on a list) that he or she could at age 18. A measurable cognitive problem that does not disrupt daily activities is often referred to as *mild cognitive impairment* (MCI). Factors that predict progression from MCI to AD include a prominent memory deficit, family history of dementia, presence of an apolipoprotein ε4 (Apo ε4) allele, small hippocampal volumes, and AD-like signature of cortical atrophy, low cerebrospinal fluid Aβ and elevated tau or positive amyloid imaging with Pittsburgh Compound-B (PiB), although the latter remains an experimental approach not yet available for routine clinical use.

The major degenerative dementias include AD, DLB, FTD and related disorders, HD, and prion diseases, including Creutzfeldt-Jakob disease (CJD). These disorders are all associated with the abnormal aggregation of a specific protein: $A\beta_{42}$ and tau in AD;

TABLE 371-1 Differential Diagnosis of Dementia

Most Common Causes of Dementia	
Alzheimer's disease	Alcoholism[a]
Vascular dementia	Parkinson's disease
Multi-infarct	Drug/medication intoxication[a]
Diffuse white matter disease (Binswanger's)	
Less Common Causes of Dementia	
Vitamin deficiencies	Toxic disorders
Thiamine (B_1): Wernicke's encephalopathy[a]	Drug, medication, and narcotic poisoning[a]
B_{12} (subacute combined degeneration)[a]	Heavy metal intoxication[a]
Nicotinic acid (pellagra)[a]	Dialysis dementia (aluminum)
Endocrine and other organ failure	Organic toxins
Hypothyroidism[a]	Psychiatric
Adrenal insufficiency and Cushing's syndrome[a]	Depression (pseudodementia)[a]
Hypo- and hyperparathyroidism[a]	Schizophrenia[a]
Renal failure[a]	Conversion reaction[a]
Liver failure[a]	Degenerative disorders
Pulmonary failure[a]	Huntington's disease
Chronic infections	Dementia with Lewy bodies
HIV	Progressive supranuclear palsy
Neurosyphilis[a]	Multisystem atrophy
Papovavirus (JC virus) (progressive multifocal leukoencephalopathy)	Hereditary ataxias (some forms)
Tuberculosis, fungal, and protozoal[a]	Motor neuron disease [amyotrophic lateral sclerosis (ALS); some forms]
Whipple's disease[a]	Frontotemporal dementia
Head trauma and diffuse brain damage	Corticobasal degeneration
Dementia pugilistica	Multiple sclerosis
Chronic subdural hematoma[a]	Adult Down syndrome with Alzheimer's disease
Postanoxia	ALS Parkinson's dementia complex of Guam
Postencephalitis	Prion (Creutzfeldt-Jakob and Gerstmann-Sträussler-Scheinker diseases)
Normal-pressure hydrocephalus[a]	Miscellaneous
Neoplastic	Sarcoidosis[a]
Primary brain tumor[a]	Vasculitis[a]
Metastatic brain tumor[a]	CADASIL, etc.
Paraneoplastic limbic encephalitis	Acute intermittent porphyria[a]
	Recurrent nonconvulsive seizures[a]
	Additional conditions in children or adolescents
	Pantothenate kinase-associated neurodegeneration
	Subacute sclerosing panencephalitis
	Metabolic disorders (e.g., Wilson's and Leigh's diseases, leukodystrophies, lipid storage diseases, mitochondrial mutations)

[a]Potentially reversible dementia.

Abbreviation: CADASIL, Cerebral autosomal dominant arteriopathy with subcortical infarcts and leukoencephalopathy.

α-synuclein in DLB; tau, TAR DNA-binding protein of 43kDa (TDP-43), or *fu*sed in *s*arcoma (FUS) in FTD; huntingtin in HD; and misfolded prion protein (PrP^{sc}) in CJD (Table 371-2).

APPROACH TO THE PATIENT: Dementias

Three major issues should be kept at the forefront: (1) What is the most accurate diagnosis? (2) Is there a treatable or reversible component to the dementia? (3) Can the physician help to alleviate the burden on caregivers? A broad overview of the approach to dementia is shown in Table 371-3. The major degenerative dementias can usually be distinguished by the initial symptoms; neuropsychological, neuropsychiatric, and neurologic findings; and neuroimaging features (Table 371-4).

HISTORY The history should concentrate on the onset, duration, and tempo of progression. An acute or subacute onset of confusion may represent delirium and should trigger the search for intoxication, infection, or metabolic derangement. An elderly person with slowly progressive memory loss over several years is likely to suffer from AD. Nearly 75% of patients with AD begin with memory symptoms, but other early symptoms include difficulty with managing money, driving, shopping, following instructions, finding words, or navigating. A personality change, disinhibition, and weight gain or compulsive eating suggest FTD, not AD. FTD is also suggested by prominent apathy, compulsivity, or progressive loss of speech fluency or word comprehension, and by a relative sparing of memory or visuospatial abilities. The diagnosis of DLB is suggested by early visual hallucinations; parkinsonism; brittle proneness to delirium or sensitivity to psychoactive medications; REM behavior disorder (RBD, the loss of skeletal muscle paralysis during dreaming); or Capgras' syndrome, the delusion that a familiar person has been replaced by an impostor.

A history of stroke with irregular stepwise progression suggests vascular dementia. Vascular dementia is also commonly seen in the setting of hypertension, atrial fibrillation, peripheral vascular disease, and diabetes. In patients suffering from cerebrovascular disease, it can be difficult to determine whether the dementia is due to AD, vascular disease, or a mixture of the two as many of the risk factors for vascular dementia, including diabetes, high cholesterol, elevated homocysteine, and low exercise, are also risk factors for AD. Rapid progression with motor rigidity and myoclonus suggests CJD. Seizures may indicate strokes or neoplasm but also occur in AD, particularly early age of onset AD. Gait disturbance is common in vascular dementia, PD/DLB, or normal-pressure hydrocephalus (NPH). A prior history of high-risk sexual behaviors or intravenous drug use should trigger a search for central nervous system (CNS) infection, especially for HIV or syphilis. A history of recurrent head trauma could indicate chronic subdural hematoma, dementia pugilistica, or NPH. Subacute onset of severe amnesia and psychosis with mesial temporal T2 hyperintensities on MRI should raise concern for paraneoplastic limbic encephalitis, especially in a long-term smoker or other patients at risk for cancer. Related nonparaneoplastic autoimmune conditions can present with a similar tempo and imaging signature. Alcoholism creates risk for malnutrition and thiamine deficiency. Veganism, bowel irradiation, an autoimmune diathesis, or a remote history of gastric surgery can result in B_{12} deficiency. Certain occupations, such as working in a battery or chemical factory, might indicate heavy metal intoxication. Careful review of medication intake, especially for sedatives and analgesics, may raise the issue of chronic drug intoxication. An autosomal dominant family

TABLE 371-2 The Molecular Basis for Degenerative Dementia

Dementia	Molecular Basis	Causal Genes and (Chromosome)	Susceptibility Genes	Pathology
AD	Aβ	<2% carry these mutations. *APP* (21), *PS-1* (14), *PS-2* (1) (most mutations are in *PS-1*)	*Apo ε4* (19)	Amyloid plaques, neurofibrillary tangles
FTD	Tau	Tau exon and intron mutations (17) (about 10% of familial cases) Progranulin (17) (10% of familial cases)	H1 tau haplotypes	Tau inclusions, Pick bodies, neurofibrillary tangles
	TDP-43 FUS			TDP-43 inclusions FUS inclusions
DLB	α-synuclein	Very rare α-synuclein (4) (dominant)	Unknown	α-synuclein inclusions (Lewy bodies)
CJD	PrP^{SC} proteins	Prion (20) (up to 15% of cases carry these dominant mutations)	Codon 129 homozygosity for methionine or valine	Tau inclusions, spongiform changes, gliosis

Abbreviations: AD, Alzheimer's disease; CJD, Creutzfeldt-Jakob disease; DLB, dementia with Lewy bodies; FTD, frontotemporal dementia.

TABLE 371-3 Evaluation of the Patient With Dementia

Routine Evaluation	Optional Focused Tests	Occasionally Helpful Tests
History	Psychometric testing	EEG
Physical examination	Chest x-ray	Parathyroid function
Laboratory tests	Lumbar puncture	Adrenal function
Thyroid function (TSH)	Liver function	Urine heavy metals
Vitamin B_{12}	Renal function	RBC sedimentation rate
Complete blood count	Urine toxin screen	Angiogram
Electrolytes	HIV	Brain biopsy
CT/MRI	Apolipoprotein E	SPECT
	RPR or VDRL	PET
Diagnostic Categories		
Reversible Causes	**Irreversible/Degenerative Dementias**	**Psychiatric Disorders**
Examples	Examples	Depression
Hypothyroidism	Alzheimer's	Schizophrenia
Thiamine deficiency	Frontotemporal dementia	Conversion reaction
Vitamin B_{12} deficiency	Huntington's	
Normal-pressure hydrocephalus	Dementia with Lewy bodies	
Subdural hematoma	Vascular	
Chronic infection	Leukoencephalopathies	
Brain tumor	Parkinson's	
Drug intoxication		
	Associated Treatable Conditions	
	Depression	Agitation
	Seizures	Caregiver "burnout"
	Insomnia	Drug side effects

Abbreviations: PET, positron emission tomography; RPR, rapid plasma reagin (test); SPECT, single-photon emission CT; VDRL, Venereal Disease Research Laboratory (test for syphilis).

TABLE 371-4 Clinical Differentiation of the Major Dementias

Disease	First Symptom	Mental Status	Neuropsychiatry	Neurology	Imaging
AD	Memory loss	Episodic memory loss	Initially normal	Initially normal	Entorhinal cortex and hippocampal atrophy
FTD	Apathy; poor judgment/insight, speech/language; hyperorality	Frontal/executive, language; spares drawing	Apathy, disinhibition, hyperorality, euphoria, depression	May have vertical gaze palsy, axial rigidity, dystonia, alien hand, or MND	Frontal, insular, and/or temporal atrophy; spares posterior parietal lobe
DLB	Visual hallucinations, REM sleep disorder, delirium, Capgras' syndrome, parkinsonism	Drawing and frontal/executive; spares memory; delirium prone	Visual hallucinations, depression, sleep disorder, delusions	Parkinsonism	Posterior parietal atrophy; hippocampi larger than in AD
CJD	Dementia, mood, anxiety, movement disorders	Variable, frontal/executive, focal cortical, memory	Depression, anxiety	Myoclonus, rigidity, parkinsonism	Cortical ribboning and basal ganglia or thalamus hyperintensity on diffusion/FLAIR MRI
Vascular	Often but not always sudden; variable; apathy, falls, focal weakness	Frontal/executive, cognitive slowing; can spare memory	Apathy, delusions, anxiety	Usually motor slowing, spasticity; can be normal	Cortical and/or subcortical infarctions, confluent white matter disease

Abbreviations: AD, Alzheimer's disease; CBD, cortical basal degeneration; CJD, Creutzfeldt-Jakob disease; DLB, dementia with Lewy bodies; FTD, frontotemporal dementia; MND, motor neuron disease; PSP, progressive supranuclear palsy.

history is found in HD and in familial forms of AD, FTD, DLB, or prion disorders. The recent death of a loved one, or depressive signs such as insomnia or weight loss, raises the possibility of depression-related cognitive impairments.

PHYSICAL AND NEUROLOGIC EXAMINATION A thorough general and neurologic examination is essential to document dementia, to look for other signs of nervous system involvement, and to search for clues suggesting a systemic disease that might be responsible for the cognitive disorder. Typical AD does not affect motor systems until later in the course. In contrast, FTD patients often develop axial rigidity, supranuclear gaze palsy, or a motor neuron disease reminiscent of amyotrophic lateral sclerosis (ALS). In DLB, the initial symptoms may include the new onset of a parkinsonian syndrome (resting tremor, cogwheel rigidity, bradykinesia, festinating gait) but often starts with visual hallucinations or dementia. Symptoms referable to the lower brainstem (RBD, gastrointestinal or autonomic problems) may arise years before parkinsonism or dementia. Corticobasal syndrome (CBS) features asymmetric akinesia and rigidity, dystonia, myoclonus, alien limb phenomena, and pyramidal or cortical sensory deficits. Associated cognitive features include nonfluent aphasia with or without motor speech impairment, executive dysfunction, apraxia, or a behavioral disorder. Progressive supranuclear palsy (PSP) is associated with unexplained falls, axial rigidity, dysphagia, and vertical gaze deficits. CJD is suggested by the presence of diffuse rigidity, an akinetic-mute state, and prominent, often startle-sensitive myoclonus.

Hemiparesis or other focal neurologic deficits suggest vascular dementia or brain tumor. Dementia with a myelopathy and peripheral neuropathy suggests vitamin B_{12} deficiency. Peripheral neuropathy could also indicate another vitamin deficiency, heavy metal intoxication, thyroid dysfunction, Lyme disease, or vasculitis. Dry, cool skin, hair loss, and bradycardia suggest hypothyroidism. Fluctuating confusion associated with repetitive stereotyped movements may indicate ongoing limbic, temporal, or frontal seizures. Hearing impairment or visual loss may produce confusion and disorientation misinterpreted as dementia. Such sensory deficits are common in the elderly but can be a manifestation of mitochondrial disorders.

COGNITIVE AND NEUROPSYCHIATRIC EXAMINATION Brief screening tools such as the mini-mental status examination (MMSE) help to confirm the presence of cognitive impairment and to follow the progression of dementia (Table 371-5). The MMSE,

TABLE 371-5 The Mini-Mental Status Examination

	Points
Orientation	
Name: season/date/day/month/year	5 (1 for each name)
Name: hospital/floor/town/state/country	5 (1 for each name)
Registration	
Identify three objects by name and ask patient to repeat	3 (1 for each object)
Attention and calculation	
Serial 7s; subtract from 100 (e.g., 93–86–79–72–65)	5 (1 for each subtraction)
Recall	
Recall the three objects presented earlier	3 (1 for each object)
Language	
Name pencil and watch	2 (1 for each object)
Repeat "No ifs, ands, or buts"	1
Follow a 3-step command (e.g., "Take this paper, fold it in half, and place it on the table")	3 (1 for each command)
Write "close your eyes" and ask patient to obey written command	1
Ask patient to write a sentence	1
Ask patient to copy a design (e.g., intersecting pentagons)	1
Total	30

a simple 30-point test of cognitive function, contains tests of orientation, working memory (e.g., spell *world* backwards), episodic memory (orientation and 3-word recall), language comprehension, naming, and figure copying. In most patients with MCI and some with clinically apparent AD, the MMSE may be normal and a more rigorous set of neuropsychological tests will be required. When the etiology for the dementia syndrome remains in doubt, a specially tailored evaluation should be performed that includes tasks of working and episodic memory, executive function, language, and visuospatial and perceptual abilities. In AD the early deficits involve episodic memory, category generation ("name as many animals as you can in one minute"), and visuoconstructive ability. Usually deficits in verbal or visual episodic memory are the first neuropsychological abnormalities detected, and tasks that require the patient to recall a long list of words or a series of pictures after a predetermined delay will demonstrate deficits in most patients. In FTD, the earliest deficits on cognitive testing involve executive or language (speech or naming) function. DLB patients have more severe deficits in visuospatial function but do better on episodic memory tasks than patients with AD. Patients with vascular dementia often demonstrate a mixture of executive and visuospatial deficits, with prominent psychomotor slowing. In delirium, the most prominent deficits involve attention, working memory, and executive function, making the assessment of other cognitive domains challenging and often uninformative.

A functional assessment should also be performed. The physician should determine the day-to-day impact of the disorder on the patient's memory, community affairs, hobbies, judgment, dressing, and eating. Knowledge of the patient's day-to-day function will help the clinician and the family to organize a therapeutic approach.

Neuropsychiatric assessment is important for diagnosis, prognosis, and treatment. In the early stages of AD, mild depressive features, social withdrawal, and irritability or anxiety are the most prominent psychiatric changes, but patients often maintain core social skills into the middle or late stages, when delusions, agitation, and sleep disturbance may emerge. In FTD, dramatic personality change featuring apathy, overeating, compulsions, disinhibition, euphoria, and loss of empathy are early and common. DLB is associated with visual hallucinations, delusions related to person or place identity, RBD, and excessive daytime sleepiness. Dramatic fluctuations occur not only in cognition but also in primary arousal, such that caregivers may seek emergency room evaluation for suspected stroke. Vascular dementia can present with psychiatric symptoms such as depression, anxiety, delusions, disinhibition, or apathy.

LABORATORY TESTS The choice of laboratory tests in the evaluation of dementia is complex. The physician must take measures to avoid missing a reversible or treatable cause, yet no single treatable etiology is common; thus, a screen must employ multiple tests, each of which has a low yield. Cost/benefit ratios are difficult to assess, and many laboratory screening algorithms for dementia discourage multiple tests. Nevertheless, even a test with only a 1–2% positive rate is probably worth undertaking if the alternative is missing a treatable cause of dementia. Table 371-3 lists most screening tests for dementia. The American Academy of Neurology recommends the routine measurement of thyroid function, a vitamin B_{12} level, and a neuroimaging study (CT or MRI).

Neuroimaging studies help to rule out primary and metastatic neoplasms, locate areas of infarction, detect subdural hematomas, and suggest NPH or diffuse white matter disease. They also help to establish a regional pattern of atrophy. Support for the diagnosis of AD includes hippocampal atrophy in addition to posterior-predominant cortical atrophy. Focal frontal and/or anterior temporal atrophy suggests FTD. DLB often features less prominent atrophy, with greater involvement of amygdala than hippocampus. In CJD, MR diffusion-weighted imaging reveals abnormalities in the cortical ribbon and basal ganglia in the majority of patients. Extensive white matter abnormalities correlate with a vascular etiology for dementia. The role of functional-metabolic imaging in the diagnosis of dementia is still under study, although the Federal Drug Administration has approved the use of positron emission tomography (PET) in dementia differential diagnosis. Single-photon emission computed tomography (SPECT) and PET scanning show temporal-parietal hypoperfusion or hypometabolism in AD and frontotemporal deficits in FTD, but these changes often reflect atrophy and can therefore be detected with MRI alone in many patients. Recently, amyloid imaging has shown promise for the diagnosis of AD, and Pittsburgh Compound-B (PiB) and ^{18}F-AV-45 appear to be reliable radioligands for detecting brain amyloid associated with amyloid angiopathy or neuritic plaques (Fig. 371-1). Because these abnormalities can be seen in cognitively normal older persons, however, amyloid imaging may detect preclinical or incidental AD in patients lacking an AD-like dementia syndrome. Once powerful disease-modifying therapies become

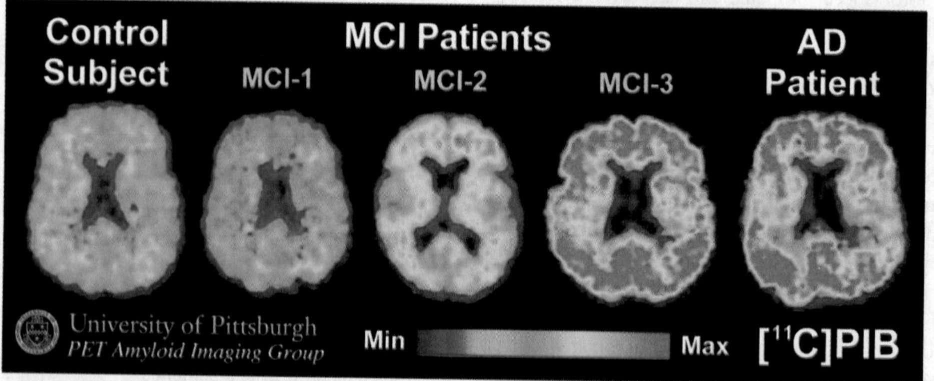

Figure 371-1 PET images obtained with the amyloid-imaging agent Pittsburgh Compound-B ([^{11}C]PIB) in a normal control (*left*); three different patients with mild cognitive impairment (MCI, *center*); and a mild AD patient (*right*). Some MCI patients have control-like levels of amyloid, some have AD-like levels of amyloid, and some have intermediate levels. AD, Alzheimer's disease; MCI, mild cognitive impairment; PET, positron emission tomography.

available, use of these biomarkers may help to identify treatment candidates before irreversible brain injury has occurred. In the meantime, however, the significance of detecting brain amyloid in an asymptomatic elder remains a topic of vigorous investigation. Similarly, MRI perfusion and functional connectivity methods are being explored as potential treatment-monitoring strategies.

Lumbar puncture need not be done routinely in the evaluation of dementia, but it is indicated when CNS infection or inflammation are credible diagnostic possibilities. Cerebrospinal fluid (CSF) levels of tau protein and Aβ_{42} show differing patterns with the various dementias; however, the sensitivity and specificity of these measures are not yet sufficiently high to warrant routine use. Formal psychometric testing, although not necessary in every patient with dementia, helps to document the severity of cognitive disturbance, suggest psychogenic causes, and provide a more formal method for following the disease course. Electroencephalogram (EEG) is rarely helpful except to suggest CJD (repetitive bursts of diffuse high-amplitude sharp waves, or "periodic complexes") or an underlying nonconvulsive seizure disorder (epileptiform discharges). Brain biopsy (including meninges) is not advised except to diagnose vasculitis, potentially treatable neoplasms, or unusual infections when the diagnosis is uncertain. Systemic disorders with CNS manifestations, such as sarcoidosis, can usually be confirmed through biopsy of lymph node or solid organ rather than brain. Angiography should be considered when cerebral vasculitis or cerebral venous thrombosis is a possible cause of the dementia.

ALZHEIMER'S DISEASE

Approximately 10% of all persons over the age of 70 have significant memory loss, and in more than half the cause is AD. It is estimated that the annual total cost of caring for a single AD patient in an advanced stage of the disease is >$50,000. The disease also exacts a heavy emotional toll on family members and caregivers. AD can occur in any decade of adulthood, but it is the most common cause of dementia in the elderly. AD most often presents with an insidious onset of memory loss followed by a slowly progressive dementia over several years. Pathologically, atrophy is distributed throughout the medial temporal lobes, as well as lateral and medial parietal lobes and lateral frontal cortex. Microscopically, there are neuritic plaques containing Aβ, neurofibrillary tangles (NFTs) composed of hyperphosphorylated tau filaments, and accumulation of amyloid in blood vessel walls in cortex and leptomeninges (see "Pathology," below). The identification of four different susceptibility genes for AD has provided a foundation for rapid progress in understanding the biologic basis of the disorder.

CLINICAL MANIFESTATIONS

The cognitive changes of AD tend to follow a characteristic pattern, beginning with memory impairment and spreading to language and visuospatial deficits. Yet, approximately 20% of patients with AD present with nonmemory complaints such as word-finding, organizational, or navigational difficulty. In the early stages of the disease, the memory loss may go unrecognized or be ascribed to benign forgetfulness. Once the memory loss becomes noticeable to the patient and spouse and falls 1.5 standard deviations below normal on standardized memory tests, the term MCI is applied. This construct provides useful prognostic information, because approximately 50% of patients with MCI (roughly 12% per year) will progress to AD over 4 years. Slowly the cognitive problems begin to interfere with daily activities, such as keeping track of finances, following instructions on the job, driving, shopping, and housekeeping. Some patients are unaware of these difficulties (*anosognosia*), while others remain acutely attuned to their deficits. Changes in environment (such as vacations or hospital stays) may be disorienting, and the patient may become lost on walks or while driving. In the middle stages of AD, the patient is unable to work, is easily lost and confused, and requires daily supervision. Social graces, routine behavior, and superficial conversation may be surprisingly intact. Language becomes impaired—first naming, then comprehension, and finally fluency. In some patients, *aphasia* is an early and prominent feature. Word-finding difficulties and circumlocution may be a problem even when formal testing demonstrates intact naming and fluency. *Apraxia* emerges, and patients have trouble performing learned sequential motor tasks. Visuospatial deficits begin to interfere with dressing, eating, or even walking, and patients fail to solve simple puzzles or copy geometric figures. Simple calculations and clock reading become difficult in parallel.

In the late stages of the disease, some persons remain ambulatory but wander aimlessly. Loss of judgment and reasoning is inevitable. Delusions are common and usually simple, with common themes of theft, infidelity, or misidentification. Approximately 10% of AD patients develop *Capgras' syndrome*, believing that a caregiver has been replaced by an impostor. In contrast to DLB, where Capgras' syndrome is an early feature, in AD this syndrome emerges later. Loss of inhibitions and aggression may occur and alternate with passivity and withdrawal. Sleep-wake patterns are disrupted, and nighttime wandering becomes disturbing to the household. Some patients develop a shuffling gait with generalized muscle rigidity associated with slowness and awkwardness of movement. Patients often look parkinsonian (Chap. 372) but rarely have a high-amplitude, rhythmic, resting tremor. In end-stage AD, patients become rigid, mute, incontinent, and bedridden. Help is needed with eating, dressing, and toileting. Hyperactive tendon reflexes and myoclonic jerks (sudden brief contractions of various muscles or the whole body) may occur spontaneously or in response to physical or auditory stimulation. Generalized seizures may also occur. Often death results from malnutrition, secondary infections, pulmonary emboli, heart disease, or, most commonly, aspiration. The typical duration of AD is 8–10 years, but the course can range from 1 to 25 years. For unknown reasons, some AD patients show a steady decline in function, while others have prolonged plateaus without major deterioration.

DIFFERENTIAL DIAGNOSIS

Early in the disease course, other etiologies of dementia should be excluded (Table 371-1). Neuroimaging studies (CT and MRI) do not show a single specific pattern with AD and may be normal early in the course of the disease. As AD progresses, more distributed but usually posterior-predominant cortical atrophy becomes apparent, along with atrophy of the medial temporal memory structures (Fig. 371-2*A*, *B*). The main purpose of imaging is to exclude other disorders, such as primary and secondary neoplasms, vascular dementia, diffuse white matter disease, and NPH; it also helps to distinguish AD from other degenerative disorders with distinctive imaging patterns such as FTD or CJD. Functional imaging studies in AD reveal hypoperfusion or hypometabolism in the posterior temporal-parietal cortex (Fig. 371-2*C*,*D*). The EEG in AD is normal or shows nonspecific slowing. Routine spinal fluid examination is also normal. CSF Aβ_{42} levels are reduced, whereas levels of hyperphosphorylated tau protein are elevated, but the considerable overlap of these levels with those of the normal aged population limits the usefulness of these measurements in diagnosis. The use of blood ApoE genotyping is discussed under "Pathology," below. *Slowly progressive decline in memory and orientation, normal results on laboratory tests, and an MRI or CT scan showing only distributed or posteriorly predominant cortical and hippocampal atrophy is highly suggestive of AD.* A clinical diagnosis of AD reached after

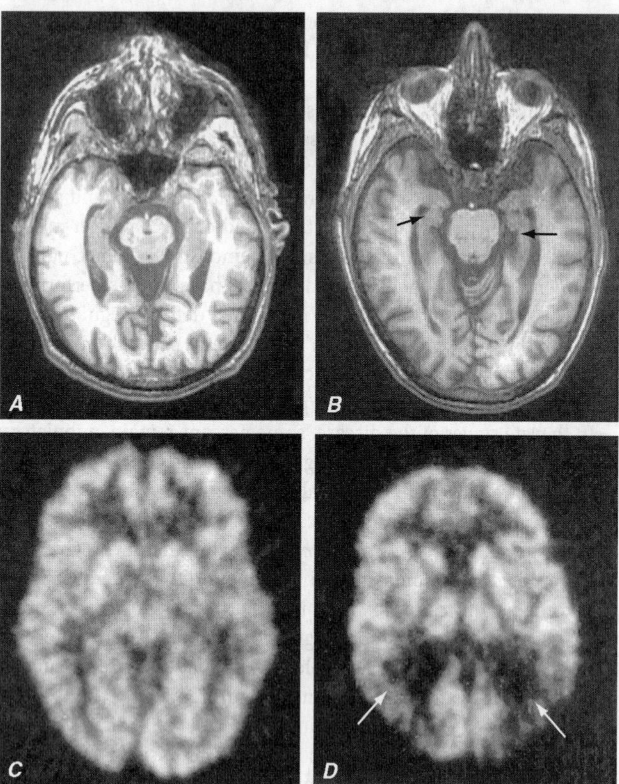

Figure 371-2 Alzheimer's disease. Axial T1-weighted MR images through the midbrain of a normal 86-year-old athlete (***A***) and a 77-year-old man with AD (***B***). Note that both individuals have mild sulcal widening and slight dilation of the temporal horns of the lateral ventricles. However, there is a reduction in hippocampal volume in the patient with AD (*arrows*) compared with the volume of the normal-for-age hippocampus (***A***). Fluorodeoxyglucose PET scans of a normal control (***C***) and a patient with AD (***D***). Note that the patient with AD shows decreased glucose metabolism in the posterior temporoparietal regions bilaterally (*arrows*), a typical finding in this condition. AD, Alzheimer's disease; PET, positron emission tomography. *(Images courtesy of TF Budinger, University of California.)*

careful evaluation is confirmed at autopsy about 90% of the time, with misdiagnosed cases usually representing one of the other dementing disorders described later in this chapter, a mixture of AD with vascular pathology, or DLB.

Simple clinical clues are useful in the differential diagnosis. Early prominent gait disturbance with only mild memory loss suggests vascular dementia or, rarely, NPH (see below). Resting tremor with stooped posture, bradykinesia, and masked facies suggest PD (Chap. 372). When dementia occurs after a well-established diagnosis of PD, PDD is usually the correct diagnosis. The early appearance of parkinsonian features in association with fluctuating alertness, visual hallucinations, or delusional misidentification suggests DLB. Chronic alcoholism should prompt the search for vitamin deficiency. Loss of sensibility to position and vibration stimuli accompanied by Babinski responses suggests vitamin B_{12} deficiency (Chap. 377). Early onset of a focal seizure suggests a metastatic or primary brain neoplasm (Chap. 379). Previous or ongoing depression raises suspicion for depression-related cognitive impairment, although AD can feature a depressive prodrome. A history of treatment for insomnia, anxiety, psychiatric disturbance, or epilepsy suggests chronic drug intoxication. Rapid progression over a few weeks or months associated with rigidity and myoclonus suggests CJD (Chap. 383). Prominent behavioral changes with intact navigation and focal anterior-predominant atrophy on brain imaging are typical of FTD. A positive family history of dementia suggests either one of the familial forms of AD or one of the other genetic disorders associated with dementia, such as HD (see below), FTD (see below), prion disease (Chap. 383), or rare hereditary ataxias (Chap. 373).

EPIDEMIOLOGY

The most important risk factors for AD are old age and a positive family history. The frequency of AD increases with each decade of adult life, reaching 20–40% of the population over the age of 85. A positive family history of dementia suggests a genetic cause of AD, although autosomal dominant inheritance occurs in only 2% of patients with AD. Female sex may also be a risk factor independent of the greater longevity of women. Some AD patients have a past history of head trauma with concussion. AD is more common in groups with low educational attainment, but education influences test-taking ability, and it is clear that AD can affect persons of all intellectual levels. One study found that the capacity to express complex written language in early adulthood correlated with a decreased risk for AD. Numerous environmental factors, including aluminum, mercury, and viruses, have been proposed as causes of AD, but none has been demonstrated to play a significant role. Similarly, several studies suggest that the use of nonsteroidal anti-inflammatory agents is associated with a decreased risk of AD, but this has not been confirmed in large prospective studies. Vascular disease, and stroke in particular, seems to lower the threshold for the clinical expression of AD. Also, in many patients with AD, amyloid angiopathy can lead to microhemorrhages, large lobar hemorrhages, or ischemic infarctions. Diabetes increases the risk of AD threefold. Elevated homocysteine and cholesterol levels; hypertension; diminished serum levels of folic acid; low dietary intake of fruits, vegetables, and red wine; and low levels of exercise are all being explored as potential risk factors for AD.

PATHOLOGY

At autopsy, the earliest and most severe degeneration is usually found in the medial temporal lobe (entorhinal/perirhinal cortex and hippocampus), lateral temporal cortex, and nucleus basalis of Meynert. The characteristic microscopic findings are neuritic plaques and NFTs. These lesions accumulate in small numbers during normal brain aging but dominate the picture in AD. Increasing evidence suggests that soluble amyloid species called *oligomers* may cause cellular dysfunction and represent the early toxic molecule in AD. Eventually, further amyloid polymerization and fibril formation lead to neuritic plaques (Fig. 371-3), which contain a central amyloid core, proteoglycans, Apo $\varepsilon4$, α-antichymotrypsin, and other proteins. Aβ is a protein of 39–42 amino acids that is derived proteolytically from a larger transmembrane protein, *amyloid precursor protein* (APP), when APP is cleaved by β and γ secretases. The normal function of Aβ is unknown. APP has neurotrophic and neuroprotective properties. The plaque core is surrounded by a halo, which contains dystrophic, tau-immunoreactive neurites and activated microglia. The accumulation of Aβ in cerebral arterioles is termed *amyloid angiopathy*. NFTs are composed of silver-staining neuronal cytoplasmic fibrils composed of abnormally phosphorylated tau (τ) protein; they appear as paired helical filaments by electron microscopy. Tau binds to and stabilizes microtubules, supporting axonal transport of organelles, glycoproteins, neurotransmitters, and other important cargoes throughout the neuron. Once hyperphosphorylated, tau can no longer bind properly to microtubules and its functions are disrupted. Finally, patients with AD often show comorbid DLB and vascular pathology.

Biochemically, AD is associated with a decrease in the cortical levels of several proteins and neurotransmitters, especially acetylcholine, its synthetic enzyme choline acetyltransferase, and nicotinic cholinergic receptors. Reduction of acetylcholine may be

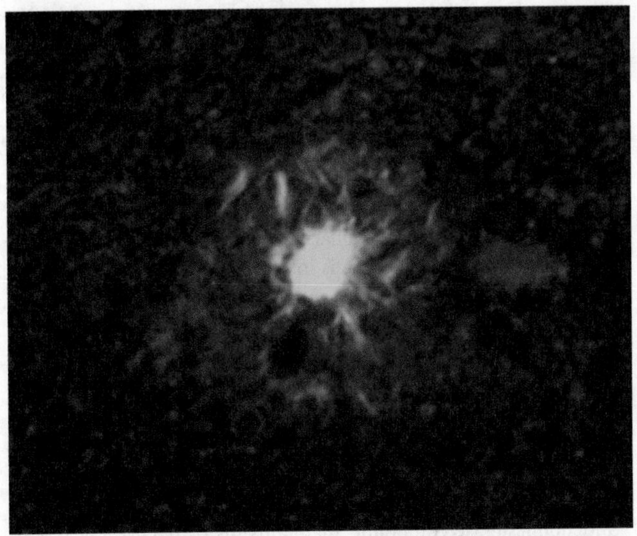

Figure 371-3 Mature neuritic plaque with a dense central amyloid core surrounded by dystrophic neurites (thioflavin S stain). *(Image courtesy of S DeArmond, University of California; with permission.)*

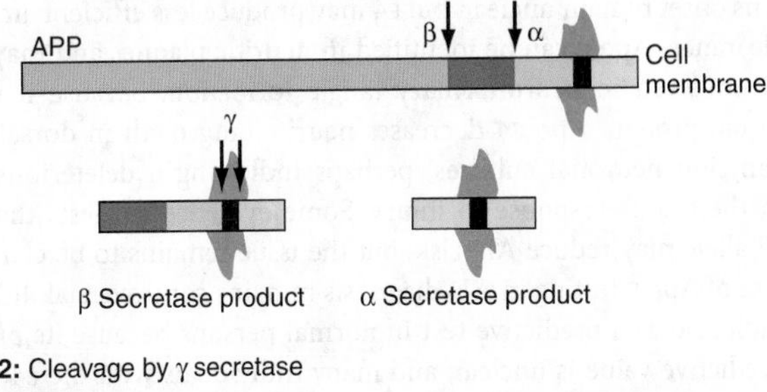

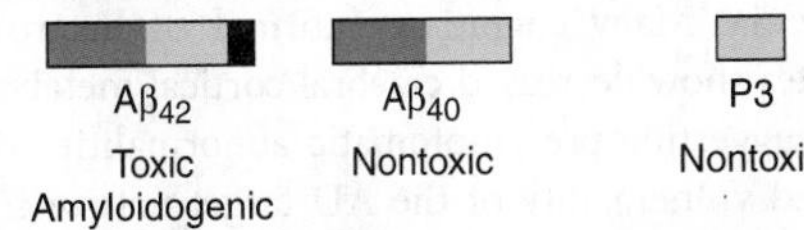

Figure 371-4 Amyloid precursor protein (APP) is catabolized by α, β, and γ secretases. A key initial step is the digestion by either β-secretase (BASE) or α secretase [ADAM10 or ADAM17 (TACE)], producing smaller non-toxic products. Cleavage of the β secretase product by γ secretase (Step 2) results in either the toxic $A\beta_{42}$ or the nontoxic $A\beta_{40}$ peptide; cleavage of the α secretase product by γ secretase produces the nontoxic P3 peptide. Excess production of $A\beta_{42}$ is a key initiator of cellular damage in Alzheimer's disease. Current AD research is focused on developing therapies designed to reduce accumulation of $A\beta_{42}$ by antagonizing β or γ secretases, promoting α secretase, or clearing $A\beta_{42}$ that has already formed by use of specific antibodies.

related in part to degeneration of cholinergic neurons in the nucleus basalis of Meynert that project throughout the cortex. There is also noradrenergic and serotonergic depletion due to degeneration of brainstem nuclei such as the locus coeruleus and dorsal raphe.

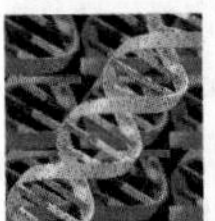

GENETIC CONSIDERATIONS

Several genes play important pathogenic roles in at least some patients with AD. One is the *APP* gene on chromosome 21. Adults with trisomy 21 (Down syndrome) consistently develop the typical neuropathologic hallmarks of AD if they survive beyond age 40. Many develop a progressive dementia superimposed on their baseline mental retardation. APP is a membrane-spanning protein that is subsequently processed into smaller units, including Aβ, which is deposited in neuritic plaques. Aβ peptide results from cleavage of APP by β and γ secretases (Fig. 371-4). Presumably, the extra dose of the *APP* gene on chromosome 21 is the initiating cause of AD in adult Down's syndrome and results in excess cerebral amyloid. Furthermore, a few families with early-onset familial Alzheimer disease (FAD) have been discovered to have point mutations in the *APP* gene. Although very rare, these families were the first examples of single-gene autosomal dominant transmission of AD.

Investigation of large families with multigenerational FAD led to the discovery of two additional AD genes, the *presenilins*. Presenilin-1 (*PS-1*) is on chromosome 14 and encodes a protein called S182. Mutations in this gene cause an early-onset AD (onset before age 60 and often before age 50) transmitted in an autosomal dominant, highly penetrant fashion. More than 100 different mutations have been found in the *PS-1* gene in families from a wide range of ethnic backgrounds. Presenilin-2 (*PS-2*) is on chromosome 1 and encodes a protein called STM2. A mutation in the *PS-2* gene was first found in a group of American families with Volga German ethnic background. Mutations in *PS-1* are much more common than those in *PS-2*. The presenilins are highly homologous and encode similar proteins that at first appeared to have seven transmembrane domains (hence the designation *STM*), but subsequent studies have suggested eight such domains, with a ninth submembrane region. Both S182 and STM2 are cytoplasmic neuronal proteins that are widely expressed throughout the nervous system. They are homologous to a cell-trafficking protein, sel 12, found in the nematode *Caenorhabditis elegans*. Patients with mutations in these genes have elevated plasma levels of $A\beta_{42}$, and *PS-1* mutations in cell cultures produce increased $A\beta_{42}$ in the media. There is evidence that *PS-1* is involved in the cleavage of APP at the gamma secretase site and mutations in either gene (*PS-1* or *APP*) may disturb this function. Mutations in *PS-1* have thus far proved to be the most common cause of early-age-of-onset FAD, representing perhaps 40–70% of this relatively rare syndrome. Mutations in *PS-1* tend to produce AD with an earlier age of onset (mean onset 45 years) and a shorter, more rapidly progressive course (mean duration 6–7 years) than the disease caused by mutations in *PS-2* (mean onset 53 years; duration 11 years). Although some carriers of uncommon *PS-2* mutations have had onset of dementia after the age of 70, mutations in the presenilins are rarely involved in the more common sporadic cases of late-onset AD occurring in the general population. Genetic testing for these uncommon mutations is now commercially available. This diagnostic avenue is likely to be revealing only in early-age-of-onset familial AD and should be performed in the context of formal genetic counseling, especially when there are asymptomatic persons at risk.

A discovery of great importance has been that the *Apo ε* gene on chromosome 19 is involved in the pathogenesis of late-onset familial and sporadic forms of AD. *Apo ε* participates in cholesterol transport (Chap. 356) and has three alleles: ε2, ε3, and ε4. The Apo ε4 allele confers increased risk of AD in the general population, including sporadic and late-age-of-onset familial forms. Approximately 24–30% of the nondemented white population has at least one ε4 allele (12–15% allele frequency), and about 2% are ε4/4 homozygotes. Among patients with AD, 40–65% have at least one ε4 allele, a highly significant difference compared with controls. Conversely, many AD patients have no ε4 allele, and ε4 carriers may never develop AD. Therefore, ε4 is neither necessary nor sufficient to cause AD. Nevertheless, the Apo ε4 allele, especially in the homozygous state, represents the most important genetic risk factor for AD and acts as a dose-dependent disease modifier, with the earliest age of onset associated with the ε4 homozygosity.

Precise mechanisms through which Apo ε4 confers AD risk or hastens onset remain unclear, but ε4 may produce less efficient amyloid clearance. Apo ε can be identified in neuritic plaques and may also be involved in neurofibrillary tangle formation, because it binds to tau protein. Apo ε4 decreases neurite outgrowth in dorsal root ganglion neuronal cultures, perhaps indicating a deleterious role in the brain's response to injury. Some evidence suggests that the ε2 allele may reduce AD risk, but the issue remains to be clarified. Use of Apo ε testing in AD diagnosis remains controversial. It is not indicated as a predictive test in normal persons because its precise predictive value is unclear, and many individuals with the ε4 allele never develop dementia. Many cognitively normal ε4 heterozygotes and homozygotes show decreased cerebral cortical metabolic function with PET, suggesting presymptomatic abnormalities due to AD or an inherited vulnerability of the AD target network. In demented persons who meet clinical criteria for AD, finding an ε4 allele increases the reliability of diagnosis however, the absence of an ε4 allele cannot be considered evidence against AD. Furthermore, all patients with dementia, including those with an ε4 allele, require a search for reversible causes of their cognitive impairment. Nevertheless, Apo ε4 remains the single most important biologic marker associated with AD risk, and studies of ε4's functional role and diagnostic utility are progressing rapidly. The ε4 allele is not associated with risk for FTD, DLB, or CJD, although some evidence suggests that ε4 may exacerbate the phenotype of non-AD degenerative disorders. Additional genes are also likely to be involved in AD, especially as minor risk alleles for sporadic forms of the disease. Recent genome-wide association studies have implicated the clusterin *(CLU)*, phosphatidylinositol-binding clathrin assembly protein *(PICALM)*, and complement component (3b/4b) receptor 1 *(CR1) genes,* and researchers are now working to understand the potential role of these genes in AD pathogenesis. CLU may play a role in synapse turnover, PICALM participates in clathrin-mediated endocytosis, and CR1 may be involved in amyloid clearance through the complement pathway.

TREATMENT Alzheimer's Disease

The management of AD is challenging and gratifying, despite the absence of a cure or a robust pharmacologic treatment. The primary focus is on long-term amelioration of associated behavioral and neurologic problems, as well as providing caregiver support.

Building rapport with the patient, family members, and other caregivers is essential to successful management. In the early stages of AD, memory aids such as notebooks and posted daily reminders can be helpful. Family members should emphasize activities that are pleasant and curtail those that are unpleasant. In other words, practicing skills that have become difficult, such as through memory games and puzzles, will often frustrate and depress the patient without proven benefits. Kitchens, bathrooms, stairways, and bedrooms need to be made safe, and eventually patients must stop driving. Loss of independence and change of environment may worsen confusion, agitation, and anger. Communication and repeated calm reassurance are necessary. Caregiver "burnout" is common, often resulting in nursing home placement of the patient or new health problems for the caregiver, and respite breaks for the caregiver help to maintain a successful long-term therapeutic milieu. Use of adult day care centers can be helpful. Local and national support groups, such as the Alzheimer's Association and the Family Caregiver Alliance, are valuable resources. Internet access to these resources has become available to clinicians and families in recent years.

Donepezil (target dose, 10 mg daily), rivastigmine (target dose, 6 mg twice daily or 9.5-mg patch daily), galantamine (target dose 24 mg daily, extended-release), memantine (target dose, 10 mg twice daily), and tacrine are the drugs presently approved by the Food and Drug Administration (FDA) for treatment of AD. Due to hepatotoxicity, tacrine is no longer used. Dose escalations for each of these medications must be carried out over 4–6 weeks to minimize side effects. The pharmacologic action of donepezil, rivastigmine, and galantamine is inhibition of the cholinesterases, primarily acetylcholinesterase, with a resulting increase in cerebral acetylcholine levels. Memantine appears to act by blocking overexcited *N*-methyl-D-aspartate (NMDA) glutamate receptors. Double-blind, placebo-controlled, crossover studies with cholinesterase inhibitors and memantine have shown them to be associated with improved caregiver ratings of patients' functioning and with an apparent decreased rate of decline in cognitive test scores over periods of up to 3 years. The average patient on an anticholinesterase compound maintains his or her MMSE score for close to a year, whereas a placebo-treated patient declines 2–3 points over the same time period. Memantine, used in conjunction with cholinesterase inhibitors or by itself, slows cognitive deterioration and decreases caregiver burden for patients with moderate to severe AD but is not approved for mild AD. Each of these compounds has only modest efficacy for AD. Cholinesterase inhibitors are relatively easy to administer, and their major side effects are gastrointestinal symptoms (nausea, diarrhea, cramps), altered sleep with unpleasant or vivid dreams, bradycardia (usually benign), and muscle cramps.

In a prospective observational study, the use of estrogen replacement therapy appeared to protect—by about 50%—against development of AD in women. This study seemed to confirm the results of two earlier case-controlled studies. Sadly, a prospective placebo-controlled study of a combined estrogen-progesterone therapy for asymptomatic postmenopausal women increased, rather than decreased, the prevalence of dementia. This study markedly dampened enthusiasm for hormonal treatments to prevent dementia. Additionally, no benefit has been found in the treatment of AD with estrogen alone.

A randomized, double-blind, placebo-controlled trial of an extract of *Ginkgo biloba* found modest improvement in cognitive function in subjects with AD and vascular dementia. Unfortunately, a comprehensive 6-year multicenter prevention study using *Ginkgo biloba* found no slowing of progression to dementia in the treated group.

Vaccination against $A\beta_{42}$ has proved highly efficacious in mouse models of AD, helping clear brain amyloid and preventing further amyloid accumulation. In human trials, this approach led to life-threatening complications, including meningoencephalitis, but modifications of the vaccine approach using passive immunization with monoclonal antibodies are currently being evaluated in phase 3 trials. Another experimental approach to AD treatment has been the use of β and γ secretase inhibitors that diminish the production of $A\beta_{42}$, but the first two placebo-controlled trials of γ secretase inhibitors, tarenflurbil and semagacestat, were negative, and semagacestat may have accelerated cognitive decline compared to placebo. Medications that modify tau phosphorylation and aggregation are beginning to be studied as possible treatments for both AD and non-AD tau-related disorders including FTD and PSP.

Several retrospective studies suggest that nonsteroidal anti-inflammatory agents and 3-hydroxy-3-methylglutaryl-coenzyme A (HMG-CoA) reductase inhibitors (statins) may have a protective effect on dementia, and controlled prospective studies are being conducted. Similarly, prospective studies with the goal of lowering serum homocysteine are underway to slow the progression to dementia, following an association of elevated homocysteine with dementia progression in epidemiologic studies. Finally, there is now a strong interest in the relationship between diabetes and AD, and insulin-regulating studies are being conducted.

Mild to moderate depression is common in the early stages of AD and may respond to antidepressants or cholinesterase inhibitors. Selective serotonin reuptake inhibitors (SSRIs) are commonly used due to their low anticholinergic side effects (escitalopram 5–10 mg daily). Generalized seizures should be treated with an appropriate anticonvulsant, such as phenytoin or carbamazepine. Agitation, insomnia, hallucinations, and belligerence are especially troublesome characteristics of some AD patients, and these behaviors can lead to nursing home placement. The newer generation of atypical antipsychotics, such as risperidone, quetiapine, and olanzapine, are being used in low doses to treat these neuropsychiatric symptoms. The few controlled studies comparing drugs against behavioral intervention in the treatment of agitation suggest mild efficacy with significant side effects related to sleep, gait, and cardiovascular complications, including an increased risk of death. All antipsychotics carry a black-box FDA warning and should be used with caution in the demented elderly however, careful, daily, nonpharmacologic behavior management is often not available, rendering medications necessary for some patients. Finally, medications with strong anticholinergic effects should be vigilantly avoided, including prescription and over-the-counter sleep aids (e.g., diphenhydramine) or incontinence therapies (e.g., oxybutynin).

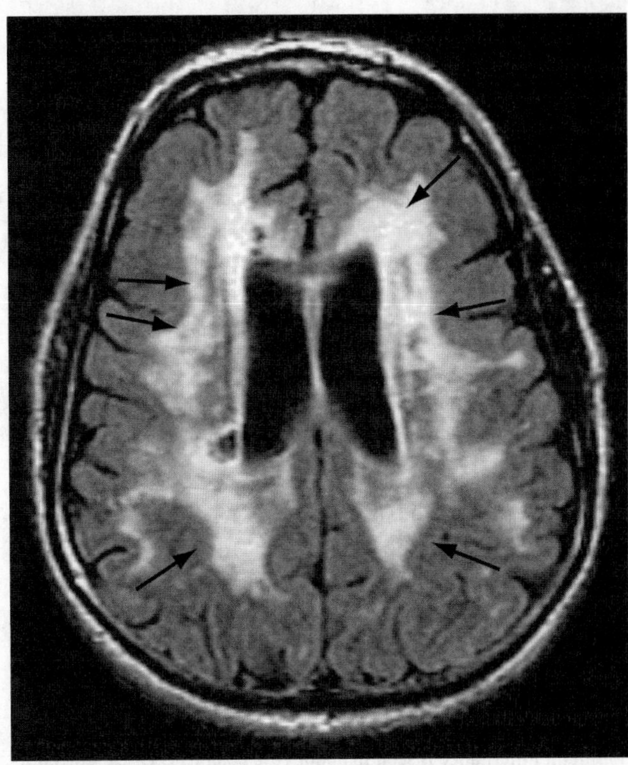

Figure 371-5 Diffuse white matter disease. Axial fluid-attenuated inversion recovery (FLAIR) MR image through the lateral ventricles reveals multiple areas of hyperintensity involving the periventricular white matter as well as the corona radiata and striatum (*arrows*). While seen in some individuals with normal cognition, this appearance is more pronounced in patients with dementia of a vascular etiology.

VASCULAR DEMENTIA

Dementia associated with cerebrovascular disease can be divided into two general categories: multi-infarct dementia and diffuse white matter disease (also called *leukoaraiosis, subcortical arteriosclerotic leukoencephalopathy,* or *Binswanger's disease*). Cerebrovascular disease appears to be a more common cause of dementia in Asia than in Europe and North America, perhaps due to the increased prevalence of intracranial atherosclerosis. Individuals who have had several strokes may develop chronic cognitive deficits, commonly called *multi-infarct dementia*. The strokes may be large or small (sometimes lacunar) and usually involve several different brain regions. The occurrence of dementia depends partly on the total volume of damaged cortex, but it is also more common in individuals with left-hemisphere lesions, independent of any language disturbance. Patients typically report previous discrete episodes of sudden neurologic deterioration. Many patients with multi-infarct dementia have a history of hypertension, diabetes, coronary artery disease, or other manifestations of widespread atherosclerosis. Physical examination usually shows focal neurologic deficits such as hemiparesis, a unilateral Babinski sign, a visual field defect, or pseudobulbar palsy. Recurrent strokes result in a stepwise disease progression. Neuroimaging reveals multiple areas of infarction. Thus, the history and neuroimaging findings differentiate this condition from AD; however, both AD and multiple infarctions are common and sometimes co-occur. With normal aging, there is also an accumulation of amyloid in cerebral blood vessels, leading to a condition called *cerebral amyloid angiopathy* (without dementia), which predisposes older persons to lobar hemorrhage and brain microhemorrhages. AD patients appear to be at increased risk for amyloid angiopathy, and this may explain some of the observed association between AD and stroke.

Some individuals with dementia are discovered on MRI to have bilateral abnormalities of subcortical white matter, termed *diffuse white matter disease*, often occurring in association with lacunar infarctions (Fig. 371-5). The dementia may be insidious in onset and progress slowly, features that distinguish it from multi-infarct dementia, but other patients show a stepwise deterioration more typical of multi-infarct dementia. Early symptoms are mild confusion, apathy, anxiety, psychosis, and memory, spatial, or executive deficits. Marked difficulties in judgment and orientation and dependence on others for daily activities develop later. Euphoria, elation, depression, or aggressive behaviors are common as the disease progresses. Both pyramidal and cerebellar signs may be present. A gait disorder is present in at least half of these patients. With advanced disease, urinary incontinence and dysarthria with or without other pseudobulbar features (e.g., dysphagia, emotional lability) are frequent. Seizures and myoclonic jerks appear in a minority of patients. This disorder appears to result from chronic ischemia due to occlusive disease of small, penetrating cerebral arteries and arterioles (microangiopathy). Any disease-causing stenosis of small cerebral vessels may be the critical underlying factor, although hypertension is the major cause. The term *Binswanger's disease* should be used with caution, because it does not clearly identify a single entity.

Other rare causes of white matter disease also present with dementia, such as adult metachromatic leukodystrophy (arylsulfatase A deficiency) and progressive multifocal leukoencephalopathy (JC virus infection). A dominantly inherited form of diffuse white matter disease is known as *cerebral autosomal dominant arteriopathy with subcortical infarcts and leukoencephalopathy* (CADASIL). Clinically, there is a progressive dementia developing in the fifth to seventh decades in multiple family members who may also have a history of migraine and recurrent lacunar stroke without hypertension. Skin biopsy may show pathognomonic osmophilic granules in the media of arterioles. The disease is caused by mutations in the *Notch 3* gene, and genetic testing is commercially available. The frequency of this disorder is unknown, and there are no effective treatments.

Mitochondrial disorders can present with stroke-like episodes and can selectively injure basal ganglia or cortex. Many such patients show other findings suggestive of a neurologic or systemic disorder such as ophthalmoplegia, retinal degeneration, deafness, myopathy, neuropathy, or diabetes. Diagnosis is difficult, but serum or (especially) CSF levels of lactate and pyruvate may be abnormal, and biopsy of affected tissue, preferably muscle, may be diagnostic.

Treatment of vascular dementia must be focused on preventing new ischemic injury by stabilizing or removing the underlying causes, such as hypertension, diabetes, smoking, or lack of exercise. Recovery of lost cognitive function is not likely, although fluctuations with periods of improvement are common.

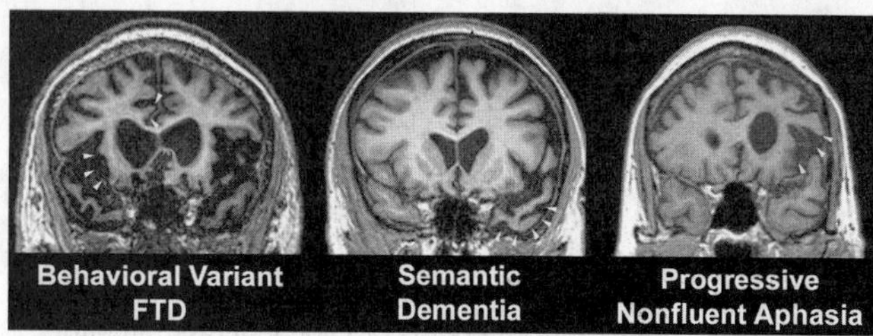

Figure 371-6 Frontotemporal dementia (FTD). Coronal MRI sections from representative patients with behavioral variant FTD (***left***), semantic dementia (***center***), and progressive nonfluent aphasia (***right***). Areas of early and severe atrophy in each syndrome are highlighted (*white arrowheads*). The behavioral variant features anterior cingulate and frontoinsular atrophy, spreading to orbital and dorsolateral prefrontal cortex. Semantic dementia shows prominent temporopolar atrophy, more often on the left. Progressive nonfluent aphasia is associated with dominant frontal opercular and dorsal insula degeneration.

FRONTOTEMPORAL DEMENTIA, PROGRESSIVE SUPRANUCLEAR PALSY, AND CORTICOBASAL DEGENERATION

Frontotemporal dementia (FTD) often begins in the fifth to seventh decades, and in this age group it is nearly as prevalent as AD. Early studies suggested that FTD may be more common in men than women, although more recent reports cast some doubt on this finding. *Unlike in AD, behavioral symptoms predominate in the early stages of FTD.* Although a family history of dementia is common, autosomal dominant inheritance is seen in about 10% of all FTD cases. The clinical heterogeneity in familial and sporadic forms of FTD is remarkable, with patients demonstrating variable mixtures of behavioral, language, movement, and motor neuron symptoms. The most common autosomal dominantly inherited mutations causing FTD involve the *MAPT* or *GRN* genes, both on chromosome 17. *MAPT* mutations lead to a change in the alternate splicing of tau or cause loss of function in the tau molecule. With *GRN*, mutations in the coding sequence of the gene encoding progranulin protein result in mRNA degradation due to nonsense-mediated decay. Progranulin appears to be a rare example of an autosomal dominant mutation that leads to haploinsufficiency, resulting in around one-half the normal level of progranulin protein. Progranulin is a growth factor that binds to tumor necrosis factor (TNF) receptors. How progranulin mutations lead to FTD is unknown. Both *MAPT* and *GRN* mutations are associated with parkinsonian features, while ALS is rare with these mutations. In contrast, familial FTD with ALS has been linked to chromosome 9. Mutations in the valosin-containing protein (chromosome 9) and the charged multivesicular body protein 2b (CHMP2b) genes (chromosome 3) also lead to rare autosomal dominant forms of familial FTD. Mutations in the TDP-43 and FUS genes (see below) cause familial ALS, sometimes in association with an FTD syndrome, although a few patients presenting with FTD alone have been reported.

In FTD, early symptoms are divided among behavioral, language, and sometimes motor abnormalities, reflecting degeneration of the anterior insular, frontal, and temporal regions, basal ganglia, and motor neurons. Cognitive testing typically reveals spared memory but impaired planning, judgment, or language. Poor business decisions and difficulty organizing work tasks are common, and speech and language deficits often emerge. Patients with FTD often show an absence of insight into their condition. Common behavioral features include apathy, disinhibition, weight gain, food fetishes, compulsions, and emotional distance or loss of empathy.

Findings at the bedside are dictated by the anatomic localization of the disorder. Asymmetric left frontal cases present with nonfluent aphasia, while left anterior temporal degeneration is characterized by loss of word meaning (semantic dementia). Nonfluent patients quickly progress to mutism, while those with semantic dementia develop features of a multimodal associative agnosia, losing the ability to recognize faces, objects, words, and the emotions of others. Visuoconstructive ability, arithmetic calculations, and navigation often remain normal late into the illness. Recently it has become apparent that many patients with nonfluent aphasia progress to clinical syndromes that overlap with PSP and corticobasal degeneration (CBD) and show these pathologies at autopsy. This left hemisphere presentation of FTD has been called *primary progressive aphasia with nonfluent and semantic variants*. In contrast, right frontal or temporal cases show profound alterations in social conduct, with loss of empathy, disinhibition, and antisocial behaviors predominating. There is a striking overlap among FTD, PSP, CBD, and motor neuron disease; ophthalmoplegia, dystonia, swallowing symptoms, and fasciculations are common at presentation of FTD or emerge during the course of the illness.

The distinguishing anatomic hallmark of FTD is a focal atrophy of frontal, insular, and/or temporal cortex, which can be visualized with neuroimaging studies and is often profound at autopsy (Figs. 371-6 and 371-7). Despite the appearance of advanced FTD,

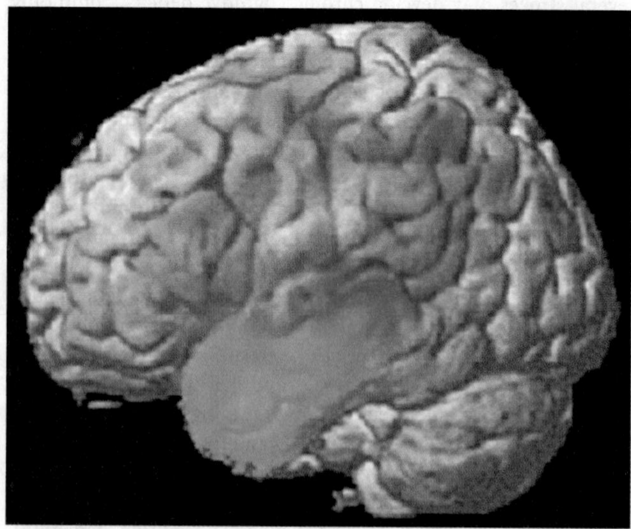

Figure 371-7 Voxel-based morphometry analysis showing differing patterns of brain atrophy in three variants of progressive aphasia, including nonfluent (*red*), semantic (*green*), and logopedic subtypes (*blue*). Voxel-based morphometry allows comparison of MRI gray matter volumes between patient groups and control subjects, as shown here. *(Image courtesy of M Gorno-Tempini, University of California at San Francisco; with permission.)*

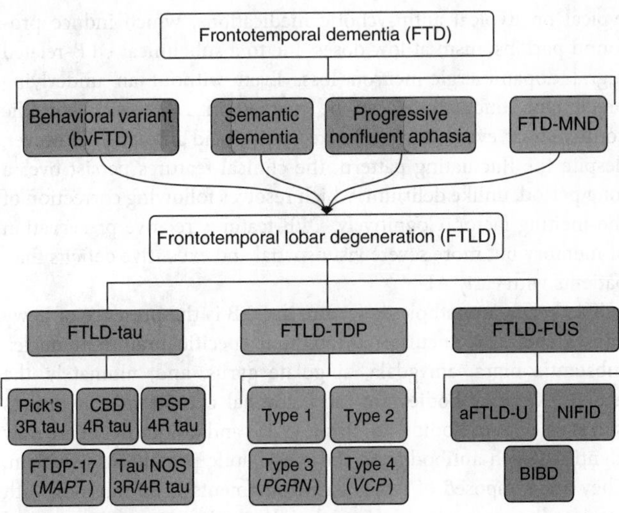

Figure 371-8 Frontotemporal dementia syndromes are united by underlying frontotemporal lobar degeneration pathology, which can be divided according to the presence of tau, TPD-43, or fused in sarcoma (FUS) inclusions in neurons and glia. Correlations between clinical syndrome and major molecular category are shown with colored shading.

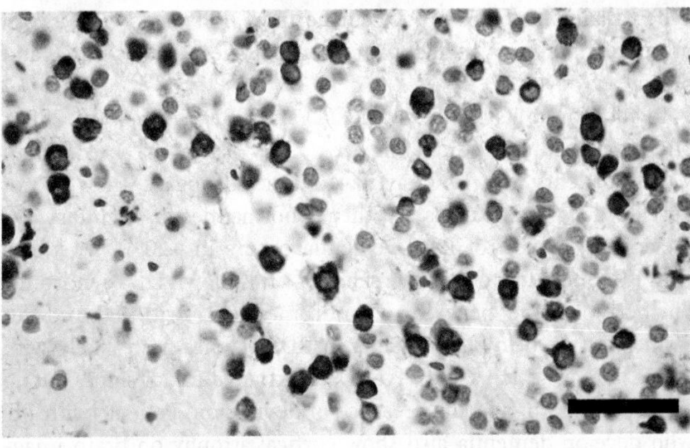

Figure 371-9 Pick's disease, a subtype of frontotemporal lobar degeneration (FTLD)-tau. Pick bodies, shown here in the dentate gyrus of a patient with advanced bvFTD, consist of loosely arranged paired helical and straight filaments and stain positively for hyperphosphorylated tau. Classical Pick's disease is seen in only 10–20% of patients with frontotemporal dementia. Scale bar represents 50 microns. *(CP-13 antibody courtesy of P. Davies.)*

however, the atrophy often begins focally in one hemisphere before spreading to anatomically interconnected regions, including basal ganglia. Microscopic findings seen across all patients with FTD include gliosis, microvacuolation, and neuronal loss, but the disease is subtyped according to the protein composition of neuronal and glial inclusions, which contain either tau or TDP-43 in at least 90% of patients, with the remaining 10% showing inclusions containing FUS (Fig. 371-8).

A toxic gain of function related to tau underlies the pathogenesis of many familial cases and is presumed to be a factor in sporadic tauopathies, although loss of tau microtubule stabilizing function may also play a role. TDP-43 and FUS, in contrast, are RNA/DNA binding proteins whose roles in neuronal function are still being actively investigated. Loss of cortical serotonergic innervation is seen in many patients. In contrast to AD, the cholinergic system is relatively spared in FTD.

Historically, *Pick's disease* was described as a progressive degenerative disorder characterized by selective involvement of the anterior frontal and temporal neocortex and pathologically by intraneuronal cytoplasmic inclusions (*Pick bodies*). Classical Pick bodies are argyrophilic, staining positively with the Bielschowsky silver method and also with immunostaining for tau (Fig. 371-9). Subsequent pathologic studies revealed a significant subset of patients with silver-negative, tau-negative inclusions, which have since been shown mainly to contain TDP-43, although a minority stain only for FUS. Although the nomenclature used to describe these patients has continued to evolve, the term *FTD* is increasingly used to refer to the clinical syndromes, while *frontotemporal lobar degeneration (FTLD)* refers to the underlying pathology, with three major subtypes recognized: FTLD-tau, FTLD-TDP, and FTLD-FUS. Despite significant progress, available data do not yet allow a reliable prediction of underlying pathology based on clinical features. Accordingly researchers continue to seek serum, CSF, or neuroimaging biomarkers that will afford greater diagnostic accuracy, defined as concordance with neuropathology.

The burden on caregivers of patients with FTD is extremely high because the illness disrupts core emotional and personality functions of the loved one. Treatment is symptomatic, and there are currently no therapies known to slow progression or improve symptoms. Many of the behaviors that accompany FTD, such as depression, hyperorality, compulsions, and irritability, can be ameliorated with antidepressants, especially SSRIs. The co-association with motor disorders such as parkinsonism necessitates the careful use of antipsychotics, which can exacerbate this problem.

Progressive supranuclear palsy (PSP) is a degenerative disease that involves the brainstem, basal ganglia, limbic structures, and selected areas of cortex. Clinically, this disorder begins with falls and executive or subtle personality changes (such as mental rigidity, impulsivity, or apathy). Shortly thereafter, a progressive oculomotor syndrome ensues that begins with square wave jerks, followed by slowed saccades (vertical worse than horizontal) before resulting in progressive supranuclear ophthalmoparesis. Dysarthria, dysphagia, and symmetric axial rigidity can be prominent features that emerge at any point in the illness. A stiff, unstable posture with hyperextension of the neck and a slow, jerky, toppling gait is characteristic. Frequent unexplained and sometimes spectacular falls are common secondary to a combination of axial rigidity, inability to look down, and bad judgment. Even once patients have severely limited voluntary eye movements, they retain oculocephalic reflexes (demonstrated using a vertical doll's head maneuver); thus, the oculomotor disorder is supranuclear. The dementia overlaps with FTD, featuring apathy, frontal-executive dysfunction, poor judgment, slowed thought processes, impaired verbal fluency, and difficulty with sequential actions and with shifting from one task to another. These features are common at presentation and often precede the motor syndrome. Some patients begin with a nonfluent aphasia or motor speech disorder and progress to classical PSP. Response to L-dopa is limited or absent; no other treatments exist. Death occurs within 5–10 years of onset. At autopsy, accumulation of hyperphosphorylated tau is seen within neurons and glia. Neuronal inclusions often take the form of neurofibrillary tangles (NFTs), which may be large, spherical, and coarse when found in brainstem oculomotor control system neurons. These characteristic tau inclusions are called globose tangles, and may be found in multiple subcortical structures (including the subthalamic nucleus, globus pallidus, substantia nigra, locus coeruleus, periaqueductal gray, superior colliculi, oculomotor nuclei, and dentate nucleus). Neocortical NFTs, like those in AD, often take on a more flame-shaped morphology, but on electron microscopy PSP tangles can be shown to consist of straight tubules rather than the paired helical filaments found in AD. Furthermore, PSP is associated with prominent tau-positive glial pathomorphologies, such as tufted and thorny astrocytes.

In addition to its overlap with FTD and CBD (see below), PSP is often confused with idiopathic *Parkinson's disease* (PD). Although elderly patients with PD may have restricted upgaze, they do not develop downgaze paresis or other abnormalities of voluntary eye movements typical of PSP. Dementia occurs in ~20% of patients with PD, often due to the emergence of a full-blown DLB syndrome. Furthermore, the behavioral syndromes seen with DLB differ from PSP (see below). Dementia in PD becomes more likely with increasing age, increasing severity of extrapyramidal signs, a long disease duration, and the presence of depression. Patients with PD who develop dementia also show cortical atrophy on brain imaging. Neuropathologically, there may be Alzheimer's disease–related changes in the cortex, DLB-related α-synuclein inclusions in both the limbic system and cortex, or no specific microscopic changes other than gliosis and neuronal loss. Parkinson's disease is discussed in detail in Chap. 372.

Corticobasal degeneration (CBD) is a slowly progressive dementing illness associated with severe gliosis and neuronal loss in both the cortex and basal ganglia (substantia nigra and striatopallidum). Some patients present with a unilateral onset with rigidity, dystonia, and apraxia of one arm and hand, sometimes called the *alien limb* when it begins to exhibit unintended motor actions, while in other instances the disease presents as a progressive behavioral, executive, or language syndrome or as progressive symmetric parkinsonism. Some patients begin with a progressive nonfluent aphasia or a progressive motor speech disorder. Eventually CBD becomes bilateral and leads to dysarthria, slow gait, action tremor, and dementia. The microscopic features include ballooned, achromatic, tau-positive neurons with astrocytic plaques and other dystrophic glial tau pathomorphologies that overlap with those seen in PSP. Most specifically, CBD features a severe tauopathy burden in the subcortical white matter, consisting of threads and oligodendroglial coiled bodies. The condition is rarely familial, the cause is unknown, and there is no specific treatment.

PARKINSON'S DISEASE DEMENTIA AND DEMENTIA WITH LEWY BODIES

The parkinsonian dementia syndromes are under increasing study, with many cases unified by Lewy body and Lewy neurite pathology that ascends from the low brainstem up through the substantia nigra, limbic system, and cortex. The DLB clinical syndrome is characterized by visual hallucinations, parkinsonism, fluctuating alertness, falls, and often RBD. Dementia can precede or follow the appearance of parkinsonism. Hence, one pathway occurs in patients with long-standing PD without cognitive impairment, who slowly develop a dementia that is associated with visual hallucinations and fluctuating alertness. When this occurs after an established diagnosis of PD, many use the term *Parkinson's disease dementia* (PDD). In others, the dementia and neuropsychiatric syndrome precede the parkinsonism, and this constellation is referred to as DLB. Both PDD and DLB may be accompanied or preceded by symptoms referable to brainstem pathology below the substantia nigra, and many researchers conceptualize these disorders as points on a spectrum of α-synuclein pathology.

Patients with PDD and DLB are highly sensitive to metabolic perturbations, and in some patients the first manifestation of illness is a delirium, often precipitated by an infection, new medicine, or other systemic disturbance. A hallucinatory delirium induced by L-dopa, prescribed for parkinsonian symptoms attributed to PD may likewise provide the initial clue to a PDD diagnosis. Conversely, patients with mild cognitive deficits and hallucinations may receive typical or atypical antipsychotic medications, which induce profound parkinsonism at low doses due to a subclinical DLB-related nigral dopaminergic neuron loss. Even without an underlying precipitant, fluctuations can be marked in DLB, with episodic confusion or even stupor admixed with lucid intervals. However, despite the fluctuating pattern, the clinical features persist over a long period, unlike delirium, which resolves following correction of the inciting factor. Cognitively, DLB features relative preservation of memory but more severe visuospatial and executive deficits than patients with early AD.

The key neuropathologic feature in DLB is the presence of Lewy bodies and Lewy neurites throughout specific brainstem nuclei, substantia nigra, amygdala, cingulate gyrus, and, ultimately, the neocortex. Lewy bodies are intraneuronal cytoplasmic inclusions that stain with periodic acid–Schiff (PAS) and ubiquitin but are now identified with antibodies to the presynaptic protein, α-synuclein. They are composed of straight neurofilaments 7–20 nm long with surrounding amorphous material and contain epitopes recognized by antibodies against phosphorylated and nonphosphorylated neurofilament proteins, ubiquitin, and α-synuclein. Lewy bodies are typically found in the substantia nigra of patients with idiopathic PD, where they can be readily seen with hematoxylin-and-eosin staining. A profound cholinergic deficit, owing to basal forebrain and pedunculopontine nucleus involvement, is present in many patients with DLB and may be a factor responsible for the fluctuations, inattention, and visual hallucinations. In patients without other pathologic features, the condition is sometimes referred to as *diffuse Lewy body disease*. In patients whose brains also contain a substantial burden of amyloid plaques and NFTs, the condition is sometimes called the *Lewy body variant of Alzheimer's disease*.

Due to the overlap with AD and the cholinergic deficit in DLB, cholinesterase inhibitors often provide significant benefit, reducing hallucinosis, stabilizing delusional symptoms, and even helping with RBD in some patients. Exercise programs maximize motor function and protect against fall-related injury. Antidepressants are often necessary. Atypical antipsychotics may be required for psychosis but can worsen extrapyramidal syndromes, even at low doses, and increase risk of death. As noted above, patients with DLB are extremely sensitive to dopaminergic medications, which must be carefully titrated; tolerability may be improved by concomitant use of a cholinesterase inhibitor.

OTHER CAUSES OF DEMENTIA

Prion diseases such as *Creutzfeldt-Jakob disease* (CJD) are rare neurodegenerative conditions (prevalence ~1 per million) that produce dementia. CJD is a rapidly progressive disorder associated with dementia, focal cortical signs, rigidity, and myoclonus, causing death <1 year after first symptoms appear. The rapidity of progression seen with CJD is uncommon in AD so that the distinction between the two disorders is usually straightforward. CBD and DLB, more rapid degenerative dementias with prominent movement abnormalities, are more likely to be mistaken for CJD. The differential diagnosis for CJD includes other rapidly progressive dementing conditions such as viral or bacterial encephalitides, Hashimoto's encephalopathy, CNS vasculitis, lymphoma, or paraneoplastic syndromes. The markedly abnormal periodic complexes on EEG and cortical ribbon and basal ganglia hyperintensities on MR diffusion-weighted imaging are highly specific diagnostic features of CJD, although rarely prolonged focal or generalized seizures can produce a similar imaging appearance. Prion diseases are discussed in detail in Chap. 383.

Huntington's disease (HD) (Chap. 372) is an autosomal dominant, degenerative brain disorder. HD clinical hallmarks include chorea, behavioral disturbance, and executive impairment. Symptoms typically begin in the fourth or fifth decade, but there is a wide range, from childhood to >70 years. Memory is frequently not impaired

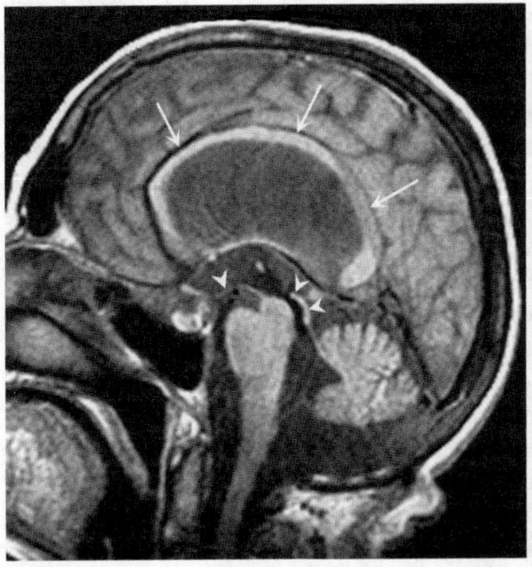

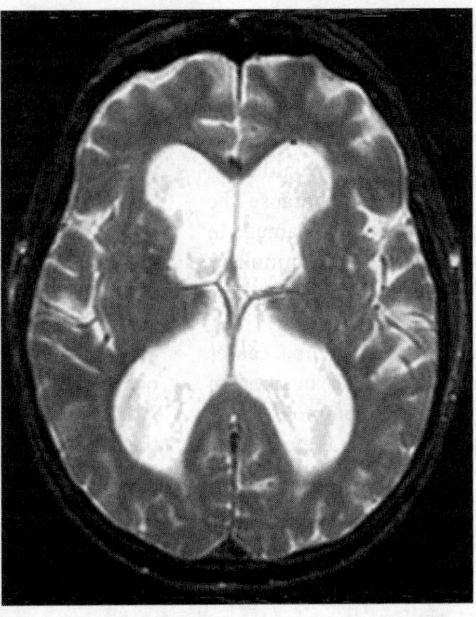

Figure 371-10 Normal-pressure hydrocephalus. ***A.*** Sagittal T1-weighted MR image demonstrates dilation of the lateral ventricle and stretching of the corpus callosum (*arrows*), depression of the floor of the third ventricle (*single arrowhead*), and enlargement of the aqueduct (*double arrowheads*). Note the diffuse dilation of the lateral, third, and fourth ventricles with a patent aqueduct, typical of communicating hydrocephalus. ***B.*** Axial T2-weighted MR images demonstrate dilation of the lateral ventricles. This patient underwent successful ventriculoperitoneal shunting.

until late in the disease, but attention, judgment, awareness, and executive functions are often deficient at an early stage. Depression, apathy, social withdrawal, irritability, and intermittent disinhibition are common. Delusions and obsessive-compulsive behavior may occur. Disease duration is typically around 15 years but is quite variable.

Normal-pressure hydrocephalus (NPH) is a relatively uncommon but treatable syndrome. The clinical, physiologic, and neuroimaging characteristics of NPH must be carefully distinguished from those of other dementias associated with gait impairment. Historically, many patients treated for NPH have suffered from other dementias, particularly AD, vascular dementia, DLB, and PSP. For NPH, the clinical triad includes an abnormal gait (ataxic or apractic), dementia (usually mild to moderate, with an emphasis on executive impairment), and urinary urgency or incontinence. Neuroimaging reveals enlarged lateral ventricles (hydrocephalus) with little or no cortical atrophy, although the sylvian fissures may appear propped open (so-called "boxcarring"), which can be mistaken for perisylvian atrophy. This syndrome is a communicating hydrocephalus with a patent aqueduct of Sylvius (Fig. 371-10), in contrast to aqueductal stenosis, in which the aqueduct is small. Lumbar puncture opening pressure falls in the high normal range, and the CSF protein, glucose, and cell counts are normal. NPH may be caused by obstruction to normal CSF flow over the cerebral convexities and delayed resorption into the venous system. The indolent nature of the process results in enlarged lateral ventricles with relatively little increase in CSF pressure. Presumed stretching and distortion of subfrontal white matter tracts may lead to clinical symptoms, but the precise underlying pathophysiology remains unclear. Some patients provide a history of conditions that produce meningeal scarring (blocking CSF resorption) such as previous meningitis, subarachnoid hemorrhage, or head trauma. Others with long-standing but asymptomatic congenital hydrocephalus may have adult-onset deterioration in gait or memory that is confused with NPH. In contrast to AD, the patient with NPH complains of an early and prominent gait disturbance without cortical atrophy on CTor MRI.

Numerous attempts to improve NPH diagnosis with various special studies and predict the success of ventricular shunting have been undertaken. These tests include radionuclide cisternography (showing a delay in CSF absorption over the convexity) and various efforts to monitor and alter CSF flow dynamics, including a constant-pressure infusion test. None has proven to be specific or consistently useful. A transient improvement in gait or cognition may follow lumbar puncture (or serial punctures) with removal of 30–50 mL of CSF, but this finding has also not proved to be consistently predictive of postshunt improvement. Perhaps the most reliable strategy is a period of close inpatient evaluation before, during, and after lumbar CSF drainage. Occasionally, when a patient with AD presents with gait impairment (at times due to comorbid subfrontal vascular injury) and absent or only mild cortical atrophy on CT or MRI, distinguishing NPH from AD can be challenging. Hippocampal atrophy on MRI favors AD, whereas a characteristic "magnetic" gait with external hip rotation, low foot clearance and short strides, along with prominent truncal sway or instability, favors NPH. The diagnosis of NPH should be avoided when hydrocephalus is not detected on imaging studies, even if the symptoms otherwise fit. Thirty to fifty percent of patients identified by careful diagnosis as having NPH will improve with ventricular shunting. Gait may improve more than cognition, but many reported failures to improve cognitively may have resulted from comorbid AD. Short-lasting improvement is common. Patients should be carefully selected for shunting, because subdural hematoma, infection, and shunt failure are known complications and can be a cause for early nursing home placement in an elderly patient with previously mild dementia.

Dementia can accompany *chronic alcoholism* (Chap. 392) and may result from associated malnutrition, especially of B vitamins, particularly thiamine. Other poorly defined aspects of chronic alcoholism may, however, also produce cerebral damage. A rare idiopathic syndrome of dementia and seizures with degeneration of the corpus callosum has been reported primarily in male Italian red wine drinkers (Marchiafava-Bignami disease).

Thiamine (vitamin B_1) deficiency causes Wernicke's encephalopathy (Chap. 275). The clinical presentation features a malnourished patient (frequently but not necessarily alcoholic) with confusion, ataxia, and diplopia resulting from inflammation and necrosis of periventricular midline structures, including dorsomedial thalamus, mammillary bodies, midline cerebellum, periaqueductal gray matter, and trochlear and abducens nuclei. Damage to the dorsomedial thalamus correlates most closely with the memory loss. Prompt administration of parenteral thiamine (100 mg intravenously for 3 days followed by daily oral dosage) may reverse the disease if given in the first days of symptom onset. However, prolonged untreated thiamine deficiency can result in an irreversible dementia/amnestic syndrome (Korsakoff's syndrome) or even death.

In *Korsakoff's syndrome*, the patient is unable to recall new information despite normal immediate memory, attention span, and level of consciousness. Memory for new events is seriously impaired, whereas knowledge acquired prior to the illness remains relatively intact. Patients are easily confused, disoriented, and cannot store information for more than a few minutes. Superficially, they may be conversant, engaging, and able to perform simple tasks and follow immediate commands. Confabulation is common, although not always present. There is no specific treatment because the previous thiamine deficiency has produced irreversible damage to the medial thalamic nuclei and mammillary bodies. Mammillary body atrophy may be visible on MRI in the chronic phase (Fig. 275-7).

Vitamin B_{12} deficiency, as can occur in pernicious anemia, causes a megaloblastic anemia and may also damage the nervous system (Chaps. 105 and 377). Neurologically, it most commonly produces a spinal cord syndrome (myelopathy) affecting the posterior columns (loss of vibration and position sense) and corticospinal tracts (hyperactive tendon reflexes with Babinski signs); it also damages peripheral nerves (neuropathy), resulting in sensory loss with depressed tendon reflexes. Damage to myelinated axons may also cause dementia. The mechanism of neurologic damage is unclear but may be related to a deficiency of *S*-adenosyl methionine (required for methylation of myelin phospholipids) due to reduced methionine synthase activity or accumulation of methylmalonate, homocysteine, and propionate, providing abnormal substrates for fatty acid synthesis in myelin. The neurologic sequelae of vitamin B_{12} deficiency may occur in the absence of hematologic manifestations, making it critical to avoid using the CBC and blood smear as a substitute for measuring B_{12} blood levels. Treatment with parenteral vitamin B_{12} (1000 μg intramuscularly daily for a week, weekly for a month, and monthly for life for pernicious anemia) stops progression of the disease if instituted promptly, but complete reversal of advanced nervous system damage will not occur.

Deficiency of nicotinic acid (*pellagra*) is associated with skin rash over sun-exposed areas, glossitis, and angular stomatitis (Chap. 74). Severe dietary deficiency of nicotinic acid along with other B vitamins such as pyridoxine may result in spastic paraparesis, peripheral neuropathy, fatigue, irritability, and dementia. This syndrome has been seen in prisoners of war and in concentration camps but should be considered in any malnourished individual. Low serum folate levels appear to be a rough index of malnutrition, but isolated folate deficiency has not been proved as a specific cause of dementia.

CNS infections usually cause delirium and other acute neurologic syndromes. However, some chronic CNS infections, particularly those associated with chronic meningitis (Chap. 382), may produce a dementing illness. The possibility of chronic infectious meningitis should be suspected in patients presenting with a dementia or behavioral syndrome, who also have headache, meningismus, cranial neuropathy, and/or radiculopathy. Between 20 and 30% of patients in the advanced stages of HIV infection become demented (Chap. 189). Cardinal features include psychomotor retardation, apathy, and impaired memory. This syndrome may result from secondary opportunistic infections but can also be caused by direct infection of CNS neurons with HIV. Neurosyphilis (Chap. 169) was a common cause of dementia in the preantibiotic era; it is now uncommon but can still be encountered in patients with multiple sex partners, particularly among patients with HIV. Characteristic CSF changes consist of pleocytosis, increased protein, and a positive venereal disease research laboratory (VDRL) test.

Primary and metastatic *neoplasms of the CNS* (Chap. 379) usually produce focal neurologic findings and seizures rather than dementia, but if tumor growth begins in the frontal or temporal lobes, the initial manifestations may be memory loss or behavioral changes. A paraneoplastic syndrome of dementia associated with occult carcinoma (often small cell lung cancer) is termed *limbic encephalitis*. In this syndrome, confusion, agitation, seizures, poor memory, emotional changes, and frank dementia may occur. Paraneoplastic *encephalitis associated with NMDA receptor antibodies* presents as a progressive psychiatric disorder with memory loss and seizures; affected patients are often young women with ovarian teratoma (Chap. 101).

A *nonconvulsive seizure disorder* may underlie a syndrome of confusion, clouding of consciousness, and garbled speech. Often, psychiatric disease is suspected, but an EEG demonstrates the epileptic nature of the illness. If recurrent or persistent, the condition may be termed *complex partial status epilepticus*. The cognitive disturbance often responds to anticonvulsant therapy. The etiology may be previous small strokes or head trauma; some cases are idiopathic.

It is important to recognize *systemic diseases* that indirectly affect the brain and produce chronic confusion or dementia. Such conditions include hypothyroidism; vasculitis; and hepatic, renal, or pulmonary disease. Hepatic encephalopathy may begin with irritability and confusion and slowly progress to agitation, lethargy, and coma.

Isolated vasculitis of the CNS (CNS granulomatous angiitis) (Chaps. 326 and 370) occasionally causes a chronic encephalopathy associated with confusion, disorientation, and clouding of consciousness. Headache is common, and strokes and cranial neuropathies may occur. Brain imaging studies may be normal or nonspecifically abnormal. CSF analysis reveals a mild pleocytosis or protein elevation. Cerebral angiography can show multifocal stenoses involving medium-caliber vessels, but some patients have only small-vessel disease that is not revealed on angiography. The angiographic appearance is not specific and may be mimicked by atherosclerosis, infection, or other causes of vascular disease. Brain or meningeal biopsy demonstrates endothelial cell proliferation and mononuclear infiltrates within blood vessel walls. The prognosis is often poor, although the disorder may remit spontaneously. Some patients respond to glucocorticoids or chemotherapy.

Chronic metal exposure represents a rare cause of dementia. The key to diagnosis is to elicit a history of exposure at work or home. Chronic lead poisoning from inadequately fire-glazed pottery has been reported. Fatigue, depression, and confusion may be associated with episodic abdominal pain and peripheral neuropathy. Gray lead lines appear in the gums, usually accompanied by an anemia with basophilic stippling of red blood cells. The clinical presentation can resemble that of acute intermittent porphyria, including elevated levels of urine porphyrins as a result of the inhibition of δ-aminolevulinic acid dehydrase. The treatment is chelation therapy with agents such as ethylenediamine tetraacetic acid (EDTA). Chronic mercury poisoning produces dementia, peripheral neuropathy, ataxia, and tremulousness that may progress to a cerebellar intention tremor or choreoathetosis. The confusion and memory loss of chronic arsenic intoxication is also associated with nausea, weight loss, peripheral neuropathy, pigmentation and scaling of the skin, and transverse white lines of the fingernails (Mees' lines). Treatment is chelation therapy with dimercaprol (BAL). Aluminum poisoning is rare but was documented with the dialysis dementia syndrome, in which water used during renal dialysis was contaminated with excessive amounts of aluminum. This poisoning resulted in a progressive encephalopathy associated with confusion, nonfluent aphasia, memory loss, agitation, and, later, lethargy and stupor. Speech arrest and myoclonic jerks were common and associated with severe and generalized EEG changes. The condition has been eliminated by the use of deionized water for dialysis.

Recurrent head trauma in professional boxers may lead to a dementia sometimes called the "punch-drunk" syndrome, or *dementia pugilistica*. The symptoms can be progressive, beginning late in a boxer's career or even long after retirement. The severity of the syndrome correlates with the length of the boxing career and number of bouts. Early in the condition, a personality change associated with social instability and sometimes paranoia and delusions occurs. Later, memory loss progresses to full-blown dementia, often associated with parkinsonian signs and ataxia or intention tremor. At autopsy, the cerebral cortex may show changes similar to AD, although NFTs are usually more prominent than amyloid plaques (which are usually diffuse rather than neuritic). Superficial layer NFT aggregates have been reported to differentiate these patients from those with more typical AD. Also, there may be loss of neurons in the substantia nigra. Chronic subdural hematoma (Chap. 378) is also occasionally associated with dementia, often in the context of underlying cortical atrophy from conditions such as AD or HD.

Transient global amnesia (TGA) is characterized by the sudden onset of a severe episodic memory deficit, usually occurring in persons over the age of 50 years. Often the amnesia occurs in the setting of an emotional stimulus or physical exertion. During the attack, the individual is alert and communicative, general cognition seems intact, and there are no other neurologic signs or symptoms. The patient may seem confused and repeatedly ask about his or her location in place and time. The ability to form new memories returns after a period of hours, and the individual returns to normal with no recall for the period of the attack. Frequently no cause is determined, but cerebrovascular disease, epilepsy (7% in one study), migraine, or cardiac arrhythmias have all been implicated. A Mayo Clinic review of 277 patients with TGA found a history of migraine in 14% and cerebrovascular disease in 11%, but these conditions were not temporally related to the TGA episodes. Approximately one-quarter of the patients had recurrent attacks, but they were not at increased risk for subsequent stroke. Rare instances of permanent memory loss after sudden onset have been reported, usually representing ischemic infarction of the hippocampus or medial thalamic nucleus bilaterally.

The *ALS/parkinsonian/dementia complex of Guam* is a rare degenerative disease that has occurred in the Chamorro natives on the island of Guam. Individuals may have any combination of parkinsonian features, dementia, and motor neuron disease. The most characteristic pathologic features are the presence of NFTs in degenerating neurons of the cortex and substantia nigra and loss of motor neurons in the spinal cord, although recent reanalysis has shown that some patients with this illness also show coexisting TDP-43 pathology. Epidemiologic evidence supports a possible environmental cause, such as exposure to a neurotoxin or an infectious agent with a long latency period. One interesting but unproven candidate neurotoxin occurs in the seed of the false palm tree, which Guamanians traditionally used to make flour. The ALS syndrome is no longer present in Guam, but a dementing illness with rigidity continues to be seen.

Rarely, adult-onset leukodystrophies, lysosomal storage diseases, and other genetic disorders can present as a dementia in middle to late life. Metachromatic leukodystrophy (MLD) causes a progressive psychiatric or dementia syndrome associated with extensive, confluent frontal white matter abnormality. MLD is diagnosed by measuring arylsulfatase A enzyme activity in white blood cells. Adult-onset presentations of adrenoleukodystrophy have been reported in female carriers, and these patients often feature spinal cord and posterior white matter involvement. Adrenoleukodystrophy is diagnosed with measurement of plasma very long chain fatty acids. CADASIL is another genetic syndrome associated with white matter disease, often frontally and temporally predominant. Diagnosis is made with skin biopsy, which shows osmophilic granules in arterioles, or, increasingly, through genetic testing for mutations in Notch 3 (see above). The neuronal ceroid lipofuscinoses are a genetically heterogeneous group of disorders associated with myoclonus, seizures, and progressive dementia. Diagnosis is made by finding curvilinear inclusions within white blood cells or neuronal tissue.

Psychogenic amnesia for personally important memories can be seen. Whether this results from deliberate avoidance of unpleasant memories, outright malingering, or from unconscious repression remains unknown and probably depends on the patient. Event-specific amnesia is more likely to occur after violent crimes such as homicide of a close relative or friend or sexual abuse. It may develop in association with severe drug or alcohol intoxication and sometimes with schizophrenia. More prolonged psychogenic amnesia occurs in fugue states that also commonly follow severe emotional stress. The patient with a fugue state suffers from a sudden loss of personal identity and may be found wandering far from home. *In contrast to neurologic amnesia, fugue states are associated with amnesia for personal identity and events closely associated with the personal past.* At the same time, memory for other recent events and the ability to learn and use new information are preserved. The episodes usually last hours or days and occasionally weeks or months while the patient takes on a new identity. On recovery, there is a residual amnesia gap for the period of the fugue. Very rarely does selective loss of autobiographic information reflect a focal injury to the brain areas involved with these functions.

Psychiatric diseases may mimic dementia. Severely depressed or anxious individuals may appear demented, a phenomenon sometimes called *pseudodementia*. Memory and language are usually intact when carefully tested, and a significant memory disturbance usually suggests an underlying dementia, even if the patient is depressed. Patients in this condition may feel confused and unable to accomplish routine tasks. Vegetative symptoms, such as insomnia, lack of energy, poor appetite, and concern with bowel function, are common. Onset is often more abrupt, and the psychosocial milieu may suggest prominent reasons for depression. Such patients respond to treatment of the underlying psychiatric illness. Schizophrenia is usually not difficult to distinguish from dementia, but occasionally the distinction can be problematic. Schizophrenia generally has a much earlier age of onset (second and third decades) than most dementing illnesses, and is associated with intact memory. The delusions and hallucinations of schizophrenia are usually more complex and bizarre than those of dementia. Some chronic schizophrenics develop an unexplained progressive dementia late in life that is not related to AD. Conversely, FTD, HD, vascular dementia, DLB, AD, or leukoencephalopathy can begin with schizophrenia-like features, leading to the misdiagnosis of a psychiatric condition. Later age of onset, significant deficits on cognitive testing, or the presence of abnormal neuroimaging point toward a degenerative condition. Memory loss may also be part of a conversion disorder. In this situation, patients commonly complain bitterly of memory loss, but careful cognitive testing either does not confirm the deficits or demonstrates inconsistent or unusual patterns of cognitive problems. The patient's behavior and "wrong" answers to questions often indicate that he or she understands the question and knows the correct answer.

Clouding of cognition by *chronic drug or medication use*, often prescribed by physicians, is an important cause of dementia. Sedatives, tranquilizers, and analgesics used to treat insomnia, pain, anxiety, or agitation may cause confusion, memory loss, and lethargy, especially in the elderly. Discontinuation of the offending medication often improves mentation.

TREATMENT Dementia

The major goals of dementia management are to treat correctable causes and to provide comfort and support to the patient and caregivers. Treatment of underlying causes might include thyroid replacement for hypothyroidism; vitamin therapy for thiamine or B_{12} deficiency or for elevated serum homocysteine; antimicrobials for opportunistic infections or antiretrovirals for HIV; ventricular shunting for NPH; or appropriate surgical, radiation, and/or chemotherapeutic treatment for CNS neoplasms. Removal of cognition-impairing drugs or medications is the most frequently useful approach employed in a dementia clinic. If the patient's cognitive complaints stem from a psychiatric disorder, vigorous treatment of this condition should seek to eliminate the cognitive complaint or confirm that it persists despite adequate resolution of the mood or anxiety symptoms. Patients with degenerative diseases may also be depressed or anxious, and those aspects of their condition may respond to therapy. Antidepressants, such as SSRIs (Chap. 391), which feature anxiolytic properties but few cognitive side effects provide the mainstay of treatment when necessary. Anticonvulsants are used to control seizures.

Agitation, hallucinations, delusions, and confusion are difficult to treat. These behavioral problems represent major causes for nursing home placement and institutionalization. Before treating these behaviors with medications, the clinician should aggressively seek out modifiable environmental or metabolic factors. Hunger, lack of exercise, toothache, constipation, urinary tract infection, or drug toxicity all represent easily correctable causes that can be remedied without psychoactive drugs. Drugs such as phenothiazines and benzodiazepines may ameliorate the behavior problems but have untoward side effects such as sedation, rigidity, dyskinesia, and occasionally paradoxical disinhibition (benzodiazepines). Despite their unfavorable side-effect profile, second-generation antipsychotics such as quetiapine (starting dose, 12.5–25 mg daily) can be used for patients with agitation, aggression, and psychosis, although the risk profile for these compounds is significant. When patients do not respond to treatment, it is usually a mistake to advance to higher doses or to use anticholinergics or sedatives (such as barbiturates or benzodiazepines). It is important to recognize and treat depression; treatment can begin with a low dose of an SSRI (e.g., escitalopram 5–10 mg daily) while monitoring for efficacy and toxicity. Sometimes apathy, visual hallucinations, depression, and other psychiatric symptoms respond to the cholinesterase inhibitors, especially in DLB, obviating the need for other more toxic therapies.

Cholinesterase inhibitors are being used to treat AD (donepezil, rivastigmine, galantamine) and PDD (rivastigmine). Other compounds, such as anti-inflammatory agents, are being investigated in the treatment or prevention of AD. These approaches are reviewed in the treatment sections for individual disorders, above. Memantine proves useful when treating some patients with moderate to severe AD; its major benefit relates to decreasing caregiver burden, most likely by decreasing resistance to dressing and grooming support.

A proactive strategy has been shown to reduce the occurrence of delirium in hospitalized patients. This strategy includes frequent orientation, cognitive activities, sleep-enhancement measures, vision and hearing aids, and correction of dehydration.

Nondrug behavior therapy has an important place in dementia management. The primary goals are to make the patient's life comfortable, uncomplicated, and safe. Preparing lists, schedules, calendars, and labels can be helpful in the early stages. It is also useful to stress familiar routines, short-term tasks, walks, and simple physical exercises. For many demented patients, memory for events is worse than for routine activities, and they may still be able to take part in physical activities such as walking, bowling, dancing, and golf. Demented patients usually object to losing control over familiar tasks such as driving, cooking, and handling finances. Attempts to help or take over may be greeted with complaints, depression, or anger. Hostile responses on the part of the caretaker are useless and sometimes harmful. Explanation, reassurance, distraction, and calm positive statements are more productive in this setting. Eventually, tasks such as finances and driving must be assumed by others, and the patient will conform and adjust. Safety is an important issue that includes not only driving but controlling the kitchen, bathroom, and sleeping area environments, as well as stairways. These areas need to be monitored, supervised, and made as safe as possible. A move to a retirement home, assisted-living center, or nursing home can initially increase confusion and agitation. Repeated reassurance, reorientation, and careful introduction to the new personnel will help to smooth the process. Providing activities that are known to be enjoyable to the patient can be of considerable benefit. The clinician must pay special attention to frustration and depression among family members and caregivers. Caregiver guilt and burnout are common. Family members often feel overwhelmed and helpless and may vent their frustrations on the patient, each other, and health care providers. Caregivers should be encouraged to take advantage of day-care facilities and respite breaks. Education and counseling about dementia are important. Local and national support groups, such as the Alzheimer's Association (*www.alz.org*), can provide considerable help.

FURTHER READINGS

KNOPMAN DS et al: Incidence and causes of nondegenerative nonvascular dementia: A population-based study. Arch Neurol 63:218, 2006

MAYEUX R: Clinical practice. Early Alzheimer's disease. N Engl J Med 362:2194, 2010

ROBERSON ED, MUCKE L: 100 years and counting: Prospects for defeating Alzheimer's disease. Science 314:781, 2006

SMALL GW et al: PET of brain amyloid and tau in mild cognitive impairment. N Engl J Med 355:2652, 2007

VAN ES MA, VAN DEN BERG LH. Alzheimer's disease beyond APOE. Nat Genet 41:1047, 2009

VAN OIJEN M et al: Atherosclerosis and risk for dementia. Ann Neurol 61:403, 2007

WHITMER RA et al: Timing of hormone therapy and dementia: The critical window theory revisited. Ann Neurol 69:163, 2011

WILLIAMS DR et al: Characteristics of two distinct clinical phenotypes in pathologically proven progressive supranuclear palsy: Richardson's syndrome and PSP-parkinsonism. Brain 128:1247, 2005

ZUCCALA G et al: Correlate of cognitive impairment among patients with heart failure: Results of a multicenter survey. Am J Med 118:496, 2005

CHAPTER 372

Parkinson's Disease and Other Movement Disorders

C. Warren Olanow
Anthony H.V. Schapira

PARKINSON'S DISEASE AND RELATED DISORDERS

Parkinson's disease (PD) is the second commonest neurodegenerative disease, exceeded only by Alzheimer's disease (AD). It is estimated that approximately 1 million persons in the United States and 5 million persons in the world suffer from this disorder. PD affects men and women of all races, all occupations, and all countries. The mean age of onset is about 60 years, but cases can be seen in patients in their 20s, and even younger. The frequency of PD increases with aging, and based on projected population demographics, it is estimated that the prevalence will dramatically increase in future decades.

Clinically, PD is characterized by rest tremor, rigidity, bradykinesia, and gait impairment, known as the "cardinal features" of the disease. Additional features can include freezing of gait, postural instability, speech difficulty, autonomic disturbances, sensory alterations, mood disorders, sleep dysfunction, cognitive impairment, and dementia (Table 372-1), all known as nondopaminergic features because they do not fully respond to dopaminergic therapy.

Pathologically, the hallmark features of PD are degeneration of dopaminergic neurons in the substantia nigra pars compacta (SNc), reduced striatal dopamine, and intracytoplasmic proteinaceous inclusions known as Lewy bodies (Fig. 372-1). While interest has primarily focused on the dopamine system, neuronal degeneration with inclusion body formation can also affect cholinergic neurons of the nucleus basalis of Meynert (NBM), norepinephrine neurons of the locus coeruleus (LC), serotonin neurons in the raphe nuclei of the brainstem, and neurons of the olfactory system, cerebral hemispheres, spinal cord, and peripheral autonomic nervous system. This "nondopaminergic" pathology is likely responsible for the nondopaminergic clinical features listed in Table 372-1. Indeed, there is evidence that pathology begins in the peripheral autonomic nervous system, olfactory system, and dorsal motor nucleus of the vagus nerve in the lower brainstem, and then spreads in a sequential manner to affect the upper brainstem and cerebral hemispheres. These studies suggest that dopamine neurons are affected in midstage disease. Indeed, several studies suggest that symptoms reflecting nondopaminergic degeneration such as constipation, anosmia, rapid eye movement (REM) behavior sleep disorder, and cardiac denervation precede the onset of the classic motor features of the illness.

DIFFERENTIAL DIAGNOSIS

Parkinsonism is a general term that is used to define a symptom complex manifest by bradykinesia with rigidity and/or tremor. It has a wide differential diagnosis (Table 372-2) and can reflect damage to different components of the basal ganglia. The basal ganglia comprise a group of subcortical nuclei that include the striatum (putamen and caudate nucleus), subthalamic nucleus (STN), globus pallidus pars externa (GPe), globus pallidus pars interna (GPi), and the SNc (Fig. 372-2). The basal ganglia play an important role in regulating normal motor behavior. It is now appreciated that basal ganglia also play a role in modulating emotional and cognitive functions. Among the different forms of parkinsonism, PD is the most common (approximately 75% of cases). Historically, PD was diagnosed based on the presence of two of three parkinsonian features (tremor, rigidity, bradykinesia). However, postmortem studies found a 24% error rate when these criteria were used. Clinicopathologic correlation studies subsequently determined that parkinsonism associated with rest tremor, asymmetry, and a good response to levodopa was more likely to predict the correct pathologic diagnosis. With these revised criteria (known as the U.K. brain bank criteria), the clinical diagnosis of PD is confirmed pathologically in 99% of cases.

Imaging of the brain dopamine system in PD with positron emission tomography (PET) or single-photon emission computed tomography (SPECT) shows reduced uptake of striatal dopaminergic markers, particularly in the posterior putamen (Fig. 372-3). Imaging can be useful in difficult cases or research studies but is rarely necessary in routine practice, as the diagnosis can usually be established on clinical criteria alone. This may change in the future when there is a disease-modifying therapy and it is important to make the diagnosis at as early a time

TABLE 372-1 Clinical Features of Parkinson's Disease

Cardinal Features	Other Motor Features	Nonmotor Features
Bradykinesia	Micrographia	Anosmia
Rest tremor	Masked facies (hypomimia) equalize	Sensory disturbances (e.g., pain)
Rigidity	Reduced eye blink	Mood disorders (e.g., depression)
Gait disturbance/ postural instability	Soft voice (hypophonia)	Sleep disturbances
	Dysphagia	Autonomic disturbances
	Freezing	Orthostatic hypotension
		Gastrointestinal disturbances
		Genitourinal disturbances
		Sexual dysfunction
		Cognitive impairment/Dementia

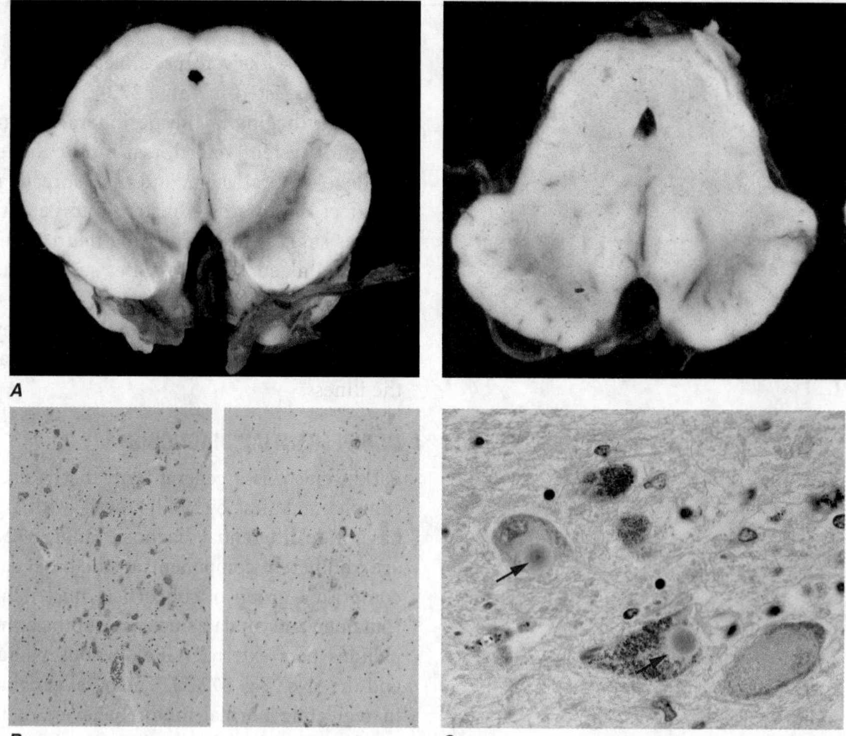

Figure 372-1 Pathologic specimens from a patient with Parkinson's disease (PD) compared to a normal control demonstrating (***A***) reduction of pigment in SNc in PD (right) vs control (left), (***B***) reduced numbers of cells in SNc in PD (right) compared to control (left), and (***C***) Lewy bodies (*arrows*) within melanized dopamine neurons in PD. SNc, substantia nigra pars compacta.

point as possible. Genetic testing is not generally employed at present, but it can be helpful for identifying at-risk individuals in a research setting. Mutations of the *LRRK2* gene (see below) have attracted particular interest as they are the commonest cause of familial PD and are responsible for approximately 1% of typical sporadic cases of the disease. Mutations in *LRRK2* are particularly common causes of PD in Ashkenazi Jews and North African Berber Arabs. The penetrance of the most common *LRRK2* mutation ranges from 28 to 74%, depending on age. Mutations in the *parkin* gene should be considered in patients with disease onset prior to 40 years.

Atypical and secondary parkinsonism

Atypical parkinsonism refers to a group of neurodegenerative conditions that usually are associated with more widespread neurodegeneration than is found in PD (often involvement of SNc and striatum and/or pallidum). As a group, they present with a parkinsonism (rigidity and bradykinesia) but typically have a slightly different clinical picture than PD, reflecting differences in underlying pathology. Parkinsonism in these conditions is often characterized by early speech and gait impairment, absence of rest tremor, no asymmetry, poor or no response to levodopa, and an aggressive clinical course. In the early stages, they may show some modest benefit from levodopa and be difficult to distinguish from PD. Neuroimaging of the dopamine system is usually not helpful, as several atypical parkinsonisms also have degeneration of dopamine neurons. Pathologically, neurodegeneration occurs without Lewy bodies (see below for individual conditions). Metabolic imaging of the basal ganglia/thalamus network may be helpful, reflecting a pattern of decreased activity in the GPi with increased activity in the thalamus, the reverse of what is seen in PD.

TABLE 372-2 Differential Diagnosis of Parkinsonism

Parkinson's Disease	Atypical Parkinsonisms	Secondary Parkinsonism	Other Neurodegenerative Disorders
Genetic	Multiple-system atrophy	Drug-induced	Wilson's disease
Sporadic	Cerebellar type (MSA-c)	Tumor	Huntington's disease
Dementia with Lewy bodies	Parkinson type (MSA-p)	Infection	Neurodegeneration with brain iron accumulation
	Progressive supranuclear palsy	Vascular	SCA 3 (spinocerebellar ataxia)
	Corticobasal ganglionic degeneration	Normal-pressure hydrocephalus	Fragile X–associated ataxia-tremor-parkinsonism
	Frontotemporal dementia	Trauma	Prion disease
		Liver failure	Dystonia-parkinsonism (DYT3)
		Toxins (e.g., carbon monoxide, manganese, MPTP, cyanide, hexane, methanol, carbon disulfide)	Alzheimer's disease with parkinsonism

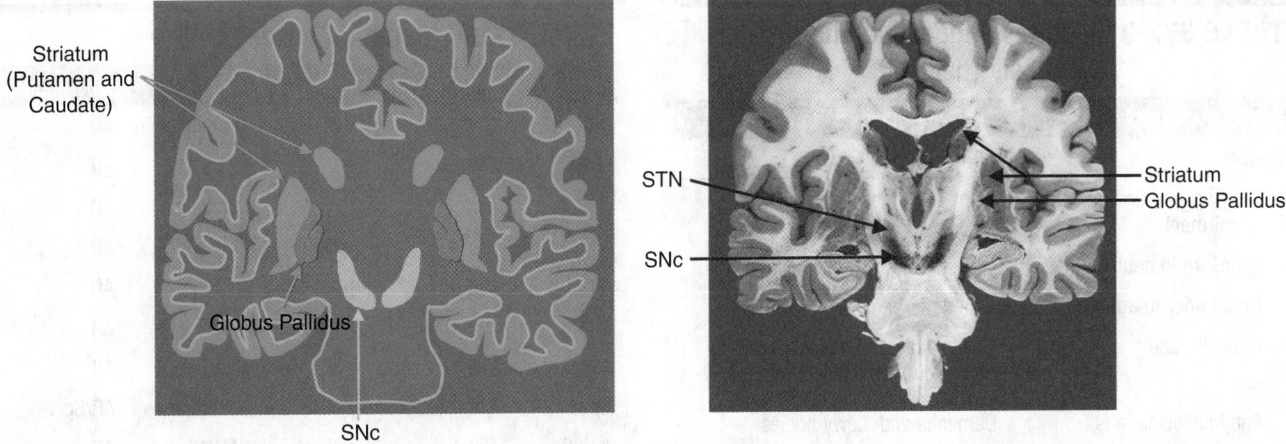

Figure 372-2 Basal ganglia nuclei. Schematic (***A***) and postmortem (***B***) coronal sections illustrating the various components of the basal ganglia. SNc, substantia nigra pars compacta; STN, subthalamic nucleus.

Multiple-system atrophy (MSA) manifests as a combination of parkinsonian, cerebellar, and autonomic features and can be divided into a predominant parkinsonian (MSA-p) or cerebellar (MSA-c) form. Clinically, MSA is suspected when a patient presents with atypical parkinsonism in conjunction with cerebellar signs and/or early and prominent autonomic dysfunction, usually orthostatic hypotension (Chap. 375). Pathologically, MSA is characterized by degeneration of the SNc, striatum, cerebellum, and inferior olivary nuclei coupled with characteristic glial cytoplasmic inclusions (GCIs) that stain for α-synuclein. MRI can show pathologic iron accumulation in the striatum on T2-weighted scans, high signal change in the region of the external surface of the putamen (putaminal rim) in MSA-p, or cerebellar and brainstem atrophy [the pontine "hot cross buns" sign (Fig. 375-2)] in MSA-c.

Progressive supranuclear palsy (PSP) is a form of atypical parkinsonism that is characterized by slow ocular saccades, eyelid apraxia, and restricted eye movements with particular impairment of downward gaze. Patients frequently experience hyperextension of the neck with early gait disturbance and falls. In later stages, speech and swallowing difficulty and dementia become evident. MRI may reveal a characteristic atrophy of the midbrain with relative preservation of the pons (the "hummingbird sign" on midsagittal images). Pathologically, PSP is characterized by degeneration of the SNc and pallidum along with neurofibrillary tangles and GCIs that stain for tau.

Corticobasal ganglionic degeneration is less common and is usually manifest by asymmetric dystonic contractions and clumsiness of one hand coupled with cortical sensory disturbances manifest as apraxia, agnosia, focal myoclonus, or alien limb phenomenon (where the limb assumes a position in space without the patient being aware of it). Dementia may occur at any stage of the disease. MRI frequently shows asymmetric cortical atrophy. Pathologic findings include achromatic neuronal degeneration with tau deposits similar to those found in PSP.

Secondary parkinsonism can be associated with drugs, stroke, tumor, infection, or exposure to toxins such as carbon monoxide or manganese. Dopamine-blocking agents such as the neuroleptics are the commonest cause of secondary parkinsonism. These drugs are most widely used in psychiatry, but physicians should be aware that drugs such as metoclopramide and chlorperazine, which are primarily used to treat gastrointestinal problems, are also neuroleptic

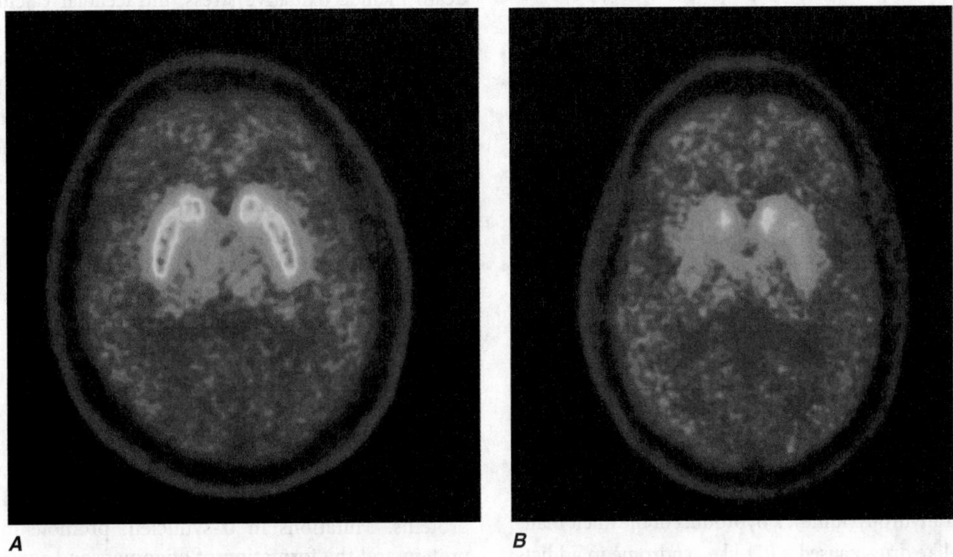

Figure 372-3 [^{11}C]dihydrotetrabenazine PET (a marker of VMAT2) in healthy control (*A*) and PD (*B*) patient. Note the reduced striatal uptake of tracer which is most pronounced in the posterior putamen and tends to be asymmetric. *(Courtesy of Dr. Jon Stoessl.)*

TABLE 372-3 Features Suggesting Alternate Diagnosis Than PD

Symptoms/Signs	Alternate Diagnosis to Consider
History	
Early speech and gait impairment	Atypical parkinsonism
Exposure to neuroleptics	Drug-induced parkinsonism
Onset prior to age 40	Genetic form of PD
Liver disease	Wilson's disease, non-Wilsonian hepatolenticular degeneration
Early hallucinations	Dementia with Lewy bodies
Diplopia	PSP
Poor or no response to an adequate trial of levodopa	Atypical or secondary parkinsonism
Physical Exam	
Dementia as first symptom	Dementia with Lewy bodies
Prominent orthostatic hypotension	MSA-p
Prominent cerebellar signs	MSA-c
Impairment of down gaze	PSP
High-frequency (8–10 Hz) symmetric postural tremor with a prominent kinetic component	Essential tremor

Abbreviations: MSA-c, multiple-system atrophy–cerebellar type; MSA-p, multiple-system atrophy–Parkinson type; PSP, progressive supranuclear palsy.

TABLE 372-4 Genetic Causes of PD

Name	Chromosome	Locus	Gene	Inheritance
Park 1	Chr 4	q21-23	α-Synuclein	AD
Park 2	Chr 6	q25-27	Parkin	AR
Park 3	Chr 2	p13	Unknown	AD
Park 4	Chr 4	q21-23	α-Synuclein	AD
Park 5	Chr 4	p14	UCHL-1	AD
Park 6	Chr 1	p35-36	PINK-1	AR
Park 7	Chr 1	p36	DJ-1	AR
Park 8	Chr 12	p11-q13	LRRK2	AR/Sp
Park 9	Chr 1	p36	ATP13A2	AR
Park 10	Chr 1	p32	Unknown	Sp
Park 11	Chr 2	q36-37	GIGYF2	AD
Park 12	Chr X	q21-25	Unknown	Sp
Park 13	Chr 2	p13	Omi/HtrA2	AD
Park 14	Chr 22	q13	PLA2G6	AR
Park 15	Chr 22	q12-13	FBX07	AR
Park 16	Chr 1	q32	Unknown	SP

Abbreviations: AD, autosomal dominant; AR, autosomal recessive; SP, sporadic.

agents and common causes of secondary parkinsonism and tardive dyskinesia. Other drugs that can cause secondary parkinsonism include tetrabenazine, amiodarone, and lithium.

Finally, parkinsonism can be seen as a feature of other degenerative disorders such as Wilson's disease, Huntington's disease (especially the juvenile form known as Westphal variant), dopa-responsive dystonia, and neurodegenerative disorders with brain iron accumulation such as pantothenate kinase (PANK)–associated neurodegeneration (formerly known as Hallervorden-Spatz disease).

Some features that suggest parkinsonism might be due to a condition other than PD are shown in Table 372-3.

ETIOLOGY AND PATHOGENESIS

Most PD cases occur sporadically (~85–90%) and are of unknown cause. Twin studies suggest that environmental factors likely play the more important role in patients older than 50 years, with genetic factors being more important in younger patients. Epidemiologic studies suggest increased risk with exposure to pesticides, rural living, and drinking well water and reduced risk with cigarette smoking and caffeine. However, no environmental factor has yet been determined to cause PD. The environmental hypothesis received a boost with the demonstration in the 1980s that MPTP (1-methyl-4-phenyl-1,2,5,6-tetrahydropyridine), a byproduct of the illicit manufacture of a heroin-like drug, caused a PD-like syndrome in addicts in northern California. MPTP is transported to the central nervous system, where it is metabolized to form MPP^+, a mitochondrial toxin that is selectively taken up by, and damages, dopamine neurons. However, MPTP or MPTP-like compounds have not been linked to sporadic PD. MPTP has, however, proved useful for generating an animal model of the disease. About 10–15% of cases are familial in origin, and multiple specific mutations and gene associations have been identified (Table 372-4). It has been proposed that most cases of PD are due to a "double hit" involving an interaction between a gene mutation that induces susceptibility coupled with exposure to a toxic environmental factor. In this scenario, both factors are required for PD to ensue, while the presence of either one alone is not sufficient to cause the disease.

Factors that have been implicated in the pathogenesis of cell death include oxidative stress, intracellular calcium accumulation with excitotoxicity, inflammation, mitochondrial dysfunction, and proteolytic stress. Whatever the pathogenic mechanism, cell death appears to occur, at least in part, by way of a signal-mediated apoptotic or "suicidal" process. Each of these mechanisms offer potential targets for neuroprotective drugs. However, it is not clear which of these factors is primary, if the cause is the same in each case, or if one or all merely represent epiphenomena unrelated to the true cause of cell death that remains undiscovered (Fig. 372-4).

Gene mutations discovered to date have been helpful in pointing to specific pathogenic mechanisms as being central to the neurodegenerative process. The most significant of these mechanisms appear to be protein misfolding and accumulation and mitochondrial dysfunction. The idea that proteins are involved in the pathogenesis of PD is not surprising, given that PD is characterized by Lewy bodies and Lewy neurites, which are composed of misfolded and aggregated proteins (**Fig. 372-1**). Protein accumulation could result from either increased formation or impaired clearance of proteins. Mutations in α-synuclein promote misfolding of the protein and the formation of oligomers and aggregates thought to be involved in the cell death process. Importantly, duplication or triplication of the wild-type α-synuclein gene can itself cause PD,

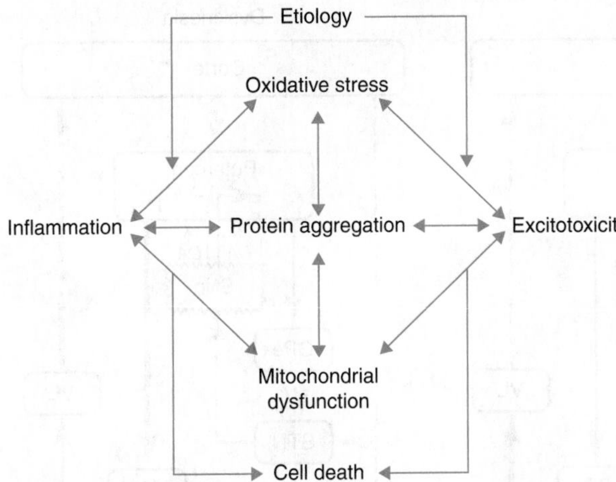

Figure 372-4 Schematic representation of how pathogenetic factors implicated in PD interact in a network manner, ultimately leading to cell death. This figure illustrates how interference with any one of these factors may not necessarily stop the cell death cascade. *(Adapted from CW Olanow: Movement Disorders, 22:S-335, 2007.)*

indicating that increased production of even the normal protein can cause PD. Increased levels of unwanted proteins could also result from impaired clearance. Proteins are normally cleared by the ubiquitin proteasome system or the autophagy/lysosome pathway. These pathways are defective in patients with sporadic PD, and interestingly α-synuclein is a prominent component of Lewy bodies in these cases. Further, mutations in parkin (a ubiquitin ligase that attaches ubiquitin to misfolded proteins to promote their transport to the proteasome for degradation) and UCH-L1 (which cleaves ubiquitin from misfolded proteins to permit their entry into the proteasome) are causative in other cases of familial PD. Collectively, these findings implicate abnormal protein accumulation in the etiology of PD. Indeed, in laboratory models both overexpression of α-synuclein or impairment of proteasomal clearance mechanisms leads to degeneration of dopamine neurons with inclusion body formation.

Mitochondrial dysfunction has also been implicated in familial PD. Several causative genes (*parkin*, *PINK1*, and *DJ1*) either localize to mitochondria and/or cause mitochondrial dysfunction in transgenic animals. Postmortem studies have also shown a defect in complex I of the respiratory chain in the SNc of patients with sporadic PD.

Six different *LRRK2* mutations have been linked to PD, with the Gly2019Ser being the commonest. The mechanism responsible for cell death with this mutation is not known but is thought to involve altered kinase activity.

Mutations in the glucocerebrosidase (GBA) gene associated with Gaucher's disease are also associated with an increased risk of idiopathic PD. Again the mechanism is not precisely known, but it is noteworthy that it is associated with altered autophagy and lysosomal function, suggesting that mutations in this gene might also impair protein clearance leading to PD.

Whole-genome association studies have provided conflicting results. Most recently, linkage to mutations in human leukocyte antigen (HLA) genes were identified in PD patients, suggesting that altered immunity or inflammation may be a causative or contributory factor.

While gene mutations account for only a small percentage of cases of PD, it is hoped that better understanding of the mechanisms whereby they cause cell death will provide insight into the nature of the cell death process in the more common sporadic form of the disease. These mutations could also permit the development of more relevant animal models of PD in which to test putative neuroprotective drugs.

PATHOPHYSIOLOGY OF PD

The classic model of basal ganglia functional organization in the normal and PD states is provided in Fig. 372-5. A series of neuronal loops link the basal ganglia nuclei with corresponding cortical motor regions in a somatotopic manner to help regulate motor function. The striatum is the major input region of the basal ganglia, while the GPi and SNr are the major output regions. The input and output regions are connected via direct and indirect pathways that have reciprocal effects on the output pathway. The output of the basal ganglia provides inhibitory tone to thalamic and brainstem neurons that in turn connect to motor systems in the cerebral cortex and spinal cord to regulate motor function. Dopaminergic projections from SNc neurons serve to modulate neuronal firing and to stabilize the basal ganglia network.

In PD, dopamine denervation leads to increased firing of neurons in the STN and GPi, resulting in excessive inhibition of the thalamus, reduced activation of cortical motor systems, and the development of parkinsonian features (**Fig. 372-5**). The current role of surgery in the treatment of PD is based upon this model, which predicted that lesions or high-frequency stimulation of the STN or GPi might reduce this neuronal overactivity and improve PD features.

TREATMENT Parkinson's Disease

LEVODOPA Since its introduction in the late 1960s, levodopa has been the mainstay of therapy for PD. Experiments in the late 1950s by Carlsson demonstrated that blocking dopamine uptake with reserpine caused rabbits to become parkinsonian; this could be reversed with the dopamine precursor, levodopa. Subsequently, Hornykiewicz demonstrated a dopamine deficiency in the striatum of PD patients and suggested the potential benefit of dopaminergic replacement therapy. Dopamine does not cross the blood-brain barrier (BBB), so clinical trials were initiated with levodopa, a precursor of dopamine. Studies over the course of the next decade confirmed the value of levodopa and revolutionized the treatment of PD.

Levodopa is routinely administered in combination with a peripheral decarboxylase inhibitor to prevent its peripheral metabolism to dopamine and the development of nausea and vomiting due to activation of dopamine receptors in the area postrema that are not protected by the BBB. In the United States, levodopa is combined with the decarboxylase inhibitor carbidopa (Sinemet), while in many other countries it is combined with benserazide (Madopar). Levodopa is also available in controlled-release formulations as well as in combination with a COMT inhibitor (see below). Levodopa remains the most effective symptomatic treatment for PD and the gold standard against which new therapies are compared. No current medical or surgical treatment provides antiparkinsonian benefits superior to what can be achieved with levodopa. Levodopa benefits the classic motor features of PD, prolongs independence and employability, improves quality of life, and increases life span. Almost all PD patients experience improvement, and failure to respond to an adequate trial should cause the diagnosis to be questioned.

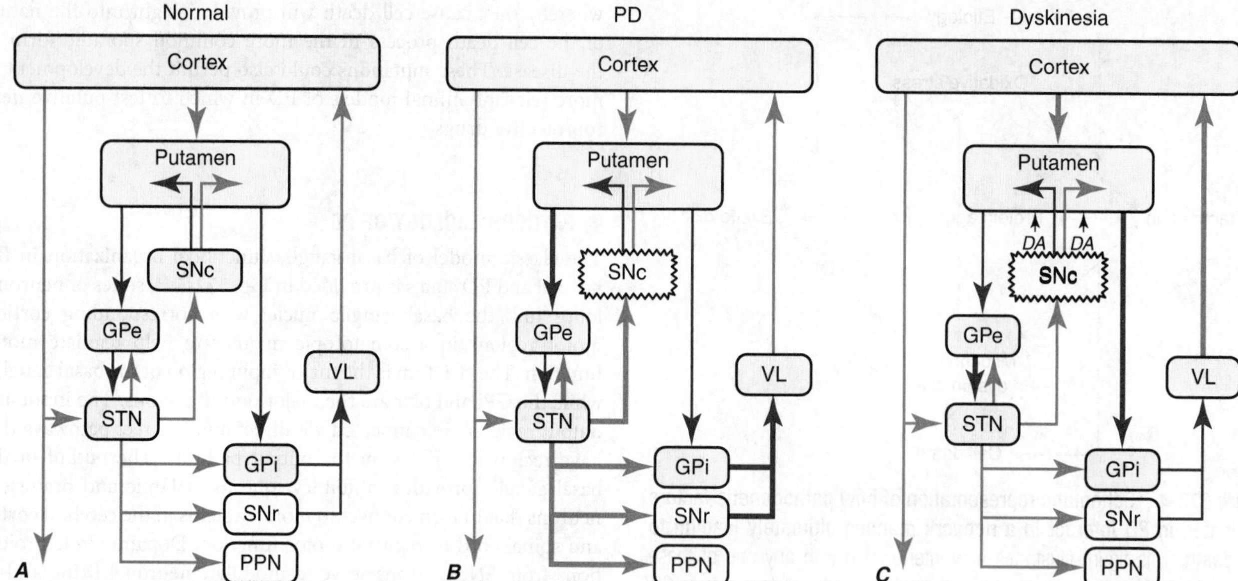

Figure 372-5 Basal ganglia organization. Classic model of the organization of the basal ganglia in the normal, PD, and levodopa-induced dyskinesia state. Inhibitory connections are shown as blue arrows and excitatory connections as red arrows. The striatum is the major input region and receives its major input from the cortex. The GPi and SNr are the major output regions and they project to the thalamocortical and brainstem motor regions. The striatum and GPi/SNr are connected by direct and indirect pathways. This model predicts that parkinsonism results from increased neuronal firing in the STN and GPi and that lesions or DBS of these targets might provide benefit. This concept led to the rationale for surgical therapies for PD. The model also predicts that dyskinesia results from decreased firing of the output regions, resulting in excessive cortical activation by the thalamus. This component of the model is not completely correct as lesions of the GPi ameliorate rather than increase dyskinesia in PD, suggesting that firing frequency is just one of the components that lead to the development of dyskinesia. DBS, deep brain stimulation; GPe, external segment of the globus pallidus; GPi, internal segment of the globus pallidus; SNr, substantia nigra, pars reticulata; SNc, substantia nigra, pars compacta; STN, subthalamic nucleus; VL, ventrolateral thalamus; PPN, pedunculopontine nucleus. *(Derived from JA Obeso et al: Trends Neurosci 23:S8, 2000.)*

There are, however, important limitations of levodopa therapy. Acute dopaminergic side effects include nausea, vomiting, and orthostatic hypotension. These are usually transient and can generally be avoided by gradual titration. If they persist, they can be treated with additional doses of a peripheral decarboxylase inhibitor (e.g., carbidopa) or a peripheral dopamine-blocking agent such as domperidone (not available in the United States). More important are motor complications (see below) that develop in the majority of patients treated long-term with levodopa therapy. In addition, features such as falling, freezing, autonomic dysfunction, sleep disorders, and dementia may emerge that are not adequately controlled by levodopa. Indeed, these nondopaminergic features are the primary source of disability and main reason for nursing home placement for patients with advanced PD.

Levodopa-induced motor complications consist of fluctuations in motor response and involuntary movements known as dyskinesias (Fig. 372-6). When patients initially take levodopa,

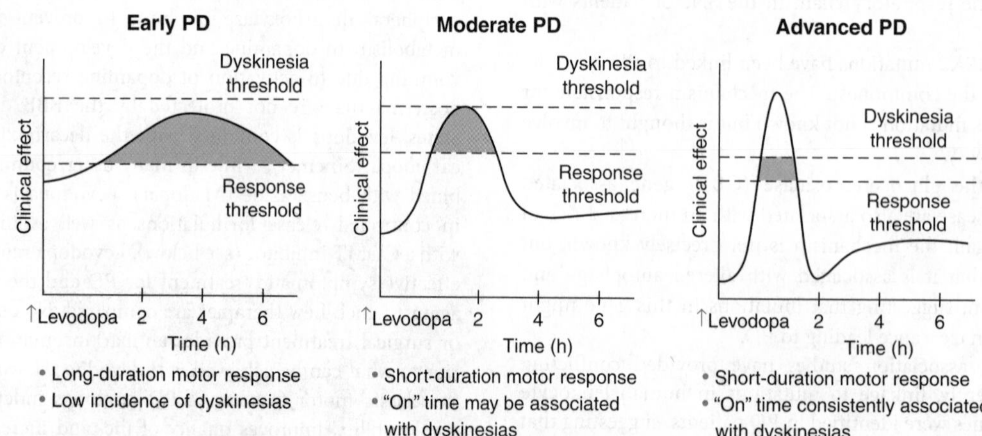

Figure 372-6 Changes in motor response associated with chronic levodopa treatment. Levodopa-induced motor complications. Schematic illustration of the gradual shortening of the duration of a beneficial motor response to levodopa (wearing off) and the appearance of dyskinesias complicating "on" time.

benefits are long-lasting (many hours) even though the drug has a relatively short half-life (60–90 minutes). With continued treatment, however, the duration of benefit following an individual dose becomes progressively shorter until it approaches the half-life of the drug. This loss of benefit is known as the *wearing-off effect*. At the same time, many patients develop dyskinesias. These tend to occur at the time of maximal clinical benefit and peak plasma concentration (peak-dose dyskinesia). They are usually choreiform in nature but can manifest as dystonia, myoclonus, or other movement disorders. They are not troublesome when mild, but can be disabling when severe and can limit the ability to fully utilize levodopa to control PD features. In more advanced states, patients may cycle between "on" periods complicated by disabling dyskinesias and "off" periods in which they suffer severe parkinsonism. Patients may also experience "diphasic dyskinesias," which occur as the levodopa dose begins to take effect and again as it wears off. These dyskinesias typically consist of transient, stereotypic, rhythmic movements that predominantly involve the lower extremities and are frequently associated with parkinsonism in other body regions. They can be relieved by increasing the dose of levodopa, although higher doses may induce more severe peak-dose dyskinesia.

The cause of levodopa-induced motor complications is not precisely known. They are more likely to occur in young individuals with severe disease and with higher doses of levodopa. The classic model of the basal ganglia has been useful for understanding the origin of motor features in PD, but has proved less valuable for understanding levodopa-induced dyskinesias (Fig. 372-5). The model predicts that dopamine replacement might excessively inhibit the pallidal output system, thereby leading to increased thalamocortical activity, enhanced stimulation of cortical motor regions, and the development of dyskinesia. However, lesions of the pallidum that completely destroy its output are associated with amelioration rather than induction of dyskinesia as suggested by the classic model. It is now thought that dyskinesia results from levodopa-induced alterations in the GPi neuronal firing pattern (pauses, bursts, synchrony, etc.) and not simply the firing frequency alone. This in turn leads to the transmission of misinformation from pallidum to thalamus/cortex, resulting in dyskinesia. Pallidotomy might thus ameliorate dyskinesia by blocking this abnormal firing pattern and preventing the transfer of misinformation to motor systems.

Current information suggests that altered neuronal firing patterns and motor complications relate to nonphysiologic levodopa replacement. Striatal dopamine levels are normally maintained at a relatively constant level. In the PD state, dopamine neurons degenerate and striatal dopamine is dependent on peripheral availability of levodopa. Intermittent doses of short-acting levodopa do not restore dopamine in a physiologic manner and cause dopamine receptors to be exposed to alternating high and low concentrations of dopamine. This intermittent or pulsatile stimulation of dopamine receptors induces molecular changes in striatal neurons and neurophysiologic changes in pallidal neurons, leading to the development of motor complications. It has been hypothesized that more continuous delivery of levodopa might prevent the development of motor complications. Indeed, continuous levodopa infusion is associated with improvement in both "off" time and dyskinesia in advanced PD patients, but this approach has not yet been proved to prevent dyskinesia in clinical trials.

Behavioral alterations can be encountered in levodopa-treated patients. A dopamine dysregulation syndrome has been described where patients have a craving for levodopa and take frequent and unnecessary doses of the drug in an addictive manner. PD patients taking high doses of levodopa can also have purposeless, stereotyped behaviors such as the meaningless assembly and disassembly or collection and sorting of objects. This is known as punding, a term taken from the Swedish description of the meaningless behaviors seen in chronic amphetamine users. Hypersexuality and other impulse-control disorders are occasionally encountered with levodopa, although these are more commonly seen with dopamine agonists.

DOPAMINE AGONISTS Dopamine agonists are a diverse group of drugs that act directly on dopamine receptors. Unlike levodopa, they do not require metabolism to an active product and do not undergo oxidative metabolism. Initial dopamine agonists were ergot derivatives (e.g., bromocriptine, pergolide, cabergoline) and were associated with ergot-related side effects, including cardiac valvular damage. They have largely been replaced by a second generation of non-ergot dopamine agonists (e.g., pramipexole, ropinirole, rotigotine). In general, dopamine agonists do not have comparable efficacy to levodopa. They were initially introduced as adjuncts to levodopa to enhance motor function and reduce "off" time in fluctuating patients. Subsequently, it was shown that dopamine agonists, possibly because they are relatively long-acting, are less prone than levodopa to induce dyskinesia. For this reason, many physicians initiate therapy with a dopamine agonist, although supplemental levodopa is eventually required in virtually all patients. Both ropinirole and pramipexole are available as orally administered immediate (tid) and extended-release (qd) formulations. Rotigotine is administered as a once-daily transdermal patch. Apomorphine is a dopamine agonist with efficacy comparable to levodopa, but it must be administered parenterally and has a very short half-life and duration of activity (45 min). It is generally administered SC as a rescue agent for the treatment of severe "off" episodes. Apomorphine can also be administered by continuous infusion and has been demonstrated to reduce both "off" time and dyskinesia in advanced patients. However, infusions are cumbersome, and this approach has not been approved in the United States.

Acute side effects of dopamine agonists include nausea, vomiting, and orthostatic hypotension. As with levodopa, these can usually be avoided by slow titration. Hallucinations and cognitive impairment are more common with dopamine agonists than with levodopa. Sedation with sudden unintended episodes of falling asleep while driving a motor vehicle have been reported. Patients should be informed about this potential problem and should not drive when tired. Injections of apomorphine and patch delivery of rotigotine can be complicated by development of skin lesions at sites of administration. Recently, it has become appreciated that dopamine agonists are associated with impulse-control disorders, including pathologic gambling, hypersexuality, and compulsive eating and shopping. The precise cause of these problems, and why they appear to occur more frequently with dopamine agonists than levodopa, remains to be resolved, but reward systems associated with dopamine and alterations in the ventral striatum have been implicated.

MAO-B INHIBITORS Inhibitors of monoamine oxidase type B (MAO-B) block central dopamine metabolism and increase synaptic concentrations of the neurotransmitter. Selegiline and rasagiline are relatively selective suicide inhibitors of the MAO-B enzyme. Clinically, MAO-B inhibitors provide modest antiparkinsonian benefits when used as monotherapy in early disease, and reduced "off" time when used as an adjunct to levodopa in patients with motor fluctuations. MAO-B inhibitors are generally safe and well tolerated. They may increase dyskinesia in levodopa-treated patients but this can usually be controlled by down-titrating the dose of levodopa. Inhibition of the MAO-A isoform prevents metabolism of tyramine in the gut, leading to a potentially fatal hypertensive reaction known as a "cheese effect" as it can be precipitated by foods rich in tyramine such as some cheeses, aged meats, and red wine. Selegiline and rasagiline do not functionally inhibit MAO-A in doses employed in clinical practice and are not associated with a cheese effect. There are theoretical risks of a serotonin reaction in patients receiving concomitant SSRI antidepressants, but these are rarely encountered.

Interest in MAO-B inhibitors has also focused on their potential to have disease-modifying effects. MPTP toxicity can be prevented by coadministration of a MAO-B inhibitor that blocks its conversion to the toxic pyridinium ion MPP^+. MAO-B inhibitors also have the potential to block the oxidative metabolism of dopamine and prevent oxidative stress. In addition, both selegiline and rasagiline incorporate a propargyl ring within their molecular structure that provides antiapoptotic effects in laboratory models. The DATATOP study showed that selegiline significantly delayed the time until the emergence of disability, necessitating the introduction of levodopa in untreated PD patients. However, it could not be determined whether this was due to a neuroprotective effect that slowed disease progression or a symptomatic effect that merely masked ongoing neurodegeneration. More recently, the ADAGIO study demonstrated that early treatment with rasagiline 1 mg/d but not 2 mg/d provided benefits that could not be achieved with delayed treatment with the same drug, consistent with a disease-modifying effect; however, the long-term significance of these findings is uncertain.

COMT INHIBITORS When levodopa is administered with a decarboxylase inhibitor, it is primarily metabolized by catechol-*O*-methyltransferase (COMT). Inhibitors of COMT increase the elimination half-life of levodopa and enhance its brain availability. Combining levodopa with a COMT inhibitor reduces "off" time and prolongs "on" time in fluctuating patients while enhancing motor scores. Two COMT inhibitors have been approved, tolcapone and entacapone. There is also a combination tablet of levodopa, carbidopa, and entacapone (Stalevo).

Side effects of COMT inhibitors are primarily dopaminergic (nausea, vomiting, increased dyskinesia) and can usually be controlled by down-titrating the dose of levodopa by 20–30%. Severe diarrhea has been described with tolcapone, and to a lesser degree with entacapone, and necessitates stopping the medication in 5–10% of individuals. Cases of fatal hepatic toxicity have been reported with tolcapone, and periodic monitoring of liver function is required. This problem has not been encountered with entacapone. Discoloration of urine can be seen with both COMT inhibitors due to accumulation of a metabolite, but it is of no clinical concern.

It has been proposed that initiating levodopa in combination with a COMT inhibitor to enhance its elimination half-life will provide more continuous levodopa delivery and reduce the risk of motor complications. While this result has been demonstrated in parkinsonian monkeys, and continuous infusion reduces "off" time and dyskinesia in advanced patients, no benefit of initiating levodopa with a COMT inhibitor compared to levodopa alone was detected in early PD patients in the STRIDE-PD study, and the main value of COMT inhibitors for now continues to be in patients who experience motor fluctuations.

OTHER MEDICAL THERAPIES Central-acting anticholinergic drugs such as trihexyphenidyl and benztropine were used historically for the treatment for PD, but they lost favor with the introduction of dopaminergic agents. Their major clinical effect is on tremor, although it is not certain that this is superior to what can be obtained with agents such as levodopa and dopamine agonists. Still, they can be helpful in individual patients. Their use is limited particularly in the elderly, due to their propensity to induce a variety of side effects including urinary dysfunction, glaucoma, and particularly cognitive impairment.

Amantadine also has historical importance. Originally introduced as an antiviral agent, it was appreciated to also have antiparkinsonian effects that are now thought to be due to NMDA-receptor antagonism. While some physicians use amantadine in patients with early disease for its mild symptomatic effects, it is most widely used as an antidyskinesia agent in patients with advanced PD. Indeed, it is the only oral agent that has been demonstrated in controlled studies to reduce dyskinesia while improving parkinsonian features, although benefits may be relatively transient. Side effects include livido reticularis, weight gain, and impaired cognitive function. Amantadine should always be discontinued gradually as patients can experience withdrawal symptoms.

A list of the major drugs and available dosage strengths is provided in Table 372-5.

NEUROPROTECTION Despite the many therapeutic agents available for the treatment of PD, patients can still experience intolerable disability due to disease progression and the emergence of features such as falling and dementia that are not controlled with dopaminergic therapies. Trials of several promising agents such as rasagiline, selegiline, coenzyme Q10, pramipexole, and ropinirole have had positive results in clinical trials consistent with disease-modifying effects. However, it is not possible to determine if the positive results are due to neuroprotection with slowed disease progression or confounding symptomatic or pharmacologic effects that mask ongoing progression. If it could be determined that a drug slowed disease progression, this would be a major advance in the treatment of PD.

SURGICAL TREATMENT Surgical treatments for PD have been employed for more than a century. Lesions placed in the motor cortex improved tremor, but were associated with motor deficits and this approach was abandoned. Subsequently, it was appreciated that lesions placed into the VIM nucleus of the thalamus reduced contralateral tremor without inducing hemiparesis, but these lesions did not meaningfully help other more disabling features of PD. Lesions placed in the GPi improved rigidity and bradykinesia as well as tremor, particularly if placed in the posteroventral portion of the nucleus. Importantly, pallidotomy was also associated with marked improvement in contralateral dyskinesia. This procedure gained favor with greater understanding of the pathophysiology of PD (see above). However, this procedure is not optimal for patients with bilateral disease, as bilateral lesions are associated with side effects such as dysphagia, dysarthria, and impaired cognition.

Most surgical procedures for PD performed today utilize deep brain stimulation (DBS). Here, an electrode is placed into the target area and connected to a stimulator inserted SC over the chest wall. DBS simulates the effects of a lesion without necessitating a brain lesion. The stimulation variables can be adjusted

TABLE 372-5 Drugs Commonly Used for Treatment of PD*

Agent	Available Dosages	Typical Dosing
Levodopa*		
Carbidopa/levodopa	10/100, 25/100, 25/250	200–1000 mg levodopa/d 2–4 times/d
Benserazide/levodopa	25/100, 50/200	
Carbidopa/ levodopa CR	25/100, 50/200	
Benserazide/ levodopa MDS	25/200, 25/250	
Parcopa	10/100, 25/100, 25/250	
Carbidopa/levodopa/ entacapone	12.5/50/200, 18.75/75/200, 25/100/200, 31.25/125/200, 37.5/150/200, 50/200/200	
Dopamine agonists		
Pramipexole	0.125, 0.25, 0.5, 1.0, 1.5 mg	0.25–1.0 mg tid
Pramipexole ER	0.375, 0.75, 1.5. 3.0, 4.5 mg	1–3 mg/d
Ropinirole	0.25, 0.5, 1.0, 3.0 mg	6–24 mg/d
Ropinirole XL	2, 4, 6, 8	6–24 mg/d
Rotigotine patch	2-, 4-, 6-mg patches	4–10 mg/d
Apomorphine SC		2–8 mg
COMT Inhibitors		
Entacapone	200 mg	200 mg with each levodopa dose
Tolcapone	100, 200 mg	100–200 mg tid
MAO-B Inhibitors		
Selegiline	5 mg	5 mg bid
Rasagiline	0.5, 1.0 mg	1.0 mg QAM

*Treatment should be individualized. Generally, drugs should be started in low doses and titrated to optimal dose.

Note: Drugs should not be withdrawn abruptly but should be gradually lowered or removed as appropriate.

Abbreviations: COMT, catechol-*O*-methyltransferase; MAO-B, monoamine oxidase type B.

with respect to electrode configuration, voltage, frequency, and pulse duration in order to maximize benefit and minimize adverse side effects. In cases with intolerable side effects, stimulation can be stopped and the system removed. The procedure has the advantage that it does not require making a lesion in the brain and is thus suitable for performing bilateral procedures with relative safety.

DBS for PD primarily targets the STN or the GPi. It provides dramatic results, particularly with respect to "off" time and dyskinesias, but does not improve features that fail to respond to levodopa and does not prevent the development or progression of nondopaminergic features such as freezing, falling, and dementia. The procedure is thus primarily indicated for patients who suffer disability resulting from levodopa-induced motor complications that cannot be satisfactorily controlled with drug manipulation. Side effects can be seen with respect to the surgical procedure (hemorrhage, infarction, infection), the DBS system (infection, lead break, lead displacement, skin ulceration), or stimulation (ocular and speech abnormalities, muscle twitches, paresthesias, depression, and rarely suicide). Recent studies indicate that benefits following DBS of the STN and GPi are comparable, but that GPi stimulation may be associated with a reduced frequency of depression. While not all PD patients are candidates, the procedure is profoundly beneficial for many. Research studies are currently examining additional targets that might benefit gait dysfunction, depression, and cognitive impairment in PD patients.

EXPERIMENTAL SURGICAL THERAPIES FOR PD There has been considerable scientific and public interest in a number of novel therapies as possible treatments for PD. These include cell-based therapies (such as transplantation of fetal nigral dopamine cells or dopamine neurons derived from stem cells), gene therapies, and trophic factors. Transplant strategies are based on implanting dopaminergic cells into the striatum to replace degenerating SNc dopamine neurons. Fetal nigral mesencephalic cells have been demonstrated to survive implantation, reinnervate the striatum in an organotypic manner, and restore motor function in PD models. Several open-label studies reported positive results. However, two double-blind, sham surgery–controlled studies failed to show significant benefit of fetal nigral transplantation in comparison to a sham operation with respect to their primary endpoints. Post hoc analyses showed possible benefits in patients aged <60 years and in those with milder disease. It is now appreciated that grafting of fetal nigral cells is associated with a previously unrecognized form of dyskinesia that persists even after lowering or stopping levodopa. In addition, there is evidence that after many years, transplanted healthy embryonic dopamine neurons from unrelated donors can develop PD pathology, suggesting that they somehow became affected by the disease process. Most importantly, it is not clear how replacing dopamine cells alone will improve nondopaminergic features such as falling and dementia, which are the major sources of disability for patients with advanced disease. These same concerns apply to dopamine neurons derived from stem cells, which have not yet been tested in PD patients, and bear the additional theoretical concern of unanticipated side effects such as tumors. The short-term future for this technology as a treatment for PD, at least in its current state, is therefore not promising.

Gene therapy involves viral vector delivery of the DNA of a therapeutic protein to specific target regions. The DNA of the therapeutic protein can then be incorporated into the genome of host cells and thereby, in principle, provide continuous and long-lasting delivery of the therapeutic molecule. The AAV2 virus has been most often used as the viral vector because it does not promote an inflammatory response, is not incorporated into the host genome, and is associated with long-lasting transgene expression. Studies performed to date in PD have delivered aromatic amino acid decarboxylase with or without tyrosine hydroxylase to the striatum to facilitate dopamine production; glutamic acid decarboxylase to the STN to inhibit overactive neuronal firing in this nucleus; and trophic factors such as GDNF (glial-derived neurotrophic factor) and neurturin to the striatum to enhance and protect residual dopamine neurons in the SNc by way of retrograde transmission. Positive results have been reported with open-label studies, but these have not yet been confirmed in double-blind trials. While gene delivery technology has great potential, this approach also carries the risk of possible unanticipated side effects, and current approaches also do not address the nondopaminergic features of the illness.

MANAGEMENT OF THE NONMOTOR AND NONDOPAMINERGIC FEATURES OF PD While most attention has focused on the dopaminergic features of PD, management of the nondopaminergic features of the illness should not be ignored. Some nonmotor features, while not thought to reflect dopaminergic pathology, nonetheless benefit from dopaminergic drugs. For example, problems such as anxiety, panic attacks, depression, sweating, sensory problems, freezing, and constipation all tend to be worse during "off" periods, and they improve with better dopaminergic control of the underlying PD state. Approximately 50% of PD patients suffer depression during the course of the disease that is frequently underdiagnosed and undertreated. Antiparkinsonian agents can help, but antidepressants should not be withheld, particularly for patients with major depression. Serotonin syndromes have been a theoretical concern with the combined use of selective serotonin reuptake inhibitors (SSRIs) and MAO-B inhibitors, but are rarely encountered. Anxiety can be treated with short-acting benzodiazepines.

Psychosis can be a major problem in PD. In contrast to AD, hallucinations are typically visual, formed, and nonthreatening and can limit the use of dopaminergic agents to adequately control PD features. Psychosis in PD often responds to low doses of atypical neuroleptics. Clozapine is the most effective, but it can be associated with agranulocytosis, and regular monitoring is required. For this reason, many physicians start with quetiapine even though it is not as effective as clozapine in controlled trials. Hallucinations in PD patients are often a harbinger of a developing dementia.

Dementia in PD (PDD) is common, affecting as many as 80% of patients. Its frequency increases with aging and, in contrast to AD, primarily affects executive functions and attention, with relative sparing of language, memory, and calculations. PDD is the commonest cause of nursing home placement for PD patients. When dementia precedes, or develops within 1 year after, the onset of motor dysfunction, it is by convention referred to as dementia with Lewy bodies (DLB; Chap. 371). These patients are particularly prone to have hallucinations and diurnal fluctuations. Pathologically, DLB is characterized by Lewy bodies distributed throughout the cerebral cortex (especially the hippocampus and amygdala). It is likely that DLB and PDD represent a PD spectrum rather than separate disease entities. Levodopa and other dopaminergic drugs can aggravate cognitive function in demented patients and should be stopped or reduced to try and provide a compromise between antiparkinsonian benefit and preserved cognitive function. Drugs are usually discontinued in the following sequence: anticholinergics, amantadine, dopamine agonists, COMT inhibitors, and MAO-B inhibitors. Eventually, patients with cognitive impairment should be managed with the lowest dose of standard levodopa that provides meaningful antiparkinsonian effects and does not aggravate mental function. Anticholinesterase agents such as rivastigmine and donepezil reduce the rate of deterioration of measures of cognitive function in controlled studies and can improve attention. Memantine, an antiglutamatergic agent, may also provide benefit for some PDD patients.

Autonomic disturbances are common and frequently require attention. Orthostatic hypotension can be problematic and contribute to falling. Initial treatment should include adding salt to the diet and elevating the head of the bed to prevent overnight sodium natriuresis. Low doses of fludrocortisol (Florinef) or midodrine control most cases. Vasopressin, erythropoietin, and the norepinephrine precursor 3-0-methylDOPS can be used in severe cases. If orthostatic hypotension is prominent in early disease, MSA should be considered. Sexual dysfunction can be helped with sildenafil or tadalafil. Urinary problems, especially in males, should be treated in consultation with a urologist to exclude prostate problems. Cholinergic agents, such as Ditropan, that promote bladder contraction may be helpful. Constipation can be a very important problem for PD patients. Mild laxatives can be useful, but physicians should first ensure that patients are drinking adequate amounts of fluid and consuming a diet rich in bulk with green leafy vegetables and bran. Agents that promote GI motility can also be helpful.

Sleep disturbances are common in PD patients, with many experiencing fragmented sleep with excess daytime sleepiness. Restless leg syndrome, sleep apnea, and other sleep disorders should be treated as appropriate. REM behavior disorder (RBD) may precede the onset of motor features. This syndrome is composed of violent movements and vocalizations during REM sleep, possibly representing acting out of dreams due to a failure of the normal inhibition of motor movements that typically accompanies REM sleep. Low doses of clonazepam are usually effective in controlling this problem. Consultation with a sleep specialist and polysomnography may be necessary to identify and optimally treat sleep problems.

NONPHARMACOLOGIC THERAPY Gait dysfunction with falling is an important cause of disability in PD. Dopaminergic therapies can help patients whose gait is worse in "off" time, but there are currently no specific therapies available. Canes and walkers may become necessary.

Freezing episodes, where patients freeze in place for seconds to minutes, are another cause of falling. Freezing during "off" periods may respond to dopaminergic therapies, but there are no specific treatments for "on" period freezing. Some patients will respond to sensory cues such as marching in place, singing a song, or stepping over an imaginary line.

Exercise, with a full range of active and passive movements, has been shown to improve and maintain function for PD patients. It is less clear that formal physical therapy is necessary, unless there is a specific indication. It is important for patients to maintain social and intellectual activities to the extent possible. Education, assistance with financial planning, social services, and attention to home safety are important elements of the overall care plan. Information is available through numerous PD foundations and on the web, but should be reviewed with physicians to ensure accuracy. The needs of the caregiver should not be neglected. Caring for a person with PD involves a substantial work effort and there is an increased incidence of depression among caregivers. Support groups for patients and caregivers may be useful.

CURRENT MANAGEMENT OF PD The management of PD should be tailored to the needs of the individual patient, and there is no single treatment approach that is universally accepted. Clearly,

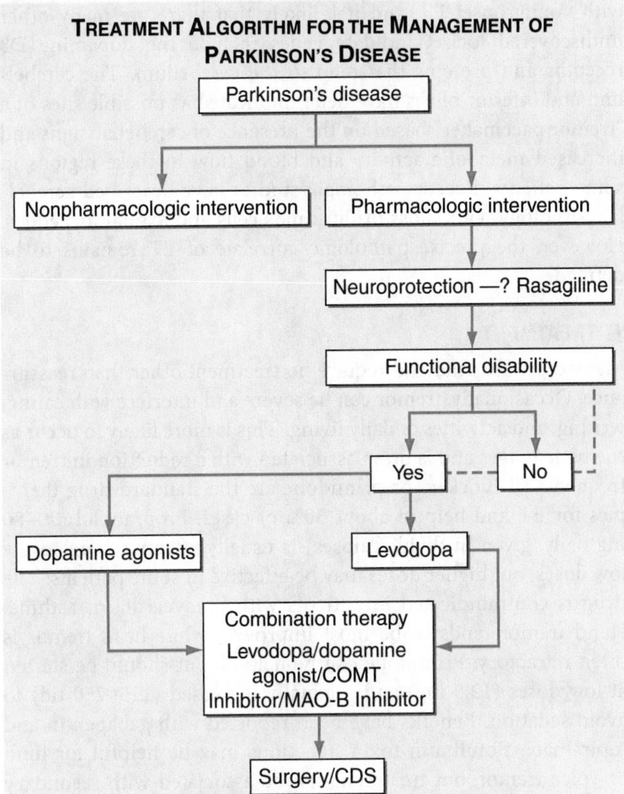

Figure 372-7 Treatment options for the management of PD. Decision points include:

a. Introduction of a neuroprotective therapy: No drug has been established to have or is currently approved for neuroprotection or disease modification, but there are several agents that have this potential based on laboratory and preliminary clinical studies (e.g., rasagiline 1 mg/d, coenzyme Q10 1200 mg/d, the dopamine agonists ropinirole and pramipexole).

b. When to initiate symptomatic therapy: There is a trend toward initiating therapy at the time of diagnosis or early in the course of the disease because patients may have some disability even at an early stage, and there is the possibility that early treatment may preserve beneficial compensatory mechanisms; however, some experts recommend waiting until there is functional disability before initiating therapy.

c. What therapy to initiate: Many experts favor starting with an MAO-B inhibitor in mildly affected patients because of the potential for a disease-modifying effect; dopamine agonists for younger patients with functionally significant disability to reduce the risk of motor complications; and levodopa for patients with more advanced disease, the elderly, or those with cognitive impairment.

d. Management of motor complications: Motor complications are typically approached with combination therapy to try and reduce dyskinesia and enhance the "on" time. When medical therapies cannot provide satisfactory control, surgical therapies can be considered.

e. Nonpharmacologic approaches: Interventions such as exercise, education, and support should be considered throughout the course of the disease.

Source: Adapted from CW Olanow et al: Neurology 72:S1, 2009.

if an agent could be demonstrated to have disease-modifying effects, it should be initiated at the time of diagnosis. Indeed, constipation, REM behavior disorder, and anosmia may represent pre-motor features of PD and could permit the initiation of a disease-modifying therapy even prior to onset of the classical motor features of the disease. However, no therapy has yet been proved to be disease-modifying. For now, physicians must use their judgment in deciding whether or not to introduce rasagiline (see above) or other drugs for their possible disease-modifying effects.

The next important issue to address is when to initiate symptomatic therapy. Several studies now suggest that it may be best to start therapy at the time of diagnosis in order to preserve beneficial compensatory mechanisms and possibly provide functional benefits even in the early stage of the disease. Levodopa remains the most effective symptomatic therapy for PD, and some recommend starting it immediately using relatively low doses, but many others prefer to delay levodopa treatment, particularly in younger patients, in order to reduce the risk of motor complications. Another approach is to begin with an MAO-B inhibitor and/or a dopamine agonist, and reserve levodopa for later stages when these drugs can no longer provide satisfactory control. In making this decision, the age, degree of disability, and side-effect profile of the drug must all be considered. In patients with more severe disability, the elderly, those with cognitive impairment, or where the diagnosis is uncertain, most physicians would initiate therapy with levodopa. Regardless of initial choice, it is important not to deny patients levodopa when they cannot be adequately controlled with alternative medications.

If motor complications develop, they can initially be treated by manipulating the frequency and dose of levodopa or by combining lower doses of levodopa with a dopamine agonist, a COMT inhibitor, or an MAO-B inhibitor. Amantadine is the only drug that has been demonstrated to treat dyskinesia without worsening parkinsonism, but benefits may be short-lasting and there are important side effects. In severe cases, it is usually necessary to consider a surgical therapy such as DBS if the patient is a suitable candidate, but as described above, these procedures have their own set of complications. There are ongoing efforts aimed at developing a long-acting oral or transdermal formulation of levodopa that mirrors the pharmacokinetic properties of a levodopa infusion. Such a formulation might provide all of the benefits of levodopa without motor complications and avoid the need for polypharmacy and surgical intervention.

A decision tree that considers the various treatment options and decision points for the management of PD is provided in Fig. 372-7.

HYPERKINETIC MOVEMENT DISORDERS

Hyperkinetic movement disorders are characterized by involuntary movements that may occur in isolation or in combination (Table 372-6). The major hyperkinetic movement disorders and the diseases with which they are associated are considered in this section.

TREMOR

CLINICAL FEATURES

Tremor consists of alternating contractions of agonist and antagonist muscles in an oscillating, rhythmic manner. It can be most prominent at rest (rest tremor), on assuming a posture (postural tremor), or on actively reaching for a target (kinetic tremor). Tremor is also assessed based on distribution, frequency, and related neurologic dysfunction.

PD is characterized by a resting tremor, essential tremor (ET) by a postural tremor, and cerebellar disease by an intention or kinetic tremor. Normal individuals can have a physiologic tremor that

TABLE 372-6 Hyperkinetic Movement Disorders

Tremor	Rhythmic oscillation of a body part due to intermittent muscle contractions
Dystonia	Involuntary patterned sustained or repeated muscle contractions often associated with twisting movements and abnormal posture.
Athetosis	Slow, distal, writhing, involuntary movements with a propensity to affect the arms and hands
Chorea	Rapid, semipurposeful, graceful, dance-like nonpatterned involuntary movements involving distal or proximal muscle groups
Myoclonus	Sudden, brief (<100 ms), jerk-like, arrhythmic muscle twitches
Tic	Brief, repeated, stereotyped muscle contractions that are often suppressible. Can be simple and involve a single muscle group or complex and affect a range of motor activities

typically manifests as a mild, high-frequency, postural or action tremor that is usually of no clinical consequence and often is only appreciated with an accelerometer. An enhanced physiologic tremor (EPT) can be seen in up to 10% of the population, often in association with anxiety, fatigue, underlying metabolic disturbance (e.g., hyperthyroidism, electrolyte abnormalities), drugs (e.g., valproate, lithium), or toxins (e.g., alcohol). Treatment is initially directed to the control of any underlying disorder and, if necessary, can often be improved with a β blocker.

ET is the commonest movement disorder, affecting approximately 5–10 million persons in the United States. It can present in childhood, but dramatically increases in prevalence over the age of 70 years. ET is characterized by a high-frequency tremor (up to 11 Hz) that predominantly affects the upper extremities. The tremor is most often manifest as a postural or kinetic tremor. It is typically bilateral and symmetric, but may begin on one side and remain asymmetric. Patients with severe ET can have an intention tremor with overshoot and slowness of movement. Tremor involves the head in ~30% of cases, voice in ~20%, tongue in ~20%, face/jaw in ~10%, and lower limbs in ~10%. The tremor is characteristically improved by alcohol and worsened by stress. Subtle impairment of coordination or tandem walking may be present. Disturbances of hearing, cognition, and even olfaction have been described, but usually the neurologic examination is normal aside from tremor. The major differential is a dystonic tremor (see below) or PD. PD can usually be differentiated from ET based on the presence of bradykinesia, rigidity, micrographia, and other parkinsonian features. However, the examiner should be aware that PD patients may have a postural tremor and ET patients may develop a rest tremor. These typically begin after a latency of a few seconds (emergent tremor). The examiner must take care to differentiate the effect of tremor on measurement of tone in ET from the cog-wheel rigidity found in PD.

ETIOLOGY AND PATHOPHYSIOLOGY

The etiology and pathophysiology of ET are not known. Approximately 50% of cases have a positive family history with an autosomal dominant pattern of inheritance. Linkage studies have detected loci at chromosomes 3q13 (ETM-1), 2p22-25 (ETM-2), and 6p23 (ETM-3). Recent genomewide studies demonstrate an association with the *LINGO1* gene, particularly in patients with young-onset ET, and it is likely that there are many other undiscovered loci. Candidate genes include the dopamine D3 receptor and proteins that map to the cerebellum. The cerebellum and inferior olives have been implicated as possible sites of a "tremor pacemaker" based on the presence of cerebellar signs and increased metabolic activity and blood flow in these regions in some patients. Recent pathologic studies have described cerebellar pathology with a loss of Purkinje's cells and axonal torpedoes. However, the precise pathologic correlate of ET remains to be defined.

TREATMENT

Many cases are mild and require no treatment other than reassurance. Occasionally, tremor can be severe and interfere with eating, writing, and activities of daily living. This is more likely to occur as the patient ages and is often associated with a reduction in tremor frequency. β Blockers or primidone are the standard drug therapies for ET and help in about 50% of cases. Propranolol (20–80 mg daily, given in divided doses) is usually effective at relatively low doses, but higher doses may be effective in some patients. The drug is contraindicated in patients with bradycardia or asthma. Hand tremor tends to be most improved, while head tremor is often refractory. Primidone can be helpful, but should be started at low doses (12.5 mg) and gradually increased (125–250 tid) to avoid sedation. Benefits have been reported with gabapentin and topiramate. Botulinum toxin injections may be helpful for limb or voice tremor, but treatment can be associated with secondary muscle weakness. Surgical therapies targeting the VIM nucleus of the thalamus can be very effective for severe and drug-resistant cases.

DYSTONIA

CLINICAL FEATURES

Dystonia is a disorder characterized by sustained or repetitive involuntary muscle contractions frequently associated with twisting or repetitive movements and abnormal postures. Dystonia can range from minor contractions in an individual muscle group to severe and disabling involvement of multiple muscle groups. The frequency is estimated at 300,000 cases in the United States, but is likely much higher as many cases may not be recognized. Dystonia is often brought out by voluntary movements (action dystonia) and can become sustained and extend to involve other body regions. It can be aggravated by stress and fatigue, and attenuated by relaxation and sensory tricks such as touching the affected body part (geste antagoniste). Dystonia can be classified according to age of onset (childhood vs adult), distribution (focal, multifocal, segmental, or generalized), or etiology (primary or secondary).

PRIMARY DYSTONIAS

Several gene mutations are associated with dystonia. Idiopathic torsion dystonia (ITD) or Oppenheim's dystonia is predominantly a childhood-onset form of dystonia with an autosomal dominant pattern of inheritance that primarily affects Ashkenazi Jewish families. The majority of patients have an age of onset younger than 26 years (mean 14 years). In young-onset patients, dystonia typically begins in the foot or the arm and in 60–70% progresses to involve other limbs as well as the head and neck. In severe cases, patients can suffer disabling postural deformities that compromise mobility. Severity can vary within a family, with some affected relatives having severe disability and others a mild dystonia that may not even be appreciated. Most childhood-onset cases are linked to a mutation in the DYT1 gene located on chromosome 9q34 resulting in a trinucleotide GAG deletion with loss of one of a pair of glutamic acid residues in the protein torsin A. DYT1 mutations are found in 90% of Ashkenazi Jewish patients with ITD and probably relate to a founder effect that occurred about 350 years ago. There is variable penetrance, with only about 30% of gene carriers expressing a clinical phenotype. Why some gene carriers express dystonia and others do not is not known. The function of torsin A is unknown, but it is a member of the AAA$^+$ (ATPase) family that resembles heat-shock proteins and may be related to protein regulation. The precise pathology responsible for dystonia is not known.

Dopa responsive dystonia (DRD) or the Segawa variant (DYT5) is a dominantly inherited form of childhood-onset dystonia due to a mutation in the gene that encodes for GTP cyclohydrolase-I, the rate-limiting enzyme for the synthesis of tetrahydrobiopterin. This mutation leads to a defect in the biochemical synthesis of tyrosine hydroxylase, the rate-limiting enzyme in the formation of dopamine. DRD typically presents in early childhood (1–12 years), and is characterized by foot dystonia that interferes with walking. Patients often experience diurnal fluctuations, with worsening of gait as the day progresses and improvement with sleep. DRD is typified by an excellent and sustained response to small doses of levodopa. Some patients may present with parkinsonian features, but can be differentiated from juvenile PD by normal striatal fluorodopa uptake on positron emission tomography and the absence of levodopa-induced dyskinesias. DRD may occasionally be confused with cerebral palsy because patients appear to have spasticity, increased reflexes, and Babinski responses (which likely reflect a dystonic contraction rather than an upper motor neuron lesion). Any patient suspected of having a childhood-onset dystonia should receive a trial of levodopa to exclude this condition.

Mutations in the *THAP1* gene (DYT6) on chromosome 8p21q22 have been identified in Amish families and are the cause of as many as 25% of cases of non-DYT1 young-onset primary torsion dystonia. Patients are more likely to have dystonia beginning in the brachial and cervical muscles, which later can become generalized and associated with speech impairment. Myoclonic dystonia (DYT11) results from a mutation in the epsilon-sarcoglycan gene on chromosome 7q21. It typically manifests as a combination of dystonia and myoclonic jerks, frequently accompanied by psychiatric disturbances.

FOCAL DYSTONIAS

These are the most common forms of dystonia. They typically present in the fourth to sixth decades and affect women more than men. The major types are (1) *blepharospasm*—dystonic contractions of the eyelids with increased blinking that can interfere with reading, watching TV, and driving. This can sometimes be so severe as to cause functional blindness. (2) *Oromandibular dystonia* (OMD)—contractions of muscles of the lower face, lips, tongue, and jaw (opening or closing). Meige syndrome is a combination of OMD and blepharospasm that predominantly affects women older than age 60 years. (3) *Spasmodic dysphonia*—dystonic contractions of the vocal cords during phonation, causing impaired speech. Most cases affect the adductor muscles and cause speech to have a choking or strained quality. Less commonly, the abductors are affected, leading to speech with a breathy or whispering quality. (4) *Cervical dystonia*—dystonic contractions of neck muscles causing the head to deviate to one side (*torticollis*), in a forward direction (*anterocollis*), or in a backward direction (*retrocollis*). Muscle contractions can be painful, and associated with a secondary cervical radiculopathy. (5) *Limb dystonias*—These can be present in either arms or legs and are often brought out by task-specific activities such as handwriting (writer's cramp), playing a musical instrument (musician's cramp), or putting (the yips). Focal dystonias can extend to involve other body regions (about 30% of cases), and are frequently misdiagnosed as psychiatric or orthopedic in origin. Their cause is not known, but genetic factors, autoimmunity, and trauma have been suggested. Focal dystonias are often associated with a high-frequency tremor that resembles ET. Dystonic tremor can usually be distinguished from ET because it tends to occur in conjunction with the dystonic contraction and disappears when the dystonia is relieved.

SECONDARY DYSTONIAS

These develop as a consequence of drugs or other neurologic disorders. Drug-induced dystonia is most commonly seen with neuroleptic drugs or after chronic levodopa treatment in PD patients. Secondary dystonia can also be observed following discrete lesions in the striatum, pallidum, thalamus, cortex, and brainstem due to infarction, anoxia, trauma, tumor, infection, or toxins such as manganese or carbon monoxide. In these cases, dystonia often assumes a segmental distribution. More rarely, dystonia can develop following peripheral nerve injury and be associated with features of chronic regional pain syndrome.

DYSTONIA PLUS SYNDROMES

Dystonia may occur as a part of neurodegenerative conditions such as HD, PD, Wilson's disease, CBGD, PSP, the Lubag form of dystonia-parkinsonism (DYT3), and mitochondrial encephalopathies. In contrast to the primary dystonias, dystonia is usually not the dominant neurologic feature in these conditions.

PATHOPHYSIOLOGY OF DYSTONIA

The pathophysiologic basis of dystonia is not known. The phenomenon is characterized by co-contracting synchronous bursts of agonist and antagonist muscle groups. This is associated with a loss of inhibition at multiple levels of the nervous system as well as increased cortical excitability and reorganization. Attention has focused on the basal ganglia as the site of origin of at least some types of dystonia as there are alterations in blood flow and metabolism in basal ganglia structures. Further, ablation or stimulation of the globus pallidus can both induce and ameliorate dystonia. The dopamine system has also been implicated, as dopaminergic therapies can both induce and treat some forms of dystonia.

TREATMENT Dystonia

Treatment of dystonia is for the most part symptomatic except in rare cases where treatment of a primary underlying condition is available. Wilson's disease should be ruled out in young patients with dystonia. Levodopa should be tried in all cases of childhood-onset dystonia to rule out DRD. High-dose anticholinergics (e.g., trihexyphenidyl 20–120 mg/d) may be beneficial in children, but adults can rarely tolerate high doses because of cognitive impairment with hallucinations. Oral baclofen (20–120 mg) may be helpful, but benefits if present are usually modest and side effects of sedation, weakness, and memory loss can be problematic. Intrathecal infusion of baclofen is more likely to be helpful particularly with leg and trunk dystonia, but benefits are frequently not sustained and complications can be serious and include infection, seizures, and coma. Tetrabenazine (the usual starting dose is 12.5 mg/d and the average treating dose is 25–75 mg/d) may be helpful in some patients, but use may be limited by sedation and the development of parkinsonism. Neuroleptics can improve as well as induce dystonia, but they are typically not recommended because of their potential to induce extrapyramidal side effects, including tardive dystonia. Clonazepam and diazepam are rarely effective.

Botulinum toxin has become the preferred treatment for patients with focal dystonia, particularly where involvement is limited to small muscle groups such as in blepharospasm, torticollis, and spasmodic dysphonia. Botulinum toxin acts by blocking the release of acetylcholine at the neuromuscular junction, leading to muscle weakness and reduced dystonia, but excessive weakness may ensue and can be troublesome particularly if it involves neck and swallowing muscles. Two serotypes of botulinum toxin are available (A and B). Both are effective, and it is not clear that there are advantages of one over the other. No systemic side effects are encountered with the doses typically employed, but benefits are transient and repeat injections are required at 2- to 5-month intervals. Some patients fail to respond after having experienced an initial benefit. This has been attributed to antibody formation, but improper muscle selection, injection technique, and inadequate dose should be excluded.

Surgical therapy is an alternative for patients with severe dystonia who are not responsive to other treatments. Peripheral procedures such as rhizotomy and myotomy were used in the past to treat cervical dystonia, but are now rarely employed. DBS of the pallidum can provide dramatic benefits for patients with primary DYT1 dystonia. This represents a major therapeutic advance as previously there was no consistently effective therapy, especially for these patients who had severe disability. Benefits tend to be obtained with a lower frequency of stimulation and often occur after a relatively long latency (weeks) in comparison to PD. Better results are typically obtained in younger patients. Recent studies suggest that DBS may also be valuable for patients with focal and secondary dystonias, although results are less consistent. Supportive treatments such as physical therapy and education are important and should be a part of the treatment regimen.

Physicians should be aware of dystonic storm, a rare but potentially fatal condition that can occur in response to a stress situation such as surgery in patients with preexisting dystonia. It consists of the acute onset of generalized and persistent dystonic contractions that can involve the vocal cords or laryngeal muscles, leading to airway obstruction. Patients may experience rhabdomyolysis with renal failure. Patients should be managed in an ICU with protection of airway if required. Treatment can be instituted with one or a combination of anticholinergics, diphenhydramine, baclofen, benzodiazepines, and dopamine agonists/antagonists. Spasms may be difficult to control, and anesthesia with muscle paralysis may be required.

CHOREAS

HUNTINGTON'S DISEASE (HD)

HD is a progressive, fatal, highly penetrant autosomal dominant disorder characterized by motor, behavioral, and cognitive dysfunction. The disease is named for George Huntington, a family physician who described cases on Long Island, New York, in the nineteenth century. Onset is typically between the ages of 25 and 45 years (range, 3–70 years) with a prevalence of 2–8 cases per 100,000 and an average age at death of 60 years. It is prevalent in Europe, North and South America, and Australia but is rare in African blacks and Asians. HD is characterized by rapid, nonpatterned, semipurposeful, involuntary choreiform movements. In the early stages, the chorea tends to be focal or segmental, but progresses over time to involve multiple body regions. Dysarthria, gait disturbance, and oculomotor abnormalities are common features. With advancing disease, there may be a reduction in chorea and emergence of dystonia, rigidity, bradykinesia, myoclonus, and spasticity. Functional decline is often predicted by progressive weight loss despite adequate calorie intake. In younger patients (about 10% of cases), HD can present as an akinetic-rigid or parkinsonian syndrome (Westphal variant). HD patients eventually develop behavioral and cognitive disturbances, and the majority progress to dementia. Depression with suicidal tendencies, aggressive behavior, and psychosis can be prominent features. HD patients may also develop non-insulin-dependent diabetes mellitus and neuroendocrine abnormalities, e.g., hypothalamic dysfunction. A clinical diagnosis of HD can be strongly suspected in cases of chorea with a positive family history. The disease predominantly strikes the striatum. Progressive atrophy of the caudate nuclei, which form the lateral margins of the lateral ventricles, can be visualized by MRI (Fig. 372-8). More diffuse cortical atrophy is seen in the middle and late stages of the disease. Supportive studies include reduced metabolic activity in the caudate nucleus and putamen. Genetic testing can be used to confirm the diagnosis and to detect at-risk individuals in the family, but this must be performed with caution and in conjunction with trained counselors, as positive results can worsen depression and generate suicidal reactions. The neuropathology of HD consists of prominent neuronal loss and gliosis in the caudate nucleus and putamen; similar changes are also widespread in the cerebral cortex. Intraneuronal inclusions containing aggregates of ubiquitin and the mutant protein huntingtin are found in the nuclei of affected neurons.

ETIOLOGY

HD is caused by an increase in the number of polyglutamine (CAG) repeats (>40) in the coding sequence of the huntingtin gene located on the short arm of chromosome 4. The larger the number of repeats, the earlier the disease is manifest. Acceleration of the process tends to occur, particularly in males, with subsequent generations having larger numbers of repeats and earlier age of disease onset, a phenomenon referred to as anticipation. The gene encodes the highly conserved cytoplasmic protein huntingtin, which is widely distributed clean in neurons throughout the CNS, but whose function is not known. Models of HD with striatal pathology can be induced by excitotoxic agents such as kainic acid and 3-nitropoprionic acid, which promote calcium entry into the cell and cytotoxicity. Mitochondrial dysfunction has been demonstrated in the striatum and skeletal muscle of symptomatic and presymptomatic individuals. Fragments of the mutant huntingtin protein can be toxic, possibly by translocating into the nucleus and interfering with transcriptional upregulation of regulatory proteins. Neuronal inclusions found in affected regions in HD may represent a protective mechanism aimed at segregating and facilitating the clearance of these toxic proteins.

TREATMENT Huntington's Disease

Treatment involves a multidisciplinary approach, with medical, neuropsychiatric, social, and genetic counseling for patients and their families. Dopamine-blocking agents may control the chorea. Tetrabenazine has recently been approved for the treatment of chorea in the United States, but it may cause secondary parkinsonism. Neuroleptics are generally not recommended because of their potential to induce other more troubling movement disorders and because HD chorea tends to be self-limited and is usually not disabling. Depression and anxiety can be

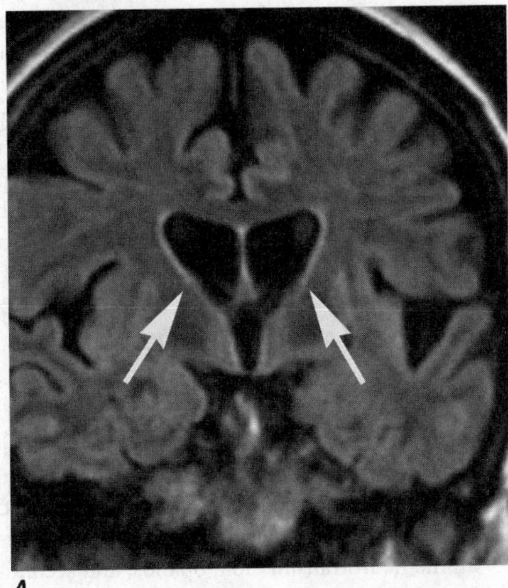

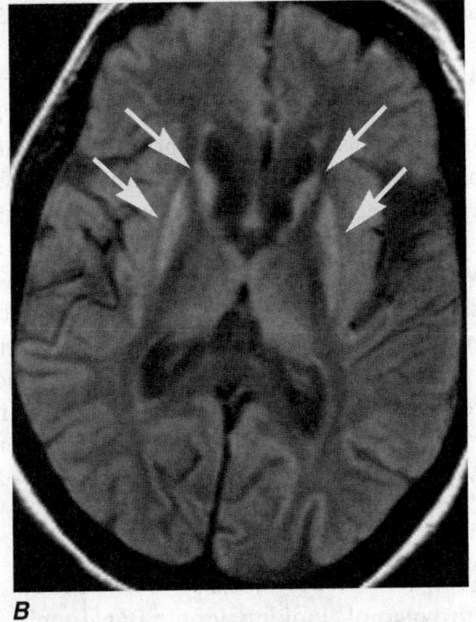

Figure 372-8 Huntington's disease. ***A.*** Coronal FLAIR MRI shows enlargement of the lateral ventricles reflecting typical atrophy (*arrows*). ***B.*** Axial FLAIR image demonstrates abnormal high signal in the caudate and putamen (*arrows*).

greater problems, and patients should be treated with appropriate antidepressant and antianxiety drugs and monitored for mania and suicidal ideations. Psychosis can be treated with atypical neuroleptics such as clozapine (50–600 mg/d), quetiapine (50–600 mg/d), and risperidone (2–8 mg/d). There is no adequate treatment for the cognitive or motor decline. A neuroprotective therapy that slows or stops disease progression is the major unmet medical need in HD. Promitochondrial agents such as ubiquinone and creatine are being tested as possible disease-modifying therapies. Antiglutamate agents, caspase inhibitors, inhibitors of protein aggregation, neurotrophic factors, and transplantation of fetal striatal cells are areas of active research, but none has as yet been demonstrated to have a disease-modifying effect.

HUNTINGTON'S DISEASE–LIKE 1 (HDL1), HUNTINGTON'S DISEASE–LIKE 2 (HDL2)

HDL1 is a rare inherited disorder due to mutations of the protein located at 20p12. Patients exhibit onset of personality change in the third or fourth decade, followed by chorea, rigidity, myoclonus, ataxia, and epilepsy. HDL2 is an autosomal dominantly inherited disorder manifesting in the third or fourth decade with a variety of movement disorders, including chorea, dystonia, or parkinsonism and dementia. Most patients, are of African descent. Acanthocytosis can sometimes be seen in these patients, and they must be differentiated from neuroacanthocytosis. HDL2 is caused by an abnormally expanded CTG/CAG trinucleotide repeat expansion in the *junctophilin-3* (*JPH3*) gene on chromosome 16q24.3. The pathology of HDL2 also demonstrates intranuclear inclusions immunoreactive for ubiquitin and expanded polyglutamine repeats.

OTHER CHOREAS

Chorea can be seen in a number of disorders. Sydenham's chorea (originally called St. Vitus' dance) is more common in females and is typically seen in childhood (5–15 years). It often develops in association with prior exposure to group A streptococcal infection and is thought to be autoimmune in nature. With the reduction in the incidence of rheumatic fever, the incidence of Sydenham's chorea has fallen, but it can still be seen in developing countries. It is characterized by the acute onset of choreiform movements, behavioral disturbances, and occasionally other motor dysfunctions. Chorea generally responds to dopamine-blocking agents, valproic acid, and carbamazepine, but is self-limited and treatment is generally restricted to those with severe chorea. Chorea may recur in later life, particularly in association with pregnancy (chorea gravidarum) or treatment with sex hormones.

Chorea-acanthocytosis (neuroacanthocytosis) is a progressive and typically fatal autosomal recessive disorder that is characterized by chorea coupled with red cell abnormalities on peripheral blood smear (acanthocytes). The chorea can be severe and associated with self-mutilating behavior, dystonia, tics, seizures, and a polyneuropathy. Mutations in the *VPS13A* gene on chromosome 9q21 encoding chorein have been described. A phenotypically similar X-linked form of the disorder has been described in older individuals who have reactivity with Kell blood group antigens (McLeod syndrome). A benign hereditary chorea of childhood (BHC1) due to mutations in the gene for thyroid transcription factor 1 and a late-onset benign senile chorea (BHC2) have also been described. It is important to ensure that patients with these types of choreas do not have HD.

A range of neurodegenerative diseases with brain iron accumulation (NBIA) manifesting with chorea and dystonia have been described including autosomal dominant neuroferritinopathy, autosomal recessive pantothenate-kinase-associated neurodegeneration (PKAN; Hallervorden-Spatz disease), and aceruloplasminemia. These disorders have excess iron accumulation on MRI and a characteristic "eye of the tiger" appearance in the globus pallidus due to iron accumulation.

Chorea may also occur in association with vascular diseases, hypo- and hyperglycemia, and a variety of infections and degenerative disorders. Systemic lupus erythematosus is the most common systemic disorder that causes chorea; the chorea can last for days to years. Choreas can also be seen with hyperthyroidism, autoimmune disorders including Sjögren's syndrome, infectious disorders including HIV disease, metabolic alterations, polycythemia rubra vera (following open-heart surgery in the pediatric population), and in association with many medications (especially anticonvulsants, cocaine, CNS stimulants, estrogens, lithium). Chorea can also be seen in paraneoplastic syndromes associated with anti-CRMP-5 or anti-Hu antibodies.

Paroxysmal dyskinesias are a group of rare disorders characterized by episodic, brief involuntary movements that can include chorea, dystonia, and ballismus. Paroxysmal kinesigenic dyskinesia (PKD) is a familial childhood-onset disorder in which chorea or chorea-dystonia is precipitated by sudden movement or running. Attacks may affect one side of the body, last seconds to minutes at a time, and recur several times a day. Prognosis is usually good, with spontaneous remission in later life. Low-dose anticonvulsant therapy (e.g., carbamazepine) is usually effective if required. Paroxysmal nonkinesigenic dyskinesia (PNKD) involves attacks of dyskinesia precipitated by alcohol, caffeine, stress, or fatigue. Like PKD, it is familial and childhood in onset and the episodes are often choreic or dystonic, but have longer duration (minutes to hours) and are less frequent (1–3/d).

TREATMENT Paroxysmal Nonkinesigenic Dyskinesia

Diagnosis and treatment of the underlying condition, where possible, is the first priority. Tetrabenazine, neuroleptics, dopamine-blocking agents, propranolol, clonazepam, and baclofen may be helpful. Treatment is not indicated if the condition is mild and self-limited. Most patients with PKND do not benefit from anticonvulsant drugs but some may respond to clonazepam.

HEMIBALLISMUS

Hemiballismus is a violent form of chorea composed of wild, flinging, large-amplitude movements on one side of the body. Proximal limb muscles tend to be predominantly affected. The movements may be so severe as to cause exhaustion, dehydration, local injury, and in extreme cases, death. The most common cause is a partial lesion (infarct or hemorrhage) in the subthalamic nucleus (STN), but rare cases can also be seen with lesions in the putamen. Fortunately, hemiballismus is usually self-limiting and tends to resolve spontaneously after weeks or months. Dopamine-blocking drugs can be helpful but can themselves lead to movement disorders. In extreme cases, pallidotomy can be very effective. Interestingly, surgically induced lesions or DBS of the STN in PD are usually not associated with hemiballismus.

TICS

TOURETTE'S SYNDROME (TS)

TS is a neurobehavioral disorder named after the French neurologist Georges Gilles de la Tourette. It predominantly affects males, and prevalence is estimated to be 0.03–1.6%, but it is likely that many mild cases do not come to medical attention. TS is characterized by multiple motor tics often accompanied by vocalizations (phonic tics). A *tic* is a brief, rapid, recurrent, and seemingly purposeless stereotyped motor contraction. Motor tics can be simple, with movement only affecting an individual muscle group (e.g., blinking, twitching of the nose, jerking of the neck), or complex, with coordinated involvement of multiple muscle groups [e.g., jumping, sniffing, head banging, and echopraxia (mimicking movements)]. Vocal tics can also be simple (e.g., grunting) or complex [e.g., echolalia (repeating other people's words), palilalia (repeating one's own words), and coprolalia (expression of obscene words)]. Patients may also experience sensory tics, composed of unpleasant focal sensations in the face, head, or neck. Patients characteristically can voluntarily suppress tics for short periods of time, but then experience an irresistible urge to express them. Tics vary in intensity and may be absent for days or weeks only to recur, occasionally in a different pattern. Tics tend to present between ages 2 and 15 years (mean 7 years) and often lessen or even disappear in adulthood. Associated behavioral disturbances include anxiety, depression, attention deficit hyperactivity disorder, and obsessive-compulsive disorder. Patients may experience personality disorders, self-destructive behaviors, difficulties in school, and impaired interpersonal relationships. Tics may present in adulthood and can be seen in association with a variety of other disorders, including PD, HD, trauma, dystonia, drugs (e.g., levodopa, neuroleptics), and toxins.

ETIOLOGY AND PATHOPHYSIOLOGY

TS is thought to be a genetic disorder, but no specific gene mutation has been identified. Current evidence supports a complex inheritance pattern, with one or more major genes, multiple loci, low penetrance, and environmental influences. The risk of a family with one affected child having a second is about 25%. The pathophysiology of TS is not known, but alterations in dopamine neurotransmission, opioids, and second-messenger systems have been proposed. Some cases of TS may be the consequence of an autoimmune response to β-hemolytic streptococcal infection [pediatric autoimmune neuropsychiatric disorder associated with streptococcal infection (PANDAS)]; however, this remains controversial.

TREATMENT Tourette's Syndrome

Patients with mild disease often only require education and counseling (for themselves and family members). Drug treatment is indicated when the tics are disabling and interfere with quality of life. Therapy is generally initiated with the α-agonist clonidine, starting at low doses and gradually increasing the dose and frequency until satisfactory control is achieved. Guanfacine (0.5–2 mg/d) is an α-agonist that is preferred by many clinicians because it only requires once-a-day dosing. If these agents are not effective, antipsychotics can be employed. Atypical neuroleptics (risperidone, olanzapine, ziprasidone) are preferred as they are thought to be associated with a reduced risk of extrapyramidal side effects. If they are not effective, low doses of classical neuroleptics such as haloperidol, fluphenazine, or pimozide can be tried. Botulinum toxin injections can be effective in controlling focal tics that involve small muscle groups. Behavioral features, and particularly anxiety and compulsions, can be a disabling feature of TS and should be treated. The potential value of DBS targeting the anterior portion of the internal capsule is currently being explored.

MYOCLONUS

Myoclonus is a brief, rapid (<100 ms) shock-like, jerky movement consisting of single or repetitive muscle discharges. Myoclonic jerks can be focal, multifocal, segmental, or generalized and can occur spontaneously, in association with voluntary movement (action myoclonus) or in response to an external stimulus (reflex or startle myoclonus). Negative myoclonus consists of a twitch due to a brief loss of muscle activity (e.g., asterixis in hepatic failure). Myoclonic jerks differ from tics in that they interfere with normal movement and are not suppressible. They can be seen in association with pathology in cortical, subcortical, or spinal cord regions and associated with hypoxemic damage (especially following cardiac arrest), encephalopathy, and neurodegeneration. Reversible myoclonus can be seen with metabolic disturbances (renal failure, electrolyte imbalance, hypocalcemia), toxins, and many medications. Essential myoclonus is a relatively benign familial condition characterized by multifocal lightning-like movements. Myoclonic jerks can be disabling when they interfere with normal movement. They can also be innocent and are commonly observed in normal people when waking up or falling asleep (hypnogogic jerks).

TREATMENT Myoclonus

Treatment primarily consists of treating the underlying condition or removing an offending agent. Pharmacologic therapy involves one or a combination of GABAergic agents such as valproic acid (800–3000 mg/d), piracetam (8–20 g/d), clonazepam (2–15 mg/d), or primidone (500–1000 mg/d). Recent studies suggest that levetiracetam may be particularly effective.

DRUG-INDUCED MOVEMENT DISORDERS

This important group of movement disorders is primarily associated with drugs that block dopamine receptors (neuroleptics) or central dopaminergic transmission. These drugs are primarily used in psychiatry, but it is important to appreciate that drugs used in the treatment of nausea or vomiting (e.g., Compazine) or gastroesophageal disorders (e.g., metoclopramide) are neuroleptic agents. Hyperkinetic movement disorders secondary to neuroleptic drugs can be divided into those that present acutely, subacutely, or after prolonged exposure (tardive syndromes). Dopamine-blocking drugs can also be associated with a reversible parkinsonian syndrome for which anticholinergics are often concomitantly prescribed, but there is concern that this may increase the risk of developing a tardive syndrome.

ACUTE

Dystonia is the most common acute hyperkinetic drug reaction. It is typically generalized in children and focal in adults (e.g., blepharospasm, torticollis, or oromandibular dystonia). The reaction can develop within minutes of exposure, and can be successfully treated in most cases with parenteral administration of anticholinergics (benztropine or diphenhydramine) or benzodiazepines (lorazepam or diazepam). Choreas, stereotypic behaviors, and tics may also be seen, particularly following acute exposure to CNS stimulants such as methylphenidate, cocaine, or amphetamines.

SUBACUTE

Akathisia is the commonest reaction in this category. It consists of motor restlessness with a need to move that is alleviated by movement. Therapy consists of removing the offending agent. When this is not possible, symptoms may be ameliorated with benzodiazepines, anticholinergics, β blockers, or dopamine agonists.

TARDIVE SYNDROMES

These disorders develop months to years after initiation of neuroleptic treatment. Tardive dyskinesia (TD) is the commonest and is typically composed of choreiform movements involving the mouth, lips, and tongue. In severe cases, the trunk, limbs, and respiratory muscles may also be affected. In approximately one-third of patients, TD remits within 3 months of stopping the drug, and most patients gradually improve over the course of several years. In contrast, abnormal movements may develop after stopping the offending agent. The movements are often mild and more upsetting to the family than to the patient, but they can be severe and disabling, particularly in the context of an underlying psychiatric disorder. Atypical antipsychotics (e.g., clozapine, risperidone, olanzapine, quetiapine, ziprasidone, and aripiprazole) are associated with a significantly lower risk of TD in comparison to traditional antipsychotics. Younger patients have a lower risk of developing neuroleptic-induced TD, whereas the elderly, females, and those with underlying organic cerebral dysfunction have been reported to be at greater risk. In addition, chronic use is associated with increased risk, and specifically, the FDA has warned that use of metoclopramide for more than 12 weeks increases the risk of TD. Since TD can be permanent and resistant to treatment, antipsychotics should be used judiciously, atypical neuroleptics should be the preferred agent whenever possible, and the need for their continued use should be regularly monitored.

Treatment primarily consists of stopping the offending agent. If the patient is receiving a traditional antipsychotic and withdrawal is not possible, replacement with an atypical antipsychotic should be tried. Abrupt cessation of a neuroleptic should be avoided as acute withdrawal can induce worsening. TD can persist after withdrawal of antipsychotics and can be difficult to treat. Benefits may be achieved with valproic acid, anticholinergics, or botulinum toxin injections. In refractory cases, catecholamine depleters such as tetrabenazine may be helpful. Tetrabenazine can be associated with dose-dependent sedation and orthostatic hypotension. Other approaches include baclofen (40–80 mg/d), clonazepam (1–8 mg/d), or valproic acid (750–3000 mg/d).

Chronic neuroleptic exposure can also be associated with tardive dystonia with preferential involvement of axial muscles and characteristic rocking movements of the trunk and pelvis. Tardive dystonia frequently persists despite stopping medication and patients are often refractory to medical therapy. Valproic acid, anticholinergics, and botulinum toxin may occasionally be beneficial. Tardive akathisia, tardive Tourette, and tardive tremor syndromes are rare but may also occur after chronic neuroleptic exposure.

Neuroleptic medications can also be associated with a neuroleptic malignant syndrome (NMS). NMS is characterized by muscle rigidity, elevated temperature, altered mental status, hyperthermia, tachycardia, labile blood pressure, renal failure, and markedly elevated creatine kinase levels. Symptoms typically evolve within days or weeks after initiating the drug. NMS can also be precipitated by the abrupt withdrawal of antiparkinsonian medications in PD patients. Treatment involves immediate cessation of the offending antipsychotic drug and the introduction of a dopaminergic agent (e.g., a dopamine agonist or levodopa), dantrolene, or a benzodiazepine. Treatment may need to be undertaken in an intensive care setting and includes supportive measures such as control of body temperature (antipyretics and cooling blankets), hydration, electrolyte replacement, and control of renal function and blood pressure.

Drugs that have serotonin-like activity (tryptophan, MDMA or "ecstasy," meperidine) or that block serotonin reuptake can induce a rare, but potentially fatal, serotonin syndrome that is characterized by confusion, hyperthermia, tachycardia, and coma as well as rigidity, ataxia, and tremor. Myoclonus is often a prominent feature, in contrast to NMS, which it resembles. Patients can be managed with propranolol, diazepam, diphenhydramine, chlorpromazine, or cyproheptadine as well as supportive measures.

A variety of drugs can also be associated with parkinsonism (see above) and hyperkinetic movement disorders. Some examples include phenytoin (chorea, dystonia, tremor, myoclonus), carbamazepine (tics and dystonia), tricyclic antidepressants (dyskinesias, tremor, myoclonus), fluoxetine (myoclonus, chorea, dystonia), oral contraceptives (dyskinesia), β adrenergics (tremor), buspirone (akathisia, dyskinesias, myoclonus), and digoxin, cimetidine, diazoxide, lithium, methadone, and fentanyl (dyskinesias).

RESTLESS LEGS SYNDROME

Restless legs syndrome (RLS) is a neurologic disorder that affects approximately 10% of the adult population (it is rare in Asians) and can cause significant morbidity in some. It was first described in the seventeenth century by an English physician (Thomas Willis), but has only recently been recognized as being a bona fide movement disorder. The four core symptoms required for diagnosis are as follows: an urge to move the legs, usually caused or accompanied by an unpleasant sensation in the legs; symptoms begin or worsen with rest; partial or complete relief by movement; worsening during the evening or night.

Symptoms most commonly begin in the legs, but can spread to or even begin in the upper limbs. The unpleasant sensation is often described as a creepy-crawly feeling, paresthesia, or burning. In about 80% of patients, RLS is associated with periodic leg movements (PLMs) during sleep and occasionally while awake. These involuntary movements are usually brief, lasting no more than a few seconds, and recur every 5–90 seconds. The restlessness and PLMs are a major cause of sleep disturbance in patients, leading to poor-quality sleep and daytime sleepiness.

RLS is a heterogeneous condition. Primary RLS is genetic, and several loci have been found with an autosomal dominant pattern of inheritance, although penetrance may be variable. The mean age of onset in genetic forms is 27 years, although pediatric cases are recognized. The severity of symptoms is variable. Secondary RLS may be associated with pregnancy or a range of underlying disorders, including anemia, ferritin deficiency, renal failure, and peripheral neuropathy. The pathogenesis probably involves disordered dopamine function, which may be peripheral or central, in association with an abnormality of iron metabolism. Diagnosis is made on clinical grounds but can be supported by polysomnography and the demonstration of PLMs. The neurologic examination is normal. Secondary RLS should be excluded and ferritin levels, glucose, and renal function should be measured.

Most RLS sufferers have mild symptoms that do not require specific treatment. General measures to improve sleep hygiene and quality should be attempted first. If symptoms remain intrusive, low doses of dopamine agonists, e.g., pramipexole (0.25–0.5 mg) and ropinirole (1–2 mg), are given 1–2 hours before bedtime. Levodopa can be effective but is frequently associated with augmentation (spread and worsening of restlessness and its appearance earlier in the day) or rebound (reappearance sometimes with worsening of symptoms at a time compatible with the drug's short half-life). Other drugs that can be effective include anticonvulsants, analgesics, and even opiates. Management of secondary RLS should be directed to correcting the underlying disorder; for example, iron replacement for anemia. Iron infusion may also be helpful for severe primary RLS but requires expert supervision.

DISORDERS THAT PRESENT WITH PARKINSONISM AND HYPERKINETIC MOVEMENTS

WILSON'S DISEASE

Wilson's disease (WD) is an autosomal recessive inherited disorder of copper metabolism that may manifest with neurologic, psychiatric, and liver disorders, alone or in combination. It is caused by mutations in the gene encoding a P-type ATPase. The disease was first comprehensively described by the English neurologist Kinnear Wilson at the beginning of the twentieth century, although at around the same time the German physicians Kayser and Fleischer separately noted the characteristic association of corneal pigmentation with hepatic and neurologic features. WD has a worldwide prevalence of approximately 1 in 30,000, with a gene carrier frequency of 1 in 90. About half of WD patients (especially younger patients) manifest with liver abnormalities. The remainder present with neurologic disease (with or without underlying liver abnormalities), and a small proportion have hematologic or psychiatric problems at disease onset.

Neurologic onset usually manifests in the second decade with tremor and rigidity. The tremor is usually in the upper limbs, bilateral, and asymmetric. Tremor can be on intention or occasionally resting and, in advanced disease, can take on a wing-beating characteristic. Other features include parkinsonism with bradykinesia, dystonia (particularly facial grimacing), dysarthria, and dysphagia. More than half of those with neurologic features have a history of psychiatric disturbances, including depression, mood swings, and overt psychosis. Kayser-Fleischer (KF) rings are seen in 80% of those with hepatic presentations and virtually all with neurologic features. KF rings represent the deposition of copper in Descemet's membrane around the cornea. They consist of a characteristic grayish rim or circle at the limbus of the cornea and are best detected by slit-lamp examination. Neuropathologic examination is characterized by neurodegeneration and astrogliosis, particularly in the basal ganglia.

WD should always be considered in the differential diagnosis of a movement disorder in a child. Low levels of blood copper and ceruloplasmin and high levels of urinary copper may be present, but normal levels do not exclude the diagnosis. CT brain scan usually reveals generalized atrophy in established cases and ~50% have hypointensity in the caudate head, globus pallidum, substantia nigra, and red nucleus. MRI shows symmetric hyperintensity on T2-weighted images in the putamen, caudate, and pallidum. However, correlation of imaging changes with clinical features is not good. It is very rare for WD patients with neurologic features not to have KF rings. Nevertheless, liver biopsy with demonstration of high copper levels remains the gold standard for the diagnosis.

In the absence of treatment, the course is progressive and leads to severe neurologic dysfunction and early death. Treatment is directed at reducing tissue copper levels and maintenance therapy to prevent reaccumulation. There is no clear consensus on treatment and all patients should be managed in a unit with expertise in WD. Penicillamine is frequently used to increase copper excretion, but it may lead to a worsening of symptoms in the initial stages of therapy. Side effects are common and can to some degree be attenuated by coadministration of pyridoxine. Tetrathiomolybdate blocks the absorption of copper and is used instead of penicillamine in many centers. Trientine and zinc are useful drugs for maintenance therapy. Effective treatment can reverse the neurologic features in most patients, particularly when started early. Some patients stabilize and a few may still progress, especially those with hepatocerebral disease. KF rings tend to decrease after 3–6 months and disappear by 2 years. Adherence to maintenance therapy is a major challenge in long-term care.

OTHER DISORDERS

Pantothenate kinase (PANK)-associated neurodegeneration, acanthocytosis, and Huntington's disease can also present with parkinsonism associated with involuntary movements.

PSYCHOGENIC DISORDERS

Virtually all movement disorders including tremor, tics, dystonia, myoclonus, chorea, ballism, and parkinsonism can be psychogenic in origin. Tremor affecting the upper limbs is the most common psychogenic movement disorder. Psychogenic movements can result from a somatoform or conversion disorder, malingering (e.g., seeking financial gain), or a factitious disorder (e.g., seeking psychological gain). Psychogenic movement disorders are common (estimated 2–3% of patients in a movement disorder clinic), more frequent in women, disabling for the patient and family, and expensive for society (estimated $20 billion annually). Clinical features suggesting a psychogenic movement disorder include an acute onset and a pattern of abnormal movement that is inconsistent with a known movement disorder. Diagnosis is based on the nonorganic quality of the movement, the absence of findings of an organic disease process, and positive features that specifically point to a psychogenic illness such as variability and distractibility. For example, the magnitude of a psychogenic tremor is increased with attention and diminishes or even disappears when the patient is distracted by being asked to perform a different task or is unaware that he or she is being observed. Other positive features suggesting a psychogenic problem include a tremor frequency that is variable or that entrains with the frequency of movement in the contralateral limb, and a positive response to placebo medication. Associated features can include nonanatomic sensory findings, give-way weakness, and astasia-abasia (an odd, gyrating gait; Chap. 24). Comorbid psychiatric problems such as anxiety, depression, and emotional trauma may be present, but are not necessary for the diagnosis of a psychogenic movement disorder to be made. Psychogenic movement disorders can occur as an isolated entity or in association with an underlying organic problem. The diagnosis can often be made based on clinical features alone and unnecessary tests or medications avoided. Underlying psychiatric problems may be present and should be identified and treated, but many patients with psychogenic movement disorders have no obvious psychiatric pathology. Psychotherapy and hypnosis may be of value for patients with conversion reaction, and cognitive behavioral therapy may be helpful for patients with somatoform disorders. Patients with hypochondriasis, factitious disorders, and malingering have a poor prognosis.

FURTHER READINGS

Emre M et al: Clinical diagnostic criteria for dementia associated with Parkinson's disease. Mov Disord 22:1689, 2007

Fahn S, Jankovic J (eds). *Principles and Practice of Movement Disorders*. Amsterdam, Elsevier, 2010

Follett KA et al: Pallidal versus subthalamic deep-brain stimulation for Parkinson's disease. N Engl J Med 362:2077, 2010

Hardy J: Genetic analysis of pathways to Parkinson disease. Neuron 68:201, 2010

Jankovic J: Treatment of hyperkinetic movement disorders. Lancet Neurol 8:844, 2009

Olanow CW et al: A double-blind delayed-start study of rasagiline in early Parkinson's Disease. N Engl J Med 361:1268, 2009

———: Non-motor and non-dopaminergic features of Parkinson's disease. Wiley Blackwell, 2001

Ross CA and Tabrizi SJ: Huntington's disease: from molecular pathogeneis to clinical treatment. Lancet Neurol 10:83, 2011

Schapira AHV, Olanow CW (eds): *Principles of Treatment for Parkinson's Disease*. Philadelphia, Butterworth Heinemann, Elsevier, 2005

Stocchi F et al: Initiating levodopa/carbidopa therapy with and without entacapone in early Parkinson's disease: The STRIDE-PD study. Ann Neurol 68:18, 2010

CHAPTER 373

Ataxic Disorders

Roger N. Rosenberg

APPROACH TO THE PATIENT: Ataxic Disorders

Symptoms and signs of ataxia consist of gait impairment, unclear ("scanning") speech, visual blurring due to nystagmus, hand incoordination, and tremor with movement. These result from the involvement of the cerebellum and its afferent and efferent pathways, including the spinocerebellar pathways, and the frontopontocerebellar pathway originating in the rostral frontal lobe. True cerebellar ataxia must be distinguished from ataxia associated with vestibular nerve or labyrinthine disease, as the latter results in a disorder of gait associated with a significant degree of dizziness, light-headedness, or the perception of movement (Chap. 21). True cerebellar ataxia is devoid of these vertiginous complaints and is clearly an unsteady gait due to imbalance. Sensory disturbances can also on occasion simulate the imbalance of cerebellar disease; with sensory ataxia, imbalance dramatically worsens when visual input is removed (Romberg sign). Rarely, weakness of proximal leg muscles mimics cerebellar disease. In the patient who presents with ataxia, the rate and pattern of the development of cerebellar symptoms help to narrow the diagnostic possibilities (Table 373-1). A gradual and progressive increase in symptoms with bilateral and symmetric involvement suggests a genetic, metabolic, immune, or toxic etiology. Conversely, focal, unilateral symptoms with headache and impaired level of consciousness accompanied by ipsilateral cranial nerve palsies and contralateral weakness imply a space-occupying cerebellar lesion.

SYMMETRIC ATAXIA Progressive and symmetric ataxia can be classified with respect to onset as acute (over hours or days), subacute (weeks or months), or chronic (months to years). Acute and reversible ataxias include those caused by intoxication with alcohol, phenytoin, lithium, barbiturates, and other drugs. Intoxication caused by toluene exposure, gasoline sniffing, glue sniffing, spray painting, or exposure to methyl mercury or bismuth are additional causes of acute or subacute ataxia, as is treatment with cytotoxic chemotherapeutic drugs such as fluorouracil and paclitaxel. Patients with a postinfectious syndrome (especially after varicella) may develop gait ataxia and mild dysarthria, both of which are reversible (Chap. 380). Rare infectious causes of acquired ataxia include poliovirus,

TABLE 373-1 Etiology of Cerebellar Ataxia

Symmetric and Progressive Signs			Focal and Ipsilateral Cerebellar Signs		
Acute (Hours to Days)	Subacute (Days to Weeks)	Chronic (Months to Years)	Acute (Hours to Days)	Subacute (Days to Weeks)	Chronic (Months to Years)
Intoxication: alcohol, lithium, phenytoin, barbiturates (positive history and toxicology screen)	Intoxication: mercury, solvents, gasoline, glue; cytotoxic chemotherapeutic, hemotherapeutic drugs	Paraneoplastic syndrome Anti-gliadin antibody syndrome Hypothyroidism	Vascular: cerebellar infarction, hemorrhage, or subdural hematoma Infectious: cerebellar abscess (mass lesion on MRI/CT, history in support of lesion)	Neoplastic: cerebellar glioma or metastatic tumor (positive for neoplasm on MRI/CT) Demyelinating: multiple sclerosis (history, CSF, and MRI are consistent)	Stable gliosis secondary to vascular lesion or demyelinating plaque (stable lesion on MRI/CT older than several months)
Acute viral cerebellitis (CSF supportive of acute viral infection) Postinfection syndrome	Alcoholic-nutritional (vitamin B_1 and B_{12} deficiency) Lyme disease	Inherited diseases Tabes dorsalis (tertiary syphilis) Phenytoin toxicity Amiodarone		AIDS-related multifocal leukoencephalopathy (positive HIV test and CD4+ cell count for AIDS)	Congenital lesion: Chiari or Dandy-Walker malformations (malformation noted on MRI/CT)

Abbreviations: CSF, cerebrospinal fluid; CT, computed tomography; MRI, magnetic resonance imaging.

coxsackievirus, echovirus, Epstein-Barr virus, toxoplasmosis, *Legionella*, and Lyme disease.

The subacute development of ataxia of gait over weeks to months (degeneration of the cerebellar vermis) may be due to the combined effects of alcoholism and malnutrition, particularly with deficiencies of vitamins B_1 and B_{12}. Hyponatremia has also been associated with ataxia. Paraneoplastic cerebellar ataxia is associated with a number of different tumors (and autoantibodies) such as breast and ovarian cancers (anti-Yo), small-cell lung cancer (anti-PQ type voltage-gated calcium channel), and Hodgkin's disease (anti-Tr) (Chap. 101). Another paraneoplastic syndrome associated with myoclonus and opsoclonus occurs with breast (anti-Ri) and lung cancers and neuroblastoma. Elevated serum anti–glutamic acid decarboxylase (GAD) antibodies have been associated with a progressive ataxic syndrome affecting speech and gait. For all of these paraneoplastic ataxias, the neurologic syndrome may be the presenting symptom of the cancer. Another immune-mediated progressive ataxia is associated with anti-gliadin (and anti-endomysium) antibodies and the human leukocyte antigen (HLA) DQB1*0201 haplotype; in some affected patients, biopsy of the small intestine reveals villus atrophy consistent with gluten-sensitive enteropathy (Chap. 294). Finally, subacute progressive ataxia may be caused by a prion disorder, especially when an infectious etiology, such as transmission from contaminated human growth hormone, is responsible (Chap. 383).

Chronic symmetric gait ataxia suggests an inherited ataxia (discussed below), a metabolic disorder, or a chronic infection. Hypothyroidism must always be considered as a readily treatable and reversible form of gait ataxia. Infectious diseases that can present with ataxia are meningovascular syphilis and tabes dorsalis due to degeneration of the posterior columns and spinocerebellar pathways in the spinal cord.

FOCAL ATAXIA Acute focal ataxia commonly results from cerebrovascular disease, usually ischemic infarction or cerebellar hemorrhage. These lesions typically produce cerebellar symptoms ipsilateral to the injured cerebellum and may be associated with an impaired level of consciousness due to brainstem compression and increased intracranial pressure; ipsilateral pontine signs, including sixth and seventh nerve palsies, may be present. Focal and worsening signs of acute ataxia should also prompt consideration of a posterior fossa subdural hematoma, bacterial abscess, or primary or metastatic cerebellar tumor. CT or MRI studies will reveal clinically significant processes of this type. Many of these lesions represent true neurologic emergencies, as sudden herniation, either rostrally through the tentorium or caudal herniation of cerebellar tonsils through the foramen magnum, can occur and is usually devastating. Acute surgical decompression may be required (Chap. 275). Lymphoma or progressive multifocal leukoencephalopathy (PML) in a patient with AIDS may present with an acute or subacute focal cerebellar syndrome. Chronic etiologies of progressive ataxia include multiple sclerosis (Chap. 380) and congenital lesions such as a Chiari malformation (Chap. 377) or a congenital cyst of the posterior fossa (Dandy-Walker syndrome).

THE INHERITED ATAXIAS

These may show autosomal dominant, autosomal recessive, or maternal (mitochondrial) modes of inheritance. A genomic classification (Table 373-2) has now largely superseded previous ones based on clinical expression alone.

Although the clinical manifestations and neuropathologic findings of cerebellar disease dominate the clinical picture, there may also be characteristic changes in the basal ganglia, brainstem, spinal cord, optic nerves, retina, and peripheral nerves. In large families with dominantly inherited ataxias, many gradations are observed from purely cerebellar manifestations to mixed cerebellar and brainstem disorders, cerebellar and basal ganglia syndromes, and spinal cord or peripheral nerve disease. Rarely, dementia is present as well. The clinical picture may be homogeneous within a family with dominantly inherited ataxia, but sometimes most affected family members show one characteristic syndrome, while one or several members have an entirely different phenotype.

■ AUTOSOMAL DOMINANT ATAXIAS

The autosomal spinocerebellar ataxias (SCAs) include SCA types 1 through SCA28, dentatorubropallidoluysian atrophy (DRPLA), and episodic ataxia (EA) types 1 and 2 (Table 373-2). SCA1, SCA2, SCA3 [Machado-Joseph disease (MJD)], SCA6, SCA7, and SCA17 are caused by CAG triplet repeat expansions in different genes. SCA8 is due to an untranslated CTG repeat expansion, SCA12 is

TABLE 373-2 Classification of the Spinocerebellar Ataxias

Name	Locus	Phenotype
SCA1 (autosomal dominant type 1)	6p22-p23 with CAG repeats (exonic); leucine-rich acidic nuclear protein (LANP), region-specific interaction protein Ataxin-1	Ataxia with ophthalmoparesis, pyramidal and extrapyramidal findings; genetic testing is available; 6% of all autosomal dominant (AD) cerebellar ataxia
SCA2 (autosomal dominant type 2)	12q23-q24.1 with CAG repeats (exonic) Ataxin-2	Ataxia with slow saccades and minimal pyramidal and extrapyramidal findings; genetic testing available; 13% of all AD cerebellar ataxia
Machado-Joseph disease/SCA3 (autosomal dominant type 3)	14q24.3-q32 with CAG repeats (exonic); codes for ubiquitin protease (inactive with polyglutamine expansion); altered turnover of cellular proteins due to proteosome dysfunction MJD–ataxin-3	Ataxia with ophthalmoparesis and variable pyramidal, extrapyramidal, and amyotrophic signs; dementia (mild); 23% of all AD cerebellar ataxia; genetic testing available
SCA4 (autosomal dominant type 4)	16q22.1-ter; pleckstrin homology domain-containing protein, family G, member 4; (PLEKHG4; puratrophin-1: Purkinje cell atrophy associated protein-1, including spectrin repeat and the guanine-nucleotide exchange factor, GEF for Rho GTPases)	Ataxia with normal eye movements, sensory axonal neuropathy, and pyramidal signs; genetic testing available
SCA5 (autosomal dominant type 5)	11p12-q12; β-III spectrin mutations; (SPTBN2); stabilizes glutamate transporter EAAT4; descendants of President Abraham Lincoln	Ataxia and dysarthria; genetic testing available
SCA6 (autosomal dominant type 6)	19p13.2 with CAG repeats in α_{1A}-voltage–dependent calcium channel gene (exonic); CACNA1A protein, P/Q type calcium channel subunit	Ataxia and dysarthria, nystagmus, mild proprioceptive sensory loss; genetic testing available
SCA7 (autosomal dominant type 7)	3p14.1-p21.1 with CAG repeats (exonic); ataxin-7; subunit of GCN5, histone acetyltransferase-containing complexes; ataxin-7 binding protein; Cbl-associated protein (CAP; SH3D5)	Ophthalmoparesis, visual loss, ataxia, dysarthria, extensor plantar response, pigmentary retinal degeneration; genetic testing available
SCA8 (autosomal dominant type 8)	13q21 with CTG repeats; noncoding; 3′ untranslated region of transcribed RNA; KLHL1AS	Gait ataxia, dysarthria, nystagmus, leg spasticity, and reduced vibratory sensation; genetic testing available;
SCA10 (autosomal dominant type 10)	22q13; pentanucleotide repeat ATTCT repeat; noncoding, intron 9	Gait ataxia, dysarthria, nystagmus; partial complex and generalized motor seizures; polyneuropathy; genetic testing available
SCA11 (autosomal dominant type 11)	15q14-q21.3 by linkage	Slowly progressive gait and extremity ataxia, dysarthria, vertical nystagmus, hyperreflexia
SCA12 (autosomal dominant type 12)	5q31-q33 by linkage; CAG repeat; protein phosphatase 2A, regulatory subunit B, (PPP2R2B); protein PP2A, serine/threonine phosphatase	Tremor, decreased movement, increased reflexes, dystonia, ataxia, dysautonomia, dementia, dysarthria; genetic testing available
SCA13 (autosomal dominant type 13)	19q13.3-q14.4	Ataxia, legs>arms; dysarthria, horizontal nystagmus; delayed motor development; mental developmental delay; tendon reflexes increased; MRI: cerebellar and pontine atrophy; genetic testing available;
SCA14 (autosomal dominant type 14)	19q-13.4; protein kinase Cγ (PRKCG), missense mutations including in-frame deletion and a splice site mutation among others; serine/threonine kinase	Gait ataxia; leg>arm ataxia; dysarthria; pure ataxia with later onset; myoclonus; tremor of head and extremities; increased deep tendon reflexes at ankles; occasional dystonia and sensory neuropathy; genetic testing available
SCA15 (autosomal dominant type 15)	3p24.2-3pter	Gait and extremity ataxia, dysarthria; nystagmus; MRI: superior vermis atrophy; sparing of hemispheres and tonsils
SCA16 (autosomal dominant type 16)	8q22.1-24.1	Pure cerebellar ataxia and head tremor, gait ataxia, and dysarthria; horizontal gaze–evoked nystagmus; MR: cerebellar atrophy; no brainstem changes

(*continued*)

TABLE 373-2 Classification of the Spinocerebellar Ataxias (*Continued*)

Name	Locus	Phenotype
SCA17 (autosomal dominant type 17)	6q27; CAG expansion in the TATA-binding protein (*TBP*) gene	Gait ataxia, dementia, parkinsonism, dystonia, chorea, seizures; hyperreflexia; dysarthria and dysphagia; MRI shows cerebral & cerebellar atrophy; genetic testing available
SCA18 (autosomal dominant type 18)	7q22-q32	Ataxia; motor/sensory neuropathy; head tremor; dysarthria; extensor plantar responses in some patients; sensory axonal neuropathy; EMG denervation; MRI: cerebellar atrophy
SCA19 (autosomal dominant type 19)	1p21-q21	Ataxia, tremor, cognitive impairment, myoclonus; MRI: atrophy of cerebellum
SCA20 (autosomal dominant)	11p13-q11	Dysarthria; gait ataxia; ocular gaze–evoked saccades; palatal tremor; dentate calcification on CT; MRI: cerebral atrophy
SCA21 (autosomal dominant)	7p21.3-p15.1	Ataxia, dysarthria, extrapyramidal features of akinesia, rigidity, tremor, cognitive defect; reduced deep tendon reflexes; MRI: cerebellar atrophy, normal basal ganglia and brainstem
SCA22 (autosomal dominant)	1p21-q23	Pure cerebellar ataxia; dysarthria; dysphagia; nystagmus; MRI: cerebellar atrophy
SCA23 (autosomal dominant)	20p13-12.3	Gait ataxia; dysarthria; extremity ataxia; ocular nystagmus, dysmetria; leg vibration loss; extensor plantar responses; MRI: cerebellar atrophy
SCA25 (autosomal dominant)	2p15-p21	Ataxia, nystagmus; vibratory loss in the feet; pain loss in some; abdominal pain; nausea and vomiting may be prominent; absent ankle reflexes; sensory nerve action potentials are absent; MRI: cerebellar atrophy, normal brainstem
SCA26 (autosomal dominant)	19p13.3	Gait ataxia; extremity ataxia; dysarthria; nystagmus; MRI: cerebellar atrophy
SCA27 (autosomal dominant)	13q34; fibroblast growth factor 14 protein; mutation F145S; produces reduced protein stability	Tremor extremities and head and orofacial dyskinesia; ataxia of arms>legs, gait ataxia; dysarthria; nystagmus; psychiatric symptoms; cognitive defect; MRI: cerebellar atrophy; genetic testing available
SCA28 (autosomal dominant)	18p11.22-q11.2	Extremity and gait ataxia; dysarthria; nystagmus; ophthalmoparesis; leg hyperreflexia and extensor plantar responses; MRI: cerebellar atrophy
SCA30 (autosomal dominant)	4q34.3-q35.1	Candidate gene *ODZ3;* gait ataxia, dysarthria, saccades; nystagmus, brisk tendon reflexes in legs; MRI: cerebellar atrophy
SCA31 (autosomal dominant)	16q22.1	Penta-nucleotide $(TGGAA)_N$ repeat insertions; previously called SCA4; gait ataxia; limb dysmetria; MRI: cerebellar atrophy
Dentatorubropallidoluysian atrophy (autosomal dominant)	12p13.31 with CAG repeats (exonic) Atrophin 1	Ataxia, choreoathetosis, dystonia, seizures, myoclonus, dementia; genetic testing available
Friedreich's ataxia (autosomal recessive)	9q13-q21.1 with intronic GAA repeats, in intron at end of exon 1 Frataxin defective; abnormal regulation of mitochondrial iron metabolism; iron accumulates in mitochondria in yeast mutants	Ataxia, areflexia, extensor plantar responses, position sense deficits, cardiomyopathy, diabetes mellitus, scoliosis, foot deformities; optic atrophy; late-onset form, as late as 50 years with preserved deep tendon reflexes, slower progression, reduced skeletal deformities, associated with an intermediate number of GAA repeats and missense mutations in one allele of frataxin; genetic testing available

(continued)

TABLE 373-2 Classification of the Spinocerebellar Ataxias (*Continued*)

Name	Locus	Phenotype
Friedreich's ataxia (autosomal recessive)	8q13.1-q13.3 (α-TTP deficiency)	Same as phenotype that maps to 9q but associated with vitamin E deficiency; genetic testing available
Sensory ataxic neuropathy and ophthalmoparesis (SANDO) with dysarthria (autosomal recessive)	15q25; mutations in DNA polymerase-gamma (POLG) gene that leads to mtDNA deletions	Young adult–onset ataxia, sensory neuropathy, ophthalmoparesis, hearing loss, gastric symptoms; a variant of progressive external ophthalmoplegia; MRI: cerebellar and thalamic abnormalities; mildly increased lactate and creatine kinase
Von Hippel-Lindau syndrome (autosomal dominant)	3p26-p25	Cerebellar hemangioblastoma; pheochromocytoma
Baltic myoclonus (Unverricht-Lundborg) (recessive)	21q22.3; cystatin B; extra repeats of 12–base pair tandem repeats	Myoclonus epilepsy; late-onset ataxia; responds to valproic acid, clonazepam; phenobarbital
Marinesco-Sjögren syndrome (recessive)	5q31; SIL 1 protein, nucleotide exchange factor for the heat-shock protein 70 (HSP70); chaperone HSPA5; homozygous 4-nucleotide duplication in exon 6; also compound heterozygote	Ataxia, dysarthria; nystagmus; retarded motor and mental maturation; rhabdomyolysis after viral illness; weakness; hypotonia; areflexia; cataracts in childhood; short stature; kyphoscoliosis; contractures; hypogonadism
Autosomal recessive spastic ataxia of Charlevoix-Saguenay (ARSACS)	Chromosome 13q12; SACS gene; loss of sacsin peptide activity	Childhood onset of ataxia, spasticity, dysarthria, distal muscle wasting, foot deformity, retinal striations, mitral valve prolapse
Kearns-Sayre syndrome (sporadic)	mtDNA deletion and duplication mutations	Ptosis, ophthalmoplegia, pigmentary retinal degeneration, cardiomyopathy, diabetes mellitus, deafness, heart block, increased CSF protein, ataxia
Myoclonic epilepsy and ragged red fiber syndrome (MERRF) (maternal inheritance)	Mutation in mtDNA of the $tRNA^{lys}$ at 8344; also mutation at 8356	Myoclonic epilepsy, ragged red fiber myopathy, ataxia
Mitochondrial encephalopathy, lactic acidosis, and stroke syndrome (MELAS) (maternal inheritance)	$tRNA^{leu}$ mutation at 3243; also at 3271 and 3252	Headache, stroke, lactic acidosis, ataxia
Neuropathy; ataxia; retinitis pigmentosa (NARP)	ATPase6 (Complex 5); mtDNA point mutation at 8993	Neuropathy; ataxia; retinitis pigmentosa; dementia; seizures
Episodic ataxia, type 1 (EA-1) (autosomal dominant)	12p13; potassium voltage-gated channel gene, *KCNA1*; Phe249Leu mutation; variable syndrome	Episodic ataxia for minutes; provoked by startle or exercise; with facial and hand myokymia; cerebellar signs are not progressive; choreoathetotic movements; responds to phenytoin; genetic testing available
Episodic ataxia, type 2 (EA-2) (autosomal dominant)	19p-13(*CACNA1A*) (allelic with SCA6) (α_{1A}-voltage–dependent calcium channel subunit); point mutations or small deletions; allelic with SCA6 and familial hemiplegic migraine	Episodic ataxia for days; provoked by stress, fatigue; with down-gaze nystagmus; vertigo; vomiting; headache; cerebellar atrophy results; progressive cerebellar signs; responds to acetazolamide; genetic testing available
Episodic ataxia, type 3 (autosomal dominant)	1q42	Episodic ataxia; 1 min to over 6 h; induced by movement; vertigo and tinnitus; headache; responds to acetazolamide
Episodic ataxia, type 4 (autosomal dominant)	Not mapped	Episodic ataxia; vertigo; diplopia; ocular slow pursuit defect; no response to acetazolamide
Episodic ataxia, type 5 (autosomal dominant)	2q22-q23; CACNB4β4 protein	Episodic ataxia; hours to weeks; seizures
Episodic ataxia, type 6	5p13; SLC1A3; glutamate transporter in astrocytes	Episodic ataxia; seizures; cognitive impairment; under 24 h
Episodic ataxia, type 7 (autosomal dominant)	19q13	Episodic ataxia; vertigo, weakness; less than 24 h

(*continued*)

TABLE 373-2 Classification of the Spinocerebellar Ataxias (*Continued*)

Name	Locus	Phenotype
Episodic ataxia with seizures, migraine, and alternating hemiplegia (autosomal dominant)	SLC1A3; 5p13; EAAT1 protein; missense mutations; glial glutamate transporter (GLAST); 1047 C to G; proline to arginine	Ataxia, duration 2–4 days; episodic hypotonia; delayed motor milestones; seizures; migraine; alternating hemiplegia; mild truncal ataxia; coma; febrile illness as a trigger; MRI: cerebellar atrophy
Fragile X tremor/ataxia syndrome (FXTAS) X-linked dominant	Xq27.3; CGG premutation expansion in FMR1 gene; expansions of 55–200 repeats in 5′ UTR of the FMR-1 mRNA; presumed dominant toxic RNA effect	Late-onset ataxia with tremor, cognitive impairment, occasional parkinsonism; males typically affected, although affected females also reported; syndrome is of high concern if affected male has grandson with mental retardation (fragile X syndrome); MRI shows increased T2 signal in middle cerebellar peduncles, cerebellar atrophy, and occasional widespread brain atrophy; genetic testing available
Ataxia telangiectasia (autosomal recessive)	11q22-23; *ATM* gene for regulation of cell cycle; mitogenic signal transduction and meiotic recombination	Telangiectasia, ataxia, dysarthria, pulmonary infections, neoplasms of lymphatic system; IgA and IgG deficiencies; diabetes mellitus, breast cancer; genetic testing available
Early-onset cerebellar ataxia with retained deep tendon reflexes (autosomal recessive)	13q11-12	Ataxia; neuropathy; preserved deep tendon reflexes; impaired cognitive and visuospatial functions; MRI, cerebellar atrophy
Ataxia with oculomotor apraxia (AOA1) (autosomal recessive)	9p13; protein is member of histidine triad superfamily, role in DNA repair	Ataxia; dysarthria; limb dysmetria; dystonia; oculomotor apraxia; optic atrophy; motor neuropathy; late sensory loss (vibration); genetic testing available
Ataxia with oculomotor apraxia 2 (AOA2) (autosomal recessive)	9q34; senataxin protein, involved in RNA maturation and termination; helicase superfamily 1	Gait ataxia; choreoathetosis; dystonia; oculomotor apraxia; neuropathy, vibration loss, position sense loss, and mild light touch loss; absent leg deep tendon reflexes; extensor plantar response; genetic testing available
Cerebellar ataxia with muscle coenzyme Q10 deficiency (autosomal recessive)	9p13	Ataxia; hypotonia; seizures; mental retardation; increased deep tendon reflexes; extensor plantar responses; coenzyme Q10 levels reduced with about 25% of patients with a block in transfer of electrons to complex 3; may respond to coenzyme 10
Joubert syndrome (autosomal recessive)	9q34.3	Ataxia; ptosis; mental retardation; oculomotor apraxia; nystagmus; retinopathy; rhythmic tongue protrusion; episodic hyperpnea or apnea; dimples at wrists and elbows; telecanthus; micrognathia
Sideroblastic anemia and spinocerebellar ataxia (X-linked recessive)	Xq13; ATP-binding cassette 7 (ABCB7; ABC7) transporter; mitochondrial inner membrane; iron homeostasis; export from matrix to the intermembrane space	Ataxia; elevated free erythrocyte protoporphyrin levels; ring sideroblasts in bone marrow; heterozygous females may have mild anemia but not ataxia
Infantile-onset spinocerebellar ataxia of Nikali et al (autosomal recessive)	10q23.3-q24.1; twinkle protein (gene); homozygous for Tyr508Cys missense mutations	Infantile ataxia, sensory neuropathy; athetosis, hearing deficit, reduced deep tendon reflexes; ophthalmoplegia, optic atrophy; seizures; primary hypogonadism in females
Hypoceruloplasminemia with ataxia and dysarthria (autosomal recessive)	Ceruloplasmin gene; 3q23-q25 (trp 858 ter)	Gait ataxia and dysarthria; hyperreflexia; cerebellar atrophy by MRI; iron deposition in cerebellum, basal ganglia, thalamus, and liver; onset in the 4th decade
Spinocerebellar ataxia with neuropathy (SCAN1) (autosomal recessive)	Tyrosyl-DNA phosphodiesterase-1 (TDP-1) 14q31-q32	Onset in 2nd decade; gait ataxia, dysarthria, seizures, cerebellar vermis atrophy on MRI, dysmetria

Abbreviations: CSF, cerebrospinal fluid; EMG, electromyogram; MRI, magnetic resonance imaging.

linked to an untranslated CAG repeat, and SCA10 is caused by an untranslated pentanucleotide repeat. The clinical phenotypes of these SCAs overlap. The genotype has become the gold standard for diagnosis and classification. CAG encodes glutamine, and these expanded CAG triplet repeat expansions result in expanded polyglutamine proteins, termed *ataxins*, that produce a toxic gain of function with autosomal dominant inheritance. Although the phenotype is variable for any given disease gene, a pattern of neuronal loss with gliosis is produced that is relatively unique for each ataxia. Immunohistochemical and biochemical studies have shown cytoplasmic (SCA2), neuronal (SCA1, MJD, SCA7), and nucleolar (SCA7) accumulation of the specific mutant polyglutamine-containing ataxin proteins. Expanded polyglutamine ataxins with more than ~40 glutamines are potentially toxic to neurons for a variety of reasons including the following: high levels of gene expression for the mutant polyglutamine ataxin in affected neurons; conformational change of the aggregated protein to a β-pleated structure; abnormal transport of the ataxin into the nucleus (SCA1, MJD, SCA7); binding to other polyglutamine proteins, including the TATA-binding transcription protein and the CREB-binding protein, impairing their functions; altering the efficiency of the ubiquitin-proteosome system of protein turnover; and inducing neuronal apoptosis. An earlier age of onset (anticipation) and more aggressive disease in subsequent generations are due to further expansion of the CAG triplet repeat and increased polyglutamine number in the mutant ataxin. The most common disorders are discussed below.

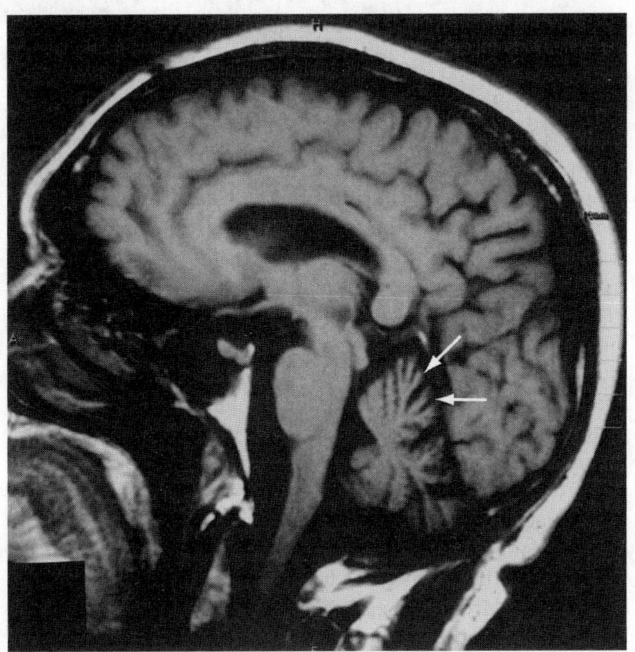

Figure 373-1 Sagittal MRI of the brain of a 60-year-old man with gait ataxia and dysarthria due to SCA1, illustrating cerebellar atrophy (*arrows*). MRI, magnetic resonance imaging; SCA1, spinocerebellar ataxia type 1.

■ SCA1

SCA1 was previously referred to as *olivopontocerebellar atrophy*, but genomic data have shown that that entity represents several different genotypes with overlapping clinical features.

Symptoms and signs

SCA1 is characterized by the development in early or middle adult life of progressive cerebellar ataxia of the trunk and limbs, impairment of equilibrium and gait, slowness of voluntary movements, scanning speech, nystagmoid eye movements, and oscillatory tremor of the head and trunk. Dysarthria, dysphagia, and oculomotor and facial palsies may also occur. Extrapyramidal symptoms include rigidity, an immobile face, and parkinsonian tremor. The reflexes are usually normal, but knee and ankle jerks may be lost, and extensor plantar responses may occur. Dementia may be noted but is usually mild. Impairment of sphincter function is common, with urinary and sometimes fecal incontinence. Cerebellar and brainstem atrophy are evident on MRI (Fig. 373-1).

Marked shrinkage of the ventral half of the pons, disappearance of the olivary eminence on the ventral surface of the medulla, and atrophy of the cerebellum are evident on gross postmortem inspection of the brain. Variable loss of Purkinje cells, reduced numbers of cells in the molecular and granular layer, demyelination of the middle cerebellar peduncle and the cerebellar hemispheres, and severe loss of cells in the pontine nuclei and olives are found on histologic examination. Degenerative changes in the striatum, especially the putamen, and loss of the pigmented cells of the substantia nigra may be found in cases with extrapyramidal features. More widespread degeneration in the central nervous system (CNS), including involvement of the posterior columns and the spinocerebellar fibers, is often present.

GENETIC CONSIDERATIONS

SCA1 encodes a gene product, called *ataxin*-1, which is a novel protein of unknown function. The mutant allele has 40 CAG repeats located within the coding region, whereas alleles from unaffected individuals have ≤36 repeats. A few patients with 38–40 CAG repeats have been described. There is a direct correlation between a larger number of repeats and a younger age of onset for SCA1. Juvenile patients have higher numbers of repeats, and anticipation is present in subsequent generations. Transgenic mice carrying SCA1 developed ataxia and Purkinje cell pathology. Nuclear localization, but not aggregation, of ataxin-1 appears to be required for cell death initiated by the mutant protein.

■ SCA2

Symptoms and signs

Another clinical phenotype, SCA2, has been described in patients from Cuba and India. Cuban patients probably are descendants of a common ancestor, and the population may be the largest homogeneous group of patients with ataxia yet described. The age of onset ranges from 2–65 years, and there is considerable clinical variability within families. Although neuropathologic and clinical findings are compatible with a diagnosis of SCA1, including slow saccadic eye movements, ataxia, dysarthria, parkinsonian rigidity, optic disc pallor, mild spasticity, and retinal degeneration, SCA2 is a unique form of cerebellar degenerative disease.

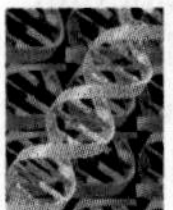

GENETIC CONSIDERATIONS

The gene in SCA2 families also contains CAG repeat expansions coding for a polyglutamine-containing protein, ataxin-2. Normal alleles contain 15–32 repeats; mutant alleles have 35–77 repeats.

■ MACHADO-JOSEPH DISEASE/SCA3

MJD was first described among the Portuguese and their descendants in New England and California. Subsequently, MJD has been found in families from Portugal, Australia, Brazil, Canada, China, England, France, India, Israel, Italy, Japan, Spain, Taiwan, and the

United States. In most populations, it is the most common autosomal dominant ataxia.

Symptoms and signs

MJD has been classified into three clinical types. In type I MJD (amyotrophic lateral sclerosis–parkinsonism–dystonia type), neurologic deficits appear in the first two decades and involve weakness and spasticity of extremities, especially the legs, often with dystonia of the face, neck, trunk, and extremities. Patellar and ankle clonus are common, as are extensor plantar responses. The gait is slow and stiff, with a slightly broadened base and lurching from side to side; this gait results from spasticity, not true ataxia. There is no truncal titubation. Pharyngeal weakness and spasticity cause difficulty with speech and swallowing. Of note is the prominence of horizontal and vertical nystagmus, loss of fast saccadic eye movements, hypermetric and hypometric saccades, and impairment of upward vertical gaze. Facial fasciculations, facial myokymia, lingual fasciculations without atrophy, ophthalmoparesis, and ocular prominence are common early manifestations.

In type II MJD (ataxic type), true cerebellar deficits of dysarthria and gait and extremity ataxia begin in the second to fourth decades along with corticospinal and extrapyramidal deficits of spasticity, rigidity, and dystonia. Type II is the most common form of MJD. Ophthalmoparesis, upward vertical gaze deficits, and facial and lingual fasciculations are also present. Type II MJD can be distinguished from the clinically similar disorders SCA1 and SCA2.

Type III MJD (ataxic-amyotrophic type) presents in the fifth to the seventh decades with a pancerebellar disorder that includes dysarthria and gait and extremity ataxia. Distal sensory loss involving pain, touch, vibration, and position senses and distal atrophy are prominent, indicating the presence of peripheral neuropathy. The deep tendon reflexes are depressed to absent, and there are no corticospinal or extrapyramidal findings.

The mean age of onset of symptoms in MJD is 25 years. Neurologic deficits invariably progress and lead to death from debilitation within 15 years of onset, especially in patients with types I and II disease. Usually, patients retain full intellectual function.

The major pathologic findings are variable loss of neurons and glial replacement in the corpus striatum and severe loss of neurons in the pars compacta of the substantia nigra. A moderate loss of neurons occurs in the dentate nucleus of the cerebellum and in the red nucleus. Purkinje cell loss and granule cell loss occur in the cerebellar cortex. Cell loss also occurs in the dentate nucleus and in the cranial nerve motor nuclei. Sparing of the inferior olives distinguishes MJD from other dominantly inherited ataxias.

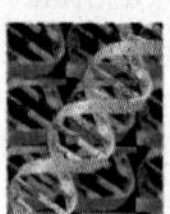

GENETIC CONSIDERATIONS

The gene for MJD maps to 14q24.3-q32. Unstable CAG repeat expansions are present in the MJD gene coding for a polyglutamine-containing protein named ataxin-3, or MJD-ataxin. An earlier age of onset is associated with longer repeats. Alleles from normal individuals have between 12 and 37 CAG repeats, while MJD alleles have 60–84 CAG repeats. Polyglutamine-containing aggregates of ataxin-3 (MJD-ataxin) have been described in neuronal nuclei undergoing degeneration. MJD-ataxin codes for a ubiquitin protease, which is inactive due to expanded polyglutamines. Proteosome function is impaired, resulting in altered clearance of proteins and cerebellar neuronal loss.

SCA6

Genomic screening for CAG repeats in other families with autosomal dominant ataxia and vibratory and proprioceptive sensory loss have yielded another locus. Of interest is that different mutations in the same gene for the α_{1A} voltage-dependent calcium channel subunit (CACNLIA4; also referred to as the *CACNA1A* gene) at 19p13 result in different clinical disorders. CAG repeat expansions (21–27 in patients; 4–16 triplets in normal individuals) result in late-onset progressive ataxia with cerebellar degeneration. Missense mutations in this gene result in familial hemiplegic migraine. Nonsense mutations resulting in termination of protein synthesis of the gene product yield hereditary paroxysmal cerebellar ataxia or EA. Some patients with familial hemiplegic migraine develop progressive ataxia and also have cerebellar atrophy.

SCA7

This disorder is distinguished from all other SCAs by the presence of retinal pigmentary degeneration. The visual abnormalities first appear as blue-yellow color blindness and proceed to frank visual loss with macular degeneration. In almost all other respects, SCA7 resembles several other SCAs in which ataxia is accompanied by various noncerebellar findings, including ophthalmoparesis and extensor plantar responses. The genetic defect is an expanded CAG repeat in the SCA7 gene at 3p14-p21.1. The expanded repeat size in SCA7 is highly variable. Consistent with this, the severity of clinical findings varies from essentially asymptomatic to mild late-onset symptoms to severe, aggressive disease in childhood with rapid progression. Marked anticipation has been recorded, especially with paternal transmission. The disease protein, ataxin-7, forms aggregates in nuclei of affected neurons, as has also been described for SCA1 and SCA3/MJD.

SCA8

This form of ataxia is caused by a CTG repeat expansion in an untranslated region of a gene on chromosome 13q21. There is marked maternal bias in transmission, perhaps reflecting contractions of the repeat during spermatogenesis. The mutation is not fully penetrant. Symptoms include slowly progressive dysarthria and gait ataxia beginning at ~40 years of age with a range between 20 and 65 years. Other features include nystagmus, leg spasticity, and reduced vibratory sensation. Severely affected individuals are nonambulatory by the fourth to sixth decades. MRI shows cerebellar atrophy. The mechanism of disease may involve a dominant "toxic" effect occurring at the RNA level, as occurs in myotonic dystrophy.

DENTATORUBROPALLIDOLUYSIAN ATROPHY

DRPLA has a variable presentation that may include progressive ataxia, choreoathetosis, dystonia, seizures, myoclonus, and dementia. DRPLA is due to unstable CAG triplet repeats in the open reading frame of a gene named *atrophin* located on chromosome 12p12-ter. Larger expansions are found in patients with earlier onset. The number of repeats is 49 in patients with DRPLA and ≤26 in normal individuals. Anticipation occurs in successive generations, with earlier onset of disease in association with an increasing CAG repeat number in children who inherit the disease from their father. One well-characterized family in North Carolina has a phenotypic variant known as the *Haw River syndrome*, now recognized to be due to the DRPLA mutation.

EPISODIC ATAXIA

EA types 1 and 2 are two rare dominantly inherited disorders that have been mapped to chromosomes 12p (a potassium channel gene) for type 1 and 19p for type 2. Patients with EA-1 have brief episodes of ataxia with myokymia and nystagmus that last only minutes. Startle, sudden change in posture, and exercise can induce episodes. Acetazolamide or anticonvulsants may be therapeutic. Patients with EA-2 have episodes of ataxia with nystagmus that can last for hours or days. Stress, exercise, or excessive fatigue may be precipitants. Acetazolamide may be therapeutic and can reverse the relative intracellular alkalosis detected by magnetic resonance spectroscopy. Stop codon, nonsense mutations causing EA-2 have been found in the *CACNA1A* gene, encoding the α_{1A} voltage-dependent calcium channel subunit (see "SCA6," above).

AUTOSOMAL RECESSIVE ATAXIAS

Friedreich's ataxia

This is the most common form of inherited ataxia, comprising one-half of all hereditary ataxias. It can occur in a classic form or in association with a genetically determined vitamin E deficiency syndrome; the two forms are clinically indistinguishable.

Symptoms and signs Friedreich's ataxia presents before 25 years of age with progressive staggering gait, frequent falling, and titubation. The lower extremities are more severely involved than the upper ones. Dysarthria occasionally is the presenting symptom; rarely, progressive scoliosis, foot deformity, nystagmus, or cardiopathy is the initial sign.

The neurologic examination reveals nystagmus, loss of fast saccadic eye movements, truncal titubation, dysarthria, dysmetria, and ataxia of trunk and limb movements. Extensor plantar responses (with normal tone in trunk and extremities), absence of deep tendon reflexes, and weakness (greater distally than proximally) are usually found. Loss of vibratory and proprioceptive sensation occurs. The median age of death is 35 years. Women have a significantly better prognosis than men.

Cardiac involvement occurs in 90% of patients. Cardiomegaly, symmetric hypertrophy, murmurs, and conduction defects are reported. Moderate mental retardation or psychiatric syndromes are present in a small percentage of patients. A high incidence of diabetes mellitus (20%) is found and is associated with insulin resistance and pancreatic β-cell dysfunction. Musculoskeletal deformities are common and include pes cavus, pes equinovarus, and scoliosis. MRI of the spinal cord shows atrophy (Fig. 373-2).

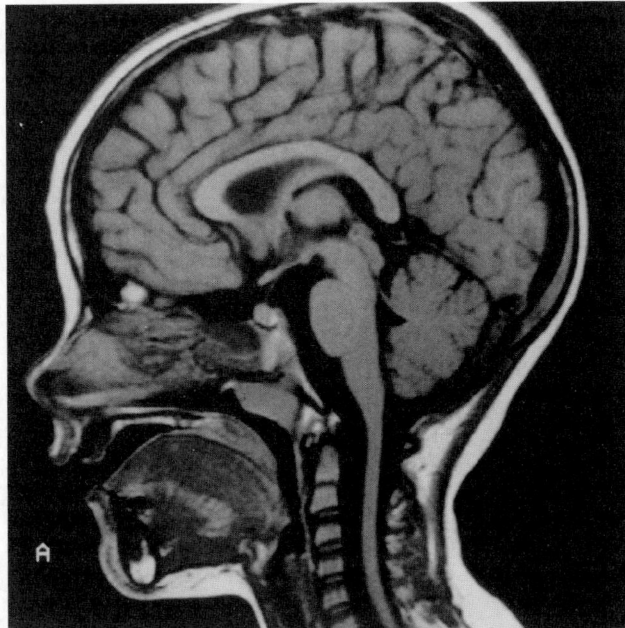

Figure 373-2 Sagittal MRI of the brain and spinal cord of a patient with Friedreich's ataxia, demonstrating spinal cord atrophy.

The primary sites of pathology are the spinal cord, dorsal root ganglion cells, and the peripheral nerves. Slight atrophy of the cerebellum and cerebral gyri may occur. Sclerosis and degeneration occur predominantly in the spinocerebellar tracts, lateral corticospinal tracts, and posterior columns. Degeneration of the glossopharyngeal, vagus, hypoglossal, and deep cerebellar nuclei is described. The cerebral cortex is histologically normal except for loss of Betz cells in the precentral gyri. The peripheral nerves are extensively involved, with a loss of large myelinated fibers. Cardiac pathology consists of myocytic hypertrophy and fibrosis, focal vascular fibromuscular dysplasia with subintimal or medial deposition of periodic acid–Schiff (PAS)-positive material, myocytopathy with unusual pleomorphic nuclei, and focal degeneration of nerves and cardiac ganglia.

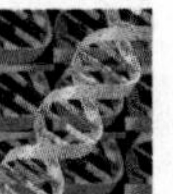

GENETIC CONSIDERATIONS

The classic form of Friedreich's ataxia has been mapped to 9q13-q21.1, and the mutant gene, *frataxin*, contains expanded GAA triplet repeats in the first intron. There is homozygosity for expanded GAA repeats in >95% of patients. Normal persons have 7–22 GAA repeats, and patients have 200–900 GAA repeats. A more varied clinical syndrome has been described in compound heterozygotes who have one copy of the GAA expansion and the other copy a point mutation in the *frataxin* gene. When the point mutation is located in the region of the gene that encodes the amino-terminal half of frataxin, the phenotype is milder, often consisting of a spastic gait, retained or exaggerated reflexes, no dysarthria, and mild or absent ataxia.

Patients with Friedreich's ataxia have undetectable or extremely low levels of *frataxin* mRNA, as compared with carriers and unrelated individuals; thus, disease appears to be caused by a loss of expression of the frataxin protein. Frataxin is a mitochondrial protein involved in iron homeostasis. Mitochondrial iron accumulation due to loss of the iron transporter coded by the mutant *frataxin* gene results in oxidized intramitochondrial iron. Excess oxidized iron results in turn in the oxidation of cellular components and irreversible cell injury.

Two forms of hereditary ataxia associated with abnormalities in the interactions of vitamin E (α-tocopherol) with very low density lipoprotein (VLDL) have been delineated. These are abetalipoproteinemia (Bassen-Kornzweig syndrome) and ataxia with vitamin E deficiency (AVED). Abetalipoproteinemia is caused by mutations in the gene coding for the larger subunit of the microsomal triglyceride transfer protein (MTP). Defects in MTP result in impairment of formation and secretion of VLDL in liver. This defect results in a deficiency of delivery of vitamin E to tissues, including the central and peripheral nervous system, as VLDL is the transport molecule for vitamin E and other fat-soluble substitutes. AVED is due to mutations in the gene for α-tocopherol transfer protein (α-TTP). These patients have an impaired ability to bind vitamin E into the VLDL produced and secreted by the liver, resulting in a deficiency of vitamin E in peripheral tissues. Hence, either absence of VLDL (abetalipoproteinemia) or impaired binding of vitamin E to VLDL (AVED) causes an ataxic syndrome. Once again, a genotype classification has proved to be essential in sorting out the various forms of the Friedreich's disease syndrome, which may be clinically indistinguishable.

Ataxia telangiectasia

Symptoms and signs Patients with ataxia telangiectasia (AT) present in the first decade of life with progressive telangiectatic lesions associated with deficits in cerebellar function and nystagmus. The neurologic manifestations correspond to those in Friedreich's disease, which should be included in the differential diagnosis. Truncal and limb ataxia, dysarthria, extensor plantar responses, myoclonic jerks, areflexia, and distal sensory deficits may develop. There is a high incidence of recurrent pulmonary infections and neoplasms of the lymphatic and reticuloendothelial system in patients with AT. Thymic hypoplasia with cellular and humoral (IgA and IgG2) immunodeficiencies, premature aging, and endocrine disorders such as Type 1 diabetes mellitus are described. There is an increased incidence of lymphomas, Hodgkin's disease, acute leukemias of the T cell type, and breast cancer.

The most striking neuropathologic changes include loss of Purkinje, granule, and basket cells in the cerebellar cortex as well as of neurons in the deep cerebellar nuclei. The inferior olives of the medulla may also have neuronal loss. There is a loss of anterior horn neurons in the spinal cord and of dorsal root ganglion cells associated with posterior column spinal cord demyelination. A poorly developed or absent thymus gland is the most consistent defect of the lymphoid system.

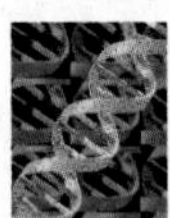

GENETIC CONSIDERATIONS

The gene for AT (the *ATM* gene) encodes a protein that is similar to several yeast and mammalian phosphatidylinositol-3′-kinases involved in mitogenic signal transduction, meiotic recombination, and cell cycle control. Defective DNA repair in AT fibroblasts exposed to ultraviolet light has been demonstrated. The discovery of *ATM* will make possible the identification of heterozygotes who are at risk for cancer (e.g., breast cancer) and permit early diagnosis.

■ MITOCHONDRIAL ATAXIAS

Spinocerebellar syndromes have been identified with mutations in mitochondrial DNA (mtDNA). Thirty pathogenic mtDNA point mutations and 60 different types of mtDNA deletions are known, several of which cause or are associated with ataxia (Chap. 387).

TREATMENT Ataxic Disorders

The most important goal in management of patients with ataxia is to identify treatable disease entities. Mass lesions must be recognized promptly and treated appropriately. Paraneoplastic disorders can often be identified by the clinical patterns of disease that they produce, measurement of specific autoantibodies, and uncovering the primary cancer; these disorders are often refractory to therapy, but some patients improve following removal of the tumor or immunotherapy (Chap. 101). Ataxia with anti-gliadin antibodies and gluten-sensitive enteropathy may improve with a gluten-free diet. Malabsorption syndromes leading to vitamin E deficiency may lead to ataxia. The vitamin E deficiency form of Friedreich's ataxia must be considered, and serum vitamin E levels measured. Vitamin E therapy is indicated for these rare patients. Vitamin B_1 and B_{12} levels in serum should be measured, and the vitamins administered to patients having deficient levels. Hypothyroidism is easily treated. The cerebrospinal fluid should be tested for a syphilitic infection in patients with progressive ataxia and other features of tabes dorsalis. Similarly, antibody titers for Lyme disease and *Legionella* should be measured and appropriate antibiotic therapy should be instituted in antibody-positive patients. Aminoacidopathies, leukodystrophies, urea-cycle abnormalities, and mitochondrial encephalomyopathies may produce ataxia, and some dietary or metabolic therapies are available for these disorders. The deleterious effects of phenytoin and alcohol on the cerebellum are well known, and these exposures should be avoided in patients with ataxia of any cause.

There is no proven therapy for any of the autosomal dominant ataxias (SCA1 to -28). There is preliminary evidence that idebenone, a free-radical scavenger, can improve myocardial hypertrophy in patients with classic Friedreich ataxia; there is no current evidence, however, that it improves neurologic function. A small preliminary study in a mixed population of patients with different inherited ataxias raised the possibility that the glutamate antagonist riluzole may offer modest benefit. Iron chelators and antioxidant drugs are potentially harmful in Friedreich's patients as they may increase heart muscle injury. Acetazolamide can reduce the duration of symptoms of episodic ataxia. At present, identification of an at-risk person's genotype, together with appropriate family and genetic counseling, can reduce the incidence of these cerebellar syndromes in future generations (Chap. 63).

FURTHER READINGS

Anheim M et al: Clinical spectrum of ataxia-telangiectasia in adulthood. Neurology 73:430, 2009

Brusse E et al: Diagnosis and management of early- and late-onset cerebellar ataxia. Clin Genet 71:12, 2007

Durr A: Autosomal dominant cerebellar ataxias: Polyglutamine expansions and beyond. Lancet Neurol 9:885, 2010

Hadjivassiliou M et al: Gluten ataxia in perspective: Epidemiology, genetic susceptibility and clinical characteristics. Brain 136:685, 2003

Ristori G et al: Riluzole in cerebellar ataxia: A randomized, double-blind, placebo-controlled pilot trial. Neurology 74:839, 2010

Rosenberg RN, Paulson HL: The inherited ataxias, in *The Molecular and Genetic Basis of Neurologic and Psychiatric Disease*, 4th ed, RN Rosenberg et al (eds). Philadelphia, Lippincott Williams & Wilkins, 2008.

Todi SV et al: Activity and cellular functions of the deubiquitinating enzyme and polyglutamine disease protein ataxin-3 are regulated by ubiquitination at lysine 117. J Biol Chem 285:39303, 2010

Cerebellar Degeneration Information Page. National Institute of Neurological Disorder and Stroke. *http://www.NINDS.NIH.gov/disorders/ataxia/ataxia.htm*

CHAPTER 374 Amyotrophic Lateral Sclerosis and Other Motor Neuron Diseases

Robert H. Brown, Jr.

AMYOTROPHIC LATERAL SCLEROSIS

Amyotrophic lateral sclerosis (ALS) is the most common form of progressive motor neuron disease. It is a prime example of a neurodegenerative disease and is arguably the most devastating of the neurodegenerative disorders.

PATHOLOGY

The pathologic hallmark of motor neuron degenerative disorders is death of lower motor neurons (consisting of anterior horn cells in the spinal cord and their brainstem homologues innervating bulbar muscles) and upper, or corticospinal, motor neurons (originating in layer five of the motor cortex and descending via the pyramidal tract to synapse with lower motor neurons, either directly or indirectly via interneurons) (Chap. 22). Although at its onset ALS may involve selective loss of function of only upper or lower motor neurons, it ultimately causes progressive loss of both categories of motor neurons. Indeed, in the absence of clear involvement of both motor neuron types, the diagnosis of ALS is questionable.

Other motor neuron diseases involve only particular subsets of motor neurons (Tables 374-1 and 374-2). Thus, in bulbar palsy and spinal muscular atrophy (SMA; also called *progressive muscular atrophy*), the lower motor neurons of brainstem and spinal cord, respectively, are most severely involved. By contrast, pseudobulbar palsy, primary lateral sclerosis (PLS), and familial spastic paraplegia (FSP) affect only upper motor neurons innervating the brainstem and spinal cord.

In each of these diseases, the affected motor neurons undergo shrinkage, often with accumulation of the pigmented lipid (lipofuscin) that normally develops in these cells with advancing age. In ALS, the motor neuron cytoskeleton is typically affected early in the illness. Focal enlargements are frequent in proximal motor axons; ultrastructurally, these "spheroids" are composed of accumulations of neurofilaments and other proteins. Also seen is proliferation of astroglia and microglia, the inevitable accompaniment of all degenerative processes in the central nervous system (CNS).

The death of the peripheral motor neurons in the brainstem and spinal cord leads to denervation and consequent atrophy of the corresponding muscle fibers. Histochemical and electrophysiologic evidence indicates that in the early phases of the illness denervated muscle can be reinnervated by sprouting of nearby distal motor nerve terminals, although reinnervation in this disease is considerably less extensive than in most other disorders affecting motor neurons (e.g., poliomyelitis, peripheral neuropathy). As denervation progresses, muscle atrophy is readily recognized in muscle biopsies and on clinical examination. This is the basis for the term *amyotrophy*. The loss of cortical motor neurons results in thinning of the corticospinal tracts that travel via the internal capsule (Fig. 374-1) and brainstem to the lateral and anterior white matter columns of the spinal cord. The loss of fibers in the lateral columns and resulting fibrillary gliosis impart a particular firmness (*lateral sclerosis*). A remarkable feature of the disease is the selectivity of neuronal cell death. By light microscopy, the entire sensory apparatus, the regulatory mechanisms for the control and coordination of movement, and the components of the brain that are needed for cognitive processes, remain intact. However, immunostaining indicates that neurons bearing ubiquitin, a marker for degeneration, are also detected in nonmotor systems. Moreover, studies of glucose metabolism in the illness also indicate that there is neuronal dysfunction outside of the motor system. Within the motor system, there is some selectivity of involvement. Thus, motor neurons required for ocular motility remain unaffected, as do the parasympathetic neurons in the sacral spinal cord (the nucleus of Onufrowicz, or Onuf) that innervate the sphincters of the bowel and bladder.

CLINICAL MANIFESTATIONS

The manifestations of ALS are somewhat variable depending on whether corticospinal neurons or lower motor neurons in the brainstem and spinal cord are more prominently involved. With lower motor neuron dysfunction and early denervation, typically the first evidence of the disease is insidiously developing asymmetric weakness, usually first evident distally in one of the limbs. A detailed history often discloses recent development of cramping with volitional movements, typically in the early hours of the morning (e.g., while stretching in bed). Weakness caused by denervation is associated with progressive wasting and atrophy of muscles and, particularly early in the illness, spontaneous twitching of motor units, or fasciculations. In the hands, a preponderance of extensor over flexor weakness is common. When the initial denervation involves bulbar rather than limb muscles, the problem at onset is difficulty with chewing, swallowing, and movements of the face and tongue. Early involvement of the muscles of respiration may lead to death before the disease is far advanced elsewhere. With prominent corticospinal involvement, there is hyperactivity of the muscle-stretch reflexes (tendon jerks) and, often, spastic resistance to passive movements of the affected limbs. Patients with significant reflex hyperactivity complain of muscle stiffness often out of proportion to weakness. Degeneration of the corticobulbar projections innervating the brainstem results in dysarthria and exaggeration of the motor expressions of emotion. The latter leads to involuntary excess in weeping or laughing (pseudobulbar affect).

Virtually any muscle group may be the first to show signs of disease, but, as time passes, more and more muscles become involved until ultimately the disorder takes on a symmetric distribution in all regions. It is characteristic of ALS that, regardless of whether the initial disease involves upper or lower motor neurons, both will eventually be implicated. Even in the late stages of the illness, sensory, bowel and bladder, and cognitive functions are preserved. Even when there is severe brainstem disease, ocular motility is spared until the very late stages of the illness. Dementia is not a component of sporadic ALS. In some families, ALS is co-inherited with frontotemporal dementia, characterized by early behavioral abnormalities with prominent behavioral features indicative of frontal lobe dysfunction.

A committee of the World Federation of Neurology has established diagnostic guidelines for ALS. Essential for the diagnosis is simultaneous upper and lower motor neuron involvement with progressive weakness, and the exclusion of all alternative diagnoses. The disorder is ranked as "definite" ALS when three or four of the following are involved: bulbar, cervical, thoracic, and lumbosacral motor neurons. When two sites are involved, the diagnosis is "probable," and when only one site is implicated, the diagnosis is "possible." An exception is made for those who have progressive

TABLE 374-1 Etiology of Motor Neuron Disorders

Diagnostic Category	Investigation
Structural lesions	MRI scan of head (including foramen magnum and cervical spine)
Parasagittal or foramen magnum tumors	
Cervical spondylosis	
Chiari malformation of syrinx	
Spinal cord arteriovenous malformation	
Infections	CSF exam, culture
Bacterial—tetanus, Lyme	Lyme titer
Viral—poliomyelitis, herpes zoster	Anti-viral antibody
Retroviral—myelopathy	HTLV-1 titers
Intoxications, physical agents	24-hour urine for heavy metals
Toxins—lead, aluminum, others	Serum lead level
Drugs—strychnine, phenytoin	
Electric shock, x-irradiation	
Immunologic mechanisms	Complete blood count[a]
Plasma cell dyscrasias	Sedimentation rate[a]
Autoimmune polyradiculopathy	Total protein[a]
Motor neuropathy with conduction block	Anti-GM1 antibodies[a]
Paraneoplastic	Anti-Hu antibody
Paracarcinomatous	MRI scan, bone marrow biopsy
Metabolic	Fasting blood sugar[a]
Hypoglycemia	Routine chemistries including calcium[a]
Hyperparathyroidism	PTH
Hyperthyroidism	Thyroid function[a]
Deficiency of folate, vitamin B_{12}, vitamin E	Vitamin B_{12}, vitamin E, folate[a]
Deficiency of copper, zinc	Serum zinc, copper[a]
Malabsorption	24-h stool fat, carotene, prothrombin time
Mitochondrial dysfunction	Fasting lactate, pyruvate, ammonia Consider mtDNA
Hyperlipidemia	Lipid electrophoresis
Hyperglycinuria	Urine and serum amino acids CSF amino acids
Hereditary disorders	WBC DNA for mutational analysis
Superoxide dismutase	
TDP43	
FUS/TLS	
Androgen receptor defect (Kennedy's disease)	
Hexosaminidase deficiency	
Infantile α-glucosidase deficiency (Pompe's)	

[a]Denotes studies that should be obtained in all cases.

Abbreviations: CSF, cerebrospinal fluid; FUS/TLS, fused in sarcoma/translocated in liposarcoma; HTLV-1, human T cell lymphotropic virus; PTH, parathyroid; WBC, white blood cell.

upper and lower motor neuron signs at only one site and a mutation in the gene encoding superoxide dismutase (SOD1; below).

EPIDEMIOLOGY

The illness is relentlessly progressive, leading to death from respiratory paralysis; the median survival is from 3–5 years. There are very rare reports of stabilization or even regression of ALS. In most societies there is an incidence of 1–3 per 100,000 and a prevalence of 3–5 per 100,000. Several endemic foci of higher prevalence exist in the western Pacific (e.g., in specific regions of Guam or Papua New Guinea). In the United States and Europe, males are somewhat more frequently affected than females. Epidemiologic studies have incriminated risk factors for this disease including exposure to pesticides and insecticides, smoking and, in one report, service in the military. While ALS is overwhelmingly a sporadic disorder, some 5–10% of cases are inherited as an autosomal dominant trait.

FAMILIAL ALS

Several forms of selective motor neuron disease are inheritable (Table 374-3). Familial ALS (FALS) involves both corticospinal and lower motor neurons. Apart from its inheritance as an autosomal dominant trait, it is clinically indistinguishable from sporadic ALS. Genetic studies have identified mutations in the genes encoding the cytosolic enzyme SOD1 (superoxide dismutase), and the RNA binding proteins TDP43 (encoded by the TAR DNA binding protein gene), and FUS/TLS (fused in sarcoma/translocated in liposarcoma), as the most common causes of FALS. Mutations in SOD1 account for about 20% of cases of FALS, while TDP43 and FUS/TLS each represent about 5% of familial cases.

Rare mutations in other genes are also clearly implicated in ALS-like diseases. Thus, a familial, dominantly inherited motor disorder that in some individuals closely mimics the ALS phenotype arises from mutations in a gene that encodes a vesicle-binding protein. A predominantly lower motor neuron disease with early hoarseness due to laryngeal dysfunction has been ascribed to mutations in the gene encoding the cellular accessory motor protein dynactin. Mutations in senataxin, a helicase, cause an early adult-onset, slowly evolving ALS variant. Kennedy's syndrome is an X-linked, adult-onset disorder that may mimic ALS, as described below.

Genetic analyses are also beginning to illuminate the pathogenesis of some childhood-onset motor neuron diseases. For example, a slowly disabling degenerative, predominantly upper motor neuron disease that starts in the first decade is caused by mutations in a gene that expresses a novel signaling molecule with properties of a guanine-exchange factor, termed *alsin*.

DIFFERENTIAL DIAGNOSIS

Because ALS is currently untreatable, it is imperative that potentially remediable causes of motor neuron dysfunction be excluded (Table 374-1). This is particularly true in cases that are atypical by virtue of (1) restriction to either upper or lower motor neurons,

TABLE 374-2 sporadic motor neuron diseases

Chronic	Entity
Upper and lower motor neuron	Amyotrophic lateral sclerosis
Predominantly upper motor neuron	Primary lateral sclerosis
Predominantly lower motor neuron	Multi focal motor neuropathy with conduction block
	Motor neuropathy with paraproteinemia or cancer
	Motor predominant peripheral neuropathies
Other	
Associated with other neurodegenerative disorders	
Secondary motor neuron disorders (see Table 374-1)	
Acute	
Poliomyelitis	
Herpes zoster	
Coxsackie virus	

(2) involvement of neurons other than motor neurons, and (3) evidence of motor neuronal conduction block on electrophysiologic testing. Compression of the cervical spinal cord or cervicomedullary junction from tumors in the cervical regions or at the foramen magnum or from cervical spondylosis with osteophytes projecting into the vertebral canal can produce weakness, wasting, and fasciculations in the upper limbs and spasticity in the legs, closely resembling ALS. The absence of cranial nerve involvement may be helpful in differentiation, although some foramen magnum lesions may

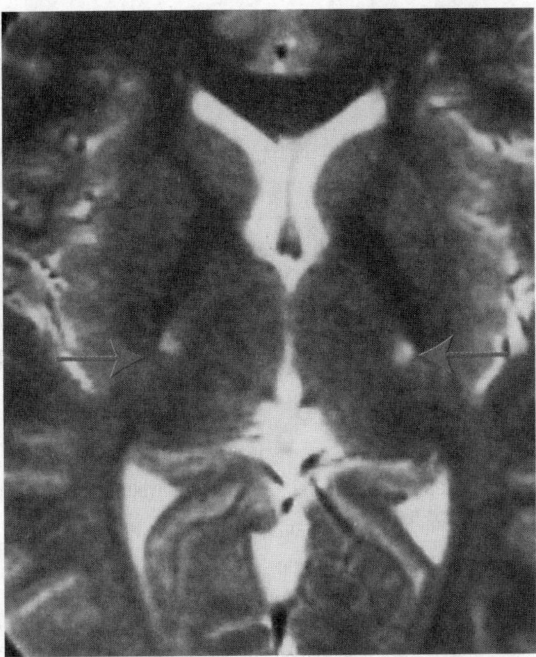

Figure 374-1 Amyotrophic lateral sclerosis. Axial T2-weighted MRI scan through the lateral ventricles of the brain reveals abnormal high signal intensity within the corticospinal tracts (*arrows*). This MRI feature represents an increase in water content in myelin tracts undergoing Wallerian degeneration secondary to cortical motor neuronal loss. This finding is commonly present in ALS, but can also be seen in AIDS-related encephalopathy, infarction, or other disease processes that produce corticospinal neuronal loss in a symmetric fashion.

compress the twelfth cranial (hypoglossal) nerve, with resulting paralysis of the tongue. Absence of pain or of sensory changes, normal bowel and bladder function, normal roentgenographic studies of the spine, and normal cerebrospinal fluid (CSF) all favor ALS. Where doubt exists, MRI scans and contrast myelography should be performed to visualize the cervical spinal cord.

Another important entity in the differential diagnosis of ALS is *multifocal motor neuropathy with conduction block* (MMCB), discussed below. A diffuse, lower motor axonal neuropathy mimicking ALS sometimes evolves in association with hematopoietic disorders such as lymphoma or multiple myeloma. In this clinical setting, the presence of an M-component in serum should prompt consideration of a bone marrow biopsy. Lyme disease (Chap. 173) may also cause an axonal, lower motor neuropathy, although typically with intense proximal limb pain and a CSF pleocytosis.

Other treatable disorders that occasionally mimic ALS are chronic lead poisoning and thyrotoxicosis. These disorders may be suggested by the patient's social or occupational history or by unusual clinical features. When the family history is positive, disorders involving the genes encoding cytosolic SOD1, TDP43, FUS/TLS, as well as adult hexosaminidase A or α-glucosidase deficiency must be excluded (Chap. 361). These are readily identified by appropriate laboratory tests. Benign fasciculations are occasionally a source of concern because on inspection they resemble the fascicular twitchings that accompany motor neuron degeneration. The absence of weakness, atrophy, or denervation phenomena on electrophysiologic examination usually excludes ALS or other serious neurologic disease. Patients who have recovered from poliomyelitis may experience a delayed deterioration of motor neurons that presents clinically with progressive weakness, atrophy, and fasciculations. Its cause is unknown, but it is thought to reflect sublethal prior injury to motor neurons by poliovirus (Chap. 191).

Rarely, ALS develops concurrently with features indicative of more widespread neurodegeneration. Thus, one infrequently encounters otherwise typical ALS patients with a parkinsonian movement disorder or dementia. It remains unclear whether this reflects the unlikely simultaneous occurrence of two disorders or a primary defect triggering two forms of neurodegeneration. The latter is suggested by the observation that multisystem neurodegenerative diseases may be inherited. For example, prominent amyotrophy has been described as a dominantly inherited disorder in individuals with bizarre behavior and a movement disorder suggestive of parkinsonism; many such cases have now been ascribed to mutations that alter the expression of tau protein in brain (Chap. 371). In other cases, ALS develops simultaneously with a striking frontotemporal dementia. These disorders may be dominantly co-inherited; in some families, this trait is linked to a locus on chromosome 9p, although the underlying genetic defect is not established. An ALS-like disorder has also been described in some individuals with chronic traumatic encephalopathy, associated with deposition of TDP43 and neurofibrillary tangles in motor neurons.

PATHOGENESIS

The cause of sporadic ALS is not well defined. Several mechanisms that impair motor neuron viability have been elucidated in mice and rats induced to develop motor neuron disease by SOD1 transgenes with ALS-associated mutations. It is evident that excitotoxic neurotransmitters such as glutamate participate in the death of motor neurons in ALS. This may be a consequence of diminished uptake of synaptic glutamate by an astroglial glutamate transporter, EAAT2. It is striking that one cellular defense against such excitotoxicity is the enzyme SOD1, which detoxifies the free radical superoxide anion (Chap. 365). Precisely why SOD1 mutations are toxic to motor nerves is not established, although it is clear the effect is not simply loss of normal scavenging of the superoxide anion. The mutant protein is conformationally unstable and prone to aberrant catalytic reactions. In turn, these features lead to

TABLE 374-3 Genetic Motor Neuron Diseases

Disease	Locus	Gene	Inheritance	Onset	Gene Function	Unusual Features
I. Upper and Lower Motor Neurons (familial ALS)						
ALS1	21q	Superoxide dismutase	AD	Adult	Protein anti oxidant	
ALS2	2q	Alsin	AR	Juvenile	GEF signalling	Severe corticobulbar, corticospinal features
ALS4	9q	Senataxin	AD	Late juvenile	DNA helicase	Late childhood onset
ALS6	16p	FUS/TLS	AD	Adult	DNA, RNA binding	
ALS8	20q	Vesicle-associated protein B	AD	Adult	Vesicular trafficking	
ALS9	14q	Angiogenin	AD	Adult	RNAse, angiogenesis	
ALS10	1q	TARDBP	AD	Adult	DNA, RNA binding	
ALS	2p	Dynactin	AD	Adult	Axonal transport	Vocal cord stridor in some families
ALS	17q	Paraoxonases 1-3	AD	Adult	Detoxify intoxicants	
ALS	mtDNA	Cytochrome c oxidase		Adult	ATP generation	
ALS	mtDNA	tRNA-isoleucine		Adult	ATP generation	
II. Lower Motor Neurons						
Spinal muscular atrophies	5q	Survival motor neuron	AR	Infancy	RNA metabolism	
GM2-gangliosidosis						
1. Sandhoff disease	5q	Hexosaminidase B	AR	Childhood	Ganglioside recycling	
2. AB variant	5q	GM2-activator protein	AR	Childhood	Ganglioside recycling	
3. Adult Tay-Sachs disease	15q	Hexosaminidase A	AR	Childhood	Ganglioside recycling	
X-linked spinobulbar muscular atrophy	Xq	Androgen receptor	XR	Adult	Nuclear signalling	
III. Upper Motor Neuron (Selected FSPs)						
SPG3A	14q	Atlastin	AD	Childhood	GTPase—vesicle recycling	Some peripheral neuropathy
SPG4	2p	Spastin	AD	Early adulthood	ATPase family—microtubule associate	± mental retardation, motor neuropathy
SPG6	15q	NIPA1	AD	Early adulthood	Membrane transporter or receptor	Deleted in Prader-Willi, Angelman
SPG8	8q	Strumpellin	AD	Early adulthood	Ubiquitous, spectrin-like	
SPG10	12q	Kinesin heavy chain KIF5A	AD	2nd–3rd decade	Motor-associated protein	± peripheral neuropathy, retardation
SPG13	2q	Heat shock protein 60	AD	Early adulthood	Chaperone protein	
SPG17	11q	Silver (BSCL2)	AD	Variable	Membrane protein in ER	Amyotrophy hands, feet
SPG31	2p	REEP1	AD	Early	Mitochondrial protein	Rarely, amyotrophy
SPG33	10q	ZFYVE27	AD	Adult	Interacts with spastin	Pes equinus
SPG42	3q	Acetyl-CoA-transporter	AD	Variable	Solute carrier	
SPG5	8q	Cytochrome P450	AR	Variable	Degrades endogenous substances	Sensory loss
SPG7	16q	Paraplegin	AR	Variable	Mitochondrial protein	Rarely, optic atrophy, ataxia, neuropathy
SPG11	15q	Spatacsin	AR	Childhood	Cytosolic, ? Membrane-associated	Some sensory loss, thin corpus callosum

(*continued*)

TABLE 374-3 Genetic Motor Neuron Diseases (*Continued*)

Disease	Locus	Gene	Inheritance	Onset	Gene Function	Unusual Features
SPG15	14q	Spastizin	AR	Childhood	Zinc finger protein	Some amyotrophy, some CNS features incl thin corpus callosum
SPG20	13q	Spartin	AR	Childhood	Endosomal-trafficking protein	Cerebellar, extrapyramidal signs, short stature, MR
SPG21	15q	Maspardin	AR	Childhood	Endosomal-trafficking protein	Cerebellar, extrapyramidal signs, short stature, MR
SPG35	16q	Fatty acid 2 hydrolase	AR	Childhood	Membrane protein	Multiple CNS features
SPG39	19p	Neuropathy target esterase	AR	Early childhood	Esterase	
SPG44	1q	Connexin 47	AR	Childhood	Gap junction protein	Possible mild CNS features
SPG2	Xq	Proteolipid protein	XR	Early childhood	Myelin protein	Sometimes multiple CNS features
SPG1	Xq	L1-CAM	XR	Infancy	Cell-adhesion molecule	
	Xq	Adrenoleukodystrophy	XR	Early adulthood	ATP-binding transporter protein	Possible adrenal insufficiency, CNS inflamation
IV. ALS-Plus Syndromes						
Amyotrophy with behavioral disorders	17q	Tau protein				
Parkinsonism						

Abbreviations: ALS, amyotrophic lateral sclerosis; BSCL2, Bernadelli-Seip congenital lipodystrophy 2B; FSP, familial spastic paraplegia; FUS/TLS, fused in sarcoma/translocated in liposarcoma; TDP43, Tar DNA binding protein 43 kd.

aggregation of SOD1 protein, impairment of axonal transport, reduced production of ATP and other perturbations of mitochondrial function, activation of neuroinflammatory cascades within the ALS spinal cord, and ultimately induction of cell death via pathways that are at least partially dependent on caspases.

It has recently been observed that mutations in the TDP43 and FUS/TLS genes also cause ALS. These multifunctional proteins bind RNA and DNA and shuttle between the nucleus and the cytoplasm, playing multiple roles in the control of cell proliferation, DNA repair and transcription, and gene translation, both in the cytoplasm and locally in dendritic spines in response to electrical activity. How mutations in FUS/TLS provoke motor neuron cell death is not clear, although this may represent loss of function of FUS/TLS in the nucleus or an acquired, toxic function of the mutant proteins in the cytosol.

Multiple recent studies have convincingly demonstrated that non-neuronal cells importantly influence the disease course, at least in ALS transgenic mice. A striking additional finding in neurodegenerative disorders is that miscreant proteins arising from gene defects in familial forms of these diseases are often implicated in sporadic forms of the same disorder. For example, germline mutations in the genes encoding beta-amyloid and alpha-synuclein cause familial forms of Alzheimer's and Parkinson's diseases (AD and PD), and posttranslational, noninherited abnormalities in these proteins are also central to sporadic AD and PD. Analogously, recent reports propose that nonheritable, post-translational modifications in SOD1 are pathogenic in sporadic ALS.

TREATMENT Amyotrophic Lateral Sclerosis

No treatment arrests the underlying pathologic process in ALS. The drug riluzole (100 mg/d) was approved for ALS because it produces a modest lengthening of survival. In one trial, the survival rate at 18 months with riluzole was similar to placebo at 15 months. The mechanism of this effect is not known with certainty; riluzole may reduce excitotoxicity by diminishing glutamate release. Riluzole is generally well tolerated; nausea, dizziness, weight loss, and elevated liver enzymes occur occasionally. Pathophysiologic studies of mutant SOD1–related ALS in mice have disclosed diverse targets for therapy; consequently, multiple therapies are presently in clinical trials for ALS. These include studies of ceftriaxone, which may augment astroglial glutamate transport and thereby be anti-excitotoxic, and pramipexole and tamoxifen, which are neuroprotective. Interventions such as antisense oligonucleotides (ASO) that diminish expression of mutant SOD1 protein prolong survival in transgenic ALS mice and rats and are also now in trial for SOD1-mediated ALS.

In the absence of a primary therapy for ALS, a variety of rehabilitative aids may substantially assist ALS patients. Foot-drop splints facilitate ambulation by obviating the need for excessive hip flexion and by preventing tripping on a floppy foot. Finger extension splints can potentiate grip. Respiratory support may be life-sustaining. For patients electing against long-term ventilation by tracheostomy, positive-pressure ventilation by mouth or nose provides transient (several weeks) relief from hypercarbia and hypoxia. Also extremely beneficial for some patients is a respiratory device (Cough Assist Device) that produces an artificial cough. This is highly effective in clearing airways and preventing aspiration pneumonia. When bulbar disease prevents normal chewing and swallowing, gastrostomy is uniformly helpful, restoring normal nutrition and hydration. Fortunately, an increasing variety of speech synthesizers are now available to augment speech when there is advanced bulbar palsy. These facilitate oral communication and may be effective for telephone use.

In contrast to ALS, several of the disorders (Tables 374-1 and 374-3) that bear some clinical resemblance to ALS are treatable. For this reason, a careful search for causes of secondary motor neuron disease is warranted.

OTHER MOTOR NEURON DISEASES

SELECTED LOWER MOTOR NEURON DISORDERS

In these motor neuron diseases, the peripheral motor neurons are affected without evidence of involvement of the corticospinal motor system (Tables 374-1 to 374-3).

X-Linked spinobulbar muscular atrophy (Kennedy's disease)

This is an X-linked lower motor neuron disorder in which progressive weakness and wasting of limb and bulbar muscles begins in males in mid-adult life and is conjoined with androgen insensitivity manifested by gynecomastia and reduced fertility (Chap. 346). In addition to gynecomastia, which may be subtle, two findings distinguishing this disorder from ALS are the absence of signs of pyramidal tract disease (spasticity) and the presence of a subtle sensory neuropathy in some patients. The underlying molecular defect is an expanded trinucleotide repeat (-CAG-) in the first exon of the androgen receptor gene on the X chromosome. DNA testing is available. An inverse correlation appears to exist between the number of -CAG- repeats and the age of onset of the disease.

Adult Tay-Sach's disease

Several reports have described adult-onset, predominantly lower motor neuropathies arising from deficiency of the enzyme β-hexosaminidase (hex A). These tend to be distinguishable from ALS because they are very slowly progressive; dysarthria and radiographically evident cerebellar atrophy may be prominent. In rare cases, spasticity may also be present, although it is generally absent (Chap. 361).

Spinal muscular atrophy

The SMAs are a family of selective lower motor neuron diseases of early onset. Despite some phenotypic variability (largely in age of onset), the defect in the majority of families with SMA maps to a locus on chromosome 5 encoding a putative motor neuron survival protein (SMN, for survival motor neuron) that is important in the formation and trafficking of RNA complexes across the nuclear membrane. Neuropathologically these disorders are characterized by extensive loss of large motor neurons; muscle biopsy reveals evidence of denervation atrophy. Several clinical forms exist.

Infantile SMA (SMA I, Werdnig-Hoffmann disease) has the earliest onset and most rapidly fatal course. In some instances it is apparent even before birth, as indicated by decreased fetal movements late in the third trimester. Though alert, afflicted infants are weak and floppy (hypotonic) and lack muscle stretch reflexes. Death generally ensues within the first year of life. *Chronic childhood SMA* (SMA II) begins later in childhood and evolves with a more slowly progressive course. *Juvenile SMA* (SMA III, Kugelberg-Welander disease) manifests during late childhood and runs a slow, indolent course. Unlike most denervating diseases, in this chronic disorder weakness is greatest in the proximal muscles; indeed, the pattern of clinical weakness can suggest a primary myopathy such as limb-girdle dystrophy. Electrophysiologic and muscle biopsy evidence of denervation distinguish SMA III from the myopathic syndromes. There is no primary therapy for SMA, although remarkable recent experimental data indicate that it may be possible to deliver the missing SMN gene to motor neurons using intravenously delivered adeno-associated viruses (e.g., AAV9) immediately after birth.

Multifocal motor neuropathy with conduction block

In this disorder lower motor neuron function is regionally and chronically disrupted by remarkably focal blocks in conduction. Many cases have elevated serum titers of mono- and polyclonal antibodies to ganglioside GM1; it is hypothesized that the antibodies produce selective, focal, paranodal demyelination of motor neurons. MMCB is not typically associated with corticospinal signs. In contrast with ALS, MMCB may respond dramatically to therapy such as IV immunoglobulin or chemotherapy; it is thus imperative that MMCB be excluded when considering a diagnosis of ALS.

Other forms of lower motor neuron disease

In individual families, other syndromes characterized by selective lower motor neuron dysfunction in an SMA-like pattern have been described. There are rare X-linked and autosomal dominant forms of apparent SMA. There is an ALS variant of juvenile onset, the Fazio-Londe syndrome, that involves mainly the musculature innervated by the brainstem. A component of lower motor neuron dysfunction is also found in degenerative disorders such as Machado-Joseph disease and the related olivopontocerebellar degenerations (Chap. 373).

SELECTED DISORDERS OF THE UPPER MOTOR NEURON

Primary lateral sclerosis

This exceedingly rare disorder arises sporadically in adults in mid- to late life. Clinically PLS is characterized by progressive spastic weakness of the limbs, preceded or followed by spastic dysarthria and dysphagia, indicating combined involvement of the corticospinal and corticobulbar tracts. Fasciculations, amyotrophy, and sensory changes are absent; neither electromyography nor muscle biopsy shows denervation. On neuropathologic examination there is selective loss of the large pyramidal cells in the precentral gyrus and degeneration of the corticospinal and corticobulbar projections. The peripheral motor neurons and other neuronal systems are spared. The course of PLS is variable; while long-term survival is documented, the course may be as aggressive as in ALS, with ~3-year survival from onset to death. Early in its course, PLS raises the question of multiple sclerosis or other demyelinating diseases such as adrenoleukodystrophy as diagnostic considerations (Chap. 380). A myelopathy suggestive of PLS is infrequently seen with infection with the retrovirus human T cell lymphotropic virus (HTLV-I) (Chap. 377). The clinical course and laboratory testing will distinguish these possibilities.

Familial spastic paraplegia

In its pure form, FSP is usually transmitted as an autosomal trait; most adult-onset cases are dominantly inherited. Symptoms usually begin in the third or fourth decade, presenting as progressive spastic weakness beginning in the distal lower extremities; however, there are variants with onset so early that the differential diagnosis includes cerebral palsy. FSP typically has a long survival, presumably because respiratory function is spared. Late in the illness there may be urinary urgency and incontinence and sometimes fecal incontinence; sexual function tends to be preserved.

In pure forms of FSP, the spastic leg weakness is often accompanied by posterior column (vibration and position) abnormalities and disturbance of bowel and bladder function. Some family members may have spasticity without clinical symptoms.

By contrast, particularly when recessively inherited, FSP may have complex or complicated forms in which altered corticospinal and dorsal column function is accompanied by significant involvement of other regions of the nervous system, including amyotrophy, mental retardation, optic atrophy, and sensory neuropathy.

Neuropathologically, in FSP there is degeneration of the corticospinal tracts, which appear nearly normal in the brainstem but show increasing atrophy at more caudal levels in the spinal cord; in effect, the pathologic picture is of a dying-back or distal axonopathy of long neuronal fibers within the CNS.

Defects at numerous loci underlie both dominantly and recessively inherited forms of FSP (Table 374-3). More than 20 FSP genes have now been identified. The gene most commonly implicated in dominantly inherited FSP is *spastin,* which encodes a microtubule interacting protein. The most common childhood-onset dominant form arises from mutations in the *atlastin* gene. A kinesin heavy-chain protein implicated in microtubule motor function was found to be defective in a family with dominantly inherited FSP of variable onset age.

An infantile-onset form of X-linked, recessive FSP arises from mutations in the gene for myelin proteolipid protein (Chap. 365). This is an example of rather striking allelic variation, as most other mutations in the same gene cause not FSP but Pelizaeus-Merzbacher disease, a widespread disorder of CNS myelin. Another recessive variant is caused by defects in the *paraplegin* gene. Paraplegin has homology to metalloproteases that are important in mitochondrial function in yeast.

WEB SITES

Several websites provide valuable information on ALS including those offered by the Muscular Dystrophy Association (*www.mdausa.org*), the Amyotrophic Lateral Sclerosis Association (*www.alsa.org*), and the World Federation of Neurology and the Neuromuscular Unit at Washington University in St. Louis (*www.neuro.wustl.edu/neuromuscular*).

FURTHER READINGS

Bosco D et al: Wild-type and mutant SOD1 share an aberrant conformation and a common pathogenic pathway in ALS. Nat Neurosci, 11:1396, 2010

Bruijn LI, Cudkowicz M: Therapeutic targets for amyotrophic lateral sclerosis: Current treatments and prospects for more effective therapies. Expert Rev Neurother 6:417, 2006

DiGiorgio et al: Non-cell autonomous effect of glia on motor neurons in an embryonic stem cell-based ALS model. Nat Neurosci 10:608, 2007

Dion PA et al: Genetics of motor neuron disorders: New insights into pathogenic mechanisms. Nat Genet 10:769, 2009

Fink JK: Hereditary spastic paraplegia. Curr Neurol Neurosci Rep 6:65, 2006

Foust K et al: Rescue of the spinal muscular atrophy phenotype in a mouse model by early postnatal delivery of SMN. Nat Biotechnol 28:271, 2010

Kiernan MC et al: Amyotrophic lateral sclerosis. Lancet 377:942, 2011

Kwiatkowski T et al: Mutations in a novel ALS gene. Science 323:1205, 2009

Lagier-Tourenne C et al: TDP-43 and FUS/TLS: Emerging roles in RNA processing and neurodegeneration. Hum Mol Gen 19:R46, 2010

McKee AC et al: TDP-43 Proteinopathy and motor neuron disease in chronic traumatic encephalopathy. J Neuropathol Exp Neurol 69:918, 2010

Smith RA et al: Antisense oligonucleotide therapy for neurodegenerative disease. J Clin Invest 116:2290, 2006

Weisskopf MG et al: Prospective study of military service and mortality from ALS. Neurology 64:32, 2005

CHAPTER 375 Disorders of the Autonomic Nervous System

Phillip A. Low
John W. Engstrom

The autonomic nervous system (ANS) innervates the entire neuraxis and permeates all organ systems. It regulates blood pressure (BP), heart rate, sleep, and bladder and bowel function. It operates automatically; its full importance becomes recognized only when ANS function is compromised, resulting in dysautonomia. Hypothalamic disorders that cause disturbances in homeostasis are discussed in Chaps. 16 and 339.

ANATOMIC ORGANIZATION

The activity of the ANS is regulated by central neurons responsive to diverse afferent inputs. After central integration of afferent information, autonomic outflow is adjusted to permit the functioning of the major organ systems in accordance with the needs of the organism as a whole. Connections between the cerebral cortex and the autonomic centers in the brainstem coordinate autonomic outflow with higher mental functions.

The preganglionic neurons of the parasympathetic nervous system leave the central nervous system (CNS) in the third, seventh, ninth, and tenth cranial nerves as well as the second and third sacral nerves, while the preganglionic neurons of the sympathetic nervous system exit the spinal cord between the first thoracic and the second lumbar segments (Fig. 375-1). These are thinly myelinated. The postganglionic neurons, located in ganglia outside the CNS, give rise to the postganglionic unmyelinated autonomic nerves that innervate organs and tissues throughout the body. Responses to sympathetic and parasympathetic stimulation are frequently antagonistic (Table 375-1), reflecting highly coordinated interactions within the CNS; the resultant changes in parasympathetic and sympathetic activity provide more precise control of autonomic responses than could be achieved by the modulation of a single system.

Acetylcholine (ACh) is the preganglionic neurotransmitter for both divisions of the ANS as well as the postganglionic neurotransmitter of the parasympathetic neurons; the preganglionic receptors are nicotinic, and the postganglionic are muscarinic in type. Norepinephrine (NE) is the neurotransmitter of the postganglionic sympathetic neurons, except for cholinergic neurons innervating the eccrine sweat glands.

CLINICAL EVALUATION

CLASSIFICATION

Disorders of the ANS may result from pathology of either the CNS or the peripheral nervous system (PNS) (Table 375-2). Signs and symptoms may result from interruption of the afferent limb, CNS processing centers, or efferent limb of reflex arcs controlling autonomic responses. For example, a lesion of the medulla produced by a posterior fossa tumor can impair BP responses to postural changes and result in orthostatic hypotension (OH). OH can also be caused by lesions of the spinal cord or peripheral vasomotor nerve fibers (e.g., diabetic autonomic neuropathy). Lesions of the efferent limb cause the most consistent and severe OH. The site of reflex interruption is usually established by the clinical context in which the dysautonomia arises, combined with judicious use of ANS testing and neuroimaging studies. The presence or absence of CNS signs, association with sensory or motor polyneuropathy, medical illnesses, medication use, and family history are often important considerations. Some syndromes do not fit easily into any classification scheme.

SYMPTOMS OF AUTONOMIC DYSFUNCTION

Clinical manifestations can result from loss of function, overactivity, or dysregulation of autonomic circuits. Disorders of autonomic function should be considered in all patients with unexplained

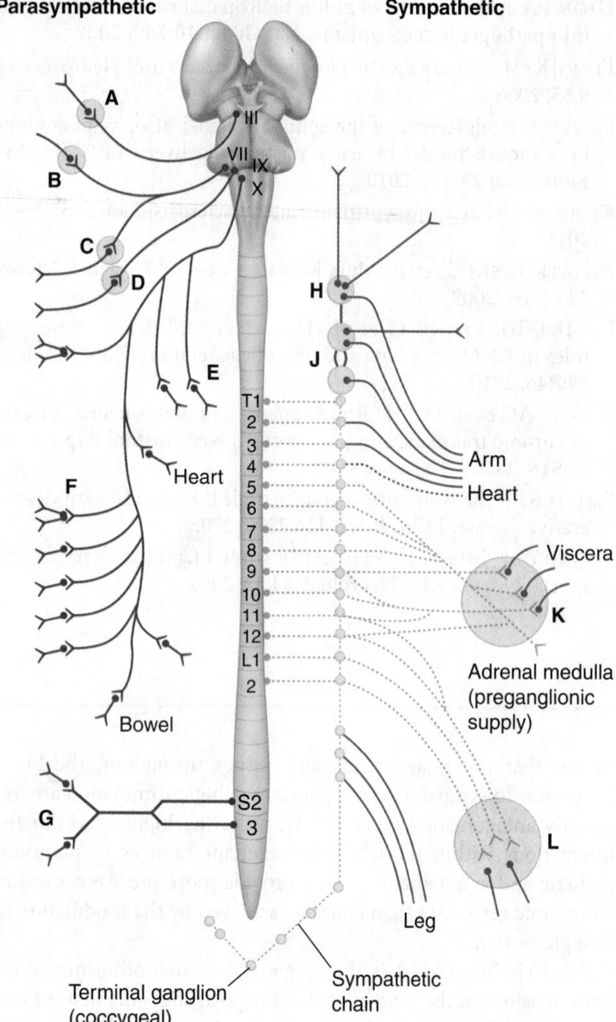

Figure 375-1 Schematic representation of the autonomic nervous system. *(From M Moskowitz: Clin Endocrinol Metab 6:77, 1977.)*

orthostatic hypotension, syncope, sleep dysfunction, altered sweating (hyperhidrosis or hypohidrosis), constipation, upper gastrointestinal symptoms (bloating, nausea, vomiting of old food), impotence, or bladder disorders (urinary frequency, hesitancy, or incontinence). Symptoms may be widespread or regional in distribution. An autonomic history focuses on systemic functions (BP, heart rate, sleep, fever, sweating) and involvement of individual organ systems (pupils, bowel, bladder, sexual function). The autonomic symptom profile is a self-report questionnaire that can be used for formal assessment. It is also important to recognize the modulating effects of age. For example, OH typically produces lightheadedness in the young, whereas cognitive slowing is more common in the elderly. Specific symptoms of orthostatic intolerance are diverse (Table 375-3). Autonomic symptoms may vary dramatically, reflecting the dynamic nature of autonomic control over homeostatic function. For example, OH might be manifest only in the early morning, following a meal, with exercise, or with raised ambient temperature, depending upon the regional vascular bed affected by dysautonomia.

TABLE 375-1 Functional Consequences of Normal ANS Activation

	Sympathetic	Parasympathetic
Heart rate	Increased	Decreased
Blood pressure	Increased	Mildly decreased
Bladder	Increased sphincter tone	Voiding (decreased tone)
Bowel motility	Decreased motility	Increased
Lung	Bronchodilation	Bronchoconstriction
Sweat glands	Sweating	—
Pupils	Dilation	Constriction
Adrenal glands	Catecholamine release	—
Sexual function	Ejaculation, orgasm	Erection
Lacrimal glands	—	Tearing
Parotid glands	—	Salivation

Early symptoms may be overlooked. Impotence, although not specific for autonomic failure, often heralds autonomic failure in men and may precede other symptoms by years (Chap. 48). A decrease in the frequency of spontaneous early morning erections may occur months before loss of nocturnal penile tumescence and development of total impotence. Bladder dysfunction may appear early in men and women, particularly in those with CNS involvement. Cold feet may indicate peripheral vasomotor constriction. Brain and spinal cord disease above the level of the lumbar spine results first in urinary frequency and small bladder volumes and eventually in incontinence (upper motor neuron or spastic bladder). By contrast, PNS disease of autonomic nerve fibers results in large bladder volumes, urinary frequency, and overflow incontinence (lower motor neuron flaccid bladder). Measurement of bladder volume (postvoid residual) is a useful bedside test for distinguishing between upper and lower motor neuron bladder dysfunction in the early stages of dysautonomia. Gastrointestinal autonomic dysfunction typically presents as severe constipation. Diarrhea occurs occasionally (as in diabetes mellitus) due to rapid transit of contents or uncoordinated small-bowel motor activity, or on an osmotic basis from bacterial overgrowth associated with small-bowel stasis. Impaired glandular secretory function may cause difficulty with food intake due to decreased salivation or eye irritation due to decreased lacrimation. Occasionally, temperature elevation and vasodilation can result from anhidrosis because sweating is normally important for heat dissipation (Chap. 16). Lack of sweating after a hot bath, during exercise, or on a hot day can suggest sudomotor failure.

OH (also called *orthostatic or postural hypotension*) is perhaps the most disabling feature of autonomic dysfunction. The prevalence of OH is relatively high, especially when OH associated

TABLE 375-2 Classification of Clinical Autonomic Disorders

I. Autonomic disorders with brain involvement
- A. Associated with multisystem degeneration
  - 1. Multisystem degeneration: autonomic failure clinically prominent
    - a. Multiple system atrophy (MSA)
    - b. Parkinson's disease with autonomic failure
    - c. Diffuse Lewy body disease (some cases)
  - 2. Multisystem degeneration: autonomic failure clinically not usually prominent
    - a. Parkinson's disease
    - b. Other extrapyramidal disorders [inherited spinocerebellar atrophies, progressive supranuclear palsy, corticobasal degeneration, Machado-Joseph disease, fragile X syndrome (FXTAS)]
- B. Unassociated with multisystem degeneration (Focal CNS disorders)
  - 1. Disorders mainly due to cerebral cortex involvement
    - a. Frontal cortex lesions causing urinary/bowel incontinence
    - b. Partial complex seizures (temporal lobe or anterior cingulate)
    - c. Cerebral infarction of the insula
  - 2. Disorders of the limbic and paralimbic circuits
    - a. Shapiro's syndrome (agenesis of corpus callosum, hyperhidrosis, hypothermia)
    - b. Autonomic seizures
    - c. Limbic encephalitis
  - 3. Disorders of the hypothalamus
    - a. Wernicke-Korsakoff syndrome
    - b. Diencephalic syndrome
    - c. Neuroleptic malignant syndrome
    - d. Serotonin syndrome
    - e. Fatal familial insomnia
    - f. Antidiuretic hormone syndromes (diabetes insipidus, inappropriate ADH secretion)
    - g. Disturbances of temperature regulation (hyperthermia, hypothermia)
    - h. Disturbances of sexual function
    - i. Disturbances of appetite
    - j. Disturbances of BP/HR and gastric function
    - k. Horner's syndrome
  - 4. Disorders of the brainstem and cerebellum
    - a. Posterior fossa tumors
    - b. Syringobulbia and Arnold-Chiari malformation
    - c. Disorders of BP control (hypertension, hypotension)
    - d. Cardiac arrhythmias
    - e. Central sleep apnea
    - f. Baroreflex failure
    - g. Horner's syndrome
    - h. Vertebrobasilar and Wallenberg syndromes
    - i. Brainstem encephalitis

II. Autonomic disorders with spinal cord involvement
- A. Traumatic quadriplegia
- B. Syringomyelia
- C. Subacute combined degeneration
- D. Multiple sclerosis and Devic disease
- E. Amyotrophic lateral sclerosis
- F. Tetanus
- G. Stiff-man syndrome
- H. Spinal cord tumors

III. Autonomic neuropathies
- A. Acute/subacute autonomic neuropathies
  - 1. Subacute autoimmune autonomic ganglionopathy (AAG)
    - a. Subacute paraneoplastic autonomic neuropathy
    - b. Guillain-Barré syndrome
    - c. Botulism
    - d. Porphyria
    - e. Drug induced autonomic neuropathies-stimulants, drug withdrawal, vasoconstrictor, vasodilators, beta-receptor antagonists, beta-agonists
    - f. Toxic autonomic neuropathies
    - g. Subacute cholinergic neuropathy
- B. Chronic peripheral autonomic neuropathies
  - 1. Distal small fiber neuropathy
  - 2. Combined sympathetic and parasympathetic failure
    - a. Amyloid
    - b. Diabetic autonomic neuropathy
    - c. Autoimmune autonomic ganglionopathy (paraneoplastic and idiopathic)
    - d. Sensory neuronopathy with autonomic failure
    - e. Familial dysautonomia (Riley-Day syndrome)
    - f. Diabetic, uremic, or nutritional deficiency
    - g. Dysautonomia of old age
  - 3. Disorders of reduced orthostatic intolerance-reflex syncope, POTS, associated with prolonged bed rest, associated with space flight, chronic fatigue

Abbreviations: BP, blood pressure; HR, heart rate; POTS, postural orthostatic tachycardia syndrome.

with aging and diabetes mellitus is included (Table 375-4). OH can cause a variety of symptoms, including dimming or loss of vision, lightheadedness, diaphoresis, diminished hearing, pallor, and weakness. Syncope results when the drop in BP impairs cerebral perfusion. Other manifestations of impaired baroreflexes are supine hypertension, a heart rate that is fixed regardless of posture, postprandial hypotension, and an excessively high nocturnal BP. Many patients with OH have a preceding diagnosis of hypertension or have concomitant supine hypertension, reflecting the great importance of baroreflexes in maintaining postural and supine normotension. The appearance of OH in patients receiving antihypertensive treatment may indicate overtreatment or the onset of an autonomic disorder. The most common causes of OH are not neurologic in origin; these must be distinguished from the neurogenic causes (Table 375-5). Neurocardiogenic and cardiac causes of syncope are considered in Chap. 20.

TABLE 375-3 Symptoms of Orthostatic Intolerance

Lightheadedness (dizziness)	88%
Weakness or tiredness	72%
Cognitive difficulty (thinking/concentrating)	47%
Blurred vision	47%
Tremulousness	38%
Vertigo	37%
Pallor	31%
Anxiety	29%
Palpitations	26%
Clammy feeling	19%
Nausea	18%

Source: From PA Low et al: Mayo Clin Proc 70:617, 1995.

APPROACH TO THE PATIENT Orthostatic Hypotension and Other ANS Disorders

The first step in the evaluation of symptomatic OH is the exclusion of treatable causes. The history should include a review of medications that may affect the autonomic system (Table 375-6). The main classes of drugs that may cause OH are diuretics, antihypertensives, antidepressants, phenothiazines, ethanol, narcotics, insulin, dopamine agonists, barbiturates, and calcium channel-blocking agents. However, the precipitation of OH by medications may also be the first sign of an underlying autonomic disorder. The history may reveal an underlying cause for symptoms (e.g., diabetes, Parkinson's disease) or specific underlying mechanisms (e.g., cardiac pump failure, reduced intravascular volume). The relationship of symptoms to meals (splanchnic pooling), standing on awakening in the morning (intravascular volume depletion), ambient warming (vasodilatation), or exercise (muscle arteriolar vasodilatation) should be sought. Standing time to first symptom and presyncope should be followed for management.

Physical examination includes measurement of supine and standing pulse and BP. OH is defined as a sustained drop in systolic (≥20 mm Hg) or diastolic (≥10 mm Hg) BP within 3 min of standing. In nonneurogenic causes of OH (such as hypovolemia), the BP drop is accompanied by a compensatory increase in heart rate of >15 beats/min. A clue that the patient

TABLE 375-4 Prevalence of Orthostatic Hypotension in Different Disorders

Disorder	Prevalence
Aging	14–20%
Diabetic neuropathy	10%
Other autonomic neuropathies	10–50 per 100,000
Multiple system atrophy	5–15 per 100,000
Pure autonomic failure	10–30 per 100,000

TABLE 375-5 Nonneurogenic Causes of Orthostatic Hypotension

Cardiac pump failure
- Myocardial infarction
- Myocarditis
- Constrictive pericarditis
- Aortic stenosis
- Tachyarrhythmias
- Bradyarrhythmias
- Salt-losing nephropathy
- Adrenal insufficiency
- Diabetes insipidus
- Venous obstruction

Reduced intravascular volume
- Straining or heavy lifting, urination, defecation
- Dehydration
- Diarrhea, emesis
- Hemorrhage
- Burns

Metabolic
- Adrenocortical insufficiency
- Hypoaldosteronism
- Pheochromocytoma
- Severe potassium depletion

Venous pooling
- Alcohol
- Postprandial dilation of splanchnic vessel beds
- Vigorous exercise with dilation of skeletal vessel beds
- Heat: hot environment, hot showers and baths, fever
- Prolonged recumbency or standing
- Sepsis

Medications
- Antihypertensives
- Diuretics
- Vasodilators: nitrates, hydralazine
- Alpha- and beta-blocking agents
- CNS sedatives: barbiturates, opiates
- Tricyclic antidepressants
- Phenothiazines

TABLE 375-6 Some Drugs That Affect Autonomic Function

Symptom	Drug Class	Specific Examples
Impotence	Opioids	Tylenol #3
	Anabolic steroids	—
	Some antiarrhythmics	Prazosin
	Some antihypertensives	Clonidine
	Some diuretics	Benazepril
	Some SSRIs	Venlafaxine
Urinary retention	Opioids	Fentanyl
	Decongestants	Brompheniramine
		Diphenhydramine
Diaphoresis	Some antihypertensives	Amlodipine
	Some SSRIs	Citalopram
	Opioids	Morphine
Hypotension	Tricyclics	Amitriptyline
	Beta blockers	Propranolol
	Diuretics	HCTZ
	CCBs	Verapamil

Abbreviations: CCBs, calcium channel blockers; HCTZ, hydrochlorothiazide; SSRIs, selective serotonin reuptake inhibitors.

TABLE 375-7 Normal Blood Pressure and Heart Rate Changes During the Valsalva Maneuver

Phase	Maneuver	Blood Pressure	Heart Rate	Comments
I	Forced expiration against a partially closed glottis	Rises; aortic compression from raised intrathoracic pressure	Decreases	Mechanical
II *early*	Continued expiration	Falls; decreased venous return to the heart	Increases (reflex tachycardia)	Reduced vagal tone
II *late*	Continued expiration	Rises; reflex increase in peripheral vascular resistance	Increases at slower rate	Requires intact efferent sympathetic response
III	End of expiration	Falls; increased capacitance of pulmonary bed	Increases further	Mechanical
IV	Recovery	Rises; persistent vasoconstriction and increased cardiac output	Compensatory bradycardia	Requires intact efferent sympathetic response

has neurogenic OH is the aggravation or precipitation of OH by autonomic stressors (such as a meal, hot tub/hot bath, and exercise). Neurologic examination should include mental status (neurodegenerative disorders), cranial nerves (impaired downgaze with progressive supranuclear palsy; abnormal pupils with Horner's or Adie's syndrome), motor tone (Parkinson's disease and parkinsonian syndromes), and reflexes and sensation (polyneuropathies). In patients without a clear diagnosis initially, follow-up evaluations may reveal the underlying cause.

Disorders of autonomic function should be considered in patients with symptoms of altered sweating (hyperhidrosis or hypohidrosis), gastroparesis (bloating, nausea, vomiting of old food), constipation, impotence, or bladder dysfunction (urinary frequency, hesitancy, or incontinence).

AUTONOMIC TESTING Autonomic function tests are helpful when the history and examination findings are inconclusive; to detect subclinical involvement; or to follow the course of an autonomic disorder.

Heart Rate Variation with Deep Breathing This is a test of the parasympathetic component of cardiovascular reflexes, via the vagus nerve. Results are influenced by multiple factors including the subject's position (recumbent, sitting or standing), rate and depth of respiration [6 breaths per minute and a forced vital capacity (FVC) >1.5 L are optimal], age, medications, weight, and degree of hypocapnia. Interpretation of results requires comparison of test data with results from age-matched controls collected under identical test conditions. For example, the lower limit of normal heart rate variation with deep breathing in persons <20 years is >15–20 beats/min, but for persons over age 60 it is 5–8 beats/min. Heart rate variation with deep breathing (respiratory sinus arrhythmia) is abolished by the muscarinic acetylcholine (ACh)-receptor antagonist atropine but is unaffected by sympathetic postganglionic blockade (e.g., propranolol).

Valsalva Response This response (Table 375-7) assesses integrity of the baroreflex control of heart rate (parasympathetic) and BP (adrenergic). Under normal conditions, increases in BP at the carotid bulb trigger a reduction in heart rate (increased vagal tone), and decreases in BP trigger an increase in heart rate (reduced vagal tone). The Valsalva response is tested in the supine position. The subject exhales against a closed glottis (or into a manometer maintaining a constant expiratory pressure of 40 mm Hg) for 15 s while measuring changes in heart rate and beat-to-beat BP. There are four phases of BP and heart rate response to the Valsalva maneuver. Phases I and III are mechanical and related to changes in intrathoracic and intraabdominal pressure. In early phase II, reduced venous return results in a fall in stroke volume and BP, counteracted by a combination of reflex tachycardia and increased total peripheral resistance. Increased total peripheral resistance arrests the BP drop ~5–8 s after the onset of the maneuver. Late phase II begins with a progressive rise in BP toward or above baseline. Venous return and cardiac output return to normal in phase IV. Persistent peripheral arteriolar vasoconstriction and increased cardiac adrenergic tone result in a temporary BP overshoot and phase IV bradycardia (mediated by the baroreceptor reflex).

Autonomic function during the Valsalva maneuver can be measured using beat-to-beat blood pressure or heart rate changes. The *Valsalva ratio* is defined as the maximum phase II tachycardia divided by the minimum phase IV bradycardia (Table 375-8). The ratio reflects the integrity of the entire baroreceptor reflex arc and of sympathetic efferents to blood vessels.

Sudomotor Function Sweating is induced by release of ACh from sympathetic postganglionic fibers. The quantitative sudomotor axon reflex test (QSART) is a measure of regional

TABLE 375-8 Neural Pathways Underlying Some Standardized Autonomic Tests

Test Evaluated	Procedure	Autonomic Function
HRDB	6 deep breaths/min	Cardiovagal function
Valsalva ratio	Expiratory pressure, 40 mm Hg for 10–15 s	Cardiovagal function
QSART	Axon-reflex test 4 limb sites	Postganglionic sudomotor function
BP_{BB} to VM	BP_{BB} response to VM	Adrenergic function: baroreflex adrenergic control of vagal and vasomotor function
HUT	BP_{BB} and heart rate response to HUT	Adrenergic and cardiovagal responses to HUT

Abbreviations: BP_{BB}, beat-to-beat blood pressure; HRDB, heart rate response to deep breathing; HUT, head-up tilt; QSART, quantitative sudomotor axon-reflex test; VM, Valsalva maneuver.

autonomic function mediated by ACh-induced sweating. A reduced or absent response indicates a lesion of the postganglionic sudomotor axon. For example, sweating may be reduced in the feet as a result of distal polyneuropathy (e.g., diabetes). The thermoregulatory sweat test (TST) is a qualitative measure of regional sweat production in response to an elevation of body temperature under controlled conditions. An indicator powder placed on the anterior surface of the body changes color with sweat production during temperature elevation. The pattern of color changes is a measure of regional sweat secretion. A postganglionic lesion is present if both QSART and TST show absent sweating. In a preganglionic lesion, QSART is normal but TST shows anhidrosis.

Orthostatic BP Recordings Beat-to-beat BP measurements determined in supine, 70° tilt, and tilt-back positions are useful to quantitate orthostatic failure of BP control. Allow a 20-min period of rest in the supine position before assessing changes in BP during tilting. The BP change combined with heart rate monitoring is useful for the evaluation of patients with suspected OH or unexplained syncope.

Tilt Table Testing for Syncope The great majority of patients with syncope do not have autonomic failure. Tilt table testing can be used to make the diagnosis of vasovagal syncope with sensitivity, specificity, and reproducibility. A standardized protocol is used that specifies the tilt apparatus, angle and duration of tilt, and procedure for provocation of vasodilation (e.g., sublingual or spray nitroglycerin). A positive nitroglycerin-stimulated test predicts recurrence of syncope. Recommendations for the performance of tilt studies for syncope have been incorporated in consensus guidelines.

SPECIFIC SYNDROMES OF ANS DYSFUNCTION

MULTIPLE SYSTEM ATROPHY (CHAP. 372)

Multiple system atrophy (MSA) is an entity that comprises autonomic failure (OH or a neurogenic bladder) *and* either parkinsonism (MSA-p) or a cerebellar syndrome (MSA-c). MSA-p is the more common form; the parkinsonism is atypical in that it is usually unassociated with significant tremor or response to levodopa. Symptomatic OH within 1 year of onset of parkinsonism predicts eventual development of MSA-p in 75% of patients. Although autonomic abnormalities are common in advanced Parkinson's disease (Chap. 372), the severity and distribution of autonomic failure is more severe and more generalized in MSA. Brain MRI is a useful diagnostic adjunct; in MSA-p, iron deposition in the striatum may be evident as T2 hypointensity, and in MSA-c cerebellar atrophy is present with a characteristic T2 hyperintense signal ("hot cross buns sign") in the pons (Fig. 375-2). Cardiac postganglionic adrenergic innervation, measured by uptake of fluorodopamine on positron emission tomography, is markedly impaired in the dysautonomia of Parkinson's disease but is usually normal in MSA.

MSA generally progresses relentlessly to death 7–10 years after onset. Neuropathologic changes include neuronal loss and gliosis in many CNS regions, including the brainstem, cerebellum, striatum, and intermediolateral cell column of the thoracolumbar spinal cord. Management is symptomatic for neurogenic OH (see below), gastrointestinal (GI), and urinary dysfunction. GI management includes frequent small meals, soft diet, stool softeners, and bulk agents. Gastroparesis is difficult to treat; metoclopramide stimulates gastric emptying but worsens parkinsonism by blocking central dopamine receptors. Domperidone has been used in other countries but is not available in the United States.

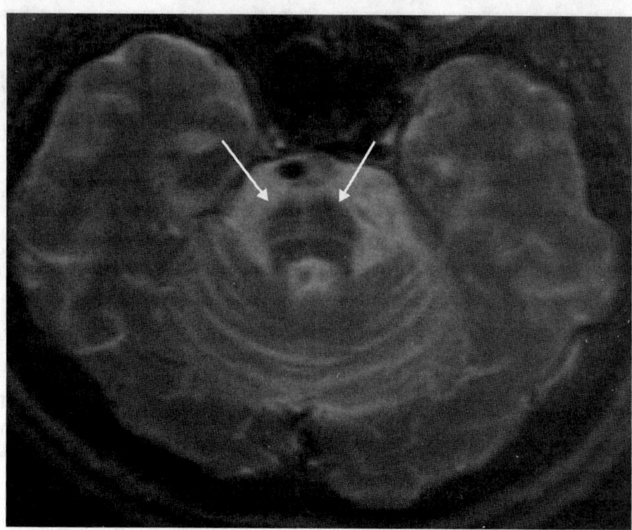

Figure 375-2 Multiple system atrophy, cerebellar type (MSA-c). Axial T2-weighted MRI at the level of the pons shows a characteristic hyperintense signal, the "hot cross buns" sign.

Autonomic dysfunction is also a common feature in dementia with Lewy bodies (Chap. 371); the severity is usually less than that found in MSA or Parkinson's disease. In multiple sclerosis (MS; Chap. 380), autonomic complications reflect the CNS location of MS involvement and generally worsen with disease duration and disability.

SPINAL CORD

Spinal cord lesions from any cause may result in focal autonomic deficits or autonomic hyperreflexia (e.g., spinal cord transection or hemisection) affecting bowel, bladder, sexual, temperature-regulation, or cardiovascular functions. Quadriparetic patients exhibit both supine hypertension and OH after upward tilting. *Autonomic dysreflexia* describes a dramatic increase in blood pressure in patients with traumatic spinal cord lesions above the C6 level, often in response to stimulation of the bladder, skin, or muscles. Suprapubic palpation of the bladder, a distended bladder, catheter insertion, catheter obstruction, or urinary infection are common triggers. Associated symptoms can include flushing, headache, or piloerection. Potential complications include intracranial vasospasm or hemorrhage, cardiac arrhythmia, and death. Awareness of the syndrome and monitoring of blood pressure during procedures in patients with acute or chronic spinal cord injury is essential. In patients with supine hypertension, BP can be lowered by tilting the head upward. Vasodilator drugs may be used to treat acute elevations in BP. Clonidine can be used prophylactically to reduce the hypertension resulting from bladder stimulation. Dangerous increases or decreases in body temperature may result from an inability to experience the sensory accompaniments of heat or cold exposure or the ability to control peripheral vasoconstriction or sweating below the level of the spinal cord injury.

PERIPHERAL NERVE AND NEUROMUSCULAR JUNCTION DISORDERS

Peripheral neuropathies (Chap. 384) are the most common cause of chronic autonomic insufficiency. Polyneuropathies that affect small myelinated and unmyelinated fibers of the sympathetic and parasympathetic nerves commonly occur in diabetes mellitus, amyloidosis, chronic alcoholism, porphyria, and Guillain-Barré syndrome.

Neuromuscular junction disorders with autonomic involvement include botulism and Lambert-Eaton syndrome (Chap. 386).

Diabetes mellitus

Autonomic neuropathy typically begins ~10 years after the onset of diabetes and is slowly progressive. Clinical features, prevention, and management are discussed in Chap. 344.

Amyloidosis

Autonomic neuropathy occurs in both sporadic and familial forms of amyloidosis (Chap. 112). The AL (immunoglobulin light chain) type is associated with primary amyloidosis or amyloidosis secondary to multiple myeloma. The ATTR type, with transthyretin as the primary protein component, is responsible for the most common form of inherited amyloidosis. Although patients usually present with a distal painful neuropathy accompanied by sensory loss, autonomic insufficiency can precede the development of the polyneuropathy or occur in isolation. Diagnosis can be made by protein electrophoresis of blood and urine, tissue biopsy (abdominal fat pad, rectal mucosa, or sural nerve) to search for amyloid deposits, and genetic testing for transthyretin mutations in familial cases. Treatment of familial cases with liver transplantation can be successful. The response of primary amyloidosis to melphalan and stem cell transplantation has been mixed. Death is usually due to cardiac or renal involvement. Postmortem studies reveal amyloid deposition in many organs, including two sites that contribute to autonomic failure: intraneural blood vessels and autonomic ganglia. Pathologic examination reveals a loss of unmyelinated and myelinated nerve fibers.

Alcoholic neuropathy

Abnormalities in parasympathetic vagal and efferent sympathetic function are usually mild in individuals with alcoholic polyneuropathy. Pathologic changes can be demonstrated in the parasympathetic (vagus) and sympathetic fibers, and in ganglia. OH is usually due to brainstem involvement. Impotence is a major problem, but concurrent gonadal hormone abnormalities may obscure the parasympathetic component. Clinical symptoms of autonomic failure generally appear when the polyneuropathy is severe, and there is usually coexisting Wernicke's encephalopathy (Chap. 275). Autonomic involvement may contribute to the high mortality rates associated with alcoholism (Chap. 392).

Porphyria (Chap. 358)

Although each of the porphyrias can cause autonomic dysfunction, the condition is most extensively documented in the acute intermittent type. Autonomic symptoms include tachycardia, sweating, urinary retention, hypertension, or (less commonly) hypotension. Other prominent symptoms include anxiety, abdominal pain, nausea, and vomiting. Abnormal autonomic function can occur both during acute attacks and during remissions. Elevated catecholamine levels during acute attacks correlate with the degree of tachycardia and hypertension that is present.

Guillain-Barré syndrome (Chap. 385)

BP fluctuations and arrhythmias can be severe. It is estimated that between 2 and 10% of patients with severe Guillain-Barré syndrome suffer fatal cardiovascular collapse. Gastrointestinal autonomic involvement, sphincter disturbances, abnormal sweating, and pupillary dysfunction also occur. Demyelination has been described in the vagus and glossopharyngeal nerves, the sympathetic chain, and the white rami communicantes. Interestingly, the degree of autonomic involvement appears to be independent of the severity of motor or sensory neuropathy.

Autoimmune autonomic neuropathy (AAN)

This disorder presents with the subacute development of autonomic disturbances with OH, enteric neuropathy (gastroparesis, ileus, constipation/diarrhea), and cholinergic failure; the latter consists of loss of sweating, sicca complex, and a tonic pupil. Autoantibodies against the ganglionic ACh receptor (A_3 AChR) are present in the serum of many patients and are now considered to be diagnostic of this syndrome. In general, the antibody titer correlates with the severity of autonomic failure. Symptoms of cholinergic failure are also associated with a high antibody titer. Onset of the neuropathy follows a viral infection in approximately half of cases. AAN is almost always monophasic; up to one-third of untreated patients experience significant functional improvement over time. There are isolated case reports of a beneficial response to plasmapheresis or intravenous immune globulin, but there are no clinical trials that systematically assess the effectiveness of immunomodulatory therapies. Symptomatic management of OH, gastroparesis, and sicca symptoms is essential. The spectrum of AAN is now broader than originally thought; some antibody-positive cases have an insidious onset and slow progression with a pure autonomic failure (see below) phenotype. A dramatic clinical response to repeated plasma exchange combined with immunosuppression was described in one patient with longstanding AAN.

AAN can have a paraneoplastic basis (Chap. 101). The clinical features of the autonomic neuropathy may be indistinguishable from a coexisting paraneoplastic syndrome, although quite often in the paraneoplastic cases, distinctive additional central features, such as cerebellar involvement or dementia, may be present (see Tables 101-1, 101-2, and 101-3). The neoplasm may be truly occult and possibly suppressed by the autoantibody.

Botulism

Botulinum toxin binds presynaptically to cholinergic nerve terminals and, after uptake into the cytosol, blocks ACh release. Manifestations consist of motor paralysis and autonomic disturbances that include blurred vision, dry mouth, nausea, unreactive or sluggishly reactive pupils, constipation, and urinary retention (Chap. 141).

■ PURE AUTONOMIC FAILURE (PAF)

This sporadic syndrome consists of postural hypotension, impotence, bladder dysfunction, and defective sweating. The disorder begins in the middle decades and occurs in women more often than men. The symptoms can be disabling, but the disease does not shorten life span. The clinical and pharmacologic characteristics suggest primary involvement of postganglionic sympathetic neurons. There is a severe reduction in the density of neurons within sympathetic ganglia that results in low supine plasma NE levels and noradrenergic supersensitivity. Some studies have questioned the specificity of PAF as a distinct clinical entity. Some cases are ganglionic antibody–positive and thus represent a type of AAN. Between 10 and 15% of cases evolve into MSA.

POSTURAL ORTHOSTATIC TACHYCARDIA SYNDROME (POTS)

This syndrome is characterized by symptomatic orthostatic intolerance (not OH) and by either an increase in heart rate to >120 beats/min or an increase of 30 beats/min with standing that subsides on sitting or lying down. Women are affected approximately five times more often than men, and most develop the syndrome between the ages of 15 and 50. Approximately half of affected patients report an antecedent viral infection. Syncopal symptoms (lightheadedness, weakness, blurred vision) combined with symptoms of autonomic overactivity (palpitations, tremulousness, nausea) are common. Recurrent unexplained episodes of dysautonomia and fatigue also occur. The pathogenesis is unclear in most cases; hypovolemia, deconditioning, venous pooling, impaired brainstem regulation, or β-receptor supersensitivity may play a role. In one affected individual, a mutation in the NE transporter, which resulted in impaired NE clearance from synapses, was responsible. Some cases are due to an underlying limited autonomic neuropathy. Although ~80% of patients improve, only one-quarter eventually resume their usual daily activities (including exercise and sports). Expansion of fluid volume and postural training (see "Treatment: Autonomic Failure") are initial approaches to treatment. If these approaches are inadequate, then midodrine, fludrocortisone, phenobarbital, beta blockers, or clonidine may be used with some success. Reconditioning and a sustained exercise program are very important.

INHERITED DISORDERS

There are five known hereditary sensory and autonomic neuropathies (HSAN I–V). The most important ones are HSAN I and HSAN III (Riley-Day syndrome; familial dysautonomia). HSAN I is dominantly inherited and often presents as a distal small-fiber neuropathy (burning feet syndrome). The responsible gene, on chromosome 9q, is designated *SPTLC1*. SPTLC is an important enzyme in the regulation of ceramide. Cells from HSAN I patients affected by mutation of *SPTLC1* produce higher-than-normal levels of glucosyl ceramide, perhaps triggering apoptosis.

HSAN III, an autosomal recessive disorder of infants and children that occurs among Ashkenazi Jews, is much less prevalent than HSAN I. Decreased tearing, hyperhidrosis, reduced sensitivity to pain, areflexia, absent fungiform papillae on the tongue, and labile BP may be present. Episodic abdominal crises and fever are common. Pathologic examination of nerves reveals a loss of small myelinated and unmyelinated nerve fibers. The defective gene, named *IKBKAP*, is also located on the long arm of chromosome 9. Pathogenic mutations may prevent normal transcription of important molecules in neural development.

PRIMARY HYPERHIDROSIS

This syndrome presents with excess sweating of the palms of the hands and soles of the feet. The disorder affects 0.6–1.0% of the population; the etiology is unclear, but there may be a genetic component. While not dangerous, the condition can be socially embarrassing (e.g., shaking hands) or disabling (e.g., inability to write without soiling the paper). Onset of symptoms is usually in adolescence; the condition tends to improve with age. Topical antiperspirants are occasionally helpful. More useful are potent anticholinergic drugs such as glycopyrrolate (1–2 mg PO tid). T2 ganglionectomy or sympathectomy is successful in >90% of patients with palmar hyperhidrosis. The advent of endoscopic transaxillary T2 sympathectomy has lowered the complication rate of the procedure. The most common postoperative complication is compensatory hyperhidrosis, which improves spontaneously over months; other potential complications include recurrent hyperhidrosis (16%), Horner's syndrome (<2%), gustatory sweating, wound infection, hemothorax, and intercostal neuralgia. Local injection of botulinum toxin has also been used to block cholinergic, postganglionic sympathetic fibers to sweat glands in patients with palmar hyperhidrosis. This approach is limited by the need for repetitive injections (the effect usually lasts 4 months before waning), pain with injection, the high cost of botulinum toxin, and the possibility of temporary intrinsic hand muscle weakness.

ACUTE AUTONOMIC SYNDROMES

The physician may be confronted occasionally with an acute autonomic syndrome, either acute autonomic failure (acute AAN syndrome) or a state of sympathetic overactivity. An *autonomic storm* is an acute state of sustained sympathetic surge that results in variable combinations of alterations in blood pressure and heart rate, body temperature, respiration, and sweating. Causes of autonomic storm are brain and spinal cord injury, toxins and drugs, autonomic neuropathy, and chemodectomas (e.g., pheochromocytoma).

Brain injury is most commonly a cause of autonomic storm following severe head trauma and in postresuscitation encephalopathy following anoxic-ischemic brain injury. Autonomic storm can also occur with other acute intracranial lesions such as hemorrhage, cerebral infarction, rapidly expanding tumors, subarachnoid hemorrhage, hydrocephalus, or (less commonly) an acute spinal cord lesion. Lesions involving the diencephalon may be more prone to present with dysautonomia, but the most consistent setting is that of an acute intracranial catastrophe of sufficient size and rapidity to produce a massive catecholaminergic surge. The surge can cause seizures, neurogenic pulmonary edema, and myocardial injury. Manifestations include fever, tachycardia, hypertension, tachypnea, hyperhidrosis, pupillary dilatation, and flushing. Lesions of the afferent limb of the baroreflex can result in milder recurrent autonomic storms; many of these follow neck irradiation.

Drugs and toxins may also be responsible, including sympathomimetics such as phenylpropanolamine, cocaine, amphetamines, and tricyclic antidepressants; tetanus; and, less often, botulinum. Phenylpropanolamine, now off the market, was in the past a potent cause of this syndrome. Cocaine, including "crack," can cause a hypertensive state with CNS hyperstimulation. Tricyclic overdose, such as amitriptyline, can cause flushing, hypertension, tachycardia, fever, mydriasis, anhidrosis, and a toxic psychosis. *Neuroleptic malignant syndrome* refers to a syndrome of muscle rigidity, hyperthermia, and hypertension in psychotic patients treated with phenothiazines.

The hyperadrenergic state with Guillain-Barré syndrome can produce a moderate autonomic storm. Pheochromocytoma presents with a paroxysmal or sustained hyperadrenergic state, headache, hyperhidrosis, palpitations, anxiety, tremulousness, and hypertension.

Management of autonomic storm includes ruling out other causes of autonomic instability, including malignant hyperthermia, porphyria, and epilepsy. Sepsis and encephalitis need to be excluded with appropriate studies. An electroencephalogram (EEG) should be done to detect epileptiform activity; MRI of the brain and spine is often necessary. The patient should be managed in an intensive care unit. Management with morphine sulphate (10 mg every 4 h) and labetalol (100–200 mg twice daily) have worked relatively well. Treatment may need to be maintained for several weeks. For chronic and milder autonomic storm, propranolol and/or clonidine can be effective.

MISCELLANEOUS

Other conditions associated with autonomic failure include infections, poisoning (organophosphates), malignancy, and aging. Disorders of the hypothalamus can affect autonomic function and produce abnormalities in temperature control, satiety, sexual function, and circadian rhythms (Chap. 339).

REFLEX SYMPATHETIC DYSTROPHY AND CAUSALGIA

The failure to identify a primary role of the ANS in the pathogenesis of these disorders has resulted in a change of nomenclature. Complex regional pain syndrome (CRPS) types I and II are now used in place of reflex sympathetic dystrophy (RSD) and causalgia, respectively.

CRPS type I is a regional pain syndrome that usually develops after tissue trauma. Examples of associated trauma include myocardial infarction, minor shoulder or limb injury, and stroke. *Allodynia* (the perception of a nonpainful stimulus as painful), *hyperpathia* (an exaggerated pain response to a painful stimulus), and spontaneous pain occur. The symptoms are unrelated to the severity of the initial trauma and are not confined to the distribution of a single peripheral nerve. CRPS type II is a regional pain syndrome that develops after injury to a specific peripheral nerve, usually a major nerve trunk. Spontaneous pain initially develops within the territory of the affected nerve but eventually may spread outside the nerve distribution.

Pain is the primary clinical feature of CRPS. Vasomotor dysfunction, sudomotor abnormalities, or focal edema may occur alone or in combination but must be present for diagnosis. Limb pain syndromes that do not meet these criteria are best classified as "limb pain—not otherwise specified." In CRPS, localized sweating (increased resting sweat output) and changes in blood flow may produce temperature differences between affected and unaffected limbs.

CRPS type I (RSD) has classically been divided into three clinical phases but is now considered to be more variable. Phase I consists of pain and swelling in the distal extremity occurring within weeks to 3 months after the precipitating event. The pain is diffuse, spontaneous, and either burning, throbbing, or aching in quality. The involved extremity is warm and edematous, and the joints are tender. Increased sweating and hair growth develop. In phase II (3–6 months after onset), thin, shiny, cool skin appears. After an additional 3–6 months (phase III), atrophy of the skin and subcutaneous tissue plus flexion contractures complete the clinical picture.

The natural history of typical CRPS may be more benign than reflected in the literature. A variety of surgical and medical treatments have been developed, with conflicting reports of efficacy. Clinical trials suggest that early mobilization with physical therapy or a brief course of glucocorticoids may be helpful for CRPS type I. Other medical treatments include the use of adrenergic blockers, nonsteroidal anti-inflammatory drugs, calcium channel blockers, phenytoin, opioids, and calcitonin. Stellate ganglion blockade is a commonly used invasive technique that often provides temporary pain relief, but the efficacy of repetitive blocks is uncertain.

TREATMENT Autonomic Failure

Management of autonomic failure is aimed at specific treatment of the cause and alleviation of symptoms. Of particular importance is the removal of drugs or amelioration of underlying conditions that cause or aggravate the autonomic symptoms, especially in the elderly. For example, OH can be caused or aggravated by angiotensin-converting enzyme inhibitors, calcium channel-blocking agents, tricyclic antidepressants, levodopa, alcohol, or insulin. A summary of drugs that can cause OH by class, putative mechanism, and magnitude of the BP drop, is shown in Table 375-6.

PATIENT EDUCATION Only a minority of patients with OH require drug treatment. All patients should be taught the mechanisms of postural normotension (volume status, resistance and capacitance bed, autoregulation) and the nature of orthostatic stressors (time of day and the influence of meals, heat, standing, and exercise). Patients should learn to recognize orthostatic symptoms early (especially subtle cognitive symptoms, weakness, and fatigue) and to modify or avoid activities that provoke episodes. Other helpful measures may include keeping a BP log and dietary education (salt/fluids). Learning physical countermaneuvers that reduce standing OH and practicing postural and resistance training are helpful measures.

SYMPTOMATIC TREATMENT Nonpharmacologic approaches are summarized in Table 375-9. Adequate intake of salt and fluids to produce a voiding volume between 1.5 and 2.5 L of urine (containing >170 meq/L of Na^+) each 24 h is essential.

TABLE 375-9 Initial Treatment of Orthostatic Hypotension (OH)

Patient education: mechanisms and stressors of OH
High-salt diet (10–20 g/d)
High-fluid intake (2 L/D)
Elevate head of bed 10 cm (4 in.)
Maintain postural stimuli
Learn physical countermaneuvers
Compression garments
Correct anemia

Sleeping with the head of the bed elevated will minimize the effects of supine nocturnal hypertension. Prolonged recumbency should be avoided when possible. Patients are advised to sit with legs dangling over the edge of the bed for several minutes before attempting to stand in the morning; other postural stresses should be similarly approached in a gradual manner. One maneuver that can reduce OH is leg-crossing with maintained contraction of leg muscles for 30 s.; this compresses leg veins and increases systemic resistance. Compressive garments, such as compression stockings and abdominal binders, are helpful on occasion but uncomfortable for some patients. Anemia should be corrected with erythropoietin, administered subcutaneously at doses of 25–75 U/kg three times per week. The hematocrit increases after 2–6 weeks. A weekly maintenance dose is usually necessary. The increased intravascular volume that accompanies the rise in hematocrit can exacerbate supine hypertension.

If these measures are not sufficient, drug treatment may be necessary. Midodrine, a directly acting α_1-agonist that does not cross the blood-brain barrier, is effective. It has a duration of action of 2–4 h. The usual dose is 5–10 mg orally tid, but some patients respond best to a decremental dose (e.g., 15 mg on awakening, 10 mg at noon, and 5 mg in the afternoon). Midodrine should not be taken after 6 p.m. Side effects include pruritus, uncomfortable piloerection, and supine hypertension especially at higher doses. Pyridostigmine appears to improve OH without aggravating supine hypertension by enhancing ganglionic transmission (maximal when orthostatic, minimal supine). Fludrocortisone will reduce OH, but it aggravates supine hypertension. At doses between 0.1 mg/d and 0.3 mg bid orally, it enhances renal sodium conservation and increases the sensitivity of arterioles to NE. Susceptible patients may develop fluid overload, congestive heart failure, supine hypertension, or hypokalemia. Potassium supplements are often necessary with chronic administration of fludrocortisone. Sustained elevations of supine BP >180/110 mm Hg should be avoided.

Postprandial OH may respond to several measures. Frequent, small, low-carbohydrate meals may diminish splanchnic shunting of blood after meals and reduce postprandial OH. Prostaglandin inhibitors (ibuprofen or indomethacin) taken with meals or midodrine (10 mg with the meal) can be helpful. The somatostatin analogue octreotide can be useful in the treatment of postprandial syncope by inhibiting the release of gastrointestinal peptides that have vasodilator and hypotensive effects. The subcutaneous dose ranges from 25 μg bid to 200 μg tid.

The patient should be taught to self-treat transient worsening of OH. Drinking two 250-mL (8-oz) glasses of water can raise standing BP 20–30 mm Hg for about 2 h, beginning ~20 min after the fluid load. The patient can increase intake of salt and fluids (bouillon treatment), increase use of physical countermaneuvers, temporarily resort to a full-body stocking (compression pressure 30–40 mm Hg), or increase the dose of midodrine. Supine hypertension (>180/110 mm Hg) can be self-treated by avoiding the supine position and reducing fludrocortisone. A daily glass of wine, if requested by the patient, can be taken shortly before bedtime. If these simple measures are not adequate, drugs to be considered include oral hydralazine (25 mg qhs), oral Procardia (10 mg qhs), or a nitroglycerin patch.

FURTHER READINGS

Low PA, Benarroch EE: *Clinical Autonomic Disorders*, 3rd ed. Philadelphia, Lippincott, 2009

Schroeder C et al: Plasma exchange for primary autoimmune autonomic failure. N Engl J Med 353:1585, 2005

Thaisetthawatkul P et al: Autonomic dysfunction in dementia with Lewy bodies. Neurology 62:1804, 2004

Thieben MJ et al: Postural orthostatic tachycardia syndrome: The Mayo Clinic experience. Mayo Clin Proc 82:308, 2007

Vinik AI, Ziegler D: Diabetic cardiovascular autonomic neuropathy. Circulation 115:387, 2007

CHAPTER 376 Trigeminal Neuralgia, Bell's Palsy, and Other Cranial Nerve Disorders

M. Flint Beal
Stephen L. Hauser

Symptoms and signs of cranial nerve pathology are common in internal medicine. They often develop in the context of a widespread neurologic disturbance, and in such situations cranial nerve involvement may represent the initial manifestation of the illness. In other disorders, involvement is largely restricted to one or several cranial nerves; these distinctive disorders are reviewed in this chapter. Disorders of ocular movement are discussed in Chap. 28, disorders of hearing in Chap. 30, and vertigo and disorders of vestibular function in Chap. 21.

FACIAL PAIN OR NUMBNESS

ANATOMIC CONSIDERATIONS

The trigeminal (fifth cranial) nerve supplies sensation to the skin of the face and anterior half of the head (Fig. 376-1). Its motor part innervates the masseter and pterygoid masticatory muscles.

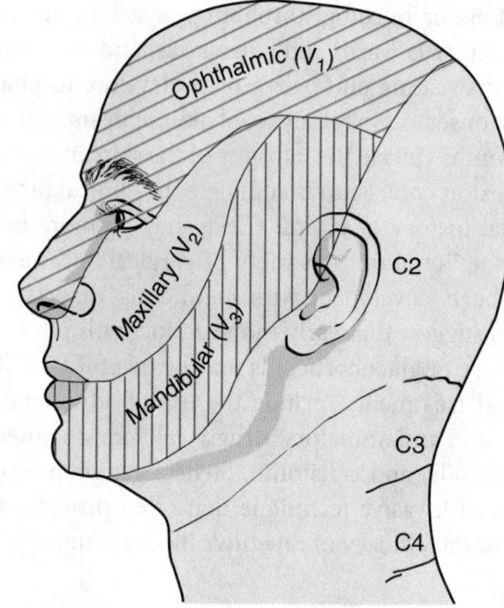

Figure 376-1 The three major sensory divisions of the trigeminal nerve consist of the ophthalmic, maxillary, and mandibular nerves.

TRIGEMINAL NEURALGIA (TIC DOULOUREUX)

Clinical manifestations

Trigeminal neuralgia is characterized by excruciating paroxysms of pain in the lips, gums, cheek, or chin and, very rarely, in the distribution of the ophthalmic division of the fifth nerve. The pain seldom lasts more than a few seconds or a minute or two but may be so intense that the patient winces, hence the term *tic*. The paroxysms, experienced as single jabs or clusters, tend to recur frequently, both day and night, for several weeks at a time. They may occur spontaneously or with movements of affected areas evoked by speaking, chewing, or smiling. Another characteristic feature is the presence of trigger zones, typically on the face, lips, or tongue, that provoke attacks; patients may report that tactile stimuli—e.g., washing the face, brushing the teeth, or exposure to a draft of air—generate excruciating pain. *An essential feature of trigeminal neuralgia is that objective signs of sensory loss cannot be demonstrated on examination.*

Trigeminal neuralgia is relatively common, with an estimated annual incidence of 4.5 per 100,000 individuals. Middle-aged and elderly persons are affected primarily, and ~60% of cases occur in women. Onset is typically sudden, and bouts tend to persist for weeks or months before remitting spontaneously. Remissions may be long-lasting, but in most patients the disorder ultimately recurs.

Pathophysiology

Symptoms result from ectopic generation of action potentials in pain-sensitive afferent fibers of the fifth cranial nerve root just before it enters the lateral surface of the pons. Compression or other pathology in the nerve leads to demyelination of large myelinated fibers that do not themselves carry pain sensation but become hyperexcitable and electrically coupled with smaller unmyelinated or poorly myelinated pain fibers in close proximity; this may explain why tactile stimuli, conveyed via the large myelinated fibers, can stimulate paroxysms of pain. Compression of the trigeminal nerve root by a blood vessel, most often the superior cerebellar artery or on occasion a tortuous vein, is the source of trigeminal neuralgia in a substantial proportion of patients. In cases of vascular compression, age-related brain sagging and increased vascular thickness and tortuosity may explain the prevalence of trigeminal neuralgia in later life.

Differential diagnosis

Trigeminal neuralgia must be distinguished from other causes of face and head pain (Chap. 14) and from pain arising from diseases of the jaw, teeth, or sinuses. Pain from migraine or cluster headache tends to be deep-seated and steady, unlike the superficial stabbing quality of trigeminal neuralgia; rarely, cluster headache is associated with trigeminal neuralgia, a syndrome known as *cluster-tic*. In temporal arteritis, superficial facial pain is present but is not typically shocklike, the patient frequently complains of myalgias and other systemic symptoms, and an elevated erythrocyte sedimentation rate (ESR) is usually present (Chap. 326). When trigeminal neuralgia develops in a young adult or is bilateral, multiple sclerosis (MS) is a key consideration, and in such cases the cause is a demyelinating plaque at the root entry zone of the fifth nerve in the pons; often, evidence of facial sensory loss can be found on careful examination. Cases that are secondary to mass lesions—such as aneurysms, neurofibromas, acoustic schwannomas, or meningiomas—usually produce objective signs of sensory loss in the trigeminal nerve distribution (trigeminal neuropathy, see below).

Laboratory evaluation

An ESR is indicated if temporal arteritis is suspected. In typical cases of trigeminal neuralgia, neuroimaging studies are usually unnecessary but may be valuable if MS is a consideration or in assessing overlying vascular lesions in order to plan for decompression surgery.

TREATMENT Trigeminal Neuralgia

Drug therapy with carbamazepine is effective in ~50–75% of patients. Carbamazepine should be started as a single daily dose of 100 mg taken with food and increased gradually (by 100 mg daily in divided doses every 1–2 days) until substantial (>50%) pain relief is achieved. Most patients require a maintenance dose of 200 mg qid. Doses >1200 mg daily provide no additional benefit. Dizziness, imbalance, sedation, and rare cases of agranulocytosis are the most important side effects of carbamazepine. If treatment is effective, it is usually continued for 1 month and then tapered as tolerated. Oxcarbazepine (300–1200 mg bid) is an alternative to carbamazepine, has less bone marrow toxicity, and probably is equally efficacious. If these agents are not well tolerated or are ineffective, lamotrigine 400 mg daily or phenytoin, 300–400 mg daily, are other options. Baclofen may also be administered, either alone or in combination with an anticonvulsant. The initial dose is 5–10 mg tid, gradually increasing as needed to 20 mg qid.

If drug treatment fails, surgical therapy should be offered. The most widely used method currently is microvascular decompression to relieve pressure on the trigeminal nerve as it exits the pons. This procedure requires a suboccipital craniotomy. Based on limited data, this procedure appears to have a >70% efficacy rate and a low rate of pain recurrence in responders; the response is better for classic tic-like symptoms than for nonlancinating facial pains. In a small number of cases, there is perioperative damage to the eighth or seventh cranial nerves or to the cerebellum, or a postoperative CSF leak syndrome. High-resolution magnetic resonance angiography is useful preoperatively to visualize the relationships between the fifth cranial nerve root and nearby blood vessels.

Gamma knife radiosurgery is also utilized for treatment and results in complete pain relief in more than two-thirds of patients and a low risk of persistent facial numbness; the response is sometimes long-lasting, but recurrent pain develops over 2–3 years in half of patients. Compared with surgical decompression, gamma knife surgery appears to be somewhat less effective but has few serious complications.

Another procedure, *radiofrequency thermal rhizotomy*, creates a heat lesion of the trigeminal (gasserian) ganglion or nerve. It is used less often now than in the past. Short-term relief is experienced by >95% of patients; however, long-term studies indicate that pain recurs in up to one-third of treated patients. Postoperatively, partial numbness of the face is common, masseter (jaw) weakness may occur especially following bilateral procedures, and corneal denervation with secondary keratitis can follow rhizotomy for first-division trigeminal neuralgia.

TRIGEMINAL NEUROPATHY

A variety of diseases may affect the trigeminal nerve (Table 376-1). Most present with sensory loss on the face or with weakness of the jaw muscles. Deviation of the jaw on opening indicates weakness of the pterygoids on the side to which the jaw deviates. Some cases are due to Sjögren's syndrome or a collagen-vascular disease such as systemic lupus erythematosus, scleroderma, or mixed connective tissue disease. Among infectious causes, herpes zoster and leprosy should be considered. Tumors of the middle cranial fossa (meningiomas), of the trigeminal nerve (schwannomas), or of the base of the skull (metastatic tumors) may cause a combination of motor and sensory signs. Lesions in the cavernous sinus can affect the first and second divisions of the trigeminal nerve, and lesions of the superior orbital fissure can affect the first (ophthalmic) division; the accompanying corneal anesthesia increases the risk of ulceration (neuro keratitis).

Loss of sensation over the chin (mental neuropathy) can be the only manifestation of systemic malignancy. Rarely, an idiopathic form of trigeminal neuropathy is observed. It is characterized by numbness and paresthesias, sometimes bilaterally, with loss of sensation in the territory of the trigeminal nerve but without weakness of the jaw. Gradual recovery is the rule. Tonic spasm of the masticatory muscles, known as *trismus*, is symptomatic of tetanus (Chap. 140) or may occur in patients treated with phenothiazine drugs.

TABLE 376-1 Trigeminal Nerve Disorders

Nuclear (brainstem) lesions	Peripheral nerve lesions
Multiple sclerosis	Nasopharyngeal carcinoma
Stroke	Trauma
Syringobulbia	Guillain-Barré syndrome
Glioma	Sjögren's syndrome
Lymphoma	Collagen-vascular diseases
Preganglionic lesions	Sarcoidosis
Acoustic neuroma	Leprosy
Meningioma	Drugs (stilbamidine, trichloroethylene)
Metastasis	Idiopathic trigeminal neuropathy
Chronic meningitis	
Cavernous carotid aneurysm	
Gasserian ganglion lesions	
Trigeminal neuroma	
Herpes zoster	
Infection (spread from otitis media or mastoiditis)	

FACIAL WEAKNESS

ANATOMIC CONSIDERATIONS

(Fig. 376-2) The seventh cranial nerve supplies all the muscles concerned with facial expression. The sensory component is small (the nervus intermedius); it conveys taste sensation from the anterior two-thirds of the tongue and probably cutaneous impulses from the anterior wall of the external auditory canal. The motor nucleus of the seventh nerve lies anterior and lateral to the abducens nucleus. After leaving the pons, the seventh nerve enters the internal auditory meatus with the acoustic nerve. The nerve continues its course in its own bony channel, the facial canal, and exits from the skull via the stylomastoid foramen. It then passes through the parotid gland and subdivides to supply the facial muscles.

A complete interruption of the facial nerve at the stylomastoid foramen paralyzes all muscles of facial expression. The corner of the mouth droops, the creases and skinfolds are effaced, the forehead is unfurrowed, and the eyelids will not close. Upon attempted closure of the lids, the eye on the paralyzed side rolls upward (*Bell's phenomenon*). The lower lid sags and falls away from the conjunctiva, permitting tears to spill over the cheek. Food collects between the teeth and lips, and saliva may dribble from the corner of the mouth. The patient complains of a heaviness or numbness in the face, but sensory loss is rarely demonstrable and taste is intact.

If the lesion is in the middle-ear portion, taste is lost over the anterior two-thirds of the tongue on the same side. If the nerve to the stapedius is interrupted, there is hyperacusis (sensitivity to loud sounds). Lesions in the internal auditory meatus may affect the adjacent auditory and vestibular nerves, causing deafness, tinnitus, or dizziness. Intrapontine lesions that paralyze the face usually affect the abducens nucleus as well, and often the corticospinal and sensory tracts.

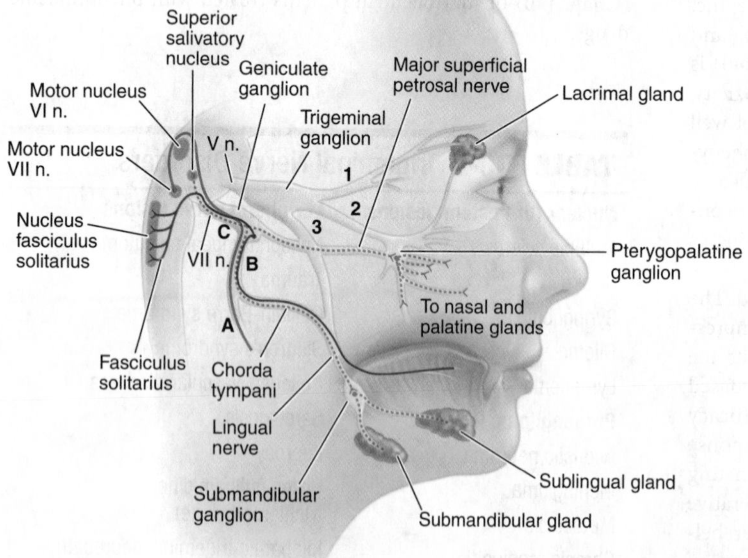

Figure 376-2 The facial nerve. A, B, and C denote lesions of the facial nerve at the stylomastoid foramen, distal and proximal to the geniculate ganglion, respectively. Green lines indicate the parasympathetic fibers, red line indicates motor fibers, and purple lines indicate visceral afferent fibers (taste). *(Adapted from MB Carpenter: Core Text of Neuroanatomy, 2nd ed. Baltimore, Williams & Wilkins, 1978.)*

If the peripheral facial paralysis has existed for some time and recovery of motor function is incomplete, a continuous diffuse contraction of facial muscles may appear. The palpebral fissure becomes narrowed, and the nasolabial fold deepens. Attempts to move one group of facial muscles may result in contraction of all (associated movements, or *synkinesis*). Facial spasms, initiated by movements of the face, may develop (*hemifacial spasm*). Anomalous regeneration of seventh nerve fibers may result in other troublesome phenomena. If fibers originally connected with the orbicularis oculi come to innervate the orbicularis oris, closure of the lids may cause a retraction of the mouth, or if fibers originally connected with muscles of the face later innervate the lacrimal gland, anomalous tearing ("crocodile tears") may occur with any activity of the facial muscles, such as eating. Another facial synkinesia is triggered by jaw opening, causing closure of the eyelids on the side of the facial palsy (jaw-winking).

BELL'S PALSY

The most common form of facial paralysis is *Bell's palsy*. The annual incidence of this idiopathic disorder is ~25 per 100,000 annually, or about 1 in 60 persons in a lifetime.

Clinical manifestations

The onset of Bell's palsy is fairly abrupt, maximal weakness being attained by 48 h as a general rule. Pain behind the ear may precede the paralysis for a day or two. Taste sensation may be lost unilaterally, and hyperacusis may be present. In some cases there is mild cerebrospinal fluid lymphocytosis. MRI may reveal swelling and uniform enhancement of the geniculate ganglion and facial nerve and, in some cases, entrapment of the swollen nerve in the temporal bone. Approximately 80% of patients recover within a few weeks or months. Electromyography may be of some prognostic value; evidence of denervation after 10 days indicates there has been axonal degeneration, that there will be a long delay (3 months as a rule) before regeneration occurs, and that it may be incomplete. The presence of incomplete paralysis in the first week is the most favorable prognostic sign.

Pathophysiology

In acute Bell's palsy there is inflammation of the facial nerve with mononuclear cells, consistent with an infectious or immune cause. Herpes simplex virus (HSV) type 1 DNA was frequently detected in endoneurial fluid and posterior auricular muscle, suggesting that a reactivation of this virus in the geniculate ganglion may be responsible for most cases. Reactivation of varicella zoster virus is associated with Bell's palsy in up to one-third of cases, and may represent the second most frequent cause. A variety of other viruses have also been implicated less commonly. An increased incidence of Bell's palsy was also reported among recipients of inactivated intranasal influenza vaccine, and it was hypothesized that this could have resulted from the *Escherichia coli* enterotoxin used as adjuvant or to reactivation of latent virus.

Differential diagnosis

There are many other causes of acute facial palsy that must be considered in the differential diagnosis of Bell's palsy. Lyme disease can cause unilateral or bilateral facial palsies; in endemic areas, 10% or more of cases of facial palsy are likely due to infection with *Borrelia burgdorferi* (Chap. 173). The *Ramsay Hunt syndrome*, caused by reactivation of herpes zoster in the geniculate ganglion, consists of a severe facial palsy associated with a vesicular eruption in the external auditory canal and sometimes in the pharynx and other parts of the cranial integument; often the eighth cranial nerve is affected as well. Facial palsy that is often bilateral occurs in sarcoidosis (Chap. 329) and in *Guillain-Barré syndrome* (Chap. 385). Leprosy frequently involves the facial nerve, and facial neuropathy may also occur in diabetes mellitus, connective tissue diseases including Sjögren's syndrome, and amyloidosis. The rare *Melkersson-Rosenthal syndrome* consists of recurrent facial paralysis; recurrent—and eventually permanent—facial (particularly labial) edema; and, less constantly, plication of the tongue. Its cause is unknown. *Acoustic neuromas* frequently involve the facial nerve by local compression. Infarcts, demyelinating lesions of multiple sclerosis, and tumors are the common pontine lesions that interrupt the facial nerve fibers; other signs of brainstem involvement are usually present. Tumors that invade the temporal bone (carotid body, cholesteatoma, dermoid) may produce a facial palsy, but the onset is insidious and the course progressive.

All these forms of nuclear or peripheral facial palsy must be distinguished from the supranuclear type. In the latter, the frontalis and orbicularis oculi muscles are involved less than those of the lower part of the face, since the upper facial muscles are innervated by corticobulbar pathways from both motor cortices, whereas the lower facial muscles are innervated only by the opposite hemisphere. In supranuclear lesions there may be a dissociation of emotional and voluntary facial movements and often some degree of paralysis of the arm and leg, or an aphasia (in dominant hemisphere lesions) is present.

Laboratory evaluation

The diagnosis of Bell's palsy can usually be made clinically in patients with (1) a typical presentation, (2) no risk factors or preexisting symptoms for other causes of facial paralysis, (3) absence of cutaneous lesions of herpes zoster in the external ear canal, and (4) a normal neurologic examination with the exception of the facial nerve. Particular attention to the eighth cranial nerve, which courses near to the facial nerve in the pontomedullary junction and in the temporal bone, and to other cranial nerves is essential. In atypical or uncertain cases, an ESR, testing for diabetes mellitus, a Lyme titer, angiotensin-converting enzyme and chest imaging studies for possible sarcoidosis, a lumbar puncture for possible Guillain-Barré syndrome, or MRI scanning may be indicated. MRI often shows swelling and enhancement of the facial nerve in idiopathic Bell's palsy (Fig. 376-3).

TREATMENT Bell's Palsy

Symptomatic measures include (1) the use of paper tape to depress the upper eyelid during sleep and prevent corneal drying, and (2) massage of the weakened muscles. A course of glucocorticoids, given as prednisone 60–80 mg daily during the first 5 days and then tapered over the next 5 days, modestly shortens the recovery period and improves the functional outcome. Although two large recently published randomized trials found no added benefit of antiviral agents valacyclovir (1000 mg daily for 5–7 days) or acyclovir (400 mg five times daily for 10 days) compared to glucocorticoids alone, the overall weight of evidence suggests that the combination therapy with prednisone plus valacyclovir may be marginally better than prednisone alone, especially in patients with severe clinical presentations.

OTHER MOTOR DISORDERS OF THE FACE

Hemifacial spasm consists of painless irregular involuntary contractions on one side of the face. Most cases appear related to vascular compression of the exiting facial nerve in the pons. Other cases develop as a sequela to Bell's palsy or are secondary to compression and/or demyelination of the nerve by tumor, infection or multiple sclerosis. Mild cases can be treated with carbamazepine, gabapentin, or, if these drugs fail, with baclofen. Local injections of botulinum toxin into affected muscles can relieve spasms for 3–4 months, and the injections can be repeated. Refractory cases due to vascular compression usually respond to surgical decompression of the facial nerve. *Blepharospasm* is an involuntary recurrent spasm of both eyelids that usually occurs in elderly persons as an isolated phenomenon or with varying degrees of spasm of other facial muscles. Severe, persistent cases of blepharospasm can be treated by local injection of botulinum toxin into the orbicularis oculi. *Facial myokymia* refers to a fine rippling activity of the facial muscles; it may be caused by multiple sclerosis or follow Guillain-Barré syndrome (Chap. 385).

Facial hemiatrophy occurs mainly in women and is characterized by a disappearance of fat in the dermal and subcutaneous tissues on one side of the face. It usually begins in adolescence or early adult years and is slowly progressive. In its advanced form, the affected side of the face is gaunt, and the skin is thin, wrinkled, and brown.

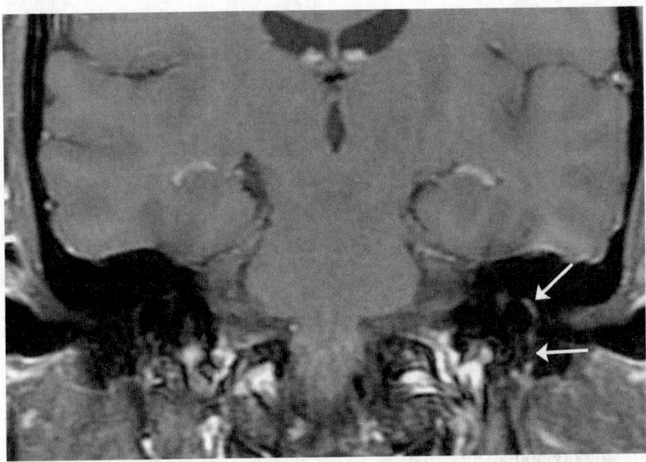

A

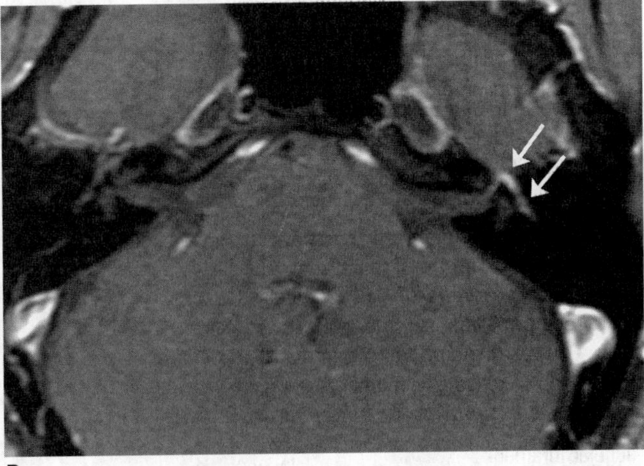

B

Figure 376-3 Axial and coronal T1-weighted images post-Gadolinium with fat suppression demonstrate diffuse smooth linear enhancement of the left facial nerve, involving the genu, tympanic, and mastoid segments within the temporal bone (*arrows*), without evidence of mass lesion. Although highly suggestive of Bell's palsy, similar findings may be seen with other etiologies such as Lyme disease, sarcoidosis, and perineural malignant spread.

The facial hair may turn white and fall out, and the sebaceous glands become atrophic. Bilateral involvement may occur. A limited form of systemic sclerosis (scleroderma) may be the cause of some cases. Treatment is cosmetic, consisting of transplantation of skin and subcutaneous fat.

OTHER CRANIAL NERVE DISORDERS

GLOSSOPHARYNGEAL NEURALGIA

This form of neuralgia involves the ninth (glossopharyngeal) and sometimes portions of the tenth (vagus) cranial nerves. It resembles trigeminal neuralgia in many respects but is much less common. The pain is intense and paroxysmal; it originates on one side of the throat, approximately in the tonsillar fossa. In some cases the pain is localized in the ear or may radiate from the throat to the ear because of involvement of the tympanic branch of the glossopharyngeal nerve. Spasms of pain may be initiated by swallowing or coughing. There is no demonstrable motor or sensory deficit; the glossopharyngeal nerve supplies taste sensation to the posterior third of the tongue and, together with the vagus nerve, sensation to the posterior pharynx. Cardiac symptoms—bradycardia or asystole, hypotension, and fainting—have been reported. Medical therapy is similar to that for trigeminal neuralgia, and carbamazepine is generally the first choice. If drug therapy is unsuccessful, surgical procedures—including microvascular decompression if vascular compression is evident—or rhizotomy of glossopharyngeal and vagal fibers in the jugular bulb is frequently successful.

Very rarely, herpes zoster involves the glossopharyngeal nerve. Glossopharyngeal neuropathy in conjunction with vagus and accessory nerve palsies may also occur with a tumor or aneurysm in the posterior fossa or in the jugular foramen. Hoarseness due to vocal cord paralysis, some difficulty in swallowing, deviation of the soft palate to the intact side, anesthesia of the posterior wall of the pharynx, and weakness of the upper part of the trapezius and sternocleidomastoid muscles make up the jugular foramen syndrome (Table 376-2).

DYSPHAGIA AND DYSPHONIA

When the intracranial portion of one vagus (tenth cranial) nerve is interrupted, the soft palate droops ipsilaterally and does not rise in phonation. There is loss of the gag reflex on the affected side, as well as of the "curtain movement" of the lateral wall of the pharynx, whereby the faucial pillars move medially as the palate rises in saying "ah." The voice is hoarse and slightly nasal, and the vocal cord lies immobile midway between abduction and adduction. Loss of sensation at the external auditory meatus and the posterior pinna may also be present.

The pharyngeal branches of both vagal nerves may be affected in diphtheria; the voice has a nasal quality, and regurgitation of liquids through the nose occurs during the act of swallowing.

The vagus nerve may be involved at the meningeal level by neoplastic and infectious processes and within the medulla by tumors, vascular lesions (e.g., the lateral medullary syndrome), and motor neuron disease. This nerve may be involved by infection with varicella zoster virus. Polymyositis and dermatomyositis, which cause hoarseness and dysphagia by direct involvement of laryngeal and pharyngeal muscles, may be confused with diseases of the vagus nerves. Dysphagia is also a symptom in some patients with myotonic dystrophy. Nonneurologic causes of dysphagia are discussed in Chap. 38.

The recurrent laryngeal nerves, especially the left, are most often damaged as a result of intrathoracic disease. Aneurysm of the aortic arch, an enlarged left atrium, and tumors of the mediastinum and bronchi are much more frequent causes of an isolated vocal cord palsy than are intracranial disorders. However, a substantial number of cases of recurrent laryngeal palsy remain idiopathic.

When confronted with a case of laryngeal palsy, the physician must attempt to determine the site of the lesion. If it is intramedullary, there are usually other signs, such as ipsilateral cerebellar dysfunction, loss of pain and temperature sensation over the ipsilateral face and contralateral arm and leg, and an ipsilateral Horner syndrome. If the lesion is extramedullary, the glossopharyngeal and spinal accessory nerves are frequently involved (jugular foramen syndrome). If it is extracranial in the posterior laterocondylar or retroparotid space, there may be a combination of ninth, tenth, eleventh, and twelfth cranial nerve palsies and a Horner syndrome (Table 376-2). If there is no sensory loss over the palate and pharynx and no palatal weakness or dysphagia, the lesion is below the origin of the pharyngeal branches, which leave the vagus nerve high in the cervical region; the usual site of disease is then the mediastinum.

NECK WEAKNESS

Isolated involvement of the accessory (eleventh cranial) nerve can occur anywhere along its route, resulting in partial or complete paralysis of the sternocleidomastoid and trapezius muscles. More commonly, involvement occurs in combination with deficits of the ninth and tenth cranial nerves in the jugular foramen or after exit from the skull (Table 376-2). An idiopathic form of accessory

TABLE 376-2 Cranial Nerve Syndromes

Site	Cranial Nerves	Usual Cause
Sphenoid fissure (superior orbital)	III, IV, first division V, VI	Invasive tumors of sphenoid bone; aneurysms
Lateral wall of cavernous sinus	III, IV, first division V, VI, often with proptosis	Infection, thrombosis, aneurysm, or fistula of cavernous sinus; invasive tumors from sinuses and sella turcica; benign granuloma responsive to glucocorticoids
Retrosphenoid space	II, III, IV, V, VI	Large tumors of middle cranial fossa
Apex of petrous bone	V, VI	Petrositis; tumors of petrous bone
Internal auditory meatus	VII, VIII	Tumors of petrous bone (dermoids, etc.); infectious processes; acoustic neuroma
Pontocerebellar angle	V, VII, VIII, and sometimes IX	Acoustic neuroma; meningioma
Jugular foramen	IX, X, XI	Tumors and aneurysms
Posterior laterocondylar space	IX, X, XI, XII	Tumors of parotid gland and carotid body and metastatic tumors
Posterior retroparotid space	IX, X, XI, XII and Horner syndrome	Tumors of parotid gland, carotid body, lymph nodes; metastatic tumor; tuberculous adenitis

neuropathy, akin to Bell's palsy, has been described, and it may be recurrent in some cases. Most but not all patients recover.

■ TONGUE PARALYSIS

The hypoglossal (twelfth cranial) nerve supplies the ipsilateral muscles of the tongue. The nucleus of the nerve or its fibers of exit may be involved by intramedullary lesions such as tumor, poliomyelitis, or most often motor neuron disease. Lesions of the basal meninges and the occipital bones (platybasia, invagination of occipital condyles, Paget's disease) may compress the nerve in its extramedullary course or in the hypoglossal canal. Isolated lesions of unknown cause can occur. Atrophy and fasciculation of the tongue develop weeks to months after interruption of the nerve.

MULTIPLE CRANIAL NERVE PALSIES

Several cranial nerves may be affected by the same disease process. In this situation, the main clinical problem is to determine whether the lesion lies within the brainstem or outside it. Lesions that lie on the surface of the brainstem are characterized by involvement of adjacent cranial nerves (often occurring in succession) and late and rather slight involvement of the long sensory and motor pathways and segmental structures lying within the brainstem. The opposite is true of primary lesions within the brainstem. The extramedullary lesion is more likely to cause bone erosion or enlargement of the foramens of exit of cranial nerves. The intramedullary lesion involving cranial nerves often produces a crossed sensory or motor paralysis (cranial nerve signs on one side of the body and tract signs on the opposite side).

Involvement of multiple cranial nerves outside the brainstem is frequently the result of trauma, localized infections including varicella zoster virus, infectious and noninfectious (especially carcinomatous) causes of meningitis (Chaps. 381 and 382), granulomatous diseases such as granulomatosis with polyangiitis (Wegener's), Behçet's disease, vascular disorders including those associated with diabetes, enlarging saccular aneurysms, or locally infiltrating tumors. Among the tumors, nasopharyngeal cancers, lymphomas, neurofibromas, meningiomas, chordomas, cholesteatomas, carcinomas, and sarcomas have all been observed to involve a succession of lower cranial nerves. Owing to their anatomic relationships, the multiple cranial nerve palsies form a number of distinctive syndromes, listed in Table 376-2. Sarcoidosis is the cause of some cases of multiple cranial neuropathy, and chronic glandular tuberculosis the cause of a few others. Platybasia, basilar invagination of the skull, and the Chiari malformation are additional causes. A purely motor disorder without atrophy always raises the question of myasthenia gravis (Chap. 386). As noted above, Guillain-Barré syndrome commonly affects the facial nerves bilaterally. In the Fisher variant of the Guillain-Barré syndrome, oculomotor paresis occurs with ataxia and areflexia in the limbs (Chap. 385). Wernicke encephalopathy can cause a severe ophthalmoplegia combined with other brainstem signs (Chap. 275).

The *cavernous sinus syndrome* (Fig. 376-4) is a distinctive and frequently life-threatening disorder. It often presents as orbital or facial pain; orbital swelling and chemosis due to occlusion of the ophthalmic veins; fever; oculomotor neuropathy affecting the third, fourth, and sixth cranial nerves; and trigeminal neuropathy affecting the ophthalmic (V_1) and occasionally the maxillary (V_2) divisions of the trigeminal nerve. Cavernous sinus thrombosis, often secondary to infection from orbital cellulitis (frequently *Staphylococcus aureus*), a cutaneous source on the face, or sinusitis (especially with mucormycosis in diabetic patients), is the most frequent cause; other etiologies include aneurysm of the carotid artery, a carotid-cavernous fistula (orbital bruit may be present), meningioma, nasopharyngeal carcinoma, other tumors, or an idiopathic granulomatous disorder (Tolosa-Hunt syndrome). The two cavernous sinuses directly communicate via intercavernous channels; thus, involvement on one side may extend to become bilateral. Early diagnosis is essential, especially when due to infection, and treatment depends on the underlying etiology.

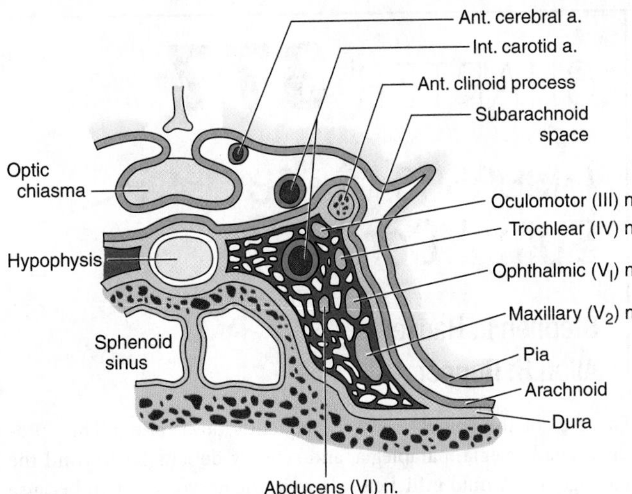

Figure 376-4 Anatomy of the cavernous sinus in coronal section, illustrating the location of the cranial nerves in relation to the vascular sinus, internal carotid artery (which loops anteriorly to the section), and surrounding structures.

In infectious cases, prompt administration of broad-spectrum antibiotics, drainage of any abscess cavities, and identification of the offending organism are essential. Anticoagulant therapy may benefit cases of primary thrombosis. Repair or occlusion of the carotid artery may be required for treatment of fistulas or aneurysms. The Tolosa-Hunt syndrome generally responds to glucocorticoids. A dramatic improvement in pain is usually evident within a few days; oral prednisone (60 mg daily) is usually continued for 2 weeks and then gradually tapered over a month, or longer if pain recurs.

An idiopathic form of multiple cranial nerve involvement on one or both sides of the face is occasionally seen. The syndrome consists of a subacute onset of boring facial pain, followed by paralysis of motor cranial nerves. The clinical features overlap those of the Tolosa-Hunt syndrome and appear to be due to idiopathic inflammation of the dura mater, which may be visualized by MRI. The syndrome is frequently responsive to glucocorticoids.

FURTHER READINGS

De Almeida JR et al: Combined corticosteroids and antiviral treatment for Bell palsy: A systematic review and meta-analysis. JAMA 302:985, 2009

Dhople AA et al: Long term outcomes of gamma knife radiosurgery for classic trigeminal neuralgia: Implications of treatment and critical review of the literature. J Neurosurg 111: 351, 2009

Gronseth G et al: Practice parameter: The diagnostic evaluation and treatment of trigeminal neuralgia (an evidence-based review): Report of the Quality Standards Subcommittee of the American Academy of Neurology and the European Federation of Neurological Societies. Neurology 71:1183, 2008

Hato N et al: Valacyclovir and prednisolone treatment for Bell's palsy: A randomized, placebo-controlled study. Otol Neurotol 28:408, 2007

Keane JR: Multiple cranial nerve palsies: Analysis of 979 cases. Arch Neurol. 62: 1714, 2005

Pearce JMS: Glossopharyngeal neuralgia. Eur Neurol 55:49, 2006

Quant EC et al: The benefits of steroids versus steroids plus antivirals for treatment of Bell's palsy: A meta-analysis. BMJ 339:b3354, 2009

CHAPTER 377 Diseases of the Spinal Cord

Stephen L. Hauser
Allan H. Ropper

Diseases of the spinal cord are frequently devastating. They produce quadriplegia, paraplegia, and sensory deficits far beyond the damage they would inflict elsewhere in the nervous system because the spinal cord contains, in a small cross-sectional area, almost the entire motor output and sensory input of the trunk and limbs. Many spinal cord diseases are reversible if recognized and treated at an early stage (Table 377-1); thus, they are among the most critical of neurologic emergencies. The efficient use of diagnostic procedures, guided by knowledge of the anatomy and the clinical features of spinal cord diseases, is required for a successful outcome.

APPROACH TO THE PATIENT Spinal Cord Disease

SPINAL CORD ANATOMY RELEVANT TO CLINICAL SIGNS The spinal cord is a thin, tubular extension of the central nervous system contained within the bony spinal canal. It originates at the medulla and continues caudally to the conus medullaris at the lumbar level; its fibrous extension, the filum terminale, terminates at the coccyx. The adult spinal cord is ~46 cm (18 in.) long, oval in shape, and enlarged in the cervical and lumbar regions, where neurons that innervate the upper and lower extremities, respectively, are located. The white matter tracts containing ascending sensory and descending motor pathways are located peripherally, whereas nerve cell bodies are clustered in an inner region shaped like a four-leaf clover that surrounds the central canal (anatomically an extension of the fourth ventricle). The membranes that cover the spinal cord—the pia, arachnoid, and dura—are continuous with those of the brain.

The spinal cord has 31 segments, each defined by a pair of exiting ventral motor roots and entering dorsal sensory roots. During embryologic development, growth of the cord lags behind that of the vertebral column, and the mature spinal cord ends at approximately the first lumbar vertebral body. The lower spinal nerves take an increasingly downward course to exit via intervertebral foramens. The first seven pairs of cervical spinal nerves exit above the same-numbered vertebral bodies, whereas all the subsequent nerves exit below the same-numbered vertebral bodies because of the presence of eight cervical spinal cord segments but only seven cervical vertebrae. The relationship between spinal cord segments and the corresponding vertebral bodies is shown in Table 377-2. These relationships assume particular importance for localization of lesions that cause spinal cord compression. Sensory loss below the circumferential level of the umbilicus, for example, corresponds to the T10 cord segment but indicates involvement of the cord adjacent to the seventh or eighth thoracic vertebral body (Figs. 23-2 and 23-3). In addition, at every level the main ascending and descending tracts are somatotopically organized with a laminated distribution that reflects the origin or destination of nerve fibers.

TABLE 377-1 Treatable Spinal Cord Disorders

Compressive
- Epidural, intradural, or intramedullary neoplasm
- Epidural abscess
- Epidural hemorrhage
- Cervical spondylosis
- Herniated disk
- Posttraumatic compression by fractured or displaced vertebra or hemorrhage

Vascular
- Arteriovenous malformation
- Antiphospholipid syndrome and other hypercoagulable states

Inflammatory
- Multiple sclerosis
- Neuromyelitis optica
- Transverse myelitis
- Sarcoidosis
- Sjögren-related myelopathy
- Systemic lupus erythematosus
- Vasculitis

Infectious
- Viral: VZV, HSV-1 and -2, CMV, HIV, HTLV-I, others
- Bacterial and mycobacterial: *Borrelia, Listeria,* syphilis, others
- *Mycoplasma pneumoniae*
- Parasitic: schistosomiasis, toxoplasmosis

Developmental
- Syringomyelia
- Meningomyelocele
- Tethered cord syndrome

Metabolic
- Vitamin B_{12} deficiency (subacute combined degeneration)
- Copper deficiency

Abbreviations: CMV, cytomegalovirus; HSV, herpes simplex virus; HTLV, human T cell lymphotropic virus; VZV, varicella-zoster virus.

Determining the Level of the Lesion The presence of a horizontally defined level below which sensory, motor, and autonomic function is impaired is a hallmark of spinal cord disease. This *sensory level* is sought by asking the patient to identify a pinprick or cold stimulus applied to the proximal legs and lower trunk and successively moved up toward the neck on each side. Sensory loss below this level is the result of damage to the spinothalamic tract on the opposite side one to two segments higher in the case of a

TABLE 377-2 Spinal Cord Levels Relative to the Vertebral Bodies

Spinal Cord Level	Corresponding Vertebral Body
Upper cervical	Same as cord level
Lower cervical	1 level higher
Upper thoracic	2 levels higher
Lower thoracic	2 to 3 levels higher
Lumbar	T10-T12
Sacral	T12-L1

unilateral spinal cord lesion, and at the level of a bilateral lesion. The discrepancy in the level of a unilateral lesion is the result of the course of the second-order sensory fibers, which originate in the dorsal horn, and ascend for one or two levels as they cross anterior to the central canal to join the opposite spinothalamic tract. Lesions that transect the descending corticospinal and other motor tracts cause paraplegia or quadriplegia with heightened deep tendon reflexes, Babinski signs, and eventual spasticity (the upper motor neuron syndrome). Transverse damage to the cord also produces autonomic disturbances consisting of absent sweating below the implicated cord level and bladder, bowel, and sexual dysfunction.

The uppermost level of a spinal cord lesion can also be localized by attention to the *segmental signs* corresponding to disturbed motor or sensory innervation by an individual cord segment. A band of altered sensation (hyperalgesia or hyperpathia) at the upper end of the sensory disturbance, fasciculations or atrophy in muscles innervated by one or several segments, or a muted or absent deep tendon reflex may be noted at this level. These signs also can occur with focal root or peripheral nerve disorders; thus, they are most useful when they occur together with signs of long tract damage. With severe and acute transverse lesions, the limbs initially may be flaccid rather than spastic. This state of "spinal shock" lasts for several days, rarely for weeks, and should not be mistaken for extensive damage to the anterior horn cells over many segments of the cord or for an acute polyneuropathy.

The main features of transverse damage at each level of the spinal cord are summarized below.

Cervical Cord Upper cervical cord lesions produce quadriplegia and weakness of the diaphragm. Lesions at C4-C5 produce quadriplegia; at C5-C6, there is loss of power and reflexes in the biceps; at C7 weakness affects finger and wrist extensors and triceps; and at C8, finger and wrist flexion are impaired. Horner's syndrome (miosis, ptosis, and facial hypohidrosis) may accompany a cervical cord lesion at any level.

Thoracic Cord Lesions here are localized by the sensory level on the trunk and by the site of midline back pain that may accompany the syndrome. Useful markers for localization are the nipples (T4) and umbilicus (T10). Leg weakness and disturbances of bladder and bowel function accompany the paralysis. Lesions at T9-T10 paralyze the lower—but not the upper—abdominal muscles, resulting in upward movement of the umbilicus when the abdominal wall contracts (*Beevor's sign*).

Lumbar Cord Lesions at the L2-L4 spinal cord levels paralyze flexion and adduction of the thigh, weaken leg extension at the knee, and abolish the patellar reflex. Lesions at L5-S1 paralyze only movements of the foot and ankle, flexion at the knee, and extension of the thigh, and abolish the ankle jerks (S1).

Sacral Cord/Conus Medullaris The conus medullaris is the tapered caudal termination of the spinal cord, comprising the lower sacral and single coccygeal segments. The distinctive conus syndrome consists of bilateral saddle anesthesia (S3-S5), prominent bladder and bowel dysfunction (urinary retention and incontinence with lax anal tone), and impotence. The bulbocavernosus (S2-S4) and anal (S4-S5) reflexes are absent (Chap. 367). Muscle strength is largely preserved. By contrast, lesions of the cauda equina, the nerve roots derived from the lower cord, are characterized by low back and radicular pain, asymmetric leg weakness and sensory loss, variable areflexia in the lower extremities, and relative sparing of bowel and bladder function. Mass lesions in the lower spinal canal often produce a mixed clinical picture with elements of both cauda equina and conus medullaris syndromes. Cauda equina syndromes are also discussed in Chap. 15.

Special Patterns of Spinal Cord Disease The location of the major ascending and descending pathways of the spinal cord are shown in Fig. 377-1. Most fiber tracts—including the posterior columns and the spinocerebellar and pyramidal tracts—are situated on the side of the body they innervate. However, afferent fibers mediating pain and temperature sensation ascend in the spinothalamic tract contralateral to the side they supply. The anatomic configurations of these tracts produce characteristic syndromes that provide clues to the underlying disease process.

Brown-Sequard Hemicord Syndrome This consists of ipsilateral weakness (corticospinal tract) and loss of joint position and vibratory sense (posterior column), with contralateral loss of pain and temperature sense (spinothalamic tract) one or two levels below the lesion. Segmental signs, such as radicular pain, muscle atrophy, or loss of a deep tendon reflex, are unilateral. Partial forms are more common than the fully developed syndrome.

Central Cord Syndrome This syndrome results from selective damage to the gray matter nerve cells and crossing spinothalamic tracts surrounding the central canal. In the cervical cord, the central cord syndrome produces arm weakness out of proportion to leg weakness and a "dissociated" sensory loss, meaning loss of pain and temperature sensations over the shoulders, lower neck, and upper trunk (cape distribution), in contrast to preservation of light touch, joint position, and vibration sense in these regions. Spinal trauma, syringomyelia, and intrinsic cord tumors are the main causes.

Anterior Spinal Artery Syndrome Infarction of the cord is generally the result of occlusion or diminished flow in this artery. The result is extensive bilateral tissue destruction that spares the posterior columns. All spinal cord functions—motor, sensory, and autonomic—are lost below the level of the lesion, with the striking exception of retained vibration and position sensation.

Foramen Magnum Syndrome Lesions in this area interrupt decussating pyramidal tract fibers destined for the legs, which cross caudal to those of the arms, resulting in weakness of the legs (*crural paresis*). Compressive lesions near the foramen magnum may produce weakness of the ipsilateral shoulder and arm followed by weakness of the ipsilateral leg, then the contralateral leg, and finally the contralateral arm, an "around-the-clock" pattern that may begin in any of the four limbs. There is typically suboccipital pain spreading to the neck and shoulders.

Intramedullary and Extramedullary Syndromes It is useful to differentiate *intramedullary* processes, arising within the substance of the cord, from *extramedullary* ones that compress the spinal cord or its vascular supply. The differentiating features are only relative and serve as clinical guides. With extramedullary lesions, radicular pain is often prominent, and there is early sacral sensory loss (lateral spinothalamic tract) and spastic weakness in the legs (corticospinal tract) due to the superficial location of leg fibers in the corticospinal tract. Intramedullary lesions tend to produce poorly localized burning pain rather than radicular pain and to spare sensation in the perineal and sacral areas ("sacral sparing"), reflecting the laminated configuration of the spinothalamic tract with sacral fibers outermost; corticospinal tract signs appear later. Regarding extramedullary lesions, a further distinction is made between extradural and intradural masses, as the former are generally malignant and the latter benign (neurofibroma being a common cause). Consequently, a long duration of symptoms favors an intradural origin.

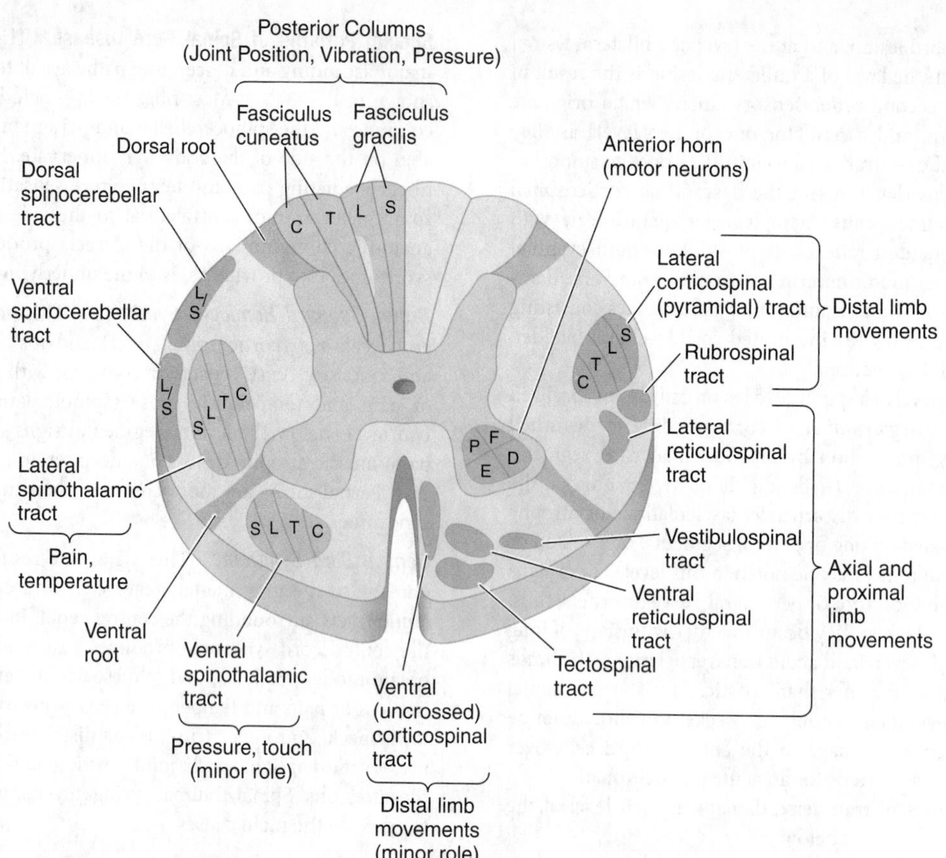

Figure 377-1 Transverse section through the spinal cord, composite representation, illustrating the principal ascending (*left*) and descending (*right*) pathways. The lateral and ventral spinothalamic tracts (*dark blue*) ascend contralateral to the side of the body that is innervated. C, cervical; D, distal; E, extensors; F, flexors; L, lumbar; P, proximal; S, sacral; T, thoracic.

ACUTE AND SUBACUTE SPINAL CORD DISEASES

The initial symptoms of disease that evolve over days or weeks are focal neck or back pain, followed by various combinations of paresthesias, sensory loss, motor weakness, and sphincter disturbance evolving over hours to several days. There may be only mild sensory symptoms or a devastating functional transection of the cord. Partial lesions selectively involve the posterior columns or anterior spinothalamic tracts or are limited to one side of the cord. Paresthesias or numbness typically begins in the feet and ascends symmetrically or asymmetrically. These symptoms initially simulate Guillain-Barré syndrome, but involvement of the trunk with a sharply demarcated spinal cord level indicates the myelopathic nature of the process. In severe and abrupt cases, areflexia reflecting spinal shock may be present, but hyperreflexia supervenes over days or weeks; persistent areflexic paralysis with a sensory level indicates necrosis over multiple segments of the spinal cord.

APPROACH TO THE PATIENT Compressive and Noncompressive Myelopathy

DISTINGUISHING COMPRESSIVE FROM NONCOMPRESSIVE MYELOPATHY The first priority is to exclude a treatable compression of the cord by a mass. The common causes are tumor, epidural abscess or hematoma, herniated disk, or vertebral pathology. Epidural compression due to malignancy or abscess often causes warning signs of neck or back pain, bladder disturbances, and sensory symptoms that precede the development of paralysis. Spinal subluxation, hemorrhage, and noncompressive etiologies such as infarction are more likely to produce myelopathy without antecedent symptoms. MRI with gadolinium infusion, centered on the clinically suspected level, is the initial diagnostic procedure; in some cases it is appropriate to image the entire spine (cervical through sacral regions) to search for additional clinically silent lesions. Once compressive lesions have been excluded, noncompressive causes of acute myelopathy that are intrinsic to the cord are considered, primarily vascular, inflammatory, and infectious etiologies.

COMPRESSIVE MYELOPATHIES

Neoplastic spinal cord compression

In adults, most neoplasms are epidural in origin, resulting from metastases to the adjacent spinal bones. The propensity of solid tumors to metastasize to the vertebral column probably reflects the high proportion of bone marrow located in the axial skeleton. Almost any malignant tumor can metastasize to the spinal column, with breast, lung, prostate, kidney, lymphoma, and plasma cell dyscrasia being particularly frequent. The thoracic spinal column is most commonly involved; exceptions are metastases from prostate and ovarian cancer, which occur disproportionately in the sacral and lumbar vertebrae, probably resulting from spread through Batson's plexus, a network of veins along the anterior epidural space. Retroperitoneal neoplasms (especially lymphomas or sarcomas) enter the spinal canal through the intervertebral foramens and produce radicular pain with signs of root weakness prior to cord compression.

Pain is usually the initial symptom of spinal metastasis; it may be aching and localized or sharp and radiating in quality and typically worsens with movement, coughing, or sneezing and characteristically

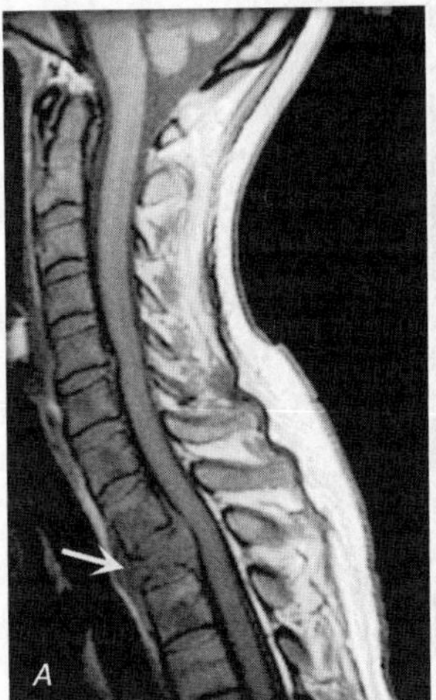

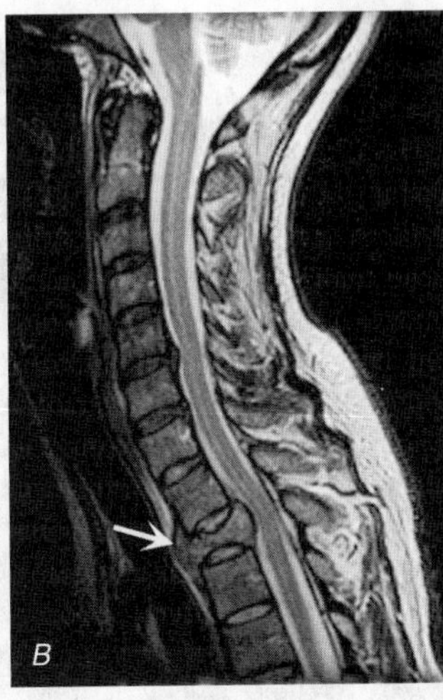

Figure 377-2 Epidural spinal cord compression due to breast carcinoma. Sagittal T1-weighted (*A*) and T2-weighted (*B*) MRI scans through the cervicothoracic junction reveal an infiltrated and collapsed second thoracic vertebral body with posterior displacement and compression of the upper thoracic spinal cord. The low-intensity bone marrow signal in *A* signifies replacement by tumor.

awakens patients at night. A recent onset of persistent back pain, particularly if in the thoracic spine (which is uncommonly involved by spondylosis), should prompt consideration of vertebral metastasis. Rarely, pain is mild or absent. Plain radiographs of the spine and radionuclide bone scans have only a limited role in diagnosis because they do not identify 15–20% of metastatic vertebral lesions and fail to detect paravertebral masses that reach the epidural space through the intervertebral foramens. MRI provides excellent anatomic resolution of the extent of spinal tumors (Fig. 377-2) and is able to distinguish between malignant lesions and other masses—epidural abscess, tuberculoma, or epidural hemorrhage, among others—that present in a similar fashion. Vertebral metastases are usually hypointense relative to a normal bone marrow signal on T1-weighted MRI scans; after the administration of gadolinium, contrast enhancement may deceptively "normalize" the appearance of the tumor by increasing its intensity to that of normal bone marrow. Infections of the spinal column (osteomyelitis and related disorders) are distinctive in that, unlike tumor, they may cross the disk space to involve the adjacent vertebral body.

If spinal cord compression is suspected, imaging should be obtained promptly. If there are radicular symptoms but no evidence of myelopathy, it is usually safe to defer imaging for 24–48 h. Up to 40% of patients who present with cord compression at one level are found to have asymptomatic epidural metastases elsewhere; thus, the length of the spine should be imaged when epidural malignancy is in question.

TREATMENT Neoplastic Spinal Cord Compression

Management of cord compression includes glucocorticoids to reduce cord edema, local radiotherapy (initiated as early as possible) to the symptomatic lesion, and specific therapy for the underlying tumor type. Glucocorticoids (dexamethasone, up to 40 mg daily) can be administered before the imaging study if the clinical suspicion is strong and continued at a lower dose until radiotherapy (generally 3000 cGy administered in 15 daily fractions) is completed. Radiotherapy appears to be effective even for most classically radioresistant metastases. A good response to radiotherapy can be expected in individuals who are ambulatory at presentation. Treatment usually prevents new weakness, and some recovery of motor function occurs in up to one-third of treated patients. Motor deficits (paraplegia or quadriplegia), once established for >12 h, do not usually improve, and beyond 48 h the prognosis for substantial motor recovery is poor. Although most patients do not experience recurrences in the months following radiotherapy, with survival beyond 2 years, recurrence becomes increasingly likely and can be managed with additional radiotherapy. New techniques, including intensity-modulated radiotherapy (IMRT), can deliver high doses of focused radiation with extreme precision, and preliminary data suggest that these methods produce similar rates of response compared to traditional radiotherapy. Biopsy of the epidural mass is unnecessary in patients with known primary cancer, but it is indicated if a history of underlying cancer is lacking. Surgery, either decompression by laminectomy or vertebral body resection, is usually considered when signs of cord compression worsen despite radiotherapy, when the maximum tolerated dose of radiotherapy has been delivered previously to the site, or when a vertebral compression fracture or spinal instability contributes to cord compression. The routine use of radiotherapy as first-line treatment for most cases of malignant spinal cord compression has recently been called into question by a randomized clinical trial indicating that surgery followed by radiotherapy is more effective than radiotherapy alone for patients with a single area of spinal cord compression by extradural tumor; patients with recurrent cord compression, brain metastases, radiosensitive tumors, or severe motor symptoms of >48 hours duration were excluded from this study.

In contrast to tumors of the epidural space, most intradural mass lesions are slow-growing and benign. Meningiomas and neurofibromas account for most of these, with occasional cases caused by chordoma, lipoma, dermoid, or sarcoma. Meningiomas (Fig. 377-3) are often located posterior to the thoracic cord or near the foramen magnum, although they can arise from the meninges anywhere along the spinal canal. Neurofibromas are benign tumors of the nerve sheath that typically arise near the posterior root; when multiple, neurofi-

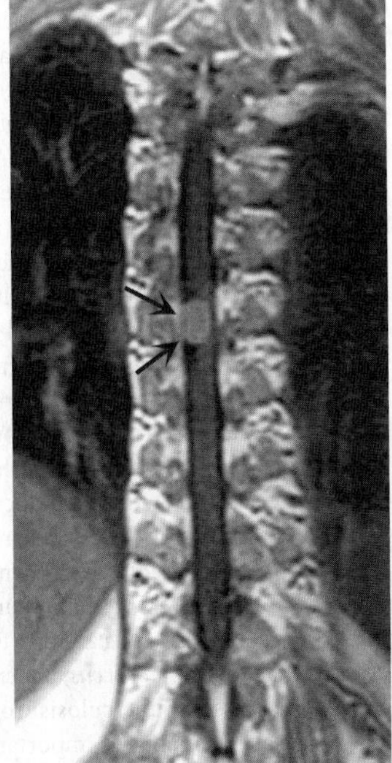

Figure 377-3 MRI of a thoracic meningioma. Coronal T1-weighted postcontrast image through the thoracic spinal cord demonstrates intense and uniform enhancement of a well-circumscribed extramedullary mass (*arrows*), which displaces the spinal cord to the left.

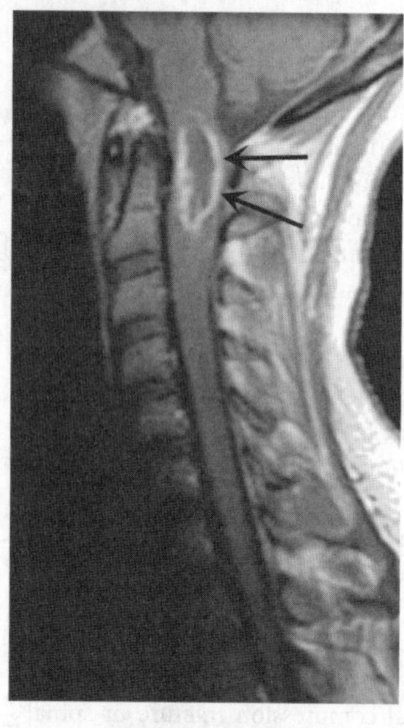

Figure 377-4 MRI of an intramedullary astrocytoma. Sagittal T1-weighted postcontrast image through the cervical spine demonstrates expansion of the upper cervical spine by a mass lesion emanating from within the spinal cord at the cervicomedullary junction. Irregular peripheral enhancement occurs within the mass (*arrows*).

bromatosis is the likely etiology. Symptoms usually begin with radicular sensory symptoms followed by an asymmetric, progressive spinal cord syndrome. Therapy is by surgical resection.

Primary intramedullary tumors of the spinal cord are uncommon. They present as central cord or hemicord syndromes, often in the cervical region; there may be poorly localized burning pain in the extremities and sparing of sacral sensation. In adults, these lesions are ependymomas, hemangioblastomas, or low-grade astrocytomas (Fig. 377-4). Complete resection of an intramedullary ependymoma is often possible with microsurgical techniques. Debulking of an intramedullary astrocytoma can also be helpful, as these are often slowly growing lesions; the value of adjunctive radiotherapy and chemotherapy is uncertain. Secondary (metastatic) intramedullary tumors also occur, especially in patients with advanced metastatic disease (Chap. 379), although these are not nearly as frequent as brain metastases.

Spinal epidural abscess

Spinal epidural abscess presents as a clinical triad of midline dorsal pain, fever, and progressive limb weakness. Prompt recognition of this distinctive process will in most cases prevent permanent sequelae. Aching pain is almost always present, either over the spine or in a radicular pattern. The duration of pain prior to presentation is generally ≤2 weeks but may on occasion be several months or longer. Fever is usual, accompanied by elevated white blood cell count, sedimentation rate, and C-reactive protein. As the abscess expands, further spinal cord damage results from venous congestion and thrombosis. Once weakness and other signs of myelopathy appear, progression may be rapid. A more chronic sterile granulomatous form of abscess is also known, usually after treatment of an acute epidural infection.

Risk factors include an impaired immune status (diabetes mellitus, renal failure, alcoholism, malignancy), intravenous drug abuse, and infections of the skin or other tissues. Two-thirds of epidural infections result from hematogenous spread of bacteria from the skin (furunculosis), soft tissue (pharyngeal or dental abscesses), or deep viscera (bacterial endocarditis). The remainder arise from direct extension of a local infection to the subdural space; examples of local predisposing conditions are vertebral osteomyelitis, decubitus ulcers, lumbar puncture, epidural anesthesia, or spinal surgery. Most cases are due to *Staphylococcus aureus*; gram-negative bacilli, *Streptococcus*, anaerobes, and fungi can also cause epidural abscesses. Tuberculosis from an adjacent vertebral source (Pott's disease) remains an important cause in the underdeveloped world (Fig. 377-5).

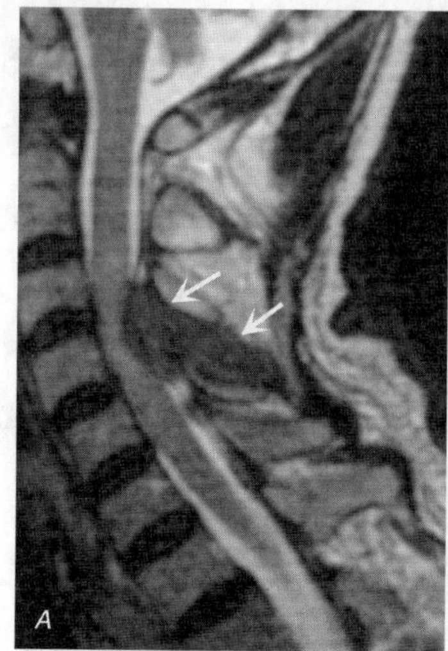

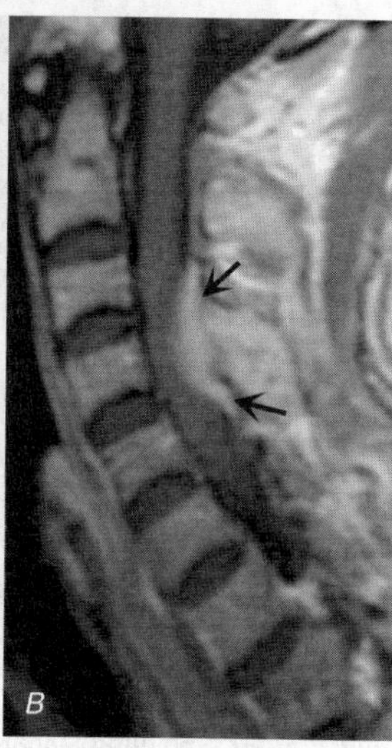

Figure 377-5 MRI of a spinal epidural abscess due to tuberculosis. ***A.*** Sagittal T2-weighted free spin-echo MR sequence. A hypointense mass replaces the posterior elements of C3 and extends epidurally to compress the spinal cord (*arrows*). ***B.*** Sagittal T1-weighted image after contrast administration reveals a diffuse enhancement of the epidural process (*arrows*) with extension into the epidural space.

MRI scans localize the abscess and exclude other causes of myelopathy. Lumbar puncture is only required if encephalopathy or other clinical signs raise the question of associated meningitis, a feature that is found in <25% of cases. The level of the puncture should be planned to minimize the risk of meningitis due to passage of the needle through infected tissue. A high cervical tap is sometimes the safest approach. CSF abnormalities in subdural abscess consist of pleocytosis with a preponderance of polymorphonuclear cells, an elevated protein level, and a reduced glucose level, but the responsible organism is not cultured unless there is associated meningitis. Blood cultures are positive in <25% of cases.

TREATMENT Spinal Epidural Abscess

Treatment is by decompressive laminectomy with debridement combined with long-term antibiotic treatment. Surgical evacuation prevents development of paralysis and may improve or reverse paralysis in evolution, but it is unlikely to improve deficits of more than several days duration. Broad-spectrum antibiotics should be started empirically before surgery and then modified on the basis of culture results; medication is continued for at least 4 weeks. If surgery is contraindicated or if there is a fixed paraplegia or quadriplegia that is unlikely to improve following surgery, long-term administration of systemic and oral antibiotics can be used; in such cases, the choice of antibiotics may be guided by results of blood cultures. However, paralysis may develop or progress during antibiotic therapy; thus, initial surgical management remains the treatment of choice unless the abscess is limited in size and causes few or no neurologic signs.

With prompt diagnosis and treatment of spinal epidural abscess, up to two-thirds of patients experience significant recovery.

Spinal epidural hematoma

Hemorrhage into the epidural (or subdural) space causes acute focal or radicular pain followed by variable signs of a spinal cord or conus medullaris disorder. Therapeutic anticoagulation, trauma, tumor, or blood dyscrasias are predisposing conditions. Rare cases complicate lumbar puncture or epidural anesthesia. MRI and CT confirm the clinical suspicion and can delineate the extent of the bleeding. Treatment consists of prompt reversal of any underlying clotting disorder and surgical decompression. Surgery may be followed by substantial recovery, especially in patients with some preservation of motor function preoperatively. Because of the risk of hemorrhage, lumbar puncture should be avoided whenever possible in patients with severe thrombocytopenia or other coagulopathies.

Hematomyelia

Hemorrhage into the substance of the spinal cord is a rare result of trauma, intraparenchymal vascular malformation (see below), vasculitis due to polyarteritis nodosa or systemic lupus erythematosus (SLE), bleeding disorders, or a spinal cord neoplasm. Hematomyelia presents as an acute painful transverse myelopathy. With large lesions, extension into the subarachnoid space results in subarachnoid hemorrhage (Chap. 275). Diagnosis is by MRI or CT. Therapy is supportive, and surgical intervention is generally not useful. An exception is hematomyelia due to an underlying vascular malformation, for which selective spinal angiography may be indicated, followed by surgery to evacuate the clot and remove the underlying vascular lesion.

NONCOMPRESSIVE MYELOPATHIES

The most frequent causes of noncompressive acute transverse myelopathy (ATM) are spinal cord infarction; systemic inflammatory disorders, including SLE and sarcoidosis; demyelinating diseases, including multiple sclerosis (MS); neuromyelitis optica (NMO); postinfectious or idiopathic transverse myelitis, which is presumed to be an immune condition related to acute disseminated encephalomyelitis (Chap. 380); and infectious (primarily viral) causes. After spinal cord compression is excluded, the evaluation generally requires a lumbar puncture and a search for underlying systemic disease (Table 377-3).

TABLE 377-3 Evaluation of Acute Transverse Myelopathy

1. MRI of spinal cord with and without contrast (exclude compressive causes).
2. CSF studies: Cell count, protein, glucose, IgG index/synthesis rate, oligoclonal bands, VDRL; Gram's stain, acid-fast bacilli, and India ink stains; PCR for VZV, HSV-2, HSV-1, EBV, CMV, HHV-6, enteroviruses, HIV; antibody for HTLV-I, *Borrelia burgdorferi, Mycoplasma pneumoniae*, and *Chlamydia pneumoniae*; viral, bacterial, mycobacterial, and fungal cultures.
3. Blood studies for infection: HIV; RPR; IgG and IgM enterovirus antibody; IgM mumps, measles, rubella, group B arbovirus, *Brucella melitensis, Chlamydia psittaci, Bartonella henselae*, schistosomal antibody; cultures for *B. melitensis*. Also consider nasal/pharyngeal/anal cultures for enteroviruses; stool O&P for *Schistosoma* ova.
4. Immune-mediated disorders: ESR; ANA; ENA; dsDNA; rheumatoid factor; anti-SSA; anti-SSB, complement levels; antiphospholipid and anticardiolipin antibodies; p-ANCA; antimicrosomal and antithyroglobulin antibodies; if Sjögren syndrome suspected, Schirmer test, salivary gland scintography, and salivary/lacrimal gland biopsy.
5. Sarcoidosis: Serum angiotensin-converting enzyme; serum Ca; 24-hour urine Ca; chest x-ray; chest CT; total body gallium scan; lymph node biopsy.
6. Demyelinating disease: Brain MRI scan, evoked potentials, CSF oligoclonal bands, neuromyelitis optica antibody (anti-aquaporin-4 [NMO] antibody).
7. Vascular causes: CT myelogram; spinal angiogram.

Abbreviations: ANA, antinuclear antibodies; CMV, cytomegalovirus; EBV, Epstein-Barr virus; ENA, epithelial neutrophil-activating peptide; ESR, erythrocyte sedimentation rate; HHV, human herpes virus; HSV, herpes simplex virus; HTLV, human T cell leukemia/lymphoma virus; O&P, ova and parasites; p-ANCA, perinuclear antineutrophilic cytoplasmic antibodies; PCR, polymerase chain reaction; RPR, rapid plasma reagin (test); VDRL, Venereal Disease Research Laboratory; VZV, varicella-zoster virus.

Spinal cord infarction

The cord is supplied by three arteries that course vertically over its surface: a single anterior spinal artery and paired posterior spinal arteries. In addition to the vertebral arteries, the anterior spinal artery is fed by radicular vessels that arise at C6, at an upper thoracic level, and, most consistently, at T11-L2 (artery of Adamkiewicz). At each segment, paired penetrating vessels branch from the anterior spinal artery to supply the anterior two-thirds of the spinal cord; the posterior spinal arteries, which often become less distinct below the midthoracic level, supply the posterior columns.

Spinal cord ischemia can occur at any level; however, the presence of the artery of Adamkiewicz creates a watershed of marginal blood flow in the upper thoracic segments. With systemic hypotension or cross-clamping of the aorta, cord infarction occurs at the level of greatest ischemic risk, usually T3-T4, and also at boundary zones between the anterior and posterior spinal artery territories which may result in a rapidly progressive syndrome (over hours) of weakness and spasticity with little sensory change.

Acute infarction in the territory of the *anterior spinal artery* produces paraplegia or quadriplegia, dissociated sensory loss affecting pain and temperature sense but sparing vibration and position sense, and loss of sphincter control ("anterior cord syndrome"). Onset may be sudden and dramatic but more typically is progressive over minutes or a few hours, quite unlike stroke in the cerebral hemispheres. Sharp midline or radiating back pain localized to the area of ischemia is frequent. Areflexia due to spinal shock is often present initially; with time, hyperreflexia and spasticity appear. Less common is infarction in the territory of the *posterior spinal arteries*, resulting in loss of posterior column function.

Spinal cord infarction results from aortic atherosclerosis, dissecting aortic aneurysm (manifest as chest or back pain with diminished pulses in legs), vertebral artery occlusion or dissection in the neck, aortic surgery, or profound hypotension from any cause. Cardiogenic emboli and vasculitis related to collagen vascular disease [particularly SLE, Sjögren's syndrome, and the antiphospholipid antibody syndrome (see below)] are other causative conditions. Occasional cases develop from *embolism of nucleus pulposus* material into spinal vessels, usually from local spine trauma. In a substantial number of cases no cause can be found, and thromboembolism in arterial feeders is suspected. The MRI may fail to demonstrate limited infarctions of the cord, especially in the first day, but as often it becomes abnormal at the affected level.

In cord infarction due to presumed thromboembolism, acute anticoagulation is probably not indicated, with the exception of the unusual transient ischemic attack or incomplete infarction with a stuttering or progressive course. The antiphospholipid antibody syndrome is treated with anticoagulation. Drainage of spinal fluid has reportedly been successful in some cases of cord infarction but has not been studied systematically.

Inflammatory and immune myelopathies (myelitis)

This broad category includes the demyelinating conditions MS, NMO, and postinfectious myelitis, as well as sarcoidosis and connective tissue disease. In approximately one-quarter of cases of myelitis, no underlying cause can be identified. Some will later manifest additional symptoms of an immune-mediated disease. *Recurrent episodes of myelitis* are usually due to one of the immune-mediated diseases or to infection with herpes simplex virus (HSV) type 2 (below).

Multiple sclerosis MS (Chap. 380) may present with acute myelitis, particularly in individuals of Asian or African ancestry. In whites, MS rarely causes a complete transverse myelopathy (i.e., acute bilateral signs), but it is among the most common causes of a partial syndrome. MRI findings in MS-associated myelitis typically consist of mild swelling and edema of the cord and diffuse or multifocal areas of abnormal signal on T2-weighted sequences. Contrast enhancement, indicating disruption in the blood-brain barrier associated with inflammation, is present in many acute cases. A brain MRI is most helpful in gauging the likelihood that a case of myelitis represents an initial attack of MS. A normal scan indicates that the risk of evolution to MS is low, ~10–15% over 5 years; in contrast, the finding of multiple periventricular T2-bright lesions indicates a much higher risk, >50% over 5 years and >90% by 14 years. The CSF may be normal, but more often there is a mild mononuclear cell pleocytosis, with normal or mildly elevated CSF protein levels; oligoclonal bands are variable, but when bands are present, a diagnosis of MS is more likely.

There are no adequate trials of therapy for MS-associated transverse myelitis. Intravenous methylprednisolone (500 mg qd for 3 days) followed by oral prednisone (1 mg/kg per day for several weeks, then gradual taper) has been used as initial treatment. A course of plasma exchange is indicated for severe cases if glucocorticoids are ineffective.

Neuromyelitis optica NMO is an immune-mediated demyelinating disorder consisting of a severe myelopathy that is typically longitudinally extensive, meaning that the lesion spans three or more vertebral segments. NMO is associated with optic neuritis that is often bilateral and may precede or follow myelitis by weeks or months, and also by brainstem and in some cases hypothalamic involvement. However, isolated recurrent myelitis without optic nerve involvemement can occur in NMO; affected individuals are usually female, and often of Asian ancestry. CSF studies reveal a variable mononuclear pleocytosis of up to several hundred cells per microliter; unlike MS, oligoclonal bands are generally absent. Diagnostic serum autoantibodies against the water channel protein aquaporin-4 are present in 60–70% of patients with NMO. NMO has also been associated with SLE and antiphospholipid antibodies (see below) as well as with other connective tissue diseases; rare cases are paraneoplastic in origin. Treatment is with glucocorticoids and, for refractory cases, plasma exchange (as for MS, above). Preliminary data suggest that treatment with azathioprine, mycophenolate, or anti-CD20 (anti–B cell) monoclonal antibody may protect against subsequent relapses; treatment for 5 years or longer is generally recommended. NMO is discussed in Chap. 380.

Systemic immune-mediated disorders Myelitis occurs in a small number of patients with SLE, many cases of which are associated with antiphospholipid antibodies. The CSF is usually normal or shows a mild lymphocytic pleocytosis; oligoclonal bands are a variable finding. Responses to glucocorticoids and/or cyclophosphamide have been reported, but there is no systematic evidence of their benefit. Other immune-mediated myelitides include cases associated with Sjögren's syndrome, mixed connective tissue disease, Behçet's syndrome, vasculitis with perinuclear antineutrophilic cytoplasmic antibodies (p-ANCA), and primary CNS vasculitis.

Another important consideration in this group is sarcoid myelopathy that may present as a slowly progressive or relapsing disorder. MRI reveals an edematous swelling of the spinal cord that may mimic tumor; there is almost always gadolinium enhancement of active lesions and in some cases of the adjacent surface of the cord; lesions may be single or multiple, and on axial images, enhancement of the central cord is usually present. The typical CSF profile consists of a variable lymphocytic pleocytosis and mildly elevated protein level; in a minority of cases reduced glucose and oligoclonal bands are found. The diagnosis is particularly difficult when systemic manifestations of sarcoid are minor or absent (nearly 50% of cases) or when other typical neurologic manifestations of the disease—such as cranial neuropathy, hypothalamic involvement, or meningeal enhancement visualized by MRI—are lacking. A slit-lamp examination of the eye to search for uveitis; chest x-ray and CT to assess pulmonary involvement; and mediastinal lymphadenopathy, serum or CSF angiotensin-converting enzyme (ACE; present in only a minority of cases), serum calcium, and a gallium scan may assist in the diagnosis. The usefulness of spinal fluid ACE is uncertain. Initial treatment is with oral glucocorticoids; immunosuppressant drugs are used for resistant cases. Sarcoidosis is discussed in Chap. 329.

Postinfectious myelitis Many cases of myelitis, termed *postinfectious* or *postvaccinal*, follow an infection or vaccination. Numerous organisms have been implicated, including Epstein-Barr virus (EBV), cytomegalovirus (CMV), mycoplasma, influenza, measles, varicella, rubeola, and mumps. As in the related disorder acute disseminated encephalomyelitis (Chap. 380), postinfectious myelitis often begins as the patient appears to be recovering from an acute febrile infection, or in the subsequent days or weeks, but an infectious agent cannot be isolated from the nervous system or spinal fluid. The presumption is that the myelitis represents an autoimmune disorder triggered by infection and is not due to direct infection of the spinal cord. No randomized controlled trials of therapy exist; treatment is usually with glucocorticoids or, in fulminant cases, plasma exchange.

Acute infectious myelitis Many viruses have been associated with an acute myelitis that is infectious in nature rather than postinfectious. Nonetheless, the two processes are often difficult to distinguish. Herpes zoster is the best characterized viral myelitis, but herpes simplex virus (HSV) types 1 and 2, EBV, CMV, and rabies virus are other well-described causes. HSV-2 (and less commonly HSV-1) produces a distinctive syndrome of recurrent sacral myelitis in association with outbreaks of genital herpes mimicking MS. Poliomyelitis is the prototypic viral myelitis, but it is more or less restricted to the gray matter of the cord. Chronic viral myelitic infections, such as that due to HIV, are discussed below.

Bacterial and mycobacterial myelitis (most are essentially abscesses) are far less common than viral causes and much less frequent than cerebral bacterial abscess. Almost any pathogenic species may be responsible, including *Listeria monocytogenes*, *Borrelia burgdorferi* (Lyme disease), and *Treponema pallidum* (syphilis). *Mycoplasma pneumoniae* may be a cause of myelitis, but its status is uncertain since many cases are more properly classified as postinfectious.

Schistosomiasis is an important cause of parasitic myelitis in endemic areas. The process is intensely inflammatory and granulomatous, caused by a local response to tissue-digesting enzymes from the ova of the parasite, typically *S. mansoni*. Toxoplasmosis can occasionally cause a focal myelopathy, and this diagnosis should be considered in patients with AIDS (Chap. 214).

In cases of suspected viral myelitis, it may be appropriate to begin specific therapy pending laboratory confirmation. Herpes zoster, HSV, and EBV myelitis are treated with intravenous acyclovir (10 mg/kg q8h) or oral valacyclovir (2 g tid) for 10–14 days; CMV with ganciclovir (5 mg/kg IV bid) plus foscarnet (60 mg/kg IV tid), or cidofovir (5 mg/kg per week for 2 weeks).

CHRONIC MYELOPATHIES

SPONDYLITIC MYELOPATHY

Spondylitic myelopathy is one of the most common causes of chronic cord compression and of gait difficulty in the elderly. Neck and shoulder pain with stiffness are early symptoms; impingement of bone and soft tissue overgrowth on nerve roots results in radicular arm pain, most often in a C5 or C6 distribution. Compression of the cervical cord, which occurs in fewer than one-third of cases, produces a slowly progressive spastic paraparesis, at times asymmetric and often accompanied by paresthesias in the feet and hands. Vibratory sense is diminished in the legs, there is a Romberg sign, and occasionally there is a sensory level for vibration on the upper thorax. In some cases, coughing or straining produces leg weakness or radiating arm or shoulder pain. Dermatomal sensory loss in the arms, atrophy of intrinsic hand muscles, increased deep-tendon reflexes in the legs, and extensor plantar responses are common. Urinary urgency or incontinence occurs in advanced cases, but there are many alternative causes of these problems in older individuals. A tendon reflex in the arms is often diminished at some level; most often at the biceps (C5-C6). In individual cases, radicular, myelopathic, or combined signs may predominate. The diagnosis should be considered in cases of progressive cervical myelopathy, paresthesias of the feet and hands, or wasting of the hands.

Diagnosis is usually made by MRI and may be suspected from CT images; plain X-rays are less helpful. Extrinsic cord compression and deformation is appreciated on axial MRI views, and T2-weighted sequences may reveal areas of high signal intensity within the cord adjacent to the site of compression. A cervical collar may be helpful in milder cases, but definitive therapy consists of surgical decompression. Posterior laminectomy or an anterior approach with resection of the protruded disk and bony material may be required. Cervical spondylosis and related degenerative diseases of the spine are discussed in Chap. 15.

VASCULAR MALFORMATIONS OF THE CORD AND DURA

Vascular malformations of the cord and overlying dura are treatable causes of progressive myelopathy. Most common are fistulas located posteriorly along the surface of the cord or within the dura. Most dural arteriovenous (AV) fistulas are located at or below the midthoracic level, usually consisting of a direct connection between a radicular feeding artery in the nerve root sleeve with dural veins. The typical presentation is a middle-aged man with a progressive myelopathy that worsens slowly or intermittently and may have periods of remission resembling MS. Acute deterioration due to hemorrhage into the spinal cord or subarachnoid space may also occur but is rare. A saltatory progression is common and is the result of local ischemia and edema from venous congestion. Most patients have incomplete sensory, motor, and bladder disturbances. The motor disorder may predominate and produce a mixture of upper and restricted lower motor neuron signs, simulating amyotrophic lateral sclerosis (ALS). Pain over the dorsal spine, dysesthesias, or radicular pain may be present. Other symptoms suggestive of arteriovenous malformation (AVM) include intermittent claudication, symptoms that change with posture, exertion such as singing, menses, or fever. Less commonly, AVM disorders are intramedullary rather than dural. One classic syndrome presents as a progressive thoracic myelopathy with paraparesis developing over weeks or several months, characterized pathologically by abnormally thick, hyalinized vessels within the cord (Foix-Alajouanine syndrome).

Spinal bruits are infrequent but should be sought at rest and after exercise in suspected cases. A vascular nevus on the overlying skin may indicate an underlying vascular malformation (Klippel-Trénaunay-Weber syndrome). High-resolution MRI with contrast administration detects many but not all AVMs (Fig. 377-6). An uncertain proportion not detected by MRI may be visualized by CT myelography as enlarged vessels along the surface of the cord. Definitive diagnosis requires selective spinal angiography, which defines the feeding vessels and the extent of the malformation. Endovascular embolization of the major feeding vessels may stabilize a progressive neurologic deficit or allow for gradual recovery.

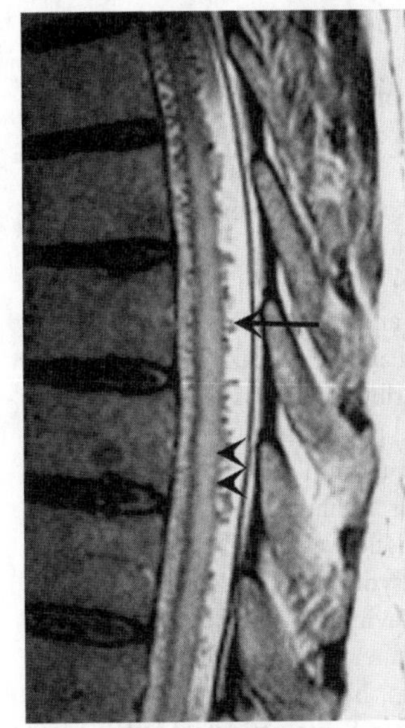
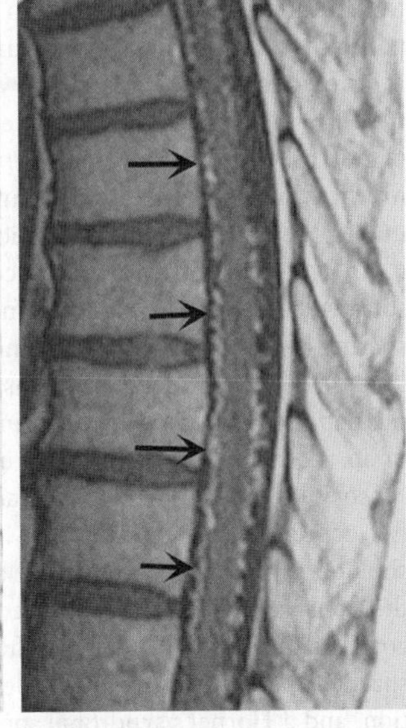

Figure 377-6 Arteriovenous malformation. Sagittal MR scans of the thoracic spinal cord: T2 fast spin-echo technique (***left***) and T1 postcontrast image (***right***). On the T2-weighted image (*left*), abnormally high signal intensity is noted in the central aspect of the spinal cord (*arrowheads*). Numerous punctate flow voids indent the dorsal and ventral spinal cord (*arrow*). These represent the abnormally dilated venous plexus supplied by a dural arteriovenous fistula. After contrast administration (*right*), multiple, serpentine, enhancing veins (*arrows*) on the ventral and dorsal aspect of the thoracic spinal cord are visualized, diagnostic of arteriovenous malformation. This patient was a 54-year-old man with a 4-year history of progressive paraparesis.

RETROVIRUS-ASSOCIATED MYELOPATHIES

The myelopathy associated with the human T cell lymphotropic virus type I (HTLV-I), formerly called *tropical spastic paraparesis*, is a slowly progressive spastic syndrome with variable sensory and bladder disturbance. Approximately half of patients have mild back or leg pain. The neurologic signs may be asymmetric, often lacking a well-defined sensory level; the only sign in the arms may be hyperreflexia after several years of illness. The onset is insidious, and the illness is slowly progressive at a variable rate; most patients are unable to walk within 10 years of onset. This presentation may resemble primary progressive MS or a thoracic AVM. Diagnosis is made by demonstration of HTLV-I–specific antibody in serum by enzyme-linked immunosorbent assay (ELISA), confirmed by radioimmunoprecipitation or Western blot analysis. There is no effective treatment, but symptomatic therapy for spasticity and bladder symptoms may be helpful.

A progressive myelopathy may also result from HIV infection (Chap. 189). It is characterized by vacuolar degeneration of the posterior and lateral tracts, resembling subacute combined degeneration (see below).

SYRINGOMYELIA

Syringomyelia is a developmental cavity of the cervical cord that is prone to enlarge and produce progressive myelopathy. Symptoms begin insidiously in adolescence or early adulthood, progress irregularly, and may undergo spontaneous arrest for several years. Many young patients acquire a cervical-thoracic scoliosis. More than half of all cases are associated with Chiari type 1 malformations in which the cerebellar tonsils protrude through the foramen magnum and into the cervical spinal canal. The pathophysiology of syrinx expansion is controversial, but some interference with the normal flow of CSF seems likely, perhaps by the Chiari malformation. Acquired cavitations of the cord in areas of necrosis are also termed *syrinx cavities*; these follow trauma, myelitis, necrotic spinal cord tumors, and chronic arachnoiditis due to tuberculosis and other etiologies.

The presentation is a central cord syndrome consisting of dissociated sensory loss (loss of pain and temperature sensation with sparing of touch and vibration) and areflexic weakness in the upper limbs. The sensory deficit has a distribution that is "suspended" over the nape of the neck, shoulders, and upper arms (cape distribution) or in the hands. Most cases begin asymmetrically with unilateral sensory loss in the hands that leads to injuries and burns that are not appreciated by the patient. Muscle wasting in the lower neck, shoulders, arms, and hands with asymmetric or absent reflexes in the arms reflects expansion of the cavity into the gray matter of the cord. As the cavity enlarges and further compresses the long tracts, spasticity and weakness of the legs, bladder and bowel dysfunction, and a Horner's syndrome appear. Some patients develop facial numbness and sensory loss from damage to the descending tract of the trigeminal nerve (C2 level or above). In cases with Chiari malformations, cough-induced headache and neck, arm, or facial pain are reported. Extension of the syrinx into the medulla, syringobulbia, causes palatal or vocal cord paralysis, dysarthria, horizontal or vertical nystagmus, episodic dizziness or vertigo, and tongue weakness with atrophy.

MRI scans accurately identify developmental and acquired syrinx cavities and their associated spinal cord enlargement (Fig. 377-7). MRI scans of the brain and the entire spinal cord should be obtained to delineate the full longitudinal extent of the syrinx, assess posterior fossa structures for the Chiari malformation, and determine whether hydrocephalus is present.

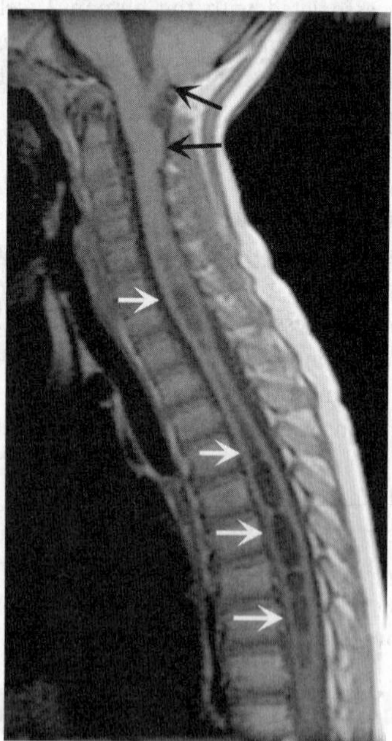

Figure 377-7 MRI of syringomyelia associated with a Chiari malformation. Sagittal T1-weighted image through the cervical and upper thoracic spine demonstrates descent of the cerebellar tonsils and vermis below the level of the foramen magnum (*black arrows*). Within the substance of the cervical and thoracic spinal cord, a CSF collection dilates the central canal (*white arrows*).

TREATMENT Syringomyelia

Treatment of syringomyelia is generally unsatisfactory. The Chiari tonsillar herniation is usually decompressed, generally by suboccipital craniectomy, upper cervical laminectomy, and placement of a dural graft. Obstruction of fourth ventricular outflow is reestablished by this procedure. If the syrinx cavity is large, some surgeons recommend direct decompression or drainage by one of a number of methods, but the added benefit of this procedure is uncertain, and morbidity is common. With Chiari malformations, shunting of hydrocephalus should generally precede any attempt to correct the syrinx. Surgery may stabilize the neurologic deficit, and some patients improve.

Syringomyelia secondary to trauma or infection is treated with a decompression and drainage procedure in which a small shunt is inserted between the syrinx cavity and the subarachnoid space; alternatively, the cavity can be fenestrated. Cases due to intramedullary spinal cord tumor are generally managed by resection of the tumor.

CHRONIC MYELOPATHY OF MULTIPLE SCLEROSIS

A chronic progressive myelopathy is the most frequent cause of disability in both primary progressive and secondary progressive forms of MS. Involvement is typically bilateral but asymmetric and produces motor, sensory, and bladder and bowel disturbances. Fixed motor disability appears to result from extensive loss of axons in the corticospinal tracts. Diagnosis is facilitated by identification of earlier attacks such as optic neuritis. MRI, CSF, and evoked-response testing are confirmatory. Therapy with interferon β, glatiramer acetate, or natalizumab is indicated for patients with progressive myelopathy, who also have coexisting MS relapses. These therapies are sometimes also offered to patients without relapses, despite the lack of evidence supporting their value in this setting. The value of anti-B cell therapy in primary progressive MS is under investigation. MS is discussed in Chap. 380.

SUBACUTE COMBINED DEGENERATION (VITAMIN B_{12} DEFICIENCY)

This treatable myelopathy presents with subacute paresthesias in the hands and feet, loss of vibration and position sensation, and a progressive spastic and ataxic weakness. Loss of reflexes due to an associated peripheral neuropathy in a patient who also has Babinski signs is an important diagnostic clue. Optic atrophy and irritability or other mental changes may be prominent in advanced cases but are rarely the presenting symptoms. The myelopathy of subacute combined degeneration tends to be diffuse rather than focal; signs are generally symmetric and reflect predominant involvement of the posterior and lateral tracts, including Romberg's sign. The diagnosis is confirmed by the finding of macrocytic red blood cells, a low serum B_{12} concentration, and elevated serum levels of homocysteine and methylmalonic acid. Treatment is by replacement therapy, beginning with 1000 μg of intramuscular vitamin B_{12} repeated at regular intervals or by subsequent oral treatment (Chap. 105).

HYPOCUPRIC MYELOPATHY

This myelopathy is virtually identical to subacute combined degeneration (above) and probably explains many cases previously described with normal serum levels of B_{12}. Low levels of serum copper are found and often there is also a low level of serum ceruloplasmin. Some cases follow gastrointestinal procedures that result in impaired copper absorption; others have been associated with excess zinc from health food supplements or, until recently, use of zinc-containing denture creams, which impair copper absorption via induction of metallothionein, a copper-binding protein. Many cases are idiopathic. Improvement or at least stabilization may be expected with reconstitution of copper stores by oral supplementation. The pathophysiology and pathology of the idiopathic form are not known.

TABES DORSALIS

The classic syndromes of tabes dorsalis and meningovascular syphilis of the spinal cord are now less frequent than in the past but must be considered in the differential diagnosis of spinal cord disorders. The characteristic symptoms of tabes are fleeting and repetitive lancinating pains, primarily in the legs or less often in the back, thorax, abdomen, arms, and face. Ataxia of the legs and gait due to loss of position sense occurs in half of patients. Paresthesias, bladder disturbances, and acute abdominal pain with vomiting (visceral crisis) occur in 15–30% of patients. The cardinal signs of tabes are loss of reflexes in the legs; impaired position and vibratory sense; Romberg's sign; and, in almost all cases, bilateral Argyll Robertson pupils, which fail to constrict to light but accommodate. Diabetic polyradiculopathy may simulate tabes.

FAMILIAL SPASTIC PARAPLEGIA

Many cases of slowly progressive myelopathy are genetic in origin (Chap. 374). More than 20 different causative loci have been identified, including autosomal dominant, autosomal recessive, and X-linked forms. Most patients present with almost imperceptibly progressive spasticity and weakness in the legs, usually but not always symmetric. Sensory symptoms and signs are absent or mild, but sphincter disturbances may be present. In some families additional neurologic signs are prominent, including nystagmus, ataxia, or optic atrophy. The onset may be as early as the first year of life or as late as middle adulthood. Only symptomatic therapies for the spasticity are currently available.

ADRENOMYELONEUROPATHY

This X-linked disorder is a variant of adrenoleukodystrophy. Affected males usually have a history of adrenal insufficiency beginning in childhood and then develop a progressive spastic (or ataxic) paraparesis beginning in early adulthood; some patients also have a mild peripheral neuropathy. Female heterozygotes may develop a slower, insidiously progressive spastic myelopathy beginning later in adulthood and without adrenal insufficiency. Diagnosis is usually made by demonstration of elevated levels of very long chain fatty acids in plasma and in cultured fibroblasts. The responsible gene encodes ADLP, a peroxisomal membrane transporter that is a member of the ATP-binding cassette (ABC) family. Steroid replacement is indicated if hypoadrenalism is present, and bone marrow transplantation and nutritional supplements have been attempted for this condition without clear evidence of efficacy.

OTHER CHRONIC MYELOPATHIES

Primary lateral sclerosis (Chap. 374) is a degenerative disorder characterized by progressive spasticity with weakness, eventually accompanied by dysarthria and dysphonia; bladder symptoms occur in approximately half of patients. Sensory function is spared. The disorder resembles ALS and is considered a variant of the motor neuron degenerations, but without the characteristic lower motor neuron disturbance. Some cases may represent familial spastic paraplegia, particularly autosomal recessive or X-linked varieties in which a family history may be absent.

Tethered cord syndrome is a developmental disorder of the lower spinal cord and nerve roots that rarely presents in adulthood as low back pain accompanied by a progressive lower spinal cord and/or nerve root syndrome. Some patients have a small leg or foot deformity indicating a long-standing process, and in others a dimple, patch of hair, or sinus tract on the skin overlying the lower back is the clue to a congenital lesion. Diagnosis is made by MRI, which demonstrates a low-lying conus medullaris and thickened filum terminale. The MRI may also reveal diastematomyelia (division of the lower spinal cord into two halves), lipomas, cysts, or other congenital abnormalities of the lower spine coexisting with the tethered cord. Treatment is with surgical release.

There are a number of rare toxic causes of spastic myelopathy, including lathyrism due to ingestion of chick peas containing the excitotoxin β-*N*-oxalylamino-L-alanine (BOAA), seen primarily in the developing world, and nitrous oxide inhalation producing a myelopathy identical to subacute combined degeneration. SLE, Sjögren's syndrome, and sarcoidosis may each cause a myelopathy without overt evidence of systemic disease. Cancer-related causes of chronic myelopathy, besides the common neoplastic compressive myelopathy discussed earlier, include radiation injury (Chap. 379) and rare paraneoplastic myelopathies. The latter are most often associated with lung or breast cancer and anti-Hu antibodies (Chap. 101); NMO can also be paraneoplastic in origin (Chap. 380). Metastases to the cord are probably more common than either of these in patients with cancer. Often, a cause of intrinsic myelopathy can be identified only through periodic reassessment.

REHABILITATION OF SPINAL CORD DISORDERS

The prospects for recovery from an acute destructive spinal cord lesion fade after ~6 months. There are currently no effective means to promote repair of injured spinal cord tissue; promising experimental approaches include the use of factors that influence reinnervation by axons of the corticospinal tract, nerve and neural sheath graft bridges, and the local introduction of stem cells. The disability associated with irreversible spinal cord damage is determined primarily by the level of the lesion and by whether the disturbance in function is complete or incomplete (Table 377-4). Even a complete high cervical cord lesion may be compatible with a productive life. The primary goals are development of a rehabilitation plan framed

TABLE 377-4 Expected Neurologic Function Following Complete Cord Lesions

Level	Self-Care	Transfers	Maximum Mobility
High quadriplegia (C1-C4)	Dependent on others; requires respiratory support	Dependent on others	Motorized wheelchair
Low quadriplegia (C5-C8)	Partially independent with adaptive equipment	May be dependent or independent	May use manual wheelchair, drive an automobile with adaptive equipment
Paraplegia (below T1)	Independent	Independent	Ambulates short distances with aids

Source: Adapted from JF Ditunno, CS Formal: N Engl J Med 330:550, 1994; with permission.

by realistic expectations and attention to the neurologic, medical, and psychological complications that commonly arise.

Many of the usual symptoms associated with medical illnesses, especially somatic and visceral pain, may be lacking because of the destruction of afferent pain pathways. Unexplained fever, worsening of spasticity, or deterioration in neurologic function should prompt a search for infection, thrombophlebitis, or an intraabdominal pathology. The loss of normal thermoregulation and inability to maintain normal body temperature can produce recurrent fever (*quadriplegic fever*), although most episodes of fever are due to infection of the urinary tract, lung, skin, or bone.

Bladder dysfunction generally results from loss of supraspinal innervation of the detrusor muscle of the bladder wall and the sphincter musculature. Detrusor spasticity is treated with anticholinergic drugs (oxybutynin, 2.5–5 mg qid) or tricyclic antidepressants that have anticholinergic properties (imipramine, 25–200 mg/d). Failure of the sphincter muscle to relax during bladder emptying (urinary dyssynergia) may be managed with the α-adrenergic blocking agent terazosin hydrochloride (1–2 mg tid or qid), with intermittent catheterization, or, if that is not feasible, by use of a condom catheter in men or a permanent indwelling catheter. Surgical options include the creation of an artificial bladder by isolating a segment of intestine that can be catheterized intermittently (enterocystoplasty) or can drain continuously to an external appliance (urinary conduit). Bladder areflexia due to acute spinal shock or conus lesions is best treated by catheterization. Bowel regimens and disimpaction are necessary in most patients to ensure at least biweekly evacuation and avoid colonic distention or obstruction.

Patients with acute cord injury are at risk for venous thrombosis and pulmonary embolism. During the first 2 weeks, use of calf-compression devices and anticoagulation with heparin (5000 U subcutaneously every 12 h) or warfarin (INR, 2–3) are recommended. In cases of persistent paralysis, anticoagulation should probably be continued for 3 months.

Prophylaxis against decubitus ulcers should involve frequent changes in position in a chair or bed, the use of special mattresses, and cushioning of areas where pressure sores often develop, such as the sacral prominence and heels. Early treatment of ulcers with careful cleansing, surgical or enzyme debridement of necrotic tissue, and appropriate dressing and drainage may prevent infection of adjacent soft tissue or bone.

Spasticity is aided by stretching exercises to maintain mobility of joints. Drug treatment is effective but may result in reduced function, as some patients depend upon spasticity as an aid to stand, transfer, or walk. Baclofen (15–240 mg/d in divided doses) is effective; it acts by facilitating γ-aminobutyric acid (GABA)-mediated inhibition of motor reflex arcs. Diazepam acts by a similar mechanism and is useful for leg spasms that interrupt sleep (2–4 mg at bedtime). Tizanidine (2–8 mg tid), an α_2-adrenergic agonist that increases presynaptic inhibition of motor neurons, is another option. For nonambulatory patients, the direct muscle inhibitor dantrolene (25–100 mg qid) may be used, but it is potentially hepatotoxic. In refractory cases, intrathecal baclofen administered via an implanted pump, botulinum toxin injections, or dorsal rhizotomy may be required to control spasticity.

Despite the loss of sensory function, many patients with spinal cord injury experience chronic pain sufficient to diminish their quality of life. Randomized controlled studies indicate that gabapentin or pregabalin are useful in this setting. Management of chronic pain is discussed in Chap. 11.

A paroxysmal autonomic hyperreflexia may occur following lesions above the major splanchnic sympathetic outflow at T6. Headache, flushing, and diaphoresis above the level of the lesion, as well as transient severe hypertension with bradycardia or tachycardia, are the major symptoms. The trigger is typically a noxious stimulus—for example, bladder or bowel distention, a urinary tract infection, or a decubitus ulcer. Treatment consists of removal of offending stimuli; ganglionic blocking agents (mecamylamine, 2.5–5 mg) or other short-acting antihypertensive drugs are useful in some patients.

Attention to these details allows longevity and a productive life for patients with complete transverse myelopathies.

FURTHER READINGS

ABRAHM JL et al: Spinal cord compression in patients with advanced metastatic cancer: "All I care about is walking and living my life." JAMA 299:937, 2008

COHEN-AUBART F et al: Spinal cord sarcoidosis: Clinical and laboratory profile and outcome of 31 patients in a case-control study. Medicine 89:133, 2010

COLE JS, PATCHELL RA: Metastatic epidural spinal cord compression. Lancet Neurol 7:459, 2008

FROHMAN EM, WINGERCHUK DM: Transverse myelitis. N Engl J Med 363: 564, 2010

GRABER JJ, NOLAN CP: Myelopathies in patients with cancer. Arch Neurol 67:298, 2010

JACOB A, WEINSHENKER BG: An approach to the diagnosis of acute transverse myelitis. Semin Neurol 28:95, 2008

KRINGS T, GEIBPRASERT S: Spinal dural arteriovenous fistulas. AJNR Am J Neuroradiol 30:639, 2009

PATCHELL RA et al: Direct decompressive surgical resection in the treatment of spinal cord compression caused by metastatic cancer: A randomized trial. Lancet 366:643, 2005

TEASELL RW et al: A systematic review of pharmacologic treatments of pain after spinal cord injury. Arch Phys Med Rehabil 91:816, 2010

TRANSVERSE MYELITIS CONSORTIUM WORKING GROUP: Proposed diagnostic criteria and nosology of acute transverse myelitis. Neurology 59:499, 2002

TRAUL DE et al: Part I: Spinal-cord neoplasms—intradural neoplasms. Lancet Oncol 8:35, 2007

YANAGAWA K et al: Pathologic and immunologic profiles of a limited form of neuromyelitis optica with myelitis. Neurology 73:1628, 2009

CHAPTER 378
Concussion and Other Head Injuries

Allan H. Ropper

Almost 10 million head injuries occur annually in the United States, about 20% of which are serious enough to cause brain damage. Among men <35 years, accidents, usually motor vehicle collisions, are the chief cause of death and >70% of these involve head injury. Furthermore, minor head injuries are so common that almost all physicians will be called upon to provide immediate care or to see patients who are suffering from various sequelae.

Medical personnel caring for head injury patients should be aware that (1) spinal injury often accompanies head injury, and care must be taken in handling the patient to prevent compression of the spinal cord due to instability of the spinal column; (2) intoxication is a common accompaniment of traumatic brain injury and, when appropriate, testing should be carried out for drugs and alcohol; and (3) additional injuries, including rupture of abdominal organs, may produce vascular collapse or respiratory distress that requires immediate attention.

TYPES OF HEAD INJURIES

CONCUSSION

This form of minor head injury refers to an immediate and transient loss of consciousness that is associated with a short period of amnesia. Many patients do not lose consciousness after a minor head injury but instead are dazed or confused, or feel stunned or "star struck." Severe concussion may precipitate a brief convulsion or autonomic signs such as facial pallor, bradycardia, faintness with mild hypotension, or sluggish pupillary reaction, but most patients are quickly neurologically normal.

The mechanics of a typical concussion involve sudden deceleration of the head when hitting a blunt object. This creates an anterior-posterior movement of the brain within the skull due to inertia and rotation of the cerebral hemispheres on the relatively fixed upper brainstem. Loss of consciousness in concussion is believed to result from a transient electrophysiologic dysfunction of the reticular activating system in the upper midbrain that is at the site of rotation (Chap. 274).

Gross and light-microscopic changes in the brain are usually absent following concussion but biochemical and ultrastructural changes, such as mitochondrial ATP depletion and local disruption of the blood-brain barrier, are transient abnormalities. CT and MRI scans are usually normal; however, a small number of patients will be found to have a skull fracture, an intracranial hemorrhage, or brain contusion.

A brief period of both retrograde and anterograde amnesia is characteristic of concussion and it recedes rapidly in alert patients. Memory loss spans the moments before impact but may encompass the previous days or weeks (rarely months). With severe injuries, the extent of retrograde amnesia roughly correlates with the severity of injury. Memory is regained from the most distant to more recent memories, with islands of amnesia occasionally remaining. The mechanism of amnesia is not known. Hysterical posttraumatic amnesia is not uncommon after head injury and should be suspected when inexplicable behavioral abnormalities occur, such as recounting events that cannot be recalled on later testing, a bizarre affect, forgetting one's own name, or a persistent anterograde deficit that is excessive in comparison with the degree of injury. Amnesia is discussed in Chap. 26.

A single, uncomplicated concussion only infrequently produces permanent neurobehavioral changes in patients who are free of preexisting psychiatric and neurologic problems. Nonetheless, residual problems in memory and concentration may have an anatomic correlate in microscopic cerebral lesions (see below).

CONTUSION, BRAIN HEMORRHAGE, AND AXONAL SHEARING LESIONS

A surface bruise of the brain, or *contusion*, consists of varying degrees of petechial hemorrhage, edema, and tissue destruction. Contusions and deeper hemorrhages result from mechanical forces that displace and compress the hemispheres forcefully and by deceleration of the brain against the inner skull, either under a point of impact (coup lesion) or, as the brain swings back, in the antipolar area (contrecoup lesion). Trauma sufficient to cause prolonged unconsciousness usually produces some degree of contusion. Blunt deceleration impact, as occurs against an automobile dashboard or from falling forward onto a hard surface, causes contusions on the orbital surfaces of the frontal lobes and the anterior and basal portions of the temporal lobes. With lateral forces, as from impact on an automobile door frame, contusions are situated on the lateral convexity of the hemisphere. The clinical signs of contusion are determined by the location and size of the lesion; often, there are no focal neurologic abnormalities, but these injured regions are later the sites of gliotic scars that may produce seizures. A hemiparesis or gaze preference is fairly typical of moderately sized contusions. Large bilateral contusions produce stupor with extensor posturing, while those limited to the frontal lobes cause a taciturn state. Contusions in the temporal lobe may cause delirium or an aggressive, combative syndrome.

Contusions are easily visible on CT and MRI scans, appearing as inhomogeneous hyperdensities on CT and as hyperintensities on MRI sequences that detect blood; there is usually localized brain edema (Fig. 378-1) and some subarachnoid bleeding. Blood in the cerebrospinal fluid (CSF) due to trauma may provoke a mild inflammatory reaction. Over a few days, contusions acquire a

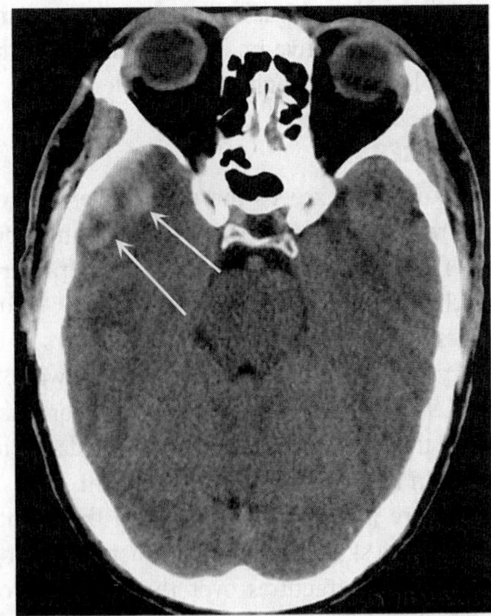

Figure 378-1 Traumatic cerebral contusion. Noncontrast CT scan demonstrating a hyperdense hemorrhagic region in the anterior temporal lobe.

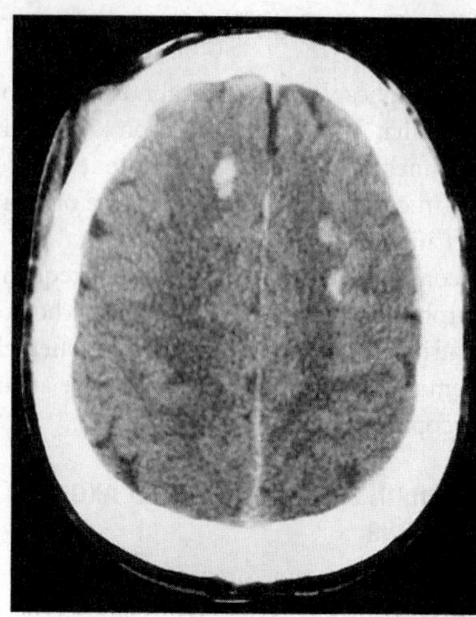

Figure 378-2 Multiple small areas of hemorrhage and tissue disruption in the white matter of the frontal lobes on noncontrast CT scan. These appear to reflect an extreme type of the diffuse axonal shearing lesions that occur with closed head injury.

surrounding contrast enhancement and edema that may be mistaken for tumor or abscess. Glial and macrophage reactions result in chronic, scarred, hemosiderin-stained depressions on the cortex (*plaques jaunes*) that are the main source of posttraumatic epilepsy.

Torsional or shearing forces within the brain cause hemorrhages of the basal ganglia and other deep regions. Large hemorrhages after minor trauma suggest that there is a bleeding diathesis or cerebrovascular amyloidosis. For unexplained reasons, deep cerebral hemorrhages may not develop until several days after injury. Sudden neurologic deterioration in a comatose patient or a sudden rise in intracranial pressure (ICP) suggests this complication and should therefore prompt investigation with a CT scan.

A special type of deep white matter lesion consists of widespread mechanical disruption, or shearing, of axons at the time of impact. Most characteristic are small areas of tissue injury in the corpus callosum and dorsolateral pons. The presence of widespread axonal damage in both hemispheres, a state called *diffuse axonal injury* (DAI), has been proposed to explain persistent coma and the vegetative state after closed head injury (Chap. 274), but small ischemic-hemorrhagic lesions in the midbrain and thalamus are as often the cause. Only severe shearing lesions that contain blood are visualized by CT, usually in the corpus callosum and centrum semiovale (Fig. 378-2); however, selective imaging sequences of the MRI can demonstrate such lesions throughout the white matter.

SKULL FRACTURES

A blow to the skull that exceeds the elastic tolerance of the bone causes a fracture. Intracranial lesions accompany roughly two-thirds of skull fractures and the presence of a fracture increases many-fold the chances of an underlying subdural or epidural hematoma. Consequently, fractures are primarily markers of the site and severity of injury. They also provide potential pathways for entry of bacteria to the CSF with a risk of meningitis and for leakage of CSF outward through the dura. Severe orthostatic headache results from lowered pressure in the spinal fluid compartment.

Most fractures are linear and extend from the point of impact toward the base of the skull. Basilar skull fractures are often extensions of adjacent linear fractures over the convexity of the skull but may occur independently owing to stresses on the floor of the middle cranial fossa or occiput. Basilar fractures are usually parallel to the petrous bone or along the sphenoid bone and directed toward the sella turcica and ethmoidal groove. Although most basilar fractures are uncomplicated, they can cause CSF leakage, pneumocephalus, and cavernous-carotid fistulas. Hemotympanum (blood behind the tympanic membrane), delayed ecchymosis over the mastoid process (Battle sign), or periorbital ecchymosis ("raccoon sign") are associated with basilar fractures. Because routine x-ray examination may fail to disclose basilar fractures, they should be suspected if these clinical signs are present.

CSF may leak through the cribriform plate or the adjacent sinus and cause CSF rhinorrhea (a watery discharge from the nose). Persistent rhinorrhea and recurrent meningitis are indications for surgical repair of torn dura underlying the fracture. The site of the leak is often difficult to determine, but useful diagnostic tests include the instillation of water-soluble contrast into the CSF followed by CT with the patient in various positions, or injection of radionuclide compounds or fluorescein into the CSF and the insertion of absorptive nasal pledgets. The location of an intermittent leak is rarely delineated, and many resolve spontaneously.

Sellar fractures, even those associated with serious neuroendocrine dysfunction, may be radiologically occult or evident only by an air-fluid level in the sphenoid sinus. Fractures of the dorsum sella cause sixth or seventh nerve palsies or optic nerve damage.

Petrous bone fractures, especially those oriented along the long axis of the bone, may be associated with facial palsy, disruption of ear ossicles, and CSF otorrhea. Transverse petrous fractures are less common; they almost always damage the cochlea or labyrinths and often the facial nerve as well. External bleeding from the ear is usually from local abrasion of the external canal but can also result from petrous fracture.

Fractures of the frontal bone are usually depressed, involving the frontal and paranasal sinuses and the orbits. Depressed skull fractures are typically compound, but they are often asymptomatic because the impact energy is dissipated in breaking the bone; some have underlying brain contusions. Debridement and exploration of compound fractures are required in order to avoid infection; simple fractures do not require surgery.

CRANIAL NERVE INJURIES

The cranial nerves most often injured with head trauma are the olfactory, optic, oculomotor, and trochlear; the first and second branches of the trigeminal nerve; and the facial and auditory nerves. Anosmia and an apparent loss of taste (actually a loss of perception of aromatic flavors, with retained elementary taste perception) occur in ~10% of persons with serious head injuries, particularly from falls on the back of the head. This is the result of displacement of the brain and shearing of the fine olfactory nerve filaments that course through the cribriform bone. At least partial recovery of olfactory and gustatory function is expected, but if bilateral anosmia persists for several months, the prognosis is poor. Partial optic nerve injuries from closed trauma result in blurring of vision, central or paracentral scotomas, or sector defects. Direct orbital injury may cause short-lived blurred vision for close objects due to reversible iridoplegia. Diplopia limited to downward gaze and corrected when the head is tilted away from the side of the affected eye indicates trochlear (fourth nerve) nerve damage. It occurs frequently as an isolated problem after minor head injury or may develop for unknown reasons after a delay of several days. Facial nerve injury caused by a basilar fracture is present immediately in up to 3% of severe injuries; it may also be delayed 5-7 days. Fractures through the petrous bone, particularly the less common transverse type, are liable to produce facial palsy. Delayed palsy, the mechanism of which is unknown, has a good prognosis. Injury to the eighth cranial nerve from a fracture of the petrous bone causes loss of hearing, vertigo, and nystagmus immediately after injury. Deafness from eighth nerve injury is rare and must be distinguished from blood in the middle ear or disruption of the middle ear ossicles. Dizziness, tinnitus, and high-tone hearing loss occur from cochlear concussion.

SEIZURES

Convulsions are surprisingly uncommon immediately after a head injury, but a brief period of tonic extensor posturing or a few clonic movements of the limbs just after the moment of impact can occur. However, the cortical scars that evolve from contusions are highly epileptogenic and may later manifest as seizures, even after many months or years (Chap. 369). The severity of injury roughly determines the risk of future seizures. It has been estimated that 17% of individuals with brain contusion, subdural hematoma, or prolonged loss of consciousness will develop a seizure disorder and that this risk extends for an indefinite period of time, whereas the risk is ≤2% after mild injury. The majority of convulsions in the latter group occur within 5 years of injury but may be delayed for decades. Penetrating injuries have a much higher rate of subsequent epilepsy.

SUBDURAL AND EPIDURAL HEMATOMAS

Hemorrhages beneath the dura (subdural) or between the dura and skull (epidural) have characteristic clinical and radiologic features. They are associated with underlying contusions and other injuries, often making it difficult to determine the relative contribution of each component to the clinical state. The mass effect and raised ICP caused by these hematomas can be life threatening, making it imperative to identify them rapidly by CT or MRI scan and to remove them when appropriate.

Acute subdural hematoma (Fig. 378-3)

Direct cranial trauma may be minor and is not required for acute subdural hemorrhage to occur, especially in the elderly and those taking anticoagulant medications. Acceleration forces alone, as from whiplash, are sometimes sufficient to produce subdural hemorrhage. Up to one-third of patients have a lucid interval lasting minutes to hours before coma supervenes, but most are drowsy or comatose from the moment of injury. A unilateral headache and slightly enlarged pupil on the side of the hematoma are frequently, but not invariably, present. Stupor or coma, hemiparesis, and unilateral pupillary enlargement are signs of larger hematomas. In an acutely deteriorating patient, burr (drainage) holes or an emergency craniotomy are required. Small subdural hematomas may be asymptomatic and usually do not require evacuation if they do not expand.

A subacutely evolving syndrome due to subdural hematoma occurs days or weeks after injury with drowsiness, headache, confusion, or mild hemiparesis, usually in alcoholics and in the elderly and often after only minor trauma. On imaging studies subdural hematomas appear as crescentic collections over the convexity of one or both hemispheres, most commonly in the frontotemporal region, and less often in the inferior middle fossa or over the occipital poles (Fig. 378-3). Interhemispheric, posterior fossa, or bilateral convexity hematomas are less frequent and are difficult to diagnose clinically, although drowsiness and the neurologic signs expected from damage in each region can usually be detected. The bleeding that causes larger hematomas is primarily venous in origin, although additional arterial bleeding sites are sometimes found at operation, and a few large hematomas have a purely arterial origin.

Epidural hematoma (Fig. 378-4)

These evolve more rapidly than subdural hematomas and are correspondingly more treacherous. They occur in up to 10% of cases of severe head injury but are associated with underlying cortical damage less often than are subdural hematomas. Most patients are unconscious when first seen. A "lucid interval" of several minutes to hours before coma supervenes is most characteristic of epidural hemorrhage, but it is still uncommon, and epidural hemorrhage is not the only cause of this temporal sequence. Rapid surgical evacuation and ligation or cautery of the damaged vessel is indicated, usually the middle meningeal artery that has been lacerated by an overlying skull fracture.

Chronic subdural hematoma (Fig. 378-5)

A history of trauma may or may not be elicited in relation to chronic subdural hematoma; the injury may have been trivial and forgotten, particularly in the elderly and those with clotting disorders. Headache is common but not invariable. Additional features may include slowed thinking, vague change in personality, seizure, or a mild hemiparesis. The headache fluctuates in severity, sometimes with changes in head position. Bilateral chronic subdural hematomas produce perplexing clinical syndromes and the initial clinical impression may be of a stroke, brain tumor, drug intoxication, depression, or a dementing illness. Drowsiness, inattentiveness,

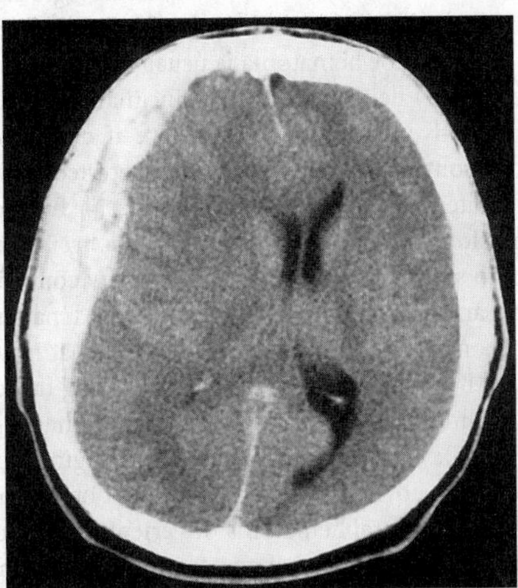

Figure 378-3 Acute subdural hematoma. Noncontrast CT scan reveals a hyperdense clot which has an irregular border with the brain and causes more horizontal displacement (mass effect) than might be expected from its thickness. The disproportionate mass effect is the result of the large rostral-caudal extent of these hematomas. Compare to Fig. 378-4.

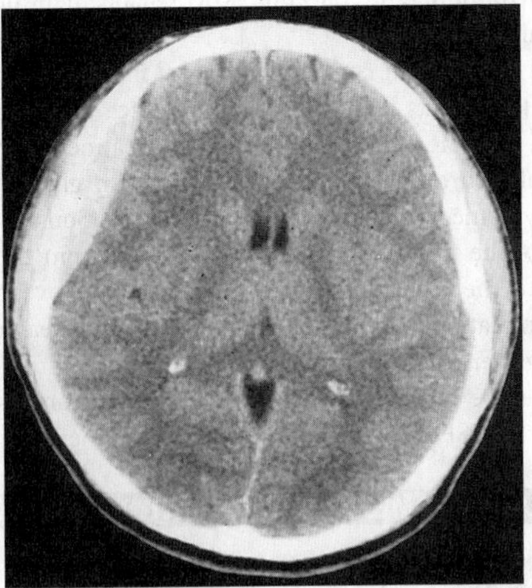

Figure 378-4 Acute epidural hematoma. The tightly attached dura is stripped from the inner table of the skull, producing a characteristic lenticular-shaped hemorrhage on noncontrast CT scan. Epidural hematomas are usually caused by tearing of the middle meningeal artery following fracture of the temporal bone.

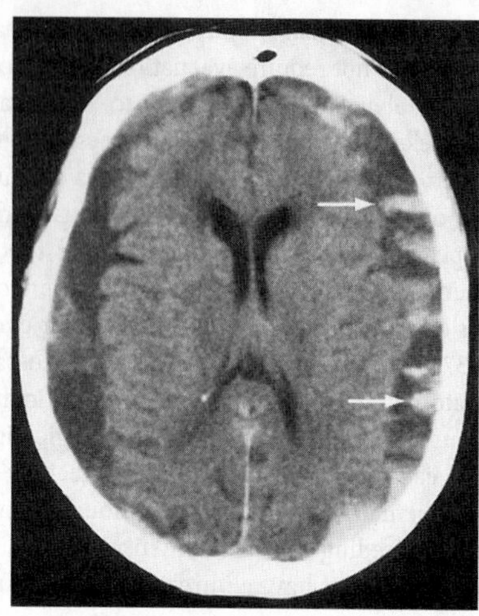

Figure 378-5 CT scan of chronic bilateral subdural hematomas of different ages. The collections began as acute hematomas and have become hypodense in comparison to the adjacent brain after a period during which they were isodense and difficult to appreciate. Some areas of resolving blood are contained on the more recently formed collection on the left (*arrows*).

and incoherence of thought are more generally prominent than focal signs such as hemiparesis. Rarely, chronic hematomas cause brief episodes of hemiparesis or aphasia that are indistinguishable from transient ischemic attacks. Patients with undetected bilateral subdural hematomas have a low tolerance for surgery, anesthesia, and drugs that depress the nervous system; drowsiness or confusion persist for long periods postoperatively.

CT without contrast initially shows a low-density mass over the convexity of the hemisphere (Fig. 378-5). Between 2 and 6 weeks after the initial bleeding the hemorrhage becomes isodense compared to adjacent brain and may be inapparent. Many subdural hematomas that are several weeks in age contain areas of blood and intermixed serous fluid. Bilateral chronic hematomas may fail to be detected because of the absence of lateral tissue shifts; this circumstance in an older patient is suggested by a "hypernormal" CT scan with fullness of the cortical sulci and small ventricles. Infusion of contrast material demonstrates enhancement of the vascular fibrous capsule surrounding the collection. MRI reliably identifies subacute and chronic hematomas.

Clinical observation coupled with serial imaging is a reasonable approach to patients with few symptoms, such as headache alone, and small chronic subdural collections. Treatment of minimally symptomatic chronic subdural hematoma with glucocorticoids is favored by some clinicians, but surgical evacuation is more often successful. The fibrous membranes that grow from the dura and encapsulate the collection require removal to prevent recurrent fluid accumulation. Small hematomas are resorbed, leaving only the organizing membranes. On imaging studies very chronic subdural hematomas are difficult to distinguish from hygromas, which are collections of CSF from a rent in the arachnoid membrane.

CLINICAL SYNDROMES AND TREATMENT OF HEAD INJURY

■ MINOR INJURY

The patient who has briefly lost consciousness or been stunned after a minor head injury usually becomes fully alert and attentive within minutes but may complain of headache, dizziness, faintness, nausea, a single episode of emesis, difficulty with concentration, a brief amnestic period, or slight blurring of vision. This typical concussion syndrome has a good prognosis with little risk of subsequent deterioration. Children are particularly prone to drowsiness, vomiting, and irritability, symptoms that are sometimes delayed for several hours after apparently minor injuries. Vasovagal syncope that follows injury may cause undue concern. Generalized or frontal headache is common in the following days. It may be migrainous (throbbing and hemicranial) in nature or aching and bilateral. After several hours of observation, patients with minor injury may be accompanied home and observed for a day by a family member or friend; written instructions to return if symptoms worsen should be provided.

Persistent severe headache and repeated vomiting in the context of normal alertness and no focal neurologic signs is usually benign, but CT should be obtained and a longer period of observation is appropriate. The decision to perform imaging tests also depends on clinical signs that indicate the impact was severe (e.g., prolonged concussion, periorbital or mastoid hematoma, repeated vomiting, palpable skull fracture), on the seriousness of other bodily injuries, and on the degree of surveillance that can be anticipated after discharge. Two studies have indicated that older age, two or more episodes of vomiting, >30 min of retrograde or persistent anterograde amnesia, seizure, and concurrent drug or alcohol intoxication are sensitive (but not specific) indicators of intracranial hemorrhage that justify CT scanning. It is appropriate to be more liberal in obtaining CT scans in children since a small number, even without loss of consciousness, will have intracranial lesions.

Concussion in sports

In the current absence of adequate data, a common sense approach to athletic concussion has been to avoid contact sports for at least several days after a mild injury, and for a longer period if there are more severe injuries or if there are protracted neurologic symptoms. The individual then undertakes a graduated program of activity until there are no further symptoms with exercise (Table 378-1). These guidelines are designed in part to avoid the extremely rare *second impact syndrome*, in which cerebral swelling follows a second minor head injury. There is some evidence that repeated concussions are associated with cumulative cognitive deficits, but this and the subsequent risk for dementia and Parkinson's disease is controversial.

■ INJURY OF INTERMEDIATE SEVERITY

Patients who are not fully alert or have persistent confusion, behavioral changes, extreme dizziness, or focal neurologic signs such as hemiparesis should be admitted to the hospital and have a CT scan. A cerebral contusion or hematoma is usually found. Common syndromes include: (1) delirium with a disinclination to be examined or moved, expletive speech, and resistance if disturbed (anterior temporal lobe contusions); (2) a quiet, disinterested, slowed mental state (abulia) alternating with irascibility (inferior frontal and frontopolar contusions); (3) a focal deficit such as aphasia or mild hemiparesis (due to subdural hematoma or convexity contusion, or, less often, carotid artery dissection); (4) confusion and inattention, poor performance on simple mental tasks, and fluctuating orientation (associated with several types of injuries, including those described above and with medial frontal contusions and interhemispheric subdural hematoma); (5) repetitive vomiting, nystagmus, drowsiness, and unsteadiness (labyrinthine concussion, but occasionally due to a posterior fossa subdural hematoma or vertebral artery dissection); and (6) diabetes insipidus (damage to the median eminence or pituitary stalk). *Injuries of this degree are often complicated by drug or alcohol intoxication, and clinically inapparent cervical spine injury may be present.*

After surgical removal of hematomas, most patients in this category improve over weeks. During the first week, the state of alertness, memory, and other cognitive functions often fluctuate, and

TABLE 378-1 Guidelines for Management of Concussion in Sports

Severity of Concussion
Grade 1: Transient confusion, no loss of consciousness (LOC), all symptoms resolve within 15 min.
Grade 2: Transient confusion, no LOC, but concussive symptoms or mental status abnormalities persist longer than 15 min.
Grade 3: Any LOC, either brief (seconds) or prolonged (minutes).
On-Site Evaluation
1. Mental status testing
a. Orientation—time, place, person, circumstances of injury
b. Concentration—digits backward, months of year in reverse order
c. Memory—names of teams, details of contest, recent events, recall of three words and objects at 0 and 5 min
2. Finger-to-nose with eyes open and closed
3. Pupillary symmetry and reaction
4. Romberg and tandem gait
5. Provocative testing—40-yard sprint, 5 push ups, 5 sit ups, 5 knee bends (development of dizziness, headaches, or other symptoms is abnormal)
Management Guidelines
Grade 1: Remove from contest. Examine immediately and at 5-min intervals. May return to contest if exam clears within 15 min. A second grade 1 concussion eliminates player for 1 week, with return contingent upon normal neurologic assessment at rest and with exertion.
Grade 2: Remove from contest, cannot return for at least 1 week. Examine at frequent intervals on sideline. Formal neurologic exam the next day. If headache or other symptoms persist for 1 week or longer, CT or MRI scan is indicated. After 1 full asymptomatic week, repeat neurologic assessment at rest and with exercise before cleared to resume play. A second grade 2 concussion eliminates player for at least 2 weeks following complete resolution of symptoms at rest or with exertion. If imaging shows abnormality, player is removed from play for the season.
Grade 3: Transport by ambulance to emergency department if still unconscious or worrisome signs are present; cervical spine stabilization may be indicated. Neurologic exam and, when indicated, CT or MRI scan will guide subsequent management. Hospital admission indicated when signs of pathology are present or if mental status remains abnormal. If findings are normal at the time of the initial medical evaluation, the athlete may be sent home, but daily exams as an outpatient are indicated. A brief (LOC for seconds) grade 3 concussion eliminates player for 1 week, and a prolonged (LOC for minutes) grade 3 concussion for 2 weeks, following complete resolution of symptoms. A second grade 3 concussion should eliminate player from sports for at least 1 month following resolution of symptoms. Any abnormality on CT or MRI scans should result in termination of the season for the athlete, and return to play at any future time should be discouraged.

Source: Modified from Quality Standards Subcommittee of the American Academy of Neurology: *The American Academy of Neurology Practice Handbook.* The American Academy of Neurology, St. Paul, MN, 1997.

agitation is common. Behavioral changes tend to be worse at night, as with many other encephalopathies, and may be treated with small doses of antipsychotic medications. Subtle abnormalities of attention, intellect, spontaneity, and memory return toward normal weeks or months after the injury, sometimes abruptly. Persistent cognitive problems are discussed below.

SEVERE INJURY

Patients who are comatose from the moment of injury require immediate neurologic attention and resuscitation. After intubation, with care taken to immobilize the cervical spine, the depth of coma, pupillary size and reactivity, limb movements, and Babinski responses are assessed. As soon as vital functions permit and cervical spine x-rays and a CT scan have been obtained, the patient should be transported to a critical care unit. Hypoxia should be reversed, and normal saline used as the resuscitation fluid in preference to albumin. The finding of an epidural or subdural hematoma or large intracerebral hemorrhage is an indication for prompt surgery and intracranial decompression in an otherwise salvageable patient. The use of prophylactic antiepileptic medications has been recommended but there is little supportive data. **Management of raised ICP, a frequent feature of severe head injury, is discussed in Chap. 275.**

GRADING AND PROGNOSIS

In severe head injury, the clinical features of eye opening, motor responses of the limbs, and verbal output have been found to be generally predictive of outcome. These three responses are assessed by the Glasgow Coma Scale; a score between 3 and 15 is assigned (Table 378-2). Over 85% of patients with aggregate scores of <5 die within 24 h. However, a number of patients with slightly higher scores, including a few without pupillary light responses, survive, suggesting that an initially aggressive approach is justified in most patients. Patients <20 years, particularly children, may make remarkable recoveries after having grave early neurologic signs. In one large study of severe head injury, 55% of children had a good outcome at 1 year, compared with 21% of adults. Older age, increased ICP, early hypoxia or hypotension, compression of the brainstem on CT or MRI, and a delay in the evacuation of large intracranial hemorrhages are indicators of a poor prognosis.

POSTCONCUSSION SYNDROME

The *postconcussion syndrome* refers to a state following minor head injury consisting of fatigue, dizziness, headache, and difficulty

TABLE 378-2 Glasgow Coma Scale for Head Injury

Eye opening (E)		Verbal response (V)	
Spontaneous	4	Oriented	5
To loud voice	3	Confused, disoriented	4
To pain	2	Inappropriate words	3
Nil	1	Incomprehensible sounds	2
		Nil	1
Best motor response (M)			
Obeys	6		
Localizes	5		
Withdraws (flexion)	4		
Abnormal flexion posturing	3		
Extension posturing	2		
Nil	1		

Note: Coma score = E + M + V. Patients scoring 3 or 4 have an 85% chance of dying or remaining vegetative, while scores >11 indicate only a 5–10% likelihood of death or vegetative state and 85% chance of moderate disability or good recovery. Intermediate scores correlate with proportional chances of recovery.

in concentration. The syndrome simulates asthenia and anxious depression. Based on experimental models, it has been proposed that subtle axonal shearing lesions or as yet undefined biochemical alterations account for the cognitive symptoms. In moderate and severe trauma, neuropsychological changes such as difficulty with attention, memory and other cognitive deficits are undoubtedly present, sometimes severe, but many problems identified by formal testing do not affect daily functioning. Test scores tend to improve rapidly during the first 6 months after injury, then more slowly for years.

Management of the postconcussive syndrome requires the identification and treatment of depression, sleeplessness, anxiety, persistent headache, and dizziness. A clear explanation of the problems that may follow concussion has been shown to reduce subsequent complaints. Care is taken to avoid prolonged use of drugs that produce dependence. Headache may initially be treated with acetaminophen and small doses of amitryptiline. Vestibular exercises (Chap. 21) and small doses of vestibular suppressants such as promethazine (Phenergan) may be helpful when dizziness is the main problem. Patients who after minor or moderate injury have difficulty with memory or with complex cognitive tasks at work may be reassured that these problems usually improve over 6–12 months. It is sometimes helpful to obtain serial and quantified neuropsychological testing in order to adjust the work environment to the patient's abilities and to document improvement over time. Whether cognitive exercises are useful in contrast to rest and a reduction in mental challenges is uncertain. Previously energetic and resilient individuals usually have the best recoveries. In patients with persistent symptoms, the possibility exists of malingering or prolongation as a result of litigation.

FURTHER READINGS

DeKosky ST et al: Traumatic brain injury—football, warfare, and long-term effects. N Engl J Med 363:1293, 2010

Dischinger PC et al: Early predictors of postconcussive syndrome in a population of trauma patients with mild traumatic brain injury. J Trauma 66:289, 2009

Lovell M: The management of sports-related concussion: Current status and future trends. Clin Sports Med 28:95, 2009

Ropper AH (ed): *Neurological and Neurosurgical Intensive Care*, 4th ed. Philadelphia, Lippincott Williams & Wilkins, 2004

———, Gorson KC: Concussion. N Engl J Med 356:166, 2007

CHAPTER 379

Primary and Metastatic Tumors of the Nervous System

Lisa M. DeAngelis
Patrick Y. Wen

INTRODUCTION

Primary brain tumors are diagnosed in approximately 52,000 people each year in the United States. At least one-half of these tumors are malignant and associated with a high mortality rate. Glial tumors account for about 60% of all primary brain tumors, and 80% of those are malignant neoplasms. Meningiomas account for 25%, vestibular schwannomas 10%, and central nervous system (CNS) lymphomas about 2%. Brain metastases are three times more common than all primary brain tumors combined and are diagnosed in approximately 150,000 people each year. Metastases to the leptomeninges and epidural space of the spinal cord each occur in approximately 3–5% of patients with systemic cancer and are also a major cause of neurologic disability in this population.

APPROACH TO THE PATIENT: Primary and Metastatic Tumors of the Nervous System

CLINICAL FEATURES Brain tumors of any type can present with a variety of symptoms and signs that fall into two categories: general and focal; patients often have a combination of the two (Table 379-1). General or nonspecific symptoms include headache, cognitive difficulties, personality change, and gait disorder. Generalized symptoms arise when the enlarging tumor and its surrounding edema cause an increase in intracranial pressure or direct compression of cerebrospinal fluid (CSF) circulation leading to hydrocephalus. The classic headache associated with a brain tumor is most evident in the morning and improves during the day, but this particular pattern is actually seen in a minority of patients. Headache may be accompanied by nausea or vomiting when intracranial pressure is elevated. Headaches are often holocephalic but can be ipsilateral to the side of a tumor. Occasionally, headaches have features of a typical migraine with unilateral throbbing pain associated with visual scotoma. Personality changes may include apathy and withdrawal from social circumstances, mimicking depression. Focal or lateralizing findings include hemiparesis, aphasia, or visual field defect. Lateralizing symptoms such as hemiparesis are typically subacute and progressive. A visual field defect is often not noticed by the patient; its presence may only be revealed after it leads to an injury such as an automobile accident occurring in the blind visual field. Language difficulties may be mistaken for confusion. Seizures are a common presentation of brain tumors, occurring in about 25% of patients with brain metastases or malignant gliomas but can be the presenting symptom in up to 90% of patients with low-grade gliomas. Most seizures have a focal signature that reflects their location in the brain and many proceed to secondary generalization. All generalized seizures that arise from a brain tumor will have a focal onset whether or not it is apparent clinically.

NEUROIMAGING Cranial MRI is the preferred diagnostic test for any patient suspected of having a brain tumor, and should be performed with gadolinium contrast administration. CT scan should be reserved for those patients unable to undergo MRI (e.g., pacemaker). Malignant brain tumors—whether primary or metastatic—typically enhance with gadolinium and may have central areas of necrosis; they are characteristically surrounded

TABLE 379-1 Symptoms and Signs at Presentation of Brain Tumors

	High-Grade Glioma (%)	Low-Grade Glioma (%)	Meningioma (%)	Metastases (%)
Generalized				
Impaired cognitive function	50	10	30	60
Hemiparesis	40	10	36	60
Headache	50	40	37	50
Lateralizing				
Seizures	20	70+	17	18
Aphasia	20	<5		18
Visual field deficit	—	—	—	7

by edema of the neighboring white matter. Low-grade gliomas typically do not enhance with gadolinium and are best appreciated on fluid-attenuated inversion recovery (FLAIR) MR images. Meningiomas have a characteristic appearance on MRI as they are dural-based with a dural tail and compress but do not invade the brain. Dural metastases or a dural lymphoma can have a similar appearance. Imaging is characteristic for many primary and metastatic tumors, but occasionally there is diagnostic uncertainty based on imaging alone. In such patients a brain biopsy may be helpful in determining a definitive diagnosis. However, when a tumor is strongly suspected, the biopsy can be obtained as an intraoperative frozen section before a definitive resection is performed.

Functional MRI is useful in presurgical planning and defining eloquent sensory, motor, and language cortex. Positron emission tomography (PET) is useful in determining the metabolic activity of the lesions seen on MRI; MR perfusion and spectroscopy can provide information on blood flow or tissue composition. These techniques may help distinguish tumor progression from necrotic tissue as a consequence of treatment with radiation and chemotherapy or identify foci of high-grade tumor in an otherwise low-grade-appearing glioma.

Neuroimaging is the only test necessary to diagnose a brain tumor. Laboratory tests are rarely useful, although patients with metastatic disease may have elevation of a tumor marker in their serum that reflects the presence of brain metastases [e.g., human chorionic gonadotropin (βhCG) from testicular cancer]. Additional testing such as cerebral angiogram, electroencephalogram (EEG), or lumbar puncture is rarely indicated or helpful.

TREATMENT Brain Tumors

Therapy of any intracranial malignancy requires both symptomatic and definitive treatments. Definitive treatment is based upon the specific tumor type and includes surgery, radiotherapy (RT), and chemotherapy. However, symptomatic treatments apply to brain tumors of any type. Most high-grade malignancies are accompanied by substantial surrounding edema, which contributes to neurologic disability and raised intracranial pressure. Glucocorticoids are highly effective at reducing perilesional edema and improving neurologic function, often within hours of administration. Dexamethasone has been the glucocorticoid of choice because of its relatively low mineralocorticoid activity. Initial doses are typically 12 mg to 16 mg a day in divided doses given orally or IV (both are equivalent). While glucocorticoids rapidly ameliorate symptoms and signs, their long-term use causes substantial toxicity including insomnia, weight gain, diabetes mellitus, steroid myopathy, and personality changes. Consequently, a taper is indicated as definitive treatment is administered and the patient improves.

Patients with brain tumors who present with seizures, require anticonvulsant drug therapy. There is no role for prophylactic anticonvulsant drugs in patients who have not had a seizure, thus their use should be restricted to those who have had a convincing ictal event. The agents of choice are those drugs that do not induce the hepatic microsomal enzyme system. These include levetiracetam, topiramate, lamotrigine, valproic acid, or lacosamide (Chap. 369). Other drugs such as phenytoin and carbamazepine are used less frequently because they are potent enzyme inducers that can interfere with both glucocorticoid metabolism and the metabolism of chemotherapeutic agents needed to treat the underlying systemic malignancy or the primary brain tumor.

Venous thromboembolic disease occurs in 20–30% of patients with high-grade gliomas and brain metastases. Therefore, anticoagulants should be used prophylactically during hospitalization and in patients who are nonambulatory. Those who have had either a deep vein thrombosis or pulmonary embolus can receive therapeutic doses of anticoagulation safely and without increasing the risk for hemorrhage into the tumor. Inferior vena cava filters are reserved for patients with absolute contraindications to anticoagulation such as recent craniotomy.

PRIMARY BRAIN TUMORS

PATHOGENESIS

No underlying cause has been identified for the majority of primary brain tumors. The only established risk factors are exposure to ionizing radiation (meningiomas, gliomas, and schwannomas) and immunosuppression (primary CNS lymphoma). Evidence for an association with exposure to electromagnetic fields including cellular telephones, head injury, foods containing *N*-nitroso compounds, or occupational risk factors, are unproven. A small minority of patients have a family history of brain tumors. Some of these familial cases are associated with genetic syndromes (Table 379-2).

As with other neoplasms, brain tumors arise as a result of a multistep process driven by the sequential acquisition of genetic alterations. These include loss of tumor suppressor genes [e.g., p53 and phosphatase and tensin homolog on chromosome 10 (PTEN)] and amplification and overexpression of protooncogenes such as the epidermal growth factor receptor (EGFR) and the platelet-derived growth factor receptors (PDGFR). The accumulation of these genetic abnormalities results in uncontrolled cell growth and tumor formation.

Important progress has been made in understanding the molecular pathogenesis of several types of brain tumors, including glioblastomas and medulloblastomas. Glioblastomas can be separated into two main subtypes based on genetic and biologic differences (Fig. 379-1). The majority are primary glioblastomas. These arise de novo and are characterized by EGFR amplification and mutations, and deletion or mutation of PTEN. Secondary glioblastomas arise in younger patients as lower-grade tumors and transform over a period of several years into glioblastomas. These tumors have inactivation of the p53 tumor suppressor gene, overexpression of PDGFR, and mutations of the isocitrate dehydrogenase 1 and 2 genes. Despite their genetic differences, primary and secondary glioblastomas

TABLE 379-2 Genetic Syndromes Associated With Primary Brain Tumors

Syndrome	Inheritance	Gene/Protein	Associated Tumors
Cowden's syndrome	AD	Mutations of PTEN (ch10p23)	**Dysplastic cerebellar gangliocytoma (Lhermitte-Duclos disease), meningioma, astrocytoma** Breast, endometrial, thyroid cancer, trichilemmomas
Familial schwannomatosis	Sporadic Hereditary	Mutations in INI1/SNF5 (ch22q11)	**Schwannomas, gliomas**
Gardner's syndrome	AD	Mutations in APC (ch5q21)	**Medulloblastoma, glioblastoma, craniopharyngioma** Familial polyposis, multiple osteomas, skin and soft tissue tumors
Gorlin syndrome (Basal cell nevus syndrome)	AD	Mutations in Patched 1 gene (ch9q22.3)	**Medulloblastomas** Basal cell carcinoma
Li-Fraumeni syndrome	AD	Mutations in p53 (ch17p13.1)	**Gliomas, medulloblastomas** Sarcomas, breast cancer, leukemias, others
Multiple Endocrine Neoplasia 1 (Werner's syndrome)	AD	Mutations in Menin (ch11q13)	**Pituitary adenoma, malignant schwannomas** Parathyroid and pancreatic islet cell tumors
Neurofibromatosis type 1 (NF1)	AD	Mutations in NF1/Neurofibromin (ch17q12-22)	**Schwannomas, astrocytomas, optic nerve gliomas, meningiomas** Neurofibromas, neurofibrosarcomas, others
Neurofibromatosis type 2 (NF2)	AD	Mutations in NF2/Merlin (ch22q12)	**Bilateral vestibular schwannomas, astrocytomas, multiple meningiomas, ependymomas**
Tuberous sclerosis (TSC) (Bourneville's disease)	AD	Mutations in TSC1/TSC2 (ch9q34/16)	**Subependymal giant cell astrocytoma, ependymomas, glioma, ganglioneuroma, hamartoma**
Turcot's syndrome	AD AR	Mutations in APC[a] (ch5) hMLH1 (ch3p21)	**Gliomas, medulloblastomas** Adenomatous colon polyps, adenocarcinoma
Von Hippel–Lindau (VHL)	AD	Mutations in VHL gene (ch3p25)	**Hemangioblastomas** Retinal angiomas, renal cell carcinoma, pheochromocytoma, pancreatic tumors and cysts, endolymphatic sac tumors of the middle ear

[a]Various DNA mismatch repair gene mutations may cause a similar clinical phenotype, also referred to as Turcot's syndrome, in which there is a predisposition to nonpolyposis colon cancer and brain tumors.

Abbreviations: AD, autosomal dominant; APC, adenomatous polyposis coli; AR, autosomal recessive; ch, chromosome; PTEN, phosphatase and tensin homologue; TSC, tuberous sclerosis complex.

are morphologically indistinguishable, although they are likely to respond differently to molecular therapies. The molecular subtypes of medulloblastomas are also being elucidated. Approximately 25% of medulloblastomas have activating mutations of the sonic hedgehog signaling pathway, raising the possibility that inhibitors of this pathway may have therapeutic potential.

The adult nervous system contains neural stem cells that are capable of self-renewal, proliferation, and differentiation into distinctive mature cell types. There is increasing evidence that neural stem cells, or related progenitor cells, can be transformed into tumor stem cells and give rise to primary brain tumors, including gliomas and medulloblastomas. These stem cells appear to be more resistant to standard therapies than the tumor cells themselves and contribute to the difficulty in eradicating these tumors. There is intense interest in developing therapeutic strategies that effectively target tumor stem cells.

INTRINSIC "MALIGNANT" TUMORS

ASTROCYTOMAS

These are infiltrative tumors with a presumptive glial cell of origin. The World Health Organization (WHO) classifies astrocytomas into four prognostic grades based on histologic features: grade I (pilocytic astrocytoma, subependymal giant cell astrocytoma); grade II (diffuse astrocytoma); grade III (anaplastic astrocytoma); and grade IV (glioblastoma). Grades I and II are considered low-grade, and grades III and IV high-grade, astrocytomas.

Low-grade astrocytoma These tumors occur predominantly in children and young adults.

Grade I astrocytomas Pilocytic astrocytomas (WHO grade I) are the most common tumor of childhood. They occur typically in the cerebellum but may also be found elsewhere in the neuraxis, including the optic nerves and brainstem. Frequently they appear as cystic lesions with an enhancing mural nodule. They are potentially curable if they can be completely resected. Giant cell subependymal astrocytomas are usually found in the ventricular wall of patients with tuberous sclerosis. They often do not require intervention but can be treated surgically or with inhibitors of the mammalian target of rapamycin (mTOR).

Grade II astrocytomas These are infiltrative tumors that usually present with seizures in young adults. They appear as nonenhancing tumors with increased T2/FLAIR signal (Fig. 379-2). If feasible, patients should undergo maximal surgical resection, although complete resection is rarely possible because of the invasive nature of the tumor. Radiotherapy is helpful, but there is no difference in overall survival between radiotherapy administered postoperatively

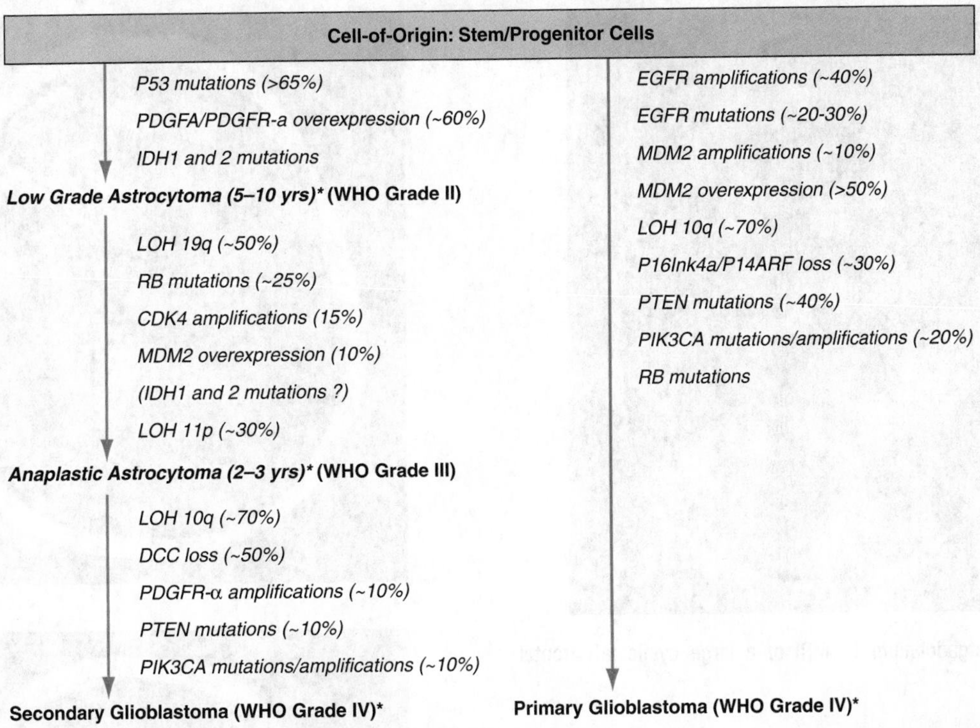

Cell-of-Origin: Stem/Progenitor Cells

P53 mutations (>65%)
PDGFA/PDGFR-a overexpression (~60%)
IDH1 and 2 mutations

Low Grade Astrocytoma (5–10 yrs)* **(WHO Grade II)**

LOH 19q (~50%)
RB mutations (~25%)
CDK4 amplifications (15%)
MDM2 overexpression (10%)
(IDH1 and 2 mutations ?)
LOH 11p (~30%)

Anaplastic Astrocytoma (2–3 yrs)* **(WHO Grade III)**

LOH 10q (~70%)
DCC loss (~50%)
PDGFR-α amplifications (~10%)
PTEN mutations (~10%)
PIK3CA mutations/amplifications (~10%)

Secondary Glioblastoma (WHO Grade IV)*

EGFR amplifications (~40%)
EGFR mutations (~20-30%)
MDM2 amplifications (~10%)
MDM2 overexpression (>50%)
LOH 10q (~70%)
P16Ink4a/P14ARF loss (~30%)
PTEN mutations (~40%)
PIK3CA mutations/amplifications (~20%)
RB mutations

Primary Glioblastoma (WHO Grade IV)*

Figure 379-1 Genetic and chromosomal alterations involved in the development of primary and secondary glioblastomas. A *slash* indicates one or the other or both. *DCC*, deleted in colorectal carcinoma; *EGFR*, epidermal growth factor receptor; *IDH*, isocitrate dehydrogenase; *LOH*, loss of heterozygosity; *MDM2*, murine double minute 2; *PDGF*, platelet-derived growth factor; *PDGFR*, platelet-derived growth factor receptor; *PIK3CA*, phosphatidylinositol 3-kinase, catalytic; *PTEN*, phosphatase and tensin homologue; *RB*, retinoblastoma; WHO, World Health Organization.

or delayed until the time of tumor progression. There is increasing evidence that chemotherapeutic agents such as temozolomide, an oral alkylating agent, can be helpful in some patients.

High-grade astrocytoma

Grade III (anaplastic) astrocytoma These account for approximately 15–20% of high-grade astrocytomas. They generally present in the fourth and fifth decades of life as variably enhancing tumors. Treatment is the same as for glioblastoma, consisting of maximal safe surgical resection followed by radiotherapy with concurrent and adjuvant temozolomide, or with radiotherapy and adjuvant temozolomide alone.

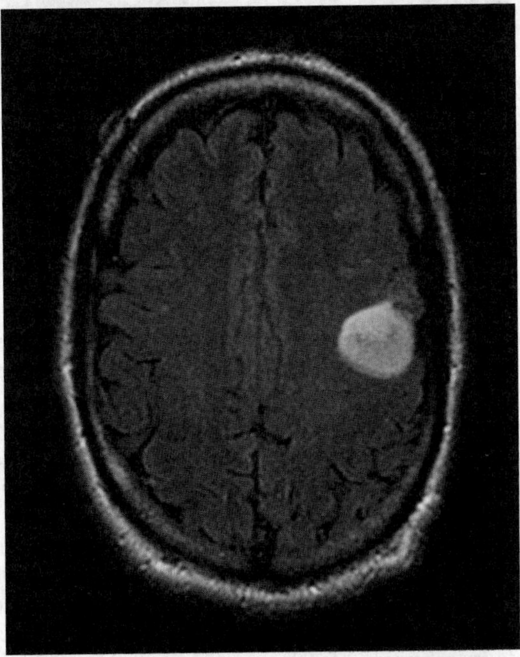

Figure 379-2 Fluid-attenuated inversion recovery (FLAIR) MRI of a left frontal low-grade astrocytoma. This lesion did not enhance.

Grade IV astrocytoma (glioblastoma) Glioblastoma accounts for the majority of high-grade astrocytomas. They are the most common cause of malignant primary brain tumors, with over 10,000 cases diagnosed each year in the United States. Patients usually present in the sixth and seventh decades of life with headache, seizures, or focal neurologic deficits. The tumors appear as ring-enhancing masses with central necrosis and surrounding edema (Fig. 379-3). These are highly infiltrative tumors, and the areas of increased T2/FLAIR signal surrounding the main tumor mass contain invading tumor cells. Treatment involves maximal surgical resection followed by partial-field external beam radiotherapy (6000 cGy in thirty 200-cGy fractions) with concomitant temozolomide, followed by 6–12 months of adjuvant temozolomide. With this regimen, median survival is increased to 14.6 months compared to only 12 months with radiotherapy alone, and 2-year survival is increased to 27%, compared to 10% with radiotherapy alone. Patients whose tumor contains the DNA repair enzyme O^6-methylguanine-DNA methyltransferase (MGMT) are relatively resistant to temozolomide and have a worse prognosis compared to those whose tumors contain low levels of MGMT as a result of silencing of the MGMT gene by promoter hypermethylation. Implantation of biodegradable polymers containing the chemotherapeutic agent carmustine into the tumor bed after resection of the tumor also produces a modest improvement in survival.

Despite optimal therapy, glioblastomas invariably recur. Treatment options for recurrent disease may include reoperation, carmustine wafers, and alternate chemotherapeutic regimens. Reirradiation is rarely helpful. Bevacizumab, a humanized vascular endothelial

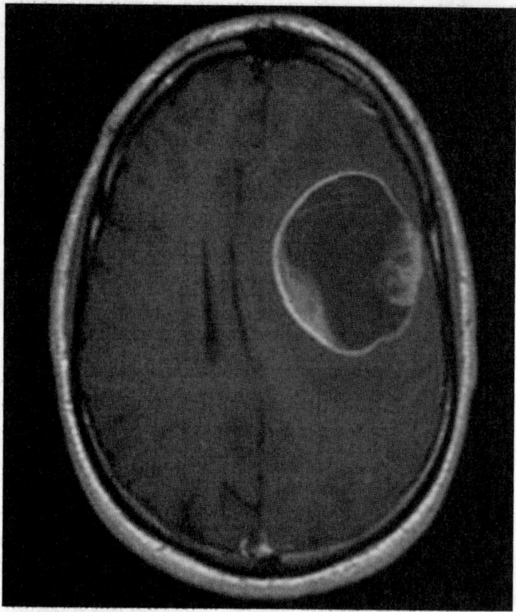

Figure 379-3 Postgadolinium T1 MRI of a large cystic left frontal glioblastoma.

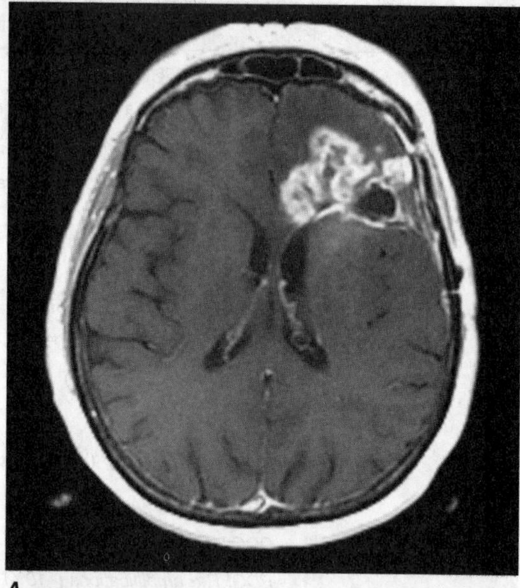

A

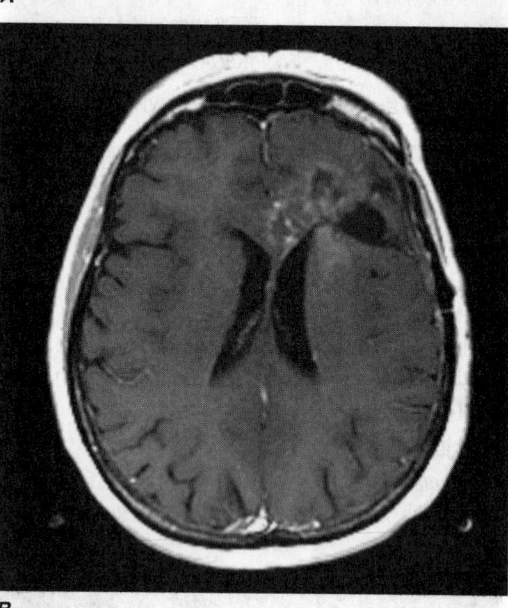

B

Figure 379-4 Postgadolinium T1 MRI of a recurrent glioblastoma before (*A*) and after (*B*) administration of bevacizumab. Note the decreased enhancement and mass effect.

growth factor (VEGF) monoclonal antibody, has activity in recurrent glioblastoma, increasing progression-free survival and reducing peritumoral edema and glucocorticoid use (Fig. 379-4). Treatment decisions for patients with recurrent glioblastoma must be made on an individual basis, taking into consideration such factors as previous therapy, time to relapse, performance status, and quality of life. Whenever feasible, patients with recurrent disease should be enrolled in clinical trials. Novel therapies undergoing evaluation in patients with glioblastoma include targeted molecular agents directed at receptor tyrosine kinases and signal transduction pathways; anti-angiogenic agents, especially those directed at the VEGF receptors; chemotherapeutic agents that cross the blood-brain barrier more effectively than currently available drugs; gene therapy; immunotherapy; and infusion of radiolabeled drugs and targeted toxins into the tumor and surrounding brain by means of convection-enhanced delivery.

The most important adverse prognostic factors in patients with high-grade astrocytomas are older age, histologic features of glioblastoma, poor Karnofsky performance status, and unresectable tumor. Patients with unmethylated MGMT promoter resulting in the presence of the repair enzyme in tumor cells and resistance to temozolomide also have a worse prognosis.

Gliomatosis cerebri Rarely, patients may present with a highly infiltrating, nonenhancing tumor involving more than two lobes. These tumors do not qualify for the histologic diagnosis of glioblastoma but behave aggressively and have a similarly poor outcome. Treatment involves radiotherapy and temozolomide chemotherapy.

Oligodendroglioma

Oligodendrogliomas account for approximately 15–20% of gliomas. They are classified by the WHO into well-differentiated oligodendrogliomas (grade II) or anaplastic oligodendrogliomas (AOs) (grade III). Tumors with oligodendroglial components have distinctive features such as perinuclear clearing—giving rise to a "fried-egg" appearance—and a reticular pattern of blood vessel growth. Some tumors have both an oligodendroglial as well as an astrocytic component. These mixed tumors, or oligoastrocytomas (OAs), are also classified into well-differentiated OA (grade II) or anaplastic oligoastrocytomas (AOAs) (grade III).

Grade II oligodendrogliomas and OAs are generally more responsive to therapy and have a better prognosis than pure astrocytic tumors. These tumors present similarly to grade II astrocytomas in young adults. The tumors are nonenhancing and often partially calcified. They should be treated with surgery and, if necessary, radiotherapy and chemotherapy. Patients with oligodendrogliomas have a median survival in excess of 10 years.

Anaplastic oligodendrogliomas and AOAs present in the fourth and fifth decades as variably enhancing tumors. They are more responsive to therapy than grade III astrocytomas. Co-deletion of chromosomes 1p and 19q, mediated by an unbalanced translocation of 19p to 1q, occurs in 61 to 89% of patients with AO and 14 to 20% of patients with AOA. Tumors with the 1p and 19q co-deletion are particularly sensitive to chemotherapy with procarbazine, lomustine [cyclohexylchloroethylnitrosourea (CCNU)], and vincristine (PCV) or temozolomide, as well as to radiotherapy. Median survival of patients with AO or AOA is approximately 3–6 years.

Ependymomas

Ependymomas are tumors derived from ependymal cells that line the ventricular surface. They account for approximately 5% of childhood tumors and frequently arise from the wall of the fourth ventricle in the posterior fossa. Although adults can have intracranial ependymomas, they occur more commonly in the spine, especially in the filum terminale of the spinal cord where they have a myxopapillary histology. Ependymomas that can be completely resected are potentially curable. Partially resected ependymomas will recur and require irradiation. The less common anaplastic ependymomas are more aggressive but can be treated in the same way as ependymomas. Subependymomas are slow-growing benign lesions arising in the wall of ventricles that often do not require treatment.

Other less common gliomas

Gangliogliomas and pleomorphic xanthoastrocytomas occur in young adults. They behave as more indolent forms of grade II gliomas and are treated in the same way. Brainstem gliomas usually occur in children or young adults. Despite treatment with radiotherapy and chemotherapy, the prognosis is poor with median survival of only 1 year. Gliosarcomas contain both an astrocytic as well as a sarcomatous component and are treated in the same way as glioblastomas.

PRIMARY CENTRAL NERVOUS SYSTEM LYMPHOMA

Primary central nervous system lymphoma (PCNSL) is a rare non-Hodgkin's lymphoma accounting for less than 3% of primary brain tumors. For unclear reasons, its incidence is increasing, particularly in immunocompetent individuals.

PCNSL in immunocompetent patients usually consists of diffuse large B-cell lymphomas. PCNSL may also occur in immunocompromised patients, usually those infected with the human immunodeficiency virus (HIV) or organ transplant recipients on immunosuppressive therapy. PCNSL in immunocompromised patients is typically large cell with immunoblastic and more aggressive features. These patients are usually severely immunocompromised with CD4 counts of less than 50/mL. The Epstein-Barr virus (EBV) frequently plays an important role in the pathogenesis of HIV-related PCNSL.

Immunocompetent patients are older (median 60 years) compared to HIV-related PCNSL (median 31 years). PCNSL usually presents as a mass lesion, with neuropsychiatric symptoms, symptoms of increased intracranial pressure, lateralizing signs, or seizures.

On contrast-enhanced MRI, PCNSL usually appears as a densely enhancing tumor (Fig. 379-5). Immunocompetent patients have solitary lesions more often than immunosuppressed patients. Frequently there is involvement of the basal ganglia, corpus callosum, or periventricular region. Although the imaging features are often characteristic, PCNSL can sometimes be difficult to differentiate from high-grade gliomas, infections, or demyelination. Stereotactic biopsy is necessary to obtain a histologic diagnosis. Whenever possible, glucocorticoids should be withheld until after the biopsy has been obtained, since they have a cytolytic effect on lymphoma cells and may lead to nondiagnostic tissue. In addition, patients should be tested for HIV and the extent of disease assessed by performing positron emission tomography (PET) or computerized tomography (CT) of the body, MRI of the spine, CSF analysis, and slit-lamp examination of the eye. Bone marrow biopsy and testicular ultrasound are occasionally performed.

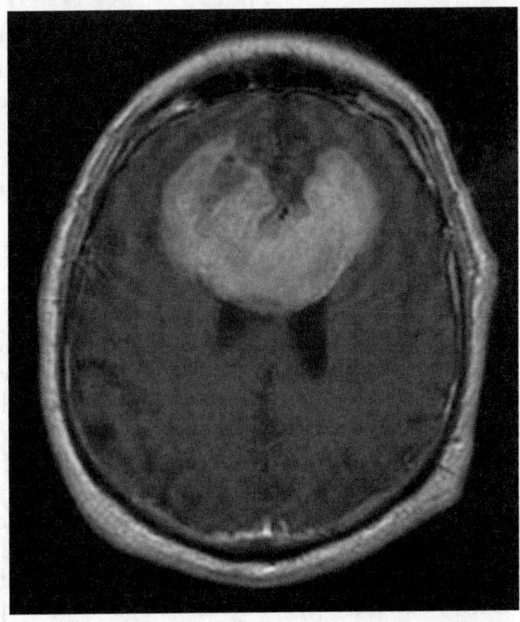

Figure 379-5 Postgadolinium T1 MRI demonstrating a large bifrontal primary central nervous system lymphoma (PCNSL). The periventricular location and diffuse enhancement pattern are characteristic of lymphoma.

TREATMENT Primary Central Nervous System Lymphoma

Unlike other primary brain tumors, PCNSL is relatively sensitive to glucocorticoids, chemotherapy, and radiotherapy. Durable complete responses and long-term survival are possible with these treatments. High-dose methotrexate, a folate antagonist that interrupts DNA synthesis, produces response rates ranging from 35 to 80% and median survival up to 50 months. Combination of methotrexate with other chemotherapeutic agents such as cytarabine, as well as whole-brain radiotherapy, increases the response rate to 70–100%. However, radiotherapy is associated with delayed neurotoxicity, especially in patients over the age of 60 years. As a result radiotherapy is frequently omitted in older patients with PCNSL. There is emerging evidence that the anti-CD20 monoclonal antibody rituximab may have activity in PCNSL, although there remain concerns about its ability to pass through the blood-brain barrier as it becomes reconstituted with therapy. For some patients, high-dose chemotherapy with autologous stem cell rescue may offer the best chance of preventing relapse.

At least 50% of patients will eventually develop recurrent disease. Treatment options include radiotherapy for patients who have not had prior irradiation, re-treatment with methotrexate, as well as other agents such as temozolomide, rituximab, procarbazine, topotecan, and pemetrexed. High-dose chemotherapy with autologous stem cell rescue may have a role in selected patients with relapsed disease.

PCNSL IN IMMUNOCOMPROMISED PATIENTS PCNSL in immunocompromised patients often produces multiple-ring enhancing lesions that can be difficult to differentiate from metastases and infections such as toxoplasmosis. The diagnosis is usually established by examination of the cerebrospinal fluid for cytology and EBV DNA, toxoplasmosis serologic testing, brain PET imaging for hypermetabolism of the lesions consistent with tumor instead of infection, and, if necessary, brain biopsy. Since the advent of highly active antiretroviral drugs, the incidence of HIV-related PCNSL has declined. These patients may be treated with whole-brain radiotherapy, high-dose methotrexate, and initiation of highly active antiretroviral therapy. In organ transplant recipients, reduction of immunosuppression may improve outcome.

MEDULLOBLASTOMAS

Medulloblastomas are the most common malignant brain tumor of childhood, accounting for approximately 20% of all primary CNS tumors among children. They arise from granule cell progenitors or from multipotent progenitors from the ventricular zone. Approximately 5% of children have inherited disorders with germ-line mutations of genes that predispose to the development of medulloblastoma. The Gorlin syndrome, the most common of these inherited disorders, is due to mutations in the patched-1 (PTCH-1) gene, a key component in the sonic hedgehog pathway. Turcot's syndrome, caused by mutations in the adenomatous polyposis coli (APC) gene and familial adenomatous polyposis, has also been associated with an increased incidence of medulloblastoma. Histologically, medulloblastomas appear as highly cellular tumors with abundant dark staining, round nuclei, and rosette formation (Homer-Wright rosettes). They present with headache, ataxia, and signs of brainstem involvement. On MRI they appear as densely enhancing tumors in the posterior fossa, sometimes associated with hydrocephalus. Seeding of the CSF is common. Treatment involves maximal surgical resection, craniospinal irradiation, and chemotherapy with agents such as cisplatin, lomustine, cyclophosphamide, and vincristine. Approximately 70% of patients have long-term survival but usually at the cost of significant neurocognitive impairment. A major goal of current research is to improve survival while minimizing long-term complications.

PINEAL REGION TUMORS

A large number of tumors can arise in the region of the pineal gland. These typically present with headache, visual symptoms, and hydrocephalus. Patients may have Parinaud's syndrome characterized by impaired upgaze and accommodation. Some pineal tumors such as pineocytomas and benign teratomas can be treated simply by surgical resection. Germinomas respond to irradiation, while pineoblastomas and malignant germ cell tumors require craniospinal radiation and chemotherapy.

EXTRINSIC "BENIGN" TUMORS

MENINGIOMAS

Meningiomas are diagnosed with increasing frequency as more people undergo neuroimaging studies for various indications. They are now the most common primary brain tumor, accounting for approximately 32% of the total. Their incidence increases with age. They tend to be more common in women and in patients with neurofibromatosis type 2. They also occur more commonly in patients with a past history of cranial irradiation.

Meningiomas arise from the dura mater and are composed of neoplastic meningothelial (arachnoidal cap) cells. They are most commonly located over the cerebral convexities, especially adjacent to the sagittal sinus, but can also occur in the skull base and along the dorsum of the spinal cord. Meningiomas are classified by the WHO into three histologic grades of increasing aggressiveness: grade I (benign meningiomas), grade II (atypical meningiomas), and grade III (malignant meningiomas).

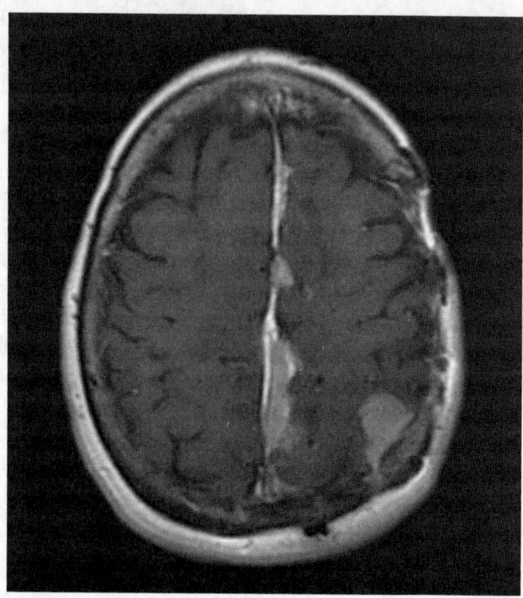

Figure 379-6 Postgadolinium T1 MRI demonstrating multiple meningiomas along the falx and left parietal cortex.

Many meningiomas are found incidentally following neuroimaging for unrelated reasons. They can also present with headaches, seizures, or focal neurologic deficits. On imaging studies they have a characteristic appearance usually consisting of a partially calcified, densely enhancing extraaxial tumor arising from the dura (Fig. 379-6). Occasionally they may have a dural tail, consisting of thickened, enhanced dura extending like a tail from the mass. The main differential diagnosis of meningioma is a dural metastasis.

If the meningioma is small and asymptomatic, no intervention is necessary and the lesion can be observed with serial MRI studies. Larger, symptomatic lesions should be resected surgically. If complete resection is achieved, the patient is cured. Incompletely resected tumors tend to recur, although the rate of recurrence can be very slow with grade I tumors. Tumors that cannot be resected, or can only be partially removed, may benefit from treatment with external beam radiotherapy or stereotactic radiosurgery (SRS). These treatments may also be helpful in patients whose tumor has recurred after surgery. Hormonal therapy and chemotherapy are currently unproven.

Rarer tumors that resemble meningiomas include hemangiopericytomas and solitary fibrous tumors. These are treated with surgery and radiotherapy but have a higher propensity to recur.

SCHWANNOMAS

These are generally benign tumors arising from the Schwann cells of cranial and spinal nerve roots. The most common schwannomas, termed *vestibular schwannomas* or *acoustic neuromas*, arise from the vestibular portion of the eighth cranial nerve and account for approximately 9% of primary brain tumors. Patients with neurofibromatosis type 2 have a high incidence of vestibular schwannomas that are frequently bilateral. Schwannomas arising from other cranial nerves, such as the trigeminal nerve (cranial nerve V), occur with much lower frequency. Neurofibromatosis type 1 is associated with an increased incidence of schwannomas of the spinal nerve roots.

Vestibular schwannomas may be found incidentally on neuroimaging or present with progressive unilateral hearing loss, dizziness, tinnitus, or less commonly, symptoms resulting from compression

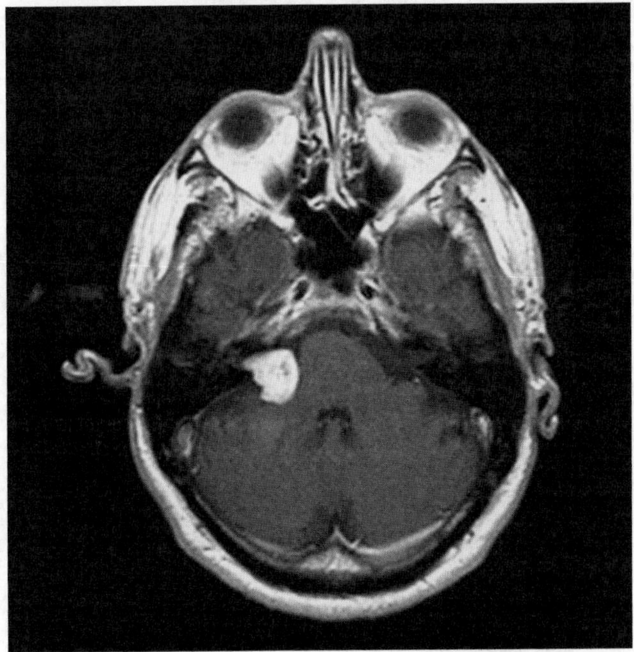

Figure 379-7 Postgadolinium MRI of a right vestibular schwannoma. The tumor can be seen to involve the internal auditory canal.

of the brainstem and cerebellum. On MRI they appear as densely enhancing lesions, enlarging the internal auditory canal and often extending into the cerebellopontine angle (Fig. 379-7). The differential diagnosis includes meningioma. Very small, asymptomatic lesions can be observed with serial MRIs. Larger lesions should be treated with surgery or stereotactic radiosurgery. The optimal treatment will depend on the size of the tumor, symptoms, and the patient's preference. In patients with small vestibular schwannomas and relatively intact hearing, early surgical intervention increases the chance of preserving hearing.

PITUITARY TUMORS (CHAP. 339)

These account for approximately 9% of primary brain tumors. They can be divided into functioning and nonfunctioning tumors. Functioning tumors are usually microadenomas (<1 cm in diameter) that secrete hormones and produce specific endocrine syndromes [e.g., acromegaly for growth hormone–secreting tumors, Cushing's syndrome for adrenocorticotropic hormone (ACTH)-secreting tumors, and galactorrhea, amenorrhea, and infertility for prolactin-secreting tumors]. Nonfunctioning pituitary tumors tend to be macroadenomas (>1 cm) that produce symptoms by mass effect, giving rise to headaches, visual impairment (such as bitemporal hemianopia), and hypopituitarism. Prolactin-secreting tumors respond well to dopamine agonists such as bromocriptine and cabergoline. Other pituitary tumors usually require treatment with surgery and sometimes radiotherapy or radiosurgery and hormonal therapy.

CRANIOPHARYNGIOMAS

Craniopharyngiomas are rare, usually suprasellar, partially calcified, solid, or mixed solid-cystic benign tumors that arise from remnants of Rathke's pouch. They have a bimodal distribution, occurring predominantly in children but also between the ages of 55 and 65 years. They present with headaches, visual impairment, and impaired growth in children and hypopituitarism in adults. Treatment involves surgery, radiotherapy, or the combination of the two.

OTHER BENIGN TUMORS

Dysembryoplastic neuroepithelial tumors (DNTs)

These are benign, supratentorial tumors, usually in the temporal lobes. They typically occur in children and young adults with a long-standing history of seizures. If the seizures are refractory, surgical resection is curative.

Epidermoid cysts

These consist of squamous epithelium surrounding a keratin-filled cyst. They are usually found in the cerebellopontine angle and the intrasellar and suprasellar regions. They may present with headaches, cranial nerve abnormalities, seizures, or hydrocephalus. Imaging studies demonstrate extraaxial lesions with characteristics that are similar to CSF but have restricted diffusion. Treatment involves surgical resection.

Dermoid cysts

Like epidermoid cysts, dermoid cysts arise from epithelial cells that are retained during closure of the neural tube. They contain both epidermal and dermal structures such as hair follicles, sweat glands, and sebaceous glands. Unlike epidermoid cysts, these tumors usually have a midline location. They occur most frequently in the posterior fossa, especially the vermis, fourth ventricle, and suprasellar cistern. Radiographically, dermoid cysts resemble lipomas, demonstrating T1 hyperintensity and variable signal on T2. Symptomatic dermoid cysts can be treated with surgery.

Colloid cysts

These usually arise in the anterior third ventricle and may present with headaches, hydrocephalus, and very rarely sudden death. Surgical resection is curative or a third ventriculostomy may relieve the obstructive hydrocephalus and be sufficient therapy.

NEUROCUTANEOUS SYNDROMES (PHAKOMATOSES)

A number of genetic disorders are characterized by cutaneous lesions and an increased risk of brain tumors. Most of these disorders have an autosomal dominance inheritance with variable penetrance.

NEUROFIBROMATOSIS TYPE 1 (NF1) (VON RECKLINGHAUSEN'S DISEASE)

NF1 is an autosomal dominant disorder with an incidence of approximately 1 in 2600–3000. Approximately half the cases are familial; the remainder are new mutations arising in patients with unaffected parents. The NF1 gene on chromosome 17q11.2 encodes a protein, neurofibromin, a guanosine triphosphatase (GTPase)-activating protein (GAP) that modulates signaling through the ras pathway. Mutations of the NF1 gene result in a large number of nervous system tumors including neurofibromas, plexiform neurofibromas, optic nerve gliomas, astrocytomas, and meningiomas. In addition to neurofibromas, which appear as multiple, soft, rubbery cutaneous tumors, other cutaneous manifestations of NF1 include café au lait spots and axillary freckling. NF1 is also associated with hamartomas of the iris termed Lisch nodules, pheochromocytomas, pseudoarthrosis of the tibia, scoliosis, epilepsy, and mental retardation.

NEUROFIBROMATOSIS TYPE 2 (NF2)

NF2 is less common than NF1, with an incidence of 1 in 25,000–40,000. It is an autosomal dominant disorder with full penetrance. As with NF1, approximately half the cases arise from new mutations. The NF2 gene on 22q encodes a cytoskeletal protein "merlin" (moesin, ezrin, radixin-like protein) that functions as a tumor suppressor. NF2 is characterized by bilateral vestibular schwannomas in over 90% of patients, multiple meningiomas, and spinal ependymomas and astrocytomas. Treatment of bilateral vestibular schwannomas can be challenging because the goal is to preserve hearing for as long as possible. These patients may also have posterior subcapsular lens opacities and retinal hamartomas.

TUBEROUS SCLEROSIS (BOURNEVILLE'S DISEASE)

This is an autosomal dominant disorder with an incidence of approximately 1 in 5000 to 10,000 live births. It is caused by mutations in either the TSC1 gene, which maps to chromosome 9q34, and encodes a protein termed hamartin, or mutations in the TSC2 gene, which maps to chromosome 16p13.3 and encodes the tuberin protein. Hamartin forms a complex with tuberin, which inhibits cellular signaling through the mammalian target of rapamycin (mTOR), and acts as a negative regulator of the cell cycle. Patients with tuberous sclerosis have seizures, mental retardation, adenoma sebaceum (facial angiofibromas), shagreen patch, hypomelanotic macules, periungual fibromas, renal angiomyolipomas, and cardiac rhabdomyomas. These patients have an increased incidence of subependymal nodules, cortical tubers, and subependymal giant cell astrocytomas (SEGA). Patients frequently require anticonvulsants for seizures. SEGAs often do not need treatment but occasionally require surgical resection. There is emerging evidence that mTOR inhibitors may have activity in SEGAs.

TUMORS METASTATIC TO THE BRAIN

Brain metastases arise from hematogenous spread and frequently arise from either a lung primary or are associated with pulmonary metastases. Most metastases develop at the gray matter–white matter junction in the watershed distribution of the brain where intravascular tumor cells lodge in terminal arterioles. The distribution of metastases in the brain approximates the proportion of blood flow such that about 85% of all metastases are supratentorial and 15% occur in the posterior fossa. The most common sources of brain metastases are lung and breast carcinomas; melanoma has the greatest propensity to metastasize to the brain, being found in 80% of patients at autopsy (Table 379-3). Other tumor types such as ovarian and esophageal carcinoma rarely metastasize to the brain. Prostate and breast cancer also have a propensity to metastasize to the dura and can mimic meningioma. Leptomeningeal metastases are common from hematologic malignancies and also breast and lung cancers. Spinal cord compression primarily arises in patients with prostate and breast cancer, tumors with a strong propensity to metastasize to the axial skeleton.

DIAGNOSIS OF METASTASES

Brain metastases are best visualized on MRI, where they usually appear as well-circumscribed lesions (Fig. 379-8). The amount of perilesional edema can be highly variable with large lesions causing minimal edema and sometimes very small lesions causing extensive edema. Enhancement may be in a ring pattern or diffuse. Occasionally, intracranial metastases will hemorrhage; although melanoma, thyroid, and kidney cancer have the greatest propensity to hemorrhage, the most common cause of a hemorrhagic metastasis is lung cancer because it accounts for

TABLE 379-3 Frequency of Nervous System Metastases by Common Primary Tumors

	Brain %	LM %	ESCC %
Lung	41	17	15
Breast	19	57	22
Melanoma	10	12	4
Prostate	1	1	10
GIT	7	—	5
Renal	3	2	7
Lymphoma	<1	10	10
Sarcoma	7	1	9
Other	11	—	18

Abbreviations: ESCC, epidural spinal cord compression; GIT, gastrointestinal tract; LM, leptomeningeal metastases.

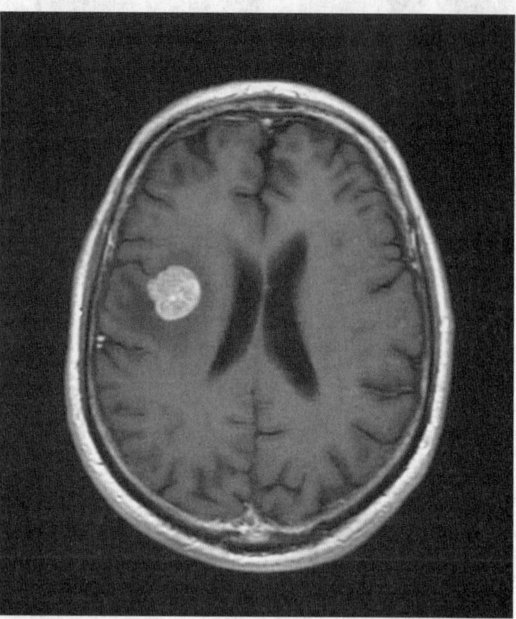
A

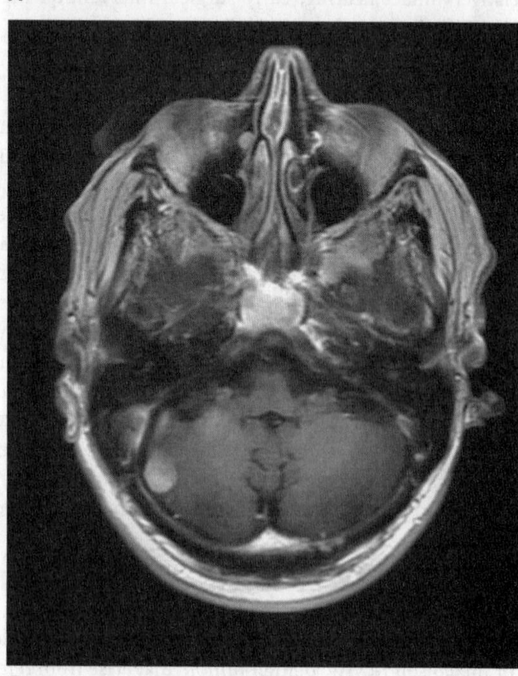
B

Figure 379-8 Postgadolinium T1 MRI of multiple brain metastases from non-small cell lung cancer involving the right frontal (***A***) and right cerebellar (***B***) hemispheres. Note the diffuse enhancement pattern and absence of central necrosis.

the majority of brain metastases. The radiographic appearance of brain metastasis is nonspecific, and similar appearing lesions can occur with infection including brain abscesses and also with demyelinating lesions, sarcoidosis, radiation necrosis in a previously treated patient, or a primary brain tumor that may be a second malignancy in a patient with systemic cancer. However, biopsy is rarely necessary for diagnosis in most patients because imaging alone in the appropriate clinical situation usually suffices. This is straightforward for the majority of patients with brain metastases because they have a known systemic cancer. However, in approximately 10% of patients a systemic cancer may present with a brain metastasis, and if there is not an easily accessible systemic site to biopsy, then a brain lesion must be removed for diagnostic purposes.

TREATMENT Tumors Metastatic to the Brain

DEFINITIVE TREATMENT The number and location of brain metastases often determine the therapeutic options. The patient's overall condition and the current or potential control of the systemic disease are also major determinants. Brain metastases are single in approximately one-half of patients and multiple in the other half.

RADIATION THERAPY The standard treatment for brain metastases has been whole-brain radiotherapy (WBRT) usually administered to a total dose of 3000 cGy in 10 fractions. This affords rapid palliation, and approximately 80% of patients improve with glucocorticoids and radiation therapy. However, it is not curative. Median survival is only 4–6 months. More recently, stereotactic radiosurgery (SRS) delivered through a variety of techniques including the gamma knife, linear accelerator, proton beam, and CyberKnife all can deliver highly focused doses of RT, usually in a single fraction. SRS can effectively sterilize the visible lesions and afford local disease control in 80–90% of patients. In addition, there are some patients who have clearly been cured of their brain metastases using SRS, whereas this is distinctly rare with WBRT. However, SRS can be used only for lesions 3 cm or less in diameter and should be confined to patients with only 1–3 metastases. The addition of WBRT to SRS improves disease control in the nervous system but does not prolong survival.

SURGERY Randomized controlled trials have demonstrated that surgical extirpation of a single brain metastasis followed by WBRT is superior to WBRT alone. Removal of two lesions or a single symptomatic mass, particularly if compressing the ventricular system, can also be useful. This is particularly useful in patients who have highly radioresistant lesions such as renal carcinoma. Surgical resection can afford rapid symptomatic improvement and prolonged survival. RT administered after complete resection of a brain metastasis improves disease control but does not prolong survival.

CHEMOTHERAPY Chemotherapy is rarely useful for brain metastases. Metastases from certain tumor types that are highly chemosensitive, such as germ cell tumors or small cell lung cancer, may respond to chemotherapeutic regimens chosen according to the underlying malignancy. Increasingly, there are data demonstrating responsiveness of brain metastases to chemotherapy including small molecule–targeted therapy when the lesion possesses the target. This has been best illustrated in patients with lung cancer harboring EGFR mutations that sensitize them to EGFR inhibitors. Antiangiogenic agents such as bevacizumab may also prove efficacious in the treatment of CNS metastases.

LEPTOMENINGEAL METASTASES

Leptomeningeal metastases are also identified as carcinomatous meningitis, meningeal carcinomatosis, or in the case of specific tumors, leukemic or lymphomatous meningitis. Among the hematologic malignancies, acute leukemia is the most common to metastasize to the subarachnoid space, and in lymphomas the aggressive diffuse lymphomas can metastasize to the subarachnoid space frequently as well. Among solid tumors, breast and lung carcinomas and melanoma most frequently spread in this fashion. Tumor cells reach the subarachnoid space via the arterial circulation or occasionally through retrograde flow in venous systems that drain metastases along the bony spine or cranium. In addition, leptomeningeal metastases may develop as a direct consequence of prior brain metastases and can develop in almost 40% of patients who have a metastasis resected from the cerebellum.

CLINICAL FEATURES

Leptomeningeal metastases are characterized clinically by multilevel symptoms and signs along the neuraxis. Combinations of lumbar and cervical radiculopathies, cranial neuropathies, seizures, confusion, and encephalopathy from hydrocephalus or raised intracranial pressure can be present. Focal deficits such as hemiparesis or aphasia are rarely due to leptomeningeal metastases unless there is direct brain infiltration and are more often associated with coexisting brain lesions. New onset limb pain in patients with breast, lung cancer, or melanoma should prompt consideration of leptomeningeal spread.

LABORATORY AND IMAGING DIAGNOSIS

Leptomeningeal metastases are particularly challenging to diagnose as identification of tumor cells in the subarachnoid compartment may be elusive. MR imaging can be definitive in patients when there are clear tumor nodules adherent to the cauda equina or spinal cord, enhancing cranial nerves, or subarachnoid enhancement on brain imaging (Fig. 379-9). Imaging is diagnostic in approximately 75% of patients and is more often positive in patients with solid tumors. Demonstration of tumor cells in the CSF is definitive and often considered the gold standard. However, CSF cytologic examination is positive in only 50% of patients on the first lumbar puncture and still misses 10% after three CSF samples. CSF cytologic examination is most useful in hematologic malignancies. Accompanying CSF abnormalities include an elevated protein concentration and an elevated white count. Hypoglycorrhachia is noted in less than 25% of patients but is useful when present. Identification of tumor markers or molecular confirmation of clonal proliferation with techniques such as flow cytometry within the CSF can also be definitive when present. Tumor markers are usually specific to solid tumors, and chromosomal or molecular markers are most useful in patients with hematologic malignancies.

TREATMENT Leptomeningeal Metastases

The treatment of leptomeningeal metastasis is palliative as there is no curative therapy. RT to the symptomatically involved areas, such as skull base for cranial neuropathy, can relieve pain and sometimes improve function. Whole neuraxis RT has extensive toxicity with myelosuppression and gastrointestinal irritation

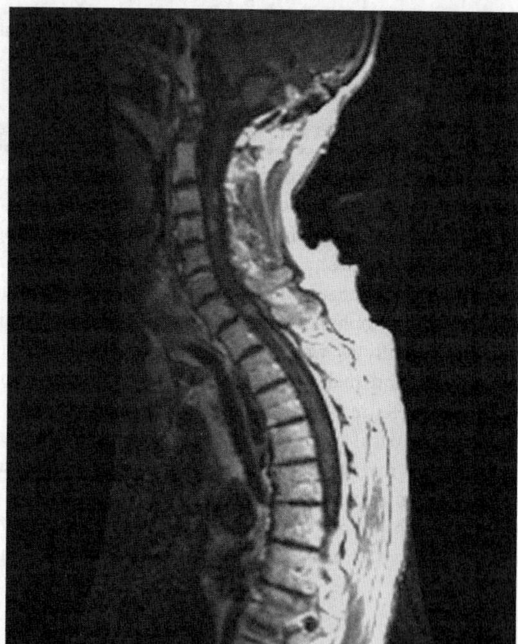

A

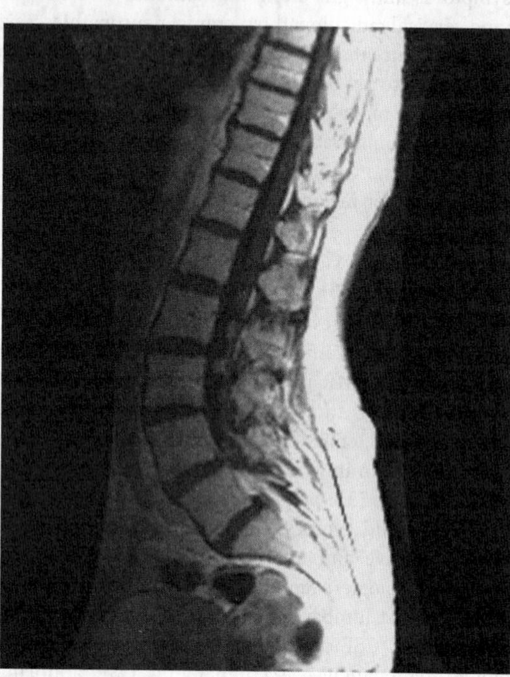

B

Figure 379-9 Postgadolinium MRI images of extensive leptomeningeal metastases from breast cancer. Nodules along the dorsal surface of the spinal cord (***A***) and cauda equina (***B***) are seen.

as well as limited effectiveness. Systemic chemotherapy with agents that can penetrate the blood-CSF barrier may be helpful. Alternatively, intrathecal chemotherapy can be effective, particularly in hematologic malignancies. This is optimally delivered through an intraventricular cannula (Ommaya reservoir) rather than by lumbar puncture. Few drugs can be delivered safely into the subarachnoid space and they have a limited spectrum of antitumor activity, perhaps accounting for the relatively poor response to this approach. In addition, impaired CSF flow dynamics can compromise intrathecal drug delivery. Surgery has a limited role in the treatment of leptomeningeal metastasis, but placement of a ventriculoperitoneal shunt can relieve raised intracranial pressure. However, it compromises delivery of chemotherapy into the CSF.

EPIDURAL METASTASIS

Epidural metastasis occurs in 3–5% of patients with a systemic malignancy and causes neurologic compromise by compressing the spinal cord or cauda equina. The most common cancers that metastasize to the epidural space are those malignancies that spread to bone, such as breast and prostate. Lymphoma can cause bone involvement and compression but it can also invade the intervertebral foramens and cause spinal cord compression without bone destruction. The thoracic spine is affected most commonly, followed by the lumbar and then cervical spine.

■ CLINICAL FEATURES

Back pain is the presenting symptom of epidural metastasis in virtually all patients; the pain may precede neurologic findings by weeks or months. The pain is usually exacerbated by lying down; by contrast, arthritic pain is often relieved by recumbency. Leg weakness is seen in about 50% of patients as is sensory dysfunction. Sphincter problems are present in about 25% of patients at diagnosis.

■ DIAGNOSIS

Diagnosis is established by imaging, with MRI of the complete spine being the best test (Fig. 379-10). Contrast is not needed to identify spinal or epidural lesions. Any patient with cancer who has severe back pain should undergo an MRI. Plain films, bone scans, or even CT scans may show bone metastases, but only MRI can reliably delineate epidural tumor. For patients unable to have an MRI, CT myelography should be performed to outline the epidural space. The differential diagnosis of epidural tumor includes epidural abscess, acute or chronic hematomas, and rarely, extramedullary hematopoiesis.

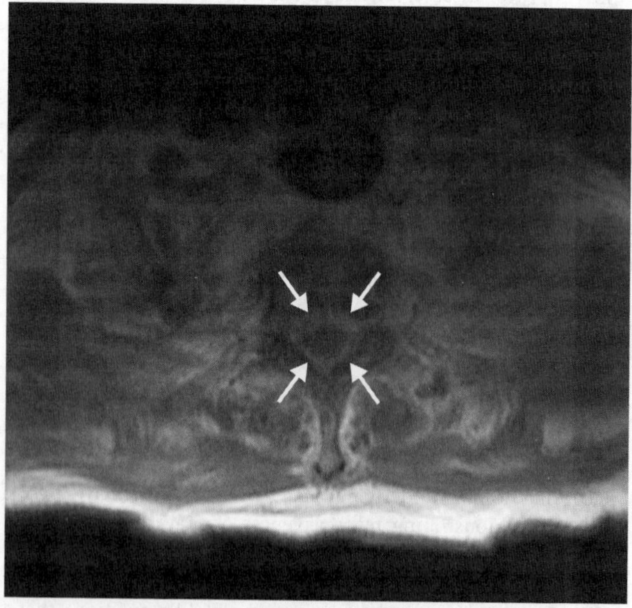

Figure 379-10 Postgadolinium T1 MRI showing circumferential epidural tumor around the thoracic spinal cord from esophageal cancer.

TREATMENT Epidural Metastasis

Epidural metastasis requires immediate treatment. A randomized controlled trial demonstrated the superiority of surgical resection followed by RT compared to RT alone. However, patients must be able to tolerate surgery, and the surgical procedure of choice is a complete removal of the mass, which is typically anterior to the spinal canal, necessitating an extensive approach and resection. Otherwise, RT is the mainstay of treatment and can be used for patients with radiosensitive tumors, such as lymphoma, or for those unable to undergo surgery. Chemotherapy is rarely used for epidural metastasis unless the patient has minimal to no neurologic deficit and a highly chemosensitive tumor such as lymphoma or germinoma. Patients generally fare well if treated before there is severe neurologic deficit. Recovery after paraparesis is better after surgery than with RT alone, but survival is often short due to widespread metastatic tumor.

NEUROLOGIC TOXICITY OF THERAPY

TOXICITY FROM RADIOTHERAPY

Radiotherapy can cause a variety of toxicities in the CNS. These are usually described based on their relationship in time to the administration of RT, e.g., they can be acute (occurring within days of RT), early delayed (months), or late delayed (years). In general, the acute and early delayed syndromes resolve and do not result in persistent deficits, whereas the late delayed toxicities are usually permanent and sometimes progressive.

Acute toxicity

Acute cerebral toxicity usually occurs during RT to the brain. RT can cause a transient disruption of the blood-brain barrier, resulting in increased edema and elevated intracranial pressure. This is usually manifest as headache, lethargy, nausea and vomiting, and can be both prevented and treated with the administration of glucocorticoids. There is no acute RT toxicity that affects the spinal cord.

Early delayed toxicity

Early delayed toxicity is usually apparent weeks to months after completion of cranial irradiation and is likely due to focal demyelination. Clinically it may be asymptomatic or take the form of worsening or reappearance of a preexisting neurologic deficit. At times a contrast-enhancing lesion can be seen on MRI/CT that can mimic the tumor for which the patient received the RT. For patients with a malignant glioma, this has been described as "pseudoprogression" because it mimics tumor recurrence on MRI but actually represents inflammation and necrotic debris engendered by effective therapy. This is seen with increased frequency when chemotherapy, particularly temozolomide, is given concurrently with RT. Pseudoprogression can resolve on its own or, if very symptomatic, may require resection. A rare form of early delayed toxicity is the somnolence syndrome that occurs primarily in children and is characterized by marked sleepiness.

In the spinal cord, early delayed RT toxicity is manifest as a Lhermitte symptom with paresthesias of the limbs or along the spine when the patient flexes the neck. Although frightening, it is benign, resolves on its own, and does not portend more serious problems.

Late delayed toxicity

Late delayed toxicities are the most serious as they are often irreversible and cause severe neurologic deficits. In the brain, late toxicities can take several forms, the most common of which include radiation necrosis and leukoencephalopathy. Radiation necrosis is a focal mass of necrotic tissue that is contrast enhancing on CT/MRI and may be associated with significant edema. This may appear identical to pseudoprogression but is seen months to years after RT and is always symptomatic. Clinical symptoms and signs include seizure and lateralizing findings referable to the location of the necrotic mass. The necrosis is caused by the effect of RT on cerebral vasculature with resultant fibrinoid necrosis and occlusion of the blood vessels. It can mimic tumor radiographically, but unlike tumor it is typically hypometabolic on a PET scan and has reduced perfusion on perfusion MR sequences. It may require resection for diagnosis and treatment unless it can be managed with glucocorticoids. There are rare reports of improvement with hyperbaric oxygen or anticoagulation but the usefulness of these approaches is questionable.

Leukoencephalopathy is seen most commonly after WBRT as opposed to focal RT. On T2 or FLAIR MR sequences there is diffuse increased signal seen throughout the hemispheric white matter, often bilaterally and symmetrically. There tends to be a periventricular predominance that may be associated with atrophy and ventricular enlargement. Clinically, patients develop cognitive impairment, gait disorder, and later urinary incontinence, all of which can progress over time. These symptoms mimic those of normal pressure hydrocephalus, and placement of a ventriculoperitoneal shunt can improve function in some patients but does not reverse the deficits completely. Increased age is a risk factor for leukoencephalopathy but not for radiation necrosis. Necrosis appears to depend on an as yet unidentified predisposition.

Other late neurologic toxicities include endocrine dysfunction if the pituitary or hypothalamus was included in the RT port. A radiation-induced neoplasm can occur many years after therapeutic RT for either a prior CNS tumor or a head and neck cancer; accurate diagnosis requires surgical resection or biopsy. In addition, RT causes accelerated atherosclerosis, which can cause stroke either from intracranial vascular disease or carotid plaque from neck irradiation.

The peripheral nervous system is relatively resistant to RT toxicities. Peripheral nerves are rarely affected by RT, but the plexus is more vulnerable. Plexopathy develops more commonly in the brachial distribution than in the lumbosacral distribution. It must be differentiated from tumor progression in the plexus, which is usually accomplished with CT/MR imaging of the area or PET scan demonstrating tumor infiltrating the region. Clinically, tumor progression is usually painful whereas radiation-induced plexopathy is painless. Radiation plexopathy is also more commonly associated with lymphedema of the affected limb. Sensory loss and weakness are seen in both.

TOXICITY FROM CHEMOTHERAPY

Neurotoxicity is second to myelosuppression as the dose-limiting toxicity of chemotherapeutic agents (Table 379-4). Chemotherapy causes peripheral neuropathy from a number of commonly used agents, and the type of neuropathy can differ, depending upon the drug. Vincristine causes paresthesias but little sensory loss and is associated with motor dysfunction, autonomic impairment (frequently ileus), and rarely cranial nerve compromise. Cisplatin causes large fiber sensory loss resulting in sensory ataxia but little cutaneous sensory loss and no weakness. The taxanes also cause a predominately sensory neuropathy. Agents such as bortezomib and thalidomide also cause neuropathy.

Encephalopathy and seizures are common toxicities from chemotherapeutic drugs. Ifosfamide can cause a severe encephalopathy, which is reversible with discontinuation of the drug and the use of methylene blue for severely affected patients. Fludarabine also causes a severe global encephalopathy that may be permanent.

TABLE 379-4 Neurologic Signs Caused by Agents Commonly Used in Patients With Cancer

Acute encephalopathy (delirium)	Seizures
Methotrexate (high-dose IV, IT)	Methotrexate
Cisplatin	Etoposide (high-dose)
Vincristine	Cisplatin
Asparaginase	Vincristine
Procarbazine	Asparaginase
5-Flourouracil (±levamisole)	Nitrogen mustard
Cytarabine (high-dose)	Carmustine
Nitrosoureas (high-dose or arterial)	Dacarbazine (intraarterial or high-dose)
Ifosfamide	Busulfan (high-dose)
Etoposide (high-dose)	
Bevacizumab (PRES)	Myelopathy (intrathecal drugs)
	Methotrexate
Chronic encephalopathy (dementia)	Cytarabine
Methotrexate	Thiotepa
Carmustine	
Cytarabine	Peripheral neuropathy
Fludarabine	Vinca alkaloids
	Cisplatin
Visual loss	Procarbazine
Tamoxifen	Etoposide
Gallium nitrate	Teniposide
Cisplatin	Cytarabine
Fludarabine	Taxanes
	Suramin
Cerebellar dysfunction/ataxia	Bortezomib
5-Fluorouracil (± levamisole)	
Cytarabine	
Procarbazine	

Abbreviations: IT, intrathecal; IV, intravenous; PRES, posterior reversible encephalopathy syndrome.

Bevacizumab and other anti-VEGF agents can cause posterior reversible encephalopathy syndrome. Cisplatin can cause hearing loss and less frequently vestibular dysfunction.

FURTHER READINGS

Clarke JL et al: Leptomeningeal metastases in the MRI era. Neurology 76:200, 2011

DeAngelis LM, Posner JB (eds): *Neurologic Complications of Cancer*, 2nd ed, New York, Oxford University Press, 2009

Elliott RE et al: Neurological complications and symptom resolution following Gamma Knife surgery for brain metastases 2 cm or smaller in relation to eloquent cortices. J Neurosurg: 113 Suppl:53, 2010

Friedman HS et al: Bevacizumab alone and in combination with irinotecan in recurrent glioblastoma. J Clin Oncol 27:4733, 2009

Lu-Emerson C, Plotkin SR: The neurofibromatoses. Part 1: NF1. Rev Neurol Dis 6:E47, 2009

________, ________: The neurofibromatoses. Part 2: NF2 and schwannomatosis. Rev Neurol Dis 6:E81, 2009

Rades D, Abrahm JL: The role of radiotherapy for metastatic epidural spinal cord compression. Nat Rev Clin Oncol 7:590, 2010

Stupp R et al: Effects of radiotherapy with concomitant and adjuvant temozolomide versus radiotherapy alone on survival in glioblastoma in a randomized phase III study: 5-Year analysis of the EORTC-NCIC trial. Lancet Oncol 10:459, 2009

Wang M et al: Cognition and quality of life after chemotherapy plus radiotherapy (RT) vs. RT for pure and mixed anaplastic oligodendrogliomas: Radiation Therapy Oncology Group Trial 9402. Int J Radiat Oncol Biol Phys 77:662, 2010

Wen PY, Kesari S: Malignant gliomas in adults. N Engl J Med 359:492, 2008

CHAPTER 380

Multiple Sclerosis and Other Demyelinating Diseases

Stephen L. Hauser
Douglas S. Goodin

Demyelinating disorders are immune-mediated conditions characterized by preferential destruction of central nervous system (CNS) myelin. The peripheral nervous system (PNS) is spared, and most patients have no evidence of an associated systemic illness. Multiple sclerosis (MS), the most common disease in this category, is second only to trauma as a cause of neurologic disability beginning in early to middle adulthood.

MULTIPLE SCLEROSIS

Multiple sclerosis (MS) is a chronic disease characterized by inflammation, demyelination, gliosis (scarring), and neuronal loss; the course can be relapsing-remitting or progressive. Lesions of MS typically occur at different times and in different CNS locations (i.e., disseminated in time and space). MS affects ~350,000 individuals in the United States and 2.5 million individuals worldwide. Manifestations of MS vary from a benign illness to a rapidly evolving and incapacitating disease requiring profound lifestyle adjustments.

PATHOGENESIS

Anatomy

New MS lesions begin with perivenular cuffing by inflammatory mononuclear cells, predominantly T cells and macrophages, which also infiltrate the surrounding white matter. At sites of inflammation, the blood-brain barrier (BBB) is disrupted, but unlike vasculitis, the vessel wall is preserved. Involvement of the humoral immune system is also evident; small numbers of B lymphocytes also infiltrate the nervous system, and myelin-specific autoantibodies are present on degenerating myelin sheaths. As lesions evolve, there is prominent astrocytic proliferation (gliosis). Surviving oligodendrocytes or those that differentiate from precursor cells can partially remyelinate the surviving naked axons, producing so-called shadow plaques. In many lesions, oligodendrocyte precursor cells are present in large numbers but fail to differentiate and remyelinate. Over time, ectopic lymphocyte follicles appear in perivascular and perimeningeal regions, consisting of aggregates of T and B cells and resembling secondary lymphoid structures. Although relative sparing of axons is typical of MS, partial or total axonal destruction can also occur, especially within highly inflammatory lesions. Thus, MS is not solely a disease of myelin, and neuronal pathology is increasingly recognized as a major contributor to irreversible neurologic disability. Inflammation and plaque formation are present in the cerebral cortex, and significant axon loss indicating death of neurons is widespread, specially in advanced cases (see "Neurodegeneration," below).

Physiology

Nerve conduction in myelinated axons occurs in a saltatory manner, with the nerve impulse jumping from one node of Ranvier to the next without depolarization of the axonal membrane underlying the myelin sheath between nodes (Fig. 380-1). This produces considerably faster conduction velocities (~70 m/s) than the slow velocities (~1 m/s) produced by continuous propagation in unmyelinated nerves. Conduction block occurs when the nerve impulse is unable to traverse the demyelinated segment. This can happen when the resting axon membrane becomes hyperpolarized due to the exposure of voltage-dependent potassium channels that are normally buried underneath the myelin sheath. A temporary conduction block often follows a demyelinating event before sodium channels (originally concentrated at the nodes) redistribute along the naked axon (Fig. 380-1). This redistribution ultimately allows continuous propagation of nerve action potentials through the demyelinated segment. Conduction block may be incomplete, affecting high- but not low-frequency volleys of impulses. Variable conduction block can occur with raised body temperature or metabolic alterations and may explain clinical fluctuations that vary from hour to hour or appear with fever or exercise. Conduction slowing occurs when the demyelinated segments of the axonal membrane is reorganized to support continuous (slow) nerve impulse propagation.

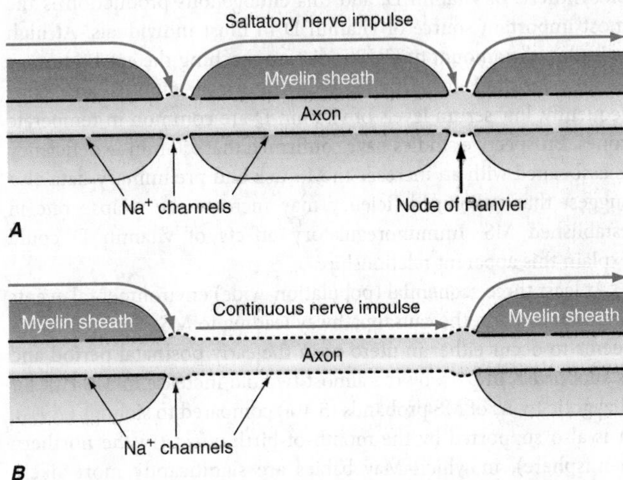

Figure 380-1 Nerve conduction in myelinated and demyelinated axons. ***A.*** Saltatory nerve conduction in myelinated axons occurs with the nerve impulse jumping from one node of Ranvier to the next. Sodium channels (shown as breaks in the solid black line) are concentrated at the nodes where axonal depolarization occurs. ***B.*** Following demyelination, additional sodium channels are redistributed along the axon itself, thereby allowing continuous propagation of the nerve action potential despite the absence of myelin.

Epidemiology

MS is approximately threefold more common in women than men. The age of onset is typically between 20 and 40 years (slightly later in men than in women), but the disease can present across the life span. In ~10% of cases it begins before age 18 years and a in a small percentage it begins before the age of 10 years.

Geographic gradients have been repeatedly observed in MS, with the highest known prevalence for MS (250 per 100,000) in the Orkney Islands, located north of Scotland. In other temperate zone areas (e.g., northern North America, northern Europe, southern Australia, and south New Zealand), the prevalence of MS is 0.1–0.2%. By contrast, in the tropics (e.g., Asia, equatorial Africa, and the Middle East), the prevalence is often ten- to twentyfold less.

One proposed explanation for the latitude effect on MS is that there is a protective effect of sun exposure. Exposure of the skin to ultraviolet-B (UVB) radiation from the sun is essential for the biosynthesis of vitamin D, and this endogenous production is the most important source of vitamin D in most individuals. At high latitudes, the amount of UVB radiation reaching the earth's surface is often insufficient, particularly during winter months, and, consequently, low serum levels of vitamin D are common in temperate zones. Prospective studies have confirmed that vitamin D deficiency is associated with an increase in MS risk and preliminary data also suggest that ongoing deficiency may increase the relapse rate in established MS. Immunoregulatory effects of vitamin D could explain this apparent relationship.

At least three sequential (population-wide) environmental events are implicated in the causal pathway leading to MS. The first factor seems to occur either in utero or in the early postnatal period and is supported, in part, by the almost twofold increase in MS risk for dizygotic twins of MS probands (5.4%) compared to siblings (2.9%). It is also supported by the month-of-birth effect (in the northern hemisphere), in which May babies are significantly more likely, and November babies less likely, to develop MS compared to babies born in other months. Importantly, a recently published population-based study in the southern hemisphere (Australia) found a similar (but inverted) month-of-birth effect with the zenith in risk occurring for November/December babies and the nadir occurring for May/June babies. This month-of-birth effect provides evidence for an early environmental event, involved in MS pathogenesis, that is both coupled to the solar cycle and time-locked to birth.

A second factor seems to occur during adolescence. Thus, several studies suggest that when individuals move (prior to their adolescent years) from an area of high MS prevalence to an area of low prevalence (or vice versa), their MS risk becomes similar to that of the region to which they moved. By contrast, when they make the same move after adolescence, their MS risk remains similar to that of the region from which they moved.

Because both of these first two factors occur well before the onset of clinically evident MS, presumably other factors are also necessary. In addition, the identification of possible point epidemics suggests a possible role for infectious agents, although the only (partially) convincing example of this occurred in the Faeroe Islands north of Denmark after the British occupation during World War II.

The prevalence of MS has increased steadily (and dramatically) in several regions around the world over the past half-century, presumably reflecting the impact of some environmental shift. Moreover, the fact that this increase has occurred primarily (or exclusively) in women indicates that women are more responsive to whatever this environmental change has been. Interestingly, recent epidemiologic data suggest that the latitude effect on MS currently may be decreasing. The reason for these changes are not known but, potentially, could be related to the increased use of sun block, which (at SPF-15) blocks 94% of the incoming UVB radiation, and which would be expected to exacerbate any population-wide vitamin D deficiency and might also mitigate the impact of differences in UVB exposure.

MS risk also correlates with high socioeconomic status, which may reflect improved sanitation and delayed initial exposures to infectious agents. By analogy, some viral infections (e.g., poliomyelitis and measles viruses) produce neurologic sequelae more frequently when the age of initial infection is delayed. Evidence of a remote Epstein-Barr virus (EBV) infection playing some role in MS is supported by a number of epidemiologic and laboratory studies. A higher risk of infectious mononucleosis (associated with relatively late EBV infection) and higher antibody titers to latency-associated EBV nuclear antigen are associated with MS. At this time, however, a causal role for EBV is not definitively established.

TABLE 380-1 Risk of Developing MS

1 in 3	If an identical twin has MS
1 in 15	If a fraternal twin has MS
1 in 25	If a sibling has MS
1 in 50	If a parent or half-sibling has MS
1 in 100	If a first cousin has MS
1 in 1000	If a spouse has MS
1 in 1000	If no one in the family has MS

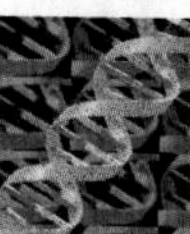

GENETIC CONSIDERATIONS

Whites are inherently at higher risk for MS than Africans or Asians, even when residing in a similar environment. MS also aggregates within some families, and adoption, half-sibling, twin, and spousal studies indicate that familial aggregation is due to genetic, and not environmental, factors (Table 380-1).

Whites to MS is polygenic, with each gene contributing a relatively small amount to the overall risk. Despite this, the influence of genetics on MS pathogenesis is substantial. The major histocompatibility complex (MHC) on chromosome 6 is by far the strongest MS susceptibility region in the genome. Fine mapping studies implicate primarily the class II region (encoding HLA molecules involved in presenting peptide antigens to T cells) and specifically the highly polymorphic *DRB1* locus, which contributes to MS risk in a allele-dependent hierarchical fashion, with the strongest association consistently found with the *DRB1*15:01* allele; a secondary signal that appears to be protective against MS is located in the class 1 region near HLA-C. Whole-genome association studies have now identified more than 50 MS susceptibility genes, each of which has only a very small effect on MS risk. *DRB1*15:01* increases MS risk by approximately threefold in the heterozygous state, and ninefold in the homozygous state; by contrast, other MS-associated variants increase risk only by 15–30%. Most MS-associated genetic variants have known roles in the immune system [i.e., genes for the interleukin (IL)-7 receptor (CD127), the IL-2 receptor (CD25), and the T cell co-stimulatory molecule LFA-3 (CD58)]; some variants also influence susceptibility to other autoimmune diseases in addition to MS. The variants identified thus far all lack specificity and sensitivity for MS, thus they are not useful for diagnosis or to predict the future course of the disease.

Immunology

Autoreactive T lymphocytes Myelin basic protein (MBP) is an important T cell antigen in experimental allergic encephalomyelitis (EAE), a laboratory model, and probably also in human MS. Activated MBP-reactive T cells have been identified in the blood, in cerebrospinal fluid (CSF), and within MS lesions. Moreover, *DRB1*15:01* may influence the autoimmune response because it binds with high affinity to a fragment of MBP (spanning amino acids 89–96), stimulating T cell responses to this self-protein. Two different populations of proinflammatory T cells are likely to mediate autoimmunity in MS. T-helper type 1 (T_H1) cells producing interferon γ (IFN-γ) are one key effector population, and more recently a role for highly proinflammatory T_H17 T cells has been established. T_H17 cells are induced by transforming growth factor β (TGF-β) and IL-6, and are amplified by IL-21 and IL-23. T_H17 cells, and levels of their corresponding cytokine IL-17, are increased in MS lesions and also in the circulation of people with active MS.

High circulating levels of IL-17 may also be a marker of a more severe course of MS. T_H1 cytokines including interleukin (IL) 2, tumor necrosis factor (TNF) α, and interferon (IFN) γ also play key roles in activating and maintaining autoimmune responses, and TNF-α and IFN-γ may directly injure oligodendrocytes or the myelin membrane.

Humoral autoimmunity B cell activation and antibody responses also appear to be necessary for the full development of demyelinating lesions to occur, both in experimental models and in human MS. Increased numbers of clonally expanded B cells with properties of postgerminal center memory or antibody-producing lymphocytes are present in MS lesions and in CSF. Myelin-specific autoantibodies, some directed against myelin oligodendrocyte glycoprotein (MOG), have been detected bound to vesiculated myelin debris in MS plaques. In the CSF, elevated levels of locally synthesized immunoglobulins and oligoclonal antibodies derived from expansion of clonally restricted plasma cells are also characteristic of MS. The pattern of oligoclonal banding is unique to each individual, and attempts to identify the targets of these antibodies have been largely unsuccessful.

Triggers Serial MRI studies in early relapsing-remitting MS reveal that bursts of focal inflammatory disease activity occur far more frequently than would have been predicted by the frequency of relapses. Thus, early in MS most disease activity is clinically silent. The triggers causing these bursts are unknown, although the fact that patients may experience relapses after nonspecific upper respiratory infections suggests that either molecular mimicry between viruses and myelin antigens or viral super-antigens activating pathogenic T cells may be responsible (Chap. 318).

Neurodegeneration

Axonal damage occurs in every newly formed MS lesion, and cumulative axonal loss is considered to be the major cause of progressive and irreversible neurologic disability in MS. As many as 70% of axons are lost from the lateral corticospinal (e.g., motor) tracts in patients with advanced paraparesis from MS, and longitudinal MRI studies suggest there is progressive axonal loss over time within established, inactive lesions. Knowledge of the mechanisms responsible for axonal injury is incomplete and, despite the fact that axonal transactions are most conspicuous in acute inflammatory lesions, it is still unclear whether demyelination is a prerequisite for axonal injury in MS. Demyelination can result in reduced trophic support for axons, redistribution of ion channels, and destabilization of action potential membrane potentials. Axons can adapt initially to these injuries; with time distal and retrograde degeneration often occurs. Therefore, promotion of remyelination and preservation of oligodendrocytes early in the disease course remain important therapeutic goals in MS. Some evidence suggests that axonal damage is mediated directly by resident and invading inflammatory cells and their toxic products, in particular by microglia, macrophages, and CD8 T lymphocytes. Activated microglia are particularly likely to cause axonal injury through the release of NO and oxygen radicals and via glutamate, which is toxic to oligodendrocytes and neurons. Interestingly, NMDA (glutamate) receptors are expressed on naked axon membranes that have undergone demyelination, perhaps providing a mechanism for glutamate-mediated calcium entry and cell death.

■ CLINICAL MANIFESTATIONS

The onset of MS may be abrupt or insidious. Symptoms may be severe or seem so trivial that a patient may not seek medical attention for months or years. Indeed, at autopsy, approximately 0.1% of individuals who were asymptomatic during life will be found, unexpectedly, to have pathologic evidence of MS. Similarly, in the modern era, an MRI scan obtained for an unrelated reason may show evidence of asymptomatic MS. Symptoms of MS are extremely varied and depend on the location and severity of lesions within the CNS (Table 380-2). Examination often reveals evidence of neurologic dysfunction, often in asymptomatic locations. For example, a patient may present with symptoms in one leg but signs in both.

TABLE 380-2 Initial Symptoms of MS

Symptom	Percent of Cases	Symptom	Percent of Cases
Sensory loss	37	Lhermitte's	3
Optic neuritis	36	Pain	3
Weakness	35	Dementia	2
Paresthesias	24	Visual loss	2
Diplopia	15	Facial palsy	1
Ataxia	11	Impotence	1
Vertigo	6	Myokymia	1
Paroxysmal attacks	4	Epilepsy	1
Bladder	4	Falling	1

Source: After WB Matthews et al, *McAlpine's Multiple Sclerosis*, New York, Churchill Livingstone, 1991.

Weakness of the limbs may manifest as loss of strength, speed, or dexterity, as fatigue, or a disturbance of gait. Exercise-induced weakness is a characteristic symptom of MS. The weakness is of the upper motor neuron type (Chap. 22) and is usually accompanied by other pyramidal signs such as spasticity, hyperreflexia, and Babinski's signs. Occasionally a tendon reflex may be lost (simulating a lower motor neuron lesion) if an MS lesion disrupts the afferent reflex fibers in the spinal cord (Fig. 22-2).

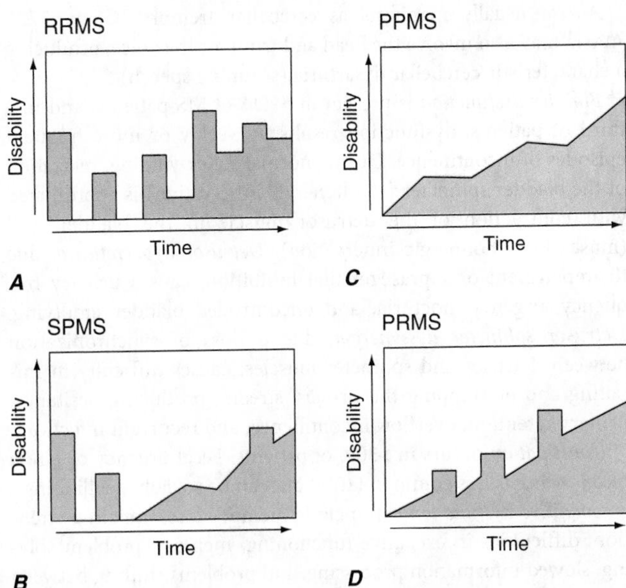

Figure 380-2 Clinical course of multiple sclerosis (MS). ***A.*** Relapsing/remitting MS. ***B.*** Secondary progressive MS. ***C.*** Primary progressive MS. ***D.*** Progressive/relapsing MS.

Spasticity (Chap. 22) is commonly associated with spontaneous and movement-induced muscle spasms. More than 30% of MS patients have moderate to severe spasticity, especially in the legs. This is often accompanied by painful spasms interfering with ambulation, work, or self-care. Occasionally spasticity provides support for the body weight during ambulation, and in these cases treatment of spasticity may actually do more harm than good.

Optic neuritis (ON) presents as diminished visual acuity, dimness, or decreased color perception (desaturation) in the central field of vision. These symptoms can be mild or may progress to severe visual loss. Rarely, there is complete loss of light perception. Visual symptoms are generally monocular but may be bilateral. Periorbital pain (aggravated by eye movement) often precedes or accompanies the visual loss. An afferent pupillary defect (Chap. 28) is usually present. Funduscopic examination may be normal or reveal optic disc swelling (papillitis). Pallor of the optic disc (optic atrophy) commonly follows ON. Uveitis is uncommon and should raise the possibility of alternative diagnoses such as sarcoid or lymphoma.

Visual blurring in MS may result from ON or diplopia (double vision); if the symptom resolves when either eye is covered, the cause is diplopia.

Diplopia may result from internuclear ophthalmoplegia (INO) or from palsy of the sixth cranial nerve (rarely the third or fourth). An INO consists of impaired adduction of one eye due to a lesion in the ipsilateral medial longitudinal fasciculus (Chap. 28). Prominent nystagmus is often observed in the abducting eye, along with a small skew deviation. A bilateral INO is particularly suggestive of MS. Other common gaze disturbances in MS include (1) a horizontal gaze palsy, (2) a "one and a half" syndrome (horizontal gaze palsy plus an INO), and (3) acquired pendular nystagmus.

Sensory symptoms are varied and include both paresthesias (e.g., tingling, prickling sensations, formications, "pins and needles," or painful burning) and hypesthesia (e.g., reduced sensation, numbness, or a "dead" feeling). Unpleasant sensations (e.g., feelings that body parts are swollen, wet, raw, or tightly wrapped) are also common. Sensory impairment of the trunk and legs below a horizontal line on the torso (a sensory level) indicates that the spinal cord is the origin of the sensory disturbance. It is often accompanied by a bandlike sensation of tightness around the torso. Pain is a common symptom of MS, experienced by >50% of patients. Pain can occur anywhere on the body and can change locations over time.

Ataxia usually manifests as cerebellar tremors (Chap. 373). Ataxia may also involve the head and trunk or the voice, producing a characteristic cerebellar dysarthria (scanning speech).

Bladder dysfunction is present in >90% of MS patients, and in a third of patients, dysfunction results in weekly or more frequent episodes of incontinence. During normal reflex voiding, relaxation of the bladder sphincter (α-adrenergic innervation) is coordinated with contraction of the detrusor muscle in the bladder wall (muscarinic cholinergic innervation). *Detrusor hyperreflexia*, due to impairment of suprasegmental inhibition, causes urinary frequency, urgency, nocturia, and uncontrolled bladder emptying. *Detrusor sphincter dyssynergia*, due to loss of synchronization between detrusor and sphincter muscles, causes difficulty in initiating and/or stopping the urinary stream, producing hesitancy, urinary retention, overflow incontinence, and recurrent infection.

Constipation occurs in >30% of patients. Fecal urgency or *bowel incontinence* is less common (15%) but can be socially debilitating.

Cognitive dysfunction can include memory loss, impaired attention, difficulties in executive functioning, memory, problem solving, slowed information processing, and problems shifting between cognitive tasks. Euphoria (elevated mood) was once thought to be characteristic of MS but is actually uncommon, occurring in <20% of patients. Cognitive dysfunction sufficient to impair activities of daily living is rare.

Depression, experienced by approximately half of patients, can be reactive, endogenous, or part of the illness itself, and can contribute to fatigue. *Fatigue* is experienced by 90% of patients; this symptom is the most common reason for work-related disability in MS. Fatigue can be exacerbated by elevated temperatures, by depression, by expending exceptional effort to accomplish basic activities of daily living, or by sleep disturbances (e.g., from frequent nocturnal awakenings to urinate).

Sexual dysfunction may manifest as decreased libido, impaired genital sensation, impotence in men, and diminished vaginal lubrication or adductor spasms in women.

Facial weakness due to a lesion in the pons may resemble idiopathic Bell's palsy (Chap. 376). Unlike Bell's palsy, facial weakness in MS is usually not associated with ipsilateral loss of taste sensation or retroauricular pain.

Vertigo may appear suddenly from a brainstem lesion, superficially resembling acute labyrinthitis (Chap. 21). *Hearing loss* may also occur in MS but is uncommon.

Ancillary symptoms

Heat sensitivity refers to neurologic symptoms produced by an elevation of the body's core temperature. For example, unilateral visual blurring may occur during a hot shower or with physical exercise (*Uhthoff's symptom*). It is also common for MS symptoms to worsen transiently, sometimes dramatically, during febrile illnesses (see "Acute Attacks or Initial Demyelinating Episodes," below). Such heat-related symptoms probably result from transient conduction block (see above).

Lhermitte's symptom is an electric shock–like sensation (typically induced by flexion or other movements of the neck) that radiates down the back into the legs. Rarely, it radiates into the arms. It is generally self-limited but may persist for years. Lhermitte's symptom can also occur with other disorders of the cervical spinal cord (e.g., cervical spondylosis).

Paroxysmal symptoms are distinguished by their brief duration (10 s to 2 min), high frequency (5–40 episodes per day), lack of any alteration of consciousness or change in background electroencephalogram during episodes, and a self-limited course (generally lasting weeks to months). They may be precipitated by hyperventilation or movement. These syndromes may include Lhermitte's symptom; tonic contractions of a limb, face, or trunk (tonic seizures); paroxysmal dysarthria and ataxia; paroxysmal sensory disturbances; and several other less well characterized syndromes. Paroxysmal symptoms probably result from spontaneous discharges, arising at the edges of demyelinated plaques and spreading to adjacent white matter tracts.

Trigeminal neuralgia, hemifacial spasm, and *glossopharyngeal neuralgia* (Chap. 376) can occur when the demyelinating lesion involves the root entry (or exit) zone of the fifth, seventh, and ninth cranial nerve, respectively. Trigeminal neuralgia (tic douloureux) is a very brief lancinating facial pain often triggered by an afferent input from the face or teeth. Most cases of trigeminal neuralgia are not MS related; however, atypical features such as onset before age 50 years, bilateral symptoms, objective sensory loss, or nonparoxysmal pain should raise concerns that MS could be responsible.

Facial myokymia consists of either persistent rapid flickering contractions of the facial musculature (especially the lower portion of the orbicularis oculi) or a contraction that slowly spreads across the face. It results from lesions of the corticobulbar tracts or brainstem course of the facial nerve.

DISEASE COURSE

Four clinical types of MS have been described (Fig. 380-2):

1 *Relapsing/remitting MS* (RRMS) accounts for 85% of MS cases at onset and is characterized by discrete attacks that

generally evolve over days to weeks (rarely over hours). There is often complete recovery over the ensuing weeks to months (Fig. 380-2A). However, when ambulation is severely impaired during an attack, approximately half will fail to improve. Between attacks, patients are neurologically stable.

2 *Secondary progressive MS* (SPMS) always begins as RRMS (Fig. 380-2B). At some point, however, the clinical course changes so that the patient experiences a steady deterioration in function unassociated with acute attacks (which may continue or cease during the progressive phase). SPMS produces a greater amount of fixed neurologic disability than RRMS. For a patient with RRMS, the risk of developing SPMS is ~2% each year, meaning that the great majority of RRMS ultimately evolves into SPMS. SPMS appears to represent a late stage of the same underlying illness as RRMS.

3 *Primary progressive MS* (PPMS) accounts for ~15% of cases. These patients do not experience attacks but only a steady functional decline from disease onset (Fig. 380-2C). Compared to RRMS, the sex distribution is more even, the disease begins later in life (mean age ~40 years), and disability develops faster (at least relative to the onset of the first clinical symptom). Despite these differences, PPMS appears to represent the same underlying illness as RRMS.

4 *Progressive/relapsing MS* (PRMS) overlaps PPMS and SPMS and accounts for ~5% of MS patients. Like patients with PPMS, these patients experience a steady deterioration in their condition from disease onset. However, like SPMS patients, they experience occasional attacks superimposed upon their progressive course (Fig. 380-2D).

DIAGNOSIS

There is no definitive diagnostic test for MS. Diagnostic criteria for clinically definite MS require documentation of two or more episodes of symptoms and two or more signs that reflect pathology in anatomically noncontiguous white matter tracts of the CNS (Table 380-3). Symptoms must last for >24 h and occur as distinct episodes that are separated by a month or more. At least one of the two required signs must be present on neurologic examination. The second may be documented by abnormal paraclinical tests such as MRI or evoked potentials (EPs). Similarly, in the most recent diagnostic scheme, the second clinical event (in time) may be supported solely by paraclinical information, usually the development of new focal white matter lesions on MRI. In patients who experience gradual progression of disability for ≥6 months without superimposed relapses, documentation of intrathecal IgG synthesis may be used to support the diagnosis.

DIAGNOSTIC TESTS

Magnetic resonance imaging

MRI has revolutionized the diagnosis and management of MS (Fig. 380-3); characteristic abnormalities are found in >95% of patients although more than 90% of the lesions visualized by MRI are asymptomatic. An increase in vascular permeability from a breakdown of the BBB is detected by leakage of intravenous gadolinium (Gd) into the parenchyma. Such leakage occurs early in the development of an MS lesion and serves as a useful marker of inflammation. Gd enhancement persists for approximately 1 month, and the residual MS plaque remains visible indefinitely as a focal area of hyperintensity (a lesion) on spin-echo (T2-weighted) and proton-density images. Lesions are frequently oriented perpendicular to the ventricular surface, corresponding to the pathologic pattern of perivenous demyelination (Dawson's fingers). Lesions are multifocal within the brain, brainstem, and spinal cord. Lesions larger than 6 mm located in the corpus callosum, periventricular white matter, brainstem, cerebellum, or spinal cord are particularly helpful diagnostically. Different criteria for the use of MRI in the diagnosis of MS have been proposed (Table 380-3).

The total volume of T2-weighted signal abnormality (the "burden of disease") shows a significant (albeit weak) correlation with clinical disability, as do measures of brain atrophy. Approximately one-third of T2-weighted lesions appear as hypointense lesions (black holes) on T1-weighted imaging. Black holes may be a marker of irreversible demyelination and axonal loss, although even this measure depends on the timing of the image acquisition (e.g., most acute Gd-enhancing T2 lesions are T1 dark).

Newer MRI measures such as magnetization transfer ratio (MTR) imaging, and proton magnetic resonance spectroscopic imaging (MRSI) may ultimately serve as surrogate markers of clinical disability. MRSI can quantitate molecules such as *N*-acetyl aspartate, which is a marker of axonal integrity, and MTR may be able to distinguish demyelination from edema.

Evoked potentials

EP testing assesses function in afferent (visual, auditory, and somatosensory) or efferent (motor) CNS pathways. EPs use computer averaging to measure CNS electric potentials evoked by repetitive stimulation of selected peripheral nerves or of the brain. These tests provide the most information when the pathways studied are clinically uninvolved. For example, in a patient with a remitting and relapsing spinal cord syndrome with sensory deficits in the legs, an abnormal somatosensory EP following posterior tibial nerve stimulation provides little new information. By contrast, an abnormal visual EP in this circumstance would permit a diagnosis of clinically definite MS (Table 380-3). Abnormalities on one or more EP modalities occur in 80–90% of MS patients. EP abnormalities are not specific to MS, although a marked delay in the latency of a specific EP component (as opposed to a reduced amplitude or distorted wave-shape) is suggestive of demyelination.

Cerebrospinal fluid

CSF abnormalities found in MS include a mononuclear cell pleocytosis and an increased level of intrathecally synthesized IgG. The total CSF protein is usually normal or slightly elevated. Various formulas distinguish intrathecally synthesized IgG from IgG that may have entered the CNS passively from the serum. One formula, the CSF IgG index, expresses the ratio of IgG to albumin in the CSF divided by the same ratio in the serum. The IgG synthesis rate uses serum and CSF IgG and albumin measurements to calculate the rate of CNS IgG synthesis. The measurement of oligoclonal banding (OCB) in the CSF also assesses intrathecal production of IgG. OCBs are detected by agarose gel electrophoresis. Two or more OCBs are found in 75–90% of patients with MS. OCBs may be absent at the onset of MS, and in individual patients the number of bands may increase with time. It is important that paired serum samples be studied to exclude a peripheral (i.e., non-CNS) origin of any OCBs detected in the CSF.

A mild CSF pleocytosis (>5 cells/μL) is present in ~25% of cases, usually in young patients with RRMS. A pleocytosis of >75 cells/μL, the presence of polymorphonuclear leukocytes, or a protein concentration >1 g/L (>100 mg/dL) in CSF should raise concern that the patient may not have MS.

DIFFERENTIAL DIAGNOSIS

No single clinical sign or test is diagnostic of MS. The diagnosis is readily made in a young adult with relapsing and remitting symptoms involving different areas of CNS white matter. The possibility of an alternative diagnosis should always be considered

TABLE 380-3 Diagnostic Criteria for MS

Clinical Presentation	Additional Data Needed for MS diagnosis
2 or more attacks; objective clinical evidence of 2 or more lesions or objective clinical evidence of 1 lesion with reasonable historical evidence of a prior attack	None
2 or more attacks; objective clinical evidence of 1 lesion	Dissemination in space, demonstrated by ▪ ≥1 T2 lesion on MRI in at least two out of four MS-typical regions of the CNS (periventricular, juxtacortical, infratentorial, or spinal cord) OR ▪ Await a further clinical attack implicating a different CNS site
1 attack; objective clinical evidence of 2 or more lesions	Dissemination in time, demonstrated by ▪ Simultaneous presence of asymptomatic gadolinium-enhancing and nonenhancing lesions at any time OR ▪ A new T2 and/or gadolinium-enhancing lesion(s) on follow-up MRI, irrespective of its timing with reference to a baseline scan OR ▪ Await a second clinical attack
1 attack; objective clinical evidence of 1 lesion (clinically isolated syndrome)	Dissemination in space and time, demonstrated by: For dissemination in space ▪ ≥1 T2 lesion in at least two out of four MS-typical regions of the CNS (periventricular, juxtacortical, infratentorial, or spinal cord) ▪ OR ▪ Await a second clinical attack implicating a different CNS site **AND** For dissemination in time ▪ Simultaneous presence of asymptomatic gadolinium-enhancing and nonenhancing lesions at any time OR ▪ A new T2 and/or gadolinium-enhancing lesion(s) on follow-up MRI, irrespective of its timing with reference to a baseline scan **OR** ▪ Await a second clinical attack
Insidious neurologic progression suggestive of MS (PPMS)	One year of disease progression (retrospectively or prospectively determined) **PLUS** Two out of the three following criteria Evidence for dissemination in space in the brain based on ≥1 T2$^+$ lesions in the MS-characteristic periventricular, juxtacortical, or infratentorial regions Evidence for dissemination in space in the spinal cord based on ≥2 T2$^+$ lesions in the cord Positive CSF (isoelectric focusing evidence of oligoclonal bands and/or elevated IgG index)

[a]***Source:*** From Polman et al.

(Table 380-4), particularly when (1) symptoms are localized exclusively to the posterior fossa, craniocervical junction, or spinal cord; (2) the patient is aged <15 or >60 years; (3) the clinical course is progressive from onset; (4) the patient has never experienced visual, sensory, or bladder symptoms; or (5) laboratory findings (e.g., MRI, CSF, or EPs) are atypical. Similarly, uncommon or rare symptoms in MS (e.g., aphasia, parkinsonism, chorea, isolated dementia, severe muscular atrophy, peripheral neuropathy, episodic loss of consciousness, fever, headache, seizures, or coma) should increase concern about an alternative diagnosis. Diagnosis is also difficult in patients with a rapid or explosive (stroke-like) onset or with mild symptoms and a normal neurologic examination. Rarely, intense inflammation and swelling may produce a mass lesion that mimics a primary or metastatic tumor. The specific tests required to exclude alternative diagnoses will vary with each clinical situation; however, an erythrocyte sedimentation rate, serum B_{12} level, ANA, and treponemal antibody should probably be obtained in all patients with suspected MS.

PROGNOSIS

Most patients with clinically evident MS ultimately experience progressive neurologic disability. In older studies, 15 years after onset, only 20% of patients had no functional limitation, and between one-third and one-half progressed to SPMS and required assistance with ambulation; furthermore, 25 years after onset, ~80% of MS

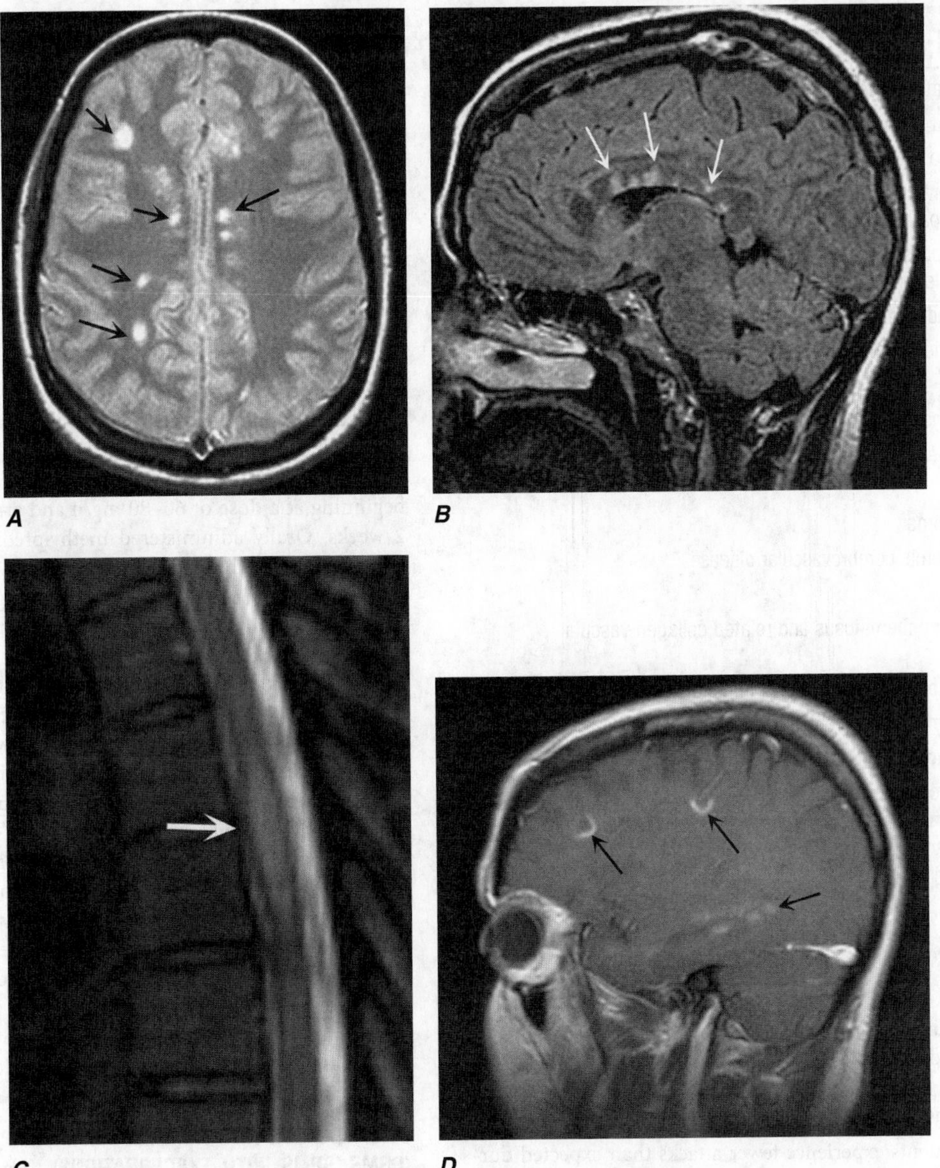

Figure 380-3 MRI findings in MS. ***A.*** Axial first-echo image from T2-weighted sequence demonstrates multiple bright signal abnormalities in white matter, typical for MS. ***B.*** Sagittal T2-weighted FLAIR (fluid attenuated inversion recovery) image in which the high signal of CSF has been suppressed. CSF appears dark, while areas of brain edema or demyelination appear high in signal as shown here in the corpus callosum (*arrows*). Lesions in the anterior corpus callosum are frequent in MS and rare in vascular disease. ***C.*** Sagittal T2-weighted fast spin echo image of the thoracic spine demonstrates a fusiform high-signal-intensity lesion in the midthoracic spinal cord. ***D.*** Sagittal T1-weighted image obtained after the intravenous administration of gadolinium DTPA reveals focal areas of blood-brain barrier disruption, identified as high-signal-intensity regions (*arrows*).

patients reached this level of disability. For unclear reasons, the long-term prognosis for untreated MS appears to have improved in recent years. In addition, the development of disease-modifying therapies for MS also appears to have favorably improved the long-term outlook. Although the prognosis in an individual is difficult to establish, certain clinical features suggest a more favorable prognosis. These include ON or sensory symptoms at onset, fewer than two relapses in the first year of illness, and minimal impairment after 5 years. By contrast, patients with truncal ataxia, action tremor, pyramidal symptoms, or a progressive disease course are more likely to become disabled. Patients with a long-term favorable course are likely to have developed fewer MRI lesions during the early years of disease, and vice versa. Importantly, some MS patients have a benign variant of MS and never develop neurologic disability. The likelihood of having benign MS is thought to be <20%. Patients with benign MS 15 years after onset who have entirely normal neurologic examinations are likely to maintain their benign course.

In patients with their first demyelinating event (i.e., a clinically isolated syndrome), the brain MRI provides prognostic information. With three or more typical T2-weighted lesions, the risk of developing MS after 20 years is ~80%. Conversely, with a normal brain MRI, the likelihood of developing MS is <20%. Similarly, two or more Gd-enhancing lesions at baseline is highly predictive of future MS, as is the appearance of either new T2-weighted lesions or new Gd enhancement ≥3 months after the initial episode.

Mortality as a direct consequence of MS is uncommon, although it has been estimated that the 25-year survival is only 85% of expected. Death can occur during an acute MS attack, although this

TABLE 380-4 Disorders That Can Mimic MS

Acute disseminated encephalomyelitis (ADEM)
Antiphospholipid antibody syndrome
Behçet's disease
Cerebral autosomal dominant arteriopathy, subcortical infarcts, and leukoencephalopathy (CADASIL)
Congenital leukodystrophies (e.g., adrenoleukodystrophy, metachromatic leukodystrophy)
Human immunodeficiency virus (HIV) infection
Ischemic optic neuropathy (arteritic and nonarteritic)
Lyme disease
Mitochondrial encephalopathy with lactic acidosis and stroke (MELAS)
Neoplasms (e.g., lymphoma, glioma, meningioma)
Sarcoid
Sjögren's syndrome
Stroke and ischemic cerebrovascular disease
Syphilis
Systemic lupus erythematosus and related collagen vascular disorders
Tropical spastic paraparesis (HTLV I/II infection)
Vascular malformations (especially spinal dural AV fistulas)
Vasculitis (primary CNS or other)
Vitamin B_{12} deficiency

Abbreviations: AV, arteriovenous; CNS, central nervous system; HTLV, human T cell lymphotropic virus.

is distinctly rare. More commonly, death occurs as a complication of MS (e.g., pneumonia in a debilitated individual). Death can also result from suicide.

Effect of pregnancy

Pregnant MS patients experience fewer attacks than expected during gestation (especially in the last trimester), but more attacks than expected in the first 3 months postpartum. When considering the pregnancy year as a whole (i.e., 9 months pregnancy plus 3 months postpartum), the overall disease course is unaffected. Decisions about childbearing should thus be made based on (1) the mother's physical state, (2) her ability to care for the child, and (3) the availability of social support. Disease-modifying therapy is generally discontinued during pregnancy, although the actual risk from the interferons and glatiramer acetate (see below) appears to be low.

TREATMENT Multiple Sclerosis

Therapy for MS can be divided into several categories: (1) treatment of acute attacks, (2) treatment with disease-modifying agents that reduce the biological activity of MS, and (3) symptomatic therapy. Treatments that promote remyelination or neural repair do not currently exist but would be highly desirable.

The Expanded Disability Status Score (EDSS) is a useful measure of neurologic impairment in MS (Table 380-5). Most patients with EDSS scores <3.5 have RRMS, walk normally, and are generally not disabled; by contrast, patients with EDSS scores >5.5 have progressive MS (SPMS or PPMS), are gait-impaired and, typically, are occupationally disabled.

ACUTE ATTACKS OR INITIAL DEMYELINATING EPISODES When patients experience acute deterioration, it is important to consider whether this change reflects new disease activity or a "pseudoexacerbation" resulting from an increase in ambient temperature, fever, or an infection. When the clinical change is thought to reflect a pseudoexacerbation, glucocorticoid treatment is inappropriate. Glucocorticoids are used to manage either first attacks or acute exacerbations. They provide short-term clinical benefit by reducing the severity and shortening the duration of attacks. Whether treatment provides any long-term benefit on the course of the illness is less clear. Therefore, mild attacks are often not treated. Physical and occupational therapy can help with mobility and manual dexterity.

Glucocorticoid treatment is usually administered as intravenous methylprednisolone, 500–1000 mg/d for 3–5 days, either without a taper or followed by a course of oral prednisone beginning at a dose of 60–80 mg/d and gradually tapered over 2 weeks. Orally administered methylprednisolone or dexamethasone (in equivalent dosages) can be substituted for the intravenous portion of the therapy, although GI complications are more common by this route. Outpatient treatment is almost always possible.

Side effects of short-term glucocorticoid therapy include fluid retention, potassium loss, weight gain, gastric disturbances, acne, and emotional lability. Concurrent use of a low-salt, potassium-rich diet and avoidance of potassium-wasting diuretics is advisable. Lithium carbonate (300 mg orally bid) may help to manage emotional lability and insomnia associated with glucocorticoid therapy. Patients with a history of peptic ulcer disease may require cimetidine (400 mg bid) or ranitidine (150 mg bid). Proton pump inhibitors such as pantoprazole (40 mg orally bid) may reduce the likelihood of gastritis, especially when large doses are administered orally. Plasma exchange (5–7 exchanges: 40–60 mL/kg per exchange, every other day for 14 days) may benefit patients with fulminant attacks of demyelination (from MS and other fulminant causes) that are unresponsive to glucocorticoids. However, the cost is high, and conclusive evidence of efficacy is lacking.

DISEASE-MODIFYING THERAPIES FOR RELAPSING FORMS OF MS (RRMS, SPMS WITH EXACERBATIONS) Seven such agents are approved by the U.S. Food and Drug Administration (FDA): (1) IFN-β-1a (Avonex), (2) IFN-β-1a (Rebif), (3) IFN-β-1b (Betaseron), (4) glatiramer acetate (Copaxone), (5) natalizumab (Tysabri), (6) fingolimod (Gilenya), and (7) mitoxantrone (Novantrone). An eighth, cladribine (Leustatin), is currently awaiting an FDA decision on its approval. Each of these treatments is also used in SPMS patients who continue to experience attacks, because SPMS can be difficult to distinguish from RRMS, and because the available clinical trials suggest that such patients also derive therapeutic benefit. In Phase III clinical trials, recipients of IFN-β-1b, IFN-β-1a, glatiramer acetate, natalizumab, and fingolimod experienced fewer clinical exacerbations and fewer new MRI lesions compared to placebo recipients (Table 380-6). Mitoxantrone (Novantrone), an immune suppressant, has also been approved in the United States, although because of its potential toxicity it is generally reserved for patients with progressive disability who have failed other treatments. When considering the data in Table 380-6, however, it is important to note that the relative efficacy of the different agents cannot be determined by cross-trial comparisons. Relative efficacy can only be determined from a non-biased head-to-head clinical trial.

Interferon-β IFN-β is a class I interferon originally identified by its antiviral properties. Efficacy in MS probably results from

TABLE 380-5 Scoring Systems for MS

Kurtzke Expanded Disability Status Score (EDSS)

0.0 = Normal neurologic exam [all grade 0 in functional status (FS)]
1.0 = No disability, minimal signs in one FS (i.e., grade 1)
1.5 = No disability, minimal signs in more than one FS (more than one grade 1)
2.0 = Minimal disability in one FS (one FS grade 2, others 0 or 1)
2.5 = Minimal disability in two FS (two FS grade 2, others 0 or 1)
3.0 = Moderate disability in one FS (one FS grade 3, others 0 or 1) or mild disability in three or four FS (three/four FS grade 2, others 0 or 1) though fully ambulatory
3.5 = Fully ambulatory but with moderate disability in one FS (one grade 3) and one or two FS grade 2; or two FS grade 3; or five FS grade 2 (others 0 or 1)
4.0 = Ambulatory without aid or rest for ~500 m
4.5 = Ambulatory without aid or rest for ~300 m
5.0 = Ambulatory without aid or rest for ~200 m
5.5 = Ambulatory without aid or rest for ~100 m
6.0 = Unilateral assistance required to walk about 100 m with or without resting
6.5 = Constant bilateral assistance required to walk about 20 m without resting
7.0 = Unable to walk beyond about 5 m even with aid; essentially restricted to wheelchair; wheels self and transfers alone
7.5 = Unable to take more than a few steps; restricted to wheelchair; may need aid to transfer
8.0 = Essentially restricted to bed or chair or perambulated in wheelchair, but out of bed most of day; retains many self-care functions; generally has effective use of arms
8.5 = Essentially restricted to bed much of the day; has some effective use of arm(s); retains some self-care functions
9.0 = Helpless bed patient; can communicate and eat
9.5 = Totally helpless bed patient; unable to communicate or eat
10.0 = Death due to MS

Functional Status (FS) Score

A. Pyramidal functions
0 = Normal
1 = Abnormal signs without disability
2 = Minimal disability
3 = Mild or moderate paraparesis or hemiparesis, or severe monoparesis
4 = Marked paraparesis or hemiparesis, moderate quadriparesis, or monoplegia
5 = Paraplegia, hemiplegia, or marked quadriparesis
6 = Quadriplegia

B. Cerebellar functions
0 = Normal
1 = Abnormal signs without disability
2 = Mild ataxia
3 = Moderate truncal or limb ataxia
4 = Severe ataxia all limbs
5 = Unable to perform coordinated movements due to ataxia

C. Brainstem functions
0 = Normal
1 = Signs only
2 = Moderate nystagmus or other mild disability
3 = Severe nystagmus, marked extraocular weakness, or moderate disability of other cranial nerves
4 = Marked dysarthria or other marked disability
5 = Inability to swallow or speak

D. Sensory functions
0 = Normal
1 = Vibration or figure-writing decrease only, in 1 or 2 limbs
2 = Mild decrease in touch or pain or position sense, and/or moderate decrease in vibration in 1 or 2 limbs, or vibratory decrease alone in 3 or 4 limbs
3 = Moderate decrease in touch or pain or position sense, and/or essentially lost vibration in 1 or 2 limbs, or mild decrease in touch or pain, and/or moderate decrease in all proprioceptive tests in 3 or 4 limbs
4 = Marked decrease in touch or pain or loss of proprioception, alone or combined, in 1 or 2 limbs or moderate decrease in touch or pain and/or severe proprioceptive decrease in more than 2 limbs
5 = Loss (essentially) of sensation in 1 or 2 limbs or moderate decrease in touch or pain and/or loss of proprioception for most of the body below the head
6 = Sensation essentially lost below the head

E. Bowel and bladder functions
0 = Normal
1 = Mild urinary hesitancy, urgency, or retention
2 = Moderate hesitancy, urgency, retention of bowel or bladder, or rare urinary incontinence
3 = Frequent urinary incontinence
4 = In need of almost constant catheterization
5 = Loss of bladder function
6 = Loss of bowel and bladder function

F. Visual (or optic) functions
0 = Normal
1 = Scotoma with visual acuity (corrected) better than 20/30
2 = Worse eye with scotoma with maximal visual acuity (corrected) of 20/30 to 20/59
3 = Worse eye with large scotoma, or moderate decrease in fields, but with maximal visual acuity (corrected) of 20/60 to 20/99
4 = Worse eye with marked decrease of fields and maximal acuity (corrected) of 20/100 to 20/200; grade 3 plus maximal acuity of better eye of 20/60 or less
5 = Worse eye with maximal visual acuity (corrected) less than 20/200; grade 4 plus maximal acuity of better eye of 20/60 or less
6 = Grade 5 plus maximal visual acuity of better eye of 20/60 or less

G. Cerebral (or mental) functions
0 = Normal
1 = Mood alteration only (does not affect EDSS score)
2 = Mild decrease in mentation
3 = Moderate decrease in mentation
4 = Marked decrease in mentation
5 = Chronic brain syndrome—severe or incompetent

Source: After JF Kurtzke: Neurology 33:1444, 1983.

TABLE 380-6 Two-Year Outcomes for FDA-Approved Therapies for Multiple Sclerosis[a]

	Clinical Outcomes[b]		MRI Outcomes[c]	
Dose, Route, and Schedule	Attack Rate, Mean	Change in Disease Severity	New T2 Lesions[d]	Total Burden of Disease
IFN-β-1b, 250 μg SC qod	−34%[e]	−29% (ns)	−83%[f]	−17%[e]
IFN-β-1a, 30 μg IM qw	−18%[g]	−37%[g]	−36%[f]	−4% (ns)
IFN-β-1a, 44 μg SC tiw	−32%[e]	−30%[g]	−78%[e]	−15%[e]
GA, 20 mg SC qd	−29%[f]	−12% (ns)	−38%[f]	−8%[f]
MTX, 12 mg/m² IV q3mo	−66%[e]	−75%[g]	−79%[g]	nr
NTZ, 300 mg IV qmo	−68%[e]	−42%[e]	−83%[e]	−18%[e]
FGM, 0.5 mg PO qd	−55%[e]	−27%[f]	−74%[e]	−23%[e]
CLD[h], 3.5 mg/kg PO qyr	−58%[e]	−33%[g]	−73%[e]	nr

[a]Percentage reductions (or increases) have been calculated by dividing the reported rates in the treated group by the comparable rates in the placebo group, except for MRI disease burden, which was calculated as the difference in the median percentage change between the treated and placebo groups.
[b]Severity = 1 point EDSS progression, sustained for 3 months (in the IFN-β-1a 30 μg qw trial, this change was sustained for 6 months; in the IFN-β-1b trial, this was over 3 years).
[c]Different studies measured these MRI measures differently, making comparisons difficult (numbers for new T2 represent the best case scenario for each trial).
[d]New lesions seen on T_2-weighted MRI.
[e]$p = .001$.
[f]$p = .01$.
[g]$p = .05$.
[h]Not FDA-approved at time of publication.
Abbreviations: IFN-β, interferon β; GA, glatiramer acetate; MTX, mitoxantrone; NTZ, natalizumab; FGM, fingolimod; CLD, Cladribine; IM, intramuscular; SC, subcutaneous; IV, intravenous; PO, oral; qod, every other day; qw, once per week; tiw, three times per week; qd, daily; q3mo, once every 3 months; qmo, once per month; qyr, once per year; ns, not significant; nr, not reported.

immunomodulatory properties, including (1) downregulating expression of MHC molecules on antigen-presenting cells, (2) inhibiting proinflammatory and increasing regulatory cytokine levels, (3) inhibition of T cell proliferation, and (4) limiting the trafficking of inflammatory cells in the CNS. IFN-β reduces the attack rate and improves disease severity measures such as EDSS progression and MRI-documented disease burden. IFN-β should be considered in patients with either RRMS or SPMS with superimposed relapses. In patients with SPMS but without relapses, efficacy has not been established. Head-to-head trials suggest that higher IFN-β doses have slightly greater efficacy but are also more likely to induce neutralizing antibodies, which may reduce the clinical benefit (see below). IFN-β-1a (Avonex), 30 μg, is administered by intramuscular injection once every week. IFN-β-1a (Rebif), 44 μg, is administered by subcutaneous injection three times per week. IFN-β-1b (Betaseron), 250 μg, is administered by subcutaneous injection every other day.

Common side effects of IFN-β therapy include flulike symptoms (e.g., fevers, chills, and myalgias) and mild abnormalities on routine laboratory evaluation (e.g., elevated liver function tests or lymphopenia). Rarely, more severe hepatotoxicity may occur. Subcutaneous IFN-β also causes reactions at the injection site (e.g., pain, redness, induration, or, rarely, skin necrosis). Side effects can usually be managed with concomitant nonsteroidal anti-inflammatory medications and with the use of an autoinjector. Depression, increased spasticity, and cognitive changes have been reported, although these symptoms can also be due to the underlying disease. In any event, side effects to IFN-β therapy usually subside with time.

Approximately 2–10% of IFN-β-1a (Avonex) recipients, 15–25% of IFN-β-1a (Rebif) recipients, and 30–40% of IFN-β-1b (Betaseron) recipients develop neutralizing antibodies to IFN-β, which may disappear over time. Two very large randomized trials (one with more than 2000 patients) provide unequivocal evidence that neutralizing antibodies reduce efficacy as determined by several MRI outcomes. Paradoxically, however, these same trials, despite abundant statistical power, failed to demonstrate any concomitant impact on the clinical outcomes of disability and relapse rate. The reason for this clinical-radiologic dissociation is unresolved. Fortunately, however, there are few situations where measurement of antibodies is necessary. Thus, for a patient doing well on therapy, the presence of antibodies should not affect treatment. Conversely, for a patient doing poorly on therapy, alternative treatment should be considered, even if there are no detectable antibodies.

Glatiramer Acetate Glatiramer acetate is a synthetic, random polypeptide composed of four amino acids (L-glutamic acid, L-lysine, L-alanine, and L-tyrosine). Its mechanism of action may include (1) induction of antigen-specific suppressor T cells; (2) binding to MHC molecules, thereby displacing bound MBP; or (3) altering the balance between proinflammatory and regulatory cytokines. Glatiramer acetate reduces the attack rate (whether measured clinically or by MRI) in RRMS. Glatiramer acetate may also benefit disease severity measures, although this is less well established than for the relapse rate. Therefore, glatiramer acetate should be considered in RRMS patients. Its usefulness in progressive disease is entirely unknown.

Head-to-head clinical trials suggest that glatiramer acetate has about equal efficacy to high IFN-β doses. Glatiramer acetate, 20 mg, is administered by subcutaneous injection every day. Injection-site reactions also occur with glatiramer acetate. Initially, these were thought to be less severe than with IFN-β-1b, although two recent head-to-head comparisons of high-dose IFN-β to glatiramer acetate did not bear out this impression. In addition, approximately 15% of patients experience one or more episodes of flushing, chest tightness, dyspnea, palpitations, and anxiety after injection. This systemic reaction is unpredictable, brief (duration <1 h), and tends not to recur. Finally, some patients experience lipoatrophy, which, on occasion, can be disfiguring and require cessation of treatment.

Natalizumab Natalizumab (Tysabri) is a humanized monoclonal antibody directed against the α_4 subunit of $\alpha_4\beta_1$ integrin, a cellular adhesion molecule expressed on the surface of lymphocytes. It prevents lymphocytes from binding to endothelial cells, thereby preventing lymphocytes from penetrating the BBB and entering the CNS. Natalizumab greatly reduces the attack rate and significantly improves all measures of disease severity in MS. Moreover, it is well tolerated and the dosing schedule of monthly intravenous infusions make it very convenient for patients. However, because of the development of progressive multifocal leukoencephalopathy (PML) in approximately 0.2% of patients treated with natalizumab for more than 2 years, natalizumab is currently recommended only for patients who have failed other therapies or who have particularly aggressive disease presentations. Its usefulness in the treatment of progressive disease has not been studied. Head-to-head data for natalizumab against low-dose (weekly) IFN-β showed a clear superiority of natalizumab in RRMS; the trial design, however, was biased against IFN-β (i.e., patients recruited could already be considered IFN-β treatment failures). Natalizumab, 300 μg, is administered by IV infusion each month. Treatment with natalizumab is, in general, well tolerated. A small percentage (<10%) of patients experience hypersensitivity reactions (including anaphylaxis) and ~6% develop neutralizing antibodies to the molecule.

The major concern with long-term treatment is the risk of PML. Because the risk is extremely low during the first year of treatment with natalizumab, we currently recommend treatment for periods of 12–18 months only for most patients; after this time, a change to another disease-modifying therapy should be considered. Recently, a blood test to detect antibodies against the PML (JC) virus has shown promise in identifying individuals who are at risk for this complication. In preliminary studies, approximately half of the adult population are antibody-positive, indicating that they experienced an asymptomatic infection with the virus at some time in the past, and to date all cases of natalizumab-associated PML have occurred in seropositive individuals.

Fingolimod Fingolimod (Gilenya) is a sphingosine-1-phosphate (S1P) inhibitor and it prevents the egress of lymphocytes from the secondary lymphoid organs such as the lymph nodes and spleen. Its mechanism of action is probably due, in part, to the trapping of lymphocytes in the periphery and the prevention, thereby, of lymphocytes reaching the brain. However, because S1P receptors are widely expressed in the CNS tissue and because fingolimod is able to cross the BBB, it may also have central effects. Fingolimod reduces the attack rate and significantly improves all measures of disease severity in MS. It is well tolerated, and the oral dosing schedule makes it very convenient for patients. Moreover, from the clinical trial data presented thus far, it seems to be a reasonably safe therapy and it is approved for first-line use by the FDA. However, as with any new therapy, long-term safety remains to be established. A large head-to-head phase III randomized study demonstrated the clear superiority of fingolimod over low dose (weekly) IFN-β. Fingolimod, 0.5 mg, is administered orally each day. Treatment with fingolimod is also, in general, well tolerated. Mild abnormalities on routine laboratory evaluation (e.g., elevated liver function tests or lymphopenia) are more common than in controls. Although rarely severe, sometimes discontinuation of the medication is necessary. First-degree heart block and bradycardia can also occur, the latter necessitating the prolonged (6-h) observation of patients receiving their first dose.

Mitoxantrone Hydrochloride Mitoxantrone (Novantrone), an anthracenedione, exerts its antineoplastic action by (1) intercalating into DNA and producing both strand breaks and interstrand cross-links, (2) interfering with RNA synthesis, and (3) inhibiting topoisomerase II (involved in DNA repair). The FDA approved mitoxantrone on the basis of a single (relatively small) phase III clinical trial in Europe, in addition to an even smaller phase II study completed earlier. Mitoxantrone received (from the FDA) the broadest indication of any current treatment for MS. Thus, mitoxantrone is indicated for use in SPMS, in PRMS, and in patients with worsening RRMS (defined as patients whose neurologic status remains significantly abnormal between MS attacks). Despite this broad indication, however, the data supporting its efficacy are weaker than for other approved therapies.

Mitoxantrone can be cardiotoxic (e.g., cardiomyopathy, reduced left ventricular ejection fraction, and irreversible congestive heart failure). As a result, a cumulative dose >140 mg/m^2 is not recommended. At currently approved doses (12 mg/m^2 every 3 months), the maximum duration of therapy can be only 2–3 years. Furthermore, >40% of women will experience amenorrhea, which may be permanent. Finally, there is risk of acute leukemia, and this complication has already been reported in several mitoxantrone-treated MS patients.

Given these risks, mitoxantrone should not be used as a first-line agent in either RRMS or relapsing SPMS. It is reasonable to consider mitoxantrone in selected patients with a progressive course who have failed other approved therapies.

Cladribine Cladribine (Leustatin) is a purine analog that inhibits DNA synthesis and repair, and acts as a general immunosuppressant. Cladribine reduces the attack rate and significantly improves several measures of disease severity in MS. It seems to be well tolerated and the easy oral dosing schedule of only taking the drug for 2 weeks/year make it very convenient for patients. Again, however, the principal concern is long-term safety, a concern that is heightened by the long-term immunosuppression that occurs in some patients and, also, by the fact that, in the pivotal RCT, 10 neoplasms and all 20 herpes zoster cases occurred in Leustatin-treated patients.

Initiating and Changing Treatment Currently, most patients with relapsing forms of MS receive IFN-β or glatiramer acetate as first-line therapy. Although approved for first-line use, the role of fingolimod in this situation has yet to be defined. Regardless of which agent is chosen first, treatment should probably be changed in patients who continue to have frequent attacks or progressive disability (Fig. 380-4). The value of combination therapy is unknown.

The long-term efficacy of these treatments remains uncertain, although several recent studies suggest that these agents can improve the long-term outcome of MS, especially when administered early in the RRMS stage of the illness. Beneficial effects seen in early MS include a reduction in the relapse rate, a reduction in CNS inflammation as measured by MRI, and a

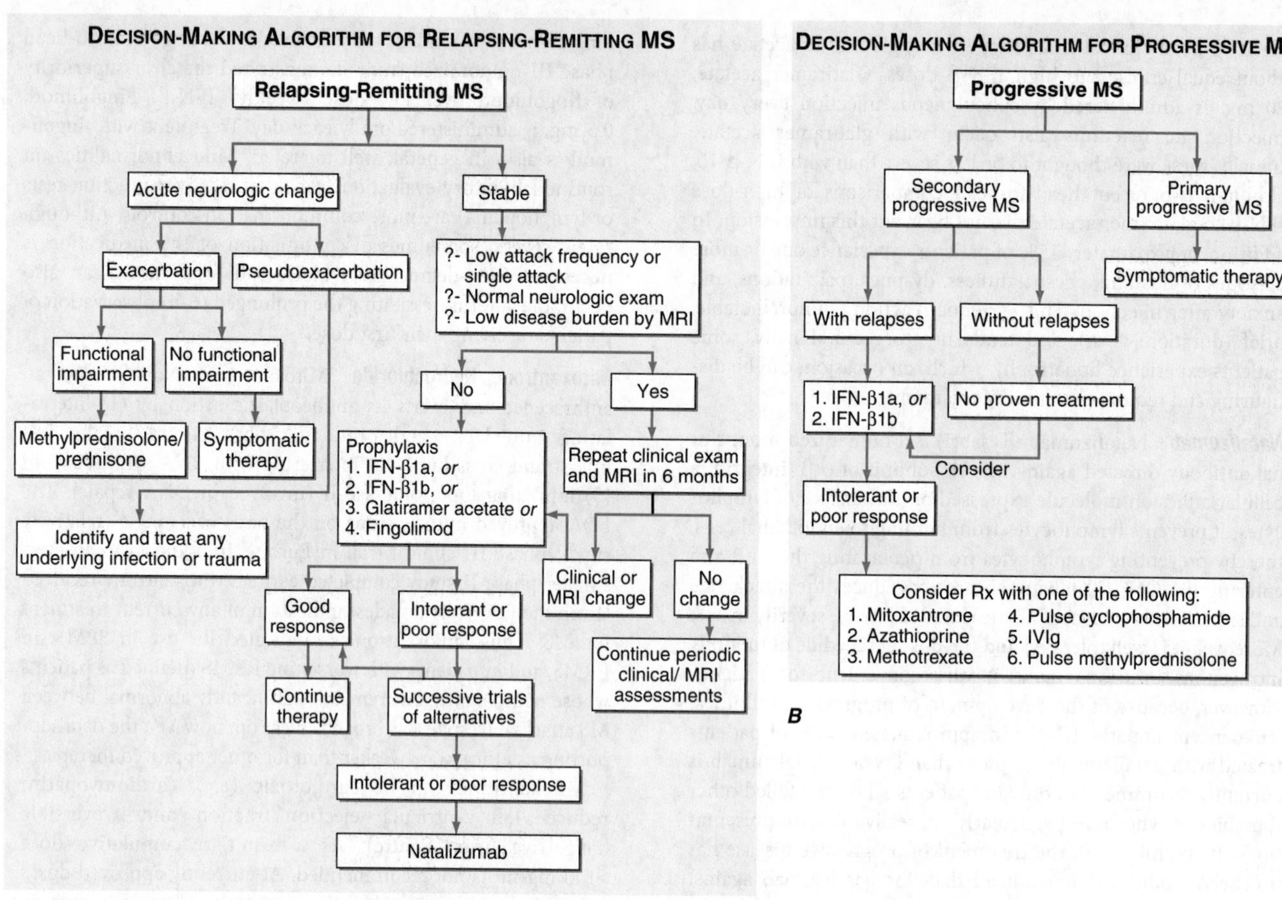

Figure 380-4 Therapeutic decision-making for MS.

prolongation in the time to reach certain disability outcomes such as SPMS and requiring assistance to ambulate. Unfortunately, however, already established progressive symptoms do not respond well to treatment with these disease-modifying therapies. Because progressive symptoms are likely to result from delayed effects of earlier focal demyelinating episodes, many experts now believe that very early treatment with a disease-modifying drug is appropriate for most MS patients. It is reasonable to delay initiating treatment in patients with (1) normal neurologic exams, (2) a single attack or a low attack frequency, and (3) a low burden of disease as assessed by brain MRI. Untreated patients, however, should be followed closely with periodic brain MRI scans; the need for therapy is reassessed if scans reveal evidence of ongoing, subclinical disease.

DISEASE-MODIFYING THERAPIES FOR PROGRESSIVE MS

SPMS High-dose IFN-β probably has a beneficial effect in patients with SPMS who are still experiencing acute relapses. IFN-β is probably ineffective in patients with SPMS who are not having acute attacks. Glatiramer acetate and natalizumab have not been studied in this patient population. Although mitoxantrone has been approved for patients with progressive MS, this is not the population studied in the pivotal trial. Therefore, no evidence-based recommendation can be made with regard to its use in this setting.

PPMS No therapies have been convincingly shown to modify the course of PPMS. A phase III clinical trial of glatiramer acetate in PPMS was stopped because of lack of efficacy. A phase II/III trial of rituximab in PPMS was also negative, but in a preplanned secondary analysis treatment appeared to slow disability progression in patients with gadolinium-enhancing lesions at entry; a follow-up trial with the humanized anti-CD20 therapy ocrelizumab will soon begin. A trial of mitoxantrone in PPMS is ongoing.

OFF-LABEL TREATMENT OPTIONS FOR RRMS AND SPMS

Azathioprine (2–3 mg/kg per day) has been used primarily in SPMS. Meta-analysis of published trials suggests that azathioprine is marginally effective at lowering relapse rates, although a benefit on disability progression has not been demonstrated.

Methotrexate (7.5–20 mg/week) was shown in one study to slow the progression of upper-extremity dysfunction in SPMS. Because of the possibility of developing irreversible liver damage, some experts recommend a blind liver biopsy after 2 years of therapy.

Cyclophosphamide (700 mg/m^2, every other month) may be helpful for treatment-refractory patients who are (1) otherwise in good health, (2) ambulatory, and (3) <40 years of age. Because cyclophosphamide can be used for periods in excess of 3 years, it may be preferable to mitoxantrone in these circumstances.

Intravenous immunoglobulin (IVIg), administered in monthly pulses (up to 1 g/kg) for up to 2 years, appears to reduce annual exacerbation rates. However, its use is limited because of its high cost, questions about optimal dose, and uncertainty about its effect on long-term disability outcome.

Methylprednisolone administered in one study as monthly high-dose intravenous pulses reduced disability progression (see above).

OTHER THERAPEUTIC CLAIMS Many purported treatments for MS have never been subjected to scientific scrutiny. These include dietary therapies (e.g., the Swank diet in addition to others), megadose vitamins, calcium orotate, bee stings, cow colostrum, hyperbaric oxygen, Procarin (a combination of histamine and caffeine), chelation, acupuncture, acupressure, various Chinese herbal remedies, and removal of mercury-amalgam tooth fillings, among many others. Patients should avoid costly or potentially hazardous unproven treatments. Many such treatments lack biologic plausibility. For example, no reliable case of mercury poisoning resembling typical MS has ever been described.

Although potential roles for EBV, HHV-6, or chlamydia have been suggested for MS, these reports are unconfirmed, and treatment with antiviral agents or antibiotics is not currently appropriate.

Most recently, chronic cerebrospinal insufficiency (CCSVI) has been proposed as a cause of multiple sclerosis and vascular-surgical intervention recommended. However, the failure of independent investigators to even approximate the initial claims of 100% sensitivity and 100% specificity for the diagnostic procedure raised considerable doubt that CCSVI is a real entity. Certainly, any potentially dangerous surgery should be avoided until more rigorous science is available.

SYMPTOMATIC THERAPY For all patients, it is useful to encourage attention to a healthy lifestyle, including maintaining an optimistic outlook, a healthy diet, and regular exercise as tolerated (swimming is often well tolerated because of the cooling effect of cold water). It is reasonable also to correct vitamin D deficiency with oral vitamin D, and to recommend dietary supplementation with long-chain (omega-3) unsaturated fatty acids (present in oily fish such as salmon) because of their immunomodulatory properties. *Ataxia/tremor* is often intractable. Clonazepam, 1.5–20 mg/d; Mysoline, 50–250 mg/d; propranolol, 40–200 mg/d; or ondansetron, 8–16 mg/d may help. Wrist weights occasionally reduce tremor in the arm or hand. Thalamotomy or deep-brain stimulation has been tried with mixed success.

Spasticity and *spasms* may improve with physical therapy, regular exercise, and stretching. Avoidance of triggers (e.g., infections, fecal impactions, bed sores) is extremely important. Effective medications include baclofen (Lioresal) (20–120 mg/d), diazepam (2–40 mg/d), tizanidine (8–32 mg/d), dantrolene (25–400 mg/d), and cyclobenzaprine hydrochloride (10–60 mg/d). For severe spasticity, a baclofen pump (delivering medication directly into the CSF) can provide substantial relief.

Weakness can sometimes be improved with the use of potassium channel blockers such as 4-amino pyridine (10–40 mg/d) and 3,4-di-aminopyridine (40–80 mg/d), particularly in the setting where lower extremity weakness interferes with the patient's ability to ambulate. The FDA has approved 4-amino pyridine (at 20 mg/day) and this can be obtained either as dalfampridine (Ampyra) or, more cheaply, through a compounding pharmacy. The principal concern with the use of these agents is the possibility of inducing seizures at high doses.

Pain is treated with anticonvulsants (carbamazepine, 100–1000 mg/d; phenytoin, 300–600 mg/d; gabapentin, 300–3600 mg/d; or pregabalin, 50–300 mg/d), antidepressants (amitriptyline, 25–150 mg/d; nortriptyline, 25–150 mg/d; desipramine, 100–300 mg/d; or venlafaxine, 75–225 mg/d), or antiarrhythmics (mexiletine, 300–900 mg/d). If these approaches fail, patients should be referred to a comprehensive pain management program.

Bladder dysfunction management is best guided by urodynamic testing. Evening fluid restriction or frequent voluntary voiding may help *detrusor hyperreflexia*. If these methods fail, propantheline bromide (10–15 mg/d), oxybutynin (5–15 mg/d), hyoscyamine sulfate (0.5–0.75 mg/d), tolterodine tartrate (2–4 mg/d), or solifenacin (5–10 mg/d) may help. Coadministration of pseudoephedrine (30–60 mg) is sometimes beneficial.

Detrusor/sphincter dyssynergia may respond to phenoxybenzamine (10–20 mg/d) or terazosin hydrochloride (1–20 mg/d). Loss of reflex bladder wall contraction may respond to bethanechol (30–150 mg/d). However, both conditions often require catheterization.

Urinary tract infections should be treated promptly. Patients with large postvoid residual urine volumes are predisposed to infections. Prevention by urine acidification (with cranberry juice or vitamin C) inhibits some bacteria. Prophylactic administration of antibiotics is sometimes necessary but may lead to colonization by resistant organisms. Intermittent catheterization may help to prevent recurrent infections.

Treatment of *constipation* includes high-fiber diets and fluids. Natural or other laxatives may help. *Fecal incontinence* may respond to a reduction in dietary fiber.

Depression should be treated. Useful drugs include the selective serotonin reuptake inhibitors (fluoxetine, 20–80 mg/d; or sertraline, 50–200 mg/d), the tricyclic antidepressants (amitriptyline, 25–150 mg/d; nortriptyline, 25–150 mg/d; or desipramine, 100–300 mg/d), and the non-tricyclic antidepressants (venlafaxine, 75–225 mg/d).

Fatigue may improve with assistive devices, help in the home, or successful management of spasticity. Patients with frequent nocturia may benefit from anticholinergic medication at bedtime. Primary MS fatigue may respond to amantadine (200 mg/d), methylphenidate (5–25 mg/d), or modafinil (100–400 mg/d).

Cognitive problems may respond to the cholinesterase inhibitor donepezil hydrochloride (10 mg/d).

Paroxysmal symptoms respond dramatically to low-dose anticonvulsants (acetazolamide, 200–600 mg/d; carbamazepine, 50–400 mg/d; phenytoin, 50–300 mg/d; or gabapentin, 600–1800 mg/d).

Heat sensitivity may respond to heat avoidance, air-conditioning, or cooling garments.

Sexual dysfunction may be helped by lubricants to aid in genital stimulation and sexual arousal. Management of pain, spasticity, fatigue, and bladder/bowel dysfunction may also help. Sildenafil (50–100 mg), tadalafil (5–20 mg), or vardenafil (5–20 mg) taken 1–2 h before sex are now the standard treatments for maintaining erections.

PROMISING EXPERIMENTAL THERAPIES Numerous clinical trials are currently underway. These include (1) combination therapies; (2) monoclonal antibodies against CD20 to deplete B cells, against the IL-2 receptor, or against CD52 to induce global lymphocyte depletion; (3) novel oral sphingosine-1-phosphate receptor antagonists to sequester lymphocytes in the secondary lymphoid organs; (4) use of MBP, or an altered peptide ligand resembling MBP, to induce antigen-specific tolerance; (5) an oral inhibitor of the enzyme dihydroorotate dehydrogenase involved in pyrimidine synthesis; (6) estriol to induce a pregnancy-like state; and (7) bone marrow transplantation.

■ CLINICAL VARIANTS OF MS

Neuromyelitis optica (NMO), or Devic's syndrome, is an aggressive inflammatory disorder consisting most typically of attacks of acute

ON and myelitis. Attacks of ON can be bilateral (rare in MS) or unilateral; myelitis can be severe and transverse (rare in MS) and is typically longitudinally extensive, involving three or more contiguous vertebral segments. Attacks of ON may be precede or follow an attack of myelitis by days, months, or years, or vice versa. In contrast to MS, progressive symptoms do not occur in NMO. The brain MRI was classically thought to be normal at the onset of NMO, but recent studies now indicate that asymptomatic lesions sometimes resembling typical MS are common. Lesions involving the hypothalamus, periaqueductal region of the brainstem, or "cloud-like" white matter lesions in the cerebral hemispheres are suggestive of NMO. Brainstem disease can present with nausea and vertigo, and large hemispheral lesions can present as encephalopathy or seizures. Spinal cord MRI typically reveals a focal enhancing region of swelling and cavitation, extending over three or more spinal cord segments and often located in central gray matter structures. Histopathology of these lesions may reveal thickening of blood-vessel walls, demyelination, deposition of antibody and complement, a characteristic loss of astrocytes, and aquaporin-4 staining not seen in MS.

NMO, which is uncommon in whites compared with Asians and Africans, is best understood as a syndrome with diverse causes. Up to 40% of patients have a systemic autoimmune disorder, often systemic lupus erythematosus, Sjögren's syndrome, p-ANCA (perinuclear antineutrophil cytoplasmic antibody)–associated vasculitis, myasthenia gravis, Hashimoto's thyroiditis, or mixed connective tissue disease. In others, onset may be associated with acute infection with varicella-zoster virus, EBV, HIV, or tuberculosis. Rare cases appear to be paraneoplastic and associated with breast, lung, or other cancers. NMO is often idiopathic, however. NMO is usually disabling over time; in one series, respiratory failure from cervical myelitis was present in one-third of patients, and 8 years after onset 60% of patients were blind and more than half had permanent paralysis of one or more limbs.

A highly specific autoantibody directed against the water channel protein aquaporin-4 is present in the sera of 60–70% of patients who have a clinical diagnosis of NMO. Seropositive patients have a very high risk for future relapses. Aquaporin-4 is localized to the foot processes of astrocytes in close apposition to endothelial surfaces. It is likely that aquaporin-4 antibodies are directly pathogenic in NMO, as passive transfer of antibodies from NMO patients into laboratory animals reproduced histologic features of the disease.

When MS affects individuals of African or Asian ancestry, there is a propensity for demyelinating lesions to involve predominantly the optic nerve and spinal cord, an MS subtype termed "opticospinal MS." Interestingly, some individuals with opticospinal MS are seropositive for aquaporin-4 antibodies, suggesting that such cases represent an NMO spectrum disorder.

Acute MS (Marburg's variant) is a fulminant demyelinating process that in some cases progresses inexorably to death within 1–2 years. Typically, there are no remissions. When acute MS presents as a solitary, usually cavitary, lesion, a brain tumor is often suspected. In such cases, a brain biopsy is usually required to establish the diagnosis. An antibody-mediated process appears to be responsible for most cases. Marburg's variant does not seem to follow infection or vaccination, and it is unclear whether this syndrome represents an extreme form of MS or another disease altogether. No controlled trials of therapy exist; high-dose glucocorticoids, plasma exchange, and cyclophosphamide have been tried, with uncertain benefit.

TREATMENT Neuromyelitis Optica

Disease-modifying therapies have not been rigorously studied in NMO. Acute attacks of NMO are usually treated with high-dose glucocorticoids (Solu-Medrol 1–2 g/d for 5–10 days followed by a prednisone taper). Because of the likelihood that NMO is antibody-mediated, plasma exchange (typically 7 qod exchanges of 1.5 plasma volumes) has also been used empirically for acute episodes that fail to respond to glucocorticoids. Prophylaxis against relapses can be achieved in some patients with one of the following regimens: mycophenolate mofetil (250 mg bid gradually increasing to 1000 mg bid); B cell depletion with anti-CD20 monoclonal antibody (Rituxan); or a combination of glucocorticoids (500 mg IV methylprednisolone daily for 5 days; then oral prednisone 1 mg/kg per day × 2 months, followed by slow taper) plus azathioprine (2 mg/kg per day started on week 3). By contrast, available evidence suggests that use of IFN-β is ineffective and paradoxically may increase the risk of NMO relapses.

ACUTE DISSEMINATED ENCEPHALOMYELITIS (ADEM)

ADEM has a monophasic course and is most frequently associated with an antecedent infection (postinfectious encephalomyelitis); approximately 5% of ADEM cases follow immunization (postvaccinal encephalomyelitis). ADEM is more common in children than adults. The hallmark of ADEM is the presence of widely scattered small foci of perivenular inflammation and demyelination in contrast to larger confluent demyelinating lesions typical of MS. In the most explosive form of ADEM, acute hemorrhagic leukoencephalitis, the lesions are vasculitic and hemorrhagic, and the clinical course is devastating.

Postinfectious encephalomyelitis is most frequently associated with the viral exanthems of childhood. Infection with measles virus is the most common antecedent (1 in 1000 cases). Worldwide, measles encephalomyelitis is still common, although use of the live measles vaccine has dramatically reduced its incidence in developed countries. An ADEM-like illness rarely follows vaccination with live measles vaccine (1–2 in 10^6 immunizations). ADEM is now most frequently associated with varicella (chickenpox) infections (1 in 4000–10,000 cases). It may also follow infection with rubella, mumps, influenza, parainfluenza, Epstein-Barr, HIV, and other viruses, and *Mycoplasma*. Some patients may have a nonspecific upper respiratory tract infection or no known antecedent illness. In addition to measles, postvaccinal encephalomyelitis may also follow the administration of smallpox (5 cases per million), the Semple rabies, and Japanese encephalitis vaccines. Modern vaccines that do not require viral culture in CNS tissue have reduced the ADEM risk.

All forms of ADEM presumably result from a cross-reactive immune response to the infectious agent or vaccine that then triggers an inflammatory demyelinating response. Autoantibodies to MBP and to other myelin antigens have been detected in the CSF from many patients with ADEM. Attempts to demonstrate direct viral invasion of the CNS have been unsuccessful.

CLINICAL MANIFESTATIONS

In severe cases, onset is abrupt and progression rapid (hours to days). In postinfectious ADEM, the neurologic syndrome generally begins late in the course of the viral illness as the exanthem is fading. Fever reappears, and headache, meningismus, and lethargy progressing to coma may develop. Seizures are common. Signs of disseminated neurologic disease are consistently present (e.g., hemiparesis or quadriparesis, extensor plantar responses, lost or hyperactive tendon reflexes, sensory loss, and brainstem involvement). In ADEM due to chickenpox, cerebellar involvement is often conspicuous. CSF protein is modestly elevated [0.5–1.5 g/L (50–150 mg/dL)]. Lymphocytic pleocytosis, generally 200 cells/μL, occurs in 80% of patients. Occasional patients have higher counts or a mixed polymorphonuclear-lymphocytic pattern during the initial days of the illness. Transient CSF oligoclonal banding has been reported. MRI usually reveals extensive changes in the brain and spinal cord, consisting of white matter hyperintensities on T2 and FLAIR sequences with gadolinium enhancement on T1-weighted sequences.

DIAGNOSIS

The diagnosis is easily established when there is a history of recent vaccination or viral exanthematous illness. In severe cases with predominantly cerebral involvement, acute encephalitis due to infection with herpes simplex or other viruses including HIV may be difficult to exclude (Chap. 381); other considerations include hypercoagulable states including the antiphospholipid antibody syndrome, vasculitis, neurosarcoid, or metastatic cancer. An explosive presentation of MS can mimic ADEM, and especially in adults it may not be possible to distinguish these conditions at onset. The simultaneous onset of disseminated symptoms and signs is common in ADEM and rare in MS. Similarly, meningismus, drowsiness, coma, or seizures suggest ADEM rather than MS. Unlike MS, in ADEM optic nerve involvement is generally bilateral and transverse myelopathy complete. MRI findings that favor ADEM include extensive and relatively symmetric white matter abnormalities, basal ganglia or cortical gray matter lesions, and Gd enhancement of all abnormal areas. By contrast, oligoclonal bands in the CSF are more common in MS. In one study of adult patients initially thought to have ADEM, 30% experienced additional relapses over a follow-up period of 3 years and they were now classified as having MS. Occasional patients with "recurrent ADEM" have also been reported especially in children; however, it is not possible to distinguish this entity from atypical MS.

TREATMENT Acute Disseminated Encephalomyelitis

Initial treatment is with high-dose glucocorticoids as for exacerbations of NMO (see above); depending on the response, treatment may need to be continued for 4–8 weeks. Patients who fail to respond within a few days may benefit from a course of plasma exchange or intravenous immunoglobulin. The prognosis reflects the severity of the underlying acute illness. Measles encephalomyelitis is associated with a mortality rate of 5–20%, and most survivors have permanent neurologic sequelae. Children who recover may have persistent seizures and behavioral and learning disorders.

FURTHER READINGS

Axtell RC et al: T helper type 1 and 17 cells determine efficacy of interferon-β in multiple sclerosis and experimental encephalomyelitis. Nat Med 16:406, 2010

Bradl M et al: Neuromyelitis optica: Pathogenicity of patient immunoglobulin in vivo. Ann Neurol 66:630, 2009

Cohen JA et al: Oral fingolimod or intramuscular interferon for relapsing multiple sclerosis. N Engl J Med 362:402, 2010

deSeze J et al: Acute fulminant demyelinating disease: A descriptive study of 60 patients. Arch Neurol 64:1426, 2007

Fisniku LK et al: Disability and T2 MRI lesions: A 20-year follow-up of patients with relapse onset of multiple sclerosis. Brain 131:808, 2008

Gorelik L et al: Anti-JC virus antibodies: Implications for PML risk stratification. Ann Neurol 68:295, 2010

Hinson SR et al: Neurological autoimmunity targeting Aquaporin-4. Neuroscience 168:1009, 2010

Kappos L et al: Effect of early vs delayed interferon beta-1b treatment on disability after a first clinical event suggestive of multiple sclerosis: A 3-year follow-up analysis of the BENEFIT study. Lancet 370:389, 2007

Miller DH, Leary SM: Primary-progressive multiple sclerosis. Lancet Neurol 6:903, 2007

Oksenberg JR, Baranzini SE: Multiple sclerosis genetics—Is the glass half full, or half empty? Nat Rev Neurol 6:429, 2010

Polman CH et al: Diagnostic criteria for multiple sclerosis: 2010 revisions to the "McDonald Criteria." Ann Neurol 69:292, 2011

Sellner J et al: EFNS guidelines on diagnosis and management of neuromyelitis optica. Eur J Neurol 17:1019, 2010

Trojano M et al: New natural history of interferon-beta-treated relapsing multiple sclerosis. Ann Neurol 61:300, 2007

Young N et al: Perivenous demyelination: Association with clinically defined acute disseminated encephalomyelitis and comparison with pathologically confirmed multiple sclerosis. Brain 133:333, 2010

CHAPTER 381

Meningitis, Encephalitis, Brain Abscess, and Empyema

Karen L. Roos
Kenneth L. Tyler

Acute infections of the nervous system are among the most important problems in medicine because early recognition, efficient decision-making, and rapid institution of therapy can be lifesaving. These distinct clinical syndromes include acute bacterial meningitis, viral meningitis, encephalitis, focal infections such as brain abscess and subdural empyema, and infectious thrombophlebitis. Each may present with a nonspecific prodrome of fever and headache, which in a previously healthy individual may initially be thought to be benign, until (with the exception of viral meningitis) altered consciousness, focal neurologic signs, or seizures appear. Key goals of early management are to emergently distinguish between these conditions, identify the responsible pathogen, and initiate appropriate antimicrobial therapy.

APPROACH TO THE PATIENT Meningitis, Encephalitis, Brain Abscess, and Empyema

(Fig. 381-1) The first task is to identify whether an infection predominantly involves the subarachnoid space (*meningitis*) or whether there is evidence of either generalized or focal involvement of brain tissue in the cerebral hemispheres, cerebellum, or brainstem. When brain tissue is directly injured by a viral infection, the disease is referred to as *encephalitis*, whereas focal infections involving brain tissue are classified as either *cerebritis* or *abscess*, depending on the presence or absence of a capsule.

Nuchal rigidity ("stiff neck") is the pathognomonic sign of meningeal irritation and is present when the neck resists passive flexion. Kernig's and Brudzinski's signs are also classic signs of meningeal irritation. *Kernig's sign* is elicited with the patient in the supine position. The thigh is flexed on the abdomen, with the knee flexed; attempts to passively extend the knee elicit pain when meningeal irritation is present. *Brudzinski's sign* is elicited with the patient in the supine position and is positive when passive flexion of the neck results in spontaneous flexion of the hips and knees. Although commonly tested on physical examinations, the sensitivity and specificity of Kernig's and Brudzinski's signs are uncertain. Both may be absent or reduced in very young or elderly patients, immunocompromised individuals, or patients with a severely depressed mental status. The high prevalence of cervical spine disease in older individuals may result in false-positive tests for nuchal rigidity.

Initial management can be guided by several considerations: (1) Empirical therapy should be initiated promptly whenever bacterial meningitis is a significant diagnostic consideration. (2) All patients who have had recent head trauma, are immunocompromised, have known malignant lesions or central nervous system (CNS) neoplasms, or have focal neurologic findings, papilledema or a depressed level of consciousness should undergo CT or MRI of the brain prior to lumbar puncture (LP). In these cases empirical antibiotic therapy should not be delayed pending test results but should be administered prior to neuroimaging and LP. (3) A significantly depressed level of consciousness (e.g., somnolence, coma), seizures, or focal neurologic deficits do not occur in viral meningitis; patients with these symptoms should be hospitalized for further evaluation and treated empirically for bacterial and viral meningoencephalitis. (4) Immunocompetent patients with a normal level of consciousness, no prior antimicrobial treatment, and a cerebrospinal fluid (CSF) profile consistent with viral meningitis (lymphocytic pleocytosis and a normal glucose concentration) can often be treated as outpatients if appropriate contact and monitoring can be ensured. Failure of a patient with suspected viral meningitis to improve within 48 h should prompt a reevaluation including follow-up neurologic and general medical examination and repeat imaging and laboratory studies, often including a second LP.

ACUTE BACTERIAL MENINGITIS

DEFINITION

Bacterial meningitis is an acute purulent infection within the subarachnoid space. It is associated with a CNS inflammatory reaction that may result in decreased consciousness, seizures, raised intracranial pressure (ICP), and stroke. The meninges, the subarachnoid space, and the brain parenchyma are all frequently involved in the inflammatory reaction (*meningoencephalitis*).

EPIDEMIOLOGY

Bacterial meningitis is the most common form of suppurative CNS infection, with an annual incidence in the United States of >2.5 cases/100,000 population. The organisms most often responsible for community-acquired bacterial meningitis are *Streptococcus pneumoniae* (~50%), *Neisseria meningitidis* (~25%), group B streptococci (~15%), and *Listeria monocytogenes* (~10%). *Haemophilus influenzae* type b accounts for <10% of cases of bacterial meningitis in most series. *N. meningitidis* is the causative organism of recurring epidemics of meningitis every 8 to 12 years.

ETIOLOGY

S. pneumoniae (Chap. 136) is the most common cause of meningitis in adults >20 years of age, accounting for nearly half the reported cases (1.1 per 100,000 persons per year). There are a number of predisposing conditions that increase the risk of pneumococcal meningitis, the most important of which is pneumococcal pneumonia. Additional risk factors include coexisting acute or chronic pneumococcal sinusitis or otitis media, alcoholism, diabetes, splenectomy, hypogammaglobulinemia, complement deficiency, and head trauma with basilar skull fracture and CSF rhinorrhea. The mortality rate remains ~20% despite antibiotic therapy.

The incidence of meningitis due to *N. meningitidis* (Chap. 143) has decreased with the routine immunization of 11- to 18-year-olds with the tetravalent (serogroups A, C, W-135, and Y) meningococcal glycoconjugate vaccine. The vaccine does not contain serogroup B, which is responsible for one-third of cases of meningococcal disease. The presence of petechial or purpuric skin lesions can provide an important clue to the diagnosis of meningococcal infection. In some patients the disease is fulminant, progressing to death within hours of symptom onset. Infection may be initiated by nasopharyngeal colonization, which can result in either an asymptomatic carrier state or invasive meningococcal disease. The risk of invasive disease following nasopharyngeal colonization depends on both bacterial virulence factors and host immune defense mechanisms, including the host's capacity to produce antimeningococcal antibodies and to lyse meningococci by both classic and alternative complement pathways. Individuals with deficiencies of any of the complement components, including properdin, are highly susceptible to meningococcal infections.

Enteric gram-negative bacilli cause meningitis in individuals with chronic and debilitating diseases such as diabetes, cirrhosis, or alcoholism and in those with chronic urinary tract infections. Gram-negative meningitis can also complicate neurosurgical procedures, particularly craniotomy.

Otitis, mastoiditis, and sinusitis are predisposing and associated conditions for meningitis due to *Streptococci* sp., gram-negative anaerobes, *S. aureus, Haemophilus* sp., and Enterobacteriaceae. Meningitis complicating endocarditis may be due to viridans streptococci, *S. aureus, S. bovis,* the HACEK group (*Haemophilus* sp., *Actinobacillus actinomycetemcomitans, Cardiobacterium hominis, Eikenella corrodens, Kingella kingae*), or enterococci.

Group B streptococcus, or *S. agalactiae*, was previously responsible for meningitis predominantly in neonates, but it has been reported with increasing frequency in individuals >50 years of age, particularly those with underlying diseases.

L. monocytogenes (Chap. 139) is an increasingly important cause of meningitis in neonates (<1 month of age), pregnant women, individuals >60 years, and immunocompromised individuals of all ages. Infection is acquired by ingesting foods contaminated by *Listeria*. Foodborne human listerial infection has been reported from contaminated coleslaw, milk, soft cheeses, and several types of "ready-to-eat" foods, including delicatessen meat and uncooked hotdogs.

The frequency of *H. influenzae* type b meningitis in children has declined dramatically since the introduction of the Hib conjugate vaccine, although rare cases of Hib meningitis in vaccinated children have been reported. More frequently, *H. influenzae* causes meningitis in unvaccinated children and older adults, and non-b *H. influenzae* is an emerging pathogen.

Staphylococcus aureus and coagulase-negative staphylococci (Chap. 135) are important causes of meningitis that occurs following invasive neurosurgical procedures, particularly shunting procedures for hydrocephalus, or as a complication of the use of subcutaneous Ommaya reservoirs for administration of intrathecal chemotherapy.

PATHOPHYSIOLOGY

The most common bacteria that cause meningitis, *S. pneumoniae* and *N. meningitidis*, initially colonize the nasopharynx by attaching to nasopharyngeal epithelial cells. Bacteria are transported across epithelial cells in membrane-bound vacuoles to the intravascular space or invade the intravascular space by creating separations in the apical tight junctions of columnar epithelial cells. Once in the bloodstream, bacteria are able to avoid phagocytosis by neutrophils and classic complement-mediated bactericidal activity because of the

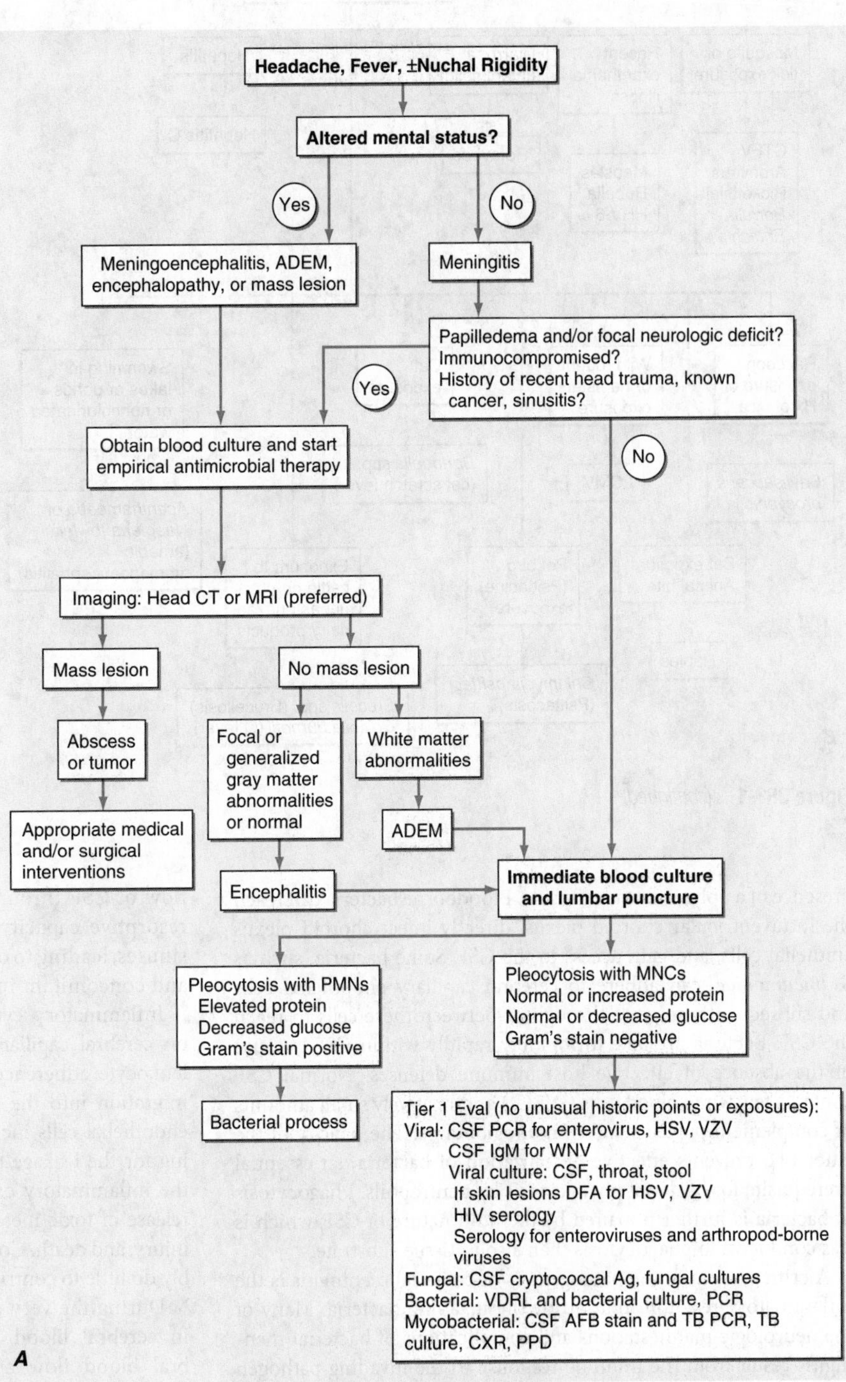

Figure 381-1 The management of patients with suspected CNS infection. ADEM, acute disseminated encephalomyelitis; AFB, acid-fast bacillus; Ag, antigen; CSF, cerebrospinal fluid; CT, computed tomography; CTFV, Colorado tick fever virus; CXR, chest x-ray; DFA, direct fluorescent antibody; EBV, Epstein-Barr virus; HHV, human herpesvirus; HSV, herpes simplex virus; LCMV, lymphocytic choriomeningitis virus; MNCs, mononuclear cells; MRI, magnetic resonance imaging; PCR, polymerase chain reaction; PMNs, polymorphonuclear leukocytes; PPD, purified protein derivative; TB, tuberculosis; VDRL, Venereal Disease Research Laboratory; VZV, varicella-zoster virus; WNV, West Nile virus.

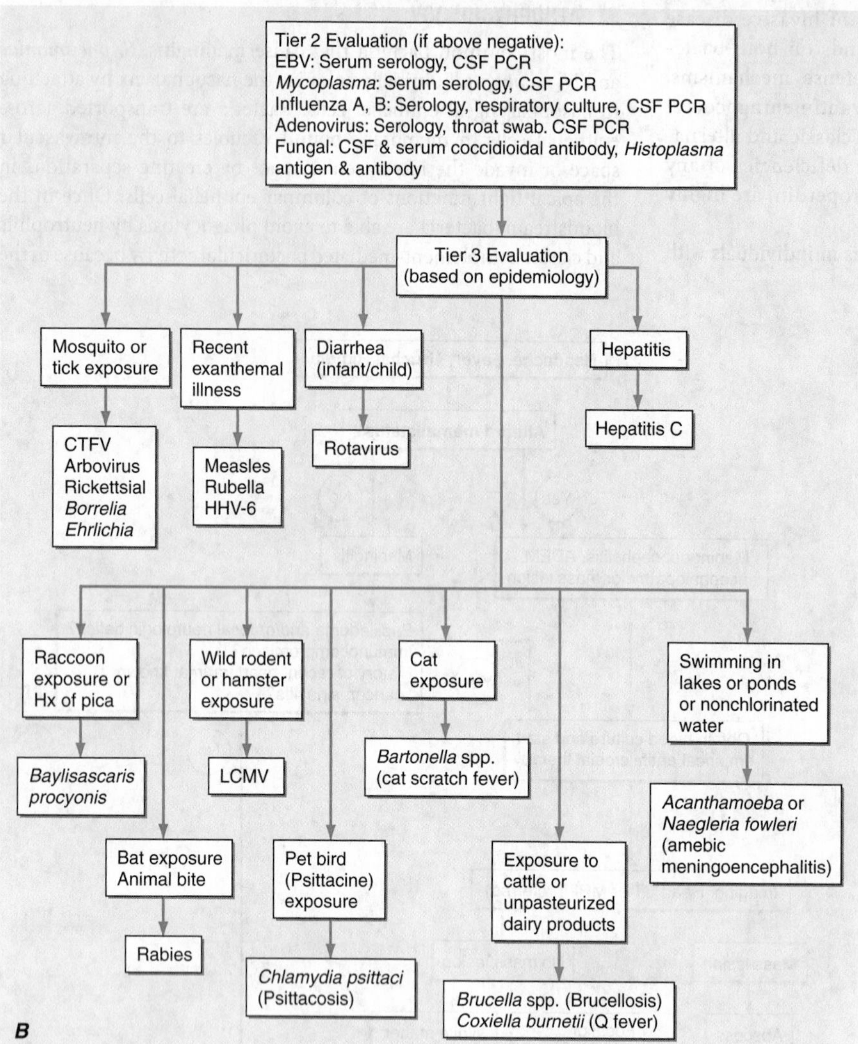

Figure 381-1 *(continued)*

presence of a polysaccharide capsule. Bloodborne bacteria can reach the intraventricular choroid plexus, directly infect choroid plexus epithelial cells, and gain access to the CSF. Some bacteria, such as *S. pneumoniae*, can adhere to cerebral capillary endothelial cells and subsequently migrate through or between these cells to reach the CSF. Bacteria are able to multiply rapidly within CSF because of the absence of effective host immune defenses. Normal CSF contains few white blood cells (WBCs) and relatively small amounts of complement proteins and immunoglobulins. The paucity of the latter two prevents effective opsonization of bacteria, an essential prerequisite for bacterial phagocytosis by neutrophils. Phagocytosis of bacteria is further impaired by the fluid nature of CSF, which is less conducive to phagocytosis than a solid tissue substrate.

A critical event in the pathogenesis of bacterial meningitis is the inflammatory reaction induced by the invading bacteria. Many of the neurologic manifestations and complications of bacterial meningitis result from the immune response to the invading pathogen rather than from direct bacteria-induced tissue injury. As a result, neurologic injury can progress even after the CSF has been sterilized by antibiotic therapy.

The lysis of bacteria with the subsequent release of cell-wall components into the subarachnoid space is the initial step in the induction of the inflammatory response and the formation of a purulent exudate in the subarachnoid space (Fig. 381-2). Bacterial cell-wall components, such as the lipopolysaccharide (LPS) molecules of gram-negative bacteria and teichoic acid and peptidoglycans of *S. pneumoniae*, induce meningeal inflammation by stimulating the production of inflammatory cytokines and chemokines by microglia, astrocytes, monocytes, microvascular endothelial cells, and CSF leukocytes. In experimental models of meningitis, cytokines including tumor necrosis factor alpha (TNF-α) and interleukin 1 β (IL-1β) are present in CSF within 1–2 h of intracisternal inoculation of LPS. This cytokine response is quickly followed by an increase in CSF protein concentration and leukocytosis. Chemokines (cytokines that induce chemotactic migration in leukocytes) and a variety of other proinflammatory cytokines are also produced and secreted by leukocytes and tissue cells that are stimulated by IL-1β and TNF-α. In addition, bacteremia and the inflammatory cytokines induce the production of excitatory amino acids, reactive oxygen and nitrogen species (free oxygen radicals, nitric oxide, and peroxynitrite), and other mediators that can induce death of brain cells, especially in the dentate gyrus of the hippocampus.

Much of the pathophysiology of bacterial meningitis is a direct consequence of elevated levels of CSF cytokines and chemokines. TNF-α and IL-1β act synergistically to increase the permeability of the blood-brain barrier, resulting in induction of vasogenic edema and the leakage of serum proteins into the subarachnoid space (Fig. 381-2). The subarachnoid exudate of proteinaceous material and leukocytes obstructs the flow of CSF through the ventricular system and diminishes the resorptive capacity of the arachnoid granulations in the dural sinuses, leading to obstructive and communicating hydrocephalus and concomitant interstitial edema.

Inflammatory cytokines upregulate the expression of selectins on cerebral capillary endothelial cells and leukocytes, promoting leukocyte adherence to vascular endothelial cells and subsequent migration into the CSF. The adherence of leukocytes to capillary endothelial cells increases the permeability of blood vessels, allowing for the leakage of plasma proteins into the CSF, which adds to the inflammatory exudate. Neutrophil degranulation results in the release of toxic metabolites that contribute to cytotoxic edema, cell injury, and death. Contrary to previous beliefs, CSF leukocytes probably do little to contribute to the clearance of CSF bacterial infection.

During the very early stages of meningitis, there is an increase in cerebral blood flow, soon followed by a decrease in cerebral blood flow and a loss of cerebrovascular autoregulation (Chap. 275). Narrowing of the large arteries at the base of the brain due to encroachment by the purulent exudate in the subarachnoid space and infiltration of the arterial wall by inflammatory cells with intimal thickening (*vasculitis*) also occur and may result in ischemia and infarction, obstruction of branches of the middle cerebral artery by thrombosis, thrombosis of the major cerebral venous sinuses, and thrombophlebitis of the cerebral cortical veins. The combination of interstitial, vasogenic, and cytotoxic edema

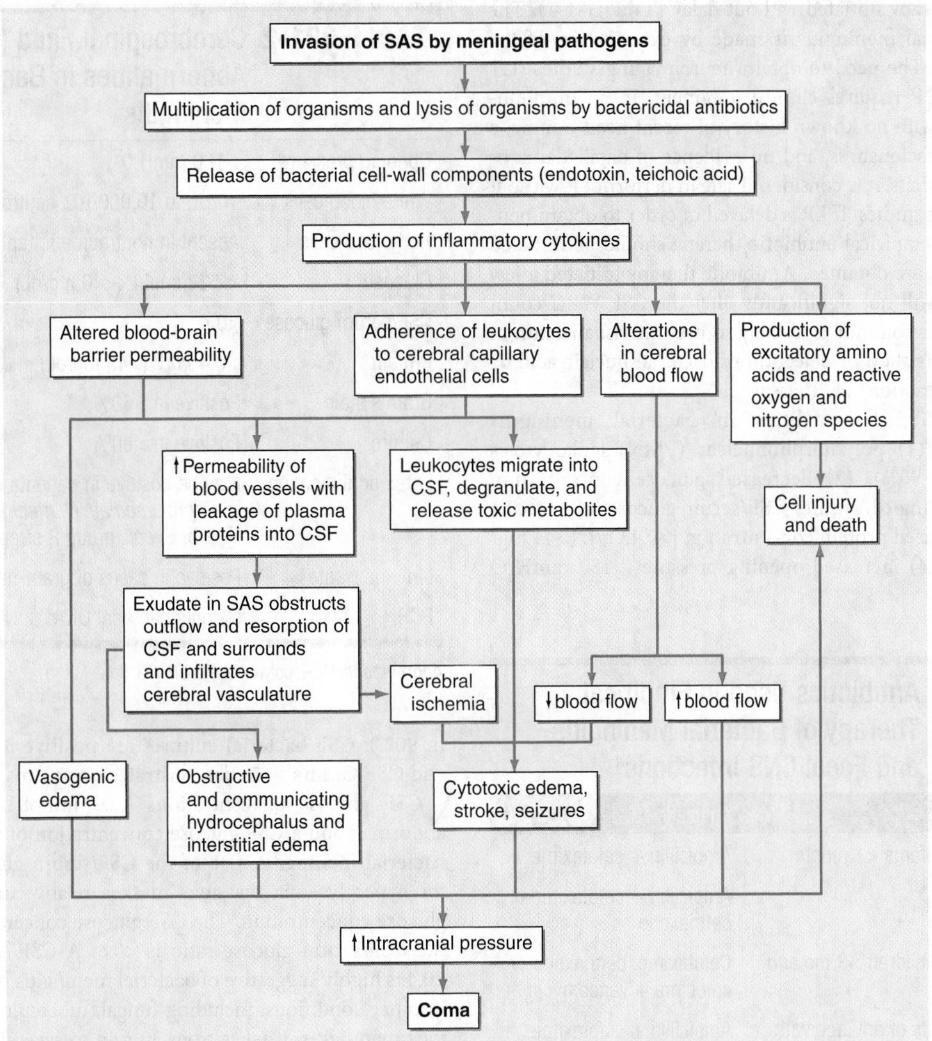

Figure 381-2 The pathophysiology of the neurologic complications of bacterial meningitis. CSF, cerebrospinal fluid; SAS, subarachnoid space.

leads to raised ICP and coma. Cerebral herniation usually results from the effects of cerebral edema, either focal or generalized; hydrocephalus and dural sinus or cortical vein thrombosis may also play a role.

CLINICAL PRESENTATION

Meningitis can present as either an acute fulminant illness that progresses rapidly in a few hours or as a subacute infection that progressively worsens over several days. The classic clinical triad of meningitis is fever, headache, and nuchal rigidity, but the classic triad may not be present. A decreased level of consciousness occurs in >75% of patients and can vary from lethargy to coma. Fever and either headache, stiff neck, or an altered level of consciousness will be present in nearly every patient with bacterial meningitis. Nausea, vomiting, and photophobia are also common complaints.

Seizures occur as part of the initial presentation of bacterial meningitis or during the course of the illness in 20–40% of patients. Focal seizures are usually due to focal arterial ischemia or infarction, cortical venous thrombosis with hemorrhage, or focal edema. Generalized seizure activity and status epilepticus may be due to hyponatremia, cerebral anoxia, or, less commonly, the toxic effects of antimicrobial agents such as high-dose penicillin.

Raised ICP is an expected complication of bacterial meningitis and the major cause of obtundation and coma in this disease. More than 90% of patients will have a CSF opening pressure >180 mmH_2O, and 20% have opening pressures >400 mmH_2O. Signs of increased ICP include a deteriorating or reduced level of consciousness, papilledema, dilated poorly reactive pupils, sixth nerve palsies, decerebrate posturing, and the Cushing reflex (bradycardia, hypertension, and irregular respirations). The most disastrous complication of increased ICP is cerebral herniation. The incidence of herniation in patients with bacterial meningitis has been reported to occur in as few as 1% to as many as 8% of cases.

Specific clinical features may provide clues to the diagnosis of individual organisms and are discussed in more detail in specific chapters devoted to individual pathogens. The most important of these clues is the rash of meningococcemia, which begins as a diffuse erythematous maculopapular rash resembling a viral exanthem; however, the skin lesions of meningococcemia rapidly become petechial. Petechiae are found on the trunk and lower extremities, in the mucous membranes and conjunctiva, and occasionally on the palms and soles.

DIAGNOSIS

When bacterial meningitis is suspected, blood cultures should be immediately obtained and empirical antimicrobial and adjunctive dexamethasone therapy initiated without delay (Table 381-1). The diagnosis of bacterial meningitis is made by examination of the CSF (Table 381-2). The need to obtain neuroimaging studies (CT or MRI) prior to LP requires clinical judgment. In an immunocompetent patient with no known history of recent head trauma, a normal level of consciousness, and no evidence of papilledema or focal neurologic deficits, it is considered safe to perform LP without prior neuroimaging studies. If LP is delayed in order to obtain neuroimaging studies, empirical antibiotic therapy should be initiated after blood cultures are obtained. Antibiotic therapy initiated a few hours prior to LP will not significantly alter the CSF WBC count or glucose concentration, nor is it likely to prevent visualization of organisms by Gram's stain or detection of bacterial nucleic acid by polymerase chain reaction (PCR) assay.

The classic CSF abnormalities in bacterial meningitis (Table 381-2) are (1) polymorphonuclear (PMN) leukocytosis (>100 cells/μL in 90%), (2) decreased glucose concentration [<2.2 mmol/L (<40 mg/dL) and/or CSF/serum glucose ratio of <0.4 in ~60%], (3) increased protein concentration [>0.45 g/L (>45 mg/dL) in 90%], and (4) increased opening pressure (>180 mmH_2O in 90%). CSF bacterial cultures are positive in >80% of patients, and CSF Gram's stain demonstrates organisms in >60%.

TABLE 381-1 Antibiotics Used in Empirical Therapy of Bacterial Meningitis and Focal CNS Infections[a]

Indication	Antibiotic
Preterm infants to infants <1 month	Ampicillin + cefotaxime
Infants 1–3 mo	Ampicillin + cefotaxime or ceftriaxone
Immunocompetent children >3 mo and adults <55	Cefotaxime, ceftriaxone or cefepime + vancomycin
Adults >55 and adults of any age with alcoholism or other debilitating illnesses	Ampicillin + cefotaxime, ceftriaxone or cefepime + vancomycin
Hospital-acquired meningitis, posttraumatic or postneurosurgery meningitis, neutropenic patients, or patients with impaired cell-mediated immunity	Ampicillin + ceftazidime or meropenem + vancomycin

Antimicrobial Agent	Total Daily Dose and Dosing Interval: Child (>1 month)	Adult
Ampicillin	200 (mg/kg)/d, q4h	12 g/d, q4h
Cefepime	150 (mg/kg)/d, q8h	6 g/d, q8h
Cefotaxime	200 (mg/kg)/d, q6h	12 g/d, q4h
Ceftriaxone	100 (mg/kg)/d, q12h	4 g/d, q12h
Ceftazidime	150 (mg/kg)/d, q8h	6 g/d, q8h
Gentamicin	7.5 (mg/kg)/d, q8h[b]	7.5 (mg/kg)/d, q8h
Meropenem	120 (mg/kg)/d, q8h	3 g/d, q8h
Metronidazole	30 (mg/kg)/d, q6h	1500–2000 mg/d, q6h
Nafcillin	100–200 (mg/kg)/d, q6h	9–12 g/d, q4h
Penicillin G	400,000 (U/kg)/d, q4h	20–24 million U/d, q4h
Vancomycin	60 (mg/kg)/d, q6h	2 g/d, q12h[b]

[a]All antibiotics are administered intravenously; doses indicated assume normal renal and hepatic function.

[b]Doses should be adjusted based on serum peak and trough levels: gentamicin therapeutic level: peak: 5–8 μg/mL; trough: <2 μg/mL; vancomycin therapeutic level: peak: 25–40 μg/mL; trough: 5–15 μg/mL.

TABLE 381-2 Cerebrospinal Fluid (CSF) Abnormalities in Bacterial Meningitis

Opening pressure	>180 mmH_2O
White blood cells	10/μL to 10,000/μL; neutrophils predominate
Red blood cells	Absent in nontraumatic tap
Glucose	<2.2 mmol/L (<40 mg/dL)
CSF/serum glucose	<0.4
Protein	>0.45 g/L (>45 mg/dL)
Gram's stain	Positive in >60%
Culture	Positive in >80%
Latex agglutination	May be positive in patients with meningitis due to *S. pneumoniae, N. meningitidis, H. influenzae* type b, *E. coli*, group B streptococci
Limulus lysate	Positive in cases of gram-negative meningitis
PCR	Detects bacterial DNA

Abbreviation: PCR, polymerase chain reaction.

CSF glucose concentrations <2.2 mmol/L (<40 mg/dL) are abnormal, and a CSF glucose concentration of zero can be seen in bacterial meningitis. Use of the CSF/serum glucose ratio corrects for hyperglycemia that may mask a relative decrease in the CSF glucose concentration. The CSF glucose concentration is low when the CSF/serum glucose ratio is <0.6. A CSF/serum glucose ratio <0.4 is highly suggestive of bacterial meningitis but may also be seen in other conditions, including fungal, tuberculous, and carcinomatous meningitis. It takes from 30 min to several hours for the concentration of CSF glucose to reach equilibrium with blood glucose levels; therefore, administration of 50 mL of 50% glucose (D50) prior to LP, as commonly occurs in emergency room settings, is unlikely to alter CSF glucose concentration significantly unless more than a few hours have elapsed between glucose administration and LP.

A 16S rRNA conserved sequence broad-based bacterial PCR can detect small numbers of viable and nonviable organisms in CSF and is expected to be useful for making a diagnosis of bacterial meningitis in patients who have been pretreated with oral or parenteral antibiotics and in whom Gram's stain and CSF culture are negative. When the broad-range PCR is positive, a PCR that uses specific bacterial primers to detect the nucleic acid of *S. pneumoniae, N. meningitidis, Escherichia coli, L. monocytogenes, H. influenzae*, and *S. agalactiae* can be obtained based on the clinical suspicion of the meningeal pathogen. The latex agglutination (LA) test for the detection of bacterial antigens of *S. pneumoniae, N. meningitidis, H. influenzae* type b, group B streptococcus, and *E. coli* K1 strains in the CSF has been useful for making a diagnosis of bacterial meningitis but is being replaced by the CSF bacterial PCR assay. The CSF LA test has a *specificity* of 95–100% for *S. pneumoniae* and *N. meningitidis*, so a positive test is virtually diagnostic of bacterial meningitis caused by these organisms. However, the *sensitivity* of the CSF LA test is only 70–100% for detection of *S. pneumoniae* and 33–70% for detection of *N. meningitidis* antigens, so a negative test does not exclude infection by these organisms. The Limulus amebocyte lysate assay is a rapid diagnostic test for the detection of gram-negative endotoxin in CSF and thus for making a diagnosis of gram-negative bacterial meningitis. The test has a specificity of 85–100% and a sensitivity approaching 100%. Thus, a positive Limulus amebocyte lysate assay occurs in virtually all patients with gram-negative bacterial meningitis, but false positives may occur.

Almost all patients with bacterial meningitis will have neuroimaging studies performed during the course of their illness. MRI is preferred over CT because of its superiority in demonstrating areas of cerebral edema and ischemia. In patients with bacterial meningitis, diffuse meningeal enhancement is often seen after the administration of gadolinium. Meningeal enhancement is not diagnostic of meningitis but occurs in any CNS disease associated with increased blood-brain barrier permeability.

Petechial skin lesions, if present, should be biopsied. The rash of meningococcemia results from the dermal seeding of organisms with vascular endothelial damage, and biopsy may reveal the organism on Gram's stain.

DIFFERENTIAL DIAGNOSIS

Viral meningoencephalitis, and particularly herpes simplex virus (HSV) encephalitis, can mimic the clinical presentation of bacterial meningitis (see "Viral Encephalitis," below). HSV encephalitis typically presents with headache, fever, altered consciousness, focal neurologic deficits (e.g., dysphasia, hemiparesis), and focal or generalized seizures. The findings on CSF studies, neuroimaging, and electroencephalogram (EEG) distinguish HSV encephalitis from bacterial meningitis. The typical CSF profile with viral CNS infections is a lymphocytic pleocytosis with a normal glucose concentration, in contrast to PMN pleocytosis and hypoglycorrhachia characteristic of bacterial meningitis. MRI abnormalities (other than meningeal enhancement) are not seen in uncomplicated bacterial meningitis. By contrast, in HSV encephalitis, on T2-weighted and fluid-attenuated inversion recovery (FLAIR) MRI images, high signal intensity lesions are seen in the orbitofrontal, anterior, and medial temporal lobes in the majority of patients within 48 h of symptom onset. Some patients with HSV encephalitis have a distinctive periodic pattern on EEG (see below).

Rickettsial disease can resemble bacterial meningitis (Chap. 174). Rocky Mountain spotted fever (RMSF) is transmitted by a tick bite and caused by the bacteria *Rickettsia rickettsii*. The disease may present acutely with high fever, prostration, myalgia, headache, nausea, and vomiting. Most patients develop a characteristic rash within 96 h of the onset of symptoms. The rash is initially a diffuse erythematous maculopapular rash that may be difficult to distinguish from that of meningococcemia. It progresses to a petechial rash, then to a purpuric rash and, if untreated, to skin necrosis or gangrene. The color of the lesions changes from bright red to very dark red, then yellowish-green to black. The rash typically begins in the wrist and ankles and then spreads distally and proximally within a matter of a few hours, involving the palms and soles. Diagnosis is made by immunofluorescent staining of skin biopsy specimens. Ehrlichioses are also transmitted by a tick bite. These are small gram-negative coccobacilli of which two species cause human disease. *Anaplasma phagocytophilum* causes human granulocytic ehrlichiosis (anaplasmosis), and *Ehrlichia chaffeensis* causes human monocytic ehrlichiosis. The clinical and laboratory manifestations of the infections are similar. Patients present with fever, headache, nausea, and vomiting. Twenty percent of patients have a maculopapular or petechial rash. There is laboratory evidence of leukopenia, thrombocytopenia, and anemia, and mild to moderate elevations in alanine aminotransferases, alkaline phosphatase, and lactate dehydrogenase. Patients with RMSF and those with ehrlichial infections may have an altered level of consciousness ranging from mild lethargy to coma, confusion, focal neurologic signs, cranial nerve palsies, hyperreflexia, and seizures.

Focal suppurative CNS infections (see below), including subdural and epidural empyema and brain abscess, should also be considered, especially when focal neurologic findings are present. MRI should be performed promptly in all patients with suspected meningitis who have focal features, both to detect the intracranial infection and to search for associated areas of infection in the sinuses or mastoid bones.

A number of noninfectious CNS disorders can mimic bacterial meningitis. Subarachnoid hemorrhage (SAH; Chap. 275) is generally the major consideration. Other possibilities include chemical meningitis due to rupture of tumor contents into the CSF (e.g., from a cystic glioma or craniopharyngioma epidermoid or dermoid cyst); drug-induced hypersensitivity meningitis; carcinomatous or lymphomatous meningitis; meningitis associated with inflammatory disorders such as sarcoid, systemic lupus erythematosus (SLE), and Behçet's syndrome; pituitary apoplexy; and uveomeningitic syndromes (Vogt-Koyanagi-Harada syndrome).

On occasion, subacutely evolving meningitis (Chap. 382) may be considered in the differential diagnosis of acute meningitis. The principal causes include *Mycobacterium tuberculosis* (Chap. 165), *Cryptococcus neoformans* (Chap. 202), *Histoplasma capsulatum* (Chap. 199), *Coccidioides immitis* (Chap. 200), and *Treponema pallidum* (Chap. 169).

TREATMENT Acute Bacterial Meningitis

EMPIRICAL ANTIMICROBIAL THERAPY (Table 381-1) Bacterial meningitis is a medical emergency. The goal is to begin antibiotic therapy within 60 min of a patient's arrival in the emergency room. Empirical antimicrobial therapy is initiated in patients with suspected bacterial meningitis before the results of CSF Gram's stain and culture are known. *S. pneumoniae* (Chap. 134) and *N. meningitidis* (Chap. 143) are the most common etiologic organisms of community-acquired bacterial meningitis. Due to the emergence of penicillin- and cephalosporin-resistant *S. pneumoniae*, empirical therapy of community-acquired suspected bacterial meningitis in children and adults should include a combination of dexamethasone, a third- or fourth-generation cephalosporin (e.g., ceftriaxone, cefotaxime, or cefepime), and vancomycin, plus acyclovir, as HSV encephalitis is the leading disease in the differential diagnosis, and doxycycline during tick season to treat tick-borne bacterial infections. Ceftriaxone or cefotaxime provide good coverage for susceptible *S. pneumoniae*, group B streptococci, and *H. influenzae* and adequate coverage for *N. meningitidis*. Cefepime is a broad-spectrum fourth-generation cephalosporin with in vitro activity similar to that of cefotaxime or ceftriaxone against *S. pneumoniae* and *N. meningitidis* and greater activity against *Enterobacter* species and *Pseudomonas aeruginosa*. In clinical trials, cefepime has been demonstrated to be equivalent to cefotaxime in the treatment of penicillin-sensitive pneumococcal and meningococcal meningitis, and it has been used successfully in some patients with meningitis due to *Enterobacter* species and *P. aeruginosa*. Ampicillin should be added to the empirical regimen for coverage of *L. monocytogenes* in individuals <3 months of age, those >55, or those with suspected impaired cell-mediated immunity because of chronic illness, organ transplantation, pregnancy, malignancy, or immunosuppressive therapy. Metronidazole is added to the empirical regimen to cover gram-negative anaerobes in patients with otitis, sinusitis, or mastoiditis. In hospital-acquired meningitis, and particularly meningitis following neurosurgical procedures, staphylococci and gram-negative organisms including *P. aeruginosa* are the most common etiologic organisms. In these patients, empirical therapy should include a combination of vancomycin and ceftazidime, cefepime, or meropenem. Ceftazidime, cefepime, or meropenem should be substituted for ceftriaxone or cefotaxime in neurosurgical patients and in neutropenic patients, as ceftriaxone and cefotaxime do not provide adequate activity against CNS infection with *P. aeruginosa*. Meropenem is a carbapenem antibiotic that is highly active in vitro against *L. monocytogenes*, has been demonstrated to be effective in cases of meningitis caused by *P. aeruginosa*, and shows good activity against penicillin-resistant pneumococci. In experimental pneumococcal meningitis, meropenem was comparable to ceftriaxone and inferior to vancomycin in sterilizing CSF cultures. The number of patients with bacterial meningitis enrolled in clinical trials of meropenem has not been sufficient to definitively assess the efficacy of this antibiotic.

SPECIFIC ANTIMICROBIAL THERAPY

Meningococcal Meningitis (Table 381-3) Although ceftriaxone and cefotaxime provide adequate empirical coverage for *N. meningitidis*, penicillin G remains the antibiotic of choice for meningococcal meningitis caused by susceptible strains. Isolates of *N. meningitidis* with moderate resistance to penicillin have been identified, but patients infected with these strains have still been successfully treated with penicillin. CSF isolates of *N. meningitidis* should be tested for penicillin and ampicillin susceptibility, and if resistance is found, cefotaxime or ceftriaxone should be substituted for penicillin. A 7-day course of intravenous antibiotic therapy is adequate for uncomplicated meningococcal meningitis. The index case and all close contacts should receive chemoprophylaxis with a 2-day regimen of rifampin (600 mg every 12 h for 2 days in adults and 10 mg/kg every 12 h for 2 days in children >1 year). Rifampin is not recommended in pregnant women. Alternatively, adults can be treated with one dose of azithromycin (500 mg), or one intramuscular dose of ceftriaxone (250 mg). Close contacts are defined as those individuals who have had contact with oropharyngeal secretions, either through kissing or by sharing toys, beverages, or cigarettes.

TABLE 381-3 Antimicrobial Therapy of CNS Bacterial Infections Based on Pathogen[a]

Organism	Antibiotic
Neisseria meningitides	
Penicillin-sensitive	Penicillin G or ampicillin
Penicillin-resistant	Ceftriaxone or cefotaxime
Streptococcus pneumoniae	
Penicillin-sensitive	Penicillin G
Penicillin-intermediate	Ceftriaxone or cefotaxime or cefepime
Penicillin-resistant	(Ceftriaxone or cefotaxime or cefepime) + vancomycin
Gram-negative bacilli (except *Pseudomonas* spp.)	Ceftriaxone or cefotaxime
Pseudomonas aeruginosa	Ceftazidime or cefepime or meropenem
Staphylococci spp.	
Methicillin-sensitive	Nafcillin
Methicillin-resistant	Vancomycin
Listeria monocytogenes	Ampicillin + gentamicin
Haemophilus influenzae	Ceftriaxone or cefotaxime or cefepime
Streptococcus agalactiae	Penicillin G or ampicillin
Bacteroides fragilis	Metronidazole
Fusobacterium spp.	Metronidazole

[a]Doses are as indicated in Table 381-1.

Pneumococcal Meningitis Antimicrobial therapy of pneumococcal meningitis is initiated with a cephalosporin (ceftriaxone, cefotaxime, or cefepime) and vancomycin. All CSF isolates of *S. pneumoniae* should be tested for sensitivity to penicillin and the cephalosporins. Once the results of antimicrobial susceptibility tests are known, therapy can be modified accordingly (Table 381-3). For *S. pneumoniae* meningitis, an isolate of *S. pneumoniae* is considered to be susceptible to penicillin with a minimal inhibitory concentration (MIC) <0.06 μg/mL, to have intermediate resistance when the MIC is 0.1–1.0 μg/mL, and to be highly resistant when the MIC >1.0 μg/mL. Isolates of *S. pneumoniae* that have cephalosporin MICs ≤0.5 μg/mL are considered sensitive to the cephalosporins (cefotaxime, ceftriaxone, cefepime). Those with MICs of 1 μg/mL are considered to have intermediate resistance, and those with MICs ≥2 μg/mL are considered resistant. For meningitis due to pneumococci, with cefotaxime or ceftriaxone MICs ≤0.5 μg/mL, treatment with cefotaxime or ceftriaxone is usually adequate. For MIC >1 μg/mL, vancomycin is the antibiotic of choice. Rifampin can be added to vancomycin for its synergistic effect but is inadequate as monotherapy because resistance develops rapidly when it is used alone.

A 2-week course of intravenous antimicrobial therapy is recommended for pneumococcal meningitis.

Patients with *S. pneumoniae* meningitis should have a repeat LP performed 24–36 h after the initiation of antimicrobial therapy to document sterilization of the CSF. Failure to sterilize the CSF after 24–36 h of antibiotic therapy should be considered presumptive evidence of antibiotic resistance. Patients with penicillin- and cephalosporin-resistant strains of *S. pneumoniae* who do not respond to intravenous vancomycin alone may benefit from the addition of intraventricular vancomycin. The intraventricular route of administration is preferred over the intrathecal route because adequate concentrations of vancomycin in the cerebral ventricles are not always achieved with intrathecal administration.

***Listeria* Meningitis** Meningitis due to *L. monocytogenes* is treated with ampicillin for at least 3 weeks (Table 381-3). Gentamicin is added in critically ill patients (2 mg/kg loading dose, then 7.5 mg/kg per day given every 8 h and adjusted for serum levels and renal function). The combination of trimethoprim (10–20 mg/kg per day) and sulfamethoxazole (50–100 mg/kg per day) given every 6 h may provide an alternative in penicillin-allergic patients.

Staphylococcal Meningitis Meningitis due to susceptible strains of *S. aureus* or coagulase-negative staphylococci is treated with nafcillin (Table 381-3). Vancomycin is the drug of choice for methicillin-resistant staphylococci and for patients allergic to penicillin. In these patients, the CSF should be monitored during therapy. If the CSF is not sterilized after 48 h of intravenous vancomycin therapy, then either intraventricular or intrathecal vancomycin, 20 mg once daily, can be added.

Gram-Negative Bacillary Meningitis The third-generation cephalosporins—cefotaxime, ceftriaxone, and ceftazidime—are equally efficacious for the treatment of gram-negative bacillary meningitis, with the exception of meningitis due to *P. aeruginosa*, which should be treated with ceftazidime, cefepime, or meropenem (Table 381-3). A 3-week course of intravenous antibiotic therapy is recommended for meningitis due to gram-negative bacilli.

ADJUNCTIVE THERAPY The release of bacterial cell-wall components by bactericidal antibiotics leads to the production of the inflammatory cytokines IL-1β and TNF-α in the subarachnoid space. Dexamethasone exerts its beneficial effect by inhibiting the synthesis of IL-1β and TNF-α at the level of mRNA, decreasing CSF outflow resistance, and stabilizing the blood-brain barrier. The rationale for giving dexamethasone 20 min before antibiotic therapy is that dexamethasone inhibits the production of TNF-α by macrophages and microglia only if it is administered before these cells are activated by endotoxin. Dexamethasone does not alter TNF-α production once it has been induced. The results of clinical trials of dexamethasone therapy in children, predominantly with meningitis due to *H. influenzae* and *S. pneumoniae*, have demonstrated its efficacy in decreasing meningeal inflammation and neurologic sequelae such as the incidence of sensorineural hearing loss.

A prospective European trial of adjunctive therapy for acute bacterial meningitis in 301 adults found that dexamethasone reduced the number of unfavorable outcomes (15 vs. 25%, p = .03) including death (7 vs. 15%, p = .04). The benefits were most striking in patients with pneumococcal meningitis. Dexamethasone (10 mg intravenously) was administered 15–20 min before the first dose of an antimicrobial agent, and the same dose was repeated every 6 h for 4 days. These results were confirmed in a second trial of dexamethasone in adults with pneumococcal meningitis. Therapy with dexamethasone should ideally be started 20 min before, or not later than concurrent with, the first dose of antibiotics. It is unlikely to be of significant benefit if started >6 h after antimicrobial therapy has been initiated. Dexamethasone may decrease the penetration of vancomycin into CSF, and it delays the sterilization of CSF in experimental models of *S. pneumoniae* meningitis. As a result, its potential benefit should be carefully weighed when vancomycin is the antibiotic of choice. Alternatively, vancomycin can be administered by the intraventricular route.

One of the concerns for using dexamethasone in adults with bacterial meningitis is that in experimental models of meningitis, dexamethasone therapy increased hippocampal cell injury and reduced learning capacity. This has not been the case in clinical series. The efficacy of dexamethasone therapy in preventing neurologic sequelae is different between high- and low-income countries. Three large randomized trials in low-income countries (sub-Saharan Africa, Southeast Asia) failed to show benefit in subgroups of patients. The lack of efficacy of dexamethasone in these trials has been attributed to late presentation to the hospital with more advanced disease, antibiotic pretreatment, malnutrition, infection with HIV, and treatment of patients with probable, but not microbiologically proven, bacterial meningitis. The results of these clinical trials suggest that patients in sub-Saharan Africa and those in low-income countries with negative CSF Gram's stain and culture should not be treated with dexamethasone.

INCREASED INTRACRANIAL PRESSURE Emergency treatment of increased ICP includes elevation of the patient's head to 30–45°, intubation and hyperventilation (Pa_{CO_2} 25–30 mm Hg), and mannitol. Patients with increased ICP should be managed in an intensive care unit; accurate ICP measurements are best obtained with an ICP monitoring device.

Treatment of increased intracranial pressure is discussed in detail in Chap. 275.

PROGNOSIS

Mortality rate is 3–7% for meningitis caused by *H. influenzae, N. meningitidis*, or group B streptococci; 15% for that due to *L. monocytogenes*; and 20% for *S. pneumoniae*. In general, the risk of death from bacterial meningitis increases with (1) decreased level of consciousness on admission, (2) onset of seizures within 24 h of admission, (3) signs of increased ICP, (4) young age (infancy) and age >50, (5) the presence of comorbid conditions including shock and/or the need for mechanical ventilation, and (6) delay in the initiation of treatment. Decreased CSF glucose concentration [<2.2 mmol/L (<40 mg/dL)] and markedly increased CSF protein concentration [>3 g/L (> 300 mg/dL)] have been predictive of increased mortality and poorer outcomes in some series. Moderate or severe sequelae occur in ~25% of survivors, although the exact incidence varies with the infecting organism. Common sequelae include decreased intellectual function, memory impairment, seizures, hearing loss and dizziness, and gait disturbances.

ACUTE VIRAL MENINGITIS

CLINICAL MANIFESTATIONS

Immunocompetent adult patients with viral meningitis usually present with headache, fever, and signs of meningeal irritation coupled with an inflammatory CSF profile (see below). Headache is almost invariably present and often characterized as frontal or retroorbital and frequently associated with photophobia and pain on moving the eyes. Nuchal rigidity is present in most cases but may be mild and present only near the limit of neck anteflexion. Constitutional signs can include malaise, myalgia, anorexia, nausea and vomiting, abdominal pain, and/or diarrhea. Patients often have mild lethargy or drowsiness; however, profound alterations in consciousness, such as stupor, coma, or marked confusion do not occur in viral meningitis and suggest the presence of encephalitis or other alternative diagnoses. Similarly, seizures or focal neurologic signs or symptoms or neuroimaging abnormalities indicative of brain parenchymal involvement are not typical of viral meningitis and suggest the presence of encephalitis or another CNS infectious or inflammatory process.

ETIOLOGY

Using a variety of diagnostic techniques, including CSF PCR, culture, and serology, a specific viral cause can be found in 75–90% of cases of viral meningitis. The most important agents are enteroviruses (including echoviruses and coxsackieviruses in addition to numbered enteroviruses), HSV type 2 (HSV-2), HIV, and arboviruses (Table 381-4). CSF cultures are positive in 30–70% of patients, the frequency of isolation depending on the specific viral agent. Approximately two-thirds of culture-negative cases of "aseptic" meningitis have a specific viral etiology identified by CSF PCR testing (see below).

EPIDEMIOLOGY

Viral meningitis is not a nationally reportable disease; however, it has been estimated that the incidence is ~75,000 cases per year. In temperate climates, there is a substantial increase in cases during the summer and early fall months, reflecting the seasonal predominance of enterovirus and arthropod-borne virus (arbovirus) infections, with a peak monthly incidence of about 1 reported case per 100,000 population.

TABLE 381-4 Viruses Causing Acute Meningitis and Encephalitis in North America

Acute Meningitis	
Common	**Less Common**
Enteroviruses (coxsackieviruses, echoviruses, and human enteroviruses 68–71)	Varicella zoster virus
Herpes simplex virus 2	Epstein-Barr virus
Arthropod-borne viruses	Lymphocytic choriomeningitis virus
HIV	
Acute Encephalitis	
Common	**Less Common**
Herpesviruses	Rabies
Herpes simplex virus 1	Eastern equine encephalitis virus
Varicella zoster virus	Western equine encephalitis virus
Epstein-Barr virus	Powassan virus
Arthropod-borne viruses	Cytomegalovirus[a]
La Crosse virus	Enteroviruses[a]
West Nile virus	Colorado tick fever
St. Louis encephalitis virus	Mumps

[a]Immunocompromised host.

LABORATORY DIAGNOSIS

CSF examination

The most important laboratory test in the diagnosis of viral meningitis is examination of the CSF. The typical profile is a lymphocytic pleocytosis (25–500 cells/μL), a normal or slightly elevated protein concentration [0.2–0.8 g/L (20–80 mg/dL)], a normal glucose concentration, and a normal or mildly elevated opening pressure (100–350 mmH_2O). Organisms are *not* seen on Gram's stain of CSF. Rarely, PMNs may predominate in the first 48 h of illness, especially with infections due to echovirus 9, West Nile virus, eastern equine encephalitis (EEE) virus, or mumps. A pleocytosis of polymorphonuclear neutrophils occurs in 45% of patients with West Nile virus (WNV) meningitis and can persist for a week or longer before shifting to a lymphocytic pleocytosis. Despite these exceptions, the presence of a CSF PMN pleocytosis in a patient with suspected viral meningitis in whom a specific diagnosis has not been established should prompt consideration of alternative diagnoses, including bacterial meningitis or parameningeal infections. The total CSF cell count in viral meningitis is typically 25–500/μL, although cell counts of several thousand/μL are occasionally seen, especially with infections due to lymphocytic choriomeningitis virus (LCMV) and mumps virus. The CSF glucose concentration is typically normal in viral infections, although it may be decreased in 10–30% of cases due to mumps or LCMV. Rare instances of decreased CSF glucose concentration occur in cases of meningitis due to echoviruses and other enteroviruses, HSV-2, and varicella-zoster virus (VZV). As a rule, a lymphocytic pleocytosis with a low glucose concentration should suggest fungal or tuberculous meningitis, *Listeria* meningoencephalitis, or noninfectious disorders (e.g., sarcoid, neoplastic meningitis).

A number of tests measuring levels of various CSF proteins, enzymes, and mediators—including C-reactive protein, lactic acid, lactate dehydrogenase, neopterin, quinolinate, IL-1β, IL-6, soluble IL-2 receptor, β_2-microglobulin, and TNF—have been proposed as potential discriminators between viral and bacterial meningitis or as markers of specific types of viral infection (e.g., infection with HIV), but they remain of uncertain sensitivity and specificity and are not widely used for diagnostic purposes.

Polymerase chain reaction amplification of viral nucleic acid

Amplification of viral-specific DNA or RNA from CSF using PCR amplification has become the single most important method for diagnosing CNS viral infections. In both enteroviral and HSV infections of the CNS, PCR has become the diagnostic procedure of choice and is substantially more sensitive than viral cultures. HSV PCR is also an important diagnostic test in patients with recurrent episodes of "aseptic" meningitis, many of whom have amplifiable HSV DNA in CSF despite negative viral cultures. CSF PCR is also used routinely to diagnose CNS viral infections caused by cytomegalovirus (CMV), Epstein-Barr virus (EBV), VZV, and human herpesvirus 6 (HHV-6). CSF PCR tests are available for WNV but are not as sensitive as detection of WNV-specific CSF IgM. PCR is also useful in the diagnosis of CNS infection caused by *Mycoplasma pneumoniae,* which can mimic viral meningitis and encephalitis.

Viral culture

The sensitivity of CSF cultures for the diagnosis of viral meningitis and encephalitis, in contrast to its utility in bacterial infections, is generally poor. In addition to CSF, specific viruses may also be isolated from throat swabs, stool, blood, and urine. Enteroviruses and adenoviruses may be found in feces; arboviruses, some enteroviruses, and LCMV in blood; mumps and CMV in urine; and enteroviruses, mumps, and adenoviruses in throat washings. During enteroviral infections, viral shedding in stool may persist for several weeks. The presence of enterovirus in stool is not diagnostic and may result from residual shedding from a previous enteroviral infection; it also occurs in some asymptomatic individuals during enteroviral epidemics.

Serologic studies

For some viruses, including many arboviruses such as WNV, serologic studies remain a crucial diagnostic tool. Serum antibody determination is less useful for viruses with high seroprevalence rates in the general population such as HSV, VZV, CMV, and EBV. For viruses with low seroprevalence rates, diagnosis of acute viral infection can be made by documenting seroconversion between acute-phase and convalescent sera (typically obtained after 2–4 weeks) or by demonstrating the presence of virus-specific IgM antibodies. Documentation of synthesis of virus-specific antibodies in CSF, as shown by an increased IgG index or the presence of CSF IgM antibodies, is more useful than serum serology alone and can provide presumptive evidence of CNS infection. Although serum and CSF IgM antibodies generally persist for only a few months after acute infection, there are exceptions to this rule. For example, WNV IgM has been shown to persist in some patients for >1 year following acute infection. Unfortunately, the delay between onset of infection and the host's generation of a virus-specific antibody response often means that serologic data are useful mainly for the retrospective establishment of a specific diagnosis, rather than in aiding acute diagnosis or management.

CSF oligoclonal gamma globulin bands occur in association with a number of viral infections. The associated antibodies are often directed against viral proteins. Oligoclonal bands also occur commonly in certain noninfectious neurologic diseases (e.g., multiple sclerosis) and may be found in nonviral infections (e.g., neurosyphilis, Lyme neuroborreliosis).

Other laboratory studies

All patients with suspected viral meningitis should have a complete blood count and differential, liver and renal function tests, erythrocyte sedimentation rate (ESR), and C-reactive protein, electrolytes, glucose, creatine kinase, aldolase, amylase, and lipase. Neuroimaging studies (MRI, CT) are not necessary in patients with uncomplicated viral meningitis but should be performed in patients with altered consciousness, seizures, focal neurologic signs or symptoms, or atypical CSF profiles.

DIFFERENTIAL DIAGNOSIS

The most important issue in the differential diagnosis of viral meningitis is to consider diseases that can mimic viral meningitis, including (1) untreated or partially treated bacterial meningitis; (2) early stages of meningitis caused by fungi, mycobacteria, or *Treponema pallidum* (neurosyphilis), in which a lymphocytic pleocytosis is common, cultures may be slow growing or negative, and hypoglycorrhachia may not be present early; (3) meningitis caused by agents such as *Mycoplasma*, *Listeria* spp., *Brucella* spp., *Coxiella* spp., *Leptospira* spp., and *Rickettsia* spp.; (4) parameningeal infections; (5) neoplastic meningitis; and (6) meningitis secondary to noninfectious inflammatory diseases, including hypersensitivity meningitis, SLE and other rheumatologic diseases, sarcoidosis, Behçet's syndrome, and the uveomeningitic syndromes. Studies in children >28 days of age suggest that the presence of CSF protein >0.5 g/L (sensitivity 89%, specificity 78%), and elevated serum procalcitonin levels >0.5 ng/m; (sensitivity 89%, specificity 89%) were clues to the presence of bacterial as opposed to "aseptic" meningitis. A variety of clinical algorithms for differentiating bacterial from aseptic meningitis have been promulgated, although none have been widely validated. One such prospectively validated system, the *bacterial meningitis score*, suggests that the probability of bacterial meningitis is 0.1% or less (negative predictive value 99.9%, 95% CI 99.6–100%) in children with CSF pleocytosis who have: (1) a negative CSF Gram's stain, (2) CSF neutrophil count <1000 cells/μL, (3) CSF protein <80 mg/dL, (4) peripheral absolute neutrophil count of <10,000 cells/μL, and (5) no prior history or current presence of seizures.

SPECIFIC VIRAL ETIOLOGIES

Enteroviruses (EV)(Chap. 191) are the most common cause of viral meningitis, accounting for >85% of cases in which a specific etiology can be identified. Cases may either be sporadic or occur in clusters. Recent outbreaks of EV meningitis in the United States have been associated with coxsackievirus B5 and echovirus strains 6, 9, and 30. Coxsackievirus strains A9, B3, and B4 are more commonly associated with individual cases. EV71 has produced large epidemics of neurologic disease outside the United States, especially in Southeast Asia, but most recently reported cases in the United States have been sporadic. Enteroviruses are the most likely cause of viral meningitis in the summer and fall months, especially in children (<15 years), although cases occur at reduced frequency year round. Although the incidence of enteroviral meningitis declines with increasing age, some outbreaks have preferentially affected older children and adults. Meningitis outside the neonatal period is usually benign. Patients present with sudden onset of fever; headache; nuchal rigidity; and often constitutional signs, including vomiting, anorexia, diarrhea, cough, pharyngitis, and myalgias. The physical examination should include a careful search for stigmata of enterovirus infection, including exanthems, hand-foot-mouth disease, herpangina, pleurodynia, myopericarditis, and hemorrhagic conjunctivitis. The CSF profile is typically a lymphocytic pleocytosis (100–1000 cells/μL) with normal glucose and normal or mildly elevated protein concentration. However, up to 15% of patients, most commonly young infants rather than older children or adults, have a normal CSF leukocyte count. In rare cases, PMNs may predominate during the first 48 h of illness. CSF reverse transcriptase PCR (RT-PCR) is the diagnostic procedure of choice and is both sensitive (>95%) and specific (>100%). CSF PCR has the highest sensitivity if performed within 48 h of symptom onset, with sensitivity declining rapidly after day 5 of symptoms. Treatment is supportive, and patients usually recover without sequelae. Chronic and severe infections can occur in neonates and in individuals with hypo- or agammaglobulinemia.

Arbovirus infections (Chap. 196) occur predominantly in the summer and early fall. Arboviral meningitis should be considered when clusters of meningitis and encephalitis cases occur in a restricted geographic region during the summer or early fall. In the United States the most important causes of arboviral meningitis and encephalitis are West Nile virus, St. Louis encephalitis virus, and the California encephalitis group of viruses. In WNV epidemics, avian deaths may serve as sentinel infections for subsequent human disease. A history of tick exposure or travel or residence in the appropriate geographic area should suggest the possibility of Colorado tick fever virus or Powassan virus infection, although nonviral tick-borne diseases, including RMSF and Lyme neuroborreliosis, may present similarly. Arbovirus meningoencephalitis is typically associated with a CSF lymphocytic pleocytosis, normal glucose concentration, and normal or mildly elevated protein concentration. However, 40–45% of patients with WNV meningoencephalitis have CSF neutrophilia, which can persist for a week or more. The rarity of hypoglycorrhachia in WNV infection as well as the absence of positive Gram's stains and the negative cultures helps distinguish these patients from those with bacterial meningitis. The presence of increased numbers of plasmacytoid cells or Mollaret-like large mononuclear cells in the CSF may be a clue to the diagnosis of WNV infection. Definitive diagnosis of arboviral meningoencephalitis is based on demonstration of viral-specific IgM in CSF or seroconversion. CSF PCR tests are available for some viruses in selected diagnostic laboratories and at the Centers for Disease Control and Prevention (CDC), but in the case of WNV, sensitivity (~70%) of CSF PCR is less than that of CSF serology.

HSV-2 meningitis (Chap. 179) has been increasingly recognized as a major cause of viral meningitis in adults, and overall it is probably second in importance to enteroviruses as a cause of viral meningitis, accounting for 5% of total cases overall and undoubtedly a higher frequency of those cases occurring in adults and/or outside of the summer-fall period when enterovirus infections are increasingly common. HSV meningitis occurs in ~25-35% of women and ~10-15% of men at the time of an initial (primary) episode of genital herpes. Of these patients, 20% go on to have recurrent attacks of meningitis. Diagnosis of HSV meningitis is usually by HSV CSF PCR as cultures may be negative, especially in patients with recurrent meningitis. Demonstration of intrathecal synthesis of HSV-specific antibody may also be useful in diagnosis, although antibody tests are less sensitive and less specific than PCR and may not become positive until after the first week of infection. In contrast to HSV encephalitis in adults in which >90% of cases are due to HSV-1, the overwhelming majority of HSV meningitis is due to HSV-2. Although a history of or the presence of HSV genital lesions is an important diagnostic clue, many patients with HSV meningitis give no history and have no evidence of active genital herpes at the time of presentation. Most cases of recurrent viral or "aseptic" meningitis, including cases previously diagnosed as Mollaret's meningitis, are likely due to HSV.

VZV meningitis should be suspected in the presence of concurrent chickenpox or shingles. However, it is important to recognize that in some series, up to 40% of VZV meningitis cases have been reported to occur in the absence of rash. The frequency of VZV as a cause of meningitis is extremely variable, ranging from as low as 3% to as high as 20% in different series. Diagnosis is usually based on CSF PCR, although the sensitivity of this test may not be as high as for the other herpesviruses. In patients with negative CSF PCR results, the diagnosis of VZV CNS infection can be made by the demonstration of VZV-specific intrathecal antibody synthesis and/or the presence of VZV CSF IgM antibodies, or by positive CSF cultures.

EBV infections may also produce aseptic meningitis, with or without associated infectious mononucleosis. The presence of atypical lymphocytes in the CSF or peripheral blood is suggestive of EBV infection but may occasionally be seen with other viral infections. EBV is almost never cultured from CSF. Serum and CSF serology can help establish the presence of acute infection, which is characterized by IgM viral capsid antibodies (VCAs), antibodies to early antigens (EAs), and the absence of antibodies to EBV-associated nuclear antigen (EBNA). CSF PCR is another important diagnostic test, although positive results may reflect viral reactivation associated with other infectious or inflammatory processes.

HIV meningitis should be suspected in any patient presenting with a viral meningitis with known or suspected risk factors for HIV infection. Meningitis may occur following primary infection with HIV in 5–10% of cases and less commonly at later stages of illness. Cranial nerve palsies, most commonly involving cranial nerves V, VII, or VIII, are more common in HIV meningitis than in other viral infections. Diagnosis can be confirmed by detection of HIV genome in blood or CSF. Seroconversion may be delayed, and patients with negative HIV serologies who are suspected of having HIV meningitis should be monitored for delayed seroconversion. For further discussion of HIV infection, see Chap. 189.

Mumps (Chap. 194) should be considered when meningitis occurs in the late winter or early spring, especially in males (male/female ratio 3:1). With the widespread use of the live attenuated mumps vaccine in the United States since 1967, the incidence of mumps meningitis has fallen by >95%; however, mumps remains a potential source of infection in nonimmunized individuals and populations. Rare cases (10–100:100,000 vaccinated individuals) of vaccine-associated mumps meningitis have been described, with onset typically 2–4 weeks after vaccination. The presence of parotitis, orchitis, oophoritis, pancreatitis, or elevations in serum lipase and amylase are suggestive of mumps meningitis; however, their absence does not exclude the diagnosis. Clinical meningitis was previously estimated to occur in 10–30% of patients with mumps parotitis; however, in a recent U.S. outbreak of nearly 2600 cases of mumps, only 11 cases of meningitis were identified, suggesting the incidence may be lower than previously suspected. Mumps infection confers lifelong immunity, so a documented history of previous infection excludes this diagnosis. Patients with meningitis have a CSF pleocytosis that can exceed 1000 cells/μL in 25%. Lymphocytes predominate in 75%, although CSF neutrophilia occurs in 25%. Hypoglycorrhachia, occurs in 10–30% of patients and may be a clue to the diagnosis when present. Diagnosis is typically made by culture of virus from CSF or by detecting IgM antibodies or seroconversion. CSF PCR is available in some diagnostic and research laboratories.

LCMV infection (Chap. 196) should be considered when aseptic meningitis occurs in the late fall or winter and in individuals with a history of exposure to house mice (*Mus musculus*), pet or laboratory rodents (e.g., hamsters, rats, mice), or their excreta. Some patients have an associated rash, pulmonary infiltrates, alopecia, parotitis, orchitis, or myopericarditis. Laboratory clues to the diagnosis of LCMV, in addition to the clinical findings noted above, may include the presence of leukopenia, thrombocytopenia, or abnormal liver function tests. Some cases present with a marked CSF pleocytosis (>1000 cells/μL) and hypoglycorrhachia (<30%). Diagnosis is based on serology and/or culture of virus from CSF.

TREATMENT Acute Viral Meningitis

Treatment of almost all cases of viral meningitis is primarily symptomatic and includes use of analgesics, antipyretics, and antiemetics. Fluid and electrolyte status should be monitored. Patients with suspected bacterial meningitis should receive appropriate empirical therapy pending culture results (see above). Hospitalization may not be required in immunocompetent patients with presumed viral meningitis and no focal signs or symptoms, no significant alteration in consciousness, and a classic CSF profile (lymphocytic pleocytosis, normal glucose, negative Gram's stain) if adequate provision for monitoring at home and medical follow-up can be ensured. Immunocompromised patients; patients with significant alteration in consciousness, seizures, or the presence of focal signs and symptoms suggesting the possibility of encephalitis or parenchymal brain involvement; and those patients who have an atypical CSF profile should be hospitalized. Oral or intravenous acyclovir may be of benefit in patients with meningitis caused by HSV-1 or -2 and in cases of severe EBV or VZV infection. Data concerning treatment of HSV, EBV, and VZV meningitis are extremely limited. Seriously ill patients should probably receive intravenous acyclovir (15–30 mg/kg per day in three divided doses), which can be followed by an oral drug such as acyclovir (800 mg, five times daily), famciclovir (500 mg tid), or valacyclovir (1000 mg tid) for a total course of 7–14 days. Patients who are less ill can be treated with oral drugs alone. Patients with HIV meningitis should receive highly active antiretroviral therapy (Chap. 189).

Patients with viral meningitis who are known to have deficient humoral immunity (e.g., X-linked agammaglobulinemia) and who are not already receiving either intramuscular gamma globulin or intravenous immunoglobulin (IVIg), should be treated with these agents. Intraventricu lar administration of immunoglobulin through an Ommaya reservoir has been tried in some patients with chronic enteroviral meningitis who have not responded to intramuscular or intravenous immunoglobulin.

An investigational drug, pleconaril, has shown efficacy against a variety of enteroviral infections and has good oral bioavailability and excellent CNS penetration. Clinical trials in patients with enteroviral meningitis indicated that pleconaril decreased the duration of symptoms compared to placebo; however, the drug is not likely to be marketed and is not generally available, due to its modest benefit in trials of non-CNS EV infections.

Vaccination is an effective method of preventing the development of meningitis and other neurologic complications associated with poliovirus, mumps, and measles infection. A live attenuated VZV vaccine (Varivax) is available in the United States. Clinical studies indicate an effectiveness rate of 70–90% for this vaccine, but a booster may be required to maintain immunity. An inactivated varicella vaccine is available for transplant recipients.

■ PROGNOSIS

In adults, the prognosis for full recovery from viral meningitis is excellent. Rare patients complain of persisting headache, mild mental impairment, incoordination, or generalized asthenia for weeks to months. The outcome in infants and neonates (<1 year) is less certain; intellectual impairment, learning disabilities, hearing loss, and other lasting sequelae have been reported in some studies.

VIRAL ENCEPHALITIS

DEFINITION

In contrast to viral meningitis, where the infectious process and associated inflammatory response are limited largely to the meninges, in encephalitis the brain parenchyma is also involved. Many patients with encephalitis also have evidence of associated meningitis (meningoencephalitis) and, in some cases, involvement of the spinal cord or nerve roots (encephalomyelitis, encephalomyeloradiculitis).

CLINICAL MANIFESTATIONS

In addition to the acute febrile illness with evidence of meningeal involvement characteristic of meningitis, the patient with encephalitis commonly has an altered level of consciousness (confusion, behavioral abnormalities), or a depressed level of consciousness ranging from mild lethargy to coma, and evidence of either focal or diffuse neurologic signs and symptoms. Patients with encephalitis may have hallucinations, agitation, personality change, behavioral disorders, and, at times, a frankly psychotic state. Focal or generalized seizures occur in many patients with encephalitis. Virtually every possible type of focal neurologic disturbance has been reported in viral encephalitis; the signs and symptoms reflect the sites of infection and inflammation. The most commonly encountered focal findings are aphasia, ataxia, upper or lower motor neuron patterns of weakness, involuntary movements (e.g., myoclonic jerks, tremor), and cranial nerve deficits (e.g., ocular palsies, facial weakness). Involvement of the hypothalamic-pituitary axis may result in temperature dysregulation, diabetes insipidus, or the development of the syndrome of inappropriate secretion of antidiuretic hormone (SIADH). Even though neurotropic viruses typically cause pathologic injury in distinct regions of the CNS, variations in clinical presentations make it impossible to reliably establish the etiology of a specific case of encephalitis on clinical grounds alone (see "Differential Diagnosis," below).

ETIOLOGY

In the United States, there are ~20,000 reported cases of encephalitis per year, although the actual number of cases is likely to be significantly larger. Despite comprehensive diagnostic efforts, the majority of cases of acute encephalitis of suspected viral etiology remain of unknown cause. Hundreds of viruses are capable of causing encephalitis, although only a limited subset is responsible for most cases in which a specific cause is identified (Table 381-4). The most commonly identified viruses causing sporadic cases of acute encephalitis in immunocompetent adults are herpesviruses (HSV, VZV, EBV). Epidemics of encephalitis are caused by arboviruses, which belong to several different viral taxonomic groups including *Alphaviruses* (e.g., EEE virus, western equine encephalitis virus), *Flaviviruses* (e.g., WNV, St. Louis encephalitis virus, Japanese encephalitis virus, Powassan virus), and *Bunyaviruses* (e.g., California encephalitis virus serogroup, LaCrosse virus). Historically, the largest number of cases of arbovirus encephalitis in the United States has been due to St. Louis encephalitis virus and the California encephalitis virus serogroup. However, since 2002, WNV has been responsible for the majority of arbovirus meningitis and encephalitis cases in the United States. The 2003 epidemic was the largest epidemic of arboviral neuroinvasive disease (encephalitis + meningitis) ever recorded in the United States, with 2866 cases and 264 deaths. In 2004–2007, WNV has accounted for between 1142 and 1459 confirmed cases of neuroinvasive disease per year in the United States and 100–177 deaths. In 2008 and 2009 there was an unexpected and dramatic decline in both the number of WNV neuroinvasive cases (2008 = 687, 2009 = 335) and the number of deaths (2008 = 44, 2009 = 30). New causes of viral CNS infections are constantly appearing, as evidenced by the recent outbreak of cases of encephalitis in Southeast Asia caused by Nipah virus, a newly identified member of the Paramyxoviridae family; of meningitis in Europe caused by Toscana virus, an arbovirus belonging to the Bunyavirus family; and of neurologic disorders associated with major epidemics of Chikungunya virus, a togavirus, in Africa, India, and Southeast Asia.

LABORATORY DIAGNOSIS

CSF examination

CSF examination should be performed in all patients with suspected viral encephalitis unless contraindicated by the presence of severely increased ICP. The characteristic CSF profile is indistinguishable from that of viral meningitis and typically consists of a lymphocytic pleocytosis, a mildly elevated protein concentration, and a normal glucose concentration. A CSF pleocytosis (>5 cells/μL) occurs in >95% of immunocompetent patients with documented viral encephalitis. In rare cases, a pleocytosis may be absent on the initial LP but present on subsequent LPs. Patients who are severely immunocompromised by HIV infection, glucocorticoid or other immunosuppressant drugs, chemotherapy, or lymphoreticular malignancies may fail to mount a CSF inflammatory response. CSF cell counts exceed 500/μL in only about 10% of patients with encephalitis. Infections with certain arboviruses (e.g., EEE virus or California encephalitis virus), mumps, and LCMV may occasionally result in cell counts >1000/μL, but this degree of pleocytosis should suggest the possibility of nonviral infections or other inflammatory processes. Atypical lymphocytes in the CSF may be seen in EBV infection and less commonly with other viruses, including CMV, HSV, and enteroviruses. Increased numbers of plasmacytoid or Mollaret-like large mononuclear cells have been reported in WNV encephalitis. Polymorphonuclear pleocytosis occurs in ~45% of patients with WNV encephalitis and is also a common feature in CMV myeloradiculitis in immunocompromised patients. Large numbers of CSF PMNs may be present in patients with encephalitis due to EEE virus, echovirus 9, and, more rarely, other enteroviruses. However, persisting CSF neutrophilia should prompt consideration of bacterial infection, leptospirosis, amebic infection, and noninfectious processes such as acute hemorrhagic leukoencephalitis. About 20% of patients with encephalitis will have a significant number of red blood cells (>500/μL) in the CSF in a nontraumatic tap. The pathologic correlate of this finding may be a hemorrhagic encephalitis of the type seen with HSV; however, CSF red blood cells occur with similar frequency and in similar numbers in patients with nonherpetic focal encephalitides. A decreased CSF glucose concentration is distinctly unusual in viral encephalitis and should suggest the possibility of bacterial, fungal, tuberculous, parasitic, leptospiral, syphilitic, sarcoid, or neoplastic meningitis. Rare patients with mumps, LCMV, or advanced HSV encephalitis and many patients with CMV myeloradiculitis have low CSF glucose concentrations.

CSF PCR

CSF PCR has become the primary diagnostic test for CNS infections caused by CMV, EBV, HHV-6, and enteroviruses (see "Viral Meningitis," above). In the case of VZV CNS infection, CSF PCR and detection of virus-specific IgM or intrathecal antibody synthesis both provide important aids to diagnosis. The sensitivity and specificity of CSF PCRs varies with the virus being tested. The sensitivity (~96%) and specificity (~99%) of HSV CSF PCR is equivalent to or exceeds that of brain biopsy. It is important to recognize that HSV CSF PCR results need to be interpreted after considering the likelihood of disease in the patient being tested, the timing of the test in relationship to onset of symptoms, and the prior use of antiviral therapy. A negative HSV CSF PCR test performed by a qualified laboratory at the appropriate time during illness in a patient with a high likelihood of HSV encephalitis based on clinical and laboratory abnormalities significantly reduces the likelihood of HSV encephalitis but does not exclude it. For example, in a patient with a pretest probability of 35% of having HSV encephalitis, a negative HSV CSF PCR reduces the posttest probability to ~2%, and for a patient with a pretest probability of 60%, a negative test reduces the posttest probability to ~6%. In both situations a positive test makes the diagnosis almost certain (98–99%). There have been several recent reports of initially negative HSV CSF PCR tests that were obtained early (≤72 h) following symptom onset and that became positive when repeated 1–3 days later. The frequency of positive HSV CSF PCRs in patients with herpes encephalitis also decreases as a function of the duration of illness, with only ~20% of cases remaining positive after ≥14 days. PCR results are generally not affected by ≤1 week of antiviral therapy. In one study, 98% of CSF specimens remained PCR-positive during the first week of initiation of antiviral therapy, but the numbers fell to ~50% by 8–14 days and to ~21% by >15 days after initiation of antiviral therapy.

The sensitivity and specificity of CSF PCR tests for viruses other than herpes simplex have not been definitively characterized. Enteroviral CSF PCR appears to have a sensitivity and specificity of >95%. The specificity of EBV CSF PCR has not been established. Positive EBV CSF PCRs associated with positive tests for other pathogens have been reported and may reflect reactivation of EBV latent in lymphocytes that enter the CNS as a result of an unrelated infectious or inflammatory process. In patients with CNS infection due to VZV, CSF antibody and PCR studies should be considered complementary, as patients may have evidence of intrathecal synthesis of VZV-specific antibodies and negative CSF PCRs. In the case of WNV infection, CSF PCR appears to be less sensitive (~70% sensitivity) than detection of WNV-specific CSF IgM, although PCR testing remains useful in immunocompromised patients who may not mount an effective anti-WNV antibody response.

CSF culture

CSF culture is generally of limited utility in the diagnosis of acute viral encephalitis. Culture may be insensitive (e.g., >95% of patients with HSV encephalitis have negative CSF cultures as do virtually all patients with EBV-associated CNS disease) and often takes too long to significantly affect immediate therapy.

Serologic studies and antigen detection

The basic approach to the serodiagnosis of viral encephalitis is identical to that discussed earlier for viral meningitis. Demonstration of WNV IgM antibodies is diagnostic of WNV encephalitis as IgM antibodies do not cross the blood-brain barrier, and their presence in CSF is therefore indicative of intrathecal synthesis. Timing of antibody collection may be important as the rate of CSF WNV IgM seropositivity increases by ~10% per day during the first week after illness onset, reaching 80% or higher on day 7 after symptom onset. In patients with HSV encephalitis, both antibodies to HSV-1 glycoproteins and glycoprotein antigens have been detected in the CSF. Optimal detection of both HSV antibodies and antigen typically occurs after the first week of illness, limiting the utility of these tests in acute diagnosis. Nonetheless, HSV CSF antibody testing is of value in selected patients whose illness is >1 week in duration and who are CSF PCR–negative for HSV. In the case of VZV infection, CSF antibody tests may be positive when PCR fails to detect viral DNA, and both tests should be considered complementary rather than mutually exclusive.

MRI, CT, EEG

Patients with suspected encephalitis almost invariably undergo neuroimaging studies and often EEG. These tests help identify or exclude alternative diagnoses and assist in the differentiation between a focal, as opposed to a diffuse, encephalitic process. Focal findings in a patient with encephalitis should always raise the possibility of HSV encephalitis. Examples of focal findings include: (1) areas of increased signal intensity in the frontotemporal, cingulate, or insular regions of the brain on T2-weighted, FLAIR, or diffusion-weighted MRI (Fig. 381-3); (2) focal areas of low absorption, mass effect, and contrast enhancement on CT; or (3) periodic focal temporal lobe spikes on a background of slow or low-amplitude ("flattened") activity on EEG. Approximately 10% of patients with PCR-documented HSV encephalitis will have a normal MRI, although nearly 80% will have abnormalities in the temporal lobe, and an additional 10% in extratemporal regions. The lesions are typically hyperintense on T2-weighted images. The addition of FLAIR and diffusion-weighted images to the standard MRI sequences enhances sensitivity. Children with HSV encephalitis may have atypical patterns of MRI lesions and often show involvement of brain regions outside the frontotemporal areas. CT is less sensitive than MRI and is normal in up to 20–35% of patients. EEG abnormalities occur in >75% of PCR-documented cases of HSV encephalitis; they typically involve the temporal lobes but are often nonspecific. Some patients with HSV encephalitis have a distinctive EEG pattern consisting of periodic, stereotyped, sharp-and-slow complexes originating in one or both temporal lobes and repeating at regular intervals of 2–3 s. The periodic complexes are typically noted between days 2 and 15 of the illness and are present in two-thirds of pathologically proven cases of HSV encephalitis.

Significant MRI abnormalities are found in only ~two-thirds of patients with WNV encephalitis, a frequency less than that with HSV encephalitis. When present, abnormalities often involve deep brain structures, including the thalamus, basal ganglia, and brainstem,

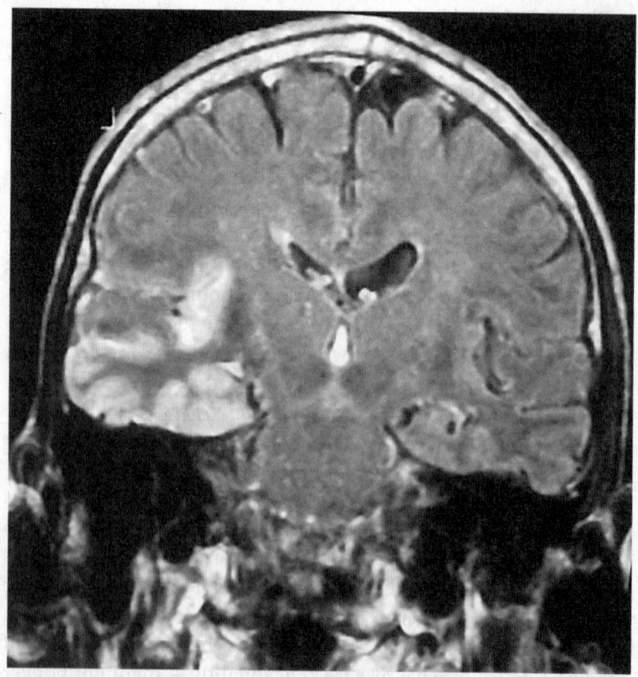

Figure 381-3 Coronal FLAIR magnetic resonance image from a patient with herpes simplex encephalitis. Note the area of increased signal in the right temporal lobe (*left side of image*) confined predominantly to the gray matter. This patient had predominantly unilateral disease; bilateral lesions are more common but may be quite asymmetric in their intensity.

rather than the cortex and may only be apparent on FLAIR images. EEGs in patients with WNV encephalitis typically show generalized slowing that may be more anteriorly prominent rather than the temporally predominant pattern of sharp or periodic discharges more characteristic of HSV encephalitis. Patients with VZV encephalitis may show multifocal areas of hemorrhagic and ischemic infarction, reflecting the tendency of this virus to produce a CNS vasculopathy rather than a true encephalitis. Immunocompromised adult patients with CMV often have enlarged ventricles with areas of increased T2 signal on MRI outlining the ventricles and sub-ependymal enhancement on T1-weighted post-contrast images. Table 381-5 highlights specific diagnostic test results that can be useful in clinical decision-making.

Brain biopsy

Brain biopsy is now generally reserved for patients in whom CSF PCR studies fail to lead to a specific diagnosis, who have focal abnormalities on MRI, and who continue to show progressive clinical deterioration despite treatment with acyclovir and supportive therapy.

TABLE 381-5 Use of Diagnostic Tests in Encephalitis

The best test for WNV encephalitis is the *CSF IgM antibody test.* The prevalence of positive CSF IgM tests increases by about 10% per day after illness onset and reaches 70–80% by the end of the first week. Serum WNV IgM can provide evidence for recent WNV infection, but in the absence of other findings does not establish the diagnosis of neuroinvasive disease (meningitis, encephalitis, acute flaccid paralysis).

Approximately 80% of patients with proven HSV encephalitis have *MRI* abnormalities involving the temporal lobes. This percentage likely increases to >90% when FLAIR and DWI MR sequences are also utilized. The absence of temporal lobe lesions on MR reduces the likelihood of HSV encephalitis and should prompt consideration of other diagnostic possibilities.

The *CSF HSV PCR* test may be negative in the first 72 h of symptoms of HSV encephalitis. A repeat study should be considered in patients with an initial early negative PCR in whom diagnostic suspicion of HSV encephalitis remains high and no alternative diagnosis has yet been established.

Detection of *intrathecal synthesis* (increased CSF/serum HSV antibody ratio corrected for breakdown of the blood-brain barrier) of *HSV-specific antibody* may be useful in diagnosis of HSV encephalitis in patients in whom only late (>1 week post-onset) CSF specimens are available and PCR studies are negative. Serum serology alone is of no value in diagnosis of HSV encephalitis due to the high seroprevalence rate in the general population.

Negative *CSF viral cultures* are of no value in excluding the diagnosis of HSV or EBV encephalitis.

VZV CSF IgM antibodies may be present in patients with a negative VZV CSF PCR. Both tests should be performed in patients with suspected VZV CNS disease.

The specificity of *EBV CSF PCR* for diagnosis of CNS infection is unknown. Positive tests may occur in patients with a CSF pleocytosis due to other causes. Detection of EBV CSF IgM or intrathecal synthesis of antibody to VCA supports the diagnosis of EBV encephalitis. Serological studies consistent with acute EBV infection (e.g., IgM VCA, presence of antibodies against EA but not against EBNA) can help support the diagnosis.

Abbreviations: CNS, central nervous system; CSF, cerebrospinal fluid; DWI, diffusion-weighted imaging; EA, early antigen; EBNA, EBV-associated nuclear antigen; EBV, Epstein-Barr virus; FLAIR, fluid-attenuated inversion recovery; HSV, herpes simplex virus; IgM, immunoglobulin M; MRI, magnetic resonance imaging; PCR, polymerase chain reaction; VCA, viral capsid antibody; VZV, varicella-zoster virus; WNV, West Nile virus.

DIFFERENTIAL DIAGNOSIS

Infection by a variety of other organisms can mimic viral encephalitis. In studies of biopsy-proven HSV encephalitis, common infectious mimics of focal viral encephalitis included mycobacteria, fungi, rickettsia, *Listeria*, *Mycoplasma*, and other bacteria (including *Bartonella* sp.).

Infection caused by the ameba *Naegleria fowleri* can also cause acute meningoencephalitis (primary amebic meningoencephalitis), whereas that caused by *Acanthamoeba* and *Balamuthia* more typically produces subacute or chronic granulomatous amebic meningoencephalitis. *Naegleria* thrive in warm, iron-rich pools of water, including those found in drains, canals, and both natural and human-made outdoor pools. Infection has typically occurred in immunocompetent children with a history of swimming in potentially infected water. The CSF, in contrast to the typical profile seen in viral encephalitis, often resembles that of bacterial meningitis with a neutrophilic pleocytosis and hypoglycorrhachia. Motile trophozoites can be seen in a wet mount of warm, fresh CSF. There have been an increasing number of cases of *Balamuthia mandrillaris* amebic encephalitis mimicking acute viral encephalitis in children and immunocompetent adults. This organism has also been associated with encephalitis in recipients of transplanted organs from a donor with unrecognized infection. No effective treatment has been identified, and mortality approaches 100%.

Encephalitis can be caused by the raccoon pinworm *Baylisascaris procyonis*. Clues to the diagnosis include a history of raccoon exposure, especially of playing in or eating dirt potentially contaminated with raccoon feces. Most patients are children, and many have an associated eosinophilia.

Once nonviral causes of encephalitis have been excluded, the major diagnostic challenge is to distinguish HSV from other viruses that cause encephalitis. This distinction is particularly important because in virtually every other instance the therapy is supportive, whereas specific and effective antiviral therapy is available for HSV, and its efficacy is enhanced when it is instituted early in the course of infection. HSV encephalitis should be considered when clinical features suggesting involvement of the inferomedial frontotemporal regions of the brain are present, including prominent olfactory or gustatory hallucinations, anosmia, unusual or bizarre behavior or personality alterations, or memory disturbance. HSV encephalitis should always be suspected in patients with signs and symptoms consistent with acute encephalitis with focal findings on clinical examination, neuroimaging studies, or EEG. The diagnostic procedure of choice in these patients is CSF PCR analysis for HSV. A positive CSF PCR establishes the diagnosis, and a negative test dramatically reduces the likelihood of HSV encephalitis (see above).

The anatomic distribution of lesions may provide an additional clue to diagnosis. Patients with rapidly progressive encephalitis and prominent brainstem signs, symptoms, or neuroimaging abnormalities may be infected by flaviviruses (WNV, St. Louis encephalitis virus, Japanese encephalitis virus), HSV, rabies, or *L. monocytogenes*. Significant involvement of deep gray matter structures, including the basal ganglia and thalamus, should also suggest possible flavivirus infection. These patients may present clinically with prominent movement disorders (tremor, myoclonus) or parkinsonian features. Patients with WNV infection can also present with a poliomyelitis-like acute flaccid paralysis, as can patients infected with enterovirus 71 and, less commonly, other enteroviruses. Acute flaccid paralysis is characterized by the acute onset of a lower motor neuron type of weakness with flaccid tone, reduced or absent reflexes, and relatively preserved sensation.

Despite an aggressive World Health Organization poliovirus eradication initiative, 1733 cases of wild-type poliovirus-induced poliomyelitis were reported worldwide in 2009, with 73% occurring in India and Nigeria. There have been recent small outbreaks of poliomyelitis associated with vaccine strains of virus that have reverted to virulence through mutation or recombination with circulating wild-type enteroviruses in Hispaniola, China, the Philippines, Indonesia, Nigeria, and Madagascar.

Epidemiologic factors may provide important clues to the diagnosis of viral meningitis or encephalitis. Particular attention should be paid to the season of the year; the geographic location and travel history; and possible exposure to animal bites or scratches, rodents, and ticks. Although transmission from the bite of an infected dog remains the most common cause of rabies worldwide, in the United States very few cases of dog rabies occur, and the most common risk factor is exposure to bats—although a clear history of a bite or scratch is often lacking. The classic clinical presentation of encephalitic (furious) rabies is of fever, fluctuating consciousness, and autonomic hyperactivity. Phobic spasms of the larynx, pharynx, neck muscles, and diaphragm can be triggered by attempts to swallow water (*hydrophobia*) or by inspiration (*aerophobia*). Patients may also present with paralytic (dumb) rabies characterized by acute ascending paralysis. Rabies due to the bite of a bat has a different clinical presentation than classic rabies due to a dog or wolf bite. Patients present with focal neurologic deficits, myoclonus, seizures, and hallucinations; phobic spasms are not a typical feature. Patients with rabies have a CSF lymphocytic pleocytosis and may show areas of increased T2 signal abnormality in the brainstem, hippocampus, and hypothalamus. Diagnosis can be made by finding rabies virus antigen in brain tissue or in the neural innervation of hair follicles at the nape of the neck. PCR amplification of viral nucleic acid from CSF and saliva or tears may also enable diagnosis. Serology is frequently negative in both serum and CSF in the first week after onset of infection, which limits its acute diagnostic utility. No specific therapy is available, and cases are almost invariably fatal, with isolated survivors having devastating neurologic sequelae.

State public health authorities provide a valuable resource concerning isolation of particular agents in individual regions. Regular updates concerning the number, type, and distribution of cases of arboviral encephalitis can be found on the CDC and U.S. Geological Survey (USGS) websites (*http://www.cdc.gov* and *http://diseasemaps.usgs.gov*).

The major noninfectious etiologies that should be included in the differential diagnosis of acute encephalitis are nonvasculitic autoimmune inflammatory meningoencephalitis, which is frequently associated with serum antithyroid microsomal and antithyroglobulin antibodies (Hashimoto's encephalopathy); paraneoplastic and non-paraneoplastic encephalitis associated with antineuronal antibodies (Chap. 101); acute disseminated encephalomyelitis and related fulminant demyelinating disorders (Chap. 380); and lymphoma. Finally, Creutzfeldt-Jakob disease (Chap. 383) can rarely present in an explosive fashion mimicking viral encephalitis.

TREATMENT Viral Encephalitis

Specific antiviral therapy should be initiated when appropriate. Vital functions, including respiration and blood pressure, should be monitored continuously and supported as required. In the initial stages of encephalitis, many patients will require care in an intensive care unit. Basic management and supportive therapy should include careful monitoring of ICP, fluid restriction, avoidance of hypotonic intravenous solutions, and suppression of fever. Seizures should be treated with standard anticonvulsant regimens, and prophylactic therapy should be considered in view of the high frequency of seizures in severe cases of encephalitis. As with all seriously ill, immobilized patients with altered levels of consciousness, encephalitis patients are at risk for aspiration pneumonia, stasis ulcers and decubiti, contractures, deep venous thrombosis and its complications, and infections of indwelling lines and catheters.

Acyclovir is of benefit in the treatment of HSV and should be started empirically in patients with suspected viral encephalitis, especially if focal features are present, while awaiting viral diagnostic studies. Treatment should be discontinued in patients found not to have HSV encephalitis, with the possible exception of patients with severe encephalitis due to VZV or EBV. HSV, VZV, and EBV all encode an enzyme, deoxypyrimidine (thymidine) kinase, that phosphorylates acyclovir to produce acyclovir-5′-monophosphate. Host cell enzymes then phosphorylate this compound to form a triphosphate derivative. It is the triphosphate that acts as an antiviral agent by inhibiting viral DNA polymerase and by causing premature termination of nascent viral DNA chains. The specificity of action depends on the fact that uninfected cells do not phosphorylate significant amounts of acyclovir to acyclovir-5′-monophosphate. A second level of specificity is provided by the fact that the acyclovir triphosphate is a more potent inhibitor of viral DNA polymerase than of the analogous host cell enzymes.

Adults should receive a dose of 10 mg/kg of acyclovir intravenously every 8 h (30 mg/kg per day total dose) for 14–21 days. CSF PCR can be repeated at the completion of this course, with PCR-positive patients receiving additional treatment, followed by a repeat CSF PCR test. Neonatal HSV CNS infection is less responsive to acyclovir therapy than HSV encephalitis in adults; it is recommended that neonates with HSV encephalitis receive 20 mg/kg of acyclovir every 8 h (60 mg/kg per day total dose) for a minimum of 21 days.

Prior to intravenous administration, acyclovir should be diluted to a concentration ≤7 mg/mL. (A 70-kg person would receive a dose of 700 mg, which would be diluted in a volume of 100 mL.) Each dose should be infused slowly over 1 h, rather than by rapid or bolus infusion, to minimize the risk of renal dysfunction. Care should be taken to avoid extravasation or intramuscular or subcutaneous administration. The alkaline pH of acyclovir can cause local inflammation and phlebitis (9%). Dose adjustment is required in patients with impaired renal glomerular filtration. Penetration into CSF is excellent, with average drug levels ~50% of serum levels. Complications of therapy include elevations in blood urea nitrogen and creatinine levels (5%), thrombocytopenia (6%), gastrointestinal toxicity (nausea, vomiting, diarrhea) (7%), and neurotoxicity (lethargy or obtundation, disorientation, confusion, agitation, hallucinations, tremors, seizures) (1%). Acyclovir resistance may be mediated by changes in either the viral deoxypyrimidine kinase or DNA polymerase. To date, acyclovir-resistant isolates have not been a significant clinical problem in immunocompetent individuals. However, there have been reports of clinically virulent acyclovir-resistant HSV isolates from sites outside the CNS in immunocompromised individuals, including those with AIDS.

Oral antiviral drugs with efficacy against HSV, VZV, and EBV, including acyclovir, famciclovir, and valacyclovir, have not been evaluated in the treatment of encephalitis either as primary therapy or as supplemental therapy following completion of a course of parenteral acyclovir. A National Institute of Allergy and Infectious Disease (NIAID)/National Institute of Neurological Disorders and Stroke–sponsored phase III trial of supplemental oral valacyclovir therapy (2 g tid for 3 months) following the initial 14- to 21-day course of therapy with parenteral acyclovir is ongoing in patients with HSV encephalitis (*www.clinicaltrials.gov*, identifier NCT00031486); this may help clarify the role of extended oral antiviral therapy.

Ganciclovir and foscarnet, either alone or in combination, are often utilized in the treatment of CMV-related CNS infections, although their efficacy remains unproven. Cidofovir (see below) may provide an alternative in patients who fail to respond to ganciclovir and foscarnet, although data concerning its use in CMV CNS infections are extremely limited.

Ganciclovir is a synthetic nucleoside analogue of 2′-deoxyguanosine. The drug is preferentially phosphorylated by virus-induced cellular kinases. Ganciclovir triphosphate acts as a competitive inhibitor of the CMV DNA polymerase, and its incorporation into nascent viral DNA results in premature chain termination. Following intravenous administration, CSF concentrations of ganciclovir are 25–70% of coincident plasma levels. The usual dose for treatment of severe neurologic illnesses is 5 mg/kg every 12 h given intravenously at a constant rate over 1 h. Induction therapy is followed by maintenance therapy of 5 mg/kg every day for an indefinite period. Induction therapy should be continued until patients show a decline in CSF pleocytosis and a reduction in CSF CMV DNA copy number on quantitative PCR testing (where available). Doses should be adjusted in patients with renal insufficiency. Treatment is often limited by the development of granulocytopenia and thrombocytopenia (20–25%), which may require reduction in or discontinuation of therapy. Gastrointestinal side effects, including nausea, vomiting, diarrhea, and abdominal pain, occur in ~20% of patients. Some patients treated with ganciclovir for CMV retinitis have developed retinal detachment, but the causal relationship to ganciclovir treatment is unclear. Valganciclovir is an orally bioavailable prodrug that can generate high serum levels of ganciclovir, although studies of its efficacy in treating CMV CNS infections are limited.

Foscarnet is a pyrophosphate analogue that inhibits viral DNA polymerases by binding to the pyrophosphate-binding site. Following intravenous infusion, CSF concentrations range from 15 to 100% of coincident plasma levels. The usual dose for serious CMV-related neurologic illness is 60 mg/kg every 8 h administered by constant infusion over 1 h. Induction therapy for 14–21 days is followed by maintenance therapy (60–120 mg/kg per day). Induction therapy may need to be extended in patients who fail to show a decline in CSF pleocytosis and a reduction in CSF CMV DNA copy number on quantitative PCR tests (where available). Approximately one-third of patients develop renal impairment during treatment, which is reversible following discontinuation of therapy in most, but not all, cases. This is often associated with elevations in serum creatinine and proteinuria and is less frequent in patients who are adequately hydrated. Many patients experience fatigue and nausea. Reduction in serum calcium, magnesium, and potassium occur in ~15% of patients and may be associated with tetany, cardiac rhythm disturbances, or seizures.

Cidofovir is a nucleotide analogue that is effective in treating CMV retinitis and equivalent to or better than ganciclovir in some experimental models of murine CMV encephalitis, although data concerning its efficacy in human CMV CNS disease are limited. The usual dose is 5 mg/kg intravenously once weekly for 2 weeks, then biweekly for two or more additional doses, depending on clinical response. Patients must be prehydrated with normal saline (e.g., 1 L over 1–2 h) prior to each dose and treated with probenecid (e.g., 1 g 3 h before cidofovir and 1 g 2 and 8 h after cidofovir). Nephrotoxicity is common; the dose should be reduced if renal function deteriorates.

Intravenous ribavirin (15–25 mg/kg per day in divided doses given every 8 h) has been reported to be of benefit in isolated cases of severe encephalitis due to California encephalitis (LaCrosse) virus. Ribavirin might be of benefit for the rare patients, typically infants or young children, with severe adenovirus or rotavirus encephalitis and in patients with encephalitis due to LCMV or other arenaviruses. However, clinical trials are lacking. Hemolysis, with resulting anemia, has been the major side effect limiting therapy.

No specific antiviral therapy of proven efficacy is currently available for treatment of WNV encephalitis. Patients have been treated with α-interferon, ribavirin, WNV-specific antisense oligonucleotides (*ClinicalTrials.gov*, identifier NCT0091845), an Israeli IVIg preparation that contains high-titer anti-WNV antibody (Omr-IgG-am) (*ClinicalTrials.gov*, identifier NCT00069316 and 0068055), and humanized monoclonal antibodies directed against the viral envelope glycoprotein (*ClinicalTrials.gov*, identifier NCT00927953 and 00515385). WNV chimeric vaccines, in which WNV envelope and premembrane proteins are inserted into the background of another flavivirus, are already undergoing human clinical testing for safety and immunogenicity (*ClinicalTrials.gov*, identifier NCT00746798 and 00442169). Both chimeric and killed inactivated WNV vaccines have been found to be safe and effective in preventing equine WNV infection, and several effective flavivirus vaccines are already in human use, creating optimism that a safe and effective human WNV vaccine can also be developed.

SEQUELAE

There is considerable variation in the incidence and severity of sequelae in patients surviving viral encephalitis. In the case of EEE virus infection, nearly 80% of survivors have severe neurologic sequelae. At the other extreme are infections due to EBV, California encephalitis virus, and Venezuelan equine encephalitis virus, where severe sequelae are unusual. For example, approximately 5–15% of children infected with LaCrosse virus have a residual seizure disorder, and 1% have persistent hemiparesis. Detailed information about sequelae in patients with HSV encephalitis treated with acyclovir is available from the NIAID-Collaborative Antiviral Study Group (CASG) trials. Of 32 acyclovir-treated patients, 26 survived (81%). Of the 26 survivors, 12 (46%) had no or only minor sequelae, 3 (12%) were moderately impaired (gainfully employed but not functioning at their previous level), and 11 (42%) were severely impaired (requiring continuous supportive care). The incidence and severity of sequelae were directly related to the age of the patient and the level of consciousness at the time of initiation of therapy. Patients with severe neurologic impairment (Glasgow coma score 6) at initiation of therapy either died or survived with severe sequelae. Young patients (<30 years) with good neurologic function at initiation of therapy did substantially better (100% survival, 62% with no or mild sequelae) compared with their older counterparts (>30 years; 64% survival, 57% no or mild sequelae). Some recent studies using quantitative HSV CSF PCR tests indicate that clinical outcome following treatment also correlates with the amount of HSV DNA present in CSF at the time of presentation. Many patients with WNV infection have sequelae, including cognitive impairment; weakness; and hyper- or hypokinetic movement disorders, including tremor, myoclonus, and parkinsonism. In a large longitudinal study of prognosis in 156 patients with WNV infection, the mean time to achieve recovery (defined as 95% of maximal predicted score on specific validated tests) was

112–148 days for fatigue, 121–175 days for physical function, 131–139 days for mood, and 302–455 days for mental function (the longer interval in each case representing patients with neuroinvasive disease).

SUBACUTE MENINGITIS

CLINICAL MANIFESTATIONS

Patients with subacute meningitis typically have an unrelenting headache, stiff neck, low-grade fever, and lethargy for days to several weeks before they present for evaluation. Cranial nerve abnormalities and night sweats may be present. This syndrome overlaps that of chronic meningitis, discussed in detail in Chap. 382.

ETIOLOGY

Common causative organisms include *M. tuberculosis, C. neoformans, H. capsulatum, C. immitis*, and *T. pallidum*. Initial infection with *M. tuberculosis* is acquired by inhalation of aerosolized droplet nuclei. Tuberculous meningitis in adults does not develop acutely from hematogenous spread of tubercle bacilli to the meninges. Rather, millet seed–sized (miliary) tubercles form in the parenchyma of the brain during hematogenous dissemination of tubercle bacilli in the course of primary infection. These tubercles enlarge and are usually caseating. The propensity for a caseous lesion to produce meningitis is determined by its proximity to the subarachnoid space (SAS) and the rate at which fibrous encapsulation develops. Subependymal caseous foci cause meningitis via discharge of bacilli and tuberculous antigens into the SAS. Mycobacterial antigens produce an intense inflammatory reaction that leads to the production of a thick exudate that fills the basilar cisterns and surrounds the cranial nerves and major blood vessels at the base of the brain.

Fungal infections are typically acquired by the inhalation of airborne fungal spores. The initial pulmonary infection may be asymptomatic or present with fever, cough, sputum production, and chest pain. The pulmonary infection is often self-limited. A localized pulmonary fungal infection can then remain dormant in the lungs until there is an abnormality in cell-mediated immunity that allows the fungus to reactivate and disseminate to the CNS. The most common pathogen causing fungal meningitis is *C. neoformans*. This fungus is found worldwide in soil and bird excreta. *H. capsulatum* is endemic to the Ohio and Mississippi River valleys of the central United States and to parts of Central and South America. *C. immitis* is endemic to the desert areas of the southwest United States, northern Mexico, and Argentina.

Syphilis is a sexually transmitted disease that is manifest by the appearance of a painless chancre at the site of inoculation. *T. pallidum* invades the CNS early in the course of syphilis. Cranial nerves VII and VIII are most frequently involved.

LABORATORY DIAGNOSIS

The classic CSF abnormalities in tuberculous meningitis are as follows: (1) elevated opening pressure, (2) lymphocytic pleocytosis (10–500 cells/μL), (3) elevated protein concentration in the range of 1–5 g/L, and (4) decreased glucose concentration in the range of 1.1–2.2 mmol/L (20–40 mg/dL). *The combination of unrelenting headache, stiff neck, fatigue, night sweats, and fever with a CSF lymphocytic pleocytosis and a mildly decreased glucose concentration is highly suspicious for tuberculous meningitis.* The last tube of fluid collected at LP is the best tube to send for a smear for acid-fast bacilli (AFB). If there is a pellicle in the CSF or a cobweb-like clot on the surface of the fluid, AFB can best be demonstrated in a smear of the clot or pellicle. Positive smears are typically reported in only 10–40% of cases of tuberculous meningitis in adults. Cultures of CSF take 4–8 weeks to identify the organism and are positive in ~50% of adults. Culture remains the gold standard to make the diagnosis of tuberculous meningitis. PCR for the detection of *M. tuberculosis* DNA should be sent on CSF if available, but the sensitivity and specificity on CSF have not been defined. The Centers for Disease Control and Prevention recommend the use of nucleic acid amplification tests for the diagnosis of pulmonary tuberculosis.

The characteristic CSF abnormalities in fungal meningitis are a mononuclear or lymphocytic pleocytosis, an increased protein concentration, and a decreased glucose concentration. There may be eosinophils in the CSF in *C. immitis* meningitis. Large volumes of CSF are often required to demonstrate the organism on india ink smear or grow the organism in culture. If spinal fluid examined by LP on two separate occasions fails to yield an organism, CSF should be obtained by high-cervical or cisternal puncture.

The cryptococcal polysaccharide antigen test is a highly sensitive and specific test for cryptococcal meningitis. A reactive CSF cryptococcal antigen test establishes the diagnosis. The detection of the histoplasma polysaccharide antigen in CSF establishes the diagnosis of a fungal meningitis but is not specific for meningitis due to *H. capsulatum*. It may be falsely positive in coccidioidal meningitis. The CSF complement fixation antibody test is reported to have a specificity of 100% and a sensitivity of 75% for coccidioidal meningitis.

The diagnosis of syphilitic meningitis is made when a reactive serum treponemal test [fluorescent treponemal antibody absorption test (FTA-ABS) or microhemagglutination assay–*T. pallidum* (MHA-TP)] is associated with a CSF lymphocytic or mononuclear pleocytosis and an elevated protein concentration, or when the CSF Venereal Disease Research Laboratory (VDRL) is positive. A reactive CSF FTA-ABS is not definitive evidence of neurosyphilis. The CSF FTA-ABS can be falsely positive from blood contamination. A negative CSF VDRL does not rule out neurosyphilis. A negative CSF FTA-ABS or MHA-TP rules out neurosyphilis.

TREATMENT Subacute Meningitis

Empirical therapy of tuberculous meningitis is often initiated on the basis of a high index of suspicion without adequate laboratory support. Initial therapy is a combination of isoniazid (300 mg/d), rifampin (10 mg/kg per day), pyrazinamide (30 mg/kg per day in divided doses), ethambutol (15–25 mg/kg per day in divided doses), and pyridoxine (50 mg/d). When the antimicrobial sensitivity of the *M. tuberculosis* isolate is known, ethambutol can be discontinued. If the clinical response is good, pyrazinamide can be discontinued after 8 weeks and isoniazid and rifampin continued alone for the next 6–12 months. A 6-month course of therapy is acceptable, but therapy should be prolonged for 9–12 months in patients who have an inadequate resolution of symptoms of meningitis or who have positive mycobacterial cultures of CSF during the course of therapy. Dexamethasone therapy is recommended for HIV-negative patients with tuberculous meningitis. The dose is 12–16 mg per day for 3 weeks, then tapered over 3 weeks.

Meningitis due to *C. neoformans* in non-HIV, nontransplant patients is treated with induction therapy with amphotericin B (AmB) (0.7 mg/kg IV per day) plus flucytosine (100 mg/kg per day in four divided doses) for at least 4 weeks if CSF culture results are negative after 2 weeks of treatment. Therapy should be extended for a total of 6 weeks in the patient with neurologic complications. Induction therapy is followed by consolidation therapy with fluconazole 400 mg per day for 8 weeks. Organ transplant recipients are treated with liposomal AmB (3–4 mg/kg per day) or AmB lipid complex (ABLC) 5 mg/kg per day plus flucytosine (100 mg/kg per day in four divided doses) for at least 2 weeks or until CSF culture is sterile. Follow CSF yeast cultures for sterilization rather than the cryptococcal antigen titer. This treatment is followed by an 8- to 10-week course of fluconazole [400–800 mg/d (6–12 mg/kg) PO]. If the CSF culture is sterile after 10 weeks of acute therapy, the dose of fluconazole is decreased to 200 mg/d for 6 months to a year. Patients with HIV infection are treated with AmB or a lipid formulation plus flucytosine for at least 2 weeks, followed by fluconazole for a minimum of 8 weeks. HIV-infected patients may require indefinite maintenance therapy with fluconazole 200 mg/day. Meningitis due to *H. capsulatum* is treated with AmB (0.7–1.0 mg/kg per day) for 4–12 weeks. A total dose of 30 mg/kg is recommended. Therapy with AmB is not discontinued until fungal cultures are sterile. After completing a course of AmB, maintenance therapy with itraconazole 200 mg twice daily is initiated and continued for at least 6 months to a year. *C. immitis* meningitis is treated with either high-dose fluconazole (1000 mg daily) as monotherapy or intravenous AmB (0.5–0.7 mg/kg per day) for >4 weeks. Intrathecal AmB (0.25–0.75 mg/d three times weekly) may be required to eradicate the infection. Lifelong therapy with fluconazole (200–400 mg daily) is recommended to prevent relapse. AmBisome (5 mg/kg per day) or AmB lipid complex (5 mg/kg per day) can be substituted for AmB in patients who have or who develop significant renal dysfunction. The most common complication of fungal meningitis is hydrocephalus. Patients who develop hydrocephalus should receive a CSF diversion device. A ventriculostomy can be used until CSF fungal cultures are sterile, at which time the ventriculostomy is replaced by a ventriculoperitoneal shunt.

Syphilitic meningitis is treated with aqueous penicillin G in a dose of 3–4 million units intravenously every 4 h for 10–14 days. An alternative regimen is 2.4 million units of procaine penicillin G intramuscularly daily with 500 mg of oral probenecid four times daily for 10–14 days. Either regimen is followed with 2.4 million units of benzathine penicillin G intramuscularly once a week for 3 weeks. The standard criterion for treatment success is reexamination of the CSF. The CSF should be reexamined at 6-month intervals for 2 years. The cell count is expected to normalize within 12 months, and the VDRL titer to decrease by two dilutions or revert to nonreactive within 2 years of completion of therapy. Failure of the CSF pleocytosis to resolve or an increase in the CSF VDRL titer by two or more dilutions requires retreatment.

CHRONIC ENCEPHALITIS

PROGRESSIVE MULTIFOCAL LEUKOENCEPHALOPATHY

Clinical features and pathology

Progressive multifocal leukoencephalopathy (PML) is characterized pathologically by multifocal areas of demyelination of varying size distributed throughout the brain but sparing the spinal cord and optic nerves. In addition to demyelination, there are characteristic cytologic alterations in both astrocytes and oligodendrocytes. Astrocytes are enlarged and contain hyperchromatic, deformed, and bizarre nuclei and frequent mitotic figures. Oligodendrocytes have enlarged, densely staining nuclei that contain viral inclusions formed by crystalline arrays of JC virus (JCV) particles. Patients often present with visual deficits (45%), typically a homonymous hemianopia; mental impairment (38%) (dementia, confusion, personality change); weakness, including hemi- or monoparesis; and ataxia. Seizures occur in ~20% of patients, predominantly in those with lesions abutting the cortex.

Almost all patients have an underlying immunosuppressive disorder. In recent series, the most common associated conditions were AIDS (80%), hematologic malignancies (13%), transplant recipients (5%), and chronic inflammatory diseases (2%). It has been estimated that up to 5% of AIDS patients will develop PML. There have been more than 30 reported cases of PML occurring in patients being treated for multiple sclerosis and inflammatory bowel disease with natalizumab, a humanized monoclonal antibody that inhibits lymphocyte trafficking into CNS and bowel mucosa by binding to α_4 integrins. Risk in these patients has been estimated at 1 PML case per 1000 treated patients after a mean of 18 months of therapy. Additional cases have been reported in patients receiving other humanized monoclonal antibodies with immunomodulatory activity including efalizumab and rituximab. The basic clinical and diagnostic features appear to be similar to those seen in PML related to HIV and other forms of immunosuppression.

Diagnostic studies

The diagnosis of PML is frequently suggested by MRI. MRI reveals multifocal asymmetric, coalescing white matter lesions located periventricularly, in the centrum semiovale, in the parietal-occipital region, and in the cerebellum. These lesions have increased signal on T2 and FLAIR images and decreased signal on T1-weighted images. PML lesions are classically nonenhancing (90%) but may rarely show ring enhancement, especially in more immunocompetent patients. PML lesions are not typically associated with edema or mass effect. CT scans, which are less sensitive than MRI for the diagnosis of PML, often show hypodense nonenhancing white matter lesions.

The CSF is typically normal, although mild elevation in protein and/or IgG may be found. Pleocytosis occurs in <25% of cases, is predominantly mononuclear, and rarely exceeds 25 cells/μL. PCR amplification of JCV DNA from CSF has become an important diagnostic tool. The presence of a positive CSF PCR for JCV DNA in association with typical MRI lesions in the appropriate clinical setting is diagnostic of PML, reflecting the assay's relatively high specificity (92–100%); however, sensitivity is variable and a negative CSF PCR does not exclude the diagnosis. In HIV-negative patients and HIV-positive patients not receiving highly active antiviral therapy (HAART), sensitivity is likely 70–90%. In HAART-treated patients, sensitivity may be closer to 60%, reflecting the lower JCV CSF viral load in this relatively more immunocompetent group. Studies with quantitative JCV CSF PCR indicate that patients with low JCV loads (<100 copies/μL) have a generally better prognosis than those with higher viral loads. Patients with negative CSF PCR studies may require brain biopsy for definitive diagnosis. In biopsy or necropsy specimens of brain, JCV antigen and nucleic acid can be detected by immunocytochemistry, in situ hybridization, or PCR amplification. Detection of JCV antigen or genomic material should only be considered diagnostic of PML if accompanied by characteristic pathologic changes, since both antigen and genomic material have been found in the brains of normal patients.

Serologic studies are of no utility in diagnosis due to high basal seroprevalence level (>80%).

TREATMENT Progressive Multifocal Leukoencephalopathy

No effective therapy for PML is available. There are case reports of potential beneficial effects of the 5-HT2a receptor antagonist mirtazapine, which may inhibit binding of JCV to its receptor on oligodendrocytes. Retrospective noncontrolled studies have also suggested a possible beneficial effect of treatment with interferon-alpha. Neither of these agents has been tested in randomized controlled clinical trials. A clinical trial to evaluate the efficacy of the antimalarial drug mefloquine, which inhibits JCV replication in cell culture, is underway (*www.clinicaltrials.gov*, identifier NCT00746941). Intravenous and/or intrathecal cytarabine were not shown to be of benefit in a randomized controlled trial in HIV-associated PML, although some experts suggest that cytarabine may have therapeutic efficacy in situations where breakdown of the blood-brain-barrier allow sufficient CSF penetration. A randomized controlled trial of cidofovir in HIV-associated PML also failed to show significant benefit. Since PML almost invariably occurs in immunocompromised individuals, any therapeutic interventions designed to enhance or restore immunocompetence should be considered. Perhaps the most dramatic demonstration of this is disease stabilization and, in rare cases, improvement associated with the improvement in the immune status of HIV-positive patients with AIDS following institution of HAART. In HIV-positive PML patients treated with HAART, 1-year survival is ~50%, although up to 80% of survivors may have significant neurologic sequelae. HIV-positive PML patients with higher CD4 counts (>300/μL^3) and low or nondetectable HIV viral loads have a better prognosis than those with lower CD4 counts and higher viral loads. Although institution of HAART enhances survival in HIV + PML patients, the associated immune reconstitution in patients with an underlying opportunistic infection such as PML may also result in a severe CNS inflammatory syndrome [immune reconstitution inflammatory syndrome (IRIS)] associated with clinical worsening, CSF pleocytosis, and the appearance of new enhancing MRI lesions. Patients receiving natalizumab or other immunomodulatory antibodies, who are suspected of having PML, should have therapy halted and circulating antibodies removed by plasma exchange.

SUBACUTE SCLEROSING PANENCEPHALITIS (SSPE)

SSPE is a rare chronic, progressive demyelinating disease of the CNS associated with a chronic nonpermissive infection of brain tissue with measles virus. The frequency has been estimated at 1 in 100,000–500,000 measles cases. An average of five cases per year are reported in the United States. The incidence has declined dramatically since the introduction of a measles vaccine. Most patients give a history of primary measles infection at an early age (2 years), which is followed after a latent interval of 6–8 years by the development of a progressive neurologic disorder. Some 85% of patients are between 5 and 15 years old at diagnosis. Initial manifestations include poor school performance and mood and personality changes. Typical signs of a CNS viral infection, including fever and headache, do not occur. As the disease progresses, patients develop progressive intellectual deterioration, focal and/or generalized seizures, myoclonus, ataxia, and visual disturbances. In the late stage of the illness, patients are unresponsive, quadriparetic, and spastic, with hyperactive tendon reflexes and extensor plantar responses.

Diagnostic studies

MRI is often normal early, although areas of increased T2 signal develop in the white matter of the brain and brainstem as disease progresses. The EEG may initially show only nonspecific slowing, but with disease progression, patients develop a characteristic periodic pattern with bursts of high-voltage, sharp, slow waves every 3–8 s, followed by periods of attenuated ("flat") background. The CSF is acellular with a normal or mildly elevated protein concentration and a markedly elevated gamma globulin level (>20% of total CSF protein). CSF antimeasles antibody levels are invariably elevated, and oligoclonal antimeasles antibodies are often present. Measles virus can be cultured from brain tissue using special cocultivation techniques. Viral antigen can be identified immunocytochemically, and viral genome can be detected by in situ hybridization or PCR amplification.

TREATMENT Subacute Sclerosing Panencephalitis

No definitive therapy for SSPE is available. Treatment with isoprinosine (Inosiplex, 100 mg/kg per day), alone or in combination with intrathecal or intraventricular alpha interferon, has been reported to prolong survival and produce clinical improvement in some patients but has never been subjected to a controlled clinical trial.

PROGRESSIVE RUBELLA PANENCEPHALITIS

This is an extremely rare disorder that primarily affects males with congenital rubella syndrome, although isolated cases have been reported following childhood rubella. After a latent period of 8–19 years, patients develop progressive neurologic deterioration. The manifestations are similar to those seen in SSPE. CSF shows a mild lymphocytic pleocytosis, slightly elevated protein concentration, markedly increased gamma globulin, and rubella virus–specific oligoclonal bands. No therapy is available. Universal prevention of both congenital and childhood rubella through the use of the available live attenuated rubella vaccine would be expected to eliminate the disease.

BRAIN ABSCESS

DEFINITION

A brain abscess is a focal, suppurative infection within the brain parenchyma, typically surrounded by a vascularized capsule. The term *cerebritis* is often employed to describe a nonencapsulated brain abscess.

EPIDEMIOLOGY

A bacterial brain abscess is a relatively uncommon intracranial infection, with an incidence of ~0.3–1.3:100,000 persons per year. Predisposing conditions include otitis media and mastoiditis, paranasal sinusitis, pyogenic infections in the chest or other body sites, penetrating head trauma or neurosurgical procedures, and dental infections. In immunocompetent individuals the most important pathogens are *Streptococcus* spp. [anaerobic, aerobic, and viridans (40%)], Enterobacteriaceae [*Proteus* spp., *E. coli* sp., *Klebsiella* spp. (25%)], anaerobes [e.g., *Bacteroides* spp., *Fusobacterium* spp. (30%)], and staphylococci (10%). In immunocompromised hosts with underlying HIV infection, organ transplantation, cancer, or immunosuppressive therapy, most brain abscesses are caused by *Nocardia* spp., *Toxoplasma gondii*, *Aspergillus* spp., *Candida* spp., and *C. neoformans*. In Latin America and in immigrants from Latin America, the most common cause of brain abscess is *Taenia solium* (neurocysticercosis). In India and the Far East, mycobacterial infection (tuberculoma) remains a major cause of focal CNS mass lesions.

ETIOLOGY

A brain abscess may develop (1) by direct spread from a contiguous cranial site of infection, such as paranasal sinusitis, otitis media, mastoiditis, or dental infection; (2) following head trauma or a neurosurgical procedure; or (3) as a result of hematogenous spread from a remote site of infection. In up to 25% of cases, no obvious primary source of infection is apparent (cryptogenic brain abscess).

Approximately one-third of brain abscesses are associated with otitis media and mastoiditis, often with an associated cholesteatoma. Otogenic abscesses occur predominantly in the temporal lobe (55–75%) and cerebellum (20–30%). In some series, up to 90% of cerebellar abscesses are otogenic. Common organisms include streptococci, *Bacteroides* spp., *Pseudomonas* spp., *Haemophilus* spp., and Enterobacteriaceae. Abscesses that develop as a result of direct spread of infection from the frontal, ethmoidal, or sphenoidal sinuses and those that occur due to dental infections are usually located in the frontal lobes. Approximately 10% of brain abscesses are associated with paranasal sinusitis, and this association is particularly strong in young males in their second and third decades of life. The most common pathogens in brain abscesses associated with paranasal sinusitis are streptococci (especially *S. milleri*), *Haemophilus* spp., *Bacteroides* spp., *Pseudomonas* spp., and *S. aureus*. Dental infections are associated with ~2% of brain abscesses, although it is often suggested that many "cryptogenic" abscesses are in fact due to dental infections. The most common pathogens in this setting are streptococci, staphylococci, *Bacteroides* spp., and *Fusobacterium* spp.

Hematogenous abscesses account for ~25% of brain abscesses. Hematogenous abscesses are often multiple, and multiple abscesses often (50%) have a hematogenous origin. These abscesses show a predilection for the territory of the middle cerebral artery (i.e., posterior frontal or parietal lobes). Hematogenous abscesses are often located at the junction of the gray and white matter and are often poorly encapsulated. The microbiology of hematogenous abscesses is dependent on the primary source of infection. For example, brain abscesses that develop as a complication of infective endocarditis are often due to viridans streptococci or *S. aureus*. Abscesses associated with pyogenic lung infections such as lung abscess or bronchiectasis are often due to streptococci, staphylococci, *Bacteroides* spp., *Fusobacterium* spp., or Enterobacteriaceae. Abscesses that follow penetrating head trauma or neurosurgical procedures are frequently due to methicillin-resistant *S. aureus* (MRSA), *S. epidermidis*, Enterobacteriaceae, *Pseudomonas* spp., and *Clostridium* spp. Enterobacteriaceae and *P. aeruginosa* are important causes of abscesses associated with urinary sepsis. Congenital cardiac malformations that produce a right-to-left shunt, such as tetralogy of Fallot, patent ductus arteriosus, and atrial and ventricular septal defects, allow bloodborne bacteria to bypass the pulmonary capillary bed and reach the brain. Similar phenomena can occur with pulmonary arteriovenous malformations. The decreased arterial oxygenation and saturation from the right-to-left shunt and polycythemia may cause focal areas of cerebral ischemia, thus providing a nidus for microorganisms that bypassed the pulmonary circulation to multiply and form an abscess. Streptococci are the most common pathogens in this setting.

PATHOGENESIS AND HISTOPATHOLOGY

Results of experimental models of brain abscess formation suggest that for bacterial invasion of brain parenchyma to occur, there must be preexisting or concomitant areas of ischemia, necrosis, or hypoxemia in brain tissue. The intact brain parenchyma is relatively resistant to infection. Once bacteria have established infection, brain abscess frequently evolves through a series of stages, influenced by the nature of the infecting organism and by the immunocompetence of the host. The early cerebritis stage (days 1–3) is characterized by a perivascular infiltration of inflammatory cells, which surround a central core of coagulative necrosis. Marked edema surrounds the lesion at this stage. In the late cerebritis stage (days 4–9), pus formation leads to enlargement of the necrotic center, which is surrounded at its border by an inflammatory infiltrate of macrophages and fibroblasts. A thin capsule of fibroblasts and reticular fibers gradually develops, and the surrounding area of cerebral edema becomes more distinct than in the previous stage. The third stage, early capsule formation (days 10–13), is characterized by the formation of a capsule that is better developed on the cortical than on the ventricular side of the lesion. This stage correlates with the appearance of a ring-enhancing capsule on neuroimaging studies. The final stage, late capsule formation (day 14 and beyond), is defined by a well-formed necrotic center surrounded by a dense collagenous capsule. The surrounding area of cerebral edema has regressed, but marked gliosis with large numbers of reactive astrocytes has developed outside the capsule. This gliotic process may contribute to the development of seizures as a sequelae of brain abscess.

CLINICAL PRESENTATION

A brain abscess typically presents as an expanding intracranial mass lesion rather than as an infectious process. Although the evolution of signs and symptoms is extremely variable, ranging from hours to weeks or even months, most patients present to the hospital 11–12 days following onset of symptoms. The classic clinical triad of headache, fever, and a focal neurologic deficit is present in <50% of cases. The most common symptom in patients with a brain abscess is headache, occurring in >75% of patients. The headache is often characterized as a constant, dull, aching sensation, either hemicranial or generalized, and it becomes progressively more severe and refractory to therapy. Fever is present in only 50% of patients at the time of diagnosis, and its absence should not exclude the diagnosis. The new onset of focal or generalized seizure activity is a presenting sign in 15–35% of patients. Focal neurologic deficits including hemiparesis, aphasia, or visual field defects are part of the initial presentation in >60% of patients.

The clinical presentation of a brain abscess depends on its location, the nature of the primary infection if present, and the level of the ICP. Hemiparesis is the most common localizing sign of a frontal lobe abscess. A temporal lobe abscess may present with a disturbance of language (dysphasia) or an upper homonymous quadrantanopia. Nystagmus and ataxia are signs of a cerebellar abscess. Signs of raised ICP—papilledema, nausea and vomiting, and drowsiness or confusion—can be the dominant presentation of some abscesses, particularly those in the cerebellum. Meningismus is not present unless the abscess has ruptured into the ventricle or the infection has spread to the subarachnoid space.

DIAGNOSIS

Diagnosis is made by neuroimaging studies. MRI (Fig. 381-4) is better than CT for demonstrating abscesses in the early (cerebritis) stages and is superior to CT for identifying abscesses in the posterior fossa. Cerebritis appears on MRI as an area of low-signal intensity on T1-weighted images with irregular postgadolinium enhancement and as an area of increased signal intensity on T2-weighted images. Cerebritis is often not visualized by CT scan but, when present, appears as an area of hypodensity. On a contrast-enhanced CT scan, a mature brain abscess appears as a focal area of hypodensity surrounded by ring enhancement with surrounding edema (hypodensity). On contrast-enhanced T1-weighted MRI, a mature brain abscess has a capsule that enhances surrounding a hypodense center and surrounded by a hypodense area of edema. On T2-weighted MRI, there is a hyperintense central area of pus surrounded by a well-defined hypointense capsule and a hyperintense surrounding area of edema. It is important to recognize that the CT and MR appearance, particularly of the capsule, may be altered by treatment with glucocorticoids. The distinction between a brain abscess and other focal CNS lesions such as primary or metastatic tumors may be facilitated by the use of diffusion-weighted imaging sequences

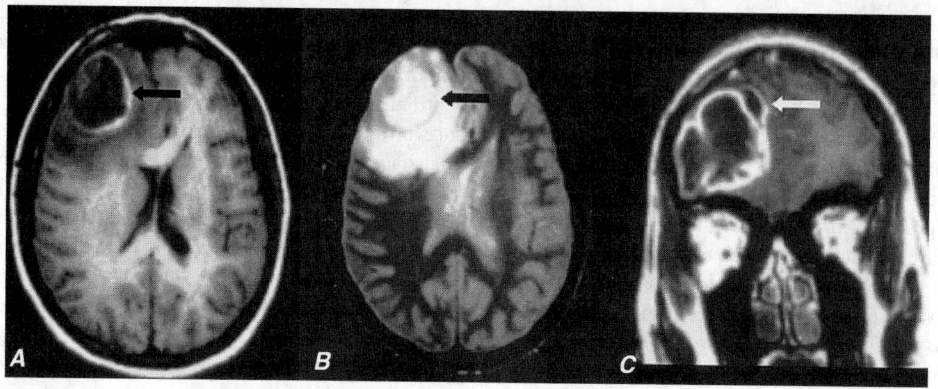

Figure 381-4 Pneumococcal brain abscess. Note that the abscess wall has hyperintense signal on the axial T1-weighted MRI (*A, black arrow*), hypointense signal on the axial proton density images (*B, black arrow*), and enhances prominently after gadolinium administration on the coronal T1-weighted image (*C*). The abscess is surrounded by a large amount of vasogenic edema and has a small "daughter" abscess (*C, white arrow*). *(Courtesy of Joseph Lurito, MD; with permission.)*

on which brain abscesses typically show increased signal due to restricted diffusion.

Microbiologic diagnosis of the etiologic agent is most accurately determined by Gram's stain and culture of abscess material obtained by CT-guided stereotactic needle aspiration. Aerobic and anaerobic bacterial cultures and mycobacterial and fungal cultures should be obtained. Up to 10% of patients will also have positive blood cultures. LP should not be performed in patients with known or suspected focal intracranial infections such as abscess or empyema; CSF analysis contributes nothing to diagnosis or therapy, and LP increases the risk of herniation.

Additional laboratory studies may provide clues to the diagnosis of brain abscess in patients with a CNS mass lesion. About 50% of patients have a peripheral leukocytosis, 60% an elevated ESR, and 80% an elevated C-reactive protein. Blood cultures are positive in ~10% of cases overall but may be positive in >85% of patients with abscesses due to *Listeria*.

DIFFERENTIAL DIAGNOSIS

Conditions that can cause headache, fever, focal neurologic signs, and seizure activity include brain abscess, subdural empyema, bacterial meningitis, viral meningoencephalitis, superior sagittal sinus thrombosis, and acute disseminated encephalomyelitis. When fever is absent, primary and metastatic brain tumors become the major differential diagnosis. Less commonly, cerebral infarction or hematoma can have an MRI or CT appearance resembling brain abscess.

TREATMENT Brain Abscess

Optimal therapy of brain abscesses involves a combination of high-dose parenteral antibiotics and neurosurgical drainage. Empirical therapy of community-acquired brain abscess in an immunocompetent patient typically includes a third- or fourth-generation cephalosporin (e.g., cefotaxime, ceftriaxone, or cefepime) and metronidazole (see Table 381-1 for antibiotic dosages). In patients with penetrating head trauma or recent neurosurgical procedures, treatment should include ceftazidime as the third-generation cephalosporin to enhance coverage of *Pseudomonas* spp. and vancomycin for coverage of staphylococci. Meropenem plus vancomycin also provides good coverage in this setting.

Aspiration and drainage of the abscess under stereotactic guidance are beneficial for both diagnosis and therapy. Empirical antibiotic coverage should be modified based on the results of Gram's stain and culture of the abscess contents. Complete excision of a bacterial abscess via craniotomy or craniectomy is generally reserved for multiloculated abscesses or those in which stereotactic aspiration is unsuccessful.

Medical therapy alone is not optimal for treatment of brain abscess and should be reserved for patients whose abscesses are neurosurgically inaccessible, for patients with small (<2–3 cm) or nonencapsulated abscesses (cerebritis), and patients whose condition is too tenuous to allow performance of a neurosurgical procedure. All patients should receive a minimum of 6–8 weeks of parenteral antibiotic therapy. The role, if any, of supplemental oral antibiotic therapy following completion of a standard course of parenteral therapy has never been adequately studied.

In addition to surgical drainage and antibiotic therapy, patients should receive prophylactic anticonvulsant therapy because of the high risk (~35%) of focal or generalized seizures. Anticonvulsant therapy is continued for at least 3 months after resolution of the abscess, and decisions regarding withdrawal are then based on the EEG. If the EEG is abnormal, anticonvulsant therapy should be continued. If the EEG is normal, anticonvulsant therapy can be slowly withdrawn, with close follow-up and repeat EEG after the medication has been discontinued.

Glucocorticoids should not be given routinely to patients with brain abscesses. Intravenous dexamethasone therapy (10 mg every 6 h) is usually reserved for patients with substantial periabscess edema and associated mass effect and increased ICP. Dexamethasone should be tapered as rapidly as possible to avoid delaying the natural process of encapsulation of the abscess.

Serial MRI or CT scans should be obtained on a monthly or twice-monthly basis to document resolution of the abscess. More frequent studies (e.g., weekly) are probably warranted in the subset of patients who are receiving antibiotic therapy alone. A small amount of enhancement may remain for months after the abscess has been successfully treated.

PROGNOSIS

The mortality rate of brain abscess has declined in parallel with the development of enhanced neuroimaging techniques, improved neurosurgical procedures for stereotactic aspiration, and improved antibiotics. In modern series, the mortality rate is typically <15%. Significant sequelae, including seizures, persisting weakness, aphasia, or mental impairment, occur in ≥20% of survivors.

NONBACTERIAL CAUSES OF INFECTIOUS FOCAL CNS LESIONS

ETIOLOGY

Neurocysticercosis is the most common parasitic disease of the CNS worldwide. Humans acquire cysticercosis by the ingestion of food contaminated with the eggs of the parasite *T. solium*. Toxoplasmosis is a parasitic disease caused by *T. gondii* and acquired from the ingestion of undercooked meat and from handling cat feces.

CLINICAL PRESENTATION

The most common manifestation of neurocysticercosis is new-onset partial seizures with or without secondary generalization. Cysticerci may develop in the brain parenchyma and cause seizures or focal neurologic deficits. When present in the subarachnoid or ventricular spaces, cysticerci can produce increased ICP by interference with CSF flow. Spinal cysticerci can mimic the presentation of intraspinal tumors. When the cysticerci first lodge in the brain, they frequently cause little in the way of an inflammatory response. As the cysticercal cyst degenerates, it elicits an inflammatory response that may present clinically as a seizure. Eventually the cyst dies, a process that may take several years and is typically associated with resolution of the inflammatory response and, often, abatement of seizures.

Primary *Toxoplasma* infection is often asymptomatic. However, during this phase parasites may spread to the CNS, where they become latent. Reactivation of CNS infection is almost exclusively associated with immunocompromised hosts, particularly those with HIV infection. During this phase patients present with headache, fever, seizures, and focal neurologic deficits.

DIAGNOSIS

The lesions of neurocysticercosis are readily visualized by MRI or CT scans. Lesions with viable parasites appear as cystic lesions. The scolex can often be visualized on MRI. Lesions may appear as contrast-enhancing lesions surrounded by edema. A very early sign of cyst death is hypointensity of the vesicular fluid on T2-weighted images when compared with CSF. Parenchymal brain calcifications are the most common finding and evidence that the parasite is no longer viable. MRI findings of toxoplasmosis consist of multiple lesions in the deep white matter, the thalamus, and basal ganglia and at the gray-white junction in the cerebral hemispheres. With contrast administration, the majority of the lesions enhance in a ringed, nodular, or homogeneous pattern and are surrounded by edema. In the presence of the characteristic neuroimaging abnormalities of *T. gondii* infection, serum IgG antibody to *T. gondii* should be obtained and, when positive, the patient should be treated.

TREATMENT Infectious Focal CNS Lesions

Anticonvulsant therapy is initiated when the patient with neurocysticercosis presents with a seizure. There is controversy about whether or not anthelmintic therapy should be given to all patients, and recommendations are based on the stage of the lesion. Cysticerci appearing as cystic lesions in the brain parenchyma with or without pericystic edema or in the subarachnoid space at the convexity of the cerebral hemispheres should be treated with anticysticidal therapy. Cysticidal drugs accelerate the destruction of the parasites, resulting in a faster resolution of the infection. Albendazole and praziquantel are used in the treatment of neurocysticercosis. Approximately 85% of parenchymal cysts are destroyed by a single course of albendazole, and ~75% are destroyed by a single course of praziquantel. The dose of albendazole is 15 mg/kg per day in two doses for 8 days. The dose of praziquantel is 50 mg/kg per day for 15 days, although a number of other dosage regimens are also frequently cited. Prednisone or dexamethasone is given with anticysticidal therapy to reduce the host inflammatory response to degenerating parasites. Many, but not all, experts recommend anticysticidal therapy for lesions that are surrounded by a contrast-enhancing ring. There is universal agreement that calcified lesions do not need to be treated with anticysticidal therapy. Antiepileptic therapy can be stopped once the follow-up CT scan shows resolution of the lesion. Long-term antiepileptic therapy is recommended when seizures occur after resolution of edema and resorption or calcification of the degenerating cyst.

CNS toxoplasmosis is treated with a combination of sulfadiazine, 1.5–2.0 g orally qid, plus pyrimethamine, 100 mg orally to load, then 75–100 mg orally qd, plus folinic acid, 10–15 mg orally qd. Folinic acid is added to the regimen to prevent megaloblastic anemia. Therapy is continued until there is no evidence of active disease on neuroimaging studies, which typically takes at least 6 weeks, and then the dose of sulfadiazine is reduced to 2–4 g/d and pyrimethamine to 50 mg/d. Clindamycin plus pyrimethamine is an alternative therapy for patients who cannot tolerate sulfadiazine, but the combination of pyrimethamine and sulfadiazine is more effective.

SUBDURAL EMPYEMA

A subdural empyema (SDE) is a collection of pus between the dura and arachnoid membranes (Fig. 381-5).

EPIDEMIOLOGY

SDE is a rare disorder that accounts for 15–25% of focal suppurative CNS infections. Sinusitis is the most common predisposing condition and typically involves the frontal sinuses, either alone or in combination with the ethmoid and maxillary sinuses. Sinusitis-associated empyema has a striking predilection for young males, possibly reflecting sex-related differences in sinus anatomy and development. It has been suggested that SDE may complicate 1–2% of cases of frontal sinusitis severe enough to require hospitalization. As a consequence of this epidemiology, SDE shows an ~3:1 male/female predominance, with 70% of cases occurring in the second and third decades of life. SDE may also develop as a complication of head trauma or neurosurgery. Secondary infection of a subdural effusion

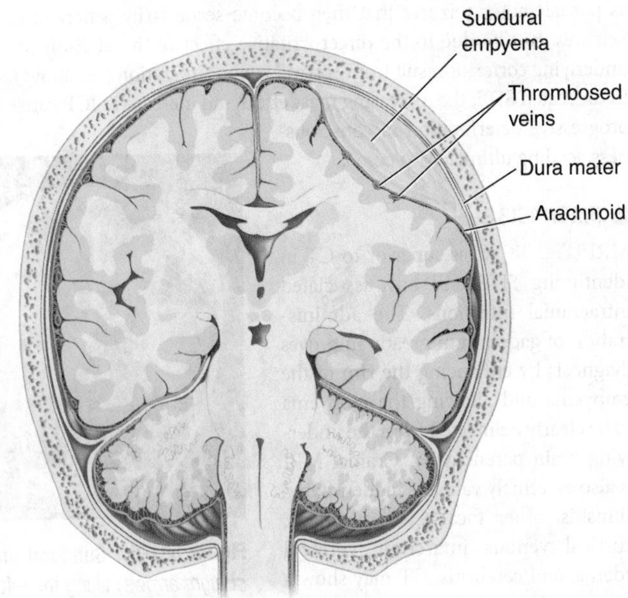

Figure 381-5 Subdural empyema.

may also result in empyema, although secondary infection of hematomas, in the absence of a prior neurosurgical procedure, is rare.

ETIOLOGY

Aerobic and anaerobic streptococci, staphylococci, Enterobacteriaceae, and anaerobic bacteria are the most common causative organisms of sinusitis-associated SDE. Staphylococci and gram-negative bacilli are often the etiologic organisms when SDE follows neurosurgical procedures or head trauma. Up to one-third of cases are culture-negative, possibly reflecting difficulty in obtaining adequate anaerobic cultures.

PATHOPHYSIOLOGY

Sinusitis-associated SDE develops as a result of either retrograde spread of infection from septic thrombophlebitis of the mucosal veins draining the sinuses or contiguous spread of infection to the brain from osteomyelitis in the posterior wall of the frontal or other sinuses. SDE may also develop from direct introduction of bacteria into the subdural space as a complication of a neurosurgical procedure. The evolution of SDE can be extremely rapid because the subdural space is a large compartment that offers few mechanical barriers to the spread of infection. In patients with sinusitis-associated SDE, suppuration typically begins in the upper and anterior portions of one cerebral hemisphere and then extends posteriorly. SDE is often associated with other intracranial infections, including epidural empyema (40%), cortical thrombophlebitis (35%), and intracranial abscess or cerebritis (>25%). Cortical venous infarction produces necrosis of underlying cerebral cortex and subcortical white matter, with focal neurologic deficits and seizures (see below).

CLINICAL PRESENTATION

A patient with SDE typically presents with fever and a progressively worsening headache. The diagnosis of SDE should always be suspected in a patient with known sinusitis who presents with new CNS signs or symptoms. Patients with underlying sinusitis frequently have symptoms related to this infection. As the infection progresses, focal neurologic deficits, seizures, nuchal rigidity, and signs of increased ICP commonly occur. Headache is the most common complaint at the time of presentation; initially it is localized to the side of the subdural infection, but then it becomes more severe and generalized. Contralateral hemiparesis or hemiplegia is the most common focal neurologic deficit and can occur from the direct effects of the SDE on the cortex or as a consequence of venous infarction. Seizures begin as partial motor seizures that then become secondarily generalized. Seizures may be due to the direct irritative effect of the SDE on the underlying cortex or result from cortical venous infarction (see above). In untreated SDE, the increasing mass effect and increase in ICP cause progressive deterioration in consciousness, leading ultimately to coma.

DIAGNOSIS

MRI (Fig. 381-6) is superior to CT in identifying SDE and any associated intracranial infections. The administration of gadolinium greatly improves diagnosis by enhancing the rim of the empyema and allowing the empyema to be clearly delineated from the underlying brain parenchyma. Cranial MRI is also extremely valuable in identifying sinusitis, other focal CNS infections, cortical venous infarction, cerebral edema, and cerebritis. CT may show a crescent-shaped hypodense lesion over one or both hemispheres or in the interhemispheric fissure. Frequently the degree of mass effect, exemplified by midline shift, ventricular compression, and sulcal effacement, is far out of proportion to the mass of the SDE.

CSF examination should be avoided in patients with known or suspected SDE as it adds no useful information and is associated with the risk of cerebral herniation.

DIFFERENTIAL DIAGNOSIS

The differential diagnosis of the combination of headache, fever, focal neurologic signs, and seizure activity that progresses rapidly to an altered level of consciousness includes subdural hematoma, bacterial meningitis, viral encephalitis, brain abscess, superior sagittal sinus thrombosis, and acute disseminated encephalomyelitis. The presence of nuchal rigidity is unusual with brain abscess or epidural empyema and should suggest the possibility of SDE when associated with significant focal neurologic signs and fever. Patients with bacterial meningitis also have nuchal rigidity but do not typically have focal deficits of the severity seen with SDE.

TREATMENT Subdural Empyema

SDE is a medical emergency. Emergent neurosurgical evacuation of the empyema, either through craniotomy, craniectomy, or burr-hole drainage, is the definitive step in the management of this infection. Empirical antimicrobial therapy for community-acquired SDE should include a combination of a third-generation cephalosporin (e.g., cefotaxime or ceftriaxone), vancomycin, and metronidazole (see Table 381-1 for dosages). Patients with hospital-acquired SDE may have infections due to *Pseudomonas* spp. or MRSA and should receive coverage with a carbapenem (e.g., meropenem) and vancomycin. Metronidazole is not necessary for anti-anaerobic therapy when meropenem is being used. Parenteral antibiotic therapy should be continued for a minimum of 3–4 weeks after SDE drainage. Patients with associated cranial osteomyelitis may require longer therapy. Specific diagnosis of the etiologic organisms is made based on Gram's stain and culture of fluid obtained via either burr holes or craniotomy; the initial empirical antibiotic coverage can be modified accordingly.

PROGNOSIS

Prognosis is influenced by the level of consciousness of the patient at the time of hospital presentation, the size of the empyema, and the speed with which therapy is instituted. Long-term neurologic sequelae, which include seizures and hemiparesis, occur in up to 50% of cases.

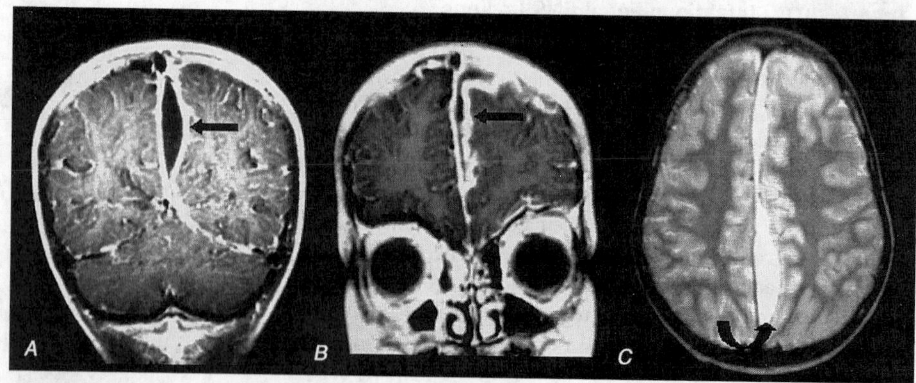

Figure 381-6 Subdural empyema. There is marked enhancement of the dura and leptomeninges (***A, B***, *straight arrows*) along the left medial hemisphere. The pus is hypointense on T1-weighted images (***A, B***) but markedly hyperintense on the proton density–weighted (***C***, *curved arrow*) image. *(Courtesy of Joseph Lurito, MD; with permission.)*

CRANIAL EPIDURAL ABSCESS

Cranial epidural abscess is a suppurative infection occurring in the potential space between the inner skull table and dura (Fig. 381-7).

ETIOLOGY AND PATHOPHYSIOLOGY

Cranial epidural abscess is less common than either brain abscess or SDE and accounts for <2% of focal suppurative CNS infections. A cranial epidural abscess develops as a complication of a craniotomy or compound skull fracture or as a result of spread of infection from the frontal sinuses, middle ear, mastoid, or orbit. An epidural abscess may develop contiguous to an area of osteomyelitis, when craniotomy is complicated by infection of the wound or bone flap, or as a result of direct infection of the epidural space. Infection in the frontal sinus, middle ear, mastoid, or orbit can reach the epidural space through retrograde spread of infection from septic thrombophlebitis in the emissary veins that drain these areas or by way of direct spread of infection through areas of osteomyelitis. Unlike the subdural space, the epidural space is really a potential rather than an actual compartment. The dura is normally tightly adherent to the inner skull table, and infection must dissect the dura away from the skull table as it spreads. As a result, epidural abscesses are often smaller than SDEs. Cranial epidural abscesses, unlike brain abscesses, only rarely result from hematogenous spread of infection from extracranial primary sites. The bacteriology of a cranial epidural abscess is similar to that of SDE (see above). The etiologic organisms of an epidural abscess that arises from frontal sinusitis, middle-ear infections, or mastoiditis are usually streptococci or anaerobic organisms. Staphylococci or gram-negative organisms are the usual cause of an epidural abscess that develops as a complication of craniotomy or compound skull fracture.

CLINICAL PRESENTATION

Patients present with fever (60%), headache (40%), nuchal rigidity (35%), seizures (10%), and focal deficits (5%). Development of symptoms may be insidious, as the empyema usually enlarges slowly in the confined anatomic space between the dura and the inner table of the skull. Periorbital edema and Potts puffy tumor, reflecting underlying associated frontal bone osteomyelitis, are present in ~40%. In patients with a recent neurosurgical procedure, wound infection is invariably present, but other symptoms may be subtle and can include altered mental status (45%), fever (35%), and headache (20%). The diagnosis should be considered when fever and headache follow recent head trauma or occur in the setting of frontal sinusitis, mastoiditis, or otitis media.

DIAGNOSIS

Cranial MRI with gadolinium enhancement is the procedure of choice to demonstrate a cranial epidural abscess. The sensitivity of CT is limited by the presence of signal artifacts arising from the bone of the inner skull table. The CT appearance of an epidural empyema is that of a lens or crescent-shaped hypodense extraaxial lesion. On MRI, an epidural empyema appears as a lentiform or crescent-shaped fluid collection that is hyperintense compared to CSF on T2-weighted images. On T1-weighted images, the fluid collection may be either isointense or hypointense compared to brain. Following the administration of gadolinium, there is linear enhancement of the dura on T1-weighted images. In distinction to subdural empyema, signs of mass effect or other parenchymal abnormalities are uncommon.

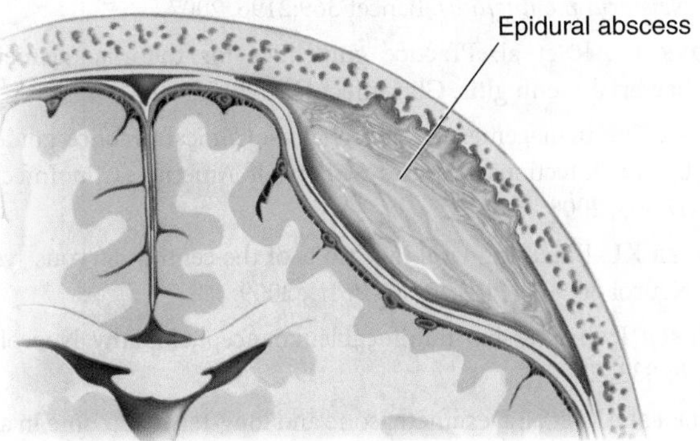

Figure 381-7 Cranial epidural abscess is a collection of pus between the dura and the inner table of the skull.

TREATMENT Epidural Abscess

Immediate neurosurgical drainage is indicated. Empirical antimicrobial therapy, pending the results of Gram's stain and culture of the purulent material obtained at surgery, should include a combination of a third-generation cephalosporin, vancomycin, and metronidazole (Table 381-1). Ceftazidime or meropenem should be substituted for ceftriaxone or cefotaxime in neurosurgical patients. Metronidazole is not necessary for anti-anaerobic coverage in patients receiving meropenem. When the organism has been identified, antimicrobial therapy can be modified accordingly. Antibiotics should be continued for 3–6 weeks after surgical drainage. Patients with associated osteomyelitis may require additional therapy.

PROGNOSIS

The mortality rate is <5% in modern series, and full recovery is the rule in most survivors.

SUPPURATIVE THROMBOPHLEBITIS

DEFINITION

Suppurative intracranial thrombophlebitis is septic venous thrombosis of cortical veins and sinuses. This may occur as a complication of bacterial meningitis; SDE; epidural abscess; or infection in the skin of the face, paranasal sinuses, middle ear, or mastoid.

ANATOMY AND PATHOPHYSIOLOGY

The cerebral veins and venous sinuses have no valves; therefore, blood within them can flow in either direction. The superior sagittal sinus is the largest of the venous sinuses (Fig. 381-8). It receives blood from the frontal, parietal, and occipital superior cerebral veins and the diploic veins, which communicate with the meningeal veins. Bacterial meningitis is a common predisposing condition for septic thrombosis of the superior sagittal sinus. The diploic veins, which drain into the superior sagittal sinus, provide a route for the spread of infection from the meninges, especially in cases where there is purulent exudate near areas of the superior sagittal sinus. Infection can also spread to the superior sagittal sinus from nearby SDE or epidural abscess. Dehydration from vomiting, hypercoagulable states, and immunologic abnormalities, including the presence of circulating antiphospholipid antibodies, also contribute to cerebral venous sinus thrombosis. Thrombosis may extend from one sinus to another, and at autopsy thrombi of different histologic ages can often be detected in several sinuses. Thrombosis of the superior sagittal sinus is often associated with thrombosis of superior cortical veins and small parenchymal hemorrhages.

The superior sagittal sinus drains into the transverse sinuses (Fig. 381-8). The transverse sinuses also receive venous drainage from small veins from both the middle ear and mastoid cells. The transverse sinus becomes the sigmoid sinus before draining into the internal jugular vein. Septic transverse/sigmoid sinus thrombosis

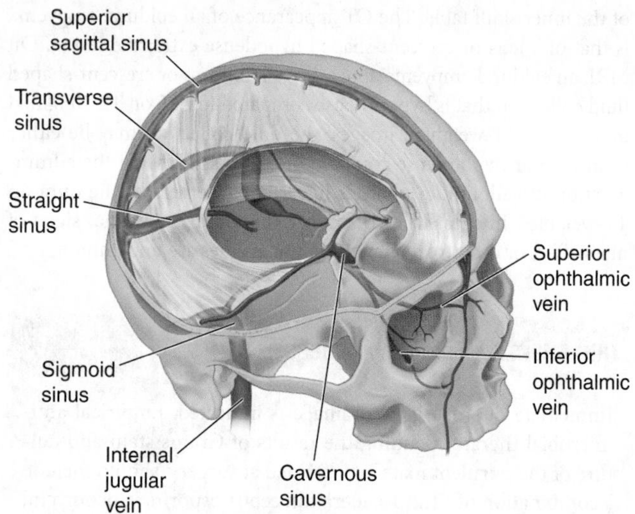

Figure 381-8 Anatomy of the cerebral venous sinuses.

can be a complication of acute and chronic otitis media or mastoiditis. Infection spreads from the mastoid air cells to the transverse sinus via the emissary veins or by direct invasion. The cavernous sinuses are inferior to the superior sagittal sinus at the base of the skull. The cavernous sinuses receive blood from the facial veins via the superior and inferior ophthalmic veins. Bacteria in the facial veins enter the cavernous sinus via these veins. Bacteria in the sphenoid and ethmoid sinuses can spread to the cavernous sinuses via the small emissary veins. The sphenoid and ethmoid sinuses are the most common sites of primary infection resulting in septic cavernous sinus thrombosis.

■ CLINICAL MANIFESTATIONS

Septic thrombosis of the superior sagittal sinus presents with headache, fever, nausea and vomiting, confusion, and focal or generalized seizures. There may be a rapid development of stupor and coma. Weakness of the lower extremities with bilateral Babinski's signs or hemiparesis is often present. When superior sagittal sinus thrombosis occurs as a complication of bacterial meningitis, nuchal rigidity and Kernig's and Brudzinski's signs may be present.

The oculomotor nerve, the trochlear nerve, the abducens nerve, the ophthalmic and maxillary branches of the trigeminal nerve, and the internal carotid artery all pass through the cavernous sinus (see Fig. 376-4). The symptoms of *septic cavernous sinus thrombosis* are fever, headache, frontal and retroorbital pain, and diplopia. The classic signs are ptosis, proptosis, chemosis, and extraocular dysmotility due to deficits of cranial nerves III, IV, and VI; hyperesthesia of the ophthalmic and maxillary divisions of the fifth cranial nerve and a decreased corneal reflex may be detected. There may be evidence of dilated, tortuous retinal veins and papilledema.

Headache and earache are the most frequent symptoms of *transverse sinus thrombosis*. A transverse sinus thrombosis may also present with otitis media, sixth nerve palsy, and retroorbital or facial pain (*Gradenigo's syndrome*). Sigmoid sinus and internal jugular vein thrombosis may present with neck pain.

■ DIAGNOSIS

The diagnosis of septic venous sinus thrombosis is suggested by an absent flow void within the affected venous sinus on MRI and confirmed by magnetic resonance venography, CT angiogram, or the venous phase of cerebral angiography. The diagnosis of thrombophlebitis of intracerebral and meningeal veins is suggested by the presence of intracerebral hemorrhage but requires cerebral angi-ography for definitive diagnosis.

TREATMENT Suppurative Thrombophlebitis

Septic venous sinus thrombosis is treated with antibiotics, hydration, and removal of infected tissue and thrombus in septic lateral or cavernous sinus thrombosis. The choice of antimicrobial therapy is based on the bacteria responsible for the predisposing or associated condition. Optimal duration of therapy is unknown, but antibiotics are usually continued for 6 weeks or until there is radiographic evidence of resolution of thrombosis. Anticoagulation with dose-adjusted intravenous heparin is recommended for aseptic venous sinus thrombosis and in the treatment of septic venous sinus thrombosis complicating bacterial meningitis in patients who have progressive neurologic deterioration despite antimicrobial therapy and intravenous fluids. The presence of a small intracerebral hemorrhage from septic thrombophlebitis is not an absolute contraindication to heparin therapy. Successful management of aseptic venous sinus thrombosis has been reported with surgical thrombectomy, catheter-directed urokinase therapy, and with a combination of intrathrombus recombinant tissue plasminogen activator (rtPA) and intravenous heparin, but there is not enough data to recommend these therapies in septic venous sinus thrombosis.

FURTHER READINGS

BROUWER MC et al: Nationwide implementation of adjunctive dexamethasone therapy for pneumococcal meningitis. Neurology 75:1533, 2010

DE GANS J, VAN DE BEEK D: Dexamethasone in adults with bacterial meningitis. N Engl J Med 347:1549, 2002

DWORKIN MS et al: The changing epidemiology of invasive *Haemophilus influenzae* disease, especially in persons ≥65 years old. Clin Infect Dis 44:810, 2007

IRANI DN: Aseptic meningitis and viral myelitis. Neurol Clin 26:635, 2008

PERFECT JR et al: Clinical practice guidelines for the management of cryptococcal disease: 2010 update by the Infectious Diseases Society of America. Clin Infect Dis 50:291, 2010

ROSENSTEIN NE et al: Meningococcal disease. N Engl J Med 344:1378, 2001

SCARBOROUGH M et al: Corticosteroids for bacterial meningitis in adults in sub-Saharan Africa. N Engl J Med 357:2441, 2007

STEPHENS DS et al: Epidemic meningitis, meningococcemia, and *Neisseria meningitidis*. Lancet 369:2196, 2007

TUNKEL AR et al: Practice guidelines for the management of bacterial meningitis. Clin Infect Dis 39:1267, 2004

———: The management of encephalitis: Clinical practice guidelines by the Infectious Diseases Society of America. Clin Infect Dis 47:303, 2008

TYLER KL: Emerging viral infections of the central nervous system. Neurol 66:939 (Pt I), 1065 (Pt II), 2009

WEBER T: Progressive multifocal leukoencephalopathy. Neurol Clin 26:833, 2008

WEISFELT M et al: Dexamethasone and long-term outcome in adults with bacterial meningitis. Ann Neurol 60:456, 2006

CHAPTER 382
Chronic and Recurrent Meningitis

Walter J. Koroshetz
Morton N. Swartz

Chronic inflammation of the meninges (pia, arachnoid, and dura) can produce profound neurologic disability and may be fatal if not successfully treated. The condition is most commonly diagnosed when a characteristic neurologic syndrome exists for >4 weeks and is associated with a persistent inflammatory response in the cerebrospinal fluid (CSF) (white blood cell count >5/μL). The causes are varied, and appropriate treatment depends on identification of the etiology. Five categories of disease account for most cases of chronic meningitis: (1) meningeal infections, (2) malignancy, (3) noninfectious inflammatory disorders, (4) chemical meningitis, and (5) parameningeal infections.

CLINICAL PATHOPHYSIOLOGY

Neurologic manifestations of chronic meningitis (Table 382-1) are determined by the anatomic location of the inflammation and its consequences. Persistent headache with or without stiff neck, hydrocephalus, cranial neuropathies, radiculopathies, and cognitive or personality changes are the cardinal features. These can occur alone or in combination. When they appear in combination, widespread dissemination of the inflammatory process along CSF pathways has occurred. In some cases, the presence of an underlying systemic illness points to a specific agent or class of agents as the probable cause. The diagnosis of chronic meningitis is usually made when the clinical presentation prompts the astute physician to examine the CSF for signs of inflammation. CSF is produced by the choroid plexus of the cerebral ventricles, exits through narrow foramina into the subarachnoid space surrounding the brain and spinal cord, circulates around the base of the brain and over the cerebral hemispheres, and is resorbed by arachnoid villi projecting into the superior sagittal sinus. CSF flow provides a pathway for rapid spread of infectious and other infiltrative processes over the brain, spinal cord, and cranial and spinal nerve roots. Spread from the subarachnoid space into brain parenchyma may occur via the arachnoid cuffs that surround blood vessels that penetrate brain tissue (Virchow-Robin spaces).

TABLE 382-1 Symptoms and Signs of Chronic Meningitis

Symptom	Sign
Chronic headache	+/– Papilledema
Neck or back pain	Brudzinski's or Kernig's sign of meningeal irritation
Change in personality	Altered mental status—drowsiness, inattention, disorientation, memory loss, frontal release signs (grasp, suck, snout), perseveration
Facial weakness	Peripheral seventh CN palsy
Double vision	Palsy of CNs III, IV, VI
Visual loss	Papilledema, optic atrophy
Hearing loss	Eighth CN palsy
Arm or leg weakness	Myelopathy or radiculopathy
Numbness in arms or legs	Myelopathy or radiculopathy
Sphincter dysfunction	Myelopathy or radiculopathy Frontal lobe dysfunction (hydrocephalus)
Clumsiness	Ataxia

Abbreviation: CN, cranial nerve.

Intracranial meningitis

Nociceptive fibers of the meninges are stimulated by the inflammatory process, resulting in headache or neck or back pain. Obstruction of CSF pathways at the foramina or arachnoid villi may produce *hydrocephalus* and symptoms of raised intracranial pressure (ICP), including headache, vomiting, apathy or drowsiness, gait instability, papilledema, visual loss, impaired upgaze, or palsy of the sixth cranial nerve (CN) (Chap. 376). Cognitive and behavioral changes during the course of chronic meningitis may also result from vascular damage, which may similarly produce seizures, stroke, or myelopathy. Inflammatory deposits seeded via the CSF circulation are often prominent around the brainstem and cranial nerves and along the undersurface of the frontal and temporal lobes. Such cases, termed *basal meningitis,* often present as multiple cranial neuropathies, with visual loss (CN II), facial weakness (CN VII), hearing loss (CN VIII), diplopia (CNs III, IV, and VI), sensory or motor abnormalities of the oropharynx (CNs IX, X, and XII), decreased olfaction (CN I), or facial sensory loss and masseter weakness (CN V).

Spinal meningitis

Injury may occur to motor and sensory roots as they traverse the subarachnoid space and penetrate the meninges. These cases present as multiple radiculopathies with combinations of radicular pain, sensory loss, motor weakness, and sphincter dysfunction. Meningeal inflammation can encircle the cord, resulting in myelopathy. Patients with slowly progressive involvement of multiple cranial nerves and/or spinal nerve roots are likely to have chronic meningitis. Electrophysiologic testing (electromyography, nerve conduction studies, and evoked response testing) may be helpful in determining whether there is involvement of cranial and spinal nerve roots.

Systemic manifestations

In some patients, evidence of systemic disease provides clues to the underlying cause of chronic meningitis. A careful history and physical examination are essential before embarking on a diagnostic workup, which may be costly, prolonged, and associated with risk from invasive procedures. A complete history of travel, sexual practice, and exposure to infectious agents should be sought. Infectious causes are often associated with fever, malaise, anorexia, and signs of localized or disseminated infection outside the nervous system. Infectious causes are of major concern in the immunosuppressed patient, especially in patients with AIDS, in whom chronic meningitis may present without headache or fever. Noninfectious inflammatory disorders often produce systemic manifestations, but meningitis may be the initial manifestation. Carcinomatous meningitis may or may not be accompanied by clinical evidence of the primary neoplasm.

APPROACH TO THE PATIENT

Chronic Meningitis

The occurrence of chronic headache, hydrocephalus, cranial neuropathy, radiculopathy, and/or cognitive decline in a patient should prompt consideration of a lumbar puncture for evidence of meningeal inflammation. On occasion, the diagnosis is made when an imaging study (CT or MRI) shows contrast enhancement of the meninges, which is always abnormal with the exception of dural enhancement after lumbar puncture, neurosurgical procedures, or spontaneous CSF leakage. Once chronic meningitis is confirmed by CSF examination, effort is focused on identifying the cause (Tables 382-2 and 382-3) by (1) further analysis of the CSF, (2) diagnosis of an underlying systemic infection or noninfectious inflammatory condition, or (3) pathologic examination of meningeal biopsy specimens.

Two clinical forms of chronic meningitis exist. In the first, the symptoms are chronic and persistent, whereas in the second there are recurrent, discrete episodes of illness. In the latter group, all symptoms, signs, and CSF parameters of meningeal inflammation resolve completely between episodes without specific therapy. In such patients, the likely etiologies include herpes simplex virus (HSV) type 2; chemical meningitis due to leakage into CSF of contents from an epidermoid tumor, craniopharyngioma, or cholesteatoma; primary inflammatory conditions, including Vogt-Koyanagi-Harada syndrome, Behçet's syndrome, systemic lupus erythematosus; and drug hypersensitivity with repeated administration of the offending agent.

The epidemiologic history is of considerable importance and may provide direction for selection of laboratory studies. Pertinent features include a history of tuberculosis or exposure to a likely case; past travel to areas endemic for fungal infections (the San Joaquin Valley in California and southwestern states for coccidioidomycosis, midwestern states for histoplasmosis, southeastern states for blastomycosis); travel to the Mediterranean

TABLE 382-2 Infectious Causes of Chronic Meningitis

Causative Agent	CSF Formula	Helpful Diagnostic Tests	Risk Factors and Systemic Manifestations
Common Bacterial Causes			
Partially treated suppurative meningitis	Mononuclear or mixed mononuclear-polymorphonuclear cells	CSF culture and Gram's stain	History consistent with acute bacterial meningitis and incomplete treatment
Parameningeal infection	Mononuclear or mixed polymorphonuclear-mononuclear cells	Contrast-enhanced CT or MRI to detect parenchymal, subdural, epidural, or sinus infection	Otitis media, pleuropulmonary infection, right-to-left cardiopulmonary shunt for brain abscess; focal neurologic signs; neck, back, ear, or sinus tenderness
Mycobacterium tuberculosis	Mononuclear cells except polymorphonuclear cells in early infection (commonly <500 WBC/μL); low CSF glucose, high protein	Tuberculin skin test may be negative; AFB culture of CSF (sputum, urine, gastric contents if indicated); tuberculostearic acid detection in CSF; identify tubercle bacillus on acid-fast stain of CSF or protein pellicle; PCR	Exposure history; previous tuberculous illness; immunosuppressed or AIDS; young children; fever, meningismus, night sweats, miliary TB on x-ray or liver biopsy; stroke due to arteritis
Lyme disease (Bannwarth's syndrome) *Borrelia burgdorferi*	Mononuclear cells; elevated protein	Serum Lyme antibody titer; Western blot confirmation; (patients with syphilis may have false-positive Lyme titer)	History of tick bite or appropriate exposure history; erythema chronicum migrans skin rash; arthritis, radiculopathy, Bell's palsy, meningoencephalitis–multiple sclerosis-like syndrome
Syphilis (secondary, tertiary) *Treponema pallidum*	Mononuclear cells; elevated protein	CSF VDRL; serum VDRL (or RPR); fluorescent treponemal antibody-absorbed (FTA) or MHA-TP; serum VDRL may be negative in tertiary syphilis	Appropriate exposure history; HIV-seropositive individuals at increased risk of aggressive infection; "dementia"; cerebral infarction due to endarteritis
Uncommon Bacterial Causes			
Actinomyces	Polymorphonuclear cells	Anaerobic culture	Parameningeal abscess or sinus tract (oral or dental focus); pneumonitis
Nocardia	Polymorphonuclear; occasionally mononuclear cells; often low glucose	Isolation may require weeks; weakly acid fast	Associated brain abscess may be present
Brucella	Mononuclear cells (rarely polymorphonuclear); elevated protein; often low glucose	CSF antibody detection; serum antibody detection	Intake of unpasteurized dairy products; exposure to goats, sheep, cows; fever, arthralgia, myalgia, vertebral osteomyelitis
Whipple's disease *Tropheryma whippelii*	Mononuclear cells	Biopsy of small bowel or lymph node; CSF PCR for *T. whippelii;* brain and meningeal biopsy (with PAS stain and EM examination)	Diarrhea, weight loss, arthralgias, fever; dementia, ataxia, paresis, ophthalmoplegia, oculomasticatory myoclonus
Rare Bacterial Causes			
Leptospirosis (occasionally if left untreated may last 3–4 weeks)			

(continued)

TABLE 382-2 Infectious Causes of Chronic Meningitis (*Continued*)

Causative Agent	CSF Formula	Helpful Diagnostic Tests	Risk Factors and Systemic Manifestations
Fungal Causes			
Cryptococcus neoformans	Mononuclear cells; count not elevated in some patients with AIDS	India ink or fungal wet mount of CSF (budding yeast); blood and urine cultures; antigen detection in CSF	AIDS and immune suppression; pigeon exposure; skin and other organ involvement due to disseminated infection
Coccidioides immitis	Mononuclear cells (sometimes 10–20% eosinophils); often low glucose	Antibody detection in CSF and serum	Exposure history—southwestern US; increased virulence in dark-skinned races
Candida sp.	Polymorphonuclear or mononuclear	Fungal stain and culture of CSF	IV drug abuse; post surgery; prolonged intravenous therapy; disseminated candidiasis
Histoplasma capsulatum	Mononuclear cells; low glucose	Fungal stain and culture of large volumes of CSF; antigen detection in CSF, serum, and urine; antibody detection in serum, CSF	Exposure history—Ohio and central Mississippi River Valley; AIDS; mucosal lesions
Blastomyces dermatitidis	Mononuclear cells	Fungal stain and culture of CSF; biopsy and culture of skin, lung lesions; antibody detection in serum	Midwestern and southeastern USA; usually systemic infection; abscesses, draining sinus, ulcers
Aspergillus sp.	Mononuclear or polymorphonuclear	CSF culture	Sinusitis; granulocytopenia or immunosuppression
Sporothrix schenckii	Mononuclear cells	Antibody detection in CSF and serum; CSF culture	Traumatic inoculation; IV drug use; ulcerated skin lesion
Rare Fungal Causes			
Xylohypha (formerly *Cladosporium*) *trichoides* and other dark-walled (demateaceous) fungi such as *Curvularia, Drechslera; Mucor*, and, after water aspiration, *Pseudoallescheria boydii*			
Protozoal Causes			
Toxoplasma gondii	Mononuclear cells	Biopsy or response to empirical therapy in clinically appropriate context (including presence of antibody in serum)	Usually with intracerebral abscesses; common in HIV-seropositive patients
Trypanosomiasis *Trypanosoma gambiense, T. rhodesiense*	Mononuclear cells, elevated protein	Elevated CSF IgM; identification of trypanosomes in CSF and blood smear	Endemic in Africa; chancre, lymphadenopathy; prominent sleep disorder
Rare Protozoal Causes			
Acanthamoeba sp. causing granulomatous amebic encephalitis and meningoencephalitis in immunocompromised and debilitated individuals. *Balamuthia mandrillaris* causing chronic meningoencephalitis in immunocompetent hosts.			
Helminthic Causes			
Cysticercosis (infection with cysts of *Taenia solium*)	Mononuclear cells; may have eosinophils; glucose level may be low	Indirect hemagglutination assay in CSF; ELISA immunoblotting in serum	Usually with multiple cysts in basal meninges and hydrocephalus; cerebral cysts, muscle calcification
Gnathostoma spinigerum	Eosinophils, mononuclear cells	Peripheral eosinophilia	History of eating raw fish; common in Thailand and Japan; subarachnoid hemorrhage; painful radiculopathy
Angiostrongylus cantonensis	Eosinophils, mononuclear cells	Recovery of worms from CSF	History of eating raw shellfish; common in tropical Pacific regions; often benign
Baylisascaris procyonis (raccoon ascarid)	Eosinophils, mononuclear cells		Infection follows accidental ingestion of *B. procyonis* eggs from raccoon feces; fatal meningoencephalitis
Rare Helminthic Causes			
Trichinella spiralis (trichinosis); *Fasciola hepatica* (liver fluke), *Echinococcus* cysts; *Schistosoma* sp. The former may produce a lymphocytic pleocytosis whereas the latter two may produce an eosinophilic response in CSF associated with cerebral cysts (*Echinococcus*) or granulomatous lesions of brain or spinal cord			

(continued)

TABLE 382-2 Infectious Causes of Chronic Meningitis (*Continued*)

Causative Agent	CSF Formula	Helpful Diagnostic Tests	Risk Factors and Systemic Manifestations
Viral causes			
Mumps	Mononuclear cells	Antibody in serum	No prior mumps or immunization; may produce meningoencephalitis; may persist for 3–4 weeks
Lymphocytic choriomeningitis	Mononuclear cells	Antibody in serum	Contact with rodents or their excreta; may persist for 3–4 weeks
Echovirus	Mononuclear cells; may have low glucose	Virus isolation from CSF	Congenital hypogammaglobulinemia; history of recurrent meningitis
HIV (acute retroviral syndrome)	Mononuclear cells	p24 antigen in serum and CSF; high level of HIV viremia	HIV risk factors; rash, fever, lymphadenopathy; lymphopenia in peripheral blood; syndrome may persist long enough to be considered as "chronic meningitis"; or chronic meningitis may develop in later stages (AIDS) due to HIV
Herpes simplex (HSV)	Mononuclear cells	PCR for HSV, CMV DNA; CSF antibody for HSV, EBV	Recurrent meningitis due to HSV-2 (rarely HSV-1) often associated with genital recurrences; EBV associated with myeloradiculopathy, CMV with polyradiculopathy

Abbreviations: AFB, acid-fast bacillus; CMV, cytomegalovirus; CSF, cerebrospinal fluid; CT, computed tomography; EBV, Epstein-Barr virus; ELISA, enzyme-linked immunosorbent assay; EM, electron microscopy; FTA, fluorescent treponemal antibody absorption test; HSV, herpes simplex virus; MHA-TP, microhemagglutination assay–*T. pallidum*; MRI, magnetic resonance imaging; PAS, periodic acid–Schiff; PCR, polymerase chain reaction; RPR, rapid plasma reagin test; TB, tuberculosis; VDRL, Venereal Disease Research Laboratories test.

region or ingestion of imported unpasteurized dairy products (*Brucella*); time spent in wooded areas endemic for Lyme disease; exposure to sexually transmitted disease (syphilis); exposure of an immunocompromised host to pigeons and their droppings (*Cryptococcus*); gardening (*Sporothrix schenkii*); ingestion of poorly cooked meat or contact with a household cat (*Toxoplasma gondii*); residence in Thailand or Japan (*Gnathostoma spinigerum*), Latin America (*Paracoccidioides brasiliiensis*), or the South Pacific (*Angiostrongylus cantonensis*); rural residence and raccoon exposure (*Baylisascaris procyonis*); and residence in Latin America, the Philippines, or Southeast Asia when eosinophilic meningitis is present (*Taenia solium*).

The presence of focal cerebral signs in a patient with chronic meningitis suggests the possibility of a brain abscess or other parameningeal infection; identification of a potential source of infection (chronic draining ear, sinusitis, right-to-left cardiac or pulmonary shunt, chronic pleuropulmonary infection) supports this diagnosis. In some cases, diagnosis may be established by recognition and biopsy of unusual skin lesions (Behçet's syndrome, cryptococcosis, blastomycosis, SLE, Lyme disease, IV drug use, sporotrichosis, trypanosomiasis) or enlarged lymph nodes (lymphoma, tuberculosis, sarcoid, infection with HIV, secondary syphilis, or Whipple's disease). A careful ophthalmologic examination may reveal uveitis [Vogt-Koyanagi-Harada syndrome, sarcoid, or central nervous system (CNS) lymphoma], keratoconjunctivitis sicca (Sjögren's syndrome), or iridocyclitis (Behçet's syndrome) and is essential to assess visual loss from papilledema. Aphthous oral lesions, genital ulcers, and hypopyon suggest Behçet's syndrome. Hepatosplenomegaly suggests lymphoma, sarcoid, tuberculosis, or brucellosis. Herpetic lesions in the genital area or on the thighs suggest HSV-2 infection. A breast nodule, a suspicious pigmented skin lesion, focal bone pain, or an abdominal mass directs attention to possible carcinomatous meningitis.

IMAGING Once the clinical syndrome is recognized as a potential manifestation of chronic meningitis, proper analysis of the CSF is essential. However, if the possibility of raised ICP exists, a brain imaging study should be performed before lumbar puncture. If ICP is elevated because of a mass lesion, brain swelling, or a block in ventricular CSF outflow (obstructive hydrocephalus), then lumbar puncture carries the potential risk of brain herniation. Obstructive hydrocephalus usually requires direct ventricular drainage of CSF. In patients with open CSF flow pathways, elevated ICP can still occur due to impaired resorption of CSF by arachnoid villi. In such patients, lumbar puncture is usually safe, but repetitive or continuous lumbar drainage may be necessary to prevent abrupt deterioration and death from raised ICP. In some patients, especially with cryptococcal meningitis, fatal levels of raised ICP can occur without enlarged ventricles.

Contrast-enhanced MRI or CT studies of the brain and spinal cord can identify meningeal enhancement, parameningeal infections (including brain abscess), encasement of the spinal cord (malignancy or inflammation and infection), or nodular deposits on the meninges or nerve roots (malignancy or sarcoidosis) (Fig. 382-1). Imaging studies are also useful to localize areas of meningeal disease prior to meningeal biopsy.

Cerebral angiography may be indicated in patients with chronic meningitis and stroke to identify cerebral arteritis (granulomatous angiitis, other inflammatory arteritides, or infectious arteritis).

CEREBROSPINAL FLUID ANALYSIS The CSF pressure should be measured and samples sent for bacterial, fungal, and tuberculous culture; Venereal Disease Research Laboratories (VDRL) test; cell count and differential; Gram's stain; and measurement of glucose and protein. Wet mount for fungus and parasites, India ink preparation and culture, culture for fastidious bacteria and fungi, assays for cryptococcal antigen and oligoclonal

TABLE 382-3 Noninfectious Causes of Chronic Meningitis

Causative Agents	CSF Formula	Helpful Diagnostic Tests	Risk Factors and Systemic Manifestations
Malignancy	Mononuclear cells, elevated protein, low glucose	Repeated cytologic examination of large volumes of CSF; CSF exam by polarizing microscopy; clonal lymphocyte markers; deposits on nerve roots or meninges seen on myelogram or contrast-enhanced MRI; meningeal biopsy	Metastatic cancer of breast, lung, stomach, or pancreas; melanoma, lymphoma, leukemia; meningeal gliomatosis; meningeal sarcoma; cerebral dysgerminoma; meningeal melanoma or B cell lymphoma
Chemical compounds (may cause recurrent meningitis)	Mononuclear or PMNs, low glucose, elevated protein; xanthochromia from subarachnoid hemorrhage in week prior to presentation with "meningitis"	Contrast-enhanced CT scan or MRI Cerebral angiogram to detect aneurysm	History of recent injection into the subarachnoid space; history of sudden onset of headache; recent resection of acoustic neuroma or craniopharyngioma; epidermoid tumor of brain or spine, sometimes with dermoid sinus tract; pituitary apoplexy
Primary Inflammation			
CNS sarcoidosis	Mononuclear cells; elevated protein; often low glucose	Serum and CSF angiotensin-converting enzyme levels; biopsy of extraneural affected tissues or brain lesion/meningeal biopsy	CN palsy, especially of CN VII; hypothalamic dysfunction, especially diabetes insipidus; abnormal chest radiograph; peripheral neuropathy or myopathy
Vogt-Koyanagi-Harada syndrome (recurrent meningitis)	Mononuclear cells		Recurrent meningoencephalitis with uveitis, retinal detachment, alopecia, lightening of eyebrows and lashes, dysacousia, cataracts, glaucoma
Isolated granulomatous angiitis of the nervous system	Mononuclear cells, elevated protein	Angiography or meningeal biopsy	Subacute dementia; multiple cerebral infarctions; recent zoster ophthalmicus
Systemic lupus erythematosus	Mononuclear or PMNs	Anti-DNA antibody, antinuclear antibodies	Encephalopathy; seizures; stroke; transverse myelopathy; rash; arthritis
Behçet's syndrome (recurrent meningitis)	Mononuclear or PMNs, elevated protein		Oral and genital aphthous ulcers; iridocyclitis; retinal hemorrhages; pathergic lesions at site of skin puncture
Chronic benign lymphocytic meningitis	Mononuclear cells		Recovery in 2–6 months, diagnosis by exclusion
Mollaret's meningitis (recurrent meningitis)	Large endothelial cells and PMNs in first hours, followed by mononuclear cells	PCR for herpes; MRI/CT to rule out epidermoid tumor or dural cyst	Recurrent meningitis; exclude HSV-2; rare cases due to HSV-1; occasional case associated with dural cyst
Drug hypersensitivity	PMNs; occasionally mononuclear cells or eosinophils	Complete blood count (eosinophilia)	Exposure to non steroidal anti-inflammatory agents, sulfonamides, isoniazid, tolmetin, ciprofloxacin, penicillin, carbamazaepine, lamotrigine, IV immunoglobulin, OKT3 antibodies, phenazopyridine; improvement after discontinuation of drug; recurrence with repeat exposure
Granulomatosis with polyangiitis (Wegener's)	Mononuclear cells	Chest and sinus radiographs; urinalysis; ANCA antibodies in serum	Associated sinus, pulmonary, or renal lesions; CN palsies; skin lesions; peripheral neuropathy
Other: multiple sclerosis, Sjögren's syndrome, neonatal-onset multisystemic inflammatory disease (NOMID), and rarer forms of vasculitis (e.g., Cogan's syndrome)			

Abbreviations: ANCA, anti-neutrophil cytoplasmic antibodies; CN, cranial nerve; CSF, cerebrospinal fluid; CT, computed tomography; HSV, herpes simplex virus; MRI, magnetic resonance imaging; PCR, polymerase chain reaction; PMNs, polymorphonuclear cells.

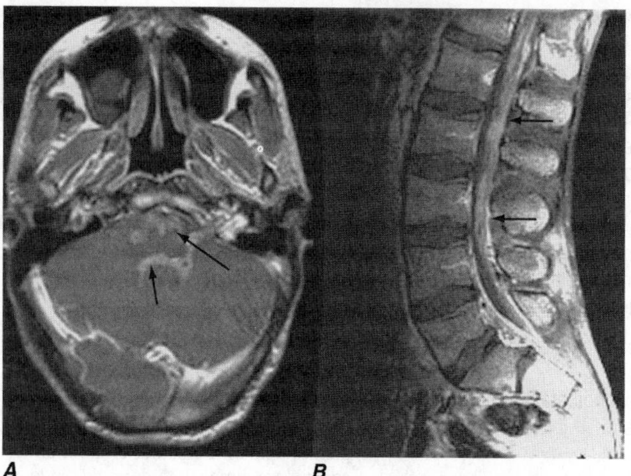

Figure 382-1 Primary central nervous system lymphoma. A 24-year-old man, immunosuppressed due to intestinal lymphangiectasia, developed multiple cranial neuropathies. CSF findings consisted of 100 lymphocytes/μL and a protein of 2.5 g/L (250 mg/dL); cytology and cultures were negative. Gadolinium-enhanced T1 MRI revealed diffuse, multifocal meningeal enhancement surrounding the brainstem (***A***), spinal cord, and cauda equina (***B***).

immunoglobulin bands, and cytology should be performed. Other specific CSF tests (Tables 382-2 and 382-3) or blood tests and cultures should be ordered as indicated on the basis of the history, physical examination, or preliminary CSF results (i.e., eosinophilic, mononuclear, or polymorphonuclear meningitis). Rapid diagnosis may be facilitated by serologic tests and polymerase chain reaction (PCR) testing to identify DNA sequences in the CSF that are specific for the suspected pathogen.

In most categories of chronic (not recurrent) meningitis, mononuclear cells predominate in the CSF. When neutrophils predominate after 3 weeks of illness, the principal etiologic considerations are *Nocardia asteroides, Actinomyces israelii, Brucella, Mycobacterium tuberculosis* (5–10% of early cases only), various fungi (*Blastomyces dermatitidis, Candida albicans, Histoplasma capsulatum, Aspergillus* spp., *Pseudallescheria boydii, Cladophialophora bantiana*), and noninfectious causes (SLE, exogenous chemical meningitis). When eosinophils predominate or are present in limited numbers in a primarily mononuclear cell response in the CSF, the differential diagnosis includes parasitic diseases (*A. cantonensis, G. spinigerum, B. procyonis*, or *Toxocara canis* infection, cysticercosis, schistosomiasis, echinococcal disease, *T. gondii* infection), fungal infections (6–20% eosinophils along with a predominantly lymphocyte pleocytosis, particularly with coccidioidal meningitis), neoplastic disease (lymphoma, leukemia, metastatic carcinoma), or other inflammatory processes (sarcoidosis, hypereosinophilic syndrome).

It is often necessary to broaden the number of diagnostic tests if the initial workup does not reveal the cause. In addition, repeated samples of large volumes of CSF may be required to diagnose certain infectious and malignant causes of chronic meningitis. For instance, lymphomatous or carcinomatous meningitis may be diagnosed by examination of sections cut from a cell block formed by spinning down the sediment from a large volume of CSF. The diagnosis of fungal meningitis may require large volumes of CSF for culture of sediment. If standard lumbar puncture is unrewarding, a cervical cisternal tap to sample CSF near to the basal meninges may be fruitful.

LABORATORY INVESTIGATION In addition to the CSF examination, an attempt should be made to uncover pertinent underlying illnesses. Tuberculin skin test, chest radiograph, urine analysis and culture, blood count and differential, renal and liver function tests, alkaline phosphatase, sedimentation rate, antinuclear antibody, anti-Ro, anti-La antibody, and serum angiotensin-converting enzyme level are often indicated. Liver or bone marrow biopsy may be diagnostic in some cases of miliary tuberculosis, disseminated fungal infection, sarcoidosis, or metastatic malignancy. Abnormalities discovered on chest radiograph or chest CT can be pursued by bronchoscopy or transthoracic needle biopsy.

MENINGEAL BIOPSY A meningeal biopsy should be strongly considered in patients who are severely disabled, who need chronic ventricular decompression, or whose illness is progressing rapidly. The activities of the surgeon, pathologist, microbiologist, and cytologist should be coordinated so that a large enough sample is obtained and the appropriate cultures and histologic and molecular studies, including electron-microscopic and PCR studies, are performed. The diagnostic yield of meningeal biopsy can be increased by targeting regions that enhance with contrast on MRI or CT. With current microsurgical techniques, most areas of the basal meninges can be accessed for biopsy via a limited craniotomy. In a series from the Mayo Clinic reported by Cheng et al., MRI demonstrated meningeal enhancement in 47% of patients undergoing meningeal biopsy. Biopsy of an enhancing region was diagnostic in 80% of cases; biopsy of nonenhancing regions was diagnostic in only 9%; sarcoid (31%) and metastatic adenocarcinoma (25%) were the most common conditions identified. Tuberculosis is the most common condition identified in many reports from outside the United States.

APPROACH TO THE ENIGMATIC CASE In approximately one-third of cases, the diagnosis is not known despite careful evaluation of CSF and potential extraneural sites of disease. A number of the organisms that cause chronic meningitis may take weeks to be identified by cultures. In enigmatic cases, several options are available, determined by the extent of the clinical deficits and rate of progression. It is prudent to wait until cultures are finalized if the patient is asymptomatic or symptoms are mild and not progressive. Unfortunately, in many cases progressive neurologic deterioration occurs, and rapid treatment is required. Ventricular-peritoneal shunts may be placed to relieve hydrocephalus, but the risk of disseminating the undiagnosed inflammatory process into the abdomen must be considered.

Empirical Treatment Diagnosis of the causative agent is essential because effective therapies exist for many etiologies of chronic meningitis, but if the condition is left untreated, progressive damage to the CNS and cranial nerves and roots is likely to occur. Occasionally, empirical therapy must be initiated when all attempts at diagnosis fail. In general, empirical therapy in the United States consists of antimycobacterial agents, amphotericin for fungal infection, or glucocorticoids for noninfectious inflammatory causes. It is important to direct empirical therapy of lymphocytic meningitis at tuberculosis, particularly if the condition is associated with hypoglycorrhachia and sixth and other CN palsies, since untreated disease is fatal in 4–8 weeks. In the Mayo Clinic series, the most useful empirical therapy was administration of glucocorticoids rather than antituberculous therapy. Carcinomatous or lymphomatous meningitis may be difficult to diagnose initially, but the diagnosis becomes evident with time.

THE IMMUNOSUPPRESSED PATIENT

Chronic meningitis is not uncommon in the course of HIV infection. Pleocytosis and mild meningeal signs often occur at the onset of HIV infection, and occasionally low-grade meningitis persists. Toxoplasmosis commonly presents as intracranial abscesses and may also be associated with meningitis. Other important causes of chronic meningitis in AIDS include infection with *Cryptococcus*, *Nocardia*, *Candida*, or other fungi; syphilis; and lymphoma (Fig. 382-1). Toxoplasmosis, cryptococcosis, nocardiosis, and other fungal infections are important etiologic considerations in individuals with immunodeficiency states other than AIDS, including those due to immunosuppressive medications. Because of the increased risk of chronic meningitis and the attenuation of clinical signs of meningeal irritation in immunosuppressed individuals, CSF examination should be performed for any persistent headache or unexplained change in mental state.

FURTHER READINGS

Cho TA, Venna N: Management of acute, recurrent, and chronic meningitides in adults. Neurol Clin 28:1061, 2010

Drake WK, Adam RD: Coccidioidal meningitis and brain abscesses: Analysis of 71 cases at a referral center. Neurology 73:1780, 2009

Gilden DH et al: Herpesvirus infections of the nervous system. Nat Clin Pract Neurol 3:82, 2007

Halperin JJ et al: Practice parameter: Treatment of nervous system Lyme disease (an evidence-based review): Report of the Quality Standards Subcommittee of the American Academy of Neurology. Neurology 69:91, 2007

Lan SH et al: Cerebral infarction in chronic meningitis: A comparison of tuberculous meningitis and cryptococcal meningitis. Q J Med 94:247, 2001

Liliang PC et al: Use of ventriculoperitoneal shunts to treat uncontrollable intracranial hypertension in patients who have cryptococcal meningitis without hydrocephalus. Clin Infect Dis 34:E64, 2002

Shapiro WR et al: Treatment modalities for leptomeningeal metastases. Semin Oncol 36:S46, 2009

Talati NJ et al: Spectrum of CNS disease caused by rapidly growing mycobacteria. Lancet Infect Dis 8:390, 2008

Vinnard C, MacGregor RR: Tuberculous meningitis in HIV-infected individuals. Curr HIV/AIDS Rep 6:139, 2009

CHAPTER 383
Prion Diseases

Stanley B. Prusiner
Bruce L. Miller

Prions are infectious proteins that cause degeneration of the central nervous system (CNS). Prion diseases are disorders of protein conformation, the most common of which in humans is called Creutzfeldt-Jakob disease (CJD). CJD typically presents with dementia and myoclonus, is relentlessly progressive, and generally causes death within a year of onset. Most CJD patients are between 50 and 75 years of age; however, patients as young as 17 and as old as 83 have been recorded.

In mammals, prions reproduce by binding to the normal, *c*ellular isoform of the *pr*ion *p*rotein (PrP^C) and stimulating conversion of PrP^C into the disease-causing isoform (PrP^{Sc}). PrP^C is rich in α-helix and has little β-structure, while PrP^{Sc} has less α-helix and a high amount of β-structure (Fig. 383-1). This α-to-β structural transition in the prion protein (PrP) is the fundamental event underlying prion diseases (Table 383-1).

Four new concepts have emerged from studies of prions: (1) Prions are the only known infectious pathogens that are devoid of nucleic acid; all other infectious agents possess genomes composed of either RNA or DNA that direct the synthesis of their progeny. (2) Prion diseases may be manifest as infectious, genetic, and sporadic disorders; no other group of illnesses with a single etiology presents with such a wide spectrum of clinical manifestations. (3) Prion diseases result from the accumulation of PrP^{Sc}, the conformation of which differs substantially from that of its precursor, PrP^C. (4) PrP^{Sc} can exist in a variety of different conformations, each of which seems to specify a particular disease phenotype. How a specific conformation of a PrP^{Sc} molecule is imparted to PrP^C during prion replication to produce nascent PrP^{Sc} with the same conformation is unknown. Additionally, it is unclear what factors determine where in the CNS a particular PrP^{Sc} molecule will be deposited.

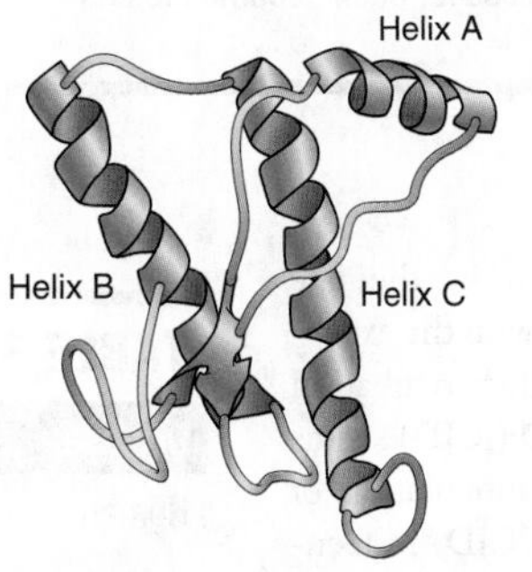

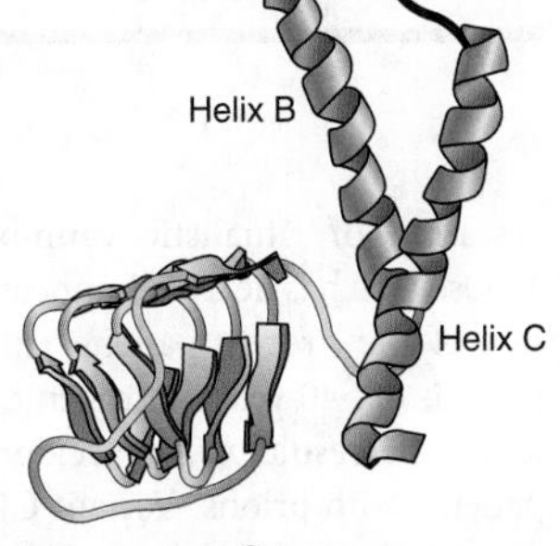

A **Recombinant PrP** ***B*** **PrP^{Sc} model**

Figure 383-1 Structures of prion proteins. *A.* NMR structure of Syrian hamster recombinant (rec) PrP(90–231). Presumably, the structure of the α-helical form of recPrP(90–231) resembles that of PrP^C. recPrP(90–231) is viewed from the interface where PrP^{Sc} is thought to bind to PrP^C. Shown are: α-helices A (residues 144–157), B (172–193), and C (200–227). Flat ribbons depict β-strands S1 (129–131) and S2 (161–163). *(**A,** from SB Prusiner: N Engl J Med 344:1516, 2001; with permission.)* ***B.*** Structural model of PrP^{Sc}. The 90–160 region has been modeled onto a β-helical architecture while the COOH terminal helices B and C are preserved as in PrP^C. *(Image prepared by C. Govaerts.)*

SPECTRUM OF PRION DISEASES

The sporadic form of CJD is the most common prion disorder in humans. Sporadic CJD (sCJD) accounts for ~85% of all cases of human prion disease, while inherited prion diseases account for 10–15% of all cases (Table 383-2). Familial CJD (fCJD), Gerstmann-Sträussler-Scheinker (GSS) disease, and fatal familial insomnia (FFI) are all dominantly inherited prion diseases that are caused by mutations in the PrP gene.

Although infectious prion diseases account for <1% of all cases and infection does not seem to play an important role in the natural history of these illnesses, the transmissibility of prions is an important biologic feature. *Kuru* of the Fore people of New Guinea is thought to have resulted from the consumption of brains from dead relatives during ritualistic cannibalism. With the

TABLE 383-1 Glossary of Prion Terminology

Prion	*Pro*teinaceous *in*fectious particle that lacks nucleic acid. Prions are composed entirely of PrP^{Sc} molecules. They can cause scrapie in sheep and goats, and related neurodegenerative diseases of humans such as Creutzfeldt-Jakob disease (CJD).
PrP^{Sc}	Di*s*ease-*c*ausing isoform of the prion protein. This protein is the only identifiable macromolecule in purified preparations of scrapie prions.
PrP^{C}	*C*ellular isoform of the prion protein. PrP^{C} is the precursor of PrP^{Sc}.
PrP 27-30	A fragment of PrP^{Sc}, generated by truncation of the NH_2-terminus by limited digestion with proteinase K. PrP 27-30 retains prion infectivity and polymerizes into amyloid.
PRNP	PrP gene located on human chromosome 20.
Prion rod	An aggregate of prions composed largely of PrP 27-30 molecules. Created by detergent extraction and limited proteolysis of PrP^{Sc}. Morphologically and histochemically indistinguishable from many amyloids.
PrP amyloid	Amyloid containing PrP in the brains of animals or humans with prion disease; often accumulates as plaques.

cessation of ritualistic cannibalism in the late 1950s, kuru has nearly disappeared, with the exception of a few recent patients exhibiting incubation periods of >40 years. Iatrogenic CJD (iCJD) seems to be the result of the accidental inoculation of patients with prions. Variant CJD (vCJD) in teenagers and young adults in Europe is the result of exposure to tainted beef from cattle with bovine spongiform encephalopathy (BSE).

Six diseases of animals are caused by prions (Table 383-2). Scrapie of sheep and goats is the prototypic prion disease. Mink encephalopathy, BSE, feline spongiform encephalopathy, and exotic ungulate encephalopathy are all thought to occur after the consumption of prion-infected foodstuffs. The BSE epidemic emerged in Britain in the late 1980s and was shown to be due to industrial cannibalism. Whether BSE began as a sporadic case of BSE in a cow or started with scrapie in sheep is unknown. The origin of chronic wasting disease (CWD), a prion disease endemic in deer and elk in regions of North America, is uncertain. In contrast to other prion diseases, CWD is highly communicable. Feces from asymptomatic, infected cervids contain prions that are likely to be responsible for the spread of CWD.

EPIDEMIOLOGY

CJD is found throughout the world. The incidence of sCJD is approximately one case per million population, and thus it accounts for about 1 in every 10,000 deaths. Because sCJD is an age-dependent neurodegenerative disease, its incidence is expected to increase steadily as older segments of populations in developed and developing countries continue to expand. Although many geographic clusters of CJD have been reported, each has been shown to segregate with a PrP gene mutation. Attempts to identify common exposure to some etiologic agent have been unsuccessful for both the sporadic and familial cases. Ingestion of scrapie-infected sheep or goat meat as a cause of CJD in humans has not been demonstrated by epidemiologic studies, although speculation about this potential route of inoculation continues. Of particular interest are deer hunters who develop CJD, because up to 90% of culled deer in some game herds have been shown to harbor CWD prions. Whether prion disease in deer or elk has passed to cows, sheep, or directly to humans remains unknown. Studies with rodents demonstrate that oral infection with prions can occur, but the process is inefficient compared to intracerebral inoculation.

PATHOGENESIS

The human prion diseases were initially classified as neurodegenerative disorders of unknown etiology on the basis of pathologic changes being confined to the CNS. With the transmission of kuru and CJD to apes, investigators began to view these diseases as infectious CNS illnesses caused by slow viruses. Even though the familial nature of a subset of CJD cases was well described, the significance of this observation became more obscure with the transmission of CJD to animals. Eventually the meaning of heritable CJD became clear with the discovery of mutations in the *PRNP* gene of these patients. The prion concept explains how a disease can manifest as a heritable as well as an infectious illness. Moreover, the hallmark of all prion

TABLE 383-2 The Prion Diseases

Disease	Host	Mechanism of Pathogenesis
Human		
Kuru	Fore people	Infection through ritualistic cannibalism
iCJD	Humans	Infection from prion-contaminated hGH, dura mater grafts, etc.
vCJD	Humans	Infection from bovine prions
fCJD	Humans	Germ-line mutations in *PRNP*
GSS	Humans	Germ-line mutations in *PRNP*
FFI	Humans	Germ-line mutation in *PRNP* (D178N, M129)
sCJD	Humans	Somatic mutation or spontaneous conversion of PrP^{C} into PrP^{Sc}?
sFI	Humans	Somatic mutation or spontaneous conversion of PrP^{C} into PrP^{Sc}?
Animal		
Scrapie	Sheep, goats	Infection in genetically susceptible sheep
BSE	Cattle	Infection with prion-contaminated MBM
TME	Mink	Infection with prions from sheep or cattle
CWD	Mule deer, elk	Unknown
FSE	Cats	Infection with prion-contaminated beef
Exotic ungulate encephalopathy	Greater kudu, nyala, or oryx	Infection with prion-contaminated MBM

Abbreviations: BSE, bovine spongiform encephalopathy; CJD, Creutzfeldt-Jakob disease; CWD, chronic wasting disease; fCJD, familial Creutzfeldt-Jakob disease; FFI, fatal familial insomnia; FSE, feline spongiform encephalopathy; GSS, Gerstmann-Sträussler-Scheinker disease; hGH, human growth hormone; iCJD, iatrogenic Creutzfeldt-Jakob disease; MBM, meat and bone meal; sCJD, sporadic Creutzfeldt-Jakob disease; sFI, sporadic fatal insomnia; TME, transmissible mink encephalopathy; vCJD, variant Creutzfeldt-Jakob disease.

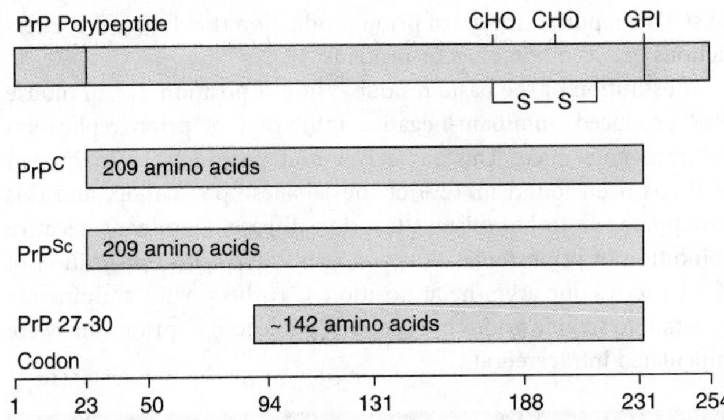

Figure 383-2 Prion protein isoforms. Bar diagram of Syrian hamster PrP, which consists of 254 amino acids. After processing of the NH_2 and COOH termini, both PrP^C and PrP^{Sc} consist of 209 residues. After limited proteolysis, the NH_2 terminus of PrP^{Sc} is truncated to form PrP 27–30 composed of ~142 amino acids.

diseases, whether sporadic, dominantly inherited, or acquired by infection, is that they involve the aberrant metabolism of PrP.

A major feature that distinguishes prions from viruses is the finding that both PrP isoforms are encoded by a chromosomal gene. In humans, the PrP gene is designated *PRNP* and is located on the short arm of chromosome 20. Limited proteolysis of PrP^{Sc} produces a smaller, protease-resistant molecule of ~142 amino acids designated PrP 27-30; PrP^C is completely hydrolyzed under the same conditions (Fig. 383-2). In the presence of detergent, PrP 27-30 polymerizes into amyloid. Prion rods formed by limited proteolysis and detergent extraction are indistinguishable from the filaments that aggregate to form PrP amyloid plaques in the CNS. Both the rods and the PrP amyloid filaments found in brain tissue exhibit similar ultrastructural morphology and green-gold birefringence after staining with Congo red dye.

Prion strains

The existence of prion strains raised the question of how heritable biologic information can be enciphered in a molecule other than nucleic acid. Various strains of prions have been defined by incubation times and the distribution of neuronal vacuolation. Subsequently, the patterns of PrP^{Sc} deposition were found to correlate with vacuolation profiles, and these patterns were also used to characterize prion strains.

Persuasive evidence that strain-specific information is enciphered in the tertiary structure of PrP^{Sc} comes from transmission of two different inherited human prion diseases to mice expressing a chimeric human-mouse PrP transgene. In FFI, the protease-resistant fragment of PrP^{Sc} after deglycosylation has a molecular mass of 19 kDa, whereas in fCJD and most sporadic prion diseases, it is 21 kDa (Table 383-3). This difference in molecular mass was shown to be due to different sites of proteolytic cleavage at the NH_2 termini of the two human PrP^{Sc} molecules, reflecting different tertiary structures. These distinct conformations were not unexpected because the amino acid sequences of the PrPs differ.

Extracts from the brains of patients with FFI transmitted disease into mice expressing a chimeric human-mouse PrP transgene and induced formation of the 19-kDa PrP^{Sc}, whereas brain extracts from fCJD and sCJD patients produced the 21-kDa PrP^{Sc} in mice expressing the same transgene. On second passage, these differences were maintained, demonstrating that chimeric PrP^{Sc} can exist in two different conformations based on the sizes of the protease-resistant fragments, even though the amino acid sequence of PrP^{Sc} is invariant.

This analysis was extended when patients with sporadic fatal insomnia (sFI) were identified. Although they did not carry a *PRNP* gene mutation, the patients demonstrated a clinical and pathologic phenotype that was indistinguishable from that of patients with FFI. Furthermore, 19-kDa PrP^{Sc} was found in their brains, and on passage of prion disease to mice expressing a chimeric human-mouse PrP transgene, 19-kDa PrP^{Sc} was also found. These findings indicate that the disease phenotype is dictated by the conformation of PrP^{Sc} and not the amino acid sequence. PrP^{Sc} acts as a template for the conversion of PrP^C into nascent PrP^{Sc}. On the passage of prions into mice expressing a chimeric hamster-mouse PrP transgene, a change in the conformation of PrP^{Sc} was accompanied by the emergence of a new strain of prions.

Many new strains of prions were generated using recombinant (rec) PrP produced in bacteria; recPrP was polymerized into amyloid fibrils and inoculated into transgenic mice expressing high levels of wild-type mouse PrP^C; about 500 days later, the mice died of prion disease. The incubation times of the "synthetic prions" in mice were dependent on the conditions used for polymerization of the amyloid fibrils. Highly stable amyloids gave rise to stable prions with long incubation times; low-stability amyloids led to prions with short incubation times. Amyloids of intermediate stability gave rise to prions with intermediate stabilities and intermediate incubation times. Such findings are consistent with earlier studies showing that the incubation times of synthetic and naturally occurring prions are directly proportional to the stability of the prion.

Species barrier

Studies on the role of the primary and tertiary structures of PrP in the transmission of prion disease have given new insights into the pathogenesis of these maladies. The amino acid sequence of PrP encodes the species of the prion, and the prion derives its PrP^{Sc} sequence from the last mammal in which it was passaged. While the primary structure of PrP is likely to be the most important or even sole determinant of the tertiary structure of PrP^C, PrP^{Sc} seems to function as a template in determining the tertiary structure of nascent PrP^{Sc} molecules as they are formed from PrP^C. In turn, prion diversity appears to be enciphered in the conformation of

TABLE 383-3 Distinct Prion Strains Generated in Humans With Inherited Prion Diseases and Transmitted to Transgenic Mice[a]

Inoculum	Host Species	Host PrP Genotype	Incubation Time [days ± SEM] (n/n_0)	PrP^{Sc} (kDa)
None	Human	FFI(D178N, M129)		19
FFI	Mouse	Tg(MHu2M)	206 ± 7 (7/7)	19
FFI → Tg(MHu2M)	Mouse	Tg(MHu2M)	136 ± 1 (6/6)	19
None	Human	fCJD(E200K)		21
fCJD	Mouse	Tg(MHu2M)	170 ± 2 (10/10)	21
fCJD → Tg(MHu2M)	Mouse	Tg(MHu2M)	167 ± 3 (15/15)	21

[a]Tg(MHu2M) mice express a chimeric mouse-human PrP gene.

Notes: Clinicopathologic phenotype is determined by the conformation of PrP^{Sc} in accord with the results of the transmission of human prions from patients with FFI to transgenic mice. fCJD, familial Creutzfeldt-Jakob disease; FFI, fatal familial insomnia.

PrP^{Sc}, and thus prion strains seem to represent different conformers of PrP^{Sc}.

In general, transmission of prion disease from one species to another is inefficient, in that not all intracerebrally inoculated animals develop disease, and those that fall ill do so only after long incubation times that can approach the natural life span of the animal. This "species barrier" to transmission is correlated with the degree of similarity between the amino acid sequences of PrP^{C} in the inoculated host and of PrP^{Sc} in the prion inoculum. The importance of sequence similarity between the host and donor PrP argues that PrP^{C} directly interacts with PrP^{Sc} in the prion conversion process.

SPORADIC AND INHERITED PRION DISEASES

Several different scenarios might explain the initiation of sporadic prion disease: (1) A somatic mutation may be the cause and thus follow a path similar to that for germ-line mutations in inherited disease. In this situation, the mutant PrP^{Sc} must be capable of targeting wild-type PrP^{C}, a process known to be possible for some mutations but less likely for others. (2) The activation energy barrier separating wild-type PrP^{C} from PrP^{Sc} could be crossed on rare occasions when viewed in the context of a population. Most individuals would be spared while presentations in the elderly with an incidence of ~1 per million would be seen. (3) PrP^{Sc} may be present at low levels in some normal cells, where it performs some important, as yet unknown, function. The level of PrP^{Sc} in such cells is hypothesized to be sufficiently low as to be not detected by routine bioassay. In some altered metabolic states, the cellular mechanisms for clearing PrP^{Sc} might become compromised and the rate of PrP^{Sc} formation would then begin to exceed the capacity of the cell to clear it. The third possible mechanism is attractive since it suggests PrP^{Sc} is not simply a misfolded protein, as proposed for the first and second mechanisms, but that it is an alternatively folded molecule with a function. Moreover, the multitude of conformational states that PrP^{Sc} can adopt, as described above, raises the possibility that PrP^{Sc} or another prion-like protein might function in a process like short-term memory where information storage occurs in the absence of new protein synthesis.

More than 40 different mutations resulting in nonconservative substitutions in the human *PRNP* gene have been found to segregate with inherited human prion diseases. Missense mutations and expansions in the octapeptide repeat region of the gene are responsible for familial forms of prion disease. Five different mutations of the *PRNP* gene have been linked genetically to heritable prion disease.

Although phenotypes may vary dramatically within families, specific phenotypes tend to be observed with certain mutations. A clinical phenotype indistinguishable from typical sCJD is usually seen with substitutions at codons 180, 183, 200, 208, 210, and 232. Substitutions at codons 102, 105, 117, 198, and 217 are associated with the GSS variant of prion disease. The normal human PrP sequence contains five repeats of an eight-amino-acid sequence. Insertions from two to nine extra octarepeats frequently cause variable phenotypes ranging from a condition indistinguishable from sCJD to a slowly progressive dementing illness of many years' duration to an early-age-of-onset disorder that is similar to Alzheimer's disease. A mutation at codon 178 resulting in substitution of asparagine for aspartic acid produces FFI if a methionine is encoded at the polymorphic 129 residue on the same allele. Typical CJD is seen if the D178N mutation occurs with a valine encoded at position 129 of the same allele.

HUMAN PRNP GENE POLYMORPHISMS

Polymorphisms influence the susceptibility to sporadic, inherited, and infectious forms of prion disease. The methionine/valine polymorphism at position 129 not only modulates the age of onset of some inherited prion diseases but can also determine the clinical phenotype. The finding that homozygosity at codon 129 predisposes to sCJD supports a model of prion production that favors PrP interactions between homologous proteins.

Substitution of the basic residue lysine at position 218 in mouse PrP produced dominant-negative inhibition of prion replication in transgenic mice. This same lysine at position 219 in human PrP has been found in 12% of the Japanese population, and this group appears to be resistant to prion disease. Dominant-negative inhibition of prion replication was also found with substitution of the basic residue arginine at position 171; sheep with arginine are resistant to scrapie prions but are susceptible to BSE prions that were inoculated intracerebrally.

INFECTIOUS PRION DISEASES

IATROGENIC CJD

Accidental transmission of CJD to humans appears to have occurred with corneal transplantation, contaminated electroencephalogram (EEG) electrode implantation, and surgical procedures. Corneas from donors with inapparent CJD have been transplanted to apparently healthy recipients who developed CJD after prolonged incubation periods. The same improperly decontaminated EEG electrodes that caused CJD in two young patients with intractable epilepsy caused CJD in a chimpanzee 18 months after their experimental implantation.

Surgical procedures may have resulted in accidental inoculation of patients with prions, presumably because some instrument or apparatus in the operating theater became contaminated when a CJD patient underwent surgery. Although the epidemiology of these studies is highly suggestive, no proof for such episodes exists.

Dura mater grafts

More than 160 cases of CJD after implantation of dura mater grafts have been recorded. All of the grafts were thought to have been acquired from a single manufacturer whose preparative procedures were inadequate to inactivate human prions. One case of CJD occurred after repair of an eardrum perforation with a pericardium graft.

Human growth hormone and pituitary gonadotropin therapy

The transmission of CJD prions from contaminated human growth hormone (hGH) preparations derived from human pituitaries has been responsible for fatal cerebellar disorders with dementia in >180 patients ranging in age from 10 to 41 years. These patients received injections of hGH every 2–4 days for 4–12 years. If it is thought that these patients developed CJD from injections of prion-contaminated hGH preparations, the possible incubation periods range from 4 to 30 years. Only recombinant hGH is now used therapeutically so that possible contamination with prions is no longer an issue. Four cases of CJD have occurred in women receiving human pituitary gonadotropin.

VARIANT CJD

The restricted geographic occurrence and chronology of vCJD raised the possibility that BSE prions had been transmitted to humans through the consumption of tainted beef. More than 190 cases of vCJD have occurred, with >90% of these in Britain. vCJD has also been reported in people either living in or originating from France, Ireland, Italy, Netherlands, Portugal, Spain, Saudi Arabia, United States, Canada, and Japan.

The steady decline in the number of vCJD cases over the past decade argues that there will not be a prion disease epidemic in Europe, similar to those seen for BSE and kuru. What is certain is that prion-tainted meat should be prevented from entering the human food supply.

The most compelling evidence that vCJD is caused by BSE prions was obtained from experiments in mice expressing the bovine PrP transgene. Both BSE and vCJD prions were efficiently transmitted to these transgenic mice and with similar incubation periods. In contrast to sCJD prions, vCJD prions did not transmit disease efficiently to mice expressing a chimeric human-mouse PrP transgene. Earlier studies with nontransgenic mice suggested that vCJD and BSE might be derived from the same source because both inocula transmitted disease with similar but very long incubation periods.

Attempts to determine the origin of BSE and vCJD prions have relied on passaging studies in mice, some of which are described above, as well as studies of the conformation and glycosylation of PrP^{Sc}. One scenario suggests that a particular conformation of bovine PrP^{Sc} was selected for heat resistance during the rendering process and was then reselected multiple times as cattle infected by ingesting prion-contaminated meat and bone meal (MBM) were slaughtered and their offal rendered into more MBM.

NEUROPATHOLOGY

Frequently the brains of patients with CJD have no recognizable abnormalities on gross examination. Patients who survive for several years have variable degrees of cerebral atrophy.

On light microscopy, the pathologic hallmarks of CJD are spongiform degeneration and astrocytic gliosis. The lack of an inflammatory response in CJD and other prion diseases is an important pathologic feature of these degenerative disorders. Spongiform degeneration is characterized by many 1- to 5-μm vacuoles in the neuropil between nerve cell bodies. Generally the spongiform changes occur in the cerebral cortex, putamen, caudate nucleus, thalamus, and molecular layer of the cerebellum. Astrocytic gliosis is a constant but nonspecific feature of prion diseases. Widespread proliferation of fibrous astrocytes is found throughout the gray matter of brains infected with CJD prions. Astrocytic processes filled with glial filaments form extensive networks.

Amyloid plaques have been found in ~10% of CJD cases. Purified CJD prions from humans and animals exhibit the ultrastructural and histochemical characteristics of amyloid when treated with detergents during limited proteolysis. In first passage from some human Japanese CJD cases, amyloid plaques have been found in mouse brains. These plaques stain with antibodies raised against PrP.

The amyloid plaques of GSS disease are morphologically distinct from those seen in kuru or scrapie. GSS plaques consist of a central dense core of amyloid surrounded by smaller globules of amyloid. Ultrastructurally, they consist of a radiating fibrillar network of amyloid fibrils, with scant or no neuritic degeneration. The plaques can be distributed throughout the brain but are most frequently found in the cerebellum. They are often located adjacent to blood vessels. Congophilic angiopathy has been noted in some cases of GSS disease.

In vCJD, a characteristic feature is the presence of "florid plaques." These are composed of a central core of PrP amyloid, surrounded by vacuoles in a pattern suggesting petals on a flower.

CLINICAL FEATURES

Nonspecific prodromal symptoms occur in about a third of patients with CJD and may include fatigue, sleep disturbance, weight loss, headache, anxiety, vertigo, malaise, and ill-defined pain. Most patients with CJD present with deficits in higher cortical function. These deficits almost always progress over weeks or months to a state of profound dementia characterized by memory loss, impaired judgment, and a decline in virtually all aspects of intellectual function. A few patients present with either visual impairment or cerebellar gait and coordination deficits. Frequently the cerebellar deficits are rapidly followed by progressive dementia. Visual problems often begin with blurred vision and diminished acuity, rapidly followed by dementia.

Other symptoms and signs include extrapyramidal dysfunction manifested as rigidity, masklike facies, or (less commonly) choreoathetoid movements; pyramidal signs (usually mild); seizures (usually major motor) and, less commonly, hypoesthesia; supranuclear gaze palsy; optic atrophy; and vegetative signs such as changes in weight, temperature, sweating, or menstruation.

Myoclonus

Most patients (~90%) with CJD exhibit myoclonus that appears at various times throughout the illness. Unlike other involuntary movements, myoclonus persists during sleep. Startle myoclonus elicited by loud sounds or bright lights is frequent. It is important to stress that myoclonus is neither specific nor confined to CJD and tends to occur later in the course of CJD. Dementia with myoclonus can also be due to Alzheimer's disease (AD) (Chap. 371), dementia with Lewy bodies (Chap. 371), corticobasal degeneration (Chap. 371), cryptococcal encephalitis (Chap. 202), or the myoclonic epilepsy disorder Unverricht-Lundborg disease (Chap. 369).

Clinical course

In documented cases of accidental transmission of CJD to humans, an incubation period of 1.5–2 years preceded the development of clinical disease. In other cases, incubation periods of up to 40 years have been suggested. Most patients with CJD live 6–12 months after the onset of clinical signs and symptoms, whereas some live for up to 5 years.

DIAGNOSIS

The constellation of dementia, myoclonus, and periodic electrical bursts in an afebrile 60-year-old patient generally indicates CJD. Clinical abnormalities in CJD are confined to the CNS. Fever, elevated sedimentation rate, leukocytosis in blood, or a pleocytosis in cerebrospinal fluid (CSF) should alert the physician to another etiology to explain the patient's CNS dysfunction.

Variations in the typical course appear in inherited and transmitted forms of the disease. fCJD has an earlier mean age of onset than sCJD. In GSS disease, ataxia is usually a prominent and presenting feature, with dementia occurring late in the disease course. GSS disease typically presents earlier than CJD (mean age 43 years) and is typically more slowly progressive than CJD; death usually occurs within 5 years of onset. FFI is characterized by insomnia and dysautonomia; dementia occurs only in the terminal phase of the illness. Rare sporadic cases have been identified. vCJD has an unusual clinical course, with a prominent psychiatric prodrome that may include visual hallucinations and early ataxia, while frank dementia is usually a late sign of vCJD.

DIFFERENTIAL DIAGNOSIS

Many conditions may mimic CJD superficially. Dementia with Lewy bodies (Chap. 371) is the most common disorder to be mistaken for CJD. It can present in a subacute fashion with delirium, myoclonus, and extrapyramidal features. Other neurodegenerative disorders (Chap. 371) to consider include AD, frontotemporal dementia, corticobasal degeneration, progressive supranuclear palsy, ceroid lipofuscinosis, and myoclonic epilepsy with Lafora bodies (Chap. 369). The absence of abnormalities on diffusion-weighted and fluid-attenuated inversion recovery (FLAIR) MRI will almost always distinguish these dementing conditions from CJD.

Hashimoto's encephalopathy, which presents as a subacute progressive encephalopathy with myoclonus and periodic triphasic complexes on the EEG, should be excluded in every case of suspected CJD. It is diagnosed by the finding of high titers of antithyroglobulin or antithyroid peroxidase (antimicrosomal) antibodies in the blood and improves with glucocorticoid therapy. Unlike CJD, fluctuations in severity typically occur in Hashimoto's encephalopathy.

Intracranial vasculitides (Chap. 326) may produce nearly all of the symptoms and signs associated with CJD, sometimes without systemic abnormalities. Myoclonus is exceptional with cerebral vasculitis, but focal seizures may confuse the picture. Prominent headache, absence of myoclonus, stepwise change in deficits, abnormal CSF, and focal white matter changes on MRI or angiographic abnormalities all favor vasculitis.

Paraneoplastic conditions, particularly limbic encephalitis and cortical encephalitis, can also mimic CJD. In many of these patients, dementia appears prior to the diagnosis of a tumor, and in some, no tumor is ever found. Detection of the paraneoplastic antibodies is often the only way to distinguish these cases from CJD.

Other diseases that can simulate CJD include neurosyphilis (Chap. 169), AIDS dementia complex (Chap. 189), progressive multifocal leukoencephalopathy (Chap. 381), subacute sclerosing panencephalitis, progressive rubella panencephalitis, herpes simplex encephalitis (Chap. 381), diffuse intracranial tumor (gliomatosis cerebri; Chap. 379), anoxic encephalopathy, dialysis dementia, uremia, hepatic encephalopathy, voltage-gated potassium channel (VGkC) autoimmune encephalopathy and lithium or bismuth intoxication.

■ LABORATORY TESTS

The only specific diagnostic tests for CJD and other human prion diseases measure PrP^{Sc}. The most widely used method involves limited proteolysis that generates PrP 27-30, which is detected by immunoassay after denaturation. The conformation-dependent immunoassay (CDI) is based on immunoreactive epitopes that are exposed in PrP^{C} but buried in PrP^{Sc}. In humans, the diagnosis of CJD can be established by brain biopsy if PrP^{Sc} is detected. If no attempt is made to measure PrP^{Sc}, but the constellation of pathologic changes frequently found in CJD is seen in a brain biopsy, then the diagnosis is reasonably secure (see "Neuropathology," above). The high sensitivity and specificity of cortical ribboning and basal ganglia hyperintensity on FLAIR and diffusion-weighted MRI for the diagnosis of CJD have greatly diminished the need for brain biopsy in patients with suspected CJD. Because PrP^{Sc} is not uniformly distributed throughout the CNS, the apparent absence of PrP^{Sc} in a limited sample such as a biopsy does not rule out prion disease. At autopsy, sufficient brain samples should be taken for both PrP^{Sc} immunoassay, preferably by CDI, and immunohistochemistry of tissue sections.

To establish the diagnosis of either sCJD or familial prion disease, sequencing the *PRNP* gene must be performed. Finding the wild-type *PRNP* gene sequence permits the diagnosis of sCJD if there is no history to suggest infection from an exogenous source of prions. The identification of a mutation in the *PRNP* gene sequence that encodes a nonconservative amino acid substitution argues for familial prion disease.

CT may be normal or show cortical atrophy. MRI is valuable for distinguishing sCJD from most other conditions. On FLAIR sequences and diffusion-weighted imaging, ~90% of patients show increased intensity in the basal ganglia and cortical ribboning (Fig. 383-3). This pattern is not seen with other neurodegenerative disorders but has been seen infrequently with viral encephalitis, paraneoplastic syndromes, or seizures. When the typical MRI pattern is present, in the proper clinical setting, diagnosis is facilitated. However, some cases of sCJD do not show this typical pattern, and other early diagnostic approaches are still needed.

CSF is nearly always normal but may show protein elevation and, rarely, mild pleocytosis. Although the stress protein 14-3-3 is elevated in the CSF of some patients with CJD, similar elevations of 14-3-3 are found in patients with other disorders; thus this elevation is not specific. Similarly, elevations of CSF neuron-specific enolase and tau occur in CJD but lack specificity for diagnosis.

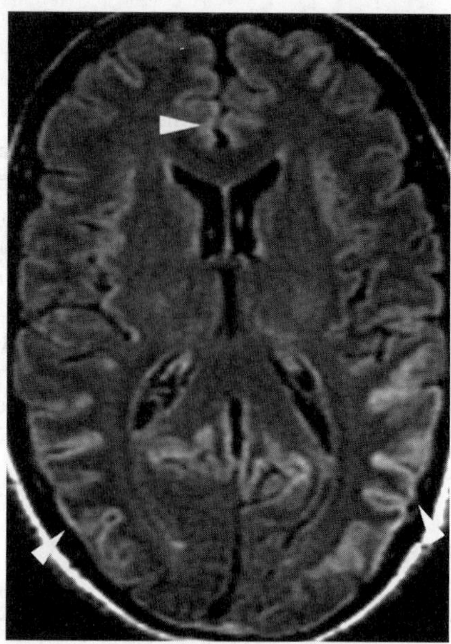

Figure 383-3 T2-weighted (FLAIR) MRI showing hyperintensity in the cortex in a patient with sporadic CJD. This so-called "cortical ribboning" along with increased intensity in the basal ganglia on T2 or diffusion-weighted imaging can aid in the diagnosis of CJD.

The EEG is often useful in the diagnosis of CJD, although only about 60% of individuals show the typical pattern. During the early phase of CJD, the EEG is usually normal or shows only scattered theta activity. In most advanced cases, repetitive, high-voltage, triphasic, and polyphasic sharp discharges are seen, but in many cases their presence is transient. The presence of these stereotyped periodic bursts of <200 ms duration, occurring every 1–2 s, makes the diagnosis of CJD very likely. These discharges are frequently but not always symmetric; there may be a one-sided predominance in amplitude. As CJD progresses, normal background rhythms become fragmentary and slower.

■ CARE OF CJD PATIENTS

Although CJD should not be considered either contagious or communicable, it is transmissible. The risk of accidental inoculation by aerosols is very small; nonetheless, procedures producing aerosols should be performed in certified biosafety cabinets. Biosafety level 2 practices, containment equipment, and facilities are recommended by the Centers for Disease Control and Prevention and the National Institutes of Health. The primary problem in caring for patients with CJD is the inadvertent infection of health care workers by needle and stab wounds. Electroencephalographic and electromyographic needles should not be reused after studies on patients with CJD have been performed.

There is no reason for pathologists or other morgue employees to resist performing autopsies on patients whose clinical diagnosis was CJD. Standard microbiologic practices outlined here, along with specific recommendations for decontamination, seem to be adequate precautions for the care of patients with CJD and the handling of infected specimens.

■ DECONTAMINATION OF CJD PRIONS

Prions are extremely resistant to common inactivation procedures, and there is some disagreement about the optimal conditions for sterilization. Some investigators recommend treating CJD-contaminated materials once with 1 *N* NaOH at room temperature, but we believe this procedure may be inadequate for sterilization. Autoclaving at 134°C for 5 h or treatment with 2 *N* NaOH for several hours is recommended for sterilization of prions. The term *sterilization* implies complete destruction of prions; any residual infectivity can be hazardous. Recent studies show that sCJD prions bound to stainless steel surfaces are resistant to inactivation by autoclaving at 134°C for 2 h; exposure of bound prions to an acidic detergent solution prior to autoclaving rendered prions susceptible to inactivation.

PREVENTION AND THERAPEUTICS

There is no known effective therapy for preventing or treating CJD. The finding that phenothiazines and acridines inhibit PrP^{Sc} formation in cultured cells led to clinical studies of quinacrine in CJD patients. Unfortunately, quinacrine failed to slow the rate of cognitive decline in CJD, possibly because therapeutic concentrations in the brain were not achieved. Although inhibition of the P-glycoprotein (Pgp) transport system resulted in substantially increased quinacrine levels in the brains of mice, the prion incubation times were not extended by treatment with the drug. Whether such an approach can be used to treat CJD remains to be established.

Like the acridines, anti-PrP antibodies have been shown to eliminate PrP^{Sc} from cultured cells. Additionally, such antibodies in mice, either administered by injection or produced from a transgene, have been shown to prevent prion disease when prions are introduced by a peripheral route, such as intraperitoneal inoculation. Unfortunately, the antibodies were ineffective in mice inoculated intracerebrally with prions. Several drugs, including pentosan polysulfate as well as porphyrin and phenylhydrazine derivatives, delay the onset of disease in animals inoculated intracerebrally with prions if the drugs are given intracerebrally beginning soon after inoculation.

PRION-LIKE PROTEINS CAUSING OTHER NEURODEGENERATIVE DISEASES

There is mounting evidence that prion-like changes in protein conformation underlie Alzheimer's (AD), Parkinson's (PD) and Huntington's (HD) diseases as well as the frontotemporal dementias (FTDs) and amyotrophic lateral sclerosis (ALS). Experimental studies have shown that transgenic mice expressing mutant amyloid precursor protein (APP) develop amyloid plaques containing fibrils composed of the amyloid beta (Aβ) peptide about a year after inoculation with extracts prepared from the brains of patients with AD. Mutant tau aggregates in transgenic mice and cultured cells can trigger the aggregation of wild-type tau into fibrils that resemble those in neurofibrillary tangles and Pick bodies that have been found in AD, FTDs, Pick's disease, and some cases of post-traumatic head injury. In patients with advanced PD who received grafts of fetal substantia nigral neurons, Lewy bodies containing β-sheet–rich α-synuclein have been identified in grafted cells about 10 years after transplantation. These findings argue for the axonal transport of misfolded α-synuclein crossing into grafted neurons, where it initiates aggregation of nascent α-synuclein into fibrils that coalesce to form Lewy bodies.

Taken together, a wealth of data argues that all neurodegenerative diseases are caused by proteins that undergo aberrant processing, which results in their assembly into amyloid fibrils. In each degenerative brain disease, prion-like protein processing is responsible for the accumulation of a particular protein in an altered state that leads to neurodegeneration. Interestingly, once these aberrant, prion-like proteins have polymerized into amyloid fibrils, they are probably inert. Amyloid plaques containing PrP^{Sc} are a nonobligatory feature of prion disease in humans and animals. Furthermore, amyloid plaques in AD do not correlate with the level of dementia; however, the level of soluble (oligomeric) Aβ peptide does correlate with memory loss and other intellectual deficits.

FURTHER READINGS

AGUZZI A et al: Molecular mechanisms of prion pathogenesis. Annu Rev Pathol 3:11, 2008

CAUGEY B et al: Getting a grip on prions: Oligomers, amyloids, and pathological membrane interactions. Annu Rev Biochem. 78:177, 2009

COLBY DW et al: Prions. Cold Spring Harb Perspect Biol 3:a006833, 2011

JUCKER M: The benefits and limitations of animal models for translation research in neurodegenerative diseases. Nat Med 16:1210, 2010

OLANOW CW et al: Is Parkinson's disease a prion disorder? Proc Natl Acad Sci USA 106:12571, 2009

PRUSINER SB: Prions, in *Fields Virology*, DM Knipe et al (eds). Philadelphia, Lippincott Willams & Wilkins, 2007, pp 3059–3092

CHAPTER 384 Peripheral Neuropathy

Anthony A. Amato
Richard J. Barohn

Peripheral nerves are composed of sensory, motor, and autonomic elements. Diseases can affect the cell body of a neuron or its peripheral processes, namely the axons or the encasing myelin sheaths. Most peripheral nerves are mixed and contain sensory and motor as well as autonomic fibers. Nerves can be subdivided into three major classes: large myelinated, small myelinated, and small unmyelinated. Motor axons are usually large myelinated fibers that conduct rapidly (approximately 50 m/s). Sensory fibers may be any of the three types. Large-diameter sensory fibers conduct proprioception and vibratory sensation to the brain, while the smaller-diameter myelinated and unmyelinated fibers transmit pain and temperature sensation. Autonomic nerves are also small in diameter. Thus, peripheral neuropathies can impair sensory, motor, or autonomic function, either singly or in combination. Peripheral neuropathies are further classified into those that primarily affect the cell body (e.g., neuronopathy or ganglionopathy), myelin (myelinopathy), and the axon (axonopathy). These different classes of peripheral neuropathies have distinct clinical and electrophysiologic features. This chapter discusses the clinical approach to a patient suspected of having a peripheral neuropathy, as well as specific neuropathies, including hereditary and acquired neuropathies. The inflammatory neuropathies are discussed in Chap. 385.

GENERAL APPROACH

In approaching a patient with a neuropathy, the clinician has three main goals: (1) identify where the lesion is, (2) identify the cause, and (3) determine the proper treatment. The first goal is accomplished by obtaining a thorough history, neurologic examination, and electrodiagnostic and other laboratory studies (Fig. 384-1). While gathering this information, seven key questions are asked (Table 384-1), the answers to which can usually identify the category of pathology that is present (Table 384-2). Despite an extensive evaluation, in approximately half of patients no etiology is ever found; these patients typically have a predominately sensory polyneuropathy and have been labeled as having idiopathic or cryptogenic sensory polyneuropathy (CSPN).

INFORMATION FROM THE HISTORY AND PHYSICAL EXAMINATION: SEVEN KEY QUESTIONS (TABLE 384-1)

1. What systems are involved?

It is important to determine if the patient's symptoms and signs are motor, sensory, autonomic, or a combination of these. If the patient has only weakness without any evidence of sensory or autonomic dysfunction, a motor neuropathy, neuromuscular junction abnormality, or myopathy should be considered. Some peripheral neuropathies are associated with significant autonomic nervous system dysfunction. Symptoms of autonomic involvement include fainting spells or orthostatic lightheadedness; heat intolerance; or any bowel, bladder, or sexual dysfunction (Chap. 375). There will typically be an orthostatic fall in blood pressure without an appropriate increase in heart rate. Autonomic dysfunction in the absence of diabetes should alert the clinician to the possibility of amyloid polyneuropathy. Rarely, a pandysautonomic syndrome can be the only manifestation of a peripheral neuropathy without other motor or sensory findings. The majority of neuropathies are predominantly sensory in nature.

2. What is the distribution of weakness?

Delineating the pattern of weakness, if present, is essential for diagnosis, and in this regard two additional questions should be answered: (1) Does the weakness only involve the distal extremity or is it both proximal and distal? and (2) Is the weakness focal and asymmetric or is it symmetric? Symmetric proximal and distal weakness is the hallmark of acquired immune demyelinating polyneuropathies, both the acute form [acute inflammatory demyelinating polyneuropathy (AIDP) also known as Guillain-Barré syndrome (GBS)] and the chronic form [chronic inflammatory demyelinating polyneuropathy (CIDP)]. The importance of finding symmetric proximal and distal weakness in a patient who presents with both motor and sensory symptoms cannot be overemphasized because this identifies the important subset of patients who may have a treatable acquired demyelinating neuropathic disorder (i.e., AIDP or CIDP).

Findings of an asymmetric or multifocal pattern of weakness narrows the differential diagnosis. Some neuropathic disorders may present with unilateral extremity weakness. In the absence of sensory symptoms and signs, such weakness evolving over weeks or months would be worrisome for motor neuron disease [e.g., amyotrophic lateral sclerosis (ALS)], but it would be important to exclude multifocal motor neuropathy that may be treatable (Chap. 374). In a patient presenting with asymmetric subacute or acute sensory and motor symptoms and signs, radiculopathies, plexopathies, compressive mononeuropathies, or multiple mononeuropathies (e.g., mononeuropathy multiplex) must be considered.

3. What is the nature of the sensory involvement?

The patient may have loss of sensation (numbness), altered sensation to touch (hyperpathia or allodynia), or uncomfortable spontaneous sensations (tingling, burning, or aching) (Chap. 23). Neuropathic pain can be burning, dull, and poorly localized (protopathic pain), presumably transmitted by polymodal C nociceptor fibers, or sharp and lancinating (epicritic pain), relayed by A-delta fibers. If pain and temperature perception are lost, while vibratory and position sense are preserved along with muscle strength, deep tendon reflexes, and normal nerve conduction studies, a small-fiber neuropathy is likely. This is important, as the most likely cause of small-fiber neuropathies, when one is identified, is diabetes mellitus or glucose intolerance. Amyloid neuropathy should be considered as well in such cases, but most of these small-fiber neuropathies remain idiopathic in nature despite extensive evaluation.

Severe proprioceptive loss also narrows the differential diagnosis. Affected patients will note imbalance, especially in the dark. A

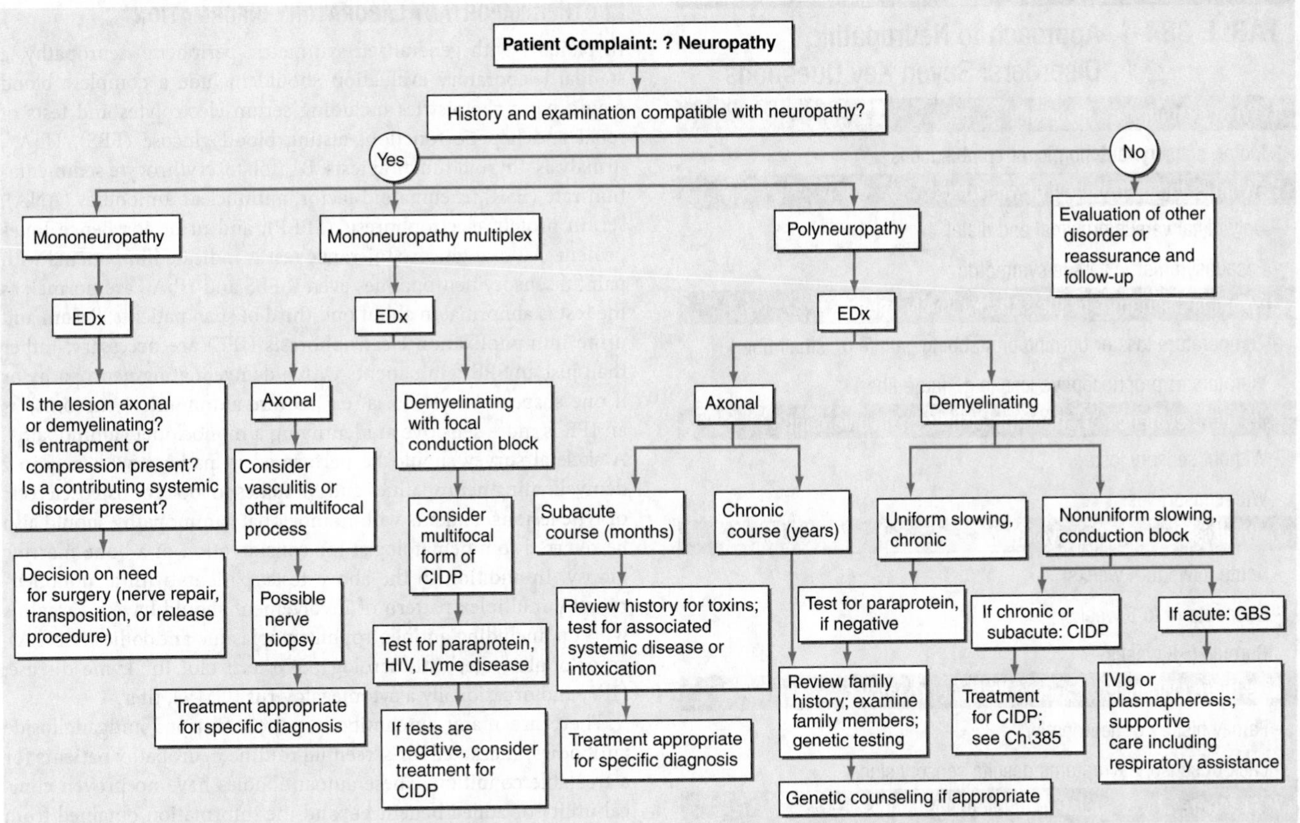

Figure 384-1 Approach to the evaluation of peripheral neuropathies. CIDP, chronic inflammatory demyelinating polyradiculoneuropathy; GBS, Guillain-Barré syndrome.

neurologic examination revealing a dramatic loss of proprioception with vibration loss and normal strength should alert the clinician to consider a sensory neuronopathy/ganglionopathy (Table 384-2, Pattern 8). In particular, if this loss is asymmetric or affects the arms more than the legs, this pattern suggests a non-length-dependent process as seen in sensory neuronopathies.

4. Is there evidence of upper motor neuron involvement?

If the patient presents with symmetric distal sensory symptoms and signs suggestive of a distal sensory neuropathy, but there is additional evidence of symmetric upper motor neuron involvement (Chap. 22), the physician should consider a disorder such as combined system degeneration with neuropathy. The most common cause for this pattern is vitamin B_{12} deficiency, but other causes of combined system degeneration with neuropathy should be considered (e.g., copper deficiency, HIV infection, severe hepatic disease, adrenomyeloneuropathy).

5. What is the temporal evolution?

It is important to determine the onset, duration, and evolution of symptoms and signs. Does the disease have an acute (days to 4 weeks), subacute (4–8 weeks), or chronic (>8 weeks) course? Is the course monophasic, progressive, or relapsing? Most neuropathies are insidious and slowly progressive in nature. Neuropathies with acute and subacute presentations include GBS, vasculitis, and radiculopathies related to diabetes or Lyme disease. A relapsing course can be present in CIDP and porphyria.

6. Is there evidence for a hereditary neuropathy?

In patients with slowly progressive distal weakness over many years with very little in the way of sensory symptoms yet with significant sensory deficits on clinical examination, the clinician should consider a hereditary neuropathy (e.g., Charcot-Marie-Tooth disease or CMT). On examination, the feet may show arch and toe abnormalities (high or flat arches, hammertoes); scoliosis may be present. In suspected cases, it may be necessary to perform both neurologic and electrophysiologic studies on family members in addition to the patient.

7. Does the patient have any other medical conditions?

It is important to inquire about associated medical conditions (e.g., diabetes mellitus, systemic lupus erythematosus); preceding or concurrent infections (e.g. diarrheal illness preceding GBS); surgeries (e.g., gastric bypass and nutritional neuropathies); medications (toxic neuropathy); including over-the-counter vitamin preparations (B_6); alcohol; dietary habits; and use of dentures (e.g., fixatives contain zinc that can lead to copper deficiency).

PATTERN RECOGNITION APPROACH TO NEUROPATHIC DISORDERS

Based upon the answers to the seven key questions, neuropathic disorders can be classified into several patterns based on the distribution or pattern of sensory, motor, and autonomic involvement (Table 384-2). Each pattern has a limited differential diagnosis. A final diagnosis is established by utilizing other clues such as the temporal course, presence of other disease states, family history, and information from laboratory studies.

ELECTRODIAGNOSTIC STUDIES

The electrodiagnostic (EDx) evaluation of patients with a suspected peripheral neuropathy consists of nerve conduction studies (NCS) and needle electromyography (EMG). In addition, studies of autonomic function can be valuable. The electrophysiologic data provides additional information about the distribution of the neuropathy that will support or refute the findings from the history and physical

TABLE 384-1 Approach to Neuropathic Disorders: Seven Key Questions

1. What systems are involved?
- Motor, sensory, autonomic, or combinations
2. What is the distribution of weakness?
- Only distal versus proximal and distal
- Focal/asymmetric versus symmetric
3. What is the nature of the sensory involvement?
- Temperature loss or burning or stabbing pain (e.g., small fiber)
- Vibratory or proprioceptive loss (e.g., large fiber)
4. Is there evidence of upper motor neuron involvement?
- Without sensory loss
- With sensory loss
5. What is the temporal evolution?
- Acute (days to 4 weeks)
- Subacute (4 to 8 weeks)
- Chronic (>8 weeks)
6. Is there evidence for a hereditary neuropathy?
- Family history of neuropathy
- Lack of sensory symptoms despite sensory signs
7. Are there any associated medical conditions?
- Cancer, diabetes mellitus, connective tissue disease or other autoimmune diseases, infection (e.g., HIV, Lyme disease, leprosy)
- Medications including over-the-counter drugs that may cause a toxic neuropathy
- Preceding events, drugs, toxins

examination; it can confirm whether the neuropathic disorder is a mononeuropathy, multiple mononeuropathy (mononeuropathy multiplex), radiculopathy, plexopathy, or generalized polyneuropathy. Similarly, EDx evaluation can ascertain whether the process involves only sensory fibers, motor fibers, autonomic fibers, or a combination of these. Finally, the electrophysiologic data can help distinguish axonopathies from myelinopathies as well as axonal degeneration secondary to ganglionopathies from the more common length-dependent axonopathies.

NCS are most helpful in classifying a neuropathy as being due to axonal degeneration or segmental demyelination (Table 384-3). In general, low-amplitude potentials with relatively preserved distal latencies, conduction velocities, and late potentials, along with fibrillations on needle EMG, suggest an axonal neuropathy. On the other hand, slow conduction velocities, prolonged distal latencies and late potentials, relatively preserved amplitudes, and the absence of fibrillations on needle EMG imply a primary demyelinating neuropathy. The presence of nonuniform slowing of conduction velocity, conduction block, or temporal dispersion further suggests an acquired demyelinating neuropathy (e.g., GBS or CIDP) as opposed to a hereditary demyelinating neuropathy (e.g., CMT type 1).

Autonomic studies are used to assess small myelinated (A-delta) or unmyelinated (C) nerve fiber involvement. Such testing includes heart rate response to deep breathing, heart rate, and blood pressure response to both the Valsalva maneuver and tilt-table testing, and quantitative sudomotor axon reflex testing (Chap. 375). These studies are particularly useful in patients who have pure small-fiber neuropathy or autonomic neuropathy in which routine NCS are normal.

OTHER IMPORTANT LABORATORY INFORMATION

In patients with generalized symmetric peripheral neuropathy, a standard laboratory evaluation should include a complete blood count, basic chemistries including serum electrolytes and tests of renal and hepatic function, fasting blood glucose (FBS), HbA_{1c}, urinalysis, thyroid function tests, B_{12}, folate, erythrocyte sedimentation rate (ESR), rheumatoid factor, antinuclear antibodies (ANA), serum protein electrophoresis (SPEP), and urine for Bence Jones protein. An oral glucose tolerance test is indicated in patients with painful sensory neuropathies even if FBS and HbA_{1c} are normal, as the test is abnormal in about one-third of such patients. Serum and urine immunofixation electrophoresis (IFE) are necessary, rather than just an SPEP, in patients with a demyelinating neuropathy or if one suspects amyloidosis (e.g., severe autonomic symptoms) as an IFE is more sensitive at identifying a monoclonal gammopathy. A skeletal survey should be performed in patients with acquired demyelinating neuropathies and M-spikes to look for osteosclerotic or lytic lesions. Patients with monoclonal gammopathy should also be referred to a hematologist for consideration of a bone marrow biopsy. In addition to the above tests, patients with a mononeuropathy multiplex pattern of involvement should have a vasculitis workup, including antineutrophil cytoplasmic antibodies (ANCA), cryoglobulins, hepatitis serology, Western blot for Lyme disease, HIV, and occasionally a cytomegalovirus (CMV), titer.

There are many autoantibody panels (various antiganglioside antibodies) marketed for screening routine neuropathy patients for a treatable condition. These autoantibodies have no proven clinical utility or added benefit beyond the information obtained from a complete clinical examination and detailed EDx. A heavy metal screen is also not necessary as a screening procedure, unless there is a history of possible exposure or suggestive features on examination (e.g., severe painful sensorimotor and autonomic neuropathy and alopecia—thallium; severe painful sensorimotor neuropathy with or without GI disturbance and Mee's lines—arsenic; wrist or finger extensor weakness and anemia with basophilic stippling of red blood cells—lead).

In patients with suspected GBS or CIDP, a lumbar puncture is indicated to look for an elevated cerebral spinal fluid (CSF) protein. In idiopathic cases of GBS and CIDP, there should not be pleocytosis in the CSF. If cells are present, one should consider HIV infection, Lyme disease, sarcoidosis, or lymphomatous or leukemic infiltration of nerve roots. Some patients with GBS and CIDP have abnormal liver function tests. In these cases, it is important to also check for hepatitis B and C, HIV, CMV, and Epstein-Barr virus (EBV) infection. In patients with an axonal GBS (by EMG/NCS) or those with a suspicious coinciding history (e.g., unexplained abdominal pain, psychiatric illness, significant autonomic dysfunction), it is reasonable to screen for porphyria.

In patients with a severe sensory ataxia, a sensory ganglionopathy or neuronopathy should be considered. The most common causes of sensory ganglionopathies are Sjögren syndrome and a paraneoplastic neuropathy. Neuropathy can be the initial manifestation of Sjögren syndrome. Thus, one should always inquire about dry eyes and mouth in patients with sensory signs and symptoms. Further, some patients can manifest sicca complex without full-blown Sjögren syndrome. Thus, patients with sensory ataxia should have an senile systemic amyloidosis (SSA) and single strand binding (SSB) in addition to the routine ANA. To workup a possible paraneoplastic sensory ganglionopathy, anti-neuronal nuclear antibodies (e.g., anti-Hu antibodies) should be obtained (Chap. 101). These antibodies are most commonly seen in patients with small cell carcinoma of the lung but are seen also in breast, ovarian, lymphoma, and other cancers. Importantly, the paraneoplastic neuropathy can precede the detection of the cancer, and detection of these autoantibodies should lead to a search for malignancy.

TABLE 384-2 Patterns of Neuropathic Disorders

Pattern 1: Symmetric proximal and distal weakness with sensory loss
Consider: inflammatory demyelinating polyneuropathy (GBS and CIDP)
Pattern 2: Symmetric distal sensory loss with or without distal weakness
Consider: cryptogenic or idiopathic sensory polyneuropathy (CSPN), diabetes mellitus and other metabolic disorders, drugs, toxins, hereditary (Charcot-Marie-Tooth, amyloidosis, and others)
Pattern 3: Asymmetric distal weakness with sensory loss
With involvement of multiple nerves
Consider: multifocal CIDP, vasculitis, cryoglobulinemia, amyloidosis, sarcoid, infectious (leprosy, Lyme, hepatitis B or C, HIV, CMV), hereditary neuropathy with liability to pressure palsies (HNPP), tumor infiltration
With involvement of single nerves/regions
Consider: may be any of the above but also could be compressive mononeuropathy, plexopathy, or radiculopathy
Pattern 4: Asymmetric proximal and distal weakness with sensory loss
Consider: polyradiculopathy or plexopathy due to diabetes mellitus, meningeal carcinomatosis or lymphomatosis, hereditary plexopathy (HNPP, HNA), idiopathic
Pattern 5: Asymmetric distal weakness without sensory loss
With upper motor neuron findings
Consider: motor neuron disease
Without upper motor neuron findings
Consider: progressive muscular atrophy, juvenile monomelic amyotrophy (Hirayama disease), multifocal motor neuropathy, multifocal acquired motor axonopathy
Pattern 6: Symmetric sensory loss and distal areflexia with upper motor neuron findings
Consider: Vitamin B_{12}, vitamin E, and copper deficiency with combined system degeneration with peripheral neuropathy, hereditary leukodystrophies (e.g., adrenomyeloneuropathy)
Pattern 7: Symmetric weakness without sensory loss
With proximal and distal weakness
Consider: spinal muscular atrophy
With distal weakness
Consider: hereditary motor neuropathy ("distal" SMA) or atypical CMT
Pattern 8: Asymmetric proprioceptive sensory loss without weakness
Consider causes of a sensory neuronopathy (ganglionopathy): Cancer (paraneoplastic) Sjögren syndrome Idiopathic sensory neuronopathy (possible GBS variant) Cisplatin and other chemotherapeutic agents Vitamin B_6 toxicity HIV-related sensory neuronopathy
Pattern 9: Autonomic Symptoms and Signs
Consider neuropathies associated with prominent autonomic dysfunction: Hereditary sensory and autonomic neuropathy Amyloidosis (familial and acquired) Diabetes mellitus Idiopathic pandysautonomia (may be a variant of Guillain-Barré syndrome) Porphyria HIV-related autonomic neuropathy Vincristine and other chemotherapeutic agents

Abbreviations: CIDP, chronic inflammatory demyelinating polyneuropathy; CMT, Charcot-Marie-Tooth disease; CMV, cytomegalovirus; GBS, Guillain-Barré syndrome; HIV, human immunodeficiency virus; HNA, hereditary neuralgic amyotrophy; SMA, spinal muscular atrophy.

TABLE 384-3 Electrophysiologic Features: Axonal Degeneration vs. Segmental Demyelination

	Axonal Degeneration	Segmental Demyelination
Motor Nerve Conduction Studies		
CMAP amplitude	Decreased	Normal (except with CB)
Distal latency	Normal	Prolonged
Conduction velocity	Normal	Slow
Conduction block	Absent	Present
Temporal dispersion	Absent	Present
F wave	Normal or absent	Prolonged or Absent
H reflex	Normal or absent	Prolonged or Absent
Sensory Nerve Conduction Studies		
SNAP amplitude	Decreased	Normal
Distal latency	Normal	Prolonged
Conduction velocity	Normal	Slow
Needle EMG		
Spontaneous activity		
Fibrillations	Present	Absent
Fasciculations	Present	Absent
Motor unit potentials		
Recruitment	Decreased	Decreased
Morphology	Long duration/polyphasic	Normal

Abbreviations: CB, conduction block; CMAP, compound motor action potential; EMG, electromyography; SNAP, sensory nerve action potential.

NERVE BIOPSIES

Nerve biopsies are now rarely indicated for evaluation of neuropathies. The primary indication for nerve biopsy is suspicion for amyloid neuropathy or vasculitis. In most instances, the abnormalities present on biopsies do not help distinguish one form of peripheral neuropathy from another (beyond what is already apparent by clinical examination and the NCS). Nerve biopsies should only be done if the NCS studies are abnormal. The sural nerve is most commonly biopsied because it is a pure sensory nerve and biopsy will not result in loss of motor function. In suspected vasculitis, a combination biopsy of a superficial peroneal nerve (pure sensory) and the underlying peroneus brevis muscle obtained from a single small incision increases the diagnostic yield. Tissue can be analyzed by frozen section and paraffin section to assess the supporting structures for evidence of inflammation, vasculitis, or amyloid deposition. Semithin plastic sections, teased fiber preparations, and electron microscopy are used to assess the morphology of the nerve fibers and to distinguish axonopathies from myelinopathies.

SKIN BIOPSIES

Skin biopsies are sometimes used to diagnose a small-fiber neuropathy. Following a punch biopsy of the skin in the distal lower extremity, immunologic staining can be used to measure the density of small unmyelinated fibers. The density of these nerve fibers is reduced in patients with small-fiber neuropathies in whom nerve conduction studies and routine nerve biopsies are often normal. This technique may allow for an objective measurement in patients with mainly subjective symptoms. However, it adds little to what one already knows from the clinical examination and EDx.

SPECIFIC DISORDERS

HEREDITARY NEUROPATHIES

Charcot-Marie-Tooth (CMT) disease is the most common type of hereditary neuropathy. Rather than one disease, CMT is a syndrome of several genetically distinct disorders (Table 384-4). The various subtypes of CMT are classified according to the nerve conduction velocities and predominant pathology (e.g., demyelination or axonal degeneration), inheritance pattern (autosomal dominant, recessive, or X-linked), and the specific mutated genes. Type 1 CMT (or CMT1) refers to inherited demyelinating sensorimotor neuropathies, while the axonal sensory neuropathies are classified as CMT2. By definition, motor conduction velocities in the arms are slowed to less than 38 m/s in CMT1 and are greater than 38 m/s in CMT2. However, most cases of CMT1 actually have motor nerve conduction velocities (NCVs) between 20 and 25 m/s. CMT1 and CMT2 usually begin in childhood or early adult life; however, onset later in life can occur, particularly in CMT2. Both are associated with autosomal dominant inheritance, with a few exceptions. CMT3 is an autosomal dominant neuropathy that appears in infancy and is associated with severe demyelination or hypomyelination. CMT4 is an autosomal recessive neuropathy that typically begins in childhood or early adult life. There are no medical therapies for any of the CMTs, but physical and occupational therapy can be beneficial as can bracing (e.g., ankle-foot orthotics for footdrop) and other orthotic devices.

CMT1

CMT1 is the most common form of hereditary neuropathy, with the ratio of CMT1:CMT2 being approximately 2:1. Affected individuals

TABLE 384-4 Classification of Charcot-Marie-Tooth Disease and Related Neuropathies

Name	Inheritance	Gene Location	Gene Product
CMT1			
CMT1A	AD	17p11.2	PMP-22 (usually duplication of gene)
CMT1B	AD	1q21-23	MPZ
CMT1C	AD	16p13.1-p12.3	LITAF
CMT1D	AD	10q21.1-22.1	ERG2
CMT1E (with deafness)	AD	17p11.2	Point mutations in PMP 22 gene
CMT1F	AD	8p13-21	Neurofilament light chain
CMT1X	X-linked dominant	Xq13	Connexin-32
HNPP	AD	17p11.2 1q21-23	PMP-22 MPZ
CMT2			
CMT2A2 (allelic to HMSN VI with optic atrophy)	AD	1p36.2	MFN2
CMT2B	AD	3q13-q22	RAB7
CMT2B1 (allelic to LGMD 1B)	AR	1q21.2	Lamin A/C
CMT2B2	AR and AD	19q13	MED25 for AR Unknown for AD
CMT2C (with vocal cord and diaphragm paralysis)	AD	12q23-24	TRPV4
CMT2D (allelic to distal SMA5)	AD	7p14	Glycine tRNA synthetase
CMT2E (allelic to CMT 1F)	AD	8p21	Neurofilament light chain
CMT2F	AD	7q11-q21	Heat-shock 27-kDa protein-1
CMT2G (may be allelic to CMT4H)	AD	12q12-q13	? (Fabrin)
CMT2H	AD	8q21.3	? (may be GDAP1)
CMT2I (allelic to CMT1B)	AD	1q22	MPZ
CMT2J	AD	1q22	MPZ
CMT2K (allelic to CMT4A)	AD	8q13-q21	GDAP1
CMT2L (allelic to distal hereditary motor neuropathy type 2)	AD	12q24	Heat-shock protein 8
CMT2M	AD	16q22	AARS
CMT2X	X-linked	Xq22-24	PRPS1
CMT3 (Dejerine-Sottas disease, congenital hypomyelinating neuropathy)	AD AD AR AR	17p11.2 1q21-23 10q21.1-22.1 19q13	PMP-22 MPZ ERG2 Periaxon

(*continued*)

TABLE 384-4 Classification of Charcot-Marie-Tooth Disease and Related Neuropathies (*Continued*)

Name	Inheritance	Gene Location	Gene Product
CMT4			
CMT4A	AR	8q13-21.1	GDAP1
CMT4B1 CMT4B2	AR AR	11q23 11p15	MTMR2 MTMR13
CMT4C	AR	5q23-33	SH3TC2
CMT4D (HMSN-Lom)	AR	8q24	NDRG1
CMT4E (Congenital hypomyelinating neuropathy)	AR	-	Probably includes PMP22, MPZ, and ERG-2
CMT4F	AR	19q13.1-13.3	Periaxin
CMT4G	AR	10q23.2	HKI
CMT4H	AR	12q12-q13	Frabin
CMT4J	AR	6q21	FIG4
HNA	AD	17q24	SEPT9
HMSN-P	AD	3q13-q14	?
HSAN1	AD; Rare AR and X-linked cases also reported	9q22	SPTLC1
HSAN2	AR	12p13.33	PRKWNK1
HSAN3	AR	9q21	IKAP
HSAN4	AR	3q	trkA/NGF receptor
HSAN5	AD or AR	1p11.2-p13.2	NGFb

Abbreviations: AARS, alanyl-tRNA synthetase; AD, autosomal dominant; AR, autosomal recessive; CMT, Charcot-Marie-Tooth; ERG2, early growth response-2 protein; FIG4, FDG1-related F actin–binding protein; GDAP1, ganglioside-induced differentiation-associated protein-1; HK1, hexokinase 1; HMSN-P, hereditary motor and sensory neuropathy-proximal; HNA, hereditary neuralgic amyotrophy; HNPP, hereditary neuropathy with liability to pressure palsies; HSAN; hereditary sensory and autonomic neuropathy; IKAP, $_{k}$B kinase complex-associated protein; LGMD, limb girdle muscular dystrophy; LITAF, lipopolysaccharide-induced tumor necrosis factor α factor; MED25, mediator 25; MFN2, mitochondrial fusion protein mitofusin 2 gene; MPZ, myelin protein zero protein; MTMR2, myotubularin-related protein-2; NDRG1, N-myc downstream regulated 1; PMP-22, peripheral myelin protein-22; PRKWNK1, protein kinase, lysine deficient 1; PRPS1, phosphoribosylpyrophosphate synthetase 1; RAB7, Ras-related protein 7; SEPT9, Septin 9; SH3TC2, SH3 domain and tetratricopeptide repeats 2; SMA, spinal muscular atrophy; SPTLC1, serine palmitoyltransferase long-chain base 1; TrkA/NGF, tyrosine kinase A/nerve growth factor; tRNA, transfer ribonucleic acid; TRPV4, transient receptor potential cation channel, subfamily V, member 4.
Source: Modified from Amato and Russell.

usually present in the first to third decade of life with distal leg weakness (e.g., footdrop), although patients may remain asymptomatic even late in life. People with CMT generally do not complain of numbness or tingling, which can be helpful in distinguishing CMT from acquired forms of neuropathy in which sensory symptoms usually predominate. Although usually asymptomatic in this regard, reduced sensation to all modalities is apparent on examination. Muscle stretch reflexes are unobtainable or reduced throughout. There is often atrophy of the muscles below the knee (particularly the anterior compartment), leading to so-called inverted champagne bottle legs.

Motor NCVs are usually in the 20–25 m/s range. Nerve biopsies usually are not performed on patients suspected of having CMT1, as the diagnosis usually can be made by less invasive testing (e.g., NCS and genetic studies). However, when done, the biopsies reveal reduction of myelinated nerve fibers with a predilection for the loss of the large-diameter fibers and Schwann cell proliferation around thinly or demyelinated fibers, forming so-called onion bulbs.

CMT1A is the most common subtype of CMT1, representing 70% of cases, and is caused by a 1.5-megabase (Mb) duplication within chromosome 17p11.2-12 wherein the gene for peripheral myelin protein-22 (PMP-22) lies. This results in patients having three copies of the PMP-22 gene rather than two. This protein accounts for 2–5% of myelin protein and is expressed in compact portions of the peripheral myelin sheath. Approximately 20% of patients with CMT1 have CMT1B, which is caused by mutations in the myelin protein zero (MPZ). CMT1B is for the most part clinically, electrophysiologically, and histologically indistinguishable from CMT1A. MPZ is an integral myelin protein and accounts for more than half of the myelin protein in peripheral nerves. Other forms of CMT1 are much less common and again indistinguishable from one another clinically and electrophysiologically.

CMT2

CMT2 tends to present later in life compared to CMT1. Affected individuals usually become symptomatic in the second decade of life; some cases present earlier in childhood, while others remain asymptomatic into late adult life. Clinically, CMT2 is for the most part indistinguishable from CMT1. NCS are helpful in this regard; in contrast to CMT1, the velocities are normal or only slightly slowed. The most common cause of CMT2 is a mutation in the gene for mitofusin 2 (MFN2), which accounts for one-third of CMT2 cases overall. MFN2 localizes to the outer mitochondrial membrane, where it regulates the mitochondrial network architecture by fusion of mitochondria. The other genes associated with CMT2 are much less common.

CMT3

CMT3 was originally described by Dejerine and Sottas as a hereditary demyelinating sensorimotor polyneuropathy presenting in infancy or early childhood. Affected children are severely weak. Motor NCVs are markedly slowed, typically 5–10 m/s or less. Most cases of CMT3 are caused by point mutations in the genes for PMP-22, MPZ, or ERG-2, which are also the genes responsible for CMT1.

CMT4

CMT4 is extremely rare and is characterized by a severe, childhood-onset sensorimotor polyneuropathy that is usually inherited in an autosomal recessive fashion. Electrophysiologic and histologic evaluations can show demyelinating or axonal features. CMT4 is genetically heterogenic (Table 384-4).

CMT1X

CMT1X is an X-linked dominant disorder with clinical features similar to CMT1 and -2, except that the neuropathy is much more severe in men than in women. CMT1X accounts for approximately 10–15% of CMT overall. Men usually present in the first two decades of life with atrophy and weakness of the distal arms and legs, areflexia, pes cavus, and hammertoes. Obligate women carriers are frequently asymptomatic, but can develop signs and symptoms. Onset in women is usually after the second decade of life, and the neuropathy is milder in severity.

NCS reveal features of both demyelination and axonal degeneration that are more severe in men compared to women. In men, motor NCVs in the arms and legs are moderately slowed (in the low to mid 30-m/s range). About 50% of men with CMT1X have motor NCVs between 15 and 35 m/s with about 80% of these falling between 25 and 35 m/s (intermediate slowing). In contrast, about 80% of women with CMT1X have NCV in the normal range and 20% had MNCV in the intermediate range. CMT1X is caused by mutations in the connexin 32 gene. Connexins are gap junction structural proteins that are important in cell-to-cell communication.

Hereditary neuropathy with liability to pressure palsies (HNPP)

HNPP is an autosomal dominant disorder related to CMT1A. While CMT1A is usually associated with a 1.5-Mb duplication in chromosome 17p11.2 that results in an extra copy of PMP-22 gene, HNPP is caused by inheritance of the chromosome with the corresponding 1.5-Mb deletion of this segment, and thus affected individuals have only one copy of the PMP-22 gene. Patients usually manifest in the second or third decade of life with painless numbness and weakness in the distribution of single peripheral nerves, although multiple mononeuropathies can occur. Symptomatic mononeuropathy or multiple mononeuropathies are often precipitated by trivial compression of nerve(s) as can occur with wearing a backpack, leaning on the elbows, or crossing one's legs for even a short period of time. These pressure-related mononeuropathies may take weeks or months to resolve. In addition, some affected individuals manifest with a progressive or relapsing, generalized and symmetric, sensorimotor peripheral neuropathy that resembles CMT.

Hereditary neuralgic amyotrophy (HNA)

HNA is an autosomal dominant disorder characterized by recurrent attacks of pain, weakness, and sensory loss in the distribution of the brachial plexus often beginning in childhood. These attacks are similar to those seen with idiopathic brachial plexitis (see below). Attacks may occur in the postpartum period, following surgery, or at other times of stress. Most patients recover over several weeks or months. Slightly dysmorphic features, including hypotelorism, epicanthal folds, cleft palate, syndactyly, micrognathia, and facial asymmetry, are evident in some individuals. EDx demonstrate an axonal process. HNA is caused by mutations in septin 9 (*SEPT9*). Septins may be important in formation of the neuronal cytoskeleton and have a role in cell division, but the mechanism of causing HNA is unclear.

Hereditary sensory and autonomic neuropathy (HSAN)

The HSANs are a very rare group of hereditary neuropathies in which sensory and autonomic dysfunction predominates over muscle weakness, unlike CMT, in which motor findings are most prominent (Table 384-4). Nevertheless, affected individuals can develop motor weakness and there can be overlap with CMT. There are no medical therapies available to treat these neuropathies, other than prevention and treatment of mutilating skin and bone lesions.

Of the HSANs, only HSAN1 typically presents in adults. The HSAN1 is the most common of the HSANs and is inherited in an autosomal dominant fashion. Affected individuals with HSAN1 usually manifest in the second through fourth decade of life. HSAN1 is associated with the degeneration of small myelinated and unmyelinated nerve fibers leading to severe loss of pain and temperature sensation, deep dermal ulcerations, recurrent osteomyelitis, Charcot joints, bone loss, gross foot and hand deformities, and amputated digits. Although most people with HSAN1 do not complain of numbness, they often describe burning, aching, or lancinating pains. Autonomic neuropathy is not a prominent feature, but bladder dysfunction and reduced sweating in the feet may occur. HSAN1A is caused by mutations in the serine palmitoyltransferase long-chain base 1 (*SPTLC1*) gene.

OTHER HEREDITARY NEUROPATHIES (TABLE 384-5)

■ FABRY DISEASE

Fabry disease (angiokeratoma corporis diffusum) is an X-linked dominant disorder. While men are more commonly and severely affected, women can also show severe signs of the disease. Angiokeratomas are reddish-purple maculopapular lesions that are usually found around the umbilicus, scrotum, inguinal region, and perineum. Burning or lancinating pain in the hands and feet often develops in males in late childhood or early adult life. However, the neuropathy is usually overshadowed by complications arising from the associated premature atherosclerosis (e.g., hypertension, renal failure, cardiac disease, and stroke) that often lead to death by the fifth decade of life. Some patients also manifest primarily with a dilated cardiomyopathy.

Fabry disease is caused by mutations in the α-galactosidase gene that leads to the accumulation of ceramide trihexoside in nerves and blood vessels. A decrease in α-galactosidase activity is evident in leukocytes and cultured fibroblasts. Glycolipid granules may be appreciated in ganglion cells of the peripheral and sympathetic nervous systems and in perineurial cells. Enzyme replacement therapy with α-galactosidase B can improve the neuropathy if patients are treated early, before irreversible nerve fiber loss.

■ ADRENOLEUKODYSTROPHY/ADRENOMYELONEUROPATHY

Adrenoleukodystrophy (ALD) and adrenomyeloneuropathy (AMN) are allelic X-linked dominant disorders caused by mutations in the

TABLE 384-5 Rare Hereditary Neuropathies

Hereditary Disorders of Lipid Metabolism
Metachromatic leukodystrophy
Krabbe disease (globoid cell leukodystrophy)
Fabry disease
Adrenoleukodystrophy/adrenomyeloneuropathy
Refsum disease
Tangier disease
Cerebrotendinous xanthomatosis
Hereditary Ataxias With Neuropathy
Friedreich ataxia
Vitamin E deficiency
Spinocerebellar ataxia
Abetalipoproteinemia (Bassen-Kornzweig disease)
Disorders of Defective DNA Repair
Ataxia-telangiectasia
Cockayne syndrome
Giant Axonal Neuropathy
Porphyria
Acute intermittent porphyria (AIP)
Hereditary coproporphyria (HCP)
Variegate porphyria (VP)
Familial Amyloid Polyneuropathy (FAP)
Transthyretin-related
Gelsolin-related
Apolipoprotein A1-related

peroxisomal transmembrane adenosine triphosphate-binding cassette (ABC) transporter gene. Patients with ALD manifest with CNS abnormalities. However, 30% with mutations in this gene present with the AMN phenotype that typically manifests in the third to fifth decade of life with mild to moderate peripheral neuropathy combined with progressive spastic paraplegia (Chap. 377). Rare patients present with an adult-onset spinocerebellar ataxia or only with adrenal insufficiency.

EDx is suggestive of a primary axonopathy with secondary demyelination. Nerve biopsies demonstrate a loss of myelinated and unmyelinated nerve fibers with lamellar inclusions in the cytoplasm of Schwann cells. Very long chain fatty acid (VLCFA) levels (C24, C25, and C26) are increased in the urine. Laboratory evidence of adrenal insufficiency is evident in approximately two-thirds of patients. The diagnosis can be confirmed by genetic testing.

Adrenal insufficiency is managed by replacement therapy; however, there is no proven effective therapy for the neurologic manifestations of ALD/AMN. Diets low in VLCFAs and supplemented with Lorenzo's oil (erucic and oleic acids) reduce the levels of VLCFAs and increase the levels of C22 in serum, fibroblasts, and liver; however, several large, open-label trials of Lorenzo's oil failed to demonstrate efficacy.

■ REFSUM DISEASE

Refsum disease can manifest in infancy to early adulthood with the classic tetrad of (1) peripheral neuropathy, (2) retinitis pigmentosa, (3) cerebellar ataxia, and (4) elevated CSF protein concentration. Most affected individuals develop progressive distal sensory loss and weakness in the legs leading to footdrop by their 20s. Subsequently, the proximal leg and arm muscles may become weak. Patients may also develop sensorineural hearing loss, cardiac conduction abnormalities, ichthyosis, and anosmia.

Serum phytanic acid levels are elevated. Sensory and motor NCS reveal reduced amplitudes, prolonged latencies, and slowed conduction velocities. Nerve biopsy demonstrates a loss of myelinated nerve fibers, with remaining axons often thinly myelinated and associated with onion bulb formation.

Refsum disease is genetically heterogeneous but autosomal recessive in nature. Classical Refsum disease with childhood or early adult onset is caused by mutations in the gene that encodes for phytanoyl-CoA α-hydroxylase (*PAHX*). Less commonly, mutations in the gene encoding peroxin 7 receptor protein (PRX 7) are responsible. These mutations lead to the accumulation of phytanic acid in the central and peripheral nervous systems. Refsum disease is treated by removing phytanic precursors (phytols: fish oils, dairy products, and ruminant fats) from the diet.

■ TANGIER DISEASE

Tangier disease is a rare autosomal recessive disorder that can present as (1) asymmetric multiple mononeuropathies, (2) a slowly progressive symmetric polyneuropathy predominantly in the legs, or (3) a pseudo-syringomyelia pattern with dissociated sensory loss (i.e., abnormal pain/temperature perception but preserved position/vibration in the arms [Chap. 377]). The tonsils may appear swollen and yellowish-orange in color, while there may also be splenomegaly and lymphadenopathy.

Tangier disease is caused by mutations in the ATP-binding cassette transporter 1 (ABC1) gene, which leads to markedly reduced levels of high-density lipoprotein (HDL) cholesterol levels while triacylglycerol levels are increased. Nerve biopsies reveal axonal degeneration with demyelination and remyelination. Electron microscopy demonstrates abnormal accumulation of lipid in Schwann cells, particularly those encompassing umyelinated and small myelinated nerves. There is no specific treatment.

■ PORPHYRIA

Porphyria is a group of inherited disorders caused by defects in heme biosynthesis (Chap. 358). Three forms of porphyria are associated with peripheral neuropathy: acute intermittent porphyria (AIP), hereditary coproporphyria (HCP), and variegate porphyria (VP). The acute neurologic manifestations are similar in each, with the exception that a photosensitive rash is seen with HCP and VP but not in AIP. Attacks of porphyria can be precipitated by certain drugs (usually those metabolized by the P450 system), hormonal changes (e.g., pregnancy, menstrual cycle), and dietary restrictions.

An acute attack of porphyria may begin with sharp abdominal pain. Subsequently, patients may develop agitation, hallucinations, or seizures. Several days later, back and extremity pain followed by weakness ensues, mimicking GBS. Weakness can involve the arms or the legs and can be asymmetric, proximal, or distal in distribution, as well as affecting the face and bulbar musculature. Dysautonomia and signs of sympathetic overactivity are common (e.g., pupillary dilation, tachycardia, and hypertension). Constipation, urinary retention, and incontinence can also be seen.

The CSF protein is typically normal or mildly elevated. Liver function tests and hematologic parameters are usually normal. Some patients are hyponatremic due to inappropriate secretion of antidiuretic hormone (Chap. 339). The urine may appear brownish in color secondary to the high concentration of porphyrin metabolites. Accumulation of intermediary precursors of heme (i.e., δ-aminolevulinic acid, porphobilinogen, uroporphobilinogen, coproporphyrinogen, and protoporphyrinogen) are found in urine. Specific enzyme activities can also be measured in erythrocytes and leukocytes. The primary abnormalities on EDx are marked reductions in CMAP amplitudes and signs of active axonal degeneration on needle EMG.

The porphyrias are inherited in an autosomal dominant fashion. AIP is associated with porphobilinogen deaminase deficiency, HCP is caused by defects in coproporphyrin oxidase, and VP is associated with protoporphyrinogen oxidase deficiency. The pathogenesis of the neuropathy is not completely understood. Treatment with glucose and hematin may reduce the accumulation of heme precursors. Intravenous glucose is started at a rate of 10–20 g/h. If there is no improvement within 24 h, intravenous hematin 2–5 mg/kg per day for 3–14 days should be given.

FAMILIAL AMYLOID POLYNEUROPATHY

Familial amyloid polyneuropathy (FAP) is phenotypically and genetically heterogeneous and is caused by mutations in the genes for transthyretin (TTR), apolipoprotein A1, or gelsolin (Chap. 112). The majority of patients with FAP have mutations in the TTR gene. Amyloid deposition may be evident in abdominal fat pad, rectal, or nerve biopsies. The clinical features, histopathology, and EDx reveal abnormalities consistent with a generalized or multifocal, predominantly axonal but occasionally demyelinating, sensorimotor polyneuropathy.

Patients with TTR-related FAP usually develop insidious onset of numbness and painful paresthesias in the distal lower limbs in the third to fourth decade of life, although some patients develop the disorder later in life. Carpal tunnel syndrome (CTS) is common. Autonomic involvement can be severe, leading to postural hypotension, constipation or persistent diarrhea, erectile dysfunction, and impaired sweating. Amyloid deposition also occurs in the heart, kidneys, liver, and the corneas. Patients usually die 10–15 years after the onset of symptoms from cardiac failure or complications from malnutrition. Because the liver produces much of the body's TTR, liver transplantation has been used to treat FAP related to TTR mutations. Serum TTR levels decrease after transplantation, and improvement in clinical and EDx features have been reported.

Patients with apolipoprotein A1–related FAP (Van Allen type) usually present in the fourth decade with numbness and painful dysesthesias in the distal limbs. Gradually, the symptoms progress, leading to proximal and distal weakness and atrophy. Although autonomic neuropathy is not severe, some patients develop diarrhea, constipation, or gastroparesis. Most patients die from systemic complications of amyloidosis (e.g., renal failure) 12–15 years after the onset of the neuropathy.

Gelsolin-related amyloidosis (Finnish type) is characterized by the combination of lattice corneal dystrophy and multiple cranial neuropathies that usually begin in the third decade of life. Over time, a mild generalized sensorimotor polyneuropathy develops. Autonomic dysfunction does not occur.

ACQUIRED NEUROPATHIES

PRIMARY OR AL AMYLOIDOSIS (SEE CHAP. 112)

Besides FAP, amyloidosis can also be acquired. In primary or AL amyloidosis, the abnormal protein deposition is composed of immunoglobulin light chains. AL amyloidosis occurs in the setting of multiple myeloma, Waldenström macroglobulinemia, lymphoma, other plasmacytomas, or lymphoproliferative disorders, or without any other identifiable disease.

Approximately 30% of patients with AL primary amyloidosis present with a polyneuropathy, most typically painful dysesthesias and burning sensations in the feet. However, the trunk can be involved and some manifest with a mononeuropathy multiplex pattern. CTS occurs in 25% of patients and may be the initial manifestation. The neuropathy is slowly progressive, and eventually weakness develops along with large-fiber sensory loss. Most patients develop autonomic involvement with postural hypertension, syncope, bowel and bladder incontinence, constipation, impotence, and impaired sweating. Patients generally die from their systemic illness (renal failure, cardiac disease).

The monoclonal protein may be composed of IgG, IgA, IgM, or only free light chain. Lambda (λ) is more common than κ light chain (>2:1) in AL amyloidosis. The CSF protein is often increased (with normal cell count), and thus the neuropathy may be mistaken for CIDP (Chap. 385). Nerve biopsies reveal axonal degeneration and amyloid deposition in either a globular or diffuse pattern infiltrating the perineurial, epineurial, and endoneurial connected tissue and in blood vessel walls.

The median survival of patients with primary amyloidosis is less than 2 years, with death usually from progressive congestive heart failure or renal failure. Chemotherapy with melphalan, prednisone, and colchicine, to reduce the concentration of monoclonal proteins, and autologous stem cell transplantation may prolong survival, but whether the neuropathy improves is controversial (Chap. 112).

DIABETIC NEUROPATHY

Diabetes mellitus (DM) is the most common cause of peripheral neuropathy in developed countries. DM is associated with several types of polyneuropathy: distal symmetric sensory or sensorimotor polyneuropathy, autonomic neuropathy, diabetic neuropathic cachexia, polyradiculoneuropathies, cranial neuropathies, and other mononeuropathies. Risk factors for the development of neuropathy include long-standing, poorly controlled DM and the presence of retinopathy and nephropathy.

Diabetic distal symmetric sensory and sensorimotor polyneuropathy (DSPN)

DSPN is the most common form of diabetic neuropathy and manifests as sensory loss beginning in the toes that gradually progresses over time up the legs and into the fingers and arms. When severe, a patient may develop sensory loss in the trunk (chest and abdomen), initially in the midline anteriorly and later extending laterally. Tingling, burning, deep aching pains may also be apparent. NCS usually show reduced amplitudes and mild to moderate slowing of conduction velocities (CVs). Nerve biopsy reveals axonal degeneration, endothelial hyperplasia, and, occasionally, perivascular inflammation. Tight control of glucose can reduce the risk of developing neuropathy or improve the underlying neuropathy. A variety of medications have been used with variable success to treat painful symptoms associated with DSPN, including antiepileptic medications, antidepressants, sodium channel blockers, and other analgesics (Table 384-6).

Diabetic autonomic neuropathy

Autonomic neuropathy is typically seen in combination with DSPN. The autonomic neuropathy can manifest as abnormal sweating, dysfunctional thermoregulation, dry eyes and mouth, pupillary abnormalities, cardiac arrhythmias, postural hypotension, gastrointestinal abnormalities (e.g., gastroparesis, postprandial bloating, chronic diarrhea or constipation), and genitourinary dysfunction (e.g., impotence, retrograde ejaculation, incontinence). Tests of autonomic function are generally abnormal, including sympathetic skin responses and quantitative sudomotor axon reflex testing. Sensory and motor NCS generally demonstrate features described above with DSPN.

TABLE 384-6 Treatment of Painful Sensory Neuropathies

Therapy	Route	Dose	Side Effects
First-Line			
Lidoderm 5% patch	Apply to painful area	Up to 3 patches qd	Skin irritation
Tricyclic antidepressants (e.g., amitriptylin, nortriptyline)	p.o.	10–100 mg qhs	Cognitive changes, sedation, dry eyes and mouth, urinary retention, constipation
Gabapentin	p.o.	300–1200 mg TID	Cognitive changes, sedation, peripheral edema
Pregabalin	p.o.	50–100 mg TID	Cognitive changes, sedation, peripheral edema
Duloxetine	p.o.	30–60 mg qd	Cognitive changes, sedation, dry eyes, diaphoresis, nausea, diarrhea, constipation
Second-Line			
Carbamazepine	p.o.	200–400 mg q 6–8 h	Cognitive changes, dizziness, leukopenia, liver dysfunction
Phenytoin	p.o.	200–400 mg qhs	Cognitive changes, dizziness, liver dysfunction
Venlafaxine	po	37.5–150 mg/d	Asthenia, sweating, nausea, constipation, anorexia, vomiting, somnolence, dry mouth, dizziness, nervousness, anxiety, tremor, and blurred vision as well as abnormal ejaculation/orgasm and impotence
Tramadol	p.o.	50 mg qid	Cognitive changes, GI upset
Third-Line			
Mexiletine	p.o.	200–300 mg tid	Arrhythmias
Other Agents			
EMLA cream 2.5% lidocaine 2.5% prilocaine	Apply cutaneously	q.i.d.	Local erythema
Capsaicin 0.025%–0.075% cream	Apply cutaneously	q.i.d.	Painful burning skin

Source: Modified from Amato and Russell.

Diabetic radiculoplexus neuropathy (diabetic amyotrophy or Bruns-Garland syndrome)

Diabetic radiculoplexus neuropathy is the presenting manifestation of DM in approximately one-third of patients. Typically, patients present with severe pain in the low back, hip, and thigh in one leg. Rarely, the diabetic polyradiculoneuropathy begins in both legs at the same time. Atrophy and weakness of proximal and distal muscles in the affected leg become apparent within a few days or weeks. The neuropathy is often accompanied or heralded by severe weight loss. Weakness usually progresses over several weeks or months, but can continue to progress for 18 months or more. Subsequently, there is slow recovery but many are left with residual weakness, sensory loss, and pain. In contrast to the more typical lumbosacral radiculoplexus neuropathy, some patients develop thoracic radiculopathy or, even less commonly, a cervical polyradiculoneuropathy. CSF protein is usually elevated, while the cell count is normal. ESR is often increased. EDx reveals evidence of active denervation in affected proximal and distal muscles in the affected limbs and in paraspinal muscles. Nerve biopsies may demonstrate axonal degeneration along with perivascular inflammation. Patients with severe pain are sometimes treated in the acute period with glucocorticoids, although a randomized controlled trial has yet to be performed, and the natural history of this neuropathy is gradual improvement.

Diabetic mononeuropathies or multiple mononeuropathies

The most common mononeuropathies are median neuropathy at the wrist and ulnar neuropathy at the elbow, but peroneal neuropathy at the fibular head, and sciatic, lateral femoral, cutaneous, or cranial neuropathies also occur. In regard to cranial mononeuropathies, seventh nerve palsies are relatively common but may have other, nondiabetic etiologies. In diabetics, a third nerve palsy is most common, followed by sixth nerve, and, less frequently, fourth nerve palsies. Diabetic third nerve palsies are characteristically pupil-sparing (Chap. 28).

■ HYPOTHYROIDISM

Hypothyroidism is more commonly associated with a proximal myopathy, but some patients develop a neuropathy, most typically carpal tunnel syndrome. Rarely, a generalized sensory polyneuropathy characterized by painful paresthesias and numbness in both the legs and hands can occur. Treatment is correction of the hypothyroidism.

■ SJÖGREN SYNDROME

Sjögren syndrome, characterized by the sicca complex of xerophthalmia, xerostomia, and dryness of other mucous membranes, can be complicated by neuropathy. Most common is a length-dependent axonal sensorimotor neuropathy characterized mainly by sensory loss in the distal extremities. A pure small-fiber neuropathy or a cranial neuropathy, particularly involving the trigeminal nerve, can also be seen. Sjögren syndrome is also associated with sensory neuronopathy/ganglionopathy. Patients with sensory ganglionopathies develop progressive numbness and tingling of the limbs, trunk, and face in a non-length-dependent manner such that symptoms can involve the face or arms more than the legs. The onset can be acute or insidious. Sensory examination demonstrates severe vibratory and proprioceptive loss leading to sensory ataxia.

Patients with neuropathy due to Sjögren syndrome may have antinuclear antibodies (ANA), SS-A/Ro, and SS-B/La antibodies in the serum but most do not. NCS demonstrate reduced amplitudes of sensory studies in the affected limbs. Nerve biopsy demonstrates axonal degeneration. Nonspecific perivascular inflammation may be present, but only rarely is there necrotizing vasculitis. There is no specific treatment for neuropathies related to Sjögren syndrome. When vasculitis is suspected, immunosuppressive agents may be beneficial. Occasionally, the sensory neuronopathy/ganglionopathy stabilizes or improves with immunotherapy, such as IVIg.

■ RHEUMATOID ARTHRITIS

Peripheral neuropathy occurs in at least 50% of patients with rheumatoid arthritis (RA) and may be vasculitic in nature (Chap. 326). Vasculitic neuropathy can present with a mononeuropathy multiplex, a generalized symmetric pattern of involvement, or a combination of these patterns. Neuropathies may also be due to drugs used to treat the RA (e.g., tumor necrosis blockers, leflunomide). Nerve biopsy often reveals thickening of the epineurial and endoneurial blood vessels as well as perivascular inflammation or vasculitis, with transmural inflammatory cell infiltration and fibrinoid necrosis of vessel walls. The neuropathy often is responsive to immunomodulating therapies.

■ SYSTEMIC LUPUS ERYTHEMATOSUS (SLE)

Between 2 and 27% of individuals with SLE develop a peripheral neuropathy. Affected patients typically present with a slowly progressive sensory loss beginning in the feet. Some patients develop burning pain and paresthesias with normal reflexes, and nerve conduction studies suggest a pure small-fiber neuropathy. Less common are multiple mononeuropathies presumably secondary to necrotizing vasculitis. Rarely, a generalized sensorimotor polyneuropathy meeting clinical, laboratory, electrophysiologic, and histologic criteria for either GBS or CIDP may occur. Immunosuppressive therapy is beneficial in SLE patients with neuropathy due to vasculitis. Immunosuppressive agents are less likely to be effective in patients with a generalized sensory or sensorimotor polyneuropathy without evidence of vasculitis. Patients with a GBS or CIDP-like neuropathy should be treated accordingly (Chap. 385).

■ SYSTEMIC SCLEROSIS (SCLERODERMA)

A distal symmetric, mainly sensory, polyneuropathy complicates 5–67% of scleroderma cases. Cranial mononeuropathies can also develop, most commonly of the trigeminal nerve, producing numbness and dysesthesias in the face. Multiple mononeuropathies also occur. The EDx and histologic features of nerve biopsy are those of an axonal sensory greater than motor polyneuropathy.

■ MIXED CONNECTIVE TISSUE DISEASE (MCTD)

A mild distal axonal sensorimotor polyneuropathy occurs in approximately 10% of patients with MCTD.

■ SARCOIDOSIS

The peripheral or central nervous systems are involved in about 5% of patients with sarcoidosis. The most common cranial nerve involved is the seventh nerve, which can be affected bilaterally. Some patients develop radiculopathy or polyradiculopathy. With a generalized root involvement, the clinical presentation can mimic GBS or CIDP. Patients can also present with multiple mononeuropathies or a generalized, slowly progressive, sensory greater than motor polyneuropathy. Some have features of a pure small-fiber neuropathy. EDx reveals an axonal neuropathy. Nerve biopsy can reveal noncaseating granulomas infiltrating the endoneurium, perineurium, and epineurium along with lymphocytic necrotizing angiitis. Neurosarcoidosis may respond to treatment with glucocorticoids or other immunosuppressive agents.

■ HYPEREOSINOPHILIC SYNDROME

Hypereosinophilic syndrome is characterized by eosinophilia associated with various skin, cardiac, hematologic, and neurologic abnormalities. A generalized peripheral neuropathy or a mononeuropathy multiplex occurs in 6–14% of patients.

■ CELIAC DISEASE (GLUTEN-INDUCED ENTEROPATHY OR NON-TROPICAL SPRUE)

Neurologic complications, particularly ataxia and peripheral neuropathy, are estimated to occur in 10% of patients with celiac disease. A generalized sensorimotor polyneuropathy, pure motor neuropathy, multiple mononeuropathies, autonomic neuropathy, small-fiber neuropathy, and neuromyotonia have all been reported in association with celiac disease or antigliadin/antiendomysial antibodies. Nerve biopsy may reveal a loss of large myelinated fibers. The neuropathy may be secondary to malabsorption of vitamins B_{12} and E. However, some patients have no appreciable vitamin deficiencies. The pathogenic basis for the neuropathy in these patients is unclear but may be autoimmune in etiology. The neuropathy does not appear to respond to a gluten-free diet. In patients with vitamin B_{12} or vitamin E deficiency, replacement therapy may improve or stabilize the neuropathy.

■ INFLAMMATORY BOWEL DISEASE

Ulcerative colitis and Crohn's disease may be complicated by GBS, CIDP, generalized axonal sensory or sensorimotor polyneuropathy, small-fiber neuropathy, or mononeuropathy. These neuropathies may be autoimmune, nutritional (e.g., vitamin B_{12} deficiency), treatment related (e.g., metronidazole), or idiopathic in nature. An acute neuropathy with demyelination resembling GBS may occur, particularly in patients treated with tumor necrosis factor α blockers.

■ UREMIC NEUROPATHY

Approximately 60% of patients with renal failure develop a polyneuropathy characterized by length-dependent numbness, tingling, allodynia, and mild distal weakness. Rarely, a rapidly progressive weakness and sensory loss very similar to GBS can occur that improves with an increase in the intensity of renal dialysis or with transplantation. Mononeuropathies can also occur, the most common of which is carpal tunnel syndrome. Ischemic monomelic neuropathy (see below) can complicate arteriovenous shunts created in the arm for dialysis. EDx in uremic patients reveals features of a length-dependent, primarily axonal, sensorimotor polyneuropathy. Sural nerve biopsies demonstrate a loss of nerve fibers (particularly large myelinated nerve fibers), active axonal degeneration, and segmental and paranodal demyelination. The sensorimotor polyneuropathy can be stabilized by hemodialysis and improved with successful renal transplantation.

■ CHRONIC LIVER DISEASE

A generalized sensorimotor neuropathy characterized by numbness, tingling, and minor weakness in the distal aspects of primarily the lower limbs commonly occurs in patients with chronic liver failure. EDx studies are consistent with a sensory greater than motor axonopathy. Sural nerve biopsy reveals both segmental demyelination and axonal loss. It is not known if hepatic failure in isolation can cause peripheral neuropathy, as the majority of patients have liver disease secondary to other disorders, such as alcoholism or viral hepatitis, which can also cause neuropathy.

CRITICAL ILLNESS POLYNEUROPATHY

The most common causes of acute generalized weakness leading to admission to a medical intensive care unit (ICU) are GBS and myasthenia gravis (Chap. 386). However, weakness developing in critically ill patients while in the ICU is usually caused by critical illness polyneuropathy (CIP) or critical illness myopathy (CIM), or much less commonly, by prolonged neuromuscular blockade. From a clinical and EDx standpoint, it can be quite difficult to distinguish these disorders. Most specialists suggest that CIM is more common. Both CIM and CIP develop as a complication of sepsis and multiple organ failure. They usually present as an inability to wean a patient from a ventilator. A coexisting encephalopathy may limit the neurologic exam, in particular the sensory examination. Muscle stretch reflexes are absent or reduced.

Serum creatine kinase (CK) is usually normal; an elevated serum CK would point to CIM as opposed to CIP. NCS reveal absent or markedly reduced amplitudes of motor and sensory studies in CIP, while sensory studies are relatively preserved in CIM. Needle EMG usually reveals profuse positive sharp waves and fibrillation potentials, and it is not unusual in patients with severe weakness to be unable to recruit motor unit action potentials. The pathogenic basis of CIP is not known. Perhaps circulating toxins and metabolic abnormalities associated with sepsis and multiorgan failure impair axonal transport or mitochondrial function, leading to axonal degeneration.

LEPROSY (HANSEN DISEASE)

Leprosy, caused by the acid-fast bacteria *Mycobacterium leprae*, is the most common cause of peripheral neuropathy in Southeast Asia, Africa, and South America (Chap. 166). Clinical manifestations range from tuberculoid leprosy at one end to lepromatous leprosy at the other end of the spectrum, with borderline leprosy in between. Neuropathies are most common in patients with borderline leprosy. Superficial cutaneous nerves of the ears and distal limbs are commonly affected. Mononeuropathies, multiple mononeuropathies, or a slowly progressive symmetric sensorimotor polyneuropathy may develop. Sensory NCS are usually absent in the lower limb and are reduced in amplitude in the arms. Motor NCS may demonstrate reduced amplitudes in affected nerves but occasionally can reveal demyelinating features. Leprosy is usually diagnosed by skin lesion biopsy. Nerve biopsy can also be diagnostic, particularly when there are no apparent skin lesions. The tuberculoid form is characterized by granulomas, and bacilli are not seen. In contrast, with lepromatous leprosy, large numbers of infiltrating bacilli, T_H2 lymphocytes, and organism-laden, foamy macrophages with minimal granulomatous infiltration are evident. The bacilli are best appreciated using the Fite stain, where they can be seen as red-staining rods often in clusters free in the endoneurium, within macrophages, or within Schwann cells.

Patients are generally treated with multiple drugs: dapsone, rifampin, and clofazimine. Other medications that are employed include thalidomide, pefloxacin, ofloxacin, sparfloxacin, minocycline, and clarithromycin. Patients are generally treated for 2 years. Treatment is sometimes complicated by the so-called reversal reaction, particularly in borderline leprosy. The reversal reaction can occur at any time during treatment and develops because of a shift to the tuberculoid end of the spectrum, with an increase in cellular immunity during treatment. The cellular response is upregulated as evidenced by an increased release of tumor necrosis factor α, interferon γ, and interleukin 2, with new granuloma formation. This can result in an exacerbation of the rash and the neuropathy as well as in appearance of new lesions. High-dose glucocorticoids blunt this adverse reaction and may be used prophylactically at treatment onset in high-risk patients. Erythema nodosum leprosum (ENL) is also treated with glucocorticoids or thalidomide.

LYME DISEASE

Lyme disease is caused by infection with *Borrelia burgdorferi*, a spirochete usually transmitted by the deer tick *Ixodes dammini* (Chap. 173). Neurologic complications may develop during the second and third stages of infection. Facial neuropathy is most common and is bilateral in about half of cases, which is rare for idiopathic Bell's palsy. Involvement of nerves is frequently asymmetric. Some patients present with a polyradiculoneuropathy or multiple mononeuropathies. EDx is suggestive of a primary axonopathy. Nerve biopsies can reveal axonal degeneration with perivascular inflammation. Treatment is with antibiotics (Chap. 173).

DIPHTHERITIC NEUROPATHY

Diphtheria is caused by the bacteria *Corynebacterium diphtheriae* (Chap. 138). Infected individuals present with flulike symptoms of generalized myalgias, headache, fatigue, low-grade fever, and irritability within a week to 10 days of the exposure. About 20–70% of patients develop a peripheral neuropathy caused by a toxin released by the bacteria. Three to 4 weeks after infection, patients may note decreased sensation in their throat and begin to develop dysphagia, dysarthria, hoarseness, and blurred vision due to impaired accommodation. A generalized polyneuropathy may manifest 2 or 3 months following the initial infection, characterized by numbness, paresthesias, and weakness of the arms and legs and occasionally ventilatory failure. CSF protein can be elevated with or without lymphocytic pleocytosis. EDx suggests a diffuse axonal sensorimotor polyneuropathy. Antitoxin and antibiotics should be given within 48 h of symptom onset (Chap. 138). Although early treatment reduces the incidence and severity of some complications (i.e., cardiomyopathy), it does not appear to alter the natural history of the associated peripheral neuropathy. The neuropathy usually resolves after several months.

HUMAN IMMUNODEFICIENCY VIRUS (HIV)

HIV infection can result in a variety of neurologic complications, including peripheral neuropathies (Chap. 189). Approximately 20% of HIV-infected individuals develop a neuropathy either as a direct result of the virus itself, other associated viral infections (e.g., cytomegalovirus), or neurotoxicity secondary to antiviral medications (see below). The major presentations of peripheral neuropathy associated with HIV infection include (1) distal symmetric polyneuropathy (DSP), (2) inflammatory demyelinating polyneuropathy (including both GBS and CIDP), (3) multiple mononeuropathies (e.g., vasculitis, CMV-related), (4) polyradiculopathy (usually CMV-related), (5) autonomic neuropathy, and (6) sensory ganglionitis.

HIV-related distal symmetric polyneuropathy (DSP)

DSP is the most common form of peripheral neuropathy associated with HIV infection and usually is seen in patients with AIDS. It is characterized by numbness and painful paresthesias involving the distal extremities. The pathogenic basis for DSP is unknown but is not due to actual infection of the peripheral nerves. The neuropathy may be immune mediated, perhaps caused by the release of cytokines from surrounding inflammatory cells. Vitamin B_{12} deficiency may contribute in some instances but is not a major cause of most cases of DSP. Some antiretroviral agents (e.g., dideoxycytidine, dideoxyinosine, stavudine) are also neurotoxic and can cause a painful sensory neuropathy.

HIV-related inflammatory demyelinating polyradiculoneuropathy

Both AIDP and CIDP can occur as a complication of HIV infection. AIDP usually develops at the time of seroconversion, while CIDP can occur any time in the course of the infection. Clinical and EDx features are indistinguishable from idiopathic AIDP or CIDP (discussed in next chapter). In addition to elevated protein levels, lymphocytic pleocytosis is evident in the CSF, a finding that helps distinguish this HIV-associated polyradiculoneuropathy from idiopathic AIDP/CIDP.

HIV-related progressive polyradiculopathy

An acute, progressive lumbosacral polyradiculoneuropathy usually secondary to cytomegalovirus (CMV) infection can develop in patients with AIDS. Patients present with severe radicular pain, numbness, and weakness in the legs, which is usually asymmetric. CSF is abnormal, demonstrating an increased protein along with reduced glucose concentration and notably a neutrophilic pleocytosis. EDx studies reveal features of active axonal degeneration. The polyradiculoneuropathy may improve with antiviral therapy.

HIV-related multiple mononeuropathies

Multiple mononeuropathies can also develop in patients with HIV infection, usually in the context of AIDS. Weakness, numbness, paresthesias, and pain occur in the distribution of affected nerves. Nerve biopsies can reveal axonal degeneration with necrotizing vasculitis or perivascular inflammation. Glucocorticoid treatment is indicated for vasculitis directly due to HIV infection.

HIV-related sensory neuronopathy/ganglionopathy

Dorsal root ganglionitis is a very rare complication of HIV infection, and neuronopathy can be the presenting manifestation. Patients develop sensory ataxia similar to idiopathic sensory neuronopathy/ganglionopathy. NCS reveal reduced amplitudes or absence of SNAPs.

HERPES VARICELLA-ZOSTER VIRUS

Peripheral neuropathy from Herpes varicella-zoster (HVZ) infection results from reactivation of latent virus or from a primary infection (Chap. 180). Two-thirds of infections in adults are characterized by dermal zoster in which severe pain and paresthesias develop in a dermatomal region followed within a week or two by a vesicular rash in the same distribution. Weakness in muscles innervated by roots corresponding to the dermatomal distribution of skin lesions occurs in 5–30% of patients. Approximately 25% of affected patients have continued pain (postherpetic neuralgia, or PHN). A large clinical trial demonstrated that vaccination against zoster reduces the incidence of HZ among vaccine recipients by 51% and reduces the incidence of PHN by 67%. Treatment of postherpetic neuralgia is symptomatic (Table 384-6).

CYTOMEGALOVIRUS

CMV can cause an acute lumbosacral polyradiculopathy and multiple mononeuropathies in patients with HIV infection and in other immune deficiency conditions (Chap. 182).

EPSTEIN-BARR VIRUS

Epstein-Barr virus (EBV) infection has been associated with GBS, cranial neuropathies, mononeuropathy multiplex, brachial plexopathy, lumbosacral radiculoplexopathy, and sensory neuronopathies (Chap. 181).

HEPATITIS VIRUSES

Hepatitis B and C can cause multiple mononeuropathies related to vasculitis, AIDP, or CIDP (Chap. 306).

NEUROPATHIES ASSOCIATED WITH MALIGNANCY

Patients with malignancy can develop neuropathies due to (1) a direct effect of the cancer by invasion or compression of the nerves, (2) remote or paraneoplastic effect, (3) a toxic effect of treatment, or (4) as a consequence of immune compromise caused by immunosuppressive medications. The most common associated malignancy is lung cancer, but neuropathies also complicate carcinoma of the breast, ovaries, stomach, colon, rectum, and other organs, including the lymphoproliferative system.

PARANEOPLASTIC SENSORY NEURONOPATHY/GANGLIONOPATHY

Paraneoplastic encephalomyelitis/sensory neuronopathy (PEM/SN) usually complicates small cell lung carcinoma (Chap. 101). Patients usually present with numbness and paresthesias in the distal extremities that are often asymmetric. The onset can be acute or insidiously progressive. Prominent loss of proprioception leads to sensory ataxia. Weakness can be present, usually secondary to an associated myelitis, motor neuronopathy, or concurrent Lambert-Eaton myasthenic syndrome (LEMS). Many patients also develop confusion, memory loss, depression, hallucinations or seizures, or cerebellar ataxia. Polyclonal antineuronal antibodies (IgG) directed against a 35- to 40-kD protein or complex of proteins, the so-called Hu antigen, are found in the sera or CSF in the majority of patients with paraneoplastic PEM/SN. CSF may be normal or may demonstrate mild lymphocytic pleocytosis and elevated protein. PEM/SN is probably the result of antigenic similarity between proteins expressed in the tumor cells and neuronal cells, leading to an immune response directed against both cell types. Treatment of the underlying cancer generally does not affect the course of PEM/SN. However, occasional patients may improve following treatment of the tumor. Unfortunately, plasmapheresis, intravenous immunoglobulin, and immunosuppressive agents have not shown benefit.

NEUROPATHY SECONDARY TO TUMOR INFILTRATION

Malignant cells, in particular leukemia and lymphoma, can infiltrate cranial and peripheral nerves, leading to mononeuropathy, mononeuropathy multiplex, polyradiculopathy, plexopathy, or even a generalized symmetric distal or proximal and distal polyneuropathy. Neuropathy related to tumor infiltration is often painful; it can be the presenting manifestation of the cancer or the heralding symptom of a relapse. The neuropathy may improve with treatment of the underlying leukemia or lymphoma or with glucocorticoids.

NEUROPATHY AS A COMPLICATION OF BONE MARROW TRANSPLANTATION

Neuropathies may develop in patients who undergo bone marrow transplantation (BMT) because of the toxic effects of chemotherapy, radiation, infection, or an autoimmune response directed against the peripheral nerves. Peripheral neuropathy in BMT is often associated with graft-versus-host disease (GVHD). Chronic GVHD shares many features with a variety of autoimmune disorders, and it is possible that an immune-mediated response directed against peripheral nerves is responsible. Patients with chronic GVHD may develop cranial neuropathies, sensorimotor polyneuropathies, multiple mononeuropathies, and severe generalized peripheral neuropathies resembling AIDP or CIDP. The neuropathy may improve by increasing the intensity of immunosuppressive or immunomodulating therapy and resolution of the GVHD.

LYMPHOMA

Lymphomas may cause neuropathy by infiltration or direct compression of nerves or by a paraneoplastic process. The neuropathy can be purely sensory or motor, but most commonly is sensorimotor. The pattern of involvement may be symmetric, asymmetric, or multifocal, and the course may be acute, gradually progressive, or relapsing and remitting. EDx can be compatible with either an axonal or demyelinating process. CSF may reveal lymphocytic pleocytosis and an elevated protein. Nerve biopsy may demonstrate endoneurial inflammatory cells in both the infiltrative and the paraneoplastic etiologies. A monoclonal population of cells favors lymphomatous invasion. The neuropathy may respond to treatment of the underlying lymphoma or immunomodulating therapies.

MULTIPLE MYELOMA

Multiple myeloma (MM) usually presents in the fifth to seventh decade of life with fatigue, bone pain, anemia, and hypercalcemia (Chap 111). Clinical and EDx features of neuropathy occur in as many as 40% of patients. The most common pattern is that of a distal, axonal, sensory, or sensorimotor polyneuropathy. Less frequently, a chronic demyelinating polyradiculoneuropathy may develop (see POEMS, Chap. 385). MM can be complicated by amyloid polyneuropathy and should be considered in patients with painful paresthesias, loss of pinprick and temperature discrimination, and autonomic dysfunction (suggestive of a small-fiber neuropathy) and carpal tunnel syndrome. Expanding plasmacytomas can compress cranial nerves and spinal roots as well. A monoclonal protein, usually composed of γ or μ heavy chains or κ light chains, may be identified in the serum or urine. EDx usually shows reduced amplitudes with normal or only mildly abnormal distal latencies and conduction velocities. A superimposed median neuropathy at the wrist is common. Abdominal fat pad, rectal, or sural nerve biopsy can be performed to look for amyloid deposition. Unfortunately, the treatment of the underlying MM does not usually affect the course of the neuropathy.

NEUROPATHIES ASSOCIATED WITH MONOCLONAL GAMMOPATHY OF UNCERTAIN SIGNIFICANCE (SEE CHAP. 375)

Toxic neuropathies secondary to chemotherapy

Many of the commonly used chemotherapy agents can cause a toxic neuropathy (Table 384-7). The mechanisms by which these agents cause toxic neuropathies vary as can the specific type of neuropathy produced. The risk of developing a toxic neuropathy or more severe neuropathy appears to be greater in patients with a preexisting neuropathy (e.g., Charcot-Marie-Tooth disease, diabetic neuropathy) and those who also take other potentially neurotoxic drugs (e.g., nitrofurantoin, isoniazid, disulfiram, pyridoxine). Chemotherapeutic agents usually cause a sensory greater than motor length-dependent axonal neuropathy or neuronopathy/ganglionopathy.

OTHER TOXIC NEUROPATHIES

Neuropathies can develop as complications of toxic effects of various drugs and other environmental exposures (Table 384-8). The more common neuropathies associated with these agents are discussed here.

CHLOROQUINE AND HYDROXYCHLOROQUINE

Chloroquine and hydroxychloroquine can cause a toxic myopathy characterized by slowly progressive, painless, proximal weakness and atrophy, which is worse in the legs than the arms. In addition, neuropathy can also develop with or without the myopathy leading to sensory loss and distal weakness. The "neuromyopathy" usually appears in patients taking 500 mg daily for a year or more but has been reported with doses as low as 200 mg/d. Serum CK levels are usually elevated due to the superimposed myopathy. NCS reveal mild slowing of motor and sensory nerve conduction velocities with a mild to moderate reduction in the amplitudes, although NCS may be normal in patients with only the myopathy. EMG demonstrates myopathic muscle action potentials (MUAPs), increased insertional activity in the form of positive sharp waves, fibrillation potentials, and occasionally myotonic potentials, particularly in the proximal muscles. Neurogenic MUAPs and reduced recruitment are found in more distal muscles. Nerve biopsy demonstrates autophagic vacuoles within Schwann cells. Vacuoles may also be evident in muscle biopsies. The pathogenic basis of the neuropathy is not known but may be related to the amphiphilic properties of the drug. These agents contain both hydrophobic and hydrophilic regions that allow them to interact with the anionic phospholipids of cell membranes and organelles. The drug-lipid complexes may be resistant to digestion by lysosomal enzymes, leading to the formation of autophagic vacuoles filled with myeloid debris that may in turn cause degeneration of nerves and muscle fibers. The signs and symptoms of the neuropathy and myopathy are usually reversible following discontinuation of medication.

AMIODARONE

Amiodarone can cause a neuromyopathy similar to chloroquine and hydroxychloroquine. The neuromyopathy typically appears after patients have taken the medication for 2–3 years. Nerve biopsy demonstrates a combination of segmental demyelination and axonal loss. Electron microscopy reveals lamellar or dense inclusions in Schwann cells, pericytes, and endothelial cells. The inclusions in muscle and nerve biopsies have persisted as long as 2 years following discontinuation of the medication.

COLCHICINE

Colchicine can also cause a neuromyopathy. Patients usually present with proximal weakness and numbness and tingling in the distal extremities. EDx reveals features of an axonal polyneuropathy. Muscle biopsy reveals a vacuolar myopathy, while sensory nerves demonstrate axonal degeneration. Colchicine inhibits the polymerization of tubulin into microtubules. The disruption of the microtubules probably leads to defective intracellular movement of important proteins, nutrients, and waste products in muscle and nerves.

THALIDOMIDE

Thalidomide is an immunomodulating agent used to treat multiple myeloma, GVHD, leprosy, and other autoimmune disorders. Thalidomide is associated with severe teratogenic effects as well as peripheral neuropathy that can be dose-limiting. Patients develop numbness, painful tingling, and burning discomfort in the feet and hands and less commonly muscle weakness and atrophy. Even after stopping the drug for 4–6 years, as many as 50% patients continue to have significant symptoms. NCS demonstrate reduced amplitudes or complete absence of sensory nerve action potentials (SNAPs), with preserved conduction velocities when obtainable. Motor NCS are usually normal. Nerve biopsy reveals a loss of large-diameter myelinated fibers and axonal degeneration. Degeneration of dorsal root ganglion cells has been reported at autopsy.

PYRIDOXINE (VITAMIN B_6) TOXICITY

Pyridoxine is an essential vitamin that serves as a coenzyme for transamination and decarboxylation. However, at high doses (116 mg/d), patients can develop a severe sensory neuropathy with dysesthesias and sensory ataxia. NCS reveal absent or markedly reduced SNAP amplitudes with relatively preserved CMAPs. Nerve biopsy

TABLE 384-7 Toxic Neuropathies Secondary to Chemotherapy

Drug	Mechanism of Neurotoxicity	Clinical Features	Nerve Histopathology	EMG/NCS
Vinca alkaloids (vincristine, vinblastine, vindesine, vinorelbine)	Interfere with axonal microtubule assembly; impairs axonal transport	Symmetric, S-M, large-/small-fiber PN; autonomic symptoms common; infrequent cranial neuropathies	Axonal degeneration of myelinated and unmyelinated fibers; regenerating clusters, minimal segmental demyelination	Axonal sensorimotor PN; distal denervation on EMG; abnormal QST, particularly vibratory perception
Cisplatin	Preferential damage to dorsal root ganglia: ? binds to and cross-links DNA ? inhibits protein synthesis ? impairs axonal transport	Predominant large-fiber sensory neuronopathy; sensory ataxia	Loss of large > small myelinated and unmyelinated fibers; axonal degeneration with small clusters of regenerating fibers; secondary segmental demyelination	Low-amplitude or unobtainable SNAPs with normal CMAPs and EMG; abnormal QST, particularly vibratory perception
Taxanes (paclitaxel, docetaxel)	Promotes axonal microtubule assembly; interferes with axonal transport	Symmetric, predominantly sensory, PN; large-fiber modalities affected more than small-fiber	Loss of large > small myelinated and unmyelinated fibers; axonal degeneration with small clusters of regenerating fibers; secondary segmental demyelination	Axonal sensorimotor PN; distal denervation on EMG; abnormal QST, particularly vibratory perception
Suramin				
Axonal PN	Unknown; ? inhibition of neurotrophic growth factor binding; ? neuronal lysosomal storage	Symmetric, length-dependent, sensory-predominant, PN	None described	Abnormalities consistent with an axonal S-M PN
Demyelinating PN	Unknown; ? immunomodulating effects	Subacute, S-M PN with diffuse proximal and distal weakness; areflexia; increased CSF protein	Loss of large and small myelinated fibers with primary demyelination and secondary axonal degeneration; occasional epi- and endoneurial inflammatory cell infiltrates	Features suggestive of an acquired demyelinating sensorimotor PN (e.g., slow CVs, prolonged distal latencies and F-wave latencies, conduction block, temporal dispersion)
ARA-C	Unknown; ? selective Schwann cell toxicity; ? immunomodulating effects	GBS-like syndrome; pure sensory neuropathy; brachial plexopathy	Loss of myelinated nerve fibers; axonal degeneration; segmental demyelination; no inflammation	Axonal, demyelinating, or mixed S-M PN; denervation on EMG
Etoposide (VP-16)	Unknown; ? selective dorsal root ganglia toxicity	Length-dependent, sensory predominant PN; autonomic neuropathy	None described	Abnormalities consistent with an axonal S-M PN
Bortezomib (Velcade)	Unknown	Length-dependent, sensory, predominantly small-fiber, PN	Not reported	Abnormalities consistent with an axonal sensory neuropathy with early small-fiber involvement (abnormal autonomic studies)

Abbreviations: CSF, cerebrospinal fluid; CVs, conduction velocities; EMG, electromyography; GBS, Guillain-Barré syndrome; NCS, nerve conduction studies; PN, polyneuropathy; QST, quantitative sensory testing; S-M, sensorimotor.

Source: From Amato and Russell.

reveals axonal loss of fiber at all diameters. Loss of dorsal root ganglion cells with subsequent degeneration of both the peripheral and central sensory tracts have been reported in animal models.

ISONIAZID

One of the most common side effects of isoniazid (INH) is peripheral neuropathy. Standard doses of INH (3–5 mg/kg per d) are associated with a 2% incidence of neuropathy, while neuropathy develops in at least 17% of patients taking in excess of 6 mg/kg per d. The elderly, malnourished, and "slow acetylators" are at increased risk for developing the neuropathy. INH inhibits pyridoxal phosphokinase, resulting in pyridoxine deficiency and the neuropathy. Prophylactic administration of pyridoxine 100 mg/d can prevent the neuropathy from developing.

TABLE 384-8 Toxic Neuropathies

Drug	Mechanism of Neurotoxicity	Clinical Features	Nerve Histopathology	EMG/NCS
Misonidazole	Unknown	Painful paresthesias and loss of large- and small-fiber sensory modalities and sometimes distal weakness in length-dependent pattern	Axonal degeneration of large myelinated fibers; axonal swellings; segmental demyelination	Low-amplitude or unobtainable SNAPs with normal or only slightly reduced CMAPs amplitudes
Metronidazole	Unknown	Painful paresthesias and loss of large- and small-fiber sensory modalities and sometimes distal weakness in length-dependent pattern	Axonal degeneration	Low-amplitude or unobtainable SNAPs with normal CMAPs
Chloroquine and hydroxychloroquine	Amphiphilic properties may lead to drug-lipid complexes that are indigestible and result in accumulation of autophagic vacuoles	Loss of large- and small-fiber sensory modalities and distal weakness in length-dependent pattern; superimposed myopathy may lead to proximal weakness	Axonal degeneration with autophagic vacuoles in nerves as well as muscle fibers	Low-amplitude or unobtainable SNAPs with normal or reduced CMAPs amplitudes; distal denervation on EMG; irritability and myopathic-appearing MUAPs proximally in patients with superimposed toxic myopathy
Amiodarone	Amphiphilic properties may lead to drug-lipid complexes that are indigestible and result in accumulation of autophagic vacuoles	Paresthesias and pain with loss of large- and small-fiber sensory modalities and distal weakness in length-dependent pattern; superimposed myopathy may lead to proximal weakness	Axonal degeneration and segmental demyelination with myeloid inclusions in nerves and muscle fibers	Low-amplitude or unobtainable SNAPs with normal or reduced CMAPs amplitudes; can also have prominent slowing of CVs; distal denervation on EMG; irritability and myopathic-appearing MUAPs proximally in patients with superimposed toxic myopathy
Colchicine	Inhibits polymerization of tubulin in microtubules and impairs axoplasmic flow	Numbness and paresthesias with loss of large-fiber modalities in a length-dependent fashion; superimposed myopathy may lead to proximal in addition to distal weakness	Nerve biopsy demonstrates axonal degeneration; muscle biopsy reveals fibers with vacuoles	Low-amplitude or unobtainable SNAPs with normal or reduced CMAPs amplitudes; irritability and myopathic-appearing MUAPs proximally in patients with superimposed toxic myopathy
Podophyllin	Binds to microtubules and impairs axoplasmic flow	Sensory loss, tingling, muscle weakness, and diminished muscle stretch reflexes in length-dependent pattern; autonomic neuropathy	Axonal degeneration	Low-amplitude or unobtainable SNAPs with normal or reduced CMAPs amplitudes
Thalidomide	Unknown	Numbness, tingling, and burning pain and weakness in a length-dependent pattern	Axonal degeneration; autopsy studies reveal degeneration of dorsal root ganglia	Low-amplitude or unobtainable SNAPs with normal or reduced CMAPs amplitudes
Disulfiram	Accumulation of neurofilaments and impaired axoplasmic flow	Numbness, tingling, and burning pain in a length-dependent pattern	Axonal degeneration with accumulation of neurofilaments in the axons	Low-amplitude or unobtainable SNAPs with normal or reduced CMAPs amplitudes
Dapsone	Unknown	Distal weakness that may progress to proximal muscles; sensory loss	Axonal degeneration and segmental demyelination	Low-amplitude or unobtainable CMAPs with normal or reduced SNAP amplitudes
Leflunomide	Unknown	Paresthesias and numbness in a length-dependent pattern	Unknown	Low-amplitude or unobtainable SNAPs with normal or reduced CMAPs amplitudes

(*continued*)

TABLE 384-8 Toxic Neuropathies (*Continued*)

Drug	Mechanism of Neurotoxicity	Clinical Features	Nerve Histopathology	EMG/NCS
Nitrofurantoin	Unknown	Numbness, painful paresthesias, and severe weakness that may resemble GBS	Axonal degeneration; autopsy studies reveal degeneration of dorsal root ganglia and anterior horn cells	Low-amplitude or unobtainable SNAPs with normal or reduced CMAPs amplitudes
Pyridoxine (vitamin B_6)	Unknown	Dysesthesias and sensory ataxia; impaired large-fiber sensory modalities on examination	Marked loss of sensory axons and cell bodies in dorsal root ganglia	Reduced amplitudes or absent SNAPs
Isoniazid	Inhibits pyridoxal phosphokinase leading to pyridoxine deficiency	Dysesthesias and sensory ataxia; impaired large-fiber sensory modalities on examination	Marked loss of sensory axons and cell bodies in dorsal root ganglia and degeneration of the dorsal columns	Reduced amplitudes or absent SNAPs and to lesser extent CMAPs
Ethambutol	Unknown	Numbness with loss of large-fiber modalities on examination	Axonal degeneration	Reduced amplitudes or absent SNAPs
Antinucleosides	Unknown	Dysesthesia and sensory ataxia; impaired large-fiber sensory modalities on examination	Axonal degeneration	Reduced amplitudes or absent SNAPs
Phenytoin	Unknown	Numbness with loss of large-fiber modalities on examination	Axonal degeneration and segmental demyelination	Low-amplitude or unobtainable SNAPs with normal or reduced CMAPs amplitudes
Lithium	Unknown	Numbness with loss of large-fiber modalities on examination	Axonal degeneration	Low-amplitude or unobtainable SNAPs with normal or reduced CMAPs amplitudes
Acrylamide	Unknown; may be caused by impaired axonal transport	Numbness with loss of large-fiber modalities on examination; sensory ataxia; mild distal weakness	Degeneration of sensory axons in peripheral nerves and posterior columns, spinocerebellar tracts, mammillary bodies, optic tracts, and corticospinal tracts in the CNS	Low-amplitude or unobtainable SNAPs with normal or reduced CMAPs amplitudes
Carbon disulfide	Unknown	Length-dependent numbness and tingling with mild distal weakness	Axonal swellings with accumulation of neurofilaments	Low-amplitude or unobtainable SNAPs with normal or reduced CMAPs amplitudes
Ethylene oxide	Unknown; may act as alkylating agent and bind DNA	Length-dependent numbness and tingling; may have mild distal weakness	Axonal degeneration	Low-amplitude or unobtainable SNAPs with normal or reduced CMAPs amplitudes
Organophosphates	Bind and inhibit neuropathy target esterase	Early features are those of neuromuscular blockade with generalized weakness; later axonal sensorimotor PN ensues	Axonal degeneration along with degeneration of gracile fasciculus and corticospinal tracts	Early: repetitive firing of CMAPs and decrement with repetitive nerve stimulation; late: axonal sensorimotor PN
Hexacarbons	Unknown; may lead to covalent cross-linking between neurofilaments	Acute, severe sensorimotor PN that may resemble GBS	Axonal degeneration and giant axons swollen with neurofilaments	Features of a mixed axonal and/or demyelinating sensorimotor axonal PN—reduced amplitudes, prolonged distal latencies, conduction block, and slowing of CVs

(*continued*)

TABLE 384-8 Toxic Neuropathies (*Continued*)

Drug	Mechanism of Neurotoxicity	Clinical Features	Nerve Histopathology	EMG/NCS
Lead	Unknown; may interfere with mitochondria	Encephalopathy; motor neuropathy (often resembles radial neuropathy with wrist and finger drop); autonomic neuropathy; bluish-black discoloration of gums	Axonal degeneration of motor axons	Reduction of CMAP amplitudes with active denervation on EMG
Mercury	Unknown; may combine with sulfhydryl groups	Abdominal pain and nephrotic syndrome; encephalopathy; ataxia; paresthesias	Axonal degeneration; degeneration of dorsal root ganglia, calcarine, and cerebellar cortex	Low-amplitude or unobtainable SNAPs with normal or reduced CMAPs amplitudes
Thallium	Unknown	Encephalopathy; painful sensory symptoms; mild loss of vibration; distal or generalized weakness may also develop; autonomic neuropathy; alopecia	Axonal degeneration	Low-amplitude or unobtainable SNAPs with normal or reduced CMAPs amplitudes
Arsenic	Unknown; may combine with sulfhydryl groups	Abdominal discomfort, burning pain and paresthesias; generalized weakness; autonomic insufficiency; can resemble GBS	Axonal degeneration	Low-amplitude or unobtainable SNAPs with normal or reduced CMAPs amplitudes; may have demyelinating features: prolonged distal latencies and slowing of CVs
Gold	Unknown	Distal paresthesias and reduction of all sensory modalities	Axonal degeneration	Low-amplitude or unobtainable SNAPs

Abbreviations: CMAP, compound motor action potential; CVs, conduction velocities; EMG, electromyography; GBS, Guillain-Barré syndrome; MUAP, muscle action potential; NCS, nerve conduction studies; PN, polyneuropathy; S-M, sensorimotor; SNAP, sensory nerve action potential.

Source: From Amato and Russell.

ANTIRETROVIRAL AGENTS

The nucleoside analogues zalcitabine (dideoxycytidine or ddC), didanosine (dideoxyinosine or ddI), stavudine (d4T), lamivudine (3TC), and antiretroviral nucleoside reverse transcriptase inhibitor (NRTI) are used to treat HIV infection. One of the major dose-limiting side effects of these medications is a predominantly sensory, length-dependent, symmetrically painful neuropathy. Zalcitabine (ddC) is the most extensively studied of the nucleoside analogues and at doses greater than 0.18 mg/kg per d is associated with a subacute onset of severe burning and lancinating pains in the feet and hands. NCS reveal decreased amplitudes of the SNAPs with normal motor studies. The nucleoside analogues inhibit mitochondrial DNA polymerase, which is the suspected pathogenic basis for the neuropathy. Because of a "coasting effect," patients can continue to worsen even 2–3 weeks after stopping the medication. Following dose reduction, improvement in the neuropathy is seen in most patients after several months (mean time about 10 weeks).

HEXACARBONS (*n*-HEXANE, METHYL *n*-BUTYL KETONE)/GLUE SNIFFER'S NEUROPATHY

n-Hexane and methyl *n*-butyl ketone are water-insoluble industrial organic solvents that are also present in some glues. Exposure through inhalation, accidentally or intentionally (glue sniffing), or through skin absorption can lead to a profound subacute sensory and motor polyneuropathy. NCS demonstrate decreased amplitudes of the SNAPs and CMAPs with slightly slow CVs. Nerve biopsy reveals a loss of myelinated fibers and giant axons that are filled with 10-nm neurofilaments. Hexacarbon exposure leads to covalent cross-linking between axonal neurofilaments that result in their aggregation, impaired axonal transport, swelling of the axons, and eventual axonal degeneration.

LEAD

Lead neuropathy is uncommon but it can be seen in children who accidentally ingest lead-based paints in older buildings and in industrial workers exposed to lead-containing products. The most common presentation of lead poisoning is an encephalopathy; however, symptoms and signs of a primarily motor neuropathy can also occur. The neuropathy is characterized by an insidious and progressive onset of weakness usually beginning in the arms, in particular involving the wrist and finger extensors, resembling a radial neuropathy. Sensation is generally preserved; however, the autonomic nervous system can be affected. Laboratory investigation can reveal a microcytic hypochromic anemia with basophilic stippling of erythrocytes, an elevated serum lead level, and an elevated serum coproporphyrin level. A 24-h urine collection demonstrates elevated levels of lead excretion. The NCS may reveal reduced CMAP amplitudes, while the SNAPs are typically normal. The pathogenic basis may be related to abnormal porphyrin metabolism. The most important principle of management is to remove the source of the exposure. Chelation therapy with calcium disodium ethylenediaminetetraacetic acid (EDTA), British anti-Lewisite (BAL), and penicillamine also demonstrates variable efficacy.

MERCURY

Mercury toxicity may occur as a result of exposure to either organic or inorganic mercurials. Mercury poisoning presents with paresthesias in hands and feet that progress proximally and may involve the face and tongue. Motor weakness can also develop. CNS symptoms often overshadow the neuropathy. EDx shows features of a primarily axonal sensorimotor polyneuropathy. The primary site of neuromuscular pathology appears to be the dorsal root ganglia. The mainstay of treatment is removing the source of exposure.

THALLIUM

Thallium can exist in a monovalent or trivalent form and is primarily used as a rodenticide. The toxic neuropathy usually manifests as burning paresthesias of the feet, abdominal pain, and vomiting. Increased thirst, sleep disturbances, and psychotic behavior may be noted. Within the first week, patients develop pigmentation of the hair, an acne-like rash in the malar area of the face, and hyperreflexia. By the second and third week, autonomic instability with labile heart rate and blood pressure may be seen. Hyporeflexia and alopecia also occur but may not be evident until the third or fourth week following exposure. With severe intoxication, proximal weakness and involvement of the cranial nerves can occur. Some patients require mechanical ventilation due to respiratory muscle involvement. The lethal dose of thallium is variable, ranging from 8 to 15 mg/kg body weight. Death can result in less than 48 h following a particularly large dose. NCS demonstrate features of a primarily axonal sensorimotor polyneuropathy. With acute intoxication, potassium ferric ferrocyanide II may be effective in preventing absorption of thallium from the gut. However, there may be no benefit once thallium has been absorbed. Unfortunately, chelating agents are not very efficacious. Adequate diuresis is essential to help eliminate thallium from the body without increasing tissue availability from the serum.

ARSENIC

Arsenic is another heavy metal that can cause a toxic sensorimotor polyneuropathy. The neuropathy manifests 5–10 days after ingestion of arsenic and progresses for several weeks, sometimes mimicking GBS. The presenting symptoms are typically an abrupt onset of abdominal discomfort, nausea, vomiting, pain, and diarrhea followed within several days by burning pain in the feet and hands. Examination of the skin can be helpful in the diagnosis as the loss of the superficial epidermal layer results in patchy regions of increased or decreased pigmentation on the skin several weeks after an acute exposure or with chronic low levels of ingestion. Mee's lines, which are transverse lines at the base of the fingernails and toenails, do not become evident until 1 or 2 months after the exposure. Multiple Mee's lines may be seen in patients with long fingernails who have had chronic exposure to arsenic. Mee's lines are not specific for arsenic toxicity as they can also be seen following thallium poisoning. Because arsenic is cleared from blood rapidly, the serum concentration of arsenic is not diagnostically helpful. However, arsenic levels are increased in the urine, hair, and fingernails of patients exposed to arsenic. Anemia with stippling of erythrocytes is common, and occasionally pancytopenia and aplastic anemia can develop. Increased CSF protein levels without pleocytosis can be seen; this can lead to misdiagnosis as GBS. NCS are usually suggestive of an axonal sensorimotor polyneuropathy; however, demyelinating features can be present. Chelation therapy with BAL has yielded inconsistent results; therefore, it is not generally recommended.

NUTRITIONAL NEUROPATHIES

COBALAMIN (VITAMIN B_{12})

Pernicious anemia is the most common cause of cobalamin deficiency. Other causes include dietary avoidance (vegetarians), gastrectomy, gastric bypass surgery, inflammatory bowel disease, pancreatic insufficiency, bacterial overgrowth, and possibly histamine-2 blockers and proton-pump inhibitors. An underappreciated cause of cobalamin deficiency is food-cobalamin malabsorption. This typically occurs in older individuals and results from an inability to adequately absorb cobalamin in food protein. No apparent cause of deficiency is identified in a significant number of patients with cobalamin deficiency. The use of nitrous oxide as an anesthetic agent or from recreational use can produce acute cobalamin deficiency neuropathy and subacute combined degeneration.

Complaints of numb hands typically appear before lower extremity paresthesias are noted. A preferential large-fiber sensory loss affecting proprioception and vibration with sparing of small-fiber modalities is present; an unsteady gait reflects sensory ataxia. These features, coupled with diffuse hyperreflexia and absent Achilles reflexes, should always focus attention on the possibility of cobalamin deficiency. Optic atrophy and, in severe cases, behavioral changes ranging from mild irritability and forgetfulness to severe dementia and frank psychosis may appear. The full clinical picture of subacute combined degeneration is uncommon. CNS manifestations, especially pyramidal tract signs, may be missing, and in fact some patients may only exhibit symptoms of peripheral neuropathy.

EDx shows an axonal sensorimotor neuropathy. CNS involvement produces abnormal somatosensory and visual evoked potential latencies. The diagnosis is confirmed by finding reduced serum cobalamin levels. In up to 40% of patients, anemia and macrocytosis are lacking. Serum methylmalonic acid and homocysteine, the metabolites that accumulate when cobalamin-dependent reactions are blocked, are elevated. Antibodies to intrinsic factor are present in approximately 60%, and antiparietal cell antibodies in about 90%, of individuals with pernicious anemia.

Cobalamin deficiency can be treated with various regimens of cobalamin. One typical regimen consists of 1000 μg cyanocobalamin IM weekly for 1 month and monthly thereafter. Patients with food cobalamin malabsorption can absorb free cobalamin and therefore can be treated with oral cobalamin supplementation. An oral cobalamin dose of 1000 μg per day should be sufficient. Treatment for cobalamin deficiency usually does not completely reverse the clinical manifestations, and at least 50% of patients exhibit some permanent neurologic deficit.

THIAMINE DEFICIENCY

Thiamine (vitamin B_1) deficiency is an uncommon cause of peripheral neuropathy in developed countries. It is now most often seen as a consequence of chronic alcohol abuse, recurrent vomiting, total parenteral nutrition, and bariatric surgery. Thiamine deficiency polyneuropathy can occur in normal, healthy young adults who do not abuse alcohol but who engage in inappropriately restrictive diets. Thiamine is water-soluble. It is present in most animal and plant tissues, but the greatest sources are unrefined cereal grains, wheat germ, yeast, soybean flour, and pork. Beriberi means "I can't, I can't" in Singhalese, the language of natives of what was once part of the Dutch East Indies (now Sri Lanka). *Dry beriberi* refers to neuropathic symptoms. The term *wet beriberi* is used when cardiac manifestations predominate (in reference to edema). Beriberi was relatively uncommon until the late 1800s when it became widespread among people for whom rice was a dietary mainstay. This epidemic was due to a new technique of processing rice that removed the germ from the rice shaft, rendering the so-called polished rice deficient in thiamine and other essential nutrients.

Symptoms of neuropathy follow prolonged deficiency. These begin with mild sensory loss and/or burning dysesthesias in the toes and feet and aching and cramping in the lower legs. Pain may be the predominant symptom. With progression, patients develop features of a nonspecific generalized polyneuropathy, with distal sensory loss in the feet and hands.

Blood and urine assays for thiamine are not reliable for diagnosis of deficiency. Erythrocyte transketolase activity and the percentage increase in activity (in vitro) following the addition of thiamine pyrophosphate (TPP) may be more accurate and reliable. EDx shows nonspecific findings of an axonal sensorimotor polyneuropathy. When a diagnosis of thiamine deficiency is made or suspected, thiamine replacement should be provided until proper nutrition is restored. Thiamine is usually given intravenously or intramuscularly at a dose of 100 mg/d. Although cardiac manifestations show a striking response to thiamine replacement, neurologic improvement is usually more variable and less dramatic.

VITAMIN E DEFICIENCY

The term *vitamin E* is usually used for α-tocopherol, the most active of the four main types of vitamin E. Because vitamin E is present in animal fat, vegetable oils, and various grains, deficiency is usually due to factors other than insufficient intake. Vitamin E deficiency usually occurs secondary to lipid malabsorption or in uncommon disorders of vitamin E transport. One hereditary disorder is abetalipoproteinemia, a rare autosomal dominant disorder characterized by steatorrhea, pigmentary retinopathy, acanthocytosis, and progressive ataxia. Patients with cystic fibrosis may also have vitamin E deficiency secondary to steatorrhea. There are genetic forms of isolated vitamin E deficiency not associated with lipid malabsorption. Vitamin E deficiency may also occur as a consequence of various cholestatic and hepatobiliary disorders as well as short-bowel syndromes resulting from the surgical treatment of intestinal disorders.

Clinical features may not appear until many years after the onset of deficiency. The onset of symptoms tends to be insidious, and progression is slow. The main clinical features are spinocerebellar ataxia and polyneuropathy, thus resembling Friedreich ataxia or other spinocerebellar ataxias. Patients manifest progressive ataxia and signs of posterior column dysfunction, such as impaired joint position and vibratory sensation. Because of the polyneuropathy, there is hyporeflexia, but plantar responses may be extensor as a result of the spinal cord involvement. Other neurologic manifestations may include ophthalmoplegia, pigmented retinopathy, night blindness, dysarthria, pseudoathetosis, dystonia, and tremor. Vitamin E deficiency may present as an isolated polyneuropathy, but this is very rare. The yield of checking serum vitamin E levels in patients with isolated polyneuropathy is extremely low, and this test should not be part of routine practice.

Diagnosis is made by measuring α-tocopherol levels in the serum. EDx shows features of an axonal neuropathy. Treatment is replacement with oral vitamin E, but high doses are not needed. For patients with isolated vitamin E deficiency, treatment consists of 1500–6000 IU/d in divided doses.

VITAMIN B_6 DEFICIENCY

Vitamin B_6, or pyridoxine, can produce neuropathic manifestations from both deficiency and toxicity. Vitamin B_6 toxicity was discussed above. Vitamin B_6 deficiency is most commonly seen in patients treated with isoniazid or hydralazine. The polyneuropathy of vitamin B_6 is nonspecific, manifesting as a generalized axonal sensorimotor polyneuropathy. Vitamin B_6 deficiency can be detected by direct assay. Vitamin B_6 supplementation with 50–100 mg/d is suggested for patients being treated with isoniazid or hydralazine. This same dose is appropriate for replacement in cases of nutritional deficiency.

PELLAGRA (NIACIN DEFICIENCY)

Pellagra is produced by deficiency of niacin. Although pellagra may be seen in alcoholics, this disorder has essentially been eradicated in most Western countries by means of enriching bread with niacin. Nevertheless, pellagra continues to be a problem in a number of underdeveloped regions, particularly in Asia and Africa, where corn is the main source of carbohydrate. Neurologic manifestations are variable; abnormalities can develop in the brain and spinal cord as well as peripheral nerves. When peripheral nerves are involved, the neuropathy is usually mild and resembles beriberi. Treatment is with niacin 40–250 mg/d.

COPPER DEFICIENCY

A syndrome that has only recently been described is myeloneuropathy secondary to copper deficiency. Most patients present with lower limb paresthesias, weakness, spasticity, and gait difficulties. Large-fiber sensory function is impaired, reflexes are brisk, and plantar responses are extensor. In some cases, light touch and pinprick sensation are affected, and nerve conduction studies indicate sensorimotor axonal polyneuropathy in addition to myelopathy.

Hematologic abnormalities are a known complication of copper deficiency; these can include microcytic anemia, neutropenia, and occasionally pancytopenia. Because copper is absorbed in the stomach and proximal jejunum, many cases of copper deficiency are in the setting of prior gastric surgery. Excess zinc is an established cause of copper deficiency. Zinc upregulates enterocyte production of metallothionine, which results in decreased absorption of copper. Excessive dietary zinc supplements or denture cream containing zinc can produce this clinical picture. Other potential causes of copper deficiency include malnutrition, prematurity, total parenteral nutrition, and ingestion of copper chelating agents.

Following oral or IV copper replacement, some patients show neurologic improvement, but this may take many months or not occur at all. Replacement consists of oral copper sulfate or gluconate 2 mg one to three times a day. If oral copper replacement is not effective, elemental copper in the copper sulfate or copper chloride forms can be given as 2 mg IV daily for 3–5 days, then weekly for 1–2 months until copper levels normalize. Thereafter, oral daily copper therapy can be resumed. In contrast to the neurologic manifestations, most of the hematologic indices completely normalize in response to copper replacement therapy.

NEUROPATHY ASSOCIATED WITH GASTRIC SURGERY

Polyneuropathy may occur following gastric surgery for ulcer, cancer, or weight reduction. This usually occurs in the context of rapid, significant weight loss and recurrent, protracted vomiting. The clinical picture is one of acute or subacute sensory loss and weakness. Neuropathy following weight loss surgery usually occurs in the first several months after surgery. Weight reduction surgical procedures include gastrojejunostomy, gastric stapling, vertical banded gastroplasty, and gastrectomy with Roux-en-Y anastomosis. The initial manifestations are usually numbness and paresthesias in the feet. In many cases, no specific nutritional deficiency factor is identified.

Management consists of parenteral vitamin supplementation, especially including thiamine. Improvement has been observed following supplementation, parenteral nutritional support, and reversal of the surgical bypass. The duration and severity of deficits before identification and treatment of neuropathy are important predictors of final outcome.

CRYPTOGENIC (IDIOPATHIC) SENSORY AND SENSORIMOTOR POLYNEUROPATHY

CSPN is a diagnosis of exclusion, established after a careful medical, family, and social history; neurologic examination; and directed laboratory testing. Despite extensive evaluation, the cause of polyneuropathy in as many as 50% of all patients is idiopathic. CSPN should be considered a distinct diagnostic subset of peripheral neuropathy. The onset of CSPN is predominantly in the sixth and seventh decades. Patients complain of distal numbness, tingling, and often burning pain that invariably begins in the feet and may eventually involve the fingers and hands. Patients exhibit a distal sensory loss to pinprick, touch, and vibration in the toes and feet, and occasionally in the fingers. It is uncommon to see significant proprioception deficits, even though patients may complain of gait unsteadiness. However, tandem gait may be abnormal in a minority of cases. Neither subjective nor objective evidence of weakness is a prominent feature. Most patients have evidence of both large- and small-fiber loss on neurologic exam and EDx. Approximately 10% of patients have only evidence of small-fiber involvement. The ankle muscle stretch reflex is frequently absent, but in cases with predominantly small-fiber loss, this may be preserved. The EDx findings range from isolated sensory nerve action potential abnormalities (usually with loss of amplitude), to evidence for an axonal sensorimotor neuropathy, to a completely normal study (if primarily small fibers are involved). Therapy primarily involves the control of neuropathic pain (Table 384-6) if present. These drugs should not be used if the patient has only numbness and tingling but no pain.

Although no treatment is available that can reverse an idiopathic distal peripheral neuropathy, the prognosis is good. Progression often does not occur or is minimal, with sensory symptoms and signs progressing proximally up to the knees and elbows. The disorder does not lead to significant motor disability over time. The relatively benign course of this disorder should be explained to patients.

MONONEUROPATHIES/PLEXOPATHIES/RADICULOPATHIES

MEDIAN NEUROPATHY

CTS is a compression of the median nerve in the carpal tunnel at the wrist. The median nerve enters the hand through the carpal tunnel by coursing under the transverse carpal ligament. The symptoms of CTS consist of numbness and paresthesias variably in the thumb, index, middle, and half of the ring finger. At times, the paresthesias can include the entire hand and extend into the forearm or upper arm or can be isolated to one or two fingers. Pain is another common symptom and can be located in the hand and forearm and, at times, in the proximal arm. CTS is common and often misdiagnosed as thoracic outlet syndrome. The signs of CTS are decreased sensation in the median nerve distribution; reproduction of the sensation of tingling when a percussion hammer is tapped over the wrist (Tinel's sign) or the wrist is flexed for 30–60 s (Phalen's sign); and weakness of thumb opposition and abduction. EDx is extremely sensitive and shows slowing of sensory and, to a lesser extent, motor median potentials across the wrist. Treatment options consist of avoidance of precipitating activities; control of underlying systemic-associated conditions if present; nonsteroidal anti-inflammatory medications; neutral (volar) position wrist splints, especially for night use; glucocorticoid/anesthetic injection into the carpal tunnel; and surgical decompression by dividing the transverse carpal ligament. The surgical option should be considered if there is a poor response to nonsurgical treatments; if there is thenar muscle atrophy and/or weakness; and if there are significant denervation potentials on EMG.

Other proximal median neuropathies are very uncommon and include the pronator teres syndrome and anterior interosseous neuropathy. These often occur as a partial form of brachial plexitis.

ULNAR NEUROPATHY AT THE ELBOW—"CUBITAL TUNNEL SYNDROME"

The ulnar nerve passes through the condylar groove between the medial epicondyle and the olecranon. Symptoms consist of paresthesias, tingling, and numbness in the medial hand and half of the fourth and the entire fifth fingers, pain at the elbow or forearm, and weakness. Signs consist of decreased sensation in an ulnar distribution, Tinel's sign at the elbow, and weakness and atrophy of ulnar-innervated hand muscles. The Froment sign indicates thumb adductor weakness and consists of flexion of the thumb at the interphalangeal joint when attempting to oppose the thumb against the lateral border of the second digit. EDx may show slowing of ulnar motor nerve conduction velocity across the elbow with prolonged ulnar sensory latencies. Treatment consists of avoiding aggravating factors, using elbow pads, and surgery to decompress the nerve in the cubital tunnel. Ulnar neuropathies can also rarely occur at the wrist in the ulnar (Guyon) canal or in the hand, usually after trauma.

RADIAL NEUROPATHY

The radial nerve winds around the proximal humerus in the spiral groove and proceeds down the lateral arm and enters the forearm, dividing into the posterior interosseous nerve and superficial nerve. The symptoms and signs consist of wristdrop; finger extension weakness; thumb abduction weakness; and sensory loss in the dorsal web between the thumb and index finger. Triceps and brachioradialis strength is often normal, and triceps reflex is often intact. Most cases of radial neuropathy are transient compressive (neuropraxic) injuries that recover spontaneously in 6–8 weeks. If there has been prolonged compression and severe axonal damage, it may take several months to recover. Treatment consists of cock-up wrist and finger splints, avoiding further compression, and physical therapy to avoid flexion contracture. If there is no improvement in 2–3 weeks, an EDx study is recommended to confirm the clinical diagnosis and determine the degree of severity.

LATERAL FEMORAL CUTANEOUS NEUROPATHY (MERALGIA PARESTHETICA)

The lateral femoral cutaneous nerve arises from the upper lumbar plexus (spinal levels L2/3), crosses through the inguinal ligament near its attachment to the iliac bone, and supplies sensation to the anterior lateral thigh. The neuropathy affecting this nerve is also known as meralgia paresthetica. Symptoms and signs consist of paresthesias, numbness, and occasionally pain in the lateral thigh. Symptoms are increased by standing or walking and are relieved by sitting. There is normal strength and knee reflexes are intact. The diagnosis is clinical, and further tests usually are not performed. EDx is only needed to rule out lumbar plexopathy, radiculopathy, or femoral neuropathy. If the symptoms and signs are classic, electromyography is not necessary. Symptoms often resolve spontaneously over weeks or months, but the patient may be left with permanent numbness. Treatment consists of weight loss and avoiding tight belts. Analgesics in the form of a lidocaine patch, nonsteroidal agents, and occasionally medications for neuropathic pain, can be used (Table 384-6). Rarely, locally injecting the nerve with an anesthetic can be tried. There is no role for surgery.

FEMORAL NEUROPATHY

Femoral neuropathies can arise as complications of retroperitoneal hematoma, lithotomy positioning, hip arthroplasty or dislocation, iliac artery occlusion, femoral arterial procedures, infiltration by hematogenous malignancy, penetrating groin trauma, pelvic surgery including hysterectomy and renal transplantation, and diabetes (a partial form of lumbosacral diabetic plexopathy); some cases are idiopathic. Patients with femoral neuropathy have difficulty extending their knee and flexing the hip. Sensory symptoms occurring either on the anterior thigh and/or medial leg occur in only half of reported cases. A prominent painful component is the exception rather than the rule, may be delayed, and is often self-limited in nature. The quadriceps (patellar) reflex is diminished.

SCIATIC NEUROPATHY

Sciatic neuropathies commonly complicate hip arthroplasty, pelvic procedures in which patients are placed in a prolonged lithotomy position, trauma, hematomas, tumor infiltration, and vasculitis. In addition, many sciatic neuropathies are idiopathic. Weakness may involve all motions of the ankles and toes as well as flexion of the leg at the knee; abduction and extension of the thigh at the hip is spared. Sensory loss occurs in the entire foot and the distal lateral leg. The ankle jerk and on occasion the internal hamstring reflex are diminished or more typically absent on the affected side. The peroneal subdivision of the sciatic nerve is typically involved disproportionately to the tibial counterpart. Thus, patients may have only ankle dorsiflexion and eversion weakness with sparing of knee flexion, ankle inversion, and plantar flexion; these features can lead to misdiagnosis of a common peroneal neuropathy.

PERONEAL NEUROPATHY

The sciatic nerve divides at the distal femur into the tibial and peroneal nerve. The common peroneal nerve passes posterior and laterally around the fibular head, under the fibular tunnel. It then divides into the superficial peroneal nerve, which supplies the ankle evertor muscles and sensation over the anterolateral distal leg and dorsum of the foot, and the deep peroneal nerve, which supplies ankle dorsiflexors and toe extensor muscles and a small area of sensation dorsally in the area of the first and second toes.

Symptoms and signs consist of footdrop (ankle dorsiflexion, toe extension, and ankle eversion weakness) and variable sensory loss, which may involve the superficial and deep peroneal pattern. There is usually no pain. Onset may be on awakening in the morning. Peroneal neuropathy needs to be distinguished from L5 radiculopathy. In L5 radiculopathy, ankle invertors and evertors are weak and needle electromyography reveals denervation. EDx can help localize the lesion. Peroneal motor conduction velocity shows slowing and amplitude drop across the fibular head. Management consists of rapid weight loss and avoiding leg crossing. Footdrop is treated with an ankle brace. A knee pad can be worn over the lateral knee to avoid further compression. Most cases spontaneously resolve over weeks or months.

RADICULOPATHIES

Radiculopathies are most often due to compression from degenerative joint disease and herniated disks, but there are a number of unusual etiologies (Table 384-9). Degenerative spine disease affects a number of different structures, which narrow the diameter of the neural foramen or canal of the spinal column and compromise nerve root integrity; these are discussed in detail in Chap. 15.

TABLE 384-9 Causes of Radiculopathy

- Herniated nucleus pulposus
- Degenerative joint disease
- Rheumatoid arthritis
- Trauma
- Vertebral body compression fracture
- Pott disease
- Compression by extradural mass (e.g., meningioma, metastatic tumor, hematoma, abscess)
- Primary nerve tumor (e.g., neurofibroma, schwannoma, neurinoma)
- Carcinomatous meningitis
- Perineurial spread of tumor (e.g., prostate cancer)
- Acute inflammatory demyelinating polyradiculopathy
- Chronic inflammatory demyelinating polyradiculopathy
- Sarcoidosis
- Amyloidoma
- Diabetic radiculopathy
- Infection (Lyme disease, herpes zoster, cytomegalovirus, syphilis, schistosomiasis, strongyloides)

PLEXOPATHIES

BRACHIAL PLEXUS

The brachial plexus is composed of three trunks (upper, middle, and lower), with two divisions (anterior and posterior) per trunk (Fig. 384-2). Subsequently, the trunks divide into three cords (medial, lateral, and posterior), and from these arise the multiple terminal nerves innervating the arm. The anterior primary rami of C5 and C6 fuse to form the upper trunk; the anterior primary ramus of C7 continues as the middle trunk, while the anterior rami of C8 and T1 join to form the lower trunk. There are several disorders commonly associated with brachial plexopathy.

Immune-mediated brachial plexus neuropathy

Immune-mediated brachial plexus neuropathy (IBPN) goes by various terms, including *acute brachial plexitis, neuralgic amyotrophy*, and *Parsonage-Turner syndrome*. IBPN usually presents with an acute onset of severe pain in the shoulder region. The intense pain usually lasts several days to a few weeks, but a dull ache can persist. Individuals who are affected may not appreciate weakness of the arm early in the course because the pain limits movement. However, as the pain dissipates, weakness and often sensory loss are appreciated. Attacks can occasionally recur.

Clinical findings are dependent on the distribution of involvement (e.g., specific trunk, divisions, cords, or terminal nerves). The most common pattern of IBPN involves the upper trunk or a single or multiple mononeuropathies primarily involving the suprascapular, long thoracic, or axillary nerves. Additionally, the phrenic and anterior interosseous nerves may be concomitantly affected. Any of these nerves may also be affected in isolation. EDx is useful to confirm and localize the site(s) of involvement. Empirical treatment of severe pain with glucocorticoids is often used in the acute period.

Brachial plexopathies associated with neoplasms

Neoplasms involving the brachial plexus may be primary nerve tumors, local cancers expanding into the plexus (e.g., Pancoast lung tumor or lymphoma), and metastatic tumors. Primary brachial plexus tumors are less common than the secondary tumors and include schwannomas, neurinomas, and neurofibromas. Secondary tumors affecting the brachial plexus are more common and are always malignant. These may arise from local tumors, expanding into the plexus. For example, a Pancoast tumor of the upper lobe of the lung may invade or compress the lower trunk, while a primary

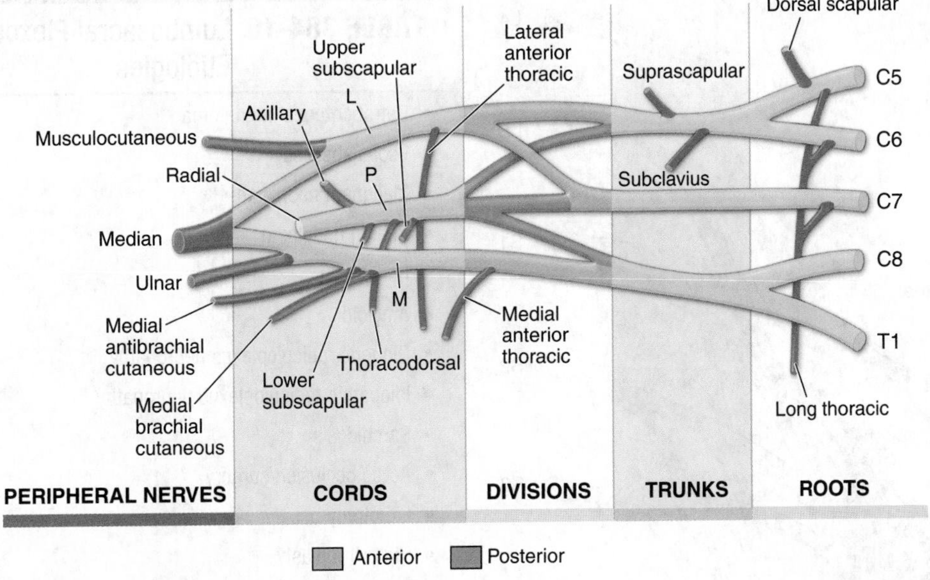

Figure 384-2 Brachial plexus anatomy. L, lateral; M, medial; P, posterior. *(From J Goodgold: Anatomical Correlates of Clinical Electromyography. Baltimore, Williams and Wilkins, 1974, p. 126, with permission.)*

lymphoma arising from the cervical or axillary lymph nodes may also infiltrate the plexus. Pancoast tumors typically present as an insidious onset of pain in the upper arm, sensory disturbance in the medial aspect of the forearm and hand, and weakness and atrophy of the intrinsic hand muscles along with an ipsilateral Horner syndrome. Chest CT scans or MRI can demonstrate extension of the tumor into the plexus. Metastatic involvement of the brachial plexus may occur with spread of breast cancer into the axillary lymph nodes with local spread into the nearby nerves.

Perioperative plexopathies (median sternotomy)

The most common surgical procedures associated with brachial plexopathy as a complication are those that involve median sternotomies (e.g., open-heart surgeries and thoracotomies). Brachial plexopathies occur in as many as 5% of patients following a median sternotomy and typically affect the lower trunk. Thus, individuals manifest with sensory disturbance affecting the medial aspect of forearm and hand along with weakness of the intrinsic hand muscles. The mechanism is related to the stretch of the lower trunk, so most individuals who are affected recover within a few months.

Lumbosacral plexus

The lumbar plexus arises from the ventral primary rami of the first to the fourth lumbar spinal nerves (Fig. 384-3). These nerves pass downward and laterally from the vertebral column within the psoas major muscle. The femoral nerve derives from the dorsal branches of the second to the fourth lumbar ventral rami. The obturator nerve arises from the ventral branches of the same lumbar rami. The lumbar plexus communicates with the sacral plexus by the lumbosacral trunk, which contains some fibers from the fourth and all of those from the fifth lumbar ventral rami (Fig. 384-4).

The sacral plexus is the part of the lumbosacral plexus that is formed by the union of the lumbosacral trunk with the ventral rami of the first to fourth sacral nerves. The plexus lies on the posterior and posterolateral wall of the pelvis with its components converging toward the sciatic notch. The lateral trunk of the sciatic nerve (which forms the common peroneal nerve) arises from the union of the dorsal branches of the lumbosacral trunk (L4, L5) and the dorsal branches of the S1 and S2 spinal nerve ventral rami. The medial trunk of the sciatic nerve (which forms the tibial nerve) derives from the ventral branches of the same ventral rami (L4-S2).

LUMBOSACRAL PLEXOPATHIES

Plexopathies are typically recognized when motor, sensory, and if applicable, reflex deficits occur in multiple nerve and segmental distributions confined to one extremity. If localization within the lumbosacral plexus can be accomplished, designation as a lumbar plexopathy, a sacral plexopathy, a lumbosacral trunk lesion, or a pan-plexopathy is the best localization that can be expected. Although lumbar plexopathies may be bilateral, usually occurring in a stepwise and chronologically dissociated manner, sacral plexopathies are more likely to behave in this manner due to their closer anatomic proximity. The differential diagnosis of plexopathy includes disorders of the conus medullaris and cauda equina (polyradiculopathy). If there is a paucity of pain and sensory involvement, motor neuron disease should be considered as well.

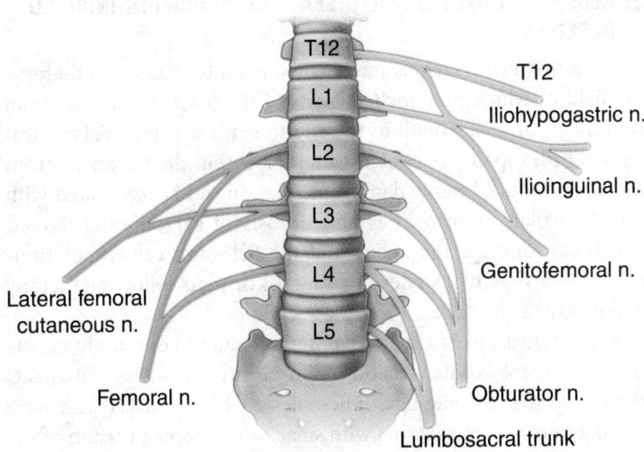

Figure 384-3 Lumbar plexus. Posterior divisions are in orange, anterior divisions are in yellow. *(From J Goodgold: Anatomical Correlates of Clinical Electromyography. Baltimore, Williams and Wilkins, 1974, p. 126, with permission.)*

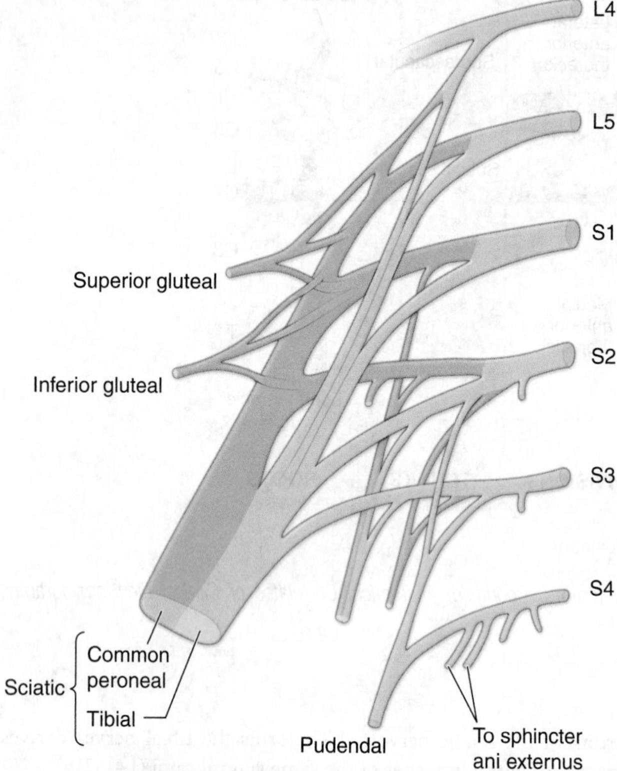

Figure 384-4 Lumbosacral plexus. Posterior divisions are in orange, anterior divisions are in yellow. *(From J Goodgold: Anatomical Correlates of Clinical Electromyography. Baltimore, Williams and Wilkins, 1974, p. 126, with permission.)*

The causes of lumbosacral plexopathies are listed in Table 384-10. Diabetic radiculopathy (discussed above) is a fairly common cause of painful leg weakness. Lumbosacral plexopathies are a well-recognized complication of retroperitoneal hemorrhage. Various primary and metastatic malignancies can affect the lumbosacral plexus as well; these include carcinoma of the cervix, endometrium, and ovary; osteosarcoma; testicular cancer; multiple myeloma; lymphoma; acute myelogenous leukemia; colon cancer; squamous cell carcinoma of the rectum; adenocarcinoma of unknown origin; and intraneural spread of prostate cancer.

RECURRENT NEOPLASTIC DISEASE OR RADIATION-INDUCED PLEXOPATHY

The treatment for various malignancies is often radiation therapy, the field of which may include parts of the brachial plexus. It can be difficult in such situations to determine if a new brachial or lumbosacral plexopathy is related to tumor within the plexus or from radiation-induced nerve damage. Radiation can be associated with microvascular abnormalities and fibrosis of surrounding tissues, which can damage the axons and the Schwann cells. Radiation-induced plexopathy can develop months or years following therapy and is dose dependent.

Tumor invasion is usually painful and more commonly affects the lower trunk, while radiation injury is often painless and affects the upper trunk. Imaging studies such as MRI and CT scans are useful but can be misleading with small microscopic invasion of the plexus. EMG can be informative if myokymic discharges are appreciated, as this finding strongly suggests radiation-induced damage.

TABLE 384-10 Lumbosacral Plexopathies: Etiologies

- Retroperitoneal hematoma
- Psoas abscess
- Malignant neoplasm
- Benign neoplasm
- Radiation
- Amyloid
- Diabetic radiculoplexus neuropathy
- Idiopathic radiculoplexus neuropathy
- Sarcoidosis
- Aortic occlusion/surgery
- Lithotomy positioning
- Hip arthroplasty
- Pelvic fracture
- Obstetric injury

EVALUATION AND TREATMENT OF PLEXOPATHIES

Most patients with plexopathies will undergo both imaging with MRI and EDx evaluations. Severe pain from acute idiopathic lumbosacral plexopathy may respond to a short course of glucocorticoids.

FURTHER READINGS

Amato AA, Russell J: *Neuromuscular Disease*. New York, McGraw-Hill, 2008

Dumitru D et al: *Electrodiagnostic Medicine*, 2nd ed. Philadelphia, Hanley & Belfus, Inc, 2002

Dyck PJ, Thomas PK (eds): *Peripheral Neuropathy*, 4th ed. Philadelphia, Elsevier Saunders, 2005

England JD et al: Evaluation of distal symmetric polyneuropathy: The role of autonomic testing, nerve biopsy, and skin biopsy (an evidence-based review). Muscle Nerve 39:106, 2009

———: Evaluation of distal symmetric polyneuropathy: The role of laboratory and genetic testing (an evidence-based review). Muscle Nerve 39:116, 2009

Jani-Acsadi A et al: Charcot-Marie-Tooth neuropathies: Diagnosis and management. Semin Neurol 28:185, 2008

Mendell JR et al: *Diagnosis and Management of Peripheral Nerve Disorders*. New York, Oxford University Press, 2001

Pascuzzi RM. Peripheral neuropathy. Med Clin North Am 93:317, 2009

Samuels MA, Ropper A (eds): *Manual of Neurologic Therapeutics*. Boston, Little, Brown, and Company, 2009

Saporta AS et al: Charcot-Marie-Tooth disease subtypes and genetic testing strategies. Ann Neurol 69:22, 2011

CHAPTER 385

Guillain-Barré Syndrome and Other Immune-Mediated Neuropathies

Stephen L. Hauser
Anthony A. Amato

GUILLAIN-BARRÉ SYNDROME

Guillain-Barré syndrome (GBS) is an acute, frequently severe, and fulminant polyradiculoneuropathy that is autoimmune in nature. It occurs year-round at a rate of between 1 and 4 cases per 100,000 annually; in the United States, ~5000–6000 cases occur per year. Males are at slightly higher risk for GBS than females, and in Western countries adults are more frequently affected than children.

Clinical manifestations

GBS manifests as a rapidly evolving areflexic motor paralysis with or without sensory disturbance. The usual pattern is an ascending paralysis that may be first noticed as rubbery legs. Weakness typically evolves over hours to a few days and is frequently accompanied by tingling dysesthesias in the extremities. The legs are usually more affected than the arms, and facial diparesis is present in 50% of affected individuals. The lower cranial nerves are also frequently involved, causing bulbar weakness with difficulty handling secretions and maintaining an airway; the diagnosis in these patients may initially be mistaken for brainstem ischemia. Pain in the neck, shoulder, back, or diffusely over the spine is also common in the early stages of GBS, occurring in ~50% of patients. Most patients require hospitalization, and in different series up to 30% require ventilatory assistance at some time during the illness. The need for mechanical ventilation is associated with more severe weakness on admission, a rapid tempo of progression, and the presence of facial and/or bulbar weakness during the first week of symptoms. Fever and constitutional symptoms are absent at the onset and, if present, cast doubt on the diagnosis. Deep tendon reflexes attenuate or disappear within the first few days of onset. Cutaneous sensory deficits (e.g., loss of pain and temperature sensation) are usually relatively mild, but functions subserved by large sensory fibers, such as deep tendon reflexes and proprioception, are more severely affected. Bladder dysfunction may occur in severe cases but is usually transient. If bladder dysfunction is a prominent feature and comes early in the course, diagnostic possibilities other than GBS should be considered, particularly spinal cord disease. Once clinical worsening stops and the patient reaches a plateau (almost always within 4 weeks of onset), further progression is unlikely.

Autonomic involvement is common and may occur even in patients whose GBS is otherwise mild. The usual manifestations are loss of vasomotor control with wide fluctuation in blood pressure, postural hypotension, and cardiac dysrhythmias. These features require close monitoring and management and can be fatal. Pain is another common feature of GBS; in addition to the acute pain described above, a deep aching pain may be present in weakened muscles that patients liken to having overexercised the previous day. Other pains in GBS include dysesthetic pain in the extremities as a manifestation of sensory nerve fiber involvement. These pains are self-limited and often respond to standard analgesics (Chap. 11).

Several subtypes of GBS are recognized, as determined primarily by electrodiagnostic (Edx) and pathologic distinctions (Table 385-1). The most common variant is acute inflammatory demyelinating polyneuropathy (AIDP). Additionally, there are two axonal variants, which are often clinically severe—the acute motor axonal neuropathy (AMAN) and acute motor sensory axonal neuropathy (AMSAN) subtypes. In addition, a range of limited or regional GBS syndromes are also encountered. Notable among these is the Miller Fisher syndrome (MFS), which presents as rapidly evolving ataxia and areflexia of limbs without weakness, and ophthalmoplegia, often with pupillary paralysis. The MFS variant accounts for ~5% of all cases and is strongly associated with antibodies to the ganglioside GQ1b (see "Immunopathogenesis," below). Other regional variants of GBS include (1) pure sensory forms; (2) ophthalmoplegia with anti-GQ1b antibodies as part of severe motor-sensory GBS; (3) GBS with severe bulbar and facial paralysis, sometimes associated with antecedent cytomegalovirus (CMV) infection and anti-GM2 antibodies; and (4) acute pandysautonomia (Chap. 375).

TABLE 385-1 Subtypes of Guillain-Barré Syndrome (GBS)

Subtype	Features	Electrodiagnosis	Pathology
Acute inflammatory demyelinating polyneuropathy (AIDP)	Adults affected more than children; 90% of cases in western world; recovery rapid; anti-GM1 antibodies (<50%)	Demyelinating	First attack on Schwann cell surface; widespread myelin damage, macrophage activation, and lymphocytic infiltration; variable secondary axonal damage
Acute motor axonal neuropathy (AMAN)	Children and young adults; prevalent in China and Mexico; may be seasonal; recovery rapid; anti-GD1a antibodies	Axonal	First attack at motor nodes of Ranvier; macrophage activation, few lymphocytes, frequent periaxonal macrophages; extent of axonal damage highly variable
Acute motor sensory axonal neuropathy (AMSAN)	Mostly adults; uncommon; recovery slow, often incomplete; closely related to AMAN	Axonal	Same as AMAN, but also affects sensory nerves and roots; axonal damage usually severe
M. Fisher syndrome (MFS)	Adults and children; uncommon; ophthalmoplegia, ataxia, and areflexia; anti-GQ1b antibodies (90%)	Demyelinating	Few cases examined; resembles AIDP

Antecedent events

Approximately 70% of cases of GBS occur 1–3 weeks after an acute infectious process, usually respiratory or gastrointestinal. Culture and seroepidemiologic techniques show that 20–30% of all cases occurring in North America, Europe, and Australia are preceded by infection or reinfection with *Campylobacter jejuni*. A similar proportion is preceded by a human herpes virus infection, often CMV or Epstein-Barr virus. Other viruses and also *Mycoplasma pneumoniae* have been identified as agents involved in antecedent infections, as have recent immunizations. The swine influenza vaccine, administered widely in the United States in 1976, is the most notable example. Influenza vaccines in use from 1992 to 1994, however, resulted in only one additional case of GBS per million persons vaccinated, and the more recent seasonal influenza vaccines appear to confer a GBS risk of <1 per million. A recent study demonstrated that there does not appear to be an increased risk of GBS with meningococcal vaccinations (Menactra) contrary to early reports. Older-type rabies vaccine, prepared in nervous system tissue, is implicated as a trigger of GBS in developing countries where it is still used; the mechanism is presumably immunization against neural antigens. GBS also occurs more frequently than can be attributed to chance alone in patients with lymphoma (including Hodgkin's disease), in HIV-seropositive individuals, and in patients with systemic lupus erythematosus (SLE). *C. jejuni* has also been implicated in summer outbreaks of AMAN among children and young adults exposed to chickens in rural China.

Immunopathogenesis

Several lines of evidence support an autoimmune basis for acute inflammatory demyelinating polyneuropathy (AIDP), the most common and best-studied type of GBS; the concept extends to all of the subtypes of GBS (Table 385-1).

It is likely that both cellular and humoral immune mechanisms contribute to tissue damage in AIDP. T cell activation is suggested by the finding that elevated levels of cytokines and cytokine receptors are present in serum [interleukin (IL) 2, soluble IL-2 receptor] and in cerebrospinal fluid (CSF) (IL-6, tumor necrosis factor α, interferon-γ). AIDP is also closely analogous to an experimental T cell–mediated immunopathy designated *experimental allergic neuritis* (EAN). EAN is induced in laboratory animals by immune sensitization against protein fragments derived from peripheral nerve proteins, and in particular against the P2 protein. Based on analogy to EAN, it was initially thought that AIDP was likely to be primarily a T cell–mediated disorder; however, abundant data now suggest that autoantibodies directed against nonprotein determinants may be central to many cases.

Circumstantial evidence suggests that all GBS results from immune responses to nonself antigens (infectious agents, vaccines) that misdirect to host nerve tissue through a resemblance-of-epitope (molecular mimicry) mechanism (Fig. 385-1). The neural targets are likely to be glycoconjugates, specifically gangliosides (Table 385-2; Fig. 385-2). Gangliosides are complex glycosphingolipids that contain one or more sialic acid residues; various gangliosides participate in cell-cell interactions (including those between axons and glia), modulation of receptors, and regulation of growth. They are typically exposed on the plasma membrane of cells, rendering them susceptible to an antibody-mediated attack. Gangliosides and other glycoconjugates are present in large quantity in human nervous tissues and in key sites, such as nodes of Ranvier. Antiganglioside antibodies, most frequently to GM1, are common in GBS (20–50% of cases), particularly in those preceded by *C. jejuni* infection. Furthermore, isolates of *C. jejuni* from stool cultures of patients with GBS have

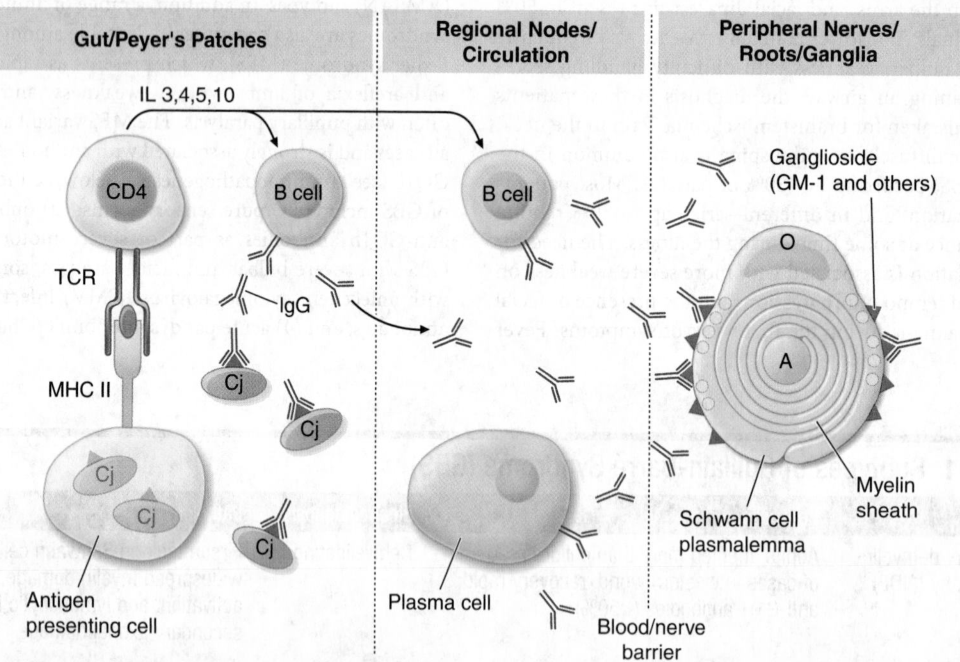

Figure 385-1 Postulated immunopathogenesis of GBS associated with *C. jejuni* infection. B cells recognize glycoconjugates on *C. jejuni* (Cj) (triangles) that cross-react with ganglioside present on Schwann cell surface and subjacent peripheral nerve myelin. Some B cells, activated via a T cell–independent mechanism, secrete primarily IgM (not shown). Other B cells (upper left side) are activated via a partially T cell–dependent route and secrete primarily IgG; T cell help is provided by CD4 cells activated locally by fragments of Cj proteins that are presented on the surface of antigen-presenting cells (APCs). A critical event in the development of GBS is the escape of activated B cells from Peyer's patches into regional lymph nodes. Activated T cells probably also function to assist in opening of the blood-nerve barrier, facilitating penetration of pathogenic autoantibodies. The earliest changes in myelin (right) consist of edema between myelin lamellae and vesicular disruption (shown as circular blebs) of the outermost myelin layers. These effects are associated with activation of the C5b-C9 membrane attack complex and probably mediated by calcium entry; it is possible that the macrophage cytokine tumor necrosis factor (TNF) also participates in myelin damage. B, B cell; MHC II, class II major histocompatibility complex molecule; TCR, T cell receptor; A, axon; O, oligodendrocyte.

TABLE 385-2 Principal Anti-Glycolipid Antibodies Implicated in Immune Neuropathies

Clinical Presentation	Antibody Target	Usual Isotype
Acute Immune Neuropathies (Guillain-Barré Syndrome)		
Acute inflammatory demyelinating polyneuropathy (AIDP)	No clear patterns GM1 most common	IgG (polyclonal)
Acute motor axonal neuropathy (AMAN)	GD1a, GM1, GM1b, GalNAc–GD1a (<50% for any)	IgG (polyclonal)
Miller Fisher syndrome (MFS)	GQ1b (>90%)	IgG (polyclonal)
Acute pharyngeal cervicobrachial neuropathy (APCBN)	GT1a (? Most)	IgG (polyclonal)
Chronic Immune Neuropathies		
Chronic inflammatory demyelinating polyneuropathy (CIDP) (75%)	Po in some	No clear pattern
CIDPa (MGUS associated) (25%)	Neural binding sites	IgG, IgA (monoclonal)
Chronic sensory > motor neuropathy	SPGP, SGLPG (on MAG) (50%)	IgM (monoclonal)
	Uncertain (50%)	IgM (monoclonal)
Multifocal motor neuropathy (MMN)	GM1, GalNAc–GD1a, others (25–50%)	IgM (polyclonal, monoclonal)
Chronic sensory ataxic neuropathy	GD1b, GQ1b, and other b-series gangliosides	IgM (monoclonal)

Abbreviations: MAG, myelin-associated glycoprotein; MGUS, monoclonal gammopathy of undetermined significance.
Source: Modified from HJ Willison, N Yuki: Brain 125:2591, 2002.

surface glycolipid structures that antigenically cross react with gangliosides, including GM1, concentrated in human nerves. Sialic acid residues from pathogenic *C. jejuni* strains can also trigger activation of dendritic cells via signaling through a toll-like receptor (TLR4), promoting B-cell differentiation and further amplifying humoral autoimmunity. Another line of evidence is derived from experience in Europe with parenteral use of purified bovine brain gangliosides for treatment of various neuropathic disorders.

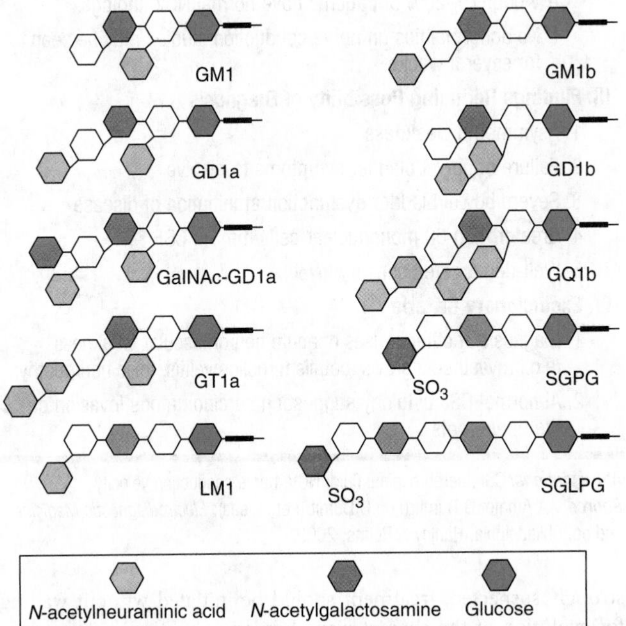

GM1 GM1b GD1a GD1b GalNAc-GD1a GQ1b GT1a SGPG SO_3 LM1 SGLPG SO_3

N-acetylneuraminic acid *N*-acetylgalactosamine Glucose *N*-acetylglucosamine Glucuronic acid Galactose Ceramide

Figure 385-2 Glycolipids implicated as antigens in immune-mediated neuropathies. *(Modified from HJ Willison, N Yuki: Brain 125:2591, 2002.)*

Between 5 and 15 days after injection, some recipients developed acute motor axonal GBS with high titers of anti-GM1 antibodies that recognized epitopes at nodes of Ranvier and motor endplates. Experimentally, anti-GM1 antibodies can trigger complement-mediated injury at paranodal axon-glial junctions, disrupting the clustering of sodium channels and likely contributing to conduction block (see "Pathophysiology," below).

Anti-GQ1b IgG antibodies are found in >90% of patients with MFS (Table 385-2; Fig. 385-2), and titers of IgG are highest early in the course. Anti-GQ1b antibodies are not found in other forms of GBS unless there is extraocular motor nerve involvement. A possible explanation for this association is that extraocular motor nerves are enriched in GQ1b gangliosides in comparison to limb nerves. In addition, a monoclonal anti-GQ1b antibody raised against *C. jejuni* isolated from a patient with MFS blocked neuromuscular transmission experimentally.

Taken together, these observations provide strong but still inconclusive evidence that autoantibodies play an important pathogenic role in GBS. Although anti-ganglioside antibodies have been studied most intensively, other antigenic targets may also be important. One report identified IgG antibodies against Schwann cells and neurons (nerve growth cone region) in some GBS cases. Proof that these antibodies are pathogenic requires that they be capable of mediating disease following direct passive transfer to naïve hosts; this has not yet been demonstrated, although one case of possible maternal-fetal transplacental transfer of GBS has been described.

In AIDP, an early step in the induction of tissue damage appears to be complement deposition along the outer surface of the Schwann cell. Activation of complement initiates a characteristic vesicular disintegration of the myelin sheath, and also leads to recruitment of activated macrophages, which participate in damage to myelin and axons. In AMAN, the pattern is different in that complement is deposited along with IgG at the nodes of Ranvier along large motor axons. Interestingly, in cases of AMAN antibodies against GD1a appear to have a fine specificity that favors binding to motor rather than sensory nerve roots, even though this ganglioside is expressed on both fiber types.

Pathophysiology

In the demyelinating forms of GBS, the basis for flaccid paralysis and sensory disturbance is conduction block. This finding, demonstrable electrophysiologically, implies that the axonal connections remain intact. Hence, recovery can take place rapidly as remyelination occurs. In severe cases of demyelinating GBS, secondary axonal degeneration usually occurs; its extent can be estimated electrophysiologically. More secondary axonal degeneration correlates with a slower rate of recovery and a greater degree of residual disability. When a severe primary axonal pattern is encountered electrophysiologically, the implication is that axons have degenerated and become disconnected from their targets, specifically the neuromuscular junctions, and must therefore regenerate for recovery to take place. In motor axonal cases in which recovery is rapid, the lesion is thought to be localized to preterminal motor branches, allowing regeneration and reinnervation to take place quickly. Alternatively, in mild cases, collateral sprouting and reinnervation from surviving motor axons near the neuromuscular junction may begin to reestablish physiologic continuity with muscle cells over a period of several months.

Laboratory features

CSF findings are distinctive, consisting of an elevated CSF protein level [1–10 g/L (100–1000 mg/dL)] without accompanying pleocytosis. The CSF is often normal when symptoms have been present for ≤48 h; by the end of the first week, the level of protein is usually elevated. A transient increase in the CSF white cell count (10–100/μL) occurs on occasion in otherwise typical GBS; however, a sustained CSF pleocytosis suggests an alternative diagnosis (viral myelitis) or a concurrent diagnosis such as unrecognized HIV infection, leukemia or lymphoma with infiltration of nerves, or neurosarcoidosis. Edx features are mild or absent in the early stages of GBS and lag behind the clinical evolution. In AIDP, the earliest features are prolonged F-wave latencies, prolonged distal latencies and reduced amplitudes of compound muscle action potentials (CMAPs), probably owing to the predilection for involvement of nerve roots and distal motor nerve terminals early in the course. Later, slowing of conduction velocity, conduction block, and temporal dispersion may be appreciated (Table 385-1). Occasionally, sensory nerve action potentials (SNAPs) may be normal in the feet (e.g., sural nerve) when abnormal in the arms. This is also a sign that the patient does not have one of the more typical "length-dependent" polyneuropathies. In cases with primary axonal pathology, the principal Edx finding is reduced amplitude of CMAPs (and also SNAPS with AMSAN) without conduction slowing or prolongation of distal latencies.

Diagnosis

GBS is a descriptive entity. The diagnosis of AIDP is made by recognizing the pattern of rapidly evolving paralysis with areflexia, absence of fever or other systemic symptoms, and characteristic antecedent events (Table 385-3). Other disorders that may enter into the differential diagnosis include acute myelopathies (especially with prolonged back pain and sphincter disturbances); diphtheria (early oropharyngeal disturbances); Lyme polyradiculitis and other tick-borne paralyses; porphyria (abdominal pain, seizures, psychosis); vasculitic neuropathy (check erythrocyte sedimentation rate, described below); poliomyelitis (fever and meningismus common); West Nile virus; CMV polyradiculitis (in immunocompromised patients); critical illness neuropathy or myopathy; neuromuscular junction disorders such as myasthenia gravis and botulism (pupillary reactivity lost early); poisonings with organophosphates, thallium, or arsenic; paralytic shellfish poisoning; or severe hypophosphatemia (rare). Laboratory tests are helpful primarily to exclude mimics of GBS. Edx features may be minimal, and the CSF protein level may not rise until the end of the first week. If the diagnosis is strongly suspected, treatment should be initiated without waiting for evolution of the characteristic Edx and CSF findings to occur. Both tau and 14-3-3 protein levels are reported to be elevated early (during the first few days of symptoms) in some cases of GBS. Tau increases in CSF may reflect axonal damage and predict a residual deficit. GBS patients with risk factors for HIV or with CSF pleocytosis should have a serologic test for HIV.

TABLE 385-3 Diagnostic Features of Acute Inflammatory Demyelinating Polyneuropathy (AIDP)

I. Required for Diagnosis

1. Progressive weakness of variable degree from mild paresis to complete paralysis
2. Generalized hypo- or areflexia

II. Supportive of Diagnosis

1. Clinical Features
   a. Symptom progression: Motor weakness rapidly progresses initially but ceases by 4 weeks. Nadir attained by 2 weeks in 50%, 3 weeks 80%, and 90% by 4 weeks.
   b. Demonstration of relative limb symmetry regarding paresis.
   c. Mild to moderate sensory signs.
   d. Frequent cranial nerve involvement: Facial (cranial nerve VII) 50% and typically bilateral but asymmetric; occasional involvement of cranial nerves XII, X, and occasionally III, IV, and VI as well as XI.
   e. Recovery typically begins 2–4 weeks following plateau phase.
   f. Autonomic dysfunction can include tachycardia, other arrhythmias, postural hypotension, hypertension, other vasomotor symptoms.
   g. A preceding gastrointestinal illness (e.g., diarrhea) or upper respiratory tract infection is common.
2. Cerebrospinal Fluid Features Supporting Diagnosis
   a. Elevated or serial elevation of CSF protein.
   b. CSF cell counts are <10 mononuclear cell/mm^3.
3. Electrodiagnostic Medicine Findings Supportive of Diagnosis
   a. 80% of patients have evidence of NCV slowing/conduction block at some time during disease process.
   b. Patchy reduction in NCV attaining values less than 60% of normal.
   c. Distal motor latency increase may reach 3 times normal values.
   d. F-waves indicate proximal NCV slowing.
   e. About 15–20% of patients have normal NCV findings.
   f. No abnormalities on nerve conduction studies may be seen for several weeks.

III. Findings Reducing Possibility of Diagnosis

1. Asymmetric weakness
2. Failure of bowel/bladder symptoms to resolve
3. Severe bowel/bladder dysfunction at initiation of disease
4. Greater than 50 mononuclear cells/mm^3 in CSF
5. Well-demarcated sensory level

IV. Exclusionary Criteria

1. Diagnosis of other causes of acute neuromuscular weakness (e.g., myasthenia gravis, botulism, poliomyelitis, toxic neuropathy).
2. Abnormal CSF cytology suggesting carcinomatous invasion of the nerve roots

Abbreviations: CSF, cerebrospinal fluid; NCV, nerve conduction velocity.
Source: AA Amato, D Dumitru, in D Dumitru et al (eds): *Electrodiagnostic Medicine*, 2nd ed, Philadelphia, Hanley & Belfus, 2002.

TREATMENT Guillain-Barré Syndrome

In the vast majority of patients with GBS, treatment should be initiated as soon after diagnosis as possible. Each day counts; ~2 weeks after the first motor symptoms, it is not known whether immunotherapy is still effective. If the patient has already reached the plateau stage, then treatment probably is no longer indicated, unless the patient has severe motor weakness and one cannot exclude the possibility that an immunologic attack is still ongoing. Either high-dose intravenous immune globulin (IVIg) or plasmapheresis can be initiated, as they are equally effective for typical GBS. A combination of the two therapies is not significantly better than either alone. IVIg is often the initial therapy chosen because of its ease of administration and good safety record. Anecdotal data has also suggested that IVIg may be preferable to PE for the AMAN and MFS variants of GBS. IVIg is administered as five daily infusions for a total dose of 2 g/kg body weight. There is some evidence that GBS autoantibodies are neutralized by anti-idiotypic antibodies present in IVIg preparations, perhaps accounting for the therapeutic effect. A course of plasmapheresis usually consists of ~40–50 mL/kg plasma exchange (PE) four to five times over a week. Meta-analysis of randomized clinical trials indicates that treatment reduces the need for mechanical ventilation by nearly half (from 27% to 14% with PE) and increases the likelihood of full recovery at 1 year (from 55% to 68%). Functionally significant improvement may occur toward the end of the first week of treatment, or may be delayed for several weeks. The lack of noticeable improvement following a course of IVIg or PE is not an indication to treat with the alternate treatment. However, there are occasional patients who are treated early in the course of GBS and improve, who then relapse within a month. Brief retreatment with the original therapy is usually effective in such cases. Glucocorticoids have not been found to be effective in GBS. Occasional patients with very mild forms of GBS, especially those who appear to have already reached a plateau when initially seen, may be managed conservatively without IVIg or PE.

In the worsening phase of GBS, most patients require monitoring in a critical care setting, with particular attention to vital capacity, heart rhythm, blood pressure, nutrition, deep vein thrombosis prophylaxis, cardiovascular status, early consideration (after 2 weeks of intubation) of tracheotomy, and chest physiotherapy. As noted, ~30% of patients with GBS require ventilatory assistance, sometimes for prolonged periods of time (several weeks or longer). Frequent turning and assiduous skin care are important, as are daily range-of-motion exercises to avoid joint contractures and daily reassurance as to the generally good outlook for recovery.

Prognosis and recovery

Approximately 85% of patients with GBS achieve a full functional recovery within several months to a year, although minor findings on examination (such as areflexia) may persist and patients often complain of continued symptoms, including fatigue. The mortality rate is <5% in optimal settings; death usually results from secondary pulmonary complications. The outlook is worst in patients with severe proximal motor and sensory axonal damage. Such axonal damage may be either primary or secondary in nature (see "Pathophysiology," above), but in either case successful regeneration cannot occur. Other factors that worsen the outlook for recovery are advanced age, a fulminant or severe attack, and a delay in the onset of treatment. Between 5 and 10% of patients with typical GBS have one or more late relapses; such cases are then classified as chronic inflammatory demyelinating polyneuropathy (CIDP).

CHRONIC INFLAMMATORY DEMYELINATING POLYNEUROPATHY

CIDP is distinguished from GBS by its chronic course. In other respects, this neuropathy shares many features with the common demyelinating form of GBS, including elevated CSF protein levels and the Edx findings of acquired demyelination. Most cases occur in adults, and males are affected slightly more often than females. The incidence of CIDP is lower than that of GBS, but due to the protracted course the prevalence is greater.

Clinical manifestations

Onset is usually gradual over a few months or longer, but in a few cases the initial attack is indistinguishable from that of GBS. An acute-onset form of CIDP should be considered when GBS deteriorates >9 weeks after onset or relapses at least three times. Symptoms are both motor and sensory in most cases. Weakness of the limbs is usually symmetric but can be strikingly asymmetric in multifocal acquired demyelinating sensory and motor (MADSAM) neuropathy variant (Lewis-Sumner syndrome) in which discrete peripheral nerves are involved. There is considerable variability from case to case. Some patients experience a chronic progressive course, whereas others, usually younger patients, have a relapsing and remitting course. Some have only motor findings, and a small proportion present with a relatively pure syndrome of sensory ataxia. Tremor occurs in ~10% and may become more prominent during periods of subacute worsening or improvement. A small proportion have cranial nerve findings, including external ophthalmoplegia. CIDP tends to ameliorate over time with treatment; the result is that many years after onset, nearly 75% of patients have reasonable functional status. Death from CIDP is uncommon.

Diagnosis

The diagnosis rests on characteristic clinical, CSF, and electrophysiologic findings. The CSF is usually acellular with an elevated protein level, sometimes several times normal. As with GBS, a CSF pleocytosis should lead to the consideration of HIV infection, leukemia or lymphoma, and neurosarcoidosis. Edx findings reveal variable degrees of conduction slowing, prolonged distal latencies, distal and temporal dispersion of CMAPs, and conduction block as the principal features. In particular, the presence of conduction block is a certain sign of an acquired demyelinating process. Evidence of axonal loss, presumably secondary to demyelination, is present in >50% of patients. Serum protein electrophoresis with immunofixation is indicated to search for monoclonal gammopathy and associated conditions (see "Monoclonal Gammopathy of Undetermined Significance," below). In all patients with presumptive CIDP, it is also reasonable to exclude vasculitis, collagen vascular disease (especially SLE), chronic hepatitis, HIV infection, amyloidosis, and diabetes mellitus. Other associated conditions include inflammatory bowel disease and lymphoma.

Pathogenesis

Although there is evidence of immune activation in CIDP, the precise mechanisms of pathogenesis are unknown. Biopsy typically reveals little inflammation and onion-bulb changes (imbricated layers of attenuated Schwann cell processes surrounding an axon) that result from recurrent demyelination and remyelination (Fig. 385-1). The response to therapy suggests that CIDP is immune-mediated; CIDP responds to glucocorticoids, whereas GBS does not. Passive transfer of demyelination into experimental animals has been accomplished using IgG purified from the serum of some patients with CIDP, lending support for a humoral autoimmune pathogenesis. Although the target antigen or antigens in CIDP have not yet been identified, the myelin protein Po has been implicated as a potential autoantigen in some patients. It is also of interest that a CIDP-like illness developed spontaneously in the nonobese diabetic (NOD) mouse when the immune co-stimulatory molecule B7-2 (CD86) was genetically deleted; this suggests that CIDP can result from altered triggering of T cells by antigen-presenting cells.

Approximately 25% of patients with clinical features of CIDP also have a monoclonal gammopathy of undetermined significance (MGUS). Cases associated with monoclonal IgA or IgG kappa usually respond to treatment as favorably as cases without a monoclonal gammopathy. Patients with IgM monoclonal gammopathy tend to have more sensory findings and a more protracted course, and usually have a less satisfactory response to treatment.

TREATMENT Chronic Inflammatory Demyelinating Polyneuropathy

Most authorities initiate treatment for CIDP when progression is rapid or walking is compromised. If the disorder is mild, management can be expectant, awaiting spontaneous remission. Controlled studies have shown that high-dose IVIg, PE, and glucocorticoids are all more effective than placebo. Initial therapy is usually with IVIg, administered as 2.0 g/kg body weight given in divided doses over 2–5 days; three monthly courses are generally recommended before concluding a patient is a treatment failure. If the patient responds, the infusion intervals can be gradually increased or the dosage decreased (e.g., 1 g/kg per month). PE, which appears to be as effective as IVIg, is initiated at two to three treatments per week for 6 weeks; periodic re-treatment may also be required. Treatment with glucocorticoids is another option (60–80 mg prednisone PO daily for 1–2 months, followed by a gradual dose reduction of 10 mg per month as tolerated), but long-term adverse effects including bone demineralization, gastrointestinal bleeding, and cushingoid changes are problematic. As many as one-third of patients with CIDP fail to respond adequately to the initial therapy chosen; a different treatment should then be tried. Patients who fail therapy with IVIg, PE, and glucocorticoids may benefit from treatment with immunosuppressive agents such as azathioprine, methotrexate, cyclosporine, and cyclophosphamide, either alone or as adjunctive therapy. Early experience with anti-CD20 (rituximab) has also shown promise. Use of these therapies requires periodic reassessment of their risks and benefits. In patients with a CIDP-like neuropathy who fail to respond to treatment it is important to evaluate for POEMS syndrome (*p*olyneuropathy, *o*rganomegaly, *e*ndocrinopathy, *m*onoclonal gammopathy, *s*kin changes; see below).

MULTIFOCAL MOTOR NEUROPATHY

Multifocal motor neuropathy (MMN) is a distinctive but uncommon neuropathy that presents as slowly progressive motor weakness and atrophy evolving over years in the distribution of selected nerve trunks, associated with sites of persistent focal motor conduction block in the same nerve trunks. Sensory fibers are relatively spared. The arms are affected more frequently than the legs, and >75% of all patients are male. Some cases have been confused with lower motor neuron forms of amyotrophic lateral sclerosis (Chap. 374). Less than 50% of patients present with high titers of polyclonal IgM antibody to the ganglioside GM1. It is uncertain how this finding relates to the discrete foci of persistent motor conduction block, but high concentrations of GM1 gangliosides are normal constituents of nodes of Ranvier in peripheral nerve fibers. Pathology reveals demyelination and mild inflammatory changes at the sites of conduction block.

Most patients with MMN respond to high-dose IVIg (dosages as for CIDP, above); periodic re-treatment is required (usually at least monthly) to maintain the benefit. Some refractory patients have responded to rituximab or cyclophosphamide. Glucocorticoids and PE are not effective.

NEUROPATHIES WITH MONOCLONAL GAMMOPATHY

MULTIPLE MYELOMA

Clinically overt polyneuropathy occurs in ~5% of patients with the commonly encountered type of multiple myeloma, which exhibits either lytic or diffuse osteoporotic bone lesions. These neuropathies are sensorimotor, are usually mild and slowly progressive but may be severe, and generally do not reverse with successful suppression of the myeloma. In most cases, Edx and pathologic features are consistent with a process of axonal degeneration.

In contrast, myeloma with osteosclerotic features, although representing only 3% of all myelomas, is associated with polyneuropathy in one-half of cases. These neuropathies, which may also occur with solitary plasmacytoma, are distinct because they (1) are usually demyelinating in nature and resemble CIDP; (2) often respond to radiation therapy or removal of the primary lesion; (3) are associated with different monoclonal proteins and light chains (almost always lambda as opposed to primarily kappa in the lytic type of multiple myeloma); (4) are typically refractory to standard treatments of CIDP; and (5) may occur in association with other systemic findings including thickening of the skin, hyperpigmentation, hypertrichosis, organomegaly, endocrinopathy, anasarca, and clubbing of fingers. These are features of the POEMS syndrome (*p*olyneuropathy, *o*rganomegaly, *e*ndocrinopathy, *M* protein, and *s*kin changes). Levels of vascular endothelial growth factor (VEGF) are increased in the serum and this factor is felt to somehow play a pathogenic role in this syndrome. Treatment of the neuropathy is best directed at the osteosclerotic myeloma using surgery, radiotherapy, chemotherapy, or autologous peripheral blood stem cell transplantation.

Neuropathies are also encountered in other systemic conditions with gammopathy, including Waldenström's macroglobulinemia, primary systemic amyloidosis, and cryoglobulinemic states (mixed essential cryoglobulinemia, some cases of hepatitis C).

MONOCLONAL GAMMOPATHY OF UNDETERMINED SIGNIFICANCE

Chronic polyneuropathies occurring in association with MGUS are usually associated with the immunoglobulin isotypes IgG, IgA, and IgM. Most patients present with isolated sensory symptoms in their distal extremities and have Edx features of an axonal sensory or sensorimotor polyneuropathy. These patients otherwise resemble idiopathic sensory polyneuropathy and the MGUS might just be coincidental. They usually do not respond to immunotherapies designed to reduce the concentration of the monoclonal protein. Some patients, however, present with generalized weakness and sensory loss and Edx studies indistinguishable from CIDP without monoclonal gammopathy (see "Chronic Inflammatory Demyelinating Polyneuropathy," above), and their response to immunosuppressive agents is also similar. An exception is the syndrome of IgM kappa monoclonal gammopathy associated with an indolent, longstanding, sometimes static sensory neuropathy, frequently with tremor and sensory ataxia. Most patients are male and older than age 50 years. In the majority, the monoclonal IgM immunoglobulin binds to a normal peripheral nerve constituent, myelin-associated glycoprotein (MAG), found in the paranodal regions of Schwann cells. Binding appears to be specific for a polysaccharide epitope that is also found in other normal peripheral nerve myelin glycoproteins, P0 and PMP22, and also in other normal nerve-related glycosphingolipids (Fig. 385-1). In the MAG-positive cases, IgM paraprotein is incorporated into the myelin sheaths of affected patients and widens the spacing of the myelin lamellae, thus producing a distinctive ultrastructural pattern. Demyelination and remyelination are the hallmarks of the lesions. The chronic demyelinating neuropathy appears to result from a destabilization of myelin metabolism rather than activation of an immune response. Therapy with chlorambucil, or cyclophosphamide combined with glucocorticoids or PE, often results in improvement of the neuropathy associated with a prolonged reduction in the levels in the circulating paraprotein; chronic use of these alkylating agents is associated with significant risks. In a small proportion of patients (30% at 10 years), MGUS will in time evolve into frankly malignant conditions such as multiple myeloma or lymphoma.

VASCULITIC NEUROPATHY

Peripheral nerve involvement is common in polyarteritis nodosa (PAN), appearing in half of all cases clinically and in 100% of cases at postmortem studies (Chap. 326). The most common pattern is multifocal (asymmetric) motor-sensory neuropathy (mononeuropathy multiplex) due to ischemic lesions of nerve trunks and roots; however, some cases of vasculitic neuropathy present as a distal, symmetric sensorimotor polyneuropathy. Symptoms of neuropathy are a common presenting complaint in patients with PAN. The Edx findings are those of an axonal process. Small- to medium-sized arteries of the vasa nervorum, particularly the epineural vessels, are affected in PAN, resulting in a widespread ischemic neuropathy. A high frequency of neuropathy occurs in allergic angiitis and granulomatosis (Churg-Strauss syndrome).

Systemic vasculitis should always be considered when a subacute or chronically evolving mononeuropathy multiplex occurs in conjunction with constitutional symptoms (fever, anorexia, weight loss, loss of energy, malaise, and nonspecific pains). Diagnosis of suspected vasculitic neuropathy is made by a combined nerve and muscle biopsy, with serial section or skip-serial techniques.

Approximately one-third of biopsy-proven cases of vasculitic neuropathy are "nonsystemic" in that the vasculitis appears to affect only peripheral nerves. Constitutional symptoms are absent, and the course is more indolent than that of PAN. The erythrocyte sedimentation rate may be elevated, but other tests for systemic disease are negative. Nevertheless, clinically silent involvement of other organs is likely, and vasculitis is frequently found in muscle biopsied at the same time as nerve.

Vasculitic neuropathy may also be seen as part of the vasculitis syndrome occurring in the course of other connective tissue disorders (Chap. 326). The most frequent is rheumatoid arthritis, but ischemic neuropathy due to involvement of vasa nervorum may also occur in mixed cryoglobulinemia, Sjögren's syndrome, granulomatosis with polyangiitis (Wegener's), hypersensitivity angiitis, systemic lupus erythematosus, and progressive systemic sclerosis. Management of these neuropathies, including the "nonsystemic" vasculitic neuropathy, consists of treatment of the underlying condition as well as the aggressive use of glucocorticoids and other immunosuppressant drugs. Use of these regimens has resulted in dramatic improvements in outcome, with 5-year survival rates now greater than 80%. One reasonable starting regimen is daily prednisone (initial dose 1 mg/kg per day PO with a gradual taper after 1 month) plus IV pulse (or daily oral) cyclophosphamide for 3–6 months.

ANTI-Hu PARANEOPLASTIC NEUROPATHY

This uncommon immune-mediated disorder manifests as a sensory neuronopathy (i.e., selective damage to sensory nerve bodies in dorsal root ganglia). The onset is often asymmetric with dysesthesias and sensory loss in the limbs that soon progress to affect all limbs, the torso, and face. Marked sensory ataxia, pseudoathetosis, and inability to walk, stand, or even sit unsupported are frequent features and are secondary to the extensive deafferentation. Subacute sensory neuronopathy may be idiopathic, but more than half of cases are paraneoplastic, primarily related to lung cancer, and most of those are small cell lung cancer (SCLC). Diagnosis of the underlying SCLC requires awareness of the association, paraneoplastic testing, and often PET scanning for the tumor. The target antigens are a family of RNA-binding proteins (HuD, HuC, and Hel-N1) that in normal tissues are only expressed by neurons. The same proteins are usually expressed by SCLC, triggering in some patients an immune response characterized by antibodies and cytotoxic T cells that cross-react with the Hu proteins of the dorsal root ganglion neurons, resulting in immune-mediated neuronal destruction. An encephalomyelitis may accompany the sensory neuronopathy and presumably has the same pathogenesis. Neurologic symptoms usually precede, by ≤6 months, the identification of SCLC. The sensory neuronopathy runs its course in a few weeks or months and stabilizes, leaving the patient disabled. Most cases are unresponsive to treatment with glucocorticoids, IVIg, PE, or immunosuppressant drugs.

FURTHER READINGS

Burns TM et al: Vasculitic neuropathies. Neurol Clin 25:89, 2007

Cats EA et al: Correlates of outcome and response to IVIg in 88 patients with multifocal motor neuropathy. Neurology 75:818, 2010

Hadden RDM et al: European Federation of Neurological Societies/Peripheral Nerve Society guideline on management of paraproteinemic demyelinating neuropathies: Report of a joint task force of the European Federation of Neurological Societies and the Peripheral Nerve Society. Eur J Neurol 13:809, 2006

Hughes RA et al: European Federation of Neurological Societies/Peripheral Nerve Society guideline on management of chronic inflammatory demyelinating polyradiculoneuropathy: Report of a joint task force of the European Federation of Neurological Societies and the Peripheral Nerve Society. Eur J Neurol 13:326, 2006

——— et al: Immunotherapy for Guillain-Barrè syndrome: A systematic review. Brain 130:2245, 2007

Kuijf ML et al: TLR4-mediated sensing of *Campylobacter jejuni* by dendritic cells is determined by sialylation. J Immunol 185:748, 2010

Latov N et al: Timing and course of clinical response to intravenous immunoglobulin in chronic inflammatory demyelinating polyradiculoneuropathy. Arch Neurol 67:802, 2010

Lopez PHH et al: Structural requirements of anti-GD1a antibodies determine their target specificity. Brain 131:1926, 2008

Lunn MP, Willison HJ: Diagnosis and treatment in inflammatory neuropathies. J Neurol Neurosurg Psychiatry 80:249, 2009

Mathew L et al: Treatment of vasculitic peripheral neuropathy: A retrospective analysis of outcome. QJM 100:41, 2007

Susuki K et al: Anti-GM1 antibodies cause complement-mediated disruption of sodium channel clusters in peripheral motor nerve fibers. J Neurosci 27:3956, 2007

Van Schaik IN et al: European Federation of Neurological Societies/Peripheral Nerve Society guideline on management of multifocal motor neuropathy. Eur J Neurol 13:802, 2006

Walgaard C et al: Prediction of respiratory insufficiency in Guillain-Barré syndrome. Ann Neurol 67:781, 2010

CHAPTER 386 Myasthenia Gravis and Other Diseases of the Neuromuscular Junction

Daniel B. Drachman

Myasthenia gravis (MG) is a neuromuscular disorder characterized by weakness and fatigability of skeletal muscles. The underlying defect is a decrease in the number of available acetylcholine receptors (AChRs) at neuromuscular junctions due to an antibody-mediated autoimmune attack. Treatment now available for MG is highly effective, although a specific cure has remained elusive.

PATHOPHYSIOLOGY

At the neuromuscular junction (Fig. 386-1), acetylcholine (ACh) is synthesized in the motor nerve terminal and stored in vesicles (quanta). When an action potential travels down a motor nerve and reaches the nerve terminal, ACh from 150 to 200 vesicles is released and combines with AChRs that are densely packed at the peaks of postsynaptic folds. The structure of the AChR has been fully elucidated; it consists of five subunits (2α, 1β, 1δ, and 1γ or ε) arranged around a central pore. When ACh combines with the binding sites on the α subunits of the AChR, the channel in the AChR opens, permitting the rapid entry of cations, chiefly sodium, which produces depolarization at the end-plate region of the muscle fiber. If the depolarization is sufficiently large, it initiates an action potential that is propagated along the muscle fiber, triggering muscle contraction. This process is rapidly terminated by hydrolysis of ACh by acetylcholinesterase (AChE), which is present within the synaptic folds, and by diffusion of ACh away from the receptor.

In MG, the fundamental defect is a decrease in the number of available AChRs at the postsynaptic muscle membrane. In addition, the postsynaptic folds are flattened, or "simplified." These changes result in decreased efficiency of neuromuscular transmission. Therefore, although ACh is released normally, it produces small end-plate potentials that may fail to trigger muscle action potentials. Failure of transmission at many neuromuscular junctions results in weakness of muscle contraction.

The amount of ACh released per impulse normally declines on repeated activity (termed *presynaptic rundown*). In the myasthenic patient, the decreased efficiency of neuromuscular transmission combined with the normal rundown results in the activation of fewer and fewer muscle fibers by successive nerve impulses and hence increasing weakness, or *myasthenic fatigue*. This mechanism also accounts for the decremental response to repetitive nerve stimulation seen on electrodiagnostic testing.

The neuromuscular abnormalities in MG are brought about by an autoimmune response mediated by specific anti-AChR antibodies. The anti-AChR antibodies reduce the number of available AChRs at neuromuscular junctions by three distinct mechanisms: (1) accelerated turnover of AChRs by a mechanism involving cross-linking and rapid endocytosis of the receptors; (2) damage to the postsynaptic muscle membrane by the antibody in collaboration with complement; and (3) blockade of the active site of the AChR, i.e., the site that normally binds ACh. An immune response to muscle-specific kinase (MuSK), a protein involved in AChR clustering at neuromuscular junctions, can also result in myasthenia gravis, with reduction of AChRs demonstrated experimentally. The pathogenic antibodies are IgG, and are T cell-dependent. Thus, immunotherapeutic strategies directed against either the antibody-producing B cells or helper T cells are effective in this antibody-mediated disease.

How the autoimmune response is initiated and maintained in MG is not completely understood, but the thymus appears to play a role in this process. The thymus is abnormal in ~75% of patients with MG; in ~65% the thymus is "hyperplastic," with the presence of active germinal centers detected histologically, though the hyperplastic thymus is not necessarily enlarged. An additional 10% of patients have thymic tumors (thymomas). Muscle-like cells within the thymus (myoid cells), which bear AChRs on their surface, may serve as a source of autoantigen and trigger the autoimmune reaction within the thymus gland.

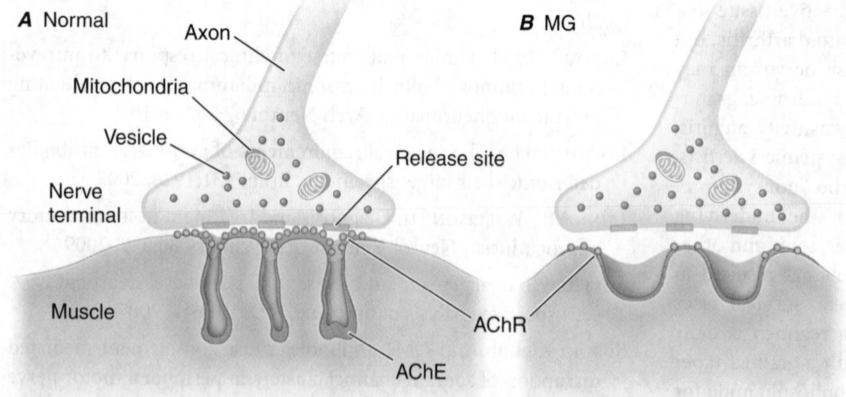

Figure 386-1 Diagrams of (*A*) normal and (*B*) myasthenic neuromuscular junctions. AChE, acetylcholinesterase. See text for description of normal neuromuscular transmission. The MG junction demonstrates a normal nerve terminal; a reduced number of AChRs (stippling); flattened, simplified postsynaptic folds; and a widened synaptic space. *(Modified from DB Drachman: N Engl J Med 330:1797, 1994; with permission.)*

CLINICAL FEATURES

MG is not rare, having a prevalence of 2–7 in 10,000. It affects individuals in all age groups, but peaks of incidence occur in women in their twenties and thirties and in men in their fifties and sixties. Overall, women are affected more frequently than men, in a ratio of ~3:2. The cardinal features are *weakness* and *fatigability* of muscles. The weakness increases during repeated use (fatigue) or late in the day, and may improve following rest or sleep. The course of MG is often variable. Exacerbations and remissions may occur, particularly during the first few years after the onset of the disease. Remissions are rarely complete or permanent. Unrelated infections or systemic disorders can lead to increased myasthenic weakness and may precipitate "crisis" (see below).

The distribution of muscle weakness often has a characteristic pattern. The cranial muscles, particularly the lids and extraocular muscles, are typically involved early in the course of MG; diplopia and ptosis are common initial complaints. Facial weakness produces a "snarling" expression when the patient attempts to smile. Weakness in chewing is most noticeable after prolonged effort, as in chewing meat. Speech may have a nasal timbre caused by weakness of the palate, or a dysarthric "mushy" quality due to tongue weakness. Difficulty in swallowing may occur as a result of weakness of the palate, tongue, or pharynx, giving rise to nasal regurgitation or aspiration of liquids or food. Bulbar weakness is especially prominent in MuSK antibody–positive MG. In ~85% of patients, the weakness becomes generalized, affecting the limb muscles as well. If weakness remains restricted to the extraocular muscles for 3 years, it is likely that it will not become generalized, and these patients are said to have *ocular MG*. The limb weakness in MG is often proximal and may be asymmetric. Despite the muscle weakness, deep tendon reflexes are preserved. If weakness of respiration becomes so severe as to require respiratory assistance, the patient is said to be in *crisis*.

DIAGNOSIS AND EVALUATION

(Table 386-1) The diagnosis is suspected on the basis of weakness and fatigability in the typical distribution described above, without loss of reflexes or impairment of sensation or other neurologic function. The suspected diagnosis should always be confirmed definitively before treatment is undertaken; this is essential because (1) other treatable conditions may closely resemble MG and (2) the treatment of MG may involve surgery and the prolonged use of drugs with potentially adverse side effects.

TABLE 386-1 Diagnosis of Myasthenia Gravis (MG)

History
Diplopia, ptosis, weakness
Weakness in characteristic distribution
Fluctuation and fatigue: worse with repeated activity, improved by rest
Effects of previous treatments
Physical examination
Ptosis, diplopia
Motor power survey: quantitative testing of muscle strength
Forward arm abduction time (5 min)
Vital capacity
Absence of other neurologic signs
Laboratory testing
Anti-AChR radioimmunoassay: ~85% positive in generalized MG; 50% in ocular MG; definite diagnosis if positive; negative result does not exclude MG. ~40% of AChR antibody–negative patients with generalized MG have anti-MuSK antibodies.
Repetitive nerve stimulation: decrement of >15% at 3 Hz: highly probable
Single-fiber electromyography: blocking and jitter, with normal fiber density; confirmatory, but not specific
Edrophonium chloride (Tensilon) 2 mg + 8 mg IV; highly probable diagnosis if unequivocally positive
For ocular or cranial MG: exclude intracranial lesions by CT or MRI

Abbreviations: AChR, acetylcholine receptor; MuSK, muscle-specific tyrosine kinase.
Source: From RT Johnson, JW Griffin (eds): *Current Therapy in Neurologic Disease*, 4th ed. St. Louis, Mosby Year Book, 1994; with permission.

Antibodies to AChR or MuSK

As noted above, anti-AChR antibodies are detectable in the serum of ~85% of all myasthenic patients but in only about 50% of patients with weakness confined to the ocular muscles. The presence of anti-AChR antibodies is virtually diagnostic of MG, but a negative test does not exclude the disease. The measured level of anti-AChR antibody does not correspond well with the severity of MG in different patients. However, in an individual patient, a treatment-induced fall in the antibody level often correlates with clinical improvement, while a rise in the level may occur with exacerbations. Antibodies to MuSK have been found to be present in ~40% of AChR antibody–negative patients with generalized MG, and their presence is a useful diagnostic test in these patients. MuSK antibodies are rarely present in AChR antibody–positive patients or in patients with MG limited to ocular muscles. These antibodies may interfere with clustering of AChRs at neuromuscular junctions, as MuSK is known to do during early development. There is also evidence that MG patients without antibodies demonstrable by standard AChR or MuSK tests may have either low-affinity antibodies, or other—as yet undefined—antibodies that impair neuromuscular transmission.

Electrodiagnostic testing

Repetitive nerve stimulation may provide helpful diagnostic evidence of MG. Anti-AChE medication is stopped 6–24 h before testing. It is best to test weak muscles or proximal muscle groups. Electric shocks are delivered at a rate of two or three per second to the appropriate nerves, and action potentials are recorded from the muscles. In normal individuals, the amplitude of the evoked muscle action potentials does not change at these rates of stimulation. However, in myasthenic patients there is a rapid reduction of >10–15% in the amplitude of the evoked responses.

Anticholinesterase test

Drugs that inhibit the enzyme AChE allow ACh to interact repeatedly with the limited number of AChRs in MG, producing improvement in muscle strength. Edrophonium is used most commonly for diagnostic testing because of the rapid onset (30 s) and short duration (~5 min) of its effect. An objective end-point must be selected to evaluate the effect of edrophonium, such as weakness of extraocular muscles, impairment of speech, or the length of time that the patient can maintain the arms in forward abduction. An initial IV dose of 2 mg of edrophonium is given. If definite improvement occurs, the test is considered positive and is terminated. If there is no change, the patient is given an additional 8 mg IV. The dose is administered in two parts because some patients react to edrophonium with side effects such as nausea, diarrhea, salivation, fasciculations, and rarely with severe symptoms of syncope or bradycardia. Atropine (0.6 mg) should be drawn up in a syringe, ready for IV administration if these symptoms become troublesome. The edrophonium test is now reserved for patients with clinical findings that are suggestive of MG but who have negative antibody and electrodiagnostic test results. False-positive tests occur in occasional patients with other neurologic disorders, such as amyotrophic lateral sclerosis, and in placebo-reactors. False-negative or equivocal tests may also occur. In some cases, it is helpful to use a longer-acting drug such as neostigmine (15 mg PO), since this permits more time for detailed evaluation of strength.

Inherited myasthenic syndromes

The congenital myasthenic syndromes (CMS) comprise a heterogeneous group of disorders of the neuromuscular junction that are not autoimmune but rather are due to genetic mutations in which virtually any component of the neuromuscular junction may be affected. Alterations in function of the presynaptic nerve terminal

TABLE 386-2 The Congenital Myasthenic Syndromes

Type	Clinical Features	Electrophysiology	Genetics	End-Plate Effects	Treatment
Slow channel	Most common; weak forearm extensors; onset 2d to 3d decade; variable severity	Repetitive muscle response on nerve stimulation; prolonged channel opening and MEPP duration	Autosomal dominant; α, β, ε AChR mutations	Excitotoxic end-plate myopathy; decreased AChRs; postsynaptic damage	Quinidine: decreases end-plate damage; made worse by anti-AChE
Low-affinity fast channel	Onset early; moderately severe; ptosis, EOM involvement; weakness and fatigue	Brief and infrequent channel openings; opposite of slow channel syndrome	Autosomal recessive; may be heteroallelic	Normal end-plate structure	3,4-DAP; anti-AChE
Severe AChR deficiencies	Early onset; variable severity; fatigue; typical MG features	Decremental response to repetitive nerve stimulation; decreased MEPP amplitudes	Autosomal recessive; ε mutations most common; many different mutations	Increased length of end plates; variable synaptic folds	Anti-AChE; ?3,4-DAP
AChE deficiency	Early onset; variable severity; scoliosis; may have normal EOM, absent pupillary responses	Decremental response to repetitive nerve stimulation	Mutant gene for AChE's collagen anchor	Small nerve terminals; degenerated junctional folds	Worse with anti-AChE drugs

Abbreviations: AChR, acetylcholine receptor; AChE, acetylcholinesterase; EOM, extraocular muscles; MEPP, miniature end-plate potentials; 3,4-DAP, 3,4-diaminopyridine.

or in the various subunits of the AChR or AChE have been identified in the different forms of CMS. These disorders share many of the clinical features of autoimmune MG, including weakness and fatigability of skeletal muscles, in some cases involving extraocular muscles (EOMs), lids, and proximal muscles, similar to the distribution in autoimmune MG. CMS should be suspected when symptoms of myasthenia have begun in infancy or childhood and AChR antibody tests are consistently negative. Features of four of the most common forms of CMS are summarized in Table 386-2. Although clinical features and electrodiagnostic and pharmacologic tests may suggest the correct diagnosis, molecular analysis is required for precise elucidation of the defect; this may lead to helpful treatment as well as genetic counseling. In the forms that involve the AChR, a wide variety of mutations have been identified in each of the subunits, but the ε subunit is affected in ~75% of these cases. In most of the recessively inherited forms of CMS, the mutations are heteroallelic; that is, different mutations affecting each of the two alleles are present.

Differential diagnosis

Other conditions that cause weakness of the cranial and/or somatic musculature include the nonautoimmune CMS discussed above, drug-induced myasthenia, Lambert-Eaton myasthenic syndrome (LEMS), neurasthenia, hyperthyroidism, botulism, intracranial mass lesions, and progressive external ophthalmoplegia. Treatment with penicillamine (used for scleroderma or rheumatoid arthritis) may result in true autoimmune MG, but the weakness is usually mild, and recovery occurs within weeks or months after discontinuing its use. Aminoglycoside antibiotics or procainamide can cause exacerbation of weakness in myasthenic patients; very large doses can cause neuromuscular weakness in normal individuals.

LEMS is a presynaptic disorder of the neuromuscular junction that can cause weakness similar to that of MG. The proximal muscles of the lower limbs are most commonly affected, but other muscles may be involved as well. Cranial nerve findings, including ptosis of the eyelids and diplopia, occur in up to 70% of patients and resemble features of MG. However, the two conditions are usually readily distinguished, since patients with LEMS have depressed or absent reflexes and experience autonomic changes such as dry mouth and impotence. Nerve stimulation produces an initial low-amplitude response and, at low rates of repetitive stimulation (2–3 Hz), decremental responses like those of MG; however, at high rates (50 Hz), or following exercise, incremental responses occur. LEMS is caused by autoantibodies directed against P/Q-type calcium channels at the motor nerve terminals, which can be detected in ~85% of LEMS patients by radioimmunoassay. These autoantibodies result in impaired release of ACh from nerve terminals. Most patients with LEMS have an associated malignancy, most commonly small cell carcinoma of the lung, which may express calcium channels that stimulate the autoimmune response. The diagnosis of LEMS may signal the presence of a tumor long before it would otherwise be detected, permitting early removal. Treatment of LEMS involves plasmapheresis and immunosuppression, as for MG. 3,4-Diaminopyridine (3,4-DAP) and pyridostigmine may also be symptomatically helpful. 3,4-DAP acts by blocking potassium channels, which results in prolonged depolarization of the motor nerve terminals and thus enhances ACh release. Pyridostigmine prolongs the action of ACh, allowing repeated interactions with AChRs.

Botulism (Chap. 141) is due to potent bacterial toxins produced by any of seven different strains of *Clostridium botulinum*. The toxins enzymatically cleave specific proteins essential for the release of acetylcholine from the motor nerve terminal, thereby interfering with neuromuscular transmission. Most commonly, botulism is caused by ingestion of improperly prepared food containing toxin. Rarely, the nearly ubiquitous spores of *C. botulinum* may germinate in wounds. In infants the spores may germinate in the GI tract, and release toxin, causing muscle weakness. Patients present with myasthenia-like bulbar weakness (e.g., diplopia, dysarthria, dysphagia) and lack sensory symptoms and signs. Weakness may generalize to the limbs and may result in respiratory failure. Reflexes are present early, but they may be diminished as the disease progresses. Mentation is normal. Autonomic findings include paralytic ileus, constipation, urinary retention, dilated or poorly reactive pupils, and dry mouth. The demonstration of toxin in serum by bioassay is definitive, but the results usually take a relatively long time to be completed and may be negative. Nerve stimulation studies reveal findings of presynaptic neuromuscular blockade with reduced compound muscle action potentials (CMAPs) that increase in amplitude following high-frequency repetitive stimulation. Treatment includes ventilatory support, and aggressive inpatient supportive care (e.g., nutrition, DVT prophylaxis) as needed. Antitoxin should be given as early as possible to be effective. A preventive vaccine is available for laboratory workers or other highly exposed individuals.

Neurasthenia is the historic term for a myasthenia-like fatigue syndrome without an organic basis. These patients may present with subjective symptoms of weakness and fatigue, but muscle testing usually reveals the "give-away weakness" characteristic of nonorganic disorders; the complaint of fatigue in these patients means tiredness or apathy rather than decreasing muscle power on repeated effort. Hyperthyroidism is readily diagnosed or excluded by tests of thyroid function, which should be carried out routinely in patients with suspected MG. Abnormalities of thyroid function (hyper- or hypothyroidism) may increase myasthenic weakness. Diplopia resembling that in MG may occasionally be due to an intracranial mass lesion that compresses nerves to the EOMs (e.g., sphenoid ridge meningioma), but MRI of the head and orbits usually reveals the lesion.

Progressive external ophthalmoplegia is a rare condition resulting in weakness of the EOMs, which may be accompanied by weakness of the proximal muscles of the limbs and other systemic features. Most patients with this condition have mitochondrial disorders that can be detected on muscle biopsy (Chap. 387).

Search for associated conditions

(Table 386-3) Myasthenic patients have an increased incidence of several associated disorders. Thymic abnormalities occur in ~75% of patients, as noted above. Neoplastic change (thymoma) may produce enlargement of the thymus, which is detected by CT scanning of the anterior mediastinum. A thymic shadow on CT scan may normally be present through young adulthood, but enlargement of the thymus in a patient aged >40 years is highly suspicious of thymoma. Hyperthyroidism occurs in 3–8% of patients and may aggravate the myasthenic weakness. Thyroid function tests should be obtained in all patients with suspected MG. Because of the association of MG with other autoimmune disorders, blood tests for rheumatoid factor and antinuclear antibodies should also be carried out. Chronic infection of any kind can exacerbate MG and should be sought carefully. Finally, measurements of ventilatory function are valuable because of the frequency and seriousness of respiratory impairment in myasthenic patients.

Because of the side effects of glucocorticoids and other immunosuppressive agents used in the treatment of MG, a thorough medical investigation should be undertaken, searching specifically for evidence of chronic or latent infection (such as tuberculosis or hepatitis), hypertension, diabetes, renal disease, and glaucoma.

TABLE 386-3 Disorders Associated With Myasthenia Gravis and Recommended Laboratory Tests

Associated disorders
Disorders of the thymus: thymoma, hyperplasia
Other autoimmune disorders: Hashimoto's thyroiditis, Graves' disease, rheumatoid arthritis, lupus erythematosus, skin disorders, family history of autoimmune disorder
Disorders or circumstances that may exacerbate myasthenia gravis: hyperthyroidism or hypothyroidism, occult infection, medical treatment for other conditions (see Table 386-4)
Disorders that may interfere with therapy: tuberculosis, diabetes, peptic ulcer, gastrointestinal bleeding, renal disease, hypertension, asthma, osteoporosis, obesity
Recommended laboratory tests or procedures
CT or MRI of mediastinum
Tests for lupus erythematosus, antinuclear antibody, rheumatoid factor, antithyroid antibodies
Thyroid-function tests
PPD skin test
Chest radiography
Fasting blood glucose measurement, hemoglobin A1c
Pulmonary-function tests
Bone densitometry in older patients

Abbreviation: PPD, purified protein derivative.

Source: From RT Johnson, JW Griffin (eds): *Current Therapy in Neurologic Disease*, 4th ed. St. Louis, Mosby Year Book, 1993, p 379; with permission.

TREATMENT Myasthenia Gravis

The prognosis has improved strikingly as a result of advances in treatment. Nearly all myasthenic patients can be returned to full productive lives with proper therapy. The most useful treatments for MG include anticholinesterase medications, immunosuppressive agents, thymectomy, and plasmapheresis or intravenous immunoglobulin (IVIg) (Fig. 386-2).

ANTICHOLINESTERASE MEDICATIONS Anticholinesterase medication produces at least partial improvement in most myasthenic patients, although improvement is complete in only a few. Pyridostigmine is the most widely used anticholinesterase drug. The beneficial action of oral pyridostigmine begins within 15–30 min and lasts for 3–4 h, but individual responses vary. Treatment is begun with a moderate dose, e.g., 30–60 mg three to four times daily. The frequency and amount of the dose should be tailored to the patient's individual requirements throughout the day. For example, patients with weakness in chewing and swallowing may benefit by taking the medication before meals so that peak strength coincides with mealtimes. Long-acting pyridostigmine may occasionally be useful to get the patient through the night but should not be used for daytime medication because of variable absorption. The maximum useful dose of pyridostigmine rarely exceeds 120 mg every 4–6 h during daytime. Overdosage with anticholinesterase medication may cause increased weakness and other side effects. In some patients, muscarinic side effects of the anticholinesterase medication (diarrhea, abdominal cramps, salivation, nausea) may limit the dose tolerated. Atropine/diphenoxylate or loperamide is useful for the treatment of gastrointestinal symptoms.

THYMECTOMY Two separate issues should be distinguished: (1) surgical removal of thymoma, and (2) thymectomy as a treatment for MG. Surgical removal of a thymoma is necessary because of the possibility of local tumor spread, although most thymomas are histologically benign. In the absence of a tumor, the available evidence suggests that up to 85% of patients experience improvement after thymectomy; of these, ~35% achieve drug-free remission. However, the improvement is typically delayed for months to years. The advantage of thymectomy is that it offers the possibility of long-term benefit, in some cases diminishing or eliminating the need for continuing medical treatment. In view of these potential benefits and of the negligible risk in skilled hands, thymectomy has gained widespread acceptance in the treatment of MG. It is the consensus that thymectomy

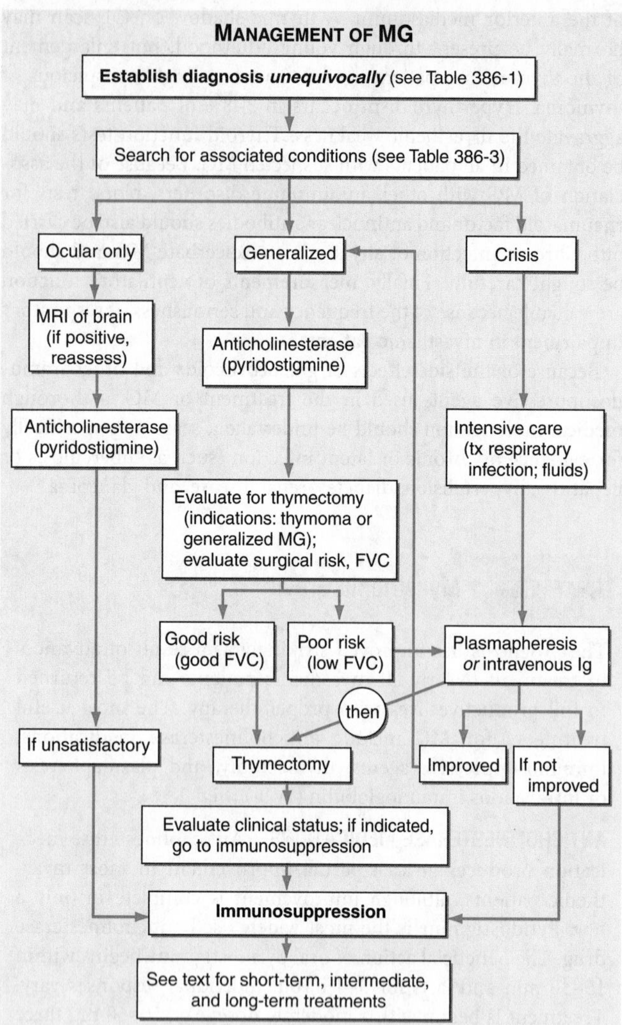

Figure 386-2 Algorithm for the management of myasthenia gravis. FVC, forced vital capacity.

should be carried out in all patients with generalized MG who are between the ages of puberty and at least 55 years. Whether thymectomy should be recommended in children, in adults >55 years of age, and in patients with weakness limited to the ocular muscles is still a matter of debate. There is also suggestive evidence that patients with MuSK antibody–positive MG may respond less well to thymectomy. Thymectomy must be carried out in a hospital where it is performed regularly and where the staff is experienced in the pre- and postoperative management, anesthesia, and surgical techniques of total thymectomy.

IMMUNOSUPPRESSION Immunosuppression using glucocorticoids, azathioprine, and other drugs is effective in nearly all patients with MG. The choice of drugs or other immunomodulatory treatments should be guided by the relative benefits and risks for the individual patient and the urgency of treatment. It is helpful to develop a treatment plan based on short-term, intermediate-term, and long-term objectives. For example, if immediate improvement is essential either because of the severity of weakness or because of the patient's need to return to activity as soon as possible, IVIg should be administered or plasmapheresis should be undertaken. For the intermediate term, glucocorticoids and cyclosporine or tacrolimus generally produce clinical improvement within a period of 1–3 months. The beneficial effects of azathioprine and mycophenolate mofetil usually begin after many months (as long as a year), but these drugs have advantages for the long-term treatment of patients with MG. For the occasional patient with MG that is genuinely refractory to optimal treatment with conventional immunosuppressive agents, a course of high-dose cyclophosphamide may induce long-lasting benefit by "rebooting" the immune system. At high doses, cyclophosphamide eliminates mature lymphocytes but spares hematopoietic precursors (stem cells), because they express the enzyme aldehyde dehydrogenase, which hydrolyzes cyclophosphamide. At present, this procedure is reserved for refractory patients and should be administered only in a facility fully familiar with this approach. We recommend maintenance immunotherapy after rebooting, to sustain the beneficial effect.

Glucocorticoid Therapy Glucocorticoids, when used properly, produce improvement in myasthenic weakness in the great majority of patients. To minimize adverse side effects, prednisone should be given in a single dose rather than in divided doses throughout the day. The initial dose should be relatively low (15–25 mg/d) to avoid the early weakening that occurs in about one-third of patients treated initially with a high-dose regimen. The dose is increased stepwise, as tolerated by the patient (usually by 5 mg/d at 2- to 3-day intervals), until there is marked clinical improvement or a dose of 50–60 mg/d is reached. This dose is maintained for 1–3 months and then is gradually modified to an alternate-day regimen over the course of an additional 1–3 months; the goal is to reduce the dose on the "off day" to zero or to a minimal level. Generally, patients begin to improve within a few weeks after reaching the maximum dose, and improvement continues to progress for months or years. The prednisone dosage may gradually be reduced, but usually months or years may be needed to determine the minimum effective dose, and close monitoring is required. Few patients are able to do without immunosuppressive agents entirely. Patients on long-term glucocorticoid therapy must be followed carefully to prevent or treat adverse side effects. The most common errors in glucocorticoid treatment of myasthenic patients include (1) insufficient persistence—improvement may be delayed and gradual; (2) tapering the dosage too early, too rapidly, or excessively; and (3) lack of attention to prevention and treatment of side effects.

The management of patients treated with glucocorticoids is discussed in Chap. 342.

Other Immunosuppressive Drugs Mycophenolate mofetil, azathioprine, cyclosporine, tacrolimus, and occasionally cyclophosphamide are effective in many patients, either alone or in various combinations.

Mycophenolate mofetil has become one of the most widely used drugs in the treatment of MG because of its effectiveness and relative lack of side effects. A dose of 1–1.5 g bid is recommended. Its mechanism of action involves inhibition of purine synthesis by the de novo pathway. Since lymphocytes lack the alternative salvage pathway that is present in all other cells, mycophenolate inhibits proliferation of lymphocytes but not proliferation of other cells. It does not kill or eliminate preexisting autoreactive lymphocytes, and therefore clinical improvement may be delayed for many months to a year, until the preexisting autoreactive lymphocytes die spontaneously. The advantage of mycophenolate lies in its relative lack of adverse side effects, with only occasional production of GI symptoms, rare development of leukopenia, and very small risks of malignancy or PML inherent in all immunosuppressive treatments. Although two published studies did not have positive outcomes, most experts attribute the negative results to flaws in the trial designs, and mycophenolate is widely used for long-term treatment of myasthenic patients. Until recently, azathioprine has been the most commonly used immunosuppressive agent for MG because of its relative safety in most patients and long track record. Its therapeutic effect may add to that of glucocorticoids and/or allow the glucocorticoid dose to be reduced. However, up to 10% of patients are unable to tolerate azathioprine because of idiosyncratic reactions consisting of flulike symptoms of fever and malaise, bone marrow suppression, or abnormalities of liver function. An initial dose of 50 mg/d should be used for several days to test for these side effects. If this dose is tolerated, it is increased gradually to about 2–3 mg/kg of total body weight, or until the white blood count falls to 3000 to 4000/μL. The beneficial effect of azathioprine takes 3–6 months to begin and even longer to peak. In patients taking azathioprine, allopurinol should never be used to treat hyperuricemia. Because the two drugs share a common degradation pathway; the result may be severe bone marrow suppression due to increased effects of the azathioprine.

The calcineurin inhibitors cyclosporine and tacrolimus (FK506) are approximately as effective as azathioprine and are being used increasingly in the management of MG. Their beneficial effect appears more rapidly than that of azathioprine. Either drug may be used alone, but they are usually used as an adjunct to glucocorticoids to permit reduction of the glucocorticoid dose. The usual dose of cyclosporine is 4–5 mg/kg per d, and the average dose of tacrolimus is 0.07–0.1 mg/kg per d, given in two equally divided doses (to minimize side effects). Side effects of these drugs include hypertension and nephrotoxicity, which must be closely monitored. "Trough" blood levels are measured 12 h after the evening dose. The therapeutic range for the trough level of cyclosporine is 150–200 ng/L, and for tacrolimus it is 5–15 ng/L.

Cyclophosphamide is reserved for occasional patients refractory to the other drugs (see above for discussion of high-dose cyclophosphamide treatment). Rituximab, a monoclonal antibody that depletes CD20 B cells, has been used with variable—sometimes dramatic—success in the treatment of MG, especially in patients with anti-MuSK antibody.

PLASMAPHERESIS AND INTRAVENOUS IMMUNOGLOBULIN Plasmapheresis has been used therapeutically in MG. Plasma, which contains the pathogenic antibodies, is mechanically separated from the blood cells, which are returned to the patient. A course of five exchanges (3–4 L per exchange) is generally administered over a 10- to 14-day period. Plasmapheresis produces a short-term reduction in anti-AChR antibodies, with clinical improvement in many patients. It is useful as a temporary expedient in seriously affected patients or to improve the patient's condition prior to surgery (e.g., thymectomy).

The indications for the use of IVIg are the same as those for plasma exchange: to produce rapid improvement to help the patient through a difficult period of myasthenic weakness or prior to surgery. This treatment has the advantages of not requiring special equipment or large-bore venous access. The usual dose is 2 g/kg, which is typically administered over 5 days (400 mg/kg per d). If tolerated, the total dose of IVIg can be given over a 3- to 4-day period. Improvement occurs in ~70% of patients, beginning during treatment, or within a week, and continuing for weeks to months. The mechanism of action of IVIg is not known; the treatment has no consistent effect on the measurable amount of circulating AChR antibody. Adverse reactions are generally not serious but include headache, fluid overload, and rarely aseptic meningitis or renal failure. IVIg should rarely be used as a long-term treatment in place of rationally managed immunosuppressive therapy. Unfortunately, there is a tendency for physicians unfamiliar with immunosuppressive treatments to rely on repeated IVIg infusions, which usually produce only intermittent benefit, do not reduce the underlying autoimmune response, and are costly. The intermediate and long-term treatment of myasthenic patients requires other methods of therapy outlined earlier in this chapter.

MANAGEMENT OF MYASTHENIC CRISIS Myasthenic crisis is defined as an exacerbation of weakness sufficient to endanger life; it usually consists of respiratory failure caused by diaphragmatic and intercostal muscle weakness. Crisis rarely occurs in properly managed patients. Treatment should be carried out in intensive care units staffed with teams experienced in the management of MG, respiratory insufficiency, infectious disease, and fluid and electrolyte therapy. The possibility that deterioration could be due to excessive anticholinesterase medication ("cholinergic crisis") is best excluded by temporarily stopping anticholinesterase drugs. The most common cause of crisis is intercurrent infection. This should be treated immediately, because the mechanical and immunologic defenses of the patient can be assumed to be compromised. The myasthenic patient with fever and early infection should be treated like other immunocompromised patients. Early and effective antibiotic therapy, respiratory assistance (preferably noninvasive, using BiPap), and pulmonary physiotherapy are essentials of the treatment program. As discussed above, plasmapheresis or IVIg is frequently helpful in hastening recovery.

DRUGS TO AVOID IN MYASTHENIC PATIENTS Many drugs have been reported to exacerbate weakness in patients with MG (Table 386-4), but not all patients react adversely to all of these. Conversely, not all "safe" drugs can be used with impunity in patients with MG. As a rule, the listed drugs should be avoided *whenever possible*, and myasthenic patients should be followed closely when *any new drug* is introduced.

■ PATIENT ASSESSMENT

To evaluate the effectiveness of treatment as well as drug-induced side effects, it is important to assess the patient's clinical status systematically at baseline and on repeated interval examinations. Because of the variability of symptoms of MG, the interval history and physical findings on examination must be taken into account. The most useful clinical tests include forward arm abduction time (up to a full 5 min), forced vital capacity, range of eye movements, and time to development of ptosis on upward gaze. Manual muscle testing or, preferably, quantitative dynamometry of limb muscles, especially proximal muscles, is also important. An interval form can provide a succinct summary of the patient's status and a guide to treatment results; an abbreviated form is shown in Fig. 386-3. A progressive reduction in the patient's AChR antibody level also provides clinically valuable confirmation of the effectiveness of treatment; conversely, a rise in AChR antibody levels during tapering of immunosuppressive medication may predict clinical exacerbation. For reliable quantitative measurement of AChR antibody levels, it is best to compare antibody levels from prior frozen serum aliquots with current serum samples in simultaneously run assays.

TABLE 386-4 Drugs With Interactions in Myasthenia Gravis (MG)

Drugs that may exacerbate MG
Antibiotics
Aminoglycosides: e.g., streptomycin, tobramycin, kanamycin
Quinolones: e.g., ciprofloxacin, levofloxacin, ofloxacin, gatifloxacin
Macrolides: e.g., erythromycin, azithromycin,
Nondepolarizing muscle relaxants for surgery
D-Tubocurarine (curare), pancuronium, vecuronium, atracurium
Beta-blocking agents
Propranolol, atenolol, metoprolol
Local anesthetics and related agents
Procaine, Xylocaine in large amounts
Procainamide (for arrhythmias)
Botulinum toxin
Botox exacerbates weakness
Quinine derivatives
Quinine, quinidine, chloroquine, mefloquine (Lariam)
Magnesium
Decreases ACh release
Penicillamine
May cause MG
Drugs with important interactions in MG
Cyclosporine
Broad range of drug interactions, which may raise or lower cyclosporine levels.
Azathioprine
Avoid allopurinol—combination may result in myelosuppression.

Myasthenia Gravis Worksheet

History				
General	Normal	Good	Fair	Poor
Diplopia	None	Rare	Occasional	Constant
Ptosis	None	Rare	Occasional	Constant
Arms	Normal	Slightly limited	Some ADL impairment	Definitely limited
Legs	Normal	Walks/runs fatigues	Can walk limited distances	Minimal walking
Speech	Normal	Dysarthric	Severely dysarthric	Unintelligible
Voice	Normal	Fades	Impaired	Severely impaired
Chew	Normal	Fatigue on normal foods	Fatigue on soft foods	Feeding tube
Swallow	Normal	Normal foods	Soft foods only	Feeding tube
Respiration	Normal	Dyspnea on unusual effort	Dyspnea on any effort	Dyspnea at rest

Examination

BP ____ Pulse ____ Wt ____	Arm abduction time R ____ L ____
Edema ____	Deltoids R ____ L ____
Vital capacity ____	Biceps R ____ L ____
Cataracts? R ____ L ____	Triceps R ____ L ____
EOMS ____	Grip R ____ L ____
Ptosis time ____	Iliopsoas R ____ L ____
Face ____	Quadriceps R ____ L ____
	Hamstrings R ____ L ____
	Other R ____ L ____

Figure 386-3 Abbreviated interval assessment form for use in evaluating treatment for myasthenia gravis.

FURTHER READINGS

DRACHMAN DB: Chapter 8. Therapy of myasthenia gravis. Handb Clin Neurol 91:253, 2008

______ et al: Rebooting the immune system with high dose cyclophosphamide for treatment of refractory myasthenia gravis. Ann NY Acad Sci 1132:305, 2008

FARRUGIA ME, VINCENT A: Autoimmune mediated neuromuscular junction defects. Curr Opin Neurol 23:489, 2010

LANG B, VINCENT A: Autoimmune disorders of the neuromuscular junction. Curr Opin Pharmacol 3:336, 2009

LEITE MI et al: IgG1 antibodies to acetylcholine receptors in "seronegative" myasthenia gravis. Brain 131:1684, 2008

OH SJ: Muscle-specific receptor tyrosine kinase antibody positive myasthenia gravis current status. J Clin Neurol 5:53, 2009

PHAN SJ et al: Mycophenolate mofetil in myasthenia gravis: The unanswered question. Expert Opin Pharmacother 14: 2545, 2008

SKEIE GO et al: Guidelines for treatment of autoimmune neuromuscular transmission disorders. Eur J Neurol 17:893, 2010

ZINMAN L et al: IV immunoglobulin in patients with myasthenia gravis: A randomized controlled trial. Neurology 68:837, 2007

CHAPTER 387

Muscular Dystrophies and Other Muscle Diseases

Anthony A. Amato
Robert H. Brown, Jr.

Skeletal muscle diseases, or myopathies, are disorders with structural changes or functional impairment of muscle. These conditions can be differentiated from other diseases of the motor unit (e.g., lower motor neuron or neuromuscular junction pathologies) by characteristic clinical and laboratory findings.

Myasthenia gravis and related disorders are discussed in Chap. 386; dermatomyositis, polymyositis, and inclusion body myositis are discussed in Chap. 388.

CLINICAL FEATURES

Most myopathies present with proximal, symmetric limb weakness (arms or legs) with preserved reflexes and sensation. However, asymmetric and predominantly distal weakness can be seen in some myopathies. An associated sensory loss suggests injury to peripheral nerve or the central nervous system (CNS) rather than myopathy. On occasion, disorders affecting the motor nerve cell bodies in the spinal cord (anterior horn cell disease), the neuromuscular junction, or peripheral nerves can mimic findings of myopathy.

Muscle weakness

Symptoms of muscle weakness can be either intermittent or persistent. Disorders causing *intermittent weakness* (Fig. 387-1) include myasthenia gravis, periodic paralyses (hypokalemic, hyperkalemic, and paramyotonia congenita), and metabolic energy deficiencies of glycolysis (especially myophosphorylase deficiency), fatty acid utilization (carnitine palmitoyltransferase deficiency), and some mitochondrial myopathies. The states of energy deficiency cause activity-related muscle breakdown accompanied by myoglobinuria, appearing as light-brown- to dark-brown-colored urine.

Most muscle disorders cause *persistent weakness* (Fig. 387-2). In the majority of these, including most types of muscular dystrophy, polymyositis, and dermatomyositis, the proximal muscles are weaker than the distal and are symmetrically affected, and the facial muscles are spared, a pattern referred to as *limb-girdle*. The differential diagnosis is more restricted for other patterns of weakness. Facial weakness (difficulty with eye closure and impaired smile) and scapular winging (Fig. 387-3) are characteristic of facioscapulohumeral dystrophy (FSHD). Facial and distal limb weakness associated with hand grip myotonia is virtually diagnostic of myotonic dystrophy type 1. When other cranial nerve muscles are weak, causing ptosis or extraocular muscle weakness, the most important disorders to consider include neuromuscular junction disorders, oculopharyngeal muscular dystrophy, mitochondrial myopathies, or some of the congenital myopathies (Table 387-1). A pathognomonic pattern characteristic of inclusion body myositis is atrophy and weakness of the flexor forearm (e.g., wrist and finger flexors) and quadriceps muscles that is often asymmetric. Less frequently, but important diagnostically, is the presence of a dropped head syndrome indicative of selective neck extensor muscle weakness. The most important neuromuscular diseases associated with this pattern of weakness include myasthenia gravis, amyotrophic lateral sclerosis, late-onset nemaline myopathy, hyperparathyroidism, focal myositis, and some forms of inclusion body myopathy. A final pattern, recognized because of preferential distal extremity weakness, is typical of a unique category of muscular dystrophy, the distal myopathies.

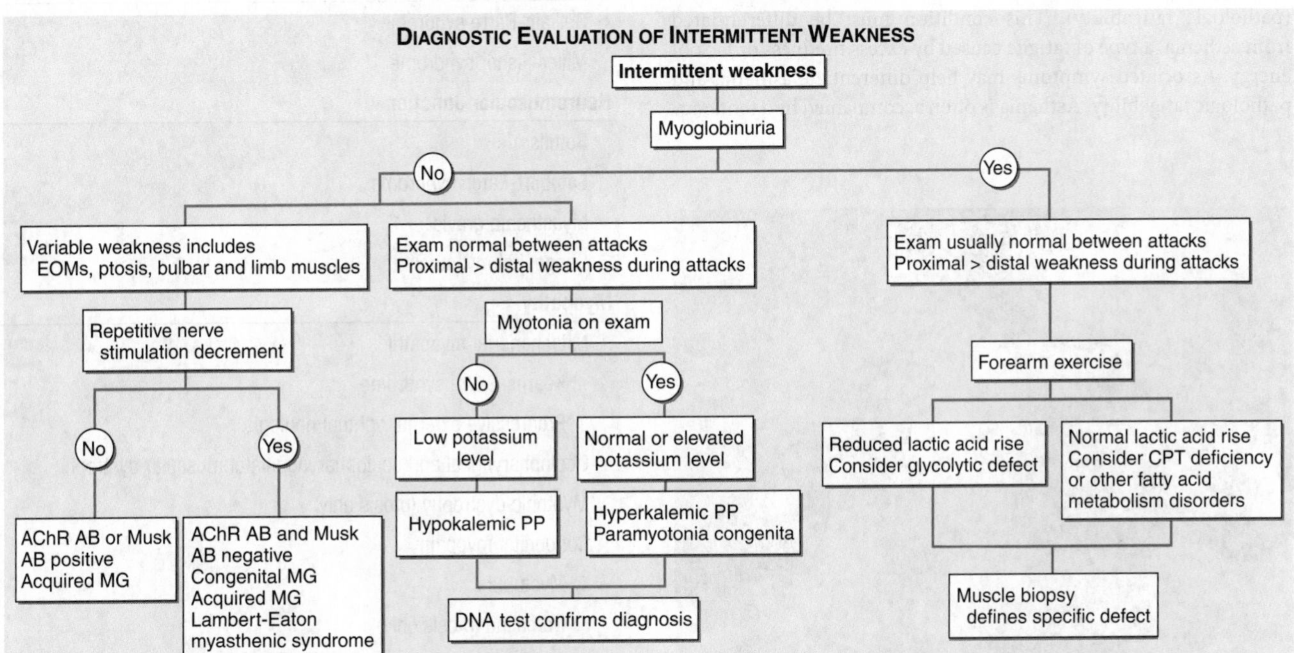

Figure 387-1 Diagnostic evaluation of intermittent weakness. AChR AB, acetylcholine receptor antibody; CPT, carnitine palmitoyltransferase; EOMs, extraocular muscles; MG, myasthenia gravis; PP, periodic paralysis.

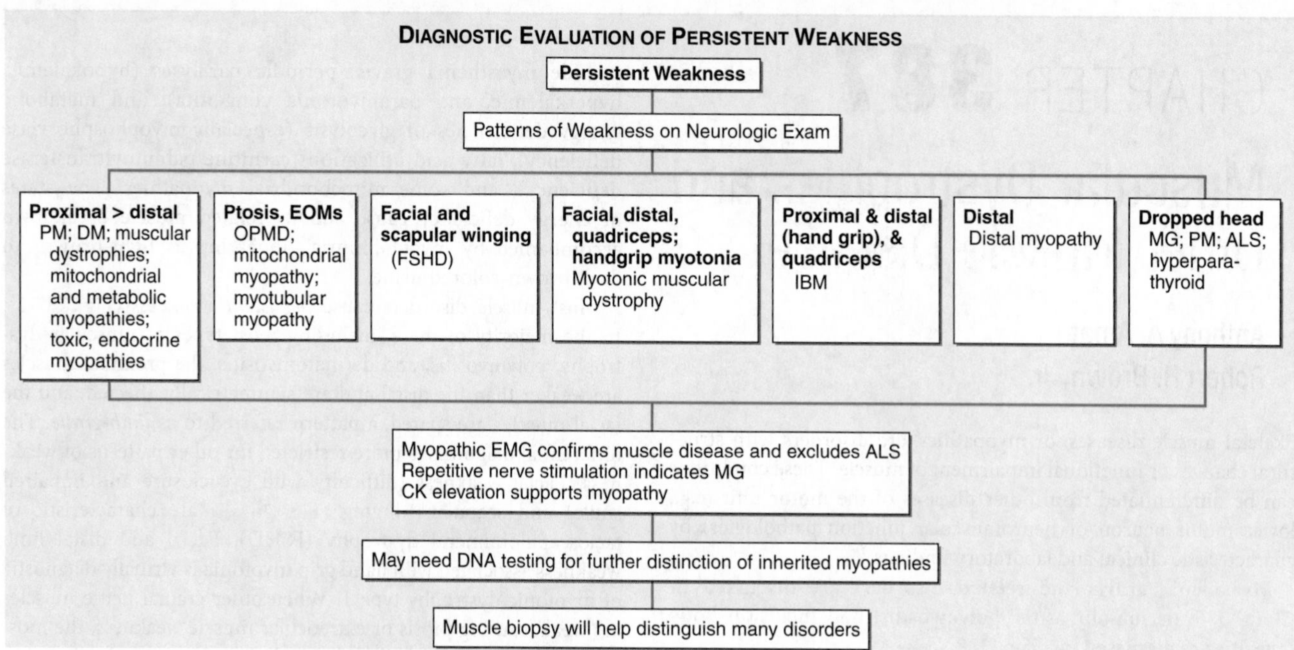

Figure 387-2 Diagnostic evaluation of persistent weakness. Examination reveals one of seven patterns of weakness. The pattern of weakness in combination with the laboratory evaluation leads to a diagnosis. EOMs, extraocular muscles; OPMD, oculopharyngeal muscular dystrophy; FSHD, facioscapulohumeral dystrophy; IBM, inclusion body myositis; DM, dermatomyositis; PM, polymyositis; MG, myasthenia gravis; ALS, amyotrophic lateral sclerosis; CK, creatine kinase; EMG, electromyography.

It is important to examine functional capabilities to help disclose certain patterns of weakness (Table 387-2). The Gowers' sign (Fig. 387-4) is particularly useful. Observing the gait of an individual may disclose a lordotic posture caused by combined trunk and hip weakness, frequently exaggerated by toe walking (Fig. 387-5). A waddling gait is caused by the inability of weak hip muscles to prevent hip drop or hip dip. Hyperextension of the knee (genu recurvatum or back-kneeing) is characteristic of quadriceps muscle weakness; and a steppage gait, due to footdrop, accompanies distal weakness.

Any disorder causing muscle weakness may be accompanied by *fatigue*, referring to an inability to maintain or sustain a force (pathologic fatigability). This condition must be differentiated from asthenia, a type of fatigue caused by excess tiredness or lack of energy. Associated symptoms may help differentiate asthenia and pathologic fatigability. Asthenia is often accompanied by a tendency to avoid physical activities, complaints of daytime sleepiness, necessity for frequent naps, and difficulty concentrating on activities such as reading. There may be feelings of overwhelming stress and depression. Thus, asthenia is not a myopathy. In contrast, pathologic fatigability occurs in disorders of neuromuscular transmission

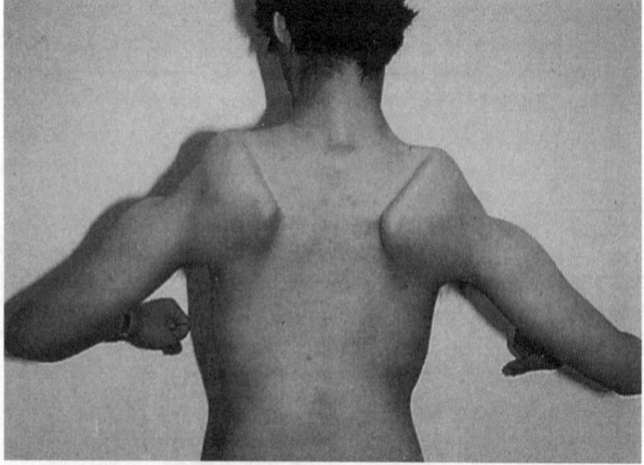

Figure 387-3 Facioscapulohumeral dystrophy with prominent scapular winging.

TABLE 387-1 Neuromuscular Causes of Ptosis or Ophthalmoplegia

Peripheral Neuropathy
Guillain-Barré syndrome
Miller-Fisher syndrome
Neuromuscular Junction
Botulism
Lambert-Eaton syndrome
Myasthenia gravis
Congenital myasthenia
Myopathy
Mitochondrial myopathies
Kearns-Sayre syndrome
Progressive external ophthalmoplegia
Oculopharyngeal and oculopharyngodistal muscular dystrophy
Myotonic dystrophy (ptosis only)
Congenital myopathy
Myotubular
Nemaline (ptosis only)
Hyperthyroidism/Graves' disease (ophthalmoplegia without ptosis)
Hereditary inclusion body myopathy type 3

TABLE 387-2 Observations on Examination That Disclose Muscle Weakness

Functional Impairment	Muscle Weakness
Inability to forcibly close eyes	Upper facial muscles
Impaired pucker	Lower facial muscles
Inability to raise head from prone position	Neck extensor muscles
Inability to raise head from supine position	Neck flexor muscles
Inability to raise arms above head	Proximal arm muscles (may be only scapular stabilizing muscles)
Inability to walk without hyperextending knee (back-kneeing or genu recurvatum)	Knee extensor muscles
Inability to walk with heels touching the floor (toe walking)	Shortening of the Achilles tendon
Inability to lift foot while walking (steppage gait or footdrop)	Anterior compartment of leg
Inability to walk without a waddling gait	Hip muscles
Inability to get up from the floor without climbing up the extremities (Gowers' sign)	Hip, thigh, and trunk muscles
Inability to get up from a chair without using arms	Hip muscles

and in disorders altering energy production, including defects in glycolysis, lipid metabolism, or mitochondrial energy production. Pathologic fatigability also occurs in chronic myopathies because of difficulty accomplishing a task with less muscle. Pathologic fatigability is accompanied by abnormal clinical or laboratory findings. Fatigue without those supportive features almost never indicates a primary muscle disease.

Muscle pain (myalgias), cramps, and stiffness

Muscle pain can be associated with cramps, spasms, contractures, and stiff or rigid muscles. In distinction, true myalgia (muscle aching), which can be localized or generalized, may be accompanied by weakness, tenderness to palpation, or swelling. Certain drugs cause true myalgia (Table 387-3).

There are two painful muscle conditions of particular importance, neither of which is associated with muscle weakness. *Fibromyalgia* is a common, yet poorly understood, type of myofascial pain syndrome. Patients complain of severe muscle pain and tenderness and have specific painful trigger points, sleep disturbances, and easy fatigability. Serum creatine kinase (CK), erythrocyte sedimentation rate (ESR), electromyography (EMG), and muscle biopsy are normal (Chap. 335). *Polymyalgia rheumatica* occurs mainly in patients >50 years and is characterized by stiffness and pain in the shoulders, lower back, hips, and thighs (Chap. 326). The ESR is elevated, while serum CK, EMG, and muscle biopsy are normal. Temporal arteritis, an inflammatory disorder of medium- and large-sized arteries, usually involving one or more branches of the carotid artery, may accompany polymyalgia rheumatica. Vision is threatened by ischemic optic neuritis. Glucocorticoids can relieve the myalgias and protect against visual loss.

Localized muscle pain is most often traumatic. A common cause of sudden abrupt-onset pain is a ruptured tendon, which leaves the muscle belly appearing rounded and shorter in appearance compared to the normal side. The biceps brachii and Achilles tendons are particularly vulnerable to rupture. Infection or neoplastic infiltration of the muscle is a rare cause of localized muscle pain.

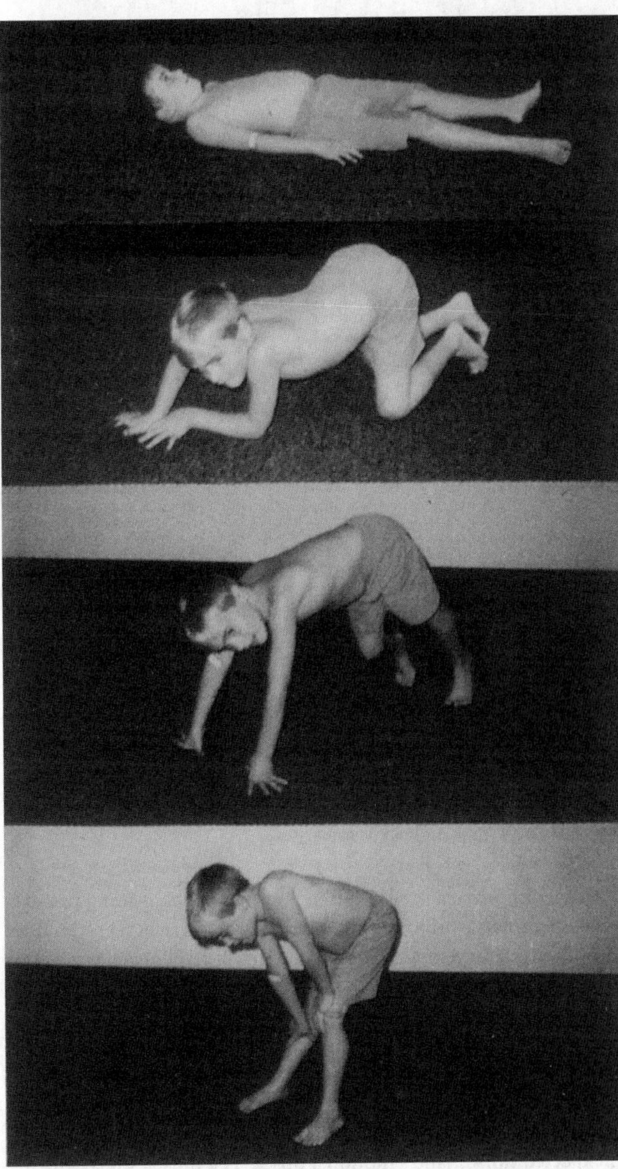

Figure 387-4 **Gowers' sign** showing a patient using arms to climb up the legs in attempting to get up from the floor.

A *muscle cramp* or *spasm* is a painful, involuntary, localized, muscle contraction with a visible or palpable hardening of the muscle. Cramps are abrupt in onset, short in duration, and may cause abnormal posturing of the joint. The EMG shows firing of motor units, reflecting an origin from spontaneous neural discharge. Muscle cramps often occur in neurogenic disorders, especially motor neuron disease (Chap. 374), radiculopathies, and polyneuropathies (Chap. 384), but are not a feature of most primary muscle diseases. Duchenne's muscular dystrophy is an exception since calf muscle complaints are a common complaint. Muscle cramps are also common during pregnancy.

A *muscle contracture* is different from a muscle cramp. In both conditions, the muscle becomes hard, but a contracture is associated with energy failure in glycolytic disorders. The muscle is unable to relax after an active muscle contraction. The EMG shows electrical silence. Confusion is created because contracture also refers to a muscle that cannot be passively stretched to its proper length (fixed contracture) because of fibrosis. In some muscle disorders, especially in Emery-Dreifuss muscular dystrophy and Bethlem's myopathy, fixed contractures occur early and represent distinctive features of the disease.

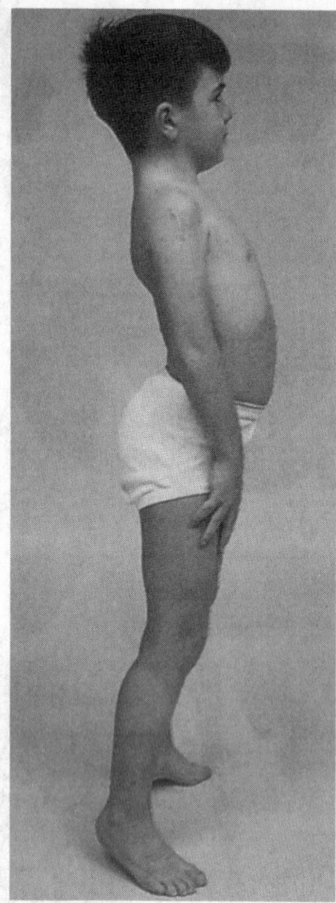

Figure 387-5 Lordotic posture, exaggerated by standing on toes, associated with trunk and hip weakness.

Muscle stiffness can refer to different phenomena. Some patients with inflammation of joints and periarticular surfaces feel stiff. This condition is different from the disorders of hyperexcitable motor nerves causing stiff or rigid muscles. In *stiff-person syndrome*, spontaneous discharges of the motor neurons of the spinal cord cause involuntary muscle contractions mainly involving the axial (trunk) and proximal lower extremity muscles. The gait becomes stiff and labored, with hyperlordosis of the lumbar spine. Superimposed episodic muscle spasms are precipitated by sudden movements, unexpected noises, and emotional upset. The muscles relax during sleep. Serum antibodies against glutamic acid decarboxylase are present in approximately two-thirds of cases. In *neuromyotonia* (*Isaac's syndrome*) there is hyperexcitability of the peripheral nerves manifesting as continuous muscle fiber activity. *Myokymia* (groups of fasciculations associated with continuous undulations of muscle) and impaired muscle relaxation are the result. Muscles of the leg are stiff, and the constant contractions of the muscle cause increased sweating of the extremities. This peripheral nerve hyperexcitability is mediated by antibodies that target voltage-gated potassium channels. The site of origin of the spontaneous nerve discharges is principally in the distal portion of the motor nerves.

Myotonia is a condition of prolonged muscle contraction followed by slow muscle relaxation. It always follows muscle activation (action myotonia), usually voluntary, but may be elicited by mechanical stimulation (percussion myotonia) of the muscle. Myotonia typically causes difficulty in releasing objects after a firm grasp. In myotonic muscular dystrophy type 1 (DM1), distal weakness usually accompanies myotonia, whereas in DM2 proximal muscles are more affected; thus the related term *proximal myotonic myopathy* (PROMM) is used to describe this condition. Myotonia also occurs with *myotonia congenita* (a chloride channel disorder), but in this condition muscle weakness is not prominent. Myotonia may also be seen in individuals with sodium channel mutations (*hyperkalemic periodic paralysis* or *potassium-sensitive myotonia*). Another sodium channelopathy, *paramyotonia congenita*, also is associated with muscle stiffness. In contrast to other disorders associated with myotonia in which the myotonia is eased by repetitive activity, paramyotonia congenita is named for a paradoxical phenomenon whereby the myotonia worsens with repetitive activity.

TABLE 387-3 Drugs That Cause True Myalgia

Cimetidine
Cocaine
Cyclosporine
Danazol
Emetine
Gold
Heroin
Labetalol
Methadone
D-Penicillamine
Statins and other cholesterol-lowering agents
L-Tryptophan
Zidovudine

Muscle enlargement and atrophy

In most myopathies muscle tissue is replaced by fat and connective tissue, but the size of the muscle is usually not affected. However, in many limb-girdle muscular dystrophies (and particularly the dystrophinopathies) enlarged calf muscles are typical. The enlargement represents true muscle hypertrophy, thus the term *pseudohypertrophy* should be avoided when referring to these patients. The calf muscles remain very strong even late in the course of these disorders. Muscle enlargement can also result from infiltration by sarcoid granulomas, amyloid deposits, bacterial and parasitic infections, and focal myositis. In contrast, muscle atrophy is characteristic of other myopathies. In dysferlinopathies (LGMD2B), there is a predilection for early atrophy of the gastrocnemius muscles, particularly the medial aspect. Atrophy of the humeral muscles is characteristic of facioscapulohumeral dystrophy (FSHD).

LABORATORY EVALUATION

A limited battery of tests can be used to evaluate a suspected myopathy. Nearly all patients require serum enzyme level measurements and electrodiagnostic studies as screening tools to differentiate muscle disorders from other motor unit diseases. The other tests described—DNA studies, the forearm exercise test, and muscle biopsy—are used to diagnose specific types of myopathies.

Serum enzymes

CK is the preferred muscle enzyme to measure in the evaluation of myopathies. Damage to muscle causes the CK to leak from the muscle fiber to the serum. The MM isoenzyme predominates in skeletal muscle, while creatine kinase-myocardial bound (CK-MB) is the marker for cardiac muscle. Serum CK can be elevated in normal individuals without provocation, presumably on a genetic basis or after strenuous activity, minor trauma (including the EMG needle), a prolonged muscle cramp, or a generalized seizure. Aspartate aminotransferase (AST), alanine aminotransferase (ALT), aldolase, and lactic dehydrogenase (LDH) are enzymes sharing an origin in both muscle and liver. Problems arise when the levels of these enzymes are found to be elevated in a routine screening battery, leading to the erroneous assumption that liver disease is present when in fact muscle could be the cause. An elevated γ-glutamyl transferase (GGT) helps to establish a liver origin since this enzyme is not found in muscle.

Electrodiagnostic studies

EMG, repetitive nerve stimulation, and nerve conduction studies (Chap. e45) are essential methods for evaluation of the patient with suspected muscle disease. In combination, they provide the information necessary to differentiate myopathies from neuropathies and neuromuscular junction diseases. Routine nerve conduction studies are typically normal in myopathies but reduced amplitudes of compound muscle action potentials may be seen in atrophied muscles. The needle EMG may reveal irritability on needle placement suggestive of a necrotizing myopathy (inflammatory myopathies, dystrophies, toxic myopathies, myotonic myopathies), whereas a lack of irritability is characteristic of long-standing myopathic disorders (muscular dystrophies, endocrine myopathies, disuse atrophy, and many of the metabolic myopathies). In addition, the EMG may demonstrate myotonic discharges that will narrow the differential diagnosis (Table 387-4). Another important EMG finding is the presence of short-duration, small-amplitude, polyphasic motor unit action potentials (MUAPs). Such MUAPs can be seen in both myopathic and neuropathic disorders; however, the recruitment or firing pattern is different. In myopathies, the MUAPs fire early but at a normal rate to compensate for the loss of individual muscle fibers, whereas in neurogenic disorders the MUAPs fire faster. The EMG is usually normal in steroid or disuse myopathy, both of which are associated with type 2 fiber atrophy; this is because the EMG preferentially assesses the physiologic function of type 1 fibers. The EMG can also be invaluable in helping to choose an appropriately affected muscle to sample for biopsy.

DNA analysis

This serves as an important tool for the definitive diagnosis of many muscle disorders. Nevertheless, there are a number of limitations in currently available molecular diagnostics. For example, in Duchenne's and Becker's dystrophies, two-thirds of patients have deletion or duplication mutations that are easy to detect, while the remainder have point mutations that are much more difficult to find. For patients without identifiable gene defects, the muscle biopsy remains the main diagnostic tool.

TABLE 387-4 Myotonic Disorders

Myotonic dystrophy type 1
Myotonic dystrophy type 2/proximal myotonic myopathy
Myotonia congenita
Paramyotonia congenita
Hyperkalemic periodic paralysis
Chondrodystrophic myotonia (Schwartz-Jampel syndrome)
Centronuclear/myotubular myopathy[a]
Drug-induced
Cholesterol-lowering agents (statin medications, fibrates)
Cyclosporine
Chloroquine
Glycogen storage disorders[a] (Pompe's disease, debrancher deficiency, branching enzyme deficiency)
Myofibrillar myopathies[a]

[a]Associated with myotonic discharges on EMG but no clinical myotonia.

Forearm exercise test

In myopathies with intermittent symptoms, and especially those associated with myoglobinuria, there may be a defect in glycolysis. Many variations of the forearm exercise test exist. For safety, the test should not be performed under ischemic conditions to avoid an unnecessary insult to the muscle, causing rhabdomyolysis. The test is performed by placing a small indwelling catheter into an antecubital vein. A baseline blood sample is obtained for lactic acid and ammonia. The forearm muscles are exercised by asking the patient to vigorously open and close the hand for 1 minute. Blood is then obtained at intervals of 1, 2, 4, 6, and 10 minutes for comparison with the baseline sample. A three- to fourfold rise of lactic acid is typical. The simultaneous measurement of ammonia serves as a control, since it should also rise with exercise. In patients with myophosphorylase deficiency or other glycolytic defects, the lactic acid rise will be absent or below normal, while the rise in ammonia will reach control values. If there is lack of effort, neither lactic acid nor ammonia will rise. Patients with selective failure to increase ammonia may have myoadenylate deaminase deficiency. This condition has been reported to be a cause of myoglobinuria, but deficiency of this enzyme in asymptomatic individuals makes interpretation controversial.

Muscle biopsy

Muscle biopsy is an important step in establishing the diagnosis of a suspected myopathy. The biopsy is usually obtained from a quadriceps or biceps brachii muscle, less commonly from a deltoid muscle. Evaluation includes a combination of techniques—light microscopy, histochemistry, immunocytochemistry with a battery of antibodies, and electron microscopy. Not all techniques are needed for every case. A specific diagnosis can be established in many disorders. Endomysial inflammatory cells surrounding and invading muscle fibers are seen in polymyositis; similar endomysial infiltrates associated with muscle fibers containing rimmed vacuoles, amyloid deposits within fibers, and TDP-43 inclusions are characteristic of inclusion body myositis; while perivascular, perimysial inflammation associated with perifascicular atrophy are features of dermatomyositis. In addition, the congenital myopathies have distinctive light and electron microscopy features essential for diagnosis. Mitochondrial and metabolic (e.g., glycogen and lipid storage diseases) myopathies also demonstrate distinctive histochemical and electron-microscopic profiles. Biopsied muscle tissue can be sent for metabolic enzyme or mitochondrial DNA analyses. A battery of antibodies is available for the identification of missing components of the dystrophin-glycoprotein complex and related proteins to help diagnose specific types of muscular dystrophies. Western blot analysis on muscle specimens can be performed to determine whether specific muscle proteins are reduced in quantity or are of abnormal size.

HEREDITARY MYOPATHIES

Muscular dystrophy refers to a group of hereditary progressive diseases each with unique phenotypic and genetic features (Tables 387-5, 387-6, and 387-7).

DUCHENNE'S MUSCULAR DYSTROPHY

This X-linked recessive disorder, sometimes also called *pseudohypertrophic muscular dystrophy*, has an incidence of ~30 per 100,000 live-born males.

Clinical features

Duchenne's dystrophy is present at birth, but the disorder usually becomes apparent between ages 3 and 5 years. The boys fall frequently and have difficulty keeping up with friends when playing.

TABLE 387-5 Progressive Muscular Dystrophies

Type	Inheritance	Defective Gene/ Protein	Onset Age	Clinical Features	Other Organ Systems Involved
Duchenne's	XR	Dystrophin	Before 5 years	Progressive weakness of girdle muscles Unable to walk after age 12 Progressive kyphoscoliosis Respiratory failure in 2d or 3d decade	Cardiomyopathy Mental impairment
Becker's	XR	Dystrophin	Early childhood to adult	Progressive weakness of girdle muscles Able to walk after age 15 Respiratory failure may develop by 4th decade	Cardiomyopathy
Limb-girdle	AD/AR	Several (Tables 387-6, 387-7)	Early childhood to early adult	Slow progressive weakness of shoulder and hip girdle muscles	± Cardiomyopathy
Emery-Dreifuss	XR/AD	Emerin/Lamins A/C Nesprin-1, Nesprin 2, *TMEM43*	Childhood to adult	Elbow contractures, humeral and peroneal weakness	Cardiomyopathy
Congenital	AR	Several	At birth or within first few months	Hypotonia, contractures, delayed milestones Progression to respiratory failure in some; static course in others	CNS abnormalities (hypomyelination, malformation) Eye abnormalities
Myotonic[a] (DM1, DM2)	AD	DM1: Expansion CTG repeat DM2: Expansion CCTG repeat	Childhood to adult Maybe infancy if mother affected (DM1 only)	Slowly progressive weakness of face, shoulder girdle, and foot dorsiflexion Preferential proximal weakness in DM2	Cardiac conduction defects Mental impairment Cataracts Frontal baldness Gonadal atrophy
Facioscapulohumeral	AD	*DUX4* 4q	Childhood to adult	Slowly progressive weakness of face, shoulder girdle, and foot dorsiflexion	Deafness Coats' (eye) disease
Oculopharyngeal	AD	Expansion, poly-A RNA binding protein	5th to 6th decade	Slowly progressive weakness of extraocular, pharyngeal, and limb muscles	—

[a]Two forms of myotonic dystrophy, DM1 and DM2 , have been identified. Many features overlap (see text).
Abbreviations: AD, autosomal dominant; AR, autosomal recessive; CNS, central nervous system; XR, X-linked recessive.

TABLE 387-6 Autosomal Dominant Limb-Girdle Muscular Dystrophies (LGMDs)

Disease	Clinical Features	Laboratory Features	Locus or Gene
LGMD1A	Onset 3rd to 4th decade Muscle weakness affects distal limb muscles, vocal cords, and pharyngeal muscles	Serum CK 2 × normal EMG mixed myopathy/neuropathy NCS normal	Myotilin
LGMD1B	Onset 1st or 2nd decade Proximal lower limb weakness and cardiomyopathy with conduction defects Some cases indistinguishable from Emery-Dreifuss muscular dystrophy with joint contractures	Serum CK 3–5 × normal NCS normal EMG myopathic	Lamin A/C
LGMD1C	Onset in early childhood Proximal weakness Gowers' sign, calf hypertrophy Exercise-related muscle cramps	Serum CK 4–25 × normal NCS normal EMG myopathic	Caveolin-3
LGMD1D	Onset 3rd to 5th decade Proximal muscle weakness Cardiomyopathy and arrhythmias	Serum CK 2–4 × normal NCS normal EMG myopathic	Linked to chromosome 7q Gene unidentified
LGMD1E	Childhood onset Proximal muscle weakness	Serum CK usually normal NCS normal EMG myopathic	Linked to chromosome 6q23 Gene unidentified

Abbreviations: CK, creatine kinase; EMG, electromyography; NCS, nerve conduction studies.

TABLE 387-7 Autosomal Recessive Limb-Girdle Muscular Dystrophies (LGMDs)

Disease	Clinical Features	Laboratory Features	Locus or Gene
LGMD2A	Onset 1st or 2nd decade Tight heel cords Contractures at elbows, wrists, and fingers; rigid spine in some Proximal and distal weakness	Serum CK 3–15 × normal NCS normal EMG myopathic	Calpain-3
LGMD2B	Onset 2nd or 3rd decade Proximal muscle weakness at onset, later distal (calf) muscles affected Miyoshi's myopathy is variant of LGMD2B with calf muscles affected at onset	Serum CK 3–100 × normal NCS normal EMG myopathic Inflammation on muscle biopsy may simulate polymyositis	Dysferlin
LGMD2C–F	Onset in childhood to teenage years Clinical condition similar to Duchenne and Becker muscular dystrophies Cardiomyopathy uncommon Cognitive function normal	Serum CK 5–100 × normal NCS normal EMG myopathic	γ, α, β, δ sarcoglycans
LGMD2G	Onset age 10 to 15 Proximal and distal muscle weakness	Serum CK 3–17 × normal NCS normal EMG myopathic	Telethonin
LGMD2H	Onset 1st to 3rd decade Proximal muscle weakness	Serum CK 2–25 × normal NCS normal EMG myopathic	TRIM32 gene
LGMD2I	Onset 1st to 3rd decade Clinical condition similar to Duchenne's or Becker's dystrophies Cardiomyopathy (some not all) Cognitive function normal	Serum CK 10–30 × normal NCS normal EMG myopathic	Fukutin-related protein
LGMD2J[a]	Onset 1st to 3rd decade Proximal lower limb weakness Mild distal weakness Progressive weakness causes loss of ambulation	Serum CK 1.5–2 × normal NCS normal EMG myopathic	Titin
LGMD2K	Usually presents in infancy as Walker-Warburg syndrome but can present in early adult life with proximal weakness and only minor CNS abnormalities	CK 10–20 × normal NCS normal EMG myopathic	POMT1
LGMD2IL	Presents in childhood or adult life. May manifest with quadriceps atrophy and myalgia Some present with early involvement of the calves in the second decade of life, resembling Miyoshi myopathy (dysferlinopathy)	CK normal to 50 × normal NCS normal EMG myopathic	Anoctamin 5
LGMD2M	Usually presents in infancy as Fukuyuma congenital muscular dystrophy but can present in early adult life with proximal weakness and only minor CNS abnormalities	CK 10–50 × normal NCS normal EMG myopathic	Fukutin
LGMD2N	Usually presents in infancy as Muscle-Eye-Brain disease but can present in early adult life with proximal weakness and only minor CNS abnormalities	CK 5–20 × normal NCS normal EMG myopathic	POMGnT1
LGMD2O	Usually presents in infancy as Walker-Warburg syndrome but can present in early adult life with proximal weakness and only minor CNS abnormalities	CK 5–20 × normal NCS normal EMG myopathic	POMT2

[a]Tibial muscular dystrophy is a form of titin deficiency with only distal muscle weakness (see Table 387-9).

Abbreviations: CK, creatine kinase; EMG, electromyography; NCS, nerve conduction studies. POMT1, protein-O-mannosyltransferase 1; POMT2, protein-O-mannosyltransferase 2; POMGNT1, O-linked mannose beta 1,2-N-acetylglucosaminyltransferase.

Running, jumping, and hopping are invariably abnormal. By age 5 years, muscle weakness is obvious by muscle testing. On getting up from the floor, the patient uses his hands to climb up himself [Gowers' maneuver (Fig. 387-4)]. Contractures of the heel cords and iliotibial bands become apparent by age 6 years, when toe walking is associated with a lordotic posture. Loss of muscle strength is progressive, with predilection for proximal limb muscles and the neck flexors; leg involvement is more severe than arm involvement. Between ages 8 and 10 years, walking may require the use of braces; joint contractures and limitations of hip flexion, knee, elbow, and wrist extension are made worse by prolonged sitting. By age 12 years, most patients are wheelchair dependent. Contractures become fixed, and a progressive scoliosis often develops that may be associated with pain. The chest deformity with scoliosis impairs pulmonary function, which is already diminished by muscle weakness. By age 16–18 years, patients are predisposed to serious, sometimes fatal pulmonary infections. Other causes of death include aspiration of food and acute gastric dilation.

A cardiac cause of death is uncommon despite the presence of a cardiomyopathy in almost all patients. Congestive heart failure seldom occurs except with severe stress such as pneumonia. Cardiac arrhythmias are rare. The typical electrocardiogram (ECG) shows an increased net RS in lead V_1; deep, narrow Q waves in the precordial leads; and tall right precordial R waves in V_1. Intellectual impairment in Duchenne's dystrophy is common; the average intelligence quotient (IQ) is ~1 SD below the mean. Impairment of intellectual function appears to be nonprogressive and affects verbal ability more than performance.

Laboratory features

Serum CK levels are invariably elevated to between 20 and 100 times normal. The levels are abnormal at birth but decline late in the disease because of inactivity and loss of muscle mass. EMG demonstrates features typical of myopathy. The muscle biopsy shows muscle fibers of varying size as well as small groups of necrotic and regenerating fibers. Connective tissue and fat replace lost muscle fibers. A definitive diagnosis of Duchenne's dystrophy can be established on the basis of dystrophin deficiency in a biopsy of muscle tissue or mutation analysis on peripheral blood leukocytes, as discussed below.

Duchenne's dystrophy is caused by a mutation of the gene that encodes dystrophin, a 427-kDa protein localized to the inner surface of the sarcolemma of the muscle fiber. The dystrophin gene is >2000 kb in size and thus is one of the largest identified human genes. It is localized to the short arm of the X chromosome at Xp21. The most common gene mutation is a deletion. The size varies but does not correlate with disease severity. Deletions are not uniformly distributed over the gene but rather are most common near the beginning (5′ end) and middle of the gene. Less often, Duchenne's dystrophy is caused by a gene duplication or point mutation. Identification of a specific mutation allows for an unequivocal diagnosis, makes possible accurate testing of potential carriers, and is useful for prenatal diagnosis.

A diagnosis of Duchenne's dystrophy can also be made by Western blot analysis of muscle biopsy specimens, revealing abnormalities on the quantity and molecular weight of dystrophin protein. In addition, immunocytochemical staining of muscle with dystrophin antibodies can be used to demonstrate absence or deficiency of dystrophin localizing to the sarcolemmal membrane. Carriers of the disease may demonstrate a mosaic pattern, butdystrophin analysis of muscle biopsy specimens for carrier detection is not reliable.

Pathogenesis

Dystrophin is part of a large complex of sarcolemmal proteins and glycoproteins (Fig. 387-6). Dystrophin binds to F-actin at its amino terminus and to β-dystroglycan at the carboxyl terminus. β-Dystroglycan complexes to α-dystroglycan, which binds to laminin in the extracellular matrix (ECM). Laminin has a heterotrimeric molecular structure arranged in the shape of a cross with one heavy chain and two light chains, β_1 and γ_1. The laminin heavy chain of skeletal muscle is designated laminin α_2. Collagen proteins IV and VI are also found in the ECM. Like β-dystroglycan, the transmembrane sarcoglycan proteins also bind to dystrophin; these five proteins (designated α- through ε-sarcoglycan) complex tightly with each other. More recently, other membrane proteins implicated in muscular dystrophy have been found to be loosely affiliated with constituents of the dystrophin complex. These include caveolin-3, α_7 integrin, and collagen VI.

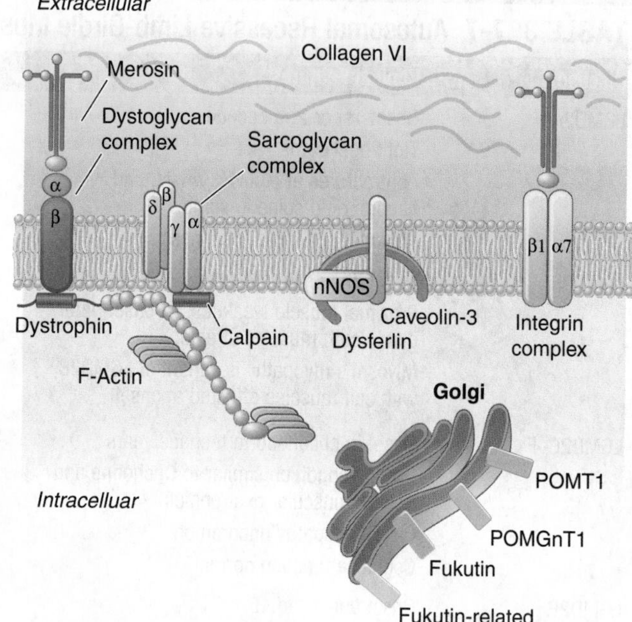

Figure 387-6 Selected muscular dystrophy–associated proteins in the cell membrane and Golgi complex.

Dystrophin localizes to the cytoplasmic face of the muscle cell membrane. It complexes with two transmembrane protein complexes, the dystroglycans and the sarcoglycans. The dystroglycans bind to the extracellular matrix protein merosin, which is also complexed with β_1 and α_7 integrins (Tables 387-5, 387-6, 387-7). Dysferlin complexes with caveolin-3 (which binds to neuronal nitric oxide synthase, or nNOS) but not with the dystrophin-associated proteins or the integrins. In some of the congenital dystrophies and limb-girdle muscular dystrophies (LGMDs), there is loss of function of different enzymes that glycosylate α-dystroglycan, which thereby inhibits proper binding to merosin: POMT1, POMT2, POMGnT1, Fukutin, Fukutin-related protein, and LARGE.

The dystrophin-glycoprotein complex appears to confer stability to the sarcolemma, although the function of each individual component of the complex is incompletely understood. Deficiency of one member of the complex may cause abnormalities in other components. For example, a primary deficiency of dystrophin (Duchenne's dystrophy) may lead to secondary loss of the sarcoglycans and dystroglycan. The primary loss of a single sarcoglycan (see "Limb-Girdle Muscular Dystrophy," below) results in a secondary loss of other sarcoglycans in the membrane without uniformly affecting dystrophin. In either instance, disruption of the dystrophin-glycoprotein complexes weakens the sarcolemma, causing membrane tears and a cascade of events leading to muscle fiber necrosis. This sequence of events occurs repeatedly during the life of a patient with muscular dystrophy.

TREATMENT Duchenne's Muscular Dystrophy

Glucocorticoids, administered as prednisone in a dose of 0.75 mg/kg per day, significantly slow progression of Duchenne's dystrophy for up to 3 years. Some patients cannot tolerate glucocorticoid therapy; weight gain and increased risk of fractures in particular represent a significant deterrent for some boys. As in other recessively inherited dystrophies presumed to arise from loss of function of a critical muscle gene, there is optimism that Duchenne's disease may benefit from novel therapies that either replace the defective gene or missing protein or implement downstream corrections (e.g., skipping mutated exons or reading through mutations that introduce stop codons).

BECKER'S MUSCULAR DYSTROPHY

This less severe form of X-linked recessive muscular dystrophy results from allelic defects of the same gene responsible for Duchenne's dystrophy. Becker's muscular dystrophy is ~10 times less frequent than Duchenne's, with an incidence of about 3 per 100,000 live-born males.

Clinical features

The pattern of muscle wasting in Becker's muscular dystrophy closely resembles that seen in Duchenne's. Proximal muscles, especially of the lower extremities, are prominently involved. As the disease progresses, weakness becomes more generalized. Significant facial muscle weakness is not a feature. Hypertrophy of muscles, particularly in the calves, is an early and prominent finding.

Most patients with Becker's dystrophy first experience difficulties between ages 5 and 15 years, although onset in the third or fourth decade or even later can occur. By definition, patients with Becker's dystrophy walk beyond age 15, while patients with Duchenne's dystrophy are typically in a wheelchair by the age of 12. Patients with Becker's dystrophy have a reduced life expectancy, but most survive into the fourth or fifth decade.

Mental retardation may occur in Becker's dystrophy, but it is not as common as in Duchenne's. Cardiac involvement occurs in Becker's dystrophy and may result in heart failure; some patients manifest with only heart failure. Other less common presentations are asymptomatic hyper-CK-emia, myalgias without weakness, and myoglobinuria.

Laboratory features

Serum CK levels, results of EMG, and muscle biopsy findings closely resemble those in Duchenne's dystrophy. The diagnosis of Becker's muscular dystrophy requires Western blot analysis of muscle biopsy samples, demonstrating a reduced amount or abnormal size of dystrophin or mutation analysis of DNA from peripheral blood leukocytes. Genetic testing reveals deletions or duplications of the dystrophin gene in 65% of patients with Becker's dystrophy, approximately the same percentage as in Duchenne's dystrophy. In both Becker's and Duchenne's dystrophies, the size of the DNA deletion does not predict clinical severity; however, in ~95% of patients with Becker's dystrophy, the DNA deletion does not alter the translational reading frame of messenger RNA. These "in-frame" mutations allow for production of some dystrophin, which accounts for the presence of altered rather than absent dystrophin on Western blot analysis.

TREATMENT Becker's Muscular Dystrophy

The use of glucocorticoids has not been adequately studied in Becker's dystrophy.

LIMB-GIRDLE MUSCULAR DYSTROPHY

The syndrome of LGMD represents more than one disorder. Both males and females are affected, with onset ranging from late in the first decade to the fourth decade. The LGMDs typically manifest with progressive weakness of pelvic and shoulder girdle musculature. Respiratory insufficiency from weakness of the diaphragm may occur, as may cardiomyopathy.

A systematic classification of LGMD is based on autosomal dominant (LGMD1) and autosomal recessive (LGMD2) inheritance. Superimposed on the backbone of LGMD1 and LGMD2, the classification employs a sequential alphabetical lettering system (LGMD1A, LGMD2A, etc.). Disorders receive letters in the order in which they are found to have chromosomal linkage. This results in an ever-expanding list of conditions. Presently there are 5 autosomal dominant and 10 autosomal recessive disorders, summarized in Tables 387-6 and 387-7. None of the conditions is as common as the dystrophinopathies; however, prevalence data for the LGMDs have not been systematically gathered for any large heterogeneous population. In referral-based clinical populations, Fukutin-related protein (FKRP) deficiency (LGMD2I), calpainopathies (LGMD2A), and to a lesser extent dysferlinopathies (LGMD2B) have emerged as the most common disorders.

EMERY-DREIFUSS MUSCULAR DYSTROPHY

There are at least five genetically distinct forms of Emery-Dreifuss muscular dystrophy (EDMD). Emerin mutations are the most common cause of X-linked EDMD, though mutations in *FHL1* may also be associated with a similar phenotype, which is X-linked as well. Mutations involving the gene for lamin A/C are the most common cause of autosomal dominant EDMD (also known as LGMD1B) and is also a common cause of hereditary cardiomyopathy. Less commonly, autosomal dominant EDMD has been reported with mutations in nesprin-1, nesprin-2, and *TMEM43*.

Clinical features

Prominent contractures can be recognized in early childhood and teenage years, often preceding muscle weakness. The contractures persist throughout the course of the disease and are present at the elbows, ankles, and neck. Muscle weakness affects humeral and peroneal muscles at first and later spreads to a limb-girdle distribution. The cardiomyopathy is potentially life threatening and may result in sudden death. A spectrum of atrial rhythm and conduction defects includes atrial fibrillation and paralysis and atrioventricular heart block. Some patients have a dilated cardiomyopathy. Female carriers of the X-linked variant may have cardiac manifestations that become clinically significant.

Laboratory features

Serum CK may be elevated two- to tenfold. EMG is myopathic. Muscle biopsy usually shows nonspecific dystrophic features, though cases associated with FHL1 mutations have features of myofibrillar myopathy. Immunohistochemistry reveals absent emerin staining of myonuclei in X-linked EDMD due to emerin mutations. ECGs demonstrate atrial and atrioventricular rhythm disturbances.

X-linked EDMD usually arises from defects in the emerin gene encoding a nuclear envelope protein. FHL1 mutations are also a cause of scapuloperoneal dystrophy, but can also present with an EDMD phenotype. The autosomal dominant disease can be caused by mutations in the *LMNA* gene encoding lamin A and C; in the synaptic nuclear envelope protein 1 (*SYNE1*) or 2 (*SYNE2*) encoding nesprin-1 and nesprin-2, respectively; and most recently in *TMEM43* encoding LUMA. These proteins are essential components of the filamentous network underlying the inner nuclear membrane. Loss of structural integrity of the nuclear envelope from defects in emerin, lamin A/C, nesprin-1, nesprin-2, and LUMA accounts for overlapping phenotypes (Fig. 387-7).

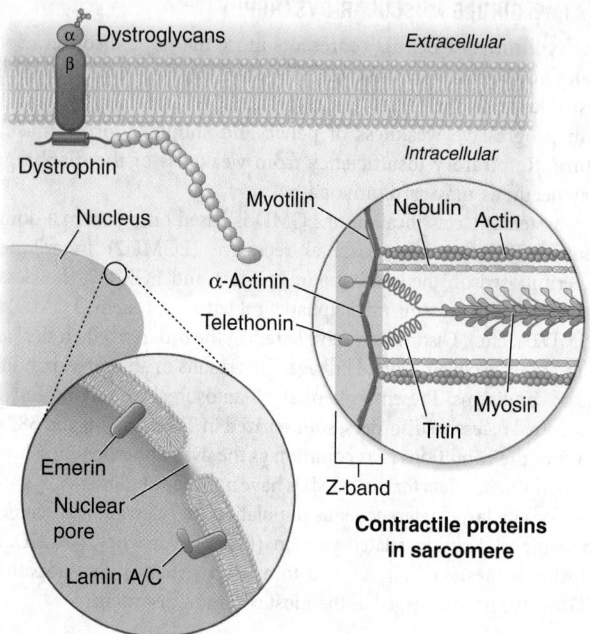

Figure 387-7 Selected muscular dystrophy–associated proteins in the nuclear membrane and sarcomere. As shown in the exploded view, emerin and lamin A/C are constituents of the inner nuclear membrane. Several dystrophy-associated proteins are represented in the sarcomere including titin, nebulin, calpain, telethonin, actinin, and myotilin. The position of the dystrophin-dystroglycan complex is also illustrated.

TREATMENT Emery-Dreifuss Muscular Dystrophy

Supportive care should be offered for neuromuscular disability, including ambulatory aids, if necessary. Stretching of contractures is difficult. Management of cardiomyopathy and arrhythmias (e.g., early use of a defibrillator or cardiac pacemaker) may be life saving.

■ CONGENITAL MUSCULAR DYSTROPHY (CMD)

This is not one entity but rather a group of disorders with varying degrees of muscle weakness, CNS impairment, and eye abnormalities.

Clinical features

As a group, CMDs present at birth or in the first few months of life with hypotonia and proximal or generalized muscle weakness. Calf muscle hypertrophy is seen in some patients. Facial muscles may be weak, but other cranial nerve–innervated muscles are spared (e.g., extraocular muscles are normal). Most patients have joint contractures of varying degrees at elbows, hips, knees, and ankles. Contractures present at birth are referred to as *arthrogryposis*. Respiratory failure may be seen in some cases.

The CNS is affected in some forms of CMD. In merosin and FKRP deficiency, cerebral hypomyelination may be seen by MRI, though only a small number of patients have mental retardation and seizures. Three forms of congenital muscular dystrophy have severe brain impairment. These include Fukuyama congenital muscular dystrophy (FCMD), muscle-eye-brain (MEB) disease, and Walker-Warburg syndrome (WWS). Patients are severely disabled in all three of these conditions. In MEB disease and WWS, but not in FCMD, ocular abnormalities impair vision. WWS is the most severe congenital muscular dystrophy, causing death by 1 year of age.

Laboratory features

Serum CK is markedly elevated in all of these conditions. The EMG is myopathic and muscle biopsies show nonspecific dystrophic features. Merosin, or laminin α_2 chain (a basal lamina protein), is deficient in surrounding muscle fibers in merosin deficiency. Skin biopsies can also demonstrate defects in laminin α_2 chain. In the other disorders (FKRP deficiency, FCMD, MEB disease, WWS), there is abnormal α-dystroglycan staining in muscle. In merosin deficiency, cerebral hypomyelination is common, and a host of brain malformations are seen in FCMD, MEB disease, and WWS.

All forms of CMD are inherited as autosomal recessive disorders. Chromosomal linkage and specific gene defects are presented in Table 387-8. With the exception of merosin, the other gene defects affect posttranslational glycosylation of α-dystroglycan. This abnormality is thought to impair binding with merosin and leads to weakening of the dystrophin-glycoprotein complex, instability of the muscle membrane, and/or abnormalities in muscle contraction. CMDs with brain and eye phenotypes probably involve defective glycosylation of additional proteins, accounting for the more extensive phenotypes.

TREATMENT Congenital Muscular Dystrophy

There is no specific treatment for CMD. Proper wheelchair seating is important. Management of epilepsy and cardiac manifestations is necessary for some patients.

■ MYOTONIC DYSTROPHY

Myotonic dystrophy is also known as *dystrophia myotonica* (DM). The condition is composed of at least two clinical disorders with overlapping phenotypes and distinct molecular genetic defects: myotonic dystrophy type 1 (DM1), the classic disease originally described by Steinert, and myotonic dystrophy type 2 (DM2), also called *proximal myotonic myopathy* (PROMM).

Clinical features

The clinical expression of DM1 varies widely and involves many systems other than muscle. Affected patients have a typical "hatchet-faced" appearance due to temporalis, masseter, and facial muscle atrophy and weakness. Frontal baldness is also characteristic of the disease. Neck muscles, including flexors and sternocleidomastoids, and distal limb muscles are involved early. Weakness of wrist extensors, finger extensors, and intrinsic hand muscles impairs function. Ankle dorsiflexor weakness may cause footdrop. Proximal muscles remain stronger throughout the course, although preferential atrophy and weakness of quadriceps muscles occur in many patients. Palatal, pharyngeal, and tongue involvement produce a dysarthric speech, nasal voice, and swallowing problems. Some patients have diaphragm and intercostal muscle weakness, resulting in respiratory insufficiency.

Myotonia, which usually appears by age 5 years, is demonstrable by percussion of the thenar eminence, the tongue, and wrist extensor muscles. Myotonia causes a slow relaxation of hand grip after a forced voluntary closure. Advanced muscle wasting makes myotonia more difficult to detect.

Cardiac disturbances occur commonly in patients with DM1. ECG abnormalities include first-degree heart block and more extensive conduction system involvement. Complete heart block and sudden death can occur. Congestive heart failure occurs infrequently but may result from cor pulmonale secondary to respiratory failure. Mitral valve prolapse also occurs commonly. Other associated features include intellectual impairment, hypersomnia,

TABLE 387-8 Congenital Muscular Dystrophies[a]

Disease	Clinical Features	Laboratory Features	Locus or Gene
Merosin deficiency	Onset at birth with hypotonia, joint contractures, delayed milestones, generalized muscle weakness Cerebral hypomyelination, less often cortical dysplasia Normal intelligence usually, some with MR (~6%) and seizures (~8%) Partial deficiency leads to milder phenotype (LGMD picture)	Serum CK 5–35 × normal EMG myopathic NCS abnormal in some cases	Laminin α_2 chain
Fukitin-related protein deficiency[b]	Onset at birth or shortly after Hypotonia and feeding problems Weakness of proximal muscles, especially shoulder girdles Hypertrophy of leg muscles Joint contractures Cognition normal	Serum CK 10–50 × normal EMG myopathic NCS normal	Fukutin-related protein
Fukuyama congenital muscular dystrophy[b]	Onset at birth Hypotonia, joint contractures Generalized muscle weakness Hypertrophy of calf muscles Seizures, mental retardation Cardiomyopathy	Serum CK 10–50 × normal EMG myopathic NCS normal MRI shows hydrocephalus and periventricular and frontal hypomyelination	Fukutin
Muscle-eye-brain disease	Onset at birth, hypotonia Eye abnormalities include: progressive myopia, cataracts, and optic nerve, glaucoma, retinal pigmentary changes Progressive muscle weakness Joint contractures Seizures, mental retardation	Serum CK 5–20 × normal MRI shows hydrocephalus, cobblestone lissencephaly, corpus callosum and cerebellar hypoplasia, cerebral hypomyelination	*N*-acetyl-glucosaminyl transferase (POMGnT1)
Walker-Warburg syndrome[b]	Onset at birth, hypotonia Generalized muscle weakness Joint contractures Microphthalmos, retinal dysplasia, buphthalmos, glaucoma, cataracts Seizures, MR	Serum CK 5–20 × normal MRI shows cobblestone lissencephaly, hydrocephalus, encephalocele, absent corpus callosum	*O*-mannoxyl-transferase-1 (POMT1)

[a]All are inherited as recessive traits.
[b]There is phenotypic overlap between disorders related to defective glycosylation. In muscle, this is a consequence of altered glycosylation of dystroglycans; in brain/eye, other glycosylated proteins are involved. Clinically, Walker-Warburg syndrome is more severe, with death by 1 year.
Abbreviations: CK, creatine kinase; EMG, electromyography; LGMD, limb-girdle muscular dystrophy; MR, mental retardation; NCS, nerve conduction studies.

posterior subcapsular cataracts, gonadal atrophy, insulin resistance, and decreased esophageal and colonic motility.

Congenital myotonic dystrophy is a more severe form of DM1 and occurs in ~25% of infants of affected mothers. It is characterized by severe facial and bulbar weakness, transient neonatal respiratory insufficiency, and mental retardation.

DM2, or PROMM, has a distinct pattern of muscle weakness affecting mainly proximal muscles. Other features of the disease overlap with DM1, including cataracts, testicular atrophy, insulin resistance, constipation, hypersomnia, and cognitive defects. Cardiac conduction defects occur but are less common, and the hatchet face and frontal baldness are less consistent features. A very striking difference is the failure to clearly identify a congenital form of DM2.

Laboratory features

The diagnosis of myotonic dystrophy can usually be made on the basis of clinical findings. Serum CK levels may be normal or mildly elevated. EMG evidence of myotonia is present in most cases of DM1 but may be more patchy in DM2. Muscle biopsy shows muscle atrophy, which selectively involves type 1 fibers in 50% of cases, and ringed fibers in DM1 but not in DM2. Typically, numerous internalized nuclei can be seen in individual muscle fibers as well as atrophic fibers with pyknotic nuclear clumps in both DM1 and DM2. Necrosis of muscle fibers and increased connective tissue, common in other muscular dystrophies, are less apparent in myotonic dystrophy.

DM1 and DM2 are both autosomal dominant disorders. New mutations do not appear to contribute to the pool of affected individuals. DM1 is transmitted by an intronic mutation consisting of an unstable expansion of a CTG trinucleotide repeat in a serine-threonine protein kinase gene (named *DMPK*) on chromosome 19q13.3. An increase in the severity of the disease phenotype in successive generations (genetic anticipation) is accompanied by an increase in the number of trinucleotide repeats. A similar type of mutation has been identified in fragile X syndrome (Chap. 61). The unstable triplet repeat in myotonic dystrophy can be used for prenatal diagnosis. Congenital disease occurs almost exclusively in infants born to affected mothers; it is possible that sperm with greatly expanded triplet repeats do not function well.

DM2 is caused by a DNA expansion mutation consisting of a CCTG repeat in intron 1 of the *ZNF9* gene located at chromosome 3q13.3-q24. The gene is believed to encode an RNA-binding protein expressed in many different tissues, including skeletal and cardiac muscle.

The DNA expansions in DM1 and DM2 almost certainly impair muscle function by a toxic gain of function of the mutant mRNA. In both DM1 and DM2, the mutant RNA appears to form intranuclear inclusions composed of aberrant RNA. These RNA inclusions sequester RNA-binding proteins essential for proper splicing of a variety of other mRNAs. This leads to abnormal transcription of multiple proteins in a variety of tissues/organ systems, in turn causing the systemic manifestations of DM1 and DM2.

TREATMENT Myotonic Dystrophy

The myotonia in DM1 rarely warrants treatment, though some patients with DM2 are significantly bothered by the discomfort related to the associated muscle stiffness. Phenytoin and mexiletine are the preferred agents for the occasional patient who requires an antimyotonia drug; other agents, particularly quinine and procainamide, may worsen cardiac conduction. A cardiac pacemaker should be considered for patients with unexplained syncope, advanced conduction system abnormalities with evidence of second-degree heart block, or trifascicular conduction disturbances with marked prolongation of the PR interval. Molded ankle-foot orthoses help stabilize gait in patients with foot drop. Excessive daytime somnolence with or without sleep apnea is not uncommon. Sleep studies, noninvasive respiratory support (biphasic positive airway pressure, BiPAP), and treatment with modafinil may be beneficial.

■ FACIOSCAPULOHUMERAL (FSH) MUSCULAR DYSTROPHY

This form of muscular dystrophy has a prevalence of ~1 in 20,000. There are two forms of FSHD that have similar pathogenesis, as will be discussed. Most patients have FSHD type 1 (95%), while approximately 5% have FSHD2. FSHD1 and FSHD2 are clinically and histopathologically identical. FSHD is not to be confused with the genetically distinct scapuloperoneal dystrophies.

Clinical features

The condition typically has an onset in childhood or young adulthood. In most cases, facial weakness is the initial manifestation, appearing as an inability to smile, whistle, or fully close the eyes. Weakness of the shoulder girdles, rather than the facial muscles, usually brings the patient to medical attention. Loss of scapular stabilizer muscles makes arm elevation difficult. Scapular winging (Fig. 387-3) becomes apparent with attempts at abduction and forward movement of the arms. Biceps and triceps muscles may be severely affected, with relative sparing of the deltoid muscles. Weakness is invariably worse for wrist extension than for wrist flexion, and weakness of the anterior compartment muscles of the legs may lead to footdrop.

In most patients, the weakness remains restricted to facial, upper extremity, and distal lower extremity muscles. In 20% of patients, weakness progresses to involve the pelvic girdle muscles, and severe functional impairment and possible wheelchair dependency result.

Characteristically, patients with FSHD do not have involvement of other organ systems, although labile hypertension is common, and there is an increased incidence of nerve deafness. *Coats' disease*, a disorder consisting of telangiectasia, exudation, and retinal detachment, also occurs.

Laboratory features

The serum CK level may be normal or mildly elevated. EMG usually indicates a myopathic pattern. The muscle biopsy shows nonspecific features of a myopathy. A prominent inflammatory infiltrate, which is often multifocal in distribution, is present in some biopsy samples. The cause or significance of this finding is unknown.

An autosomal dominant inheritance pattern with almost complete penetrance has been established, but each family member should be examined for the presence of the disease, since ~30% of those affected are unaware of involvement. FSHD1 is associated with deletions of tandem 3.3-kb repeats at 4q35. The deletion reduces the number of repeats to a fragment of <35 kb in most patients. Within these repeats lies the *DUX4* gene, which usually is not expressed. In patients with FSHD1 these deletions in the setting of a specific polymorphism leads to hypomethylation of the region and toxic expression of the *DUX 4* gene. Interestingly, in patients with FSHD2, there is no deletion but in the setting of the same polymorphism there again is seen hypomethylation of the region and the permissive expression of the *DUX4* gene. In either instance, the permissive polymorphism introduces a polyadenylation signal that results in an aberrant, toxic *DUX4* transcript.

TREATMENT Facioscapulohumeral Muscular Dystrophy

No specific treatment is available; ankle-foot orthoses are helpful for footdrop. Scapular stabilization procedures improve scapular winging but may not improve function.

■ OCULOPHARYNGEAL DYSTROPHY

This form of muscular dystrophy represents one of several disorders characterized by progressive external ophthalmoplegia, which consists of slowly progressive ptosis and limitation of eye movements with sparing of pupillary reactions for light and accommodation. Patients usually do not complain of diplopia, in contrast to patients having conditions with a more acute onset of ocular muscle weakness (e.g., myasthenia gravis).

Clinical features

Oculopharyngeal muscular dystrophy has a late onset; it usually presents in the fourth to sixth decade with ptosis and/or dysphagia. The extraocular muscle impairment is less prominent in the early phase but may be severe later. The swallowing problem may become debilitating and result in pooling of secretions and repeated episodes of aspiration. Mild weakness of the neck and extremities also occurs.

Laboratory features

The serum CK level may be two to three times normal. Myopathic EMG findings are typical. On biopsy, muscle fibers are found to contain rimmed vacuoles, which by electron microscopy are shown to contain membranous whorls, accumulation of glycogen, and other nonspecific debris related to lysosomes. A distinct feature of oculopharyngeal dystrophy is the presence of tubular filaments, 8.5 nm in diameter, in muscle cell nuclei.

Oculopharyngeal dystrophy has an autosomal dominant inheritance pattern with complete penetrance. The incidence is high in French-Canadians and in Spanish-American families of the southwestern United States. Large kindreds of Italian and of eastern European Jewish descent have been reported. The molecular defect in oculopharyngeal muscular dystrophy is a subtle expansion of a modest polyalanine repeat tract in a poly-RNA-binding protein (PABP2) in muscle.

TREATMENT Oculopharyngeal Dystrophy

Dysphagia can lead to significant undernourishment and inanition, making oculopharyngeal muscular dystrophy a potentially life-threatening disease. Cricopharyngeal myotomy may improve swallowing, although it does not prevent aspiration. Eyelid crutches can improve vision when ptosis obstructs vision; candidates for ptosis surgery must be carefully selected—those with severe facial weakness are not suitable.

DISTAL MYOPATHIES

A group of muscle diseases, the distal myopathies, are notable for their preferential distal distribution of muscle weakness in contrast to most muscle conditions associated with proximal weakness. The major distal myopathies are summarized in Table 387-9.

Clinical features

Welander's, *Udd's*, and *Markesbery-Griggs distal myopathies* are all late onset, dominantly inherited disorders of distal limb muscles, usually beginning after age 40 years. Welander's distal myopathy preferentially involves the wrist and finger extensors, whereas the others are associated with anterior tibial weakness leading to progressive footdrop. *Laing's distal myopathy* is also a dominantly inherited disorder heralded by tibial weakness; however, it is distinguished by onset in childhood or early adult life. *Nonaka's distal myopathy* and *Miyoshi's myopathy* are distinguished by autosomal recessive inheritance and onset in the late teens or twenties. Nonaka's myopathy entails anterior tibial weakness, whereas Miyoshi's myopathy is unique in that gastrocnemius muscles are preferentially affected at onset. Finally, the *myofibrillar myopathies* (MFMs) are a clinically and genetically heterogeneous group of disorders that can be associated with prominent distal weakness; they can be inherited in an autosomal dominant or recessive pattern. Of note, Markesbery-Griggs myopathy (caused by mutations in ZASP) and LGMD1B (caused by mutations in myotilin) are in fact subtypes of myofibrillar myopathy.

Laboratory features

Serum CK level is particularly helpful in diagnosing Miyoshi's myopathy since it is very elevated. In the other conditions, serum CK is only slightly increased. EMGs are myopathic. In the MFMs, myotonic or pseudomyotonic discharges are common. Muscle biopsy shows nonspecific dystrophic features and, with the exception of Laing's and Miyoshi's myopathies, often shows rimmed vacuoles. MFM is associated with the accumulation of dense inclusions, as well as amorphous material best seen on Gomori's trichrome and myofibrillar disruption on electron microscopy. Immune staining sometimes demonstrates accumulation of desmin and other proteins in MFM, large deposits of myosin heavy chain in the subsarcolemmal region of type 1 muscle fibers in Laing's myopathy, and reduced or absent dysferlin in Miyoshi's myopathy.

The affected genes and their gene products are listed in Table 387-9. The gene for Welander's disease awaits identification.

TREATMENT Distal Myopathies

Occupational therapy is offered for loss of hand function; ankle-foot orthoses can support distal lower limb muscles. The MFMs can be associated with cardiomyopathy (congestive heart failure or arrhythmias) and respiratory failure that may require medical management. Laing's-type distal myopathy can also be associated with a cardiomyopathy.

CONGENITAL MYOPATHIES

These rare disorders are distinguished from muscular dystrophies by the presence of specific histochemical and structural abnormalities in muscle. Although primarily disorders of infancy or childhood, three forms that may present in adulthood are described here: central core disease, nemaline (rod) myopathy, and centronuclear (myotubular) myopathy. Sarcotubular myopathy is caused by mutations in TRIM-32 and is identical to LGMD2H. Other types, such as minicore myopathy (multi-minicore disease), fingerprint body myopathy, and cap myopathy, are not discussed.

CENTRAL CORE DISEASE

Patients with central core disease may have decreased fetal movements and breech presentation. Hypotonia and delay in motor milestones, particularly in walking, are common. Later in childhood, patients develop problems with stair climbing, running, and getting up from the floor. On examination, there is mild facial, neck-flexor, and proximal-extremity muscle weakness. Legs are more affected than arms. Skeletal abnormalities include congenital hip dislocation, scoliosis, and pes cavus; clubbed feet also occur. Most cases are nonprogressive, but exceptions are well documented. Susceptibility to malignant hyperthermia must be considered as a potential risk factor for patients with central core disease.

The serum CK level is usually normal. Needle EMG demonstrates a myopathic pattern. Muscle biopsy shows fibers with single or multiple central or eccentric discrete zones (*cores*) devoid of oxidative enzymes. Cores occur preferentially in type 1 fibers and represent poorly aligned sarcomeres associated with Z disk streaming.

Autosomal dominant inheritance is characteristic; sporadic cases also occur. The disease is caused by point mutations of the ryanodine receptor gene on chromosome 19q, encoding the calcium-release channel of the sarcoplasmic reticulum of skeletal muscle; mutations of this gene also account for some cases of inherited malignant hyperthermia (Chap. 16). Malignant hyperthermia is an allelic condition; C-terminal mutations of the *RYR1* gene predispose to this complication.

Specific treatment is not required, but establishing a diagnosis of central core disease is extremely important because these patients have a known predisposition to malignant hyperthermia during anesthesia.

NEMALINE MYOPATHY

The term *nemaline* refers to the distinctive presence in muscle fibers of rods or threadlike structures (Greek *nema*, "thread"). Nemaline myopathy is clinically heterogeneous. A severe neonatal form presents with hypotonia and feeding and respiratory difficulties, leading to early death. Nemaline myopathy usually presents in infancy or childhood with delayed motor milestones. The course is

TABLE 387-9 Distal Myopathies

Disease	Clinical Features	Laboratory Features	Inheritance/Locus or Gene
Welander's distal myopathy	Onset in 5th decade Weakness begins in hands Slow progression with spread to distal lower extremities Lifespan normal	Serum CK 2–3 × normal EMG myopathic NCS normal Muscle biopsy shows dystrophic features	AD Chromosome 2p13
Tibial muscular dystrophy (Udd's)	Onset 4th to 8th decade Distal lower extremity weakness (tibial distribution) Upper extremities usually normal Lifespan normal	Serum CK 2–4 × normal EMG myopathic NCS normal Muscle biopsy shows dystrophic features Titin absent in M-line of muscle	AD Titin AR (associated with more proximal weakness—LGMD2J)
Markesbery-Griggs distal myopathy	Onset 4th to 8th decade Distal lower extremity weakness (tibial distribution) with progression to distal arms and proximal muscles	Serum CK is usually mildly elevated EMG reveals irritative myopathy Muscle biopsies demonstrate rimmed vacuoles and features of myofibrillar myopathy	AD Z-band alternatively spliced PDX motif-containing protein (ZASP)
Laing's distal myopathy	Onset childhood to 3rd decade Distal lower extremity weakness (tibial distribution) and neck flexors affected early May have cardiomyopathy	Serum CK is normal or slightly elevated Muscle biopsies do not show rimmed vacuoles Large deposits of myosin heavy chain are seen in type 1 muscle fibers	AD Myosin heavy chain 7
Nonaka's distal myopathy (autosomal recessive hereditary inclusion body myopathy)	Onset: 2nd to 3rd decade Lower extremity distal weakness Mild distal upper limb weakness may be present early Progression to other muscles sparing quadriceps Ambulation may be lost in 10–15 y	Serum CK 3–10 × normal EMG myopathic NCS normal Dystrophic features on muscle biopsy plus rimmed vacuoles and 15- to 19-nm filaments within vacuoles	AR *GNE* gene: UDP-*N*-acetylglucosamine 2-epimerase/*N*-acetylmannosamine kinase Allelic to hereditary inclusion body myopathy
Miyoshi's myopathy	Onset: 2nd to 3rd decade Lower extremity weakness in posterior compartment muscles Progression leads to weakness in other muscle groups Ambulation lost after 10–15 years in about one-third of cases	Serum CK 20–100 × normal EMG myopathic NCS normal Muscle biopsy shows nonspecific dystrophic features often with prominent inflammatory cell infiltration; no rimmed vacuoles	AR Allelic to LGMD2B (see Table 387-7) Dysferlin
Myofibrillar myopathies	Onset from early childhood to late adult life Weakness may be distal, proximal, or generalized Cardiomyopathy and respiratory involvement is not uncommon	Serum CKs can be normal or moderately elevated EMG is myopathic and often associated with myotonic discharges Muscle biopsy demonstrates abnormal accumulation of desmin and other proteins, rimmed vacuoles, and myofibrillar degeneration	Genetically heterogeneous AD Myotilin (also known as LGMD 1A) ZASP (see Markesbery-Griggs distal myopathy) Filamin-C Desmin Alpha B crystallin Bag3 FHL-1 AR Desmin Selenoprotein N1

Abbreviations: AD, autosomal dominant; AR, autosomal recessive; CK, creatine kinase; EMG, electromyography; NCS, nerve conduction studies.

nonprogressive or slowly progressive. The physical appearance is striking because of the long, narrow facies, high-arched palate, and open-mouthed appearance due to a prognathous jaw. Other skeletal abnormalities include pectus excavatum, kyphoscoliosis, pes cavus, and clubfoot deformities. Facial and generalized muscle weakness, including respiratory muscle weakness, is common. An adult-onset disorder with progressive proximal weakness may be seen. Myocardial involvement is occasionally present in both the childhood and adult-onset forms. The serum CK level is usually normal or slightly elevated. The EMG demonstrates a myopathic pattern. Muscle biopsy shows clusters of small rods (nemaline bodies), which occur preferentially, but not exclusively, in the sarcoplasm of type 1 muscle fibers. Occasionally, the rods are also apparent in myonuclei. The muscle often shows type 1 muscle fiber predominance. Rods originate from the Z disk material of the muscle fiber.

Six genes have been associated with nemaline myopathy. Five of these code for thin filament–associated proteins, suggesting disturbed assembly or interplay of these structures as a pivotal mechanism. Mutations of the nebulin (*NEB*) gene account for most cases, including both severe neonatal and early childhood forms, inherited as autosomal recessive disorders. Neonatal and childhood cases, inherited as predominantly autosomal dominant disorders, are caused by mutations of the skeletal muscle α-actinin (*ACTA1*) gene. In milder forms of the disease with autosomal dominant inheritance, mutations have been identified in both the slow α-tropomyosin (*TPM3*) and β-tropomyosin (*TPM2*) genes accounting for <3% of cases. Muscle troponin T (*TNNT1*) gene mutations appear to be limited to the Amish population in North America. Mutations in a sixth nemaline myopathy gene, *NEM6*, have recently been reported; this gene encodes a putative BTB/Kelch protein. No specific treatment is available.

■ CENTRONUCLEAR (MYOTUBULAR) MYOPATHY

Three distinct variants of centronuclear myopathy occur. A neonatal form, also known as *myotubular myopathy*, presents with severe hypotonia and weakness at birth. The late infancy–early childhood form presents with delayed motor milestones. Later, difficulty with running and stair climbing becomes apparent. A marfanoid, slender body habitus, long narrow face, and high-arched palate are typical. Scoliosis and clubbed feet may be present. Most patients exhibit progressive weakness, some requiring wheelchairs. Progressive external ophthalmoplegia with ptosis and varying degrees of extraocular muscle impairment are characteristic of both the neonatal and the late-infantile forms. A third variant, the late childhood–adult form, has an onset in the second or third decade. Patients have full extraocular muscle movements and rarely exhibit ptosis. There is mild, slowly progressive limb weakness that may be distally predominant [some of these patients have been classified as having Charcot-Marie-Tooth disease type 2 (CMT2; Chap. 384)].

Normal or slightly elevated CK levels occur in each of the forms. Nerve conduction studies may reveal reduced amplitudes of distal compound muscle action potentials, in particular in adult-onset cases that resemble CMT2. EMG studies often give distinctive results, showing positive sharp waves and fibrillation potentials, complex and repetitive discharges, and rarely myotonic discharges. Muscle biopsy specimens in longitudinal section demonstrate rows of central nuclei, often surrounded by a halo. In transverse sections, central nuclei are found in 25–80% of muscle fibers.

A gene for the neonatal form of centronuclear myopathy has been localized to Xq28; this gene encodes myotubularin, a protein tyrosine phosphatase. Missense, frameshift, and splice-site mutations predict loss of myotubularin function in affected individuals. Carrier identification and prenatal diagnosis are possible. Autosomal recessive forms are caused by mutations in *BIB1* that encodes for amphyphysin-2, while some autosomal dominant cases, which are allelic to a form of CMT2, are associated with mutations in the gene that encodes dynamin-2. No specific medical treatments are available at this time.

DISORDERS OF MUSCLE ENERGY METABOLISM

There are two principal sources of energy for skeletal muscle—fatty acids and glucose. Abnormalities in either glucose or lipid utilization can be associated with distinct clinical presentations that can range from an acute, painful syndrome with rhabdomyolysis and myoglobinuria to a chronic, progressive muscle weakness simulating muscular dystrophy.

■ GLYCOGEN STORAGE AND GLYCOLYTIC DEFECTS

Disorders of glycogen storage causing progressive weakness

α-Glucosidase, or acid maltase, deficiency (Pompe's disease) Three clinical forms of α-glucosidase, or acid maltase, deficiency (*type II glycogenosis*) can be distinguished. The infantile form is the most common, with onset of symptoms in the first 3 months of life. Infants develop severe muscle weakness, cardiomegaly, hepatomegaly, and respiratory insufficiency. Glycogen accumulation in motor neurons of the spinal cord and brainstem contributes to muscle weakness. Death usually occurs by 1 year of age. In the childhood form, the picture resembles muscular dystrophy. Delayed motor milestones result from proximal limb muscle weakness and involvement of respiratory muscles. The heart may be involved, but the liver and brain are unaffected. The adult form usually begins in the third or fourth decade but can present as late as the seventh decade. Respiratory failure and diaphragmatic weakness are often initial manifestations, heralding progressive proximal muscle weakness. The heart and liver are not involved.

The serum CK level is 2 to 10 times normal in infantile or childhood-onset Pompe's disease but can be normal in adult-onset cases. EMG examination demonstrates a myopathic pattern, but other features are especially distinctive, including myotonic discharges, trains of fibrillation and positive waves, and complex repetitive discharges. EMG discharges are very prominent in the paraspinal muscles. The muscle biopsy in infants typically reveals vacuoles containing glycogen and the lysosomal enzyme acid phosphatase. Electron microscopy reveals membrane-bound and free tissue glycogen. However, muscle biopsies in late-onset Pompe's disease may demonstrate only nonspecific abnormalities. Enzyme analysis of dried blood spots is a sensitive technique to screen for Pompe's disease. A definitive diagnosis is established by enzyme assay in muscle or cultured fibroblasts or by genetic testing.

Pompe's disease is inherited as an autosomal recessive disorder caused by mutations of the α-glucosidase gene. Enzyme replacement therapy (ERT) with IV recombinant human α-glucosidase has been shown to be beneficial in infantile-onset Pompe's disease. Clinical benefits in the infantile disease include reduced heart size, improved muscle function, reduced need for ventilatory support, and longer life. In late-onset cases, ERT has not been associated with the dramatic response that can be seen in classic infantile Pompe's disease, yet it appears to stabilize the disease process.

Other glycogen storage diseases with progressive weakness In *debranching enzyme deficiency* (*type III glycogenosis*), a slowly progressive form of muscle weakness can develop after puberty. Rarely, myoglobinuria may be seen. Patients are usually diagnosed in infancy, however, because of hypotonia and delayed motor milestones, hepatomegaly, growth retardation, and hypoglycemia. *Branching enzyme deficiency* (*type IV glycogenosis*) is a rare and fatal glycogen storage disease characterized by failure to thrive and hepatomegaly. Hypotonia and muscle wasting may be present, but the skeletal muscle manifestations are minor compared to liver failure.

Disorders of glycolysis causing exercise intolerance

Several glycolytic defects are associated with recurrent myoglobinuria: *myophosphorylase deficiency (type V glycogenosis), phosphofructokinase deficiency (type VII glycogenosis), phosphoglycerate kinase deficiency (type IX glycogenosis), phosphoglycerate mutase deficiency (type X glycogenosis), lactate dehydrogenase deficiency (glycogenosis type XI)*, and *β-enolase deficiency*. Myophosphorylase deficiency, also known as *McArdle's disease*, is by far the most common of the glycolytic defects associated with exercise intolerance. These glycolytic defects result in a common failure to support energy production at the initiation of exercise, although the exact site of energy failure remains controversial.

Clinical muscle manifestations in these conditions usually begin in adolescence. Symptoms are precipitated by brief bursts of high-intensity exercise such as running or lifting heavy objects. A history of myalgia and muscle stiffness usually precedes the intensely painful muscle contractures, which may be followed by myoglobinuria. Acute renal failure accompanies significant pigmenturia.

Certain features help distinguish some enzyme defects. In McArdle's disease, exercise tolerance can be enhanced by a slow induction phase (warm-up) or brief periods of rest, allowing for the start of the "second-wind" phenomenon (switching to utilization of fatty acids). Varying degrees of hemolytic anemia accompany deficiencies of both phosphofructokinase (mild) and phosphoglycerate kinase (severe). In phosphoglycerate kinase deficiency, the usual clinical presentation is a seizure disorder associated with mental retardation; exercise intolerance is an infrequent manifestation.

In all of these conditions, the serum CK levels fluctuate widely and may be elevated even during symptom-free periods. CK levels >100 times normal are expected, accompanying myoglobinuria. All patients with suspected glycolytic defects leading to exercise intolerance should undergo a forearm exercise test. An impaired rise in venous lactate is highly indicative of a glycolytic defect. In lactate dehydrogenase deficiency, venous levels of lactate do not increase, but pyruvate rises to normal. A definitive diagnosis of glycolytic disease is made by muscle biopsy and subsequent enzyme analysis or by genetic testing.

Myophosphorylase deficiency, phosphofructokinase deficiency, and phosphoglycerate mutase deficiency are inherited as autosomal recessive disorders. Phosphoglycerate kinase deficiency is X-linked recessive. Mutations can be found in the respective genes encoding the abnormal proteins in each of these disorders.

Training may enhance exercise tolerance, perhaps by increasing perfusion to muscle. Dietary intake of free glucose or fructose prior to activity may improve function but care must be taken to avoid obesity from ingesting too many calories.

LIPID AS AN ENERGY SOURCE AND ASSOCIATED DEFECTS

Lipid is an important muscle energy source during rest and during prolonged, submaximal exercise. Fatty acids are derived from circulating very low-density lipoprotein (VLDL) in the blood or from triglycerides stored in muscle fibers. Oxidation of fatty acids occurs in the mitochondria. To enter the mitochondria, a fatty acid must first be converted to an "activated fatty acid," acyl-CoA. The acyl-CoA must be linked with carnitine by the enzyme carnitine palmitoyltransferase (CPT) I for transport into the mitochondria. CPT I is present on the inner side of the outer mitochondrial membrane. Carnitine is removed by CPT II, an enzyme attached to the inside of the inner mitochondrial membrane, allowing transport of acyl-CoA into the mitochondrial matrix for β-oxidation.

Carnitine palmitoyltransferase deficiency

CPT II deficiency is the most common recognizable cause of recurrent myoglobinuria, more common than the glycolytic defects. Onset is usually in the teenage years or early twenties. Muscle pain and myoglobinuria typically occur after prolonged exercise but can also be precipitated by fasting or infections; up to 20% of patients do not exhibit myoglobinuria, however. Strength is normal between attacks. In contrast to disorders caused by defects in glycolysis, in which muscle cramps follow short, intense bursts of exercise, the muscle pain in CPT II deficiency does not occur until the limits of utilization have been exceeded and muscle breakdown has already begun. Episodes of rhabdomyolysis may produce severe weakness. In young children and newborns, CPT II deficiency can present with a very severe clinical picture including hypoketotic hypoglycemia, cardiomyopathy, liver failure, and sudden death.

Serum CK levels and EMG findings are both usually normal between episodes. A normal rise of venous lactate during forearm exercise distinguishes this condition from glycolytic defects, especially myophosphorylase deficiency. Muscle biopsy does not show lipid accumulation and is usually normal between attacks. The diagnosis requires direct measurement of muscle CPT or genetic testing.

CPT II deficiency is much more common in men than women (5:1); nevertheless, all evidence indicates autosomal recessive inheritance. A mutation in the gene for CPT II (chromosome 1p36) causes the disease in some individuals. Attempts to improve exercise tolerance with frequent meals and a low-fat, high-carbohydrate diet, or by substituting medium-chain triglycerides in the diet, have not proven to be beneficial.

Myoadenylate deaminase deficiency

The muscle enzyme myoadenylate deaminase converts adenosine-5′-monophosphate (5′-AMP) to inosine monophosphate (IMP) with liberation of ammonia. Myoadenylate deaminase may play a role in regulating adenosine triphosphate (ATP) levels in muscles. Most individuals with myoadenylate deaminase deficiency have no symptoms. There have been a few reports of patients with this disorder who have exercise-exacerbated myalgia and myoglobinuria. Many questions have been raised about the clinical effects of myoadenylate deaminase deficiency, and, specifically, its relationship to exertional myalgia and fatigability, but there is no consensus.

MITOCHONDRIAL MYOPATHIES

In 1972, Olson and colleagues recognized that muscle fibers with significant numbers of abnormal mitochondria could be highlighted with the modified trichrome stain; the term *ragged red fibers* was coined. By electron microscopy, the mitochondria in ragged red fibers are enlarged and often bizarrely shaped and have crystalline inclusions. Since that seminal observation, the understanding of these disorders of muscle and other tissues has expanded (Chap. 61).

Mitochondria play a key role in energy production. Oxidation of the major nutrients derived from carbohydrate, fat, and protein leads to the generation of reducing equivalents. The latter are transported through the respiratory chain in the process known as *oxidative phosphorylation*. The energy generated by the oxidation-reduction reactions of the respiratory chain is stored in an electrochemical gradient coupled to ATP synthesis.

A novel feature of mitochondria is their genetic composition. Each mitochondrion possesses a DNA genome that is distinct from that of the nuclear DNA. Human mitochondrial DNA (mtDNA) consists of a double-strand, circular molecule comprising 16,569 base pairs. It codes for 22 transfer RNAs, 2 ribosomal RNAs, and 13 polypeptides of the respiratory chain enzymes. The genetics of mitochondrial diseases differ from the genetics of chromosomal disorders. The DNA of mitochondria is directly inherited from the cytoplasm of the gametes, mainly from the oocyte. The sperm contributes very little of its mitochondria to the offspring at the time of fertilization. Thus, mitochondrial genes are derived almost exclusively from the mother, accounting for maternal inheritance of some mitochondrial disorders.

Patients with mitochondrial myopathies have clinical manifestations that usually fall into three groups: chronic progressive external ophthalmoplegia (CPEO), skeletal muscle–CNS syndromes, and pure myopathy simulating muscular dystrophy or metabolic myopathy.

PROGRESSIVE EXTERNAL OPHTHALMOPLEGIA SYNDROMES WITH RAGGED RED FIBERS

The single most common sign of a mitochondrial myopathy is CPEO, occurring in >50% of all mitochondrial myopathies. Varying degrees of ptosis and weakness of extraocular muscles are seen, usually in the absence of diplopia, a point of distinction from disorders with fluctuating eye weakness (e.g., myasthenia gravis).

KEARNS-SAYRE SYNDROME (KSS)

KSS is a widespread multiorgan system disorder with a defined triad of clinical findings: onset before age 20, CPEO, and pigmentary retinopathy, plus one or more of the following features: complete heart block, cerebrospinal fluid (CSF) protein >1 g/L (100 mg/dL), or cerebellar ataxia. Some patients with CPEO and ragged red fibers may not fulfill all of the criteria for KSS. The cardiac disease includes syncopal attacks and cardiac arrest related to the abnormalities in the cardiac conduction system: prolonged intraventricular conduction time, bundle branch block, and complete atrioventricular block. Death attributed to heart block occurs in ~20% of the patients. Varying degrees of progressive limb muscle weakness and easy fatigability affect activities of daily living. Endocrine abnormalities are common, including gonadal dysfunction in both sexes with delayed puberty, short stature, and infertility. Diabetes mellitus is a cardinal sign of mitochondrial disorders and is estimated to occur in 13% of KSS patients. Other less common endocrine disorders include thyroid disease, hyperaldosteronism, Addison's disease, and hypoparathyroidism. Both mental retardation and dementia are common accompaniments to this disorder. Serum CK levels are normal or slightly elevated. Serum lactate and pyruvate levels may be elevated. EMG is myopathic. Nerve conduction studies may be abnormal related to an associated neuropathy. Muscle biopsies reveal ragged red fibers, highlighted in oxidative enzyme stains, many showing defects in cytochrome oxidase. By electron microscopy there are increased numbers of mitochondria that often appear enlarged and contain paracrystalline inclusions.

KSS is a sporadic disorder. The disease is caused by single mtDNA deletions presumed to arise spontaneously in the ovum or zygote. The most common deletion, occurring in about one-third of patients, removes 4,977 bp of contiguous mtDNA. Monitoring for cardiac conduction defects is critical. Prophylactic pacemaker implantation is indicated when ECGs demonstrate a bifascicular block. In KSS, no benefit has been shown for supplementary therapies, including multivitamins or coenzyme Q10. Of all the proposed options, exercise might be the most applicable but must be approached cautiously because of defects in the cardiac conduction system.

PROGRESSIVE EXTERNAL OPHTHALMOPLEGIA (PEO)

This condition is caused by nuclear DNA mutations affecting mtDNA copy number and integrity and is thus inherited in a Mendelian fashion. Onset is usually after puberty. Fatigue, exercise intolerance, and complaints of muscle weakness are typical. Some patients notice swallowing problems. The neurologic examination confirms the ptosis and ophthalmoplegia, usually asymmetric in distribution. A sensorineural hearing loss may be encountered. Mild facial, neck flexor, and proximal weakness are typical. Rarely, respiratory muscles may be progressively affected and may be the direct cause of death. Serum CK is normal or mildly elevated. The resting lactate level is normal or slightly elevated but may rise excessively after exercise. CSF protein is normal. The EMG is myopathic, and nerve conduction studies are usually normal. Ragged red fibers are prominently displayed in the muscle biopsy. Southern blots of muscle reveal a normal mtDNA band at 16.6 kb and several additional mtDNA deletion bands with genomes varying from 0.5 to 10 kb.

This autosomal dominant form of CPEO has been linked to loci on three chromosomes: 4q35, 10q24, and 15q22–26. In the chromosome 4q-related form of disease, mutations of the gene encoding the heart and skeletal muscle–specific isoform of the adenine nucleotide translocator 1 (*ANT1*) gene are found. This highly abundant mitochondrial protein forms a homodimeric inner mitochondrial channel through which adenosine diphosphate (ADP) enters and ATP leaves the mitochondrial matrix. In the chromosome 10q–related disorder, mutations of the gene *C10orf2* are found. Its gene product, *twinkle*, co-localizes with the mtDNA and is named for its punctate, starlike staining properties. The function of twinkle is presumed to be critical for lifetime maintenance of mitochondrial integrity. In the cases mapped to chromosome 15q, a mutation affects the gene encoding mtDNA polymerase (*POLG*), an enzyme important in mtDNA replication. Autosomal recessive PEO has also been described with mutations in the *POLG* gene. Point mutations have been identified within various mitochondrial tRNA (Leu, Ile, Asn, Trp) genes in families with maternal inheritance of PEO.

Exercise may improve function but will depend on the patient's ability to participate.

MITOCHONDRIAL DNA SKELETAL MUSCLE–CENTRAL NERVOUS SYSTEM SYNDROMES

Myoclonic epilepsy with ragged red fibers (MERRF)

The onset of MERRF is variable, ranging from late childhood to middle adult life. Characteristic features include myoclonic epilepsy, cerebellar ataxia, and progressive muscle weakness. The seizure disorder is an integral part of the disease and may be the initial symptom. Cerebellar ataxia precedes or accompanies epilepsy. It is slowly progressive and generalized. The third major feature of the disease is muscle weakness in a limb-girdle distribution. Other more variable features include dementia, peripheral neuropathy, optic atrophy, hearing loss, and diabetes mellitus.

Serum CK levels are normal or slightly increased. The serum lactate may be elevated. EMG is myopathic, and in some patients nerve conduction studies show a neuropathy. The electroencephalogram is abnormal, corroborating clinical findings of epilepsy. Typical ragged red fibers are seen on muscle biopsy. MERRF is caused by maternally inherited point mutations of mitochondrial tRNA genes. The most common mutation found in 80% of MERRF patients is an A to G substitution at nucleotide 8344 of tRNA lysine (A8344G $tRNA^{lys}$). Other $tRNA^{lys}$ mutations include base-pair substitutions T8356C and G8363A. Only supportive treatment is possible, with special attention to epilepsy.

Mitochondrial myopathy, encephalopathy, lactic acidosis, and strokelike episodes (MELAS)

MELAS is the most common mitochondrial encephalomyopathy. The term *strokelike* is appropriate because the cerebral lesions do not conform to a strictly vascular distribution. The onset in the majority of patients is before age 20. Seizures, usually partial motor or generalized, are common and may represent the first clearly recognizable sign of disease. The cerebral insults that resemble strokes cause hemiparesis, hemianopia, and cortical blindness. A presumptive stroke occurring before age 40 should place this mitochondrial encephalomyopathy high in the differential diagnosis. Associated conditions include hearing loss, diabetes mellitus, hypothalamic pituitary dysfunction causing growth hormone deficiency, hypothyroidism, and absence of secondary sexual characteristics. In its full expression, MELAS leads to dementia, a bedridden state, and a fatal outcome. Serum lactic acid is typically elevated. The CSF protein is also increased but is usually ≤1 g/L (100 mg/dL). Muscle biopsies show ragged red fibers. Neuroimaging demonstrates basal ganglia calcification in a high percentage of cases. Focal lesions that mimic infarction are present predominantly in the occipital and parietal lobes. Strict vascular territories are not respected, and cerebral angiography fails to demonstrate lesions of the major cerebral blood vessels.

MELAS is caused by maternally inherited point mutations of mitochondrial tRNA genes. Most of the tRNA mutations are lethal, accounting for the paucity of multigeneration families with this syndrome. The A3243G point mutation in $tRNA^{Leu(UUR)}$ is the most common, occurring in ~80% of MELAS cases. About 10% of MELAS patients have other mutations of the $tRNA^{Leu(UUR)}$ gene, including 3252G, 3256T, 3271C, and 3291C. Other tRNA gene mutations have also been reported in MELAS, including G583A $tRNA^{Phe}$, G1642A $tRNA^{Val}$, G4332A $tRNA^{Glu}$, and T8316C $tRNA^{Lys}$. Mutations have also been reported in mtDNA polypeptide-coding genes. Two mutations were found in the ND5 subunit of complex I of the respiratory chain. A missense mutation has been reported at mtDNA position 9957 in the gene for subunit III of cytochrome C oxidase. No specific treatment is available. Supportive treatment is essential for the strokelike episodes, seizures, and endocrinopathies.

PURE MYOPATHY SYNDROMES

Muscle weakness and fatigue can be the predominant manifestations of mtDNA mutations. When the condition affects exclusively muscle (pure myopathy), the disorder becomes difficult to recognize. Occasionally, mitochondrial myopathies can present with recurrent myoglobinuria without fixed weakness and thus resemble a glycogen storage disorder or CPT deficiency.

Mitochondrial DNA depletion syndromes

Mitochondrial DNA depletion syndrome (MDS) is a heterogeneous group of disorders that are inherited in an autosomal recessive fashion and can present in infancy or adults. MDS can be caused by mutations in genes (*TK2, DGUOK, RRM2B, TYMP, SUCLA1,* and *SUCLA2*) that lead to depletion of pools of mitochondrial deoxyribonucleotide (dNTP) pools necessary for mtDNA replication The other major cause of MDS is a set of mutations in genes essential for mtDNA replication (e.g., *POLG1* and *C10orf2*). The clinical phenotypes associated with MDS vary. Patients may develop a severe encephalopathy (e.g., Leigh's syndrome), PEO, an isolated myopathy, myo-neuro-gastrointestinal-encephalopathy (MNGIE), and a sensory neuropathy with ataxia.

DISORDERS OF MUSCLE MEMBRANE EXCITABILITY

Muscle membrane excitability is affected in a group of disorders referred to as *channelopathies.* The heart may also be involved, resulting in life-threatening complications (Table 387-10).

CALCIUM CHANNEL DISORDERS OF MUSCLE

Hypokalemic periodic paralysis (HypoKPP)

Onset occurs at adolescence. Men are more often affected because of decreased penetrance in women. Episodic weakness with onset after age 25 is almost never due to periodic paralyses, with the exception of thyrotoxic periodic paralysis (see below). Attacks are often provoked by meals high in carbohydrates or sodium and may accompany rest following prolonged exercise. Weakness usually affects proximal limb muscles more than distal. Ocular and bulbar muscles are less likely to be affected. Respiratory muscles are usually spared but when they are involved, the condition may prove fatal. Weakness may take as long as 24 hours to resolve. Life-threatening cardiac arrhythmias related to hypokalemia may occur during attacks. As a late complication, patients commonly develop severe, disabling proximal lower extremity weakness.

TABLE 387-10 Clinical Features of Periodic Paralysis and Nondystrophic Myotonias

	Calcium Channel	Sodium Channel		Potassium Channel
Feature	Hypokalemic PP	Hyperkalemic PP	Paramyotonia Congenita	Andersen-Tawil Syndrome[a]
Mode of inheritance	AD	AD	AD	AD
Age of onset	Adolescence	Early childhood	Early childhood	Early childhood
Myotonia[b]	No	Yes	Yes	No
Episodic weakness	Yes	Yes	Yes	Yes
Frequency of attacks of weakness	Daily to yearly	May be 2–3/d	With cold, usually rare	Daily to yearly
Duration of attacks of weakness	2–12 h	From 1–2 h to >1 d	2–24 h	2–24 h
Serum K^+ level during attacks of weakness	Decreased	Increased or normal	Usually normal	Variable
Effect of K^+ loading	No change	Increased myotonia, then weakness	Increased myotonia	No change
Effect of muscle cooling	No change	Increased myotonia	Increased myotonia, then weakness	No change
Fixed weakness	Yes	Yes	Yes	Yes

[a]Dysmorphic features and cardiac arrhythmias are distinguishing features (see text).
[b]May be paradoxical in paramyotonia congenita.
Abbreviations: AD, autosomal dominant; PP, periodic paralysis.

Attacks of thyrotoxic periodic paralysis resemble those of primary HypoKPP. Despite a higher incidence of thyrotoxicosis in women, men, particularly those of Asian descent, are more likely to manifest this complication. Attacks abate with treatment of the underlying thyroid condition.

A low serum potassium level during an attack, excluding secondary causes, establishes the diagnosis. Interattack muscle biopsies show the presence of single or multiple centrally placed vacuoles or tubular aggregates. Provocative tests with glucose and insulin to establish a diagnosis are usually not necessary and are potentially hazardous.

In the midst of an attack of weakness, motor conduction studies may demonstrate reduced amplitudes, whereas EMG may show electrical silence in severely weak muscles. In between attacks, the EMG and nerve conduction studies are normal, with the exception that myopathic MUAPs may be seen in patients with fixed weakness.

HypoKPP is caused by mutations in either of two genes. HypoKPP type 1, the most common form, is inherited as an autosomal dominant disorder with incomplete penetrance. These patients have mutations in the voltage-sensitive, skeletal muscle calcium channel gene, *CALCL1A3* (Fig. 387-8). Approximately 10% of cases are HypoKPP type 2, arising from mutations in the voltage-sensitive sodium channel gene (*SCN4A*). In either instance, the mutations lead to an abnormal gating pore current that predisposes the muscle cell to depolarize when potassium levels are low. It is also now recognized that some cases of thyrotoxic HypoKPP are caused by genetic variants in a potassium channel (Kir 2.6), whose expression is regulated by thyroid hormone.

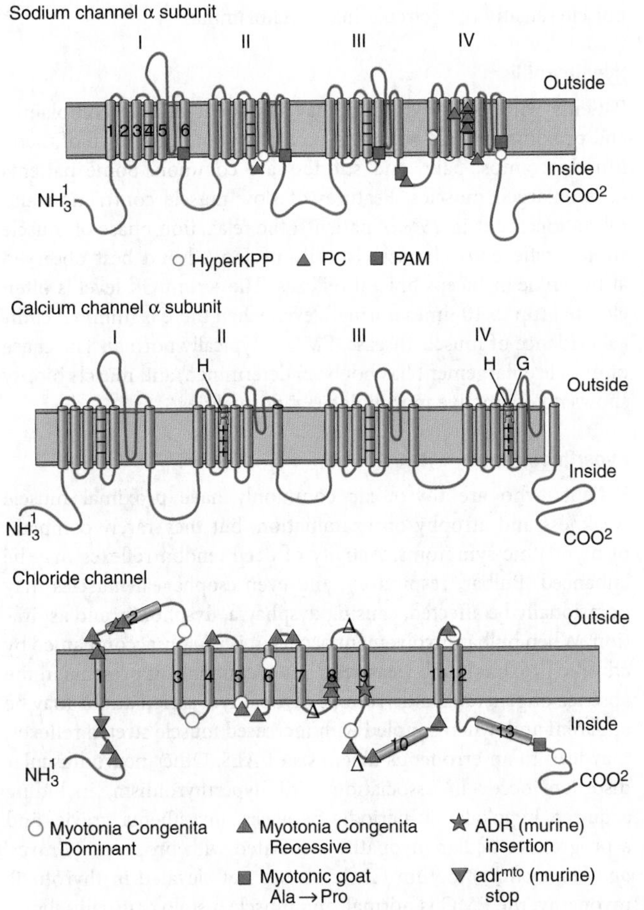

Figure 387-8 The sodium and calcium channels are depicted here as containing four homologous domains, each with six membrane-spanning segments. The fourth segment of each domain bears positive charges and acts as the "voltage sensor" for the channel. The association of the four domains is thought to form a pore through which ions pass. Sodium channel mutations are shown along with the phenotype that they confer. HyperKPP, hyperkalemic periodic paralysis; PC, paramyotonia congenita; PAM, potassium-aggravated myotonia. See text for details. **The chloride channel** is envisioned to have 10 membrane-spanning domains. The positions of mutations causing dominantly and recessively inherited myotonia congenita are indicated, along with mutations that cause this disease in mice and goats.

TREATMENT Hypokalemic Periodic Paralysis

The acute paralysis improves after the administration of potassium. Muscle strength and ECG should be monitored. Oral KCl (0.2–0.4 mmol/kg) should be given every 30 minutes. Only rarely is IV therapy necessary (e.g., when swallowing problems or vomiting is present). Administration of potassium in a glucose solution should be avoided because it may further reduce serum potassium levels. Mannitol is the preferred vehicle for administration of IV potassium. The long-term goal of therapy is to avoid attacks. This may reduce late-onset, fixed weakness. Patients should be made aware of the importance of a low-carbohydrate, low-sodium diet and consequences of intense exercise. Prophylactic administration of acetazolamide (125–1000 mg/d in divided doses) reduces or may abolish attacks in HypoKPP type 1. Paradoxically the potassium is lowered, but this is offset by the beneficial effect of metabolic acidosis. If attacks persist on acetazolamide, oral KCl should be added. Some patients require treatment with triamterine (25–100 mg/d) or spironolactone (25–100 mg/d). However, in patients with HypoKPP type 2, attacks of weakness can be exacerbated with acetazolamide.

SODIUM CHANNEL DISORDERS OF MUSCLE

Hyperkalemic periodic paralysis (HyperKPP)

The term *hyperkalemic* is misleading since patients are often normokalemic during attacks. The fact that attacks are precipitated by potassium administration best defines the disease. The onset is in the first decade; males and females are affected equally. Attacks are brief and mild, usually lasting 30 minutes to 4 hours. Weakness affects proximal muscles, sparing bulbar muscles. Attacks are precipitated by rest following exercise and fasting. In a variant of this disorder, the predominant symptom is myotonia without weakness (*potassium-aggravated myotonia*). The symptoms are aggravated by cold, and myotonia makes the muscles stiff and painful. This disorder can be confused with paramyotonia congenita, myotonia congenita, and proximal myotonic myopathy (DM2).

Potassium may be slightly elevated but may also be normal during an attack. As in HypoKPP, nerve conduction studies in HyperKPP muscle may demonstrate reduced motor amplitudes and the EMG may be silent in very weak muscles. In between attacks of weakness, the conduction studies are normal. The EMG will often demonstrate myotonic discharges during and between attacks.

The muscle biopsy shows vacuoles that are smaller, less numerous, and more peripheral compared to the hypokalemic form or tubular aggregates. Provocative tests by administration of potassium can induce weakness but are usually not necessary to establish the diagnosis. HyperKPP and potassium-aggravated myotonia are inherited as autosomal dominant disorders. Mutations of the voltage-gated sodium channel *SCN4A* gene (Fig. 387-8) cause these conditions. For patients with frequent attacks, acetazolamide

(125–1000 mg/d) is helpful. We have found mexiletine to be helpful in patients with significant myotonia.

Paramyotonia congenita

In paramyotonia congenita (PC), the attacks of weakness are cold-induced or occur spontaneously and are mild. Myotonia is a prominent feature but worsens with muscle activity (paradoxical myotonia). This is in contrast to classic myotonia in which exercise alleviates the condition. Attacks of weakness are seldom severe enough to require emergency room treatment. Over time patients develop interattack weakness as they do in other forms of periodic paralysis. PC is usually associated with normokalemia or hyperkalemia.

Serum CK is usually mildly elevated. Routine sensory and motor nerve conduction studies are normal. Cooling of the muscle often dramatically reduces the amplitude of the compound muscle action potentials. EMG reveals diffuse myotonic potentials in PC. Upon local cooling of the muscle, the myotonic discharges disappear as the patient becomes unable to activate MUAPs.

PC is inherited as an autosomal dominant condition; voltage-gated sodium channel mutations (Fig. 387-8) are responsible and thus this disorder is allelic with HyperKPP and potassium-aggravated myotonia. Patients with PC seldom seek treatment during attacks. Oral administration of glucose or other carbohydrates hastens recovery. Since interattack weakness may develop after repeated episodes, prophylactic treatment is usually indicated. Thiazide diuretics (e.g., chlorothiazide, 250–1000 mg/d) and mexiletine (slowly increase dose from 450 mg/d) are reported to be helpful. Patients should be advised to increase carbohydrates in their diet.

■ POTASSIUM CHANNEL DISORDERS

Andersen-Tawil syndrome

This rare disease is characterized by episodic weakness, cardiac arrhythmias, and dysmorphic features (short stature, scoliosis, clinodactyly, hypertelorism, small or prominent low-set ears, micrognathia, and broad forehead). The cardiac arrhythmias are potentially serious and life threatening. They include long QT, ventricular ectopy, bidirectional ventricular arrhythmias, and tachycardia. For many years the classification of this disorder was uncertain because episodes of weakness are associated with elevated, normal, or reduced levels of potassium during an attack. In addition, the potassium levels differ among kindreds but are consistent within a family. Inheritance is autosomal dominant, with incomplete penetrance and variable expressivity. The disease is caused by mutations of the inwardly rectifying potassium channel (*Kir 2.1*) gene that heighten muscle cell excitability. The treatment is similar to that for other forms of periodic paralysis and must include cardiac monitoring. The episodes of weakness may differ between patients because of potassium variability. Acetazolamide may decrease the attack frequency and severity.

■ CHLORIDE CHANNEL DISORDERS

Two forms of this disorder, autosomal dominant (*Thomsen's disease*) and autosomal recessive (*Becker's disease*), are related to the same gene abnormality. Symptoms are noted in infancy and early childhood. The severity lessens in the third to fourth decade. Myotonia is worsened by cold and improved by activity. The gait may appear slow and labored at first but improves with walking. In Thomsen's disease muscle strength is normal, but in Becker's disease, which is usually more severe, there may be muscle weakness. Muscle hypertrophy is usually present. Myotonic discharges are prominently displayed by EMG recordings.

Serum CK is normal or mildly elevated. The muscle biopsy shows hypertrophied fibers. The disease is inherited as dominant or recessive and is caused by mutations of the chloride channel gene (Fig. 387-8) that increase muscle cell excitability. Many patients will not require treatment and learn that the symptoms improve with activity. Medications that can be used to decrease myotonia include quinine, phenytoin, and mexiletine.

ENDOCRINE AND METABOLIC MYOPATHIES

Many endocrine disorders cause weakness. Muscle fatigue is more common than true weakness. The cause of weakness in these disorders is not well defined. It is not even clear that weakness results from disease of muscle as opposed to another part of the motor unit, since the serum CK level is often normal (except in hypothyroidism) and the muscle histology is characterized by atrophy rather than destruction of muscle fibers. Nearly all endocrine myopathies respond to treatment.

■ THYROID DISORDERS

(See also Chap. 341) Abnormalities of thyroid function can cause a wide array of muscle disorders. These conditions relate to the important role of thyroid hormones in regulating the metabolism of carbohydrates and lipids as well as the rate of protein synthesis and enzyme production. Thyroid hormones also stimulate calorigenesis in muscle, increase muscle demand for vitamins, and enhance muscle sensitivity to circulating catecholamines.

Hypothyroidism

Patients with hypothyroidism have frequent muscle complaints, and proximal muscle weakness occurs in about one-third of them. Muscle cramps, pain, and stiffness are common. Some patients have enlarged muscles. Features of slow muscle contraction and relaxation occur in 25% of patients; the relaxation phase of muscle stretch reflexes is characteristically prolonged and best observed at the ankle or biceps brachii reflexes. The serum CK level is often elevated (up to 10 times normal), even when there is minimal clinical evidence of muscle disease. EMG is typically normal. The cause of muscle enlargement has not been determined, and muscle biopsy shows no distinctive morphologic abnormalities.

Hyperthyroidism

Patients who are thyrotoxic commonly have proximal muscle weakness and atrophy on examination, but they rarely complain of myopathic symptoms. Activity of deep tendon reflexes may be enhanced. Bulbar, respiratory, and even esophageal muscles may occasionally be affected, causing dysphagia, dysphonia, and aspiration. When bulbar involvement occurs, it is usually accompanied by chronic proximal limb weakness, but occasionally it presents in the absence of generalized thyrotoxic myopathy. Fasciculations may be apparent and, when coupled with increased muscle stretch reflexes, may lead to an erroneous diagnosis of ALS. Other neuromuscular disorders occur in association with hyperthyroidism, including acquired hypokalemic periodic paralysis, myasthenia gravis, and a progressive ocular myopathy associated with proptosis (*Graves' ophthalmopathy*). Serum CK levels are not elevated in thyrotoxic myopathy, the EMG is normal, and muscle histology usually shows only atrophy of muscle fibers.

■ PARATHYROID DISORDERS

(See also Chap. 353)

Hyperparathyroidism

Muscle weakness is an integral part of primary and secondary hyperparathyroidism. Proximal muscle weakness, muscle wasting, and brisk muscle stretch reflexes are the main features of this endocrinopathy. Some patients develop neck extensor weakness (part of the dropped head syndrome). Serum CK levels are usually normal or slightly elevated. Serum parathyroid hormone levels are elevated. Serum calcium and phosphorus levels show no correlation with the clinical neuromuscular manifestations. Muscle biopsies show only varying degrees of atrophy without muscle fiber degeneration.

Hypoparathyroidism

An overt myopathy due to hypocalcemia rarely occurs. Neuromuscular symptoms are usually related to localized or generalized tetany. Serum CK levels may be increased secondary to muscle damage from sustained tetany. Hyporeflexia or areflexia is usually present and contrasts with the hyperreflexia in hyperparathyroidism.

■ ADRENAL DISORDERS

(See also Chap. 342) Conditions associated with glucocorticoid excess cause a myopathy; in fact, steroid myopathy is the most commonly diagnosed endocrine muscle disease. Glucocorticoid excess, either endogenous or exogenous (see "Drug-Induced Myopathies," below), produces various degrees of proximal limb weakness. Muscle wasting may be striking. A cushingoid appearance usually accompanies clinical signs of myopathy. Histologic sections demonstrate muscle fiber atrophy, preferentially affecting type 2b fibers, rather than degeneration or necrosis of muscle fibers. Adrenal insufficiency commonly causes muscle fatigue. The degree of weakness may be difficult to assess but is typically mild. In primary hyperaldosteronism (*Conn's syndrome*), neuromuscular complications are due to potassium depletion. The clinical picture is one of persistent muscle weakness. Long-standing hyperaldosteronism may lead to proximal limb weakness and wasting. Serum CK levels may be elevated, and a muscle biopsy may demonstrate degenerating fibers, some with vacuoles. These changes relate to hypokalemia and are not a direct effect of aldosterone on skeletal muscle.

■ PITUITARY DISORDERS

(See also Chap. 339) Patients with acromegaly usually have mild proximal weakness without muscle atrophy. Muscles often appear enlarged but exhibit decreased force generation. The duration of acromegaly, rather than the serum growth hormone levels, correlates with the degree of myopathy.

■ DIABETES MELLITUS

(See also Chap. 344) Neuromuscular complications of diabetes mellitus are most often related to neuropathy, with cranial and peripheral nerve palsies or distal sensorimotor polyneuropathy. *Diabetic amyotrophy* is a clumsy term since the condition represents a neuropathy affecting the proximal major nerve trunks and lumbosacral plexus. More appropriate terms for this disorder include *diabetic proximal neuropathy* and *lumbosacral radiculoplexus neuropathy*.

The only notable myopathy of diabetes mellitus is ischemic infarction of leg muscles, usually involving one of the thigh muscles but on occasion affecting the distal leg. This condition occurs in patients with poorly controlled diabetes and presents with abrupt onset of pain, tenderness, and edema of one thigh. The area of muscle infarction is hard and indurated. The muscles most often affected include the vastus lateralis, thigh adductors, and biceps femoris. CT or MRI can demonstrate focal abnormalities in the affected muscle. Diagnosis by imaging is preferable to muscle biopsy, if possible, as hemorrhage into the biopsy site can occur.

■ VITAMIN DEFICIENCY

Vitamin D deficiency (Chap. 74) due to either decreased intake, decreased absorption, or impaired vitamin D metabolism (as occurs in renal disease) may lead to chronic muscle weakness. Pain reflects the underlying bone disease (*osteomalacia*). Vitamin E deficiency may result from malabsorption. Clinical manifestations include ataxic neuropathy due to loss of proprioception and myopathy with proximal weakness. Progressive external ophthalmoplegia is a distinctive finding. It has not been established that deficiency of other vitamins causes a myopathy.

MYOPATHIES OF SYSTEMIC ILLNESS

Systemic illnesses such as chronic respiratory, cardiac, or hepatic failure are frequently associated with severe muscle wasting and complaints of weakness. Fatigue is usually a more significant problem than weakness, which is typically mild.

Myopathy may be a manifestation of chronic renal failure (CRF), independent of the better known uremic polyneuropathy. Abnormalities of calcium and phosphorus homeostasis and bone metabolism in chronic renal failure result from a reduction in 1,25-dihydroxyvitamin D, leading to decreased intestinal absorption of calcium. Hypocalcemia, further accentuated by hyperphosphatemia due to decreased renal phosphate clearance, leads to secondary hyperparathyroidism. Renal osteodystrophy results from the compensatory hyperparathyroidism, which leads to osteomalacia from reduced calcium availability and to osteitis fibrosa from the parathyroid hormone excess. The clinical picture of the myopathy of CRF is identical to that of primary hyperparathyroidism and osteomalacia. There is proximal limb weakness with bone pain.

Gangrenous calcification represents a separate, rare, and sometimes fatal complication of CRF. In this condition, widespread arterial calcification occurs and results in ischemia. Extensive skin necrosis may occur, along with painful myopathy and even myoglobinuria.

DRUG-INDUCED MYOPATHIES

Drug-induced myopathies are relatively uncommon in clinical practice with the exception of those caused by the cholesterol-lowering agents and glucocorticoids. Others impact practice to a lesser degree but are important to consider in specific situations. Table 387-11 provides a comprehensive list of drug-induced myopathies with their distinguishing features.

■ MYOPATHY FROM LIPID-LOWERING AGENTS

All classes of lipid-lowering agents have been implicated in muscle toxicity, including fibrates (clofibrate, gemfibrozil), HMG-CoA reductase inhibitors (referred to as *statins*), niacin (nicotinic acid), and ezetimibe. Myalgia, malaise, and muscle tenderness are the most common manifestations. Muscle pain may be related to exercise. Patients may exhibit proximal weakness. Varying degrees of muscle necrosis are seen, and in severe reactions rhabdomyolysis and myoglobinuria occur. Concomitant use of statins with fibrates and cyclosporine is more likely to cause adverse reactions than use of one agent alone. Elevated serum CK is an important indication of toxicity. Muscle weakness is accompanied by a myopathic EMG, and muscle necrosis is observed by muscle biopsy. Severe myalgias, muscle weakness, significant elevations in serum CK (>three times baseline), and myoglobinuria are indications for stopping the drug. Patients usually improve with drug cessation, although this may take several weeks. Rare cases continue to progress after the offending agent is discontinued. It is possible that in such cases the statin may have triggered an immune-mediated necrotizing myopathy, as these individuals require immunotherapy (e.g., prednisone and sometimes other agents) to improve and often relapse when

TABLE 387-11 Drug-Induced Myopathies

Drugs	Major Toxic Reaction
Lipid-lowering agents Fibric acid derivatives HMG-CoA reductase inhibitors Niacin (nicotinic acid)	Drugs belonging to all three of the major classes of lipid-lowering agents can produce a spectrum of toxicity: asymptomatic serum creatine kinase elevation, myalgias, exercise-induced pain, rhabdomyolysis, and myoglobinuria.
Glucocorticoids	Acute, high-dose glucocorticoid treatment can cause acute quadriplegic myopathy. These high doses of steroids are often combined with nondepolarizing neuromuscular blocking agents but the weakness can occur without their use. Chronic steroid administration produces predominantly proximal weakness.
Nondepolarizing neuromuscular blocking agents	Acute quadriplegic myopathy can occur with or without concomitant glucocorticoids.
Zidovudine	Mitochondrial myopathy with ragged red fibers.
Drugs of abuse Alcohol Amphetamines Cocaine Heroin Phencyclidine Meperidine	All drugs in this group can lead to widespread muscle breakdown, rhabdomyolysis, and myoglobinuria. Local injections cause muscle necrosis, skin induration, and limb contractures.
Autoimmune toxic myopathy D-Penicillamine	Use of this drug may cause polymyositis and myasthenia gravis.
Amphophilic cationic drugs Amiodarone Chloroquine Hydroxychloroquine	All amphophilic drugs have the potential to produce painless, proximal weakness associated with autophagic vacuoles in the muscle biopsy.
Antimicrotubular drugs Colchicine	This drug produces painless, proximal weakness especially in the setting of renal failure. Muscle biopsy shows autophagic vacuoles.

these therapies are discontinued. Interestingly, antibodies directed against the 100-kD HMG-CoA reductase receptor on muscle fibers has been identified in many of these cases.

GLUCOCORTICOID-RELATED MYOPATHIES

Glucocorticoid myopathy occurs with chronic treatment or as "acute quadriplegic" myopathy secondary to high-dose IV glucocorticoid use. Chronic administration produces proximal weakness accompanied by cushingoid manifestations, which can be quite debilitating; the chronic use of prednisone at a daily dose of ≥30 mg/d is most often associated with toxicity. Patients taking fluorinated glucocorticoids (triamcinolone, betamethasone, dexamethasone) appear to be at especially high risk for myopathy. In chronic steroid myopathy, the serum CK is usually normal. Serum potassium may be low. The muscle biopsy in chronic cases shows preferential type 2 muscle fiber atrophy; this is not reflected in the EMG, which is usually normal.

Patients receiving high-dose IV glucocorticoids for status asthmaticus, chronic obstructive pulmonary disease, organ transplantation, or other indications may develop severe generalized weakness (critical illness myopathy). This myopathy, also known as acute quadriplegic myopathy, can also occur in the setting of sepsis. Involvement of the diaphragm and intercostal muscles causes respiratory failure and requires ventilatory support. In these settings, the use of glucocorticoids in combination with nondepolarizing neuromuscular blocking agents potentiate this complication. In critical illness myopathy, the muscle biopsy is abnormal, showing a distinctive loss of thick filaments (myosin) by electron microscopy. By light microscopy, there is focal loss of ATPase staining in central or paracentral areas of the muscle fiber. Calpain stains show diffusely reactive atrophic fibers. Withdrawal of glucocorticoids will improve the chronic myopathy. In acute quadriplegic myopathy, recovery is slow. Patients require supportive care and rehabilitation.

DRUG-INDUCED MITOCHONDRIAL MYOPATHY

Zidovudine, used in the treatment of HIV infection, is a thymidine analogue that inhibits viral replication by interrupting reverse transcriptase. Myopathy is a well-established complication of this agent. Patients present with myalgias, muscle weakness, and atrophy affecting the thigh and calf muscles. The complication occurs in about 17% of patients treated with doses of 1200 mg/d for 6 months. The introduction of protease inhibitors for treatment of HIV infection has led to lower doses of zidovudine therapy and a decreased incidence of myopathy. Serum CK is elevated and EMG is myopathic. Muscle biopsy shows ragged red fibers with minimal inflammation; the lack of inflammation serves to distinguish zidovudine toxicity from HIV-related myopathy. If the myopathy is thought to be drug related, the medication should be stopped or the dosage reduced.

DRUGS OF ABUSE AND RELATED MYOPATHIES

Myotoxicity is a potential consequence of addiction to alcohol and illicit drugs. Ethanol is one of the most commonly abused substances with potential to damage muscle. Other potential toxins include cocaine, heroin, and amphetamines. The most deleterious reactions occur from overdosing leading to coma and seizures, causing rhabdomyolysis, myoglobinuria, and renal failure. Direct toxicity can occur from cocaine, heroin, and amphetamines causing muscle breakdown and varying degrees of weakness. The effects of alcohol are more controversial. Direct muscle damage is less certain, since toxicity usually occurs in the setting of poor nutrition and possible contributing factors such as hypokalemia and hypophosphatemia. Alcoholics are also prone to neuropathy (Chap. 392).

Focal myopathies from self-administration of meperidine, heroin, and pentazocine can cause pain, swelling, muscle necrosis, and hemorrhage. The cause is multifactorial; needle trauma, direct toxicity of the drug or vehicle, and infection may all play a role. When severe, there may be overlying skin induration and contractures with replacement of muscle by connective tissue. Elevated serum CK and myopathic EMG are characteristic of these reactions. The muscle biopsy shows widespread or focal areas of necrosis. In conditions leading to rhabdomyolysis, patients need adequate hydration to reduce serum myoglobin and protect renal function. In all of these conditions, counseling is essential to limit drug abuse.

DRUG-INDUCED AUTOIMMUNE MYOPATHIES

The most consistent drug-related inflammatory or antibody-mediated myopathy is caused by D-penicillamine. This drug chelates copper and is used in the treatment of Wilson's disease.

It is also used to treat other disorders including scleroderma, rheumatoid arthritis, and primary biliary cirrhosis. Adverse events include drug-induced polymyositis, indistinguishable from the spontaneous disease. The incidence of this inflammatory muscle disease is about 1%. Myasthenia gravis is also induced by D-penicillamine, with a higher incidence estimated at 7%. These disorders resolve with drug withdrawal, although immunosuppressive therapy may be warranted in severe cases.

Scattered reports of other drugs causing an inflammatory myopathy are rare and include a heterogeneous group of agents: cimetidine, phenytoin, procainamide, and propylthiouracil. In most cases, a cause-and-effect relationship is uncertain. A complication of interest was related to L-tryptophan. In 1989 an epidemic of eosinophilia-myalgia syndrome (EMS) in the United States was caused by a contaminant in the product from one manufacturer. The product was withdrawn, and incidence of EMS diminished abruptly following this action.

OTHER DRUG-INDUCED MYOPATHIES

Certain drugs produce painless, largely proximal, muscle weakness. These drugs include the amphophilic cationic drugs (amiodarone, chloroquine, hydroxychloroquine) and antimicrotubular drugs (colchicine) (Table 387-11). Muscle biopsy can be useful in the identification of toxicity since autophagic vacuoles are prominent pathologic features of these toxins.

FURTHER READINGS

Abu-Baker A, Rouleau GA: Oculopharyngeal muscular dystrophy: Recent advances in the understanding of the molecular pathogenic mechanisms and treatment strategies. Biochim Biophys Acta 772:173, 2007

Berardo A et al: A diagnostic algorithm for metabolic myopathies. Curr Neurol Neurosci Rep 10:118, 2010

Bushby K: Diagnosis and management of the limb girdle muscular dystrophies. Pract Neurol 9:314, 2009

Cannon SC: Voltage sensor mutations in channelopathies of skeletal muscle. J Physiol 588:1887, 2010

Christopher-Stine L et al: A novel autoantibody recognizing 200-kD and 100-kD proteins is associated with an immune-mediated necrotizing myopathy. Arthritis Rheum 62:2757, 2010

Glover L, Brown RH Jr: Dysferlin in membrane trafficking and patch repair. Traffic 8:785, 2007

Grable-Esposito P et al: Immune-mediated necrotizing myopathy associated with statins. Muscle Nerve 41:185, 2010

Kishnani PS et al: Recombinant human acid α-glucosidase: Major clinical benefits in infantile-onset Pompe disease. Neurology 68:99, 2007

Lemmers RJ et al: A unifying genetic model for facioscapulohumeral muscular dystrophy. Science 329:1650, 2010

Matthews E et al: The non-dystrophic myotonias: Molecular pathogenesis, diagnosis and treatment. Brain 133:9, 2010

Osborne RJ et al: Transcriptional and post-transcriptional impact of toxic RNA in myotonic dystrophy. Hum Mol Genet 18:1471, 2009

Rodino-Klapac LR et al: Gene therapy for Duchenne muscular dystrophy: Expectations and challenges. Arch Neurol 64:1236, 2007

Suomalainen A, Isohanni P: Mitochondrial depletion syndromes—Many genes, common mechanisms. Neuromuscular Dis 20:429, 2010

van der Ploeg AT et al: A randomized study of alglucosidase alfa in late-onset Pompe's disease. N Engl J Med 362:1396, 2010

Venance SL et al: The primary periodic paralyses: Diagnosis, pathogenesis and treatment. Brain 129:8, 2006

CHAPTER 388

Polymyositis, Dermatomyositis, and Inclusion Body Myositis

Marinos C. Dalakas

The inflammatory myopathies represent the largest group of acquired and potentially treatable causes of skeletal muscle weakness. They are classified into three major groups: polymyositis (PM), dermatomyositis (DM), and inclusion body myositis (IBM).

CLINICAL FEATURES

The prevalence of the inflammatory myopathies is estimated at 1 in 100,000. PM as a stand-alone entity is a rare disease. DM affects both children and adults and women more often than men. IBM is three times more frequent in men than in women, more common in whites than blacks, and is most likely to affect persons aged >50 years.

These disorders present as progressive and symmetric muscle weakness except for IBM, which can have an asymmetric pattern. Patients usually report increasing difficulty with everyday tasks requiring the use of proximal muscles, such as getting up from a chair, climbing steps, stepping onto a curb, lifting objects, or combing hair. Fine-motor movements that depend on the strength of distal muscles, such as buttoning a shirt, sewing, knitting, or writing, are affected only late in the course of PM and DM, but fairly early in IBM. Falling is common in IBM because of early involvement of the quadriceps muscle, with buckling of the knees. Ocular muscles are spared, even in advanced, untreated cases; if these muscles are affected, the diagnosis of inflammatory myopathy should be questioned. Facial muscles are unaffected in PM and DM, but mild facial muscle weakness is common in patients with IBM. In all forms of inflammatory myopathy, pharyngeal and neck-flexor muscles are often involved, causing dysphagia or difficulty in holding up the head (*head drop*). In advanced and rarely in acute cases, respiratory muscles may also be affected. Severe weakness, if untreated, is almost always associated with muscle wasting. Sensation remains normal. The tendon reflexes are preserved but may be absent in severely weakened or atrophied muscles, especially in IBM, where atrophy of the quadriceps and the distal muscles is common. Myalgia and muscle tenderness may occur in a small number of patients, usually early in the disease, and particularly in DM associated with connective tissue disorders. Weakness in PM and DM progresses subacutely over a period of weeks or months and rarely acutely; by contrast, IBM progresses very slowly, over years, simulating a late-life muscular dystrophy (Chap. 387) or slowly progressive motor neuron disorder (Chap. 374).

■ SPECIFIC FEATURES

(Table 388-1)

Polymyositis

The actual onset of PM is often not easily determined, and patients typically delay seeking medical advice for several weeks or even months. This is in contrast to DM, in which the rash facilitates early recognition (see below). PM mimics many other myopathies and is a diagnosis of exclusion. It is a subacute inflammatory myopathy affecting adults, and rarely children, who *do not have* any of the following: rash, involvement of the extraocular and facial muscles, family history of a neuromuscular disease, history of exposure to myotoxic drugs or toxins, endocrinopathy, neurogenic disease, muscular dystrophy, biochemical muscle disorder (deficiency of a muscle enzyme), or IBM as excluded by muscle biopsy analysis (see below). As an isolated entity, PM is a rare (and overdiagnosed) disorder; more commonly, PM occurs in association with a systemic autoimmune or connective tissue disease, or with a known viral or bacterial infection. Drugs, especially D-penicillamine, statins, or zidovudine (AZT), may also trigger an inflammatory myopathy similar to PM.

TABLE 388-1 Features Associated with Inflammatory Myopathies

Characteristic	Polymyositis	Dermatomyositis	Inclusion Body Myositis
Age at onset	>18 years	Adulthood and childhood	>50 years
Familial association	No	No	Yes, in some cases
Extramuscular manifestations	Yes	Yes	Yes
Associated conditions			
Connective tissue diseases	Yes[a]	Scleroderma and mixed connective tissue disease (overlap syndromes)	Yes, in up to 20% of cases[a]
Systemic autoimmune diseases[b]	Frequent	Infrequent	Infrequent
Malignancy	No	Yes, in up to 15% of cases	No
Viruses	Yes[c]	Unproven	Yes[c]
Drugs[d]	Yes	Yes, rarely	No
Parasites and bacteria[e]	Yes	No	No

[a]Systemic lupus erythematosus, rheumatoid arthritis, Sjögren's syndrome, systemic sclerosis, mixed connective tissue disease.

[b]Crohn's disease, vasculitis, sarcoidosis, primary biliary cirrhosis, adult celiac disease, chronic graft-versus-host disease, discoid lupus, ankylosing spondylitis, Behçet's syndrome, myasthenia gravis, acne fulminans, dermatitis herpetiformis, psoriasis, Hashimoto's disease, granulomatous diseases, agammaglobulinemia, monoclonal gammopathy, hypereosinophilic syndrome, Lyme disease, Kawasaki disease, autoimmune thrombocytopenia, hypergammaglobulinemic purpura, hereditary complement deficiency, IgA deficiency.

[c]HIV (human immunodeficiency virus) and HTLV-I (human T cell lymphotropic virus type I).

[d]Drugs include penicillamine (dermatomyositis and polymyositis), zidovudine (polymyositis), and contaminated tryptophan (dermatomyositis-like illness). Other myotoxic drugs may cause myopathy but not an inflammatory myopathy (see text for details).

[e]Parasites (protozoa, cestodes, nematodes), tropical and bacterial myositis (pyomyositis).

Dermatomyositis

DM is a distinctive entity identified by a characteristic rash accompanying, or more often preceding, muscle weakness. The rash may consist of a blue-purple discoloration on the upper eyelids with edema (heliotrope rash; see Fig. 54-3), a flat red rash on the face and upper trunk, and erythema of the knuckles with a raised violaceous scaly eruption (*Gottron's sign*; see Fig. 54-4). The erythematous rash can also occur on other body surfaces, including the knees, elbows, malleoli, neck and anterior chest (often in a *V sign*), or back and shoulders (*shawl sign*), and may worsen after sun exposure. In some patients, the rash is pruritic, especially on the scalp, chest, and back. Dilated capillary loops at the base of the fingernails are also characteristic. The cuticles may be irregular, thickened, and distorted, and the lateral and palmar areas of the fingers may become rough and cracked, with irregular, "dirty" horizontal lines, resembling *mechanic's hands*. The weakness can be mild, moderate, or severe enough to lead to quadriparesis. At times, the muscle strength appears normal, hence the term *dermatomyositis sine myositis*. When muscle biopsy is performed in such cases, however, significant perivascular and perimysial inflammation is often seen.

DM usually occurs alone but may overlap with scleroderma and mixed connective tissue disease. Fasciitis and thickening of the skin, similar to that seen in chronic cases of DM, have occurred in patients with the *eosinophilia-myalgia syndrome* associated with the ingestion of contaminated L-tryptophan.

Inclusion body myositis

In patients ≥50 years of age, IBM is the most common of the inflammatory myopathies. It is often misdiagnosed as PM and is suspected only later when a patient with presumed PM does not respond to therapy. Weakness and atrophy of the distal muscles, especially foot extensors and deep finger flexors, occur in almost all cases of IBM and may be a clue to early diagnosis. Some patients present with falls because their knees collapse due to early quadriceps weakness. Others present with weakness in the small muscles of the hands, especially finger flexors, and complain of inability to hold objects such as golf clubs or perform tasks such as turning keys or tying knots. On occasion, the weakness and accompanying atrophy can be asymmetric and selectively involve the quadriceps, iliopsoas, triceps, biceps, and finger flexors, resembling a lower motor neuron disease. Dysphagia is common, occurring in up to 60% of IBM patients, and may lead to episodes of choking. Sensory examination is generally normal; some patients have mildly diminished vibratory sensation at the ankles that presumably is age-related. The pattern of distal weakness, which superficially resembles motor neuron or peripheral nerve disease, results from the myopathic process affecting distal muscles selectively. Disease progression is slow but steady, and most patients require an assistive device such as cane, walker, or wheelchair within several years of onset.

In at least 20% of cases, IBM is associated with systemic autoimmune or connective tissue diseases. Familial aggregation of typical IBM may occur; such cases have been designated as *familial inflammatory IBM*. This disorder is distinct from *hereditary inclusion body myopathy* (h-IBM), which describes a heterogeneous group of recessive, and less frequently dominant, inherited syndromes; the h-IBMs are noninflammatory myopathies. A subset of h-IBM that spares the quadriceps muscles has emerged as a distinct entity. This disorder, originally described in Iranian Jews and now seen in many ethnic groups, is linked to chromosome 9p1 and results from mutations in the UDP-*N*-acetylglucosamine 2-epimerase/*N*-acetylmannosamine kinase (*GNE*) gene.

■ ASSOCIATED CLINICAL FINDINGS

Extramuscular manifestations

These may be present to a varying degree in patients with PM or DM, and include:

1. *Systemic symptoms*, such as fever, malaise, weight loss, arthralgia, and Raynaud's phenomenon, especially when inflammatory myopathy is associated with a connective tissue disorder.
2. *Joint contractures*, mostly in DM and especially in children.
3. *Dysphagia and gastrointestinal symptoms*, due to involvement of oropharyngeal striated muscles and upper esophagus, especially in DM and IBM.
4. *Cardiac disturbances*, including atrioventricular conduction defects, tachyarrhythmias, dilated cardiomyopathy, a low ejection fraction, and congestive heart failure, may rarely occur, either from the disease itself or from hypertension associated with long-term use of glucocorticoids.
5. *Pulmonary dysfunction*, due to weakness of the thoracic muscles, interstitial lung disease, or drug-induced pneumonitis (e.g., from methotrexate), which may cause dyspnea, nonproductive cough, and aspiration pneumonia. Interstitial lung disease may precede myopathy or occur early in the disease and develops in up to 10% of patients with PM or DM, most of whom have antibodies to t-RNA synthetases, as described below.
6. *Subcutaneous calcifications*, in DM, sometimes extruding on the skin and causing ulcerations and infections.
7. *Arthralgias*, synovitis, or deforming arthropathy with subluxation in the interphalangeal joints can occur in some patients with DM and PM who have Jo-1 antibodies (see below).

Association with malignancies

Although all the inflammatory myopathies can have a chance association with malignant lesions, especially in older age groups, the incidence of malignant conditions appears to be specifically increased only in patients with DM and not in those with PM or IBM. The most common tumors associated with DM are ovarian cancer, breast cancer, melanoma, colon cancer, and non-Hodgkin lymphoma. The extent of the search that should be conducted for an occult neoplasm in adults with DM depends on the clinical circumstances. Tumors in these patients are usually uncovered by abnormal findings in the medical history and physical examination and not through an extensive blind search. The weight of evidence argues against performing expensive, invasive, and nondirected tumor searches. A complete annual physical examination with pelvic, breast (mammogram, if indicated), and rectal examinations (with colonoscopy according to age and family history); urinalysis; complete blood count; blood chemistry tests; and a chest film should suffice in most cases. In Asians, nasopharyngeal cancer is common, and a careful examination of ears, nose, and throat is indicated. If malignancy is clinically suspected, screening with whole-body PET scan should be considered.

Overlap syndromes

These describe the association of inflammatory myopathies with connective tissue diseases. A well-characterized overlap syndrome occurs in patients with DM who also have manifestations of systemic sclerosis or mixed connective tissue disease, such as sclerotic thickening of the dermis, contractures, esophageal hypomotility, microangiopathy, and calcium deposits (Table 388-1). By contrast, signs of rheumatoid arthritis, systemic lupus erythematosus, or Sjögren's syndrome are very rare in patients with DM. Patients with the overlap syndrome of DM and systemic sclerosis may have a specific antinuclear antibody, the anti-PM/Scl, directed against a nucleolar-protein complex.

■ PATHOGENESIS

An autoimmune etiology of the inflammatory myopathies is indirectly supported by an association with other autoimmune or connective tissue diseases; the presence of various autoantibodies; an association with specific major histocompatibility complex (MHC) genes; demonstration of T cell–mediated myocytotoxicity or complement-mediated microangiopathy; and a response to immunotherapy.

Autoantibodies and immunogenetics

Various autoantibodies against nuclear antigens (antinuclear antibodies) and cytoplasmic antigens are found in up to 20% of patients with inflammatory myopathies. The antibodies to cytoplasmic antigens are directed against ribonucleoproteins involved in protein synthesis (antisynthetases) or translational transport (anti-signal-recognition particles). The antibody directed against the histidyl-transfer RNA synthetase, called *anti-Jo-1*, accounts for 75% of all the antisynthetases and is clinically useful because up to 80% of patients with anti-Jo-1 antibodies have interstitial lung disease. Some patients with the anti-Jo-1 antibody also have Raynaud's phenomenon, nonerosive arthritis, and the MHC molecules DR3 and DRw52. DR3 haplotypes (molecular designation DRB1*0301, DQB1*0201) occur in up to 75% of patients with PM and IBM, whereas in juvenile DM there is an increased frequency of DQA1*0501 (Chap. 315).

Immunopathologic mechanisms

In DM, humoral immune mechanisms are implicated, resulting in a microangiopathy and muscle ischemia (Fig. 388-1). Endomysial inflammatory infiltrates are composed of B cells located in proximity to CD4 T cells, plasmacytoid dendritic cells, and macrophages; there is a relative absence of lymphocytic invasion of nonnecrotic muscle fibers. Activation of the complement C5b-9 membranolytic attack complex is thought to be a critical early event that triggers release of proinflammatory cytokines and chemokines, induces expression of vascular cell adhesion molecule (VCAM) 1 and intercellular adhesion molecule (ICAM) 1 on endothelial cells, and facilitates migration of activated lymphoid cells to the perimysial and endomysial spaces. Necrosis of the endothelial cells, reduced numbers of endomysial capillaries, ischemia, and muscle-fiber destruction resembling microinfarcts occur. The remaining capillaries often have dilated lumens in response to the ischemic process. Larger intramuscular blood vessels may also be affected in the same pattern. Residual perifascicular atrophy reflects the endofascicular hypoperfusion that is prominent in the periphery of muscle fascicles. Increased expression of type I interferon-inducible proteins is also noted in these regions.

By contrast, in PM and IBM a mechanism of T cell–mediated cytotoxicity is likely. CD8 T cells, along with macrophages, initially surround and eventually invade and destroy healthy, nonnecrotic muscle fibers that aberrantly express class I MHC molecules. MHC-I expression, absent from the sarcolemma of normal muscle fibers, is probably induced by cytokines secreted by activated

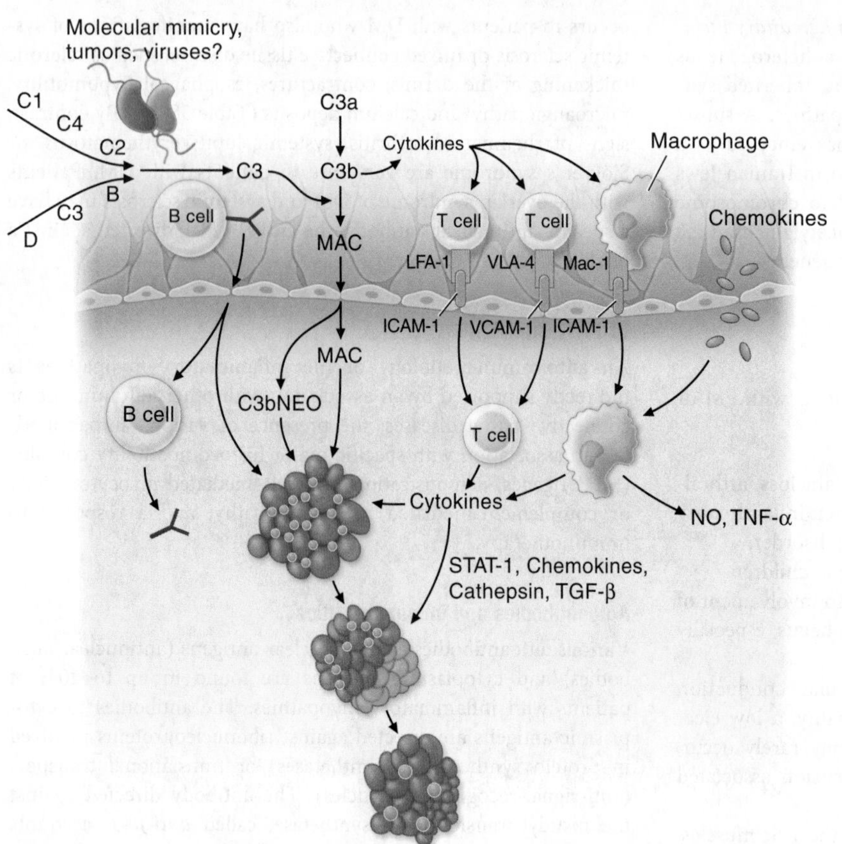

Figure 388-1 Immunopathogenesis of dermatomyositis. Activation of complement, possibly by autoantibodies (Y), against endothelial cells and formation of C3 via the classic or alternative pathway. Activated C3 leads to formation of C3b, C3bNEO, and membrane attack complexes (MAC), which are deposited in and around the endothelial cell wall of the endomysial capillaries. Deposition of MAC leads to destruction of capillaries, ischemia, or microinfarcts, most prominent in the periphery of the fascicles, and perifascicular atrophy. B cells, plasmacytoid dendritic cells, CD4 T cells, and macrophages traffic from the circulation to the muscle. Endothelial expression of vascular cell adhesion molecule (VCAM) and intercellular adhesion molecule (ICAM) is induced by cytokines released by the mononuclear cells. Integrins, specifically very late activation antigen (VLA)-4 and lymphocyte function–associated antigen (LFA)-1, bind VCAM and ICAM and promote T cell and macrophage infiltration of muscle through the endothelial cell wall.

T cells and macrophages. The CD8/MHC-I complex is characteristic of PM and IBM; its detection can aid in confirming the histologic diagnosis of PM, as discussed below. The cytotoxic CD8 T cells contain perforin and granzyme granules directed toward the surface of the muscle fibers and capable of inducing myonecrosis. Analysis of T cell receptor molecules expressed by the infiltrating CD8 cells has revealed clonal expansion and conserved sequences in the antigen-binding region, both suggesting an antigen-driven T cell response. Whether the putative antigens are endogenous (e.g., muscle) or exogenous (e.g., viral) sequences is unknown. Viruses have not been identified within the muscle fibers. Co-stimulatory molecules and their counterreceptors, which are fundamental for T cell activation and antigen recognition, are strongly upregulated in PM and IBM. Key molecules involved in T cell–mediated cytotoxicity are depicted in Fig. 388-2.

The role of nonimmune factors in IBM

In IBM, the presence of Congo red–positive amyloid deposits within some vacuolated muscle fibers and abnormal mitochondria with cytochrome oxidase–negative fibers suggest that, in addition to the autoimmune component, there is also a degenerative process. Similar to Alzheimer's disease, the intracellular amyloid deposits in IBM are immunoreactive against amyloid precursor protein (APP), β-amyloid, chymotrypsin, apolipoprotein E, presenilin, ubiquitin, and phosphorylated tau, but it is unclear whether these deposits, which are also seen in other vacuolar myopathies, are directly pathogenic or represent secondary phenomena. The same is true for the mitochondrial abnormalities, which may also be secondary to the effects of aging or a bystander effect of upregulated cytokines. Expression of cytokines and upregulation of MHC class I by the muscle fibers may cause an endoplasmic reticulum stress response resulting in intracellular accumulation of stressor molecules or misfolded glycoproteins and activation of nuclear factor κB (NF-κB), leading to further cytokine activation.

Association with viral infections and the role of retroviruses

Several viruses, including coxsackieviruses, influenza, paramyxoviruses, mumps, cytomegalovirus, and Epstein-Barr virus, have been indirectly associated with myositis. For the coxsackieviruses, an autoimmune myositis triggered by molecular mimicry has been proposed because of structural homology between histidyl-transfer RNA synthetase that is the target of the Jo-1 antibody (see above) and genomic RNA of an animal picornavirus, the encephalomyocarditis virus. Sensitive polymerase chain reaction (PCR) studies, however, have repeatedly failed to confirm the presence of such viruses in muscle biopsies.

The best evidence of a viral connection in PM and IBM is with the retroviruses. Some individuals infected with HIV or with human T cell lymphotropic virus I (HTLV-I) develop PM or IBM; a similar disorder has been described in nonhuman primates infected with the simian immunodeficiency virus. The inflammatory myopathy may occur as the initial manifestation of a retroviral infection, or myositis may develop later in the disease course. Retroviral antigens have been detected only in occasional endomysial macrophages and not within the muscle fibers themselves, suggesting that persistent infection and viral replication within the muscle do not occur. Histologic findings are identical to retroviral-negative PM or IBM. The infiltrating T cells in the muscle are clonally driven and a number of them are retroviral-specific. This disorder should be distinguished from a toxic myopathy related to long-term therapy with AZT, characterized by fatigue, myalgia, mild muscle weakness, and mild elevation of creatine kinase (CK). AZT-induced myopathy, which generally improves when the drug is discontinued, is a mitochondrial disorder characterized histologically by "ragged-red" fibers. AZT inhibits γ-DNA polymerase, an enzyme found solely in the mitochondrial matrix.

DIFFERENTIAL DIAGNOSIS

The clinical picture of the typical skin rash and proximal or diffuse muscle weakness has few causes other than DM. However, proximal muscle weakness without skin involvement can be due to many conditions other than PM or IBM.

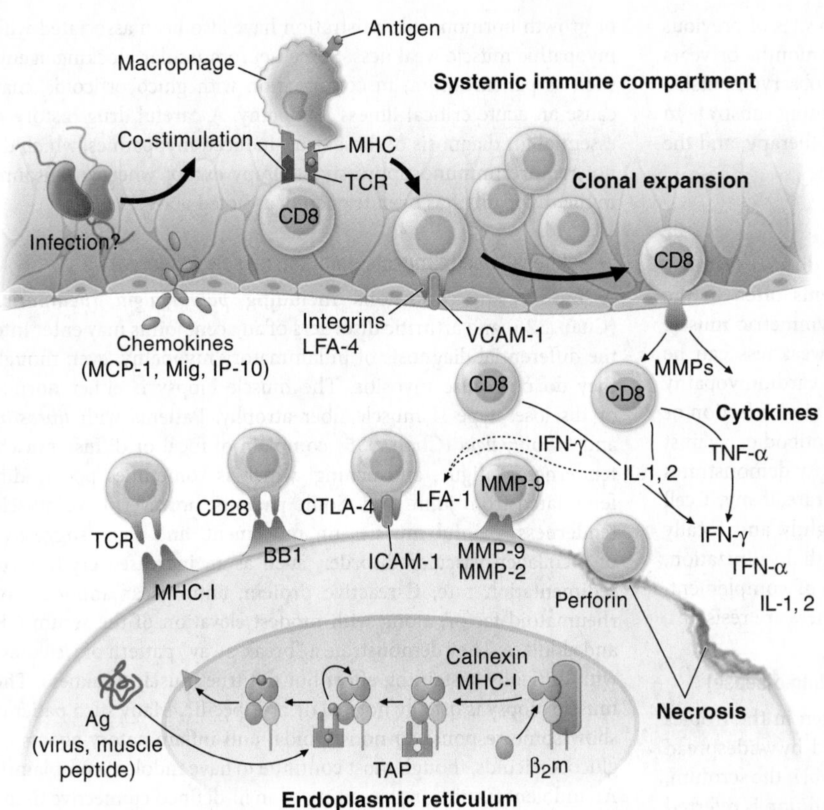

Figure 388-2 Cell-mediated mechanisms of muscle damage in polymyositis (PM) and inclusion body myositis (IBM). Antigen-specific CD8 cells are expanded in the periphery, cross the endothelial barrier, and bind directly to muscle fibers via T cell receptor (TCR) molecules that recognize aberrantly expressed MHC-I. Engagement of co-stimulatory molecules (BB1 and ICOSL) with their ligands (CD28, CTLA-4, and ICOS), along with ICAM-1/LFA-1, stabilize the CD8–muscle fiber interaction. Metalloproteinases (MMPs) facilitate the migration of T cells and their attachment to the muscle surface. Muscle fiber necrosis occurs via perforin granules released by the autoaggressive T cells. A direct myocytotoxic effect exerted by the cytokines interferon (IFN) γ, interleukin (IL) 1, or tumor necrosis factor (TNF) α may also play a role. Death of the muscle fiber is mediated by necrosis. MHC class I molecules consist of a heavy chain and a light chain [β_2 microglobulin (β_2m)] complexed with an antigenic peptide that is transported into the endoplasmic reticulum by TAP proteins (Chap. 315).

Subacute or chronic progressive muscle weakness

This may be due to denervating conditions such as the spinal muscular atrophies or amyotrophic lateral sclerosis (Chap. 374). In addition to the muscle weakness, upper motor neuron signs in the latter and signs of denervation detected by electromyography (EMG) aid in the diagnosis. The muscular dystrophies (Chap. 387) may be additional considerations; however, these disorders usually develop over years rather than weeks or months and rarely present after the age of 30 years. It may be difficult, even with a muscle biopsy, to distinguish chronic PM from a rapidly advancing muscular dystrophy. This is particularly true of facioscapulohumeral muscular dystrophy, dysferlin myopathy, and the dystrophinopathies where inflammatory cell infiltration is often found early in the disease. Such doubtful cases should always be given an adequate trial of glucocorticoid therapy and undergo genetic testing to exclude muscular dystrophy. Identification of the MHC/CD8 lesion by muscle biopsy is helpful to identify cases of PM. Some metabolic myopathies, including glycogen storage disease due to myophosphorylase or acid maltase deficiency, lipid storage myopathies due to carnitine deficiency, and mitochondrial diseases produce weakness that is often associated with other characteristic clinical signs; diagnosis rests upon histochemical and biochemical studies of the muscle biopsy. The endocrine myopathies such as those due to hypercorticosteroidism, hyper- and hypothyroidism, and hyper- and hypoparathyroidism require the appropriate laboratory investigations for diagnosis. Muscle wasting in patients with an underlying neoplasm may be due to disuse, cachexia, or rarely to a paraneoplastic neuromyopathy (Chap. 101).

Diseases of the neuromuscular junction, including myasthenia gravis or the Lambert-Eaton myasthenic syndrome, cause fatiguing weakness that also affects ocular and other cranial muscles (Chap. 386). Repetitive nerve stimulation and single-fiber EMG studies aid in diagnosis.

Acute muscle weakness

This may be caused by an acute neuropathy such as Guillain-Barré syndrome (Chap. 385), transverse myelitis (Chap. 377), a neurotoxin (Chap. 387), or a neurotropic viral infection such as poliomyelitis or West Nile virus (Chap. 381). When acute weakness is associated with very high levels of serum creatine kinase (CK) (often in the thousands), painful muscle cramps, rhabdomyolysis, and myoglobinuria, it may be due to a viral infection or a metabolic disorder such as myophosphorylase deficiency or carnitine palmitoyltransferase deficiency (Chap. 387). Several animal parasites, including protozoa (*Toxoplasma*, *Trypanosoma*), cestodes (cysticerci), and nematodes (trichinae), may produce a focal or diffuse inflammatory myopathy known as *parasitic polymyositis*. *Staphylococcus aureus*, *Yersinia*, *Streptococcus*, or anaerobic bacteria may produce a suppurative myositis, known as *tropical polymyositis*, or *pyomyositis*. Pyomyositis, previously rare in the west, is now occasionally seen in AIDS patients. Other bacteria, such as *Borrelia burgdorferi* (Lyme disease) and *Legionella pneumophila* (Legionaire's disease), may infrequently cause myositis.

Patients with periodic paralysis experience recurrent episodes of acute muscle weakness without pain, always beginning in childhood. Chronic alcoholics may develop painful myopathy with myoglobinuria after a bout of heavy drinking. Acute painless muscle weakness with myoglobinuria may occur with prolonged hypokalemia, or hypophosphatemia and hypomagnesemia, usually in chronic alcoholics or in patients on nasogastric suction receiving parenteral hyperalimentation.

Myofasciitis

This distinctive inflammatory disorder affecting muscle and fascia presents as diffuse myalgias, skin induration, fatigue, and mild muscle weakness; mild elevations of serum CK are usually present. The most common form is eosinophilic myofasciitis characterized by peripheral blood eosinophilia and eosinophilic infiltrates in the endomysial tissue. In some patients, the eosinophilic myositis/fasciitis occurs in the context of parasitic infections, vasculitis, mixed connective tissue disease, hypereosinophilic syndrome, or toxic exposures (e.g., toxic oil syndrome, contaminated L-tryptophan) or with mutations in the calpain gene. A distinct subset of myofasciitis is characterized by pronounced infiltration of the connective tissue around the muscle by sheets of periodic acid–Schiff-positive macrophages and occasional CD8 T cells (macrophagic myofasciitis).

Such histologic involvement is focal and limited to sites of previous vaccinations, which may have been administered months or years earlier. This disorder, which to date has not been observed outside of France, has been linked to an aluminum-containing substrate in vaccines. Most patients respond to glucocorticoid therapy, and the overall prognosis seems favorable.

Necrotizing myositis

This is an increasingly recognized entity that has distinct features, even though it is often labeled as PM. It presents often in the fall or winter as an acute or subacute onset of symmetric muscle weakness; CK is typically extremely high. The weakness can be severe. Coexisting interstitial lung disease and cardiomyopathy may be present. The disorder may develop after a viral infection or in association with cancer. Some patients have antibodies against signal recognition particle (SRP). The muscle biopsy demonstrates necrotic fibers infiltrated by macrophages but only rare, if any, T cell infiltrates. Muscle MHC-I expression is only slightly and focally upregulated. The capillaries may be swollen with hyalinization, thickening of the capillary wall, and deposition of complement. Some patients respond to immunotherapy, but others are resistant.

Hyperacute necrotizing fasciitis/myositis (flesh-eating disease)

This a fulminant infectious disease, seen most often in the tropics or in conditions with poor hygiene, characterized by widespread necrosis of the superficial fascia and muscle of a limb; if the scrotum, perineum, and abdominal wall are affected, the condition is referred to as Fournier's gangrene. It may be caused by group A β-hemolytic streptococcus, methicillin-sensitive *S. aureus*, *Pseudomonas aeruginosa*, *Vibrio vulnificus*, clostridial species (gas gangrene; Chap. 142), or polymicrobial infection with anaerobes and facultative bacteria (Chap. 164); toxins from these bacteria may act as superantigens (Chap. 314). The port of bacterial entry is usually a trivial cut or skin abrasion and the source is contact with carriers of the organism. Individuals with diabetes mellitus, immunodeficiency states, or systemic illnesses such as liver failure are most susceptible. Systemic varicella is a predisposing factor in children.

The disease presents with swelling, pain, and redness in the involved area followed by a rapid tissue necrosis of fascia and muscle that progresses at an estimated rate of 3 cm/h. Emergency debridement, antibiotics, as well as IVIg, or even hyperbaric oxygen have been recommended. In progressive or advanced cases, amputation of the affected limb may be necessary to avoid a fatal outcome.

Drug-induced myopathies

D-Penicillamine, procainamide, and statins may produce a true myositis resembling PM, and a DM-like illness had been associated with the contaminated preparations of L-tryptophan. As noted above, AZT causes a mitochondrial myopathy. Other drugs may elicit a toxic noninflammatory myopathy that is histologically different from DM, PM, or IBM. These include cholesterol-lowering agents such as clofibrate, lovastatin, simvastatin, or provastatin, especially when combined with cyclosporine, amiodarone, or gemfibrozil. Statin-induced necrotizing myopathy or asymptomatic elevations of CK usually improve after discontinuation of the drug. In rare patients, however, muscle weakness continues to progress even after the statin is withdrawn; in these cases, a diagnostic muscle biopsy is indicated, and if evidence of inflammation and MHC-I upregulation is present, immunotherapy for PM should be considered. Rhabdomyolysis and myoglobinuria have been rarely associated with amphotericin B, ε-aminocaproic acid, fenfluramine, heroin, and phencyclidine. The use of amiodarone, chloroquine, colchicine, carbimazole, emetine, etretinate, ipecac syrup, chronic laxative or licorice use resulting in hypokalemia, and glucocorticoids or growth hormone administration have also been associated with myopathic muscle weakness. Some neuromuscular blocking agents such as pancuronium, in combination with glucocorticoids, may cause an acute critical illness myopathy. A careful drug history is essential for diagnosis of these drug-induced myopathies, which do not require immunosuppressive therapy except when an autoimmune myopathy has been triggered, as noted above.

"Weakness" due to muscle pain and muscle tenderness

A number of conditions including *polymyalgia rheumatica* (Chap. 326) and arthritic disorders of adjacent joints may enter into the differential diagnosis of inflammatory myopathy, even though they do not cause myositis. The muscle biopsy is either normal or discloses type II muscle fiber atrophy. Patients with *fibrositis* and *fibromyalgia* (Chap. 335) complain of focal or diffuse muscle tenderness, fatigue, and aching, which is sometimes poorly differentiated from joint pain. Some patients, however, have muscle tenderness, painful muscles on movement, and signs suggestive of a collagen vascular disorder, such as an increased erythrocyte sedimentation rate, C-reactive protein, antinuclear antibody, or rheumatoid factor, along with modest elevation of the serum CK and aldolase. They demonstrate a "break-away" pattern of weakness with difficulty sustaining effort but not true muscle weakness. The muscle biopsy is usually normal or nonspecific. Many such patients show some response to nonsteroidal anti-inflammatory agents or glucocorticoids, though most continue to have indolent complaints. An indolent fasciitis in the setting of an ill-defined connective tissue disorder may be present, and these patients should not be labeled as having a psychosomatic disorder. *Chronic fatigue syndrome*, which may follow a viral infection, can present with debilitating fatigue, fever, sore throat, painful lymphadenopathy, myalgia, arthralgia, sleep disorder, and headache (Chap. 389). These patients do not have muscle weakness, and the muscle biopsy is normal.

■ DIAGNOSIS

The clinically suspected diagnosis of PM, DM, or IBM is confirmed by analysis of serum muscle enzymes, EMG findings, and muscle biopsy (Table 388-2).

The most sensitive enzyme is CK, which in active disease can be elevated as much as fiftyfold. Although the CK level usually parallels disease activity, it can be normal in some patients with active IBM or DM, especially when associated with a connective tissue disease. The CK is always elevated in patients with active PM. Along with the CK, the serum glutamic-oxaloacetic and glutamate pyruvate transaminases, lactate dehydrogenase, and aldolase may be elevated.

Needle EMG shows myopathic potentials characterized by short-duration, low-amplitude polyphasic units on voluntary activation and increased spontaneous activity with fibrillations, complex repetitive discharges, and positive sharp waves. Mixed potentials (polyphasic units of short and long duration) indicating a chronic process and muscle fiber regeneration are often present in IBM. These EMG findings are not diagnostic of an inflammatory myopathy but are useful to identify the presence of active or chronic myopathy and to exclude neurogenic disorders.

MRI is not routinely used for the diagnosis of PM, DM, or IBM. However, it may provide information or guide the location of the muscle biopsy in certain clinical settings.

Muscle biopsy—in spite of occasional variability in demonstrating all of the typical pathologic findings—is the most sensitive and specific test for establishing the diagnosis of inflammatory myopathy and for excluding other neuromuscular diseases. Inflammation is the histologic hallmark for these diseases; however, additional features are characteristic of each subtype (Figs. 388-3, 388-4, and 388-5).

TABLE 388-2 Criteria for Diagnosis of Inflammatory Myopathies

Criterion	Polymyositis: Definite	Polymyositis: Probable	Dermatomyositis	Inclusion Body Myositis
Myopathic muscle weakness[a]	Yes	Yes	Yes[b]	Yes; slow onset, early involvement of distal muscles, frequent falls
Electromyographic findings	Myopathic	Myopathic	Myopathic	Myopathic with mixed potentials
Muscle enzymes	Elevated (up to fiftyfold)	Elevated (up to fiftyfold)	Elevated (up to fiftyfold) or normal	Elevated (up to tenfold) or normal
Muscle biopsy findings[c]	"Primary" inflammation with the CD8/MHC-I complex and no vacuoles	Ubiquitous MHC-I expression but minimal inflammation and no vacuoles[d]	Perifascicular, perimysial, or perivascular infiltrates, perifascicular atrophy	Primary inflammation with CD8/MHC-I complex; vacuolated fibers with β-amyloid deposits; cytochrome oxygenase–negative fibers; signs of chronic myopathy[e]
Rash or calcinosis	Absent	Absent	Present[f]	Absent

[a]Myopathic muscle weakness, affecting proximal muscles more than distal ones and sparing eye and facial muscles, is characterized by a subacute onset (weeks to months) and rapid progression in patients who have no family history of neuromuscular disease, no endocrinopathy, no exposure to myotoxic drugs or toxins, and no biochemical muscle disease (excluded on the basis of muscle-biopsy findings).

[b]In some cases with the typical rash, the muscle strength is seemingly normal (dermatomyositis sine myositis); these patients often have new onset of easy fatigue and reduced endurance. Careful muscle testing may reveal mild muscle weakness.

[c]See text for details.

[d]An adequate trial of prednisone or other immunosuppressive drugs is warranted in probable cases. If, in retrospect, the disease is unresponsive to therapy, another muscle biopsy should be considered to exclude other diseases or possible evolution in inclusion body myositis.

[e]If the muscle biopsy does not contain vacuolated fibers but shows chronic myopathy with hypertrophic fibers, primary inflammation with the CD8/MHC-I complex and cytochrome oxygenase–negative fibers, the diagnosis is probable inclusion body myositis.

[f]If rash is absent but muscle biopsy findings are characteristic of dermatomyositis, the diagnosis is probable dermatomyositis.

In PM the inflammation is *primary*, a term used to indicate that the inflammation is not reactive and the T cell infiltrates, located primarily within the muscle fascicles (endomysially), surround individual, healthy muscle fibers and result in phagocytosis and necrosis (Fig. 388-3). The MHC-I molecule is ubiquitously expressed on the sarcolemma, even in fibers not invaded by CD8+ cells. The CD8/MHC-I lesion is characteristic and essential to confirm or establish the diagnosis and to exclude disorders with secondary, nonspecific, inflammation, such as in some muscular dystrophies. When the disease is chronic, connective tissue is increased and may react positively with alkaline phosphatase.

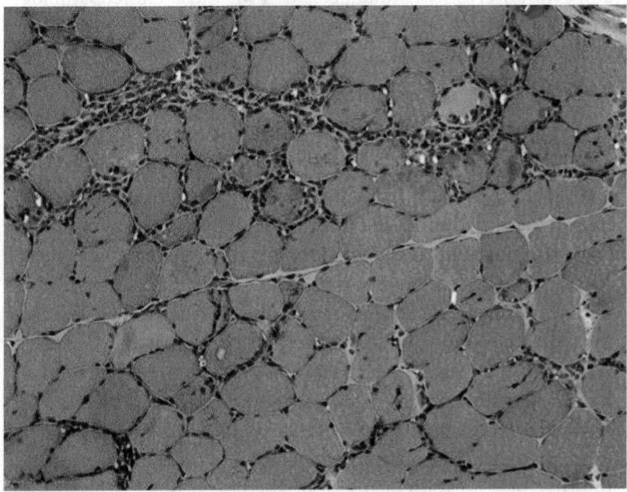

Figure 388-3 Cross-section of a muscle biopsy from a patient with polymyositis demonstrates scattered inflammatory foci with lymphocytes invading or surrounding muscle fibers. Note lack of chronic myopathic features (increased connective tissue, atrophic or hypertrophic fibers) as seen in inclusion body myositis.

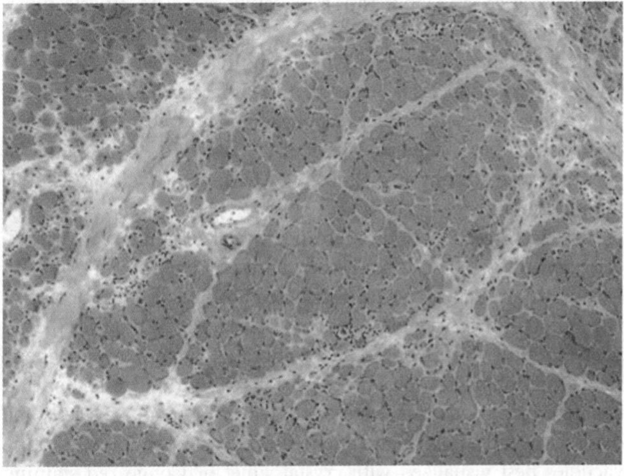

Figure 388-4 Cross-section of a muscle biopsy from a patient with dermatomyositis demonstrates atrophy of the fibers at the periphery of the fascicle (perifascicular atrophy).

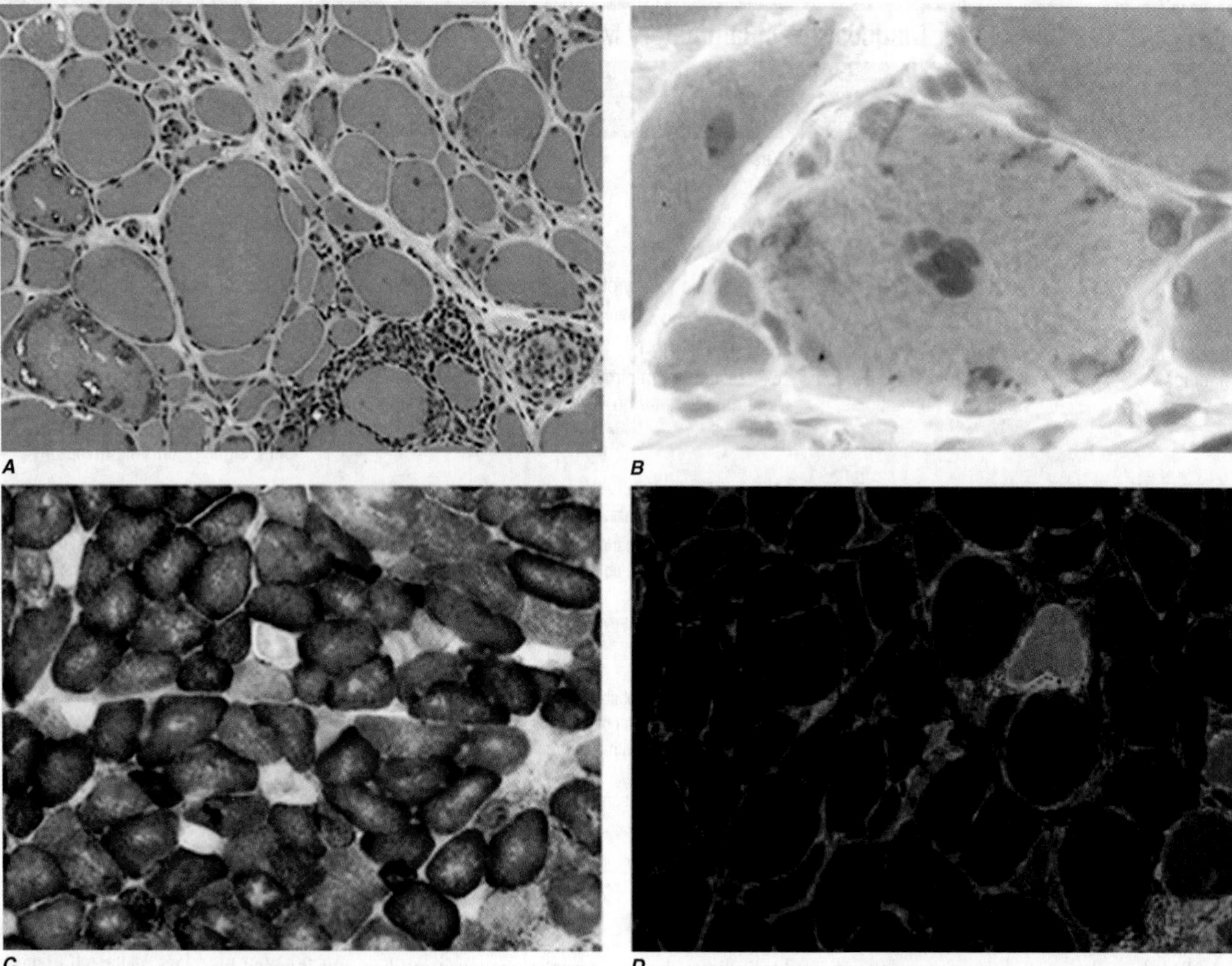

Figure 388-5 Cross-sections of a muscle biopsy from a patient with inclusion body myositis demonstrate the typical features of vacuoles with lymphocytic infiltrates surrounding nonvacuolated or necrotic fibers (***A***), tiny endomysial deposits of amyloid visualized with crystal violet (***B***), cytochrome oxidase–negative fibers, indicative of mitochondrial dysfunction (***C***), and ubiquitous MHC-I expression at the periphery of all fibers (***D***).

In DM the endomysial inflammation is predominantly perivascular or in the interfascicular septae and around—rather than within—the muscle fascicles (Fig. 388-4). The intramuscular blood vessels show endothelial hyperplasia with tubuloreticular profiles, fibrin thrombi, and obliteration of capillaries. The muscle fibers undergo necrosis, degeneration, and phagocytosis, often in groups involving a portion of a muscle fasciculus in a wedgelike shape or at the periphery of the fascicle, due to microinfarcts within the muscle. This results in perifascicular atrophy, characterized by 2–10 layers of atrophic fibers at the periphery of the fascicles. The presence of perifascicular atrophy is diagnostic of DM, *even in the absence of inflammation.*

In IBM (Fig. 388-5), there is endomysial inflammation with T cells invading MHC-I-expressing nonvacuolated muscle fibers; basophilic granular deposits distributed around the edge of slitlike vacuoles (rimmed vacuoles); loss of fibers, replaced by fat and connective tissue, hypertrophic fibers, and angulated or round fibers; rare eosinophilic cytoplasmic inclusions; abnormal mitochondria characterized by the presence of ragged-red fibers or cytochrome oxidase–negative fibers; and amyloid deposits within or next to the vacuoles best visualized with crystal violet or Congo-red staining viewed with fluorescent optics. Electron microscopy demonstrates filamentous inclusions in the vicinity of the rimmed vacuoles. In at least 15% of patients with the typical clinical phenotype of IBM, no vacuoles or amyloid deposits can be identified in muscle biopsy, leading to an erroneous diagnosis of PM. Close clinicopathologic correlations are essential; if uncertain, a repeat muscle biopsy from another site is often helpful.

TREATMENT Therapy of Inflammatory Myopathies

The goal of therapy is to improve muscle strength, thereby improving function in activities of daily living, and ameliorate the extramuscular manifestations (rash, dysphagia, dyspnea, fever). When strength improves, the serum CK falls concurrently; however, the reverse is not always true. Unfortunately, there is a common tendency to "chase" or treat the CK level instead of the muscle weakness, a practice that has led to prolonged and unnecessary use of immunosuppressive drugs and erroneous assessment of their efficacy. It is prudent to discontinue these drugs if, after an adequate trial, there is no objective improvement in muscle strength whether or not CK levels are reduced. Agents used in the treatment of PM and DM include the following:

1. *Glucocorticoids.* Oral prednisone is the initial treatment of choice; the effectiveness and side effects of this therapy determine the

future need for stronger immunosuppressive drugs. High-dose prednisone, at least 1 mg/kg per day, is initiated as early in the disease as possible. After 3–4 weeks, prednisone is tapered slowly over a period of 10 weeks to 1 mg/kg every other day. If there is evidence of efficacy and no serious side effects, the dosage is then further reduced by 5 or 10 mg every 3–4 weeks until the lowest possible dose that controls the disease is reached. The efficacy of prednisone is determined by an objective increase in muscle strength and activities of daily living, which almost always occurs by the third month of therapy. A feeling of increased energy or a reduction of the CK level without a concomitant increase in muscle strength is not a reliable sign of improvement. If prednisone provides no objective benefit after ~3 months of high-dose therapy, the disease is probably unresponsive to the drug and tapering should be accelerated while the next-in-line immunosuppressive drug is started. Although controlled trials have not been performed, almost all patients with true PM or DM respond to glucocorticoids to *some degree and for some period of time*; in general, DM responds better than PM.

The long-term use of prednisone may cause increased weakness associated with a normal or unchanged CK level; this effect is referred to as *steroid myopathy*. In a patient who previously responded to high doses of prednisone, the development of new weakness may be related to steroid myopathy or to disease activity that either will respond to a higher dose of glucocorticoids or has become glucocorticoid-resistant. In uncertain cases, the prednisone dosage can be steadily increased or decreased as desired: the cause of the weakness is usually evident in 2–8 weeks.

2. *Other immunosuppressive drugs*. Approximately 75% of patients ultimately require additional treatment. This occurs when a patient fails to respond adequately to glucocorticoids after a 3-month trial, the patient becomes glucocorticoid-resistant, glucocorticoid-related side effects appear, attempts to lower the prednisone dose repeatedly result in a new relapse, or rapidly progressive disease with evolving severe weakness and respiratory failure develops.

The following drugs are commonly used but have never been tested in controlled studies: (1) *Azathioprine* is well tolerated, has few side effects, and appears to be as effective for long-term therapy as other drugs. The dose is up to 3 mg/kg daily. (2) *Methotrexate* has a faster onset of action than azathioprine. It is given orally starting at 7.5 mg weekly for the first 3 weeks (2.5 mg every 12 h for 3 doses), with gradual dose escalation by 2.5 mg per week to a total of 25 mg weekly. A rare side effect is methotrexate pneumonitis, which can be difficult to distinguish from the interstitial lung disease of the primary myopathy associated with Jo-1 antibodies (described above). (3) *Mycophenolate mofetil* also has a faster onset of action than azathioprine. At doses up to 2.5 or 3 gm/d in two divided doses, it is well tolerated for long-term use. (4) Monoclonal anti-CD20 antibody (rituximab) has been shown in a small uncontrolled series to benefit patients with DM and PM. (5) *Cyclosporine* has inconsistent and mild benefit. (6) *Cyclophosphamide* (0.5–1 g/m^2 IV monthly for 6 months) has limited success and significant toxicity. (7) Tacrolimus (formerly known as Fk506) has been effective in some difficult cases of PM.

3. *Immunomodulation*. In a controlled trial of patients with refractory DM, intravenous immunoglobulin (IVIg) improved not only strength and rash but also the underlying immunopathology. The benefit is often short-lived (≤8 weeks), and repeated infusions every 6–8 weeks are generally required to maintain improvement. A dose of 2 g/kg divided over 2–5 days per course is recommended. Uncontrolled observations suggest that IVIg may also be beneficial for patients with PM. Neither plasmapheresis nor leukapheresis appears to be effective in PM and DM.

The following sequential empirical approach to the treatment of PM and DM is suggested: *Step 1*: high-dose prednisone; *Step 2*: azathioprine, mycophenolate, or methotrexate for steroid-sparing effect; *Step 3*: IVIg; *Step 4*: a trial, with guarded optimism, of one of the following agents, chosen according to the patient's age, degree of disability, tolerance, experience with the drug, and general health: rituximab, cyclosporine, cyclophosphamide, or tacrolimus. Patients with interstitial lung disease may benefit from aggressive treatment with cyclophosphamide or tacrolimus.

A patient with presumed PM who has not responded to any form of immunotherapy most likely has IBM or another disease, usually a metabolic myopathy, a muscular dystrophy, a drug-induced myopathy, or an endocrinopathy. In these cases, a repeat muscle biopsy and a renewed search for another cause of the myopathy is indicated.

Calcinosis, a manifestation of DM, is difficult to treat; however, new calcium deposits may be prevented if the primary disease responds to the available therapies. Bisphosphonates, aluminum hydroxide, probenecid, colchicine, low doses of warfarin, calcium blockers, and surgical excision have all been tried without success.

IBM is generally resistant to immunosuppressive therapies. Prednisone together with azathioprine or methotrexate is often tried for a few months in newly diagnosed patients, although results are generally disappointing. Because occasional patients may feel subjectively weaker after these drugs are discontinued, some clinicians prefer to maintain these patients on low-dose, every-other-day prednisone along with mycophenolate in an effort to slow disease progression, even though there is no objective evidence or controlled study to support this practice. In two controlled studies of IVIg in IBM, minimal benefit in up to 30% of patients was found; the strength gains, however, were not of sufficient magnitude to justify its routine use. Another trial of IVIg combined with prednisone was ineffective. Nonetheless, many experts believe that a 2- to 3-month trial with IVIg may be reasonable for selected patients with IBM who experience rapid progression of muscle weakness or choking episodes due to worsening dysphagia.

PROGNOSIS

The 5-year survival rate for treated patients with PM and DM is ~95% and the 10-year survival rate is 84%; death is usually due to pulmonary, cardiac, or other systemic complications. The prognosis is worse for patients who are severely affected at presentation, when initial treatment is delayed, and in cases with severe dysphagia or respiratory difficulties. Older patients, and those with associated cancer also have a worse prognosis. DM responds more favorably to therapy than PM and thus has a better prognosis. Most patients improve with therapy, and many make a full functional recovery, which is often sustained with maintenance therapy. Up to 30% may be left with some residual muscle weakness. Relapses may occur at any time.

IBM has the least favorable prognosis of the inflammatory myopathies. Most patients will require the use of an assistive device such as a cane, walker, or wheelchair within 5–10 years of onset. In general, the older the age of onset in IBM, the more rapidly progressive is the course.

FURTHER READINGS

ASKANAS V et al: Inclusion body myositis: A degenerative muscle disease associated with intra-muscle fiber multi-protein aggregates, proteasome inhibition, endoplasmic reticulum stress and decreased lysosomal degradation. Brain Pathol 19:493, 2009

CHANIN N, ENGEL AG: Correlation of muscle biopsy, clinical course and outcome in polymyositis and sporadic IBM. Neurology 70:418, 2008

DALAKAS MC: Signaling pathways and immunobiology of inflammatory myopathies. Nat Clin Pract Rheumatol 2:219, 2006

———: Sporadic inclusion body myositis: Diagnosis, pathogenesis and therapeutic strategies. Nat Clin Pract Neurol 2:437, 2006

———: Toxic and drug-induced myopathies. J Neurol Neurosurg Psych 80:832, 2009

———: Immunotherapy of myositis: Issues, concerns and future prospects. Nat Rev Rheumatol 6:129, 2010

———: Review: An update on inflammatory and autoimmune myopathies. Neuropathol Appl Neurobiol 37:226, 2011

——— et al: Inclusion body myositis with human immunodeficiency virus infection: Four cases with clonal expansion of viral-specific T cells. Ann Neurol 61:466, 2007

ENGEL AG et al: The polymyositis and dermatomyositis syndrome, in *Myology*, AG Engel, C Franzini-Armstrong (eds). New York, McGraw-Hill, 2008, pp 1335–1383

MARIE I et al: Polymyositis and dermatomyositis: Short-term and long-term outcome and predictive factors of prognosis. J Rheumatol 28:2230, 2001

MASTAGLIA FL: Inflammatory myopathies: Clinical, diagnostic and therapeutic aspects. Muscle Nerve 27:407, 2003

MIKOL J, ENGEL AG: Inclusion body myositis, in: *Myology*, 3rd ed, AG Engel, C Franzini-Armstrong (eds). New York, McGraw-Hill, 2004, pp 1367–1388

NEEDHAM M, MASTAGLIA FL: Inclusion body myositis: Current pathogenic concepts and diagnostic and therapeutic approaches. Lancet Neurol 6:620, 2007

SONTHEIMER RD: Dermatomyositis: An overview of recent progress with emphasis on dermatologic aspects. Dermatol Clin 20:387, 2002

CHAPTER 389 Chronic Fatigue Syndrome

Gijs Bleijenberg
Jos W.M. van der Meer

DEFINITION

Chronic fatigue syndrome (CFS) is a disorder characterized by persistent and unexplained fatigue resulting in severe impairment in daily functioning. Besides intense fatigue, most patients with CFS report concomitant symptoms such as pain, cognitive dysfunction, and unrefreshing sleep. Additional symptoms can include headache, sore throat, tender lymph nodes, muscle aches, joint aches, feverishness, difficulty sleeping, psychiatric problems, allergies, and abdominal cramps. Criteria for the diagnosis of CFS have been developed by the U.S. Centers for Disease Control and Prevention (Table 389-1).

TABLE 389-1 Diagnostic Criteria for Chronic Fatigue Syndrome

Characterized by Persistent or Relapsing Unexplained Chronic Fatigue
Fatigue lasts for at least 6 months
Fatigue is of new or definite onset
Fatigue is not the result of an organic disease or of continuing exertion
Fatigue is not alleviated by rest
Fatigue results in a substantial reduction in previous occupational, educational, social, and personal activities
Four or more of the following symptoms, concurrently present for 6 months:
Impaired memory or concentration, sore throat, tender cervical or axillary lymph nodes, muscle pain, pain in several joints, new headaches, unrefreshing sleep, or malaise after exertion
Exclusion Criteria
Medical condition explaining fatigue
Major depressive disorder (psychotic features) or bipolar disorder
Schizophrenia, dementia, or delusional disorder
Anorexia nervosa, bulimia nervosa
Alcohol or substance abuse
Severe obesity (BMI >40)

EPIDEMIOLOGY

CFS is seen worldwide, with adult prevalence rates varying between 0.2 and 0.4%. In the United States, the prevalence is higher in women, members of minority groups (African and Native Americans), and individuals with lower levels of education and occupational status. Approximately 75% of all CFS patients are women. The mean age of onset is between 29 and 35 years. It is probable that many patients go undiagnosed and/or do not seek help.

ETIOLOGY

There are numerous hypotheses about the etiology of CFS; there is no definitively indentified cause. Distinguishing between predisposing, precipitating, and perpetuating factors in CFS helps to provide a framework for understanding this complex condition (Table 389-2).

Predisposing factors

Physical inactivity and trauma in childhood tend to increase the risk of CFS in adults. Neuroendocrine dysfunction may be associated with childhood trauma, reflecting a biological correlate of vulnerability. Psychiatric illness and physical hyperactivity in adulthood raise the risk of CFS in later life. Twin studies suggest a familial predisposition to CFS, but no causative genes have been identified.

TABLE 389-2 Predisposing, Precipitating, and Perpetuating Factors in Chronic Fatigue Syndrome

TIME
Predisposing Factors
Childhood trauma (sexual, physical, emotional abuse; emotional and physical neglect)
Physical inactivity during childhood
Premorbid psychiatric illness or psychopathology
Premorbid hyperactivity
↓
Precipitating Factors
Somatic events: infection (mononucleosis, Q fever, Lyme disease), surgery, pregnancy
Psychosocial stress, life events
↓
Perpetuating Factors
(Non)acknowledgment by physician
Negative self-efficacy
Strong physical attributions
Strong focus on bodily symptoms
Fear of fatigue
(Lack of) social support
Low physical activity pattern

Precipitating factors

Physical or psychological stress may elicit the onset of CFS. Most patients report an infection (usually a flulike illness or infectious mononucleosis) as the trigger of their fatigue. Relatively high percentages of CFS follow Q fever and Lyme disease. However, no differences were found in Epstein-Barr virus load and immunologic reactivity in individuals who developed CFS and those who did not. While antecedent infections are associated with CFS, a direct microbial causality is unproven and unlikely. A recent study identified a murine leukemia virus-related retrovirus (XMRV); however, several subsequent studies have failed to confirm this result. Patients also often report other precipitating somatic events such as serious injury, surgery, pregnancy, or childbirth. Serious life events such as the loss of a loved one or a job, military combat, and other stressful situations may also precipitate CFS. A third of all patients cannot recall a trigger.

Perpetuating factors

Once CFS has developed, numerous factors may impede recovery. Physicians may contribute to chronicity by ordering unnecessary diagnostic procedures, by persistently suggesting psychological causes, and by not acknowledging CFS as a diagnosis.

A patient's focus on illness and avoidance of activities may perpetuate symptoms. A firm belief in a physical cause, a strong focus on bodily sensations, and a poor sense of control over symptoms may also prolong or exacerbate the fatigue and functional impairment. In most patients, inactivity is caused by negative illness perceptions rather than by poor physical fitness. Solicitous behavior of others may reinforce a patient's illness-related perceptions and behavior. A lack of social support is another known perpetuating factor.

■ PATHOPHYSIOLOGY

The pathophysiology of CFS is unclear. Neuroimaging studies have reported that CFS is associated with reduced gray matter volume, associated with a decline in physical activity; these changes were partially reversed following cognitive behavioral therapy (CBT). In addition, functional MRI data have suggested that abnormal patterns of activation correlate with self-reported problems with information processing. Neurophysiologic studies have shown altered CNS activation patterns during muscle contraction.

Evidence for immunologic dysfunction is inconsistent. Modest elevations in titers of antinuclear antibodies, reductions in immunoglobulin subclasses, deficiencies in mitogen-driven lymphocyte proliferation, reductions in natural killer cell activity, disturbances in cytokine production, and shifts in lymphocyte subsets have been described. None of these immune findings appear in most patients, nor do any correlate with the severity of CFS. In theory, symptoms of CFS could result from excessive production of a cytokine, such as interleukin 1, that induces asthenia and other flulike symptoms; however, compelling data in support of this hypothesis are lacking.

There is some evidence that CFS patients have mild hypocortisolism, the degree of which is associated with a poorer response to CBT.

Discrepancies in perceived and actual cognitive performance are a consistent finding in patients with CFS.

■ DIAGNOSIS

In addition to a thorough history, a systematic physical examination is warranted to exclude disorders causing fatigue (e.g. endocrine disorders, neoplasms, heart failure, etc.). The heart rate of CFS patients is often slightly above normal. Laboratory tests primarily serve to exclude other diagnoses; there is no test that can diagnose CFS. The following laboratory screen usually suffices: complete blood count; ESR, CRP; serum creatinine, electrolytes, calcium and iron; blood glucose; creatine kinase; liver function tests; TSH; anti-gliadin antibodies; urinalysis. Serology for viral or bacterial infections is usually not helpful. No specific abnormalities have been identified on MRI or CT scans. CFS is a constellation of symptoms without any pathognomonic features, and remains a diagnosis of exclusion.

Bipolar disorders, schizophrenia, and substance abuse exclude a diagnosis of CFS, as do eating disorders, unless these have been resolved 5 years or longer before symptom onset. Also, CFS is excluded if the chronic fatigue developed immediately after a depressive episode. Depression developing in the course of the fatigue, however, does not preclude CFS. Co-occurring psychiatric disorder, especially anxiety and mood disorders, is seen in 30–60% of all cases.

■ INITIAL MANAGEMENT

In cases of suspected CFS, the clinician should acknowledge the impact of the patient's symptoms on daily functioning. Disbelief or denial can provoke an exacerbation of genuine symptoms, which in turn strengthens the clinician's disbelief, leading to an unfortunate cycle of miscommunication. The possibility of CFS should be considered if a patient fulfils all criteria (Table 389-1), and if other diagnoses have been excluded.

The patient should be asked to describe the symptoms (fatigue and accompanying symptoms) and their duration as well as the consequences (reduction in daily activities). To assess symptom severity and the extent of daily-life impairment, the patient should describe a typical day, from waking to retiring, and to contrast this with an average day prior to symptom onset. Next, potential fatigue-precipitating factors are sought. The severity of fatigue is difficult to assess quantitatively; a brief questionnaire is often helpful (Fig. 389-1).

The patient should be informed of the current understanding of precipitating and perpetuating factors and effective treatments, and be offered general advice about disease management. If CBT for CFS is not available as an initial treatment option (see below) and depression and anxiety are present, these symptoms should be treated. For patients with headache, diffuse pain, and feverishness, nonsteroidal anti-inflammatory drugs may be helpful. Even modest improvements in symptoms can make an important difference in the patient's degree of self-sufficiency and ability to appreciate life's pleasures.

Controlled therapeutic trials have established that acyclovir, fludrocortisone, galantamine, modafinil, and IV immunoglobulin, among other agents, offer no significant benefit in CFS. Countless anecdotes circulate regarding other traditional and nontraditional therapies. It is important to guide patients away from those therapeutic modalities that are toxic, expensive, or unreasonable.

The patient should be encouraged to maintain regular sleep patterns, to remain as active as possible, and to gradually return to previous exercise and activity (work) levels.

TREATMENT Chronic Fatigue Syndrome

CBT and graded exercise therapy (GET) have been found to be the only beneficial interventions in CFS. Some patient groups argue against these approaches because of the implication that CFS is a purely mental disorder. CBT is a psychotherapeutic approach directed at changing condition-related cognitions and behaviors. CBT for CFS aims at changing a patient's perpetuating factors by exploiting various techniques and components. It includes educating the patient about the etiologic model, setting goals, restoring fixed bedtime and wake-up time, challenging and changing fatigue- and activity-related cognitions, reducing

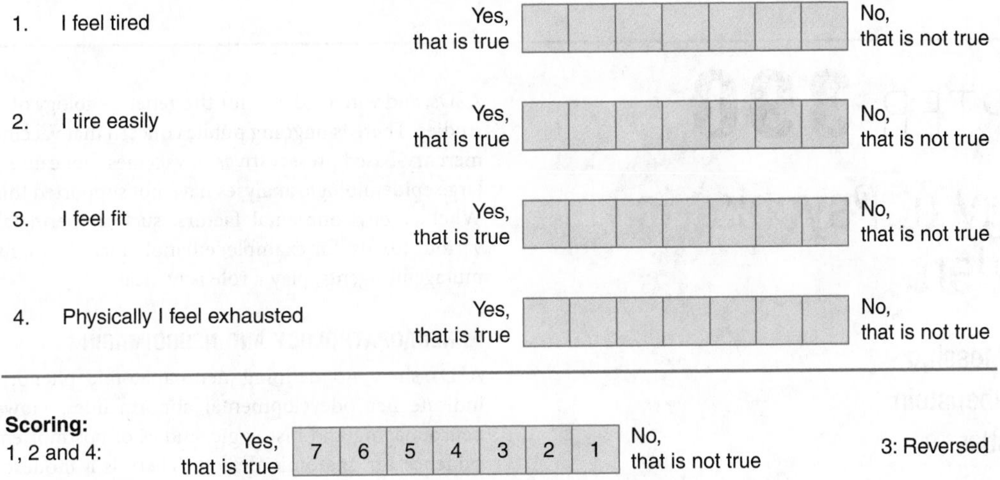

How have you felt during the last two weeks?
Please rate all four statements and per statement check the box that reflects your situation best.
1. I feel tired
Yes, that is true
No, that is not true
2. I tire easily
Yes, that is true
No, that is not true
3. I feel fit
Yes, that is true
No, that is not true
4. Physically I feel exhausted
Yes, that is true
No, that is not true
Scoring:
1, 2 and 4:
Yes, that is true
7 6 5 4 3 2 1
No, that is not true
3: Reversed
Sum scores >18 indicate severe fatigue

Figure 389-1 Shortened fatigue questionnaire (SFQ).

symptom focusing, spreading activities evenly throughout the day, gradually increasing physical activity, planning a return to work, and resuming other activities. The intervention, which typically consists of 12–14 sessions spread over 6 months, helps CFS patients gain control over their symptoms.

GET is based on the model of deconditioning and exercise intolerance and usually involves a home exercise program that continues for 3–5 months. Walking or cycling is systematically increased, with set target heart rates. Evidence that deconditioning is the basis for symptoms in CFS is lacking, however. The primary component of CBT and GET that results in a reduction in fatigue is the change in the patient's perception of fatigue and focus on symptoms.

CBT is generally the more complex treatment, which might explain why CBT studies tend to yield better improvement rates than GET trials.

Not all patients benefit from CBT or GET. Predictors of poor outcome are somatic comorbidity, current disability claims, and severe pain. CBT offered in an early stage of the illness reduces the burden of CFS for the patient as well as society in terms of decreased medical and disability-related costs.

PROGNOSIS

Full recovery from untreated CFS is rare: the median annual recovery rate is 5% (range 0–31%) and the improvement rate 39% (range 8–63%). Patients with an underlying psychiatric disorder and those who continue to attribute their symptoms to an undiagnosed medical condition have poorer outcomes.

FURTHER READINGS

Baker R, Shaw EJ: Diagnosis and management of chronic fatigue syndrome or myalgic encephalitis (or encephalopathy): Summary of NICE guidance. BMJ 335:446, 2007

Presson AP et al: Integrated weighted gene co-expression network analysis with an application to chronic fatigue syndrome. BMC Syst Biol 2:95, 2008

Price JR et al: Cognitive behaviour therapy for chronic fatigue syndrome in adults. Cochrane Database Syst Rev (3):CD001027, 2008

Prins JB et al: Chronic fatigue syndrome. Lancet 367:346, 2006

Satterfield BC et al: Serologic and PCR testing of persons with chronic fatigue syndrome in the United States shows no association with xenotropic or polytropic murine leukemia virus-related viruses. Retrovirology 8:12, 2011

Tak LM et al: Meta-analysis and meta-regression of hypothalamic-pituitary-adrenal axis activity in functional somatic disorders. Biol Psychol 87:183, 2011

SECTION 5 Psychiatric Disorders

CHAPTER 390 Biology of Psychiatric Disorders

Robert O. Messing
John H. Rubenstein
Eric J. Nestler

Psychiatric disorders are central nervous system diseases characterized by disturbances in emotion, cognition, motivation, and socialization. As a result of their high prevalence, early onset, and persistence, they contribute substantially to the burden of illness worldwide. Most psychiatric disorders are heterogeneous syndromes that currently lack well-defined neuropathology and bona fide biological markers. Therefore, diagnoses continue to be made solely from clinical observations using criteria in the *Diagnostic and Statistical Manual of Mental Disorders* of the American Psychiatric Association (2000), 4th edition, text revision (DSM-IVTR). Recent advances in neuroimaging are beginning to provide evidence of brain pathology, which may one day be used for diagnosis and for following treatment. Family, twin, and adoption studies have shown that all common psychiatric syndromes are highly heritable, with genetic risk comprising 20–90% of disease vulnerability. The epidemiology, genetics, and biology of four common psychiatric disorders—autism, schizophrenia, mood disorders, and drug addiction—are presented below. A detailed discussion of the clinical manifestations and treatment of schizophrenia and mood disorders can be found in Chap. 391. Further discussion of alcoholism can be found in Chap. 392, opiate addiction in Chap. 393, cocaine and other drugs of abuse in Chap. 394, and nicotine addiction in Chap. 395.

AUTISM SPECTRUM DISORDERS

The DSM-IVTR criteria for Autism Spectrum Disorders (ASDs) require delays or abnormal functioning in social interactions, language as used in social communication, and symbolic or imaginative play, with onset prior to age 3. In addition to abnormal social behavior, ASDs are frequently, but not always, associated with reduced IQ and epilepsy. Individuals who exhibit some autism-like symptoms with relatively preserved cognitive functioning and language skills are described as having Asperger's syndrome.

EPIDEMIOLOGY

There has been a dramatic increase in the diagnosis of ASDs, from ~1/1000 (1950s–1990s) to a current level of ~1/150. Whether this increase reflects increased disease prevalence remains uncertain; ongoing studies are searching for genetic, environmental, and sociologic mechanisms that may have contributed to this change. In the 1950s–1960s, psychological factors were held to underlie autism. This conception was largely debunked by the 1970s, with the demonstration that prenatal rubella and phenylketonuria can cause ASDs, and with evidence for the genetic etiology of ASDs from twin studies. There is ongoing public concern that vaccines in general, or mercury-based preservatives in vaccines, can cause ASDs; however, large epidemiologic analyses have not supported this as an etiology. Whether environmental factors, such as perinatal infection and various toxins, for example, ethanol, illicit drugs, medications, and mutagenic agents, play a role is unclear.

NEUROPATHOLOGY AND NEUROIMAGING

ASDs show no defining neuroanatomic phenotype that would indicate neurodevelopmental abnormalities. However, structural neuroimaging and histologic studies of postmortem brain provide evidence for anatomic defects. There is a modest increase in cerebrum growth (~10%; affecting both the white and grey matter) during early childhood (years 1–3), with the largest effect in the frontal lobes; the growth rate then decreases with age. Cerebellar size is increased by about 7% in children under age 5 years, but is decreased in older patients, and there are reduced (~30%) numbers of cerebellar Purkinje neurons. Finally, there is reduced cell size and increased cell density in the limbic areas of the brain.

GENETICS

ASDs are highly heritable; concordance rates in monozygotic twins (~60–90%) are roughly tenfold higher than in dizygotic twins and siblings, and first-degree relatives show about fiftyfold increased risk for autism compared with prevalence in the general population. For unknown reasons, ASDs affect four times as many boys as girls. ASDs are also genetically heterogeneous. More than 20 known mutations, including copy number variations, account for about 10–20% of all cases, though none of these causes individually accounts for more than 1–2% (Table 390-1). Many of the genes linked to ASDs can also cause other illnesses. For instance, mutations in MeCP2, FMR1, and TSC1&2 (see Table 390-1 for abbreviations) can cause mental retardation without ASDs, and alleles of certain genes, for example, neurexin 1, are associated with both ASDs and schizophrenia. It is likely that many cases of ASDs result from more complex genetic mechanisms, including inheritance of multiple genetic variants or epigenetic modifications.

PATHOGENESIS

Despite the genetic heterogeneity of ASDs, there are some common themes that may explain pathogenesis. These include mutations in proteins involved in the formation and function of synapses, control over the size and projections of neurons, production and signaling of neurotransmitters and neuromodulators, the function of ion channels, general cell metabolism, gene expression, and protein synthesis (see Table 390-1). Many of these mutations have a clear relationship to activity-dependent neural responses and can affect the development of neural systems that underlie cognition and social behaviors. They may be detrimental by altering the balance of excitatory vs. inhibitory synaptic signaling in local and extended circuits, and by altering the mechanisms that control brain growth. Another class of mutations affects genes (e.g., PTEN and Tsc) that negatively regulate signaling from several types of extracellular stimuli, including those transduced by receptor tyrosine kinases. Their dysregulation can have pleiotropic effects, including altering brain and

TABLE 390-1 Examples of Genes Implicated in Autism

Gene Symbol	Gene Name	Function
PTEN	Phosphatase and tensin homolog	Signal transduction Synaptic function
TSC1	Tuberous sclerosis 1	Signal transduction Translation and protein stability Synaptic function
TSC2	Tuberous sclerosis 2	Signal transduction Translation and protein stability Synaptic function
FMR1	Fragile X mental retardation 1	Translation and protein stability Synaptic function
UBE3A	Ubiquitin protein ligase E3A	Translation and protein stability Synaptic function
CNTN3	Contactin 3	Synaptic function
CNTN4	Contactin 4	Synaptic function
CNTNAP2	Contactin-associated protein-like 2	Synaptic function
NLGN3	Neuroligin 3	Synaptic function
NLGN4	Neuroligin 4	Synaptic function
NRXN1	Neurexin 1	Synaptic function
PCDH10	Protocadherin 10	Synaptic function
SHANK3	Shank 3	Synaptic function
SLC6A4	Serotonin transporter	Neurotransmitter signaling
AVPR1	Arginine vasopressin receptor 1	Neurotransmitter signaling
OXTR	Oxytosin receptor	Neurotransmitter signaling
CACNA1C	Voltage-gated calcium channel–alpha 1C subunit	Ion channel
CACNA1H	Voltage-gated calcium channel–alpha 1H subunit	Ion channel
SCN1A	Sodium channel, voltage-gated, type I, alpha subunit	Ion channel
SCN2A	Sodium channel, voltage-gated, type II, alpha subunit	Ion channel
SLC9A9	Sodium/hydrogen exchanger	Ion channel
DHCR7	7-Dehydrocholesterol reductase	Metabolism
PAH	Phenylalanine hydroxylase	Metabolism
ARX	Arx transcription factor	Gene expression
En2	Engrailed 2 transcription factor	Gene expression
MeCP2	Methyl CpG–binding protein 2 (Rett syndrome)	Gene expression
RNF8	Ring finger protein 8	Gene expression

neuronal growth as well as synaptic development and function. With further understanding of pathogenesis and the definition of specific ASD subtypes, there is reason to believe that effective therapies will be identified, as in the case of dietary treatments for phenylketonuria. In addition, work in mouse models (e.g., with fragile X or Rett syndrome mutations) has suggested that autism-like behavioral abnormalities can be reversed even in fully developed adult animals by reversing the underlying pathology, which holds out hope for many affected individuals.

SCHIZOPHRENIA

Schizophrenia appears to be a heterogeneous collection of many distinct diseases, which remain poorly defined but linked by common clinical features. Three major symptom clusters are seen in schizophrenia: positive, negative, and cognitive symptoms. Positive symptoms include hallucinations and delusions, experiences that are not characteristic of normal mental life. Negative symptoms represent deficits in normal functions such as blunted affect, impoverished speech, asocial behavior, and diminished motivation. Cognitive symptoms include deficits in working memory and cognitive control of behavior that often prove extremely disabling. Current antipsychotic drugs are efficacious for positive symptoms only and generally lack efficacy for negative and cognitive symptoms.

■ EPIDEMIOLOGY

Schizophrenia is common, affecting males and females roughly equally, with a worldwide prevalence of approximately 1%. Environmental risks are thought to include prenatal exposure to viral infection (influenza), prenatal poor nutrition, perinatal hypoxia, psychotropic drug use (in particular, cannabis), and psychological stress. Advanced paternal age, birth order, and season of birth have also been implicated. However, none of these environmental influences has a specific or strong association with most cases of schizophrenia.

■ NEUROPATHOLOGY AND NEUROIMAGING

The best-established neuropathologic finding in schizophrenia is enlargement of the lateral ventricles of the cerebral hemispheres. This is accompanied by a reduction in cortical thickness. These abnormalities are not specific to schizophrenia and are seen in many other conditions, including many neurodegenerative disorders. However, there is a general consensus that the reduction in cortical thickness in schizophrenia is associated with increased cell packing density and reduced neuropil (defined as axons, dendrites, and glial cell processes) without an overt change in neuronal cell number. Specific classes of interneurons in prefrontal cortex consistently show reduced expression of the gene encoding the enzyme glutamic acid decarboxylase 1 (*GAD1*), which synthesizes γ-aminobutyric acid (GABA), the principal inhibitory neurotransmitter in the brain. Functional imaging studies, by positron emission tomography (PET) or functional magnetic resonance imaging (MRI), show evidence of reduced metabolic or neural activity in the dorsolateral prefrontal cortex at rest and when performing psychological tests of executive function, including working memory. Alleles of two candidate risk genes [catechol-*O*-methyltransferase (COMT) and metabotropic glutamate receptor 3 (mGluR3)] are reported to affect dorsolateral prefrontal cortex activity, but these findings need to be replicated in larger samples. Similar pathologic and brain imaging abnormalities are seen in several other brain regions, in particular, the hippocampus. There are also numerous reports of abnormalities in myelin and oligodendrocytes in the cerebral cortex of patients with schizophrenia.

■ GENETICS

Twins studies establish the heritability of schizophrenia, with co-inheritance at ~50% for monozygotic twins and ~10% for dizygotic twins. Genomewide linkage and association studies, and studies of copy number variation, have identified many regions and alleles that confer increased disease risk, particularly near genes on chromosome 22 [disrupted in schizophrenia 1 (DISC1), COMT, neuregulin 1, the neuregulin receptor ERBB4, and the DiGeorge (or velocardiofacial syndrome) region], and on chromosome 16p. The DiGeorge region deletions produce, in heterozygous form, a psychotic disorder with variable clinical features and a moderate to strong degree of penetrance. In contrast, the contribution of each of the individual genes to schizophrenia remains to be established with certainty. Moreover, the responsible genes within the DiGeorge region have not yet been identified. What is clear is that none of these other alleles produce schizophrenia with a high degree of penetrance. The current view in the field is that multiple rare alleles, many or most with limited penetrance, likely contribute to risk of schizophrenia. As for ASDs, the same allele may be a risk factor for multiple disorders. For instance, duplication of chromosome 16p is associated with both schizophrenia and autism, while DiGeorge region deletions and the *DISC1* locus on chromosome 22 are associated with schizophrenia, autism, and bipolar disorder.

■ PATHOGENESIS

There are several prevailing hypotheses about neurochemical mechanisms underlying schizophrenia. A reduction in the function of cortical and perhaps hippocampal GABAergic interneurons fits with reduced expression of glutamic acid decarboxylase. However, it is unknown whether this is a primary or compensatory feature of the disorder. Nevertheless, defects in parvalbumin-expressing GABAergic interneurons are known to reduce gamma-frequency activity on the EEG, which is a feature of many people with schizophrenia. Reduced excitatory neurotransmitter (glutamate) function is posited based on psychotic and cognitive symptoms generated in humans exposed to ketamine or phencyclidine, which are noncompetitive antagonists of the NMDA subtype of glutamate receptors. There are reports of altered levels of glutamate receptors or associated proteins in the brains of individuals with schizophrenia examined postmortem, but no findings have yet been widely replicated. Finally, overactivity of dopamine neurotransmission at D_2-type dopamine receptors is proposed based on the ability of D_2 antagonists (an action common to all current antipsychotic agents; see Chap. 391) to ameliorate the positive symptoms of schizophrenia. Excessive dopamine release in the striatum elicited by an acute dose of amphetamine has been demonstrated by PET imaging in some patients with schizophrenia. However, it is unclear whether this abnormality reflects the underlying illness or a lasting effect of antipsychotic medications. In contrast, reduced activity of dopamine at D_1 dopamine receptors in the prefrontal cortex has been implicated in working memory deficits based on the cognitive effects of D_1 receptor agonists and antagonists in the illness. Nevertheless, inferring something about disease pathogenesis from the actions of psychotropic drugs, for example, as with the glutamate and dopamine hypotheses, is fraught with artifact.

Efforts to understand how defects in these neurotransmitter systems might generate similar behavioral phenotypes have led to intriguing hypotheses. For instance, in the hippocampus, reduced glutamate transmission (based on a hypothesized deficit in glutamate release or glutamate receptors) onto GABAergic interneurons could lead to reduced glutamic acid decarboxylase expression, reduced gamma oscillations, and reduced inhibition onto excitatory neurons. These events in turn could lead to increased dopamine release from the ventral tegmental area, with dopamine antagonists thereby helping to reset the system to its nonpathologic state. It must be emphasized that these are working models only, and a true pathophysiology (or pathophysiologies) for schizophrenia remains to be established.

Overlaid on these neurotransmitter-based hypotheses is speculation as to how mutations in any of several genes implicated, however tentatively, in schizophrenia lead to the associated pathologic and behavioral abnormalities. DISC1 was originally discovered based on its association with schizophrenia in an Icelandic family. However, as stated earlier, DISC1 has since been variably associated with other neuropsychiatric conditions and its role in schizophrenia remains uncertain. The DISC1 protein has been implicated in several cellular functions, including neuronal growth and maturation, neurite outgrowth, and even the proliferation of new neurons during development. Neuregulin 1 (NRG1), a member of the EGF family of growth factors, and its receptor ERBB4 have also been implicated in schizophrenia in several genetic studies. Interestingly, NRG1 and ERBB4 play important roles in the maturation of GABAergic interneurons in cerebral cortex, and regulate dopamine transmission to several limbic brain regions. Moreover, loss of NRG1-ERBB4 in mice leads to reduced neuropil, thus phenocopying a pathologic finding in schizophrenia. Another gene of potential interest encodes Reelin, a secreted extracellular matrix serine protease. There are unconfirmed reports of association of schizophrenia with the Reelin locus on chromosome 7, and of reduced Reelin expression in the cerebral cortex of schizophrenic subjects, possibly related to increased methylation of the Reelin gene promoter. Reelin is important during development in the migration of newly born neurons to their appropriate layers of cerebral cortex. In the adult brain, the protein is enriched in cortical GABAergic interneurons and has been implicated in regulating NMDA glutamate receptor function. It is, therefore, easy to imagine how abnormalities in DISC1, NRG1, or Reelin may be related to GABAergic, glutamatergic, and dopaminergic mechanisms in schizophrenia, and to associated pathologic abnormalities, but all such connections are currently speculative.

MOOD DISORDERS

Mood disorders are divided into depressive and bipolar disorders. Depressive disorders include the major depressive disorders, dysthymia, and more minor forms of depression. These disorders are heterogeneous syndromes, each composed of several diseases with presumably distinct pathophysiologies that remain to be elucidated.

■ EPIDEMIOLOGY

Mood disorders are common, with a prevalence of ~1–2% for bipolar disorder, ~5% for major depression, and ~15–20% for milder forms of depression. Between 40–50% of the risk for depression appears to be genetic. Nongenetic factors as diverse as stress and emotional trauma, viral infections, and even stochastic (random) processes during brain development have been implicated in the etiology. Depressive syndromes can occur in the context of general medical conditions such as endocrine disturbances (hyper- or hypocortisolemia, hyper- or hypothyroidism), autoimmune diseases, Parkinson's disease, traumatic brain injury, certain cancers, asthma, diabetes, and stroke. Depression and obesity/metabolic syndrome are important risk factors for each other. In predisposed individuals, stressful life events can lead to clear-cut depressive episodes, while severe stress can induce posttraumatic stress disorder (PTSD), instead of depression. Bipolar disorder is characterized by episodes of mania and depression and is one of the most heritable of psychiatric illnesses, with genetic risk of ~80%. Stress and disrupted circadian rhythms can promote the manic episodes, during which patients exhibit extremely elevated mood, abnormal thought patterns, and sometimes psychosis. Several of these clinical signs can resemble certain features of schizophrenia; indeed, recent epidemiologic and genetic research has questioned the DSM-IVTR designations of bipolar disorder, schizophrenia, and schizoaffective disorder as distinct syndromes.

NEUROPATHOLOGY AND NEUROIMAGING

Brain imaging studies in humans are defining the neural circuitry of mood within the brain's limbic system (Fig. 390-1). Integral to this system are the nucleus accumbens (important for brain reward—see below under Substance Use Disorders), amygdala, hippocampus, and regions of prefrontal cortex. Given that many symptoms of depression (so-called neurovegetative symptoms) involve physiologic functions, a key role for the hypothalamus is also presumed. Depressed individuals show a small reduction in hippocampal size. PET and functional MRI have revealed increased activation of the amygdala by negative stimuli and reduced activation of the nucleus accumbens by rewarding stimuli. There is also evidence for altered activity in prefrontal cortex, for example, hyperactivity of subgenual area 25 in anterior cingulate cortex. Deep brain stimulation (DBS) of either the nucleus accumbens or subgenual area 25 elevates mood in normal and depressed individuals. While there are numerous reports of pathologic findings within these various regions postmortem, there is to date no defined neuropathology of depression.

GENETICS

Although depression and bipolar disorder are highly heritable, the specific genes that comprise this risk remain unknown. As noted above, some of the genes implicated in autism or schizophrenia seem to cause bipolar disorder in some families. Large genomewide association studies have identified genes for diacylglycerol kinase η (*DGKH*), ankyrin G (*ANK3*), an L-type voltage-gated calcium channel (*CACNA1C*), and a gene-rich region on chromosome 16p12 as being associated with bipolar disorder, but these findings await confirmation by additional studies. Numerous susceptibility genes have also been implicated in linkage and association studies, but none has yet been definitively established as a bona fide depression gene. However, a few genes with variants that may modify depression risk are worthy of mention since they may be linked to mechanisms of pathogenesis (see below). These include genes for the type 1 receptor for corticotrophin-releasing factor (*CRHR1*); the glucocorticoid receptor gene (*GR*); *FKBP5*, which encodes a chaperone protein for the glucocorticoid receptor; the serotonin transporter gene (*SLA6A4*); the catechol-O-methyltransferase gene (*COMT*); and brain-derived neurotrophic factor (*BDNF*).

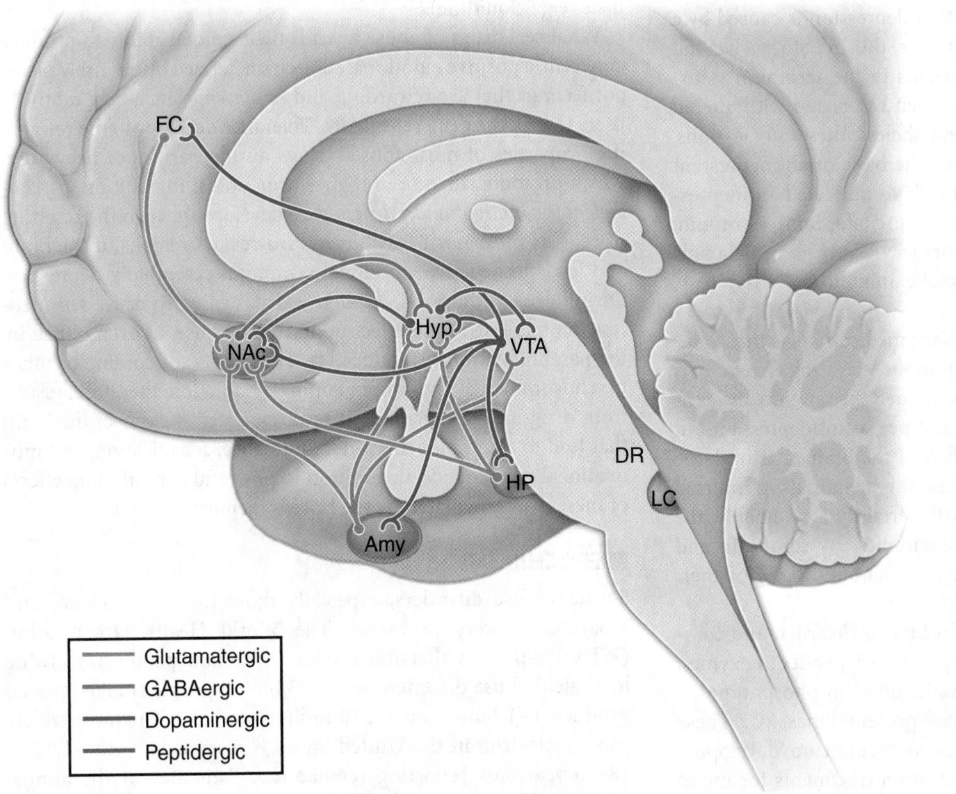

Figure 390-1 Neural circuitry of depression and addiction. The figure shows a simplified summary of a series of limbic circuits in brain that regulate mood and motivation and are implicated in depression and addiction. Shown in the figure are the hippocampus (HP) and amygdala (Amy), regions of prefrontal cortex, nucleus accumbens (NAc), and hypothalamus (Hyp). Only a subset of the known interconnections among these brain regions is shown. Also shown is the innervation of several of these brain regions by monoaminergic neurons. The ventral tegmental area (VTA) provides dopaminergic input to each of the limbic structures. Norepinephrine (from the locus coeruleus or LC) and serotonin [from the dorsal raphe (DR) and other raphe nuclei] innervate all of the regions shown. In addition, there are strong connections between the hypothalamus and the VTA-NAc pathway. Important peptidergic projections from the hypothalamus include those from the arcuate nucleus that release β-endorphin and melanocortin and from the lateral hypothalamus that release orexin.

PATHOGENESIS

Human and animal research in depression has focused on the long-term effects of chronic stress on the brain and their reversal by antidepressant medications; prominent examples are discussed here. A subset of depressed patients show elevated levels of cortisol associated with increased production of corticotrophin-releasing factor from the hypothalamus and perhaps other brain regions (e.g., amygdala). In animals, sustained elevations in glucocorticoids impair hippocampal function, in part via direct damage to hippocampal neurons, which is consistent with reduced hippocampal volumes seen in some depressed humans. As the hippocampus exerts the major inhibitory influence over the hypothalamic-pituitary-adrenal axis, impairment of hippocampal function would lead to still further increases in glucocorticoid secretion, establishing a pathologic feed-forward loop.

Stress-induced damage to the hippocampus, and perhaps other limbic regions (e.g., amygdala), in animals is also mediated in part by reduced levels of BDNF and other growth factors and cytokines. Furthermore, stress leads to a decrease in the birth of new neurons in the adult hippocampus. Interestingly, antidepressant treatments reverse these effects of stress, and the antidepressant effects of these medications seem to depend, in part, on their ability to promote hippocampal neurogenesis in animal models of depression. The clinical ramifications of such observations are unproven, although similar regulation of adult hippocampal neurogenesis may be important for certain forms of learning and memory.

Another important target of stress in animals is the nucleus accumbens, where stress regulation of numerous signaling events (dopaminergic transmission and BDNF signaling are two examples) exert potent effects on depression-like behavioral abnormalities. While a reduction in BDNF in the hippocampus promotes depression-like behaviors, an induction of BDNF in the nucleus accumbens promotes depression; similar changes in BDNF expression have been observed in postmortem brains of depressed patients. Thus the role of BDNF in regulating mood is highly brain-region specific.

In contrast to depression, animal models of mania as well as bipolar disorder have proved much more elusive. Mice with loss-of-function mutations in the *Clock* or *GluR6* glutamate receptor genes or transgenic mice that overexpress glycogen synthase kinase 3β (GSK3β) show manic-like behavioral abnormalities, although the relevance of these observations to human mania remains unknown.

The observation that tricyclic antidepressants (e.g., imipramine) inhibit serotonin and/or norepinephrine reuptake, and that monoamine oxidase inhibitors (e.g., tranylcypromine) are effective antidepressants, initially led to the view that depression is caused by a deficiency of these monoamines. However, this hypothesis has not been well substantiated, although variants in the serotonin transporter, and in the *COMT* gene, have been associated with altered mood states in some individuals. Nevertheless, these medications, particularly the tricyclics, have formed the basis of antidepressant discovery efforts, with virtually all of today's marketed antidepressants being SSRIs (e.g., fluoxetine, sertraline, citalopram), serotonin, and norepinephrine reuptake inhibitors (SNRIs) (e.g., venlafaxine, duloxetine), or norepinephrine reuptake inhibitors (NRIs) (e.g., atomoxetine).

A cardinal feature of all antidepressant medications is that long-term administration is needed for their mood-elevating effects. This means that their short-term actions, namely promotion of serotonin or norepinephrine function, is not per se antidepressant but rather induces a cascade of adaptations in the brain that underlie their clinical effects. The nature of these therapeutic drug-induced adaptations has not been identified with certainty. Presumably, the rich innervation of the brain's limbic circuitry by serotonin and norepinephrine (Fig. 390-1) provide the anatomic basis of their therapeutic actions.

Lithium is a highly effective drug for bipolar disorder, and competes with magnesium to inhibit magnesium-dependent enzymes, including GSK3β and several enzymes involved in phosphoinositide signaling leading to activation of protein kinase C. These findings have led to discovery programs focused on developing GSK3 and PKC inhibitors as potential novel treatments for mood disorders. Another commonly prescribed drug for bipolar disorder is valproic acid, which has pleiotropic effects, including inhibition of histone deacetylases (HDACs). Histone acetylation promotes transcriptional activation through posttranslational modification of N-terminal lysine residues in histones and thereby causes chromatin decondensation. HDAC inhibitors have shown some antidepressant effects in animal models of depression. Another form of epigenetic control of gene expression is methylation of cytosine residues in DNA, which inhibits gene transcription. DNA methylation has been shown to be important for inherited maternal effects on emotional behavior. Thus, rats born to mothers that exhibit low levels of nurturing behavior show increased anxiety and reduced expression of hippocampal glucocorticoid receptors due to increased methylation of the receptor gene. They pass these traits on to their offspring, but cross-fostering by mothers that display high levels of nurturing reverses them. As research into epigenetic mechanisms progresses, there is hope that it may become possible to identify specific depression-associated alterations in human chromatin.

SUBSTANCE USE DISORDERS

The DSM-IVTR uses the terms *substance dependence* and *substance abuse* to describe substance use disorders. It is unfortunate that the term *substance dependence* instead of addiction is used, because dependence can develop without addiction, and addiction involves much more than dependence per se. *Physical dependence* develops through resetting of homeostatic cellular mechanisms to permit normal function despite the continued presence of a drug; when drug intake is terminated abruptly, a withdrawal syndrome emerges. Withdrawal from alcohol or other sedative-hypnotics causes nervous system hyperactivity, whereas withdrawal from psychostimulants produces fatigue and sedation. *Tolerance* is a reduction in response to a drug, which like dependence, develops after repeated use. It results from a change in drug metabolism (pharmacokinetic tolerance) or cell signaling (pharmacodynamic tolerance). It is important to recognize that many nonaddictive medications induce tolerance and physical dependence, including β-adrenergic antagonists (e.g., propranolol) and α_2-adrenergic agonists (e.g., clonidine).

What sets drugs of abuse apart is their unique ability to produce *euphoria*, a positive emotional state characterized by intensely pleasant feelings that are rewarding and *reinforcing* since they motivate users to take the drug repeatedly. Tolerance develops to the rewarding properties of most abused drugs during periods of heavy use, which promotes the use of higher drug doses. In addition, *psychological* (or *motivational) dependence* develops through the resetting of cellular mechanisms within reward-related regions of the brain and leads to negative emotional symptoms resembling depression during drug withdrawal. Addictive drugs can also cause *sensitization*, an increased drug effect upon repeated use, as exemplified by the paranoid psychosis induced by chronic use of cocaine or other psychostimulants (e.g., amphetamine). Addiction, therefore, results from drug-induced changes in reward-related regions of the brain that lead to a complex mixture of tolerance, sensitization, and motivational dependence, in addition to powerful conditioning effects of these drugs mediated by the brain's memory circuits.

EPIDEMIOLOGY

Substance use disorders, especially those involving alcohol and tobacco, are very prevalent. The World Health Organization (WHO) estimates that more than 76 million people worldwide have alcohol use disorders and ~1.3 billion people smoke tobacco products (~1 billion men, 250 million women). The most widely used illicit drug in the United States is marijuana, with ~17% of 18–25-year-olds reporting regular use. Estimates of the annual economic burden of substance use disorders in the United States, including health- and crime-related costs and losses in productivity, exceed $500 billion.

NEUROPATHOLOGY AND NEUROIMAGING

Imaging studies in humans demonstrate that addictive drugs, as well as craving for them, activate the brain's reward circuitry (see below). However, there is no established pathology associated with addiction risk. Patients who abuse alcohol or psychostimulants show reduced gray matter in the prefrontal cortex. Functional MRI or PET studies show reduced activity in anterior cingulate and orbitofrontal cortex during tasks of attention and inhibitory control. Damage to these cortical areas may contribute to addiction by impairing decision making and increasing impulsivity.

GENETICS

Substance use disorders are highly heritable, with genetic risk estimated to be 0.4 to 0.7; however, the specific genes that comprise this risk remain largely unknown. The best-established genetic contribution to addiction is the protective effect that mutations in alcohol-metabolizing enzymes have on risk for alcoholism. Mutations that increase alcohol dehydrogenase (ADH) activity and decrease aldehyde dehydrogenase (ALDH) activity are additive and promote accumulation of acetaldehyde following ingestion of alcohol. This produces intoxication at low doses and a flushing reaction that is unpleasant, resembling the reaction to disulfiram, a drug used to prevent relapse. These variants are common among people of East Asian descent, and individuals expressing these variants rarely abuse alcohol.

Genes that promote risk for addiction have begun to emerge from large family and population studies, but all genes identified to date represent only a very small fraction of the overall genetic risk for addiction. The best established susceptibility loci are regions on chromosomes 4 and 5 containing $GABA_A$ receptor gene clusters linked to alcohol use disorders and the nicotinic acetylcholine receptor gene cluster on chromosome 15 associated with nicotine and alcohol dependence. There are reports of numerous other addiction susceptibility genes (e.g., variants in COMT, the μ-opioid receptor, and the serotonin transporter), but further work is needed to validate these findings. In addition, several genes have been implicated in impulsivity, which is strongly associated with substance abuse. These include variants in genes for the D_4 dopamine receptor, the dopamine transporter, monoamine oxidase A, COMT, and the 5-HT1B serotonin receptor.

PATHOGENESIS

Work in rodents and nonhuman primates has established the brain's reward regions as key neural substrates for the acute actions of drugs of abuse and for addiction induced by repeated drug administration (Fig. 390-1). Midbrain dopamine neurons in the ventral tegmental area (VTA) function normally as rheostats of reward: They are activated by natural rewards (food, sex, social interaction) or even by the expectation of such rewards, and many are suppressed by the absence of an expected reward or by aversive stimuli. These neurons thereby transmit crucial survival signals to the rest of the limbic brain to promote reward-related behavior, including motor responses to seek and obtain the rewards (nucleus accumbens), memories of reward-related cues (amygdala, hippocampus), and executive control of obtaining rewards (prefrontal cortex).

Drugs of abuse alter neurotransmission through initial actions at different classes of ion channels, neurotransmitter receptors, or neurotransmitter transporters (Table 390-2). Although the initial targets differ, the actions of these drugs converge on the brain's reward circuitry by promoting dopamine neurotransmission in the nucleus accumbens and other limbic targets of the VTA. In addition, some drugs promote activation of opioid and cannabinoid receptors, which modulate this reward circuitry. By these mechanisms, drugs of abuse produce powerful rewarding signals, which, after repeated drug administration, corrupt the brain's reward circuitry in ways that promote addiction. Three major pathologic adaptations have been described. First, drugs produce tolerance and dependence in reward circuits, which promote escalating drug intake and a negative emotional state during drug withdrawal that promotes relapse. Second, sensitization to the rewarding effects of the drugs and associated cues is seen during prolonged abstinence and also triggers relapse. Third, executive function is impaired in such a way as to increase impulsivity and compulsivity, both of which promote relapse.

Repeated intake of abused drugs induces specific changes in cellular signal transduction, synaptic strength (long-term potentiation or depression), and neuronal structure (altered dendritic branching or cell soma size) within the brain's reward circuitry. These modifications are mediated in part by changes in gene expression, achieved by drug regulation of transcription factors [e.g., CREB (cAMP response element binding protein) and ΔFosB] and their target genes. Together, these drug-induced adaptations underlie alterations in numerous neurotransmitter systems (e.g., glutamate, GABA, dopamine), growth factors (e.g., BDNF), neuropeptides (e.g. corticotrophin releasing factor), and intracellular signaling cascades. These adaptations provide opportunities for developing treatments targeted to drug-addicted individuals. The fact that the spectrum of these adaptations partly differ depending on the particular addictive substance used creates opportunities for treatments that are specific for different classes of addictive drugs and that may, therefore, be less likely to disturb basic mechanisms that govern motivation and reward.

Increasingly, causal relationships are being established between individual molecular-cellular adaptations and specific behavioral abnormalities that characterize the addicted state. For example,

TABLE 390-2 Initial Actions of Drugs of Abuse

Drug	Neurotransmitter Affected	Drug Target (Action)
Opiates	Endorphins, enkephalins	μ- and δ-opioid receptors (agonist)
Psychostimulants (cocaine, amphetamine methamphetamine)	Dopamine	Dopamine transporter (antagonist—cocaine; reverse transport—amphetamine, methamphetamine)
Nicotine	Acetylcholine	Nicotinic cholinergic receptors (agonist)
Ethanol	GABA	$GABA_A$ receptors (positive allosteric modulator)
	Glutamate	NMDA glutamate receptors (antagonist)
	Acetylcholine	Nicotinic cholinergic receptors (allosteric modulator)
	Serotonin	5HT-3 receptor (positive allosteric modulator)
	—	Calcium-activated K^+ channel (acivator)
Marijuana	Endocannabinoids (anandamide, 2-arachidonoylglycerol)	CB_1 receptor (agonist)
Phencyclidine	Glutamate	NMDA glutamate receptor (antagonist)

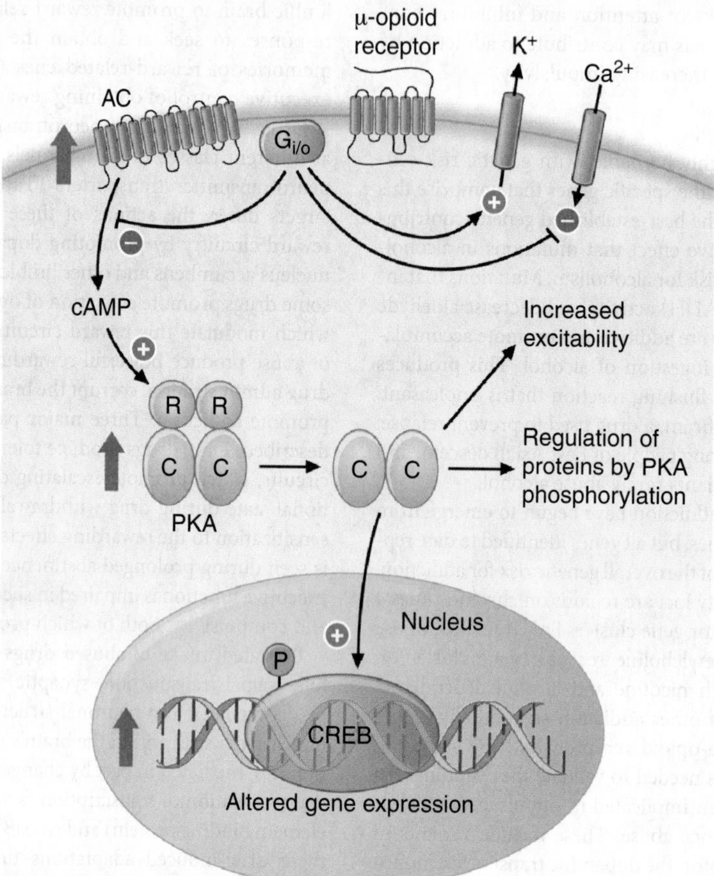

Figure 390-2 Opiate action in the locus coeruleus (LC). Binding of opiate agonists to μ-opioid receptors catalyzes nucleotide exchange on G_i and G_o proteins, leading to inhibition of adenylyl cyclase, neuronal hyperpolarization via activation of K^+ channels, and inhibition of neurotransmitter release *via* inhibition of Ca^{2+} channels. Activation of $G_{i/o}$ also inhibits adenylyl cyclase (AC), reducing protein kinase A (PKA) activity and phosphorylation of several PKA substrate proteins, thereby altering their function. For example, opiates reduce phosphorylation of the cAMP response element-binding protein (CREB), which appears to initiate long-term changes in neuronal function. Chronic administration of opiates increases levels of AC isoforms, PKA catalytic (C) and regulatory (R) subunits, and the phosphorylation of several proteins, including CREB (indicated by red arrows). These changes contribute to the altered phenotype of the drug-addicted state. For example, the excitability of LC neurons is increased by enhanced cAMP signaling, although the ionic basis of this effect remains unknown. Activation of CREB causes upregulation of AC isoforms and tyrosine hydroxylase, the rate-limiting enzyme in catecholamine biosynthesis.

acute activation of μ-opioid receptors by morphine or other opiates activates $G_{i/o}$ proteins leading to inhibition of adenylyl cyclase, resulting in reduced cAMP production, protein kinase A (PKA) activation, and activation of the transcription factor CREB. Repeated administration of these drugs (Fig. 390-2) evokes a homeostatic response resulting in upregulation of adenylyl cyclases, increased production of cAMP, and increased activation of PKA and CREB. Such upregulation of cAMP signaling has been identified in the locus coeruleus, periaqueductal gray, VTA, and nucleus accumbens and contributes to opiate craving and signs of opiate withdrawal. The fact that endogenous opioid peptides do not produce tolerance and dependence while morphine and heroin do may relate to the recent observation that, unlike endogenous opioids, morphine and heroin are weak inducers of μ-opioid receptor desensitization and endocytosis. Therefore, these drugs cause prolonged receptor activation and inhibition of adenylyl cyclases, which provides a powerful stimulus for the upregulation of cAMP signaling that characterizes the opiate-dependent state.

FURTHER READINGS

Abrahams BS, Geschwind DH: Advances in autism genetics: On the threshold of a new neurobiology. Nat Rev Genet 9:341, 2008

Jaaro-Peled H et al: Review of pathological hallmarks of schizophrenia: Comparison of genetic models with patients and nongenetic models. Schizophr Bull 36:301, 2010

Koob GF, Le Moal M: Neurobiological mechanisms for opponent motivational processes in addiction. Philos Trans R Soc London B Biol Sci 363:3113, 2008

———, Volkow ND: Neurocircuitry of addiction. Neuropsychopharmacology 35:217, 2010

Krishnan V, Nestler EJ: The molecular neurobiology of depression. Nature 455:894, 2008

Maia TV, Frank MJ: From reinforcement learning models to psychiatric and neurological disorders. Nat Neurosci 14:154, 2011

Martinowich K et al: Bipolar disorder: From genes to behavior pathways. J Clin Invest 119:726, 2009

Ressler KJ, Mayberg HS: Targeting abnormal neural circuits in mood and anxiety disorders: From the laboratory to the clinic. Nat Neurosci 10:1116, 2007

Spanagel R: Alcoholism: A systems approach from molecular physiology to addictive behavior. Physiol Rev 89:649, 2009

Walsh CA et al: Autism and brain development. Cell 135:396, 2008

CHAPTER 391 Mental Disorders

Victor I. Reus

Mental disorders are common in medical practice and may present either as a primary disorder or as a comorbid condition. The prevalence of mental or substance use disorders in the United States is approximately 30%, only one-third of whom are currently receiving treatment. Global burden of disease statistics indicate that 4 of the 10 most important causes of disease worldwide are psychiatric in origin.

The revised fourth edition for use by primary care physicians of the *Diagnostic and Statistical Manual* (DSM-IV-PC) provides a useful synopsis of mental disorders most likely to be seen in primary care practice. The current system of classification is multiaxial and includes the presence or absence of a major mental disorder (axis I), any underlying personality disorder (axis II), general medical condition (axis III), psychosocial and environmental problems (axis IV), and overall rating of general psychosocial functioning (axis V).

Changes in health care delivery underscore the need for primary care physicians to assume responsibility for the initial diagnosis and treatment of the most common mental disorders. Prompt diagnosis is essential to ensure that patients have access to appropriate medical services and to maximize the clinical outcome. Validated patient-based questionnaires have been developed that systematically probe for signs and symptoms associated with the most prevalent psychiatric diagnoses and guide the clinician into targeted assessment. Prime MD (and a self-report form, the PHQ) and the Symptom-Driven Diagnostic System for Primary Care (SDDS-PC) are inventories that require only 10 minutes to complete and link patient responses to the formal diagnostic criteria of anxiety, mood, somatoform, and eating disorders and to alcohol abuse or dependence.

A physician who refers patients to a psychiatrist should know not only when doing so is appropriate but also how to refer, since societal misconceptions and the stigma of mental illness impede the process. Primary care physicians should base referrals to a psychiatrist on the presence of signs and symptoms of a mental disorder and not simply on the absence of a physical explanation for a patient's complaint. The physician should discuss with the patient the reasons for requesting the referral or consultation and provide reassurance that he or she will continue to provide medical care and work collaboratively with the mental health professional. Consultation with a psychiatrist or transfer of care is appropriate when physicians encounter evidence of psychotic symptoms, mania, severe depression, or anxiety; symptoms of posttraumatic stress disorder (PTSD); suicidal or homicidal preoccupation; or a failure to respond to first-order treatment. Eating disorders are discussed in Chap. 79, and the biology of psychiatric and addictive disorders in Chap. 390.

ANXIETY DISORDERS

Anxiety disorders, the most prevalent psychiatric illnesses in the general community, are present in 15–20% of medical clinic patients. Anxiety, defined as a subjective sense of unease, dread, or foreboding, can indicate a primary psychiatric condition or can be a component of, or reaction to, a primary medical disease. The primary anxiety disorders are classified according to their duration and course and the existence and nature of precipitants.

When evaluating the anxious patient, the clinician must first determine whether the anxiety antedates or postdates a medical illness or is due to a medication side effect. Approximately one-third of patients presenting with anxiety have a medical etiology for their psychiatric symptoms, but an anxiety disorder can also present with somatic symptoms in the absence of a diagnosable medical condition.

PANIC DISORDER

Clinical manifestations

Panic disorder is defined by the presence of recurrent and unpredictable panic attacks, which are distinct episodes of intense fear and discomfort associated with a variety of physical symptoms, including palpitations, sweating, trembling, shortness of breath, chest pain, dizziness, and a fear of impending doom or death (Table 391-1). Paresthesias, gastrointestinal distress, and feelings of unreality are also common. Diagnostic criteria require at least 1 month of concern or worry about the attacks or a change in behavior related to them. The lifetime prevalence of panic disorder is 1–3%. Panic attacks have a sudden onset, developing within 10 minutes and usually resolving over the course of an hour, and they occur in an unexpected fashion. The frequency and severity of panic attacks vary, ranging from once a week to clusters of attacks separated by months of well-being. The first attack is usually outside the home, and onset is typically in late adolescence to early adulthood. In some individuals, anticipatory anxiety develops over time and results in a generalized fear and a progressive avoidance of places or situations in which a panic attack might recur. *Agoraphobia*, which occurs commonly in patients with panic disorder, is an acquired irrational fear of being in places where one might feel trapped or unable to escape (Table 391-2). Typically, it leads the patient into a progressive restriction in lifestyle and, in a literal sense, in geography.

TABLE 391-1 Diagnostic Criteria for Panic Attack

A discrete period of intense fear or discomfort, in which four or more of the following symptoms developed abruptly and reached a peak within 10 minutes:

1. Palpitations, pounding heart, or accelerated heart rate
2. Sweating
3. Trembling or shaking
4. Sensations of shortness of breath or smothering
5. Feeling of choking
6. Chest pain or discomfort
7. Nausea or abdominal distress
8. Feeling dizzy, unsteady, lightheaded, or faint
9. Derealization (feelings of unreality) or depersonalization (being detached from oneself)
10. Fear of losing control or going crazy
11. Fear of dying
12. Paresthesias (numbness or tingling sensations)
13. Chills or hot flushes

Source: *Diagnostic and Statistical Manual of Mental Disorders*, 4th ed. Washington, DC, American Psychiatric Association, 2000.

TABLE 391-2 Diagnostic Criteria for Agoraphobia

1. Anxiety about being in places or situations from which escape might be difficult (or embarrassing) or in which help may not be available in the event of having an unexpected or situationally predisposed panic attack or panic-like symptoms. Agoraphobic fears typically involve characteristic clusters of situations that include being outside the home alone; being in a crowd or standing in a line; being on a bridge; and traveling in a bus, train, or automobile.
2. The situations are avoided (e.g., travel is restricted) or else are endured with marked distress or with anxiety about having a panic attack or panic-like symptoms, or require the presence of a companion.
3. The anxiety or phobic avoidance is not better accounted for by another mental disorder such as social phobia (e.g., avoidance limited to social situations because of fear of embarrassment), specific phobia (e.g., avoidance limited to a single situation like elevators), obsessive-compulsive disorder (e.g., avoidance of dirt in someone with an obsession about contamination), posttraumatic stress disorder (e.g., avoidance of stimuli associated with a severe stressor), or separation anxiety disorder (e.g., avoidance of leaving home or relatives).

Source: *Diagnostic and Statistical Manual of Mental Disorders*, 4th ed. Washington, DC, American Psychiatric Association, 2000.

Frequently, patients are embarrassed that they are housebound and dependent on the company of others to go out into the world and do not volunteer this information; thus physicians will fail to recognize the syndrome if direct questioning is not pursued.

Differential diagnosis

A diagnosis of panic disorder is made after a medical etiology for the panic attacks has been ruled out. A variety of cardiovascular, respiratory, endocrine, and neurologic conditions can present with anxiety as the chief complaint. Patients with true panic disorder will often focus on one specific feature to the exclusion of others. For example, 20% of patients who present with syncope as a primary medical complaint have a primary diagnosis of a mood, anxiety, or substance-abuse disorder, the most common being panic disorder. The differential diagnosis of panic disorder is complicated by a high rate of comorbidity with other psychiatric conditions, especially alcohol and benzodiazepine abuse, which patients initially use in an attempt at self-medication. Some 75% of panic disorder patients will also satisfy criteria for major depression at some point in their illness.

When the history is nonspecific, physical examination and focused laboratory testing must be used to rule out anxiety states resulting from medical disorders such as pheochromocytoma, thyrotoxicosis, or hypoglycemia. Electrocardiogram (ECG) and echocardiogram may detect some cardiovascular conditions associated with panic such as paroxysmal atrial tachycardia and mitral valve prolapse. In two studies, panic disorder was the primary diagnosis in 43% of patients with chest pain who had normal coronary angiograms and was present in 9% of all outpatients referred for cardiac evaluation. Panic disorder has also been diagnosed in many patients referred for pulmonary function testing or with symptoms of irritable bowel syndrome.

Etiology and pathophysiology

The etiology of panic disorder is unknown but appears to involve a genetic predisposition, altered autonomic responsivity, and social learning. Panic disorder shows familial aggregation; the disorder is concordant in 30–45% of monozygotic twins, and genomewide screens have identified suggestive risk loci. Acute panic attacks appear to be associated with increased noradrenergic discharges in the locus coeruleus. Intravenous infusion of sodium lactate evokes an attack in two-thirds of panic disorder patients, as do the α_2-adrenergic antagonist yohimbine, cholecystokinin tetrapeptide (CCK-4), and carbon dioxide inhalation. It is hypothesized that each of these stimuli activates a pathway involving noradrenergic neurons in the locus coeruleus and serotonergic neurons in the dorsal raphe. Agents that block serotonin reuptake can prevent attacks. Panic-disorder patients have a heightened sensitivity to somatic symptoms, which triggers increasing arousal, setting off the panic attack; accordingly, therapeutic intervention involves altering the patient's cognitive interpretation of anxiety-producing experiences as well as preventing the attack itself.

TREATMENT Panic Disorder

Achievable goals of treatment are to decrease the frequency of panic attacks and to reduce their intensity. The cornerstone of drug therapy is antidepressant medication (Tables 391-3 through 391-5). Selective serotonin reuptake inhibitors (SSRIs) benefit the majority of panic disorder patients and do not have the adverse effects of tricyclic antidepressants (TCAs). Fluoxetine, paroxetine, sertraline, and the selective serotonin-norepinephrine reuptake inhibitor (SNRI) venlafaxine have received approval from the U.S. Food and Drug Administration (FDA) for this indication. These drugs should be started at one-third to one-half of their usual antidepressant dose (e.g., 5–10 mg fluoxetine, 25–50 mg sertraline, 10 mg paroxetine, venlafaxine 37.5 mg). Monoamine oxidase inhibitors (MAOIs) are also effective and may specifically benefit patients who have comorbid features of atypical depression (i.e., hypersomnia and weight gain). Insomnia, orthostatic hypotension, and the need to maintain a low-tyramine diet (avoidance of cheese and wine) have limited their use, however. Antidepressants typically take 2–6 weeks to become effective, and doses may need to be adjusted based upon the clinical response.

Because of anticipatory anxiety and the need for immediate relief of panic symptoms, benzodiazepines are useful early in the course of treatment and sporadically thereafter (Table 391-6). For example, alprazolam, starting at 0.5 mg qid and increasing to 4 mg/d in divided doses, is effective, but patients must be monitored closely, as some develop dependence and begin to escalate the dose of this medication. Clonazepam, at a final maintenance dose of 2–4 mg/d, is also helpful; its longer half-life permits twice-daily dosing, and patients appear less likely to develop dependence on this agent.

Early psychotherapeutic intervention and education aimed at symptom control enhances the effectiveness of drug treatment. Patients can be taught breathing techniques, be educated about physiologic changes that occur with panic, and learn to expose themselves voluntarily to precipitating events in a treatment program spanning 12–15 sessions. Homework assignments and monitored compliance are important components of successful treatment. Once patients have achieved a satisfactory response, drug treatment should be maintained for 1–2 years to prevent relapse. Controlled trials indicate a success rate of 75–85%, although the likelihood of complete remission is somewhat lower.

GENERALIZED ANXIETY DISORDER

Clinical manifestations

Patients with generalized anxiety disorder (GAD) have persistent, excessive, and/or unrealistic worry associated with muscle

TABLE 391-3 Antidepressants

Name	Usual Daily Dose, mg	Side Effects	Comments
SSRIs			
Fluoxetine (Prozac)	10–80	Headache; nausea and other GI effects; jitteriness; insomnia; sexual dysfunction; can affect plasma levels of other medicines (except sertraline); akathisia rare	Once-daily dosing, usually in the morning; fluoxetine has very long half-life; must not be combined with MAOIs
Sertraline (Zoloft)	50–200		
Paroxetine (Paxil)	20–60		
Fluvoxamine (Luvox)	100–300		
Citalopram (Celexa)	20–60		
Escitalopram (Lexapro)	10–30		
TCAs			
Amitriptyline (Elavil)	150–300	Anticholinergic (dry mouth, tachycardia, constipation, urinary retention, blurred vision); sweating; tremor; postural hypotension; cardiac conduction delay; sedation; weight gain	Once-daily dosing, usually qhs; blood levels of most TCAs available; can be lethal in O.D. (lethal dose = 2 g); nortriptyline best tolerated, especially by elderly
Nortriptyline (Pamelor)	50–200		
Imipramine (Tofranil)	150–300		
Desipramine (Norpramin)	150–300		
Doxepin (Sinequan)	150–300		
Clomipramine (Anafranil)	150–300		
Mixed Norepinephrine/Serotonin Reuptake Inhibitors and Receptor Blockers			
Venlafaxine (Effexor)	75–375	Nausea; dizziness; dry mouth; headaches; increased blood pressure; anxiety and insomnia	Bid-tid dosing (extended release available); lower potential for drug interactions than SSRIs; contraindicated with MAOIs
Desvenlafaxine, (Pristiq)	50–400	Nausea, dizziness, insomnia	Primary metabolite of venlafaxine. No increased efficacy with higher dosing
Duloxetine (Cymbalta)	40–60	Nausea, dizziness, headache, insomnia, constipation	May have utility in treatment of neuropathic pain and stress incontinence
Mirtazapine (Remeron)	15–45	Somnolence; weight gain; neutropenia rare	Once daily dosing
Mixed-action Drugs			
Bupropion (Wellbutrin)	250–450	Jitteriness; flushing; seizures in at-risk patients; anorexia; tachycardia; psychosis	Tid dosing, but sustained release also available; fewer sexual side effects than SSRIs or TCAs; may be useful for adult ADD
Trazodone (Desyrel)	200–600	Sedation; dry mouth; ventricular irritability; postural hypotension; priapism rare	Useful in low doses for sleep because of sedating effects with no anticholinergic side effects
Nefazodone (Serzone)	300–600	Sedation; headache; dry mouth; nausea; constipation	Discontinued sale in United States and several other countries due to risk of liver failure
Amoxapine (Asendin)	200–600	Sexual dysfunction	Lethality in overdose; EPS possible
MAOIs			
Phenelzine (Nardil)	45–90	Insomnia; hypotension; anorgasmia; weight gain; hypertensive crisis; toxic reactions with SSRIs; narcotics	May be more effective in patients with atypical features or treatment-refractory depression
Tranylcypromine (Parnate)	20–50		
Isocarboxazid (Marplan)	20–60		
Transdermal selegiline (Emsam)	6–12	Local skin reaction hypertension	No dietary restrictions with 6 mg dose

Abbreviations: ADD, attention deficit disorder; EPS, extrapyramidal symptoms; MAOIs, monoamine oxidase inhibitors; SSRIs, selective serotonin reuptake inhibitors; TCAs, tricyclic antidepressants.

tension, impaired concentration, autonomic arousal, feeling "on edge" or restless, and insomnia (Table 391-7). Onset is usually before age 20 years, and a history of childhood fears and social inhibition may be present. The lifetime prevalence of GAD is 5–6%; the risk is higher in first-degree relatives of patients with the diagnosis. Interestingly, family studies indicate that GAD and panic disorder segregate independently. More than 80% of patients with GAD also suffer from major depression, dysthymia, or social phobia. Comorbid substance abuse is common in these patients, particularly alcohol and/or sedative/hypnotic abuse. Patients with GAD worry excessively over minor matters, with life-disrupting effects; unlike in panic disorder, complaints

TABLE 391-4 Management of Antidepressant Side Effects

Symptoms	Comments and Management Strategies
Gastrointestinal	
Nausea, loss of appetite	Usually short-lived and dose-related; consider temporary dose reduction or administration with food and antacids
Diarrhea	Famotidine, 20–40 mg/d
Constipation	Wait for tolerance; try diet change, stool softener, exercise; avoid laxatives
Sexual dysfunction	Consider dose reduction; drug holiday
Anorgasmia/impotence; impaired ejaculation	Bethanechol, 10–20 mg, 2 h before activity, or cyproheptadine, 4–8 mg 2 h before activity, or bupropion, 100 mg bid or amantadine, 100 mg bid/tid
Orthostasis	Tolerance unlikely; increase fluid intake, use calf exercises/support hose; fludrocortisone, 0.025 mg/d
Anticholinergic	Wait for tolerance
Dry mouth, eyes	Maintain good oral hygiene; use artificial tears, sugar-free gum
Tremor/jitteriness	Antiparkinsonian drugs not effective; use dose reduction/slow increase; lorazepam, 0.5 mg bid, or propranolol, 10–20 mg bid
Insomnia	Schedule all doses for the morning; trazodone, 50–100 mg qhs
Sedation	Caffeine; schedule all dosing for bedtime; bupropion, 75–100 mg in afternoon
Headache	Evaluate diet, stress, other drugs; try dose reduction; amitriptyline, 50 mg/d
Weight gain	Decrease carbohydrates; exercise; consider fluoxetine
Loss of therapeutic benefit over time	Related to tolerance? Increase dose or drug holiday; add amantadine, 100 mg bid, buspirone, 10 mg tid, or pindolol, 2.5 mg bid

of shortness of breath, palpitations, and tachycardia are relatively rare.

Etiology and pathophysiology

All anxiogenic agents act on the γ-aminobutyric acid $(\text{GABA})_A$ receptor/chloride ion channel complex, implicating this neurotransmitter system in the pathogenesis of anxiety and panic attacks. Benzodiazepines are thought to bind two separate GABA_A receptor sites: type I, which has a broad neuroanatomic distribution, and type II, which is concentrated in the hippocampus, striatum, and neocortex. The antianxiety effects of the various benzodiazepines and side effects such as sedation and memory impairment are influenced by their relative binding to type I and type II receptor sites. Serotonin [5-hydroxytryptamine (5HT)] and 3α-reduced neuractive steroids (allosteric modulators of GABA_A) also appear to have a role in anxiety, and buspirone, a partial 5HT_{1A} receptor agonist, and certain 5HT_{2A} and 5HT_{2C} receptor antagonists (e.g., nefazodone) may have beneficial effects.

TABLE 391-5 Possible Drug Interactions With Selective Serotonin Reuptake Inhibitors

Agent	Effect
Monoamine oxidase inhibitors	Serotonin syndrome—absolute contraindication
Serotonergic agonists, e.g., tryptophan, fenfluramine	Potential serotonin syndrome
Drugs that are metabolized by P450 isoenzymes: tricyclics, other SSRIs, antipsychotics, beta blockers, codeine, triazolobenzodiazepines, calcium channel blockers	Delayed metabolism resulting in increased blood levels and potential toxicity
Drugs that are bound tightly to plasma proteins, e.g., warfarin	Increased bleeding secondary to displacement
Drugs that inhibit the metabolism of SSRIs by P450 isoenzymes, e.g., quinidine	Increased SSRI side effects

Abbreviation: SSRIs, selective serotonin reuptake inhibitors.

TREATMENT Generalized Anxiety Disorder

A combination of pharmacologic and psychotherapeutic interventions is most effective in GAD, but complete symptomatic relief is rare. A short course of a benzodiazepine is usually indicated, preferably lorazepam, oxazepam, or temazepam. (The first two of these agents are metabolized via conjugation rather than oxidation and thus do not accumulate if hepatic function is impaired.) Treatment should be initiated at the lowest dose possible and prescribed on an as-needed basis as symptoms warrant. Benzodiazepines differ in their milligram per kilogram potency, half-life, lipid solubility, metabolic pathways, and presence of active metabolites. Agents that are absorbed rapidly and are lipid soluble, such as diazepam, have a rapid onset of action and a higher abuse potential. Benzodiazepines should generally not be prescribed for >4–6 weeks because of the development of tolerance and the risk of abuse and dependence. Withdrawal must be closely monitored as relapses can occur. It is important to warn patients that concomitant use of alcohol or other sedating drugs may be neurotoxic and impair their ability to function. An optimistic approach that encourages the patient to clarify environmental precipitants, anticipate his or her reactions, and plan effective response strategies is an essential element of therapy.

Adverse effects of benzodiazepines generally parallel their relative half-lives. Longer-acting agents, such as diazepam, chlordiazepoxide, flurazepam, and clonazepam, tend to accumulate active metabolites, with resultant sedation, impairment of cognition, and poor psychomotor performance. Shorter-acting compounds, such as alprazolam and oxazepam, can produce daytime anxiety, early morning insomnia, and, with discontinuation, rebound anxiety and insomnia. Although patients develop tolerance to the sedative effects of benzodiazepines, they are less likely to habituate to the adverse psychomotor effects. Withdrawal from the longer half-life benzodiazepines can be accomplished through gradual, stepwise dose reduction (by 10% every 1–2 weeks) over 6–12 weeks. It is usually more difficult to taper patients off shorter-acting benzodiazepines. Physicians

TABLE 391-6 Anxiolytics

Name	Equivalent PO Dose, mg	Onset of Action	Half-life, h	Comments
Benzodiazepines				
Diazepam (Valium)	5	Fast	20–70	Active metabolites; quite sedating
Flurazepam (Dalmane)	15	Fast	30–100	Flurazepam is a prodrug; metabolites are active; quite sedating
Triazolam (Halcion)	0.25	Intermediate	1.5–5	No active metabolites; can induce confusion and delirium, especially in elderly
Lorazepam (Ativan)	1	Intermediate	10–20	No active metabolites; direct hepatic glucuronide conjugation; quite sedating
Alprazolam (Xanax)	0.5	Intermediate	12–15	Active metabolites; not too sedating; may have specific antidepressant and antipanic activity; tolerance and dependence develop easily
Chlordiazepoxide (Librium)	10	Intermediate	5–30	Active metabolites; moderately sedating
Oxazepam (Serax)	15	Slow	5–15	No active metabolites; direct glucuronide conjugation; not too sedating
Temazepam (Restoril)	15	Slow	9–12	No active metabolites; moderately sedating
Clonazepam (Klonopin)	0.5	Slow	18–50	No active metabolites; moderately sedating
Nonbenzodiazepines				
Buspirone (BuSpar)	7.5	2 weeks	2–3	Active metabolites; tid dosing—usual daily dose 10–20 mg tid; nonsedating; no additive effects with alcohol; useful for controlling agitation in demented or brain-injured patients

TABLE 391-7 Diagnostic Criteria for Generalized Anxiety Disorder

A. Excessive anxiety and worry (apprehensive expectation), occurring more days than not for at least 6 months, about a number of events or activities (such as work or school performance).

B. The person finds it difficult to control the worry.

C. The anxiety and worry are associated with three (or more) of the following six symptoms (with at least some symptoms present for more days than not for the past 6 months): (1) restlessness or feeling keyed up or on edge; (2) being easily fatigued; (3) difficulty concentrating or mind going blank; (4) irritability; (5) muscle tension; (6) sleep disturbance (difficulty falling or staying asleep, or restless unsatisfying sleep).

D. The focus of the anxiety and worry is not confined to features of an axis I disorder [e.g., the anxiety or worry is not about having a panic attack (as in panic disorder), being embarrassed in public (as in social phobia), being contaminated (as in obsessive-compulsive disorder), being away from home or close relatives (as in separation anxiety disorder), gaining weight (as in anorexia nervosa), having multiple physical complaints (as in somatization disorder), or having a serious illness (as in hypochondriasis)], and the anxiety and worry do not occur exclusively during posttraumatic stress disorder.

E. The anxiety, worry, or physical symptoms cause clinically significant distress or impairment in social, occupational, or other important areas of functioning.

F. The disturbance is not due to the direct physiologic effects of a substance (e.g., a drug of abuse, a medication) or a general medical condition (e.g., hyperthyroidism) and does not occur exclusively during a mood disorder, a psychotic disorder, or a pervasive developmental disorder.

Source: *Diagnostic and Statistical Manual of Mental Disorders*, 4th ed. Washington, DC, American Psychiatric Association, 2000.

may need to switch the patient to a benzodiazepine with a longer half-life or use an adjunctive medication such as a beta blocker or carbamazepine, before attempting to discontinue the benzodiazepine. Withdrawal reactions vary in severity and duration; they can include depression, anxiety, lethargy, diaphoresis, autonomic arousal, and, rarely, seizures.

Buspirone is a nonbenzodiazepine anxiolytic agent. It is nonsedating, does not produce tolerance or dependence, does not interact with benzodiazepine receptors or alcohol, and has no abuse or disinhibition potential. However, it requires several weeks to take effect and requires thrice-daily dosing. Patients who were previously responsive to a benzodiazepine are unlikely to rate buspirone as equally effective, but patients with head injury or dementia who have symptoms of anxiety and/or agitation may do well with this agent. Escitalopram, paroxetine, and venlafaxine are FDA approved for the treatment of GAD, usually at doses that are comparable to their efficacy in major depression. Benzodiazepines are contraindicated during pregnancy and breast-feeding.

Anticonvulsants with GABAergic properties may also be effective against anxiety. Gabapentin, oxcarbazepine, tiagabine, pregabalin, and divalproex have all shown some degree of benefit in a variety of anxiety-related syndromes. Agents that selectively target $GABA_A$ receptor subtypes are currently under development, and it is hoped that these will lack the sedating, memory-impairing, and addicting properties of benzodiazepines.

PHOBIC DISORDERS

Clinical manifestations

The cardinal feature of phobic disorders is a marked and persistent fear of objects or situations, exposure to which results in an immediate anxiety reaction. The patient avoids the phobic stimulus, and this avoidance usually impairs occupational or social functioning. Panic attacks may be triggered by the phobic stimulus or may occur spontaneously. Unlike patients with other anxiety disorders, individuals with phobias usually experience anxiety only in specific situations. Common phobias include fear of closed spaces (claustrophobia), fear of blood, and fear of flying. Social phobia is distinguished by a specific fear of social or performance situations in which the individual is exposed to unfamiliar individuals or to possible examination and evaluation by others. Examples include having to converse at a party, use public restrooms, and meet strangers. In each case, the affected individual is aware that the experienced fear is excessive and unreasonable given the circumstance. The specific content of a phobia may vary across gender, ethnic, and cultural boundaries.

Phobic disorders are common, affecting ~10% of the population. Full criteria for diagnosis are usually satisfied first in early adulthood, but behavioral avoidance of unfamiliar people, situations, or objects dating from early childhood is common.

In one study of female twins, concordance rates for agoraphobia, social phobia, and animal phobia were found to be 23% for monozygotic twins and 15% for dizygotic twins. A twin study of fear conditioning, a model for the acquisition of phobias, demonstrated a heritability of 35–45%, and a genomewide linkage scan identified a risk locus on chromosome 14 in a region previously implicated in a mouse model of fear. Animal studies of fear conditioning have indicated that processing of the fear stimulus occurs through the lateral nucleus of the amygdala, extending through the central nucleus and projecting to the periaqueductal gray region, lateral hypothalamus, and paraventricular hypothalamus.

TREATMENT Phobic Disorders

Beta blockers (e.g., propranolol, 20–40 mg orally 2 hours before the event) are particularly effective in the treatment of "performance anxiety" (but not general social phobia) and appear to work by blocking the peripheral manifestations of anxiety such as perspiration, tachycardia, palpitations, and tremor. MAOIs alleviate social phobia independently of their antidepressant activity, and paroxetine, sertraline, and venlafaxine have received FDA approval for treatment of social anxiety. Benzodiazepines can be helpful in reducing fearful avoidance, but the chronic nature of phobic disorders limits their usefulness.

Behaviorally focused psychotherapy is an important component of treatment, as relapse rates are high when medication is used as the sole treatment. Cognitive-behavioral strategies are based upon the finding that distorted perceptions and interpretations of fear-producing stimuli play a major role in perpetuation of phobias. Individual and group therapy sessions teach the patient to identify specific negative thoughts associated with the anxiety-producing situation and help to reduce the patient's fear of loss of control. In desensitization therapy, hierarchies of feared situations are constructed and the patient is encouraged to pursue and master gradual exposure to the anxiety-producing stimuli.

Patients with social phobia, in particular, have a high rate of comorbid alcohol abuse, as well as of other psychiatric conditions (e.g., eating disorders), necessitating the need for parallel management of each disorder if anxiety reduction is to be achieved.

STRESS DISORDERS

Clinical manifestations

Patients may develop anxiety after exposure to extreme traumatic events such as the threat of personal death or injury or the death of a loved one. The reaction may occur shortly after the trauma (*acute stress disorder*) or be delayed and subject to recurrence (PTSD) (Table 391-8). In both syndromes, individuals experience associated symptoms of detachment and loss of emotional responsivity. The patient may feel depersonalized and unable to recall specific aspects of the trauma, though typically it is reexperienced through intrusions in thought, dreams, or flashbacks, particularly when cues of the original event are present. Patients often actively avoid

TABLE 391-8 Diagnostic Criteria for Posttraumatic Stress Disorder

A. The person has been exposed to a traumatic event in which both of the following were present:
   1. The person experienced, witnessed, or was confronted with an event or events that involved actual or threatened death or serious injury, or a threat to the physical integrity of self or others.
   2. The person's response involved intense fear, helplessness, or horror.

B. The traumatic event is persistently reexperienced in one (or more) of the following ways:
   1. Recurrent and intrusive distressing recollections of the event, including images, thoughts, or perceptions.
   2. Recurrent distressing dreams of the event.
   3. Acting or feeling as if the traumatic event were recurring (includes a sense of reliving the experience, illusions, hallucinations, and dissociative flashback episodes, including those that occur on awakening or when intoxicated).
   4. Intense psychological distress at exposure to internal or external cues that symbolize or resemble an aspect of the traumatic event.
   5. Physiologic reactivity on exposure to internal or external cues that symbolize or resemble an aspect of the traumatic event.

C. Persistent avoidance of stimuli associated with the trauma and numbing of general responsiveness (not present before the trauma), as indicated by three or more of the following:
   1. Efforts to avoid thoughts, feelings, or conversations associated with the trauma
   2. Efforts to avoid activities, places, or people that arouse recollections of the trauma
   3. Inability to recall an important aspect of the trauma
   4. Markedly diminished interest or participation in significant activities
   5. Feeling of detachment or estrangement from others
   6. Restricted range of affect (e.g., unable to have loving feelings)
   7. Sense of a foreshortened future (e.g., does not expect to have a career, marriage, children, or a normal life span)

D. Persistent symptoms of increased arousal (not present before the trauma), as indicated by two (or more) of the following:
   1. Difficulty falling or staying asleep
   2. Irritability or outbursts of anger
   3. Difficulty concentrating
   4. Hypervigilance
   5. Exaggerated startle response

E. Duration of the disturbance (symptoms in criteria B, C, and D) is more than 1 month

F. The disturbance causes clinically significant distress or impairment in social, occupational, or other important areas of functioning.

Source: *Diagnostic and Statistical Manual of Mental Disorders*, 4th ed. Washington, DC, American Psychiatric Association, 2000.

stimuli that precipitate recollections of the trauma and demonstrate a resulting increase in vigilance, arousal, and startle response. Patients with stress disorders are at risk for the development of other disorders related to anxiety, mood, and substance abuse (especially alcohol). Between 5 and 10% of Americans will at some time in their life satisfy criteria for PTSD, with women more likely to be affected than men.

Risk factors for the development of PTSD include a past psychiatric history and personality characteristics of high neuroticism and extroversion. Twin studies show a substantial genetic influence on all symptoms associated with PTSD, with less evidence for an environmental effect.

Etiology and pathophysiology

It is hypothesized that in PTSD there is excessive release of norepinephrine from the locus coeruleus in response to stress and increased noradrenergic activity at projection sites in the hippocampus and amygdala. These changes theoretically facilitate the encoding of fear-based memories. Greater sympathetic responses to cues associated with the traumatic event occur in PTSD, although pituitary adrenal responses are blunted.

TREATMENT Stress Disorders

Acute stress reactions are usually self-limited, and treatment typically involves the short-term use of benzodiazepines and supportive/expressive psychotherapy. The chronic and recurrent nature of PTSD, however, requires a more complex approach employing drug and behavioral treatments. PTSD is highly correlated with peritraumatic dissociative symptoms and the development of an acute stress disorder at the time of the trauma. TCAs such as imipramine and amitriptyline, the MAOI phenelzine, and the SSRIs can all reduce anxiety, symptoms of intrusion, and avoidance behaviors, as can prazosin, an α_1 antagonist. Propranolol and opiates such as morphine, given during the acute stress period may have beneficial effects in preventing the development of PTSD. Trazodone, a sedating antidepressant, is frequently used at night to help with insomnia (50–150 mg qhs). Carbamazepine, valproic acid, or alprazolam have also independently produced improvement in uncontrolled trials. Psychotherapeutic strategies for PTSD help the patient overcome avoidance behaviors and demoralization and master fear of recurrence of the trauma; therapies that encourage the patient to dismantle avoidance behaviors through stepwise focusing on the experience of the traumatic event are the most effective.

OBSESSIVE-COMPULSIVE DISORDER

Clinical manifestations

Obsessive-compulsive disorder (OCD) is characterized by obsessive thoughts and compulsive behaviors that impair everyday functioning. Fears of contamination and germs are common, as are handwashing, counting behaviors, and having to check and recheck such actions as whether a door is locked. The degree to which the disorder is disruptive for the individual varies, but in all cases obsessive-compulsive activities take up >1 hour per day and are undertaken to relieve the anxiety triggered by the core fear. Patients often conceal their symptoms, usually because they are embarrassed by the content of their thoughts or the nature of their actions. Physicians must ask specific questions regarding recurrent thoughts and behaviors, particularly if physical clues such as chafed and reddened hands or patchy hair loss (from repetitive hair pulling, or trichotillomania) are present. Comorbid conditions are common, the most frequent being depression, other anxiety disorders, eating disorders, and tics. OCD has a lifetime prevalence of 2–3% worldwide. Onset is usually gradual, beginning in early adulthood, but childhood onset is not rare. The disorder usually has a waxing and waning course, but some cases may show a steady deterioration in psychosocial functioning.

Etiology and pathophysiology

A genetic contribution to OCD is suggested by twin studies. A genomewide association study (GWAS) reported linkage to chromosome 2p23.2; however, no susceptibility gene for OCD has been identified to date. Family studies show an aggregation of OCD with Tourette's disorder, and both are more common in males and in first-born children.

The anatomy of obsessive-compulsive behavior is thought to include the orbital frontal cortex, caudate nucleus, and globus pallidus. The caudate nucleus appears to be involved in the acquisition and maintenance of habit and skill learning, and interventions that are successful in reducing obsessive-compulsive behaviors also decrease metabolic activity measured in the caudate.

TREATMENT Obsessive-Compulsive Disorder

Clomipramine, fluoxetine, fluvoxamine, and sertraline are approved for the treatment of OCD. Clomipramine is a TCA that is often tolerated poorly owing to anticholinergic and sedative side effects at the doses required to treat the illness (25–250 mg/d); its efficacy in OCD is unrelated to its antidepressant activity. Fluoxetine (5–60 mg/d), fluvoxamine (25–300 mg/d), and sertraline (50–150 mg/d) are as effective as clomipramine and have a more benign side effect profile. Only 50–60% of patients with OCD show adequate improvement with pharmacotherapy alone. In treatment-resistant cases, augmentation with other serotonergic agents such as buspirone, or with a neuroleptic or benzodiazepine may be beneficial and in severe cases deep brain stimulation has been found to be effective. When a therapeutic response is achieved, long-duration maintenance therapy is usually indicated.

For many individuals, particularly those with time-consuming compulsions, behavior therapy will result in as much improvement as that afforded by medication. Effective techniques include the gradual increase in exposure to stressful situations, maintenance of a diary to clarify stressors, and homework assignments that substitute new activities for compulsive behaviors.

MOOD DISORDERS

Mood disorders are characterized by a disturbance in the regulation of mood, behavior, and affect. Mood disorders are subdivided into (1) depressive disorders, (2) bipolar disorders, and (3) depression in association with medical illness or alcohol and substance abuse (Chaps. 392 through 394). Major depressive disorder (MDD) is differentiated from bipolar disorder by the absence of a manic or hypomanic episode. The relationship between pure depressive syndromes and bipolar disorders is not well understood; MDD is more frequent in families of bipolar individuals, but the reverse is not true. In the Global Burden of Disease Study conducted by the World Health Organization, unipolar major depression ranked fourth among all diseases in terms of disability-adjusted life-years and was projected to rank second by the year 2020. In the United States, lost productivity directly related to mood disorders has been estimated at $55.1 billion per year.

DEPRESSION IN ASSOCIATION WITH MEDICAL ILLNESS

Depression occurring in the context of medical illness is difficult to evaluate. Depressive symptomatology may reflect the psychological stress of coping with the disease, may be caused by the disease process itself or by the medications used to treat it, or may simply coexist in time with the medical diagnosis.

Virtually every class of *medication* includes some agent that can induce depression. Antihypertensive drugs, anticholesterolemic agents, and antiarrhythmic agents are common triggers of depressive symptoms. Iatrogenic depression should also be considered in patients receiving glucocorticoids, antimicrobials, systemic analgesics, antiparkinsonian medications, and anticonvulsants. To decide whether a causal relationship exists between pharmacologic therapy and a patient's change in mood, it may sometimes be necessary to undertake an empirical trial of an alternative medication.

Between 20 and 30% of *cardiac* patients manifest a depressive disorder; an even higher percentage experience depressive symptomatology when self-reporting scales are used. Depressive symptoms following unstable angina, myocardial infarction, cardiac bypass surgery, or heart transplant impair rehabilitation and are associated with higher rates of mortality and medical morbidity. Depressed patients often show decreased variability in heart rate (an index of reduced parasympathetic nervous system activity); which may predispose individuals to ventricular arrhythmia and increased morbidity. Depression also appears to increase the risk of developing coronary heart disease, possibly through increased platelet aggregation. TCAs are contraindicated in patients with bundle branch block, and TCA-induced tachycardia is an additional concern in patients with congestive heart failure. SSRIs appear not to induce ECG changes or adverse cardiac events and thus are reasonable first-line drugs for patients at risk for TCA-related complications. SSRIs may interfere with hepatic metabolism of anticoagulants, however, causing increased anticoagulation.

In patients with *cancer*, the mean prevalence of depression is 25%, but depression occurs in 40–50% of patients with cancers of the pancreas or oropharynx. This association is not due to the effect of cachexia alone, as the higher prevalence of depression in patients with pancreatic cancer persists when compared to those with advanced gastric cancer. Initiation of antidepressant medication in cancer patients has been shown to improve quality of life as well as mood. Psychotherapeutic approaches, particularly group therapy, may have some effect on short-term depression, anxiety, and pain symptoms.

Depression occurs frequently in patients with *neurologic disorders*, particularly cerebrovascular disorders, Parkinson's disease, dementia, multiple sclerosis, and traumatic brain injury. One in five patients with left-hemisphere stroke involving the dorsolateral frontal cortex experiences major depression. Late-onset depression in otherwise cognitively normal individuals increases the risk of a subsequent diagnosis of Alzheimer's disease. Both TCA and SSRI agents are effective against these depressions, as are stimulant compounds and, in some patients, MAOIs.

The reported prevalence of depression in patients with *diabetes mellitus* varies from 8 to 27%, with the severity of the mood state correlating with the level of hyperglycemia and the presence of diabetic complications. Treatment of depression may be complicated by effects of antidepressive agents on glycemic control. MAOIs can induce hypoglycemia and weight gain, while TCAs can produce hyperglycemia and carbohydrate craving. SSRIs, like MAOIs, may reduce fasting plasma glucose, but they are easier to use and may also improve dietary and medication compliance.

Hypothyroidism is frequently associated with features of depression, most commonly depressed mood and memory impairment. Hyperthyroid states may also present in a similar fashion, usually in geriatric populations. Improvement in mood usually follows normalization of thyroid function, but adjunctive antidepressant medication is sometimes required. Patients with subclinical hypothyroidism can also experience symptoms of depression and cognitive difficulty that respond to thyroid replacement.

The lifetime prevalence of depression in *HIV-positive* individuals has been estimated at 22–45%. The relationship between depression and disease progression is multifactorial and likely to involve psychological and social factors, alterations in immune function, and central nervous system (CNS) disease. Chronic hepatitis C infection is also associated with depression, which may worsen with interferon-α treatment.

Some chronic disorders of uncertain etiology such as chronic fatigue syndrome (Chap. 389) and fibromyalgia (Chap. 335), are strongly associated with depression and anxiety; patients may benefit from antidepressant treatment or anticonvulsant agents such as pregabalin,

DEPRESSIVE DISORDERS

Clinical manifestations

Major depression is defined as depressed mood on a daily basis for a minimum duration of 2 weeks (Table 391-9). An episode may be characterized by sadness, indifference, apathy, or irritability and is usually associated with changes in sleep patterns, appetite, and weight; motor agitation or retardation; fatigue; impaired concentration and decision making; feelings of shame or guilt; and thoughts of death or dying. Patients with depression have a profound loss of pleasure in all enjoyable activities, exhibit early morning awakening, feel that the dysphoric mood state is qualitatively different from sadness, and often notice a diurnal variation in mood (worse in morning hours).

Approximately 15% of the population experiences a major depressive episode at some point in life, and 6–8% of all outpatients in primary care settings satisfy diagnostic criteria for the disorder. Depression is often undiagnosed, and, even more frequently, it is treated inadequately. If a physician suspects the presence of a major depressive episode, the initial task is to determine whether it represents unipolar or bipolar depression or is one of the 10–15% of cases that are secondary to general medical illness or substance abuse. Physicians should also assess the risk of suicide by direct questioning, as patients are often reluctant to verbalize such thoughts without prompting. If specific plans are uncovered or if significant risk factors exist (e.g., a past history of suicide attempts, profound hopelessness, concurrent medical illness, substance abuse, or social isolation), the patient must be referred to a mental health specialist for immediate care. The physician should specifically probe each of these areas in an empathic and hopeful manner, being sensitive to denial and possible minimization of distress. The presence of anxiety, panic, or agitation significantly increases near-term suicidal risk. Approximately 4–5% of all depressed patients will commit suicide; most will have sought help from physicians within 1 month of their deaths.

In some depressed patients, the mood disorder does not appear to be episodic and is not clearly associated with either psychosocial dysfunction or change from the individual's usual experience in life. *Dysthymic disorder* consists of a pattern of chronic (at least 2 years), ongoing, mild depressive symptoms that are less severe and less disabling than those found in major depression; the two conditions are sometimes difficult to separate, however, and can occur together ("double depression"). Many patients who exhibit a profile of pessimism, disinterest, and low self-esteem respond to antidepressant treatment. Dysthymic disorder exists in ~5% of primary care patients. The term *minor depression* is used for individuals who experience at least two depressive symptoms for 2 weeks but who

TABLE 391-9 Criteria for a Major Depressive Episode
A. Five (or more) of the following symptoms have been present during the same 2-week period and represent a change from previous functioning; at least one of the symptoms is either (1) depressed mood or (2) loss of interest or pleasure. **Note:** Do not include symptoms that are clearly due to a general medical condition, or mood-incongruent delusions or hallucinations.
1. Depressed mood most of the day, nearly every day, as indicated by either subjective report (e.g., feels sad or empty) or observation made by others (e.g., appears tearful)
2. Markedly diminished interest or pleasure in all, or almost all, activities most of the day, nearly every day (as indicated by either subjective account or observation made by others)
3. Significant weight loss when not dieting or weight gain (e.g., a change of >5% of body weight in a month), or decrease or increase in appetite nearly every day
4. Insomnia or hypersomnia nearly every day
5. Psychomotor agitation or retardation nearly every day (observable by others, not merely subjective feelings of restlessness or being slowed down)
6. Fatigue or loss of energy nearly every day
7. Feelings of worthlessness or excessive or inappropriate guilt (which may be delusional) nearly every day (not merely self-reproach or guilt about being sick)
8. Diminished ability to think or concentrate, or indecisiveness, nearly every day (either by subjective account or as observed by others)
9. Recurrent thoughts of death (not just fear of dying), recurrent suicidal ideation without a specific plan, or a suicide attempt or a specific plan for committing suicide
B. The symptoms do not meet criteria for a mixed episode
C. The symptoms cause clinically significant distress or impairment in social, occupational, or other important areas of functioning
D. The symptoms are not due to the direct physiologic effects of a substance (e.g., a drug of abuse, a medication) or a general medical condition (e.g., hypothyroidism)
E. The symptoms are not better accounted for by bereavement (i.e., after the loss of a loved one), the symptoms persist for >2 months or are characterized by marked functional impairment, morbid preoccupation with worthlessness, suicidal ideation, psychotic symptoms, or psychomotor retardation

Source: *Diagnostic and Statistical Manual of Mental Disorders*, 4th ed. Washington, DC, American Psychiatric Association, 2000.

do not meet the full criteria for major depression. Despite its name, minor depression is associated with significant morbidity and disability and also responds to pharmacologic treatment.

Depression is approximately twice as common in women as in men, and the incidence increases with age in both sexes. Twin studies indicate that the liability to major depression of early onset (before age 25) is largely genetic in origin. Negative life events can precipitate and contribute to depression, but genetic factors influence the sensitivity of individuals to these stressful events. In most cases, both biologic and psychosocial factors are involved in the precipitation and unfolding of depressive episodes. The most potent stressors appear to involve death of a relative, assault, or severe marital or relationship problems.

Unipolar depressive disorders usually begin in early adulthood and recur episodically over the course of a lifetime. The best predictor of future risk is the number of past episodes; 50–60% of patients who have a first episode have at least one or two recurrences. Some patients experience multiple episodes that become more severe and frequent over time. The duration of an untreated episode varies greatly, ranging from a few months to ≥1 year. The pattern of recurrence and clinical progression in a developing episode are also variable. Within an individual, the nature of episodes (e.g., specific presenting symptoms, frequency and duration) may be similar over time. In a minority of patients, a severe depressive episode may progress to a psychotic state; in elderly patients, depressive symptoms may be associated with cognitive deficits mimicking dementia ("pseudodementia"). A seasonal pattern of depression, called *seasonal affective disorder*, may manifest with onset and remission of episodes at predictable times of the year. This disorder is more common in women, whose symptoms are anergy, fatigue, weight gain, hypersomnia, and episodic carbohydrate craving. The prevalence increases with distance from the equator, and improvement may occur by altering light exposure.

Etiology and pathophysiology

Although evidence for genetic transmission of unipolar depression is not as strong as in bipolar disorder, monozygotic twins have a higher concordance rate (46%) than dizygotic siblings (20%), with little support for any effect of a shared family environment.

Neuroendocrine abnormalities that reflect the neurovegetative signs and symptoms of depression include: (1) increased cortisol and corticotropin-releasing hormone (CRH) secretion, (2) an increase in adrenal size, (3) a decreased inhibitory response of glucocorticoids to dexamethasone, and (4) a blunted response of thyroid-stimulating hormone (TSH) level to infusion of thyroid-releasing hormone (TRH). Antidepressant treatment leads to normalization of these abnormalities. Major depression is also associated with an upregulation of proinflammatory cytokines, which also normalizes with antidepressant treatment.

Diurnal variations in symptom severity and alterations in circadian rhythmicity of a number of neurochemical and neurohumoral factors suggest that biologic differences may be secondary to a primary defect in regulation of biologic rhythms. Patients with major depression show consistent findings of a decrease in rapid eye movement (REM) sleep onset (REM latency), an increase in REM density, and, in some subjects, a decrease in stage IV delta slow-wave sleep.

Although antidepressant drugs inhibit neurotransmitter uptake within hours, their therapeutic effects typically emerge over several weeks, implicating adaptive changes in second messenger systems and transcription factors as possible mechanisms of action.

The pathogenesis of depression is discussed in detail in Chap. 390.

TREATMENT Depressive Disorders

Treatment planning requires coordination of short-term strategies to induce remission combined with longer term maintenance designed to prevent recurrence. The most effective intervention for achieving remission and preventing relapse is medication, but combined treatment, incorporating psychotherapy to help the patient cope with decreased self-esteem and demoralization, improves outcome (Fig. 391-1). Approximately 40% of primary care patients with depression drop out of treatment and discontinue medication if symptomatic improvement is not noted within a month, unless additional support is provided. Outcome improves with (1) increased intensity and frequency of visits during the first 4–6 weeks of treatment, (2) supplemental educational materials, and (3) psychiatric consultation as indicated. Despite the widespread use of SSRIs

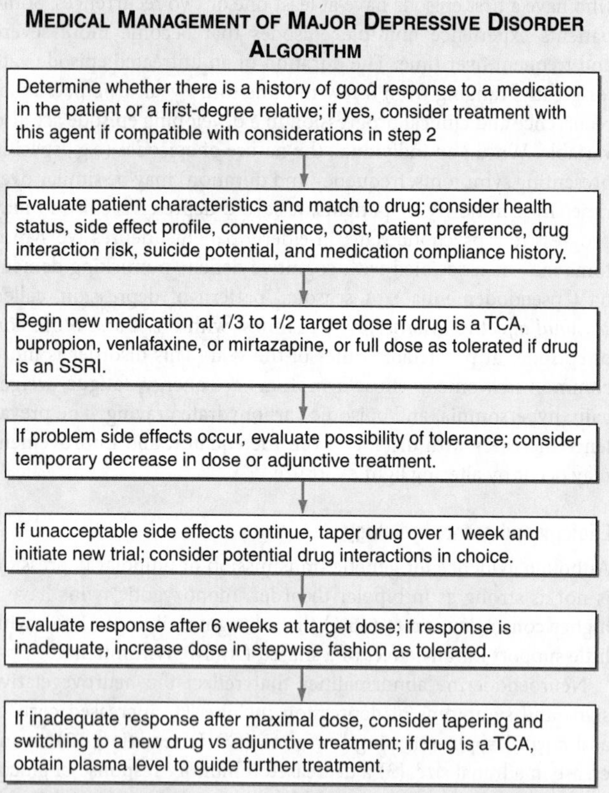

MEDICAL MANAGEMENT OF MAJOR DEPRESSIVE DISORDER ALGORITHM

Determine whether there is a history of good response to a medication in the patient or a first-degree relative; if yes, consider treatment with this agent if compatible with considerations in step 2

↓

Evaluate patient characteristics and match to drug; consider health status, side effect profile, convenience, cost, patient preference, drug interaction risk, suicide potential, and medication compliance history.

↓

Begin new medication at 1/3 to 1/2 target dose if drug is a TCA, bupropion, venlafaxine, or mirtazapine, or full dose as tolerated if drug is an SSRI.

↓

If problem side effects occur, evaluate possibility of tolerance; consider temporary decrease in dose or adjunctive treatment.

↓

If unacceptable side effects continue, taper drug over 1 week and initiate new trial; consider potential drug interactions in choice.

↓

Evaluate response after 6 weeks at target dose; if response is inadequate, increase dose in stepwise fashion as tolerated.

↓

If inadequate response after maximal dose, consider tapering and switching to a new drug vs adjunctive treatment; if drug is a TCA, obtain plasma level to guide further treatment.

Figure 391-1 A guideline for the medical management of major depressive disorder. SSRI, selective serotonin reuptake inhibitor; TCA, tricyclic antidepressant.

and other second-generation antidepressant drugs, there is no convincing evidence that this class of antidepressant is more efficacious than TCAs. Between 60 and 70% of all depressed patients respond to any drug chosen, if it is given in a sufficient dose for 6–8 weeks. There is no ideal antidepressant; no current compound combines rapid onset of action, moderate half-life, a meaningful relationship between dose and blood level, a low side effect profile, minimal interaction with other drugs, and safety in overdose.

A rational approach to selecting which antidepressant to use involves matching the patient's preference and medical history with the metabolic and side effect profile of the drug (Tables 391-4 and 391-5). A previous response, or a family history of a positive response, to a specific antidepressant often suggests that that drug be tried first. Before initiating antidepressant therapy, the physician should evaluate the possible contribution of comorbid illnesses and consider their specific treatment. In individuals with suicidal ideation, particular attention should be paid to choosing a drug with low toxicity if taken in overdose. The SSRIs, and other newer antidepressant drugs are distinctly safer in this regard; nevertheless, the advantages of TCAs have not been completely superseded. The existence of generic equivalents make TCAs relatively cheap, and for secondary tricyclics, particularly nortriptyline and desipramine, well-defined relationships among dose, plasma level, and therapeutic response exist. The steady-state plasma level achieved for a given drug dose can vary more than tenfold between individuals and plasma levels may help in interpreting apparent resistance to treatment and/or unexpected drug toxicity. The principal side effects of TCAs are antihistamine (sedation) and anticholinergic (constipation, dry mouth, urinary hesitancy, blurred vision). TCAs are contraindicated in patients with serious cardiovascular risk factors and overdoses of tricyclic agents can be lethal, with desipramine carrying the greatest risk. It is judicious to prescribe only a 10-day supply when suicide is a risk. Most patients require a daily dose of 150–200 mg of imipramine or amitriptyline or its equivalent to achieve a therapeutic blood level of 150–300 ng/mL and a satisfactory remission; some patients show a partial effect at lower doses. Geriatric patients may require a low starting dose and slow escalation. Ethnic differences in drug metabolism are significant, with Hispanic, Asian, and black patients generally requiring lower doses than whites to achieve a comparable blood level. P450 profiling using genetic chip technology may be clinically useful in predicting individual sensitivity.

Second-generation antidepressants include amoxapine, maprotiline, trazodone, and bupropion. Amoxapine is a dibenzoxazepine derivative that blocks norepinephrine and serotonin reuptake and has a metabolite that shows a degree of dopamine blockade. Long-term use of this drug carries a risk of tardive dyskinesia. Maprotiline is a potent noradrenergic reuptake blocker that has little anticholinergic effect but may produce seizures. Bupropion is a novel antidepressant whose mechanism of action is thought to involve enhancement of noradrenergic function. It has no anticholinergic, sedating, or orthostatic side effects and has a low incidence of sexual side effects. It may, however, be associated with stimulant-like side effects, may lower seizure threshold, and has an exceptionally short half-life, requiring frequent dosing. An extended-release preparation is available.

SSRIs such as fluoxetine, sertraline, paroxetine, citalopram, and escitalopram cause a lower frequency of anticholinergic, sedating, and cardiovascular side effects but a possibly greater incidence of gastrointestinal complaints, sleep impairment, and sexual dysfunction than do TCAs. Akathisia, involving an inner sense of restlessness and anxiety in addition to increased motor activity, may also be more common, particularly during the first week of treatment. One concern is the risk of "serotonin syndrome," thought to result from hyperstimulation of brainstem $5HT_{1A}$ receptors and characterized by myoclonus, agitation, abdominal cramping, hyperpyrexia, hypertension, and potentially death. Serotonergic agonists taken in combination should be monitored closely for this reason. Considerations such as half-life, compliance, toxicity, and drug-drug interactions may guide the choice of a particular SSRI. Fluoxetine and its principal active metabolite, norfluoxetine, for example, have a combined half-life of almost 7 days, resulting in a delay of 5 weeks before steady-state levels are achieved and a similar delay for complete drug excretion once its use is discontinued. All the SSRIs may impair sexual function, resulting in diminished libido, impotence, or difficulty in achieving orgasm. Sexual dysfunction frequently results in noncompliance and should be asked about specifically. Sexual dysfunction can sometimes be ameliorated by lowering the dose, by instituting weekend drug holidays (two or three times a month), or by treatment with amantadine (100 mg tid), bethanechol (25 mg tid), buspirone (10 mg tid), or bupropion (100–150 mg/d). Paroxetine appears to be more anticholinergic than either fluoxetine or sertraline, and sertraline carries a lower risk of producing an adverse drug interaction than the other two. Rare side effects of SSRIs include angina due to vasospasm and prolongation of the prothrombin time. Escitalopram is the most specific of currently available SSRIs and appears to have no specific inhibitory effects on the P450 system.

Venlafaxine, desvenlafaxine, and duloxetine block the reuptake of both norepinephrine and serotonin but produce relatively little in the way of traditional tricyclic side effects. Unlike the SSRIs, venlafaxine has a relatively linear dose-response curve. Patients should be monitored for a possible increase in diastolic blood pressure, and multiple daily dosing is required because of the drug's short half-life. An extended-release form is available and has a somewhat lower incidence of gastrointestinal side effects. Mirtazapine is a TCA that has a unique spectrum of activity. It increases noradrenergic and serotonergic neurotransmission through a blockade of central α_2-adrenergic receptors and postsynaptic $5HT_2$ and $5HT_3$ receptors. It is also strongly antihistaminic and, as such, may produce sedation.

With the exception of citalopram and escitalopram, each of the SSRIs may inhibit one or more cytochrome P450 enzymes. Depending on the specific isoenzyme involved, the metabolism of a number of concomitantly administered medications can be dramatically affected. Fluoxetine and paroxetine, for example, by inhibiting 2D6, can cause dramatic increases in the blood level of type 1C antiarrhythmics, while sertraline, by acting on 3A4, may alter blood levels of carbamazepine, or digoxin.

The MAOIs are highly effective, particularly in atypical depression, but the risk of hypertensive crisis following intake of tyramine-containing food or sympathomimetic drugs makes them inappropriate as first-line agents. Transdermal selegiline may avert this risk at low dose. Common side effects include orthostatic hypotension, weight gain, insomnia, and sexual dysfunction. MAOIs should not be used concomitantly with SSRIs, because of the risk of serotonin syndrome, or with TCAs, because of possible hyperadrenergic effects.

Electroconvulsive therapy is at least as effective as medication, but its use is reserved for treatment-resistant cases and delusional depressions. Transcranial magnetic stimulation (TMS) is approved for treatment-resistant depression and has been shown to have efficacy in several controlled trials. Vagus nerve stimulation (VNS) has also recently been approved for treatment-resistant depression, but its degree of efficacy is controversial. Deep brain stimulation is another treatment that is being used experimentally in treatment resistant cases.

Regardless of the treatment undertaken, the response should be evaluated after ~2 months. Three-quarters of patients show improvement by this time, but if remission is inadequate the patient should be questioned about compliance and an increase in medication dose should be considered if side effects are not troublesome. If this approach is unsuccessful, referral to a mental health specialist is advised. Strategies for treatment then include selection of an alternative drug, combinations of antidepressants, and/or adjunctive treatment with other classes of drugs, including lithium, thyroid hormone, atypical antipsychotic agents, and dopamine agonists. A large randomized trial (STAR-D) was unable to show preferential efficacy, but the addition of atypical antipsychotic drugs has received FDA approval. Patients whose response to an SSRI wanes over time may benefit from the addition of buspirone (10 mg tid) or pindolol (2–5 mg tid) or small amounts of a TCA such as desipramine (25 mg bid or tid). Most patients will show some degree of response but aggressive treatment should be pursued until remission is achieved, and drug treatment should be continued for at least 6–9 more months to prevent relapse. In patients who have had two or more episodes of depression, indefinite maintenance treatment should be considered.

It is essential to educate patients both about depression and the benefits and side effects of medications they are receiving. Advice about stress reduction and cautions that alcohol may exacerbate depressive symptoms and impair drug response are helpful. Patients should be given time to describe their experience, their outlook, and the impact of the depression on them and their families. Occasional empathic silence may be as helpful for the treatment alliance as verbal reassurance. Controlled trials have shown that cognitive-behavioral and interpersonal therapies are effective in improving psychological and social adjustment and that a combined treatment approach is more successful than medication alone for many patients.

BIPOLAR DISORDER

Clinical manifestations

Bipolar disorder is characterized by unpredictable swings in mood from mania (or hypomania) to depression. Some patients suffer only from recurrent attacks of *mania*, which in its pure form is associated with increased psychomotor activity; excessive social extroversion; decreased need for sleep; impulsivity and impairment in judgment; and expansive, grandiose, and sometimes irritable mood (Table 391-10). In severe mania, patients may experience delusions and paranoid thinking indistinguishable from schizophrenia.

TABLE 391-10 Criteria for a Manic Episode

A. A distinct period of abnormally and persistently elevated, expansive, or irritable mood, lasting at least 1 week (or any duration if hospitalization is necessary)

B. During the period of mood disturbance, three (or more) of the following symptoms have persisted (four if the mood is only irritable) and have been present to a significant degree:

1. Inflated self-esteem or grandiosity
2. Decreased need for sleep (e.g., feels rested after only 3 hours of sleep)
3. More talkative than usual or pressure to keep talking
4. Flight of ideas or subjective experience that thoughts are racing
5. Distractibility (i.e., attention too easily drawn to unimportant or irrelevant external stimuli)
6. Increase in goal-directed activity (either socially, at work or school, or sexually) or psychomotor agitation
7. Excessive involvement in pleasurable activities that have a high potential for painful consequences (e.g., engaging in unrestrained buying sprees, sexual indiscretions, or foolish business investments)

C. The symptoms do not meet criteria for a mixed episode.

D. The mood disturbance is sufficiently severe to cause marked impairment in occupational functioning or in usual social activities or relationships with others, or to necessitate hospitalization to prevent harm to self or others, or there are psychotic features.

E. The symptoms are not due to the direct physiologic effects of a substance (e.g., a drug of abuse, a medication, or other treatment) or a general medical condition (e.g., hyperthyroidism).

Note: Manic-like episodes that are clearly caused by somatic antidepressant treatment (e.g., medication, electroconvulsive therapy, light therapy) should not count toward a diagnosis of bipolar I disorder.

Source: *Diagnostic and Statistical Manual of Mental Disorders*, 4th ed. Washington, DC, American Psychiatric Association, 2000.

One-half of patients with bipolar disorder present with a mixture of psychomotor agitation and activation with dysphoria, anxiety, and irritability. It may be difficult to distinguish *mixed mania* from *agitated depression*. In some bipolar patients (*bipolar II disorder*), the full criteria for mania are lacking, and the requisite recurrent depressions are separated by periods of mild activation and increased energy (hypomania). In *cyclothymic disorder*, there are numerous hypomanic periods, usually of relatively short duration, alternating with clusters of depressive symptoms that fail, either in severity or duration, to meet the criteria of major depression. The mood fluctuations are chronic and should be present for at least 2 years before the diagnosis is made.

Manic episodes typically emerge over a period of days to weeks, but onset within hours is possible, usually in the early morning hours. An untreated episode of either depression or mania can be as short as several weeks or last as long as 8–12 months, and rare patients have an unremitting chronic course. The term *rapid cycling* is used for patients who have four or more episodes of either depression or mania in a given year. This pattern occurs in 15% of all patients, almost all of whom are women. In some cases, rapid cycling is linked to an underlying thyroid dysfunction and, in others, it is iatrogenically triggered by prolonged antidepressant treatment. Approximately one-half of patients have sustained difficulties in work performance and psychosocial functioning, with depressive phases being more responsible for impairment than mania.

Bipolar disorder is common, affecting ~1.5% of the population in the United States. Onset is typically between 20 and 30 years of age, but many individuals report premorbid symptoms in late childhood or early adolescence. The prevalence is similar for men and women; women are likely to have more depressive and men more manic episodes over a lifetime.

Differential diagnosis

The differential diagnosis of mania includes secondary mania induced by stimulant or sympathomimetic drugs, hyperthyroidism, AIDS, neurologic disorders, such as Huntington's or Wilson's disease, and cerebrovascular accidents. Comorbidity with alcohol and substance abuse is common, either because of poor judgment and increased impulsivity or because of an attempt to self-treat the underlying mood symptoms and sleep disturbances.

Etiology and pathophysiology

Genetic predisposition to bipolar disorder is evident from family studies; the concordance rate for monozygotic twins approaches 80%. Patients with bipolar disorder also appear to have altered circadian rhythmicity, and lithium may exert its therapeutic benefit through a resynchronization of intrinsic rhythms keyed to the light/dark cycle. A detailed discussion of the pathogenesis of bipolar disorder is presented in Chap. 390.

TREATMENT Bipolar Disorder

(Table 391-11) Lithium carbonate is the mainstay of treatment in bipolar disorder, although sodium valproate and olanzapine are equally effective in acute mania, as is lamotrigine in the depressed phase. The response rate to lithium carbonate is 70–80% in acute mania, with beneficial effects appearing in 1–2 weeks. Lithium also has a prophylactic effect in prevention of recurrent mania and, to a lesser extent, in the prevention of recurrent depression. A simple cation, lithium is rapidly absorbed from the gastrointestinal tract and remains unbound to plasma or tissue proteins. Some 95% of a given dose is excreted unchanged through the kidneys within 24 hours.

TABLE 391-11 Clinical Pharmacology of Mood Stabilizers

Agent and Dosing	Side Effects and Other Effects
Lithium	**Common Side Effects**
Starting dose: 300 mg bid or tid Therapeutic blood level: 0.8–1.2 meq/L	Nausea/anorexia/diarrhea, fine tremor, thirst, polyuria, fatigue, weight gain, acne, folliculitis, neutrophilia, hypothyroidism Blood level is increased by thiazides, tetracyclines, and NSAIDs Blood level is decreased by bronchodilators, verapamil, and carbonic anhydrase inhibitors *Rare side effects:* Neurotoxicity, renal toxicity, hypercalcemia, ECG changes
Valproic Acid	**Common Side Effects**
Starting dose: 250 mg tid Therapeutic blood level: 50–125 μg/mL	Nausea/anorexia, weight gain, sedation, tremor, rash, alopecia Inhibits hepatic metabolism of other medications *Rare side effects:* Pancreatitis, hepatotoxicity, Stevens-Johnson syndrome
Carbamazepine/ Oxcarbazepine	**Common Side Effects**
Starting dose: 200 mg bid for carbamazepine, 150 mg bid for oxcarbazepine Therapeutic blood level: 4–12 μg/mL for carbamazepine	Nausea/anorexia, sedation, rash, dizziness/ataxia Carbamazepine, but not oxcarbazepine, induces hepatic metabolism of other medications *Rare side effects:* Hyponatremia, agranulocytosis, Stevens-Johnson syndrome
Lamotrigine	**Common Side Effects**
Starting dose: 25 mg/d	Rash, dizziness, headache, tremor, sedation, nausea *Rare side effect:* Stevens-Johnson syndrome

Abbreviations: NSAIDs, nonsteroidal anti-inflammatory drugs; ECG, electrocardiogram.

Serious side effects from lithium are rare, but minor complaints such as gastrointestinal discomfort, nausea, diarrhea, polyuria, weight gain, skin eruptions, alopecia, and edema are common. Over time, urine-concentrating ability may be decreased, but significant nephrotoxicity does not usually occur. Lithium exerts an antithyroid effect by interfering with the synthesis and release of thyroid hormones. More serious side effects include tremor, poor concentration and memory, ataxia, dysarthria, and incoordination. There is suggestive, but not conclusive, evidence that lithium is teratogenic, inducing cardiac malformations in the first trimester.

In the treatment of acute mania, lithium is initiated at 300 mg bid or tid, and the dose is then increased by 300 mg every 2–3 days to achieve blood levels of 0.8–1.2 meq/L. Because the therapeutic effect of lithium may not appear until after 7–10 days of treatment, adjunctive usage of lorazepam (1–2 mg every 4 hours) or clonazepam (0.5–1 mg every 4 hours) may be beneficial to control agitation. Antipsychotics are indicated in patients with severe agitation who respond only partially to benzodiazepines. Patients using lithium should be monitored closely, since the blood levels required to achieve a therapeutic benefit are close to those associated with toxicity.

Valproic acid may be better than lithium for patients who experience rapid cycling (i.e., more than four episodes a year) or who present with a mixed or dysphoric mania. Tremor and weight gain are the most common side effects; hepatotoxicity and pancreatitis are rare toxicities.

Carbamazepine and oxcarbazepine, although not formally approved by the FDA for bipolar disorder, have clinical efficacy in the treatment of acute mania. Second-generation antipsychotic drugs (olanzapine, quetiapine, risperidone, ziprasidone, aripiprazole, and asenapine) have also been shown to be effective, either alone or in combination with a mood stabilizer. An increased risk of weight gain and other metabolic abnormalities is a concern with these agents.

The recurrent nature of bipolar mood disorder necessitates maintenance treatment. A sustained blood lithium level of at least 0.8 mEq/L is important for optimal prophylaxis and has been shown to reduce risk of suicide, a finding not yet apparent for other mood stabilizers. Compliance is frequently an issue and often requires enlistment and education of concerned family members. Efforts to identify and modify psychosocial factors that may trigger episodes are important, as is an emphasis on lifestyle regularity. Antidepressant medications are sometimes required for the treatment of severe breakthrough depressions, but their use should generally be avoided during maintenance treatment because of the risk of precipitating mania or accelerating the cycle frequency. Loss of efficacy over time may be observed with any of the mood-stabilizing agents. In such situations, an alternative agent or combination therapy is usually helpful.

Consensus guidelines for the treatment of acute mania and bipolar depression are described in Table 391-12.

TABLE 391-12 Consensus Guidelines on the Drug Treatment of Acute Mania and Bipolar Depression

Condition	Preferred Agents
Euphoric mania	Lithium
Mixed/dysphoric mania	Valproic acid
Mania with psychosis	Valproic acid with olanzapine, aripiprazole, conventional antipsychotic, or risperidone
Hypomania	Lithium, lamotrigine, or valproic acid alone
Severe depression with psychosis	Venlafaxine, bupropion, or paroxetine *plus* lithium *plus* olanzapine, *or* risperidone; consider ECT
Severe depression without psychosis	Bupropion, paroxetine, sertraline, venlafaxine, *or* citalopram *plus* lithium
Mild to moderate depression	Lithium *or* lamotrigine alone; add bupropion if needed

Abbreviation: ECT, electroconvulsive therapy.
Source: From GS Sachs et al: Postgrad Med April, 2000.

SOMATOFORM DISORDERS

CLINICAL MANIFESTATIONS

Patients with multiple somatic complaints that cannot be explained by a known medical condition or by the effects of alcohol or of recreational or prescription drugs are commonly seen in primary care practice; one survey indicated a prevalence of such complaints of 5%. In *somatization disorder*, the patient presents with multiple physical complaints referable to different organ systems (Table 391-13). Onset is usually before age 30 years, and the disorder is persistent. Formal diagnostic criteria require the recording of at least four pain, two gastrointestinal, one sexual, and one pseudoneurologic symptom. Patients with somatization disorder often present with dramatic complaints, but the complaints are inconsistent. Symptoms of comorbid anxiety and mood disorder are common and may be the result of drug interactions due to regimens initiated independently by different physicians. Patients with somatization disorder may be impulsive and demanding and

TABLE 391-13 Diagnostic Criteria for Somatization Disorder

A. A history of many physical complaints beginning before age 30 years that occur over a period of several years and result in treatment being sought or significant impairment in social, occupational, or other important areas of functioning.

B. Each of the following criteria must have been met, with individual symptoms occurring at any time during the course of the disturbance:
   1. *Four pain symptoms:* a history of pain related to at least four different sites or functions (e.g., head, abdomen, back, joints, extremities, chest, rectum, during menstruation, during sexual intercourse, or during urination)
   2. *Two gastrointestinal symptoms:* a history of at least two gastrointestinal symptoms other than pain (e.g., nausea, bloating, vomiting other than during pregnancy, diarrhea, or intolerance of several different foods)
   3. *One sexual symptom:* a history of at least one sexual or reproductive symptom other than pain (e.g., sexual indifference, erectile or ejaculatory dysfunction, irregular menses, excessive menstrual bleeding, vomiting throughout pregnancy)
   4. *One pseudoneurologic symptom:* a history of at least one symptom or deficit suggesting a neurologic condition not limited to pain (conversion symptoms such as impaired coordination or balance, paralysis or localized weakness, difficulty swallowing or lump in throat, aphonia, urinary retention, hallucinations, loss of touch or pain sensation, double vision, blindness, deafness, seizures; dissociative symptoms such as amnesia; or loss of consciousness other than fainting)

C. Either of the following:
   1. After appropriate investigation, each of the symptoms in criterion B cannot be fully explained by a known general medical condition or the direct effects of a substance (e.g., a drug of abuse, a medication)
   2. When there is a related general medical condition, the physical complaints or resulting social or occupational impairment are in excess of what would be expected from the history, physical examination, or laboratory findings

D. The symptoms are not intentionally produced or feigned (as in factitious disorder or malingering).

Source: *Diagnostic and Statistical Manual of Mental Disorders*, 4th ed. Washington, DC, American Psychiatric Association, 2000.

frequently qualify for a formal comorbid psychiatric diagnosis. In *conversion disorder*, the symptoms focus on deficits that involve motor or sensory function and on psychological factors that initiate or exacerbate the medical presentation. Like somatization disorder, the deficit is not intentionally produced or simulated, as is the case in factitious disorder (malingering). In *hypochondriasis*, the essential feature is a belief of serious medical illness that persists despite reassurance and appropriate medical evaluation. As with somatization disorder, patients with hypochondriasis have a history of poor relationships with physicians stemming from their sense that they have been evaluated and treated inappropriately or inadequately. Hypochondriasis can be disabling in intensity and is persistent, with waxing and waning symptomatology.

In *factitious illnesses*, the patient consciously and voluntarily produces physical symptoms of illness. The term *Munchausen's syndrome* is reserved for individuals with particularly dramatic, chronic, or severe factitious illness. In true factitious illness, the sick role itself is gratifying. A variety of signs, symptoms, and diseases have been either simulated or caused by factitious behavior, the most common including chronic diarrhea, fever of unknown origin, intestinal bleeding or hematuria, seizures, and hypoglycemia. Factitious disorder is usually not diagnosed until 5–10 years after its onset, and it can produce significant social and medical costs. In *malingering*, the fabrication derives from a desire for some external reward such as a narcotic medication or disability reimbursement.

TREATMENT Somatoform Disorders

Patients with somatization disorders are frequently subjected to many diagnostic tests and exploratory surgeries in an attempt to find their "real" illness. Such an approach is doomed to failure and does not address the core issue. Successful treatment is best achieved through behavior modification, in which access to the physician is tightly regulated and adjusted to provide a sustained and predictable level of support that is less clearly contingent on the patient's level of presenting distress. Visits can be brief and should not be associated with a need for a diagnostic or treatment action. Although the literature is limited, some patients with somatization disorder may benefit from antidepressant treatment.

Any attempt to confront the patient usually creates a sense of humiliation and causes the patient to abandon treatment from that caregiver. A better strategy is to introduce psychological causation as one of a number of possible explanations and to include factitious illness as an option in the differential diagnoses that are discussed. Without directly linking psychotherapeutic intervention to the diagnosis, the patient can be offered a face-saving means by which the pathologic relationship with the health care system can be examined and alternative approaches to life stressors developed.

PERSONALITY DISORDERS

Clinical manifestations

Personality disorders are characteristic patterns of thinking, feeling, and interpersonal behavior that are relatively inflexible and cause significant functional impairment or subjective distress for the individual. The observed behaviors are not secondary to another mental disorder, nor are they precipitated by substance abuse or a general medical condition. This distinction is often difficult to make in clinical practice, as personality change may be the first sign of serious neurologic, endocrine, or other medical illness. Patients with frontal lobe tumors, for example, can present with changes in motivation and personality while the results of the neurologic examination remain within normal limits. Individuals with personality disorders are often regarded as "difficult patients" in clinical medical practice because they are seen as excessively demanding and/or unwilling to follow recommended treatment plans. Although DSM-IV portrays personality disorders as qualitatively distinct categories, there is an alternative perspective that personality characteristics vary as a continuum between normal functioning and formal mental disorder.

Personality disorders have been grouped into three overlapping clusters. *Cluster A* includes paranoid, schizoid, and schizotypal personality disorders. It includes individuals who are odd and eccentric and who maintain an emotional distance from others. Individuals have a restricted emotional range and remain socially isolated. Patients with schizotypal personality disorder frequently have unusual perceptual experiences and express magical beliefs about the external world. The essential feature of paranoid personality disorder is a pervasive mistrust and suspiciousness of others to an extent that is unjustified by available evidence. *Cluster B* disorders include antisocial, borderline, histrionic, and narcissistic types and describe individuals whose behavior is impulsive, excessively emotional, and erratic. *Cluster C* incorporates avoidant, dependent, and obsessive-compulsive personality types; enduring traits are anxiety and fear. The boundaries between cluster types are to some extent artificial, and many patients who meet criteria for one personality disorder also meet criteria for aspects of another. The risk of a comorbid major mental disorder is increased in patients who qualify for a diagnosis of personality disorder.

TREATMENT Personality Disorders

Dialectical behavior therapy (DBT) is a cognitive-behavioral approach that focuses on behavioral change while providing acceptance, compassion, and validation of the patient. Several randomized trials have demonstrated the efficacy of DBT in the treatment of personality disorders. Antidepressant medications and low-dose antipsychotic drugs have some efficacy in cluster A personality disorders, while anticonvulsant mood-stabilizing agents and MAOIs may be considered for patients with cluster B diagnoses who show marked mood reactivity, behavioral dyscontrol, and/or rejection hypersensitivity. Anxious or fearful cluster C patients often respond to medications used for axis I anxiety disorders (see above). It is important that the physician and the patient have reasonable expectations vis-à-vis the possible benefit of any medication used and its side effects. Improvement may be subtle and observable only over time.

SCHIZOPHRENIA

Clinical manifestations

Schizophrenia is a heterogeneous syndrome characterized by perturbations of language, perception, thinking, social activity, affect, and volition. There are no pathognomonic features. The syndrome commonly begins in late adolescence, has an insidious (and less commonly acute) onset, and, often, a poor outcome, progressing from social withdrawal and perceptual distortions to recurrent delusions and hallucinations. Patients may present with positive symptoms (such as conceptual disorganization, delusions, or hallucinations) or negative symptoms (loss of function, anhedonia, decreased emotional expression, impaired concentration, and diminished social engagement) and must have at least two of these for a 1-month period and continuous signs for at least 6 months to meet formal diagnostic criteria. As individuals age, positive psychotic symptoms tend to attenuate and some measure of social and occupational function may be regained. "Negative" symptoms predominate in one-third of the schizophrenic population and are associated with a poor long-term outcome and a poor response to drug treatment. However, marked variability in the course and individual character of symptoms is typical.

The four main subtypes of schizophrenia are catatonic, paranoid, disorganized, and residual. Many individuals have symptoms of more than one type. *Catatonic-type* describes patients whose clinical presentation is dominated by profound changes in motor activity, negativism, and echolalia or echopraxia. *Paranoid-type* describes patients who have a prominent preoccupation with a specific delusional system and who otherwise do not qualify as having *disorganized-type* disease, in which disorganized speech and behavior are accompanied by a superficial or silly affect. In *residual-type* disease, negative symptomatology exists in the absence of delusions, hallucinations, or motor disturbance. The term *schizophreniform disorder* describes patients who meet the symptom requirements but not the duration requirements for schizophrenia, and *schizoaffective disorder* is used for those who manifest symptoms of schizophrenia and independent periods of mood disturbance. Prognosis depends not on symptom severity but on the response to antipsychotic medication. A permanent remission without recurrence does occasionally occur. About 10% of schizophrenic patients commit suicide.

Schizophrenia is present in 0.85% of individuals worldwide, with a lifetime prevalence of ~1–1.5%. An estimated 300,000 episodes of acute schizophrenia occur annually in the United States, resulting in direct and indirect costs of $62.7 billion.

Differential diagnosis

The diagnosis is principally one of exclusion, requiring the absence of significant associated mood symptoms, any relevant medical condition, and substance abuse. Drug reactions that cause hallucinations, paranoia, confusion, or bizarre behavior may be dose-related or idiosyncratic; parkinsonian medications, clonidine, quinacrine, and procaine derivatives are the most common prescription medications associated with these symptoms. Drug causes should be ruled out in any case of newly emergent psychosis. The general neurologic examination in patients with schizophrenia is usually normal, but motor rigidity, tremor, and dyskinesias are noted in one-quarter of untreated patients.

Epidemiology and pathophysiology

Epidemiologic surveys identify several risk factors for schizophrenia, including genetic susceptibility, early developmental insults, winter birth, and increasing parental age. Genetic factors are involved in at least a subset of individuals who develop schizophrenia. Schizophrenia is observed in ~6.6% of all first-degree relatives of an affected proband. If both parents are affected, the risk for offspring is 40%. The concordance rate for monozygotic twins is 50%, compared to 10% for dizygotic twins. Schizophrenia-prone families are also at risk for other psychiatric disorders, including schizoaffective disorder and *schizotypal* and *schizoid personality disorders*, the latter terms designating individuals who show a lifetime pattern of social and interpersonal deficits characterized by an inability to form close interpersonal relationships, eccentric behavior, and mild perceptual distortions. The pathogenesis of schizophrenia is discussed in detail in Chap. 390.

TREATMENT Schizophrenia

Antipsychotic agents (Table 391-14) are the cornerstone of acute and maintenance treatment of schizophrenia and are effective in the treatment of hallucinations, delusions, and thought disorders, regardless of etiology. The mechanism of action involves, at least in part, binding to dopamine D_2/D_3 receptors in the ventral striatum; the clinical potencies of traditional antipsychotic drugs parallel their affinities for the D_2 receptor, and even the newer "atypical" agents exert some degree of D_2 receptor blockade. All neuroleptics induce expression of the immediate-early gene *c-fos* in the nucleus accumbens, a dopaminergic site connecting prefrontal and limbic cortices. The clinical efficacy of newer atypical neuroleptics, however, may involve *N*-methyl-D-aspartate (NMDA) receptor blockade, α_1- and α_2-noradrenergic activity, altering the relationship between $5HT_2$ and D_2 receptor activity, as well as faster dissociation of D_2 binding and effects on neuroplasticity.

Conventional neuroleptics differ in their potency and side-effect profile. Older agents such as chlorpromazine and thioridazine, are more sedating and anticholinergic and more likely to cause orthostatic hypotension, while higher potency antipsychotics such as haloperidol, perphenazine, and thiothixene, are more likely to induce extrapyramidal side effects. The model "atypical" antipsychotic agent is *clozapine*, a dibenzodiazepine that has a greater potency in blocking the $5HT_2$ than the D_2 receptor and a much higher affinity for the D_4 than the D_2 receptor. Its principal disadvantage is a risk of blood dyscrasias. Paliperidone is a recently approved agent that is a metabolite of risperidone and shares many of its properties. Unlike other antipsychotics, clozapine does not cause a rise in prolactin level. Approximately 30% of patients who do not benefit from conventional antipsychotic agents will have a better response to this drug, which also has a demonstrated superiority to other antipsychotic agents in preventing suicide; however, its side-effect profile makes it most appropriate for treatment-resistant cases. *Risperidone*, a benzisoxazole derivative, is more potent at $5HT_2$ than D_2 receptor sites, like clozapine, but it also exerts significant α_2 antagonism, a property that may contribute to its perceived ability to improve mood and increase motor activity. Risperidone is not as effective as clozapine in treatment-resistant cases but does not carry a risk of blood dyscrasias. *Olanzapine* is similar neurochemically to clozapine but has a significant risk of inducing weight gain. *Quetiapine* is distinct in having a weak D_2 effect but potent α_1 and histamine blockade. *Ziprasidone* causes minimal weight gain and is unlikely to increase prolactin but may increase QT prolongation. *Aripiprazole* also has little risk of weight gain or prolactin increase but may increase anxiety, nausea, and insomnia as a result of its partial agonist properties.

Antipsychotic agents are effective in 70% of patients presenting with a first episode. Improvement may be observed within hours or days, but full remission usually requires 6–8 weeks. The choice of agent depends principally on the side effect profile and cost of treatment or on a past personal or family history of a favorable response to the drug in question. Atypical agents appear to be more effective in treating negative symptoms and improving cognitive function. An equivalent treatment response can usually be achieved with relatively low doses of any drug selected (i.e., 4–6 mg/d of haloperidol, 10–15 mg of olanzapine, or 4–6 mg/d of risperidone). Doses in this range result in >80% D_2 receptor blockade, and there is little evidence that higher doses increase either the rapidity or degree of response. Maintenance treatment requires careful attention to the possibility of relapse and monitoring for the development of a movement disorder. Intermittent drug treatment is less effective than regular dosing, but gradual dose reduction is likely to improve social functioning in many schizophrenic patients who have been maintained at high doses. If medications are completely discontinued, however, the relapse rate is 60% within 6 months.

TABLE 391-14 Antipsychotic Agents

Name	Usual PO Daily Dose, mg	Side Effects	Sedation	Comments
First-Generation Antipsychotics				
Low-potency				
Chlorpromazine (Thorazine)	100–1000	Anticholinergic effects; orthostasis; photosensitivity; cholestasis; QT prolongation	+ + +	EPSEs usually not prominent; can cause anticholinergic delirium in elderly patients
Thioridazine (Mellaril)	100–600			
Midpotency				
Trifluoperazine (Stelazine)	2–50	Fewer anticholinergic side effects	+ +	Well tolerated by most patients
Perphenazine (Trilafon)	4–64	Fewer EPSEs than with higher potency agents.	++	
Loxapine (Loxitane)	30–100	Frequent EPSEs	+ +	
Molindone (Moban)	30–100	Frequent EPSEs	0	Little weight gain
High potency				
Haloperidol (Haldol)	5–20	No anticholinergic side effects; EPSEs often prominent	0/+	Often prescribed in doses that are too high; long-acting injectable forms of haloperidol and fluphenazine available
Fluphenazine (Prolixin)	1–20	Frequent EPSEs	0/+	
Thiothixene (Navane)	2–50	Frequent EPSEs	0/+	
Second-Generation Antipsychotics				
Clozapine (Clozaril)	150–600	Agranulocytosis (1%); weight gain; seizures; drooling; hyperthermia	+ +	Requires weekly WBC count for first 6 months, then biweekly if stable
Risperidone (Risperdal)	2–8	Orthostasis	+	Requires slow titration; EPSEs observed with doses >6 mg qd
Olanzapine (Zyprexa)	10–30	Weight gain	+ +	Mild prolactin elevation
Quetiapine (Seroquel)	350–800	Sedation; weight gain; anxiety	+ + +	Bid dosing
Ziprasidone (Geodon)	120–200	Orthostatic hypotension	+/++	Minimal weight gain; increases QT interval
Aripiprazole (Abilify)	10–30	Nausea, anxiety, insomnia	0/+	Mixed agonist/antagonist
Paliperidone (Invega)	3–12	Restlessness, EPSEs	+	Active metabolite of risperidone
Iloperidone (Fanapt)	12–24	Dizziness, hypotension	0/+	Requires dose titration
Asenapine (Saphris)	10–20	Dizziness, EPSEs, weight gain	++	Sublingual tablets; bid dosing
Lurasidone (Latuda)	40–80	Nausea, EPSEs	++	Uses CYP3A4

Abbreviations: EPSEs, extrapyramidal side effects; WBC, white blood cell.

Long-acting injectable preparations (risperidone) are considered when noncompliance with oral therapy leads to relapses. In treatment-resistant patients, a transition to clozapine usually results in rapid improvement, but a prolonged delay in response in some cases necessitates a 6- to 9-month trial for maximal benefit to occur.

Antipsychotic medications can cause a broad range of side effects, including lethargy, weight gain, postural hypotension, constipation, and dry mouth. Extrapyramidal symptoms such as dystonia, akathisia, and akinesia are also frequent with first-generation agents and may contribute to poor adherence if not specifically addressed. Anticholinergic and parkinsonian symptoms respond well to trihexyphenidyl, 2 mg bid, or benztropine mesylate, 1–2 mg bid. Akathisia may respond to beta blockers. In rare cases, more serious and occasionally life-threatening side effects may emerge, including hyperprolactinemia, ventricular arrhythmias, gastrointestinal obstruction, retinal pigmentation, obstructive jaundice, and neuroleptic malignant syndrome (characterized by hyperthermia, autonomic dysfunction, muscular rigidity, and elevated creatine phosphokinase levels). The most serious adverse effects of clozapine are agranulocytosis, which has an incidence of 1%, and induction of seizures, which has an incidence of 10%. Weekly white blood cell counts are required, particularly during the first 3 months of treatment.

The risk of type 2 diabetes mellitus appears to be increased in schizophrenia, and second-generation agents as a group produce greater adverse effects on glucose regulation, independent of effects on obesity, than traditional agents. Clozapine, olanzapine, and quetiapine seem more likely to cause hyperglycemia, weight gain, and hypertriglyceridemia than other atypical antipsychotic drugs. Close monitoring of plasma glucose and lipid levels are indicated with the use of these agents.

A serious side effect of long-term use of first generation antipsychotic agents is *tardive dyskinesia*, characterized by repetitive, involuntary, and potentially irreversible movements of the tongue and lips (bucco-linguo-masticatory triad), and, in approximately half of cases, choreoathetosis. Tardive dyskinesia has an incidence of 2–4% per year of exposure, and a prevalence of 20% in chronically treated patients. The prevalence increases with age, total dose, and duration of drug administration. The risk associated with second-generation agents appears to be much lower. The cause may involve formation of free radicals and perhaps mitochondrial energy failure. Vitamin E may reduce abnormal involuntary movements if given early in the syndrome.

The CATIE study, a large-scale investigation of the effectiveness of antipsychotic agents in "real world" patients, revealed a high rate of discontinuation of treatment over 18 months. Olanzapine showed greater effectiveness than quetiapine, risperidone, perphenazine, or ziprasidone but also a higher discontinuation rate due to weight gain and metabolic effects. Surprisingly, perphenazine, a first-generation agent, showed little evidence of inferiority to newer drugs.

Drug treatment of schizophrenia is by itself insufficient. Educational efforts directed toward families and relevant community resources have proved to be necessary to maintain stability and optimize outcome. A treatment model involving a multidisciplinary case-management team that seeks out and closely follows the patient in the community has proved particularly effective.

ASSESSMENT AND EVALUATION OF VIOLENCE

Primary care physicians may encounter situations in which family, domestic, or societal violence is discovered or suspected. Such an awareness can carry legal and moral obligations; many state laws mandate reporting of child, spousal, and elder abuse. Physicians are frequently the first point of contact for both victim and abuser. Approximately 2 million older Americans and 1.5 million U.S. children are thought to experience some form of physical maltreatment each year. Spousal abuse is thought to be even more prevalent. An interview study of 24,000 women in 10 countries found a lifetime prevalence of physical or sexual violence that ranged from 15 to 71%; these individuals are more likely to suffer from depression, anxiety, somatization disorder, and substance abuse and to have attempted suicide. In addition, abused individuals frequently express low self-esteem, vague somatic symptomatology, social isolation, and a passive feeling of loss of control. Although it is essential to treat these elements in the victim, the first obligation is to ensure that the perpetrator has taken responsibility for preventing any further violence. Substance abuse and/or dependence and serious mental illness in the abuser may contribute to the risk of harm and require direct intervention. Depending on the situation, law enforcement agencies, community resources such as support groups and shelters, and individual and family counseling can be appropriate components of a treatment plan. A safety plan should be formulated with the victim, in addition to providing information about abuse, its likelihood of recurrence, and its tendency to increase in severity and frequency. Antianxiety and antidepressant medications may sometimes be useful in treating the acute symptoms, but only if independent evidence for an appropriate psychiatric diagnosis exists.

MENTAL HEALTH PROBLEMS IN THE HOMELESS

There is a high prevalence of mental disorders and substance abuse among homeless and impoverished individuals. Depending on the definition used, estimates of the total number of homeless individuals in the United States range from 800,000 to 2 million, one-third of whom qualify as having a serious mental disorder. Poor hygiene and nutrition, substance abuse, psychiatric illness, physical trauma, and exposure to the elements combine to make the provision of medical care challenging. Only a minority of these individuals receive formal mental health care; the main points of contact are outpatient medical clinics and emergency departments. Primary care settings represent a critical site in which housing needs, treatment of substance dependence, and evaluation and treatment of psychiatric illness can most efficiently take place. Successful intervention is dependent on breaking down traditional administrative barriers to health care and recognizing the physical constraints and emotional costs imposed by homelessness. Simplifying health care instructions and follow-up, allowing frequent visits, and dispensing medications in limited amounts that require ongoing contact are possible techniques for establishing a successful therapeutic relationship.

FURTHER READINGS

Allgulander C: Generalized anxiety disorder: Between now and DSM-V. Psychiatr Clin North Am 32:611, 2009

American Psychiatric Association: American Psychiatric Association Practice Guidelines for the Treatment of Psychiatric Disorders: *http://www.Psychiatryonline.com/Pracguide*

Buchanan RW et al: Schizophrenia Patient Outcomes Research Team (PORT): The 2009 schizophrenia PORT psychopharmacological treatment recommendations and summary statements. Schizophr Bull 1:71, 2010

Figueredo VM: The time has come for physicians to take notice: The impact of psychosocial stressors on the heart. Am J Med 8:704, 2009

Frye MA: Bipolar disorder—A focus on depression. N Engl J Med 364:51, 2011

Grunze H et al: The World Federation of Societies of Biological Psychiatry (WFSBP) Guidelines for the Biological Treatment of Bipolar Disorders: Update 2010 on the treatment of acute bipolar depression. World J Biol Psychiatry 2:81, 2010

Laugharne J et al: Role of psychological trauma in the cause and treatment of anxiety and depressive disorders. Curr Opin Psychiatry 1:25, 2010

Nutt DJ et al: International consensus statement on major depressive disorder. J Clin Psychiatry 71 Suppl E1:e08, 2010

Ravindran LN: Pharmacotherapy of PTSD: Premises, principles, and priorities. Brain Res 1293:24, 2009

Reid S, Barbui C: Long term treatment of depression with selective serotonin reuptake inhibitors and newer antidepressants. BMJ 340:c1468. doi:10.1136/bmj.c1468, 2010

Schanzer B et al: Homelessness, health status, and health care use. Am J Public Health 97:464, 2007

SECTION 6 Alcoholism and Drug Dependency

CHAPTER 392 Alcohol and Alcoholism

Marc A. Schuckit

INTRODUCTION

Alcohol (beverage ethanol) distributes throughout the body, affecting almost all systems and altering nearly every neurochemical process in the brain. This drug is likely to exacerbate most medical conditions, affect almost any medication metabolized in the liver, and temporarily mimic many medical (e.g., diabetes) and psychiatric (e.g., depression) conditions. Because ~80% of people in Western countries have consumed alcohol, and two-thirds have been drunk in the prior year, the lifetime risk for serious, repetitive alcohol problems is almost 20% for men and 10% for women, regardless of a person's education or income. While low doses of alcohol have some healthful benefits, the intake of more than three standard drinks per day on a regular basis enhances the risk for cancer and vascular disease, and alcohol use disorders decrease the life span by about 10 years. Unfortunately, most clinicians have had only limited education regarding these conditions. This chapter presents a brief overview of clinically useful information about alcohol use, abuse, and dependence.

PHARMACOLOGY AND NUTRITIONAL IMPACT OF ETHANOL

Blood levels of ethanol are expressed as milligrams or grams of ethanol per deciliter (e.g., 100 mg/dL = 0.10 g/dL), with values of ~0.02 g/dL resulting from the ingestion of one typical drink. In round figures, 340 mL (12 oz) of beer, 115 mL (4 oz) of nonfortified wine, and 43 mL (1.5 oz) (a shot) of 80-proof beverage such as whisky, gin, or vodka each contain ~10–15 g of ethanol and represent a standard drink; 0.5 L (1 pint) of 80-proof beverage contains ~160 g (about 16 standard drinks), and 750 mL of wine contains ~60 g of ethanol. These beverages also have additional components known as *congeners* that affect the drink's taste and might contribute to adverse effects on the body. Congeners include methanol, butanol, acetaldehyde, histamine, tannins, iron, and lead. Alcohol acutely decreases neuronal activity and has similar behavioral effects and cross-tolerance with other depressants, including benzodiazepines and barbiturates.

Alcohol is absorbed from mucous membranes of the mouth and esophagus (in small amounts), from the stomach and large bowel (in modest amounts), and from the proximal portion of the small intestine (the major site). The rate of absorption is increased by rapid gastric emptying (as can be induced by carbonated beverages); by the absence of proteins, fats, or carbohydrates (which interfere with absorption); and by dilution to a modest percentage of ethanol (maximum at ~20% by volume).

Between 2% (at low blood alcohol concentrations) and 10% (at high blood alcohol concentrations) of ethanol is excreted directly through the lungs, urine, or sweat, but the greater part is metabolized to acetaldehyde, primarily in the liver. The most important pathway occurs in the cell cytosol where alcohol dehydrogenase (ADH) produces acetaldehyde, which is then rapidly destroyed by aldehyde dehydrogenase (ALDH) in the cytosol and mitochondria (Fig. 392-1). A second pathway in the microsomes of the smooth endoplasmic reticulum (the microsomal ethanol-oxidizing system, or MEOS) is responsible for ≥10% of ethanol oxidation at high blood alcohol concentrations.

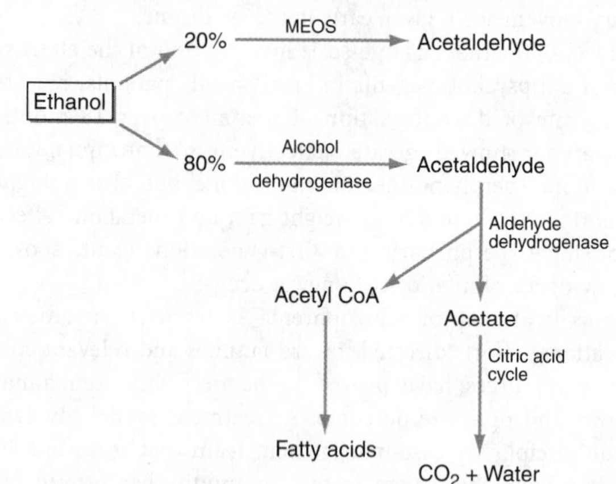

Figure 392-1 The metabolism of alcohol. MEOS, microsomal ethanol-oxidizing system.

While alcohol supplies calories (a drink contains ~300 kJ, or 70–100 kcal), these are devoid of nutrients such as minerals, proteins, and vitamins. In addition, alcohol can also interfere with absorption of vitamins in the small intestine and decreases their storage in the liver with modest effects on folate (folacin or folic acid), pyridoxine (B_6), thiamine (B_1), nicotinic acid (niacin, B_3), and vitamin A.

A heavy ethanol load in a fasting, healthy individual is likely to produce transient hypoglycemia within 6–36 h, secondary to the acute actions of ethanol on gluconeogenesis. This can result in temporary abnormal glucose tolerance tests (with a resulting erroneous diagnosis of diabetes mellitus) until the alcoholic has abstained for 2–4 weeks. Alcohol ketoacidosis, probably reflecting a decrease in fatty acid oxidation coupled with poor diet or recurrent vomiting, can be misdiagnosed as diabetic ketosis. With the former, patients show an increase in serum ketones along with a mild increase in glucose but a large anion gap, a mild to moderate increase in serum lactate, and a β-hydroxybutyrate/lactate ratio of between 2:1 and 9:1 (with normal being 1:1).

In the brain, alcohol affects almost all neurotransmitter systems, with acute actions that are often the opposite of those seen following desistance after a period of heavy drinking. The most prominent actions relate to boosting gamma aminobutyric acid (GABA) activity, especially in $GABA_A$ receptors. Enhancement of this complex chloride channel system contributes to anticonvulsant, sleep-inducing, antianxiety, and muscle relaxation effects of all GABA-boosting drugs. Acutely administered alcohol produces a release of GABA, and continued use of this drug increases density of $GABA_A$ receptors, while alcohol withdrawal states are characterized by decreases in GABA-related activity. Equally important is the ability of acute alcohol to inhibit postsynaptic *N*-methyl-D-aspartate (NMDA) excitatory glutamate receptors, while chronic drinking and desistance are associated with an upregulation of these excitatory receptor subunits. The relationships between greater GABA and diminished NMDA receptor activity during acute intoxication and diminished

GABA with enhanced NMDA actions during alcohol withdrawal explain much of intoxication and withdrawal phenomena.

As with all pleasurable activities, drinking alcohol acutely increases dopamine levels in the brain, especially in the ventral tegmentum and related brain regions, and this effect plays an important role in continued alcohol use, craving, and relapse. The changes in dopamine pathways are also linked to increases in "stress hormones," including cortisol and adrenocorticotropic hormone (ACTH) during intoxication and decreases in these hormones during withdrawal. Such alterations are likely to contribute to both feelings of reward during intoxication and depression during falling blood alcohol concentrations. Also closely linked to alterations in dopamine (especially in the nucleus accumbens) are alcohol-induced changes in opioid receptors, with acute alcohol also causing release of beta endorphins.

Additional important neurochemical changes include increases in synaptic levels of serotonin during acute intoxication, and subsequent upregulation of serotonin receptors. Acute increases in nicotinic acetylcholine systems also contribute to the impact of alcohol in the ventral tegmental region, which occur in concert with enhanced dopamine activity. In the same regions, alcohol impacts on cannabinol receptors, with resulting release of dopamine, GABA, and glutamate as well as subsequent effects on brain reward circuits.

■ BEHAVIORAL EFFECTS, TOLERANCE, AND DEPENDENCE

The acute effects of a drug depend on the dose, the rate of increase in plasma, the concomitant presence of other drugs, and the past experience with the agent. "Legal intoxication" with alcohol in most states requires a blood alcohol concentration of 0.08 g/dL, while levels of 0.04 or even lower are cited in other countries. However, behavioral, psychomotor, and cognitive changes are seen at levels as low as 0.02–0.03 g/dL (i.e., after one to two drinks) (Table 392-1). Deep but disturbed sleep can be seen at twice the legal intoxication level, and death can occur with levels between 0.30 and 0.40 g/dL. Beverage alcohol is probably responsible for more overdose deaths than any other drug.

Repeated use of alcohol contributes to acquired tolerance, a complex phenomenon involving at least three types of compensatory mechanisms. (1) After 1–2 weeks of daily drinking, *metabolic or pharmacokinetic tolerance* can be seen, with up to 30% increase in the rate of hepatic ethanol metabolism. This alteration disappears almost as rapidly as it develops. (2) *Cellular or pharmacodynamic tolerance* develops through neurochemical changes that maintain relatively normal physiologic functioning despite the presence of alcohol. Subsequent decreases in blood levels contribute to symptoms of withdrawal. (3) Individuals learn to adapt their behavior so that they can function better than expected under influence of the drug (*learned or behavioral tolerance*).

TABLE 392-1 Effects of Blood Alcohol Levels in the Absence of Tolerance

Blood Level, g/dL	Usual Effect
0.02	Decreased inhibitions, a slight feeling of intoxication
0.08	Decrease in complex cognitive functions and motor performance
0.20	Obvious slurred speech, motor incoordination, irritability, and poor judgment
0.30	Light coma and depressed vital signs
0.40	Death

The cellular changes caused by chronic ethanol exposure may not resolve for several weeks or longer following cessation of drinking. Rapid decreases in blood alcohol levels before that time can result in a withdrawal syndrome, which is most intense during the first 5 days, but some symptoms (e.g., disturbed sleep and anxiety) can take up to 4–6 months to resolve.

THE EFFECTS OF ETHANOL ON ORGAN SYSTEMS

Relatively low doses of alcohol (one or two drinks per day) have potential beneficial effects of increasing high-density lipoprotein cholesterol and decreasing aggregation of platelets, with a resulting decrease in risk for occlusive coronary disease and embolic strokes. Red wine has additional potential health-promoting qualities at relatively low doses due to flavinols and related substances, which may work by inhibiting platelet activation. Modest drinking might also decrease the risk for vascular dementia and, possibly, Alzheimer's disease. However, any potential healthful effects disappear with the regular consumption of three or more drinks per day, and knowledge about the deleterious effects of alcohol can both help the physician to identify patients with alcohol abuse and dependence, and to supply them with information that might help motivate a change in behavior.

■ NERVOUS SYSTEM

Approximately 35% of drinkers (and a much higher proportion of alcoholics) experience a *blackout*, an episode of temporary anterograde amnesia, in which the person forgets all or part of what occurred during a drinking evening. Another common problem, one seen after as few as one or two drinks shortly before bedtime, is disturbed sleep. Although alcohol might initially help a person to fall asleep, it disrupts sleep throughout the rest of the night. The stages of sleep are also altered, and time spent in rapid eye movement (REM) and deep sleep is reduced. Alcohol relaxes muscles in the pharynx, which can cause snoring and exacerbate sleep apnea; symptoms of the latter occur in 75% of alcoholic men older than age 60 years. Patients may also experience prominent and sometimes disturbing dreams. All of these sleep problems are more pronounced in alcoholics, and their persistence may contribute to relapse.

Another common consequence of alcohol use is impaired judgment and coordination, increasing the risk of accidents and injury. In the United States, ~40% of drinkers have at some time driven while intoxicated. Heavy drinking can also be associated with headache, thirst, nausea, vomiting, and fatigue the following day, a hangover syndrome that is responsible for much missed time and temporary cognitive deficits at work and school.

The effect of alcohol on the *nervous system* is even more pronounced among alcohol-dependent individuals. Chronic high doses cause *peripheral neuropathy* in ~10% of alcoholics: similar to diabetes, patients experience bilateral limb numbness, tingling, and paresthesias, all of which are more pronounced distally. Approximately 1% of alcoholics develop *cerebellar degeneration or atrophy*. This is a syndrome of progressive unsteady stance and gait often accompanied by mild nystagmus; neuroimaging studies reveal atrophy of the cerebellar vermis. Fortunately, very few alcoholics (perhaps as few as 1 in 500 for the full syndrome) develop *Wernicke's* (ophthalmoparesis, ataxia, and encephalopathy) and *Korsakoff's* (retrograde and anterograde amnesia) *syndromes*, although a higher proportion have one or more neuropathologic findings related to these syndromes. These occur as the result of low levels of thiamine, especially in predisposed individuals, e.g., those with transketolase deficiency. Alcoholics can manifest *cognitive problems* and temporary memory impairment lasting for weeks to months after drinking very heavily for days or weeks. Brain atrophy, evident as ventricular enlargement and widened cortical sulci on MRI and CT scans, occurs in ~50% of chronic alcoholics; these changes are usually reversible if abstinence is maintained. There is no single alcoholic dementia syndrome; rather, this label is used to describe patients who have apparently irreversible cognitive changes (possibly from diverse causes) in the context of chronic alcoholism.

Psychiatric comorbidity

As many as two-thirds of alcohol-dependent individuals meet the criteria for a psychiatric syndrome in the fourth edition of the *Diagnostic and Statistical Manual of Mental Disorders* (DSM-IV) of the American Psychiatric Association (Chap. 391). Half of these relate to a preexisting antisocial personality manifesting as impulsivity and disinhibition that contribute to both alcohol and drug dependence. The lifetime risk is 3% in males, and ≥80% of such individuals demonstrate alcohol and/or drug dependence. Another common comorbidity occurs with dependence on illicit substances. The remainder of alcoholics with psychiatric syndromes have preexisting conditions such as schizophrenia or manic-depressive disease and anxiety disorders such as panic disorder. The comorbidities of alcoholism with independent psychiatric disorders might represent an overlap in genetic vulnerabilities, impaired judgment in the use of alcohol from the independent psychiatric condition, or an attempt to use alcohol to alleviate some of the symptoms of the disorder or side effects of medications.

Many psychiatric syndromes can be seen *temporarily* during heavy drinking and subsequent withdrawal. These alcohol-induced conditions include an intense *sadness* lasting for days to weeks in the midst of heavy drinking seen in 40% of alcoholics, which tends to disappear over several weeks of abstinence (alcohol-induced mood disorder); temporary severe *anxiety* in 10–30% of alcoholics, often beginning during alcohol withdrawal, which can persist for a month or more after cessation of drinking (alcohol-induced anxiety disorder); and auditory *hallucinations* and/or paranoid delusions in a person who is alert and oriented, seen in 3–5% of alcoholics (*alcohol-induced psychotic disorder*).

Treatment of all forms of alcohol-induced psychopathology includes helping patients achieve abstinence and offering supportive care, as well as reassurance and "talk therapy" such as cognitive-behavioral approaches. However, with the exception of short-term antipsychotics or similar drugs for substance-induced psychoses, substance-induced psychiatric conditions only rarely require medications. Recovery is likely within several days to 4 weeks of abstinence. Conversely, because alcohol-induced conditions are temporary and do not indicate a need for long-term pharmacotherapy, a history of alcohol intake is an important part of the workup for any patient with one of these psychiatric symptoms.

THE GASTROINTESTINAL SYSTEM

Esophagus and stomach

Alcohol intake can result in inflammation of the esophagus and stomach causing epigastric distress and gastrointestinal bleeding, making alcohol one of the most common causes of hemorrhagic gastritis. Violent vomiting can produce severe bleeding through a Mallory-Weiss lesion, a longitudinal tear in the mucosa at the gastroesophageal junction.

Pancreas and liver

The incidence of acute pancreatitis (~25 per 1000 per year) is almost threefold higher in alcoholics than in the general population, accounting for an estimated 10% or more of the total cases. Alcohol impairs gluconeogenesis in the liver, resulting in a fall in the amount of glucose produced from glycogen, increased lactate production, and decreased oxidation of fatty acids. This contributes to an increase in fat accumulation in liver cells. In healthy individuals these changes are reversible, but with repeated exposure to ethanol, especially daily heavy drinking, more severe changes in the liver occur, including alcohol-induced hepatitis, perivenular sclerosis, and cirrhosis, with the latter observed in an estimated 15% of alcoholics (Chap. 307). Perhaps through an enhanced vulnerability to infections, alcoholics have an elevated rate of hepatitis C, and drinking in the context of that disease is associated with more severe liver deterioration.

CANCER

As few as 1.5 drinks per day increases a woman's risk of breast cancer 1.4-fold. For both genders, four drinks per day increases the risk for oral and esophageal cancers approximately threefold and rectal cancers by a factor of 1.5; seven to eight or more drinks per day enhances approximately fivefold the risks for many cancers. These consequences may result directly from cancer-promoting effects of alcohol and acetaldehyde or indirectly by interfering with immune homeostasis.

HEMATOPOIETIC SYSTEM

Ethanol causes an increase in red blood cell size [mean corpuscular volume (MCV)], which reflects its effects on stem cells. If heavy drinking is accompanied by folic acid deficiency, there can also be hypersegmented neutrophils, reticulocytopenia, and a hyperplastic bone marrow; if malnutrition is present, sideroblastic changes can be observed. Chronic heavy drinking can decrease production of white blood cells, decrease granulocyte mobility and adherence, and impair delayed-hypersensitivity responses to novel antigens (with a possible false-negative tuberculin skin test). Associated immune deficiencies can contribute to vulnerability toward infections, including hepatitis and HIV, and interfere with their treatment. Finally, many alcoholics have mild thrombocytopenia, which usually resolves within a week of abstinence unless there is hepatic cirrhosis or congestive splenomegaly.

CARDIOVASCULAR SYSTEM

Acutely, ethanol decreases myocardial contractility and causes peripheral vasodilation, with a resulting mild decrease in blood pressure and a compensatory increase in cardiac output. Exercise-induced increases in cardiac oxygen consumption are higher after alcohol intake. These acute effects have little clinical significance for the average healthy drinker but can be problematic when persisting cardiac disease is present.

The consumption of three or more drinks per day results in a dose-dependent increase in blood pressure, which returns to normal within weeks of abstinence. Thus, heavy drinking is an important factor in mild to moderate hypertension. Chronic heavy drinkers also have a sixfold increased risk for coronary artery disease, related, in part, to increased low-density lipoprotein cholesterol, and carry an increased risk for cardiomyopathy through direct effects of alcohol on heart muscle. Symptoms of the latter include unexplained arrhythmias in the presence of left ventricular impairment, heart failure, hypocontractility of heart muscle, and dilation of all four heart chambers with associated mural thrombi and mitral valve regurgitation. Atrial or ventricular arrhythmias, especially paroxysmal tachycardia, can also occur temporarily after heavy drinking in individuals showing no other evidence of heart disease—a syndrome known as the "holiday heart."

GENITOURINARY SYSTEM CHANGES, SEXUAL FUNCTIONING, AND FETAL DEVELOPMENT

Drinking in adolescence can affect normal sexual development and reproductive onset. At any age, modest ethanol doses (e.g., blood alcohol concentrations of 0.06 gm/dL) can increase sexual drive but also decrease erectile capacity in men. Even in the absence of liver impairment, a significant minority of chronic alcoholic men show irreversible testicular atrophy with shrinkage of the seminiferous tubules, decreases in ejaculate volume, and a lower sperm count (Chap. 346).

The repeated ingestion of high doses of ethanol by women can result in amenorrhea, a decrease in ovarian size, absence of corpora lutea with associated infertility, and an increased risk of spontaneous abortion. Heavy drinking during pregnancy results in the rapid placental transfer of both ethanol and acetaldehyde, which may have serious consequences for fetal development. One severe result is the *fetal alcohol syndrome* (FAS), seen in ~5% of children born to heavy-drinking mothers, which can include any of the following: facial changes with epicanthal eye folds; poorly formed ear concha; small teeth with faulty enamel; cardiac atrial or ventricular septal defects; an aberrant palmar crease and limitation in joint movement; and microcephaly with mental retardation. A less severe condition is the *fetal alcohol spectrum disorder* (FASD), which can include low birth weight, a lower IQ, hyperactive behavior, and some modest cognitive deficits. The amount of ethanol required and the time of vulnerability during pregnancy have not been defined, making it advisable for pregnant women to abstain completely.

OTHER EFFECTS

Between one-half and two-thirds of alcoholics have skeletal muscle weakness caused by acute *alcoholic myopathy*, a condition that improves but which might not fully remit with abstinence. Effects of repeated heavy drinking on the *skeletal system* include changes in calcium metabolism, lower bone density, and decreased growth in the epiphyses, leading to an increased risk for fractures and osteonecrosis of the femoral head. *Hormonal changes* include an increase in cortisol levels, which can remain elevated during heavy drinking; inhibition of vasopressin secretion at rising blood alcohol concentrations and enhanced secretion at falling blood alcohol concentrations (with the final result that most alcoholics are likely to be slightly overhydrated); a modest and reversible decrease in serum thyroxine (T_4); and a more marked decrease in serum triiodothyronine (T_3). Hormone irregularities should be reevaluated as they may disappear after a month of abstinence.

ALCOHOLISM (ALCOHOL ABUSE OR DEPENDENCE)

Because many drinkers occasionally imbibe to excess, temporary alcohol-related pathology is common in nonalcoholics, especially in the late teens to the late twenties. When repeated problems in multiple life areas develop, the individual is likely to meet criteria for alcohol abuse or dependence.

DEFINITIONS AND EPIDEMIOLOGY

Alcohol dependence is defined in DSM-IV as repeated alcohol-related difficulties in at least three of seven life areas that cluster together at about the same time (e.g., over the same 12-month period). Two of these seven items, tolerance and withdrawal, may have special importance as they are associated with a more severe clinical course. Dependence predicts a course of recurrent problems with the use of alcohol and the consequent shortening of the life span by a decade.

Alcohol abuse is defined as repetitive problems with alcohol in any one of four life areas—social, interpersonal, legal, and occupational—or repeated use in hazardous situations such as driving while intoxicated in an individual who is not alcohol dependent. About 50% of those with alcohol abuse continue to have alcohol problems 2–5 years later, but only ~10% of these patients—including adolescents—go on to develop alcohol dependence.

The lifetime risk for alcohol dependence in most Western countries is about 10–15% for men and 5–8% for women. Rates are generally similar in the United States, Canada, Germany, Australia, and the United Kingdom; tend to be lower in most Mediterranean countries, such as Italy, Greece, and Israel; and may be higher in Ireland, France, and Scandinavia. An even higher lifetime prevalence has been reported for most native cultures, including American Indians, Eskimos, Maori groups, and aboriginal tribes of Australia. These differences reflect both cultural and genetic influences, as described below. In Western countries, the typical alcoholic is more often a blue- or white-collar worker or homemaker. The lifetime risk for alcoholism among physicians is similar to that of the general population.

GENETICS

Approximately 60% of the risk for alcohol use disorders is attributed to genes, as indicated by the fourfold higher risk for alcohol abuse and dependence in children of alcoholics (even if these children were adopted early in life and raised by nonalcoholics) and a higher risk in identical twins as compared to fraternal twins of alcoholics. The genetic variations appear to operate primarily through intermediate characteristics that subsequently relate to the environment in altering the risk for heavy drinking and alcohol problems. These include genes relating to a high risk for all substance use disorders that operate through impulsivity, schizophrenia, and bipolar disorder. Another characteristic, an intense flushing response when drinking, decreases the risk for only alcohol use disorders through gene variations for several alcohol-metabolizing enzymes, especially aldehyde dehydrogenase (a mutation only seen in Asians), and to a lesser extent, variations in alcohol dehydrogenase.

An additional genetically influenced characteristic, a low sensitivity to alcohol, affects the risk for heavy drinking and may operate, in part, through variations in genes relating to potassium channels, GABA, nicotinic, and serotonin systems. A low response per drink is observed early in the drinking career and before alcohol use disorders have developed. All follow-up studies have demonstrated that this need for higher doses of alcohol to achieve desired effects predicts future heavy drinking, alcohol problems, and alcohol use disorders. The impact of a low response to alcohol on adverse drinking outcomes is mediated, at least in part, by a range of environmental influences, including the selection of heavier-drinking friends, the development of more positive expectations of the effects of high doses of alcohol, and suboptimal ways of coping with stress.

NATURAL HISTORY

Although the age of the first drink (~15 years) is similar in most alcoholics and nonalcoholics, a slightly earlier onset of regular drinking and drunkenness, especially in the context of conduct problems, is associated with a higher risk for later alcohol use disorders. By the early to midtwenties, most nonalcoholic men and women moderate their drinking (perhaps learning from more minor problems), whereas alcoholics are likely to escalate their patterns of drinking despite difficulties. The first major life problem from alcohol often appears in the late teens to early twenties, and a pattern of multiple alcohol difficulties by the midtwenties. Once established, the course of alcoholism is likely to be one of exacerbations and remissions, with little difficulty in temporarily stopping or controlling alcohol use when problems develop, but without help, desistance usually gives way to escalations in alcohol intake and subsequent problems. Following treatment, between half and two-thirds of alcoholics maintain abstinence for years, and often permanently. Even without formal treatment or self-help groups there is also at least a 20% chance of spontaneous remission with long-term abstinence. However, should the alcoholic continue to drink, the life span is shortened by ~10 years on average, with the leading causes of death, heart disease, cancer, accidents, and suicide.

TREATMENT

The approach to treating alcohol-related conditions is relatively straightforward: (1) recognize that at least 20% of all patients have alcohol abuse or dependence; (2) learn how to identify and treat acute alcohol-related conditions; (3) know how to help patients begin to address their alcohol problems; and (4) know enough about treating alcoholism to appropriately refer patients for additional help.

IDENTIFICATION OF THE ALCOHOLIC

Even in affluent locales, ~20% of patients have an alcohol use disorder. These men and women can be identified by asking questions about *alcohol problems* and noting laboratory test results that are likely to be abnormal in the context of regular consumption of six to eight or more drinks per day. The two blood tests with ≥60% sensitivity and specificity for heavy alcohol consumption are γ-glutamyl transferase (GGT) (>35 U) and carbohydrate-deficient transferrin (CDT) (>20 U/L or >2.6%); the combination of the two is likely to be more accurate than either alone. The values for these serologic markers are likely to return toward normal within several weeks of abstinence. Other useful blood tests include high-normal MCVs (≥91 μm^3) and serum uric acid (>416 mol/L, or 7 mg/dL).

The diagnosis of alcohol abuse or dependence ultimately rests on the documentation of a pattern of repeated difficulties associated with alcohol use. Thus, in screening it is important to probe for marital or job problems, legal difficulties, histories of accidents, medical problems, evidence of tolerance, etc., and then attempt to tie in use of alcohol or another substance. Some standardized questionnaires can be helpful, including the 10-item Alcohol Use Disorders Identification Test (AUDIT) (Table 392-2), but these are only screening tools, and a face-to-face interview is still required for a meaningful diagnosis.

TABLE 392-2 The Alcohol Use Disorders Identification Test (AUDIT)[a]

Item	5-Point Scale (Least to Most)
1. How often do you have a drink containing alcohol?	Never (0) to 4+ per week (4)
2. How many drinks containing alcohol do you have on a typical day?	1 or 2 (0) to 10+ (4)
3. How often do you have six or more drinks on one occasion?	Never (0) to daily or almost daily (4)
4. How often during the last year have you found that you were not able to stop drinking once you had started?	Never (0) to daily or almost daily (4)
5. How often during the last year have you failed to do what was normally expected from you because of drinking?	Never (0) to daily or almost daily (4)
6. How often during the last year have you needed a first drink in the morning to get yourself going after a heavy drinking session?	Never (0) to daily or almost daily (4)
7. How often during the last year have you had a feeling of guilt or remorse after drinking?	Never (0) to daily or almost daily (4)
8. How often during the last year have you been unable to remember what happened the night before because you had been drinking?	Never (0) to daily or almost daily (4)
9. Have you or someone else been injured as a result of your drinking?	No (0) to yes, during the last year (4)
10. Has a relative, friend, doctor or other health worker been concerned about your drinking or suggested that you should cut down?	No (0) to yes, during the last year (4)

[a]The AUDIT is scored by simply summing the values associated with the endorsed response.

Source: Adapted from DF Reinert, GP Allen: *Alcoholism: Clinical & Experimental Research* 26:272, 2002, and from MA Schuckit, 2006.

TREATMENT Alcohol-Related Conditions

Acute Intoxication The first priority in treating severe intoxication is to assess vital signs and manage respiratory depression, cardiac arrhythmia, or blood pressure instability, if present. The possibility of intoxication with other drugs should be considered by obtaining toxicology screens for opioids or other CNS depressants such as benzodiazepines. Aggressive behavior should be handled by offering reassurance but also by considering the possibility of a show of force with an intervention team. If the aggressive behavior continues, relatively low doses of a short-acting benzodiazepine such as lorazepam (e.g., 1–2 mg PO or IV) may be used and can be repeated as needed, but care must be taken not to destabilize vital signs or worsen confusion. An alternative approach is to use an antipsychotic medication (e.g., 0.5–5 mg of haloperidol PO or IM every 4–8 h as needed, or olanzapine 2.5–10 mg IM repeated at 2 and 6 h, if needed).

Intervention There are two main elements to intervention in a person with alcoholism: motivational interviewing and brief interventions. During motivational interviewing, the clinician helps the patient to think through the assets (e.g., comfort in social situations) and liabilities (e.g., health and interpersonal related problems) of the current pattern of drinking. The patient's responses are key, and the clinician should listen empathetically, helping to weigh options and encouraging the patient to take responsibility for changes that need to be made. Patients should be reminded that only they can decide to avoid the consequences that will occur without changes in drinking. The process of motivational interviewing has been summarized by the acronym FRAMES: Feedback to the patient; Responsibility to be taken by the patient; Advice, rather than orders, on what needs to be done; Menus of options that might be considered; Empathy for understanding of the patient's thoughts and feelings; and Self-efficacy, i.e., offering support for the capacity of the patient to succeed in making changes.

Once the patient begins to consider change, the emphasis shifts to brief interventions designed to help the patient understand more about potential action. Discussions focus on consequences of high alcohol consumption, suggested approaches to stopping drinking, and help in recognizing and avoiding situations likely to lead to heavy drinking. Both motivational interviewing and brief interventions can be carried out in 15-min sessions, but because patients do not always change behavior right away, multiple meetings are often required to explain the problem, discuss optimal treatments, and explain the benefits of abstinence.

Alcohol Withdrawal If the patient agrees to stop drinking, sudden decreases in alcohol intake can produce withdrawal symptoms, many of which are the opposite of those produced by intoxication. Features include tremor of the hands (shakes); agitation and anxiety; autonomic nervous system overactivity including an increase in pulse, respiratory rate, and body temperature; and insomnia. These symptoms usually begin within 5–10 h of decreasing ethanol intake, peak on day 2 or 3, and improve by day 4 or 5, although mild levels of these problems may persist for 4–6 months as a protracted abstinence syndrome.

About 2–5% of alcoholics experience a withdrawal seizure, with the risk increasing in the context of concomitant medical problems, misuse of additional drugs, and higher alcohol quantities. The same risk factors also contribute to a similar rate of *delirium tremens* (DTs), where the withdrawal includes delirium (mental confusion, agitation, and fluctuating levels of consciousness) associated with a tremor and autonomic overactivity (e.g., marked increases in pulse, blood pressure, and respirations). The risks for seizures and DTs can be diminished by identifying and treating any underlying medical conditions early in the course of withdrawal.

The first step in treating withdrawal is to perform a thorough physical examination in all alcoholics who are considering stopping drinking, including a search for evidence of liver failure, gastrointestinal bleeding, cardiac arrhythmia, infection, and glucose or electrolyte imbalance. It is also important to offer adequate nutrition and oral multiple B vitamins, including 50–100 mg of thiamine daily for a week or more. Because most alcoholics who enter withdrawal are either normally hydrated or mildly overhydrated, IV fluids should be avoided unless there is a relevant medical problem or significant recent bleeding, vomiting, or diarrhea.

The next step is to recognize that because withdrawal symptoms reflect the rapid removal of a CNS depressant, alcohol, the symptoms can be controlled by administering any depressant in doses that decrease the agitation and then gradually tapering the dose over 3–5 days. While most CNS depressants are effective, benzodiazepines (Chap. 391) have the highest margin of safety and lowest cost and are, therefore, the preferred class of drugs. Short-half-life benzodiazepines can be considered for patients with serious liver impairment or evidence of brain damage, but they must be given every 4 h to avoid abrupt blood-level fluctuations that may increase the risk for seizures. Therefore, most clinicians use drugs with longer half-lives (e.g., chlordiazepoxide), adjusting the dose if signs of withdrawal escalate, and withholding the drug if the patient is sleeping or has evidence of orthostatic hypotension. The average patient requires doses of 25–50 mg of chlordiazepoxide or 10 mg of diazepam given PO every 4–6 h on the first day, with doses then decreased to zero over the next 5 days. While alcohol withdrawal can be treated in a hospital, patients in good physical condition who demonstrate mild signs of withdrawal despite low blood alcohol concentrations and who have no prior history of DTs or withdrawal seizures can be considered for outpatient detoxification. These patients should return daily for evaluation of vital signs and can be hospitalized if signs and symptoms of withdrawal escalate.

Treatment of the patient with DTs can be challenging, and the condition is likely to run a course of 3–5 days regardless of the therapy employed. The focus of care is to identify and correct medical problems and to control behavior and prevent injuries. Many clinicians recommend the use of high doses of a benzodiazepine (as much as 800 mg/d of chlordiazepoxide has been reported), a treatment that will decrease agitation and raise the seizure threshold but probably does little to improve the confusion. Other clinicians recommend the use of antipsychotic medications, such as haloperidol or olanzapine as discussed above, although these drugs have not been directly evaluated for DTs. Antipsychotics are less likely to exacerbate confusion but may increase the risk of seizures; they have no place in the treatment of mild withdrawal symptoms.

Generalized withdrawal seizures rarely require more than giving an adequate dose of benzodiazepines. There is little evidence that anticonvulsants such as phenytoin or gabapentin are more effective in drug-withdrawal seizures, and the risk of seizures has usually passed by the time effective drug levels are reached. The rare patient with status epilepticus must be treated aggressively (Chap. 369).

REHABILITATION OF ALCOHOLICS

An Overview After completing alcoholic rehabilitation, ≥60% of alcoholics, especially middle-class patients, maintain abstinence for at least a year, and many achieve lifetime sobriety. The core of treatment uses cognitive-behavioral approaches to help patients recognize the need to change, while working with them to alter their behaviors to enhance compliance. A key step is to optimize motivation toward abstinence through education about alcoholism and instructions to family members to stop protecting the patient from problems caused by alcohol. After years of heavy drinking, patients also need counseling, vocational rehabilitation, and self-help groups such as Alcoholics Anonymous (AA) to help them learn how to deal with life's stresses while sober. A third component, *relapse prevention*, helps the patient to identify situations in which a return to drinking is likely, formulate ways of managing these risks, and develop coping strategies that increase the chances of a return to abstinence if a slip occurs.

While many patients can be treated as outpatients, more intense interventions work better, and some alcoholics do not respond to AA or outpatient groups. Whatever the setting, subsequent contact with outpatient treatment staff should be maintained for a minimum of 6 months and preferably a full year after abstinence. Counseling focuses on areas of improved functioning in the absence of alcohol (i.e., why it is a good idea to continue to abstain) and helping the patient to manage free time without alcohol, develop a nondrinking peer group, and handle stresses on the job.

The physician serves an important role in identifying the alcoholic, diagnosing and treating associated medical or psychiatric syndromes, overseeing detoxification, referring the patient to rehabilitation programs, providing counseling, and, if appropriate, selecting which (if any) medication might be needed. For insomnia, patients should be reassured that troubled sleep is normal after alcohol withdrawal and will improve over subsequent weeks. They should be taught the basic elements of "sleep hygiene" including maintaining consistent schedules for bedtime and awakening. Sleep medications have the danger of being misused and of rebound insomnia when stopped. Sedating antidepressants (e.g., trazodone) should not be used as they interfere with cognitive functioning the next morning and disturb the normal sleep architecture, but occasional use of over-the-counter sleeping medications (sedating antihistamines) can be considered. Anxiety can be addressed by helping the person to gain insight into the temporary nature of the symptoms and to develop strategies to achieve relaxation as well as by using forms of cognitive therapy.

Medications for Rehabilitation Several medications have modest benefits when used for the first 6 months of recovery. The opioid-antagonist, naltrexone, 50–150 mg/d orally, appears to shorten subsequent relapses, whether used in the oral form or as a once-per-month 380-mg injection, especially in individuals with the G allele of the AII8G polymorphism of the μ opioid receptor. By blocking opioid receptors, naltrexone may decrease activity in the dopamine-rich ventral tegmental reward system, and decrease the feeling of pleasure or reward if alcohol is imbibed. A second medication, acamprosate (Campral) at ~2 g/d divided into three oral doses, has similar modest effects; acamprosate inhibits NMDA receptors, decreasing mild symptoms of protracted withdrawal. Several trials of combined naltrexone and acamprosate using doses similar to those noted above have reported that the combination may be superior to either drug alone, although not all studies agree.

It is more difficult to establish the asset-to-liability ratio of a third drug, disulfiram, an ALDH inhibitor, used at doses of 250 mg/d. This drug produces vomiting and autonomic nervous system instability in the presence of alcohol as a result of rapidly rising blood levels of the first metabolite of alcohol, acetaldehyde. This reaction can be dangerous, especially for patients with heart disease, stroke, diabetes mellitus, or hypertension. The drug itself carries potential risks of depression, psychotic symptoms, peripheral neuropathy, and liver damage. Disulfiram is best given under supervision of another individual (such as a spouse), especially during discrete periods identified as representing high-risk drinking situations (such as the Christmas holiday). Other relevant drugs under investigation include the nicotinic receptor agonist varenicline, the serotonin antagonist ondansetron, the α-adrenergic agonist prazosin, the GABA-B receptor agonist baclofen, the anticonvulsant topiramate, and cannabinol receptor antagonists. At present, there are insufficient data to determine the asset-to-liability ratio for these medications in treating alcoholism and, therefore, no data to offer solid support for their use in clinical settings.

FURTHER READINGS

Apodaca TR, Longabaugh R: Mechanisms of change in motivational interviewing: A review and preliminary evaluation of the evidence. Addiction 104:705, 2009

Donovan DM et al: Combined pharmacotherapies and behavioral interventions for alcohol dependence (the COMBINE study): Examination of posttreatment drinking outcomes. J Stud Alcohol Drugs 69:5, 2008

Koob GF, Volkow ND: Neurocircuitry of addiction. Neuropsychopharmacology 35: 217, 2010

Russell M et al: Drinking patterns and myocardial infarction: A linear dose-response model. Alcohol Clin Exp Res 33:324, 2009

Schuckit MA: Alcohol-use disorders. Lancet 373:492, 2009

———: An overview of genetic influences in alcoholism. J Subst Abuse Treat 36:S5, 2009

Spanagel R, Kiefer F: Drugs for relapse prevention of alcoholism: Ten years of progress. Trends Pharmacol Sci 29:109, 2008

Taylor B et al: Alcohol and hypertension: Gender differences in dose-response relationships determined through systematic review and meta-analysis. Addiction 104:1981, 2009

Thygesen LC et al: Cancer incidence among patients with alcohol use disorders—Long-term follow-up. Alcohol Alcohol 44:387, 2009

Vengeliene V: Neuropharmacology of alcohol addiction. Br J Pharmacol 154:299, 2008

Verrill C et al: Alcohol-related cirrhosis—Early abstinence is a key factor in prognosis, even in the most severe cases. Addiction 104:768, 2009

CHAPTER 393

Opioid Drug Abuse and Dependence

Thomas R. Kosten

INTRODUCTION

Opiate analgesics are some of the oldest and most common medications in clinical practice, but have also been abused since at least 300 B.C. Nepenthe (Greek "free from sorrow") helped the hero of the *Odyssey*, but widespread opium smoking in China and the Near East has caused harm for centuries. Since the first chemical isolation of opium and codeine 200 years ago, a wide range of synthetic opioids have been developed, and endogenous opioid peptides were discovered in 1995. Two of the most important adverse effects of all these agents are overdose and dependence. The 0.14% annual prevalence of heroin dependence in the United States is only about one-third the rate of prescription opiate abuse and is substantially lower than the 2% rate of morphine dependence in Southeast and Southwest Asia. While these rates are low relative to other abused substances, their disease burden is substantial, with high rates of morbidity and mortality; disease transmission; increased health care, crime, and law enforcement costs; and less tangible costs of family distress and lost productivity.

The diagnosis of opiate dependence in the *Fourth Diagnostic and Statistical Manual* (DSM-IV) requires the repeated use of the drug while producing problems in three or more areas in a 12-month period. The areas include tolerance, withdrawal, use of greater amounts of opiates than intended, and use despite adverse consequences. The abuse diagnosis is related to legal problems, inability to meet obligations, use in hazardous situations, and continued use despite problems. The most striking aspect of opiate abuse has been its marked increase as the gateway to illicit drugs in the United States. Since 2007, prescription opiates have surpassed marijuana as the most common illicit drug that adolescents initially abuse.

The most commonly abused opiates are diverted prescriptions for oxycodone, followed by heroin and morphine, and—among health professionals—meperidine and fentanyl. Two opiate maintenance treatment agents—methadone and buprenorphine—are also abused, but at substantially lower rates, and the partial opiate agonists such as butorphanol, tramadol, and pentazocine are infrequently abused. The chemistry and general pharmacology of these agents are covered in major pharmacology texts, and this chapter focuses on the neurobiology and pharmacology relevant to abuse, dependence, and their treatments.

NEUROBIOLOGY

During the past 30 years, substantial progress has been made in elucidating the neurobiology of opiates and their effects not only on the three types of opiate receptors (mu, kappa, and delta) but also on the cascade of second, third, and fourth intracellular messenger systems and on neuronal action potentials. The different functional activities of these three receptors are summarized in Table 393-1, and abuse liability is primarily associated with the mu receptor. A fourth type of opiate receptor, the orphanin receptor, also modulates pain but is not affected by opiate drugs. These opiate receptors are all G protein–linked and coupled to the cyclic adenosine monophosphate (cyclic AMP) second messenger system and to potassium channels. Opiates are inhibitory and block the potassium channels from opening and depolarizing the neuron, which would produce an action potential. Thus, opiates acutely inhibit neuronal activity. Analgesia and sedation are induced through this inhibition of specific brain pathways, while the "high" from opiates involves an indirect activation of a different brain pathway—the mesolimbic dopamine pathway.

The various effects of opiates are related to the specific neuroanatomic locations of mu receptors. Reinforcing and euphoric effects of opiates occur in the dopaminegic pathway from the ventral tegmental area (VTA) to the nucleus accumbens, where opiates increase synaptic levels of dopamine. This increase is due to inhibition of GABAergic neurons that inhibit both the VTA and nucleus accumbens activity. However, the "high" only occurs when the *rate of change* in dopamine is fast. Large, rapidly administered doses of opiates block GABA inhibition and produce a burst of nucleus accumbens activity that is associated with "high" in all abused drugs. Therefore, routes of administration that slowly increase opiate blood and brain levels, such as oral and transdermal routes, are effective for analgesia and sedation but do not produce an opiate "high" that follows smoking and intravenous routes. Other acute effects such as analgesia and respiratory depression leading to overdose are due to stimulation of opiate receptors located in other areas such as the locus coeruleus.

Opiate dependence and withdrawal are chronic effects related to the cyclic AMP system. This second messenger phosphorylates various intracellular proteins and produces a cascade of changes reaching into the nucleus and DNA. Immediate early gene products such as c-*fos* and c-*jun* are activated followed by regulation of other genes with more sustained protein transcription such as *delta c-fos*. With these sustained gene activations, several receptor-level changes occur, including downregulation of receptor numbers, reduced neuronal cell-surface receptor trafficking, uncoupling of G proteins from the mu opiate receptors, and upregulation of cyclic AMP second messenger systems. These effects are also reflective of genetic risk factors for drug dependence, with estimates of up to 50% of the risk for dependence due to polygenic inheritance. Specific functional genetic polymorphisms in the mu opiate receptor gene appear associated with this risk for opiate abuse, including one producing a threefold increase in this receptor's affinity for opiates and the endogenous ligand beta endorphin. Epigenetic methylation changes also occur on the DNA of the mu receptor gene of opiate addicts. DNA methylation inhibits gene transcription.

This molecular cascade links acute intoxication and sedation to chronic opiate dependence and withdrawal within the specific neuroanatomic structure of the locus coeruleus. The locus coeruleus is the brain's largest concentration of noradrenergic neurons and is responsible for a large proportion of brain cortical activation. When large opiate doses saturate and activate all of its mu receptors, its steady rate of action potentials can cease due to the inactivation of potassium channels. When this direct inhibitory effect is sustained over weeks and months of opiate use, a secondary set of regulatory effects take place in the cyclic AMP system that leads to tolerance, dependence, and withdrawal symptoms.

Opiate withdrawal symptoms reflect overactivity of adrenergic neurons that are located in the locus ceruleus. Opiates suppress the activity of these neurons, and when this suppression continues chronically from daily opiate use, a secondary upregulation occurs in adenyl cyclase enzyme capacity and the production of cyclic AMP from ATP. This upregulation is a homeostatic response to the chronic opiate suppression, but when that suppression is terminated by discontinuing the opiate, this enhanced adenyl cyclase activity leads to a marked increase in cyclic AMP. The now very high levels of cyclic AMP activate the sodium-potassium channels and produce a high level of action potentials in these adrenergic neurons. This adrenergic arousal is one basis for the symptoms of opiate withdrawal and takes about 7 days to readjust to normal levels of adenyl cyclase activity and the associated resolution of opiate withdrawal symptoms. This molecular model of adrenergic neuronal activation during withdrawal has had important treatment implications, such as the use of clonidine for opioid withdrawal.

TABLE 393-1 Actions of Opioid Receptors

Receptor Type	Actions
Mu (μ) (e.g., morphine)	Analgesia, reinforcement euphoria, cough and appetite suppression, decreased respirations, decreased GI motility, sedation, hormone changes, dopamine and acetylcholine release
Kappa (κ) (e.g., butorphanol)	Dysphoria, decreased GI motility, decreased appetite, decreased respiration, psychotic symptoms, sedation, diuresis, analgesia
Delta (Δ) (e.g., etorphine)	Hormone changes, appetite suppression, dopamine release

Abbreviation: GI, gastrointestinal.

PHARMACOLOGY

Tolerance and withdrawal commonly occur with chronic daily use as quickly as 6–8 weeks depending on the dose and frequency of dosing. Tolerance appears to be primarily a pharmacodynamic rather than pharmacokinetic effect, with relatively limited induction of the cytochrome P450 or other liver enzymes. The metabolism of opiates occurs in the liver primarily through the cytochrome P450 systems of 2D6 and 3A4. They then are conjugated to glucuronic acid and excreted in small amounts in feces. The plasma half-lives generally range from 2.5 to 3 h for morphine and more than 22 h for methadone. The shortest half-lives of several minutes are for fentanyl-related opiates and the longest are for buprenorphine and its active metabolites, which can block opiate withdrawal for up to 3 days after a single dose. Tolerance to the mental effects of opioids leads to the need for ever-increasing amounts of drugs to sustain the desired euphoriant effects—as well as to avoid the discomfort of withdrawal. This combination has the expected consequence of strongly reinforcing dependence once it has started. The role of endogenous opioid peptides in opioid dependence is uncertain.

The clinical aspects of abuse are tied to route of administration and the rapidity of an opiate bolus in reaching the brain. Intravenous and smoked administration is routine not only because it is the most efficient route but also because it rapidly produces a bolus of high drug concentration in the brain. This bolus produces a "rush," followed by euphoria, a feeling of tranquility, and sleepiness ("the nod"). Heroin produces effects that last 3–5 h, and several doses a day are required to forestall manifestations of withdrawal in dependent persons. Symptoms of opioid withdrawal begin 8–10 h after the last dose. Many of these symptoms reflect increased activity of the autonomic nervous system. Lacrimation, rhinorrhea, yawning, and sweating appear first. Restless sleep followed by weakness, chills, gooseflesh ("cold turkey"), nausea and vomiting, muscle aches, and involuntary movements ("kicking the habit"), hyperpnea, hyperthermia, and hypertension occur in later stages of the withdrawal syndrome. The acute course of withdrawal may last 7–10 days. A secondary phase of protracted abstinence lasts for 26–30 weeks and is characterized by hypotension, bradycardia, hypothermia, mydriasis, and decreased responsiveness of the respiratory center to carbon dioxide.

Opioid effects on organs

Besides the brain effects of opioids on sedation and euphoria and the combined brain and peripheral nervous system effects on analgesia, a wide range of other organs can be affected. The cough reflex is inhibited through the brain, leading to the use of some opiates as an antitussive, and nausea and vomiting are due to brainstem effects on the medulla. The release of several hormones is inhibited including corticotropin-releasing factor (CRF) and luteinizing hormone, which reduce cortisol and sex hormone levels, respectively. The clinical manifestations of these reductions can involve poor responses to stress and reductions in sex drive. An increase in prolactin also contributes to the reduced sex drive in males. Two other hormones affected are decreased thyrotropin and increased growth hormone. Respiratory depression results from opiate-induced insensitivity of brainstem neurons to increases in carbon dioxide. This depression contributes to overdose, but in patients with pulmonary disease even opiate doses well below those typical of overdose can produce clinically significant complications. In overdoses, aspiration pneumonia is a common complication due to loss of the choking reflex. Opiates reduce gut motility, which is helpful for diarrhea, but can lead to nausea, constipation, and anorexia with weight loss. Deaths have occurred in early methadone maintenance programs due to severe constipation and toxic megacolon. Opiates may prolong QT intervals and lead to sudden death in some patients. Two opiates particularly noted for this complication are methadone and a long-acting form of methadone called LAAM that was withdrawn from the market. Orthostatic hypotension may occur due to histamine release and peripheral blood vessel dilation, which is an opiate effect usefully applied to managing acute myocardial infarction.

Heroin users in particular tend to use opiates intravenously and be polydrug users, also using alcohol, sedatives, cannabinoids, and stimulants. None of these other drugs serve as substitutes for opioids, but they have desired additive effects. One needs to be sure that the person undergoing a withdrawal reaction is not also withdrawing from alcohol or sedatives, which might be more dangerous and more difficult to manage.

Besides the ever-present risk of fatal overdose, hepatitis B and AIDS are among the many potential complications of sharing contaminated hypodermic syringes. Bacterial infections lead to septic complications such as meningitis, osteomyelitis, and abscesses in various organs. Attempts to illicitly manufacture meperidine in the 1980s resulted in the production of a highly specific neurotoxin, MPTP, which produced parkinsonism in users.

Toxicity and overdose

Lethal overdose is a relatively common complication of opiate dependence and must be rapidly recognized and treated because naloxone provides a highly specific reversal agent that is relatively free of complications. The diagnosis generally does not rely on blood or urine toxicology results but on clinical signs and symptoms. The presentation involves shallow and slow respirations, pupillary miosis (mydriasis does not occur until significant brain anoxia supervenes), bradycardia, hypothermia, and stupor or coma. If naloxone is not administered, progression to respiratory and cardiovascular collapse leading to death occurs. At autopsy, cerebral edema and sometimes frothy pulmonary edema are generally found, but those pulmonary effects are most likely from allergic reactions to adulterants mixed with the heroin. Opiates generally do not produce seizures except for unusual cases of mixed drug abuse with the opiate meperidine or with high doses of tramadol.

TREATMENT Opioid Overdose

Beyond the acute treatment of opiate overdose with naloxone, clinicians have two general treatment paths: opioid maintenance treatment or detoxification. Most opioid-dependent individuals engage in multiple episodes of all three categories of treatment during the course of their drug-using careers. Agonist and partial agonist medications are commonly utilized for both maintenance and detoxification purposes. Alpha-2-adrenergic agonists are primarily used for detoxification. Antagonists are used to accelerate detoxification and then continued postdetoxification to prevent relapse. Only the residential medication-free programs have had success that comes close to matching that of the medication-based programs. Success of the various treatment approaches is assessed as retention in treatment, reduced opioid and other drug use, as well as secondary outcomes such as HIV risk behaviors, crime, psychiatric symptoms, and medical co-morbidity.

Stopping opiates is like stopping most drugs of abuse—it is much easier to stop than to prevent relapses. Long-term relapse prevention for opioid-dependent persons requires combined pharmacologic and psychosocial approaches. Chronic users tend to prefer pharmacologic approaches; those with shorter histories of drug abuse are more amenable to detoxification and psychosocial interventions.

Opiate Overdose Treatment Managing overdose requires naloxone and support of vital functions, including intubation if needed. The opiate antagonist naloxone is given at 0.4–2 mg IV or IM, with an expected response within 1–2 min. If the overdose is due to buprenorphine, then naloxone might be required at total doses of 10 mg or greater, but primary buprenorphine overdose is nearly impossible because this agent is a partial opiate agonist. Partial agonism means that as the dose of buprenorphine is increased, it has greater opiate antagonist than agonist activity. Thus, a 0.2-mg buprenorphine dose leads to analgesia and sedation, while a hundred times greater 20-mg dose produces profound opiate antagonism, precipitating opiate withdrawal in a person who was opiate dependent on morphine or methadone. When 10 mg of naloxone fails to produce arousal in the patient, another cause of toxicity must be found. Before reaching such large naloxone doses, however, it is important to recognize that the goal is to reverse the respiratory depression and not to administer so much naloxone that it precipitates opiate withdrawal. Because naloxone only lasts a few hours and most opiates last considerably longer, close monitoring and an IV naloxone drip is frequently employed to provide a continuous level of antagonism for 24–72 h depending on the opiate used in the overdose (e.g., morphine vs. methadone). Other sedative drugs that produce significant overdoses must also be considered if naloxone has only a limited effect. The most common are benzodiazepines, which have produced overdoses and deaths in combination with buprenorphine. A specific antagonist for benzodiazepines—flumazenil at 0.2 mg/min—can be given to a maximum of 3 g/h, but it may precipitate seizures and increase intracranial pressure. Like naloxone, administration for a prolonged period is usually required since most benzodiazepines remain active for considerably longer than flumazenil.

Support of vital functions may include oxygen and positive-pressure breathing, IV fluids, pressor agents for hypotension, and cardiac monitoring to detect QT prolongation, which might require treatment. Activated charcoal and gastric lavage may be helpful for oral ingestions, but intubation will be needed if the patient is stuporous.

Opiate Withdrawal Treatment The principles of detoxification are the same for all drugs: to substitute a longer-acting, orally active, pharmacologically equivalent drug for the abused drug, stabilize the patient on that drug, and then gradually withdraw the substituted drug. Methadone is admirably suited for such use in opioid-dependent persons, and the partial mu agonist buprenorphine is another option. Clonidine, a centrally acting sympatholytic agent, has also been used for detoxification. By reducing central sympathetic outflow, clonidine mitigates many of the signs of sympathetic overactivity. Clonidine has no narcotic action and is not addictive. Lofexidine, a clonidine analogue with less hypotensive effect, is being developed for use.

Methadone for Detoxification Methadone dose tapering regimens for detoxification range from 2 to 3 weeks to as long as 180 days, but this approach is controversial given the relative effectiveness of methadone maintenance and the low success rates of detoxification. Unfortunately, the vast majority of patients tend to relapse to heroin or other opiates during or after the detoxification period, indicative of the chronic and relapsing nature of opioid dependence.

Buprenorphine for Detoxification Because it is a partial agonist, buprenorphine produces fewer withdrawal symptoms and may allow briefer detoxifications compared with full agonists like methadone, but it does not appear to have better outcomes than methadone tapering. Buprenorphine is superior to the alpha-2-adrenergic agonist clonidine in reducing symptoms of withdrawal, retaining patients in a withdrawal protocol, and in treatment completion.

Alpha-2-Adrenergic Agonists for Detoxification Several alpha-2-adrenergic agonists have relieved opioid withdrawal by suppressing central noradrenergic hyperactivity. Alpha-2-adrenergic agonists moderate the symptoms of noradrenergic hyperactivity via actions in the central nervous system. Clonidine relieves some signs and symptoms of opiate withdrawal such as lacrimation, rhinorrhea, muscle pain, joint pain, restlessness, and gastrointestinal symptoms, but it is not a drug of abuse or dependence. Unfortunately, clonidine is associated with significant hypotension, which has stimulated investigation of lofexidine, guanfacine, and guanabenz acetate. Lofexidine can be dosed up to ~2 mg/d and appears to be associated with fewer adverse effects, and it is therefore likely to replace clonidine as the leading opioid withdrawal treatment in this drug class. Clonidine or lofexidine are typically administered orally, in three or four doses per day, with dizziness, sedation, lethargy, and dry mouth as the primary adverse side effects. Completion rates of managed withdrawal assisted with clonidine and other alpha-2-adrenergic agents vs. methadone have been comparable.

Rapid and Ultrarapid Opiate Detoxification The opioid antagonist naltrexone typically combined with an alpha-2-adrenergic agonist has been purported to shorten the duration of withdrawal without significantly increasing patient discomfort. Another benefit to rapid opiate detoxification (ROD) is the reduced time between opioid use and the commencement of sustained naltrexone treatment for prevention of relapse (see below). ROD completion rates using naltrexone and clonidine range from 75 to 81% compared to 40–65% for methadone or clonidine alone. Buprenorphine in combination with naltrexone and clonidine reduced ROD from 3 to 1 day of detoxification. Ultrarapid opiate detoxification is an extension of ROD using anesthetics, but is highly controversial due to the medical risks and mortality associated with it.

Agonist medications for opioid dependence

Methadone maintenance substitutes a once-daily oral opioid dose for three-to-four times daily heroin. Methadone saturates the opioid receptors, and by inducing a high level of opiate tolerance, blocks the desired euphoria from additional opiates. Buprenorphine, a partial opioid agonist, also can be given once daily at sublingual doses of 4–32 mg daily, and in contrast to methadone it can be given in an office-based primary care setting.

Methadone maintenance Methadone's slow onset of action when taken orally, long elimination half-life (24–36 h), and production of cross-tolerance at doses from 80 to 150 mg are the basis for its efficacy in treatment retention and reductions in IV drug use, criminal activity, and HIV risk behaviors and mortality. Methadone can prolong the QT interval at rates as high as 16% above the rates in non-methadone-maintained, drug-injecting patients, but it has been used safely in the treatment of opioid dependence for 40 years.

Buprenorphine maintenance While France and Australia have had sublingual buprenorphine maintenance since 1996, the USFDA approved it as a Schedule III drug in 2002 for managing opiate dependence. Unlike the full agonist methadone, buprenorphine is a partial agonist of mu-opioid receptors with a slow onset and long duration of action, allowing for alternate-day dosing. Its partial agonism reduces the risk of unintentional overdose but limits its efficacy to patients who need the equivalent of only 60–70 mg of methadone, and many patients in methadone maintenance require higher doses up to 150 mg daily. Buprenorphine is combined with naloxone at a 4:1 ratio in order to reduce its abuse liability. A subcutaneous buprenorphine implant has also been tested, but results are not yet available.

In the United States, the ability of primary care physicians to prescribe buprenorphine for opioid dependence presents an important and far-reaching opportunity to improve access and quality of treatment as well as reduce social harm. Europe, Asia, and Australia have found reduced opioid-related deaths and drug-injection-related medical morbidity with buprenorphine available in primary care. Retention in office-based buprenorphine treatment has been greater than 70% at 6-month follow-ups.

Antagonist medications for opioid dependence

The rationale for using narcotic antagonist therapy is that blocking the action of self-administered opioids should eventually extinguish the habit, but this therapy is poorly accepted by patients. Naltrexone, a long-acting orally active pure opioid antagonist, can be given three times a week at doses of 100–150 mg and a depot form for monthly administration is available. Because it is an antagonist, the patient must first be detoxified from opioid dependence before starting naltrexone. When taken chronically for even years, it is safe, associated with few side effects (headache, nausea, abdominal pain), and can be given to patients infected with hepatitis B or C without producing hepatotoxicity. However, most providers refrain from prescribing it if liver function tests are 3–5 times above normal levels. Naltrexone maintenance combined with psychosocial therapy is effective in reducing heroin use, but medication adherence is low. Depot injection formulations lasting up to 4 weeks markedly improve adherence, retention, and drug use. Subcutaneous naltrexone implants in Russia, China, and Australia have doubled treatment retention and reduced relapse to half that of oral naltrexone.

Medication-free treatment

Most opiate addicts enter medication-free treatments in inpatient, residential, or outpatient settings, but 1- to 5-year outcomes are very poor compared to pharmacotherapy except for residential settings lasting 6 to 18 months. The residential programs require full immersion in a regimented system that has progressively increasing levels of independence and responsibility within a controlled community of fellow drug abusers. These medication-free programs, as well as the pharmacotherapy programs, also include counseling and behavioral treatments designed to teach interpersonal and cognitive skills for coping with stress and for avoiding situations leading to easy access to drugs or to craving. Relapse is prevented by having the individual very gradually reintroduced to greater responsibilities and to the working environment outside of the protected therapeutic community.

PREVENTION

Preventing opiate abuse represents a critically important challenge for physicians. Opiate prescriptions are the most common source of drugs accessed by adolescents who begin a pattern of illicit drug abuse; in the United States, 9000 adolescents become opiate abusers every day. The major sources of these drugs are family members, not drug dealers or the Internet. Pain management involves giving sufficient opiates to relieve the pain over as short a period of time as the pain warrants. The patient then needs to dispose of any remaining opiates, not save them in the medicine cabinet, because this behavior leads to diversion to adolescents. Finally, physicians should never prescribe opiates for themselves.

FURTHER READINGS

Johnston LD et al: *Monitoring the Future: National Results on Adolescent Drug Use: Overview of Key Findings 2008*. Bethesda, Maryland, National Institute on Drug Abuse, 2008

Nestler EJ: Transcriptional mechanisms of addiction: Role of DeltaFosB. Philos Trans R Soc Lond B Biol Sci 363:3245, 2008

Ries R et al (eds): *Principles of Addiction Medicine,* 4th ed. Philadelphia, Lippincott Williams & Wilkins, 2009

CHAPTER 394 Cocaine and Other Commonly Abused Drugs

Nancy K. Mello
Jack H. Mendelson[†]

The abuse of cocaine and other psychostimulant drugs reflects a complex interaction between the pharmacologic properties of each drug, the personality and expectations of the user, and the environmental context in which the drug is used. Polydrug abuse involving the concurrent use of several drugs with different pharmacologic effects is increasingly common. Some forms of polydrug abuse, such as the combined use of heroin and cocaine intravenously, are especially dangerous and are a major problem in hospital emergency rooms. Sometimes one drug is used to enhance the effects of another, as with the combined use of benzodiazepines and methadone, or cocaine and heroin in methadone-maintained patients.

Chronic cocaine and psychostimulant abuse may cause a number of adverse health consequences, and preexisting disorders such as hypertension and cardiac disease may be exacerbated by drug abuse. The combined use of two or more drugs may accentuate medical complications associated with abuse of one of them. Chronic drug abuse is often associated with immune system dysfunction and increased vulnerability to infections, which in turn contributes to the risk for HIV infection. In addition, concurrent use of cocaine and opiates (the "speedball") is frequently associated with needle sharing by IV drug users. Intravenous drug abusers continue to represent the largest single group of persons with HIV infection in several major metropolitan areas in the United States as well as in many parts of Europe and Asia.

COCAINE

Cocaine is a stimulant and a local anesthetic with potent vasoconstrictor properties. The leaves of the *coca* plant (*Erythroxylon coca*) contain ~0.5–1% cocaine. The drug produces physiologic and behavioral effects when administered orally, intranasally, intravenously, or via inhalation following pyrolysis (smoking). The reinforcing effects of cocaine appear to be related to activation of dopaminergic neurons in the mesolimbic system. Cocaine increases synaptic concentrations of the monamine neurotransmitters dopamine, norepinephrine, and serotonin by binding to transporter proteins in presynaptic neurons and blocking reuptake.

Prevalence of cocaine use

Cocaine is widely available throughout the United States, and cocaine abuse occurs in virtually all social and economic strata of society. The prevalence of cocaine abuse in the general population has been accompanied by an increase in cocaine abuse by heroin-dependent persons, including those in methadone maintenance programs. Intravenous cocaine is often used concurrently with IV heroin. This combination purportedly attenuates the postcocaine "crash" and substitutes a cocaine "high" for the heroin "high" blocked by methadone.

Acute and chronic intoxication

There has been an increase in both IV administration and inhalation of pyrolyzed cocaine via smoking. Following intranasal administration, changes in mood and sensation are perceived within 3–5 min, and peak effects occur at 10–20 min. The effects rarely last more than 1 h. Inhalation of pyrolyzed materials includes inhaling crack/cocaine or smoking coca paste, a product made by extracting cocaine preparations with flammable solvents, and cocaine freebase smoking. Freebase cocaine, including the freebase prepared with sodium bicarbonate (crack), has become increasingly popular because of the relative high potency of the compound and its rapid onset of action (8–10 s following smoking).

Cocaine produces a brief, dose-related stimulation and enhancement of mood and an increase in cardiac rate and blood pressure. Body temperature usually increases following cocaine administration, and high doses of cocaine may induce lethal pyrexia or hypertension. Because cocaine inhibits reuptake of catecholamines at adrenergic nerve endings, the drug potentiates sympathetic nervous system activity. Cocaine has a short plasma half-life of approximately 45–60 min. It is metabolized by plasma esterases, and cocaine metabolites are excreted in urine. The very short duration of the euphorigenic effects of cocaine observed in chronic abusers is probably due to both acute and chronic tolerance. Frequent self-administration of the drug (two to three times

[†]Deceased

per hour) is often reported by chronic cocaine abusers. Alcohol is often used to modulate both the cocaine high and the dysphoria associated with the abrupt disappearance of cocaine's effects. A metabolite of cocaine, cocaethylene, has been detected in the blood and urine of persons who concurrently abuse alcohol and cocaine. Cocaethylene induces changes in cardiovascular function similar to those of cocaine alone, and the pathophysiologic consequences of alcohol abuse plus cocaine abuse may be additive when both are used together.

The prevalent assumption that cocaine inhalation or IV administration is relatively safe is contradicted by reports of death from respiratory depression, cardiac arrhythmias, and convulsions associated with cocaine use. In addition to generalized seizures, neurologic complications may include headache, ischemic or hemorrhagic stroke, or subarachnoid hemorrhage. Disorders of cerebral blood flow and perfusion in cocaine-dependent persons have been detected with magnetic resonance spectroscopy (MRS) studies. Severe pulmonary disease may develop in individuals who inhale crack cocaine; this effect is attributed both to the direct effects of cocaine and to residual contaminants in the smoked material. Hepatic necrosis may occur following chronic crack/cocaine use. Protracted cocaine abuse may also cause paranoid ideation and visual and auditory hallucinations, a state that resembles alcoholic hallucinosis.

Although men and women who abuse cocaine may report that the drug enhances libidinal drive, chronic cocaine use causes significant loss of libido and adversely affects sexual function. Impotence and gynecomastia have been observed in male cocaine abusers, and these abnormalities often persist for long periods following cessation of drug use. Women who abuse cocaine may have major derangements in menstrual cycle function, including galactorrhea, amenorrhea, and infertility. Chronic cocaine abuse may cause persistent hyperprolactinemia as a consequence of disordered dopaminergic inhibition of prolactin secretion by the anterior pituitary. Cocaine abuse by pregnant women, particularly crack smoking, has been associated with both an increased risk of congenital malformations in the fetus and perinatal cardiovascular and cerebrovascular disease in the mother. However, cocaine abuse per se is probably not the sole cause of these perinatal disorders, because maternal cocaine abuse is often associated with poor nutrition and prenatal health care as well as polydrug abuse that may contribute to the risk for perinatal disease.

Psychological dependence on cocaine, indicated by inability to abstain from frequent compulsive use, has also been reported. Although the occurrence of withdrawal syndromes involving psychomotor agitation and autonomic hyperactivity remains controversial, severe depression ("crashing") following cocaine intoxication may accompany drug withdrawal.

TREATMENT Cocaine Overdose and Chronic Abuse

Treatment of cocaine overdose is a medical emergency that is best managed in an intensive care unit. Cocaine toxicity produces a hyperadrenergic state characterized by hypertension, tachycardia, tonic-clonic seizures, dyspnea, and ventricular arrhythmias. Intravenous diazepam in doses up to 0.5 mg/kg administered over an 8-h period has been shown to be effective for control of seizures. Ventricular arrhythmias have been managed successfully by administration of 0.5–1 mg of propranolol IV. Since many instances of cocaine-related mortality have been associated with concurrent use of other illicit drugs (particularly heroin), the physician must be prepared to institute effective emergency treatment for multiple drug toxicities.

Treatment of chronic cocaine abuse requires the combined efforts of primary care physicians, psychiatrists, and psychosocial care providers. Early abstinence from cocaine use is often complicated by symptoms of depression and guilt, insomnia, and anorexia, which may be as severe as those observed in major affective disorders. Individual and group psychotherapy, family therapy, and peer group assistance programs are often useful for inducing prolonged remission from drug use. A number of medications used for the treatment of various medical and psychiatric disorders have been administered to reduce the duration and severity of cocaine abuse and dependence. The search for a medication that is both safe and highly effective for cocaine detoxification or maintenance of abstinence is continuing. Although psychotherapy may be effective, no specific form of psychotherapy or behavioral modification is uniquely beneficial.

MARIJUANA AND CANNABIS COMPOUNDS

Cannabis sativa contains >400 compounds in addition to the psychoactive substance, delta-9-tetrahydrocannabinol (THC). Marijuana cigarettes are prepared from the leaves and flowering tops of the plant, and a typical marijuana cigarette contains 0.5–1 g of plant material. The usual THC concentration varies between 10 and 40 mg, but concentrations >100 mg per cigarette have been detected. Hashish is prepared from concentrated resin of *C. sativa* and contains a THC concentration of between 8 and 12% by weight. "Hash oil," a lipid-soluble plant extract, may contain THC between 25 and 60% and may be added to marijuana or hashish to enhance its THC concentration. Smoking is the most common mode of marijuana or hashish use. During pyrolysis, >150 compounds in addition to THC are released in the smoke. Although most of these compounds do not have psychoactive properties, they may have physiologic effects.

THC is quickly absorbed from the lungs into blood, and then rapidly sequestered in tissues. THC is metabolized primarily in the liver, where it is converted to 11-hydroxy-THC, a psychoactive compound, and >20 other metabolites. Many THC metabolites are excreted through the feces at a relatively slow rate of clearance in comparison to most other psychoactive drugs.

Specific cannabinoid receptors (CB_1 and CB_2) have been identified in the central and peripheral nervous system. High densities of cannabinoid receptors have been found in the cerebral cortex, basal ganglia, and hippocampus. T and B lymphocytes also contain cannabinoid receptors, and these appear to mediate the anti-inflammatory and immunoregulatory properties of cannabinoids. A naturally occurring THC-like ligand has been identified and is widely distributed in the nervous system.

Prevalence of use

Marijuana is the most commonly used illegal drug in the United States, and its use is particularly prevalent among adolescents. Marijuana is relatively inexpensive and is often considered to be less hazardous than other controlled drugs and substances. Very potent forms of marijuana (sinsemilla) are now available in many locations, and concurrent use of marijuana with crack/cocaine and phencyclidine is not uncommon.

Acute and chronic intoxication

Acute intoxication from marijuana and cannabis compounds is related to both the dose of THC and the route of administration. THC is absorbed more rapidly from marijuana smoking than from orally ingested cannabis compounds. Acute marijuana intoxication may produce a perception of relaxation and mild euphoria resembling mild to moderate alcohol intoxication. This condition is usually accompanied by some impairment in thinking, concentration, and perceptual and psychomotor function. Higher doses of cannabis may produce more pronounced impairment in concentration and perception, as well as greater sedation. Although the acute effects of marijuana intoxication are relatively benign in normal users, the drug can precipitate severe emotional disorders in individuals who have antecedent psychotic or neurotic problems. Like other psychoactive compounds, both the user's expectations and the environmental context are important determinants of the type and severity of the effects of marijuana intoxication.

As with abuse of cocaine, opioids, and alcohol, chronic marijuana abusers may lose interest in common socially desirable goals and steadily devote more time to drug acquisition and use. However, THC does not cause a specific and unique "amotivational syndrome." The range of symptoms sometimes attributed to marijuana use is difficult to distinguish from mild to moderate depression and the maturational dysfunctions often associated with protracted adolescence. Chronic marijuana use has also been reported to increase the risk of psychotic symptoms in individuals with a past history of schizophrenia. Persons who initiate marijuana smoking before the age of 17 may exhibit more pronounced cognitive deficits and they may also be at higher risk for polydrug and alcohol abuse problems in later life, but the role of marijuana in this causal sequence is uncertain.

Physical effects

Conjunctival injection and tachycardia are the most frequent immediate physical concomitants of smoking marijuana. Tolerance for marijuana-induced tachycardia develops rapidly among regular users. However, marijuana smoking may precipitate angina in persons with a history of coronary insufficiency. Exercise-induced angina may be increased after marijuana use to a greater extent than after tobacco cigarette smoking. Patients with cardiac disease should be strongly advised not to smoke marijuana or use cannabis compounds.

Significant decrements in pulmonary vital capacity have been found in regular daily marijuana smokers. Because marijuana smoking typically involves deep inhalation and prolonged retention of marijuana smoke, marijuana smokers may develop chronic bronchial irritation. Impairment of single-breath carbon monoxide diffusion capacity (DL_{CO}) is greater in persons who smoke both marijuana and tobacco than in tobacco smokers.

Although marijuana has also been associated with a number of other adverse effects, many of these studies await replication and confirmation. A reported correlation between chronic marijuana use and decreased testosterone levels in males has not been confirmed. Decreased sperm count and sperm motility and morphologic abnormalities of spermatozoa following marijuana use have been reported. Prospective studies demonstrated a correlation between impaired fetal growth and development and heavy marijuana use during pregnancy. Marijuana has also been implicated in derangements of the immune system; in chromosomal abnormalities; and in inhibition of DNA, RNA, and protein synthesis; however, these findings have not been confirmed or related to any specific physiologic effect in humans.

Tolerance and physical dependence

Habitual marijuana users rapidly develop tolerance to the psychoactive effects of marijuana, then smoke more frequently and try to acquire more potent cannabis compounds. Tolerance for the physiologic effects of marijuana develops at different rates; e.g., tolerance develops rapidly for marijuana-induced tachycardia but more slowly for marijuana-induced conjunctival injection. Tolerance for both behavioral and physiologic effects of marijuana decreases rapidly upon cessation of marijuana use.

Withdrawal signs and symptoms have been reported in chronic cannabis users, and the severity of symptoms is related to dosage and duration of use. These symptoms typically reach their peak several days after cessation of chronic use and include irritability, anorexia, and sleep disturbances. Withdrawal signs and symptoms observed in chronic marijuana users are usually relatively mild in comparison to those observed in heavy opiate or alcohol users and rarely require medical or pharmacologic intervention. However, more severe and protracted abstinence syndromes may occur after sustained use of high-potency cannabis compounds.

Therapeutic use of marijuana

Marijuana, administered as cigarettes or as a synthetic oral cannabinoid (dronabinol), has been proposed to have a number of medicinal properties that may be clinically useful in some situations. These include antiemetic effects in chemotherapy recipients, appetite-promoting effects in AIDS patients, reduction of intraocular pressure in glaucoma, and reduction of spasticity in multiple sclerosis and other neurologic disorders. With the possible exception of AIDS-related cachexia, none of these attributes of marijuana compounds is clearly superior to other readily available therapies.

METHAMPHETAMINE

Methamphetamine is also referred to as "meth," "speed," "crank," "chalk," "ice," "glass," or "crystal." Methamphetamine is a mixed-action monoamine releaser with activity at dopamine, serotonin, and norepinephrine systems. Despite drug seizures, closures of clandestine laboratories that produce methamphetamine illegally, and an increase in methamphetamine abuse prevention programs, methamphetamine was considered second only to cocaine as a drug threat to society by the U.S. Department of Justice in 2009. Hospital admissions for methamphetamine treatment more than doubled between 1998 and 2007, and young adults (aged 18–25 years) have the highest use rates.

Methamphetamine can be used by smoking, snorting, IV injection, or oral administration. Methamphetamine abusers report that drug use induces feelings of euphoria and decreased fatigue. Adverse consequences of methamphetamine abuse include headache, difficulty concentrating, diminished appetite, abdominal pain, vomiting or diarrhea, disordered sleep, paranoid or aggressive behavior, and psychosis. Chronic methamphetamine abuse can result in severe dental caries, described as blackened, rotting, crumbling teeth. Severe, life-threatening methamphetamine toxicity may include hypertension, cardiac arrhythmia or cardiac failure, subarachnoid hemorrhage, ischemic stroke, intracerebral hemorrhage, convulsions, or coma. Methamphetamines increase the release of monoamine neurotransmitters (dopamine, norepinephrine, and serotonin) from presynaptic neurons. It is thought that the euphoric and reinforcing effects of this class of drugs are mediated through dopamine and the mesolimbic system, whereas the cardiovascular effects are related to norepinephrine. MRS studies of the brain suggest that chronic abusers have neuronal damage in the frontal areas and basal ganglia.

Therapy of acute methamphetamine overdose is largely symptomatic. Ammonium chloride may be useful to acidify the urine and enhance clearance of the drug. Hypertension may respond to sodium nitroprusside or α-adrenergic antagonists. Sedatives may reduce agitation and other signs of central nervous system hyperactivity. Treatment of chronic methamphetamine dependence may be accomplished in either an inpatient or outpatient setting using strategies similar to those described above for cocaine abuse.

MDMA (3,4-methylenedioxymethamphetamine), or *ecstasy*, is a derivative of methamphetamine. Ecstasy is usually taken orally but may be injected or inhaled; its effects last for 3–6 h. In addition to amphetamine-like effects, MDMA can induce hyperthermia and vivid hallucinations and other perceptual distortions. Recent studies have revealed that MDMA use is associated with cognitive and memory impairment and a mild withdrawal syndrome after cessation of use. The long-term consequences of recreational use of MDMA by young persons are poorly understood.

LYSERGIC ACID DIETHYLAMIDE (LSD)

The discovery of the psychedelic effects of LSD led to an epidemic of LSD abuse during the 1960s. Imposition of stringent constraints on the manufacture and distribution of LSD (classified as a Schedule I substance by the U.S. Food and Drug Administration), as well as public recognition that psychedelic experiences induced by LSD were a health hazard, have resulted in a reduction in LSD abuse. LSD still remains popular among adolescents and young adults, and there are indications that LSD use among young persons has been increasing in some areas in the United States.

LSD is a very potent hallucinogen; oral doses as low as 20 μg may induce profound psychological and physiologic effects. Tachycardia, hypertension, pupillary dilation, tremor, and hyperpyrexia occur within minutes following oral administration of 0.5–2 μg/kg. A variety of bizarre and often conflicting perceptual and mood changes, including visual illusions, synesthesias, and extreme lability of mood, usually occur within 30 min after LSD intake. These effects of LSD may persist for 12–18 h, even though the half-life of the drug is only 3 h.

The most frequent acute medical emergency associated with LSD use is a panic episode (the "bad trip"), which may persist up to 24 h. Management of this problem is best accomplished by supportive reassurance ("talking down") and, if necessary, administration of small doses of anxiolytic drugs. Adverse consequences of chronic LSD use include enhanced risk for schizophreniform psychosis and derangements in memory function, problem solving, and abstract thinking. Treatment of these disorders is best carried out in specialized psychiatric facilities.

Tolerance develops rapidly for LSD-induced changes in psychological function when the drug is used one or more times per day for >4 days. Abrupt abstinence following continued use does not produce withdrawal signs or symptoms. There have been no clinical reports of death caused by the direct effects of LSD.

PHENCYCLIDINE (PCP)

Phencyclidine (PCP), a cyclohexylamine derivative, is widely used in veterinary medicine to briefly immobilize large animals and is sometimes described as a dissociative anesthetic. PCP binds to ionotropic *N*-methyl-D-aspartate (NMDA) receptors in the nervous system, blocking ion current through these channels. PCP is easily synthesized; its abusers are primarily young people and polydrug users. It is used orally, by smoking, by snorting, or by IV injection. It is also used as an adulterant in THC, LSD, amphetamine, or cocaine. The most common street preparation, *angel dust*, is a white granular powder that contains 50–100% percent of the drug. Low doses (5 mg) produce agitation, excitement, impaired motor coordination, dysarthria, and analgesia. Physical signs of intoxication may include horizontal or vertical nystagmus, flushing, diaphoresis, and hyperacusis. Behavioral changes include distortions of body image, disorganization of thinking, and feelings of estrangement. Higher doses of PCP (5–10 mg) may produce profuse salivation, vomiting, myoclonus, fever, stupor, or coma. PCP doses of ≥10 mg cause convulsions, opisthotonus, and decerebrate posturing, which may be followed by prolonged coma.

The diagnosis of PCP overdose is difficult because the patient's initial symptoms (anxiety, paranoia, delusions, hallucinations) may suggest an acute schizophrenic reaction. Confirmation of PCP use is possible by determination of PCP levels in serum or urine. PCP assays are available at most toxicologic centers. PCP remains in urine for 1–5 days following high-dose intake.

PCP overdose requires life-support measures, including treatment of coma, convulsions, and respiratory depression in an intensive care unit. There is no specific antidote or antagonist for PCP. PCP excretion from the body can be enhanced by gastric lavage and acidification of urine. Death from PCP overdose may occur as a consequence of some combination of pharyngeal hypersecretion, hyperthermia, respiratory depression, severe hypertension, seizures, hypertensive encephalopathy, and intracerebral hemorrhage.

Acute psychosis associated with PCP use is a psychiatric emergency since patients may be at high risk for suicide or extreme violence toward others. Phenothiazines should not be used for treatment because these drugs potentiate PCP's anticholinergic effects. Haloperidol (5 mg IM) has been administered on an hourly basis to induce suppression of psychotic behavior. PCP, like LSD and mescaline, produces vasospasm of cerebral arteries at relatively low doses. Chronic PCP use has been shown to induce insomnia, anorexia, severe social and behavioral changes, and, in some cases, chronic schizophrenia.

OTHER DRUGS OF ABUSE

A number of other pharmacologically diverse drugs of abuse are often referred to as "club drugs" because these are frequently used in bars, at concerts, and rave parties. Commonly abused club drugs include flunitrazepam, GHB, and ketamine and are described below. Methamphetamine, MDMA, and LSD are also considered club drugs and were described earlier in this chapter. Abuse of club drugs at high doses, especially in combination with alcohol, can be lethal and should be treated as a medical emergency. GHB and ketamine can be identified in blood, and flunitrazepam can be identified in urine and hair samples. Flunitrazepam and GHB toxicity can be treated with antagonists at benzodiazepine and $GABA_B$ receptors, respectively.

Flunitrazepam

Flunitrazepam (Rohypnol) is a benzodiazepine derivative primarily used for treatment of insomnia, but it has significant abuse potential because of its strong hypnotic, anxiolytic and amnesia-producing effects. It is a club drug commonly referred to as a "date-rape drug" or "roofies." The drug enhances $GABA_A$ receptor activity, and overdose can be treated with flumazenil, a benzodiazepine receptor antagonist. Flunitrazepam is typically used orally but can be snorted or injected. Concomitant use of alcohol or opiates is common, and this enhances the sedative and hypnotic effects of flunitrazepam and also the risk of motor vehicle accidents. Overdose can produce life-threatening respiratory depression and coma. Abrupt cessation after chronic use may result in a benzodiazepine withdrawal syndrome consisting of anxiety, insomnia, disordered thinking, and seizures.

GHB

Gamma-hydroxybutyric acid (Xyrem) is a sedative drug that is FDA-approved for the treatment of narcolepsy. It is classified as a club drug, is sometimes used in combination with alcohol or other drugs of abuse, and has been implicated in cases of date rape. GHB is usually taken orally and has no distinctive color or odor. Its stimulant properties are attributed to agonist activity at the GHB receptor, but it also has sedative effects at high doses that reflect its activity at $GABA_B$ receptors. $GABA_B$ antagonists can reverse GHB's sedative effects, and opioid antagonists (naloxone, naltrexone) can attenuate GHB effects on dopamine release. Low doses of GHB may produce euphoria and disinhibition, whereas high doses result in nausea, agitation, convulsions, and sedation that can lead to unconsciousness and death from respiratory depression.

Ketamine

Ketamine (Ketaset, Ketalar) is a dissociative anesthetic, similar to phencyclidine (PCP). In veterinary medicine, it is used for brief immobilization. In clinical medicine, it is used for sedation, analgesia, and to supplement anesthesia. Ketamine increases heart rate and blood pressure, with less respiratory depression than other anesthetics. Ketamine's popularity as a club drug appears to reflect its ability to induce a dissociative state and feelings of depersonalization, accompanied by intense hallucinations and subsequent amnesia. It can be administered orally, by smoking (usually in combination with tobacco and/or marijuana), or by IV or IM injection. Like PCP, it binds to NMDA receptors and acts as an uncompetitive NMDA antagonist. Ketamine has a complex profile of action and appears to be useful as an antidepressant in treatment-resistant patients and as an analgesic in chronic-pain patients. The extent to which chronic recreational use leads to memory impairment remains controversial.

POLYDRUG ABUSE

Although some drug abusers may prefer a particular drug, the concurrent use of multiple drugs is often reported. Polydrug abuse often involves substances that may have different pharmacologic effects from the preferred drug. For example, concurrent use of such dissimilar compounds as stimulants and opiates or stimulants and alcohol is common. The diversity of reported drug use combinations suggests that achieving a subjective change in state, rather than any particular direction of change (stimulation or sedation), may be the primary reinforcer in polydrug abuse. There is also evidence that intoxication with alcohol, opiates, and cocaine is associated with increased tobacco smoking. There are relatively few controlled studies of multiple drug interactions. However, the combined use of cocaine, heroin, and alcohol increases the risk for toxic effects and adverse medical consequences. One determinant of polydrug use patterns is the relative availability and cost of the drugs. For example, alcohol abuse, with its attendant medical complications, is one of the most serious problems encountered in former heroin addicts participating in methadone maintenance programs.

The physician must recognize that perpetuation of polydrug abuse and drug dependence is not necessarily a symptom of an underlying emotional disorder. Neither alleviation of anxiety nor reduction of depression accounts for initiation and perpetuation of polydrug abuse. Severe depression and anxiety are the consequences of polydrug abuse as frequently as they are the antecedents. Interestingly, some adverse consequences of drug use may be reinforcing and contribute to the continuation of polydrug abuse.

Adequate treatment of polydrug abuse, as well as other forms of drug abuse, requires innovative intervention programs. The first step in successful treatment is detoxification, a process that may be difficult when several drugs with different pharmacologic actions (e.g., alcohol, opiates, and cocaine) have been abused. Since patients may not recall or may deny simultaneous multiple drug use, diagnostic evaluation should always include urinalysis for qualitative detection of psychoactive substances and their metabolites. Treatment of polydrug abuse often requires hospitalization or inpatient residential care during detoxification and the initial phase of drug abstinence. When possible, specialized facilities for the care and treatment of drug-dependent persons should be used. Outpatient detoxification of polydrug abuse patients is likely to be ineffective and may be dangerous.

Drug abuse disorders often respond to effective treatment, but episodes of relapse may occur unpredictably. The physician should continue to assist patients during relapse and recognize that occasional recurrent drug use is not unusual in this complex behavioral disorder.

FURTHER READINGS

BRADY KT et al (eds): *Women & Addiction: A Comprehensive Handbook*. New York, Guilford Press, 2009

HABER PS et al: Management of injecting drug users admitted to hospital. Lancet 384:1284, 2009

HERIN DV et al: Agonist-like pharmacotherapy for stimulant dependence: Preclinical, human laboratory, and clinical studies. Ann N Y Acad Sci 1187:76, 2010

LOWINSON JH et al (eds): *Substance Abuse: A Comprehensive Textbook*. Baltimore, Williams & Wilkins, 2005

MELLO NK, MENDELSON JH: Cocaine, hormones and behavior: Clinical and preclinical studies, in *Hormones, Brain and Behavior*, 2nd ed, DW Pfaff et al (eds). San Diego, Academic Press 2009, pp 3081–3139

Principles of Drug Addiction Treatment: A Research-Based Guide, 2nd ed. National Institute on Drug Abuse, NIH Publication No. 09-4180, U.S. Department of Health and Human Services, 2009

CHAPTER 395

Nicotine Addiction

David M. Burns

The use of tobacco leaf to create and satisfy nicotine addiction was introduced to Columbus by Native Americans and spread rapidly to Europe. Use of tobacco as cigarettes, however, only became popular in the twentieth century and so is a modern phenomenon, as is the epidemic of disease caused by this form of tobacco use.

Nicotine is the principal constituent of tobacco responsible for its addictive character, but other smoke constituents and behavioral associations contribute to the strength of the addiction. Addicted smokers regulate their nicotine intake by adjusting the frequency and intensity of their tobacco use both to obtain the desired psychoactive effects and avoid withdrawal.

Unburned cured tobacco used orally contains nicotine, carcinogens, and other toxicants capable of causing gum disease, oral and pancreatic cancers, and an increase in the risk of heart disease. When tobacco is burned, the resultant smoke contains, in addition to nicotine, more than 4000 other compounds that result from volatilization, pyrolysis, and pyrosynthesis of tobacco and various chemical additives used in making different tobacco products. The smoke is composed of a fine aerosol and a vapor phase; aerosolized particles are of a size range that results in deposition in the airways and alveolar surfaces of the lungs. The aggregate of particulate matter, after subtracting nicotine and moisture, is referred to as tar.

The alkaline pH of smoke from blends of tobacco utilized for pipes and cigars allows sufficient absorption of nicotine across the oral mucosa to satisfy the smoker's need for this drug. Therefore, smokers of pipes and cigars tend not to inhale the smoke into the lung, confining the toxic and carcinogenic exposure (and the increased rates of disease) largely to the upper airway for most users of these products. The acidic pH of smoke generated by the tobacco used in cigarettes dramatically reduces absorption of nicotine in the mouth, necessitating inhalation of the smoke into the larger surface of the lungs in order to absorb quantities of nicotine sufficient to satisfy the smoker's addiction. The shift to using tobacco as cigarettes, with resultant increased deposition of smoke in the lung, has created the epidemic of heart disease, lung disease, and lung cancer that dominates the current disease manifestations of tobacco use.

Several genes have been associated with nicotine addiction. Some reduce the clearance of nicotine, and others have been associated with an increased likelihood of becoming dependent on tobacco and other drugs as well as a higher incidence of depression. Rates of smoking cessation have increased, and rates of nicotine addiction have decreased dramatically, since the mid-1950s, suggesting that factors other than genetics are important. It is likely that genetic susceptibility can influence the probability that adolescent experimentation with tobacco will lead to addiction as an adult.

Adult cigarette smoking prevalence has declined to about 20% in the United States, with similar declines in Canada and most European countries. Male smoking prevalence is falling but remains high in most Asian countries, with increasing smoking prevalence among women in those countries. The highest rates of smoking and least cessation are observed in eastern European countries. Of particular concern is the rapidly rising smoking rate observed in the developing world. The recently ratified World Health Organization Framework Convention on Tobacco Control is encouraging effective tobacco control approaches in these countries with the hope of preventing a future epidemic of tobacco-related illness.

DISEASE MANIFESTATIONS OF CIGARETTE SMOKING

More than 400,000 individuals die prematurely each year in the United States from cigarette use; this represents almost one of every five deaths in the United States. Approximately 40% of cigarette smokers will die prematurely due to cigarette smoking unless they are able to quit.

The major diseases caused by cigarette smoking are listed in Table 395-1. The ratio of smoking-related disease rates in smokers compared to never smokers (relative risk) is greater at younger ages, particularly for coronary artery disease and stroke. At older ages, the background rate of disease in nonsmokers increases, diminishing the fractional contribution of smoking and the relative risk; however, absolute excess rates of disease mortality found in smokers compared to nonsmokers increase with increasing age. The organ damage caused by smoking and the number of smokers who die from smoking are both greater among the elderly, as one would expect from a process of cumulative injury.

TABLE 395-1 Relative Risks for Current Smokers of Cigarettes

Disease or Condition	Current Smokers Males	Current Smokers Females
Coronary Heart Disease		
Age 35–64	2.8	3.1
Age ≥65	1.5	1.6
Cerebrovascular Disease		
Age 35–64	3.3	4
Age ≥65	1.6	1.5
Aortic aneurysm	6.2	7.1
Chronic airway obstruction	10.6	13.1
Cancer		
Lung	23.3	12.7
Larynx	14.6	13
Lip, oral cavity, pharynx	10.9	5.1
Esophagus	6.8	7.8
Bladder, other urinary organs	3.3	2.2
Kidney	2.7	1.3
Pancreas	2.3	2.3
Stomach	2	1.4
Cervix		1.6
Acute myeloid leukemia	1.4	1.4
Sudden infant death syndrome		2.3
Infant respiratory distress syndrome		1.3
Low birth weight at delivery		1.8

CARDIOVASCULAR DISEASES

Cigarette smokers are more likely than nonsmokers to develop both large-vessel atherosclerosis and small-vessel disease. Approximately 90% of peripheral vascular disease in the nondiabetic population can be attributed to cigarette smoking, as can ~50% of aortic aneurysms. In contrast, 20–30% of coronary artery disease and ~10% of occlusive cerebrovascular disease are caused by cigarette smoking. There is a multiplicative interaction between cigarette smoking and other cardiac risk factors such that the increment in risk produced by smoking among individuals with hypertension or elevated serum lipids is substantially greater than the increment in risk produced by smoking for individuals without these risk factors.

In addition to its role in promoting atherosclerosis, cigarette smoking also increases the likelihood of myocardial infarction and sudden cardiac death by promoting platelet aggregation and vascular occlusion. Reversal of these effects on coagulation may explain the rapid benefit of smoking cessation for a new coronary event demonstrable among those who have survived a first myocardial infarction. This effect may also explain the substantially higher rates of graft occlusion among continuing smokers following vascular bypass surgery for cardiac or peripheral vascular disease.

Cessation of cigarette smoking reduces the risk of a second coronary event within 6–12 months; rates of first myocardial infarction and death from coronary heart disease also decline within the first few years following cessation. After 15 years of abstinence, the risk of a new myocardial infarction or death from coronary heart disease in former smokers is similar to that for those who have never smoked.

CANCER

Tobacco smoking causes cancer of the lung; oral cavity; naso-, oro-, and hypopharynx; nasal cavity and paranasal sinuses; larynx; esophagus; stomach; pancreas; liver; kidney (body and pelvis); ureter; urinary bladder; and uterine cervix and also causes myeloid leukemia. There is evidence suggesting that cigarette smoking may play a role in increasing the risk of colorectal, hepatocellular, and possibly premenopausal breast cancer. There is no association with postmenopausal breast cancer. There does not appear to be a causal link between cigarette smoking and cancer of the endometrium, and there is a lower risk of uterine cancer among postmenopausal women who smoke. The risks of cancer increase with the increasing number of cigarettes smoked per day and with increasing duration of smoking. Additionally, there are synergistic interactions between cigarette smoking and alcohol use for cancer of the oral cavity, esophagus, and possibly lung. Several occupational exposures synergistically increase lung cancer risk among cigarette smokers, most notably occupational asbestos and radon exposure.

Cessation of cigarette smoking reduces the risk of developing cancer relative to continuing smoking, but even 20 years after cessation there is a modest persistent increased risk of developing lung cancer.

RESPIRATORY DISEASE

Cigarette smoking is responsible for 90% of chronic obstructive pulmonary disease. Within 1–2 years of beginning to smoke regularly, many young smokers will develop inflammatory changes in their small airways, although lung function measures of these changes do not predict development of chronic airflow obstruction. After 20 years of smoking, pathophysiologic changes in the lungs develop and progress proportional to smoking intensity and duration. Chronic mucous hyperplasia of the larger airways results in a chronic productive cough in as many as 80% of smokers >60 years. Chronic inflammation and narrowing of the small airways and/or enzymatic digestion of alveolar walls resulting in pulmonary emphysema can result in reduced expiratory airflow sufficient to produce clinical symptoms of respiratory limitation in ~15–25% of smokers.

Changes in the small airways of young smokers will reverse after 1–2 years of cessation. There may also be a small increase in measures of expiratory airflow following cessation among individuals who have developed chronic airflow obstruction, but the major change following cessation is a slowing of the rate of decline in lung function with advancing age rather than a return of lung function toward normal.

PREGNANCY

Cigarette smoking is associated with several maternal complications of pregnancy: premature rupture of membranes, abruptio placentae, and placenta previa; there is also a small increase in the risk of spontaneous abortion among smokers. Infants of smoking mothers are more likely to experience preterm delivery, have a higher perinatal mortality rate, be small for their gestational age, and have higher rates of infant respiratory distress syndrome; they are more likely to die of sudden infant death syndrome, and appear to have a developmental lag for at least the first several years of life.

OTHER CONDITIONS

Smoking delays healing of peptic ulcers; increases the risk of osteoporosis, senile cataracts, and macular degeneration; and results in premature menopause, wrinkling of the skin, gallstones and cholecystitis in women, and male impotence.

ENVIRONMENTAL TOBACCO SMOKE

Long-term exposure to environmental tobacco smoke increases the risk of lung cancer and coronary artery disease among nonsmokers. It also increases the incidence of respiratory infections, chronic otitis media, and asthma in children as well as causing exacerbation of asthma in children. Some evidence suggests that environmental tobacco smoke exposure may increase the risk of premenopausal breast cancer, but this relationship remains controversial.

PHARMACOLOGIC INTERACTIONS

Cigarette smoking may interact with a variety of other drugs (Table 395-2). Cigarette smoking induces the cytochrome P450 system, which may alter the metabolic clearance of drugs such as theophylline. This may result in inadequate serum levels in smokers as outpatients when the dosage is established in the hospital under nonsmoking conditions. Correspondingly, serum levels may rise when smokers are hospitalized and not allowed to smoke. Smokers may also have higher first-pass clearance for drugs such as lidocaine, and the stimulant effects of nicotine may reduce the effect of benzodiazepines or beta blockers.

TABLE 395-2 Interactions of Smoking and Prescription Drugs

Drug	Interaction
Benzodiazepines	Less sedation
Beta blockers	Reduced lowering of heart rate and blood pressure
Caffeine	Faster metabolic clearance
Chlorpromazine	Decreased serum concentrations[a]
Clomipramine	Decreased serum concentrations[a]
Clozapine	Decreased serum concentrations[a]
Dextropropoxyphene	Less analgesia
Estrogens (oral)	Increased hepatic clearance
Flecainide	Increased first-pass clearance
Fluphenazine	Decreased serum concentrations[a]
Fluvoxamine	Decreased serum concentrations[a]
Haloperidol	Decreased serum concentrations[a]
Heparin	Faster clearance
Imipramine	Decreased serum concentrations[a]
Insulin	Delayed absorption due to skin vasoconstriction
Lidocaine	Increased first-pass clearance
Mexiletine	Increased first-pass clearance
Olanzapine	Faster clearance
Pentazocine	Less analgesia, possible increased clearance
Propranolol	Increased first-pass clearance
Tacrine	Faster metabolic clearance
Theophylline	Faster metabolic clearance
Thiothixene	Faster metabolic clearance
Trazodone	Decreased serum concentrations[a]

[a]Clinical implications uncertain.

OTHER FORMS OF TOBACCO USE

Other major forms of tobacco use are moist snuff deposited between the cheek and gum, chewing tobacco, pipes and cigars, and recently bidi (tobacco wrapped in tendu or temburni leaf; commonly used in India), clove cigarettes, and water pipes. Oral tobacco use leads to gum disease and can result in oral and pancreatic cancer as well as heart disease, with dramatic differences in the risks evident for products used in Africa and Asia as compared to those in the U.S. and Europe.

All forms of burned tobacco generate toxic and carcinogenic smoke similar to that of cigarette smoke. The differences in disease consequences of use relate to frequency of use and depth of inhalation. The risk of upper airway cancers is similar among cigarette and cigar smokers, while those who have smoked only cigars have a much lower risk of lung cancer, heart disease, and chronic obstructive pulmonary disease. However, cigarette smokers who switch to pipes or cigars do tend to inhale the smoke, increasing their risk; and it is likely that comparable inhalation and frequency of exposure to tobacco smoke from any of these forms of tobacco use will lead to comparable disease outcomes.

A resurgence of cigar, bidi, and water pipe use among adolescents of both genders has raised concerns that these older forms of tobacco use are once again causing a public health problem. A variety of devices are currently sold that deliver nicotine by electronically heating materials containing nicotine, the so-called electronic cigarettes. While these devices are marketed as substitutes for cigarettes and as cessation tools, little is known about their composition and evidence suggests that users may not absorb much nicotine from these devices.

LOWER TAR AND NICOTINE CIGARETTES

Filtered cigarettes with lower machine-measured yields of tar and nicotine commonly use ventilation holes in the filters and other engineering designs to artificially lower the machine measurements. Smokers compensate for the lowered nicotine delivery by changing the manner in which they puff on the cigarette or the number of cigarettes smoked per day and preserve their intake of nicotine (and tar). There is no meaningful disease-reduction benefit for smokers who switch to lower-yield cigarettes, and smokers should be discouraged from thinking of low-yield cigarettes as an alternative to cessation.

CESSATION

The process of stopping smoking is often a cyclical one, with the smoker sometimes making multiple attempts to quit and failing before finally being successful. Approximately 70–80% of smokers would like to quit smoking, approximately one-third of current smokers attempt to quit each year, and 90% of these unassisted attempts fail. Clinician-based smoking interventions should encourage smokers to try to quit and to use different forms of cessation assistance with each new cessation attempt rather than focusing exclusively on immediate cessation at the time of the first visit.

Advice from a physician to quit smoking, particularly around an acute illness, is a powerful trigger for cessation attempts, with up to half of patients who are advised to quit making a cessation effort. Other triggers include the cost of cigarettes, media campaigns, and changes in rules to restrict smoking in the workplace.

PHYSICIAN INTERVENTION (Table 395-3)

All patients should be asked whether they smoke, their past experience with quitting, and whether they are currently interested in quitting. Even those who are not interested in quitting should be encouraged and motivated to quit; provided a clear, strong, and personalized physician message that smoking is an important health concern; and offered assistance if they become interested in quitting in the future. There is a relationship between the amount of assistance a patient is willing to accept and the success of the cessation attempt. For those interested in quitting, a quit date should be negotiated, usually not the day of the visit but within the next few weeks, and a follow-up contact by office staff around the time of the quit date should be provided.

There are a variety of nicotine-replacement products, including over-the-counter nicotine patches, gum, and lozenges, as well as nicotine nasal and oral inhalers available by prescription. These products can be used for up to 3–6 months, and some products are formulated to allow a gradual step-down in dosage with increasing duration of abstinence. Antidepressants such as bupropion (300 mg in divided doses for up to 6 months) have also been shown to be effective, as has varenicline, a partial agonist for the nicotinic acetylcholine receptor (initial dose 0.5 mg daily increasing to 1 mg twice daily at day 8; treatment duration up to 6 months). Severe psychiatric symptoms, including suicidal ideation, have been reported with varenicline, resulting in an FDA-mandated warning and a recommendation for closer therapeutic supervision, but evidence to establish the frequency of these responses and the specificity of their association with varenicline remains unclear. Some evidence supports the combined use of nicotine-replacement therapy (NRT) and antidepressants as well as the use of gum or lozenges for acute cravings in patients using patches. Pretreatment with antidepressants or varenicline is recommended for 1–2 weeks prior to the quit date, and pretreatment with nicotine-replacement products is also being explored. NRT is provided in different dosages, with higher doses being recommended for more intense smokers. Clonidine or nortriptyline may be useful for patients who have failed on first-line pharmacologic treatment or who are unable to use other therapies. Antidepressants are more effective in those with a history of depression symptoms.

TABLE 395-3 Clinical Practice Guidelines

Physician Actions
Ask: Systematically identify all tobacco users at every visit
Advise: Strongly urge all smokers to quit
Identify smokers willing to quit
Assist the patient in quitting
Arrange follow-up contact
Effective Pharmacologic Interventions[a]
First-line therapies
Nicotine gum (1.5)
Nicotine patch (1.9)
Nicotine nasal inhaler (2.7)
Nicotine oral inhaler (2.5)
Nicotine lozenge (2.0)
Bupropion (2.1)
Varenicline (2.7)
Second-line therapies
Clonidine (2.1)
Nortriptyline (3.2)
Other Effective Interventions[a]
Physician or other medical personnel counseling (10 min) (1.3)
Intensive smoking cessation programs (at least 4–7 sessions of 20- to 30-min duration lasting at least 2 and preferably 8 weeks) (2.3)
Clinic-based smoking status identification system (3.1)
Counseling by nonclinicians and social support by family and friends
Telephone counseling (1.2)

[a]Numerical value following the intervention is the multiple for cessation success compared to no intervention.

Current recommendations are to offer pharmacologic treatment, usually with NRT or varenicline, to all who will accept it and to provide counseling and other support as a part of the cessation attempt. Currently, indications approved by the U.S. Food and Drug Administration for NRT products limit them to short-term use in conjunction with a cessation attempt. Nevertheless, it is not uncommon for individual smokers to use these products, particularly the products available over the counter, for longer durations and sometimes with no intent to stop. There are some data to suggest that longer-term use of NRT may enable cessation in some smokers who are unable to quit with shorter duration use and that some individuals are able to achieve abstinence from tobacco through use of NRT chronically. It is useful for the practicing physician to recognize that these patterns of use exist among smokers trying to quit and that they may contribute to successful abstinence in some smokers. Cessation advice alone by a physician or his or her staff is likely to increase success compared with no intervention; a more comprehensive approach with advice, pharmacologic assistance, and counseling can increase cessation success by almost threefold.

Incorporation of cessation assistance into a practice requires a change of the care delivery infrastructure. Simple changes include (1) adding questions about smoking and interest in cessation on patient-intake questionnaires, (2) asking patients whether they smoke as part of the initial vital sign measurements made by office staff, (3) listing smoking as a problem in the medical record, and (4) automating follow-up contact with the patient on the quit date. These changes are essential to institutionalizing smoking intervention within the practice setting; without this institutionalization, the best intentions of physicians to intervene with their patients who smoke are often lost in the time crush of a busy practice.

PREVENTION

Approximately 90% of individuals who become cigarette smokers initiate the behavior during adolescence. Factors that promote adolescent initiation are parental or older-generation cigarette smoking, tobacco advertising and promotional activities, the availability of cigarettes, and the social acceptability of smoking. The need for an enhanced self-image and to imitate adult behavior is greatest for those adolescents who have the least external validation of their self-worth, which may explain in part the enormous differences in adolescent smoking prevalence by socioeconomic and school performance strata.

Prevention of smoking initiation must begin early, preferably in the elementary school years. Physicians who treat adolescents should be sensitive to the prevalence of this problem. Physicians should ask all adolescents whether they have experimented with tobacco or currently use tobacco, reinforce the fact that most adolescents and adults do not smoke, and explain that all forms of tobacco are both addictive and harmful.

FURTHER READINGS

Agency for Health Research and Quality: *Treating Tobacco Use and Dependence: 2008 Update*. Clinical Practice Guideline, Public Health Service, DHHS, 2008 *http://www.ncbi.nlm.nih.gov/bookshelf/br.fcgi?book=hsahcpr&part=A28163*

Benowitz N: Nicotine addiction. NEJM 362:2295, 2010

International Agency for Research on Cancer: *Reversal of Risk After Quitting Smoking*. IARC Handbooks of Cancer Prevention, Tobacco Control, Vol 11. Lyon, France, IARC, 2006

US Department of Health and Human Services: *The Health Consequences of Tobacco Use: A Report of the Surgeon General*. National Center for Chronic Disease Prevention and Health Promotion, Office on Smoking and Health, 2004

———: *How Tobacco Smoke Causes Disease—The Biology and Behavioral Basis for Tobacco Attributable Disease: A Report of the Surgeon General*. National Center for Chronic Disease Prevention and Health Promotion, Office on Smoking and Health, 2010

PART 18
Poisoning, Drug Overdose, and Envenomation

CHAPTER 396

Disorders Caused by Venomous Snakebites and Marine Animal Exposures

Paul S. Auerbach
Robert L. Norris

This chapter outlines general principles for the evaluation and management of victims of envenomation and poisoning by venomous snakes and marine creatures. Because the incidence of serious bites and stings is relatively low in developed nations, there is a paucity of relevant clinical research; as a result, therapeutic decision-making often is based on anecdotal information.

VENOMOUS SNAKEBITE

EPIDEMIOLOGY

Venomous snakes belong to the families Viperidae (subfamily Viperinae: Old World vipers; subfamily Crotalinae: New World and Asian pit vipers), Elapidae (including cobras, kraits, coral snakes, and all Australian venomous snakes), Hydrophiidae (sea snakes), Atractaspididae (burrowing asps), and Colubridae (a large family in which most species are nonvenomous and only a few are dangerously toxic to humans). Bite rates are highest in temperate and tropical regions where populations subsist by manual agriculture. Recent estimates indicate somewhere between 1.2 million and 5.5 million snakebites worldwide each year, with 421,000–1,841,000 envenomations and 20,000–94,000 deaths. Such wide-ranging estimates bear testimony to two facts: collection of data is problematic in the regions most affected by venomous snakes (the "developing world"), and what constitutes a "snakebite" varies among researchers. Some count all snakebites (a figure that may include bites by nonvenomous snakes), whereas others count only apparent envenomations.

SNAKE ANATOMY/IDENTIFICATION

The typical snake-venom apparatus consists of bilateral venom glands situated below and behind the eye and connected by ducts to hollow anterior maxillary teeth. In viperids (vipers and pit vipers), those teeth are long mobile fangs that retract against the roof of the mouth when the animal is at rest. In elapids and sea snakes, the fangs are smaller and are relatively fixed in an erect position. In ~20% of pit viper bites and higher percentages of other snakebites (up to 75% for sea snakes), no venom is released ("dry" bites). Significant envenomation probably occurs in ~50% of all venomous snakebites.

Differentiation of venomous from nonvenomous snake species can be difficult. Viperids are characterized by somewhat triangular heads (a feature shared with many harmless snakes), elliptical pupils (also seen in some nonvenomous snakes, such as boas and pythons), enlarged maxillary fangs, and, in pit vipers, paired heat-sensing pits (foveal organs) on each side of the head. The New World rattlesnakes generally have a series of interlocking keratin plates (the rattle) on the tip of the tail; this rattle is used to dissuade potential threats. Color pattern is notoriously misleading in identifying most venomous snakes. Many harmless snakes have color patterns that closely mimic those of venomous snakes found in the same region.

VENOMS AND CLINICAL MANIFESTATIONS

Snake venoms are complex mixtures of enzymes, low-molecular-weight polypeptides, glycoproteins, metal ions, and other constituents. Among the deleterious components are hemorrhagins that promote vascular leakage and cause both local and systemic bleeding. Proteolytic enzymes cause local tissue necrosis, affect the coagulation pathway at various steps, and impair organ function. Myocardial depressant factors reduce cardiac output, and neurotoxins act either pre- or postsynaptically to inhibit peripheral nerve impulses. Most snake venoms have multisystem effects on their victims.

Envenomations by most viperids and some elapids with necrotizing venoms cause progressive local swelling, pain, ecchymosis (Fig. 396-1), and (over a period of hours or days) hemorrhagic bullae and serum-filled vesicles. In serious bites, tissue loss can be significant (Fig. 396-2). Systemic findings can include changes in taste, mouth numbness, muscle fasciculations, tachycardia or bradycardia, hypotension, pulmonary edema, hemorrhage (from essentially any anatomic site), and renal dysfunction. Envenomations by neurotoxic elapids such as kraits (*Bungarus* spp.), many Australian elapids [e.g., death adders (*Atractaspis* spp.)

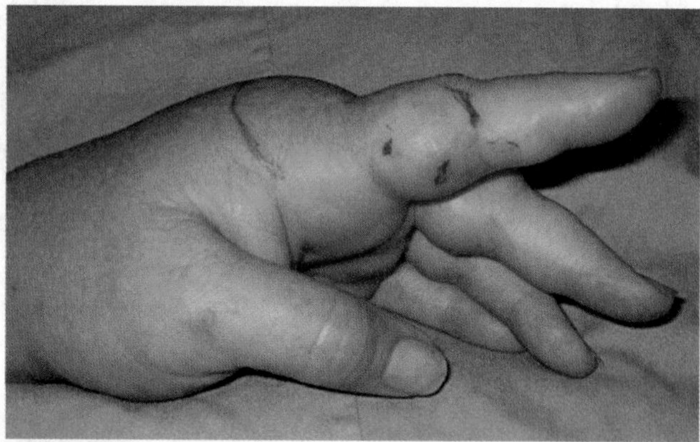

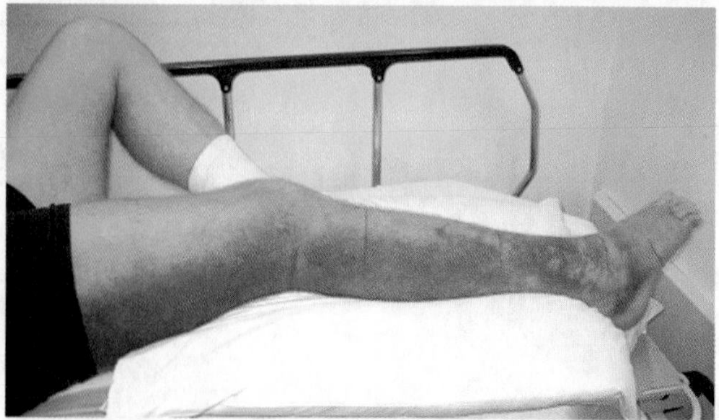

Figure 396-1 Northern Pacific rattlesnake (*Crotalus oreganus oreganus*) envenomations. ***Top:*** Moderately severe envenomation. Note edema and early ecchymosis 2 h after a bite to the finger. ***Bottom:*** Severe envenomation. Note extensive ecchymosis 5 days after a bite to the ankle.

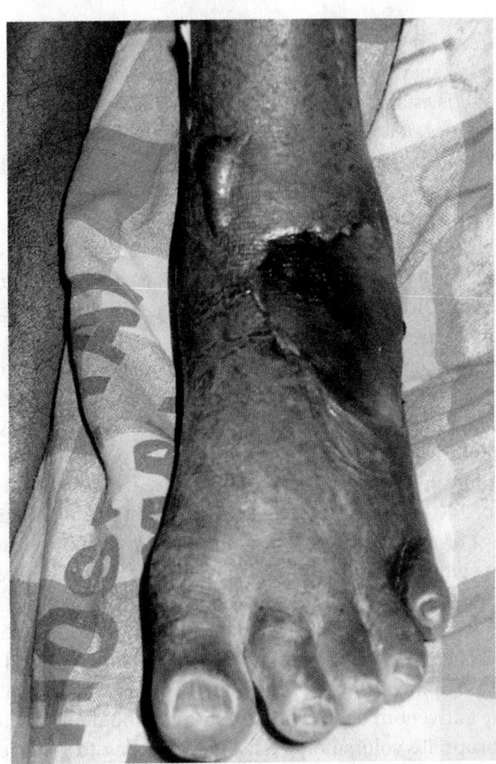

Figure 396-2 Early stages of severe, full-thickness necrosis 5 days after a **Russell's viper *(Daboia russelii)* bite** in southwestern India.

and tiger snakes (*Notechis* spp.)], some cobras (*Naja* spp.), and some viperids [e.g., the South American rattlesnake (*Crotalus durissus*) and some Indian Russell's vipers (*Daboia russelii*)] cause neurologic dysfunction. Early findings may consist of cranial nerve weakness (e.g., manifested by ptosis) and altered mental status. Severe envenomation may result in paralysis, including the muscles of respiration, and lead to death from respiratory failure and aspiration. After elapid bites, the time of onset of venom intoxication varies from minutes to hours, depending on the species involved, the anatomic location of the bite, and the amount of venom injected. Sea snake envenomation usually causes local pain (variable), myalgias, rhabdomyolysis, and neurotoxicity; these manifestations occasionally are delayed for hours.

TREATMENT Venomous Snakebite

Field Management The most important aspect of prehospital care of a person bitten by a venomous snake is rapid delivery to a medical facility equipped to provide supportive care (airway, breathing, and circulation) and antivenom administration. Most of the first-aid recommendations made in the past are of little benefit, and some actually worsen outcome. It is reasonable to apply a splint to the bitten extremity to lessen bleeding and discomfort and, if possible, to keep the extremity at approximately heart level. In developing regions, indigenous people should be encouraged to seek care quickly at health care facilities equipped with antivenoms as opposed to consulting traditional healers and thus incurring significant delays in reaching appropriate care.

Incising wounds and/or applying suction to the bite should be avoided, as these measures are ineffective and exacerbate local tissue damage. Similarly ineffective and potentially damaging are the application of poultices, ice, and electric shock. Techniques or devices used in an effort to limit venom spread (e.g., lymphoocclusive bandages or tourniquets) are ineffective and may result in greater local-tissue damage, particularly that due to necrotic venoms. Tourniquet use can result in amputation and loss of function even in the absence of envenomation.

Elapid venoms that are primarily neurotoxic and have no significant effects on local tissue may be localized by pressure-immobilization, a technique in which the entire limb is wrapped immediately with a bandage (e.g., crepe or elastic) and then immobilized. For this technique to be effective, the wrap pressure must be precise (40–70 mmHg in upper extremity application and 55–70 mmHg in lower extremity application), and the victim must be carried from the scene of the bite to avoid muscle-pump action that—regardless of the anatomic site of the bite—will disperse venom if the victim walks. Pressure-immobilization should be used only in cases in which the offending snake is reliably identified and known to be primarily neurotoxic, the rescuer is skilled in pressure-wrap application, the necessary supplies are readily available, and the victim can be carried to medical care—an uncommon combination of conditions, particularly in regions where such bites are most common.

Hospital Management In the hospital, the victim should be closely monitored (vital signs, cardiac rhythm, oxygen saturation, urine output) while a history is obtained quickly and a rapid, thorough physical examination is performed. For objective evaluation of the progression of local envenomation, the level of swelling in the bitten extremity should be marked and limb circumferences measured every 15 min until swelling has stabilized. During this period of observation/monitoring, the extremity should be positioned at approximately heart level. Measures applied in the field (such as constriction bands or tourniquets) should be removed once IV access has been obtained, with cognizance that the release of such ligatures may result in hypotension or dysrhythmias when stagnant acidotic blood is released to the central circulation. Large-bore IV access in one or two unaffected extremities should be established. Early hypotension is due to pooling of blood in the pulmonary and splanchnic vascular beds. Later, systemic bleeding, hemolysis, and loss of intravascular volume into soft tissues may play important roles. Fluid resuscitation with isotonic saline (20–40 mL/kg IV) should be initiated if there is any evidence of hemodynamic instability, and a trial of 5% albumin (10–20 mL/kg) may be given when patients fail to respond to saline infusion. Only after aggressive volume resuscitation and antivenom administration (see below) should vasopressors (e.g., dopamine) be added. Invasive hemodynamic monitoring (central venous and/or pulmonary arterial pressures) can be helpful in such cases, although obtaining access is risky if coagulopathy has developed.

Blood should be drawn for typing and cross-matching and for laboratory evaluation as soon as possible. Important studies include a complete blood count to evaluate the degree of hemorrhage or hemolysis and to identify thrombocytopenia, studies of renal and hepatic function, coagulation studies to diagnose consumptive coagulopathy, and testing of urine for blood or myoglobin. In developing regions, the 20-min whole-blood clotting test can be used for reliable diagnosis of coagulopathy. A few milliliters of fresh blood are placed in a new, clean, plain glass receptacle (e.g., a test tube) and left undisturbed for 20 min. The tube then is tipped once to 45° to determine whether a clot has formed. If it has not, coagulopathy is diagnosed. Arterial blood gas studies, electrocardiography, and chest radiography may be helpful in severe envenomations or when there is significant comorbidity. Any arterial puncture in the setting of coagulopathy, however, requires great caution and must be performed at an anatomic site amenable to direct-pressure tamponade. After antivenom therapy (see below), laboratory values should be rechecked every 6 h until clinical stability is achieved. If initial laboratory values are normal, the complete blood count and coagulation studies should be repeated every hour until it is clear that no systemic envenomation has occurred. Victims of neurotoxic envenomation should be watched carefully for evidence of cranial nerve dysfunction (e.g., ptosis) that may precede the onset of difficulty swallowing or respiratory insufficiency and necessitate definitive securing of the airway by endotracheal intubation.

The key to management of venomous snakebite resulting in significant envenomation is the administration of specific antivenom. Antivenoms are produced by the injection of venoms from medically important snakes into animals, generally horses or sheep. Once the stock animals develop antibodies to the venoms, their serum is harvested and the antibodies are isolated for antivenom preparation, which may involve varying degrees of digestion and purification of the IgG molecules. The goal of antivenom administration is to allow antibodies (or antibody fragments) to bind up circulating venom components before they can attach to target tissues and cause deleterious effects. Antivenoms may be monospecific (for a particular snake species) or polyspecific (covering several medically important species in the region) but rarely offer cross-protection against snake species other than those used in their production unless the species are known to have homologous venoms. Thus, antivenom selection must be specific for the offending snake; if the antivenom chosen does not contain antibodies to that snake's venom components, it will be of no value and may lead to unnecessary complications (see below). In the United States, assistance in finding appropriate antivenom can be obtained from regional poison control centers.

Indications for antivenom administration to victims of bites by viperids or cytotoxic elapids include any evidence of systemic envenomation (systemic symptoms or signs, laboratory abnormalities) and significant progressive local findings (e.g., soft tissue swelling crossing a joint or involving more than half the bitten limb). Care must be used in determining the significance of isolated soft tissue swelling after the bite of an unidentified snake because the saliva of some relatively harmless species can cause mild edema at the bite site. In such bites, antivenoms are useless and potentially harmful. The efficacy of antivenoms in preventing tissue damage caused by necrotizing venoms is limited. It may be impossible to prevent necrosis completely, as venom components bind to local tissues very quickly—before antivenom administration can be instituted. Nevertheless, antivenom administration should begin as soon as the need for it is identified to limit further tissue damage and systemic effects. Antivenom administration after the bites of neurotoxic elapids is indicated at the first sign of any evidence of neurotoxicity [cranial nerve dysfunction (e.g., ptosis) or peripheral neuropathy].

Specific comments related to the management of venomous snake bite in the United States and Canada appear in Table 396-1. The package insert for the selected antivenom can be consulted regarding species covered, method of administration, starting dose, and need (if any) for redosing. The information in antivenom package inserts, however, is not always accurate and reliable. Whenever possible, it is advisable for treating physicians to seek advice from experts in snakebite management regarding indications for and dosing of antivenom. For viperid bites, antivenom administration generally should be continued as needed until the victim shows definite improvement (e.g., stabilized vital signs, reduced pain, restored coagulation). Neurotoxicity from elapid bites may be harder to reverse with antivenom. Once neurotoxicity is established and endotracheal intubation is required, further doses of antivenom are unlikely to be beneficial. In such cases, the victim must be maintained on mechanical ventilation until recovery, which may take days or weeks.

Use of any heterologous serum product carries a risk of acute nonallergic (and, less commonly, allergic) anaphylaxis and delayed-type hypersensitivity reactions (serum sickness). Skin testing for potential allergy, although recommended by some antivenom manufacturers, is insensitive and nonspecific and should be omitted. Worldwide, the quality of antivenoms is highly variable. Rates of acute nonallergic anaphylactic reactions to some of these products exceed 50%. For this reason, some authorities have recommended pretreatment with IV antihistamines (e.g., diphenhydramine, 1 mg/kg to a maximum of 100 mg, and cimetidine, 5–10 mg/kg to a maximum of 300 mg) or even a prophylactic subcutaneous or intramuscular dose of epinephrine (0.01 mg/kg, up to 0.3 mg). Further research is necessary, however, to determine whether any pretreatment measures are truly beneficial. Modest expansion of the patient's intravascular volume with crystalloids may blunt acute adverse reactions. Epinephrine should always be immediately available, and the antivenom dose to be administered should be diluted in an appropriate volume of crystalloid according to the package insert. Antivenom should be given only by the IV route, and the infusion should be started slowly, with the physician at the bedside during the initial period to intervene immediately at the first signs of an acute reaction (which may be heralded by a single hive or mild itching or may present as bronchospasm or acute cardiovascular collapse). The rate of infusion can be increased gradually in the absence of a reaction until the full starting dose has been administered (over a total period of ~1 h). Further antivenom may be necessary if the patient's acute clinical condition worsens or fails to stabilize. There is some evidence that smaller-molecular-weight Fab-fragment antivenoms are cleared more quickly from the circulation than are whole-IgG or $F(ab)_2$ antivenoms and thus may require redosing if venom effects that were controlled initially begin to recur. The decision to administer further antivenom to a stabilized patient generally should be based on clinical evidence of persistent circulation of unbound venom components. Antivenom is effective only in reversing active venom toxicity; it is of no benefit in reversing effects that already have been established (e.g., renal failure, established paralysis, necrosis) and that will improve only with time and other therapies.

If the patient develops an acute reaction to antivenom, the infusion should be temporarily stopped and the reaction immediately treated with IM epinephrine and IV antihistamines and glucocorticoids (Chap. 317). Once the reaction is controlled, if the severity of envenomation warrants additional antivenom, the dose should be diluted further in isotonic saline and restarted as soon as possible. Rarely, in recalcitrant cases, a concomitant IV infusion of epinephrine may be required to hold allergic sequelae at bay while further antivenom is administered. The patient must be monitored very closely, preferably in an intensive care setting, during such therapy.

Blood products are rarely necessary in the management of an envenomated patient. The venoms of many snake species can cause a drop in platelet count or hematocrit and depletion of coagulation factors. Nevertheless, these components usually rebound within hours after administration of adequate antivenom. If the need for blood products is thought to be great (e.g., for a dangerously low platelet count in a hemorrhaging

TABLE 396-1 Management of Venomous Snakebite in the United States and Canada[a]

Pit viper bites [rattlesnakes (*Crotalus* and *Sistrurus* spp.), cottonmouth water moccasins (*Agkistrodon piscivorus*), and copperheads (*A. contortrix*)]

- Stabilize airway, breathing, and circulation.
- Institute monitoring (cardiac and pulse oximetry).
- Establish two large-bore IV lines with normal saline infusion (administer a bolus of 20–40 mL/kg of body weight if the patient is hypotensive; if hypotension persists, consider albumin).
- Take rapid history and perform rapid physical examination (including vital signs).
- Measure/record circumferences of the bitten extremity every 15 min until swelling has stabilized.
- Identify the offending reptile if possible.
- Send laboratory studies (CBC, metabolic panel, PT/INR/PTT, fibrinogen level, FDP, blood type and screening, urinalysis).
  - If normal, repeat CBC, PT/INR/PTT, fibrinogen level, and FDP every hour until it is clear that no systemic envenomation has occurred.
  - If abnormal, repeat 6 h after antivenom administration (see below).
- Determine severity of envenomation.
  - None ("dry bite"): fang marks only
  - Mild: local findings only (e.g., pain, local ecchymosis, nonprogressive swelling)
  - Moderate: swelling that is clearly progressing, systemic signs or symptoms, and/or laboratory abnormalities
  - Severe: respiratory distress, neurologic dysfunction, and/or cardiovascular instability/shock
- Locate and administer antivenom as indicated: Crotalidae Polyvalent Immune Fab (CroFab) (Ovine) (Protherics US Inc., Brentwood, TN).
  - Starting dose
    - Based on severity of envenomation
      - None or mild: none
      - Moderate: 4–6 vials
      - Severe: 6 vials
    - Mix reconstituted vials in 250 mL of normal saline.
    - No pretesting for potential allergy; no premedication
    - Give IV over 1 h (with physician in close attendance).
  - If acute reaction to antivenom
    - Stop infusion.
    - Treat with standard doses of epinephrine (IM or IV; the latter route only in the setting of severe hypotension), antihistamines (IV), and glucocorticoids (IV).
    - When reaction is controlled, restart antivenom as soon as possible (may further dilute in a larger volume of normal saline).
  - Monitor clinical status over 1 h.
    - Stabilized, improved: hospital admission
    - Progressing or unimproved: repetition of starting dose (this pattern continued until patient's condition is stable or improved)
- Pain management: acetaminophen and/or narcotics as needed (avoid salicylates and nonsteroidal anti-inflammatory agents)
- Update tetanus immunization as needed.
- Prophylactic antibiotics are unnecessary unless prehospital care included incisions or mouth suction.
- Blood products and coagulation factors are rarely needed; if required, they should be given only after antivenom administration.
- Admit to hospital. (If no evidence of envenomation, monitor for 8 h before discharge.)
  - Give further CroFab (two vials q6h for three additional doses; close monitoring).
  - Monitor for evidence of rising intracompartmental pressures (see text).
  - Provide wound care (see text).
  - Begin physical therapy (see text).
- At discharge, warn patient of possible recurrent coagulopathy and signs/symptoms of delayed serum sickness.

Coral snakebites (*Micrurus* spp. and *Micruroides euryxanthus*)

- Stabilize airway, breathing, and circulation as needed.
- Institute monitoring (cardiac and pulse oximetry).
- Establish one large-bore IV line with normal saline infusion.
- Take rapid history and perform rapid physical examination (including vital signs).
- Identify the offending reptile if possible.
- Laboratory studies are unlikely to be helpful.

(*continued*)

TABLE 396-1 Management of Venomous Snakebite in the United States and Canada[a] (*Continued*)

- If any evidence of neurologic dysfunction (e.g., any cranial nerve abnormalities such as ptosis):
  - Trial of anticholinesterase inhibitors (see Table 396-2)
  - With any evidence of difficulty swallowing or breathing, proceed with endotracheal intubation and ventilatory support (may be required for days or weeks).
- Update tetanus immunization as needed.
- Prophylactic antibiotics are unnecessary unless prehospital care included incisions or mouth suction.
- Admit to hospital (intensive care unit) even if there is no evidence of envenomation (monitor for at least 24 h).
- At the time of this publication, no coral snake antivenom is commercially available for routine use in the United States.

[a]These recommendations are specific to the care of victims of venomous snakebite in the United States and Canada and should not be applied to bites in other regions of the world.

Abbreviations: CBC, complete blood count; FDP, fibrin degradation products; PT/INR/PTT, prothrombin time/international normalized ratio/activated partial thromboplastin time.

patient), these products should be given only after adequate antivenom administration to avoid adding fuel to an ongoing consumptive coagulopathy.

Rhabdomyolysis and hemolysis should be managed in standard fashion. Victims who develop acute renal failure should be evaluated by a nephrologist and referred for peritoneal dialysis or hemodialysis as needed. Such renal failure, which usually is due to acute tubular necrosis, is frequently reversible. If bilateral cortical necrosis occurs, however, the prognosis for renal recovery is grimmer, and long-term dialysis with possible renal transplantation may be necessary.

Acetylcholinesterase inhibitors (e.g., edrophonium and neostigmine) may promote neurologic improvement in patients bitten by snakes with postsynaptic neurotoxins. Victims with objective evidence of neurologic dysfunction after snakebite should receive a trial of acetylcholinesterase inhibitors, as outlined in Table 396-2. If they respond, additional doses of long-acting neostigmine can be continued as needed. Special vigilance is required to prevent aspiration if repetitive dosing of neostigmine is used in an attempt to obviate endotracheal intubation.

Care of the bite wound includes application of a dry, sterile dressing and splinting of the extremity with padding between the digits. Once the administration of antivenom has been initiated, the extremity should be elevated above heart level to relieve edema. Tetanus immunization should be updated as appropriate. Prophylactic antibiotics are generally unnecessary after bites by North American snakes, as the incidence of secondary infection is low. Antibiotics can be considered, however, if misguided first aid efforts have included incisions or mouth suction. In some regions, secondary bacterial infection is more common and the consequences are dire. In these regions, prophylactic antibiotics (e.g., cephalosporins) are used commonly. Pain control should be achieved with acetaminophen or narcotic analgesics. Salicylates and nonsteroidal anti-inflammatory agents should be avoided because of their effects on blood clotting.

Most snake envenomations involve subcutaneous deposition of venom. On occasion, however, venom can be injected more deeply into muscle compartments, particularly if the offending snake was large and the bite occurred to the lower leg or the forearm or hand. If swelling in the bitten extremity raises concern that subfascial muscle edema may be impeding tissue perfusion (muscle-compartment syndrome), intracompartmental pressures (ICPs) should be checked by any minimally invasive technique—e.g., wick catheter or ICP monitor (Stryker Instruments, Kalamazoo, MI). If any ICP is high (>30–40 mmHg), the extremity should be kept elevated while further antivenom is given. A dose of IV mannitol (1 g/kg) can be given in an effort to reduce muscle edema if the patient's hemodynamic status is stable. If, after 1 h of such therapy, the ICP remains elevated, a surgical consultation for possible fasciotomy should be obtained. Although preliminary evidence from studies in animals suggests that fasciotomy actually may worsen myonecrosis, compartmental decompression is still required to preserve nerve function. Fortunately, the incidence of muscle-compartment syndrome is very low after snakebite, with fasciotomies required in <1% of cases. Nevertheless, vigilance is required; if a fasciotomy is deemed necessary, it should be undertaken with the patient's informed consent whenever possible.

Wound care in the days after the bite may require careful aseptic debridement of clearly necrotic tissue once coagulation has been restored. Intact serum-filled vesicles or hemorrhagic blebs should be left undisturbed. If ruptured, they should be debrided with sterile technique. Any debridement of damaged muscle should be conservative, as there is evidence that such muscle may recover to a significant degree.

Physical therapy should be started when pain allows so that the victim can return to a functional state. The incidence of long-term loss of function (e.g., reduced range of motion, impaired sensory function) is unclear but is probably quite high (>30%), particularly after viperid bites.

TABLE 396-2 Use of Acetylcholinesterase Inhibitors in Neurotoxic Snake Envenomation

1. Patients with clear, objective evidence of neurotoxicity after snakebite (e.g., ptosis or inability to maintain upward gaze) should receive a trial of edrophonium (if available) or neostigmine.
   a. Pretreat with atropine: 0.6 mg IV (children, 0.02 mg/kg; minimum of 0.1 mg)
   b. Follow with:
      Edrophonium: 10 mg IV (children, 0.25 mg/kg)
      or
      Neostigmine: 1.5–2.0 mg IM (children, 0.025–0.08 mg/kg)
2. If objective improvement is evident at 5 min, continue neostigmine at a dose of 0.5 mg (children, 0.01 mg/kg) IV or SC every 30 min as needed, with continued administration of atropine by continuous infusion of 0.6 mg over 8 h (children, 0.02 mg/kg over 8 h).
3. Maintain vigilance regarding aspiration risk and secure the airway with endotracheal intubation as needed.

Any patient with signs of envenomation should be observed in the hospital for at least 24 h. In North America, a patient with an apparently "dry" viperid bite should be watched for at least 8 h before discharge, as significant toxicity occasionally develops after a delay of several hours. The onset of systemic symptoms commonly is delayed for a number of hours after bites by several of the elapids (including coral snakes, *Micrurus* spp.), some non–North American viperids [e.g., the hump-nosed pit viper (*Hypnale hypnale*)], and sea snakes. Patients bitten by these reptiles should be observed in the hospital for at least 24 h. Patients whose condition is not stable should be admitted to an intensive care setting.

At discharge, victims of venomous snakebite should be warned about signs and symptoms of wound infection, antivenom-related serum sickness, and potential long-term sequelae, such as pituitary insufficiency in Russell's viper (*D. russelii*) bites. If coagulopathy developed in the acute stages of envenomation, it can recur during the first 2–3 weeks after the bite. In such cases, victims should be warned to avoid elective surgery or activities posing a high risk of trauma during this period. Outpatient analgesic treatment and physical therapy should be continued.

In the event of serum sickness (fever, chills, urticaria, myalgias, arthralgias, and possibly renal or neurologic dysfunction developing 1–2 weeks after antivenom administration), the victim should be treated with systemic glucocorticoids (e.g., oral prednisone, 1–2 mg/kg daily) until all findings resolve; the dose is then tapered over 1–2 weeks. Oral antihistamines and analgesics provide additional relief of symptoms.

■ MORBIDITY AND MORTALITY

The overall mortality rates for venomous snakebite are low in areas with rapid access to medical care and appropriate antivenoms. In the United States, for example, the mortality rate is <1% for victims who receive antivenom. Eastern and western diamondback rattlesnakes (*Crotalus adamanteus* and *C. atrox*, respectively) are responsible for the majority of snakebite deaths in the United States. Snakes responsible for large numbers of deaths in other countries include cobras (*Naja* spp.), carpet and saw-scaled vipers (*Echis* spp.), Russell's vipers (*D. russelii*), large African vipers (*Bitis* spp.), lancehead pit vipers (*Bothrops* spp.), and tropical rattlesnakes (*C. durissus*).

The incidence of morbidity—defined as permanent functional loss in a bitten extremity—is difficult to estimate but is substantial. Morbidity may be due to muscle, nerve, or vascular injury or to scar contracture. Such morbidity can have devastating consequences for victims in the developing world when their ability to work and provide for their families is lost. In the United States, functional loss tends to be more common and severe after rattlesnake bites than after bites by copperheads (*Agkistrodon contortrix*) or water moccasins (*A. piscivorus*).

The global crisis

In many developing countries where snakebite is common, scarce access to medical care and antivenom resources contributes to high rates of morbidity and death. In many countries, the available antivenoms are inappropriate and ineffective against the venoms of medically important indigenous snakes. In those regions, further research is necessary to determine the actual impact of venomous snakebite and the specific antivenom needs in terms of both quantity and spectrum of coverage. Without accurate statistics, it is difficult to persuade antivenom manufacturers to begin and sustain production of appropriate antisera in developing nations. There is evidence that antivenoms can be produced in much more cost-effective ways than those currently being used. Just as important as getting the correct antivenoms into underserved regions is the need to educate populations about the prevention of snakebite and train medical care providers in proper management approaches. Local protocols written with significant input from experienced providers in the region of concern should be developed and distributed. Appropriate antivenoms must be available at the likely first point of medical contact for patients (e.g., primary health centers) to minimize the common practice of referring victims to more distant, higher levels of care for the initiation of antivenom therapy. Those who care for snakebite victims in these often remote clinics must have the skills and confidence required to begin antivenom treatment (and to treat possible reactions) as soon as possible when needed.

MARINE ENVENOMATIONS

Much of the management of envenomation by marine creatures is supportive in nature. A specific marine antivenom can be used when appropriate.

■ INVERTEBRATES

Cnidarians

The Golgi apparatus of the cnidoblast cells within cnidarians such as hydroids, fire coral, jellyfish, Portuguese men-of-war, and sea anemones secretes specialized living stinging organelles called *cnidae* (also referred to as *cnidocysts*, a term that encompasses nematocysts, ptychocysts, and spirocysts). Within each organelle resides a stinging mechanism ("thread tube") and venom. In the stinging process, cnidocysts are released and discharged upon mechanosensory stimulation. The venoms from these organisms are mixtures of proteins, carbohydrates, and other components. Victims usually report immediate prickling or burning, pruritus, paresthesias, and painful throbbing with radiation. The skin becomes reddened, darkened, edematous, and/or blistered. A legion of neurologic, cardiovascular, respiratory, rheumatologic, gastrointestinal, renal, and ocular symptoms have been described. Anaphylaxis is possible. *Irukandji syndrome*, associated with the Australian jellyfish *Carukia barnesi* and other species, is a potentially fatal condition that most commonly is characterized by severe back, chest, and abdominal pain; nausea and vomiting; headache; sweating; and, in the most serious cases, myocardial troponin leak and pulmonary edema. This syndrome is thought to be mediated, at least in part, by the release of endogenous catecholamines.

Rescuers should note that envenomations by different cnidarians (typified by jellyfish) may respond differently to similar therapies; thus, the recommendations in this chapter must be tailored to local species and clinical practices. During stabilization, the skin should be decontaminated immediately with a generous application of vinegar (5% acetic acid), which is the all-purpose agent useful for inactivating the nematocysts in the greatest number of species. Rubbing alcohol (40–70% isopropyl alcohol), baking soda (sodium bicarbonate), papain (unseasoned meat tenderizer), fresh lemon or lime juice, household ammonia, olive oil, or sugar may be effective, depending on the species of stinging creature. For the sting of the venomous box-jellyfish (*Chironex fleckeri*), vinegar should be used. Local application of heat (up to 45°C/113°F), commonly by immersion in hot water, may be as effective. Commercial (chemical) cold packs or real ice packs applied over a thin dry cloth or plastic membrane have been shown to be effective in alleviating mild or moderate *Physalia utriculus* (bluebottle jellyfish) stings but may be less effective than application of heat. Perfume, aftershave lotion, and high-proof ethanol are not efficacious and may be detrimental; formalin, ether, gasoline, and other organic solvents should not be used. Shaving the skin helps remove remaining nematocysts.

Freshwater irrigation and rubbing lead to further stinging by adherent nematocysts and should be avoided. After decontamination, topical application of an anesthetic ointment (lidocaine, benzocaine), an antihistamine (diphenhydramine), or a glucocorticoid (hydrocortisone) may be helpful. Persistent severe pain after decontamination may be treated with morphine, meperidine, fentanyl, or another narcotic analgesic. Muscle spasms may respond to diazepam (2–5 mg, titrated upward as necessary) or 10% calcium gluconate (5–10 mL) given IV. An ovine-derived antivenom is available from Commonwealth Serum Laboratories (see the section on antivenom sources, below) for stings from the box-jellyfish found in Australian and Indo-Pacific waters. Ongoing discussion about its efficacy centers on the notion that *C. fleckeri* venom acts more rapidly than the antivenom can bind to the venom. As of this writing, this antivenom has not been used to treat envenomation by the box-shaped jellyfish (possibly of the genus *Chiropsalmus*) that has been found in Florida waters. Treatment for Irukandji syndrome may require the administration of $MgSO_4$ and aggressive antihypertensive treatment.

The pressure-immobilization technique is no longer recommended for venom containment in the setting of a jellyfish sting. Safe Sea, a "jellyfish-safe" sunblock (*www.nidaria.com*) applied to the skin before an individual enters the water, inactivates the recognition and discharge mechanisms of nematocysts, has been tested successfully against a number of marine stingers, and may prevent or diminish the effects of coelenterate stings. Whenever possible, a dive skin or wet suit should be worn when entering ocean waters.

Sea sponges

Touching a sea sponge may result in dermatitis. The afflicted skin should be gently dried and adhesive tape used to remove embedded spicules. Vinegar should be applied immediately and then for 10–30 min three or four times a day. Rubbing alcohol may be used if vinegar is unavailable. After spicule removal and skin decontamination, steroid or antihistamine cream may be applied to the skin. Severe vesiculation should be treated with a 2-week course of systemic glucocorticoids.

Annelid worms

Annelid worms (bristleworms) possess rows of soft, cactus-like spines capable of inflicting painful stings. Contact results in symptoms similar to those of nematocyst envenomation. Without treatment, pain usually subsides over several hours, but inflammation may persist for up to a week. Victims should resist the urge to scratch, since scratching may fracture retrievable spines. Visible bristles should be removed with forceps and adhesive tape or a commercial facial peel; alternatively, a thin layer of rubber cement can be used to entrap the spines. Use of vinegar, rubbing alcohol, or dilute ammonia or a brief application of unseasoned meat tenderizer (papain) may provide additional relief. Local inflammation should be treated with topical or systemic glucocorticoids.

Sea urchins

Sea urchins possess either hollow, venom-filled calcified spines or triple-jawed, globiferous pedicellariae with venom glands. The venom contains toxic components, including steroid glycosides, hemolysins, proteases, serotonin, and cholinergic substances. Contact with either venom apparatus produces immediate and intensely painful stings. The affected part should be immersed immediately in hot water (see below). Accessible embedded spines should be removed but may break off and remain lodged in the victim. Residual dye from the surface of a spine remaining after the spine's removal may mimic a retained spine but is otherwise of no consequence. Soft tissue radiography or MRI can confirm the presence of retained spines, which may warrant referral for attempted surgical removal if the spines are near vital structures (e.g., joints, neurovascular bundles). Retained spines may cause the formation of granulomas that are amenable to excision or to intralesional injection with triamcinolone hexacetonide (5 mg/mL). Chronic granulomatous arthritis of the proximal interphalangeal joints has been treated with synovectomy and removal of granulation tissue. Erbium-YAG laser ablation has been deployed to destroy multiple sea urchin spines embedded in the foot and identified visually at surface level without causing thermal necrosis of the adjacent tissues. Eosinophilic pneumonia and local and diffuse neuropathies have been observed separately after penetration by multiple spines of the black sea urchin (presumed *Diadema* spp.). The pathophysiology of this phenomenon has not been determined.

Octopuses

Serious envenomations and deaths have followed bites of Australian blue-ringed octopuses (*Octopus maculosus* and *O. lunulata*). Although these animals rarely exceed 20 cm in length, their venom contains a potent neurotoxin (maculotoxin) that inhibits peripheral nerve transmission by blocking sodium conductance. Oral numbness and facial numbness develop within several minutes of a serious envenomation and rapidly progress to total flaccid paralysis, including failure of respiratory muscles. Immediately after envenomation, a circumferential pressure-immobilization dressing 15 cm wide should be applied over a gauze pad (~7 × 7 × 2 cm) that has been placed directly over the sting. The dressing should be applied at venous-lymphatic pressure, with the preservation of distal arterial pulses. The limb should then be splinted. Once the victim has been transported to the nearest medical facility, the bandage can be released. Since there is no antidote, treatment is supportive. If respirations are assisted, the victim may remain awake although completely paralyzed. Even with serious envenomations, significant recovery often takes place within 4–10 h. Sequelae are uncommon unless related to hypoxia.

■ VERTEBRATES

Stingrays

A stingray injury is both an envenomation and a traumatic wound. Thoracic and cardiac penetration, major vessel laceration, and compartment syndrome have all been observed. The venom, which contains serotonin, 5′-nucleotidase, and phosphodiesterase, causes immediate, intense pain that may last up to 48 h. The wound often becomes ischemic in appearance and heals poorly, with adjacent soft tissue swelling and prolonged disability. Systemic effects include weakness, diaphoresis, nausea, vomiting, diarrhea, dysrhythmias, syncope, hypotension, muscle cramps, fasciculations, paralysis, and (in rare cases) death. Because of the differences in toxins present on the tissues covering the stingers, freshwater stingrays may cause more severe injuries than do marine stingrays.

Scorpionfish

The designation *scorpionfish* encompasses members of the family Scorpaenidae and includes not only scorpionfish but also lionfish and stonefish. A complex venom with neuromuscular toxicity is delivered through 12 or 13 dorsal, 2 pelvic, and 3 anal spines. In general, the sting of a stonefish is regarded as the most serious (severe to life-threatening); that of the scorpionfish is of intermediate seriousness; and that of the lionfish is the least serious. Like that of a stingray, the sting of a scorpionfish is immediately and intensely painful. Pain from a stonefish envenomation may last for days. Systemic manifestations of scorpionfish stings are similar to those of stingray envenomations but may be more pronounced, particularly in the case of a stonefish sting. The rare deaths that follow stonefish envenomation usually occur within 6–8 h.

Other fish

Two species of marine catfish—*Plotosus lineatus* (the oriental catfish) and *Galeichthys felis* (the common sea catfish)—as well as several species of freshwater catfish are capable of stinging humans. Venom is delivered through a single dorsal spine and two pectoral spines. Clinically, a catfish sting is comparable to that of a stingray, although marine catfish envenomations are generally more severe than those of their freshwater counterparts. Surgeonfish (doctorfish, tang), weeverfish, ratfish, and horned venomous sharks have also envenomated humans.

TREATMENT Marine Vertebrate Stings

The stings of all marine vertebrates are treated in a similar fashion. Except for stonefish and serious scorpionfish envenomations (see below), no antivenom is available. The affected part should be immersed immediately in nonscalding hot water (45°C/113°F) for 30–90 min or until there is significant relief of pain. Recurrent pain may respond to repeated hot-water treatment. Cryotherapy is contraindicated. Opiates will help alleviate the pain, as will local wound infiltration or regional nerve block with 1% lidocaine, 0.5% bupivacaine, and sodium bicarbonate mixed in a 5:5:1 ratio. After soaking and anesthetic administration, the wound must be explored and debrided. Radiography (in particular, MRI) may be helpful in identification of foreign bodies. After exploration and debridement, the wound should be irrigated vigorously with warm sterile water, saline, or 1% povidone-iodine in solution. Bleeding usually can be controlled by sustained local pressure for 10–15 min. In general, wounds should be left open to heal by secondary intention or treated by delayed primary closure. Tetanus immunization should be updated. Antibiotic treatment should be considered for serious wounds and for envenomation in immunocompromised hosts. The initial antibiotics should cover *Staphylococcus* and *Streptococcus* spp. If the victim is immunocompromised, if a wound is primarily repaired and is more than minor, or if an infection develops, antibiotic coverage should be broadened to include *Vibrio* spp. Infection with *Aeromonas* spp. is of similar concern for wounds associated with natural freshwater.

APPROACH TO THE PATIENT Marine Envenomations

It is useful to be familiar with the local marine fauna and to recognize patterns of injury.

A large puncture wound or jagged laceration (particularly on the lower extremity) that is more painful than one would expect from the size and configuration of the wound is likely to be a stingray envenomation. Smaller punctures, as described above, represent the activity of a sea urchin or starfish. Stony corals cause rough abrasions and, in rare instances, lacerations or puncture wounds.

Coelenterate (marine invertebrate) stings sometimes create diagnostic skin patterns. A diffuse urticarial rash on exposed skin is often indicative of exposure to fragmented hydroids or larval anemones. A linear, whiplike print pattern appears where a jellyfish tentacle has contacted the skin. In the case of the dreaded box-jellyfish (Fig. 396-3), a cross-hatched appearance, followed by development of dark purple coloration within a few hours of the sting, heralds skin necrosis. A frosted appearance may be created by aluminum salt–based remedies applied to the wound. An encounter with fire coral causes immediate pain and swollen red skin irritation in the pattern of contact, similar to but more severe than the imprint left by exposure to an intact feather hydroid. Seabather's eruption, caused by thimble jellyfishes and larval anemones, may produce a diffuse rash that consists of clusters of erythematous macules or raised papules and is accompanied by intense itching (Fig. 396-4). Toxic sponges create a burning and painful red rash on exposed skin, which may blister and later desquamate. Virtually all marine stingers invoke the sequelae of inflammation, so that local erythema, swelling, and adenopathy are fairly nonspecific.

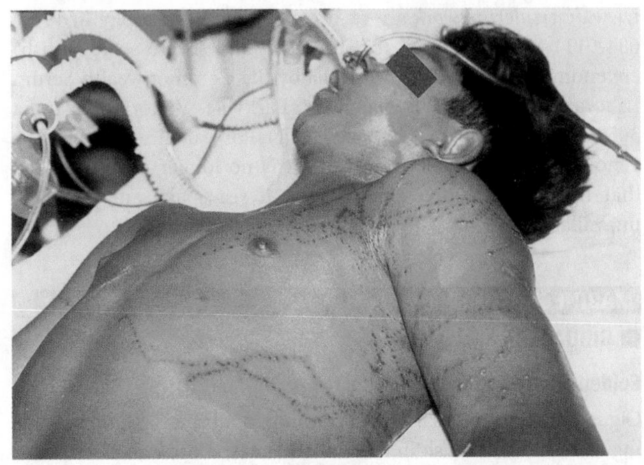

Figure 396-3 Skin lesions caused by *Chironex fleckeri* sting. *(Courtesy of Dr. V. Pranava Murthy; with permission.)*

SOURCES OF ANTIVENOMS AND OTHER ASSISTANCE

The best way to locate a specific antivenom in the United States is to call a regional poison control center and ask for assistance. Divers Alert Network, a nonprofit organization designed to assist in the care of injured divers, also may help with the treatment of marine injuries. The network can be reached on the Internet at

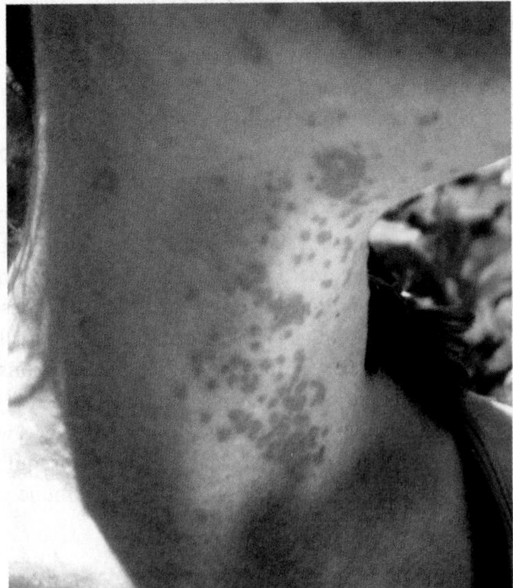

Figure 396-4 Erythematous, papular rash typical of seabather's eruption caused by thimble jellyfish and larval anemones.

www.diversalertnetwork.org or by telephone 24 h a day at (919) 684-9111. An antivenom for stonefish (and severe scorpionfish) envenomation is made in Australia by the Commonwealth Serum Laboratories (CSL; 45 Poplar Road, Parkville, Victoria, Australia 3052; *www.csl.com.au*; 61-3-9389-1911). Polyvalent sea snake antivenom is also available from CSL. It is no longer recommended that tiger snake antivenom be used if sea snake antivenom is unavailable.

MARINE POISONINGS

CIGUATERA

Epidemiology and pathogenesis

Ciguatera poisoning is the most common nonbacterial food poisoning associated with fish in the United States; most U.S. cases occur in Florida and Hawaii. The poisoning almost exclusively involves tropical and semitropical marine coral reef fish common in the Indian Ocean, the South Pacific, and the Caribbean Sea. Among reported cases, 75% (except in Hawaii) involve the barracuda, snapper, jack, or grouper. The ciguatera syndrome is associated with at least five polyether sodium channel activator toxins that originate in photosynthetic dinoflagellates (such as *Gambierdiscus toxicus*) and accumulate in the food chain. Three major ciguatoxins are found in the flesh and viscera of ciguateric fishes: CTX-1, -2, and -3. TRPV1, a nonselective cation channel expressed in nociceptive neurons, may play a role in the unique neurologic disturbances in ciguatera poisoning. Most, if not all, ciguatoxins are unaffected by freeze-drying, heat, cold, and gastric acid. None of the toxins affects the odor, color, or taste of fish. Cooking methods may alter the relative concentrations of the various toxins.

Clinical manifestations

The onset of symptoms may come within 15–30 min of ingestion and typically takes place within 2–6 h. Symptoms increase in severity over the ensuing 4–6 h. Most victims develop symptoms within 12 h of ingestion, and virtually all are afflicted within 24 h. The >150 symptoms reported include abdominal pain, nausea, vomiting, diarrhea, chills, paresthesias, pruritus, tongue and throat numbness or burning, sensation of "carbonation" during swallowing, odontalgia or dental dysesthesias, dysphagia, dysuria, dyspnea, weakness, fatigue, tremor, fasciculations, athetosis, meningismus, aphonia, ataxia, vertigo, pain and weakness in the lower extremities, visual blurring, transient blindness, hyporeflexia, seizures, nasal congestion and dryness, conjunctivitis, maculopapular rash, skin vesiculations, dermatographism, sialorrhea, diaphoresis, headache, arthralgias, myalgias, insomnia, bradycardia, hypotension, central respiratory failure, and coma. Death is rare.

Diarrhea, vomiting, and abdominal pain usually develop 3–6 h after ingestion of a ciguatoxic fish. Symptoms may persist for 48 h and then generally resolve (even without treatment). A pathognomonic symptom is the reversal of hot and cold tactile perception, which develops in some persons after 3–5 days and may last for months. Tachycardia and hypertension have been described, in some cases after potentially severe transient bradycardia and hypotension. More severe reactions tend to occur in persons previously stricken with the disease. Persons who have ingested parrotfish (scaritoxin) may develop classic ciguatera poisoning as well as a "second-phase" syndrome (after 5–10 days' delay) of disequilibrium with locomotor ataxia, dysmetria, and resting or kinetic tremor. This syndrome may persist for 2–6 weeks.

Diagnosis

The differential diagnosis of ciguatera includes paralytic shellfish poisoning, eosinophilic meningitis, type E botulism, organophosphate insecticide poisoning, tetrodotoxin poisoning, and psychogenic hyperventilation. At present, the diagnosis of ciguatera poisoning is made on clinical grounds because no routinely used laboratory test detects ciguatoxin in human blood. High-performance liquid chromatography (HPLC) is available for ciguatoxins and okadaic acid but is of limited clinical value because most health care institutions do not have the equipment needed to perform the test. A ciguatoxin enzyme immunoassay or radioimmunoassay may be used to test small portions of the suspected fish, but even these tests may not detect the very small amount of toxin (0.1 ppb) necessary to render fish flesh toxic.

TREATMENT Ciguatera Poisoning

Therapy is supportive and is based on symptoms. Nausea and vomiting may be controlled with an antiemetic such as ondansetron (4–8 mg IV). Hypotension may require the administration of IV crystalloid and, in rare cases, a pressor drug. Bradyarrhythmias that lead to cardiac insufficiency and hypotension generally respond well to atropine (0.5 mg IV, up to 2 mg). Cool showers or the administration of hydroxyzine (25 mg PO every 6–8 h) may relieve pruritus. Amitriptyline (25 mg PO twice a day) reportedly alleviates pruritus and dysesthesias. In three cases unresponsive to amitriptyline, tocainide appeared to be efficacious. Nifedipine has been used to treat headache. IV infusion of mannitol may be beneficial in moderate or severe cases, particularly for the relief of distressing neurologic or cardiovascular symptoms, although the efficacy of this therapy has been challenged and has not been definitively proved. The infusion is rendered initially as 1 g/kg per day over 45–60 min during the acute phase (days 1–5). If symptoms improve, a second dose may be given within 3–4 h and repeated on the next day. Care must be taken to avoid dehydration in a treated patient. The mechanism of the benefit against ciguatera intoxication is perhaps hyperosmotic water-drawing action, which reverses ciguatoxin-induced Schwann cell edema. Mannitol may also act in some fashion as a "hydroxyl scavenger" or may competitively inhibit ciguatoxin at the cell membrane.

During recovery from ciguatera poisoning, the victim should exclude the following from the diet: fish (fresh or preserved), fish sauces, shellfish, shellfish sauces, alcoholic beverages, nuts, and nut oils. Consumption of fish in ciguatera-endemic regions should be avoided. All oversized fish of any predacious reef species should be suspected of harboring ciguatoxin. Neither moray eels nor the viscera of tropical marine fish should ever be eaten.

PARALYTIC SHELLFISH POISONING

Paralytic shellfish poisoning is induced by ingestion of any of a variety of feral or aquacultured filter-feeding organisms, including clams, oysters, scallops, mussels, chitons, limpets, starfish, and sand crabs. The origin of their toxicity is the chemical toxin they accumulate and concentrate by feeding on various planktonic dinoflagellates (e.g., *Protogonyaulax*, *Ptychodiscus*, and *Gymnodinium*) and protozoan organisms. The unicellular phytoplanktonic organisms form the foundation of the food chain, and in warm summer months these organisms "bloom" in nutrient-rich coastal temperate and semitropical waters. These planktonic species can release massive amounts of toxic metabolites into the water and cause mortality in bird and marine populations. The paralytic shellfish toxins are water-soluble as well as heat- and acid-stable; they cannot be destroyed by ordinary cooking. The best-characterized and most frequently identified paralytic shellfish toxin is saxitoxin, which takes its name from the Alaska butter clam *Saxidomus giganteus*. A toxin concentration of >75 μg/100 g of foodstuff is considered hazardous to humans. In the 1972 New England "red tide," the concentration of saxitoxin in blue mussels exceeded 9000 μg/100 g of foodstuff. Saxitoxin appears to block sodium conductance, inhibiting neuromuscular transmission at the axonal and muscle membrane levels.

The onset of intraoral and perioral paresthesias (notably of the lips, tongue, and gums) comes within minutes to a few hours after ingestion of contaminated shellfish, and these paresthesias progress rapidly to involve the neck and distal extremities. The tingling or burning sensation later changes to numbness. Other symptoms rapidly develop and include light-headedness, disequilibrium, incoordination, weakness, hyperreflexia, incoherence, dysarthria, sialorrhea, dysphagia, thirst, diarrhea, abdominal pain, nausea, vomiting, nystagmus, dysmetria, headache, diaphoresis, loss of vision, chest pain, and tachycardia. Flaccid paralysis and respiratory insufficiency may follow 2–12 h after ingestion. In the absence of hypoxia, the victim often remains alert but paralyzed.

TREATMENT Paralytic Shellfish Poisoning

Treatment is supportive and is based on symptoms. If the victim comes to medical attention within the first few hours after poison ingestion, the stomach should be emptied by gastric lavage and then irrigated with 2 L (in 200-mL aliquots) of a solution of 2% sodium bicarbonate; this intervention has not been proved to be of benefit but is based on the notion that gastric acidity may enhance the potency of saxitoxin. Because breathing difficulty can be rapid in onset, induction of emesis is not advised. The administration of activated charcoal (50–100 g) and a cathartic (sorbitol, 20–50 g) makes empirical sense since these shellfish toxins are believed to bind well to charcoal. Some authors advise against administration of magnesium-based solutions (e.g., certain cathartics), cautioning that hypermagnesemia may contribute to suppression of nerve conduction.

The most serious problem is respiratory paralysis. The victim should be closely observed in a hospital for at least 24 h for respiratory distress. With prompt recognition of ventilatory failure, endotracheal intubation and assisted ventilation prevent anoxic myocardial and brain injury.

A direct human serum assay to identify the toxin responsible for paralytic shellfish poisoning is not yet clinically available; the mouse bioassay in widespread use may be replaced by an automated tissue culture bioassay. A polyclonal enzyme-linked immunosorbent assay (ELISA) to measure specific toxins is under development, as is fluorimetric HPLC.

DOMOIC ACID INTOXICATION (AMNESTIC SHELLFISH POISONING)

In late 1987 in eastern Canada, an outbreak of gastrointestinal and neurologic symptoms (amnestic shellfish poisoning) was documented in persons who had consumed mussels found to be contaminated with domoic acid. In this outbreak, the source of the toxin was *Nitzschia pungens*, a diatom ingested by the mussels. In 1991, an epidemic of domoic acid poisoning in the state of Washington was attributed to the consumption of razor clams. A heat-stable neuroexcitatory amino acid whose biochemical analogues are kainic acid and glutamic acid, domoic acid binds to the kainate type of glutamate receptor with three times the affinity of kainic acid and is 20 times as powerful a toxin. Shellfish can be tested for domoic acid by mouse bioassay and HPLC. The regulatory limit for domoic acid in shellfish is 20 parts per million.

The abnormalities noted within 24 h of ingesting contaminated mussels (*Mytilus edulis*) include arousal, confusion, disorientation, and memory loss. The median time of onset is 5.5 h. Other prominent symptoms include severe headache, nausea, vomiting, diarrhea, abdominal cramps, hiccups, arrhythmias, hypotension, seizures, ophthalmoplegia, pupillary dilation, piloerection, hemiparesis, mutism, grimacing, agitation, emotional lability, coma, copious bronchial secretions, and pulmonary edema. Histologic study of brain tissue taken at autopsy has shown neuronal necrosis or cell loss and astrocytosis, most prominently in the hippocampus and the amygdaloid nucleus—findings similar to those in animals poisoned with kainic acid. Several months after the primary intoxication, victims still display chronic residual memory deficits and motor neuronopathy or axonopathy. Nonneurologic illness does not persist.

TREATMENT Domoic Acid Intoxication

Therapy is supportive and is based on symptoms. Since kainic acid neuropathology seems to be nearly entirely seizure-mediated, the emphasis should be on anticonvulsive therapy, for which diazepam appears to be as effective as any other drug.

SCOMBROID POISONING

Scombroid (mackerel-like) fish include the albacore, bluefin, and yellowfin tuna; mackerel; saury; needlefish; wahoo; skipjack; and bonito. Nonscombroid fish that produce scombroid poisoning include the dolphinfish (Hawaiian mahimahi, *Coryphaena hippurus*), kahawai, sardine, black marlin, pilchard, anchovy, herring, amberjack, and Australian ocean salmon. In the northeastern and mid-Atlantic United States, bluefish (*Pomatomus saltatrix*) has been linked to scombroid poisoning. Because greater numbers of nonscombroid fish are being recognized as scombrotoxic, the syndrome may more appropriately be called pseudoallergic fish poisoning.

Under conditions of inadequate preservation or refrigeration, the musculature of these dark- or red-fleshed fish undergoes bacterial decomposition, which includes decarboxylation of the amino acid L-histidine to histamine, histamine phosphate, and histamine hydrochloride. Histamine levels of 20–50 mg/100 g are noted in toxic fish, with levels >400 mg/100 g on occasion. However, it is possible that some other compound may be responsible for this intoxication, since large doses of oral histamine do not reproduce the affliction. Whatever toxin or toxins are involved are heat-stable and are not destroyed by domestic or commercial cooking. Affected fish typically have a sharply metallic or peppery taste; however, they may be normal in appearance, color, and flavor. Not all persons who eat a contaminated fish necessarily become ill, perhaps because of uneven distribution of decay within the fish.

Symptoms develop within 15–90 min of ingestion and include flushing (sharply demarcated; exacerbated by ultraviolet exposure; particularly pronounced on the face, neck, and upper trunk), a sensation of warmth without elevated core temperature, conjunctival hyperemia, pruritus, urticaria, angioneurotic edema, bronchospasm, nausea, vomiting, diarrhea, epigastric pain, abdominal cramps, dysphagia, headache, thirst, pharyngitis, gingival burning, palpitations, tachycardia, dizziness, and hypotension. Without treatment, the symptoms generally resolve within 8–12 h. Because of blockade of gastrointestinal tract histaminase, the reaction may be more severe in a person who is concurrently ingesting isoniazid.

TREATMENT Scombroid Poisoning

Therapy is directed at reversing the histamine effect with antihistamines, either H-1 or H-2. If bronchospasm is severe, an inhaled bronchodilator—or in rare, extremely severe circumstances, injected epinephrine—may be used. Glucocorticoids are of no proven benefit. Protracted nausea and vomiting, which may empty the stomach of toxin, may be controlled with a specific antiemetic, such as prochlorperazine. The persistent headache of scombroid poisoning may respond to cimetidine or a similar antihistamine if standard analgesics are not effective.

FURTHER READINGS

Auerbach PS (ed): *Wilderness Medicine*, 5th ed, St. Louis, Mosby, 2007

Bush SP: Snakebite suction devices don't remove venom: They just suck. Ann Emerg Med 43:187, 2004

Dart RC et al: A randomized multicenter trial of Crotalinae polyvalent immune Fab (ovine) antivenom for the treatment for crotaline snakebite in the United States. Arch Intern Med 161:2030, 2001

Gold BS et al: Bites of venomous snakes. N Engl J Med 347:347, 2002

Lavonas EJ et al: Crotaline Fab antivenom appears to be effective in cases of severe North American pit viper envenomation: An integrative review. BMC Emerg Med 9:13, 2009

Mebs D: *Venomous and Poisonous Animals.* Boca Raton, FL, CRC Press, 2002

Meier J, White J (eds): *Handbook of Clinical Toxicology of Animal Venoms and Poisons.* Boca Raton, FL, CRC Press, 1996, pp 89–176

Pearn J: Neurology of ciguatera. J Neurol Neurosurg Psychiatry 70:4, 2001

Sharma H et al: An effective alternative management for multiple sea urchin spine injury: Erbium-YAG laser ablation. Foot Ankle Surg 12:51, 2006

Simpson ID, Jacobsen IM: Antisnake venom production crisis—who told us it was uneconomic and unsustainable? Wilderness Environ Med 20:144, 2009

———, Norris RL: The global snakebite crisis—a public health issue misunderstood, not neglected. Wilderness Environ Med 20:43, 2009

Winter KL et al: An examination of the cardiovascular effects of an "Irukandji" jellyfish, *Alatina nr mordens.* Toxicol Lett 179:18, 2008

———: An in vivo comparison of the efficacy of CSL box jellyfish antivenom with antibodies raised against nematocyst-derived *Chironex fleckeri* venom. Toxicol Lett 187:94, 2009

CHAPTER 397 Ectoparasite Infestations and Arthropod Bites and Stings

Richard J. Pollack

Ectoparasites are arthropods or helminths that infest the skin or hair of other animals, from which they derive sustenance and shelter. They may penetrate beneath the surface of the host or attach superficially by their mouthparts and specialized claws. These organisms damage their hosts by inflicting direct injury, eliciting a hypersensitivity reaction, inoculating toxins or pathogens, and inciting fear. The main medically important ectoparasites are arachnids (including mites and ticks), insects (including lice, fleas, bedbugs, and flies), pentastomes (tongue worms), and leeches. Arthropods also may harm humans through brief encounters during which they take a blood meal or attempt to defend themselves by biting, stinging, or exuding venoms. Various arachnids (spiders, scorpions), insects (bees, hornets, wasps, ants, flies, bugs, caterpillars, and beetles), millipedes, and centipedes produce ill effects in these manners, as do certain ectoparasites of animals, including ticks, biting mites, and fleas. In the United States, more people die each year from arthropod stings than from the bites of poisonous snakes. Lesions resulting from the bites and stings of arthropods are so diverse and variable that it is rarely possible to identify precisely what kind of insect or tick is involved without a bona fide specimen and entomologic expertise.

SCABIES

The human itch mite, *Sarcoptes scabiei*, is a common cause of itching dermatosis, infesting ~300 million persons worldwide. Gravid female mites that measure ~0.3 mm in length burrow superficially beneath the stratum corneum, depositing three or fewer eggs per day. Nymphs mature in ~2 weeks and then emerge as adults to the surface of the skin, where they mate and (re)invade the skin of the same or another host. Transfer of newly fertilized female mites from person to person occurs mainly by intimate contact and is facilitated by crowding, poor hygiene, and multiple sexual partners. Generally, these mites die within a day or so in the absence of host contact. Transmission via sharing of contaminated bedding or clothing therefore occurs infrequently. In the United States, scabies may account for up to 5% of visits to dermatologists. Outbreaks occur in nursing homes, mental institutions, and hospitals.

The itching and rash associated with scabies derive from a sensitization reaction directed against the excreta that the mite deposits in its burrow. An initial infestation remains asymptomatic for up to 6 weeks, and a reinfestation produces a hypersensitivity reaction without delay. Burrows become surrounded by infiltrates of eosinophils, lymphocytes, and histiocytes, and a generalized hypersensitivity rash later develops in remote sites. Immunity and associated scratching limit most infestations to <15 mites per person. Hyperinfestation with thousands of mites, a condition known as *crusted scabies* or *Norwegian scabies*, may result from glucocorticoid use, immunodeficiency, and neurologic and psychiatric illnesses that limit itching and scratching.

Intense itching worsens at night and after a hot shower. Typical burrows may be difficult to find because they are few in number and may be obscured by excoriations. Burrows appear as dark wavy lines in the epidermis and measure up to 15 mm. Lesions occur most frequently on the volar wrists, between the fingers, on the elbows, and on the penis. Small papules and vesicles, often accompanied by eczematous plaques, pustules, or nodules, are distributed symmetrically in those sites and in skinfolds under the breasts and around the navel, axillae, belt line, buttocks, upper thighs, and scrotum. Except in infants, the face, scalp, neck, palms, and soles are spared. Crusted scabies resembles psoriasis in its typical widespread erythema, thick keratotic crusts, scaling, and dystrophic nails. Characteristic burrows are not seen in crusted scabies, and patients usually do not itch, although their infestations are highly contagious and have been responsible for outbreaks of classic scabies in hospitals.

Scabies should be considered in patients with pruritus and symmetric polymorphic skin lesions in characteristic locations, particularly if there is a history of household contact with an affected person. Burrows should be sought and unroofed with a sterile needle or scalpel blade, and the scrapings should be examined microscopically for the mite, its eggs, and its fecal pellets. Biopsies (including superficial cyanoacrylate biopsy), scrapings, and dermascopic imaging of papulovesicular lesions as well as microscopic inspection of clear adhesive tape lifted from lesions also may be diagnostic. In the absence of identifiable mites or mite products, the diagnosis is based on clinical presentation and history. Diverse kinds of dermatitis due to other causes frequently are misdiagnosed as scabies.

TREATMENT Scabies

Permethrin cream (5%) is less toxic than 1% lindane preparations and is effective against lindane-tolerant infestations. Scabicides are applied thinly but thoroughly behind the ears and from the neck down after bathing and are removed 8 h later with soap and water. Successful treatment of crusted scabies requires preapplication of a keratolytic agent such as 6% salicylic acid and then of scabicides to the scalp, face, and ears. Repeated treatments or the sequential use of several agents may be necessary. Ivermectin has not been approved by the U.S. Food and Drug Administration (FDA) for use against any form of scabies, but a single oral dose (200 μg/kg) effectively treats scabies in otherwise healthy persons; patients with crusted scabies may require two doses separated by an interval of 1–2 weeks.

Although effectively treated scabies infestations become noninfectious within a day, itching and rash due to hypersensitivity to the dead mites and their excreted and secreted products frequently persist for weeks or months. Unnecessary re-treatment with topical agents may provoke contact dermatitis. Antihistamines, salicylates, and calamine lotion relieve itching during treatment, and topical glucocorticoids are useful for pruritus that lingers after effective treatment. To prevent reinfestations, bedding and clothing should be washed and/or dried on high heat or heat-pressed, and close contacts, even if asymptomatic, should be treated simultaneously.

■ CHIGGERS AND OTHER BITING MITES

Chiggers are the larvae of trombiculid (harvest) mites that normally feed on mice in grassy or brush-covered sites in the tropics and subtropics and less frequently in temperate areas during warm months. They wait for hosts on low vegetation and attach themselves to passing animals or humans. The larva pierces the skin of its host and produces a secreted tubelike structure (*stylostome*) in the dermis through which it imbibes tissue fluids. The stylostome is highly antigenic and causes an exceptionally pruritic papular, papulovesicular, or papulourticarial lesion (≤2 cm in diameter) that develops within hours of attachment in persons previously sensitized to mite antigen. Feeding mites appear as tiny red vesicles adjacent to hair follicles. Scratching invariably destroys the body of a mite. Generally, lesions vesiculate and develop a hemorrhagic base. Itching and burning persist for weeks. The rash is common on the ankles and areas where clothing obstructs the further wanderings of the mites. Repellents are useful for preventing chigger bites.

Diverse mites associated with birds and rodents can be particularly bothersome when they invade homes and bite human inhabitants. In North America, the northern fowl mite, the chicken mite, the tropical rat mite, and the house mouse mite normally feed on poultry, various songbirds, and small mammals and are abundant in and near their hosts' nests. These mites invade homes after their natural hosts die or leave their nests. Although the mites often are not seen because of their small size, their bites can be painful and pruritic. Painful bitelike sensations associated only with certain rooms of a home may be due to biting mites. Rodent- and bird-associated mites are best eliminated by excluding hosts, removing nests, and cleaning and treating the nesting area with appropriate acaricides. *Pyemotes* and other mites that infest grain, straw, cheese, hay, or other products occasionally produce similar episodes of rash and discomfort.

Diagnosis of mite-induced dermatitides (including those caused by chiggers) relies on confirmation of the mite's identity or elicitation of a history of exposure to the mite's source. Antihistamines or topical steroids effectively reduce mite-induced pruritus.

■ TICK BITES AND TICK PARALYSIS

Ticks attach and feed painlessly; blood is their only food. Their secretions produce local reactions, a febrile illness, or paralysis and transmit diverse pathogens. Generally, soft ticks attach for <1 h and may produce erythematous macular lesions ≤3 cm in diameter. Some species in Africa, the western United States, and Mexico produce painful hemorrhagic lesions. In contrast, hard ticks attach and feed for several days or sometimes for >1 week. At the site of hard-tick bites, small areas of induration with surrounding erythema and occasionally necrotic ulcers develop. Chronic nodules (tick granulomas) reach several centimeters in diameter and may require surgical excision. Tick-induced fever, associated with headache, nausea, and malaise, usually resolves ≤36 h after the tick is removed.

Tick paralysis, an acute ascending flaccid paralysis, is believed to be caused by one or more toxins in tick saliva that produce neuromuscular block, decreased nerve conduction, and sometimes hypertension. Throughout the world, this rare complication has followed the bites of >60 kinds of ticks; in the United States, dog and wood ticks are most commonly involved. Weakness begins in the lower extremities ≤6 days after the tick's attachment and ascends symmetrically over several days to result in complete paralysis of the extremities and cranial nerves. Deep tendon reflexes are diminished or lacking altogether, but sensory examination and findings on lumbar puncture are typically normal. Removal of the tick generally results in improvement within a few hours and complete recovery after several days, although the patient's condition may continue to deteriorate for up to 1 day. Failure to remove the tick may lead to dysarthria, dysphagia, and ultimately death from aspiration or respiratory paralysis. Diagnosis depends on finding the tick, which is often hidden beneath hair. An antiserum to the saliva of *Ixodes holocyclus*, the usual cause of tick paralysis in Australia, effectively reverses paralysis caused by these ticks.

Ticks should be removed by firm traction with fine-tipped forceps placed near the point of attachment. Use of occlusive dressings, heat, or other substances merely delays tick removal. The site of attachment should be disinfected. Tick mouthparts remaining in the skin generally are shed within days without excision. Removal of ticks during the first 36 h of attachment nearly always prevents transmission of the agents of Lyme disease, babesiosis, anaplasmosis, and ehrlichiosis. Gentle handling (to avoid rupture of ticks) and use of gloves may avert accidental contamination with tick fluids

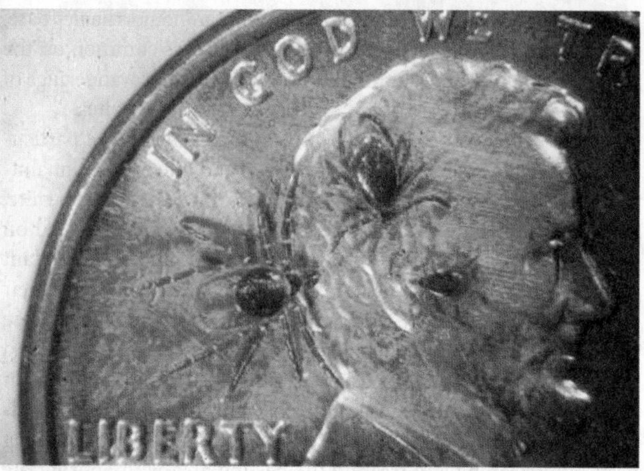

Figure 397-1 **Deer ticks** (*Ixodes scapularis*, black-legged ticks) on a U.S. penny: larva (*below ear*), nymph (*right*), adult male (*above*), and adult female (*left*).

containing pathogens. Rather than awaiting results of tick testing or seroconversion to Lyme disease, adult patients with bites thought to be associated with deer ticks (Fig. 397-1) in Lyme disease–endemic areas from Maryland to Maine and in Wisconsin and Minnesota may be treated presumptively with a single oral dose of doxycycline (200 mg) within 72 h of tick removal.

LOUSE INFESTATION (PEDICULIASIS AND PTHIRIASIS)

Nymphs and adults of all three kinds of human lice feed at least once a day, ingesting human blood exclusively. Head lice (*Pediculus capitis*) infest mainly the hair of the scalp, body lice (*Pediculus humanus*) the clothing, and crab or pubic lice (*Pthirus pubis*) mainly the hair of the pubis. The saliva of lice produces an irritating maculopapular or urticarial rash in certain sensitized persons. Female head and pubic lice cement their eggs firmly to hair, and female body lice cement their eggs to clothing. A nymph hatches after ~10 days of development. The empty egg (nit) may remain affixed for months thereafter.

In North America, head lice infest ~1% of elementary school–age children. Head lice are transmitted mainly by direct head-to-head contact rather than by fomites (shared headgear, grooming implements, bedding). Infestations by head lice tend to be asymptomatic. Pruritus, due mainly to hypersensitivity to the louse's saliva, generally is transient and mild. Head lice removed from a person succumb to desiccation and starvation within ~1 day. Head lice are unimportant as vectors of pathogenic agents.

Body lice remain on clothing except when feeding and generally succumb in ≤2 days if separated from their host. These lice mainly infest disaster victims or indigent people who are in close contact with other infested individuals. Body lice are acquired by direct contact or by sharing of clothing and bedding. These lice are vectors for the agents of louse-borne typhus (Chap. 174), louse-borne relapsing fever (Chap. 172), and trench fever (Chap. 160). Pruritic lesions from their bites are particularly common around the neckline. Chronic infestations result in a postinflammatory hyperpigmentation and thickening of skin known as *vagabonds' disease*.

The crab or pubic louse is transmitted mainly by sexual contact. These lice occur mainly on pubic hair and less frequently on hair of the axillae and the face, including the eyelashes. Children and adults may acquire pubic lice by sexual or close nonsexual contact. Intensely pruritic lesions and blue macules ~3 mm in diameter (*maculae ceruleae*) develop at the site of bites. Blepharitis commonly accompanies infestations of the eyelashes.

Pediculiasis may be suspected upon the detection of nits on hairs or in clothing, but confirmation should be based on discovery of a live louse.

TREATMENT Louse Infestation

Generally, treatment is warranted only if live lice are discovered. The presence of nits alone is evidence of former—not current—infestation. Mechanical removal of lice and their eggs by means of a fine-toothed louse or nit comb (Fig. 397-2) often fails to eliminate infestations. Treatment of newly identified active infestations generally relies on a 10-min application of ~1% permethrin or pyrethrins, with a second application 10 days later. Lice persisting after this treatment may be resistant to pyrethroids (see below). Chronic infestations may be treated for ≤12 h with 0.5% malathion. Lindane is applied for just 4 min but seems less effective and may pose a greater risk of adverse reactions, particularly when misused. Resistance of head lice to permethrin, malathion, and lindane has been reported. Newer pediculicides contain benzyl alcohol, dimethicone, or spinosad. Although children infested by head lice are frequently isolated or excluded from school, this practice increasingly is seen as unjustified.

Body lice usually are eliminated by bathing and by changing to laundered clothes. Application of topical pediculicides from head to foot may be necessary for hirsute patients. Clothes and bedding are effectively deloused by heating in a clothes dryer at ≥55°C (131°F) for 30 min or by heat-pressing. Emergency mass delousing of persons and clothing may be warranted during periods of civil strife and after natural disasters to reduce the risk of pathogen transmission by body lice.

Pubic louse infestations are treated with topical pediculicides except for eyelid infestations (*pthiriasis palpebrum*), which generally respond to a coating of petrolatum applied for 3–4 days.

MYIASIS (FLY INFESTATION)

Myiasis refers to infestations by diverse kinds of fly larvae (maggots) that invade living or necrotic tissue or body cavities and produce different clinical syndromes, depending on the species of fly.

In forested parts of Central and South America, larvae of the human botfly *Dermatobia hominis* produce boil-like subcutaneous nodules ≤3 cm in diameter. The adult female captures a mosquito or another bloodsucking insect and deposits her eggs on its abdomen. When the carrier insect attacks a human or bovine host

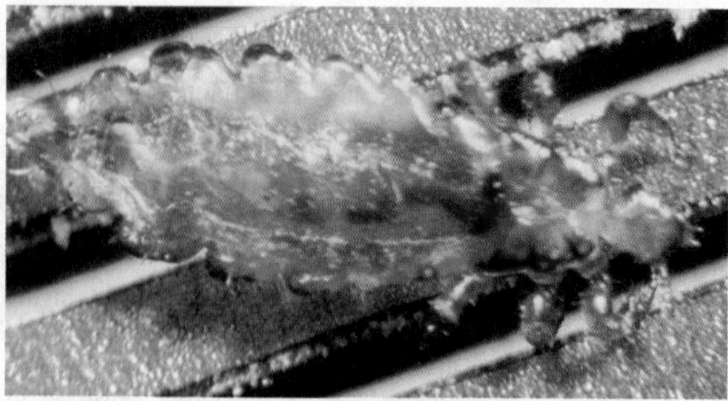

Figure 397-2 Adult female human head louse (*Pediculus capitis*) on a nit (louse-egg) comb.

several days later, the warmth and moisture of the host's surface stimulate the larvae to hatch. The larvae promptly penetrate intact skin. After 6–12 weeks of development, mature larvae emerge from the skin and drop to the ground. The African tumbu fly *Cordylobia anthropophaga* deposits its eggs on sand or drying laundry contaminated with urine or sweat. Larvae hatch on contact with the body, penetrate the skin, and produce boils from which they emerge ~9 days later. Furuncular myiasis is suggested by uncomfortable lesions with a central breathing pore that emits bubbles when submerged in water. A sensation of movement under the patient's skin may lead to severe emotional distress. Botfly larvae may be induced to emerge if the air pore is coated with petrolatum or another occlusive substance. Removal may be facilitated by injection of a local anesthetic into the surrounding tissue, but surgical excision is often necessary because upward-pointing spines of some species hold the larva firmly in place.

Larvae of the horse botfly *Gasterophilus intestinalis* do not mature after penetrating human skin but migrate for weeks in the epidermis. The resulting pruritic and serpiginous eruption resembles cutaneous larva migrans caused by hookworms (Chap. 216). Horseback riders become infested when eggs deposited on the flank of the horse hatch against their bare legs. The larvae of the cattle botfly invade more deeply and produce boil-like swellings, and larvae of rabbit and rodent *Cuterebra* occasionally cause dermal or tracheopulmonary myiasis.

Certain flies are attracted to blood and pus, and their newly hatched larvae enter wounds or diseased skin. Larvae of the green bottle fly usually remain superficial and confined to necrotic tissue, but specially prepared "surgical maggots" sometimes are used intentionally for wound debridement. Larvae of screwworm flies and the flesh fly invade viable tissue more deeply and produce large suppurating lesions. Larvae that infest wounds also may infest body cavities such as the mouth, nose, ears, sinuses, anus, vagina, and lower urinary tract, particularly in unconscious or otherwise debilitated patients. The consequences range from harmless colonization to destruction of the nose, meningitis, and deafness. Treatment involves removal of maggots and debridement of tissue.

The maggots responsible for furuncular and wound myiasis also may cause ophthalmomyiasis. Sequelae include nodules in the eyelid, retinal detachment, and destruction of the globe. Most instances in which maggots are found in human feces result from larviposition by flesh flies on recently passed stools.

PENTASTOMIASIS

Pentastomids (tongue worms) inhabit the respiratory passages of reptiles and carnivorous mammals. Human infestation by *Linguatula serrata* is common in the Middle East and results from the ingestion of encysted larval stages in raw liver or lymph nodes of sheep and goats—the intermediate hosts. Larvae migrate to the nasopharynx and produce an acute self-limiting syndrome known as *Halzoun* or *Marrara*, which is characterized by pain and itching of the throat and ears, coughing, hoarseness, dysphagia, and dyspnea. Severe edema may cause obstruction that necessitates tracheostomy; ocular invasion has been described. Diagnostic larvae measuring ≤10 mm in length appear in copious nasal discharge or vomitus. Individuals become infected with *Armillifer armillatus* by ingesting eggs in contaminated food or drink or after handling the definitive host, the African python. Larvae encyst in various organs but rarely cause symptoms. Cysts occasionally require surgical removal as they enlarge during molting, but they usually are encountered as an incidental finding at autopsy. Parasite-induced lesions may be misinterpreted as a malignancy, with the correct diagnosis confirmed by histopathologic findings. Cutaneous larva migrans syndromes due to other pentastomes have been reported from Southeast Asia and Central America.

LEECH INFESTATIONS

Medically important leeches are annelid worms that attach to their hosts with chitinous cutting jaws and draw blood through muscular suckers. The medicinal leech *Hirudo medicinalis* is still used occasionally to reduce venous congestion in surgical flaps or replanted body parts. This practice has been complicated by intractable bleeding, wound infections, myonecrosis, and sepsis due to *Aeromonas hydrophila*, which colonizes the gullets of commercially available leeches.

Ubiquitous aquatic leeches that parasitize fish, frogs, and turtles readily attach to the skin of humans and avidly suck blood. More notorious are the land leeches that live among moist vegetation of tropical rain forests. Attachment is usually painless. Hirudinin, a powerful anticoagulant secreted by the leech, causes continued bleeding after the leech has detached. Healing of the wound is slow, and bacterial infections are not uncommon. Several kinds of aquatic leeches in Africa, Asia, and southern Europe can enter through the mouth, nose, and genitourinary tract and attach to mucosal surfaces at sites as deep as the esophagus and trachea. Externally attached leeches generally drop off after they have engorged, but removal is hastened by gentle scraping aside of the anterior and posterior suckers and traction or by application of alcohol, salt, vinegar, insect repellent, or a flame or heated instrument to the leech. Internally attached leeches may detach on exposure to gargled saline or may be removed by forceps.

SPIDER BITES

Of the >30,000 recognized species of spiders, only ~100 defend themselves aggressively and have fangs sufficiently long to penetrate human skin. The venom that spiders use to immobilize and digest their prey can cause necrosis of skin and systemic toxicity. Whereas the bites of most spiders are painful but not harmful, envenomations by recluse or fiddle spiders (*Loxosceles* species) and widow spiders (*Latrodectus* species) may be life-threatening. Identification of the offending spider should be attempted both because specific treatments exist for bites of widow and brown recluse spiders and because injuries attributed to spiders are frequently due to other causes. Except in cases where the patient actually observes a spider immediately associated with the bite or fleeing from the site, lesions reported to be due to spider bites are most often due to other injuries or to infections with bacteria such as methicillin-resistant *Staphylococcus aureus*.

Recluse spider bites and necrotic arachnidism

Brown recluse spiders occur mainly in the southern and midwestern United States, and their close relatives are found in the Americas, Africa, and the Middle East. Most bites by the brown recluse spider result in only minor injury with edema and erythema. Envenomation, however, may cause severe necrosis of skin and subcutaneous tissue and systemic hemolysis. These spiders are not aggressive toward human beings and bite only if threatened or pressed against the skin. They hide under rocks and logs or in caves and animal burrows. They invade homes and seek dark and undisturbed hiding spots in closets, in folds of clothing, or under furniture and rubbish in storage rooms, garages, and attics. Despite their impressive abundance in some homes, these spiders only infrequently bite humans. Bites tend to occur while the victim is dressing and are sustained primarily on the arms, neck, and lower abdomen.

The venoms of these spiders contain an esterase, alkaline phosphatase, proteases, and other enzymes that produce tissue necrosis and hemolysis. Sphingomyelinase D, the most important dermonecrotic factor, binds cell membranes and promotes chemotaxis of neutrophils, leading to vascular thrombosis and an Arthus-like reaction. Initially, the bite is painless or produces a stinging sensation. Within the next few hours, the site becomes painful and pruritic, with central induration surrounded by a pale zone of ischemia and a zone of erythema. In most cases, the lesion resolves without treatment in just a few days. In severe cases, the erythema spreads, and the center of the lesion becomes hemorrhagic and necrotic with an overlying bulla. A black eschar forms and sloughs several weeks later, leaving an ulcer that eventually may result in a depressed scar. Healing usually takes place in ≤6 months but may take as long as 3 years if adipose tissue is involved. Local complications include injury to nerves and secondary infection. Fever, chills, weakness, headache, nausea, vomiting, myalgia, arthralgia, maculopapular rash, and leukocytosis may develop ≤72 h after the bite. In rare instances, acute complications such as hemolytic anemia, hemoglobinuria, and renal failure are fatal.

TREATMENT Recluse Spider Bites

Initial management includes RICE (rest, ice, compression, elevation). Analgesics, antihistamines, antibiotics, and tetanus prophylaxis should be administered if indicated. Debridement and later skin grafting may be necessary after signs of acute inflammation have subsided, but immediate surgical excision of the wound is detrimental. Patients should be monitored closely for signs of hemolysis, renal failure, and other systemic complications.

Widow spider bites

The black widow, which is best known and most abundant in the southeastern United States, measures ≤1 cm in body length and 5 cm in leg span and is shiny black with a red hourglass marking on the ventral abdomen. Other dangerous *Latrodectus* species occur elsewhere in temperate and subtropical parts of the world. The bites of the female widow spiders are notorious for their potent neurotoxins.

Widow spiders spin their webs under stones, logs, plants, or rock piles and in dark spaces in barns, garages, and outhouses. Bites are most common in the summer and early autumn and occur when the web is disturbed or when the spider is trapped or provoked. The initial bite goes unnoticed or is perceived as a sharp pinprick. Fang puncture marks are uncommon. The venom that is injected does not produce local necrosis, and some persons experience no other symptoms. α-Latrotoxin, the most active component of the venom, binds irreversibly to nerves and causes release and eventual depletion of acetylcholine, norepinephrine, and other neurotransmitters from presynaptic terminals. Painful cramps may spread within 60 min from the bite site to large muscles of the extremities and trunk. Extreme rigidity of the abdominal muscles and excruciating pain may suggest peritonitis, but the abdomen is not tender on palpation. The pain begins to subside during the first 12 h but may recur during several days or weeks before resolving spontaneously. Other features include salivation, diaphoresis, vomiting, hypertension, tachycardia, labored breathing, anxiety, headache, weakness, fasciculations, paresthesia, hyperreflexia, urinary retention, uterine contractions, and premature labor. Rhabdomyolysis and renal failure have been reported, and respiratory arrest, cerebral hemorrhage, or cardiac failure may end fatally, especially in very young, elderly, or debilitated persons.

TREATMENT Widow Spider Bites

Treatment consists of RICE and tetanus prophylaxis. Hypertension that does not respond to analgesics and antispasmodics (e.g., benzodiazepines or methocarbamol) requires specific antihypertensive medication. The efficacy of antivenom is controversial. Because of the risk of anaphylaxis and serum sickness, antivenom should be reserved for severe cases involving respiratory arrest, uncontrollable hypertension, seizures, or pregnancy.

Tarantulas and other spiders

Tarantulas are hairy spiders of which 30 species are found in the United States, mainly in the Southwest. The tarantulas that have become popular household pets are usually imported species. Tarantulas bite only when threatened and cause no more harm than a bee sting, but the venom occasionally provokes deep pain and swelling. Tarantulas of several species are covered with urticating hairs that are brushed off in the thousands when a threatened spider rubs its hind legs across its dorsal abdomen. These hairs penetrate human skin and produce pruritic papules that may persist for weeks. Failure to wear gloves or to wash the hands after handling the Chilean Rose tarantula, a popular pet spider, has resulted in transfer of hairs to the eye and devastating ocular inflammation. Treatment of bites includes local washing and elevation of the bitten area, tetanus prophylaxis, and analgesic administration. Antihistamines and topical or systemic glucocorticoids are given for exposure to urticating hairs.

Atrax robustus, a funnel-web spider of Australia, and *Phoneutria* species, the South American banana spiders, are among the most dangerous spiders in the world because of their aggressive behavior and potent neurotoxins. Envenomation by *A. robustus* causes a rapidly progressive neuromotor syndrome that can be fatal within 2 h. The bite of a banana spider causes severe local pain followed by profound systemic symptoms and respiratory paralysis that can lead to death within 2–6 h. Specific antivenoms for envenomation by each of these spiders are available. Yellow sac spiders (*Cheiracanthium*) are common in homes worldwide. Their bites, though painful, generally lead to only minor erythema, edema, and pruritus.

SCORPION STINGS

Scorpions are arachnids that feed on ground-dwelling arthropods and small lizards, which they paralyze by injecting venom from a stinger on the tip of the tail. Painful but relatively harmless scorpion stings need to be distinguished from the potentially lethal envenomations that are produced by ~30 of the ~1000 known species and that cause >5000 deaths worldwide each year. Scorpions feed at night and remain hidden during the day in crevices or burrows or under wood, loose bark, or rocks on the ground. They seek cool spots under buildings and often enter houses, where they hide in shoes, clothing, or bedding or enter bathtubs and sinks in search of water. Scorpions sting human beings only when disturbed.

Of the 40 or so scorpion species in the United States, only the bark scorpion (*Centruroides sculpturatus* or *C. exilicauda*) produces venom that can be lethal. This venom contains neurotoxins that cause sodium channels to remain open and neurons to fire repetitively. Such envenomations usually are associated with little swelling, but prominent pain, paresthesia, and hyperesthesia can be accentuated by tapping on the affected area (the tap test). These symptoms soon spread to other locations; dysfunction of cranial nerves and hyperexcitability of skeletal muscles develop within hours. Patients present with restlessness, blurred vision, abnormal eye movements, profuse salivation, lacrimation, rhinorrhea, slurred speech, difficulty in handling secretions, diaphoresis, nausea, and vomiting. Muscle twitching, jerking, and shaking may be mistaken for a seizure. Complications include tachycardia, arrhythmias, hypertension, hyperthermia, rhabdomyolysis, and acidosis. Symptoms progress to maximal severity in ~5 h and subside within a day or two, although pain and paresthesia can last for weeks. Fatal respiratory arrest is most common among young children and the elderly.

Envenomations by *Leiurus quinquestriatus* in the Middle East and North Africa, by *Mesobuthus tamulus* in India, by *Androctonus* species along the Mediterranean littoral and in North Africa and the Middle East, and by *Tityus serrulatus* in Brazil cause massive release of endogenous catecholamines with hypertensive crises, arrhythmias, pulmonary edema, and myocardial damage. Acute pancreatitis occurs with stings of *Tityus trinitatis* in Trinidad, and central nervous toxicity complicates stings of *Parabuthus* and *Buthotus* scorpions of South Africa. Tissue necrosis and hemolysis may follow stings of the Iranian *Hemiscorpius lepturus*.

Stings of most other species cause immediate sharp local pain followed by edema, ecchymosis, and a burning sensation. Symptoms typically resolve within a few hours, and skin does not slough. Allergic reactions to the venom sometimes develop.

TREATMENT Scorpion Stings

Identification of the offending scorpion aids in planning therapy. Stings of nonlethal species require at most ice packs, analgesics, or antihistamines. Because most victims experience only local discomfort, they can be managed at home with instructions to return to the emergency department if signs of cranial-nerve or neuromuscular dysfunction develop. Aggressive supportive care and judicious use of antivenom can reduce or eliminate deaths from more severe envenomations. Keeping the patient calm and applying pressure dressings and cold packs to the sting site are measures that decrease the absorption of venom. A continuous IV infusion of midazolam controls the agitation, flailing, and involuntary muscle movements produced by scorpion stings. Close monitoring during treatment with this drug and other sedatives or narcotics is necessary for persons with neuromuscular symptoms because of the risk of respiratory arrest. Hypertension and pulmonary edema respond to nifedipine, nitroprusside, hydralazine, or prazosin, and bradyarrhythmias can be controlled with atropine.

Commercially prepared antivenoms are available in several countries for some of the most dangerous species. A *C. sculpturatus* antivenom (not yet approved by the FDA) is available as an investigational drug only in Arizona. IV administration of antivenom rapidly reverses cranial-nerve dysfunction and muscular symptoms but does not affect pain and paresthesia. The benefit of scorpion antivenom has not been established in controlled trials.

HYMENOPTERA STINGS

Insects that sting to defend their colonies or subdue their prey belong to the order Hymenoptera, which includes bees, wasps, hornets, yellow jackets, and ants. Their venoms contain a wide array of amines, peptides, and enzymes that cause local and systemic reactions. Although the toxic effect of multiple stings can be fatal, nearly all of the ≥100 deaths due to hymenopteran stings in the United States each year result from allergic reactions.

Bee and wasp stings

Honeybees often lose their stinging apparatus and the attached venom sac in the act of stinging and subsequently die, whereas other bees, ants, and vespids can sting numerous times in succession. The familiar honeybees (*Apis mellifera*) and bumblebees (*Bombus* and other genera) generally attack only when a colony is disturbed. Africanized honeybees, however, respond to minimal intrusions more aggressively. Since their introduction into Brazil in 1957, these "killer bees" have spread through South and Central America to the southern and western United States.

In bees and wasps, venom is produced in glands at the posterior end of the abdomen and is expelled rapidly by contraction of muscles of the venom sac, which has a capacity of up to 0.1 mL. The venoms of different species of hymenopterans are biochemically and immunologically distinct. Direct toxic effects are mediated by mixtures of low-molecular-weight compounds such as serotonin, histamine, and acetylcholine and several kinins. Polypeptide toxins in honeybee venom include mellitin, which damages cell membranes; mast cell–degranulating protein, which causes histamine release; apamin, a neurotoxin; and adolapin, which has anti-inflammatory activity. Enzymes in venom include hyaluronidase, which allows the spread of other venom components, and phospholipases, which may be among the major venom allergens. There appears to be little cross-sensitization between honeybee and wasp venoms.

Uncomplicated stings cause immediate pain, a wheal-and-flare reaction, and local edema and swelling that subside in a few hours. Stings from accidentally swallowed insects may induce life-threatening edema of the upper airways. Multiple stings can lead to vomiting, diarrhea, generalized edema, dyspnea, hypotension, and collapse. Rhabdomyolysis and intravascular hemolysis may cause renal failure. Death from the direct effects of venom has followed 300–500 honeybee stings.

Large local reactions that spread ≥10 cm around the sting site over 24–48 h are not uncommon. These reactions may resemble cellulitis but are caused by hypersensitivity rather than secondary infection. Such reactions tend to recur on subsequent exposure but are seldom accompanied by anaphylaxis and are not prevented by venom immunotherapy.

An estimated 0.4–4.0% of the U.S. population exhibits clinical immediate-type hypersensitivity to insect stings, and 15% may have asymptomatic sensitization manifested by positive skin tests. Persons who experience severe allergic reactions are likely to have similar reactions after subsequent stings; occasionally, adults who have had mild reactions later experience serious reactions. Mild anaphylactic reactions from insect stings, as from other causes, consist of nausea, abdominal cramping, generalized urticaria, flushing, and angioedema. Serious reactions, including upper airway edema, bronchospasm, hypotension, and shock, may be rapidly fatal. Severe reactions usually begin within 10 min of the sting and only rarely develop after 5 h.

TREATMENT Bee and Wasp Stings

Honeybee stingers embedded in the skin should be removed as promptly as possible to limit the quantity of venom delivered. The stinger and venom sac may be scraped off with a blade or a fingernail or grasped with forceps. The site should be cleansed and disinfected and ice packs applied to slow the spread of venom. Elevation of the affected site and administration of analgesics, oral antihistamines, and topical calamine lotion relieve symptoms. Large local reactions may require a short course of oral therapy with glucocorticoids. Patients with numerous stings should be monitored for 24 h for evidence of renal failure or coagulopathy.

Anaphylaxis is treated with subcutaneous (SC) injection of 0.3–0.5 mL of epinephrine hydrochloride in a 1:1000 dilution; treatment is repeated every 20–30 min as necessary. IV epinephrine (2–5 mL of a 1:10,000 solution administered by slow push) is indicated for profound shock. A tourniquet may slow the spread of venom. Parenteral antihistamines, fluid resuscitation, bronchodilators, oxygen, intubation, and vasopressors may be required. Patients should be observed for 24 h for recurrent anaphylaxis.

Persons with a history of allergy to insect stings should carry a sting kit with a preloaded syringe containing epinephrine for self-administration. These patients should seek medical attention immediately after using the kit.

Repeated injections of purified venom produce a blocking IgG antibody response to venom and reduce the incidence of recurrent anaphylaxis. Honeybee, wasp, yellow jacket, and mixed vespid venoms are commercially available for desensitization and for skin testing. Results of skin tests and venom-specific radioallergosorbent tests aid in the selection of patients for immunotherapy and guide the design of such treatment.

Stinging ants

Stinging fire ants are an important medical problem in the United States. Imported fire ants infest southern states from Texas to North Carolina, with colonies in California, New Mexico, Arizona, and Virginia. Slight disturbances of their mound nests have provoked massive outpourings of ants and as many as 10,000 stings on a single person. Elderly and immobile persons are at high risk for attacks when fire ants invade dwellings.

Fire ants attach to skin with powerful mandibles and rotate their bodies while repeatedly injecting venom with posteriorly situated stingers. The alkaloid venom consists of cytotoxic and hemolytic piperidines and several proteins with enzymatic activity. The initial wheal-and-flare reaction, burning, and itching resolve in ~30 min, and a sterile pustule develops within 24 h. The pustule ulcerates over the next 48 h and then heals in ≥1 week. Large areas of erythema and edema lasting several days are not uncommon and in extreme cases may compress nerves and blood vessels. Anaphylaxis occurs in ≤2% of persons, and seizures and mononeuritis have been reported. Stings are treated with ice packs, topical glucocorticoids, and oral antihistamines. Covering pustules with bandages and antibiotic ointment may prevent bacterial infection. Epinephrine and supportive measures are indicated for anaphylactic reactions. Whole-body extracts are available for skin testing and immunotherapy, which appears to lower the rate of anaphylactic reactions.

The western United States is home to harvester ants. The painful local reaction that follows harvester ant stings often extends to lymph nodes and may be accompanied by anaphylaxis.

DIPTERAN (FLY AND MOSQUITO) BITES

In the process of feeding on vertebrate blood, adults of certain fly species inflict painful bites, produce local allergic reactions, or transmit pathogenic agents. Bites of mosquitoes, tiny "no-see-um" midges, and phlebotomine sand flies typically produce a wheal and a pruritic papule. Nodular lesions at the site of midge bites may last for months. Bites of small humpbacked black flies (simuliids) leave a bleeding laceration and a painful and pruritic sore that are slow to heal; regional lymphadenopathy, fever, or anaphylaxis occasionally ensues. The widely distributed deer and horse flies as well as the tsetse flies of Africa are stout flies measuring ≤25 mm in length that attack during the day and produce large and painful bleeding punctures.

TREATMENT Fly and Mosquito Bites

Treatment of fly bites is symptom-based. Topical application of antipruritic agents, glucocorticoids, or antiseptic lotions may relieve itching and pain. Allergic reactions may require oral antihistamines. Antibiotics may be necessary for the treatment of large bite wounds that become secondarily infected.

FLEA BITES

Common human-biting fleas include the dog and cat fleas (*Ctenocephalides* species) and the rat flea (*Xenopsylla cheopis*), which inhabit the nests and resting sites of their hosts. Sensitized persons develop erythematous pruritic papules, urticaria, and occasionally vesicles and bacterial superinfection at the site of the bite. Treatment consists of antihistamines and antipruritics.

Flea infestations are eliminated by frequent cleaning of nesting sites and of the host's bedding and by application of contact insecticides. Flea infestations in the home may abate if pets are treated with veterinary antiparasitic agents and insect growth regulators.

Tunga penetrans, like other fleas, is a wingless, laterally flattened insect that feeds on blood. Also known as the chigoe flea, sand flea, or jigger, it occurs in tropical regions of Africa and the Americas. Adults live in sandy soil and burrow under the skin between toes, under nails, or on the soles of bare feet. Chigoes engorge on blood and grow from pinpoint to pea size during a 2-week period. The lesions they produce resemble a white pustule with a central black depression and may be pruritic or painful. Occasional complications include tetanus, bacterial infections, and autoamputation of toes. Tungiasis is treated by removal of the intact flea with a sterile needle or scalpel, tetanus vaccination, and topical application of antibiotics.

HEMIPTERAN (TRUE BUG) BITES

Several true bugs of the family Reduviidae inflict bites that produce allergic reactions and are sometimes painful. The cone-nose bugs, so called because of their elongated heads, include the assassin and wheel bugs, which feed on other insects and bite vertebrates only in self-defense, and the kissing bugs, which routinely feed on vertebrate blood. The bites of the nocturnally feeding kissing bugs are painless. Reactions to such bites depend on prior sensitization and include tender and pruritic papules, vesicular or bullous lesions, giant urticaria, fever, lymphadenopathy, and anaphylaxis. Bug bites are treated with topical antipruritics or oral antihistamines. Persons with anaphylactic reactions to reduviid bites should keep an epinephrine kit available. The cosmopolitan bedbugs (*Cimex* species) hide in crevices of mattresses, bed frames and other furniture, walls, and picture frames and under loose wallpaper. Bedbugs have become resurgent, recently attaining populations and spreading to an extent not encountered since the mid-twentieth century. These bugs are now a fairly common nuisance in homes, dormitories, and hotels and on cruise ships. The bugs hide during the day and take their blood meal at night. Their bite is painless, but sensitized persons develop erythema, itching, and wheals around a central hemorrhagic punctum. Bedbugs are not known to transmit pathogens.

CENTIPEDE BITES AND MILLIPEDE DERMATITIS

The fangs of centipedes of the genus *Scolopendra* can penetrate human skin and deliver a venom that produces intense burning pain, swelling, erythema, and lymphangitis. Dizziness, nausea, and anxiety occasionally are described, and rhabdomyolysis and renal failure have been reported. Treatment includes washing of the site, application of cold dressings, oral analgesic administration or local lidocaine infiltration, and tetanus prophylaxis.

Millipedes, unlike centipedes, do not bite, but some secrete defensive fluids that burn and discolor human skin. Affected skin turns brown overnight and may blister and exfoliate. Secretions in the eye cause intense pain and inflammation that may lead to corneal ulceration and blindness. Management includes irrigation with copious amounts of water or saline, use of analgesics, and local care of denuded skin.

CATERPILLAR STINGS AND DERMATITIS

The surface of caterpillars of several moth species is covered with hairs or spines that produce mechanical irritation and may contain or be coated with venom. Contact with these caterpillars causes an immediate burning sensation followed by local swelling and erythema and occasionally by regional lymphadenopathy, nausea, vomiting, and headache; shock, seizures, and coagulopathy are rare complications. In the United States, dermatitis most often is associated with io, puss, saddleback, and brown-tail moths. Contact with even detached hairs of other caterpillars, such as gypsy moth larvae, can later produce a pruritic urticarial or papular rash. Spines may be deposited on tree trunks and drying laundry or may be airborne and cause irritation of the eyes and upper airways. Treatment of caterpillar stings consists of repeated application of adhesive or cellophane tape to remove the hairs, which can then be identified microscopically. Local ice packs, topical steroids, and oral antihistamines relieve symptoms.

BEETLE VESICATION

When disturbed, blister beetles extrude cantharidin, a low-molecular-weight toxin that produces thin-walled blisters measuring ≤5 cm in diameter 2–5 h after contact. The blisters are not painful or pruritic unless broken and resolve without treatment in ≤10 days. Nephritis may follow unusually heavy cantharidin exposure. Contact occurs when individuals sit on the ground, work in the garden, or deliberately handle the beetles. The hemolymph of certain rove beetles contains paederin, a potent vesicant. When these beetles are crushed or brushed against the skin, the released fluid may provoke erythematous and bullous lesions. These beetles occur worldwide but are most numerous and problematic in parts of Africa and Asia. Ocular lesions are common from impacts with the flying beetles at night or transfer of the vesicant on the fingers. Treatment is rarely necessary, although ruptured blisters should be kept clean and bandaged.

DELUSIONAL INFESTATIONS

The groundless conviction that one is infested with arthropods or other parasites is an extremely difficult disorder to treat and unfortunately is not rare. Patients report infestations of their skin, clothing, or homes and describe sensations of something moving in or on their skin. Excoriations often accompany reports of pruritus or insect bites. Frequently, patients submit as evidence of infestation specimens that consist of plant-feeding and nonbiting peridomestic arthropods, pieces of skin, vegetable matter, or inanimate objects. It is imperative to rule out true infestations and bites by arthropods, endocrinopathies, neuropathies, drug use, environmental irritants (e.g., fragments or threads of glass insulation), and other causes of tingling or prickling sensations. Frequently, such patients repeatedly seek medical consultations, resist alternative explanations for their symptoms, and exacerbate their discomfort by self-treatment. Pharmacotherapy with pimozide or other psychotropic agents has been more helpful than psychotherapy in treating this disorder.

ACKNOWLEDGMENT

The substantial contributions of James H. Maguire to this chapter in previous editions are gratefully acknowledged.

FURTHER READINGS

Clark RP, Hu LT: Prevention of Lyme disease and other tick-borne infections. Infect Dis Clin North Am 22:381, 2008

Goddard J: *Physician's Guide to Arthropods of Medical Importance*, 5th ed. Boca Raton, FL, CRC Press, 2007

Hicks MI, Elston DM: Scabies. Dermatol Ther 22:279, 2009

Hinkle N: Ekbom syndrome: The challenge of "invisible bug" infestations. Annu Rev Entomol 55:77, 2010

McGraw TA, Turiansky MC: Cutaneous myiasis. J Am Acad Dermatol 58:907, 2008

Mullen G, Durden L: *Medical and Veterinary Entomology*, 2nd ed. Amsterdam, Academic Press, 2009

Pollack RJ, Marcus L: A travel medicine guide to arthropods of medical importance. Infect Dis Clin North Am 19:169, 2005

Saucier JR: Arachnid envenomation. Emerg Med Clin North Am 22:405, 2004

Steen CJ et al: Insect sting reactions to bees, wasps, and ants. Int J Dermatol 44:91, 2005

Vetter RS, Isbister GK: Medical aspects of spider bites. Annu Rev Entomol 53:409, 2008

APPENDIX: Laboratory Values of Clinical Importance

Alexander Kratz
Michael A. Pesce
Robert C. Basner
Andrew J. Einstein

This Appendix contains tables of reference values for laboratory tests, special analytes, and special function tests. A variety of factors can influence reference values. Such variables include the population studied, the duration and means of specimen transport, laboratory methods and instrumentation, and even the type of container used for the collection of the specimen. The reference or "normal" ranges given in this appendix may therefore not be appropriate for all laboratories, and these values should only be used as general guidelines. Whenever possible, reference values provided by the laboratory performing the testing should be utilized in the interpretation of laboratory data. Values supplied in this Appendix reflect typical reference ranges in adults. Pediatric reference ranges may vary significantly from adult values.

In preparing the Appendix, the authors have taken into account the fact that the system of international units (SI, système international d'unités) is used in most countries and in some medical journals. However, clinical laboratories may continue to report values in "traditional" or conventional units. Therefore, both systems are provided in the Appendix. The dual system is also used in the text except for (1) those instances in which the numbers remain the same but only the terminology is changed (mmol/L for meq/L or IU/L for mIU/mL), when only the SI units are given; and (2) most pressure measurements (e.g., blood and cerebrospinal fluid pressures), when the traditional units (mmHg, mmH$_2$O) are used. In all other instances in the text the SI unit is followed by the traditional unit in parentheses.

REFERENCE VALUES FOR LABORATORY TESTS

TABLE 1 Hematology and Coagulation

Analyte	Specimen	SI Units	Conventional Units
Activated clotting time	WB	70–180 s	70–180 s
Activated protein C resistance (factor V Leiden)	P	Not applicable	Ratio >2.1
ADAMTS13 activity	P	≥0.67	≥67%
ADAMTS13 inhibitor activity	P	Not applicable	≤0.4 U
ADAMTS13 antibody	P	Not applicable	≤18 U
Alpha$_2$ antiplasmin	P	0.87–1.55	87–155%
Antiphospholipid antibody panel			
PTT-LA (lupus anticoagulant screen)	P	Negative	Negative
Platelet neutralization procedure	P	Negative	Negative
Dilute viper venom screen	P	Negative	Negative
Anticardiolipin antibody	S		
IgG		0–15 arbitrary units	0–15 GPL
IgM		0–15 arbitrary units	0–15 MPL
Antithrombin III	P		
Antigenic		220–390 mg/L	22–39 mg/dL
Functional		0.7–1.30 U/L	70–130 %
Anti-Xa assay (heparin assay)	P		
Unfractionated heparin		0.3–0.7 kIU/L	0.3–0.7 IU/mL
Low-molecular-weight heparin		0.5–1.0 kIU/L	0.5–1.0 IU/mL
Danaparoid (Orgaran)		0.5–0.8 kIU/L	0.5–0.8 IU/mL
Autohemolysis test	WB	0.004–0.045	0.4–4.50%
Autohemolysis test with glucose	WB	0.003–0.007	0.3–0.7%
Bleeding time (adult)		<7.1 min	<7.1 min
Bone marrow: See Table 7			
Clot retraction	WB	0.50–1.00/2 h	50–100%/2 h
Cryofibrinogen	P	Negative	Negative

(continued)

TABLE 1 Hematology and Coagulation (*Continued*)

Analyte	Specimen	SI Units	Conventional Units
D-dimer	P	220–740 ng/mL FEU	220–740 ng/mL FEU
Differential blood count	WB		
Relative counts:			
Neutrophils		0.40–0.70	40–70%
Bands		0.0–0.05	0–5%
Lymphocytes		0.20–0.50	20–50%
Monocytes		0.04–0.08	4–8%
Eosinophils		0.0–0.6	0–6%
Basophils		0.0–0.02	0–2%
Absolute counts:			
Neutrophils		$1.42–6.34 \times 10^9$/L	1420–6340/mm^3
Bands		$0–0.45 \times 10^9$/L	0–450/mm^3
Lymphocytes		$0.71–4.53 \times 10^9$/L	710–4530/mm^3
Monocytes		$0.14–0.72 \times 10^9$/L	140–720/mm^3
Eosinophils		$0–0.54 \times 10^9$/L	0–540/mm^3
Basophils		$0–0.18 \times 10^9$/L	0–180/mm^3
Erythrocyte count	WB		
Adult males		$4.30–5.60 \times 10^{12}$/L	$4.30–5.60 \times 10^6/mm^3$
Adult females		$4.00–5.20 \times 10^{12}$/L	$4.00–5.20 \times 10^6/mm^3$
Erythrocyte life span	WB		
Normal survival		120 days	120 days
Chromium labeled, half-life ($t_{1/2}$)		25–35 days	25–35 days
Erythrocyte sedimentation rate	WB		
Females		0–20 mm/h	0–20 mm/h
Males		0–15 mm/h	0–15 mm/h
Euglobulin lysis time	P	7200–14400 s	120–240 min
Factor II, prothrombin	P	0.50–1.50	50–150%
Factor V	P	0.50–1.50	50–150%
Factor VII	P	0.50–1.50	50–150%
Factor VIII	P	0.50–1.50	50–150%
Factor IX	P	0.50–1.50	50–150%
Factor X	P	0.50–1.50	50–150%
Factor XI	P	0.50–1.50	50–150%
Factor XII	P	0.50–1.50	50–150 %
Factor XIII screen	P	Not applicable	Present
Factor inhibitor assay	P	<0.5 Bethesda Units	<0.5 Bethesda Units
Fibrin(ogen) degradation products	P	0–1 mg/L	0–1 µg/mL
Fibrinogen	P	2.33–4.96 g/L	233–496 mg/dL
Glucose-6-phosphate dehydrogenase (erythrocyte)	WB	<2400 s	<40 min
Ham's test (acid serum)	WB	Negative	Negative
Hematocrit	WB		
Adult males		0.388–0.464	38.8–46.4
Adult females		0.354–0.444	35.4–44.4
Hemoglobin			
Plasma	P	6–50 mg/L	0.6–5.0 mg/dL
Whole blood:	WB		
Adult males		133–162 g/L	13.3–16.2 g/dL
Adult females		120–158 g/L	12.0–15.8 g/dL

(*continued*)

TABLE 1 Hematology and Coagulation (*Continued*)

Analyte	Specimen	SI Units	Conventional Units
Hemoglobin electrophoresis	WB		
Hemoglobin A		0.95–0.98	95–98%
Hemoglobin A_2		0.015–0.031	1.5–3.1%
Hemoglobin F		0–0.02	0–2.0%
Hemoglobins other than A, A_2, or F		Absent	Absent
Heparin-induced thrombocytopenia antibody	P	Negative	Negative
Immature platelet fraction (IPF)	WB	0.011–0.061	1.1–6.1%
Joint fluid crystal	JF	Not applicable	No crystals seen
Joint fluid mucin	JF	Not applicable	Only type I mucin present
Leukocytes			
Alkaline phosphatase (LAP)	WB	0.2–1.6 µkat/L	13–100 µ/L
Count (WBC)	WB	$3.54–9.06 \times 10^9$/L	$3.54–9.06 \times 10^3$/mm^3
Mean corpuscular hemoglobin (MCH)	WB	26.7–31.9 pg/cell	26.7–31.9 pg/cell
Mean corpuscular hemoglobin concentration (MCHC)	WB	323–359 g/L	32.3–35.9 g/dL
Mean corpuscular hemoglobin of reticulocytes (CH)	WB	24–36 pg	24–36 pg
Mean corpuscular volume (MCV)	WB	79–93.3 fL	79–93.3 µm^3
Mean platelet volume (MPV)	WB	9.00–12.95 fL	9.00–12.95
Osmotic fragility of erythrocytes	WB		
Direct		0.0035–0.0045	0.35–0.45%
Indirect		0.0030–0.0065	0.30–0.65%
Partial thromboplastin time, activated	P	26.3–39.4 s	26.3–39.4 s
Plasminogen	P		
Antigen		84–140 mg/L	8.4–14.0 mg/dL
Functional		0.70–1.30	70–130%
Plasminogen activator inhibitor 1	P	4–43 µg/L	4–43 ng/mL
Platelet aggregation	PRP	Not applicable	>65% aggregation in response to adenosine diphosphate, epinephrine, collagen, ristocetin, and arachidonic acid
Platelet count	WB	$165–415 \times 10^9$/L	$165–415 \times 10^3$/mm^3
Platelet, mean volume	WB	6.4–11 fL	6.4–11.0 µm^3
Prekallikrein assay	P	0.50–1.5	50–150%
Prekallikrein screen	P		No deficiency detected
Protein C	P		
Total antigen		0.70–1.40	70–140%
Functional		0.70–1.30	70–130%
Protein S	P		
Total antigen		0.70–1.40	70–140%
Functional		0.65–1.40	65–140%
Free antigen		0.70–1.40	70–140%
Prothrombin gene mutation G20210A	WB	Not applicable	Not present
Prothrombin time	P	12.7–15.4 s	12.7–15.4 s
Protoporphyrin, free erythrocyte	WB	0.28–0.64 µmol/L of red blood cells	16–36 µg/dL of red blood cells
Red cell distribution width	WB	<0.145	<14.5%
Reptilase time	P	16–23.6 s	16–23.6 s

(*continued*)

APPENDIX Laboratory Values of Clinical Importance

TABLE 1 Hematology and Coagulation (*Continued*)

Analyte	Specimen	SI Units	Conventional Units
Reticulocyte count	WB		
Adult males		0.008–0.023 red cells	0.8–2.3% red cells
Adult females		0.008–0.020 red cells	0.8–2.0% red cells
Reticulocyte hemoglobin content	WB	>26 pg/cell	>26 pg/cell
Ristocetin cofactor (functional von Willebrand factor)	P		
Blood group O		0.75 mean of normal	75% mean of normal
Blood group A		1.05 mean of normal	105% mean of normal
Blood group B		1.15 mean of normal	115% mean of normal
Blood group AB		1.25 mean of normal	125% mean of normal
Serotonin release assay	S	<0.2 release	<20% release
Sickle cell test	WB	Negative	Negative
Sucrose hemolysis	WB	<0.1	<10% hemolysis
Thrombin time	P	15.3–18.5 s	15.3–18.5 s
Total eosinophils	WB	150–300 $\times 10^6$/L	150–300/mm^3
Transferrin receptor	S, P	9.6–29.6 nmol/L	9.6–29.6 nmol/L
Viscosity			
Plasma	P	1.7–2.1	1.7–2.1
Serum	S	1.4–1.8	1.4–1.8
von Willebrand factor (vWF) antigen (factor VIII:R antigen)	P		
Blood group O		0.75 mean of normal	75% mean of normal
Blood group A		1.05 mean of normal	105% mean of normal
Blood group B		1.15 mean of normal	115% mean of normal
Blood group AB		1.25 mean of normal	125% mean of normal
von Willebrand factor multimers	P	Normal distribution	Normal distribution
White blood cells: see "Leukocytes"			

Abbreviations: JF, joint fluid; P, plasma; PRP, platelet-rich plasma; S, serum; WB, whole blood.

TABLE 2 Clinical Chemistry and Immunology

Analyte	Specimen[a]	SI Units	Conventional Units
Acetoacetate	P	49–294 μmol/L	0.5–3.0 mg/dL
Adrenocorticotropin (ACTH)	P	1.3–16.7 pmol/L	6.0–76.0 pg/mL
Alanine aminotransferase (ALT, SGPT)	S	0.12–0.70 μkat/L	7–41 U/L
Albumin	S	40–50 g/L	4.0–5.0 mg/dL
Aldolase	S	26–138 nkat/L	1.5–8.1 U/L
Aldosterone (adult)			
Supine, normal sodium diet	S, P	<443 pmol/L	<16 ng/dL
Upright, normal	S, P	111–858 pmol/L	4–31 ng/dL
Alpha fetoprotein (adult)	S	0–8.5 μg/L	0–8.5 ng/mL
Alpha$_1$ antitrypsin	S	1.0–2.0 g/L	100–200 mg/dL
Ammonia, as NH_3	P	11–35 μmol/L	19–60 μg/dL
Amylase (method dependent)	S	0.34–1.6 μkat/L	20–96 U/L

(*continued*)

TABLE 2 Clinical Chemistry and Immunology (*Continued*)

Analyte	Specimen[a]	SI Units	Conventional Units
Androstendione (adult)	S		
Males		0.81–3.1 nmol/L	23–89 ng/dL
Females			
Premenopausal		0.91–7.5 nmol/L	26–214 ng/dL
Postmenopausal		0.46–2.9 nmol/L	13–82 ng/dL
Angiotensin-converting enzyme (ACE)	S	0.15–1.1 μkat/L	9–67 U/L
Anion gap	S	7–16 mmol/L	7–16 mmol/L
Apolipoprotein A-1	S		
Male		0.94–1.78 g/L	94–178 mg/dL
Female		1.01–1.99 g/L	101–199 mg/dL
Apolipoprotein B	S		
Male		0.55–1.40 g/L	55–140 mg/dL
Female		0.55–1.25 g/L	55–125 mg/dL
Arterial blood gases	WB		
$[HCO_3^-]$		22–30 mmol/L	22–30 meq/L
P_{CO_2}		4.3–6.0 kPa	32–45 mmHg
pH		7.35–7.45	7.35–7.45
P_{O_2}		9.6–13.8 kPa	72–104 mmHg
Aspartate aminotransferase (AST, SGOT)	S	0.20–0.65 μkat/L	12–38 U/L
Autoantibodies	S		
Anti-centromere antibody IgG		≤29 AU/mL	≤29 AU/mL
Anti-double-strand (native) DNA		<25 IU/L	<25 IU/L
Anti-glomerular basement membrane antibodies			
Qualitative IgG, IgA		Negative	Negative
Quantitative IgG antibody		≤19 AU/mL	≤19 AU/mL
Anti-histone antibodies		<1.0 U	<1.0 U
Anti-Jo-1 antibody		≤29 AU/mL	≤29 AU/mL
Anti-mitochondrial antibody		Not applicable	<20 Units
Anti-neutrophil cytoplasmic autoantibodies		Not applicable	<1:20
Serine proteinase 3 antibodies		≤19 AU/mL	≤19 AU/mL
Myeloperoxidase antibodies		≤19 AU/mL	≤19 AU/mL
Antinuclear antibody		Not applicable	Negative at 1:40
Anti-parietal cell antibody		Not applicable	None detected
Anti-RNP antibody		Not applicable	<1.0 U
Anti-Scl 70 antibody		Not applicable	<1.0 U
Anti-Smith antibody		Not applicable	<1.0 U
Anti–smooth muscle antibody		Not applicable	<1.0 U
Anti-SSA antibody		Not applicable	<1.0 U
Anti-SSB antibody		Not applicable	Negative
Anti-thyroglobulin antibody		<40 KIU/L	<40 IU/mL
Anti-thyroid peroxidase antibody		<35 KIU/L	<35 IU/mL
B-type natriuretic peptide (BNP)	P	Age and gender specific: <100 ng/L	Age and gender specific: <100 pg/mL
Bence Jones protein, serum qualitative	S	Not applicable	None detected
Bence Jones protein, serum quantitative	S		
Free kappa		3.3–19.4 mg/L	0.33–1.94 mg/dL
Free lambda		5.7–26.3 mg/L	0.57–2.63 mg/dL
K/L ratio		0.26–1.65	0.26–1.65
Beta-2-microglobulin	S	1.1–2.4 mg/L	1.1–2.4 mg/L

(*continued*)

TABLE 2 Clinical Chemistry and Immunology (*Continued*)

Analyte	Specimen[a]	SI Units	Conventional Units
Bilirubin	S		
Total		5.1–22 μmol/L	0.3–1.3 mg/dL
Direct		1.7–6.8 μmol/L	0.1–0.4 mg/dL
Indirect		3.4–15.2 μmol/L	0.2–0.9 mg/dL
C peptide	S	0.27–1.19 nmol/L	0.8–3.5 ng/mL
C1-esterase-inhibitor protein	S	210–390 mg/L	21–39 mg/dL
CA 125	S	<35 kU/L	<35 U/mL
CA 19-9	S	<37 kU/L	<37 U/mL
CA 15-3	S	<33 kU/L	<33 U/mL
CA 27-29	S	0–40 kU/L	0–40 U/mL
Calcitonin	S		
Male		0–7.5 ng/L	0–7.5 pg/mL
Female		0–5.1 ng/L	0–5.1 pg/mL
Calcium	S	2.2–2.6 mmol/L	8.7–10.2 mg/dL
Calcium, ionized	WB	1.12–1.32 mmol/L	4.5–5.3 mg/dL
Carbon dioxide content (TCO_2)	P (sea level)	22–30 mmol/L	22–30 meq/L
Carboxyhemoglobin (carbon monoxide content)	WB		
Nonsmokers		0.0–0.015	0–1.5%
Smokers		0.04–0.09	4–9%
Loss of consciousness and death		>0.50	>50%
Carcinoembryonic antigen (CEA)	S		
Nonsmokers		0.0–3.0 μg/L	0.0–3.0 ng/mL
Smokers		0.0–5.0 μg/L	0.0–5.0 ng/mL
Ceruloplasmin	S	250–630 mg/L	25–63 mg/dL
Chloride	S	102–109 mmol/L	102–109 meq/L
Cholesterol: see Table 5			
Cholinesterase	S	5–12 kU/L	5–12 U/mL
Chromogranin A	S	0–50 μg/L	0–50 ng/mL
Complement	S		
C3		0.83–1.77 g/L	83–177 mg/dL
C4		0.16–0.47 g/L	16–47 mg/dL
Complement total		60–144 CAE units	60–144 CAE units
Cortisol			
Fasting, 8 A.M.–12 noon	S	138–690 nmol/L	5–25 μg/dL
12 noon–8 P.M.		138–414 nmol/L	5–15 μg/dL
8 P.M.–8 A.M.		0–276 nmol/L	0–10 μg/dL
C-reactive protein	S	<10 mg/L	<10 mg/L
C-reactive protein, high sensitivity	S	Cardiac risk Low: <1.0 mg/L Average: 1.0–3.0 mg/L High: >3.0 mg/L	Cardiac risk Low: <1.0 mg/L Average: 1.0–3.0 mg/L High: >3.0 mg/L
Creatine kinase (total)	S		
Females		0.66–4.0 μkat/L	39–238 U/L
Males		0.87–5.0 μkat/L	51–294 U/L

(*continued*)

TABLE 2 Clinical Chemistry and Immunology (*Continued*)

Analyte	Specimen[a]	SI Units	Conventional Units
Creatine kinase-MB	S		
Mass		0.0–5.5 μg/L	0.0–5.5 ng/mL
Fraction of total activity (by electrophoresis)		0–0.04	0–4.0%
Creatinine	S		
Female		44–80 μmol/L	0.5–0.9 mg/dL
Male		53–106 μmol/L	0.6–1.2 mg/dL
Cryoglobulins	S	Not applicable	None detected
Cystatin C	S	0.5–1.0 mg/L	0.5–1.0 mg/L
Dehydroepiandrosterone (DHEA) (adult)			
Male	S	6.2–43.4 nmol/L	180–1250 ng/dL
Female		4.5–34.0 nmol/L	130–980 ng/dL
Dehydroepiandrosterone (DHEA) sulfate	S		
Male (adult)		100–6190 μg/L	10–619 μg/dL
Female (adult, premenopausal)		120–5350 μg/L	12–535 μg/dL
Female (adult, postmenopausal)		300–2600 μg/L	30–260 μg/dL
11-Deoxycortisol (adult)(compound S)	S	0.34–4.56 nmol/L	12–158 ng/dL
Dihydrotestosterone			
Male	S, P	1.03–2.92 nmol/L	30–85 ng/dL
Female		0.14–0.76 nmol/L	4–22 ng/dL
Dopamine	P	0–130 pmol/L	0–20 pg/mL
Epinephrine	P		
Supine (30 min)		<273 pmol/L	<50 pg/mL
Sitting		<328 pmol/L	<60 pg/mL
Standing (30 min)		<491pmol/L	<90 pg/mL
Erythropoietin	S	4–27 U/L	4–27 U/L
Estradiol	S, P		
Female			
Menstruating:			
Follicular phase		74–532 pmol/L	<20–145 pg/mL
Midcycle peak		411–1626 pmol/L	112–443 pg/mL
Luteal phase		74–885 pmol/L	<20–241 pg/mL
Postmenopausal		217 pmol/L	<59 pg/mL
Male		74 pmol/L	<20 pg/mL
Estrone	S, P		
Female			
Menstruating:			
Follicular phase		<555 pmol/L	<150 pg/mL
Luteal phase		<740 pmol/L	<200 pg/mL
Postmenopausal		11–118 pmol/L	3–32 pg/mL
Male		33–133 pmol/L	9–36 pg/mL
Fatty acids, free (nonesterified)	P	0.1–0.6 mmol/L	2.8–16.8 mg/dL
Ferritin	S		
Female		10–150 μg/L	10–150 ng/mL
Male		29–248 μg/L	29–248 ng/mL

(*continued*)

TABLE 2 Clinical Chemistry and Immunology (*Continued*)

Analyte	Specimen*	SI Units	Conventional Units
Follicle-stimulating hormone (FSH)	S, P		
Female			
Menstruating		3.0–20.0 IU/L	3.0–20.0 mIU/mL
Follicular phase		9.0–26.0 IU/L	9.0–26.0 mIU/mL
Ovulatory phase		1.0–12.0 IU/L	1.0–12.0 mIU/mL
Luteal phase		18.0–153.0 IU/L	18.0–153.0 mIU/mL
Postmenopausal			
Male		1.0–12.0 IU/L	1.0–12.0 mIU/mL
Fructosamine	S	<285 umol/L	<285 umol/L
Gamma glutamyltransferase	S	0.15–0.99 μkat/L	9–58 U/L
Gastrin	S	<100 ng/L	<100 pg/mL
Glucagon	P	40–130 ng/L	40–130 pg/mL
Glucose	WB	3.6–5.3 mmol/L	65–95 mg/dL
Glucose (fasting)	P		
Normal		4.2–5.6 mmol/L	75–100 mg/dL
Increased risk for diabetes		5.6–6.9 mmol/L	100–125 mg/dL
Diabetes mellitus		Fasting ≥7.0 mmol/L	Fasting ≥126 mg/dL
		A 2-hour level of ≥11.1 mmol/L during an oral glucose tolerance test	A 2-hour level of ≥200 mg/dL during an oral glucose tolerance test
		A random glucose level of ≥11.1 mmol/L in patients with symptoms of hyperglycemia	A random glucose level of ≥200 mg/dL in patients with symptoms of hyperglycemia
Growth hormone	S	0–5 μg/L	0–5 ng/mL
Hemoglobin A_{1c}	WB	0.04–0.06 HgB fraction	4.0–5.6%
Pre-diabetes		0.057-0.064 HgB fraction	5.7–6.4%
Diabetes mellitus		A hemoglobin A_{1c} level of ≥0.065 Hgb fraction as suggested by the American Diabetes Association	A hemoglobin A_{1c} level of ≥6.5% as suggested by the American Diabetes Association
Hemoglobin A_{1c} with estimated average glucose (eAg)	WB	eAg mmoL/L = $1.59 \times HbA_{1c} - 2.59$	eAg (mg/dL) = $28.7 \times HbA_{1c} - 46.7$
High-density lipoprotein (HDL) (see Table 5)			
Homocysteine	P	4.4–10.8 μmol/L	4.4–10.8 μmol/L
Human chorionic gonadotropin (HCG)	S		
Nonpregnant female		<5 IU/L	<5 mIU/ml
1–2 weeks postconception		9–130 IU/L	9–130 mIU/mL
2–3 weeks postconception		75–2600 IU/L	75–2600 mIU/mL
3–4 weeks postconception		850–20,800 IU/L	850–20,800 mIU/mL
4–5 weeks postconception		4000–100,200 IU/L	4000–100,200 mIU/mL
5–10 weeks postconception		11,500–289,000 IU/L	11,500–289,000 mIU/mL
10–14 weeks post conception		18,300–137,000 IU/L	18,300–137,000 mIU/mL
Second trimester		1400–53,000 IU/L	1400–53,000 mIU/mL
Third trimester		940–60,000 IU/L	940–60,000 mIU/mL
β-Hydroxybutyrate	P	60–170 μmol/L	0.6–1.8 mg/dL

(*continued*)

TABLE 2 Clinical Chemistry and Immunology (*Continued*)

Analyte	Specimen*	SI Units	Conventional Units
17-Hydroxyprogesterone (adult)	S		
Male		<4.17 nmol/L	<139 ng/dL
Female			
Follicular phase		0.45–2.1 nmol/L	15–70 ng/dL
Luteal phase		1.05–8.7 nmol/L	35–290 ng/dL
Immunofixation	S	Not applicable	No bands detected
Immunoglobulin, quantitation (adult)			
IgA	S	0.70–3.50 g/L	70–350 mg/dL
IgD	S	0–140 mg/L	0–14 mg/dL
IgE	S	1–87 KIU/L	1–87 IU/mL
IgG	S	7.0–17.0 g/L	700–1700 mg/dL
IgG_1	S	2.7–17.4 g/L	270–1740 mg/dL
IgG_2	S	0.3–6.3 g/L	30–630 mg/dL
IgG_3	S	0.13–3.2 g/L	13–320 mg/dL
IgG_4	S	0.11–6.2 g/L	11–620 mg/dL
IgM	S	0.50–3.0 g/L	50–300 mg/dL
Insulin	S, P	14.35–143.5 pmol/L	2–20 μU/mL
Iron	S	7–25 μmol/L	41–141 μg/dL
Iron-binding capacity	S	45–73 μmol/L	251–406 μg/dL
Iron-binding capacity saturation	S	0.16–0.35	16–35%
Ischemia modified albumin	S	<85 KU/L	<85 U/mL
Joint fluid crystal	JF	Not applicable	No crystals seen
Joint fluid mucin	JF	Not applicable	Only type I mucin present
Ketone (acetone)	S	Negative	Negative
Lactate	P, arterial	0.5–1.6 mmol/L	4.5–14.4 mg/dL
	P, venous	0.5–2.2 mmol/L	4.5–19.8 mg/dL
Lactate dehydrogenase	S	2.0–3.8 μkat/L	115–221 U/L
Lipase	S	0.51–0.73 μkat/L	3–43 U/L
Lipids: see Table 5			
Lipoprotein (a)	S	0–300 mg/L	0–30 mg/dL
Low-density lipoprotein (LDL) (see Table 5)			
Luteinizing hormone (LH)	S, P		
Female			
Menstruating			
Follicular phase		2.0–15.0 U/L	2.0–15.0 mIU/mL
Ovulatory phase		22.0–105.0 U/L	22.0–105.0 mIU/mL
Luteal phase		0.6–19.0 U/L	0.6–19.0 mIU/mL
Postmenopausal		16.0–64.0 U/L	16.0–64.0 mIU/mL
Male		2.0–12.0 U/L	2.0–12.0 mIU/mL
Magnesium	S	0.62–0.95 mmol/L	1.5–2.3 mg/dL
Metanephrine	P	<0.5 nmol/L	<100 pg/mL
Methemoglobin	WB	0.0–0.01	0–1%
Myoglobin	S		
Male		20–71 μg/L	20–71 μg/L
Female		25–58 μg/L	25–58 μg/L

(*continued*)

APPENDIX

Laboratory Values of Clinical Importance

TABLE 2 Clinical Chemistry and Immunology (*Continued*)

Analyte	Specimen	SI Units	Conventional Units
Norepinephrine	P		
Supine (30 min)		650–2423 pmol/L	110–410 pg/mL
Sitting		709–4019 pmol/L	120–680 pg/mL
Standing (30 min)		739–4137 pmol/L	125–700 pg/mL
N-telopeptide (cross-linked), NTx	S		
Female, premenopausal		6.2–19.0 nmol BCE	6.2–19.0 nmol BCE
Male		5.4–24.2 nmol BCE	5.4–24.2 nmol BCE
BCE = bone collagen equivalent			
NT-Pro BNP	S, P	<125 ng/L up to 75 years <450 ng/L >75 years	<125 pg/mL up to 75 years <450 pg/mL >75 years
5′ Nucleotidase	S	0.00–0.19 μkat/L	0–11 U/L
Osmolality	P	275–295 mOsmol/kg serum water	275–295 mOsmol/kg serum water
Osteocalcin	S	11–50 μg/L	11–50 ng/mL
Oxygen content	WB		
Arterial (sea level)		17–21	17–21 vol%
Venous (sea level)		10–16	10–16 vol%
Oxygen saturation (sea level)	WB	Fraction:	Percent:
Arterial		0.94–1.0	94–100%
Venous, arm		0.60–0.85	60–85%
Parathyroid hormone (intact)	S	8–51 ng/L	8–51 pg/mL
Phosphatase, alkaline	S	0.56–1.63 μkat/L	33–96 U/L
Phosphorus, inorganic	S	0.81–1.4 mmol/L	2.5–4.3 mg/dL
Potassium	S	3.5–5.0 mmol/L	3.5–5.0 meq/L
Prealbumin	S	170–340 mg/L	17–34 mg/dL
Procalcitonin	S	<0.1 μg/L	<0.1 ng/mL
Progesterone	S, P		
Female: Follicular		<3.18 nmol/L	<1.0 ng/mL
Midluteal		9.54–63.6 nmol/L	3–20 ng/mL
Male		<3.18 nmol/L	<1.0 ng/mL
Prolactin	S		
Male		53–360 mIU/L	2.5–17 ng/mL
Female		40–530 mIU/L	1.9–25 ng/mL
Prostate-specific antigen (PSA)	S	0.0–4.0 μg/L	0.0–4.0 ng/mL
Prostate-specific antigen, free	S	With total PSA between 4 and 10 μg/L and when the free PSA is: >0.25 decreased risk of prostate cancer <0.10 increased risk of prostate cancer	With total PSA between 4 and 10 ng/mL and when the free PSA is: >25% decreased risk of prostate cancer <10% increased risk of prostate cancer
Protein fractions:	S		
Albumin		35–55 g/L	3.5–5.5 g/dL (50–60%)
Globulin		20–35 g/L	2.0–3.5 g/dL (40–50%)
$Alpha_1$		2–4 g/L	0.2–0.4 g/dL (4.2–7.2%)
$Alpha_2$		5–9 g/L	0.5–0.9 g/dL (6.8–12%)
Beta		6–11 g/L	0.6–1.1 g/dL (9.3–15%)
Gamma		7–17 g/L	0.7–1.7 g/dL (13–23%)

(*continued*)

TABLE 2 Clinical Chemistry and Immunology (*Continued*)

Analyte	Specimen*	SI Units	Conventional Units
Protein, total	S	67–86 g/L	6.7–8.6 g/dL
Pyruvate	P	40–130 μmol/L	0.35–1.14 mg/dL
Rheumatoid factor	S	<15 kIU/L	<15 IU/mL
Serotonin	WB	0.28–1.14 umol/L	50–200 ng/mL
Serum protein electrophoresis	S	Not applicable	Normal pattern
Sex hormone–binding globulin (adult)	S		
Male		11–80 nmol/L	11–80 nmol/L
Female		30–135 nmol/L	30–135 nmol/L
Sodium	S	136–146 mmol/L	136–146 meq/L
Somatomedin-C (IGF-1)(adult)	S		
16 years		226–903 μg/L	226–903 ng/mL
17 years		193–731 μg/L	193–731 ng/mL
18 years		163–584 μg/L	163–584 ng/mL
19 years		141–483 μg/L	141–483 ng/mL
20 years		127–424 μg/L	127–424 ng/mL
21–25 years		116–358 μg/L	116–358 ng/mL
26–30 years		117–329 μg/L	117–329 ng/mL
31–35 years		115–307 μg/L	115–307 ng/mL
36–40 years		119–204 μg/L	119–204 ng/mL
41–45 years		101–267 μg/L	101–267 ng/mL
46–50 years		94–252 μg/L	94–252 ng/mL
51–55 years		87–238 μg/L	87–238 ng/mL
56–60 years		81–225 μg/L	81–225 ng/mL
61–65 years		75–212 μg/L	75–212 ng/mL
66–70 years		69–200 μg/L	69–200 ng/mL
71–75 years		64–188 μg/L	64–188 ng/mL
76–80 years		59–177 μg/L	59–177 ng/mL
81–85 years		55–166 μg/L	55–166 ng/mL
Somatostatin	P	<25 ng/L	<25 pg/mL
Testosterone, free			
Female, adult	S	10.4–65.9 pmol/L	3–19 pg/mL
Male, adult		312–1041 pmol/L	90–300 pg/mL
Testosterone, total,	S		
Female		0.21–2.98 nmol/L	6–86 ng/dL
Male		9.36–37.10 nmol/L	270–1070 ng/dL
Thyroglobulin	S	1.3–31.8 μg/L	1.3–31.8 ng/mL
Thyroid-binding globulin	S	13–30 mg/L	1.3–3.0 mg/dL
Thyroid-stimulating hormone	S	0.34–4.25 mIU/L	0.34–4.25 μIU/mL
Thyroxine, free (fT4)	S	9.0–16 pmol/L	0.7–1.24 ng/dL
Thyroxine, total (T4)	S	70–151 nmol/L	5.4–11.7 μg/dL
Thyroxine index (free)	S	6.7–10.9	6.7–10.9
Transferrin	S	2.0–4.0 g/L	200–400 mg/dL
Triglycerides (see Table 5)	S	0.34–2.26 mmol/L	30–200 mg/dL
Triiodothyronine, free (fT3)	S	3.7–6.5 pmol/L	2.4–4.2 pg/mL
Triiodothyronine, total (T3)	S	1.2–2.1 nmol/L	77–135 ng/dL
Troponin I (method dependent)	S,P		
99th percentile of a healthy population		0–0.04 μg/L	0–0.04 ng/mL

(*continued*)

TABLE 2 Clinical Chemistry and Immunology (*Continued*)

Analyte	Specimen*	SI Units	Conventional Units
Troponin T	S,P		
99th percentile of a healthy population		0–0.01 μg/L	0–0.01 ng/mL
Urea nitrogen	S	2.5–7.1 mmol/L	7–20 mg/dL
Uric acid	S		
Females		0.15–0.33 mmol/L	2.5–5.6 mg/dL
Males		0.18–0.41 mmol/L	3.1–7.0 mg/dL
Vasoactive intestinal polypeptide	P	0–60 ng/L	0–60 pg/mL
Zinc protoporphyrin	WB	0–400 μg/L	0–40 μg/dL
Zinc protoporphyrin (ZPP)-to-heme ratio	WB	0–69 μmol ZPP/mol heme	0–69 μmol ZPP/mol heme

Abbreviations: P, plasma; S, serum; WB, whole blood.

TABLE 3 Toxicology and Therapeutic Drug Monitoring

	Therapeutic Range		Toxic Level	
Drug	SI Units	Conventional Units	SI Units	Conventional Units
Acetaminophen	66–199 μmol/L	10–30 μg/mL	>1320 μmol/L	>200 μg/mL
Amikacin				
Peak	34–51 μmol/L	20–30 μg/mL	>60 μmol/L	>35 μg/mL
Trough	0–17 μmol/L	0–10 μg/mL	>17 μmol/L	>10 μg/mL
Amitriptyline/nortriptyline (total drug)	430–900 nmol/L	120–250 ng/mL	>1800 nmol/L	>500 ng/mL
Amphetamine	150–220 nmol/L	20–30 ng/mL	>1500 nmol/L	>200 ng/mL
Bromide	9.4–18.7 mmol/L	75–150 mg/dL	>18.8 mmol/L	>150 mg/dL
Mild toxicity			6.4–18.8 mmol/L	51–150 mg/dL
Severe toxicity			>18.8 mmol/L	>150 mg/dL
Lethal			>37.5 mmol/L	>300 mg/dL
Caffeine	25.8–103 μmol/L	5–20 μg/ml	>206 μmol/L	>40 μg/mL
Carbamazepine	17–42 μmol/L	4–10 μg/mL	> 85 μmol/L	>20 μg/mL
Chloramphenicol				
Peak	31–62 μmol/L	10–20 μg/mL	>77 μmol/L	>25 μg/mL
Trough	15–31 μmol/L	5–10 μg/mL	>46 μmol/L	>15 μg/mL
Chlordiazepoxide	1.7–10 μmol/L	0.5–3.0 μg/mL	>17 μmol/L	>5.0 μg/mL
Clonazepam	32–240 nmol/L	10–75 ng/mL	>320 nmol/L	>100 ng/mL
Clozapine	0.6–2.1 μmol/L	200–700 ng/mL	>3.7 μmol/L	>1200 ng/mL
Cocaine			>3.3 μmol/L	>1.0 μg/mL
Codeine	43–110 nmol/mL	13–33 ng/mL	>3700 nmol/mL	>1100 ng/mL (lethal)
Cyclosporine				
Renal transplant				
0–6 months	208–312 nmol/L	250–375 ng/mL	>312 nmol/L	>375 ng/mL
6–12 months after transplant	166–250 nmol/L	200–300 ng/mL	>250 nmol/L	>300 ng/mL
>12 months	83–125 nmol/L	100–150 ng/mL	>125 nmol/L	>150 ng/mL
Cardiac transplant				
0–6 months	208–291 nmol/L	250–350 ng/mL	>291 nmol/L	>350 ng/mL
6–12 months after transplant	125–208 nmol/L	150–250 ng/mL	>208 nmol/L	>250 ng/mL
>12 months	83–125 nmol/L	100–150 ng/mL	>125 nmol/L	150 ng/mL

(*continued*)

TABLE 3 Toxicology and Therapeutic Drug Monitoring (*Continued*)

Drug	Therapeutic Range		Toxic Level	
	SI Units	Conventional Units	SI Units	Conventional Units
Cyclosporine (Continued)				
Lung transplant				
0–6 months	250–374 nmol/L	300–450 ng/mL	>374 nmol/L	>450 ng/mL
Liver transplant				
Initiation	208–291 nmol/L	250–350 ng/mL	>291 nmol/L	>350 ng/mL
Maintenance	83–166 nmol/L	100–200 ng/mL	>166 nmol/L	>200 ng/mL
Desipramine	375–1130 nmol/L	100–300 ng/mL	>1880 nmol/L	>500 ng/mL
Diazepam (and metabolite)				
Diazepam	0.7 –3.5 μmol/L	0.2–1.0 μg/mL	>7.0 μmol/L	>2.0 μg/mL
Nordiazepam	0.4– 6.6 μmol/L	0.1–1.8 μg/mL	>9.2 μmol/L	>2.5 μg/mL
Digoxin	0.64–2.6 nmol/L	0.5–2.0 ng/mL	>5.0 nmol/L	>3.9 ng/mL
Disopyramide	5.3–14.7 μmol/L	2–5 μg/mL	>20.6 μmol/L	>7 μg/mL
Doxepin and nordoxepin				
Doxepin	0.36–0.98 μmol/L	101–274 ng/mL	>1.8 μmol/L	>503 ng/mL
Nordoxepin	0.38–1.04 μmol/L	106–291 ng/mL	>1.9 μmol/L	>531 ng/mL
Ethanol				
Behavioral changes			>4.3 mmol/L	>20 mg/dL
Legal limit			≥17 mmol/L	≥80 mg/dL
Critical with acute exposure			>54 mmol/L	>250 mg/dL
Ethylene glycol				
Toxic			>2 mmol/L	>12 mg/dL
Lethal			>20 mmol/L	>120 mg/dL
Ethosuximide	280–700 μmol/L	40–100 μg/mL	>700 μmol/L	>100 μg/mL
Everolimus	3.13–8.35 nmol/L	3–8 ng/mL	>12.5 nmol/L	>12 ng/mL
Flecainide	0.5–2.4 μmol/L	0.2–1.0 μg/mL	>3.6 μmol/L	>1.5 μg/mL
Gentamicin				
Peak	10–21 μmol/mL	5–10 μg/mL	>25 μmol/mL	>12 μg/mL
Trough	0–4.2 μmol/mL	0–2 μg/mL	>4.2 μmol/mL	>2 μg/mL
Heroin (diacetyl morphine)			>700 μmol/L	>200 ng/mL (as morphine)
Ibuprofen	49–243 μmol/L	10–50 μg/mL	>970 μmol/L	>200 μg/mL
Imipramine (and metabolite)				
Desimipramine	375–1130 nmol/L	100–300 ng/mL	>1880 nmol/L	>500 ng/mL
Total imipramine + desimipramine	563–1130 nmol/L	150–300 ng/mL	>1880 nmol/L	>500 ng/mL
Lamotrigine	11.7–54.7 μmol/L	3–14 μg/mL	>58.7 μmol/L	>15 μg/mL
Lidocaine	5.1–21.3 μmol/L	1.2–5.0 μg/mL	>38.4 μmol/L	>9.0 μg/mL
Lithium	0.5–1.3 mmol/L	0.5–1.3 meq/L	>2 mmol/L	>2 meq/L
Methadone	1.0–3.2 μmol/L	0.3–1.0 μg/mL	>6.5 μmol/L	>2 μg/mL
Methamphetamine	0.07–0.34 μmol/L	0.01–0.05 μg/mL	>3.35 μmol/L	>0.5 μg/mL
Methanol			>6 mmol/L	>20 mg/dL
Methotrexate				
Low-dose	0.01–0.1 μmol/L	0.01–0.1 μmol/L	>0.1 mmol/L	>0.1 mmol/L
High-dose (24h)	<5.0 μmol/L	<5.0 μmol/L	>5.0 μmol/L	>5.0 μmol/L
High-dose (48h)	<0.50 μmol/L	<0.50 μmol/L	>0.5 μmol/L	>0.5 μmol/L
High-dose (72h)	<0.10 μmol/L	<0.10 μmol/L	>0.1 μmol/L	>0.1 μmol/L

(*continued*)

TABLE 3 Toxicology and Therapeutic Drug Monitoring (*Continued*)

Drug	Therapeutic Range		Toxic Level	
	SI Units	Conventional Units	SI Units	Conventional Units
Morphine	232–286 µmol/L	65–80 ng/mL	>720 µmol/L	>200 ng/mL
Mycophenolic acid	3.1–10.9 µmol/L	1.0–3.5 ng/mL	>37 µmol/L	>12 ng/mL
Nitroprusside (as thiocyanate)	103–499 µmol/L	6–29 µg/mL	860 µmol/L	>50 µg/mL
Nortriptyline	190–569 nmol/L	50–150 ng/mL	>1900 nmol/L	>500 ng/mL
Phenobarbital	65–172 µmol/L	15–40 µg/mL	>258 µmol/L	>60 µg/mL
Phenytoin	40–79 µmol/L	10–20 µg/mL	>158 µmol/L	>40 µg/mL
Phenytoin, free	4.0–7.9 µg/mL	1–2 µg/mL	>13.9 µg/mL	>3.5 µg/mL
% Free	0.08–0.14	8–14%		
Primidone and metabolite				
Primidone	23–55 µmol/L	5–12 µg/mL	>69 µmol/L	>15 µg/mL
Phenobarbital	65–172 µmol/L	15–40 µg/mL	>215 µmol/L	>50 µg/mL
Procainamide				
Procainamide	17–42 µmol/L	4–10 µg/mL	>43 µmol/L	>10 µg/mL
NAPA (*N*-acetylprocainamide)	22–72 µmol/L	6–20 µg/mL	>126 µmol/L	>35 µg/mL
Quinidine	6.2–15.4 µmol/L	2.0–5.0 µg/mL	>19 µmol/L	>6 µg/mL
Salicylates	145–2100 µmol/L	2–29 mg/dL	>2900 µmol/L	>40 mg/dL
Sirolimus (trough level)				
Kidney transplant	4.4–15.4 nmol/L	4–14 ng/mL	>16 nmol/L	>15 ng/mL
Tacrolimus (FK506) (trough)				
Kidney and liver	12–19 nmol/L	10–15 ng/mL	>25 nmol/L	>20 ng/mL
Initiation				
Maintenance	6–12 nmol/L	5–10 ng/mL	>25 nmol/L	>20 ng/mL
Heart				
Initiation	19–25 nmol/L	15–20 ng/mL		
Maintenance	6–12 nmol/L	5–10 ng/mL		
Theophylline	56–111 µg/mL	10–20 µg/mL	>168 µg/mL	>30 µg/mL
Thiocyanate				
After nitroprusside infusion	103–499 µmol/L	6–29 µg/mL	860 µmol/L	>50 µg/mL
Nonsmoker				
Smoker	17–69 µmol/L	1–4 µg/mL		
	52–206 µmol/L	3–12 µg/mL		
Tobramycin				
Peak	11–22 µg/L	5–10 µg/mL	>26 µg/L	>12 µg/mL
Trough	0–4.3 µg/L	0–2 µg/mL	>4.3 µg/L	>2 µg/mL
Valproic acid	346–693 µmol/L	50–100 µg/mL	>693 µmol/L	>100 µg/mL
Vancomycin				
Peak	14–28 µmol/L	20–40 µg/mL	>55 µmol/L	>80 µg/mL
Trough	3.5–10.4 µmol/L	5–15 µg/mL	>14 µmol/L	>20 µg/mL

TABLE 4 Vitamins and Selected Trace Minerals

Specimen	Analyte	Reference Range	
		SI Units	Conventional Units
Aluminum	S	<0.2 μmol/L	<5.41 μg/L
Arsenic	WB	0.03–0.31 μmol/L	2–23 μg/L
Cadmium	WB	<44.5 nmol/L	<5.0 μg/L
Coenzyme Q10 (ubiquinone)	P	433–1532 μg/L	433–1532 μg/L
β-Carotene	S	0.07–1.43 μmol/L	4–77 μg/dL
Copper	S	11–22 μmol/L	70–140 μg/dL
Folic acid	RC	340–1020 nmol/L cells	150–450 ng/mL cells
Folic acid	S	12.2–40.8 nmol/L	5.4–18.0 ng/mL
Lead (adult)	S	<0.5 μmol/L	<10 μg/dL
Mercury	WB	3.0–294 nmol/L	0.6–59 μg/L
Selenium	S	0.8–2.0 umol/L	63–160 μg/L
Vitamin A	S	0.7–3.5 μmol/L	20–100 μg/dL
Vitamin B_1 (thiamine)	S	0–75 nmol/L	0–2 μg/dL
Vitamin B_2 (riboflavin)	S	106–638 nmol/L	4–24 μg/dL
Vitamin B_6	P	20–121 nmol/L	5–30 ng/mL
Vitamin B_{12}	S	206–735 pmol/L	279–996 pg/mL
Vitamin C (ascorbic acid)	S	23–57 μmol/L	0.4–1.0 mg/dL
Vitamin D_3,1,25-dihydroxy, total	S, P	36–180 pmol/L	15–75 pg/mL
Vitamin D_3,25-hydroxy, total	P	75–250 nmol/L	30–100 ng/mL
Vitamin E	S	12–42 μmol/L	5–18 μg/mL
Vitamin K	S	0.29–2.64 nmol/L	0.13–1.19 ng/mL
Zinc	S	11.5–18.4 μmol/L	75–120 μg/dL

Abbreviations: P, plasma; RC, red cells; S, serum; WB, whole blood.

TABLE 5 Classification of LDL, Total, and HDL Cholesterol

LDL Cholesterol	
<70 mg/dL	Therapeutic option for very high risk patients
<100 mg/dL	Optimal
100–129 mg/dL	Near optimal/above optimal
130–159 mg/dL	Borderline high
160–189 mg/dL	High
≥190 mg/dL	Very high
Total Cholesterol	
<200 mg/dL	Desirable
200–239 mg/dL	Borderline high
≥240 mg/dL	High
HDL Cholesterol	
<40 mg/dL	Low
≥60 mg/dL	High

Abbreviations: LDL, low-density lipoprotein; HDL, high-density lipoprotein.
Source: Executive summary of the third report of the National Cholesterol Education Program (NCEP) expert panel on detection, evaluation, and treatment of high blood cholesterol in adults (adult treatment panel III). JAMA 2001; 285:2486–97. Implications of Recent Clinical Trials for the National Cholesterol Education Program Adult Treatment Panel III Guidelines. SM Grundy et al for the Coordinating Committee of the National Cholesterol Education Program: Circulation 110:227, 2004.

TABLE 6 Cerebrospinal Fluid[a]

	Reference Range	
Constituent	SI Units	Conventional Units
Osmolarity	292–297 mmol/kg water	292–297 mOsm/L
Electrolytes		
Sodium	137–145 mmol/L	137–145 meq/L
Potassium	2.7–3.9 mmol/L	2.7–3.9 meq/L
Calcium	1.0–1.5 mmol/L	2.1–3.0 meq/L
Magnesium	1.0–1.2 mmol/L	2.0–2.5 meq/L
Chloride	116–122 mmol/L	116–122 meq/L
CO_2 content	20–24 mmol/L	20–24 meq/L
Pco_2	6–7 kPa	45–49 mmHg
pH	7.31–7.34	
Glucose	2.22–3.89 mmol/L	40–70 mg/dL
Lactate	1–2 mmol/L	10–20 mg/dL
Total protein:		
Lumbar	0.15–0.5 g/L	15–50 mg/dL
Cisternal	0.15–0.25 g/L	15–25 mg/dL
Ventricular	0.06–0.15 g/L	6–15 mg/dL
Albumin	0.066–0.442 g/L	6.6–44.2 mg/dL
IgG	0.009–0.057 g/L	0.9–5.7 mg/dL
IgG index[b]	0.29–0.59	
Oligoclonal bands (OGB)	<2 bands not present in matched serum sample	
Ammonia	15–47 μmol/L	25–80 μg/dL
Creatinine	44–168 μmol/L	0.5–1.9 mg/dL
Myelin basic protein	<4 μg/L	
CSF pressure		50–180 mmH_2O
CSF volume (adult)	~150 mL	
Red blood cells	0	0
Leukocytes		
Total	0–5 mononuclear cells per μL	
Differential		
Lymphocytes	60–70%	
Monocytes	30–50%	
Neutrophils	None	

[a]Since cerebrospinal fluid concentrations are equilibrium values, measurements of the same parameters in blood plasma obtained at the same time are recommended. However, there is a time lag in attainment of equilibrium, and cerebrospinal levels of plasma constituents that can fluctuate rapidly (such as plasma glucose) may not achieve stable values until after a significant lag phase.
[b]IgG index = CSF IgG (mg/dL) × serum albumin (g/dL)/serum IgG (g/dL) × CSF albumin (mg/dL).

TABLE 7A Differential Nucleated Cell Counts of Bone Marrow Aspirates[a] (See Chaps. 57, e17)

	Observed Range (%)	95% Range (%)	Mean (%)
Blast cells	0–3.2	0–3.0	1.4
Promyelocytes	3.6–13.2	3.2–12.4	7.8
Neutrophil myelocytes	4–21.4	3.7–10.0	7.6
Eosinophil myelocytes	0–5.0	0–2.8	1.3
Metamyelocytes	1–7.0	2.3–5.9	4.1
Neutrophils			
Males	21.0–45.6	21.9–42.3	32.1
Females	29.6–46.6	28.8–45.9	37.4
Eosinophils	0.4–4.2	0.3–4.2	2.2
Eosinophils plus eosinophil myelocytes	0.9–7.4	0.7–6.3	3.5
Basophils	0–0.8	0–0.4	0.1
Erythroblasts			
Male	18.0–39.4	16.2–40.1	28.1
Females	14.0–31.8	13.0–32.0	22.5
Lymphocytes	4.6–22.6	6.0–20.0	13.1
Plasma cells	0–1.4	0–1.2	0.6
Monocytes	0–3.2	0–2.6	1.3
Macrophages	0–1.8	0–1.3	0.4
M:E ratio			
Males	1.1–4.0	1.1–4.1	2.1
Females	1.6–5.4	1.6–5.2	2.8

[a]Based on bone marrow aspirate from 50 healthy volunteers (30 men, 20 women).
Abbreviation: M:E, myeloid to erythroid ratio.
Source: BJ Bain: Br J Haematol 94:206, 1996.

TABLE 7B Bone Marrow Cellularity

Age	Observed Range	95% Range	Mean
Under 10 years	59.0–95.1%	72.9–84.7%	78.8%
10–19 years	41.5–86.6%	59.2–69.4%	64.3%
20–29 years	32.0–83.7%	54.1–61.9%	58.0%
30–39 years	30.3–81.3%	41.1–54.1%	47.6%
40–49 years	16.3–75.1%	43.5–52.9%	48.2%
50–59 years	19.7–73.6%	41.2–51.4%	46.3%
60–69 years	16.3–65.7%	40.8–50.6%	45.7%
70–79 years	11.3–47.1%	22.6–35.2%	28.9%

Source: From RJ Hartsock et al: Am J Clin Pathol 1965; 43:326, 1965.

TABLE 8 Stool Analysis

	Reference Range	
	SI Units	Conventional Units
Alpha-1-antitrypsin	≤540 mg/L	≤54 mg/dL
Amount	0.1–0.2 kg/d	100–200 g/24 h
Coproporphyrin	611–1832 nmol/d	400–1200 μg/24 h
Fat		
Adult		<7 g/d
Adult on fat-free diet		<4 g/d
Fatty acids	0–21 mmol/d	0–6 g/24 h
Leukocytes	None	None
Nitrogen	<178 mmol/d	<2.5 g/24 h
pH	7.0–7.5	
Potassium	14–102 mmol/L	14–102 mmol/L
Occult blood	Negative	Negative
Osmolality	280–325 mOsm	280–325 mOsm
Sodium	7–72 mmol/L	7–72 mmol/L
Trypsin		20–95 U/g
Urobilinogen	85–510 μmol/d	50–300 mg/24 h
Uroporphyrins	12–48 nmol/d	10–40 μg/24 h
Water	<0.75	<75%

Source: Modified from: FT Fishbach, MB Dunning III: *A Manual of Laboratory and Diagnostic Tests*, 7th ed. Philadelphia, Lippincott Williams & Wilkins, 2004.

TABLE 9 Urine Analysis and Renal Function Tests

	Reference Range	
	SI Units	Conventional Units
Acidity, titratable	20–40 mmol/d	20–40 meq/d
Aldosterone	Normal diet: 6–25 μg/d Low-salt diet: 17–44 μg/d High-salt diet: 0–6 μg/d	Normal diet: 6–25 μg/d Low-salt diet: 17–44 μg/d High-salt diet: 0–6 μg/d
Aluminum	0.19–1.11 μmol/L	5–30 μg/L
Ammonia	30–50 mmol/d	30–50 meq/d
Amylase		4–400 U/L
Amylase/creatinine clearance ratio [(Cl_{am}/Cl_{cr}) × 100]	1–5	1–5
Arsenic	0.07–0.67 μmol/d	5–50 μg/d
Bence Jones protein, urine, qualitative	Not applicable	None detected
Bence Jones protein, urine, quantitative		
Free Kappa	1.4–24.2 mg/L	0.14–2.42 mg/dL
Free Lambda	0.2–6.7 mg/L	0.02–0.67 mg/dL
K/L ratio	2.04–10.37	2.04–10.37
Calcium (10 meq/d or 200 mg/d dietary calcium)	<7.5 mmol/d	<300 mg/d
Chloride	140–250 mmol/d	140–250 mmol/d
Citrate	320–1240 mg/d	320–1240 mg/d
Copper	<0.95 μmol/d	<60 μg/d
Coproporphyrins (types I and III)	0–20 μmol/mol creatinine	0–20 μmol/mol creatinine
Cortisol, free	55–193 nmol/d	20–70 μg/d
Creatine, as creatinine		
Female	<760 μmol/d	<100 mg/d
Male	<380 μmol/d	<50 mg/d
Creatinine	8.8–14 mmol/d	1.0–1.6 g/d
Dopamine	392–2876 nmol/d	60–440 μg/d
Eosinophils	<100 eosinophils/mL	<100 eosinophils/mL
Epinephrine	0–109 nmol/day	0–20 μg/day
Glomerular filtration rate	>60 mL/min/1.73 m^2 For African Americans multiply the result by 1.21	>60 mL/min/1.73 m^2 For African Americans multiply the result by 1.21
Glucose (glucose oxidase method)	0.3–1.7 mmol/d	50–300 mg/d
5-Hydroindoleacetic acid [5-HIAA]	0–78.8 μmol/d	0–15 mg/d
Hydroxyproline	53–328 μmol/d	53–328 μmol/d
Iodine, spot urine		
WHO classification of iodine deficiency:		
Not iodine deficient	>100 μg/L	>100 μg/L
Mild iodine deficiency	50–100 μg/L	50–100 μg/L
Moderate iodine deficiency	20–49 μg/L	20–49 μg/L
Severe iodine deficiency	<20 μg/L	<20 μg/L
Ketone (acetone)	Negative	Negative
17 Ketosteroids	3–12 mg/d	3–12 mg/d
Metanephrines		
Metanephrine	30–350 μg/d	30–350 μg/d
Normetanephrine	50–650 μg/d	50–650 μg/d

(continued)

TABLE 9 Urine Analysis and Renal Function Tests (*Continued*)

	Reference Range	
	SI Units	Conventional Units
Microalbumin		
Normal	0.0–0.03 g/d	0–30 mg/d
Microalbuminuria	0.03–0.30 g/d	30–300 mg/d
Clinical albuminuria	>0.3 g/d	>300 mg/d
Microalbumin/creatinine ratio		
Normal	0–3.4 g/mol creatinine	0–30 μg/mg creatinine
Microalbuminuria	3.4–34 g/mol creatinine	30–300 μg/mg creatinine
Clinical albuminuria	>34 g/mol creatinine	>300 μg/mg creatinine
β_2-Microglobulin	0–160 μg/L	0–160 μg/L
Norepinephrine	89–473 nmol/d	15–80 μg/d
N-telopeptide (cross-linked), NTx		
Female, premenopausal	17–94 nmol BCE/mmol creatinine	17–94 nmol BCE/mmol creatinine
Female, postmenopausal	26–124 nmol BCE/mmol creatinine	26–124 nmol BCE/mmol creatinine
Male	21–83 nmol BCE/mmol creatinine	21–83 nmol BCE/mmol creatinine
BCE = bone collagen equivalent		
Osmolality	500–800 mOsmol/kg water	500–800 mOsmol/kg water
Oxalate		
Male	80–500 μmol/d	7–44 mg/d
Female	45–350 μmol/d	4–31 mg/d
pH	5.0–9.0	5.0–9.0
Phosphate (phosphorus) (varies with intake)	12.9–42.0 mmol/d	400–1300 mg/d
Porphobilinogen	None	None
Potassium (varies with intake)	25–100 mmol/d	25–100 meq/d
Protein	<0.15 g/d	<150 mg/d
Protein/creatinine ratio	Male: 15–68 mg/g Female: 10–107 mg/g	Male: 15–68 mg/g Female: 10–107 mg/g
Sediment		
Red blood cells	0–2/high-power field	
White blood cells	0–2/high-power field	
Bacteria	None	
Crystals	None	
Bladder cells	None	
Squamous cells	None	
Tubular cells	None	
Broad casts	None	
Epithelial cell casts	None	
Granular casts	None	
Hyaline casts	0–5/low-power field	
Red blood cell casts	None	
Waxy casts	None	
White cell casts	None	
Sodium (varies with intake)	100–260 mmol/d	100–260 meq/d
Specific gravity:		
After 12-h fluid restriction	>1.025	>1.025
After 12-h deliberate water intake	≤1.003	≤1.003
Tubular reabsorption, phosphorus	0.79–0.94 of filtered load	79–94% of filtered load
Urea nitrogen	214–607 mmol/d	6–17 g/d
Uric acid (normal diet)	1.49–4.76 mmol/d	250–800 mg/d
Vanillylmandelic acid (VMA)	<30 μmol/d	<6 mg/d

TABLE 10 Normal Pressures in Heart and Great Vessels

Pressure (mmHg)	Average	Range
Right Atrium		
Mean	2.8	1–5
a wave	5.6	2.5–7
c wave	3.8	1.5–6
x wave	1.7	0–5
v wave	4.6	2–7.5
y wave	2.4	0–6
Right Ventricle		
Peak systolic	25	17–32
End-diastolic	4	1–7
Pulmonary Artery		
Mean	15	9–19
Peak systolic	25	17–32
End-diastolic	9	4–13
Pulmonary Artery Wedge		
Mean	9	4.5–13
Left Atrium		
Mean	7.9	2–12
a wave	10.4	4–16
v wave	12.8	6–21
Left Ventricle		
Peak systolic	130	90–140
End-diastolic	8.7	5–12
Brachial Artery		
Mean	85	70–105
Peak systolic	130	90–140
End-diastolic	70	60–90

Source: Reproduced from: MJ Kern *The Cardiac Catheterization Handbook*, 4th ed., Philadelphia, Mosby, 2003.

TABLE 11 Circulatory Function Tests

Test	Results: Reference Range	
	SI Units (Range)	Conventional Units (Range)
Arteriovenous oxygen difference	30–50 mL/L	30–50 mL/L
Cardiac output (Fick)	2.5–3.6 L/m² of body surface area per min	2.5–3.6 L/m² of body surface area per min
Contractility indexes		
Max. left ventricular *dp/dt* (*dp/dt*)	220 kPa/s (176–250 kPa/s)	1650 mmHg/s (1320–1880 mmHg/s)
DP when DP = 5.3 kPa (40 mmHg) (DP, developed LV pressure)	(37.6 ± 12.2)/s	(37.6 ± 12.2)/s
	3.32 ± 0.84 end-diastolic volumes per second	3.32 ± 0.84 end-diastolic volumes per second
Mean normalized systolic ejection rate (angiography)	1.83 ± 0.56 circumferences per second	1.83 ± 0.56 circumferences per second
Mean velocity of circumferential fiber shortening (angiography)		
Ejection fraction: stroke volume/end-diastolic volume (SV/EDV)	0.67 ± 0.08 (0.55–0.78)	0.67 ± 0.08 (0.55–0.78)
End-diastolic volume	70 ± 20.0 mL/m² (60–88 mL/m²)	70 ± 20.0 mL/m² (60–88 mL/m²)
End-systolic volume	25 ± 5.0 mL/m² (20–33 mL/m²)	25 ± 5.0 mL/m² (20–33 mL/m²)
Left ventricular work		
Stroke work index	50 ± 20.0 (g·m)/m² (30–110)	50 ± 20.0 (g·m)/m² (30–110)
Left ventricular minute work index	1.8–6.6 [(kg·m)/m²]/min	1.8–6.6 [(kg·m)/m²]/min
Oxygen consumption index	110–150 mL	110–150 mL
Maximum oxygen uptake	35 mL/min (20–60 mL/min)	35 mL/min (20–60 mL/min)
Pulmonary vascular resistance	2–12 (kPa·s)/L	20–130 (dyn·s)/cm⁵
Systemic vascular resistance	77–150 (kPa·s)/L	770–1600 (dyn·s)/cm⁵

Source: E Braunwald et al: *Heart Disease*, 6th ed. Philadelphia, W.B. Saunders Co., 2001.

TABLE 12 Normal Echocardiographic Reference Limits and Partition Values in Adults

	Women Reference Range	Mildly Abnormal	Moderately Abnormal	Severely Abnormal	Men Reference Range	Mildly Abnormal	Moderately Abnormal	Severely Abnormal
Left ventricular dimensions								
Septal thickness, cm	0.6–0.9	1.0–1.2	1.3–1.5	≥1.6	0.6–1.0	1.1–1.3	1.4–1.6	≥1.7
Posterior wall thickness, cm	0.6–0.9	1.0–1.2	1.3–1.5	≥1.6	0.6–1.0	1.1–1.3	1.4–1.6	≥1.7
Diastolic diameter, cm	3.9–5.3	5.4–5.7	5.8–6.1	≥6.2	4.2–5.9	6.0–6.3	6.4–6.8	≥6.9
Diastolic diameter/BSA, cm/m²	2.4–3.2	3.3–3.4	3.5–3.7	≥3.8	2.2–3.1	3.2–3.4	3.5–3.6	≥3.7
Diastolic diameter/height, cm/m	2.5–3.2	3.3–3.4	3.5–3.6	≥3.7	2.4–3.3	3.4–3.5	3.6–3.7	≥3.8
Left ventricular volumes								
Diastolic, mL	56–104	105–117	118–130	≥131	67–155	156–178	179–201	≥202
Diastolic/BSA, mL/m²	35–75	76–86	87–96	≥97	35–75	76–86	87–96	≥97
Systolic, mL	19–49	50–59	60–69	≥70	22–58	59–70	71–82	≥83
Systolic/BSA, mL/m²	12–30	31–36	37–42	≥43	12–30	31–36	37–42	≥43
Left ventricular mass, 2D method								
Mass, g	66–150	151–171	172–182	≥183	96–200	201–227	228–254	≥255
Mass/BSA, g/m²	44–88	89–100	101–112	≥113	50–102	103–116	117–130	≥131
Left ventricular function								
Endocardial fractional shortening (%)	27–45	22–26	17–21	≤16	25–43	20–24	15–19	≤14
Midwall fractional shortening (%)	15–23	13–14	11–12	≤10	14–22	12–13	10–11	≤9
Ejection fraction, 2D method (%)	≥55	45–54	30–44	≤29	≥55	45–54	30–44	≤29
Right heart dimensions (cm)								
Basal RV diameter	2.0–2.8	2.9–3.3	3.4–3.8	≥3.9	2.0–2.8	2.9–3.3	3.4–3.8	≥3.9
Mid-RV diameter	2.7–3.3	3.4–3.7	3.8–4.1	≥4.2	2.7–3.3	3.4–3.7	3.8–4.1	≥4.2

(continued)

TABLE 12 Normal Echocardiographic Reference Limits and Partition Values in Adults *(Continued)*

	Women Reference Range	Mildly Abnormal	Moderately Abnormal	Severely Abnormal	Men Reference Range	Mildly Abnormal	Moderately Abnormal	Severely Abnormal
Base-to-apex length	7.1–7.9	8.0–8.5	8.6–9.1	≥9.2	7.1–7.9	8.0–8.5	8.6–9.1	≥9.2
RVOT diameter above aortic valve	2.5–2.9	3.0–3.2	3.3–3.5	≥3.6	2.5–2.9	3.0–3.2	3.3–3.5	≥3.6
RVOT diameter above pulmonic valve	1.7–2.3	2.4–2.7	2.8–3.1	≥3.2	1.7–2.3	2.4–2.7	2.8–3.1	≥3.2
Pulmonary artery diameter below pulmonic valve	1.5–2.1	2.2–2.5	2.6–2.9	≥3.0	1.5–2.1	2.2–2.5	2.6–2.9	≥3.0
Right ventricular size and function in 4-chamber view								
Diastolic area, cm^2	11–28	29–32	33–37	≥38	11–28	29–32	33–37	≥38
Systolic area, cm^2	7.5–16	17–19	20–22	≥23	7.5–16	17–19	20–22	≥23
Fractional area change, %	32–60	25–31	18–24	≤17	32–60	25–31	18–24	≤17
Atrial sizes								
LA diameter, cm	2.7–3.8	3.9–4.2	4.3–4.6	≥4.7	3.0–4.0	4.1–4.6	4.7–5.2	≥5.3
LA diameter/BSA, cm/m^2	1.5–2.3	2.4–2.6	2.7–2.9	≥3.0	1.5–2.3	2.4–2.6	2.7–2.9	≥3.0
RA minor axis, cm	2.9–4.5	4.6–4.9	5.0–5.4	≥5.5	2.9–4.5	4.6–4.9	5.0–5.4	≥5.5
RA minor axis/BSA, cm/m^2	1.7–2.5	2.6–2.8	2.9–3.1	≥3.2	1.7–2.5	2.6–2.8	2.9–3.1	≥3.2
LA area, cm^2	<20	20–30	30–40	≥41	<20	20–30	30–40	≥41
LA volume, mL	22–52	53–62	63–72	≥73	18–58	59–68	69–78	≥79
LA volume/BSA, mL/m^2	16–28	29–33	34–39	≥40	16–28	29–33	34–39	≥40
Aortic stenosis, classification of severity								
Aortic jet velocity, m/s		2.6–2.9	3.0–4.0	>4.0		2.6–2.9	3.0–4.0	>4.0
Mean gradient, mmHg		<20	20–40	>40		<20	20–40	>40
Valve area, cm^2		>1.5	1.0–1.5	<1.0		>1.5	1.0–1.5	<1.0
Indexed valve area, cm^2/m^2		>0.85	0.60–0.85	<0.6		>0.85	0.60–0.85	<0.6
Velocity ratio		>0.50	0.25–0.50	<0.25		>0.50	0.25–0.50	<0.25
Mitral stenosis, classification of severity								
Valve area, cm^2		>1.5	1.0–1.5	<1.0		>1.5	1.0–1.5	<1.0
Mean gradient, mmHg		<5	5–10	>10		<5	5–10	>10
Pulmonary artery pressure, mmHg		<30	30–50	>50		<30	30–50	>50
Aortic regurgitation, indices of severity								
Vena contracta width, cm		<0.30	0.30–0.60	≥0.60		<0.30	0.30–0.60	≥0.60
Jet width/LVOT width, %		<25	25–64	≥65		<25	25–64	≥65
Jet CSA/LVOT CSA, %		<5	5–59	≥60		<5	5–59	≥60
Regurgitant volume, mL/beat		<30	30–59	≥60		<30	30–59	≥60
Regurgitant fraction, %		<30	30–49	≥50		<30	30–49	≥50
Effective regurgitant orifice area, cm^2		<0.10	0.10–0.29	≥0.30		<0.10	0.10–0.29	≥0.30
Mitral regurgitation, indices of severity								
Vena contracta width, cm		<0.30	0.30–0.69	≥0.70		<0.30	0.30–0.69	≥0.70
Regurgitant volume, mL/beat		<30	30–59	≥60		<30	30–59	≥60
Regurgitant fraction, %		<30	30–49	≥50		<30	30–49	≥50
Effective regurgitant orifice area, cm^2		<0.20	0.20–0.39	≥0.40		<0.20	0.20–0.39	≥0.40

Abbreviations: BSA, body surface area; CSA, cross-sectional area; LA, left atrium; LVOT, left ventricular outflow tract; RA, right atrium; RV, right ventricle; RVOT, right ventricular outflow tract; 2D, 2-dimensional.

Source: Values adapted from: American Society of Echocardiography, Guidelines and Standards. *http://www.asecho.org/i4a/pages/index.cfm?pageid=3317*. Accessed Feb 23, 2010.

TABLE 13 Summary of Values Useful in Pulmonary Physiology

	Symbol	Typical Values: Man Aged 40, 75 kg, 175 cm Tall	Typical Values: Woman Aged 40, 60 kg, 160 cm Tall
Pulmonary Mechanics			
Spirometry—volume-time curves			
Forced vital capacity	FVC	5.0 L	3.4 L
Forced expiratory volume in 1 s	FEV_1	4.0 L	2.8 L
FEV_1/FVC	FEV_1%	80%	78%
Maximal midexpiratory flow rate	MMEF (FEF 25–75)	4.1 L/s	3.2L/s
Maximal expiratory flow rate	MEFR (FEF 200–1200)	9.0 L/s	6.1 L/s
Spirometry—flow-volume curves			
Maximal expiratory flow at 50% of expired vital capacity	V_{max} 50 (FEF 50%)	5.0 L/s	4.0 L/s
Maximal expiratory flow at 75% of expired vital capacity	V_{max} 75 (FEF 75%)	2.1 L/s	2.0 L/s
Resistance to airflow:			
Pulmonary resistance	RL (R_L)	<3.0 (cmH_2O/s)/L	
Airway resistance	Raw	<2.5 (cmH_2O/s)/L	
Specific conductance	SGaw	>0.13 cmH_2O/s	
Pulmonary compliance			
Static recoil pressure at total lung capacity	Pst TLC	25 ± 5 cmH_2O	
Compliance of lungs (static)	CL	0.2 L cmH_2O	
Compliance of lungs and thorax	C(L + T)	0.1 L cmH_2O	
Dynamic compliance of 20 breaths per minute	C dyn 20	0.25 ± 0.05 L/cmH_2O	
Maximal static respiratory pressures:			
Maximal inspiratory pressure	MIP	>110 cmH_2O	>70 cmH_2O
Maximal expiratory pressure	MEP	>200 cmH_2O	>140 cmH_2O
Lung Volumes			
Total lung capacity	TLC	6.9 L	4.9 L
Functional residual capacity	FRC	3.3 L	2.6 L
Residual volume	RV	1.9 L	1.5 L
Inspiratory capacity	IC	3.7 L	2.3 L
Expiratory reserve volume	ERV	1.4 L	1.1 L
Vital capacity	VC	5.0 L	3.4 L
Gas Exchange (Sea Level)			
Arterial O_2 tension	Pa_{O_2}	12.7 ± 0.7 kPa (95 ± 5 mmHg)	
Arterial CO_2 tension	Pa_{CO_2}	5.3 ± 0.3 kPa (40 ± 2 mmHg)	
Arterial O_2 saturation	Sa_{O_2}	0.97 ± 0.02 (97 ± 2%)	
Arterial blood pH	pH	7.40 ± 0.02	
Arterial bicarbonate	HCO_3^-	24 + 2 meq/L	
Base excess	BE	0 ± 2 meq/L	
Diffusing capacity for carbon monoxide (single breath)	DL_{CO}	37 mL CO/min/mmHg 27 mL CO/min/mmHg	
Dead space volume	V_D	2 mL/kg body wt	
Physiologic dead space; dead space-tidal volume ratio	V_D/V_T		
Rest		≤35% V_T	
Exercise		≤20% V_T	
Alveolar-arterial difference for O_2	$P(A - a)_{O_2}$	≤2.7 kPa ≤20 kPa (≤24 mmHg)	

Source: Based on: AH Morris et al: *Clinical Pulmonary Function Testing. A Manual of Uniform Laboratory Procedures*, 2nd ed. Salt Lake City, Utah, Intermountain Thoracic Society, 1984.

TABLE 14 Gastrointestinal Tests

Test	Results	
	SI Units	Conventional Units
Absorption tests		
D-Xylose: after overnight fast, 25 g xylose given in oral aqueous solution		
Urine, collected for following 5 h	25% of ingested dose	25% of ingested dose
Serum, 2 h after dose	2.0–3.5 mmol/L	30–52 mg/dL
Vitamin A: a fasting blood specimen is obtained and 200,000 units of vitamin A in oil is given orally	Serum level should rise to twice fasting level in 3–5 h	Serum level should rise to twice fasting level in 3–5 h
Bentiromide test (pancreatic function): 500 mg bentiromide (chymex) orally; *p*-aminobenzoic acid (PABA) measured		
Plasma		>3.6 (±1.1) μg/mL at 90 min
Urine	>50% recovered in 6 h	>50% recovered in 6 h
Gastric juice		
Volume		
24 h	2–3 L	2–3 L
Nocturnal	600–700 mL	600–700 mL
Basal, fasting	30–70 mL/h	30–70 mL/h
Reaction		
pH	1.6–1.8	1.6–1.8
Titratable acidity of fasting juice	4–9 μmol/s	15–35 meq/h
Acid output		
Basal		
Females (mean ± 1 SD)	0.6 ± 0.5 μmol/s	2.0 ± 1.8 meq/h
Males (mean ± 1 SD)	0.8 ± 0.6 μmol/s	3.0 ± 2.0 meq/h
Maximal (after SC histamine acid phosphate, 0.004 mg/kg body weight, and preceded by 50 mg promethazine, or after betazole, 1.7 mg/kg body weight, or pentagastrin, 6 μg/kg body weight)		
Females (mean ± 1 SD)	4.4 ± 1.4 μmol/s	16 ± 5 meq/h
Males (mean ± 1 SD)	6.4 ± 1.4 μmol/s	23 ± 5 meq/h
Basal acid output/maximal acid output ratio	≤0.6	≤0.6
Gastrin, serum	0–200 μg/L	0–200 pg/mL
Secretin test (pancreatic exocrine function): 1 unit/kg body weight, IV		
Volume (pancreatic juice) in 80 min	>2.0 mL/kg	>2.0 mL/kg
Bicarbonate concentration	>80 mmol/L	>80 meq/L
Bicarbonate output in 30 min	>10 mmol	>10 meq

TABLE 15 Body Fluids and Other Mass Data

	Reference Range	
	SI Units	Conventional Units
Ascitic fluid: See Chap. 43		
Body fluid,		
Total volume (lean) of body weight	50% (in obese) to 70%	
Intracellular	0.3–0.4 of body weight	
Extracellular	0.2–0.3 of body weight	
Blood		
Total volume		
Males	69 mL/kg body weight	
Females	65 mL/kg body weight	
Plasma volume		
Males	39 mL/kg body weight	
Females	40 mL/kg body weight	
Red blood cell volume		
Males	30 mL/kg body weight	1.15–1.21 L/m^2 of body surface area
Females	25 mL/kg body weight	0.95–1.00 L/m^2 of body surface area
Body mass index	18.5–24.9 kg/m^2	18.5–24.9 kg/m^2

TABLE 16 Radiation-Derived Units

Quantity	Measures	Old Unit	SI Unit	Special Name for SI Unit (Abbreviation)	Conversion
Activity	Rate of radioactive decay	curie (Ci)	Disintegrations per second (dps)	becquerel (Bq)	1 Ci = 3.7×10^{10} Bq 1 mCi = 37 MBq 1 Bq = 2.703×10^{-11} Ci
Exposure	Amount of ionizations produced in dry air by x-rays or gamma rays, per unit of mass	roentgen (R)	Coulomb per kilogram (C/kg)	none	1 C/kg = 3876 R 1 R = 2.58×10^{-4} C/kg 1 mR = 258 pC/kg
Air kerma	Sum of initial energies of charged particles liberated by ionizing radiation in air, per unit of mass	rad	Joule per kilogram (J/kg)	gray (Gy)	1 Gy = 100 rad 1 rad = 0.01 Gy 1 mrad = 10 μGy
Absorbed dose	Energy deposited per unit of mass in a medium, e.g. an organ/tissue	rad	Joule per kilogram (J/kg)	gray (Gy)	1 Gy = 100 rad 1 rad = 0.01 Gy 1 mrad = 10 μGy
Equivalent dose	Energy deposited per unit of mass in a medium, e.g. an organ/tissue, weighted to reflect type(s) of radiation	rem	Joule per kilogram (J/kg)	sievert (Sv)	1 Sv = 100 rem 1 rem = 0.01 Sv 1 mrem = 10 μSv
Effective dose	Energy deposited per unit of mass in a reference individual, doubly weighted to reflect type(s) of radiation and organ(s) irradiated	rem	Joule per kilogram (J/kg)	sievert (Sv)	1 Sv = 100 rem 1 rem = 0.01 Sv 1 mrem = 10 μSv

ACKNOWLEDGMENT

The contributions of Drs. Daniel J. Fink, Patrick M. Sluss, James L. Januzzi, and Kent B. Lewandrowski to this chapter in previous editions are gratefully acknowledged. We also express our gratitude to Drs. Amudha Palanisamy and Scott Fink for careful review of tables and helpful suggestions.

FURTHER READINGS

Hickman PE, Koerbin G: Methods in Clinical Chemistry. An accessory work to the fifth edition of Kaplan and Pesce's: *Clinical Chemistry: Theory, Analysis, Correlation*, 5th ed, LA Kaplan, AJ Pesce (eds). Philadelphia, Elsevier Mosby, 2009

Kratz A et al: Case records of the Massachusetts General Hospital. Weekly clinicopathological exercises. Laboratory reference values. N Engl J Med 351:1548, 2004

Lehman HP, Henry JB: SI Units, in *Henry's Clinical Diagnosis and Management by Laboratory Methods,* 21st ed, RC McPherson, MR Pincus (eds). Philadelphia, Elsevier Saunders, 2007, pp 1404–1418

Pesce MA: Reference ranges for laboratory tests and procedures, in *Nelson's Textbook of Pediatrics*, 18th ed, RM Klegman et al (eds). Philadelphia, Elsevier Saunders, 2007, pp 2943–2949

Roberts WL et al: Reference information of the clinical laboratory, in *Tietz Textbook of Clinical Chemistry and Molecular Diagnostics*, 4th ed, CA Burtis et al (eds). Philadelphia, Elsevier Saunders, 2006, pp 2251–2318

INDEX

Bold numbers indicate the start of the main discussion of a topic; numbers followed by "f" or "t" refer to figures and tables; numbers preceded by "e" refer to the e-chapter pages on the DVD; "V" refers to the videos on the DVD.

INDEX

INDEX

INDEX

INDEX

INDEX

INDEX

INDEX

INDEX

INDEX

INDEX

INDEX

INDEX

INDEX

INDEX

INDEX

INDEX

INDEX

INDEX

INDEX

INDEX

INDEX

INDEX

INDEX

INDEX

D

INDEX

INDEX

INDEX

INDEX

INDEX

INDEX

INDEX

INDEX

INDEX

INDEX

INDEX

INDEX

INDEX

INDEX

INDEX

INDEX

INDEX

INDEX

INDEX

INDEX

INDEX

INDEX

INDEX

INDEX

INDEX

INDEX

INDEX

INDEX

INDEX

INDEX

INDEX

INDEX

INDEX

INDEX

INDEX

INDEX

INDEX

INDEX

INDEX

INDEX

INDEX

INDEX

INDEX

INDEX

INDEX

P

INDEX

INDEX

INDEX

INDEX

INDEX

INDEX

INDEX

INDEX

INDEX

INDEX

INDEX

INDEX

INDEX

INDEX

INDEX

INDEX

INDEX

INDEX

INDEX

INDEX

INDEX

INDEX

INDEX

INDEX

INDEX

INDEX

INDEX

INDEX

INDEX

INDEX

INDEX

INDEX